Optum

ICD-10-CM Professional for Physicians

The complete official code set

Codes valid from October 1, 2022
through September 30, 2023

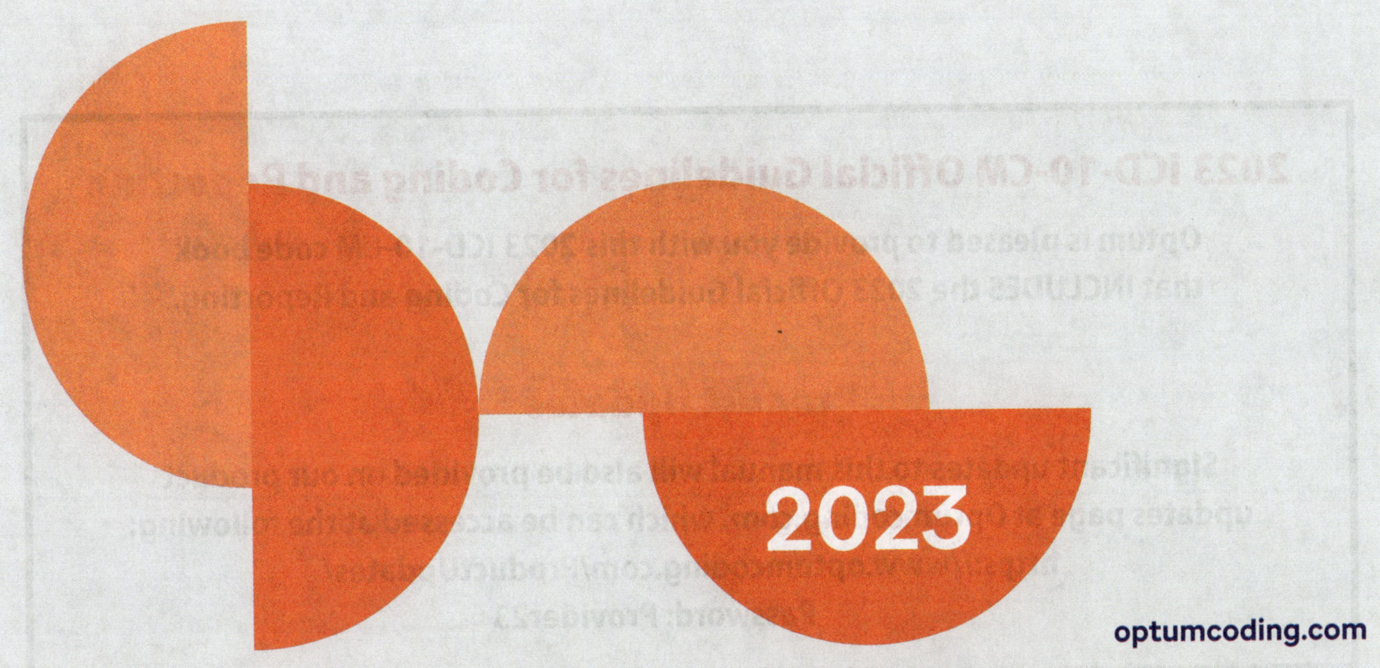

optumcoding.com

Publisher's Notice

Acknowledgments

Marianne Randall, CPC, *Product Manager*
Anita Schmidt, BS, RHIA, AHIMA-approved ICD-10-CM/PCS Trainer, *Subject Matter Expert*
Leanne Patterson, CPC, *Subject Matter Expert*
LaJuana Green, RHIA, CCS, *Subject Matter Expert*
Jacqueline R. Petersen, BS, RHIA, CHDA, CPC, *Subject Matter Expert*
Stacy Perry, *Manager, Desktop Publishing*
Tracy Betzler, *Senior Desktop Publishing Specialist*
Hope M. Dunn, *Senior Desktop Publishing Specialist*
Katie Russell, *Desktop Publishing Specialist*
Kate Holden, *Editor*

Our Commitment to Accuracy

Optum is committed to producing accurate and reliable materials.

To report corrections, please email customerassistance@optum.com. You can also reach customer service by calling 1.800.464.3649, option 1.

Copyright

Made in the USA
ISBN 978-1-62254-836-1

Leanne Patterson, CPC

Ms. Patterson has more than 15 years of experience in the healthcare profession. She has an extensive background in professional component coding, with expertise in E/M coding and auditing, and HIPAA compliance. Her experience includes general surgery coding, serving as Director of Compliance, conducting chart-to-claim audits, and physician education. She has been responsible for coding and denial management in large multi-specialty physician practices, and most recently has been part of a team developing content for educational products related to ICD-10-CM. Ms. Patterson is credentialed by the American Academy of Professional Coders (AAPC) as a Certified Professional Coder (CPC).

LaJuana Green, RHIA, CCS

Ms. Green is a Registered Health Information Administrator with over 35 years of experience in multiple areas of information management. She has proven expertise in the analysis of medical record documentation, assignment of ICD-10-CM and PCS codes, DRG validation, and CPT code assignment in ambulatory surgery units and the hospital outpatient setting. Her experience includes serving as a director of a health information management department, clinical technical editing, new technology research and writing, medical record management, utilization review activities, quality assurance, tumor registry, medical library services, and chargemaster maintenance. Ms. Green is an active member of the American Health Information Management Association (AHIMA).

2023 ICD-10-CM Official Guidelines for Coding and Reporting

Optum is pleased to provide you with this 2023 ICD-10-CM code book that INCLUDES the 2023 Official Guidelines for Coding and Reporting.

Product Updates

Significant updates to this manual will also be provided on our product updates page at Optumcoding.com, which can be accessed at the following:
https://www.optumcoding.com/ProductUpdates/
Password: Provider23

Contents

How to Use ICD-10-CM Professional for Physicians 2023.. iii
- Introduction ... iii
- What's New for 2023 ... iii
- Conversion Table ... iii
- 10 Steps to Correct Coding ... iii
- Official ICD-10-CM Guidelines for Coding and Reporting ... iii
- Indexes ... iii
  - Index to Diseases and Injuries ... iii
  - Neoplasm Table ... iii
  - Table of Drugs and Chemicals ... iii
  - External Causes Index ... iii
  - Index Notations ... iv
- Tabular List of Diseases ... iv
  - Code and Code Descriptions ... iv
  - Tabular Notations ... v
  - Official Notations ... v
  - Optum Notations ... vi
  - Icons ... vi
  - Color Bars ... vii
  - Footnotes ... vii
- Chapter-Level Notations ... viii
- Illustrations ... viii

What's New for 2023 ... ix
- Official Updates ... ix
- Proprietary Updates ... xi

Conversion Table of ICD-10-CM Codes ... xiii

10 Steps to Correct Coding ... xvii

ICD-10-CM Official Guidelines for Coding and Reporting ... Coding Guidelines–1

ICD-10-CM Index to Diseases and Injuries ... 1

ICD-10-CM Neoplasm Table ... 342

ICD-10-CM Table of Drugs and Chemicals ... 361

ICD-10-CM Index to External Causes ... 411

ICD-10-CM Tabular List of Diseases and Injuries ... 447
- Chapter 1. Certain Infectious and Parasitic Diseases (AØØ-B99) ... 447
- Chapter 2. Neoplasms (CØØ-D49) ... 473
- Chapter 3. Diseases of the Blood and Blood-forming Organs and Certain Disorders Involving the Immune Mechanism (D5Ø-D89) ... 515
- Chapter 4. Endocrine, Nutritional and Metabolic Diseases (EØØ-E89) ... 529
- Chapter 5. Mental, Behavioral, and Neurodevelopmental Disorders (FØ1-F99) ... 553
- Chapter 6. Diseases of the Nervous System (GØØ-G99) ... 587
- Chapter 7. Diseases of the Eye and Adnexa (HØØ-H59) ... 611
- Chapter 8. Diseases of the Ear and Mastoid Process (H6Ø-H95) ... 647
- Chapter 9. Diseases of the Circulatory System (IØØ-I99) ... 659
- Chapter 10. Diseases of the Respiratory System (JØØ-J99) ... 705
- Chapter 11. Diseases of the Digestive System (KØØ-K95) ... 723
- Chapter 12. Diseases of the Skin and Subcutaneous Tissue (LØØ-L99) ... 749
- Chapter 13. Diseases of the Musculoskeletal System and Connective Tissue (MØØ-M99) ... 773
- Chapter 14. Diseases of the Genitourinary System (NØØ-N99) ... 865
- Chapter 15. Pregnancy, Childbirth, and the Puerperium (OØØ-O9A) ... 887
- Chapter 16. Certain Conditions Originating in the Perinatal Period (PØØ-P96) ... 929
- Chapter 17. Congenital Malformations, Deformations and Chromosomal Abnormalities (QØØ-Q99) ... 943
- Chapter 18. Symptoms, Signs and Abnormal Clinical and Laboratory Findings (RØØ-R99) ... 963
- Chapter 19. Injury, Poisoning and Certain Other Consequences of External Causes (SØØ-T88) ... 985
- Chapter 20. External Causes of Morbidity (VØØ-Y99) ... 1191
- Chapter 21. Factors Influencing Health Status and Contact With Health Services (ZØØ-Z99) ... 1259
- Chapter 22. Codes for Special Purposes (UØØ-U85) ... 1297

Illustrations ... Illustrations–1
- Chapter 3. Diseases of the Blood and Blood-forming Organs and Certain Disorders Involving the Immune Mechanism (D5Ø–D89) ... Illustrations–1
  - Red Blood Cells ... Illustrations–1
  - White Blood Cell ... Illustrations–1
  - Platelet ... Illustrations–2
  - Coagulation ... Illustrations–2
  - Spleen Anatomical Location and External Structures ... Illustrations–3
  - Spleen Interior Structures ... Illustrations–3
- Chapter 4. Endocrine, Nutritional and Metabolic Diseases (EØØ–E89) ... Illustrations–4
  - Endocrine System ... Illustrations–4
  - Thyroid ... Illustrations–5
  - Thyroid and Parathyroid Glands ... Illustrations–5
  - Pancreas ... Illustrations–6
  - Anatomy of the Adrenal Gland ... Illustrations–6
  - Structure of an Ovary ... Illustrations–7
  - Testis and Associated Structures ... Illustrations–7
  - Thymus ... Illustrations–8
- Chapter 6. Diseases of the Nervous System (GØØ–G99) ... Illustrations–9
  - Brain ... Illustrations–9
  - Cranial Nerves ... Illustrations–9
  - Peripheral Nervous System ... Illustrations–10
  - Spinal Cord and Spinal Nerves ... Illustrations–11
  - Nerve Cell ... Illustrations–12
  - Trigeminal and Facial Nerve Branches ... Illustrations–12

Chapter 7. Diseases of the Eye and Adnexa (HØØ–H59) Illustrations–13
- Eye Illustrations–13
- Posterior Pole of Globe/Flow of Aqueous Humor Illustrations–13
- Lacrimal System Illustrations–14
- Eye Musculature Illustrations–14
- Eyelid Structures Illustrations–14

Chapter 8. Diseases of the Ear and Mastoid Process (H6Ø–H95) Illustrations–15
- Ear Anatomy Illustrations–15

Chapter 9. Diseases of the Circulatory System (IØØ–I99) Illustrations–16
- Anatomy of the Heart Illustrations–16
- Heart Cross Section Illustrations–16
- Heart Valves Illustrations–17
- Heart Conduction System Illustrations–17
- Coronary Arteries Illustrations–18
- Arteries Illustrations–19
- Veins Illustrations–20
- Internal Carotid and Vertebral Arteries and Branches Illustrations–21
- External Carotid Artery and Branches Illustrations–21
- Branches of Abdominal Aorta Illustrations–22
- Portal Venous Circulation Illustrations–22
- Lymphatic System Illustrations–23
- Axillary Lymph Nodes Illustrations–24
- Lymphatic System of Head and Neck Illustrations–24
- Lymphatic Capillaries Illustrations–25
- Lymphatic Drainage Illustrations–25

Chapter 10. Diseases of the Respiratory System (JØØ–J99) Illustrations–26
- Respiratory System Illustrations–26
- Upper Respiratory System Illustrations–27
- Lower Respiratory System Illustrations–27
- Paranasal Sinuses Illustrations–27
- Lung Segments Illustrations–28
- Alveoli Illustrations–28

Chapter 11. Diseases of the Digestive System (KØØ–K95) Illustrations–29
- Digestive System Illustrations–29
- Omentum and Mesentery Illustrations–30
- Peritoneum and Retroperitoneum .. Illustrations–30

Chapter 12. Diseases of the Skin and Subcutaneous Tissue (LØØ–L99) Illustrations–31
- Nail Anatomy Illustrations–31
- Skin and Subcutaneous Tissue Illustrations–31

Chapter 13. Diseases of the Musculoskeletal System and Connective Tissue (MØØ–M99) Illustrations–32
- Bones and Joints Illustrations–32
- Shoulder Anterior View Illustrations–33
- Shoulder Posterior View Illustrations–33
- Elbow Anterior View Illustrations–33
- Elbow Posterior View Illustrations–33
- Hand Illustrations–33
- Hip Anterior View Illustrations–34
- Hip Posterior View Illustrations–34
- Knee Anterior View Illustrations–34
- Knee Posterior View Illustrations–34
- Foot Illustrations–34
- Muscles Illustrations–35

Chapter 14. Diseases of the Genitourinary System (NØØ–N99) Illustrations–36
- Urinary System Illustrations–36
- Male Genitourinary System Illustrations–37
- Female Internal Genitalia Illustrations–37
- Female Genitourinary Tract Lateral View Illustrations–37

Chapter 15. Pregnancy, Childbirth and the Puerperium (OØØ–O9A) Illustrations–38
- Term Pregnancy – Single Gestation Illustrations–38
- Twin Gestation–Dichorionic–Diamniotic (DI-DI) Illustrations–38
- Twin Gestation–Monochorionic–Diamniotic (MO-DI) Illustrations–39
- Twin Gestation–Monochorionic–Monoamniotic (MO-MO) Illustrations–39

Chapter 19. Injury, Poisoning and Certain Other Consequences of External Causes (SØØ-T88) Illustrations–40
- Types of Fractures Illustrations–40
- Salter-Harris Fracture Types Illustrations–40

How to Use ICD-10-CM Professional for Physicians 2023

Introduction

ICD-10-CM Professional for Physicians: The Complete Official Code Set is your definitive coding resource, combining the work of the National Center for Health Statistics (NCHS), Centers for Medicare and Medicaid Services (CMS), American Hospital Association (AHA), and Optum experts to provide the information you need for coding accuracy.

The International Classification of Diseases, 10th Revision, Clinical Modification (ICD-10-CM), is an adaptation of ICD-10, copyrighted by the World Health Organization (WHO). The development and maintenance of this clinical modification (CM) is the responsibility of the NCHS as authorized by WHO. Any new concepts added to ICD-10-CM are based on an established update process through the collaboration of WHO's Update and Revision Committee and the ICD-10-CM Coordination and Maintenance Committee.

In addition to the ICD-10-CM classification, other official government source information has been included in this manual. Depending on the source, updates to information may be annual or quarterly. This manual provides the most current information that was available at the time of publication. For updates to the source documents that may have occurred after this manual was published, please refer to the following:

- **NCHS, International Classification of Diseases, Tenth Revision, Clinical Modification (ICD-10-CM)**

  https://www.cms.gov/medicare/icd-10/2023-icd-10-cm
- **CMS Integrated Outpatient Code Editor (IOCE), version 23.2**

  https://www.cms.gov/Medicare/Coding/OutpatientCodeEdit/OCEQtrReleaseSpecs.html
- **CMS-HCC Risk Adjustment Model, version 24**
- **CMS ESRD-HCC Risk Adjustment Model, version 24**
- **CMS RxHCC Risk Adjustment Model, version 08**

  https://www.cms.gov/Medicare/Health-Plans/MedicareAdvtgSpecRateStats/Risk-Adjustors.html
- **HHS-HCC Commercial Risk Adjustment Model, version 07**

  https://www.cms.gov/CCIIO/Resources/Regulations-and-Guidance
- **CMS Quality Payment Program (QPP)**

  https://qpp.cms.gov/mips/explore-measures/quality-measures?tab=qualityMeasures&py=2022
- **AHA Coding Clinics**

  https://www.codingclinicadvisor.com/

The official NCHS ICD-10-CM classification includes three main sections: the guidelines, the indexes, and the tabular list, all of which make up the bulk of this coding manual. To complement the classification, Optum's coding experts have incorporated Medicare-related coding edits and proprietary features, such as supplementary notations, coding tools, and appendixes, into a comprehensive and easy-to-use reference. This publication is organized as follows:

What's New for 2023

This section provides a high-level overview of the code changes made for fiscal 2023. The list of codes provided identifies new, revised, and deleted codes. Asterisked codes identify prior midyear changes that were made to the classification, effective April 1, 2022. All changes are based on official addenda, provided by the National Center for Health Statistics (NCHS), the agency charged with maintaining and updating ICD-10-CM. NCHS is part of the Centers for Disease Control and Prevention (CDC).

Conversion Table

The conversion table was developed by National Center for Healthcare Statistics (NCHS) to help facilitate data retrieval as new codes are added to the ICD-10-CM classification. This table provides a crosswalk from each fiscal 2023 new code to the equivalent code(s) assigned, prior to October 1, 2022, for that diagnosis or condition. Asterisked codes identify prior midyear additions, effective April 1, 2022. For the full conversion table, refer to the Conversion Table zip file at https://www.cms.gov/medicare/icd-10/2023-icd-10-cm.

10 Steps to Correct Coding

This step-by-step tutorial walks the coder through the process of finding the correct code — from locating the code in the official indexes to verifying the code in the tabular section — while following applicable conventions, guidelines, and instructional notes. Specific examples are provided with detailed explanations of each coding step along with advice for proper sequencing.

Official ICD-10-CM Guidelines for Coding and Reporting

This section provides the full official conventions and guidelines regulating the appropriate assignment and reporting of ICD-10-CM codes. These conventions and guidelines are published by the U.S. Department of Health and Human Services (DHHS) and approved by the cooperating parties (American Health Information Management Association [AHIMA], National Center for Health Statistics [NCHS], Centers for Disease Control and Prevention [CDC], and the American Hospital Association [AHA]).

Indexes

Index to Diseases and Injuries

The Index to Diseases and Injuries is arranged in alphabetic order by terms specific to a disease, condition, illness, injury, eponym, or abbreviation as well as terms that describe circumstances other than a disease or injury that may require attention from a health care professional.

Neoplasm Table

The Neoplasm Table is arranged in alphabetic order by anatomical site. Codes are then listed in individual columns based upon the histological behavior (malignant, in situ, benign, uncertain, or unspecified) of the neoplasm.

Table of Drugs and Chemicals

The Table of Drugs and Chemicals is arranged in alphabetic order by the specific drug or chemical name. Codes are listed in individual columns based upon the associated intent (poisoning, adverse effect, or underdosing). Drugs with an asterisk identify substances added to the table by Optum subject matter experts.

External Causes Index

The External Causes Index is arranged in alphabetic order by main terms that describe the cause, the intent, the place of occurrence, the activity, and the status of the patient at the time the injury occurred or health condition arose.

Index Notations

With

The word "with" or "in" should be interpreted to mean "associated with" or "due to." The classification presumes a causal relationship between the two conditions linked by these terms in the index. These conditions should be coded as related even in the absence of provider documentation explicitly linking them unless the documentation clearly states the conditions are unrelated or when another guideline specifically requires a documented linkage between two conditions (e.g., the sepsis guideline for "acute organ dysfunction that is not clearly associated with the sepsis"). For conditions not specifically linked by these relational terms in the classification or when a guideline requires explicit documentation of a linkage between two conditions, provider documentation must link the conditions to code them as related.

The word "with" in the index is sequenced immediately following the main term, not in alphabetical order.

Dermatopolymyositis M33.9Ø
- with
  - myopathy M33.92
  - respiratory involvement M33.91
  - specified organ involvement NEC M33.99
- amyopathic M33.93

See

When the instruction "see" follows a term in the index, it indicates that another term must be referenced to locate the correct code.

Hematoperitoneum *see* Hemoperitoneum

See Also

The instructional note "see also" simply provides alternative terms the coder may reference that may be useful in determining the correct code but are not necessary to follow if the main term supplies the appropriate code.

Hematinuria — *see also* Hemaglobinuria
- malarial B5Ø.8

Default Codes

In the index, the default code is the code listed next to the main term and represents the condition most commonly associated with that main term. This code may be assigned when documentation does not support reporting a more specific code. Alternatively, it may provide an unspecified code for the condition.

Hemiatrophy R68.89
- cerebellar G31.9
- face, facial, progressive (Romberg) G51.8
- tongue K14.8

Parentheses

Parentheses in the indexes enclose nonessential modifiers, supplementary words that may be present or absent in the statement of a disease without affecting the code.

Pseudomeningocele (cerebral) (infective) (post-traumatic) G96.198
- postprocedural (spinal) G97.82

Brackets

ICD-10-CM has a coding convention addressing code assignment for manifestations that occur as a result of an underlying condition. This convention requires the underlying condition to be sequenced first, followed by the code or codes for the associated manifestation. In the index, italicized codes in brackets identify manifestation codes.

Polyneuropathy (peripheral) G62.9
- alcoholic G62.1
- amyloid (Portuguese) E85.1 *[G63]*
  - transthyretin-related (ATTR) familial E85.1 *[G63]*

Shaded Guides

Exclusive vertical shaded guides in the Index to Diseases and Injuries and External Causes Index help the user easily follow the indent levels for the subentries under a main term. Sequencing rules may apply depending on the level of indent for separate subentries.

Hemicrania
- congenital malformation QØØ.Ø
- continua G44.51
- meaning migraine — *see also* Migraine G43.9Ø9
- paroxysmal G44.Ø39
  - chronic G44.Ø49
    - intractable G44.Ø41
    - not intractable G44.Ø49
  - episodic G44.Ø39
    - intractable G44.Ø31
    - not intractable G44.Ø39
  - intractable G44.Ø31
  - not intractable G44.Ø39

Following References

The Index to Diseases and Injuries includes "following" references to assist in locating out-of-sequence codes in the tabular list. Out-of-sequence codes contain an alphabetic character (letter) in the third- or fourth-character position. These codes are placed according to the classification rules — according to condition — not according to alphabetic or numeric sequencing rules.

Carcinoma (malignant) — *see also* Neoplasm, by site, malignant
- neuroendocrine — *see also* Tumor, neuroendocrine
  - high grade, any site C7A.1 (*following* C75)
  - poorly differentiated, any site C7A.1 (*following* C75)

Additional Character Required

The Index to Diseases and Injuries, Neoplasm Table, and External Causes Index provide an icon after certain codes to signify to the user that additional characters are required to make the code valid. The tabular list should be consulted for appropriate character selection.

Fall, falling (accidental) W19 ☑
- building W2Ø.1 ☑

Tabular List of Diseases

ICD-10-CM codes and descriptions are arranged numerically within the tabular list of diseases with 19 separate chapters providing codes associated with a particular body system or nature of injury or disease. There is also a chapter providing codes for external causes of an injury or health conditions, a chapter for codes that address encounters with healthcare facilities for circumstances other than a disease or injury, and finally, a chapter for codes that capture special circumstances such as new diseases of uncertain etiology or emergency use codes..

Code and Code Descriptions

ICD-10-CM is an alphanumeric classification system that contains categories, subcategories, and valid codes. The first character is always a letter with any additional characters represented by either a letter or number. A three-character category without further subclassification is equivalent to a valid three-character code. Valid codes may be three, four, five, six, or seven characters in length, with each level of subdivision after a three-character category representing a subcategory. The final level of subdivision is a valid code.

Boldface

Boldface type is used for all codes and descriptions in the tabular list.

Italics

Italicized type is used to identify manifestation codes, those codes that should not be reported as first-listed diagnoses.

Deleted Text

~~Strikethrough~~ on a code and code description indicates a deletion from the classification for the current year.

Key Word

Green font is used throughout the Tabular List of Diseases to differentiate the key words that appear in similar code descriptions in a given category or subcategory. The key word convention is used only in those categories in which there are multiple codes with very similar descriptions with only a few words that differentiate them.

For example, refer to the list of codes below from category H55:

> ✓4th **H55 Nystagmus and other irregular eye movements**
> ✓5th **H55.Ø Nystagmus**
> **H55.ØØ Unspecified nystagmus**
> **H55.Ø1 Congenital nystagmus**
> **H55.Ø2 Latent nystagmus**
> **H55.Ø3 Visual deprivation nystagmus**
> **H55.Ø4 Dissociated nystagmus**
> **H55.Ø9 Other forms of nystagmus**

The portion of the code description that appears in **green font** in the tabular list helps the coder quickly identify the key terms and the correct code. This convention is especially useful when the codes describe laterality, such as the following codes from subcategory H4Ø.22:

> ✓6th **H4Ø.22 Chronic angle-closure glaucoma**
> Chronic primary angle closure glaucoma
> ✓7th **H4Ø.221 Chronic angle-closure glaucoma, right eye**
> ✓7th **H4Ø.222 Chronic angle-closure glaucoma, left eye**
> ✓7th **H4Ø.223 Chronic angle-closure glaucoma, bilateral**
> ✓7th **H4Ø.229 Chronic angle-closure glaucoma, unspecified eye**

Tabular Notations

Official parenthetical notes as well as Optum's supplementary notations are provided at the chapter, code block, category, subcategory, and individual code level to help the user assign proper codes. The information in the notation can apply to one or more codes depending on where the citation is placed.

Official Notations

Includes Notes

The word INCLUDES appears immediately under certain categories to further define, clarify, or give examples of the content of a code category.

Inclusion Terms

Lists of inclusion terms are included under certain codes. These terms indicate some of the conditions for which that code number may be used. Inclusion terms may be synonyms with the code title, or, in the case of "other specified" codes, the terms may also provide a list of various conditions included within a classification code. The inclusion terms are not exhaustive. The index may provide additional terms that may also be assigned to a given code.

Excludes Notes

ICD-10-CM has two types of excludes notes. Each note has a different definition for use. However, they are similar in that they both indicate that codes excluded from each other are independent of each other.

Excludes 1

An EXCLUDES 1 note is a "pure" excludes. It means "NOT CODED HERE!" An Excludes 1 note indicates mutually exclusive codes: two conditions that cannot be reported together. An Excludes1 note indicates that the code excluded should never be used at the same time as the code above the Excludes1 note. An Excludes1 is used when two conditions cannot occur together, such as a congenital form versus an acquired form of the same condition.

An exception to the Excludes 1 definition is when the two conditions are unrelated to each other. If it is not clear whether the two conditions involving an Excludes 1 note are related or not, query the provider. For example, code F45.8 Other somatoform disorders, has an Excludes 1 note for "sleep related teeth grinding (G47.63)" because "teeth grinding" is an inclusion term under F45.8. Only one of these two codes should be assigned for teeth grinding. However psychogenic dysmenorrhea is also an inclusion term under F45.8, and a patient could have both this condition and sleep-related teeth grinding. In this case, the two conditions are clearly unrelated to each other, so it would be appropriate to report F45.8 and G47.63 together.

Excludes 2

An EXCLUDES 2 note means "NOT INCLUDED HERE." An Excludes 2 note indicates that although the excluded condition is not part of the condition it is excluded from, a patient may have both conditions at the same time. Therefore, when an Excludes 2 note appears under a code, it may be acceptable to use both the code and the excluded code together if supported by the medical documentation.

Note

The term "NOTE" appears as an icon and precedes the instructional information. These notes function as alerts to highlight coding instructions within the text.

Code First/Use additional code

These instructional notes provide sequencing instruction. They may appear independently of each other or to designate certain etiology/manifestation paired codes. These instructions signal the coder that an additional code should be reported to provide a more complete picture of that diagnosis.

In etiology/manifestation coding, ICD-10-CM requires the underlying condition to be sequenced first, followed by the manifestation. In these situations, codes with "In diseases classified elsewhere" in the code description are never permitted as a first-listed or principal diagnosis code and must be sequenced following the underlying condition code.

Code Also

A "code also" note alerts the coder that more than one code may be required to fully describe the condition. The sequencing depends on the circumstances of the encounter. Factors that may determine sequencing include severity and reason for the encounter.

Revised Text

The revised text ▶◀ "bow ties" alert the user to changes in official notations for the current year. Revised text may include the following:

- A change in a current parenthetical description
- A change in the code(s) associated with a current parenthetical note
- A change in how a current parenthetical note is classified (e.g., an Excludes 1 note that changed to an Excludes 2 note)
- Addition of a new parenthetical note(s) to a code

Deleted Text

~~Strikethrough~~ on official notations indicate a deletion from the classification for the current year.

Optum Notations

AHA Coding Clinic Citations

Coding Clinics are official American Hospital Association (AHA) publications that provide coding advice specific to ICD-10-CM and ICD-10-PCS.

Coding Clinic citations included in this manual are current up to the second quarter of 2022.

These citations identify the year, quarter, and page number of one or more *Coding Clinic* publications that may have coding advice relevant to a particular code or group of codes. With the most current citation listed first, these notations are preceded by the symbol **AHA:** and appear in purple type.

> **I15.1 Hypertension secondary to other renal disorders**
> AHA: 2016, 3Q, 22

Definitions

Definitions explain a specific term, condition, or disease process in layman's terms. These notations are preceded by the symbol **DEF:** and appear in purple type.

> ✓5th **M51.4 Schmorl's nodes**
> DEF: Irregular bone defect in the margin of the vertebral body that causes herniation into the end plate of the vertebral body.

Coding Tips

The tips in the tabular list offer coding advice that is not readily available within the ICD-10-CM classification. It may relate official coding guidelines, indexing nuances, or advice from *AHA's Coding Clinic for ICD-10-CM/PCS*. These notations are preceded by the symbol **TIP:** and appear in brown type.

> ✓5th **B97.2 Coronavirus as the cause of diseases classified elsewhere**
> TIP: Do not report a code from this subcategory for COVID-19, refer to U07.1.

Icons

Note: The following icons are placed to the left of the code.

Changes to ICD-10-CM codes, since the last published edition of this manual, are highlighted in two ways:

The following green icons identify new or revised codes effective April 1, 2022:

- ● **New Code – Midyear**
- ▲ **Revised Code – Midyear**

The following black icons identify new or revised codes effective October 1, 2022:

- ● **New Code**
- ▲ **Revised Code**
- ✓ **Additional Characters Required**
  - ✓4th This symbol indicates that the code requires a 4th character.
  - ✓5th This symbol indicates that the code requires a 5th character.
  - ✓6th This symbol indicates that the code requires a 6th character.
  - ✓7th This symbol indicates that the code requires a 7th character.

> ✓5th **H60.3 Other infective otitis externa**
> ✓6th **H60.31 Diffuse otitis externa**
> **H60.311 Diffuse otitis externa, right ear**
> **H60.312 Diffuse otitis externa, left ear**
> **H60.313 Diffuse otitis externa, bilateral**
> **H60.319 Diffuse otitis externa, unspecified ear**

✓x7th **Placeholder Alert**

This symbol indicates that the code requires a 7th character following the placeholder "X". Codes with fewer than six characters that require a 7th character must contain placeholder "X" to fill in the empty character(s).

> ✓x7th **T16.1 Foreign body in right ear**

This manual provides the most current information that was available at the time of publication. Except where otherwise noted, the icons and/or color bars reflect edits provided in the Integrated Outpatient Code Editor (IOCE) quarterly files utilized under the outpatient prospective payment system (OPPS). Because the October 2022 quarterly files were not available at the time this book was printed, the edits in this manual are based on the July 2022 quarterly files.

Note: In an effort to provide the most current edit information, Optum has provided a searchable data file that includes the final edit designations for all ICD-10-CM codes based on the IOCE October 2022 quarterly files. The edits included in the data file are as follows:

- Age
- Sex
- Manifestation
- Unacceptable principal diagnosis

This data file can be accessed at the following:

https://www.optumcoding.com/ProductUpdates/

Title: "2023 ICD-10-CM Outpatient Edits Data File"

Password: Provider23

Note: The following icons are placed at the end of the code description.

Age Edits

N **Newborn Age: 0**

These diagnoses are intended for newborns and neonates and the patient's age must be 0 years.

> **N47.0 Adherent prepuce, newborn** N♂

P **Pediatric Age: 0-17**

These diagnoses are intended for children and the patient's age must be between 0 and 17 years.

> **L21.1 Seborrheic infantile dermatitis** P

M **Maternity Age: 9-64**

These diagnoses are intended for childbearing patients between the age of 9 and 64 years.

> **O02.9 Abnormal product of conception, unspecified** M♀

A **Adult Age: 15-124**

These diagnoses are intended for patients between the age of 15 and 124 years.

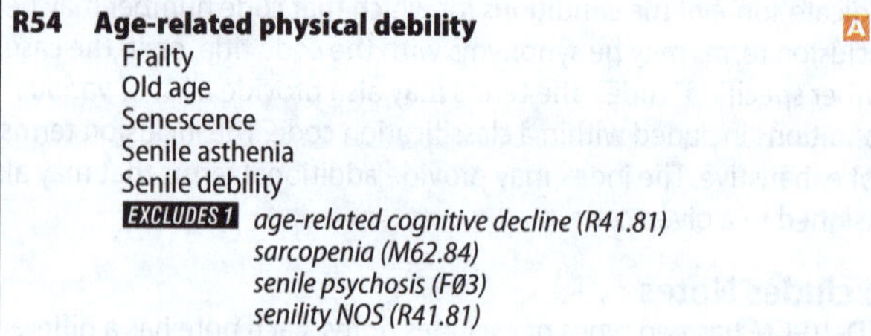

> **R54 Age-related physical debility** A
> Frailty
> Old age
> Senescence
> Senile asthenia
> Senile debility
> EXCLUDES 1 *age-related cognitive decline (R41.81)*
> *sarcopenia (M62.84)*
> *senile psychosis (F03)*
> *senility NOS (R41.81)*

Sex Edits

♂ **Male diagnosis only**

Q98.Ø	Klinefelter syndrome karyotype 47, XXY ♂

♀ **Female diagnosis only**

N35.12	Postinfective urethral stricture, not elsewhere classified, female ♀

UPD **Unacceptable Principal Diagnosis**

This icon identifies codes that are not appropriate as a first-listed code for *outpatient* encounters. These codes describe circumstances that influence an individual's health status but are not a current illness or injury, or that are not specifically manifestations but may be due to an underlying cause.

7th T48.5X5	Adverse effect of other anti-common-cold drugs UPD

HCC **CMS-HCC Condition**

This icon identifies codes that are considered a CMS-HCC (hierarchical condition category) diagnosis.

The HCC codes represented in this manual have been updated to reflect the 2022 Initial ICD-10-CM Mappings for CMS-HCC Model v24.

Y62.2	Failure of sterile precautions during kidney dialysis and other perfusion HCC

Rx **Rx-HCC Condition**

This icon identifies codes that are included in the Rx-HCC risk-adjustment model, which covers the Part D (prescription drug) benefit.

The Rx-HCC codes represented in this manual have been updated to reflect the 2023 Initial ICD-10-CM Mappings for CMS Rx-HCC Model v08..

Z21	Asymptomatic human immunodeficiency virus [HIV] infection status HCC Rx ESR COM

ESR **ESRD HCC Condition**

This icon identifies codes that are included in the end-stage renal disease (ESRD) HCC risk-adjustment model.

The ESRD HCC codes represented in this manual have been updated to reflect the 2023 Initial ICD-10-CM Mappings for CMS ESRD HCC Model v24.

Z21	Asymptomatic human immunodeficiency virus [HIV] infection status HCC Rx ESR COM

COM **Commercial HCC Condition**

This icon identifies codes that are included in the commercial HHS-HCC risk-adjustment model.

The commercial HCC codes represented in this manual are based on the commercial HCC Model v07.

Z21	Asymptomatic human immunodeficiency virus [HIV] infection status HCC Rx ESR COM

Note: Finalized ICD-10-CM to HCC mappings for CMS-HCC, Rx-HCC, ESRD HCC, and Commercial HCC have been provided in an easily searchable data file that can be accessed at the following:

https://www.optumcoding.com/ProductUpdates/

Title: "2023 Final ICD-10-CM to HCC Mappings Data File"

Password: Provider23

Q **QPP Condition**

This icon identifies codes recognized as a quality measure for claims-based reporting under CMS's Merit-based Incentive Payment System (MIPS) Claims Single Source v6.0.

G44.52	New daily persistent headache (NDPH) Q

PDx **Z-code as First-Listed Diagnosis**

Section IV of the official guidelines states that the term "first-listed diagnosis" is used instead of principal diagnosis in the outpatient setting and represents the diagnosis that is chiefly responsible for the services provided during the encounter. This icon identifies Z codes that, in general, may be reported only as a first-listed diagnosis. According to guideline I.C.21.c.16, these are the only Z codes that are specifically meant to be utilized as a first-listed diagnosis; all other Z codes may be either first-listed or secondary diagnoses, depending upon the circumstances of the encounter, coding instructions, and guidelines.

Note: The codes identified with this icon may be used as a secondary diagnosis if the patient has multiple encounters on the same day and those medical records are combined.

Z51.12	Encounter for antineoplastic immunotherapy PDx

Color Bars

Manifestation Code

Codes defined as manifestation codes appear in italic type, with a blue color bar over the code description. A manifestation cannot be reported as a first-listed code; it is sequenced as a secondary diagnosis with the underlying disease code listed first.

G32.89	***Other specified degenerative disorders of nervous system in diseases classified elsewhere*** Degenerative encephalopathy in diseases classified elsewhere

Unspecified Diagnosis

Codes that appear with a gray color bar over the alphanumeric code identify unspecified diagnoses. These codes should be used in limited circumstances, when neither the diagnostic statement nor the documentation provides enough information to assign a more specific diagnosis code. The abbreviation NOS, "not otherwise specified," in the tabular list may be interpreted as "unspecified."

G03.9	Meningitis, unspecified Arachnoiditis (spinal) NOS

Footnotes

Certain codes in the tabular section have a numerical superscript located to the upper left of the code. This numerical superscript corresponds to a specific footnote description.

For example:

[1] 7th M48.51	Collapsed vertebra, not elsewhere classified, occipito-atlanto-axial region HCC

For convenience, the footnote descriptions are

The following list also provides the footnote descriptions of all numerical superscripts found in the Tabular List of Diseases:

1. These codes are considered an HCC when reported as an initial encounter (7th character A, B, or C).
2. These codes are considered an HCC when reported as an initial encounter (7th character A or B) OR sequela (7th character S).
3. These codes are considered an HCC when reported as a sequela (7th character S).

Chapter-Level Notations

Chapter-specific Guidelines with Coding Examples

Each chapter begins with the Official Guidelines for Coding and Reporting specific to that chapter, where provided. Coding examples specific to outpatient care settings have been provided to illustrate the coding and/or sequencing guidance in these guidelines.

Muscle and Tendon Table

ICD-10-CM categorizes certain muscles and tendons in the upper and lower extremities by their action (e.g., extension or flexion) as well as their anatomical location. The Muscle/Tendon table is provided at the beginning of chapter 13 and chapter 19 to help users when code selection depends on the action of the muscle and/or tendon.

Note: This table is not all-inclusive, and proper code assignment should be based on the provider's documentation.

Illustrations

This section includes illustrations of normal anatomy with ICD-10-CM-specific terminology.

What's New for 2023

Official Updates

A summary of changes to the official ICD-10-CM code set is provided below, identifying changes made for fiscal 2023, effective October 1, 2022, to September 30, 2023. Asterisked codes identify prior midyear changes that were made to the classification, effective April 1, 2022. All code changes were made by the agency charged with maintaining and updating the ICD-10-CM code set, the National Center for Health Statistics (NCHS), a section of the Centers for Disease Control and Prevention (CDC).

1179 New Codes

B37.31 B37.32 D59.30 D59.31 D59.32
D59.39 D68.00 D68.01 D68.020 D68.021
D68.022 D68.023 D68.029 D68.03 D68.04
D68.09 D75.821 D75.822 D75.828 D75.829
D75.84 D81.82 E34.30 E34.31 E34.321
E34.322 E34.328 E34.329 E34.39 E87.20
E87.21 E87.22 E87.29 F01.511 F01.518
F01.52 F01.53 F01.54 F01.A0 F01.A11
F01.A18 F01.A2 F01.A3 F01.A4 F01.B0
F01.B11 F01.B18 F01.B2 F01.B3 F01.B4
F01.C0 F01.C11 F01.C18 F01.C2 F01.C3
F01.C4 F02.811 F02.818 F02.82 F02.83
F02.84 F02.A0 F02.A11 F02.A18 F02.A2
F02.A3 F02.A4 F02.B0 F02.B11 F02.B18
F02.B2 F02.B3 F02.B4 F02.C0 F02.C11
F02.C18 F02.C2 F02.C3 F02.C4 F03.911
F03.918 F03.92 F03.93 F03.94 F03.A0
F03.A11 F03.A18 F03.A2 F03.A3 F03.A4
F03.B0 F03.B11 F03.B18 F03.B2 F03.B3
F03.B4 F03.C0 F03.C11 F03.C18 F03.C2
F03.C3 F03.C4 F06.70 F06.71 F10.90
F10.91 F11.91 F12.91 F13.91 F14.91
F15.91 F16.91 F18.91 F19.91 F43.81
F43.89 G71.031 G71.032 G71.033 G71.0340
G71.0341 G71.0342 G71.0349 G71.035 G71.038
G71.039 G90.A G93.31 G93.32 G93.39
I20.2 I25.112 I25.702 I25.712 I25.722
I25.732 I25.752 I25.762 I25.792 I31.31
I31.39 I34.81 I34.89 I47.20 I47.21
I47.29 I71.010 I71.011 I71.012 I71.019
I71.10 I71.11 I71.12 I71.13 I71.20
I71.21 I71.22 I71.23 I71.30 I71.31
I71.32 I71.33 I71.40 I71.41 I71.42
I71.43 I71.50 I71.51 I71.52 I71.60
I71.61 I71.62 I77.82 J95.87 K76.82
M51.A0 M51.A1 M51.A2 M51.A3 M51.A4
M51.A5 M62.5A0 M62.5A1 M62.5A2 M62.5A9
M93.004 M93.014 M93.024 M93.034 M93.041
M93.042 M93.043 M93.044 M93.051 M93.052
M93.053 M93.054 M93.061 M93.062 M93.063
M93.064 M93.071 M93.072 M93.073 M93.074
M96.A1 M96.A2 M96.A3 M96.A4 M96.A9
N14.11 N14.19 N76.82 N80.00 N80.01
N80.02 N80.03 N80.101 N80.102 N80.103
N80.109 N80.111 N80.112 N80.113 N80.119
N80.121 N80.122 N80.123 N80.129 N80.201
N80.202 N80.203 N80.209 N80.211 N80.212
N80.213 N80.219 N80.221 N80.222 N80.223
N80.229 N80.30 N80.311 N80.312 N80.319
N80.321 N80.322 N80.329 N80.331 N80.332
N80.333 N80.339 N80.341 N80.342 N80.343
N80.349 N80.351 N80.352 N80.353 N80.359
N80.361 N80.362 N80.363 N80.369 N80.371
N80.372 N80.373 N80.379 N80.381 N80.382
N80.383 N80.389 N80.391 N80.392 N80.399
N80.3A1 N80.3A2 N80.3A3 N80.3A9 N80.3B1
N80.3B2 N80.3B3 N80.3B9 N80.3C1 N80.3C2
N80.3C3 N80.3C9 N80.40 N80.41 N80.42
N80.50 N80.511 N80.512 N80.519 N80.521
N80.522 N80.529 N80.531 N80.532 N80.539
N80.541 N80.542 N80.549 N80.551 N80.552
N80.559 N80.561 N80.562 N80.569 N80.A0
N80.A1 N80.A2 N80.A41 N80.A42 N80.A43
N80.A49 N80.A51 N80.A52 N80.A53 N80.A59
N80.A61 N80.A62 N80.A63 N80.A69 N80.B1
N80.B2 N80.B31 N80.B32 N80.B39 N80.B4
N80.B5 N80.B6 N80.C0 N80.C10 N80.C11
N80.C19 N80.C2 N80.C3 N80.C4 N80.C9
N80.D0 N80.D1 N80.D2 N80.D3 N80.D4
N80.D5 N80.D6 N80.D9 N85.A O35.00X0
O35.00X1 O35.00X2 O35.00X3 O35.00X4 O35.00X5
O35.00X9 O35.01X0 O35.01X1 O35.01X2 O35.01X3
O35.01X4 O35.01X5 O35.01X9 O35.02X0 O35.02X1
O35.02X2 O35.02X3 O35.02X4 O35.02X5 O35.02X9
O35.03X0 O35.03X1 O35.03X2 O35.03X3 O35.03X4
O35.03X5 O35.03X9 O35.04X0 O35.04X1 O35.04X2
O35.04X3 O35.04X4 O35.04X5 O35.04X9 O35.05X0
O35.05X1 O35.05X2 O35.05X3 O35.05X4 O35.05X5
O35.05X9 O35.06X0 O35.06X1 O35.06X2 O35.06X3
O35.06X4 O35.06X5 O35.06X9 O35.07X0 O35.07X1
O35.07X2 O35.07X3 O35.07X4 O35.07X5 O35.07X9
O35.08X0 O35.08X1 O35.08X2 O35.08X3 O35.08X4
O35.08X5 O35.08X9 O35.09X0 O35.09X1 O35.09X2
O35.09X3 O35.09X4 O35.09X5 O35.09X9 O35.10X0
O35.10X1 O35.10X2 O35.10X3 O35.10X4 O35.10X5
O35.10X9 O35.11X0 O35.11X1 O35.11X2 O35.11X3
O35.11X4 O35.11X5 O35.11X9 O35.12X0 O35.12X1
O35.12X2 O35.12X3 O35.12X4 O35.12X5 O35.12X9
O35.13X0 O35.13X1 O35.13X2 O35.13X3 O35.13X4
O35.13X5 O35.13X9 O35.14X0 O35.14X1 O35.14X2
O35.14X3 O35.14X4 O35.14X5 O35.14X9 O35.15X0
O35.15X1 O35.15X2 O35.15X3 O35.15X4 O35.15X5
O35.15X9 O35.19X0 O35.19X1 O35.19X2 O35.19X3
O35.19X4 O35.19X5 O35.19X9 O35.AXX0 O35.AXX1
O35.AXX2 O35.AXX3 O35.AXX4 O35.AXX5 O35.AXX9
O35.BXX0 O35.BXX1 O35.BXX2 O35.BXX3 O35.BXX4
O35.BXX5 O35.BXX9 O35.CXX0 O35.CXX1 O35.CXX2
O35.CXX3 O35.CXX4 O35.CXX5 O35.CXX9 O35.DXX0
O35.DXX1 O35.DXX2 O35.DXX3 O35.DXX4 O35.DXX5
O35.DXX9 O35.EXX0 O35.EXX1 O35.EXX2 O35.EXX3
O35.EXX4 O35.EXX5 O35.EXX9 O35.FXX0 O35.FXX1
O35.FXX2 O35.FXX3 O35.FXX4 O35.FXX5 O35.FXX9
O35.GXX0 O35.GXX1 O35.GXX2 O35.GXX3 O35.GXX4
O35.GXX5 O35.GXX9 O35.HXX0 O35.HXX1 O35.HXX2
O35.HXX3 O35.HXX4 O35.HXX5 O35.HXX9 P28.30
P28.31 P28.32 P28.33 P28.39 P28.40
P28.41 P28.42 P28.43 P28.49 Q21.10
Q21.11 Q21.12 Q21.13 Q21.14 Q21.15
Q21.16 Q21.19 Q21.20 Q21.21 Q21.22
Q21.23 Q85.81 Q85.82 Q85.83 Q85.89
S06.0XAA S06.0XAD S06.0XAS S06.1XAA S06.1XAD
S06.1XAS S06.2XAA S06.2XAD S06.2XAS S06.30AA
S06.30AD S06.30AS S06.31AA S06.31AD S06.31AS
S06.32AA S06.32AD S06.32AS S06.33AA S06.33AD
S06.33AS S06.34AA S06.34AD S06.34AS S06.35AA
S06.35AD S06.35AS S06.36AA S06.36AD S06.36AS
S06.37AA S06.37AD S06.37AS S06.38AA S06.38AD
S06.38AS S06.4XAA S06.4XAD S06.4XAS S06.5XAA

S06.5XAD S06.5XAS S06.6XAA S06.6XAD S06.6XAS
S06.81AA S06.81AD S06.81AS S06.82AA S06.82AD
S06.82AS S06.89AA S06.89AD S06.89AS S06.8A0A
S06.8A0D S06.8A0S S06.8A1A S06.8A1D S06.8A1S
S06.8A2A S06.8A2D S06.8A2S S06.8A3A S06.8A3D
S06.8A3S S06.8A4A S06.8A4D S06.8A4S S06.8A5A
S06.8A5D S06.8A5S S06.8A6A S06.8A6D S06.8A6S
S06.8A7A S06.8A8A S06.8A9A S06.8A9D S06.8A9S
S06.8AAA S06.8AAD S06.8AAS S06.9XAA S06.9XAD
S06.9XAS T43.651A T43.651D T43.651S T43.652A
T43.652D T43.652S T43.653A T43.653D T43.653S
T43.654A T43.654D T43.654S T43.655A T43.655D
T43.655S T43.656A T43.656D T43.656S V20.01XA
V20.01XD V20.01XS V20.09XA V20.09XD V20.09XS
V20.11XA V20.11XD V20.11XS V20.19XA V20.19XD
V20.19XS V20.21XA V20.21XD V20.21XS V20.29XA
V20.29XD V20.29XS V20.31XA V20.31XD V20.31XS
V20.39XA V20.39XD V20.39XS V20.41XA V20.41XD
V20.41XS V20.49XA V20.49XD V20.49XS V20.51XA
V20.51XD V20.51XS V20.59XA V20.59XD V20.59XS
V20.91XA V20.91XD V20.91XS V20.99XA V20.99XD
V20.99XS V21.01XA V21.01XD V21.01XS V21.09XA
V21.09XD V21.09XS V21.11XA V21.11XD V21.11XS
V21.19XA V21.19XD V21.19XS V21.21XA V21.21XD
V21.21XS V21.29XA V21.29XD V21.29XS V21.31XA
V21.31XD V21.31XS V21.39XA V21.39XD V21.39XS
V21.41XA V21.41XD V21.41XS V21.49XA V21.49XD
V21.49XS V21.51XA V21.51XD V21.51XS V21.59XA
V21.59XD V21.59XS V21.91XA V21.91XD V21.91XS
V21.99XA V21.99XD V21.99XS V22.01XA V22.01XD
V22.01XS V22.09XA V22.09XD V22.09XS V22.11XA
V22.11XD V22.11XS V22.19XA V22.19XD V22.19XS
V22.21XA V22.21XD V22.21XS V22.29XA V22.29XD
V22.29XS V22.31XA V22.31XD V22.31XS V22.39XA
V22.39XD V22.39XS V22.41XA V22.41XD V22.41XS
V22.49XA V22.49XD V22.49XS V22.51XA V22.51XD
V22.51XS V22.59XA V22.59XD V22.59XS V22.91XA
V22.91XD V22.91XS V22.99XA V22.99XD V22.99XS
V23.01XA V23.01XD V23.01XS V23.09XA V23.09XD
V23.09XS V23.11XA V23.11XD V23.11XS V23.19XA
V23.19XD V23.19XS V23.21XA V23.21XD V23.21XS
V23.29XA V23.29XD V23.29XS V23.31XA V23.31XD
V23.31XS V23.39XA V23.39XD V23.39XS V23.41XA
V23.41XD V23.41XS V23.49XA V23.49XD V23.49XS
V23.51XA V23.51XD V23.51XS V23.59XA V23.59XD
V23.59XS V23.91XA V23.91XD V23.91XS V23.99XA
V23.99XD V23.99XS V24.01XA V24.01XD V24.01XS
V24.09XA V24.09XD V24.09XS V24.11XA V24.11XD
V24.11XS V24.19XA V24.19XD V24.19XS V24.21XA
V24.21XD V24.21XS V24.29XA V24.29XD V24.29XS
V24.31XA V24.31XD V24.31XS V24.39XA V24.39XD
V24.39XS V24.41XA V24.41XD V24.41XS V24.49XA
V24.49XD V24.49XS V24.51XA V24.51XD V24.51XS
V24.59XA V24.59XD V24.59XS V24.91XA V24.91XD
V24.91XS V24.99XA V24.99XD V24.99XS V25.01XA
V25.01XD V25.01XS V25.09XA V25.09XD V25.09XS
V25.11XA V25.11XD V25.11XS V25.19XA V25.19XD
V25.19XS V25.21XA V25.21XD V25.21XS V25.29XA
V25.29XD V25.29XS V25.31XA V25.31XD V25.31XS
V25.39XA V25.39XD V25.39XS V25.41XA V25.41XD
V25.41XS V25.49XA V25.49XD V25.49XS V25.51XA
V25.51XD V25.51XS V25.59XA V25.59XD V25.59XS
V25.91XA V25.91XD V25.91XS V25.99XA V25.99XD
V25.99XS V26.01XA V26.01XD V26.01XS V26.09XA
V26.09XD V26.09XS V26.11XA V26.11XD V26.11XS
V26.19XA V26.19XD V26.19XS V26.21XA V26.21XD
V26.21XS V26.29XA V26.29XD V26.29XS V26.31XA
V26.31XD V26.31XS V26.39XA V26.39XD V26.39XS
V26.41XA V26.41XD V26.41XS V26.49XA V26.49XD
V26.49XS V26.51XA V26.51XD V26.51XS V26.59XA
V26.59XD V26.59XS V26.91XA V26.91XD V26.91XS
V26.99XA V26.99XD V26.99XS V27.01XA V27.01XD
V27.01XS V27.09XA V27.09XD V27.09XS V27.11XA
V27.11XD V27.11XS V27.19XA V27.19XD V27.19XS
V27.21XA V27.21XD V27.21XS V27.29XA V27.29XD
V27.29XS V27.31XA V27.31XD V27.31XS V27.39XA
V27.39XD V27.39XS V27.41XA V27.41XD V27.41XS
V27.49XA V27.49XD V27.49XS V27.51XA V27.51XD
V27.51XS V27.59XA V27.59XD V27.59XS V27.91XA
V27.91XD V27.91XS V27.99XA V27.99XD V27.99XS
V28.01XA V28.01XD V28.01XS V28.09XA V28.09XD
V28.09XS V28.11XA V28.11XD V28.11XS V28.19XA
V28.19XD V28.19XS V28.21XA V28.21XD V28.21XS
V28.29XA V28.29XD V28.29XS V28.31XA V28.31XD
V28.31XS V28.39XA V28.39XD V28.39XS V28.41XA
V28.41XD V28.41XS V28.49XA V28.49XD V28.49XS
V28.51XA V28.51XD V28.51XS V28.59XA V28.59XD
V28.59XS V28.91XA V28.91XD V28.91XS V28.99XA
V28.99XD V28.99XS V29.001A V29.001D V29.001S
V29.008A V29.008D V29.008S V29.091A V29.091D
V29.091S V29.098A V29.098D V29.098S V29.101A
V29.101D V29.101S V29.108A V29.108D V29.108S
V29.191A V29.191D V29.191S V29.198A V29.198D
V29.198S V29.201A V29.201D V29.201S V29.208A
V29.208D V29.208S V29.291A V29.291D V29.291S
V29.298A V29.298D V29.298S V29.31XA V29.31XD
V29.31XS V29.39XA V29.39XD V29.39XS V29.401A
V29.401D V29.401S V29.408A V29.408D V29.408S
V29.491A V29.491D V29.491S V29.498A V29.498D
V29.498S V29.501A V29.501D V29.501S V29.508A
V29.508D V29.508S V29.591A V29.591D V29.591S
V29.598A V29.598D V29.598S V29.601A V29.601D
V29.601S V29.608A V29.608D V29.608S V29.691A
V29.691D V29.691S V29.698A V29.698D V29.698S
V29.811A V29.811D V29.811S V29.818A V29.818D
V29.818S V29.881A V29.881D V29.881S V29.888A
V29.888D V29.888S V29.91XA V29.91XD V29.91XS
V29.99XA V29.99XD V29.99XS W23.2XXA W23.2XXD
W23.2XXS Z03.83 *Z28.310 *Z28.311 *Z28.39
Z59.82 Z59.86 Z59.87 Z71.87 Z71.88
Z72.823 Z79.60 Z79.61 Z79.620 Z79.621
Z79.622 Z79.623 Z79.624 Z79.630 Z79.631
Z79.632 Z79.633 Z79.634 Z79.64 Z79.69
Z79.85 Z87.61 Z87.68 Z87.731 Z87.732
Z87.760 Z87.761 Z87.762 Z87.763 Z87.768
Z91.110 Z91.118 Z91.119 Z91.190 Z91.198
Z91.199 Z91.A10 Z91.A18 Z91.A20 Z91.A28
Z91.A3 Z91.A4 Z91.A5 Z91.A9

28 Revised Codes

Note: Each code is listed with its revised description only.

C84.40 Peripheral T-cell lymphoma, not elsewhere classified, unspecified site

C84.41 Peripheral T-cell lymphoma, not elsewhere classified, lymph nodes of head, face, and neck

C84.42 Peripheral T-cell lymphoma, not elsewhere classified, intrathoracic lymph nodes

C84.43 Peripheral T-cell lymphoma, not elsewhere classified, intra-abdominal lymph nodes

C84.44 Peripheral T-cell lymphoma, not elsewhere classified, lymph nodes of axilla and upper limb

C84.45 Peripheral T-cell lymphoma, not elsewhere classified, lymph nodes of inguinal region and lower limb

C84.46 Peripheral T-cell lymphoma, not elsewhere classified, intrapelvic lymph nodes

C84.47 Peripheral T-cell lymphoma, not elsewhere classified, spleen

C84.48 Peripheral T-cell lymphoma, not elsewhere classified, lymph nodes of multiple sites

C84.49 Peripheral T-cell lymphoma, not elsewhere classified, extranodal and solid organ sites

C94.6 Myelodysplastic disease, not elsewhere classified

FØ1.5Ø Vascular dementia, unspecified severity, without behavioral disturbance, psychotic disturbance, mood disturbance, and anxiety

FØ2.8Ø Dementia in other diseases classified elsewhere, unspecified severity, without behavioral disturbance, psychotic disturbance, mood disturbance, and anxiety

FØ3.9Ø Unspecified dementia, unspecified severity, without behavioral disturbance, psychotic disturbance, mood disturbance, and anxiety

G31.Ø9 Other frontotemporal neurocognitive disorder

G31.83 Neurocognitive disorder with Lewy bodies

G31.84 Mild cognitive impairment of uncertain or unknown etiology

K35.32 Acute appendicitis with perforation, localized peritonitis, and gangrene, without abscess

K35.33 Acute appendicitis with perforation, localized peritonitis, and gangrene, with abscess

M93.Ø11 Acute slipped upper femoral epiphysis, stable (nontraumatic), right hip

M93.Ø12 Acute slipped upper femoral epiphysis, stable (nontraumatic), left hip

M93.Ø13 Acute slipped upper femoral epiphysis, stable (nontraumatic), unspecified hip

M93.Ø21 Chronic slipped upper femoral epiphysis, stable (nontraumatic), right hip

M93.Ø22 Chronic slipped upper femoral epiphysis, stable (nontraumatic), left hip

M93.Ø23 Chronic slipped upper femoral epiphysis, stable (nontraumatic), unspecified hip

M93.Ø31 Acute on chronic slipped upper femoral epiphysis, stable (nontraumatic), right hip

M93.Ø32 Acute on chronic slipped upper femoral epiphysis, stable (nontraumatic), left hip

M93.Ø33 Acute on chronic slipped upper femoral epiphysis, stable (nontraumatic), unspecified hip

251 Deleted Codes

O35.ØXXØ O35.ØXX1 O35.ØXX2 O35.ØXX3 O35.ØXX4
O35.ØXX5 O35.ØXX9 O35.1XXØ O35.1XX1 O35.1XX2
O35.1XX3 O35.1XX4 O35.1XX5 O35.1XX9 V2Ø.ØXXA
V2Ø.ØXXD V2Ø.ØXXS V2Ø.1XXA V2Ø.1XXD V2Ø.1XXS
V2Ø.2XXA V2Ø.2XXD V2Ø.2XXS V2Ø.3XXA V2Ø.3XXD
V2Ø.3XXS V2Ø.4XXA V2Ø.4XXD V2Ø.4XXS V2Ø.5XXA
V2Ø.5XXD V2Ø.5XXS V2Ø.9XXA V2Ø.9XXD V2Ø.9XXS
V21.ØXXA V21.ØXXD V21.ØXXS V21.1XXA V21.1XXD
V21.1XXS V21.2XXA V21.2XXD V21.2XXS V21.3XXA
V21.3XXD V21.3XXS V21.4XXA V21.4XXD V21.4XXS
V21.5XXA V21.5XXD V21.5XXS V21.9XXA V21.9XXD
V21.9XXS V22.ØXXA V22.ØXXD V22.ØXXS V22.1XXA
V22.1XXD V22.1XXS V22.2XXA V22.2XXD V22.2XXS
V22.3XXA V22.3XXD V22.3XXS V22.4XXA V22.4XXD
V22.4XXS V22.5XXA V22.5XXD V22.5XXS V22.9XXA
V22.9XXD V22.9XXS V23.ØXXA V23.ØXXD V23.ØXXS
V23.1XXA V23.1XXD V23.1XXS V23.2XXA V23.2XXD
V23.2XXS V23.3XXA V23.3XXD V23.3XXS V23.4XXA
V23.4XXD V23.4XXS V23.5XXA V23.5XXD V23.5XXS
V23.9XXA V23.9XXD V23.9XXS V24.ØXXA V24.ØXXD
V24.ØXXS V24.1XXA V24.1XXD V24.1XXS V24.2XXA
V24.2XXD V24.2XXS V24.3XXA V24.3XXD V24.3XXS
V24.4XXA V24.4XXD V24.4XXS V24.5XXA V24.5XXD
V24.5XXS V24.9XXA V24.9XXD V24.9XXS V25.ØXXA
V25.ØXXD V25.ØXXS V25.1XXA V25.1XXD V25.1XXS
V25.2XXA V25.2XXD V25.2XXS V25.3XXA V25.3XXD
V25.3XXS V25.4XXA V25.4XXD V25.4XXS V25.5XXA
V25.5XXD V25.5XXS V25.9XXA V25.9XXD V25.9XXS
V26.ØXXA V26.ØXXD V26.ØXXS V26.1XXA V26.1XXD
V26.1XXS V26.2XXA V26.2XXD V26.2XXS V26.3XXA
V26.3XXD V26.3XXS V26.4XXA V26.4XXD V26.4XXS
V26.5XXA V26.5XXD V26.5XXS V26.9XXA V26.9XXD
V26.9XXS V27.ØXXA V27.ØXXD V27.ØXXS V27.1XXA
V27.1XXD V27.1XXS V27.2XXA V27.2XXD V27.2XXS
V27.3XXA V27.3XXD V27.3XXS V27.4XXA V27.4XXD
V27.4XXS V27.5XXA V27.5XXD V27.5XXS V27.9XXA
V27.9XXD V27.9XXS V28.ØXXA V28.ØXXD V28.ØXXS
V28.1XXA V28.1XXD V28.1XXS V28.2XXA V28.2XXD
V28.2XXS V28.3XXA V28.3XXD V28.3XXS V28.4XXA
V28.4XXD V28.4XXS V28.5XXA V28.5XXD V28.5XXS
V28.9XXA V28.9XXD V28.9XXS V29.ØØXA V29.ØØXD
V29.ØØXS V29.Ø9XA V29.Ø9XD V29.Ø9XS V29.1ØXA
V29.1ØXD V29.1ØXS V29.19XA V29.19XD V29.19XS
V29.2ØXA V29.2ØXD V29.2ØXS V29.29XA V29.29XD
V29.29XS V29.3XXA V29.3XXD V29.3XXS V29.4ØXA
V29.4ØXD V29.4ØXS V29.49XA V29.49XD V29.49XS
V29.5ØXA V29.5ØXD V29.5ØXS V29.59XA V29.59XD
V29.59XS V29.6ØXA V29.6ØXD V29.6ØXS V29.69XA
V29.69XD V29.69XS V29.81XA V29.81XD V29.81XS
V29.88XA V29.88XD V29.88XS V29.9XXA V29.9XXD
V29.9XXS

Proprietary Updates

The following proprietary features have also been added:

- New definitions that describe, in lay terms, a specific condition or disease process
- New coding tips that provide coding advice beyond the code classification
- Updated *AHA Coding Clinic* references through second quarter 2022

Conversion Table of ICD-10-CM Codes

The fiscal 2023 (October 1, 2022 - September 30, 2023) Conversion Table for new ICD-10-CM codes is provided to assist users in data retrieval. For each new code the table shows its previously assigned code equivalent. Asterisks identify new codes added to the classification April 1, 2022.

Code Assignment Beginning 10/1/2022	Previous Code(s) Assignment
B37.31	B37.3
B37.32	B37.3
D59.30	D59.3
D59.31	D59.3
D59.32	D59.3
D59.39	D59.3
D68.00	D68.0
D68.01	D68.0
D68.020	D68.0
D68.021	D68.0
D68.022	D68.0
D68.023	D68.0
D68.029	D68.0
D68.03	D68.0
D68.04	D68.0
D68.09	D68.0
D75.821	D75.82
D75.822	D75.82
D75.828	D75.82
D75.829	D75.82
D75.84	D75.89
D81.82	D81.89
E34.30	E34.3
E34.31	E34.3
E34.321	E34.3
E34.322	E34.3
E34.328	E34.3
E34.329	E34.3
E34.39	E34.3
E87.20	E87.2
E87.21	E87.2
E87.22	E87.2
E87.29	E87.2
F01.511	F01.51
F01.518	F01.51
F01.52	F01.51
F01.53	F01.51
F01.54	F01.51
F01.A0	F01.50
F01.A11	F01.51
F01.A18	F01.51
F01.A2	F01.51
F01.A3	F01.51
F01.A4	F01.51
F01.B0	F01.50
F01.B11	F01.51
F01.B18	F01.51
F01.B2	F01.51
F01.B3	F01.51
F01.B4	F01.51
F01.C0	F01.50
F01.C11	F01.51
F01.C18	F01.51
F01.C2	F01.51
F01.C3	F01.51
F01.C4	F01.51
F02.811	F02.81
F02.818	F02.81
F02.82	F02.81
F02.83	F02.81
F02.84	F02.81
F02.A0	F02.80
F02.A11	F02.81
F02.A18	F02.81
F02.A2	F02.81
F02.A3	F02.81
F02.A4	F02.81
F02.B0	F02.80
F02.B11	F02.81
F02.B18	F02.81
F02.B2	F02.81
F02.B3	F02.81
F02.B4	F02.81
F02.C0	F02.80
F02.C11	F02.81
F02.C18	F02.81
F02.C2	F02.81
F02.C3	F02.81
F02.C4	F02.81
F03.911	F03.91
F03.918	F03.91
F03.92	F03.91
F03.93	F03.91
F03.94	F03.91
F03.A0	F03.90
F03.A11	F03.91
F03.A18	F03.91
F03.A2	F03.91
F03.A3	F03.91
F03.A4	F03.91
F03.B0	F03.90
F03.B11	F03.91
F03.B18	F03.91
F03.B2	F03.91
F03.B3	F03.91
F03.B4	F03.91
F03.C0	F03.90
F03.C11	F03.91
F03.C18	F03.91
F03.C2	F03.91
F03.C3	F03.91
F03.C4	F03.91
F06.70	G31.84
F06.71	G31.84
F10.90	Z72.89
F10.91	Z72.89
F11.91	F11.90
F12.91	F12.90
F13.91	F13.90
F14.91	F14.90
F15.91	F15.90
F16.91	F16.90
F18.91	F18.90
F19.91	F19.90
F43.81	F43.8
F43.89	F43.8
G71.031	G71.09
G71.032	G71.09
G71.033	G71.09
G71.0340	G71.09
G71.0341	G71.09
G71.0342	G71.09
G71.0349	G71.09
G71.035	G71.09
G71.038	G71.09
G71.039	G71.09
G90.A	I49.8
G93.31	G93.3
G93.32	G93.3; R53.82
G93.39	G93.3
I20.2	I20.0-I20.1; I20.8
I25.112	I25.110-I25.111; I25.118
I25.702	I25.700-I25.701; I25.708
I25.712	I25.710-I25.711; I25.718
I25.722	I25.720-I25.721; I25.728
I25.732	I25.730-I25.731; I25.738
I25.752	I25.750-I25.751; I25.758
I25.762	I25.760-I25.761; I25.768
I25.792	I25.790-I25.791; I25.798
I31.31	I31.3
I31.39	I31.3
I34.81	I34.8
I34.89	I34.8
I47.20	I47.2
I47.21	I47.2
I47.29	I47.2
I71.010	I71.01
I71.011	I71.01
I71.012	I71.01
I71.019	I71.01
I71.10	I71.1
I71.11	I71.1
I71.12	I71.1
I71.13	I71.1
I71.20	I71.2
I71.21	I71.2
I71.22	I71.2
I71.23	I71.2
I71.30	I71.3
I71.31	I71.3
I71.32	I71.3
I71.33	I71.3
I71.40	I71.4
I71.41	I71.4
I71.42	I71.4
I71.43	I71.4
I71.50	I71.5
I71.51	I71.5
I71.52	I71.5
I71.60	I71.6
I71.61	I71.6
I71.62	I71.6
I77.82	I77.89
J95.87	J95.89
K76.82	K72.90-K72.91
M51.A0	M51.86
M51.A1	M51.86
M51.A2	M51.86
M51.A3	M51.87
M51.A4	M51.87
M51.A5	M51.87
M62.5A0	M62.58
M62.5A1	M62.58
M62.5A2	M62.58
M62.5A9	M62.58
M93.004	M93.001 & M93.002
M93.014	M93.011 & M93.012
M93.024	M93.021 & M93.022
M93.034	M93.031 & M93.032
M93.041	M93.011
M93.042	M93.012
M93.043	M93.013
M93.044	M93.011 & M93.012
M93.051	M93.031
M93.052	M93.032
M93.053	M93.033
M93.054	M93.031 & M93.032
M93.061	M93.011
M93.062	M93.012
M93.063	M93.013
M93.064	M93.011 & M93.012
M93.071	M93.031
M93.072	M93.032
M93.073	M93.033
M93.074	M93.031 & M93.032
M96.A1	M96.89 & Y84.8
M96.A2	M96.89 & Y84.8
M96.A3	M96.89 & Y84.8
M96.A4	M96.89 & Y84.8
M96.A9	M96.89 & Y84.8
N14.11	N14.1
N14.19	N14.1
N76.82	N76.89
N80.00	N80.0
N80.01	N80.0
N80.02	N80.0
N80.03	N80.0
N80.101	N80.1
N80.102	N80.1
N80.103	N80.1
N80.109	N80.1
N80.111	N80.1
N80.112	N80.1
N80.113	N80.1
N80.119	N80.1
N80.121	N80.1
N80.122	N80.1
N80.123	N80.1
N80.129	N80.1
N80.201	N80.2
N80.202	N80.2
N80.203	N80.2
N80.209	N80.2
N80.211	N80.2
N80.212	N80.2
N80.213	N80.2
N80.219	N80.2
N80.221	N80.2
N80.222	N80.2
N80.223	N80.2
N80.229	N80.2
N80.30	N80.3
N80.311	N80.3
N80.312	N80.3
N80.319	N80.3
N80.321	N80.3
N80.322	N80.3
N80.329	N80.3
N80.331	N80.3
N80.332	N80.3
N80.333	N80.3
N80.339	N80.3
N80.341	N80.3
N80.342	N80.3
N80.343	N80.3
N80.349	N80.3
N80.351	N80.3
N80.352	N80.3
N80.353	N80.3
N80.359	N80.3
N80.361	N80.3
N80.362	N80.3
N80.363	N80.3
N80.369	N80.3
N80.371	N80.3
N80.372	N80.3
N80.373	N80.3
N80.379	N80.3
N80.381	N80.3
N80.382	N80.3
N80.383	N80.3
N80.389	N80.3
N80.3A1	N80.3
N80.3A2	N80.3
N80.3A3	N80.3
N80.3A9	N80.3
N80.3B1	N80.3
N80.3B2	N80.3
N80.3B3	N80.3
N80.3B9	N80.3
N80.3C1	N80.3
N80.3C2	N80.3
N80.3C3	N80.3
N80.3C9	N80.3
N80.391	N80.3
N80.392	N80.3
N80.399	N80.3
N80.40	N80.3
N80.41	N80.4
N80.42	N80.4
N80.50	N80.5
N80.511	N80.5
N80.512	N80.5
N80.519	N80.5
N80.521	N80.5
N80.522	N80.5
N80.529	N80.5
N80.531	N80.5
N80.532	N80.5
N80.539	N80.5

Code Assignment Beginning 10/1/2022	Previous Code(s) Assignment	Code Assignment Beginning 10/1/2022	Previous Code(s) Assignment	Code Assignment Beginning 10/1/2022	Previous Code(s) Assignment	Code Assignment Beginning 10/1/2022	Previous Code(s) Assignment	Code Assignment Beginning 10/1/2022	Previous Code(s) Assignment	Code Assignment Beginning 10/1/2022	Previous Code(s) Assignment
N8Ø.541	N8Ø.5	O35.Ø1X3	O35.ØXX3	O35.Ø9X9	O35.ØXX9	O35.BXX2	O35.8XX2	Q21.12	Q21.1	SØ6.81AA	SØ6.819A
N8Ø.542	N8Ø.5	O35.Ø1X4	O35.ØXX4	O35.1ØXØ	O35.1XXØ	O35.BXX3	O35.8XX3	Q21.13	Q21.1	SØ6.81AD	SØ6.819D
N8Ø.549	N8Ø.5	O35.Ø1X5	O35.ØXX5	O35.1ØX1	O35.1XX1	O35.BXX4	O35.8XX4	Q21.14	Q21.1	SØ6.81AS	SØ6.819S
N8Ø.551	N8Ø.5	O35.Ø1X9	O35.ØXX9	O35.1ØX2	O35.1XX2	O35.BXX5	O35.8XX5	Q21.15	Q21.1	SØ6.82AA	SØ6.829A
N8Ø.552	N8Ø.5	O35.Ø2XØ	O35.ØXXØ	O35.1ØX3	O35.1XX3	O35.BXX9	O35.8XX9	Q21.16	Q21.1	SØ6.82AD	SØ6.829D
N8Ø.559	N8Ø.5	O35.Ø2X1	O35.ØXX1	O35.1ØX4	O35.1XX4	O35.CXXØ	O35.8XXØ	Q21.19	Q21.1	SØ6.82AS	SØ6.829S
N8Ø.561	N8Ø.5	O35.Ø2X2	O35.ØXX2	O35.1ØX5	O35.1XX5	O35.CXX1	O35.8XX1	Q21.2Ø	Q21.2	SØ6.8AØA	SØ6.ØXØA
N8Ø.562	N8Ø.5	O35.Ø2X3	O35.ØXX3	O35.1ØX9	O35.1XX9	O35.CXX2	O35.8XX2	Q21.21	Q21.2	SØ6.8AØD	SØ6.ØXØD
N8Ø.569	N8Ø.5	O35.Ø2X4	O35.ØXX4	O35.11XØ	O35.1XXØ	O35.CXX3	O35.8XX3	Q21.22	Q21.2	SØ6.8AØS	SØ6.ØXØS
N8Ø.AØ	N8Ø.8	O35.Ø2X5	O35.ØXX5	O35.11X1	O35.1XX1	O35.CXX4	O35.8XX4	Q21.23	Q21.2	SØ6.8A1A	SØ6.ØX9A
N8Ø.A1	N8Ø.8	O35.Ø2X9	O35.ØXX9	O35.11X2	O35.1XX2	O35.CXX5	O35.8XX5	Q85.81	Q85.8	SØ6.8A1D	SØ6.ØX9D
N8Ø.A2	N8Ø.8	O35.Ø3XØ	O35.ØXXØ	O35.11X3	O35.1XX3	O35.CXX9	O35.8XX9	Q85.82	Q85.8	SØ6.8A1S	SØ6.ØX9S
N8Ø.A41	N8Ø.8	O35.Ø3X1	O35.ØXX1	O35.11X4	O35.1XX4	O35.DXXØ	O35.8XXØ	Q85.83	Q85.8	SØ6.8A2A	SØ6.ØX9A
N8Ø.A42	N8Ø.8	O35.Ø3X2	O35.ØXX2	O35.11X5	O35.1XX5	O35.DXX1	O35.8XX1	Q85.89	Q85.8	SØ6.8A2D	SØ6.ØX9D
N8Ø.A43	N8Ø.8	O35.Ø3X3	O35.ØXX3	O35.11X9	O35.1XX9	O35.DXX2	O35.8XX2	SØ6.ØXAA	SØ6.ØX9A	SØ6.8A2S	SØ6.ØX9S
N8Ø.A49	N8Ø.8	O35.Ø3X4	O35.ØXX4	O35.12XØ	O35.1XXØ	O35.DXX3	O35.8XX3	SØ6.ØXAD	SØ6.ØX9D	SØ6.8A3A	SØ6.ØX9A
N8Ø.A51	N8Ø.8	O35.Ø3X5	O35.ØXX5	O35.12X1	O35.1XX1	O35.DXX4	O35.8XX4	SØ6.ØXAS	SØ6.ØX9S	SØ6.8A3D	SØ6.ØX9D
N8Ø.A52	N8Ø.8	O35.Ø3X9	O35.ØXX9	O35.12X2	O35.1XX2	O35.DXX5	O35.8XX5	SØ6.1XAA	SØ6.1X9A	SØ6.8A3S	SØ6.ØX9S
N8Ø.A53	N8Ø.8	O35.Ø4XØ	O35.ØXXØ	O35.12X3	O35.1XX3	O35.DXX9	O35.8XX9	SØ6.1XAD	SØ6.1X9D	SØ6.8A4A	SØ6.ØX9A
N8Ø.A59	N8Ø.8	O35.Ø4X1	O35.ØXX1	O35.12X4	O35.1XX4	O35.EXXØ	O35.8XXØ	SØ6.1XAS	SØ6.1X9S	SØ6.8A4D	SØ6.ØX9D
N8Ø.A61	N8Ø.8	O35.Ø4X2	O35.ØXX2	O35.12X5	O35.1XX5	O35.EXX1	O35.8XX1	SØ6.2XAA	SØ6.2X9A	SØ6.8A4S	SØ6.ØX9S
N8Ø.A62	N8Ø.8	O35.Ø4X3	O35.ØXX3	O35.12X9	O35.1XX9	O35.EXX2	O35.8XX2	SØ6.2XAD	SØ6.2X9D	SØ6.8A5A	SØ6.ØX9A
N8Ø.A63	N8Ø.8	O35.Ø4X4	O35.ØXX4	O35.13XØ	O35.1XXØ	O35.EXX3	O35.8XX3	SØ6.2XAS	SØ6.2X9S	SØ6.8A5D	SØ6.ØX9D
N8Ø.A69	N8Ø.8	O35.Ø4X5	O35.ØXX5	O35.13X1	O35.1XX1	O35.EXX4	O35.8XX4	SØ6.3ØAA	SØ6.3Ø9A	SØ6.8A5S	SØ6.ØX9S
N8Ø.B1	N8Ø.8	O35.Ø4X9	O35.ØXX9	O35.13X2	O35.1XX2	O35.EXX5	O35.8XX5	SØ6.3ØAD	SØ6.3Ø9D	SØ6.8A6A	SØ6.ØX9A
N8Ø.B2	N8Ø.8	O35.Ø5XØ	O35.ØXXØ	O35.13X3	O35.1XX3	O35.EXX9	O35.8XX9	SØ6.3ØAS	SØ6.3Ø9S	SØ6.8A6D	SØ6.ØX9D
N8Ø.B31	N8Ø.8	O35.Ø5X1	O35.ØXX1	O35.13X4	O35.1XX4	O35.FXXØ	O35.8XXØ	SØ6.31AA	SØ6.319A	SØ6.8A6S	SØ6.ØX9S
N8Ø.B32	N8Ø.8	O35.Ø5X2	O35.ØXX2	O35.13X5	O35.1XX5	O35.FXX1	O35.8XX1	SØ6.31AD	SØ6.319D	SØ6.8A7A	SØ6.ØX9A
N8Ø.B39	N8Ø.8	O35.Ø5X3	O35.ØXX3	O35.13X9	O35.1XX9	O35.FXX2	O35.8XX2	SØ6.31AS	SØ6.319S	SØ6.8A8A	SØ6.ØX9A
N8Ø.B4	N8Ø.8	O35.Ø5X4	O35.ØXX4	O35.14XØ	O35.1XXØ	O35.FXX3	O35.8XX3	SØ6.32AA	SØ6.329A	SØ6.8AAA	SØ6.ØX9A
N8Ø.B5	N8Ø.8	O35.Ø5X5	O35.ØXX5	O35.14X1	O35.1XX1	O35.FXX4	O35.8XX4	SØ6.32AD	SØ6.329D	SØ6.8AAD	SØ6.ØX9D
N8Ø.B6	N8Ø.8	O35.Ø5X9	O35.ØXX9	O35.14X2	O35.1XX2	O35.FXX5	O35.8XX5	SØ6.32AS	SØ6.329S	SØ6.8AAS	SØ6.ØX9S
N8Ø.CØ	N8Ø.8	O35.Ø6XØ	O35.ØXXØ	O35.14X3	O35.1XX3	O35.FXX9	O35.8XX9	SØ6.33AA	SØ6.339A	SØ6.8A9A	SØ6.ØX9A
N8Ø.C1Ø	N8Ø.8	O35.Ø6X1	O35.ØXX1	O35.14X4	O35.1XX4	O35.GXXØ	O35.8XXØ	SØ6.33AD	SØ6.339D	SØ6.8A9D	SØ6.ØX9D
N8Ø.C11	N8Ø.8	O35.Ø6X2	O35.ØXX2	O35.14X5	O35.1XX5	O35.GXX1	O35.8XX1	SØ6.33AS	SØ6.339S	SØ6.8A9S	SØ6.ØX9S
N8Ø.C19	N8Ø.8	O35.Ø6X3	O35.ØXX3	O35.14X9	O35.1XX9	O35.GXX2	O35.8XX2	SØ6.34AA	SØ6.349A	SØ6.89AA	SØ6.ØX9A
N8Ø.C2	N8Ø.8	O35.Ø6X4	O35.ØXX4	O35.15XØ	O35.1XXØ	O35.GXX3	O35.8XX3	SØ6.34AD	SØ6.349D	SØ6.89AD	SØ6.ØX9D
N8Ø.C3	N8Ø.8	O35.Ø6X5	O35.ØXX5	O35.15X1	O35.1XX1	O35.GXX4	O35.8XX4	SØ6.34AS	SØ6.349S	SØ6.89AS	SØ6.ØX9S
N8Ø.C4	N8Ø.8	O35.Ø6X9	O35.ØXX9	O35.15X2	O35.1XX2	O35.GXX5	O35.8XX5	SØ6.35AA	SØ6.359A	SØ6.9XAA	SØ6.9X9A
N8Ø.C9	N8Ø.8	O35.Ø7XØ	O35.ØXXØ	O35.15X3	O35.1XX3	O35.GXX9	O35.8XX9	SØ6.35AD	SØ6.359D	SØ6.9XAD	SØ6.9X9D
N8Ø.DØ	N8Ø.8	O35.Ø7X1	O35.ØXX1	O35.15X4	O35.1XX4	O35.HXXØ	O35.8XXØ	SØ6.35AS	SØ6.359S	SØ6.9XAS	SØ6.9X9S
N8Ø.D1	N8Ø.8	O35.Ø7X2	O35.ØXX2	O35.15X5	O35.1XX5	O35.HXX1	O35.8XX1	SØ6.36AA	SØ6.369A	T43.651A	T43.621A
N8Ø.D2	N8Ø.8	O35.Ø7X3	O35.ØXX3	O35.15X9	O35.1XX9	O35.HXX2	O35.8XX2	SØ6.36AD	SØ6.369D	T43.651D	T43.621D
N8Ø.D3	N8Ø.8	O35.Ø7X4	O35.ØXX4	O35.19XØ	O35.1XXØ	O35.HXX3	O35.8XX3	SØ6.36AS	SØ6.369S	T43.651S	T43.621S
N8Ø.D4	N8Ø.8	O35.Ø7X5	O35.ØXX5	O35.19X1	O35.1XX1	O35.HXX4	O35.8XX4	SØ6.37AA	SØ6.379A	T43.652A	T43.622A
N8Ø.D5	N8Ø.8	O35.Ø7X9	O35.ØXX9	O35.19X2	O35.1XX2	O35.HXX5	O35.8XX5	SØ6.37AD	SØ6.379D	T43.652D	T43.621D
N8Ø.D6	N8Ø.8	O35.Ø8XØ	O35.ØXXØ	O35.19X3	O35.1XX3	O35.HXX9	O35.8XX9	SØ6.37AS	SØ6.379S	T43.652S	T43.621S
N8Ø.D9	N8Ø.8	O35.Ø8X1	O35.ØXX1	O35.19X4	O35.1XX4	P28.3Ø	P28.3	SØ6.38AA	SØ6.389A	T43.653A	T43.623A
N85.A	N85.8	O35.Ø8X2	O35.ØXX2	O35.19X5	O35.1XX5	P28.31	P28.3	SØ6.38AD	SØ6.389D	T43.653D	T43.623D
O35.ØØXØ	O35.ØXXØ	O35.Ø8X3	O35.ØXX3	O35.19X9	O35.1XX9	P28.32	P28.3	SØ6.38AS	SØ6.389S	T43.653S	T43.623S
O35.ØØX1	O35.ØXX1	O35.Ø8X4	O35.ØXX4	O35.AXXØ	O35.8XXØ	P28.33	P28.3	SØ6.4XAA	SØ6.4X9A	T43.654A	T43.624A
O35.ØØX2	O35.ØXX2	O35.Ø8X5	O35.ØXX5	O35.AXX1	O35.8XX1	P28.39	P28.3	SØ6.4XAD	SØ6.4X9D	T43.654D	T43.624D
O35.ØØX3	O35.ØXX3	O35.Ø8X9	O35.ØXX9	O35.AXX2	O35.8XX2	P28.4Ø	P28.4	SØ6.4XAS	SØ6.4X9S	T43.654S	T43.624S
O35.ØØX4	O35.ØXX4	O35.Ø9XØ	O35.ØXXØ	O35.AXX3	O35.8XX3	P28.41	P28.4	SØ6.5XAA	SØ6.5X9A	T43.655A	T43.625A
O35.ØØX5	O35.ØXX5	O35.Ø9X1	O35.ØXX1	O35.AXX4	O35.8XX4	P28.42	P28.4	SØ6.5XAD	SØ6.5X9D	T43.655D	T43.625D
O35.ØØX9	O35.ØXX9	O35.Ø9X2	O35.ØXX2	O35.AXX5	O35.8XX5	P28.43	P28.4	SØ6.5XAS	SØ6.5X9S	T43.655S	T43.625S
O35.Ø1XØ	O35.ØXXØ	O35.Ø9X3	O35.ØXX3	O35.AXX9	O35.8XX9	P28.49	P28.4	SØ6.6XAA	SØ6.6X9A	T43.656A	T43.626A
O35.Ø1X1	O35.ØXX1	O35.Ø9X4	O35.ØXX4	O35.BXXØ	O35.8XXØ	Q21.1Ø	Q21.1	SØ6.6XAD	SØ6.6X9D	T43.656D	T43.626D
O35.Ø1X2	O35.ØXX2	O35.Ø9X5	O35.ØXX5	O35.BXX1	O35.8XX1	Q21.11	Q21.1	SØ6.6XAS	SØ6.6X9S	T43.656S	T43.626S

Code Assignment Beginning 10/1/2022	Previous Code(s) Assignment
V20.01XA	V20.0XXA
V20.01XD	V20.0XXD
V20.01XS	V20.0XXS
V20.09XA	V20.0XXA
V20.09XD	V20.0XXD
V20.09XS	V20.0XXS
V20.11XA	V20.1XXA
V20.11XD	V20.1XXD
V20.11XS	V20.1XXS
V20.19XA	V20.1XXA
V20.19XD	V20.1XXD
V20.19XS	V20.1XXS
V20.21XA	V20.2XXA
V20.21XD	V20.2XXD
V20.21XS	V20.2XXS
V20.29XA	V20.2XXA
V20.29XD	V20.2XXD
V20.29XS	V20.2XXS
V20.31XA	V20.3XXA
V20.31XD	V20.3XXD
V20.31XS	V20.3XXS
V20.39XA	V20.3XXA
V20.39XD	V20.3XXD
V20.39XS	V20.3XXS
V20.41XA	V20.4XXA
V20.41XD	V20.4XXD
V20.41XS	V20.4XXS
V20.49XA	V20.4XXA
V20.49XD	V20.4XXD
V20.49XS	V20.4XXS
V20.51XA	V20.5XXA
V20.51XD	V20.5XXD
V20.51XS	V20.5XXS
V20.59XA	V20.5XXA
V20.59XD	V20.5XXD
V20.59XS	V20.5XXS
V20.91XA	V20.9XXA
V20.91XD	V20.9XXD
V20.91XS	V20.9XXS
V20.99XA	V20.9XXA
V20.99XD	V20.9XXD
V20.99XS	V20.9XXS
V21.01XA	V21.0XXA
V21.01XD	V21.0XXD
V21.01XS	V21.0XXS
V21.09XA	V21.0XXA
V21.09XD	V21.0XXD
V21.09XS	V21.0XXS
V21.11XA	V21.1XXA
V21.11XD	V21.1XXD
V21.11XS	V21.1XXS
V21.19XA	V21.1XXA
V21.19XD	V21.1XXD
V21.19XS	V21.1XXS
V21.21XA	V21.2XXA
V21.21XD	V21.2XXD
V21.21XS	V21.2XXS
V21.29XA	V21.2XXA
V21.29XD	V21.2XXD
V21.29XS	V21.2XXS
V21.31XA	V21.3XXA
V21.31XD	V21.3XXD
V21.31XS	V21.3XXS
V21.39XA	V21.3XXA
V21.39XD	V21.3XXD
V21.39XS	V21.3XXS
V21.41XA	V21.4XXA
V21.41XD	V21.4XXD
V21.41XS	V21.4XXS
V21.49XA	V21.4XXA
V21.49XD	V21.4XXD
V21.49XS	V21.4XXS
V21.51XA	V21.5XXA
V21.51XD	V21.5XXD
V21.51XS	V21.5XXS
V21.59XA	V21.5XXA
V21.59XD	V21.5XXD
V21.59XS	V21.5XXS
V21.91XA	V21.9XXA
V21.91XD	V21.9XXD
V21.91XS	V21.9XXS
V21.99XA	V21.9XXA
V21.99XD	V21.9XXD
V21.99XS	V21.9XXS
V22.01XA	V22.0XXA
V22.01XD	V22.0XXD
V22.01XS	V22.0XXS
V22.09XA	V22.0XXA
V22.09XD	V22.0XXD
V22.09XS	V22.0XXS
V22.11XA	V22.1XXA
V22.11XD	V22.1XXD
V22.11XS	V22.1XXS
V22.19XA	V22.1XXA
V22.19XD	V22.1XXD
V22.19XS	V22.1XXS
V22.21XA	V22.2XXA
V22.21XD	V22.2XXD
V22.21XS	V22.2XXS
V22.29XA	V22.2XXA
V22.29XD	V22.2XXD
V22.29XS	V22.2XXS
V22.31XA	V22.3XXA
V22.31XD	V22.3XXD
V22.31XS	V22.3XXS
V22.39XA	V22.3XXA
V22.39XD	V22.3XXD
V22.39XS	V22.3XXS
V22.41XA	V22.4XXA
V22.41XD	V22.4XXD
V22.41XS	V22.4XXS
V22.49XA	V22.4XXA
V22.49XD	V22.4XXD
V22.49XS	V22.4XXS
V22.51XA	V22.5XXA
V22.51XD	V22.5XXD
V22.51XS	V22.5XXS
V22.59XA	V22.5XXA
V22.59XD	V22.5XXD
V22.59XS	V22.5XXS
V22.91XA	V22.9XXA
V22.91XD	V22.9XXD
V22.91XS	V22.9XXS
V22.99XA	V22.9XXA
V22.99XD	V22.9XXD
V22.99XS	V22.9XXS
V23.01XA	V23.0XXA
V23.01XD	V23.0XXD
V23.01XS	V23.0XXS
V23.09XA	V23.0XXA
V23.09XD	V23.0XXD
V23.09XS	V23.0XXS
V23.11XA	V23.1XXA
V23.11XD	V23.1XXD
V23.11XS	V23.1XXS
V23.19XA	V23.1XXA
V23.19XD	V23.1XXD
V23.19XS	V23.1XXS
V23.21XA	V23.2XXA
V23.21XD	V23.2XXD
V23.21XS	V23.2XXS
V23.29XA	V23.2XXA
V23.29XD	V23.2XXD
V23.29XS	V23.2XXS
V23.31XA	V23.3XXA
V23.31XD	V23.3XXD
V23.31XS	V23.3XXS
V23.39XA	V23.3XXA
V23.39XD	V23.3XXD
V23.39XS	V23.3XXS
V23.41XA	V23.4XXA
V23.41XD	V23.4XXD
V23.41XS	V23.4XXS
V23.49XA	V23.4XXA
V23.49XD	V23.4XXD
V23.49XS	V23.4XXS
V23.51XA	V23.5XXA
V23.51XD	V23.5XXD
V23.51XS	V23.5XXS
V23.59XA	V23.5XXA
V23.59XD	V23.5XXD
V23.59XS	V23.5XXS
V23.91XA	V23.9XXA
V23.91XD	V23.9XXD
V23.91XS	V23.9XXS
V23.99XA	V23.9XXA
V23.99XD	V23.9XXD
V23.99XS	V23.9XXS
V24.01XA	V24.0XXA
V24.01XD	V24.0XXD
V24.01XS	V24.0XXS
V24.09XA	V24.0XXA
V24.09XD	V24.0XXD
V24.09XS	V24.0XXS
V24.11XA	V24.1XXA
V24.11XD	V24.1XXD
V24.11XS	V24.1XXS
V24.19XA	V24.1XXA
V24.19XD	V24.1XXD
V24.19XS	V24.1XXS
V24.21XA	V24.2XXA
V24.21XD	V24.2XXD
V24.21XS	V24.2XXS
V24.29XA	V24.2XXA
V24.29XD	V24.2XXD
V24.29XS	V24.2XXS
V24.31XA	V24.3XXA
V24.31XD	V24.3XXD
V24.31XS	V24.3XXS
V24.39XA	V24.3XXA
V24.39XD	V24.3XXD
V24.39XS	V24.3XXS
V24.41XA	V24.4XXA
V24.41XD	V24.4XXD
V24.41XS	V24.4XXS
V24.49XA	V24.4XXA
V24.49XD	V24.4XXD
V24.49XS	V24.4XXS
V24.51XA	V24.5XXA
V24.51XD	V24.5XXD
V24.51XS	V24.5XXS
V24.59XA	V24.5XXA
V24.59XD	V24.5XXD
V24.59XS	V24.5XXS
V24.91XA	V24.9XXA
V24.91XD	V24.9XXD
V24.91XS	V24.9XXS
V24.99XA	V24.9XXA
V24.99XD	V24.9XXD
V24.99XS	V24.9XXS
V25.01XA	V25.0XXA
V25.01XD	V25.0XXD
V25.01XS	V25.0XXS
V25.09XA	V25.0XXA
V25.09XD	V25.0XXD
V25.09XS	V25.0XXS
V25.11XA	V25.1XXA
V25.11XD	V25.1XXD
V25.11XS	V25.1XXS
V25.19XA	V25.1XXA
V25.19XD	V25.1XXD
V25.19XS	V25.1XXS
V25.21XA	V25.2XXA
V25.21XD	V25.2XXD
V25.21XS	V25.2XXS
V25.29XA	V25.2XXA
V25.29XD	V25.2XXD
V25.29XS	V25.2XXS
V25.31XA	V25.3XXA
V25.31XD	V25.3XXD
V25.31XS	V25.3XXS
V25.39XA	V25.3XXA
V25.39XD	V25.3XXD
V25.39XS	V25.3XXS
V25.41XA	V25.4XXA
V25.41XD	V25.4XXD
V25.41XS	V25.4XXS
V25.49XA	V25.4XXA
V25.49XD	V25.4XXD
V25.49XS	V25.4XXS
V25.51XA	V25.5XXA
V25.51XD	V25.5XXD
V25.51XS	V25.5XXS
V25.59XA	V25.5XXA
V25.59XD	V25.5XXD
V25.59XS	V25.5XXS
V25.91XA	V25.9XXA
V25.91XD	V25.9XXD
V25.91XS	V25.9XXS
V25.99XA	V25.9XXA
V25.99XD	V25.9XXD
V25.99XS	V25.9XXS
V26.01XA	V26.0XXA
V26.01XD	V26.0XXD
V26.01XS	V26.0XXS
V26.09XA	V26.0XXA
V26.09XD	V26.0XXD
V26.09XS	V26.0XXS
V26.11XA	V26.1XXA
V26.11XD	V26.1XXD
V26.11XS	V26.1XXS
V26.19XA	V26.1XXA
V26.19XD	V26.1XXD
V26.19XS	V26.1XXS
V26.21XA	V26.2XXA
V26.21XD	V26.2XXD
V26.21XS	V26.2XXS
V26.29XA	V26.2XXA
V26.29XD	V26.2XXD
V26.29XS	V26.2XXS
V26.31XA	V26.3XXA
V26.31XD	V26.3XXD
V26.31XS	V26.3XXS
V26.39XA	V26.3XXA
V26.39XD	V26.3XXD
V26.39XS	V26.3XXS
V26.41XA	V26.4XXA
V26.41XD	V26.4XXD
V26.41XS	V26.4XXS
V26.49XA	V26.4XXA
V26.49XD	V26.4XXD
V26.49XS	V26.4XXS
V26.51XA	V26.5XXA
V26.51XD	V26.5XXD
V26.51XS	V26.5XXS
V26.59XA	V26.5XXA
V26.59XD	V26.5XXD
V26.59XS	V26.5XXS
V26.91XA	V26.9XXA
V26.91XD	V26.9XXD
V26.91XS	V26.9XXS
V26.99XA	V26.9XXA
V26.99XD	V26.9XXD
V26.99XS	V26.9XXS
V27.01XA	V27.0XXA
V27.01XD	V27.0XXD
V27.01XS	V27.0XXS
V27.09XA	V27.0XXA
V27.09XD	V27.0XXD
V27.09XS	V27.0XXS
V27.11XA	V27.1XXA
V27.11XD	V27.1XXD
V27.11XS	V27.1XXS
V27.19XA	V27.1XXA
V27.19XD	V27.1XXD
V27.19XS	V27.1XXS
V27.21XA	V27.2XXA
V27.21XD	V27.2XXD
V27.21XS	V27.2XXS
V27.29XA	V27.2XXA
V27.29XD	V27.2XXD
V27.29XS	V27.2XXS
V27.31XA	V27.3XXA
V27.31XD	V27.3XXD
V27.31XS	V27.3XXS
V27.39XA	V27.3XXA
V27.39XD	V27.3XXD
V27.39XS	V27.3XXS
V27.41XA	V27.4XXA
V27.41XD	V27.4XXD
V27.41XS	V27.4XXS
V27.49XA	V27.4XXA
V27.49XD	V27.4XXD
V27.49XS	V27.4XXS
V27.51XA	V27.5XXA
V27.51XD	V27.5XXD
V27.51XS	V27.5XXS
V27.59XA	V27.5XXA
V27.59XD	V27.5XXD
V27.59XS	V27.5XXS
V27.91XA	V27.9XXA
V27.91XD	V27.9XXD
V27.91XS	V27.9XXS
V27.99XA	V27.9XXA
V27.99XD	V27.9XXD
V27.99XS	V27.9XXS
V28.01XA	V28.0XXA
V28.01XD	V28.0XXD
V28.01XS	V28.0XXS
V28.09XA	V28.0XXA
V28.09XD	V28.0XXD
V28.09XS	V28.0XXS
V28.11XA	V28.1XXA
V28.11XD	V28.1XXD
V28.11XS	V28.1XXS
V28.19XA	V28.1XXA
V28.19XD	V28.1XXD
V28.19XS	V28.1XXS
V28.21XA	V28.2XXA
V28.21XD	V28.2XXD
V28.21XS	V28.2XXS
V28.29XA	V28.2XXA
V28.29XD	V28.2XXD
V28.29XS	V28.2XXS

Code Assignment Beginning 10/1/2022	Previous Code(s) Assignment
V28.31XA	V28.3XXA
V28.31XD	V28.3XXD
V28.31XS	V28.3XXS
V28.39XA	V28.3XXA
V28.39XD	V28.3XXD
V28.39XS	V28.3XXS
V28.41XA	V28.4XXA
V28.41XD	V28.4XXD
V28.41XS	V28.4XXS
V28.49XA	V28.4XXA
V28.49XD	V28.4XXD
V28.49XS	V28.4XXS
V28.51XA	V28.5XXA
V28.51XD	V28.5XXD
V28.51XS	V28.5XXS
V28.59XA	V28.5XXA
V28.59XD	V28.5XXD
V28.59XS	V28.5XXS
V28.91XA	V28.9XXA
V28.91XD	V28.9XXD
V28.91XS	V28.9XXS
V28.99XA	V28.9XXA
V28.99XD	V28.9XXD
V28.99XS	V28.9XXS
V29.ØØ1A	V29.ØØXA
V29.ØØ1D	V29.ØØXD
V29.ØØ1S	V29.ØØXS
V29.ØØ8A	V29.ØØXA
V29.ØØ8D	V29.ØØXD
V29.ØØ8S	V29.ØØXS
V29.Ø91A	V29.Ø9XA
V29.Ø91D	V29.Ø9XD
V29.Ø91S	V29.Ø9XS

Code Assignment Beginning 10/1/2022	Previous Code(s) Assignment
V29.Ø98A	V29.Ø9XA
V29.Ø98D	V29.Ø9XD
V29.Ø98S	V29.Ø9XS
V29.1Ø1A	V29.1ØXA
V29.1Ø1D	V29.1ØXD
V29.1Ø1S	V29.1ØXS
V29.1Ø8A	V29.1ØXA
V29.1Ø8D	V29.1ØXD
V29.1Ø8S	V29.1ØXS
V29.191A	V29.19XA
V29.191D	V29.19XD
V29.191S	V29.19XS
V29.198A	V29.19XA
V29.198D	V29.19XD
V29.198S	V29.19XS
V29.2Ø1A	V29.2ØXA
V29.2Ø1D	V29.2ØXD
V29.2Ø1S	V29.2ØXS
V29.2Ø8A	V29.2ØXA
V29.2Ø8D	V29.2ØXD
V29.2Ø8S	V29.2ØXS
V29.291A	V29.29XA
V29.291D	V29.29XD
V29.291S	V29.29XS
V29.298A	V29.29XA
V29.298D	V29.29XD
V29.298S	V29.29XS
V29.31XA	V29.3XXA
V29.31XD	V29.3XXD
V29.31XS	V29.3XXS
V29.39XA	V29.3XXA
V29.39XD	V29.3XXD
V29.39XS	V29.3XXS

Code Assignment Beginning 10/1/2022	Previous Code(s) Assignment
V29.4Ø1A	V29.4ØXA
V29.4Ø1D	V29.4ØXD
V29.4Ø1S	V29.4ØXS
V29.4Ø8A	V29.4ØXA
V29.4Ø8D	V29.4ØXD
V29.4Ø8S	V29.4ØXS
V29.491A	V29.49XA
V29.491D	V29.49XD
V29.491S	V29.49XS
V29.498A	V29.49XA
V29.498D	V29.49XD
V29.498S	V29.49XS
V29.5Ø1A	V29.5ØXA
V29.5Ø1D	V29.5ØXD
V29.5Ø1S	V29.5ØXS
V29.5Ø8A	V29.5ØXA
V29.5Ø8D	V29.5ØXD
V29.5Ø8S	V29.5ØXS
V29.591A	V29.59XA
V29.591D	V29.59XD
V29.591S	V29.59XS
V29.598A	V29.59XA
V29.598D	V29.59XD
V29.598S	V29.59XS
V29.6Ø1A	V29.6ØXA
V29.6Ø1D	V29.6ØXD
V29.6Ø1S	V29.6ØXS
V29.6Ø8A	V29.6ØXA
V29.6Ø8D	V29.6ØXD
V29.6Ø8S	V29.6ØXS
V29.691A	V29.69XA
V29.691D	V29.69XD
V29.691S	V29.69XS

Code Assignment Beginning 10/1/2022	Previous Code(s) Assignment
V29.698A	V29.69XA
V29.698D	V29.69XD
V29.698S	V29.69XS
V29.811A	V29.8ØXA
V29.811D	V29.8ØXD
V29.811S	V29.8ØXS
V29.818A	V29.8ØXA
V29.818D	V29.8ØXD
V29.818S	V29.8ØXS
V29.881A	V29.89XA
V29.881D	V29.89XD
V29.881S	V29.89XS
V29.888A	V29.89XA
V29.888D	V29.89XD
V29.888S	V29.89XS
V29.91XA	V29.9XXA
V29.91XD	V29.9XXD
V29.91XS	V29.9XXS
V29.99XA	V29.9XXA
V29.99XD	V29.9XXD
V29.99XS	V29.9XXS
W23.2XXA	W23.ØXXA & W23.1XXA
W23.2XXD	W23.ØXXD & W23.1XXD
W23.2XXS	W23.ØXXS & W23.1XXS
ZØ3.83	ZØ3.89
*Z28.31Ø	Z28.3
*Z28.311	Z28.3
*Z28.39	Z28.3
Z59.82	Z59.89

Code Assignment Beginning 10/1/2022	Previous Code(s) Assignment
Z59.86	Z59.89
Z59.87	Z59.89
Z71.87	Z71.89
Z71.88	Z71.89
Z72.823	Z72.89
Z79.6Ø	Z79.899
Z79.61	Z79.899
Z79.62Ø	Z79.899
Z79.621	Z79.899
Z79.622	Z79.899
Z79.623	Z79.899
Z79.624	Z79.899
Z79.63Ø	Z79.899
Z79.631	Z79.899
Z79.632	Z79.899
Z79.633	Z79.899
Z79.634	Z79.899
Z79.64	Z79.899
Z79.69	Z79.899
Z79.85	Z79.899
Z87.61	Z87.898
Z87.68	Z87.898
Z87.731	Z87.738
Z87.732	Z87.738
Z87.76Ø	Z87.76
Z87.761	Z87.76
Z87.762	Z87.76
Z87.763	Z87.76
Z87.768	Z87.76
Z91.11Ø	Z91.11
Z91.118	Z91.11
Z91.119	Z91.11
Z91.19Ø	Z91.19

Code Assignment Beginning 10/1/2022	Previous Code(s) Assignment
Z91.198	Z91.19
Z91.199	Z91.19
Z91.A1Ø	Z91.19
Z91.A18	Z91.19
Z91.A2Ø	Z91.19
Z91.A28	Z91.19
Z91.A3	Z91.19
Z91.A4	Z91.19
Z91.A5	Z91.19
Z91.A9	Z91.19

10 Steps to Correct Coding

Follow the 10 steps below to correctly code encounters for health care services.

Step 1: Identify the reason for the visit or encounter (i.e., a sign, symptom, diagnosis and/or condition).

The medical record documentation should accurately reflect the patient's condition, using terminology that includes specific diagnoses and symptoms or clearly states the reasons for the encounter.

Choosing the main term that best describes the reason chiefly responsible for the service provided is the most important step in coding. If symptoms are present and documented but a definitive diagnosis has not yet been determined, code the symptoms. *For outpatient cases, do not code conditions that are referred to as "rule out," "suspected," "probable," or "questionable."* Diagnoses often are not established at the time of the initial encounter/visit and may require two or more visits to be established. Code only what is documented in the available outpatient records and only to the highest degree of certainty known at the time of the patient's visit. For inpatient medical records, uncertain diagnoses may be reported if documented at the time of discharge.

Step 2: After selecting the reason for the encounter, consult the alphabetic index.

The most critical rule is to begin code selection in the alphabetic index. Never turn first to the tabular list. The index provides cross-references, essential and nonessential modifiers, and other instructional notations that may not be found in the tabular list.

Step 3: Locate the main term entry.

The alphabetic index lists conditions, which may be expressed as nouns or eponyms, with critical use of adjectives. Some conditions known by several names have multiple main entries. Reasons for encounters may be located under general terms such as admission, encounter, and examination. Other general terms such as history, status (post), or presence (of) can be used to locate other factors influencing health.

Step 4: Scan subterm entries.

Scan the subterm entries, as appropriate, being sure to review continued lines and additional subterms that may appear in the next column or on the next page. Shaded vertical guidelines in the index indicate the indentation level for each subterm in relation to the main terms.

Step 5: Pay close attention to index instructions.

- Parentheses ( ) enclose nonessential modifiers, terms that are supplementary words or explanatory information that may or may not appear in the diagnostic statement and do not affect code selection.
- Brackets [ ] enclose manifestation codes that can be used only as secondary codes to the underlying condition code immediately preceding it. If used, manifestation codes must be reported with the appropriate etiology codes.
- Default codes are listed next to the main term and represent the condition most commonly associated with the main term or the unspecified code for the main term.
- "*See*" cross-references, identified by italicized type and "code by" cross-references indicate that another term *must be referenced* to locate the correct code.
- "*See also*" cross-references, identified by italicized type, provide alternative terms that may be useful to look up but *are not mandatory*.
- "Omit code" cross-references identify instances when a code is not applicable depending on the condition being coded.
- "With" subterms are listed out of alphabetic order and identify a presumed causal relationship between the two conditions they link.
- "Due to" subterms identify a relationship between the two conditions they link.
- "NEC," abbreviation for "not elsewhere classified," follows some main terms or subterms and indicates that there is no specific code for the condition even though the medical documentation may be very specific.
- "NOS," abbreviation for "not otherwise specified," follows some main terms or subterms and is the equivalent of unspecified; NOS signifies that the information in the medical record is insufficient for assigning a more specific code.
- *Following* references help coders locate alphanumeric codes that are out of sequence in the tabular section.
- Check-additional-character symbols flag codes that require additional characters to make the code valid; the characters available to complete the code should be verified in the tabular section.

Step 6: Choose a potential code and locate it in the tabular list.

To prevent coding errors, always use both the alphabetic index (to identify a code) and the tabular list (to verify a code), as the index does not include the important instructional notes found in the tabular list. An added benefit of using the tabular list, which groups like things together, is that while looking at one code in the list, a coder might see a more specific one that would have been missed had the coder relied solely on the alphabetic index. Additionally, many of the codes require a fourth, fifth, sixth, or seventh character to be valid, and many of these characters can be found only in the tabular list.

Step 7: Read all instructional material in the tabular section.

The coder must follow any Includes, Excludes 1 and Excludes 2 notes, and other instructional notes, such as "Code first" and "Use additional code," listed in the tabular list for the chapter, category, subcategory, and subclassification levels of code selection that direct the coder to use a different or additional code. Any codes in the tabular range AØØ.Ø- through T88.9- may be used to identify the diagnostic reason for the encounter. The tabular list encompasses many codes describing disease and injury classifications (e.g., infectious and parasitic diseases, neoplasms, symptoms, nervous and circulatory system, etc.).

Codes that describe symptoms and signs, as opposed to definitive diagnoses, should be reported when an established diagnosis has not been made (confirmed) by the physician. Chapter 18 of the ICD-10-CM code book, "Symptoms, Signs, and Abnormal Clinical and Laboratory Findings, Not Elsewhere Classified" (codes RØØ–R99), contains many, but not all, codes for symptoms.

ICD-10-CM classifies encounters with health care providers for circumstances other than a disease or injury in chapter 21, "Factors Influencing Health Status and Contact with Health Services" (codes ZØØ–Z99). Circumstances other than a disease or injury often are recorded as chiefly responsible for the encounter.

A code is invalid if it does not include the full number of characters (greatest level of specificity) required. Codes in ICD-10-CM can contain from three to seven alphanumeric characters. A three-character code is to be used only if the category is not further subdivided into four-, five-, six-, or seven-character codes. Placeholder character X is used as part of an alphanumeric code to allow for future expansion and as a placeholder for empty characters in a code that requires a seventh character but has no fourth, fifth, or sixth character. Note that certain categories require seventh characters that apply to all codes in that category. Always check the category level for applicable seventh characters for that category.

Step 8: Consult the official ICD-10-CM conventions and guidelines.

The *ICD-10-CM Official Guidelines for Coding and Reporting* govern the use of certain codes. These guidelines provide both general and chapter-specific coding guidance.

Step 9: Confirm and assign the code.

Having reviewed all relevant information concerning the possible code choices, assign the code that most completely describes the condition.

Repeat steps 1 through 9 for all additional documented conditions that meet the following criteria:

- They exist at the time of the visit *AND*
- They require or affect patient care, treatment, or management

Step 10: Sequence codes correctly.

Sequencing is the order in which the codes are listed on the claim. List first the ICD-10-CM code for the diagnosis, condition, problem, or other reason for the encounter/visit that is shown in the medical record to be chiefly responsible for the services provided. List additional codes that describe any coexisting conditions. Follow the official coding guidelines (see the guidelines, section II, "Selection of Principal Diagnosis"; section III, "Reporting Additional Diagnoses"; and section IV, "Diagnostic Coding and Reporting Guidelines for Outpatient Services") on proper sequencing of codes.

Coding Examples

Diagnosis: Anorexia

Step 1: The reason for the encounter was the condition, anorexia.

Step 2: Consult the alphabetic index.

Step 3: Locate the main term "Anorexia."

Step 4: Two possible subterms are available, "hysterical" and "nervosa." Neither is documented in this instance, however, so they cannot be used in code selection.

Step 5: The code listed next to the main term is called the default code selection. Because the two subentries (essential modifiers) do not apply in this instance, the default code (R63.Ø) should be used.

Step 6: Turn to code R63.Ø in the tabular list and read all instructional notes.

Step 7: The Excludes 1 note at code R63.Ø indicates that anorexia nervosa and loss of appetite determined to be of nonorganic origin should be reported with a code from chapter 5. The diagnostic statement does not describe the condition as anorexia nervosa, however, and does not indicate that the anorexia is of a nonorganic origin. There is no further division of the category past the fourth-character subcategory. Therefore, code R63.Ø is at the highest level of specificity.

Step 8: Review of official guideline I.C.18 indicates that a symptom code is appropriate when a more definitive diagnosis is not documented.

Step 9: The default code, R63.Ø Anorexia, is the correct code selection.

Repeat steps 1 through 9 for any concomitant diagnoses.

Step 10: Since anorexia is listed as the chief reason for the health care encounter, the first-listed, or principal, diagnosis is R63.Ø. Note that this is a chapter 18 symptom code but can be assigned for both inpatient and outpatient records since the provider did not establish a more definitive diagnosis, according to sections II.A and IV.D.

Diagnosis: Acute bronchitis

Step 1: The reason for the encounter was the condition, acute bronchitis.

Step 2: Consult the alphabetic index.

Step 3: Locate the main term "Bronchitis."

Step 4: There is a subterm for "acute or subacute." Additional subterms are not included in the diagnostic statement.

Step 5: Nonessential modifiers (with bronchospasm or obstruction) are terms that do not affect code assignment. Since no other subterms indented under "acute" apply here, the code listed next to this subentry—in this case J2Ø.9—should be chosen.

Step 6: Turn to code J2Ø.9 in the tabular list and read all instructional notes.

Step 7: The Includes note under category J2Ø lists alternative terms for acute bronchitis. Note that the list is not exhaustive but is only a representative selection of diagnoses that are included in the subcategory. The Excludes 1 note refers to category J4Ø for bronchitis and tracheobronchitis NOS. There are several conditions in the Excludes 2 notes that, if applicable, can be coded in addition to this code.

Note that the codes included in J2Ø represent acute bronchitis due to various infectious organisms that could be selected if identified in the documentation. In this case, the organism was not identified and there is no further division of the category past the fourth character subcategory. Therefore, code J2Ø.9 is at the highest level of specificity.

Step 8: Review of official guideline I.C.10 provides no additional information affecting the code selected.

Step 9: Assign code J2Ø.9 Acute bronchitis, unspecified.

Repeat steps 1 through 9 for any concomitant diagnoses.

Step 10: In the absence of additional diagnoses that may affect sequencing, code J2Ø.9 should be sequenced as the first-listed, or principal, diagnosis.

Diagnosis: Cerebellar ataxia in myxedema

Step 1: The reason for the encounter was the condition, cerebellar ataxia.

Step 2: Consult the alphabetic index.

Step 3: Locate the main term "Ataxia."

Step 4: Available subterms include "cerebellar (hereditary)," with additional indented subterms for "in" and "myxedema," all essential modifiers that are included in the diagnostic statement. Two codes are provided, EØ3.9 and G13.2, the latter of which is in brackets.

Step 5: Note the nonessential modifier (in parentheses) after the subterm cerebellar includes the term "hereditary." Because it is in parentheses, this term is not required in the diagnostic statement for this subentry to apply. The brackets around G13.2 identify this code as a manifestation of the condition described by code EØ3.9 and indicate that the two must be reported together and sequencing rules apply.

Step 6: Locate codes EØ3.9 and G13.2 in the tabular list, and read all instructional notes.

Step 7: For code EØ3.9, there are no instructional notes in the tabular list at the category EØ3 or code level that indicate that this condition should be coded elsewhere in the classification or that additional codes are required. Without further information from the diagnostic statement, myxedema, not otherwise specified (NOS), is appropriately reported with code EØ3.9 Hypothyroidism, unspecified, according to the inclusion term at this code.

Code G13.2 in the tabular list has an instructional note to "Code first underlying disease," which includes conditions found in category EØ3.-. Based on this note, codes EØ3.9 and G13.2 are to be coded together, with G13.2 listed only as a secondary diagnosis. This correlates with what the alphabetic index indicated. As there is no further division of codes in category G13 beyond the fourth character, G13.2 is at the highest level of specificity.

Step 8: Although there are some general conventions, such as how to interpret brackets in the alphabetic index, no chapter-specific guidelines apply to this coding scenario.

Step 9: Assign codes EØ3.9 Hypothyroidism, unspecified, and G13.2 Systemic atrophy primarily affecting the central nervous system in myxedema.

Repeat steps 1 through 9 for any concomitant diagnoses.

Step 10: Based on the alphabetic index and tabular instructional notations, code EØ3.9 should be sequenced as the first-listed, or principal, diagnosis followed by G13.2 as a secondary diagnosis.

Diagnosis: Decubitus ulcer of right elbow with skin loss and necrosis of subcutaneous tissue

Step 1: The reason for the encounter was the condition, decubitus ulcer.

Step 2: Consult the alphabetic index.

Step 3: Locate the main term "Ulcer."

Step 4: For the subterm "decubitus," there is no code provided or additional subterms indented, but a cross-reference is listed.

Step 5: The italicized cross-reference instructs the coder to "*see* Ulcer, pressure, by site."

Repeat steps 3 through 5 for the cross-reference:

Step 3: Locate the main term "Ulcer."

Step 4: Review the subentries for the subterm "pressure." The next level of indent lists either the site of the ulcer or the specific stage of the ulcer (stage 1–4, unstageable, and unspecified stages). The diagnostic statement provides the site, right elbow, and the extent of tissue damage (skin loss and necrosis of subcutaneous tissue) but does not specifically state that the ulcer is stage 1, stage 2, etc. Nonessential modifiers (in parentheses) at each stage include a description of the typical extent of damage at each stage. For example, stage 1 describes "pre-ulcer skin changes limited to persistent focal edema." Based on the documentation in the record, the coder can correlate the documentation to the nonessential modifiers and choose the specific stage from the index. The coder can also go directly to the body site, choosing the stage of the ulcer after reviewing the code options and instructional notations in the tabular list.

The diagnostic statement indicates that the extent of the damage to the elbow includes skin loss and necrosis of subcutaneous tissue, coinciding with the nonessential modifier next to the subentry "stage 3." The body site of elbow (L89.Ø-) is listed as another level of indent with other body sites.

Step 5: Note that code L89.Ø is followed by a dash and an additional-character-required icon, which indicate that more characters are needed to complete the code. From here, the tabular listing for L89.Ø- can be consulted.

Step 6: Locate code L89.Ø- in the tabular list and read all instructional notes.

Step 7: The tabular listing at category L89 has an Includes note for "decubitus ulcer," which confirms that category L89 is the appropriate category to represent what is documented in the diagnostic statement.

Several Excludes 2 notes are also listed at the category level. Excludes 2 notes represent conditions that can occur concomitantly with the decubitus ulcer and can be coded in addition to code L89, if supported by the documentation.

The subcategory codes under L89.Ø indicate that the fifth character describes laterality. Locate the right elbow at subcategory L89.Ø1. See that an additional sixth character to specify the stage of the ulcer is now needed to complete the code. The stage can be determined either by the specific documentation of the stage (e.g., stage 1, stage 2) or, in this case, a description that matches one of the inclusion terms that follow each stage code. For example, the diagnostic description in this case of "skin loss and necrosis of the subcutaneous tissue" matches the inclusion term under L89.Ø13 Pressure ulcer of right elbow, stage 3. No additional characters are required because code L89.Ø13 is at its highest level of specificity.

Step 8: The official guidelines contain quite a bit of information relating to pressure ulcers in chapter-specific guideline I.C.12 as well as information in general guideline I.B.14. These and any other pertinent guidelines should be reviewed to ensure appropriate code assignment.

Step 9: Assign code L89.Ø13 Pressure ulcer of right elbow, stage 3.

Repeat steps 1 through 9 for any concomitant diagnoses.

Step 10: Since the decubitus ulcer is listed as the chief reason for the health care encounter, the first-listed, or principal, diagnosis is L89.Ø13. However, according to the code first instructional note at the L89 category level, gangrene (I96) would be sequenced before the pressure ulcer if it were documented.

Diagnosis: Emergency department visit for bimalleolar fracture of the right ankle due to trauma

Step 1: The reason for the encounter was the condition, bimalleolar fracture.

Step 2: Consult the alphabetic index.

Step 3: Locate the main term "Fracture." Note that many main terms represent fractures: "Fracture, burst," "Fracture, chronic," "Fracture, insufficiency," "Fracture, nontraumatic NEC," "Fracture, pathological," and "Fracture, traumatic." Since the diagnostic statement specifically states that this fracture was the result of trauma, the main term "Fracture, traumatic" should be used.

Step 4: Subterms that should be referenced are "ankle" and "bimalleolar (displaced)," which lists code S82.84-.

Step 5: A nonessential modifier (in parentheses) next to the term bimalleolar for "displaced" indicates that S82.84- is the default category unless the fracture is specifically identified as "nondisplaced."

Note that code S82.84- is followed by a dash and an additional-character icon, both of which indicate that more characters are required. From here, the tabular list can be consulted.

Step 6: Locate code S82.84- in the tabular list and read all instructional notes.

Step: 7: The instructional notes at category S82 indicate that fractures not specified as displaced or nondisplaced default to displaced and that fractures not designated as open or closed default to closed. Additional instructional notes can be found at the category level but none pertain to the current scenario.

Read through the subcategory codes under S82.84, and note that the sixth character specifies displaced or nondisplaced and laterality. Based on the index nonessential modifier (displaced) and the code note at category S82, code selection should identify a displaced fracture of the right side. A displaced bimalleolar fracture of the right lower leg is coded to S82.841.

To complete the code, a seventh character must be assigned to identify the type of encounter (initial, subsequent, or sequela) and whether the fracture is open or closed. Most of the codes in category S82 require a seventh character represented in the list at the category level. However, it is important to note that some subcategories have their own specific set of seventh characters. In this instance, subcategory S82.84- does not have a unique set of seventh characters and the list provided at the category level should be used. Without documentation of the fracture being open, the tabular notation indicates that the default is closed. Character A, representing "initial encounter for closed fracture," listed in the box at the category level is the most appropriate option.

Step 8: Assign code S82.841A Displaced bimalleolar fracture of right lower leg, initial encounter for closed fracture.

Repeat steps 1 through 9 for any concomitant diagnoses.

Step 9: Review chapter-specific guideline I.C.19. and any other official conventions or guidelines to ensure appropriate code assignment.

Step 10: Additional codes can be applied to relate the specific cause of the injury, the place of occurrence, the activity of the patient at the time of the injury, and the patient's status, when this information is available in the record. However, coding this information is voluntary and reporting requirements depend on state mandates and/or facility-specific reporting requirements. If assigned, the external cause codes should be reported as secondary diagnoses only with the injury (fracture) sequenced first. Most codes in chapter 20, "External Causes of Morbidity," require a seventh character to identify the type of encounter. The seventh character assigned to an external cause code should match the seventh character of the code assigned for the associated injury or condition for the encounter.

2023 ICD-10-CM Official Guidelines for Coding and Reporting

Narrative changes effective October 1, 2022 appear in **bold** text

Narrative changes effective April 1, 2022 appear in shaded text

Items underlined have been moved within the guidelines since the FY 2022 version

Italics are used to indicate revisions to heading changes

The Centers for Medicare and Medicaid Services (CMS) and the National Center for Health Statistics (NCHS), two departments within the U.S. Federal Government's Department of Health and Human Services (DHHS) provide the following guidelines for coding and reporting using the International Classification of Diseases, 10th Revision, Clinical Modification (ICD-10-CM). These guidelines should be used as a companion document to the official version of the ICD-10-CM as published on the NCHS website. The ICD-10-CM is a morbidity classification published by the United States for classifying diagnoses and reason for visits in all health care settings. The ICD-10-CM is based on the ICD-10, the statistical classification of disease published by the World Health Organization (WHO).

These guidelines have been approved by the four organizations that make up the Cooperating Parties for the ICD-10-CM: the American Hospital Association (AHA), the American Health Information Management Association (AHIMA), CMS, and NCHS.

These guidelines are a set of rules that have been developed to accompany and complement the official conventions and instructions provided within the ICD-10-CM itself. The instructions and conventions of the classification take precedence over guidelines. These guidelines are based on the coding and sequencing instructions in the Tabular List and Alphabetic Index of ICD-10-CM, but provide additional instruction. Adherence to these guidelines when assigning ICD-10-CM diagnosis codes is required under the Health Insurance Portability and Accountability Act (HIPAA). The diagnosis codes (Tabular List and Alphabetic Index) have been adopted under HIPAA for all healthcare settings. A joint effort between the healthcare provider and the coder is essential to achieve complete and accurate documentation, code assignment, and reporting of diagnoses and procedures. These guidelines have been developed to assist both the healthcare provider and the coder in identifying those diagnoses that are to be reported. The importance of consistent, complete documentation in the medical record cannot be overemphasized. Without such documentation accurate coding cannot be achieved. The entire record should be reviewed to determine the specific reason for the encounter and the conditions treated.

The term encounter is used for all settings, including hospital admissions. In the context of these guidelines, the term provider is used throughout the guidelines to mean physician or any qualified health care practitioner who is legally accountable for establishing the patient's diagnosis. Only this set of guidelines, approved by the Cooperating Parties, is official.

The guidelines are organized into sections. Section I includes the structure and conventions of the classification and general guidelines that apply to the entire classification, and chapter-specific guidelines that correspond to the chapters as they are arranged in the classification. Section II includes guidelines for selection of principal diagnosis for non-outpatient settings. Section III includes guidelines for reporting additional diagnoses in non-outpatient settings. Section IV is for outpatient coding and reporting. It is necessary to review all sections of the guidelines to fully understand all of the rules and instructions needed to code properly.

Section I. Conventions, general coding guidelines and chapter specific guidelines 3

- A. Conventions for the ICD-10-CM 3
  - 1. The Alphabetic Index and Tabular List 3
  - 2. Format and Structure: 3
  - 3. Use of codes for reporting purposes 3
  - 4. Placeholder character 3
  - 5. 7th Characters 3
  - 6. Abbreviations 3
    - a. Alphabetic Index abbreviations 3
    - b. Tabular List abbreviations 3
  - 7. Punctuation 3
  - 8. Use of "and" 3
  - 9. Other and Unspecified codes 3
    - a. "Other" codes 3
    - b. "Unspecified" codes 3
  - 10. Includes Notes 3
  - 11. Inclusion terms 3
  - 12. Excludes Notes 3
    - a. Excludes1 3
    - b. Excludes2 3
  - 13. Etiology/manifestation convention ("code first", "use additional code" and "in diseases classified elsewhere" notes) 3
  - 14. "And" 4
  - 15. "With" 4
  - 16. "See" and "See Also" 4
  - 17. "Code also" note 4
  - 18. Default codes 4
  - 19. Code assignment and Clinical Criteria 4
- B. General Coding Guidelines 4
  - 1. Locating a code in the ICD-10-CM 4
  - 2. Level of Detail in Coding 4
  - 3. Code or codes from A00.0 through T88.9, Z00-Z99.8, U00-U85 4
  - 4. Signs and symptoms 4
  - 5. Conditions that are an integral part of a disease process 4
  - 6. Conditions that are not an integral part of a disease process 4
  - 7. Multiple coding for a single condition 4
  - 8. Acute and Chronic Conditions 5
  - 9. Combination Code 5
  - 10. Sequela (Late Effects) 5
  - 11. Impending or Threatened Condition 5
  - 12. Reporting Same Diagnosis Code More than Once 5
  - 13. Laterality 5
  - 14. Documentation by Clinicians Other than the Patient's Provider 5
  - 15. Syndromes 5
  - 16. Documentation of Complications of Care 5
  - 17. Borderline Diagnosis 5
  - 18. Use of Sign/Symptom/Unspecified Codes 6
  - 19. Coding for Healthcare Encounters in Hurricane Aftermath 6
    - a. Use of External Cause of Morbidity Codes 6
    - b. Sequencing of External Causes of Morbidity Codes 6
    - c. Other External Causes of Morbidity Code Issues 6
    - d. Use of Z codes 6
- C. Chapter-Specific Coding Guidelines 6
  - 1. Chapter 1: Certain Infectious and Parasitic Diseases (A00-B99), U07.1, U09.9 6
    - a. Human Immunodeficiency Virus (HIV) Infections 6
    - b. Infectious agents as the cause of diseases classified to other chapters 7
    - c. Infections resistant to antibiotics 7
    - d. Sepsis, Severe Sepsis, and Septic Shock Infections resistant to antibiotics 7
    - e. Methicillin Resistant Staphylococcus aureus (MRSA) Conditions 8
    - f. Zika virus infections 8
    - g. Coronavirus infections 9
  - 2. Chapter 2: Neoplasms (C00-D49) 10
    - a. *Admission/Encounter for treatment of primary site* 10
    - b. *Admission/Encounter for* treatment of secondary site 10
    - c. Coding and sequencing of complications 10
    - d. Primary malignancy previously excised 10
    - e. Admissions/Encounters involving chemotherapy, immunotherapy and radiation therapy 10
    - f. Admission/encounter to determine extent of malignancy 11
    - g. Symptoms, signs, and abnormal findings listed in Chapter 18 associated with neoplasms 11
    - h. Admission/encounter for pain control/management 11
    - i. Malignancy in two or more noncontiguous sites 11
    - j. Disseminated malignant neoplasm, unspecified 11
    - k. Malignant neoplasm without specification of site 11
    - l. Sequencing of neoplasm codes 11
    - m. Current malignancy versus personal history of malignancy 11
    - n. Leukemia, Multiple Myeloma, and Malignant Plasma Cell Neoplasms in remission versus personal history 11
    - o. Aftercare following surgery for neoplasm 11
    - p. Follow-up care for completed treatment of a malignancy 11
    - q. Prophylactic organ removal for prevention of malignancy 11
    - r. Malignant neoplasm associated with transplanted organ 11
    - s. Breast Implant Associated Anaplastic Large Cell Lymphoma 12
    - t. Secondary malignant neoplasm of lymphoid tissue 12
  - 3. Chapter 3: Disease of the blood and blood-forming organs and certain disorders involving the immune mechanism (D50-D89) 12
  - 4. Chapter 4: Endocrine, Nutritional, and Metabolic Diseases (E00-E89) .. 12
    - a. Diabetes mellitus 12
  - 5. Chapter 5: Mental, Behavioral and Neurodevelopmental disorders (F01-F99) 12
    - a. Pain disorders related to psychological factors 12
    - b. Mental and behavioral disorders due to psychoactive substance use 13
    - c. Factitious Disorder 13
    - d. Dementia 13
  - 6. Chapter 6: Diseases of the Nervous System (G00-G99) 13
    - a. Dominant/nondominant side 13
    - b. Pain - Category G89 13

7. Chapter 7: Diseases of the Eye and Adnexa (HØØ-H59) 14
   a. Glaucoma 14
   b. Blindness 14
8. Chapter 8: Diseases of the Ear and Mastoid Process (H6Ø-H95) 14
9. Chapter 9: Diseases of the Circulatory System (IØØ-I99) 14
   a. Hypertension 14
   b. Atherosclerotic Coronary Artery Disease and Angina 15
   c. Intraoperative and Postprocedural Cerebrovascular Accident 15
   d. Sequelae of Cerebrovascular Disease 15
   e. Acute myocardial infarction (AMI) 15
10. Chapter 10: Diseases of the Respiratory System (JØØ-J99), UØ7.Ø 16
   a. Chronic Obstructive Pulmonary Disease [COPD] and Asthma 16
   b. Acute Respiratory Failure 16
   c. Influenza due to certain identified influenza viruses 16
   d. Ventilator associated Pneumonia 16
   e. Vaping-related disorders 17
11. Chapter 11: Diseases of the Digestive System (KØØ-K95) 17
12. Chapter 12: Diseases of the Skin and Subcutaneous Tissue (LØØ-L99) 17
   a. Pressure ulcer stage codes 17
   b. Non-Pressure Chronic Ulcers 17
13. Chapter 13: Diseases of the Musculoskeletal System and Connective Tissue (MØØ-M99) 17
   a. Site and laterality 17
   b. Acute traumatic versus chronic or recurrent musculoskeletal conditions 17
   c. Coding of Pathologic Fractures 17
   d. Osteoporosis 17
   e. Multisystem Inflammatory Syndrome 18
14. Chapter 14: Diseases of Genitourinary System (NØØ-N99) 18
   a. Chronic kidney disease 18
15. Chapter 15: Pregnancy, Childbirth, and the Puerperium (OØØ-O9A) 18
   a. General Rules for Obstetric Cases 18
   b. Selection of OB Principal or First-listed Diagnosis 18
   c. Pre-existing conditions versus conditions due to the pregnancy 19
   d. Pre-existing hypertension in pregnancy 19
   e. Fetal Conditions Affecting the Management of the Mother 19
   f. HIV Infection in Pregnancy, Childbirth and the Puerperium 19
   g. Diabetes mellitus in pregnancy 19
   h. Long term use of insulin and oral hypoglycemics 19
   i. Gestational (pregnancy induced) diabetes 19
   j. Sepsis and septic shock complicating abortion, pregnancy, childbirth and the puerperium 19
   k. Puerperal sepsis 19
   l. Alcohol, tobacco and drug use during pregnancy, childbirth and the puerperium 19
   m. Poisoning, toxic effects, adverse effects and underdosing in a pregnant patient 20
   n. Normal Delivery, Code O8Ø 20
   o. The Peripartum and Postpartum Periods 20
   p. Code O94, Sequelae of complication of pregnancy, childbirth, and the puerperium 20
   q. Termination of Pregnancy and Spontaneous abortions 20
   r. Abuse in a pregnant patient 20
   s. COVID-19 infection in pregnancy, childbirth, and the puerperium 20
16. Chapter 16: Certain Conditions Originating in the Perinatal Period (PØØ-P96) 20
   a. General Perinatal Rules 20
   b. Observation and Evaluation of Newborns for Suspected Conditions not Found 21
   c. Coding Additional Perinatal Diagnoses 21
   d. Prematurity and Fetal Growth Retardation 21
   e. Low birth weight and immaturity status 21
   f. Bacterial Sepsis of Newborn 21
   g. Stillbirth 21
   h. COVID-19 Infection in Newborn 21
17. Chapter 17: Congenital malformations, deformations, and chromosomal abnormalities (QØØ-Q99) 21
18. Chapter 18: Symptoms, signs, and abnormal clinical and laboratory findings, not elsewhere classified (RØØ-R99) 21
   a. Use of symptom codes 21
   b. Use of a symptom code with a definitive diagnosis code 21
   c. Combination codes that include symptoms 22
   d. Repeated falls 22
   e. Coma 22
   f. Functional quadriplegia 22
   g. SIRS due to Non-Infectious Process 22
   h. Death NOS 22
   i. NIHSS Stroke Scale 22
19. Chapter 19: Injury, poisoning, and certain other consequences of external causes (SØØ-T88) 22
   a. Application of 7th Characters in Chapter 19 22
   b. Coding of Injuries 22
   c. Coding of Traumatic Fractures 22
   d. Coding of Burns and Corrosions 23
   e. Adverse Effects, Poisoning, Underdosing and Toxic Effects 23
   f. Adult and child abuse, neglect and other maltreatment 24
   g. Complications of care 24
20. Chapter 20: External Causes of Morbidity (VØØ-Y99) 25
   a. General External Cause Coding Guidelines 25
   b. Place of Occurrence Guideline 25
   c. Activity Code 25
   d. Place of Occurrence, Activity, and Status Codes Used with other External Cause Code 25
   e. If the Reporting Format Limits the Number of External Cause Codes 25
   f. Multiple External Cause Coding Guidelines 25
   g. Child and Adult Abuse Guideline 26
   h. Unknown or Undetermined Intent Guideline 26
   i. Sequelae (Late Effects) of External Cause Guidelines 26
   j. Terrorism Guidelines 26
   k. External Cause Status 26
21. Chapter 21: Factors influencing health status and contact with health services (ZØØ-Z99) 26
   a. Use of Z Codes in Any Healthcare Setting 26
   b. Z Codes Indicate a Reason for an Encounter or Provide Additional Information about a Patient Encounter 26
   c. Categories of Z Codes 26
22. Chapter 22: Codes for Special Purposes (UØØ-U85) 31

Section II. Selection of Principal Diagnosis 31

A. Codes for symptoms, signs, and ill-defined conditions 31
B. Two or more interrelated conditions, each potentially meeting the definition for principal diagnosis 31
C. Two or more diagnoses that equally meet the definition for principal diagnosis 31
D. Two or more comparative or contrasting conditions 31
E. A symptom(s) followed by contrasting/comparative diagnoses 31
F. Original treatment plan not carried out 31
G. Complications of surgery and other medical care 31
H. Uncertain Diagnosis 31
I. Admission from Observation Unit 31
   1. Admission Following Medical Observation 31
   2. Admission Following Post-Operative Observation 31
J. Admission from Outpatient Surgery 31
K. Admissions/Encounters for Rehabilitation 31

Section III. Reporting Additional Diagnoses 31

A. Previous conditions 32
B. Abnormal findings 32
C. Uncertain Diagnosis 32

Section IV. Diagnostic Coding and Reporting Guidelines for Outpatient Services 32

A. Selection of first-listed condition 32
   1. Outpatient Surgery 32
   2. Observation Stay 32
B. Codes from AØØ.Ø through T88.9, ZØØ-Z99, UØØ-U85 32
C. Accurate reporting of ICD-10-CM diagnosis codes 32
D. Codes that describe symptoms and signs 32
E. Encounters for circumstances other than a disease or injury 32
F. Level of Detail in Coding 32
   1. ICD-10-CM codes with 3, 4, 5, 6 or 7 characters 32
   2. Use of full number of characters required for a code 32
   3. Highest level of specificity 32
G. ICD-10-CM code for the diagnosis, condition, problem, or other reason for encounter/visit 32
H. Uncertain diagnosis 32
I. Chronic diseases 32
J. Code all documented conditions that coexist 33
K. Patients receiving diagnostic services only 33
L. Patients receiving therapeutic services only 33
M. Patients receiving preoperative evaluations only 33
N. Ambulatory surgery 33
O. Routine outpatient prenatal visits 33
P. Encounters for general medical examinations with abnormal findings 33
Q. Encounters for routine health screenings 33

Appendix I. Present on Admission Reporting Guidelines 33

Section I. Conventions, general coding guidelines and chapter specific guidelines

The conventions, general guidelines and chapter-specific guidelines are applicable to all health care settings unless otherwise indicated. The conventions and instructions of the classification take precedence over guidelines.

A. Conventions for the ICD-10-CM

The conventions for the ICD-10-CM are the general rules for use of the classification independent of the guidelines. These conventions are incorporated within the Alphabetic Index and Tabular List of the ICD-10-CM as instructional notes.

1. **The Alphabetic Index and Tabular List**
   The ICD-10-CM is divided into the Alphabetic Index, an alphabetical list of terms and their corresponding code, and the Tabular List, a structured list of codes divided into chapters based on body system or condition. The Alphabetic Index consists of the following parts: the Index of Diseases and Injury, the Index of External Causes of Injury, the Table of Neoplasms and the Table of Drugs and Chemicals.

   See Section I.C.2. ***Neoplasms***

   See Section I.C.19. Adverse effects, poisoning, underdosing and toxic effects
2. **Format and Structure:**
   The ICD-10-CM Tabular List contains categories, subcategories and codes. Characters for categories, subcategories and codes may be either a letter or a number. All categories are 3 characters. A three-character category that has no further subdivision is equivalent to a code. Subcategories are either 4 or 5 characters. Codes may be 3, 4, 5, 6 or 7 characters. That is, each level of subdivision after a category is a subcategory. The final level of subdivision is a code. Codes that have applicable 7th characters are still referred to as codes, not subcategories. A code that has an applicable 7th character is considered invalid without the 7th character.

   The ICD-10-CM uses an indented format for ease in reference.
3. **Use of codes for reporting purposes**
   For reporting purposes only codes are permissible, not categories or subcategories, and any applicable 7th character is required.
4. **Placeholder character**
   The ICD-10-CM utilizes a placeholder character "X". The "X" is used as a placeholder at certain codes to allow for future expansion. An example of this is at the poisoning, adverse effect and underdosing codes, categories T36-T5Ø. Where a placeholder exists, the X must be used in order for the code to be considered a valid code.
5. **7th Characters**
   Certain ICD-10-CM categories have applicable 7th characters. The applicable 7th character is required for all codes within the category, or as the notes in the Tabular List instruct. The 7th character must always be the 7th character in the data field. If a code that requires a 7th character is not 6 characters, a placeholder X must be used to fill in the empty characters.
6. **Abbreviations**
   a. **Alphabetic Index abbreviations**
      NEC "Not elsewhere classifiable"
      This abbreviation in the Alphabetic Index represents "other specified." When a specific code is not available for a condition, the Alphabetic Index directs the coder to the "other specified" code in the Tabular List.
      NOS "Not otherwise specified"
      This abbreviation is the equivalent of unspecified.
   b. **Tabular List abbreviations**
      NEC "Not elsewhere classifiable"
      This abbreviation in the Tabular List represents "other specified". When a specific code is not available for a condition, the Tabular List includes an NEC entry under a code to identify the code as the "other specified" code.
      NOS "Not otherwise specified"
      This abbreviation is the equivalent of unspecified.
7. **Punctuation**
   [ ] Brackets are used in the Tabular List to enclose synonyms, alternative wording or explanatory phrases. Brackets are used in the Alphabetic Index to identify manifestation codes.

   ( ) Parentheses are used in both the Alphabetic Index and Tabular List to enclose supplementary words that may be present or absent in the statement of a disease or procedure without affecting the code number to which it is assigned. The terms within the parentheses are referred to as nonessential modifiers. The nonessential modifiers in the Alphabetic Index to Diseases apply to subterms following a main term except when a nonessential modifier and a subentry are mutually exclusive, the subentry takes precedence. For example, in the ICD-10-CM Alphabetic Index under the main term Enteritis, "acute" is a nonessential modifier and "chronic" is a subentry. In this case, the nonessential modifier "acute" does not apply to the subentry "chronic".

   : Colons are used in the Tabular List after an incomplete term which needs one or more of the modifiers following the colon to make it assignable to a given category.
8. **Use of "and".**
   See Section I.A.14. Use of the term "And"
9. **Other and Unspecified codes**
   a. **"Other" codes**
      Codes titled "other" or "other specified" are for use when the information in the medical record provides detail for which a specific code does not exist. Alphabetic Index entries with NEC in the line designate "other" codes in the Tabular List. These Alphabetic Index entries represent specific disease entities for which no specific code exists, so the term is included within an "other" code.
   b. **"Unspecified" codes**
      Codes titled "unspecified" are for use when the information in the medical record is insufficient to assign a more specific code. For those categories for which an unspecified code is not provided, the "other specified" code may represent both other and unspecified.
      See Section I.B.18. Use of Signs/Symptom/Unspecified Codes
10. **Includes Notes**
    This note appears immediately under a three-character code title to further define, or give examples of, the content of the category.
11. **Inclusion terms**
    List of terms is included under some codes. These terms are the conditions for which that code is to be used. The terms may be synonyms of the code title, or, in the case of "other specified" codes, the terms are a list of the various conditions assigned to that code. The inclusion terms are not necessarily exhaustive. Additional terms found only in the Alphabetic Index may also be assigned to a code.
12. **Excludes Notes**
    The ICD-10-CM has two types of excludes notes. Each type of note has a different definition for use, but they are all similar in that they indicate that codes excluded from each other are independent of each other.
    a. **Excludes1**
       A type 1 Excludes note is a pure excludes note. It means "NOT CODED HERE!" An Excludes1 note indicates that the code excluded should never be used at the same time as the code above the Excludes1 note. An Excludes1 is used when two conditions cannot occur together, such as a congenital form versus an acquired form of the same condition.

       An exception to the Excludes1 definition is the circumstance when the two conditions are unrelated to each other. If it is not clear whether the two conditions involving an Excludes1 note are related or not, query the provider. For example, code F45.8, Other somatoform disorders, has an Excludes1 note for "sleep related teeth grinding (G47.63)," because "teeth grinding" is an inclusion term under F45.8. Only one of these two codes should be assigned for teeth grinding. However psychogenic dysmenorrhea is also an inclusion term under F45.8, and a patient could have both this condition and sleep related teeth grinding. In this case, the two conditions are clearly unrelated to each other, and so it would be appropriate to report F45.8 and G47.63 together.
    b. **Excludes2**
       A type 2 Excludes note represents "Not included here." An excludes2 note indicates that the condition excluded is not part of the condition represented by the code, but a patient may have both conditions at the same time. When an Excludes2 note appears under a code, it is acceptable to use both the code and the excluded code together, when appropriate.
13. **Etiology/manifestation convention ("code first", "use additional code" and "in diseases classified elsewhere" notes)**
    Certain conditions have both an underlying etiology and multiple body system manifestations due to the underlying etiology. For such conditions, the ICD-10-CM has a coding convention that requires the underlying condition be sequenced first, if applicable, followed by the manifestation. Wherever such a combination exists, there is a "use additional code" note at the etiology code, and a "code first" note at the manifestation code. These instructional notes indicate the proper sequencing order of the codes, etiology followed by manifestation.

    In most cases the manifestation codes will have in the code title, "in diseases classified elsewhere." Codes with this title are a component of the etiology/ manifestation convention. The code title indicates that it is a manifestation code. "In diseases classified elsewhere" codes are never permitted to be used as first listed or principal diagnosis codes. They must be used in conjunction with an underlying condition code and they must be listed following the underlying condition. See category FØ2, Dementia in other diseases classified elsewhere, for an example of this convention.

There are manifestation codes that do not have "in diseases classified elsewhere" in the title. For such codes, there is a "use additional code" note at the etiology code and a "code first" note at the manifestation code, and the rules for sequencing apply.

In addition to the notes in the Tabular List, these conditions also have a specific Alphabetic Index entry structure. In the Alphabetic Index both conditions are listed together with the etiology code first followed by the manifestation codes in brackets. The code in brackets is always to be sequenced second.

An example of the etiology/manifestation convention is dementia **with** Parkinson's disease. In the Alphabetic Index, code G2Ø is listed first, followed by code FØ2.8Ø or FØ2.81- in brackets. Code G2Ø represents the underlying etiology, Parkinson's disease, and must be sequenced first, whereas code**s** FØ2.8Ø and FØ2.81- represent the manifestation of dementia in diseases classified elsewhere, with or without behavioral disturbance.

"Code first" and "Use additional code" notes are also used as sequencing rules in the classification for certain codes that are not part of an etiology/ manifestation combination.

See Section I.B.7. Multiple coding for a single condition.

14. "And"

The word "and" should be interpreted to mean either "and" or "or" when it appears in a title.

For example, cases of "tuberculosis of bones", "tuberculosis of joints" and "tuberculosis of bones and joints" are classified to subcategory A18.Ø, Tuberculosis of bones and joints.

15. "With"

The word "with" or "in" should be interpreted to mean "associated with" or "due to" when it appears in a code title, the Alphabetic Index (either under a main term or subterm), or an instructional note in the Tabular List. The classification presumes a causal relationship between the two conditions linked by these terms in the Alphabetic Index or Tabular List. These conditions should be coded as related even in the absence of provider documentation explicitly linking them, unless the documentation clearly states the conditions are unrelated or when another guideline exists that specifically requires a documented linkage between two conditions (e.g., sepsis guideline for "acute organ dysfunction that is not clearly associated with the sepsis").

For conditions not specifically linked by these relational terms in the classification or when a guideline requires that a linkage between two conditions be explicitly documented, provider documentation must link the conditions in order to code them as related.

The word "with" in the Alphabetic Index is sequenced immediately following the main term or subterm, not in alphabetical order.

16. "See" and "See Also"

The "see" instruction following a main term in the Alphabetic Index indicates that another term should be referenced. It is necessary to go to the main term referenced with the "see" note to locate the correct code.

A "see also" instruction following a main term in the Alphabetic Index instructs that there is another main term that may also be referenced that may provide additional Alphabetic Index entries that may be useful. It is not necessary to follow the "see also" note when the original main term provides the necessary code.

17. "Code also" note

A "code also" note instructs that two codes may be required to fully describe a condition, but this note does not provide sequencing direction. The sequencing depends on the circumstances of the encounter.

18. Default codes

A code listed next to a main term in the ICD-10-CM Alphabetic Index is referred to as a default code. The default code represents that condition that is most commonly associated with the main term or is the unspecified code for the condition. If a condition is documented in a medical record (for example, appendicitis) without any additional information, such as acute or chronic, the default code should be assigned.

19. Code assignment and Clinical Criteria

The assignment of a diagnosis code is based on the provider's diagnostic statement that the condition exists. The provider's statement that the patient has a particular condition is sufficient. Code assignment is not based on clinical criteria used by the provider to establish the diagnosis. **If there is conflicting medical record documentation, query the provider.**

B. General Coding Guidelines

1. Locating a code in the ICD-10-CM

To select a code in the classification that corresponds to a diagnosis or reason for visit documented in a medical record, first locate the term in the Alphabetic Index, and then verify the code in the Tabular List. Read and be guided by instructional notations that appear in both the Alphabetic Index and the Tabular List.

It is essential to use both the Alphabetic Index and Tabular List when locating and assigning a code. The Alphabetic Index does not always provide the full code. Selection of the full code, including laterality and any applicable 7th character can only be done in the Tabular List. A dash (-) at the end of an Alphabetic Index entry indicates that additional characters are required. Even if a dash is not included at the Alphabetic Index entry, it is necessary to refer to the Tabular List to verify that no 7th character is required.

2. Level of Detail in Coding

Diagnosis codes are to be used and reported at their highest number of characters available and to the highest level of specificity documented in the medical record.

ICD-10-CM diagnosis codes are composed of codes with 3, 4, 5, 6 or 7 characters. Codes with three characters are included in ICD-10-CM as the heading of a category of codes that may be further subdivided by the use of fourth and/or fifth characters and/or sixth characters, which provide greater detail.

A three-character code is to be used only if it is not further subdivided. A code is invalid if it has not been coded to the full number of characters required for that code, including the 7th character, if applicable.

3. Code or codes from AØØ.Ø through T88.9, ZØØ-Z99.8, UØØ-U85

The appropriate code or codes from AØØ.Ø through T88.9, ZØØ-Z99.8, and UØØ-U85 must be used to identify diagnoses, symptoms, conditions, problems, complaints or other reason(s) for the encounter/visit.

4. Signs and symptoms

Codes that describe symptoms and signs, as opposed to diagnoses, are acceptable for reporting purposes when a related definitive diagnosis has not been established (confirmed) by the provider. Chapter 18 of ICD-10-CM, Symptoms, Signs, and Abnormal Clinical and Laboratory Findings, Not Elsewhere Classified (codes RØØ.Ø-R99) contains many, but not all, codes for symptoms.

See Section I.B.18. Use of Signs/Symptom/Unspecified Codes

5. Conditions that are an integral part of a disease process

Signs and symptoms that are associated routinely with a disease process should not be assigned as additional codes, unless otherwise instructed by the classification.

6. Conditions that are not an integral part of a disease process

Additional signs and symptoms that may not be associated routinely with a disease process should be coded when present.

7. Multiple coding for a single condition

In addition to the etiology/manifestation convention that requires two codes to fully describe a single condition that affects multiple body systems, there are other single conditions that also require more than one code. "Use additional code" notes are found in the Tabular List at codes that are not part of an etiology/manifestation pair where a secondary code is useful to fully describe a condition. The sequencing rule is the same as the etiology/manifestation pair, "use additional code" indicates that a secondary code should be added, if known.

For example, for bacterial infections that are not included in chapter 1, a secondary code from category B95, Streptococcus, Staphylococcus, and Enterococcus, as the cause of diseases classified elsewhere, or B96, Other bacterial agents as the cause of diseases classified elsewhere, may be required to identify the bacterial organism causing the infection. A "use additional code" note will normally be found at the infectious disease code, indicating a need for the organism code to be added as a secondary code.

"Code first" notes are also under certain codes that are not specifically manifestation codes but may be due to an underlying cause. When there is a "code first" note and an underlying condition is present, the underlying condition should be sequenced first, if known.

"Code, if applicable, any causal condition first" notes indicate that this code may be assigned as a principal diagnosis when the causal condition is unknown or not applicable. If a causal condition is known, then the code for that condition should be sequenced as the principal or first-listed diagnosis.

Multiple codes may be needed for sequela, complication codes and obstetric codes to more fully describe a condition. See the specific guidelines for these conditions for further instruction.

8. Acute and Chronic Conditions

If the same condition is described as both acute (subacute) and chronic, and separate subentries exist in the Alphabetic Index at the same indentation level, code both and sequence the acute (subacute) code first.

9. Combination Code

A combination code is a single code used to classify:

Two diagnoses, or

A diagnosis with an associated secondary process (manifestation)

A diagnosis with an associated complication

Combination codes are identified by referring to subterm entries in the Alphabetic Index and by reading the inclusion and exclusion notes in the Tabular List.

Assign only the combination code when that code fully identifies the diagnostic conditions involved or when the Alphabetic Index so directs. Multiple coding should not be used when the classification provides a combination code that clearly identifies all of the elements documented in the diagnosis. When the combination code lacks necessary specificity in describing the manifestation or complication, an additional code should be used as a secondary code.

10. Sequela (Late Effects)

A sequela is the residual effect (condition produced) after the acute phase of an illness or injury has terminated. There is no time limit on when a sequela code can be used. The residual may be apparent early, such as in cerebral infarction, or it may occur months or years later, such as that due to a previous injury. Examples of sequela include: scar formation resulting from a burn, deviated septum due to a nasal fracture, and infertility due to tubal occlusion from old tuberculosis. Coding of sequela generally requires two codes sequenced in the following order: the condition or nature of the sequela is sequenced first. The sequela code is sequenced second.

An exception to the above guidelines are those instances where the code for the sequela is followed by a manifestation code identified in the Tabular List and title, or the sequela code has been expanded (at the fourth, fifth or sixth character levels) to include the manifestation(s). The code for the acute phase of an illness or injury that led to the sequela is never used with a code for the late effect.

See Section I.C.9. Sequelae of cerebrovascular disease

See Section I.C.15. Sequelae of complication of pregnancy, childbirth and the puerperium

See Section I.C.19. Application of 7th characters for Chapter 19

11. Impending or Threatened Condition

Code any condition described at the time of discharge as "impending" or "threatened" as follows:

If it did occur, code as confirmed diagnosis.

If it did not occur, reference the Alphabetic Index to determine if the condition has a subentry term for "impending" or "threatened" and also reference main term entries for "Impending" and for "Threatened."

If the subterms are listed, assign the given code.

If the subterms are not listed, code the existing underlying condition(s) and not the condition described as impending or threatened.

12. Reporting Same Diagnosis Code More than Once

Each unique ICD-10-CM diagnosis code may be reported only once for an encounter. This applies to bilateral conditions when there are no distinct codes identifying laterality or two different conditions classified to the same ICD-10-CM diagnosis code.

13. Laterality

Some ICD-10-CM codes indicate laterality, specifying whether the condition occurs on the left, right or is bilateral. If no bilateral code is provided and the condition is bilateral, assign separate codes for both the left and right side. If the side is not identified in the medical record, assign the code for the unspecified side.

When a patient has a bilateral condition and each side is treated during separate encounters, assign the "bilateral" code (as the condition still exists on both sides), including for the encounter to treat the first side. For the second encounter for treatment after one side has previously been treated and the condition no longer exists on that side, assign the appropriate unilateral code for the side where the condition still exists (e.g., cataract surgery performed on each eye in separate encounters). The bilateral code would not be assigned for the subsequent encounter, as the patient no longer has the condition in the previously-treated site. If the treatment on the first side did not completely resolve the condition, then the bilateral code would still be appropriate.

When laterality is not documented by the patient's provider, code assignment for the affected side may be based on medical record documentation from other clinicians. If there is conflicting medical record documentation regarding the affected side, the patient's attending provider should be queried for clarification. Codes for "unspecified" side should rarely be used, such as when the documentation in the record is insufficient to determine the affected side and it is not possible to obtain clarification.

14. Documentation by Clinicians Other than the Patient's Provider

Code assignment is based on the documentation by the patient's provider (i.e., physician or other qualified healthcare practitioner legally accountable for establishing the patient's diagnosis). There are a few exceptions when code assignment may be based on medical record documentation from clinicians who are not the patient's provider (i.e., physician or other qualified healthcare practitioner legally accountable for establishing the patient's diagnosis). In this context, "clinicians" other than the patient's provider refer to healthcare professionals permitted, based on regulatory or accreditation requirements or internal hospital policies, to document in a patient's official medical record.

These exceptions include codes for:

- Body Mass Index (BMI)
- Depth of non-pressure chronic ulcers
- Pressure ulcer stage
- Coma scale
- NIH stroke scale (NIHSS)
- Social determinants of health (SDOH)
- Laterality
- Blood alcohol level
- **Underimmunization status**

This information is typically, or may be, documented by other clinicians involved in the care of the patient (e.g., a dietitian often documents the BMI, a nurse often documents the pressure ulcer stages, and an emergency medical technician often documents the coma scale). However, the associated diagnosis (such as overweight, obesity, acute stroke, pressure ulcer, or a condition classifiable to category F1Ø, Alcohol related disorders) must be documented by the patient's provider. If there is conflicting medical record documentation, either from the same clinician or different clinicians, the patient's attending provider should be queried for clarification.

The BMI, coma scale, NIHSS, blood alcohol level codes, codes for social determinants of health **and underimmunization status** should only be reported as secondary diagnoses.

See Section I.C.21.c.17. for additional information regarding coding social determinants of health.

15. Syndromes

Follow the Alphabetic Index guidance when coding syndromes. In the absence of Alphabetic Index guidance, assign codes for the documented manifestations of the syndrome. Additional codes for manifestations that are not an integral part of the disease process may also be assigned when the condition does not have a unique code.

16. Documentation of Complications of Care

Code assignment is based on the provider's documentation of the relationship between the condition and the care or procedure, unless otherwise instructed by the classification. The guideline extends to any complications of care, regardless of the chapter the code is located in. It is important to note that not all conditions that occur during or following medical care or surgery are classified as complications. There must be a cause-and-effect relationship between the care provided and the condition, and **the documentation must support that the condition is clinically significant. It is not necessary for the provider to explicitly document the term "complication." For example, if the condition alters the course of the surgery as documented in the operative report, then it would be appropriate to report a complication code.** Query the provider for clarification **if the documentation is not clear as to the relationship between the condition and the care or procedure.**

17. Borderline Diagnosis

If the provider documents a "borderline" diagnosis at the time of discharge, the diagnosis is coded as confirmed, unless the classification provides a specific entry (e.g., borderline diabetes). If a borderline condition has a specific index entry in ICD-10-CM, it should be coded as such. Since borderline conditions are not uncertain diagnoses, no distinction is made between the care setting (inpatient versus outpatient). Whenever the documentation is unclear regarding a borderline condition, coders are encouraged to query for clarification.

18. Use of Sign/Symptom/Unspecified Codes

Sign/symptom and "unspecified" codes have acceptable, even necessary, uses. While specific diagnosis codes should be reported when they are supported by the available medical record documentation and clinical knowledge of the patient's health condition, there are instances when signs/symptoms or unspecified codes are the best choices for accurately reflecting the healthcare encounter. Each healthcare encounter should be coded to the level of certainty known for that encounter.

As stated in the introductory section of these official coding guidelines, a joint effort between the healthcare provider and the coder is essential to achieve complete and accurate documentation, code assignment, and reporting of diagnoses and procedures. The importance of consistent, complete documentation in the medical record cannot be overemphasized. Without such documentation accurate coding cannot be achieved. The entire record should be reviewed to determine the specific reason for the encounter and the conditions treated.

If a definitive diagnosis has not been established by the end of the encounter, it is appropriate to report codes for sign(s) and/or symptom(s) in lieu of a definitive diagnosis. When sufficient clinical information isn't known or available about a particular health condition to assign a more specific code, it is acceptable to report the appropriate "unspecified" code (e.g., a diagnosis of pneumonia has been determined, but not the specific type). Unspecified codes should be reported when they are the codes that most accurately reflect what is known about the patient's condition at the time of that particular encounter. It would be inappropriate to select a specific code that is not supported by the medical record documentation or conduct medically unnecessary diagnostic testing in order to determine a more specific code.

19. Coding for Healthcare Encounters in Hurricane Aftermath

a. Use of External Cause of Morbidity Codes

An external cause of morbidity code should be assigned to identify the cause of the injury(ies) incurred as a result of the hurricane. The use of external cause of morbidity codes is supplemental to the application of ICD-10-CM codes. External cause of morbidity codes are never to be recorded as a principal diagnosis (first-listed in non-inpatient settings). The appropriate injury code should be sequenced before any external cause codes. The external cause of morbidity codes capture how the injury or health condition happened (cause), the intent (unintentional or accidental; or intentional, such as suicide or assault), the place where the event occurred, the activity of the patient at the time of the event, and the person's status (e.g., civilian, military). They should not be assigned for encounters to treat hurricane victims' medical conditions when no injury, adverse effect or poisoning is involved. External cause of morbidity codes should be assigned for each encounter for care and treatment of the injury. External cause of morbidity codes may be assigned in all health care settings. For the purpose of capturing complete and accurate ICD-10-CM data in the aftermath of the hurricane, a healthcare setting should be considered as any location where medical care is provided by licensed healthcare professionals.

b. Sequencing of External Causes of Morbidity Codes

Codes for cataclysmic events, such as a hurricane, take priority over all other external cause codes except child and adult abuse and terrorism and should be sequenced before other external cause of injury codes. Assign as many external cause of morbidity codes as necessary to fully explain each cause. For example, if an injury occurs as a result of a building collapse during the hurricane, external cause codes for both the hurricane and the building collapse should be assigned, with the external causes code for hurricane being sequenced as the first external cause code. For injuries incurred as a direct result of the hurricane, assign the appropriate code(s) for the injuries, followed by the code X37.Ø-, Hurricane (with the appropriate 7th character), and any other applicable external cause of injury codes. Code X37.Ø- also should be assigned when an injury is incurred as a result of flooding caused by a levee breaking related to the hurricane. Code X38.-, Flood (with the appropriate 7th character), should be assigned when an injury is from flooding resulting directly from the storm. Code X36.Ø.-, Collapse of dam or man-made structure, should not be assigned when the cause of the collapse is due to the hurricane. Use of code X36.Ø- is limited to collapses of man-made structures due to earth surface movements, not due to storm surges directly from a hurricane.

c. Other External Causes of Morbidity Code Issues

For injuries that are not a direct result of the hurricane, such as an evacuee that has incurred an injury as a result of a motor vehicle accident, assign the appropriate external cause of morbidity code(s) to describe the cause of the injury, but do not assign code X37.Ø-, Hurricane. If it is not clear whether the injury was a direct result of the hurricane, assume the injury is due to the hurricane and assign code X37.Ø-, Hurricane, as well as any other applicable external cause of morbidity codes. In addition to code X37.Ø-, Hurricane, other possible applicable external cause of morbidity codes include:

X3Ø-, Exposure to excessive natural heat
X31-, Exposure to excessive natural cold
X38-, Flood

d. Use of Z codes

Z codes (other reasons for healthcare encounters) may be assigned as appropriate to further explain the reasons for presenting for healthcare services, including transfers between healthcare facilities, or provide additional information relevant to a patient encounter. The ICD-10-CM Official Guidelines for Coding and Reporting identify which codes maybe assigned as principal or first-listed diagnosis only, secondary diagnosis only, or principal/first-listed or secondary (depending on the circumstances). Possible applicable Z codes include:

Z59.Ø-, Homelessness
Z59.1, Inadequate housing
Z59.5, Extreme poverty
Z75.1, Person awaiting admission to adequate facility elsewhere
Z75.3, Unavailability and inaccessibility of health-care facilities
Z75.4, Unavailability and inaccessibility of other helping agencies
Z76.2, Encounter for health supervision and care of other healthy infant and child
Z99.12, Encounter for respirator [ventilator] dependence during power failure

The external cause of morbidity codes and the Z codes listed above are not an all-inclusive list. Other codes may be applicable to the encounter based upon the documentation. Assign as many codes as necessary to fully explain each healthcare encounter. Since patient history information may be very limited, use any available documentation to assign the appropriate external cause of morbidity and Z codes.

C. Chapter-Specific Coding Guidelines

In addition to general coding guidelines, there are guidelines for specific diagnoses and/or conditions in the classification. Unless otherwise indicated, these guidelines apply to all health care settings. Please refer to Section II for guidelines on the selection of principal diagnosis.

1. Chapter 1: Certain Infectious and Parasitic Diseases (AØØ-B99), UØ7.1, UØ9.9

a. Human Immunodeficiency Virus (HIV) Infections

1) Code only confirmed cases

Code only confirmed cases of HIV infection/illness. This is an exception to the hospital inpatient guideline Section II, H.

In this context, "confirmation" does not require documentation of positive serology or culture for HIV; the provider's diagnostic statement that the patient is HIV positive or has an HIV-related illness is sufficient.

2) Selection and sequencing of HIV codes

(a) Patient admitted for HIV-related condition

If a patient is admitted for an HIV-related condition, the principal diagnosis should be B2Ø, Human immunodeficiency virus [HIV] disease followed by additional diagnosis codes for all reported HIV-related conditions.

An exception to this guideline is if the reason for admission is hemolytic-uremic syndrome associated with HIV disease. Assign code D59.31, Infection-associated hemolytic-uremic syndrome, followed by code B2Ø, Human immunodeficiency virus [HIV] disease.

(b) Patient with HIV disease admitted for unrelated condition

If a patient with HIV disease is admitted for an unrelated condition (such as a traumatic injury), the code for the unrelated condition (e.g., the nature of injury code) should be the principal diagnosis. Other diagnoses would be B2Ø followed by additional diagnosis codes for all reported HIV-related conditions.

(c) Whether the patient is newly diagnosed

Whether the patient is newly diagnosed or has had previous admissions/encounters for HIV conditions is irrelevant to the sequencing decision.

(d) Asymptomatic human immunodeficiency virus

Z21, Asymptomatic human immunodeficiency virus [HIV] infection status, is to be applied when the patient without any documentation of symptoms is listed as being "HIV positive," "known HIV," "HIV test positive," or similar terminology. Do not use this code if the term "AIDS" or "HIV disease" is used or if the patient is treated for any HIV-related illness or is described as having any condition(s) resulting from his/her HIV positive status; use B2Ø in these cases.

(e) Patients with inconclusive HIV serology
Patients with inconclusive HIV serology, but no definitive diagnosis or manifestations of the illness, may be assigned code R75, Inconclusive laboratory evidence of human immunodeficiency virus [HIV].

(f) Previously diagnosed HIV-related illness
Patients with any known prior diagnosis of an HIV-related illness should be coded to B2Ø. Once a patient has developed an HIV-related illness, the patient should always be assigned code B2Ø on every subsequent admission/encounter. Patients previously diagnosed with any HIV illness (B2Ø) should never be assigned to R75 or Z21, Asymptomatic human immunodeficiency virus [HIV] infection status.

(g) HIV Infection in Pregnancy, Childbirth and the Puerperium
During pregnancy, childbirth or the puerperium, a patient admitted (or presenting for a health care encounter) because of an HIV-related illness should receive a principal diagnosis code of O98.7-, Human immunodeficiency [HIV] disease complicating pregnancy, childbirth and the puerperium, followed by B2Ø and the code(s) for the HIV-related illness(es). Codes from Chapter 15 always take sequencing priority.

Patients with asymptomatic HIV infection status admitted (or presenting for a health care encounter) during pregnancy, childbirth, or the puerperium should receive codes of O98.7- and Z21.

(h) Encounters for testing for HIV
If a patient is being seen to determine his/her HIV status, use code Z11.4, Encounter for screening for human immunodeficiency virus [HIV]. Use additional codes for any associated high-risk behavior, if applicable.

If a patient with signs or symptoms is being seen for HIV testing, code the signs and symptoms. An additional counseling code Z71.7, Human immunodeficiency virus [HIV] counseling, may be used if counseling is provided during the encounter for the test.

When a patient returns to be informed of his/her HIV test results and the test result is negative, use code Z71.7, Human immunodeficiency virus [HIV] counseling.

If the results are positive, see previous guidelines and assign codes as appropriate.

(i) HIV managed by antiretroviral medication
If a patient with documented HIV disease, **HIV-related illness or AIDS** is currently managed on antiretroviral medications, assign code B2Ø, Human immunodeficiency virus [HIV] disease. Code Z79.899, Other long term (current) drug therapy, may be assigned as an additional code to identify the long-term (current) use of antiretroviral medications.

b. Infectious agents as the cause of diseases classified to other chapters
Certain infections are classified in chapters other than Chapter 1 and no organism is identified as part of the infection code. In these instances, it is necessary to use an additional code from Chapter 1 to identify the organism. A code from category B95, Streptococcus, Staphylococcus, and Enterococcus as the cause of diseases classified to other chapters, B96, Other bacterial agents as the cause of diseases classified to other chapters, or B97, Viral agents as the cause of diseases classified to other chapters, is to be used as an additional code to identify the organism. An instructional note will be found at the infection code advising that an additional organism code is required.

c. Infections resistant to antibiotics
Many bacterial infections are resistant to current antibiotics. It is necessary to identify all infections documented as antibiotic resistant. Assign a code from category Z16, Resistance to antimicrobial drugs, following the infection code only if the infection code does not identify drug resistance.

d. Sepsis, Severe Sepsis, and Septic Shock Infections resistant to antibiotics

1) Coding of Sepsis and Severe Sepsis

(a) Sepsis
For a diagnosis of sepsis, assign the appropriate code for the underlying systemic infection. If the type of infection or causal organism is not further specified, assign code A41.9, Sepsis, unspecified organism.

A code from subcategory R65.2, Severe sepsis, should not be assigned unless severe sepsis or an associated acute organ dysfunction is documented.

(i) Negative or inconclusive blood cultures and sepsis
Negative or inconclusive blood cultures do not preclude a diagnosis of sepsis in patients with clinical evidence of the condition; however, the provider should be queried.

(ii) Urosepsis
The term urosepsis is a nonspecific term. It is not to be considered synonymous with sepsis. It has no default code in the Alphabetic Index. Should a provider use this term, he/she must be queried for clarification.

(iii) Sepsis with organ dysfunction
If a patient has sepsis and associated acute organ dysfunction or multiple organ dysfunction (MOD), follow the instructions for coding severe sepsis.

(iv) Acute organ dysfunction that is not clearly associated with the sepsis
If a patient has sepsis and an acute organ dysfunction, but the medical record documentation indicates that the acute organ dysfunction is related to a medical condition other than the sepsis, do not assign a code from subcategory R65.2, Severe sepsis. An acute organ dysfunction must be associated with the sepsis in order to assign the severe sepsis code. If the documentation is not clear as to whether an acute organ dysfunction is related to the sepsis or another medical condition, query the provider.

(b) Severe sepsis
The coding of severe sepsis requires a minimum of 2 codes: first a code for the underlying systemic infection, followed by a code from subcategory R65.2, Severe sepsis. If the causal organism is not documented, assign code A41.9, Sepsis, unspecified organism, for the infection. Additional code(s) for the associated acute organ dysfunction are also required.

Due to the complex nature of severe sepsis, some cases may require querying the provider prior to assignment of the codes.

2) Septic shock
Septic shock generally refers to circulatory failure associated with severe sepsis, and therefore, it represents a type of acute organ dysfunction.

For cases of septic shock, the code for the systemic infection should be sequenced first, followed by code R65.21, Severe sepsis with septic shock or code T81.12, Postprocedural septic shock. Any additional codes for the other acute organ dysfunctions should also be assigned. As noted in the sequencing instructions in the Tabular List, the code for septic shock cannot be assigned as a principal diagnosis.

3) Sequencing of severe sepsis
If severe sepsis is present on admission, and meets the definition of principal diagnosis, the underlying systemic infection should be assigned as principal diagnosis followed by the appropriate code from subcategory R65.2 as required by the sequencing rules in the Tabular List. A code from subcategory R65.2 can never be assigned as a principal diagnosis.

When severe sepsis develops during an encounter (it was not present on admission), the underlying systemic infection and the appropriate code from subcategory R65.2 should be assigned as secondary diagnoses.

Severe sepsis may be present on admission, but the diagnosis may not be confirmed until sometime after admission. If the documentation is not clear whether severe sepsis was present on admission, the provider should be queried.

For infection-associated hemolytic-uremic syndrome with severe sepsis, see guideline I.C.1.d.9.

4) Sepsis or severe sepsis with a localized infection

If the reason for admission is sepsis or severe sepsis and a localized infection, such as pneumonia or cellulitis, a code(s) for the underlying systemic infection should be assigned first and the code for the localized infection should be assigned as a secondary diagnosis. If the patient has severe sepsis, a code from subcategory R65.2 should also be assigned as a secondary diagnosis. If the patient is admitted with a localized infection, such as pneumonia, and sepsis/severe sepsis doesn't develop until after admission, the localized infection should be assigned first, followed by the appropriate sepsis/severe sepsis codes.

For hemolytic-uremic syndrome associated with sepsis, see guideline I.C.1.d.9.

5) Sepsis due to a postprocedural infection

(a) Documentation of causal relationship

As with all postprocedural complications, code assignment is based on the provider's documentation of the relationship between the infection and the procedure.

(b) Sepsis due to a postprocedural infection

For infections following a procedure, a code from T81.4Ø, to T81.43 Infection following a procedure, or a code from O86.ØØ to O86.Ø3, Infection of obstetric surgical wound, that identifies the site of the infection should be coded first, if known. Assign an additional code for sepsis following a procedure (T81.44) or sepsis following an obstetrical procedure (O86.Ø4). Use an additional code to identify the infectious agent. If the patient has severe sepsis, the appropriate code from subcategory R65.2 should also be assigned with the additional code(s) for any acute organ dysfunction.

For infections following infusion, transfusion, therapeutic injection, or immunization, a code from subcategory T8Ø.2, Infections following infusion, transfusion, and therapeutic injection, or code T88.Ø-, Infection following immunization, should be coded first, followed by the code for the specific infection. If the patient has severe sepsis, the appropriate code from subcategory R65.2 should also be assigned, with the additional codes(s) for any acute organ dysfunction.

(c) Postprocedural infection and postprocedural septic shock

If a postprocedural infection has resulted in postprocedural septic shock, assign the codes indicated above for sepsis due to a postprocedural infection, followed by code T81.12-, Postprocedural septic shock. Do not assign code R65.21, Severe sepsis with septic shock. Additional code(s) should be assigned for any acute organ dysfunction.

6) Sepsis and severe sepsis associated with a noninfectious process (condition)

In some cases, a noninfectious process (condition) such as trauma, may lead to an infection which can result in sepsis or severe sepsis. If sepsis or severe sepsis is documented as associated with a noninfectious condition, such as a burn or serious injury, and this condition meets the definition for principal diagnosis, the code for the noninfectious condition should be sequenced first, followed by the code for the resulting infection. If severe sepsis is present, a code from subcategory R65.2 should also be assigned with any associated organ dysfunction(s) codes. It is not necessary to assign a code from subcategory R65.1, Systemic inflammatory response syndrome (SIRS) of non-infectious origin, for these cases.

If the infection meets the definition of principal diagnosis, it should be sequenced before the non-infectious condition. When both the associated non-infectious condition and the infection meet the definition of principal diagnosis, either may be assigned as principal diagnosis.

Only one code from category R65, Symptoms and signs specifically associated with systemic inflammation and infection, should be assigned. Therefore, when a non-infectious condition leads to an infection resulting in severe sepsis, assign the appropriate code from subcategory R65.2, Severe sepsis. Do not additionally assign a code from subcategory R65.1, Systemic inflammatory response syndrome (SIRS) of non-infectious origin.

See Section I.C.18. SIRS due to non-infectious process

7) Sepsis and septic shock complicating abortion, pregnancy, childbirth, and the puerperium

See Section I.C.15. Sepsis and septic shock complicating abortion, pregnancy, childbirth and the puerperium

8) Newborn sepsis

See Section I.C.16. f. Bacterial sepsis of Newborn

9) Hemolytic-uremic syndrome associated with sepsis

If the reason for admission is hemolytic-uremic syndrome that is associated with sepsis, assign code D59.31, Infection-associated hemolytic-uremic syndrome, as the principal diagnosis. Codes for the underlying systemic infection and any other conditions (such as severe sepsis) should be assigned as secondary diagnoses.

e. Methicillin Resistant Staphylococcus aureus (MRSA) Conditions

1) Selection and sequencing of MRSA codes

(a) Combination codes for MRSA infection

When a patient is diagnosed with an infection that is due to methicillin resistant *Staphylococcus aureus* (MRSA), and that infection has a combination code that includes the causal organism (e.g., sepsis, pneumonia) assign the appropriate combination code for the condition (e.g., code A41.Ø2, Sepsis due to Methicillin resistant Staphylococcus aureus or code J15.212, Pneumonia due to Methicillin resistant Staphylococcus aureus). Do not assign code B95.62, Methicillin resistant Staphylococcus aureus infection as the cause of diseases classified elsewhere, as an additional code, because the combination code includes the type of infection and the MRSA organism. Do not assign a code from subcategory Z16.11, Resistance to penicillins, as an additional diagnosis.

See Section C.1. for instructions on coding and sequencing of sepsis and severe sepsis.

(b) Other codes for MRSA infection

When there is documentation of a current infection (e.g., wound infection, stitch abscess, urinary tract infection) due to MRSA, and that infection does not have a combination code that includes the causal organism, assign the appropriate code to identify the condition along with code B95.62, Methicillin resistant Staphylococcus aureus infection as the cause of diseases classified elsewhere for the MRSA infection. Do not assign a code from subcategory Z16.11, Resistance to penicillins.

(c) Methicillin susceptible Staphylococcus aureus (MSSA) and MRSA colonization

The condition or state of being colonized or carrying MSSA or MRSA is called colonization or carriage, while an individual person is described as being colonized or being a carrier.

Colonization means that MSSA or MSRA is present on or in the body without necessarily causing illness. A positive MRSA colonization test might be documented by the provider as "MRSA screen positive" or "MRSA nasal swab positive".

Assign code Z22.322, Carrier or suspected carrier of Methicillin resistant Staphylococcus aureus, for patients documented as having MRSA colonization. Assign code Z22.321, Carrier or suspected carrier of Methicillin susceptible Staphylococcus aureus, for patients documented as having MSSA colonization. Colonization is not necessarily indicative of a disease process or as the cause of a specific condition the patient may have unless documented as such by the provider.

(d) MRSA colonization and infection

If a patient is documented as having both MRSA colonization and infection during a hospital admission, code Z22.322, Carrier or suspected carrier of Methicillin resistant Staphylococcus aureus, and a code for the MRSA infection may both be assigned.

f. Zika virus infections

1) Code only confirmed cases

Code only a confirmed diagnosis of Zika virus (A92.5, Zika virus disease) as documented by the provider. This is an exception to the hospital inpatient guideline Section II, H. In this context, "confirmation" does not require documentation of the type of test performed; the provider's diagnostic statement that the condition is confirmed is sufficient. This code should be assigned regardless of the stated mode of transmission.

If the provider documents "suspected", "possible" or "probable" Zika, do not assign code A92.5. Assign a code(s) explaining the reason for encounter (such as fever, rash, or joint pain) or Z2Ø.821, Contact with and (suspected) exposure to Zika virus.

g. Coronavirus infections

1) COVID-19 infection (infection due to SARS-CoV-2)

(a) Code only confirmed cases

Code only a confirmed diagnosis of the 2019 novel coronavirus disease (COVID-19) as documented by the provider, or documentation of a positive COVID-19 test result. For a confirmed diagnosis, assign code U07.1, COVID-19. This is an exception to the hospital inpatient guideline Section II, H. In this context, "confirmation" does not require documentation of a positive test result for COVID-19; the provider's documentation that the individual has COVID-19 is sufficient.

If the provider documents "suspected," "possible," "probable," or "inconclusive" COVID-19, do not assign code U07.1. Instead, code the signs and symptoms reported. See guideline I.C.1.g.1.g.

(b) Sequencing of codes

When COVID-19 meets the definition of principal diagnosis, code U07.1, COVID-19, should be sequenced first, followed by the appropriate codes for associated manifestations, except when another guideline requires that certain codes be sequenced first, such as obstetrics, sepsis, or transplant complications.

For a COVID-19 infection that progresses to sepsis, see Section I.C.1.d. Sepsis, Severe Sepsis, and Septic Shock

See Section I.C.15.s. for COVID-19 infection in pregnancy, childbirth, and the puerperium

See Section I.C.16.h. for COVID-19 infection in newborn

For a COVID-19 infection in a lung transplant patient, see Section I.C.19.g.3.a. Transplant complications other than kidney.

(c) Acute respiratory manifestations of COVID-19

When the reason for the encounter/admission is a respiratory manifestation of COVID-19, assign code U07.1, COVID-19, as the principal/first-listed diagnosis and assign code(s) for the respiratory manifestation(s) as additional diagnoses.

The following conditions are examples of common respiratory manifestations of COVID-19.

(i) Pneumonia

For a patient with pneumonia confirmed as due to COVID-19, assign codes U07.1, COVID-19, and J12.82, Pneumonia due to coronavirus disease 2019.

(ii) Acute bronchitis

For a patient with acute bronchitis confirmed as due to COVID-19, assign codes U07.1, and J20.8, Acute bronchitis due to other specified organisms.

Bronchitis not otherwise specified (NOS) due to COVID-19 should be coded using code U07.1 and J40, Bronchitis, not specified as acute or chronic.

(iii) Lower respiratory infection

If the COVID-19 is documented as being associated with a lower respiratory infection, not otherwise specified (NOS), or an acute respiratory infection, NOS, codes U07.1 and J22, Unspecified acute lower respiratory infection, should be assigned.

If the COVID-19 is documented as being associated with a respiratory infection, NOS, codes U07.1 and J98.8, Other specified respiratory disorders, should be assigned.

(iv) Acute respiratory distress syndrome

For acute respiratory distress syndrome (ARDS) due to COVID-19, assign codes U07.1, and J80, Acute respiratory distress syndrome.

(v) Acute respiratory failure

For acute respiratory failure due to COVID-19, assign code U07.1, and code J96.0-, Acute respiratory failure.

(d) Non-respiratory manifestations of COVID-19

When the reason for the encounter/admission is a non-respiratory manifestation (e.g., viral enteritis) of COVID-19, assign code U07.1, COVID-19, as the principal/first-listed diagnosis and assign code(s) for the manifestation(s) as additional diagnoses.

(e) Exposure to COVID-19

For asymptomatic individuals with actual or suspected exposure to COVID-19, assign code Z20.822, Contact with and (suspected) exposure to COVID-19.

For symptomatic individuals with actual or suspected exposure to COVID-19 and the infection has been ruled out, or test results are inconclusive or unknown, assign code Z20.822, Contact with and (suspected) exposure to COVID-19. See guideline I.C.21.c.1, Contact/Exposure, for additional guidance regarding the use of category Z20 codes.

If COVID-19 is confirmed, see guideline I.C.1.g.1.a.

(f) Screening for COVID-19

During the COVID-19 pandemic, a screening code is generally not appropriate. Do not assign code Z11.52, Encounter for screening for COVID-19. For encounters for COVID-19 testing, including preoperative testing, code as exposure to COVID-19 (guideline I.C.1.g.1.e).

Coding guidance will be updated as new information concerning any changes in the pandemic status becomes available.

(g) Signs and symptoms without definitive diagnosis of COVID-19

For patients presenting with any signs/symptoms associated with COVID-19 (such as fever, etc.) but a definitive diagnosis has not been established, assign the appropriate code(s) for each of the presenting signs and symptoms such as:

- R05.1, Acute cough, or R05.9, Cough, unspecified
- R06.02 Shortness of breath
- R50.9 Fever, unspecified

If a patient with signs/symptoms associated with COVID-19 also has an actual or suspected contact with or exposure to COVID-19, assign Z20.822, Contact with and (suspected) exposure to COVID-19, as an additional code.

(h) Asymptomatic individuals who test positive for COVID-19

For asymptomatic individuals who test positive for COVID-19, see guideline I.C.1.g.1.a. Although the individual is asymptomatic, the individual has tested positive and is considered to have the COVID-19 infection.

(i) Personal history of COVID-19

For patients with a history of COVID-19, assign code Z86.16, Personal history of COVID-19.

(j) Follow-up visits after COVID-19 infection has resolved

For individuals who previously had COVID-19, without residual symptom(s) or condition(s), and are being seen for follow-up evaluation, and COVID-19 test results are negative, assign codes Z09, Encounter for follow-up examination after completed treatment for conditions other than malignant neoplasm, and Z86.16, Personal history of COVID-19.

For follow-up visits for individuals with symptom(s) or condition(s) related to a previous COVID-19 infection, see guideline I.C.1.g.1.m.

See Section I.C.21.c.8, Factors influencing health states and contact with health services, Follow-up

(k) Encounter for antibody testing

For an encounter for antibody testing that is not being performed to confirm a current COVID-19 infection, nor is a follow-up test after resolution of COVID-19, assign Z01.84, Encounter for antibody response examination.

Follow the applicable guidelines above if the individual is being tested to confirm a current COVID-19 infection.

For follow-up testing after a COVID-19 infection, see guideline I.C.1.g.1.j.

(l) Multisystem Inflammatory Syndrome

For individuals with multisystem inflammatory syndrome (MIS) and COVID-19, assign code U07.1, COVID-19, as the principal/first-listed diagnosis and assign code M35.81, Multisystem inflammatory syndrome, as an additional diagnosis.

If an individual with a history of COVID-19 develops MIS, assign codes M35.81, Multisystem inflammatory syndrome, and U09.9, Post COVID-19 condition, unspecified.

If an individual with a known or suspected exposure to COVID-19, and no current COVID-19 infection or history of

COVID-19, develops MIS, assign codes M35.81, Multisystem inflammatory syndrome, and Z20.822, Contact with and (suspected) exposure to COVID-19.

Additional codes should be assigned for any associated complications of MIS.

(m) Post COVID-19 Condition

For sequela of COVID-19, or associated symptoms or conditions that develop following a previous COVID-19 infection, assign a code(s) for the specific symptom(s) or condition(s) related to the previous COVID-19 infection, if known, and code U09.9, Post COVID-19 condition, unspecified.

Code U09.9 should not be assigned for manifestations of an active (current) COVID-19 infection.

If a patient has a condition(s) associated with a previous COVID-19 infection and develops a new active (current) COVID-19 infection, code U09.9 may be assigned in conjunction with code U07.1, COVID-19, to identify that the patient also has a condition(s) associated with a previous COVID-19 infection. Code(s) for the specific condition(s) associated with the previous COVID-19 infection and code(s) for manifestation(s) of the new active (current) COVID-19 infection should also be assigned.

(n) Underimmunization for COVID-19 Status

Code Z28.310, Unvaccinated for COVID-19, may be assigned when the patient has not received **a** COVID-19 vaccine **of any type.** Code Z28.311, Partially vaccinated for COVID-19, may be assigned when the patient has **been partially vaccinated for COVID-19 as per the recommendations of** the Centers for Disease Control and Prevention (CDC) in place at the time of the encounter. For information, visit the CDC's website https://www.cdc.gov/coronavirus/2019-ncov/vaccines/.

See Section I.B.14. for underimmunization documentation by clinicians other than patient's provider.

2. Chapter 2: Neoplasms (C00-D49)

General Guidelines

Chapter 2 of the ICD-10-CM contains the codes for most benign and all malignant neoplasms. Certain benign neoplasms, such as prostatic adenomas, may be found in the specific body system chapters. To properly code a neoplasm, it is necessary to determine from the record if the neoplasm is benign, in-situ, malignant, or of uncertain histologic behavior. If malignant, any secondary (metastatic) sites should also be determined.

Primary malignant neoplasms overlapping site boundaries

A primary malignant neoplasm that overlaps two or more contiguous (next to each other) sites should be classified to the subcategory/code .8 ('overlapping lesion'), unless the combination is specifically indexed elsewhere. For multiple neoplasms of the same site that are not contiguous such as tumors in different quadrants of the same breast, codes for each site should be assigned.

Malignant neoplasm of ectopic tissue

Malignant neoplasms of ectopic tissue are to be coded to the site of origin mentioned, e.g., ectopic pancreatic malignant neoplasms involving the stomach are coded to malignant neoplasm of pancreas, unspecified (C25.9).

The neoplasm table in the Alphabetic Index should be referenced first. However, if the histological term is documented, that term should be referenced first, rather than going immediately to the Neoplasm Table, in order to determine which column in the Neoplasm Table is appropriate. For example, if the documentation indicates "adenoma," refer to the term in the Alphabetic Index to review the entries under this term and the instructional note to "see also neoplasm, by site, benign." The table provides the proper code based on the type of neoplasm and the site. It is important to select the proper column in the table that corresponds to the type of neoplasm. The Tabular List should then be referenced to verify that the correct code has been selected from the table and that a more specific site code does not exist.

See Section I.C.21. Factors influencing health status and contact with health services, Status, for information regarding Z15.0, codes for genetic susceptibility to cancer.

a. *Admission/Encounter for treatment of primary site*

If the malignancy **is chiefly responsible for occasioning the patient admission/encounter and treatment is directed at the primary site**, designate the **primary** malignancy as the principal/**first-listed** diagnosis.

The only exception to this guideline is if the administration of chemotherapy, immunotherapy or external beam radiation therapy **is chiefly responsible for occasioning the admission/encounter. In that case**, assign the appropriate Z51.-- code as the first-listed or principal diagnosis, and the **underlying** diagnosis or problem for which the service is being performed as a secondary diagnosis.

b. *Admission/Encounter for* treatment of secondary site

When a patient is admitted because of a primary neoplasm with metastasis and treatment is directed toward the secondary site only, the secondary neoplasm is designated as the principal diagnosis even though the primary malignancy is still present.

c. Coding and sequencing of complications

Coding and sequencing of complications associated with the malignancies or with the therapy thereof are subject to the following guidelines:

1) Anemia associated with malignancy

When admission/encounter is for management of an anemia associated with the malignancy, and the treatment is only for anemia, the appropriate code for the malignancy is sequenced as the principal or first-listed diagnosis followed by the appropriate code for the anemia (such as code D63.0, Anemia in neoplastic disease).

2) Anemia associated with chemotherapy, immunotherapy and radiation therapy

When the admission/encounter is for management of an anemia associated with an adverse effect of the administration of chemotherapy or immunotherapy and the only treatment is for the anemia, the anemia code is sequenced first followed by the appropriate codes for the neoplasm and the adverse effect (T45.1X5-, Adverse effect of antineoplastic and immunosuppressive drugs).

When the admission/encounter is for management of an anemia associated with an adverse effect of radiotherapy, the anemia code should be sequenced first, followed by the appropriate neoplasm code and code Y84.2, Radiological procedure and radiotherapy as the cause of abnormal reaction of the patient, or of later complication, without mention of misadventure at the time of the procedure.

3) Management of dehydration due to the malignancy

When the admission/encounter is for management of dehydration due to the malignancy and only the dehydration is being treated (intravenous rehydration), the dehydration is sequenced first, followed by the code(s) for the malignancy.

4) Treatment of a complication resulting from a surgical procedure

When the admission/encounter is for treatment of a complication resulting from a surgical procedure, designate the complication as the principal or first-listed diagnosis if treatment is directed at resolving the complication.

d. Primary malignancy previously excised

When a primary malignancy has been previously excised or eradicated from its site and there is no further treatment directed to that site and there is no evidence of any existing primary malignancy at that site, a code from category Z85, Personal history of malignant neoplasm, should be used to indicate the former site of the malignancy. Any mention of extension, invasion, or metastasis to another site is coded as a secondary malignant neoplasm to that site. The secondary site may be the principal or first-listed diagnosis with the Z85 code used as a secondary code.

See section I.C.2.t. Secondary malignant neoplasm of lymphoid tissue.

e. Admissions/Encounters involving chemotherapy, immunotherapy and radiation therapy

1) Episode of care involves surgical removal of neoplasm

When an episode of care involves the surgical removal of a neoplasm, primary or secondary site, followed by adjunct chemotherapy or radiation treatment during the same episode of care, the code for the neoplasm should be assigned as principal or first-listed diagnosis.

2) Patient admission/encounter solely for administration of chemotherapy, immunotherapy and radiation therapy

If a patient admission/encounter is solely for the administration of chemotherapy, immunotherapy or external beam radiation therapy assign code Z51.0, Encounter for antineoplastic radiation therapy, or Z51.11, Encounter for antineoplastic chemotherapy, or Z51.12, Encounter for antineoplastic immunotherapy as the first-listed or principal diagnosis. If a patient receives more than one of these therapies during the same admission more than one of these codes may be assigned, in any sequence.

The malignancy for which the therapy is being administered should be assigned as a secondary diagnosis.

If a patient admission/encounter is for the insertion or implantation of radioactive elements (e.g., brachytherapy) the appropriate code for the malignancy is sequenced as the principal or first-listed diagnosis. Code Z51.Ø should not be assigned.

3) Patient admitted for radiation therapy, chemotherapy or immunotherapy and develops complications

When a patient is admitted for the purpose of external beam radiotherapy, immunotherapy or chemotherapy and develops complications such as uncontrolled nausea and vomiting or dehydration, the principal or first-listed diagnosis is Z51.Ø, Encounter for antineoplastic radiation therapy, or Z51.11, Encounter for antineoplastic chemotherapy, or Z51.12, Encounter for antineoplastic immunotherapy followed by any codes for the complications.

When a patient is admitted for the purpose of insertion or implantation of radioactive elements (e.g., brachytherapy) and develops complications such as uncontrolled nausea and vomiting or dehydration, the principal or first-listed diagnosis is the appropriate code for the malignancy followed by any codes for the complications.

f. Admission/encounter to determine extent of malignancy

When the reason for admission/encounter is to determine the extent of the malignancy, or for a procedure such as paracentesis or thoracentesis, the primary malignancy or appropriate metastatic site is designated as the principal or first-listed diagnosis, even though chemotherapy or radiotherapy is administered.

g. Symptoms, signs, and abnormal findings listed in Chapter 18 associated with neoplasms

Symptoms, signs, and ill-defined conditions listed in Chapter 18 characteristic of, or associated with, an existing primary or secondary site malignancy cannot be used to replace the malignancy as principal or first-listed diagnosis, regardless of the number of admissions or encounters for treatment and care of the neoplasm.

See section I.C.21. Factors influencing health status and contact with health services, Encounter for prophylactic organ removal.

h. Admission/encounter for pain control/management

See Section I.C.6. for information on coding admission/encounter for pain control/management.

i. Malignancy in two or more noncontiguous sites

A patient may have more than one malignant tumor in the same organ. These tumors may represent different primaries or metastatic disease, depending on the site. Should the documentation be unclear, the provider should be queried as to the status of each tumor so that the correct codes can be assigned.

j. Disseminated malignant neoplasm, unspecified

Code C8Ø.Ø, Disseminated malignant neoplasm, unspecified, is for use only in those cases where the patient has advanced metastatic disease and no known primary or secondary sites are specified. It should not be used in place of assigning codes for the primary site and all known secondary sites.

k. Malignant neoplasm without specification of site

Code C8Ø.1, Malignant (primary) neoplasm, unspecified, equates to Cancer, unspecified. This code should only be used when no determination can be made as to the primary site of a malignancy. This code should rarely be used in the inpatient setting.

l. Sequencing of neoplasm codes

1) Encounter for treatment of primary malignancy

If the reason for the encounter is for treatment of a primary malignancy, assign the malignancy as the principal/first-listed diagnosis. The primary site is to be sequenced first, followed by any metastatic sites.

2) Encounter for treatment of secondary malignancy

When an encounter is for a primary malignancy with metastasis and treatment is directed toward the metastatic (secondary) site(s) only, the metastatic site(s) is designated as the principal/first-listed diagnosis. The primary malignancy is coded as an additional code.

3) Malignant neoplasm in a pregnant patient

When a pregnant patient has a malignant neoplasm, a code from subcategory O9A.1-, Malignant neoplasm complicating pregnancy, childbirth, and the puerperium, should be sequenced first, followed by the appropriate code from Chapter 2 to indicate the type of neoplasm.

4) Encounter for complication associated with a neoplasm

When an encounter is for management of a complication associated with a neoplasm, such as dehydration, and the treatment is only for the complication, the complication is coded first, followed by the appropriate code(s) for the neoplasm.

The exception to this guideline is anemia. When the admission/encounter is for management of an anemia associated with the malignancy, and the treatment is only for anemia, the appropriate code for the malignancy is sequenced as the principal or first-listed diagnosis followed by code D63.Ø, Anemia in neoplastic disease.

5) Complication from surgical procedure for treatment of a neoplasm

When an encounter is for treatment of a complication resulting from a surgical procedure performed for the treatment of the neoplasm, designate the complication as the principal/first-listed diagnosis. See the guideline regarding the coding of a current malignancy versus personal history to determine if the code for the neoplasm should also be assigned.

6) Pathologic fracture due to a neoplasm

When an encounter is for a pathological fracture due to a neoplasm, and the focus of treatment is the fracture, a code from subcategory M84.5, Pathological fracture in neoplastic disease, should be sequenced first, followed by the code for the neoplasm.

If the focus of treatment is the neoplasm with an associated pathological fracture, the neoplasm code should be sequenced first, followed by a code from M84.5 for the pathological fracture.

m. Current malignancy versus personal history of malignancy

When a primary malignancy has been excised but further treatment, such as an additional surgery for the malignancy, radiation therapy or chemotherapy is directed to that site, the primary malignancy code should be used until treatment is completed.

When a primary malignancy has been previously excised or eradicated from its site, there is no further treatment (of the malignancy) directed to that site, and there is no evidence of any existing primary malignancy at that site, a code from category Z85, Personal history of malignant neoplasm, should be used to indicate the former site of the malignancy.

Codes from subcategories Z85.Ø – Z85.85 should only be assigned for the former site of a primary malignancy, not the site of a secondary malignancy. Code Z85.89 may be assigned for the former site(s) of either a primary or secondary malignancy.

See Section I.C.21. Factors influencing health status and contact with health services, History (of)

n. Leukemia, Multiple Myeloma, and Malignant Plasma Cell Neoplasms in remission versus personal history

The categories for leukemia, and category C9Ø, Multiple myeloma and malignant plasma cell neoplasms, have codes indicating whether or not the leukemia has achieved remission. There are also codes Z85.6, Personal history of leukemia, and Z85.79, Personal history of other malignant neoplasms of lymphoid, hematopoietic and related tissues. If the documentation is unclear as to whether the leukemia has achieved remission, the provider should be queried.

See Section I.C.21. Factors influencing health status and contact with health services, History (of)

o. Aftercare following surgery for neoplasm

See Section I.C.21. Factors influencing health status and contact with health services, Aftercare

p. Follow-up care for completed treatment of a malignancy

See Section I.C.21. Factors influencing health status and contact with health services, Follow-up

q. Prophylactic organ removal for prevention of malignancy

See Section I.C. 21, Factors influencing health status and contact with health services, Prophylactic organ removal

r. Malignant neoplasm associated with transplanted organ

A malignant neoplasm of a transplanted organ should be coded as a transplant complication. Assign first the appropriate code from category T86.-, Complications of transplanted organs and tissue, followed by code C8Ø.2, Malignant neoplasm associated with transplanted organ. Use an additional code for the specific malignancy.

s. Breast Implant Associated Anaplastic Large Cell Lymphoma

Breast implant associated anaplastic large cell lymphoma (BIA-ALCL) is a type of lymphoma that can develop around breast implants. Assign code C84.7A, Anaplastic large cell lymphoma, ALK-negative, breast, for BIA-ALCL. Do not assign a complication code from chapter 19.

t. Secondary malignant neoplasm of lymphoid tissue

When a malignant neoplasm of lymphoid tissue metastasizes beyond the lymph nodes, a code from categories C81-C85 with a final character "9" should be assigned identifying "extranodal and solid organ sites" rather than a code for the secondary neoplasm of the affected solid organ. For example, for metastasis of B-cell lymphoma to the lung, brain and left adrenal gland, assign code C83.39, Diffuse large B-cell lymphoma, extranodal and solid organ sites.

3. Chapter 3: Disease of the blood and blood-forming organs and certain disorders involving the immune mechanism (D5Ø-D89)

Reserved for future guideline expansion

4. Chapter 4: Endocrine, Nutritional, and Metabolic Diseases (EØØ-E89)

a. Diabetes mellitus

The diabetes mellitus codes are combination codes that include the type of diabetes mellitus, the body system affected, and the complications affecting that body system. As many codes within a particular category as are necessary to describe all of the complications of the disease may be used. They should be sequenced based on the reason for a particular encounter. Assign as many codes from categories EØ8 – E13 as needed to identify all of the associated conditions that the patient has.

1) Type of diabetes

The age of a patient is not the sole determining factor, though most type 1 diabetics develop the condition before reaching puberty. For this reason, type 1 diabetes mellitus is also referred to as juvenile diabetes.

2) Type of diabetes mellitus not documented

If the type of diabetes mellitus is not documented in the medical record the default is E11.-, Type 2 diabetes mellitus.

3) Diabetes mellitus and the use of insulin, oral hypoglycemics, and injectable non-insulin drugs

If the documentation in a medical record does not indicate the type of diabetes but does indicate that the patient uses insulin, code E11-, Type 2 diabetes mellitus, should be assigned. Additional code(s) should be assigned from category Z79 to identify the long-term (current) use of insulin, oral hypoglycemic drugs, or injectable non-insulin antidiabetic, as follows:

If the patient is treated with both oral **hypoglycemic drugs** and insulin, both code Z79.4, Long term (current) use of insulin, and code Z79.84, Long term (current) use of oral hypoglycemic drugs, should be assigned.

If the patient is treated with both insulin and an injectable non-insulin antidiabetic drug, assign codes Z79.4, Long term (current) use of insulin, and **Z79.85, Long-term (current) use of injectable non-insulin antidiabetic drugs.**

If the patient is treated with both oral hypoglycemic drugs and an injectable non-insulin antidiabetic drug, assign codes Z79.84, Long term (current) use of oral hypoglycemic drugs, and **Z79.85, Long-term (current) use of injectable non-insulin antidiabetic drugs.**

Code Z79.4 should not be assigned if insulin is given temporarily to bring a type 2 patient's blood sugar under control during an encounter.

4) Diabetes mellitus in pregnancy and gestational diabetes

See Section I.C.15. Diabetes mellitus in pregnancy.

See Section I.C.15. Gestational (pregnancy induced) diabetes

5) Complications due to insulin pump malfunction

(a) Underdose of insulin due to insulin pump failure

An underdose of insulin due to an insulin pump failure should be assigned to a code from subcategory T85.6, Mechanical complication of other specified internal and external prosthetic devices, implants and grafts, that specifies the type of pump malfunction, as the principal or first-listed code, followed by code T38.3X6-, Underdosing of insulin and oral hypoglycemic [antidiabetic] drugs. Additional codes for the type of diabetes mellitus and any associated complications due to the underdosing should also be assigned.

(b) Overdose of insulin due to insulin pump failure

The principal or first-listed code for an encounter due to an insulin pump malfunction resulting in an overdose of insulin, should also be T85.6-, Mechanical complication of other specified internal and external prosthetic devices, implants and grafts, followed by code T38.3X1-, Poisoning by insulin and oral hypoglycemic [antidiabetic] drugs, accidental (unintentional).

6) Secondary diabetes mellitus

Codes under categories EØ8, Diabetes mellitus due to underlying condition, EØ9, Drug or chemical induced diabetes mellitus, and E13, Other specified diabetes mellitus, identify complications/manifestations associated with secondary diabetes mellitus. Secondary diabetes is always caused by another condition or event (e.g., cystic fibrosis, malignant neoplasm of pancreas, pancreatectomy, adverse effect of drug, or poisoning).

(a) Secondary diabetes mellitus and the use of insulin, oral hypoglycemic drugs, or injectable non-insulin drugs

For patients with secondary diabetes mellitus who routinely use insulin, oral hypoglycemic drugs, or injectable non-insulin drugs, additional code(s) from category Z79 should be assigned to identify the long-term (current) use of insulin, oral hypoglycemic drugs, or non-injectable non-insulin drugs as follows:

If the patient is treated with both oral **hypoglycemic drugs** and insulin, both code Z79.4, Long term (current) use of insulin, and code Z79.84, Long term (current) use of oral hypoglycemic drugs, should be assigned.

If the patient is treated with both insulin and an injectable non-insulin antidiabetic drug, assign codes Z79.4, Long-term (current) use of insulin, and **Z79.85, Long-term (current) use of injectable non-insulin antidiabetic drugs.**

If the patient is treated with both oral hypoglycemic drugs and an injectable non-insulin antidiabetic drug, assign codes Z79.84, Long-term (current) use of oral hypoglycemic drugs, and **Z79.85, Long-term (current) use of injectable non-insulin antidiabetic drugs.**

Code Z79.4 should not be assigned if insulin is given temporarily to bring a secondary diabetic patient's blood sugar under control during an encounter.

(b) Assigning and sequencing secondary diabetes codes and its causes

The sequencing of the secondary diabetes codes in relationship to codes for the cause of the diabetes is based on the Tabular List instructions for categories EØ8, EØ9 and E13.

(i) Secondary diabetes mellitus due to pancreatectomy

For postpancreatectomy diabetes mellitus (lack of insulin due to the surgical removal of all or part of the pancreas), assign code E89.1, Postprocedural hypoinsulinemia.

Assign a code from category E13 and a code from subcategory Z9Ø.41, Acquired absence of pancreas, as additional codes.

(ii) Secondary diabetes due to drugs

Secondary diabetes may be caused by an adverse effect of correctly administered medications, poisoning or sequela of poisoning.

See section I.C.19.e. for coding of adverse effects and poisoning, and section I.C.20 for external cause code reporting.

5. Chapter 5: Mental, Behavioral and Neurodevelopmental disorders (FØ1-F99)

a. Pain disorders related to psychological factors

Assign code F45.41, for pain that is exclusively related to psychological disorders. As indicated by the Excludes 1 note under category G89, a code from category G89 should not be assigned with code F45.41.

Code F45.42, Pain disorders with related psychological factors, should be used with a code from category G89, Pain, not elsewhere classified, if there is documentation of a psychological component for a patient with acute or chronic pain.

See Section I.C.6. Pain

b. Mental and behavioral disorders due to psychoactive substance use

1) In Remission

Selection of codes **describing** "in remission" for categories F1Ø-F19, Mental and behavioral disorders due to psychoactive substance use (categories F1Ø-F19 with -.11, -.21, **-.91**) requires the provider's clinical judgment **and** are assigned only on the basis of provider documentation (as defined in the Official Guidelines for Coding and Reporting), unless otherwise instructed by the classification.

Mild substance use disorders in early or sustained remission are classified to the appropriate codes for substance abuse in remission, and moderate or severe substance use disorders in early or sustained remission are classified to the appropriate codes for substance dependence in remission.

2) Psychoactive Substance Use, Abuse and Dependence

When the provider documentation refers to use, abuse and dependence of the same substance (e.g. alcohol, opioid, cannabis, etc.), only one code should be assigned to identify the pattern of use based on the following hierarchy:

- If both use and abuse are documented, assign only the code for abuse
- If both abuse and dependence are documented, assign only the code for dependence
- If use, abuse and dependence are all documented, assign only the code for dependence
- If both use and dependence are documented, assign only the code for dependence.

3) Psychoactive Substance Use, Unspecified

As with all other unspecified diagnoses, the codes for unspecified psychoactive substance use (F1Ø.9-, F11.9-, F12.9-, F13.9-, F14.9-, F15.9-, F16.9-, F18.9-, F19.9-) should only be assigned based on provider documentation and when they meet the definition of a reportable diagnosis (see Section III, Reporting Additional Diagnoses). These codes are to be used only when the psychoactive substance use is associated with a substance related disorder (chapter 5 disorders such as sexual dysfunction, sleep disorder, or a mental or behavioral disorder) or medical condition, and such a relationship is documented by the provider.

4) Medical Conditions Due to Psychoactive Substance Use, Abuse and Dependence

Medical conditions due to substance use, abuse, and dependence are not classified as substance-induced disorders. Assign the diagnosis code for the medical condition as directed by the Alphabetical Index along with the appropriate psychoactive substance use, abuse or dependence code. For example, for alcoholic pancreatitis due to alcohol dependence, assign the appropriate code from subcategory K85.2, Alcohol induced acute pancreatitis, and the appropriate code from subcategory F1Ø.2, such as code F1Ø.2Ø, Alcohol dependence, uncomplicated. It would not be appropriate to assign code F1Ø.288, Alcohol dependence with other alcohol-induced disorder.

5) Blood Alcohol Level

A code from category Y9Ø, Evidence of alcohol involvement determined by blood alcohol level, may be assigned when this information is documented and the patient's provider has documented a condition classifiable to category F1Ø, Alcohol related disorders. The blood alcohol level does not need to be documented by the patient's provider in order for it to be coded.

See Section I.B.14. for blood alcohol level documentation by clinicians other than patient's provider.

c. Factitious Disorder

Factitious disorder imposed on self or Munchausen's syndrome is a disorder in which a person falsely reports or causes his or her own physical or psychological signs or symptoms. For patients with documented factitious disorder on self or Munchausen's syndrome, assign the appropriate code from subcategory F68.1-, Factitious disorder imposed on self.

Munchausen's syndrome by proxy (MSBP) is a disorder in which a caregiver (perpetrator) falsely reports or causes an illness or injury in another person (victim) under his or her care, such as a child, an elderly adult, or a person who has a disability. The condition is also referred to as "factitious disorder imposed on another" or "factitious disorder by proxy." The perpetrator, not the victim, receives this diagnosis. Assign code F68.A, Factitious disorder imposed on another, to the perpetrator's record. For the victim of a patient suffering from MSBP, assign the appropriate code from categories T74, Adult and child abuse, neglect and other maltreatment, confirmed, or T76, Adult and child abuse, neglect and other maltreatment, suspected.

See Section I.C.19.f. Adult and child abuse, neglect and other maltreatment

d. Dementia

The ICD-10-CM classifies dementia (categories FØ1, FØ2, and FØ3) on the basis of the etiology and severity (unspecified, mild, moderate or severe). Selection of the appropriate severity level requires the provider's clinical judgment and codes should be assigned only on the basis of provider documentation (as defined in the *Official Guidelines for Coding and Reporting*), unless otherwise instructed by the classification. If the documentation does not provide information about the severity of the dementia, assign the appropriate code for unspecified severity.

If a patient is admitted to an inpatient acute care hospital or other inpatient facility setting with dementia at one severity level and it progresses to a higher severity level, assign one code for the highest severity level reported during the stay.

6. Chapter 6: Diseases of the Nervous System (GØØ-G99)

a. Dominant/nondominant side

Codes from category G81, Hemiplegia and hemiparesis, and subcategories G83.1, Monoplegia of lower limb, G83.2, Monoplegia of upper limb, and G83.3, Monoplegia, unspecified, identify whether the dominant or nondominant side is affected. Should the affected side be documented, but not specified as dominant or nondominant, and the classification system does not indicate a default, code selection is as follows:

- For ambidextrous patients, the default should be dominant.
- If the left side is affected, the default is non-dominant.
- If the right side is affected, the default is dominant.

b. Pain - Category G89

1) General coding information

Codes in category G89, Pain, not elsewhere classified, may be used in conjunction with codes from other categories and chapters to provide more detail about acute or chronic pain and neoplasm-related pain, unless otherwise indicated below.

If the pain is not specified as acute or chronic, post-thoracotomy, postprocedural, or neoplasm-related, do not assign codes from category G89.

A code from category G89 should not be assigned if the underlying (definitive) diagnosis is known, unless the reason for the encounter is pain control/ management and not management of the underlying condition.

When an admission or encounter is for a procedure aimed at treating the underlying condition (e.g., spinal fusion, kyphoplasty), a code for the underlying condition (e.g., vertebral fracture, spinal stenosis) should be assigned as the principal diagnosis. No code from category G89 should be assigned.

(a) Category G89 Codes as Principal or First-Listed Diagnosis

Category G89 codes are acceptable as principal diagnosis or the first-listed code:

- When pain control or pain management is the reason for the admission/encounter (e.g., a patient with displaced intervertebral disc, nerve impingement and severe back pain presents for injection of steroid into the spinal canal). The underlying cause of the pain should be reported as an additional diagnosis, if known.
- When a patient is admitted for the insertion of a neurostimulator for pain control, assign the appropriate pain code as the principal or first-listed diagnosis. When an admission or encounter is for a procedure aimed at treating the underlying condition and a neurostimulator is inserted for pain control during the same admission/encounter, a code for the underlying condition should be assigned as the principal diagnosis and the appropriate pain code should be assigned as a secondary diagnosis.

(b) Use of Category G89 Codes in Conjunction with Site Specific Pain Codes

(i) Assigning Category G89 and Site-Specific Pain Codes

Codes from category G89 may be used in conjunction with codes that identify the site of pain (including codes from chapter 18) if the category G89 code provides additional information. For example, if the code describes the site of the pain, but does not fully describe whether the pain is acute or chronic, then both codes should be assigned.

(ii) Sequencing of Category G89 Codes with Site-Specific Pain Codes

The sequencing of category G89 codes with site-specific pain codes (including chapter 18 codes), is dependent on the circumstances of the encounter/admission as follows:

- If the encounter is for pain control or pain management, assign the code from category G89 followed by the code identifying the specific site of pain (e.g., encounter for pain management for acute neck pain from trauma is assigned code G89.11, Acute pain due to trauma, followed by code M54.2, Cervicalgia, to identify the site of pain).
- If the encounter is for any other reason except pain control or pain management, and a related definitive diagnosis has not been established (confirmed) by the provider, assign the code for the specific site of pain first, followed by the appropriate code from category G89.

2) Pain due to devices, implants and grafts

See Section I.C.19. Pain due to medical devices

3) Postoperative Pain

The provider's documentation should be used to guide the coding of postoperative pain, as well as *Section III. Reporting Additional Diagnoses* and *Section IV. Diagnostic Coding and Reporting in the Outpatient Setting.*

The default for post-thoracotomy and other postoperative pain not specified as acute or chronic is the code for the acute form.

Routine or expected postoperative pain immediately after surgery should not be coded.

(a) Postoperative pain not associated with specific postoperative complication

Postoperative pain not associated with a specific postoperative complication is assigned to the appropriate postoperative pain code in category G89.

(b) Postoperative pain associated with specific postoperative complication

Postoperative pain associated with a specific postoperative complication (such as painful wire sutures) is assigned to the appropriate code(s) found in Chapter 19, Injury, poisoning, and certain other consequences of external causes. If appropriate, use additional code(s) from category G89 to identify acute or chronic pain (G89.18 or G89.28).

4) Chronic pain

Chronic pain is classified to subcategory G89.2. There is no time frame defining when pain becomes chronic pain. The provider's documentation should be used to guide use of these codes.

5) Neoplasm Related Pain

Code G89.3 is assigned to pain documented as being related, associated or due to cancer, primary or secondary malignancy, or tumor. This code is assigned regardless of whether the pain is acute or chronic.

This code may be assigned as the principal or first-listed code when the stated reason for the admission/encounter is documented as pain control/pain management. The underlying neoplasm should be reported as an additional diagnosis.

When the reason for the admission/encounter is management of the neoplasm and the pain associated with the neoplasm is also documented, code G89.3 may be assigned as an additional diagnosis. It is not necessary to assign an additional code for the site of the pain.

See Section I.C.2. for instructions on the sequencing of neoplasms for all other stated reasons for the admission/encounter (except for pain control/pain management).

6) Chronic pain syndrome

Central pain syndrome (G89.Ø) and chronic pain syndrome (G89.4) are different than the term "chronic pain," and therefore codes should only be used when the provider has specifically documented this condition.

See Section I.C.5. Pain disorders related to psychological factors

7. Chapter 7: Diseases of the Eye and Adnexa (HØØ-H59)

a. Glaucoma

1) Assigning Glaucoma Codes

Assign as many codes from category H4Ø, Glaucoma, as needed to identify the type of glaucoma, the affected eye, and the glaucoma stage.

2) Bilateral glaucoma with same type and stage

When a patient has bilateral glaucoma and both eyes are documented as being the same type and stage, and there is a code for bilateral glaucoma, report only the code for the type of glaucoma, bilateral, with the seventh character for the stage.

When a patient has bilateral glaucoma and both eyes are documented as being the same type and stage, and the classification does not provide a code for bilateral glaucoma (i.e. subcategories H4Ø.1Ø, and H4Ø.2Ø) report only one code for the type of glaucoma with the appropriate seventh character for the stage.

3) Bilateral glaucoma stage with different types or stages

When a patient has bilateral glaucoma and each eye is documented as having a different type or stage, and the classification distinguishes laterality, assign the appropriate code for each eye rather than the code for bilateral glaucoma.

When a patient has bilateral glaucoma and each eye is documented as having a different type, and the classification does not distinguish laterality (i.e., subcategories H4Ø.1Ø, and H4Ø.2Ø), assign one code for each type of glaucoma with the appropriate seventh character for the stage.

When a patient has bilateral glaucoma and each eye is documented as having the same type, but different stage, and the classification does not distinguish laterality (i.e., subcategories H4Ø.1Ø and H4Ø.2Ø), assign a code for the type of glaucoma for each eye with the seventh character for the specific glaucoma stage documented for each eye.

4) Patient admitted with glaucoma and stage evolves during the admission

If a patient is admitted with glaucoma and the stage progresses during the admission, assign the code for highest stage documented.

5) Indeterminate stage glaucoma

Assignment of the seventh character "4" for "indeterminate stage" should be based on the clinical documentation. The seventh character "4" is used for glaucomas whose stage cannot be clinically determined. This seventh character should not be confused with the seventh character "Ø", unspecified, which should be assigned when there is no documentation regarding the stage of the glaucoma.

b. Blindness

If "blindness" or "low vision" of both eyes is documented but the visual impairment category is not documented, assign code H54.3, Unqualified visual loss, both eyes. If "blindness" or "low vision" in one eye is documented but the visual impairment category is not documented, assign a code from H54.6-, Unqualified visual loss, one eye. If "blindness" or "visual loss" is documented without any information about whether one or both eyes are affected, assign code H54.7, Unspecified visual loss.

8. Chapter 8: Diseases of the Ear and Mastoid Process (H6Ø-H95)

Reserved for future guideline expansion

9. Chapter 9: Diseases of the Circulatory System (IØØ-I99)

a. Hypertension

The classification presumes a causal relationship between hypertension and heart involvement and between hypertension and kidney involvement, as the two conditions are linked by the term "with" in the Alphabetic Index. These conditions should be coded as related even in the absence of provider documentation explicitly linking them, unless the documentation clearly states the conditions are unrelated.

For hypertension and conditions not specifically linked by relational terms such as "with," "associated with" or "due to" in the classification, provider documentation must link the conditions in order to code them as related.

1) **Hypertension with Heart Disease**
Hypertension with heart conditions classified to I5Ø.- or I51.4-I51.7, I51.89, I51.9, are assigned to a code from category I11, Hypertensive heart disease. Use additional code(s) from category I5Ø, Heart failure, to identify the type(s) of heart failure in those patients with heart failure.

The same heart conditions (I5Ø.-, I51.4-I51.7, I51.89, I51.9) with hypertension are coded separately if the provider has documented they are unrelated to the hypertension. Sequence according to the circumstances of the admission/encounter.

2) **Hypertensive Chronic Kidney Disease**
Assign codes from category I12, Hypertensive chronic kidney disease, when both hypertension and a condition classifiable to category N18, Chronic kidney disease (CKD), are present. CKD should not be coded as hypertensive if the provider indicates the CKD is not related to the hypertension.

The appropriate code from category N18 should be used as a secondary code with a code from category I12 to identify the stage of chronic kidney disease.

See Section I.C.14. Chronic kidney disease.

If a patient has hypertensive chronic kidney disease and acute renal failure, the acute renal failure should also be coded. Sequence according to the circumstances of the admission/encounter.

3) **Hypertensive Heart and Chronic Kidney Disease**
Assign codes from combination category I13, Hypertensive heart and chronic kidney disease, when there is hypertension with both heart and kidney involvement. If heart failure is present, assign an additional code from category I5Ø to identify the type of heart failure.

The appropriate code from category N18, Chronic kidney disease, should be used as a secondary code with a code from category I13 to identify the stage of chronic kidney disease.

See Section I.C.14. Chronic kidney disease.

The codes in category I13, Hypertensive heart and chronic kidney disease, are combination codes that include hypertension, heart disease and chronic kidney disease. The Includes note at I13 specifies that the conditions included at I11 and I12 are included together in I13. If a patient has hypertension, heart disease and chronic kidney disease, then a code from I13 should be used, not individual codes for hypertension, heart disease and chronic kidney disease, or codes from I11 or I12.

For patients with both acute renal failure and chronic kidney disease, the acute renal failure should also be coded. Sequence according to the circumstances of the admission/encounter.

4) **Hypertensive Cerebrovascular Disease**
For hypertensive cerebrovascular disease, first assign the appropriate code from categories I6Ø-I69, followed by the appropriate hypertension code.

5) **Hypertensive Retinopathy**
Subcategory H35.Ø, Background retinopathy and retinal vascular changes, should be used along with a code from categories I1Ø-I15, in the Hypertensive diseases section, to include the systemic hypertension. The sequencing is based on the reason for the encounter.

6) **Hypertension, Secondary**
Secondary hypertension is due to an underlying condition. Two codes are required: one to identify the underlying etiology and one from category I15 to identify the hypertension. Sequencing of codes is determined by the reason for admission/encounter.

7) **Hypertension, Transient**
Assign code RØ3.Ø, Elevated blood pressure reading without diagnosis of hypertension, unless patient has an established diagnosis of hypertension. Assign code O13.-, Gestational [pregnancy-induced] hypertension without significant proteinuria, or O14.-, Pre-eclampsia, for transient hypertension of pregnancy.

8) **Hypertension, Controlled**
This diagnostic statement usually refers to an existing state of hypertension under control by therapy. Assign the appropriate code from categories I1Ø-I15, Hypertensive diseases.

9) **Hypertension, Uncontrolled**
Uncontrolled hypertension may refer to untreated hypertension or hypertension not responding to current therapeutic regimen. In either case, assign the appropriate code from categories I1Ø-I15, Hypertensive diseases.

10) **Hypertensive Crisis**
Assign a code from category I16, Hypertensive crisis, for documented hypertensive urgency, hypertensive emergency or unspecified hypertensive crisis. Code also any identified hypertensive disease (I1Ø-I15). The sequencing is based on the reason for the encounter.

11) **Pulmonary Hypertension**
Pulmonary hypertension is classified to category I27, Other pulmonary heart diseases. For secondary pulmonary hypertension (I27.1, I27.2-), code also any associated conditions or adverse effects of drugs or toxins. The sequencing is based on the reason for the encounter, except for adverse effects of drugs (See Section I.C.19.e.).

b. **Atherosclerotic Coronary Artery Disease and Angina**
ICD-10-CM has combination codes for atherosclerotic heart disease with angina pectoris. The subcategories for these codes are I25.11, Atherosclerotic heart disease of native coronary artery with angina pectoris and I25.7, Atherosclerosis of coronary artery bypass graft(s) and coronary artery of transplanted heart with angina pectoris. When using one of these combination codes it is not necessary to use an additional code for angina pectoris. A causal relationship can be assumed in a patient with both atherosclerosis and angina pectoris, unless the documentation indicates the angina is due to something other than the atherosclerosis.

If a patient with coronary artery disease is admitted due to an acute myocardial infarction (AMI), the AMI should be sequenced before the coronary artery disease.

See Section I.C.9. Acute myocardial infarction (AMI)

c. **Intraoperative and Postprocedural Cerebrovascular Accident**
Medical record documentation should clearly specify the cause-and-effect relationship between the medical intervention and the cerebrovascular accident in order to assign a code for intraoperative or postprocedural cerebrovascular accident.

Proper code assignment depends on whether it was an infarction or hemorrhage and whether it occurred intraoperatively or postoperatively. If it was a cerebral hemorrhage, code assignment depends on the type of procedure performed.

d. **Sequelae of Cerebrovascular Disease**

1) **Category I69, Sequelae of Cerebrovascular disease**
Category I69 is used to indicate conditions classifiable to categories I6Ø-I67 as the causes of sequela (neurologic deficits), themselves classified elsewhere. These "late effects" include neurologic deficits that persist after initial onset of conditions classifiable to categories I6Ø-I67. The neurologic deficits caused by cerebrovascular disease may be present from the onset or may arise at any time after the onset of the condition classifiable to categories I6Ø-I67.

Codes from category I69, Sequelae of cerebrovascular disease, that specify hemiplegia, hemiparesis and monoplegia identify whether the dominant or nondominant side is affected. Should the affected side be documented, but not specified as dominant or nondominant, and the classification system does not indicate a default, code selection is as follows:

- For ambidextrous patients, the default should be dominant.
- If the left side is affected, the default is non-dominant.
- If the right side is affected, the default is dominant.

2) **Codes from category I69 with codes from I6Ø-I67**
Codes from category I69 may be assigned on a health care record with codes from I6Ø-I67, if the patient has a current cerebrovascular disease and deficits from an old cerebrovascular disease.

3) **Codes from category I69 and Personal history of transient ischemic attack (TIA) and cerebral infarction (Z86.73)**
Codes from category I69 should not be assigned if the patient does not have neurologic deficits.

See Section I.C.21.4. History (of) for use of personal history codes

e. **Acute myocardial infarction (AMI)**

1) **Type 1 ST elevation myocardial infarction (STEMI) and non-ST elevation myocardial infarction (NSTEMI)**
The ICD-10-CM codes for type 1 acute myocardial infarction (AMI) identify the site, such as anterolateral wall or true posterior wall. Subcategories I21.Ø-I21.2 and code I21.3 are used for type 1 ST elevation myocardial infarction (STEMI). Code I21.4, Non-ST

elevation (NSTEMI) myocardial infarction, is used for type 1 non-ST elevation myocardial infarction (NSTEMI) and nontransmural MIs.

If a type 1 NSTEMI evolves to STEMI, assign the STEMI code. If a type 1 STEMI converts to NSTEMI due to thrombolytic therapy, it is still coded as STEMI.

For encounters occurring while the myocardial infarction is equal to, or less than, four weeks old, including transfers to another acute setting or a postacute setting, and the myocardial infarction meets the definition for "other diagnoses" (see Section III, Reporting Additional Diagnoses), codes from category I21 may continue to be reported. For encounters after the 4-week time frame and the patient is still receiving care related to the myocardial infarction, the appropriate aftercare code should be assigned, rather than a code from category I21. For old or healed myocardial infarctions not requiring further care, code I25.2, Old myocardial infarction, may be assigned.

2) Acute myocardial infarction, unspecified

Code I21.9, Acute myocardial infarction, unspecified, is the default for unspecified acute myocardial infarction or unspecified type. If only type 1 STEMI or transmural MI without the site is documented, assign code I21.3, ST elevation (STEMI) myocardial infarction of unspecified site.

3) AMI documented as nontransmural or subendocardial but site provided

If an AMI is documented as nontransmural or subendocardial, but the site is provided, it is still coded as a subendocardial AMI.

See Section I.C.21.3. for information on coding status post administration of tPA in a different facility within the last 24 hours.

4) Subsequent acute myocardial infarction

A code from category I22, Subsequent ST elevation (STEMI) and non-ST elevation (NSTEMI) myocardial infarction, is to be used when a patient who has suffered a type 1 or unspecified AMI has a new AMI within the 4 week time frame of the initial AMI. A code from category I22 must be used in conjunction with a code from category I21. The sequencing of the I22 and I21 codes depends on the circumstances of the encounter.

Do not assign code I22 for subsequent myocardial infarctions other than type 1 or unspecified. For subsequent type 2 AMI assign only code I21.A1. For subsequent type 4 or type 5 AMI, assign only code I21.A9.

If a subsequent myocardial infarction of one type occurs within 4 weeks of a myocardial infarction of a different type, assign the appropriate codes from category I21 to identify each type. Do not assign a code from I22. Codes from category I22 should only be assigned if both the initial and subsequent myocardial infarctions are type 1 or unspecified.

5) Other Types of Myocardial Infarction

The ICD-10-CM provides codes for different types of myocardial infarction. Type 1 myocardial infarctions are assigned to codes I21.Ø-I21.4.

Type 2 myocardial infarction (myocardial infarction due to demand ischemia or secondary to ischemic imbalance) is assigned to code I21.A1, Myocardial infarction type 2 with the underlying cause coded first. Do not assign code I24.8, Other forms of acute ischemic heart disease, for the demand ischemia. If a type 2 AMI is described as NSTEMI or STEMI, only assign code I21.A1. Codes I21.Ø1-I21.4 should only be assigned for type 1 AMIs.

Acute myocardial infarctions type 3, 4a, 4b, 4c and 5 are assigned to code I21.A9, Other myocardial infarction type.

The "Code also" and "Code first" notes should be followed related to complications, and for coding of postprocedural myocardial infarctions during or following cardiac surgery.

10. Chapter 10: Diseases of the Respiratory System (JØØ-J99), UØ7.Ø

a. Chronic Obstructive Pulmonary Disease [COPD] and Asthma

1) Acute exacerbation of chronic obstructive bronchitis and asthma

The codes in categories J44 and J45 distinguish between uncomplicated cases and those in acute exacerbation. An acute exacerbation is a worsening or a decompensation of a chronic condition. An acute exacerbation is not equivalent to an infection superimposed on a chronic condition, though an exacerbation may be triggered by an infection.

b. Acute Respiratory Failure

1) Acute respiratory failure as principal diagnosis

A code from subcategory J96.Ø, Acute respiratory failure, or subcategory J96.2, Acute and chronic respiratory failure, may be assigned as a principal diagnosis when it is the condition established after study to be chiefly responsible for occasioning the admission to the hospital, and the selection is supported by the Alphabetic Index and Tabular List. However, chapter-specific coding guidelines (such as obstetrics, poisoning, HIV, newborn) that provide sequencing direction take precedence.

2) Acute respiratory failure as secondary diagnosis

Respiratory failure may be listed as a secondary diagnosis if it occurs after admission, or if it is present on admission, but does not meet the definition of principal diagnosis.

3) Sequencing of acute respiratory failure and another acute condition

When a patient is admitted with respiratory failure and another acute condition, (e.g., myocardial infarction, cerebrovascular accident, aspiration pneumonia), the principal diagnosis will not be the same in every situation. This applies whether the other acute condition is a respiratory or nonrespiratory condition. Selection of the principal diagnosis will be dependent on the circumstances of admission. If both the respiratory failure and the other acute condition are equally responsible for occasioning the admission to the hospital, and there are no chapter-specific sequencing rules, the guideline regarding two or more diagnoses that equally meet the definition for principal diagnosis (Section II, C.) may be applied in these situations.

If the documentation is not clear as to whether acute respiratory failure and another condition are equally responsible for occasioning the admission, query the provider for clarification.

c. Influenza due to certain identified influenza viruses

Code only confirmed cases of influenza due to certain identified influenza viruses (category JØ9), and due to other identified influenza virus (category J1Ø). This is an exception to the hospital inpatient guideline Section II, H. (Uncertain Diagnosis).

In this context, "confirmation" does not require documentation of positive laboratory testing specific for avian or other novel influenza A or other identified influenza virus. However, coding should be based on the provider's diagnostic statement that the patient has avian influenza, or other novel influenza A, for category JØ9, or has another particular identified strain of influenza, such as H1N1 or H3N2, but not identified as novel or variant, for category J1Ø.

If the provider records "suspected" or "possible" or "probable" avian influenza, or novel influenza, or other identified influenza, then the appropriate influenza code from category J11, Influenza due to unidentified influenza virus, should be assigned. A code from category JØ9, Influenza due to certain identified influenza viruses, should not be assigned nor should a code from category J1Ø, Influenza due to other identified influenza virus.

d. Ventilator associated Pneumonia

1) Documentation of Ventilator associated Pneumonia

As with all procedural or postprocedural complications, code assignment is based on the provider's documentation of the relationship between the condition and the procedure.

Code J95.851, Ventilator associated pneumonia, should be assigned only when the provider has documented ventilator associated pneumonia (VAP). An additional code to identify the organism (e.g., Pseudomonas aeruginosa, code B96.5) should also be assigned. Do not assign an additional code from categories J12-J18 to identify the type of pneumonia.

Code J95.851 should not be assigned for cases where the patient has pneumonia and is on a mechanical ventilator and the provider has not specifically stated that the pneumonia is ventilator-associated pneumonia. If the documentation is unclear as to whether the patient has a pneumonia that is a complication attributable to the mechanical ventilator, query the provider.

2) Ventilator associated Pneumonia Develops after Admission

A patient may be admitted with one type of pneumonia (e.g., code J13, Pneumonia due to Streptococcus pneumonia) and subsequently develop VAP. In this instance, the principal diagnosis would be the appropriate code from categories J12-J18 for the pneumonia diagnosed at the time of admission. Code J95.851, Ventilator associated pneumonia, would be assigned as an additional diagnosis when the provider has also documented the presence of ventilator associated pneumonia.

e. Vaping-related disorders

For patients presenting with condition(s) related to vaping, assign code U07.0, Vaping-related disorder, as the principal diagnosis. For lung injury due to vaping, assign only code U07.0. Assign additional codes for other manifestations, such as acute respiratory failure (subcategory J96.0-) or pneumonitis (code J68.0).

Associated respiratory signs and symptoms due to vaping, such as cough, shortness of breath, etc., are not coded separately, when a definitive diagnosis has been established. However, it would be appropriate to code separately any gastrointestinal symptoms, such as diarrhea and abdominal pain.

See Section I.C.1.g.1.c.i. for Pneumonia confirmed as due to COVID-19

11. Chapter 11: Diseases of the Digestive System (K00-K95)

Reserved for future guideline expansion

12. Chapter 12: Diseases of the Skin and Subcutaneous Tissue (L00-L99)

a. Pressure ulcer stage codes

1) Pressure ulcer stages

Codes in category L89, Pressure ulcer, identify the site and stage of the pressure ulcer.

The ICD-10-CM classifies pressure ulcer stages based on severity, which is designated by stages 1-4, deep tissue pressure injury, unspecified stage, and unstageable.

Assign as many codes from category L89 as needed to identify all the pressure ulcers the patient has, if applicable.

See Section I.B.14. for pressure ulcer stage documentation by clinicians other than patient's provider.

2) Unstageable pressure ulcers

Assignment of the code for unstageable pressure ulcer (L89.--0) should be based on the clinical documentation. These codes are used for pressure ulcers whose stage cannot be clinically determined (e.g., the ulcer is covered by eschar or has been treated with a skin or muscle graft). This code should not be confused with the codes for unspecified stage (L89.--9). When there is no documentation regarding the stage of the pressure ulcer, assign the appropriate code for unspecified stage (L89.-- 9).

If during an encounter, the stage of an unstageable pressure ulcer is revealed after debridement, assign only the code for the stage revealed following debridement.

3) Documented pressure ulcer stage

Assignment of the pressure ulcer stage code should be guided by clinical documentation of the stage or documentation of the terms found in the Alphabetic Index. For clinical terms describing the stage that are not found in the Alphabetic Index, and there is no documentation of the stage, the provider should be queried.

4) Patients admitted with pressure ulcers documented as healed

No code is assigned if the documentation states that the pressure ulcer is completely healed at the time of admission.

5) Pressure ulcers documented as healing

Pressure ulcers described as healing should be assigned the appropriate pressure ulcer stage code based on the documentation in the medical record. If the documentation does not provide information about the stage of the healing pressure ulcer, assign the appropriate code for unspecified stage.

If the documentation is unclear as to whether the patient has a current (new) pressure ulcer or if the patient is being treated for a healing pressure ulcer, query the provider.

For ulcers that were present on admission but healed at the time of discharge, assign the code for the site and stage of the pressure ulcer at the time of admission.

6) Patient admitted with pressure ulcer evolving into another stage during the admission

If a patient is admitted to an inpatient hospital with a pressure ulcer at one stage and it progresses to a higher stage, two separate codes should be assigned: one code for the site and stage of the ulcer on admission and a second code for the same ulcer site and the highest stage reported during the stay.

7) Pressure-induced deep tissue damage

For pressure-induced deep tissue damage or deep tissue pressure injury, assign only the appropriate code for pressure-induced deep tissue damage (L89.--6).

b. Non-Pressure Chronic Ulcers

1) Patients admitted with non-pressure ulcers documented as healed

No code is assigned if the documentation states that the non-pressure ulcer is completely healed at the time of admission.

2) Non-pressure ulcers documented as healing

Non-pressure ulcers described as healing should be assigned the appropriate non-pressure ulcer code based on the documentation in the medical record. If the documentation does not provide information about the severity of the healing non-pressure ulcer, assign the appropriate code for unspecified severity.

If the documentation is unclear as to whether the patient has a current (new) non-pressure ulcer or if the patient is being treated for a healing non-pressure ulcer, query the provider.

For ulcers that were present on admission but healed at the time of discharge, assign the code for the site and severity of the non-pressure ulcer at the time of admission.

3) Patient admitted with non-pressure ulcer that progresses to another severity level during the admission

If a patient is admitted to an inpatient hospital with a non-pressure ulcer at one severity level and it progresses to a higher severity level, two separate codes should be assigned: one code for the site and severity level of the ulcer on admission and a second code for the same ulcer site and the highest severity level reported during the stay.

See Section I.B.14. for pressure ulcer stage documentation by clinicians other than patient's provider

13. Chapter 13: Diseases of the Musculoskeletal System and Connective Tissue (M00-M99)

a. Site and laterality

Most of the codes within Chapter 13 have site and laterality designations. The site represents the bone, joint or the muscle involved. For some conditions where more than one bone, joint or muscle is usually involved, such as osteoarthritis, there is a "multiple sites" code available. For categories where no multiple site code is provided and more than one bone, joint or muscle is involved, multiple codes should be used to indicate the different sites involved.

1) Bone versus joint

For certain conditions, the bone may be affected at the upper or lower end, (e.g., avascular necrosis of bone, M87, Osteoporosis, M80, M81). Though the portion of the bone affected may be at the joint, the site designation will be the bone, not the joint.

b. Acute traumatic versus chronic or recurrent musculoskeletal conditions

Many musculoskeletal conditions are a result of previous injury or trauma to a site, or are recurrent conditions. Bone, joint or muscle conditions that are the result of a healed injury are usually found in chapter 13. Recurrent bone, joint or muscle conditions are also usually found in chapter 13. Any current, acute injury should be coded to the appropriate injury code from chapter 19. Chronic or recurrent conditions should generally be coded with a code from chapter 13. If it is difficult to determine from the documentation in the record which code is best to describe a condition, query the provider.

c. Coding of Pathologic Fractures

7th character A is for use as long as the patient is receiving active treatment for the fracture. While the patient may be seen by a new or different provider over the course of treatment for a pathological fracture, assignment of the 7th character is based on whether the patient is undergoing active treatment and not whether the provider is seeing the patient for the first time.

7th character D is to be used for encounters after the patient has completed active treatment for the fracture and is receiving routine care for the fracture during the healing or recovery phase. The other 7th characters, listed under each subcategory in the Tabular List, are to be used for subsequent encounters for treatment of problems associated with the healing, such as malunions, nonunions, and sequelae.

Care for complications of surgical treatment for fracture repairs during the healing or recovery phase should be coded with the appropriate complication codes.

See Section I.C.19. Coding of traumatic fractures.

d. Osteoporosis

Osteoporosis is a systemic condition, meaning that all bones of the musculoskeletal system are affected. Therefore, site is not a component of the codes under category M81, Osteoporosis without current pathological fracture. The site codes under category M8Ø, Osteoporosis with current pathological fracture, identify the site of the fracture, not the osteoporosis.

1) Osteoporosis without pathological fracture

Category M81, Osteoporosis without current pathological fracture, is for use for patients with osteoporosis who do not currently have a pathologic fracture due to the osteoporosis, even if they have had a fracture in the past. For patients with a history of osteoporosis fractures, status code Z87.31Ø, Personal history of (healed) osteoporosis fracture, should follow the code from M81.

2) Osteoporosis with current pathological fracture

Category M8Ø, Osteoporosis with current pathological fracture, is for patients who have a current pathologic fracture at the time of an encounter. The codes under M8Ø identify the site of the fracture. A code from category M8Ø, not a traumatic fracture code, should be used for any patient with known osteoporosis who suffers a fracture, even if the patient had a minor fall or trauma, if that fall or trauma would not usually break a normal, healthy bone.

e. Multisystem Inflammatory Syndrome

See Section I.C.1.g.1.l. for Multisystem Inflammatory Syndrome

14. Chapter 14: Diseases of Genitourinary System (NØØ-N99)

a. Chronic kidney disease

1) Stages of chronic kidney disease (CKD)

The ICD-10-CM classifies CKD based on severity. The severity of CKD is designated by stages 1-5. Stage 2, code N18.2, equates to mild CKD; stage 3, codes N18.3Ø-N18.32, equate to moderate CKD; and stage 4, code N18.4, equates to severe CKD. Code N18.6, End stage renal disease (ESRD), is assigned when the provider has documented end-stage renal disease (ESRD).

If both a stage of CKD and ESRD are documented, assign code N18.6 only.

2) Chronic kidney disease and kidney transplant status

Patients who have undergone kidney transplant may still have some form of chronic kidney disease (CKD) because the kidney transplant may not fully restore kidney function. Therefore, the presence of CKD alone does not constitute a transplant complication. Assign the appropriate N18 code for the patient's stage of CKD and code Z94.Ø, Kidney transplant status. If a transplant complication such as failure or rejection or other transplant complication is documented, see section I.C.19.g for information on coding complications of a kidney transplant. If the documentation is unclear as to whether the patient has a complication of the transplant, query the provider.

3) Chronic kidney disease with other conditions

Patients with CKD may also suffer from other serious conditions, most commonly diabetes mellitus and hypertension. The sequencing of the CKD code in relationship to codes for other contributing conditions is based on the conventions in the Tabular List.

See I.C.9. Hypertensive chronic kidney disease.

See I.C.19. Chronic kidney disease and kidney transplant complications.

15. Chapter 15: Pregnancy, Childbirth, and the Puerperium (OØØ-O9A)

a. General Rules for Obstetric Cases

1) Codes from chapter 15 and sequencing priority

Obstetric cases require codes from chapter 15, codes in the range OØØ-O9A, Pregnancy, Childbirth, and the Puerperium. Chapter 15 codes have sequencing priority over codes from other chapters. Additional codes from other chapters may be used in conjunction with chapter 15 codes to further specify conditions. Should the provider document that the pregnancy is incidental to the encounter, then code Z33.1, Pregnant state, incidental, should be used in place of any chapter 15 codes. It is the provider's responsibility to state that the condition being treated is not affecting the pregnancy.

2) Chapter 15 codes used only on the maternal record

Chapter 15 codes are to be used only on the maternal record, never on the record of the newborn.

3) Final character for trimester

The majority of codes in Chapter 15 have a final character indicating the trimester of pregnancy. The timeframes for the trimesters are indicated at the beginning of the chapter. If trimester is not a component of a code, it is because the condition always occurs in a specific trimester, or the concept of trimester of pregnancy is not applicable. Certain codes have characters for only certain trimesters because the condition does not occur in all trimesters, but it may occur in more than just one.

Assignment of the final character for trimester should be based on the provider's documentation of the trimester (or number of weeks) for the current admission/encounter. This applies to the assignment of trimester for pre-existing conditions as well as those that develop during or are due to the pregnancy. The provider's documentation of the number of weeks may be used to assign the appropriate code identifying the trimester.

Whenever delivery occurs during the current admission, and there is an "in childbirth" option for the obstetric complication being coded, the "in childbirth" code should be assigned. When the classification does not provide an obstetric code with an "in childbirth" option, it is appropriate to assign a code describing the current trimester.

4) Selection of trimester for inpatient admissions that encompass more than one trimester

In instances when a patient is admitted to a hospital for complications of pregnancy during one trimester and remains in the hospital into a subsequent trimester, the trimester character for the antepartum complication code should be assigned on the basis of the trimester when the complication developed, not the trimester of the discharge. If the condition developed prior to the current admission/encounter or represents a pre-existing condition, the trimester character for the trimester at the time of the admission/encounter should be assigned.

5) Unspecified trimester

Each category that includes codes for trimester has a code for "unspecified trimester." The "unspecified trimester" code should rarely be used, such as when the documentation in the record is insufficient to determine the trimester and it is not possible to obtain clarification.

6) 7th character for fetus identification

Where applicable, a 7th character is to be assigned for certain categories (O31, O32, O33.3-O33.6, O35, O36, O4Ø, O41, O6Ø.1, O6Ø.2, O64, and O69) to identify the fetus for which the complication code applies.

Assign 7th character "Ø":

- For single gestations
- When the documentation in the record is insufficient to determine the fetus affected and it is not possible to obtain clarification.
- When it is not possible to clinically determine which fetus is affected.

7) Completed weeks of gestation

In ICD-10-CM, "completed" weeks of gestation refers to full weeks. For example, if the provider documents gestation at 39 weeks and 6 days, the code for 39 weeks of gestation should be assigned, as the patient has not yet reached 40 completed weeks.

b. Selection of OB Principal or First-listed Diagnosis

1) Routine outpatient prenatal visits

For routine outpatient prenatal visits when no complications are present, a code from category Z34, Encounter for supervision of normal pregnancy, should be used as the first-listed diagnosis. These codes should not be used in conjunction with chapter 15 codes.

2) Supervision of High-Risk Pregnancy

Codes from category OØ9, Supervision of high-risk pregnancy, are intended for use only during the prenatal period. For complications during the labor or delivery episode as a result of a high-risk pregnancy, assign the applicable complication codes from Chapter 15. If there are no complications during the labor or delivery episode, assign code O8Ø, Encounter for full-term uncomplicated delivery.

For routine prenatal outpatient visits for patients with high-risk pregnancies, a code from category OØ9, Supervision of high-risk pregnancy, should be used as the first-listed diagnosis. Secondary chapter 15 codes may be used in conjunction with these codes if appropriate.

3) Episodes when no delivery occurs

In episodes when no delivery occurs, the principal diagnosis should correspond to the principal complication of the pregnancy which necessitated the encounter. Should more than one complication exist, all of which are treated or monitored, any of the complication codes may be sequenced first.

4) When a delivery occurs

When an obstetric patient is admitted and delivers during that admission, the condition that prompted the admission should be sequenced as the principal diagnosis. If multiple conditions prompted the admission, sequence the one most related to the delivery as the principal diagnosis. A code for any complication of the delivery should be assigned as an additional diagnosis. In cases of cesarean delivery, if the patient was admitted with a condition that resulted in the performance of a cesarean procedure, that condition should be selected as the principal diagnosis. If the reason for the admission was unrelated to the condition resulting in the cesarean delivery, the condition related to the reason for the admission should be selected as the principal diagnosis.

5) Outcome of delivery

A code from category Z37, Outcome of delivery, should be included on every maternal record when a delivery has occurred. These codes are not to be used on subsequent records or on the newborn record.

c. Pre-existing conditions versus conditions due to the pregnancy

Certain categories in Chapter 15 distinguish between conditions of the mother that existed prior to pregnancy (pre-existing) and those that are a direct result of pregnancy. When assigning codes from Chapter 15, it is important to assess if a condition was pre-existing prior to pregnancy or developed during or due to the pregnancy in order to assign the correct code.

Categories that do not distinguish between pre-existing and pregnancy-related conditions may be used for either. It is acceptable to use codes specifically for the puerperium with codes complicating pregnancy and childbirth if a condition arises postpartum during the delivery encounter.

d. Pre-existing hypertension in pregnancy

Category O1Ø, Pre-existing hypertension complicating pregnancy, childbirth and the puerperium, includes codes for hypertensive heart and hypertensive chronic kidney disease. When assigning one of the O1Ø codes that includes hypertensive heart disease or hypertensive chronic kidney disease, it is necessary to add a secondary code from the appropriate hypertension category to specify the type of heart failure or chronic kidney disease.

See Section I.C.9. Hypertension.

e. Fetal Conditions Affecting the Management of the Mother

1) Codes from categories O35 and O36

Codes from categories O35, Maternal care for known or suspected fetal abnormality and damage, and O36, Maternal care for other fetal problems, are assigned only when the fetal condition is actually responsible for modifying the management of the mother, i.e., by requiring diagnostic studies, additional observation, special care, or termination of pregnancy. The fact that the fetal condition exists does not justify assigning a code from this series to the mother's record.

2) In utero surgery

In cases when surgery is performed on the fetus, a diagnosis code from category O35, Maternal care for known or suspected fetal abnormality and damage, should be assigned identifying the fetal condition. Assign the appropriate procedure code for the procedure performed.

No code from Chapter 16, the perinatal codes, should be used on the mother's record to identify fetal conditions. Surgery performed in utero on a fetus is still to be coded as an obstetric encounter.

f. HIV Infection in Pregnancy, Childbirth and the Puerperium

During pregnancy, childbirth or the puerperium, a patient admitted because of an HIV-related illness should receive a principal diagnosis from subcategory O98.7-, Human immunodeficiency [HIV] disease complicating pregnancy, childbirth and the puerperium, followed by the code(s) for the HIV-related illness(es).

Patients with asymptomatic HIV infection status admitted during pregnancy, childbirth, or the puerperium should receive codes of O98.7- and Z21, Asymptomatic human immunodeficiency virus [HIV] infection status.

g. Diabetes mellitus in pregnancy

Diabetes mellitus is a significant complicating factor in pregnancy. Pregnant patients who are diabetic should be assigned a code from category O24, Diabetes mellitus in pregnancy, childbirth, and the puerperium, first, followed by the appropriate diabetes code(s) (EØ8-E13) from Chapter 4.

h. Long term use of insulin and oral hypoglycemics

See section I.C.4.a.3 for information on the long-term use of insulin and oral hypoglycemics.

i. Gestational (pregnancy induced) diabetes

Gestational (pregnancy induced) diabetes can occur during the second and third trimester of pregnancy in patients who were not diabetic prior to pregnancy. Gestational diabetes can cause complications in the pregnancy similar to those of pre-existing diabetes mellitus. It also puts the patient at greater risk of developing diabetes after the pregnancy.

Codes for gestational diabetes are in subcategory O24.4, Gestational diabetes mellitus. No other code from category O24, Diabetes mellitus in pregnancy, childbirth, and the puerperium, should be used with a code from O24.4.

The codes under subcategory O24.4 include diet controlled, insulin controlled, and controlled by oral hypoglycemic drugs. If a patient with gestational diabetes is treated with both diet and insulin, only the code for insulin-controlled is required. If a patient with gestational diabetes is treated with both diet and oral hypoglycemic medications, only the code for "controlled by oral hypoglycemic drugs" is required. Codes Z79.4, Long-term (current) use of insulin, Z79.84, Long-term (current) use of oral hypoglycemic drugs, **and Z79.85, Long-term (current) use of injectable non-insulin antidiabetic drugs,** should not be assigned with codes from subcategory O24.4.

An abnormal glucose tolerance in pregnancy is assigned a code from subcategory O99.81, Abnormal glucose complicating pregnancy, childbirth, and the puerperium.

j. Sepsis and septic shock complicating abortion, pregnancy, childbirth and the puerperium

When assigning a chapter 15 code for sepsis complicating abortion, pregnancy, childbirth, and the puerperium, a code for the specific type of infection should be assigned as an additional diagnosis. If severe sepsis is present, a code from subcategory R65.2, Severe sepsis, and code(s) for associated organ dysfunction(s) should also be assigned as additional diagnoses.

k. Puerperal sepsis

Code O85, Puerperal sepsis, should be assigned with a secondary code to identify the causal organism (e.g., for a bacterial infection, assign a code from category B95-B96, Bacterial infections in conditions classified elsewhere). A code from category A4Ø, Streptococcal sepsis, or A41, Other sepsis, should not be used for puerperal sepsis. If applicable, use additional codes to identify severe sepsis (R65.2-) and any associated acute organ dysfunction.

Code O85 should not be assigned for sepsis following an obstetrical procedure (See Section I.C.1.d.5.b., Sepsis due to a postprocedural infection).

l. Alcohol, tobacco and drug use during pregnancy, childbirth and the puerperium

1) Alcohol use during pregnancy, childbirth and the puerperium

Codes under subcategory O99.31, Alcohol use complicating pregnancy, childbirth, and the puerperium, should be assigned for any pregnancy case when a patient uses alcohol during the pregnancy or postpartum. A secondary code from category F1Ø, Alcohol related disorders, should also be assigned to identify manifestations of the alcohol use.

2) Tobacco use during pregnancy, childbirth and the puerperium

Codes under subcategory O99.33, Smoking (tobacco) complicating pregnancy, childbirth, and the puerperium, should be assigned for any pregnancy case when a patient uses any type of tobacco product during the pregnancy or postpartum.

A secondary code from category F17, Nicotine dependence, should also be assigned to identify the type of nicotine dependence.

3) Drug use during pregnancy, childbirth and the puerperium

Codes under subcategory O99.32, Drug use complicating pregnancy, childbirth, and the puerperium, should be assigned for any pregnancy case when a patient uses drugs during the pregnancy or postpartum. This can involve illegal drugs, or inappropriate use or abuse of prescription drugs. Secondary code(s) from categories F11-F16 and F18-F19 should also be assigned to identify manifestations of the drug use.

m. Poisoning, toxic effects, adverse effects and underdosing in a pregnant patient

A code from subcategory O9A.2, Injury, poisoning and certain other consequences of external causes complicating pregnancy, childbirth, and the puerperium, should be sequenced first, followed by the appropriate injury, poisoning, toxic effect, adverse effect or underdosing code, and then the additional code(s) that specifies the condition caused by the poisoning, toxic effect, adverse effect or underdosing.

See Section I.C.19. Adverse effects, poisoning, underdosing and toxic effects.

n. Normal Delivery, Code O80

1) Encounter for full term uncomplicated delivery

Code O80 should be assigned when a patient is admitted for a full-term normal delivery and delivers a single, healthy infant without any complications antepartum, during the delivery, or postpartum during the delivery episode. Code O80 is always a principal diagnosis. It is not to be used if any other code from chapter 15 is needed to describe a current complication of the antenatal, delivery, or postnatal period. Additional codes from other chapters may be used with code O80 if they are not related to or are in any way complicating the pregnancy.

2) Uncomplicated delivery with resolved antepartum complication

Code O80 may be used if the patient had a complication at some point during the pregnancy, but the complication is not present at the time of the admission for delivery.

3) Outcome of delivery for O80

Z37.0, Single live birth, is the only outcome of delivery code appropriate for use with O80.

o. The Peripartum and Postpartum Periods

1) Peripartum and Postpartum periods

The postpartum period begins immediately after delivery and continues for six weeks following delivery. The peripartum period is defined as the last month of pregnancy to five months postpartum.

2) Peripartum and postpartum complication

A postpartum complication is any complication occurring within the six-week period.

3) Pregnancy-related complications after 6-week period

Chapter 15 codes may also be used to describe pregnancy-related complications after the peripartum or postpartum period if the provider documents that a condition is pregnancy related.

4) Admission for routine postpartum care following delivery outside hospital

When the mother delivers outside the hospital prior to admission and is admitted for routine postpartum care and no complications are noted, code Z39.0, Encounter for care and examination of mother immediately after delivery, should be assigned as the principal diagnosis.

5) Pregnancy associated cardiomyopathy

Pregnancy associated cardiomyopathy, code O90.3, is unique in that it may be diagnosed in the third trimester of pregnancy but may continue to progress months after delivery. For this reason, it is referred to as peripartum cardiomyopathy. Code O90.3 is only for use when the cardiomyopathy develops as a result of pregnancy in a patient who did not have pre-existing heart disease.

p. Code O94, Sequelae of complication of pregnancy, childbirth, and the puerperium

1) Code O94

Code O94, Sequelae of complication of pregnancy, childbirth, and the puerperium, is for use in those cases when an initial complication of a pregnancy develops a sequela or sequelae requiring care or treatment at a future date.

2) After the initial postpartum period

This code may be used at any time after the initial postpartum period.

3) Sequencing of Code O94

This code, like all sequela codes, is to be sequenced following the code describing the sequelae of the complication.

q. Termination of Pregnancy and Spontaneous abortions

1) Abortion with Liveborn Fetus

When an attempted termination of pregnancy results in a liveborn fetus, assign code Z33.2, Encounter for elective termination of pregnancy and a code from category Z37, Outcome of Delivery.

2) Retained Products of Conception following an abortion

Subsequent encounters for retained products of conception following a spontaneous abortion or elective termination of pregnancy, without complications are assigned O03.4, Incomplete spontaneous abortion without complication, or code O07.4, Failed attempted termination of pregnancy without complication. This advice is appropriate even when the patient was discharged previously with a discharge diagnosis of complete abortion. If the patient has a specific complication associated with the spontaneous abortion or elective termination of pregnancy in addition to retained products of conception, assign the appropriate complication code (e.g., O03.-, O04.-, O07.-) instead of code O03.4 or O07.4.

3) Complications leading to abortion

Codes from Chapter 15 may be used as additional codes to identify any documented complications of the pregnancy in conjunction with codes in categories in O04, O07 and O08.

4) Hemorrhage following elective abortion

For hemorrhage post elective abortion, assign code O04.6, Delayed or excessive hemorrhage following (induced) termination of pregnancy. Do not assign code O72.1, Other immediate postpartum hemorrhage, as this code should not be assigned for post abortion conditions. Do not assign code Z33.2, Encounter for elective termination of pregnancy, when the patient experiences a complication post elective abortion.

r. Abuse in a pregnant patient

For suspected or confirmed cases of abuse of a pregnant patient, a code(s) from subcategories O9A.3, Physical abuse complicating pregnancy, childbirth, and the puerperium, O9A.4, Sexual abuse complicating pregnancy, childbirth, and the puerperium, and O9A.5, Psychological abuse complicating pregnancy, childbirth, and the puerperium, should be sequenced first, followed by the appropriate codes (if applicable) to identify any associated current injury due to physical abuse, sexual abuse, and the perpetrator of abuse.

See Section I.C.19. Adult and child abuse, neglect and other maltreatment.

s. COVID-19 infection in pregnancy, childbirth, and the puerperium

During pregnancy, childbirth or the puerperium, when COVID-19 is the reason for admission/encounter , code O98.5-, Other viral diseases complicating pregnancy, childbirth and the puerperium, should be sequenced as the principal/first-listed diagnosis, and code U07.1, COVID-19, and the appropriate codes for associated manifestation(s) should be assigned as additional diagnoses. Codes from Chapter 15 always take sequencing priority.

If the reason for admission/encounter is unrelated to COVID-19 but the patient tests positive for COVID-19 during the admission/encounter, the appropriate code for the reason for admission/encounter should be sequenced as the principal/first-listed diagnosis, and codes O98.5- and U07.1, as well as the appropriate codes for associated COVID-19 manifestations, should be assigned as additional diagnoses.

16. Chapter 16: Certain Conditions Originating in the Perinatal Period (P00-P96)

For coding and reporting purposes the perinatal period is defined as before birth through the 28th day following birth. The following guidelines are provided for reporting purposes.

a. General Perinatal Rules

1) Use of Chapter 16 Codes

Codes in this chapter are <u>never</u> for use on the maternal record. Codes from Chapter 15, the obstetric chapter, are never permitted on the newborn record. Chapter 16 codes may be used throughout the life of the patient if the condition is still present.

2) Principal Diagnosis for Birth Record

When coding the birth episode in a newborn record, assign a code from category Z38, Liveborn infants according to place of birth and type of delivery, as the principal diagnosis. A code from category Z38 is assigned only once, to a newborn at the time of birth. If a newborn is transferred to another institution, a code from category Z38 should not be used at the receiving hospital.

A code from category Z38 is used only on the newborn record, not on the mother's record.

3) **Use of Codes from other Chapters with Codes from Chapter 16**
Codes from other chapters may be used with codes from chapter 16 if the codes from the other chapters provide more specific detail. Codes for signs and symptoms may be assigned when a definitive diagnosis has not been established. If the reason for the encounter is a perinatal condition, the code from chapter 16 should be sequenced first.

4) **Use of Chapter 16 Codes after the Perinatal Period**
Should a condition originate in the perinatal period, and continue throughout the life of the patient, the perinatal code should continue to be used regardless of the patient's age.

5) **Birth process or community acquired conditions**
If a newborn has a condition that may be either due to the birth process or community acquired and the documentation does not indicate which it is, the default is due to the birth process and the code from Chapter 16 should be used. If the condition is community-acquired, a code from Chapter 16 should not be assigned.

For COVID-19 infection in a newborn, see guideline I.C.16.h.

6) **Code all clinically significant conditions**
All clinically significant conditions noted on routine newborn examination should be coded. A condition is clinically significant if it requires:

- clinical evaluation; or
- therapeutic treatment; or
- diagnostic procedures; or
- extended length of hospital stay; or
- increased nursing care and/or monitoring; or
- has implications for future health care needs

Note: The perinatal guidelines listed above are the same as the general coding guidelines for "additional diagnoses," except for the final point regarding implications for future health care needs. Codes should be assigned for conditions that have been specified by the provider as having implications for future health care needs.

b. **Observation and Evaluation of Newborns for Suspected Conditions not Found**

1) **Use of Z05 codes**
Assign a code from category Z05, Observation and evaluation of newborn for suspected **diseases and** conditions ruled out, to identify those instances when a healthy newborn is evaluated for a suspected condition/**disease** that is determined after study not to be present. Do not use a code from category Z05 when the patient **is documented to have** signs or symptoms of a suspected problem; in such cases code the sign or symptom.

2) **Z05 on other than the birth record**
A code from category Z05 may also be assigned as a principal or first-listed code for readmissions or encounters when the code from category Z38 code no longer applies. Codes from category Z05 are for use only for healthy newborns and infants for which no condition after study is found to be present.

3) **Z05 on a birth record**
A code from category Z05 is to be used as a secondary code after the code from category Z38, Liveborn infants according to place of birth and type of delivery.

c. **Coding Additional Perinatal Diagnoses**

1) **Assigning codes for conditions that require treatment**
Assign codes for conditions that require treatment or further investigation, prolong the length of stay, or require resource utilization.

2) **Codes for conditions specified as having implications for future health care needs**
Assign codes for conditions that have been specified by the provider as having implications for future health care needs.
Note: This guideline should not be used for adult patients.

d. **Prematurity and Fetal Growth Retardation**
Providers utilize different criteria in determining prematurity. A code for prematurity should not be assigned unless it is documented. Assignment of codes in categories P05, Disorders of newborn related to slow fetal growth and fetal malnutrition, and P07, Disorders of newborn related to short gestation and low birth weight, not elsewhere classified, should be based on the recorded birth weight and estimated gestational age.

When both birth weight and gestational age are available, two codes from category P07 should be assigned, with the code for birth weight sequenced before the code for gestational age.

e. **Low birth weight and immaturity status**
Codes from category P07, Disorders of newborn related to short gestation and low birth weight, not elsewhere classified, are for use for a child or adult who was premature or had a low birth weight as a newborn and this is affecting the patient's current health status.

See Section I.C.21. Factors influencing health status and contact with health services, Status.

f. **Bacterial Sepsis of Newborn**
Category P36, Bacterial sepsis of newborn, includes congenital sepsis. If a perinate is documented as having sepsis without documentation of congenital or community acquired, the default is congenital and a code from category P36 should be assigned. If the P36 code includes the causal organism, an additional code from category B95, Streptococcus, Staphylococcus, and Enterococcus as the cause of diseases classified elsewhere, or B96, Other bacterial agents as the cause of diseases classified elsewhere, should not be assigned. If the P36 code does not include the causal organism, assign an additional code from category B96. If applicable, use additional codes to identify severe sepsis (R65.2-) and any associated acute organ dysfunction.

g. **Stillbirth**
Code P95, Stillbirth, is only for use in institutions that maintain separate records for stillbirths. No other code should be used with P95. Code P95 should not be used on the mother's record.

h. **COVID-19 Infection in Newborn**
For a newborn that tests positive for COVID-19, assign code U07.1, COVID-19, and the appropriate codes for associated manifestation(s) in neonates/newborns in the absence of documentation indicating a specific type of transmission. For a newborn that tests positive for COVID-19 and the provider documents the condition was contracted in utero or during the birth process, assign codes P35.8, Other congenital viral diseases, and U07.1, COVID-19. When coding the birth episode in a newborn record, the appropriate code from category Z38, Liveborn infants according to place of birth and type of delivery, should be assigned as the principal diagnosis.

17. **Chapter 17: Congenital malformations, deformations, and chromosomal abnormalities (Q00-Q99)**
Assign an appropriate code(s) from categories Q00-Q99, Congenital malformations, deformations, and chromosomal abnormalities when a malformation/deformation or chromosomal abnormality is documented. A malformation/deformation/or chromosomal abnormality may be the principal/first-listed diagnosis on a record or a secondary diagnosis.

When a malformation/deformation or chromosomal abnormality does not have a unique code assignment, assign additional code(s) for any manifestations that may be present.

When the code assignment specifically identifies the malformation/deformation or chromosomal abnormality, manifestations that are an inherent component of the anomaly should not be coded separately. Additional codes should be assigned for manifestations that are not an inherent component.

Codes from Chapter 17 may be used throughout the life of the patient. If a congenital malformation or deformity has been corrected, a personal history code should be used to identify the history of the malformation or deformity. Although present at birth, a malformation/deformation/or chromosomal abnormality may not be identified until later in life. Whenever the condition is diagnosed by the provider, it is appropriate to assign a code from codes Q00-Q99. For the birth admission, the appropriate code from category Z38, Liveborn infants, according to place of birth and type of delivery, should be sequenced as the principal diagnosis, followed by any congenital anomaly codes, Q00-Q99.

18. **Chapter 18: Symptoms, signs, and abnormal clinical and laboratory findings, not elsewhere classified (R00-R99)**
Chapter 18 includes symptoms, signs, abnormal results of clinical or other investigative procedures, and ill-defined conditions regarding which no diagnosis classifiable elsewhere is recorded. Signs and symptoms that point to a specific diagnosis have been assigned to a category in other chapters of the classification.

a. **Use of symptom codes**
Codes that describe symptoms and signs are acceptable for reporting purposes when a related definitive diagnosis has not been established (confirmed) by the provider.

b. **Use of a symptom code with a definitive diagnosis code**
Codes for signs and symptoms may be reported in addition to a related definitive diagnosis when the sign or symptom is not routinely

associated with that diagnosis, such as the various signs and symptoms associated with complex syndromes. The definitive diagnosis code should be sequenced before the symptom code.

Signs or symptoms that are associated routinely with a disease process should not be assigned as additional codes, unless otherwise instructed by the classification.

c. Combination codes that include symptoms

ICD-10-CM contains a number of combination codes that identify both the definitive diagnosis and common symptoms of that diagnosis. When using one of these combination codes, an additional code should not be assigned for the symptom.

d. Repeated falls

Code R29.6, Repeated falls, is for use for encounters when a patient has recently fallen and the reason for the fall is being investigated.

Code Z91.81, History of falling, is for use when a patient has fallen in the past and is at risk for future falls. When appropriate, both codes R29.6 and Z91.81 may be assigned together.

e. Coma

Code R40.20, Unspecified coma, may be assigned in conjunction with codes for any medical condition.

Do not report codes for unspecified coma, individual or total Glasgow coma scale scores for a patient with a medically induced coma or a sedated patient.

1) Coma Scale

The coma scale codes (R40.21- to R40.24-) can be used in conjunction with traumatic brain injury codes. These codes are primarily for use by trauma registries, but they may be used in any setting where this information is collected. The coma scale codes should be sequenced after the diagnosis code(s).

These codes, one from each subcategory, are needed to complete the scale. The 7th character indicates when the scale was recorded. The 7th character should match for all three codes.

At a minimum, report the initial score documented on presentation at your facility. This may be a score from the emergency medicine technician (EMT) or in the emergency department. If desired, a facility may choose to capture multiple coma scale scores.

Assign code R40.24-, Glasgow coma scale, total score, when only the total score is documented in the medical record and not the individual score(s).

If multiple coma scores are captured within the first 24 hours after hospital admission, assign only the code for the score at the time of admission. ICD-10-CM does not classify coma scores that are reported after admission but less than 24 hours later.

See Section I.B.14. for coma scale documentation by clinicians other than patient's provider

f. Functional quadriplegia

GUIDELINE HAS BEEN DELETED EFFECTIVE OCTOBER 1, 2017

g. SIRS due to Non-Infectious Process

The systemic inflammatory response syndrome (SIRS) can develop as a result of certain non-infectious disease processes, such as trauma, malignant neoplasm, or pancreatitis. When SIRS is documented with a noninfectious condition, and no subsequent infection is documented, the code for the underlying condition, such as an injury, should be assigned, followed by code R65.10, Systemic inflammatory response syndrome (SIRS) of non-infectious origin without acute organ dysfunction, or code R65.11, Systemic inflammatory response syndrome (SIRS) of non-infectious origin with acute organ dysfunction. If an associated acute organ dysfunction is documented, the appropriate code(s) for the specific type of organ dysfunction(s) should be assigned in addition to code R65.11. If acute organ dysfunction is documented, but it cannot be determined if the acute organ dysfunction is associated with SIRS or due to another condition (e.g., directly due to the trauma), the provider should be queried.

h. Death NOS

Code R99, Ill-defined and unknown cause of mortality, is only for use in the very limited circumstance when a patient who has already died is brought into an emergency department or other healthcare facility and is pronounced dead upon arrival. It does not represent the discharge disposition of death.

i. NIHSS Stroke Scale

The NIH stroke scale (NIHSS) codes (R29.7- -) can be used in conjunction with acute stroke codes (I63) to identify the patient's neurological status and the severity of the stroke. The stroke scale codes should be sequenced after the acute stroke diagnosis code(s).

At a minimum, report the initial score documented. If desired, a facility may choose to capture multiple stroke scale scores.

See Section I.B.14. for NIHSS stroke scale documentation by clinicians other than patient's provider

19. Chapter 19: Injury, poisoning, and certain other consequences of external causes (S00-T88)

a. Application of 7th Characters in Chapter 19

Most categories in chapter 19 have a 7th character requirement for each applicable code. Most categories in this chapter have three 7th character values (with the exception of fractures): A, initial encounter, D, subsequent encounter and S, sequela. Categories for traumatic fractures have additional 7th character values. While the patient may be seen by a new or different provider over the course of treatment for an injury, assignment of the 7th character is based on whether the patient is undergoing active treatment and not whether the provider is seeing the patient for the first time.

For complication codes, active treatment refers to treatment for the condition described by the code, even though it may be related to an earlier precipitating problem. For example, code T84.50XA, Infection and inflammatory reaction due to unspecified internal joint prosthesis, initial encounter, is used when active treatment is provided for the infection, even though the condition relates to the prosthetic device, implant or graft that was placed at a previous encounter.

7th character "A", initial encounter is used for each encounter where the patient is receiving active treatment for the condition.

7th character "D" subsequent encounter is used for encounters after the patient has completed active treatment of the condition and is receiving routine care for the condition during the healing or recovery phase.

The aftercare Z codes should not be used for aftercare for conditions such as injuries or poisonings, where 7th characters are provided to identify subsequent care. For example, for aftercare of an injury, assign the acute injury code with the 7th character "D" (subsequent encounter).

7th character "S", sequela, is for use for complications or conditions that arise as a direct result of a condition, such as scar formation after a burn. The scars are sequelae of the burn. When using 7th character "S", it is necessary to use both the injury code that precipitated the sequela and the code for the sequela itself. The "S" is added only to the injury code, not the sequela code. The 7th character "S" identifies the injury responsible for the sequela. The specific type of sequela (e.g. scar) is sequenced first, followed by the injury code.

See Section I.B.10. Sequelae, (Late Effects)

b. Coding of Injuries

When coding injuries, assign separate codes for each injury unless a combination code is provided, in which case the combination code is assigned. Codes from category T07, Unspecified multiple injuries should not be assigned in the inpatient setting unless information for a more specific code is not available. Traumatic injury codes (S00-T14.9) are not to be used for normal, healing surgical wounds or to identify complications of surgical wounds.

The code for the most serious injury, as determined by the provider and the focus of treatment, is sequenced first.

1) Superficial injuries

Superficial injuries such as abrasions or contusions are not coded when associated with more severe injuries of the same site.

2) Primary injury with damage to nerves/blood vessels

When a primary injury results in minor damage to peripheral nerves or blood vessels, the primary injury is sequenced first with additional code(s) for injuries to nerves and spinal cord (such as category S04), and/or injury to blood vessels (such as category S15). When the primary injury is to the blood vessels or nerves, that injury should be sequenced first.

3) Iatrogenic injuries

Injury codes from Chapter 19 should not be assigned for injuries that occur during, or as a result of, a medical intervention. Assign the appropriate complication code(s).

c. Coding of Traumatic Fractures

The principles of multiple coding of injuries should be followed in coding fractures. Fractures of specified sites are coded individually by site in accordance with both the provisions within categories S02, S12, S22, S32, S42, S49, S52, S59, S62, S72, S79, S82, S89, S92 and the level of detail furnished by medical record content.

A fracture not indicated as open or closed should be coded to closed. A fracture not indicated whether displaced or not displaced should be coded to displaced.

More specific guidelines are as follows:

1) Initial vs. subsequent encounter for fractures

Traumatic fractures are coded using the appropriate 7th character for initial encounter (A, B, C) for each encounter where the patient is receiving active treatment for the fracture. The appropriate 7th character for initial encounter should also be assigned for a patient who delayed seeking treatment for the fracture or nonunion.

Fractures are coded using the appropriate 7th character for subsequent care for encounters after the patient has completed active treatment of the fracture and is receiving routine care for the fracture during the healing or recovery phase.

Care for complications of surgical treatment for fracture repairs during the healing or recovery phase should be coded with the appropriate complication codes.

Care of complications of fractures, such as malunion and nonunion, should be reported with the appropriate 7th character for subsequent care with nonunion (K, M, N,) or subsequent care with malunion (P, Q, R).

Malunion/nonunion: The appropriate 7th character for initial encounter should also be assigned for a patient who delayed seeking treatment for the fracture or nonunion.

The open fracture designations in the assignment of the 7th character for fractures of the forearm, femur and lower leg, including ankle are based on the Gustilo open fracture classification. When the Gustilo classification type is not specified for an open fracture, the 7th character for open fracture type I or II should be assigned (B, E, H, M, Q).

A code from category M8Ø, not a traumatic fracture code, should be used for any patient with known osteoporosis who suffers a fracture, even if the patient had a minor fall or trauma, if that fall or trauma would not usually break a normal, healthy bone.

See Section I.C.13. Osteoporosis.

The aftercare Z codes should not be used for aftercare for traumatic fractures. For aftercare of a traumatic fracture, assign the acute fracture code with the appropriate 7th character.

2) Multiple fractures sequencing

Multiple fractures are sequenced in accordance with the severity of the fracture.

3) Physeal fractures

For physeal fractures, assign only the code identifying the type of physeal fracture. Do not assign a separate code to identify the specific bone that is fractured.

d. Coding of Burns and Corrosions

The ICD-10-CM makes a distinction between burns and corrosions. The burn codes are for thermal burns, except sunburns, that come from a heat source, such as a fire or hot appliance. The burn codes are also for burns resulting from electricity and radiation. Corrosions are burns due to chemicals. The guidelines are the same for burns and corrosions.

Current burns (T2Ø-T25) are classified by depth, extent and by agent (X code). Burns are classified by depth as first degree (erythema), second degree (blistering), and third degree (full-thickness involvement). Burns of the eye and internal organs (T26-T28) are classified by site, but not by degree.

1) Sequencing of burn and related condition codes

Sequence first the code that reflects the highest degree of burn when more than one burn is present.

a. When the reason for the admission or encounter is for treatment of external multiple burns, sequence first the code that reflects the burn of the highest degree.

b. When a patient has both internal and external burns, the circumstances of admission govern the selection of the principal diagnosis or first-listed diagnosis.

c. When a patient is admitted for burn injuries and other related conditions such as smoke inhalation and/or respiratory failure, the circumstances of admission govern the selection of the principal or first-listed diagnosis.

2) Burns of the same anatomic site

Classify burns of the same anatomic site and on the same side but of different degrees to the subcategory identifying the highest degree recorded in the diagnosis (e.g., for second and third degree burns of right thigh, assign only code T24.311-).

3) Non-healing burns

Non-healing burns are coded as acute burns.

Necrosis of burned skin should be coded as a non-healed burn.

4) Infected burn

For any documented infected burn site, use an additional code for the infection.

5) Assign separate codes for each burn site

When coding burns, assign separate codes for each burn site. Category T3Ø, Burn and corrosion, body region unspecified is extremely vague and should rarely be used.

Codes for burns of "multiple sites" should only be assigned when the medical record documentation does not specify the individual sites.

6) Burns and corrosions classified according to extent of body surface involved

Assign codes from category T31, Burns classified according to extent of body surface involved, or T32, Corrosions classified according to extent of body surface involved, for acute burns or corrosions when the site of the burn or corrosion is not specified or when there is a need for additional data. It is advisable to use category T31 as additional coding when needed to provide data for evaluating burn mortality, such as that needed by burn units. It is also advisable to use category T31 as an additional code for reporting purposes when there is mention of a third-degree burn involving 20 percent or more of the body surface. Codes from categories T31 and T32 should not be used for sequelae of burns or corrosions.

Categories T31 and T32 are based on the classic "rule of nines" in estimating body surface involved: head and neck are assigned nine percent, each arm nine percent, each leg 18 percent, the anterior trunk 18 percent, posterior trunk 18 percent, and genitalia one percent. Providers may change these percentage assignments where necessary to accommodate infants and children who have proportionately larger heads than adults, and patients who have large buttocks, thighs, or abdomen that involve burns.

7) Encounters for treatment of sequela of burns

Encounters for the treatment of the late effects of burns or corrosions (i.e., scars or joint contractures) should be coded with a burn or corrosion code with the 7th character "S" for sequela.

8) Sequelae with a late effect code and current burn

When appropriate, both a code for a current burn or corrosion with 7th character "A" or "D" and a burn or corrosion code with 7th character "S" may be assigned on the same record (when both a current burn and sequelae of an old burn exist). Burns and corrosions do not heal at the same rate and a current healing wound may still exist with sequela of a healed burn or corrosion.

See Section I.B.10. Sequela (Late Effects)

9) Use of an external cause code with burns and corrosions

An external cause code should be used with burns and corrosions to identify the source and intent of the burn, as well as the place where it occurred.

e. Adverse Effects, Poisoning, Underdosing and Toxic Effects

Codes in categories T36-T65 are combination codes that include the substance that was taken as well as the intent. No additional external cause code is required for poisonings, toxic effects, adverse effects and underdosing codes.

1) Do not code directly from the Table of Drugs

Do not code directly from the Table of Drugs and Chemicals. Always refer back to the Tabular List.

2) Use as many codes as necessary to describe

Use as many codes as necessary to describe completely all drugs, medicinal or biological substances.

3) If the same code would describe the causative agent

If the same code would describe the causative agent for more than one adverse reaction, poisoning, toxic effect or underdosing, assign the code only once.

4) If two or more drugs, medicinal or biological substances

If two or more drugs, medicinal or biological substances are taken, code each individually unless a combination code is listed in the Table of Drugs and Chemicals.

If multiple unspecified drugs, medicinal or biological substances were taken, assign the appropriate code from subcategory

T5Ø.91, Poisoning by, adverse effect of and underdosing of multiple unspecified drugs, medicaments and biological substances.

5) **The occurrence of drug toxicity is classified in ICD-10-CM as follows:**

(a) **Adverse Effect**

When coding an adverse effect of a drug that has been correctly prescribed and properly administered, assign the appropriate code for the nature of the adverse effect followed by the appropriate code for the adverse effect of the drug (T36-T5Ø). The code for the drug should have a 5th or 6th character "5" (for example T36.ØX5-) Examples of the nature of an adverse effect are tachycardia, delirium, gastrointestinal hemorrhaging, vomiting, hypokalemia, hepatitis, renal failure, or respiratory failure.

(b) **Poisoning**

When coding a poisoning or reaction to the improper use of a medication (e.g., overdose, wrong substance given or taken in error, wrong route of administration), first assign the appropriate code from categories T36-T5Ø. The poisoning codes have an associated intent as their 5th or 6th character (accidental, intentional self-harm, assault and undetermined). If the intent of the poisoning is unknown or unspecified, code the intent as accidental intent. The undetermined intent is only for use if the documentation in the record specifies that the intent cannot be determined. Use additional code(s) for all manifestations of poisonings.

If there is also a diagnosis of abuse or dependence of the substance, the abuse or dependence is assigned as an additional code.

Examples of poisoning include:

(i) Error was made in drug prescription
Errors made in drug prescription or in the administration of the drug by provider, nurse, patient, or other person.

(ii) Overdose of a drug intentionally taken
If an overdose of a drug was intentionally taken or administered and resulted in drug toxicity, it would be coded as a poisoning.

(iii) Nonprescribed drug taken with correctly prescribed and properly administered drug
If a nonprescribed drug or medicinal agent was taken in combination with a correctly prescribed and properly administered drug, any drug toxicity or other reaction resulting from the interaction of the two drugs would be classified as a poisoning.

(iv) Interaction of drug(s) and alcohol
When a reaction results from the interaction of a drug(s) and alcohol, this would be classified as poisoning.

See Section I.C.4. if poisoning is the result of insulin pump malfunctions.

(c) **Underdosing**

Underdosing refers to taking less of a medication than is prescribed by a provider or a manufacturer's instruction. Discontinuing the use of a prescribed medication on the patient's own initiative (not directed by the patient's provider) is also classified as an underdosing. For underdosing, assign the code from categories T36-T5Ø (fifth or sixth character "6"). **Documentation of a change in the patient's condition is not required in order to assign an underdosing code. Documentation that the patient is taking less of a medication than is prescribed or discontinued the prescribed medication is sufficient for code assignment.**

Codes for underdosing should never be assigned as principal or first-listed codes. If a patient has a relapse or exacerbation of the medical condition for which the drug is prescribed because of the reduction in dose, then the medical condition itself should be coded.

Noncompliance (Z91.12-, Z91.13- and Z91.14-) or complication of care (Y63.6-Y63.9) codes are to be used with an underdosing code to indicate intent, if known.

(d) **Toxic Effects**

When a harmful substance is ingested or comes in contact with a person, this is classified as a toxic effect. The toxic effect codes are in categories T51-T65.

Toxic effect codes have an associated intent: accidental, intentional self-harm, assault and undetermined.

f. **Adult and child abuse, neglect and other maltreatment**

Sequence first the appropriate code from categories T74, Adult and child abuse, neglect and other maltreatment, confirmed, or T76, Adult and child abuse, neglect and other maltreatment, suspected, for abuse, neglect and other maltreatment, followed by any accompanying mental health or injury code(s).

If the documentation in the medical record states abuse or neglect, it is coded as confirmed (T74.-). It is coded as suspected if it is documented as suspected (T76.-).

For cases of confirmed abuse or neglect an external cause code from the assault section (X92-YØ9) should be added to identify the cause of any physical injuries. A perpetrator code (YØ7) should be added when the perpetrator of the abuse is known. For suspected cases of abuse or neglect, do not report external cause or perpetrator code.

If a suspected case of abuse, neglect or mistreatment is ruled out during an encounter code ZØ4.71, Encounter for examination and observation following alleged physical adult abuse, ruled out, or code ZØ4.72, Encounter for examination and observation following alleged child physical abuse, ruled out, should be used, not a code from T76.

If a suspected case of alleged rape or sexual abuse is ruled out during an encounter code ZØ4.41, Encounter for examination and observation following alleged adult rape or code ZØ4.42, Encounter for examination and observation following alleged child rape, should be used, not a code from T76.

If a suspected case of forced sexual exploitation or forced labor exploitation is ruled out during an encounter, code ZØ4.81, Encounter for examination and observation of victim following forced sexual exploitation, or code ZØ4.82, Encounter for examination and observation of victim following forced labor exploitation, should be used, not a code from T76.

See Section I.C.15. Abuse in a pregnant patient.

g. **Complications of care**

1) **General guidelines for complications of care**

(a) **Documentation of complications of care**

See Section I.B.16. for information on documentation of complications of care.

2) **Pain due to medical devices**

Pain associated with devices, implants or grafts left in a surgical site (for example painful hip prosthesis) is assigned to the appropriate code(s) found in Chapter 19, Injury, poisoning, and certain other consequences of external causes. Specific codes for pain due to medical devices are found in the T code section of the ICD-10-CM. Use additional code(s) from category G89 to identify acute or chronic pain due to presence of the device, implant or graft (G89.18 or G89.28).

3) **Transplant complications**

(a) **Transplant complications other than kidney**

Codes under category T86, Complications of transplanted organs and tissues, are for use for both complications and rejection of transplanted organs. A transplant complication code is only assigned if the complication affects the function of the transplanted organ. Two codes are required to fully describe a transplant complication: the appropriate code from category T86 and a secondary code that identifies the complication.

Pre-existing conditions or conditions that develop after the transplant are not coded as complications unless they affect the function of the transplanted organs.

See I.C.21. for transplant organ removal status

See I.C.2. for malignant neoplasm associated with transplanted organ.

(b) **Kidney transplant complications**

Patients who have undergone kidney transplant may still have some form of chronic kidney disease (CKD) because the kidney transplant may not fully restore kidney function. Code T86.1- should be assigned for documented complications of a kidney transplant, such as transplant failure or rejection or other transplant complication. Code T86.1- should not be assigned for post kidney transplant patients who have chronic kidney (CKD) unless a transplant complication such as transplant failure or rejection is documented. If the documentation is unclear as to whether the patient has a complication of the transplant, query the provider.

Conditions that affect the function of the transplanted kidney, other than CKD, should be assigned a code from subcategory T86.1, Complications of transplanted organ, Kidney, and a secondary code that identifies the complication.

For patients with CKD following a kidney transplant, but who do not have a complication such as failure or rejection, *see section I.C.14. Chronic kidney disease and kidney transplant status.*

4) **Complication codes that include the external cause**
As with certain other T codes, some of the complications of care codes have the external cause included in the code. The code includes the nature of the complication as well as the type of procedure that caused the complication. No external cause code indicating the type of procedure is necessary for these codes.

5) **Complications of care codes within the body system chapters**
Intraoperative and postprocedural complication codes are found within the body system chapters with codes specific to the organs and structures of that body system. These codes should be sequenced first, followed by a code(s) for the specific complication, if applicable.

Complication codes from the body system chapters should be assigned for intraoperative and postprocedural complications (e.g., the appropriate complication code from chapter 9 would be assigned for a vascular intraoperative or postprocedural complication) unless the complication is specifically indexed to a T code in chapter 19.

20. Chapter 20: External Causes of Morbidity (VØØ-Y99)

The external causes of morbidity codes should never be sequenced as the first-listed or principal diagnosis.

External cause codes are intended to provide data for injury research and evaluation of injury prevention strategies. These codes capture how the injury or health condition happened (cause), the intent (unintentional or accidental; or intentional, such as suicide or assault), the place where the event occurred the activity of the patient at the time of the event, and the person's status (e.g., civilian, military).

There is no national requirement for mandatory ICD-10-CM external cause code reporting. Unless a provider is subject to a state-based external cause code reporting mandate or these codes are required by a particular payer, reporting of ICD-10-CM codes in Chapter 20, External Causes of Morbidity, is not required. In the absence of a mandatory reporting requirement, providers are encouraged to voluntarily report external cause codes, as they provide valuable data for injury research and evaluation of injury prevention strategies.

a. **General External Cause Coding Guidelines**

1) **Used with any code in the range of AØØ.Ø-T88.9, ZØØ-Z99**
An external cause code may be used with any code in the range of AØØ.Ø-T88.9, ZØØ-Z99, classification that represents a health condition due to an external cause. Though they are most applicable to injuries, they are also valid for use with such things as infections or diseases due to an external source, and other health conditions, such as a heart attack that occurs during strenuous physical activity.

2) **External cause code used for length of treatment**
Assign the external cause code, with the appropriate 7th character (initial encounter, subsequent encounter or sequela) for each encounter for which the injury or condition is being treated.

Most categories in chapter 20 have a 7th character requirement for each applicable code. Most categories in this chapter have three 7th character values: A, initial encounter, D, subsequent encounter and S, sequela. While the patient may be seen by a new or different provider over the course of treatment for an injury or condition, assignment of the 7th character for external cause should match the 7th character of the code assigned for the associated injury or condition for the encounter.

3) **Use the full range of external cause codes**
Use the full range of external cause codes to completely describe the cause, the intent, the place of occurrence, and if applicable, the activity of the patient at the time of the event, and the patient's status, for all injuries, and other health conditions due to an external cause.

4) **Assign as many external cause codes as necessary**
Assign as many external cause codes as necessary to fully explain each cause. If only one external code can be recorded, assign the code most related to the principal diagnosis.

5) **The selection of the appropriate external cause code**
The selection of the appropriate external cause code is guided by the Alphabetic Index of External Causes and by Inclusion and Exclusion notes in the Tabular List.

6) **External cause code can never be a principal diagnosis**
An external cause code can never be a principal (first-listed) diagnosis.

7) **Combination external cause codes**
Certain of the external cause codes are combination codes that identify sequential events that result in an injury, such as a fall which results in striking against an object. The injury may be due to either event or both. The combination external cause code used should correspond to the sequence of events regardless of which caused the most serious injury.

8) **No external cause code needed in certain circumstances**
No external cause code from Chapter 20 is needed if the external cause and intent are included in a code from another chapter (e.g., T36.ØX1-, Poisoning by penicillins, accidental (unintentional)).

b. **Place of Occurrence Guideline**

Codes from category Y92, Place of occurrence of the external cause, are secondary codes for use after other external cause codes to identify the location of the patient at the time of injury or other condition.

Generally, a place of occurrence code is assigned only once, at the initial encounter for treatment. However, in the rare instance that a new injury occurs during hospitalization, an additional place of occurrence code may be assigned. No 7th characters are used for Y92.

Do not use place of occurrence code Y92.9 if the place is not stated or is not applicable.

c. **Activity Code**

Assign a code from category Y93, Activity code, to describe the activity of the patient at the time the injury or other health condition occurred.

An activity code is used only once, at the initial encounter for treatment. Only one code from Y93 should be recorded on a medical record.

The activity codes are not applicable to poisonings, adverse effects, misadventures or sequela.

Do not assign Y93.9, Unspecified activity, if the activity is not stated.

A code from category Y93 is appropriate for use with external cause and intent codes if identifying the activity provides additional information about the event.

d. **Place of Occurrence, Activity, and Status Codes Used with other External Cause Code**

When applicable, place of occurrence, activity, and external cause status codes are sequenced after the main external cause code(s). Regardless of the number of external cause codes assigned, generally there should be only one place of occurrence code, one activity code, and one external cause status code assigned to an encounter. However, in the rare instance that a new injury occurs during hospitalization, an additional place of occurrence code may be assigned.

e. **If the Reporting Format Limits the Number of External Cause Codes**

If the reporting format limits the number of external cause codes that can be used in reporting clinical data, report the code for the cause/intent most related to the principal diagnosis. If the format permits capture of additional external cause codes, the cause/intent, including medical misadventures, of the additional events should be reported rather than the codes for place, activity, or external status.

f. **Multiple External Cause Coding Guidelines**

More than one external cause code is required to fully describe the external cause of an illness or injury. The assignment of external cause codes should be sequenced in the following priority:

If two or more events cause separate injuries, an external cause code should be assigned for each cause. The first-listed external cause code will be selected in the following order:

External codes for child and adult abuse take priority over all other external cause codes.

See Section I.C.19., Child and Adult abuse guidelines.

External cause codes for terrorism events take priority over all other external cause codes except child and adult abuse.

External cause codes for cataclysmic events take priority over all other external cause codes except child and adult abuse and terrorism.

External cause codes for transport accidents take priority over all other external cause codes except cataclysmic events, child and adult abuse and terrorism.

Activity and external cause status codes are assigned following all causal (intent) external cause codes.

The first-listed external cause code should correspond to the cause of the most serious diagnosis due to an assault, accident, or self-harm, following the order of hierarchy listed above.

g. Child and Adult Abuse Guideline

Adult and child abuse, neglect and maltreatment are classified as assault. Any of the assault codes may be used to indicate the external cause of any injury resulting from the confirmed abuse.

For confirmed cases of abuse, neglect and maltreatment, when the perpetrator is known, a code from YØ7, Perpetrator of maltreatment and neglect, should accompany any other assault codes.

See Section I.C.19. Adult and child abuse, neglect and other maltreatment

h. Unknown or Undetermined Intent Guideline

If the intent (accident, self-harm, assault) of the cause of an injury or other condition is unknown or unspecified, code the intent as accidental intent. All transport accident categories assume accidental intent.

1) Use of undetermined intent

External cause codes for events of undetermined intent are only for use if the documentation in the record specifies that the intent cannot be determined.

i. Sequelae (Late Effects) of External Cause Guidelines

1) Sequelae external cause codes

Sequela are reported using the external cause code with the 7th character "S" for sequela. These codes should be used with any report of a late effect or sequela resulting from a previous injury.

See Section I.B.10. Sequela (Late Effects)

2) Sequela external cause code with a related current injury

A sequela external cause code should never be used with a related current nature of injury code.

3) Use of sequela external cause codes for subsequent visits

Use a late effect external cause code for subsequent visits when a late effect of the initial injury is being treated. Do not use a late effect external cause code for subsequent visits for follow-up care (e.g., to assess healing, to receive rehabilitative therapy) of the injury when no late effect of the injury has been documented.

j. Terrorism Guidelines

1) Cause of injury identified by the Federal Government (FBI) as terrorism

When the cause of an injury is identified by the Federal Government (FBI) as terrorism, the first-listed external cause code should be a code from category Y38, Terrorism. The definition of terrorism employed by the FBI is found at the inclusion note at the beginning of category Y38. Use additional code for place of occurrence (Y92.-). More than one Y38 code may be assigned if the injury is the result of more than one mechanism of terrorism.

2) Cause of an injury is suspected to be the result of terrorism

When the cause of an injury is suspected to be the result of terrorism a code from category Y38 should not be assigned. Suspected cases should be classified as assault.

3) Code Y38.9, Terrorism, secondary effects

Assign code Y38.9, Terrorism, secondary effects, for conditions occurring subsequent to the terrorist event. This code should not be assigned for conditions that are due to the initial terrorist act.

It is acceptable to assign code Y38.9 with another code from Y38 if there is an injury due to the initial terrorist event and an injury that is a subsequent result of the terrorist event.

k. External Cause Status

A code from category Y99, External cause status, should be assigned whenever any other external cause code is assigned for an encounter, including an Activity code, except for the events noted below. Assign a code from category Y99, External cause status, to indicate the work status of the person at the time the event occurred. The status code indicates whether the event occurred during military activity, whether a non-military person was at work, whether an individual including a student or volunteer was involved in a non-work activity at the time of the causal event.

A code from Y99, External cause status, should be assigned, when applicable, with other external cause codes, such as transport accidents and falls. The external cause status codes are not applicable to poisonings, adverse effects, misadventures or late effects.

Do not assign a code from category Y99 if no other external cause codes (cause, activity) are applicable for the encounter.

An external cause status code is used only once, at the initial encounter for treatment. Only one code from Y99 should be recorded on a medical record.

Do not assign code Y99.9, Unspecified external cause status, if the status is not stated.

21. Chapter 21: Factors influencing health status and contact with health services (ZØØ-Z99)

Note: The chapter specific guidelines provide additional information about the use of Z codes for specified encounters.

a. Use of Z Codes in Any Healthcare Setting

Z codes are for use in any healthcare setting. Z codes may be used as either a first-listed (principal diagnosis code in the inpatient setting) or secondary code, depending on the circumstances of the encounter. Certain Z codes may only be used as first-listed or principal diagnosis.

b. Z Codes Indicate a Reason for an Encounter or Provide Additional Information about a Patient Encounter

Z codes are not procedure codes. A corresponding procedure code must accompany a Z code to describe any procedure performed.

c. Categories of Z Codes

1) Contact/Exposure

Category Z2Ø indicates contact with, and suspected exposure to, communicable diseases. These codes are for patients who are suspected to have been exposed to a disease by close personal contact with an infected individual or are in an area where a disease is epidemic.

Category Z77, Other contact with and (suspected) exposures hazardous to health, indicates contact with and suspected exposures hazardous to health.

Contact/exposure codes may be used as a first-listed code to explain an encounter for testing, or, more commonly, as a secondary code to identify a potential risk.

2) Inoculations and vaccinations

Code Z23 is for encounters for inoculations and vaccinations. It indicates that a patient is being seen to receive a prophylactic inoculation against a disease. Procedure codes are required to identify the actual administration of the injection and the type(s) of immunizations given. Code Z23 may be used as a secondary code if the inoculation is given as a routine part of preventive health care, such as a well-baby visit.

3) Status

Status codes indicate that a patient is either a carrier of a disease or has the sequelae or residual of a past disease or condition. This includes such things as the presence of prosthetic or mechanical devices resulting from past treatment. A status code is informative, because the status may affect the course of treatment and its outcome. A status code is distinct from a history code. The history code indicates that the patient no longer has the condition.

A status code should not be used with a diagnosis code from one of the body system chapters, if the diagnosis code includes the information provided by the status code. For example, code Z94.1, Heart transplant status, should not be used with a code from subcategory T86.2, Complications of heart transplant. The status code does not provide additional information. The complication code indicates that the patient is a heart transplant patient.

For encounters for weaning from a mechanical ventilator, assign a code from subcategory J96.1, Chronic respiratory failure, followed by code Z99.11, Dependence on respirator [ventilator] status.

The status Z codes/categories are:

Z14 Genetic carrier

Genetic carrier status indicates that a person carries a gene, associated with a particular disease, which may be passed to offspring who may develop that disease. The person does not have the disease and is not at risk of developing the disease.

Z15 Genetic susceptibility to disease

Genetic susceptibility indicates that a person has a gene that increases the risk of that person developing the disease.

Codes from category Z15 should not be used as principal or first-listed codes. If the patient has the condition to which he/she is susceptible, and that condition is the reason for the encounter, the code for the current condition should be sequenced first. If the patient is being seen for follow-up after completed treatment for this condition, and the condition no longer exists, a follow-up code should be sequenced first, followed by the appropriate personal history and genetic susceptibility codes. If the purpose of the encounter is genetic counseling associated with procreative management, code Z31.5, Encounter for genetic counseling, should be assigned as the first-listed code, followed by a code from category Z15. Additional codes should be assigned for any applicable family or personal history.

Z16 Resistance to antimicrobial drugs
This code indicates that a patient has a condition that is resistant to antimicrobial drug treatment. Sequence the infection code first.

Z17 Estrogen receptor status

Z18 Retained foreign body fragments

Z19 Hormone sensitivity malignancy status

Z21 Asymptomatic HIV infection status
This code indicates that a patient has tested positive for HIV but has manifested no signs or symptoms of the disease.

Z22 Carrier of infectious disease
Carrier status indicates that a person harbors the specific organisms of a disease without manifest symptoms and is capable of transmitting the infection.

Z28.3 Underimmunization status
See Section I.B.14. for underimmunization documentation by clinicians other than the patient's provider.

Z33.1 Pregnant state, incidental
This code is a secondary code only for use when the pregnancy is in no way complicating the reason for visit. Otherwise, a code from the obstetric chapter is required.

Z66 Do not resuscitate
This code may be used when it is documented by the provider that a patient is on do not resuscitate status at any time during the stay.

Z67 Blood type

Z68 Body mass index (BMI)
BMI codes should only be assigned when there is an associated, reportable diagnosis (such as obesity). Do not assign BMI codes during pregnancy.
See Section I.B.14. for BMI documentation by clinicians other than the patient's provider.

Z74.Ø1 Bed confinement status

Z76.82 Awaiting organ transplant status

Z78 Other specified health status
Code Z78.1, Physical restraint status, may be used when it is documented by the provider that a patient has been put in restraints during the current encounter. Please note that this code should not be reported when it is documented by the provider that a patient is temporarily restrained during a procedure.

Z79 Long-term (current) drug therapy
Codes from this category indicate a patient's continuous use of a prescribed drug (including such things as aspirin therapy) for the long-term treatment of a condition or for prophylactic use. It is not for use for patients who have addictions to drugs. This subcategory is not for use of medications for detoxification or maintenance programs to prevent withdrawal symptoms (e.g., methadone maintenance for opiate dependence). Assign the appropriate code for the drug use, abuse, or dependence instead.
Assign a code from Z79 if the patient is receiving a medication for an extended period as a prophylactic measure (such as for the prevention of deep vein thrombosis) or as treatment of a chronic condition (such as arthritis) or a disease requiring a lengthy course of treatment (such as cancer). Do not assign a code from category Z79 for medication being administered for a brief period of time to treat an acute illness or injury (such as a course of antibiotics to treat acute bronchitis).

Z88 Allergy status to drugs, medicaments and biological substances
Except: Z88.9, Allergy status to unspecified drugs, medicaments and biological substances status

Z89 Acquired absence of limb

Z9Ø Acquired absence of organs, not elsewhere classified

Z91.Ø- Allergy status, other than to drugs and biological substances

Z92.82 Status post administration of tPA (rtPA) in a different facility within the last 24 hours prior to admission to a current facility
Assign code Z92.82, Status post administration of tPA (rtPA) in a different facility within the last 24 hours prior to admission to current facility, as a secondary diagnosis when a patient is received by transfer into a facility and documentation indicates they were administered tissue plasminogen activator (tPA) within the last 24 hours prior to admission to the current facility.
This guideline applies even if the patient is still receiving the tPA at the time they are received into the current facility.
The appropriate code for the condition for which the tPA was administered (such as cerebrovascular disease or myocardial infarction) should be assigned first.
Code Z92.82 is only applicable to the receiving facility record and not to the transferring facility record.

Z93 Artificial opening status

Z94 Transplanted organ and tissue status

Z95 Presence of cardiac and vascular implants and grafts

Z96 Presence of other functional implants

Z97 Presence of other devices

Z98 Other postprocedural states
Assign code Z98.85, Transplanted organ removal status, to indicate that a transplanted organ has been previously removed. This code should not be assigned for the encounter in which the transplanted organ is removed. The complication necessitating removal of the transplant organ should be assigned for that encounter.
See section I.C.19. for information on the coding of organ transplant complications.

Z99 Dependence on enabling machines and devices, not elsewhere classified
Note: Categories Z89-Z9Ø and Z93-Z99 are for use only if there are no complications or malfunctions of the organ or tissue replaced, the amputation site or the equipment on which the patient is dependent.

4) History (of)

There are two types of history Z codes, personal and family. Personal history codes explain a patient's past medical condition that no longer exists and is not receiving any treatment, but that has the potential for recurrence, and therefore may require continued monitoring.

Family history codes are for use when a patient has a family member(s) who has had a particular disease that causes the patient to be at higher risk of also contracting the disease.

Personal history codes may be used in conjunction with follow-up codes and family history codes may be used in conjunction with screening codes to explain the need for a test or procedure. History codes are also acceptable on any medical record regardless of the reason for visit. A history of an illness, even if no longer present, is important information that may alter the type of treatment ordered.

The reason for the encounter (for example, screening or counseling) should be sequenced first and the appropriate personal and/or family history code(s) should be assigned as additional diagnos(es).

The history Z code categories are:

Z8Ø Family history of primary malignant neoplasm

Z81 Family history of mental and behavioral disorders

Z82 Family history of certain disabilities and chronic diseases (leading to disablement)

Z83 Family history of other specific disorders

Z84 Family history of other conditions

Z85 Personal history of malignant neoplasm

Z86 Personal history of certain other diseases

Z87 Personal history of other diseases and conditions

Z91.4- Personal history of psychological trauma, not elsewhere classified

Z91.5- Personal history of self-harm

Z91.81 History of falling

Z91.82 Personal history of military deployment

Z92 Personal history of medical treatment
Except: Z92.Ø, Personal history of contraception
Except: Z92.82, Status post administration of tPA (rtPA) in a different facility within the last 24 hours prior to admission to a current facility

5) Screening

Screening is the testing for disease or disease precursors in seemingly well individuals so that early detection and treatment can be provided for those who test positive for the disease (e.g., screening mammogram).

The testing of a person to rule out or confirm a suspected diagnosis because the patient has some sign or symptom is a diagnostic examination, not a screening. In these cases, the sign or symptom is used to explain the reason for the test.

A screening code may be a first-listed code if the reason for the visit is specifically the screening exam. It may also be used as an additional code if the screening is done during an office visit for other health problems. A screening code is not necessary if the screening is inherent to a routine examination, such as a pap smear done during a routine pelvic examination.

Should a condition be discovered during the screening then the code for the condition may be assigned as an additional diagnosis.

The Z code indicates that a screening exam is planned. A procedure code is required to confirm that the screening was performed.

The screening Z codes/categories:

Z11 Encounter for screening for infectious and parasitic diseases

Z12 Encounter for screening for malignant neoplasms

Z13 Encounter for screening for other diseases and disorders
Except: Z13.9, Encounter for screening, unspecified

Z36 Encounter for antenatal screening for mother

6) Observation

There are three observation Z code categories. They are for use in very limited circumstances when a person is being observed for a suspected condition that is ruled out. The observation codes are not for use if an injury or illness or any signs or symptoms related to the suspected condition are present. In such cases the diagnosis/symptom code is used with the corresponding external cause code.

The observation codes are primarily to be used as a principal/first-listed diagnosis. An observation code may be assigned as a secondary diagnosis code when the patient is being observed for a condition that is ruled out and is unrelated to the principal/first-listed diagnosis. Also, when the principal diagnosis is required to be a code from category Z38, Liveborn infants according to place of birth and type of delivery, then a code from category ZØ5, Encounter for observation and evaluation of newborn for suspected diseases and conditions ruled out, is sequenced after the Z38 code. Additional codes may be used in addition to the observation code, but only if they are unrelated to the suspected condition being observed.

Codes from subcategory ZØ3.7, Encounter for suspected maternal and fetal conditions ruled out, may either be used as a first-listed or as an additional code assignment depending on the case. They are for use in very limited circumstances on a maternal record when an encounter is for a suspected maternal or fetal condition that is ruled out during that encounter (for example, a maternal or fetal condition may be suspected due to an abnormal test result). These codes should not be used when the condition is confirmed. In those cases, the confirmed condition should be coded. In addition, these codes are not for use if an illness or any signs or symptoms related to the suspected condition or problem are present. In such cases the diagnosis/symptom code is used.

Additional codes may be used in addition to the code from subcategory ZØ3.7, but only if they are unrelated to the suspected condition being evaluated.

Codes from subcategory ZØ3.7 may not be used for encounters for antenatal screening of mother. *See Section I.C.21. Screening.*

For encounters for suspected fetal condition that are inconclusive following testing and evaluation, assign the appropriate code from category O35, O36, O4Ø or O41.

The observation Z code categories:

ZØ3 Encounter for medical observation for suspected diseases and conditions ruled out

ZØ4 Encounter for examination and observation for other reasons Except: ZØ4.9, Encounter for examination and observation for unspecified reason

ZØ5 Encounter for observation and evaluation of newborn for suspected diseases and conditions ruled out

7) Aftercare

Aftercare visit codes cover situations when the initial treatment of a disease has been performed and the patient requires continued care during the healing or recovery phase, or for the long-term consequences of the disease. The aftercare Z code should not be used if treatment is directed at a current, acute disease. The diagnosis code is to be used in these cases. Exceptions to this rule are codes Z51.Ø, Encounter for antineoplastic radiation therapy, and codes from subcategory Z51.1, Encounter for antineoplastic chemotherapy and immunotherapy. These codes are to be first listed, followed by the diagnosis code when a patient's encounter is solely to receive radiation therapy, chemotherapy, or immunotherapy for the treatment of a neoplasm. If the reason for the encounter is more than one type of antineoplastic therapy, code Z51.Ø and a code from subcategory Z51.1 may be assigned together, in which case one of these codes would be reported as a secondary diagnosis.

The aftercare Z codes should also not be used for aftercare for injuries. For aftercare of an injury, assign the acute injury code with the appropriate 7th character (for subsequent encounter).

The aftercare codes are generally first listed to explain the specific reason for the encounter. An aftercare code may be used as an additional code when some type of aftercare is provided in addition to the reason for admission and no diagnosis code is applicable. An example of this would be the closure of a colostomy during an encounter for treatment of another condition.

Aftercare codes should be used in conjunction with other aftercare codes or diagnosis codes to provide better detail on the specifics of an aftercare encounter visit, unless otherwise directed by the classification. The sequencing of multiple aftercare codes depends on the circumstances of the encounter.

Certain aftercare Z code categories need a secondary diagnosis code to describe the resolving condition or sequelae. For others, the condition is included in the code title.

Additional Z code aftercare category terms include fitting and adjustment, and attention to artificial openings.

Status Z codes may be used with aftercare Z codes to indicate the nature of the aftercare. For example, code Z95.1, Presence of aortocoronary bypass graft, may be used with code Z48.812, Encounter for surgical aftercare following surgery on the circulatory system, to indicate the surgery for which the aftercare is being performed. A status code should not be used when the aftercare code indicates the type of status, such as using Z43.Ø, Encounter for attention to tracheostomy, with Z93.Ø, Tracheostomy status.

The aftercare Z category/codes:

Z42 Encounter for plastic and reconstructive surgery following medical procedure or healed injury

Z43 Encounter for attention to artificial openings

Z44 Encounter for fitting and adjustment of external prosthetic device

Z45 Encounter for adjustment and management of implanted device

Z46 Encounter for fitting and adjustment of other devices

Z47 Orthopedic aftercare

Z48 Encounter for other postprocedural aftercare

Z49 Encounter for care involving renal dialysis

Z51 Encounter for other aftercare and medical care

8) Follow-up

The follow-up codes are used to explain continuing surveillance following completed treatment of a disease, condition, or injury. They imply that the condition has been fully treated and no longer exists. They should not be confused with aftercare codes, or injury codes with a 7th character for subsequent encounter, that explain ongoing care of a healing condition or its sequelae. Follow-up codes may be used in conjunction with history codes to provide the full picture of the healed condition and its treatment. The follow-up code is sequenced first, followed by the history code.

A follow-up code may be used to explain multiple visits. Should a condition be found to have recurred on the follow-up visit, then the diagnosis code for the condition should be assigned in place of the follow-up code.

The follow-up Z code categories:

Z08 Encounter for follow-up examination after completed treatment for malignant neoplasm

Z09 Encounter for follow-up examination after completed treatment for conditions other than malignant neoplasm

Z39 Encounter for maternal postpartum care and examination

9) Donor

Codes in category Z52, Donors of organs and tissues, are used for living individuals who are donating blood or other body tissue. These codes are for individuals donating for others, as well as for self-donations. They are not used to identify cadaveric donations.

10) Counseling

Counseling Z codes are used when a patient or family member receives assistance in the aftermath of an illness or injury, or when support is required in coping with family or social problems.

The counseling Z codes/categories:

Z30.0- Encounter for general counseling and advice on contraception

Z31.5 Encounter for procreative genetic counseling

Z31.6- Encounter for general counseling and advice on procreation

Z32.2 Encounter for childbirth instruction

Z32.3 Encounter for childcare instruction

Z69 Encounter for mental health services for victim and perpetrator of abuse

Z70 Counseling related to sexual attitude, behavior and orientation

Z71 Persons encountering health services for other counseling and medical advice, not elsewhere classified

Note: Code Z71.84, Encounter for health counseling related to travel, is to be used for health risk and safety counseling for future travel purposes.

Code Z71.85, Encounter for immunization safety counseling, is to be used for counseling of the patient or caregiver regarding the safety of a vaccine. This code should not be used for the provision of general information regarding risks and potential side effects during routine encounters for the administration of vaccines.

Code Z71.87, Encounter for pediatric-to-adult transition counseling, should be assigned when pediatric to adult transition counseling is the sole reason for the encounter or when this counseling is provided in addition to other services, such as treatment of a chronic condition. If both transition counseling and treatment of a medical condition are provided during the same encounter, the code(s) for the medical condition(s) treated and code Z71.87 should be assigned, with sequencing depending on the circumstances of the encounter.

Z76.81 Expectant mother prebirth pediatrician visit

11) Encounters for Obstetrical and Reproductive Services

See Section I.C.15. Pregnancy, Childbirth, and the Puerperium, for further instruction on the use of these codes.

Z codes for pregnancy are for use in those circumstances when none of the problems or complications included in the codes from the Obstetrics chapter exist (a routine prenatal visit or postpartum care). Codes in category Z34, Encounter for supervision of normal pregnancy, are always first listed and are not to be used with any other code from the OB chapter.

Codes in category Z3A, Weeks of gestation, may be assigned to provide additional information about the pregnancy. Category Z3A codes should not be assigned for pregnancies with abortive outcomes (categories O00-O08), elective termination of pregnancy (code Z33.2), nor for postpartum conditions, as category Z3A is not applicable to these conditions. The date of the admission should be used to determine weeks of gestation for inpatient admissions that encompass more than one gestational week.

The outcome of delivery, category Z37, should be included on all maternal delivery records. It is always a secondary code.

Codes in category Z37 should not be used on the newborn record.

Z codes for family planning (contraceptive) or procreative management and counseling should be included on an obstetric record either during the pregnancy or the postpartum stage, if applicable.

Z codes/categories for obstetrical and reproductive services:

Z30 Encounter for contraceptive management

Z31 Encounter for procreative management

Z32.2 Encounter for childbirth instruction

Z32.3 Encounter for childcare instruction

Z33 Pregnant state

Z34 Encounter for supervision of normal pregnancy

Z36 Encounter for antenatal screening of mother

Z3A Weeks of gestation

Z37 Outcome of delivery

Z39 Encounter for maternal postpartum care and examination

Z76.81 Expectant mother prebirth pediatrician visit

12) Newborns and Infants

See Section I.C.16. Newborn (Perinatal) Guidelines, for further instruction on the use of these codes.

Newborn Z codes/categories:

Z76.1 Encounter for health supervision and care of foundling

Z00.1- Encounter for routine child health examination

Z38 Liveborn infants according to place of birth and type of delivery

13) Routine and Administrative Examinations

The Z codes allow for the description of encounters for routine examinations, such as, a general check-up, or, examinations for administrative purposes, such as, a pre-employment physical. The codes are not to be used if the examination is for diagnosis of a suspected condition or for treatment purposes. In such cases the diagnosis code is used. During a routine exam, should a diagnosis or condition be discovered, it should be coded as an additional code. Pre-existing and chronic conditions and history codes may also be included as additional codes as long as the examination is for administrative purposes and not focused on any particular condition.

Some of the codes for routine health examinations distinguish between "with" and "without" abnormal findings. Code assignment depends on the information that is known at the time the encounter is being coded. For example, if no abnormal findings were found during the examination, but the encounter is being coded before test results are back, it is acceptable to assign the code for "without abnormal findings." When assigning a code for "with abnormal findings," additional code(s) should be assigned to identify the specific abnormal finding(s).

Pre-operative examination and pre-procedural laboratory examination Z codes are for use only in those situations when a patient is being cleared for a procedure or surgery and no treatment is given.

The Z codes/categories for routine and administrative examinations:

Z00 Encounter for general examination without complaint, suspected or reported diagnosis

Z01 Encounter for other special examination without complaint, suspected or reported diagnosis

Z02 Encounter for administrative examination
Except: Z02.9, Encounter for administrative examinations, unspecified

Z32.0- Encounter for pregnancy test

14) Miscellaneous Z Codes

The miscellaneous Z codes capture a number of other health care encounters that do not fall into one of the other categories. Some of these codes identify the reason for the encounter; others are for use as additional codes that provide useful information on circumstances that may affect a patient's care and treatment.

Prophylactic Organ Removal

For encounters specifically for prophylactic removal of an organ (such as prophylactic removal of breasts due to a genetic susceptibility to cancer or a family history of cancer), the principal or first-listed code should be a code from category Z4Ø, Encounter for prophylactic surgery, followed by the appropriate codes to identify the associated risk factor (such as genetic susceptibility or family history).

If the patient has a malignancy of one site and is having prophylactic removal at another site to prevent either a new primary malignancy or metastatic disease, a code for the malignancy should also be assigned in addition to a code from subcategory Z4Ø.Ø, Encounter for prophylactic surgery for risk factors related to malignant neoplasms. A Z4Ø.Ø code should not be assigned if the patient is having organ removal for treatment of a malignancy, such as the removal of the testes for the treatment of prostate cancer.

Miscellaneous Z codes/categories:

Z28 Immunization not carried out
Except: Z28.3-, Underimmunization status

Z29 Encounter for other prophylactic measures

Z4Ø Encounter for prophylactic surgery

Z41 Encounter for procedures for purposes other than remedying health state
Except: Z41.9, Encounter for procedure for purposes other than remedying health state, unspecified

Z53 Persons encountering health services for specific procedures and treatment, not carried out

Z72 Problems related to lifestyle
Note: These codes should be assigned only when the documentation specifies that the patient has an associated problem

Z73 Problems related to life management difficulty
Note: These codes should be assigned only when the documentation specifies that the patient has an associated problem.

Z74 Problems related to care provider dependency
Except: Z74.Ø1, Bed confinement status

Z75 Problems related to medical facilities and other health care

Z76.Ø Encounter for issue of repeat prescription

Z76.3 Healthy person accompanying sick person

Z76.4 Other boarder to healthcare facility

Z76.5 Malingerer [conscious simulation]

Z91.1- Patient's noncompliance with medical treatment and regimen

Z91.83 Wandering in diseases classified elsewhere

Z91.84- Oral health risk factors

Z91.89 Other specified personal risk factors, not elsewhere classified

See Section I.B.14. for Z55-Z65 Persons with potential health hazards related to socioeconomic and psychosocial circumstances, documentation by clinicians other than the patient's provider

15) Nonspecific Z Codes

Certain Z codes are so non-specific, or potentially redundant with other codes in the classification, that there can be little justification for their use in the inpatient setting. Their use in the outpatient setting should be limited to those instances when there is no further documentation to permit more precise coding. Otherwise, any sign or symptom or any other reason for visit that is captured in another code should be used.

Nonspecific Z codes/categories:

Z02.9 Encounter for administrative examinations, unspecified

ZØ4.9 Encounter for examination and observation for unspecified reason

Z13.9 Encounter for screening, unspecified

Z41.9 Encounter for procedure for purposes other than remedying health state, unspecified

Z52.9 Donor of unspecified organ or tissue

Z86.59 Personal history of other mental and behavioral disorders

Z88.9 Allergy status to unspecified drugs, medicaments and biological substances status

Z92.Ø Personal history of contraception

16) Z Codes That May Only be Principal/First-Listed Diagnosis

The following Z codes/categories may only be reported as the principal/first-listed diagnosis, except when there are multiple encounters on the same day and the medical records for the encounters are combined:

ZØØ Encounter for general examination without complaint, suspected or reported diagnosis
Except: ZØØ.6

ZØ1 Encounter for other special examination without complaint, suspected or reported diagnosis

ZØ2 Encounter for administrative examination

ZØ4 Encounter for examination and observation for other reasons

Z33.2 Encounter for elective termination of pregnancy

Z31.81 Encounter for male factor infertility in female patient

Z31.83 Encounter for assisted reproductive fertility procedure cycle

Z31.84 Encounter for fertility preservation procedure

Z34 Encounter for supervision of normal pregnancy

Z39 Encounter for maternal postpartum care and examination

Z38 Liveborn infants according to place of birth and type of delivery

Z4Ø Encounter for prophylactic surgery

Z42 Encounter for plastic and reconstructive surgery following medical procedure or healed injury

Z51.Ø Encounter for antineoplastic radiation therapy

Z51.1- Encounter for antineoplastic chemotherapy and immunotherapy

Z52 Donors of organs and tissues
Except: Z52.9, Donor of unspecified organ or tissue

Z76.1 Encounter for health supervision and care of foundling

Z76.2 Encounter for health supervision and care of other healthy infant and child

Z99.12 Encounter for respirator [ventilator] dependence during power failure

17) Social Determinants of Health

Codes describing **problems or risk factors related to** social determinants of health (SDOH) should be assigned when this information is documented. **Assign as many SDOH codes as are necessary to describe all of the problems or risk factors. These codes should be assigned only when the documentation specifies that the patient has an associated problem or risk factor. For example, not every individual living alone would be assigned code Z6Ø.2, Problems related to living alone.**

For social determinants of health, such as information found in categories Z55-Z65, Persons with potential health hazards related to socioeconomic and psychosocial circumstances, code assignment may be based on medical record documentation from clinicians involved in the care of the patient who are not the patient's provider since this information represents social information, rather than medical diagnoses.

For example, coding professionals may utilize documentation of social information from social workers, community health workers, case managers, or nurses, if their documentation is included in the official medical record.

Patient self-reported documentation may be used to assign codes for social determinants of health, as long as the patient self-reported information is signed-off by and incorporated into the medical record by either a clinician or provider.

Social determinants of health codes are located primarily in these Z code categories:

Z55 Problems related to education and literacy

Z56 Problems related to employment and unemployment

Z57 Occupational exposure to risk factors

Z58 Problems related to physical environment

Z59 Problems related to housing and economic circumstances

Z6Ø Problems related to social environment

Z62 Problems related to upbringing

Z63 Other problems related to primary support group, including family circumstances

Z64 Problems related to certain psychosocial circumstances

Z65 Problems related to other psychosocial circumstances

See Section I.B.14. Documentation by Clinicians Other than the Patient's Provider.

22. **Chapter 22: Codes for Special Purposes (UØØ-U85)**
    - UØ7.Ø Vaping-related disorder (see Section I.C.1Ø.e., Vaping-related disorders)
    - UØ7.1 COVID-19 (see Section I.C.1.g.1., COVID-19 infection)
    - UØ9.9 Post COVID-19 condition, unspecified (see Section I.C.1.g.1.m.)

Section II. Selection of Principal Diagnosis

The circumstances of inpatient admission always govern the selection of principal diagnosis. The principal diagnosis is defined in the Uniform Hospital Discharge Data Set (UHDDS) as "that condition established after study to be chiefly responsible for occasioning the admission of the patient to the hospital for care."

The UHDDS definitions are used by hospitals to report inpatient data elements in a standardized manner. These data elements and their definitions can be found in the July 31, 1985, Federal Register (Vol. 50, No, 147), pp. 31038-40.

Since that time, the application of the UHDDS definitions has been expanded to include all non-outpatient settings (acute care, short term, long term care and psychiatric hospitals; home health agencies; rehab facilities; nursing homes, etc.). The UHDDS definitions also apply to hospice services (all levels of care).

In determining principal diagnosis, coding conventions in the ICD-10-CM, the Tabular List and Alphabetic Index take precedence over these official coding guidelines.

(See Section I.A., Conventions for the ICD-10-CM)

The importance of consistent, complete documentation in the medical record cannot be overemphasized. Without such documentation the application of all coding guidelines is a difficult, if not impossible, task.

A. Codes for symptoms, signs, and ill-defined conditions

Codes for symptoms, signs, and ill-defined conditions from Chapter 18 are not to be used as principal diagnosis when a related definitive diagnosis has been established.

B. Two or more interrelated conditions, each potentially meeting the definition for principal diagnosis.

When there are two or more interrelated conditions (such as diseases in the same ICD-10-CM chapter or manifestations characteristically associated with a certain disease) potentially meeting the definition of principal diagnosis, either condition may be sequenced first, unless the circumstances of the admission, the therapy provided, the Tabular List, or the Alphabetic Index indicate otherwise.

C. Two or more diagnoses that equally meet the definition for principal diagnosis

In the unusual instance when two or more diagnoses equally meet the criteria for principal diagnosis as determined by the circumstances of admission, diagnostic workup and/or therapy provided, and the Alphabetic Index, Tabular List, or another coding guidelines does not provide sequencing direction, any one of the diagnoses may be sequenced first.

D. Two or more comparative or contrasting conditions

In those rare instances when two or more contrasting or comparative diagnoses are documented as "either/or" (or similar terminology), they are coded as if the diagnoses were confirmed and the diagnoses are sequenced according to the circumstances of the admission. If no further determination can be made as to which diagnosis should be principal, either diagnosis may be sequenced first.

E. A symptom(s) followed by contrasting/comparative diagnoses

GUIDELINE HAS BEEN DELETED EFFECTIVE OCTOBER 1, 2014

F. Original treatment plan not carried out

Sequence as the principal diagnosis the condition, which after study occasioned the admission to the hospital, even though treatment may not have been carried out due to unforeseen circumstances.

G. Complications of surgery and other medical care

When the admission is for treatment of a complication resulting from surgery or other medical care, the complication code is sequenced as the principal diagnosis. If the complication is classified to the T8Ø-T88 series and the code lacks the necessary specificity in describing the complication, an additional code for the specific complication should be assigned.

H. Uncertain Diagnosis

If the diagnosis documented at the time of discharge is qualified as "probable," "suspected," "likely," "questionable," "possible," or "still to be ruled out," "compatible with," "consistent with," or other similar terms indicating uncertainty, code the condition as if it existed or was established. The bases for these guidelines are the diagnostic workup, arrangements for further workup or observation, and initial therapeutic approach that correspond most closely with the established diagnosis.

Note: This guideline is applicable only to inpatient admissions to short-term, acute, long-term care and psychiatric hospitals.

I. Admission from Observation Unit

1. Admission Following Medical Observation

When a patient is admitted to an observation unit for a medical condition, which either worsens or does not improve, and is subsequently admitted as an inpatient of the same hospital for this same medical condition, the principal diagnosis would be the medical condition which led to the hospital admission.

2. Admission Following Post-Operative Observation

When a patient is admitted to an observation unit to monitor a condition (or complication) that develops following outpatient surgery, and then is subsequently admitted as an inpatient of the same hospital, hospitals should apply the Uniform Hospital Discharge Data Set (UHDDS) definition of principal diagnosis as "that condition established after study to be chiefly responsible for occasioning the admission of the patient to the hospital for care."

J. Admission from Outpatient Surgery

When a patient receives surgery in the hospital's outpatient surgery department and is subsequently admitted for continuing inpatient care at the same hospital, the following guidelines should be followed in selecting the principal diagnosis for the inpatient admission:

- If the reason for the inpatient admission is a complication, assign the complication as the principal diagnosis.
- If no complication, or other condition, is documented as the reason for the inpatient admission, assign the reason for the outpatient surgery as the principal diagnosis.
- If the reason for the inpatient admission is another condition unrelated to the surgery, assign the unrelated condition as the principal diagnosis.

K. Admissions/Encounters for Rehabilitation

When the purpose for the admission/encounter is rehabilitation, sequence first the code for the condition for which the service is being performed. For example, for an admission/encounter for rehabilitation for right-sided dominant hemiplegia following a cerebrovascular infarction, report code I69.351, Hemiplegia and hemiparesis following cerebral infarction affecting right dominant side, as the first-listed or principal diagnosis.

If the condition for which the rehabilitation service is being provided is no longer present, report the appropriate aftercare code as the first-listed or principal diagnosis, unless the rehabilitation service is being provided following an injury. For rehabilitation services following active treatment of an injury, assign the injury code with the appropriate seventh character for subsequent encounter as the first-listed or principal diagnosis. For example, if a patient with severe degenerative osteoarthritis of the hip, underwent hip replacement and the current encounter/admission is for rehabilitation, report code Z47.1, Aftercare following joint replacement surgery, as the first-listed or principal diagnosis. If the patient requires rehabilitation post hip replacement for right intertrochanteric femur fracture, report code S72.141D, Displaced intertrochanteric fracture of right femur, subsequent encounter for closed fracture with routine healing, as the first-listed or principal diagnosis.

See Section I.C.21.c.7., Factors influencing health states and contact with health services, Aftercare.

See Section I.C.19.a., for additional information about the use of 7th characters for injury codes.

Section III. Reporting Additional Diagnoses

GENERAL RULES FOR OTHER (ADDITIONAL) DIAGNOSES

For reporting purposes, the definition for "other diagnoses" is interpreted as additional conditions that affect patient care in terms of requiring:

clinical evaluation; or

therapeutic treatment; or

diagnostic procedures; or

extended length of hospital stay; or

increased nursing care and/or monitoring.

The UHDDS item #11-b defines Other Diagnoses as "all conditions that coexist at the time of admission, that develop subsequently, or that affect the treatment received and/or the length of stay. Diagnoses that relate to an earlier episode which have no bearing on the current hospital stay are to be excluded." UHDDS definitions apply to inpatients in acute care, short-term, long term care and psychiatric hospital setting. The UHDDS definitions are used by acute care short-term hospitals to report inpatient data elements in a standardized manner. These data elements and their definitions can be found in the July 31, 1985, Federal Register (Vol. 50, No, 147), pp. 31038-40.

Since that time, the application of the UHDDS definitions has been expanded to include all non-outpatient settings (acute care, short term, long term care and psychiatric hospitals; home health agencies; rehab facilities; nursing homes, etc.). The UHDDS definitions also apply to hospice services (all levels of care).

The following guidelines are to be applied in designating "other diagnoses" when neither the Alphabetic Index nor the Tabular List in ICD-10-CM provide direction. The listing of the diagnoses in the patient record is the responsibility of the attending provider.

A. Previous conditions

If the provider has included a diagnosis in the final diagnostic statement, such as the discharge summary or the face sheet, it should ordinarily be coded. Some providers include in the diagnostic statement resolved conditions or diagnoses and status-post procedures from previous admissions that have no bearing on the current stay. Such conditions are not to be reported and are coded only if required by hospital policy.

However, history codes (categories Z80-Z87) may be used as secondary codes if the historical condition or family history has an impact on current care or influences treatment.

B. Abnormal findings

Abnormal findings (laboratory, x-ray, pathologic, and other diagnostic results) are not coded and reported unless the provider indicates their clinical significance. If the findings are outside the normal range and the attending provider has ordered other tests to evaluate the condition or prescribed treatment, it is appropriate to ask the provider whether the abnormal finding should be added.

Please note: This differs from the coding practices in the outpatient setting for coding encounters for diagnostic tests that have been interpreted by a provider.

C. Uncertain Diagnosis

If the diagnosis documented at the time of discharge is qualified as "probable," "suspected," "likely," "questionable," "possible," or "still to be ruled out," "compatible with," "consistent with," or other similar terms indicating uncertainty, code the condition as if it existed or was established. The bases for these guidelines are the diagnostic workup, arrangements for further workup or observation, and initial therapeutic approach that correspond most closely with the established diagnosis.

Note: This guideline is applicable only to inpatient admissions to short-term, acute, long-term care and psychiatric hospitals.

Section IV. Diagnostic Coding and Reporting Guidelines for Outpatient Services

These coding guidelines for outpatient diagnoses have been approved for use by hospitals/ providers in coding and reporting hospital-based outpatient services and provider-based office visits. Guidelines in Section I, Conventions, general coding guidelines and chapter-specific guidelines, should also be applied for outpatient services and office visits.

Information about the use of certain abbreviations, punctuation, symbols, and other conventions used in the ICD-10-CM Tabular List (code numbers and titles), can be found in Section IA of these guidelines, under "Conventions Used in the Tabular List." Section I.B. contains general guidelines that apply to the entire classification. Section I.C. contains chapter-specific guidelines that correspond to the chapters as they are arranged in the classification. Information about the correct sequence to use in finding a code is also described in Section I.

The terms encounter and visit are often used interchangeably in describing outpatient service contacts and, therefore, appear together in these guidelines without distinguishing one from the other.

Though the conventions and general guidelines apply to all settings, coding guidelines for outpatient and provider reporting of diagnoses will vary in a number of instances from those for inpatient diagnoses, recognizing that:

The Uniform Hospital Discharge Data Set (UHDDS) definition of principal diagnosis does not apply to hospital-based outpatient services and provider-based office visits.

Coding guidelines for inconclusive diagnoses (probable, suspected, rule out, etc.) were developed for inpatient reporting and do not apply to outpatients.

A. Selection of first-listed condition

In the outpatient setting, the term first-listed diagnosis is used in lieu of principal diagnosis.

In determining the first-listed diagnosis the coding conventions of ICD-10-CM, as well as the general and disease specific guidelines take precedence over the outpatient guidelines.

Diagnoses often are not established at the time of the initial encounter/visit. It may take two or more visits before the diagnosis is confirmed.

The most critical rule involves beginning the search for the correct code assignment through the Alphabetic Index. Never begin searching initially in the Tabular List as this will lead to coding errors.

1. **Outpatient Surgery**

   When a patient presents for outpatient surgery (same day surgery), code the reason for the surgery as the first-listed diagnosis (reason for the encounter), even if the surgery is not performed due to a contraindication.

2. **Observation Stay**

   When a patient is admitted for observation for a medical condition, assign a code for the medical condition as the first-listed diagnosis.

   When a patient presents for outpatient surgery and develops complications requiring admission to observation, code the reason for the surgery as the first reported diagnosis (reason for the encounter), followed by codes for the complications as secondary diagnoses.

B. Codes from A00.0 through T88.9, Z00-Z99, U00-U85

The appropriate code(s) from A00.0 through T88.9, Z00-Z99 and U00-U85 must be used to identify diagnoses, symptoms, conditions, problems, complaints, or other reason(s) for the encounter/visit.

C. Accurate reporting of ICD-10-CM diagnosis codes

For accurate reporting of ICD-10-CM diagnosis codes, the documentation should describe the patient's condition, using terminology which includes specific diagnoses as well as symptoms, problems, or reasons for the encounter. There are ICD-10-CM codes to describe all of these.

D. Codes that describe symptoms and signs

Codes that describe symptoms and signs, as opposed to diagnoses, are acceptable for reporting purposes when a diagnosis has not been established (confirmed) by the provider. Chapter 18 of ICD-10-CM, Symptoms, Signs, and Abnormal Clinical and Laboratory Findings Not Elsewhere Classified (codes R00-R99) contain many, but not all codes for symptoms.

E. Encounters for circumstances other than a disease or injury

ICD-10-CM provides codes to deal with encounters for circumstances other than a disease or injury. The Factors Influencing Health Status and Contact with Health Services codes (Z00-Z99) are provided to deal with occasions when circumstances other than a disease or injury are recorded as diagnosis or problems.

See Section I.C.21. Factors influencing health status and contact with health services.

F. Level of Detail in Coding

1. **ICD-10-CM codes with 3, 4, 5, 6 or 7 characters**

   ICD-10-CM is composed of codes with 3, 4, 5, 6 or 7 characters. Codes with three characters are included in ICD-10-CM as the heading of a category of codes that may be further subdivided by the use of fourth, fifth, sixth or seventh characters to provide greater specificity.

2. **Use of full number of characters required for a code**

   A three-character code is to be used only if it is not further subdivided. A code is invalid if it has not been coded to the full number of characters required for that code, including the 7th character, if applicable.

3. **Highest level of specificity**

   Code to the highest level of specificity when supported by the medical record documentation.

G. ICD-10-CM code for the diagnosis, condition, problem, or other reason for encounter/visit

List first the ICD-10-CM code for the diagnosis, condition, problem, or other reason for encounter/visit shown in the medical record to be chiefly responsible for the services provided. List additional codes that describe any coexisting conditions. In some cases, the first-listed diagnosis may be a symptom when a diagnosis has not been established (confirmed) by the provider.

H. Uncertain diagnosis

Do not code diagnoses documented as "probable", "suspected," "questionable," "rule out," "compatible with," "consistent with," or "working diagnosis" or other similar terms indicating uncertainty. Rather, code the condition(s) to the highest degree of certainty for that encounter/visit, such as symptoms, signs, abnormal test results, or other reason for the visit.

Please note: This differs from the coding practices used by short-term, acute care, long-term care and psychiatric hospitals.

I. Chronic diseases

Chronic diseases treated on an ongoing basis may be coded and reported as many times as the patient receives treatment and care for the condition(s)

J. Code all documented conditions that coexist

Code all documented conditions that coexist at the time of the encounter/visit and that require or affect patient care, treatment or management. Do not code conditions that were previously treated and no longer exist. However, history codes (categories Z80-Z87) may be used as secondary codes if the historical condition or family history has an impact on current care or influences treatment.

K. Patients receiving diagnostic services only

For patients receiving diagnostic services only during an encounter/visit, sequence first the diagnosis, condition, problem, or other reason for encounter/visit shown in the medical record to be chiefly responsible for the outpatient services provided during the encounter/visit. Codes for other diagnoses (e.g., chronic conditions) may be sequenced as additional diagnoses.

For encounters for routine laboratory/radiology testing in the absence of any signs, symptoms, or associated diagnosis, assign Z01.89, Encounter for other specified special examinations. If routine testing is performed during the same encounter as a test to evaluate a sign, symptom, or diagnosis, it is appropriate to assign both the Z code and the code describing the reason for the non-routine test.

For outpatient encounters for diagnostic tests that have been interpreted by a physician, and the final report is available at the time of coding, code any confirmed or definitive diagnosis(es) documented in the interpretation. Do not code related signs and symptoms as additional diagnoses.

Please note: This differs from the coding practice in the hospital inpatient setting regarding abnormal findings on test results.

L. Patients receiving therapeutic services only

For patients receiving therapeutic services only during an encounter/visit, sequence first the diagnosis, condition, problem, or other reason for encounter/visit shown in the medical record to be chiefly responsible for the outpatient services provided during the encounter/visit. Codes for other diagnoses (e.g., chronic conditions) may be sequenced as additional diagnoses.

The only exception to this rule is that when the primary reason for the admission/encounter is chemotherapy or radiation therapy, the appropriate Z code for the service is listed first, and the diagnosis or problem for which the service is being performed listed second.

M. Patients receiving preoperative evaluations only

For patients receiving preoperative evaluations only, sequence first a code from subcategory Z01.81, Encounter for pre-procedural examinations, to describe the pre-op consultations. Assign a code for the condition to describe the reason for the surgery as an additional diagnosis. Code also any findings related to the pre-op evaluation.

N. Ambulatory surgery

For ambulatory surgery, code the diagnosis for which the surgery was performed. If the postoperative diagnosis is known to be different from the preoperative diagnosis at the time the diagnosis is confirmed, select the postoperative diagnosis for coding, since it is the most definitive.

O. Routine outpatient prenatal visits

See Section I.C.15. Routine outpatient prenatal visits.

P. Encounters for general medical examinations with abnormal findings

The subcategories for encounters for general medical examinations, Z00.0- and encounter for routine child health examination, Z00.12-, provide codes for with and without abnormal findings. Should a general medical examination result in an abnormal finding, the code for general medical examination with abnormal finding should be assigned as the first-listed diagnosis. An examination with abnormal findings refers to a condition/diagnosis that is newly identified or a change in severity of a chronic condition (such as uncontrolled hypertension, or an acute exacerbation of chronic obstructive pulmonary disease) during a routine physical examination. A secondary code for the abnormal finding should also be coded.

Q. Encounters for routine health screenings

See Section I.C.21. Factors influencing health status and contact with health services, Screening

Appendix I. Present on Admission Reporting Guidelines

Introduction

These guidelines are to be used as a supplement to the *ICD-10-CM Official Guidelines for Coding and Reporting* to facilitate the assignment of the Present on Admission (POA) indicator for each diagnosis and external cause of injury code reported on claim forms (UB-04 and 837 Institutional).

These guidelines are not intended to replace any guidelines in the main body of the *ICD-10-CM Official Guidelines for Coding and Reporting*. The POA guidelines are not intended to provide guidance on when a condition should be coded, but rather, how to apply the POA indicator to the final set of diagnosis codes that have been assigned in accordance with Sections I, II, and III of the official coding guidelines. Subsequent to the assignment of the ICD-10-CM codes, the POA indicator should then be assigned to those conditions that have been coded.

As stated in the Introduction to the *ICD-10-CM Official Guidelines for Coding and Reporting*, a joint effort between the healthcare provider and the coder is essential to achieve complete and accurate documentation, code assignment, and reporting of diagnoses and procedures. The importance of consistent, complete documentation in the medical record cannot be overemphasized. Medical record documentation from any provider involved in the care and treatment of the patient may be used to support the determination of whether a condition was present on admission or not. In the context of the official coding guidelines, the term "provider" means a physician or any qualified healthcare practitioner who is legally accountable for establishing the patient's diagnosis.

These guidelines are not a substitute for the provider's clinical judgment as to the determination of whether a condition was/was not present on admission. The provider should be queried regarding issues related to the linking of signs/symptoms, timing of test results, and the timing of findings.

Please see the CDC website for the detailed list of ICD-10-CM codes that do not require the use of a POA indicator (https://www.cdc.gov/nchs/icd/icd10cm.htm). The codes and categories on this exempt list are for circumstances regarding the healthcare encounter or factors influencing health status that do not represent a current disease or injury or that describe conditions that are always present on admission.

General Reporting Requirements

All claims involving inpatient admissions to general acute care hospitals or other facilities that are subject to a law or regulation mandating collection of present on admission information.

Present on admission is defined as present at the time the order for inpatient admission occurs -- conditions that develop during an outpatient encounter, including emergency department, observation, or outpatient surgery, are considered as present on admission.

POA indicator is assigned to principal and secondary diagnoses (as defined in Section II of the Official Guidelines for Coding and Reporting) and the external cause of injury codes.

Issues related to inconsistent, missing, conflicting or unclear documentation must still be resolved by the provider.

If a condition would not be coded and reported based on UHDDS definitions and current official coding guidelines, then the POA indicator would not be reported.

Reporting Options

- Y – Yes
- N – No
- U – Unknown
- W – Clinically undetermined
- Unreported/Not used – (Exempt from POA reporting)

Reporting Definitions

- Y = present at the time of inpatient admission
- N = not present at the time of inpatient admission
- U = documentation is insufficient to determine if condition is present on admission
- W = provider is unable to clinically determine whether condition was present on admission or not

Timeframe for POA Identification and Documentation

There is no required timeframe as to when a provider (per the definition of "provider" used in these guidelines) must identify or document a condition to be present on admission. In some clinical situations, it may not be possible for a provider to make a definitive diagnosis (or a condition may not be recognized or reported by the patient) for a period of time after admission. In some cases, it may be several days before the provider arrives at a definitive diagnosis. This does not mean that the condition was not present on admission. Determination of whether the condition was present on admission or not will be based on the applicable POA guideline as identified in this document, or on the provider's best clinical judgment.

If at the time of code assignment the documentation is unclear as to whether a condition was present on admission or not, it is appropriate to query the provider for clarification.

Assigning the POA Indicator

Condition is on the "Exempt from Reporting" list

Leave the "present on admission" field blank if the condition is on the list of ICD-10-CM codes for which this field is not applicable. This is the only circumstance in which the field may be left blank.

POA Explicitly Documented

Assign Y for any condition the provider explicitly documents as being present on admission.

Assign N for any condition the provider explicitly documents as not present at the time of admission.

Conditions diagnosed prior to inpatient admission

Assign "Y" for conditions that were diagnosed prior to admission (example: hypertension, diabetes mellitus, asthma)

Conditions diagnosed during the admission but clearly present before admission

Assign "Y" for conditions diagnosed during the admission that were clearly present but not diagnosed until after admission occurred.

Diagnoses subsequently confirmed after admission are considered present on admission if at the time of admission they are documented as suspected, possible, rule out, differential diagnosis, or constitute an underlying cause of a symptom that is present at the time of admission.

Condition develops during outpatient encounter prior to inpatient admission

Assign Y for any condition that develops during an outpatient encounter prior to a written order for inpatient admission.

Documentation does not indicate whether condition was present on admission

Assign "U" when the medical record documentation is unclear as to whether the condition was present on admission. "U" should not be routinely assigned and used only in very limited circumstances. Coders are encouraged to query the providers when the documentation is unclear.

Documentation states that it cannot be determined whether the condition was or was not present on admission

Assign "W" when the medical record documentation indicates that it cannot be clinically determined whether or not the condition was present on admission.

Chronic condition with acute exacerbation during the admission

If a single code identifies both the chronic condition and the acute exacerbation, see POA guidelines pertaining to codes that contain multiple clinical concepts.

If a single code only identifies the chronic condition and not the acute exacerbation (e.g., acute exacerbation of chronic leukemia), assign "Y."

Conditions documented as possible, probable, suspected, or rule out at the time of discharge

If the final diagnosis contains a possible, probable, suspected, or rule out diagnosis, and this diagnosis was based on signs, symptoms or clinical findings suspected at the time of inpatient admission, assign "Y."

If the final diagnosis contains a possible, probable, suspected, or rule out diagnosis, and this diagnosis was based on signs, symptoms or clinical findings that were not present on admission, assign "N".

Conditions documented as impending or threatened at the time of discharge

If the final diagnosis contains an impending or threatened diagnosis, and this diagnosis is based on symptoms or clinical findings that were present on admission, assign "Y".

If the final diagnosis contains an impending or threatened diagnosis, and this diagnosis is based on symptoms or clinical findings that were not present on admission, assign "N".

Acute and Chronic Conditions

Assign "Y" for acute conditions that are present at time of admission and N for acute conditions that are not present at time of admission.

Assign "Y" for chronic conditions, even though the condition may not be diagnosed until after admission.

If a single code identifies both an acute and chronic condition, see the POA guidelines for codes that contain multiple clinical concepts.

Codes That Contain Multiple Clinical Concepts

Assign "N" if at least one of the clinical concepts included in the code was not present on admission (e.g., COPD with acute exacerbation and the exacerbation was not present on admission; gastric ulcer that does not start bleeding until after admission; asthma patient develops status asthmaticus after admission).

Assign "Y" if all of the clinical concepts included in the code were present on admission (e.g., duodenal ulcer that perforates prior to admission).

For infection codes that include the causal organism, assign "Y" if the infection (or signs of the infection) were present on admission, even though the culture results may not be known until after admission (e.g., patient is admitted with pneumonia and the provider documents Pseudomonas as the causal organism a few days later).

Same Diagnosis Code for Two or More Conditions

When the same ICD-10-CM diagnosis code applies to two or more conditions during the same encounter (e.g. two separate conditions classified to the same ICD-10-CM diagnosis code):

Assign "Y" if all conditions represented by the single ICD-10-CM code were present on admission (e.g. bilateral unspecified age-related cataracts).

Assign "N" if any of the conditions represented by the single ICD-10-CM code was not present on admission (e.g. traumatic secondary and recurrent hemorrhage and seroma is assigned to a single code T79.2, but only one of the conditions was present on admission).

Obstetrical conditions

Whether or not the patient delivers during the current hospitalization does not affect assignment of the POA indicator. The determining factor for POA assignment is whether the pregnancy complication or obstetrical condition described by the code was present at the time of admission or not.

If the pregnancy complication or obstetrical condition was present on admission (e.g., patient admitted in preterm labor), assign "Y".

If the pregnancy complication or obstetrical condition was not present on admission (e.g., 2nd degree laceration during delivery, postpartum hemorrhage that occurred during current hospitalization, fetal distress develops after admission), assign "N".

If the obstetrical code includes more than one diagnosis and any of the diagnoses identified by the code were not present on admission assign "N". (e.g., Category O11, Pre-existing hypertension with pre-eclampsia)

Perinatal conditions

Newborns are not considered to be admitted until after birth. Therefore, any condition present at birth or that developed in utero is considered present at admission and should be assigned "Y". This includes conditions that occur during delivery (e.g., injury during delivery, meconium aspiration, exposure to streptococcus B in the vaginal canal).

Congenital conditions and anomalies

Assign "Y" for congenital conditions and anomalies except for categories Q00-Q99, Congenital anomalies, which are on the exempt list. Congenital conditions are always considered present on admission.

External cause of injury codes

Assign "Y" for any external cause code representing an external cause of morbidity that occurred prior to inpatient admission (e.g., patient fell out of bed at home, patient fell out of bed in emergency room prior to admission)

Assign "N" for any external cause code representing an external cause of morbidity that occurred during inpatient hospitalization (e.g., patient fell out of hospital bed during hospital stay, patient experienced an adverse reaction to a medication administered after inpatient admission).

ICD-10-CM Index to Diseases and Injuries

A

- **Aarskog's syndrome** Q87.19
- **Abandonment** — *see* Maltreatment
- **Abasia** (-astasia) (hysterical) F44.4
- **Abderhalden-Kaufmann-Lignac syndrome** (cystinosis) E72.Ø4
- **Abdomen, abdominal** — *see also* condition
  - muscle deficiency syndrome Q79.4
  - angina K55.1
  - acute R1Ø.Ø
- **Abdominalgia** — *see* Pain, abdominal
- **Abduction contracture, hip or other joint** — *see* Contraction, joint
- **Aberrant** (congenital) — *see also* Malposition, congenital
  - adrenal gland Q89.1
  - artery (peripheral) Q27.8
    - basilar NEC Q28.1
    - cerebral Q28.3
    - coronary Q24.5
    - digestive system Q27.8
    - eye Q15.8
    - lower limb Q27.8
    - precerebral Q28.1
    - pulmonary Q25.79
    - renal Q27.2
    - retina Q14.1
    - specified site NEC Q27.8
    - subclavian Q27.8
    - upper limb Q27.8
    - vertebral Q28.1
  - breast Q83.8
  - endocrine gland NEC Q89.2
  - hepatic duct Q44.5
  - pancreas Q45.3
  - parathyroid gland Q89.2
  - pituitary gland Q89.2
  - sebaceous glands, mucous membrane, mouth, congenital Q38.6
  - spleen Q89.Ø9
  - subclavian artery Q27.8
  - thymus (gland) Q89.2
  - thyroid gland Q89.2
  - vein (peripheral) NEC Q27.8
    - cerebral Q28.3
    - digestive system Q27.8
    - lower limb Q27.8
    - precerebral Q28.1
    - specified site NEC Q27.8
    - upper limb Q27.8
- **Aberration**
  - distantial — *see* Disturbance, visual
  - mental F99
- **Abetalipoproteinemia** E78.6
- **Abiotrophy** R68.89
- **Ablatio, ablation**
  - retinae — *see* Detachment, retina
- **Ablepharia, ablepharon** Q1Ø.3
- **Abnormal, abnormality, abnormalities** — *see also* Anomaly
  - acid-base balance (mixed) E87.4
  - albumin R77.Ø
  - alphafetoprotein R77.2
  - alveolar ridge KØ8.9
  - anatomical relationship Q89.9
  - apertures, congenital, diaphragm Q79.1
  - atrial septal, specified NEC Q21.19
  - auditory perception H93.29- ☑
    - diplacusis — *see* Diplacusis
    - hyperacusis — *see* Hyperacusis
    - recruitment — *see* Recruitment, auditory
    - threshold shift — *see* Shift, auditory threshold
  - autosomes Q99.9
    - fragile site Q95.5
  - basal metabolic rate R94.8
  - biosynthesis, testicular androgen E29.1
  - bleeding time R79.1
  - blood amino-acid level R79.83
  - blood level (of)
    - cobalt R79.Ø
    - copper R79.Ø
    - iron R79.Ø

Abnormal, abnormality, abnormalities — *continued*

  - blood level — *continued*
    - lithium R78.89
    - magnesium R79.Ø
    - mineral NEC R79.Ø
    - zinc R79.Ø
  - blood pressure
    - elevated RØ3.Ø
    - low reading (nonspecific) RØ3.1
  - blood sugar R73.Ø9
  - blood-gas level R79.81
  - bowel sounds R19.15
    - absent R19.11
    - hyperactive R19.12
  - brain scan R94.Ø2
  - breathing RØ6.9
  - caloric test R94.138
  - cerebrospinal fluid R83.9
    - cytology R83.6
    - drug level R83.2
    - enzyme level R83.Ø
    - hormones R83.1
    - immunology R83.4
    - microbiology R83.5
    - nonmedicinal level R83.3
    - specified type NEC R83.8
  - chemistry, blood R79.9
    - C-reactive protein R79.82
    - drugs — *see* Findings, abnormal, in blood
    - gas level R79.81
    - minerals R79.Ø
    - pancytopenia D61.818
    - PTT R79.1
    - specified NEC R79.89
    - toxins — *see* Findings, abnormal, in blood
  - chest sounds (friction) (rales) RØ9.89
  - chromosome, chromosomal Q99.9
    - with more than three X chromosomes, female Q97.1
    - analysis result R89.8
      - bronchial washings R84.8
      - cerebrospinal fluid R83.8
      - cervix uteri NEC R87.89
      - nasal secretions R84.8
      - nipple discharge R89.8
      - peritoneal fluid R85.89
      - pleural fluid R84.8
      - prostatic secretions R86.8
      - saliva R85.89
      - seminal fluid R86.8
      - sputum R84.8
      - synovial fluid R89.8
      - throat scrapings R84.8
      - vagina R87.89
      - vulva R87.89
      - wound secretions R89.8
    - dicentric replacement Q93.2
    - ring replacement Q93.2
    - sex Q99.8
      - female phenotype Q97.9
        - specified NEC Q97.8
      - male phenotype Q98.9
        - specified NEC Q98.8
      - structural male Q98.6
    - specified NEC Q99.8
  - clinical findings NEC R68.89
  - coagulation D68.9
    - newborn, transient P61.6
    - profile R79.1
    - time R79.1
  - communication — *see* Fistula
  - conjunctiva, vascular H11.41- ☑
  - coronary artery Q24.5
  - cortisol-binding globulin E27.8
  - course, eustachian tube Q17.8
  - creatinine clearance R94.4
  - cytology
    - anus R85.619
      - atypical squamous cells cannot exclude high grade squamous intraepithelial lesion (ASC-H) R85.611
      - atypical squamous cells of undetermined significance (ASC-US) R85.61Ø

Abnormal, abnormality, abnormalities — *continued*

  - cytology — *continued*
    - anus — *continued*
      - cytologic evidence of malignancy R85.614
      - high grade squamous intraepithelial lesion (HGSIL) R85.613
      - human papillomavirus (HPV) DNA test
        - high risk positive R85.81
        - low risk postive R85.82
      - inadequate smear R85.615
      - low grade squamous intraepithelial lesion (LGSIL) R85.612
      - satisfactory anal smear but lacking transformation zone R85.616
      - specified NEC R85.618
      - unsatisfactory smear R85.615
    - female genital organs — *see* Abnormal, Papanicolaou (smear)
  - dark adaptation curve H53.61
  - dentofacial NEC — *see* Anomaly, dentofacial
  - development, developmental Q89.9
    - central nervous system QØ7.9
  - diagnostic imaging
    - abdomen, abdominal region NEC R93.5
    - biliary tract R93.2
    - bladder R93.41
    - breast R92.8
    - central nervous system NEC R9Ø.89
    - cerebrovascular NEC R9Ø.89
    - coronary circulation R93.1
    - digestive tract NEC R93.3
    - gastrointestinal (tract) R93.3
    - genitourinary organs R93.89
    - head R93.Ø
    - heart R93.1
    - intrathoracic organ NEC R93.89
    - kidney R93.42- ☑
    - limbs R93.6
    - liver R93.2
    - lung (field) R91.8
    - musculoskeletal system NEC R93.7
    - renal pelvis R93.41
    - retroperitoneum R93.5
    - site specified NEC R93.89
    - skin and subcutaneous tissue R93.89
    - skull R93.Ø
    - testis R93.81- ☑
    - ureter R93.41
    - urinary organs specified NEC R93.49
  - direction, teeth, fully erupted M26.3Ø
  - ear ossicles, acquired NEC H74.39- ☑
    - ankylosis — *see* Ankylosis, ear ossicles
    - discontinuity — *see* Discontinuity, ossicles, ear
    - partial loss — *see* Loss, ossicles, ear (partial)
  - Ebstein Q22.5
  - echocardiogram R93.1
  - echoencephalogram R9Ø.81
  - echogram — *see* Abnormal, diagnostic imaging
  - electrocardiogram [ECG] [EKG] R94.31
  - electroencephalogram [EEG] R94.Ø1
  - electrolyte — *see* Imbalance, electrolyte
  - electromyogram [EMG] R94.131
  - electro-oculogram [EOG] R94.11Ø
  - electrophysiological intracardiac studies R94.39
  - electroretinogram [ERG] R94.111
  - erythrocytes
    - congenital, with perinatal jaundice D58.9
  - feces (color) (contents) (mucus) R19.5
  - finding — *see* Findings, abnormal, without diagnosis
  - fluid
    - amniotic — *see* Abnormal, specimen, specified
    - cerebrospinal — *see* Abnormal, cerebrospinal fluid
    - peritoneal — *see* Abnormal, specimen, digestive organs
    - pleural — *see* Abnormal, specimen, respiratory organs
    - synovial — *see* Abnormal, specimen, specified
    - thorax (bronchial washings) (pleural fluid) — *see* Abnormal, specimen, respiratory organs
    - vaginal — *see* Abnormal, specimen, female genital organs

- **Abnormal, abnormality, abnormalities** — *continued*
  - form
    - teeth KØØ.2
    - uterus — *see* Anomaly, uterus
  - function studies
    - auditory R94.12Ø
    - bladder R94.8
    - brain R94.Ø9
    - cardiovascular R94.3Ø
    - ear R94.128
    - endocrine NEC R94.7
    - eye NEC R94.118
    - kidney R94.4
    - liver R94.5
    - nervous system
      - central NEC R94.Ø9
      - peripheral NEC R94.138
    - pancreas R94.8
    - placenta R94.8
    - pulmonary R94.2
    - special senses NEC R94.128
    - spleen R94.8
    - thyroid R94.6
    - vestibular R94.121
  - gait — *see* Gait
    - hysterical F44.4
  - gastrin secretion E16.4
  - globulin R77.1
    - cortisol-binding E27.8
    - thyroid-binding EØ7.89
  - glomerular, minor — *see also* NØØ-NØ7 with fourth character .Ø NØ5.Ø
  - glucagon secretion E16.3
  - glucose tolerance (test) (non-fasting) R73.Ø9
  - gravitational (G) forces or states (effect of) T75.81 ☑
  - hair (color) (shaft) L67.9
    - specified NEC L67.8
  - hard tissue formation in pulp (dental) KØ4.3
  - head movement R25.Ø
  - heart
    - rate RØØ.9
      - specified NEC RØØ.8
    - shadow R93.1
    - sounds NEC RØ1.2
  - hemoglobin (disease) — *see also* Disease, hemoglobin D58.2
    - trait — *see* Trait, hemoglobin, abnormal
  - histology NEC R89.7
  - immunological findings R89.4
    - in serum R76.9
      - specified NEC R76.8
  - increase in appetite R63.2
  - involuntary movement — *see* Abnormal, movement, involuntary
  - jaw closure M26.51
  - karyotype R89.8
  - kidney function test R94.4
  - knee jerk R29.2
  - leukocyte (cell) (differential) NEC D72.9
  - liver function test — *see also* Elevated, liver function, test R79.89
  - loss of
    - height R29.89Ø
    - weight R63.4
  - mammogram NEC R92.8
    - calcification (calculus) R92.1
    - microcalcification R92.Ø
  - Mantoux test R76.11
  - movement (disorder) — *see also* Disorder, movement
    - head R25.Ø
    - involuntary R25.9
      - fasciculation R25.3
      - of head R25.Ø
      - spasm R25.2
      - specified type NEC R25.8
      - tremor R25.1
  - myoglobin (Aberdeen) (Annapolis) R89.7
  - neonatal screening PØ9.9
    - for
      - congenital adrenal hyperplasia PØ9.2
      - congenital endocrine disease PØ9.2
      - congenital hematologic disorders PØ9.3
      - critical congenital heart disease PØ9.5
      - cystic fibrosis PØ9.4
      - hemoglobinothies PØ9.3
      - hypothyroidism PØ9.2
      - inborn errors of metabolism PØ9.1

- **Abnormal, abnormality, abnormalities** — *continued*
  - neonatal screening — *continued*
    - for — *continued*
      - neonatal hearing loss PØ9.6
      - red cell membrane defects PØ9.3
      - sickle cell PØ9.3
      - specified NEC PØ9.8
  - oculomotor study R94.113
  - palmar creases Q82.8
  - Papanicolaou (smear)
    - anus R85.619
      - atypical squamous cells cannot exclude high grade squamous intraepithelial lesion (ASC-H) R85.611
      - atypical squamous cells of undetermined significance (ASC-US) R85.61Ø
      - cytologic evidence of malignancy R85.614
      - high grade squamous intraepithelial lesion (HGSIL) R85.613
      - human papillomavirus (HPV) DNA test
        - high risk positive R85.81
        - low risk postive R85.82
      - inadequate smear R85.615
      - low grade squamous intraepithelial lesion (LGSIL) R85.612
      - satisfactory anal smear but lacking transformation zone R85.616
      - specified NEC R85.618
      - unsatisfactory smear R85.615
    - bronchial washings R84.6
    - cerebrospinal fluid R83.6
    - cervix R87.619
      - atypical squamous cells cannot exclude high grade squamous intraepithelial lesion (ASC-H) R87.611
      - atypical squamous cells of undetermined significance (ASC-US) R87.61Ø
      - cytologic evidence of malignancy R87.614
      - high grade squamous intraepithelial lesion (HGSIL) R87.613
      - inadequate smear R87.615
      - low grade squamous intraepithelial lesion (LGSIL) R87.612
      - non-atypical endometrial cells R87.618
      - satisfactory cervical smear but lacking transformation zone R87.616
      - specified NEC R87.618
      - thin preparaton R87.619
      - unsatisfactory smear R87.615
    - nasal secretions R84.6
    - nipple discharge R89.6
    - peritoneal fluid R85.69
    - pleural fluid R84.6
    - prostatic secretions R86.6
    - saliva R85.69
    - seminal fluid R86.6
    - sites NEC R89.6
    - sputum R84.6
    - synovial fluid R89.6
    - throat scrapings R84.6
    - vagina R87.629
      - atypical squamous cells cannot exclude high grade squamous intraepithelial lesion (ASC-H) R87.621
      - atypical squamous cells of undetermined significance (ASC-US) R87.62Ø
      - cytologic evidence of malignancy R87.624
      - high grade squamous intraepithelial lesion (HGSIL) R87.623
      - inadequate smear R87.625
      - low grade squamous intraepithelial lesion (LGSIL) R87.622
      - specified NEC R87.628
      - thin preparation R87.629
      - unsatisfactory smear R87.625
    - vulva R87.69
    - wound secretions R89.6
  - partial thromboplastin time (PTT) R79.1
  - pelvis (bony) — *see* Deformity, pelvis
  - percussion, chest (tympany) RØ9.89
  - periods (grossly) — *see* Menstruation
  - phonocardiogram R94.39
  - plantar reflex R29.2
  - plasma
    - protein R77.9
      - specified NEC R77.8
    - viscosity R7Ø.1
  - pleural (folds) Q34.Ø

- **Abnormal, abnormality, abnormalities** — *continued*
  - posture R29.3
  - product of conception OØ2.9
    - specified type NEC OØ2.89
  - prothrombin time (PT) R79.1
  - pulmonary
    - artery, congenital Q25.79
    - function, newborn P28.89
    - test results R94.2
  - pulsations in neck RØØ.2
  - pupillary H21.56- ☑
    - function (reaction) (reflex) — *see* Anomaly, pupil, function
  - radiological examination — *see* Abnormal, diagnostic imaging
  - red blood cell(s) (morphology) (volume) R71.8
  - reflex — *see* Reflex
  - renal function test R94.4
  - response to nerve stimulation R94.13Ø
  - retinal correspondence H53.31
  - retinal function study R94.111
  - rhythm, heart — *see also* Arrhythmia
  - saliva — *see* Abnormal, specimen, digestive organs
  - scan
    - kidney R94.4
    - liver R93.2
    - thyroid R94.6
  - secretion
    - gastrin E16.4
    - glucagon E16.3
  - semen, seminal fluid — *see* Abnormal, specimen, male genital organs
  - serum level (of)
    - acid phosphatase R74.8
    - alkaline phosphatase R74.8
    - amylase R74.8
    - enzymes R74.9
      - specified NEC R74.8
    - lipase R74.8
    - triacylglycerol lipase R74.8
  - shape
    - gravid uterus — *see* Anomaly, uterus
  - sinus venosus Q21.16
  - size, tooth, teeth KØØ.2
  - spacing, tooth, teeth, fully erupted M26.3Ø
  - specimen
    - digestive organs (peritoneal fluid) (saliva) R85.9
      - cytology R85.69
      - drug level R85.2
      - enzyme level R85.Ø
      - histology R85.7
      - hormones R85.1
      - immunology R85.4
      - microbiology R85.5
      - nonmedicinal level R85.3
      - specified type NEC R85.89
    - female genital organs (secretions) (smears) R87.9
      - cytology R87.69
        - cervix R87.619
          - human papillomavirus (HPV) DNA test
            - high risk positive R87.81Ø
            - low risk positive R87.82Ø
          - inadequate (unsatisfactory) smear R87.615
          - non-atypical endometrial cells R87.618
          - specified NEC R87.618
        - vagina R87.629
          - human papillomavirus (HPV) DNA test
            - high risk positive R87.811
            - low risk positive R87.821
          - inadequate (unsatisfactory) smear R87.625
        - vulva R87.69
      - drug level R87.2
      - enzyme level R87.Ø
      - histological R87.7
      - hormones R87.1
      - immunology R87.4
      - microbiology R87.5
      - nonmedicinal level R87.3
      - specified type NEC R87.89
    - male genital organs (prostatic secretions) (semen) R86.9
      - cytology R86.6
      - drug level R86.2
      - enzyme level R86.Ø
      - histological R86.7

- **Abnormal, abnormality, abnormalities** — *continued*
  - specimen — *continued*
    - male genital organs — *continued*
      - hormones R86.1
      - immunology R86.4
      - microbiology R86.5
      - nonmedicinal level R86.3
      - specified type NEC R86.8
    - nipple discharge — *see* Abnormal, specimen, specified
    - respiratory organs (bronchial washings) (nasal secretions) (pleural fluid) (sputum) R84.9
      - cytology R84.6
      - drug level R84.2
      - enzyme level R84.Ø
      - histology R84.7
      - hormones R84.1
      - immunology R84.4
      - microbiology R84.5
      - nonmedicinal level R84.3
      - specified type NEC R84.8
    - specified organ, system and tissue NOS R89.9
      - cytology R89.6
      - drug level R89.2
      - enzyme level R89.Ø
      - histology R89.7
      - hormones R89.1
      - immunology R89.4
      - microbiology R89.5
      - nonmedicinal level R89.3
      - specified type NEC R89.8
    - synovial fluid — *see* Abnormal, specimen, specified
    - thorax (bronchial washings) (pleural fluids) — *see* Abnormal, specimen, respiratory organs
    - vagina (secretion) (smear) R87.629
    - vulva (secretion) (smear) R87.69
    - wound secretion — *see* Abnormal, specimen, specified
  - spermatozoa — *see* Abnormal, specimen, male genital organs
  - sputum (amount) (color) (odor) RØ9.3
  - stool (color) (contents) (mucus) R19.5
    - bloody K92.1
    - guaiac positive R19.5
  - synchondrosis Q78.8
  - thermography — *see also* Abnormal, diagnostic imaging R93.89
  - thyroid-binding globulin EØ7.89
  - tooth, teeth (form) (size) KØØ.2
  - toxicology (findings) R78.9
  - transport protein E88.Ø9
  - tumor marker NEC R97.8
  - ultrasound results — *see* Abnormal, diagnostic imaging
  - umbilical cord complicating delivery O69.9 ☑
  - urination NEC R39.198
  - urine (constituents) R82.9Ø
    - bile R82.2
    - cytological examination R82.89
    - drugs R82.5
    - fat R82.Ø
    - glucose R81
    - heavy metals R82.6
    - hemoglobin R82.3
    - histological examination R82.89
    - ketones R82.4
    - microbiological examination (culture) R82.79
    - myoglobin R82.1
    - positive culture R82.79
    - protein — *see* Proteinuria
    - specified substance NEC R82.998
      - chromoabnormality NEC R82.91
    - substances nonmedical R82.6
  - uterine hemorrhage — *see* Hemorrhage, uterus
  - vectorcardiogram R94.39
  - visually evoked potential (VEP) R94.112
  - white blood cells D72.9
    - specified NEC D72.89
  - X-ray examination — *see* Abnormal, diagnostic imaging
- **Abnormity** (any organ or part) — *see* Anomaly
- **Abocclusion** M26.29
  - hemolytic disease (newborn) P55.1
  - incompatibility reaction ABO — *see* Complication(s), transfusion, incompatibility reaction, ABO
- **Abolition, language** R48.8
- **Aborter, habitual or recurrent** — *see* Loss (of), pregnancy, recurrent
- **Abortion** (complete) (spontaneous) OØ3.9
- **Abortion** — *continued*
  - with
    - retained products of conception — *see* Abortion, incomplete
  - attempted (elective) (failed) OØ7.4
    - complicated by OØ7.3Ø
      - afibrinogenemia OØ7.1
      - cardiac arrest OØ7.36
      - chemical damage of pelvic organ(s) OØ7.34
      - circulatory collapse OØ7.31
      - cystitis OØ7.38
      - defibrination syndrome OØ7.1
      - electrolyte imbalance OØ7.33
      - embolism (air) (amniotic fluid) (blood clot) (fat) (pulmonary) (septic) (soap) OØ7.2
      - endometritis OØ7.Ø
      - genital tract and pelvic infection OØ7.Ø
      - hemolysis OØ7.1
      - hemorrhage (delayed) (excessive) OØ7.1
      - infection
        - genital tract or pelvic OØ7.Ø
        - urinary tract tract OØ7.38
      - intravascular coagulation OØ7.1
      - laceration of pelvic organ(s) OØ7.34
      - metabolic disorder OØ7.33
      - oliguria OØ7.32
      - oophoritis OØ7.Ø
      - parametritis OØ7.Ø
      - pelvic peritonitis OØ7.Ø
      - perforation of pelvic organ(s) OØ7.34
      - renal failure or shutdown OØ7.32
      - salpingitis or salpingo-oophoritis OØ7.Ø
      - sepsis OØ7.37
      - shock OØ7.31
      - specified condition NEC OØ7.39
      - tubular necrosis (renal) OØ7.32
      - uremia OØ7.32
      - urinary tract infection OØ7.38
      - venous complication NEC OØ7.35
        - embolism (air) (amniotic fluid) (blood clot) (fat) (pulmonary) (septic) (soap) OØ7.2
  - complicated (by) (following) OØ3.8Ø
    - afibrinogenemia OØ3.6
    - cardiac arrest OØ3.86
    - chemical damage of pelvic organ(s) OØ3.84
    - circulatory collapse OØ3.81
    - cystitis OØ3.88
    - defibrination syndrome OØ3.6
    - electrolyte imbalance OØ3.83
    - embolism (air) (amniotic fluid) (blood clot) (fat) (pulmonary) (septic) (soap) OØ3.7
    - endometritis OØ3.5
    - genital tract and pelvic infection OØ3.5
    - hemolysis OØ3.6
    - hemorrhage (delayed) (excessive) OØ3.6
    - infection
      - genital tract or pelvic OØ3.5
      - urinary tract OØ3.88
    - intravascular coagulation OØ3.6
    - laceration of pelvic organ(s) OØ3.84
    - metabolic disorder OØ3.83
    - oliguria OØ3.82
    - oophoritis OØ3.5
    - parametritis OØ3.5
    - pelvic peritonitis OØ3.5
    - perforation of pelvic organ(s) OØ3.84
    - renal failure or shutdown OØ3.82
    - salpingitis or salpingo-oophoritis OØ3.5
    - sepsis OØ3.87
    - shock OØ3.81
    - specified condition NEC OØ3.89
    - tubular necrosis (renal) OØ3.82
    - uremia OØ3.82
    - urinary tract infection OØ3.88
    - venous complication NEC OØ3.85
      - embolism (air) (amniotic fluid) (blood clot) (fat) (pulmonary) (septic) (soap) OØ3.7
  - failed — *see* Abortion, attempted
  - habitual or recurrent N96
    - with current abortion — *see* categories OØ3-OØ4
    - without current pregnancy N96
    - care in current pregnancy O26.2- ☑
  - incomplete (spontaneous) OØ3.4
    - complicated (by) (following) OØ3.3Ø
      - afibrinogenemia OØ3.1
      - cardiac arrest OØ3.36
      - chemical damage of pelvic organ(s) OØ3.34
      - circulatory collapse OØ3.31
      - cystitis OØ3.38
- **Abortion** — *continued*
  - incomplete — *continued*
    - complicated — *continued*
      - defibrination syndrome OØ3.1
      - electrolyte imbalance OØ3.33
      - embolism (air) (amniotic fluid) (blood clot) (fat) (pulmonary) (septic) (soap) OØ3.2
      - endometritis OØ3.Ø
      - genital tract and pelvic infection OØ3.Ø
      - hemolysis OØ3.1
      - hemorrhage (delayed) (excessive) OØ3.1
      - infection
        - genital tract or pelvic OØ3.Ø
        - urinary tract OØ3.38
      - intravascular coagulation OØ3.1
      - laceration of pelvic organ(s) OØ3.34
      - metabolic disorder OØ3.33
      - oliguria OØ3.32
      - oophoritis OØ3.Ø
      - parametritis OØ3.Ø
      - pelvic peritonitis OØ3.Ø
      - perforation of pelvic organ(s) OØ3.34
      - renal failure or shutdown OØ3.32
      - salpingitis or salpingo-oophoritis OØ3.Ø
      - sepsis OØ3.37
      - shock OØ3.31
      - specified condition NEC OØ3.39
      - tubular necrosis (renal) OØ3.32
      - uremia OØ3.32
      - urinary infection OØ3.38
      - venous complication NEC OØ3.35
        - embolism (air) (amniotic fluid) (blood clot) (fat) (pulmonary) (septic) (soap) OØ3.2
  - induced (encounter for) Z33.2
    - complicated by OØ4.8Ø
      - afibrinogenemia OØ4.6
      - cardiac arrest OØ4.86
      - chemical damage of pelvic organ(s) OØ4.84
      - circulatory collapse OØ4.81
      - cystitis OØ4.88
      - defibrination syndrome OØ4.6
      - electrolyte imbalance OØ4.83
      - embolism (air) (amniotic fluid) (blood clot) (fat) (pulmonary) (septic) (soap) OØ4.7
      - endometritis OØ4.5
      - genital tract and pelvic infection OØ4.5
      - hemolysis OØ4.6
      - hemorrhage (delayed) (excessive) OØ4.6
      - infection
        - genital tract or pelvic OØ4.5
        - urinary tract OØ4.88
      - intravascular coagulation OØ4.6
      - laceration of pelvic organ(s) OØ4.84
      - metabolic disorder OØ4.83
      - oliguria OØ4.82
      - oophoritis OØ4.5
      - parametritis OØ4.5
      - pelvic peritonitis OØ4.5
      - perforation of pelvic organ(s) OØ4.84
      - renal failure or shutdown OØ4.82
      - salpingitis or salpingo-oophoritis OØ4.5
      - sepsis OØ4.87
      - shock OØ4.81
      - specified condition NEC OØ4.89
      - tubular necrosis (renal) OØ4.82
      - uremia OØ4.82
      - urinary tract infection OØ4.88
      - venous complication NEC OØ4.85
        - embolism (air) (amniotic fluid) (blood clot) (fat) (pulmonary) (septic) (soap) OØ4.7
  - inevitable OØ3.4
  - missed OØ2.1
  - spontaneous — *see* Abortion (complete) (spontaneous)
    - threatened O2Ø.Ø
  - threatened (spontaneous) O2Ø.Ø
  - tubal OØØ.1Ø- ☑
    - with intrauterine pregnancy OØØ.11- ☑
- **Abortus fever** A23.1
- **Aboulomania** F6Ø.7
- **Abrami's disease** D59.8
- **Abramov-Fiedler myocarditis** (acute isolated myocarditis) I4Ø.1
- **Abrasion** T14.8 ☑
  - abdomen, abdominal (wall) S3Ø.811 ☑
  - alveolar process SØØ.512 ☑
  - ankle S9Ø.51- ☑
  - antecubital space — *see* Abrasion, elbow
  - anus S3Ø.817 ☑

- **Abrasion** — *continued*
  - arm (upper) S40.81- ☑
  - auditory canal — *see* Abrasion, ear
  - auricle — *see* Abrasion, ear
  - axilla — *see* Abrasion, arm
  - back, lower S30.810 ☑
  - breast S20.11- ☑
  - brow S00.81 ☑
  - buttock S30.810 ☑
  - calf — *see* Abrasion, leg
  - canthus — *see* Abrasion, eyelid
  - cheek S00.81 ☑
    - internal S00.512 ☑
  - chest wall — *see* Abrasion, thorax
  - chin S00.81 ☑
  - clitoris S30.814 ☑
  - cornea S05.0- ☑
  - costal region — *see* Abrasion, thorax
  - dental K03.1
  - digit(s)
    - foot — *see* Abrasion, toe
    - hand — *see* Abrasion, finger
  - ear S00.41- ☑
  - elbow S50.31- ☑
  - epididymis S30.813 ☑
  - epigastric region S30.811 ☑
  - epiglottis S10.11 ☑
  - esophagus (thoracic) S27.818 ☑
    - cervical S10.11 ☑
  - eyebrow — *see* Abrasion, eyelid
  - eyelid S00.21- ☑
  - face S00.81 ☑
  - finger(s) S60.41- ☑
    - index S60.41- ☑
    - little S60.41- ☑
    - middle S60.41- ☑
    - ring S60.41- ☑
  - flank S30.811 ☑
  - foot (except toe(s) alone) S90.81- ☑
    - toe — *see* Abrasion, toe
  - forearm S50.81- ☑
    - elbow only — *see* Abrasion, elbow
  - forehead S00.81 ☑
  - genital organs, external
    - female S30.816 ☑
    - male S30.815 ☑
  - groin S30.811 ☑
  - gum S00.512 ☑
  - hand S60.51- ☑
  - head S00.91 ☑
    - ear — *see* Abrasion, ear
    - eyelid — *see* Abrasion, eyelid
    - lip S00.511 ☑
    - nose S00.31 ☑
    - oral cavity S00.512 ☑
    - scalp S00.01 ☑
    - specified site NEC S00.81 ☑
  - heel — *see* Abrasion, foot
  - hip S70.21- ☑
  - inguinal region S30.811 ☑
  - interscapular region S20.419 ☑
  - jaw S00.81 ☑
  - knee S80.21- ☑
  - labium (majus) (minus) S30.814 ☑
  - larynx S10.11 ☑
  - leg (lower) S80.81- ☑
    - knee — *see* Abrasion, knee
    - upper — *see* Abrasion, thigh
  - lip S00.511 ☑
  - lower back S30.810 ☑
  - lumbar region S30.810 ☑
  - malar region S00.81 ☑
  - mammary — *see* Abrasion, breast
  - mastoid region S00.81 ☑
  - mouth S00.512 ☑
  - nail
    - finger — *see* Abrasion, finger
    - toe — *see* Abrasion, toe
  - nape S10.81 ☑
  - nasal S00.31 ☑
  - neck S10.91 ☑
    - specified site NEC S10.81 ☑
    - throat S10.11 ☑
  - nose S00.31 ☑
  - occipital region S00.01 ☑
  - oral cavity S00.512 ☑

- **Abrasion** — *continued*
  - orbital region — *see* Abrasion, eyelid
  - palate S00.512 ☑
  - palm — *see* Abrasion, hand
  - parietal region S00.01 ☑
  - pelvis S30.810 ☑
  - penis S30.812 ☑
  - perineum
    - female S30.814 ☑
    - male S30.810 ☑
  - periocular area — *see* Abrasion, eyelid
  - phalanges
    - finger — *see* Abrasion, finger
    - toe — *see* Abrasion, toe
  - pharynx S10.11 ☑
  - pinna — *see* Abrasion, ear
  - popliteal space — *see* Abrasion, knee
  - prepuce S30.812 ☑
  - pubic region S30.810 ☑
  - pudendum
    - female S30.816 ☑
    - male S30.815 ☑
  - sacral region S30.810 ☑
  - scalp S00.01 ☑
  - scapular region — *see* Abrasion, shoulder
  - scrotum S30.813 ☑
  - shin — *see* Abrasion, leg
  - shoulder S40.21- ☑
  - skin NEC T14.8 ☑
  - sternal region S20.319 ☑
  - submaxillary region S00.81 ☑
  - submental region S00.81 ☑
  - subungual
    - finger(s) — *see* Abrasion, finger
    - toe(s) — *see* Abrasion, toe
  - supraclavicular fossa S10.81 ☑
  - supraorbital S00.81 ☑
  - temple S00.81 ☑
  - temporal region S00.81 ☑
  - testis S30.813 ☑
  - thigh S70.31- ☑
  - thorax, thoracic (wall) S20.91 ☑
    - back S20.41- ☑
    - front S20.31- ☑
  - throat S10.11 ☑
  - thumb S60.31- ☑
  - toe(s) (lesser) S90.416 ☑
    - great S90.41- ☑
  - tongue S00.512 ☑
  - tooth, teeth (dentifrice) (habitual) (hard tissues) (occupational) (ritual) (traditional) K03.1
  - trachea S10.11 ☑
  - tunica vaginalis S30.813 ☑
  - tympanum, tympanic membrane — *see* Abrasion, ear
  - uvula S00.512 ☑
  - vagina S30.814 ☑
  - vocal cords S10.11 ☑
  - vulva S30.814 ☑
  - wrist S60.81- ☑
- **Abrism** — *see* Poisoning, food, noxious, plant
- **Abruptio placentae** O45.9- ☑
  - with
    - afibrinogenemia O45.01- ☑
    - coagulation defect O45.00- ☑
      - specified NEC O45.09- ☑
    - disseminated intravascular coagulation O45.02- ☑
    - hypofibrinogenemia O45.01- ☑
  - specified NEC O45.8- ☑
- **Abruption, placenta** — *see* Abruptio placentae
- **Abscess** (connective tissue) (embolic) (fistulous) (infective) (metastatic) (multiple) (pernicious) (pyogenic) (septic) L02.91
  - with
    - diverticular disease (intestine) K57.80
      - with bleeding K57.81
      - large intestine K57.20
        - with
          - bleeding K57.21
          - small intestine K57.40
            - with bleeding K57.41
      - small intestine K57.00
        - with
          - bleeding K57.01
          - large intestine K57.40
            - with bleeding K57.41

- **Abscess** — *continued*
  - with — *continued*
    - lymphangitis — *code by* site under Abscess
  - abdomen, abdominal
    - cavity K65.1
    - wall L02.211
  - abdominopelvic K65.1
  - accessory sinus — *see* Sinusitis
  - adrenal (capsule) (gland) E27.8
  - alveolar K04.7
    - with sinus K04.6
  - amebic A06.4
    - brain (and liver or lung abscess) A06.6
    - genitourinary tract A06.82
    - liver (without mention of brain or lung abscess) A06.4
    - lung (and liver) (without mention of brain abscess) A06.5
    - specified site NEC A06.89
    - spleen A06.89
  - anerobic A48.0
  - ankle — *see* Abscess, lower limb
  - anorectal K61.2
  - antecubital space — *see* Abscess, upper limb
  - antrum (chronic) (Highmore) — *see* Sinusitis, maxillary
  - anus K61.0
  - apical (tooth) K04.7
    - with sinus (alveolar) K04.6
  - appendix K35.33
  - areola (acute) (chronic) (nonpuerperal) N61.1
    - puerperal, postpartum or gestational — *see* Infection, nipple
  - arm (any part) — *see* Abscess, upper limb
  - artery (wall) I77.89
  - atheromatous I77.2
  - auricle, ear — *see* Abscess, ear, external
  - axilla (region) L02.41- ☑
    - lymph gland or node L04.2
  - back (any part, except buttock) L02.212
  - Bartholin's gland N75.1
    - with
      - abortion — *see* Abortion, by type complicated by, sepsis
      - ectopic or molar pregnancy O08.0
    - following ectopic or molar pregnancy O08.0
  - Bezold's — *see* Mastoiditis, acute
  - bilharziasis B65.1
  - bladder (wall) — *see* Cystitis, specified type NEC
  - bone (subperiosteal) — *see also* Osteomyelitis, specified type NEC
    - accessory sinus (chronic) — *see* Sinusitis
    - chronic or old — *see* Osteomyelitis, chronic
    - jaw (lower) (upper) M27.2
    - mastoid — *see* Mastoiditis, acute, subperiosteal
    - petrous — *see* Petrositis
    - spinal (tuberculous) A18.01
      - nontuberculous — *see* Osteomyelitis, vertebra
  - bowel K63.0
  - brain (any part) (cystic) (otogenic) G06.0
    - amebic (with abscess of any other site) A06.6
    - gonococcal A54.82
    - pheomycotic (chromomycotic) B43.1
    - tuberculous A17.81
  - breast (acute) (chronic) (nonpuerperal) N61.1
    - newborn P39.0
    - puerperal, postpartum, gestational — *see* Mastitis, obstetric, purulent
  - broad ligament N73.2
    - acute N73.0
    - chronic N73.1
  - Brodie's (localized) (chronic) M86.8X- ☑
  - bronchi J98.09
  - buccal cavity K12.2
  - bulbourethral gland N34.0
  - bursa M71.00
    - ankle M71.07- ☑
    - elbow M71.02- ☑
    - foot M71.07- ☑
    - hand M71.04- ☑
    - hip M71.05- ☑
    - knee M71.06- ☑
    - multiple sites M71.09
    - pharyngeal J39.1
    - shoulder M71.01- ☑
    - specified site NEC M71.08
    - wrist M71.03- ☑
  - buttock L02.31
  - canthus — *see* Blepharoconjunctivitis

- **Abscess** — *continued*
  - cartilage — *see* Disorder, cartilage, specified type NEC
  - cecum K35.33
  - cerebellum, cerebellar G06.0
    - sequelae G09
  - cerebral (embolic) G06.0
    - sequelae G09
  - cervical (meaning neck) L02.11
    - lymph gland or node L04.0
  - cervix (stump) (uteri) — *see* Cervicitis
  - cheek (external) L02.01
    - inner K12.2
  - chest J86.9
    - with fistula J86.0
    - wall L02.213
  - chin L02.01
  - choroid — *see* Inflammation, chorioretinal
  - circumtonsillar J36
  - cold (lung) (tuberculous) — *see also* Tuberculosis, abscess, lung
    - articular — *see* Tuberculosis, joint
  - colon (wall) K63.0
  - colostomy K94.02
  - conjunctiva — *see* Conjunctivitis, acute
  - cornea H16.31- ☑
  - corpus
    - cavernosum N48.21
    - luteum — *see* Oophoritis
  - Cowper's gland N34.0
  - cranium G06.0
  - cul-de-sac (Douglas') (posterior) — *see* Peritonitis, pelvic, female
  - cutaneous — *see* Abscess, by site
  - dental K04.7
    - with sinus (alveolar) K04.6
  - dentoalveolar K04.7
    - with sinus K04.6
  - diaphragm, diaphragmatic K65.1
  - Douglas' cul-de-sac or pouch — *see* Peritonitis, pelvic, female
  - Dubois A50.59
  - ear (middle) — *see also* Otitis, media, suppurative
    - acute — *see* Otitis, media, suppurative, acute
    - external H60.0- ☑
  - entamebic — *see* Abscess, amebic
  - enterostomy K94.12
  - epididymis N45.4
  - epidural G06.2
    - brain G06.0
    - spinal cord G06.1
  - epiglottis J38.7
  - epiploon, epiploic K65.1
  - erysipelatous — *see* Erysipelas
  - esophagus K20.80
  - ethmoid (bone) (chronic) (sinus) J32.2
  - external auditory canal — *see* Abscess, ear, external
  - extradural G06.2
    - brain G06.0
      - sequelae G09
    - spinal cord G06.1
  - extraperitoneal K68.19
  - eye — *see* Endophthalmitis, purulent
  - eyelid H00.03- ☑
  - face (any part, except ear, eye and nose) L02.01
  - fallopian tube — *see* Salpingitis
  - fascia M72.8
  - fauces J39.1
  - fecal K63.0
  - femoral (region) — *see* Abscess, lower limb
  - filaria, filarial — *see* Infestation, filarial
  - finger (any) — *see also* Abscess, hand
    - nail — *see* Cellulitis, finger
  - foot L02.61- ☑
  - forehead L02.01
  - frontal sinus (chronic) J32.1
  - gallbladder K81.0
  - genital organ or tract
    - female (external) N76.4
    - male N49.9
      - multiple sites N49.8
      - specified NEC N49.8
  - gestational mammary O91.11- ☑
  - gestational subareolar O91.11- ☑
  - gingival
    - aggressive K05.20
      - generalized K05.229
        - moderate K05.222
        - severe K05.223

- **Abscess** — *continued*
  - gingival — *continued*
    - aggressive — *continued*
      - generalized — *continued*
        - slight K05.221
      - localized K05.219
        - moderate K05.212
        - severe K05.213
        - slight K05.211
  - gland, glandular (lymph) (acute) — *see* Lymphadenitis, acute
  - gluteal (region) L02.31
  - gonorrheal — *see* Gonococcus
  - groin L02.214
  - gum
    - aggressive K05.20
      - generalized K05.229
        - moderate K05.222
        - severe K05.223
        - slight K05.221
      - localized K05.219
        - moderate K05.212
        - severe K05.213
        - slight K05.211
  - hand L02.51- ☑
  - head NEC L02.811
    - face (any part, except ear, eye and nose) L02.01
  - heart — *see* Carditis
  - heel — *see* Abscess, foot
  - helminthic — *see* Infestation, helminth
  - hepatic (cholangitic) (hematogenic) (lymphogenic) (pylephlebitic) K75.0
    - amebic A06.4
  - hip (region) — *see* Abscess, lower limb
  - horseshoe K61.31
  - ileocecal K35.33
  - ileostomy (bud) K94.12
  - iliac (region) L02.214
    - fossa K35.33
  - infraclavicular (fossa) — *see* Abscess, upper limb
  - inguinal (region) L02.214
    - lymph gland or node L04.1
  - intersphincteric K61.4
  - intestine, intestinal NEC K63.0
    - rectal K61.1
  - intra-abdominal — *see also* Abscess, peritoneum K65.1
    - following procedure T81.43 ☑
      - obstetrical O86.03
    - postprocedural T81.43 ☑
      - retroperitoneal K68.11
  - intracranial G06.0
  - intramammary — *see* Abscess, breast
  - intramuscular, following procedure T81.42 ☑
    - obstetrical O86.02
  - intraorbital — *see* Abscess, orbit
  - intraperitoneal K65.1
  - intrasphincteric (anus) K61.4
  - intraspinal G06.1
  - intratonsillar J36
  - ischiorectal (fossa) (specified NEC) K61.39
  - jaw (bone) (lower) (upper) M27.2
  - joint — *see* Arthritis, pyogenic or pyemic
    - spine (tuberculous) A18.01
      - nontuberculous — *see* Spondylopathy, infective
  - kidney N15.1
    - with calculus N20.0
      - with hydronephrosis N13.6
    - puerperal (postpartum) O86.21
  - knee — *see also* Abscess, lower limb
    - joint M00.9
  - labium (majus) (minus) N76.4
  - lacrimal
    - caruncle — *see* Inflammation, lacrimal, passages, acute
    - gland — *see* Dacryoadenitis
    - passages (duct) (sac) — *see* Inflammation, lacrimal, passages, acute
  - lacunar N34.0
  - larynx J38.7
  - lateral (alveolar) K04.7
    - with sinus K04.6
  - leg (any part) — *see* Abscess, lower limb
  - lens H27.8
  - lingual K14.0
    - tonsil J36
  - lip K13.0
  - Littre's gland N34.0

- **Abscess** — *continued*
  - liver (cholangitic) (hematogenic) (lymphogenic) (pylephlebitic) (pyogenic) K75.0
    - amebic (due to Entamoeba histolytica) (dysenteric) (tropical) A06.4
      - with
        - brain abscess (and liver or lung abscess) A06.6
        - lung abscess A06.5
  - loin (region) L02.211
  - lower limb L02.41- ☑
  - lumbar (tuberculous) A18.01
    - nontuberculous L02.212
  - lung (miliary) (putrid) J85.2
    - with pneumonia J85.1
      - due to specified organism (see Pneumonia, in (due to))
    - amebic (with liver abscess) A06.5
      - with
        - brain abscess A06.6
        - pneumonia A06.5
  - lymph, lymphatic, gland or node (acute) — *see also* Lymphadenitis, acute
    - mesentery I88.0
  - malar M27.2
  - mammary gland — *see* Abscess, breast
  - marginal, anus K61.0
  - mastoid — *see* Mastoiditis, acute
  - maxilla, maxillary M27.2
    - molar (tooth) K04.7
      - with sinus K04.6
    - premolar K04.7
    - sinus (chronic) J32.0
  - mediastinum J85.3
  - meibomian gland — *see* Hordeolum
  - meninges G06.2
  - mesentery, mesenteric K65.1
  - mesosalpinx — *see* Salpingitis
  - mons pubis L02.215
  - mouth (floor) K12.2
  - muscle — *see* Myositis, infective
  - myocardium I40.0
  - nabothian (follicle) — *see* Cervicitis
  - nasal J32.9
  - nasopharyngeal J39.1
  - navel L02.216
    - newborn P38.9
      - with mild hemorrhage P38.1
      - without hemorrhage P38.9
  - neck (region) L02.11
    - lymph gland or node L04.0
  - nephritic — *see* Abscess, kidney
  - nipple N61.1
    - associated with
      - lactation — *see* Pregnancy, complicated by
      - pregnancy — *see* Pregnancy, complicated by
  - nose (external) (fossa) (septum) J34.0
    - sinus (chronic) — *see* Sinusitis
  - omentum K65.1
  - operative wound T81.49 ☑
  - orbit, orbital — *see* Cellulitis, orbit
  - otogenic G06.0
  - ovary, ovarian (corpus luteum) — *see* Oophoritis
  - oviduct — *see* Oophoritis
  - palate (soft) K12.2
    - hard M27.2
  - palmar (space) — *see* Abscess, hand
  - pancreas (duct) — *see* Pancreatitis, acute
  - parafrenal N48.21
  - parametric, parametrium N73.2
    - acute N73.0
    - chronic N73.1
  - paranephric N15.1
  - parapancreatic — *see* Pancreatitis, acute
  - parapharyngeal J39.0
  - pararectal K61.1
  - parasinus — *see* Sinusitis
  - parauterine — *see also* Disease, pelvis, inflammatory N73.2
  - paravaginal — *see* Vaginitis
  - parietal region (scalp) L02.811
  - parodontal — *see* Periodontitis, aggressive, localized
  - parotid (duct) (gland) K11.3
    - region K12.2
  - pectoral (region) L02.213
  - pelvis, pelvic
    - female — *see* Disease, pelvis, inflammatory
    - male, peritoneal K65.1
  - penis N48.21

Index

Abscess — Abscess

Abscess — *continued*
  penis — *continued*
    gonococcal (accessory gland) (periurethral) A54.1
  perianal K61.Ø
  periapical KØ4.7
    with sinus (alveolar) KØ4.6
  periappendicular K35.33
  pericardial I3Ø.1
  pericecal K35.33
  pericemental — *see* Periodontitis, aggressive, localized
  pericholecystic — *see* Cholecystitis, acute
  pericoronal — *see* Periodontitis, aggressive, localized
  peridental — *see* Periodontitis, aggressive, localized
  perimetric — *see also* Disease, pelvis, inflammatory N73.2
  perinephric, perinephritic — *see* Abscess, kidney
  perineum, perineal (superficial) LØ2.215
    urethra N34.Ø
  periodontal (parietal) — *see* Periodontitis, aggressive, localized
    apical KØ4.7
  periosteum, periosteal — *see also* Osteomyelitis, specified type NEC
    with osteomyelitis — *see also* Osteomyelitis, specified type NEC
      acute — *see* Osteomyelitis, acute
      chronic — *see* Osteomyelitis, chronic
  peripharyngeal J39.Ø
  peripleuritic J86.9
    with fistula J86.Ø
  periprostatic N41.2
  perirectal K61.1
  perirenal (tissue) — *see* Abscess, kidney
  perisinuous (nose) — *see* Sinusitis
  peritoneum, peritoneal (perforated) (ruptured) K65.1
    with appendicitis — *see also* Appendicitis K35.33
    pelvic
      female — *see* Peritonitis, pelvic, female
      male K65.1
    postoperative T81.43 ☑
    puerperal, postpartum, childbirth O85
    tuberculous A18.31
  peritonsillar J36
  perityphlic K35.33
  periureteral N28.89
  periurethral N34.Ø
    gonococcal (accessory gland) (periurethral) A54.1
  periuterine — *see also* Disease, pelvis, inflammatory N73.2
  perivesical — *see* Cystitis, specified type NEC
  petrous bone — *see* Petrositis
  phagedenic NOS LØ2.91
    chancroid A57
  pharynx, pharyngeal (lateral) J39.1
  pilonidal LØ5.Ø1
  pituitary (gland) E23.6
  pleura J86.9
    with fistula J86.Ø
  popliteal — *see* Abscess, lower limb
  postcecal K35.33
  postlaryngeal J38.7
  postnasal J34.Ø
  postoperative (any site) — *see also* Infection, postoperative wound T81.49 ☑
    retroperitoneal K68.11
  postpharyngeal J39.Ø
  posttonsillar J36
  post-typhoid AØ1.Ø9
  pouch of Douglas — *see* Peritonitis, pelvic, female
  premammary — *see* Abscess, breast
  prepatellar — *see* Abscess, lower limb
  presacral K68.19
  prostate N41.2
    gonococcal (acute) (chronic) A54.22
  psoas muscle K68.12
  puerperal — *code by* site under Puerperal, abscess
  pulmonary — *see* Abscess, lung
  pulp, pulpal (dental) KØ4.Ø1
    irreversible KØ4.Ø2
    reversible KØ4.Ø1
  rectovaginal septum K63.Ø
  rectovesical — *see* Cystitis, specified type NEC
  rectum K61.1
  renal — *see* Abscess, kidney
  retina — *see* Inflammation, chorioretinal
  retrobulbar — *see* Abscess, orbit
  retrocecal K65.1
  retrolaryngeal J38.7
  retromammary — *see* Abscess, breast
  retroperitoneal NEC K68.19
    postprocedural K68.11
  retropharyngeal J39.Ø
  retrouterine — *see* Peritonitis, pelvic, female
  retrovesical — *see* Cystitis, specified type NEC
  root, tooth KØ4.7
    with sinus (alveolar) KØ4.6
  round ligament — *see also* Disease, pelvis, inflammatory N73.2
  rupture (spontaneous) NOS LØ2.91
  sacrum (tuberculous) A18.Ø1
    nontuberculous M46.28
  salivary (duct) (gland) K11.3
  scalp (any part) LØ2.811
  scapular — *see* Osteomyelitis, specified type NEC
  sclera — *see* Scleritis
  scrofulous (tuberculous) A18.2
  scrotum N49.2
  seminal vesicle N49.Ø
  septal, dental KØ4.7
    with sinus (alveolar) KØ4.6
  serous — *see* Periostitis
  shoulder (region) — *see* Abscess, upper limb
  sigmoid K63.Ø
  sinus (accessory) (chronic) (nasal) — *see also* Sinusitis
    intracranial venous (any) GØ6.Ø
  Skene's duct or gland N34.Ø
  skin — *see* Abscess, by site
  specified site NEC LØ2.818
  spermatic cord N49.1
  sphenoidal (sinus) (chronic) J32.3
  spinal cord (any part) (staphylococcal) GØ6.1
    tuberculous A17.81
  spine (column) (tuberculous) A18.Ø1
    epidural GØ6.1
    nontuberculous — *see* Osteomyelitis, vertebra
  spleen D73.3
    amebic AØ6.89
  stitch T81.41 ☑
    following an obstetrical procedure O86.Ø1
  subarachnoid GØ6.2
    brain GØ6.Ø
    spinal cord GØ6.1
  subareolar — *see* Abscess, breast
  subcecal K35.33
  subcutaneous — *see also* Abscess, by site
    following procedure T81.41 ☑
      obstetrical O86.Ø1
    pheomycotic (chromomycotic) B43.2
  subdiaphragmatic K65.1
  subdural GØ6.2
    brain GØ6.Ø
      sequelae GØ9
    spinal cord GØ6.1
  sub-fascial, following an obstetrical procedure O86.Ø2
  subgaleal LØ2.811
  subhepatic K65.1
  sublingual K12.2
    gland K11.3
  submammary — *see* Abscess, breast
  submandibular (region) (space) (triangle) K12.2
    gland K11.3
  submaxillary (region) LØ2.Ø1
    gland K11.3
  submental LØ2.Ø1
    gland K11.3
  subperiosteal — *see* Osteomyelitis, specified type NEC
  subphrenic K65.1
    following an obstetrical procedure O86.Ø3
    postoperative T81.43 ☑
  suburethral N34.Ø
  sudoriparous L75.8
  supraclavicular (fossa) — *see* Abscess, upper limb
  supralevator K61.5
  suprapelvic, acute N73.Ø
  suprarenal (capsule) (gland) E27.8
  sweat gland L74.8
  tear duct — *see* Inflammation, lacrimal, passages, acute
  temple LØ2.Ø1
  temporal region LØ2.Ø1
  temporosphenoidal GØ6.Ø
  tendon (sheath) M65.ØØ
    ankle M65.Ø7- ☑
    foot M65.Ø7- ☑
    forearm M65.Ø3- ☑
    hand M65.Ø4- ☑

Abscess — *continued*
  tendon — *continued*
    lower leg M65.Ø6- ☑
    pelvic region M65.Ø5- ☑
    shoulder region M65.Ø1- ☑
    specified site NEC M65.Ø8
    thigh M65.Ø5- ☑
    upper arm M65.Ø2- ☑
  testis N45.4
  thigh — *see* Abscess, lower limb
  thorax J86.9
    with fistula J86.Ø
  throat J39.1
  thumb — *see also* Abscess, hand
    nail — *see* Cellulitis, finger
  thymus (gland) E32.1
  thyroid (gland) EØ6.Ø
  toe (any) — *see also* Abscess, foot
    nail — *see* Cellulitis, toe
  tongue (staphylococcal) K14.Ø
  tonsil(s) (lingual) J36
  tonsillopharyngeal J36
  tooth, teeth (root) KØ4.7
    with sinus (alveolar) KØ4.6
    supporting structures NEC — *see* Periodontitis, aggressive, localized
  trachea J39.8
  trunk LØ2.219
    abdominal wall LØ2.211
    back LØ2.212
    chest wall LØ2.213
    groin LØ2.214
    perineum LØ2.215
    umbilicus LØ2.216
  tubal — *see* Salpingitis
  tuberculous — *see* Tuberculosis, abscess
  tubo-ovarian — *see* Salpingo-oophoritis
  tunica vaginalis N49.1
  umbilicus LØ2.216
  upper
    limb LØ2.41- ☑
    respiratory J39.8
  urethral (gland) N34.Ø
  urinary N34.Ø
  uterus, uterine (wall) — *see also* Endometritis
    ligament — *see also* Disease, pelvis, inflammatory N73.2
    neck — *see* Cervicitis
  uvula K12.2
  vagina (wall) — *see* Vaginitis
  vaginorectal — *see* Vaginitis
  vas deferens N49.1
  vermiform appendix K35.33
  vertebra (column) (tuberculous) A18.Ø1
    nontuberculous — *see* Osteomyelitis, vertebra
  vesical — *see* Cystitis, specified type NEC
  vesico-uterine pouch — *see* Peritonitis, pelvic, female
  vitreous (humor) — *see* Endophthalmitis, purulent
  vocal cord J38.3
  von Bezold's — *see* Mastoiditis, acute
  vulva N76.4
  vulvovaginal gland N75.1
  web space — *see* Abscess, hand
  wound T81.49 ☑
  wrist — *see* Abscess, upper limb
Absence (of) (organ or part) (complete or partial)
  adrenal (gland) (congenital) Q89.1
    acquired E89.6
  albumin in blood E88.Ø9
  alimentary tract (congenital) Q45.8
    upper Q4Ø.8
  alveolar process (acquired) — *see* Anomaly, alveolar
  ankle (acquired) Z89.44- ☑
  anus (congenital) Q42.3
    with fistula Q42.2
  aorta (congenital) Q25.41
  appendix, congenital Q42.8
  arm (acquired) Z89.2Ø- ☑
    above elbow Z89.22- ☑
      congenital (with hand present) — *see* Agenesis, arm, with hand present
        and hand — *see* Agenesis, forearm, and hand
    below elbow Z89.21- ☑
      congenital (with hand present) — *see* Agenesis, arm, with hand present
        and hand — *see* Agenesis, forearm, and hand
    congenital — *see* Defect, reduction, upper limb

Absence — *continued*
- arm — *continued*
  - shoulder (following explantation of shoulder joint prosthesis) (joint) (with or without presence of antibiotic-impregnated cement spacer) Z89.23- ☑
  - congenital (with hand present) — *see* Agenesis, arm, with hand present
- artery (congenital) (peripheral) Q27.8
  - brain Q28.3
  - coronary Q24.5
  - pulmonary Q25.79
  - specified NEC Q27.8
  - umbilical Q27.0
- atrial septum (congenital) Q21.19
- auditory canal (congenital) (external) Q16.1
- auricle (ear), congenital Q16.0
- bile, biliary duct, congenital Q44.5
- bladder (acquired) Z90.6
  - congenital Q64.5
- bowel sounds R19.11
- brain Q00.0
  - part of Q04.3
- breast(s) (and nipple(s)) (acquired) Z90.1- ☑
  - congenital Q83.8
- broad ligament Q50.6
- bronchus (congenital) Q32.4
- canaliculus lacrimalis, congenital Q10.4
- cerebellum (vermis) Q04.3
- cervix (acquired) (with uterus) Z90.710
  - with remaining uterus Z90.712
  - congenital Q51.5
- chin, congenital Q18.8
- cilia (congenital) Q10.3
  - acquired — *see* Madarosis
- clitoris (congenital) Q52.6
- coccyx, congenital Q76.49
- cold sense R20.8
- congenital
  - lumen — *see* Atresia
  - organ or site NEC — *see* Agenesis
  - septum — *see* Imperfect, closure
- corpus callosum Q04.0
- cricoid cartilage, congenital Q31.8
- diaphragm (with hernia), congenital Q79.1
- digestive organ(s) or tract, congenital Q45.8
  - acquired NEC Z90.49
  - upper Q40.8
- ductus arteriosus Q28.8
- duodenum (acquired) Z90.49
  - congenital Q41.0
- ear, congenital Q16.9
  - acquired H93.8- ☑
  - auricle Q16.0
  - external Q16.0
  - inner Q16.5
  - lobe, lobule Q17.8
  - middle, except ossicles Q16.4
    - ossicles Q16.3
  - ossicles Q16.3
- ejaculatory duct (congenital) Q55.4
- endocrine gland (congenital) NEC Q89.2
  - acquired E89.89
- epididymis (congenital) Q55.4
  - acquired Z90.79
- epiglottis, congenital Q31.8
- esophagus (congenital) Q39.8
  - acquired (partial) Z90.49
- eustachian tube (congenital) Q16.2
- extremity (acquired) Z89.9
  - congenital Q73.0
  - knee (following explantation of knee joint prosthesis) (joint) (with or without presence of antibiotic-impregnated cement spacer) Z89.52- ☑
  - lower (above knee) Z89.619
    - below knee Z89.51- ☑
  - upper — *see* Absence, arm
- eye (acquired) Z90.01
  - congenital Q11.1
  - muscle (congenital) Q10.3
- eyeball (acquired) Z90.01
- eyelid (fold) (congenital) Q10.3
  - acquired Z90.01
- face, specified part NEC Q18.8
- fallopian tube(s) (acquired) Z90.79
  - congenital Q50.6
- family member (causing problem in home) NEC — *see also* Disruption, family Z63.32

Absence — *continued*
- femur, congenital — *see* Defect, reduction, lower limb, longitudinal, femur
- fibrinogen (congenital) D68.2
  - acquired D65
- finger(s) (acquired) Z89.02- ☑
  - congenital — *see* Agenesis, hand
- foot (acquired) Z89.43- ☑
  - congenital — *see* Agenesis, foot
- forearm (acquired) — *see* Absence, arm, below elbow
- gallbladder (acquired) Z90.49
  - congenital Q44.0
- gamma globulin in blood D80.1
  - hereditary D80.0
- genital organs
  - acquired (female) (male) Z90.79
  - female, congenital Q52.8
    - external Q52.71
    - internal NEC Q52.8
  - male, congenital Q55.8
- genitourinary organs, congenital NEC
  - female Q52.8
  - male Q55.8
- globe (acquired) Z90.01
  - congenital Q11.1
- glottis, congenital Q31.8
- hand and wrist (acquired) Z89.11- ☑
  - congenital — *see* Agenesis, hand
- head, part (acquired) NEC Z90.09
- heat sense R20.8
- hip (following explantation of hip joint prosthesis) (joint) (with or without presence of antibiotic-impregnated cement spacer) Z89.62- ☑
- hymen (congenital) Q52.4
- ileum (acquired) Z90.49
  - congenital Q41.2
- immunoglobulin, isolated NEC D80.3
  - IgA D80.2
  - IgG D80.3
  - IgM D80.4
- incus (acquired) — *see* Loss, ossicles, ear
  - congenital Q16.3
- inner ear, congenital Q16.5
- intestine (acquired) (small) Z90.49
  - congenital Q41.9
    - specified NEC Q41.8
  - large Z90.49
    - congenital Q42.9
      - specified NEC Q42.8
- iris, congenital Q13.1
- jejunum (acquired) Z90.49
  - congenital Q41.1
- joint
  - acquired
    - hip (following explantation of hip joint prosthesis) (with or without presence of antibiotic-impregnated cement spacer) Z89.62- ☑
    - knee (following explantation of knee joint prosthesis) (with or without presence of antibiotic-impregnated cement spacer) Z89.52- ☑
    - shoulder (following explantation of shoulder joint prosthesis) (with or without presence of antibiotic-impregnated cement spacer) Z89.23- ☑
  - congenital NEC Q74.8
- kidney(s) (acquired) Z90.5
  - congenital Q60.2
    - bilateral Q60.1
    - unilateral Q60.0
- knee (following explantation of knee joint prosthesis) (joint) (with or without presence of antibiotic-impregnated cement spacer) Z89.52- ☑
- labyrinth, membranous Q16.5
- larynx (congenital) Q31.8
  - acquired Z90.02
- leg (acquired) (above knee) Z89.61- ☑
  - below knee (acquired) Z89.51- ☑
  - congenital — *see* Defect, reduction, lower limb
- lens (acquired) — *see also* Aphakia
  - congenital Q12.3
  - post cataract extraction Z98.4- ☑
- limb (acquired) — *see* Absence, extremity
- lip Q38.6
- liver (congenital) Q44.7
- lung (fissure) (lobe) (bilateral) (unilateral) (congenital) Q33.3
  - acquired (any part) Z90.2

Absence — *continued*
- menstruation — *see* Amenorrhea
- muscle (congenital) (pectoral) Q79.8
  - ocular Q10.3
- neck, part Q18.8
- neutrophil — *see* Agranulocytosis
- nipple(s) (with breast(s)) (acquired) Z90.1- ☑
  - congenital Q83.2
- nose (congenital) Q30.1
  - acquired Z90.09
- organ
  - of Corti, congenital Q16.5
  - or site, congenital NEC Q89.8
    - acquired NEC Z90.89
- osseous meatus (ear) Q16.4
- ovary (acquired)
  - bilateral Z90.722
  - congenital
    - bilateral Q50.02
    - unilateral Q50.01
  - unilateral Z90.721
- oviduct (acquired)
  - bilateral Z90.722
  - congenital Q50.6
  - unilateral Z90.721
- pancreas (congenital) Q45.0
  - acquired Z90.410
    - complete Z90.410
    - partial Z90.411
    - total Z90.410
- parathyroid gland (acquired) E89.2
  - congenital Q89.2
- patella, congenital Q74.1
- penis (congenital) Q55.5
  - acquired Z90.79
- pericardium (congenital) Q24.8
- pituitary gland (congenital) Q89.2
  - acquired E89.3
- prostate (acquired) Z90.79
  - congenital Q55.4
- pulmonary valve Q22.0
- punctum lacrimale (congenital) Q10.4
- radius, congenital — *see* Defect, reduction, upper limb, longitudinal, radius
- rectum (congenital) Q42.1
  - with fistula Q42.0
  - acquired Z90.49
- respiratory organ NOS Q34.9
- rib (acquired) Z90.89
  - congenital Q76.6
- sacrum, congenital Q76.49
- salivary gland(s), congenital Q38.4
- scrotum, congenital Q55.29
- seminal vesicles (congenital) Q55.4
  - acquired Z90.79
- septum
  - atrial (congenital) Q21.19
  - between aorta and pulmonary artery Q21.4
  - ventricular (congenital) Q20.4
- sex chromosome
  - female phenotype Q97.8
  - male phenotype Q98.8
- skull bone (congenital) Q75.8
  - with
    - anencephaly Q00.0
    - encephalocele — *see* Encephalocele
    - hydrocephalus Q03.9
      - with spina bifida — *see* Spina bifida, by site, with hydrocephalus
    - microcephaly Q02
- spermatic cord, congenital Q55.4
- spine, congenital Q76.49
- spleen (congenital) Q89.01
  - acquired Z90.81
- sternum, congenital Q76.7
- stomach (acquired) (partial) Z90.3
  - congenital Q40.2
- superior vena cava, congenital Q26.8
- teeth, tooth (congenital) K00.0
  - acquired (complete) K08.109
    - class I K08.101
    - class II K08.102
    - class III K08.103
    - class IV K08.104
    - due to
      - caries K08.139
        - class I K08.131
        - class II K08.132
        - class III K08.133

- **Absence** — *continued*
  - teeth, tooth — *continued*
    - acquired — *continued*
      - due to — *continued*
        - caries — *continued*
          - class IV KØ8.134
        - periodontal disease KØ8.129
          - class I KØ8.121
          - class II KØ8.122
          - class III KØ8.123
          - class IV KØ8.124
        - specified NEC KØ8.199
          - class I KØ8.191
          - class II KØ8.192
          - class III KØ8.193
          - class IV KØ8.194
        - trauma KØ8.119
          - class I KØ8.111
          - class II KØ8.112
          - class III KØ8.113
          - class IV KØ8.114
      - partial KØ8.4Ø9
        - class I KØ8.4Ø1
        - class II KØ8.4Ø2
        - class III KØ8.4Ø3
        - class IV KØ8.4Ø4
        - due to
          - caries KØ8.439
            - class I KØ8.431
            - class II KØ8.432
            - class III KØ8.433
            - class IV KØ8.434
          - periodontal disease KØ8.429
            - class I KØ8.421
            - class II KØ8.422
            - class III KØ8.423
            - class IV KØ8.424
          - specified NEC KØ8.499
            - class I KØ8.491
            - class II KØ8.492
            - class III KØ8.493
            - class IV KØ8.494
          - trauma KØ8.419
            - class I KØ8.411
            - class II KØ8.412
            - class III KØ8.413
            - class IV KØ8.414
  - tendon (congenital) Q79.8
  - testis (congenital) Q55.Ø
    - acquired Z9Ø.79
  - thumb (acquired) Z89.Ø1- ☑
    - congenital — *see* Agenesis, hand
  - thymus gland Q89.2
  - thyroid (gland) (acquired) E89.Ø
    - cartilage, congenital Q31.8
    - congenital EØ3.1
  - toe(s) (acquired) Z89.42- ☑
    - with foot — *see* Absence, foot and ankle
    - congenital — *see* Agenesis, foot
    - great Z89.41- ☑
  - tongue, congenital Q38.3
  - trachea (cartilage), congenital Q32.1
  - transverse aortic arch, congenital Q25.49
  - tricuspid valve Q22.4
  - umbilical artery, congenital Q27.Ø
  - upper arm and forearm with hand present, congenital — *see* Agenesis, arm, with hand present
  - ureter (congenital) Q62.4
    - acquired Z9Ø.6
  - urethra, congenital Q64.5
  - uterus (acquired) Z9Ø.71Ø
    - with cervix Z9Ø.71Ø
    - with remaining cervical stump Z9Ø.711
    - congenital Q51.Ø
  - uvula, congenital Q38.5
  - vagina, congenital Q52.Ø
  - vas deferens (congenital) Q55.4
    - acquired Z9Ø.79
  - vein (peripheral) congenital NEC Q27.8
    - cerebral Q28.3
    - digestive system Q27.8
    - great Q26.8
    - lower limb Q27.8
    - portal Q26.5
    - precerebral Q28.1
    - specified site NEC Q27.8
    - upper limb Q27.8
  - vena cava (inferior) (superior), congenital Q26.8

- **Absence** — *continued*
  - ventricular septum Q2Ø.4
  - vertebra, congenital Q76.49
  - von Willebrand factor, complete (near) — *see also* Disease, von Willebrand D68.Ø3
  - vulva, congenital Q52.71
  - wrist (acquired) Z89.12- ☑
- **Absorbent system disease** I87.8
- **Absorption**
  - carbohydrate, disturbance K9Ø.49
  - chemical — *see* Table of Drugs and Chemicals
    - through placenta (newborn) PØ4.9
      - environmental substance PØ4.6
      - nutritional substance PØ4.5
      - obstetric anesthetic or analgesic drug PØ4.Ø
  - drug NEC — *see* Table of Drugs and Chemicals
    - addictive
      - through placenta (newborn) — *see also* Newborn, affected by, maternal, use of PØ4.4Ø
        - cocaine PØ4.41
        - hallucinogens PØ4.42
        - specified drug NEC PØ4.49
    - medicinal
      - through placenta (newborn) PØ4.19
    - through placenta (newborn) PØ4.19
      - obstetric anesthetic or analgesic drug PØ4.Ø
  - fat, disturbance K9Ø.49
    - pancreatic K9Ø.3
  - noxious substance — *see* Table of Drugs and Chemicals
  - protein, disturbance K9Ø.49
  - starch, disturbance K9Ø.49
  - toxic substance — *see* Table of Drugs and Chemicals
  - uremic — *see* Uremia
- **Abstinence symptoms, syndrome**
  - alcohol F1Ø.239
    - with delirium F1Ø.231
  - cocaine F14.23
  - neonatal P96.1
  - nicotine — *see* Dependence, drug, nicotine, with, withdrawal
  - opioid F11.93
    - with dependence F11.23
  - psychoactive NEC F19.939
    - with
      - delirium F19.931
      - dependence F19.239
        - with
          - delirium F19.231
          - perceptual disturbance F19.232
        - uncomplicated F19.23Ø
      - perceptual disturbance F19.932
    - uncomplicated F19.93Ø
  - sedative F13.939
    - with
      - delirium F13.931
      - dependence F13.239
        - with
          - delirium F13.231
          - perceptual disturbance F13.232
        - uncomplicated F13.23Ø
      - perceptual disturbance F13.932
    - uncomplicated F13.93Ø
  - stimulant NEC F15.93
    - with dependence F15.23
- **Abulia** R68.89
- **Abulomania** F6Ø.7
- **Abuse**
  - adult — *see* Maltreatment, adult
    - as reason for
      - couple seeking advice (including offender) Z63.Ø
  - alcohol (non-dependent) F1Ø.1Ø
    - with
      - anxiety disorder F1Ø.18Ø
      - intoxication F1Ø.129
        - with delirium F1Ø.121
        - uncomplicated F1Ø.12Ø
      - mood disorder F1Ø.14
      - other specified disorder F1Ø.188
      - psychosis F1Ø.159
        - delusions F1Ø.15Ø
        - hallucinations F1Ø.151
      - sexual dysfunction F1Ø.181
      - sleep disorder F1Ø.182
      - unspecified disorder F1Ø.19
      - withdrawal F1Ø.139
        - with
          - perceptual disturbance F1Ø.132
        - delirium F1Ø.131

- **Abuse** — *continued*
  - alcohol — *continued*
    - with — *continued*
      - withdrawal — *continued*
        - uncomplicated F1Ø.13Ø
    - counseling and surveillance Z71.41
    - in remission (early) (sustained) F1Ø.11
  - amphetamine (or related substance) — *see also* Abuse, drug, stimulant NEC
    - stimulant NEC F15.1Ø
      - with
        - anxiety disorder F15.18Ø
        - intoxication F15.129
          - with
            - delirium F15.121
            - perceptual disturbance F15.122
        - withdrawal F15.13
  - analgesics (non-prescribed) (over the counter) F55.8
  - antacids F55.Ø
  - antidepressants — *see* Abuse, drug, psychoactive NEC
  - anxiolytic — *see* Abuse, drug, sedative
  - barbiturates — *see* Abuse, drug, sedative
  - caffeine — *see* Abuse, drug, stimulant NEC
  - cannabis, cannabinoids — *see* Abuse, drug, cannabis
  - child — *see* Maltreatment, child
  - cocaine — *see* Abuse, drug, cocaine
  - drug NEC (non-dependent) F19.1Ø
    - with sleep disorder F19.182
    - amphetamine type — *see* Abuse, drug, stimulant NEC
    - analgesics (non-prescribed) (over the counter) F55.8
    - antacids F55.Ø
    - antidepressants — *see* Abuse, drug, psychoactive NEC
    - anxiolytics — *see* Abuse, drug, sedative
    - barbiturates — *see* Abuse, drug, sedative
    - caffeine — *see* Abuse, drug, stimulant NEC
    - cannabis F12.1Ø
      - with
        - anxiety disorder F12.18Ø
        - intoxication F12.129
          - with
            - delirium F12.121
            - perceptual disturbance F12.122
          - uncomplicated F12.12Ø
        - other specified disorder F12.188
        - psychosis F12.159
          - delusions F12.15Ø
          - hallucinations F12.151
        - unspecified disorder F12.19
        - withdrawal F12.13
      - in remission (early) (sustained) F12.11
    - cocaine F14.1Ø
      - with
        - anxiety disorder F14.18Ø
        - intoxication F14.129
          - with
            - delirium F14.121
            - perceptual disturbance F14.122
          - uncomplicated F14.12Ø
        - mood disorder F14.14
        - other specified disorder F14.188
        - psychosis F14.159
          - delusions F14.15Ø
          - hallucinations F14.151
        - sexual dysfunction F14.181
        - sleep disorder F14.182
        - unspecified disorder F14.19
        - withdrawal F14.13
      - in remission (early) (sustained) F14.11
    - counseling and surveillance Z71.51
    - hallucinogen F16.1Ø
      - with
        - anxiety disorder F16.18Ø
        - flashbacks F16.183
        - intoxication F16.129
          - with
            - delirium F16.121
            - perceptual disturbance F16.122
          - uncomplicated F16.12Ø
        - mood disorder F16.14
        - other specified disorder F16.188
        - perception disorder, persisting F16.183
        - psychosis F16.159
          - delusions F16.15Ø
          - hallucinations F16.151
        - unspecified disorder F16.19
      - in remission (early) (sustained) F16.11

Abuse — *continued*
  drug — *continued*
    hashish — *see* Abuse, drug, cannabis
    herbal or folk remedies F55.1
    hormones F55.3
    hypnotics — *see* Abuse, drug, sedative
    in remission (early) (sustained) F19.11
    inhalant F18.1Ø
      with
        anxiety disorder F18.18Ø
        dementia, persisting F18.17
        intoxication F18.129
          with delirium F18.121
          uncomplicated F18.12Ø
        mood disorder F18.14
        other specified disorder F18.188
        psychosis F18.159
          delusions F18.15Ø
          hallucinations F18.151
        unspecified disorder F18.19
      in remission (early) (sustained) F18.11
    laxatives F55.2
    LSD — *see* Abuse, drug, hallucinogen
    marihuana — *see* Abuse, drug, cannabis
    morphine type (opioids) — *see* Abuse, drug, opioid
    opioid F11.1Ø
      with
        intoxication F11.129
          with
            delirium F11.121
            perceptual disturbance F11.122
          uncomplicated F11.12Ø
        mood disorder F11.14
        other specified disorder F11.188
        psychosis F11.159
          delusions F11.15Ø
          hallucinations F11.151
        sexual dysfunction F11.181
        sleep disorder F11.182
        unspecified disorder F11.19
        withdrawal F11.13
      in remission (early) (sustained) F11.11
    PCP (phencyclidine) (or related substance) — *see* Abuse, drug, hallucinogen
    psychoactive NEC F19.1Ø
      with
        amnestic disorder F19.16
        anxiety disorder F19.18Ø
        dementia F19.17
        intoxication F19.129
          with
            delirium F19.121
            perceptual disturbance F19.122
          uncomplicated F19.12Ø
        mood disorder F19.14
        other specified disorder F19.188
        psychosis F19.159
          delusions F19.15Ø
          hallucinations F19.151
        sexual dysfunction F19.181
        sleep disorder F19.182
        unspecified disorder F19.19
        withdrawal F19.139
          with
            perceptual disturbance F19.132
          delirium F19.131
          uncomplicated F19.13Ø
    sedative, hypnotic or anxiolytic F13.1Ø
      with
        anxiety disorder F13.18Ø
        intoxication F13.129
          with delirium F13.121
          uncomplicated F13.12Ø
        mood disorder F13.14
        other specified disorder F13.188
        psychosis F13.159
          delusions F13.15Ø
          hallucinations F13.151
        sexual dysfunction F13.181
        sleep disorder F13.182
        unspecified disorder F13.19
        withdrawal F13.139
          with
            perceptual disturbance F13.132
          delirium F13.131
          uncomplicated F13.13Ø
      in remission (early) (sustained) F13.11
    solvent — *see* Abuse, drug, inhalant

Abuse — *continued*
  drug — *continued*
    steroids F55.3
    stimulant NEC F15.1Ø
      with
        anxiety disorder F15.18Ø
        intoxication F15.129
          with
            delirium F15.121
            perceptual disturbance F15.122
          uncomplicated F15.12Ø
        mood disorder F15.14
        other specified disorder F15.188
        psychosis F15.159
          delusions F15.15Ø
          hallucinations F15.151
        sexual dysfunction F15.181
        sleep disorder F15.182
        unspecified disorder F15.19
        withdrawal F15.13
      in remission (early) (sustained) F15.11
    tranquilizers — *see* Abuse, drug, sedative
    vitamins F55.4
  hallucinogens — *see* Abuse, drug, hallucinogen
  hashish — *see* Abuse, drug, cannabis
  herbal or folk remedies F55.1
  hormones F55.3
  hypnotic — *see* Abuse, drug, sedative
  inhalant — *see* Abuse, drug, inhalant
  laxatives F55.2
  LSD — *see* Abuse, drug, hallucinogen
  marihuana — *see* Abuse, drug, cannabis
  morphine type (opioids) — *see* Abuse, drug, opioid
  non-psychoactive substance NEC F55.8
    antacids F55.Ø
    folk remedies F55.1
    herbal remedies F55.1
    hormones F55.3
    laxatives F55.2
    steroids F55.3
    vitamins F55.4
  opioids — *see* Abuse, drug, opioid
  PCP (phencyclidine) (or related substance) — *see* Abuse, drug, hallucinogen
  physical (adult) (child) — *see* Maltreatment
  psychoactive substance — *see* Abuse, drug, psychoactive NEC
  psychological (adult) (child) — *see* Maltreatment
  sedative — *see* Abuse, drug, sedative
  sexual — *see* Maltreatment
  solvent — *see* Abuse, drug, inhalant
  steroids F55.3
  vitamins F55.4
Acalculia R48.8
  developmental F81.2
Acanthamebiasis (with) B6Ø.1Ø
  conjunctiva B6Ø.12
  keratoconjunctivitis B6Ø.13
  meningoencephalitis B6Ø.11
  other specified B6Ø.19
Acanthocephaliasis B83.8
Acanthocheilonemiasis B74.4
Acanthocytosis E78.6
Acantholysis L11.9
Acanthosis (acquired) (nigricans) L83
  benign Q82.8
  congenital Q82.8
  seborrheic L82.1
    inflamed L82.Ø
  tongue K14.3
Acapnia E87.3
Acarbia E87.29
Acardia, acardius Q89.8
Acardiacus amorphus Q89.8
Acardiotrophia I51.4
Acariasis B88.Ø
  scabies B86
Acarodermatitis (urticarioides) B88.Ø
Acarophobia F4Ø.218
Acatalasemia, acatalasia E8Ø.3
Acathisia (drug induced) G25.71
Accelerated atrioventricular conduction I45.6
Accentuation of personality traits (type A) Z73.1
Accessory (congenital)
  adrenal gland Q89.1
  anus Q43.4
  appendix Q43.4
  atrioventricular conduction I45.6

Accessory — *continued*
  auditory ossicles Q16.3
  auricle (ear) Q17.Ø
  biliary duct or passage Q44.5
  bladder Q64.79
  blood vessels NEC Q27.9
    coronary Q24.5
  bone NEC Q79.8
  breast tissue, axilla Q83.1
  carpal bones Q74.Ø
  cecum Q43.4
  chromosome(s) NEC (nonsex) Q92.9
    with complex rearrangements NEC Q92.5
      seen only at prometaphase Q92.8
    13 — *see* Trisomy, 13
    18 — *see* Trisomy, 18
    21 — *see* Trisomy, 21
    partial Q92.9
    sex
      female phenotype Q97.8
  coronary artery Q24.5
  cusp(s), heart valve NEC Q24.8
    pulmonary Q22.3
  cystic duct Q44.5
  digit(s) Q69.9
  ear (auricle) (lobe) Q17.Ø
  endocrine gland NEC Q89.2
  eye muscle Q1Ø.3
  eyelid Q1Ø.3
  face bone(s) Q75.8
  fallopian tube (fimbria) (ostium) Q5Ø.6
  finger(s) Q69.Ø
  foreskin N47.8
  frontonasal process Q75.8
  gallbladder Q44.1
  genital organ(s)
    female Q52.8
      external Q52.79
      internal NEC Q52.8
    male Q55.8
  genitourinary organs NEC Q89.8
    female Q52.8
    male Q55.8
  hallux Q69.2
  heart Q24.8
    valve NEC Q24.8
      pulmonary Q22.3
  hepatic ducts Q44.5
  hymen Q52.4
  intestine (large) (small) Q43.4
  kidney Q63.Ø
  lacrimal canal Q1Ø.6
  leaflet, heart valve NEC Q24.8
  ligament, broad Q5Ø.6
  liver Q44.7
    duct Q44.5
  lobule (ear) Q17.Ø
  lung (lobe) Q33.1
  muscle Q79.8
  navicular of carpus Q74.Ø
  nervous system, part NEC QØ7.8
  nipple Q83.3
  nose Q3Ø.8
  organ or site not listed — *see* Anomaly, by site
  ovary Q5Ø.31
  oviduct Q5Ø.6
  pancreas Q45.3
  parathyroid gland Q89.2
  parotid gland (and duct) Q38.4
  pituitary gland Q89.2
  preauricular appendage Q17.Ø
  prepuce N47.8
  renal arteries (multiple) Q27.2
  rib Q76.6
    cervical Q76.5
  roots (teeth) KØØ.2
  salivary gland Q38.4
  sesamoid bones Q74.8
    foot Q74.2
    hand Q74.Ø
  skin tags Q82.8
  spleen Q89.Ø9
  sternum Q76.7
  submaxillary gland Q38.4
  tarsal bones Q74.2
  teeth, tooth KØØ.1
  tendon Q79.8
  thumb Q69.1
  thymus gland Q89.2

Accessory — *continued*
- thyroid gland Q89.2
- toes Q69.2
- tongue Q38.3
- tooth, teeth KØØ.1
- tragus Q17.Ø
- ureter Q62.5
- urethra Q64.79
- urinary organ or tract NEC Q64.8
- uterus Q51.28
- vagina Q52.1Ø
- valve, heart NEC Q24.8
  - pulmonary Q22.3
- vertebra Q76.49
- vocal cords Q31.8
- vulva Q52.79

Accident
- birth — *see* Birth, injury
- cardiac — *see* Infarct, myocardium
- cerebral I63.9
- cerebrovascular (embolic) (ischemic) (thrombotic) I63.9
  - aborted I63.9
  - hemorrhagic — *see* Hemorrhage, intracranial, intracerebral
  - old (without sequelae) Z86.73
    - with sequelae (of) — *see* Sequelae, infarction, cerebral
- coronary — *see* Infarct, myocardium
- craniovascular I63.9
- vascular, brain I63.9

Accidental — *see* condition

Accommodation (disorder) — *see also* condition
- hysterical paralysis of F44.89
- insufficiency of H52.4
- paresis — *see* Paresis, of accommodation
- spasm — *see* Spasm, of accommodation

Accouchement — *see* Delivery

Accreta placenta O43.21- ☑

Accretio cordis (nonrheumatic) I31.Ø

Accretions, tooth, teeth KØ3.6

Acculturation difficulty Z6Ø.3

Accumulation secretion, prostate N42.89

Acephalia, acephalism, acephalus, acephaly QØØ.Ø

Acephalobrachia monster Q89.8

Acephalochirus monster Q89.8

Acephalogaster Q89.8

Acephalostomus monster Q89.8

Acephalothorax Q89.8

Acerophobia F4Ø.298

Acetonemia R79.89
- in Type 1 diabetes E1Ø.1Ø
  - with coma E1Ø.11

Acetonuria R82.4

Achalasia (cardia) (esophagus) K22.Ø
- congenital Q39.5
- pylorus Q4Ø.Ø
- sphincteral NEC K59.89

Ache(s) — *see* Pain

Acheilia Q38.6

Achilloburstis — *see* Tendinitis, Achilles

Achillodynia — *see* Tendinitis, Achilles

Achlorhydria, achlorhydric (neurogenic) K31.83
- anemia D5Ø.8
- diarrhea K31.83
- psychogenic F45.8
- secondary to vagotomy K91.1

Achluophobia F4Ø.228

Acholia K82.8

Acholuric jaundice (familial) (splenomegalic) — *see also* Spherocytosis
- acquired D59.8

Achondrogenesis Q77.Ø

Achondroplasia (osteosclerosis congenita) Q77.4

Achroma, cutis L8Ø

Achromat (ism), achromatopsia (acquired) (congenital) H53.51

Achromia, congenital — *see* Albinism

Achromia parasitica B36.Ø

Achylia gastrica K31.89
- psychogenic F45.8

Acid
- burn — *see* Corrosion
- deficiency
  - amide nicotinic E52
  - ascorbic E54
  - folic E53.8
  - nicotinic E52

Acid — *continued*
- deficiency — *continued*
  - pantothenic E53.8
- intoxication — *see also* Acidosis E87.29
- peptic disease K3Ø
- phosphatase deficiency E83.39
- stomach K3Ø
  - psychogenic F45.8

Acidemia — *see also* Acidosis E87.2Ø
- argininosuccinic E72.22
- isovaleric E71.11Ø
- metabolic (newborn) P19.9
  - first noted before onset of labor P19.Ø
  - first noted during labor P19.1
  - noted at birth P19.2
- methylmalonic E71.12Ø
- pipecolic E72.3
- propionic E71.121

Acidity, gastric (high) K3Ø
- psychogenic F45.8

Acidocytopenia — *see* Agranulocytosis

Acidocytosis D72.1Ø

Acidopenia — *see* Agranulocytosis

Acidosis (lactic) E87.2Ø
- in Type 1 diabetes E1Ø.1Ø
  - with coma E1Ø.11
- kidney, tubular N25.89
- lactic E87.2Ø
  - acute E87.21
  - chronic E87.22
- metabolic NEC E87.2Ø
  - with respiratory acidosis E87.4
  - acute E87.21
  - chronic E87.22
  - hyperchloremic, of newborn P74.421
  - late, of newborn P74.Ø
- mixed metabolic and respiratory, newborn P84
- newborn P84
- renal (hyperchloremic) (tubular) N25.89
- respiratory E87.29
  - acute J96.Ø2
  - chronic J96.12
  - complicated by
    - metabolic
      - acidosis E87.4
      - alkalosis E87.4
- specified NEC E87.29

Aciduria
- 4-hydroxybutyric E72.81
- argininosuccinic E72.22
- gamma-hydroxybutyric E72.81
- glutaric (type I) E72.3
  - type II E71.313
  - type III E71.5- ☑
- orotic (congenital) (hereditary) (pyrimidine deficiency) E79.8
  - anemia D53.Ø

Acladiosis (skin) B36.Ø

Aclasis, diaphyseal Q78.6

Acleistocardia Q21.19

Aclusion — *see* Anomaly, dentofacial, malocclusion

Acne L7Ø.9
- artificialis L7Ø.8
- atrophica L7Ø.2
- cachecticorum (Hebra) L7Ø.8
- conglobata L7Ø.1
- cystic L7Ø.Ø
- decalvans L66.2
- excoriée (des jeunes filles) L7Ø.5
- frontalis L7Ø.2
- indurata L7Ø.Ø
- infantile L7Ø.4
- keloid L73.Ø
- lupoid L7Ø.2
- necrotic, necrotica (miliaris) L7Ø.2
- neonatal L7Ø.4
- nodular L7Ø.Ø
- occupational L7Ø.8
- picker's L7Ø.5
- pustular L7Ø.Ø
- rodens L7Ø.2
- rosacea L71.9
- specified NEC L7Ø.8
- tropica L7Ø.3
- varioliformis L7Ø.2
- vulgaris L7Ø.Ø

Acnitis (primary) A18.4

Acosta's disease T7Ø.29 ☑

Acoustic — *see* condition

Acousticophobia F4Ø.298

ACPO (acute colonic pseudo-obstruction) K59.81

Acquired — *see also* condition
- immunodeficiency syndrome (AIDS) B2Ø

Acrania QØØ.Ø

Acroangiodermatitis I78.9

Acroasphyxia, chronic I73.89

Acrobystitis N47.7

Acrocephalopolysyndactyly Q87.Ø

Acrocephalosyndactyly Q87.Ø

Acrocephaly Q75.Ø

Acrochondrohyperplasia — *see* Syndrome, Marfan's

Acrocyanosis I73.89
- newborn P28.2
  - meaning transient blue hands and feet — *omit code*

Acrodermatitis L3Ø.8
- atrophicans (chronica) L9Ø.4
- continua (Hallopeau) L4Ø.2
- enteropathica (hereditary) E83.2
- Hallopeau's L4Ø.2
- infantile papular L44.4
- perstans L4Ø.2
- pustulosa continua L4Ø.2
- recalcitrant pustular L4Ø.2

Acrodynia — *see* Poisoning, mercury

Acromegaly, acromegalia E22.Ø

Acromelalgia I73.81

Acromicria, acromikria Q79.8

Acronyx L6Ø.Ø

Acropachy, thyroid — *see* Thyrotoxicosis

Acroparesthesia (simple) (vasomotor) I73.89

Acropathy, thyroid — *see* Thyrotoxicosis

Acrophobia F4Ø.241

Acroposthitis N47.7

Acroscleriasis, acroscleroderma, acrosclerosis — *see* Sclerosis, systemic

Acrosphacelus I96

Acrospiroma, eccrine — *see* Neoplasm, skin, benign

Acrostealgia — *see* Osteochondropathy

Acrotrophodynia — *see* Immersion

ACTH ectopic syndrome E24.3

Actinic — *see* condition

Actinobacillosis, actinobacillus A28.8
- mallei A24.Ø
- muris A25.1

Actinomyces israelii (infection) — *see* Actinomycosis

Actinomycetoma (foot) B47.1

Actinomycosis, actinomycotic A42.9
- with pneumonia A42.Ø
- abdominal A42.1
- cervicofacial A42.2
- cutaneous A42.89
- gastrointestinal A42.1
- pulmonary A42.Ø
- sepsis A42.7
- specified site NEC A42.89

Actinoneuritis G62.82

Action, heart
- disorder I49.9
- irregular I49.9
  - psychogenic F45.8

Activated protein C resistance D68.51

Activation
- mast cell (disorder) (syndrome) D89.4Ø
  - idiopathic D89.42
  - monoclonal D89.41
  - secondary D89.43
  - specified type NEC D89.49

Active — *see* condition

Acute — *see also* condition
- abdomen R1Ø.Ø
- gallbladder — *see* Cholecystitis, acute

Acyanotic heart disease (congenital) Q24.9

Acystia Q64.5

Adair-Dighton syndrome (brittle bones and blue sclera, deafness) Q78.Ø

Adamantinoblastoma — *see* Ameloblastoma

Adamantinoma — *see also* Cyst, calcifying odontogenic
- long bones C4Ø.9Ø
  - lower limb C4Ø.2- ☑
  - upper limb C4Ø.Ø- ☑
- malignant C41.1
  - jaw (bone) (lower) C41.1
    - upper C41.Ø
- tibial C4Ø.2- ☑

Adamantoblastoma — *see* Ameloblastoma

- **Adams-Stokes** (-Morgagni) disease or syndrome I45.9
- **Adaption reaction** — *see* Disorder, adjustment
- **Addiction** — *see also* Dependence F19.2Ø
  - alcohol, alcoholic (ethyl) (methyl) (wood) (without remission) F1Ø.2Ø
    - with remission F1Ø.21
  - drug — *see* Dependence, drug
  - ethyl alcohol (without remission) F1Ø.2Ø
    - with remission F1Ø.21
  - heroin — *see* Dependence, drug, opioid
  - methyl alcohol (without remission) F1Ø.2Ø
    - with remission F1Ø.21
  - methylated spirit (without remission) F1Ø.2Ø
    - with remission F1Ø.21
  - morphine (-like substances) — *see* Dependence, drug, opioid
  - nicotine — *see* Dependence, drug, nicotine
  - opium and opioids — *see* Dependence, drug, opioid
  - tobacco — *see* Dependence, drug, nicotine
- **Addison-Biermer anemia** (pernicious) D51.Ø
- **Addisonian crisis** E27.2
- **Addison's**
  - anemia (pernicious) D51.Ø
  - disease (bronze) or syndrome E27.1
    - tuberculous A18.7
  - keloid L94.Ø
- **Addison-Schilder complex** E71.528
- **Additional** — *see also* Accessory
  - chromosome(s) Q99.8
    - 21 — *see* Trisomy, 21
    - sex — *see* Abnormal, chromosome, sex
- **Adduction contracture, hip or other joint** — *see* Contraction, joint
- **Adenitis** — *see also* Lymphadenitis
  - acute, unspecified site LØ4.9
  - axillary I88.9
    - acute LØ4.2
    - chronic or subacute I88.1
  - Bartholin's gland N75.8
  - bulbourethral gland — *see* Urethritis
  - cervical I88.9
    - acute LØ4.Ø
    - chronic or subacute I88.1
  - chancroid (Hemophilus ducreyi) A57
  - chronic, unspecified site I88.1
  - Cowper's gland — *see* Urethritis
  - due to Pasteurella multocida (P. septica) A28.Ø
  - epidemic, acute B27.Ø9
  - gangrenous LØ4.9
  - gonorrheal NEC A54.89
  - groin I88.9
    - acute LØ4.1
    - chronic or subacute I88.1
  - infectious (acute) (epidemic) B27.Ø9
  - inguinal I88.9
    - acute LØ4.1
    - chronic or subacute I88.1
  - lymph gland or node, except mesenteric I88.9
    - acute — *see* Lymphadenitis, acute
    - chronic or subacute I88.1
  - mesenteric (acute) (chronic) (nonspecific) (subacute) I88.Ø
  - parotid gland (suppurative) — *see* Sialoadenitis
  - salivary gland (any) (suppurative) — *see* Sialoadenitis
  - scrofulous (tuberculous) A18.2
  - Skene's duct or gland — *see* Urethritis
  - strumous, tuberculous A18.2
  - subacute, unspecified site I88.1
  - sublingual gland (suppurative) — *see* Sialoadenitis
  - submandibular gland (suppurative) — *see* Sialoadenitis
  - submaxillary gland (suppurative) — *see* Sialoadenitis
  - tuberculous — *see* Tuberculosis, lymph gland
  - urethral gland — *see* Urethritis
  - Wharton's duct (suppurative) — *see* Sialoadenitis
- **Adenoacanthoma** — *see* Neoplasm, malignant, by site
- **Adenoameloblastoma** — *see* Cyst, calcifying odontogenic
- **Adenocarcinoid** (tumor) — *see* Neoplasm, malignant, by site
- **Adenocarcinoma** — *see also* Neoplasm, malignant, by site
  - acidophil
    - specified site — *see* Neoplasm, malignant, by site
    - unspecified site C75.1
  - adrenal cortical C74.Ø- ☑
  - alveolar — *see* Neoplasm, lung, malignant
  - apocrine
    - breast — *see* Neoplasm, breast, malignant

Adenocarcinoma — *continued*

  - apocrine — *continued*
    - in situ
      - breast DØ5.8- ☑
      - specified site NEC — *see* Neoplasm, skin, in situ
      - unspecified site DØ4.9
    - specified site NEC — *see* Neoplasm, skin, malignant
    - unspecified site C44.99
  - basal cell
    - specified site — *see* Neoplasm, skin, malignant
    - unspecified site CØ8.9
  - basophil
    - specified site — *see* Neoplasm, malignant, by site
    - unspecified site C75.1
  - bile duct type C22.1
    - liver C22.1
    - specified site NEC — *see* Neoplasm, malignant, by site
    - unspecified site C22.1
  - bronchiolar — *see* Neoplasm, lung, malignant
  - bronchioloalveolar — *see* Neoplasm, lung, malignant
  - ceruminous C44.29- ☑
  - cervix, in situ — *see also* Carcinoma, cervix uteri, in situ DØ6.9
  - chromophobe
    - specified site — *see* Neoplasm, malignant, by site
    - unspecified site C75.1
  - diffuse type
    - specified site — *see* Neoplasm, malignant, by site
    - unspecified site C16.9
  - duct
    - infiltrating
      - with Paget's disease — *see* Neoplasm, breast, malignant
      - specified site — *see* Neoplasm, malignant, by site
      - unspecified site (female) C5Ø.91- ☑
        - male C5Ø.92- ☑
    - specified site — *see* Neoplasm, malignant, by site
    - unspecified site
      - female C56.9
      - male C61
  - eosinophil
    - specified site — *see* Neoplasm, malignant, by site
    - unspecified site C75.1
  - follicular
    - with papillary C73
    - moderately differentiated C73
    - specified site — *see* Neoplasm, malignant, by site
    - trabecular C73
    - unspecified site C73
    - well differentiated C73
  - Hurthle cell C73
  - in
    - adenomatous
      - polyposis coli C18.9
  - infiltrating duct
    - with Paget's disease — *see* Neoplasm, breast, malignant
    - specified site — *see* Neoplasm, by site, malignant
    - unspecified site (female) C5Ø.91- ☑
      - male C5Ø.92- ☑
  - inflammatory
    - specified site — *see* Neoplasm, by site, malignant
    - unspecified site (female) C5Ø.91- ☑
      - male C5Ø.92- ☑
  - intestinal type
    - specified site — *see* Neoplasm, by site, malignant
    - unspecified site C16.9
  - intracystic papillary
  - intraductal
    - breast DØ5.1- ☑
    - noninfiltrating
      - breast DØ5.1- ☑
      - papillary
        - with invasion
          - specified site — *see* Neoplasm, by site, malignant
          - unspecified site (female) C5Ø.91- ☑
            - male C5Ø.92- ☑
        - breast DØ5.1- ☑
        - specified site NEC — *see* Neoplasm, in situ, by site
        - unspecified site DØ5.1- ☑
      - specified site NEC — *see* Neoplasm, in situ, by site
      - unspecified site DØ5.1- ☑

Adenocarcinoma — *continued*

  - intraductal — *continued*
    - papillary
      - with invasion
        - specified site — *see* Neoplasm, malignant, by site
        - unspecified site (female) C5Ø.91- ☑
          - male C5Ø.92- ☑
      - breast DØ5.1- ☑
      - specified site — *see* Neoplasm, in situ, by site
      - unspecified site DØ5.1- ☑
    - specified site NEC — *see* Neoplasm, in situ, by site
    - unspecified site DØ5.1- ☑
  - islet cell
    - with exocrine, mixed
      - specified site — *see* Neoplasm, malignant, by site
      - unspecified site C25.9
    - pancreas C25.4
    - specified site NEC — *see* Neoplasm, malignant, by site
    - unspecified site C25.4
  - lobular
    - in situ
      - breast DØ5.Ø- ☑
      - specified site NEC — *see* Neoplasm, in situ, by site
      - unspecified site DØ5.Ø- ☑
    - specified site — *see* Neoplasm, malignant, by site
    - unspecified site (female) C5Ø.91- ☑
      - male C5Ø.92- ☑
  - mucoid — *see also* Neoplasm, malignant, by site
    - cell
      - specified site — *see* Neoplasm, malignant, by site
      - unspecified site C75.1
  - nonencapsulated sclerosing C73
  - papillary
    - with follicular C73
    - follicular variant C73
    - intraductal (noninfiltrating)
      - with invasion
        - specified site — *see* Neoplasm, malignant, by site
        - unspecified site (female) C5Ø.91- ☑
          - male C5Ø.92- ☑
      - breast DØ5.1- ☑
      - specified site NEC — *see* Neoplasm, in situ, by site
      - unspecified site DØ5.1- ☑
    - serous
      - specified site — *see* Neoplasm, malignant, by site
      - unspecified site C56.9
  - papillocystic
    - specified site — *see* Neoplasm, malignant, by site
    - unspecified site C56.9
  - pseudomucinous
    - specified site — *see* Neoplasm, malignant, by site
    - unspecified site C56.9
  - renal cell C64- ☑
  - sebaceous — *see* Neoplasm, skin, malignant
  - serous — *see also* Neoplasm, malignant, by site
    - papillary
      - specified site — *see* Neoplasm, malignant, by site
      - unspecified site C56.9
  - sweat gland — *see* Neoplasm, skin, malignant
  - water-clear cell C75.Ø
- **Adenocarcinoma-in-situ** — *see also* Neoplasm, in situ, by site
  - breast DØ5.9- ☑
- **Adenofibroma**
  - clear cell — *see* Neoplasm, benign, by site
  - endometrioid D27.9
    - borderline malignancy D39.1Ø
    - malignant C56- ☑
  - mucinous
    - specified site — *see* Neoplasm, benign, by site
    - unspecified site D27.9
  - papillary
    - specified site — *see* Neoplasm, benign, by site
    - unspecified site D27.9
  - prostate — *see* Enlargement, enlarged, prostate
  - serous
    - specified site — *see* Neoplasm, benign, by site
    - unspecified site D27.9

Adenofibroma — *continued*
specified site — *see* Neoplasm, benign, by site
unspecified site D27.9
Adenofibrosis
breast — *see* Fibroadenosis, breast
endometrioid N80.00
Adenoiditis (chronic) J35.02
with tonsillitis J35.03
acute J03.90
recurrent J03.91
specified organism NEC J03.80
recurrent J03.81
staphylococcal J03.80
recurrent J03.81
streptococcal J03.00
recurrent J03.01
Adenoids — *see* condition
Adenolipoma — *see* Neoplasm, benign, by site
Adenolipomatosis, Launois-Bensaude E88.89
Adenolymphoma
specified site — *see* Neoplasm, benign, by site
unspecified site D11.9
Adenoma — *see also* Neoplasm, benign, by site
acidophil
specified site — *see* Neoplasm, benign, by site
unspecified site D35.2
acidophil-basophil, mixed
specified site — *see* Neoplasm, benign, by site
unspecified site D35.2
adrenal (cortical) D35.00
clear cell D35.00
compact cell D35.00
glomerulosa cell D35.00
heavily pigmented variant D35.00
mixed cell D35.00
alpha-cell
pancreas D13.7
specified site NEC — *see* Neoplasm, benign, by site
unspecified site D13.7
alveolar D14.30
apocrine
breast D24- ☑
specified site NEC — *see* Neoplasm, skin, benign, by site
unspecified site D23.9
basal cell D11.9
basophil
specified site — *see* Neoplasm, benign, by site
unspecified site D35.2
basophil-acidophil, mixed
specified site — *see* Neoplasm, benign, by site
unspecified site D35.2
beta-cell
pancreas D13.7
specified site NEC — *see* Neoplasm, benign, by site
unspecified site D13.7
bile duct D13.4
common D13.5
extrahepatic D13.5
intrahepatic D13.4
specified site NEC — *see* Neoplasm, benign, by site
unspecified site D13.4
black D35.00
bronchial D38.1
cylindroid type — *see* Neoplasm, lung, malignant
ceruminous D23.2- ☑
chief cell D35.1
chromophobe
specified site — *see* Neoplasm, benign, by site
unspecified site D35.2
colloid
specified site — *see* Neoplasm, benign, by site
unspecified site D34
eccrine, papillary — *see* Neoplasm, skin, benign
endocrine, multiple
single specified site — *see* Neoplasm, uncertain behavior, by site
two or more specified sites D44- ☑
unspecified site D44.9
endometrioid — *see also* Neoplasm, benign
borderline malignancy — *see* Neoplasm, uncertain behavior, by site
eosinophil
specified site — *see* Neoplasm, benign, by site
unspecified site D35.2
fetal
specified site — *see* Neoplasm, benign, by site
unspecified site D34

Adenoma — *continued*
follicular
specified site — *see* Neoplasm, benign, by site
unspecified site D34
hepatocellular D13.4
Hurthle cell D34
islet cell
pancreas D13.7
specified site NEC — *see* Neoplasm, benign, by site
unspecified site D13.7
liver cell D13.4
macrofollicular
specified site — *see* Neoplasm, benign, by site
unspecified site D34
malignant, malignum — *see* Neoplasm, malignant, by site
microcystic
pancreas D13.6
specified site NEC — *see* Neoplasm, benign, by site
unspecified site D13.6
microfollicular
specified site — *see* Neoplasm, benign, by site
unspecified site D34
mucoid cell
specified site — *see* Neoplasm, benign, by site
unspecified site D35.2
multiple endocrine
single specified site — *see* Neoplasm, uncertain behavior, by site
two or more specified sites D44- ☑
unspecified site D44.9
nipple D24- ☑
papillary — *see also* Neoplasm, benign, by site
eccrine — *see* Neoplasm, skin, benign, by site
Pick's tubular
specified site — *see* Neoplasm, benign, by site
unspecified site
female D27.9
male D29.20
pleomorphic
carcinoma in — *see* Neoplasm, salivary gland, malignant
specified site — *see* Neoplasm, malignant, by site
unspecified site C08.9
polypoid — *see also* Neoplasm, benign
adenocarcinoma in — *see* Neoplasm, malignant, by site
adenocarcinoma in situ — *see* Neoplasm, in situ, by site
prostate — *see* Neoplasm, benign, prostate
rete cell D29.20
sebaceous — *see* Neoplasm, skin, benign
Sertoli cell
specified site — *see* Neoplasm, benign, by site
unspecified site
female D27.9
male D29.20
skin appendage — *see* Neoplasm, skin, benign
sudoriferous gland — *see* Neoplasm, skin, benign
sweat gland — *see* Neoplasm, skin, benign
testicular
specified site — *see* Neoplasm, benign, by site
unspecified site
female D27.9
male D29.20
tubular — *see also* Neoplasm, benign, by site
adenocarcinoma in — *see* Neoplasm, malignant, by site
adenocarcinoma in situ — *see* Neoplasm, in situ, by site
Pick's
specified site — *see* Neoplasm, benign, by site
unspecified site
female D27.9
male D29.20
tubulovillous — *see also* Neoplasm, benign, by site
adenocarcinoma in — *see* Neoplasm, malignant, by site
adenocarcinoma in situ — *see* Neoplasm, in situ, by site
villous — *see* Neoplasm, uncertain behavior, by site
adenocarcinoma in — *see* Neoplasm, malignant, by site
adenocarcinoma in situ — *see* Neoplasm, in situ, by site
water-clear cell D35.1

Adenomatosis
endocrine (multiple) E31.20
single specified site — *see* Neoplasm, uncertain behavior, by site
erosive of nipple D24- ☑
pluriendocrine — *see* Adenomatosis, endocrine
pulmonary D38.1
malignant — *see* Neoplasm, lung, malignant
specified site — *see* Neoplasm, benign, by site
unspecified site D12.6
Adenomatous
goiter (nontoxic) E04.9
with hyperthyroidism — *see* Hyperthyroidism, with, goiter, nodular
toxic — *see* Hyperthyroidism, with, goiter, nodular
Adenomyoma — *see also* Neoplasm, benign, by site
prostate — *see* Enlarged, prostate
Adenomyometritis N80.00
Adenomyosis (uterus) N80.03
Adenopathy (lymph gland) R59.9
generalized R59.1
inguinal R59.0
localized R59.0
mediastinal R59.0
mesentery R59.0
syphilitic (secondary) A51.49
tracheobronchial R59.0
tuberculous A15.4
primary (progressive) A15.7
tuberculous — *see also* Tuberculosis, lymph gland
tracheobronchial A15.4
primary (progressive) A15.7
Adenosalpingitis — *see* Salpingitis
Adenosarcoma — *see* Neoplasm, malignant, by site
Adenosclerosis I88.8
Adenosis (sclerosing) breast — *see* Fibroadenosis, breast
Adenovirus, as cause of disease classified elsewhere B97.0
Adentia (complete) (partial) — *see* Absence, teeth
Adherent — *see also* Adhesions
labia (minora) N90.89
pericardium (nonrheumatic) I31.0
rheumatic I09.2
placenta (with hemorrhage) O72.0
without hemorrhage O73.0
prepuce, newborn N47.0
scar (skin) L90.5
tendon in scar L90.5
Adhesions, adhesive (postinfective) K66.0
with intestinal obstruction K56.50
complete K56.52
incomplete K56.51
partial K56.51
abdominal (wall) — *see* Adhesions, peritoneum
appendix K38.8
bile duct (common) (hepatic) K83.8
bladder (sphincter) N32.89
bowel — *see* Adhesions, peritoneum
cardiac I31.0
rheumatic I09.2
cecum — *see* Adhesions, peritoneum
cervicovaginal N88.1
congenital Q52.8
postpartal O90.89
old N88.1
cervix N88.1
ciliary body NEC — *see* Adhesions, iris
clitoris N90.89
colon — *see* Adhesions, peritoneum
common duct K83.8
congenital — *see also* Anomaly, by site
fingers — *see* Syndactylism, complex, fingers
omental, anomalous Q43.3
peritoneal Q43.3
tongue (to gum or roof of mouth) Q38.3
conjunctiva (acquired) H11.21- ☑
congenital Q15.8
cystic duct K82.8
diaphragm — *see* Adhesions, peritoneum
due to foreign body — *see* Foreign body
duodenum — *see* Adhesions, peritoneum
ear
middle H74.1- ☑
epididymis N50.89
epidural — *see* Adhesions, meninges
epiglottis J38.7
eyelid H02.59
female pelvis N73.6

Adhesions, adhesive — *continued*
- gallbladder K82.8
- globe H44.89
- heart I31.Ø
  - rheumatic IØ9.2
- ileocecal (coil) — *see* Adhesions, peritoneum
- ileum — *see* Adhesions, peritoneum
- intestine — *see also* Adhesions, peritoneum
  - with obstruction K56.5Ø
    - complete K56.52
    - incomplete K56.51
    - partial K56.51
- intra-abdominal — *see* Adhesions, peritoneum
- iris H21.5Ø- ☑
  - anterior H21.51- ☑
  - goniosynechiae H21.52- ☑
  - posterior H21.54- ☑
  - to corneal graft T85.898 ☑
- joint — *see* Ankylosis
  - knee M23.8X ☑
  - temporomandibular M26.61- ☑
- labium (majus) (minus), congenital Q52.5
- liver — *see* Adhesions, peritoneum
- lung J98.4
- mediastinum J98.59
- meninges (cerebral) (spinal) G96.12
  - congenital QØ7.8
  - tuberculous (cerebral) (spinal) A17.Ø
- mesenteric — *see* Adhesions, peritoneum
- nasal (septum) (to turbinates) J34.89
- ocular muscle — *see* Strabismus, mechanical
- omentum — *see* Adhesions, peritoneum
- ovary N73.6
  - congenital (to cecum, kidney or omentum) Q5Ø.39
- paraovarian N73.6
- pelvic (peritoneal)
  - female N73.6
    - postprocedural N99.4
  - male — *see* Adhesions, peritoneum
  - postpartal (old) N73.6
  - tuberculous A18.17
- penis to scrotum (congenital) Q55.8
- periappendiceal — *see also* Adhesions, peritoneum
- pericardium (nonrheumatic) I31.Ø
  - focal I31.8
  - rheumatic IØ9.2
  - tuberculous A18.84
- pericholecystic K82.8
- perigastric — *see* Adhesions, peritoneum
- periovarian N73.6
- periprostatic N42.89
- perirectal — *see* Adhesions, peritoneum
- perirenal N28.89
- peritoneum, peritoneal (postinfective) K66.Ø
  - with obstruction (intestinal) K56.5Ø
    - complete K56.52
    - incomplete K56.51
    - partial K56.51
  - congenital Q43.3
  - pelvic, female N73.6
    - postprocedural N99.4
  - postpartal, pelvic N73.6
  - postprocedural K66.Ø
  - to uterus N73.6
- peritubal N73.6
- periureteral N28.89
- periuterine N73.6
- perivesical N32.89
- perivesicular (seminal vesicle) N5Ø.89
- pleura, pleuritic J94.8
  - tuberculous NEC A15.6
- pleuropericardial J94.8
- postoperative (gastrointestinal tract) K66.Ø
  - with obstruction — *see also* Obstruction, intestine, postoperative K91.3Ø
  - due to foreign body accidentally left in wound — *see* Foreign body, accidentally left during a procedure
  - pelvic peritoneal N99.4
  - urethra — *see* Stricture, urethra, postprocedural
  - vagina N99.2
- postpartal, old (vulva or perineum) N9Ø.89
- preputial, prepuce N47.5
- pulmonary J98.4
- pylorus — *see* Adhesions, peritoneum
- sciatic nerve — *see* Lesion, nerve, sciatic
- seminal vesicle N5Ø.89
- shoulder (joint) — *see* Capsulitis, adhesive

Adhesions, adhesive — *continued*
- sigmoid flexure — *see* Adhesions, peritoneum
- spermatic cord (acquired) N5Ø.89
  - congenital Q55.4
- spinal canal G96.12
- stomach — *see* Adhesions, peritoneum
- subscapular — *see* Capsulitis, adhesive
- temporomandibular M26.61- ☑
- tendinitis (*see also* Tenosynovitis, specified type NEC)
  - shoulder — *see* Capsulitis, adhesive
- testis N44.8
- tongue, congenital (to gum or roof of mouth) Q38.3
  - acquired K14.8
- trachea J39.8
- tubo-ovarian N73.6
- tunica vaginalis N44.8
- uterus N73.6
  - internal N85.6
  - to abdominal wall N73.6
- vagina (chronic) N89.5
  - postoperative N99.2
- vitreomacular H43.82- ☑
- vitreous H43.89
- vulva N9Ø.89

Adiaspiromycosis B48.8

Adie (-Holmes) **pupil or syndrome** — *see* Anomaly, pupil, function, tonic pupil

Adiponecrosis neonatorum P83.88

Adiposis — *see also* Obesity
- cerebralis E23.6
- dolorosa E88.2

Adiposity — *see also* Obesity
- heart — *see* Degeneration, myocardial
- localized E65

Adiposogenital dystrophy E23.6

Adjustment
- disorder — *see* Disorder, adjustment
- implanted device — *see* Encounter (for), adjustment (of)
- prosthesis, external — *see* Fitting
- reaction — *see* Disorder, adjustment

Administration of tPA (rtPA) in a different facility within the last 24 hours prior to admission to current facility Z92.82

Admission (for) — *see also* Encounter (for)
- adjustment (of)
  - artificial
    - arm Z44.ØØ- ☑
      - complete Z44.Ø1- ☑
      - partial Z44.Ø2- ☑
    - eye Z44.2 ☑
    - leg Z44.1Ø- ☑
      - complete Z44.11- ☑
      - partial Z44.12- ☑
  - brain neuropacemaker Z46.2
    - implanted Z45.42
  - breast
    - implant Z45.81 ☑
    - prosthesis (external) Z44.3 ☑
  - colostomy belt Z46.89
  - contact lenses Z46.Ø
  - cystostomy device Z46.6
  - dental prosthesis Z46.3
  - device NEC
    - abdominal Z46.89
    - implanted Z45.89
      - cardiac Z45.Ø9
        - defibrillator (with synchronous cardiac pacemaker) Z45.Ø2
        - pacemaker (cardiac resynchronization therapy (CRT-P)) Z45.Ø18
          - pulse generator Z45.Ø1Ø
        - resynchronization therapy defibrillator (CRT-D) Z45.Ø2
      - hearing device Z45.328
        - bone conduction Z45.32Ø
        - cochlear Z45.321
      - infusion pump Z45.1
      - nervous system Z45.49
        - CSF drainage Z45.41
        - hearing device — *see* Admission, adjustment, device, implanted, hearing device
        - neuropacemaker Z45.42
        - visual substitution Z45.31
      - specified NEC Z45.89
      - vascular access Z45.2
      - visual substitution Z45.31

Admission — *continued*
- adjustment — *continued*
  - device — *continued*
    - nervous system Z46.2
      - implanted — *see* Admission, adjustment, device, implanted, nervous system
    - orthodontic Z46.4
    - prosthetic Z44.9
      - arm — *see* Admission, adjustment, artificial, arm
      - breast Z44.3 ☑
      - dental Z46.3
      - eye Z44.2 ☑
      - leg — *see* Admission, adjustment, artificial, leg
      - specified type NEC Z44.8
    - substitution
      - auditory Z46.2
        - implanted — *see* Admission, adjustment, device, implanted, hearing device
      - nervous system Z46.2
        - implanted — *see* Admission, adjustment, device, implanted, nervous system
      - visual Z46.2
        - implanted Z45.31
    - urinary Z46.6
  - hearing aid Z46.1
    - implanted — *see* Admission, adjustment, device, implanted, hearing device
  - ileostomy device Z46.89
  - intestinal appliance or device NEC Z46.89
  - neuropacemaker (brain) (peripheral nerve) (spinal cord) Z46.2
    - implanted Z45.42
  - orthodontic device Z46.4
  - orthopedic (brace) (cast) (device) (shoes) Z46.89
  - pacemaker (cardiac resynchronization therapy (CRT-P))
    - cardiac Z45.Ø18
      - pulse generator Z45.Ø1Ø
    - nervous system Z46.2
      - implanted Z45.42
  - portacath (port-a-cath) Z45.2
  - prosthesis Z44.9
    - arm — *see* Admission, adjustment, artificial, arm
    - breast Z44.3 ☑
    - dental Z46.3
    - eye Z44.2 ☑
    - leg — *see* Admission, adjustment, artificial, leg
    - specified NEC Z44.8
  - spectacles Z46.Ø
- aftercare — *see also* Aftercare Z51.89
  - postpartum
    - immediately after delivery Z39.Ø
    - routine follow-up Z39.2
  - radiation therapy (antineoplastic) Z51.Ø
- attention to artificial opening (of) Z43.9
  - artificial vagina Z43.7
  - colostomy Z43.3
  - cystostomy Z43.5
  - enterostomy Z43.4
  - gastrostomy Z43.1
  - ileostomy Z43.2
  - jejunostomy Z43.4
  - nephrostomy Z43.6
  - specified site NEC Z43.8
    - intestinal tract Z43.4
    - urinary tract Z43.6
  - tracheostomy Z43.Ø
  - ureterostomy Z43.6
  - urethrostomy Z43.6
- breast augmentation or reduction Z41.1
- breast reconstruction following mastectomy Z42.1
- change of
  - dressing (nonsurgical) Z48.ØØ
  - neuropacemaker device (brain) (peripheral nerve) (spinal cord) Z46.2
    - implanted Z45.42
  - surgical dressing Z48.Ø1
- circumcision, ritual or routine (in absence of diagnosis) Z41.2
- clinical research investigation (control) (normal comparison) (participant) ZØØ.6
- contraceptive management Z3Ø.9
- cosmetic surgery NEC Z41.1
- counseling — *see also* Counseling
  - dietary Z71.3
  - gestational carrier Z31.7

Admission — *continued*
- counseling — *see also* Counseling — *continued*
  - HIV Z71.7
  - human immunodeficiency virus Z71.7
  - nonattending third party Z71.Ø
  - procreative management NEC Z31.69
- delivery, full-term, uncomplicated O8Ø
  - cesarean, without indication O82
- desensitization to allergens Z51.6
- dietary surveillance and counseling Z71.3
- ear piercing Z41.3
- examination at health care facility (adult) — *see also* Examination ZØØ.ØØ
  - with abnormal findings ZØØ.Ø1
  - clinical research investigation (control) (normal comparison) (participant) ZØØ.6
  - dental ZØ1.2Ø
    - with abnormal findings ZØ1.21
  - donor (potential) ZØØ.5
  - ear ZØ1.1Ø
    - with abnormal findings NEC ZØ1.118
  - eye ZØ1.ØØ
    - with abnormal findings ZØ1.Ø1
    - following failed vision screening ZØ1.Ø2Ø
      - with abnormal findings ZØ1.Ø21
  - general, specified reason NEC ZØØ.8
  - hearing ZØ1.1Ø
    - with abnormal findings NEC ZØ1.118
    - infant or child (over 28 days old) ZØØ.129
      - with abnormal findings ZØØ.121
  - postpartum checkup Z39.2
  - psychiatric (general) ZØØ.8
    - requested by authority ZØ4.6
  - vision ZØ1.ØØ
    - with abnormal findings ZØ1.Ø1
    - following failed vision screening ZØ1.Ø2Ø
      - with abnormal findings ZØ1.Ø21
    - infant or child (over 28 days old) ZØØ.129
      - with abnormal findings ZØØ.121
- fitting (of)
  - artificial
    - arm — *see* Admission, adjustment, artificial, arm
    - eye Z44.2 ☑
    - leg — *see* Admission, adjustment, artificial, leg
  - brain neuropacemaker Z46.2
    - implanted Z45.42
  - breast prosthesis (external) Z44.3 ☑
  - colostomy belt Z46.89
  - contact lenses Z46.Ø
  - cystostomy device Z46.6
  - dental prosthesis Z46.3
  - dentures Z46.3
  - device NEC
    - abdominal Z46.89
    - nervous system Z46.2
      - implanted — *see* Admission, adjustment, device, implanted, nervous system
    - orthodontic Z46.4
    - prosthetic Z44.9
      - breast Z44.3 ☑
      - dental Z46.3
      - eye Z44.2 ☑
    - substitution
      - auditory Z46.2
        - implanted — *see* Admission, adjustment, device, implanted, hearing device
      - nervous system Z46.2
        - implanted — *see* Admission, adjustment, device, implanted, nervous system
      - visual Z46.2
        - implanted Z45.31
  - hearing aid Z46.1
  - ileostomy device Z46.89
  - intestinal appliance or device NEC Z46.89
  - neuropacemaker (brain) (peripheral nerve) (spinal cord) Z46.2
    - implanted Z45.42
  - orthodontic device Z46.4
  - orthopedic device (brace) (cast) (shoes) Z46.89
  - prosthesis Z44.9
    - arm — *see* Admission, adjustment, artificial, arm
    - breast Z44.3 ☑
    - dental Z46.3
    - eye Z44.2 ☑
    - leg — *see* Admission, adjustment, artificial, leg
    - specified type NEC Z44.8
  - spectacles Z46.Ø
- follow-up examination ZØ9

Admission — *continued*
- intrauterine device management Z3Ø.431
  - initial prescription Z3Ø.Ø14
- mental health evaluation ZØØ.8
  - requested by authority ZØ4.6
- observation — *see* Observation
- Papanicolaou smear, cervix Z12.4
  - for suspected malignant neoplasm Z12.4
- plastic and reconstructive surgery following medical procedure or healed injury NEC Z42.8
- plastic surgery, cosmetic NEC Z41.1
- postpartum observation
  - immediately after delivery Z39.Ø
  - routine follow-up Z39.2
- poststerilization (for restoration) Z31.Ø
  - aftercare Z31.42
- procreative management Z31.9
- prophylactic (measure) — *see also* Encounter, prophylactic measures
  - organ removal Z4Ø.ØØ
    - breast Z4Ø.Ø1
    - fallopian tube(s) Z4Ø.Ø3
      - with ovary(s) Z4Ø.Ø2
    - ovary(s) Z4Ø.Ø2
    - specified organ NEC Z4Ø.Ø9
    - testes Z4Ø.Ø9
  - vaccination Z23
- psychiatric examination (general) ZØØ.8
  - requested by authority ZØ4.6
- radiation therapy (antineoplastic) Z51.Ø
- reconstructive surgery following medical procedure or healed injury NEC Z42.8
- removal of
  - cystostomy catheter Z43.5
  - drains Z48.Ø3
  - dressing (nonsurgical) Z48.ØØ
  - implantable subdermal contraceptive Z3Ø.46
  - intrauterine contraceptive device Z3Ø.432
  - neuropacemaker (brain) (peripheral nerve) (spinal cord) Z46.2
    - implanted Z45.42
  - staples Z48.Ø2
  - surgical dressing Z48.Ø1
  - sutures Z48.Ø2
  - ureteral stent Z46.6
- respirator [ventilator] use during power failure Z99.12
- restoration of organ continuity (poststerilization) Z31.Ø
  - aftercare Z31.42
- sensitivity test — *see also* Test, skin
  - allergy NEC ZØ1.82
  - Mantoux Z11.1
- tuboplasty following previous sterilization Z31.Ø
  - aftercare Z31.42
- vasoplasty following previous sterilization Z31.Ø
  - aftercare Z31.42
- vision examination ZØ1.ØØ
  - with abnormal findings ZØ1.Ø1
  - following failed vision screening ZØ1.Ø2Ø
    - with abnormal findings ZØ1.Ø21
  - infant or child (over 28 days old) ZØØ.129
    - with abnormal findings ZØØ.121
- waiting period for admission to other facility Z75.1

Adnexitis (suppurative) — *see* Salpingo-oophoritis

Adolescent X-linked adrenoleukodystrophy E71.521

Adrenal (gland) — *see* condition

Adrenalism, tuberculous A18.7

Adrenalitis, adrenitis E27.8
- autoimmune E27.1
- meningococcal, hemorrhagic A39.1

Adrenarche, premature E27.Ø

Adrenocortical syndrome — *see* Cushing's, syndrome

Adrenogenital syndrome E25.9
- acquired E25.8
- congenital E25.Ø
- salt loss E25.Ø

Adrenogenitalism, congenital E25.Ø

Adrenoleukodystrophy E71.529
- neonatal E71.511
- X-linked E71.529
  - Addison only phenotype E71.528
  - Addison-Schilder E71.528
  - adolescent E71.521
  - adrenomyeloneuropathy E71.522
  - childhood cerebral E71.52Ø
  - other specified E71.528

Adrenomyeloneuropathy E71.522

Adventitious bursa — *see* Bursopathy, specified type NEC

Adverse effect — *see* Table of Drugs and Chemicals, categories T36-T5Ø, with 6th character 5

Advice — *see* Counseling

Adynamia (episodica) (hereditary) (periodic) G72.3

Aeration lung imperfect, newborn — *see* Atelectasis

Aerobullosis T7Ø.3 ☑

Aerocele — *see* Embolism, air

Aerodermectasia
- subcutaneous (traumatic) T79.7 ☑

Aerodontalgia T7Ø.29 ☑

Aeroembolism T7Ø.3 ☑

Aerogenes capsulatus infection A48.Ø

Aero-otitis media T7Ø.Ø ☑

Aerophagy, aerophagia (psychogenic) F45.8

Aerophobia F4Ø.228

Aerosinusitis T7Ø.1 ☑

Aerotitis T7Ø.Ø ☑

Affection — *see* Disease

Afibrinogenemia — *see also* Defect, coagulation D68.8
- acquired D65
- congenital D68.2
- following ectopic or molar pregnancy OØ8.1
- in abortion — *see* Abortion, by type, complicated by, afibrinogenemia
- puerperal O72.3

African
- sleeping sickness B56.9
- tick fever A68.1
- trypanosomiasis B56.9
  - gambian B56.Ø
  - rhodesian B56.1

Aftercare — *see also* Care Z51.89
- following surgery (for) (on)
  - amputation Z47.81
  - attention to
    - drains Z48.Ø3
    - dressings (nonsurgical) Z48.ØØ
      - surgical Z48.Ø1
    - sutures Z48.Ø2
  - circulatory system Z48.812
  - delayed (planned) wound closure Z48.1
  - digestive system Z48.815
  - explantation of joint prosthesis (staged procedure)
    - hip Z47.32
    - knee Z47.33
    - shoulder Z47.31
  - genitourinary system Z48.816
  - joint replacement Z47.1
  - neoplasm Z48.3
  - nervous system Z48.811
  - oral cavity Z48.814
  - organ transplant
    - bone marrow Z48.29Ø
    - heart Z48.21
    - heart-lung Z48.28Ø
    - kidney Z48.22
    - liver Z48.23
    - lung Z48.24
    - multiple organs NEC Z48.288
    - specified NEC Z48.298
  - orthopedic NEC Z47.89
  - planned wound closure Z48.1
  - removal of internal fixation device Z47.2
  - respiratory system Z48.813
  - scoliosis Z47.82
  - sense organs Z48.81Ø
  - skin and subcutaneous tissue Z48.817
  - specified body system
    - circulatory Z48.812
    - digestive Z48.815
    - genitourinary Z48.816
    - nervous Z48.811
    - oral cavity Z48.814
    - respiratory Z48.813
    - sense organs Z48.81Ø
    - skin and subcutaneous tissue Z48.817
    - teeth Z48.814
  - specified NEC Z48.89
  - spinal Z47.89
  - teeth Z48.814
- fracture — *code to* fracture with seventh character D
- involving
  - removal of
    - drains Z48.Ø3
    - dressings (nonsurgical) Z48.ØØ
    - staples Z48.Ø2
    - surgical dressings Z48.Ø1
    - sutures Z48.Ø2

Aftercare — *continued*
- neuropacemaker (brain) (peripheral nerve) (spinal cord) Z46.2
  - implanted Z45.42
- orthopedic NEC Z47.89
- postprocedural — *see* Aftercare, following surgery

After-cataract — *see* Cataract, secondary

Agalactia (primary) O92.3
- elective, secondary or therapeutic O92.5

Agammaglobulinemia (acquired (secondary) (nonfamilial) D8Ø.1
- with
  - immunoglobulin-bearing B-lymphocytes D8Ø.1
  - lymphopenia D81.9
- autosomal recessive (Swiss type) D8Ø.Ø
- Bruton's X-linked D8Ø.Ø
- common variable (CVAgamma) D8Ø.1
- congenital sex-linked D8Ø.Ø
- hereditary D8Ø.Ø
- lymphopenic D81.9
- Swiss type (autosomal recessive) D8Ø.Ø
- X-linked (with growth hormone deficiency) (Bruton) D8Ø.Ø

Aganglionosis (bowel) (colon) Q43.1

Age (old) — *see* Senility

Agenesis
- adrenal (gland) Q89.1
- alimentary tract (complete) (partial) NEC Q45.8
  - upper Q4Ø.8
- anus, anal (canal) Q42.3
  - with fistula Q42.2
- aorta Q25.41
- appendix Q42.8
- arm (complete) Q71.Ø- ☑
  - with hand present Q71.1- ☑
- artery (peripheral) Q27.9
  - brain Q28.3
  - coronary Q24.5
  - pulmonary Q25.79
  - specified NEC Q27.8
  - umbilical Q27.Ø
- auditory (canal) (external) Q16.1
- auricle (ear) Q16.Ø
- bile duct or passage Q44.5
- bladder Q64.5
- bone Q79.9
- brain QØØ.Ø
  - part of QØ4.3
- breast (with nipple present) Q83.8
  - with absent nipple Q83.Ø
- bronchus Q32.4
- canaliculus lacrimalis Q1Ø.4
- carpus — *see* Agenesis, hand
- cartilage Q79.9
- cecum Q42.8
- cerebellum QØ4.3
- cervix Q51.5
- chin Q18.8
- cilia Q1Ø.3
- circulatory system, part NOS Q28.9
- clavicle Q74.Ø
- clitoris Q52.6
- coccyx Q76.49
- colon Q42.9
  - specified NEC Q42.8
- corpus callosum QØ4.Ø
- cricoid cartilage Q31.8
- diaphragm (with hernia) Q79.1
- digestive organ(s) or tract (complete) (partial) NEC Q45.8
  - upper Q4Ø.8
- ductus arteriosus Q28.8
- duodenum Q41.Ø
- ear Q16.9
  - auricle Q16.Ø
  - lobe Q17.8
- ejaculatory duct Q55.4
- endocrine (gland) NEC Q89.2
- epiglottis Q31.8
- esophagus Q39.8
- eustachian tube Q16.2
- eye Q11.1
  - adnexa Q15.8
- eyelid (fold) Q1Ø.3
- face
  - bones NEC Q75.8
  - specified part NEC Q18.8
- fallopian tube Q5Ø.6

Agenesis — *continued*
- femur — *see* Defect, reduction, lower limb, longitudinal, femur
- fibula — *see* Defect, reduction, lower limb, longitudinal, fibula
- finger (complete) (partial) — *see* Agenesis, hand
- foot (and toes) (complete) (partial) Q72.3- ☑
- forearm (with hand present) — *see* Agenesis, arm, with hand present
  - and hand Q71.2- ☑
- gallbladder Q44.Ø
- gastric Q4Ø.2
- genitalia, genital (organ(s))
  - female Q52.8
    - external Q52.71
    - internal NEC Q52.8
  - male Q55.8
- glottis Q31.8
- hair Q84.Ø
- hand (and fingers) (complete) (partial) Q71.3- ☑
- heart Q24.8
  - valve NEC Q24.8
    - pulmonary Q22.Ø
- hepatic Q44.7
- humerus — *see* Defect, reduction, upper limb
- hymen Q52.4
- ileum Q41.2
- incus Q16.3
- intestine (small) Q41.9
  - large Q42.9
    - specified NEC Q42.8
- iris (dilator fibers) Q13.1
- jaw M26.Ø9
- jejunum Q41.1
- kidney(s) (partial) Q6Ø.2
  - bilateral Q6Ø.1
  - unilateral Q6Ø.Ø
- labium (majus) (minus) Q52.71
- labyrinth, membranous Q16.5
- lacrimal apparatus Q1Ø.4
- larynx Q31.8
- leg (complete) Q72.Ø- ☑
  - with foot present Q72.1- ☑
  - lower leg (with foot present) — *see* Agenesis, leg, with foot present
    - and foot Q72.2- ☑
- lens Q12.3
- limb (complete) Q73.Ø
  - lower — *see* Agenesis, leg
  - upper — *see* Agenesis, arm
- lip Q38.Ø
- liver Q44.7
- lung (fissure) (lobe) (bilateral) (unilateral) Q33.3
- mandible, maxilla M26.Ø9
- metacarpus — *see* Agenesis, hand
- metatarsus — *see* Agenesis, foot
- muscle Q79.8
  - eyelid Q1Ø.3
  - ocular Q15.8
- musculoskeletal system NEC Q79.8
- nail(s) Q84.3
- neck, part Q18.8
- nerve QØ7.8
- nervous system, part NEC QØ7.8
- nipple Q83.2
- nose Q3Ø.1
- nuclear QØ7.8
- organ
  - of Corti Q16.5
  - or site not listed — *see* Anomaly, by site
- osseous meatus (ear) Q16.1
- ovary
  - bilateral Q5Ø.Ø2
  - unilateral Q5Ø.Ø1
- oviduct Q5Ø.6
- pancreas Q45.Ø
- parathyroid (gland) Q89.2
- parotid gland(s) Q38.4
- patella Q74.1
- pelvic girdle (complete) (partial) Q74.2
- penis Q55.5
- pericardium Q24.8
- pituitary (gland) Q89.2
- prostate Q55.4
- punctum lacrimale Q1Ø.4
- radioulnar — *see* Defect, reduction, upper limb
- radius — *see* Defect, reduction, upper limb, longitudinal, radius

Agenesis — *continued*
- rectum Q42.1
  - with fistula Q42.Ø
- renal Q6Ø.2
  - bilateral Q6Ø.1
  - unilateral Q6Ø.Ø
- respiratory organ NEC Q34.8
- rib Q76.6
- roof of orbit Q75.8
- round ligament Q52.8
- sacrum Q76.49
- salivary gland Q38.4
- scapula Q74.Ø
- scrotum Q55.29
- seminal vesicles Q55.4
- septum
  - atrial Q21.19
  - between aorta and pulmonary artery Q21.4
  - ventricular Q2Ø.4
- shoulder girdle (complete) (partial) Q74.Ø
- skull (bone) Q75.8
  - with
    - anencephaly QØØ.Ø
    - encephalocele — *see* Encephalocele
    - hydrocephalus QØ3.9
      - with spina bifida — *see* Spina bifida, by site, with hydrocephalus
    - microcephaly QØ2
- spermatic cord Q55.4
- spinal cord QØ6.Ø
- spine Q76.49
- spleen Q89.Ø1
- sternum Q76.7
- stomach Q4Ø.2
- submaxillary gland(s) (congenital) Q38.4
- tarsus — *see* Agenesis, foot
- tendon Q79.8
- testicle Q55.Ø
- thymus (gland) Q89.2
- thyroid (gland) EØ3.1
  - cartilage Q31.8
- tibia — *see* Defect, reduction, lower limb, longitudinal, tibia
- tibiofibular — *see* Defect, reduction, lower limb, specified type NEC
- toe (and foot) (complete) (partial) — *see* Agenesis, foot
- tongue Q38.3
- trachea (cartilage) Q32.1
- ulna — *see* Defect, reduction, upper limb, longitudinal, ulna
- upper limb — *see* Agenesis, arm
- ureter Q62.4
- urethra Q64.5
- urinary tract NEC Q64.8
- uterus Q51.Ø
- uvula Q38.5
- vagina Q52.Ø
- vas deferens Q55.4
- vein(s) (peripheral) Q27.9
  - brain Q28.3
  - great NEC Q26.8
  - portal Q26.5
- vena cava (inferior) (superior) Q26.8
- vermis of cerebellum QØ4.3
- vertebra Q76.49
- vulva Q52.71

Ageusia R43.2

Agitated — *see* condition

Agitation R45.1

Aglossia (congenital) Q38.3

Aglossia-adactylia syndrome Q87.Ø

Aglycogenosis E74.ØØ

Agnosia (body image) (other senses) (tactile) R48.1
- developmental F88
- verbal R48.1
  - auditory R48.1
    - developmental F8Ø.2
  - developmental F8Ø.2
- visual (object) R48.3

Agoraphobia F4Ø.ØØ
- with panic disorder F4Ø.Ø1
- without panic disorder F4Ø.Ø2

Agrammatism R48.8

Agranulocytopenia — *see* Agranulocytosis

Agranulocytosis (chronic) (cyclical) (genetic) (infantile) (periodic) (pernicious) — *see also* Neutropenia D7Ø.9
- congenital D7Ø.Ø

Index

Aftercare — Agranulocytosis

- **Agranulocytosis** — *continued*
  - cytoreductive cancer chemotherapy sequela D7Ø.1
  - drug-induced D7Ø.2
    - due to cytoreductive cancer chemotherapy D7Ø.1
  - due to infection D7Ø.3
  - secondary D7Ø.4
    - drug-induced D7Ø.2
      - due to cytoreductive cancer chemotherapy D7Ø.1
- **Agraphia** (absolute) R48.8
  - with alexia R48.Ø
  - developmental F81.81
- **Ague** (dumb) — *see* Malaria
- **Agyria** QØ4.3
- **Ahumada-del Castillo syndrome** E23.Ø
- **Aichomophobia** F4Ø.298
- **AIDS** (related complex) B2Ø
- **Ailment heart** — *see* Disease, heart
- **Ailurophobia** F4Ø.218
- **AIN** — *see* Neoplasia, intraepithelial, anal
- **Ainhum** (disease) L94.6
- **AIPHI** (acute idiopathic pulmonary hemorrhage in infants (over 28 days old)) RØ4.81
- **Air**
  - anterior mediastinum J98.2
  - compressed, disease T7Ø.3 ☑
  - conditioner lung or pneumonitis J67.7
  - embolism (artery) (cerebral) (any site) T79.Ø ☑
    - with ectopic or molar pregnancy OØ8.2
    - due to implanted device NEC — *see* Complications, by site and type, specified NEC
    - following
      - abortion — *see* Abortion by type, complicated by, embolism
      - ectopic or molar pregnancy OØ8.2
      - infusion, therapeutic injection or transfusion T8Ø.Ø ☑
    - in pregnancy, childbirth or puerperium — *see* Embolism, obstetric
    - traumatic T79.Ø ☑
  - hunger, psychogenic F45.8
  - rarefied, effects of — *see* Effect, adverse, high altitude
  - sickness T75.3 ☑
- **Airplane sickness** T75.3 ☑
- **Akathisia** (drug-induced) (treatment-induced) G25.71
  - neuroleptic induced (acute) G25.71
  - tardive G25.71
- **Akinesia** R29.898
- **Akinetic mutism** R41.89
- **Akureyri's disease** G93.39
- **Alactasia, congenital** E73.Ø
- **Alagille's syndrome** Q44.7
- **Alastrim** BØ3
- **Albers-Schönberg syndrome** Q78.2
- **Albert's syndrome** — *see* Tendinitis, Achilles
- **Albinism, albino** E7Ø.3Ø
  - with hematologic abnormality E7Ø.339
    - Chédiak-Higashi syndrome E7Ø.33Ø
    - Hermansky-Pudlak syndrome E7Ø.331
    - other specified E7Ø.338
  - I E7Ø.32Ø
  - II E7Ø.321
  - ocular E7Ø.319
    - autosomal recessive E7Ø.311
    - other specified E7Ø.318
    - X-linked E7Ø.31Ø
  - oculocutaneous E7Ø.329
    - other specified E7Ø.328
    - tyrosinase (ty) negative E7Ø.32Ø
    - tyrosinase (ty) positive E7Ø.321
  - other specified E7Ø.39
- **Albinismus** E7Ø.3Ø
- **Albright** (-McCune)(-Sternberg) syndrome Q78.1
- **Albuminous** — *see* condition
- **Albuminuria, albuminuric** (acute) (chronic) (subacute) — *see also* Proteinuria R8Ø.9
  - complicating pregnancy — *see* Proteinuria, gestational
    - with
      - gestational hypertension — *see* Pre-eclampsia
      - pre-existing hypertension — *see* Hypertension, complicating pregnancy, pre-existing, with, pre-eclampsia
  - gestational — *see* Proteinuria, gestational
    - with
      - gestational hypertension — *see* Pre-eclampsia
      - pre-existing hypertension — *see* Hypertension, complicating pregnancy, pre-existing, with, pre-eclampsia
- **Albuminuria, albuminuric** — *continued*
  - orthostatic R8Ø.2
  - postural R8Ø.2
  - pre-eclamptic — *see* Pre-eclampsia
  - scarlatinal A38.8
- **Albuminurophobia** F4Ø.298
- **Alcaptonuria** E7Ø.29
- **Alcohol, alcoholic, alcohol-induced**
  - addiction (without remission) F1Ø.2Ø
    - with remission F1Ø.21
  - amnestic disorder, persisting F1Ø.96
    - with dependence F1Ø.26
  - anxiety disorder F1Ø.98Ø
  - bipolar and related disorder F1Ø.94
  - brain syndrome, chronic F1Ø.97
    - with dependence F1Ø.27
  - cardiopathy I42.6
  - counseling and surveillance Z71.41
    - family member Z71.42
  - delirium (acute) (tremens) (withdrawal) F1Ø.921
    - with intoxication F1Ø.921
    - in
      - abuse F1Ø.121
      - dependence F1Ø.221
    - dependence (acute) (tremens) (withdrawal) F1Ø.231
  - dementia F1Ø.97
    - with dependence F1Ø.27
  - depressive disorder F1Ø.94
  - deterioration F1Ø.97
    - with dependence F1Ø.27
  - hallucinosis (acute) F1Ø.951
    - in
      - abuse F1Ø.151
      - dependence F1Ø.251
  - insanity F1Ø.959
  - intoxication (acute) (without dependence) F1Ø.129
    - with
      - delirium F1Ø.121
      - dependence F1Ø.229
        - with delirium F1Ø.221
        - uncomplicated F1Ø.22Ø
    - uncomplicated F1Ø.12Ø
  - jealousy F1Ø.988
  - Korsakoff's, Korsakov's, Korsakow's F1Ø.26
  - liver K7Ø.9
    - acute — *see* Disease, liver, alcoholic, hepatitis
  - major neurocognitive disorder, amnestic-confabulatory type F1Ø.96
  - major neurocognitive disorder, nonamnestic-confabulatory type F1Ø.97
  - mania (acute) (chronic) F1Ø.959
  - mild neurocognitive disorder F1Ø.988
  - paranoia, paranoid (type) psychosis F1Ø.95Ø
  - pellagra E52
  - poisoning, accidental (acute) NEC — *see* Table of Drugs and Chemicals, alcohol, poisoning
  - psychosis — *see* Psychosis, alcoholic
  - psychotic disorder F1Ø.959
  - sexual dysfunction F1Ø.981
  - sleep disorder F1Ø.982
  - withdrawal (without convulsions) F1Ø.239
    - with delirium F1Ø.231
- **Alcoholism** (chronic) (without remission) F1Ø.2Ø
  - with
    - psychosis — *see* Psychosis, alcoholic
    - remission F1Ø.21
  - Korsakov's F1Ø.96
    - with dependence F1Ø.26
- **Alder** (-Reilly) **anomaly or syndrome** (leukocyte granulation) D72.Ø
- **Aldosteronism** E26.9
  - familial (type I) E26.Ø2
  - glucocorticoid-remediable E26.Ø2
  - primary (due to (bilateral) adrenal hyperplasia) E26.Ø9
  - primary NEC E26.Ø9
  - secondary E26.1
  - specified NEC E26.89
- **Aldosteronoma** D44.1Ø
- **Aldrich** (-Wiskott) **syndrome** (eczema-thrombocytopenia) D82.Ø
- **Alektorophobia** F4Ø.218
- **Aleppo boil** B55.1
- **Aleukemic** — *see* condition
- **Aleukia**
  - congenital D7Ø.Ø
  - hemorrhagica D61.9
    - congenital D61.Ø9
  - splenica D73.1
- **Alexia** R48.Ø
  - developmental F81.Ø
  - secondary to organic lesion R48.Ø
- **Algoneurodystrophy** M89.ØØ
  - ankle M89.Ø7- ☑
  - foot M89.Ø7- ☑
  - forearm M89.Ø3- ☑
  - hand M89.Ø4- ☑
  - lower leg M89.Ø6- ☑
  - multiple sites M89.Ø- ☑
  - shoulder M89.Ø1- ☑
  - specified site NEC M89.Ø8
  - thigh M89.Ø5- ☑
  - upper arm M89.Ø2- ☑
- **Algophobia** F4Ø.298
- **Alienation, mental** — *see* Psychosis
- **Alkalemia** E87.3
- **Alkalosis** E87.3
  - metabolic E87.3
    - with respiratory acidosis E87.4
    - of newborn P74.41
  - respiratory E87.3
- **Alkaptonuria** E7Ø.29
- **Allen-Masters syndrome** N83.8
- **Allergy, allergic** (reaction) (to) T78.4Ø ☑
  - air-borne substance NEC (rhinitis) J3Ø.89
  - alveolitis (extrinsic) J67.9
    - due to
      - Aspergillus clavatus J67.4
      - Cryptostroma corticale J67.6
      - organisms (fungal, thermophilic actinomycete) growing in ventilation (air conditioning) systems J67.7
    - specified type NEC J67.8
  - anaphylactic reaction or shock T78.2 ☑
  - angioneurotic edema T78.3 ☑
  - animal (dander) (epidermal) (hair) (rhinitis) J3Ø.81
  - bee sting (anaphylactic shock) — *see* Toxicity, venom, arthropod, bee
  - biological — *see* Allergy, drug
  - colitis — *see also* Colitis, allergic K52.29
  - dander (animal) (rhinitis) J3Ø.81
  - dandruff (rhinitis) J3Ø.81
  - dental restorative material (existing) KØ8.55
  - dermatitis — *see* Dermatitis, contact, allergic
  - diathesis — *see* History, allergy
  - drug, medicament & biological (any) (external) (internal) T78.4Ø ☑
    - correct substance properly administered — *see* Table of Drugs and Chemicals, by drug, adverse effect
    - wrong substance given or taken NEC (by accident) — *see* Table of Drugs and Chemicals, by drug, poisoning
  - due to pollen J3Ø.1
  - dust (house) (stock) (rhinitis) J3Ø.89
    - with asthma — *see* Asthma, allergic extrinsic
  - eczema — *see* Dermatitis, contact, allergic
  - epidermal (animal) (rhinitis) J3Ø.81
  - feathers (rhinitis) J3Ø.89
  - food (any) (ingested) NEC T78.1 ☑
    - anaphylactic shock — *see* Shock, anaphylactic, due to food
    - dermatitis — *see* Dermatitis, due to, food
    - dietary counseling and surveillance Z71.3
    - in contact with skin L23.6
    - rhinitis J3Ø.5
    - status (without reaction) Z91.Ø18
      - beef Z91.Ø14
      - eggs Z91.Ø12
      - lamb Z91.Ø14
      - mammalian meats Z91.Ø14
      - milk products Z91.Ø11
      - peanuts Z91.Ø1Ø
      - pork Z91.Ø14
      - red meats Z91.Ø14
      - seafood Z91.Ø13
      - specified NEC Z91.Ø18
  - gastrointestinal — *see also* specific type of allergic reaction
    - meaning colitis — *see also* Colitis, allergic K52.29
    - meaning gastroenteritis — *see also* Gastroenteritis, allergic K52.29
    - meaning other adverse food reaction not elsewhere classified T78.1 ☑
  - grain J3Ø.1
  - grass (hay fever) (pollen) J3Ø.1

Allergy, allergic — *continued*
  grass — *continued*
    asthma — *see* Asthma, allergic extrinsic
  hair (animal) (rhinitis) J3Ø.81
  history (of) — *see* History, allergy
  horse serum — *see* Allergy, serum
  inhalant (rhinitis) J3Ø.89
    pollen J3Ø.1
  kapok (rhinitis) J3Ø.89
  medicine — *see* Allergy, drug
  milk protein — *see also* Allergy, food Z91.Ø11
    anaphylactic reaction T78.Ø7 ☑
    dermatitis L27.2
    enterocolitis syndrome K52.21
    enteropathy K52.22
    gastroenteritis K52.29
    gastroesophageal reflux — *see also* Reaction, adverse, food K21.9
      with esophagitis (without bleeding) K21.ØØ
        with bleeding K21.Ø1
    proctocolitis K52.29
  nasal, seasonal due to pollen J3Ø.1
  pneumonia J82.89
  pollen (any) (hay fever) J3Ø.1
    asthma — *see* Asthma, allergic extrinsic
  primrose J3Ø.1
  primula J3Ø.1
  proctocolitis K52.29
  purpura D69.Ø
  ragweed (hay fever) (pollen) J3Ø.1
    asthma — *see* Asthma, allergic extrinsic
  rose (pollen) J3Ø.1
  seasonal NEC J3Ø.2
  Senecio jacobae (pollen) J3Ø.1
  serum — *see also* Reaction, serum T8Ø.69 ☑
    anaphylactic shock T8Ø.59 ☑
  shock (anaphylactic) T78.2 ☑
    due to
      administration of blood and blood products T8Ø.51 ☑
      adverse effect of correct medicinal substance properly administered T88.6 ☑
      immunization T8Ø.52 ☑
      serum NEC T8Ø.59 ☑
      vaccination T8Ø.52 ☑
  specific NEC T78.49 ☑
  tree (any) (hay fever) (pollen) J3Ø.1
    asthma — *see* Asthma, allergic extrinsic
  upper respiratory J3Ø.9
  urticaria L5Ø.Ø
  vaccine — *see* Allergy, serum
  wheat — *see* Allergy, food
Allescheriasis B48.2
Alligator skin disease Q8Ø.9
Allocheiria, allochiria R2Ø.8
Almeida's disease — *see* Paracoccidioidomycosis
Alopecia (hereditaria) (seborrheica) L65.9
  androgenic L64.9
    drug-induced L64.Ø
    specified NEC L64.8
  areata L63.9
    ophiasis L63.2
    specified NEC L63.8
    totalis L63.Ø
    universalis L63.1
  cicatricial L66.9
    specified NEC L66.8
  circumscripta L63.9
  congenital, congenitalis Q84.Ø
  due to cytotoxic drugs NEC L65.8
  mucinosa L65.2
  postinfective NEC L65.8
  postpartum L65.Ø
  premature L64.8
  specific (syphilitic) A51.32
  specified NEC L65.8
  syphilitic (secondary) A51.32
  totalis (capitis) L63.Ø
  universalis (entire body) L63.1
  X-ray L58.1
Alpers' disease G31.81
Alpine sickness T7Ø.29 ☑
Alport syndrome Q87.81
ALTE (apparent life threatening event) **in newborn and infant** R68.13
Alteration (of), **Altered**
  awareness
    transient R4Ø.4
Alteration (of), **Altered** — *continued*
  awareness — *continued*
    unintended under general anesthesia, during procedure T88.53 ☑
  mental status R41.82
  pattern of family relationships affecting child Z62.898
  sensation
    following
      cerebrovascular disease I69.998
        cerebral infarction I69.398
        intracerebral hemorrhage I69.198
        nontraumatic intracranial hemorrhage NEC I69.298
        specified disease NEC I69.898
        subarachnoid hemorrhage I69.Ø98
Alternating — *see* condition
Altitude, high (effects) — *see* Effect, adverse, high altitude
Aluminosis (of lung) J63.Ø
Alveolitis
  allergic (extrinsic) — *see* Pneumonitis, hypersensitivity
  due to
    Aspergillus clavatus J67.4
    Cryptostroma corticale J67.6
  fibrosing (cryptogenic) (idiopathic) J84.112
  jaw M27.3
  sicca dolorosa M27.3
Alveolus, alveolar — *see* condition
Alymphocytosis D72.81Ø
  thymic (with immunodeficiency) D82.1
Alymphoplasia, thymic D82.1
Alzheimer's disease or sclerosis — *see* Disease, Alzheimer's
Amastia (with nipple present) Q83.8
  with absent nipple Q83.Ø
Amathophobia F4Ø.228
Amaurosis (acquired) (congenital) — *see also* Blindness
  fugax G45.3
  hysterical F44.6
  Leber's congenital H35.5Ø
  uremic — *see* Uremia
Amaurotic idiocy (infantile) (juvenile) (late) E75.4
Amaxophobia F4Ø.248
Ambiguous genitalia Q56.4
Amblyopia (congenital) (ex anopsia) (partial) (suppression) H53.ØØ- ☑
  anisometropic — *see* Amblyopia, refractive
  deprivation H53.Ø1- ☑
  hysterical F44.6
  nocturnal — *see also* Blindness, night
    vitamin A deficiency E5Ø.5
  refractive H53.Ø2- ☑
  strabismic H53.Ø3- ☑
  suspect H53.Ø4- ☑
  tobacco H53.8
  toxic NEC H53.8
  uremic — *see* Uremia
Ameba, amebic (histolytica) — *see also* Amebiasis
  abscess (liver) AØ6.4
Amebiasis AØ6.9
  with abscess — *see* Abscess, amebic
  acute AØ6.Ø
  chronic (intestine) AØ6.1
    with abscess — *see* Abscess, amebic
  cutaneous AØ6.7
  cutis AØ6.7
  cystitis AØ6.81
  genitourinary tract NEC AØ6.82
  hepatic — *see* Abscess, liver, amebic
  intestine AØ6.Ø
  nondysenteric colitis AØ6.2
  skin AØ6.7
  specified site NEC AØ6.89
Ameboma (of intestine) AØ6.3
Amelia Q73.Ø
  lower limb — *see* Agenesis, leg
  upper limb — *see* Agenesis, arm
Ameloblastoma — *see also* Cyst, calcifying odontogenic
  long bones C4Ø.9- ☑
    lower limb C4Ø.2- ☑
    upper limb C4Ø.Ø- ☑
  malignant C41.1
    jaw (bone) (lower) C41.1
      upper C41.Ø
  tibial C4Ø.2- ☑
Amelogenesis imperfecta KØØ.5
  nonhereditaria (segmentalis) KØØ.4
Amenorrhea N91.2
  hyperhormonal E28.8
  primary N91.Ø
  secondary N91.1
Amentia — *see* Disability, intellectual
  Meynert's (nonalcoholic) FØ4
American
  leishmaniasis B55.2
  mountain tick fever A93.2
Ametropia — *see* Disorder, refraction
AMH (asymptomatic microscopic hematuria) R31.21
Amianthosis J61
Amimia R48.8
Amino-acid disorder E72.9
  anemia D53.Ø
Aminoacidopathy E72.9
Aminoaciduria E72.9
Amnesia R41.3
  anterograde R41.1
  auditory R48.8
  dissociative F44.Ø
    with dissociative fugue F44.1
  hysterical F44.Ø
  postictal in epilepsy — *see* Epilepsy
  psychogenic F44.Ø
  retrograde R41.2
  transient global G45.4
Amnes(t)ic syndrome (post-traumatic) FØ4
  induced by
    alcohol F1Ø.96
      with dependence F1Ø.26
    psychoactive NEC F19.96
      with
        abuse F19.16
        dependence F19.26
    sedative F13.96
      with dependence F13.26
Amnion, amniotic — *see* condition
Amnionitis — *see* Pregnancy, complicated by
Amok F68.8
Amoral traits F6Ø.89
Amphetamine (or other stimulant) **-induced**
  anxiety disorder F15.98Ø
  bipolar and related disorder F15.94
  delirium F15.921
  depressive disorder F15.94
  obsessive-compulsive and related disorder F15.988
  psychotic disorder F15.959
  sexual dysfunction F15.981
  sleep disorder F15.982
  stimulant withdrawal F15.23
Ampulla
  lower esophagus K22.89
  phrenic K22.89
Amputation — *see also* Absence, by site, acquired
  neuroma (postoperative) (traumatic) — *see* Complications, amputation stump, neuroma
  stump (surgical)
    abnormal, painful, or with complication (late) — *see* Complications, amputation stump
    healed or old NOS Z89.9
  traumatic (complete) (partial)
    arm (upper) (complete) S48.91- ☑
      at
        elbow S58.Ø1- ☑
          partial S58.Ø2- ☑
        shoulder joint (complete) S48.Ø1- ☑
          partial S48.Ø2- ☑
      between
        elbow and wrist (complete) S58.11- ☑
          partial S58.12- ☑
        shoulder and elbow (complete) S48.11- ☑
          partial S48.12- ☑
      partial S48.92- ☑
    breast (complete) S28.21- ☑
      partial S28.22- ☑
    clitoris (complete) S38.211 ☑
      partial S38.212 ☑
    ear (complete) SØ8.11- ☑
      partial SØ8.12- ☑
    finger (complete) (metacarpophalangeal) S68.11- ☑
      index S68.11- ☑
      little S68.11- ☑
      middle S68.11- ☑
      partial S68.12- ☑
        index S68.12- ☑
        little S68.12- ☑

- **Amputation** — *continued*
  - traumatic — *continued*
    - finger — *continued*
      - partial — *continued*
        - middle S68.12- ☑
        - ring S68.12- ☑
      - ring S68.11- ☑
      - thumb — *see* Amputation, traumatic, thumb
      - transphalangeal (complete) S68.61- ☑
        - index S68.61- ☑
        - little S68.61- ☑
        - middle S68.61- ☑
        - partial S68.62- ☑
          - index S68.62- ☑
          - little S68.62- ☑
          - middle S68.62- ☑
          - ring S68.62- ☑
        - ring S68.61- ☑
    - foot (complete) S98.91- ☑
      - at ankle level S98.Ø1- ☑
        - partial S98.Ø2- ☑
      - midfoot S98.31- ☑
        - partial S98.32- ☑
      - partial S98.92- ☑
    - forearm (complete) S58.91- ☑
      - at elbow level (complete) S58.Ø1- ☑
        - partial S58.Ø2- ☑
      - between elbow and wrist (complete) S58.11- ☑
        - partial S58.12- ☑
      - partial S58.92- ☑
    - genital organ(s) (external)
      - female (complete) S38.211 ☑
        - partial S38.212 ☑
      - male
        - penis (complete) S38.221 ☑
          - partial S38.222 ☑
        - scrotum (complete) S38.231 ☑
          - partial S38.232 ☑
        - testes (complete) S38.231 ☑
          - partial S38.232 ☑
    - hand (complete) (wrist level) S68.41- ☑
      - finger(s) alone — *see* Amputation, traumatic, finger
      - partial S68.42- ☑
      - thumb alone — *see* Amputation, traumatic, thumb
      - transmetacarpal (complete) S68.71- ☑
        - partial S68.72- ☑
    - head
      - ear — *see* Amputation, traumatic, ear
      - nose (partial) SØ8.812 ☑
        - complete SØ8.811 ☑
      - part SØ8.89 ☑
      - scalp SØ8.Ø ☑
    - hip (and thigh) (complete) S78.91- ☑
      - at hip joint (complete) S78.Ø1- ☑
        - partial S78.Ø2- ☑
      - between hip and knee (complete) S78.11- ☑
        - partial S78.12- ☑
      - partial S78.92- ☑
    - labium (majus) (minus) (complete) S38.21- ☑
      - partial S38.21- ☑
    - leg (lower) S88.91- ☑
      - at knee level S88.Ø1- ☑
        - partial S88.Ø2- ☑
      - between knee and ankle S88.11- ☑
        - partial S88.12- ☑
      - partial S88.92- ☑
    - nose (partial) SØ8.812 ☑
      - complete SØ8.811 ☑
    - penis (complete) S38.221 ☑
      - partial S38.222 ☑
    - scrotum (complete) S38.231 ☑
      - partial S38.232 ☑
    - shoulder — *see* Amputation, traumatic, arm
      - at shoulder joint — *see* Amputation, traumatic, arm, at shoulder joint
    - testes (complete) S38.231 ☑
      - partial S38.232 ☑
    - thigh — *see* Amputation, traumatic, hip
    - thorax, part of S28.1 ☑
      - breast — *see* Amputation, traumatic, breast
    - thumb (complete) (metacarpophalangeal) S68.Ø1- ☑
      - partial S68.Ø2- ☑
      - transphalangeal (complete) S68.51- ☑

- **Amputation** — *continued*
  - traumatic — *continued*
    - thumb — *continued*
      - transphalangeal — *continued*
        - partial S68.52- ☑
    - toe (lesser) S98.13- ☑
      - great S98.11- ☑
        - partial S98.12- ☑
      - more than one S98.21- ☑
        - partial S98.22- ☑
      - partial S98.14- ☑
    - vulva (complete) S38.211 ☑
      - partial S38.212 ☑
- **Amputee** (bilateral) (old) Z89.9
- **Amsterdam dwarfism** Q87.19
- **Amusia** R48.8
  - developmental F8Ø.89
- **Amyelencephalus, amyelencephaly** QØØ.Ø
- **Amyelia** QØ6.Ø
- **Amygdalitis** — *see* Tonsillitis
- **Amygdalolith** J35.8
- **Amyloid heart** (disease) E85.4 *[I43]*
- **Amyloidosis** (generalized) (primary) E85.9
  - with lung involvement E85.4 *[J99]*
  - familial E85.2
  - genetic E85.2
  - heart E85.4 *[I43]*
  - hemodialysis-associated E85.3
  - light chain (AL) E85.81
  - liver E85.4 *[K77]*
  - localized E85.4
  - neuropathic heredofamilial E85.1
  - non-neuropathic heredofamilial E85.Ø
  - organ limited E85.4
  - Portuguese E85.1
  - pulmonary E85.4 *[J99]*
  - secondary systemic E85.3
  - senile systemic (SSA) E85.82
  - skin (lichen) (macular) E85.4 *[L99]*
  - specified NEC E85.89
  - subglottic E85.4 *[J99]*
  - wild-type transthyretin-related (ATTR) E85.82
- **Amylopectinosis** (brancher enzyme deficiency) E74.Ø3
- **Amylophagia** — *see* Pica
- **Amyoplasia congenita** Q79.8
- **Amyotonia** M62.89
  - congenita G7Ø.2
- **Amyotrophia, amyotrophy, amyotrophic** G71.8
  - congenita Q79.8
  - diabetic — *see* Diabetes, amyotrophy
  - lateral sclerosis G12.21
  - neuralgic G54.5
  - spinal progressive G12.25
- **Anacidity, gastric** K31.83
  - psychogenic F45.8
- **Anaerosis of newborn** P28.89
- **Analbuminemia** E88.Ø9
- **Analgesia** — *see* Anesthesia
- **Analphalipoproteinemia** E78.6
- **Anaphylactic**
  - purpura D69.Ø
  - shock or reaction — *see* Shock, anaphylactic
- **Anaphylactoid shock or reaction** — *see* Shock, anaphylactic
- **Anaphylactoid syndrome of pregnancy** O88.Ø1- ☑
- **Anaphylaxis** — *see* Shock, anaphylactic
- **Anaplasia cervix** — *see also* Dysplasia, cervix N87.9
- **Anaplasmosis** [A. phagocytophilum] (transfusion transmitted) A79.82
  - human A77.49
- **Anarthria** R47.1
- **Anasarca** R6Ø.1
  - cardiac — *see* Failure, heart, congestive
  - lung J18.2
  - newborn P83.2
  - nutritional E43
  - pulmonary J18.2
  - renal NØ4.9
- **Anastomosis**
  - aneurysmal — *see* Aneurysm
  - arteriovenous ruptured brain I6Ø.8
    - intracerebral I61.8
    - intraparenchymal I61.8
    - intraventricular I61.5
    - subarachnoid I6Ø.8
  - intestinal K63.89
    - complicated NEC K91.89

- **Anastomosis** — *continued*
  - intestinal — *continued*
    - complicated — *continued*
      - involving urinary tract N99.89
  - retinal and choroidal vessels (congenital) Q14.8
- **Anatomical narrow angle** H4Ø.Ø3- ☑
- **Ancylostoma, ancylostomiasis** (braziliense) (caninum) (ceylanicum) (duodenale) B76.Ø
  - Necator americanus B76.1
- **Andersen's disease** (glycogen storage) E74.Ø9
- **Anderson-Fabry disease** E75.21
- **Andes disease** T7Ø.29 ☑
- **Andrews' disease** (bacterid) LØ8.89
- **Androblastoma**
  - benign
    - specified site — *see* Neoplasm, benign, by site
    - unspecified site
      - female D27.9
      - male D29.2Ø
  - malignant
    - specified site — *see* Neoplasm, malignant, by site
    - unspecified site
      - female C56.9
      - male C62.9Ø
  - specified site — *see* Neoplasm, uncertain behavior, by site
  - tubular
    - with lipid storage
      - specified site — *see* Neoplasm, benign, by site
      - unspecified site
        - female D27.9
        - male D29.2Ø
    - specified site — *see* Neoplasm, benign, by site
    - unspecified site
      - female D27.9
      - male D29.2Ø
  - unspecified site
    - female D39.1Ø
    - male D4Ø.1Ø
- **Androgen insensitivity syndrome** — *see also* Syndrome, androgen insensitivity E34.5Ø
- **Androgen resistance syndrome** — *see also* Syndrome, androgen insensitivity E34.5Ø
- **Android pelvis** Q74.2
  - with disproportion (fetopelvic) O33.3 ☑
    - causing obstructed labor O65.3
- **Androphobia** F4Ø.29Ø
- **Anectasis, pulmonary** (newborn) — *see* Atelectasis
- **Anemia** (essential) (general) (hemoglobin deficiency) (infantile) (primary) (profound) D64.9
  - with (due to) (in)
    - disorder of
      - anaerobic glycolysis D55.29
      - pentose phosphate pathway D55.1
    - koilonychia D5Ø.9
  - achlorhydric D5Ø.8
  - achrestic D53.1
  - Addison (-Biermer) (pernicious) D51.Ø
  - agranulocytic — *see* Agranulocytosis
  - amino-acid-deficiency D53.Ø
  - aplastic D61.9
    - congenital D61.Ø9
    - drug-induced D61.1
    - due to
      - drugs D61.1
      - external agents NEC D61.2
      - infection D61.2
      - radiation D61.2
    - idiopathic D61.3
    - red cell (pure) D6Ø.9
      - chronic D6Ø.Ø
      - congenital D61.Ø1
      - specified type NEC D6Ø.8
      - transient D6Ø.1
    - specified type NEC D61.89
    - toxic D61.2
  - aregenerative
    - congenital D61.Ø9
  - asiderotic D5Ø.9
  - atypical (primary) D64.9
  - Baghdad spring D55.Ø
  - Balantidium coli AØ7.Ø
  - Biermer's (pernicious) D51.Ø
  - blood loss (chronic) D5Ø.Ø
    - acute D62
  - bothriocephalus B7Ø.Ø *[D63.8]*
  - brickmaker's B76.9 *[D63.8]*
  - cerebral I67.89

Anemia — *continued*
  childhood D58.9
  chlorotic D5Ø.8
  chronic
    blood loss D5Ø.Ø
    hemolytic D58.9
      idiopathic D59.9
    simple D53.9
  chronica congenita aregenerativa D61.Ø9
  combined system disease NEC D51.Ø *[G32.Ø]*
    due to dietary vitamin B12 deficiency D51.3 *[G32.Ø]*
  complicating pregnancy, childbirth or puerperium — *see* Pregnancy, complicated by (management affected by), anemia
  congenital P61.4
    aplastic D61.Ø9
    due to isoimmunization NOS P55.9
    dyserythropoietic, dyshematopoietic D64.4
    following fetal blood loss P61.3
    Heinz body D58.2
    hereditary hemolytic NOS D58.9
    pernicious D51.Ø
    spherocytic D58.Ø
  Cooley's (erythroblastic) D56.1
  cytogenic D51.Ø
  deficiency D53.9
    2, 3 diphosphoglycurate mutase D55.29
    2, 3 PG D55.29
    6 phosphogluconate dehydrogenase D55.1
    6-PGD D55.1
    amino-acid D53.Ø
    combined B12 and folate D53.1
    enzyme D55.9
      drug-induced (hemolytic) D59.2
      glucose-6-phosphate dehydrogenase (G6PD) D55.Ø
      glycolytic D55.29
      nucleotide metabolism D55.3
      related to hexose monophosphate (HMP) shunt pathway NEC D55.1
      specified type NEC D55.8
    erythrocytic glutathione D55.1
    folate D52.9
      dietary D52.Ø
      drug-induced D52.1
    folic acid D52.9
      dietary D52.Ø
      drug-induced D52.1
    G SH D55.1
    G6PD D55.Ø
    GGS-R D55.1
    glucose-6-phosphate dehydrogenase D55.Ø
    glutathione reductase D55.1
    glyceraldehyde phosphate dehydrogenase D55.29
    hexokinase D55.29
    iron D5Ø.9
      secondary to blood loss (chronic) D5Ø.Ø
    nutritional D53.9
      with
        poor iron absorption D5Ø.8
        specified deficiency NEC D53.8
    phosphofructo-aldolase D55.29
    phosphoglycerate kinase D55.29
    PK D55.21
    protein D53.Ø
    pyruvate kinase D55.21
    transcobalamin II D51.2
    triose-phosphate isomerase D55.29
    vitamin B12 NOS D51.9
      dietary D51.3
      due to
        intrinsic factor deficiency D51.Ø
        selective vitamin B12 malabsorption with proteinuria D51.1
      pernicious D51.Ø
      specified type NEC D51.8
  Diamond-Blackfan (congenital hypoplastic) D61.Ø1
  dibothriocephalus B7Ø.Ø *[D63.8]*
  dimorphic D53.1
  diphasic D53.1
  Diphyllobothrium (Dibothriocephalus) B7Ø.Ø *[D63.8]*
  due to (in) (with)
    antineoplastic chemotherapy D64.81
    blood loss (chronic) D5Ø.Ø
      acute D62
    chemotherapy, antineoplastic D64.81
    chronic disease classified elsewhere NEC D63.8
    chronic kidney disease D63.1

Anemia — *continued*
  due to — *continued*
    deficiency
      amino-acid D53.Ø
      copper D53.8
      folate (folic acid) D52.9
        dietary D52.Ø
        drug-induced D52.1
      molybdenum D53.8
      protein D53.Ø
      zinc D53.8
    dietary vitamin B12 deficiency D51.3
    disorder of
      glutathione metabolism D55.1
      nucleotide metabolism D55.3
    drug — *see* Anemia, by type — *see also* Table of Drugs and Chemicals
    end stage renal disease D63.1
    enzyme disorder D55.9
    fetal blood loss P61.3
    fish tapeworm (D.latum) infestation B7Ø.Ø *[D63.8]*
    hemorrhage (chronic) D5Ø.Ø
      acute D62
    impaired absorption D5Ø.9
    loss of blood (chronic) D5Ø.Ø
      acute D62
    myxedema EØ3.9 *[D63.8]*
    Necator americanus B76.1 *[D63.8]*
    prematurity P61.2
    selective vitamin B12 malabsorption with proteinuria D51.1
    transcobalamin II deficiency D51.2
  Dyke-Young type (secondary) (symptomatic) D59.19
  dyserythropoietic (congenital) D64.4
  dyshematopoietic (congenital) D64.4
  Egyptian B76.9 *[D63.8]*
  elliptocytosis — *see* Elliptocytosis
  enzyme-deficiency, drug-induced D59.2
  epidemic — *see also* Ancylostomiasis B76.9 *[D63.8]*
  erythroblastic
    familial D56.1
    newborn — *see also* Disease, hemolytic P55.9
    of childhood D56.1
  erythrocytic glutathione deficiency D55.1
  erythropoietin-resistant anemia (EPO resistant anemia) D63.1
  Faber's (achlorhydric anemia) D5Ø.9
  factitious (self-induced blood letting) D5Ø.Ø
  familial erythroblastic D56.1
  Fanconi's (congenital pancytopenia) D61.Ø9
  favism D55.Ø
  fish tapeworm (D. latum) infestation B7Ø.Ø *[D63.8]*
  folate (folic acid) deficiency D52.9
  glucose-6-phosphate dehydrogenase (G6PD) deficiency D55.Ø
  glutathione-reductase deficiency D55.1
  goat's milk D52.Ø
  granulocytic — *see* Agranulocytosis
  Heinz body, congenital D58.2
  hemolytic D58.9
    acquired D59.9
      with hemoglobinuria NEC D59.6
      autoimmune NEC D59.19
      infectious D59.4
      specified type NEC D59.8
      toxic D59.4
    acute D59.9
      due to enzyme deficiency specified type NEC D55.8
      Lederer's D59.19
    autoimmune D59.1Ø
      cold D59.12
      drug-induced D59.Ø
      mixed D59.13
      warm D59.11
    chronic D58.9
      idiopathic D59.9
    cold type (primary) (secondary) (symptomatic) D59.12
    congenital (spherocytic) — *see* Spherocytosis
    due to
      cardiac conditions D59.4
      drugs (nonautoimmune) D59.2
        autoimmune D59.Ø
      enzyme disorder D55.9
        drug-induced D59.2
      presence of shunt or other internal prosthetic device D59.4

Anemia — *continued*
  hemolytic — *continued*
    familial D58.9
    hereditary D58.9
      due to enzyme disorder D55.9
        specified type NEC D55.8
      specified type NEC D58.8
    idiopathic (chronic) D59.9
    mechanical D59.4
    microangiopathic D59.4
    mixed type (primary) (secondary) (symptomatic) D59.13
    nonautoimmune D59.4
      drug-induced D59.2
    nonspherocytic
      congenital or hereditary NEC D55.8
        glucose-6-phosphate dehydrogenase deficiency D55.Ø
        pyruvate kinase deficiency D55.21
        type
          I D55.1
          II D55.29
      type
        I D55.1
        II D55.29
    primary
      autoimmune
        cold type D59.12
        mixed type D59.13
        warm type D59.11
    secondary D59.4
      autoimmune
        cold type D59.12
        mixed type D59.13
        warm type D59.11
    specified (hereditary) type NEC D58.8
    Stransky-Regala type — *see also* Hemoglobinopathy D58.8
    symptomatic D59.4
      autoimmune
        cold type D59.12
        mixed type D59.13
        warm type D59.11
    toxic D59.4
    warm type (primary) (secondary) (symptomatic) D59.11
  hemorrhagic (chronic) D5Ø.Ø
    acute D62
  Herrick's D57.1
  hexokinase deficiency D55.29
  hookworm B76.9 *[D63.8]*
  hypochromic (idiopathic) (microcytic) (normoblastic) D5Ø.9
    due to blood loss (chronic) D5Ø.Ø
      acute D62
    familial sex-linked D64.Ø
    pyridoxine-responsive D64.3
    sideroblastic, sex-linked D64.Ø
  hypoplasia, red blood cells D61.9
    congenital or familial D61.Ø1
  hypoplastic (idiopathic) D61.9
    congenital or familial (of childhood) D61.Ø1
  hypoproliferative (refractive) D61.9
  idiopathic D64.9
    aplastic D61.3
    hemolytic, chronic D59.9
  in (due to) (with)
    chronic kidney disease D63.1
    end stage renal disease D63.1
    failure, kidney (renal) D63.1
    neoplastic disease — *see also* Neoplasm D63.Ø
  intertropical — *see also* Ancylostomiasis D63.8
  iron deficiency D5Ø.9
    secondary to blood loss (chronic) D5Ø.Ø
      acute D62
    specified type NEC D5Ø.8
  Joseph-Diamond-Blackfan (congenital hypoplastic) D61.Ø1
  Lederer's (hemolytic) D59.19
  leukoerythroblastic D61.82
  macrocytic D53.9
    nutritional D52.Ø
    tropical D52.8
  malarial — *see also* Malaria B54 *[D63.8]*
  malignant (progressive) D51.Ø
  malnutrition D53.9
  marsh — *see also* Malaria B54 *[D63.8]*
  Mediterranean (with other hemoglobinopathy) D56.9
  megaloblastic D53.1

- **Anemia** — *continued*
  - megaloblastic — *continued*
    - combined B12 and folate deficiency D53.1
    - hereditary D51.1
    - nutritional D52.Ø
    - orotic aciduria D53.Ø
    - refractory D53.1
    - specified type NEC D53.1
  - megalocytic D53.1
  - microcytic (hypochromic) D5Ø.9
    - due to blood loss (chronic) D5Ø.Ø
      - acute D62
    - familial D56.8
  - microdrepanocytosis D57.4Ø
  - microelliptopoikilocytic (Rietti-Greppi- Micheli) D56.9
  - miner's B76.9 *[D63.8]*
  - myelodysplastic D46.9
  - myelofibrosis D75.81
  - myelogenous D64.89
  - myelopathic D64.89
  - myelophthisic D61.82
  - myeloproliferative D47.Z9 (*following* D47.4)
  - newborn P61.4
    - due to
      - ABO (antibodies, isoimmunization, maternal/fetal incompatibility) P55.1
      - Rh (antibodies, isoimmunization, maternal/fetal incompatibility) P55.Ø
    - following fetal blood loss P61.3
    - posthemorrhagic (fetal) P61.3
  - nonspherocytic hemolytic — *see* Anemia, hemolytic, nonspherocytic
  - normocytic (infectional) D64.9
    - due to blood loss (chronic) D5Ø.Ø
      - acute D62
    - myelophthisic D61.82
  - nutritional (deficiency) D53.9
    - with
      - poor iron absorption D5Ø.8
      - specified deficiency NEC D53.8
    - megaloblastic D52.Ø
  - of prematurity P61.2
  - orotaciduric (congenital) (hereditary) D53.Ø
  - osteosclerotic D64.89
  - ovalocytosis (hereditary) — *see* Elliptocytosis
  - paludal — *see also* Malaria B54 *[D63.8]*
  - pernicious (congenital) (malignant) (progressive) D51.Ø
  - pleochromic D64.89
    - of sprue D52.8
  - posthemorrhagic (chronic) D5Ø.Ø
    - acute D62
    - newborn P61.3
  - postoperative (postprocedural)
    - due to (acute) blood loss D62
      - chronic blood loss D5Ø.Ø
    - specified NEC D64.89
  - postpartum O9Ø.81
  - pressure D64.89
  - progressive D64.9
    - malignant D51.Ø
    - pernicious D51.Ø
  - protein-deficiency D53.Ø
  - pseudoleukemica infantum D64.89
  - pure red cell D6Ø.9
    - congenital D61.Ø1
  - pyridoxine-responsive D64.3
  - pyruvate kinase deficiency D55.21
  - refractory D46.4
    - with
      - excess of blasts D46.2Ø
        - 1 (RAEB 1) D46.21
        - 2 (RAEB 2) D46.22
        - in transformation (RAEB T) — *see* Leukemia, acute myeloblastic
      - hemochromatosis D46.1
      - sideroblasts (ring) (RARS) D46.1
    - megaloblastic D53.1
    - sideroblastic D46.1
    - sideropenic D5Ø.9
    - without ring sideroblasts, so stated D46.Ø
    - without sideroblasts without excess of blasts D46.Ø
  - Rietti-Greppi-Micheli D56.9
  - scorbutic D53.2
  - secondary to
    - blood loss (chronic) D5Ø.Ø
      - acute D62
    - hemorrhage (chronic) D5Ø.Ø
      - acute D62
  - semiplastic D61.89
  - sickle-cell — *see* Disease, sickle-cell
  - sideroblastic D64.3
    - hereditary D64.Ø
    - hypochromic, sex-linked D64.Ø
    - pyridoxine-responsive NEC D64.3
    - refractory D46.1
    - secondary (due to)
      - disease D64.1
      - drugs and toxins D64.2
    - specified type NEC D64.3
  - sideropenic (refractory) D5Ø.9
    - due to blood loss (chronic) D5Ø.Ø
      - acute D62
  - simple chronic D53.9
  - specified type NEC D64.89
  - spherocytic (hereditary) — *see* Spherocytosis
  - splenic D64.89
  - splenomegalic D64.89
  - stomatocytosis D58.8
  - syphilitic (acquired) (late) A52.79 *[D63.8]*
  - target cell D64.89
  - thalassemia D56.9
  - thrombocytopenic — *see* Thrombocytopenia
  - toxic D61.2
  - tropical B76.9 *[D63.8]*
    - macrocytic D52.8
  - tuberculous A18.89 *[D63.8]*
  - vegan D51.3
  - vitamin
    - B12 deficiency (dietary) pernicious D51.Ø
    - B6-responsive D64.3
  - von Jaksch's D64.89
  - Witts' (achlorhydric anemia) D5Ø.8
- **Anemophobia** F4Ø.228
- **Anencephalus, anencephaly** QØØ.Ø
- **Anergasia** — *see* Psychosis, organic
- **Anesthesia, anesthetic** R2Ø.Ø
  - complication or reaction NEC — *see also* Complications, anesthesia T88.59 ☑
    - due to
      - correct substance properly administered — *see* Table of Drugs and Chemicals, by drug, adverse effect
      - overdose or wrong substance given — *see* Table of Drugs and Chemicals, by drug, poisoning
    - unintended awareness under general anesthesia during procedure T88.53 ☑
      - personal history of Z92.84
  - cornea H18.81- ☑
  - dissociative F44.6
  - functional (hysterical) F44.6
  - hyperesthetic, thalamic G89.Ø
  - hysterical F44.6
  - local skin lesion R2Ø.Ø
  - sexual (psychogenic) F52.1
  - shock (due to) T88.2 ☑
  - skin R2Ø.Ø
  - testicular N5Ø.9
- **Anetoderma** (maculosum) (of) L9Ø.8
  - Jadassohn-Pellizzari L9Ø.2
  - Schweniger-Buzzi L9Ø.1
- **Aneurin deficiency** E51.9
- **Aneurysm** (anastomotic) (artery) (cirsoid) (diffuse) (false) (fusiform) (multiple) (saccular) I72.9
  - abdominal (aorta) I71.4Ø
    - infrarenal I71.43
      - ruptured I71.33
    - juxtarenal I71.42
      - ruptured I71.32
    - pararenal I71.41
      - ruptured I71.31
    - ruptured I71.3Ø
    - syphilitic A52.Ø1
  - aorta, aortic (nonsyphilitic) I71.9
    - abdominal I71.4Ø
      - dissecting — *see* Dissection, aorta, abdominal
      - ruptured I71.3Ø
    - arch I71.22
      - ruptured I71.12
    - arteriosclerotic I71.9
      - ruptured I71.8
    - ascending I71.21
      - ruptured I71.11
    - congenital Q25.43
    - descending I71.9
      - abdominal I71.4Ø
- **Aneurysm** — *continued*
  - aorta, aortic — *continued*
    - descending — *continued*
      - abdominal — *continued*
        - ruptured I71.3Ø
      - ruptured I71.8
      - thoracic I71.23
        - ruptured I71.13
    - dissecting — *see* Dissection, aorta
    - root Q25.43
    - ruptured I71.8
    - sinus, congenital Q25.43
    - syphilitic A52.Ø1
    - thoracic I71.2Ø
      - ruptured I71.1Ø
    - thoracoabdominal I71.6Ø
      - paravisceral I71.62
        - ruptured I71.52
      - ruptured I71.5Ø
      - supraceliac I71.61
        - ruptured I71.51
    - thorax, thoracic I71.2Ø
      - arch I71.22
        - ruptured I71.12
      - ascending I71.21
        - ruptured I71.11
      - descending I71.23
        - ruptured I71.13
      - ruptured I71.1Ø
        - arch I71.12
        - ascending I71.11
        - descending I71.13
    - transverse I71.22
      - ruptured I71.12
    - valve (heart) — *see also* Endocarditis, aortic I35.8
  - arteriosclerotic I72.9
    - cerebral I67.1
      - ruptured — *see* Hemorrhage, intracranial, subarachnoid
  - arteriovenous (congenital) — *see also* Malformation, arteriovenous
    - acquired I77.Ø
      - brain I67.1
        - ruptured — *see* Aneurysm, arteriovenous, brain, ruptured
      - coronary I25.41
      - pulmonary I28.Ø
    - brain Q28.2
      - ruptured I6Ø.8
        - intracerebral I61.8
        - intraparenchymal I61.8
        - intraventricular I61.5
        - subarachnoid I6Ø.8
    - peripheral — *see* Malformation, arteriovenous, peripheral
    - precerebral vessels Q28.Ø
    - specified site NEC — *see also* Malformation, arteriovenous
      - acquired I77.Ø
  - basal — *see* Aneurysm, brain
  - basilar (trunk) I72.5
  - berry (congenital) (nonruptured) I67.1
    - ruptured I6Ø.7
  - brain I67.1
    - arteriosclerotic I67.1
      - ruptured — *see* Hemorrhage, intracranial, subarachnoid
    - arteriovenous (congenital) (nonruptured) Q28.2
      - acquired I67.1
        - ruptured — *see* Aneurysm, arteriovenous, brain, ruptured I6Ø.8-
      - ruptured — *see* Aneurysm, arteriovenous, brain, ruptured I6Ø.8-
    - berry (congenital) (nonruptured) I67.1
      - ruptured — *see also* Hemorrhage, intracranial, subarachnoid I6Ø.7
    - congenital Q28.3
      - ruptured I6Ø.7
    - meninges I67.1
      - ruptured I6Ø.8
    - miliary (congenital) (nonruptured) I67.1
      - ruptured — *see also* Hemorrhage, intracranial, subarachnoid I6Ø.7
    - mycotic I33.Ø
    - ruptured — *see* Aneurysm, arteriovenous, brain, ruptured I6Ø.8
    - syphilitic (hemorrhage) A52.Ø5
  - cardiac (false) — *see also* Aneurysm, heart I25.3

Aneurysm — *continued*
carotid artery (common) (external) I72.Ø
internal (intracranial) I67.1
extracranial portion I72.Ø
ruptured into brain I6Ø.Ø- ☑
syphilitic A52.Ø9
intracranial A52.Ø5
cavernous sinus I67.1
arteriovenous (congenital) (nonruptured) Q28.3
ruptured I6Ø.8
celiac I72.8
central nervous system, syphilitic A52.Ø5
cerebral — *see* Aneurysm, brain
chest — *see* Aneurysm, thorax
circle of Willis I67.1
congenital Q28.3
ruptured I6Ø.6
ruptured I6Ø.6
common iliac artery I72.3
congenital (peripheral) Q27.8
aorta (root) (sinus) Q25.43
brain Q28.3
ruptured I6Ø.7
coronary Q24.5
digestive system Q27.8
lower limb Q27.8
pulmonary Q25.79
retina Q14.1
specified site NEC Q27.8
upper limb Q27.8
conjunctiva — *see* Abnormality, conjunctiva, vascular
conus arteriosus — *see* Aneurysm, heart
coronary (arteriosclerotic) (artery) I25.41
arteriovenous, congenital Q24.5
congenital Q24.5
ruptured — *see* Infarct, myocardium
syphilitic A52.Ø6
vein I25.89
cylindroid (aorta) I71.9
ruptured I71.8
syphilitic A52.Ø1
ductus arteriosus Q25.Ø
endocardial, infective (any valve) I33.Ø
femoral (artery) (ruptured) I72.4
gastroduodenal I72.8
gastroepiploic I72.8
heart (wall) (chronic or with a stated duration of over 4 weeks) I25.3
valve — *see* Endocarditis
hepatic I72.8
iliac (common) (artery) (ruptured) I72.3
infective I72.9
endocardial (any valve) I33.Ø
innominate (nonsyphilitic) I72.8
syphilitic A52.Ø9
interauricular septum — *see* Aneurysm, heart
interventricular septum — *see* Aneurysm, heart
intrathoracic (nonsyphilitic) — *see also* Aneurysm, aorta, thorax I71.2Ø
ruptured — *see also* Aneurysm, aorta, thorax, ruptured I71.1Ø
syphilitic A52.Ø1
lower limb I72.4
lung (pulmonary artery) I28.1
mediastinal (nonsyphilitic) I72.8
syphilitic A52.Ø9
miliary (congenital) I67.1
ruptured — *see* Hemorrhage, intracerebral, subarachnoid, intracranial
mitral (heart) (valve) I34.89
mural — *see* Aneurysm, heart
mycotic I72.9
endocardial (any valve) I33.Ø
ruptured, brain — *see* Hemorrhage, intracerebral, subarachnoid
myocardium — *see* Aneurysm, heart
neck I72.Ø
pancreaticoduodenal I72.8
patent ductus arteriosus Q25.Ø
peripheral NEC I72.8
congenital Q27.8
digestive system Q27.8
lower limb Q27.8
specified site NEC Q27.8
upper limb Q27.8
popliteal (artery) (ruptured) I72.4
precerebral
congenital (nonruptured) Q28.1

Aneurysm — *continued*
precerebral — *continued*
specified site, NEC I72.5
pulmonary I28.1
arteriovenous Q25.72
acquired I28.Ø
syphilitic A52.Ø9
valve (heart) — *see* Endocarditis, pulmonary
racemose (peripheral) I72.9
congenital — *see* Aneurysm, congenital
radial I72.1
Rasmussen NEC A15.Ø
renal (artery) I72.2
retina — *see also* Disorder, retina, microaneurysms
congenital Q14.1
diabetic — *see* EØ8-E13 with .3-
sinus of Valsalva Q25.49
specified NEC I72.8
spinal (cord) I72.8
syphilitic (hemorrhage) A52.Ø9
splenic I72.8
subclavian (artery) (ruptured) I72.8
syphilitic A52.Ø9
superior mesenteric I72.8
syphilitic (aorta) A52.Ø1
central nervous system A52.Ø5
congenital (late) A5Ø.54 *[I79.Ø]*
spine, spinal A52.Ø9
thoracoabdominal (aorta) I71.6Ø
ruptured I71.5Ø
syphilitic A52.Ø1
thorax, thoracic (aorta) (arch) (nonsyphilitic) — *see* Aneurysm, aorta, thorax
ruptured — *see* Aneurysm, aorta, thorax, ruptured
syphilitic A52.Ø1
traumatic (complication) (early), specified site — *see* Injury, blood vessel
tricuspid (heart) (valve) IØ7.8
ulnar I72.1
upper limb (ruptured) I72.1
valve, valvular — *see* Endocarditis
venous — *see also* Varix I86.8
congenital Q27.8
digestive system Q27.8
lower limb Q27.8
specified site NEC Q27.8
upper limb Q27.8
ventricle — *see* Aneurysm, heart
vertebral artery I72.6
visceral NEC I72.8
Angelman syndrome Q93.51
Anger R45.4
Angiectasis, angiectopia I99.8
Angiitis I77.6
allergic granulomatous M3Ø.1
hypersensitivity M31.Ø
necrotizing M31.9
specified NEC M31.8
nervous system, granulomatous I67.7
Angina (attack) (cardiac) (chest) (heart) (pectoris) (syndrome) (vasomotor) I2Ø.9
with
atherosclerotic heart disease — *see* Arteriosclerosis, coronary (artery),
documented spasm I2Ø.1
abdominal K55.1
accelerated — *see* Angina, unstable
agranulocytic — *see* Agranulocytosis
angiospastic — *see* Angina, with documented spasm
aphthous BØ8.5
crescendo — *see* Angina, unstable
croupous JØ5.Ø
cruris I73.9
de novo effort — *see* Angina, unstable
diphtheritic, membranous A36.Ø
equivalent I2Ø.8
exudative, chronic J37.Ø
following acute myocardial infarction I23.7
gangrenous diphtheritic A36.Ø
intestinal K55.1
Ludovici K12.2
Ludwig's K12.2
malignant diphtheritic A36.Ø
membranous JØ5.Ø
diphtheritic A36.Ø
Vincent's A69.1
mesenteric K55.1
monocytic — *see* Mononucleosis, infectious

Angina — *continued*
of effort — *see* Angina, specified NEC
phlegmonous J36
diphtheritic A36.Ø
post-infarctional I23.7
pre-infarctional — *see* Angina, unstable
Prinzmetal — *see* Angina, with documented spasm
progressive — *see* Angina, unstable
pseudomembranous A69.1
pultaceous, diphtheritic A36.Ø
refractory I2Ø.2
spasm-induced — *see* Angina, with documented spasm
specified NEC I2Ø.8
stable I2Ø.8
stenocardia — *see* Angina, specified NEC
stridulous, diphtheritic A36.2
tonsil J36
trachealis JØ5.Ø
unstable I2Ø.Ø
variant — *see* Angina, with documented spasm
Vincent's A69.1
worsening effort — *see* Angina, unstable
Angioblastoma — *see* Neoplasm, connective tissue, uncertain behavior
Angiocholecystitis — *see* Cholecystitis, acute
Angiocholitis — *see also* Cholecystitis, acute K83.Ø9
Angiodysgenesis spinalis G95.19
Angiodysplasia (cecum) (colon) K55.2Ø
with bleeding K55.21
duodenum (and stomach) K31.819
with bleeding K31.811
stomach (and duodenum) K31.819
with bleeding K31.811
Angioedema (allergic) (any site) (with urticaria) T78.3 ☑
episodic, with eosinophilia D72.118
hereditary D84.1
Angioendothelioma — *see* Neoplasm, uncertain behavior, by site
benign D18.ØØ
intra-abdominal D18.Ø3
intracranial D18.Ø2
skin D18.Ø1
specified site NEC D18.Ø9
bone — *see* Neoplasm, bone, malignant
Ewing's — *see* Neoplasm, bone, malignant
Angioendotheliomatosis C85.8- ☑
Angiofibroma — *see also* Neoplasm, benign, by site
juvenile
specified site — *see* Neoplasm, benign, by site
unspecified site D1Ø.6
Angiohemophilia (A) (B) — *see* Disease, von Willebrand
Angioid streaks (choroid) (macula) (retina) H35.33
Angiokeratoma — *see* Neoplasm, skin, benign
corporis diffusum E75.21
Angioleiomyoma — *see* Neoplasm, connective tissue, benign
Angiolipoma — *see also* Lipoma
infiltrating — *see* Lipoma
Angioma — *see also* Hemangioma, by site
capillary I78.1
hemorrhagicum hereditaria I78.Ø
intra-abdominal D18.Ø3
intracranial D18.Ø2
malignant — *see* Neoplasm, connective tissue, malignant
plexiform D18.ØØ
intra-abdominal D18.Ø3
intracranial D18.Ø2
skin D18.Ø1
specified site NEC D18.Ø9
senile I78.1
serpiginosum L81.7
skin D18.Ø1
specified site NEC D18.Ø9
spider I78.1
stellate I78.1
venous Q28.3
Angiomatosis Q82.8
bacillary A79.89
encephalotrigeminal Q85.89
hemorrhagic familial I78.Ø
hereditary familial I78.Ø
liver K76.4
Angiomyolipoma — *see* Lipoma
Angiomyoliposarcoma — *see* Neoplasm, connective tissue, malignant
Angiomyoma — *see* Neoplasm, connective tissue, benign

Index Aneurysm — Angiomyoma

- **Angiomyosarcoma** — *see* Neoplasm, connective tissue, malignant
- **Angiomyxoma** — *see* Neoplasm, connective tissue, uncertain behavior
- **Angioneurosis** F45.8
- **Angioneurotic edema** (allergic) (any site) (with urticaria) T78.3 ☑
  - hereditary D84.1
- **Angiopathia, angiopathy** I99.9
  - cerebral I67.9
    - amyloid E85.4 *[I68.Ø]*
  - diabetic (peripheral) — *see* Diabetes, angiopathy
  - peripheral I73.9
    - diabetic — *see* Diabetes, angiopathy
    - specified type NEC I73.89
  - retinae syphilitica A52.Ø5
  - retinalis (juvenilis)
    - diabetic — *see* Diabetes, retinopathy
    - proliferative — *see* Retinopathy, proliferative
- **Angiosarcoma** — *see also* Neoplasm, connective tissue, malignant
  - liver C22.3
- **Angiosclerosis** — *see* Arteriosclerosis
- **Angiospasm** (peripheral) (traumatic) (vessel) I73.9
  - brachial plexus G54.Ø
  - cerebral G45.9
  - cervical plexus G54.2
  - nerve
    - arm — *see* Mononeuropathy, upper limb
      - axillary G54.Ø
      - median — *see* Lesion, nerve, median
      - ulnar — *see* Lesion, nerve, ulnar
    - axillary G54.Ø
    - leg — *see* Mononeuropathy, lower limb
    - median — *see* Lesion, nerve, median
    - plantar — *see* Lesion, nerve, plantar
    - ulnar — *see* Lesion, nerve, ulnar
- **Angiospastic disease or edema** I73.9
- **Angiostrongyliasis**
  - due to
    - Parastrongylus
      - cantonensis B83.2
      - costaricensis B81.3
  - intestinal B81.3
- **Anguillulosis** — *see* Strongyloidiasis
- **Angulation**
  - cecum — *see* Obstruction, intestine
  - coccyx (acquired) — *see also* subcategory M43.8 ☑
    - congenital NEC Q76.49
  - femur (acquired) — *see also* Deformity, limb, specified type NEC, thigh
    - congenital Q74.2
  - intestine (large) (small) — *see* Obstruction, intestine
  - sacrum (acquired) — *see also* subcategory M43.8 ☑
    - congenital NEC Q76.49
  - sigmoid (flexure) — *see* Obstruction, intestine
  - spine — *see* Dorsopathy, deforming, specified NEC
  - tibia (acquired) — *see also* Deformity, limb, specified type NEC, lower leg
    - congenital Q74.2
  - ureter N13.5
    - with infection N13.6
  - wrist (acquired) — *see also* Deformity, limb, specified type NEC, forearm
    - congenital Q74.Ø
- **Angulus infectiosus** (lips) K13.Ø
- **Anhedonia** R45.84
  - sexual F52.Ø
- **Anhidrosis** L74.4
- **Anhydration** E86.Ø
- **Anhydremia** E86.Ø
- **Anidrosis** L74.4
- **Aniridia** (congenital) Q13.1
- **Anisakiasis** (infection) (infestation) B81.Ø
- **Anisakis larvae infestation** B81.Ø
- **Aniseikonia** H52.32
- **Anisocoria** (pupil) H57.Ø2
  - congenital Q13.2
- **Anisocytosis** R71.8
- **Anisometropia** (congenital) H52.31
- **Ankle** — *see* condition
- **Ankyloblepharon** (eyelid) (acquired) — *see also* Blepharophimosis
  - filiforme (adnatum) (congenital) Q1Ø.3
  - total Q1Ø.3
- **Ankyloglossia** Q38.1
- **Ankylosis** (fibrous) (osseous) (joint) M24.6Ø
- **Ankylosis** — *continued*
  - ankle M24.67- ☑
  - arthrodesis status Z98.1
  - cricoarytenoid (cartilage) (joint) (larynx) J38.7
  - dental KØ3.5
  - ear ossicles H74.31- ☑
  - elbow M24.62- ☑
  - foot M24.67- ☑
  - hand M24.64- ☑
  - hip M24.65- ☑
  - incostapedial joint (infectional) — *see* Ankylosis, ear ossicles
  - jaw (temporomandibular) M26.61- ☑
  - knee M24.66- ☑
  - lumbosacral (joint) M43.27
  - postoperative (status) Z98.1
  - produced by surgical fusion, status Z98.1
  - sacro-iliac (joint) M43.28
  - shoulder M24.61- ☑
  - specified site NEC M24.69
  - spine (joint) — *see also* Fusion, spine
    - spondylitic — *see* Spondylitis, ankylosing
  - surgical Z98.1
  - temporomandibular M26.61- ☑
  - tooth, teeth (hard tissues) KØ3.5
  - wrist M24.63- ☑
- **Ankylostoma** — *see* Ancylostoma
- **Ankylostomiasis** — *see* Ancylostomiasis
- **Ankylurethria** — *see* Stricture, urethra
- **Annular** — *see also* condition
  - detachment, cervix N88.8
  - organ or site, congenital NEC — *see* Distortion
  - pancreas (congenital) Q45.1
- **Anoctaminopathy** G71.Ø35
- **Anodontia** (complete) (partial) (vera) KØØ.Ø
  - acquired KØ8.1Ø ☑
- **Anomaly, anomalous** (congenital) (unspecified type) Q89.9
  - abdominal wall NEC Q79.59
  - acoustic nerve QØ7.8
  - adrenal (gland) Q89.1
  - Alder (-Reilly) (leukocyte granulation) D72.Ø
  - alimentary tract Q45.9
    - upper Q4Ø.9
  - alveolar M26.7Ø
    - hyperplasia M26.79
      - mandibular M26.72
      - maxillary M26.71
    - hypoplasia M26.79
      - mandibular M26.74
      - maxillary M26.73
    - ridge (process) M26.79
    - specified NEC M26.79
  - ankle (joint) Q74.2
  - anus Q43.9
  - aorta (arch) NEC Q25.4Ø
    - coarctation (preductal) (postductal) Q25.1
  - aortic cusp or valve Q23.9
  - appendix Q43.8
  - apple peel syndrome Q41.1
  - aqueduct of Sylvius QØ3.Ø
    - with spina bifida — *see* Spina bifida, with hydrocephalus
  - arm Q74.Ø
  - arteriovenous NEC
    - coronary Q24.5
    - gastrointestinal Q27.33
      - acquired — *see* Angiodysplasia
  - artery (peripheral) Q27.9
    - basilar NEC Q28.1
    - cerebral Q28.3
    - coronary Q24.5
    - digestive system Q27.8
    - eye Q15.8
    - great Q25.9
      - specified NEC Q25.8
    - lower limb Q27.8
    - peripheral Q27.9
      - specified NEC Q27.8
    - pulmonary NEC Q25.79
    - renal Q27.2
    - retina Q14.1
    - specified site NEC Q27.8
    - subclavian Q27.8
      - origin Q25.48
    - umbilical Q27.Ø
    - upper limb Q27.8
    - vertebral NEC Q28.1
- **Anomaly, anomalous** — *continued*
  - aryteno-epiglottic folds Q31.8
  - atrial
    - bands or folds Q2Ø.8
    - septa Q21.1Ø
  - atrioventricular
    - excitation I45.6
    - septum Q21.Ø
  - auditory canal Q17.8
  - auricle
    - ear Q17.8
      - causing impairment of hearing Q16.9
    - heart Q2Ø.8
  - Axenfeld's Q15.Ø
  - back Q89.9
  - band
    - atrial Q2Ø.8
    - heart Q24.8
    - ventricular Q24.8
  - Bartholin's duct Q38.4
  - biliary duct or passage Q44.5
  - bladder Q64.7Ø
    - absence Q64.5
    - diverticulum Q64.6
    - exstrophy Q64.1Ø
      - cloacal Q64.12
      - extroversion Q64.19
      - specified type NEC Q64.19
      - supravesical fissure Q64.11
    - neck obstruction Q64.31
    - specified type NEC Q64.79
  - bone Q79.9
    - arm Q74.Ø
    - face Q75.9
    - leg Q74.2
    - pelvic girdle Q74.2
    - shoulder girdle Q74.Ø
    - skull Q75.9
      - with
        - anencephaly QØØ.Ø
        - encephalocele — *see* Encephalocele
        - hydrocephalus QØ3.9
          - with spina bifida — *see* Spina bifida, by site, with hydrocephalus
        - microcephaly QØ2
  - brain (multiple) QØ4.9
    - vessel Q28.3
  - breast Q83.9
  - broad ligament Q5Ø.6
  - bronchus Q32.4
  - bulbus cordis Q21.9
  - bursa Q79.9
  - canal of Nuck Q52.4
  - canthus Q1Ø.3
  - capillary Q27.9
  - cardiac Q24.9
    - chambers Q2Ø.9
      - specified NEC Q2Ø.8
    - septal closure Q21.9
      - specified NEC Q21.8
    - valve NEC Q24.8
      - pulmonary Q22.3
  - cardiovascular system Q28.8
  - carpus Q74.Ø
  - caruncle, lacrimal Q1Ø.6
  - cascade stomach Q4Ø.2
  - cauda equina QØ6.3
  - cecum Q43.9
  - cerebral QØ4.9
    - vessels Q28.3
  - cervix Q51.9
  - Chédiak-Higashi (-Steinbrinck) (congenital gigantism of peroxidase granules) E7Ø.33Ø
  - cheek Q18.9
  - chest wall Q67.8
    - bones Q76.9
  - chin Q18.9
  - chordae tendineae Q24.8
  - choroid Q14.3
    - plexus QØ7.8
  - chromosomes, chromosomal Q99.9
    - D (1) — *see* condition, chromosome 13
    - E (3) — *see* condition, chromosome 18
    - G — *see* condition, chromosome 21
    - sex
      - female phenotype Q97.8
      - gonadal dysgenesis (pure) Q99.1
      - Klinefelter's Q98.4
      - male phenotype Q98.9

Anomaly, anomalous — *continued*
chromosomes, chromosomal — *continued*
sex — *continued*
Turner's Q96.9
specified NEC Q99.8
cilia Q10.3
circulatory system Q28.9
clavicle Q74.0
clitoris Q52.6
coccyx Q76.49
colon Q43.9
common duct Q44.5
communication
coronary artery Q24.5
left ventricle with right atrium Q21.0
concha (ear) Q17.3
connection
portal vein Q26.5
pulmonary venous Q26.4
partial Q26.3
total Q26.2
renal artery with kidney Q27.2
cornea (shape) Q13.4
coronary artery or vein Q24.5
cranium — *see* Anomaly, skull
cricoid cartilage Q31.8
cystic duct Q44.5
dental
alveolar — *see* Anomaly, alveolar
arch relationship M26.20
specified NEC M26.29
dentofacial M26.9
alveolar — *see* Anomaly, alveolar
dental arch relationship M26.20
specified NEC M26.29
functional M26.50
specified NEC M26.59
jaw size M26.00
macrogenia M26.05
mandibular
hyperplasia M26.03
hypoplasia M26.04
maxillary
hyperplasia M26.01
hypoplasia M26.02
microgenia M26.06
specified type NEC M26.09
jaw-cranial base relationship M26.10
asymmetry M26.12
maxillary M26.11
specified type NEC M26.19
malocclusion M26.4
dental arch relationship NEC M26.29
jaw size — *see* Anomaly, dentofacial, jaw size
jaw-cranial base relationship — *see* Anomaly, dentofacial, jaw-cranial base relationship
specified type NEC M26.89
temporomandibular joint M26.60- ☑
adhesions M26.61- ☑
ankylosis M26.61- ☑
arthralgia M26.62- ☑
articular disc M26.63- ☑
specified type NEC M26.69
tooth position, fully erupted M26.30
specified NEC M26.39
dermatoglyphic Q82.8
diaphragm (apertures) NEC Q79.1
digestive organ(s) or tract Q45.9
lower Q43.9
upper Q40.9
distance, interarch (excessive) (inadequate) M26.25
distribution, coronary artery Q24.5
ductus
arteriosus Q25.0
botalli Q25.0
duodenum Q43.9
dura (brain) Q04.9
spinal cord Q06.9
ear (external) Q17.9
causing impairment of hearing Q16.9
inner Q16.5
middle (causing impairment of hearing) Q16.4
ossicles Q16.3
Ebstein's (heart) (tricuspid valve) Q22.5
ectodermal Q82.9
Eisenmenger's (ventricular septal defect) Q21.8
ejaculatory duct Q55.4
elbow Q74.0

Anomaly, anomalous — *continued*
endocrine gland NEC Q89.2
epididymis Q55.4
epiglottis Q31.8
esophagus Q39.9
eustachian tube Q17.8
eye Q15.9
anterior segment Q13.9
specified NEC Q13.89
posterior segment Q14.9
specified NEC Q14.8
ptosis (eyelid) Q10.0
specified NEC Q15.8
eyebrow Q18.8
eyelid Q10.3
ptosis Q10.0
face Q18.9
bone(s) Q75.9
fallopian tube Q50.6
fascia Q79.9
femur NEC Q74.2
fibula NEC Q74.2
finger Q74.0
fixation, intestine Q43.3
flexion (joint) NOS Q74.9
hip or thigh Q65.89
foot NEC Q74.2
varus (congenital) Q66.3- ☑
foramen
Botalli Q21.12
ovale Q21.12
forearm Q74.0
forehead Q75.8
form, teeth K00.2
fovea centralis Q14.1
frontal bone — *see* Anomaly, skull
gallbladder (position) (shape) (size) Q44.1
Gartner's duct Q52.4
gastrointestinal tract Q45.9
genitalia, genital organ(s) or system
female Q52.9
external Q52.70
internal NOS Q52.9
male Q55.9
hydrocele P83.5
specified NEC Q55.8
genitourinary NEC
female Q52.9
male Q55.9
Gerbode Q21.0
glottis Q31.8
granulation or granulocyte, genetic (constitutional) (leukocyte) D72.0
gum Q38.6
gyri Q07.9
hair Q84.2
hand Q74.0
hard tissue formation in pulp K04.3
head — *see* Anomaly, skull
heart Q24.9
auricle Q20.8
bands or folds Q24.8
fibroelastosis cordis I42.4
obstructive NEC Q22.6
patent ductus arteriosus (Botalli) Q25.0
septum Q21.9
auricular Q21.19
interatrial Q21.19
interventricular Q21.0
with pulmonary stenosis or atresia, dextraposition of aorta and hypertrophy of right ventricle Q21.3
specified NEC Q21.8
ventricular Q21.0
with pulmonary stenosis or atresia, dextraposition of aorta and hypertrophy of right ventricle Q21.3
tetralogy of Fallot Q21.3
valve NEC Q24.8
aortic
bicuspid valve Q23.1
insufficiency Q23.1
stenosis Q23.0
subaortic Q24.4
mitral
insufficiency Q23.3
stenosis Q23.2
pulmonary Q22.3
atresia Q22.0

Anomaly, anomalous — *continued*
heart — *continued*
valve — *continued*
pulmonary — *continued*
insufficiency Q22.2
stenosis Q22.1
infundibular Q24.3
subvalvular Q24.3
tricuspid
atresia Q22.4
stenosis Q22.4
ventricle Q20.8
heel NEC Q74.2
Hegglin's D72.0
hemianencephaly Q00.0
hemicephaly Q00.0
hemicrania Q00.0
hepatic duct Q44.5
hip NEC Q74.2
hourglass stomach Q40.2
humerus Q74.0
hydatid of Morgagni
female Q50.5
male (epididymal) Q55.4
testicular Q55.29
hymen Q52.4
hypersegmentation of neutrophils, hereditary D72.0
hypophyseal Q89.2
ileocecal (coil) (valve) Q43.9
ileum Q43.9
ilium NEC Q74.2
integument Q84.9
specified NEC Q84.8
interarch distance (excessive) (inadequate) M26.25
intervertebral cartilage or disc Q76.49
intestine (large) (small) Q43.9
with anomalous adhesions, fixation or malrotation Q43.3
iris Q13.2
ischium NEC Q74.2
jaw — *see* Anomaly, dentofacial
alveolar — *see* Anomaly, alveolar
jaw-cranial base relationship — *see* Anomaly, dentofacial, jaw-cranial base relationship
jejunum Q43.8
joint Q74.9
specified NEC Q74.8
Jordan's D72.0
kidney(s) (calyx) (pelvis) Q63.9
artery Q27.2
specified NEC Q63.8
Klippel-Feil (brevicollis) Q76.1
knee Q74.1
labium (majus) (minus) Q52.70
labyrinth, membranous Q16.5
lacrimal apparatus or duct Q10.6
larynx, laryngeal (muscle) Q31.9
web (bed) Q31.0
lens Q12.9
leukocytes, genetic D72.0
granulation (constitutional) D72.0
lid (fold) Q10.3
ligament Q79.9
broad Q50.6
round Q52.8
limb Q74.9
lower NEC Q74.2
reduction deformity — *see* Defect, reduction, lower limb
upper Q74.0
lip Q38.0
liver Q44.7
duct Q44.5
lower limb NEC Q74.2
lumbosacral (joint) (region) Q76.49
kyphosis — *see* Kyphosis, congenital
lordosis — *see* Lordosis, congenital
lung (fissure) (lobe) Q33.9
mandible — *see* Anomaly, dentofacial
maxilla — *see* Anomaly, dentofacial
May (-Hegglin) D72.0
meatus urinarius NEC Q64.79
meningeal bands or folds Q07.9
constriction of Q07.8
spinal Q06.9
meninges Q07.9
cerebral Q04.8
spinal Q06.9

Anomaly, anomalous — *continued*
meningocele Q05.9
mesentery Q45.9
metacarpus Q74.0
metatarsus NEC Q74.2
middle ear Q16.4
ossicles Q16.3
mitral (leaflets) (valve) Q23.9
insufficiency Q23.3
specified NEC Q23.8
stenosis Q23.2
mouth Q38.6
Müllerian — *see also* Anomaly, by site
uterus NEC Q51.818
multiple NEC Q89.7
muscle Q79.9
eyelid Q10.3
musculoskeletal system, except limbs Q79.9
myocardium Q24.8
nail Q84.6
narrowness, eyelid Q10.3
nasal sinus (wall) Q30.8
neck (any part) Q18.9
nerve Q07.9
acoustic Q07.8
optic Q07.8
nervous system (central) Q07.9
nipple Q83.9
nose, nasal (bones) (cartilage) (septum) (sinus) Q30.9
specified NEC Q30.8
ocular muscle Q15.8
omphalomesenteric duct Q43.0
opening, pulmonary veins Q26.4
optic
disc Q14.2
nerve Q07.8
opticociliary vessels Q13.2
orbit (eye) Q10.7
organ Q89.9
of Corti Q16.5
origin
artery
innominate Q25.8
pulmonary Q25.79
renal Q27.2
subclavian Q25.48
osseous meatus (ear) Q16.1
ovary Q50.39
oviduct Q50.6
palate (hard) (soft) NEC Q38.5
pancreas or pancreatic duct Q45.3
papillary muscles Q24.8
parathyroid gland Q89.2
paraurethral ducts Q64.79
parotid (gland) Q38.4
patella Q74.1
Pelger-Huët (hereditary hyposegmentation) D72.0
pelvic girdle NEC Q74.2
pelvis (bony) NEC Q74.2
rachitic E64.3
penis (glans) Q55.69
pericardium Q24.8
peripheral vascular system Q27.9
Peter's Q13.4
pharynx Q38.8
pigmentation L81.9
congenital Q82.8
pituitary (gland) Q89.2
pleural (folds) Q34.0
portal vein Q26.5
connection Q26.5
position, tooth, teeth, fully erupted M26.30
specified NEC M26.39
precerebral vessel Q28.1
prepuce Q55.69
prostate Q55.4
pulmonary Q33.9
artery NEC Q25.79
valve Q22.3
atresia Q22.0
insufficiency Q22.2
specified type NEC Q22.3
stenosis Q22.1
infundibular Q24.3
subvalvular Q24.3
venous connection Q26.4
partial Q26.3
total Q26.2
pupil Q13.2

Anomaly, anomalous — *continued*
pupil — *continued*
function H57.00
anisocoria H57.02
Argyll Robertson pupil H57.01
miosis H57.03
mydriasis H57.04
specified type NEC H57.09
tonic pupil H57.05- ☑
pylorus Q40.3
radius Q74.0
rectum Q43.9
reduction (extremity) (limb)
femur (longitudinal) — *see* Defect, reduction, lower limb, longitudinal, femur
fibula (longitudinal) — *see* Defect, reduction, lower limb, longitudinal, fibula
lower limb — *see* Defect, reduction, lower limb
radius (longitudinal) — *see* Defect, reduction, upper limb, longitudinal, radius
tibia (longitudinal) — *see* Defect, reduction, lower limb, longitudinal, tibia
ulna (longitudinal) — *see* Defect, reduction, upper limb, longitudinal, ulna
upper limb — *see* Defect, reduction, upper limb
refraction — *see* Disorder, refraction
renal Q63.9
artery Q27.2
pelvis Q63.9
specified NEC Q63.8
respiratory system Q34.9
specified NEC Q34.8
retina Q14.1
rib Q76.6
cervical Q76.5
Rieger's Q13.81
rotation — *see* Malrotation
hip or thigh Q65.89
round ligament Q52.8
sacroiliac (joint) NEC Q74.2
sacrum NEC Q76.49
kyphosis — *see* Kyphosis, congenital
lordosis — *see* Lordosis, congenital
saddle nose, syphilitic A50.57
salivary duct or gland Q38.4
scapula Q74.0
scrotum — *see* Malformation, testis and scrotum
sebaceous gland Q82.9
seminal vesicles Q55.4
sense organs NEC Q07.8
sex chromosomes NEC — *see also* Anomaly, chromosomes
female phenotype Q97.8
male phenotype Q98.9
shoulder (girdle) (joint) Q74.0
sigmoid (flexure) Q43.9
simian crease Q82.8
sinus of Valsalva Q25.49
skeleton generalized Q78.9
skin (appendage) Q82.9
skull Q75.9
with
anencephaly Q00.0
encephalocele — *see* Encephalocele
hydrocephalus Q03.9
with spina bifida — *see* Spina bifida, by site, with hydrocephalus
microcephaly Q02
specified organ or site NEC Q89.8
spermatic cord Q55.4
spine, spinal NEC Q76.49
column NEC Q76.49
kyphosis — *see* Kyphosis, congenital
lordosis — *see* Lordosis, congenital
cord Q06.9
nerve root Q07.8
spleen Q89.09
agenesis Q89.01
stenonian duct Q38.4
sternum NEC Q76.7
stomach Q40.3
submaxillary gland Q38.4
tarsus NEC Q74.2
tendon Q79.9
testis — *see* Malformation, testis and scrotum
thigh NEC Q74.2
thorax (wall) Q67.8
bony Q76.9

Anomaly, anomalous — *continued*
throat Q38.8
thumb Q74.0
thymus gland Q89.2
thyroid (gland) Q89.2
cartilage Q31.8
tibia NEC Q74.2
saber A50.56
toe Q74.2
tongue Q38.3
tooth, teeth K00.9
eruption K00.6
position, fully erupted M26.30
spacing, fully erupted M26.30
trachea (cartilage) Q32.1
tragus Q17.9
tricuspid (leaflet) (valve) Q22.9
atresia or stenosis Q22.4
Ebstein's Q22.5
Uhl's (hypoplasia of myocardium, right ventricle) Q24.8
ulna Q74.0
umbilical artery Q27.0
union
cricoid cartilage and thyroid cartilage Q31.8
thyroid cartilage and hyoid bone Q31.8
trachea with larynx Q31.8
upper limb Q74.0
urachus Q64.4
ureter Q62.8
obstructive NEC Q62.39
cecoureterocele Q62.32
orthotopic ureterocele Q62.31
urethra Q64.70
absence Q64.5
double Q64.74
fistula to rectum Q64.73
obstructive Q64.39
stricture Q64.32
prolapse Q64.71
specified type NEC Q64.79
urinary tract Q64.9
uterus Q51.9
with only one functioning horn Q51.4
uvula Q38.5
vagina Q52.4
valleculae Q31.8
valve (heart) NEC Q24.8
coronary sinus Q24.5
inferior vena cava Q24.8
pulmonary Q22.3
sinus coronario Q24.5
venae cavae inferioris Q24.8
vas deferens Q55.4
vascular Q27.9
brain Q28.3
ring Q25.45
vein(s) (peripheral) Q27.9
brain Q28.3
cerebral Q28.3
coronary Q24.5
developmental Q28.3
great Q26.9
specified NEC Q26.8
vena cava (inferior) (superior) Q26.9
venous — *see* Anomaly, vein(s)
venous return Q26.8
ventricular
bands or folds Q24.8
septa Q21.0
vertebra Q76.49
kyphosis — *see* Kyphosis, congenital
lordosis — *see* Lordosis, congenital
vesicourethral orifice Q64.79
vessel(s) Q27.9
optic papilla Q14.2
precerebral Q28.1
vitelline duct Q43.0
vitreous body or humor Q14.0
vulva Q52.70
wrist (joint) Q74.0
Anomia R48.8
Anonychia (congenital) Q84.3
acquired L60.8
Anophthalmos, anophthalmus (congenital) (globe) Q11.1
acquired Z90.01
Anopia, anopsia H53.46- ☑
quadrant H53.46- ☑

Anorchia, anorchism, anorchidism Q55.Ø
Anorexia R63.Ø
hysterical F44.89
nervosa F5Ø.ØØ
atypical F5Ø.9
binge-eating type F5Ø.2
with purging F5Ø.Ø2
restricting type F5Ø.Ø1
Anorgasmy, psychogenic (female) F52.31
male F52.32
Anosmia R43.Ø
hysterical F44.6
postinfectional J39.8
Anosognosia R41.89
Anosteoplasia Q78.9
Anovulatory cycle N97.Ø
Anoxemia RØ9.Ø2
newborn P84
Anoxia (pathological) RØ9.Ø2
altitude T7Ø.29 ☑
cerebral G93.1
complicating
anesthesia (general) (local) or other sedation T88.59 ☑
in labor and delivery O74.3
in pregnancy O29.21- ☑
postpartum, puerperal O89.2
delivery (cesarean) (instrumental) O75.4
during a procedure G97.81
newborn P84
resulting from a procedure G97.82
due to
drowning T75.1 ☑
high altitude T7Ø.29 ☑
heart — *see* Insufficiency, coronary
intrauterine P84
myocardial — *see* Insufficiency, coronary
newborn P84
spinal cord G95.11
systemic (by suffocation) (low content in atmosphere) — *see* Asphyxia, traumatic
Anteflexion — *see* Anteversion
Antenatal
care (normal pregnancy) Z34.9Ø
screening (encounter for) of mother — *see also* Encounter, antenatal screening Z36.9
Antepartum — *see* condition
Anterior — *see* condition
Antero-occlusion M26.22Ø
Anteversion
cervix — *see* Anteversion, uterus
femur (neck), congenital Q65.89
uterus, uterine (cervix) (postinfectional) (postpartal, old) N85.4
congenital Q51.818
in pregnancy or childbirth — *see* Pregnancy, complicated by
Anthophobia F4Ø.228
Anthracosilicosis J6Ø
Anthracosis (lung) (occupational) J6Ø
lingua K14.3
Anthrax A22.9
with pneumonia A22.1
cerebral A22.8
colitis A22.2
cutaneous A22.Ø
gastrointestinal A22.2
inhalation A22.1
intestinal A22.2
meningitis A22.8
pulmonary A22.1
respiratory A22.1
sepsis A22.7
specified manifestation NEC A22.8
Anthropoid pelvis Q74.2
with disproportion (fetopelvic) O33.Ø
Anthropophobia F4Ø.1Ø
generalized F4Ø.11
Antibodies, maternal (blood group) — *see* Isoimmunization, affecting management of pregnancy
anti-D — *see* Isoimmunization, affecting management of pregnancy, Rh
newborn P55.Ø
Antibody
anticardiolipin R76.Ø
with
hemorrhagic disorder D68.312
hypercoagulable state D68.61
Antibody — *continued*
antiphosphatidylglycerol R76.Ø
with
hemorrhagic disorder D68.312
hypercoagulable state D68.61
antiphosphatidylinositol R76.Ø
with
hemorrhagic disorder D68.312
hypercoagulable state D68.61
antiphosphatidylserine R76.Ø
with
hemorrhagic disorder D68.312
hypercoagulable state D68.61
antiphospholipid R76.Ø
with
hemorrhagic disorder D68.312
hypercoagulable state D68.61
Anticardiolipin syndrome D68.61
Anticoagulant, circulating (intrinsic) — *see also* Disorder, hemorrhagic D68.318
drug-induced (extrinsic) — *see also* Disorder, hemorrhagic D68.32
iatrogenic D68.32
Antidiuretic hormone syndrome E22.2
Antimonial cholera — *see* Poisoning, antimony
Antiphospholipid
antibody
with hemorrhagic disorder D68.312
syndrome D68.61
Antisocial personality F6Ø.2
Antithrombinemia — *see* Circulating anticoagulants
Antithromboplastinemia D68.318
Antithromboplastinogenemia D68.318
Antitoxin complication or reaction — *see* Complications, vaccination
Antlophobia F4Ø.228
Antritis J32.Ø
maxilla J32.Ø
acute JØ1.ØØ
recurrent JØ1.Ø1
stomach K29.5Ø
with bleeding K29.51
Antrum, antral — *see* condition
Anuria R34
calculous (impacted) (recurrent) — *see also* Calculus, urinary N2Ø.9
following
abortion — *see* Abortion by type complicated by, renal failure
ectopic or molar pregnancy OØ8.4
newborn P96.Ø
postprocedural N99.Ø
postrenal N13.8
traumatic (following crushing) T79.5 ☑
Anus, anal — *see* condition
Anusitis K62.89
Anxiety F41.9
depression F41.8
episodic paroxysmal F41.Ø
generalized F41.1
hysteria F41.8
neurosis F41.1
panic type F41.Ø
reaction F41.1
separation, abnormal (of childhood) F93.Ø
specified NEC F41.8
state F41.1
Aorta, aortic — *see* condition
Aortectasia — *see* Ectasia, aorta
with aneurysm — *see* Aneurysm, aorta
Aortitis (nonsyphilitic) (calcific) I77.6
arteriosclerotic I7Ø.Ø
Doehle-Heller A52.Ø2
luetic A52.Ø2
rheumatic — *see* Endocarditis, acute, rheumatic
specific (syphilitic) A52.Ø2
syphilitic A52.Ø2
congenital A5Ø.54 *[I79.1]*
Apathetic thyroid storm — *see* Thyrotoxicosis
Apathy R45.3
Apeirophobia F4Ø.228
Apepsia K3Ø
psychogenic F45.8
Aperistalsis, esophagus K22.Ø
Apertognathia M26.29
Apert's syndrome Q87.Ø
Aphagia R13.Ø
psychogenic F5Ø.9
Aphakia (acquired) (postoperative) H27.Ø- ☑
congenital Q12.3
Aphasia (amnestic) (global) (nominal) (semantic) (syntactic) R47.Ø1
acquired, with epilepsy (Landau-Kleffner syndrome) — *see* Epilepsy, specified NEC
auditory (developmental) F8Ø.2
developmental (receptive type) F8Ø.2
expressive type F8Ø.1
Wernicke's F8Ø.2
following
cerebrovascular disease I69.92Ø
cerebral infarction I69.32Ø
intracerebral hemorrhage I69.12Ø
nontraumatic intracranial hemorrhage NEC I69.22Ø
specified disease NEC I69.82Ø
subarachnoid hemorrhage I69.Ø2Ø
primary progressive — *see also* Dementia, in, diseases specified elsewhere G31.Ø1 *[FØ2.8Ø]*
with behavioral disturbance — *see also* Dementia, in, diseases specified elsewhere G31.Ø1 *[FØ2.81-]* ☑
progressive isolated — *see also* Dementia, in, diseases specified elsewhere G31.Ø1 *[FØ2.8Ø]*
with behavioral disturbance — *see also* Dementia, in, diseases specified elsewhere G31.Ø1 *[FØ2.81-]* ☑
sensory F8Ø.2
syphilis, tertiary A52.19
Wernicke's (developmental) F8Ø.2
Aphonia (organic) R49.1
hysterical F44.4
psychogenic F44.4
Aphthae, aphthous — *see also* condition
Bednar's K12.Ø
cachectic K14.Ø
epizootic BØ8.8
fever BØ8.8
oral (recurrent) K12.Ø
stomatitis (major) (minor) K12.Ø
thrush B37.Ø
ulcer (oral) (recurrent) K12.Ø
genital organ(s) NEC
female N76.6
male N5Ø.89
larynx J38.7
Apical — *see* condition
Apiphobia F4Ø.218
Aplasia — *see also* Agenesis
abdominal muscle syndrome Q79.4
alveolar process (acquired) — *see* Anomaly, alveolar
congenital Q38.6
aorta (congenital) Q25.41
axialis extracorticalis (congenita) E75.29
bone marrow (myeloid) D61.9
congenital D61.Ø1
brain QØØ.Ø
part of QØ4.3
bronchus Q32.4
cementum KØØ.4
cerebellum QØ4.3
cervix (congenital) Q51.5
congenital pure red cell D61.Ø1
corpus callosum QØ4.Ø
cutis congenita Q84.8
erythrocyte congenital D61.Ø1
extracortical axial E75.29
eye Q11.1
fovea centralis (congenital) Q14.1
gallbladder, congenital Q44.Ø
iris Q13.1
labyrinth, membranous Q16.5
limb (congenital) Q73.8
lower — *see* Defect, reduction, lower limb
upper — *see* Agenesis, arm
lung, congenital (bilateral) (unilateral) Q33.3
pancreas Q45.Ø
parathyroid-thymic D82.1
Pelizaeus-Merzbacher E75.29
penis Q55.5
prostate Q55.4
red cell (with thymoma) D6Ø.9
acquired D6Ø.9
due to drugs D6Ø.9
adult D6Ø.9
chronic D6Ø.Ø
congenital D61.Ø1

- **Aplasia** — *continued*
  - red cell — *continued*
    - constitutional D61.01
    - due to drugs D60.9
    - hereditary D61.01
    - of infants D61.01
    - primary D61.01
    - pure D61.01
      - due to drugs D60.9
    - specified type NEC D60.8
    - transient D60.1
  - round ligament Q52.8
  - skin Q84.8
  - spermatic cord Q55.4
  - spleen Q89.01
  - testicle Q55.0
  - thymic, with immunodeficiency D82.1
  - thyroid (congenital) (with myxedema) E03.1
  - uterus Q51.0
  - ventral horn cell Q06.1
- **Apnea, apneic** (of) (spells) R06.81
  - newborn P28.40
    - central P28.41
    - mixed P28.43
    - obstructive P28.42
    - sleep
      - primary P28.30
        - central P28.31
        - mixed P28.33
        - obstructive P28.32
        - specified NEC P28.39
    - specified NEC P28.49
  - prematurity P28.49
  - sleep G47.30
    - central (primary) G47.31
      - idiopathic G47.31
      - in conditions classified elsewhere G47.37
    - obstructive (adult) (pediatric) G47.33
      - hypopnea G47.33
    - primary central G47.31
    - specified NEC G47.39
- **Apneumatosis, newborn** P28.0
- **Apocrine metaplasia** (breast) — *see* Dysplasia, mammary, specified type NEC
- **Apophysitis** (bone) — *see also* Osteochondropathy
  - calcaneus M92.8
  - juvenile M92.9
- **Apoplectiform convulsions** (cerebral ischemia) I67.82
- **Apoplexia, apoplexy, apoplectic**
  - adrenal A39.1
  - heart (auricle) (ventricle) — *see* Infarct, myocardium
  - heat T67.01 ☑
  - hemorrhagic (stroke) — *see* Hemorrhage, intracranial
  - meninges, hemorrhagic — *see* Hemorrhage, intracranial, subarachnoid
  - uremic N18.9 *[I68.8]*
- **Appearance**
  - bizarre R46.1
  - specified NEC R46.89
  - very low level of personal hygiene R46.0
- **Appendage**
  - epididymal (organ of Morgagni) Q55.4
  - intestine (epiploic) Q43.8
  - preauricular Q17.0
  - testicular (organ of Morgagni) Q55.29
- **Appendicitis** (pneumococcal) (retrocecal) K37
  - with
    - gangrene K35.891
      - with localized peritonitis K35.31
    - perforation NOS K35.32
    - peritoneal abscess K35.33
    - peritonitis NEC K35.33
      - generalized (with perforation or rupture) K35.20
        - with abscess K35.21
      - localized K35.30
        - with
          - gangrene K35.31
          - perforation K35.32
            - and abscess K35.33
    - rupture (with localized peritonitis) K35.32
  - acute (catarrhal) (fulminating) (obstructive) (retrocecal) (suppurative) K35.80
    - with
      - gangrene K35.891
      - peritoneal abscess K35.33
      - peritonitis NEC K35.33
        - generalized (with perforation or rupture) K35.20
- **Appendicitis** — *continued*
  - acute — *continued*
    - with — *continued*
      - peritonitis — *continued*
        - generalized — *continued*
          - with abscess K35.21
        - localized K35.30
          - with
            - gangrene K35.31
            - perforation K35.32
              - and abscess K35.33
    - specified NEC K35.890
      - with gangrene K35.891
        - with localized peritonitis K35.31
  - amebic A06.89
  - chronic (recurrent) K36
  - exacerbation — *see* Appendicitis, with, gangrene
  - gangrenous — *see* Appendicitis, acute
  - healed (obliterative) K36
  - interval K36
  - neurogenic K36
  - obstructive K36
  - recurrent K36
  - relapsing K36
  - ruptured NOS (with localized peritonitis) K35.32
  - subacute (adhesive) K36
  - subsiding K36
  - suppurative — *see* Appendicitis, acute
  - tuberculous A18.32
- **Appendicopathia oxyurica** B80
- **Appendix, appendicular** — *see also* condition
  - epididymis Q55.4
  - Morgagni
    - female Q50.5
    - male (epididymal) Q55.4
      - testicular Q55.29
  - testis Q55.29
- **Appetite**
  - depraved — *see* Pica
  - excessive R63.2
  - lack or loss — *see also* Anorexia R63.0
    - nonorganic origin F50.89
    - psychogenic F50.89
  - perverted (hysterical) — *see* Pica
- **Apple peel syndrome** Q41.1
- **Apprehension state** F41.1
- **Apprehensiveness, abnormal** F41.9
- **Approximal wear** K03.0
- **Apraxia** (classic) (ideational) (ideokinetic) (ideomotor) (motor) (verbal) R48.2
  - following
    - cerebrovascular disease I69.990
      - cerebral infarction I69.390
      - intracerebral hemorrhage I69.190
      - nontraumatic intracranial hemorrhage NEC I69.290
      - specified disease NEC I69.890
      - subarachnoid hemorrhage I69.090
  - oculomotor, congenital H51.8
- **Aptyalism** K11.7
- **Apudoma** — *see* Neoplasm, uncertain behavior, by site
- **Aqueous misdirection** H40.83- ☑
- **Arabicum elephantiasis** — *see* Infestation, filarial
- **Arachnitis** — *see* Meningitis
- **Arachnodactyly** — *see* Syndrome, Marfan's
- **Arachnoiditis** (acute) (adhesive) (basal) (brain) (cerebrospinal) — *see* Meningitis
- **Arachnophobia** F40.210
- **Arboencephalitis, Australian** A83.4
- **Arborization block** (heart) I45.5
- **ARC** (AIDS-related complex) B20
- **Arch**
  - aortic Q25.49
  - bovine Q25.49
- **Arches** — *see* condition
- **Arcuate uterus** Q51.810
- **Arcuatus uterus** Q51.810
- **Arcus** (cornea) senilis — *see* Degeneration, cornea, senile
- **Arc-welder's lung** J63.4
- **Areflexia** R29.2
- **Areola** — *see* condition
- **Argentaffinoma** — *see also* Neoplasm, uncertain behavior, by site
  - malignant — *see* Neoplasm, malignant, by site
  - syndrome E34.0
- **Argininemia** E72.21
- **Arginosuccinic aciduria** E72.22
- **Argyll Robertson phenomenon, pupil or syndrome** (syphilitic) A52.19
  - atypical H57.09
  - nonsyphilitic H57.09
- **Argyria, argyriasis**
  - conjunctival H11.13- ☑
  - from drug or medicament — *see* Table of Drugs and Chemicals, by substance
- **Argyrosis, conjunctival** H11.13- ☑
- **Arhinencephaly** Q04.1
- **Ariboflavinosis** E53.0
- **Arm** — *see* condition
- **Arnold-Chiari disease, obstruction or syndrome** (type II) Q07.00
  - with
    - hydrocephalus Q07.02
      - with spina bifida Q07.03
    - spina bifida Q07.01
      - with hydrocephalus Q07.03
  - type III — *see* Encephalocele
  - type IV Q04.8
- **Aromatic amino-acid metabolism disorder** E70.9
  - specified NEC E70.89
- **Arousals, confusional** G47.51
- **Arrest, arrested**
  - cardiac I46.9
    - complicating
      - abortion — *see* Abortion, by type, complicated by, cardiac arrest
      - anesthesia (general) (local) or other sedation — *see* Table of Drugs and Chemicals, by drug
        - in labor and delivery O74.2
        - in pregnancy O29.11- ☑
        - postpartum, puerperal O89.1
      - delivery (cesarean) (instrumental) O75.4
    - due to
      - cardiac condition I46.2
      - specified condition NEC I46.8
    - intraoperative I97.71- ☑
    - newborn P29.81
    - personal history, successfully resuscitated Z86.74
    - postprocedural I97.12- ☑
      - obstetric procedure O75.4
  - cardiorespiratory — *see* Arrest, cardiac
  - circulatory — *see* Arrest, cardiac
  - deep transverse O64.0 ☑
  - development or growth
    - bone — *see* Disorder, bone, development or growth
    - child R62.50
    - tracheal rings Q32.1
  - epiphyseal
    - complete
      - femur M89.15- ☑
      - humerus M89.12- ☑
      - tibia M89.16- ☑
      - ulna M89.13- ☑
    - forearm M89.13- ☑
      - specified NEC M89.13- ☑
      - ulna — *see* Arrest, epiphyseal, by type, ulna
    - lower leg M89.16- ☑
      - specified NEC M89.168
      - tibia — *see* Arrest, epiphyseal, by type, tibia
    - partial
      - femur M89.15- ☑
      - humerus M89.12- ☑
      - tibia M89.16- ☑
      - ulna M89.13- ☑
    - specified NEC M89.18
  - granulopoiesis — *see* Agranulocytosis
  - growth plate — *see* Arrest, epiphyseal
  - heart — *see* Arrest, cardiac
  - legal, anxiety concerning Z65.3
  - physeal — *see* Arrest, epiphyseal
  - respiratory R09.2
    - newborn P28.81
  - sinus I45.5
  - spermatogenesis (complete) — *see* Azoospermia
    - incomplete — *see* Oligospermia
  - transverse (deep) O64.0 ☑
- **Arrhenoblastoma**
  - benign
    - specified site — *see* Neoplasm, benign, by site
    - unspecified site
      - female D27.9
      - male D29.20
  - malignant
    - specified site — *see* Neoplasm, malignant, by site

Arrhenoblastoma — *continued*
  malignant — *continued*
    unspecified site
      female C56.9
      male C62.9Ø
  specified site — *see* Neoplasm, uncertain behavior, by site
  unspecified site
    female D39.1Ø
    male D4Ø.1Ø
Arrhythmia (auricle) (cardiac) (juvenile) (nodal) (reflex) (supraventricular) (transitory) (ventricle) I49.9
  block I45.9
  extrasystolic I49.49
  newborn
    bradycardia P29.12
    occurring before birth PØ3.819
      before onset of labor PØ3.81Ø
      during labor PØ3.811
    tachycardia P29.11
  psychogenic F45.8
  sinus I49.8
  specified NEC I49.8
  vagal R55
  ventricular re-entry I47.Ø
Arrillaga-Ayerza syndrome (pulmonary sclerosis with pulmonary hypertension) I27.Ø
Arsenical pigmentation L81.8
  from drug or medicament — *see* Table of Drugs and Chemicals
Arsenism — *see* Poisoning, arsenic
Arterial — *see* condition
Arteriofibrosis — *see* Arteriosclerosis
Arteriolar sclerosis — *see* Arteriosclerosis
Arteriolith — *see* Arteriosclerosis
Arteriolitis I77.6
  necrotizing, kidney I77.5
  renal — *see* Hypertension, kidney
Arteriolosclerosis — *see* Arteriosclerosis
Arterionephrosclerosis — *see* Hypertension, kidney
Arteriopathy I77.9
  cerebral autosomal dominant, with subcortical infarcts and leukoencephalopathy (CADASIL) I67.85Ø
Arteriosclerosis, arteriosclerotic (diffuse) (obliterans) (of) (senile) (with calcification) I7Ø.9Ø
  with
    chronic limb-threatening ischemia — *see* Arteriosclerosis, with critical limb ischemia
    critical limb ischemia
      bypass graft I7Ø.329
        autologous vein graft I7Ø.429
          leg I7Ø.429
            with
              gangrene (and intermittent claudication, rest pain, and ulcer) I7Ø.469
              rest pain (and intermittent claudication) I7Ø.429
            bilateral I7Ø.423
              with
                gangrene (and intermittent claudication, rest pain, and ulcer) I7Ø.463
                rest pain (and intermittent claudication) I7Ø.423
            left I7Ø.422
              with
                gangrene (and intermittent claudication, rest pain, and ulcer) I7Ø.462
                rest pain (and intermittent claudication) I7Ø.422
                ulceration (and intermittent claudication and rest pain) I7Ø.449
                  ankle I7Ø.443
                  calf I7Ø.442
                  foot site NEC I7Ø.445
                  heel I7Ø.444
                  lower leg NEC I7Ø.448
                  mid foot I7Ø.444
                  thigh I7Ø.441
            right I7Ø.421
              with
                gangrene (and intermittent claudication, rest pain, and ulcer) I7Ø.461

Arteriosclerosis, arteriosclerotic — *continued*
  with — *continued*
    critical limb ischemia — *continued*
      bypass graft — *continued*
        autologous vein graft — *continued*
          leg — *continued*
            right — *continued*
              with — *continued*
                rest pain (and intermittent claudication) I7Ø.421
                ulceration (and intermittent claudication and rest pain) I7Ø.439
                  ankle I7Ø.433
                  calf I7Ø.432
                  foot site NEC I7Ø.435
                  heel I7Ø.434
                  lower leg NEC I7Ø.438
                  midfoot I7Ø.434
                  thigh I7Ø.431
        leg I7Ø.329
          with
            gangrene (and intermittent claudication, rest pain, and ulcer) I7Ø.369
            rest pain (and intermittent claudication) I7Ø.329
          bilateral I7Ø.323
            with
              gangrene (and intermittent claudication, rest pain, and ulcer) I7Ø.363
              rest pain (and intermittent claudication) I7Ø.323
          left I7Ø.322
            with
              gangrene (and intermittent claudication, rest pain, and ulcer) I7Ø.362
              rest pain (and intermittent claudication) I7Ø.322
              ulceration (and intermittent claudication and rest pain) I7Ø.349
                ankle I7Ø.343
                calf I7Ø.342
                foot site NEC I7Ø.345
                heel I7Ø.344
                lower leg NEC I7Ø.348
                midfoot I7Ø.344
                thigh I7Ø.341
          right I7Ø.321
            with
              gangrene (and intermittent claudication, rest pain, and ulcer) I7Ø.361
              rest pain (and intermittent claudication) I7Ø.321
              ulceration (and intermittent claudication and rest pain) I7Ø.339
                ankle I7Ø.333
                calf I7Ø.332
                foot site NEC I7Ø.335
                heel I7Ø.334
                lower leg NEC I7Ø.338
                midfoot I7Ø.334
                thigh I7Ø.331
        nonautologous biological graft I7Ø.529
          leg I7Ø.529
            with
              gangrene (and intermittent claudication, rest pain, and ulcer) I7Ø.569
              rest pain (and intermittent claudication) I7Ø.529
            bilateral I7Ø.523
              with
                gangrene (and intermittent claudication, rest pain, and ulcer) I7Ø.563
                rest pain (and intermittent claudication) I7Ø.523
            left I7Ø.522
              with
                gangrene (and intermittent claudication, rest pain, and ulcer) I7Ø.562
                rest pain (and intermittent claudication) I7Ø.522

Arteriosclerosis, arteriosclerotic — *continued*
  with — *continued*
    critical limb ischemia — *continued*
      bypass graft — *continued*
        nonautologous biological graft — *continued*
          leg — *continued*
            left — *continued*
              with — *continued*
                ulceration (and intermittent claudication and rest pain) I7Ø.549
                  ankle I7Ø.543
                  calf I7Ø.542
                  foot site NEC I7Ø.545
                  heel I7Ø.544
                  lower leg NEC I7Ø.548
                  midfoot I7Ø.544
                  thigh I7Ø.541
            right I7Ø.521
              with
                gangrene (and intermittent claudication, rest pain, and ulcer) I7Ø.561
                rest pain (and intermittent claudication) I7Ø.521
                ulceration (and intermittent claudication and rest pain) I7Ø.539
                  ankle I7Ø.533
                  calf I7Ø.532
                  foot site NEC I7Ø.535
                  heel I7Ø.534
                  lower leg NEC I7Ø.538
                  midfoot I7Ø.534
                  thigh I7Ø.531
        nonbiological graft I7Ø.629
          leg I7Ø.629
            with
              gangrene (and intermittent claudication, rest pain, and ulcer) I7Ø.669
              rest pain (and intermittent claudication) I7Ø.629
            bilateral I7Ø.623
              with
                gangrene (and intermittent claudication, rest pain, and ulcer) I7Ø.663
                rest pain (intermittent claudication) I7Ø.623
            left I7Ø.622
              with
                gangrene (and intermittent claudication, rest pain, and ulcer) I7Ø.662
                rest pain (and intermittent claudication) I7Ø.622
                ulceration (and intermittent claudication and rest pain) I7Ø.649
                  ankle I7Ø.643
                  calf I7Ø.642
                  foot site NEC I7Ø.645
                  heel I7Ø.644
                  lower leg NEC I7Ø.648
                  midfoot I7Ø.644
                  thigh I7Ø.641
            right I7Ø.621
              with
                gangrene (and intermittent claudication, rest pain, and ulcer) I7Ø.661
                rest pain (and intermittent claudication) I7Ø.621
                ulceration (and intermittent claudication and rest pain) I7Ø.639
                  ankle I7Ø.633
                  calf I7Ø.632
                  foot site NEC I7Ø.635
                  heel I7Ø.634
                  lower leg NEC I7Ø.638
                  midfoot I7Ø.634
                  thigh I7Ø.631
        specified graft NEC I7Ø.729
          leg I7Ø.729

Arteriosclerosis, arteriosclerotic — *continued*
with — *continued*
critical limb ischemia — *continued*
bypass graft — *continued*
specified graft — *continued*
leg — *continued*
with
gangrene (and intermittent claudication, rest pain, and ulcer) I70.769
rest pain (and intermittent claudication) I70.729
bilateral I70.723
with
gangrene (and intermittent claudication, rest pain, and ulcer) I70.763
rest pain (and intermittent claudication) I70.723
left I70.722
with
gangrene (and intermittent claudication, rest pain, and ulcer) I70.762
rest pain (and intermittent claudication) I70.722
ulceration (and intermittent claudication and rest pain) I70.749
ankle I70.743
calf I70.742
foot site NEC I70.745
heel I70.744
lower leg NEC I70.748
midfoot I70.744
thigh I70.741
right I70.721
with
gangrene (and intermittent claudication, rest pain, and ulcer) I70.761
rest pain (and intermittent claudication) I70.721
ulceration (and intermittent claudication and rest pain) I70.739
ankle I70.733
calf I70.732
foot site NEC I70.735
heel I70.734
lower leg NEC I70.738
midfoot I70.734
thigh I70.731
leg I70.229
with
gangrene (and intermittent claudication, rest pain, and ulcer) I70.269
rest pain (and intermittent claudication) I70.229
bilateral I70.223
with
gangrene (and intermittent claudication, rest pain, and ulcer) I70.263
rest pain (and intermittent claudication) I70.223
left I70.222
with
gangrene (and intermittent claudication, rest pain, and ulcer) I70.262
rest pain (and intermittent claudication) I70.222
ulceration (and intermittent claudication and rest pain) I70.249
ankle I70.243
calf I70.242
foot site NEC I70.245
heel I70.244
lower leg NEC I70.248
midfoot I70.244
thigh I70.241
right I70.221
with
gangrene (and intermittent claudication, rest pain, and ulcer) I70.261
rest pain (and intermittent claudication) I70.221

Arteriosclerosis, arteriosclerotic — *continued*
with — *continued*
critical limb ischemia — *continued*
leg — *continued*
right — *continued*
with — *continued*
ulceration (and intermittent claudication and rest pain) I70.239
ankle I70.233
calf I70.232
foot site NEC I70.235
heel I70.234
lower leg NEC I70.238
midfoot I70.234
thigh I70.231
aorta I70.0
arteries of extremities — *see* Arteriosclerosis, extremities
with
chronic limb-threatening ischemia — *see* Arteriosclerosis, with critical limb ischemia
critical limb ischemia — *see* Arteriosclerosis, with critical limb ischemia
brain I67.2
bypass graft
with
chronic limb-threatening ischemia — *see* Arteriosclerosis, with critical limb ischemia
critical limb ischemia — *see* Arteriosclerosis, with critical limb ischemia
coronary — *see* Arteriosclerosis, coronary, bypass graft
extremities — *see* Arteriosclerosis, extremities, bypass graft
cardiac — *see* Disease, heart, ischemic, atherosclerotic
cardiopathy — *see* Disease, heart, ischemic, atherosclerotic
cardiorenal — *see* Hypertension, cardiorenal
cardiovascular — *see* Disease, heart, ischemic, atherosclerotic
carotid — *see also* Occlusion, artery, carotid I65.2- ☑
central nervous system I67.2
cerebral I67.2
cerebrovascular I67.2
coronary (artery) I25.10
due to
calcified coronary lesion (severely) I25.84
lipid rich plaque I25.83
bypass graft I25.810
with
angina pectoris I25.709
with documented spasm I25.701
refractory I25.702
specified type NEC I25.708
unstable I25.700
ischemic chest pain I25.709
autologous artery I25.810
with
angina pectoris I25.729
with documented spasm I25.721
refractory I25.722
specified type I25.728
unstable I25.720
ischemic chest pain I25.729
autologous vein I25.810
with
angina pectoris I25.719
with documented spasm I25.711
refractory I25.712
specified type I25.718
unstable I25.710
ischemic chest pain I25.719
nonautologous biological I25.810
with
angina pectoris I25.739
with documented spasm I25.731
refractory I25.732
specified type I25.738
unstable I25.730
ischemic chest pain I25.739
specified type NEC I25.810
with
angina pectoris I25.799
with documented spasm I25.791
refractory I25.792
specified type I25.798
unstable I25.790
ischemic chest pain I25.799

Arteriosclerosis, arteriosclerotic — *continued*
coronary — *continued*
native vessel
with
angina pectoris I25.119
with documented spasm I25.111
refractory I25.112
specified type NEC I25.118
unstable I25.110
ischemic chest pain I25.119
transplanted heart I25.811
bypass graft I25.812
with
angina pectoris I25.769
with documented spasm I25.761
refractory I25.762
specified type I25.768
unstable I25.760
ischemic chest pain I25.769
native coronary artery I25.811
with
angina pectoris I25.759
with documented spasm I25.751
refractory I25.752
specified type I25.758
unstable I25.750
ischemic chest pain I25.759
extremities (native arteries) I70.209
with
chronic limb-threatening ischemia — *see* Arteriosclerosis, with critical limb ischemia
critical limb ischemia — *see* Arteriosclerosis, with critical limb ischemia
bypass graft I70.309
with
chronic limb-threatening ischemia — *see* Arteriosclerosis, with critical limb ischemia
critical limb ischemia — *see* Arteriosclerosis, with critical limb ischemia
autologous vein graft I70.409
leg I70.409
with
gangrene (and intermittent claudication, rest pain and ulcer) I70.469
intermittent claudication I70.419
rest pain (and intermittent claudication) I70.429
bilateral I70.403
with
gangrene (and intermittent claudication, rest pain and ulcer) I70.463
intermittent claudication I70.463
rest pain (and intermittent claudication) I70.423
specified type NEC I70.493
left I70.402
with
gangrene (and intermittent claudication, rest pain and ulcer) I70.462
intermittent claudication I70.412
rest pain (and intermittent claudication) I70.422
ulceration (and intermittent claudication and rest pain) I70.449
ankle I70.443
calf I70.442
foot site NEC I70.445
heel I70.444
lower leg NEC I70.448
midfoot I70.444
thigh I70.441
specified type NEC I70.492
right I70.401
with
gangrene (and intermittent claudication, rest pain and ulcer) I70.461
intermittent claudication I70.411
rest pain (and intermittent claudication) I70.421
ulceration (and intermittent claudication and rest pain) I70.439
ankle I70.433
calf I70.432
foot site NEC I70.435
heel I70.434
lower leg NEC I70.438

- **Arteriosclerosis, arteriosclerotic** — *continued*
  - extremities — *continued*
    - bypass graft — *continued*
      - autologous vein graft — *continued*
        - leg — *continued*
          - right — *continued*
            - with — *continued*
              - ulceration — *continued*
                - midfoot I70.434
                - thigh I70.431
              - specified type NEC I70.491
            - specified type NEC I70.499
        - specified NEC I70.408
          - with
            - gangrene (and intermittent claudication, rest pain and ulcer) I70.468
            - intermittent claudication I70.418
            - rest pain (and intermittent claudication) I70.428
            - ulceration (and intermittent claudication and rest pain) I70.45
          - specified type NEC I70.498
      - leg I70.309
        - with
          - gangrene (and intermittent claudication, rest pain and ulcer) I70.369
          - intermittent claudication I70.319
          - rest pain (and intermittent claudication) I70.329
        - bilateral I70.303
          - with
            - gangrene (and intermittent claudication, rest pain and ulcer) I70.363
            - intermittent claudication I70.313
            - rest pain (and intermittent claudication) I70.323
          - specified type NEC I70.393
        - left I70.302
          - with
            - gangrene (and intermittent claudication, rest pain and ulcer) I70.362
            - intermittent claudication I70.312
            - rest pain (and intermittent claudication) I70.322
            - ulceration (and intermittent claudication and rest pain) I70.349
              - ankle I70.343
              - calf I70.342
              - foot site NEC I70.345
              - heel I70.344
              - lower leg NEC I70.348
              - midfoot I70.344
              - thigh I70.341
          - specified type NEC I70.392
        - right I70.301
          - with
            - gangrene (and intermittent claudication, rest pain and ulcer) I70.361
            - intermittent claudication I70.311
            - rest pain (and intermittent claudication) I70.321
            - ulceration (and intermittent claudication and rest pain I70.339
              - ankle I70.333
              - calf I70.332
              - foot site NEC I70.335
              - heel I70.334
              - lower leg NEC I70.338
              - midfoot I70.334
              - thigh I70.331
          - specified type NEC I70.391
        - specified type NEC I70.399
      - nonautologous biological graft I70.509
        - leg I70.509
          - with
            - gangrene (and intermittent claudication, rest pain and ulcer) I70.569
            - intermittent claudication I70.519
            - rest pain (and intermittent claudication) I70.529
          - bilateral I70.503
            - with
              - gangrene (and intermittent claudication, rest pain and ulcer) I70.563
              - intermittent claudication I70.513
              - rest pain (and intermittent claudication) I70.523
            - specified type NEC I70.593

- **Arteriosclerosis, arteriosclerotic** — *continued*
  - extremities — *continued*
    - bypass graft — *continued*
      - nonautologous biological graft — *continued*
        - leg — *continued*
          - left I70.502
            - with
              - gangrene (and intermittent claudication, rest pain and ulcer) I70.562
              - intermittent claudication I70.512
              - rest pain (and intermittent claudication) I70.522
              - ulceration (and intermittent claudication and rest pain) I70.549
                - ankle I70.543
                - calf I70.542
                - foot site NEC I70.545
                - heel I70.544
                - lower leg NEC I70.548
                - midfoot I70.544
                - thigh I70.541
            - specified type NEC I70.592
          - right I70.501
            - with
              - gangrene (and intermittent claudication, rest pain and ulcer) I70.561
              - intermittent claudication I70.511
              - rest pain (and intermittent claudication) I70.521
              - ulceration (and intermittent claudication and rest pain) I70.539
                - ankle I70.533
                - calf I70.532
                - foot site NEC I70.535
                - heel I70.534
                - lower leg NEC I70.538
                - midfoot I70.534
                - thigh I70.531
            - specified type NEC I70.591
          - specified type NEC I70.599
        - specified NEC I70.508
          - with
            - gangrene (and intermittent claudication, rest pain and ulcer) I70.568
            - intermittent claudication I70.518
            - rest pain (and intermittent claudication) I70.528
            - ulceration (and intermittent claudication and rest pain) I70.55
          - specified type NEC I70.598
      - nonbiological graft I70.609
        - leg I70.609
          - with
            - gangrene (and intermittent claudication, rest pain and ulcer) I70.669
            - intermittent claudication I70.619
            - rest pain (and intermittent claudication) I70.629
          - bilateral I70.603
            - with
              - gangrene (and intermittent claudication, rest pain and ulcer) I70.663
              - intermittent claudication I70.613
              - rest pain (and intermittent claudication) I70.623
            - specified type NEC I70.693
          - left I70.602
            - with
              - gangrene (and intermittent claudication, rest pain and ulcer) I70.662
              - intermittent claudication I70.612
              - rest pain (and intermittent claudication) I70.622
              - ulceration (and intermittent claudication and rest pain) I70.649
                - ankle I70.643
                - calf I70.642
                - foot site NEC I70.645
                - heel I70.644
                - lower leg NEC I70.648
                - midfoot I70.644
                - thigh I70.641
            - specified type NEC I70.692
          - right I70.601

- **Arteriosclerosis, arteriosclerotic** — *continued*
  - extremities — *continued*
    - bypass graft — *continued*
      - nonbiological graft — *continued*
        - leg — *continued*
          - right — *continued*
            - with
              - gangrene (and intermittent claudication, rest pain and ulcer) I70.661
              - intermittent claudication I70.611
              - rest pain (and intermittent claudication) I70.621
              - ulceration (and intermittent claudication and rest pain) I70.639
                - ankle I70.633
                - calf I70.632
                - foot site NEC I70.635
                - heel I70.634
                - lower leg NEC I70.638
                - midfoot I70.634
                - thigh I70.631
            - specified type NEC I70.691
          - specified type NEC I70.699
        - specified NEC I70.608
          - with
            - gangrene (and intermittent claudication, rest pain and ulcer) I70.668
            - intermittent claudication I70.618
            - rest pain (and intermittent claudication) I70.628
            - ulceration (and intermittent claudication and rest pain) I70.65
          - specified type NEC I70.698
      - specified graft NEC I70.709
        - leg I70.709
          - with
            - gangrene (and intermittent claudication, rest pain and ulcer) I70.769
            - intermittent claudication I70.719
            - rest pain (and intermittent claudication) I70.729
          - bilateral I70.703
            - with
              - gangrene (and intermittent claudication, rest pain and ulcer) I70.763
              - intermittent claudication I70.713
              - rest pain (and intermittent claudication) I70.723
            - specified type NEC I70.793
          - left I70.702
            - with
              - gangrene (and intermittent claudication, rest pain and ulcer) I70.762
              - intermittent claudication I70.712
              - rest pain (and intermittent claudication) I70.722
              - ulceration (and intermittent claudication and rest pain) I70.749
                - ankle I70.743
                - calf I70.742
                - foot site NEC I70.745
                - heel I70.744
                - lower leg NEC I70.748
                - midfoot I70.744
                - thigh I70.741
            - specified type NEC I70.792
          - right I70.701
            - with
              - gangrene (and intermittent claudication, rest pain and ulcer) I70.761
              - intermittent claudication I70.711
              - rest pain (and intermittent claudication) I70.721
              - ulceration (and intermittent claudication and rest pain) I70.739
                - ankle I70.733
                - calf I70.732
                - foot site NEC I70.735
                - heel I70.734
                - lower leg NEC I70.738
                - midfoot I70.734
                - thigh I70.731
            - specified type NEC I70.791
          - specified type NEC I70.799
        - specified NEC I70.708

- **Arteriosclerosis, arteriosclerotic** — *continued*
  - extremities — *continued*
    - bypass graft — *continued*
      - specified graft — *continued*
        - specified — *continued*
          - with
            - gangrene (and intermittent claudication, rest pain and ulcer) I7Ø.768
            - intermittent claudication I7Ø.718
            - rest pain (and intermittent claudication) I7Ø.728
            - ulceration (and intermittent claudication and rest pain) I7Ø.75
          - specified type NEC I7Ø.798
      - specified NEC I7Ø.3Ø8
        - with
          - gangrene (and intermittent claudication, rest pain and ulcer) I7Ø.368
          - intermittent claudication I7Ø.318
          - rest pain (and intermittent claudication) I7Ø.328
          - ulceration (and intermittent claudication and rest pain) I7Ø.35
        - specifiec type NEC I7Ø.398
    - leg I7Ø.2Ø9
      - with
        - gangrene (and intermittent claudication, rest pain and ulcer) I7Ø.269
        - intermittent claudication I7Ø.219
        - rest pain (and intermittent claudication) I7Ø.229
      - bilateral I7Ø.2Ø3
        - with
          - gangrene (and intermittent claudication, rest pain and ulcer) I7Ø.263
          - intermittent claudication I7Ø.213
          - rest pain (and intermittent claudication) I7Ø.223
        - specified type NEC I7Ø.293
      - left I7Ø.2Ø2
        - with
          - gangrene (and intermittent claudication, rest pain and ulcer) I7Ø.262
          - intermittent claudication I7Ø.212
          - rest pain (and intermittent claudication) I7Ø.222
          - ulceration (and intermittent claudication and rest pain) I7Ø.249
            - ankle I7Ø.243
            - calf I7Ø.242
            - foot site NEC I7Ø.245
            - heel I7Ø.244
            - lower leg NEC I7Ø.248
            - midfoot I7Ø.244
            - thigh I7Ø.241
        - specified type NEC I7Ø.292
      - right I7Ø.2Ø1
        - with
          - gangrene (and intermittent claudication, rest pain and ulcer) I7Ø.261
          - intermittent claudication I7Ø.211
          - rest pain (and intermittent claudication) I7Ø.221
          - ulceration (and intermittent claudication and rest pain) I7Ø.239
            - ankle I7Ø.233
            - calf I7Ø.232
            - foot site NEC I7Ø.235
            - heel I7Ø.234
            - lower leg NEC I7Ø.238
            - midfoot I7Ø.234
            - thigh I7Ø.231
        - specified type NEC I7Ø.291
      - specified type NEC I7Ø.299
    - specified site NEC I7Ø.2Ø8
      - with
        - gangrene (and intermittent claudication, rest pain and ulcer) I7Ø.268
        - intermittent claudication I7Ø.218
        - rest pain (and intermittent claudication) I7Ø.228
        - ulceration (and intermittent claudication and rest pain) I7Ø.25
      - specified type NEC I7Ø.298
  - generalized I7Ø.91
  - heart (disease) — *see* Arteriosclerosis, coronary (artery),
  - kidney — *see* Hypertension, kidney
  - medial — *see* Arteriosclerosis, extremities
  - mesenteric (artery) K55.1

- **Arteriosclerosis, arteriosclerotic** — *continued*
  - Mönckeberg's — *see* Arteriosclerosis, extremities
  - myocarditis I51.4
  - peripheral (of extremities) — *see* Arteriosclerosis, extremities
  - pulmonary (idiopathic) I27.Ø
  - renal (arterioles) — *see also* Hypertension, kidney artery I7Ø.1
  - retina (vascular) I7Ø.8 *[H35.Ø-]* ☑
  - specified artery NEC I7Ø.8
  - spinal (cord) G95.19
  - vertebral (artery) I67.2
- **Arteriospasm** I73.9
- **Arteriovenous** — *see* condition
- **Arteritis** I77.6
  - allergic M31.Ø
  - aorta (nonsyphilitic) I77.6
    - syphilitic A52.Ø2
  - aortic arch M31.4
  - brachiocephalic M31.4
  - brain I67.7
    - syphilitic A52.Ø4
  - cerebral I67.7
    - in systemic lupus erythematosus M32.19
    - listerial A32.89
    - syphilitic A52.Ø4
    - tuberculous A18.89
  - coronary (artery) I25.89
    - rheumatic IØ1.8
      - chronic IØ9.89
    - syphilitic A52.Ø6
  - cranial (left) (right), giant cell M31.6
  - deformans — *see* Arteriosclerosis
  - giant cell NEC M31.6
    - with polymyalgia rheumatica M31.5
  - necrosing or necrotizing M31.9
    - specified NEC M31.8
  - nodosa M3Ø.Ø
  - obliterans — *see* Arteriosclerosis
  - pulmonary I28.8
  - rheumatic — *see* Fever, rheumatic
  - senile — *see* Arteriosclerosis
  - suppurative I77.2
  - syphilitic (general) A52.Ø9
    - brain A52.Ø4
    - coronary A52.Ø6
    - spinal A52.Ø9
  - temporal, giant cell M31.6
  - young female aortic arch syndrome M31.4
- **Artery, arterial** — *see also* condition
  - abscess I77.89
  - single umbilical Q27.Ø
- **Arthralgia** (allergic) — *see also* Pain, joint
  - in caisson disease T7Ø.3 ☑
  - temporomandibular M26.62- ☑
- **Arthritis, arthritic** (acute) (chronic) (nonpyogenic) (subacute) M19.9Ø
  - allergic — *see* Arthritis, specified form NEC
  - ankylosing (crippling) (spine) — *see also* Spondylitis, ankylosing
    - sites other than spine — *see* Arthritis, specified form NEC
  - atrophic — *see* Osteoarthritis
    - spine — *see* Spondylitis, ankylosing
  - back — *see* Spondylopathy, inflammatory
  - blennorrhagic (gonococcal) A54.42
  - Charcot's — *see* Arthropathy, neuropathic
    - diabetic — *see* Diabetes, arthropathy, neuropathic
    - syringomyelic G95.Ø
  - chylous (filarial) — *see also* category MØ1 B74.9
  - climacteric (any site) NEC — *see* Arthritis, specified form NEC
  - crystal (-induced) — *see* Arthritis, in, crystals
  - deformans — *see* Osteoarthritis
  - degenerative — *see* Osteoarthritis
  - due to or associated with
    - acromegaly E22.Ø
    - brucellosis — *see* Brucellosis
    - caisson disease T7Ø.3 ☑
    - diabetes — *see* Diabetes, arthropathy
    - dracontiasis — *see also* category MØ1 B72
    - enteritis NEC
      - regional — *see* Enteritis, regional
    - erysipelas — *see also* category MØ1 A46
    - erythema
      - epidemic A25.1
      - nodosum L52
    - filariasis NOS B74.9

- **Arthritis, arthritic** — *continued*
  - due to or associated with — *continued*
    - glanders A24.Ø
    - helminthiasis — *see also* category MØ1 B83.9
    - hemophilia D66 *[M36.2]*
    - Henoch- (Schönlein) purpura D69.Ø *[M36.4]*
    - human parvovirus — *see also* category MØ1 B97.6
    - infectious disease NEC MØ1 ☑
    - leprosy (see also category MØ1) — *see also* Leprosy A3Ø.9
    - Lyme disease A69.23
    - mycobacteria — *see also* category MØ1 A31.8
    - parasitic disease NEC — *see also* category MØ1 B89
    - paratyphoid fever (see also category MØ1) — *see also* Fever, paratyphoid AØ1.4
    - rat bite fever — *see also* category MØ1 A25.1
    - regional enteritis — *see* Enteritis, regional
    - respiratory disorder NOS J98.9
    - serum sickness — *see also* Reaction, serum T8Ø.69 ☑
    - syringomyelia G95.Ø
    - typhoid fever AØ1.Ø4
  - epidemic erythema A25.1
  - facet joint — *see also* Spondylosis M47.819
  - febrile — *see* Fever, rheumatic
  - gonococcal A54.42
  - gouty (acute) — *see* Gout
  - in (due to)
    - acromegaly — *see also* subcategory M14.8- E22.Ø
    - amyloidosis — *see also* subcategory M14.8- E85.4
    - bacterial disease — *see also* subcategory MØ1 A49.9
    - Behçet's syndrome M35.2
    - caisson disease — *see also* subcategory M14.8- T7Ø.3 ☑
    - coliform bacilli (Escherichia coli) — *see* Arthritis, in, pyogenic organism NEC
    - crystals M11.9
      - dicalcium phosphate — *see* Arthritis, in, crystals, specified type NEC
      - hydroxyapatite M11.Ø- ☑
      - pyrophosphate — *see* Arthritis, in, crystals, specified type NEC
      - specified type NEC M11.8Ø
        - ankle M11.87- ☑
        - elbow M11.82- ☑
        - foot joint M11.87- ☑
        - hand joint M11.84- ☑
        - hip M11.85- ☑
        - knee M11.86- ☑
        - multiple sites M11.8- ☑
        - shoulder M11.81- ☑
        - vertebrae M11.88
        - wrist M11.83- ☑
    - dermatoarthritis, lipoid E78.81
    - dracontiasis (dracunculiasis) — *see also* category MØ1 B72
    - endocrine disorder NEC — *see also* subcategory M14.8- E34.9
    - enteritis, infectious NEC — *see also* category MØ1 AØ9
      - specified organism NEC — *see also* category MØ1 AØ8.8
    - erythema
      - multiforme — *see also* subcategory M14.8- L51.9
      - nodosum — *see also* subcategory M14.8- L52
    - gout — *see* Gout
    - helminthiasis NEC — *see also* category MØ1 B83.9
    - hemochromatosis — *see also* subcategory M14.8- E83.118
    - hemoglobinopathy NEC D58.2 *[M36.3]*
    - hemophilia NEC D66 *[M36.2]*
    - Hemophilus influenzae MØØ.8- ☑ *[B96.3]*
    - Henoch (-Schönlein) purpura D69.Ø *[M36.4]*
    - hyperparathyroidism NEC — *see also* subcategory M14.8- E21.3
    - hypersensitivity reaction NEC T78.49 ☑ *[M36.4]*
    - hypogammaglobulinemia — *see also* subcategory M14.8- D8Ø.1
    - hypothyroidism NEC — *see also* subcategory M14.8- EØ3.9
    - infection — *see* Arthritis, pyogenic or pyemic
      - spine — *see* Spondylopathy, infective
    - infectious disease NEC MØ1 ☑
    - leprosy — *see also* category MØ1 A3Ø.9
    - leukemia NEC C95.9- ☑ *[M36.1]*
    - lipoid dermatoarthritis E78.81
    - Lyme disease A69.23

- **Arthritis, arthritic** — *continued*
  - in — *continued*
    - Mediterranean fever, familial — *see also* subcategory M14.8- MØ4.1
    - Meningococcus A39.83
    - metabolic disorder NEC — *see also* subcategory M14.8- E88.9
    - multiple myelomatosis C9Ø.Ø- ☑ *[M36.1]*
    - mumps B26.85
    - mycosis NEC — *see also* category MØ1 B49
    - myelomatosis (multiple) C9Ø.Ø- ☑ *[M36.1]*
    - neurological disorder NEC G98.Ø
    - ochronosis — *see also* subcategory M14.8- E7Ø.29
    - O'nyong-nyong — *see also* category MØ1 A92.1
    - parasitic disease NEC — *see also* category MØ1 B89
    - paratyphoid fever — *see also* category MØ1 AØ1.4
    - Pseudomonas — *see* Arthritis, pyogenic, bacterial NEC
    - psoriasis L4Ø.5Ø
    - pyogenic organism NEC — *see* Arthritis, pyogenic, bacterial NEC
    - Reiter's disease — *see* Reiter's disease
    - respiratory disorder NEC — *see also* subcategory M14.8- J98.9
    - reticulosis, malignant — *see also* subcategory M14.8- C86.Ø
    - rubella BØ6.82
    - Salmonella (arizonae) (cholerae-suis) (enteritidis) (typhimurium) AØ2.23
    - sarcoidosis D86.86
    - specified bacteria NEC — *see* Arthritis, pyogenic, bacterial NEC
    - sporotrichosis B42.82
    - syringomyelia G95.Ø
    - thalassemia NEC D56.9 *[M36.3]*
    - tuberculosis — *see* Tuberculosis, arthritis
    - typhoid fever AØ1.Ø4
    - urethritis, Reiter's — *see* Reiter's disease
    - viral disease NEC — *see also* category MØ1 B34.9
  - infectious or infective — *see also* Arthritis, pyogenic or pyemic
    - spine — *see* Spondylopathy, infective
  - juvenile MØ8.9Ø
    - with systemic onset — *see* Still's disease
    - ankle MØ8.97- ☑
    - elbow MØ8.92- ☑
    - foot joint MØ8.97- ☑
    - hand joint MØ8.94- ☑
    - hip MØ8.95- ☑
    - knee MØ8.96- ☑
    - multiple site MØ8.99
    - pauciarticular MØ8.4Ø
      - ankle MØ8.47- ☑
      - elbow MØ8.42- ☑
      - foot joint MØ8.47- ☑
      - hand joint MØ8.44- ☑
      - hip MØ8.45- ☑
      - knee MØ8.46- ☑
      - shoulder MØ8.41- ☑
      - specified site NEC MØ8.4A
      - vertebrae MØ8.48
      - wrist MØ8.43- ☑
    - psoriatic L4Ø.54
    - rheumatoid — *see* Arthritis, rheumatoid, juvenile
    - shoulder MØ8.91- ☑
    - specified site NEC MØ8.9A
    - specified type NEC MØ8.8Ø
      - ankle MØ8.87- ☑
      - elbow MØ8.82- ☑
      - foot joint MØ8.87- ☑
      - hand joint MØ8.84- ☑
      - hip MØ8.85- ☑
      - knee MØ8.86- ☑
      - multiple site MØ8.89
      - shoulder MØ8.81- ☑
      - specified joint NEC MØ8.88
      - vertebrae MØ8.88
      - wrist MØ8.83- ☑
    - wrist MØ8.93- ☑
  - meaning osteoarthritis — *see* Osteoarthritis
  - meningococcal A39.83
  - menopausal (any site) NEC — *see* Arthritis, specified form NEC
  - mutilans (psoriatic) L4Ø.52
  - mycotic NEC — *see also* category MØ1 B49
  - neuropathic (Charcot) — *see* Arthropathy, neuropathic
    - diabetic — *see* Diabetes, arthropathy, neuropathic

- **Arthritis, arthritic** — *continued*
  - neuropathic — *see* Arthropathy, neuropathic — *continued*
    - nonsyphilitic NEC G98.Ø
    - syringomyelic G95.Ø
  - ochronotic — *see also* subcategory M14.8- E7Ø.29
  - palindromic (any site) — *see* Rheumatism, palindromic
  - pneumococcal MØØ.1Ø
    - ankle MØØ.17- ☑
    - elbow MØØ.12- ☑
    - foot joint — *see* Arthritis, pneumococcal, ankle
    - hand joint MØØ.14- ☑
    - hip MØØ.15- ☑
    - knee MØØ.16- ☑
    - multiple site MØØ.19
    - shoulder MØØ.11- ☑
    - vertebra MØØ.18
    - wrist MØØ.13- ☑
  - postdysenteric — *see* Arthropathy, postdysenteric
  - postmeningococcal A39.84
  - postrheumatic, chronic — *see* Arthropathy, postrheumatic, chronic
  - primary progressive — *see also* Arthritis, specified form NEC
    - spine — *see* Spondylitis, ankylosing
  - psoriatic L4Ø.5Ø
  - purulent (any site except spine) — *see* Arthritis, pyogenic or pyemic
    - spine — *see* Spondylopathy, infective
  - pyogenic or pyemic (any site except spine) MØØ.9
    - bacterial NEC MØØ.8Ø
      - ankle MØØ.87- ☑
      - elbow MØØ.82- ☑
      - foot joint — *see* Arthritis, pyogenic, bacterial NEC, ankle
      - hand joint MØØ.84- ☑
      - hip MØØ.85- ☑
      - knee MØØ.86- ☑
      - multiple site MØØ.89
      - shoulder MØØ.81- ☑
      - vertebra MØØ.88
      - wrist MØØ.83- ☑
    - pneumococcal — *see* Arthritis, pneumococcal
    - spine — *see* Spondylopathy, infective
    - staphylococcal — *see* Arthritis, staphylococcal
    - streptococcal — *see* Arthritis, streptococcal NEC
      - pneumococcal — *see* Arthritis, pneumococcal
  - reactive — *see* Reiter's disease
  - rheumatic — *see also* Arthritis, rheumatoid
    - acute or subacute — *see* Fever, rheumatic
  - rheumatoid MØ6.9
    - with
      - carditis — *see* Rheumatoid, carditis
      - endocarditis — *see* Rheumatoid, carditis
      - heart involvement NEC — *see* Rheumatoid, carditis
      - lung involvement — *see* Rheumatoid, lung
      - myocarditis — *see* Rheumatoid, carditis
      - myopathy — *see* Rheumatoid, myopathy
      - pericarditis — *see* Rheumatoid, carditis
      - polyneuropathy — *see* Rheumatoid, polyneuropathy
      - rheumatoid factor — *see* Arthritis, rheumatoid, seropositive
      - splenoadenomegaly and leukopenia — *see* Felty's syndrome
      - vasculitis — *see* Rheumatoid, vasculitis
      - visceral involvement NEC — *see* Rheumatoid, arthritis, with involvement of organs NEC
    - juvenile (with or without rheumatoid factor) MØ8.ØØ
      - with systemic onset — *see* Still's disease
      - ankle MØ8.Ø7- ☑
      - elbow MØ8.Ø2- ☑
      - foot joint MØ8.Ø7- ☑
      - hand joint MØ8.Ø4- ☑
      - hip MØ8.Ø5- ☑
      - knee MØ8.Ø6- ☑
      - multiple site MØ8.Ø9
      - shoulder MØ8.Ø1- ☑
      - specified site NEC MØ8.ØA
      - vertebra MØ8.Ø8
      - wrist MØ8.Ø3- ☑
    - seronegative MØ6.ØØ
      - ankle MØ6.Ø7- ☑
      - elbow MØ6.Ø2- ☑
      - foot joint MØ6.Ø7- ☑
      - hand joint MØ6.Ø4- ☑

- **Arthritis, arthritic** — *continued*
  - rheumatoid — *continued*
    - seronegative — *continued*
      - hip MØ6.Ø5- ☑
      - knee MØ6.Ø6- ☑
      - multiple site MØ6.Ø9
      - shoulder MØ6.Ø1- ☑
      - specified site NEC MØ6.ØA
      - vertebra MØ6.Ø8
      - wrist MØ6.Ø3- ☑
    - seropositive MØ5.9
      - specified NEC MØ5.8Ø
        - ankle MØ5.87- ☑
        - elbow MØ5.82- ☑
        - foot joint MØ5.87- ☑
        - hand joint MØ5.84- ☑
        - hip MØ5.85- ☑
        - knee MØ5.86- ☑
        - multiple sites MØ5.89
        - shoulder MØ5.81- ☑
        - specified site NEC MØ5.8A
        - vertebra — *see* Spondylitis, ankylosing
        - wrist MØ5.83- ☑
      - without organ involvement MØ5.7Ø
        - ankle MØ5.77- ☑
        - elbow MØ5.72- ☑
        - foot joint MØ5.77- ☑
        - hand joint MØ5.74- ☑
        - hip MØ5.75- ☑
        - knee MØ5.76- ☑
        - multiple sites MØ5.79
        - shoulder MØ5.71- ☑
        - specified site NEC MØ5.7A
        - vertebra — *see* Spondylitis, ankylosing
        - wrist MØ5.73- ☑
    - specified type NEC MØ6.8Ø
      - ankle MØ6.87- ☑
      - elbow MØ6.82- ☑
      - foot joint MØ6.87- ☑
      - hand joint MØ6.84- ☑
      - hip MØ6.85- ☑
      - knee MØ6.86- ☑
      - multiple site MØ6.89
      - shoulder MØ6.81- ☑
      - specified site NEC MØ6.8A
      - vertebra MØ6.88
      - wrist MØ6.83- ☑
    - spine — *see* Spondylitis, ankylosing
  - rubella BØ6.82
  - scorbutic — *see also* subcategory M14.8- E54
  - senile or senescent — *see* Osteoarthritis
  - septic (any site except spine) — *see* Arthritis, pyogenic or pyemic
    - spine — *see* Spondylopathy, infective
  - serum (nontherapeutic) (therapeutic) — *see* Arthropathy, postimmunization
  - specified form NEC M13.8Ø
    - ankle M13.87- ☑
    - elbow M13.82- ☑
    - foot joint M13.87- ☑
    - hand joint M13.84- ☑
    - hip M13.85- ☑
    - knee M13.86- ☑
    - multiple site M13.89
    - shoulder M13.81- ☑
    - specified joint NEC M13.88
    - wrist M13.83- ☑
  - spine — *see also* Spondylosis
    - infectious or infective NEC — *see* Spondylopathy, infective
    - Marie-Strümpell — *see* Spondylitis, ankylosing
    - pyogenic — *see* Spondylopathy, infective
    - rheumatoid — *see* Spondylitis, ankylosing
    - traumatic (old) — *see* Spondylopathy, traumatic
    - tuberculous A18.Ø1
  - staphylococcal MØØ.ØØ
    - ankle MØØ.Ø7- ☑
    - elbow MØØ.Ø2- ☑
    - foot joint — *see* Arthritis, staphylococcal, ankle
    - hand joint MØØ.Ø4- ☑
    - hip MØØ.Ø5- ☑
    - knee MØØ.Ø6- ☑
    - multiple site MØØ.Ø9
    - shoulder MØØ.Ø1- ☑
    - vertebra MØØ.Ø8
    - wrist MØØ.Ø3- ☑
  - streptococcal NEC MØØ.2Ø

Arthritis, arthritic — *continued*
- streptococcal — *continued*
  - ankle M00.27- ☑
  - elbow M00.22- ☑
  - foot joint — *see* Arthritis, streptococcal, ankle
  - hand joint M00.24- ☑
  - hip M00.25- ☑
  - knee M00.26- ☑
  - multiple site M00.29
  - shoulder M00.21- ☑
  - vertebra M00.28
  - wrist M00.23- ☑
- suppurative — *see* Arthritis, pyogenic or pyemic
- syphilitic (late) A52.16
  - congenital A50.55 *[M12.80]*
- syphilitica deformans (Charcot) A52.16
- temporomandibular joint M26.64- ☑
- toxic of menopause (any site) — *see* Arthritis, specified form NEC
- transient — *see* Arthropathy, specified form NEC
- traumatic (chronic) — *see* Arthropathy, traumatic
- tuberculous A18.02
  - spine A18.01
- uratic — *see* Gout
- urethritica (Reiter's) — *see* Reiter's disease
- vertebral — *see* Spondylopathy, inflammatory
- villous (any site) — *see* Arthropathy, specified form NEC

Arthrocele — *see* Effusion, joint

Arthrodesis status Z98.1

Arthrodynia — *see also* Pain, joint

Arthrodysplasia Q74.9

Arthrofibrosis, joint — *see* Ankylosis

Arthrogryposis (congenital) Q68.8
- multiplex congenita Q74.3

Arthrokatadysis M24.7

Arthropathy — *see also* Arthritis M12.9
- Charcot's — *see* Arthropathy, neuropathic
  - diabetic — *see* Diabetes, arthropathy, neuropathic
  - syringomyelic G95.0
- cricoarytenoid J38.7
- crystal (-induced) — *see* Arthritis, in, crystals
- diabetic NEC — *see* Diabetes, arthropathy
- distal interphalangeal, psoriatic L40.51
- enteropathic M07.60
  - ankle M07.67- ☑
  - elbow M07.62- ☑
  - foot joint M07.67- ☑
  - hand joint M07.64- ☑
  - hip M07.65- ☑
  - knee M07.66- ☑
  - multiple site M07.69
  - shoulder M07.61- ☑
  - vertebra M07.68
  - wrist M07.63- ☑
- facet joint — *see also* Spondylosis M47.819
- following intestinal bypass M02.00
  - ankle M02.07- ☑
  - elbow M02.02- ☑
  - foot joint M02.07- ☑
  - hand joint M02.04- ☑
  - hip M02.05- ☑
  - knee M02.06- ☑
  - multiple site M02.09
  - shoulder M02.01- ☑
  - vertebra M02.08
  - wrist M02.03- ☑
- gouty — *see also* Gout
  - in (due to)
    - Lesch-Nyhan syndrome E79.1 *[M14.8-]* ☑
    - sickle-cell disorders D57- ☑ *[M14.8-]* ☑
- hemophilic NEC D66 *[M36.2]*
  - in (due to)
    - hyperparathyroidism NEC E21.3 *[M14.8-]* ☑
    - metabolic disease NOS E88.9 *[M14.8-]* ☑
- in (due to)
  - acromegaly E22.0 *[M14.8-]* ☑
  - amyloidosis E85.4 *[M14.8-]* ☑
  - blood disorder NOS D75.9 *[M36.3]*
  - diabetes — *see* Diabetes, arthropathy
  - endocrine disease NOS E34.9 *[M14.8-]* ☑
  - erythema
    - multiforme L51.9 *[M14.8-]* ☑
    - nodosum L52 *[M14.8-]* ☑
  - hemochromatosis E83.118 *[M14.8-]* ☑
  - hemoglobinopathy NEC D58.2 *[M36.3]*

Arthropathy — *continued*
- in — *continued*
  - hemophilia NEC D66 *[M36.2]*
  - Henoch-Schönlein purpura D69.0 *[M36.4]*
  - hyperthyroidism E05.90 *[M14.8-]* ☑
  - hypothyroidism E03.9 *[M14.8-]* ☑
  - infective endocarditis I33.0 *[M12.80]*
  - leukemia NEC C95.9- ☑ *[M36.1]*
  - malignant histiocytosis C96.A *[M36.1]*
  - metabolic disease NOS E88.9 *[M14.8-]* ☑
  - multiple myeloma C90.0- ☑ *[M36.1]*
  - neoplastic disease NOS (*see also* Neoplasm) D49.9 *[M36.1]*
  - nutritional deficiency — *see also* subcategory M14.8- E63.9
  - psoriasis NOS L40.50
  - sarcoidosis D86.86
  - syphilis (late) A52.77
    - congenital A50.55 *[M12.80]*
  - thyrotoxicosis — *see also* subcategory M14.8- E05.90
  - ulcerative colitis K51.90 *[M07.60]*
  - viral hepatitis (postinfectious) NEC B19.9 *[M12.80]*
  - Whipple's disease — *see also* subcategory M14.8- K90.81
- Jaccoud — *see* Arthropathy, postrheumatic, chronic
- juvenile — *see* Arthritis, juvenile
  - psoriatic L40.54
- mutilans (psoriatic) L40.52
- neuropathic (Charcot) M14.60
  - ankle M14.67- ☑
  - diabetic — *see* Diabetes, arthropathy, neuropathic
  - elbow M14.62- ☑
  - foot joint M14.67- ☑
  - hand joint M14.64- ☑
  - hip M14.65- ☑
  - knee M14.66- ☑
  - multiple site M14.69
  - nonsyphilitic NEC G98.0
  - shoulder M14.61- ☑
  - syringomyelic G95.0
  - vertebra M14.68
  - wrist M14.63- ☑
- osteopulmonary — *see* Osteoarthropathy, hypertrophic, specified NEC
- postdysenteric M02.10
  - ankle M02.17- ☑
  - elbow M02.12- ☑
  - foot joint M02.17- ☑
  - hand joint M02.14- ☑
  - hip M02.15- ☑
  - knee M02.16- ☑
  - multiple site M02.19
  - shoulder M02.11- ☑
  - vertebra M02.18
  - wrist M02.13- ☑
- postimmunization M02.20
  - ankle M02.27- ☑
  - elbow M02.22- ☑
  - foot joint M02.27- ☑
  - hand joint M02.24- ☑
  - hip M02.25- ☑
  - knee M02.26- ☑
  - multiple site M02.29
  - shoulder M02.21- ☑
  - vertebra M02.28
  - wrist M02.23- ☑
- postinfectious NEC B99 ☑ *[M12.80]*
  - in (due to)
    - enteritis due to Yersinia enterocolitica A04.6 *[M12.80]*
    - syphilis A52.77
    - viral hepatitis NEC B19.9 *[M12.80]*
- postrheumatic, chronic (Jaccoud) M12.00
  - ankle M12.07- ☑
  - elbow M12.02- ☑
  - foot joint M12.07- ☑
  - hand joint M12.04- ☑
  - hip M12.05- ☑
  - knee M12.06- ☑
  - multiple site M12.09
  - shoulder M12.01- ☑
  - specified joint NEC M12.08
  - vertebrae M12.08
  - wrist M12.03- ☑
- psoriatic NEC L40.59
  - interphalangeal, distal L40.51

Arthropathy — *continued*
- reactive M02.9
  - in (due to)
    - infective endocarditis I33.0 *[M02.9]*
  - specified type NEC M02.80
    - ankle M02.87- ☑
    - elbow M02.82- ☑
    - foot joint M02.87- ☑
    - hand joint M02.84- ☑
    - hip M02.85- ☑
    - knee M02.86- ☑
    - multiple site M02.89
    - shoulder M02.81- ☑
    - vertebra M02.88
    - wrist M02.83- ☑
- specified form NEC M12.80
  - ankle M12.87- ☑
  - elbow M12.82- ☑
  - foot joint M12.87- ☑
  - hand joint M12.84- ☑
  - hip M12.85- ☑
  - knee M12.86- ☑
  - multiple site M12.89
  - shoulder M12.81- ☑
  - specified joint NEC M12.88
  - vertebrae M12.88
  - wrist M12.83- ☑
- syringomyelic G95.0
- tabes dorsalis A52.16
- tabetic A52.16
- temporomandibular joint M26.65- ☑
- transient — *see* Arthropathy, specified form NEC
- traumatic M12.50
  - ankle M12.57- ☑
  - elbow M12.52- ☑
  - foot joint M12.57- ☑
  - hand joint M12.54- ☑
  - hip M12.55- ☑
  - knee M12.56- ☑
  - multiple site M12.59
  - shoulder M12.51- ☑
  - specified joint NEC M12.58
  - vertebrae M12.58
  - wrist M12.53- ☑

Arthropyosis — *see* Arthritis, pyogenic or pyemic

Arthrosis (deformans) (degenerative) (localized) — *see also* Osteoarthritis M19.90
- spine — *see* Spondylosis

Arthus' phenomenon or reaction T78.41 ☑
- due to
  - drug — *see* Table of Drugs and Chemicals, by drug

Articular — *see* condition

Articulation, reverse (teeth) M26.24

Artificial
- insemination complication — *see* Complications, artificial, fertilization
- opening status (functioning) (without complication) Z93.9
  - anus (colostomy) Z93.3
  - colostomy Z93.3
  - cystostomy Z93.50
    - appendico-vesicostomy Z93.52
    - cutaneous Z93.51
    - specified NEC Z93.59
  - enterostomy Z93.4
  - gastrostomy Z93.1
  - ileostomy Z93.2
  - intestinal tract NEC Z93.4
  - jejunostomy Z93.4
  - nephrostomy Z93.6
  - specified site NEC Z93.8
  - tracheostomy Z93.0
  - ureterostomy Z93.6
  - urethrostomy Z93.6
  - urinary tract NEC Z93.6
  - vagina Z93.8
- vagina status Z93.8

Arytenoid — *see* condition

Asbestosis (occupational) J61

Ascariasis B77.9
- with
  - complications NEC B77.89
  - intestinal complications B77.0
  - pneumonia, pneumonitis B77.81

Ascaridosis, ascaridiasis — *see* Ascariasis

Ascaris (infection) (infestation) (lumbricoides) — *see* Ascariasis

- **Ascending** — *see* condition
- **ASC-H** (atypical squamous cells cannot exclude high grade squamous intraepithelial lesion on cytologic smear)
  - anus R85.611
  - cervix R87.611
  - vagina R87.621
- **Aschoff's bodies** — *see* Myocarditis, rheumatic
- **Ascites** (abdominal) R18.8
  - cardiac — *see also* Failure, heart, right I50.810
  - chylous (nonfilarial) I89.8
    - filarial — *see* Infestation, filarial
  - due to
    - cirrhosis, alcoholic K70.31
    - hepatitis
      - alcoholic K70.11
      - chronic active K71.51
    - S. japonicum B65.2
  - heart — *see also* Failure, heart, right I50.810
  - malignant R18.0
  - pseudochylous R18.8
  - syphilitic A52.74
  - tuberculous A18.31
- **ASC-US** (atypical squamous cells of undetermined significance on cytologic smear)
  - anus R85.610
  - cervix R87.610
  - vagina R87.620
- **Aseptic** — *see* condition
- **Asherman's syndrome** N85.6
- **Asialia** K11.7
- **Asiatic cholera** — *see* Cholera
- **Asimultagnosia** (simultanagnosia) R48.3
- **Askin's tumor** — *see* Neoplasm, connective tissue, malignant
- **Asocial personality** F60.2
- **Asomatognosia** R41.4
- **Aspartylglucosaminuria** E77.1
- **Asperger's disease or syndrome** F84.5
- **Aspergilloma** — *see* Aspergillosis
- **Aspergillosis** (with pneumonia) B44.9
  - bronchopulmonary, allergic B44.81
  - disseminated B44.7
  - generalized B44.7
  - pulmonary NEC B44.1
    - allergic B44.81
    - invasive B44.0
  - specified NEC B44.89
  - tonsillar B44.2
- **Aspergillus** (flavus) (fumigatus) (infection) (terreus) — *see* Aspergillosis
- **Aspermatogenesis** — *see* Azoospermia
- **Aspermia** (testis) — *see* Azoospermia
- **Asphyxia, asphyxiation** (by) R09.01
  - antenatal P84
  - birth P84
  - bunny bag — *see* Asphyxia, due to, mechanical threat to breathing, trapped in bed clothes
  - crushing S28.0 ☑
  - drowning T75.1 ☑
  - gas, fumes, or vapor — *see* Table of Drugs and Chemicals
  - inhalation — *see* Inhalation
  - intrauterine P84
  - local I73.00
    - with gangrene I73.01
  - mucus — *see also* Foreign body, respiratory tract, causing asphyxia
    - newborn P84
  - pathological R09.01
  - postnatal P84
    - mechanical — *see* Asphyxia, due to, mechanical threat to breathing
  - prenatal P84
  - reticularis R23.1
  - strangulation — *see* Asphyxia, due to, mechanical threat to breathing
  - submersion T75.1 ☑
  - traumatic T71.9 ☑
    - due to
      - crushed chest S28.0 ☑
      - foreign body (in) — *see* Foreign body, respiratory tract, causing asphyxia
      - low oxygen content of ambient air T71.20 ☑
        - due to
          - being trapped in
            - low oxygen environment T71.29 ☑
              - in car trunk T71.221 ☑

Asphyxia, asphyxiation — *continued*
  - traumatic — *continued*
    - due to — *continued*
      - low oxygen content of ambient air — *continued*
        - due to — *continued*
          - being trapped in — *continued*
            - low oxygen environment — *continued*
              - in car trunk — *continued*
                - circumstances undetermined T71.224 ☑
                - done with intent to harm by
                  - another person T71.223 ☑
                  - self T71.222 ☑
              - in refrigerator T71.231 ☑
                - circumstances undetermined T71.234 ☑
                - done with intent to harm by
                  - another person T71.233 ☑
                  - self T71.232 ☑
          - cave-in T71.21 ☑
      - mechanical threat to breathing (accidental) T71.191 ☑
        - circumstances undetermined T71.194 ☑
        - done with intent to harm by
          - another person T71.193 ☑
          - self T71.192 ☑
        - hanging T71.161 ☑
          - circumstances undetermined T71.164 ☑
          - done with intent to harm by
            - another person T71.163 ☑
            - self T71.162 ☑
        - plastic bag T71.121 ☑
          - circumstances undetermined T71.124 ☑
          - done with intent to harm by
            - another person T71.123 ☑
            - self T71.122 ☑
        - smothering
          - in furniture T71.151 ☑
            - circumstances undetermined T71.154 ☑
            - done with intent to harm by
              - another person T71.153 ☑
              - self T71.152 ☑
          - under
            - another person's body T71.141 ☑
              - circumstances undetermined T71.144 ☑
              - done with intent to harm T71.143 ☑
            - pillow T71.111 ☑
              - circumstances undetermined T71.114 ☑
              - done with intent to harm by
                - another person T71.113 ☑
                - self T71.112 ☑
        - trapped in bed clothes T71.131 ☑
          - circumstances undetermined T71.134 ☑
          - done with intent to harm by
            - another person T71.133 ☑
            - self T71.132 ☑
  - vomiting, vomitus — *see* Foreign body, respiratory tract, causing asphyxia
- **Aspiration**
  - amniotic (clear) fluid (newborn) P24.10
    - with
      - pneumonia (pneumonitis) P24.11
      - respiratory symptoms P24.11
  - blood
    - newborn (without respiratory symptoms) P24.20
      - with
        - pneumonia (pneumonitis) P24.21
        - respiratory symptoms P24.21
    - specified age NEC — *see* Foreign body, respiratory tract
  - bronchitis J69.0
  - food or foreign body — *see* Foreign body, by site
  - liquor (amnii) (newborn) P24.10
    - with
      - pneumonia (pneumonitis) P24.11
      - respiratory symptoms P24.11
  - meconium (newborn) (without respiratory symptoms) P24.00
    - with
      - pneumonitis (pneumonitis) P24.01
      - respiratory symptoms P24.01
  - milk (newborn) (without respiratory symptoms) P24.30

Aspiration — *continued*
  - milk — *continued*
    - with
      - pneumonia (pneumonitis) P24.31
      - respiratory symptoms P24.31
    - specified age NEC — *see* Foreign body, respiratory tract
  - mucus — *see also* Foreign body, by site, causing asphyxia
    - newborn P24.10
      - with
        - pneumonia (pneumonitis) P24.11
        - respiratory symptoms P24.11
  - neonatal P24.9
    - specific NEC (without respiratory symptoms) P24.80
      - with
        - pneumonia (pneumonitis) P24.81
        - respiratory symptoms P24.81
  - newborn P24.9
    - specific NEC (without respiratory symptoms) P24.80
      - with
        - pneumonia (pneumonitis) P24.81
        - respiratory symptoms P24.81
  - pneumonia J69.0
  - pneumonitis J69.0
  - syndrome of newborn — *see* Aspiration, by substance, with pneumonia
  - vernix caseosa (newborn) P24.80
    - with
      - pneumonia (pneumonitis) P24.81
      - respiratory symptoms P24.81
  - vomitus — *see also* Foreign body, respiratory tract
    - newborn (without respiratory symptoms) P24.30
      - with
        - pneumonia (pneumonitis) P24.31
        - respiratory symptoms P24.31
- **Asplenia** (congenital) Q89.01
  - postsurgical Z90.81
- **Assam fever** B55.0
- **Assault, sexual** — *see* Maltreatment
- **Assmann's focus NEC** A15.0
- **Astasia** (-abasia) (hysterical) F44.4
- **Asteatosis cutis** L85.3
- **Astereognosia, astereognosis** R48.1
- **Asterixis** R27.8
  - in liver disease K71.3
- **Asteroid hyalitis** — *see* Deposit, crystalline
- **Asthenia, asthenic** R53.1
  - cardiac — *see also* Failure, heart I50.9
    - psychogenic F45.8
  - cardiovascular — *see also* Failure, heart I50.9
    - psychogenic F45.8
  - heart — *see also* Failure, heart I50.9
    - psychogenic F45.8
  - hysterical F44.4
  - myocardial — *see also* Failure, heart I50.9
    - psychogenic F45.8
  - nervous F48.8
  - neurocirculatory F45.8
  - neurotic F48.8
  - psychogenic F48.8
  - psychoneurotic F48.8
  - psychophysiologic F48.8
  - reaction (psychophysiologic) F48.8
  - senile R54
- **Asthenopia** — *see also* Discomfort, visual
  - hysterical F44.6
  - psychogenic F44.6
- **Asthenospermia** — *see* Abnormal, specimen, male genital organs
- **Asthma, asthmatic** (bronchial) (catarrh) (spasmodic) J45.909
  - with
    - chronic obstructive bronchitis J44.9
      - with
        - acute lower respiratory infection J44.0
        - exacerbation (acute) J44.1
    - chronic obstructive pulmonary disease J44.9
      - with
        - acute lower respiratory infection J44.0
        - exacerbation (acute) J44.1
    - exacerbation (acute) J45.901
    - hay fever — *see* Asthma, allergic extrinsic
    - rhinitis, allergic — *see* Asthma, allergic extrinsic
    - status asthmaticus J45.902
  - allergic extrinsic J45.909
    - with
      - exacerbation (acute) J45.901

- **Asthma, asthmatic** — *continued*
  - allergic extrinsic — *continued*
    - with — *continued*
      - status asthmaticus J45.9Ø2
  - atopic — *see* Asthma, allergic extrinsic
  - cardiac — *see* Failure, ventricular, left
  - cardiobronchial I5Ø.1
  - childhood J45.9Ø9
    - with
      - exacerbation (acute) J45.9Ø1
      - status asthmaticus J45.9Ø2
  - chronic obstructive J44.9
    - with
      - acute lower respiratory infection J44.Ø
      - exacerbation (acute) J44.1
  - collier's J6Ø
  - cough variant J45.991
  - detergent J69.8
  - due to
    - detergent J69.8
    - inhalation of fumes J68.3
  - eosinophilic J82.83
  - extrinsic, allergic — *see* Asthma, allergic extrinsic
  - grinder's J62.8
  - hay — *see* Asthma, allergic extrinsic
  - heart I5Ø.1
  - idiosyncratic — *see* Asthma, nonallergic
  - intermittent (mild) J45.2Ø
    - with
      - exacerbation (acute) J45.21
      - status asthmaticus J45.22
  - intrinsic, nonallergic — *see* Asthma, nonallergic
  - Kopp's E32.8
  - late-onset J45.9Ø9
    - with
      - exacerbation (acute) J45.9Ø1
      - status asthmaticus J45.9Ø2
  - mild intermittent J45.2Ø
    - with
      - exacerbation (acute) J45.21
      - status asthmaticus J45.22
  - mild persistent J45.3Ø
    - with
      - exacerbation (acute) J45.31
      - status asthmaticus J45.32
  - Millar's (laryngismus stridulus) J38.5
  - miner's J6Ø
  - mixed J45.9Ø9
    - with
      - exacerbation (acute) J45.9Ø1
      - status asthmaticus J45.9Ø2
  - moderate persistent J45.4Ø
    - with
      - exacerbation (acute) J45.41
      - status asthmaticus J45.42
  - nervous — *see* Asthma, nonallergic
  - nonallergic (intrinsic) J45.9Ø9
    - with
      - exacerbation (acute) J45.9Ø1
      - status asthmaticus J45.9Ø2
  - persistent
    - mild J45.3Ø
      - with
        - exacerbation (acute) J45.31
        - status asthmaticus J45.32
    - moderate J45.4Ø
      - with
        - exacerbation (acute) J45.41
        - status asthmaticus J45.42
    - severe J45.5Ø
      - with
        - exacerbation (acute) J45.51
        - status asthmaticus J45.52
  - platinum J45.998
  - pneumoconiotic NEC J64
  - potter's J62.8
  - predominantly allergic J45.9Ø9
  - psychogenic F54
  - pulmonary eosinophilic J82.83
  - red cedar J67.8
  - Rostan's I5Ø.1
  - sandblaster's J62.8
  - sequoiosis J67.8
  - severe persistent J45.5Ø
    - with
      - exacerbation (acute) J45.51
      - status asthmaticus J45.52
  - specified NEC J45.998

- **Asthma, asthmatic** — *continued*
  - stonemason's J62.8
  - thymic E32.8
  - tuberculous — *see* Tuberculosis, pulmonary
  - Wichmann's (laryngismus stridulus) J38.5
  - wood J67.8
- **Astigmatism** (compound) (congenital) H52.2Ø- ☑
  - irregular H52.21- ☑
  - regular H52.22- ☑
- **Astraphobia** F4Ø.22Ø
- **Astroblastoma**
  - specified site — *see* Neoplasm, malignant, by site
  - unspecified site C71.9
- **Astrocytoma** (cystic)
  - anaplastic
    - specified site — *see* Neoplasm, malignant, by site
    - unspecified site C71.9
  - fibrillary
    - specified site — *see* Neoplasm, malignant, by site
    - unspecified site C71.9
  - fibrous
    - specified site — *see* Neoplasm, malignant, by site
    - unspecified site C71.9
  - gemistocytic
    - specified site — *see* Neoplasm, malignant, by site
    - unspecified site C71.9
  - juvenile
    - specified site — *see* Neoplasm, malignant, by site
    - unspecified site C71.9
  - pilocytic
    - specified site — *see* Neoplasm, malignant, by site
    - unspecified site C71.9
  - piloid
    - specified site — *see* Neoplasm, malignant, by site
    - unspecified site C71.9
  - protoplasmic
    - specified site — *see* Neoplasm, malignant, by site
    - unspecified site C71.9
  - specified site NEC — *see* Neoplasm, malignant, by site
  - subependymal D43.2
    - giant cell
      - specified site — *see* Neoplasm, uncertain behavior, by site
      - unspecified site D43.2
    - specified site — *see* Neoplasm, uncertain behavior, by site
    - unspecified site D43.2
  - unspecified site C71.9
- **Astroglioma**
  - specified site — *see* Neoplasm, malignant, by site
  - unspecified site C71.9
- **Asymbolia** R48.8
- **Asymmetry** — *see also* Distortion
  - between native and reconstructed breast N65.1
  - face Q67.Ø
  - jaw (lower) — *see* Anomaly, dentofacial, jaw-cranial base relationship, asymmetry
- **Asynergia, asynergy** R27.8
  - ventricular I51.89
- **Asystole** (heart) — *see* Arrest, cardiac
- **At risk**
  - for
    - dental caries Z91.849
      - high Z91.843
      - low Z91.841
      - moderate Z91.842
    - falling Z91.81
- **Ataxia, ataxy, ataxic** R27.Ø
  - acute R27.8
  - autosomal recessive Friedreich G11.11
  - brain (hereditary) G11.9
  - cerebellar (hereditary) G11.9
    - with defective DNA repair G11.3
    - alcoholic G31.2
    - early-onset G11.1Ø
    - with
      - essential tremor G11.19
      - myoclonus [Hunt's ataxia] G11.19
      - retained tendon reflexes G11.19
    - in
      - alcoholism G31.2
      - myxedema EØ3.9 *[G13.2]*
      - neoplastic disease — *see also* Neoplasm D49.9 *[G32.81]*
      - specified disease NEC G32.81
    - late-onset (Marie's) G11.2
  - cerebral (hereditary) G11.9
  - congenital nonprogressive G11.Ø

- **Ataxia, ataxy, ataxic** — *continued*
  - family, familial — *see* Ataxia, hereditary
  - following
    - cerebrovascular disease I69.993
      - cerebral infarction I69.393
      - intracerebral hemorrhage I69.193
      - nontraumatic intracranial hemorrhage NEC I69.293
      - specified disease NEC I69.893
      - subarachnoid hemorrhage I69.Ø93
  - Friedreich's (heredofamilial) (cerebellar) (spinal) (with retained reflexes) G11.11
  - gait R26.Ø
    - hysterical F44.4
  - general R27.8
  - gluten M35.9 *[G32.81]*
    - with celiac disease K9Ø.Ø *[G32.81]*
  - hereditary G11.9
    - with neuropathy G6Ø.2
    - cerebellar — *see* Ataxia, cerebellar
    - spastic G11.4
    - specified NEC G11.8
    - spinal (Friedreich's) G11.11
  - heredofamilial — *see* Ataxia, hereditary
  - Hunt's G11.19
  - hysterical F44.4
  - locomotor (progressive) (syphilitic) (partial) (spastic) A52.11
    - diabetic — *see* Diabetes, ataxia
  - Marie's (cerebellar) (heredofamilial) (late- onset) G11.2
  - nonorganic origin F44.4
  - nonprogressive, congenital G11.Ø
  - psychogenic F44.4
  - Roussy-Lévy G6Ø.Ø
  - Sanger-Brown's (hereditary) G11.2
  - spastic hereditary G11.4
  - spinal
    - hereditary (Friedreich's) G11.11
    - progressive (syphilitic) A52.11
  - spinocerebellar, X-linked recessive G11.19
  - telangiectasia (Louis-Bar) G11.3
- **Ataxia-telangiectasia** (Louis-Bar) G11.3
- **Atelectasis** (massive) (partial) (pressure) (pulmonary) J98.11
  - newborn P28.1Ø
    - due to resorption P28.11
    - partial P28.19
    - primary P28.Ø
    - secondary P28.19
  - primary (newborn) P28.Ø
  - tuberculous — *see* Tuberculosis, pulmonary
- **Atelocardia** Q24.9
- **Atelomyelia** QØ6.1
- **Atheroembolism**
  - of
    - extremities
      - lower I75.Ø2- ☑
      - upper I75.Ø1- ☑
    - kidney I75.81
    - specified NEC I75.89
- **Atheroma, atheromatous** — *see also* Arteriosclerosis I7Ø.9Ø
  - aorta, aortic I7Ø.Ø
    - valve — *see also* Endocarditis, aortic I35.8
  - aorto-iliac I7Ø.Ø
  - artery — *see* Arteriosclerosis
  - basilar (artery) I67.2
  - carotid (artery) (common) (internal) I67.2
  - cerebral (arteries) I67.2
  - coronary (artery) I25.1Ø
    - with angina pectoris — *see* Arteriosclerosis, coronary (artery),
  - degeneration — *see* Arteriosclerosis
  - heart, cardiac — *see* Disease, heart, ischemic, atherosclerotic
  - mitral (valve) I34.89
  - myocardium, myocardial — *see* Disease, heart, ischemic, atherosclerotic
  - pulmonary valve (heart) — *see also* Endocarditis, pulmonary I37.8
  - tricuspid (heart) (valve) I36.8
  - valve, valvular — *see* Endocarditis
  - vertebral (artery) I67.2
- **Atheromatosis** — *see* Arteriosclerosis
- **Atherosclerosis** — *see also* Arteriosclerosis
  - coronary
    - artery I25.1Ø

Atherosclerosis — *continued*
  coronary — *continued*
    artery — *continued*
      with angina pectoris — *see* Arteriosclerosis, coronary (artery),
      due to
        calcified coronary lesion (severely) I25.84
        lipid rich plaque I25.83
  transplanted heart I25.811
    bypass graft I25.812
      with angina pectoris — *see* Arteriosclerosis, coronary (artery),
    native coronary artery I25.811
      with angina pectoris — *see* Arteriosclerosis, coronary (artery),
Athetosis (acquired) R25.8
  bilateral (congenital) G80.3
  congenital (bilateral) (double) G80.3
  double (congenital) G80.3
  unilateral R25.8
Athlete's
  foot B35.3
  heart I51.7
Athrepsia E41
Athyrea (acquired) — *see also* Hypothyroidism
  congenital E03.1
Atonia, atony, atonic
  bladder (sphincter) (neurogenic) N31.2
  capillary I78.8
  cecum K59.89
    psychogenic F45.8
  colon — *see* Atony, intestine
  congenital P94.2
  esophagus K22.89
  intestine K59.89
    psychogenic F45.8
  stomach K31.89
    neurotic or psychogenic F45.8
  uterus (during labor) O62.2
    with hemorrhage (postpartum) O72.1
    postpartum (with hemorrhage) O72.1
      without hemorrhage O75.89
Atopy — *see* History, allergy
Atransferrinemia, congenital E88.09
Atresia, atretic
  alimentary organ or tract NEC Q45.8
    upper Q40.8
  ani, anus, anal (canal) Q42.3
    with fistula Q42.2
  aorta (ring) Q25.29
  aortic (orifice) (valve) Q23.0
    arch Q25.21
    congenital with hypoplasia of ascending aorta and defective development of left ventricle (with mitral stenosis) Q23.4
    in hypoplastic left heart syndrome Q23.4
  aqueduct of Sylvius Q03.0
    with spina bifida — *see* Spina bifida, with hydrocephalus
  artery NEC Q27.8
    cerebral Q28.3
    coronary Q24.5
    digestive system Q27.8
    eye Q15.8
    lower limb Q27.8
    pulmonary Q25.5
    specified site NEC Q27.8
    umbilical Q27.0
    upper limb Q27.8
  auditory canal (external) Q16.1
  bile duct (common) (congenital) (hepatic) Q44.2
    acquired — *see* Obstruction, bile duct
  bladder (neck) Q64.39
    obstruction Q64.31
  bronchus Q32.4
  cecum Q42.8
  cervix (acquired) N88.2
    congenital Q51.828
    in pregnancy or childbirth — *see* Anomaly, cervix, in pregnancy or childbirth
      causing obstructed labor O65.5
  choana Q30.0
  colon Q42.9
    specified NEC Q42.8
  common duct Q44.2
  cricoid cartilage Q31.8
  cystic duct Q44.2
    acquired K82.8

Atresia, atretic — *continued*
  cystic duct — *continued*
    acquired — *continued*
      with obstruction K82.0
  digestive organs NEC Q45.8
  duodenum Q41.0
  ear canal Q16.1
  ejaculatory duct Q55.4
  epiglottis Q31.8
  esophagus Q39.0
    with tracheoesophageal fistula Q39.1
  eustachian tube Q17.8
  fallopian tube (congenital) Q50.6
    acquired N97.1
  follicular cyst N83.0- ☑
  foramen of
    Luschka Q03.1
      with spina bifida — *see* Spina bifida, with hydrocephalus
    Magendie Q03.1
      with spina bifida — *see* Spina bifida, with hydrocephalus
  gallbladder Q44.1
  genital organ
    external
      female Q52.79
      male Q55.8
    internal
      female Q52.8
      male Q55.8
  glottis Q31.8
  gullet Q39.0
    with tracheoesophageal fistula Q39.1
  heart valve NEC Q24.8
    pulmonary Q22.0
    tricuspid Q22.4
  hymen Q52.3
    acquired (postinfective) N89.6
  ileum Q41.2
  intestine (small) Q41.9
    large Q42.9
      specified NEC Q42.8
  iris, filtration angle Q15.0
  jejunum Q41.1
  lacrimal apparatus Q10.4
  larynx Q31.8
  meatus urinarius Q64.33
  mitral valve Q23.2
    in hypoplastic left heart syndrome Q23.4
  nares (anterior) (posterior) Q30.0
  nasopharynx Q34.8
  nose, nostril Q30.0
    acquired J34.89
  organ or site NEC Q89.8
  osseous meatus (ear) Q16.1
  oviduct (congenital) Q50.6
    acquired N97.1
  parotid duct Q38.4
    acquired K11.8
  pulmonary (artery) Q25.5
    valve Q22.0
  pulmonic Q22.0
  pupil Q13.2
  rectum Q42.1
    with fistula Q42.0
  salivary duct Q38.4
    acquired K11.8
  sublingual duct Q38.4
    acquired K11.8
  submandibular duct Q38.4
    acquired K11.8
  submaxillary duct Q38.4
    acquired K11.8
  thyroid cartilage Q31.8
  trachea Q32.1
  tricuspid valve Q22.4
  ureter Q62.10
    pelvic junction Q62.11
    vesical orifice Q62.12
  ureteropelvic junction Q62.11
  ureterovesical orifice Q62.12
  urethra (valvular) Q64.39
    stricture Q64.32
  urinary tract NEC Q64.8
  uterus Q51.818
    acquired N85.8
  vagina (congenital) Q52.4
    acquired (postinfectional) (senile) N89.5
  vas deferens Q55.3

Atresia, atretic — *continued*
  vascular NEC Q27.8
    cerebral Q28.3
    digestive system Q27.8
    lower limb Q27.8
    specified site NEC Q27.8
    upper limb Q27.8
  vein NEC Q27.8
    digestive system Q27.8
    great Q26.8
    lower limb Q27.8
    portal Q26.5
    pulmonary Q26.4
      partial Q26.3
      total Q26.2
    specified site NEC Q27.8
    upper limb Q27.8
  vena cava (inferior) (superior) Q26.8
  vesicourethral orifice Q64.31
  vulva Q52.79
    acquired N90.5
Atrichia, atrichosis — *see* Alopecia
Atrophia — *see also* Atrophy
  cutis senilis L90.8
    due to radiation L57.8
  gyrata of choroid and retina H31.23
  senilis R54
    dermatological L90.8
      due to radiation (nonionizing) (solar) L57.8
  unguium L60.3
    congenita Q84.6
Atrophie blanche (en plaque) (de Milian) L95.0
Atrophoderma, atrophodermia (of) L90.9
  diffusum (idiopathic) L90.4
  maculatum L90.8
    et striatum L90.8
      due to syphilis A52.79
    syphilitic A51.39
  neuriticum L90.8
  Pasini and Pierini L90.3
  pigmentosum Q82.1
  reticulatum symmetricum faciei L66.4
  senile L90.8
    due to radiation (nonionizing) (solar) L57.8
  vermiculata (cheeks) L66.4
Atrophy, atrophic (of)
  adrenal (capsule) (gland) E27.49
    primary (autoimmune) E27.1
  alveolar process or ridge (edentulous) K08.20
  anal sphincter (disuse) N81.84
  appendix K38.8
  arteriosclerotic — *see* Arteriosclerosis
  bile duct (common) (hepatic) K83.8
  bladder N32.89
    neurogenic N31.8
  blanche (en plaque) (of Milian) L95.0
  bone (senile) NEC — *see also* Disorder, bone, specified type NEC
    due to
      tabes dorsalis (neurogenic) A52.11
  brain (cortex) (progressive) G31.9
    frontotemporal circumscribed — *see also* Dementia, in, diseases specified elsewhere G31.01 *[F02.80]*
      with behavioral disturbance — *see also* Dementia, in, diseases specified elsewhere G31.01 *[F02.81-]* ☑
    senile NEC G31.1
  breast N64.2
    obstetric — *see* Disorder, breast, specified type NEC
  buccal cavity K13.79
  cardiac — *see* Degeneration, myocardial
  cartilage (infectional) (joint) — *see* Disorder, cartilage, specified NEC
  cerebellar — *see* Atrophy, brain
  cerebral — *see* Atrophy, brain
  cervix (mucosa) (senile) (uteri) N88.8
    menopausal N95.8
  Charcot-Marie-Tooth G60.0
  choroid (central) (macular) (myopic) (retina) H31.10- ☑
    diffuse secondary H31.12- ☑
    gyrate H31.23
    senile H31.11- ☑
  ciliary body — *see* Atrophy, iris
  conjunctiva (senile) H11.89
  corpus cavernosum N48.89
  cortical — *see* Atrophy, brain
  cystic duct K82.8

Atrophy, atrophic — *continued*
- Déjérine-Thomas G23.8
- disuse NEC — *see* Atrophy, muscle
- Duchenne-Aran G12.21
- ear H93.8- ☑
- edentulous alveolar ridge KØ8.2Ø
- endometrium (senile) N85.8
  - cervix N88.8
- enteric K63.89
- epididymis N5Ø.89
- eyeball — *see* Disorder, globe, degenerated condition, atrophy
- eyelid (senile) — *see* Disorder, eyelid, degenerative
- facial (skin) L9Ø.9
- fallopian tube (senile) N83.32- ☑
  - with ovary N83.33- ☑
- fascioscapulohumeral (Landouzy- Déjérine) G71.Ø2
- fatty, thymus (gland) E32.8
- gallbladder K82.8
- gastric K29.4Ø
  - with bleeding K29.41
- gastrointestinal K63.89
- glandular I89.8
- globe H44.52- ☑
- gum — *see* Recession, gingival
- hair L67.8
- heart (brown) — *see* Degeneration, myocardial
- hemifacial Q67.4
  - Romberg G51.8
- infantile E41
  - paralysis, acute — *see* Poliomyelitis, paralytic
- intestine K63.89
- iris (essential) (progressive) H21.26- ☑
  - specified NEC H21.29
- kidney (senile) (terminal) — *see also* Sclerosis, renal N26.1
  - congenital or infantile Q6Ø.5
    - bilateral Q6Ø.4
    - unilateral Q6Ø.3
  - hydronephrotic — *see* Hydronephrosis
- lacrimal gland (primary) HØ4.14- ☑
  - secondary HØ4.15- ☑
- Landouzy-Déjérine G71.Ø2
- laryngitis, infective J37.Ø
- larynx J38.7
- Leber's optic (hereditary) H47.22
- lip K13.Ø
- liver (yellow) K72.9Ø
  - with coma K72.91
  - acute, subacute K72.ØØ
    - with coma K72.Ø1
  - chronic K72.1Ø
    - with coma K72.11
- lung (senile) J98.4
- macular (dermatological) L9Ø.8
  - syphilitic, skin A51.39
    - striated A52.79
- mandible (edentulous) KØ8.2Ø
  - minimal KØ8.21
  - moderate KØ8.22
  - severe KØ8.23
- maxilla KØ8.2Ø
  - minimal KØ8.24
  - moderate KØ8.25
  - severe KØ8.26
- muscle, muscular (diffuse) (general) (idiopathic) (primary) M62.5Ø
  - ankle M62.57- ☑
  - back M62.5A9
    - cervical M62.5AØ
    - lumbosacral M62.5A2
    - thoracic M62.5A1
  - Duchenne-Aran G12.21
  - foot M62.57- ☑
  - forearm M62.53- ☑
  - hand M62.54- ☑
  - infantile spinal G12.Ø
  - lower leg M62.56- ☑
  - multiple sites M62.59
  - myelopathic — *see* Atrophy, muscle, spinal
  - myotonic G71.11
  - neuritic G58.9
  - neuropathic (peroneal) (progressive) G6Ø.Ø
  - pelvic (disuse) N81.84
  - peroneal G6Ø.Ø
  - progressive (bulbar) G12.21
    - adult G12.1
    - infantile (spinal) G12.Ø

Atrophy, atrophic — *continued*
- muscle, muscular — *continued*
  - progressive — *continued*
    - spinal G12.25
      - adult G12.1
      - infantile G12.Ø
  - pseudohypertrophic G71.Ø2
  - shoulder region M62.51- ☑
  - specified site NEC M62.58
  - spinal G12.9
    - adult form G12.1
    - Aran-Duchenne G12.21
    - childhood form, type II G12.1
    - distal G12.1
    - hereditary NEC G12.1
    - infantile, type I (Werdnig-Hoffmann) G12.Ø
    - juvenile form, type III (Kugelberg- Welander) G12.1
    - progressive G12.25
    - scapuloperoneal form G12.1
    - specified NEC G12.8
  - syphilitic A52.78
  - thigh M62.55- ☑
  - upper arm M62.52- ☑
- myocardium — *see* Degeneration, myocardial
- myometrium (senile) N85.8
  - cervix N88.8
- myopathic NEC — *see* Atrophy, muscle
- myotonia G71.11
- nail L6Ø.3
- nasopharynx J31.1
- nerve — *see also* Disorder, nerve
  - abducens — *see* Strabismus, paralytic, sixth nerve
  - accessory G52.8
  - acoustic or auditory H93.3 ☑
  - cranial G52.9
    - eighth (auditory) H93.3 ☑
    - eleventh (accessory) G52.8
    - fifth (trigeminal) G5Ø.8
    - first (olfactory) G52.Ø
    - fourth (trochlear) — *see* Strabismus, paralytic, fourth nerve
    - second (optic) H47.2Ø
    - sixth (abducens) — *see* Strabismus, paralytic, sixth nerve
    - tenth (pneumogastric) (vagus) G52.2
    - third (oculomotor) — *see* Strabismus, paralytic, third nerve
    - twelfth (hypoglossal) G52.3
  - hypoglossal G52.3
  - oculomotor — *see* Strabismus, paralytic, third nerve
  - olfactory G52.Ø
  - optic (papillomacular bundle)
    - syphilitic (late) A52.15
      - congenital A5Ø.44
  - pneumogastric G52.2
  - trigeminal G5Ø.8
  - trochlear — *see* Strabismus, paralytic, fourth nerve
  - vagus (pneumogastric) G52.2
- neurogenic, bone, tabetic A52.11
- nutritional E43
  - with marasmus E41
- old age R54
- olivopontocerebellar G23.8
- optic (nerve) H47.2Ø
  - glaucomatous H47.23- ☑
  - hereditary H47.22
  - primary H47.21- ☑
  - specified type NEC H47.29- ☑
  - syphilitic (late) A52.15
    - congenital A5Ø.44
- orbit HØ5.31- ☑
- ovary (senile) N83.31- ☑
  - with fallopian tube N83.33- ☑
- oviduct (senile) — *see* Atrophy, fallopian tube
- palsy, diffuse (progressive) G12.22
- pancreas (duct) (senile) K86.89
- parotid gland K11.Ø
- pelvic muscle N81.84
- penis N48.89
- pharynx J39.2
- pluriglandular E31.8
  - autoimmune E31.Ø
- polyarthritis M15.9
- prostate N42.89
- pseudohypertrophic (muscle) G71.Ø2
- renal — *see also* Sclerosis, renal N26.1
- retina, retinal (postinfectional) H35.89

Atrophy, atrophic — *continued*
- rhinitis J31.Ø
- salivary gland K11.Ø
- scar L9Ø.5
- sclerosis, lobar (of brain) — *see also* Dementia, in, diseases specified elsewhere G31.Ø9 *[FØ2.8Ø]*
  - with behavioral disturbance — *see also* Dementia, in, diseases specified elsewhere G31.Ø9 *[FØ2.81-]* ☑
- scrotum N5Ø.89
- seminal vesicle N5Ø.89
- senile R54
  - due to radiation (nonionizing) (solar) L57.8
- skin (patches) (spots) L9Ø.9
  - degenerative (senile) L9Ø.8
  - due to radiation (nonionizing) (solar) L57.8
  - senile L9Ø.8
- spermatic cord N5Ø.89
- spinal (acute) (cord) G95.89
  - muscular — *see* Atrophy, muscle, spinal
  - paralysis G12.2Ø
    - acute — *see* Poliomyelitis, paralytic
    - meaning progressive muscular atrophy G12.25
- spine (column) — *see* Spondylopathy, specified NEC
- spleen (senile) D73.Ø
- stomach K29.4Ø
  - with bleeding K29.41
- striate (skin) L9Ø.6
  - syphilitic A52.79
- subcutaneous L9Ø.9
- sublingual gland K11.Ø
- submandibular gland K11.Ø
- submaxillary gland K11.Ø
- Sudeck's — *see* Algoneurodystrophy
- suprarenal (capsule) (gland) E27.49
  - primary E27.1
- systemic affecting central nervous system
  - in
    - myxedema EØ3.9 *[G13.2]*
    - neoplastic disease — *see also* Neoplasm D49.9 *[G13.1]*
    - specified disease NEC G13.8
- tarso-orbital fascia, congenital Q1Ø.3
- testis N5Ø.Ø
- thenar, partial — *see* Syndrome, carpal tunnel
- thymus (fatty) E32.8
- thyroid (gland) (acquired) EØ3.4
  - with cretinism EØ3.1
  - congenital (with myxedema) EØ3.1
- tongue (senile) K14.8
  - papillae K14.4
- trachea J39.8
- tunica vaginalis N5Ø.89
- turbinate J34.89
- tympanic membrane (nonflaccid) H73.82- ☑
  - flaccid H73.81- ☑
- upper respiratory tract J39.8
- uterus, uterine (senile) N85.8
  - cervix N88.8
  - due to radiation (intended effect) N85.8
    - adverse effect or misadventure N99.89
- vagina (senile) N95.2
- vas deferens N5Ø.89
- vascular I99.8
- vertebra (senile) — *see* Spondylopathy, specified NEC
- vulva (senile) N9Ø.5
- Werdnig-Hoffmann G12.Ø
- yellow — *see* Failure, hepatic

Attack, attacks
- with alteration of consciousness (with automatisms) — *see* Epilepsy, localization-related, symptomatic, with complex partial seizures
- Adams-Stokes I45.9
- akinetic — *see* Epilepsy, generalized, specified NEC
- angina — *see* Angina
- atonic — *see* Epilepsy, generalized, specified NEC
- benign shuddering G25.83
- cataleptic — *see* Catalepsy
- coronary — *see* Infarct, myocardium
- cyanotic, newborn P28.2
- drop NEC R55
- epileptic — *see* Epilepsy
- heart — *see* infarct, myocardium
- hysterical F44.9
- jacksonian — *see* Epilepsy, localization-related, symptomatic, with simple partial seizures
- myocardium, myocardial — *see* Infarct, myocardium
- myoclonic — *see* Epilepsy, generalized, specified NEC

- **Attack, attacks** — *continued*
  - panic F41.Ø
  - psychomotor — *see* Epilepsy, localization-related, symptomatic, with complex partial seizures
  - salaam — *see* Epilepsy, spasms
  - schizophreniform, brief F23
  - shuddering, benign G25.83
  - Stokes-Adams I45.9
  - syncope R55
  - transient ischemic (TIA) G45.9
    - specified NEC G45.8
  - unconsciousness R55
    - hysterical F44.89
  - vasomotor R55
  - vasovagal (paroxysmal) (idiopathic) R55
  - without alteration of consciousness — *see* Epilepsy, localization-related, symptomatic, with simple partial seizures
- **Attention** (to)
  - artificial
    - opening (of) Z43.9
      - digestive tract NEC Z43.4
        - colon Z43.3
        - ilium Z43.2
        - stomach Z43.1
      - specified NEC Z43.8
      - trachea Z43.Ø
      - urinary tract NEC Z43.6
        - cystostomy Z43.5
        - nephrostomy Z43.6
        - ureterostomy Z43.6
        - urethrostomy Z43.6
    - vagina Z43.7
  - colostomy Z43.3
  - cystostomy Z43.5
  - deficit disorder or syndrome F98.8
    - with hyperactivity — *see* Disorder, attention-deficit hyperactivity
  - gastrostomy Z43.1
  - ileostomy Z43.2
  - jejunostomy Z43.4
  - nephrostomy Z43.6
  - surgical dressings Z48.Ø1
  - sutures Z48.Ø2
  - tracheostomy Z43.Ø
  - ureterostomy Z43.6
  - urethrostomy Z43.6
- **Attrition**
  - gum — *see* Recession, gingival
  - tooth, teeth (excessive) (hard tissues) KØ3.Ø
- **Atypical, atypism** — *see also* condition
  - cells (on cytolgocial smear) (endocervical) (endometrial) (glandular)
    - cervix R87.619
    - vagina R87.629
  - cervical N87.9
  - endometrium N85.9
    - hyperplasia N85.ØØ
  - parenting situation Z62.9
- **Auditory** — *see* condition
- **Aujeszky's disease** B33.8
- **Aurantiasis, cutis** E67.1
- **Auricle, auricular** — *see also* condition
  - cervical Q18.2
- **Auriculotemporal syndrome** G5Ø.8
- **Austin Flint murmur** (aortic insufficiency) I35.1
- **Australian**
  - Q fever A78
  - X disease A83.4
- **Autism, autistic** (childhood) (infantile) F84.Ø
  - atypical F84.9
  - spectrum disorder F84.Ø
- **Autodigestion** R68.89
- **Autoerythrocyte sensitization** (syndrome) D69.2
- **Autographism** L5Ø.3
- **Autoimmune**
  - disease (systemic) M35.9
  - inhibitors to clotting factors D68.311
  - lymphoproliferative syndrome [ALPS] D89.82
  - thyroiditis EØ6.3
- **Autointoxication** R68.89
- **Automatism** G93.89
  - with temporal sclerosis G93.81
  - epileptic — *see* Epilepsy, localization-related, symptomatic, with complex partial seizures
  - paroxysmal, idiopathic — *see* Epilepsy, localization-related, symptomatic, with complex partial seizures
- **Autonomic, autonomous**
  - bladder (neurogenic) N31.2
  - hysteria seizure F44.5
- **Autosensitivity, erythrocyte** D69.2
- **Autosensitization, cutaneous** L3Ø.2
- **Autosome** — *see* condition by chromosome involved
- **Autotopagnosia** R48.1
- **Autotoxemia** R68.89
- **Autumn** — *see* condition
- **Avellis' syndrome** G46.8
- **Aversion**
  - oral R63.39
    - newborn P92.- ☑
    - nonorganic origin F98.2 ☑
  - sexual F52.1
- **Aviator's**
  - disease or sickness — *see* Effect, adverse, high altitude
  - ear T7Ø.Ø ☑
- **Avitaminosis** (multiple) — *see also* Deficiency, vitamin E56.9
  - B E53.9
    - with
      - beriberi E51.11
      - pellagra E52
  - B2 E53.Ø
  - B6 E53.1
  - B12 E53.8
  - D E55.9
    - with rickets E55.Ø
  - G E53.Ø
  - K E56.1
  - nicotinic acid E52
- **AVNRT** (atrioventricular nodal re-entrant tachycardia) I47.1
- **AVRT** (atrioventricular nodal re-entrant tachycardia) I47.1
- **Avulsion** (traumatic)
  - blood vessel — *see* Injury, blood vessel
  - bone — *see* Fracture, by site
  - cartilage — *see also* Dislocation, by site
    - symphyseal (inner), complicating delivery O71.6
  - external site other than limb — *see* Wound, open, by site
  - eye SØ5.7- ☑
  - head (intracranial)
    - external site NEC SØ8.89 ☑
    - scalp SØ8.Ø ☑
  - internal organ or site — *see* Injury, by site
  - joint — *see also* Dislocation, by site
    - capsule — *see* Sprain, by site
  - kidney S37.Ø6- ☑
  - ligament — *see* Sprain, by site
  - limb — *see also* Amputation, traumatic, by site
    - skin and subcutaneous tissue — *see* Wound, open, by site
  - muscle — *see* Injury, muscle
  - nerve (root) — *see* Injury, nerve
  - scalp SØ8.Ø ☑
  - skin and subcutaneous tissue — *see* Wound, open, by site
  - spleen S36.Ø32 ☑
  - symphyseal cartilage (inner), complicating delivery O71.6
  - tendon — *see* Injury, muscle
  - tooth SØ3.2 ☑
- **Awareness of heart beat** RØØ.2
- **Axenfeld's**
  - anomaly or syndrome Q15.Ø
  - degeneration (calcareous) Q13.4
- **Axilla, axillary** — *see also* condition
  - breast Q83.1
- **Axonotmesis** — *see* Injury, nerve
- **Ayerza's disease or syndrome** (pulmonary artery sclerosis with pulmonary hypertension) I27.Ø
- **Azoospermia** (organic) N46.Ø1
  - due to
    - drug therapy N46.Ø21
    - efferent duct obstruction N46.Ø23
    - infection N46.Ø22
    - radiation N46.Ø24
    - specified cause NEC N46.Ø29
    - systemic disease N46.Ø25
- **Azotemia** R79.89
  - meaning uremia N19
- **Aztec ear** Q17.3
- **Azygos**
  - continuation inferior vena cava Q26.8
  - lobe (lung) Q33.1

B

- **Baastrup's disease** — *see* Kissing spine
- **Babesiosis** B6Ø.ØØ
  - due to
    - Babesia
      - divergens B6Ø.Ø3
      - duncani B6Ø.Ø2
      - KO-1 B6Ø.Ø9
      - microti B6Ø.Ø1
      - MO-1 B6Ø.Ø3
      - species
        - unspecified B6Ø.ØØ
      - venatorum B6Ø.Ø9
    - specified NEC B6Ø.Ø9
- **Babington's disease** (familial hemorrhagic telangiectasia) I78.Ø
- **Babinski's syndrome** A52.79
- **Baby**
  - crying constantly R68.11
  - floppy (syndrome) P94.2
- **Bacillary** — *see* condition
- **Bacilluria** R82.71
- **Bacillus** — *see also* Infection, bacillus
  - abortus infection A23.1
  - anthracis infection A22.9
  - coli infection — *see also* Escherichia coli B96.2Ø
  - Flexner's AØ3.1
  - mallei infection A24.Ø
  - Shiga's AØ3.Ø
  - suipestifer infection — *see* Infection, salmonella
- **Back** — *see* condition
- **Backache** (postural) M54.9
  - sacroiliac M53.3
  - specified NEC M54.89
- **Backflow** — *see* Reflux
- **Backward reading** (dyslexia) F81.Ø
- **Bacteremia** R78.81
  - with sepsis — *see* Sepsis
- **Bactericholia** — *see* Cholecystitis, acute
- **Bacterid, bacteride** (pustular) L4Ø.3
- **Bacterium, bacteria, bacterial**
  - agent NEC, as cause of disease classified elsewhere B96.89
  - in blood — *see* Bacteremia
  - in urine — *see* Bacteriuria
- **Bacteriuria, bacteruria** R82.71
  - asymptomatic R82.71
- **Bacteroides**
  - fragilis, as cause of disease classified elsewhere B96.6
- **Bad**
  - heart — *see* Disease, heart
  - trip
    - due to drug abuse — *see* Abuse, drug, hallucinogen
    - due to drug dependence — *see* Dependence, drug, hallucinogen
- **Baelz's disease** (cheilitis glandularis apostematosa) K13.Ø
- **Baerensprung's disease** (eczema marginatum) B35.6
- **Bagasse disease or pneumonitis** J67.1
- **Bagassosis** J67.1
- **Baker's cyst** — *see* Cyst, Baker's
- **Bakwin-Krida syndrome** (metaphyseal dysplasia) Q78.5
- **Balancing side interference** M26.56
- **Balanitis** (circinata) (erosiva) (gangrenosa) (phagedenic) (vulgaris) N48.1
  - amebic AØ6.82
  - candidal B37.42
  - due to Haemophilus ducreyi A57
  - gonococcal (acute) (chronic) A54.23
  - xerotica obliterans N48.Ø
- **Balanoposthitis** N47.6
  - gonococcal (acute) (chronic) A54.23
  - ulcerative (specific) A63.8
- **Balanorrhagia** — *see* Balanitis
- **Balantidiasis, balantidiosis** AØ7.Ø
- **Bald tongue** K14.4
- **Baldness** — *see also* Alopecia
  - male-pattern — *see* Alopecia, androgenic
- **Balkan grippe** A78
- **Balloon disease** — *see* Effect, adverse, high altitude
- **Balo's disease** (concentric sclerosis) G37.5
- **Bamberger-Marie disease** — *see* Osteoarthropathy, hypertrophic, specified type NEC
- **Bancroft's filariasis** B74.Ø
- **Band**(s)
  - adhesive — *see* Adhesions, peritoneum

Band(s) — *continued*
- anomalous or congenital — *see also* Anomaly, by site
  - heart (atrial) (ventricular) Q24.8
  - intestine Q43.3
  - omentum Q43.3
- cervix N88.1
- constricting, congenital Q79.8
- gallbladder (congenital) Q44.1
- intestinal (adhesive) — *see* Adhesions, peritoneum
- obstructive
  - intestine K56.50
    - complete K56.52
    - incomplete K56.51
    - partial K56.51
  - peritoneum K56.50
    - complete K56.52
    - incomplete K56.51
    - partial K56.51
- periappendiceal, congenital Q43.3
- peritoneal (adhesive) — *see* Adhesions, peritoneum
- uterus N73.6
  - internal N85.6
- vagina N89.5

Bandemia D72.825
Bandl's ring (contraction), complicating delivery O62.4
Bangkok hemorrhagic fever A91
Bang's disease (brucella abortus) A23.1
Bankruptcy (anxiety concerning) Z59.86
Bannister's disease T78.3 ☑
- hereditary D84.1

Banti's disease or syndrome (with cirrhosis) (with portal hypertension) K76.6
Bar, median, prostate — *see* Enlargement, enlarged, prostate
Barcoo disease or rot — *see* Ulcer, skin
Barlow's disease E54
Barodontalgia T70.29 ☑
Baron Münchausen syndrome — *see* Disorder, factitious
Barosinusitis T70.1 ☑
Barotitis T70.0 ☑
Barotrauma T70.29 ☑
- odontalgia T70.29 ☑
- otitic T70.0 ☑
- sinus T70.1 ☑

Barraquer (-Simons) **disease or syndrome** (progressive lipodystrophy) E88.1
Barré-Guillain disease or syndrome G61.0
Barrel chest M95.4
Barré-Liéou syndrome (posterior cervical sympathetic) M53.0
Barrett's
- disease — *see* Barrett's, esophagus
- esophagus K22.70
  - with dysplasia K22.719
    - high grade K22.711
    - low grade K22.710
  - without dysplasia K22.70
- syndrome — *see* Barrett's, esophagus
- ulcer K22.10
  - with bleeding K22.11
  - without bleeding K22.10

Bársony (-Polgár) (-Teschendorf) **syndrome** (corkscrew esophagus) K22.4
Barth syndrome E78.71
Bartholinitis (suppurating) N75.8
- gonococcal (acute) (chronic) (with abscess) A54.1

Bartonellosis A44.9
- cutaneous A44.1
- mucocutaneous A44.1
- specified NEC A44.8
- systemic A44.0

Barton's fracture S52.56- ☑
Bartter's syndrome E26.81
Basal — *see* condition
Basan's (hidrotic) ectodermal dysplasia Q82.4
Baseball finger — *see* Dislocation, finger
Basedow's disease (exophthalmic goiter) — *see* Hyperthyroidism, with, goiter
Basic — *see* condition
Basilar — *see* condition
Bason's (hidrotic) ectodermal dysplasia Q82.4
Basopenia — *see* Agranulocytosis
Basophilia D72.824
Basophilism (cortico-adrenal) (Cushing's) (pituitary) E24.0
Bassen-Kornzweig disease or syndrome E78.6
Bat ear Q17.5
Bateman's
- disease B08.1
- purpura (senile) D69.2

Bathing cramp T75.1 ☑
Bathophobia F40.248
Batten (-Mayou) **disease** E75.4
- retina E75.4 *[H36]*

Batten-Steinert syndrome G71.11
Battered — *see* Maltreatment
Battey Mycobacterium infection A31.0
Battle exhaustion F43.0
Battledore placenta O43.19- ☑
Baumgarten-Cruveilhier cirrhosis, disease or syndrome K74.69
Bauxite fibrosis (of lung) J63.1
Bayle's disease (general paresis) A52.17
Bazin's disease (primary) (tuberculous) A18.4
Beach ear — *see* Swimmer's, ear
Beaded hair (congenital) Q84.1
Béal conjunctivitis or syndrome B30.2
Beard's disease (neurasthenia) F48.8
Beat(s)
- atrial, premature I49.1
- ectopic I49.49
- elbow — *see* Bursitis, elbow
- escaped, heart I49.49
- hand — *see* Bursitis, hand
- knee — *see* Bursitis, knee
- premature I49.40
  - atrial I49.1
  - auricular I49.1
  - supraventricular I49.1

Beau's
- disease or syndrome — *see* Degeneration, myocardial
- lines (transverse furrows on fingernails) L60.4

Bechterev's syndrome — *see* Spondylitis, ankylosing
Becker's
- cardiomyopathy I42.8
- disease
  - idiopathic mural endomyocardial disease I42.3
  - myotonia congenita, recessive form G71.12
- dystrophy G71.01
- pigmented hairy nevus D22.5

Beck's syndrome (anterior spinal artery occlusion) I65.8
Beckwith-Wiedemann syndrome Q87.3
Bed confinement status Z74.01
Bed sore — *see* Ulcer, pressure, by site
Bedbug bite(s) — *see* Bite(s), by site, superficial, insect
Bedclothes, asphyxiation or suffocation by — *see* Asphyxia, traumatic, due to, mechanical, trapped
Bednar's
- aphthae K12.0
- tumor — *see* Neoplasm, malignant, by site

Bedridden Z74.01
Bed-sharing, infant Z72.823
Bedsore — *see* Ulcer, pressure, by site
Bedwetting — *see* Enuresis
Bee sting (with allergic or anaphylactic shock) — *see* Toxicity, venom, arthropod, bee
Beer drinker's heart (disease) I42.6
Begbie's disease (exophthalmic goiter) — *see* Hyperthyroidism, with, goiter
Behavior
- antisocial
  - adult Z72.811
  - child or adolescent Z72.810
- disorder, disturbance — *see* Disorder, conduct
- disruptive — *see* Disorder, conduct
- drug seeking Z76.5
- inexplicable R46.2
- marked evasiveness R46.5
- obsessive-compulsive R46.81
- overactivity R46.3
- poor responsiveness R46.4
- self-damaging (life-style) Z72.89
- sleep-incompatible Z72.821
- slowness R46.4
- specified NEC R46.89
- strange (and inexplicable) R46.2
- suspiciousness R46.5
- type A pattern Z73.1
- undue concern or preoccupation with stressful events R46.6
- verbosity and circumstantial detail obscuring reason for contact R46.7

Behçet's disease or syndrome M35.2
Behr's disease — *see* Degeneration, macula
Beigel's disease or morbus (white piedra) B36.2
Bejel A65
Bekhterev's syndrome — *see* Spondylitis, ankylosing
Belching — *see* Eructation
Bell's
- mania F30.8
- palsy, paralysis G51.0
  - infant or newborn P11.3
- spasm G51.3- ☑

Bence Jones albuminuria or proteinuria NEC R80.3
Bends T70.3 ☑
Benedikt's paralysis or syndrome G46.3
Benign — *see also* condition
- prostatic hyperplasia — *see* Hyperplasia, prostate

Bennett's fracture (displaced) S62.21- ☑
Benson's disease — *see* Deposit, crystalline
Bent
- back (hysterical) F44.4
- nose M95.0
  - congenital Q67.4

Bereavement (uncomplicated) Z63.4
Bergeron's disease (hysterical chorea) F44.4
Berger's disease — *see* Nephropathy, IgA
Beriberi (dry) E51.11
- heart (disease) E51.12
- polyneuropathy E51.11
- wet E51.12
  - involving circulatory system E51.11

Berlin's disease or edema (traumatic) S05.8X- ☑
Berlock (berloque) **dermatitis** L56.2
Bernard-Horner syndrome G90.2
Bernard-Soulier disease or thrombopathia D69.1
Bernhardt (-Roth) **disease** — *see* Mononeuropathy, lower limb, meralgia paresthetica
Bernheim's syndrome — *see* Failure, heart, right
Bertielliasis B71.8
Berylliosis (lung) J63.2
Besnier-Boeck (-Schaumann) **disease** — *see* Sarcoidosis
Besnier's
- lupus pernio D86.3
- prurigo L20.0

Bestiality F65.89
Best's disease H35.50
Betalipoproteinemia, broad or floating E78.2
Beta-mercaptolactate-cysteine disulfiduria E72.09
Betting and gambling Z72.6
- pathological (compulsive) F63.0

Bezoar T18.9 ☑
- intestine T18.3 ☑
- stomach T18.2 ☑

Bezold's abscess — *see* Mastoiditis, acute
Bianchi's syndrome R48.8
Bicornate or bicornis uterus Q51.3
- in pregnancy or childbirth O34.00
  - causing obstructed labor O65.5

Bicuspid aortic valve Q23.1
Biedl-Bardet syndrome Q87.89
Bielschowsky (-Jansky) disease E75.4
Biermer's (pernicious) anemia or disease D51.0
Biett's disease L93.0
Bifid (congenital)
- apex, heart Q24.8
- clitoris Q52.6
- kidney Q63.8
- nose Q30.2
- patella Q74.1
- scrotum Q55.29
- toe NEC Q74.2
- tongue Q38.3
- ureter Q62.8
- uterus Q51.3
- uvula Q35.7

Biforis uterus (suprasimplex) Q51.3
Bifurcation (congenital)
- gallbladder Q44.1
- kidney pelvis Q63.8
- renal pelvis Q63.8
- rib Q76.6
- tongue, congenital Q38.3
- trachea Q32.1
- ureter Q62.8
- urethra Q64.74
- vertebra Q76.49

Big spleen syndrome D73.1
Bigeminal pulse R00.8
Bilateral — *see* condition

- **Bile**
  - duct — *see* condition
  - pigments in urine R82.2
- **Bilharziasis** — *see also* Schistosomiasis
  - chyluria B65.Ø
  - cutaneous B65.3
  - galacturia B65.Ø
  - hematochyluria B65.Ø
  - intestinal B65.1
  - lipemia B65.9
  - lipuria B65.Ø
  - oriental B65.2
  - piarhemia B65.9
  - pulmonary NOS B65.9 *[J99]*
    - pneumonia B65.9 *[J17]*
  - tropical hematuria B65.Ø
  - vesical B65.Ø
- **Biliary** — *see* condition
- **Bilirubin metabolism disorder** E8Ø.7
  - specified NEC E8Ø.6
- **Bilirubinemia, familial nonhemolytic** E8Ø.4
- **Bilirubinuria** R82.2
- **Biliuria** R82.2
- **Bilocular stomach** K31.2
- **Binswanger's disease** I67.3
- **Biparta, bipartite**
  - carpal scaphoid Q74.Ø
  - patella Q74.1
  - vagina Q52.1Ø
- **Bird**
  - face Q75.8
  - fancier's disease or lung J67.2
- **Birth**
  - complications in mother — *see* Delivery, complicated
  - compression during NOS P15.9
  - defect — *see* Anomaly
  - immature (less than 37 completed weeks) — *see* Preterm, newborn
    - extremely (less than 28 completed weeks) — *see* Immaturity, extreme
  - inattention, at or after — *see* Maltreatment, child, neglect
  - injury NOS P15.9
    - basal ganglia P11.1
    - brachial plexus NEC P14.3
    - brain (compression) (pressure) P11.2
    - central nervous system NOS P11.9
    - cerebellum P11.1
    - cerebral hemorrhage P1Ø.1
    - external genitalia P15.5
    - eye P15.3
    - face P15.4
    - fracture
      - bone P13.9
        - specified NEC P13.8
      - clavicle P13.4
      - femur P13.2
      - humerus P13.3
      - long bone, except femur P13.3
      - radius and ulna P13.3
      - skull P13.Ø
      - spine P11.5
      - tibia and fibula P13.3
    - intracranial P11.2
      - laceration or hemorrhage P1Ø.9
        - specified NEC P1Ø.8
    - intraventricular hemorrhage P1Ø.2
    - laceration
      - brain P1Ø.1
      - by scalpel P15.8
      - peripheral nerve P14.9
    - liver P15.Ø
    - meninges
      - brain P11.1
      - spinal cord P11.5
    - nerve
      - brachial plexus P14.3
      - cranial NEC (except facial) P11.4
      - facial P11.3
      - peripheral P14.9
      - phrenic (paralysis) P14.2
    - paralysis
      - facial nerve P11.3
      - spinal P11.5
    - penis P15.5
    - rupture
      - spinal cord P11.5
    - scalp P12.9

- **Birth** — *continued*
  - injury — *continued*
    - scalpel wound P15.8
    - scrotum P15.5
    - skull NEC P13.1
      - fracture P13.Ø
    - specified type NEC P15.8
    - spinal cord P11.5
    - spine P11.5
    - spleen P15.1
    - sternomastoid (hematoma) P15.2
    - subarachnoid hemorrhage P1Ø.3
    - subcutaneous fat necrosis P15.6
    - subdural hemorrhage P1Ø.Ø
    - tentorial tear P1Ø.4
    - testes P15.5
    - vulva P15.5
  - lack of care, at or after — *see* Maltreatment, child, neglect
  - neglect, at or after — *see* Maltreatment, child, neglect
  - palsy or paralysis, newborn, NOS (birth injury) P14.9
  - premature (infant) — *see* Preterm, newborn
  - shock, newborn P96.89
  - trauma — *see* Birth, injury
  - weight
    - low (2499 grams or less) — *see* Low, birthweight
      - extremely (999 grams or less) — *see* Low, birthweight, extreme
    - 4ØØØ grams to 4499 grams PØ8.1
    - 45ØØ grams or more PØ8.Ø
- **Birthmark** Q82.5
- **Birt-Hogg-Dube syndrome** Q87.89
- **Bisalbuminemia** E88.Ø9
- **Biskra's button** B55.1
- **Bite**(s) (animal) (human)
  - abdomen, abdominal
    - wall S31.159 ☑
      - with penetration into peritoneal cavity S31.659 ☑
      - epigastric region S31.152 ☑
        - with penetration into peritoneal cavity S31.652 ☑
      - left
        - lower quadrant S31.154 ☑
          - with penetration into peritoneal cavity S31.654 ☑
        - upper quadrant S31.151 ☑
          - with penetration into peritoneal cavity S31.651 ☑
      - periumbilic region S31.155 ☑
        - with penetration into peritoneal cavity S31.655 ☑
      - right
        - lower quadrant S31.153 ☑
          - with penetration into peritoneal cavity S31.653 ☑
        - upper quadrant S31.15Ø ☑
          - with penetration into peritoneal cavity S31.65Ø ☑
      - superficial NEC S3Ø.871 ☑
        - insect S3Ø.861 ☑
  - alveolar (process) — *see* Bite, oral cavity
  - amphibian (venomous) — *see* Venom, bite, amphibian
  - animal — *see also* Bite, by site
    - venomous — *see* Venom
  - ankle S91.Ø5- ☑
    - superficial NEC S9Ø.57- ☑
      - insect S9Ø.56- ☑
  - antecubital space — *see* Bite, elbow
  - anus S31.835 ☑
    - superficial NEC S3Ø.877 ☑
      - insect S3Ø.867 ☑
  - arm (upper) S41.15- ☑
    - lower — *see* Bite, forearm
    - superficial NEC S4Ø.87- ☑
      - insect S4Ø.86- ☑
  - arthropod NEC — *see* Venom, bite, arthropod
  - auditory canal (external) (meatus) — *see* Bite, ear
  - auricle, ear — *see* Bite, ear
  - axilla — *see* Bite, arm
  - back — *see also* Bite, thorax, back
    - lower S31.Ø5Ø ☑
      - with penetration into retroperitoneal space S31.Ø51 ☑
    - superficial NEC S3Ø.87Ø ☑
      - insect S3Ø.86Ø ☑
  - bedbug — *see* Bite(s), by site, superficial, insect

- **Bite**(s) — *continued*
  - breast S21.Ø5- ☑
    - superficial NEC S2Ø.17- ☑
      - insect S2Ø.16- ☑
  - brow — *see* Bite, head, specified site NEC
  - buttock S31.8Ø5 ☑
    - left S31.825 ☑
    - right S31.815 ☑
    - superficial NEC S3Ø.87Ø ☑
      - insect S3Ø.86Ø ☑
  - calf — *see* Bite, leg
  - canaliculus lacrimalis — *see* Bite, eyelid
  - canthus, eye — *see* Bite, eyelid
  - centipede — *see* Toxicity, venom, arthropod, centipede
  - cheek (external) SØ1.45- ☑
    - internal — *see* Bite, oral cavity
    - superficial NEC SØØ.87 ☑
      - insect SØØ.86 ☑
  - chest wall — *see* Bite, thorax
  - chigger B88.Ø
  - chin — *see* Bite, head, specified site NEC
  - clitoris — *see* Bite, vulva
  - costal region — *see* Bite, thorax
  - digit(s)
    - hand — *see* Bite, finger
    - toe — *see* Bite, toe
  - ear (canal) (external) SØ1.35- ☑
    - superficial NEC SØØ.47- ☑
      - insect SØØ.46- ☑
  - elbow S51.Ø5- ☑
    - superficial NEC S5Ø.37- ☑
      - insect S5Ø.36- ☑
  - epididymis — *see* Bite, testis
  - epigastric region — *see* Bite, abdomen
  - epiglottis — *see* Bite, neck, specified site NEC
  - esophagus, cervical S11.25 ☑
    - superficial NEC S1Ø.17 ☑
      - insect S1Ø.16 ☑
  - eyebrow — *see* Bite, eyelid
  - eyelid SØ1.15- ☑
    - superficial NEC SØØ.27- ☑
      - insect SØØ.26- ☑
  - face NEC — *see* Bite, head, specified site NEC
  - finger(s) S61.259 ☑
    - with
      - damage to nail S61.359 ☑
    - index S61.258 ☑
      - with
        - damage to nail S61.358 ☑
      - left S61.251 ☑
        - with
          - damage to nail S61.351 ☑
      - right S61.25Ø ☑
        - with
          - damage to nail S61.35Ø ☑
      - superficial NEC S6Ø.478 ☑
        - insect S6Ø.46- ☑
    - little S61.25- ☑
      - with
        - damage to nail S61.35- ☑
      - superficial NEC S6Ø.47- ☑
        - insect S6Ø.46- ☑
    - middle S61.25- ☑
      - with
        - damage to nail S61.35- ☑
      - superficial NEC S6Ø.47- ☑
        - insect S6Ø.46- ☑
    - ring S61.25- ☑
      - with
        - damage to nail S61.35- ☑
      - superficial NEC S6Ø.47- ☑
        - insect S6Ø.46- ☑
    - superficial NEC S6Ø.479 ☑
      - insect S6Ø.469 ☑
    - thumb — *see* Bite, thumb
  - flank — *see* Bite, abdomen, wall
  - flea — *see* Bite, by site, superficial, insect
  - foot (except toe(s) alone) S91.35- ☑
    - superficial NEC S9Ø.87- ☑
      - insect S9Ø.86- ☑
    - toe — *see* Bite, toe
  - forearm S51.85- ☑
    - elbow only — *see* Bite, elbow
    - superficial NEC S5Ø.87- ☑
      - insect S5Ø.86- ☑
  - forehead — *see* Bite, head, specified site NEC

- **Bite**(s) — *continued*
  - genital organs, external
    - female S31.552 ☑
      - superficial NEC S3Ø.876 ☑
        - insect S3Ø.866 ☑
      - vagina and vulva — *see* Bite, vulva
    - male S31.551 ☑
      - penis — *see* Bite, penis
      - scrotum — *see* Bite, scrotum
      - superficial NEC S3Ø.875 ☑
        - insect S3Ø.865 ☑
      - testes — *see* Bite, testis
  - groin — *see* Bite, abdomen, wall
  - gum — *see* Bite, oral cavity
  - hand S61.45- ☑
    - finger — *see* Bite, finger
    - superficial NEC S6Ø.57- ☑
      - insect S6Ø.56- ☑
    - thumb — *see* Bite, thumb
  - head SØ1.95 ☑
    - cheek — *see* Bite, cheek
    - ear — *see* Bite, ear
    - eyelid — *see* Bite, eyelid
    - lip — *see* Bite, lip
    - nose — *see* Bite, nose
    - oral cavity — *see* Bite, oral cavity
    - scalp — *see* Bite, scalp
    - specified site NEC SØ1.85 ☑
      - superficial NEC SØØ.87 ☑
        - insect SØØ.86 ☑
    - superficial NEC SØØ.97 ☑
      - insect SØØ.96 ☑
    - temporomandibular area — *see* Bite, cheek
  - heel — *see* Bite, foot
  - hip S71.Ø5- ☑
    - superficial NEC S7Ø.27- ☑
      - insect S7Ø.26- ☑
  - hymen S31.45 ☑
  - hypochondrium — *see* Bite, abdomen, wall
  - hypogastric region — *see* Bite, abdomen, wall
  - inguinal region — *see* Bite, abdomen, wall
  - insect — *see* Bite, by site, superficial, insect
  - instep — *see* Bite, foot
  - interscapular region — *see* Bite, thorax, back
  - jaw — *see* Bite, head, specified site NEC
  - knee S81.Ø5- ☑
    - superficial NEC S8Ø.27- ☑
      - insect S8Ø.26- ☑
  - labium (majus) (minus) — *see* Bite, vulva
  - lacrimal duct — *see* Bite, eyelid
  - larynx S11.Ø15 ☑
    - superficial NEC S1Ø.17 ☑
      - insect S1Ø.16 ☑
  - leg (lower) S81.85- ☑
    - ankle — *see* Bite, ankle
    - foot — *see* Bite, foot
    - knee — *see* Bite, knee
    - superficial NEC S8Ø.87- ☑
      - insect S8Ø.86- ☑
    - toe — *see* Bite, toe
    - upper — *see* Bite, thigh
  - lip SØ1.551 ☑
    - superficial NEC SØØ.571 ☑
      - insect SØØ.561 ☑
  - lizard (venomous) — *see* Venom, bite, reptile
  - loin — *see* Bite, abdomen, wall
  - lower back — *see* Bite, back, lower
  - lumbar region — *see* Bite, back, lower
  - malar region — *see* Bite, head, specified site NEC
  - mammary — *see* Bite, breast
  - marine animals (venomous) — *see* Toxicity, venom, marine animal
  - mastoid region — *see* Bite, head, specified site NEC
  - mouth — *see* Bite, oral cavity
  - nail
    - finger — *see* Bite, finger
    - toe — *see* Bite, toe
  - nape — *see* Bite, neck, specified site NEC
  - nasal (septum) (sinus) — *see* Bite, nose
  - nasopharynx — *see* Bite, head, specified site NEC
  - neck S11.95 ☑
    - involving
      - cervical esophagus — *see* Bite, esophagus, cervical
      - larynx — *see* Bite, larynx
      - pharynx — *see* Bite, pharynx

- **Bite**(s) — *continued*
  - neck — *continued*
    - involving — *continued*
      - thyroid gland S11.15 ☑
      - trachea — *see* Bite, trachea
    - specified site NEC S11.85 ☑
      - superficial NEC S1Ø.87 ☑
        - insect S1Ø.86 ☑
    - superficial NEC S1Ø.97 ☑
      - insect S1Ø.96 ☑
    - throat S11.85 ☑
      - superficial NEC S1Ø.17 ☑
        - insect S1Ø.16 ☑
  - nose (septum) (sinus) SØ1.25 ☑
    - superficial NEC SØØ.37 ☑
      - insect SØØ.36 ☑
  - occipital region — *see* Bite, scalp
  - oral cavity SØ1.552 ☑
    - superficial NEC SØØ.572 ☑
      - insect SØØ.562 ☑
  - orbital region — *see* Bite, eyelid
  - palate — *see* Bite, oral cavity
  - palm — *see* Bite, hand
  - parietal region — *see* Bite, scalp
  - pelvis S31.Ø5Ø ☑
    - with penetration into retroperitoneal space S31.Ø51 ☑
    - superficial NEC S3Ø.87Ø ☑
      - insect S3Ø.86Ø ☑
  - penis S31.25 ☑
    - superficial NEC S3Ø.872 ☑
      - insect S3Ø.862 ☑
  - perineum
    - female — *see* Bite, vulva
    - male — *see* Bite, pelvis
  - periocular area (with or without lacrimal passages) — *see* Bite, eyelid
  - phalanges
    - finger — *see* Bite, finger
    - toe — *see* Bite, toe
  - pharynx S11.25 ☑
    - superficial NEC S1Ø.17 ☑
      - insect S1Ø.16 ☑
  - pinna — *see* Bite, ear
  - poisonous — *see* Venom
  - popliteal space — *see* Bite, knee
  - prepuce — *see* Bite, penis
  - pubic region — *see* Bite, abdomen, wall
  - rectovaginal septum — *see* Bite, vulva
  - red bug B88.Ø
  - reptile NEC — *see also* Venom, bite, reptile
    - nonvenomous — *see* Bite, by site
    - snake — *see* Venom, bite, snake
  - sacral region — *see* Bite, back, lower
  - sacroiliac region — *see* Bite, back, lower
  - salivary gland — *see* Bite, oral cavity
  - scalp SØ1.Ø5 ☑
    - superficial NEC SØØ.Ø7 ☑
      - insect SØØ.Ø6 ☑
  - scapular region — *see* Bite, shoulder
  - scrotum S31.35 ☑
    - superficial NEC S3Ø.873 ☑
      - insect S3Ø.863 ☑
  - sea-snake (venomous) — *see* Toxicity, venom, snake, sea snake
  - shin — *see* Bite, leg
  - shoulder S41.Ø5- ☑
    - superficial NEC S4Ø.27- ☑
      - insect S4Ø.26- ☑
  - snake — *see also* Venom, bite, snake
    - nonvenomous — *see* Bite, by site
  - spermatic cord — *see* Bite, testis
  - spider (venomous) — *see* Toxicity, venom, spider
    - nonvenomous — *see* Bite, by site, superficial, insect
  - sternal region — *see* Bite, thorax, front
  - submaxillary region — *see* Bite, head, specified site NEC
  - submental region — *see* Bite, head, specified site NEC
  - subungual
    - finger(s) — *see* Bite, finger
    - toe — *see* Bite, toe
  - superficial — *see* Bite, by site, superficial
  - supraclavicular fossa S11.85 ☑
  - supraorbital — *see* Bite, head, specified site NEC
  - temple, temporal region — *see* Bite, head, specified site NEC

- **Bite**(s) — *continued*
  - temporomandibular area — *see* Bite, cheek
  - testis S31.35 ☑
    - superficial NEC S3Ø.873 ☑
      - insect S3Ø.863 ☑
  - thigh S71.15- ☑
    - superficial NEC S7Ø.37- ☑
      - insect S7Ø.36- ☑
  - thorax, thoracic (wall) S21.95 ☑
    - back S21.25- ☑
      - with penetration into thoracic cavity S21.45- ☑
    - breast — *see* Bite, breast
    - front S21.15- ☑
      - with penetration into thoracic cavity S21.35- ☑
    - superficial NEC S2Ø.97 ☑
      - back S2Ø.47- ☑
      - front S2Ø.37- ☑
      - insect S2Ø.96 ☑
        - back S2Ø.46- ☑
        - front S2Ø.36- ☑
  - throat — *see* Bite, neck, throat
  - thumb S61.Ø5- ☑
    - with
      - damage to nail S61.15- ☑
    - superficial NEC S6Ø.37- ☑
      - insect S6Ø.36- ☑
  - thyroid S11.15 ☑
    - superficial NEC S1Ø.87 ☑
      - insect S1Ø.86 ☑
  - toe(s) S91.15- ☑
    - with
      - damage to nail S91.25- ☑
    - great S91.15- ☑
      - with
        - damage to nail S91.25- ☑
    - lesser S91.15- ☑
      - with
        - damage to nail S91.25- ☑
    - superficial NEC S9Ø.47- ☑
      - great S9Ø.47- ☑
      - insect S9Ø.46- ☑
        - great S9Ø.46- ☑
  - tongue SØ1.552 ☑
  - trachea S11.Ø25 ☑
    - superficial NEC S1Ø.17 ☑
      - insect S1Ø.16 ☑
  - tunica vaginalis — *see* Bite, testis
  - tympanum, tympanic membrane — *see* Bite, ear
  - umbilical region S31.155 ☑
  - uvula — *see* Bite, oral cavity
  - vagina — *see* Bite, vulva
  - venomous — *see* Venom
  - vocal cords S11.Ø35 ☑
    - superficial NEC S1Ø.17 ☑
      - insect S1Ø.16 ☑
  - vulva S31.45 ☑
    - superficial NEC S3Ø.874 ☑
      - insect S3Ø.864 ☑
  - wrist S61.55- ☑
    - superficial NEC S6Ø.87- ☑
      - insect S6Ø.86- ☑
- **Biting, cheek or lip** K13.1
- **Biventricular failure** (heart) I5Ø.82
- **Björck** (-Thorson) **syndrome** (malignant carcinoid) E34.Ø
- **Black**
  - death A2Ø.9
  - eye SØØ.1- ☑
  - hairy tongue K14.3
  - heel (foot) S9Ø.3- ☑
  - lung (disease) J6Ø
  - palm (hand) S6Ø.22- ☑
- **Blackfan-Diamond anemia or syndrome** (congenital hypoplastic anemia) D61.Ø1
- **Blackhead** L7Ø.Ø
- **Blackout** R55
- **Bladder** — *see* condition
- **Blast** (air) (hydraulic) (immersion) (underwater)
  - blindness SØ5.8X- ☑
  - injury
    - abdomen or thorax — *see* Injury, by site
    - ear (acoustic nerve trauma) — *see* Injury, nerve, acoustic, specified type NEC
  - syndrome NEC T7Ø.8 ☑
- **Blastoma** — *see* Neoplasm, malignant, by site
  - pulmonary — *see* Neoplasm, lung, malignant
- **Blastomycosis, blastomycotic** B4Ø.9

Blastomycosis, blastomycotic — *continued*
  Brazilian — *see* Paracoccidioidomycosis
  cutaneous B4Ø.3
  disseminated B4Ø.7
  European — *see* Cryptococcosis
  generalized B4Ø.7
  keloidal B48.Ø
  North American B4Ø.9
  primary pulmonary B4Ø.Ø
  pulmonary B4Ø.2
    acute B4Ø.Ø
    chronic B4Ø.1
  skin B4Ø.3
  South American — *see* Paracoccidioidomycosis
  specified NEC B4Ø.89
Bleb(s) R23.8
  emphysematous (lung) (solitary) J43.9
  endophthalmitis H59.43
  filtering (vitreous), after glaucoma surgery Z98.83
  inflammed (infected), postprocedural H59.4Ø
    stage 1 H59.41
    stage 2 H59.42
    stage 3 H59.43
  lung (ruptured) J43.9
    congenital — *see* Atelectasis
    newborn P25.8
  subpleural (emphysematous) J43.9
Blebitis, postprocedural H59.4Ø
  stage 1 H59.41
  stage 2 H59.42
  stage 3 H59.43
Bleeder (familial) (hereditary) — *see* Hemophilia
Bleeding — *see also* Hemorrhage
  anal K62.5
  anovulatory N97.Ø
  atonic, following delivery O72.1
  capillary I78.8
    puerperal O72.2
  contact (postcoital) N93.Ø
  due to uterine subinvolution N85.3
  ear — *see* Otorrhagia
  excessive, associated with menopausal onset N92.4
  familial — *see* Defect, coagulation
  following intercourse N93.Ø
  gastrointestinal K92.2
  hemorrhoids — *see* Hemorrhoids
  intermenstrual (regular) N92.3
    irregular N92.1
  intraoperative — *see* Complication, intraoperative, hemorrhage
  irregular N92.6
  menopausal N92.4
  newborn, intraventricular — *see* Newborn, affected by, hemorrhage, intraventricular
  nipple N64.59
  nose RØ4.Ø
  ovulation N92.3
  perimenopausal N92.4
  postclimacteric N95.Ø
  postcoital N93.Ø
  postmenopausal N95.Ø
  postoperative — *see* Complication, postprocedural, hemorrhage
  preclimacteric N92.4
  pre-pubertal vaginal N93.1
  puberty (excessive, with onset of menstrual periods) N92.2
  rectum, rectal K62.5
    newborn P54.2
  tendencies — *see* Defect, coagulation
  throat RØ4.1
  tooth socket (post-extraction) K91.84Ø
  umbilical stump P51.9
  uterus, uterine NEC N93.9
    climacteric N92.4
    dysfunctional or functional N93.8
    menopausal N92.4
    preclimacteric or premenopausal N92.4
    unrelated to menstrual cycle N93.9
  vagina, vaginal (abnormal) N93.9
    dysfunctional or functional N93.8
    newborn P54.6
    pre-pubertal N93.1
  vicarious N94.89
Blennorrhagia, blennorrhagic — *see* Gonorrhea
Blennorrhea (acute) (chronic) — *see also* Gonorrhea
  inclusion (neonatal) (newborn) P39.1
  lower genitourinary tract (gonococcal) A54.ØØ
Blennorrhea — *continued*
  neonatorum (gonococcal ophthalmia) A54.31
Blepharelosis — *see* Entropion
Blepharitis (angularis) (ciliaris) (eyelid) (marginal) (nonulcerative) HØ1.ØØ9
  herpes zoster BØ2.39
  left HØ1.ØØ6
    lower HØ1.ØØ5
    upper HØ1.ØØ4
    upper and lower HØ1.ØØB
  right HØ1.ØØ3
    lower HØ1.ØØ2
    upper HØ1.ØØ1
    upper and lower HØ1.ØØA
  squamous HØ1.Ø29
    left HØ1.Ø26
      lower HØ1.Ø25
      upper HØ1.Ø24
      upper and lower HØ1.Ø2B
    right HØ1.Ø23
      lower HØ1.Ø22
      upper HØ1.Ø21
      upper and lower HØ1.Ø2A
  ulcerative HØ1.Ø19
    left HØ1.Ø16
      lower HØ1.Ø15
      upper HØ1.Ø14
      upper and lower HØ1.Ø1B
    right HØ1.Ø13
      lower HØ1.Ø12
      upper HØ1.Ø11
      upper and lower HØ1.Ø1A
Blepharochalasis HØ2.3Ø
  congenital Q1Ø.Ø
  left HØ2.36
    lower HØ2.35
    upper HØ2.34
  right HØ2.33
    lower HØ2.32
    upper HØ2.31
Blepharoclonus HØ2.59
Blepharoconjunctivitis H1Ø.5Ø- ☑
  angular H1Ø.52- ☑
  contact H1Ø.53- ☑
  ligneous H1Ø.51- ☑
Blepharophimosis (eyelid) HØ2.529
  congenital Q1Ø.3
  left HØ2.526
    lower HØ2.525
    upper HØ2.524
  right HØ2.523
    lower HØ2.522
    upper HØ2.521
Blepharoptosis HØ2.4Ø- ☑
  congenital Q1Ø.Ø
  mechanical HØ2.41- ☑
  myogenic HØ2.42- ☑
  neurogenic HØ2.43- ☑
  paralytic HØ2.43- ☑
Blepharopyorrhea, gonococcal A54.39
Blepharospasm G24.5
  drug induced G24.Ø1
Blighted ovum OØ2.Ø
Blind — *see also* Blindness
  bronchus (congenital) Q32.4
  loop syndrome K9Ø.2
    congenital Q43.8
  sac, fallopian tube (congenital) Q5Ø.6
  spot, enlarged — *see* Defect, visual field, localized, scotoma, blind spot area
  tract or tube, congenital NEC — *see* Atresia, by site
Blindness (acquired) (congenital) (both eyes) H54.ØX- ☑
  blast SØ5.8X- ☑
  color — *see* Deficiency, color vision
  concussion SØ5.8X- ☑
  cortical H47.619
    left brain H47.612
    right brain H47.611
  day H53.11
  due to injury (current episode) SØ5.9- ☑
    sequelae — *code to* injury with seventh character S
  eclipse (total) — *see* Retinopathy, solar
  emotional (hysterical) F44.6
  face H53.16
  hysterical F44.6
  legal (both eyes) (USA definition) H54.8
  mind R48.8
Blindness — *continued*
  night H53.6Ø
    abnormal dark adaptation curve H53.61
    acquired H53.62
    congenital H53.63
    specified type NEC H53.69
    vitamin A deficiency E5Ø.5
  one eye (other eye normal) H54.4Ø
    left (normal vision on right) H54.42- ☑
      low vision on right H54.12- ☑
    low vision, other eye H54.1Ø
    right (normal vision on left) H54.41- ☑
      low vision on left H54.11- ☑
  psychic R48.8
  river B73.Ø1
  snow — *see* Photokeratitis
  sun, solar — *see* Retinopathy, solar
  transient — *see* Disturbance, vision, subjective, loss, transient
  traumatic (current episode) SØ5.9- ☑
  word (developmental) F81.Ø
    acquired R48.Ø
    secondary to organic lesion R48.Ø
Blister (nonthermal)
  abdominal wall S3Ø.821 ☑
  alveolar process SØØ.522 ☑
  ankle S9Ø.52- ☑
  antecubital space — *see* Blister, elbow
  anus S3Ø.827 ☑
  arm (upper) S4Ø.82- ☑
  auditory canal — *see* Blister, ear
  auricle — *see* Blister, ear
  axilla — *see* Blister, arm
  back, lower S3Ø.82Ø ☑
  beetle dermatitis L24.89
  breast S2Ø.12- ☑
  brow SØØ.82 ☑
  calf — *see* Blister, leg
  canthus — *see* Blister, eyelid
  cheek SØØ.82 ☑
    internal SØØ.522 ☑
  chest wall — *see* Blister, thorax
  chin SØØ.82 ☑
  costal region — *see* Blister, thorax
  digit(s)
    foot — *see* Blister, toe
    hand — *see* Blister, finger
  due to burn — *see* Burn, by site, second degree
  ear SØØ.42- ☑
  elbow S5Ø.32- ☑
  epiglottis S1Ø.12 ☑
  esophagus, cervical S1Ø.12 ☑
  eyebrow — *see* Blister, eyelid
  eyelid SØØ.22- ☑
  face SØØ.82 ☑
  fever BØØ.1
  finger(s) S6Ø.429 ☑
    index S6Ø.42- ☑
    little S6Ø.42- ☑
    middle S6Ø.42- ☑
    ring S6Ø.42- ☑
  foot (except toe(s) alone) S9Ø.82- ☑
    toe — *see* Blister, toe
  forearm S5Ø.82- ☑
    elbow only — *see* Blister, elbow
  forehead SØØ.82 ☑
  fracture — *omit code*
  genital organ
    female S3Ø.826 ☑
    male S3Ø.825 ☑
  gum SØØ.522 ☑
  hand S6Ø.52- ☑
  head SØØ.92 ☑
    ear — *see* Blister, ear
    eyelid — *see* Blister, eyelid
    lip SØØ.521 ☑
    nose SØØ.32 ☑
    oral cavity SØØ.522 ☑
    scalp SØØ.Ø2 ☑
    specified site NEC SØØ.82 ☑
  heel — *see* Blister, foot
  hip S7Ø.22- ☑
  interscapular region S2Ø.429 ☑
  jaw SØØ.82 ☑
  knee S8Ø.22- ☑
  larynx S1Ø.12 ☑

- **Blister** — *continued*
  - leg (lower) S8Ø.82- ☑
    - knee — *see* Blister, knee
    - upper — *see* Blister, thigh
  - lip SØØ.521 ☑
  - malar region SØØ.82 ☑
  - mammary — *see* Blister, breast
  - mastoid region SØØ.82 ☑
  - mouth SØØ.522 ☑
  - multiple, skin, nontraumatic R23.8
  - nail
    - finger — *see* Blister, finger
    - toe — *see* Blister, toe
  - nasal SØØ.32 ☑
  - neck S1Ø.92 ☑
    - specified site NEC S1Ø.82 ☑
    - throat S1Ø.12 ☑
  - nose SØØ.32 ☑
  - occipital region SØØ.Ø2 ☑
  - oral cavity SØØ.522 ☑
  - orbital region — *see* Blister, eyelid
  - palate SØØ.522 ☑
  - palm — *see* Blister, hand
  - parietal region SØØ.Ø2 ☑
  - pelvis S3Ø.82Ø ☑
  - penis S3Ø.822 ☑
  - periocular area — *see* Blister, eyelid
  - phalanges
    - finger — *see* Blister, finger
    - toe — *see* Blister, toe
  - pharynx S1Ø.12 ☑
  - pinna — *see* Blister, ear
  - popliteal space — *see* Blister, knee
  - scalp SØØ.Ø2 ☑
  - scapular region — *see* Blister, shoulder
  - scrotum S3Ø.823 ☑
  - shin — *see* Blister, leg
  - shoulder S4Ø.22- ☑
  - sternal region S2Ø.329 ☑
  - submaxillary region SØØ.82 ☑
  - submental region SØØ.82 ☑
  - subungual
    - finger(s) — *see* Blister, finger
    - toe(s) — *see* Blister, toe
  - supraclavicular fossa S1Ø.82 ☑
  - supraorbital SØØ.82 ☑
  - temple SØØ.82 ☑
  - temporal region SØØ.82 ☑
  - testis S3Ø.823 ☑
  - thermal — *see* Burn, second degree, by site
  - thigh S7Ø.32- ☑
  - thorax, thoracic (wall) S2Ø.92 ☑
    - back S2Ø.42- ☑
    - front S2Ø.32- ☑
  - throat S1Ø.12 ☑
  - thumb S6Ø.32- ☑
  - toe(s) S9Ø.42- ☑
    - great S9Ø.42- ☑
  - tongue SØØ.522 ☑
  - trachea S1Ø.12 ☑
  - tympanum, tympanic membrane — *see* Blister, ear
  - upper arm — *see* Blister, arm (upper)
  - uvula SØØ.522 ☑
  - vagina S3Ø.824 ☑
  - vocal cords S1Ø.12 ☑
  - vulva S3Ø.824 ☑
  - wrist S6Ø.82- ☑
- **Bloating** R14.Ø
- **Bloch-Sulzberger disease or syndrome** Q82.3
- **Block, blocked**
  - alveolocapillary J84.1Ø
  - arborization (heart) I45.5
  - arrhythmic I45.9
  - atrioventricular (incomplete) (partial) I44.3Ø
    - with atrioventricular dissociation I44.2
    - complete I44.2
      - congenital Q24.6
    - congenital Q24.6
    - first degree I44.Ø
    - second degree (types I and II) I44.1
    - specified NEC I44.39
    - third degree I44.2
    - types I and II I44.1
  - auriculoventricular — *see* Block, atrioventricular
  - bifascicular (cardiac) I45.2
  - bundle-branch (complete) (false) (incomplete) I45.4
- **Block, blocked** — *continued*
  - bundle-branch — *continued*
    - bilateral I45.2
    - left I44.7
      - with right bundle branch block I45.2
      - hemiblock I44.6Ø
        - anterior I44.4
        - posterior I44.5
      - incomplete I44.7
        - with right bundle branch block I45.2
    - right I45.1Ø
      - with
        - left bundle branch block I45.2
        - left fascicular block I45.2
      - specified NEC I45.19
    - Wilson's type I45.19
  - cardiac I45.9
  - conduction I45.9
    - complete I44.2
  - fascicular (left) I44.6Ø
    - anterior I44.4
    - posterior I44.5
    - right I45.Ø
    - specified NEC I44.69
  - foramen Magendie (acquired) G91.1
    - congenital QØ3.1
      - with spina bifida — *see* Spina bifida, by site, with hydrocephalus
  - heart I45.9
    - bundle branch I45.4
      - bilateral I45.2
    - complete (atrioventricular) I44.2
    - congenital Q24.6
    - first degree (atrioventricular) I44.Ø
    - second degree (atrioventricular) I44.1
    - specified type NEC I45.5
    - third degree (atrioventricular) I44.2
  - hepatic vein I82.Ø
  - intraventricular (nonspecific) I45.4
    - bundle branch
      - bilateral I45.2
  - kidney N28.9
    - postcystoscopic or postprocedural N99.Ø
  - Mobitz (types I and II) I44.1
  - myocardial — *see* Block, heart
  - nodal I45.5
  - organ or site, congenital NEC — *see* Atresia, by site
  - portal (vein) I81
  - second degree (types I and II) I44.1
  - sinoatrial I45.5
  - sinoauricular I45.5
  - third degree I44.2
  - trifascicular I45.3
  - tubal N97.1
  - vein NOS I82.9Ø
  - Wenckebach (types I and II) I44.1
- **Blockage** — *see* Obstruction
- **Blocq's disease** F44.4
- **Blood**
  - constituents, abnormal R78.9
  - disease D75.9
  - donor — *see* Donor, blood
  - dyscrasia D75.9
    - with
      - abortion — *see* Abortion, by type, complicated by, hemorrhage
      - ectopic pregnancy OØ8.1
      - molar pregnancy OØ8.1
    - following ectopic or molar pregnancy OØ8.1
    - newborn P61.9
    - puerperal, postpartum O72.3
  - flukes NEC — *see* Schistosomiasis
  - in
    - feces K92.1
      - occult R19.5
    - urine — *see* Hematuria
  - mole OØ2.Ø
  - occult in feces R19.5
  - pressure
    - decreased, due to shock following injury T79.4 ☑
    - examination only ZØ1.3Ø
    - fluctuating I99.8
    - high — *see* Hypertension
      - borderline RØ3.Ø
      - incidental reading, without diagnosis of hypertension RØ3.Ø
    - low — *see also* Hypotension
- **Blood** — *continued*
  - pressure — *continued*
    - low — *see also* Hypotension — *continued*
      - incidental reading, without diagnosis of hypotension RØ3.1
  - spitting — *see* Hemoptysis
  - staining cornea — *see* Pigmentation, cornea, stromal
  - transfusion
    - reaction or complication — *see* Complications, transfusion
  - type
    - A (Rh positive) Z67.1Ø
      - Rh negative Z67.11
    - AB (Rh positive) Z67.3Ø
      - Rh negative Z67.31
    - B (Rh positive) Z67.2Ø
      - Rh negative Z67.21
    - O (Rh positive) Z67.4Ø
      - Rh negative Z67.41
    - Rh (positive) Z67.9Ø
      - negative Z67.91
  - vessel rupture — *see* Hemorrhage
  - vomiting — *see* Hematemesis
- **Blood-forming organs, disease** D75.9
- **Bloodgood's disease** — *see* Mastopathy, cystic
- **Bloom** (-Machacek)(-Torre) **syndrome** Q82.8
- **Blount disease or osteochondrosis** M92.51- ☑
- **Blue**
  - baby Q24.9
  - diaper syndrome E72.Ø9
  - dome cyst (breast) — *see* Cyst, breast
  - dot cataract Q12.Ø
  - nevus D22.9
  - sclera Q13.5
    - with fragility of bone and deafness Q78.Ø
  - toe syndrome I75.Ø2- ☑
- **Blueness** — *see* Cyanosis
- **Blues, postpartal** O9Ø.6
  - baby O9Ø.6
- **Blurring, visual** H53.8
- **Blushing** (abnormal) (excessive) R23.2
- **BMI** — *see* Body, mass index
- **Boarder, hospital NEC** Z76.4
  - accompanying sick person Z76.3
  - healthy infant or child Z76.2
    - foundling Z76.1
- **Bockhart's impetigo** LØ1.Ø2
- **Bodechtel-Guttman disease** (subacute sclerosing panencephalitis) A81.1
- **Boder-Sedgwick syndrome** (ataxia-telangiectasia) G11.3
- **Body, bodies**
  - Aschoff's — *see* Myocarditis, rheumatic
  - asteroid, vitreous — *see* Deposit, crystalline
  - cytoid (retina) — *see* Occlusion, artery, retina
  - drusen (degenerative) (macula) (retinal) — *see also* Degeneration, macula, drusen
    - optic disc — *see* Drusen, optic disc
  - foreign — *see* Foreign body
  - loose
    - joint, except knee — *see* Loose, body, joint
      - knee M23.4- ☑
    - sheath, tendon — *see* Disorder, tendon, specified type NEC
  - mass index (BMI)
    - adult
      - 19.9 or less Z68.1
      - 2Ø.Ø-2Ø.9 Z68.2Ø
      - 21.Ø-21.9 Z68.21
      - 22.Ø-22.9 Z68.22
      - 23.Ø-23.9 Z68.23
      - 24.Ø-24.9 Z68.24
      - 25.Ø-25.9 Z68.25
      - 26.Ø-26.9 Z68.26
      - 27.Ø-27.9 Z68.27
      - 28.Ø-28.9 Z68.28
      - 29.Ø-29.9 Z68.29
      - 3Ø.Ø-3Ø.9 Z68.3Ø
      - 31.Ø-31.9 Z68.31
      - 32.Ø-32.9 Z68.32
      - 33.Ø-33.9 Z68.33
      - 34.Ø-34.9 Z68.34
      - 35.Ø-35.9 Z68.35
      - 36.Ø-36.9 Z68.36
      - 37.Ø-37.9 Z68.37
      - 38.Ø-38.9 Z68.38
      - 39.Ø-39.9 Z68.39
      - 4Ø.Ø-44.9 Z68.41
      - 45.Ø-49.9 Z68.42

Body, bodies — *continued*
- mass index — *continued*
  - adult — *continued*
    - 5Ø.Ø-59.9 Z68.43
    - 6Ø.Ø-69.9 Z68.44
    - 7Ø and over Z68.45
  - pediatric
    - 5th percentile to less than 85th percentile for age Z68.52
    - 85th percentile to less than 95th percentile for age Z68.53
    - greater than or equal to ninety-fifth percentile for age Z68.54
    - less than fifth percentile for age Z68.51
- Mooser's A75.2
- rice — *see also* Loose, body, joint
  - knee M23.4- ☑
- rocking F98.4

Boeck's
- disease or sarcoid — *see* Sarcoidosis
- lupoid (miliary) D86.3

Boerhaave's syndrome (spontaneous esophageal rupture) K22.3

Boggy
- cervix N88.8
- uterus N85.8

Boil — *see also* Furuncle, by site
- Aleppo B55.1
- Baghdad B55.1
- Delhi B55.1
- lacrimal
  - gland — *see* Dacryoadenitis
  - passages (duct) (sac) — *see* Inflammation, lacrimal, passages, acute
- Natal B55.1
- orbit, orbital — *see* Abscess, orbit
- tropical B55.1

Bold hives — *see* Urticaria

Bombé, iris — *see* Membrane, pupillary

Bone — *see* condition

Bonnevie-Ullrich syndrome — *see also* Turner's syndrome Q87.19

Bonnier's syndrome H81.8 ☑

Bonvale dam fever T73.3 ☑

Bony block of joint — *see* Ankylosis

BOOP (bronchiolitis obliterans organized pneumonia) J84.89

Borderline
- diabetes mellitus R73.Ø3
- hypertension RØ3.Ø
- osteopenia M85.8- ☑
- pelvis, with obstruction during labor O65.1
- personality F6Ø.3

Borna disease A83.9

Bornholm disease B33.Ø

Boston exanthem A88.Ø

Botalli, ductus (patent) (persistent) Q25.Ø

Bothriocephalus latus infestation B7Ø.Ø

Botulism (foodborne intoxication) AØ5.1
- infant A48.51
- non foodborne A48.52
- wound A48.52

Bouba — *see* Yaws

Bouchard's nodes (with arthropathy) M15.2

Bouffée délirante F23

Bouillaud's disease or syndrome (rheumatic heart disease) IØ1.9

Bourneville's disease Q85.1

Boutonniere deformity (finger) — *see* Deformity, finger, boutonniere

Bouveret (-Hoffmann) **syndrome** (paroxysmal tachycardia) I47.9

Bovine heart — *see* Hypertrophy, cardiac

Bowel — *see* condition

Bowen's
- dermatosis (precancerous) — *see* Neoplasm, skin, in situ
- disease — *see* Neoplasm, skin, in situ
- epithelioma — *see* Neoplasm, skin, in situ
- type
  - epidermoid carcinoma-in-situ — *see* Neoplasm, skin, in situ
  - intraepidermal squamous cell carcinoma — *see* Neoplasm, skin, in situ

Bowing
- femur — *see also* Deformity, limb, specified type NEC, thigh

Bowing — *continued*
- femur — *see also* Deformity, limb, specified type NEC, thigh — *continued*
  - congenital Q68.3
- fibula — *see also* Deformity, limb, specified type NEC, lower leg
  - congenital Q68.4
- forearm — *see* Deformity, limb, specified type NEC, forearm
- leg(s), long bones, congenital Q68.5
- radius — *see* Deformity, limb, specified type NEC, forearm
- tibia — *see also* Deformity, limb, specified type NEC, lower leg
  - congenital Q68.4

Bowleg(s) (acquired) M21.16- ☑
- congenital Q68.5
- rachitic E64.3

Boyd's dysentery AØ3.2

Brachial — *see* condition

Brachycardia RØØ.1

Brachycephaly Q75.Ø

Bradley's disease AØ8.19

Bradyarrhythmia, cardiac I49.8

Bradycardia (sinoatrial) (sinus) (vagal) RØØ.1
- neonatal P29.12
- reflex G9Ø.Ø9
- tachycardia syndrome I49.5

Bradykinesia R25.8

Bradypnea RØ6.89

Bradytachycardia I49.5

Brailsford's disease or osteochondrosis — *see* Osteochondrosis, juvenile, radius

Brain — *see also* condition
- death G93.82
- syndrome — *see* Syndrome, brain

Branched-chain amino-acid disorder E71.2

Branchial — *see* condition
- cartilage, congenital Q18.2

Branchiogenic remnant (in neck) Q18.Ø

Brandt's syndrome (acrodermatitis enteropathica) E83.2

Brash (water) R12

Bravais-jacksonian epilepsy — *see* Epilepsy, localization-related, symptomatic, with simple partial seizures

Braxton Hicks contractions — *see* False, labor

Brazilian leishmaniasis B55.2

BRBPR K62.5

Break, retina (without detachment) H33.3Ø- ☑
- with retinal detachment — *see* Detachment, retina
- horseshoe tear H33.31- ☑
- multiple H33.33- ☑
- round hole H33.32- ☑

Breakdown
- device, graft or implant — *see also* Complications, by site and type, mechanical T85.618 ☑
  - arterial graft NEC — *see* Complication, cardiovascular device, mechanical, vascular
  - breast (implant) T85.41 ☑
  - catheter NEC T85.618 ☑
    - cystostomy T83.Ø1Ø ☑
    - dialysis (renal) T82.41 ☑
      - intraperitoneal T85.611 ☑
    - Hopkins T83.Ø18 ☑
    - ileostomy T83.Ø18 ☑
    - infusion NEC T82.514 ☑
      - cranial T85.61Ø- ☑
      - epidural T85.61Ø ☑
      - intrathecal T85.61Ø ☑
      - spinal T85.61Ø ☑
      - subarachnoid T85.61Ø ☑
      - subdural T85.61Ø ☑
    - nephrostomy T83.Ø12 ☑
    - urethral indwelling T83.Ø11 ☑
    - urinary NEC T83.Ø18 ☑
    - urostomy T83.Ø18 ☑
  - electronic (electrode) (pulse generator) (stimulator)
    - bone T84.31Ø ☑
    - cardiac T82.119 ☑
      - electrode T82.11Ø ☑
      - pulse generator T82.111 ☑
      - specified type NEC T82.118 ☑
    - nervous system — *see* Complication, prosthetic device, mechanical, electronic nervous system stimulator
    - urinary — *see* Complication, genitourinary, device, urinary, mechanical

Breakdown — *continued*
- device, graft or implant — *see also* Complications, by site and type, mechanical — *continued*
  - fixation, internal (orthopedic) NEC — *see* Complication, fixation device, mechanical
  - gastrointestinal — *see* Complications, prosthetic device, mechanical, gastrointestinal device
  - genital NEC T83.418 ☑
    - intrauterine contraceptive device T83.31 ☑
    - penile prosthesis (cylinder) (implanted) (pump) (resevoir) T83.41Ø ☑
    - testicular prosthesis T83.411 ☑
  - heart NEC — *see* Complication, cardiovascular device, mechanical
  - intrathecal infusion pump T85.615 ☑
  - joint prosthesis — *see* Complications, joint prosthesis, internal, mechanical, by site
  - nervous system, specified device NEC T85.615 ☑
  - ocular NEC — *see* Complications, prosthetic device, mechanical, ocular device
  - orthopedic NEC — *see* Complication, orthopedic, device, mechanical
  - specified NEC T85.618 ☑
  - subcutaneous device pocket
    - nervous system prosthetic device, implant, or graft T85.89Ø ☑
    - other internal prosthetic device, implant, or graft T85.898 ☑
  - sutures, permanent T85.612 ☑
    - used in bone repair — *see* Complications, fixation device, internal (orthopedic), mechanical
  - urinary NEC T83.118 ☑
    - graft T83.21 ☑
    - sphincter, implanted T83.111 ☑
    - stent (ileal conduit) (nephroureteral) T83.113 ☑
      - ureteral indwelling T83.112 ☑
  - vascular NEC — *see* Complication, cardiovascular device, mechanical
  - ventricular intracranial shunt T85.Ø1 ☑
- nervous F48.8
- perineum O9Ø.1
- respirator J95.85Ø
  - specified NEC J95.859
- ventilator J95.85Ø
  - specified NEC J95.859

Breast — *see also* condition
- buds E3Ø.1
  - in newborn P96.89
- dense R92.2
- nodule — *see also* Lump, breast N63.Ø

Breath
- foul R19.6
- holder, child RØ6.89
- holding spell RØ6.89
- shortness RØ6.Ø2

Breathing
- labored — *see* Hyperventilation
- mouth RØ6.5
  - causing malocclusion M26.5 ☑
- periodic RØ6.3
  - high altitude G47.32

Breathlessness RØ6.81

Breda's disease — *see* Yaws

Breech presentation (mother) O32.1 ☑
- causing obstructed labor O64.1 ☑
- footling O32.8 ☑
  - causing obstructed labor O64.8 ☑
- incomplete O32.8 ☑
  - causing obstructed labor O64.8 ☑

Breisky's disease N9Ø.4

Brennemann's syndrome I88.Ø

Brenner
- tumor (benign) D27.9
  - borderline malignancy D39.1- ☑
  - malignant C56 ☑
  - proliferating D39.1- ☑

Bretonneau's disease or angina A36.Ø

Breus' mole OØ2.Ø

Brevicollis Q76.49

Brickmakers' anemia B76.9 *[D63.8]*

Bridge, myocardial Q24.5

Bright red blood per rectum (BRBPR) K62.5

Bright's disease — *see also* Nephritis
- arteriosclerotic — *see* Hypertension, kidney

Brill (-Zinsser) **disease** (recrudescent typhus) A75.1

Brill-Symmers' disease C82.9Ø

Brion-Kayser disease — *see* Fever, parathyroid

Briquet's disorder or syndrome F45.Ø
Brissaud's
- infantilism or dwarfism E23.Ø
- motor-verbal tic F95.2

Brittle
- bones disease Q78.Ø
- nails L6Ø.3
  - congenital Q84.6

Broad — *see also* condition
- beta disease E78.2
- ligament laceration syndrome N83.8

Broad- or floating-betalipoproteinemia E78.2
Brock's syndrome (atelectasis due to enlarged lymph nodes) J98.19
Brocq-Duhring disease (dermatitis herpetiformis) L13.Ø
Brodie's abscess or disease M86.8X- ☑
Broken
- arches — *see also* Deformity, limb, flat foot
- arm (meaning upper limb) — *see* Fracture, arm
- back — *see* Fracture, vertebra
- bone — *see* Fracture
- implant or internal device — *see* Complications, by site and type, mechanical
- leg (meaning lower limb) — *see* Fracture, leg
- nose SØ2.2 ☑
- tooth, teeth — *see* Fracture, tooth

Bromhidrosis, bromidrosis L75.Ø
Bromidism, bromism G92.8
- due to
  - correct substance properly administered — *see* Table of Drugs and Chemicals, by drug, adverse effect
  - overdose or wrong substance given or taken — *see* Table of Drugs and Chemicals, by drug, poisoning
- chronic (dependence) F13.2Ø

Bromidrosiphobia F4Ø.298
Bronchi, bronchial — *see* condition
Bronchiectasis (cylindrical) (diffuse) (fusiform) (localized) (saccular) J47.9
- with
  - acute
    - bronchitis J47.Ø
    - lower respiratory infection J47.Ø
  - exacerbation (acute) J47.1
- congenital Q33.4
- tuberculous NEC — *see* Tuberculosis, pulmonary

Bronchiolectasis — *see* Bronchiectasis
Bronchiolitis (acute) (infective) (subacute) J21.9
- with
  - bronchospasm or obstruction J21.9
  - influenza, flu or grippe — *see* Influenza, with, respiratory manifestations NEC
- chemical (chronic) J68.4
  - acute J68.Ø
- chronic (fibrosing) (obliterative) J44.9
- due to
  - external agent — *see* Bronchitis, acute, due to
  - human metapneumovirus J21.1
  - respiratory syncytial virus (RSV) J21.Ø
  - specified organism NEC J21.8
- fibrosa obliterans J44.9
- influenzal — *see* Influenza, with, respiratory manifestations NEC
- obliterans J42
  - with organizing pneumonia (BOOP) J84.89
- obliterative (chronic) (subacute) J44.9
  - due to fumes or vapors J68.4
  - due to chemicals, gases, fumes or vapors (inhalation) J68.4
- respiratory, interstitial lung disease J84.115

Bronchitis (diffuse) (fibrinous) (hypostatic) (infective) (membranous) J4Ø
- with
  - influenza, flu or grippe — *see* Influenza, with, respiratory manifestations NEC
  - obstruction (airway) (lung) J44.9
  - tracheitis (15 years of age and above) J4Ø
    - acute or subacute J2Ø.9
    - chronic J42
    - under 15 years of age J2Ø.9
- acute or subacute (with bronchospasm or obstruction) J2Ø.9
  - with
    - bronchiectasis J47.Ø
    - chronic obstructive pulmonary disease J44.Ø
  - chemical (due to gases, fumes or vapors) J68.Ø

Bronchitis — *continued*
- acute or subacute — *continued*
  - due to
    - fumes or vapors J68.Ø
    - Haemophilus influenzae J2Ø.1
    - Mycoplasma pneumoniae J2Ø.Ø
    - radiation J7Ø.Ø
    - specified organism NEC J2Ø.8
    - Streptococcus J2Ø.2
    - virus
      - coxsackie J2Ø.3
      - echovirus J2Ø.7
      - parainfluenzae J2Ø.4
      - respiratory syncytial (RSV) J2Ø.5
      - rhinovirus J2Ø.6
  - viral NEC J2Ø.8
- allergic (acute) J45.9Ø9
  - with
    - exacerbation (acute) J45.9Ø1
    - status asthmaticus J45.9Ø2
- arachidic T17.528 ☑
- aspiration (due to food and vomit) J69.Ø
- asthmatic J45.9 ☑
  - chronic J44.9
    - with
      - acute lower respiratory infection J44.Ø
      - exacerbation (acute) J44.1
- capillary — *see* Pneumonia, broncho
- caseous (tuberculous) A15.5
- Castellani's A69.8
- catarrhal (15 years of age and above) J4Ø
  - acute — *see* Bronchitis, acute
  - chronic J41.Ø
  - under 15 years of age J2Ø.9
- chemical (acute) (subacute) J68.Ø
  - chronic J68.4
  - due to fumes or vapors J68.Ø
    - chronic J68.4
- chronic J42
  - with
    - airways obstruction J44.9
    - tracheitis (chronic) J42
  - asthmatic (obstructive) J44.9
  - catarrhal J41.Ø
  - chemical (due to fumes or vapors) J68.4
  - due to
    - chemicals, gases, fumes or vapors (inhalation) J68.4
    - radiation J7Ø.1
    - tobacco smoking J41.Ø
  - emphysematous J44.9
  - mucopurulent J41.1
  - non-obstructive J41.Ø
  - obliterans J44.9
  - obstructive J44.9
  - purulent J41.1
  - simple J41.Ø
- croupous — *see* Bronchitis, acute
- due to gases, fumes or vapors (chemical) J68.Ø
- emphysematous (obstructive) J44.9
- exudative — *see* Bronchitis, acute
- fetid J41.1
- grippal — *see* Influenza, with, respiratory manifestations NEC
- in those under 15 years age — *see* Bronchitis, acute
  - chronic — *see* Bronchitis, chronic
- influenzal — *see* Influenza, with, respiratory manifestations NEC
- mixed simple and mucopurulent J41.8
- moulder's J62.8
- mucopurulent (chronic) (recurrent) J41.1
  - acute or subacute J2Ø.9
  - simple (mixed) J41.8
- obliterans (chronic) J44.9
- obstructive (chronic) (diffuse) J44.9
- pituitous J41.1
- pneumococcal, acute or subacute J2Ø.2
- pseudomembranous, acute or subacute — *see* Bronchitis, acute
- purulent (chronic) (recurrent) J41.1
  - acute or subacute — *see* Bronchitis, acute
- putrid J41.1
- senile (chronic) J42
- simple and mucopurulent (mixed) J41.8
- smokers' J41.Ø
- spirochetal NEC A69.8
- subacute — *see* Bronchitis, acute
- suppurative (chronic) J41.1

Bronchitis — *continued*
- suppurative — *continued*
  - acute or subacute — *see* Bronchitis, acute
- tuberculous A15.5
- under 15 years of age — *see* Bronchitis, acute
  - chronic — *see* Bronchitis, chronic
- viral NEC, acute or subacute — *see also* Bronchitis, acute J2Ø.8

Bronchoalveolitis J18.Ø
Bronchoaspergillosis B44.1
Bronchocele meaning goiter EØ4.Ø
Broncholithiasis J98.Ø9
- tuberculous NEC A15.5

Bronchomalacia J98.Ø9
- congenital Q32.2

Bronchomycosis NOS B49 *[J99]*
- candidal B37.1

Bronchopleuropneumonia — *see* Pneumonia, broncho
Bronchopneumonia — *see* Pneumonia, broncho
Bronchopneumonitis — *see* Pneumonia, broncho
Bronchopulmonary — *see* condition
Bronchopulmonitis — *see* Pneumonia, broncho
Bronchorrhagia (see Hemoptysis)
Bronchorrhea J98.Ø9
- acute J2Ø.9
- chronic (infective) (purulent) J42

Bronchospasm (acute) J98.Ø1
- with
  - bronchiolitis, acute J21.9
  - bronchitis, acute (conditions in J2Ø) — *see* Bronchitis, acute
- due to external agent — *see* condition, respiratory, acute, due to
- exercise induced J45.99Ø

Bronchospirochetosis A69.8
- Castellani A69.8

Bronchostenosis J98.Ø9
Bronchus — *see* condition
Brontophobia F4Ø.22Ø
Bronze baby syndrome P83.88
Brooke's tumor — *see* Neoplasm, skin, benign
Brown enamel of teeth (hereditary) KØØ.5
Brown's sheath syndrome H5Ø.61- ☑
Brown-Séquard disease, paralysis or syndrome G83.81
Bruce sepsis A23.Ø
Brucellosis (infection) A23.9
- abortus A23.1
- canis A23.3
- dermatitis A23.9
- melitensis A23.Ø
- mixed A23.8
- sepsis A23.9
  - melitensis A23.Ø
  - specified NEC A23.8
- suis A23.2

Bruck-de Lange disease Q87.19
Bruck's disease — *see* Deformity, limb
BRUE (brief resolved unexplained event) R68.13
Brugsch's syndrome Q82.8
Bruise (skin surface intact) — *see also* Contusion
- with
  - open wound — *see* Wound, open
- internal organ — *see* Injury, by site
- newborn P54.5
  - scalp, due to birth injury, newborn P12.3
- umbilical cord O69.5 ☑

Bruit (arterial) RØ9.89
- cardiac RØ1.1

Brush burn — *see* Abrasion, by site
Bruton's X-linked agammaglobulinemia D8Ø.Ø
Bruxism
- psychogenic F45.8
- sleep related G47.63

Bubbly lung syndrome P27.Ø
Bubo I88.8
- blennorrhagic (gonococcal) A54.89
- chancroidal A57
- climatic A55
- due to Haemophilus ducreyi A57
- gonococcal A54.89
- indolent (nonspecific) I88.8
- inguinal (nonspecific) I88.8
  - chancroidal A57
  - climatic A55
  - due to H. ducreyi A57
  - infective I88.8

- **Bubo** — *continued*
  - scrofulous (tuberculous) A18.2
  - soft chancre A57
  - suppurating — *see* Lymphadenitis, acute
  - syphilitic (primary) A51.Ø
    - congenital A5Ø.Ø7
  - tropical A55
  - virulent (chancroidal) A57
- **Bubonic plague** A2Ø.Ø
- **Bubonocele** — *see* Hernia, inguinal
- **Buccal** — *see* condition
- **Buchanan's disease or osteochondrosis** M91.Ø
- **Buchem's syndrome** (hyperostosis corticalis) M85.2
- **Bucket-handle fracture or tear** (semilunar cartilage) — *see* Tear, meniscus
- **Budd-Chiari syndrome** (hepatic vein thrombosis) I82.Ø
- **Budgerigar fancier's disease or lung** J67.2
- **Buds**
  - breast E3Ø.1
    - in newborn P96.89
- **Buerger's disease** (thromboangiitis obliterans) I73.1
- **Bulbar** — *see* condition
- **Bulbus cordis** (left ventricle) (persistent) Q21.8
- **Bulimia** (nervosa) F5Ø.2
  - atypical F5Ø.9
  - normal weight F5Ø.9
- **Bulky**
  - stools R19.5
  - uterus N85.2
- **Bulla** (e) R23.8
  - lung (emphysematous) (solitary) J43.9
    - newborn P25.8
- **Bullet wound** — *see also* Puncture
  - fracture — *code as* Fracture, by site
  - internal organ — *see* Injury, by site
- **Bundle**
  - branch block (complete) (false) (incomplete) — *see* Block, bundle-branch
  - of His — *see* condition
- **Bunion** M21.61- ☑
  - tailor's M21.62- ☑
- **Bunionette** M21.62- ☑
- **Buphthalmia, buphthalmos** (congenital) Q15.Ø
- **Burdwan fever** B55.Ø
- **Bürger-Grütz disease or syndrome** E78.3
- **Buried**
  - penis (congenital) Q55.64
    - acquired N48.83
  - roots KØ8.3
- **Burke's syndrome** K86.89
- **Burkitt**
  - cell leukemia C91.Ø- ☑
  - lymphoma (malignant) C83.7- ☑
    - small noncleaved, diffuse C83.7- ☑
    - spleen C83.77
    - undifferentiated C83.7- ☑
  - tumor C83.7- ☑
  - type
    - acute lymphoblastic leukemia C91.Ø- ☑
    - undifferentiated C83.7- ☑
- **Burn** (electricity) (flame) (hot gas, liquid or hot object) (radiation) (steam) (thermal) T3Ø.Ø
  - abdomen, abdominal (muscle) (wall) T21.Ø2 ☑
    - first degree T21.12 ☑
    - second degree T21.22 ☑
    - third degree T21.32 ☑
  - above elbow T22.Ø39 ☑
    - first degree T22.139 ☑
    - left T22.Ø32 ☑
      - first degree T22.132 ☑
      - second degree T22.232 ☑
      - third degree T22.332 ☑
    - right T22.Ø31 ☑
      - first degree T22.131 ☑
      - second degree T22.231 ☑
      - third degree T22.331 ☑
    - second degree T22.239 ☑
    - third degree T22.339 ☑
  - acid (caustic) (external) (internal) — *see* Corrosion, by site
  - alimentary tract NEC T28.2 ☑
    - esophagus T28.1 ☑
    - mouth T28.Ø ☑
    - pharynx T28.Ø ☑
  - alkaline (caustic) (external) (internal) — *see* Corrosion, by site

- **Burn** — *continued*
  - ankle T25.Ø19 ☑
    - first degree T25.119 ☑
    - left T25.Ø12 ☑
      - first degree T25.112 ☑
      - second degree T25.212 ☑
      - third degree T25.312 ☑
    - multiple with foot — *see* Burn, lower, limb, multiple, ankle and foot
    - right T25.Ø11 ☑
      - first degree T25.111 ☑
      - second degree T25.211 ☑
      - third degree T25.311 ☑
    - second degree T25.219 ☑
    - third degree T25.319 ☑
  - anus — *see* Burn, buttock
  - arm (lower) (upper) — *see* Burn, upper, limb
  - axilla T22.Ø49 ☑
    - first degree T22.149 ☑
    - left T22.Ø42 ☑
      - first degree T22.142 ☑
      - second degree T22.242 ☑
      - third degree T22.342 ☑
    - right T22.Ø41 ☑
      - first degree T22.141 ☑
      - second degree T22.241 ☑
      - third degree T22.341 ☑
    - second degree T22.249 ☑
    - third degree T22.349 ☑
  - back (lower) T21.Ø4 ☑
    - first degree T21.14 ☑
    - second degree T21.24 ☑
    - third degree T21.34 ☑
    - upper T21.Ø3 ☑
      - first degree T21.13 ☑
      - second degree T21.23 ☑
      - third degree T21.33 ☑
  - blisters — *code as* Burn, second degree, by site
  - breast(s) — *see* Burn, chest wall
  - buttock(s) T21.Ø5 ☑
    - first degree T21.15 ☑
    - second degree T21.25 ☑
    - third degree T21.35 ☑
  - calf T24.Ø39 ☑
    - first degree T24.139 ☑
    - left T24.Ø32 ☑
      - first degree T24.132 ☑
      - second degree T24.232 ☑
      - third degree T24.332 ☑
    - right T24.Ø31 ☑
      - first degree T24.131 ☑
      - second degree T24.231 ☑
      - third degree T24.331 ☑
    - second degree T24.239 ☑
    - third degree T24.339 ☑
  - canthus (eye) — *see* Burn, eyelid
  - caustic acid or alkaline — *see* Corrosion, by site
  - cervix T28.3 ☑
  - cheek T2Ø.Ø6 ☑
    - first degree T2Ø.16 ☑
    - second degree T2Ø.26 ☑
    - third degree T2Ø.36 ☑
  - chemical (acids) (alkalines) (caustics) (external) (internal) — *see* Corrosion, by site
  - chest wall T21.Ø1 ☑
    - first degree T21.11 ☑
    - second degree T21.21 ☑
    - third degree T21.31 ☑
  - chin T2Ø.Ø3 ☑
    - first degree T2Ø.13 ☑
    - second degree T2Ø.23 ☑
    - third degree T2Ø.33 ☑
  - colon T28.2 ☑
  - conjunctiva (and cornea) — *see* Burn, cornea
  - cornea (and conjunctiva) T26.1- ☑
    - chemical — *see* Corrosion, cornea
  - corrosion (external) (internal) — *see* Corrosion, by site
  - deep necrosis of underlying tissue — *code as* Burn, third degree, by site
  - dorsum of hand T23.Ø69 ☑
    - first degree T23.169 ☑
    - left T23.Ø62 ☑
      - first degree T23.162 ☑
      - second degree T23.262 ☑
      - third degree T23.362 ☑
    - right T23.Ø61 ☑

- **Burn** — *continued*
  - dorsum of hand — *continued*
    - right — *continued*
      - first degree T23.161 ☑
      - second degree T23.261 ☑
      - third degree T23.361 ☑
    - second degree T23.269 ☑
    - third degree T23.369 ☑
  - due to ingested chemical agent — *see* Corrosion, by site
  - ear (auricle) (external) (canal) T2Ø.Ø1 ☑
    - first degree T2Ø.11 ☑
    - second degree T2Ø.21 ☑
    - third degree T2Ø.31 ☑
  - elbow T22.Ø29 ☑
    - first degree T22.129 ☑
    - left T22.Ø22 ☑
      - first degree T22.122 ☑
      - second degree T22.222 ☑
      - third degree T22.322 ☑
    - right T22.Ø21 ☑
      - first degree T22.121 ☑
      - second degree T22.221 ☑
      - third degree T22.321 ☑
    - second degree T22.229 ☑
    - third degree T22.329 ☑
  - epidermal loss — *code as* Burn, second degree, by site
  - erythema, erythematous — *code as* Burn, first degree, by site
  - esophagus T28.1 ☑
  - extent (percentage of body surface)
    - less than 1Ø percent T31.Ø
    - 1Ø-19 percent T31.1Ø
      - with Ø-9 percent third degree burns T31.1Ø
      - with 1Ø-19 percent third degree burns T31.11
    - 2Ø-29 percent T31.2Ø
      - with Ø-9 percent third degree burns T31.2Ø
      - with 1Ø-19 percent third degree burns T31.21
      - with 2Ø-29 percent third degree burns T31.22
    - 3Ø-39 percent T31.3Ø
      - with Ø-9 percent third degree burns T31.3Ø
      - with 1Ø-19 percent third degree burns T31.31
      - with 2Ø-29 percent third degree burns T31.32
      - with 3Ø-39 percent third degree burns T31.33
    - 4Ø-49 percent T31.4Ø
      - with Ø-9 percent third degree burns T31.4Ø
      - with 1Ø-19 percent third degree burns T31.41
      - with 2Ø-29 percent third degree burns T31.42
      - with 3Ø-39 percent third degree burns T31.43
      - with 4Ø-49 percent third degree burns T31.44
    - 5Ø-59 percent T31.5Ø
      - with Ø-9 percent third degree burns T31.5Ø
      - with 1Ø-19 percent third degree burns T31.51
      - with 2Ø-29 percent third degree burns T31.52
      - with 3Ø-39 percent third degree burns T31.53
      - with 4Ø-49 percent third degree burns T31.54
      - with 5Ø-59 percent third degree burns T31.55
    - 6Ø-69 percent T31.6Ø
      - with Ø-9 percent third degree burns T31.6Ø
      - with 1Ø-19 percent third degree burns T31.61
      - with 2Ø-29 percent third degree burns T31.62
      - with 3Ø-39 percent third degree burns T31.63
      - with 4Ø-49 percent third degree burns T31.64
      - with 5Ø-59 percent third degree burns T31.65
      - with 6Ø-69 percent third degree burns T31.66
    - 7Ø-79 percent T31.7Ø
      - with Ø-9 percent third degree burns T31.7Ø
      - with 1Ø-19 percent third degree burns T31.71
      - with 2Ø-29 percent third degree burns T31.72
      - with 3Ø-39 percent third degree burns T31.73
      - with 4Ø-49 percent third degree burns T31.74
      - with 5Ø-59 percent third degree burns T31.75
      - with 6Ø-69 percent third degree burns T31.76
      - with 7Ø-79 percent third degree burns T31.77
    - 8Ø-89 percent T31.8Ø
      - with Ø-9 percent third degree burns T31.8Ø
      - with 1Ø-19 percent third degree burns T31.81
      - with 2Ø-29 percent third degree burns T31.82
      - with 3Ø-39 percent third degree burns T31.83
      - with 4Ø-49 percent third degree burns T31.84
      - with 5Ø-59 percent third degree burns T31.85
      - with 6Ø-69 percent third degree burns T31.86
      - with 7Ø-79 percent third degree burns T31.87
      - with 8Ø-89 percent third degree burns T31.88
    - 9Ø percent or more T31.9Ø
      - with Ø-9 percent third degree burns T31.9Ø
      - with 1Ø-19 percent third degree burns T31.91
      - with 2Ø-29 percent third degree burns T31.92

- **Burn** — *continued*
  - extent — *continued*
    - 90 percent or more — *continued*
      - with 30-39 percent third degree burns T31.93
      - with 40-49 percent third degree burns T31.94
      - with 50-59 percent third degree burns T31.95
      - with 60-69 percent third degree burns T31.96
      - with 70-79 percent third degree burns T31.97
      - with 80-89 percent third degree burns T31.98
      - with 90 percent or more third degree burns T31.99
  - extremity — *see* Burn, limb
  - eye(s) and adnexa T26.4- ☑
    - with resulting rupture and destruction of eyeball T26.2- ☑
    - conjunctival sac — *see* Burn, cornea
    - cornea — *see* Burn, cornea
    - lid — *see* Burn, eyelid
    - periocular area — *see* Burn, eyelid
    - specified site NEC T26.3- ☑
  - eyeball — *see* Burn, eye
  - eyelid(s) T26.0- ☑
    - chemical — *see* Corrosion, eyelid
  - face — *see* Burn, head
  - finger T23.029 ☑
    - first degree T23.129 ☑
    - left T23.022 ☑
      - first degree T23.122 ☑
      - second degree T23.222 ☑
      - third degree T23.322 ☑
    - multiple sites (without thumb) T23.039 ☑
      - with thumb T23.049 ☑
        - first degree T23.149 ☑
        - left T23.042 ☑
          - first degree T23.142 ☑
          - second degree T23.242 ☑
          - third degree T23.342 ☑
        - right T23.041 ☑
          - first degree T23.141 ☑
          - second degree T23.241 ☑
          - third degree T23.341 ☑
        - second degree T23.249 ☑
        - third degree T23.349 ☑
      - first degree T23.139 ☑
      - left T23.032 ☑
        - first degree T23.132 ☑
        - second degree T23.232 ☑
        - third degree T23.332 ☑
      - right T23.031 ☑
        - first degree T23.131 ☑
        - second degree T23.231 ☑
        - third degree T23.331 ☑
      - second degree T23.239 ☑
      - third degree T23.339 ☑
    - right T23.021 ☑
      - first degree T23.121 ☑
      - second degree T23.221 ☑
      - third degree T23.321 ☑
    - second degree T23.229 ☑
    - third degree T23.329 ☑
  - flank — *see* Burn, abdominal wall
  - foot T25.029 ☑
    - first degree T25.129 ☑
    - left T25.022 ☑
      - first degree T25.122 ☑
      - second degree T25.222 ☑
      - third degree T25.322 ☑
    - multiple with ankle — *see* Burn, lower, limb, multiple, ankle and foot
    - right T25.021 ☑
      - first degree T25.121 ☑
      - second degree T25.221 ☑
      - third degree T25.321 ☑
    - second degree T25.229 ☑
    - third degree T25.329 ☑
  - forearm T22.019 ☑
    - first degree T22.119 ☑
    - left T22.012 ☑
      - first degree T22.112 ☑
      - second degree T22.212 ☑
      - third degree T22.312 ☑
    - right T22.011 ☑
      - first degree T22.111 ☑
      - second degree T22.211 ☑
      - third degree T22.311 ☑
    - second degree T22.219 ☑

- **Burn** — *continued*
  - forearm — *continued*
    - third degree T22.319 ☑
  - forehead T20.06 ☑
    - first degree T20.16 ☑
    - second degree T20.26 ☑
    - third degree T20.36 ☑
  - fourth degree — *code as* Burn, third degree, by site
  - friction — *see* Burn, by site
  - from swallowing caustic or corrosive substance NEC — *see* Corrosion, by site
  - full thickness skin loss — *code as* Burn, third degree, by site
  - gastrointestinal tract NEC T28.2 ☑
    - from swallowing caustic or corrosive substance T28.7 ☑
  - genital organs
    - external
      - female T21.07 ☑
        - first degree T21.17 ☑
        - second degree T21.27 ☑
        - third degree T21.37 ☑
      - male T21.06 ☑
        - first degree T21.16 ☑
        - second degree T21.26 ☑
        - third degree T21.36 ☑
    - internal T28.3 ☑
      - from caustic or corrosive substance T28.8 ☑
  - groin — *see* Burn, abdominal wall
  - hand(s) T23.009 ☑
    - back — *see* Burn, dorsum of hand
    - finger — *see* Burn, finger
    - first degree T23.109 ☑
    - left T23.002 ☑
      - first degree T23.102 ☑
      - second degree T23.202 ☑
      - third degree T23.302 ☑
    - multiple sites with wrist T23.099 ☑
      - first degree T23.199 ☑
      - left T23.092 ☑
        - first degree T23.192 ☑
        - second degree T23.292 ☑
        - third degree T23.392 ☑
      - right T23.091 ☑
        - first degree T23.191 ☑
        - second degree T23.291 ☑
        - third degree T23.391 ☑
      - second degree T23.299 ☑
      - third degree T23.399 ☑
    - palm — *see* Burn, palm
    - right T23.001 ☑
      - first degree T23.101 ☑
      - second degree T23.201 ☑
      - third degree T23.301 ☑
    - second degree T23.209 ☑
    - third degree T23.309 ☑
    - thumb — *see* Burn, thumb
  - head (and face) (and neck) T20.00 ☑
    - cheek — *see* Burn, cheek
    - chin — *see* Burn, chin
    - ear — *see* Burn, ear
    - eye(s) only — *see* Burn, eye
    - first degree T20.10 ☑
    - forehead — *see* Burn, forehead
    - lip — *see* Burn, lip
    - multiple sites T20.09 ☑
      - first degree T20.19 ☑
      - second degree T20.29 ☑
      - third degree T20.39 ☑
    - neck — *see* Burn, neck
    - nose — *see* Burn, nose
    - scalp — *see* Burn, scalp
    - second degree T20.20 ☑
    - third degree T20.30 ☑
  - hip(s) — *see* Burn, thigh
  - inhalation — *see* Burn, respiratory tract
    - caustic or corrosive substance (fumes) — *see* Corrosion, respiratory tract
  - internal organ(s) T28.40 ☑
    - alimentary tract T28.2 ☑
      - esophagus T28.1 ☑
    - eardrum T28.41 ☑
    - esophagus T28.1 ☑
    - from caustic or corrosive substance (swallowing) NEC — *see* Corrosion, by site
    - genitourinary T28.3 ☑

- **Burn** — *continued*
  - internal organ(s) — *continued*
    - mouth T28.0 ☑
    - pharynx T28.0 ☑
    - respiratory tract — *see* Burn, respiratory tract
    - specified organ NEC T28.49 ☑
  - interscapular region — *see* Burn, back, upper
  - intestine (large) (small) T28.2 ☑
  - knee T24.029 ☑
    - first degree T24.129 ☑
    - left T24.022 ☑
      - first degree T24.122 ☑
      - second degree T24.222 ☑
      - third degree T24.322 ☑
    - right T24.021 ☑
      - first degree T24.121 ☑
      - second degree T24.221 ☑
      - third degree T24.321 ☑
    - second degree T24.229 ☑
    - third degree T24.329 ☑
  - labium (majus) (minus) — *see* Burn, genital organs, external, female
  - lacrimal apparatus, duct, gland or sac — *see* Burn, eye, specified site NEC
  - larynx T27.0 ☑
    - with lung T27.1 ☑
  - leg(s) (lower) (upper) — *see* Burn, lower, limb
  - lightning — *see* Burn, by site
  - limb(s)
    - lower (except ankle or foot alone) — *see* Burn, lower, limb
    - upper — *see* Burn, upper limb
  - lip(s) T20.02 ☑
    - first degree T20.12 ☑
    - second degree T20.22 ☑
    - third degree T20.32 ☑
  - lower
    - back — *see* Burn, back
    - limb T24.009 ☑
      - ankle — *see* Burn, ankle
      - calf — *see* Burn, calf
      - first degree T24.109 ☑
      - foot — *see* Burn, foot
      - hip — *see* Burn, thigh
      - knee — *see* Burn, knee
      - left T24.002 ☑
        - first degree T24.102 ☑
        - second degree T24.202 ☑
        - third degree T24.302 ☑
      - multiple sites, except ankle and foot T24.099 ☑
        - ankle and foot T25.099 ☑
          - first degree T25.199 ☑
          - left T25.092 ☑
            - first degree T25.192 ☑
            - second degree T25.292 ☑
            - third degree T25.392 ☑
          - right T25.091 ☑
            - first degree T25.191 ☑
            - second degree T25.291 ☑
            - third degree T25.391 ☑
          - second degree T25.299 ☑
          - third degree T25.399 ☑
        - first degree T24.199 ☑
        - left T24.092 ☑
          - first degree T24.192 ☑
          - second degree T24.292 ☑
          - third degree T24.392 ☑
        - right T24.091 ☑
          - first degree T24.191 ☑
          - second degree T24.291 ☑
          - third degree T24.391 ☑
        - second degree T24.299 ☑
        - third degree T24.399 ☑
      - right T24.001 ☑
        - first degree T24.101 ☑
        - second degree T24.201 ☑
        - third degree T24.301 ☑
      - second degree T24.209 ☑
      - thigh — *see* Burn, thigh
      - third degree T24.309 ☑
      - toe — *see* Burn, toe
  - lung (with larynx and trachea) T27.1 ☑
  - mouth T28.0 ☑
  - neck T20.07 ☑
    - first degree T20.17 ☑
    - second degree T20.27 ☑

- **Burn** — *continued*
  - neck — *continued*
    - third degree T2Ø.37 ☑
  - nose (septum) T2Ø.Ø4 ☑
    - first degree T2Ø.14 ☑
    - second degree T2Ø.24 ☑
    - third degree T2Ø.34 ☑
  - ocular adnexa — *see* Burn, eye
  - orbit region — *see* Burn, eyelid
  - palm T23.Ø59 ☑
    - first degree T23.159 ☑
    - left T23.Ø52 ☑
      - first degree T23.152 ☑
      - second degree T23.252 ☑
      - third degree T23.352 ☑
    - right T23.Ø51 ☑
      - first degree T23.151 ☑
      - second degree T23.251 ☑
      - third degree T23.351 ☑
    - second degree T23.259 ☑
    - third degree T23.359 ☑
  - partial thickness — *code as* Burn, by site, second degree
  - pelvis — *see* Burn, trunk
  - penis — *see* Burn, genital organs, external, male
  - perineum
    - female — *see* Burn, genital organs, external, female
    - male — *see* Burn, genital organs, external, male
  - periocular area — *see* Burn, eyelid
  - pharynx T28.Ø
  - rectum T28.2 ☑
  - respiratory tract T27.3 ☑
    - larynx — *see* Burn, larynx
    - specified part NEC T27.2 ☑
    - trachea — *see* Burn, trachea
  - sac, lacrimal — *see* Burn, eye, specified site NEC
  - scalp T2Ø.Ø5 ☑
    - first degree T2Ø.15 ☑
    - second degree T2Ø.25 ☑
    - third degree T2Ø.35 ☑
  - scapular region T22.Ø69 ☑
    - first degree T22.169 ☑
    - left T22.Ø62 ☑
      - first degree T22.162 ☑
      - second degree T22.262 ☑
      - third degree T22.362 ☑
    - right T22.Ø61 ☑
      - first degree T22.161 ☑
      - second degree T22.261 ☑
      - third degree T22.361 ☑
    - second degree T22.269 ☑
    - third degree T22.369 ☑
  - sclera — *see* Burn, eye, specified site NEC
  - scrotum — *see* Burn, genital organs, external, male
  - shoulder T22.Ø59 ☑
    - first degree T22.159 ☑
    - left T22.Ø52 ☑
      - first degree T22.152 ☑
      - second degree T22.252 ☑
      - third degree T22.352 ☑
    - right T22.Ø51 ☑
      - first degree T22.151 ☑
      - second degree T22.251 ☑
      - third degree T22.351 ☑
    - second degree T22.259 ☑
    - third degree T22.359 ☑
  - stomach T28.2 ☑
  - temple — *see* Burn, head
  - testis — *see* Burn, genital organs, external, male
  - thigh T24.Ø19 ☑
    - first degree T24.119 ☑
    - left T24.Ø12 ☑
      - first degree T24.112 ☑
      - second degree T24.212 ☑
      - third degree T24.312 ☑
    - right T24.Ø11 ☑
      - first degree T24.111 ☑
      - second degree T24.211 ☑
      - third degree T24.311 ☑
    - second degree T24.219 ☑
    - third degree T24.319 ☑
  - thorax (external) — *see* Burn, trunk
  - throat (meaning pharynx) T28.Ø ☑
  - thumb(s) T23.Ø19 ☑
    - first degree T23.119 ☑
    - left T23.Ø12 ☑
      - first degree T23.112 ☑

- **Burn** — *continued*
  - thumb(s) — *continued*
    - left — *continued*
      - second degree T23.212 ☑
      - third degree T23.312 ☑
    - multiple sites with fingers T23.Ø49 ☑
      - first degree T23.149 ☑
      - left T23.Ø42 ☑
        - first degree T23.142 ☑
        - second degree T23.242 ☑
        - third degree T23.342 ☑
      - right T23.Ø41 ☑
        - first degree T23.141 ☑
        - second degree T23.241 ☑
        - third degree T23.341 ☑
      - second degree T23.249 ☑
      - third degree T23.349 ☑
    - right T23.Ø11 ☑
      - first degree T23.111 ☑
      - second degree T23.211 ☑
      - third degree T23.311 ☑
    - second degree T23.219 ☑
    - third degree T23.319 ☑
  - toe T25.Ø39 ☑
    - first degree T25.139 ☑
    - left T25.Ø32 ☑
      - first degree T25.132 ☑
      - second degree T25.232 ☑
      - third degree T25.332 ☑
    - right T25.Ø31 ☑
      - first degree T25.131 ☑
      - second degree T25.231 ☑
      - third degree T25.331 ☑
    - second degree T25.239 ☑
    - third degree T25.339 ☑
  - tongue T28.Ø ☑
  - tonsil(s) T28.Ø ☑
  - trachea T27.Ø ☑
    - with lung T27.1 ☑
  - trunk T21.ØØ ☑
    - abdominal wall — *see* Burn, abdominal wall
    - anus — *see* Burn, buttock
    - axilla — *see* Burn, upper limb
    - back — *see* Burn, back
    - breast — *see* Burn, chest wall
    - buttock — *see* Burn, buttock
    - chest wall — *see* Burn, chest wall
    - first degree T21.1Ø ☑
    - flank — *see* Burn, abdominal wall
    - genital
      - female — *see* Burn, genital organs, external, female
      - male — *see* Burn, genital organs, external, male
    - groin — *see* Burn, abdominal wall
    - interscapular region — *see* Burn, back, upper
    - labia — *see* Burn, genital organs, external, female
    - lower back — *see* Burn, back
    - penis — *see* Burn, genital organs, external, male
    - perineum
      - female — *see* Burn, genital organs, external, female
      - male — *see* Burn, genital organs, external, male
    - scapula region — *see* Burn, scapular region
    - scrotum — *see* Burn, genital organs, external, male
    - second degree T21.2Ø ☑
    - specified site NEC T21.Ø9 ☑
      - first degree T21.19 ☑
      - second degree T21.29 ☑
      - third degree T21.39 ☑
    - testes — *see* Burn, genital organs, external, male
    - third degree T21.3Ø ☑
    - upper back — *see* Burn, back, upper
    - vulva — *see* Burn, genital organs, external, female
  - unspecified site with extent of body surface involved specified
    - less than 1Ø percent T31.Ø
    - 1Ø-19 percent (Ø-9 percent third degree) T31.1Ø
      - with 1Ø-19 percent third degree T31.11
    - 2Ø-29 percent (Ø-9 percent third degree) T31.2Ø
      - with
        - 1Ø-19 percent third degree T31.21
        - 2Ø-29 percent third degree T31.22
    - 3Ø-39 percent (Ø-9 percent third degree) T31.3Ø
      - with
        - 1Ø-19 percent third degree T31.31
        - 2Ø-29 percent third degree T31.32

- **Burn** — *continued*
  - unspecified site with extent of body surface involved specified — *continued*
    - 3Ø-39 percent — *continued*
      - with — *continued*
        - 3Ø-39 percent third degree T31.33
    - 4Ø-49 percent (Ø-9 percent third degree) T31.4Ø
      - with
        - 1Ø-19 percent third degree T31.41
        - 2Ø-29 percent third degree T31.42
        - 3Ø-39 percent third degree T31.43
        - 4Ø-49 percent third degree T31.44
    - 5Ø-59 percent (Ø-9 percent third degree) T31.5Ø
      - with
        - 1Ø-19 percent third degree T31.51
        - 2Ø-29 percent third degree T31.52
        - 3Ø-39 percent third degree T31.53
        - 4Ø-49 percent third degree T31.54
        - 5Ø-59 percent third degree T31.55
    - 6Ø-69 percent (Ø-9 percent third degree) T31.6Ø
      - with
        - 1Ø-19 percent third degree T31.61
        - 2Ø-29 percent third degree T31.62
        - 3Ø-39 percent third degree T31.63
        - 4Ø-49 percent third degree T31.64
        - 5Ø-59 percent third degree T31.65
        - 6Ø-69 percent third degree T31.66
    - 7Ø-79 percent (Ø-9 percent third degree) T31.7Ø
      - with
        - 1Ø-19 percent third degree T31.71
        - 2Ø-29 percent third degree T31.72
        - 3Ø-39 percent third degree T31.73
        - 4Ø-49 percent third degree T31.74
        - 5Ø-59 percent third degree T31.75
        - 6Ø-69 percent third degree T31.76
        - 7Ø-79 percent third degree T31.77
    - 8Ø-89 percent (Ø-9 percent third degree) T31.8Ø
      - with
        - 1Ø-19 percent third degree T31.81
        - 2Ø-29 percent third degree T31.82
        - 3Ø-39 percent third degree T31.83
        - 4Ø-49 percent third degree T31.84
        - 5Ø-59 percent third degree T31.85
        - 6Ø-69 percent third degree T31.86
        - 7Ø-79 percent third degree T31.87
        - 8Ø-89 percent third degree T31.88
    - 9Ø percent or more (Ø-9 percent third degree) T31.9Ø
      - with
        - 1Ø-19 percent third degree T31.91
        - 2Ø-29 percent third degree T31.92
        - 3Ø-39 percent third degree T31.93
        - 4Ø-49 percent third degree T31.94
        - 5Ø-59 percent third degree T31.95
        - 6Ø-69 percent third degree T31.96
        - 7Ø-79 percent third degree T31.97
        - 8Ø-89 percent third degree T31.98
        - 9Ø-99 percent third degree T31.99
  - upper limb T22.ØØ ☑
    - above elbow — *see* Burn, above elbow
    - axilla — *see* Burn, axilla
    - elbow — *see* Burn, elbow
    - first degree T22.1Ø ☑
    - forearm — *see* Burn, forearm
    - hand — *see* Burn, hand
    - interscapular region — *see* Burn, back, upper
    - multiple sites T22.Ø99 ☑
      - first degree T22.199 ☑
      - left T22.Ø92 ☑
        - first degree T22.192 ☑
        - second degree T22.292 ☑
        - third degree T22.392 ☑
      - right T22.Ø91 ☑
        - first degree T22.191 ☑
        - second degree T22.291 ☑
        - third degree T22.391 ☑
      - second degree T22.299 ☑
      - third degree T22.399 ☑
    - scapular region — *see* Burn, scapular region
    - second degree T22.2Ø ☑
    - shoulder — *see* Burn, shoulder
    - third degree T22.3Ø ☑
    - wrist — *see* Burn, wrist
  - uterus T28.3 ☑
  - vagina T28.3 ☑
  - vulva — *see* Burn, genital organs, external, female
  - wrist T23.Ø79 ☑
    - first degree T23.179 ☑
    - left T23.Ø72 ☑

Burn — *continued*
  wrist — *continued*
    left — *continued*
      first degree T23.172 ☑
      second degree T23.272 ☑
      third degree T23.372 ☑
    multiple sites with hand T23.Ø99 ☑
      first degree T23.199 ☑
      left T23.Ø92 ☑
        first degree T23.192 ☑
        second degree T23.292 ☑
        third degree T23.392 ☑
      right T23.Ø91 ☑
        first degree T23.191 ☑
        second degree T23.291 ☑
        third degree T23.391 ☑
      second degree T23.299 ☑
      third degree T23.399 ☑
    right T23.Ø71 ☑
      first degree T23.171 ☑
      second degree T23.271 ☑
      third degree T23.371 ☑
    second degree T23.279 ☑
    third degree T23.379 ☑
Burnett's syndrome E83.52
Burning
  feet syndrome E53.9
  sensation R2Ø.8
  tongue K14.6
Burn-out (state) Z73.Ø
Burns' disease or osteochondrosis — *see* Osteochondrosis, juvenile, ulna
Bursa — *see* condition
Bursitis M71.9
  Achilles — *see* Tendinitis, Achilles
  adhesive — *see* Bursitis, specified NEC
  ankle — *see* Enthesopathy, lower limb, ankle, specified type NEC
  calcaneal — *see* Enthesopathy, foot, specified type NEC
  collateral ligament, tibial — *see* Bursitis, tibial collateral
  due to use, overuse, pressure — *see also* Disorder, soft tissue, due to use, specified type NEC
    specified NEC — *see* Disorder, soft tissue, due to use, specified NEC
  Duplay's M75.Ø ☑
  elbow NEC M7Ø.3- ☑
    olecranon M7Ø.2- ☑
  finger — *see* Disorder, soft tissue, due to use, specified type NEC, hand
  foot — *see* Enthesopathy, foot, specified type NEC
  gonococcal A54.49
  gouty — *see* Gout
  hand M7Ø.1- ☑
  hip NEC M7Ø.7- ☑
    trochanteric M7Ø.6- ☑
  infective NEC M71.1Ø
    abscess — *see* Abscess, bursa
    ankle M71.17- ☑
    elbow M71.12- ☑
    foot M71.17- ☑
    hand M71.14- ☑
    hip M71.15- ☑
    knee M71.16- ☑
    multiple sites M71.19
    shoulder M71.11- ☑
    specified site NEC M71.18
    wrist M71.13- ☑
  ischial — *see* Bursitis, hip
  knee NEC M7Ø.5- ☑
    prepatellar M7Ø.4- ☑
  occupational NEC — *see also* Disorder, soft tissue, due to, use
  olecranon — *see* Bursitis, elbow, olecranon
  pharyngeal J39.1
  popliteal — *see* Bursitis, knee
  prepatellar M7Ø.4- ☑
  radiohumeral M7Ø.3- ☑
  rheumatoid MØ6.2Ø
    ankle MØ6.27- ☑
    elbow MØ6.22- ☑
    foot joint MØ6.27- ☑
    hand joint MØ6.24- ☑
    hip MØ6.25- ☑
    knee MØ6.26- ☑
    multiple site MØ6.29
    shoulder MØ6.21- ☑
Bursitis — *continued*
  rheumatoid — *continued*
    vertebra MØ6.28
    wrist MØ6.23- ☑
  scapulohumeral — *see* Bursitis, shoulder
  semimembranous muscle (knee) — *see* Bursitis, knee
  shoulder M75.5- ☑
    adhesive — *see* Capsulitis, adhesive
  specified NEC M71.5Ø
    ankle M71.57- ☑
    due to use, overuse or pressure — *see* Disorder, soft tissue, due to, use
    elbow M71.52- ☑
    foot M71.57- ☑
    hand M71.54- ☑
    hip M71.55- ☑
    knee M71.56- ☑
    shoulder — *see* Bursitis, shoulder
    specified site NEC M71.58
    tibial collateral M76.4- ☑
    wrist M71.53- ☑
  subacromial — *see* Bursitis, shoulder
  subcoracoid — *see* Bursitis, shoulder
  subdeltoid — *see* Bursitis, shoulder
  syphilitic A52.78
  Thornwaldt, Tornwaldt J39.2
  tibial collateral M76.4- ☑
  toe — *see* Enthesopathy, foot, specified type NEC
  trochanteric (area) — *see* Bursitis, hip, trochanteric
  wrist — *see* Bursitis, hand
Bursopathy M71.9
  specified type NEC M71.8Ø
    ankle M71.87- ☑
    elbow M71.82- ☑
    foot M71.87- ☑
    hand M71.84- ☑
    hip M71.85- ☑
    knee M71.86- ☑
    multiple sites M71.89
    shoulder M71.81- ☑
    specified site NEC M71.88
    wrist M71.83- ☑
Burst stitches or sutures (complication of surgery) T81.31 ☑
  external operation wound T81.31 ☑
  internal operation wound T81.32 ☑
Buruli ulcer A31.1
Bury's disease L95.1
Buschke's
  disease — *see* Cryptococcosis by site
  scleredema — *see* Sclerosis, systemic
Busse-Buschke disease — *see* Cryptococcosis by site
Buttock — *see* condition
Button
  Biskra B55.1
  Delhi B55.1
  oriental B55.1
Buttonhole deformity (finger) — *see* Deformity, finger, boutonniere
Bwamba fever A92.8
Byssinosis J66.Ø
Bywaters' syndrome T79.5 ☑

C

Cachexia R64
  cancerous R64
  cardiac — *see* Disease, heart
  dehydration E86.Ø
  due to malnutrition R64
  exophthalmic — *see* Hyperthyroidism
  heart — *see* Disease, heart
  hypophyseal E23.Ø
  hypopituitary E23.Ø
  lead — *see* Poisoning, lead
  malignant R64
  marsh — *see* Malaria
  nervous F48.8
  old age R54
  paludal — *see* Malaria
  pituitary E23.Ø
  pulmonary R64
  renal N28.9
  saturnine — *see* Poisoning, lead
  senile R54
  Simmonds' E23.Ø
  splenica D73.Ø
Cachexia — *continued*
  strumipriva EØ3.4
  tuberculous NEC — *see* Tuberculosis
CADASIL (cerebral autosomal dominant arteriopathy with subcortical infarcts and leukoencephalopathy) I67.85Ø
Café, au lait spots L81.3
Caffeine-induced
  anxiety disorder F15.98Ø
  sleep disorder F15.982
Caffey's syndrome Q78.8
Caisson disease T7Ø.3 ☑
Cake kidney Q63.1
Caked breast (puerperal, postpartum) O92.79
Calabar swelling B74.3
Calcaneal spur — *see* Spur, bone, calcaneal
Calcaneo-apophysitis M92.8
Calcareous — *see* condition
Calcicosis J62.8
Calciferol (vitamin D) deficiency E55.9
  with rickets E55.Ø
Calcification
  adrenal (capsule) (gland) E27.49
    tuberculous B9Ø.8 *[E35]*
  aorta I7Ø.Ø
  artery (annular) — *see* Arteriosclerosis
  auricle (ear) — *see* Disorder, pinna, specified type NEC
  basal ganglia G23.8
  bladder N32.89
    due to Schistosoma hematobium B65.Ø
  brain (cortex) — *see* Calcification, cerebral
  bronchus J98.Ø9
  bursa M71.4Ø
    ankle M71.47- ☑
    elbow M71.42- ☑
    foot M71.47- ☑
    hand M71.44- ☑
    hip M71.45- ☑
    knee M71.46- ☑
    multiple sites M71.49
    shoulder M75.3- ☑
    specified site NEC M71.48
    wrist M71.43- ☑
  cardiac — *see* Degeneration, myocardial
  cerebral (cortex) G93.89
    artery I67.2
  cervix (uteri) N88.8
  choroid plexus G93.89
  conjunctiva — *see* Concretion, conjunctiva
  corpora cavernosa (penis) N48.89
  cortex (brain) — *see* Calcification, cerebral
  dental pulp (nodular) KØ4.2
  dentinal papilla KØØ.4
  fallopian tube N83.8
  falx cerebri G96.198
  gallbladder K82.8
  general E83.59
  heart — *see also* Degeneration, myocardial
    valve — *see also* Endocarditis
      mitral — *see* Calcification, mitral
  idiopathic infantile arterial (IIAC) Q28.8
  intervertebral cartilage or disc (postinfective) — *see* Disorder, disc, specified NEC
  intracranial — *see* Calcification, cerebral
  joint — *see* Disorder, joint, specified type NEC
  kidney N28.89
    tuberculous N29 *[B9Ø.1]*
  larynx (senile) J38.7
  lens — *see* Cataract, specified NEC
  lung (active) (postinfectional) J98.4
    tuberculous B9Ø.9
  lymph gland or node (postinfectional) I89.8
    tuberculous — *see also* Tuberculosis, lymph gland B9Ø.8
  mammographic R92.1
  massive (paraplegic) — *see* Myositis, ossificans, in, quadriplegia
  medial — *see* Arteriosclerosis, extremities
  meninges (cerebral) (spinal) G96.198
  metastatic E83.59
  mitral (valve)
    annular I34.81
      nonrheumatic I34.81
      rheumatic IØ5.8
    annulus I34.81
      nonrheumatic I34.81
      rheumatic IØ5.8

Calcification — *continued*
  Mönckeberg's — *see* Arteriosclerosis, extremities
  muscle M61.9
    due to burns — *see* Myositis, ossificans, in, burns
    paralytic — *see* Myositis, ossificans, in, quadriplegia
    specified type NEC M61.4Ø
      ankle M61.47- ☑
      foot M61.47- ☑
      forearm M61.43- ☑
      hand M61.44- ☑
      lower leg M61.46- ☑
      multiple sites M61.49
      pelvic region M61.45- ☑
      shoulder region M61.41- ☑
      specified site NEC M61.48
      thigh M61.45- ☑
      upper arm M61.42- ☑
  myocardium, myocardial — *see* Degeneration, myocardial
  ovary N83.8
  pancreas K86.89
  penis N48.89
  periarticular — *see* Disorder, joint, specified type NEC
  pericardium — *see also* Pericarditis I31.1
  pineal gland E34.8
  pleura J94.8
    postinfectional J94.8
    tuberculous NEC B9Ø.9
  pulpal (dental) (nodular) KØ4.2
  sclera H15.89
  spleen D73.89
  subcutaneous L94.2
  suprarenal (capsule) (gland) E27.49
  tendon (sheath) — *see also* Tenosynovitis, specified type NEC
    with bursitis, synovitis or tenosynovitis — *see* Tendinitis, calcific
  trachea J39.8
  ureter N28.89
  uterus N85.8
  vitreous — *see* Deposit, crystalline
Calcified — *see* Calcification
Calcinosis (interstitial) (tumoral) (universalis) E83.59
  with Raynaud's phenomenon, esophageal dysfunction, sclerodactyly, telangiectasia (CREST syndrome) M34.1
  circumscripta (skin) L94.2
  cutis L94.2
Calciphylaxis — *see also* Calcification, by site E83.59
Calcium
  deposits — *see* Calcification, by site
  metabolism disorder E83.5Ø
  salts or soaps in vitreous — *see* Deposit, crystalline
Calciuria R82.994
Calculi — *see* Calculus
Calculosis, intrahepatic — *see* Calculus, bile duct
Calculus, calculi, calculous
  ampulla of Vater — *see* Calculus, bile duct
  anuria (impacted) (recurrent) — *see also* Calculus, urinary N2Ø.9
  appendix K38.1
  bile duct (common) (hepatic) K8Ø.5Ø
    with
      calculus of gallbladder — *see* Calculus, gallbladder and bile duct
      cholangitis K8Ø.3Ø
        with
          cholecystitis — *see* Calculus, bile duct, with cholecystitis
        obstruction K8Ø.31
        acute K8Ø.32
          with
            chronic cholangitis K8Ø.36
              with obstruction K8Ø.37
          obstruction K8Ø.33
        chronic K8Ø.34
          with
            acute cholangitis K8Ø.36
              with obstruction K8Ø.37
          obstruction K8Ø.35
      cholecystitis (with cholangitis) K8Ø.4Ø
        with obstruction K8Ø.41
        acute K8Ø.42
          with
            chronic cholecystitis K8Ø.46
              with obstruction K8Ø.47
          obstruction K8Ø.43
        chronic K8Ø.44

Calculus, calculi, calculous — *continued*
  bile duct — *continued*
    with — *continued*
      cholecystitis — *continued*
        chronic — *continued*
          with
            acute cholecystitis K8Ø.46
              with obstruction K8Ø.47
          obstruction K8Ø.45
  biliary — *see also* Calculus, gallbladder
    specified NEC K8Ø.8Ø
      with obstruction K8Ø.81
  bilirubin, multiple — *see* Calculus, gallbladder
  bladder (encysted) (impacted) (urinary) (diverticulum) N21.Ø
  bronchus J98.Ø9
  calyx (kidney) (renal) — *see* Calculus, kidney
  cholesterol (pure) (solitary) — *see* Calculus, gallbladder
  common duct (bile) — *see* Calculus, bile duct
  conjunctiva — *see* Concretion, conjunctiva
  cystic N21.Ø
    duct — *see* Calculus, gallbladder
  dental (subgingival) (supragingival) KØ3.6
  diverticulum
    bladder N21.Ø
    kidney N2Ø.Ø
  epididymis N5Ø.89
  gallbladder K8Ø.2Ø
    with
      bile duct calculus — *see* Calculus, gallbladder and bile duct
      cholecystitis K8Ø.1Ø
        with obstruction K8Ø.11
        acute K8Ø.ØØ
          with
            chronic cholecystitis K8Ø.12
              with obstruction K8Ø.13
          obstruction K8Ø.Ø1
        chronic K8Ø.1Ø
          with
            acute cholecystitis K8Ø.12
              with obstruction K8Ø.13
          obstruction K8Ø.11
        specified NEC K8Ø.18
          with obstruction K8Ø.19
      obstruction K8Ø.21
  gallbladder and bile duct K8Ø.7Ø
    with
      cholecystitis K8Ø.6Ø
        with obstruction K8Ø.61
        acute K8Ø.62
          with
            chronic cholecystitis K8Ø.66
              with obstruction K8Ø.67
          obstruction K8Ø.63
        chronic K8Ø.64
          with
            acute cholecystitis K8Ø.66
              with obstruction K8Ø.67
          obstruction K8Ø.65
      obstruction K8Ø.71
  hepatic (duct) — *see* Calculus, bile duct
  ileal conduit N21.8
  intestinal (impaction) (obstruction) K56.49
  kidney (impacted) (multiple) (pelvis) (recurrent) (staghorn) N2Ø.Ø
    with calculus, ureter N2Ø.2
    congenital Q63.8
  lacrimal passages — *see* Dacryolith
  liver (impacted) — *see* Calculus, bile duct
  lung J98.4
  mammographic R92.1
  nephritic (impacted) (recurrent) — *see* Calculus, kidney
  nose J34.89
  pancreas (duct) K86.89
  parotid duct or gland K11.5
  pelvis, encysted — *see* Calculus, kidney
  prostate N42.Ø
  pulmonary J98.4
  pyelitis (impacted) (recurrent) N2Ø.Ø
    with hydronephrosis N13.6
  pyelonephritis (impacted) (recurrent) — *see* category N2Ø ☑
    with hydronephrosis N13.6
  renal (impacted) (recurrent) — *see* Calculus, kidney
  salivary (duct) (gland) K11.5
  seminal vesicle N5Ø.89
  staghorn — *see* Calculus, kidney

Calculus, calculi, calculous — *continued*
  Stensen's duct K11.5
  stomach K31.89
  sublingual duct or gland K11.5
    congenital Q38.4
  submandibular duct, gland or region K11.5
  submaxillary duct, gland or region K11.5
  suburethral N21.8
  tonsil J35.8
  tooth, teeth (subgingival) (supragingival) KØ3.6
  tunica vaginalis N5Ø.89
  ureter (impacted) (recurrent) N2Ø.1
    with calculus, kidney N2Ø.2
      with hydronephrosis N13.2
        with infection N13.6
  ureteropelvic junction N2Ø.1
  urethra (impacted) N21.1
  urinary (duct) (impacted) (passage) (tract) N2Ø.9
    with hydronephrosis N13.2
      with infection N13.6
    in (due to)
    lower N21.9
      specified NEC N21.8
  vagina N89.8
  vesical (impacted) N21.Ø
  Wharton's duct K11.5
  xanthine E79.8 *[N22]*
Calicectasis N28.89
Caliectasis N28.89
California
  disease B38.9
  encephalitis A83.5
Caligo cornea — *see* Opacity, cornea, central
Callositas, callosity (infected) L84
Callus (infected) L84
  bone — *see* Osteophyte
    excessive, following fracture — *code as* Sequelae of fracture
CALME (childhood asymmetric labium majus enlargement) N9Ø.61
Calorie deficiency or malnutrition — *see also* Malnutrition E46
Calpainopathy (primary) G71.Ø32
  autosomal dominant G71.Ø31
  autosomal recessive G71.Ø32
Calvé-Perthes disease — *see* Legg-Calvé-Perthes disease
Calvé's disease — *see* Osteochondrosis, juvenile, spine
Calvities — *see* Alopecia, androgenic
Cameroon fever — *see* Malaria
Camptocormia (hysterical) F44.4
Camurati-Engelmann syndrome Q78.3
Canal — *see also* condition
  atrioventricular Q21.2Ø
    common Q21.23
    incomplete Q21.21
    intermediate Q21.22
    partial Q21.21
    transitional Q21.22
Canaliculitis (lacrimal) (acute) (subacute) HØ4.33- ☑
  Actinomyces A42.89
  chronic HØ4.42- ☑
Canavan's disease E75.29
Canceled procedure (surgical) Z53.9
  because of
    contraindication Z53.Ø9
      smoking Z53.Ø1
    left against medical advice (AMA) Z53.29
    patient's decision Z53.2Ø
      for reasons of belief or group pressure Z53.1
      specified reason NEC Z53.29
    specified reason NEC Z53.8
Cancer — *see also* Neoplasm, by site, malignant
  bile duct type liver C22.1
  blood — *see* Leukemia
  breast — *see also* Neoplasm, breast, malignant C5Ø.91- ☑
  hepatocellular C22.Ø
  lung — *see also* Neoplasm, lung, malignant C34.9Ø
  ovarian — *see also* Neoplasm ovary, malignant C56.9
  unspecified site (primary) C8Ø.1
Cancer (o) phobia F45.29
Cancerous — *see* Neoplasm, malignant, by site
Cancrum oris A69.Ø
Candidiasis, candidal B37.9
  balanitis B37.42
  bronchitis B37.1
  cheilitis B37.83

- **Candidiasis, candidal** — *continued*
  - congenital P37.5
  - cystitis B37.41
  - disseminated B37.7
  - endocarditis B37.6
  - enteritis B37.82
  - esophagitis B37.81
  - intertrigo B37.2
  - lung B37.1
  - meningitis B37.5
  - mouth B37.Ø
  - nails B37.2
  - neonatal P37.5
  - onychia B37.2
  - oral B37.Ø
  - osteomyelitis B37.89
  - otitis externa B37.84
  - paronychia B37.2
  - perionyxis B37.2
  - pneumonia B37.1
  - proctitis B37.82
  - pulmonary B37.1
  - pyelonephritis B37.49
  - sepsis B37.7
  - skin B37.2
  - specified site NEC B37.89
  - stomatitis B37.Ø
  - systemic B37.7
  - urethritis B37.41
  - urogenital site NEC B37.49
  - vagina (acute) B37.31
    - chronic (recurrent) B37.32
  - vulva (acute) B37.31
    - chronic (recurrent) B37.32
  - vulvovaginitis (acute) B37.31
    - chronic (recurrent) B37.32
- **Candidid** L3Ø.2
- **Candidosis** — *see* Candidiasis
- **Candiru infection or infestation** B88.8
- **Canities** (premature) L67.1
  - congenital Q84.2
- **Canker** (mouth) (sore) K12.Ø
  - rash A38.9
- **Cannabinosis** J66.2
- **Cannabis induced**
  - anxiety disorder F12.98Ø
  - psychotic disorder F12.959
  - sleep disorder F12.988
- **Canton fever** A75.9
- **Cantrell's syndrome** Q87.89
- **Capillariasis** (intestinal) B81.1
  - hepatic B83.8
- **Capillary** — *see* condition
- **Caplan's syndrome** — *see* Rheumatoid, lung
- **Capsule** — *see* condition
- **Capsulitis** (joint) — *see also* Enthesopathy
  - adhesive (shoulder) M75.Ø- ☑
  - hepatic K65.8
  - labyrinthine — *see* Otosclerosis, specified NEC
  - thyroid EØ6.9
- **Caput**
  - crepitus Q75.8
  - medusae I86.8
  - succedaneum P12.81
- **Car sickness** T75.3 ☑
- **Carapata** (disease) A68.Ø
- **Carate** — *see* Pinta
- **Carbon lung** J6Ø
- **Carbuncle** LØ2.93
  - abdominal wall LØ2.231
  - anus K61.Ø
  - auditory canal, external — *see* Abscess, ear, external
  - auricle ear — *see* Abscess, ear, external
  - axilla LØ2.43- ☑
  - back (any part) LØ2.232
  - breast N61.1
  - buttock LØ2.33
  - cheek (external) LØ2.Ø3
  - chest wall LØ2.233
  - chin LØ2.Ø3
  - corpus cavernosum N48.21
  - ear (any part) (external) (middle) — *see* Abscess, ear, external
  - external auditory canal — *see* Abscess, ear, external
  - eyelid — *see* Abscess, eyelid
  - face NEC LØ2.Ø3
  - femoral (region) — *see* Carbuncle, lower limb
  - finger — *see* Carbuncle, hand
- **Carbuncle** — *continued*
  - flank LØ2.231
  - foot LØ2.63- ☑
  - forehead LØ2.Ø3
  - genital — *see* Abscess, genital
  - gluteal (region) LØ2.33
  - groin LØ2.234
  - hand LØ2.53- ☑
  - head NEC LØ2.831
  - heel — *see* Carbuncle, foot
  - hip — *see* Carbuncle, lower limb
  - kidney — *see* Abscess, kidney
  - knee — *see* Carbuncle, lower limb
  - labium (majus) (minus) N76.4
  - lacrimal
    - gland — *see* Dacryoadenitis
    - passages (duct) (sac) — *see* Inflammation, lacrimal, passages, acute
  - leg — *see* Carbuncle, lower limb
  - lower limb LØ2.43- ☑
  - malignant A22.Ø
  - navel LØ2.236
  - neck LØ2.13
  - nose (external) (septum) J34.Ø
  - orbit, orbital — *see* Abscess, orbit
  - palmar (space) — *see* Carbuncle, hand
  - partes posteriores LØ2.33
  - pectoral region LØ2.233
  - penis N48.21
  - perineum LØ2.235
  - pinna — *see* Abscess, ear, external
  - popliteal — *see* Carbuncle, lower limb
  - scalp LØ2.831
  - seminal vesicle N49.Ø
  - shoulder — *see* Carbuncle, upper limb
  - specified site NEC LØ2.838
  - temple (region) LØ2.Ø3
  - thumb — *see* Carbuncle, hand
  - toe — *see* Carbuncle, foot
  - trunk LØ2.239
    - abdominal wall LØ2.231
    - back LØ2.232
    - chest wall LØ2.233
    - groin LØ2.234
    - perineum LØ2.235
    - umbilicus LØ2.236
  - umbilicus LØ2.236
  - upper limb LØ2.43- ☑
  - urethra N34.Ø
  - vulva N76.4
- **Carbunculus** — *see* Carbuncle
- **Carcinoid** (tumor) — *see* Tumor, carcinoid
- **Carcinoidosis** E34.Ø
- **Carcinoma** (malignant) — *see also* Neoplasm, by site, malignant
  - acidophil
    - specified site — *see* Neoplasm, malignant, by site
    - unspecified site C75.1
  - acidophil-basophil, mixed
    - specified site — *see* Neoplasm, malignant, by site
    - unspecified site C75.1
  - adnexal (skin) — *see* Neoplasm, skin, malignant
  - adrenal cortical C74.Ø- ☑
  - alveolar — *see* Neoplasm, lung, malignant
    - cell — *see* Neoplasm, lung, malignant
  - ameloblastic C41.1
    - upper jaw (bone) C41.Ø
  - apocrine
    - breast — *see* Neoplasm, breast, malignant
    - specified site NEC — *see* Neoplasm, skin, malignant
    - unspecified site C44.99
  - basal cell (pigmented) (*see also* Neoplasm, skin, malignant) C44.91
    - fibro-epithelial — *see* Neoplasm, skin, malignant
    - morphea — *see* Neoplasm, skin, malignant
    - multicentric — *see* Neoplasm, skin, malignant
  - basaloid
  - basal-squamous cell, mixed — *see* Neoplasm, skin, malignant
  - basophil
    - specified site — *see* Neoplasm, malignant, by site
    - unspecified site C75.1
  - basophil-acidophil, mixed
    - specified site — *see* Neoplasm, malignant, by site
    - unspecified site C75.1
  - basosquamous — *see* Neoplasm, skin, malignant
- **Carcinoma** — *continued*
  - bile duct
    - with hepatocellular, mixed C22.Ø
    - liver C22.1
    - specified site NEC — *see* Neoplasm, malignant, by site
    - unspecified site C22.1
  - branchial or branchiogenic C1Ø.4
  - bronchial or bronchogenic — *see* Neoplasm, lung, malignant
  - bronchiolar — *see* Neoplasm, lung, malignant
  - bronchioloalveolar — *see* Neoplasm, lung, malignant
  - C cell
    - specified site — *see* Neoplasm, malignant, by site
    - unspecified site C73
  - ceruminous C44.29- ☑
  - cervix uteri
    - in situ DØ6.9
      - endocervix DØ6.Ø
      - exocervix DØ6.1
      - specified site NEC DØ6.7
  - chorionic
    - specified site — *see* Neoplasm, malignant, by site
    - unspecified site
      - female C58
      - male C62.9Ø
  - chromophobe
    - specified site — *see* Neoplasm, malignant, by site
    - unspecified site C75.1
  - cloacogenic
    - specified site — *see* Neoplasm, malignant, by site
    - unspecified site C21.2
  - diffuse type
    - specified site — *see* Neoplasm, malignant, by site
    - unspecified site C16.9
  - duct (cell)
    - with Paget's disease — *see* Neoplasm, breast, malignant
    - infiltrating
      - with lobular carcinoma (in situ)
        - specified site — *see* Neoplasm, malignant, by site
        - unspecified site (female) C5Ø.91- ☑
          - male C5Ø.92- ☑
      - specified site — *see* Neoplasm, malignant, by site
      - unspecified site (female) C5Ø.91- ☑
        - male C5Ø.92- ☑
  - ductal
    - with lobular
      - specified site — *see* Neoplasm, malignant, by site
      - unspecified site (female) C5Ø.91- ☑
        - male C5Ø.92- ☑
  - ductular, infiltrating
    - specified site — *see* Neoplasm, malignant, by site
    - unspecified site (female) C5Ø.91- ☑
      - male C5Ø.92- ☑
  - embryonal
    - liver C22.7
  - endometrioid
    - specified site — *see* Neoplasm, malignant, by site
    - unspecified site
      - female C56.9
      - male C61
  - eosinophil
    - specified site — *see* Neoplasm, malignant, by site
    - unspecified site C75.1
  - epidermoid — *see also* Neoplasm, skin, malignant
    - in situ, Bowen's type — *see* Neoplasm, skin, in situ
  - fibroepithelial, basal cell — *see* Neoplasm, skin, malignant
  - follicular
    - with papillary (mixed) C73
    - moderately differentiated C73
    - pure follicle C73
    - specified site — *see* Neoplasm, malignant, by site
    - trabecular C73
    - unspecified site C73
    - well differentiated C73
  - generalized, with unspecified primary site C8Ø.Ø
  - glycogen-rich — *see* Neoplasm, breast, malignant
  - granulosa cell C56- ☑
  - hepatic cell C22.Ø
  - hepatocellular C22.Ø
    - with bile duct, mixed C22.Ø
    - fibrolamellar C22.Ø
  - hepatocholangiolitic C22.Ø

Carcinoma — *continued*
  Hurthle cell C73
  in
    adenomatous
      polyposis coli C18.9
    pleomorphic adenoma — *see* Neoplasm, salivary glands, malignant
    situ — *see* Carcinoma-in-situ
  infiltrating
    duct
      with lobular
        specified site — *see* Neoplasm, malignant, by site
        unspecified site (female) C5Ø.91- ☑
          male C5Ø.92- ☑
      with Paget's disease — *see* Neoplasm, breast, malignant
      specified site — *see* Neoplasm, malignant
      unspecified site (female) C5Ø.91- ☑
        male C5Ø.92- ☑
    ductular
      specified site — *see* Neoplasm, malignant
      unspecified site (female) C5Ø.91- ☑
        male C5Ø.92- ☑
    lobular
      specified site — *see* Neoplasm, malignant
      unspecified site (female) C5Ø.91- ☑
        male C5Ø.92- ☑
  inflammatory
    specified site — *see* Neoplasm, malignant
    unspecified site (female) C5Ø.91- ☑
      male C5Ø.92- ☑
  intestinal type
    specified site — *see* Neoplasm, malignant, by site
    unspecified site C16.9
  intracystic
    noninfiltrating — *see* Neoplasm, in situ, by site
  intraductal (noninfiltrating)
    with Paget's disease — *see* Neoplasm, breast, malignant
    breast DØ5.1- ☑
    papillary
      with invasion
        specified site — *see* Neoplasm, malignant, by site
        unspecified site (female) C5Ø.91- ☑
          male C5Ø.92- ☑
      breast DØ5.1- ☑
      specified site NEC — *see* Neoplasm, in situ, by site
      unspecified site (female) DØ5.1- ☑
    specified site NEC — *see* Neoplasm, in situ, by site
    unspecified site (female) DØ5.1- ☑
  intraepidermal — *see* Neoplasm, in situ
    squamous cell, Bowen's type — *see* Neoplasm, skin, in situ
  intraepithelial — *see* Neoplasm, in situ, by site
    squamous cell — *see* Neoplasm, in situ, by site
  intraosseous C41.1
    upper jaw (bone) C41.Ø
  islet cell
    with exocrine, mixed
      specified site — *see* Neoplasm, malignant, by site
      unspecified site C25.9
    pancreas C25.4
    specified site NEC — *see* Neoplasm, malignant, by site
    unspecified site C25.4
  juvenile, breast — *see* Neoplasm, breast, malignant
  large cell
    small cell
      specified site — *see* Neoplasm, malignant, by site
      unspecified site C34.9Ø
  Leydig cell (testis)
    specified site — *see* Neoplasm, malignant, by site
    unspecified site
      female C56.9
      male C62.9Ø
  lipid-rich (female) C5Ø.91- ☑
    male C5Ø.92- ☑
  liver cell C22.Ø
  liver NEC C22.7

Carcinoma — *continued*
  lobular (infiltrating)
    with intraductal
      specified site — *see* Neoplasm, malignant, by site
      unspecified site (female) C5Ø.91- ☑
        male C5Ø.92- ☑
    noninfiltrating
      breast DØ5.Ø- ☑
      specified site NEC — *see* Neoplasm, in situ, by site
      unspecified site DØ5.Ø- ☑
    specified site — *see* Neoplasm, malignant, by site
    unspecified site (female) C5Ø.91- ☑
      male C5Ø.92- ☑
  medullary
    with
      amyloid stroma
        specified site — *see* Neoplasm, malignant, by site
        unspecified site C73
      lymphoid stroma
        specified site — *see* Neoplasm, malignant, by site
        unspecified site (female) C5Ø.91- ☑
          male C5Ø.92- ☑
  Merkel cell C4A.9 (*following* C43)
    anal margin C4A.51 (*following* C43)
    anal skin C4A.51 (*following* C43)
    canthus C4A.1- ☑ (*following* C43)
    ear and external auricular canal C4A.2- ☑ (*following* C43)
    external auricular canal C4A.2- ☑ (*following* C43)
    eyelid, including canthus C4A.1- ☑ (*following* C43)
    face C4A.3Ø (*following* C43)
      specified NEC C4A.39 (*following* C43)
    hip C4A.7- ☑ (*following* C43)
    lip C4A.Ø (*following* C43)
    lower limb, including hip C4A.7- ☑ (*following* C43)
    neck C4A.4 (*following* C43)
    nodal presentation C7B.1 (*following* C75)
    nose C4A.31 (*following* C43)
    overlapping sites C4A.8 (*following* C43)
    perianal skin C4A.51 (*following* C43)
    scalp C4A.4 (*following* C43)
    secondary C7B.1 (*following* C75)
    shoulder C4A.6- ☑ (*following* C43)
    skin of breast C4A.52 (*following* C43)
    trunk NEC C4A.59 (*following* C43)
    upper limb, including shoulder C4A.6- ☑ (*following* C43)
    visceral metastatic C7B.1 (*following* C75)
  metastatic — *see* Neoplasm, secondary, by site
  metatypical — *see* Neoplasm, skin, malignant
  morphea, basal cell — *see* Neoplasm, skin, malignant
  mucoid
    cell
      specified site — *see* Neoplasm, malignant, by site
      unspecified site C75.1
  neuroendocrine — *see also* Tumor, neuroendocrine
    high grade, any site C7A.1 (*following* C75)
    poorly differentiated, any site C7A.1 (*following* C75)
  nonencapsulated sclerosing C73
  noninfiltrating
    intracystic — *see* Neoplasm, in situ, by site
    intraductal
      breast DØ5.1- ☑
      papillary
        breast DØ5.1- ☑
        specified site NEC — *see* Neoplasm, in situ, by site
        unspecified site DØ5.1- ☑
      specified site — *see* Neoplasm, in situ, by site
      unspecified site DØ5.1- ☑
    lobular
      breast DØ5.Ø- ☑
      specified site NEC — *see* Neoplasm, in situ, by site
      unspecified site (female) DØ5.Ø- ☑
  oat cell
    specified site — *see* Neoplasm, malignant, by site
    unspecified site C34.9Ø
  odontogenic C41.1
    upper jaw (bone) C41.Ø
  papillary
    with follicular (mixed) C73

Carcinoma — *continued*
  papillary — *continued*
    follicular variant C73
    intraductal (noninfiltrating)
      with invasion
        specified site — *see* Neoplasm, malignant, by site
        unspecified site (female) C5Ø.91- ☑
          male C5Ø.92- ☑
      breast DØ5.1- ☑
      specified site NEC — *see* Neoplasm, in situ, by site
      unspecified site DØ5.1- ☑
    serous
      specified site — *see* Neoplasm, malignant, by site
      surface
        specified site — *see* Neoplasm, malignant, by site
        unspecified site C56.9
      unspecified site C56.9
  papillocystic
    specified site — *see* Neoplasm, malignant, by site
    unspecified site C56.9
  parafollicular cell
    specified site — *see* Neoplasm, malignant, by site
    unspecified site C73
  pilomatrix — *see* Neoplasm, skin, malignant
  pseudomucinous
    specified site — *see* Neoplasm, malignant, by site
    unspecified site C56.9
  renal cell C64- ☑
  Schmincke — *see* Neoplasm, nasopharynx, malignant
  Schneiderian
    specified site — *see* Neoplasm, malignant, by site
    unspecified site C3Ø.Ø
  sebaceous — *see* Neoplasm, skin, malignant
  secondary — *see also* Neoplasm, secondary, by site
    Merkel cell C7B.1 (*following* C75)
  secretory, breast — *see* Neoplasm, breast, malignant
  serous
    papillary
      specified site — *see* Neoplasm, malignant, by site
      unspecified site C56.9
    surface, papillary
      specified site — *see* Neoplasm, malignant, by site
      unspecified site C56.9
  Sertoli cell
    specified site — *see* Neoplasm, malignant, by site
    unspecified site C62.9Ø
      female C56.9
      male C62.9Ø
  skin appendage — *see* Neoplasm, skin, malignant
  small cell
    fusiform cell
      specified site — *see* Neoplasm, malignant, by site
      unspecified site C34.9Ø
    intermediate cell
      specified site — *see* Neoplasm, malignant, by site
      unspecified site C34.9Ø
    large cell
      specified site — *see* Neoplasm, malignant, by site
      unspecified site C34.9Ø
  solid
    with amyloid stroma
      specified site — *see* Neoplasm, malignant, by site
      unspecified site C73
    microinvasive
      specified site — *see* Neoplasm, malignant, by site
      unspecified site C53.9
  sweat gland — *see* Neoplasm, skin, malignant
  theca cell C56.- ☑
  thymic C37
  unspecified site (primary) C8Ø.1
  water-clear cell C75.Ø
Carcinoma-in-situ — *see also* Neoplasm, in situ, by site
  breast NOS DØ5.9- ☑
    specified type NEC DØ5.8- ☑
  epidermoid — *see also* Neoplasm, in situ, by site
    with questionable stromal invasion
      cervix DØ6.9

- **Carcinoma-in-situ** — *continued*
  - epidermoid — *see also* Neoplasm, in situ, by site — *continued*
    - with questionable stromal invasion — *continued*
      - specified site NEC — *see* Neoplasm, in situ, by site
      - unspecified site DØ6.9
    - Bowen's type — *see* Neoplasm, skin, in situ
  - intraductal
    - breast DØ5.1- ☑
    - specified site NEC — *see* Neoplasm, in situ, by site
    - unspecified site DØ5.1- ☑
  - lobular
    - with
      - infiltrating duct
        - breast (female) C5Ø.91- ☑
          - male C5Ø.92- ☑
        - specified site NEC — *see* Neoplasm, malignant
        - unspecified site (female) C5Ø.91- ☑
          - male C5Ø.92- ☑
      - intraductal
        - breast DØ5.8- ☑
        - specified site NEC — *see* Neoplasm, in situ, by site
        - unspecified site (female) DØ5.8- ☑
    - breast DØ5.Ø- ☑
    - specified site NEC — *see* Neoplasm, in situ, by site
    - unspecified site DØ5.Ø- ☑
  - squamous cell — *see also* Neoplasm, in situ, by site
    - with questionable stromal invasion
      - cervix DØ6.9
      - specified site NEC — *see* Neoplasm, in situ, by site
      - unspecified site DØ6.9
- **Carcinomaphobia** F45.29
- **Carcinomatosis** C8Ø.Ø
  - peritonei C78.6
  - unspecified site (primary) (secondary) C8Ø.Ø
- **Carcinosarcoma** — *see* Neoplasm, malignant, by site
  - embryonal — *see* Neoplasm, malignant, by site
- **Cardia, cardial** — *see* condition
- **Cardiac** — *see also* condition
  - death, sudden — *see* Arrest, cardiac
  - pacemaker
    - in situ Z95.Ø
    - management or adjustment Z45.Ø18
  - tamponade I31.4
- **Cardialgia** — *see* Pain, precordial
- **Cardiectasis** — *see* Hypertrophy, cardiac
- **Cardiochalasia** K21.9
- **Cardiomalacia** I51.5
- **Cardiomegalia glycogenica diffusa** E74.Ø2 *[I43]*
- **Cardiomegaly** — *see also* Hypertrophy, cardiac
  - congenital Q24.8
  - glycogen E74.Ø2 *[I43]*
  - idiopathic I51.7
- **Cardiomyoliposis** I51.5
- **Cardiomyopathy** (familial) (idiopathic) I42.9
  - alcoholic I42.6
  - amyloid E85.4 *[I43]*
    - transthyretin-related (ATTR) familial E85.4 *[I43]*
  - arteriosclerotic — *see* Disease, heart, ischemic, atherosclerotic
  - beriberi E51.12
  - cobalt-beer I42.6
  - congenital I42.4
  - congestive I42.Ø
  - constrictive NOS I42.5
  - dilated I42.Ø
  - due to
    - alcohol I42.6
    - beriberi E51.12
    - cardiac glycogenosis E74.Ø2 *[I43]*
    - drugs I42.7
    - external agents NEC I42.7
    - Friedreich's ataxia G11.11
    - myotonia atrophica G71.11 *[I43]*
    - progressive muscular dystrophy — *see also* Dystrophy, muscular, by type G71.Ø9 *[I43]*
  - glycogen storage E74.Ø2 *[I43]*
  - hypertensive — *see* Hypertension, heart
  - hypertrophic (nonobstructive) I42.2
    - obstructive I42.1
      - congenital Q24.8
  - in
    - Chagas' disease (chronic) B57.2
      - acute B57.Ø
- **Cardiomyopathy** — *continued*
  - in — *continued*
    - sarcoidosis D86.85
  - ischemic I25.5
  - metabolic E88.9 *[I43]*
    - thyrotoxic EØ5.9Ø *[I43]*
      - with thyroid storm EØ5.91 *[I43]*
  - newborn I42.8
    - congenital I42.4
  - non-ischemic — *see also* by cause I42.8
  - nutritional E63.9 *[I43]*
    - beriberi E51.12
  - obscure of Africa I42.8
  - peripartum O9Ø.3
  - postpartum O9Ø.3
  - restrictive NEC I42.5
  - rheumatic IØ9.Ø
  - secondary I42.9
  - specified NEC I42.8
  - stress induced I51.81
  - takotsubo I51.81
  - thyrotoxic EØ5.9Ø *[I43]*
    - with thyroid storm EØ5.91 *[I43]*
  - toxic NEC I42.7
  - transthyretin-related (ATTR) familial amyloid E85.4
  - tuberculous A18.84
  - viral B33.24
- **Cardionephritis** — *see* Hypertension, cardiorenal
- **Cardionephropathy** — *see* Hypertension, cardiorenal
- **Cardionephrosis** — *see* Hypertension, cardiorenal
- **Cardiopathia nigra** I27.Ø
- **Cardiopathy** — *see also* Disease, heart I51.9
  - idiopathic I42.9
  - mucopolysaccharidosis E76.3 *[I52]*
- **Cardiopericarditis** — *see* Pericarditis
- **Cardiophobia** F45.29
- **Cardiorenal** — *see* condition
- **Cardiorrhexis** — *see* Infarct, myocardium
- **Cardiosclerosis** — *see* Disease, heart, ischemic, atherosclerotic
- **Cardiosis** — *see* Disease, heart
- **Cardiospasm** (esophagus) (reflex) (stomach) K22.Ø
  - congenital Q39.5
    - with megaesophagus Q39.5
- **Cardiostenosis** — *see* Disease, heart
- **Cardiosymphysis** I31.Ø
- **Cardiovascular** — *see* condition
- **Carditis** (acute) (bacterial) (chronic) (subacute) I51.89
  - meningococcal A39.5Ø
  - rheumatic — *see* Disease, heart, rheumatic
  - rheumatoid — *see* Rheumatoid, carditis
  - viral B33.2Ø
- **Care** (of) (for) (following)
  - child (routine) Z76.2
  - family member (handicapped) (sick)
    - creating problem for family Z63.6
    - provided away from home for holiday relief Z75.5
    - unavailable, due to
      - absence (person rendering care) (sufferer) Z74.2
      - inability (any reason) of person rendering care Z74.2
  - foundling Z76.1
  - holiday relief Z75.5
  - improper — *see* Maltreatment
  - lack of (at or after birth) (infant) — *see* Maltreatment, child, neglect
  - lactating mother Z39.1
  - palliative Z51.5
  - postpartum
    - immediately after delivery Z39.Ø
    - routine follow-up Z39.2
  - respite Z75.5
  - unavailable, due to
    - absence of person rendering care Z74.2
    - inability (any reason) of person rendering care Z74.2
  - well-baby Z76.2
- **Caries**
  - bone NEC A18.Ø3
  - dental (dentino enamel junction) (early childhood) (of dentine) (pre-eruptive) (recurrent) (to the pulp) KØ2.9
    - arrested (coronal) (root) KØ2.3
    - chewing surface
      - limited to enamel KØ2.51
      - penetrating into dentin KØ2.52
      - penetrating into pulp KØ2.53
- **Caries** — *continued*
  - dental — *continued*
    - coronal surface
      - chewing surface
        - limited to enamel KØ2.51
        - penetrating into dentin KØ2.52
        - penetrating into pulp KØ2.53
      - pit and fissure surface
        - limited to enamel KØ2.51
        - penetrating into dentin KØ2.52
        - penetrating into pulp KØ2.53
      - smooth surface
        - limited to enamel KØ2.61
        - penetrating into dentin KØ2.62
        - penetrating into pulp KØ2.63
    - pit and fissure surface
      - limited to enamel KØ2.51
      - penetrating into dentin KØ2.52
      - penetrating into pulp KØ2.53
    - primary, cervical origin KØ2.52
    - root KØ2.7
    - smooth surface
      - limited to enamel KØ2.61
      - penetrating into dentin KØ2.62
      - penetrating into pulp KØ2.63
  - external meatus — *see* Disorder, ear, external, specified type NEC
  - hip (tuberculous) A18.Ø2
  - initial (tooth)
    - chewing surface KØ2.51
    - pit and fissure surface KØ2.51
    - smooth surface KØ2.61
  - knee (tuberculous) A18.Ø2
  - labyrinth H83.8 ☑
  - limb NEC (tuberculous) A18.Ø3
  - mastoid process (chronic) — *see* Mastoiditis, chronic
    - tuberculous A18.Ø3
  - middle ear H74.8 ☑
  - nose (tuberculous) A18.Ø3
  - orbit (tuberculous) A18.Ø3
  - ossicles, ear — *see* Abnormal, ear ossicles
  - petrous bone — *see* Petrositis
  - root (dental) (tooth) KØ2.7
  - sacrum (tuberculous) A18.Ø1
  - spine, spinal (column) (tuberculous) A18.Ø1
  - syphilitic A52.77
    - congenital (early) A5Ø.Ø2 *[M9Ø.8Ø]*
  - tooth, teeth — *see* Caries, dental
  - tuberculous A18.Ø3
  - vertebra (column) (tuberculous) A18.Ø1
- **Carious teeth** — *see* Caries, dental
- **Carneous mole** OØ2.Ø
- **Carnitine insufficiency** E71.4Ø
- **Carotenemia** (dietary) E67.1
- **Carotenosis** (cutis) (skin) E67.1
- **Carotid body or sinus syndrome** G9Ø.Ø1
- **Carotidynia** G9Ø.Ø1
- **Carpal tunnel syndrome** — *see* Syndrome, carpal tunnel
- **Carpenter's syndrome** Q87.Ø
- **Carpopedal spasm** — *see* Tetany
- **Carr-Barr-Plunkett syndrome** Q97.1
- **Carrier** (suspected) of
  - amebiasis Z22.1
  - bacterial disease NEC Z22.39
    - diphtheria Z22.2
    - intestinal infectious NEC Z22.1
      - typhoid Z22.Ø
    - meningococcal Z22.31
    - sexually transmitted Z22.4
    - specified NEC Z22.39
    - staphylococcal (Methicillin susceptible) Z22.321
      - Methicillin resistant Z22.322
    - streptococcal Z22.338
      - group B Z22.33Ø
        - complicating pregnancy or delivery O99.82- ☑
    - typhoid Z22.Ø
  - cholera Z22.1
  - diphtheria Z22.2
  - gastrointestinal pathogens NEC Z22.1
  - genetic Z14.8
    - cystic fibrosis Z14.1
    - hemophilia A (asymptomatic) Z14.Ø1
      - symptomatic Z14.Ø2
  - gestational, pregnant Z33.1
  - gonorrhea Z22.4
  - HAA (hepatitis Australian-antigen) B18.8
  - HB (c)(s)-AG B18.1

Carrier of — *continued*
  hepatitis (viral) B18.9
    Australia-antigen (HAA) B18.8
    B surface antigen (HBsAg) B18.1
      with acute delta- (super)infection B17.Ø
    C B18.2
    specified NEC B18.8
  human T-cell lymphotropic virus type-1 (HTLV-1) infection Z22.6
  infectious organism Z22.9
    specified NEC Z22.8
  meningococci Z22.31
  Salmonella typhosa Z22.Ø
  serum hepatitis — *see* Carrier, hepatitis
  staphylococci (Methicillin susceptible) Z22.321
    Methicillin resistant Z22.322
  streptococci Z22.338
    group B Z22.33Ø
      complicating pregnancy or delivery O99.82- ☑
  syphilis Z22.4
  typhoid Z22.Ø
  venereal disease NEC Z22.4
Carrion's disease A44.Ø
Carter's relapsing fever (Asiatic) A68.1
Cartilage — *see* condition
Caruncle (inflamed)
  conjunctiva (acute) — *see* Conjunctivitis, acute
  labium (majus) (minus) N9Ø.89
  lacrimal — *see* Inflammation, lacrimal, passages
  myrtiform N89.8
  urethral (benign) N36.2
Cascade stomach K31.2
Caseation lymphatic gland (tuberculous) A18.2
Cassidy (-Scholte) syndrome (malignant carcinoid) E34.Ø
Castellani's disease A69.8
Castration, traumatic, male S38.231 ☑
Casts in urine R82.998
Cat
  cry syndrome Q93.4
  ear Q17.3
  eye syndrome Q92.8
Catabolism, senile R54
Catalepsy (hysterical) F44.2
  schizophrenic F2Ø.2
Cataplexy (idiopathic) — *see* Narcolepsy
Cataract (cortical) (immature) (incipient) H26.9
  with
    neovascularization — *see* Cataract, complicated
  age-related — *see* Cataract, senile
  anterior
    and posterior axial embryonal Q12.Ø
    pyramidal Q12.Ø
  associated with
    galactosemia E74.21 *[H28]*
    myotonic disorders G71.19 *[H28]*
  blue Q12.Ø
  central Q12.Ø
  cerulean Q12.Ø
  complicated H26.2Ø
    with
      neovascularization H26.21- ☑
      ocular disorder H26.22- ☑
    glaucomatous flecks H26.23- ☑
  congenital Q12.Ø
  coraliform Q12.Ø
  coronary Q12.Ø
  crystalline Q12.Ø
  diabetic — *see* Diabetes, cataract
  drug-induced H26.3- ☑
  due to
    ocular disorder — *see* Cataract, complicated
    radiation H26.8
  electric H26.8
  extraction status Z98.4- ☑
  glass-blower's H26.8
  heat ray H26.8
  heterochromic — *see* Cataract, complicated
  hypermature — *see* Cataract, senile, morgagnian type
  in (due to)
    chronic iridocyclitis — *see* Cataract, complicated
    diabetes — *see* Diabetes, cataract
    endocrine disease E34.9 *[H28]*
    eye disease — *see* Cataract, complicated
    hypoparathyroidism E2Ø.9 *[H28]*
    malnutrition-dehydration E46 *[H28]*
    metabolic disease E88.9 *[H28]*
    myotonic disorders G71.19 *[H28]*

Cataract — *continued*
  in — *continued*
    nutritional disease E63.9 *[H28]*
  infantile — *see* Cataract, presenile
  irradiational — *see* Cataract, specified NEC
  juvenile — *see* Cataract, presenile
  malnutrition-dehydration E46 *[H28]*
  morgagnian — *see* Cataract, senile, morgagnian type
  myotonic G71.19 *[H28]*
  myxedema EØ3.9 *[H28]*
  nuclear
    embryonal Q12.Ø
    sclerosis — *see* Cataract, senile, nuclear
  presenile H26.ØØ- ☑
    combined forms H26.Ø6- ☑
    cortical H26.Ø1- ☑
    lamellar — *see* Cataract, presenile, cortical
    nuclear H26.Ø3- ☑
    specified NEC H26.Ø9
    subcapsular polar (anterior) H26.Ø4- ☑
      posterior H26.Ø5- ☑
    zonular — *see* Cataract, presenile, cortical
  secondary H26.4Ø
    Soemmering's ring H26.41- ☑
    specified NEC H26.49- ☑
    to eye disease — *see* Cataract, complicated
  senile H25.9
    brunescens — *see* Cataract, senile, nuclear
    combined forms H25.81- ☑
    coronary — *see* Cataract, senile, incipient
    cortical H25.Ø1- ☑
    hypermature — *see* Cataract, senile, morgagnian type
    incipient (mature) (total) H25.Ø9- ☑
      cortical — *see* Cataract, senile, cortical
      subcapsular — *see* Cataract, senile, subcapsular
    morgagnian type (hypermature) H25.2- ☑
    nuclear (sclerosis) H25.1- ☑
    polar subcapsular (anterior) (posterior) — *see* Cataract, senile, incipient
    punctate — *see* Cataract, senile, incipient
    specified NEC H25.89
    subcapsular polar (anterior) H25.Ø3- ☑
      posterior H25.Ø4- ☑
  snowflake — *see* Diabetes, cataract
  specified NEC H26.8
  toxic — *see* Cataract, drug-induced
  traumatic H26.1Ø- ☑
    localized H26.11- ☑
    partially resolved H26.12- ☑
    total H26.13- ☑
  zonular (perinuclear) Q12.Ø
Cataracta — *see also* Cataract
  brunescens — *see* Cataract, senile, nuclear
  centralis pulverulenta Q12.Ø
  cerulea Q12.Ø
  complicata — *see* Cataract, complicated
  congenita Q12.Ø
  coralliformis Q12.Ø
  coronaria Q12.Ø
  diabetic — *see* Diabetes, cataract
  membranacea
    accreta — *see* Cataract, secondary
    congenita Q12.Ø
  nigra — *see* Cataract, senile, nuclear
  sunflower — *see* Cataract, complicated
Catarrh, catarrhal (acute) (febrile) (infectious) (inflammation) — *see also* condition JØØ
  bronchial — *see* Bronchitis
  chest — *see* Bronchitis
  chronic J31.Ø
  due to congenital syphilis A5Ø.Ø3
  enteric — *see* Enteritis
  eustachian H68.ØØ9
  fauces — *see* Pharyngitis
  gastrointestinal — *see* Enteritis
  gingivitis KØ5.ØØ
    nonplaque induced KØ5.Ø1
    plaque induced KØ5.ØØ
  hay — *see* Fever, hay
  intestinal — *see* Enteritis
  larynx, chronic J37.Ø
  liver B15.9
    with hepatic coma B15.Ø
  lung — *see* Bronchitis
  middle ear, chronic — *see* Otitis, media, nonsuppurative, chronic, serous

Catarrh, catarrhal — *continued*
  mouth K12.1
  nasal (chronic) — *see* Rhinitis
  nasobronchial J31.1
  nasopharyngeal (chronic) J31.1
    acute JØØ
  pulmonary — *see* Bronchitis
  spring (eye) (vernal) — *see* Conjunctivitis, acute, atopic
  summer (hay) — *see* Fever, hay
  throat J31.2
  tubotympanal — *see also* Otitis, media, nonsuppurative
    chronic — *see* Otitis, media, nonsuppurative, chronic, serous
Catatonia (schizophrenic) F2Ø.2
Catatonic
  disorder due to known physiologic condition FØ6.1
  schizophrenia F2Ø.2
  stupor R4Ø.1
Cat-scratch — *see also* Abrasion
  disease or fever A28.1
Cauda equina — *see* condition
Cauliflower ear M95.1- ☑
Causalgia (upper limb) G56.4- ☑
  lower limb G57.7- ☑
Cause
  external, general effects T75.89 ☑
Caustic burn — *see* Corrosion, by site
Cavare's disease (familial periodic paralysis) G72.3
Cave-in, injury
  crushing (severe) — *see* Crush
  suffocation — *see* Asphyxia, traumatic, due to low oxygen, due to cave-in
Cavernitis (penis) N48.29
Cavernositis N48.29
Cavernous — *see* condition
Cavitation of lung — *see also* Tuberculosis, pulmonary
  nontuberculous J98.4
Cavities, dental — *see* Caries, dental
Cavity
  lung — *see* Cavitation of lung
  optic papilla Q14.2
  pulmonary — *see* Cavitation of lung
Cavovarus foot, congenital Q66.1- ☑
Cavus foot (congenital) Q66.7- ☑
  acquired — *see* Deformity, limb, foot, specified NEC
Cazenave's disease L1Ø.2
CDKL5 (Cyclin-Dependent Kinase-Like 5 Deficiency Disorder) G4Ø.42
Cecitis K52.9
  with perforation, peritonitis, or rupture K65.8
Cecoureterocele Q62.32
Cecum — *see* condition
Celiac
  artery compression syndrome I77.4
  disease (with steatorrhea) K9Ø.Ø
  infantilism K9Ø.Ø
Cell(s), cellular — *see also* condition
  in urine R82.998
Cellulitis (diffuse) (phlegmonous) (septic) (suppurative) LØ3.9Ø
  abdominal wall LØ3.311
  anaerobic A48.Ø
  ankle — *see* Cellulitis, lower limb
  anus K61.Ø
  arm — *see* Cellulitis, upper limb
  auricle (ear) — *see* Cellulitis, ear
  axilla LØ3.11- ☑
  back (any part) LØ3.312
  breast (acute) (nonpuerperal) (subacute) N61.Ø
    nipple N61.Ø
  broad ligament
    acute N73.Ø
  buttock LØ3.317
  cervical (meaning neck) LØ3.221
  cervix (uteri) — *see* Cervicitis
  cheek (external) LØ3.211
    internal K12.2
  chest wall LØ3.313
  chronic LØ3.9Ø
  clostridial A48.Ø
  corpus cavernosum N48.22
  digit
    finger — *see* Cellulitis, finger
    toe — *see* Cellulitis, toe
  Douglas' cul-de-sac or pouch
    acute N73.Ø
  drainage site (following operation) T81.49 ☑

- **Cellulitis** — *continued*
  - ear (external) H6Ø.1- ☑
  - eosinophilic (granulomatous) L98.3
  - erysipelatous — *see* Erysipelas
  - external auditory canal — *see* Cellulitis, ear
  - eyelid — *see* Abscess, eyelid
  - face NEC LØ3.211
  - finger (intrathecal) (periosteal) (subcutaneous) (subcuticular) LØ3.Ø1- ☑
  - foot — *see* Cellulitis, lower limb
  - gangrenous — *see* Gangrene
  - genital organ NEC
    - female (external) N76.4
    - male N49.9
      - multiple sites N49.8
      - specified NEC N49.8
  - gluteal (region) LØ3.317
  - gonococcal A54.89
  - groin LØ3.314
  - hand — *see* Cellulitis, upper limb
  - head NEC LØ3.811
    - face (any part, except ear, eye and nose) LØ3.211
  - heel — *see* Cellulitis, lower limb
  - hip — *see* Cellulitis, lower limb
  - jaw (region) LØ3.211
  - knee — *see* Cellulitis, lower limb
  - labium (majus) (minus) — *see* Vulvitis
  - lacrimal passages — *see* Inflammation, lacrimal, passages
  - larynx J38.7
  - leg — *see* Cellulitis, lower limb
  - lip K13.Ø
  - lower limb LØ3.11- ☑
    - toe — *see* Cellulitis, toe
  - mouth (floor) K12.2
  - multiple sites, so stated LØ3.9Ø
  - nasopharynx J39.1
  - navel LØ3.316
    - newborn P38.9
      - with mild hemorrhage P38.1
      - without hemorrhage P38.9
  - neck (region) LØ3.221
  - nipple (acute) (nonpuerperal) (subacute) N61.Ø
  - nose (septum) (external) J34.Ø
  - orbit, orbital HØ5.Ø1- ☑
  - palate (soft) K12.2
  - pectoral (region) LØ3.313
  - pelvis, pelvic (chronic)
    - female — *see also* Disease, pelvis, inflammatory N73.2
      - acute N73.Ø
    - following ectopic or molar pregnancy OØ8.Ø
    - male K65.Ø
  - penis N48.22
  - perineal, perineum LØ3.315
  - periorbital LØ3.213
  - perirectal K61.1
  - peritonsillar J36
  - periurethral N34.Ø
  - periuterine — *see also* Disease, pelvis, inflammatory N73.2
    - acute N73.Ø
  - pharynx J39.1
  - preseptal LØ3.213
  - rectum K61.1
  - retroperitoneal K68.9
  - round ligament
    - acute N73.Ø
  - scalp (any part) LØ3.811
  - scrotum N49.2
  - seminal vesicle N49.Ø
  - shoulder — *see* Cellulitis, upper limb
  - specified site NEC LØ3.818
  - submandibular (region) (space) (triangle) K12.2
    - gland K11.3
  - submaxillary (region) K12.2
    - gland K11.3
  - thigh — *see* Cellulitis, lower limb
  - thumb (intrathecal) (periosteal) (subcutaneous) (subcuticular) — *see* Cellulitis, finger
  - toe (intrathecal) (periosteal) (subcutaneous) (subcuticular) LØ3.Ø3- ☑
  - tonsil J36
  - trunk LØ3.319
    - abdominal wall LØ3.311
    - back (any part) LØ3.312
    - buttock LØ3.317
    - chest wall LØ3.313

- **Cellulitis** — *continued*
  - trunk — *continued*
    - groin LØ3.314
    - perineal, perineum LØ3.315
    - umbilicus LØ3.316
  - tuberculous (primary) A18.4
  - umbilicus LØ3.316
  - upper limb LØ3.11- ☑
    - axilla — *see* Cellulitis, axilla
    - finger — *see* Cellulitis, finger
    - thumb — *see* Cellulitis, finger
  - vaccinal T88.Ø ☑
  - vocal cord J38.3
  - vulva — *see* Vulvitis
  - wrist — *see* Cellulitis, upper limb
- **Cementoblastoma, benign** — *see* Cyst, calcifying odontogenic
- **Cementoma** — *see* Cyst, calcifying odontogenic
- **Cementoperiostitis** — *see* Periodontitis
- **Cementosis** KØ3.4
- **Central auditory processing disorder** H93.25
- **Central pain syndrome** G89.Ø
- **Cephalematocele, cephal** (o)hematocele
  - newborn P52.8
    - birth injury P1Ø.8
  - traumatic — *see* Hematoma, brain
- **Cephalematoma, cephalhematoma** (calcified)
  - newborn (birth injury) P12.Ø
  - traumatic — *see* Hematoma, brain
- **Cephalgia, cephalalgia** — *see also* Headache
  - histamine G44.ØØ9
    - intractable G44.ØØ1
    - not intractable G44.ØØ9
  - trigeminal autonomic (TAC) NEC G44.Ø99
    - intractable G44.Ø91
    - not intractable G44.Ø99
- **Cephalic** — *see* condition
- **Cephalitis** — *see* Encephalitis
- **Cephalocele** — *see* Encephalocele
- **Cephalomenia** N94.89
- **Cephalopelvic** — *see* condition
- **Cerclage** (with cervical incompetence) in pregnancy — *see* Incompetence, cervix, in pregnancy
- **Cerebellitis** — *see* Encephalitis
- **Cerebellum, cerebellar** — *see* condition
- **Cerebral** — *see* condition
- **Cerebritis** — *see* Encephalitis
- **Cerebro-hepato-renal syndrome** Q87.89
- **Cerebromalacia** — *see* Softening, brain
  - sequelae of cerebrovascular disease I69.398
- **Cerebroside lipidosis** E75.22
- **Cerebrospasticity** (congenital) G8Ø.1
- **Cerebrospinal** — *see* condition
- **Cerebrum** — *see* condition
- **Ceroid-lipofuscinosis, neuronal** E75.4
- **Cerumen** (accumulation) (impacted) H61.2- ☑
- **Cervical** — *see also* condition
  - auricle Q18.2
  - dysplasia in pregnancy — *see* Abnormal, cervix, in pregnancy or childbirth
  - erosion in pregnancy — *see* Abnormal, cervix, in pregnancy or childbirth
  - fibrosis in pregnancy — *see* Abnormal, cervix, in pregnancy or childbirth
  - fusion syndrome Q76.1
  - rib Q76.5
  - shortening (complicating pregnancy) O26.87- ☑
- **Cervicalgia** M54.2
- **Cervicitis** (acute) (atrophic) (chronic) (nonvenereal) (senile) (subacute) (with ulceration) N72
  - with
    - abortion — *see* Abortion, by type complicated by genital tract and pelvic infection
    - ectopic pregnancy OØ8.Ø
    - molar pregnancy OØ8.Ø
  - chlamydial A56.Ø9
  - gonococcal A54.Ø3
  - herpesviral A6Ø.Ø3
  - puerperal (postpartum) O86.11
  - syphilitic A52.76
  - trichomonal A59.Ø9
  - tuberculous A18.16
- **Cervicocolpitis** (emphysematosa) — *see also* Cervicitis N72
- **Cervix** — *see* condition
- **Cesarean delivery, previous, affecting management of pregnancy** O34.219

- **Cesarean delivery, previous, affecting management of pregnancy** — *continued*
  - classical (vertical) scar O34.212
  - isthmocele (non-pregnant state) N85.A
    - maternal care for O34.22
  - low transverse scar O34.211
  - mid-transverse T incision O34.218
  - scar
    - defect (non-pregnant state) N85.A
      - maternal care for O34.22
    - specified type NEC O34.218
- **Céstan** (-Chenais) paralysis or syndrome G46.3
- **Céstan-Raymond syndrome** I65.8
- **Cestode infestation** B71.9
  - specified type NEC B71.8
- **Cestodiasis** B71.9
- **Chabert's disease** A22.9
- **Chacaleh** E53.8
- **Chafing** L3Ø.4
- **Chagas'** (-Mazza) disease (chronic) B57.2
  - with
    - cardiovascular involvement NEC B57.2
    - digestive system involvement B57.3Ø
      - megacolon B57.32
      - megaesophagus B57.31
      - other specified B57.39
    - megacolon B57.32
    - megaesophagus B57.31
    - myocarditis B57.2
    - nervous system involvement B57.4Ø
      - meningitis B57.41
      - meningoencephalitis B57.42
      - other specified B57.49
    - specified organ involvement NEC B57.5
  - acute (with) B57.1
    - cardiovascular NEC B57.Ø
    - myocarditis B57.Ø
- **Chagres fever** B5Ø.9
- **Chairridden** Z74.Ø9
- **Chalasia** (cardiac sphincter) K21.9
- **Chalazion** HØØ.19
  - left HØØ.16
    - lower HØØ.15
    - upper HØØ.14
  - right HØØ.13
    - lower HØØ.12
    - upper HØØ.11
- **Chalcosis** — *see also* Disorder, globe, degenerative, chalcosis
  - cornea — *see* Deposit, cornea
  - crystalline lens — *see* Cataract, complicated
  - retina H35.89
- **Chalicosis** (pulmonum) J62.8
- **Chancre** (any genital site) (hard) (hunterian) (mixed) (primary) (seronegative) (seropositive) (syphilitic) A51.Ø
  - congenital A5Ø.Ø7
  - conjunctiva NEC A51.2
  - Ducrey's A57
  - extragenital A51.2
  - eyelid A51.2
  - lip A51.2
  - nipple A51.2
  - Nisbet's A57
  - of
    - carate A67.Ø
    - pinta A67.Ø
    - yaws A66.Ø
  - palate, soft A51.2
  - phagedenic A57
  - simple A57
  - soft A57
    - bubo A57
    - palate A51.2
  - urethra A51.Ø
  - yaws A66.Ø
- **Chancroid** (anus) (genital) (penis) (perineum) (rectum) (urethra) (vulva) A57
- **Chandler's disease** (osteochondritis dissecans, hip) — *see* Osteochondritis, dissecans, hip
- **Change**(s) (in) (of) — *see also* Removal
  - arteriosclerotic — *see* Arteriosclerosis
  - bone — *see also* Disorder, bone
    - diabetic — *see* Diabetes, bone change
  - bowel habit R19.4
  - cardiorenal (vascular) — *see* Hypertension, cardiorenal
  - cardiovascular — *see* Disease, cardiovascular
  - circulatory I99.9

Change(s) — *continued*
- cognitive (mild) (organic) R41.89
- color, tooth, teeth
  - during formation KØØ.8
  - posteruptive KØ3.7
- contraceptive device Z3Ø.433
- corneal membrane H18.3Ø
  - Bowman's membrane fold or rupture H18.31- ☑
  - Descemet's membrane
    - fold H18.32- ☑
    - rupture H18.33- ☑
- coronary — *see* Disease, heart, ischemic
- degenerative, spine or vertebra — *see* Spondylosis
- dental pulp, regressive KØ4.2
- dressing (nonsurgical) Z48.ØØ
  - surgical Z48.Ø1
- heart — *see* Disease, heart
- hip joint — *see* Derangement, joint, hip
- hyperplastic larynx J38.7
- hypertrophic
  - nasal sinus J34.89
  - turbinate, nasal J34.3
  - upper respiratory tract J39.8
- indwelling catheter Z46.6
- inflammatory — *see also* Inflammation
  - sacroiliac M46.1
- job, anxiety concerning Z56.1
- joint — *see* Derangement, joint
- life — *see* Menopause
- mental status R41.82
- minimal (glomerular) — *see also* NØØ-NØ7 with fourth character .Ø NØ5.Ø
- myocardium, myocardial — *see* Degeneration, myocardial
- of life — *see* Menopause
- pacemaker Z45.Ø18
  - pulse generator Z45.Ø1Ø
- personality (enduring) F68.8
  - due to (secondary to)
    - general medical condition FØ7.Ø
  - secondary (nonspecific) F6Ø.89
- regressive, dental pulp KØ4.2
- renal — *see* Disease, renal
- retina H35.9
  - myopic — *see also* Myopia, degenerative H44.2- ☑
- sacroiliac joint M53.3
- senile — *see also* condition R54
- sensory R2Ø.8
- skin R23.9
  - acute, due to ultraviolet radiation L56.9
    - specified NEC L56.8
  - chronic, due to nonionizing radiation L57.9
    - specified NEC L57.8
  - cyanosis R23.Ø
  - flushing R23.2
  - pallor R23.1
  - petechiae R23.3
  - specified change NEC R23.8
  - swelling — *see* Mass, localized
  - texture R23.4
- trophic
  - arm — *see* Mononeuropathy, upper limb
  - leg — *see* Mononeuropathy, lower limb
- vascular I99.9
- vasomotor I73.9
- voice R49.9
  - psychogenic F44.4
  - specified NEC R49.8

Changing sleep-work schedule, affecting sleep G47.26
Changuinola fever A93.1
Chapping skin T69.8 ☑
Charcot-Marie-Tooth disease, paralysis or syndrome G6Ø.Ø
Charcot's
- arthropathy — *see* Arthropathy, neuropathic
- cirrhosis K74.3
- disease (tabetic arthropathy) A52.16
- joint (disease) (tabetic) A52.16
  - diabetic — *see* Diabetes, with, arthropathy
  - syringomyelic G95.Ø
- syndrome (intermittent claudication) I73.9

CHARGE association Q89.8
Charley-horse (quadriceps) M62.831
- traumatic (quadriceps) S76.11- ☑

Charlouis' disease — *see* Yaws
Cheadle's disease E54
Checking (of)
- cardiac pacemaker (battery) (electrode(s)) Z45.Ø18
  - pulse generator Z45.Ø1Ø
- implantable subdermal contraceptive Z3Ø.46
- intrauterine contraceptive device Z3Ø.431
- wound Z48.Ø- ☑
  - due to injury — code to Injury, by site, using appropriate seventh character for subsequent encounter

Check-up — *see* Examination
Chédiak-Higashi (-Steinbrinck) **syndrome** (congenital gigantism of peroxidase granules) E7Ø.33Ø
Cheek — *see* condition
Cheese itch B88.Ø
Cheese-washer's lung J67.8
Cheese-worker's lung J67.8
Cheilitis (acute) (angular) (catarrhal) (chronic) (exfoliative) (gangrenous) (glandular) (infectional) (suppurative) (ulcerative) (vesicular) K13.Ø
- actinic (due to sun) L56.8
  - other than from sun L59.8
- candidal B37.83

Cheilodynia K13.Ø
Cheiloschisis — *see* Cleft, lip
Cheilosis (angular) K13.Ø
- with pellagra E52
- due to
  - vitamin B2 (riboflavin) deficiency E53.Ø

Cheiromegaly M79.89
Cheiropompholyx L3Ø.1
Cheloid — *see* Keloid
Chemical burn — *see* Corrosion, by site
Chemodectoma — *see* Paraganglioma, nonchromaffin
Chemosis, conjunctiva — *see* Edema, conjunctiva
Chemotherapy (session) (for)
- cancer Z51.11
- neoplasm Z51.11

Cherubism M27.8
Chest — *see* condition
Cheyne-Stokes breathing (respiration) RØ6.3
Chiari's
- disease or syndrome (hepatic vein thrombosis) I82.Ø
- malformation
  - type I G93.5
  - type II — *see* Spina bifida
- net Q24.8

Chicago disease B4Ø.9
Chickenpox — *see* Varicella
Chiclero ulcer or sore B55.1
Chigger (infestation) B88.Ø
Chignon (disease) B36.8
- newborn (from vacuum extraction) (birth injury) P12.1

Chilaiditi's syndrome (subphrenic displacement, colon) Q43.3
Chilblain(s) (lupus) T69.1 ☑
Child
- custody dispute Z65.3

Childbirth — *see* Delivery
Childhood
- cerebral X-linked adrenoleukodystrophy E71.52Ø
- period of rapid growth ZØØ.2

Chill(s) R68.83
- with fever R5Ø.9
- congestive in malarial regions B54
- without fever R68.83

Chilomastigiasis AØ7.8
Chimera 46,XX/46,XY Q99.Ø
Chin — *see* condition
Chinese dysentery AØ3.9
Chionophobia F4Ø.228
Chitral fever A93.1
Chlamydia, chlamydial A74.9
- cervicitis A56.Ø9
- conjunctivitis A74.Ø
- cystitis A56.Ø1
- endometritis A56.11
- epididymitis A56.19
- female
  - pelvic inflammatory disease A56.11
  - pelviperitonitis A56.11
- orchitis A56.19
- peritonitis A74.81
- pharyngitis A56.4
- proctitis A56.3
- psittaci (infection) A7Ø
- salpingitis A56.11
- sexually-transmitted infection NEC A56.8

Chlamydia, chlamydial — *continued*
- specified NEC A74.89
- urethritis A56.Ø1
- vulvovaginitis A56.Ø2

Chlamydiosis — *see* Chlamydia
Chloasma (skin) (idiopathic) (symptomatic) L81.1
- eyelid HØ2.719
  - hyperthyroid EØ5.9Ø *[HØ2.719]*
    - with thyroid storm EØ5.91 *[HØ2.719]*
  - left HØ2.716
    - lower HØ2.715
    - upper HØ2.714
  - right HØ2.713
    - lower HØ2.712
    - upper HØ2.711

Chloroma C92.3- ☑
Chlorosis D5Ø.9
- Egyptian B76.9 *[D63.8]*
- miner's B76.9 *[D63.8]*

Chlorotic anemia D5Ø.8
Chocolate cyst (ovary) N8Ø.1Ø- ☑
Choked
- disc or disk — *see* Papilledema
- on food, phlegm, or vomitus NOS — *see* Foreign body, by site
- while vomiting NOS — *see* Foreign body, by site

Chokes (resulting from bends) T7Ø.3 ☑
Choking sensation RØ9.89
Cholangiectasis K83.8
Cholangiocarcinoma
- with hepatocellular carcinoma, combined C22.Ø
- liver C22.1
- specified site NEC — *see* Neoplasm, malignant, by site
- unspecified site C22.1

Cholangiohepatitis K83.8
- due to fluke infestation B66.1

Cholangiohepatoma C22.Ø
Cholangiolitis (acute) (chronic) (extrahepatic) (gangrenous) (intrahepatic) K83.Ø9
- paratyphoidal — *see* Fever, paratyphoid
- typhoidal AØ1.Ø9

Cholangioma D13.4
- malignant — *see* Cholangiocarcinoma

Cholangitis (ascending) (recurrent) (secondary) (stenosing) (suppurative) K83.Ø9
- with calculus, bile duct — *see* Calculus, bile duct, with cholangitis
- chronic nonsuppurative destructive K74.3
- primary K83.Ø9
  - sclerosing K83.Ø1
- sclerosing K83.Ø9

Cholecystectasia K82.8
Cholecystitis K81.9
- with
  - calculus, stones in
    - bile duct (common) (hepatic) — *see* Calculus, bile duct, with cholecystitis
    - cystic duct — *see* Calculus, gallbladder, with cholecystitis
    - gallbladder — *see* Calculus, gallbladder, with cholecystitis
  - choledocholithiasis — *see* Calculus, bile duct, with cholecystitis
  - cholelithiasis — *see* Calculus, gallbladder, with cholecystitis
  - gangrene of gallbladder K82.A1
  - perforation of gallbladder K82.A2
- acute (emphysematous) (gangrenous) (suppurative) K81.Ø
  - with
    - calculus, stones in
      - cystic duct — *see* Calculus, gallbladder, with cholecystitis, acute
      - gallbladder — *see* Calculus, gallbladder, with cholecystitis, acute
    - choledocholithiasis — *see* Calculus, bile duct, with cholecystitis, acute
    - cholelithiasis — *see* Calculus, gallbladder, with cholecystitis, acute
    - chronic cholecystitis K81.2
      - with gallbladder calculus K8Ø.12
        - with obstruction K8Ø.13
- chronic K81.1
  - with acute cholecystitis K81.2
    - with gallbladder calculus K8Ø.12
      - with obstruction K8Ø.13
- emphysematous (acute) — *see* Cholecystitis, acute

- **Cholecystitis** — *continued*
  - gangrenous — *see* Cholecystitis, acute
  - paratyphoidal, current AØ1.4
  - suppurative — *see* Cholecystitis, acute
  - typhoidal AØ1.Ø9
- **Cholecystolithiasis** — *see* Calculus, gallbladder
- **Choledochitis** (suppurative) K83.Ø9
- **Choledocholith** — *see* Calculus, bile duct
- **Choledocholithiasis** (common duct) (hepatic duct) — *see* Calculus, bile duct
  - cystic — *see* Calculus, gallbladder
  - typhoidal AØ1.Ø9
- **Cholelithiasis** (cystic duct) (gallbladder) (impacted) (multiple) — *see* Calculus, gallbladder
  - bile duct (common) (hepatic) — *see* Calculus, bile duct
  - hepatic duct — *see* Calculus, bile duct
  - specified NEC K8Ø.8Ø
    - with obstruction K8Ø.81
- **Cholemia** — *see also* Jaundice
  - familial (simple) (congenital) E8Ø.4
  - Gilbert's E8Ø.4
- **Choleperitoneum, choleperitonitis** K65.3
- **Cholera** (Asiatic) (epidemic) (malignant) AØØ.9
  - antimonial — *see* Poisoning, antimony
  - classical AØØ.Ø
  - due to Vibrio cholerae Ø1 AØØ.9
    - biovar cholerae AØØ.Ø
    - biovar eltor AØØ.1
    - el tor AØØ.1
  - el tor AØØ.1
- **Cholerine** — *see* Cholera
- **Cholestasis NEC** K83.1
  - with hepatocyte injury K71.Ø
  - due to total parenteral nutrition (TPN) K76.89
  - pure K71.Ø
- **Cholesteatoma** (ear) (middle) (with reaction) H71.9- ☑
  - attic H71.Ø- ☑
  - external ear (canal) H6Ø.4- ☑
  - mastoid H71.2- ☑
  - postmastoidectomy cavity (recurrent) — *see* Complications, postmastoidectomy, recurrent cholesteatoma
  - recurrent (postmastoidectomy) — *see* Complications, postmastoidectomy, recurrent cholesteatoma
  - tympanum H71.1- ☑
- **Cholesteatosis, diffuse** H71.3- ☑
- **Cholesteremia** E78.ØØ
- **Cholesterin in vitreous** — *see* Deposit, crystalline
- **Cholesterol**
  - deposit
    - retina H35.89
    - vitreous — *see* Deposit, crystalline
  - elevated (high) E78.ØØ
    - with elevated (high) triglycerides E78.2
    - screening for Z13.22Ø
  - imbibition of gallbladder K82.4
- **Cholesterolemia** (essential) (pure) E78.ØØ
  - familial E78.Ø1
  - hereditary E78.Ø1
- **Cholesterolosis, cholesterosis** (gallbladder) K82.4
  - cerebrotendinous E75.5
- **Cholocolic fistula** K82.3
- **Choluria** R82.2
- **Chondritis** M94.8X9
  - aurical H61.Ø3- ☑
  - costal (Tietze's) M94.Ø
  - external ear H61.Ø3- ☑
  - patella, posttraumatic — *see* Chondromalacia, patella
  - pinna H61.Ø3- ☑
  - purulent M94.8X- ☑
  - tuberculous NEC A18.Ø2
    - intervertebral A18.Ø1
- **Chondroblastoma** — *see also* Neoplasm, bone, benign
  - malignant — *see* Neoplasm, bone, malignant
- **Chondrocalcinosis** M11.2Ø
  - ankle M11.27- ☑
  - elbow M11.22- ☑
  - familial M11.1Ø
    - ankle M11.17- ☑
    - elbow M11.12- ☑
    - foot joint M11.17- ☑
    - hand joint M11.14- ☑
    - hip M11.15- ☑
    - knee M11.16- ☑
    - multiple site M11.19
    - shoulder M11.11- ☑
    - vertebrae M11.18
- **Chondrocalcinosis** — *continued*
  - familial — *continued*
    - wrist M11.13- ☑
  - foot joint M11.27- ☑
  - hand joint M11.24- ☑
  - hip M11.25- ☑
  - knee M11.26- ☑
  - multiple site M11.29
  - shoulder M11.21- ☑
  - specified type NEC M11.2Ø
    - ankle M11.27- ☑
    - elbow M11.22- ☑
    - foot joint M11.27- ☑
    - hand joint M11.24- ☑
    - hip M11.25- ☑
    - knee M11.26- ☑
    - multiple site M11.29
    - shoulder M11.21- ☑
    - vertebrae M11.28
    - wrist M11.23- ☑
  - vertebrae M11.28
  - wrist M11.23- ☑
- **Chondrodermatitis nodularis helicis or anthelicis** — *see* Perichondritis, ear
- **Chondrodysplasia** Q78.9
  - with hemangioma Q78.4
  - calcificans congenita Q77.3
  - fetalis Q77.4
  - metaphyseal (Jansen's) (McKusick's) (Schmid's) Q78.8
  - punctata Q77.3
- **Chondrodystrophy, chondrodystrophia** (familial) (fetalis) (hypoplastic) Q78.9
  - calcificans congenita Q77.3
  - myotonic (congenital) G71.13
  - punctata Q77.3
- **Chondroectodermal dysplasia** Q77.6
- **Chondrogenesis imperfecta** Q77.4
- **Chondrolysis** M94.35- ☑
- **Chondroma** — *see also* Neoplasm, cartilage, benign
  - juxtacortical — *see* Neoplasm, bone, benign
  - periosteal — *see* Neoplasm, bone, benign
- **Chondromalacia** (systemic) M94.2Ø
  - acromioclavicular joint M94.21- ☑
  - ankle M94.27- ☑
  - elbow M94.22- ☑
  - foot joint M94.27- ☑
  - glenohumeral joint M94.21- ☑
  - hand joint M94.24- ☑
  - hip M94.25- ☑
  - knee M94.26- ☑
    - patella M22.4- ☑
  - multiple sites M94.29
  - patella M22.4- ☑
  - rib M94.28
  - sacroiliac joint M94.259
  - shoulder M94.21- ☑
  - sternoclavicular joint M94.21- ☑
  - vertebral joint M94.28
  - wrist M94.23- ☑
- **Chondromatosis** — *see also* Neoplasm, cartilage, uncertain behavior
  - internal Q78.4
- **Chondromyxosarcoma** — *see* Neoplasm, cartilage, malignant
- **Chondro-osteodysplasia** (Morquio-Brailsford type) E76.219
- **Chondro-osteodystrophy** E76.29
- **Chondro-osteoma** — *see* Neoplasm, bone, benign
- **Chondropathia tuberosa** M94.Ø
- **Chondrosarcoma** — *see* Neoplasm, cartilage, malignant
  - juxtacortical — *see* Neoplasm, bone, malignant
  - mesenchymal — *see* Neoplasm, connective tissue, malignant
  - myxoid — *see* Neoplasm, cartilage, malignant
- **Chordee** (nonvenereal) N48.89
  - congenital Q54.4
  - gonococcal A54.Ø9
- **Chorditis** (fibrinous) (nodosa) (tuberosa) J38.2
- **Chordoma** — *see* Neoplasm, vertebral (column), malignant
- **Chorea** (chronic) (gravis) (posthemiplegic) (senile) (spasmodic) G25.5
  - with
    - heart involvement IØ2.Ø
      - active or acute (conditions in IØ1-) IØ2.Ø
      - rheumatic IØ2.9
        - with valvular disorder IØ2.Ø
- **Chorea** — *continued*
  - with — *continued*
    - rheumatic heart disease (chronic) (inactive) (quiescent) — *code to* rheumatic heart condition involved
  - drug-induced G25.4
  - habit F95.8
  - hereditary G1Ø
  - Huntington's G1Ø
  - hysterical F44.4
  - minor IØ2.9
    - with heart involvement IØ2.Ø
  - progressive G25.5
    - hereditary G1Ø
  - rheumatic (chronic) IØ2.9
    - with heart involvement IØ2.Ø
  - Sydenham's IØ2.9
    - with heart involvement — *see* Chorea, with rheumatic heart disease
    - nonrheumatic G25.5
- **Choreoathetosis** (paroxysmal) G25.5
- **Chorioadenoma** (destruens) D39.2
- **Chorioamnionitis** O41.12- ☑
- **Chorioangioma** D26.7
- **Choriocarcinoma** — *see* Neoplasm, malignant, by site
  - combined with
    - embryonal carcinoma — *see* Neoplasm, malignant, by site
    - other germ cell elements — *see* Neoplasm, malignant, by site
    - teratoma — *see* Neoplasm, malignant, by site
  - specified site — *see* Neoplasm, malignant, by site
  - unspecified site
    - female C58
    - male C62.9Ø
- **Chorioencephalitis** (acute) (lymphocytic) (serous) A87.2
- **Chorioepithelioma** — *see* Choriocarcinoma
- **Choriomeningitis** (acute) (lymphocytic) (serous) A87.2
- **Chorionepithelioma** — *see* Choriocarcinoma
- **Chorioretinitis** — *see also* Inflammation, chorioretinal
  - disseminated — *see also* Inflammation, chorioretinal, disseminated
    - in neurosyphilis A52.19
  - Egyptian B76.9 *[D63.8]*
  - focal — *see also* Inflammation, chorioretinal, focal
  - histoplasmic B39.9 *[H32]*
  - in (due to)
    - histoplasmosis B39.9 *[H32]*
    - syphilis (secondary) A51.43
      - late A52.71
    - toxoplasmosis (acquired) B58.Ø1
      - congenital (active) P37.1 *[H32]*
    - tuberculosis A18.53
  - juxtapapillary, juxtapapillaris — *see* Inflammation, chorioretinal, focal, juxtapapillary
  - leprous A3Ø.9 *[H32]*
  - miner's B76.9 *[D63.8]*
  - progressive myopia (degeneration) — *see also* Myopia, degenerative H44.2- ☑
  - syphilitic (secondary) A51.43
    - congenital (early) A5Ø.Ø1 *[H32]*
      - late A5Ø.32
    - late A52.71
  - tuberculous A18.53
- **Chorioretinopathy, central serous** H35.71- ☑
- **Choroid** — *see* condition
- **Choroideremia** H31.21
- **Choroiditis** — *see* Chorioretinitis
- **Choroidopathy** — *see* Disorder, choroid
- **Choroidoretinitis** — *see* Chorioretinitis
- **Choroidoretinopathy, central serous** — *see* Chorioretinopathy, central serous
- **Christian-Weber disease** M35.6
- **Christmas disease** D67
- **Chromaffinoma** — *see also* Neoplasm, benign, by site
  - malignant — *see* Neoplasm, malignant, by site
- **Chromatopsia** — *see* Deficiency, color vision
- **Chromhidrosis, chromidrosis** L75.1
- **Chromoblastomycosis** — *see* Chromomycosis
- **Chromoconversion** R82.91
- **Chromomycosis** B43.9
  - brain abscess B43.1
  - cerebral B43.1
  - cutaneous B43.Ø
  - skin B43.Ø
  - specified NEC B43.8
  - subcutaneous abscess or cyst B43.2

Chromophytosis B36.Ø
Chromosome — *see* Anomaly, by chromosome involved
D (1) — *see* Anomaly, chromosome 13
E (3) — *see* Anomaly, chromosome 18
G — *see* Anomaly, chromosome 21
Chromotrichomycosis B36.8
Chronic — *see* condition
fracture — *see* Fracture, pathological
Churg-Strauss syndrome M3Ø.1
Chyle cyst, mesentery I89.8
Chylocele (nonfilarial) I89.8
filarial — *see also* Infestation, filarial B74.9 *[N51]*
tunica vaginalis N5Ø.89
filarial — *see also* Infestation, filarial B74.9 *[N51]*
Chylomicronemia (fasting) (with hyperprebetalipoproteinemia) E78.3
Chylopericardium I31.39
acute I3Ø.9
Chylothorax (nonfilarial) J94.Ø
filarial — *see also* Infestation, filarial B74.9 *[J91.8]*
Chylous — *see* condition
Chyluria (nonfilarial) R82.Ø
due to
bilharziasis B65.Ø
Brugia (malayi) B74.1
timori B74.2
schistosomiasis (bilharziasis) B65.Ø
Wuchereria (bancrofti) B74.Ø
filarial — *see* Infestation, filarial
Cicatricial (deformity) — *see* Cicatrix
Cicatrix (adherent) (contracted) (painful) (vicious) — *see also* Scar L9Ø.5
adenoid (and tonsil) J35.8
alveolar process M26.79
anus K62.89
auricle — *see* Disorder, pinna, specified type NEC
bile duct (common) (hepatic) K83.8
bladder N32.89
bone — *see* Disorder, bone, specified type NEC
brain G93.89
cervix (postoperative) (postpartal) N88.1
common duct K83.8
cornea H17.9
tuberculous A18.59
duodenum (bulb), obstructive K31.5
esophagus K22.2
eyelid — *see* Disorder, eyelid function
hypopharynx J39.2
lacrimal passages — *see* Obstruction, lacrimal
larynx J38.7
lung J98.4
middle ear H74.8 ☑
mouth K13.79
muscle M62.89
with contracture — *see* Contraction, muscle NEC
nasopharynx J39.2
palate (soft) K13.79
penis N48.89
pharynx J39.2
prostate N42.89
rectum K62.89
retina — *see* Scar, chorioretinal
semilunar cartilage — *see* Derangement, meniscus
seminal vesicle N5Ø.89
skin L9Ø.5
infected LØ8.89
postinfective L9Ø.5
tuberculous B9Ø.8
specified site NEC L9Ø.5
throat J39.2
tongue K14.8
tonsil (and adenoid) J35.8
trachea J39.8
tuberculous NEC B9Ø.9
urethra N36.8
uterus N85.8
vagina N89.8
postoperative N99.2
vocal cord J38.3
wrist, constricting (annular) L9Ø.5
CIDP (chronic inflammatory demyelinating polyneuropathy) G61.81
CIN — *see* Neoplasia, intraepithelial, cervix
CINCA (chronic infantile neurological, cutaneous and articular syndrome) MØ4.2
Cinchonism — *see* Deafness, ototoxic
correct substance properly administered — *see* Table of Drugs and Chemicals, by drug, adverse effect
Cinchonism — *continued*
overdose or wrong substance given or taken — *see* Table of Drugs and Chemicals, by drug, poisoning
Circle of Willis — *see* condition
Circular — *see* condition
Circulating anticoagulants — *see also* Disorder, hemorrhagic D68.318
due to drugs — *see also* Disorder, hemorrhagic D68.32
following childbirth O72.3
Circulation
collateral, any site I99.8
defective (lower extremity) I99.9
congenital Q28.9
embryonic Q28.9
failure (peripheral) R57.9
newborn P29.89
fetal, persistent P29.38
heart, incomplete Q28.9
Circulatory system — *see* condition
Circulus senilis (cornea) — *see* Degeneration, cornea, senile
Circumcision (in absence of medical indication) (ritual) (routine) Z41.2
Circumscribed — *see* condition
Circumvallate placenta O43.11- ☑
Cirrhosis, cirrhotic (hepatic) (liver) K74.6Ø
alcoholic K7Ø.3Ø
with ascites K7Ø.31
atrophic — *see* Cirrhosis, liver
Baumgarten-Cruveilhier K74.69
biliary (cholangiolitic) (cholangitic) (hypertrophic) (obstructive) (pericholangiolitic) K74.5
due to
Clonorchiasis B66.1
flukes B66.3
primary K74.3
secondary K74.4
cardiac (of liver) K76.1
Charcot's K74.3
cholangiolitic, cholangitic, cholostatic (primary) K74.3
congestive K76.1
Cruveilhier-Baumgarten K74.69
cryptogenic (liver) K74.69
due to
hepatolenticular degeneration E83.Ø1
Wilson's disease E83.Ø1
xanthomatosis E78.2
fatty K76.Ø
alcoholic K7Ø.Ø
Hanot's (hypertrophic) K74.3
hepatic — *see* Cirrhosis, liver
hypertrophic K74.3
Indian childhood K74.69
kidney — *see* Sclerosis, renal
Laennec's K7Ø.3Ø
with ascites K7Ø.31
alcoholic K7Ø.3Ø
with ascites K7Ø.31
nonalcoholic K74.69
liver K74.6Ø
alcoholic K7Ø.3Ø
with ascites K7Ø.31
fatty K7Ø.Ø
congenital P78.81
syphilitic A52.74
lung (chronic) J84.1Ø
macronodular K74.69
alcoholic K7Ø.3Ø
with ascites K7Ø.31
micronodular K74.69
alcoholic K7Ø.3Ø
with ascites K7Ø.31
mixed type K74.69
monolobular K74.3
nephritis — *see* Sclerosis, renal
nutritional K74.69
alcoholic K7Ø.3Ø
with ascites K7Ø.31
obstructive — *see* Cirrhosis, biliary
ovarian N83.8
pancreas (duct) K86.89
pigmentary E83.11Ø
portal K74.69
alcoholic K7Ø.3Ø
with ascites K7Ø.31
postnecrotic K74.69
alcoholic K7Ø.3Ø
with ascites K7Ø.31
Cirrhosis, cirrhotic — *continued*
pulmonary J84.1Ø
renal — *see* Sclerosis, renal
spleen D73.2
stasis K76.1
Todd's K74.3
unilobar K74.3
xanthomatous (biliary) K74.5
due to xanthomatosis (familial) (metabolic) (primary) E78.2
Cistern, subarachnoid R93.Ø
Citrullinemia E72.23
Citrullinuria E72.23
Civatte's disease or poikiloderma L57.3
Clam digger's itch B65.3
Clammy skin R23.1
Clap — *see* Gonorrhea
Clarke-Hadfield syndrome (pancreatic infantilism) K86.89
Clark's paralysis G8Ø.9
Clastothrix L67.8
Claude Bernard-Horner syndrome G9Ø.2
traumatic — *see* Injury, nerve, cervical sympathetic
Claude's disease or syndrome G46.3
Claudicatio venosa intermittens I87.8
Claudication (intermittent) I73.9
cerebral (artery) G45.9
spinal cord (arteriosclerotic) G95.19
syphilitic A52.Ø9
venous (axillary) I87.8
Claustrophobia F4Ø.24Ø
Clavus (infected) L84
Clawfoot (congenital) Q66.89
acquired — *see* Deformity, limb, clawfoot
Clawhand (acquired) — *see also* Deformity, limb, clawhand
congenital Q68.1
Clawtoe (congenital) Q66.89
acquired — *see* Deformity, toe, specified NEC
Clay eating — *see* Pica
Cleansing of artificial opening — *see* Attention to, artificial, opening
Cleft (congenital) — *see also* Imperfect, closure
alveolar process M26.79
branchial (persistent) Q18.2
cyst Q18.Ø
fistula Q18.Ø
sinus Q18.Ø
cricoid cartilage, posterior Q31.8
cyst Q18.Ø
fistula Q18.Ø
sinus Q18.Ø
foot Q72.7 ☑
hand Q71.6 ☑
lip (unilateral) Q36.9
with cleft palate Q37.9
hard Q37.1
with soft Q37.5
soft Q37.3
with hard Q37.5
bilateral Q36.Ø
with cleft palate Q37.8
hard Q37.Ø
with soft Q37.4
soft Q37.2
with hard Q37.4
median Q36.1
nose Q3Ø.2
palate Q35.9
with cleft lip (unilateral) Q37.9
bilateral Q37.8
hard Q35.1
with
cleft lip (unilateral) Q37.1
bilateral Q37.Ø
soft Q35.5
with cleft lip (unilateral) Q37.5
bilateral Q37.4
medial Q35.5
soft Q35.3
with
cleft lip (unilateral) Q37.3
bilateral Q37.2
hard Q35.5
with cleft lip (unilateral) Q37.5
bilateral Q37.4
penis Q55.69
scrotum Q55.29

- **Cleft** — *continued*
  - thyroid cartilage Q31.8
  - uvula Q35.7
- **Cleidocranial dysostosis** Q74.Ø
- **Cleptomania** F63.2
- **Clicking hip** (newborn) R29.4
- **Climacteric** (female) — *see also* Menopause
  - arthritis (any site) NEC — *see* Arthritis, specified form NEC
  - depression (single episode) F32.89
    - recurrent episode F33.8
  - male (symptoms) (syndrome) NEC N5Ø.89
  - melancholia (single episode) F32.89
    - recurrent episode F33.8
  - paranoid state F22
  - polyarthritis NEC — *see* Arthritis, specified form NEC
  - symptoms (female) N95.1
- **Clinical research investigation** (clinical trial) (control subject) (normal comparison) (participant) ZØØ.6
- **Clitoris** — *see* condition
- **Cloaca** (persistent) Q43.7
- **Clonorchiasis, clonorchis infection** (liver) B66.1
- **Clonus** R25.8
- **Closed bite** M26.29
- **Clostridium** (C.) **perfringens, as cause of disease classified elsewhere** B96.7
- **Closure**
  - congenital, nose Q3Ø.Ø
  - cranial sutures, premature Q75.Ø
  - defective or imperfect NEC — *see* Imperfect, closure
  - fistula, delayed — *see* Fistula
  - foramen ovale, imperfect Q21.12
  - hymen N89.6
  - interauricular septum, defective Q21.19
  - interventricular septum, defective Q21.Ø
  - lacrimal duct — *see also* Stenosis, lacrimal, duct
    - congenital Q1Ø.5
  - nose (congenital) Q3Ø.Ø
    - acquired M95.Ø
  - of artificial opening — *see* Attention to, artificial, opening
  - vagina N89.5
  - valve — *see* Endocarditis
  - vulva N9Ø.5
- **Clot** (blood) — *see also* Embolism
  - artery (obstruction) (occlusion) — *see* Embolism
  - bladder N32.89
  - brain (intradural or extradural) — *see* Occlusion, artery, cerebral
  - circulation I74.9
  - heart — *see also* Infarct, myocardium
    - not resulting in infarction I51.3
  - vein — *see* Thrombosis
- **Clouded state** R4Ø.1
  - epileptic — *see* Epilepsy, specified NEC
  - paroxysmal — *see* Epilepsy, specified NEC
- **Cloudy antrum, antra** J32.Ø
- **Clouston's** (hidrotic) **ectodermal dysplasia** Q82.4
- **Clubbed nail pachydermoperiostosis** M89.4Ø *[L62]*
- **Clubbing of finger**(s) (nails) R68.3
- **Clubfinger** R68.3
  - congenital Q68.1
- **Clubfoot** (congenital) Q66.89
  - acquired — *see* Deformity, limb, clubfoot
  - equinovarus Q66.Ø- ☑
  - paralytic — *see* Deformity, limb, clubfoot
- **Clubhand** (congenital) (radial) Q71.4- ☑
  - acquired — *see* Deformity, limb, clubhand
- **Clubnail** R68.3
  - congenital Q84.6
- **Clump, kidney** Q63.1
- **Clumsiness, clumsy child syndrome** F82
- **Cluttering** F8Ø.81
- **Clutton's joints** A5Ø.51 *[M12.8Ø]*
- **Coagulation, intravascular** (diffuse) (disseminated) — *see also* Defibrination syndrome
  - complicating abortion — *see* Abortion, by type, complicated by, intravascular coagulation
  - following ectopic or molar pregnancy OØ8.1
- **Coagulopathy** — *see also* Defect, coagulation
  - consumption D65
  - intravascular D65
    - newborn P6Ø
- **Coalition**
  - calcaneo-scaphoid Q66.89
  - tarsal Q66.89
- **Coalminer's**
  - elbow — *see* Bursitis, elbow, olecranon
  - lung or pneumoconiosis J6Ø
- **Coalworker's lung or pneumoconiosis** J6Ø
- **Coarctation**
  - aorta (preductal) (postductal) Q25.1
  - pulmonary artery Q25.71
- **Coated tongue** K14.3
- **Coats' disease** (exudative retinopathy) — *see* Retinopathy, exudative
- **Cocaine-induced**
  - anxiety disorder F14.98Ø
  - bipolar and related disorder F14.94
  - depressive disorder F14.94
  - obsessive-compulsive and related disorder F14.988
  - psychotic disorder F14.959
  - sexual dysfunction F14.981
  - sleep disorder F14.982
- **Cocainism** — *see* Disorder, cocaine use
- **Coccidioidomycosis** B38.9
  - cutaneous B38.3
  - disseminated B38.7
  - generalized B38.7
  - meninges B38.4
  - prostate B38.81
  - pulmonary B38.2
    - acute B38.Ø
    - chronic B38.1
  - skin B38.3
  - specified NEC B38.89
- **Coccidioidosis** — *see* Coccidioidomycosis
- **Coccidiosis** (intestinal) AØ7.3
- **Coccydynia, coccygodynia** M53.3
- **Coccyx** — *see* condition
- **Cochin-China diarrhea** K9Ø.1
- **Cockayne's syndrome** Q87.19
- **Cocked up toe** — *see* Deformity, toe, specified NEC
- **Cock's peculiar tumor** L72.3
- **Codman's tumor** — *see* Neoplasm, bone, benign
- **Coenurosis** B71.8
- **Coffee-worker's lung** J67.8
- **Cogan's syndrome** H16.32- ☑
  - oculomotor apraxia H51.8
- **Coitus, painful** (female) N94.1Ø
  - male N53.12
  - psychogenic F52.6
- **Cold** JØØ
  - with influenza, flu, or grippe — *see* Influenza, with, respiratory manifestations NEC
  - agglutinin disease or hemoglobinuria (chronic) D59.12
  - bronchial — *see* Bronchitis
  - chest — *see* Bronchitis
  - common (head) JØØ
  - effects of T69.9 ☑
    - specified effect NEC T69.8 ☑
  - excessive, effects of T69.9 ☑
    - specified effect NEC T69.8 ☑
  - exhaustion from T69.8 ☑
  - exposure to T69.9 ☑
    - specified effect NEC T69.8 ☑
  - head JØØ
  - injury syndrome (newborn) P8Ø.Ø
  - on lung — *see* Bronchitis
  - rose J3Ø.1
  - sensitivity, auto-immune D59.12
  - symptoms JØØ
  - virus JØØ
- **Coldsore** BØØ.1
- **Colibacillosis** A49.8
  - as the cause of other disease — *see also* Escherichia coli B96.2Ø
  - generalized A41.5Ø
- **Colic** (bilious) (infantile) (intestinal) (recurrent) (spasmodic) R1Ø.83
  - abdomen R1Ø.83
    - psychogenic F45.8
  - appendix, appendicular K38.8
  - bile duct — *see* Calculus, bile duct
  - biliary — *see* Calculus, bile duct
  - common duct — *see* Calculus, bile duct
  - cystic duct — *see* Calculus, gallbladder
  - Devonshire NEC — *see* Poisoning, lead
  - gallbladder — *see* Calculus, gallbladder
  - gallstone — *see* Calculus, gallbladder
    - gallbladder or cystic duct — *see* Calculus, gallbladder
  - hepatic (duct) — *see* Calculus, bile duct
- **Colic** — *continued*
  - hysterical F45.8
  - kidney N23
  - lead NEC — *see* Poisoning, lead
  - mucous K58.9
    - with diarrhea K58.Ø
    - psychogenic F54
  - nephritic N23
  - painter's NEC — *see* Poisoning, lead
  - pancreas K86.89
  - psychogenic F45.8
  - renal N23
  - saturnine NEC — *see* Poisoning, lead
  - ureter N23
  - urethral N36.8
    - due to calculus N21.1
  - uterus NEC N94.89
    - menstrual — *see* Dysmenorrhea
  - worm NOS B83.9
- **Colicystitis** — *see* Cystitis
- **Colitis** (acute) (catarrhal) (chronic) (noninfective) (hemorrhagic) — *see also* Enteritis K52.9
  - allergic K52.29
    - with
      - food protein-induced enterocolitis syndrome K52.21
      - proctocolitis K52.29
  - amebic (acute) — *see also* Amebiasis AØ6.Ø
    - nondysenteric AØ6.2
  - anthrax A22.2
  - bacillary — *see* Infection, Shigella
  - balantidial AØ7.Ø
  - Clostridium difficile
    - not specified as recurrent AØ4.72
    - recurrent AØ4.71
  - coccidial AØ7.3
  - collagenous K52.831
  - cystica superficialis K52.89
  - dietary counseling and surveillance (for) Z71.3
  - dietetic — *see also* Colitis, allergic K52.29
  - drug-induced K52.1
  - due to radiation K52.Ø
  - eosinophilic K52.82
  - food hypersensitivity — *see also* Colitis, allergic K52.29
  - giardial AØ7.1
  - granulomatous — *see* Enteritis, regional, large intestine
  - indeterminate, so stated K52.3
  - infectious — *see* Enteritis, infectious
  - ischemic K55.9
    - acute (subacute) — *see also* Ischemia, intestine, acute K55.Ø39
    - chronic K55.1
    - due to mesenteric artery insufficiency K55.1
    - fulminant (acute) — *see also* Ischemia, intestine, acute K55.Ø39
  - left sided K51.5Ø
    - with
      - abscess K51.514
      - complication K51.519
        - specified NEC K51.518
      - fistula K51.513
      - obstruction K51.512
      - rectal bleeding K51.511
  - lymphocytic K52.832
  - membranous
    - psychogenic F54
  - microscopic K52.839
    - specified NEC K52.838
  - mucous — *see* Syndrome, irritable, bowel
    - psychogenic F54
  - noninfective K52.9
    - specified NEC K52.89
  - polyposa — *see* Polyp, colon, inflammatory
  - protozoal AØ7.9
  - pseudomembranous
    - not specified as recurrent AØ4.72
    - recurrent AØ4.71
  - pseudomucinous — *see* Syndrome, irritable, bowel
  - regional — *see* Enteritis, regional, large intestine
    - infectious AØ9
  - segmental — *see* Enteritis, regional, large intestine
  - septic — *see* Enteritis, infectious
  - spastic K58.9
    - with diarrhea K58.Ø
    - psychogenic F54
  - staphylococcal AØ4.8
    - foodborne AØ5.Ø

Colitis — *continued*
- subacute ischemic — *see also* Ischemia, intestine, acute K55.Ø39
- thromboulcerative — *see also* Ischemia, intestine, acute K55.Ø39
- toxic NEC K52.1
  - due to Clostridium difficile
    - not specified as recurrent AØ4.72
    - recurrent AØ4.71
- transmural — *see* Enteritis, regional, large intestine
- trichomonal AØ7.8
- tuberculous (ulcerative) A18.32
- ulcerative (chronic) K51.9Ø
  - with
    - complication K51.919
      - abscess K51.914
      - fistula K51.913
      - obstruction K51.912
      - rectal bleeding K51.911
      - specified complication NEC K51.918
  - enterocolitis — *see* Enterocolitis, ulcerative
  - ileocolitis — *see* Ileocolitis, ulcerative
  - mucosal proctocolitis — *see* Proctocolitis, mucosal
  - proctitis — *see* Proctitis, ulcerative
  - pseudopolyposis — *see* Polyp, colon, inflammatory
  - psychogenic F54
  - rectosigmoiditis — *see* Rectosigmoiditis, ulcerative
  - specified type NEC K51.8Ø
    - with
      - complication K51.819
        - abscess K51.814
        - fistula K51.813
        - obstruction K51.812
        - rectal bleeding K51.811
        - specified complication NEC K51.818

Collagenosis, collagen disease (nonvascular) (vascular) M35.9
- cardiovascular I42.8
- reactive perforating L87.1
- specified NEC M35.89

Collapse R55
- adrenal E27.2
- cardiorespiratory R57.Ø
- cardiovascular R57.Ø
  - newborn P29.89
- circulatory (peripheral) R57.9
  - during or after labor and delivery O75.1
  - following ectopic or molar pregnancy OØ8.3
  - newborn P29.89
- during or
  - after labor and delivery O75.1
  - resulting from a procedure, not elsewhere classified T81.1Ø ☑
- external ear canal — *see* Stenosis, external ear canal
- general R55
- heart — *see* Disease, heart
- heat T67.1 ☑
- hysterical F44.89
- labyrinth, membranous (congenital) Q16.5
- lung (massive) — *see also* Atelectasis J98.19
  - pressure due to anesthesia (general) (local) or other sedation T88.2 ☑
    - during labor and delivery O74.1
    - in pregnancy O29.Ø2- ☑
    - postpartum, puerperal O89.Ø9
- myocardial — *see* Disease, heart
- nervous F48.8
- neurocirculatory F45.8
- nose M95.Ø
- postoperative T81.1Ø ☑
- pulmonary — *see also* Atelectasis J98.19
  - newborn — *see* Atelectasis
- trachea J39.8
- tracheobronchial J98.Ø9
- valvular — *see* Endocarditis
- vascular (peripheral) R57.9
  - during or after labor and delivery O75.1
  - following ectopic or molar pregnancy OØ8.3
  - newborn P29.89
- vertebra M48.5Ø- ☑
  - cervical region M48.52- ☑
  - cervicothoracic region M48.53- ☑
  - in (due to)
    - neoplasm (metastasis) M84.58- ☑
    - osteoporosis — *see also* Osteoporosis M8Ø.88 ☑
      - cervical region M8Ø.88 ☑
      - cervicothoracic region M8Ø.88 ☑
      - lumbar region M8Ø.88 ☑

Collapse — *continued*
- vertebra — *continued*
  - in — *continued*
    - osteoporosis — *see also* Osteoporosis — *continued*
      - lumbosacral region M8Ø.88 ☑
      - multiple sites M8Ø.88 ☑
      - occipito-atlanto-axial region M8Ø.88 ☑
      - sacrococcygeal region M8Ø.88 ☑
      - thoracic region M8Ø.88 ☑
      - thoracolumbar region M8Ø.88 ☑
    - specified disease NEC M48.5Ø- ☑
      - cervical region M48.52- ☑
      - cervicothoracic region M48.53- ☑
      - lumbar region M48.56- ☑
      - lumbosacral region M48.57- ☑
      - occipito-atlanto-axial region M48.51- ☑
      - sacrococcygeal region M48.58- ☑
      - thoracic region M48.54- ☑
      - thoracolumbar region M48.55- ☑
  - lumbar region M48.56- ☑
  - lumbosacral region M48.57- ☑
  - occipito-atlanto-axial region M48.51- ☑
  - sacrococcygeal region M48.58- ☑
  - thoracic region M48.54- ☑
  - thoracolumbar region M48.55- ☑

Collateral — *see also* condition
- circulation (venous) I87.8
- dilation, veins I87.8

Colles' fracture S52.53- ☑

Collet (-Sicard) syndrome G52.7

Collier's asthma or lung J6Ø

Collodion baby Q8Ø.2

Colloid nodule (of thyroid) (cystic) EØ4.1

Coloboma (iris) Q13.Ø
- eyelid Q1Ø.3
- fundus Q14.8
- lens Q12.2
- optic disc (congenital) Q14.2
  - acquired H47.31- ☑

Coloenteritis — *see* Enteritis

Colon — *see* condition

Colonization
- MRSA (Methicillin resistant Staphylococcus aureus) Z22.322
- MSSA (Methicillin susceptible Staphylococcus aureus) Z22.321
- status — *see* Carrier (suspected) of

Coloptosis K63.4

Color blindness — *see* Deficiency, color vision

Colostomy
- attention to Z43.3
- fitting or adjustment Z46.89
- malfunctioning K94.Ø3
- status Z93.3

Colpitis (acute) — *see* Vaginitis

Colpocele N81.5

Colpocystitis — *see* Vaginitis

Colpospasm N94.2

Column, spinal, vertebral — *see* condition

Coma R4Ø.2Ø
- with
  - motor response (none) R4Ø.231 ☑
    - abnormal extensor posturing to pain or noxious stimuli (< 2 years of age) R4Ø.232 ☑
    - abnormal flexure posturing to pain or noxious stimuli (Ø-5 years of age) R4Ø.233 ☑
    - extensor posturing to pain or noxious stimuli (2-5 years of age) R4Ø.232 ☑
    - flexion/decorticate posturing (< 2 years of age) R4Ø.233 ☑
    - localizes pain (2-5 years of age) R4Ø.235 ☑
    - normal or spontaneous movement (< 2 years of age) R4Ø.236 ☑
    - obeys commands (2-5 years of age) R4Ø.236 ☑
    - score of
      - 1 R4Ø.231 ☑
      - 2 R4Ø.232 ☑
      - 3 R4Ø.233 ☑
      - 4 R4Ø.234 ☑
      - 5 R4Ø.235 ☑
      - 6 R4Ø.236 ☑
    - withdraws from pain or noxious stimuli (Ø-5 years of age) R4Ø.234 ☑
    - withdraws to touch (< 2 years of age) R4Ø.235 ☑
  - opening of eyes (never) R4Ø.211 ☑

Coma — *continued*
- with — *continued*
  - opening of eyes — *continued*
    - in response to
      - pain R4Ø.212 ☑
      - sound R4Ø.213 ☑
    - score of
      - 1 R4Ø.211 ☑
      - 2 R4Ø.212 ☑
      - 3 R4Ø.213 ☑
      - 4 R4Ø.214 ☑
    - spontaneous R4Ø.214 ☑
  - verbal response (none) R4Ø.221 ☑
    - confused conversation R4Ø.224 ☑
    - cooing or babbling or crying appropriately (<2 years of age) R4Ø.225 ☑
    - inappropriate crying or screaming (< 2 years of age) R4Ø.223 ☑
    - inappropriate words (2-5 years of age) R4Ø.224 ☑
    - inappropriate words R4Ø.223 ☑
    - incomprehensible sounds (2-5 years of age) R4Ø.222 ☑
    - incomprehensible words R4Ø.222 ☑
    - irritable cries (< 2 years of age) R4Ø.224 ☑
    - moans/grunts to pain; restless (< 2 years old) R4Ø.222 ☑
    - oriented R4Ø.225 ☑
    - score of
      - 1 R4Ø.221 ☑
      - 2 R4Ø.222 ☑
      - 3 R4Ø.223 ☑
      - 4 R4Ø.224 ☑
      - 5 R4Ø.225 ☑
    - screaming (2-5 years of age) R4Ø.223 ☑
    - uses appropriate words (2-5 years of age) R4Ø.225 ☑
- eclamptic — *see* Eclampsia
- epileptic — *see* Epilepsy
- Glasgow, scale score — *see* Glasgow coma scale
- hepatic — *see* Failure, hepatic, by type, with coma
- hyperglycemic (diabetic) — *see* Diabetes, by type, with hyperosmolarity, with coma
- hyperosmolar (diabetic) — *see* Diabetes, by type, with hyperosmolarity, with coma
- hypoglycemic (diabetic) — *see* Diabetes, by type, with hypoglycemia, with coma
  - nondiabetic E15
- in diabetes — *see* Diabetes, coma
- insulin-induced — *see* Coma, hypoglycemic
- ketoacidotic (diabetic) — *see* Diabetes, by type, with ketoacidosis, with coma
- myxedematous EØ3.5
- newborn P91.5
- persistent vegetative state R4Ø.3
- specified NEC, without documented Glasgow coma scale score, or with partial Glasgow coma scale score reported R4Ø.244 ☑

Comatose — *see* Coma

Combat fatigue F43.Ø

Combined — *see* condition

Comedo, comedones (giant) L7Ø.Ø

Comedocarcinoma — *see also* Neoplasm, breast, malignant
- noninfiltrating
  - breast DØ5.8- ☑
  - specified site — *see* Neoplasm, in situ, by site
  - unspecified site DØ5.8- ☑

Comedomastitis — *see* Ectasia, mammary duct

Comminuted fracture — *code as* Fracture, closed

Common
- arterial trunk Q2Ø.Ø
- atrioventricular canal Q21.23
- atrium Q21.19
- cold (head) JØØ
- truncus (arteriosus) Q2Ø.Ø
- variable immunodeficiency — *see* Immunodeficiency, common variable
- ventricle Q2Ø.4

Commotio, commotion (current)
- brain — *see* Injury, intracranial, concussion
- cerebri — *see* Injury, intracranial, concussion
- retinae SØ5.8X- ☑
- spinal cord — *see* Injury, spinal cord, by region
- spinalis — *see* Injury, spinal cord, by region

- **Communication**
  - between
    - base of aorta and pulmonary artery Q21.4
    - left ventricle and right atrium Q2Ø.5
    - pericardial sac and pleural sac Q34.8
    - pulmonary artery and pulmonary vein, congenital Q25.72
  - congenital between uterus and digestive or urinary tract Q51.7
- **Compartment syndrome** (deep) (posterior) (traumatic) T79.AØ ☑ (*following* T79.7)
  - abdomen T79.A3 ☑ (*following* T79.7)
  - lower extremity (hip, buttock, thigh, leg, foot, toes) T79.A2 ☑ (*following* T79.7)
  - nontraumatic
    - abdomen M79.A3 (*following* M79.7)
    - lower extremity (hip, buttock, thigh, leg, foot, toes) M79.A2- ☑ (*following* M79.7)
    - specified site NEC M79.A9 (*following* M79.7)
    - upper extremity (shoulder, arm, forearm, wrist, hand, fingers) M79.A1- ☑ (*following* M79.7)
  - specified site NEC T79.A9 ☑ (*following* T79.7)
  - upper extremity (shoulder, arm, forearm, wrist, hand, fingers) T79.A1- ☑ (*following* T79.7)
- **Compensation**
  - failure — *see* Disease, heart
  - neurosis, psychoneurosis — *see* Disorder, factitious
- **Complaint** — *see also* Disease
  - bowel, functional K59.9
    - psychogenic F45.8
  - intestine, functional K59.9
    - psychogenic F45.8
  - kidney — *see* Disease, renal
  - miners' J6Ø
- **Complete** — *see* condition
- **Complex**
  - Addison-Schilder E71.528
  - cardiorenal — *see* Hypertension, cardiorenal
  - Costen's M26.69
  - disseminated mycobacterium avium- intracellulare (DMAC) A31.2
  - Eisenmenger's (ventricular septal defect) I27.83
  - hypersexual F52.8
  - jumped process, spine — *see* Dislocation, vertebra
  - primary, tuberculous A15.7
  - Schilder-Addison E71.528
  - subluxation (vertebral) M99.19
    - abdomen M99.19
    - acromioclavicular M99.17
    - cervical region M99.11
    - cervicothoracic M99.11
    - costochondral M99.18
    - costovertebral M99.18
    - head region M99.1Ø
    - hip M99.15
    - lower extremity M99.16
    - lumbar region M99.13
    - lumbosacral M99.13
    - occipitocervical M99.1Ø
    - pelvic region M99.15
    - pubic M99.15
    - rib cage M99.18
    - sacral region M99.14
    - sacrococcygeal M99.14
    - sacroiliac M99.14
    - specified NEC M99.19
    - sternochondral M99.18
    - sternoclavicular M99.17
    - thoracic region M99.12
    - thoracolumbar M99.12
    - upper extremity M99.17
  - Taussig-Bing (transposition, aorta and overriding pulmonary artery) Q2Ø.1
- **Complication**(s) (from) (of)
  - accidental puncture or laceration during a procedure (of) — *see* Complications, intraoperative (intraprocedural), puncture or laceration
  - amputation stump (surgical) (late) NEC T87.9
    - dehiscence T87.81
    - infection or inflammation T87.4Ø
      - lower limb T87.4- ☑
      - upper limb T87.4- ☑
    - necrosis T87.5Ø
      - lower limb T87.5- ☑
      - upper limb T87.5- ☑
    - neuroma T87.3Ø
      - lower limb T87.3- ☑
      - upper limb T87.3- ☑

Complication(s) — *continued*

- amputation stump — *continued*
  - specified type NEC T87.89
- anastomosis (and bypass) — *see also* Complications, prosthetic device or implant
  - intestinal (internal) NEC K91.89
    - involving urinary tract N99.89
  - urinary tract (involving intestinal tract) N99.89
  - vascular — *see* Complications, cardiovascular device or implant
- anesthesia, anesthetic — *see also* Anesthesia, complication T88.59 ☑
  - brain, postpartum, puerperal O89.2
  - cardiac
    - in
      - labor and delivery O74.2
      - pregnancy O29.19- ☑
    - postpartum, puerperal O89.1
  - central nervous system
    - in
      - labor and delivery O74.3
      - pregnancy O29.29- ☑
    - postpartum, puerperal O89.2
  - difficult or failed intubation T88.4 ☑
    - in pregnancy O29.6- ☑
  - failed sedation (conscious) (moderate) during procedure T88.52 ☑
  - general, unintended awareness during procedure T88.53 ☑
  - hyperthermia, malignant T88.3 ☑
  - hypothermia T88.51 ☑
  - intubation failure T88.4 ☑
  - malignant hyperthermia T88.3 ☑
  - pulmonary
    - in
      - labor and delivery O74.1
      - pregnancy NEC O29.Ø9- ☑
    - postpartum, puerperal O89.Ø9
  - shock T88.2 ☑
  - spinal and epidural
    - in
      - labor and delivery NEC O74.6
        - headache O74.5
      - pregnancy NEC O29.5X- ☑
    - postpartum, puerperal NEC O89.5
      - headache O89.4
  - unintended awareness under general anesthesia during procedure T88.53 ☑
- anti-reflux device — *see* Complications, esophageal anti-reflux device
- aortic (bifurcation) graft — *see* Complications, graft, vascular
- aortocoronary (bypass) graft — *see* Complications, coronary artery (bypass) graft
- aortofemoral (bypass) graft — *see* Complications, extremity artery (bypass) graft
- arteriovenous
  - fistula, surgically created T82.9 ☑
    - embolism T82.818 ☑
    - fibrosis T82.828 ☑
    - hemorrhage T82.838 ☑
    - infection or inflammation T82.7 ☑
    - mechanical
      - breakdown T82.51Ø ☑
      - displacement T82.52Ø ☑
      - leakage T82.53Ø ☑
      - malposition T82.52Ø ☑
      - obstruction T82.59Ø ☑
      - perforation T82.59Ø ☑
      - protrusion T82.59Ø ☑
    - pain T82.848 ☑
    - specified type NEC T82.898 ☑
    - stenosis T82.858 ☑
    - thrombosis T82.868 ☑
  - shunt, surgically created T82.9 ☑
    - embolism T82.818 ☑
    - fibrosis T82.828 ☑
    - hemorrhage T82.838 ☑
    - infection or inflammation T82.7 ☑
    - mechanical
      - breakdown T82.511 ☑
      - displacement T82.521 ☑
      - leakage T82.531 ☑
      - malposition T82.521 ☑
      - obstruction T82.591 ☑
      - perforation T82.591 ☑
      - protrusion T82.591 ☑

Complication(s) — *continued*

- arteriovenous — *continued*
  - shunt, surgically created — *continued*
    - pain T82.848 ☑
    - specified type NEC T82.898 ☑
    - stenosis T82.858 ☑
    - thrombosis T82.868 ☑
- arthroplasty — *see* Complications, joint prosthesis
- artificial
  - fertilization or insemination N98.9
    - attempted introduction (of)
      - embryo in embryo transfer N98.3
      - ovum following in vitro fertilization N98.2
    - hyperstimulation of ovaries N98.1
    - infection N98.Ø
    - specified NEC N98.8
  - heart T82.9 ☑
    - embolism T82.817 ☑
    - fibrosis T82.827 ☑
    - hemorrhage T82.837 ☑
    - infection or inflammation T82.7 ☑
    - mechanical
      - breakdown T82.512 ☑
      - displacement T82.522 ☑
      - leakage T82.532 ☑
      - malposition T82.522 ☑
      - obstruction T82.592 ☑
      - perforation T82.592 ☑
      - protrusion T82.592 ☑
    - pain T82.847 ☑
    - specified type NEC T82.897 ☑
    - stenosis T82.857 ☑
    - thrombosis T82.867 ☑
  - opening
    - cecostomy — *see* Complications, colostomy
    - colostomy — *see* Complications, colostomy
    - cystostomy — *see* Complications, cystostomy
    - enterostomy — *see* Complications, enterostomy
    - gastrostomy — *see* Complications, gastrostomy
    - ileostomy — *see* Complications, enterostomy
    - jejunostomy — *see* Complications, enterostomy
    - nephrostomy — *see* Complications, stoma, urinary tract
    - tracheostomy — *see* Complications, tracheostomy
    - ureterostomy — *see* Complications, stoma, urinary tract
    - urethrostomy — *see* Complications, stoma, urinary tract
- balloon implant or device
  - gastrointestinal T85.9 ☑
    - embolism T85.818 ☑
    - fibrosis T85.828 ☑
    - hemorrhage T85.838 ☑
    - infection and inflammation T85.79 ☑
    - pain T85.848 ☑
    - specified type NEC T85.898 ☑
    - stenosis T85.858 ☑
    - thrombosis T85.868 ☑
  - vascular (counterpulsation) T82.9 ☑
    - embolism T82.818 ☑
    - fibrosis T82.828 ☑
    - hemorrhage T82.838 ☑
    - infection or inflammation T82.7 ☑
    - mechanical
      - breakdown T82.513 ☑
      - displacement T82.523 ☑
      - leakage T82.533 ☑
      - malposition T82.523 ☑
      - obstruction T82.593 ☑
      - perforation T82.593 ☑
      - protrusion T82.593 ☑
    - pain T82.848 ☑
    - specified type NEC T82.898 ☑
    - stenosis T82.858 ☑
    - thrombosis T82.868 ☑
- bariatric procedure
  - gastric band procedure K95.Ø9
    - infection K95.Ø1
  - specified procedure NEC K95.89
    - infection K95.81
- bile duct implant (prosthetic) T85.9 ☑
  - embolism T85.818 ☑
  - fibrosis T85.828 ☑
  - hemorrhage T85.838 ☑
  - infection and inflammation T85.79 ☑

Complication(s) — *continued*
bile duct implant — *continued*
mechanical
breakdown T85.51Ø ☑
displacement T85.52Ø ☑
malfunction T85.51Ø ☑
malposition T85.52Ø ☑
obstruction T85.59Ø ☑
perforation T85.59Ø ☑
protrusion T85.59Ø ☑
specified NEC T85.59Ø ☑
pain T85.848 ☑
specified type NEC T85.898 ☑
stenosis T85.858 ☑
thrombosis T85.868 ☑
bladder device (auxiliary) — *see* Complications, genitourinary, device or implant, urinary system
bleeding (postoperative) — *see* Complication, postoperative, hemorrhage
intraoperative — *see* Complication, intraoperative, hemorrhage
blood vessel graft — *see* Complications, graft, vascular
bone
device NEC T84.9 ☑
embolism T84.81 ☑
fibrosis T84.82 ☑
hemorrhage T84.83 ☑
infection or inflammation T84.7 ☑
mechanical
breakdown T84.318 ☑
displacement T84.328 ☑
malposition T84.328 ☑
obstruction T84.398 ☑
perforation T84.398 ☑
protrusion T84.398 ☑
pain T84.84 ☑
specified type NEC T84.89 ☑
stenosis T84.85 ☑
thrombosis T84.86 ☑
graft — *see* Complications, graft, bone
growth stimulator (electrode) — *see* Complications, electronic stimulator device, bone
marrow transplant — *see* Complications, transplant, bone, marrow
brain neurostimulator (electrode) — *see* Complications, electronic stimulator device, brain
breast implant (prosthetic) T85.9 ☑
capsular contracture T85.44 ☑
embolism T85.818 ☑
fibrosis T85.828 ☑
hemorrhage T85.838 ☑
infection and inflammation T85.79 ☑
mechanical
breakdown T85.41 ☑
displacement T85.42 ☑
leakage T85.43 ☑
malposition T85.42 ☑
obstruction T85.49 ☑
perforation T85.49 ☑
protrusion T85.49 ☑
specified NEC T85.49 ☑
pain T85.848 ☑
specified type NEC T85.898 ☑
stenosis T85.858 ☑
thrombosis T85.868 ☑
bypass — *see also* Complications, prosthetic device or implant
aortocoronary — *see* Complications, coronary artery (bypass) graft
arterial — *see also* Complications, graft, vascular
extremity — *see* Complications, extremity artery (bypass) graft
cardiac — *see also* Disease, heart
device, implant or graft T82.9 ☑
embolism T82.817 ☑
fibrosis T82.827 ☑
hemorrhage T82.837 ☑
infection or inflammation T82.7 ☑
valve prosthesis T82.6 ☑
mechanical
breakdown T82.519 ☑
specified device NEC T82.518 ☑
displacement T82.529 ☑
specified device NEC T82.528 ☑
leakage T82.539 ☑
specified device NEC T82.538 ☑

Complication(s) — *continued*
cardiac — *see also* Disease, heart — *continued*
device, implant or graft — *continued*
mechanical — *continued*
malposition T82.529 ☑
specified device NEC T82.528 ☑
obstruction T82.599 ☑
specified device NEC T82.598 ☑
perforation T82.599 ☑
specified device NEC T82.598 ☑
protrusion T82.599 ☑
specified device NEC T82.598 ☑
pain T82.847 ☑
specified type NEC T82.897 ☑
stenosis T82.857 ☑
thrombosis T82.867 ☑
cardiovascular device, graft or implant T82.9 ☑
aortic graft — *see* Complications, graft, vascular
arteriovenous
fistula, artificial — *see* Complication, arteriovenous, fistula, surgically created
shunt — *see* Complication, arteriovenous, shunt, surgically created
artificial heart — *see* Complication, artificial, heart
balloon (counterpulsation) device — *see* Complication, balloon implant, vascular
carotid artery graft — *see* Complications, graft, vascular
coronary bypass graft — *see* Complication, coronary artery (bypass) graft
dialysis catheter (vascular) — *see* Complication, catheter, dialysis
electronic T82.9 ☑
electrode T82.9 ☑
embolism T82.817 ☑
fibrosis T82.827 ☑
hemorrhage T82.837 ☑
infection T82.7 ☑
mechanical
breakdown T82.11Ø ☑
displacement T82.12Ø ☑
leakage T82.19Ø ☑
obstruction T82.19Ø ☑
perforation T82.19Ø ☑
protrusion T82.19Ø ☑
specified type NEC T82.19Ø ☑
pain T82.847 ☑
specified NEC T82.897 ☑
stenosis T82.857 ☑
thrombosis T82.867 ☑
embolism T82.817 ☑
fibrosis T82.827 ☑
hemorrhage T82.837 ☑
infection T82.7 ☑
mechanical
breakdown T82.119 ☑
displacement T82.129 ☑
leakage T82.199 ☑
obstruction T82.199 ☑
perforation T82.199 ☑
protrusion T82.199 ☑
specified type NEC T82.199 ☑
pain T82.847 ☑
pulse generator T82.9 ☑
embolism T82.817 ☑
fibrosis T82.827 ☑
hemorrhage T82.837 ☑
infection T82.7 ☑
mechanical
breakdown T82.111 ☑
displacement T82.121 ☑
leakage T82.191 ☑
obstruction T82.191 ☑
perforation T82.191 ☑
protrusion T82.191 ☑
specified type NEC T82.191 ☑
pain T82.847 ☑
specified NEC T82.897 ☑
stenosis T82.857 ☑
thrombosis T82.867 ☑
specified condition NEC T82.897 ☑
specified device NEC T82.9 ☑
embolism T82.817 ☑
fibrosis T82.827 ☑
hemorrhage T82.837 ☑
infection T82.7 ☑

Complication(s) — *continued*
cardiovascular device, graft or implant — *continued*
electronic — *continued*
specified device — *continued*
mechanical
breakdown T82.118 ☑
displacement T82.128 ☑
leakage T82.198 ☑
obstruction T82.198 ☑
perforation T82.198 ☑
protrusion T82.198 ☑
specified type NEC T82.198 ☑
pain T82.847 ☑
specified NEC T82.897 ☑
stenosis T82.857 ☑
thrombosis T82.867 ☑
stenosis T82.857 ☑
thrombosis T82.867 ☑
extremity artery graft — *see* Complication, extremity artery (bypass) graft
femoral artery graft — *see* Complication, extremity artery (bypass) graft
heart
transplant — *see* Complication, transplant, heart
valve — *see* Complication, prosthetic device, heart valve
graft — *see* Complication, heart, valve, graft
heart-lung transplant — *see* Complication, transplant, heart, with lung
infection or inflammation T82.7 ☑
umbrella device — *see* Complication, umbrella device, vascular
vascular graft (or anastomosis) — *see* Complication, graft, vascular
carotid artery (bypass) graft — *see* Complications, graft, vascular
catheter (device) NEC — *see also* Complications, prosthetic device or implant
cranial infusion
infection and inflammation T85.735 ☑
mechanical
breakdown T85.61Ø ☑
displacement T85.62Ø ☑
leakage T85.63Ø ☑
malfunction T85.69Ø ☑
malposition T85.62Ø ☑
obstruction T85.69Ø ☑
perforation T85.69Ø ☑
protrusion T85.69Ø ☑
specified NEC T85.69Ø ☑
cystostomy T83.9 ☑
embolism T83.81 ☑
fibrosis T83.82 ☑
hemorrhage T83.83 ☑
infection and inflammation T83.51Ø ☑
mechanical
breakdown T83.Ø1Ø ☑
displacement T83.Ø2Ø ☑
leakage T83.Ø3Ø ☑
malposition T83.Ø2Ø ☑
obstruction T83.Ø9Ø ☑
perforation T83.Ø9Ø ☑
protrusion T83.Ø9Ø ☑
specified NEC T83.Ø9Ø ☑
pain T83.84 ☑
specified type NEC T83.89 ☑
stenosis T83.85 ☑
thrombosis T83.86 ☑
dialysis (vascular) T82.9 ☑
embolism T82.818 ☑
fibrosis T82.828 ☑
hemorrhage T82.838 ☑
infection and inflammation T82.7 ☑
intraperitoneal — *see* Complications, catheter, intraperitoneal
mechanical
breakdown T82.41 ☑
displacement T82.42 ☑
leakage T82.43 ☑
malposition T82.42 ☑
obstruction T82.49 ☑
perforation T82.49 ☑
protrusion T82.49 ☑
pain T82.848 ☑
specified type NEC T82.898 ☑
stenosis T82.858 ☑

Complication(s) — *continued*
- catheter — *see also* Complications, prosthetic device or implant — *continued*
  - dialysis — *continued*
    - thrombosis T82.868 ☑
  - epidural infusion T85.9 ☑
    - embolism T85.81Ø ☑
    - fibrosis T85.82Ø ☑
    - hemorrhage T85.83Ø ☑
    - infection and inflammation T85.735 ☑
    - mechanical
      - breakdown T85.61Ø ☑
      - displacement T85.62Ø ☑
      - leakage T85.63Ø ☑
      - malfunction T85.61Ø ☑
      - malposition T85.62Ø ☑
      - obstruction T85.69Ø ☑
      - perforation T85.69Ø ☑
      - protrusion T85.69Ø ☑
      - specified NEC T85.69Ø ☑
    - pain T85.84Ø ☑
    - specified type NEC T85.89Ø ☑
    - stenosis T85.85Ø ☑
    - thrombosis T85.86Ø ☑
  - intraperitoneal dialysis T85.9 ☑
    - embolism T85.818 ☑
    - fibrosis T85.828 ☑
    - hemorrhage T85.838 ☑
    - infection and inflammation T85.71 ☑
    - mechanical
      - breakdown T85.611 ☑
      - displacement T85.621 ☑
      - leakage T85.631 ☑
      - malfunction T85.611 ☑
      - malposition T85.621 ☑
      - obstruction T85.691 ☑
      - perforation T85.691 ☑
      - protrusion T85.691 ☑
      - specified NEC T85.691 ☑
    - pain T85.848 ☑
    - specified type NEC T85.898 ☑
    - stenosis T85.858 ☑
    - thrombosis T85.868 ☑
  - intrathecal infusion
    - infection and inflammation T85.735 ☑
    - mechanical
      - breakdown T85.61Ø ☑
      - displacement T85.62Ø ☑
      - leakage T85.63Ø ☑
      - malfunction T85.69Ø ☑
      - malposition T85.62Ø ☑
      - obstruction T85.69Ø ☑
      - perforation T85.69Ø ☑
      - protrusion T85.69Ø ☑
      - specified NEC T85.69Ø ☑
  - intravenous infusion T82.9 ☑
    - embolism T82.818 ☑
    - fibrosis T82.828 ☑
    - hemorrhage T82.838 ☑
    - infection or inflammation T82.7 ☑
    - mechanical
      - breakdown T82.514 ☑
      - displacement T82.524 ☑
      - leakage T82.534 ☑
      - malposition T82.524 ☑
      - obstruction T82.594 ☑
      - perforation T82.594 ☑
      - protrusion T82.594 ☑
    - pain T82.848 ☑
    - specified type NEC T82.898 ☑
    - stenosis T82.858 ☑
    - thrombosis T82.868 ☑
  - spinal infusion
    - infection and inflammation T85.735 ☑
    - mechanical
      - breakdown T85.61Ø ☑
      - displacement T85.62Ø ☑
      - leakage T85.63Ø ☑
      - malfunction T85.69Ø ☑
      - malposition T85.62Ø ☑
      - obstruction T85.69Ø ☑
      - perforation T85.69Ø ☑
      - protrusion T85.69Ø ☑
      - specified NEC T85.69Ø ☑
  - subarachnoid infusion
    - infection and inflammation T85.735 ☑

Complication(s) — *continued*
- catheter — *see also* Complications, prosthetic device or implant — *continued*
  - subarachnoid infusion — *continued*
    - mechanical
      - breakdown T85.61Ø ☑
      - displacement T85.62Ø ☑
      - leakage T85.63Ø ☑
      - malfunction T85.69Ø ☑
      - malposition T85.62Ø ☑
      - obstruction T85.69Ø ☑
      - perforation T85.69Ø ☑
      - protrusion T85.69Ø ☑
      - specified NEC T85.69Ø ☑
  - subdural infusion T85.9 ☑
    - embolism T85.81Ø ☑
    - fibrosis T85.82Ø ☑
    - hemorrhage T85.83Ø ☑
    - infection and inflammation T85.735 ☑
    - mechanical
      - breakdown T85.61Ø ☑
      - displacement T85.62Ø ☑
      - leakage T85.63Ø ☑
      - malfunction T85.61Ø ☑
      - malposition T85.62Ø ☑
      - obstruction T85.69Ø ☑
      - perforation T85.69Ø ☑
      - protrusion T85.69Ø ☑
      - specified NEC T85.69Ø ☑
    - pain T85.84Ø ☑
    - specified type NEC T85.89Ø ☑
    - stenosis T85.85Ø ☑
    - thrombosis T85.86Ø ☑
  - urethral T83.9 ☑
    - displacement T83.Ø28 ☑
    - embolism T83.81 ☑
    - fibrosis T83.82 ☑
    - hemorrhage T83.83 ☑
    - indwelling
      - breakdown T83.Ø11 ☑
      - displacement T83.Ø21 ☑
      - infection and inflammation T83.511 ☑
      - leakage T83.Ø31 ☑
      - specified complication NEC T83.Ø91 ☑
    - infection and inflammation T83.511 ☑
    - leakage T83.Ø38 ☑
    - malposition T83.Ø28 ☑
    - mechanical
      - breakdown T83.Ø11 ☑
    - obstruction (mechanical) T83.Ø91 ☑
    - pain T83.84 ☑
    - perforation T83.Ø91 ☑
    - protrusion T83.Ø91 ☑
    - specified type NEC T83.Ø91 ☑
    - stenosis T83.85 ☑
    - thrombosis T83.86 ☑
  - urinary NEC
    - breakdown T83.Ø18 ☑
    - displacement T83.Ø28 ☑
    - infection and inflammation T83.518 ☑
    - leakage T83.Ø38 ☑
    - specified complication NEC T83.Ø98 ☑
- cecostomy (stoma) — *see* Complications, colostomy
- cesarean delivery wound NEC O9Ø.89
  - disruption O9Ø.Ø
  - hematoma O9Ø.2
  - infection (following delivery) O86.ØØ
- chemotherapy (antineoplastic) NEC T88.7 ☑
- chimeric antigen receptor (CAR-T) cell therapy T8Ø.82 ☑
- chin implant (prosthetic) — *see* Complication, prosthetic device or implant, specified NEC
- circulatory system I99.8
  - intraoperative I97.88
  - postprocedural I97.89
    - following cardiac surgery — *see also* Infarct, myocardium, associated with revascularization procedure I97.19- ☑
      - postcardiotomy syndrome I97.Ø
    - hypertension I97.3
    - lymphedema after mastectomy I97.2
    - postcardiotomy syndrome I97.Ø
    - specified NEC I97.89
- colostomy (stoma) K94.ØØ
  - hemorrhage K94.Ø1
  - infection K94.Ø2

Complication(s) — *continued*
- colostomy — *continued*
  - malfunction K94.Ø3
  - mechanical K94.Ø3
  - specified complication NEC K94.Ø9
- contraceptive device, intrauterine — *see* Complications, intrauterine, contraceptive device
- cord (umbilical) — *see* Complications, umbilical cord
- corneal graft — *see* Complications, graft, cornea
- coronary artery (bypass) graft T82.9 ☑
  - atherosclerosis — *see* Arteriosclerosis, coronary (artery)
  - embolism T82.817 ☑
  - fibrosis T82.827 ☑
  - hemorrhage T82.837 ☑
  - infection and inflammation T82.7 ☑
  - mechanical
    - breakdown T82.211 ☑
    - displacement T82.212 ☑
    - leakage T82.213 ☑
    - malposition T82.212 ☑
    - obstruction T82.218 ☑
    - perforation T82.218 ☑
    - protrusion T82.218 ☑
    - specified NEC T82.218 ☑
  - pain T82.847 ☑
  - specified type NEC T82.898 ☑
  - stenosis T82.857 ☑
  - thrombosis T82.867 ☑
- counterpulsation device (balloon), intra- aortic — *see* Complications, balloon implant, vascular
- cystostomy (stoma) N99.518
  - catheter — *see* Complications, catheter, cystostomy
  - hemorrhage N99.51Ø
  - infection N99.511
  - malfunction N99.512
  - specified type NEC N99.518
- delivery — *see also* Complications, obstetric O75.9
  - procedure (instrumental) (manual) (surgical) O75.4
  - specified NEC O75.89
- dialysis (peritoneal) (renal) — *see also* Complications, infusion
  - catheter (vascular) — *see* Complication, catheter, dialysis
  - peritoneal, intraperitoneal — *see* Complications, catheter, intraperitoneal
- dorsal column (spinal) neurostimulator — *see* Complications, electronic stimulator device, spinal cord
- drug NEC T88.7 ☑
- ear procedure — *see also* Disorder, ear
  - intraoperative H95.88
    - hematoma — *see* Complications, intraoperative, hemorrhage (hematoma) (of), ear
    - hemorrhage — *see* Complications, intraoperative, hemorrhage (hematoma) (of), ear
    - laceration — *see* Complications, intraoperative, puncture or laceration, ear
    - specified NEC H95.88
  - postoperative H95.89
    - external ear canal stenosis H95.81- ☑
    - hematoma — *see* Complications, postprocedural, hematoma (of), ear
    - hemorrhage — *see* Complications, postprocedural, hemorrhage (of), ear
    - postmastoidectomy — *see* Complications, postmastoidectomy
    - seroma — *see* Complications, postprocedural, seroma (of), mastoid process
    - specified NEC H95.89
- ectopic pregnancy OØ8.9
  - damage to pelvic organs OØ8.6
  - embolism OØ8.2
  - genital infection OØ8.Ø
  - hemorrhage (delayed) (excessive) OØ8.1
  - metabolic disorder OØ8.5
  - renal failure OØ8.4
  - shock OØ8.3
  - specified type NEC OØ8.Ø
  - venous complication NEC OØ8.7
- electronic stimulator device
  - bladder (urinary) — *see* Complications, electronic stimulator device, urinary
  - bone T84.9 ☑
    - breakdown T84.31Ø ☑
    - displacement T84.32Ø ☑
    - embolism T84.81 ☑
    - fibrosis T84.82 ☑

Complication(s) — *continued*
electronic stimulator device — *continued*
bone — *continued*
hemorrhage T84.83 ☑
infection or inflammation T84.7 ☑
malfunction T84.310 ☑
malposition T84.320 ☑
mechanical NEC T84.390 ☑
obstruction T84.390 ☑
pain T84.84 ☑
perforation T84.390 ☑
protrusion T84.390 ☑
specified type NEC T84.89 ☑
stenosis T84.85 ☑
thrombosis T84.86 ☑
brain T85.9 ☑
embolism T85.810 ☑
fibrosis T85.820 ☑
hemorrhage T85.830 ☑
infection and inflammation T85.731 ☑
mechanical
breakdown T85.110 ☑
displacement T85.120 ☑
leakage T85.190 ☑
malposition T85.120 ☑
obstruction T85.190 ☑
perforation T85.190 ☑
protrusion T85.190 ☑
specified NEC T85.190 ☑
pain T85.840 ☑
specified type NEC T85.890 ☑
stenosis T85.850 ☑
thrombosis T85.860 ☑
cardiac (defibrillator) (pacemaker) — *see* Complications, cardiovascular device or implant, electronic
generator (brain) (gastric) (peripheral) (sacral) (spinal)
breakdown T85.113 ☑
displacement T85.123 ☑
leakage T85.193 ☑
malposition T85.123 ☑
obstruction T85.193 ☑
perforation T85.193 ☑
protrusion T85.193 ☑
specified type NEC T85.193 ☑
muscle T84.9 ☑
breakdown T84.418 ☑
displacement T84.428 ☑
embolism T84.81 ☑
fibrosis T84.82 ☑
hemorrhage T84.83 ☑
infection or inflammation T84.7 ☑
mechanical NEC T84.498 ☑
pain T84.84 ☑
specified type NEC T84.89 ☑
stenosis T84.85 ☑
thrombosis T84.86 ☑
nervous system T85.9 ☑
brain — *see* Complications, electronic stimulator device, brain
cranial nerve — *see* Complications, electronic stimulator device, peripheral nerve
embolism T85.810 ☑
fibrosis T85.820 ☑
gastric nerve — *see* Complications, electronic stimulator device, peripheral nerve
hemorrhage T85.830 ☑
infection and inflammation T85.738 ☑
mechanical
breakdown T85.118 ☑
displacement T85.128 ☑
leakage T85.199 ☑
malposition T85.128 ☑
obstruction T85.199 ☑
perforation T85.199 ☑
protrusion T85.199 ☑
specified NEC T85.199 ☑
pain T85.840 ☑
peripheral nerve — *see* Complications, electronic stimulator device, peripheral nerve
sacral nerve — *see* Complications, electronic stimulator device, peripheral nerve
specified type NEC T85.890 ☑
spinal cord — *see* Complications, electronic stimulator device, spinal cord

Complication(s) — *continued*
electronic stimulator device — *continued*
nervous system — *continued*
stenosis T85.850 ☑
thrombosis T85.860 ☑
vagal nerve — *see* Complications, electronic stimulator device, peripheral nerve
peripheral nerve T85.9 ☑
embolism T85.810 ☑
fibrosis T85.820 ☑
hemorrhage T85.830 ☑
infection and inflammation T85.732 ☑
mechanical
breakdown T85.111 ☑
displacement T85.121 ☑
leakage T85.191 ☑
malposition T85.121 ☑
obstruction T85.191 ☑
perforation T85.191 ☑
protrusion T85.191 ☑
specified NEC T85.191 ☑
pain T85.840 ☑
specified type NEC T85.890 ☑
stenosis T85.850 ☑
thrombosis T85.860 ☑
spinal cord T85.9 ☑
embolism T85.810 ☑
fibrosis T85.820 ☑
hemorrhage T85.830 ☑
infection and inflammation T85.733 ☑
mechanical
breakdown T85.112 ☑
displacement T85.122 ☑
leakage T85.192 ☑
malposition T85.122 ☑
obstruction T85.192 ☑
perforation T85.192 ☑
protrusion T85.192 ☑
specified NEC T85.192 ☑
pain T85.840 ☑
specified type NEC T85.890 ☑
stenosis T85.850 ☑
thrombosis T85.860 ☑
urinary T83.9 ☑
embolism T83.81 ☑
fibrosis T83.82 ☑
hemorrhage T83.83 ☑
infection and inflammation T83.598 ☑
mechanical
breakdown T83.110 ☑
displacement T83.120 ☑
malposition T83.120 ☑
perforation T83.190 ☑
protrusion T83.190 ☑
specified NEC T83.190 ☑
pain T83.84 ☑
specified type NEC T83.89 ☑
stenosis T83.85 ☑
thrombosis T83.86 ☑
electroshock therapy T88.9 ☑
specified NEC T88.8 ☑
endocrine E34.9
postprocedural
adrenal hypofunction E89.6
hypoinsulinemia E89.1
hypoparathyroidism E89.2
hypopituitarism E89.3
hypothyroidism E89.0
ovarian failure E89.40
asymptomatic E89.40
symptomatic E89.41
specified NEC E89.89
testicular hypofunction E89.5
endodontic treatment NEC M27.59
enterostomy (stoma) K94.10
hemorrhage K94.11
infection K94.12
malfunction K94.13
mechanical K94.13
specified complication NEC K94.19
episiotomy, disruption O90.1
esophageal anti-reflux device T85.9 ☑
embolism T85.818 ☑
fibrosis T85.828 ☑
hemorrhage T85.838 ☑
infection and inflammation T85.79 ☑

Complication(s) — *continued*
esophageal anti-reflux device — *continued*
mechanical
breakdown T85.511 ☑
displacement T85.521 ☑
malfunction T85.511 ☑
malposition T85.521 ☑
obstruction T85.591 ☑
perforation T85.591 ☑
protrusion T85.591 ☑
specified NEC T85.591 ☑
pain T85.848 ☑
specified type NEC T85.898 ☑
stenosis T85.858 ☑
thrombosis T85.868 ☑
esophagostomy K94.30
hemorrhage K94.31
infection K94.32
malfunction K94.33
mechanical K94.33
specified complication NEC K94.39
extracorporeal circulation T80.90 ☑
extremity artery (bypass) graft T82.9 ☑
arteriosclerosis — *see* Arteriosclerosis, extremities, bypass graft
embolism T82.818 ☑
fibrosis T82.828 ☑
hemorrhage T82.838 ☑
infection and inflammation T82.7 ☑
mechanical
breakdown T82.318 ☑
femoral artery T82.312 ☑
displacement T82.328 ☑
femoral artery T82.322 ☑
leakage T82.338 ☑
femoral artery T82.332 ☑
malposition T82.328 ☑
femoral artery T82.322 ☑
obstruction T82.398 ☑
femoral artery T82.392 ☑
perforation T82.398 ☑
femoral artery T82.392 ☑
protrusion T82.398 ☑
femoral artery T82.392 ☑
pain T82.848 ☑
specified type NEC T82.898 ☑
stenosis T82.858 ☑
thrombosis T82.868 ☑
eye H57.9
corneal graft — *see* Complications, graft, cornea
implant (prosthetic) T85.9 ☑
embolism T85.818 ☑
fibrosis T85.828 ☑
hemorrhage T85.838 ☑
infection and inflammation T85.79 ☑
mechanical
breakdown T85.318 ☑
displacement T85.328 ☑
leakage T85.398 ☑
malposition T85.328 ☑
obstruction T85.398 ☑
perforation T85.398 ☑
protrusion T85.398 ☑
specified NEC T85.398 ☑
pain T85.848 ☑
specified type NEC T85.898 ☑
stenosis T85.858 ☑
thrombosis T85.868 ☑
intraocular lens — *see* Complications, intraocular lens
orbital prosthesis — *see* Complications, orbital prosthesis
female genital N94.9
device, implant or graft NEC — *see* Complications, genitourinary, device or implant, genital tract
femoral artery (bypass) graft — *see* Complication, extremity artery (bypass) graft
fixation device, internal (orthopedic) T84.9 ☑
infection and inflammation T84.60 ☑
arm T84.61- ☑
humerus T84.61- ☑
radius T84.61- ☑
ulna T84.61- ☑
leg T84.629 ☑
femur T84.62- ☑
fibula T84.62- ☑

- **Complication**(s) — *continued*
  - fixation device, internal — *continued*
    - infection and inflammation — *continued*
      - leg — *continued*
        - tibia T84.62- ☑
      - specified site NEC T84.89 ☑
      - spine T84.63 ☑
    - mechanical
      - breakdown
        - limb T84.119 ☑
          - carpal T84.21Ø ☑
          - femur T84.11- ☑
          - fibula T84.11- ☑
          - humerus T84.11- ☑
          - metacarpal T84.21Ø ☑
          - metatarsal T84.213 ☑
          - phalanx
            - foot T84.213 ☑
            - hand T84.21Ø ☑
          - radius T84.11- ☑
          - tarsal T84.213 ☑
          - tibia T84.11- ☑
          - ulna T84.11- ☑
        - specified bone NEC T84.218 ☑
        - spine T84.216 ☑
      - displacement
        - limb T84.129 ☑
          - carpal T84.22Ø ☑
          - femur T84.12- ☑
          - fibula T84.12- ☑
          - humerus T84.12- ☑
          - metacarpal T84.22Ø ☑
          - metatarsal T84.223 ☑
          - phalanx
            - foot T84.223 ☑
            - hand T84.22Ø ☑
          - radius T84.12- ☑
          - tarsal T84.223 ☑
          - tibia T84.12- ☑
          - ulna T84.12- ☑
        - specified bone NEC T84.228 ☑
        - spine T84.226 ☑
      - malposition — *see* Complications, fixation device, internal, mechanical, displacement
      - obstruction — *see* Complications, fixation device, internal, mechanical, specified type NEC
      - perforation — *see* Complications, fixation device, internal, mechanical, specified type NEC
      - protrusion — *see* Complications, fixation device, internal, mechanical, specified type NEC
      - specified type NEC
        - limb T84.199 ☑
          - carpal T84.29Ø ☑
          - femur T84.19- ☑
          - fibula T84.19- ☑
          - humerus T84.19- ☑
          - metacarpal T84.29Ø ☑
          - metatarsal T84.293 ☑
          - phalanx
            - foot T84.293 ☑
            - hand T84.29Ø ☑
          - radius T84.19- ☑
          - tarsal T84.293 ☑
          - tibia T84.19- ☑
          - ulna T84.19- ☑
        - specified bone NEC T84.298 ☑
        - vertebra T84.296 ☑
    - specified type NEC T84.89 ☑
      - embolism T84.81 ☑
      - fibrosis T84.82 ☑
      - hemorrhage T84.83 ☑
      - pain T84.84 ☑
      - specified complication NEC T84.89 ☑
      - stenosis T84.85 ☑
      - thrombosis T84.86 ☑
  - following
    - acute myocardial infarction NEC I23.8
      - aneurysm (false) (of cardiac wall) (of heart wall) (ruptured) I23.3
      - angina I23.7
      - atrial
        - septal defect I23.1
        - thrombosis I23.6
      - cardiac wall rupture I23.3
      - chordae tendinae rupture I23.4

- **Complication**(s) — *continued*
  - following — *continued*
    - acute myocardial infarction — *continued*
      - defect
        - septal
          - atrial (heart) I23.1
          - ventricular (heart) I23.2
      - hemopericardium I23.Ø
      - papillary muscle rupture I23.5
      - rupture
        - cardiac wall I23.3
          - with hemopericardium I23.Ø
        - chordae tendineae I23.4
        - papillary muscle I23.5
      - specified NEC I23.8
      - thrombosis
        - atrium I23.6
        - auricular appendage I23.6
        - ventricle (heart) I23.6
      - ventricular
        - septal defect I23.2
        - thrombosis I23.6
    - ectopic or molar pregnancy OØ8.9
      - cardiac arrest OØ8.81
      - sepsis OØ8.82
      - specified type NEC OØ8.89
      - urinary tract infection OØ8.83
    - termination of pregnancy — *see* Abortion
  - gastrointestinal K92.9
    - bile duct prosthesis — *see* Complications, bile duct implant
    - esophageal anti-reflux device — *see* Complications, esophageal anti-reflux device
    - postoperative
      - colostomy — *see* Complications, colostomy
      - dumping syndrome K91.1
      - enterostomy — *see* Complications, enterostomy
      - gastrostomy — *see* Complications, gastrostomy
      - malabsorption NEC K91.2
      - obstruction — *see also* Obstruction, intestine, postoperative K91.3Ø
      - postcholecystectomy syndrome K91.5
      - specified NEC K91.89
      - vomiting after GI surgery K91.Ø
    - prosthetic device or implant
      - bile duct prosthesis — *see* Complications, bile duct implant
      - esophageal anti-reflux device — *see* Complications, esophageal anti-reflux device
      - specified type NEC
        - embolism T85.818 ☑
        - fibrosis T85.828 ☑
        - hemorrhage T85.838 ☑
        - mechanical
          - breakdown T85.518 ☑
          - displacement T85.528 ☑
          - malfunction T85.518 ☑
          - malposition T85.528 ☑
          - obstruction T85.598 ☑
          - perforation T85.598 ☑
          - protrusion T85.598 ☑
          - specified NEC T85.598 ☑
        - pain T85.848 ☑
        - specified complication NEC T85.898 ☑
        - stenosis T85.858 ☑
        - thrombosis T85.868 ☑
  - gastrostomy (stoma) K94.2Ø
    - hemorrhage K94.21
    - infection K94.22
    - malfunction K94.23
    - mechanical K94.23
    - specified complication NEC K94.29
  - genitourinary
    - device or implant T83.9 ☑
      - genital tract T83.9 ☑
        - infection or inflammation T83.69 ☑
        - intrauterine contraceptive device — *see* Complications, intrauterine, contraceptive device
        - mechanical — *see* Complications, by device, mechanical
        - mesh — *see* Complications, prosthetic device or implant, mesh
        - penile prosthesis — *see* Complications, prosthetic device, penile
        - specified type NEC T83.89 ☑
          - embolism T83.81 ☑

- **Complication**(s) — *continued*
  - genitourinary — *continued*
    - device or implant — *continued*
      - genital tract — *continued*
        - specified type — *continued*
          - fibrosis T83.82 ☑
          - hemorrhage T83.83 ☑
          - pain T83.84 ☑
          - specified complication NEC T83.89 ☑
          - stenosis T83.85 ☑
          - thrombosis T83.86 ☑
        - vaginal mesh — *see* Complications, prosthetic device or implant, mesh
      - urinary system T83.9 ☑
        - cystostomy catheter — *see* Complication, catheter, cystostomy
        - electronic stimulator — *see* Complications, electronic stimulator device, urinary
        - indwelling urethral catheter — *see* Complications, catheter, urethral, indwelling
        - infection or inflammation T83.598 ☑
          - indwelling urethral catheter T83.511 ☑
        - kidney transplant — *see* Complication, transplant, kidney
        - organ graft — *see* Complication, graft, urinary organ
        - specified type NEC T83.89 ☑
          - embolism T83.81 ☑
          - fibrosis T83.82 ☑
          - hemorrhage T83.83 ☑
          - mechanical T83.198 ☑
            - breakdown T83.118 ☑
            - displacement T83.128 ☑
            - malfunction T83.118 ☑
            - malposition T83.128 ☑
            - obstruction T83.198 ☑
            - perforation T83.198 ☑
            - protrusion T83.198 ☑
            - specified NEC T83.198 ☑
        - sphincter implant — *see* Complications, implant, urinary sphincter
        - sphincter, implanted T83.191 ☑
        - stent (ileal conduit) (nephroureteral) T83.193 ☑
          - pain T83.84 ☑
          - specified complication NEC T83.89 ☑
          - stenosis T83.85 ☑
          - thrombosis T83.86 ☑
          - ureteral indwelling T83.192 ☑
    - postprocedural
      - pelvic peritoneal adhesions N99.4
      - renal failure N99.Ø
      - specified NEC N99.89
      - stoma — *see* Complications, stoma, urinary tract
      - urethral stricture — *see* Stricture, urethra, postprocedural
      - vaginal
        - adhesions N99.2
        - vault prolapse N99.3
  - graft (bypass) (patch) — *see also* Complications, prosthetic device or implant
    - aorta — *see* Complications, graft, vascular
    - arterial — *see* Complication, graft, vascular
    - bone T86.839
      - failure T86.831
      - infection T86.832
      - mechanical T84.318 ☑
        - breakdown T84.318 ☑
        - displacement T84.328 ☑
        - protrusion T84.398 ☑
        - specified type NEC T84.398 ☑
      - rejection T86.83Ø
      - specified type NEC T86.838
    - carotid artery — *see* Complications, graft, vascular
    - cornea T86.849- ☑
      - failure T86.841- ☑
      - infection T86.842- ☑
      - mechanical T85.398 ☑
        - breakdown T85.318 ☑
        - displacement T85.328 ☑
        - protrusion T85.398 ☑
        - specified type NEC T85.398 ☑
      - rejection T86.84Ø- ☑
      - retroprosthetic membrane T85.398 ☑
      - specified type NEC T86.848- ☑
    - femoral artery (bypass) — *see* Complication, extremity artery (bypass) graft

Complication(s) — *continued*
graft — *see also* Complications, prosthetic device or implant — *continued*
genital organ or tract — *see* Complications, genitourinary, device or implant, genital tract
muscle T84.9 ☑
breakdown T84.41Ø ☑
displacement T84.42Ø ☑
embolism T84.81 ☑
fibrosis T84.82 ☑
hemorrhage T84.83 ☑
infection and inflammation T84.7 ☑
mechanical NEC T84.49Ø ☑
pain T84.84 ☑
specified type NEC T84.89 ☑
stenosis T84.85 ☑
thrombosis T84.86 ☑
nerve — *see* Complication, prosthetic device or implant, specified NEC
skin — *see* Complications, prosthetic device or implant, skin graft
tendon T84.9 ☑
breakdown T84.41Ø ☑
displacement T84.42Ø ☑
embolism T84.81 ☑
fibrosis T84.82 ☑
hemorrhage T84.83 ☑
infection and inflammation T84.7 ☑
mechanical NEC T84.49Ø ☑
pain T84.84 ☑
specified type NEC T84.89 ☑
stenosis T84.85 ☑
thrombosis T84.86 ☑
urinary organ T83.9 ☑
embolism T83.81 ☑
fibrosis T83.82 ☑
hemorrhage T83.83 ☑
infection and inflammation T83.598 ☑
indwelling urethral catheter T83.511 ☑
mechanical
breakdown T83.21 ☑
displacement T83.22 ☑
erosion T83.24 ☑
exposure T83.25 ☑
leakage T83.23 ☑
malposition T83.22 ☑
obstruction T83.29 ☑
perforation T83.29 ☑
protrusion T83.29 ☑
specified NEC T83.29 ☑
pain T83.84 ☑
specified type NEC T83.89 ☑
stenosis T83.85 ☑
thrombosis T83.86 ☑
vascular T82.9 ☑
embolism T82.818 ☑
femoral artery — *see* Complication, extremity artery (bypass) graft
fibrosis T82.828 ☑
hemorrhage T82.838 ☑
mechanical
breakdown T82.319 ☑
aorta (bifurcation) T82.31Ø ☑
carotid artery T82.311 ☑
specified vessel NEC T82.318 ☑
displacement T82.329 ☑
aorta (bifurcation) T82.32Ø ☑
carotid artery T82.321 ☑
specified vessel NEC T82.328 ☑
leakage T82.339 ☑
aorta (bifurcation) T82.33Ø ☑
carotid artery T82.331 ☑
specified vessel NEC T82.338 ☑
malposition T82.329 ☑
aorta (bifurcation) T82.32Ø ☑
carotid artery T82.321 ☑
specified vessel NEC T82.328 ☑
obstruction T82.399 ☑
aorta (bifurcation) T82.39Ø ☑
carotid artery T82.391 ☑
specified vessel NEC T82.398 ☑
perforation T82.399 ☑
aorta (bifurcation) T82.39Ø ☑
carotid artery T82.391 ☑
specified vessel NEC T82.398 ☑
protrusion T82.399 ☑

Complication(s) — *continued*
graft — *see also* Complications, prosthetic device or implant — *continued*
vascular — *continued*
mechanical — *continued*
protrusion — *continued*
aorta (bifurcation) T82.39Ø ☑
carotid artery T82.391 ☑
specified vessel NEC T82.398 ☑
pain T82.848 ☑
specified complication NEC T82.898 ☑
stenosis T82.858 ☑
thrombosis T82.868 ☑
heart I51.9
assist device
infection and inflammation T82.7 ☑
following acute myocardial infarction — *see* Complications, following, acute myocardial infarction
postoperative — *see* Complications, circulatory system
transplant — *see* Complication, transplant, heart and lung(s) — *see* Complications, transplant, heart, with lung
valve
graft (biological) T82.9 ☑
embolism T82.817 ☑
fibrosis T82.827 ☑
hemorrhage T82.837 ☑
infection and inflammation T82.7 ☑
mechanical T82.228 ☑
breakdown T82.221 ☑
displacement T82.222 ☑
leakage T82.223 ☑
malposition T82.222 ☑
obstruction T82.228 ☑
perforation T82.228 ☑
protrusion T82.228 ☑
pain T82.847 ☑
specified type NEC T82.897 ☑
stenosis T82.857 ☑
thrombosis T82.867 ☑
prosthesis T82.9 ☑
embolism T82.817 ☑
fibrosis T82.827 ☑
hemorrhage T82.837 ☑
infection or inflammation T82.6 ☑
mechanical T82.Ø9 ☑
breakdown T82.Ø1 ☑
displacement T82.Ø2 ☑
leakage T82.Ø3 ☑
malposition T82.Ø2 ☑
obstruction T82.Ø9 ☑
perforation T82.Ø9 ☑
protrusion T82.Ø9 ☑
pain T82.847 ☑
specified type NEC T82.897 ☑
mechanical T82.Ø9 ☑
stenosis T82.857 ☑
thrombosis T82.867 ☑
hematoma
intraoperative — *see* Complication, intraoperative, hemorrhage
postprocedural — *see* Complication, postprocedural, hematoma
hemodialysis — *see* Complications, dialysis
hemorrhage
intraoperative — *see* Complication, intraoperative, hemorrhage
postprocedural — *see* Complication, postprocedural, hemorrhage
IEC (immune effector cellular) therapy T8Ø.82 ☑
ileostomy (stoma) — *see* Complications, enterostomy
immune effector cellular (IEC) therapy T8Ø.82 ☑
immunization (procedure) — *see* Complications, vaccination
implant — *see also* Complications, by site and type
urinary sphincter T83.9 ☑
embolism T83.81 ☑
fibrosis T83.82 ☑
hemorrhage T83.83 ☑
infection and inflammation T83.591 ☑
mechanical
breakdown T83.111 ☑
displacement T83.121 ☑
leakage T83.191 ☑

Complication(s) — *continued*
implant — *see also* Complications, by site and type — *continued*
urinary sphincter — *continued*
mechanical — *continued*
malposition T83.121 ☑
obstruction T83.191 ☑
perforation T83.191 ☑
protrusion T83.191 ☑
specified NEC T83.191 ☑
pain T83.84 ☑
specified type NEC T83.89 ☑
stenosis T83.85 ☑
thrombosis T83.86 ☑
infusion (procedure) T8Ø.9Ø ☑
air embolism T8Ø.Ø ☑
blood — *see* Complications, transfusion
catheter — *see* Complications, catheter
infection T8Ø.29 ☑
pump — *see* Complications, cardiovascular, device or implant
sepsis T8Ø.29 ☑
serum reaction — *see also* Reaction, serum T8Ø.69 ☑
anaphylactic shock — *see also* Shock, anaphylactic T8Ø.59 ☑
specified type NEC T8Ø.89 ☑
inhalation therapy NEC T81.81 ☑
injection (procedure) T8Ø.9Ø ☑
drug reaction — *see* Reaction, drug
infection T8Ø.29 ☑
sepsis T8Ø.29 ☑
serum (prophylactic) (therapeutic) — *see* Complications, vaccination
specified type NEC T8Ø.89 ☑
vaccine (any) — *see* Complications, vaccination
inoculation (any) — *see* Complications, vaccination
insulin pump
infection and inflammation T85.72 ☑
mechanical
breakdown T85.614 ☑
displacement T85.624 ☑
leakage T85.633 ☑
malposition T85.624 ☑
obstruction T85.694 ☑
perforation T85.694 ☑
protrusion T85.694 ☑
specified NEC T85.694 ☑
intestinal pouch NEC K91.858
intraocular lens (prosthetic) T85.9 ☑
embolism T85.818 ☑
fibrosis T85.828 ☑
hemorrhage T85.838 ☑
infection and inflammation T85.79 ☑
mechanical
breakdown T85.21 ☑
displacement T85.22 ☑
malposition T85.22 ☑
obstruction T85.29 ☑
perforation T85.29 ☑
protrusion T85.29 ☑
specified NEC T85.29 ☑
pain T85.848 ☑
specified type NEC T85.898 ☑
stenosis T85.858 ☑
thrombosis T85.868 ☑
intraoperative (intraprocedural)
cardiac arrest — *see also* Infarct, myocardium, associated with revascularization procedure
during cardiac surgery I97.71Ø
during other surgery I97.711
cardiac functional disturbance NEC — *see also* Infarct, myocardium, associated with revascularization procedure
during cardiac surgery I97.79Ø
during other surgery I97.791
hemorrhage (hematoma) (of)
circulatory system organ or structure
during cardiac bypass I97.411
during cardiac catheterization I97.41Ø
during other circulatory system procedure I97.418
during other procedure I97.42
digestive system organ
during procedure on digestive system K91.61
during procedure on other organ K91.62

Complication(s) — *continued*
- intraoperative — *continued*
  - hemorrhage — *continued*
    - ear
      - during procedure on ear and mastoid process H95.21
      - during procedure on other organ H95.22
    - endocrine system organ or structure
      - during procedure on endocrine system organ or structure E36.Ø1
      - during procedure on other organ E36.Ø2
    - eye and adnexa
      - during ophthalmic procedure H59.11- ☑
      - during other procedure H59.12- ☑
    - genitourinary organ or structure
      - during procedure on genitourinary organ or structure N99.61
      - during procedure on other organ N99.62
    - mastoid process
      - during procedure on ear and mastoid process H95.21
      - during procedure on other organ H95.22
    - musculoskeletal structure
      - during musculoskeletal surgery M96.81Ø
      - during non-orthopedic surgery M96.811
      - during orthopedic surgery M96.81Ø
    - nervous system
      - during a nervous system procedure G97.31
      - during other procedure G97.32
    - respiratory system
      - during other procedure J95.62
      - during procedure on respiratory system organ or structure J95.61
    - skin and subcutaneous tissue
      - during a dermatologic procedure L76.Ø1
      - during a procedure on other organ L76.Ø2
    - spleen
      - during a procedure on other organ D78.Ø2
      - during a procedure on the spleen D78.Ø1
  - puncture or laceration (accidental) (unintentional) (of)
    - brain
      - during a nervous system procedure G97.48
      - during other procedure G97.49
    - circulatory system organ or structure
      - during circulatory system procedure I97.51
      - during other procedure I97.52
    - digestive system
      - during procedure on digestive system K91.71
      - during procedure on other organ K91.72
    - ear
      - during procedure on ear and mastoid process H95.31
      - during procedure on other organ H95.32
    - endocrine system organ or structure
      - during procedure on endocrine system organ or structure E36.11
      - during procedure on other organ E36.12
    - eye and adnexa
      - during ophthalmic procedure H59.21- ☑
      - during other procedure H59.22- ☑
    - genitourinary organ or structure
      - during procedure on genitourinary organ or structure N99.71
      - during procedure on other organ N99.72
    - mastoid process
      - during procedure on ear and mastoid process H95.31
      - during procedure on other organ H95.32
    - musculoskeletal structure
      - during musculoskeletal surgery M96.82Ø
      - during non-orthopedic surgery M96.821
      - during orthopedic surgery M96.82Ø
    - nervous system
      - during a nervous system procedure G97.48
      - during other procedure G97.49
    - respiratory system
      - during other procedure J95.72
      - during procedure on respiratory system organ or structure J95.71
    - skin and subcutaneous tissue
      - during a dermatologic procedure L76.11
      - during a procedure on other organ L76.12
    - spleen
      - during a procedure on other organ D78.12
      - during a procedure on the spleen D78.11
  - specified NEC
    - circulatory system I97.88
    - digestive system K91.81
    - ear H95.88
    - endocrine system E36.8
    - eye and adnexa H59.88
    - genitourinary system N99.81
    - mastoid process H95.88
    - musculoskeletal structure M96.89
    - nervous system G97.81
    - respiratory system J95.88
    - skin and subcutaneous tissue L76.81
    - spleen D78.81
- intraperitoneal catheter (dialysis) (infusion) — *see* Complication(s), catheter, intraperitoneal dialysis
- intrathecal infusion pump
  - infection and inflammation T85.738 ☑
  - mechanical
    - breakdown T85.615 ☑
    - displacement T85.625 ☑
    - leakage T85.635 ☑
    - malfunction T85.695 ☑
    - malposition T85.625 ☑
    - obstruction T85.695 ☑
    - perforation T85.695 ☑
    - protrusion T85.695 ☑
    - specified NEC T85.695 ☑
- intrauterine
  - contraceptive device
    - embolism T83.81 ☑
    - fibrosis T83.82 ☑
    - hemorrhage T83.83 ☑
    - infection and inflammation T83.69 ☑
    - mechanical
      - breakdown T83.31 ☑
      - displacement T83.32 ☑
      - malposition T83.32 ☑
      - obstruction T83.39 ☑
      - perforation T83.39 ☑
      - protrusion T83.39 ☑
      - specified NEC T83.39 ☑
    - pain T83.84 ☑
    - specified type NEC T83.89 ☑
    - stenosis T83.85 ☑
    - thrombosis T83.86 ☑
  - procedure (fetal), to newborn P96.5
- jejunostomy (stoma) — *see* Complications, enterostomy
- joint prosthesis, internal T84.9 ☑
  - breakage (fracture) T84.Ø1- ☑
  - dislocation T84.Ø2- ☑
  - fracture T84.Ø1- ☑
  - infection or inflammation T84.5Ø ☑
    - hip T84.5- ☑
    - knee T84.5- ☑
    - specified joint NEC T84.59 ☑
  - instability T84.Ø2- ☑
  - malposition — *see* Complications, joint prosthesis, mechanical, displacement
  - mechanical
    - breakage, broken T84.Ø1- ☑
    - dislocation T84.Ø2- ☑
    - fracture T84.Ø1- ☑
    - instability T84.Ø2- ☑
    - leakage — *see* Complications, joint prosthesis, mechanical, specified NEC
    - loosening T84.Ø39 ☑
      - hip T84.Ø3- ☑
      - knee T84.Ø3- ☑
      - specified joint NEC T84.Ø38 ☑
    - obstruction — *see* Complications, joint prosthesis, mechanical, specified NEC
    - perforation — *see* Complications, joint prosthesis, mechanical, specified NEC
      - osteolysis T84.Ø59 ☑
        - hip T84.Ø5- ☑
        - knee T84.Ø5- ☑
        - other specified joint T84.Ø58 ☑
    - periprosthetic osteolysis, by site T84.Ø5- ☑
    - protrusion — *see* Complications, joint prosthesis, mechanical, specified NEC
    - specified complication NEC T84.Ø99 ☑
      - hip T84.Ø9- ☑
      - knee T84.Ø9- ☑
      - other specified joint T84.Ø98 ☑
    - subluxation T84.Ø2- ☑
    - wear of articular bearing surface T84.Ø69 ☑
      - hip T84.Ø6- ☑
      - knee T84.Ø6- ☑
      - other specified joint T84.Ø68 ☑
  - specified joint NEC T84.89 ☑
    - embolism T84.81 ☑
    - fibrosis T84.82 ☑
    - hemorrhage T84.83 ☑
    - pain T84.84 ☑
    - specified complication NEC T84.89 ☑
    - stenosis T84.85 ☑
    - thrombosis T84.86 ☑
  - subluxation T84.Ø2- ☑
- kidney transplant — *see* Complications, transplant, kidney
- labor O75.9
  - specified NEC O75.89
- liver transplant (immune or nonimmune) — *see* Complications, transplant, liver
- lumbar puncture G97.1
  - cerebrospinal fluid leak G97.Ø
  - headache or reaction G97.1
- lung transplant — *see* Complications, transplant, lung
  - and heart — *see* Complications, transplant, lung, with heart
- male genital N5Ø.9
  - device, implant or graft — *see* Complications, genitourinary, device or implant, genital tract
  - postprocedural or postoperative — *see* Complications, genitourinary, postprocedural
  - specified NEC N99.89
- mastoid (process) procedure
  - intraoperative H95.88
    - hematoma — *see* Complications, intraoperative, hemorrhage (hematoma) (of), mastoid process
    - hemorrhage — *see* Complications, intraoperative, hemorrhage (hematoma) (of), mastoid process
    - laceration — *see* Complications, intraoperative, puncture or laceration, mastoid process
    - specified NEC H95.88
  - postmastoidectomy — *see* Complications, postmastoidectomy
  - postoperative H95.89
    - external ear canal stenosis H95.81 ☑
    - hematoma — *see* Complications, postprocedural, hematoma (of), mastoid process
    - hemorrhage — *see* Complications, postprocedural, hemorrhage (of), mastoid process
    - postmastoidectomy — *see* Complications, postmastoidectomy
    - seroma — *see* Complications, postprocedural, seroma (of), mastoid process
    - specified NEC H95.89
- mastoidectomy cavity — *see* Complications, postmastoidectomy
- mechanical — *see* Complications, by site and type, mechanical
- medical procedures — *see also* Complication(s), intraoperative T88.9 ☑
- metabolic E88.9
  - postoperative E89.89
    - specified NEC E89.89
- molar pregnancy NOS OØ8.9
  - damage to pelvic organs OØ8.6
  - embolism OØ8.2
  - genital infection OØ8.Ø
  - hemorrhage (delayed) (excessive) OØ8.1
  - metabolic disorder OØ8.5
  - renal failure OØ8.4
  - shock OØ8.3
  - specified type NEC OØ8.Ø
  - venous complication NEC OØ8.7
- musculoskeletal system — *see also* Complication, intraoperative (intraprocedural), by site
  - device, implant or graft NEC — *see* Complications, orthopedic, device or implant
  - internal fixation (nail) (plate) (rod) — *see* Complications, fixation device, internal
  - joint prosthesis — *see* Complications, joint prosthesis
  - post radiation M96.89
    - kyphosis M96.2

Complication(s) — *continued*
  musculoskeletal system — *see also* Complication, intraoperative, by site — *continued*
    post radiation — *continued*
      scoliosis M96.5
      specified complication NEC M96.89
    postoperative (postprocedural) M96.89
      with osteoporosis — *see* Osteoporosis
      fracture following insertion of device — *see* Fracture, following insertion of orthopedic implant, joint prosthesis or bone plate
      joint instability after prosthesis removal M96.89
      lordosis M96.4
      postlaminectomy syndrome NEC M96.1
        kyphosis M96.3
      pseudarthrosis M96.Ø
      specified complication NEC M96.89
  nephrostomy (stoma) — *see* Complications, stoma, urinary tract, external NEC
  nervous system G98.8
    central G96.9
    device, implant or graft — *see also* Complication, prosthetic device or implant, specified NEC
      electronic stimulator (electrode(s)) — *see* Complications, electronic stimulator device
      specified NEC
        infection and inflammation T85.738 ☑
        mechanical T85.695 ☑
          breakdown T85.615 ☑
          displacement T85.625 ☑
          leakage T85.635 ☑
          malfunction T85.695 ☑
          malposition T85.625 ☑
          obstruction T85.695 ☑
          perforation T85.695 ☑
          protrusion T85.695 ☑
          specified NEC T85.695 ☑
      ventricular shunt — *see* Complications, ventricular shunt
    electronic stimulator (electrode(s)) — *see* Complications, electronic stimulator device
    postprocedural G97.82
      intracranial hypotension G97.2
      specified NEC G97.82
      spinal fluid leak G97.Ø
  newborn, due to intrauterine (fetal) procedure P96.5
  nonabsorbable (permanent) sutures — *see* Complication, sutures, permanent
  obstetric O75.9
    procedure (instrumental) (manual) (surgical) specified NEC O75.4
    specified NEC O75.89
    surgical wound NEC O9Ø.89
      hematoma O9Ø.2
      infection O86.ØØ
  ocular lens implant — *see* Complications, intraocular lens
  ophthalmologic
    postprocedural bleb — *see* Blebitis
  orbital prosthesis T85.9 ☑
    embolism T85.818 ☑
    fibrosis T85.828 ☑
    hemorrhage T85.838 ☑
    infection and inflammation T85.79 ☑
    mechanical
      breakdown T85.31- ☑
      displacement T85.32- ☑
      malposition T85.32- ☑
      obstruction T85.39- ☑
      perforation T85.39- ☑
      protrusion T85.39- ☑
      specified NEC T85.39- ☑
    pain T85.848 ☑
    specified type NEC T85.898 ☑
    stenosis T85.858 ☑
    thrombosis T85.868 ☑
  organ or tissue transplant (partial) (total) — *see* Complications, transplant
  orthopedic — *see also* Disorder, soft tissue
    device or implant T84.9 ☑
      bone
        device or implant — *see* Complication, bone, device NEC
        graft — *see* Complication, graft, bone
      breakdown T84.418 ☑
      displacement T84.428 ☑

Complication(s) — *continued*
  orthopedic — *see also* Disorder, soft tissue — *continued*
    device or implant — *continued*
      electronic bone stimulator — *see* Complications, electronic stimulator device, bone
      embolism T84.81 ☑
      fibrosis T84.82 ☑
      fixation device — *see* Complication, fixation device, internal
      hemorrhage T84.83 ☑
      infection or inflammation T84.7 ☑
      joint prosthesis — *see* Complication, joint prosthesis, internal
      malfunction T84.418 ☑
      malposition T84.428 ☑
      mechanical NEC T84.498 ☑
      muscle graft — *see* Complications, graft, muscle
      obstruction T84.498 ☑
      pain T84.84 ☑
      perforation T84.498 ☑
      protrusion T84.498 ☑
      specified complication NEC T84.89 ☑
      stenosis T84.85 ☑
      tendon graft — *see* Complications, graft, tendon
      thrombosis T84.86 ☑
    fracture (following insertion of device) — *see* Fracture, following insertion of orthopedic implant, joint prosthesis or bone plate
    postprocedural M96.89
      fracture — *see* Fracture, following insertion of orthopedic implant, joint prosthesis or bone plate
      postlaminectomy syndrome NEC M96.1
        kyphosis M96.3
        lordosis M96.4
      postradiation
        kyphosis M96.2
        scoliosis M96.5
      pseudarthrosis post-fusion M96.Ø
      specified type NEC M96.89
  pacemaker (cardiac) — *see* Complications, cardiovascular device or implant, electronic
  pancreas transplant — *see* Complications, transplant, pancreas
  penile prosthesis (implant) — *see* Complications, prosthetic device, penile
  perfusion NEC T8Ø.9Ø ☑
  perineal repair (obstetrical) NEC O9Ø.89
    disruption O9Ø.1
    hematoma O9Ø.2
    infection (following delivery) O86.Ø9
  phototherapy T88.9 ☑
    specified NEC T88.8 ☑
  postmastoidectomy NEC H95.19- ☑
    cyst, mucosal H95.13- ☑
    granulation H95.12- ☑
    inflammation, chronic H95.11- ☑
    recurrent cholesteatoma H95.Ø- ☑
  postoperative — *see* Complications, postprocedural
    circulatory — *see* Complications, circulatory system
    ear — *see* Complications, ear
    endocrine — *see* Complications, endocrine
    eye — *see* Complications, eye
    lumbar puncture G97.1
      cerebrospinal fluid leak G97.Ø
    nervous system (central) (peripheral) — *see* Complications, nervous system
    respiratory system — *see* Complications, respiratory system
  postprocedural — *see also* Complications, surgical procedure
    cardiac arrest — *see also* Infarct, myocardium, associated with revascularization procedure
      following cardiac surgery I97.12Ø
      following other surgery I97.121
    cardiac functional disturbance NEC — *see also* Infarct, myocardium, associated with revascularization procedure
      following cardiac surgery I97.19Ø
      following other surgery I97.191
    cardiac insufficiency
      following cardiac surgery I97.11Ø
      following other surgery I97.111
    chorioretinal scars following retinal surgery H59.81- ☑

Complication(s) — *continued*
  postprocedural — *see also* Complications, surgical procedure — *continued*
    following cataract surgery
      cataract (lens) fragments H59.Ø2- ☑
      cystoid macular edema H59.Ø3- ☑
      specified NEC H59.Ø9- ☑
      vitreous (touch) syndrome H59.Ø1- ☑
    heart failure
      following cardiac surgery I97.13Ø
      following other surgery I97.131
    hematoma (of)
      circulatory system organ or structure
        following cardiac bypass I97.631
        following cardiac catheterization I97.63Ø
        following other circulatory system procedure I97.638
        following other procedure I97.621
      digestive system
        following procedure on digestive system K91.87Ø
        following procedure on other organ K91.871
      ear
        following other procedure H95.52
        following procedure on ear and mastoid process H95.51
      endocrine system
        following endocrine system procedure E89.82Ø
        following other procedure E89.821
      eye and adnexa
        following ophthalmic procedure H59.33- ☑
        following other procedure H59.34- ☑
      genitourinary organ or structure
        following procedure on genitourinary organ or structure N99.84Ø
        following procedure on other organ N99.841
      mastoid process
        following other procedure H95.52
        following procedure on ear and mastoid process H95.51
      musculoskeletal structure
        following musculoskeletal surgery M96.84Ø
        following non-orthopedic surgery M96.841
        following orthopedic surgery M96.84Ø
      nervous system
        following nervous system procedure G97.61
        following other procedure G97.62
      respiratory system
        following other procedure J95.861
        following procedure on respiratory system organ or structure J95.86Ø
      skin and subcutaneous tissue
        following dermatologic procedure L76.31
        following procedure on other organ L76.32
      spleen
        following procedure on other organ D78.32
        following procedure on the spleen D78.31
    hemorrhage (of)
      circulatory system organ or structure
        following cardiac bypass I97.611
        following cardiac catheterization I97.61Ø
        following other circulatory system procedure I97.618
        following other procedure I97.62Ø
      digestive system
        following procedure on digestive system K91.84Ø
        following procedure on other organ K91.841
      ear
        following other procedure H95.42
        following procedure on ear and mastoid process H95.41
      endocrine system
        following endocrine system procedure E89.81Ø
        following other procedure E89.811
      eye and adnexa
        following ophthalmic procedure H59.31- ☑
        following other procedure H59.32- ☑
      genitourinary organ or structure
        following procedure on genitourinary organ or structure N99.82Ø
        following procedure on other organ N99.821
      mastoid process
        following other procedure H95.42
        following procedure on ear and mastoid process H95.41

Complication(s) — *continued*
  postprocedural — *see also* Complications, surgical procedure — *continued*
    hemorrhage — *continued*
      musculoskeletal structure
        following musculoskeletal surgery M96.830
        following non-orthopedic surgery M96.831
        following orthopedic surgery M96.830
      nervous system
        following nervous system procedure G97.51
        following other procedure G97.52
      respiratory system
        following a respiratory system procedure J95.830
        following other procedure J95.831
      skin and subcutaneous tissue
        following a procedure on other organ L76.22
        following dermatologic procedure L76.21
      spleen
        following procedure on other organ D78.22
        following procedure on the spleen D78.21
    seroma (of)
      circulatory system organ or structure
        following cardiac bypass I97.641
        following cardiac catheterization I97.640
        following other circulatory system procedure I97.648
        following other procedure I97.622
      digestive system
        following procedure on digestive system K91.872
        following procedure on other organ K91.873
      ear
        following other procedure H95.54
        following procedure on ear and mastoid process H95.53
      endocrine system
        following endocrine system procedure E89.822
        following other procedure E89.823
      eye and adnexa
        following ophthalmic procedure H59.35- ☑
        following other procedure H59.36- ☑
      genitourinary organ or structure
        following procedure on genitourinary organ or structure N99.842
        following procedure on other organ N99.843
      mastoid process
        following other procedure H95.54
        following procedure on ear and mastoid process H95.53
      musculoskeletal structure
        following musculoskeletal surgery M96.842
        following non-orthopedic surgery M96.843
        following orthopedic surgery M96.842
      nervous system
        following nervous system procedure G97.63
        following other procedure G97.64
      respiratory system
        following other procedure J95.863
        following procedure on respiratory system organ or structure J95.862
      skin and subcutaneous tissue
        following dermatologic procedure L76.33
        following procedure on other organ L76.34
      spleen
        following procedure on other organ D78.34
        following procedure on the spleen D78.33
    specified NEC
      circulatory system I97.89
      digestive K91.89
      ear H95.89
      endocrine E89.89
      eye and adnexa H59.89
      genitourinary N99.89
      mastoid process H95.89
      metabolic E89.89
      musculoskeletal structure M96.89
      nervous system G97.82
      respiratory system J95.89
      skin and subcutaneous tissue L76.82
      spleen D78.89
  pregnancy NEC — *see* Pregnancy, complicated by
  prosthetic device or implant T85.9 ☑
    bile duct — *see* Complications, bile duct implant
    breast — *see* Complications, breast implant

Complication(s) — *continued*
  prosthetic device or implant — *continued*
    bulking agent
      ureteral
        erosion T83.714 ☑
        exposure T83.724 ☑
      urethral
        erosion T83.713 ☑
        exposure T83.723 ☑
    cardiac and vascular NEC — *see* Complications, cardiovascular device or implant
    corneal transplant — *see* Complications, graft, cornea
    electronic nervous system stimulator — *see* Complications, electronic stimulator device
    epidural infusion catheter — *see* Complications, catheter, epidural
    esophageal anti-reflux device — *see* Complications, esophageal anti-reflux device
    genital organ or tract — *see* Complications, genitourinary, device or implant, genital tract
      specified NEC T83.79- ☑
    heart valve — *see* Complications, heart, valve, prosthesis
    infection or inflammation T85.79 ☑
      intestine transplant T86.852
      liver transplant T86.43
      lung transplant T86.812
      pancreas transplant T86.892
      skin graft T86.822
    intraocular lens — *see* Complications, intraocular lens
    intraperitoneal (dialysis) catheter — *see* Complication(s), catheter, intraperitoneal dialysis
    joint — *see* Complications, joint prosthesis, internal
    mechanical NEC T85.698 ☑
      dialysis catheter (vascular) — *see also* Complication, catheter, dialysis, mechanical
        peritoneal — *see* Complication(s), catheter, intraperitoneal dialysis
      gastrointestinal device T85.598 ☑
      ocular device T85.398 ☑
      subdural (infusion) catheter T85.690 ☑
      suture, permanent T85.692 ☑
        that for bone repair — *see* Complications, fixation device, internal (orthopedic), mechanical
      ventricular shunt
        breakdown T85.01 ☑
        displacement T85.02 ☑
        leakage T85.03 ☑
        malposition T85.02 ☑
        obstruction T85.09 ☑
        perforation T85.09 ☑
        protrusion T85.09 ☑
        specified NEC T85.09 ☑
    mesh
      erosion (to surrounding organ or tissue) T83.718 ☑
        urethral (into pelvic floor muscles) T83.712 ☑
        vaginal (into pelvic floor muscles) T83.711 ☑
      exposure (into surrounding organ or tissue) T83.728 ☑
        urethral (through urethral wall) T83.722 ☑
        vaginal (into vagina) (through vaginal wall) T83.721 ☑
    orbital — *see* Complications, orbital prosthesis
    penile T83.9 ☑
      embolism T83.81 ☑
      fibrosis T83.82 ☑
      hemorrhage T83.83 ☑
      infection and inflammation T83.61 ☑
      mechanical
        breakdown T83.410 ☑
        displacement T83.420 ☑
        leakage T83.490 ☑
        malposition T83.420 ☑
        obstruction T83.490 ☑
        perforation T83.490 ☑
        protrusion T83.490 ☑
        specified NEC T83.490 ☑
      pain T83.84 ☑
      specified type NEC T83.89 ☑
      stenosis T83.85 ☑
      thrombosis T83.86 ☑

Complication(s) — *continued*
  prosthetic device or implant — *continued*
    prosthetic materials NEC
      erosion (to surrounding organ or tissue) T83.718 ☑
      exposure (into surrounding organ or tissue) T83.728 ☑
    skin graft T86.829
      artificial skin or decellularized allodermis
        embolism T85.818 ☑
        fibrosis T85.828 ☑
        hemorrhage T85.838 ☑
        infection and inflammation T85.79 ☑
        mechanical
          breakdown T85.613 ☑
          displacement T85.623 ☑
          malfunction T85.613 ☑
          malposition T85.623 ☑
          obstruction T85.693 ☑
          perforation T85.693 ☑
          protrusion T85.693 ☑
          specified NEC T85.693 ☑
        pain T85.848 ☑
        specified type NEC T85.898 ☑
        stenosis T85.858 ☑
        thrombosis T85.868 ☑
      failure T86.821
      infection T86.822
      rejection T86.820
      specified NEC T86.828
    sling
      urethral (female) (male)
        erosion T83.712 ☑
        exposure T83.722 ☑
    specified NEC T85.9 ☑
      embolism T85.818 ☑
      fibrosis T85.828 ☑
      hemorrhage T85.838 ☑
      infection and inflammation T85.79 ☑
      mechanical
        breakdown T85.618 ☑
        displacement T85.628 ☑
        leakage T85.638 ☑
        malfunction T85.618 ☑
        malposition T85.628 ☑
        obstruction T85.698 ☑
        perforation T85.698 ☑
        protrusion T85.698 ☑
        specified NEC T85.698 ☑
      pain T85.848 ☑
      specified type NEC T85.898 ☑
      stenosis T85.858 ☑
      thrombosis T85.868 ☑
    subdural infusion catheter — *see* Complications, catheter, subdural
    sutures — *see* Complications, sutures
    urinary organ or tract NEC — *see* Complications, genitourinary, device or implant, urinary system
    vascular — *see* Complications, cardiovascular device or implant
    ventricular shunt — *see* Complications, ventricular shunt (device)
  puerperium — *see* Puerperal
  puncture, spinal G97.1
    cerebrospinal fluid leak G97.0
    headache or reaction G97.1
  pyelogram N99.89
  radiation
    kyphosis M96.2
    scoliosis M96.5
  reattached
    extremity (infection) (rejection)
      lower T87.1X- ☑
      upper T87.0X- ☑
    specified body part NEC T87.2
  reconstructed breast
    asymmetry between native and reconstructed breast N65.1
    deformity N65.0
    disproportion between native and reconstructed breast N65.1
    excess tissue N65.0
    misshappen N65.0
  reimplant NEC — *see also* Complications, prosthetic device or implant

Complication(s) — *continued*
- reimplant — *see also* Complications, prosthetic device or implant — *continued*
  - limb (infection) (rejection) — *see* Complications, reattached, extremity
  - organ (partial) (total) — *see* Complications, transplant
  - prosthetic device NEC — *see* Complications, prosthetic device
- renal N28.9
  - allograft — *see* Complications, transplant, kidney
  - dialysis — *see* Complications, dialysis
- respirator
  - mechancial J95.85Ø
    - specified NEC J95.859
- respiratory system J98.9
  - device, implant or graft — *see* Complication, prosthetic device or implant, specified NEC
  - lung transplant — *see* Complications, prosthetic device or implant, lung transplant
  - postoperative J95.89
    - air leak J95.812
    - Mendelson's syndrome (chemical pneumonitis) J95.4
    - pneumothorax J95.811
    - pulmonary insufficiency (acute) (after nonthoracic surgery) J95.2
      - chronic J95.3
      - following thoracic surgery J95.1
    - respiratory failure (acute) J95.821
      - acute and chronic J95.822
    - specified NEC J95.89
    - subglottic stenosis J95.5
    - tracheostomy complication — *see* Complications, tracheostomy
  - therapy T81.89 ☑
- sedation during labor and delivery O74.9
  - cardiac O74.2
  - central nervous system O74.3
  - pulmonary NEC O74.1
- shunt — *see also* Complications, prosthetic device or implant
  - arteriovenous — *see* Complications, arteriovenous, shunt
  - ventricular (communicating) — *see* Complications, ventricular shunt
- skin
  - graft T86.829
    - failure T86.821
    - infection T86.822
    - rejection T86.82Ø
    - specified type NEC T86.828
- spinal
  - anesthesia — *see* Complications, anesthesia, spinal
  - catheter (epidural) (subdural) — *see* Complications, catheter
  - puncture or tap G97.1
    - cerebrospinal fluid leak G97.Ø
    - headache or reaction G97.1
- stent
  - bile duct — *see* Complications, bile duct prosthesis
  - ureteral indwelling
    - breakdown T83.112 ☑
    - displacement T83.122 ☑
    - leakage T83.192 ☑
    - malposition T83.122 ☑
    - obstruction T83.192 ☑
    - perforation T83.192 ☑
    - protrusion T83.192 ☑
    - specified NEC T83.192 ☑
  - urinary NEC (ileal conduit) (nephroureteral) T83.193 ☑
    - embolism T83.81 ☑
    - fibrosis T83.82 ☑
    - hemorrhage T83.83 ☑
    - infection and inflammation T83.593 ☑
    - mechanical
      - breakdown T83.113 ☑
      - displacement T83.123 ☑
      - leakage T83.193 ☑
      - malposition T83.123 ☑
      - obstruction T83.193 ☑
      - perforation T83.193 ☑
      - protrusion T83.193 ☑
      - specified NEC T83.193 ☑
    - pain T83.84 ☑
    - specified type NEC T83.89 ☑

Complication(s) — *continued*
- stent — *continued*
  - urinary — *continued*
    - stenosis T83.85 ☑
    - thrombosis T83.86 ☑
  - vascular
    - end stent stenosis — *see* Restenosis, stent
    - in stent stenosis — *see* Restenosis, stent
- stoma
  - digestive tract
    - colostomy — *see* Complications, colostomy
    - enterostomy — *see* Complications, enterostomy
    - esophagostomy — *see* Complications, esophagostomy
    - gastrostomy — *see* Complications, gastrostomy
  - urinary tract N99.528
    - continent N99.538
      - hemorrhage N99.53Ø
      - herniation N99.533
      - infection N99.531
      - malfunction N99.532
      - specified type NEC N99.538
      - stenosis N99.534
    - cystostomy — *see* Complications, cystostomy
    - external NOS N99.528
    - hemorrhage N99.52Ø
    - herniation N99.523
    - incontinent N99.528
      - hemorrhage N99.52Ø
      - herniation N99.523
      - infection N99.521
      - malfunction N99.522
      - specified type NEC N99.528
      - stenosis N99.524
    - infection N99.521
    - malfunction N99.522
    - specified type NEC N99.528
    - stenosis N99.524
- stomach banding — *see* Complication(s), bariatric procedure
- stomach stapling — *see* Complication(s), bariatric procedure
- surgical material, nonabsorbable — *see* Complication, suture, permanent
- surgical procedure (on) T81.9 ☑
  - amputation stump (late) — *see* Complications, amputation stump
  - cardiac — *see* Complications, circulatory system
  - cholesteatoma, recurrent — *see* Complications, postmastoidectomy, recurrent cholesteatoma
  - circulatory (early) — *see* Complications, circulatory system
  - digestive system — *see* Complications, gastrointestinal
  - dumping syndrome (postgastrectomy) K91.1
  - ear — *see* Complications, ear
  - elephantiasis or lymphedema I97.89
    - postmastectomy I97.2
  - emphysema (surgical) T81.82 ☑
  - endocrine — *see* Complications, endocrine
  - eye — *see* Complications, eye
  - fistula (persistent postoperative) T81.83 ☑
  - foreign body inadvertently left in wound (sponge) (suture) (swab) — *see* Foreign body, accidentally left during a procedure
  - gastrointestinal — *see* Complications, gastrointestinal
  - genitourinary NEC N99.89
  - hematoma
    - intraoperative — *see* Complication, intraoperative, hemorrhage
    - postprocedural — *see* Complication, postprocedural, hematoma
  - hemorrhage
    - intraoperative — *see* Complication, intraoperative, hemorrhage
    - postprocedural — *see* Complication, postprocedural, hemorrhage
  - hepatic failure K91.82
  - hyperglycemia (postpancreatectomy) E89.1
  - hypoinsulinemia (postpancreatectomy) E89.1
  - hypoparathyroidism (postparathyroidectomy) E89.2
  - hypopituitarism (posthypophysectomy) E89.3
  - hypothyroidism (post-thyroidectomy) E89.Ø
  - intestinal obstruction — *see also* Obstruction, intestine, postoperative K91.3Ø
  - intracranial hypotension following ventricular shunting (ventriculostomy) G97.2

Complication(s) — *continued*
- surgical procedure — *continued*
  - lymphedema I97.89
    - postmastectomy I97.2
  - malabsorption (postsurgical) NEC K91.2
    - osteoporosis — *see* Osteoporosis, postsurgical malabsorption
  - mastoidectomy cavity NEC — *see* Complications, postmastoidectomy
  - metabolic E89.89
    - specified NEC E89.89
  - musculoskeletal — *see* Complications, musculoskeletal system
  - nervous system (central) (peripheral) — *see* Complications, nervous system
  - ovarian failure E89.4Ø
    - asymptomatic E89.4Ø
    - symptomatic E89.41
  - peripheral vascular — *see* Complications, surgical procedure, vascular
  - postcardiotomy syndrome I97.Ø
  - postcholecystectomy syndrome K91.5
  - postcommissurotomy syndrome I97.Ø
  - postgastrectomy dumping syndrome K91.1
  - postlaminectomy syndrome NEC M96.1
    - kyphosis M96.3
  - postmastectomy lymphedema syndrome I97.2
  - postmastoidectomy cholesteatoma — *see* Complications, postmastoidectomy, recurrent cholesteatoma
  - postvagotomy syndrome K91.1
  - postvalvulotomy syndrome I97.Ø
  - pulmonary insufficiency (acute) J95.2
    - chronic J95.3
    - following thoracic surgery J95.1
  - reattached body part — *see* Complications, reattached
  - respiratory — *see* Complications, respiratory system
  - shock (hypovolemic) T81.19 ☑
  - spleen (postoperative) D78.89
    - intraoperative D78.81
  - stitch abscess T81.41 ☑
  - subglottic stenosis (postsurgical) J95.5
  - testicular hypofunction E89.5
  - transplant — *see* Complications, organ or tissue transplant
  - urinary NEC N99.89
  - vaginal vault prolapse (posthysterectomy) N99.3
  - vascular (peripheral)
    - artery T81.719 ☑
      - mesenteric T81.71Ø ☑
      - renal T81.711 ☑
      - specified NEC T81.718 ☑
    - vein T81.72 ☑
  - wound infection T81.49 ☑
- suture, permanent (wire) NEC T85.9 ☑
  - with repair of bone — *see* Complications, fixation device, internal
  - embolism T85.818 ☑
  - fibrosis T85.828 ☑
  - hemorrhage T85.838 ☑
  - infection and inflammation T85.79 ☑
  - mechanical
    - breakdown T85.612 ☑
    - displacement T85.622 ☑
    - malfunction T85.612 ☑
    - malposition T85.622 ☑
    - obstruction T85.692 ☑
    - perforation T85.692 ☑
    - protrusion T85.692 ☑
    - specified NEC T85.692 ☑
  - pain T85.848 ☑
  - specified type NEC T85.898 ☑
  - stenosis T85.858 ☑
  - thrombosis T85.868 ☑
- tracheostomy J95.ØØ
  - granuloma J95.Ø9
  - hemorrhage J95.Ø1
  - infection J95.Ø2
  - malfunction J95.Ø3
  - mechanical J95.Ø3
  - obstruction J95.Ø3
  - specified type NEC J95.Ø9
  - tracheo-esophageal fistula J95.Ø4
- transfusion (blood) (lymphocytes) (plasma) T8Ø.92 ☑
  - air emblism T8Ø.Ø ☑
  - circulatory overload E87.71

- **Complication**(s) — *continued*
  - transfusion — *continued*
    - febrile nonhemolytic transfusion reaction R50.84
    - hemochromatosis E83.111
    - hemolysis T80.89 ☑
    - hemolytic reaction (antigen unspecified) T80.919 ☑
    - incompatibility reaction (antigen unspecified) T80.919 ☑
      - ABO T80.30 ☑
        - delayed serologic (DSTR) T80.39 ☑
        - hemolytic transfusion reaction (HTR) (unspecified time after transfusion) T80.319 ☑
          - acute (AHTR) (less than 24 hours after transfusion) T80.310 ☑
          - delayed (DHTR) (24 hours or more after transfusion) T80.311 ☑
        - specified NEC T80.39 ☑
      - acute (antigen unspecified) T80.910 ☑
      - delayed (antigen unspecified) T80.911 ☑
      - delayed serologic (DSTR) T80.89 ☑
      - non-ABO (minor antigens (Duffy) (K) (Kell) (Kidd) (Lewis) (M) (N) (P) (S)) T80.A0 ☑ (*following* T80.4)
        - delayed serologic (DSTR) T80.A9 ☑ (*following* T80.4)
        - hemolytic transfusion reaction (HTR) (unspecified time after transfusion) T80.A19 ☑ (*following* T80.4)
          - acute (AHTR) (less than 24 hours after transfusion) T80.A10 ☑ (*following* T80.4)
          - delayed (DHTR) (24 hours or more after transfusion) T80.A11 ☑ (*following* T80.4)
        - specified NEC T80.A9 ☑ (*following* T80.4)
      - Rh (antigens (C) (c) (D) (E) (e)) (factor) T80.40 ☑
        - delayed serologic (DSTR) T80.49 ☑
        - hemolytic transfusion reaction (HTR) (unspecified time after transfusion) T80.419 ☑
          - acute (AHTR) (less than 24 hours after transfusion) T80.410 ☑
          - delayed (DHTR) (24 hours or more after transfusion) T80.411 ☑
        - specified NEC T80.49 ☑
    - infection T80.29 ☑
      - acute T80.22- ☑
    - reaction NEC T80.89 ☑
    - sepsis T80.29 ☑
    - shock T80.89 ☑
  - transplant T86.90
    - bone T86.839
      - failure T86.831
      - infection T86.832
      - rejection T86.830
      - specified type NEC T86.838
    - bone marrow T86.00
      - failure T86.02
      - infection T86.03
      - rejection T86.01
      - specified type NEC T86.09
    - cornea T86.849- ☑
      - failure T86.841- ☑
      - infection T86.842- ☑
      - rejection T86.840- ☑
      - specified type NEC T86.848- ☑
    - failure T86.92
    - heart T86.20
      - with lung T86.30
      - cardiac allograft vasculopathy T86.290
        - failure T86.32
        - infection T86.33
        - rejection T86.31
        - specified type NEC T86.39
      - failure T86.22
      - infection T86.23
      - rejection T86.21
      - specified type NEC T86.298
    - infection T86.93
    - intestine T86.859
      - failure T86.851
      - infection T86.852
      - rejection T86.850
      - specified type NEC T86.858
    - kidney T86.10
      - failure T86.12
      - infection T86.13
      - rejection T86.11

- **Complication**(s) — *continued*
  - transplant — *continued*
    - kidney — *continued*
      - specified type NEC T86.19
    - liver T86.40
      - failure T86.42
      - infection T86.43
      - rejection T86.41
      - specified type NEC T86.49
    - lung T86.819
      - with heart T86.30
        - failure T86.32
        - infection T86.33
        - rejection T86.31
        - specified type NEC T86.39
      - failure T86.811
      - infection T86.812
      - rejection T86.810
      - specified type NEC T86.818
    - malignant neoplasm C80.2
    - pancreas T86.899
      - failure T86.891
      - infection T86.892
      - rejection T86.890
      - specified type NEC T86.898
    - peripheral blood stem cells T86.5
    - post-transplant lymphoproliferative disorder (PTLD) D47.Z1 (*following* D47.4)
    - rejection T86.91
    - skin T86.829
      - failure T86.821
      - infection T86.822
      - rejection T86.820
      - specified type NEC T86.828
    - specified
      - tissue T86.899
        - failure T86.891
        - infection T86.892
        - rejection T86.890
        - specified type NEC T86.898
      - type NEC T86.99
    - stem cell (from peripheral blood) (from umbilical cord) T86.5
    - umbilical cord stem cells T86.5
  - trauma (early) T79.9 ☑
    - specified NEC T79.8 ☑
  - ultrasound therapy NEC T88.9 ☑
  - umbilical cord NEC
    - complicating delivery O69.9 ☑
      - specified NEC O69.89 ☑
  - umbrella device, vascular T82.9 ☑
    - embolism T82.818 ☑
    - fibrosis T82.828 ☑
    - hemorrhage T82.838 ☑
    - infection or inflammation T82.7 ☑
    - mechanical
      - breakdown T82.515 ☑
      - displacement T82.525 ☑
      - leakage T82.535 ☑
      - malposition T82.525 ☑
      - obstruction T82.595 ☑
      - perforation T82.595 ☑
      - protrusion T82.595 ☑
    - pain T82.848 ☑
    - specified type NEC T82.898 ☑
    - stenosis T82.858 ☑
    - thrombosis T82.868 ☑
  - urethral catheter — *see* Complications, catheter, urethral, indwelling
  - vaccination T88.1 ☑
    - anaphylaxis NEC T80.52 ☑
    - arthropathy — *see* Arthropathy, postimmunization
    - cellulitis T88.0 ☑
    - encephalitis or encephalomyelitis G04.02
    - infection (general) (local) NEC T88.0 ☑
    - meningitis G03.8
    - myelitis G04.02
    - protein sickness T80.62 ☑
    - rash T88.1 ☑
    - reaction (allergic) T88.1 ☑
      - serum T80.62 ☑
    - sepsis T88.0 ☑
    - serum intoxication, sickness, rash, or other serum reaction NEC T80.62 ☑
      - anaphylactic shock T80.52 ☑
    - shock (allergic) (anaphylactic) T80.52 ☑
    - vaccinia (generalized) (localized) T88.1 ☑

- **Complication**(s) — *continued*
  - vas deferens device or implant — *see* Complications, genitourinary, device or implant, genital tract
  - vascular I99.9
    - device or implant T82.9 ☑
      - embolism T82.818 ☑
      - fibrosis T82.828 ☑
      - hemorrhage T82.838 ☑
      - infection or inflammation T82.7 ☑
      - mechanical
        - breakdown T82.519 ☑
          - specified device NEC T82.518 ☑
        - displacement T82.529 ☑
          - specified device NEC T82.528 ☑
        - leakage T82.539 ☑
          - specified device NEC T82.538 ☑
        - malposition T82.529 ☑
          - specified device NEC T82.528 ☑
        - obstruction T82.599 ☑
          - specified device NEC T82.598 ☑
        - perforation T82.599 ☑
          - specified device NEC T82.598 ☑
        - protrusion T82.599 ☑
          - specified device NEC T82.598 ☑
      - pain T82.848 ☑
      - specified type NEC T82.898 ☑
      - stenosis T82.858 ☑
      - thrombosis T82.868 ☑
    - dialysis catheter — *see* Complication, catheter, dialysis
    - following infusion, therapeutic injection or transfusion T80.1 ☑
    - graft T82.9 ☑
      - embolism T82.818 ☑
      - fibrosis T82.828 ☑
      - hemorrhage T82.838 ☑
      - mechanical
        - breakdown T82.319 ☑
          - aorta (bifurcation) T82.310 ☑
          - carotid artery T82.311 ☑
          - specified vessel NEC T82.318 ☑
        - displacement T82.329 ☑
          - aorta (bifurcation) T82.320 ☑
          - carotid artery T82.321 ☑
          - specified vessel NEC T82.328 ☑
        - leakage T82.339 ☑
          - aorta (bifurcation) T82.330 ☑
          - carotid artery T82.331 ☑
          - femoral artery T82.332 ☑
          - specified vessel NEC T82.338 ☑
        - malposition T82.329 ☑
          - aorta (bifurcation) T82.320 ☑
          - carotid artery T82.321 ☑
          - specified vessel NEC T82.328 ☑
        - obstruction T82.399 ☑
          - aorta (bifurcation) T82.390 ☑
          - carotid artery T82.391 ☑
          - specified vessel NEC T82.398 ☑
        - perforation T82.399 ☑
          - aorta (bifurcation) T82.390 ☑
          - carotid artery T82.391 ☑
          - specified vessel NEC T82.398 ☑
        - protrusion T82.399 ☑
          - aorta (bifurcation) T82.390 ☑
          - carotid artery T82.391 ☑
          - specified vessel NEC T82.398 ☑
      - pain T82.848 ☑
      - specified complication NEC T82.898 ☑
      - stenosis T82.858 ☑
      - thrombosis T82.868 ☑
    - postoperative — *see* Complications, postoperative, circulatory
  - vena cava device (filter) (sieve) (umbrella) — *see* Complications, umbrella device, vascular
  - ventilation therapy NEC T81.81 ☑
  - ventilator
    - mechanical J95.850
      - specified NEC J95.859
  - ventricular (communicating) shunt (device) T85.9 ☑
    - embolism T85.810 ☑
    - fibrosis T85.820 ☑
    - hemorrhage T85.830 ☑
    - infection and inflammation T85.730 ☑
    - mechanical
      - breakdown T85.01 ☑
      - displacement T85.02 ☑

- **Complication**(s) — *continued*
  - ventricular shunt — *continued*
    - mechanical — *continued*
      - leakage T85.Ø3 ☑
      - malposition T85.Ø2 ☑
      - obstruction T85.Ø9 ☑
      - perforation T85.Ø9 ☑
      - protrusion T85.Ø9 ☑
      - specified NEC T85.Ø9 ☑
    - pain T85.84Ø ☑
    - specified type NEC T85.89Ø ☑
    - stenosis T85.85Ø ☑
    - thrombosis T85.86Ø ☑
  - wire suture, permanent (implanted) — *see* Complications, suture, permanent
- **Compressed air disease** T7Ø.3 ☑
- **Compression**
  - with injury — *code by* Nature of injury
  - artery I77.1
    - celiac, syndrome I77.4
  - brachial plexus G54.Ø
  - brain (stem) G93.5
    - due to
      - contusion (diffuse) — *see also* Injury, intracranial, diffuse SØ6.AØ ☑
        - with herniation SØ6.A1 ☑
        - focal — *see also* Injury, intracranial, focal SØ6.AØ ☑
          - with herniation SØ6.A1 ☑
      - injury NEC — *see also* Injury, intracranial, diffuse SØ6.AØ ☑
    - nontraumatic G93.5
    - traumatic — *see also* Injury, intracranial, diffuse SØ6.AØ ☑
      - with herniation SØ6.A1 ☑
  - bronchus J98.Ø9
  - cauda equina G83.4
  - celiac (artery) (axis) I77.4
  - cerebral — *see* Compression, brain
  - cervical plexus G54.2
  - cord
    - spinal — *see* Compression, spinal
    - umbilical — *see* Compression, umbilical cord
  - cranial nerve G52.9
    - eighth H93.3 ☑
    - eleventh G52.8
    - fifth G5Ø.8
    - first G52.Ø
    - fourth — *see* Strabismus, paralytic, fourth nerve
    - ninth G52.1
    - second — *see* Disorder, nerve, optic
    - seventh G51.8
    - sixth — *see* Strabismus, paralytic, sixth nerve
    - tenth G52.2
    - third — *see* Strabismus, paralytic, third nerve
    - twelfth G52.3
  - diver's squeeze T7Ø.3 ☑
  - during birth (newborn) P15.9
  - esophagus K22.2
  - eustachian tube — *see* Obstruction, eustachian tube, cartilaginous
  - facies Q67.1
  - fracture
    - nontraumatic NOS — *see* Collapse, vertebra
    - pathological — *see* Fracture, pathological
    - traumatic — *see* Fracture, traumatic
  - heart — *see* Disease, heart
  - intestine — *see* Obstruction, intestine
  - laryngeal nerve, recurrent G52.2
    - with paralysis of vocal cords and larynx J38.ØØ
      - bilateral J38.Ø2
      - unilateral J38.Ø1
  - lumbosacral plexus G54.1
  - lung J98.4
  - lymphatic vessel I89.Ø
  - medulla — *see* Compression, brain
  - nerve — *see also* Disorder, nerve G58.9
    - arm NEC — *see* Mononeuropathy, upper limb
    - axillary G54.Ø
    - cranial — *see* Compression, cranial nerve
    - leg NEC — *see* Mononeuropathy, lower limb
    - median (in carpal tunnel) — *see* Syndrome, carpal tunnel
    - optic — *see* Disorder, nerve, optic
    - plantar — *see* Lesion, nerve, plantar
    - posterior tibial (in tarsal tunnel) — *see* Syndrome, tarsal tunnel
- **Compression** — *continued*
  - nerve — *see also* Disorder, nerve — *continued*
    - root or plexus NOS (in) G54.9
      - intervertebral disc disorder NEC — *see* Disorder, disc, with, radiculopathy
        - with myelopathy — *see* Disorder, disc, with, myelopathy
      - neoplastic disease — *see also* Neoplasm D49.9 *[G55]*
      - spondylosis — *see* Spondylosis, with radiculopathy
    - sciatic (acute) — *see* Lesion, nerve, sciatic
    - sympathetic G9Ø.8
    - traumatic — *see* Injury, nerve
    - ulnar — *see* Lesion, nerve, ulnar
    - upper extremity NEC — *see* Mononeuropathy, upper limb
  - spinal (cord) G95.2Ø
    - by displacement of intervertebral disc NEC — *see also* Disorder, disc, with, myelopathy
    - nerve root NOS G54.9
      - due to displacement of intervertebral disc NEC — *see* Disorder, disc, with, radiculopathy
        - with myelopathy — *see* Disorder, disc, with, myelopathy
    - specified NEC G95.29
    - spondylogenic (cervical) (lumbar, lumbosacral) (thoracic) — *see* Spondylosis, with myelopathy NEC
      - anterior — *see* Syndrome, anterior, spinal artery, compression
    - traumatic — *see* Injury, spinal cord, by region
  - subcostal nerve (syndrome) — *see* Mononeuropathy, upper limb, specified NEC
  - sympathetic nerve NEC G9Ø.8
  - syndrome T79.5 ☑
  - trachea J39.8
  - ulnar nerve (by scar tissue) — *see* Lesion, nerve, ulnar
  - umbilical cord
    - complicating delivery O69.2 ☑
      - cord around neck O69.1 ☑
      - prolapse O69.Ø ☑
      - specified NEC O69.2 ☑
  - ureter N13.5
  - vein I87.1
  - vena cava (inferior) (superior) I87.1
- **Compulsion, compulsive**
  - gambling F63.Ø
  - neurosis F42.8
  - personality F6Ø.5
  - states F42.8
  - swearing F42.8
    - in Gilles de la Tourette's syndrome F95.2
  - tics and spasms F95.9
- **Concato's disease** (pericardial polyserositis) A19.9
  - nontubercular I31.1
  - pleural — *see* Pleurisy, with effusion
- **Concavity chest wall** M95.4
- **Concealed penis** Q55.64
- **Concern** (normal) **about sick person in family** Z63.6
- **Concrescence** (teeth) KØØ.2
- **Concretio cordis** I31.1
  - rheumatic IØ9.2
- **Concretion** — *see also* Calculus
  - appendicular K38.1
  - canaliculus — *see* Dacryolith
  - clitoris N9Ø.89
  - conjunctiva H11.12- ☑
  - eyelid — *see* Disorder, eyelid, specified type NEC
  - lacrimal passages — *see* Dacryolith
  - prepuce (male) N47.8
  - salivary gland (any) K11.5
  - seminal vesicle N5Ø.89
  - tonsil J35.8
- **Concussion** (brain) (cerebral) (current) SØ6.ØX9 ☑
  - with
    - loss of consciousness
      - 3Ø minutes or less SØ6.ØX1 ☑
      - brief SØ6.ØX1 ☑
      - status unknown SØ6.ØXA ☑
      - unspecified duration SØ6.ØX9 ☑
    - no loss of consciousness SØ6.ØXØ ☑
  - blast (air) (hydraulic) (immersion) (underwater)
    - abdomen or thorax — *see* Injury, blast, by site
    - ear with acoustic nerve injury — *see* Injury, nerve, acoustic, specified type NEC
  - cauda equina S34.3 ☑
- **Concussion** — *continued*
  - conus medullaris S34.Ø2 ☑
  - ocular SØ5.8X- ☑
  - spinal (cord)
    - cervical S14.Ø ☑
    - lumbar S34.Ø1 ☑
    - sacral S34.Ø2 ☑
    - thoracic S24.Ø ☑
  - syndrome FØ7.81
  - without loss of consciousness SØ6.ØXØ ☑
- **Condition** — *see also* Disease
  - post COVID-19 UØ9.9
- **Conditions arising in the perinatal period** — *see* Newborn, affected by
- **Conduct disorder** — *see* Disorder, conduct
- **Condyloma** A63.Ø
  - acuminatum A63.Ø
  - gonorrheal A54.Ø9
  - latum A51.31
  - syphilitic A51.31
    - congenital A5Ø.Ø7
  - venereal, syphilitic A51.31
- **Conflagration** — *see also* Burn
  - asphyxia (by inhalation of gases, fumes or vapors) — *see also* Table of Drugs and Chemicals T59.9- ☑
- **Conflict** (with) — *see also* Discord
  - family Z73.9
  - marital Z63.Ø
    - involving divorce or estrangement Z63.5
  - parent-child Z62.82Ø
    - parent-adopted child Z62.821
    - parent-biological child Z62.82Ø
    - parent-foster child Z62.822
  - social role NEC Z73.5
- **Confluent** — *see* condition
- **Confusion, confused** R41.Ø
  - epileptic FØ5
  - mental state (psychogenic) F44.89
  - psychogenic F44.89
  - reactive (from emotional stress, psychological trauma) F44.89
- **Confusional arousals** G47.51
- **Congelation** T69.9 ☑
- **Congenital** — *see also* condition
  - aortic septum Q25.49
  - intrinsic factor deficiency D51.Ø
  - malformation — *see* Anomaly
- **Congestion, congestive**
  - bladder N32.89
  - bowel K63.89
  - brain G93.89
  - breast N64.59
  - bronchial J98.Ø9
  - catarrhal J31.Ø
  - chest RØ9.89
  - chill, malarial — *see* Malaria
  - circulatory NEC I99.8
  - duodenum K31.89
  - eye — *see* Hyperemia, conjunctiva
  - facial, due to birth injury P15.4
  - general R68.89
  - glottis J37.Ø
  - heart — *see* Failure, heart, congestive
  - hepatic K76.1
  - hypostatic (lung) — *see* Edema, lung
  - intestine K63.89
  - kidney N28.89
  - labyrinth H83.8 ☑
  - larynx J37.Ø
  - liver K76.1
  - lung RØ9.89
    - active or acute — *see* Pneumonia
  - malaria, malarial — *see* Malaria
  - nasal RØ9.81
  - nose RØ9.81
  - orbit, orbital — *see also* Exophthalmos
    - inflammatory (chronic) — *see* Inflammation, orbit
  - ovary N83.8
  - pancreas K86.89
  - pelvic, female N94.89
  - pleural J94.8
  - prostate (active) N42.1
  - pulmonary — *see* Congestion, lung
  - renal N28.89
  - retina H35.81
  - seminal vesicle N5Ø.1
  - spinal cord G95.19
  - spleen (chronic) D73.2

Congestion, congestive — *continued*
stomach K31.89
trachea — *see* Tracheitis
urethra N36.8
uterus N85.8
with subinvolution N85.3
venous (passive) I87.8
viscera R68.89
Congestive — *see* Congestion
Conical
cervix (hypertrophic elongation) N88.4
cornea — *see* Keratoconus
teeth KØØ.2
Conjoined twins Q89.4
Conjugal maladjustment Z63.Ø
involving divorce or estrangement Z63.5
Conjunctiva — *see* condition
Conjunctivitis (staphylococcal) (streptococcal) NOS H1Ø.9
Acanthamoeba B6Ø.12
acute H1Ø.3- ☑
atopic H1Ø.1- ☑
chemical — *see also* Corrosion, cornea H1Ø.21- ☑
mucopurulent H1Ø.Ø2- ☑
follicular H1Ø.Ø1- ☑
pseudomembranous H1Ø.22- ☑
serous except viral H1Ø.23- ☑
viral — *see* Conjunctivitis, viral
toxic H1Ø.21- ☑
adenoviral (acute) (follicular) B3Ø.1
allergic (acute) — *see* Conjunctivitis, acute, atopic
chronic H1Ø.45
vernal H1Ø.44
anaphylactic — *see* Conjunctivitis, acute, atopic
Apollo B3Ø.3
atopic (acute) — *see* Conjunctivitis, acute, atopic
Béal's B3Ø.2
blennorrhagic (gonococcal) (neonatorum) A54.31
chemical (acute) — *see also* Corrosion, cornea H1Ø.21- ☑
chlamydial A74.Ø
due to trachoma A71.1
neonatal P39.1
chronic (nodosa) (petrificans) (phlyctenular) H1Ø.4Ø- ☑
allergic H1Ø.45
vernal H1Ø.44
follicular H1Ø.43- ☑
giant papillary H1Ø.41- ☑
simple H1Ø.42- ☑
vernal H1Ø.44
coxsackievirus 24 B3Ø.3
diphtheritic A36.86
due to
dust — *see* Conjunctivitis, acute, atopic
filariasis B74.9
mucocutaneous leishmaniasis B55.2
enterovirus type 7Ø (hemorrhagic) B3Ø.3
epidemic (viral) B3Ø.9
hemorrhagic B3Ø.3
gonococcal (neonatorum) A54.31
granular (trachomatous) A71.1
sequelae (late effect) B94.Ø
hemorrhagic (acute) (epidemic) B3Ø.3
herpes zoster BØ2.31
in (due to)
Acanthamoeba B6Ø.12
adenovirus (acute) (follicular) B3Ø.1
Chlamydia A74.Ø
coxsackievirus 24 B3Ø.3
diphtheria A36.86
enterovirus type 7Ø (hemorrhagic) B3Ø.3
filariasis B74.9
gonococci A54.31
herpes (simplex) virus BØØ.53
zoster BØ2.31
infectious disease NEC B99 ☑
meningococci A39.89
mucocutaneous leishmaniasis B55.2
rosacea H1Ø.82- ☑
syphilis (late) A52.71
zoster BØ2.31
inclusion A74.Ø
infantile P39.1
gonococcal A54.31
Koch-Weeks' — *see* Conjunctivitis, acute, mucopurulent
light — *see* Conjunctivitis, acute, atopic
ligneous — *see* Blepharoconjunctivitis, ligneous
meningococcal A39.89

Conjunctivitis — *continued*
mucopurulent — *see* Conjunctivitis, acute, mucopurulent
neonatal P39.1
gonococcal A54.31
Newcastle B3Ø.8
of Béal B3Ø.2
parasitic
filariasis B74.9
mucocutaneous leishmaniasis B55.2
Parinaud's H1Ø.89
petrificans H1Ø.89
rosacea H1Ø.82- ☑
specified NEC H1Ø.89
swimming-pool B3Ø.1
trachomatous A71.1
acute A71.Ø
sequelae (late effect) B94.Ø
traumatic NEC H1Ø.89
tuberculous A18.59
tularemic A21.1
tularensis A21.1
viral B3Ø.9
due to
adenovirus B3Ø.1
enterovirus B3Ø.3
specified NEC B3Ø.8
Conjunctivochalasis H11.82- ☑
Connective tissue — *see* condition
Conn's syndrome E26.Ø1
Conradi (-Hunermann) **disease** Q77.3
Consanguinity Z84.3
counseling Z71.89
Conscious simulation (of illness) Z76.5
Consecutive — *see* condition
Consolidation lung (base) — *see* Pneumonia, lobar
Constipation (atonic) (neurogenic) (simple) (spastic) K59.ØØ
chronic K59.Ø9
idiopathic K59.Ø4
drug-induced K59.Ø3
functional K59.Ø4
outlet dysfunction K59.Ø2
psychogenic F45.8
slow transit K59.Ø1
specified NEC K59.Ø9
Constitutional — *see also* condition
substandard F6Ø.7
Constitutionally substandard F6Ø.7
Constriction — *see also* Stricture
auditory canal — *see* Stenosis, external ear canal
bronchial J98.Ø9
duodenum K31.5
esophagus K22.2
external
abdomen, abdominal (wall) S3Ø.841 ☑
alveolar process SØØ.542 ☑
ankle S9Ø.54- ☑
antecubital space — *see* Constriction, external, forearm
arm (upper) S4Ø.84- ☑
auricle — *see* Constriction, external, ear
axilla — *see* Constriction, external, arm
back, lower S3Ø.84Ø ☑
breast S2Ø.14- ☑
brow SØØ.84 ☑
buttock S3Ø.84Ø ☑
calf — *see* Constriction, external, leg
canthus — *see* Constriction, external, eyelid
cheek SØØ.84 ☑
internal SØØ.542 ☑
chest wall — *see* Constriction, external, thorax
chin SØØ.84 ☑
clitoris S3Ø.844 ☑
costal region — *see* Constriction, external, thorax
digit(s)
foot — *see* Constriction, external, toe
hand — *see* Constriction, external, finger
ear SØØ.44- ☑
elbow S5Ø.34- ☑
epididymis S3Ø.843 ☑
epigastric region S3Ø.841 ☑
esophagus, cervical S1Ø.14 ☑
eyebrow — *see* Constriction, external, eyelid
eyelid SØØ.24- ☑
face SØØ.84 ☑
finger(s) S6Ø.44- ☑

Constriction — *continued*
external — *continued*
finger(s) — *continued*
index S6Ø.44- ☑
little S6Ø.44- ☑
middle S6Ø.44- ☑
ring S6Ø.44- ☑
flank S3Ø.841 ☑
foot (except toe(s) alone) S9Ø.84- ☑
toe — *see* Constriction, external, toe
forearm S5Ø.84- ☑
elbow only — *see* Constriction, external, elbow
forehead SØØ.84 ☑
genital organs, external
female S3Ø.846 ☑
male S3Ø.845 ☑
groin S3Ø.841 ☑
gum SØØ.542 ☑
hand S6Ø.54- ☑
head SØØ.94 ☑
ear — *see* Constriction, external, ear
eyelid — *see* Constriction, external, eyelid
lip SØØ.541 ☑
nose SØØ.34 ☑
oral cavity SØØ.542 ☑
scalp SØØ.Ø4 ☑
specified site NEC SØØ.84 ☑
heel — *see* Constriction, external, foot
hip S7Ø.24- ☑
inguinal region S3Ø.841 ☑
interscapular region S2Ø.449 ☑
jaw SØØ.84 ☑
knee S8Ø.24- ☑
labium (majus) (minus) S3Ø.844 ☑
larynx S1Ø.14 ☑
leg (lower) S8Ø.84- ☑
knee — *see* Constriction, external, knee
upper — *see* Constriction, external, thigh
lip SØØ.541 ☑
lower back S3Ø.84Ø ☑
lumbar region S3Ø.84Ø ☑
malar region SØØ.84 ☑
mammary — *see* Constriction, external, breast
mastoid region SØØ.84 ☑
mouth SØØ.542 ☑
nail
finger — *see* Constriction, external, finger
toe — *see* Constriction, external, toe
nasal SØØ.34 ☑
neck S1Ø.94 ☑
specified site NEC S1Ø.84 ☑
throat S1Ø.14 ☑
nose SØØ.34 ☑
occipital region SØØ.Ø4 ☑
oral cavity SØØ.542 ☑
orbital region — *see* Constriction, external, eyelid
palate SØØ.542 ☑
palm — *see* Constriction, external, hand
parietal region SØØ.Ø4 ☑
pelvis S3Ø.84Ø ☑
penis S3Ø.842 ☑
perineum
female S3Ø.844 ☑
male S3Ø.84Ø ☑
periocular area — *see* Constriction, external, eyelid
phalanges
finger — *see* Constriction, external, finger
toe — *see* Constriction, external, toe
pharynx S1Ø.14 ☑
pinna — *see* Constriction, external, ear
popliteal space — *see* Constriction, external, knee
prepuce S3Ø.842 ☑
pubic region S3Ø.84Ø ☑
pudendum
female S3Ø.846 ☑
male S3Ø.845 ☑
sacral region S3Ø.84Ø ☑
scalp SØØ.Ø4 ☑
scapular region — *see* Constriction, external, shoulder
scrotum S3Ø.843 ☑
shin — *see* Constriction, external, leg
shoulder S4Ø.24- ☑
sternal region S2Ø.349 ☑
submaxillary region SØØ.84 ☑
submental region SØØ.84 ☑

Index

Congestion, congestive — Constriction

Constriction — *continued*
external — *continued*
subungual
finger(s) — *see* Constriction, external, finger
toe(s) — *see* Constriction, external, toe
supraclavicular fossa S10.84 ☑
supraorbital S00.84 ☑
temple S00.84 ☑
temporal region S00.84 ☑
testis S30.843 ☑
thigh S70.34- ☑
thorax, thoracic (wall) S20.94 ☑
back S20.44- ☑
front S20.34- ☑
throat S10.14 ☑
thumb S60.34- ☑
toe(s) (lesser) S90.44- ☑
great S90.44- ☑
tongue S00.542 ☑
trachea S10.14 ☑
tunica vaginalis S30.843 ☑
uvula S00.542 ☑
vagina S30.844 ☑
vulva S30.844 ☑
wrist S60.84- ☑
gallbladder — *see* Obstruction, gallbladder
intestine — *see* Obstruction, intestine
larynx J38.6
congenital Q31.8
specified NEC Q31.8
subglottic Q31.1
organ or site, congenital NEC — *see* Atresia, by site
prepuce (acquired) (congenital) N47.1
pylorus (adult hypertrophic) K31.1
congenital or infantile Q40.0
newborn Q40.0
ring dystocia (uterus) O62.4
spastic — *see also* Spasm
ureter N13.5
ureter N13.5
with infection N13.6
urethra — *see* Stricture, urethra
visual field (peripheral) (functional) — *see* Defect, visual field
Constrictive — *see* condition
Consultation
medical — *see* Counseling, medical
religious Z71.81
specified reason NEC Z71.89
spiritual Z71.81
without complaint or sickness Z71.9
feared complaint unfounded Z71.1
specified reason NEC Z71.89
Consumption — *see* Tuberculosis
Contact (with) — *see also* Exposure (to)
acariasis Z20.7
AIDS virus Z20.6
air pollution Z77.110
algae and algae toxins Z77.121
algae bloom Z77.121
anthrax Z20.810
aromatic amines Z77.020
aromatic (hazardous) compounds NEC Z77.028
aromatic dyes NOS Z77.028
arsenic Z77.010
asbestos Z77.090
bacterial disease NEC Z20.818
benzene Z77.021
blue-green algae bloom Z77.121
body fluids (potentially hazardous) Z77.21
brown tide Z77.121
chemicals (chiefly nonmedicinal) (hazardous) NEC Z77.098
cholera Z20.09
chromium compounds Z77.018
communicable disease Z20.9
bacterial NEC Z20.818
specified NEC Z20.89
viral NEC Z20.828
Zika virus Z20.821
coronavirus (disease) (novel) 2019 Z20.822
COVID-19 Z20.822
cyanobacteria bloom Z77.121
dyes Z77.098
Escherichia coli (E. coli) Z20.01
fiberglass — *see* Table of Drugs and Chemicals, fiberglass
German measles Z20.4

Contact — *continued*
gonorrhea Z20.2
hazardous metals NEC Z77.018
hazardous substances NEC Z77.29
hazards in the physical environment NEC Z77.128
hazards to health NEC Z77.9
HIV Z20.6
HTLV-III/LAV Z20.6
human immunodeficiency virus (HIV) Z20.6
infection Z20.9
specified NEC Z20.89
infestation (parasitic) NEC Z20.7
intestinal infectious disease NEC Z20.09
Escherichia coli (E. coli) Z20.01
lead Z77.011
meningococcus Z20.811
mold (toxic) Z77.120
nickel dust Z77.018
noise Z77.122
parasitic disease Z20.7
pediculosis Z20.7
pfiesteria piscicida Z77.121
poliomyelitis Z20.89
pollution
air Z77.110
environmental NEC Z77.118
soil Z77.112
water Z77.111
polycyclic aromatic hydrocarbons Z77.028
positive maternal group B streptococcus P00.82
rabies Z20.3
radiation, naturally occurring NEC Z77.123
radon Z77.123
red tide (Florida) Z77.121
rubella Z20.4
SARS-CoV-2 Z20.822
sexually-transmitted disease Z20.2
smallpox (laboratory) Z20.89
syphilis Z20.2
tuberculosis Z20.1
uranium Z77.012
varicella Z20.820
venereal disease Z20.2
viral disease NEC Z20.828
viral hepatitis Z20.5
water pollution Z77.111
Zika virus Z20.821
Contamination, food — *see* Intoxication, foodborne
Contraception, contraceptive
advice Z30.09
counseling Z30.09
device (intrauterine) (in situ) Z97.5
causing menorrhagia T83.83 ☑
checking Z30.431
complications — *see* Complications, intrauterine, contraceptive device
in place Z97.5
initial prescription Z30.014
reinsertion Z30.433
removal Z30.432
replacement Z30.433
emergency (postcoital) Z30.012
initial prescription Z30.019
barrier Z30.018
diaphragm Z30.018
injectable Z30.013
intrauterine device Z30.014
pills Z30.011
postcoital (emergency) Z30.012
specified type NEC Z30.018
subdermal implantable Z30.017
transdermal patch hormonal Z30.016
vaginal ring hormonal Z30.015
maintenance Z30.40
barrier Z30.49
diaphragm Z30.49
examination Z30.8
injectable Z30.42
intrauterine device Z30.431
pills Z30.41
specified type NEC Z30.49
subdermal implantable Z30.46
transdermal patch hormonal Z30.45
vaginal ring hormonal Z30.44
management Z30.9
specified NEC Z30.8
postcoital (emergency) Z30.012
prescription Z30.019
repeat Z30.40

Contraception, contraceptive — *continued*
sterilization Z30.2
surveillance (drug) — *see* Contraception, maintenance
Contraction(s), contracture, contracted
Achilles tendon — *see also* Short, tendon, Achilles
congenital Q66.89
amputation stump (surgical) (flexion) (late) (next proximal joint) T87.89
anus K59.89
bile duct (common) (hepatic) K83.8
bladder N32.89
neck or sphincter N32.0
bowel, cecum, colon or intestine, any part — *see* Obstruction, intestine
Braxton Hicks — *see* False, labor
breast implant, capsular T85.44 ☑
bronchial J98.09
burn (old) — *see* Cicatrix
cervix — *see* Stricture, cervix
cicatricial — *see* Cicatrix
conjunctiva, trachomatous, active A71.1
sequelae (late effect) B94.0
Dupuytren's M72.0
eyelid — *see* Disorder, eyelid function
fascia (lata) (postural) M72.8
Dupuytren's M72.0
palmar M72.0
plantar M72.2
finger NEC — *see also* Deformity, finger
congenital Q68.1
joint — *see* Contraction, joint, hand
flaccid — *see* Contraction, paralytic
gallbladder K82.0
heart valve — *see* Endocarditis
hip — *see* Contraction, joint, hip
hourglass
bladder N32.89
congenital Q64.79
gallbladder K82.0
congenital Q44.1
stomach K31.89
congenital Q40.2
psychogenic F45.8
uterus (complicating delivery) O62.4
hysterical F44.4
internal os — *see* Stricture, cervix
joint (abduction) (acquired) (adduction) (flexion) (rotation) M24.50
ankle M24.57- ☑
congenital NEC Q68.8
hip Q65.89
elbow M24.52- ☑
foot joint M24.57- ☑
hand joint M24.54- ☑
hip M24.55- ☑
congenital Q65.89
hysterical F44.4
knee M24.56- ☑
shoulder M24.51- ☑
specified site NEC M24.59
wrist M24.53- ☑
kidney (granular) (secondary) N26.9
congenital Q63.8
hydronephritic — *see* Hydronephrosis
Page N26.2
pyelonephritic — *see* Pyelitis, chronic
tuberculous A18.11
ligament — *see also* Disorder, ligament
congenital Q79.8
muscle (postinfective) (postural) NEC M62.40
with contracture of joint — *see* Contraction, joint
ankle M62.47- ☑
congenital Q79.8
sternocleidomastoid Q68.0
extraocular — *see* Strabismus
eye (extrinsic) — *see* Strabismus
foot M62.47- ☑
forearm M62.43- ☑
hand M62.44- ☑
hysterical F44.4
ischemic (Volkmann's) T79.6 ☑
lower leg M62.46- ☑
multiple sites M62.49
pelvic region M62.45- ☑
posttraumatic — *see* Strabismus, paralytic
psychogenic F45.8
conversion reaction F44.4

- **Contraction(s), contracture, contracted** — *continued*
  - muscle — *continued*
    - shoulder region M62.41- ☑
    - specified site NEC M62.48
    - thigh M62.45- ☑
    - upper arm M62.42- ☑
  - neck — *see* Torticollis
  - ocular muscle — *see* Strabismus
  - organ or site, congenital NEC — *see* Atresia, by site
  - outlet (pelvis) — *see* Contraction, pelvis
  - palmar fascia M72.Ø
  - paralytic
    - joint — *see* Contraction, joint
    - muscle — *see also* Contraction, muscle NEC
      - ocular — *see* Strabismus, paralytic
  - pelvis (acquired) (general) M95.5
    - with disproportion (fetopelvic) O33.1
      - causing obstructed labor O65.1
      - inlet O33.2
      - mid-cavity O33.3 ☑
      - outlet O33.3 ☑
  - plantar fascia M72.2
  - premature
    - atrium I49.1
    - auriculoventricular I49.49
    - heart I49.49
    - junctional I49.2
    - supraventricular I49.1
    - ventricular I49.3
  - prostate N42.89
  - pylorus NEC — *see also* Pylorospasm
    - psychogenic F45.8
  - rectum, rectal (sphincter) K59.89
  - ring (Bandl's) (complicating delivery) O62.4
  - scar — *see* Cicatrix
  - spine — *see* Dorsopathy, deforming
  - sternocleidomastoid (muscle), congenital Q68.Ø
  - stomach K31.89
    - hourglass K31.89
      - congenital Q4Ø.2
      - psychogenic F45.8
    - psychogenic F45.8
  - tendon (sheath) M62.4Ø
    - with contracture of joint — *see* Contraction, joint
    - Achilles — *see* Short, tendon, Achilles
    - ankle M62.47- ☑
      - Achilles — *see* Short, tendon, Achilles
    - foot M62.47- ☑
    - forearm M62.43- ☑
    - hand M62.44- ☑
    - lower leg M62.46- ☑
    - multiple sites M62.49
    - neck M62.48
    - pelvic region M62.45- ☑
    - shoulder region M62.41- ☑
    - specified site NEC M62.48
    - thigh M62.45- ☑
    - thorax M62.48
    - trunk M62.48
    - upper arm M62.42- ☑
  - toe — *see* Deformity, toe, specified NEC
  - ureterovesical orifice (postinfectional) N13.5
    - with infection N13.6
  - urethra — *see also* Stricture, urethra
    - orifice N32.Ø
  - uterus N85.8
    - abnormal NEC O62.9
    - clonic (complicating delivery) O62.4
    - dyscoordinate (complicating delivery) O62.4
    - hourglass (complicating delivery) O62.4
    - hypertonic O62.4
    - hypotonic NEC O62.2
    - inadequate
      - primary O62.Ø
      - secondary O62.1
    - incoordinate (complicating delivery) O62.4
    - poor O62.2
    - tetanic (complicating delivery) O62.4
  - vagina (outlet) N89.5
  - vesical N32.89
    - neck or urethral orifice N32.Ø
  - visual field — *see* Defect, visual field, generalized
  - Volkmann's (ischemic) T79.6 ☑
- **Contusion** (skin surface intact) T14.8 ☑
  - abdomen, abdominal (muscle) (wall) S3Ø.1 ☑
  - adnexa, eye NEC SØ5.8X- ☑
  - adrenal gland S37.812 ☑
  - alveolar process SØØ.532 ☑
  - ankle S9Ø.Ø- ☑
  - antecubital space — *see* Contusion, forearm
  - anus S3Ø.3 ☑
  - arm (upper) S4Ø.Ø2- ☑
    - lower (with elbow) — *see* Contusion, forearm
  - auditory canal — *see* Contusion, ear
  - auricle — *see* Contusion, ear
  - axilla — *see* Contusion, arm, upper
  - back — *see also* Contusion, thorax, back
    - lower S3Ø.Ø ☑
  - bile duct S36.13 ☑
  - bladder S37.22 ☑
  - bone NEC T14.8 ☑
  - brain (diffuse) — *see* Injury, intracranial, diffuse
    - focal — *see* Injury, intracranial, focal
  - brainstem SØ6.38- ☑
  - breast S2Ø.Ø- ☑
  - broad ligament S37.892 ☑
  - brow SØØ.83 ☑
  - buttock S3Ø.Ø ☑
  - canthus, eye SØØ.1- ☑
  - cauda equina S34.3 ☑
  - cerebellar, traumatic SØ6.37- ☑
  - cerebral SØ6.33- ☑
    - left side SØ6.32- ☑
    - right side SØ6.31- ☑
  - cheek SØØ.83 ☑
    - internal SØØ.532 ☑
  - chest (wall) — *see* Contusion, thorax
  - chin SØØ.83 ☑
  - clitoris S3Ø.23 ☑
  - colon — *see* Injury, intestine, large, contusion
  - common bile duct S36.13 ☑
  - conjunctiva SØ5.1- ☑
    - with foreign body (in conjunctival sac) — *see* Foreign body, conjunctival sac
  - conus medullaris (spine) S34.139 ☑
  - cornea — *see* Contusion, eyeball
    - with foreign body — *see* Foreign body, cornea
  - corpus cavernosum S3Ø.21 ☑
  - cortex (brain) (cerebral) — *see* Injury, intracranial, diffuse
    - focal — *see* Injury, intracranial, focal
  - costal region — *see* Contusion, thorax
  - cystic duct S36.13 ☑
  - diaphragm S27.8Ø2 ☑
  - duodenum S36.42Ø ☑
  - ear SØØ.43- ☑
  - elbow S5Ø.Ø- ☑
    - with forearm — *see* Contusion, forearm
  - epididymis S3Ø.22 ☑
  - epigastric region S3Ø.1 ☑
  - epiglottis S1Ø.Ø ☑
  - esophagus (thoracic) S27.812 ☑
    - cervical S1Ø.Ø ☑
  - eyeball SØ5.1- ☑
  - eyebrow SØØ.1- ☑
  - eyelid (and periocular area) SØØ.1- ☑
  - face NEC SØØ.83 ☑
  - fallopian tube S37.529 ☑
    - bilateral S37.522 ☑
    - unilateral S37.521 ☑
  - femoral triangle S3Ø.1 ☑
  - finger(s) S6Ø.ØØ ☑
    - with damage to nail (matrix) S6Ø.1Ø ☑
    - index S6Ø.Ø2- ☑
      - with damage to nail S6Ø.12- ☑
    - little S6Ø.Ø5- ☑
      - with damage to nail S6Ø.15- ☑
    - middle S6Ø.Ø3- ☑
      - with damage to nail S6Ø.13- ☑
    - ring S6Ø.Ø4- ☑
      - with damage to nail S6Ø.14- ☑
    - thumb — *see* Contusion, thumb
  - flank S3Ø.1 ☑
  - foot (except toe(s) alone) S9Ø.3- ☑
    - toe — *see* Contusion, toe
  - forearm S5Ø.1- ☑
    - elbow only — *see* Contusion, elbow
  - forehead SØØ.83 ☑
  - gallbladder S36.122 ☑
  - genital organs, external
    - female S3Ø.2Ø2 ☑
    - male S3Ø.2Ø1 ☑
  - globe (eye) — *see* Contusion, eyeball
  - groin S3Ø.1 ☑
  - gum SØØ.532 ☑
  - hand S6Ø.22- ☑
    - finger(s) — *see* Contusion, finger
    - wrist — *see* Contusion, wrist
  - head SØØ.93 ☑
    - ear — *see* Contusion, ear
    - eyelid — *see* Contusion, eyelid
    - lip SØØ.531 ☑
    - nose SØØ.33 ☑
    - oral cavity SØØ.532 ☑
    - scalp SØØ.Ø3 ☑
    - specified part NEC SØØ.83 ☑
  - heart — *see also* Injury, heart S26.91 ☑
  - heel — *see* Contusion, foot
  - hepatic duct S36.13 ☑
  - hip S7Ø.Ø- ☑
  - ileum S36.428 ☑
  - iliac region S3Ø.1 ☑
  - inguinal region S3Ø.1 ☑
  - interscapular region S2Ø.229 ☑
  - intra-abdominal organ S36.92 ☑
    - colon — *see* Injury, intestine, large, contusion
    - liver S36.112 ☑
    - pancreas — *see* Contusion, pancreas
    - rectum S36.62 ☑
    - small intestine — *see* Injury, intestine, small, contusion
    - specified organ NEC S36.892 ☑
    - spleen — *see* Contusion, spleen
    - stomach S36.32 ☑
  - iris (eye) — *see* Contusion, eyeball
  - jaw SØØ.83 ☑
  - jejunum S36.428 ☑
  - kidney S37.Ø1- ☑
    - major (greater than 2 cm) S37.Ø2- ☑
    - minor (less than 2 cm) S37.Ø1- ☑
  - knee S8Ø.Ø- ☑
  - labium (majus) (minus) S3Ø.23 ☑
  - lacrimal apparatus, gland or sac SØ5.8X- ☑
  - larynx S1Ø.Ø ☑
  - leg (lower) S8Ø.1- ☑
    - knee — *see* Contusion, knee
  - lens — *see* Contusion, eyeball
  - lip SØØ.531 ☑
  - liver S36.112 ☑
  - lower back S3Ø.Ø ☑
  - lumbar region S3Ø.Ø ☑
  - lung S27.329 ☑
    - bilateral S27.322 ☑
    - unilateral S27.321 ☑
  - malar region SØØ.83 ☑
  - mastoid region SØØ.83 ☑
  - membrane, brain — *see* Injury, intracranial, diffuse
    - focal — *see* Injury, intracranial, focal
  - mesentery S36.892 ☑
  - mesosalpinx S37.892 ☑
  - mouth SØØ.532 ☑
  - muscle — *see* Contusion, by site
  - nail
    - finger — *see* Contusion, finger, with damage to nail
    - toe — *see* Contusion, toe, with damage to nail
  - nasal SØØ.33 ☑
  - neck S1Ø.93 ☑
    - specified site NEC S1Ø.83 ☑
    - throat S1Ø.Ø ☑
  - nerve — *see* Injury, nerve
  - newborn P54.5
  - nose SØØ.33 ☑
  - occipital
    - lobe (brain) — *see* Injury, intracranial, diffuse
      - focal — *see* Injury, intracranial, focal
    - region (scalp) SØØ.Ø3 ☑
  - orbit (region) (tissues) SØ5.1- ☑
  - ovary S37.429 ☑
    - bilateral S37.422 ☑
    - unilateral S37.421 ☑
  - palate SØØ.532 ☑
  - pancreas S36.229 ☑
    - body S36.221 ☑
    - head S36.22Ø ☑
    - tail S36.222 ☑

Contusion — *continued*
- parietal
  - lobe (brain) — *see* Injury, intracranial, diffuse
    - focal — *see* Injury, intracranial, focal
  - region (scalp) S00.03 ☑
- pelvic organ S37.92 ☑
  - adrenal gland S37.812 ☑
  - bladder S37.22 ☑
  - fallopian tube — *see* Contusion, fallopian tube
  - kidney — *see* Contusion, kidney
  - ovary — *see* Contusion, ovary
  - prostate S37.822 ☑
  - specified organ NEC S37.892 ☑
  - ureter S37.12 ☑
  - urethra S37.32 ☑
  - uterus S37.62 ☑
- pelvis S30.0 ☑
- penis S30.21 ☑
- perineum
  - female S30.23 ☑
  - male S30.0 ☑
- periocular area S00.1- ☑
- peritoneum S36.81 ☑
- periurethral tissue — *see* Contusion, urethra
- pharynx S10.0 ☑
- pinna — *see* Contusion, ear
- popliteal space — *see* Contusion, knee
- prepuce S30.21 ☑
- prostate S37.822 ☑
- pubic region S30.1 ☑
- pudendum
  - female S30.202 ☑
  - male S30.201 ☑
- quadriceps femoris — *see* Contusion, thigh
- rectum S36.62 ☑
- retroperitoneum S36.892 ☑
- round ligament S37.892 ☑
- sacral region S30.0 ☑
- scalp S00.03 ☑
  - due to birth injury P12.3
- scapular region — *see* Contusion, shoulder
- sclera — *see* Contusion, eyeball
- scrotum S30.22 ☑
- seminal vesicle S37.892 ☑
- shoulder S40.01- ☑
- skin NEC T14.8 ☑
- small intestine — *see* Injury, intestine, small, contusion
- spermatic cord S30.22 ☑
- spinal cord — *see* Injury, spinal cord, by region
  - cauda equina S34.3 ☑
  - conus medullaris S34.139 ☑
- spleen S36.029 ☑
  - major S36.021 ☑
  - minor S36.020 ☑
- sternal region S20.219 ☑
- stomach S36.32 ☑
- subconjunctival S05.1- ☑
- subcutaneous NEC T14.8 ☑
- submaxillary region S00.83 ☑
- submental region S00.83 ☑
- subperiosteal NEC T14.8 ☑
- subungual
  - finger — *see* Contusion, finger, with damage to nail
  - toe — *see* Contusion, toe, with damage to nail
- supraclavicular fossa S10.83 ☑
- supraorbital S00.83 ☑
- suprarenal gland S37.812 ☑
- temple (region) S00.83 ☑
- temporal
  - lobe (brain) — *see* Injury, intracranial, diffuse
    - focal — *see* Injury, intracranial, focal
  - region S00.83 ☑
- testis S30.22 ☑
- thigh S70.1- ☑
- thorax (wall) S20.20 ☑
  - back S20.22- ☑
  - front S20.21- ☑
- throat S10.0 ☑
- thumb S60.01- ☑
  - with damage to nail S60.11- ☑
- toe(s) (lesser) S90.12- ☑
  - with damage to nail S90.22- ☑
  - great S90.11- ☑
    - with damage to nail S90.21- ☑
- tongue S00.532 ☑
- trachea (cervical) S10.0 ☑

Contusion — *continued*
- trachea — *continued*
  - thoracic S27.52 ☑
- tunica vaginalis S30.22 ☑
- tympanum, tympanic membrane — *see* Contusion, ear
- ureter S37.12 ☑
- urethra S37.32 ☑
- urinary organ NEC S37.892 ☑
- uterus S37.62 ☑
- uvula S00.532 ☑
- vagina S30.23 ☑
- vas deferens S37.892 ☑
- vesical S37.22 ☑
- vocal cord(s) S10.0 ☑
- vulva S30.23 ☑
- wrist S60.21- ☑

Conus (congenital) (any type) Q14.8
- cornea — *see* Keratoconus
- medullaris syndrome G95.81

Conversion hysteria, neurosis or reaction F44.9

Converter, tuberculosis (test reaction) R76.11

Conviction (legal), **anxiety concerning** Z65.0
- with imprisonment Z65.1

Convulsions (idiopathic) — *see also* Seizure(s) R56.9
- apoplectiform (cerebral ischemia) I67.82
- dissociative F44.5
- epileptic — *see* Epilepsy
- epileptiform, epileptoid — *see* Seizure, epileptiform
- ether (anesthetic) — *see* Table of Drugs and Chemicals, by drug
- febrile R56.00
  - with status epilepticus G40.901
  - complex R56.01
    - with status epilepticus G40.901
  - simple R56.00
- hysterical F44.5
- infantile P90
  - epilepsy — *see* Epilepsy
- jacksonian — *see* Epilepsy, localization-related, symptomatic, with simple partial seizures
- myoclonic G25.3
- newborn P90
- obstetrical (nephritic) (uremic) — *see* Eclampsia
- paretic A52.17
- post traumatic R56.1
- psychomotor — *see* Epilepsy, localization-related, symptomatic, with complex partial seizures
- recurrent R56.9
- reflex R25.8
- scarlatinal A38.8
- tetanus, tetanic — *see* Tetanus
- thymic E32.8

Convulsive — *see also* Convulsions

Cooley's anemia D56.1

Coolie itch B76.9

Cooper's
- disease — *see* Mastopathy, cystic
- hernia — *see* Hernia, abdomen, specified site NEC

Copra itch B88.0

Coprophagy F50.89

Coprophobia F40.298

Coproporphyria, hereditary E80.29

Cor
- biloculare Q20.8
- bovis, bovinum — *see* Hypertrophy, cardiac
- pulmonale (chronic) I27.81
  - acute I26.09
- triatriatum, triatrium Q24.2
- triloculare Q20.8
  - biatrium Q20.4
  - biventriculare Q21.19

Corbus' disease (gangrenous balanitis) N48.1

Cord — *see also* condition
- around neck
  - complicating delivery O69.81 ☑
    - with compression O69.1 ☑
- bladder G95.89
  - tabetic A52.19

Cordis ectopia Q24.8

Corditis (spermatic) N49.1

Corectopia Q13.2

Cori's disease (glycogen storage) E74.03

Corkhandler's disease or lung J67.3

Corkscrew esophagus K22.4

Corkworker's disease or lung J67.3

Corn (infected) L84

Cornea — *see also* condition
- donor Z52.5
- plana Q13.4

Cornelia de Lange syndrome Q87.19

Cornu cutaneum L85.8

Cornual gestation or pregnancy O00.80
- with intrauterine pregnancy O00.81

Coronary (artery) — *see* condition

Coronavirus (infection)
- 2019 — *see also* COVID-19 U07.1
- as cause of diseases classified elsewhere B97.29
- coronavirus-19 — *see also* COVID-19 U07.1
- COVID-19 — *see also* COVID-19 U07.1
- SARS-associated B97.21

Corpora — *see also* condition
- amylacea, prostate N42.89
- cavernosa — *see* condition

Corpulence — *see* Obesity

Corpus — *see* condition

Corrected transposition Q20.5

Corrosion (injury) (acid) (caustic) (chemical) (lime) (external) (internal) T30.4
- abdomen, abdominal (muscle) (wall) T21.42 ☑
  - first degree T21.52 ☑
  - second degree T21.62 ☑
  - third degree T21.72 ☑
- above elbow T22.439 ☑
  - first degree T22.539 ☑
  - left T22.432 ☑
    - first degree T22.532 ☑
    - second degree T22.632 ☑
    - third degree T22.732 ☑
  - right T22.431 ☑
    - first degree T22.531 ☑
    - second degree T22.631 ☑
    - third degree T22.731 ☑
  - second degree T22.639 ☑
  - third degree T22.739 ☑
- alimentary tract NEC T28.7 ☑
- ankle T25.419 ☑
  - first degree T25.519 ☑
  - left T25.412 ☑
    - first degree T25.512 ☑
    - second degree T25.612 ☑
    - third degree T25.712 ☑
  - multiple with foot — *see* Corrosion, lower, limb, multiple, ankle and foot
  - right T25.411 ☑
    - first degree T25.511 ☑
    - second degree T25.611 ☑
    - third degree T25.711 ☑
  - second degree T25.619 ☑
  - third degree T25.719 ☑
- anus — *see* Corrosion, buttock
- arm(s) (meaning upper limb(s)) — *see* Corrosion, upper limb
- axilla T22.449 ☑
  - first degree T22.549 ☑
  - left T22.442 ☑
    - first degree T22.542 ☑
    - second degree T22.642 ☑
    - third degree T22.742 ☑
  - right T22.441 ☑
    - first degree T22.541 ☑
    - second degree T22.641 ☑
    - third degree T22.741 ☑
  - second degree T22.649 ☑
  - third degree T22.749 ☑
- back (lower) T21.44 ☑
  - first degree T21.54 ☑
  - second degree T21.64 ☑
  - third degree T21.74 ☑
  - upper T21.43 ☑
    - first degree T21.53 ☑
    - second degree T21.63 ☑
    - third degree T21.73 ☑
- blisters — *code as* Corrosion, second degree, by site
- breast(s) — *see* Corrosion, chest wall
- buttock(s) T21.45 ☑
  - first degree T21.55 ☑
  - second degree T21.65 ☑
  - third degree T21.75 ☑
- calf T24.439 ☑
  - first degree T24.539 ☑
  - left T24.432 ☑
    - first degree T24.532 ☑

Corrosion — *continued*
- calf — *continued*
  - left — *continued*
    - second degree T24.632 ☑
    - third degree T24.732 ☑
  - right T24.431 ☑
    - first degree T24.531 ☑
    - second degree T24.631 ☑
    - third degree T24.731 ☑
  - second degree T24.639 ☑
  - third degree T24.739 ☑
- canthus (eye) — *see* Corrosion, eyelid
- cervix T28.8 ☑
- cheek T20.46 ☑
  - first degree T20.56 ☑
  - second degree T20.66 ☑
  - third degree T20.76 ☑
- chest wall T21.41 ☑
  - first degree T21.51 ☑
  - second degree T21.61 ☑
  - third degree T21.71 ☑
- chin T20.43 ☑
  - first degree T20.53 ☑
  - second degree T20.63 ☑
  - third degree T20.73 ☑
- colon T28.7 ☑
- conjunctiva (and cornea) — *see* Corrosion, cornea
- cornea (and conjunctiva) T26.6- ☑
- deep necrosis of underlying tissue — *code as* Corrosion, third degree, by site
- dorsum of hand T23.469 ☑
  - first degree T23.569 ☑
  - left T23.462 ☑
    - first degree T23.562 ☑
    - second degree T23.662 ☑
    - third degree T23.762 ☑
  - right T23.461 ☑
    - first degree T23.561 ☑
    - second degree T23.661 ☑
    - third degree T23.761 ☑
  - second degree T23.669 ☑
  - third degree T23.769 ☑
- ear (auricle) (external) (canal) T20.41 ☑
  - drum T28.91 ☑
  - first degree T20.51 ☑
  - second degree T20.61 ☑
  - third degree T20.71 ☑
- elbow T22.429 ☑
  - first degree T22.529 ☑
  - left T22.422 ☑
    - first degree T22.522 ☑
    - second degree T22.622 ☑
    - third degree T22.722 ☑
  - right T22.421 ☑
    - first degree T22.521 ☑
    - second degree T22.621 ☑
    - third degree T22.721 ☑
  - second degree T22.629 ☑
  - third degree T22.729 ☑
- entire body — *see* Corrosion, multiple body regions
- epidermal loss — *code as* Corrosion, second degree, by site
- epiglottis T27.4 ☑
- erythema, erythematous — *code as* Corrosion, first degree, by site
- esophagus T28.6 ☑
- extent (percentage of body surface)
  - less than 10 percent T32.0
  - 10-19 percent (0-9 percent third degree) T32.10
    - with 10-19 percent third degree T32.11
  - 20-29 percent (0-9 percent third degree) T32.20
    - with
      - 10-19 percent third degree T32.21
      - 20-29 percent third degree T32.22
  - 30-39 percent (0-9 percent third degree) T32.30
    - with
      - 10-19 percent third degree T32.31
      - 20-29 percent third degree T32.32
      - 30-39 percent third degree T32.33
  - 40-49 percent (0-9 percent third degree) T32.40
    - with
      - 10-19 percent third degree T32.41
      - 20-29 percent third degree T32.42
      - 30-39 percent third degree T32.43
      - 40-49 percent third degree T32.44
  - 50-59 percent (0-9 percent third degree) T32.50

Corrosion — *continued*
- extent — *continued*
  - 50-59 percent — *continued*
    - with
      - 10-19 percent third degree T32.51
      - 20-29 percent third degree T32.52
      - 30-39 percent third degree T32.53
      - 40-49 percent third degree T32.54
      - 50-59 percent third degree T32.55
  - 60-69 percent (0-9 percent third degree) T32.60
    - with
      - 10-19 percent third degree T32.61
      - 20-29 percent third degree T32.62
      - 30-39 percent third degree T32.63
      - 40-49 percent third degree T32.64
      - 50-59 percent third degree T32.65
      - 60-69 percent third degree T32.66
  - 70-79 percent (0-9 percent third degree) T32.70
    - with
      - 10-19 percent third degree T32.71
      - 20-29 percent third degree T32.72
      - 30-39 percent third degree T32.73
      - 40-49 percent third degree T32.74
      - 50-59 percent third degree T32.75
      - 60-69 percent third degree T32.76
      - 70-79 percent third degree T32.77
  - 80-89 percent (0-9 percent third degree) T32.80
    - with
      - 10-19 percent third degree T32.81
      - 20-29 percent third degree T32.82
      - 30-39 percent third degree T32.83
      - 40-49 percent third degree T32.84
      - 50-59 percent third degree T32.85
      - 60-69 percent third degree T32.86
      - 70-79 percent third degree T32.87
      - 80-89 percent third degree T32.88
  - 90 percent or more (0-9 percent third degree) T32.90
    - with
      - 10-19 percent third degree T32.91
      - 20-29 percent third degree T32.92
      - 30-39 percent third degree T32.93
      - 40-49 percent third degree T32.94
      - 50-59 percent third degree T32.95
      - 60-69 percent third degree T32.96
      - 70-79 percent third degree T32.97
      - 80-89 percent third degree T32.98
      - 90-99 percent third degree T32.99
- extremity — *see* Corrosion, limb
- eye(s) and adnexa T26.9- ☑
  - with resulting rupture and destruction of eyeball T26.7- ☑
  - conjunctival sac — *see* Corrosion, cornea
  - cornea — *see* Corrosion, cornea
  - lid — *see* Corrosion, eyelid
  - periocular area — *see* Corrosion eyelid
  - specified site NEC T26.8- ☑
- eyeball — *see* Corrosion, eye
- eyelid(s) T26.5- ☑
- face — *see* Corrosion, head
- finger T23.429 ☑
  - first degree T23.529 ☑
  - left T23.422 ☑
    - first degree T23.522 ☑
    - second degree T23.622 ☑
    - third degree T23.722 ☑
  - multiple sites (without thumb) T23.439 ☑
    - with thumb T23.449 ☑
      - first degree T23.549 ☑
      - left T23.442 ☑
        - first degree T23.542 ☑
        - second degree T23.642 ☑
        - third degree T23.742 ☑
      - right T23.441 ☑
        - first degree T23.541 ☑
        - second degree T23.641 ☑
        - third degree T23.741 ☑
      - second degree T23.649 ☑
      - third degree T23.749 ☑
    - first degree T23.539 ☑
    - left T23.432 ☑
      - first degree T23.532 ☑
      - second degree T23.632 ☑
      - third degree T23.732 ☑
    - right T23.431 ☑
      - first degree T23.531 ☑
      - second degree T23.631 ☑
      - third degree T23.731 ☑

Corrosion — *continued*
- finger — *continued*
  - multiple sites — *continued*
    - second degree T23.639 ☑
    - third degree T23.739 ☑
  - right T23.421 ☑
    - first degree T23.521 ☑
    - second degree T23.621 ☑
    - third degree T23.721 ☑
  - second degree T23.629 ☑
  - third degree T23.729 ☑
- flank — *see* Corrosion, abdomen
- foot T25.429 ☑
  - first degree T25.529 ☑
  - left T25.422 ☑
    - first degree T25.522 ☑
    - second degree T25.622 ☑
    - third degree T25.722 ☑
  - multiple with ankle — *see* Corrosion, lower, limb, multiple, ankle and foot
  - right T25.421 ☑
    - first degree T25.521 ☑
    - second degree T25.621 ☑
    - third degree T25.721 ☑
  - second degree T25.629 ☑
  - third degree T25.729 ☑
- forearm T22.419 ☑
  - first degree T22.519 ☑
  - left T22.412 ☑
    - first degree T22.512 ☑
    - second degree T22.612 ☑
    - third degree T22.712 ☑
  - right T22.411 ☑
    - first degree T22.511 ☑
    - second degree T22.611 ☑
    - third degree T22.711 ☑
  - second degree T22.619 ☑
  - third degree T22.719 ☑
- forehead T20.46 ☑
  - first degree T20.56 ☑
  - second degree T20.66 ☑
  - third degree T20.76 ☑
- fourth degree — *code as* Corrosion, third degree, by site
- full thickness skin loss — *code as* Corrosion, third degree, by site
- gastrointestinal tract NEC T28.7 ☑
- genital organs
  - external
    - female T21.47 ☑
      - first degree T21.57 ☑
      - second degree T21.67 ☑
      - third degree T21.77 ☑
    - male T21.46 ☑
      - first degree T21.56 ☑
      - second degree T21.66 ☑
      - third degree T21.76 ☑
  - internal T28.8 ☑
- groin — *see* Corrosion, abdominal wall
- hand(s) T23.409 ☑
  - back — *see* Corrosion, dorsum of hand
  - finger — *see* Corrosion, finger
  - first degree T23.509 ☑
  - left T23.402 ☑
    - first degree T23.502 ☑
    - second degree T23.602 ☑
    - third degree T23.702 ☑
  - multiple sites with wrist T23.499 ☑
    - first degree T23.599 ☑
    - left T23.492 ☑
      - first degree T23.592 ☑
      - second degree T23.692 ☑
      - third degree T23.792 ☑
    - right T23.491 ☑
      - first degree T23.591 ☑
      - second degree T23.691 ☑
      - third degree T23.791 ☑
    - second degree T23.699 ☑
    - third degree T23.799 ☑
  - palm — *see* Corrosion, palm
  - right T23.401 ☑
    - first degree T23.501 ☑
    - second degree T23.601 ☑
    - third degree T23.701 ☑
  - second degree T23.609 ☑
  - third degree T23.709 ☑

Corrosion — *continued*
hand(s) — *continued*
thumb — *see* Corrosion, thumb
head (and face) (and neck) T20.40 ☑
cheek — *see* Corrosion, cheek
chin — *see* Corrosion, chin
ear — *see* Corrosion, ear
eye(s) only — *see* Corrosion, eye
first degree T20.50 ☑
forehead — *see* Corrosion, forehead
lip — *see* Corrosion, lip
multiple sites T20.49 ☑
first degree T20.59 ☑
second degree T20.69 ☑
third degree T20.79 ☑
neck — *see* Corrosion, neck
nose — *see* Corrosion, nose
scalp — *see* Corrosion, scalp
second degree T20.60 ☑
third degree T20.70 ☑
hip(s) — *see* Corrosion, lower, limb
inhalation — *see* Corrosion, respiratory tract
internal organ(s) — *see also* Corrosion, by site T28.90 ☑
alimentary tract T28.7 ☑
esophagus T28.6 ☑
esophagus T28.6 ☑
genitourinary T28.8 ☑
mouth T28.5 ☑
pharynx T28.5 ☑
specified organ NEC T28.99 ☑
interscapular region — *see* Corrosion, back, upper
intestine (large) (small) T28.7 ☑
knee T24.429 ☑
first degree T24.529 ☑
left T24.422 ☑
first degree T24.522 ☑
second degree T24.622 ☑
third degree T24.722 ☑
right T24.421 ☑
first degree T24.521 ☑
second degree T24.621 ☑
third degree T24.721 ☑
second degree T24.629 ☑
third degree T24.729 ☑
labium (majus) (minus) — *see* Corrosion, genital organs, external, female
lacrimal apparatus, duct, gland or sac — *see* Corrosion, eye, specified site NEC
larynx T27.4 ☑
with lung T27.5 ☑
leg(s) (meaning lower limb(s)) — *see* Corrosion, lower limb
limb(s)
lower — *see* Corrosion, lower, limb
upper — *see* Corrosion, upper limb
lip(s) T20.42 ☑
first degree T20.52 ☑
second degree T20.62 ☑
third degree T20.72 ☑
lower
back — *see* Corrosion, back
limb T24.409 ☑
ankle — *see* Corrosion, ankle
calf — *see* Corrosion, calf
first degree T24.509 ☑
foot — *see* Corrosion, foot
knee — *see* Corrosion, knee
left T24.402 ☑
first degree T24.502 ☑
second degree T24.602 ☑
third degree T24.702 ☑
multiple sites, except ankle and foot T24.499 ☑
ankle and foot T25.499 ☑
first degree T25.599 ☑
left T25.492 ☑
first degree T25.592 ☑
second degree T25.692 ☑
third degree T25.792 ☑
right T25.491 ☑
first degree T25.591 ☑
second degree T25.691 ☑
third degree T25.791 ☑
second degree T25.699 ☑
third degree T25.799 ☑
first degree T24.599 ☑

Corrosion — *continued*
lower — *continued*
limb — *continued*
multiple sites, except ankle and foot — *continued*
left T24.492 ☑
first degree T24.592 ☑
second degree T24.692 ☑
third degree T24.792 ☑
right T24.491 ☑
first degree T24.591 ☑
second degree T24.691 ☑
third degree T24.791 ☑
second degree T24.699 ☑
third degree T24.799 ☑
right T24.401 ☑
first degree T24.501 ☑
second degree T24.601 ☑
third degree T24.701 ☑
second degree T24.609 ☑
thigh — *see* Corrosion, thigh
third degree T24.709 ☑
lung (with larynx and trachea) T27.5 ☑
mouth T28.5 ☑
neck T20.47 ☑
first degree T20.57 ☑
second degree T20.67 ☑
third degree T20.77 ☑
nose (septum) T20.44 ☑
first degree T20.54 ☑
second degree T20.64 ☑
third degree T20.74 ☑
ocular adnexa — *see* Corrosion, eye
orbit region — *see* Corrosion, eyelid
palm T23.459 ☑
first degree T23.559 ☑
left T23.452 ☑
first degree T23.552 ☑
second degree T23.652 ☑
third degree T23.752 ☑
right T23.451 ☑
first degree T23.551 ☑
second degree T23.651 ☑
third degree T23.751 ☑
second degree T23.659 ☑
third degree T23.759 ☑
partial thickness — *code as* Corrosion, unspecified degree, by site
pelvis — *see* Corrosion, trunk
penis — *see* Corrosion, genital organs, external, male
perineum
female — *see* Corrosion, genital organs, external, female
male — *see* Corrosion, genital organs, external, male
periocular area — *see* Corrosion, eyelid
pharynx T28.5 ☑
rectum T28.7 ☑
respiratory tract T27.7 ☑
larynx — *see* Corrosion, larynx
specified part NEC T27.6 ☑
trachea — *see* Corrosion, larynx
sac, lacrimal — *see* Corrosion, eye, specified site NEC
scalp T20.45 ☑
first degree T20.55 ☑
second degree T20.65 ☑
third degree T20.75 ☑
scapular region T22.469 ☑
first degree T22.569 ☑
left T22.462 ☑
first degree T22.562 ☑
second degree T22.662 ☑
third degree T22.762 ☑
right T22.461 ☑
first degree T22.561 ☑
second degree T22.661 ☑
third degree T22.761 ☑
second degree T22.669 ☑
third degree T22.769 ☑
sclera — *see* Corrosion, eye, specified site NEC
scrotum — *see* Corrosion, genital organs, external, male
shoulder T22.459 ☑
first degree T22.559 ☑
left T22.452 ☑
first degree T22.552 ☑
second degree T22.652 ☑

Corrosion — *continued*
shoulder — *continued*
left — *continued*
third degree T22.752 ☑
right T22.451 ☑
first degree T22.551 ☑
second degree T22.651 ☑
third degree T22.751 ☑
second degree T22.659 ☑
third degree T22.759 ☑
stomach T28.7 ☑
temple — *see* Corrosion, head
testis — *see* Corrosion, genital organs, external, male
thigh T24.419 ☑
first degree T24.519 ☑
left T24.412 ☑
first degree T24.512 ☑
second degree T24.612 ☑
third degree T24.712 ☑
right T24.411 ☑
first degree T24.511 ☑
second degree T24.611 ☑
third degree T24.711 ☑
second degree T24.619 ☑
third degree T24.719 ☑
thorax (external) — *see* Corrosion, trunk
throat (meaning pharynx) T28.5 ☑
thumb(s) T23.419 ☑
first degree T23.519 ☑
left T23.412 ☑
first degree T23.512 ☑
second degree T23.612 ☑
third degree T23.712 ☑
multiple sites with fingers T23.449 ☑
first degree T23.549 ☑
left T23.442 ☑
first degree T23.542 ☑
second degree T23.642 ☑
third degree T23.742 ☑
right T23.441 ☑
first degree T23.541 ☑
second degree T23.641 ☑
third degree T23.741 ☑
second degree T23.649 ☑
third degree T23.749 ☑
right T23.411 ☑
first degree T23.511 ☑
second degree T23.611 ☑
third degree T23.711 ☑
second degree T23.619 ☑
third degree T23.719 ☑
toe T25.439 ☑
first degree T25.539 ☑
left T25.432 ☑
first degree T25.532 ☑
second degree T25.632 ☑
third degree T25.732 ☑
right T25.431 ☑
first degree T25.531 ☑
second degree T25.631 ☑
third degree T25.731 ☑
second degree T25.639 ☑
third degree T25.739 ☑
tongue T28.5 ☑
tonsil(s) T28.5 ☑
total body — *see* Corrosion, multiple body regions
trachea T27.4 ☑
with lung T27.5 ☑
trunk T21.40 ☑
abdominal wall — *see* Corrosion, abdominal wall
anus — *see* Corrosion, buttock
axilla — *see* Corrosion, upper limb
back — *see* Corrosion, back
breast — *see* Corrosion, chest wall
buttock — *see* Corrosion, buttock
chest wall — *see* Corrosion, chest wall
first degree T21.50 ☑
flank — *see* Corrosion, abdominal wall
genital
female — *see* Corrosion, genital organs, external, female
male — *see* Corrosion, genital organs, external, male
groin — *see* Corrosion, abdominal wall
interscapular region — *see* Corrosion, back, upper

Corrosion — *continued*
- trunk — *continued*
  - labia — *see* Corrosion, genital organs, external, female
  - lower back — *see* Corrosion, back
  - penis — *see* Corrosion, genital organs, external, male
  - perineum
    - female — *see* Corrosion, genital organs, external, female
    - male — *see* Corrosion, genital organs, external, male
  - scapular region — *see* Corrosion, upper limb
  - scrotum — *see* Corrosion, genital organs, external, male
  - second degree T21.60 ☑
  - shoulder — *see* Corrosion, upper limb
  - specified site NEC T21.49 ☑
    - first degree T21.59 ☑
    - second degree T21.69 ☑
    - third degree T21.79 ☑
  - testes — *see* Corrosion, genital organs, external, male
  - third degree T21.70 ☑
  - upper back — *see* Corrosion, back, upper
  - vagina T28.8 ☑
  - vulva — *see* Corrosion, genital organs, external, female
- unspecified site with extent of body surface involved specified
  - less than 10 percent T32.0
  - 10-19 percent (0-9 percent third degree) T32.10
    - with 10-19 percent third degree T32.11
  - 20-29 percent (0-9 percent third degree) T32.20
    - with
      - 10-19 percent third degree T32.21
      - 20-29 percent third degree T32.22
  - 30-39 percent (0-9 percent third degree) T32.30
    - with
      - 10-19 percent third degree T32.31
      - 20-29 percent third degree T32.32
      - 30-39 percent third degree T32.33
  - 40-49 percent (0-9 percent third degree) T32.40
    - with
      - 10-19 percent third degree T32.41
      - 20-29 percent third degree T32.42
      - 30-39 percent third degree T32.43
      - 40-49 percent third degree T32.44
  - 50-59 percent (0-9 percent third degree) T32.50
    - with
      - 10-19 percent third degree T32.51
      - 20-29 percent third degree T32.52
      - 30-39 percent third degree T32.53
      - 40-49 percent third degree T32.54
      - 50-59 percent third degree T32.55
  - 60-69 percent (0-9 percent third degree) T32.60
    - with
      - 10-19 percent third degree T32.61
      - 20-29 percent third degree T32.62
      - 30-39 percent third degree T32.63
      - 40-49 percent third degree T32.64
      - 50-59 percent third degree T32.65
      - 60-69 percent third degree T32.66
  - 70-79 percent (0-9 percent third degree) T32.70
    - with
      - 10-19 percent third degree T32.71
      - 20-29 percent third degree T32.72
      - 30-39 percent third degree T32.73
      - 40-49 percent third degree T32.74
      - 50-59 percent third degree T32.75
      - 60-69 percent third degree T32.76
      - 70-79 percent third degree T32.77
  - 80-89 percent (0-9 percent third degree) T32.80
    - with
      - 10-19 percent third degree T32.81
      - 20-29 percent third degree T32.82
      - 30-39 percent third degree T32.83
      - 40-49 percent third degree T32.84
      - 50-59 percent third degree T32.85
      - 60-69 percent third degree T32.86
      - 70-79 percent third degree T32.87
      - 80-89 percent third degree T32.88
  - 90 percent or more (0-9 percent third degree) T32.90
    - with
      - 10-19 percent third degree T32.91
      - 20-29 percent third degree T32.92
      - 30-39 percent third degree T32.93
      - 40-49 percent third degree T32.94

Corrosion — *continued*
- unspecified site with extent of body surface involved specified — *continued*
  - 90 percent or more — *continued*
    - with — *continued*
      - 50-59 percent third degree T32.95
      - 60-69 percent third degree T32.96
      - 70-79 percent third degree T32.97
      - 80-89 percent third degree T32.98
      - 90-99 percent third degree T32.99
- upper limb (axilla) (scapular region) T22.40 ☑
  - above elbow — *see* Corrosion, above elbow
  - axilla — *see* Corrosion, axilla
  - elbow — *see* Corrosion, elbow
  - first degree T22.50 ☑
  - forearm — *see* Corrosion, forearm
  - hand — *see* Corrosion, hand
  - interscapular region — *see* Corrosion, back, upper
  - multiple sites T22.499 ☑
    - first degree T22.599 ☑
    - left T22.492 ☑
      - first degree T22.592 ☑
      - second degree T22.692 ☑
      - third degree T22.792 ☑
    - right T22.491 ☑
      - first degree T22.591 ☑
      - second degree T22.691 ☑
      - third degree T22.791 ☑
    - second degree T22.699 ☑
    - third degree T22.799 ☑
  - scapular region — *see* Corrosion, scapular region
  - second degree T22.60 ☑
  - shoulder — *see* Corrosion, shoulder
  - third degree T22.70 ☑
  - wrist — *see* Corrosion, hand
- uterus T28.8 ☑
- vagina T28.8 ☑
- vulva — *see* Corrosion, genital organs, external, female
- wrist T23.479 ☑
  - first degree T23.579 ☑
  - left T23.472 ☑
    - first degree T23.572 ☑
    - second degree T23.672 ☑
    - third degree T23.772 ☑
  - multiple sites with hand T23.499 ☑
    - first degree T23.599 ☑
    - left T23.492 ☑
      - first degree T23.592 ☑
      - second degree T23.692 ☑
      - third degree T23.792 ☑
    - right T23.491 ☑
      - first degree T23.591 ☑
      - second degree T23.691 ☑
      - third degree T23.791 ☑
    - second degree T23.699 ☑
    - third degree T23.799 ☑
  - right T23.471 ☑
    - first degree T23.571 ☑
    - second degree T23.671 ☑
    - third degree T23.771 ☑
  - second degree T23.679 ☑
  - third degree T23.779 ☑

Corrosive burn — *see* Corrosion

Corsican fever — *see* Malaria

Cortical — *see* condition

Cortico-adrenal — *see* condition

Coryza (acute) J00
- with grippe or influenza — *see* Influenza, with, respiratory manifestations NEC
- syphilitic
  - congenital (chronic) A50.05

Co-sleeping, child-caregiver Z72.823

Costen's syndrome or complex M26.69

Costiveness — *see* Constipation

Costochondritis M94.0

Cot death R99

Cotard's syndrome F22

Cotia virus B08.8

Cotton wool spots (retinal) H35.81

Cotungo's disease — *see* Sciatica

Cough (affected) (epidemic) (nervous) R05.9
- with hemorrhage — *see* Hemoptysis
- acute R05.1
- bronchial R05.8
  - with grippe or influenza — *see* Influenza, with, respiratory manifestations NEC

Cough — *continued*
- chronic R05.3
- functional F45.8
- hysterical F45.8
- laryngeal, spasmodic R05.8
- paroxysmal, due to Bordetella pertussis (without pneumonia) A37.00
  - with pneumonia A37.01
- persistent R05.3
- psychogenic F45.8
- refractory R05.3
- smokers' J41.0
- specified NEC R05.8
- subacute R05.2
- syncope R05.4
- tea taster's B49
- unexplained R05.3

Counseling (for) Z71.9
- abuse NEC
  - perpetrator Z69.82
  - victim Z69.81
- alcohol abuser Z71.41
  - family Z71.42
- child abuse
  - nonparental
    - perpetrator Z69.021
    - victim Z69.020
  - parental
    - perpetrator Z69.011
    - victim Z69.010
- consanguinity Z71.89
- contraceptive Z30.09
- dietary Z71.3
- drug abuser Z71.51
  - family member Z71.52
- exercise Z71.82
- family Z71.89
- fertility preservation (prior to cancer therapy) (prior to removal of gonads) Z31.62
- for non-attending third party Z71.0
  - related to sexual behavior or orientation Z70.2
- genetic
  - nonprocreative Z71.83
  - procreative NEC Z31.5
- gestational carrier Z31.7
- health (advice) (education) (instruction) — *see* Counseling, medical
  - risk for travel (international) Z71.84
- human immunodeficiency virus (HIV) Z71.7
- immunization safety Z71.85
- impotence Z70.1
- insulin pump use Z46.81
- medical (for) Z71.9
  - boarding school resident Z59.3
  - consanguinity Z71.89
  - feared complaint and no disease found Z71.1
  - human immunodeficiency virus (HIV) Z71.7
  - institutional resident Z59.3
  - on behalf of another Z71.0
    - related to sexual behavior or orientation Z70.2
  - person living alone Z60.2
  - specified reason NEC Z71.89
- natural family planning
  - procreative Z31.61
  - to avoid pregnancy Z30.02
- pediatric-to-adult transition Z71.87
- perpetrator (of)
  - abuse NEC Z69.82
  - child abuse
    - non-parental Z69.021
    - parental Z69.011
  - rape NEC Z69.82
  - spousal abuse Z69.12
- procreative NEC Z31.69
  - fertility preservation (prior to cancer therapy) (prior to removal of gonads) Z31.62
  - using natural family planning Z31.61
- promiscuity Z70.1
- rape victim Z69.81
- religious Z71.81
- safety for travel (international) Z71.84
- sex, sexual (related to) Z70.9
  - attitude(s) Z70.0
  - behavior or orientation Z70.1
  - combined concerns Z70.3
  - non-responsiveness Z70.1
  - on behalf of third party Z70.2
  - specified reason NEC Z70.8
- socioeconomic factors Z71.88

Counseling — *continued*
- specified reason NEC Z71.89
- spiritual Z71.81
- spousal abuse (perpetrator) Z69.12
  - victim Z69.11
- substance abuse Z71.89
  - alcohol Z71.41
  - drug Z71.51
  - tobacco Z71.6
- tobacco use Z71.6
- travel (international) Z71.84
- use (of)
  - insulin pump Z46.81
- vaccine product safety Z71.85
- victim (of)
  - abuse Z69.81
  - child abuse
    - by parent Z69.Ø1Ø
    - non-parental Z69.Ø2Ø
  - rape NEC Z69.81

Coupled rhythm RØØ.8

Couvelaire syndrome or uterus (complicating delivery) O45.8X- ☑

COVID-19 UØ7.1
- condition post UØ9.9
- contact (with) Z2Ø.822
- exposure (to) Z2Ø.822
- history of (personal) Z86.16
- long (haul) UØ9.9
- partially vaccinated (for) Z28.311
- pneumonia J12.82
- screening Z11.52
- sequelae (post acute) UØ9.9
- unvaccinated (for) Z28.31Ø

Cowperitis — *see* Urethritis

Cowper's gland — *see* condition

Cowpox BØ8.Ø1Ø
- due to vaccination T88.1 ☑

Coxa
- magna M91.4- ☑
- plana M91.2- ☑
- valga (acquired) — *see also* Deformity, limb, specified type NEC, thigh
  - congenital Q65.81
  - sequelae (late effect) of rickets E64.3
- vara (acquired) — *see also* Deformity, limb, specified type NEC, thigh
  - congenital Q65.82
  - sequelae (late effect) of rickets E64.3

Coxalgia, coxalgic (nontuberculous) — *see also* Pain, joint, hip
- tuberculous A18.Ø2

Coxitis — *see* Monoarthritis, hip

Coxsackie (virus) (infection) B34.1
- as cause of disease classified elsewhere B97.11
- carditis B33.2Ø
- central nervous system NEC A88.8
- endocarditis B33.21
- enteritis AØ8.39
- meningitis (aseptic) A87.Ø
- myocarditis B33.22
- pericarditis B33.23
- pharyngitis BØ8.5
- pleurodynia B33.Ø
- specific disease NEC B33.8

Crabs, meaning pubic lice B85.3

Crack baby PØ4.41

Cracked nipple N64.Ø
- associated with
  - lactation O92.13
  - pregnancy O92.11- ☑
  - puerperium O92.12

Cracked tooth KØ3.81

Cradle cap L21.Ø

Craft neurosis F48.8

Cramp(s) R25.2
- abdominal — *see* Pain, abdominal
- bathing T75.1 ☑
- colic R1Ø.83
  - psychogenic F45.8
- due to immersion T75.1 ☑
- fireman T67.2 ☑
- heat T67.2 ☑
- immersion T75.1 ☑
- intestinal — *see* Pain, abdominal
  - psychogenic F45.8
- leg, sleep related G47.62
- limb (lower) (upper) NEC R25.2

Cramp(s) — *continued*
- limb — *continued*
  - sleep related G47.62
- linotypist's F48.8
  - organic G25.89
- muscle (limb) (general) R25.2
  - due to immersion T75.1 ☑
  - psychogenic F45.8
- occupational (hand) F48.8
  - organic G25.89
- salt-depletion E87.1
- sleep related, leg G47.62
- stoker's T67.2 ☑
- swimmer's T75.1 ☑
- telegrapher's F48.8
  - organic G25.89
- typist's F48.8
  - organic G25.89
- uterus N94.89
  - menstrual — *see* Dysmenorrhea
- writer's F48.8
  - organic G25.89

Cranial — *see* condition

Craniocleidodysostosis Q74.Ø

Craniofenestria (skull) Q75.8

Craniolacunia (skull) Q75.8

Craniopagus Q89.4

Craniopathy, metabolic M85.2

Craniopharyngeal — *see* condition

Craniopharyngioma D44.4

Craniorachischisis (totalis) QØØ.1

Cranioschisis Q75.8

Craniostenosis Q75.Ø

Craniosynostosis Q75.Ø

Craniotabes (cause unknown) M83.8
- neonatal P96.3
- rachitic E64.3
- syphilitic A5Ø.56

Cranium — *see* condition

Craw-craw — *see* Onchocerciasis

Creaking joint — *see* Derangement, joint, specified type NEC

Creeping
- eruption B76.9
- palsy or paralysis G12.22

Crenated tongue K14.8

Creotoxism AØ5.9

Crepitus
- caput Q75.8
- joint — *see* Derangement, joint, specified type NEC

Crescent or conus choroid, congenital Q14.3

CREST syndrome M34.1

Cretin, cretinism (congenital) (endemic) (nongoitrous) (sporadic) EØØ.9
- pelvis
  - with disproportion (fetopelvic) O33.Ø
    - causing obstructed labor O65.Ø
- type
  - hypothyroid EØØ.1
  - mixed EØØ.2
  - myxedematous EØØ.1
  - neurological EØØ.Ø

Creutzfeldt-Jakob disease or syndrome (with dementia) A81.ØØ
- familial A81.Ø9
- iatrogenic A81.Ø9
- specified NEC A81.Ø9
- sporadic A81.Ø9
- variant (vCJD) A81.Ø1

Crib death R99

Cribriform hymen Q52.3

Cri-du-chat syndrome Q93.4

Crigler-Najjar disease or syndrome E8Ø.5

Crime, victim of Z65.4

Crimean hemorrhagic fever A98.Ø

Criminalism F6Ø.2

Crisis
- abdomen R1Ø.Ø
- acute reaction F43.Ø
- addisonian E27.2
- adrenal (cortical) E27.2
- celiac K9Ø.Ø
- Dietl's N13.8
- emotional — *see also* Disorder, adjustment
  - acute reaction to stress F43.Ø
  - specific to childhood and adolescence F93.8

Crisis — *continued*
- glaucomatocyclitic — *see* Glaucoma, secondary, inflammation
- heart — *see* Failure, heart
- nitritoid I95.2
  - correct substance properly administered — *see* Table of Drugs and Chemicals, by drug, adverse effect
  - overdose or wrong substance given or taken — *see* Table of Drugs and Chemicals, by drug, poisoning
- oculogyric H51.8
  - psychogenic F45.8
- Pel's (tabetic) A52.11
- psychosexual identity F64.2
- renal N28.Ø
- sickle-cell — *see also* Disease, sickle-cell, by type, with crisis D57.ØØ
  - with
    - acute chest syndrome D57.Ø1
    - cerebral vascular involvement D57.Ø3
    - complication specified NEC D57.Ø9
    - splenic sequestration D57.Ø2
    - vasoocclusive pain D57.ØØ
- state (acute reaction) F43.Ø
- tabetic A52.11
- thyroid — *see* Thyrotoxicosis with thyroid storm
- thyrotoxic — *see* Thyrotoxicosis with thyroid storm

Crocq's disease (acrocyanosis) I73.89

Crohn's disease — *see* Enteritis, regional

Crooked septum, nasal J34.2

Cross syndrome E7Ø.328

Crossbite (anterior) (posterior) M26.24

Cross-eye — *see* Strabismus, convergent concomitant

Croup, croupous (catarrhal) (infectious) (inflammatory) (nondiphtheritic) JØ5.Ø
- bronchial J2Ø.9
- diphtheritic A36.2
- false J38.5
- spasmodic J38.5
  - diphtheritic A36.2
- stridulous J38.5
  - diphtheritic A36.2

Crouzon's disease Q75.1

Crowding, tooth, teeth, fully erupted M26.31

CRST syndrome M34.1

Cruchet's disease A85.8

Cruelty in children — *see also* Disorder, conduct

Crural ulcer — *see* Ulcer, lower limb

Crush, crushed, crushing T14.8 ☑
- abdomen S38.1 ☑
- ankle S97.Ø- ☑
- arm (upper) (and shoulder) S47.- ☑
- axilla — *see* Crush, arm
- back, lower S38.1 ☑
- buttock S38.1 ☑
- cheek SØ7.Ø ☑
- chest S28.Ø ☑
- cranium SØ7.1 ☑
- ear SØ7.Ø ☑
- elbow S57.Ø- ☑
- extremity
  - lower
    - ankle — *see* Crush, ankle
    - below knee — *see* Crush, leg
    - foot — *see* Crush, foot
    - hip — *see* Crush, hip
    - knee — *see* Crush, knee
    - thigh — *see* Crush, thigh
    - toe — *see* Crush, toe
  - upper
    - below elbow S67.9- ☑
    - elbow — *see* Crush, elbow
    - finger — *see* Crush, finger
    - forearm — *see* Crush, forearm
    - hand — *see* Crush, hand
    - thumb — *see* Crush, thumb
    - upper arm — *see* Crush, arm
    - wrist — *see* Crush, wrist
- face SØ7.Ø ☑
- finger(s) S67.1- ☑
  - with hand (and wrist) — *see* Crush, hand, specified site NEC
  - index S67.19- ☑
  - little S67.19- ☑
  - middle S67.19- ☑
  - ring S67.19- ☑

Crush, crushed, crushing — *continued*
- finger(s) — *continued*
  - thumb — *see* Crush, thumb
- foot S97.8- ☑
  - toe — *see* Crush, toe
- forearm S57.8- ☑
- genitalia, external
  - female S38.ØØ2 ☑
    - vagina S38.Ø3 ☑
    - vulva S38.Ø3 ☑
  - male S38.ØØ1 ☑
    - penis S38.Ø1 ☑
    - scrotum S38.Ø2 ☑
    - testis S38.Ø2 ☑
- hand (except fingers alone) S67.2- ☑
  - with wrist S67.4- ☑
- head SØ7.9 ☑
  - specified NEC SØ7.8 ☑
- heel — *see* Crush, foot
- hip S77.Ø- ☑
  - with thigh S77.2- ☑
- internal organ (abdomen, chest, or pelvis) NEC T14.8 ☑
- knee S87.Ø- ☑
- labium (majus) (minus) S38.Ø3 ☑
- larynx S17.Ø ☑
- leg (lower) S87.8- ☑
  - knee — *see* Crush, knee
- lip SØ7.Ø ☑
- lower
  - back S38.1 ☑
  - leg — *see* Crush, leg
- neck S17.9 ☑
- nerve — *see* Injury, nerve
- nose SØ7.Ø ☑
- pelvis S38.1 ☑
- penis S38.Ø1 ☑
- scalp SØ7.8 ☑
- scapular region — *see* Crush, arm
- scrotum S38.Ø2 ☑
- severe, unspecified site T14.8 ☑
- shoulder (and upper arm) — *see* Crush, arm
- skull SØ7.1 ☑
- syndrome (complication of trauma) T79.5 ☑
- testis S38.Ø2 ☑
- thigh S77.1- ☑
  - with hip S77.2- ☑
- throat S17.8 ☑
- thumb S67.Ø- ☑
  - with hand (and wrist) — *see* Crush, hand, specified site NEC
- toe(s) S97.1Ø- ☑
  - great S97.11- ☑
  - lesser S97.12- ☑
- trachea S17.Ø ☑
- vagina S38.Ø3 ☑
- vulva S38.Ø3 ☑
- wrist S67.3- ☑
  - with hand S67.4- ☑

Crusta lactea L21.Ø

Crusts R23.4

Crutch paralysis — *see* Injury, brachial plexus

Cruveilhier-Baumgarten cirrhosis, disease or syndrome K74.69

Cruveilhier's atrophy or disease G12.8

Crying (constant) (continuous) (excessive)
- child, adolescent, or adult R45.83
- infant (baby) (newborn) R68.11

Cryofibrinogenemia D89.2

Cryoglobulinemia (essential) (idiopathic) (mixed) (primary) (purpura) (secondary) (vasculitis) D89.1
- with lung involvement D89.1 *[J99]*

Cryptitis (anal) (rectal) K62.89

Cryptococcosis, cryptococcus (infection) (neoformans) B45.9
- bone B45.3
- cerebral B45.1
- cutaneous B45.2
- disseminated B45.7
- generalized B45.7
- meningitis B45.1
- meningocerebralis B45.1
- osseous B45.3
- pulmonary B45.Ø
- skin B45.2
- specified NEC B45.8

Cryptopapillitis (anus) K62.89

Cryptophthalmos Q11.2
- syndrome Q87.Ø

Cryptorchid, cryptorchism, cryptorchidism Q53.9
- bilateral Q53.2Ø
  - abdominal Q53.211
  - perineal Q53.22
- unilateral Q53.1Ø
  - abdominal Q53.111
  - perineal Q53.12

Cryptosporidiosis AØ7.2
- hepatobiliary B88.8
- respiratory B88.8

Cryptostromosis J67.6

Crystalluria R82.998

Cubitus
- congenital Q68.8
- valgus (acquired) M21.Ø- ☑
  - congenital Q68.8
  - sequelae (late effect) of rickets E64.3
- varus (acquired) M21.1- ☑
  - congenital Q68.8
  - sequelae (late effect) of rickets E64.3

Cultural deprivation or shock Z6Ø.3

Curling esophagus K22.4

Curling's ulcer — *see* Ulcer, peptic, acute

Curschmann (-Batten) (-Steinert) **disease or syndrome** G71.11

Curse, Ondine's — *see* Apnea, sleep

Curvature
- organ or site, congenital NEC — *see* Distortion
- penis (lateral) Q55.61
- Pott's (spinal) A18.Ø1
- radius, idiopathic, progressive (congenital) Q74.Ø
- spine (acquired) (angular) (idiopathic) (incorrect) (postural) — *see* Dorsopathy, deforming
  - congenital Q67.5
  - due to or associated with
    - Charcot-Marie-Tooth disease — *see also* subcategory M49.8 G6Ø.Ø
    - osteitis
      - deformans M88.88
      - fibrosa cystica — *see also* subcategory M49.8 E21.Ø
    - tuberculosis (Pott's curvature) A18.Ø1
  - sequelae (late effect) of rickets E64.3
  - tuberculous A18.Ø1

Cushingoid due to steroid therapy E24.2
- correct substance properly administered — *see* Table of Drugs and Chemicals, by drug, adverse effect
- overdose or wrong substance given or taken — *see* Table of Drugs and Chemicals, by drug, poisoning

Cushing's
- syndrome or disease E24.9
  - drug-induced E24.2
  - iatrogenic E24.2
  - pituitary-dependent E24.Ø
  - specified NEC E24.8
- ulcer — *see* Ulcer, peptic, acute

Cusp, Carabelli — *omit code*

Cut (external) — *see also* Laceration
- muscle — *see* Injury, muscle

Cutaneous — *see also* condition
- hemorrhage R23.3
- larva migrans B76.9

Cutis — *see also* condition
- hyperelastica Q82.8
  - acquired L57.4
- laxa (hyperelastica) — *see* Dermatolysis
- marmorata R23.8
- osteosis L94.2
- pendula — *see* Dermatolysis
- rhomboidalis nuchae L57.2
- verticis gyrata Q82.8
  - acquired L91.8

Cyanosis R23.Ø
- due to
  - patent foramen botalli Q21.12
  - persistent foramen ovale Q21.12
- enterogenous D74.8
- paroxysmal digital — *see* Raynaud's disease
  - with gangrene I73.Ø1
- retina, retinal H35.89

Cyanotic heart disease I24.9
- congenital Q24.9

Cycle
- anovulatory N97.Ø
- menstrual, irregular N92.6

Cyclencephaly QØ4.9

Cyclical vomiting, in migraine — *see also* Vomiting, cyclical G43.AØ *(following G43.7)*
- psychogenic F5Ø.89

Cyclitis — *see also* Iridocyclitis H2Ø.9
- chronic — *see* Iridocyclitis, chronic
- Fuchs' heterochromic H2Ø.81- ☑
- granulomatous — *see* Iridocyclitis, chronic
- lens-induced — *see* Iridocyclitis, lens-induced
- posterior H3Ø.2- ☑

Cycloid personality F34.Ø

Cyclophoria H5Ø.54

Cyclopia, cyclops Q87.Ø

Cyclopism Q87.Ø

Cyclosporiasis AØ7.4

Cyclothymia F34.Ø

Cyclothymic personality F34.Ø

Cyclotropia H5Ø.41- ☑

Cylindroma — *see also* Neoplasm, malignant, by site
- eccrine dermal — *see* Neoplasm, skin, benign
- skin — *see* Neoplasm, skin, benign

Cylindruria R82.998

Cynanche
- diphtheritic A36.2
- tonsillaris J36

Cynophobia F4Ø.218

Cynorexia R63.2

Cyphosis — *see* Kyphosis

Cyprus fever — *see* Brucellosis

Cyst (colloid) (mucous) (simple) (retention)
- adenoid (infected) J35.8
- adrenal gland E27.8
  - congenital Q89.1
- air, lung J98.4
- allantoic Q64.4
- alveolar process (jaw bone) M27.4Ø
- amnion, amniotic O41.8X- ☑
- aneurysmal M27.49
- anterior
  - chamber (eye) — *see* Cyst, iris
  - nasopalatine KØ9.1
- antrum J34.1
- anus K62.89
- apical (tooth) (periodontal) KØ4.8
- appendix K38.8
- arachnoid, brain (acquired) G93.Ø
  - congenital QØ4.6
- arytenoid J38.7
- Baker's M71.2- ☑
  - ruptured M66.Ø
  - tuberculous A18.Ø2
- Bartholin's gland N75.Ø
- bile duct (common) (hepatic) K83.5
- bladder (multiple) (trigone) N32.89
- blue dome (breast) — *see* Cyst, breast
- bone (local) NEC M85.6Ø
  - aneurysmal M85.5Ø
    - ankle M85.57- ☑
    - foot M85.57- ☑
    - forearm M85.53- ☑
    - hand M85.54- ☑
    - jaw M27.49
    - lower leg M85.56- ☑
    - multiple site M85.59
    - neck M85.58
    - rib M85.58
    - shoulder M85.51- ☑
    - skull M85.58
    - specified site NEC M85.58
    - thigh M85.55- ☑
    - toe M85.57- ☑
    - upper arm M85.52- ☑
    - vertebra M85.58
  - solitary M85.4Ø
    - ankle M85.47- ☑
    - fibula M85.46- ☑
    - foot M85.47- ☑
    - hand M85.44- ☑
    - humerus M85.42- ☑
    - jaw M27.49
    - neck M85.48
    - pelvis M85.45- ☑
    - radius M85.43- ☑
    - rib M85.48
    - shoulder M85.41- ☑
    - skull M85.48
    - specified site NEC M85.48
    - tibia M85.46- ☑

Cyst — *continued*
bone — *continued*
solitary — *continued*
toe M85.47- ☑
ulna M85.43- ☑
vertebra M85.48
specified type NEC M85.6Ø
ankle M85.67- ☑
foot M85.67- ☑
forearm M85.63- ☑
hand M85.64- ☑
jaw M27.4Ø
developmental (nonodontogenic) KØ9.1
odontogenic KØ9.Ø
latent M27.Ø
lower leg M85.66- ☑
multiple site M85.69
neck M85.68
rib M85.68
shoulder M85.61- ☑
skull M85.68
specified site NEC M85.68
thigh M85.65- ☑
toe M85.67- ☑
upper arm M85.62- ☑
vertebra M85.68
brain (acquired) G93.Ø
congenital QØ4.6
hydatid B67.99 *[G94]*
third ventricle (colloid), congenital QØ4.6
branchial (cleft) Q18.Ø
branchiogenic Q18.Ø
breast (benign) (blue dome) (pedunculated) (solitary) N6Ø.Ø- ☑
involution — *see* Dysplasia, mammary, specified type NEC
sebaceous — *see* Dysplasia, mammary, specified type NEC
broad ligament (benign) N83.8
bronchogenic (mediastinal) (sequestration) J98.4
congenital Q33.Ø
buccal KØ9.8
bulbourethral gland N36.8
bursa, bursal NEC M71.3Ø
with rupture — *see* Rupture, synovium
ankle M71.37- ☑
elbow M71.32- ☑
foot M71.37- ☑
hand M71.34- ☑
hip M71.35- ☑
multiple sites M71.39
pharyngeal J39.2
popliteal space — *see* Cyst, Baker's
shoulder M71.31- ☑
specified site NEC M71.38
wrist M71.33- ☑
calcifying odontogenic D16.5
upper jaw (bone) (maxilla) D16.4
canal of Nuck (female) N94.89
congenital Q52.4
canthus — *see* Cyst, conjunctiva
carcinomatous — *see* Neoplasm, malignant, by site
cauda equina G95.89
cavum septi pellucidi — *see* Cyst, brain
celomic (pericardium) Q24.8
cerebellopontine (angle) — *see* Cyst, brain
cerebellum — *see* Cyst, brain
cerebral — *see* Cyst, brain
cervical lateral Q18.Ø
cervix NEC N88.8
embryonic Q51.6
nabothian N88.8
chiasmal optic NEC — *see* Disorder, optic, chiasm
chocolate (ovary) N8Ø.1Ø- ☑
choledochus, congenital Q44.4
chorion O41.8X- ☑
choroid plexus G93.Ø
congenital QØ4.6
ciliary body — *see* Cyst, iris
clitoris N9Ø.7
colon K63.89
common (bile) duct K83.5
congenital NEC Q89.8
adrenal gland Q89.1
epiglottis Q31.8
esophagus Q39.8
fallopian tube Q5Ø.4

Cyst — *continued*
congenital — *continued*
kidney Q61.ØØ
more than one (multiple) Q61.Ø2
specified as polycystic Q61.3
adult type Q61.2
infantile type NEC Q61.19
collecting duct dilation Q61.11
solitary Q61.Ø1
larynx Q31.8
liver Q44.6
lung Q33.Ø
mediastinum Q34.1
ovary Q5Ø.1
oviduct Q5Ø.4
periurethral (tissue) Q64.79
prepuce Q55.69
salivary gland (any) Q38.4
sublingual Q38.6
submaxillary gland Q38.6
thymus (gland) Q89.2
tongue Q38.3
ureterovesical orifice Q62.8
vulva Q52.79
conjunctiva H11.44- ☑
cornea H18.89- ☑
corpora quadrigemina G93.Ø
corpus
albicans N83.29- ☑
luteum (hemorrhagic) (ruptured) N83.1- ☑
Cowper's gland (benign) (infected) N36.8
cranial meninges G93.Ø
craniobuccal pouch E23.6
craniopharyngeal pouch E23.6
cystic duct K82.8
Cysticercus — *see* Cysticercosis
Dandy-Walker QØ3.1
with spina bifida — *see* Spina bifida
dental (root) KØ4.8
developmental KØ9.Ø
eruption KØ9.Ø
primordial KØ9.Ø
dentigerous (mandible) (maxilla) KØ9.Ø
dermoid — *see* Neoplasm, benign, by site
with malignant transformation C56.- ☑
implantation
external area or site (skin) NEC L72.Ø
iris — *see* Cyst, iris, implantation
vagina N89.8
vulva N9Ø.7
mouth KØ9.8
oral soft tissue KØ9.8
sacrococcygeal — *see* Cyst, pilonidal
developmental KØ9.1
odontogenic KØ9.Ø
oral region (nonodontogenic) KØ9.1
ovary, ovarian Q5Ø.1
dura (cerebral) G93.Ø
spinal G96.198
ear (external) Q18.1
echinococcal — *see* Echinococcus
embryonic
cervix uteri Q51.6
fallopian tube Q5Ø.4
vagina Q52.4
endometrium, endometrial (uterus) N85.8
ectopic — *see* Endometriosis
enterogenous Q43.8
epidermal, epidermoid (inclusion) (*see also* Cyst, skin) L72.Ø
mouth KØ9.8
oral soft tissue KØ9.8
epididymis N5Ø.3
epiglottis J38.7
epiphysis cerebri E34.8
epithelial (inclusion) L72.Ø
epoophoron Q5Ø.5
eruption KØ9.Ø
esophagus K22.89
ethmoid sinus J34.1
external female genital organs NEC N9Ø.7
eyelid (sebaceous) HØ2.829
infected — *see* Hordeolum
left HØ2.826
lower HØ2.825
upper HØ2.824
right HØ2.823
lower HØ2.822

Cyst — *continued*
eyelid — *continued*
right — *continued*
upper HØ2.821
eye NEC H57.89
congenital Q15.8
fallopian tube N83.8
congenital Q5Ø.4
fimbrial (twisted) Q5Ø.4
fissural (oral region) KØ9.1
follicle (graafian) (hemorrhagic) N83.Ø- ☑
nabothian N88.8
follicular (atretic) (hemorrhagic) (ovarian) N83.Ø- ☑
dentigerous KØ9.Ø
odontogenic KØ9.Ø
skin L72.9
specified NEC L72.8
frontal sinus J34.1
gallbladder K82.8
ganglion — *see* Ganglion
Gartner's duct Q52.4
gingiva KØ9.Ø
gland of Moll — *see* Cyst, eyelid
globulomaxillary KØ9.1
graafian follicle (hemorrhagic) N83.Ø- ☑
granulosal lutein (hemorrhagic) N83.1- ☑
hemangiomatous D18.ØØ
intra-abdominal D18.Ø3
intracranial D18.Ø2
skin D18.Ø1
specified site NEC D18.Ø9
hemorrhagic M27.49
hydatid — *see also* Echinococcus B67.9Ø
brain B67.99 *[G94]*
liver — *see also* Cyst, liver, hydatid B67.8
lung NEC B67.99 *[J99]*
Morgagni
female Q5Ø.5
male (epididymal) Q55.4
testicular Q55.29
specified site NEC B67.99
hymen N89.8
embryonic Q52.4
hypopharynx J39.2
hypophysis, hypophyseal (duct) (recurrent) E23.6
cerebri E23.6
implantation (dermoid)
external area or site (skin) NEC L72.Ø
iris — *see* Cyst, iris, implantation
vagina N89.8
vulva N9Ø.7
incisive canal KØ9.1
inclusion (epidermal) (epithelial) (epidermoid) (squamous) L72.Ø
not of skin — *code under* Cyst, by site
intestine (large) (small) K63.89
intracranial — *see* Cyst, brain
intraligamentous — *see also* Disorder, ligament
knee — *see* Derangement, knee
intrasellar E23.6
iris H21.3Ø9
exudative H21.31- ☑
idiopathic H21.3Ø- ☑
implantation H21.32- ☑
parasitic H21.33- ☑
pars plana (primary) H21.34- ☑
exudative H21.35- ☑
jaw (bone) M27.4Ø
aneurysmal M27.49
developmental (odontogenic) KØ9.Ø
fissural KØ9.1
hemorrhagic M27.49
traumatic M27.49
joint NEC — *see* Disorder, joint, specified type NEC
kidney N28.1
acquired N28.1
calyceal — *see* Hydronephrosis
congenital Q61.ØØ
more than one (multiple) Q61.Ø2
specified as polycystic Q61.3
adult type (autosomal dominant) Q61.2
infantile type (autosomal recessive) NEC Q61.19
collecting duct dilation Q61.11
pyelogenic — *see* Hydronephrosis
simple N28.1
solitary (single) N28.1
acquired N28.1

Cyst — *continued*
  kidney — *continued*
    solitary — *continued*
      congenital Q61.Ø1
  labium (majus) (minus) N9Ø.7
    sebaceous N9Ø.7
  lacrimal — *see also* Disorder, lacrimal system, specified NEC
    gland HØ4.13- ☑
    passages or sac — *see* Disorder, lacrimal system, specified NEC
  larynx J38.7
  lateral periodontal KØ9.Ø
  lens H27.8
    congenital Q12.8
  lip (gland) K13.Ø
  liver (idiopathic) (simple) K76.89
    congenital Q44.6
    hydatid B67.8
      granulosus B67.Ø
      multilocularis B67.5
  lung J98.4
    congenital Q33.Ø
    giant bullous J43.9
  lutein N83.1- ☑
  lymphangiomatous D18.1
  lymphoepithelial, oral soft tissue KØ9.8
  macula — *see* Degeneration, macula, hole
  malignant — *see* Neoplasm, malignant, by site
  mammary gland — *see* Cyst, breast
  mandible M27.4Ø
    dentigerous KØ9.Ø
    radicular KØ4.8
  maxilla M27.4Ø
    dentigerous KØ9.Ø
    radicular KØ4.8
  medial, face and neck Q18.8
  median
    anterior maxillary KØ9.1
    palatal KØ9.1
  mediastinum, congenital Q34.1
  meibomian (gland) — *see* Chalazion
    infected — *see* Hordeolum
  membrane, brain G93.Ø
  meninges (cerebral) G93.Ø
    spinal G96.198
  meniscus, knee — *see* Derangement, knee, meniscus, cystic
  mesentery, mesenteric K66.8
    chyle I89.8
  mesonephric duct
    female Q5Ø.5
    male Q55.4
  milk N64.89
  Morgagni (hydatid)
    female Q5Ø.5
    male (epididymal) Q55.4
      testicular Q55.29
  mouth KØ9.8
  Müllerian duct Q5Ø.4
    appendix testis Q55.29
    cervix Q51.6
    fallopian tube Q5Ø.4
    female Q5Ø.4
    male Q55.29
    prostatic utricle Q55.4
    vagina (embryonal) Q52.4
  multilocular (ovary) D39.1Ø
    benign — *see* Neoplasm, benign, by site
  myometrium N85.8
  nabothian (follicle) (ruptured) N88.8
  nasoalveolar KØ9.1
  nasolabial KØ9.1
  nasopalatine (anterior) (duct) KØ9.1
  nasopharynx J39.2
  neoplastic — *see* Neoplasm, uncertain behavior, by site
    benign — *see* Neoplasm, benign, by site
  nerve root
    cervical G96.191
    lumbar G96.191
    sacral G96.191
    thoracic G96.191
  nervous system NEC G96.89
  neuroenteric (congenital) QØ6.8
  nipple — *see* Cyst, breast
  nose (turbinates) J34.1
    sinus J34.1

Cyst — *continued*
  odontogenic, developmental KØ9.Ø
  omentum (lesser) K66.8
    congenital Q45.8
  ora serrata — *see* Cyst, retina, ora serrata
  oral
    region KØ9.9
      developmental (nonodontogenic) KØ9.1
      specified NEC KØ9.8
    soft tissue KØ9.9
      specified NEC KØ9.8
  orbit HØ5.81- ☑
  ovary, ovarian (twisted) N83.2Ø- ☑
    adherent N83.2Ø- ☑
    chocolate N8Ø.1Ø- ☑
    corpus
      albicans N83.29- ☑
      luteum (hemorrhagic) N83.1- ☑
    dermoid D27.9
    developmental Q5Ø.1
    due to failure of involution NEC N83.2Ø- ☑
    endometrial N8Ø.1Ø- ☑
    follicular (graafian) (hemorrhagic) N83.Ø- ☑
    hemorrhagic N83.2Ø- ☑
    in pregnancy or childbirth O34.8- ☑
      with obstructed labor O65.5
    multilocular D39.1Ø
    pseudomucinous D27.9
    retention N83.29- ☑
    serous N83.2Ø- ☑
    specified NEC N83.29- ☑
    theca lutein (hemorrhagic) N83.1- ☑
    tuberculous A18.18
  oviduct N83.8
  palate (median) (fissural) KØ9.1
  palatine papilla (jaw) KØ9.1
  pancreas, pancreatic (hemorrhagic) (true) K86.2
    congenital Q45.2
    false K86.3
  paralabral
    hip M24.85- ☑
    shoulder S43.43- ☑
  paramesonephric duct Q5Ø.4
    female Q5Ø.4
    male Q55.29
  paranephric N28.1
  paraphysis, cerebri, congenital QØ4.6
  parasitic B89
  parathyroid (gland) E21.4
  paratubal N83.8
  paraurethral duct N36.8
  paroophoron Q5Ø.5
  parotid gland K11.6
  parovarian Q5Ø.5
  pelvis, female N94.89
    in pregnancy or childbirth O34.8- ☑
      causing obstructed labor O65.5
  penis (sebaceous) N48.89
  periapical KØ4.8
  pericardial (congenital) Q24.8
    acquired (secondary) I31.8
  pericoronal KØ9.Ø
  perineural G96.191
  periodontal KØ4.8
    lateral KØ9.Ø
  peripelvic (lymphatic) N28.1
  peritoneum K66.8
    chylous I89.8
  periventricular, acquired, newborn P91.1
  pharynx (wall) J39.2
  pilar L72.11
  pilonidal (infected) (rectum) LØ5.91
    with abscess LØ5.Ø1
    malignant C44.59- ☑
  pituitary (duct) (gland) E23.6
  placenta O43.19- ☑
  pleura J94.8
  popliteal — *see* Cyst, Baker's
  porencephalic QØ4.6
    acquired G93.Ø
  postanal (infected) — *see* Cyst, pilonidal
  postmastoidectomy cavity (mucosal) — *see* Complications, postmastoidectomy, cyst
  preauricular Q18.1
  prepuce N47.4
    congenital Q55.69
  primordial (jaw) KØ9.Ø
  prostate N42.83

Cyst — *continued*
  pseudomucinous (ovary) D27.9
  pupillary, miotic H21.27- ☑
  radicular (residual) KØ4.8
  radiculodental KØ4.8
  ranular K11.8
  Rathke's pouch E23.6
  rectum (epithelium) (mucous) K62.89
  renal — *see* Cyst, kidney
  residual (radicular) KØ4.8
  retention (ovary) N83.29- ☑
    salivary gland K11.6
  retina H33.19- ☑
    ora serrata H33.11- ☑
    parasitic H33.12- ☑
  retroperitoneal K68.9
  sacrococcygeal (dermoid) — *see* Cyst, pilonidal
  salivary gland or duct (mucous extravasation or retention) K11.6
  Sampson's N8Ø.1Ø- ☑
  sclera H15.89
  scrotum L72.9
    sebaceous L72.3
  sebaceous (duct) (gland) L72.3
    breast — *see* Dysplasia, mammary, specified type NEC
    eyelid — *see* Cyst, eyelid
    genital organ NEC
      female N94.89
      male N5Ø.89
    scrotum L72.3
  semilunar cartilage (knee) (multiple) — *see* Derangement, knee, meniscus, cystic
  seminal vesicle N5Ø.89
  serous (ovary) N83.2Ø- ☑
  sinus (accessory) (nasal) J34.1
  Skene's gland N36.8
  skin L72.9
    breast — *see* Dysplasia, mammary, specified type NEC
    epidermal, epidermoid L72.Ø
    epithelial L72.Ø
    eyelid — *see* Cyst, eyelid
    genital organ NEC
      female N9Ø.7
      male N5Ø.89
    inclusion L72.Ø
    scrotum L72.9
    sebaceous L72.3
    sweat gland or duct L74.8
  solitary
    bone — *see* Cyst, bone, solitary
    jaw M27.4Ø
    kidney N28.1
  spermatic cord N5Ø.89
  sphenoid sinus J34.1
  spinal meninges G96.198
  spleen NEC D73.4
    congenital Q89.Ø9
    hydatid — *see also* Echinococcus B67.99 *[D77]*
  Stafne's M27.Ø
  subarachnoid intrasellar R93.Ø
  subcutaneous, pheomycotic (chromomycotic) B43.2
  subdural (cerebral) G93.Ø
    spinal cord G96.198
  sublingual gland K11.6
  submandibular gland K11.6
  submaxillary gland K11.6
  suburethral N36.8
  suprarenal gland E27.8
  suprasellar — *see* Cyst, brain
  sweat gland or duct L74.8
  synovial — *see also* Cyst, bursa
    ruptured — *see* Rupture, synovium
  Tarlov G96.191
  tarsal — *see* Chalazion
  tendon (sheath) — *see* Disorder, tendon, specified type NEC
  testis N44.2
    tunica albuginea N44.1
  theca lutein (ovary) N83.1- ☑
  Thornwaldt's J39.2
  thymus (gland) E32.8
  thyroglossal duct (infected) (persistent) Q89.2
  thyroid (gland) EØ4.1
  thyrolingual duct (infected) (persistent) Q89.2
  tongue K14.8
  tonsil J35.8

Cyst — *continued*
tooth — *see* Cyst, dental
Tornwaldt's J39.2
trichilemmal (proliferating) L72.12
trichodermal L72.12
tubal (fallopian) N83.8
inflammatory — *see* Salpingitis, chronic
tubo-ovarian N83.8
inflammatory N70.13
tunica
albuginea testis N44.1
vaginalis N50.89
turbinate (nose) J34.1
Tyson's gland N48.89
urachus, congenital Q64.4
ureter N28.89
ureterovesical orifice N28.89
urethra, urethral (gland) N36.8
uterine ligament N83.8
uterus (body) (corpus) (recurrent) N85.8
embryonic Q51.818
cervix Q51.6
vagina, vaginal (implantation) (inclusion) (squamous cell) (wall) N89.8
embryonic Q52.4
vallecula, vallecular (epiglottis) J38.7
vesical (orifice) N32.89
vitreous body H43.89
vulva (implantation) (inclusion) N90.7
congenital Q52.79
sebaceous gland N90.7
vulvovaginal gland N90.7
wolffian
female Q50.5
male Q55.4
Cystadenocarcinoma — *see* Neoplasm, malignant, by site
bile duct C22.1
endometrioid — *see* Neoplasm, malignant, by site
specified site — *see* Neoplasm, malignant, by site
unspecified site
female C56.9
male C61
mucinous
papillary
specified site — *see* Neoplasm, malignant, by site
unspecified site C56.9
specified site — *see* Neoplasm, malignant, by site
unspecified site C56.9
papillary
mucinous
specified site — *see* Neoplasm, malignant, by site
unspecified site C56.9
pseudomucinous
specified site — *see* Neoplasm, malignant, by site
unspecified site C56.9
serous
specified site — *see* Neoplasm, malignant, by site
unspecified site C56.9
specified site — *see* Neoplasm, malignant, by site
unspecified site C56.9
pseudomucinous
papillary
specified site — *see* Neoplasm, malignant, by site
unspecified site C56.9
specified site — *see* Neoplasm, malignant, by site
unspecified site C56.9
serous
papillary
specified site — *see* Neoplasm, malignant, by site
unspecified site C56.9
specified site — *see* Neoplasm, malignant, by site
unspecified site C56.9
Cystadenofibroma
clear cell — *see* Neoplasm, benign, by site
endometrioid D27.9
borderline malignancy D39.1- ☑
malignant C56.- ☑
mucinous
specified site — *see* Neoplasm, benign, by site
unspecified site D27.9
Cystadenofibroma — *continued*
serous
specified site — *see* Neoplasm, benign, by site
unspecified site D27.9
specified site — *see* Neoplasm, benign, by site
unspecified site D27.9
Cystadenoma — *see also* Neoplasm, benign, by site
bile duct D13.4
endometrioid — *see* Neoplasm, benign, by site
borderline malignancy — *see* Neoplasm, uncertain behavior, by site
malignant — *see* Neoplasm, malignant, by site
mucinous
borderline malignancy
ovary C56.- ☑
specified site NEC — *see* Neoplasm, uncertain behavior, by site
unspecified site C56.9
papillary
borderline malignancy
ovary C56.- ☑
specified site NEC — *see* Neoplasm, uncertain behavior, by site
unspecified site C56.9
specified site — *see* Neoplasm, benign, by site
unspecified site D27.9
specified site — *see* Neoplasm, benign, by site
unspecified site D27.9
papillary
borderline malignancy
ovary C56.- ☑
specified site NEC — *see* Neoplasm, uncertain behavior, by site
unspecified site C56.9
lymphomatosum
specified site — *see* Neoplasm, benign, by site
unspecified site D11.9
mucinous
borderline malignancy
ovary C56.- ☑
specified site NEC — *see* Neoplasm, uncertain behavior, by site
unspecified site C56.9
specified site — *see* Neoplasm, benign, by site
unspecified site D27.9
pseudomucinous
borderline malignancy
ovary C56.- ☑
specified site NEC — *see* Neoplasm, uncertain behavior, by site
unspecified site C56.9
specified site — *see* Neoplasm, benign, by site
unspecified site D27.9
serous
borderline malignancy
ovary C56.- ☑
specified site NEC — *see* Neoplasm, uncertain behavior, by site
unspecified site C56.9
specified site — *see* Neoplasm, benign, by site
unspecified site D27.9
specified site — *see* Neoplasm, benign, by site
unspecified site D27.9
pseudomucinous
borderline malignancy
ovary C56.- ☑
specified site NEC — *see* Neoplasm, uncertain behavior, by site
unspecified site C56.9
papillary
borderline malignancy
ovary C56.- ☑
specified site NEC — *see* Neoplasm, uncertain behavior, by site
unspecified site C56.9
specified site — *see* Neoplasm, benign, by site
unspecified site D27.9
specified site — *see* Neoplasm, benign, by site
unspecified site D27.9
serous
borderline malignancy
ovary C56.- ☑
specified site NEC — *see* Neoplasm, uncertain behavior, by site
unspecified site C56.9
papillary
borderline malignancy
ovary C56.- ☑
Cystadenoma — *continued*
serous — *continued*
papillary — *continued*
borderline malignancy — *continued*
specified site NEC — *see* Neoplasm, uncertain behavior, by site
unspecified site C56.9
specified site — *see* Neoplasm, benign, by site
unspecified site D27.9
specified site — *see* Neoplasm, benign, by site
unspecified site D27.9
Cystathionine synthase deficiency E72.11
Cystathioninemia E72.19
Cystathioninuria E72.19
Cystic — *see also* condition
breast (chronic) — *see* Mastopathy, cystic
corpora lutea (hemorrhagic) N83.1- ☑
duct — *see* condition
eyeball (congenital) Q11.0
fibrosis — *see* Fibrosis, cystic
kidney (congenital) Q61.9
adult type Q61.2
infantile type NEC Q61.19
collecting duct dilatation Q61.11
medullary Q61.5
liver, congenital Q44.6
lung disease J98.4
congenital Q33.0
mastitis, chronic — *see* Mastopathy, cystic
medullary, kidney Q61.5
meniscus — *see* Derangement, knee, meniscus, cystic
ovary N83.20- ☑
Cysticercosis, cysticerciasis B69.9
with
epileptiform fits B69.0
myositis B69.81
brain B69.0
central nervous system B69.0
cerebral B69.0
ocular B69.1
specified NEC B69.89
Cysticercus cellulose infestation — *see* Cysticercosis
Cystinosis (malignant) E72.04
Cystinuria E72.01
Cystitis (exudative) (hemorrhagic) (septic) (suppurative) N30.90
with
fibrosis — *see* Cystitis, chronic, interstitial
hematuria N30.91
leukoplakia — *see* Cystitis, chronic, interstitial
malakoplakia — *see* Cystitis, chronic, interstitial
metaplasia — *see* Cystitis, chronic, interstitial
prostatitis N41.3
acute N30.00
with hematuria N30.01
of trigone N30.30
with hematuria N30.31
allergic — *see* Cystitis, specified type NEC
amebic A06.81
bilharzial B65.9 *[N33]*
blennorrhagic (gonococcal) A54.01
bullous — *see* Cystitis, specified type NEC
calculous N21.0
chlamydial A56.01
chronic N30.20
with hematuria N30.21
interstitial N30.10
with hematuria N30.11
of trigone N30.30
with hematuria N30.31
specified NEC N30.20
with hematuria N30.21
cystic (a) — *see* Cystitis, specified type NEC
diphtheritic A36.85
echinococcal
granulosus B67.39
multilocularis B67.69
emphysematous — *see* Cystitis, specified type NEC
encysted — *see* Cystitis, specified type NEC
eosinophilic — *see* Cystitis, specified type NEC
follicular — *see* Cystitis, of trigone
gangrenous — *see* Cystitis, specified type NEC
glandularis — *see* Cystitis, specified type NEC
gonococcal A54.01
incrusted — *see* Cystitis, specified type NEC
interstitial (chronic) — *see* Cystitis, chronic, interstitial
irradiation N30.40
with hematuria N30.41

Cystitis — *continued*
irritation — *see* Cystitis, specified type NEC
malignant — *see* Cystitis, specified type NEC
of trigone N30.30
with hematuria N30.31
panmural — *see* Cystitis, chronic, interstitial
polyposa — *see* Cystitis, specified type NEC
prostatic N41.3
puerperal (postpartum) O86.22
radiation — *see* Cystitis, irradiation
specified type NEC N30.80
with hematuria N30.81
subacute — *see* Cystitis, chronic
submucous — *see* Cystitis, chronic, interstitial
syphilitic (late) A52.76
trichomonal A59.03
tuberculous A18.12
ulcerative — *see* Cystitis, chronic, interstitial
Cystocele (-urethrocele)
female N81.10
with prolapse of uterus — *see* Prolapse, uterus
lateral N81.12
midline N81.11
paravaginal N81.12
Cystocele — *continued*
in pregnancy or childbirth O34.8- ☑
causing obstructed labor O65.5
male N32.89
Cystolithiasis N21.0
Cystoma — *see also* Neoplasm, benign, by site
endometrial, ovary N80.10- ☑
mucinous
specified site — *see* Neoplasm, benign, by site
unspecified site D27.9
serous
specified site — *see* Neoplasm, benign, by site
unspecified site D27.9
simple (ovary) N83.29- ☑
Cystoplegia N31.2
Cystoptosis N32.89
Cystopyelitis — *see* Pyelonephritis
Cystorrhagia N32.89
Cystosarcoma phyllodes D48.6- ☑
benign D24- ☑
malignant — *see* Neoplasm, breast, malignant
Cystostomy
attention to Z43.5
complication — *see* Complications, cystostomy
Cystostomy — *continued*
status Z93.50
appendico-vesicostomy Z93.52
cutaneous Z93.51
specified NEC Z93.59
Cystourethritis — *see* Urethritis
Cystourethrocele — *see also* Cystocele
female N81.10
with uterine prolapse — *see* Prolapse, uterus
lateral N81.12
midline N81.11
paravaginal N81.12
male N32.89
Cytomegalic inclusion disease
congenital P35.1
Cytomegalovirus infection B25.9
Cytomycosis (reticuloendothelial) B39.4
Cytopenia D75.9
refractory
with multilineage dysplasia D46.A (*following* D46.2)
and ring sideroblasts (RCMD RS) D46.B (*following* D46.2)
Czerny's disease (periodic hydrarthrosis of the knee) — *see* Effusion, joint, knee

D

- **Da Costa's syndrome** F45.8
- **Daae** (-Finsen) **disease** (epidemic pleurodynia) B33.0
- **Dabney's grip** B33.0
- **Dacryoadenitis, dacryadenitis** H04.00- ☑
  - acute H04.01- ☑
  - chronic H04.02- ☑
- **Dacryocystitis** H04.30- ☑
  - acute H04.32- ☑
  - chronic H04.41- ☑
  - neonatal P39.1
  - phlegmonous H04.31- ☑
  - syphilitic A52.71
    - congenital (early) A50.01
  - trachomatous, active A71.1
    - sequelae (late effect) B94.0
- **Dacryocystoblenorrhea** — *see* Inflammation, lacrimal, passages, chronic
- **Dacryocystocele** — *see* Disorder, lacrimal system, changes
- **Dacryolith, dacryolithiasis** H04.51- ☑
- **Dacryoma** — *see* Disorder, lacrimal system, changes
- **Dacryopericystitis** — *see* Dacryocystitis
- **Dacryops** H04.11- ☑
- **Dacryostenosis** — *see also* Stenosis, lacrimal
  - congenital Q10.5
- **Dactylitis**
  - bone — *see* Osteomyelitis
  - sickle-cell D57.00
    - Hb C D57.219
    - Hb SS D57.00
    - specified NEC D57.819
  - skin L08.9
  - syphilitic A52.77
  - tuberculous A18.03
- **Dactylolysis spontanea** (ainhum) L94.6
- **Dactylosymphysis** Q70.9
  - fingers — *see* Syndactylism, complex, fingers
  - toes — *see* Syndactylism, complex, toes
- **Damage**
  - arteriosclerotic — *see* Arteriosclerosis
  - brain (nontraumatic) G93.9
    - anoxic, hypoxic G93.1
      - resulting from a procedure G97.82
    - child NEC G80.9
    - due to birth injury P11.2
  - cardiorenal (vascular) — *see* Hypertension, cardiorenal
  - cerebral NEC — *see* Damage, brain
  - coccyx, complicating delivery O71.6
  - coronary — *see* Disease, heart, ischemic
  - deep tissue, pressure-induced — *see also* L89 with final character .6
  - eye, birth injury P15.3
  - liver (nontraumatic) K76.9
    - alcoholic K70.9
    - due to drugs — *see* Disease, liver, toxic
    - toxic — *see* Disease, liver, toxic
  - lung
    - dabbing (related) U07.0
    - electronic cigarette (related) U07.0
    - vaping (associated) (device) (product) (use) U07.0
  - medication T88.7 ☑
  - organ
    - dabbing (related) U07.0
    - electronic cigarette (related) U07.0
    - vaping (associated) (device) (product) (use) U07.0
  - pelvic
    - joint or ligament, during delivery O71.6
    - organ NEC
      - during delivery O71.5
      - following ectopic or molar pregnancy O08.6
  - renal — *see* Disease, renal
  - subendocardium, subendocardial — *see* Degeneration, myocardial
  - vascular I99.9
- **Dana-Putnam syndrome** (subacute combined sclerosis with pernicious anemia) — *see* Degeneration, combined
- **Danbolt** (-Cross) **syndrome** (acrodermatitis enteropathica) E83.2
- **Dandruff** L21.0
- **Dandy-Walker syndrome** Q03.1
  - with spina bifida — *see* Spina bifida
- **Danlos' syndrome** — *see also* Syndrome, Ehlers-Danlos Q79.60
- **Darier** (-White) **disease** (congenital) Q82.8
  - meaning erythema annulare centrifugum L53.1
- **Darier-Roussy sarcoid** D86.3
- **Darling's disease or histoplasmosis** B39.4
- **Darwin's tubercle** Q17.8
- **Dawson's** (inclusion body) **encephalitis** A81.1
- **De Beurmann** (-Gougerot) **disease** B42.1
- **De la Tourette's syndrome** F95.2
- **De Lange's syndrome** Q87.19
- **De Morgan's spots** (senile angiomas) I78.1
- **De Quervain's**
  - disease (tendon sheath) M65.4
  - syndrome E34.51
  - thyroiditis (subacute granulomatous thyroiditis) E06.1
- **De Toni-Fanconi** (-Debré) **syndrome** E72.09
  - with cystinosis E72.04
- **Dead**
  - fetus, retained (mother) O36.4 ☑
    - early pregnancy O02.1
  - labyrinth H83.2 ☑
  - ovum, retained O02.0
- **Deaf nonspeaking NEC** H91.3
- **Deafmutism** (acquired) (congenital) NEC H91.3
  - hysterical F44.6
  - syphilitic, congenital — *see also* subcategory H94.8 A50.09
- **Deafness** (acquired) (complete) (hereditary) (partial) H91.9- ☑
  - with blue sclera and fragility of bone Q78.0
  - auditory fatigue — *see* Deafness, specified type NEC
  - aviation T70.0 ☑
    - nerve injury — *see* Injury, nerve, acoustic, specified type NEC
  - boilermaker's H83.3 ☑
  - central — *see* Deafness, sensorineural
  - conductive H90.2
    - and sensorineural
      - mixed H90.8
        - bilateral H90.6
    - bilateral H90.0
    - unilateral H90.1- ☑
      - with restricted hearing on the contralateral side H90.A- ☑
  - congenital H90.5
    - with blue sclera and fragility of bone Q78.0
  - due to toxic agents — *see* Deafness, ototoxic
  - emotional (hysterical) F44.6
  - functional (hysterical) F44.6
  - high frequency H91.9- ☑
  - hysterical F44.6
  - low frequency H91.9- ☑
  - mental R48.8
  - mixed conductive and sensorineural H90.8
    - bilateral H90.6
    - unilateral H90.7- ☑
  - nerve — *see* Deafness, sensorineural
  - neural — *see* Deafness, sensorineural
  - noise-induced — *see also* subcategory H83.3 ☑
    - nerve injury — *see* Injury, nerve, acoustic, specified type NEC
  - nonspeaking H91.3
  - ototoxic H91.0 ☑
  - perceptive — *see* Deafness, sensorineural
  - psychogenic (hysterical) F44.6
  - sensorineural H90.5
    - and conductive
      - bilateral H90.6
      - mixed H90.8
        - bilateral H90.6
    - bilateral H90.3
    - unilateral H90.4- ☑
      - with restricted hearing on the contralateral side H90.A- ☑
  - sensory — *see* Deafness, sensorineural
  - specified type NEC H91.8 ☑
  - sudden (idiopathic) H91.2- ☑
  - syphilitic A52.15
  - transient ischemic H93.01- ☑
  - traumatic — *see* Injury, nerve, acoustic, specified type NEC
  - word (developmental) H93.25
- **Death** (cause unknown) (of) (unexplained) (unspecified cause) R99
  - brain G93.82
  - cardiac (sudden) (with successful resuscitation) — *see* Arrest, cardiac
    - family history of Z82.41

Death — *continued*
  - cardiac — *see* Arrest, cardiac — *continued*
    - personal history of Z86.74
  - family member (assumed) Z63.4
- **Debility** (chronic) (general) (nervous) R53.81
  - congenital or neonatal NOS P96.9
  - nervous R53.81
  - old age R54
  - senile R54
- **Débove's disease** (splenomegaly) R16.1
- **Debt, burdensome** Z59.86
- **Decalcification**
  - bone — *see* Osteoporosis
  - teeth K03.89
- **Decapsulation, kidney** N28.89
- **Decay**
  - dental — *see* Caries, dental
  - senile R54
  - tooth, teeth — *see* Caries, dental
- **Deciduitis** (acute)
  - following ectopic or molar pregnancy O08.0
- **Decline** (general) — *see* Debility
  - cognitive, age-associated R41.81
- **Decompensation**
  - cardiac (acute) (chronic) — *see* Disease, heart
  - cardiovascular — *see* Disease, cardiovascular
  - heart — *see* Disease, heart
  - hepatic — *see* Failure, hepatic
  - myocardial (acute) (chronic) — *see* Disease, heart
  - respiratory J98.8
- **Decompression sickness** T70.3 ☑
- **Decrease** (d)
  - absolute neutrophile count — *see* Neutropenia
  - blood
    - platelets — *see* Thrombocytopenia
    - pressure R03.1
      - due to shock following
        - injury T79.4 ☑
        - operation T81.19 ☑
  - estrogen E28.39
    - postablative E89.40
      - asymptomatic E89.40
      - symptomatic E89.41
  - fragility of erythrocytes D58.8
  - function
    - lipase (pancreatic) K90.3
    - ovary in hypopituitarism E23.0
    - parenchyma of pancreas K86.89
    - pituitary (gland) (anterior) (lobe) E23.0
      - posterior (lobe) E23.0
  - functional activity R68.89
  - glucose R73.09
  - hematocrit R71.0
  - hemoglobin R71.0
  - leukocytes D72.819
    - specified NEC D72.818
  - libido R68.82
  - lymphocytes D72.810
  - platelets D69.6
  - respiration, due to shock following injury T79.4 ☑
  - sexual desire R68.82
  - tear secretion NEC — *see* Syndrome, dry eye
  - tolerance
    - fat K90.49
    - glucose R73.09
    - pancreatic K90.3
    - salt and water E87.8
  - vision NEC H54.7
  - white blood cell count D72.819
    - specified NEC D72.818
- **Decubitus** (ulcer) — *see* Ulcer, pressure, by site
  - cervix N86
- **Deepening acetabulum** — *see* Derangement, joint, specified type NEC, hip
- **Defect, defective** Q89.9
  - 3-beta-hydroxysteroid dehydrogenase E25.0
  - 11-hydroxylase E25.0
  - 21-hydroxylase E25.0
  - abdominal wall, congenital Q79.59
  - antibody immunodeficiency D80.9
  - aorticopulmonary septum Q21.4
  - atrial septal Q21.10
    - coronary sinus Q21.13
    - following acute myocardial infarction (current complication) I23.1
    - ostium primum type (type I) Q21.20

Defect, defective — *continued*
- atrial septal — *continued*
  - ostium primum type — *continued*
    - with
      - common atrioventricular valves and moderate or larger inlet VSD Q21.23
      - separate atrioventricular valves Q21.21
        - and small or restrictive inlet VSD Q21.22
  - ostium secundum type (patent persistent) (type II) Q21.11
  - sinus venosus Q21.16
    - inferior Q21.15
    - superior Q21.14
  - specified NEC Q21.19
  - vena cava type
    - inferior Q21.15
    - superior Q21.14
- atrioventricular
  - canal Q21.2Ø
  - septal
    - common Q21.23
    - complete Q21.23
    - incomplete Q21.21
    - intermediate Q21.22
    - partial Q21.21
    - transitional Q21.22
    - unspecified as to partial or complete Q21.2Ø
  - septum Q21.2Ø
- auricular septal Q21.1Ø
- bilirubin excretion NEC E8Ø.6
- biosynthesis, androgen (testicular) E29.1
- bulbar septum Q21.Ø
- catalase E8Ø.3
- cell membrane receptor complex (CR3) D71
- circulation I99.9
  - congenital Q28.9
  - newborn Q28.9
- coagulation (factor) — *see also* Deficiency, factor D68.9
  - with
    - ectopic pregnancy OØ8.1
    - molar pregnancy OØ8.1
  - acquired D68.4
  - antepartum with hemorrhage — *see* Hemorrhage, antepartum, with coagulation defect
  - due to
    - liver disease D68.4
    - vitamin K deficiency D68.4
  - hereditary NEC D68.2
  - intrapartum O67.Ø
  - newborn, transient P61.6
  - postpartum O99.13
    - with hemorrhage O72.3
  - specified type NEC D68.8
- complement system D84.1
- conduction (heart) I45.9
  - bone — *see* Deafness, conductive
- congenital, organ or site not listed — *see* Anomaly, by site
- coronary sinus Q21.13
- cushion, endocardial Q21.2Ø
  - common Q21.23
  - incomplete Q21.21
  - intermediate Q21.22
  - transitional Q21.22
- degradation, glycoprotein E77.1
- dental bridge, crown, fillings — *see* Defect, dental restoration
- dental restoration KØ8.5Ø
  - specified NEC KØ8.59
- dentin (hereditary) KØØ.5
- Descemet's membrane, congenital Q13.89
- developmental — *see also* Anomaly
  - cauda equina QØ6.3
- diaphragm
  - with elevation, eventration or hernia — *see* Hernia, diaphragm
  - congenital Q79.1
    - with hernia Q79.Ø
    - gross (with hernia) Q79.Ø
- ectodermal, congenital Q82.9
- Eisenmenger's Q21.8
- enzyme
  - catalase E8Ø.3
  - peroxidase E8Ø.3
- esophagus, congenital Q39.9
- extensor retinaculum M62.89
- fibrin polymerization D68.2

Defect, defective — *continued*
- filling
  - bladder R93.41
  - kidney R93.42- ☑
  - renal pelvis R93.41
  - stomach R93.3
  - ureter R93.41
  - urinary organs, specified NEC R93.49
- GABA (gamma aminobutyric acid) metabolic E72.81
- Gerbode Q21.Ø
- glucose transport, blood-brain barrier E74.81Ø
- glycoprotein degradation E77.1
- Hageman (factor) D68.2
- hearing — *see* Deafness
- high grade F7Ø
- interatrial septal Q21.19
- interauricular septal Q21.19
- interventricular septal Q21.Ø
  - with dextroposition of aorta, pulmonary stenosis and hypertrophy of right ventricle Q21.3
  - in tetralogy of Fallot Q21.3
- intervertebral annular fibrosis — *see also* Disease, intervertebral disc, by site M51.9
  - lumbar M51.AØ
    - large M51.A2
    - small M51.A1
  - lumbosacral M51.A3
    - large M51.A5
    - small M51.A4
- learning (specific) — *see* Disorder, learning
- lymphocyte function antigen-1 (LFA-1) D84.Ø
- lysosomal enzyme, post-translational modification E77.Ø
- major osseous M89.7Ø
  - ankle M89.77- ☑
  - carpus M89.74- ☑
  - clavicle M89.71- ☑
  - femur M89.75- ☑
  - fibula M89.76- ☑
  - fingers M89.74- ☑
  - foot M89.77- ☑
  - forearm M89.73- ☑
  - hand M89.74- ☑
  - humerus M89.72- ☑
  - lower leg M89.76- ☑
  - metacarpus M89.74- ☑
  - metatarsus M89.77- ☑
  - multiple sites M89.79
  - pelvic region M89.75- ☑
  - pelvis M89.75- ☑
  - radius M89.73- ☑
  - scapula M89.71- ☑
  - shoulder region M89.71- ☑
  - specified NEC M89.78
  - tarsus M89.77- ☑
  - thigh M89.75- ☑
  - tibia M89.76- ☑
  - toes M89.77- ☑
  - ulna M89.73- ☑
- mental — *see* Disability, intellectual
- modification, lysosomal enzymes, post-translational E77.Ø
- obstructive, congenital
  - renal pelvis Q62.39
  - ureter Q62.39
    - atresia — *see* Atresia, ureter
    - cecoureterocele Q62.32
    - megaureter Q62.2
    - orthotopic ureterocele Q62.31
- osseous, major M89.7Ø
  - ankle M89.77- ☑
  - carpus M89.74- ☑
  - clavicle M89.71- ☑
  - femur M89.75- ☑
  - fibula M89.76- ☑
  - fingers M89.74- ☑
  - foot M89.77- ☑
  - forearm M89.73- ☑
  - hand M89.74- ☑
  - humerus M89.72- ☑
  - lower leg M89.76- ☑
  - metacarpus M89.74- ☑
  - metatarsus M89.77- ☑
  - multiple sites M89.9
  - pelvic region M89.75- ☑
  - pelvis M89.75- ☑
  - radius M89.73- ☑

Defect, defective — *continued*
- osseous, major — *continued*
  - scapula M89.71- ☑
  - shoulder region M89.71- ☑
  - specified NEC M89.78
  - tarsus M89.77- ☑
  - thigh M89.75- ☑
  - tibia M89.76- ☑
  - toes M89.77- ☑
  - ulna M89.73- ☑
- osteochondral NEC — *see also* Deformity M95.8
- ostium
  - primum Q21.2Ø
  - secundum Q21.11
- peroxidase E8Ø.3
- placental blood supply — *see* Insufficiency, placental
- platelets, qualitative D69.1
  - constitutional — *see* Disease, von Willebrand
- postural NEC, spine — *see* Dorsopathy, deforming
- qualitative, of von Willebrand factor
  - with
    - decreased platelet adhesion and selective deficiency of high-molecular-weight multimers — *see also* Disease, von Willebrand D68.Ø2Ø
    - defective platelet adhesion with a normal size distribution of von Willebrand factor multimers — *see also* Disease, von Willebrand D68.Ø22
    - defective von Willebrand factor to factor VIII binding — *see also* Disease, von Willebrand D68.Ø23
    - high-molecular-weight von Willebrand factor loss — *see also* Disease, von Willebrand D68.Ø21
    - hyper-adhesive forms — *see also* Disease, von Willebrand D68.Ø21
    - increased affinity for platelet glycoprotein Ib — *see also* Disease, von Willebrand D68.Ø21
    - markedly decreased affinity for factor VIII — *see also* Disease, von Willebrand D68.Ø23
  - in von Willebrand factor function, with no further subtyping — *see also* Disease, von Willebrand D68.Ø29
- reduction
  - limb Q73.8
    - lower Q72.9- ☑
      - absence — *see* Agenesis, leg
        - foot — *see* Agenesis, foot
      - longitudinal
        - femur Q72.4- ☑
        - fibula Q72.6- ☑
        - tibia Q72.5- ☑
      - specified type NEC Q72.89- ☑
      - split foot Q72.7- ☑
    - specified type NEC Q73.8
    - upper Q71.9- ☑
      - absence — *see* Agenesis, arm
        - forearm — *see* Agenesis, forearm
        - hand — *see* Agenesis, hand
      - lobster-claw hand Q71.6- ☑
      - longitudinal
        - radius Q71.4- ☑
        - ulna Q71.5- ☑
      - specified type NEC Q71.89- ☑
- renal pelvis Q63.8
  - obstructive Q62.39
- respiratory system, congenital Q34.9
- restoration, dental KØ8.5Ø
  - specified NEC KØ8.59
- retinal nerve bundle fibers H35.89
- septal (heart) NOS Q21.9
  - acquired (atrial) (auricular) (ventricular) (old) I51.Ø
  - atrial — *see also* Defect, atrial septal Q21.1Ø
    - concurrent with acute myocardial infarction — *see* Infarct, myocardium
    - following acute myocardial infarction (current complication) I23.1
  - ventricular — *see also* Defect, ventricular septal Q21.Ø
- sinus venosus — *see also* Defect, atrial septal, sinus venosus Q21.16
- speech — *see* Disorder, speech
  - developmental F8Ø.9
  - specified NEC R47.89
- Taussig-Bing (aortic transposition and overriding pulmonary artery) Q2Ø.1

Defect, defective — *continued*
- teeth, wedge KØ3.1
- vascular (local) I99.9
  - congenital Q27.9
- ventricular septal Q21.Ø
  - concurrent with acute myocardial infarction — *see* Infarct, myocardium
  - following acute myocardial infarction (current complication) I23.2
  - in tetralogy of Fallot Q21.3
- vision NEC H54.7
- visual field H53.4Ø
  - bilateral
    - heteronymous H53.47
    - homonymous H53.46- ☑
  - generalized contraction H53.48- ☑
  - localized
    - arcuate H53.43- ☑
    - scotoma (central area) H53.41- ☑
      - blind spot area H53.42- ☑
    - sector H53.43- ☑
    - specified type NEC H53.45- ☑
- voice R49.9
  - specified NEC R49.8
- wedge, tooth, teeth (abrasion) KØ3.1

Deferentitis N49.1
- gonorrheal (acute) (chronic) A54.23

Defibrination (syndrome) D65
- antepartum — *see* Hemorrhage, antepartum, with coagulation defect, disseminated intravascular coagulation
- following ectopic or molar pregnancy OØ8.1
- intrapartum O67.Ø
- newborn P6Ø
- postpartum O72.3

Deficiency, deficient
- 3-beta hydroxysteroid dehydrogenase E25.Ø
- 5-alpha reductase (with male pseudohermaphroditism) E29.1
- 11-hydroxylase E25.Ø
- 21-hydroxylase E25.Ø
- AADC (aromatic L-amino acid decarboxylase) E7Ø.81
- abdominal muscle syndrome Q79.4
- AC globulin (congenital) (hereditary) D68.2
  - acquired D68.4
- accelerator globulin (Ac G) (blood) D68.2
- acid phosphatase E83.39
- acid sphingomyelinase (ASMD) E75.249
  - type
    - A E75.24Ø
    - A/B E75.244
    - B E75.241
- activating factor (blood) D68.2
- ADA2 (adenosine deaminase 2) D81.32
- adenosine deaminase (ADA) D81.3Ø
  - with severe combined immunodeficiency (SCID) D81.31
  - partial (type 1) D81.39
  - specified NEC D81.39
  - type 1 (without SCID) (without severe combined immunodeficiency) D81.39
  - type 2 D81.32
- aldolase (hereditary) E74.19
- alpha-1-antitrypsin E88.Ø1
- amino-acids E72.9
- anemia — *see* Anemia
- aneurin E51.9
- antibody with
  - hyperimmunoglobulinemia D8Ø.6
  - near-normal immunoglobins D8Ø.6
- antidiuretic hormone E23.2
- anti-hemophilic
  - factor (A) D66
    - B D67
    - C D68.1
  - globulin (AHG) NEC D66
- antithrombin (antithrombin III) D68.59
- aromatic L-amino acid decarboxylase (AADC) E7Ø.81
- ascorbic acid E54
- attention (disorder) (syndrome) F98.8
  - with hyperactivity — *see* Disorder, attention-deficit hyperactivity
- autoprothrombin
  - I D68.2
  - II D67
  - C D68.2
- beta-glucuronidase E76.29
- biotin E53.8

Deficiency, deficient — *continued*
- biotin-dependent carboxylase D81.819
- biotinidase D81.81Ø
- brancher enzyme (amylopectinosis) E74.Ø3
- C1 esterase inhibitor (C1-INH) D84.1
- calciferol E55.9
  - with
    - adult osteomalacia M83.8
    - rickets — *see* Rickets
- calcium (dietary) E58
- calorie, severe E43
  - with marasmus E41
    - and kwashiorkor E42
- cardiac — *see* Insufficiency, myocardial
- carnitine E71.4Ø
  - due to
    - hemodialysis E71.43
    - inborn errors of metabolism E71.42
    - Valproic acid therapy E71.43
  - iatrogenic E71.43
  - muscle palmityltransferase E71.314
  - primary E71.41
  - secondary E71.448
- carotene E5Ø.9
- central nervous system G96.89
- ceruloplasmin (Wilson) E83.Ø1
- choline E53.8
- Christmas factor D67
- chromium E61.4
- chronic neurovisceral acid sphingomyelinase E75.244
- chronic visceral acid sphingomyelinase E75.241
- clotting (blood) — *see also* Deficiency, coagulation factor D68.9
- clotting factor NEC (hereditary) — *see also* Deficiency, factor D68.2
- coagulation NOS D68.9
  - with
    - ectopic pregnancy OØ8.1
    - molar pregnancy OØ8.1
  - acquired (any) D68.4
  - antepartum hemorrhage — *see* Hemorrhage, antepartum, with coagulation defect
  - clotting factor NEC — *see also* Deficiency, factor D68.2
  - due to
    - hyperprothrombinemia D68.4
    - liver disease D68.4
    - vitamin K deficiency D68.4
  - newborn, transient P61.6
  - postpartum O72.3
  - specified NEC D68.8
- cognitive FØ9
- color vision H53.5Ø
  - achromatopsia H53.51
  - acquired H53.52
  - deuteranomaly H53.53
  - protanomaly H53.54
  - specified type NEC H53.59
  - tritanomaly H53.55
- combined glucocorticoid and mineralocorticoid E27.49
- contact factor D68.2
- copper (nutritional) E61.Ø
- corticoadrenal E27.4Ø
  - primary E27.1
- craniofacial axis Q75.Ø
- cyanocobalamin E53.8
- debrancher enzyme (limit dextrinosis) E74.Ø3
- dehydrogenase
  - long chain/very long chain acyl CoA E71.31Ø
  - medium chain acyl CoA E71.311
  - short chain acyl CoA E71.312
- diet E63.9
- dihydropyrimidine dehydrogenase (DPD) E88.89
- disaccharidase E73.9
- edema — *see* Malnutrition, severe
- endocrine E34.9
- energy-supply — *see* Malnutrition
- enzymes, circulating NEC E88.Ø9
- ergosterol E55.9
  - with
    - adult osteomalacia M83.8
    - rickets — *see* Rickets
- essential fatty acid (EFA) E63.Ø
- eye movements
  - saccadic H55.81
  - smooth pursuit H55.82
- factor — *see also* Deficiency, coagulation
  - Hageman D68.2

Deficiency, deficient — *continued*
- factor — *see also* Deficiency, coagulation — *continued*
  - I (congenital) (hereditary) D68.2
  - II (congenital) (hereditary) D68.2
  - IX (congenital) (functional) (hereditary) (with functional defect) D67
  - multiple (congenital) D68.8
    - acquired D68.4
  - V (congenital) (hereditary) D68.2
  - VII (congenital) (hereditary) D68.2
  - VIII (congenital) (functional) (hereditary) (with functional defect) D66
    - with vascular defect — *see* Disease, von Willebrand
  - X (congenital) (hereditary) D68.2
  - XI (congenital) (hereditary) D68.1
  - XII (congenital) (hereditary) D68.2
  - XIII (congenital) (hereditary) D68.2
- femoral, proximal focal (congenital) — *see* Defect, reduction, lower limb, longitudinal, femur
- fibrinase D68.2
- fibrinogen (congenital) (hereditary) D68.2
  - acquired D65
- fibrin-stabilizing factor (congenital) (hereditary) D68.2
  - acquired D68.4
- folate E53.8
- folic acid E53.8
- foreskin N47.3
- fructokinase E74.11
- fructose 1,6-diphosphatase E74.19
- fructose-1-phosphate aldolase E74.19
- GABA (gamma aminobutyric acid) transaminase E72.81
- GABA-T (gamma aminobutyric acid transaminase) E72.81
- galactokinase E74.29
- galactose-1-phosphate uridyl transferase E74.29
- gammaglobulin in blood D8Ø.1
  - hereditary D8Ø.Ø
- glass factor D68.2
- glucocorticoid E27.49
  - mineralocorticoid E27.49
- glucose transporter protein type 1 E74.81Ø
- glucose-6-phosphatase E74.Ø1
- glucose-6-phosphate dehydrogenase
  - anemia D55.Ø
  - without anemia D75.A
- glucuronyl transferase E8Ø.5
- Glut1 E74.81Ø
- glycogen synthetase E74.Ø9
- gonadotropin (isolated) E23.Ø
- growth hormone (idiopathic) (isolated) E23.Ø
- Hageman factor D68.2
- hemoglobin D64.9
- hepatophosphorylase E74.Ø9
- homogentisate 1,2-dioxygenase E7Ø.29
- hormone
  - anterior pituitary (partial) NEC E23.Ø
    - growth E23.Ø
  - growth (isolated) E23.Ø
  - pituitary E23.Ø
  - testicular E29.1
- hypoxanthine- (guanine)-phosphoribosyltransferase (HG- PRT) (total H-PRT) E79.1
- immunity D84.9
  - cell-mediated D84.89
    - with thrombocytopenia and eczema D82.Ø
  - combined D81.9
  - humoral D8Ø.9
  - IgA (secretory) D8Ø.2
  - IgG D8Ø.3
  - IgM D8Ø.4
- immuno — *see* Immunodeficiency
- immunoglobulin, selective
  - A (IgA) D8Ø.2
  - G (IgG) (subclasses) D8Ø.3
  - M (IgM) D8Ø.4
- infantile neurovisceral acid sphingomyelinase E75.24Ø
- inositol (B complex) E53.8
- intrinsic
  - factor (congenital) D51.Ø
  - sphincter N36.42
    - with urethral hypermobility N36.43
- iodine E61.8
  - congenital syndrome — *see* Syndrome, iodine-deficiency, congenital
- iron E61.1
  - anemia D5Ø.9
- kalium E87.6

Deficiency, deficient — *continued*
- kappa-light chain D8Ø.8
- labile factor (congenital) (hereditary) D68.2
  - acquired D68.4
- lacrimal fluid (acquired) — *see also* Syndrome, dry eye
  - congenital Q1Ø.6
- lactase
  - congenital E73.Ø
  - secondary E73.1
- Laki-Lorand factor D68.2
- lecithin cholesterol acyltransferase E78.6
- lipocaic K86.89
- lipoprotein (familial) (high density) E78.6
- liver phosphorylase E74.Ø9
- lysosomal alpha-1, 4 glucosidase E74.Ø2
- magnesium E61.2
- major histocompatibility complex
  - class I D81.6
  - class II D81.7
- manganese E61.3
- menadione (vitamin K) E56.1
  - newborn P53
- mental (familial) (hereditary) — *see* Disability, intellectual
- methylenetetrahydrofolate reductase (MTHFR) E72.12
- mevalonate kinase MØ4.1
- mineralocorticoid E27.49
  - with glucocorticoid E27.49
- mineral NEC E61.8
- molybdenum (nutritional) E61.5
- moral F6Ø.2
- multiple nutrient elements E61.7
- multiple sulfatase (MSD) E75.26
- muscle
  - carnitine (palmityltransferase) E71.314
  - phosphofructokinase E74.Ø9
- myoadenylate deaminase E79.2
- myocardial — *see* Insufficiency, myocardial
- myophosphorylase E74.Ø4
- NADH diaphorase or reductase (congenital) D74.Ø
- NADH-methemoglobin reductase (congenital) D74.Ø
- natrium E87.1
- niacin (amide) (-tryptophan) E52
- nicotinamide E52
- nicotinic acid E52
- number of teeth — *see* Anodontia
- nutrient element E61.9
  - multiple E61.7
  - specified NEC E61.8
- nutrition, nutritional — *see also* Nutrition deficient E63.9
  - sequelae — *see* Sequelae, nutritional deficiency
  - specified NEC E63.8
- of interleukin 1 receptor antagonist [DIRA] MØ4.8
- ornithine transcarbamylase E72.4
- ovarian E28.39
- oxygen — *see* Anoxia
- pantothenic acid E53.8
- parathyroid (gland) E2Ø.9
- perineum (female) N81.89
- phenylalanine hydroxylase E7Ø.1
- phosphoenolpyruvate carboxykinase E74.4
- phosphofructokinase E74.19
- phosphomannomutuse E74.818
- phosphomannose isomerase E74.818
- phosphomannosyl mutase E74.818
- phosphorylase kinase, liver E74.Ø9
- pituitary hormone (isolated) E23.Ø
- plasma thromboplastin
  - antecedent (PTA) D68.1
  - component (PTC) D67
- plasminogen (type 1) (type 2) E88.Ø2
- platelet NEC D69.1
  - constitutional — *see* Disease, von Willebrand
- polyglandular E31.8
  - autoimmune E31.Ø
- potassium (K) E87.6
- prepuce N47.3
- proaccelerin (congenital) (hereditary) D68.2
  - acquired D68.4
- proconvertin factor (congenital) (hereditary) D68.2
  - acquired D68.4
- protein — *see also* Malnutrition E46
  - anemia D53.Ø
  - C D68.59
  - S D68.59
- prothrombin (congenital) (hereditary) D68.2
  - acquired D68.4

Deficiency, deficient — *continued*
- Prower factor D68.2
- pseudocholinesterase E88.Ø9
- PTA (plasma thromboplastin antecedent) D68.1
- PTC (plasma thromboplastin component) D67
- purine nucleoside phosphorylase (PNP) D81.5
- pyracin (alpha) (beta) E53.1
- pyridoxal E53.1
- pyridoxamine E53.1
- pyridoxine (derivatives) E53.1
- pyruvate
  - carboxylase E74.4
  - dehydrogenase E74.4
- riboflavin (vitamin B2) E53.Ø
- salt E87.1
- secretion
  - ovary E28.39
  - salivary gland (any) K11.7
  - urine R34
- selenium (dietary) E59
- serum antitrypsin, familial E88.Ø1
- short stature homeobox gene (SHOX)
  - with
    - dyschondrosteosis Q78.8
    - short stature (idiopathic) E34.328
    - Turner's syndrome Q96.9
- sodium (Na) E87.1
- SPCA (factor VII) D68.2
- sphincter, intrinsic N36.42
  - with urethral hypermobility N36.43
- stable factor (congenital) (hereditary) D68.2
  - acquired D68.4
- Stuart-Prower (factor X) D68.2
- succinic semialdehyde dehydrogenase E72.81
- sucrase E74.39
- sulfatase E75.26
- sulfite oxidase E72.19
- thiamin, thiaminic (chloride) E51.9
  - beriberi (dry) E51.11
    - wet E51.12
- thrombokinase D68.2
  - newborn P53
- thyroid (gland) — *see* Hypothyroidism
- tocopherol E56.Ø
- tooth bud KØØ.Ø
- transcobalamine II (anemia) D51.2
- vanadium E61.6
- vascular I99.9
- vasopressin E23.2
- vertical ridge KØ6.8
- viosterol — *see* Deficiency, calciferol
- vitamin (multiple) NOS E56.9
  - A E5Ø.9
    - with
      - Bitot's spot (corneal) E5Ø.1
      - follicular keratosis E5Ø.8
      - keratomalacia E5Ø.4
      - manifestations NEC E5Ø.8
      - night blindness E5Ø.5
      - scar of cornea, xerophthalmic E5Ø.6
      - xeroderma E5Ø.8
      - xerophthalmia E5Ø.7
      - xerosis
        - conjunctival E5Ø.Ø
          - and Bitot's spot E5Ø.1
        - cornea E5Ø.2
          - and ulceration E5Ø.3
    - sequelae E64.1
  - B (complex) NOS E53.9
    - with
      - beriberi (dry) E51.11
        - wet E51.12
      - pellagra E52
  - B1 NOS E51.9
    - beriberi (dry) E51.11
      - with circulatory system manifestations E51.11
      - wet E51.12
  - B12 E53.8
  - B2 (riboflavin) E53.Ø
  - B6 E53.1
  - C E54
    - sequelae E64.2
  - D E55.9
    - with
      - adult osteomalacia M83.8
      - rickets — *see* Rickets
    - 25-hydroxylase E83.32
  - E E56.Ø
  - folic acid E53.8

Deficiency, deficient — *continued*
- vitamin — *continued*
  - G E53.Ø
  - group B E53.9
    - specified NEC E53.8
  - H (biotin) E53.8
  - K E56.1
    - of newborn P53
  - nicotinic E52
  - P E56.8
  - PP (pellagra-preventing) E52
  - specified NEC E56.8
  - thiamin E51.9
    - beriberi — *see* Beriberi
- von Willebrand factor
  - partial quantitative — *see also* Disease, von Willebrand D68.Ø1
  - total quantitative — *see also* Disease, von Willebrand D68.Ø3
- zinc, dietary E6Ø

Deficit — *see also* Deficiency
- attention and concentration R41.84Ø
  - disorder — *see* Attention, deficit
  - following
    - cerebral infarction I69.31Ø
    - cerebrovascular disease I69.91Ø
      - specified disease NEC I69.81Ø
    - nontraumatic
      - intracerebral hemorrhage I69.11Ø
      - specified intracranial hemorrhage NEC I69.21Ø
      - subarachnoid hemorrhage I69.Ø1Ø
- cognitive
  - communication R41.841
  - emotional
    - following
      - cerebral infarction I69.315
      - cerebrovascular disease I69.915
        - specified disease NEC I69.815
      - nontraumatic
        - intracerebral hemorrhage I69.115
        - specified intracranial hemorrhage NEC I69.215
        - subarachnoid hemorrhage I69.Ø15
  - following
    - cerebral infarction I69.319
    - cerebrovascular disease I69.919
      - specified disease NEC I69.819
    - nontraumatic
      - intracerebral hemorrhage I69.119
      - specified intracranial hemorrhage NEC I69.219
      - subarachnoid hemorrhage I69.Ø19
  - social
    - following
      - cerebral infarction I69.315
      - cerebrovascular disease I69.915
        - specified disease NEC I69.815
      - nontraumatic
        - intracerebral hemorrhage I69.115
        - specified intracranial hemorrhage NEC I69.215
        - subarachnoid hemorrhage I69.Ø15
- cognitive NEC R41.89
  - following
    - cerebral infarction I69.318
    - cerebrovascular disease I69.918
      - specified disease NEC I69.818
    - nontraumatic
      - intracerebral hemorrhage I69.118
      - specified intracranial hemorrhage NEC I69.218
      - subarachnoid hemorrhage I69.Ø18
- concentration R41.84Ø
- executive function R41.844
  - following
    - cerebral infarction I69.314
    - cerebrovascular disease I69.914
      - specified disease NEC I69.814
    - nontraumatic
      - intracerebral hemorrhage I69.114
      - specified intracranial hemorrhage NEC I69.214
      - subarachnoid hemorrhage I69.Ø14
- frontal lobe R41.844
  - following
    - cerebral infarction I69.314
    - cerebrovascular disease I69.914
      - specified disease NEC I69.814
    - nontraumatic
      - intracerebral hemorrhage I69.114
      - specified intracranial hemorrhage NEC I69.214
      - subarachnoid hemorrhage I69.Ø14

Deficit — *continued*
memory
following
cerebral infarction I69.311
cerebrovascular disease I69.911
specified disease NEC I69.811
nontraumatic
intracerebral hemorrhage I69.111
specified intracranial hemorrhage NEC I69.211
subarachnoid hemorrhage I69.Ø11
neurologic NEC R29.818
ischemic
reversible (RIND) I63.9
prolonged (PRIND) I63.9
oxygen RØ9.Ø2
prolonged reversible ischemic neurologic (PRIND) I63.9
psychomotor R41.843
following
cerebral infarction I69.313
cerebrovascular disease I69.913
specified disease NEC I69.813
nontraumatic
intracerebral hemorrhage I69.113
specified intracranial hemorrhage NEC I69.213
subarachnoid hemorrhage I69.Ø13
visuospatial R41.842
following
cerebral infarction I69.312
cerebrovascular disease I69.912
specified disease NEC I69.812
nontraumatic
intracerebral hemorrhage I69.112
specified intracranial hemorrhage NEC I69.212
subarachnoid hemorrhage I69.Ø12
Deflection
radius — *see* Deformity, limb, specified type NEC, forearm
septum (acquired) (nasal) (nose) J34.2
spine — *see* Curvature, spine
turbinate (nose) J34.2
Defluvium
capillorum — *see* Alopecia
ciliorum — *see* Madarosis
unguium L6Ø.8
Deformity Q89.9
abdomen, congenital Q89.9
abdominal wall
acquired M95.8
congenital Q79.59
acquired (unspecified site) M95.9
adrenal gland Q89.1
alimentary tract, congenital Q45.9
upper Q4Ø.9
ankle (joint) (acquired) — *see also* Deformity, limb, lower leg
abduction — *see* Contraction, joint, ankle
congenital Q68.8
contraction — *see* Contraction, joint, ankle
specified type NEC — *see* Deformity, limb, foot, specified NEC
anus (acquired) K62.89
congenital Q43.9
aorta (arch) (congenital) Q25.4Ø
acquired I77.89
aortic
arch, acquired I77.89
cusp or valve (congenital) Q23.8
acquired — *see also* Endocarditis, aortic I35.8
arm (acquired) (upper) — *see also* Deformity, limb, upper arm
congenital Q68.8
forearm — *see* Deformity, limb, forearm
artery (congenital) (peripheral) NOS Q27.9
acquired I77.89
coronary (acquired) I25.9
congenital Q24.5
umbilical Q27.Ø
atrial septal — *see also* Defect, atrial septal Q21.1Ø
auditory canal (external) (congenital) — *see also* Malformation, ear, external
acquired — *see* Disorder, ear, external, specified type NEC
auricle
ear (congenital) — *see also* Malformation, ear, external
acquired — *see* Disorder, pinna, deformity
back — *see* Dorsopathy, deforming
bile duct (common) (congenital) (hepatic) Q44.5
Deformity — *continued*
bile duct — *continued*
acquired K83.8
biliary duct or passage (congenital) Q44.5
acquired K83.8
bladder (neck) (trigone) (sphincter) (acquired) N32.89
congenital Q64.79
bone (acquired) NOS M95.9
congenital Q79.9
turbinate M95.Ø
brain (congenital) QØ4.9
acquired G93.89
reduction QØ4.3
breast (acquired) N64.89
congenital Q83.9
reconstructed N65.Ø
bronchus (congenital) Q32.4
acquired NEC J98.Ø9
bursa, congenital Q79.9
canaliculi (lacrimalis) (acquired) — *see also* Disorder, lacrimal system, changes
congenital Q1Ø.6
canthus, acquired — *see* Disorder, eyelid, specified type NEC
capillary (acquired) I78.8
cardiovascular system, congenital Q28.9
caruncle, lacrimal (acquired) — *see also* Disorder, lacrimal system, changes
congenital Q1Ø.6
cascade, stomach K31.2
cecum (congenital) Q43.9
acquired K63.89
cerebral, acquired G93.89
congenital QØ4.9
cervix (uterus) (acquired) NEC N88.8
congenital Q51.9
cheek (acquired) M95.2
congenital Q18.9
chest (acquired) (wall) M95.4
congenital Q67.8
sequelae (late effect) of rickets E64.3
chin (acquired) M95.2
congenital Q18.9
choroid (congenital) Q14.3
acquired H31.8
plexus QØ7.8
acquired G96.198
cicatricial — *see* Cicatrix
cilia, acquired — *see* Disorder, eyelid, specified type NEC
clavicle (acquired) M95.8
congenital Q68.8
clitoris (congenital) Q52.6
acquired N9Ø.89
clubfoot — *see* Clubfoot
coccyx (acquired) — *see* subcategory M43.8 ☑
colon (congenital) Q43.9
acquired K63.89
concha (ear), congenital — *see also* Malformation, ear, external
acquired — *see* Disorder, pinna, deformity
cornea (acquired) H18.7Ø
congenital Q13.4
descemetocele — *see* Descemetocele
ectasia — *see* Ectasia, cornea
specified NEC H18.79- ☑
staphyloma — *see* Staphyloma, cornea
coronary artery (acquired) I25.9
congenital Q24.5
cranium (acquired) — *see* Deformity, skull
cricoid cartilage (congenital) Q31.8
acquired J38.7
cystic duct (congenital) Q44.5
acquired K82.8
Dandy-Walker QØ3.1
with spina bifida — *see* Spina bifida
diaphragm (congenital) Q79.1
acquired J98.6
digestive organ NOS Q45.9
ductus arteriosus Q25.Ø
duodenal bulb K31.89
duodenum (congenital) Q43.9
acquired K31.89
dura — *see* Deformity, meninges
ear (acquired) — *see also* Disorder, pinna, deformity
congenital (external) Q17.9
internal Q16.5
middle Q16.4
Deformity — *continued*
ear — *see also* Disorder, pinna, deformity — *continued*
congenital — *continued*
middle — *continued*
ossicles Q16.3
ossicles Q16.3
ectodermal (congenital) NEC Q84.9
ejaculatory duct (congenital) Q55.4
acquired N5Ø.89
elbow (joint) (acquired) — *see also* Deformity, limb, upper arm
congenital Q68.8
contraction — *see* Contraction, joint, elbow
endocrine gland NEC Q89.2
epididymis (congenital) Q55.4
acquired N5Ø.89
epiglottis (congenital) Q31.8
acquired J38.7
esophagus (congenital) Q39.9
acquired K22.89
eustachian tube (congenital) NEC Q17.8
eye, congenital Q15.9
eyebrow (congenital) Q18.8
eyelid (acquired) — *see also* Disorder, eyelid, specified type NEC
congenital Q1Ø.3
face (acquired) M95.2
congenital Q18.9
fallopian tube, acquired N83.8
femur (acquired) — *see* Deformity, limb, specified type NEC, thigh
fetal
with fetopelvic disproportion O33.7 ☑
causing obstructed labor O66.3
finger (acquired) M2Ø.ØØ- ☑
boutonniere M2Ø.Ø2- ☑
congenital Q68.1
flexion contracture — *see* Contraction, joint, hand
mallet finger M2Ø.Ø1- ☑
specified NEC M2Ø.Ø9- ☑
swan-neck M2Ø.Ø3- ☑
flexion (joint) (acquired) — *see also* Deformity, limb, flexion M21.2Ø
congenital NOS Q74.9
hip Q65.89
foot (acquired) — *see also* Deformity, limb, lower leg
cavovarus (congenital) Q66.1- ☑
congenital NOS Q66.9- ☑
specified type NEC Q66.89
specified type NEC — *see* Deformity, limb, foot, specified NEC
valgus (congenital) Q66.6
acquired — *see* Deformity, valgus, ankle
varus (congenital) NEC Q66.3- ☑
acquired — *see* Deformity, varus, ankle
forearm (acquired) — *see also* Deformity, limb, forearm
congenital Q68.8
forehead (acquired) M95.2
congenital Q75.8
frontal bone (acquired) M95.2
congenital Q75.8
gallbladder (congenital) Q44.1
acquired K82.8
gastrointestinal tract (congenital) NOS Q45.9
acquired K63.89
genitalia, genital organ(s) or system NEC
female (congenital) Q52.9
acquired N94.89
external Q52.7Ø
male (congenital) Q55.9
acquired N5Ø.89
globe (eye) (congenital) Q15.8
acquired H44.89
gum, acquired NEC KØ6.8
hand (acquired) — *see* Deformity, limb, hand
congenital Q68.1
head (acquired) M95.2
congenital Q75.8
heart (congenital) Q24.9
septum Q21.9
auricular — *see also* Defect, atrial septal Q21.1Ø
ventricular Q21.Ø
valve (congenital) NEC Q24.8
acquired — *see* Endocarditis
heel (acquired) — *see* Deformity, foot
hepatic duct (congenital) Q44.5
acquired K83.8

Deformity — *continued*
hip (joint) (acquired) (*see also* Deformity, limb, thigh)
congenital Q65.9
due to (previous) juvenile osteochondrosis — *see* Coxa, plana
flexion — *see* Contraction, joint, hip
hourglass — *see* Contraction, hourglass
humerus (acquired) M21.82- ☑
congenital Q74.Ø
hypophyseal (congenital) Q89.2
ileocecal (coil) (valve) (acquired) K63.89
congenital Q43.9
ileum (congenital) Q43.9
acquired K63.89
ilium (acquired) M95.5
congenital Q74.2
integument (congenital) Q84.9
intervertebral cartilage or disc (acquired) — *see* Disorder, disc, specified NEC
intestine (large) (small) (congenital) NOS Q43.9
acquired K63.89
intrinsic minus or plus (hand) — *see* Deformity, limb, specified type NEC, forearm
iris (acquired) H21.89
congenital Q13.2
ischium (acquired) M95.5
congenital Q74.2
jaw (acquired) (congenital) M26.9
joint (acquired) NEC M21.9Ø
congenital Q68.8
elbow M21.92- ☑
hand M21.94- ☑
hip M21.95- ☑
knee M21.96- ☑
shoulder M21.92- ☑
wrist M21.93- ☑
kidney(s) (calyx) (pelvis) (congenital) Q63.9
acquired N28.89
artery (congenital) Q27.2
acquired I77.89
Klippel-Feil (brevicollis) Q76.1
knee (acquired) NEC — *see also* Deformity, limb, lower leg
congenital Q68.2
labium (majus) (minus) (congenital) Q52.79
acquired N9Ø.89
lacrimal passages or duct (congenital) NEC Q1Ø.6
acquired — *see* Disorder, lacrimal system, changes
larynx (muscle) (congenital) Q31.8
acquired J38.7
web (glottic) Q31.Ø
leg (upper) (acquired) NEC — *see also* Deformity, limb, thigh
congenital Q68.8
lower leg — *see* Deformity, limb, lower leg
lens (acquired) H27.8
congenital Q12.9
lid (fold) (acquired) — *see also* Disorder, eyelid, specified type NEC
congenital Q1Ø.3
ligament (acquired) — *see* Disorder, ligament
congenital Q79.9
limb (acquired) M21.9Ø
clawfoot M21.53- ☑
clawhand M21.51- ☑
congenital Q68.1
clubfoot M21.54- ☑
clubhand M21.52- ☑
congenital, except reduction deformity Q74.9
flat foot M21.4- ☑
flexion M21.2Ø
ankle M21.27- ☑
elbow M21.22- ☑
finger M21.24- ☑
hip M21.25- ☑
knee M21.26- ☑
shoulder M21.21- ☑
toe M21.27- ☑
wrist M21.23- ☑
foot
claw — *see* Deformity, limb, clawfoot
club — *see* Deformity, limb, clubfoot
drop M21.37- ☑
flat — *see* Deformity, limb, flat foot
specified NEC M21.6X- ☑
forearm M21.93- ☑
hand M21.94- ☑

Deformity — *continued*
limb — *continued*
lower leg M21.96- ☑
specified type NEC M21.8Ø
forearm M21.83- ☑
lower leg M21.86- ☑
thigh M21.85- ☑
upper arm M21.82- ☑
thigh M21.95- ☑
unequal length M21.7Ø
short site is
femur M21.75- ☑
fibula M21.76- ☑
humerus M21.72- ☑
radius M21.73- ☑
tibia M21.76- ☑
ulna M21.73- ☑
upper arm M21.92- ☑
valgus — *see* Deformity, valgus
varus — *see* Deformity, varus
wrist drop M21.33- ☑
lip (acquired) NEC K13.Ø
congenital Q38.Ø
liver (congenital) Q44.7
acquired K76.89
lumbosacral (congenital) (joint) (region) Q76.49
acquired — *see* subcategory M43.8 ☑
kyphosis — *see* Kyphosis, congenital
lordosis — *see* Lordosis, congenital
lung (congenital) Q33.9
acquired J98.4
lymphatic system, congenital Q89.9
Madelung's (radius) Q74.Ø
mandible (acquired) (congenital) M26.9
maxilla (acquired) (congenital) M26.9
meninges or membrane (congenital) QØ7.9
cerebral QØ4.8
acquired G96.198
spinal cord (congenital) QØ6.- ☑
acquired G96.198
metacarpus (acquired) — *see* Deformity, limb, forearm
congenital Q74.Ø
metatarsus (acquired) — *see* Deformity, foot
congenital Q66.9- ☑
middle ear (congenital) Q16.4
ossicles Q16.3
mitral (leaflets) (valve) IØ5.8
parachute Q23.2
stenosis, congenital Q23.2
mouth (acquired) K13.79
congenital Q38.6
multiple, congenital NEC Q89.7
muscle (acquired) M62.89
congenital Q79.9
sternocleidomastoid Q68.Ø
musculoskeletal system (acquired) M95.9
congenital Q79.9
specified NEC M95.8
nail (acquired) L6Ø.8
congenital Q84.6
nasal — *see* Deformity, nose
neck (acquired) M95.3
congenital Q18.9
sternocleidomastoid Q68.Ø
nervous system (congenital) QØ7.9
nipple (congenital) Q83.9
acquired N64.89
nose (acquired) (cartilage) M95.Ø
bone (turbinate) M95.Ø
congenital Q3Ø.9
bent or squashed Q67.4
saddle M95.Ø
syphilitic A5Ø.57
septum (acquired) J34.2
congenital Q3Ø.8
sinus (wall) (congenital) Q3Ø.8
acquired M95.Ø
syphilitic (congenital) A5Ø.57
late A52.73
ocular muscle (congenital) Q1Ø.3
acquired — *see* Strabismus, mechanical
opticociliary vessels (congenital) Q13.2
orbit (eye) (acquired) HØ5.3Ø
atrophy — *see* Atrophy, orbit
congenital Q1Ø.7
due to
bone disease NEC HØ5.32- ☑
trauma or surgery HØ5.33- ☑

Deformity — *continued*
orbit — *continued*
enlargement — *see* Enlargement, orbit
exostosis — *see* Exostosis, orbit
organ of Corti (congenital) Q16.5
ovary (congenital) Q5Ø.39
acquired N83.8
oviduct, acquired N83.8
palate (congenital) Q38.5
acquired M27.8
cleft (congenital) — *see* Cleft, palate
pancreas (congenital) Q45.3
acquired K86.89
parathyroid (gland) Q89.2
parotid (gland) (congenital) Q38.4
acquired K11.8
patella (acquired) — *see* Disorder, patella, specified NEC
pelvis, pelvic (acquired) (bony) M95.5
with disproportion (fetopelvic) O33.Ø
causing obstructed labor O65.Ø
congenital Q74.2
rachitic sequelae (late effect) E64.3
penis (glans) (congenital) Q55.69
acquired N48.89
pericardium (congenital) Q24.8
acquired — *see* Pericarditis
pharynx (congenital) Q38.8
acquired J39.2
pinna, acquired — *see also* Disorder, pinna, deformity
congenital Q17.9
pituitary (congenital) Q89.2
posture — *see* Dorsopathy, deforming
prepuce (congenital) Q55.69
acquired N47.8
prostate (congenital) Q55.4
acquired N42.89
pupil (congenital) Q13.2
acquired — *see* Abnormality, pupillary
pylorus (congenital) Q4Ø.3
acquired K31.89
rachitic (acquired), old or healed E64.3
radius (acquired) — *see also* Deformity, limb, forearm
congenital Q68.8
rectum (congenital) Q43.9
acquired K62.89
reduction (extremity) (limb), congenital — *see also* condition and site Q73.8
brain QØ4.3
lower — *see* Defect, reduction, lower limb
upper — *see* Defect, reduction, upper limb
renal — *see* Deformity, kidney
respiratory system (congenital) Q34.9
rib (acquired) M95.4
congenital Q76.6
cervical Q76.5
rotation (joint) (acquired) — *see* Deformity, limb, specified site NEC
congenital Q74.9
hip — *see* Deformity, limb, specified type NEC, thigh
congenital Q65.89
sacroiliac joint (congenital) — *see* subcategory Q74.2
acquired — *see* subcategory M43.8 ☑
sacrum (acquired) — *see* subcategory M43.8 ☑
saddle
back — *see* Lordosis
nose M95.Ø
syphilitic A5Ø.57
salivary gland or duct (congenital) Q38.4
acquired K11.8
scapula (acquired) M95.8
congenital Q68.8
scrotum (congenital) — *see also* Malformation, testis and scrotum
acquired N5Ø.89
seminal vesicles (congenital) Q55.4
acquired N5Ø.89
septum, nasal (acquired) J34.2
shoulder (joint) (acquired) — *see* Deformity, limb, upper arm
congenital Q74.Ø
contraction — *see* Contraction, joint, shoulder
sigmoid (flexure) (congenital) Q43.9
acquired K63.89
skin (congenital) Q82.9
skull (acquired) M95.2
congenital Q75.8

- **Deformity** — *continued*
  - skull — *continued*
    - congenital — *continued*
      - with
        - anencephaly QØØ.Ø
        - encephalocele — *see* Encephalocele
        - hydrocephalus QØ3.9
          - with spina bifida — *see* Spina bifida, by site, with hydrocephalus
        - microcephaly QØ2
  - soft parts, organs or tissues (of pelvis)
    - in pregnancy or childbirth NEC O34.8- ☑
      - causing obstructed labor O65.5
  - spermatic cord (congenital) Q55.4
    - acquired N5Ø.89
      - torsion — *see* Torsion, spermatic cord
  - spinal — *see* Dorsopathy, deforming
    - column (acquired) — *see* Dorsopathy, deforming
      - congenital Q67.5
    - cord (congenital) QØ6.9
      - acquired G95.89
    - nerve root (congenital) QØ7.9
  - spine (acquired) — *see also* Dorsopathy, deforming
    - congenital Q67.5
    - rachitic E64.3
    - specified NEC — *see* Dorsopathy, deforming, specified NEC
  - spleen
    - acquired D73.89
    - congenital Q89.Ø9
  - Sprengel's (congenital) Q74.Ø
  - sternocleidomastoid (muscle), congenital Q68.Ø
  - sternum (acquired) M95.4
    - congenital NEC Q76.7
  - stomach (congenital) Q4Ø.3
    - acquired K31.89
  - submandibular gland (congenital) Q38.4
  - submaxillary gland (congenital) Q38.4
    - acquired K11.8
  - talipes — *see* Talipes
  - testis (congenital) — *see also* Malformation, testis and scrotum
    - acquired N44.8
      - torsion — *see* Torsion, testis
  - thigh (acquired) — *see also* Deformity, limb, thigh
    - congenital NEC Q68.8
  - thorax (acquired) (wall) M95.4
    - congenital Q67.8
    - sequelae of rickets E64.3
  - thumb (acquired) — *see also* Deformity, finger
    - congenital NEC Q68.1
  - thymus (tissue) (congenital) Q89.2
  - thyroid (gland) (congenital) Q89.2
    - cartilage Q31.8
      - acquired J38.7
  - tibia (acquired) — *see also* Deformity, limb, specified type NEC, lower leg
    - congenital NEC Q68.8
    - saber (syphilitic) A5Ø.56
  - toe (acquired) M2Ø.6- ☑
    - congenital Q66.9- ☑
    - hallux rigidus M2Ø.2- ☑
    - hallux valgus M2Ø.1- ☑
    - hallux varus M2Ø.3- ☑
    - hammer toe M2Ø.4- ☑
    - specified NEC M2Ø.5X- ☑
  - tongue (congenital) Q38.3
    - acquired K14.8
  - tooth, teeth KØØ.2
  - trachea (rings) (congenital) Q32.1
    - acquired J39.8
  - transverse aortic arch (congenital) Q25.49
  - tricuspid (leaflets) (valve) IØ7.8
    - atresia or stenosis Q22.4
    - Ebstein's Q22.5
  - trunk (acquired) M95.8
    - congenital Q89.9
  - ulna (acquired) — *see also* Deformity, limb, forearm
    - congenital NEC Q68.8
  - urachus, congenital Q64.4
  - ureter (opening) (congenital) Q62.8
    - acquired N28.89
  - urethra (congenital) Q64.79
    - acquired N36.8
  - urinary tract (congenital) Q64.9
    - urachus Q64.4
  - uterus (congenital) Q51.9
    - acquired N85.8

- **Deformity** — *continued*
  - uvula (congenital) Q38.5
  - vagina (acquired) N89.8
    - congenital Q52.4
  - valgus NEC M21.ØØ
    - ankle M21.Ø7- ☑
    - elbow M21.Ø2- ☑
    - hip M21.Ø5- ☑
    - knee M21.Ø6- ☑
  - valve, valvular (congenital) (heart) Q24.8
    - acquired — *see* Endocarditis
  - varus NEC M21.1Ø
    - ankle M21.17- ☑
    - elbow M21.12- ☑
    - hip M21.15 ☑
    - knee M21.16- ☑
    - tibia — *see* Osteochondrosis, juvenile, tibia
  - vas deferens (congenital) Q55.4
    - acquired N5Ø.89
  - vein (congenital) Q27.9
    - great Q26.9
  - vertebra — *see* Dorsopathy, deforming
  - vertical talus (congenital) Q66.8Ø
    - left foot Q66.82
    - right foot Q66.81
  - vesicourethral orifice (acquired) N32.89
    - congenital NEC Q64.79
  - vessels of optic papilla (congenital) Q14.2
  - visual field (contraction) — *see* Defect, visual field
  - vitreous body, acquired H43.89
  - vulva (congenital) Q52.79
    - acquired N9Ø.89
  - wrist (joint) (acquired) — *see also* Deformity, limb, forearm
    - congenital Q68.8
    - contraction — *see* Contraction, joint, wrist

- **Degeneration, degenerative**
  - adrenal (capsule) (fatty) (gland) (hyaline) (infectional) E27.8
  - amyloid — *see also* Amyloidosis E85.9
  - anterior cornua, spinal cord G12.29
  - anterior labral S43.49- ☑
  - aorta, aortic I7Ø.Ø
    - fatty I77.89
  - aortic valve (heart) — *see* Endocarditis, aortic
  - arteriovascular — *see* Arteriosclerosis
  - artery, arterial (atheromatous) (calcareous) — *see also* Arteriosclerosis
    - cerebral, amyloid E85.4 *[I68.Ø]*
    - medial — *see* Arteriosclerosis, extremities
  - articular cartilage NEC — *see* Derangement, joint, articular cartilage, by site
  - atheromatous — *see* Arteriosclerosis
  - basal nuclei or ganglia G23.9
    - specified NEC G23.8
  - bone NEC — *see* Disorder, bone, specified type NEC
  - brachial plexus G54.Ø
  - brain (cortical) (progressive) G31.9
    - alcoholic G31.2
    - arteriosclerotic I67.2
    - childhood G31.9
      - specified NEC G31.89
    - cystic G31.89
      - congenital QØ4.6
    - in
      - alcoholism G31.2
      - beriberi E51.2
      - cerebrovascular disease I67.9
      - congenital hydrocephalus QØ3.9
        - with spina bifida — *see also* Spina bifida
      - Fabry-Anderson disease E75.21
      - Gaucher's disease E75.22
      - Hunter's syndrome E76.1
      - lipidosis
        - cerebral E75.4
        - generalized E75.6
      - mucopolysaccharidosis — *see* Mucopolysaccharidosis
      - myxedema EØ3.9 *[G32.89]*
      - neoplastic disease — *see also* Neoplasm D49.6 *[G32.89]*
      - Niemann-Pick disease E75.249 *[G32.89]*
      - sphingolipidosis E75.3 *[G32.89]*
      - vitamin B12 deficiency E53.8 *[G32.89]*
    - senile NEC G31.1
  - breast N64.89
  - Bruch's membrane — *see* Degeneration, choroid
  - capillaries (fatty) I78.8

- **Degeneration, degenerative** — *continued*
  - capillaries — *continued*
    - amyloid E85.89 *[I79.8]*
  - cardiac — *see also* Degeneration, myocardial
    - valve, valvular — *see* Endocarditis
  - cardiorenal — *see* Hypertension, cardiorenal
  - cardiovascular — *see also* Disease, cardiovascular
    - renal — *see* Hypertension, cardiorenal
  - cerebellar NOS G31.9
    - alcoholic G31.2
    - primary (hereditary) (sporadic) G11.9
  - cerebral — *see* Degeneration, brain
  - cerebrovascular I67.9
    - due to hypertension I67.4
  - cervical plexus G54.2
  - cervix N88.8
    - due to radiation (intended effect) N88.8
      - adverse effect or misadventure N99.89
  - chamber angle H21.21- ☑
  - changes, spine or vertebra — *see* Spondylosis
  - chorioretinal — *see also* Degeneration, choroid
    - hereditary H31.2Ø
  - choroid (colloid) (drusen) H31.1Ø- ☑
    - atrophy — *see* Atrophy, choroidal
    - hereditary — *see* Dystrophy, choroidal, hereditary
  - ciliary body H21.22- ☑
  - cochlear — *see* subcategory H83.8 ☑
  - combined (spinal cord) (subacute) E53.8 *[G32.Ø]*
    - with anemia (pernicious) D51.Ø *[G32.Ø]*
      - due to dietary vitamin B12 deficiency D51.3 *[G32.Ø]*
    - in (due to)
      - vitamin B12 deficiency E53.8 *[G32.Ø]*
        - anemia D51.9 *[G32.Ø]*
  - conjunctiva H11.1Ø
    - concretions — *see* Concretion, conjunctiva
    - deposits — *see* Deposit, conjunctiva
    - pigmentations — *see* Pigmentation, conjunctiva
    - pinguecula — *see* Pinguecula
    - xerosis — *see* Xerosis, conjunctiva
  - cornea H18.4Ø
    - calcerous H18.43
      - band keratopathy H18.42- ☑
    - familial, hereditary — *see* Dystrophy, cornea
    - hyaline (of old scars) H18.49
    - keratomalacia — *see* Keratomalacia
    - nodular H18.45- ☑
    - peripheral H18.46- ☑
    - senile H18.41- ☑
    - specified type NEC H18.49
  - cortical (cerebellar) (parenchymatous) G31.89
    - alcoholic G31.2
    - diffuse, due to arteriopathy I67.2
  - corticobasal G31.85
  - cutis L98.8
    - amyloid E85.4 *[L99]*
  - dental pulp KØ4.2
  - disc disease — *see* Degeneration, intervertebral disc, by site
  - dorsolateral (spinal cord) — *see* Degeneration, combined
  - extrapyramidal G25.9
  - eye, macular — *see also* Degeneration, macula
    - congenital or hereditary — *see* Dystrophy, retina
  - facet joints — *see* Spondylosis
  - fatty
    - liver NEC K76.Ø
      - alcoholic K7Ø.Ø
  - grey matter (brain) (Alpers') G31.81
  - heart — *see also* Degeneration, myocardial
    - amyloid E85.4 *[I43]*
    - atheromatous — *see* Disease, heart, ischemic, atherosclerotic
    - ischemic — *see* Disease, heart, ischemic
  - hepatolenticular (Wilson's) E83.Ø1
  - hepatorenal K76.7
  - hyaline (diffuse) (generalized)
    - localized — *see* Degeneration, by site
  - infrapatellar fat pad M79.4
  - intervertebral disc NOS
    - with
      - myelopathy — *see* Disorder, disc, with, myelopathy
      - radiculitis or radiculopathy — *see* Disorder, disc, with, radiculopathy
    - cervical, cervicothoracic — *see* Disorder, disc, cervical, degeneration

- **Degeneration, degenerative** — *continued*
  - intervertebral disc — *continued*
    - cervical, cervicothoracic — *see* Disorder, disc, cervical, degeneration — *continued*
      - with
        - myelopathy — *see* Disorder, disc, cervical, with myelopathy
        - neuritis, radiculitis or radiculopathy — *see* Disorder, disc, cervical, with neuritis
    - lumbar region M51.36
      - with
        - myelopathy M51.06
        - neuritis, radiculitis, radiculopathy or sciatica M51.16
    - lumbosacral region M51.37
      - with
        - neuritis, radiculitis, radiculopathy or sciatica M51.17
    - sacrococcygeal region M53.3
    - thoracic region M51.34
      - with
        - myelopathy M51.04
        - neuritis, radiculitis, radiculopathy M51.14
    - thoracolumbar region M51.35
      - with
        - myelopathy M51.05
        - neuritis, radiculitis, radiculopathy M51.15
  - intestine, amyloid E85.4
  - iris (pigmentary) H21.23- ☑
  - ischemic — *see* Ischemia
  - joint disease — *see* Osteoarthritis
  - kidney N28.89
    - amyloid E85.4 *[N29]*
    - cystic, congenital Q61.9
    - fatty N28.89
    - polycystic Q61.3
      - adult type (autosomal dominant) Q61.2
      - infantile type (autosomal recessive) NEC Q61.19
        - collecting duct dilatation Q61.11
  - Kuhnt-Junius — *see also* Degeneration, macula H35.32- ☑
  - lens — *see* Cataract
  - lenticular (familial) (progressive) (Wilson's) (with cirrhosis of liver) E83.01
  - liver (diffuse) NEC K76.89
    - amyloid E85.4 *[K77]*
    - cystic K76.89
      - congenital Q44.6
    - fatty NEC K76.0
      - alcoholic K70.0
    - hypertrophic K76.89
    - parenchymatous, acute or subacute K72.00
      - with coma K72.01
    - pigmentary K76.89
    - toxic (acute) K71.9
  - lung J98.4
  - lymph gland I89.8
    - hyaline I89.8
  - macula, macular (acquired) (age-related) (senile) H35.30
    - angioid streaks H35.33
    - atrophic age-related H35.31- ☑
    - congenital or hereditary — *see* Dystrophy, retina
    - cystoid H35.35- ☑
    - drusen H35.36- ☑
    - dry age-related H35.31- ☑
    - exudative H35.32- ☑
    - hole H35.34- ☑
    - nonexudative H35.31- ☑
    - puckering H35.37- ☑
    - toxic H35.38- ☑
    - wet age-related H35.32- ☑
  - membranous labyrinth, congenital (causing impairment of hearing) Q16.5
  - meniscus — *see* Derangement, meniscus
  - mitral — *see* Insufficiency, mitral
  - Mönckeberg's — *see* Arteriosclerosis, extremities
  - motor centers, senile G31.1
  - multi-system G90.3
  - mural — *see* Degeneration, myocardial
  - muscle (fatty) (fibrous) (hyaline) (progressive) M62.89
    - heart — *see* Degeneration, myocardial
  - myelin, central nervous system G37.9
  - myocardial, myocardium (fatty) (hyaline) (senile) I51.5
    - with rheumatic fever (conditions in I00) I09.0
      - active, acute or subacute I01.2
        - with chorea I02.0
      - inactive or quiescent (with chorea) I09.0

- **Degeneration, degenerative** — *continued*
  - myocardial, myocardium — *continued*
    - hypertensive — *see* Hypertension, heart
    - rheumatic — *see* Degeneration, myocardial, with rheumatic fever
    - syphilitic A52.06
  - nasal sinus (mucosa) J32.9
    - frontal J32.1
    - maxillary J32.0
  - nerve — *see* Disorder, nerve
  - nervous system G31.9
    - alcoholic G31.2
    - amyloid E85.4 *[G99.8]*
    - autonomic G90.9
    - fatty G31.89
    - specified NEC G31.89
  - nipple N64.89
  - olivopontocerebellar (hereditary) (familial) G23.8
  - osseous labyrinth — *see* subcategory H83.8 ☑
  - ovary N83.8
    - cystic N83.20- ☑
    - microcystic N83.20- ☑
  - pallidal pigmentary (progressive) G23.0
  - pancreas K86.89
    - tuberculous A18.83
  - penis N48.89
  - pigmentary (diffuse) (general)
    - localized — *see* Degeneration, by site
    - pallidal (progressive) G23.0
  - pineal gland E34.8
  - pituitary (gland) E23.6
  - popliteal fat pad M79.4
  - posterolateral (spinal cord) — *see* Degeneration, combined
  - pulmonary valve (heart) I37.8
  - pulp (tooth) K04.2
  - pupillary margin H21.24- ☑
  - renal — *see* Degeneration, kidney
  - retina H35.9
    - hereditary (cerebroretinal) (congenital) (juvenile) (macula) (peripheral) (pigmentary) — *see* Dystrophy, retina
    - Kuhnt-Junius — *see also* Degeneration, macula H35.32- ☑
    - macula (cystic) (exudative) (hole) (nonexudative) (pseudohole) (senile) (toxic) — *see* Degeneration, macula
    - peripheral H35.40
      - lattice H35.41- ☑
      - microcystoid H35.42- ☑
      - paving stone H35.43- ☑
      - secondary
        - pigmentary H35.45- ☑
        - vitreoretinal H35.46- ☑
      - senile reticular H35.44- ☑
    - pigmentary (primary) — *see also* Dystrophy, retina
      - secondary — *see* Degeneration, retina, peripheral, secondary
    - posterior pole — *see* Degeneration, macula
  - saccule, congenital (causing impairment of hearing) Q16.5
  - senile R54
    - brain G31.1
    - cardiac, heart or myocardium — *see* Degeneration, myocardial
    - motor centers G31.1
    - vascular — *see* Arteriosclerosis
  - sinus (cystic) — *see also* Sinusitis
    - polypoid J33.1
  - skin L98.8
    - amyloid E85.4 *[L99]*
    - colloid L98.8
  - spinal (cord) G31.89
    - amyloid E85.4 *[G32.89]*
    - combined (subacute) — *see* Degeneration, combined
    - dorsolateral — *see* Degeneration, combined
    - familial NEC G31.89
    - fatty G31.89
    - funicular — *see* Degeneration, combined
    - posterolateral — *see* Degeneration, combined
    - subacute combined — *see* Degeneration, combined
    - tuberculous A17.81
  - spleen D73.0
    - amyloid E85.4 *[D77]*
  - stomach K31.89
  - striatonigral G23.2
  - suprarenal (capsule) (gland) E27.8

- **Degeneration, degenerative** — *continued*
  - synovial membrane (pulpy) — *see* Disorder, synovium, specified type NEC
  - tapetoretinal — *see* Dystrophy, retina
  - thymus (gland) E32.8
    - fatty E32.8
  - thyroid (gland) E07.89
  - tricuspid (heart) (valve) I07.9
  - tuberculous NEC — *see* Tuberculosis
  - turbinate J34.89
  - uterus (cystic) N85.8
  - vascular (senile) — *see* Arteriosclerosis
    - hypertensive — *see* Hypertension
  - vitreoretinal, secondary — *see* Degeneration, retina, peripheral, secondary, vitreoretinal
  - vitreous (body) H43.81- ☑
  - Wallerian — *see* Disorder, nerve
  - Wilson's hepatolenticular E83.01
- **Deglutition**
  - paralysis R13.0
    - hysterical F44.4
  - pneumonia J69.0
- **Degos' disease** I77.89
- **Dehiscence** (of)
  - amputation stump T87.81
  - cesarean wound O90.0
  - closure of
    - cornea T81.31 ☑
    - craniotomy T81.32 ☑
    - fascia (muscular) (superficial) T81.32 ☑
    - internal organ or tissue T81.32 ☑
    - laceration (external) (internal) T81.33 ☑
    - ligament T81.32 ☑
    - mucosa T81.31 ☑
    - muscle or muscle flap T81.32 ☑
    - ribs or rib cage T81.32 ☑
    - skin and subcutaneous tissue (full-thickness) (superficial) T81.31 ☑
    - skull T81.32 ☑
    - sternum (sternotomy) T81.32 ☑
    - tendon T81.32 ☑
    - traumatic laceration (external) (internal) T81.33 ☑
  - episiotomy O90.1
  - operation wound NEC T81.31 ☑
    - external operation wound (superficial) T81.31 ☑
    - internal operation wound (deep) T81.32 ☑
  - perineal wound (postpartum) O90.1
  - traumatic injury wound repair T81.33 ☑
  - wound T81.30 ☑
    - traumatic repair T81.33 ☑
- **Dehydration** E86.0
  - newborn P74.1
- **Déjérine-Roussy syndrome** G89.0
- **Déjérine-Sottas disease or neuropathy** (hypertrophic) G60.0
- **Déjérine-Thomas atrophy** G23.8
- **Delay, delayed**
  - any plane in pelvis
    - complicating delivery O66.9
  - birth or delivery NOS O63.9
  - closure, ductus arteriosus (Botalli) P29.38
  - coagulation — *see* Defect, coagulation
  - conduction (cardiac) (ventricular) I45.9
  - delivery, second twin, triplet, etc O63.2
  - development R62.50
    - global F88
    - intellectual (specific) F81.9
    - language F80.9
      - due to hearing loss F80.4
    - learning F81.9
    - milestone R62.0
    - pervasive F84.9
    - physiological R62.50
      - specified stage NEC R62.0
    - reading F81.0
    - sexual E30.0
    - speech F80.9
      - due to hearing loss F80.4
    - spelling F81.81
  - ejaculation F52.32
  - gastric emptying K30
  - menarche E30.0
  - menstruation (cause unknown) N91.0
  - milestone R62.0
  - passage of meconium (newborn) P76.0
  - primary respiration P28.9
  - puberty (constitutional) E30.0

Delay, delayed — *continued*
- separation of umbilical cord P96.82
- sexual maturation, female E30.0
- sleep phase syndrome G47.21
- union, fracture — *see* Fracture, by site
- vaccination Z28.9

Deletion(s)
- autosome Q93.9
  - identified by fluorescence in situ hybridization (FISH) Q93.89
  - identified by in situ hybridization (ISH) Q93.89
- chromosome
  - with complex rearrangements NEC Q93.7
  - part of NEC Q93.59
  - seen only at prometaphase Q93.89
  - short arm
    - 22q11.2 Q93.81
    - 4 Q93.3
    - 5p Q93.4
  - specified NEC Q93.89
- long arm chromosome 18 or 21 Q93.89
  - with complex rearrangements NEC Q93.7
- microdeletions NEC Q93.88

Delhi boil or button B55.1

Delinquency (juvenile) (neurotic) F91.8
- group Z72.810

Delinquent immunization status Z28.39
- COVID-19 Z28.31- ☑

Delirium, delirious (acute or subacute) (not alcohol- or drug-induced) (with dementia) R41.0
- alcoholic (acute) (tremens) (withdrawal) F10.921
  - with intoxication F10.921
    - in
      - abuse F10.121
      - dependence F10.221
- due to (secondary to)
  - alcohol
    - intoxication F10.921
      - in
        - abuse F10.121
        - dependence F10.221
    - withdrawal F10.231
  - amphetamine intoxication F15.921
    - in
      - abuse F15.121
      - dependence F15.221
  - anxiolytic
    - intoxication F13.921
      - in
        - abuse F13.121
        - dependence F13.221
    - withdrawal F13.231
  - cannabis intoxication (acute) F12.921
    - in
      - abuse F12.121
      - dependence F12.221
  - cocaine intoxication (acute) F14.921
    - in
      - abuse F14.121
      - dependence F14.221
  - general medical condition F05
  - hallucinogen intoxication F16.921
    - in
      - abuse F16.121
      - dependence F16.221
  - hypnotic
    - intoxication F13.921
      - in
        - abuse F13.121
        - dependence F13.221
    - withdrawal F13.231
  - inhalant intoxication (acute) F18.921
    - in
      - abuse F18.121
      - dependence F18.221
  - multiple etiologies F05
  - opioid intoxication (acute) F11.921
    - in
      - abuse F11.121
      - dependence F11.221
  - other (or unknown) substance F19.921
  - phencyclidine intoxication (acute) F16.921
    - in
      - abuse F16.121
      - dependence F16.221
  - psychoactive substance NEC intoxication (acute) F19.921

Delirium, delirious — *continued*
- due to — *continued*
  - psychoactive substance intoxication — *continued*
    - in
      - abuse F19.121
      - dependence F19.221
  - sedative
    - intoxication F13.921
      - in
        - abuse F13.121
        - dependence F13.221
    - withdrawal F13.231
  - unknown etiology R41.0
- exhaustion F43.0
- hysterical F44.89
- postprocedural (postoperative) F05
- puerperal F05
- thyroid — *see* Thyrotoxicosis with thyroid storm
- traumatic — *see* Injury, intracranial
- tremens (alcohol-induced) F10.231
  - sedative-induced F13.231

Delivery (childbirth) (labor)
- arrested active phase O62.1
- cesarean (for)
  - abnormal
    - pelvis (bony) (deformity) (major) NEC with disproportion (fetopelvic) O33.0
      - with obstructed labor O65.0
    - presentation or position O32.9 ☑
  - abruptio placentae — *see also* Abruptio placentae O45.9- ☑
  - acromion presentation O32.2 ☑
  - atony, uterus O62.2
  - breech presentation O32.1 ☑
    - incomplete O32.8 ☑
  - brow presentation O32.3 ☑
  - cephalopelvic disproportion O33.9
  - cerclage O34.3- ☑
  - chin presentation O32.3 ☑
  - cicatrix of cervix O34.4- ☑
  - contracted pelvis (general)
    - inlet O33.2
    - outlet O33.3 ☑
  - cord presentation or prolapse O69.0 ☑
  - cystocele O34.8- ☑
  - deformity (acquired) (congenital)
    - pelvic organs or tissues NEC O34.8- ☑
    - pelvis (bony) NEC O33.0
  - disproportion NOS O33.9
  - eclampsia — *see* Eclampsia
  - face presentation O32.3 ☑
  - failed
    - forceps O66.5
    - induction of labor O61.9
      - instrumental O61.1
      - mechanical O61.1
      - medical O61.0
      - specified NEC O61.8
      - surgical O61.1
    - trial of labor NOS O66.40
      - following previous cesarean delivery O66.41
    - vacuum extraction O66.5
    - ventouse O66.5
  - fetal-maternal hemorrhage O43.01- ☑
  - hemorrhage (intrapartum) O67.9
    - with coagulation defect O67.0
    - specified cause NEC O67.8
  - high head at term O32.4 ☑
  - hydrocephalic fetus O33.6 ☑
  - incarceration of uterus O34.51- ☑
  - incoordinate uterine action O62.4
  - increased size, fetus O33.5 ☑
  - inertia, uterus O62.2
    - primary O62.0
    - secondary O62.1
  - isthmocele O34.22
  - lateroversion, uterus O34.59- ☑
  - mal lie O32.9 ☑
  - malposition
    - fetus O32.9 ☑
    - pelvic organs or tissues NEC O34.8- ☑
    - uterus NEC O34.59- ☑
  - malpresentation NOS O32.9 ☑
  - oblique presentation O32.2 ☑
  - occurring after 37 completed weeks of gestation but before 39 completed weeks gestation due to (spontaneous) onset of labor O75.82

Delivery — *continued*
- cesarean — *continued*
  - oversize fetus O33.5 ☑
  - pelvic tumor NEC O34.8- ☑
  - placenta previa O44.0- ☑
    - complete O44.0- ☑
      - with hemorrhage O44.1- ☑
  - placental insufficiency O36.51- ☑
  - planned, occurring after 37 completed weeks of gestation but before 39 completed weeks gestation due to (spontaneous) onset of labor O75.82
  - polyp, cervix O34.4- ☑
    - causing obstructed labor O65.5
  - poor dilatation, cervix O62.0
  - pre-eclampsia O14.94
    - mild O14.04
    - moderate O14.04
    - severe O14.14
      - with hemolysis, elevated liver enzymes and low platelet count (HELLP) O14.24
  - previous
    - cesarean delivery O34.219
      - classical (vertical) scar O34.212
      - isthmocele O34.22
      - low transverse scar O34.211
      - mid-transverse T incision O34.218
      - scar
        - defect (isthmocele) O34.22
        - specified type NEC O34.218
    - surgery (to)
      - cervix O34.4- ☑
      - gynecological NEC O34.8- ☑
      - rectum O34.7- ☑
      - uterus O34.29
      - vagina O34.6- ☑
  - prolapse
    - arm or hand O32.2 ☑
    - uterus O34.52- ☑
  - prolonged labor NOS O63.9
  - rectocele O34.8- ☑
  - retroversion
    - uterus O34.53- ☑
  - rigid
    - cervix O34.4- ☑
    - pelvic floor O34.8- ☑
    - perineum O34.7- ☑
    - vagina O34.6- ☑
    - vulva O34.7- ☑
  - sacculation, pregnant uterus O34.59- ☑
  - scar(s)
    - cervix O34.4- ☑
    - cesarean delivery O34.219
      - classical (vertical) O34.212
      - isthmocele O34.22
      - low transverse O34.211
      - mid-transverse T incision O34.218
      - scar
        - defect (isthmocele) O34.22
        - specified type NEC O34.218
    - defect (isthmocele) O34.22
    - transmural uterine O34.29
    - uterus O34.29
  - Shirodkar suture in situ O34.3- ☑
  - shoulder presentation O32.2 ☑
  - stenosis or stricture, cervix O34.4- ☑
  - streptococcus group B (GBS) carrier state O99.824
  - transmural uterine scar O34.29
  - transverse presentation or lie O32.2 ☑
  - tumor, pelvic organs or tissues NEC O34.8- ☑
    - cervix O34.4- ☑
  - umbilical cord presentation or prolapse O69.0 ☑
  - without indication O82
- completely normal case O80
- complicated O75.9
  - by
    - abnormal, abnormality (of)
      - forces of labor O62.9
        - specified type NEC O62.8
      - glucose O99.814
      - uterine contractions NOS O62.9
    - abruptio placentae — *see also* Abruptio placentae O45.9- ☑
    - abuse
      - physical O9A.32 (*following* O99)
      - psychological O9A.52 (*following* O99)
      - sexual O9A.42 (*following* O99)

- **Delivery** — *continued*
  - complicated — *continued*
    - by — *continued*
      - adherent placenta O72.Ø
        - without hemorrhage O73.Ø
      - alcohol use O99.314
      - anemia (pre-existing) O99.Ø2
      - anesthetic death O74.8
      - annular detachment of cervix O71.3
      - atony, uterus O62.2
      - attempted vacuum extraction and forceps O66.5
      - Bandl's ring O62.4
      - bariatric surgery status O99.844
      - biliary tract disorder O26.62
      - bleeding — *see* Delivery, complicated by, hemorrhage
      - blood disorder NEC O99.12
      - cervical dystocia (hypotonic) O62.2
        - primary O62.Ø
        - secondary O62.1
      - circulatory system disorder O99.42
      - compression of cord (umbilical) NEC O69.2 ☑
      - condition NEC O99.892
      - contraction, contracted ring O62.4
      - cord (umbilical)
        - around neck
          - with compression O69.1 ☑
          - without compression O69.81 ☑
        - bruising O69.5 ☑
        - complication O69.9 ☑
          - specified NEC O69.89 ☑
        - compression NEC O69.2 ☑
        - entanglement O69.2 ☑
          - without compression O69.82 ☑
        - hematoma O69.5 ☑
        - presentation O69.Ø ☑
        - prolapse O69.Ø ☑
        - short O69.3 ☑
        - thrombosis (vessels) O69.5 ☑
        - vascular lesion O69.5 ☑
      - Couvelaire uterus O45.8X- ☑
      - damage to (injury to) NEC
        - perineum O71.82
        - periurethral tissue O71.82
        - vulva O71.82
      - delay following rupture of membranes (spontaneous) — *see* Pregnancy, complicated by, premature rupture of membranes
      - depressed fetal heart tones O76
      - diabetes O24.92
        - gestational O24.429
          - diet controlled O24.42Ø
          - insulin controlled O24.424
          - oral drug controlled (antidiabetic) (hypoglycemic) O24.425
        - pre-existing O24.32
          - specified NEC O24.82
          - type 1 O24.Ø2
          - type 2 O24.12
      - diastasis recti (abdominis) O71.89
      - dilatation
        - bladder O66.8
        - cervix incomplete, poor or slow O62.Ø
      - disease NEC O99.892
      - disruptio uteri — *see* Delivery, complicated by, rupture, uterus
      - drug use O99.324
      - dysfunction, uterus NOS O62.9
        - hypertonic O62.4
        - hypotonic O62.2
          - primary O62.Ø
          - secondary O62.1
        - incoordinate O62.4
      - eclampsia O15.1
      - embolism (pulmonary) — *see* Embolism, obstetric
      - endocrine, nutritional or metabolic disease NEC O99.284
      - failed
        - attempted vaginal birth after previous cesarean delivery O66.41
        - induction of labor O61.9
          - instrumental O61.1
          - mechanical O61.1
          - medical O61.Ø
          - specified NEC O61.8
          - surgical O61.1
        - trial of labor O66.4Ø

- **Delivery** — *continued*
  - complicated — *continued*
    - by — *continued*
      - female genital mutilation O65.5
      - fetal
        - abnormal acid-base balance O68
        - acidemia O68
        - acidosis O68
        - alkalosis O68
        - death, early OØ2.1
        - deformity O66.3
        - heart rate or rhythm (abnormal) (non-reassuring) O76
        - hypoxia O77.8
        - stress O77.9
          - due to drug administration O77.1
          - electrocardiographic evidence of O77.8
          - specified NEC O77.8
          - ultrasound evidence of O77.8
      - fever during labor O75.2
      - gastric banding status O99.844
      - gastric bypass status O99.844
      - gastrointestinal disease NEC O99.62
      - gestational
        - diabetes O24.429
          - diet controlled O24.42Ø
          - insulin (and diet) controlled O24.424
          - oral drug controlled (antidiabetic) (hypoglycemic) O24.425
        - edema O12.Ø4
          - with proteinuria O12.24
        - proteinuria O12.14
      - gonorrhea O98.22
      - hematoma O71.7
        - ischial spine O71.7
        - pelvic O71.7
        - vagina O71.7
        - vulva or perineum O71.7
      - hemorrhage (uterine) O67.9
        - associated with
          - afibrinogenemia O67.Ø
          - coagulation defect O67.Ø
          - hyperfibrinolysis O67.Ø
          - hypofibrinogenemia O67.Ø
        - due to
          - low implantation of placenta O44.5- ☑
          - low-lying placenta O44.5- ☑
          - placenta previa O44.1- ☑
            - marginal O44.3- ☑
            - partial O44.3- ☑
          - premature separation of placenta (normally implanted) — *see also* Abruptio placentae O45.9- ☑
          - retained placenta O72.Ø
          - uterine leiomyoma O67.8
        - placenta NEC O67.8
        - postpartum NEC (atonic) (immediate) O72.1
          - with retained or trapped placenta O72.Ø
          - delayed O72.2
          - secondary O72.2
          - third stage O72.Ø
      - hourglass contraction, uterus O62.4
      - hypertension, hypertensive (pre-existing) — *see* Hypertension, complicated by, childbirth (labor)
      - hypotension O26.5- ☑
      - incomplete dilatation (cervix) O62.Ø
      - incoordinate uterus contractions O62.4
      - inertia, uterus O62.2
        - during latent phase of labor O62.Ø
        - primary O62.Ø
        - secondary O62.1
      - infection (maternal) O98.92
        - carrier state NEC O99.834
        - gonorrhea O98.22
        - human immunodeficiency virus (HIV) O98.72
        - sexually transmitted NEC O98.32
        - specified NEC O98.82
        - syphilis O98.12
        - tuberculosis O98.Ø2
        - viral hepatitis O98.42
        - viral NEC O98.52
      - injury (to mother) — *see also* Delivery, complicated, by, damage to O71.9
        - nonobstetric O9A.22 (*following* O99)
          - caused by abuse — *see* Delivery, complicated by, abuse
      - intrauterine fetal death, early OØ2.1

- **Delivery** — *continued*
  - complicated — *continued*
    - by — *continued*
      - inversion, uterus O71.2
      - laceration (perineal) O7Ø.9
        - anus (sphincter) O7Ø.4
          - with third degree laceration — *see also* Delivery, complicated, by, laceration, perineum, third degree O7Ø.2Ø
            - with mucosa O7Ø.3
          - without third degree laceration O7Ø.2 ☑
        - bladder (urinary) O71.5
        - bowel O71.5
        - cervix (uteri) O71.3
        - fourchette O7Ø.Ø
        - hymen O7Ø.Ø
        - labia O7Ø.Ø
        - pelvic
          - floor O7Ø.1
          - organ NEC O71.5
        - perineum, perineal O7Ø.9
          - first degree O7Ø.Ø
          - fourth degree O7Ø.3
          - muscles O7Ø.1
          - second degree O7Ø.1
          - skin O7Ø.Ø
          - slight O7Ø.Ø
          - third degree O7Ø.2Ø
            - with
              - both external anal sphincter (EAS) and internal anal sphincter (IAS) torn (IIIc) O7Ø.23
              - less than 5Ø% of external anal sphincter (EAS) thickness torn (IIIa) O7Ø.21
              - more than 5Ø% external anal sphincter (EAS) thickness torn (IIIb) O7Ø.22
            - IIIa O7Ø.21
            - IIIb O7Ø.22
            - IIIc O7Ø.23
        - peritoneum (pelvic) O71.5
        - rectovaginal (septum) (without perineal laceration) O71.4
          - with perineum — *see also* Delivery, complicated, by, laceration, perineum, third degree O7Ø.2Ø
            - with anal or rectal mucosa O7Ø.3
        - specified NEC O71.89
        - sphincter ani — *see* Delivery, complicated, by, laceration, anus (sphincter)
        - urethra O71.5
        - uterus O71.81
          - before labor O71.81
        - vagina, vaginal (deep) (high) (without perineal laceration) O71.4
          - with perineum O7Ø.Ø
          - muscles, with perineum O7Ø.1
        - vulva O7Ø.Ø
      - liver disorder O26.62
      - malignancy O9A.12 (*following* O99)
      - malnutrition O25.2
      - malposition, malpresentation
        - uterus or cervix O65.5
        - placenta O44.Ø- ☑
          - with hemorrhage O44.1- ☑
        - without obstruction — *see also* Delivery, complicated by, obstruction O32.9 ☑
          - breech O32.1 ☑
          - compound O32.6 ☑
          - face (brow) (chin) O32.3 ☑
          - footling O32.8 ☑
          - high head O32.4 ☑
          - oblique O32.2 ☑
          - specified NEC O32.8 ☑
          - transverse O32.2 ☑
          - unstable lie O32.Ø ☑
      - meconium in amniotic fluid O77.Ø
      - mental disorder NEC O99.344
      - metrorrhexis — *see* Delivery, complicated by, rupture, uterus
      - nervous system disorder O99.354
      - obesity (pre-existing) O99.214
      - obesity surgery status O99.844
      - obstetric trauma O71.9
        - specified NEC O71.89

Delivery — *continued*
- complicated — *continued*
  - by — *continued*
    - obstructed labor
      - due to
        - breech (complete) (frank) presentation O64.1 ☑
          - incomplete O64.8 ☑
        - brow presentation O64.3 ☑
        - buttock presentation O64.1 ☑
        - chin presentation O64.2 ☑
        - compound presentation O64.5 ☑
        - contracted pelvis O65.1
        - deep transverse arrest O64.Ø ☑
        - deformed pelvis O65.Ø
        - dystocia (fetal) O66.9
          - due to
            - conjoined twins O66.3
            - fetal
              - abnormality NEC O66.3
              - ascites O66.3
              - hydrops O66.3
              - meningomyelocele O66.3
              - sacral teratoma O66.3
              - tumor O66.3
            - hydrocephalic fetus O66.3
          - shoulder O66.Ø
        - face presentation O64.2 ☑
        - fetopelvic disproportion O65.4
        - footling presentation O64.8 ☑
        - impacted shoulders O66.Ø
        - incomplete rotation of fetal head O64.Ø ☑
        - large fetus O66.2
        - locked twins O66.1
        - malposition O64.9 ☑
          - specified NEC O64.8 ☑
        - malpresentation O64.9 ☑
          - specified NEC O64.8 ☑
        - multiple fetuses NEC O66.6
        - pelvic
          - abnormality (maternal) O65.9
          - organ O65.5
          - specified NEC O65.8
          - contraction
            - inlet O65.2
            - mid-cavity O65.3
            - outlet O65.3
        - persistent (position)
          - occipitoiliac O64.Ø ☑
          - occipitoposterior O64.Ø ☑
          - occipitosacral O64.Ø ☑
          - occipitotransverse O64.Ø ☑
        - prolapsed arm O64.4 ☑
        - shoulder presentation O64.4 ☑
      - specified NEC O66.8
    - pathological retraction ring, uterus O62.4
    - penetration, pregnant uterus by instrument O71.1
    - perforation — *see* Delivery, complicated by, laceration
    - placenta, placental
      - ablatio — *see also* Abruptio placentae O45.9- ☑
      - abnormality O43.9- ☑
        - specified NEC O43.89- ☑
      - abruptio — *see also* Abruptio placentae O45.9- ☑
      - accreta O43.21- ☑
      - adherent (with hemorrhage) O72.Ø
        - without hemorrhage O73.Ø
      - detachment (premature) — *see also* Abruptio placentae O45.9- ☑
      - disorder O43.9- ☑
        - specified NEC O43.89- ☑
      - hemorrhage NEC O67.8
      - increta O43.22- ☑
      - low (implantation) (lying) O44.4- ☑
        - with hemorrhage O44.5- ☑
      - malformation O43.1Ø- ☑
      - malposition O44.Ø- ☑
        - without hemorrhage O44.1- ☑
      - percreta O43.23- ☑
      - previa (central) (complete) (lateral) (total) O44.Ø- ☑
        - with hemorrhage O44.1- ☑
        - marginal O44.2- ☑

Delivery — *continued*
- complicated — *continued*
  - by — *continued*
    - placenta, placental — *continued*
      - previa — *continued*
        - marginal — *continued*
          - with hemorrhage O44.3- ☑
        - partial O44.2- ☑
          - with hemorrhage O44.3- ☑
      - retained (with hemorrhage) O72.Ø
        - without hemorrhage O73.Ø
      - separation (premature) O45.9- ☑
        - specified NEC O45.8X- ☑
      - vicious insertion O44.1- ☑
    - precipitate labor O62.3
    - premature rupture, membranes — *see also* Pregnancy, complicated by, premature rupture of membranes O42.9Ø
    - prolapse
      - arm or hand O32.2 ☑
      - cord (umbilical) O69.Ø ☑
      - foot or leg O32.8 ☑
      - uterus O34.52- ☑
    - prolonged labor O63.9
      - first stage O63.Ø
      - second stage O63.1
    - protozoal disease (maternal) O98.62
    - respiratory disease NEC O99.52
    - retained membranes or portions of placenta O72.2
      - without hemorrhage O73.1
    - retarded birth O63.9
    - retention of secundines (with hemorrhage) O72.Ø
      - without hemorrhage O73.Ø
      - partial O72.2
        - without hemorrhage O73.1
    - rupture
      - bladder (urinary) O71.5
      - cervix O71.3
      - pelvic organ NEC O71.5
      - urethra O71.5
      - uterus (during or after labor) O71.1
        - before labor O71.Ø- ☑
    - separation, pubic bone (symphysis pubis) O71.6
    - shock O75.1
    - shoulder presentation O64.4 ☑
    - skin disorder NEC O99.72
    - spasm, cervix O62.4
    - stenosis or stricture, cervix O65.5
    - streptococcus group B (GBS) carrier state O99.824
    - subluxation of symphysis (pubis) O26.72
    - syphilis (maternal) O98.12
    - tear — *see* Delivery, complicated by, laceration
    - tetanic uterus O62.4
    - trauma (obstetrical) — *see also* Delivery, complicated, by, damage to O71.9
      - non-obstetric O9A.22 (*following* O99)
      - periurethral O71.82
      - specified NEC O71.89
    - tuberculosis (maternal) O98.Ø2
    - tumor, pelvic organs or tissues NEC O65.5
    - umbilical cord around neck
      - with compression O69.1 ☑
      - without compression O69.81 ☑
    - uterine inertia O62.2
      - during latent phase of labor O62.Ø
      - primary O62.Ø
      - secondary O62.1
    - vasa previa O69.4 ☑
    - velamentous insertion of cord O43.12- ☑
  - specified complication NEC O75.89
- delayed NOS O63.9
  - following rupture of membranes
    - artificial O75.5
  - second twin, triplet, etc. O63.2
- forceps, low following failed vacuum extraction O66.5
- missed (at or near term) O36.4 ☑
- normal O8Ø
- obstructed — *see* Delivery, complicated by, obstructed labor
- precipitate O62.3
- preterm — *see also* Pregnancy, complicated by, preterm labor O6Ø.1Ø ☑
- spontaneous O8Ø
- term pregnancy NOS O8Ø
- uncomplicated O8Ø
- vaginal, following previous cesarean delivery O34.219
  - classical (vertical) scar O34.212

Delivery — *continued*
- vaginal, following previous cesarean delivery — *continued*
  - low transverse scar O34.211
  - mid-transverse T incision O34.218
  - scar
    - defect (isthmocele) O34.22
    - specified type NEC O34.218

Delusions (paranoid) — *see* Disorder, delusional

Dementia (degenerative (primary)) (old age) (persisting) (unspecified severity) (without behavioral disturbance, psychotic disturbance, mood disturbance, and anxiety) FØ3.9Ø
- with
  - aberrant motor behavior (exit-seeking) (pacing) (restlessness) (rocking) FØ3.911
  - agitation FØ3.911
  - anxiety FØ3.94
  - behavioral disturbances (sexual disinhibition) (sleep disturbance) (social disinhibition) FØ3.918
    - specified NEC FØ3.918
  - Lewy bodies — *see also* Dementia, in, diseases specified elsewhere G31.83 *[FØ2.8Ø]*
    - with behavioral disturbance — *see also* Dementia, in, diseases specified elsewhere G31.83 *[FØ2.81-]* ☑
  - mood disturbance (anhedonia) (apathy) (depression) FØ3.93
  - Parkinsonism — *see also* Dementia, in, diseases specified elsewhere G2Ø *[FØ2.8Ø]*
    - with behavioral disturbance — *see also* Dementia, in, diseases specified elsewhere G2Ø *[FØ2.81-]* ☑
  - Parkinson's disease — *see also* Dementia, in, diseases specified elsewhere G2Ø *[FØ2.8Ø]*
    - with behavioral disturbance — *see also* Dementia, in, diseases specified elsewhere G2Ø *[FØ2.81-]* ☑
  - psychotic disturbance (delusional state) (hallucinations) (paranoia) (suspiciousness) FØ3.92
  - verbal or physical behaviors (anger) (aggression) (combativeness) (profanity) (shouting) (threatening) (violence) FØ3.911
- alcoholic F1Ø.97
  - with dependence F1Ø.27
- Alzheimer's type — *see* Disease, Alzheimer's
- arteriosclerotic — *see* Dementia, vascular
- atypical, Alzheimer's type — *see* Disease, Alzheimer's, specified NEC
- congenital — *see* Disability, intellectual
- frontal (lobe) — *see also* Dementia, in, diseases specified elsewhere G31.Ø9 *[FØ2.8Ø]*
  - with behavioral disturbance — *see also* Dementia, in, diseases specified elsewhere G31.Ø9 *[FØ2.81-]* ☑
- frontotemporal G31.Ø9 *[FØ2.8Ø]*
  - with behavioral disturbance G31.Ø9 *[FØ2.81]* ☑
  - specified NEC — *see also* Dementia, in, diseases specified elsewhere G31.Ø9 *[FØ2.8Ø]*
    - with behavioral disturbance — *see also* Dementia, in, diseases specified elsewhere G31.Ø9 *[FØ2.81-]* ☑
- in (due to)
  - alcohol F1Ø.97
    - with dependence F1Ø.27
  - Alzheimer's disease — *see* Disease, Alzheimer's
  - arteriosclerotic brain disease — *see* Dementia, vascular
  - cerebral lipidoses — *see also* Dementia, in, diseases specified elsewhere E75.- ☑ *[FØ2.8Ø]*
    - with behavioral disturbance — *see also* Dementia, in, diseases specified elsewhere E75.- ☑ *[FØ2.81-]* ☑
  - Creutzfeldt-Jakob disease — *see also* Creutzfeldt-Jakob disease or syndrome (with dementia) A81.ØØ
  - diseases specified elsewhere (unspecified severity) (without behavioral disturbance, psychotic disturbance, mood disturbance, and anxiety) FØ2.8Ø
    - with
      - aberrant motor behavior (exit-seeking) (pacing) (restlessness) (rocking) FØ2.811
      - agitation FØ2.811
      - anxiety FØ2.84

Index

Delivery — Dementia

Dementia — *continued*
in — *continued*
diseases specified elsewhere — *continued*
with — *continued*
behavioral disturbances (sexual disinhibition) (sleep disturbance) (social disinhibition) FØ2.818
specified NEC FØ2.818
mood disturbance (anhedonia) (apathy) (depression) FØ2.83
psychotic disturbance (delusional state) (hallucinations) (paranoia) (suspiciousness) FØ2.82
verbal or physical behaviors (anger) (aggression) (combativeness) (profanity) (shouting) (threatening) (violence) FØ2.811
mild FØ2.AØ
with
aberrant motor behavior (exit-seeking) (pacing) (restlessness) (rocking) FØ2.A11
agitation FØ2.A11
anxiety FØ2.A4
behavioral disturbances (sexual disinhibition) (sleep disturbance) (social disinhibition) FØ2.A18
specified NEC FØ2.A18
mood disturbance (anhedonia) (apathy) (depression) FØ2.A3
psychotic disturbance (delusional state) (hallucinations) (paranoia) (suspiciousness) FØ2.A2
verbal or physical behaviors (anger) (aggression) (combativeness) (profanity) (shouting) (threatening) (violence) FØ2.A11
moderate FØ2.BØ
with
aberrant motor behavior (exit-seeking) (pacing) (restlessness) (rocking) FØ2.B11
agitation FØ2.B11
anxiety FØ2.B4
behavioral disturbances (sexual disinhibition) (sleep disturbance) (social disinhibition) FØ2.B18
specified NEC FØ2.B18
mood disturbance (anhedonia) (apathy) (depression) FØ2.B3
psychotic disturbance (delusional state) (hallucinations) (paranoia) (suspiciousness) FØ2.B2
verbal or physical behaviors (anger) (aggression) (combativeness) (profanity) (shouting) (threatening) (violence) FØ2.B11
severe FØ2.CØ
with
aberrant motor behavior (exit-seeking) (pacing) (restlessness) (rocking) FØ2.C11
agitation FØ2.C11
anxiety FØ2.C4
behavioral disturbances (sexual disinhibition) (sleep disturbance) (social disinhibition) FØ2.C18
specified NEC FØ2.C18
mood disturbance (anhedonia) (apathy) (depression) FØ2.C3
psychotic disturbance (delusional state) (hallucinations) (paranoia) (suspiciousness) FØ2.C2
verbal or physical behaviors (anger) (aggression) (combativeness) (profanity) (shouting) (threatening) (violence) FØ2.C11
epilepsy — *see also* Dementia, in, diseases specified elsewhere G4Ø.- ☑ *[FØ2.8Ø]*
with behavioral disturbance — *see also* Dementia, in, diseases specified elsewhere G4Ø.- ☑ *[FØ2.81-]* ☑
hepatolenticular degeneration — *see also* Dementia, in, diseases specified elsewhere E83.Ø1 *[FØ2.8Ø]*
with behavioral disturbance — *see also* Dementia, in, diseases specified elsewhere E83.Ø1 *[FØ2.81-]* ☑

Dementia — *continued*
in — *continued*
human immunodeficiency virus (HIV) disease — *see also* Dementia, in, diseases specified elsewhere B2Ø *[FØ2.8Ø]*
with behavioral disturbance — *see also* Dementia, in, diseases specified elsewhere B2Ø *[FØ2.81-]* ☑
Huntington's disease or chorea — *see also* Dementia, in, diseases specified elsewhere G1Ø *[FØ2.8Ø]*
with behavioral disturbance — *see also* Dementia, in, diseases specified elsewhere G1Ø *[FØ2.81-]* ☑
hypercalcemia — *see also* Dementia, in, diseases specified elsewhere E83.52 *[FØ2.8Ø]*
with behavioral disturbance — *see also* Dementia, in, diseases specified elsewhere E83.52 *[FØ2.81-]* ☑
hypothyroidism, acquired — *see also* Dementia, in, diseases specified elsewhere EØ3.9 *[FØ2.8Ø]*
with behavioral disturbance — *see also* Dementia, in, diseases specified elsewhere EØ3.9 *[FØ2.81-]* ☑
due to iodine deficiency — *see also* Dementia, in, diseases specified elsewhere EØ1.8 *[FØ2.8Ø]*
with behavioral disturbance — *see also* Dementia, in, diseases specified elsewhere EØ1.8 *[FØ2.81-]* ☑
inhalants F18.97
with dependence F18.27
multiple
etiologies FØ3 ☑
sclerosis — *see also* Dementia, in, diseases specified elsewhere G35 *[FØ2.8Ø]*
with behavioral disturbance — *see also* Dementia, in, diseases specified elsewhere G35 *[FØ2.81-]* ☑
neurosyphilis — *see also* Dementia, in, diseases specified elsewhere A52.17 *[FØ2.8Ø]*
with behavioral disturbance — *see also* Dementia, in, diseases specified elsewhere A52.17 *[FØ2.81-]* ☑
juvenile — *see also* Dementia, in, diseases specified elsewhere A5Ø.49 *[FØ2.8Ø]*
with behavioral disturbance — *see also* Dementia, in, diseases specified elsewhere A5Ø.49 *[FØ2.81-]* ☑
niacin deficiency — *see also* Dementia, in, diseases specified elsewhere E52 *[FØ2.8Ø]*
with behavioral disturbance — *see also* Dementia, in, diseases specified elsewhere E52 *[FØ2.81-]* ☑
paralysis agitans — *see also* Dementia, in, diseases specified elsewhere G2Ø *[FØ2.8Ø]*
with behavioral disturbance — *see also* Dementia, in, diseases specified elsewhere G2Ø *[FØ2.81-]* ☑
Parkinson's disease — *see also* Dementia, in, diseases specified elsewhere G2Ø *[FØ2.8Ø]*
pellagra — *see also* Dementia, in, diseases specified elsewhere E52 *[FØ2.8Ø]*
with behavioral disturbance — *see also* Dementia, in, diseases specified elsewhere E52 *[FØ2.81-]* ☑
Pick's — *see also* Dementia, in, diseases specified elsewhere G31.Ø1 *[FØ2.8Ø]*
with behavioral disturbance — *see also* Dementia, in, diseases specified elsewhere G31.Ø1 *[FØ2.81-]* ☑
polyarteritis nodosa — *see also* Dementia, in, diseases specified elsewhere M3Ø.Ø *[FØ2.8Ø]*
with behavioral disturbance — *see also* Dementia, in, diseases specified elsewhere M3Ø.Ø *[FØ2.81-]* ☑
psychoactive drug F19.97
with dependence F19.27
inhalants F18.97
with dependence F18.27
sedatives, hypnotics or anxiolytics F13.97
with dependence F13.27
sedatives, hypnotics or anxiolytics F13.97
with dependence F13.27
systemic lupus erythematosus — *see also* Dementia, in, diseases specified elsewhere M32.- ☑ *[FØ2.8Ø]*

Dementia — *continued*
in — *continued*
systemic lupus erythematosus — *see also* Dementia, in, diseases specified elsewhere — *continued*
with behavioral disturbance — *see also* Dementia, in, diseases specified elsewhere M32.- ☑ *[FØ2.81-]* ☑
trypanosomiasis
African — *see also* Dementia, in, diseases specified elsewhere B56.9 *[FØ2.8Ø]*
with behavioral disturbance — *see also* Dementia, in, diseases specified elsewhere B56.9 *[FØ2.81-]* ☑
unknown etiology FØ3.- ☑
vitamin B12 deficiency — *see also* Dementia, in, diseases specified elsewhere E53.8 *[FØ2.8Ø]*
with behavioral disturbance — *see also* Dementia, in, diseases specified elsewhere E53.8 *[FØ2.81-]* ☑
volatile solvents F18.97
with dependence F18.27
infantile, infantilis F84.3
Lewy body — *see also* Dementia, in, diseases specified elsewhere G31.83 *[FØ2.8Ø]*
with behavioral disturbance — *see also* Dementia, in, diseases specified elsewhere G31.83 *[FØ2.81-]* ☑
mild FØ3.AØ
with
aberrant motor behavior (exit-seeking) (pacing) (restlessness) (rocking) FØ3.A11
agitation FØ3.A11
anxiety FØ3.A4
behavioral disturbances (sexual disinhibition) (sleep disturbance) (social disinhibition) FØ3.A18
specified NEC FØ3.A18
mood disturbance (anhedonia) (apathy) (depression) FØ3.A3
psychotic disturbance (delusional state) (hallucinations) (paranoia) (suspiciousness) FØ3.A2
verbal or physical behaviors (anger) (aggression) (combativeness) (profanity) (shouting) (threatening) (violence) FØ3.A11
moderate FØ3.BØ
with
aberrant motor behavior (exit-seeking) (pacing) (restlessness) (rocking) FØ3.B11
agitation FØ3.B11
anxiety FØ3.B4
behavioral disturbances (sexual disinhibition) (sleep disturbance) (social disinhibition) FØ3.B18
specified NEC FØ3.B18
mood disturbance (anhedonia) (apathy) (depression) FØ3.B3
psychotic disturbance (delusional state) (hallucinations) (paranoia) (suspiciousness) FØ3.B2
verbal or physical behaviors (anger) (aggression) (combativeness) (profanity) (shouting) (threatening) (violence) FØ3.B11
multi-infarct — *see* Dementia, vascular
paralytica, paralytic (syphilitic) — *see also* Dementia, in, diseases specified elsewhere A52.17 *[FØ2.8Ø]*
with behavioral disturbance — *see also* Dementia, in, diseases specified elsewhere A52.17 *[FØ2.81-]* ☑
juvenilis A5Ø.45
paretic A52.17
praecox — *see* Schizophrenia
presenile FØ3 ☑
Alzheimer's type — *see* Disease, Alzheimer's, early onset
primary degenerative FØ3 ☑
progressive, syphilitic A52.17
senile FØ3 ☑
with acute confusional state FØ5
Alzheimer's type — *see* Disease, Alzheimer's, late onset
depressed or paranoid type FØ3 ☑
severe FØ3.CØ
with
aberrant motor behavior (exit-seeking) (pacing) (restlessness) (rocking) FØ3.C11
agitation FØ3.C11
anxiety FØ3.C4

Dementia — *continued*
severe — *continued*
with — *continued*
behavioral disturbances (sexual disinhibition) (sleep disturbance) (social disinhibition) FØ3.C18
specified NEC FØ3.C18
mood disturbance (anhedonia) (apathy) (depression) FØ3.C3
psychotic disturbance (delusional state) (hallucinations) (paranoia) (suspiciousness) FØ3.C2
verbal or physical behaviors (anger) (aggression) (combativeness) (profanity) (shouting) (threatening) (violence) FØ3.C11
vascular (acute onset) (mixed) (multi-infarct) (subcortical) (unspecified severity) (without behavioral disturbance, psychotic disturbance, mood disturbance, and anxiety) FØ1.5Ø
with
aberrant motor behavior (exit-seeking) (pacing) (restlessness) (rocking) FØ1.511
agitation FØ1.511
anxiety FØ1.54
behavioral disturbances (sleep disturbance) (sexual disinhibition) (social disinhibition) FØ1.518
specified NEC FØ1.518
mood disturbance (anhedonia) (apathy) (depression) FØ1.53
psychotic disturbance (delusional state) (hallucinations) (paranoia) (suspiciousness) FØ1.52
verbal or physical behaviors (anger) (aggression) (combativeness) (profanity) (shouting) (threatening) (violence) FØ1.511
mild FØ1.AØ
with
aberrant motor behavior (exit-seeking) (pacing) (restlessness) (rocking) FØ1.A11
agitation FØ1.A11
anxiety FØ1.A4
behavioral disturbances (sleep disturbance) (sexual disinhibition) (social disinhibition) FØ1.A18
specified NEC FØ1.A18
mood disturbance (anhedonia) (apathy) (depression) FØ1.A3
psychotic disturbance (delusional state) (hallucinations) (paranoia) (suspiciousness) FØ1.A2
verbal or physical behaviors (anger) (aggression) (combativeness) (profanity) (shouting) (threatening) (violence) FØ1.A11
moderate FØ1.BØ
with
aberrant motor behavior (exit-seeking) (pacing) (restlessness) (rocking) FØ1.B11
agitation FØ1.B11
anxiety FØ1.B4
behavioral disturbances (sleep disturbance) (sexual disinhibition) (social disinhibition) FØ1.B18
specified NEC FØ1.B18
mood disturbance (anhedonia) (apathy) (depression) FØ1.B3
psychotic disturbance (delusional state) (hallucinations) (paranoia) (suspiciousness) FØ1.B2
verbal or physical behaviors (anger) (aggression) (combativeness) (profanity) (shouting) (threatening) (violence) FØ1.B11
severe FØ1.CØ
with
aberrant motor behavior (exit-seeking) (pacing) (restlessness) (rocking) FØ1.C11
agitation FØ1.C11
anxiety FØ1.C4
behavioral disturbances (sleep disturbance) (sexual disinhibition) (social disinhibition) FØ1.C18
specified NEC FØ1.C18
mood disturbance (anhedonia) (apathy) (depression) FØ1.C3
psychotic disturbance (delusional state) (hallucinations) (paranoia) (suspiciousness) FØ1.C2

Dementia — *continued*
vascular — *continued*
severe — *continued*
with — *continued*
verbal or physical behaviors (anger) (aggression) (combativeness) (profanity) (shouting) (threatening) (violence) FØ1.C11
Demineralization, bone — *see* Osteoporosis
Demodex folliculorum (infestation) B88.Ø
Demophobia F4Ø.248
Demoralization R45.3
Demyelination, demyelinization
central nervous system G37.9
specified NEC G37.8
corpus callosum (central) G37.1
disseminated, acute G36.9
specified NEC G36.8
global G35
in optic neuritis G36.Ø
Dengue (classical) (fever) A9Ø
hemorrhagic A91
sandfly A93.1
Dennie-Marfan syphilitic syndrome A5Ø.45
Dens evaginatus, in dente or invaginatus KØØ.2
Dense breasts R92.2
Density
increased, bone (disseminated) (generalized) (spotted) — *see* Disorder, bone, density and structure, specified type NEC
lung (nodular) J98.4
Dental — *see also* condition
examination ZØ1.2Ø
with abnormal findings ZØ1.21
restoration
aesthetically inadequate or displeasing KØ8.56
defective KØ8.5Ø
specified NEC KØ8.59
failure of marginal integrity KØ8.51
failure of periodontal anatomical integrity KØ8.54
Dentia praecox KØØ.6
Denticles (pulp) KØ4.2
Dentigerous cyst KØ9.Ø
Dentin
irregular (in pulp) KØ4.3
opalescent KØØ.5
secondary (in pulp) KØ4.3
sensitive KØ3.89
Dentinogenesis imperfecta KØØ.5
Dentinoma — *see* Cyst, calcifying odontogenic
Dentition (syndrome) KØØ.7
delayed KØØ.6
difficult KØØ.7
precocious KØØ.6
premature KØØ.6
retarded KØØ.6
Dependence (on) (syndrome) F19.2Ø
with remission F19.21
alcohol (ethyl) (methyl) (without remission) F1Ø.2Ø
with
amnestic disorder, persisting F1Ø.26
anxiety disorder F1Ø.28Ø
dementia, persisting F1Ø.27
intoxication F1Ø.229
with delirium F1Ø.221
uncomplicated F1Ø.22Ø
mood disorder F1Ø.24
psychotic disorder F1Ø.259
with
delusions F1Ø.25Ø
hallucinations F1Ø.251
remission F1Ø.21
sexual dysfunction F1Ø.281
sleep disorder F1Ø.282
specified disorder NEC F1Ø.288
withdrawal F1Ø.239
with
delirium F1Ø.231
perceptual disturbance F1Ø.232
uncomplicated F1Ø.23Ø
counseling and surveillance Z71.41
in remission F1Ø.21
amobarbital — *see* Dependence, drug, sedative
amphetamine(s) (type) — *see* Dependence, drug, stimulant NEC
amytal (sodium) — *see* Dependence, drug, sedative
analgesic NEC F55.8

Dependence — *continued*
anesthetic (agent) (gas) (general) (local) NEC — *see* Dependence, drug, psychoactive NEC
anxiolytic NEC — *see* Dependence, drug, sedative
barbital(s) — *see* Dependence, drug, sedative
barbiturate(s) (compounds) (drugs classifiable to T42) — *see* Dependence, drug, sedative
benzedrine — *see* Dependence, drug, stimulant NEC
bhang — *see* Dependence, drug, cannabis
bromide(s) NEC — *see* Dependence, drug, sedative
caffeine — *see* Dependence, drug, stimulant NEC
cannabis (sativa) (indica) (resin) (derivatives) (type) — *see* Dependence, drug, cannabis
chloral (betaine) (hydrate) — *see* Dependence, drug, sedative
chlordiazepoxide — *see* Dependence, drug, sedative
coca (leaf) (derivatives) — *see* Dependence, drug, cocaine
cocaine — *see* Dependence, drug, cocaine
codeine — *see* Dependence, drug, opioid
combinations of drugs F19.2Ø
dagga — *see* Dependence, drug, cannabis
demerol — *see* Dependence, drug, opioid
dexamphetamine — *see* Dependence, drug, stimulant NEC
dexedrine — *see* Dependence, drug, stimulant NEC
dextromethorphan — *see* Dependence, drug, opioid
dextromoramide — *see* Dependence, drug, opioid
dextro-nor-pseudo-ephedrine — *see* Dependence, drug, stimulant NEC
dextrorphan — *see* Dependence, drug, opioid
diazepam — *see* Dependence, drug, sedative
dilaudid — *see* Dependence, drug, opioid
D-lysergic acid diethylamide — *see* Dependence, drug, hallucinogen
drug NEC F19.2Ø
with sleep disorder F19.282
cannabis F12.2Ø
with
anxiety disorder F12.28Ø
intoxication F12.229
with
delirium F12.221
perceptual disturbance F12.222
uncomplicated F12.22Ø
other specified disorder F12.288
psychosis F12.259
delusions F12.25Ø
hallucinations F12.251
unspecified disorder F12.29
withdrawal F12.23
in remission F12.21
cocaine F14.2Ø
with
anxiety disorder F14.28Ø
intoxication F14.229
with
delirium F14.221
perceptual disturbance F14.222
uncomplicated F14.22Ø
mood disorder F14.24
other specified disorder F14.288
psychosis F14.259
delusions F14.25Ø
hallucinations F14.251
sexual dysfunction F14.281
sleep disorder F14.282
unspecified disorder F14.29
withdrawal F14.23
in remission F14.21
withdrawal symptoms in newborn P96.1
counseling and surveillance Z71.51
hallucinogen F16.2Ø
with
anxiety disorder F16.28Ø
flashbacks F16.283
intoxication F16.229
with delirium F16.221
uncomplicated F16.22Ø
mood disorder F16.24
other specified disorder F16.288
perception disorder, persisting F16.283
psychosis F16.259
delusions F16.25Ø
hallucinations F16.251
unspecified disorder F16.29
in remission F16.21
in remission F19.21

- **Dependence** — *continued*
  - drug — *continued*
    - inhalant F18.2Ø
      - with
        - anxiety disorder F18.28Ø
        - dementia, persisting F18.27
        - intoxication F18.229
          - with delirium F18.221
          - uncomplicated F18.22Ø
        - mood disorder F18.24
        - other specified disorder F18.288
        - psychosis F18.259
          - delusions F18.25Ø
          - hallucinations F18.251
        - unspecified disorder F18.29
      - in remission F18.21
    - nicotine F17.2ØØ
      - with disorder F17.2Ø9
        - in remission F17.2Ø1
        - specified disorder NEC F17.2Ø8
        - withdrawal F17.2Ø3
      - chewing tobacco F17.22Ø
        - with disorder F17.229
          - in remission F17.221
          - specified disorder NEC F17.228
          - withdrawal F17.223
      - cigarettes F17.21Ø
        - with disorder F17.219
          - in remission F17.211
          - specified disorder NEC F17.218
          - withdrawal F17.213
      - specified product NEC F17.29Ø
        - with disorder F17.299
          - remission F17.291
          - specified disorder NEC F17.298
          - withdrawal F17.293
    - opioid F11.2Ø
      - with
        - intoxication F11.229
          - with
            - delirium F11.221
            - perceptual disturbance F11.222
          - uncomplicated F11.22Ø
        - mood disorder F11.24
        - other specified disorder F11.288
        - psychosis F11.259
          - delusions F11.25Ø
          - hallucinations F11.251
        - sexual dysfunction F11.281
        - sleep disorder F11.282
        - unspecified disorder F11.29
        - withdrawal F11.23
      - in remission F11.21
    - psychoactive NEC F19.2Ø
      - with
        - amnestic disorder F19.26
        - anxiety disorder F19.28Ø
        - dementia F19.27
        - intoxication F19.229
          - with
            - delirium F19.221
            - perceptual disturbance F19.222
          - uncomplicated F19.22Ø
        - mood disorder F19.24
        - other specified disorder F19.288
        - psychosis F19.259
          - delusions F19.25Ø
          - hallucinations F19.251
        - sexual dysfunction F19.281
        - sleep disorder F19.282
        - unspecified disorder F19.29
        - withdrawal F19.239
          - with
            - delirium F19.231
            - perceptual disturbance F19.232
          - uncomplicated F19.23Ø
    - sedative, hypnotic or anxiolytic F13.2Ø
      - with
        - amnestic disorder F13.26
        - anxiety disorder F13.28Ø
        - dementia, persisting F13.27
        - intoxication F13.229
          - with delirium F13.221
          - uncomplicated F13.22Ø
        - mood disorder F13.24
        - other specified disorder F13.288
        - psychosis F13.259
          - delusions F13.25Ø
          - hallucinations F13.251

- **Dependence** — *continued*
  - drug — *continued*
    - sedative, hypnotic or anxiolytic — *continued*
      - with — *continued*
        - sexual dysfunction F13.281
        - sleep disorder F13.282
        - unspecified disorder F13.29
        - withdrawal F13.239
          - with
            - delirium F13.231
            - perceptual disturbance F13.232
          - uncomplicated F13.23Ø
      - in remission F13.21
    - stimulant NEC F15.2Ø
      - with
        - anxiety disorder F15.28Ø
        - intoxication F15.229
          - with
            - delirium F15.221
            - perceptual disturbance F15.222
          - uncomplicated F15.22Ø
        - mood disorder F15.24
        - other specified disorder F15.288
        - psychosis F15.259
          - delusions F15.25Ø
          - hallucinations F15.251
        - sexual dysfunction F15.281
        - sleep disorder F15.282
        - unspecified disorder F15.29
        - withdrawal F15.23
      - in remission F15.21
  - ethyl
    - alcohol (without remission) F1Ø.2Ø
      - with remission F1Ø.21
    - bromide — *see* Dependence, drug, sedative
    - carbamate F19.2Ø
    - chloride F19.2Ø
    - morphine — *see* Dependence, drug, opioid
  - ganja — *see* Dependence, drug, cannabis
  - glue (airplane) (sniffing) — *see* Dependence, drug, inhalant
  - glutethimide — *see* Dependence, drug, sedative
  - hallucinogenics — *see* Dependence, drug, hallucinogen
  - hashish — *see* Dependence, drug, cannabis
  - hemp — *see* Dependence, drug, cannabis
  - heroin (salt) (any) — *see* Dependence, drug, opioid
  - hypnotic NEC — *see* Dependence, drug, sedative
  - Indian hemp — *see* Dependence, drug, cannabis
  - inhalants — *see* Dependence, drug, inhalant
  - khat — *see* Dependence, drug, stimulant NEC
  - laudanum — *see* Dependence, drug, opioid
  - LSD (-25) (derivatives) — *see* Dependence, drug, hallucinogen
  - luminal — *see* Dependence, drug, sedative
  - lysergic acid — *see* Dependence, drug, hallucinogen
  - maconha — *see* Dependence, drug, cannabis
  - marihuana — *see* Dependence, drug, cannabis
  - meprobamate — *see* Dependence, drug, sedative
  - mescaline — *see* Dependence, drug, hallucinogen
  - methadone — *see* Dependence, drug, opioid
  - methamphetamine(s) — *see* Dependence, drug, stimulant NEC
  - methaqualone — *see* Dependence, drug, sedative
  - methyl
    - alcohol (without remission) F1Ø.2Ø
      - with remission F1Ø.21
    - bromide — *see* Dependence, drug, sedative
    - morphine — *see* Dependence, drug, opioid
    - phenidate — *see* Dependence, drug, stimulant NEC
    - sulfonal — *see* Dependence, drug, sedative
  - morphine (sulfate) (sulfite) (type) — *see* Dependence, drug, opioid
  - narcotic (drug) NEC — *see* Dependence, drug, opioid
  - nembutal — *see* Dependence, drug, sedative
  - neraval — *see* Dependence, drug, sedative
  - neravan — *see* Dependence, drug, sedative
  - neurobarb — *see* Dependence, drug, sedative
  - nicotine — *see* Dependence, drug, nicotine
  - nitrous oxide F19.2Ø
  - nonbarbiturate sedatives and tranquilizers with similar effect — *see* Dependence, drug, sedative
  - on
    - artificial heart (fully implantable) (mechanical) Z95.812
    - aspirator Z99.Ø
    - care provider (because of) Z74.9
      - impaired mobility Z74.Ø9

- **Dependence** — *continued*
  - on — *continued*
    - care provider — *continued*
      - need for
        - assistance with personal care Z74.1
        - continuous supervision Z74.3
        - no other household member able to render care Z74.2
      - specified reason NEC Z74.8
    - machine Z99.89
      - enabling NEC Z99.89
      - specified type NEC Z99.89
    - renal dialysis (hemodialysis) (peritoneal) Z99.2
    - respirator Z99.11
    - ventilator Z99.11
    - wheelchair Z99.3
  - opiate — *see* Dependence, drug, opioid
  - opioids — *see* Dependence, drug, opioid
  - opium (alkaloids) (derivatives) (tincture) — *see* Dependence, drug, opioid
  - oxygen (long-term) (supplemental) Z99.81
  - paraldehyde — *see* Dependence, drug, sedative
  - paregoric — *see* Dependence, drug, opioid
  - PCP (phencyclidine) (or related substance) — *see* Dependence, drug, hallucinogen
  - pentobarbital — *see* Dependence, drug, sedative
  - pentobarbitone (sodium) — *see* Dependence, drug, sedative
  - pentothal — *see* Dependence, drug, sedative
  - peyote — *see* Dependence, drug, hallucinogen
  - phencyclidine (PCP) (or related substance) — *see* Dependence, drug, hallucinogen
  - phenmetrazine — *see* Dependence, drug, stimulant NEC
  - phenobarbital — *see* Dependence, drug, sedative
  - polysubstance F19.2Ø
  - psilocibin, psilocin, psilocyn, psilocyline — *see* Dependence, drug, hallucinogen
  - psychostimulant NEC — *see* Dependence, drug, stimulant NEC
  - secobarbital — *see* Dependence, drug, sedative
  - seconal — *see* Dependence, drug, sedative
  - sedative NEC — *see* Dependence, drug, sedative
  - specified drug NEC — *see* Dependence, drug
  - stimulant NEC — *see* Dependence, drug, stimulant NEC
  - substance NEC — *see* Dependence, drug
  - supplemental oxygen Z99.81
  - tobacco — *see* Dependence, drug, nicotine
    - counseling and surveillance Z71.6
  - tranquilizer NEC — *see* Dependence, drug, sedative
  - vitamin B6 E53.1
  - volatile solvents — *see* Dependence, drug, inhalant
- **Dependency**
  - care-provider Z74.9
  - passive F6Ø.7
  - reactions (persistent) F6Ø.7
- **Depersonalization** (in neurotic state) (neurotic) (syndrome) F48.1
- **Depletion**
  - extracellular fluid E86.9
  - plasma E86.1
  - potassium E87.6
    - nephropathy N25.89
  - salt or sodium E87.1
    - causing heat exhaustion or prostration T67.4 ☑
    - nephropathy N28.9
  - volume NOS E86.9
- **Deployment** (current) (military) status Z56.82
  - in theater or in support of military war, peacekeeping and humanitarian operations Z56.82
  - personal history of Z91.82
    - military war, peacekeeping and humanitarian deployment (current or past conflict) Z91.82
  - returned from Z91.82
- **Depolarization, premature** I49.4Ø
  - atrial I49.1
  - junctional I49.2
  - specified NEC I49.49
  - ventricular I49.3
- **Deposit**
  - bone in Boeck's sarcoid D86.89
  - calcareous, calcium — *see* Calcification
  - cholesterol
    - retina H35.89
    - vitreous (body) (humor) — *see* Deposit, crystalline
  - conjunctiva H11.11- ☑
  - cornea H18.ØØ- ☑
    - argentous H18.Ø2- ☑

Deposit — *continued*
- cornea — *continued*
  - due to metabolic disorder H18.Ø3- ☑
  - Kayser-Fleischer ring H18.Ø4- ☑
  - pigmentation — *see* Pigmentation, cornea
- crystalline, vitreous (body) (humor) H43.2- ☑
- hemosiderin in old scars of cornea — *see* Pigmentation, cornea, stromal
- metallic in lens — *see* Cataract, specified NEC
- skin R23.8
- tooth, teeth (betel) (black) (green) (materia alba) (orange) (tobacco) KØ3.6
- urate, kidney — *see* Calculus, kidney

Depraved appetite — *see* Pica

Depressed
- HDL cholesterol E78.6

Depression (acute) (mental) F32.A
- agitated (single episode) F32.2
- anaclitic — *see* Disorder, adjustment
- anxiety F41.8
  - persistent F34.1
- arches — *see also* Deformity, limb, flat foot
- atypical (single episode) F32.89
  - recurrent episode F33.8
- basal metabolic rate R94.8
- bone marrow D75.89
- central nervous system RØ9.2
- cerebral R29.818
  - newborn P91.4
- cerebrovascular I67.9
- chest wall M95.4
- climacteric (single episode) F32.89
  - recurrent episode F33.8
- endogenous (without psychotic symptoms) F33.2
  - with psychotic symptoms F33.3
- functional activity R68.89
- hysterical F44.89
- involutional (single episode) F32.89
  - recurrent episode F33.8
- major F32.9
  - with psychotic symptoms F32.3
  - recurrent — *see* Disorder, depressive, recurrent
- manic-depressive — *see* Disorder, depressive, recurrent
- masked (single episode) F32.89
- medullary G93.89
- menopausal (single episode) F32.89
  - recurrent episode F33.8
- metatarsus — *see* Depression, arches
- monopolar F33.9
- nervous F34.1
- neurotic F34.1
- nose M95.Ø
- postnatal (NOS) F53.Ø
- postpartum (NOS) F53.Ø
- post-psychotic of schizophrenia F32.89
- post-schizophrenic F32.89
- psychogenic (reactive) (single episode) F32.9
- psychoneurotic F34.1
- psychotic (single episode) F32.3
  - recurrent F33.3
- reactive (psychogenic) (single episode) F32.9
  - psychotic (single episode) F32.3
- recurrent — *see* Disorder, depressive, recurrent
- respiratory center G93.89
- seasonal — *see* Disorder, depressive, recurrent
- senile FØ3 ☑
- severe, single episode F32.2
- situational F43.21
- skull Q67.4
- specified NEC (single episode) F32.89
- sternum M95.4
- visual field — *see* Defect, visual field
- vital (recurrent) (without psychotic symptoms) F33.2
  - with psychotic symptoms F33.3
  - single episode F32.2

Deprivation
- cultural Z6Ø.3
- effects NOS T73.9 ☑
  - specified NEC T73.8 ☑
- emotional NEC Z65.8
  - affecting infant or child — *see* Maltreatment, child, psychological
- food T73.Ø ☑
- material Z59.87
- protein — *see* Malnutrition
- sleep Z72.82Ø
- social Z6Ø.4

Deprivation — *continued*
- social — *continued*
  - affecting infant or child — *see* Maltreatment, child, psychological
- specified NEC T73.8 ☑
- vitamins — *see* Deficiency, vitamin
- water T73.1 ☑

Derangement
- ankle (internal) — *see* Derangement, joint, articular cartilage, ankle
- cartilage (articular) NEC — *see* Derangement, joint, articular cartilage, by site
  - recurrent — *see* Dislocation, recurrent
- cruciate ligament, anterior, current injury — *see* Sprain, knee, cruciate, anterior
- elbow (internal) — *see* Derangement, joint, articular cartilage, elbow
- hip (joint) (internal) (old) — *see* Derangement, joint, articular cartilage, hip
- joint (internal) M24.9
  - ankylosis — *see* Ankylosis
  - articular cartilage M24.1Ø
    - ankle M24.17- ☑
    - elbow M24.12- ☑
    - foot M24.17- ☑
    - hand M24.14- ☑
    - hip M24.15- ☑
    - knee NEC M23.9- ☑
    - loose body — *see* Loose, body
    - shoulder M24.11- ☑
    - specified site NEC M24.19
    - wrist M24.13- ☑
  - contracture — *see* Contraction, joint
  - current injury — *see also* Dislocation
    - knee, meniscus or cartilage — *see* Tear, meniscus
  - dislocation
    - pathological — *see* Dislocation, pathological
    - recurrent — *see* Dislocation, recurrent
  - knee — *see* Derangement, knee
  - ligament — *see* Disorder, ligament
  - loose body — *see* Loose, body
  - recurrent — *see* Dislocation, recurrent
  - specified type NEC M24.8Ø
    - ankle M24.87- ☑
    - elbow M24.82- ☑
    - foot joint M24.87- ☑
    - hand joint M24.84- ☑
    - hip M24.85- ☑
    - shoulder M24.81- ☑
    - specified site NEC M24.89
    - wrist M24.83- ☑
  - temporomandibular M26.69
- knee (recurrent) M23.9- ☑
  - ligament disruption, spontaneous M23.6Ø- ☑
    - anterior cruciate M23.61- ☑
    - capsular M23.67- ☑
    - instability, chronic M23.5- ☑
    - lateral collateral M23.64- ☑
    - medial collateral M23.63- ☑
    - posterior cruciate M23.62- ☑
  - loose body M23.4- ☑
  - meniscus M23.3Ø- ☑
    - cystic M23.ØØ- ☑
      - lateral M23.ØØ2
        - anterior horn M23.Ø4- ☑
        - posterior horn M23.Ø5- ☑
        - specified NEC M23.Ø6- ☑
      - medial M23.ØØ5
        - anterior horn M23.Ø1- ☑
        - posterior horn M23.Ø2- ☑
        - specified NEC M23.Ø3- ☑
    - degenerate — *see* Derangement, knee, meniscus, specified NEC
    - detached — *see* Derangement, knee, meniscus, specified NEC
    - due to old tear or injury M23.2Ø- ☑
      - lateral M23.2Ø- ☑
        - anterior horn M23.24- ☑
        - posterior horn M23.25- ☑
        - specified NEC M23.26- ☑
      - medial M23.2Ø- ☑
        - anterior horn M23.21- ☑
        - posterior horn M23.22- ☑
        - specified NEC M23.23- ☑
    - retained — *see* Derangement, knee, meniscus, specified NEC

Derangement — *continued*
- knee — *continued*
  - meniscus — *continued*
    - specified NEC M23.3Ø- ☑
      - lateral M23.3Ø- ☑
        - anterior horn M23.34- ☑
        - posterior horn M23.35- ☑
        - specified NEC M23.36- ☑
      - medial M23.3Ø- ☑
        - anterior horn M23.31- ☑
        - posterior horn M23.32- ☑
        - specified NEC M23.33- ☑
  - old M23.8X- ☑
  - specified NEC — *see* subcategory M23.8 ☑
- low back NEC — *see* Dorsopathy, specified NEC
- meniscus — *see* Derangement, knee, meniscus
- mental — *see* Psychosis
- patella, specified NEC — *see* Disorder, patella, derangement NEC
- semilunar cartilage (knee) — *see* Derangement, knee, meniscus, specified NEC
- shoulder (internal) — *see* Derangement, joint, shoulder

Dercum's disease E88.2

Derealization (neurotic) F48.1

Dermal — *see* condition

Dermaphytid — *see* Dermatophytosis

Dermatitis (eczematous) L3Ø.9
- ab igne L59.Ø
- acarine B88.Ø
- actinic (due to sun) L57.8
  - other than from sun L59.8
- allergic — *see* Dermatitis, contact, allergic
- ambustionis, due to burn or scald — *see* Burn
- amebic AØ6.7
- ammonia L22
- arsenical (ingested) L27.8
- artefacta L98.1
  - psychogenic F54
- atopic L2Ø.9
  - psychogenic F54
  - specified NEC L2Ø.89
- autoimmune progesterone L3Ø.8
- berlock, berloque L56.2
- blastomycotic B4Ø.3
- blister beetle L24.89
- bullous, bullosa L13.9
  - mucosynechial, atrophic L12.1
  - seasonal L3Ø.8
  - specified NEC L13.8
- calorica L59.Ø
  - due to burn or scald — *see* Burn
- caterpillar L24.89
- cercarial B65.3
- combustionis L59.Ø
  - due to burn or scald — *see* Burn
- congelationis T69.1 ☑
- contact (occupational) L25.9
  - allergic L23.9
    - due to
      - adhesives L23.1
      - cement L23.5
      - chemical products NEC L23.5
      - chromium L23.Ø
      - cosmetics L23.2
      - dander (cat) (dog) L23.81
      - drugs in contact with skin L23.3
      - dyes L23.4
      - food in contact with skin L23.6
      - hair (cat) (dog) L23.81
      - insecticide L23.5
      - metals L23.Ø
      - nickel L23.Ø
      - plants, non-food L23.7
      - plastic L23.5
      - rubber L23.5
      - specified agent NEC L23.89
  - due to
    - cement L25.3
    - chemical products NEC L25.3
    - cosmetics L25.Ø
    - dander (cat) (dog) L23.81
    - drugs in contact with skin L25.1
    - dyes L25.2
    - food in contact with skin L25.4
    - hair (cat) (dog) L23.81
    - plants, non-food L25.5
    - specified agent NEC L25.8
  - irritant L24.9

- **Dermatitis** — *continued*
  - contact — *continued*
    - irritant — *continued*
      - due to
        - body fluids L24.AØ
          - incontinence (dual) (fecal) (urinary) L24.A2
          - saliva L24.A1
          - specified NEC L24.A9
        - cement L24.5
        - chemical products NEC L24.5
        - cosmetics L24.3
        - detergents L24.Ø
        - drugs in contact with skin L24.4
        - food in contact with skin L24.6
        - oils and greases L24.1
        - plants, non-food L24.7
        - solvents L24.2
        - specified agent NEC L24.89
      - related to
        - colostomy L24.B3
        - endotracheal tube L24.A9
        - enterocutaneous fistula L24.B3
        - gastrostomy L24.B1
        - ileostomy L24.B3
        - jejunostomy L24.B1
        - saliva or spit fistula L24.B1
        - stoma or fistula L24.BØ
          - digestive L24.B1
          - fecal or urinary L24.B3
          - respiratory L24.B2
        - tracheostomy L24.B2
  - contusiformis L52
  - desquamative L3Ø.8
  - diabetic — *see* EØ8-E13 with .62Ø
  - diaper L22
  - diphtheritica A36.3
  - dry skin L85.3
  - due to
    - acetone (contact) (irritant) L24.2
    - acids (contact) (irritant) L24.5
    - adhesive(s) (allergic) (contact) (plaster) L23.1
      - irritant L24.5
    - alcohol (irritant) (skin contact) (substances in category T51) L24.2
      - taken internally L27.8
    - alkalis (contact) (irritant) L24.5
    - arsenic (ingested) L27.8
    - carbon disulfide (contact) (irritant) L24.2
    - caustics (contact) (irritant) L24.5
    - cement (contact) L25.3
    - cereal (ingested) L27.2
    - chemical(s) NEC L25.3
      - taken internally L27.8
    - chlorocompounds L24.2
    - chromium (contact) (irritant) L24.81
    - coffee (ingested) L27.2
    - cold weather L3Ø.8
    - cosmetics (contact) L25.Ø
      - allergic L23.2
      - irritant L24.3
    - cyclohexanes L24.2
    - dander (cat) (dog) L23.81
    - Demodex species B88.Ø
    - Dermanyssus gallinae B88.Ø
    - detergents (contact) (irritant) L24.Ø
    - dichromate L24.81
    - drugs and medicaments (generalized) (internal use) L27.Ø
      - external — *see* Dermatitis, due to, drugs, in contact with skin
      - in contact with skin L25.1
        - allergic L23.3
        - irritant L24.4
      - localized skin eruption L27.1
      - specified substance — *see* Table of Drugs and Chemicals
    - dyes (contact) L25.2
      - allergic L23.4
      - irritant L24.89
    - epidermophytosis — *see* Dermatophytosis
    - esters L24.2
    - external irritant NEC L24.9
    - fish (ingested) L27.2
    - flour (ingested) L27.2
    - food (ingested) L27.2
      - in contact with skin L25.4
    - fruit (ingested) L27.2
    - furs (allergic) (contact) L23.81

- **Dermatitis** — *continued*
  - due to — *continued*
    - glues — *see* Dermatitis, due to, adhesives
    - glycols L24.2
    - greases NEC (contact) (irritant) L24.1
    - hair (cat) (dog) L23.81
    - hot
      - objects and materials — *see* Burn
      - weather or places L59.Ø
    - hydrocarbons L24.2
    - infrared rays L59.8
    - ingestion, ingested substance L27.9
      - chemical NEC L27.8
      - drugs and medicaments — *see* Dermatitis, due to, drugs
      - food L27.2
      - specified NEC L27.8
    - insecticide in contact with skin L24.5
    - internal agent L27.9
      - drugs and medicaments (generalized) — *see* Dermatitis, due to, drugs
      - food L27.2
    - irradiation — *see* Dermatitis, due to, radioactive substance
    - ketones L24.2
    - lacquer tree (allergic) (contact) L23.7
    - light (sun) NEC L57.8
      - acute L56.8
      - other L59.8
    - Liponyssoides sanguineus B88.Ø
    - low temperature L3Ø.8
    - meat (ingested) L27.2
    - metals, metal salts (contact) (irritant) L24.81
    - milk (ingested) L27.2
    - nickel (contact) (irritant) L24.81
    - nylon (contact) (irritant) L24.5
    - oils NEC (contact) (irritant) L24.1
    - paint solvent (contact) (irritant) L24.2
    - petroleum products (contact) (irritant) (substances in T52.Ø) L24.2
    - plants NEC (contact) L25.5
      - allergic L23.7
      - irritant L24.7
    - plasters (adhesive) (any) (allergic) (contact) L23.1
      - irritant L24.5
    - plastic (contact) L25.3
    - preservatives (contact) — *see* Dermatitis, due to, chemical, in contact with skin
    - primrose (allergic) (contact) L23.7
    - primula (allergic) (contact) L23.7
    - radiation L59.8
      - nonionizing (chronic exposure) L57.8
      - sun NEC L57.8
        - acute L56.8
    - radioactive substance L58.9
      - acute L58.Ø
      - chronic L58.1
    - radium L58.9
      - acute L58.Ø
      - chronic L58.1
    - ragweed (allergic) (contact) L23.7
    - Rhus (allergic) (contact) (diversiloba) (radicans) (toxicodendron) (venenata) (verniciflua) L23.7
    - rubber (contact) L24.5
    - Senecio jacobaea (allergic) (contact) L23.7
    - solvents (contact) (irritant) (substances in category T52) L24.2
    - specified agent NEC (contact) L25.8
      - allergic L23.89
      - irritant L24.89
    - sunshine NEC L57.8
      - acute L56.8
    - tetrachlorethylene (contact) (irritant) L24.2
    - toluene (contact) (irritant) L24.2
    - turpentine (contact) L24.2
    - ultraviolet rays (sun NEC) (chronic exposure) L57.8
      - acute L56.8
    - vaccine or vaccination L27.Ø
      - specified substance — *see* Table of Drugs and Chemicals
    - varicose veins — *see* Varix, leg, with, inflammation
    - X-rays L58.9
      - acute L58.Ø
      - chronic L58.1
  - dyshydrotic L3Ø.1
  - dysmenorrheica N94.6
  - escharotica — *see* Burn
  - exfoliative, exfoliativa (generalized) L26

- **Dermatitis** — *continued*
  - exfoliative, exfoliativa — *continued*
    - neonatorum LØØ
  - eyelid — *see also* Dermatosis, eyelid HØ1.9
    - allergic HØ1.119
      - left HØ1.116
        - lower HØ1.115
        - upper HØ1.114
      - right HØ1.113
        - lower HØ1.112
        - upper HØ1.111
    - contact — *see* Dermatitis, eyelid, allergic
    - due to
      - Demodex species B88.Ø
      - herpes (zoster) BØ2.39
        - simplex BØØ.59
    - eczematous HØ1.139
      - left HØ1.136
        - lower HØ1.135
        - upper HØ1.134
      - right HØ1.133
        - lower HØ1.132
        - upper HØ1.131
    - specified NEC HØ1.8
  - facta, factitia, factitial L98.1
    - psychogenic F54
  - flexural NEC L2Ø.82
  - friction L3Ø.4
  - fungus B36.9
    - specified type NEC B36.8
  - gangrenosa, gangrenous infantum LØ8.Ø
  - harvest mite B88.Ø
  - heat L59.Ø
  - herpesviral, vesicular (ear) (lip) BØØ.1
  - herpetiformis (bullous) (erythematous) (pustular) (vesicular) L13.Ø
    - juvenile L12.2
    - senile L12.Ø
  - hiemalis L3Ø.8
  - hypostatic, hypostatica — *see* Varix, leg, with, inflammation
  - infectious eczematoid L3Ø.3
  - infective L3Ø.3
  - irritant — *see* Dermatitis, contact, irritant
  - Jacquet's (diaper dermatitis) L22
  - Leptus B88.Ø
  - lichenified NEC L28.Ø
  - medicamentosa (generalized) (internal use) — *see* Dermatitis, due to drugs
  - mite B88.Ø
  - multiformis L13.Ø
    - juvenile L12.2
  - napkin L22
  - neurotica L13.Ø
  - nummular L3Ø.Ø
  - papillaris capillitii L73.Ø
  - pellagrous E52
  - perioral L71.Ø
  - photocontact L56.2
  - polymorpha dolorosa L13.Ø
  - pruriginosa L13.Ø
  - pruritic NEC L3Ø.8
  - psychogenic F54
  - purulent LØ8.Ø
  - pustular
    - contagious BØ8.Ø2
    - subcorneal L13.1
  - pyococcal LØ8.Ø
  - pyogenica LØ8.Ø
  - repens L4Ø.2
  - Ritter's (exfoliativa) LØØ
  - Schamberg's L81.7
  - schistosome B65.3
  - seasonal bullous L3Ø.8
  - seborrheic L21.9
    - infantile L21.1
    - specified NEC L21.8
  - sensitization NOS L23.9
  - septic LØ8.Ø
  - solare L57.8
  - specified NEC L3Ø.8
  - stasis I87.2
    - with
      - varicose ulcer — *see* Varix, leg, with ulcer, with inflammation
      - varicose veins — *see* Varix, leg, with, inflammation

Dermatitis — *continued*
- stasis — *continued*
  - due to postthrombotic syndrome — *see* Syndrome, postthrombotic
- suppurative L08.Ø
- traumatic NEC L3Ø.4
- trophoneurotica L13.Ø
- ultraviolet (sun) (chronic exposure) L57.8
  - acute L56.8
- varicose — *see* Varix, leg, with, inflammation
- vegetans L1Ø.1
- verrucosa B43.Ø
- vesicular, herpesviral BØØ.1

Dermatoarthritis, lipoid E78.81

Dermatochalasis, eyelid HØ2.839
- left HØ2.836
  - lower HØ2.835
  - upper HØ2.834
- right HØ2.833
  - lower HØ2.832
  - upper HØ2.831

Dermatofibroma (lenticulare) — *see* Neoplasm, skin, benign
- protuberans — *see* Neoplasm, skin, uncertain behavior

Dermatofibrosarcoma (pigmented) (protuberans) — *see* Neoplasm, skin, malignant

Dermatographia L5Ø.3

Dermatolysis (exfoliativa) (congenital) Q82.8
- acquired L57.4
- eyelids — *see* Blepharochalasis
- palpebrarum — *see* Blepharochalasis
- senile L57.4

Dermatomegaly NEC Q82.8

Dermatomucosomyositis — *see also* Dermatomyositis M33.1Ø
- with
  - myopathy M33.12
  - respiratory involvement M33.11
  - specified organ involvement NEC M33.19

Dermatomycosis B36.9
- furfuracea B36.Ø
- specified type NEC B36.8

Dermatomyositis (acute) (chronic) — *see also* Dermatopolymyositis
- adult — *see also* Dermatomyositis, specified NEC M33.1Ø
- in (due to) neoplastic disease — *see also* Neoplasm D49.9 *[M36.Ø]*
- juvenile M33.ØØ
  - with
    - myopathy M33.Ø2
    - respiratory involvement M33.Ø1
    - specified organ involvement NEC M33.Ø9
  - amyopathic M33.Ø3
  - without myopathy M33.Ø3
- specified NEC M33.1Ø
  - with
    - myopathy M33.12
    - respiratory involvement M33.11
    - specified organ involvement NEC M33.19
  - amyopathic M33.13
  - without myopathy M33.13

Dermatoneuritis of children — *see* Poisoning, mercury

Dermatophilosis A48.8

Dermatophytid L3Ø.2

Dermatophytide — *see* Dermatophytosis

Dermatophytosis (epidermophyton) (infection) (Microsporum) (tinea) (Trichophyton) B35.9
- beard B35.Ø
- body B35.4
- capitis B35.Ø
- corporis B35.4
- deep-seated B35.8
- disseminated B35.8
- foot B35.3
- granulomatous B35.8
- groin B35.6
- hand B35.2
- nail B35.1
- perianal (area) B35.6
- scalp B35.Ø
- specified NEC B35.8

Dermatopolymyositis M33.9Ø
- with
  - myopathy M33.92
  - respiratory involvement M33.91
  - specified organ involvement NEC M33.99
- amyopathic M33.93

Dermatopolymyositis — *continued*
- in neoplastic disease — *see also* Neoplasm D49.9 *[M36.Ø]*
- juvenile M33.ØØ
  - with
    - myopathy M33.Ø2
    - respiratory involvement M33.Ø1
    - specified organ involvement NEC M33.Ø9
  - amyopathic M33.Ø3
  - without myopathy M33.Ø3
- specified NEC M33.1Ø
  - amyopathic M33.13
  - myopathy M33.12
  - respiratory involvement M33.11
  - specified organ involvement NEC M33.19
  - without myopathy M33.13
- without myopathy M33.93

Dermatopolyneuritis — *see* Poisoning, mercury

Dermatorrhexis — *see also* Syndrome, Ehlers-Danlos Q79.6Ø
- acquired L57.4

Dermatosclerosis — *see also* Scleroderma
- localized L94.Ø

Dermatosis L98.9
- Andrews' LØ8.89
- Bowen's — *see* Neoplasm, skin, in situ
- bullous L13.9
  - specified NEC L13.8
- exfoliativa L26
- eyelid (noninfectious) — *see also* Dermatitis, eyelid HØ1.9
  - discoid lupus erythematosus — *see* Lupus, erythematosus, eyelid
  - xeroderma — *see* Xeroderma, acquired, eyelid
- factitial L98.1
- febrile neutrophilic L98.2
- gonococcal A54.89
- herpetiformis L13.Ø
  - juvenile L12.2
- linear IgA L13.8
- menstrual NEC L98.8
- neutrophilic, febrile L98.2
- occupational — *see* Dermatitis, contact
- papulosa nigra L82.1
- pigmentary L81.9
  - progressive L81.7
  - Schamberg's L81.7
- psychogenic F54
- purpuric, pigmented L81.7
- pustular, subcorneal L13.1
- transient acantholytic L11.1

Dermographia, dermographism L5Ø.3

Dermoid (cyst) — *see also* Neoplasm, benign, by site
- with malignant transformation C56- ☑
- due to radiation (nonionizing) L57.8

Dermopathy
- infiltrative with thyrotoxicosis — *see* Thyrotoxicosis
- nephrogenic fibrosing L9Ø.8

Dermophytosis — *see* Dermatophytosis

Descemetocele H18.73- ☑

Descemet's membrane — *see* condition

Descending — *see* condition

Descensus uteri — *see* Prolapse, uterus

Desert
- rheumatism B38.Ø
- sore — *see* Ulcer, skin

Desertion (newborn) — *see* Maltreatment

Desmoid (extra-abdominal) (tumor) — *see* Neoplasm, connective tissue, uncertain behavior
- abdominal D48.1

Despondency F32.A

Desquamation, skin R23.4

Destruction, destructive — *see also* Damage
- articular facet — *see also* Derangement, joint, specified type NEC
  - knee M23.8X- ☑
  - vertebra — *see* Spondylosis
- bone — *see also* Disorder, bone, specified type NEC
  - syphilitic A52.77
- joint — *see also* Derangement, joint, specified type NEC
  - sacroiliac M53.3
- rectal sphincter K62.89
- septum (nasal) J34.89
- tuberculous NEC — *see* Tuberculosis
- tympanum, tympanic membrane (nontraumatic) — *see* Disorder, tympanic membrane, specified NEC
- vertebral disc — *see* Degeneration, intervertebral disc

Destructiveness — *see also* Disorder, conduct
- adjustment reaction — *see* Disorder, adjustment

Desultory labor O62.2

Detachment
- cartilage — *see* Sprain
- cervix, annular N88.8
  - complicating delivery O71.3
- choroid (old) (postinfectional) (simple) (spontaneous) H31.4Ø- ☑
  - hemorrhagic H31.41- ☑
  - serous H31.42- ☑
- ligament — *see* Sprain
- meniscus (knee) — *see also* Derangement, knee, meniscus, specified NEC
  - current injury — *see* Tear, meniscus
  - due to old tear or injury — *see* Derangement, knee, meniscus, due to old tear
- retina (without retinal break) (serous) H33.2- ☑
  - with retinal:
    - break H33.ØØ- ☑
      - giant H33.Ø3- ☑
      - multiple H33.Ø2- ☑
      - single H33.Ø1- ☑
    - dialysis H33.Ø4- ☑
  - pigment epithelium — *see* Degeneration, retina, separation of layers, pigment epithelium detachment
  - rhegmatogenous — *see* Detachment, retina, with retinal, break
  - specified NEC H33.8
  - total H33.Ø5- ☑
  - traction H33.4- ☑
- vitreous (body) H43.81 ☑

Detergent asthma J69.8

Deterioration
- epileptic FØ6.8
- general physical R53.81
- heart, cardiac — *see* Degeneration, myocardial
- mental — *see* Psychosis
- myocardial, myocardium — *see* Degeneration, myocardial
- senile (simple) R54

Deuteranomaly (anomalous trichromat) H53.53

Deuteranopia (complete) (incomplete) H53.53

Development
- abnormal, bone Q79.9
- arrested R62.5Ø
  - bone — *see* Arrest, development or growth, bone
  - child R62.5Ø
  - due to malnutrition E45
- defective, congenital — *see also* Anomaly, by site
  - cauda equina QØ6.3
  - left ventricle Q24.8
    - in hypoplastic left heart syndrome Q23.4
  - valve Q24.8
    - pulmonary Q22.3
- delayed — *see also* Delay, development R62.5Ø
  - arithmetical skills F81.2
  - language (skills) (expressive) F8Ø.1
  - learning skill F81.9
  - mixed skills F88
  - motor coordination F82
  - reading F81.Ø
  - specified learning skill NEC F81.89
  - speech F8Ø.9
  - spelling F81.81
  - written expression F81.81
- imperfect, congenital — *see also* Anomaly, by site
  - heart Q24.9
  - lungs Q33.6
- incomplete
  - bronchial tree Q32.4
  - organ or site not listed — *see* Hypoplasia, by site
  - respiratory system Q34.9
- sexual, precocious NEC E3Ø.1
- tardy, mental — *see also* Disability, intellectual F79

Developmental — *see* condition
- testing, infant or child — *see* Examination, child

Devergie's disease (pityriasis rubra pilaris) L44.Ø

Deviation (in)
- conjugate palsy (eye) (spastic) H51.Ø
- esophagus (acquired) K22.89
- eye, skew H51.8
- midline (jaw) (teeth) (dental arch) M26.29
  - specified site NEC — *see* Malposition
- nasal septum J34.2
  - congenital Q67.4

- **Deviation** — *continued*
  - opening and closing of the mandible M26.53
  - organ or site, congenital NEC — *see* Malposition, congenital
  - septum (nasal) (acquired) J34.2
    - congenital Q67.4
  - sexual F65.9
    - bestiality F65.89
    - erotomania F52.8
    - exhibitionism F65.2
    - fetishism, fetishistic F65.Ø
      - transvestism F65.1
    - frotteurism F65.81
    - masochism F65.51
    - multiple F65.89
    - necrophilia F65.89
    - nymphomania F52.8
    - pederosis F65.4
    - pedophilia F65.4
    - sadism, sadomasochism F65.52
    - satyriasis F52.8
    - specified type NEC F65.89
    - transvestism F64.1
    - voyeurism F65.3
  - teeth, midline M26.29
  - trachea J39.8
  - ureter, congenital Q62.61
- **Device**
  - cerebral ventricle (communicating) in situ Z98.2
  - contraceptive — *see* Contraceptive, device
  - drainage, cerebrospinal fluid, in situ Z98.2
- **Devic's disease** G36.Ø
- **Devil's**
  - grip B33.Ø
  - pinches (purpura simplex) D69.2
- **Devitalized tooth** KØ4.99
- **Devonshire colic** — *see* Poisoning, lead
- **Dextraposition, aorta** Q2Ø.3
  - in tetralogy of Fallot Q21.3
- **Dextrinosis, limit** (debrancher enzyme deficiency) E74.Ø3
- **Dextrocardia** (true) Q24.Ø
  - with
    - complete transposition of viscera Q89.3
    - situs inversus Q89.3
- **Dextrotransposition, aorta** Q2Ø.3
- **d-glycericacidemia** E72.59
- **Dhat syndrome** F48.8
- **Dhobi itch** B35.6
- **Di George's syndrome** D82.1
- **Di Guglielmo's disease** C94.Ø- ☑
- **Diabetes, diabetic** (mellitus) (sugar) E11.9
  - with
    - amyotrophy E11.44
    - arthropathy NEC E11.618
    - autonomic (poly)neuropathy E11.43
    - cataract E11.36
    - Charcot's joints E11.61Ø
    - chronic kidney disease E11.22
    - circulatory complication NEC E11.59
    - coma due to
      - hyperosmolarity E11.Ø1
      - hypoglycemia E11.641
      - ketoacidosis E11.11
    - complication E11.8
      - specified NEC E11.69
    - dermatitis E11.62Ø
    - foot ulcer E11.621
    - gangrene E11.52
    - gastroparalysis E11.43
    - gastroparesis E11.43
    - glomerulonephrosis, intracapillary E11.21
    - glomerulosclerosis, intercapillary E11.21
    - hyperglycemia E11.65
    - hyperosmolarity E11.ØØ
      - with coma E11.Ø1
    - hypoglycemia E11.649
      - with coma E11.641
    - ketoacidosis E11.1Ø
      - with coma E11.11
    - kidney complications NEC E11.29
    - Kimmelstiel-Wilson disease E11.21
    - loss of protective sensation (LOPS) — *see* Diabetes, by type, with neuropathy
    - mononeuropathy E11.41
    - myasthenia E11.44
    - necrobiosis lipoidica E11.62Ø
    - nephropathy E11.21
    - neuralgia E11.42

- **Diabetes, diabetic** — *continued*
  - with — *continued*
    - neurologic complication NEC E11.49
    - neuropathic arthropathy E11.61Ø
    - neuropathy E11.4Ø
    - ophthalmic complication NEC E11.39
    - oral complication NEC E11.638
    - osteomyelitis E11.69
    - periodontal disease E11.63Ø
    - peripheral angiopathy E11.51
      - with gangrene E11.52
    - polyneuropathy E11.42
    - renal complication NEC E11.29
    - renal tubular degeneration E11.29
    - retinopathy E11.319
      - with macular edema E11.311
        - resolved following treatment E11.37- ☑
      - nonproliferative E11.329 ☑
        - with macular edema E11.321 ☑
        - mild E11.329 ☑
          - with macular edema E11.321 ☑
        - moderate E11.339 ☑
          - with macular edema E11.331 ☑
        - severe E11.349 ☑
          - with macular edema E11.341 ☑
      - proliferative E11.359 ☑
        - with
          - combined traction retinal detachment and rhegmatogenous retinal detachment E11.354 ☑
          - macular edema E11.351 ☑
          - stable proliferative diabetic retinopathy E11.355 ☑
          - traction retinal detachment involving the macula E11.352 ☑
          - traction retinal detachment not involving the macula E11.353 ☑
    - skin complication NEC E11.628
    - skin ulcer NEC E11.622
  - brittle — *see* Diabetes, type 1
  - bronzed E83.11Ø
  - complicating pregnancy — *see* Pregnancy, complicated by, diabetes
  - dietary counseling and surveillance Z71.3
  - due to
    - autoimmune process — *see* Diabetes, type 1
    - immune mediated pancreatic islet beta-cell destruction — *see* Diabetes, type 1
  - due to drug or chemical EØ9.9
    - with
      - amyotrophy EØ9.44
      - arthropathy NEC EØ9.618
      - autonomic (poly)neuropathy EØ9.43
      - cataract EØ9.36
      - Charcot's joints EØ9.61Ø
      - chronic kidney disease EØ9.22
      - circulatory complication NEC EØ9.59
      - complication EØ9.8
        - specified NEC EØ9.69
      - dermatitis EØ9.62Ø
      - foot ulcer EØ9.621
      - gangrene EØ9.52
      - gastroparalysis EØ9.43
      - gastroparesis EØ9.43
      - glomerulonephrosis, intracapillary EØ9.21
      - glomerulosclerosis, intercapillary EØ9.21
      - hyperglycemia EØ9.65
      - hyperosmolarity EØ9.ØØ
        - with coma EØ9.Ø1
      - hypoglycemia EØ9.649
        - with coma EØ9.641
      - ketoacidosis EØ9.1Ø
        - with coma EØ9.11
      - kidney complications NEC EØ9.29
      - Kimmelstiel-Wilson disease EØ9.21
      - mononeuropathy EØ9.41
      - myasthenia EØ9.44
      - necrobiosis lipoidica EØ9.62Ø
      - nephropathy EØ9.21
      - neuralgia EØ9.42
      - neurologic complication NEC EØ9.49
      - neuropathic arthropathy EØ9.61Ø
      - neuropathy EØ9.4Ø
      - ophthalmic complication NEC EØ9.39
      - oral complication NEC EØ9.638
      - periodontal disease EØ9.63Ø
      - peripheral angiopathy EØ9.51
        - with gangrene EØ9.52

- **Diabetes, diabetic** — *continued*
  - due to drug or chemical — *continued*
    - with — *continued*
      - polyneuropathy EØ9.42
      - renal complication NEC EØ9.29
      - renal tubular degeneration EØ9.29
      - retinopathy EØ9.319
        - with macular edema EØ9.311
          - resolved following treatment EØ9.37 ☑
        - nonproliferative EØ9.329 ☑
          - with macular edema EØ9.321 ☑
          - mild EØ9.329 ☑
            - with macular edema EØ9.321 ☑
          - moderate EØ9.339 ☑
            - with macular edema EØ9.331 ☑
          - severe EØ9.349 ☑
            - with macular edema EØ9.341 ☑
        - proliferative EØ9.359 ☑
          - with
            - combined traction retinal detachment and rhegmatogenous retinal detachment EØ9.354 ☑
            - macular edema EØ9.351 ☑
            - stable proliferative diabetic retinopathy EØ9.355 ☑
            - traction retinal detachment involving the macula EØ9.352 ☑
            - traction retinal detachment not involving the macula EØ9.353 ☑
      - skin complication NEC EØ9.628
      - skin ulcer NEC EØ9.622
  - due to underlying condition EØ8.9
    - with
      - amyotrophy EØ8.44
      - arthropathy NEC EØ8.618
      - autonomic (poly)neuropathy EØ8.43
      - cataract EØ8.36
      - Charcot's joints EØ8.61Ø
      - chronic kidney disease EØ8.22
      - circulatory complication NEC EØ8.59
      - complication EØ8.8
        - specified NEC EØ8.69
      - dermatitis EØ8.62Ø
      - foot ulcer EØ8.621
      - gangrene EØ8.52
      - gastroparalysis EØ8.43
      - gastroparesis EØ8.43
      - glomerulonephrosis, intracapillary EØ8.21
      - glomerulosclerosis, intercapillary EØ8.21
      - hyperglycemia EØ8.65
      - hyperosmolarity EØ8.ØØ
        - with coma EØ8.Ø1
      - hypoglycemia EØ8.649
        - with coma EØ8.641
      - ketoacidosis EØ8.1Ø
        - with coma EØ8.11
      - kidney complications NEC EØ8.29
      - Kimmelstiel-WIlson disease EØ8.21
      - mononeuropathy EØ8.41
      - myasthenia EØ8.44
      - necrobiosis lipoidica EØ8.62Ø
      - nephropathy EØ8.21
      - neuralgia EØ8.42
      - neurologic complication NEC EØ8.49
      - neuropathic arthropathy EØ8.61Ø
      - neuropathy EØ8.4Ø
      - ophthalmic complication NEC EØ8.39
      - oral complication NEC EØ8.638
      - periodontal disease EØ8.63Ø
      - peripheral angiopathy EØ8.51
        - with gangrene EØ8.52
      - polyneuropathy EØ8.42
      - renal complication NEC EØ8.29
      - renal tubular degeneration EØ8.29
      - retinopathy EØ8.319
        - with macular edema EØ8.311
          - resolved following treatment EØ8.37 ☑
        - nonproliferative EØ8.329 ☑
          - with macular edema EØ8.321 ☑
          - mild EØ8.329 ☑
            - with macular edema EØ8.321 ☑
          - moderate EØ8.339 ☑
            - with macular edema EØ8.331 ☑
          - severe EØ8.349 ☑
            - with macular edema EØ8.341 ☑
        - proliferative EØ8.359 ☑

- **Diabetes, diabetic** — *continued*
  - due to underlying condition — *continued*
    - with — *continued*
      - retinopathy — *continued*
        - proliferative — *continued*
          - with
            - combined traction retinal detachment and rhegmatogenous retinal detachment E08.354 ☑
            - macular edema E08.351 ☑
            - stable proliferative diabetic retinopathy E08.355 ☑
            - traction retinal detachment involving the macula E08.352 ☑
            - traction retinal detachment not involving the macula E08.353 ☑
      - skin complication NEC E08.628
      - skin ulcer NEC E08.622
  - gestational (in pregnancy) O24.419
    - affecting newborn P70.0
    - diet controlled O24.410
    - in childbirth O24.429
      - diet controlled O24.420
      - insulin (and diet) controlled O24.424
      - oral drug controlled (antidiabetic) (hypoglycemic) O24.425
    - insulin (and diet) controlled O24.414
    - oral drug controlled (antidiabetic) (hypoglycemic) O24.415
    - puerperal O24.439
      - diet controlled O24.430
      - insulin (and diet) controlled O24.434
      - oral drug controlled (antidiabetic) (hypoglycemic) O24.435
  - hepatogenous E13.9
  - idiopathic — *see* Diabetes, type 1
  - inadequately controlled — *see* Diabetes, by type, with hyperglycemia
  - insipidus E23.2
    - nephrogenic N25.1
    - pituitary E23.2
    - vasopressin resistant N25.1
  - insulin dependent — *code to* type of diabetes
  - juvenile-onset — *see* Diabetes, type 1
  - ketosis-prone — *see* Diabetes, type 1
  - latent R73.03
  - neonatal (transient) P70.2
  - non-insulin dependent — *code to* type of diabetes
  - out of control — *see* Diabetes, by type, with hyperglycemia
  - phosphate E83.39
  - poorly controlled — *see* Diabetes, by type, with hyperglycemia
  - postpancreatectomy — *see* Diabetes, specified type NEC
  - postprocedural — *see* Diabetes, specified type NEC
  - retina, hemorrhage E13.39
  - secondary diabetes mellitus NEC — *see* Diabetes, specified type NEC
  - specified type NEC E13.9
    - with
      - amyotrophy E13.44
      - arthropathy NEC E13.618
      - autonomic (poly)neuropathy E13.43
      - cataract E13.36
      - Charcot's joints E13.610
      - chronic kidney disease E13.22
      - circulatory complication NEC E13.59
      - complication E13.8
        - specified NEC E13.69
      - dermatitis E13.620
      - foot ulcer E13.621
      - gangrene E13.52
      - gastroparalysis E13.43
      - gastroparesis E13.43
      - glomerulonephrosis, intracapillary E13.21
      - glomerulosclerosis, intercapillary E13.21
      - hyperglycemia E13.65
      - hyperosmolarity E13.00
        - with coma E13.01
      - hypoglycemia E13.649
        - with coma E13.641
      - ketoacidosis E13.10
        - with coma E13.11
      - kidney complications NEC E13.29
      - Kimmelsteil-Wilson disease E13.21
      - mononeuropathy E13.41
      - myasthenia E13.44

- **Diabetes, diabetic** — *continued*
  - specified type — *continued*
    - with — *continued*
      - necrobiosis lipoidica E13.620
      - nephropathy E13.21
      - neuralgia E13.42
      - neurologic complication NEC E13.49
      - neuropathic arthropathy E13.610
      - neuropathy E13.40
      - ophthalmic complication NEC E13.39
      - oral complication NEC E13.638
      - periodontal disease E13.630
      - peripheral angiopathy E13.51
        - with gangrene E13.52
      - polyneuropathy E13.42
      - renal complication NEC E13.29
      - renal tubular degeneration E13.29
      - retinopathy E13.319
        - with macular edema E13.311
        - resolved following treatment E13.37 ☑
        - nonproliferative E13.329 ☑
          - with macular edema E13.321 ☑
          - mild E13.329 ☑
            - with macular edema E13.321 ☑
          - moderate E13.339 ☑
            - with macular edema E13.331 ☑
          - severe E13.349 ☑
            - with macular edema E13.341 ☑
        - proliferative E13.359 ☑
          - with
            - combined traction retinal detachment and rhegmatogenous retinal detachment E13.354 ☑
            - macular edema E13.351 ☑
            - stable proliferative diabetic retinopathy E13.355 ☑
            - traction retinal detachment involving the macula E13.352 ☑
            - traction retinal detachment not involving the macula E13.353 ☑
      - skin complication NEC E13.628
      - skin ulcer NEC E13.622
  - steroid-induced — *see* Diabetes, due to, drug or chemical
  - type 1 E10.9
    - with
      - amyotrophy E10.44
      - arthropathy NEC E10.618
      - autonomic (poly)neuropathy E10.43
      - cataract E10.36
      - Charcot's joints E10.610
      - chronic kidney disease E10.22
      - circulatory complication NEC E10.59
      - coma due to
        - hyperosmolarity E11.01
        - hypoglycemia E11.641
        - ketoacidosis E10.11
      - complication E10.8
        - specified NEC E10.69
      - dermatitis E10.620
      - foot ulcer E10.621
      - gangrene E10.52
      - gastroparalysis E10.43
      - gastroparesis E10.43
      - glomerulonephrosis, intracapillary E10.21
      - glomerulosclerosis, intercapillary E10.21
      - hyperglycemia E10.65
      - hypoglycemia E10.649
        - with coma E10.641
      - ketoacidosis E10.10
        - with coma E10.11
      - kidney complications NEC E10.29
      - Kimmelsteil-Wilson disease E10.21
      - mononeuropathy E10.41
      - myasthenia E10.44
      - necrobiosis lipoidica E10.620
      - nephropathy E10.21
      - neuralgia E10.42
      - neurologic complication NEC E10.49
      - neuropathic arthropathy E10.610
      - neuropathy E10.40
      - ophthalmic complication NEC E10.39
      - oral complication NEC E10.638
      - osteomyelitis E10.69
      - periodontal disease E10.630
      - peripheral angiopathy E10.51
        - with gangrene E10.52
      - polyneuropathy E10.42

- **Diabetes, diabetic** — *continued*
  - type 1 — *continued*
    - with — *continued*
      - renal complication NEC E10.29
      - renal tubular degeneration E10.29
      - retinopathy E10.319
        - with macular edema E10.311
        - resolved following treatment E10.37 ☑
        - nonproliferative E10.329 ☑
          - with macular edema E10.321 ☑
          - mild E10.329 ☑
            - with macular edema E10.321 ☑
          - moderate E10.339 ☑
            - with macular edema E10.331 ☑
          - severe E10.349 ☑
            - with macular edema E10.341 ☑
        - proliferative E10.359 ☑
          - with
            - combined traction retinal detachment and rhegmatogenous retinal detachment E10.354 ☑
            - macular edema E10.351 ☑
            - stable proliferative diabetic retinopathy E10.355 ☑
            - traction retinal detachment involving the macula E10.352 ☑
            - traction retinal detachment not involving the macula E10.353 ☑
      - skin complication NEC E10.628
      - skin ulcer NEC E10.622
  - type 2 E11.9
    - with
      - amyotrophy E11.44
      - arthropathy NEC E11.618
      - autonomic (poly)neuropathy E11.43
      - cataract E11.36
      - Charcot's joints E11.610
      - chronic kidney disease E11.22
      - circulatory complication NEC E11.59
      - coma due to
        - hyperosmolarity E11.01
        - hypoglycemia E11.641
        - ketoacidosis E11.1- ☑
      - complication E11.8
        - specified NEC E11.69
      - dermatitis E11.620
      - foot ulcer E11.621
      - gangrene E11.52
      - gastroparalysis E11.43
      - gastroparesis E11.43
      - glomerulonephrosis, intracapillary E11.21
      - glomerulosclerosis, intercapillary E11.21
      - hyperglycemia E11.65
      - hyperosmolarity E11.00
        - with coma E11.01
      - hypoglycemia E11.649
        - with coma E11.641
      - ketoacidosis E11.10
        - with coma E11.11
      - kidney complications NEC E11.29
      - Kimmelsteil-Wilson disease E11.21
      - mononeuropathy E11.41
      - myasthenia E11.44
      - necrobiosis lipoidica E11.620
      - nephropathy E11.21
      - neuralgia E11.42
      - neurologic complication NEC E11.49
      - neuropathic arthropathy E11.610
      - neuropathy E11.40
      - ophthalmic complication NEC E11.39
      - oral complication NEC E11.638
      - osteomyelitis E11.69
      - periodontal disease E11.630
      - peripheral angiopathy E11.51
        - with gangrene E11.52
      - polyneuropathy E11.42
      - renal complication NEC E11.29
      - renal tubular degeneration E11.29
      - retinopathy E11.319
        - with macular edema E11.311
        - resolved following treatment E11.37 ☑
        - nonproliferative E11.329 ☑
          - with macular edema E11.321 ☑
          - mild E11.329 ☑
            - with macular edema E11.321 ☑
          - moderate E11.339 ☑
            - with macular edema E11.331 ☑
          - severe E11.349 ☑

Diabetes, diabetic — *continued*
- type 2 — *continued*
  - with — *continued*
    - retinopathy — *continued*
      - nonproliferative — *continued*
        - severe — *continued*
          - with macular edema E11.341 ☑
      - proliferative E11.359 ☑
        - with
          - combined traction retinal detachment and rhegmatogenous retinal detachment E11.354 ☑
          - macular edema E11.351 ☑
          - stable proliferative diabetic retinopathy E11.355 ☑
          - traction retinal detachment involving the macula E11.352 ☑
          - traction retinal detachment not involving the macula E11.353 ☑
    - skin complication NEC E11.628
      - skin ulcer NEC E11.622
- uncontrolled
  - meaning
    - hyperglycemia — *see* Diabetes, by type, with, hyperglycemia
    - hypoglycemia — *see* Diabetes, by type, with, hypoglycemia

Diacyclothrombopathia D69.1

Diagnosis deferred R69

Dialysis (intermittent) (treatment)
- noncompliance (with) Z91.15
- renal (hemodialysis) (peritoneal), status Z99.2
- retina, retinal — *see* Detachment, retina, with retinal, dialysis

Diamond-Blackfan anemia (congenital hypoplastic) D61.Ø1

Diamond-Gardener syndrome (autoerythrocyte sensitization) D69.2

Diaper rash L22

Diaphoresis (excessive) R61

Diaphragm — *see* condition

Diaphragmalgia RØ7.1

Diaphragmatitis, diaphragmitis J98.6

Diaphysial aclasis Q78.6

Diaphysitis — *see* Osteomyelitis, specified type NEC

Diarrhea, diarrheal (disease) (infantile) (inflammatory) R19.7
- achlorhydric K31.83
- allergic K52.29
  - due to
    - colitis — *see* Colitis, allergic
    - enteritis — *see* Enteritis, allergic
- amebic — *see also* Amebiasis AØ6.Ø
  - with abscess — *see* Abscess, amebic
  - acute AØ6.Ø
  - chronic AØ6.1
  - nondysenteric AØ6.2
- bacillary — *see* Dysentery, bacillary
- balantidial AØ7.Ø
- cachectic NEC K52.89
- Chilomastix AØ7.8
- choleriformis AØØ.1
- chronic (noninfectious) K52.9
- coccidial AØ7.3
- Cochin-China K9Ø.1
  - strongyloidiasis B78.Ø
- Dientamoeba AØ7.8
- dietetic — *see also* Diarrhea, allergic K52.29
- drug-induced K52.1
- due to
  - bacteria AØ4.9
    - specified NEC AØ4.8
  - Campylobacter AØ4.5
  - Capillaria philippinensis B81.1
  - Clostridium difficile
    - not specified as recurrent AØ4.72
    - recurrent AØ4.71
  - Clostridium perfringens (C) (F) AØ4.8
  - Cryptosporidium AØ7.2
  - drugs K52.1
  - Escherichia coli AØ4.4
    - enteroaggregative AØ4.4
    - enterohemorrhagic AØ4.3
    - enteroinvasive AØ4.2
    - enteropathogenic AØ4.Ø
    - enterotoxigenic AØ4.1
    - specified NEC AØ4.4

Diarrhea, diarrheal — *continued*
- due to — *continued*
  - food hypersensitivity — *see also* Diarrhea, allergic K52.29
  - Necator americanus B76.1
  - S. japonicum B65.2
  - specified organism NEC AØ8.8
    - bacterial AØ4.8
    - viral AØ8.39
  - Staphylococcus AØ4.8
  - Trichuris trichiuria B79
  - virus — *see* Enteritis, viral
  - Yersinia enterocolitica AØ4.6
- dysenteric AØ9
- endemic AØ9
- epidemic AØ9
- flagellate AØ7.9
- Flexner's (ulcerative) AØ3.1
- functional K59.1
  - following gastrointestinal surgery K91.89
  - psychogenic F45.8
- Giardia lamblia AØ7.1
- giardial AØ7.1
- hill K9Ø.1
- infectious AØ9
- malarial — *see* Malaria
- mite B88.Ø
- mycotic NEC B49
- neonatal (noninfectious) P78.3
- nervous F45.8
- neurogenic K59.1
- noninfectious K52.9
- postgastrectomy K91.1
- postvagotomy K91.1
- protozoal AØ7.9
  - specified NEC AØ7.8
- psychogenic F45.8
- specified
  - bacterium NEC AØ4.8
  - virus NEC AØ8.39
- strongyloidiasis B78.Ø
- toxic K52.1
- trichomonal AØ7.8
- tropical K9Ø.1
- tuberculous A18.32
- viral — *see* Enteritis, viral

Diastasis
- cranial bones M84.88
  - congenital NEC Q75.8
- joint (traumatic) — *see* Dislocation
- muscle M62.ØØ
  - ankle M62.Ø7- ☑
  - congenital Q79.8
  - foot M62.Ø7- ☑
  - forearm M62.Ø3- ☑
  - hand M62.Ø4- ☑
  - lower leg M62.Ø6- ☑
  - pelvic region M62.Ø5- ☑
  - shoulder region M62.Ø1- ☑
  - specified site NEC M62.Ø8
  - thigh M62.Ø5- ☑
  - upper arm M62.Ø2- ☑
- recti (abdomen)
  - complicating delivery O71.89
  - congenital Q79.59

Diastema, tooth, teeth, fully erupted M26.32

Diastematomyelia QØ6.2

Diataxia, cerebral G8Ø.4

Diathesis
- allergic — *see* History, allergy
- bleeding (familial) D69.9
- cystine (familial) E72.ØØ
- gouty — *see* Gout
- hemorrhagic (familial) D69.9
  - newborn NEC P53
- spasmophilic R29.Ø

Diaz's disease or osteochondrosis (juvenile) (talus) — *see* Osteochondrosis, juvenile, tarsus

Dibothriocephalus, dibothriocephaliasis (latus) (infection) (infestation) B7Ø.Ø
- larval B7Ø.1

Dicephalus, dicephaly Q89.4

Dichotomy, teeth KØØ.2

Dichromat, dichromatopsia (congenital) — *see* Deficiency, color vision

Dichuchwa A65

Dicroceliasis B66.2

Didelphia, didelphys — *see* Double uterus

Didymytis N45.1
- with orchitis N45.3

Dietary
- inadequacy or deficiency E63.9
- surveillance and counseling Z71.3

Dietl's crisis N13.8

Dieulafoy lesion (hemorrhagic)
- duodenum K31.82
- esophagus K22.89
- intestine (colon) K63.81
- stomach K31.82

Difficult, difficulty (in)
- acculturation Z6Ø.3
- feeding R63.3Ø
  - newborn P92.9
    - breast P92.5
    - specified NEC P92.8
  - nonorganic (infant or child) F98.29
  - specified NEC R63.39
- intubation, in anesthesia T88.4 ☑
- mechanical, gastroduodenal stoma K91.89
  - causing obstruction — *see also* Obstruction, intestine, postoperative K91.3Ø
- micturition
  - need to immediately re-void R39.191
  - position dependent R39.192
  - specified NEC R39.198
- reading (developmental) F81.Ø
  - secondary to emotional disorders F93.9
- spelling (specific) F81.81
  - with reading disorder F81.89
  - due to inadequate teaching Z55.8
- swallowing — *see* Dysphagia
- walking R26.2
- work
  - conditions NEC Z56.5
  - schedule Z56.3

Diffuse — *see* condition

Digestive — *see* condition

Dihydropyrimidine dehydrogenase disease (DPD) E88.89

Diktyoma — *see* Neoplasm, malignant, by site

Dilaceration, tooth KØØ.4

Dilatation
- anus K59.89
  - venule — *see* Hemorrhoids
- aorta (focal) (general) — *see* Ectasia, aorta
  - with aneuysm — *see* Aneurysm, aorta
  - congenital Q25.44
- artery — *see* Aneurysm
- bladder (sphincter) N32.89
  - congenital Q64.79
- blood vessel I99.8
- bronchial J47.9
  - with
    - exacerbation (acute) J47.1
    - lower respiratory infection J47.Ø
- calyx N28.89
  - due to obstruction — *see* Hydronephrosis
- capillaries I78.8
- cardiac (acute) (chronic) — *see also* Hypertrophy, cardiac
  - congenital Q24.8
    - valve NEC Q24.8
      - pulmonary Q22.3
  - valve — *see* Endocarditis
- cavum septi pellucidi QØ6.8
- cervix (uteri) — *see also* Incompetency, cervix
  - incomplete, poor, slow complicating delivery O62.Ø
- colon K59.39
  - congenital Q43.1
  - psychogenic F45.8
  - toxic K59.31
- common duct (acquired) K83.8
  - congenital Q44.5
- cystic duct (acquired) K82.8
  - congenital Q44.5
- duct, mammary — *see* Ectasia, mammary duct
- duodenum K59.89
- esophagus K22.89
  - congenital Q39.5
  - due to achalasia K22.Ø
- eustachian tube, congenital Q17.8
- gallbladder K82.8
- gastric — *see* Dilatation, stomach
- heart (acute) (chronic) — *see also* Hypertrophy, cardiac
  - congenital Q24.8
  - valve — *see* Endocarditis

Index

Diabetes, diabetic — Dilatation

Dilatation — *continued*
ileum K59.89
psychogenic F45.8
jejunum K59.89
psychogenic F45.8
kidney (calyx) (collecting structures) (cystic) (parenchyma) (pelvis) (idiopathic) N28.89
due to obstruction — *see* Hydronephrosis
lacrimal passages or duct — *see* Disorder, lacrimal system, changes
lymphatic vessel I89.Ø
mammary duct — *see* Ectasia, mammary duct
Meckel's diverticulum (congenital) Q43.Ø
malignant — *see* Table of Neoplasms, small intestine, malignant
myocardium (acute) (chronic) — *see* Hypertrophy, cardiac
organ or site, congenital NEC — *see* Distortion
pancreatic duct K86.89
pericardium — *see* Pericarditis
pharynx J39.2
prostate N42.89
pulmonary
artery (idiopathic) I28.8
valve, congenital Q22.3
pupil H57.Ø4
rectum K59.39
saccule, congenital Q16.5
salivary gland (duct) K11.8
sphincter ani K62.89
stomach K31.89
acute K31.Ø
psychogenic F45.8
submaxillary duct K11.8
trachea, congenital Q32.1
ureter (idiopathic) N28.82
congenital Q62.2
due to obstruction N13.4
urethra (acquired) N36.8
vasomotor I73.9
vein I86.8
ventricular, ventricle (acute) (chronic) — *see also* Hypertrophy, cardiac
cerebral, congenital QØ4.8
venule NEC I86.8
vesical orifice N32.89
Dilated, dilation — *see* Dilatation
Diminished, diminution
hearing (acuity) — *see* Deafness
sense or sensation (cold) (heat) (tactile) (vibratory) R2Ø.8
vision NEC H54.7
vital capacity R94.2
Diminuta taenia B71.Ø
Dimitri-Sturge-Weber disease Q85.89
Dimple
congenital sacral Q82.6
parasacral Q82.6
pilonidal or postanal — *see* Cyst, pilonidal
Dioctophyme renalis (infection) (infestation) B83.8
Dipetalonemiasis B74.4
Diphallus Q55.69
Diphtheria, diphtheritic (gangrenous) (hemorrhagic) A36.9
carrier (suspected) Z22.2
cutaneous A36.3
faucial A36.Ø
infection of wound A36.3
laryngeal A36.2
myocarditis A36.81
nasal, anterior A36.89
nasopharyngeal A36.1
neurological complication A36.89
pharyngeal A36.Ø
specified site NEC A36.89
tonsillar A36.Ø
Diphyllobothriasis (intestine) B7Ø.Ø
larval B7Ø.1
Diplacusis H93.22- ☑
Diplegia (upper limbs) G83.Ø
congenital (cerebral) G8Ø.8
facial G51.Ø
lower limbs G82.2Ø
spastic G8Ø.1
Diplococcus, diplococcal — *see* condition
Diplopia H53.2
Dipsomania F1Ø.2Ø
Dipsomania — *continued*
with
psychosis — *see* Psychosis, alcoholic
remission F1Ø.21
Dipylidiasis B71.1
DIRA (deficiency of interleukin 1 receptor antagonist) MØ4.8
Direction, teeth, abnormal, fully erupted M26.3Ø
Dirofilariasis B74.8
Dirt-eating child F98.3
Disability, disabilities
heart — *see* Disease, heart
intellectual F79
with
autistic features F84.9
pathogenic CHAMP1 (genetic) (variant) F78.A9
pathogenic HNRNPH2 (genetic) (variant) F78.A9
pathogenic SATB2 (genetic) (variant) F78.A9
pathogenic SETBP1 (genetic) (variant) F78.A9
pathogenic STXBP1 (genetic) (variant) F78.A9
pathogenic SYNGAP1 (genetic) (variant) F78.A1
autosomal dominant F78.A9
autosomal recessive F78.A9
genetic related F78.A9
with
pathogenic CHAMP1 (variant) F78.A9
pathogenic HNRNPH2 (variant) F78.A9
pathogenic SATB2 (variant) F78.A9
pathogenic SETBP1 (variant) F78.A9
pathogenic STXBP1 (variant) F78.A9
pathogenic SYNGAP1 (variant) F78.A1
specified NEC F78.A9
SYNGAP1-related F78.A1
in
autosomal dominant mental retardation F78.A9
autosomal recessive mental retardation F78.A9
SATB2-associated syndrome F78.A9
SETBP1 disorder F78.A9
STXBP1 encephalopathy with epilepsy — *see also* Encephalopathy; and — *see also* Epilepsy
X-linked mental retardation (syndromic) (Bain type) F78.A9
mild (I.Q. 5Ø-69) F7Ø
moderate (I.Q. 35-49) F71
profound (I.Q. under 2Ø) F73
severe (I.Q. 2Ø-34) F72
specified level NEC F78.A9
SYNGAP1-related F78.A1
X-linked (syndromic) (Bain type) F78.A9
knowledge acquisition F81.9
learning F81.9
limiting activities Z73.6
spelling, specific F81.81
Disappearance of family member Z63.4
Disarticulation — *see* Amputation
meaning traumatic amputation — *see* Amputation, traumatic
Discharge (from)
abnormal finding in — *see* Abnormal, specimen
breast (female) (male) N64.52
diencephalic autonomic idiopathic — *see* Epilepsy, specified NEC
ear — *see also* Otorrhea
blood — *see* Otorrhagia
excessive urine R35.89
nipple N64.52
penile R36.9
postnasal RØ9.82
prison, anxiety concerning Z65.2
urethral R36.9
without blood R36.Ø
hematospermia R36.1
vaginal N89.8
Discitis, diskitis M46.4Ø
cervical region M46.42
cervicothoracic region M46.43
lumbar region M46.46
lumbosacral region M46.47
multiple sites M46.49
occipito-atlanto-axial region M46.41
pyogenic — *see* Infection, intervertebral disc, pyogenic
sacrococcygeal region M46.48
thoracic region M46.44
thoracolumbar region M46.45
Discoid
meniscus (congenital) Q68.6
Discoid — *continued*
semilunar cartilage (congenital) — *see* Derangement, knee, meniscus, specified NEC
Discoloration
nails L6Ø.8
teeth (posteruptive) KØ3.7
during formation KØØ.8
Discomfort
chest RØ7.89
visual H53.14- ☑
Discontinuity, ossicles, ear H74.2- ☑
Discord (with)
boss Z56.4
classmates Z55.4
counselor Z64.4
employer Z56.4
family Z63.8
fellow employees Z56.4
in-laws Z63.1
landlord Z59.2
lodgers Z59.2
neighbors Z59.2
probation officer Z64.4
social worker Z64.4
teachers Z55.4
workmates Z56.4
Discordant connection
atrioventricular (congenital) Q2Ø.5
ventriculoarterial Q2Ø.3
Discrepancy
centric occlusion maximum intercuspation M26.55
leg length (acquired) — *see* Deformity, limb, unequal length
congenital — *see* Defect, reduction, lower limb
uterine size date O26.84- ☑
Discrimination
ethnic Z6Ø.5
political Z6Ø.5
racial Z6Ø.5
religious Z6Ø.5
sex Z6Ø.5
Disease, diseased — *see also* Syndrome
absorbent system I87.8
acid-peptic K3Ø
Acosta's T7Ø.29 ☑
Adams-Stokes (-Morgagni) (syncope with heart block) I45.9
Addison's anemia (pernicious) D51.Ø
adenoids (and tonsils) J35.9
adrenal (capsule) (cortex) (gland) (medullary) E27.9
hyperfunction E27.Ø
specified NEC E27.8
ainhum L94.6
airway
obstructive, chronic J44.9
due to
cotton dust J66.Ø
specific organic dusts NEC J66.8
reactive — *see* Asthma
akamushi (scrub typhus) A75.3
Albers-Schönberg (marble bones) Q78.2
Albert's — *see* Tendinitis, Achilles
alimentary canal K63.9
alligator-skin Q8Ø.9
acquired L85.Ø
alpha heavy chain C88.3
alpine T7Ø.29 ☑
altitude T7Ø.2Ø ☑
alveolar ridge
edentulous KØ6.9
specified NEC KØ6.8
alveoli, teeth KØ8.9
Alzheimer's — *see also* Dementia, in, diseases specified elsewhere G3Ø.9 *[FØ2.8Ø]*
with behavioral disturbance — *see also* Dementia, in, diseases specified elsewhere G3Ø.9 *[FØ2.81-]* ☑
early onset — *see also* Dementia, in, diseases specified elsewhere G3Ø.Ø *[FØ2.8Ø]*
with behavioral disturbance — *see also* Dementia, in, diseases specified elsewhere G3Ø.Ø *[FØ2.81-]* ☑
late onset — *see also* Dementia, in, diseases specified elsewhere G3Ø.1 *[FØ2.8Ø]*
with behavioral disturbance — *see also* Dementia, in, diseases specified elsewhere G3Ø.1 *[FØ2.81-]* ☑

Disease, diseased — *continued*
- Alzheimer's — *see also* Dementia, in, diseases specified elsewhere — *continued*
  - specified NEC — *see also* Dementia, in, diseases specified elsewhere G3Ø.8 *[FØ2.8Ø]*
    - with behavioral disturbance — *see also* Dementia, in, diseases specified elsewhere G3Ø.8 *[FØ2.81]* ☑
- amyloid — *see* Amyloidosis
- Andersen's (glycogenosis IV) E74.Ø9
- Andes T7Ø.29 ☑
- Andrews' (bacterid) LØ8.89
- angiospastic I73.9
  - cerebral G45.9
  - vein I87.8
- anterior
  - chamber H21.9
  - horn cell G12.29
- antiglomerular basement membrane (anti- GBM) antibody M31.Ø
  - tubulo-interstitial nephritis N12
- antral — *see* Sinusitis, maxillary
- anus K62.9
  - specified NEC K62.89
- aorta (nonsyphilitic) I77.9
  - syphilitic NEC A52.Ø2
- aortic (heart) (valve) I35.9
  - rheumatic IØ6.9
- Apollo B3Ø.3
- aponeuroses — *see* Enthesopathy
- appendix K38.9
  - specified NEC K38.8
- aqueous (chamber) H21.9
- Arnold-Chiari *see* Arnold-Chiari disease
- arterial I77.9
  - occlusive — *see* Occlusion, by site
    - due to stricture or stenosis I77.1
  - peripheral I73.9
- arteriocardiorenal — *see* Hypertension, cardiorenal
- arteriolar (generalized) (obliterative) I77.9
- arteriorenal — *see* Hypertension, kidney
- arteriosclerotic — *see also* Arteriosclerosis
  - cardiovascular — *see* Disease, heart, ischemic, atherosclerotic
  - coronary (artery) — *see* Disease, heart, ischemic, atherosclerotic
  - heart — *see* Disease, heart, ischemic, atherosclerotic
- artery I77.9
  - cerebral I67.9
  - coronary I25.1Ø
    - with angina pectoris — *see* Arteriosclerosis, coronary (artery)
  - peripheral I73.9
- arthropod-borne NOS (viral) A94
  - specified type NEC A93.8
- atticoantral, chronic H66.2Ø
  - left H66.22
    - with right H66.23
  - right H66.21
    - with left H66.23
- auditory canal — *see* Disorder, ear, external
- auricle, ear NEC — *see* Disorder, pinna
- Australian X A83.4
- autoimmune (systemic) NOS M35.9
  - hemolytic D59.1Ø
    - cold type (primary) (secondary) (symptomatic) D59.12
    - drug-induced D59.Ø
    - mixed type (primary) (secondary) (symptomatic) D59.13
    - warm type (primary) (secondary) (symptomatic) D59.11
  - thyroid EØ6.3
- autoinflammatory MØ4.9
  - NOD2-associated MØ4.8
  - specified type NEC MØ4.8
- aviator's — *see* Effect, adverse, high altitude
- Ayerza's (pulmonary artery sclerosis with pulmonary hypertension) I27.Ø
- Babington's (familial hemorrhagic telangiectasia) I78.Ø
- bacterial A49.9
  - specified NEC A48.8
  - zoonotic A28.9
    - specified type NEC A28.8
- Baelz's (cheilitis glandularis apostematosa) K13.Ø
- bagasse J67.1
- balloon — *see* Effect, adverse, high altitude
- Bang's (brucella abortus) A23.1

Disease, diseased — *continued*
- Bannister's T78.3 ☑
- barometer makers' — *see* Poisoning, mercury
- Barraquer (-Simons') (progressive lipodystrophy) E88.1
- Barrett's — *see* Barrett's, esophagus
- Bartholin's gland N75.9
- basal ganglia G25.9
  - degenerative G23.9
    - specified NEC G23.8
  - specified NEC G25.89
- Basedow's (exophthalmic goiter) — *see* Hyperthyroidism, with, goiter (diffuse)
- Bateman's BØ8.1
- Batten-Steinert G71.11
- Battey A31.Ø
- Beard's (neurasthenia) F48.8
- Becker
  - idiopathic mural endomyocardial I42.3
  - myotonia congenita G71.12
- Begbie's (exophthalmic goiter) — *see* Hyperthyroidism, with, goiter (diffuse)
- behavioral, organic FØ7.9
- Beigel's (white piedra) B36.2
- Benson's — *see* Deposit, crystalline
- Bernard-Soulier (thrombopathy) D69.1
- Bernhardt (-Roth) — *see* Mononeuropathy, lower limb, meralgia paresthetica
- Biermer's (pernicious anemia) D51.Ø
- bile duct (common) (hepatic) K83.9
  - with calculus, stones — *see* Calculus, bile duct
  - specified NEC K83.8
- biliary (tract) K83.9
  - specified NEC K83.8
- Billroth's — *see* Spina bifida
- bird fancier's J67.2
- black lung J6Ø
- bladder N32.9
  - in (due to)
    - schistosomiasis (bilharziasis) B65.Ø *[N33]*
  - specified NEC N32.89
- bleeder's D66
- blood D75.9
  - forming organs D75.9
  - vessel I99.9
- Bloodgood's — *see* Mastopathy, cystic
- Blount M92.51- ☑
- Bodechtel-Guttmann (subacute sclerosing panencephalitis) A81.1
- bone — *see also* Disorder, bone
  - aluminum M83.4
  - fibrocystic NEC
    - jaw M27.49
- bone-marrow D75.9
- Borna A83.9
- Bornholm (epidemic pleurodynia) B33.Ø
- Bouchard's (myopathic dilatation of the stomach) K31.Ø
- Bouillaud's (rheumatic heart disease) IØ1.9
- Bourneville (-Brissaud) (tuberous sclerosis) Q85.1
- Bouveret (-Hoffmann) (paroxysmal tachycardia) I47.9
- bowel K63.9
  - functional K59.9
    - psychogenic F45.8
- brain — *see also* Dementia, in, diseases specified elsewhere G93.9
  - arterial, artery I67.9
  - arteriosclerotic I67.2
  - congenital QØ4.9
  - degenerative — *see* Degeneration, brain
  - inflammatory — *see* Encephalitis
  - organic G93.9
    - arteriosclerotic I67.2
  - parasitic NEC B71.9 *[G94]*
  - senile NEC G31.1
  - specified NEC G93.89
- breast — *see also* Disorder, breast N64.9
  - cystic (chronic) — *see* Mastopathy, cystic
  - fibrocystic — *see* Mastopathy, cystic
  - Paget's
    - female, unspecified side C5Ø.91- ☑
    - male, unspecified side C5Ø.92- ☑
  - specified NEC N64.89
- Breda's — *see* Yaws
- Bretonneau's (diphtheritic malignant angina) A36.Ø
- Bright's — *see* Nephritis
  - arteriosclerotic — *see* Hypertension, kidney
- Brill's (recrudescent typhus) A75.1
- Brill-Zinsser (recrudescent typhus) A75.1
- Brion-Kayser — *see* Fever, paratyphoid

Disease, diseased — *continued*
- broad
  - beta E78.2
  - ligament (noninflammatory) N83.9
    - inflammatory — *see* Disease, pelvis, inflammatory
    - specified NEC N83.8
- Brocq-Duhring (dermatitis herpetiformis) L13.Ø
- Brocq's
  - meaning
    - dermatitis herpetiformis L13.Ø
    - prurigo L28.2
- bronchopulmonary J98.4
- bronchus NEC J98.Ø9
- bronze Addison's E27.1
  - tuberculous A18.7
- budgerigar fancier's J67.2
- Buerger's (thromboangiitis obliterans) I73.1
- bullous L13.9
  - chronic of childhood L12.2
  - specified NEC L13.8
- Bürger-Grütz (essential familial hyperlipemia) E78.3
- bursa — *see* Bursopathy
- caisson T7Ø.3 ☑
- California — *see* Coccidioidomycosis
- capillaries I78.9
  - specified NEC I78.8
- Carapata A68.Ø
- cardiac — *see* Disease, heart
- cardiopulmonary, chronic I27.9
- cardiorenal (hepatic) (hypertensive) (vascular) — *see* Hypertension, cardiorenal
- cardiovascular (atherosclerotic) I25.1Ø
  - with angina pectoris — *see* Arteriosclerosis, coronary (artery),
  - congenital Q28.9
  - hypertensive — *see* Hypertension, heart
  - newborn P29.9
    - specified NEC P29.89
  - renal (hypertensive) — *see* Hypertension, cardiorenal
  - syphilitic (asymptomatic) A52.ØØ
- cartilage — *see* Disorder, cartilage
- Castellani's A69.8
- Castleman (unicentric) (multicentric) D47.Z2
  - HHV-8-associated — *see also* Herpesvirus, human, 8 D47.Z2
- cat-scratch A28.1
- Cavare's (familial periodic paralysis) G72.3
- cecum K63.9
- celiac (adult) (infantile) (with steatorrhea) K9Ø.Ø
- cellular tissue L98.9
- central core G71.29
- cerebellar, cerebellum — *see* Disease, brain
- cerebral — *see also* Disease, brain
  - degenerative — *see* Degeneration, brain
- cerebrospinal G96.9
- cerebrovascular I67.9
  - acute I67.89
    - embolic I63.4- ☑
    - thrombotic I63.3- ☑
  - arteriosclerotic I67.2
  - hereditary NEC I67.858
  - specified NEC I67.89
- cervix (uteri) (noninflammatory) N88.9
  - inflammatory — *see* Cervicitis
  - specified NEC N88.8
- Chabert's A22.9
- Chandler's (osteochondritis dissecans, hip) — *see* Osteochondritis, dissecans, hip
- Charlouis — *see* Yaws
- Chédiak-Steinbrinck (-Higashi) (congenital gigantism of peroxidase granules) E7Ø.33Ø
- chest J98.9
- Chiari's (hepatic vein thrombosis) I82.Ø
- Chicago B4Ø.9
- Chignon B36.8
- chigo, chigoe B88.1
- childhood granulomatous D71
- Chinese liver fluke B66.1
- chlamydial A74.9
  - specified NEC A74.89
- cholecystic K82.9
- choroid H31.9
  - specified NEC H31.8
- Christmas D67
- chronic bullous of childhood L12.2
- chylomicron retention E78.3

Disease, diseased — *continued*
  ciliary body H21.9
    specified NEC H21.89
  circulatory (system) NEC I99.8
    newborn P29.9
    syphilitic A52.ØØ
      congenital A5Ø.54
  coagulation factor deficiency (congenital) — *see* Defect, coagulation
  coccidioidal — *see* Coccidioidomycosis
  cold
    agglutinin or hemoglobinuria D59.12
      paroxysmal D59.6
    hemagglutinin (chronic) D59.12
  collagen NOS (nonvascular) (vascular) M35.9
    specified NEC M35.89
  colon K63.9
    functional K59.9
      congenital Q43.2
    ischemic — *see also* Ischemia, intestine, acute K55.Ø39
  colonic inflammatory bowel, unclassified (IBDU) K52.3
  combined system — *see* Degeneration, combined
  compressed air T7Ø.3 ☑
  Concato's (pericardial polyserositis) A19.9
    nontubercular I31.1
    pleural — *see* Pleurisy, with effusion
  conjunctiva H11.9
    chlamydial A74.Ø
    specified NEC H11.89
    viral B3Ø.9
      specified NEC B3Ø.8
  connective tissue, systemic (diffuse) M35.9
    in (due to)
      hypogammaglobulinemia D8Ø.1 *[M36.8]*
      ochronosis E7Ø.29 *[M36.8]*
    specified NEC M35.89
  Conor and Bruch's (boutonneuse fever) A77.1
  Cooper's — *see* Mastopathy, cystic
  Cori's (glycogenosis III) E74.Ø3
  corkhandler's or corkworker's J67.3
  cornea H18.9
    specified NEC H18.89- ☑
  coronary (artery) — *see* Disease, heart, ischemic, atherosclerotic
    congenital Q24.5
    ostial, syphilitic (aortic) (mitral) (pulmonary) A52.Ø3
  corpus cavernosum N48.9
    specified NEC N48.89
  Cotugno's — *see* Sciatica
  COVID-19 UØ7.1
  coxsackie (virus) NEC B34.1
  cranial nerve NOS G52.9
  Creutzfeldt-Jakob — *see* Creutzfeldt-Jakob disease or syndrome
  Crocq's (acrocyanosis) I73.89
  Crohn's — *see* Enteritis, regional
  Curschmann G71.11
  cystic
    breast (chronic) — *see* Mastopathy, cystic
    kidney, congenital Q61.9
    liver, congenital Q44.6
    lung J98.4
      congenital Q33.Ø
  cytomegalic inclusion (generalized) B25.9
    with pneumonia B25.Ø
    congenital P35.1
  cytomegaloviral B25.9
    specified NEC B25.8
  Czerny's (periodic hydrarthrosis of the knee) — *see* Effusion, joint, knee
  Daae (-Finsen) (epidemic pleurodynia) B33.Ø
  Darling's — *see* Histoplasmosis capsulati
  de Quervain's (tendon sheath) M65.4
    thyroid (subacute granulomatous thyroiditis) EØ6.1
  Débove's (splenomegaly) R16.1
  deer fly — *see* Tularemia
  Degos' I77.89
  demyelinating, demyelinizating (nervous system) G37.9
    multiple sclerosis G35
    specified NEC G37.8
  dense deposit — *see also* NØØ-NØ7 with fourth character .6 NØ5.6
  deposition, hydroxyapatite — *see* Disease, hydroxyapatite deposition
  Devergie's (pityriasis rubra pilaris) L44.Ø
  Devic's G36.Ø
  diaphorase deficiency D74.Ø

Disease, diseased — *continued*
  diaphragm J98.6
  diarrheal, infectious NEC AØ9
  digestive system K92.9
    specified NEC K92.89
  disc, degenerative — *see* Degeneration, intervertebral disc
  discogenic — *see also* Displacement, intervertebral disc NEC
    with myelopathy — *see* Disorder, disc, with, myelopathy
  diverticular — *see* Diverticula
  Dubois (thymus) A5Ø.59 *[E35]*
  Duchenne-Griesinger G71.Ø1
  Duchenne's
    muscular dystrophy G71.Ø1
    pseudohypertrophy, muscles G71.Ø1
  ductless glands E34.9
  Duhring's (dermatitis herpetiformis) L13.Ø
  duodenum K31.9
    specified NEC K31.89
  Dupré's (meningism) R29.1
  Dupuytren's (muscle contracture) M72.Ø
  Durand-Nicholas-Favre (climatic bubo) A55
  Duroziez's (congenital mitral stenosis) Q23.2
  ear — *see* Disorder, ear
  Eberth's — *see* Fever, typhoid
  Ebola (virus) A98.4
  Ebstein's heart Q22.5
  Echinococcus — *see* Echinococcus
  echovirus NEC B34.1
  Eddowes' (brittle bones and blue sclera) Q78.Ø
  edentulous (alveolar) ridge KØ6.9
    specified NEC KØ6.8
  Edsall's T67.2 ☑
  Eichstedt's (pityriasis versicolor) B36.Ø
  Eisenmenger's (irreversible) I27.83
  Ellis-van Creveld (chondroectodermal dysplasia) Q77.6
  end stage renal (ESRD) N18.6
    due to hypertension I12.Ø
  endocrine glands or system NEC E34.9
  endomyocardial (eosinophilic) I42.3
  English (rickets) E55.Ø
  enteroviral, enterovirus NEC B34.1
    central nervous system NEC A88.8
  epidemic B99.9
    specified NEC B99.8
  epididymis N5Ø.9
  Erb (-Landouzy) G71.Ø2
  Erdheim-Chester (ECD) E88.89
  esophagus K22.9
    functional K22.4
    psychogenic F45.8
    specified NEC K22.89
  Eulenburg's (congenital paramyotonia) G71.19
  eustachian tube — *see* Disorder, eustachian tube
  external
    auditory canal — *see* Disorder, ear, external
    ear — *see* Disorder, ear, external
  extrapyramidal G25.9
    specified NEC G25.89
  eye H57.9
    anterior chamber H21.9
    inflammatory NEC H57.89
    muscle (external) — *see* Strabismus
    specified NEC H57.89
    syphilitic — *see* Oculopathy, syphilitic
  eyeball H44.9
    specified NEC H44.89
  eyelid — *see* Disorder, eyelid
    specified NEC — *see* Disorder, eyelid, specified type NEC
  eyeworm of Africa B74.3
  facial nerve (seventh) G51.9
    newborn (birth injury) P11.3
  Fahr (of brain) G23.8
  Fahr Volhard (of kidney) I12.- ☑
  fallopian tube (noninflammatory) N83.9
    inflammatory — *see* Salpingo-oophoritis
    specified NEC N83.8
  familial periodic paralysis G72.3
  Fanconi's (congenital pancytopenia) D61.Ø9
  fascia NEC — *see also* Disorder, muscle
    inflammatory — *see* Myositis
    specified NEC M62.89
  Fauchard's (periodontitis) — *see* Periodontitis
  Favre-Durand-Nicolas (climatic bubo) A55
  Fede's K14.Ø

Disease, diseased — *continued*
  Feer's — *see* Poisoning, mercury
  female pelvic inflammatory — *see also* Disease, pelvis, inflammatory N73.9
    syphilitic (secondary) A51.42
    tuberculous A18.17
  Fernels' (aortic aneurysm) I71.9
  fibrocaseous of lung — *see* Tuberculosis, pulmonary
  fibrocystic — *see* Fibrocystic disease
  Fiedler's (leptospiral jaundice) A27.Ø
  fifth BØ8.3
  file-cutter's — *see* Poisoning, lead
  fish-skin Q8Ø.9
    acquired L85.Ø
  Flajani (-Basedow) (exophthalmic goiter) — *see* Hyperthyroidism, with, goiter (diffuse)
  flax-dresser's J66.1
  fluke — *see* Infestation, fluke
  foot and mouth BØ8.8
  foot process NØ4.9
  Forbes' (glycogenosis III) E74.Ø3
  Fordyce-Fox (apocrine miliaria) L75.2
  Fordyce's (ectopic sebaceous glands) (mouth) Q38.6
  Forestier's (rhizomelic pseudopolyarthritis) M35.3
    meaning ankylosing hyperostosis — *see* Hyperostosis, ankylosing
  Fothergill's
    neuralgia — *see* Neuralgia, trigeminal
    scarlatina anginosa A38.9
  Fournier (gangrene) N49.3
    female N76.82
    vagina and vulva N76.82
  fourth BØ8.8
  Fox (-Fordyce) (apocrine miliaria) L75.2
  Francis' — *see* Tularemia
  Franklin C88.2
  Frei's (climatic bubo) A55
  Friedreich's
    combined systemic or ataxia G11.11
    myoclonia G25.3
  frontal sinus — *see* Sinusitis, frontal
  fungus NEC B49
  Gaisböck's (polycythemia hypertonica) D75.1
  gallbladder K82.9
    calculus — *see* Calculus, gallbladder
    cholecystitis — *see* Cholecystitis
    cholesterolosis K82.4
    fistula — *see* Fistula, gallbladder
    hydrops K82.1
    obstruction — *see* Obstruction, gallbladder
    perforation K82.2
    specified NEC K82.8
  gamma heavy chain C88.2
  Gamna's (siderotic splenomegaly) D73.2
  Gamstorp's (adynamia episodica hereditaria) G72.3
  Gandy-Nanta (siderotic splenomegaly) D73.2
  ganister J62.8
  gastric — *see* Disease, stomach
  gastroesophageal reflux (GERD) K21.9
    with esophagitis (without bleeding) K21.ØØ
      with bleeding K21.Ø1
  gastrointestinal (tract) K92.9
    amyloid E85.4
    functional K59.9
      psychogenic F45.8
    specified NEC K92.89
  Gee (-Herter) (-Heubner) (-Thaysen) (nontropical sprue) K9Ø.Ø
  genital organs
    female N94.9
    male N5Ø.9
  Gerhardt's (erythromelalgia) I73.81
  Gibert's (pityriasis rosea) L42
  Gierke's (glycogenosis I) E74.Ø1
  Gilles de la Tourette's (motor-verbal tic) F95.2
  gingiva KØ6.9
    plaque induced KØ5.ØØ
    specified NEC KØ6.8
  gland (lymph) I89.9
  Glanzmann's (hereditary hemorrhagic thrombasthenia) D69.1
  glass-blower's (cataract) — *see* Cataract, specified NEC
    salivary gland hypertrophy K11.1
  Glisson's — *see* Rickets
  globe H44.9
    specified NEC H44.89
  glomerular — *see also* Glomerulonephritis
    with edema — *see* Nephrosis

Disease, diseased — *continued*
- glomerular — *see also* Glomerulonephritis — *continued*
  - acute — *see* Nephritis, acute
  - chronic — *see* Nephritis, chronic
  - minimal change NØ5.Ø
  - rapidly progressive NØ1.9
- glycogen storage E74.ØØ
  - Andersen's E74.Ø9
  - Cori's E74.Ø3
  - Forbes' E74.Ø3
  - generalized E74.ØØ
  - glucose-6-phosphatase deficiency E74.Ø1
  - heart E74.Ø2 *[I43]*
  - hepatorenal E74.Ø9
  - Hers' E74.Ø9
  - liver and kidney E74.Ø9
  - McArdle's E74.Ø4
  - muscle phosphofructokinase E74.Ø9
  - myocardium E74.Ø2 *[I43]*
  - Pompe's E74.Ø2
  - Tauri's E74.Ø9
  - type Ø E74.Ø9
  - type I E74.Ø1
  - type II E74.Ø2
  - type III E74.Ø3
  - type IV E74.Ø9
  - type V E74.Ø4
  - type VI-XI E74.Ø9
  - Von Gierke's E74.Ø1
- Goldstein's (familial hemorrhagic telangiectasia) I78.Ø
- gonococcal NOS A54.9
- graft-versus-host (GVH) D89.813
  - acute D89.81Ø
  - acute on chronic D89.812
  - chronic D89.811
- grainhandler's J67.8
- granulomatous (childhood) (chronic) D71
- Graves' (exophthalmic goiter) — *see* Hyperthyroidism, with, goiter (diffuse)
- Griesinger's — *see* Ancylostomiasis
- Grisel's M43.6
- Gruby's (tinea tonsurans) B35.Ø
- Guillain-Barré G61.Ø
- Guinon's (motor-verbal tic) F95.2
- gum KØ6.9
- gynecological N94.9
- H (Hartnup's) E72.Ø2
- Haff — *see* Poisoning, mercury
- Hageman (congenital factor XII deficiency) D68.2
- hair (color) (shaft) L67.9
  - follicles L73.9
    - specified NEC L73.8
- Hamman's (spontaneous mediastinal emphysema) J98.2
- hand, foot and mouth BØ8.4
- Hansen's — *see* Leprosy
- Hantavirus, with pulmonary manifestations B33.4
  - with renal manifestations A98.5
- Harada's H3Ø.81- ☑
- Hartnup (pellagra-cerebellar ataxia-renal aminoaciduria) E72.Ø2
- Hart's (pellagra-cerebellar ataxia-renal aminoaciduria) E72.Ø2
- Hashimoto's (struma lymphomatosa) EØ6.3
- Hb — *see* Disease, hemoglobin
- heart (organic) I51.9
  - with
    - pulmonary edema (acute) — *see also* Failure, ventricular, left I5Ø.1
    - rheumatic fever (conditions in IØØ)
      - active IØ1.9
        - with chorea IØ2.Ø
        - specified NEC IØ1.8
      - inactive or quiescent (with chorea) IØ9.9
        - specified NEC IØ9.89
  - amyloid E85.4 *[I43]*
  - aortic (valve) I35.9
  - arteriosclerotic or sclerotic (senile) — *see* Disease, heart, ischemic, atherosclerotic
  - artery, arterial — *see* Disease, heart, ischemic, atherosclerotic
  - beer drinkers' I42.6
  - beriberi (wet) E51.12
  - black I27.Ø
  - congenital Q24.9
    - cyanotic Q24.9
    - specified NEC Q24.8

Disease, diseased — *continued*
- heart — *continued*
  - coronary — *see* Disease, heart, ischemic
  - cryptogenic I51.9
  - fibroid — *see* Myocarditis
  - functional I51.89
    - psychogenic F45.8
  - glycogen storage E74.Ø2 *[I43]*
  - gonococcal A54.83
  - hypertensive — *see* Hypertension, heart
  - hyperthyroid — *see also* Hyperthyroidism EØ5.9Ø *[I43]*
    - with thyroid storm EØ5.91 *[I43]*
  - ischemic (chronic or with a stated duration of over 4 weeks) I25.9
    - atherosclerotic (of) I25.1Ø
      - with angina pectoris — *see* Arteriosclerosis, coronary (artery)
      - coronary artery bypass graft — *see* Arteriosclerosis, coronary (artery),
    - cardiomyopathy I25.5
    - diagnosed on ECG or other special investigation, but currently presenting no symptoms I25.6
    - silent I25.6
    - specified form NEC I25.89
  - kyphoscoliotic I27.1
  - meningococcal A39.5Ø
    - endocarditis A39.51
    - myocarditis A39.52
    - pericarditis A39.53
  - mitral IØ5.9
    - specified NEC IØ5.8
  - muscular — *see* Degeneration, myocardial
  - psychogenic (functional) F45.8
  - pulmonary (chronic) I27.9
    - in schistosomiasis B65.9 *[I52]*
    - specified NEC I27.89
  - rheumatic (chronic) (inactive) (old) (quiescent) (with chorea) IØ9.9
    - active or acute IØ1.9
      - with chorea (acute) (rheumatic) (Sydenham's) IØ2.Ø
    - specified NEC IØ9.89
  - senile — *see* Myocarditis
  - syphilitic A52.Ø6
    - aortic A52.Ø3
      - aneurysm A52.Ø1
    - congenital A5Ø.54 *[I52]*
  - thyrotoxic — *see also* Thyrotoxicosis EØ5.9Ø *[I43]*
    - with thyroid storm EØ5.91 *[I43]*
  - valve, valvular (obstructive) (regurgitant) — *see also* Endocarditis
    - congenital NEC Q24.8
      - pulmonary Q22.3
  - vascular — *see* Disease, cardiovascular
- heavy chain NEC C88.2
  - alpha C88.3
  - gamma C88.2
  - mu C88.2
- Hebra's
  - pityriasis
    - maculata et circinata L42
    - rubra pilaris L44.Ø
  - prurigo L28.2
- hematopoietic organs D75.9
- hemoglobin or Hb
  - abnormal (mixed) NEC D58.2
    - with thalassemia D56.9
  - AS genotype D57.3
  - Bart's D56.Ø
  - C (Hb-C) D58.2
    - with other abnormal hemoglobin NEC D58.2
    - elliptocytosis D58.1
    - Hb-S D57.2- ☑
    - sickle-cell D57.2- ☑
    - thalassemia D56.8
  - Constant Spring D58.2
  - D (Hb-D) D58.2
  - E (Hb-E) D58.2
  - E-beta thalassemia D56.5
  - elliptocytosis D58.1
  - H (Hb-H) (thalassemia) D56.Ø
    - with other abnormal hemoglobin NEC D56.9
    - Constant Spring D56.Ø
  - I thalassemia D56.9
  - M D74.Ø
  - S or SS D57.1

Disease, diseased — *continued*
- hemoglobin or Hb — *continued*
  - S or SS — *continued*
    - with
      - acute chest syndrome D57.Ø1
      - cerebral vascular involvement D57.Ø3
      - crisis (painful) D57.ØØ
        - with complication specified NEC D57.Ø9
      - splenic sequestration D57.Ø2
      - vasoocclusive pain D57.ØØ
    - beta plus D57.44
      - with
        - acute chest syndrome D57.451
        - cerebral vascular involvement D57.453
        - crisis D57.459
          - with specified complication NEC D57.458
        - splenic sequestration D57.452
        - vasoocclusive pain D57.459
      - without crisis D57.44
    - beta zero D57.42
      - with
        - acute chest syndrome D57.431
        - cerebral vascular involvement D57.433
        - crisis D57.439
          - with specified complication NEC D57.438
        - splenic sequestration D57.432
        - vasoocclusive pain
      - without crisis D57.42
  - SC D57.2- ☑
  - SD D57.8- ☑
  - SE D57.8- ☑
  - spherocytosis D58.Ø
  - unstable, hemolytic D58.2
- hemolytic (newborn) P55.9
  - autoimmune D59.1Ø
    - cold type (primary) (secondary) (symptomatic) D59.12
    - mixed type (primary) (secondary) (symptomatic) D59.13
    - warm type (primary) (secondary) (symptomatic) D59.11
  - drug-induced D59.Ø
  - due to or with
    - incompatibility
      - ABO (blood group) P55.1
      - blood (group) (Duffy) (K) (Kell) (Kidd) (Lewis) (M) (S) NEC P55.8
      - Rh (blood group) (factor) P55.Ø
    - Rh negative mother P55.Ø
  - specified type NEC P55.8
  - unstable hemoglobin D58.2
- hemorrhagic D69.9
  - newborn P53
- Henoch (-Schönlein) (purpura nervosa) D69.Ø
- hepatic — *see* Disease, liver
- hepatolenticular E83.Ø1
- heredodegenerative NEC
  - spinal cord G95.89
- herpesviral, disseminated BØØ.7
- Hers' (glycogenosis VI) E74.Ø9
- Herter (-Gee) (-Heubner) (nontropical sprue) K9Ø.Ø
- Heubner-Herter (nontropical sprue) K9Ø.Ø
- high fetal gene or hemoglobin thalassemia D56.9
- Hildenbrand's — *see* Typhus
- hip (joint) M25.9
  - congenital Q65.89
  - suppurative MØØ.9
  - tuberculous A18.Ø2
- His (-Werner) (trench fever) A79.Ø
- Hodgson's — *see also* Aneurysm, aorta, thorax I71.2Ø
  - ruptured — *see also* Aneurysm, aorta, thorax, ruptured I71.1Ø
- Holla — *see* Spherocytosis
- hookworm B76.9
  - specified NEC B76.8
- host-versus-graft D89.813
  - acute D89.81Ø
  - acute on chronic D89.812
  - chronic D89.811
- human immunodeficiency virus (HIV) B2Ø
- Huntington's G1Ø
  - with dementia — *see also* Dementia, in, diseases specified elsewhere G1Ø *[FØ2.8Ø]*
- Hutchinson's (cheiropompholyx) — *see* Hutchinson's disease
- hyaline (diffuse) (generalized)

- **Disease, diseased** — *continued*
  - hyaline — *continued*
    - membrane (lung) (newborn) P22.Ø
      - adult J8Ø
  - hydatid — *see* Echinococcus
  - hydroxyapatite deposition M11.ØØ
    - ankle M11.Ø7- ☑
    - elbow M11.Ø2- ☑
    - foot joint M11.Ø7- ☑
    - hand joint M11.Ø4- ☑
    - hip M11.Ø5- ☑
    - knee M11.Ø6- ☑
    - multiple site M11.Ø9
    - shoulder M11.Ø1- ☑
    - vertebra M11.Ø8
    - wrist M11.Ø3- ☑
  - hyperkinetic — *see* Hyperkinesia
  - hypertensive — *see* Hypertension
  - hypophysis E23.7
  - Iceland G93.39
  - I-cell E77.Ø
  - immune D89.9
  - immunoproliferative (malignant) C88.9
    - small intestinal C88.3
    - specified NEC C88.8
  - inclusion B25.9
    - salivary gland B25.9
  - infectious, infective B99.9
    - congenital P37.9
      - specified NEC P37.8
      - viral P35.9
        - specified type NEC P35.8
    - specified NEC B99.8
  - inflammatory
    - penis N48.29
      - abscess N48.21
      - cellulitis N48.22
    - prepuce N47.7
      - balanoposthitis N47.6
    - tubo-ovarian — *see* Salpingo-oophoritis
  - intervertebral disc — *see also* Disorder, disc
    - with myelopathy — *see* Disorder, disc, with, myelopathy
    - cervical, cervicothoracic — *see* Disorder, disc, cervical
      - with
        - myelopathy — *see* Disorder, disc, cervical, with myelopathy
        - neuritis, radiculitis or radiculopathy — *see* Disorder, disc, cervical, with neuritis
      - specified NEC — *see* Disorder, disc, cervical, specified type NEC
    - lumbar (with)
      - myelopathy M51.Ø6
      - neuritis, radiculitis, radiculopathy or sciatica M51.16
      - specified NEC M51.86
    - lumbosacral (with)
      - neuritis, radiculitis, radiculopathy or sciatica M51.17
      - specified NEC M51.87
    - specified NEC — *see* Disorder, disc, specified NEC
    - thoracic (with)
      - myelopathy M51.Ø4
      - neuritis, radiculitis or radiculopathy M51.14
      - specified NEC M51.84
    - thoracolumbar (with)
      - myelopathy M51.Ø5
      - neuritis, radiculitis or radiculopathy M51.15
      - specified NEC M51.85
  - intestine K63.9
    - functional K59.9
      - psychogenic F45.8
      - specified NEC K59.89
    - organic K63.9
    - protozoal AØ7.9
    - specified NEC K63.89
  - iris H21.9
    - specified NEC H21.89
  - iron metabolism or storage E83.1Ø
  - island (scrub typhus) A75.3
  - itai-itai — *see* Poisoning, cadmium
  - Jakob-Creutzfeldt — *see* Creutzfeldt-Jakob disease or syndrome
  - jaw M27.9
    - fibrocystic M27.49
    - specified NEC M27.8
  - jigger B88.1

- **Disease, diseased** — *continued*
  - joint — *see also* Disorder, joint
    - Charcot's — *see* Arthropathy, neuropathic (Charcot)
    - degenerative — *see* Osteoarthritis
      - multiple M15.9
      - spine — *see* Spondylosis
    - facet joint — *see also* Spondylosis M47.819
    - hypertrophic — *see* Osteoarthritis
    - sacroiliac M53.3
    - specified NEC — *see* Disorder, joint, specified type NEC
    - spine NEC — *see* Dorsopathy
    - suppurative — *see* Arthritis, pyogenic or pyemic
  - Jourdain's (acute gingivitis) KØ5.ØØ
    - nonplaque induced KØ5.Ø1
    - plaque induced KØ5.ØØ
  - Kaschin-Beck (endemic polyarthritis) M12.1Ø
    - ankle M12.17- ☑
    - elbow M12.12- ☑
    - foot joint M12.17- ☑
    - hand joint M12.14- ☑
    - hip M12.15- ☑
    - knee M12.16- ☑
    - multiple site M12.19
    - shoulder M12.11- ☑
    - vertebra M12.18
    - wrist M12.13- ☑
  - Katayama B65.2
  - Kedani (scrub typhus) A75.3
  - Keshan E59
  - kidney (functional) (pelvis) N28.9
    - chronic N18.9
      - hypertensive — *see* Hypertension, kidney
      - stage 1 N18.1
      - stage 2 (mild) N18.2
      - stage 3 (moderate) N18.3Ø
      - stage 3a N18.31
      - stage 3b N18.32
      - stage 4 (severe) N18.4
      - stage 5 N18.5
    - complicating pregnancy — *see* Pregnancy, complicated by, renal disease
    - cystic (congenital) Q61.9
    - fibrocystic (congenital) Q61.8
    - hypertensive — *see* Hypertension, kidney
    - in (due to)
      - schistosomiasis (bilharziasis) B65.9 *[N29]*
    - multicystic Q61.4
    - polycystic Q61.3
      - adult type Q61.2
      - childhood type NEC Q61.19
        - collecting duct dilatation Q61.11
  - Kimmelstiel (-Wilson) (intercapillary polycystic (congenital) glomerulosclerosis) — *see* EØ8-E13 with .21
  - Kinnier Wilson's (hepatolenticular degeneration) E83.Ø1
  - kissing — *see* Mononucleosis, infectious
  - Klebs' — *see also* Glomerulonephritis NØ5- ☑
  - Klippel-Feil (brevicollis) Q76.1
  - Köhler-Pellegrini-Stieda (calcification, knee joint) — *see* Bursitis, tibial collateral
  - Kok Q89.8
  - König's (osteochondritis dissecans) — *see* Osteochondritis, dissecans
  - Korsakoff's (nonalcoholic) FØ4
    - alcoholic F1Ø.96
      - with dependence F1Ø.26
  - Kostmann's (infantile genetic agranulocytosis) D7Ø.Ø
  - kuru A81.81
  - Kyasanur Forest A98.2
  - labyrinth, ear — *see* Disorder, ear, inner
  - lacrimal system — *see* Disorder, lacrimal system
  - Lafora's — *see* Epilepsy, generalized, idiopathic
  - Lancereaux-Mathieu (leptospiral jaundice) A27.Ø
  - Landry's G61.Ø
  - Larrey-Weil (leptospiral jaundice) A27.Ø
  - larynx J38.7
  - legionnaires' A48.1
    - nonpneumonic A48.2
  - Lenegre's I44.2
  - lens H27.9
    - specified NEC H27.8
  - Lev's (acquired complete heart block) I44.2
  - Lewy body (dementia) — *see also* Dementia, in, diseases specified elsewhere G31.83 *[FØ2.8Ø]*
    - with behavioral disturbance — *see also* Dementia, in, diseases specified elsewhere G31.83 *[FØ2.81-]* ☑

- **Disease, diseased** — *continued*
  - Lichtheim's (subacute combined sclerosis with pernicious anemia) D51.Ø
  - Lightwood's (renal tubular acidosis) N25.89
  - Lignac's (cystinosis) E72.Ø4
  - lip K13.Ø
  - lipid-storage E75.6
    - specified NEC E75.5
  - Lipschütz's N76.6
  - liver (chronic) (organic) K76.9
    - alcoholic (chronic) K7Ø.9
      - acute — *see* Disease, liver, alcoholic, hepatitis
      - cirrhosis K7Ø.3Ø
        - with ascites K7Ø.31
      - failure K7Ø.4Ø
        - with coma K7Ø.41
      - fatty liver K7Ø.Ø
      - fibrosis K7Ø.2
      - hepatitis K7Ø.1Ø
        - with ascites K7Ø.11
      - sclerosis K7Ø.2
    - cystic, congenital Q44.6
    - drug-induced (idiosyncratic) (toxic) (predictable) (unpredictable) — *see* Disease, liver, toxic
    - end stage K72.1- ☑
      - due to hepatitis — *see* Hepatitis
      - with coma K72.11
    - fatty, nonalcoholic (NAFLD) K76.Ø
      - alcoholic K7Ø.Ø
    - fibrocystic (congenital) Q44.6
    - fluke
      - Chinese B66.1
      - oriental B66.1
      - sheep B66.3
    - gestational alloimmune (GALD) P78.84
    - glycogen storage E74.Ø9 *[K77]*
    - in (due to)
      - schistosomiasis (bilharziasis) B65.9 *[K77]*
    - inflammatory K75.9
      - alcoholic K7Ø.1 ☑
      - specified NEC K75.89
    - polycystic (congenital) Q44.6
    - toxic K71.9
      - with
        - cholestasis K71.Ø
        - cirrhosis (liver) K71.7
        - fibrosis (liver) K71.7
        - focal nodular hyperplasia K71.8
        - hepatic granuloma K71.8
        - hepatic necrosis K71.1Ø
          - with coma K71.11
        - hepatitis NEC K71.6
          - acute K71.2
          - chronic
            - active K71.5Ø
              - with ascites K71.51
            - lobular K71.4
            - persistent K71.3
          - lupoid K71.5Ø
            - with ascites K71.51
        - peliosis hepatis K71.8
        - veno-occlusive disease (VOD) of liver K71.8
    - veno-occlusive K76.5
  - Lobo's (keloid blastomycosis) B48.Ø
  - Lobstein's (brittle bones and blue sclera) Q78.Ø
  - Ludwig's (submaxillary cellulitis) K12.2
  - lumbosacral region M53.87
  - lung J98.4
    - black J6Ø
    - congenital Q33.9
    - cystic J98.4
      - congenital Q33.Ø
    - dabbing (related) UØ7.Ø
    - electronic cigarette (related) UØ7.Ø
    - fibroid (chronic) — *see* Fibrosis, lung
    - fluke B66.4
      - oriental B66.4
    - in
      - amyloidosis E85.4 *[J99]*
      - sarcoidosis D86.Ø
      - Sjögren's syndrome M35.Ø2
      - systemic
        - lupus erythematosus M32.13
        - sclerosis M34.81
    - interstitial J84.9
      - of childhood, specified NEC J84.848
      - respiratory bronchiolitis J84.115
      - specified NEC J84.89

- **Disease, diseased** — *continued*
  - lung — *continued*
    - interstitial — *continued*
      - with progressive fibrotic phenotype, in diseases classified elsewhere J84.17Ø
    - obstructive (chronic) J44.9
      - with
        - acute
          - bronchitis J44.Ø
          - exacerbation NEC J44.1
          - lower respiratory infection J44.Ø
        - alveolitis, allergic J67.9
        - asthma J44.9
        - bronchiectasis J47.9
          - with
            - exacerbation (acute) J47.1
            - lower respiratory infection J47.Ø
        - bronchitis J44.9
          - with
            - exacerbation (acute) J44.1
            - lower respiratory infection J44.Ø
        - emphysema J43.9
        - hypersensitivity pneumonitis J67.9
      - decompensated J44.1
        - with
          - exacerbation (acute) J44.1
    - polycystic J98.4
      - congenital Q33.Ø
    - rheumatoid (diffuse) (interstitial) — *see* Rheumatoid, lung
    - vaping (associated) (device) (product) (use) UØ7.Ø
  - Lutembacher's (atrial septal defect with mitral stenosis) Q21.19
  - Lyme A69.2Ø
  - lymphatic (gland) (system) (channel) (vessel) I89.9
  - lymphoproliferative D47.9
    - specified NEC D47.Z9 (*following* D47.4)
    - T-gamma D47.Z9 (*following* D47.4)
    - X-linked D82.3
  - Magitot's M27.2
  - malarial — *see* Malaria
  - malignant — *see also* Neoplasm, malignant, by site
  - Manson's B65.1
  - maple bark J67.6
  - maple-syrup-urine E71.Ø
  - Marburg (virus) A98.3
  - Marion's (bladder neck obstruction) N32.Ø
  - Marsh's (exophthalmic goiter) — *see* Hyperthyroidism, with, goiter (diffuse)
  - mastoid (process) — *see* Disorder, ear, middle
  - Mathieu's (leptospiral jaundice) A27.Ø
  - Maxcy's A75.2
  - McArdle (-Schmid-Pearson) (glycogenosis V) E74.Ø4
  - mediastinum J98.59
  - medullary center (idiopathic) (respiratory) G93.89
  - Meige's (chronic hereditary edema) Q82.Ø
  - meningococcal — *see* Infection, meningococcal
  - mental F99
    - organic FØ9
  - mesenchymal M35.9
  - mesenteric embolic — *see also* Ischemia, intestine, acute K55.Ø39
  - metabolic, metabolism E88.9
    - bilirubin E8Ø.7
  - metal-polisher's J62.8
  - metastatic — *see also* Neoplasm, secondary, by site C79.9
  - microvascular - code to condition
  - microvillus
    - atrophy Q43.8
    - inclusion (MVD) Q43.8
  - middle ear — *see* Disorder, ear, middle
  - Mikulicz' (dryness of mouth, absent or decreased lacrimation) K11.8
  - Milroy's (chronic hereditary edema) Q82.Ø
  - Minamata — *see* Poisoning, mercury
  - minicore G71.29
  - Minor's G95.19
  - Minot's (hemorrhagic disease, newborn) P53
  - Minot-von Willebrand-Jürgens (angiohemophilia) — *see* Disease, von Willebrand
  - Mitchell's (erythromelalgia) I73.81
  - mitral (valve) IØ5.9
    - nonrheumatic I34.9
  - mixed connective tissue M35.1
  - moldy hay J67.Ø
  - Monge's T7Ø.29 ☑
  - Morgagni-Adams-Stokes (syncope with heart block) I45.9
  - Morgagni's (syndrome) (hyperostosis frontalis interna) M85.2
  - Morton's (with metatarsalgia) — *see* Lesion, nerve, plantar
  - Morvan's G6Ø.8
  - motor neuron (bulbar) (mixed type) (spinal) G12.2Ø
    - amyotrophic lateral sclerosis G12.21
    - familial G12.24
    - progressive bulbar palsy G12.22
    - specified NEC G12.29
  - moyamoya I67.5
  - mu heavy chain disease C88.2
  - multicore G71.29
  - multiminicore G71.29
  - muscle — *see also* Disorder, muscle
    - inflammatory — *see* Myositis
    - ocular (external) — *see* Strabismus
  - musculoskeletal system, soft tissue — *see also* Disorder, soft tissue
    - specified NEC — *see* Disorder, soft tissue, specified type NEC
  - mushroom workers' J67.5
  - mycotic B49
  - myelodysplastic — *see also* Syndrome, myelodysplasia C94.6
  - myelodysplastic/myeloproliferative neoplasm, unclassifiable C94.6
  - myeloproliferative D47.1
    - chronic D47.1
    - not classified C94.6
    - specified NEC C94.6
    - unclassifiable C94.6
  - myocardium, myocardial — *see also* Degeneration, myocardial I51.5
    - primary (idiopathic) I42.9
  - myoneural G7Ø.9
  - Naegeli's D69.1
  - nails L6Ø.9
    - specified NEC L6Ø.8
  - Nairobi (sheep virus) A93.8
  - nasal J34.9
  - nemaline body G71.21
  - nerve — *see* Disorder, nerve
  - nervous system G98.8
    - autonomic G9Ø.9
    - central G96.9
      - specified NEC G96.89
    - congenital QØ7.9
    - parasympathetic G9Ø.9
    - specified NEC G98.8
    - sympathetic G9Ø.9
    - vegetative G9Ø.9
  - neuromuscular system G7Ø.9
  - Newcastle B3Ø.8
  - Nicolas (-Durand)-Favre (climatic bubo) A55
  - nipple N64.9
    - Paget's C5Ø.Ø1- ☑
      - female C5Ø.Ø1- ☑
      - male C5Ø.Ø2- ☑
  - Nishimoto (-Takeuchi) I67.5
  - nonarthropod-borne NOS (viral) B34.9
    - enterovirus NEC B34.1
  - nonautoimmune hemolytic D59.4
    - drug-induced D59.2
  - Nonne-Milroy-Meige (chronic hereditary edema) Q82.Ø
  - nose J34.9
  - nucleus pulposus — *see* Disorder, disc
  - nutritional E63.9
  - oast-house-urine E72.19
    - ocular
      - herpesviral BØØ.5Ø
      - zoster BØ2.3Ø
  - obliterative vascular I77.1
  - Ohara's — *see* Tularemia
  - Opitz's (congestive splenomegaly) D73.2
  - Oppenheim-Urbach (necrobiosis lipoidica diabeticorum) — *see* EØ8-E13 with .62Ø
  - optic nerve NEC — *see* Disorder, nerve, optic
  - orbit — *see* Disorder, orbit
  - organ
    - dabbing (related) UØ7.Ø
    - electronic cigarette (related) UØ7.Ø
    - vaping (associated) (device) (product) (use) UØ7.Ø
  - Oriental liver fluke B66.1
  - Oriental lung fluke B66.4
  - Ormond's N13.5
  - Oropouche virus A93.Ø
  - Osler-Rendu (familial hemorrhagic telangiectasia) I78.Ø
  - osteofibrocystic E21.Ø
  - Otto's M24.7
  - outer ear — *see* Disorder, ear, external
  - ovary (noninflammatory) N83.9
    - cystic N83.2Ø- ☑
    - inflammatory — *see* Salpingo-oophoritis
    - polycystic E28.2
    - specified NEC N83.8
  - Owren's (congenital) — *see* Defect, coagulation
  - p11Ød-activating mutation causing senescent T cells, lymphadenopathy, and immunodeficiency [PASLI] D81.82
  - pancreas K86.9
    - cystic K86.2
    - fibrocystic E84.9
    - specified NEC K86.89
  - panvalvular IØ8.9
    - specified NEC IØ8.8
  - parametrium (noninflammatory) N83.9
  - parasitic B89
    - cerebral NEC B71.9 *[G94]*
    - intestinal NOS B82.9
    - mouth B37.Ø
    - skin NOS B88.9
    - specified type — *see* Infestation
    - tongue B37.Ø
  - parathyroid (gland) E21.5
    - specified NEC E21.4
  - Parkinson's G2Ø
  - parodontal KØ5.6
  - Parrot's (syphilitic osteochondritis) A5Ø.Ø2
  - Parry's (exophthalmic goiter) — *see* Hyperthyroidism, with, goiter (diffuse)
  - Parson's (exophthalmic goiter) — *see* Hyperthyroidism, with, goiter (diffuse)
  - Paxton's (white piedra) B36.2
  - pearl-worker's — *see* Osteomyelitis, specified type NEC
  - Pellegrini-Stieda (calcification, knee joint) — *see* Bursitis, tibial collateral
  - pelvis, pelvic
    - female NOS N94.9
      - specified NEC N94.89
    - gonococcal (acute) (chronic) A54.24
    - inflammatory (female) N73.9
      - acute N73.Ø
      - chlamydial A56.11
      - chronic N73.1
      - specified NEC N73.8
      - syphilitic (secondary) A51.42
        - late A52.76
      - tuberculous A18.17
    - organ, female N94.9
    - peritoneum, female NEC N94.89
  - penis N48.9
    - inflammatory N48.29
      - abscess N48.21
      - cellulitis N48.22
    - specified NEC N48.89
  - periapical tissues NOS KØ4.9Ø
  - periodontal KØ5.6
    - specified NEC KØ5.5
  - periosteum — *see* Disorder, bone, specified type NEC
  - peripheral
    - arterial I73.9
    - autonomic nervous system G9Ø.9
    - nerves — *see* Polyneuropathy
    - vascular NOS I73.9
  - peritoneum K66.9
    - pelvic, female NEC N94.89
    - specified NEC K66.8
  - persistent mucosal (middle ear) H66.2Ø
    - left H66.22
      - with right H66.23
    - right H66.21
      - with left H66.23
  - Petit's — *see* Hernia, abdomen, specified site NEC
  - pharynx J39.2
    - specified NEC J39.2
  - Phocas' — *see* Mastopathy, cystic
  - photochromogenic (acid-fast bacilli) (pulmonary) A31.Ø
    - nonpulmonary A31.9
  - Pick's — *see also* Dementia, in, diseases specified elsewhere G31.Ø1 *[FØ2.8Ø]*

Disease, diseased — *continued*

- Pick's — *see also* Dementia, in, diseases specified elsewhere — *continued*
  - with behavioral disturbance — *see also* Dementia, in, diseases specified elsewhere G31.01 *[F02.81-]* ☑
  - brain G31.01 *[F02.80]*
    - with behavioral disturbance — *see also* Dementia, in, diseases specified elsewhere G31.01 *[F02.81-]* ☑
  - of pericardium (pericardial pseudocirrhosis of liver) I31.1
- pigeon fancier's J67.2
- pineal gland E34.8
- pink — *see* Poisoning, mercury
- Pinkus' (lichen nitidus) L44.1
- pinworm B80
- Piry virus A93.8
- pituitary (gland) E23.7
- pituitary-snuff-taker's J67.8
- pleura (cavity) J94.9
  - specified NEC J94.8
- pneumatic drill (hammer) T75.21 ☑
- Pollitzer's (hidradenitis suppurativa) L73.2
- polycystic
  - kidney or renal Q61.3
    - adult type Q61.2
    - childhood type NEC Q61.19
      - collecting duct dilatation Q61.11
  - liver or hepatic Q44.6
  - lung or pulmonary J98.4
    - congenital Q33.0
  - ovary, ovaries E28.2
  - spleen Q89.09
- polyethylene T84.05- ☑
- Pompe's (glycogenosis II) E74.02
- Posadas-Wernicke B38.9
- Potain's (pulmonary edema) — *see* Edema, lung
- prepuce N47.8
  - inflammatory N47.7
    - balanoposthitis N47.6
- Pringle's (tuberous sclerosis) Q85.1
- prion, central nervous system A81.9
  - specified NEC A81.89
- prostate N42.9
  - specified NEC N42.89
- protozoal B64
  - acanthamebiasis — *see* Acanthamebiasis
  - African trypanosomiasis — *see* African trypanosomiasis
  - babesiosis — *see also* Babesiosis B60.00
  - Chagas disease — *see* Chagas disease
  - intestine, intestinal A07.9
  - leishmaniasis — *see* Leishmaniasis
  - malaria — *see* Malaria
  - naegleriasis B60.2
  - pneumocystosis B59
  - specified organism NEC B60.8
  - toxoplasmosis — *see* Toxoplasmosis
- pseudo-Hurler's E77.0
- psychiatric F99
- psychotic — *see* Psychosis
- Puente's (simple glandular cheilitis) K13.0
- puerperal — *see also* Puerperal O90.89
- pulmonary — *see also* Disease, lung
  - artery I28.9
  - chronic obstructive J44.9
    - with
      - acute bronchitis J44.0
      - exacerbation (acute) J44.1
      - lower respiratory infection (acute) J44.0
    - decompensated J44.1
      - with
        - exacerbation (acute) J44.1
  - heart I27.9
    - specified NEC I27.89
  - hypertensive (vascular) — *see also* Hypertension, pulmonary I27.20
    - NEC I27.2 ☑
    - primary (idiopathic) I27.0
  - valve I37.9
    - rheumatic I09.89
- pulp (dental) NOS K04.90
- pulseless M31.4
- Putnam's (subacute combined sclerosis with pernicious anemia) D51.0
- Pyle (-Cohn) (metaphyseal dysplasia) Q78.5
- ragpicker's or ragsorter's A22.1
- Raynaud's — *see* Raynaud's disease
- reactive airway — *see* Asthma
- Reclus' (cystic) — *see* Mastopathy, cystic
- rectum K62.9
  - specified NEC K62.89
- Refsum's (heredopathia atactica polyneuritiformis) G60.1
- renal (functional) (pelvis) — *see also* Disease, kidney N28.9
  - with
    - edema — *see* Nephrosis
    - glomerular lesion — *see* Glomerulonephritis
      - with edema — *see* Nephrosis
    - interstitial nephritis N12
  - acute N28.9
  - chronic — *see also* Disease, kidney, chronic N18.9
  - cystic, congenital Q61.9
  - diabetic — *see* E08-E13 with .22
  - end-stage (failure) N18.6
    - due to hypertension I12.0
  - fibrocystic (congenital) Q61.8
  - hypertensive — *see* Hypertension, kidney
  - lupus M32.14
  - phosphate-losing (tubular) N25.0
  - polycystic (congenital) Q61.3
    - adult type Q61.2
    - childhood type NEC Q61.19
      - collecting duct dilatation Q61.11
  - rapidly progressive N01.9
  - subacute N01.9
- Rendu-Osler-Weber (familial hemorrhagic telangiectasia) I78.0
- renovascular (arteriosclerotic) — *see* Hypertension, kidney
- respiratory (tract) J98.9
  - acute or subacute NOS J06.9
    - due to
      - chemicals, gases, fumes or vapors (inhalation) J68.3
      - external agent J70.9
        - specified NEC J70.8
      - radiation J70.0
      - smoke inhalation J70.5
    - noninfectious J39.8
  - chronic NOS J98.9
    - due to
      - chemicals, gases, fumes or vapors J68.4
      - external agent J70.9
        - specified NEC J70.8
      - radiation J70.1
    - newborn P27.9
      - specified NEC P27.8
  - due to
    - chemicals, gases, fumes or vapors J68.9
      - acute or subacute NEC J68.3
      - chronic J68.4
    - external agent J70.9
      - specified NEC J70.8
  - newborn P28.9
    - specified type NEC P28.89
  - upper J39.9
    - acute or subacute J06.9
    - noninfectious NEC J39.8
    - specified NEC J39.8
    - streptococcal J06.9
- retina, retinal H35.9
  - Batten's or Batten-Mayou E75.4 *[H36]*
  - specified NEC H35.89
- rheumatoid — *see* Arthritis, rheumatoid
- rickettsial NOS A79.9
  - specified type NEC A79.89
- Riga (-Fede) (cachectic aphthae) K14.0
- Riggs' (compound periodontitis) — *see* Periodontitis
- Ritter's L00
- Rivalta's (cervicofacial actinomycosis) A42.2
- Robles' (onchocerciasis) B73.01
- rod body G71.21
- Roger's (congenital interventricular septal defect) Q21.0
- Rosenthal's (factor XI deficiency) D68.1
- Ross River B33.1
- Rossbach's (hyperchlorhydria) K31.89
  - psychogenic F45.8
- Rotes Quérol — *see* Hyperostosis, ankylosing
- Roth (-Bernhardt) — *see* Mononeuropathy, lower limb, meralgia paresthetica
- Runeberg's (progressive pernicious anemia) D51.0
- sacroiliac NEC M53.3
- salivary gland or duct K11.9
  - inclusion B25.9
  - specified NEC K11.8
  - virus B25.9
- sandworm B76.9
- Schimmelbusch's — *see* Mastopathy, cystic
- Schmorl's — *see* Schmorl's disease or nodes
- Schönlein (-Henoch) (purpura rheumatica) D69.0
- Schottmüller's — *see* Fever, paratyphoid
- Schultz's (agranulocytosis) — *see* Agranulocytosis
- Schwalbe-Ziehen-Oppenheim G24.1
- Schwartz-Jampel G71.13
- sclera H15.9
  - specified NEC H15.89
- scrofulous (tuberculous) A18.2
- scrotum N50.9
- sebaceous glands L73.9
- semilunar cartilage, cystic — *see also* Derangement, knee, meniscus, cystic
- seminal vesicle N50.9
- serum NEC — *see also* Reaction, serum T80.69 ☑
- sexually transmitted A64
  - anogenital
    - herpesviral infection — *see* Herpes, anogenital
    - warts A63.0
  - chancroid A57
  - chlamydial infection — *see* Chlamydia
  - gonorrhea — *see* Gonorrhea
  - granuloma inguinale A58
  - specified organism NEC A63.8
  - syphilis — *see* Syphilis
  - trichomoniasis — *see* Trichomoniasis
- Sézary C84.1- ☑
- shimamushi (scrub typhus) A75.3
- shipyard B30.0
- sickle-cell D57.1
  - with
    - acute chest syndrome D57.01
    - cerebral vascular involvement D57.03
    - crisis (painful) D57.00
      - with complication specified NEC D57.09
    - splenic sequestration D57.02
    - vasoocclusive pain D57.00
  - elliptocytosis D57.8- ☑
  - Hb-C D57.20
    - with
      - acute chest syndrome D57.211
      - cerebral vascular involvement D57.213
      - crisis D57.219
        - with specified complication NEC D57.218
      - splenic sequestration D57.212
      - vasoocclusive pain D57.219
    - without crisis D57.20
  - Hb-SD D57.80
    - with
      - acute chest syndrome D57.811
      - cerebral vascular involvement D57.813
      - crisis D57.819
        - with complication specified NEC D57.818
      - splenic sequestration D57.812
      - vasoocclusive pain D57.819
    - without crisis D57.80
  - Hb-SE D57.80
    - with
      - acute chest syndrome D57.811
      - cerebral vascular involvement D57.813
      - crisis D57.819
        - with complication specified NEC D57.818
      - splenic sequestration D57.812
      - vasoocclusive pain D57.819
    - without crisis D57.80
  - specified NEC D57.80
    - with
      - acute chest syndrome D57.811
      - cerebral vascular involvement D57.813
      - crisis D57.819
        - with complication specified NEC D57.818
      - splenic sequestration D57.812
      - vasoocclusive pain D57.819
    - without crisis D57.80
  - spherocytosis D57.80
    - with
      - acute chest syndrome D57.811
      - cerebral vascular involvement D57.813
      - crisis D57.819
        - with complication specified NEC D57.818
      - splenic sequestration D57.812

Disease, diseased — *continued*
sickle-cell — *continued*
spherocytosis — *continued*
with — *continued*
vasoocclusive pain D57.819
without crisis D57.80
thalassemia D57.40
with
acute chest syndrome D57.411
cerebral vascular involvement D57.413
crisis (painful) D57.419
with specified complication NEC D57.418
splenic sequestration D57.412
vasoocclusive pain D57.419
beta plus D57.44
with
acute chest syndrome D57.451
cerebral vascular involvement D57.453
crisis D57.459
with specified complication NEC D57.458
splenic sequestration D57.452
vasoocclusive pain D57.459
without crisis D57.44
beta zero D57.42
with
acute chest syndrome D57.431
cerebral vascular involvement D57.433
crisis D57.439
with specified complication NEC D57.438
splenic sequestration D57.432
vasoocclusive pain D57.439
without crisis D57.42
silo-filler's J68.8
bronchitis J68.0
pneumonitis J68.0
pulmonary edema J68.1
simian B B00.4
Simons' (progressive lipodystrophy) E88.1
sin nombre virus B33.4
sinus — *see* Sinusitis
Sirkari's B55.0
sixth B08.20
due to human herpesvirus 6 B08.21
due to human herpesvirus 7 B08.22
skin L98.9
due to metabolic disorder NEC E88.9 *[L99]*
specified NEC L98.8
slim (HIV) B20
small vessel I73.9
Sneddon-Wilkinson (subcorneal pustular dermatosis) L13.1
South African creeping B88.0
spinal (cord) G95.9
congenital Q06.9
specified NEC G95.89
spine — *see also* Spondylopathy
joint — *see* Dorsopathy
tuberculous A18.01
spinocerebellar (hereditary) G11.9
specified NEC G11.8
spleen D73.9
amyloid E85.4 *[D77]*
organic D73.9
polycystic Q89.09
postinfectional D73.89
sponge-diver's — *see* Toxicity, venom, marine animal, sea anemone
Startle Q89.8
Steinert's G71.11
Sticker's (erythema infectiosum) B08.3
Stieda's (calcification, knee joint) — *see* Bursitis, tibial collateral
Stokes' (exophthalmic goiter) — *see* Hyperthyroidism, with, goiter (diffuse)
Stokes-Adams (syncope with heart block) I45.9
stomach K31.9
functional, psychogenic F45.8
specified NEC K31.89
stonemason's J62.8
storage
glycogen — *see* Disease, glycogen storage
mucopolysaccharide — *see* Mucopolysaccharidosis
striatopallidal system NEC G25.89
Stuart-Prower (congenital factor X deficiency) D68.2
Stuart's (congenital factor X deficiency) D68.2
subcutaneous tissue — *see* Disease, skin

Disease, diseased — *continued*
supporting structures of teeth K08.9
specified NEC K08.89
suprarenal (capsule) (gland) E27.9
hyperfunction E27.0
specified NEC E27.8
sweat glands L74.9
specified NEC L74.8
Sweeley-Klionsky E75.21
Swift (-Feer) — *see* Poisoning, mercury
swimming-pool granuloma A31.1
Sylvest's (epidemic pleurodynia) B33.0
sympathetic nervous system G90.9
synovium — *see* Disorder, synovium
syphilitic — *see* Syphilis
systemic tissue mast cell D47.02
tanapox (virus) B08.71
Tangier E78.6
Tarral-Besnier (pityriasis rubra pilaris) L44.0
Tauri's E74.09
tear duct — *see* Disorder, lacrimal system
tendon, tendinous — *see also* Disorder, tendon
nodular — *see* Trigger finger
terminal vessel I73.9
testis N50.9
thalassemia Hb-S — *see* Disease, sickle-cell, thalassemia
Thaysen-Gee (nontropical sprue) K90.0
Thomsen G71.12
throat J39.2
septic J02.0
thromboembolic — *see* Embolism
thymus (gland) E32.9
specified NEC E32.8
thyroid (gland) E07.9
heart — *see also* Hyperthyroidism E05.90 *[I43]*
with thyroid storm E05.91 *[I43]*
specified NEC E07.89
Tietze's M94.0
tongue K14.9
specified NEC K14.8
tonsils, tonsillar (and adenoids) J35.9
tooth, teeth K08.9
hard tissues K03.9
specified NEC K03.89
pulp NEC K04.99
specified NEC K08.89
Tourette's F95.2
trachea NEC J39.8
tricuspid I07.9
nonrheumatic I36.9
triglyceride-storage E75.5
trophoblastic — *see* Mole, hydatidiform
tsutsugamushi A75.3
tube (fallopian) (noninflammatory) N83.9
inflammatory — *see* Salpingitis
specified NEC N83.8
tuberculous NEC — *see* Tuberculosis
tubo-ovarian (noninflammatory) N83.9
inflammatory — *see* Salpingo-oophoritis
specified NEC N83.8
tubotympanic, chronic — *see* Otitis, media, suppurative, chronic, tubotympanic
tubulo-interstitial N15.9
specified NEC N15.8
tympanum — *see* Disorder, tympanic membrane
Uhl's Q24.8
Underwood's (sclerema neonatorum) P83.0
Unverricht (-Lundborg) — *see* Epilepsy, generalized, idiopathic
Urbach-Oppenheim (necrobiosis lipoidica diabeticorum) — *see* E08-E13 with .620
ureter N28.9
in (due to)
schistosomiasis (bilharziasis) B65.0 *[N29]*
urethra N36.9
specified NEC N36.8
urinary (tract) N39.9
bladder N32.9
specified NEC N32.89
specified NEC N39.8
uterus (noninflammatory) N85.9
infective — *see* Endometritis
inflammatory — *see* Endometritis
specified NEC N85.8
uveal tract (anterior) H21.9
posterior H31.9
vagabond's B85.1
vagina, vaginal (noninflammatory) N89.9

Disease, diseased — *continued*
vagina, vaginal — *continued*
inflammatory NEC N76.89
specified NEC N89.8
valve, valvular I38
multiple I08.9
specified NEC I08.8
van Creveld-von Gierke (glycogenosis I) E74.01
vas deferens N50.9
vascular I99.9
arteriosclerotic — *see* Arteriosclerosis
ciliary body NEC — *see* Disorder, iris, vascular
hypertensive — *see* Hypertension
iris NEC — *see* Disorder, iris, vascular
obliterative I77.1
peripheral I73.9
occlusive I99.8
peripheral (occlusive) I73.9
in diabetes mellitus — *see* E08-E13 with .51
vasomotor I73.9
vasospastic I73.9
vein I87.9
venereal — *see also* Disease, sexually transmitted A64
chlamydial NEC A56.8
anus A56.3
genitourinary NOS A56.2
pharynx A56.4
rectum A56.3
fifth A55
sixth A55
specified nature or type NEC A63.8
vertebra, vertebral — *see also* Spondylopathy
disc — *see* Disorder, disc
vibration — *see* Vibration, adverse effects
viral, virus — *see also* Disease, by type of virus B34.9
arbovirus NOS A94
arthropod-borne NOS A94
congenital P35.9
specified NEC P35.8
Hanta (with renal manifestations) (Dobrava) (Puumala) (Seoul) A98.5
with pulmonary manifestations (Andes) (Bayou) (Bermejo) (Black Creek Canal) (Choclo) (Juquitiba) (Laguna negra) (Lechiguanas) (New York) (Oran) (Sin nombre) B33.4
Hantaan (Korean hemorrhagic fever) A98.5
human immunodeficiency (HIV) B20
Kunjin A83.4
nonarthropod-borne NOS B34.9
Powassan A84.81
Rocio (encephalitis) A83.6
Sin nombre (Hantavirus) (cardio)-pulmonary syndrome) B33.4
Tahyna B33.8
vesicular stomatitis A93.8
vitreous H43.9
specified NEC H43.89
vocal cord J38.3
Volkmann's, acquired T79.6 ☑
von Eulenburg's (congenital paramyotonia) G71.19
von Gierke's (glycogenosis I) E74.01
von Graefe's — *see* Strabismus, paralytic, ophthalmoplegia, progressive
von Willebrand (-Jürgens) (angiohemophilia) D68.00
acquired D68.04
platelet-type D68.09
pseudo D68.09
specified NEC D68.09
type 1 D68.01
type 1C D68.01
type 2 D68.029
type 2A D68.020
type 2B D68.021
type 2M D68.022
type 2N D68.023
type 3 D68.03
Vrolik's (osteogenesis imperfecta) Q78.0
vulva (noninflammatory) N90.9
inflammatory NEC N76.89
specified NEC N90.89
Wallgren's (obstruction of splenic vein with collateral circulation) I87.8
Wassilieff's (leptospiral jaundice) A27.0
wasting NEC R64
due to malnutrition E43
with marasmus E41
Waterhouse-Friderichsen A39.1
Wegner's (syphilitic osteochondritis) A50.02

Disease, diseased — *continued*
Weil's (leptospiral jaundice of lung) A27.Ø
Weir Mitchell's (erythromelalgia) I73.81
Werdnig-Hoffmann G12.Ø
Wermer's E31.21
Werner-His (trench fever) A79.Ø
Werner-Schultz (neutropenic splenomegaly) D73.81
Wernicke-Posadas B38.9
whipworm B79
white blood cells D72.9
specified NEC D72.89
white matter R9Ø.82
white-spot, meaning lichen sclerosus et atrophicus L9Ø.Ø
penis N48.Ø
vulva N9Ø.4
Wilkie's K55.1
Wilkinson-Sneddon (subcorneal pustular dermatosis) L13.1
Willis' — *see* Diabetes
Wilson's (hepatolenticular degeneration) E83.Ø1
woolsorter's A22.1
yaba monkey tumor BØ8.72
yaba pox (virus) BØ8.72
Zika virus A92.5
congenital P35.4
zoonotic, bacterial A28.9
specified type NEC A28.8
Disfigurement (due to scar) L9Ø.5
Disgerminoma — *see* Dysgerminoma
DISH (diffuse idiopathic skeletal hyperostosis) — *see* Hyperostosis, ankylosing
Disinsertion, retina — *see* Detachment, retina
Dislocatable hip, congenital Q65.6
Dislocation (articular)
with fracture — *see* Fracture
acromioclavicular (joint) S43.1Ø- ☑
with displacement
1ØØ%-2ØØ% S43.12- ☑
more than 2ØØ% S43.13- ☑
inferior S43.14- ☑
posterior S43.15- ☑
ankle S93.Ø- ☑
astragalus — *see* Dislocation, ankle
atlantoaxial S13.121 ☑
atlantooccipital S13.111 ☑
atloidooccipital S13.111 ☑
breast bone S23.29 ☑
capsule, joint — *code by* site under Dislocation
carpal (bone) — *see* Dislocation, wrist
carpometacarpal (joint) NEC S63.Ø5- ☑
thumb S63.Ø4- ☑
cartilage (joint) — *code by* site under Dislocation
cervical spine (vertebra) — *see* Dislocation, vertebra, cervical
chronic — *see* Dislocation, recurrent
clavicle — *see* Dislocation, acromioclavicular joint
coccyx S33.2 ☑
congenital NEC Q68.8
coracoid — *see* Dislocation, shoulder
costal cartilage S23.29 ☑
costochondral S23.29 ☑
cricoarytenoid articulation S13.29 ☑
cricothyroid articulation S13.29 ☑
dorsal vertebra — *see* Dislocation, vertebra, thoracic
ear ossicle — *see* Discontinuity, ossicles, ear
elbow S53.1Ø- ☑
congenital Q68.8
pathological — *see* Dislocation, pathological NEC, elbow
radial head alone — *see* Dislocation, radial head
recurrent — *see* Dislocation, recurrent, elbow
traumatic S53.1Ø- ☑
anterior S53.11- ☑
lateral S53.14- ☑
medial S53.13- ☑
posterior S53.12- ☑
specified type NEC S53.19- ☑
eye, nontraumatic — *see* Luxation, globe
eyeball, nontraumatic — *see* Luxation, globe
femur
distal end — *see* Dislocation, knee
proximal end — *see* Dislocation, hip
fibula
distal end — *see* Dislocation, ankle
proximal end — *see* Dislocation, knee
finger S63.25- ☑

Dislocation — *continued*
finger — *continued*
index S63.25- ☑
interphalangeal S63.27- ☑
distal S63.29- ☑
index S63.29- ☑
little S63.29- ☑
middle S63.29- ☑
ring S63.29- ☑
index S63.27- ☑
little S63.27- ☑
middle S63.27- ☑
proximal S63.28- ☑
index S63.28- ☑
little S63.28- ☑
middle S63.28- ☑
ring S63.28- ☑
ring S63.27- ☑
little S63.25- ☑
metacarpophalangeal S63.26- ☑
index S63.26- ☑
little S63.26- ☑
middle S63.26- ☑
ring S63.26- ☑
middle S63.25- ☑
recurrent — *see* Dislocation, recurrent, finger
ring S63.25- ☑
thumb — *see* Dislocation, thumb
foot S93.3Ø- ☑
recurrent — *see* Dislocation, recurrent, foot
specified site NEC S93.33- ☑
tarsal joint S93.31- ☑
tarsometatarsal joint S93.32- ☑
toe — *see* Dislocation, toe
fracture — *see* Fracture
glenohumeral (joint) — *see* Dislocation, shoulder
glenoid — *see* Dislocation, shoulder
habitual — *see* Dislocation, recurrent
hip S73.ØØ- ☑
anterior S73.Ø3- ☑
obturator S73.Ø2- ☑
central S73.Ø4- ☑
congenital (total) Q65.2
bilateral Q65.1
partial Q65.5
bilateral Q65.4
unilateral Q65.3- ☑
unilateral Q65.Ø- ☑
developmental M24.85- ☑
pathological — *see* Dislocation, pathological NEC, hip
posterior S73.Ø1- ☑
recurrent — *see* Dislocation, recurrent, hip
humerus, proximal end — *see* Dislocation, shoulder
incomplete — *see* Subluxation, by site
incus — *see* Discontinuity, ossicles, ear
infracoracoid — *see* Dislocation, shoulder
innominate (pubic junction) (sacral junction) S33.39 ☑
acetabulum — *see* Dislocation, hip
interphalangeal (joint(s))
finger S63.279 ☑
distal S63.29- ☑
index S63.29- ☑
little S63.29- ☑
middle S63.29- ☑
ring S63.29- ☑
index S63.27- ☑
little S63.27- ☑
middle S63.27- ☑
proximal S63.28- ☑
index S63.28- ☑
little S63.28- ☑
middle S63.28- ☑
ring S63.28- ☑
ring S63.27- ☑
foot or toe — *see* Dislocation, toe
thumb S63.12- ☑
jaw (cartilage) (meniscus) SØ3.Ø- ☑
joint prosthesis — *see* Complications, joint prosthesis, mechanical, displacement, by site
knee S83.1Ø6 ☑
cap — *see* Dislocation, patella
congenital Q68.2
old M23.8X- ☑
patella — *see* Dislocation, patella

Dislocation — *continued*
knee — *continued*
pathological — *see* Dislocation, pathological NEC, knee
proximal tibia
anteriorly S83.11- ☑
laterally S83.14- ☑
medially S83.13- ☑
posteriorly S83.12- ☑
recurrent — *see also* Derangement, knee, specified NEC
specified type NEC S83.19- ☑
lacrimal gland HØ4.16- ☑
lens (complete) H27.1Ø
anterior H27.12- ☑
congenital Q12.1
ocular implant — *see* Complications, intraocular lens
partial H27.11- ☑
posterior H27.13- ☑
traumatic SØ5.8X- ☑
ligament — *code by* site under Dislocation
lumbar (vertebra) — *see* Dislocation, vertebra, lumbar
lumbosacral (vertebra) — *see also* Dislocation, vertebra, lumbar
congenital Q76.49
mandible SØ3.Ø- ☑
meniscus (knee) — *see* Tear, meniscus
other sites - code by site under Dislocation
metacarpal (bone)
distal end — *see* Dislocation, finger
proximal end S63.Ø6- ☑
metacarpophalangeal (joint)
finger S63.26- ☑
index S63.26- ☑
little S63.26- ☑
middle S63.26- ☑
ring S63.26- ☑
thumb S63.11- ☑
metatarsal (bone) — *see* Dislocation, foot
metatarsophalangeal (joint(s)) — *see* Dislocation, toe
midcarpal (joint) S63.Ø3- ☑
midtarsal (joint) — *see* Dislocation, foot
neck S13.2Ø ☑
specified site NEC S13.29 ☑
vertebra — *see* Dislocation, vertebra, cervical
nose (septal cartilage) SØ3.1 ☑
occipitoatloid S13.111 ☑
old — *see* Derangement, joint, specified type NEC
ossicles, ear — *see* Discontinuity, ossicles, ear
partial — *see* Subluxation, by site
patella S83.ØØ6 ☑
congenital Q74.1
lateral S83.Ø1- ☑
recurrent (nontraumatic) M22.Ø- ☑
incomplete M22.1- ☑
specified type NEC S83.Ø9- ☑
pathological NEC M24.3Ø
ankle M24.37- ☑
elbow M24.32- ☑
foot joint M24.37- ☑
hand joint M24.34- ☑
hip M24.35- ☑
knee M24.36- ☑
lumbosacral joint — *see* subcategory M53.2 ☑
pelvic region — *see* Dislocation, pathological, hip
sacroiliac — *see* subcategory M53.2 ☑
shoulder M24.31- ☑
specified site NEC M24.39
wrist M24.33- ☑
pelvis NEC S33.3Ø ☑
specified NEC S33.39 ☑
phalanx
finger or hand — *see* Dislocation, finger
foot or toe — *see* Dislocation, toe
prosthesis, internal — *see* Complications, prosthetic device, by site, mechanical
radial head S53.ØØ6 ☑
anterior S53.Ø1- ☑
posterior S53.Ø2- ☑
specified type NEC S53.Ø9- ☑
radiocarpal (joint) S63.Ø2- ☑
radiohumeral (joint) — *see* Dislocation, radial head
radioulnar (joint)
distal S63.Ø1- ☑
proximal — *see* Dislocation, elbow

Dislocation — *continued*
radius
distal end — *see* Dislocation, wrist
proximal end — *see* Dislocation, radial head
recurrent M24.4Ø
ankle M24.47- ☑
elbow M24.42- ☑
finger M24.44- ☑
foot joint M24.47- ☑
hand joint M24.44- ☑
hip M24.45- ☑
knee M24.46- ☑
patella — *see* Dislocation, patella, recurrent
patella — *see* Dislocation, patella, recurrent
sacroiliac — *see* subcategory M53.2 ☑
shoulder M24.41- ☑
specified site NEC M24.49
toe M24.47- ☑
vertebra — *see also* subcategory M43.5 ☑
atlantoaxial M43.4
with myelopathy M43.3
wrist M24.43- ☑
rib (cartilage) S23.29 ☑
sacrococcygeal S33.2 ☑
sacroiliac (joint) (ligament) S33.2 ☑
congenital Q74.2
recurrent — *see* subcategory M53.2 ☑
sacrum S33.2 ☑
scaphoid (bone) (hand) (wrist) — *see* Dislocation, wrist
foot — *see* Dislocation, foot
scapula — *see* Dislocation, shoulder, girdle, scapula
semilunar cartilage, knee — *see* Tear, meniscus
septal cartilage (nose) SØ3.1 ☑
septum (nasal) (old) J34.2
sesamoid bone — *code by* site under Dislocation
shoulder (blade) (ligament) (joint) (traumatic) S43.ØØ6 ☑
acromioclavicular — *see* Dislocation, acromioclavicular
chronic — *see* Dislocation, recurrent, shoulder
congenital Q68.8
girdle S43.3Ø- ☑
scapula S43.31- ☑
specified site NEC S43.39- ☑
humerus S43.ØØ- ☑
anterior S43.Ø1- ☑
inferior S43.Ø3- ☑
posterior S43.Ø2- ☑
pathological — *see* Dislocation, pathological NEC, shoulder
recurrent — *see* Dislocation, recurrent, shoulder
specified type NEC S43.Ø8- ☑
spine
cervical — *see* Dislocation, vertebra, cervical
congenital Q76.49
due to birth trauma P11.5
lumbar — *see* Dislocation, vertebra, lumbar
thoracic — *see* Dislocation, vertebra, thoracic
spontaneous — *see* Dislocation, pathological
sternoclavicular (joint) S43.2Ø6 ☑
anterior S43.21- ☑
posterior S43.22- ☑
sternum S23.29 ☑
subglenoid — *see* Dislocation, shoulder
symphysis pubis S33.4 ☑
talus — *see* Dislocation, ankle
tarsal (bone(s)) (joint(s)) — *see* Dislocation, foot
tarsometatarsal (joint(s)) — *see* Dislocation, foot
temporomandibular (joint) SØ3.Ø- ☑
thigh, proximal end — *see* Dislocation, hip
thorax S23.2Ø ☑
specified site NEC S23.29 ☑
vertebra — *see* Dislocation, vertebra
thumb S63.1Ø- ☑
interphalangeal joint — *see* Dislocation, interphalangeal (joint), thumb
metacarpophalangeal joint — *see* Dislocation, metacarpophalangeal (joint), thumb
thyroid cartilage S13.29 ☑
tibia
distal end — *see* Dislocation, ankle
proximal end — *see* Dislocation, knee
tibiofibular (joint)
distal — *see* Dislocation, ankle
superior — *see* Dislocation, knee
toe(s) S93.1Ø6 ☑

Dislocation — *continued*
toe(s) — *continued*
great S93.1Ø- ☑
interphalangeal joint S93.11- ☑
metatarsophalangeal joint S93.12- ☑
interphalangeal joint S93.119 ☑
lesser S93.1Ø6 ☑
interphalangeal joint S93.11- ☑
metatarsophalangeal joint S93.12- ☑
metatarsophalangeal joint S93.12- ☑
tooth SØ3.2 ☑
trachea S23.29 ☑
ulna
distal end S63.Ø7- ☑
proximal end — *see* Dislocation, elbow
ulnohumeral (joint) — *see* Dislocation, elbow
vertebra (articular process) (body) (traumatic)
cervical S13.1Ø1 ☑
atlantoaxial joint S13.121 ☑
atlantooccipital joint S13.111 ☑
atloidooccipital joint S13.111 ☑
joint between
CØ and C1 S13.111 ☑
C1 and C2 S13.121 ☑
C2 and C3 S13.131 ☑
C3 and C4 S13.141 ☑
C4 and C5 S13.151 ☑
C5 and C6 S13.161 ☑
C6 and C7 S13.171 ☑
C7 and T1 S13.181 ☑
occipitoatloid joint S13.111 ☑
congenital Q76.49
lumbar S33.1Ø1 ☑
joint between
L1 and L2 S33.111 ☑
L2 and L3 S33.121 ☑
L3 and L4 S33.131 ☑
L4 and L5 S33.141 ☑
nontraumatic — *see* Displacement, intervertebral disc
partial — *see* Subluxation, by site
recurrent NEC — *see* subcategory M43.5 ☑
thoracic S23.1Ø1 ☑
joint between
T1 and T2 S23.111 ☑
T2 and T3 S23.121 ☑
T3 and T4 S23.123 ☑
T4 and T5 S23.131 ☑
T5 and T6 S23.133 ☑
T6 and T7 S23.141 ☑
T7 and T8 S23.143 ☑
T8 and T9 S23.151 ☑
T9 and T1Ø S23.153 ☑
T1Ø and T11 S23.161 ☑
T11 and T12 S23.163 ☑
T12 and L1 S23.171 ☑
wrist (carpal bone) S63.ØØ6 ☑
carpometacarpal joint — *see* Dislocation, carpometacarpal (joint)
distal radioulnar joint — *see* Dislocation, radioulnar (joint), distal
metacarpal bone, proximal — *see* Dislocation, metacarpal (bone), proximal end
midcarpal — *see* Dislocation, midcarpal (joint)
radiocarpal joint — *see* Dislocation, radiocarpal (joint)
recurrent — *see* Dislocation, recurrent, wrist
specified site NEC S63.Ø9- ☑
ulna — *see* Dislocation, ulna, distal end
xiphoid cartilage S23.29 ☑
Disorder (of) — *see also* Disease
acantholytic L11.9
specified NEC L11.8
acute
psychotic — *see* Psychosis, acute
stress F43.Ø
adjustment (grief) F43.2Ø
with
anxiety F43.22
with depressed mood F43.23
conduct disturbance F43.24
with emotional disturbance F43.25
depressed mood F43.21
with anxiety F43.23
other specified symptom F43.29
adrenal (capsule) (gland) (medullary) E27.9

Disorder — *continued*
adrenal — *continued*
specified NEC E27.8
adrenogenital — *see also* Adrenogenital syndrome E25.9
drug-induced E25.8
iatrogenic E25.8
idiopathic E25.8
adult personality (and behavior) F69
specified NEC F68.8
affective (mood) — *see* Disorder, mood
aggressive, unsocialized F91.1
alcohol use
mild F1Ø.1Ø
with
alcohol intoxication F1Ø.129
delirium F1Ø.121
alcohol-induced
anxiety disorder F1Ø.18Ø
bipolar and related disorder F1Ø.14
depressive disorder F1Ø.14
psychotic disorder F1Ø.159
sexual dysfunction F1Ø.181
sleep disorder F1Ø.182
in remission (early) (sustained) F1Ø.11
moderate or severe F1Ø.2Ø
with
alcohol intoxication F1Ø.229
delirium F1Ø.221
alcohol-induced
anxiety disorder F1Ø.28Ø
bipolar and related disorder F1Ø.24
depressive disorder F1Ø.24
major neurocognitive disorder, amnestic-confabulatory type F1Ø.26
major neurocognitive disorder, non-amnestic-confabulatory type F1Ø.27
mild neurocognitive disorder F1Ø.288
psychotic disorder F1Ø.259
sexual dysfunction F1Ø.281
sleep disorder F1Ø.282
in remission (early) (sustained) F1Ø.21
alcohol-related F1Ø.99
with
amnestic disorder, persisting F1Ø.96
anxiety disorder F1Ø.98Ø
dementia, persisting F1Ø.97
intoxication F1Ø.929
with delirium F1Ø.921
uncomplicated F1Ø.92Ø
mood disorder F1Ø.94
other specified F1Ø.988
psychotic disorder F1Ø.959
with
delusions F1Ø.95Ø
hallucinations F1Ø.951
sexual dysfunction F1Ø.981
sleep disorder F1Ø.982
allergic — *see* Allergy
alveolar NEC J84.Ø9
amino-acid
cystathioninuria E72.19
cystinosis E72.Ø4
cystinuria E72.Ø1
glycinuria E72.Ø9
homocystinuria E72.11
metabolism — *see* Disturbance, metabolism, amino-acid
specified NEC E72.89
neonatal, transitory P74.8
renal transport NEC E72.Ø9
transport NEC E72.Ø9
amnesic, amnestic
alcohol-induced F1Ø.96
with dependence F1Ø.26
due to (secondary to) general medical condition FØ4
psychoactive NEC-induced F19.96
with
abuse F19.16
dependence F19.26
sedative, hypnotic or anxiolytic-induced F13.96
with dependence F13.26
amphetamine (or other stimulant) use
mild
with
amphetamine, cocaine, or other stimulant intoxication
with perceptual disturbances F15.122

- **Disorder** — *continued*
  - amphetamine use — *continued*
    - mild — *continued*
      - with — *continued*
        - amphetamine, cocaine, or other stimulant intoxication — *continued*
          - without perceptual disturbances F15.129
        - amphetamine (or other stimulant) -induced
          - anxiety disorder F15.180
          - bipolar and related disorder F15.14
          - depressive disorder F15.14
          - obsessive-compulsive and related disorder F15.188
          - psychotic disorder F15.159
          - sexual dysfunction F15.181
        - intoxication delirium F15.121
    - moderate or severe
      - with
        - amphetamine, cocaine, or other stimulant intoxication
          - with perceptual disturbances F15.222
          - without perceptual disturbances F15.229
        - amphetamine (or other stimulant) -induced
          - anxiety disorder F15.280
          - bipolar and related disorder F15.24
          - depressive disorder F15.24
          - obsessive-compulsive and related disorder F15.288
          - psychotic disorder F15.259
          - sexual dysfunction F15.281
        - intoxication delirium F15.221
  - amphetamine-type substance use
    - mild F15.10
      - in remission (early) (sustained) F15.11
    - moderate F15.20
      - in remission (early) (sustained) F15.21
    - severe F15.20
      - in remission (early) (sustained) F15.21
  - anaerobic glycolysis with anemia D55.29
  - anxiety F41.9
    - due to (secondary to)
      - alcohol F10.980
        - in
          - abuse F10.180
          - dependence F10.280
      - amphetamine F15.980
        - in
          - abuse F15.180
          - dependence F15.280
      - anxiolytic F13.980
        - in
          - abuse F13.180
          - dependence F13.280
      - caffeine F15.980
        - in
          - abuse F15.180
          - dependence F15.280
      - cannabis F12.980
        - in
          - abuse F12.180
          - dependence F12.280
      - cocaine F14.980
        - in
          - abuse F14.180
          - dependence F14.180
      - general medical condition F06.4
      - hallucinogen F16.980
        - in
          - abuse F16.180
          - dependence F16.280
      - hypnotic F13.980
        - in
          - abuse F13.180
          - dependence F13.280
      - inhalant F18.980
        - in
          - abuse F18.180
          - dependence F18.280
      - phencyclidine F16.980
        - in
          - abuse F16.180
          - dependence F16.280
      - psychoactive substance NEC F19.980
        - in
          - abuse F19.180
          - dependence F19.280
      - sedative F13.980
        - in
          - abuse F13.180

- **Disorder** — *continued*
  - anxiety — *continued*
    - due to — *continued*
      - sedative — *continued*
        - in — *continued*
          - dependence F13.280
      - volatile solvents F18.980
        - in
          - abuse F18.180
          - dependence F18.280
    - generalized F41.1
    - illness F45.21
    - mixed
      - with depression (mild) F41.8
      - specified NEC F41.3
    - organic F06.4
    - phobic F40.9
      - of childhood F40.8
    - specified NEC F41.8
  - aortic valve — *see* Endocarditis, aortic
  - aromatic amino-acid metabolism E70.9
    - specified NEC E70.89
  - arteriole NEC I77.89
  - artery NEC I77.89
  - articulation — *see* Disorder, joint
  - attachment (childhood)
    - disinhibited F94.2
    - reactive F94.1
  - attention-deficit hyperactivity (adolescent) (adult) (child) F90.9
    - combined
      - presentation F90.2
      - type F90.2
    - hyperactive
      - impulsive presentation F90.1
      - type F90.1
    - inattentive
      - presentation F90.0
      - type F90.0
    - specified type NEC F90.8
  - attention-deficit without hyperactivity (adolescent) (adult) (child) F98.8
  - auditory processing (central) H93.25
  - autism spectrum F84.0
  - autistic F84.0
  - autoimmune D89.89
  - autonomic nervous system G90.9
    - specified NEC G90.8
  - avoidant
    - child or adolescent F40.10
    - restrictive food intake F50.82
  - balance
    - acid-base E87.8
      - mixed E87.4
    - electrolyte E87.8
    - fluid NEC E87.8
  - behavioral (disruptive) — *see* Disorder, conduct
  - bereavement, persistent complex F43.81
  - beta-amino-acid metabolism E72.89
  - bile acid and cholesterol metabolism E78.70
    - Barth syndrome E78.71
    - other specified E78.79
    - Smith-Lemli-Opitz syndrome E78.72
  - bilirubin excretion E80.6
  - binge eating F50.81
  - binocular
    - movement H51.9
      - convergence
        - excess H51.12
        - insufficiency H51.11
      - internuclear ophthalmoplegia — *see* Ophthalmoplegia, internuclear
      - palsy of conjugate gaze H51.0
      - specified type NEC H51.8
    - vision NEC — *see* Disorder, vision, binocular
  - bipolar (I) seasonal) (type I) F31.9
    - and related due to a known physiological condition
      - with
        - manic features F06.33
        - manic- or hypomanic-like episodes F06.33
        - mixed features F06.34
    - current (or most recent) episode
      - depressed F31.9
        - with psychotic features F31.5
        - without psychotic features F31.30
          - mild F31.31
          - moderate F31.32
          - severe (without psychotic features) F31.4
            - with psychotic features F31.5

- **Disorder** — *continued*
  - bipolar seasonal — *continued*
    - current episode — *continued*
      - hypomanic F31.0
      - manic F31.9
        - with psychotic features F31.2
        - without psychotic features F31.10
          - mild F31.11
          - moderate F31.12
          - severe (without psychotic features) F31.13
            - with psychotic features F31.2
      - mixed F31.60
        - mild F31.61
        - moderate F31.62
        - severe (without psychotic features) F31.63
          - with psychotic features F31.64
      - severe depression (without psychotic features) F31.4
        - with psychotic features F31.5
    - II (type 2) F31.81
    - in remission (currently) F31.70
      - in full remission
        - most recent episode
          - depressed F31.76
          - hypomanic F31.72
          - manic F31.74
          - mixed F31.78
      - in partial remission
        - most recent episode
          - depressed F31.75
          - hypomanic F31.71
          - manic F31.73
          - mixed F31.77
    - organic F06.30
    - single manic episode F30.9
      - mild F30.11
      - moderate F30.12
      - severe (without psychotic symptoms) F30.13
        - with psychotic symptoms F30.2
    - specified NEC F31.89
  - bladder N32.9
    - functional NEC N31.9
    - in schistosomiasis B65.0 *[N33]*
    - specified NEC N32.89
  - bleeding D68.9
  - blood D75.9
    - in congenital early syphilis A50.09 *[D77]*
  - body dysmorphic F45.22
  - bone M89.9
    - continuity M84.9
      - specified type NEC M84.80
        - ankle M84.87- ☑
        - fibula M84.86- ☑
        - foot M84.87- ☑
        - hand M84.84- ☑
        - humerus M84.82- ☑
        - neck M84.88
        - pelvis M84.859
        - radius M84.83- ☑
        - rib M84.88
        - shoulder M84.81- ☑
        - skull M84.88
        - thigh M84.85- ☑
        - tibia M84.86- ☑
        - ulna M84.83- ☑
        - vertebra M84.88
    - density and structure M85.9
      - cyst — *see also* Cyst, bone, specified type NEC
        - aneurysmal — *see* Cyst, bone, aneurysmal
        - solitary — *see* Cyst, bone, solitary
      - diffuse idiopathic skeletal hyperostosis — *see* Hyperostosis, ankylosing
      - fibrous dysplasia (monostotic) — *see* Dysplasia, fibrous, bone
      - fluorosis — *see* Fluorosis, skeletal
      - hyperostosis of skull M85.2
      - osteitis condensans — *see* Osteitis, condensans
      - specified type NEC M85.8- ☑
        - ankle M85.87- ☑
        - foot M85.87- ☑
        - forearm M85.83- ☑
        - hand M85.84- ☑
        - lower leg M85.86- ☑
        - multiple sites M85.89
        - neck M85.88
        - rib M85.88
        - shoulder M85.81- ☑

- **Disorder** — *continued*
  - bone — *continued*
    - density and structure — *continued*
      - specified type — *continued*
        - skull M85.88
        - thigh M85.85- ☑
        - upper arm M85.82- ☑
        - vertebra M85.88
    - development and growth NEC M89.2Ø
      - carpus M89.24- ☑
      - clavicle M89.21- ☑
      - femur M89.25- ☑
      - fibula M89.26- ☑
      - finger M89.24- ☑
      - humerus M89.22- ☑
      - ilium M89.259
      - ischium M89.259
      - metacarpus M89.24- ☑
      - metatarsus M89.27- ☑
      - multiple sites M89.29
      - neck M89.28
      - radius M89.23- ☑
      - rib M89.28
      - scapula M89.21- ☑
      - skull M89.28
      - tarsus M89.27- ☑
      - tibia M89.26- ☑
      - toe M89.27- ☑
      - ulna M89.23- ☑
      - vertebra M89.28
    - specified type NEC M89.8X- ☑
  - brachial plexus G54.Ø
  - branched-chain amino-acid metabolism E71.2
    - specified NEC E71.19
  - breast N64.9
    - agalactia — *see* Agalactia
    - associated with
      - lactation O92.7Ø
        - specified NEC O92.79
      - pregnancy O92.2Ø
        - specified NEC O92.29
      - puerperium O92.2Ø
        - specified NEC O92.29
    - cracked nipple — *see* Cracked nipple
    - galactorrhea — *see* Galactorrhea
    - hypogalactia O92.4
    - lactation disorder NEC O92.79
    - mastitis — *see* Mastitis
    - nipple infection — *see* Infection, nipple
    - retracted nipple — *see* Retraction, nipple
    - specified type NEC N64.89
  - Briquet's F45.Ø
  - bullous, in diseases classified elsewhere L14
  - caffeine use
    - mild
      - with
        - caffeine-induced
          - anxiety disorder F15.18Ø
          - sleep disorder F15.182
    - moderate or severe
      - with
        - caffeine-induced
          - anxiety disorder F15.28Ø
          - sleep disorder F15.282
  - cannabis use
    - mild F12.1Ø
      - with
        - cannabis intoxication delirium F12.121
          - with perceptual disturbances F12.122
          - without perceptual disturbances F12.129
        - cannabis-induced
          - anxiety disorder F12.18Ø
          - psychotic disorder F12.159
          - sleep disorder F12.188
      - in remission (early) (sustained) F12.11
    - moderate or severe F12.2Ø
      - with
        - cannabis intoxication
          - with perceptual disturbances F12.222
          - without perceptual disturbances F12.229
        - cannabis-induced
          - anxiety disorder F12.28Ø
          - psychotic disorder F12.259
          - sleep disorder F12.288
        - delirium F12.221
      - in remission (early) (sustained) F12.21
  - carbohydrate
    - absorption, intestinal NEC E74.39

- **Disorder** — *continued*
  - carbohydrate — *continued*
    - metabolism (congenital) E74.9
      - specified NEC E74.89
  - cardiac, functional I51.89
  - carnitine metabolism E71.4Ø
  - cartilage M94.9
    - articular NEC — *see* Derangement, joint, articular cartilage
      - chondrocalcinosis — *see* Chondrocalcinosis
    - specified type NEC M94.8X- ☑
      - articular — *see* Derangement, joint, articular cartilage
      - multiple sites M94.8XØ
  - catatonia (due to known physiological condition) (with another mental disorder) FØ6.1
  - catatonic
    - due to (secondary to) known physiological condition FØ6.1
    - organic FØ6.1
  - central auditory processing H93.25
  - cervical
    - region NEC M53.82
    - root (nerve) NEC G54.2
  - character NOS F6Ø.9
  - childhood disintegrative NEC F84.3
  - cholesterol and bile acid metabolism E78.7Ø
    - Barth syndrome E78.71
    - other specified E78.79
    - Smith-Lemli-Opitz syndrome E78.72
  - choroid H31.9
    - atrophy — *see* Atrophy, choroid
    - degeneration — *see* Degeneration, choroid
    - detachment — *see* Detachment, choroid
    - dystrophy — *see* Dystrophy, choroid
    - hemorrhage — *see* Hemorrhage, choroid
    - rupture — *see* Rupture, choroid
    - scar — *see* Scar, chorioretinal
    - solar retinopathy — *see* Retinopathy, solar
    - specified type NEC H31.8
  - ciliary body — *see* Disorder, iris
    - degeneration — *see* Degeneration, ciliary body
  - coagulation (factor) — *see also* Defect, coagulation D68.9
    - newborn, transient P61.6
  - cocaine use
    - mild F14.1Ø
      - with
        - amphetamine, cocaine, or other stimulant intoxication
          - with perceptual disturbances F14.122
          - without perceptual disturbances F14.129
        - cocaine intoxication delirium F14.121
        - cocaine-induced
          - anxiety disorder F14.18Ø
          - bipolar and related disorder F14.14
          - depressive disorder F14.14
          - obsessive-compulsive and related disorder F14.188
          - psychotic disorder F14.159
          - sexual dysfunction F14.181
          - sleep disorder F14.182
      - in remission (early) (sustained) F14.11
    - moderate or severe F14.2Ø
      - with
        - amphetamine, cocaine, or other stimulant intoxication
          - with perceptual disturbances F14.222
          - without perceptual disturbances F14.229
        - cocaine intoxication delirium F14.221
        - cocaine-induced
          - anxiety disorder F14.28Ø
          - bipolar and related disorder F14.24
          - depressive disorder F14.24
          - obsessive-compulsive and related disorder F14.288
          - psychotic disorder F14.259
          - sexual dysfunction F14.281
          - sleep disorder F14.282
      - in remission (early) (sustained) F14.21
  - coccyx NEC M53.3
  - cognitive FØ9
    - due to (secondary to) general medical condition FØ9
    - persisting R41.89
      - due to
        - alcohol F1Ø.97
          - with dependence F1Ø.27
        - anxiolytics F13.97

- **Disorder** — *continued*
  - cognitive — *continued*
    - persisting — *continued*
      - due to — *continued*
        - anxiolytics — *continued*
          - with dependence F13.27
        - hypnotics F13.97
          - with dependence F13.27
        - sedatives F13.97
          - with dependence F13.27
        - specified substance NEC F19.97
          - with
            - abuse F19.17
            - dependence F19.27
  - communication F8Ø.9
    - social pragmatic F8Ø.82
  - conduct (childhood) F91.9
    - adjustment reaction — *see* Disorder, adjustment
    - adolescent onset type F91.2
    - childhood onset type F91.1
    - compulsive F63.9
    - confined to family context F91.Ø
    - depressive F91.8
    - group type F91.2
    - hyperkinetic — *see* Disorder, attention-deficit hyperactivity
    - oppositional defiance F91.3
    - socialized F91.2
    - solitary aggressive type F91.1
    - specified NEC F91.8
    - unsocialized (aggressive) F91.1
  - conduction, heart I45.9
  - congenital glycosylation (CDG) E74.89
  - conjunctiva H11.9
    - infection — *see* Conjunctivitis
  - connective tissue, localized L94.9
    - specified NEC L94.8
  - conversion (functional neurological symptom disorder)
    - with
      - abnormal movement F44.4
      - anesthesia or sensory loss F44.6
      - attacks or seizures F44.5
      - mixed symptoms F44.7
      - special sensory symptoms F44.6
      - speech symptoms F44.4
      - swallowing symptoms F44.4
      - weakness or paralysis F44.4
  - convulsive (secondary) — *see* Convulsions
  - cornea H18.9
    - deformity — *see* Deformity, cornea
    - degeneration — *see* Degeneration, cornea
    - deposits — *see* Deposit, cornea
    - due to contact lens H18.82- ☑
      - specified as edema — *see* Edema, cornea
    - edema — *see* Edema, cornea
    - keratitis — *see* Keratitis
    - keratoconjunctivitis — *see* Keratoconjunctivitis
    - membrane change — *see* Change, corneal membrane
    - neovascularization — *see* Neovascularization, cornea
    - scar — *see* Opacity, cornea
    - specified type NEC H18.89- ☑
    - ulcer — *see* Ulcer, cornea
  - corpus cavernosum N48.9
  - cranial nerve — *see* Disorder, nerve, cranial
  - Cyclin-Dependent Kinase-Like 5 Deficiency (CDKL5) G4Ø.42
  - cyclothymic F34.Ø
  - defiant oppositional F91.3
  - delusional (persistent) (systematized) F22
    - induced F24
  - depersonalization F48.1
  - depressive F32.A
    - due to known physiological condition
      - with
        - depressive features FØ6.31
        - major depressive-like episode FØ6.32
        - mixed features FØ6.34
    - major F32.9
      - with psychotic symptoms F32.3
      - in remission (full) F32.5
        - partial F32.4
      - recurrent F33.9
        - with psychotic features F33.3
      - single episode F32.9
        - mild F32.Ø
        - moderate F32.1

- **Disorder** — *continued*
  - depressive — *continued*
    - major — *continued*
      - single episode — *continued*
        - severe (without psychotic symptoms) F32.2
          - with psychotic symptoms F32.3
    - organic FØ6.31
    - persistent F34.1
    - recurrent F33.9
      - current episode
        - mild F33.Ø
        - moderate F33.1
        - severe (without psychotic symptoms) F33.2
          - with psychotic symptoms F33.3
      - in remission F33.4Ø
        - full F33.42
        - partial F33.41
      - specified NEC F33.8
    - single episode — *see* Episode, depressive
    - specified NEC F32.89
  - developmental F89
    - arithmetical skills F81.2
    - coordination (motor) F82
    - expressive writing F81.81
    - language F8Ø.9
      - expressive F8Ø.1
      - mixed receptive and expressive F8Ø.2
      - receptive type F8Ø.2
      - specified NEC F8Ø.89
    - learning F81.9
      - arithmetical F81.2
      - reading F81.Ø
    - mixed F88
    - motor coordination or function F82
    - pervasive F84.9
      - specified NEC F84.8
    - phonological F8Ø.Ø
    - reading F81.Ø
    - scholastic skills — *see also* Disorder, learning
      - mixed F81.89
    - specified NEC F88
    - speech F8Ø.9
      - articulation F8Ø.Ø
      - specified NEC F8Ø.89
    - written expression F81.81
  - diaphragm J98.6
  - digestive (system) K92.9
    - newborn P78.9
      - specified NEC P78.89
    - postprocedural — *see* Complication, gastrointestinal
    - psychogenic F45.8
  - disc (intervertebral) M51.9
    - with
      - myelopathy
        - cervical region M5Ø.ØØ
        - cervicothoracic region M5Ø.Ø3
        - high cervical region M5Ø.Ø1
        - lumbar region M51.Ø6
        - mid-cervical region M5Ø.Ø2Ø
        - sacrococcygeal region M53.3
        - thoracic region M51.Ø4
        - thoracolumbar region M51.Ø5
      - radiculopathy
        - cervical region M5Ø.1Ø
        - cervicothoracic region M5Ø.13
        - high cervical region M5Ø.11
        - lumbar region M51.16
        - lumbosacral region M51.17
        - mid-cervical region M5Ø.12Ø
        - sacrococcygeal region M53.3
        - thoracic region M51.14
        - thoracolumbar region M51.15
    - cervical M5Ø.9Ø
      - with
        - myelopathy M5Ø.ØØ
          - C2-C3 M5Ø.Ø1
          - C3-C4 M5Ø.Ø1
          - C4-C5 M5Ø.Ø21
          - C5-C6 M5Ø.Ø22
          - C6-C7 M5Ø.Ø23
          - C7-T1 M5Ø.Ø3
          - cervicothoracic region M5Ø.Ø3
          - high cervical region M5Ø.Ø1
          - mid-cervical region M5Ø.Ø2Ø
        - neuritis, radiculitis or radiculopathy M5Ø.1Ø
          - C2-C3 M5Ø.11
          - C3-C4 M5Ø.11
          - C4-C5 M5Ø.121
          - C5-C6 M5Ø.122
- **Disorder** — *continued*
  - disc — *continued*
    - cervical — *continued*
      - with — *continued*
        - neuritis, radiculitis or radiculopathy — *continued*
          - C6-C7 M5Ø.123
          - C7-T1 M5Ø.13
          - cervicothoracic region M5Ø.13
          - high cervical region M5Ø.11
          - mid-cervical region M5Ø.12Ø
      - C2-C3 M5Ø.91
      - C3-C4 M5Ø.91
      - C4-C5 M5Ø.921
      - C5-C6 M5Ø.922
      - C6-C7 M5Ø.923
      - C7-T1 M5Ø.93
      - cervicothoracic region M5Ø.93
      - degeneration M5Ø.3Ø
        - C2-C3 M5Ø.31
        - C3-C4 M5Ø.31
        - C4-C5 M5Ø.321
        - C5-C6 M5Ø.322
        - C6-C7 M5Ø.323
        - C7-T1 M5Ø.33
        - cervicothoracic region M5Ø.33
        - high cervical region M5Ø.31
        - mid-cervical region M5Ø.32Ø
      - displacement M5Ø.2Ø
        - C2-C3 M5Ø.21
        - C3-C4 M5Ø.21
        - C4-C5 M5Ø.221
        - C5-C6 M5Ø.222
        - C6-C7 M5Ø.223
        - C7-T1 M5Ø.23
        - cervicothoracic region M5Ø.23
        - high cervical region M5Ø.21
        - mid-cervical region M5Ø.22Ø
      - high cervical region M5Ø.91
      - mid-cervical region M5Ø.92Ø
      - specified type NEC M5Ø.8Ø
        - C2-C3 M5Ø.81
        - C3-C4 M5Ø.81
        - C4-C5 M5Ø.821
        - C5-C6 M5Ø.822
        - C6-C7 M5Ø.823
        - C7-T1 M5Ø.83
        - cervicothoracic region M5Ø.83
        - high cervical region M5Ø.81
        - mid-cervical region M5Ø.82Ø
    - specified NEC
      - lumbar region M51.86
      - lumbosacral region M51.87
      - sacrococcygeal region M53.3
      - thoracic region M51.84
      - thoracolumbar region M51.85
  - disinhibited attachment (childhood) F94.2
  - disintegrative, childhood NEC F84.3
  - disruptive F91.9
    - mood dysregulation F34.81
    - specified NEC F91.8
  - disruptive behavior — *see* Disorder, conduct
  - dissocial personality F6Ø.2
  - dissociative F44.9
    - affecting
      - motor function F44.4
        - and sensation F44.7
      - sensation F44.6
        - and motor function F44.7
    - brief reactive F43.Ø
    - due to (secondary to) general medical condition FØ6.8
    - mixed F44.7
    - organic FØ6.8
    - other specified NEC F44.89
  - double heterozygous sickling — *see* Disease, sickle-cell
  - dream anxiety F51.5
  - drug induced hemorrhagic D68.32
  - drug related F19.99
    - abuse — *see* Abuse, drug
    - dependence — *see* Dependence, drug
  - dysmorphic body F45.22
  - dysthymic F34.1
  - ear H93.9- ☑
    - bleeding — *see* Otorrhagia
    - deafness — *see* Deafness
    - degenerative H93.Ø9- ☑
    - discharge — *see* Otorrhea
- **Disorder** — *continued*
  - ear — *continued*
    - external H61.9- ☑
      - auditory canal stenosis — *see* Stenosis, external ear canal
      - exostosis — *see* Exostosis, external ear canal
      - impacted cerumen — *see* Impaction, cerumen
      - otitis — *see* Otitis, externa
      - perichondritis — *see* Perichondritis, ear
      - pinna — *see* Disorder, pinna
      - specified type NEC H61.89- ☑
    - inner H83.9- ☑
      - vestibular dysfunction — *see* Disorder, vestibular function
    - middle H74.9- ☑
      - adhesive H74.1- ☑
      - ossicle — *see* Abnormal, ear ossicles
      - polyp — *see* Polyp, ear (middle)
      - specified NEC, in diseases classified elsewhere H75.8- ☑
    - postprocedural — *see* Complications, ear, procedure
    - specified NEC, in diseases classified elsewhere H94.8- ☑
  - eating (adult) (psychogenic) F5Ø.9
    - anorexia — *see* Anorexia
    - binge F5Ø.81
    - bulimia F5Ø.2
    - child F98.29
      - pica F98.3
      - rumination disorder F98.21
    - pica F5Ø.89
      - childhood F98.3
  - electrolyte (balance) NEC E87.8
    - with
      - abortion — *see* Abortion by type complicated by specified condition NEC
      - ectopic pregnancy OØ8.5
      - molar pregnancy OØ8.5
    - acidosis (lactic) (metabolic) E87.2Ø
      - acute E87.21
      - chronic E87.22
      - respiratory E87.29
      - specified NEC E87.29
    - alkalosis (metabolic) (respiratory) E87.3
  - elimination, transepidermal L87.9
    - specified NEC L87.8
  - emotional (persistent) F34.9
    - of childhood F93.9
      - specified NEC F93.8
  - endocrine E34.9
    - postprocedural E89.89
      - specified NEC E89.89
  - erectile (male) (organic) — *see also* Dysfunction, sexual, male, erectile N52.9
    - nonorganic F52.21
  - erythematous — *see* Erythema
  - esophagus K22.9
    - functional K22.4
    - psychogenic F45.8
  - eustachian tube H69.9- ☑
    - infection — *see* Salpingitis, eustachian
    - obstruction — *see* Obstruction, eustachian tube
    - patulous — *see* Patulous, eustachian tube
    - specified NEC H69.8- ☑
  - exhibitionistic F65.2
  - extrapyramidal G25.9
    - in deseases classified elsewhere — *see* category G26
    - specified type NEC G25.89
  - eye H57.9
    - postprocedural — *see* Complication, postprocedural, eye
  - eyelid HØ2.9
    - cyst — *see* Cyst, eyelid
    - degenerative HØ2.7Ø
      - chloasma — *see* Chloasma, eyelid
      - madarosis — *see* Madarosis
      - specified type NEC HØ2.79
      - vitiligo — *see* Vitiligo, eyelid
      - xanthelasma — *see* Xanthelasma
    - dermatochalasis — *see* Dermatochalasis
    - edema — *see* Edema, eyelid
    - elephantiasis — *see* Elephantiasis, eyelid
    - foreign body, retained — *see* Foreign body, retained, eyelid
    - function HØ2.59

- **Disorder** — *continued*
  - eyelid — *continued*
    - function — *continued*
      - abnormal innervation syndrome — *see* Syndrome, abnormal innervation
      - blepharochalasis — *see* Blepharochalasis
      - blepharoclonus — *see* Blepharoclonus
      - blepharophimosis — *see* Blepharophimosis
      - blepharoptosis — *see* Blepharoptosis
      - lagophthalmos — *see* Lagophthalmos
      - lid retraction — *see* Retraction, lid
    - hypertrichosis — *see* Hypertrichosis, eyelid
    - specified type NEC HØ2.89
    - vascular HØ2.879
      - left HØ2.876
        - lower HØ2.875
        - upper HØ2.874
      - right HØ2.873
        - lower HØ2.872
        - upper HØ2.871
  - factitious
    - by proxy F68.A
    - imposed on another F68.A
    - imposed on self F68.1Ø
      - with predominantly
        - psychological symptoms F68.11
          - with physical symptoms F68.13
        - physical symptoms F68.12
          - with psychological symptoms F68.13
  - factor, coagulation — *see* Defect, coagulation
  - fatty acid
    - metabolism E71.3Ø
      - specified NEC E71.39
    - oxidation
      - LCAD E71.31Ø
      - MCAD E71.311
      - SCAD E71.312
      - specified deficiency NEC E71.318
  - feeding (infant or child) — *see also* Disorder, eating R63.3Ø
    - or eating disorder F5Ø.9
    - pediatric
      - acute R63.31
      - chronic R63.32
    - specified NEC F5Ø.9
  - feigned (with obvious motivation) Z76.5
    - without obvious motivation — *see* Disorder, factitious
  - female
    - hypoactive sexual desire F52.Ø
    - orgasmic F52.31
    - sexual interest/arousal F52.22
  - fetishistic F65.Ø
  - fibroblastic M72.9
    - specified NEC M72.8
  - fluency
    - adult onset F98.5
    - childhood onset F8Ø.81
    - following
      - cerebral infarction I69.323
      - cerebrovascular disease I69.923
        - specified disease NEC I69.823
      - intracerebral hemorrhage I69.123
      - nontraumatic intracranial hemorrhage NEC I69.223
      - subarachnoid hemorrhage I69.Ø23
    - in conditions classified elsewhere R47.82
  - fluid balance E87.8
  - follicular (skin) L73.9
    - specified NEC L73.8
  - frotteuristic F65.81
  - fructose metabolism E74.1Ø
    - essential fructosuria E74.11
    - fructokinase deficiency E74.11
    - fructose-1, 6-diphosphatase deficiency E74.19
    - hereditary fructose intolerance E74.12
    - other specified E74.19
  - functional polymorphonuclear neutrophils D71
  - gallbladder, biliary tract and pancreas in diseases classified elsewhere K87
  - gambling F63.Ø
  - gamma aminobutyric acid (GABA) metabolism E72.81
  - gamma-glutamyl cycle E72.89
  - gastric (functional) K31.9
    - motility K3Ø
    - psychogenic F45.8
    - secretion K3Ø
  - gastrointestinal (functional) NOS K92.9

- **Disorder** — *continued*
  - gastrointestinal — *continued*
    - newborn P78.9
    - psychogenic F45.8
  - gender-identity or -role F64.9
    - childhood F64.2
    - effect on relationship F66
    - of adolescence or adulthood F64.Ø
      - nontranssexual F64.8
    - specified NEC F64.8
    - uncertainty F66
  - genito-pelvic pain penetration F52.6
  - genitourinary system
    - female N94.9
    - male N5Ø.9
    - psychogenic F45.8
  - globe H44.9
    - degenerated condition H44.5Ø
      - absolute glaucoma H44.51- ☑
      - atrophy H44.52- ☑
      - leucocoria H44.53- ☑
    - degenerative H44.3Ø
      - chalcosis H44.31- ☑
      - myopia — *see also* Myopia, degenerative H44.2- ☑
      - siderosis H44.32- ☑
      - specified type NEC H44.39- ☑
    - endophthalmitis — *see* Endophthalmitis
    - foreign body, retained — *see* Foreign body, intraocular, old, retained
    - hemophthalmos — *see* Hemophthalmos
    - hypotony H44.4Ø
      - due to
        - ocular fistula H44.42- ☑
        - specified disorder NEC H44.43- ☑
      - flat anterior chamber H44.41- ☑
      - primary H44.44- ☑
    - luxation — *see* Luxation, globe
    - specified type NEC H44.89
  - glomerular (in) NØ5.9
    - amyloidosis E85.4 *[NØ8]*
    - cryoglobulinemia D89.1 *[NØ8]*
    - disseminated intravascular coagulation D65 *[NØ8]*
    - Fabry's disease E75.21 *[NØ8]*
    - familial lecithin cholesterol acyltransferase deficiency E78.6 *[NØ8]*
    - Goodpasture's syndrome M31.Ø
    - hemolytic-uremic syndrome — *see* Syndrome, hemolytic-uremic
    - Henoch (-Schönlein) purpura D69.Ø *[NØ8]*
    - malariae malaria B52.Ø
    - microscopic polyangiitis M31.7 *[NØ8]*
    - multiple myeloma C9Ø.Ø- ☑ *[NØ8]*
    - mumps B26.83
    - schistosomiasis B65.9 *[NØ8]*
    - sepsis NEC A41.- ☑ *[NØ8]*
      - streptococcal A4Ø.- ☑ *[NØ8]*
    - sickle-cell disorders D57.- ☑ *[NØ8]*
    - strongyloidiasis B78.9 *[NØ8]*
    - subacute bacterial endocarditis I33.Ø *[NØ8]*
    - syphilis A52.75
    - systemic lupus erythematosus M32.14
    - thrombotic thrombocytopenic purpura M31.19 *[NØ8]*
    - Waldenström macroglobulinemia C88.Ø *[NØ8]*
    - Wegener's granulomatosis M31.31
  - gluconeogenesis E74.4
  - glucosaminoglycan metabolism — *see* Disorder, metabolism, glucosaminoglycan
  - glucose transport E74.819
    - specified NEC E74.818
  - glycine metabolism E72.5Ø
    - d-glycericacidemia E72.59
    - hyperhydroxyprolinemia E72.59
    - hyperoxaluria R82.992
      - primary E72.53
    - hyperprolinemia E72.59
    - non-ketotic hyperglycinemia E72.51
    - oxalosis E72.53
    - oxaluria E72.53
    - sarcosinemia E72.59
    - trimethylaminuria E72.52
  - glycoprotein metabolism E77.9
    - specified NEC E77.8
  - grief
    - complicated F43.81
    - prolonged F43.81
  - habit (and impulse) F63.9

- **Disorder** — *continued*
  - habit — *continued*
    - involving sexual behavior NEC F65.9
    - specified NEC F63.89
  - hallucinogen use
    - mild F16.1Ø
      - with
        - hallucinogen intoxication delirium F16.121
        - hallucinogen-induced
          - anxiety disorder F16.18Ø
          - bipolar and related disorder F16.14
          - depressive disorder F16.14
          - psychotic disorder F16.159
        - other hallucinogen intoxication F16.129
      - in remission (early) (sustained) F16.11
    - moderate or severe F16.2Ø
      - with
        - hallucinogen intoxication delirium F16.221
        - hallucinogen-induced
          - anxiety disorder F16.28Ø
          - bipolar and related disorder F16.24
          - depressive disorder F16.24
          - psychotic disorder F16.259
        - other hallucinogen intoxication F16.229
      - in remission (early) (sustained) F16.21
  - heart action I49.9
  - hematological D75.9
    - newborn (transient) P61.9
      - specified NEC P61.8
  - hematopoietic organs D75.9
  - hemorrhagic NEC D69.9
    - drug-induced D68.32
    - due to
      - extrinsic circulating anticoagulants D68.32
      - increase in
        - anti-IIa D68.32
        - anti-Xa D68.32
      - intrinsic
        - circulating anticoagulants D68.318
        - increase in
          - anti-IXa D68.318
          - antithrombin D68.318
          - anti-VIIIa D68.318
          - anti-XIa D68.318
    - following childbirth O72.3
  - hemostasis — *see* Defect, coagulation
  - histidine metabolism E7Ø.4Ø
    - histidinemia E7Ø.41
    - other specified E7Ø.49
  - hoarding F42.3
  - hyperkinetic — *see* Disorder, attention-deficit hyperactivity
  - hyperleucine-isoleucinemia E71.19
  - hypervalinemia E71.19
  - hypoactive sexual desire F52.Ø
  - hypochondriacal F45.2Ø
    - body dysmorphic F45.22
    - neurosis F45.21
    - other specified F45.29
  - identity
    - dissociative F44.81
    - illness anxiety F45.21
    - of childhood F93.8
  - immune mechanism (immunity) D89.9
    - specified type NEC D89.89
  - impaired renal tubular function N25.9
    - specified NEC N25.89
  - impulse (control) F63.9
  - inflammatory
    - pelvic, in diseases classified elsewhere — *see* category N74
    - penis N48.29
      - abscess N48.21
      - cellulitis N48.22
  - inhalant use
    - mild F18.1Ø
      - with
        - inhalant intoxication F18.129
        - inhalant intoxication delirium F18.121
        - inhalant-induced
          - anxiety disorder F18.18Ø
          - depressive disorder F18.14
          - major neurocognitive disorder F18.17
          - mild neurocognitive disorder F18.188
          - psychotic disorder F18.159
      - in remission (early) (sustained) F18.11
    - moderate or severe F18.2Ø
      - with
        - inhalant intoxication F18.229

- **Disorder** — *continued*
  - inhalant use — *continued*
    - moderate or severe — *continued*
      - with — *continued*
        - inhalant intoxication delirium F18.221
        - inhalant-induced
          - anxiety disorder F18.28Ø
          - depressive disorder F18.24
          - major neurocognitive disorder F18.27
          - mild neurocognitive disorder F18.288
          - psychotic disorder F18.259
      - in remission (early) (sustained) F18.21
  - integument, newborn P83.9
    - specified NEC P83.88
  - intermittent explosive F63.81
  - internal secretion pancreas — *see* Increased, secretion, pancreas, endocrine
  - intestine, intestinal
    - carbohydrate absorption NEC E74.39
      - postoperative K91.2
    - functional NEC K59.9
      - postoperative K91.89
    - psychogenic F45.8
    - vascular K55.9
      - chronic K55.1
      - specified NEC K55.8
  - intraoperative (intraprocedural) — *see* Complications, intraoperative
  - involuntary emotional expression (IEED) FØ7.89
  - iris H21.9
    - adhesions — *see* Adhesions, iris
    - atrophy — *see* Atrophy, iris
    - chamber angle recession — *see* Recession, chamber angle
    - cyst — *see* Cyst, iris
    - degeneration — *see* Degeneration, iris
    - in diseases classified elsewhere H22
    - iridodialysis — *see* Iridodialysis
    - iridoschisis — *see* Iridoschisis
    - miotic pupillary cyst — *see* Cyst, pupillary
    - pupillary
      - abnormality — *see* Abnormality, pupillary
      - membrane — *see* Membrane, pupillary
    - specified type NEC H21.89
    - vascular NEC H21.1X- ☑
  - iron metabolism E83.1Ø
    - specified NEC E83.19
  - isovaleric acidemia E71.11Ø
  - jaw, developmental M27.Ø
    - temporomandibular — *see also* Anomaly, dentofacial, temporomandibular joint M26.6Ø- ☑
  - joint M25.9
    - derangement — *see* Derangement, joint
    - effusion — *see* Effusion, joint
    - fistula — *see* Fistula, joint
    - hemarthrosis — *see* Hemarthrosis
    - instability — *see* Instability, joint
    - osteophyte — *see* Osteophyte
    - pain — *see* Pain, joint
    - psychogenic F45.8
    - specified type NEC M25.8Ø
      - ankle M25.87- ☑
      - elbow M25.82- ☑
      - foot joint M25.87- ☑
      - hand joint M25.84- ☑
      - hip M25.85- ☑
      - knee M25.86- ☑
      - shoulder M25.81- ☑
      - wrist M25.83- ☑
    - stiffness — *see* Stiffness, joint
  - ketone metabolism E71.32
  - kidney N28.9
    - functional (tubular) N25.9
    - in
      - schistosomiasis B65.9 *[N29]*
    - tubular function N25.9
      - specified NEC N25.89
  - lacrimal system HØ4.9
    - changes HØ4.69
      - fistula — *see* Fistula, lacrimal
    - gland HØ4.19
      - atrophy — *see* Atrophy, lacrimal gland
      - cyst — *see* Cyst, lacrimal, gland
      - dacryops — *see* Dacryops
      - dislocation — *see* Dislocation, lacrimal gland
      - dry eye syndrome — *see* Syndrome, dry eye
      - infection — *see* Dacryoadenitis

- **Disorder** — *continued*
  - lacrimal system — *continued*
    - granuloma — *see* Granuloma, lacrimal
    - inflammation — *see* Inflammation, lacrimal
    - obstruction — *see* Obstruction, lacrimal
    - specified NEC HØ4.89
  - lactation NEC O92.79
  - language (developmental) F8Ø.9
    - expressive F8Ø.1
    - mixed receptive and expressive F8Ø.2
    - receptive F8Ø.2
  - late luteal phase dysphoric N94.89
  - learning (specific) F81.9
    - acalculia R48.8
    - alexia R48.Ø
    - mathematics F81.2
    - reading F81.Ø
    - specified
      - with impairment in
        - mathematics F81.2
        - reading F81.Ø
        - written expression F81.81
    - specified NEC F81.89
    - spelling F81.81
    - written expression F81.81
  - lens H27.9
    - aphakia — *see* Aphakia
    - cataract — *see* Cataract
    - dislocation — *see* Dislocation, lens
    - specified type NEC H27.8
  - ligament M24.2Ø
    - ankle M24.27- ☑
    - attachment, spine — *see* Enthesopathy, spinal
    - elbow M24.22- ☑
    - foot joint M24.27- ☑
    - hand joint M24.24- ☑
    - hip M24.25- ☑
    - knee — *see* Derangement, knee, specified NEC
    - shoulder M24.21- ☑
    - specified site NEC M24.29
    - vertebra M24.28
    - wrist M24.23- ☑
  - ligamentous attachments — *see also* Enthesopathy
    - spine — *see* Enthesopathy, spinal
  - lipid
    - metabolism, congenital E78.9
    - storage E75.6
      - specified NEC E75.5
  - lipoprotein
    - deficiency (familial) E78.6
    - metabolism E78.9
      - specified NEC E78.89
  - liver K76.9
    - malarial B54 *[K77]*
  - low back — *see also* Dorsopathy, specified NEC
  - lumbosacral
    - plexus G54.1
    - root (nerve) NEC G54.4
  - lung, interstitial, drug-induced J7Ø.4
    - acute J7Ø.2
    - chronic J7Ø.3
    - dabbing (related) UØ7.Ø
    - e-cigarette (related) UØ7.Ø
    - electronic cigarette (related) UØ7.Ø
    - vaping (associated) (device) (product) (related) (use) UØ7.Ø
  - lymphoproliferative, post-transplant (PTLD) D47.Z1 (*following* D47.4)
  - lysine and hydroxylysine metabolism E72.3
  - major neurocognitive — *see also* Dementia, in (due to) FØ3- ☑
  - male
    - erectile (organic) — *see also* Dysfunction, sexual, male, erectile N52.9
      - nonorganic F52.21
    - hypoactive sexual desire F52.Ø
    - orgasmic F52.32
  - manic F3Ø.9
    - organic FØ6.33
  - mast cell activation — *see* Activation, mast cell
  - mastoid — *see also* Disorder, ear, middle
    - postprocedural — *see* Complications, ear, procedure
  - meninges, specified type NEC G96.198
  - meniscus — *see* Derangement, knee, meniscus
  - menopausal N95.9
    - specified NEC N95.8
  - menstrual N92.6
    - psychogenic F45.8

- **Disorder** — *continued*
  - menstrual — *continued*
    - specified NEC N92.5
  - mental (or behavioral) (nonpsychotic) F99
    - due to (secondary to)
      - amphetamine
        - due to drug abuse — *see* Abuse, drug, stimulant
        - due to drug dependence — *see* Dependence, drug, stimulant
      - brain disease, damage and dysfunction FØ9
      - caffeine use
        - due to drug abuse — *see* Abuse, drug, stimulant
        - due to drug dependence — *see* Dependence, drug, stimulant
      - cannabis use
        - due to drug abuse — *see* Abuse, drug, cannabis
        - due to drug dependence — *see* Dependence, drug, cannabis
      - general medical condition FØ9
      - sedative or hypnotic use
        - due to drug abuse — *see* Abuse, drug, sedative
        - due to drug dependence — *see* Dependence, drug, sedative
      - tobacco (nicotine) use — *see* Dependence, drug, nicotine
    - following organic brain damage FØ7.9
      - frontal lobe syndrome FØ7.Ø
      - personality change FØ7.Ø
      - postconcussional syndrome FØ7.81
      - specified NEC FØ7.89
    - infancy, childhood or adolescence F98.9
    - neurotic — *see* Neurosis
    - organic or symptomatic FØ9
    - presenile, psychotic FØ3 ☑
    - problem NEC
      - psychoneurotic — *see* Neurosis
      - psychotic — *see* Psychosis
    - puerperal F53.Ø
    - senile, psychotic NEC FØ3 ☑
  - metabolic, amino acid, transitory, newborn P74.8
  - metabolism NOS E88.9
    - amino-acid E72.9
      - aromatic E7Ø.9
        - albinism — *see* Albinism
        - histidine E7Ø.4Ø
          - histidinemia E7Ø.41
          - other specified E7Ø.49
        - hyperphenylalaninemia E7Ø.1
          - classical phenylketonuria E7Ø.Ø
        - other specified E7Ø.89
        - tryptophan E7Ø.5
        - tyrosine E7Ø.2Ø
          - hypertyrosinemia E7Ø.21
          - other specified E7Ø.29
      - branched chain E71.2
        - 3-methylglutaconic aciduria E71.111
        - hyperleucine-isoleucinemia E71.19
        - hypervalinemia E71.19
        - isovaleric acidemia E71.11Ø
        - maple syrup urine disease E71.Ø
        - methylmalonic acidemia E71.12Ø
        - organic aciduria NEC E71.118
        - other specified E71.19
        - proprionate NEC E71.128
        - proprionic acidemia E71.121
      - glycine E72.5Ø
        - d-glycericacidemia E72.59
        - hyperhydroxyprolinemia E72.59
        - hyperoxaluria R82.992
          - primary E72.53
        - hyperprolinemia E72.59
        - non-ketotic hyperglycinemia E72.51
        - other specified E72.59
        - sarcosinemia E72.59
        - trimethylaminuria E72.52
      - hydroxylysine E72.3
      - lysine E72.3
      - ornithine E72.4
      - other specified E72.89
        - beta-amino acid E72.89
        - gamma-glutamyl cycle E72.89
      - straight-chain E72.89
      - sulfur-bearing E72.1Ø
        - homocystinuria E72.11

Index — Disorder

Disorder — *continued*
metabolism — *continued*
amino-acid — *continued*
sulfur-bearing — *continued*
methylenetetrahydrofolate reductase deficiency E72.12
other specified E72.19
bile acid and cholesterol metabolism E78.70
bilirubin E80.7
specified NEC E80.6
calcium E83.50
hypercalcemia E83.52
hypocalcemia E83.51
other specified E83.59
carbohydrate E74.9
specified NEC E74.89
cholesterol and bile acid metabolism E78.70
congenital E88.9
copper E83.00
specified type NEC E83.09
Wilson's disease E83.01
cystinuria E72.01
fructose E74.10
galactose E74.20
glucosaminoglycan E76.9
mucopolysaccharidosis — *see* Mucopolysaccharidosis
specified NEC E76.8
glutamine E72.89
glycine E72.50
glycogen storage (hepatorenal) E74.09
glycoprotein E77.9
specified NEC E77.8
glycosaminoglycan E76.9
specified NEC E76.8
in labor and delivery O75.89
iron E83.10
isoleucine E71.19
leucine E71.19
lipoid E78.9
lipoprotein E78.9
specified NEC E78.89
magnesium E83.40
hypermagnesemia E83.41
hypomagnesemia E83.42
other specified E83.49
mineral E83.9
specified NEC E83.89
mitochondrial E88.40
MELAS syndrome E88.41
MERRF syndrome (myoclonic epilepsy associated with ragged-red fibers) E88.42
other specified E88.49
ornithine E72.4
phosphatases E83.30
phosphorus E83.30
acid phosphatase deficiency E83.39
hypophosphatasia E83.39
hypophosphatemia E83.39
familial E83.31
other specified E83.39
pseudovitamin D deficiency E83.32
plasma protein NEC E88.09
porphyrin — *see* Porphyria
postprocedural E89.89
specified NEC E89.89
purine E79.9
specified NEC E79.8
pyrimidine E79.9
specified NEC E79.8
pyruvate E74.4
serine E72.89
sodium E87.8
specified NEC E88.89
threonine E72.89
valine E71.19
zinc E83.2
methylmalonic acidemia E71.120
micturition NEC — *see also* Difficulty, micturition R39.198
feeling of incomplete emptying R39.14
hesitancy R39.11
poor stream R39.12
psychogenic F45.8
split stream R39.13
straining R39.16
urgency R39.15
mild neurocognitive G31.84

Disorder — *continued*
mild neurocognitive — *continued*
due to known physiological condition (without behavioral disturbance) F06.70
with behavioral disturbance F06.71
mitochondrial metabolism E88.40
mitral (valve) — *see* Endocarditis, mitral
mixed
anxiety and depressive F41.8
of scholastic skills (developmental) F81.89
receptive expressive language F80.2
mood F39
bipolar — *see* Disorder, bipolar
depressive — *see* Disorder, depressive
due to (secondary to)
alcohol F10.94
amphetamine F15.94
in
abuse F15.14
dependence F15.24
anxiolytic F13.94
in
abuse F13.14
dependence F13.24
cocaine F14.94
in
abuse F14.14
dependence F14.24
general medical condition F06.30
hallucinogen F16.94
in
abuse F16.14
dependence F16.24
hypnotic F13.94
in
abuse F13.14
dependence F13.24
inhalant F18.94
in
abuse F18.14
dependence F18.24
opioid F11.94
in
abuse F11.14
dependence F11.24
phencyclidine (PCP) F16.94
in
abuse F16.14
dependence F16.24
physiological condition F06.30
with
depressive features F06.31
major depressive-like episode F06.32
manic features F06.33
mixed features F06.34
psychoactive substance NEC F19.94
in
abuse F19.14
dependence F19.24
sedative F13.94
in
abuse F13.14
dependence F13.24
volatile solvents F18.94
in
abuse F18.14
dependence F18.24
manic episode F30.9
with psychotic symptoms F30.2
in remission (full) F30.4
partial F30.3
specified type NEC F30.8
without psychotic symptoms F30.10
mild F30.11
moderate F30.12
severe F30.13
organic F06.30
right hemisphere F07.89
persistent F34.9
cyclothymia F34.0
dysthymia F34.1
specified type NEC F34.89
recurrent F39
right hemisphere organic F07.89
movement G25.9
drug-induced G25.70
akathisia G25.71
specified NEC G25.79
hysterical F44.4

Disorder — *continued*
movement — *continued*
in diseases classified elsewhere — *see* category G26
periodic limb G47.61
sleep related G47.61
sleep related NEC G47.69
specified NEC G25.89
stereotyped F98.4
treatment-induced G25.9
multiple personality F44.81
muscle M62.9
attachment, spine — *see* Enthesopathy, spinal
in trichinellosis — *see* Trichinellosis, with muscle disorder
psychogenic F45.8
specified type NEC M62.89
tone, newborn P94.9
specified NEC P94.8
muscular
attachments — *see also* Enthesopathy
spine — *see* Enthesopathy, spinal
urethra N36.44
musculoskeletal system, soft tissue — *see* Disorder, soft tissue
postprocedural M96.89
psychogenic F45.8
myoneural G70.9
due to lead G70.1
specified NEC G70.89
toxic G70.1
myotonic NEC G71.19
nail, in diseases classified elsewhere L62
neck region NEC — *see* Dorsopathy, specified NEC
neonatal onset multisystemic inflammatory (NOMID) M04.2
nerve G58.9
abducent NEC — *see* Strabismus, paralytic, sixth nerve
accessory G52.8
acoustic *see* subcategory H93.3 ☑
auditory — *see* subcategory H93.3 ☑
auriculotemporal G50.8
axillary G54.0
cerebral — *see* Disorder, nerve, cranial
cranial G52.9
eighth — *see* subcategory H93.3 ☑
eleventh G52.8
fifth G50.9
first G52.0
fourth NEC — *see* Strabismus, paralytic, fourth nerve
multiple G52.7
ninth G52.1
second NEC — *see* Disorder, nerve, optic
seventh NEC G51.8
sixth NEC — *see* Strabismus, paralytic, sixth nerve
specified NEC G52.8
tenth G52.2
third NEC — *see* Strabismus, paralytic, third nerve
twelfth G52.3
entrapment — *see* Neuropathy, entrapment
facial G51.9
specified NEC G51.8
femoral — *see* Lesion, nerve, femoral
glossopharyngeal NEC G52.1
hypoglossal G52.3
intercostal G58.0
lateral
cutaneous of thigh — *see* Mononeuropathy, lower limb, meralgia paresthetica
popliteal — *see* Lesion, nerve, popliteal
lower limb — *see* Mononeuropathy, lower limb
medial popliteal — *see* Lesion, nerve, popliteal, medial
median NEC — *see* Lesion, nerve, median
multiple G58.7
oculomotor NEC — *see* Strabismus, paralytic, third nerve
olfactory G52.0
optic NEC H47.09- ☑
hemorrhage into sheath — *see* Hemorrhage, optic nerve
ischemic H47.01- ☑
peroneal — *see* Lesion, nerve, popliteal
phrenic G58.8
plantar — *see* Lesion, nerve, plantar
pneumogastric G52.2
posterior tibial — *see* Syndrome, tarsal tunnel

- **Disorder** — *continued*
  - nerve — *continued*
    - radial — *see* Lesion, nerve, radial
    - recurrent laryngeal G52.2
    - root G54.9
      - cervical G54.2
      - lumbosacral G54.1
      - specified NEC G54.8
      - thoracic G54.3
    - sciatic NEC — *see* Lesion, nerve, sciatic
    - specified NEC G58.8
      - lower limb — *see* Mononeuropathy, lower limb, specified NEC
      - upper limb — *see* Mononeuropathy, upper limb, specified NEC
    - sympathetic G90.9
    - tibial — *see* Lesion, nerve, popliteal, medial
    - trigeminal G50.9
      - specified NEC G50.8
    - trochlear NEC — *see* Strabismus, paralytic, fourth nerve
    - ulnar — *see* Lesion, nerve, ulnar
    - upper limb — *see* Mononeuropathy, upper limb
    - vagus G52.2
  - nervous system G98.8
    - autonomic (peripheral) G90.9
      - specified NEC G90.8
    - central G96.9
      - specified NEC G96.89
    - parasympathetic G90.9
    - specified NEC G98.8
    - sympathetic G90.9
    - vegetative G90.9
  - neurocognitive R41.9
    - with Lewy bodies — *see also* Dementia, in, diseases specified elsewhere G31.83 *[F02.-]* ☑
    - frontotemporal, specified NEC — *see also* Dementia, in, diseases specified elsewhere G31.09 *[F02.-]* ☑
    - major — *see also* Dementia F03.- ☑
      - due to vascular disease — *see* Dementia, vascular
        - mild — *see* Dementia, vascular, mild
        - moderate — *see* Dementia, vascular, moderate
        - severe — *see* Dementia, vascular, severe
      - in (due to) (other diseases classified elsewhere) — *see also* Dementia, in (due to) F02.80
        - with
          - aggressive behavior — *see also* Dementia, in (due to) F02.81- ☑
          - combative behavior — *see also* Dementia, in (due to) F02.81- ☑
          - violent behavior — *see also* Dementia, in (due to) F02.81- ☑
    - mild (of uncertain or unknown etiology) — *see also* Disorder, mild neurocognitive G31.84
  - neurodevelopmental F89
    - specified NEC F88
  - neurohypophysis NEC E23.3
  - neurological NEC R29.818
  - neuromuscular G70.9
    - hereditary NEC G71.9
    - specified NEC G70.89
    - toxic G70.1
  - neurotic F48.9
    - specified NEC F48.8
  - neutrophil, polymorphonuclear D71
  - nicotine use — *see* Dependence, drug, nicotine
  - nightmare F51.5
  - non-rapid eye movement sleep arousal
    - sleep terror type F51.4
    - sleepwalking type F51.3
  - nose J34.9
    - specified NEC J34.89
  - obsessive-compulsive F42.9
    - and related disorder due to a known physiological condition F06.8
  - odontogenesis NOS K00.9
  - opioid use
    - with
      - opioid-induced psychotic disorder F11.959
        - with
          - delusions F11.950
          - hallucinations F11.951
    - due to drug abuse — *see* Abuse, drug, opioid
    - due to drug dependence — *see* Dependence, drug, opioid
    - mild F11.10
- **Disorder** — *continued*
  - opioid use — *continued*
    - mild — *continued*
      - with
        - opioid-induced
          - anxiety disorder F11.188
          - depressive disorder F11.14
          - sexual dysfunction F11.181
        - opioid intoxication
          - with perceptual disturbances F11.122
          - delirium F11.121
          - without perceptual disturbances F11.129
      - in remission (early) (sustained) F11.11
    - moderate or severe F11.20
      - with
        - opioid-induced
          - anxiety disorder F11.288
          - anxiety disorder F11.988
          - depressive disorder F11.24
          - depressive disorder F11.94
          - sexual dysfunction F11.281
          - sexual dysfunction F11.981
        - opioid intoxication
          - with perceptual disturbances F11.222
          - delirium F11.221
          - without perceptual disturbances F11.229
      - in remission (early) (sustained) F11.21
  - oppositional defiant F91.3
  - optic
    - chiasm H47.49
      - due to
        - inflammatory disorder H47.41
        - neoplasm H47.42
        - vascular disorder H47.43
    - disc H47.39- ☑
      - coloboma — *see* Coloboma, optic disc
      - drusen — *see* Drusen, optic disc
      - pseudopapilledema — *see* Pseudopapilledema
    - radiations — *see* Disorder, visual, pathway
    - tracts — *see* Disorder, visual, pathway
  - orbit H05.9
    - cyst — *see* Cyst, orbit
    - deformity — *see* Deformity, orbit
    - edema — *see* Edema, orbit
    - enophthalmos — *see* Enophthalmos
    - exophthalmos — *see* Exophthalmos
    - hemorrhage — *see* Hemorrhage, orbit
    - inflammation — *see* Inflammation, orbit
    - myopathy — *see* Myopathy, extraocular muscles
    - retained foreign body — *see* Foreign body, orbit, old
    - specified type NEC H05.89
  - organic
    - anxiety F06.4
    - catatonic F06.1
    - delusional F06.2
    - dissociative F06.8
    - emotionally labile (asthenic) F06.8
    - mood (affective) F06.30
    - schizophrenia-like F06.2
  - orgasmic (female) F52.31
    - male F52.32
  - ornithine metabolism E72.4
  - overanxious F41.1
    - of childhood F93.8
  - pain
    - with related psychological factors F45.42
    - exclusively related to psychological factors F45.41
    - genito-pelvic penetration disorder F52.6
  - pancreatic internal secretion E16.9
    - specified NEC E16.8
  - panic F41.0
    - with agoraphobia F40.01
  - papulosquamous L44.9
    - in diseases classified elsewhere L45
    - specified NEC L44.8
  - paranoid F22
    - induced F24
    - shared F24
  - paraphilic F65.9
    - specified NEC F65.89
  - parathyroid (gland) E21.5
    - specified NEC E21.4
  - parietoalveolar NEC J84.09
  - paroxysmal, mixed R56.9
  - patella M22.9- ☑
    - chondromalacia — *see* Chondromalacia, patella
    - derangement NEC M22.3X- ☑
- **Disorder** — *continued*
  - patella — *continued*
    - recurrent
      - dislocation — *see* Dislocation, patella, recurrent
      - subluxation — *see* Dislocation, patella, recurrent, incomplete
    - specified NEC M22.8X- ☑
  - patellofemoral M22.2X- ☑
  - pedophilic F65.4
  - pentose phosphate pathway with anemia D55.1
  - perception, due to hallucinogens F16.983
    - in
      - abuse F16.183
      - dependence F16.283
  - peripheral nervous system NEC G64
  - peroxisomal E71.50
    - biogenesis
      - neonatal adrenoleukodystrophy E71.511
      - specified disorder NEC E71.518
      - Zellweger syndrome E71.510
    - rhizomelic chondrodysplasia punctata E71.540
    - specified form NEC E71.548
      - group 1 E71.518
      - group 2 E71.53
      - group 3 E71.542
    - X-linked adrenoleukodystrophy E71.529
      - adolescent E71.521
      - adrenomyeloneuropathy E71.522
      - childhood E71.520
      - specified form NEC E71.528
    - Zellweger-like syndrome E71.541
  - persistent
    - (somatoform) pain F45.41
    - affective (mood) F34.9
  - personality — *see also* Personality F60.9
    - affective F34.0
    - aggressive F60.3
    - amoral F60.2
    - anankastic F60.5
    - antisocial F60.2
    - anxious F60.6
    - asocial F60.2
    - asthenic F60.7
    - avoidant F60.6
    - borderline F60.3
    - change (secondary) due to general medical condition F07.0
    - compulsive F60.5
    - cyclothymic F34.0
    - dependent (passive) F60.7
    - depressive F34.1
    - dissocial F60.2
    - emotional instability F60.3
    - expansive paranoid F60.0
    - explosive F60.3
    - following organic brain damage F07.9
    - histrionic F60.4
    - hyperthymic F34.0
    - hypothymic F34.1
    - hysterical F60.4
    - immature F60.89
    - inadequate F60.7
    - labile F60.3
    - mixed (nonspecific) F60.89
    - moral deficiency F60.2
    - narcissistic F60.81
    - negativistic F60.89
    - obsessional F60.5
    - obsessive (-compulsive) F60.5
    - organic F07.9
    - overconscientious F60.5
    - paranoid F60.0
    - passive (-dependent) F60.7
    - passive-aggressive F60.89
    - pathological NEC F60.9
    - pseudosocial F60.2
    - psychopathic F60.2
    - schizoid F60.1
    - schizotypal F21
    - self-defeating F60.7
    - specified NEC F60.89
    - type A F60.5
    - unstable (emotional) F60.3
  - pervasive, developmental F84.9
  - phencyclidine use
    - mild F16.10
      - with
        - phencyclidine intoxication F16.129
        - phencyclidine intoxication delirium F16.121

- **Disorder** — *continued*
  - phencyclidine use — *continued*
    - mild — *continued*
      - with — *continued*
        - phencyclidine-induced
          - anxiety disorder F16.18Ø
          - bipolar and related disorder F16.14
          - depressive disorder F16.14
          - psychotic disorder F16.159
      - in remission (early) (sustained) F16.11
    - moderate or severe F16.2Ø
      - with
        - phencyclidine intoxication F16.229
        - phencyclidine intoxication delirium F16.221
        - phencyclidine-induced
          - anxiety disorder F16.28Ø
          - bipolar and related disorder F16.14
          - depressive disorder F16.24
          - psychotic disorder F16.259
      - in remission (early) (sustained) F16.21
  - phobic anxiety, childhood F4Ø.8
  - phosphate-losing tubular N25.Ø
  - pigmentation L81.9
    - choroid, congenital Q14.3
    - diminished melanin formation L81.6
    - iron L81.8
    - specified NEC L81.8
  - pinna (noninfective) H61.1Ø- ☑
    - deformity, acquired H61.11- ☑
    - hematoma H61.12- ☑
    - perichondritis — *see* Perichondritis, ear
    - specified type NEC H61.19- ☑
  - pituitary gland E23.7
    - iatrogenic (postprocedural) E89.3
    - specified NEC E23.6
  - platelet-activating anti-PF4, specified NEC D75.84
  - platelets D69.1
  - plexus G54.9
    - specified NEC G54.8
  - polymorphonuclear neutrophils D71
  - porphyrin metabolism — *see* Porphyria
  - postconcussional FØ7.81
  - posthallucinogen perception F16.983
    - in
      - abuse F16.183
      - dependence F16.283
  - postmenopausal N95.9
    - specified NEC N95.8
  - postprocedural (postoperative) — *see* Complications, postprocedural
  - post-transplant lymphoproliferative D47.Z1 (*following* D47.4)
  - post-traumatic stress (PTSD) F43.1Ø
    - acute F43.11
    - chronic F43.12
  - premenstrual dysphoric (PMDD) F32.81
  - prepuce N47.8
  - propionic acidemia E71.121
  - prostate N42.9
    - specified NEC N42.89
  - psychogenic NOS — *see also* condition F45.9
    - anxiety F41.8
    - appetite F5Ø.9
    - asthenic F48.8
    - cardiovascular (system) F45.8
    - compulsive F42.8
    - cutaneous F54
    - depressive F32.9
    - digestive (system) F45.8
    - dysmenorrheic F45.8
    - dyspneic F45.8
    - endocrine (system) F54
    - eye NEC F45.8
    - feeding — *see* Disorder, eating
    - functional NEC F45.8
    - gastric F45.8
    - gastrointestinal (system) F45.8
    - genitourinary (system) F45.8
    - heart (function) (rhythm) F45.8
    - hyperventilatory F45.8
    - hypochondriacal — *see* Disorder, hypochondriacal
    - intestinal F45.8
    - joint F45.8
    - learning F81.9
    - limb F45.8
    - lymphatic (system) F45.8
    - menstrual F45.8
    - micturition F45.8
- **Disorder** — *continued*
  - psychogenic — *see also* condition — *continued*
    - monoplegic NEC F44.4
    - motor F44.4
    - muscle F45.8
    - musculoskeletal F45.8
    - neurocirculatory F45.8
    - obsessive F42.8
    - occupational F48.8
    - organ or part of body NEC F45.8
    - paralytic NEC F44.4
    - phobic F4Ø.9
    - physical NEC F45.8
    - rectal F45.8
    - respiratory (system) F45.8
    - rheumatic F45.8
    - sexual (function) F52.9
    - skin (allergic) (eczematous) F54
    - sleep F51.9
    - specified part of body NEC F45.8
    - stomach F45.8
  - psychological F99
    - associated with
      - disease classified elsewhere F54
      - sexual
        - development F66
        - relationship F66
      - uncertainty about gender identity F64.9
  - psychomotor NEC F44.4
    - hysterical F44.4
  - psychoneurotic — *see also* Neurosis
    - mixed NEC F48.8
  - psychophysiologic — *see* Disorder, somatoform
  - psychosexual F65.9
    - development F66
    - identity of childhood F64.2
  - psychosomatic NOS — *see* Disorder, somatoform
    - multiple F45.Ø
    - undifferentiated F45.1
  - psychotic — *see* Psychosis
    - transient (acute) F23
  - puberty E3Ø.9
    - specified NEC E3Ø.8
  - pulmonary (valve) — *see* Endocarditis, pulmonary
  - purine metabolism E79.9
  - pyrimidine metabolism E79.9
  - pyruvate metabolism E74.4
  - reactive attachment (childhood) F94.1
  - reading R48.Ø
    - developmental (specific) F81.Ø
  - receptive language F8Ø.2
  - receptor, hormonal, peripheral — *see also* Syndrome, androgen insensitivity E34.5Ø
  - recurrent brief depressive F33.8
  - reflex R29.2
  - refraction H52.7
    - aniseikonia H52.32
    - anisometropia H52.31
    - astigmatism — *see* Astigmatism
    - hypermetropia — *see* Hypermetropia
    - myopia — *see* Myopia
    - presbyopia H52.4
    - specified NEC H52.6
  - relationship F68.8
    - due to sexual orientation F66
  - REM sleep behavior G47.52
  - renal function, impaired (tubular) N25.9
  - resonance R49.9
    - specified NEC R49.8
  - respiratory function, impaired — *see also* Failure, respiration
    - postprocedural — *see* Complication, postoperative, respiratory system
    - psychogenic F45.8
  - retina H35.9
    - angioid streaks H35.33
    - changes in vascular appearance H35.Ø1- ☑
    - degeneration — *see* Degeneration, retina
    - dystrophy (hereditary) — *see* Dystrophy, retina
    - edema H35.81
    - hemorrhage — *see* Hemorrhage, retina
    - ischemia H35.82
    - macular degeneration — *see* Degeneration, macula
    - microaneurysms H35.Ø4- ☑
    - microvascular abnormality NEC H35.Ø9
    - neovascularization — *see* Neovascularization, retina
    - retinopathy — *see* Retinopathy
    - separation of layers H35.7Ø
- **Disorder** — *continued*
  - retina — *continued*
    - separation of layers — *continued*
      - central serous chorioretinopathy H35.71- ☑
      - pigment epithelium detachment (serous) H35.72- ☑
        - hemorrhagic H35.73- ☑
    - specified type NEC H35.89
    - telangiectasis — *see* Telangiectasis, retina
    - vasculitis — *see* Vasculitis, retina
  - retroperitoneal K68.9
  - right hemisphere organic affective FØ7.89
  - rumination (infant or child) F98.21
  - sacrum, sacrococcygeal NEC M53.3
  - schizoaffective F25.9
    - bipolar type F25.Ø
    - depressive type F25.1
    - manic type F25.Ø
    - mixed type F25.Ø
    - specified NEC F25.8
  - schizoid of childhood F84.5
  - schizophrenia spectrum and other psychotic disorder F29
    - specified NEC F28
  - schizophreniform F2Ø.81
    - brief F23
  - schizotypal (personality) F21
  - seasonal affective, recurrent episodes F33.- ☑
  - secretion, thyrocalcitonin EØ7.Ø
  - sedative, hypnotic, or anxiolytic use
    - mild F13.1Ø
      - with
        - sedative, hypnotic, or anxiolytic intoxication F13.129
        - sedative, hypnotic, or anxiolytic intoxication delirium F13.121
        - sedative, hypnotic, or anxiolytic-induced
          - anxiety disorder F13.18Ø
          - bipolar and related disorder F13.14
          - depressive disorder F13.14
          - psychotic disorder F13.159
          - sexual dysfunction F13.181
      - in remission (early) (sustained) F13.11
    - moderate or severe F13.2Ø
      - with
        - sedative, hypnotic, or anxiolytic intoxication F13.229
        - sedative, hypnotic, or anxiolytic intoxication delirium F13.221
        - sedative, hypnotic, or anxiolytic-induced
          - anxiety disorder F13.28Ø
          - bipolar and related disorder F13.24
          - depressive disorder F13.24
          - major neurocognitive disorder F13.27
          - mild neurocognitive disorder F13.288
          - psychotic disorder F13.259
          - sexual dysfunction F13.281
      - in remission (early) (sustained) F13.21
  - seizure — *see also* Epilepsy G4Ø.9Ø9
    - intractable G4Ø.919
      - with status epilepticus G4Ø.911
  - semantic pragmatic F8Ø.89
    - with autism F84.Ø
  - sense of smell R43.1
    - psychogenic F45.8
  - separation anxiety, of childhood F93.Ø
  - sexual
    - aversion F52.1
    - function, psychogenic F52.9
    - interest/arousal, female F52.22
    - masochism F65.51
    - maturation F66
    - nonorganic F52.9
    - preference — *see also* Deviation, sexual F65.9
      - fetishistic transvestism F65.1
    - relationship F66
    - sadism F65.52
  - shyness, of childhood and adolescence F4Ø.1Ø
  - sibling rivalry F93.8
  - sickle-cell (sickling) (homozygous) — *see* Disease, sickle-cell
    - heterozygous D57.3
    - specified type NEC D57.8- ☑
    - trait D57.3
  - sinus (nasal) J34.9
    - specified NEC J34.89
  - skin L98.9
    - atrophic L9Ø.9

- **Disorder** — *continued*
  - skin — *continued*
    - atrophic — *continued*
      - specified NEC L90.8
    - granulomatous L92.9
      - specified NEC L92.8
    - hypertrophic L91.9
      - specified NEC L91.8
    - infiltrative NEC L98.6
    - newborn P83.9
      - specified NEC P83.88
    - picking F42.4
    - psychogenic (allergic) (eczematous) F54
  - sleep G47.9
    - breathing-related — *see* Apnea, sleep
    - circadian rhythm G47.20
      - advance sleep phase type G47.22
      - delayed sleep phase type G47.21
      - due to
        - alcohol
          - abuse F10.182
          - dependence F10.282
          - use F10.982
        - amphetamines
          - abuse F15.182
          - dependence F15.282
          - use F15.982
        - caffeine
          - abuse F15.182
          - dependence F15.282
          - use F15.982
        - cocaine
          - abuse F14.182
          - dependence F14.282
          - use F14.982
        - drug NEC
          - abuse F19.182
          - dependence F19.282
          - use F19.982
        - opioid
          - abuse F11.182
          - dependence F11.282
          - use F11.982
        - psychoactive substance NEC
          - abuse F19.182
          - dependence F19.282
          - use F19.982
        - sedative, hypnotic, or anxiolytic
          - abuse F13.182
          - dependence F13.282
          - use F13.982
        - stimulant NEC
          - abuse F15.182
          - dependence F15.282
          - use F15.982
      - free running type G47.24
      - in conditions classified elsewhere G47.27
      - irregular sleep wake type G47.23
      - jet lag type G47.25
      - non-24-hour sleep-wake type G47.24
      - shift work type G47.26
      - specified NEC G47.29
    - due to
      - alcohol
        - abuse F10.182
        - dependence F10.282
        - use F10.982
      - amphetamine
        - abuse F15.182
        - dependence F15.282
        - use F15.982
      - anxiolytic
        - abuse F13.182
        - dependence F13.282
        - use F13.982
      - caffeine
        - abuse F15.182
        - dependence F15.282
        - use F15.982
      - cocaine
        - abuse F14.182
        - dependence F14.282
        - use F14.982
      - drug NEC
        - abuse F19.182
        - dependence F19.282
        - use F19.982
      - hypnotic
        - abuse F13.182

- **Disorder** — *continued*
  - sleep — *continued*
    - due to — *continued*
      - hypnotic — *continued*
        - dependence F13.282
        - use F13.982
      - opioid
        - abuse F11.182
        - dependence F11.282
        - use F11.982
      - psychoactive substance NEC
        - abuse F19.182
        - dependence F19.282
        - use F19.982
      - sedative
        - abuse F13.182
        - dependence F13.282
        - use F13.982
      - stimulant NEC
        - abuse F15.182
        - dependence F15.282
        - use F15.982
    - emotional F51.9
    - excessive somnolence — *see* Hypersomnia
    - hypersomnia type — *see* Hypersomnia
    - initiating or maintaining — *see* Insomnia
    - nightmares F51.5
    - nonorganic F51.9
      - specified NEC F51.8
    - parasomnia type G47.50
    - specified NEC G47.8
    - terrors F51.4
    - walking F51.3
  - sleep-wake pattern or schedule — *see also* Disorder, sleep, circadian rhythm G47.9
    - specified NEC G47.8
  - social
    - anxiety (of childhood) F40.10
      - generalized F40.11
    - functioning in childhood F94.9
      - specified NEC F94.8
    - pragmatic F80.82
  - soft tissue M79.9
    - ankle M79.9
    - due to use, overuse and pressure M70.90
      - ankle M70.97- ☑
      - bursitis — *see* Bursitis
      - foot M70.97- ☑
      - forearm M70.93- ☑
      - hand M70.94- ☑
      - lower leg M70.96- ☑
      - multiple sites M70.99
      - pelvic region M70.95- ☑
      - shoulder region M70.91- ☑
      - specified site NEC M70.98
      - specified type NEC M70.80
        - ankle M70.87- ☑
        - foot M70.87- ☑
        - forearm M70.83- ☑
        - hand M70.84- ☑
        - lower leg M70.86- ☑
        - multiple sites M70.89
        - pelvic region M70.85- ☑
        - shoulder region M70.81- ☑
        - specified site NEC M70.88
        - thigh M70.85- ☑
        - upper arm M70.82- ☑
      - thigh M70.95- ☑
      - upper arm M70.92- ☑
    - foot M79.9
    - forearm M79.9
    - hand M79.9
    - lower leg M79.9
    - multiple sites M79.9
    - occupational — *see* Disorder, soft tissue, due to use, overuse and pressure
    - pelvic region M79.9
    - shoulder region M79.9
    - specified type NEC M79.89
    - thigh M79.9
    - upper arm M79.9
  - somatic symptom F45.1
  - somatization F45.0
  - somatoform F45.9
    - pain (persistent) F45.41
    - somatization (multiple) (long-lasting) F45.0
    - specified NEC F45.8
    - undifferentiated F45.1

- **Disorder** — *continued*
  - somnolence, excessive — *see* Hypersomnia
  - specific
    - arithmetical F81.2
    - developmental, of motor F82
    - reading F81.0
    - speech and language F80.9
    - spelling F81.81
    - written expression F81.81
  - speech R47.9
    - articulation (functional) (specific) F80.0
    - developmental F80.9
    - specified NEC R47.89
  - speech-sound F80.0
  - spelling (specific) F81.81
  - spine — *see also* Dorsopathy
    - ligamentous or muscular attachments, peripheral — *see* Enthesopathy, spinal
    - specified NEC — *see* Dorsopathy, specified NEC
  - stereotyped, habit or movement F98.4
  - stimulant use (other) (unspecified)
    - mild F15.10
      - in remission (early) (sustained) F15.11
    - moderate or severe F15.20
      - in remission (early) (sustained) F15.21
  - stomach (functional) — *see* Disorder, gastric
  - stress F43.9
    - acute F43.0
    - post-traumatic F43.10
      - acute F43.11
      - chronic F43.12
  - substance use (other) (unknown)
    - mild F19.10
      - with substance-induced
        - anxiety disorder F19.180
        - bipolar and related disorder F19.14
        - depressive disorder F19.14
        - major neurocognitive disorder F19.17
        - mild neurocognitive disorder F19.188
        - obsessive-compulsive and related disorder F19.188
        - sexual dysfunction F19.181
      - substance intoxication F19.129
      - substance intoxication delirium F19.121
    - moderate or severe F19.20
      - with substance-induced
        - anxiety disorder F19.280
        - bipolar and related disorder F19.24
        - depressive disorder F19.24
        - major neurocognitive disorder F19.27
        - mild neurocognitive disorder F19.288
        - obsessive-compulsive and related disorder F19.288
        - sexual dysfunction F19.281
      - in remission (early) (sustained) F19.21
      - substance intoxication F19.229
      - substance intoxication delirium F19.221
  - sulfur-bearing amino-acid metabolism E72.10
  - sweat gland (eccrine) L74.9
    - apocrine L75.9
      - specified NEC L75.8
    - specified NEC L74.8
  - synovium M67.90
    - acromioclavicular M67.91- ☑
    - ankle M67.97- ☑
    - elbow M67.92- ☑
    - foot M67.97- ☑
    - forearm M67.93- ☑
    - hand M67.94- ☑
    - hip M67.95- ☑
    - knee M67.96- ☑
    - multiple sites M67.99
    - rupture — *see* Rupture, synovium
    - shoulder M67.91- ☑
    - specified type NEC M67.80
      - acromioclavicular M67.81- ☑
      - ankle M67.87- ☑
      - elbow M67.82- ☑
      - foot M67.87- ☑
      - hand M67.84- ☑
      - hip M67.85- ☑
      - knee M67.86- ☑
      - multiple sites M67.89
      - wrist M67.83- ☑
    - synovitis — *see* Synovitis
    - upper arm M67.92- ☑
    - wrist M67.93- ☑
  - temperature regulation, newborn P81.9

Disorder — *continued*
- temperature regulation, newborn — *continued*
  - specified NEC P81.8
- temporomandibular joint M26.6Ø- ☑
- tendon M67.9Ø
  - acromioclavicular M67.91- ☑
  - ankle M67.97- ☑
  - contracture — *see* Contracture, tendon
  - elbow M67.92- ☑
  - foot M67.97- ☑
  - forearm M67.93- ☑
  - hand M67.94- ☑
  - hip M67.95- ☑
  - knee M67.96- ☑
  - multiple sites M67.99
  - rupture — *see* Rupture, tendon
  - shoulder M67.91- ☑
  - specified type NEC M67.8Ø
    - acromioclavicular M67.81- ☑
    - ankle M67.87- ☑
    - elbow M67.82- ☑
    - foot M67.87- ☑
    - hand M67.84- ☑
    - hip M67.85- ☑
    - knee M67.86- ☑
    - multiple sites M67.89
    - trunk M67.88
    - wrist M67.83- ☑
  - synovitis — *see* Synovitis
  - tendinitis — *see* Tendinitis
  - tenosynovitis — *see* Tenosynovitis
  - trunk M67.98
  - upper arm M67.92- ☑
  - wrist M67.93- ☑
- thoracic root (nerve) NEC G54.3
- thyrocalcitonin hypersecretion EØ7.Ø
- thyroid (gland) EØ7.9
  - function NEC, neonatal, transitory P72.2
  - iodine-deficiency related EØ1.8
  - specified NEC EØ7.89
- tic — *see* Tic
- tobacco use
  - chewing tobacco (mild) (moderate) (severe)
    - in remission (early) (sustained) F17.221
  - cigarettes (mild) (moderate) (severe)
    - in remission (early) (sustained) F17.211
  - mild F17.2ØØ
    - in remission (early) (sustained) F17.2Ø1
  - moderate F17.2ØØ
    - in remission (early) (sustained) F17.2Ø1
  - severe F17.2ØØ
    - in remission (early) (sustained) F17.2Ø1
  - specified product NEC (mild) (moderate) (severe)
    - in remission (early) (sustained) F17.291
- tooth KØ8.9
  - development KØØ.9
    - specified NEC KØØ.8
  - eruption KØØ.6
- Tourette's F95.2
- trance and possession F44.89
- transvestic F65.1
- trauma and stressor-related NOS F43.9
  - other specified F43.89
  - unspecified F43.9
- tricuspid (valve) — *see* Endocarditis, tricuspid
- tryptophan metabolism E7Ø.5
- tubular, phosphate-losing N25.Ø
- tubulo-interstitial (in)
  - brucellosis A23.9 *[N16]*
  - cystinosis E72.Ø4
  - diphtheria A36.84
  - glycogen storage disease E74.ØØ *[N16]*
  - leukemia NEC C95.9- ☑ *[N16]*
  - lymphoma NEC C85.9- ☑ *[N16]*
  - mixed cryoglobulinemia D89.1 *[N16]*
  - multiple myeloma C9Ø.Ø- ☑ *[N16]*
  - Salmonella infection AØ2.25
  - sarcoidosis D86.84
  - sepsis A41.9 *[N16]*
    - streptococcal A4Ø.9 *[N16]*
  - systemic lupus erythematosus M32.15
  - toxoplasmosis B58.83
  - transplant rejection T86.91 *[N16]*
  - Wilson's disease E83.Ø1 *[N16]*
- tubulo-renal function, impaired N25.9
  - specified NEC N25.89
- tympanic membrane H73.9- ☑

Disorder — *continued*
- tympanic membrane — *continued*
  - atrophy — *see* Atrophy, tympanic membrane
  - infection — *see* Myringitis
  - perforation — *see* Perforation, tympanum
  - specified NEC H73.89- ☑
- unsocialized aggressive F91.1
- urea cycle metabolism E72.2Ø
  - argininemia E72.21
  - arginosuccinic aciduria E72.22
  - citrullinemia E72.23
  - ornithine transcarbamylase deficiency E72.4
  - other specified E72.29
- ureter (in) N28.9
  - schistosomiasis B65.Ø *[N29]*
  - tuberculosis A18.11
- urethra N36.9
  - specified NEC N36.8
- urinary system N39.9
  - specified NEC N39.8
- valve, heart
  - aortic — *see* Endocarditis, aortic
  - mitral — *see* Endocarditis, mitral
  - pulmonary — *see* Endocarditis, pulmonary
  - rheumatic
    - aortic — *see* Endocarditis, aortic, rheumatic
    - mitral — *see* Endocarditis, mitral
    - pulmonary — *see* Endocarditis, pulmonary, rheumatic
    - tricuspid — *see* Endocarditis, tricuspid
  - tricuspid — *see* Endocarditis, tricuspid
- vestibular function H81.9- ☑
  - specified NEC — *see* subcategory H81.8 ☑
    - in diseases classified elsewhere H82.- ☑
  - vertigo — *see* Vertigo
- vision, binocular H53.3Ø
  - abnormal retinal correspondence H53.31
  - diplopia H53.2
  - fusion with defective stereopsis H53.32
  - simultaneous perception H53.33
  - suppression H53.34
- visual
  - cortex
    - blindness H47.619
      - left brain H47.612
      - right brain H47.611
    - due to
      - inflammatory disorder H47.629
        - left brain H47.622
        - right brain H47.621
      - neoplasm H47.639
        - left brain H47.632
        - right brain H47.631
      - vascular disorder H47.649
        - left brain H47.642
        - right brain H47.641
  - pathway H47.9
    - due to
      - inflammatory disorder H47.51- ☑
      - neoplasm H47.52- ☑
      - vascular disorder H47.53- ☑
    - optic chiasm — *see* Disorder, optic, chiasm
- vitreous body H43.9
  - crystalline deposits — *see* Deposit, crystalline
  - degeneration — *see* Degeneration, vitreous
  - hemorrhage — *see* Hemorrhage, vitreous
  - opacities — *see* Opacity, vitreous
  - prolapse — *see* Prolapse, vitreous
  - specified type NEC H43.89
- voice R49.9
  - specified type NEC R49.8
- volatile solvent use
  - due to drug abuse — *see* Abuse, drug, inhalant
  - due to drug dependence — *see* Dependence, drug, inhalant
- voyeuristic F65.3
- white blood cells D72.9
  - specified NEC D72.89
- withdrawing, child or adolescent F4Ø.1Ø

Disorientation R41.Ø

Displacement, displaced
- acquired traumatic of bone, cartilage, joint, tendon NEC — *see* Dislocation
- adrenal gland (congenital) Q89.1
- appendix, retrocecal (congenital) Q43.8
- auricle (congenital) Q17.4
- bladder (acquired) N32.89
  - congenital Q64.19

Displacement, displaced — *continued*
- brachial plexus (congenital) QØ7.8
- brain stem, caudal (congenital) QØ4.8
- canaliculus (lacrimalis), congenital Q1Ø.6
- cardia through esophageal hiatus (congenital) Q4Ø.1
- cerebellum, caudal (congenital) QØ4.8
- cervix — *see* Malposition, uterus
- colon (congenital) Q43.3
- device, implant or graft — *see also* Complications, by site and type, mechanical T85.628 ☑
  - arterial graft NEC — *see* Complication, cardiovascular device, mechanical, vascular
  - breast (implant) T85.42 ☑
  - catheter NEC T85.628 ☑
    - dialysis (renal) T82.42 ☑
      - intraperitoneal T85.621 ☑
    - infusion NEC T82.524 ☑
      - spinal (epidural) (subdural) T85.62Ø ☑
    - urinary
      - cystostomy T83.Ø2Ø ☑
      - Hopkins T83.Ø28 ☑
      - ileostomy T83.Ø28 ☑
      - indwelling T83.Ø21 ☑
      - nephrostomy T83.Ø22 ☑
      - specified NEC T83.Ø28 ☑
      - urostomy T83.Ø28 ☑
  - electronic (electrode) (pulse generator) (stimulator) — *see* Complication, electronic stimulator
  - fixation, internal (orthopedic) NEC — *see* Complication, fixation device, mechanical
  - gastrointestinal — *see* Complications, prosthetic device, mechanical, gastrointestinal device
  - genital NEC T83.428 ☑
    - intrauterine contraceptive device (string) T83.32 ☑
    - penile prosthesis (cylinder) (implanted) (pump) (reservoir) T83.42Ø ☑
    - testicular prosthesis T83.421 ☑
  - heart NEC — *see* Complication, cardiovascular device, mechanical
  - joint prosthesis — *see* Complications, joint prosthesis, mechanical
  - ocular — *see* Complications, prosthetic device, mechanical, ocular device
  - orthopedic NEC — *see* Complication, orthopedic, device or graft, mechanical
  - specified NEC T85.628 ☑
  - urinary NEC T83.128 ☑
    - graft T83.22 ☑
    - sphincter, implanted T83.121 ☑
    - stent (ileal conduit) (nephroureteral) T83.123 ☑
      - ureteral indwelling T83.122 ☑
  - vascular NEC — *see* Complication, cardiovascular device, mechanical
  - ventricular intracranial shunt T85.Ø2 ☑
- electronic stimulator
  - bone T84.32Ø ☑
  - cardiac — *see* Complications, cardiac device, electronic
  - nervous system — *see* Complication, prosthetic device, mechanical, electronic nervous system stimulator
  - urinary — *see* Complications, electronic stimulator, urinary
- esophageal mucosa into cardia of stomach, congenital Q39.8
- esophagus (acquired) K22.89
  - congenital Q39.8
- eyeball (acquired) (lateral) (old) — *see* Displacement, globe
  - congenital Q15.8
  - current — *see* Avulsion, eye
- fallopian tube (acquired) N83.4- ☑
  - congenital Q5Ø.6
  - opening (congenital) Q5Ø.6
- gallbladder (congenital) Q44.1
- gastric mucosa (congenital) Q4Ø.2
- globe (acquired) (old) (lateral) HØ5.21- ☑
  - current — *see* Avulsion, eye
- heart (congenital) Q24.8
  - acquired I51.89
- hymen (upward) (congenital) Q52.4
- intervertebral disc NEC
  - with myelopathy — *see* Disorder, disc, with, myelopathy
  - cervical, cervicothoracic (with) M5Ø.2Ø

- **Displacement, displaced** — *continued*
  - intervertebral disc — *continued*
    - cervical, cervicothoracic — *continued*
      - myelopathy — *see* Disorder, disc, cervical, with myelopathy
      - neuritis, radiculitis or radiculopathy — *see* Disorder, disc, cervical, with neuritis
    - due to trauma — *see* Dislocation, vertebra
    - lumbar region M51.26
      - with
        - myelopathy M51.Ø6
        - neuritis, radiculitis, radiculopathy or sciatica M51.16
    - lumbosacral region M51.27
      - with
        - neuritis, radiculitis, radiculopathy or sciatica M51.17
    - sacrococcygeal region M53.3
    - thoracic region M51.24
      - with
        - myelopathy M51.Ø4
        - neuritis, radiculitis, radiculopathy M51.14
    - thoracolumbar region M51.25
      - with
        - myelopathy M51.Ø5
        - neuritis, radiculitis, radiculopathy M51.15
  - intrauterine device (string) T83.32 ☑
  - kidney (acquired) N28.83
    - congenital Q63.2
  - lachrymal, lacrimal apparatus or duct (congenital) Q1Ø.6
  - lens, congenital Q12.1
  - macula (congenital) Q14.1
  - Meckel's diverticulum Q43.Ø
    - malignant — *see* Table of Neoplasms, small intestine, malignant
  - nail (congenital) Q84.6
    - acquired L6Ø.8
  - opening of Wharton's duct in mouth Q38.4
  - organ or site, congenital NEC — *see* Malposition, congenital
  - ovary (acquired) N83.4- ☑
    - congenital Q5Ø.39
    - free in peritoneal cavity (congenital) Q5Ø.39
    - into hernial sac N83.4- ☑
  - oviduct (acquired) N83.4- ☑
    - congenital Q5Ø.6
  - parathyroid (gland) E21.4
  - parotid gland (congenital) Q38.4
  - punctum lacrimale (congenital) Q1Ø.6
  - sacro-iliac (joint) (congenital) Q74.2
    - current injury S33.2 ☑
    - old — *see* subcategory M53.2 ☑
  - salivary gland (any) (congenital) Q38.4
  - spleen (congenital) Q89.Ø9
  - stomach, congenital Q4Ø.2
  - sublingual duct Q38.4
  - tongue (downward) (congenital) Q38.3
  - tooth, teeth, fully erupted M26.3Ø
    - horizontal M26.33
    - vertical M26.34
  - trachea (congenital) Q32.1
  - ureter or ureteric opening or orifice (congenital) Q62.62
  - uterine opening of oviducts or fallopian tubes Q5Ø.6
  - uterus, uterine — *see* Malposition, uterus
  - ventricular septum Q21.Ø
    - with rudimentary ventricle Q2Ø.4
- **Disproportion**
  - between native and reconstructed breast N65.1
  - fiber-type G71.2Ø
    - congenital G71.29
- **Disruptio uteri** — *see* Rupture, uterus
- **Disruption** (of)
  - ciliary body NEC H21.89
  - closure of
    - cornea T81.31 ☑
    - craniotomy T81.32 ☑
    - fascia (muscular) (superficial) T81.32 ☑
    - internal organ or tissue T81.32 ☑
    - laceration (external) (internal) T81.33 ☑
    - ligament T81.32 ☑
    - mucosa T81.31 ☑
    - muscle or muscle flap T81.32 ☑
    - ribs or rib cage T81.32 ☑
    - skin and subcutaneous tissue (full-thickness) (superficial) T81.31 ☑
    - skull T81.32 ☑
    - sternum (sternotomy) T81.32 ☑
    - tendon T81.32 ☑
- **Disruption** — *continued*
  - closure of — *continued*
    - traumatic laceration (external) (internal) T81.33 ☑
  - family Z63.8
    - due to
      - absence of family member due to military deployment Z63.31
      - absence of family member NEC Z63.32
      - alcoholism and drug addiction in family Z63.72
      - bereavement Z63.4
      - death (assumed) or disappearance of family member Z63.4
      - divorce or separation Z63.5
      - drug addiction in family Z63.72
      - return of family member from military deployment (current or past conflict) Z63.71
      - stressful life events NEC Z63.79
  - iris NEC H21.89
  - ligament(s) — *see also* Sprain
    - knee
      - current injury — *see* Dislocation, knee
      - old (chronic) — *see* Derangement, knee, instability
      - spontaneous NEC — *see* Derangement, knee, disruption ligament
  - ossicular chain — *see* Discontinuity, ossicles, ear
  - pelvic ring (stable) S32.81Ø ☑
    - unstable S32.811 ☑
  - traumatic injury wound repair T81.33 ☑
  - wound T81.3Ø ☑
    - episiotomy O9Ø.1
    - operation T81.31 ☑
      - cesarean O9Ø.Ø
      - external operation wound (superficial) T81.31 ☑
      - internal operation wound (deep) T81.32 ☑
    - perineal (obstetric) O9Ø.1
    - traumatic injury repair T81.33 ☑
- **Dissatisfaction with**
  - employment Z56.9
  - school environment Z55.4
- **Dissecting** — *see* condition
- **Dissection**
  - aorta I71.ØØ
    - abdominal I71.Ø2
    - thoracic I71.Ø19
      - aortic arch I71.Ø11
      - ascending aorta I71.Ø1Ø
      - descending thoracic aorta I71.Ø12
    - thoracoabdominal I71.Ø3
  - artery I77.7Ø
    - basilar (trunk) I77.75
    - carotid I77.71
    - cerebral (nonruptured) I67.Ø
      - ruptured — *see* Hemorrhage, intracranial, subarachnoid
    - coronary I25.42
    - extremity
      - lower I77.77
      - upper I77.76
    - iliac I77.72
    - precerebral
      - congenital (nonruptured) Q28.1
      - specified site NEC I77.75
    - renal I77.73
    - specified NEC I77.79
    - vertebral I77.74
  - precerebral artery, congenital (nonruptured) Q28.1
    - Heartland A93.8
  - traumatic — *see* Wound, open, by site
  - vascular I99.8
  - wound — *see* Wound, open
- **Disseminated** — *see* condition
- **Dissociation**
  - auriculoventricular or atrioventricular (AV) (any degree) (isorhythmic) I45.89
    - with heart block I44.2
  - interference I45.89
- **Dissociative reaction, state** F44.9
- **Dissolution, vertebra** — *see* Osteoporosis
- **Distension, distention**
  - abdomen R14.Ø
  - bladder N32.89
  - cecum K63.89
  - colon K63.89
  - gallbladder K82.8
  - intestine K63.89
  - kidney N28.89
  - liver K76.89
- **Distension, distention** — *continued*
  - seminal vesicle N5Ø.89
  - stomach K31.89
    - acute K31.Ø
    - psychogenic F45.8
  - ureter — *see* Dilatation, ureter
  - uterus N85.8
- **Distoma hepaticum infestation** B66.3
- **Distomiasis** B66.9
  - bile passages B66.3
  - hemic B65.9
  - hepatic B66.3
    - due to Clonorchis sinensis B66.1
  - intestinal B66.5
  - liver B66.3
    - due to Clonorchis sinensis B66.1
  - lung B66.4
  - pulmonary B66.4
- **Distomolar** (fourth molar) KØØ.1
- **Disto-occlusion** (Division I) (Division II) M26.212
- **Distortion**(s) (congenital)
  - adrenal (gland) Q89.1
  - arm NEC Q68.8
  - bile duct or passage Q44.5
  - bladder Q64.79
  - brain QØ4.9
  - cervix (uteri) Q51.9
  - chest (wall) Q67.8
    - bones Q76.8
  - clavicle Q74.Ø
  - clitoris Q52.6
  - coccyx Q76.49
  - common duct Q44.5
  - coronary Q24.5
  - cystic duct Q44.5
  - ear (auricle) (external) Q17.3
    - inner Q16.5
    - middle Q16.4
      - ossicles Q16.3
  - endocrine NEC Q89.2
  - eustachian tube Q17.8
  - eye (adnexa) Q15.8
  - face bone(s) NEC Q75.8
  - fallopian tube Q5Ø.6
  - femur NEC Q68.8
  - fibula NEC Q68.8
  - finger(s) Q68.1
  - foot Q66.9- ☑
  - genitalia, genital organ(s)
    - female Q52.8
      - external Q52.79
      - internal NEC Q52.8
  - gyri QØ4.8
  - hand bone(s) Q68.1
  - heart (auricle) (ventricle) Q24.8
    - valve (cusp) Q24.8
  - hepatic duct Q44.5
  - humerus NEC Q68.8
  - hymen Q52.4
  - intrafamilial communications Z63.8
  - jaw NEC M26.89
  - labium (majus) (minus) Q52.79
  - leg NEC Q68.8
  - lens Q12.8
  - liver Q44.7
  - lumbar spine Q76.49
    - with disproportion O33.8
      - causing obstructed labor O65.Ø
  - lumbosacral (joint) (region) Q76.49
    - kyphosis — *see* Kyphosis, congenital
    - lordosis — *see* Lordosis, congenital
  - nerve QØ7.8
  - nose Q3Ø.8
  - organ
    - of Corti Q16.5
    - or site not listed — *see* Anomaly, by site
  - ossicles, ear Q16.3
  - oviduct Q5Ø.6
  - pancreas Q45.3
  - parathyroid (gland) Q89.2
  - pituitary (gland) Q89.2
  - radius NEC Q68.8
  - sacroiliac joint Q74.2
  - sacrum Q76.49
  - scapula Q74.Ø
  - shoulder girdle Q74.Ø
  - skull bone(s) NEC Q75.8

Distortion(s) — *continued*
  skull bone(s) — *continued*
    with
      anencephalus QØØ.Ø
      encephalocele — *see* Encephalocele
      hydrocephalus QØ3.9
        with spina bifida — *see* Spina bifida, with hydrocephalus
      microcephaly QØ2
  spinal cord QØ6.8
  spine Q76.49
    kyphosis — *see* Kyphosis, congenital
    lordosis — *see* Lordosis, congenital
  spleen Q89.Ø9
  sternum NEC Q76.7
  thorax (wall) Q67.8
    bony Q76.8
  thymus (gland) Q89.2
  thyroid (gland) Q89.2
  tibia NEC Q68.8
  toe(s) Q66.9- ☑
  tongue Q38.3
  trachea (cartilage) Q32.1
  ulna NEC Q68.8
  ureter Q62.8
  urethra Q64.79
    causing obstruction Q64.39
  uterus Q51.9
  vagina Q52.4
  vertebra Q76.49
    kyphosis — *see* Kyphosis, congenital
    lordosis — *see* Lordosis, congenital
  visual — *see also* Disturbance, vision
    shape and size H53.15
  vulva Q52.79
  wrist (bones) (joint) Q68.8
Distress
  abdomen — *see* Pain, abdominal
  acute respiratory RØ6.Ø3
    syndrome (adult) (child) J8Ø
  epigastric R1Ø.13
  fetal P84
    complicating pregnancy — *see* Stress, fetal
  gastrointestinal (functional) K3Ø
    psychogenic F45.8
  intestinal (functional) NOS K59.9
    psychogenic F45.8
  maternal, during labor and delivery O75.Ø
  relationship, with spouse or intimate partner Z63.Ø
  respiratory (adult) (child) RØ6.Ø3
    newborn P22.9
      specified NEC P22.8
    orthopnea RØ6.Ø1
    psychogenic F45.8
    shortness of breath RØ6.Ø2
    specified type NEC RØ6.Ø9
Distribution vessel, atypical Q27.9
  coronary artery Q24.5
  precerebral Q28.1
Districhiasis L68.8
Disturbance(s) — *see also* Disease
  absorption K9Ø.9
    calcium E58
    carbohydrate K9Ø.49
    fat K9Ø.49
      pancreatic K9Ø.3
    protein K9Ø.49
    starch K9Ø.49
    vitamin — *see* Deficiency, vitamin
  acid-base equilibrium E87.8
    mixed E87.4
  activity and attention (with hyperkinesis) — *see* Disorder, attention-deficit hyperactivity
  amino acid transport E72.ØØ
  assimilation, food K9Ø.9
  auditory nerve, except deafness — *see* subcategory H93.3 ☑
  behavior — *see* Disorder, conduct
  blood clotting (mechanism) — *see also* Defect, coagulation D68.9
  cerebral
    nerve — *see* Disorder, nerve, cranial
    status, newborn P91.9
      specified NEC P91.88
  circulatory I99.9
  conduct — *see also* Disorder, conduct F91.9
    adjustment reaction — *see* Disorder, adjustment
    compulsive F63.9

Disturbance(s) — *continued*
  conduct — *see also* Disorder, conduct — *continued*
    disruptive F91.9
    hyperkinetic — *see* Disorder, attention-deficit hyperactivity
    socialized F91.2
    specified NEC F91.8
    unsocialized F91.1
  coordination R27.8
  cranial nerve — *see* Disorder, nerve, cranial
  deep sensibility — *see* Disturbance, sensation
  digestive K3Ø
    psychogenic F45.8
  electrolyte — *see also* Imbalance, electrolyte
    newborn, transitory P74.49
      hyperammonemia P74.6
      hyperchloremia P74.421
      hyperchloremic metabolic acidosis P74.421
      hypochloremia P74.422
      potassium balance
        hyperkalemia P74.31
        hypokalemia P74.32
      sodium balance
        hypernatremia P74.21
        hyponatremia P74.22
      specified type NEC P74.49
  emotions specific to childhood and adolescence F93.9
    with
      anxiety and fearfulness NEC F93.8
      elective mutism F94.Ø
      oppositional disorder F91.3
      sensitivity (withdrawal) F4Ø.1Ø
      shyness F4Ø.1Ø
      social withdrawal F4Ø.1Ø
    involving relationship problems F93.8
    mixed F93.8
    specified NEC F93.8
  endocrine (gland) E34.9
    neonatal, transitory P72.9
      specified NEC P72.8
  equilibrium R42
  fructose metabolism E74.1Ø
  gait — *see* Gait
    hysterical F44.4
    psychogenic F44.4
  gastrointestinal (functional) K3Ø
    psychogenic F45.8
  habit, child F98.9
  hearing, except deafness and tinnitus — *see* Abnormal, auditory perception
  heart, functional (conditions in I44-I5Ø)
    due to presence of (cardiac) prosthesis I97.19- ☑
    postoperative I97.89
      cardiac surgery — *see also* Infarct, myocardium, associated with revascularization procedure I97.19- ☑
  hormones E34.9
  innervation uterus (parasympathetic) (sympathetic) N85.8
  keratinization NEC
    gingiva KØ5.1Ø
      nonplaque induced KØ5.11
      plaque induced KØ5.1Ø
    lip K13.Ø
    oral (mucosa) (soft tissue) K13.29
    tongue K13.29
  learning (specific) — *see* Disorder, learning
  memory — *see* Amnesia
    mild, following organic brain damage FØ6.8
  mental F99
    associated with diseases classified elsewhere F54
  metabolism E88.9
    with
      abortion — *see* Abortion, by type with other specified complication
      ectopic pregnancy OØ8.5
      molar pregnancy OØ8.5
    amino-acid E72.9
      aromatic E7Ø.9
      branched-chain E71.2
      straight-chain E72.89
      sulfur-bearing E72.1Ø
    ammonia E72.2Ø
    arginine E72.21
    arginosuccinic acid E72.22
    carbohydrate E74.9
    cholesterol E78.9
    citrulline E72.23

Disturbance(s) — *continued*
  metabolism — *continued*
    cystathionine E72.19
    general E88.9
    glutamine E72.89
    histidine E7Ø.4Ø
    homocystine E72.19
    hydroxylysine E72.3
    in labor or delivery O75.89
    iron E83.1Ø
    lipoid E78.9
    lysine E72.3
    methionine E72.19
    neonatal, transitory P74.9
      calcium and magnesium P71.9
        specified type NEC P71.8
      carbohydrate metabolism P7Ø.9
        specified type NEC P7Ø.8
      specified NEC P74.8
    ornithine E72.4
    phosphate E83.39
    sodium NEC E87.8
    threonine E72.89
    tryptophan E7Ø.5
    tyrosine E7Ø.2Ø
    urea cycle E72.2Ø
  motor R29.2
  nervous, functional R45.Ø
  neuromuscular mechanism (eye), due to syphilis A52.15
  nutritional E63.9
    nail L6Ø.3
  ocular motion H51.9
    psychogenic F45.8
  oculogyric H51.8
    psychogenic F45.8
  oculomotor H51.9
    psychogenic F45.8
  olfactory nerve R43.1
  optic nerve NEC — *see* Disorder, nerve, optic
  oral epithelium, including tongue NEC K13.29
  perceptual due to
    alcohol withdrawal F1Ø.232
    amphetamine intoxication F15.922
      in
        abuse F15.122
        dependence F15.222
    anxiolytic withdrawal F13.232
    cannabis intoxication (acute) F12.922
      in
        abuse F12.122
        dependence F12.222
    cocaine intoxication (acute) F14.922
      in
        abuse F14.122
        dependence F14.222
    hypnotic withdrawal F13.232
    opioid intoxication (acute) F11.922
      in
        abuse F11.122
        dependence F11.222
    phencyclidine intoxication (acute) F16.122
    sedative withdrawal F13.232
  personality (pattern) (trait) — *see also* Disorder, personality F6Ø.9
    following organic brain damage FØ7.9
  polyglandular E31.9
    specified NEC E31.8
  potassium balance, newborn
    hyperkalemia P74.31
    hypokalemia P74.32
  psychogenic F45.9
  psychomotor F44.4
  psychophysical visual H53.16
  pupillary — *see* Anomaly, pupil, function
  reflex R29.2
  rhythm, heart I49.9
  salivary secretion K11.7
  sensation (cold) (heat) (localization) (tactile discrimination) (texture) (vibratory) NEC R2Ø.9
    hysterical F44.6
    skin R2Ø.9
      anesthesia R2Ø.Ø
      hyperesthesia R2Ø.3
      hypoesthesia R2Ø.1
      paresthesia R2Ø.2
      specified type NEC R2Ø.8
    smell R43.9
      and taste (mixed) R43.8
      anosmia R43.Ø

Disturbance(s) — *continued*
- sensation — *continued*
  - smell — *continued*
    - parosmia R43.1
    - specified NEC R43.8
  - taste R43.9
    - and smell (mixed) R43.8
    - parageusia R43.2
    - specified NEC R43.8
- sensory — *see* Disturbance, sensation
- situational (transient) — *see also* Disorder, adjustment
  - acute F43.0
- sleep G47.9
  - nonorganic origin F51.9
- smell — *see* Disturbance, sensation, smell
- sociopathic F60.2
- sodium balance, newborn
  - hypernatremia P74.21
  - hyponatremia P74.22
- speech R47.9
  - developmental F80.9
  - specified NEC R47.89
- stomach (functional) K31.9
- sympathetic (nerve) G90.9
- taste — *see* Disturbance, sensation, taste
- temperature
  - regulation, newborn P81.9
    - specified NEC P81.8
  - sense R20.8
    - hysterical F44.6
- tooth
  - eruption K00.6
  - formation K00.4
  - structure, hereditary NEC K00.5
- touch — *see* Disturbance, sensation
- vascular I99.9
  - arteriosclerotic — *see* Arteriosclerosis
- vasomotor I73.9
- vasospastic I73.9
- vision, visual H53.9
  - following
    - cerebral infarction I69.398
    - cerebrovascular disease I69.998
      - specified NEC I69.898
    - intracerebral hemorrhage I69.198
    - nontraumatic intracranial hemorrhage NEC I69.298
    - specified disease NEC I69.898
    - subarachnoid hemorrhage I69.098
  - psychophysical H53.16
  - specified NEC H53.8
  - subjective H53.10
    - day blindness H53.11
    - discomfort H53.14- ☑
    - distortions of shape and size H53.15
    - loss
      - sudden H53.13- ☑
      - transient H53.12- ☑
    - specified type NEC H53.19
- voice R49.9
  - psychogenic F44.4
  - specified NEC R49.8

Diuresis R35.89

Diver's palsy, paralysis or squeeze T70.3 ☑

Diverticulitis (acute) K57.92
- bladder — *see* Cystitis
- ileum — *see* Diverticulitis, intestine, small
- intestine K57.92
  - with
    - abscess, perforation K57.80
      - with bleeding K57.81
    - bleeding K57.93
  - congenital Q43.8
  - large K57.32
    - with
      - abscess, perforation K57.20
        - with bleeding K57.21
      - bleeding K57.33
      - small intestine K57.52
        - with
          - abscess, perforation K57.40
            - with bleeding K57.41
          - bleeding K57.53
  - small K57.12
    - with
      - abscess, perforation K57.00
        - with bleeding K57.01
      - bleeding K57.13

Diverticulitis — *continued*
- intestine — *continued*
  - small — *continued*
    - with — *continued*
      - large intestine K57.52
        - with
          - abscess, perforation K57.40
            - with bleeding K57.41
          - bleeding K57.53

Diverticulosis K57.90
- with bleeding K57.91
- large intestine K57.30
  - with
    - bleeding K57.31
    - small intestine K57.50
      - with bleeding K57.51
- small intestine K57.10
  - with
    - bleeding K57.11
    - large intestine K57.50
      - with bleeding K57.51

Diverticulum, diverticula (multiple) K57.90
- appendix (noninflammatory) K38.2
- bladder (sphincter) N32.3
  - congenital Q64.6
- bronchus (congenital) Q32.4
  - acquired J98.09
- calyx, calyceal (kidney) N28.89
- cardia (stomach) K31.4
- cecum — *see* Diverticulosis, intestine, large
  - congenital Q43.8
- colon — *see* Diverticulosis, intestine, large
  - congenital Q43.8
- duodenum — *see* Diverticulosis, intestine, small
  - congenital Q43.8
- epiphrenic (esophagus) K22.5
- esophagus (congenital) Q39.6
  - acquired (epiphrenic) (pulsion) (traction) K22.5
- eustachian tube — *see* Disorder, eustachian tube, specified NEC
- fallopian tube N83.8
- gastric K31.4
- heart (congenital) Q24.8
- ileum — *see* Diverticulosis, intestine, small
- jejunum — *see* Diverticulosis, intestine, small
- kidney (pelvis) (calyces) N28.89
  - with calculus — *see* Calculus, kidney
- Meckel's (displaced) (hypertrophic) Q43.0
  - malignant — *see* Table of Neoplasms, small intestine, malignant
- midthoracic K22.5
- organ or site, congenital NEC — *see* Distortion
- pericardium (congenital) (cyst) Q24.8
  - acquired I31.8
- pharyngoesophageal (congenital) Q39.6
  - acquired K22.5
- pharynx (congenital) Q38.7
- rectosigmoid — *see* Diverticulosis, intestine, large
  - congenital Q43.8
- rectum — *see* Diverticulosis, intestine, large
- Rokitansky's K22.5
- seminal vesicle N50.89
- sigmoid — *see* Diverticulosis, intestine, large
  - congenital Q43.8
- stomach (acquired) K31.4
  - congenital Q40.2
- trachea (acquired) J39.8
- ureter (acquired) N28.89
  - congenital Q62.8
- ureterovesical orifice N28.89
- urethra (acquired) N36.1
  - congenital Q64.79
- ventricle, left (congenital) Q24.8
- vesical N32.3
  - congenital Q64.6
- Zenker's (esophagus) K22.5

Division
- cervix uteri (acquired) N88.8
- glans penis Q55.69
- labia minora (congenital) Q52.79
- ligament (partial or complete) (current) — *see also* Sprain
  - with open wound — *see* Wound, open
- muscle (partial or complete) (current) — *see also* Injury, muscle
  - with open wound — *see* Wound, open
- nerve (traumatic) — *see* Injury, nerve
- spinal cord — *see* Injury, spinal cord, by region

Division — *continued*
- vein I87.8

Divorce, causing family disruption Z63.5

Dix-Hallpike neurolabyrinthitis — *see* Neuronitis, vestibular

Dizziness R42
- hysterical F44.89
- psychogenic F45.8

DMAC (disseminated mycobacterium avium-intracellulare complex) A31.2

DNR (do not resuscitate) Z66

Doan-Wiseman syndrome (primary splenic neutropenia) — *see* Agranulocytosis

Doehle-Heller aortitis A52.02

Dog bite — *see* Bite

Dohle body panmyelopathic syndrome D72.0

Dolichocephaly Q67.2

Dolichocolon Q43.8

Dolichostenomelia — *see* Syndrome, Marfan's

Donohue's syndrome E34.8

Donor (organ or tissue) Z52.9
- blood (whole) Z52.000
  - autologous Z52.010
  - specified component (lymphocytes) (platelets) NEC Z52.008
    - autologous Z52.018
    - specified donor NEC Z52.098
  - specified donor NEC Z52.090
  - stem cells Z52.001
    - autologous Z52.011
    - specified donor NEC Z52.091
- bone Z52.20
  - autologous Z52.21
  - marrow Z52.3
  - specified type NEC Z52.29
- cornea Z52.5
- egg (Oocyte) Z52.819
  - age 35 and over Z52.812
    - anonymous recipient Z52.812
    - designated recipient Z52.813
  - under age 35 Z52.810
    - anonymous recipient Z52.810
    - designated recipient Z52.811
- kidney Z52.4
- liver Z52.6
- lung Z52.89
- lymphocyte — *see* Donor, blood, specified components NEC
- Oocyte — *see* Donor, egg
- platelets Z52.008
- potential, examination of Z00.5
- semen Z52.89
- skin Z52.10
  - autologous Z52.11
  - specified type NEC Z52.19
- specified organ or tissue NEC Z52.89
- sperm Z52.89

Donovanosis A58

Dorsalgia M54.9
- psychogenic F45.41
- specified NEC M54.89

Dorsopathy M53.9
- deforming M43.9
  - specified NEC — *see* subcategory M43.8 ☑
- specified NEC M53.80
  - cervical region M53.82
  - cervicothoracic region M53.83
  - lumbar region M53.86
  - lumbosacral region M53.87
  - occipito-atlanto-axial region M53.81
  - sacrococcygeal region M53.88
  - thoracic region M53.84
  - thoracolumbar region M53.85

Double
- albumin E88.09
- aortic arch Q25.45
- auditory canal Q17.8
- auricle (heart) Q20.8
- bladder Q64.79
- cervix Q51.820
  - with doubling of uterus (and vagina) Q51.10
    - with obstruction Q51.11
- inlet ventricle Q20.4
- kidney with double pelvis (renal) Q63.0
- meatus urinarius Q64.75
- monster Q89.4
- outlet
  - left ventricle Q20.2

- **Double** — *continued*
  - outlet — *continued*
    - right ventricle Q2Ø.1
  - pelvis (renal) with double ureter Q62.5
  - tongue Q38.3
  - ureter (one or both sides) Q62.5
    - with double pelvis (renal) Q62.5
  - urethra Q64.74
  - urinary meatus Q64.75
  - uterus Q51.28
    - with
      - doubling of cervix (and vagina) Q51.1Ø
        - with obstruction Q51.11
    - complete Q51.21
    - in pregnancy or childbirth O34.Ø- ☑
      - causing obstructed labor O65.5
    - partial Q51.22
    - specified NEC Q51.28
  - vagina Q52.1Ø
    - with doubling of uterus (and cervix) Q51.1Ø
      - with obstruction Q51.11
  - vision H53.2
  - vulva Q52.79
- **Doubled up** Z59.Ø1
- **Douglas' pouch, cul-de-sac** — *see* condition
- **Down syndrome** Q9Ø.9
  - meiotic nondisjunction Q9Ø.Ø
  - mitotic nondisjunction Q9Ø.1
  - mosaicism Q9Ø.1
  - translocation Q9Ø.2
- **DPD** (dihydropyrimidine dehydrogenase deficiency) E88.89
- **Dracontiasis** B72
- **Dracunculiasis, dracunculosis** B72
- **Dream state, hysterical** F44.89
- **Drepanocytic anemia** — *see* Disease, sickle-cell
- **Dresbach's syndrome** (elliptocytosis) D58.1
- **Dreschlera** (hawaiiensis) (infection) B43.8
- **Dressler's syndrome** I24.1
- **Drift, ulnar** — *see* Deformity, limb, specified type NEC, forearm
- **Drinking** (alcohol)
  - excessive, to excess NEC (without dependence) F1Ø.1Ø
    - habitual (continual) (without remission) F1Ø.2Ø
      - with remission F1Ø.21
- **Drip, postnasal** (chronic) RØ9.82
  - due to
    - allergic rhinitis — *see* Rhinitis, allergic
    - common cold JØØ
    - gastroesophageal reflux — *see* Reflux, gastroesophageal
    - nasopharyngitis — *see* Nasopharyngitis
    - other known condition — *code to* condition
    - sinusitis — *see* Sinusitis
- **Droop**
  - facial R29.81Ø
    - cerebrovascular disease I69.992
      - cerebral infarction I69.392
      - intracerebral hemorrhage I69.192
      - nontraumatic intracranial hemorrhage NEC I69.292
      - specified disease NEC I69.892
      - subarachnoid hemorrhage I69.Ø92
- **Drop** (in)
  - attack NEC R55
  - finger — *see* Deformity, finger
  - foot — *see* Deformity, limb, foot, drop
  - hematocrit (precipitous) R71.Ø
  - hemoglobin R71.Ø
  - toe — *see* Deformity, toe, specified NEC
  - wrist — *see* Deformity, limb, wrist drop
- **Dropped heart beats** I45.9
- **Dropsy, dropsical** — *see also* Hydrops
  - abdomen R18.8
  - brain — *see* Hydrocephalus
  - cardiac, heart — *see* Failure, heart, congestive
  - gangrenous — *see* Gangrene
  - heart — *see* Failure, heart, congestive
  - kidney — *see* Nephrosis
  - lung — *see* Edema, lung
  - newborn due to isoimmunization P56.Ø
  - pericardium — *see* Pericarditis
- **Drowned, drowning** (near) T75.1 ☑
- **Drowsiness** R4Ø.Ø
- **Drug**
  - abuse counseling and surveillance Z71.51
  - addiction — *see* Dependence
- **Drug** — *continued*
  - dependence — *see* Dependence
  - habit — *see* Dependence
  - harmful use — *see* Abuse, drug
  - induced fever R5Ø.2
  - overdose — *see* Table of Drugs and Chemicals, by drug, poisoning
  - poisoning — *see* Table of Drugs and Chemicals, by drug, poisoning
  - resistant organism infection — *see also* Resistant, organism, to, drug Z16.3Ø
  - therapy
    - long term (current) (prophylactic) — *see* Therapy, drug long-term (current) (prophylactic)
    - short term — *omit code*
  - wrong substance given or taken in error — *see* Table of Drugs and Chemicals, by drug, poisoning
- **Drunkenness** (without dependence) F1Ø.129
  - acute in alcoholism F1Ø.229
  - chronic (without remission) F1Ø.2Ø
    - with remission F1Ø.21
  - pathological (without dependence) F1Ø.129
    - with dependence F1Ø.229
  - sleep F51.9
- **Drusen**
  - macula (degenerative) (retina) — *see* Degeneration, macula, drusen
  - optic disc H47.32- ☑
- **Dry, dryness** — *see also* condition
  - larynx J38.7
  - mouth R68.2
    - due to dehydration E86.Ø
  - nose J34.89
  - socket (teeth) M27.3
  - throat J39.2
- **DSAP** L56.5
- **Duane's syndrome** H5Ø.81- ☑
- **Dubin-Johnson disease or syndrome** E8Ø.6
- **Dubois' disease** (thymus gland) A5Ø.59 *[E35]*
- **Dubowitz' syndrome** Q87.19
- **Duchenne-Aran muscular atrophy** G12.21
- **Duchenne-Griesinger disease** G71.Ø1
- **Duchenne's**
  - disease or syndrome
    - motor neuron disease G12.22
    - muscular dystrophy G71.Ø1
  - locomotor ataxia (syphilitic) A52.11
  - paralysis
    - birth injury P14.Ø
    - due to or associated with
      - motor neuron disease G12.22
      - muscular dystrophy G71.Ø1
- **Ducrey's chancre** A57
- **Duct, ductus** — *see* condition
- **Duhring's disease** (dermatitis herpetiformis) L13.Ø
- **Dullness, cardiac** (decreased) (increased) RØ1.2
- **Dumb ague** — *see* Malaria
- **Dumbness** — *see* Aphasia
- **Dumdum fever** B55.Ø
- **Dumping syndrome** (postgastrectomy) K91.1
- **Duodenitis** (nonspecific) (peptic) K29.8Ø
  - with bleeding K29.81
- **Duodenocholangitis** — *see* Cholangitis
- **Duodenum, duodenal** — *see* condition
- **Duplay's bursitis or periarthritis** M75.Ø ☑
- **Duplication, duplex** — *see also* Accessory
  - alimentary tract Q45.8
  - anus Q43.4
  - appendix (and cecum) Q43.4
  - biliary duct (any) Q44.5
  - bladder Q64.79
  - cecum (and appendix) Q43.4
  - cervix Q51.82Ø
  - chromosome NEC
    - with complex rearrangements NEC Q92.5
    - seen only at prometaphase Q92.8
  - cystic duct Q44.5
  - digestive organs Q45.8
  - esophagus Q39.8
  - frontonasal process Q75.8
  - intestine (large) (small) Q43.4
  - kidney Q63.Ø
  - liver Q44.7
  - pancreas Q45.3
  - penis Q55.69
  - respiratory organs NEC Q34.8
  - salivary duct Q38.4
  - spinal cord (incomplete) QØ6.2
- **Duplication, duplex** — *continued*
  - stomach Q4Ø.2
- **Dupré's disease** (meningism) R29.1
- **Dupuytren's contraction or disease** M72.Ø
- **Durand-Nicolas-Favre disease** A55
- **Durotomy** (inadvertent) (incidental) G97.41
- **Duroziez's disease** (congenital mitral stenosis) Q23.2
- **Dutton's relapsing fever** (West African) A68.1
- **Dwarfism** — *see also* Stature, short E34.328
  - achondroplastic Q77.4
  - congenital — *see also* Stature, short E34.328
  - constitutional E34.31
  - hypochondroplastic Q77.4
  - hypophyseal E23.Ø
  - infantile — *see also* Stature, short E34.328
  - Laron-type — *see also* Stature, short E34.321
  - Lorain (-Levi) type E23.Ø
  - metatropic Q77.8
  - nephrotic-glycosuric (with hypophosphatemic rickets) E72.Ø9
  - nutritional E45
  - pancreatic K86.89
  - pituitary E23.Ø
  - renal N25.Ø
  - thanatophoric Q77.1
- **Dyke-Young anemia** (secondary) (symptomatic) D59.19
- **Dysacusis** — *see* Abnormal, auditory perception
- **Dysadrenocortism** E27.9
  - hyperfunction E27.Ø
- **Dysarthria** R47.1
  - following
    - cerebral infarction I69.322
    - cerebrovascular disease I69.922
      - specified disease NEC I69.822
    - intracerebral hemorrhage I69.122
    - nontraumatic intracranial hemorrhage NEC I69.222
    - subarachnoid hemorrhage I69.Ø22
- **Dysautonomia** (familial) G9Ø.1
- **Dysbarism** T7Ø.3 ☑
- **Dysbasia** R26.2
  - angiosclerotica intermittens I73.9
  - hysterical F44.4
  - lordotica (progressiva) G24.1
  - nonorganic origin F44.4
  - psychogenic F44.4
- **Dysbetalipoproteinemia** (familial) E78.2
- **Dyscalculia** R48.8
  - developmental F81.2
- **Dyschezia** K59.ØØ
- **Dyschondroplasia** (with hemangiomata) Q78.4
- **Dyschromia** (skin) L81.9
- **Dyscollagenosis** M35.9
- **Dyscranio-pygo-phalangy** Q87.Ø
- **Dyscrasia**
  - blood (with) D75.9
    - antepartum hemorrhage — *see* Hemorrhage, antepartum, with coagulation defect
    - intrapartum hemorrhage O67.Ø
    - newborn P61.9
      - specified type NEC P61.8
    - puerperal, postpartum O72.3
  - polyglandular, pluriglandular E31.9
- **Dysendocrinism** E34.9
- **Dysentery, dysenteric** (catarrhal) (diarrhea) (epidemic) (hemorrhagic) (infectious) (sporadic) (tropical) AØ9
  - abscess, liver AØ6.4
  - amebic — *see also* Amebiasis AØ6.Ø
    - with abscess — *see* Abscess, amebic
    - acute AØ6.Ø
    - chronic AØ6.1
  - arthritis — *see also* category MØ1 AØ9
    - bacillary (*see also* category MØ1) AØ3.9
  - bacillary AØ3.9
    - arthritis — *see also* category MØ1 AØ3.9
    - Boyd AØ3.2
    - Flexner AØ3.1
    - Schmitz (-Stutzer) AØ3.Ø
    - Shiga (-Kruse) AØ3.Ø
    - Shigella AØ3.9
      - boydii AØ3.2
      - dysenteriae AØ3.Ø
      - flexneri AØ3.1
      - group A AØ3.Ø
      - group B AØ3.1
      - group C AØ3.2
      - group D AØ3.3
      - sonnei AØ3.3
      - specified type NEC AØ3.8

Dysentery, dysenteric — *continued*
bacillary — *continued*
Sonne A03.3
specified type NEC A03.8
balantidial A07.0
Balantidium coli A07.0
Boyd's A03.2
candidal B37.82
Chilomastix A07.8
Chinese A03.9
coccidial A07.3
Dientamoeba (fragilis) A07.8
Embadomonas A07.8
Entamoeba, entamebic — *see* Dysentery, amebic
Flexner-Boyd A03.2
Flexner's A03.1
Giardia lamblia A07.1
Hiss-Russell A03.1
Lamblia A07.1
leishmanial B55.0
malarial — *see* Malaria
metazoal B82.0
monilial B37.82
protozoal A07.9
Salmonella A02.0
schistosomal B65.1
Schmitz (-Stutzer) A03.0
Shiga (-Kruse) A03.0
Shigella NOS — *see* Dysentery, bacillary
Sonne A03.3
strongyloidiasis B78.0
trichomonal A07.8
viral — *see also* Enteritis, viral A08.4
Dysequilibrium R42
Dysesthesia R20.8
hysterical F44.6
Dysferlinopathy G71.033
Dysfibrinogenemia (congenital) D68.2
Dysfunction
adrenal E27.9
hyperfunction E27.0
autonomic
due to alcohol G31.2
somatoform F45.8
bladder N31.9
neurogenic NOS — *see* Dysfunction, bladder, neuromuscular
neuromuscular NOS N31.9
atonic (motor) (sensory) N31.2
autonomous N31.2
flaccid N31.2
nonreflex N31.2
reflex N31.1
specified NEC N31.8
uninhibited N31.0
bleeding, uterus N93.8
cerebral G93.89
colon K59.9
psychogenic F45.8
colostomy K94.03
cystic duct K82.8
cystostomy (stoma) — *see* Complications, cystostomy
ejaculatory N53.19
anejaculatory orgasm N53.13
painful N53.12
premature F52.4
retarded N53.11
endocrine NOS E34.9
endometrium N85.8
enterostomy K94.13
erectile — *see* Dysfunction, sexual, male, erectile
feeding, pediatric
acute R63.31
chronic R63.32
gallbladder K82.8
gastrostomy (stoma) K94.23
gland, glandular NOS E34.9
meibomian, of eyelid — *see* Dysfunction, meibomian gland
heart I51.89
hemoglobin D75.89
hepatic K76.89
hypophysis E23.7
hypothalamic NEC E23.3
ileostomy (stoma) K94.13
jejunostomy (stoma) K94.13
kidney — *see* Disease, renal
labyrinthine — *see* subcategory H83.2 ☑

Dysfunction — *continued*
left ventricular, following sudden emotional stress I51.81
liver K76.89
male — *see* Dysfunction, sexual, male
meibomian gland, of eyelid H02.889
left H02.886
lower H02.885
upper H02.884
upper and lower eyelids H02.88B
right H02.883
lower H02.882
upper H02.881
upper and lower eyelids H02.88A
orgasmic (female) F52.31
male F52.32
ovary E28.9
specified NEC E28.8
papillary muscle I51.89
parathyroid E21.4
physiological NEC R68.89
psychogenic F59
pineal gland E34.8
pituitary (gland) E23.3
platelets D69.1
polyglandular E31.9
specified NEC E31.8
psychophysiologic F59
psychosexual F52.9
with
dyspareunia F52.6
premature ejaculation F52.4
vaginismus F52.5
pylorus K31.9
rectum K59.9
psychogenic F45.8
reflex (sympathetic) — *see* Syndrome, pain, complex regional I
segmental — *see* Dysfunction, somatic
senile R54
sexual (due to) R37
alcohol F10.981
amphetamine F15.981
in
abuse F15.181
dependence F15.281
anxiolytic F13.981
in
abuse F13.181
dependence F13.281
cocaine F14.981
in
abuse F14.181
dependence F14.281
excessive sexual drive F52.8
failure of genital response (male) F52.21
female F52.22
female N94.9
aversion F52.1
dyspareunia N94.10
psychogenic F52.6
frigidity F52.22
nymphomania F52.8
orgasmic F52.31
psychogenic F52.9
aversion F52.1
dyspareunia F52.6
frigidity F52.22
nymphomania F52.8
orgasmic F52.31
vaginismus F52.5
vaginismus N94.2
psychogenic F52.5
hypnotic F13.981
in
abuse F13.181
dependence F13.281
inhibited orgasm (female) F52.31
male F52.32
lack
of sexual enjoyment F52.1
or loss of sexual desire F52.0
male N53.9
anejaculatory orgasm N53.13
ejaculatory N53.19
painful N53.12
premature F52.4
retarded N53.11
erectile N52.9

Dysfunction — *continued*
sexual — *continued*
male — *continued*
erectile — *continued*
drug induced N52.2
due to
disease classified elsewhere N52.1
drug N52.2
postoperative (postprocedural) N52.39
following
cryotherapy N52.37
interstitial seed therapy N52.36
prostate ablative therapy N52.37
prostatectomy N52.34
radical N52.31
radiation therapy N52.35
radical cystectomy N52.32
ultrasound ablative therapy N52.37
urethral surgery N52.33
psychogenic F52.21
specified cause NEC N52.8
vasculogenic
arterial insufficiency N52.01
with corporo-venous occlusive N52.03
corporo-venous occlusive N52.02
with arterial insufficiency N52.03
impotence — *see* Dysfunction, sexual, male, erectile
psychogenic F52.9
aversion F52.1
erectile F52.21
orgasmic F52.32
premature ejaculation F52.4
satyriasis F52.8
specified type NEC F52.8
specified type NEC N53.8
nonorganic F52.9
specified NEC F52.8
opioid F11.981
in
abuse F11.181
dependence F11.281
orgasmic dysfunction (female) F52.31
male F52.32
premature ejaculation F52.4
psychoactive substances NEC F19.981
in
abuse F19.181
dependence F19.281
psychogenic F52.9
sedative F13.981
in
abuse F13.181
dependence F13.281
sexual aversion F52.1
vaginismus (nonorganic) (psychogenic) F52.5
sinoatrial node I49.5
somatic M99.09
abdomen M99.09
acromioclavicular M99.07
cervical region M99.01
cervicothoracic M99.01
costochondral M99.08
costovertebral M99.08
head region M99.00
hip M99.05
lower extremity M99.06
lumbar region M99.03
lumbosacral M99.03
occipitocervical M99.00
pelvic region M99.05
pubic M99.05
rib cage M99.08
sacral region M99.04
sacrococcygeal M99.04
sacroiliac M99.04
specified NEC M99.09
sternochondral M99.08
sternoclavicular M99.07
thoracic region M99.02
thoracolumbar M99.02
upper extremity M99.07
somatoform autonomic F45.8
stomach K31.89
psychogenic F45.8
suprarenal E27.9
hyperfunction E27.0
symbolic R48.9
specified type NEC R48.8

- **Dysfunction** — *continued*
  - temporomandibular (joint) M26.69
    - joint-pain syndrome M26.62- ☑
  - testicular (endocrine) E29.9
    - specified NEC E29.8
  - thymus E32.9
  - thyroid EØ7.9
  - ureterostomy (stoma) — *see* Complications, stoma, urinary tract
  - urethrostomy (stoma) — *see* Complications, stoma, urinary tract
  - uterus, complicating delivery O62.9
    - hypertonic O62.4
    - hypotonic O62.2
      - primary O62.Ø
      - secondary O62.1
  - ventricular I51.9
    - with congestive heart failure — *see also* Failure, heart I5Ø.9
    - left, reversible, following sudden emotional stress I51.81
- **Dysgenesis**
  - gonadal (due to chromosomal anomaly) Q96.9
    - pure Q99.1
  - renal Q6Ø.5
    - bilateral Q6Ø.4
    - unilateral Q6Ø.3
  - reticular D72.Ø
  - tidal platelet D69.3
- **Dysgerminoma**
  - specified site — *see* Neoplasm, malignant, by site
  - unspecified site
    - female C56.9
    - male C62.9Ø
- **Dysgeusia** R43.2
- **Dysgraphia** R27.8
- **Dyshidrosis, dysidrosis** L3Ø.1
- **Dyskaryotic cervical smear** R87.619
- **Dyskeratosis** L85.8
  - cervix — *see* Dysplasia, cervix
  - congenital Q82.8
  - uterus NEC N85.8
- **Dyskinesia** G24.9
  - biliary (cystic duct or gallbladder) K82.8
  - drug induced
    - orofacial G24.Ø1
  - esophagus K22.4
  - hysterical F44.4
  - intestinal K59.89
  - nonorganic origin F44.4
  - orofacial (idiopathic) G24.4
    - drug induced G24.Ø1
  - psychogenic F44.4
  - subacute, drug induced G24.Ø1
  - tardive G24.Ø1
    - neuroleptic induced G24.Ø1
  - trachea J39.8
  - tracheobronchial J98.Ø9
- **Dyslalia** (developmental) F8Ø.Ø
- **Dyslexia** R48.Ø
  - developmental F81.Ø
- **Dyslipidemia** E78.5
  - depressed HDL cholesterol E78.6
  - elevated fasting triglycerides E78.1
- **Dysmaturity** — *see also* Light for dates
  - pulmonary (newborn) (Wilson-Mikity) P27.Ø
- **Dysmenorrhea** (essential) (exfoliative) N94.6
  - congestive (syndrome) N94.6
  - primary N94.4
  - psychogenic F45.8
  - secondary N94.5
- **Dysmetabolic syndrome X** E88.81
- **Dysmetria** R27.8
- **Dysmorphism** (due to)
  - alcohol Q86.Ø
  - exogenous cause NEC Q86.8
  - hydantoin Q86.1
  - warfarin Q86.2
- **Dysmorphophobia** (nondelusional) F45.22
  - delusional F22
- **Dysnomia** R47.Ø1
- **Dysorexia** R63.Ø
  - psychogenic F5Ø.89
- **Dysostosis**
  - cleidocranial, cleidocranialis Q74.Ø
  - craniofacial Q75.1
  - Fairbank's (idiopathic familial generalized osteophytosis) Q78.9
- **Dysostosis** — *continued*
  - mandibulofacial (incomplete) Q75.4
  - multiplex E76.Ø1
  - oculomandibular Q75.5
- **Dyspareunia** (female) N94.1Ø
  - deep N94.12
  - male N53.12
  - nonorganic F52.6
  - psychogenic F52.6
  - secondary N94.19
  - specified NEC N94.19
  - superficial (introital) N94.11
- **Dyspepsia** R1Ø.13
  - atonic K3Ø
  - functional (allergic) (congenital) (gastrointestinal) (occupational) (reflex) K3Ø
  - intestinal K59.89
  - nervous F45.8
  - neurotic F45.8
  - psychogenic F45.8
- **Dysphagia** R13.1Ø
  - cervical R13.19
  - following
    - cerebral infarction I69.391
    - cerebrovascular disease I69.991
      - specified NEC I69.891
    - intracerebral hemorrhage I69.191
    - nontraumatic intracranial hemorrhage NEC I69.291
    - specified disease NEC I69.891
    - subarachnoid hemorrhage I69.Ø91
  - functional (hysterical) F45.8
  - hysterical F45.8
  - nervous (hysterical) F45.8
  - neurogenic R13.19
  - oral phase R13.11
  - oropharyngeal phase R13.12
  - pharyngeal phase R13.13
  - pharyngoesophageal phase R13.14
  - psychogenic F45.8
  - sideropenic D5Ø.1
  - spastica K22.4
  - specified NEC R13.19
- **Dysphagocytosis, congenital** D71
- **Dysphasia** R47.Ø2
  - developmental
    - expressive type F8Ø.1
    - receptive type F8Ø.2
  - following
    - cerebrovascular disease I69.921
      - cerebral infarction I69.321
      - intracerebral hemorrhage I69.121
      - nontraumatic intracranial hemorrhage NEC I69.221
      - specified disease NEC I69.821
      - subarachnoid hemorrhage I69.Ø21
- **Dysphonia** R49.Ø
  - functional F44.4
  - hysterical F44.4
  - psychogenic F44.4
  - spastica J38.3
- **Dysphoria**
  - gender F64.9
    - in
      - adolescence and adulthood F64.Ø
      - children F64.2
    - specified NEC F64.8
  - postpartal O9Ø.6
- **Dyspituitarism** E23.3
- **Dysplasia** — *see also* Anomaly
  - acetabular, congenital Q65.89
  - alveolar capillary, with vein misalignment J84.843
  - anus (histologically confirmed) (mild) (moderate) K62.82
    - severe DØ1.3
  - arrhythmogenic right ventricular I42.8
  - arterial, fibromuscular I77.3
  - asphyxiating thoracic (congenital) Q77.2
  - brain QØ7.9
  - bronchopulmonary, perinatal P27.1
  - cervix (uteri) N87.9
    - mild N87.Ø
    - moderate N87.1
    - severe DØ6.9
  - chondroectodermal Q77.6
  - colon D12.6
  - craniometaphyseal Q78.8
  - dentinal KØØ.5
  - diaphyseal, progressive Q78.3
- **Dysplasia** — *continued*
  - dystrophic Q77.5
  - ectodermal (anhidrotic) (congenital) (hereditary) Q82.4
    - hydrotic Q82.8
  - epithelial, uterine cervix — *see* Dysplasia, cervix
  - eye (congenital) Q11.2
  - fibrous
    - bone NEC (monostotic) M85.ØØ
      - ankle M85.Ø7- ☑
      - foot M85.Ø7- ☑
      - forearm M85.Ø3- ☑
      - hand M85.Ø4- ☑
      - lower leg M85.Ø6- ☑
      - multiple site M85.Ø9
      - neck M85.Ø8
      - rib M85.Ø8
      - shoulder M85.Ø1- ☑
      - skull M85.Ø8
      - specified site NEC M85.Ø8
      - thigh M85.Ø5- ☑
      - toe M85.Ø7- ☑
      - upper arm M85.Ø2- ☑
      - vertebra M85.Ø8
    - diaphyseal, progressive Q78.3
    - jaw M27.8
    - polyostotic Q78.1
  - florid osseous — *see also* Cyst, calcifying odontogenic
  - high grade, focal D12.6
  - hip, congenital Q65.89
  - joint, congenital Q74.8
  - kidney Q61.4
    - multicystic Q61.4
  - leg Q74.2
  - lung, congenital (not associated with short gestation) Q33.6
  - mammary (gland) (benign) N6Ø.9- ☑
    - cyst (solitary) — *see* Cyst, breast
    - cystic — *see* Mastopathy, cystic
    - duct ectasia — *see* Ectasia, mammary duct
    - fibroadenosis — *see* Fibroadenosis, breast
    - fibrosclerosis — *see* Fibrosclerosis, breast
    - specified type NEC N6Ø.8- ☑
  - metaphyseal Q78.5
  - muscle Q79.8
  - oculodentodigital Q87.Ø
  - periapical (cemental) (cemento-osseous) — *see* Cyst, calcifying odontogenic
  - periosteum — *see* Disorder, bone, specified type NEC
  - polyostotic fibrous Q78.1
  - prostate — *see also* Neoplasia, intraepithelial, prostate N42.3Ø
    - severe DØ7.5
    - specified NEC N42.39
  - renal Q61.4
    - multicystic Q61.4
  - retinal, congenital Q14.1
  - right ventricular, arrhythmogenic I42.8
  - septo-optic QØ4.4
  - skin L98.8
  - spinal cord QØ6.1
  - spondyloepiphyseal Q77.7
  - thymic, with immunodeficiency D82.1
  - vagina N89.3
    - mild N89.Ø
    - moderate N89.1
    - severe NEC DØ7.2
  - vulva N9Ø.3
    - mild N9Ø.Ø
    - moderate N9Ø.1
    - severe NEC DØ7.1
- **Dysplasminogenemia** E88.Ø2
- **Dyspnea** (nocturnal) (paroxysmal) RØ6.ØØ
  - asthmatic (bronchial) J45.9Ø9
    - with
      - bronchitis J45.9Ø9
        - with
          - exacerbation (acute) J45.9Ø1
          - status asthmaticus J45.9Ø2
        - chronic J44.9
      - exacerbation (acute) J45.9Ø1
      - status asthmaticus J45.9Ø2
    - cardiac — *see* Failure, ventricular, left
  - cardiac — *see* Failure, ventricular, left
  - functional F45.8
  - hyperventilation RØ6.4
  - hysterical F45.8
  - newborn P28.89
  - orthopnea RØ6.Ø1

Dyspnea — *continued*
- psychogenic F45.8
- shortness of breath R06.02
- specified type NEC R06.09
- transfusion-associated [TAD] J95.87

Dyspraxia R27.8
- developmental (syndrome) F82

Dysproteinemia E88.09

Dysreflexia, autonomic G90.4

Dysrhythmia
- cardiac I49.9
  - newborn
    - bradycardia P29.12
    - occurring before birth P03.819
      - before onset of labor P03.810
      - during labor P03.811
    - tachycardia P29.11
  - postoperative I97.89
- cerebral or cortical — *see* Epilepsy

Dyssomnia — *see* Disorder, sleep

Dyssynergia
- biliary K83.8
- bladder sphincter N36.44
- cerebellaris myoclonica (Hunt's ataxia) G11.19

Dysthymia F34.1

Dysthyroidism E07.9

Dystocia O66.9
- affecting newborn P03.1
- cervical (hypotonic) O62.2
  - affecting newborn P03.6
  - primary O62.0
  - secondary O62.1
- contraction ring O62.4
- fetal O66.9
  - abnormality NEC O66.3
  - conjoined twins O66.3
  - oversize O66.2
- maternal O66.9
- positional O64.9 ☑
- shoulder (girdle) O66.0
  - causing obstructed labor O66.0
- uterine NEC O62.4

Dystonia G24.9
- cervical G24.3
- deformans progressiva G24.1
- drug induced NEC G24.09
  - acute G24.02
  - specified NEC G24.09
- familial G24.1
- idiopathic G24.1
  - familial G24.1
  - nonfamilial G24.2
  - orofacial G24.4
- lenticularis G24.8
- musculorum deformans G24.1
- neuroleptic induced (acute) G24.02
- orofacial (idiopathic) G24.4
- oromandibular G24.4
  - due to drug G24.01
- specified NEC G24.8
- torsion (familial) (idiopathic) G24.1
  - acquired G24.8
  - genetic G24.1
  - symptomatic (nonfamilial) G24.2

Dystonic movements R25.8

Dystrophy, dystrophia
- adiposogenital E23.6
- autosomal recessive, childhood type, muscular dystrophy resembling Duchenne or Becker G71.01
- Becker's type G71.01
- cervical sympathetic G90.2
- choroid (hereditary) H31.20
  - central areolar H31.22
  - choroideremia H31.21
  - gyrate atrophy H31.23
  - specified type NEC H31.29
- cornea (hereditary) H18.50- ☑
  - endothelial H18.51- ☑
  - epithelial H18.52- ☑
  - granular H18.53- ☑
  - lattice H18.54- ☑
  - macular H18.55- ☑
  - specified type NEC H18.59- ☑
- Duchenne's type G71.01
- due to malnutrition E45
- Erb's G71.02
- Fuchs' H18.51- ☑
- Gower's muscular G71.01

Dystrophy, dystrophia — *continued*
- hair L67.8
- infantile neuraxonal G31.89
- Landouzy-Déjérine G71.02
- Leyden-Möbius — *see also* Dystrophy, muscular, limb-girdle, by type G71.039
  - meaning Limb girdle muscular dystrophy NOS G71.039
  - meaning Limb girdle muscular dystrophy, other specified type — *see* by type
  - meaning Limb girdle muscular dystrophy, specified type NEC G71.038
  - meaning Limb girdle muscular dystrophy type 2A (autosomal recessive) G71.032
- muscular G71.00
  - autosomal recessive, childhood type, muscular dystrophy resembling Duchenne or Becker G71.01
  - benign (Becker type) G71.01
    - scapuloperoneal with early contractures [Emery-Dreifuss] G71.09
  - congenital (hereditary) (progressive) (with specific morphological abnormalities of the muscle fiber) G71.09
    - myotonic G71.11
  - distal G71.09
  - Duchenne type G71.01
  - Emery-Dreifuss G71.09
  - Erb type G71.02
  - facioscapulohumeral G71.02
  - Gower's G71.01
  - hereditary (progressive) — *see also* Dystrophy, muscular, by type G71.09
  - Landouzy-Déjérine type G71.02
  - limb-girdle G71.039
    - alpha-sarcoglycan-relate G71.0341
    - anoctamin-5-related autosomal recessive (R12) G71.035
    - autosomal recessive NEC G71.038
    - beta-sarcoglycan-related G71.0342
    - calpain-3-related G71.032
      - autosomal dominant G71.031
      - autosomal recessive G71.032
    - collagen VI related
      - autosomal dominant G71.031
      - autosomal recessive G71.038
    - D1 (autosomal dominant) G71.031
    - D2 (autosomal dominant) G71.031
    - D3 (autosomal dominant) G71.031
    - D4 (autosomal dominant) G71.031
    - D5 (autosomal dominant) G71.031
    - delta-sarcoglycan-related G71.0349
    - due to
      - alpha sarcoglycan dysfunction G71.0341
      - anoctamin-5 dysfunction G71.035
      - beta sarcoglycan dysfunction G71.0342
      - fukutin related protein dysfunction G71.038
      - sarcoglycan dysfunction, specified NEC G71.0349
    - FKRP-related autosomal recessive G71.038
    - gamma-sarcoglycan-related G71.0349
    - R1 (autosomal recessive) G71.032
    - R2 (autosomal recessive) G71.033
    - R3 (autosomal recessive) G71.0341
    - R4 (autosomal recessive) G71.0342
    - R5 (autosomal recessive) G71.0349
    - R6 (autosomal recessive) G71.0349
    - R7 (autosomal recessive) G71.038
    - R8 (autosomal recessive) G71.038
    - R9 (autosomal recessive) G71.038
    - R10 (autosomal recessive) G71.038
    - R11 (autosomal recessive) G71.038
    - R12 (autosomal recessive) G71.035
    - R13 (autosomal recessive) G71.038
    - R14 (autosomal recessive) G71.038
    - R15 (autosomal recessive) G71.038
    - R16 (autosomal recessive) G71.038
    - R17 (autosomal recessive) G71.038
    - R18 (autosomal recessive) G71.038
    - R19 (autosomal recessive) G71.038
    - R20 (autosomal recessive) G71.038
    - R21 (autosomal recessive) G71.038
    - R22 (autosomal recessive) G71.038
    - R23 (autosomal recessive) G71.038
    - R24 (autosomal recessive) G71.038
    - type 1 (autosomal dominant) G71.031
    - type 1A (autosomal dominant) G71.031
    - type 1B (autosomal dominant) G71.031
    - type 1C (autosomal dominant) G71.031

Dystrophy, dystrophia — *continued*
- muscular — *continued*
  - limb-girdle — *continued*
    - type 1E (autosomal dominant) G71.031
    - type 1H (autosomal dominant) G71.031
    - type 1I (autosomal dominant) G71.031
    - type 2 (autosomal recessive) G71.038
      - specified NEC G71.038
    - type 2A (autosomal recessive) G71.032
    - type 2B (autosomal recessive) G71.033
    - type 2C (autosomal recessive) G71.0349
    - type 2D (autosomal recessive) G71.0341
    - type 2E (autosomal recessive) G71.0342
    - type 2F (autosomal recessive) G71.0349
    - type 2I (autosomal recessive) G71.038
    - type 2L (autosomal recessive) G71.035
  - myotonic G71.11
  - progressive (hereditary) — *see also* Dystrophy, muscular, by type G71.09
    - Charcot-Marie (-Tooth) type G60.0
  - pseudohypertrophic (infantile) G71.01
  - scapulohumeral G71.02
  - scapuloperoneal G71.09
  - severe (Duchenne type) G71.01
  - specified type NEC G71.09
- myocardium, myocardial — *see* Degeneration, myocardial
- nail L60.3
  - congenital Q84.6
- nutritional E45
- ocular G71.09
- oculocerebrorenal E72.03
- oculopharyngeal G71.09
- ovarian N83.8
- polyglandular E31.8
- reflex (neuromuscular) (sympathetic) — *see* Syndrome, pain, complex regional I
- retinal (hereditary) H35.50
  - in
    - lipid storage disorders E75.6 *[H36]*
    - systemic lipidoses E75.6 *[H36]*
  - involving
    - pigment epithelium H35.54
    - sensory area H35.53
  - pigmentary H35.52
  - vitreoretinal H35.51
- Salzmann's nodular — *see* Degeneration, cornea, nodular
- scapuloperoneal G71.09
- skin NEC L98.8
- sympathetic (reflex) — *see* Syndrome, pain, complex regional I
  - cervical G90.2
- tapetoretinal H35.54
- thoracic, asphyxiating Q77.2
- unguium L60.3
  - congenital Q84.6
- vitreoretinal H35.51
- vulva N90.4
- yellow (liver) — *see* Failure, hepatic

Dysuria R30.0
- psychogenic F45.8

E

Eales' disease H35.06- ☑

Ear — *see also* condition
- piercing Z41.3
- tropical NEC B36.9 *[H62.40]*
  - in
    - aspergillosis B44.89
    - candidiasis B37.84
    - moniliasis B37.84
- wax (impacted) H61.20
  - left H61.22
    - with right H61.23
  - right H61.21
    - with left H61.23

Earache — *see* subcategory H92.0 ☑

Early satiety R68.81

Eaton-Lambert syndrome — *see* Syndrome, Lambert-Eaton

Eberth's disease (typhoid fever) A01.00

Ebola virus disease A98.4

Ebstein's anomaly or syndrome (heart) Q22.5

Eccentro-osteochondrodysplasia E76.29

Ecchondroma — *see* Neoplasm, bone, benign

Ecchondrosis D48.0

Ecchymosis R58
conjunctiva — *see* Hemorrhage, conjunctiva
eye (traumatic) — *see* Contusion, eyeball
eyelid (traumatic) — *see* Contusion, eyelid
newborn P54.5
spontaneous R23.3
traumatic — *see* Contusion
Echinococciasis — *see* Echinococcus
Echinococcosis — *see* Echinococcus
Echinococcus (infection) B67.9Ø
granulosus B67.4
bone B67.2
liver B67.Ø
lung B67.1
multiple sites B67.32
specified site NEC B67.39
thyroid B67.31
liver NOS B67.8
granulosus B67.Ø
multilocularis B67.5
lung NEC B67.99
granulosus B67.1
multilocularis B67.69
multilocularis B67.7
liver B67.5
multiple sites B67.61
specified site NEC B67.69
specified site NEC B67.99
granulosus B67.39
multilocularis B67.69
thyroid NEC B67.99
granulosus B67.31
multilocularis B67.69 *[E35]*
Echinorhynchiasis B83.8
Echinostomiasis B66.8
Echolalia R48.8
Echovirus, as cause of disease classified elsewhere B97.12
Eclampsia, eclamptic (coma) (convulsions) (delirium) (with hypertension) NEC O15.9
complicating
labor and delivery O15.1
postpartum O15.2
pregnancy O15.Ø- ☑
puerperium O15.2
Economic circumstances affecting care Z59.9
Economo's disease A85.8
Ectasia, ectasis
annuloaortic I35.8
aorta I77.819
with aneurysm — *see* Aneurysm, aorta
abdominal I77.811
thoracic I77.81Ø
thoracoabdominal I77.812
breast — *see* Ectasia, mammary duct
capillary I78.8
cornea H18.71- ☑
gastric antral vascular (GAVE) K31.819
with hemorrhage K31.811
without hemorrhage K31.819
mammary duct N6Ø.4- ☑
salivary gland (duct) K11.8
sclera — *see* Sclerectasia
Ecthyma LØ8.Ø
contagiosum BØ8.Ø2
gangrenosum LØ8.Ø
infectiosum BØ8.Ø2
Ectocardia Q24.8
Ectodermal dysplasia (anhidrotic) Q82.4
Ectodermosis erosiva pluriorificialis L51.1
Ectopic, ectopia (congenital)
abdominal viscera Q45.8
due to defect in anterior abdominal wall Q79.59
ACTH syndrome E24.3
adrenal gland Q89.1
anus Q43.5
atrial beats I49.1
beats I49.49
atrial I49.1
ventricular I49.3
bladder Q64.1Ø
bone and cartilage in lung Q33.5
brain QØ4.8
breast tissue Q83.8
cardiac Q24.8
cerebral QØ4.8
cordis Q24.8
endometrium — *see* Endometriosis
Ectopic, ectopia — *continued*
gastric mucosa Q4Ø.2
gestation — *see* Pregnancy, by site
heart Q24.8
hormone secretion NEC E34.2
kidney (crossed) (pelvis) Q63.2
lens, lentis Q12.1
mole — *see* Pregnancy, by site
organ or site NEC — *see* Malposition, congenital
pancreas Q45.3
pregnancy — *see* Pregnancy, ectopic
pupil — *see* Abnormality, pupillary
renal Q63.2
sebaceous glands of mouth Q38.6
spleen Q89.Ø9
testis Q53.ØØ
bilateral Q53.Ø2
unilateral Q53.Ø1
thyroid Q89.2
tissue in lung Q33.5
ureter Q62.63
ventricular beats I49.3
vesicae Q64.1Ø
Ectromelia Q73.8
lower limb — *see* Defect, reduction, limb, lower, specified type NEC
upper limb — *see* Defect, reduction, limb, upper, specified type NEC
Ectropion HØ2.1Ø9
cervix N86
with cervicitis N72
congenital Q1Ø.1
eyelid HØ2.1Ø9
cicatricial HØ2.119
left HØ2.116
lower HØ2.115
upper HØ2.114
right HØ2.113
lower HØ2.112
upper HØ2.111
congenital Q1Ø.1
left HØ2.1Ø6
lower HØ2.1Ø5
upper HØ2.1Ø4
mechanical HØ2.129
left HØ2.126
lower HØ2.125
upper HØ2.124
right HØ2.123
lower HØ2.122
upper HØ2.121
paralytic HØ2.159
left HØ2.156
lower HØ2.155
upper HØ2.154
right HØ2.153
lower HØ2.152
upper HØ2.151
right HØ2.1Ø3
lower HØ2.1Ø2
upper HØ2.1Ø1
senile HØ2.139
left HØ2.136
lower HØ2.135
upper HØ2.134
right HØ2.133
lower HØ2.132
upper HØ2.131
spastic HØ2.149
left HØ2.146
lower HØ2.145
upper HØ2.144
right HØ2.143
lower HØ2.142
upper HØ2.141
iris H21.89
lip (acquired) K13.Ø
congenital Q38.Ø
urethra N36.8
uvea H21.89
Eczema (acute) (chronic) (erythematous) (fissum) (rubrum) (squamous) — *see also* Dermatitis L3Ø.9
contact — *see* Dermatitis, contact
dyshydrotic L3Ø.1
external ear — *see* Otitis, externa, acute, eczematoid
flexural L2Ø.82
herpeticum BØØ.Ø
hypertrophicum L28.Ø
Eczema — *continued*
hypostatic — *see* Varix, leg, with, inflammation
impetiginous LØ1.1
infantile (due to any substance) L2Ø.83
intertriginous L21.1
seborrheic L21.1
intertriginous NEC L3Ø.4
infantile L21.1
intrinsic (allergic) L2Ø.84
lichenified NEC L28.Ø
marginatum (hebrae) B35.6
pustular L3Ø.3
stasis I87.2
with varicose veins — *see* Varix, leg, with, inflammation
vaccination, vaccinatum T88.1 ☑
varicose — *see* Varix, leg, with, inflammation
Eczematid L3Ø.2
Eddowes (-Spurway) **syndrome** Q78.Ø
Edema, edematous (infectious) (pitting) (toxic) R6Ø.9
with nephritis — *see* Nephrosis
allergic T78.3 ☑
amputation stump (surgical) (sequelae (late effect)) T87.89
angioneurotic (allergic) (any site) (with urticaria) T78.3 ☑
hereditary D84.1
angiospastic I73.9
Berlin's (traumatic) SØ5.8X- ☑
brain (cytotoxic) (vasogenic) G93.6
due to birth injury P11.Ø
newborn (anoxia or hypoxia) P52.4
birth injury P11.Ø
traumatic — *see* Injury, intracranial, cerebral edema
cardiac — *see* Failure, heart, congestive
cardiovascular — *see* Failure, heart, congestive
cerebral — *see* Edema, brain
cerebrospinal — *see* Edema, brain
cervix (uteri) (acute) N88.8
puerperal, postpartum O9Ø.89
chronic hereditary Q82.Ø
circumscribed, acute T78.3 ☑
hereditary D84.1
conjunctiva H11.42- ☑
cornea H18.2- ☑
idiopathic H18.22- ☑
secondary H18.23- ☑
due to contact lens H18.21- ☑
due to
lymphatic obstruction I89.Ø
salt retention E87.Ø
epiglottis — *see* Edema, glottis
essential, acute T78.3 ☑
hereditary D84.1
extremities, lower — *see* Edema, legs
eyelid NEC HØ2.849
left HØ2.846
lower HØ2.845
upper HØ2.844
right HØ2.843
lower HØ2.842
upper HØ2.841
familial, hereditary Q82.Ø
famine — *see* Malnutrition, severe
generalized R6Ø.1
glottis, glottic, glottidis (obstructive) (passive) J38.4
allergic T78.3 ☑
hereditary D84.1
heart — *see* Failure, heart, congestive
heat T67.7 ☑
hereditary Q82.Ø
inanition — *see* Malnutrition, severe
intracranial G93.6
iris H21.89
joint — *see* Effusion, joint
larynx — *see* Edema, glottis
legs R6Ø.Ø
due to venous obstruction I87.1
hereditary Q82.Ø
localized R6Ø.Ø
due to venous obstruction I87.1
lower limbs — *see* Edema, legs
lung J81.1
with heart condition or failure — *see* Failure, ventricular, left
acute J81.Ø
chemical (acute) J68.1
chronic J68.1

Edema, edematous — *continued*
- lung — *continued*
  - chronic J81.1
    - due to
      - chemicals, gases, fumes or vapors (inhalation) J68.1
      - external agent J7Ø.9
        - specified NEC J7Ø.8
      - radiation J7Ø.1
  - due to
    - chemicals, fumes or vapors (inhalation) J68.1
    - external agent J7Ø.9
      - specified NEC J7Ø.8
    - high altitude T7Ø.29 ☑
    - near drowning T75.1 ☑
    - radiation J7Ø.Ø
  - meaning failure, left ventricle I5Ø.1
- lymphatic I89.Ø
  - due to mastectomy I97.2
- macula H35.81
  - cystoid, following cataract surgery — *see* Complications, postprocedural, following cataract surgery
  - diabetic — *see* Diabetes, by type, with, retinopathy, with macular edema
- malignant — *see* Gangrene, gas
- Milroy's Q82.Ø
- nasopharynx J39.2
- newborn P83.3Ø
  - hydrops fetalis — *see* Hydrops, fetalis
  - specified NEC P83.39
- nutritional — *see also* Malnutrition, severe
  - with dyspigmentation, skin and hair E4Ø
- optic disc or nerve — *see* Papilledema
- orbit HØ5.22- ☑
- pancreas K86.89
- papilla, optic — *see* Papilledema
- penis N48.89
- periodic T78.3 ☑
  - hereditary D84.1
- pharynx J39.2
- pulmonary — *see* Edema, lung
- Quincke's T78.3 ☑
  - hereditary D84.1
- renal — *see* Nephrosis
- retina H35.81
  - diabetic — *see* Diabetes, by type, with, retinopathy, with macular edema
- salt E87.Ø
- scrotum N5Ø.89
- seminal vesicle N5Ø.89
- spermatic cord N5Ø.89
- spinal (cord) (vascular) (nontraumatic) G95.19
- starvation — *see* Malnutrition, severe
- stasis — *see* Hypertension, venous, (chronic)
- subglottic — *see* Edema, glottis
- supraglottic — *see* Edema, glottis
- testis N44.8
- tunica vaginalis N5Ø.89
- vas deferens N5Ø.89
- vulva (acute) N9Ø.89

Edentulism — *see* Absence, teeth, acquired

Edsall's disease T67.2 ☑

Educational handicap Z55.9
- less than a high school diploma Z55.5
- no general equivalence degree (GED) Z55.5
- specified NEC Z55.8

Edward's syndrome — *see* Trisomy, 18

Effect(s) (of) (from) — *see* Effect, adverse NEC

Effect, adverse
- abnormal gravitational (G) forces or states T75.81 ☑
- abuse — *see* Maltreatment
- air pressure T7Ø.9 ☑
  - specified NEC T7Ø.8 ☑
- altitude (high) — *see* Effect, adverse, high altitude
- anesthesia — *see also* Anesthesia T88.59 ☑
  - in labor and delivery O74.9
  - local, toxic
    - in labor and delivery O74.4
    - in pregnancy NEC O29.3- ☑
    - postpartum, puerperal O89.3
  - postpartum, puerperal O89.9
  - specified NEC T88.59 ☑
    - in labor and delivery O74.8
    - postpartum, puerperal O89.8
  - spinal and epidural T88.59 ☑
    - headache T88.59 ☑

Effect, adverse — *continued*
- anesthesia — *see also* Anesthesia — *continued*
  - spinal and epidural — *continued*
    - headache — *continued*
      - in labor and delivery O74.5
      - postpartum, puerperal O89.4
    - specified NEC
      - in labor and delivery O74.6
      - postpartum, puerperal O89.5
- antitoxin — *see* Complications, vaccination
- atmospheric pressure T7Ø.9 ☑
  - due to explosion T7Ø.8 ☑
  - high T7Ø.3 ☑
  - low — *see* Effect, adverse, high altitude
  - specified effect NEC T7Ø.8 ☑
- biological, correct substance properly administered — *see* Effect, adverse, drug
- blood (derivatives) (serum) (transfusion) — *see* Complications, transfusion
- chemical substance — *see* Table of Drugs and Chemicals
- cold (temperature) (weather) T69.9 ☑
  - chilblains T69.1 ☑
  - frostbite — *see* Frostbite
  - specified effect NEC T69.8 ☑
- drugs and medicaments T88.7 ☑
  - specified drug — *see* Table of Drugs and Chemicals, by drug, adverse effect
  - specified effect — *code to* condition
- electric current, electricity (shock) T75.4 ☑
  - burn — *see* Burn
- exertion (excessive) T73.3 ☑
- exposure — *see* Exposure
- external cause NEC T75.89 ☑
- foodstuffs T78.1 ☑
  - allergic reaction — *see* Allergy, food
    - causing anaphylaxis — *see* Shock, anaphylactic, due to food
  - noxious — *see* Poisoning, food, noxious
- gases, fumes, or vapors T59.9- ☑
  - specified agent — *see* Table of Drugs and Chemicals
- glue (airplane) sniffing
  - due to drug abuse — *see* Abuse, drug, inhalant
  - due to drug dependence — *see* Dependence, drug, inhalant
- heat — *see* Heat
- high altitude NEC T7Ø.29 ☑
  - anoxia T7Ø.29 ☑
  - on
    - ears T7Ø.Ø ☑
    - sinuses T7Ø.1 ☑
  - polycythemia D75.1
- high pressure fluids T7Ø.4 ☑
- hot weather — *see* Heat
- hunger T73.Ø ☑
- immersion, foot — *see* Immersion
- immunization — *see* Complications, vaccination
- immunological agents — *see* Complications, vaccination
- infrared (radiation) (rays) NOS T66 ☑
  - dermatitis or eczema L59.8
- infusion — *see* Complications, infusion
- lack of care of infants — *see* Maltreatment, child
- lightning — *see* Lightning
- medical care T88.9 ☑
  - specified NEC T88.8 ☑
- medicinal substance, correct, properly administered — *see* Effect, adverse, drug
- motion T75.3 ☑
- noise, on inner ear — *see* subcategory H83.3 ☑
- overheated places — *see* Heat
- psychosocial, of work environment Z56.5
- radiation (diagnostic) (infrared) (natural source) (therapeutic) (ultraviolet) (X-ray) NOS T66 ☑
  - dermatitis or eczema — *see* Dermatitis, due to, radiation
  - fibrosis of lung J7Ø.1
  - pneumonitis J7Ø.Ø
  - pulmonary manifestations
    - acute J7Ø.Ø
    - chronic J7Ø.1
  - skin L59.9
- radioactive substance NOS
  - dermatitis or eczema — *see* Radiodermatitis
- reduced temperature T69.9 ☑
  - immersion foot or hand — *see* Immersion
  - specified effect NEC T69.8 ☑

Effect, adverse — *continued*
- serum NEC — *see also* Reaction, serum T8Ø.69 ☑
- specified NEC T78.8 ☑
  - external cause NEC T75.89 ☑
- strangulation — *see* Asphyxia, traumatic
- submersion T75.1 ☑
- thirst T73.1 ☑
- toxic — *see* Toxicity
- transfusion — *see* Complications, transfusion
- ultraviolet (radiation) (rays) NOS T66 ☑
  - burn — *see* Burn
  - dermatitis or eczema — *see* Dermatitis, due to, ultraviolet rays
    - acute L56.8
- vaccine (any) — *see* Complications, vaccination
- vibration — *see* Vibration, adverse effects
- water pressure NEC T7Ø.9 ☑
  - specified NEC T7Ø.8 ☑
- weightlessness T75.82 ☑
- whole blood — *see* Complications, transfusion
- work environment Z56.5

Effects, late — *see* Sequelae

Effluvium
- anagen L65.1
- telogen L65.Ø

Effort syndrome (psychogenic) F45.8

Effusion
- amniotic fluid — *see* Pregnancy, complicated by, premature rupture of membranes
- brain (serous) G93.6
- bronchial — *see* Bronchitis
- cerebral G93.6
- cerebrospinal — *see also* Meningitis
  - vessel G93.6
- chest — *see* Effusion, pleura
- chylous, chyliform (pleura) J94.Ø
- intracranial G93.6
- joint M25.4Ø
  - ankle M25.47- ☑
  - elbow M25.42- ☑
  - foot joint M25.47- ☑
  - hand joint M25.44- ☑
  - hip M25.45- ☑
  - knee M25.46- ☑
  - shoulder M25.41- ☑
  - specified joint NEC M25.48
  - wrist M25.43- ☑
- malignant pleural J91.Ø
- meninges — *see* Meningitis
- pericardium, pericardial (noninflammatory) I31.39
  - acute — *see* Pericarditis, acute
  - malignant, in disease classified elsewhere I31.31
  - specified type, NEC I31.39
- peritoneal (chronic) R18.8
- pleura, pleurisy, pleuritic, pleuropericardial J9Ø
  - chylous, chyliform J94.Ø
  - due to systemic lupus erythematosis M32.13
  - in conditions classified elsewhere J91.8
  - influenzal — *see* Influenza, with, respiratory manifestations NEC
  - malignant J91.Ø
  - newborn P28.89
  - tuberculous NEC A15.6
    - primary (progressive) A15.7
- spinal — *see* Meningitis
- thorax, thoracic — *see* Effusion, pleura

Egg shell nails L6Ø.3
- congenital Q84.6

EGPA (eosinophilic granulomatosis with polyangiitis) M3Ø.1

Egyptian splenomegaly B65.1

Ehlers-Danlos syndrome — *see also* Syndrome, Ehlers-Danlos Q79.6Ø

Ehrlichiosis A77.4Ø
- due to
  - E. chafeensis A77.41
  - E. ewingii A77.49
  - E. muris euclairensis A77.49
  - E. sennetsu A79.81
  - specified organism NEC A77.49

Eichstedt's disease B36.Ø

Eisenmenger's
- complex or syndrome I27.83
- defect Q21.8

Ejaculation
- delayed F52.32
- painful N53.12

☑ **Additional Character Required — Refer to the Tabular List for Character Selection**

Ejaculation — *continued*
- premature F52.4
- retarded N53.11
- retrograde N53.14
- semen, painful N53.12
  - psychogenic F52.6

Ekbom's syndrome (restless legs) G25.81
Ekman's syndrome (brittle bones and blue sclera) Q78.Ø
Elastic skin Q82.8
- acquired L57.4

Elastofibroma — *see* Neoplasm, connective tissue, benign
Elastoma (juvenile) Q82.8
- Miescher's L87.2

Elastomyofibrosis I42.4
Elastosis
- actinic, solar L57.8
- atrophicans (senile) L57.4
- perforans serpiginosa L87.2
- senilis L57.4

Elbow — *see* condition
Electric current, electricity, effects (concussion) (fatal) (nonfatal) (shock) T75.4 ☑
- burn — *see* Burn

Electric feet syndrome E53.8
Electrocution T75.4 ☑
- from electroshock gun (taser) T75.4 ☑

Electrolyte imbalance E87.8
- with
  - abortion — *see* Abortion by type, complicated by, electrolyte imbalance
  - ectopic pregnancy OØ8.5
  - molar pregnancy OØ8.5

Elephantiasis (nonfilarial) I89.Ø
- arabicum — *see* Infestation, filarial
- bancroftian B74.Ø
- congenital (any site) (hereditary) Q82.Ø
- due to
  - Brugia (malayi) B74.1
    - timori B74.2
  - mastectomy I97.2
  - Wuchereria (bancrofti) B74.Ø
- eyelid HØ2.859
  - left HØ2.856
    - lower HØ2.855
    - upper HØ2.854
  - right HØ2.853
    - lower HØ2.852
    - upper HØ2.851
- filarial, filariensis — *see* Infestation, filarial
- glandular I89.Ø
- graecorum A3Ø.9
- lymphangiectatic I89.Ø
- lymphatic vessel I89.Ø
  - due to mastectomy I97.2
- scrotum (nonfilarial) I89.Ø
- streptococcal I89.Ø
- surgical I97.89
  - postmastectomy I97.2
- telangiectodes I89.Ø
- vulva (nonfilarial) N9Ø.89

Elevated, elevation
- alanine transaminase (ALT) R74.Ø1
- ALT (alanine transaminase) R74.Ø1
- antibody titer R76.Ø
- aspartate transaminase (AST) R74.Ø1
- AST (aspartate transaminase) R74.Ø1
- basal metabolic rate R94.8
- blood pressure — *see also* Hypertension
  - reading (incidental) (isolated) (nonspecific), no diagnosis of hypertension RØ3.Ø
- blood sugar R73.9
- body temperature (of unknown origin) R5Ø.9
- cancer antigen 125 [CA 125] R97.1
- carcinoembryonic antigen [CEA] R97.Ø
- cholesterol E78.ØØ
  - with high triglycerides E78.2
- conjugate, eye H51.Ø
- C-reactive protein (CRP) R79.82
- diaphragm, congenital Q79.1
- erythrocyte sedimentation rate R7Ø.Ø
- fasting glucose R73.Ø1
- fasting triglycerides E78.1
- finding on laboratory examination — *see* Findings, abnormal, inconclusive, without diagnosis, by type of exam

Elevated, elevation — *continued*
- GFR (glomerular filtration rate) — *see* Findings, abnormal, inconclusive, without diagnosis, by type of exam
- glucose tolerance (oral) R73.Ø2
- immunoglobulin level R76.8
- indoleacetic acid R82.5
- lactic acid dehydrogenase (LDH) level R74.Ø2
- leukocytes D72.829
- lipoprotein a (Lp(a)) level E78.41
- liver function
  - study R94.5
  - test R79.89
    - alkaline phosphatase R74.8
    - aminotransferase R74.Ø1
    - bilirubin R17
    - hepatic enzyme R74.8
    - lactate dehydrogenase R74.Ø2
- Lp(a) (lipoprotein(a)) E78.41
- lymphocytes D72.82Ø
- prostate specific antigen [PSA] R97.2Ø
- Rh titer — *see* Complication(s), transfusion, incompatibility reaction, Rh (factor)
- scapula, congenital Q74.Ø
- sedimentation rate R7Ø.Ø
- SGOT R74.Ø1
- SGPT R74.Ø1
- transaminase level R74.Ø1
- triglycerides E78.1
  - with high cholesterol E78.2
- troponin R77.8
- tumor associated antigens [TAA] NEC R97.8
- tumor specific antigens [TSA] NEC R97.8
- urine level of
  - 17-ketosteroids R82.5
  - catecholamine R82.5
  - indoleacetic acid R82.5
  - steroids R82.5
  - vanillylmandelic acid (VMA) R82.5
- venous pressure I87.8
- white blood cell count D72.829
  - specified NEC D72.828

Elliptocytosis (congenital) (hereditary) D58.1
- Hb C (disease) D58.1
- hemoglobin disease D58.1
- sickle-cell (disease) D57.8- ☑
  - trait D57.3

Ellison-Zollinger syndrome E16.4
Ellis-van Creveld syndrome (chondroectodermal dysplasia) Q77.6
Elongated, elongation (congenital) — *see also* Distortion
- bone Q79.9
- cervix (uteri) Q51.828
  - acquired N88.4
  - hypertrophic N88.4
- colon Q43.8
- common bile duct Q44.5
- cystic duct Q44.5
- frenulum, penis Q55.69
- labia minora (acquired) N9Ø.69
- ligamentum patellae Q74.1
- petiolus (epiglottidis) Q31.8
- tooth, teeth KØØ.2
- uvula Q38.6

Eltor cholera AØØ.1
Emaciation R64
- due to malnutrition E43

Embadomoniasis AØ7.8
Embedded tooth, teeth KØ1.Ø
- root only KØ8.3

Embolic — *see* condition
Embolism (multiple) (paradoxical) I74.9
- air (any site) (traumatic) T79.Ø ☑
  - following
    - abortion — *see* Abortion by type complicated by embolism
    - ectopic pregnancy OØ8.2
    - infusion, therapeutic injection or transfusion T8Ø.Ø ☑
    - molar pregnancy OØ8.2
    - procedure NEC
      - artery T81.719 ☑
        - mesenteric T81.71Ø ☑
        - renal T81.711 ☑
        - specified NEC T81.718 ☑
      - vein T81.72 ☑

Embolism — *continued*
- air — *continued*
  - in pregnancy, childbirth or puerperium — *see* Embolism, obstetric
- amniotic fluid (pulmonary) — *see also* Embolism, obstetric
  - following
    - abortion — *see* Abortion by type complicated by embolism
    - ectopic pregnancy OØ8.2
    - molar pregnancy OØ8.2
- aorta, aortic I74.1Ø
  - abdominal I74.Ø9
    - saddle I74.Ø1
  - bifurcation I74.Ø9
  - saddle I74.Ø1
  - thoracic I74.11
- artery I74.9
  - auditory, internal I65.8
  - basilar — *see* Occlusion, artery, basilar
  - carotid (common) (internal) — *see* Occlusion, artery, carotid
  - cerebellar (anterior inferior) (posterior inferior) (superior) I66.3
  - cerebral — *see* Occlusion, artery, cerebral
  - choroidal (anterior) I65.8
  - communicating posterior I65.8
  - coronary — *see also* Infarct, myocardium
    - not resulting in infarction I24.Ø
  - extremity I74.4
    - lower I74.3
    - upper I74.2
  - hypophyseal I65.8
  - iliac I74.5
  - limb I74.4
    - lower I74.3
    - upper I74.2
  - mesenteric (with gangrene) — *see also* Ischemia, intestine, acute K55.Ø59
  - ophthalmic — *see* Occlusion, artery, retina
  - peripheral I74.4
  - pontine I65.8
  - precerebral — *see* Occlusion, artery, precerebral
  - pulmonary — *see* Embolism, pulmonary
  - renal N28.Ø
  - retinal — *see* Occlusion, artery, retina
  - septic I76
  - specified NEC I74.8
  - vertebral — *see* Occlusion, artery, vertebral
- basilar (artery) I65.1
- blood clot
  - following
    - abortion — *see* Abortion by type complicated by embolism
    - ectopic or molar pregnancy OØ8.2
  - in pregnancy, childbirth or puerperium — *see* Embolism, obstetric
- brain — *see also* Occlusion, artery, cerebral
  - following
    - abortion — *see* Abortion by type complicated by embolism
    - ectopic or molar pregnancy OØ8.2
  - puerperal, postpartum, childbirth — *see* Embolism, obstetric
- capillary I78.8
- cardiac — *see also* Infarct, myocardium
  - not resulting in infarction I51.3
- carotid (artery) (common) (internal) — *see* Occlusion, artery, carotid
- cavernous sinus (venous) — *see* Embolism, intracranial venous sinus
- cerebral — *see* Occlusion, artery, cerebral
- cholesterol — *see* Atheroembolism
- coronary (artery or vein) (systemic) — *see* Occlusion, coronary
- due to device, implant or graft — *see also* Complications, by site and type, specified NEC
  - arterial graft NEC T82.818 ☑
  - breast (implant) T85.818 ☑
  - catheter NEC T85.818 ☑
    - dialysis (renal) T82.818 ☑
      - intraperitoneal T85.818 ☑
    - infusion NEC T82.818 ☑
      - spinal (epidural) (subdural) T85.81Ø ☑
    - urinary (indwelling) T83.81 ☑
  - electronic (electrode) (pulse generator) (stimulator)
    - bone T84.81 ☑
    - cardiac T82.817 ☑

Embolism — *continued*
due to device, implant or graft — *see also* Complications, by site and type, specified — *continued*
electronic — *continued*
nervous system (brain) (peripheral nerve) (spinal) T85.81Ø ☑
urinary T83.81 ☑
fixation, internal (orthopedic) NEC T84.81 ☑
gastrointestinal (bile duct) (esophagus) T85.818 ☑
genital NEC T83.81 ☑
heart (graft) (valve) T82.817 ☑
joint prosthesis T84.81 ☑
ocular (corneal graft) (orbital implant) T85.818 ☑
orthopedic (bone graft) NEC T86.838
specified NEC T85.818 ☑
urinary (graft) NEC T83.81 ☑
vascular NEC T82.818 ☑
ventricular intracranial shunt T85.81Ø ☑
extremities
lower — *see* Embolism, vein, lower extremity
arterial I74.3
upper I74.2
eye H34.9
fat (cerebral) (pulmonary) (systemic) T79.1 ☑
complicating delivery — *see* Embolism, obstetric
following
abortion — *see* Abortion by type complicated by embolism
ectopic or molar pregnancy OØ8.2
following
abortion — *see* Abortion by type complicated by embolism
ectopic or molar pregnancy OØ8.2
infusion, therapeutic injection or transfusion
air T8Ø.Ø ☑
heart (fatty) — *see also* Infarct, myocardium
not resulting in infarction I51.3
hepatic (vein) I82.Ø
in pregnancy, childbirth or puerperium — *see* Embolism, obstetric
intestine (artery) (vein) (with gangrene) — *see also* Ischemia, intestine, acute K55.Ø39
intracranial — *see also* Occlusion, artery, cerebral
venous sinus (any) GØ8
nonpyogenic I67.6
intraspinal venous sinuses or veins GØ8
nonpyogenic G95.19
kidney (artery) N28.Ø
lateral sinus (venous) — *see* Embolism, intracranial, venous sinus
leg — *see* Embolism, vein, lower extremity
arterial I74.3
longitudinal sinus (venous) — *see* Embolism, intracranial, venous sinus
lung (massive) — *see* Embolism, pulmonary
meninges I66.8
mesenteric (artery) (vein) (with gangrene) — *see also* Ischemia, intestine, acute K55.Ø59
obstetric (in) (pulmonary)
childbirth O88.22
air O88.Ø2
amniotic fluid O88.12
blood clot O88.22
fat O88.82
pyemic O88.32
septic O88.32
specified type NEC O88.82
pregnancy O88.21- ☑
air O88.Ø1- ☑
amniotic fluid O88.11- ☑
blood clot O88.21- ☑
fat O88.81- ☑
pyemic O88.31- ☑
septic O88.31- ☑
specified type NEC O88.81- ☑
puerperal O88.23
air O88.Ø3
amniotic fluid O88.13
blood clot O88.23
fat O88.83
pyemic O88.33
septic O88.33
specified type NEC O88.83
ophthalmic — *see* Occlusion, artery, retina
penis N48.81
peripheral artery NOS I74.4
pituitary E23.6

Embolism — *continued*
popliteal (artery) I74.3
portal (vein) I81
postoperative, postprocedural
artery T81.719 ☑
mesenteric T81.71Ø ☑
renal T81.711 ☑
specified NEC T81.718 ☑
vein T81.72 ☑
precerebral artery — *see* Occlusion, artery, precerebral
puerperal — *see* Embolism, obstetric
pulmonary (acute) (artery) (vein) I26.99
with acute cor pulmonale I26.Ø9
chronic I27.82
following
abortion — *see* Abortion by type complicated by embolism
ectopic or molar pregnancy OØ8.2
healed or old Z86.711
in pregnancy, childbirth or puerperium — *see* Embolism, obstetric
multiple subsegmental without acute cor pulmonale I26.94
personal history of Z86.711
saddle I26.92
with acute cor pulmonale I26.Ø2
septic I26.9Ø
with acute cor pulmonale I26.Ø1
single subsegmental without acute cor pulmonale I26.93
subsegmental NOS I26.93
pyemic (multiple) I76
following
abortion — *see* Abortion by type complicated by embolism
ectopic or molar pregnancy OØ8.2
Hemophilus influenzae A41.3
pneumococcal A4Ø.3
with pneumonia J13
puerperal, postpartum, childbirth (any organism) — *see* Embolism, obstetric
specified organism NEC A41.89
staphylococcal A41.2
streptococcal A4Ø.9
renal (artery) N28.Ø
vein I82.3
retina, retinal — *see* Occlusion, artery, retina
saddle
abdominal aorta I74.Ø1
pulmonary artery I26.92
with acute cor pulmonale I26.Ø2
septic (arterial) I76
complicating abortion — *see* Abortion, by type, complicated by, embolism
sinus — *see* Embolism, intracranial, venous sinus
soap complicating abortion — *see* Abortion, by type, complicated by, embolism
spinal cord G95.19
pyogenic origin GØ6.1
spleen, splenic (artery) I74.8
upper extremity I74.2
vein (acute) I82.9Ø
antecubital I82.61- ☑
chronic I82.71- ☑
axillary I82.A1- ☑ (*following* I82.7)
chronic I82.A2- ☑ (*following* I82.7)
basilic I82.61- ☑
chronic I82.71- ☑
brachial I82.62- ☑
chronic I82.72- ☑
brachiocephalic (innominate) I82.29Ø
chronic I82.291
calf, muscle I82.46- ☑
chronic I82.56- ☑
cephalic I82.61- ☑
chronic I82.71- ☑
chronic I82.91
deep (DVT) I82.4Ø- ☑
calf I82.4Z- ☑
chronic I82.5Z- ☑
lower leg I82.4Z- ☑
chronic I82.5Z- ☑
thigh I82.4Y- ☑
chronic I82.5Y- ☑
upper leg I82.4Y ☑
chronic I82.5Y-
femoral I82.41- ☑

Embolism — *continued*
vein — *continued*
femoral — *continued*
chronic I82.51- ☑
gastrocnemial I82.46- ☑
chronic I82.56- ☑
iliac (iliofemoral) I82.42- ☑
chronic I82.52- ☑
innominate I82.29Ø
chronic I82.291
internal jugular I82.C1- ☑ (*following* I82.7)
chronic I82.C2- ☑ (*following* I82.7)
lower extremity
deep I82.4Ø- ☑
chronic I82.5Ø- ☑
specified NEC I82.49- ☑
chronic NEC I82.59- ☑
distal
deep I82.4Z- ☑
proximal
deep I82.4Y- ☑
chronic I82.5Y- ☑
superficial I82.81- ☑
peroneal I82.45- ☑
chronic I82.55- ☑
popliteal I82.43- ☑
chronic I82.53- ☑
radial I82.62- ☑
chronic I82.72- ☑
renal I82.3
saphenous (greater) (lesser) I82.81- ☑
soleal I82.46- ☑
chronic I82.56- ☑
specified NEC I82.89Ø
chronic NEC I82.891
subclavian I82.B1- ☑ (*following* I82.7)
chronic I82.B2- ☑ (*following* I82.7)
thoracic NEC I82.29Ø
chronic I82.291
tibial I82.44- ☑
chronic I82.54- ☑
ulnar I82.62- ☑
chronic I82.72- ☑
upper extremity I82.6Ø- ☑
chronic I82.7Ø- ☑
deep I82.62- ☑
chronic I82.72- ☑
superficial I82.61- ☑
chronic I82.71- ☑
vena cava
inferior (acute) I82.22Ø
chronic I82.221
superior (acute) I82.21Ø
chronic I82.211
venous sinus GØ8
vessels of brain — *see* Occlusion, artery, cerebral
Embolus — *see* Embolism
Embryoma — *see also* Neoplasm, uncertain behavior, by site
benign — *see* Neoplasm, benign, by site
kidney C64.- ☑
liver C22.Ø
malignant — *see also* Neoplasm, malignant, by site
kidney C64.- ☑
liver C22.Ø
testis C62.9- ☑
descended (scrotal) C62.1- ☑
undescended C62.Ø- ☑
testis C62.9- ☑
descended (scrotal) C62.1- ☑
undescended C62.Ø- ☑
Embryonic
circulation Q28.9
heart Q28.9
vas deferens Q55.4
Embryopathia NOS Q89.9
Embryotoxon Q13.4
Emesis — *see* Vomiting
Emotional lability R45.86
Emotionality, pathological F6Ø.3
Emotogenic disease — *see* Disorder, psychogenic
Emphysema (atrophic) (bullous) (chronic) (interlobular) (lung) (obstructive) (pulmonary) (senile) (vesicular) J43.9
cellular tissue (traumatic) T79.7 ☑
surgical T81.82 ☑

- **Emphysema** — *continued*
  - centrilobular J43.2
  - compensatory J98.3
  - congenital (interstitial) P25.Ø
  - conjunctiva H11.89
  - connective tissue (traumatic) T79.7 ☑
    - surgical T81.82 ☑
  - due to chemicals, gases, fumes or vapors J68.4
  - eyelid(s) — *see* Disorder, eyelid, specified type NEC
    - surgical T81.82 ☑
    - traumatic T79.7 ☑
  - interstitial J98.2
    - congenital P25.Ø
    - perinatal period P25.Ø
  - laminated tissue T79.7 ☑
    - surgical T81.82 ☑
  - mediastinal J98.2
    - newborn P25.2
  - orbit, orbital — *see* Disorder, orbit, specified type NEC
  - panacinar J43.1
  - panlobular J43.1
  - specified NEC J43.8
  - subcutaneous (traumatic) T79.7 ☑
    - nontraumatic J98.2
    - postprocedural T81.82 ☑
    - surgical T81.82 ☑
  - surgical T81.82 ☑
  - thymus (gland) (congenital) E32.8
  - traumatic (subcutaneous) T79.7 ☑
  - unilateral J43.Ø
- **Empty nest syndrome** Z6Ø.Ø
- **Empyema** (acute) (chest) (double) (pleura) (supradiaphragmatic) (thorax) J86.9
  - with fistula J86.Ø
  - accessory sinus (chronic) — *see* Sinusitis
  - antrum (chronic) — *see* Sinusitis, maxillary
  - brain (any part) — *see* Abscess, brain
  - ethmoidal (chronic) (sinus) — *see* Sinusitis, ethmoidal
  - extradural — *see* Abscess, extradural
  - frontal (chronic) (sinus) — *see* Sinusitis, frontal
  - gallbladder K81.Ø
  - mastoid (process) (acute) — *see* Mastoiditis, acute
  - maxilla, maxillary M27.2
    - sinus (chronic) — *see* Sinusitis, maxillary
  - nasal sinus (chronic) — *see* Sinusitis
  - sinus (accessory) (chronic) (nasal) — *see* Sinusitis
  - sphenoidal (sinus) (chronic) — *see* Sinusitis, sphenoidal
  - subarachnoid — *see* Abscess, extradural
  - subdural — *see* Abscess, subdural
  - tuberculous A15.6
  - ureter — *see* Ureteritis
  - ventricular — *see* Abscess, brain
- **En coup de sabre lesion** L94.1
- **Enamel pearls** KØØ.2
- **Enameloma** KØØ.2
- **Enanthema, viral** BØ9
- **Encephalitis** (chronic) (hemorrhagic) (idiopathic) (nonepidemic) (spurious) (subacute) GØ4.9Ø
  - acute — *see also* Encephalitis, viral A86
    - disseminated GØ4.ØØ
      - infectious GØ4.Ø1
      - noninfectious GØ4.81
      - postimmunization (postvaccination) GØ4.Ø2
      - postinfectious GØ4.Ø1
    - inclusion body A85.8
    - necrotizing hemorrhagic GØ4.3Ø
      - postimmunization GØ4.32
      - postinfectious GØ4.31
      - specified NEC GØ4.39
  - arboviral, arbovirus NEC A85.2
  - arthropod-borne NEC (viral) A85.2
  - Australian A83.4
  - California (virus) A83.5
  - Central European (tick-borne) A84.1
  - Czechoslovakian A84.1
  - Dawson's (inclusion body) A81.1
  - diffuse sclerosing A81.1
  - disseminated, acute GØ4.ØØ
  - due to
    - cat scratch disease A28.1
    - human immunodeficiency virus (HIV) disease B2Ø *[GØ5.3]*
    - malaria — *see* Malaria
    - rickettsiosis — *see* Rickettsiosis
    - smallpox inoculation GØ4.Ø2
    - typhus — *see* Typhus
  - Eastern equine A83.2
- **Encephalitis** — *continued*
  - endemic (viral) A86
  - epidemic NEC (viral) A86
  - equine (acute) (infectious) (viral) A83.9
    - Eastern A83.2
    - Venezuelan A92.2
    - Western A83.1
  - Far Eastern (tick-borne) A84.Ø
  - following vaccination or other immunization procedure GØ4.Ø2
  - herpes zoster BØ2.Ø
  - herpesviral BØØ.4
    - due to herpesvirus 6 B1Ø.Ø1
    - due to herpesvirus 7 B1Ø.Ø9
    - specified NEC B1Ø.Ø9
  - Ilheus (virus) A83.8
  - in (due to)
    - actinomycosis A42.82
    - adenovirus A85.1
    - African trypanosomiasis B56.9 *[GØ5.3]*
    - Chagas' disease (chronic) B57.42
    - cytomegalovirus B25.8
    - enterovirus A85.Ø
    - herpes (simplex) virus BØØ.4
      - due to herpesvirus 6 B1Ø.Ø1
      - due to herpesvirus 7 B1Ø.Ø9
      - specified NEC B1Ø.Ø9
    - infectious disease NEC B99 ☑ *[GØ5.3]*
    - influenza — *see* Influenza, with, encephalopathy
    - listeriosis A32.12
    - measles BØ5.Ø
    - mumps B26.2
    - naegleriasis B6Ø.2
    - parasitic disease NEC B89 *[GØ5.3]*
    - poliovirus A8Ø.9 *[GØ5.3]*
    - rubella BØ6.Ø1
    - syphilis
      - congenital A5Ø.42
      - late A52.14
    - systemic lupus erythematosus M32.19
    - toxoplasmosis (acquired) B58.2
      - congenital P37.1
    - tuberculosis A17.82
    - zoster BØ2.Ø
  - inclusion body A81.1
  - infectious (acute) (virus) NEC A86
  - Japanese (B type) A83.Ø
  - La Crosse A83.5
  - lead — *see* Poisoning, lead
  - lethargica (acute) (infectious) A85.8
  - louping ill A84.89
  - lupus erythematosus, systemic M32.19
  - lymphatica A87.2
  - Mengo A85.8
  - meningococcal A39.81
  - Murray Valley A83.4
  - otitic NEC H66.4Ø *[GØ5.3]*
  - parasitic NOS B71.9
  - periaxial G37.Ø
  - periaxialis (concentrica) (diffuse) G37.5
  - postchickenpox BØ1.11
  - postexanthematous NEC BØ9
  - postimmunization GØ4.Ø2
  - postinfectious NEC GØ4.Ø1
  - postmeasles BØ5.Ø
  - postvaccinal GØ4.Ø2
  - postvaricella BØ1.11
  - postviral NEC A86
  - Powassan A84.81
  - Rasmussen GØ4.81
  - Rio Bravo A85.8
  - Russian
    - autumnal A83.Ø
    - spring-summer (taiga) A84.Ø
  - saturnine — *see* Poisoning, lead
  - specified NEC GØ4.81
  - St. Louis A83.3
  - subacute sclerosing A81.1
  - summer A83.Ø
  - suppurative GØ4.81
  - tick-borne A84.9
  - Torula, torular (cryptococcal) B45.1
  - toxic NEC G92.8
  - trichinosis B75 *[GØ5.3]*
  - type
    - B A83.Ø
    - C A83.3
  - van Bogaert's A81.1
- **Encephalitis** — *continued*
  - Venezuelan equine A92.2
  - Vienna A85.8
  - viral, virus A86
    - arthropod-borne NEC A85.2
      - mosquito-borne A83.9
        - Australian X disease A83.4
        - California virus A83.5
        - Eastern equine A83.2
        - Japanese (B type) A83.Ø
        - Murray Valley A83.4
        - specified NEC A83.8
        - St. Louis A83.3
        - type B A83.Ø
        - type C A83.3
        - Western equine A83.1
      - tick-borne A84.9
        - biundulant A84.1
        - central European A84.1
        - Czechoslovakian A84.1
        - diphasic meningoencephalitis A84.1
        - Far Eastern A84.Ø
        - Russian spring-summer (taiga) A84.Ø
        - specified NEC A84.89
    - specified type NEC A85.8
    - tick-borne, specified NEC A84.89
  - Western equine A83.1
- **Encephalocele** QØ1.9
  - frontal QØ1.Ø
  - nasofrontal QØ1.1
  - occipital QØ1.2
  - specified NEC QØ1.8
- **Encephalocystocele** — *see* Encephalocele
- **Encephaloduroarteriomyosynangiosis** (EDAMS) I67.5
- **Encephalomalacia** (brain) (cerebellar) (cerebral) — *see* Softening, brain
- **Encephalomeningitis** — *see* Meningoencephalitis
- **Encephalomeningocele** — *see* Encephalocele
- **Encephalomeningomyelitis** — *see* Meningoencephalitis
- **Encephalomyelitis** — *see also* Encephalitis GØ4.9Ø
  - acute disseminated GØ4.ØØ
    - infectious GØ4.Ø1
    - noninfectious GØ4.81
    - postimmunization GØ4.Ø2
    - postinfectious GØ4.Ø1
  - acute necrotizing hemorrhagic GØ4.3Ø
    - postimmunization GØ4.32
    - postinfectious GØ4.31
    - specified NEC GØ4.39
  - equine A83.9
    - Eastern A83.2
    - Venezuelan A92.2
    - Western A83.1
  - in diseases classified elsewhere GØ5.3
  - myalgic G93.32
    - chronic fatigue syndrome [ME/CFS] G93.32
  - postchickenpox BØ1.11
  - postinfectious NEC GØ4.Ø1
  - postmeasles BØ5.Ø
  - postvaccinal GØ4.Ø2
  - postvaricella BØ1.11
  - rubella BØ6.Ø1
  - specified NEC GØ4.81
  - Venezuelan equine A92.2
- **Encephalomyelocele** — *see* Encephalocele
- **Encephalomyelomeningitis** — *see* Meningoencephalitis
- **Encephalomyelopathy** G96.9
- **Encephalomyeloradiculitis** (acute) G61.Ø
- **Encephalomyeloradiculoneuritis** (acute) (Guillain-Barré) G61.Ø
- **Encephalomyeloradiculopathy** G96.9
- **Encephalopathia hyperbilirubinemica, newborn** P57.9
  - due to isoimmunization (conditions in P55) P57.Ø
- **Encephalopathy** (acute) G93.4Ø
  - acute necrotizing hemorrhagic GØ4.3Ø
    - postimmunization GØ4.32
    - postinfectious GØ4.31
    - specified NEC GØ4.39
  - alcoholic G31.2
  - anoxic — *see* Damage, brain, anoxic
  - arteriosclerotic I67.2
  - centrolobar progressive (Schilder) G37.Ø
  - congenital QØ7.9
  - degenerative, in specified disease NEC G32.89
  - demyelinating callosal G37.1

Encephalopathy — *continued*
  due to
    drugs — *see also* Table of Drugs and Chemicals G92.8
  hepatic (without coma) K76.82
  hyperbilirubinemic, newborn P57.9
    due to isoimmunization (conditions in P55) P57.0
  hypertensive I67.4
  hypoglycemic E16.2
  hypoxic — *see* Damage, brain, anoxic
  hypoxic ischemic P91.60
    mild P91.61
    moderate P91.62
    severe P91.63
  in (due to) (with)
    birth injury P11.1
    hyperinsulinism E16.1 *[G94]*
    influenza — *see* Influenza, with, encephalopathy
    lack of vitamin — *see also* Deficiency, vitamin E56.9 *[G32.89]*
    neoplastic disease — *see also* Neoplasm D49.9 *[G13.1]*
    serum — *see also* Reaction, serum T80.69 ☑
    syphilis A52.17
    trauma (postconcussional) F07.81
      current injury — *see* Injury, intracranial
    vaccination G04.02
  lead — *see* Poisoning, lead
  metabolic G93.41
    drug induced G92.8
    toxic G92.8
  myoclonic, early, symptomatic — *see* Epilepsy, generalized, specified NEC
  necrotizing, subacute (Leigh) G31.82
  neonatal P91.819
    in diseases classified elsewhere P91.811
  pellagrous E52 *[G32.89]*
  portal-systemic K76.82
  postcontusional F07.81
    current injury — *see* Injury, intracranial, diffuse
  posthypoglycemic (coma) E16.1 *[G94]*
  postradiation G93.89
  saturnine — *see* Poisoning, lead
  septic G93.41
  specified NEC G93.49
  spongioform, subacute (viral) A81.09
  toxic G92.9
    metabolic G92.8
  traumatic (postconcussional) F07.81
    current injury — *see* Injury, intracranial
  vitamin B deficiency NEC E53.9 *[G32.89]*
    vitamin B1 E51.2
  Wernicke's E51.2
Encephalorrhagia — *see* Hemorrhage, intracranial, intracerebral
Encephalosis, posttraumatic F07.81
Enchondroma — *see also* Neoplasm, bone, benign
Enchondromatosis (cartilaginous) (multiple) Q78.4
Encopresis R15.9
  functional F98.1
  nonorganic origin F98.1
  psychogenic F98.1
Encounter (with health service) (for) Z76.89
  adjustment and management (of)
    breast implant Z45.81 ☑
    implanted device NEC Z45.89
    myringotomy device (stent) (tube) Z45.82
    neurostimulator (brain) (gastric) (peripheral nerve) (sacral nerve) (spinal cord) (vagus nerve) Z45.42
  administrative purpose only Z02.9
    examination for
      adoption Z02.82
      armed forces Z02.3
      disability determination Z02.71
      driving license Z02.4
      employment Z02.1
      insurance Z02.6
      medical certificate NEC Z02.79
      paternity testing Z02.81
      residential institution admission Z02.2
      school admission Z02.0
      sports Z02.5
    specified reason NEC Z02.89
  aftercare — *see* Aftercare
  antenatal screening Z36.9
    cervical length Z36.86
    chromosomal anomalies Z36.0

Encounter — *continued*
  antenatal screening — *continued*
    congenital cardiac abnormalities Z36.83
    elevated maternal serum alphafetoprotein Z36.1
    fetal growth retardation Z36.4
    fetal lung maturity Z36.84
    fetal macrosomia Z36.88
    hydrops fetalis Z36.81
    intrauterine growth restriction (IUGR) /small-for-dates Z36.4
    isoimmunization Z36.5
    large-for-dates Z36.88
    malformations Z36.3
    non-visualized anatomy on a previous scan Z36.2
    nuchal translucency Z36.82
    raised alphafetoprotein level Z36.1
    risk of pre-term labor Z36.86
    specified follow-up NEC Z36.2
    specified genetic defects NEC Z36.8A
    specified type NEC Z36.89
    Streptococcus B Z36.85
    suspected anomaly Z36.3
    uncertain dates Z36.87
  assisted reproductive fertility procedure cycle Z31.83
  blood typing Z01.83
    Rh typing Z01.83
  breast augmentation or reduction Z41.1
  breast implant exchange (different material) (different size) Z45.81 ☑
  breast reconstruction following mastectomy Z42.1
  check-up — *see* Examination
  chemotherapy for neoplasm Z51.11
  colonoscopy, screening Z12.11
  counseling — *see* Counseling
  delivery, full-term, uncomplicated O80
    cesarean, without indication O82
  desensitization to allergens Z51.6
  ear piercing Z41.3
  examination — *see* Examination
  expectant parent(s) (adoptive) pre-birth pediatrician visit Z76.81
  fertility preservation procedure (prior to cancer therapy) (prior to removal of gonads) Z31.84
  fitting (of) — *see* Fitting (and adjustment) (of)
  genetic
    counseling
      nonprocreative Z71.83
      procreative Z31.5
    testing — *see* Test, genetic
  hearing conservation and treatment Z01.12
  immunotherapy for neoplasm Z51.12
  in vitro fertilization cycle Z31.83
  instruction (in)
    child care (postpartal) (prenatal) Z32.3
    childbirth Z32.2
    natural family planning
      procreative Z31.61
      to avoid pregnancy Z30.02
  insulin pump titration Z46.81
  joint prosthesis insertion following prior explantation of joint prosthesis (staged procedure)
    hip Z47.32
    knee Z47.33
    shoulder Z47.31
  laboratory (as part of a general medical examination) Z00.00
    with abnormal findings Z00.01
  mental health services (for)
    abuse NEC
      perpetrator Z69.82
      victim Z69.81
    child abuse
      nonparental
        perpetrator Z69.021
        victim Z69.020
      parental
        perpetrator Z69.011
        victim Z69.010
    child neglect
      nonparental
        perpetrator Z69.021
        victim Z69.020
      parental
        perpetrator Z69.011
        victim Z69.010
    child psychological abuse
      nonparental
        perpetrator Z69.021
        victim Z69.020

Encounter — *continued*
  mental health services — *continued*
    child psychological abuse — *continued*
      parental
        perpetrator Z69.011
        victim Z69.010
    child sexual abuse
      nonparental
        perpetrator Z69.021
        victim Z69.020
      parental
        perpetrator Z69.011
        victim Z69.010
    non-spousal adult abuse
      perpetrator Z69.82
      victim Z69.81
    spousal or partner
      abuse
        perpetrator Z69.12
        victim Z69.11
      neglect
        perpetrator Z69.12
        victim Z69.11
      psychological abuse
        perpetrator Z69.12
        victim Z69.11
      violence
        perpetrator (physical) (sexual) Z69.12
        victim (physical) Z69.11
          sexual Z69.81
  observation (for) (ruled out)
    alarm, without findings
      apnea Z03.83
      bradycardia Z03.83
      oximeter Z03.83
    condition suspected related to home physiologic monitoring device Z03.83
    exposure to (suspected)
      anthrax Z03.810
      biological agent NEC Z03.818
    malfunction of home cardiorespiratory monitor Z03.83
    non-specific findings home physiologic monitoring device Z03.83
  pediatrician visit, by expectant parent(s) (adoptive) Z76.81
  placental sample (taken vaginally) — *see also* Encounter, antenatal screening Z36.9
  plastic and reconstructive surgery following medical procedure or healed injury NEC Z42.8
  pregnancy
    supervision of — *see* Pregnancy, supervision of
    test Z32.00
      result negative Z32.02
      result positive Z32.01
  procreative management and counseling for gestational carrier Z31.7
  prophylactic measures Z29.9
    antivenin Z29.12
    fluoride administration Z29.3
    immunotherapy for respiratory syncytial virus (RSV) Z29.11
    rabies immune globin Z29.14
    Rho (D) immune globulin Z29.13
    specified NEC Z29.8
  radiation therapy (antineoplastic) Z51.0
  radiological (as part of a general medical examination) Z00.00
    with abnormal findings Z00.01
  reconstructive surgery following medical procedure or healed injury NEC Z42.8
  removal (of) — *see also* Removal
    artificial
      arm Z44.00- ☑
        complete Z44.01- ☑
        partial Z44.02- ☑
      eye Z44.2- ☑
      leg Z44.10- ☑
        complete Z44.11- ☑
        partial Z44.12- ☑
    breast implant Z45.81 ☑
      tissue expander (with or without synchronous insertion of permanent implant) Z45.81 ☑
    device Z46.9
      specified NEC Z46.89

- **Encounter** — *continued*
  - removal — *see also* Removal — *continued*
    - external
      - fixation device — *code to* fracture with seventh character D
      - prosthesis, prosthetic device Z44.9
        - breast Z44.3- ☑
        - specified NEC Z44.8
    - implanted device NEC Z45.89
    - insulin pump Z46.81
    - internal fixation device Z47.2
    - myringotomy device (stent) (tube) Z45.82
    - nervous system device NEC Z46.2
      - brain neuropacemaker Z46.2
      - visual substitution device Z46.2
        - implanted Z45.31
    - non-vascular catheter Z46.82
    - orthodontic device Z46.4
    - stent
      - ureteral Z46.6
    - urinary device Z46.6
  - repeat cervical smear to confirm findings of recent normal smear following initial abnormal smear ZØ1.42
  - respirator [ventilator] use during power failure Z99.12
  - Rh typing ZØ1.83
  - screening — *see* Screening
  - specified NEC Z76.89
  - sterilization Z3Ø.2
  - suspected condition, ruled out
    - amniotic cavity and membrane ZØ3.71
    - cervical shortening ZØ3.75
    - fetal anomaly ZØ3.73
    - fetal growth ZØ3.74
    - maternal and fetal conditions NEC ZØ3.79
    - oligohydramnios ZØ3.71
    - placental problem ZØ3.72
    - polyhydramnios ZØ3.71
  - suspected exposure (to), ruled out
    - anthrax ZØ3.81Ø
    - biological agents NEC ZØ3.818
  - termination of pregnancy, elective Z33.2
  - testing — *see* Test
  - therapeutic drug level monitoring Z51.81
  - titration, insulin pump Z46.81
  - to determine fetal viability of pregnancy O36.8Ø ☑
  - training
    - insulin pump Z46.81
  - X-ray of chest (as part of a general medical examination) ZØØ.ØØ
    - with abnormal findings ZØØ.Ø1
- **Encystment** — *see* Cyst
- **Endarteritis** (bacterial, subacute) (infective) I77.6
  - brain I67.7
  - cerebral or cerebrospinal I67.7
  - deformans — *see* Arteriosclerosis
  - embolic — *see* Embolism
  - obliterans — *see also* Arteriosclerosis
    - pulmonary I28.8
  - pulmonary I28.8
  - retina — *see* Vasculitis, retina
  - senile — *see* Arteriosclerosis
  - syphilitic A52.Ø9
    - brain or cerebral A52.Ø4
    - congenital A5Ø.54 *[I79.8]*
  - tuberculous A18.89
- **Endemic** — *see* condition
- **Endocarditis** (chronic) (marantic) (nonbacterial) (thrombotic) (valvular) I38
  - with rheumatic fever (conditions in IØØ)
    - active — *see* Endocarditis, acute, rheumatic
    - inactive or quiescent (with chorea) IØ9.1
  - acute or subacute I33.9
    - infective I33.Ø
    - rheumatic (aortic) (mitral) (pulmonary) (tricuspid) IØ1.1
      - with chorea (acute) (rheumatic) (Sydenham's) IØ2.Ø
  - aortic (heart) (nonrheumatic) (valve) I35.8
    - with
      - mitral disease IØ8.Ø
        - with tricuspid (valve) disease IØ8.3
        - active or acute IØ1.1
          - with chorea (acute) (rheumatic) (Sydenham's) IØ2.Ø
      - rheumatic fever (conditions in IØØ)
        - active — *see* Endocarditis, acute, rheumatic
        - inactive or quiescent (with chorea) IØ6.9

- **Endocarditis** — *continued*
  - aortic — *continued*
    - with — *continued*
      - tricuspid (valve) disease IØ8.2
        - with mitral (valve) disease IØ8.3
    - acute or subacute I33.9
    - arteriosclerotic I35.8
    - rheumatic IØ6.9
      - with mitral disease IØ8.Ø
        - with tricuspid (valve) disease IØ8.3
        - active or acute IØ1.1
          - with chorea (acute) (rheumatic) (Sydenham's) IØ2.Ø
      - active or acute IØ1.1
        - with chorea (acute) (rheumatic) (Sydenham's) IØ2.Ø
      - specified NEC IØ6.8
    - specified cause NEC I35.8
    - syphilitic A52.Ø3
  - arteriosclerotic I38
  - atypical verrucous (Libman-Sacks) M32.11
  - bacterial (acute) (any valve) (subacute) I33.Ø
  - candidal B37.6
  - congenital Q24.8
  - constrictive I33.Ø
  - Coxiella burnetii A78 *[I39]*
  - Coxsackie B33.21
  - due to
    - prosthetic cardiac valve T82.6 ☑
    - Q fever A78 *[I39]*
    - Serratia marcescens I33.Ø
    - typhoid (fever) AØ1.Ø2
  - gonococcal A54.83
  - infectious or infective (acute) (any valve) (subacute) I33.Ø
  - lenta (acute) (any valve) (subacute) I33.Ø
  - Libman-Sacks M32.11
  - listerial A32.82
  - Löffler's I42.3
  - malignant (acute) (any valve) (subacute) I33.Ø
  - meningococcal A39.51
  - mitral (chronic) (double) (fibroid) (heart) (inactive) (valve) (with chorea) IØ5.9
    - with
      - aortic (valve) disease IØ8.Ø
        - with tricuspid (valve) disease IØ8.3
        - active or acute IØ1.1
          - with chorea (acute) (rheumatic) (Sydenham's) IØ2.Ø
      - rheumatic fever (conditions in IØØ)
        - active — *see* Endocarditis, acute, rheumatic
        - inactive or quiescent (with chorea) IØ5.9
      - tricuspid (valve) disease IØ8.1
        - with aortic (valve) disease IØ8.3
    - active or acute IØ1.1
      - with chorea (acute) (rheumatic) (Sydenham's) IØ2.Ø
      - bacterial I33.Ø
    - arteriosclerotic I34.89
    - nonrheumatic I34.89
      - acute or subacute I33.9
    - specified NEC IØ5.8
  - monilial B37.6
  - multiple valves IØ8.9
    - specified disorders IØ8.8
  - mycotic (acute) (any valve) (subacute) I33.Ø
  - pneumococcal (acute) (any valve) (subacute) I33.Ø
  - pulmonary (chronic) (heart) (valve) I37.8
    - with rheumatic fever (conditions in IØØ)
      - active — *see* Endocarditis, acute, rheumatic
      - inactive or quiescent (with chorea) IØ9.89
        - with aortic, mitral or tricuspid disease IØ8.8
    - acute or subacute I33.9
      - rheumatic IØ1.1
        - with chorea (acute) (rheumatic) (Sydenham's) IØ2.Ø
    - arteriosclerotic I37.8
    - congenital Q22.2
    - rheumatic (chronic) (inactive) (with chorea) IØ9.89
      - active or acute IØ1.1
        - with chorea (acute) (rheumatic) (Sydenham's) IØ2.Ø
    - syphilitic A52.Ø3
  - purulent (acute) (any valve) (subacute) I33.Ø
  - Q fever A78 *[I39]*
  - rheumatic (chronic) (inactive) (with chorea) IØ9.1
    - active or acute (aortic) (mitral) (pulmonary) (tricuspid) IØ1.1

- **Endocarditis** — *continued*
  - rheumatic — *continued*
    - active or acute — *continued*
      - with chorea (acute) (rheumatic) (Sydenham's) IØ2.Ø
  - rheumatoid — *see* Rheumatoid, carditis
  - septic (acute) (any valve) (subacute) I33.Ø
  - streptococcal (acute) (any valve) (subacute) I33.Ø
  - subacute — *see* Endocarditis, acute
  - suppurative (acute) (any valve) (subacute) I33.Ø
  - syphilitic A52.Ø3
  - toxic I33.9
  - tricuspid (chronic) (heart) (inactive) (rheumatic) (valve) (with chorea) IØ7.9
    - with
      - aortic (valve) disease IØ8.2
        - mitral (valve) disease IØ8.3
      - mitral (valve) disease IØ8.1
        - aortic (valve) disease IØ8.3
      - rheumatic fever (conditions in IØØ)
        - active — *see* Endocarditis, acute, rheumatic
        - inactive or quiescent (with chorea) IØ7.8
    - active or acute IØ1.1
      - with chorea (acute) (rheumatic) (Sydenham's) IØ2.Ø
    - arteriosclerotic I36.8
    - nonrheumatic I36.8
      - acute or subacute I33.9
    - specified cause, except rheumatic I36.8
  - tuberculous — *see* Tuberculosis, endocarditis
  - typhoid AØ1.Ø2
  - ulcerative (acute) (any valve) (subacute) I33.Ø
  - vegetative (acute) (any valve) (subacute) I33.Ø
  - verrucous (atypical) (nonbacterial) (nonrheumatic) M32.11
- **Endocardium, endocardial** — *see also* condition
  - cushion defect Q21.2Ø
- **Endocervicitis** — *see also* Cervicitis
  - due to intrauterine (contraceptive) device T83.69 ☑
  - hyperplastic N72
- **Endocrine** — *see* condition
- **Endocrinopathy, pluriglandular** E31.9
- **Endodontic**
  - overfill M27.52
  - underfill M27.53
- **Endodontitis** KØ4.Ø1
  - irreversible KØ4.Ø2
  - reversible KØ4.Ø1
- **Endomastoiditis** — *see* Mastoiditis
- **Endometrioma** N8Ø.12- ☑
- **Endometriosis** N8Ø.9
  - abdomen, abdominal N8Ø.CØ
    - specified site, NEC N8Ø.C9
    - wall N8Ø.C19
      - fascia and muscular layers N8Ø.C11
      - subcutaneous tissue N8Ø.C1Ø
      - unspecified depth N8Ø.C19
  - appendix N8Ø.549
    - deep N8Ø.542
    - superficial N8Ø.541
  - bladder (unspecified depth) N8Ø.AØ
    - deep N8Ø.A2
    - superficial N8Ø.A1
  - bowel N8Ø.5Ø
  - broad ligament N8Ø.3C ☑
  - cardiothoracic space N8Ø.B6
  - cecum N8Ø.539
    - deep N8Ø.532
    - superficial N8Ø.531
  - cervix N8Ø.Ø- ☑
  - colon N8Ø.559
    - descending N8Ø.559
      - deep N8Ø.552
      - superficial N8Ø.551
    - sigmoid N8Ø.529
      - deep N8Ø.522
      - superficial N8Ø.521
    - transverse N8Ø.559
      - deep N8Ø.552
      - superficial N8Ø.551
  - cul-de-sac (Douglas')
    - anterior (unspecified depth) N8Ø.319
      - deep N8Ø.312
      - superficial N8Ø.311
    - posterior (unspecified depth) N8Ø.329
      - deep N8Ø.322
      - superficial N8Ø.321

Endometriosis — *continued*
- deep
  - involving muscular wall of fallopian tube N80.22 ☑
  - retrocervical N80.02
- diaphragm N80.B39
  - deep N80.B32
  - superficial N80.B31
  - unspecified depth N80.B39
- exocervix N80.01
- extra-pelvic abdominal peritoneum N80.C4
- fallopian tube (unspecified depth) N80.20- ☑
  - deep N80.22- ☑
  - superficial N80.21- ☑
- female genital organ NEC N80.8
- gallbladder N80.8
- in scar of skin N80.6
- inguinal canal N80.C3
- internal N80.02
- intestine N80.50
- lung N80.B2
- mediastinal space N80.B5
- myometrium N80.03
- nerve
  - femoral N80.D6
  - obturator N80.D3
  - pelvic N80.D0
    - splanchnic N80.D1
  - pudendal N80.D5
  - retroperitoneum, NEC N80.D9
  - sacral splanchnic N80.D1
  - sciatic N80.D4
  - specified, NEC N80.D9
- ovary (unspecified depth) N80.10- ☑
  - deep N80.12- ☑
  - superficial N80.11- ☑
- parametrium N80.399
- pelvic
  - brim N80.38- ☑
    - deep N80.37- ☑
    - superficial N80.36- ☑
  - peritoneum N80.30
    - specified sites, NEC N80.399
      - deep N80.392
      - superficial N80.391
  - sidewall N80.35- ☑
    - deep N80.34- ☑
    - superficial N80.33- ☑
- pericardial space N80.B4
- peritoneal (pelvic) N80.30
- pleura N80.B1
- rectovaginal septum N80.40
  - with involvement of vagina N80.42
  - without involvement of vagina N80.41
- rectum N80.519
  - deep (multifocal) N80.512
  - superficial N80.511
- retroperitoneum N80.30
- round ligament N80.3C9
- sacral nerve roots N80.D2
- skin (scar) N80.6
- small N80.569
  - deep (multifocal) N80.562
  - superficial N80.561
- specified site NEC N80.8
- stromal D39.0
- thorax N80.B- ☑
- umbilicus N80.C2
- ureter N80.A69
  - deep N80.A5- ☑
  - extrinsic N80.A4- ☑
  - intrinsic N80.A5- ☑
  - superficial N80.A4- ☑
  - unspecified depth N80.A6- ☑
- uterosacral ligament(s) N80.3C- ☑
  - deep N80.3B- ☑
  - superficial N80.3A- ☑
- uterus N80.00
  - deep N80.02
  - internal N80.02
  - superficial N80.01
- vagina N80.42
- vulva N80.8

Endometritis (decidual) (nonspecific) (purulent) (senile) (atrophic) (suppurative) N71.9
- with ectopic pregnancy O08.0
- acute N71.0
- blenorrhagic (gonococcal) (acute) (chronic) A54.24

Endometritis — *continued*
- cervix, cervical (with erosion or ectropion) — *see also* Cervicitis
  - hyperplastic N72
- chlamydial A56.11
- chronic N71.1
- following
  - abortion — *see* Abortion by type complicated by genital infection
  - ectopic or molar pregnancy O08.0
- gonococcal, gonorrheal (acute) (chronic) A54.24
- hyperplastic — *see also* Hyperplasia, endometrial N85.00
  - cervix N72
- puerperal, postpartum, childbirth O86.12
- subacute N71.0
- tuberculous A18.17

Endometrium — *see* condition
Endomyocardiopathy, South African I42.3
Endomyocarditis — *see* Endocarditis
Endomyofibrosis I42.3
Endomyometritis — *see* Endometritis
Endopericarditis — *see* Endocarditis
Endoperineuritis — *see* Disorder, nerve
Endophlebitis — *see* Phlebitis
Endophthalmia — *see* Endophthalmitis, purulent
Endophthalmitis (acute) (infective) (metastatic) (subacute) H44.009
- bleb associated — *see also* Bleb, inflamed (infected), postprocedural H59.4 ☑
- gonorrheal A54.39
- in (due to)
  - cysticercosis B69.1
  - onchocerciasis B73.01
  - toxocariasis B83.0
- panuveitis — *see* Panuveitis
- parasitic H44.12- ☑
- purulent H44.00- ☑
  - panophthalmitis — *see* Panophthalmitis
  - vitreous abscess H44.02- ☑
- specified NEC H44.19
- sympathetic — *see* Uveitis, sympathetic

Endosalpingioma D28.2
Endosalpingiosis N94.89
Endosteitis — *see* Osteomyelitis
Endothelioma, bone — *see* Neoplasm, bone, malignant
Endotheliosis (hemorrhagic infectional) D69.8
Endotoxemia — code to condition
Endotrachelitis — *see* Cervicitis
Engelmann (-Camurati) **syndrome** Q78.3
English disease — *see* Rickets
Engman's disease L30.3
Engorgement
- breast N64.59
  - newborn P83.4
  - puerperal, postpartum O92.79
- lung (passive) — *see* Edema, lung
- pulmonary (passive) — *see* Edema, lung
- stomach K31.89
- venous, retina — *see* Occlusion, retina, vein, engorgement

Enlargement, enlarged — *see also* Hypertrophy
- adenoids J35.2
  - with tonsils J35.3
- alveolar ridge K08.89
  - congenital — *see* Anomaly, alveolar
- apertures of diaphragm (congenital) Q79.1
- gingival K06.1
- heart, cardiac — *see* Hypertrophy, cardiac
- labium majus, childhood asymmetric (CALME) N90.61
- lacrimal gland, chronic H04.03- ☑
- liver — *see* Hypertrophy, liver
- lymph gland or node R59.9
  - generalized R59.1
  - localized R59.0
- orbit H05.34- ☑
- organ or site, congenital NEC — *see* Anomaly, by site
- parathyroid (gland) E21.0
- pituitary fossa R93.0
- prostate N40.0
  - with lower urinary tract symptoms (LUTS) N40.1
  - without lower urinary tract symtpoms (LUTS) N40.0
- sella turcica R93.0
- spleen — *see* Splenomegaly
- thymus (gland) (congenital) E32.0
- thyroid (gland) — *see* Goiter
- tongue K14.8

Enlargement, enlarged — *continued*
- tonsils J35.1
  - with adenoids J35.3
- uterus N85.2
- vestibular aqueduct Q16.5

Enophthalmos H05.40- ☑
- due to
  - orbital tissue atrophy H05.41- ☑
  - trauma or surgery H05.42- ☑

Enostosis M27.8
Entamebic, entamebiasis — *see* Amebiasis
Entanglement
- umbilical cord(s) O69.82 ☑
  - with compression O69.2 ☑
  - around neck (with compression) O69.81 ☑
    - with compression O69.1 ☑
    - without compression O69.81 ☑
  - of twins in monoamniotic sac O69.2 ☑
  - without compression O69.82 ☑

Enteralgia — *see* Pain, abdominal
Enteric — *see* condition
Enteritis (acute) (diarrheal) (hemorrhagic) (noninfective) K52.9
- adenovirus A08.2
- aertrycke infection A02.0
- allergic K52.29
  - with
    - eosinophilic gastritis or gastroenteritis K52.81
    - food protein-induced enterocolitis syndrome K52.21
    - food protein-induced enteropathy K52.22
    - FPIES K52.21
- amebic (acute) A06.0
  - with abscess — *see* Abscess, amebic
  - chronic A06.1
    - with abscess — *see* Abscess, amebic
    - nondysenteric A06.2
  - nondysenteric A06.2
- astrovirus A08.32
- bacillary NOS A03.9
- bacterial A04.9
  - specified NEC A04.8
- calicivirus A08.31
- candidal B37.82
- Chilomastix A07.8
- choleriformis A00.1
- chronic (noninfectious) K52.9
  - ulcerative — *see* Colitis, ulcerative
- cicatrizing (chronic) — *see* Enteritis, regional, small intestine
- Clostridium
  - botulinum (food poisoning) A05.1
  - difficile
    - not specified as recurrent A04.72
    - recurrent A04.71
- coccidial A07.3
- coxsackie virus A08.39
- dietetic — *see also* Enteritis, allergic K52.29
- drug-induced K52.1
- due to
  - astrovirus A08.32
  - calicivirus A08.31
  - coxsackie virus A08.39
  - drugs K52.1
  - echovirus A08.39
  - enterovirus NEC A08.39
  - food hypersensitivity — *see also* Enteritis, allergic K52.29
  - infectious organism (bacterial) (viral) — *see* Enteritis, infectious
  - torovirus A08.39
  - Yersinia enterocolitica A04.6
- echovirus A08.39
- eltor A00.1
- enterovirus NEC A08.39
- eosinophilic K52.81
- epidemic (infectious) A09
- fulminant — *see also* Ischemia, intestine, acute K55.019
- gangrenous — *see* Enteritis, infectious
- giardial A07.1
- infectious NOS A09
  - due to
    - adenovirus A08.2
    - Aerobacter aerogenes A04.8
    - Arizona (bacillus) A02.0
    - bacteria NOS A04.9
      - specified NEC A04.8
    - Campylobacter A04.5

- **Enteritis** — *continued*
  - infectious — *continued*
    - due to — *continued*
      - Clostridium difficile
        - not specified as recurrent AØ4.72
        - recurrent AØ4.71
      - Clostridium perfringens AØ4.8
      - Enterobacter aerogenes AØ4.8
      - enterovirus AØ8.39
      - Escherichia coli AØ4.4
        - enteroaggregative AØ4.4
        - enterohemorrhagic AØ4.3
        - enteroinvasive AØ4.2
        - enteropathogenic AØ4.Ø
        - enterotoxigenic AØ4.1
        - specified NEC AØ4.4
      - specified
        - bacteria NEC AØ4.8
        - virus NEC AØ8.39
      - Staphylococcus AØ4.8
      - virus NEC AØ8.4
        - specified type NEC AØ8.39
      - Yersinia enterocolitica AØ4.6
    - specified organism NEC AØ8.8
  - influenzal — *see* Influenza, with, digestive manifestations
  - ischemic K55.9
    - acute — *see also* Ischemia, intestine, acute K55.Ø19
    - chronic K55.1
  - microsporidial AØ7.8
  - mucomembranous, myxomembranous — *see* Syndrome, irritable bowel
  - mucous — *see* Syndrome, irritable bowel
  - necroticans AØ5.2
  - necrotizing of newborn — *see* Enterocolitis, necrotizing, in newborn
  - neurogenic — *see* Syndrome, irritable bowel
  - newborn necrotizing — *see* Enterocolitis, necrotizing, in newborn
  - noninfectious K52.9
  - norovirus AØ8.11
  - parasitic NEC B82.9
  - paratyphoid (fever) — *see* Fever, paratyphoid
  - protozoal AØ7.9
    - specified NEC AØ7.8
  - radiation K52.Ø
  - regional (of) K5Ø.9Ø
    - with
      - complication K5Ø.919
        - abscess K5Ø.914
        - fistula K5Ø.913
        - intestinal obstruction K5Ø.912
        - rectal bleeding K5Ø.911
        - specified complication NEC K5Ø.918
    - colon — *see* Enteritis, regional, large intestine
    - duodenum — *see* Enteritis, regional, small intestine
    - ileum — *see* Enteritis, regional, small intestine
    - jejunum — *see* Enteritis, regional, small intestine
    - large bowel — *see* Enteritis, regional, large intestine
    - large intestine (colon) (rectum) K5Ø.1Ø
      - with
        - complication K5Ø.119
          - abscess K5Ø.114
          - fistula K5Ø.113
          - intestinal obstruction K5Ø.112
          - rectal bleeding K5Ø.111
          - small intestine (duodenum) (ileum) (jejunum) involvement K5Ø.8Ø
            - with
              - complication K5Ø.819
                - abscess K5Ø.814
                - fistula K5Ø.813
                - intestinal obstruction K5Ø.812
                - rectal bleeding K5Ø.811
                - specified complication NEC K5Ø.818
          - specified complication NEC K5Ø.118
    - rectum — *see* Enteritis, regional, large intestine
    - small intestine (duodenum) (ileum) (jejunum) K5Ø.ØØ
      - with
        - complication K5Ø.Ø19
          - abscess K5Ø.Ø14
          - fistula K5Ø.Ø13
          - intestinal obstruction K5Ø.Ø12
          - large intestine (colon) (rectum) involvement K5Ø.8Ø
- **Enteritis** — *continued*
  - regional — *continued*
    - small intestine — *continued*
      - with — *continued*
        - complication — *continued*
          - large intestine involvement — *continued*
            - with
              - complication K5Ø.819
                - abscess K5Ø.814
                - fistula K5Ø.813
                - intestinal obstruction K5Ø.812
                - rectal bleeding K5Ø.811
                - specified complication NEC K5Ø.818
          - rectal bleeding K5Ø.Ø11
          - specified complication NEC K5Ø.Ø18
  - rotaviral AØ8.Ø
  - Salmonella, salmonellosis (arizonae) (cholerae-suis) (enteritidis) (typhimurium) AØ2.Ø
  - segmental — *see* Enteritis, regional
  - septic AØ9
  - Shigella — *see* Infection, Shigella
  - small round structured NEC AØ8.19
  - spasmodic, spastic — *see* Syndrome, irritable bowel
  - staphylococcal AØ4.8
    - due to food AØ5.Ø
  - torovirus AØ8.39
  - toxic NEC K52.1
    - due to Clostridium difficile
      - not specified as recurrent AØ4.72
      - recurrent AØ4.71
  - trichomonal AØ7.8
  - tuberculous A18.32
  - typhosa AØ1.ØØ
  - ulcerative (chronic) — *see* Colitis, ulcerative
  - viral AØ8.4
    - adenovirus AØ8.2
    - enterovirus AØ8.39
    - Rotavirus AØ8.Ø
    - small round structured NEC AØ8.19
    - specified NEC AØ8.39
    - virus specified NEC AØ8.39
- **Enterobiasis** B8Ø
- **Enterobius vermicularis** (infection) (infestation) B8Ø
- **Enterocele** — *see also* Hernia, abdomen
  - pelvic, pelvis (acquired) (congenital) N81.5
  - vagina, vaginal (acquired) (congenital) NEC N81.5
- **Enterocolitis** — *see also* Enteritis K52.9
  - due to Clostridium difficile
    - not specified as recurrent AØ4.72
    - recurrent AØ4.71
  - fulminant ischemic — *see also* Ischemia, intestine, acute K55.Ø59
  - granulomatous — *see* Enteritis, regional
  - hemorrhagic (acute) — *see also* Ischemia, intestine, acute K55.Ø59
    - chronic K55.1
  - infectious NEC AØ9
  - ischemic K55.9
  - necrotizing K55.3Ø
    - with
      - perforation K55.33
      - pneumatosis K55.32
        - and perforation K55.33
    - due to Clostridium difficile
      - not specified as recurrent AØ4.72
      - recurrent AØ4.71
    - in non-newborn K55.3Ø
      - stage 1 (without pneumatosis, without perforation) K55.31
      - stage 2 (with pneumatosis, without perforation) K55.32
      - stage 3 (with pneumatosis, with perforation) K55.33
    - in newborn P77.9
      - stage 1 (without pneumatosis, without perforation) P77.1
      - stage 2 (with pneumatosis, without perforation) P77.2
      - stage 3 (with pneumatosis, with perforation) P77.3
    - without pneumatosis or perforation K55.31
  - noninfectious K52.9
    - newborn — *see* Enterocolitis, necrotizing, in newborn
  - pseudomembranous (newborn)
    - not specified as recurrent AØ4.72
- **Enterocolitis** — *continued*
  - pseudomembranous — *continued*
    - recurrent AØ4.71
  - radiation K52.Ø
    - newborn — *see* Enterocolitis, necrotizing, in newborn
  - ulcerative (chronic) — *see* Pancolitis, ulcerative (chronic)
- **Enterogastritis** — *see* Enteritis
- **Enteropathy** K63.9
  - celiac-gluten-sensitive K9Ø.Ø
    - non-celiac K9Ø.41
  - food protein-induced K52.22
  - hemorrhagic, terminal — *see also* Ischemia, intestine, acute K55.Ø59
  - protein-losing K9Ø.49
- **Enteroperitonitis** — *see* Peritonitis
- **Enteroptosis** K63.4
- **Enterorrhagia** K92.2
- **Enterospasm** — *see also* Syndrome, irritable, bowel
  - psychogenic F45.8
- **Enterostenosis** — *see also* Obstruction, intestine, specified NEC K56.699
- **Enterostomy**
  - complication — *see* Complication, enterostomy
  - status Z93.4
- **Enterovirus, as cause of disease classified elsewhere** B97.1Ø
  - coxsackievirus B97.11
  - echovirus B97.12
  - other specified B97.19
- **Enthesopathy** (peripheral) M77.9
  - Achilles tendinitis — *see* Tendinitis, Achilles
  - ankle and tarsus M77.5- ☑
    - specified type NEC — *see* Enthesopathy, foot, specified type NEC
  - anterior tibial syndrome M76.81- ☑
  - calcaneal spur — *see* Spur, bone, calcaneal
  - elbow region M77.8
    - lateral epicondylitis — *see* Epicondylitis, lateral
    - medial epicondylitis — *see* Epicondylitis, medial
  - foot NEC M77.8
    - metatarsalgia — *see* Metatarsalgia
    - specified type NEC M77.5- ☑
  - forearm M77.8
  - gluteal tendinitis — *see* Tendinitis, gluteal
  - hand M77.8
  - hip — *see* Enthesopathy, lower limb, specified type NEC
  - iliac crest spur — *see* Spur, bone, iliac crest
  - iliotibial band syndrome — *see* Syndrome, iliotibial band
  - knee — *see* Enthesopathy, lower limb, lower leg, specified type NEC
  - lateral epicondylitis — *see* Epicondylitis, lateral
  - lower limb (excluding foot) M76.9
    - Achilles tendinitis — *see* Tendinitis, Achilles
    - ankle and tarsus M77.5- ☑
      - specified type NEC — *see* Enthesopathy, foot, specified type NEC
    - anterior tibial syndrome M76.81- ☑
    - gluteal tendinitis — *see* Tendinitis, gluteal
    - iliac crest spur — *see* Spur, bone, iliac crest
    - iliotibial band syndrome — *see* Syndrome, iliotibial band
    - patellar tendinitis — *see* Tendinitis, patellar
    - pelvic region — *see* Enthesopathy, lower limb, specified type NEC
    - peroneal tendinitis — *see* Tendinitis, peroneal
    - posterior tibial syndrome M76.82- ☑
    - psoas tendinitis — *see* Tendinitis, psoas
    - specified type NEC M76.89- ☑
    - tibial collateral bursitis — *see* Bursitis, tibial collateral
  - medial epicondylitis — *see* Epicondylitis, medial
  - metatarsalgia — *see* Metatarsalgia
  - multiple sites M77.8
  - patellar tendinitis — *see* Tendinitis, patellar
  - pelvis M77.8
  - periarthritis of wrist — *see* Periarthritis, wrist
  - peroneal tendinitis — *see* Tendinitis, peroneal
  - posterior tibial syndrome M76.82- ☑
  - psoas tendinitis — *see* Tendinitis, psoas
  - shoulder M77.8
  - shoulder region — *see* Lesion, shoulder
  - specified type NEC M77.8
  - spinal M46.ØØ

- **Enthesopathy** — *continued*
  - spinal — *continued*
    - cervical region M46.Ø2
    - cervicothoracic region M46.Ø3
    - lumbar region M46.Ø6
    - lumbosacral region M46.Ø7
    - multiple sites M46.Ø9
    - occipito-atlanto-axial region M46.Ø1
    - sacrococcygeal region M46.Ø8
    - thoracic region M46.Ø4
    - thoracolumbar region M46.Ø5
  - tibial collateral bursitis — *see* Bursitis, tibial collateral
  - upper arm M77.8
  - wrist and carpus NEC M77.8
    - calcaneal spur — *see* Spur, bone, calcaneal
    - periarthritis of wrist — *see* Periarthritis, wrist
- **Entomophobia** F4Ø.218
- **Entomophthoromycosis** B46.8
- **Entrance, air into vein** — *see* Embolism, air
- **Entrapment, nerve** — *see* Neuropathy, entrapment
- **Entropion** (eyelid) (paralytic) HØ2.ØØ9
  - cicatricial HØ2.Ø19
    - left HØ2.Ø16
      - lower HØ2.Ø15
      - upper HØ2.Ø14
    - right HØ2.Ø13
      - lower HØ2.Ø12
      - upper HØ2.Ø11
  - congenital Q1Ø.2
  - left HØ2.ØØ6
    - lower HØ2.ØØ5
    - upper HØ2.ØØ4
  - mechanical HØ2.Ø29
    - left HØ2.Ø26
      - lower HØ2.Ø25
      - upper HØ2.Ø24
    - right HØ2.Ø23
      - lower HØ2.Ø22
      - upper HØ2.Ø21
  - right HØ2.ØØ3
    - lower HØ2.ØØ2
    - upper HØ2.ØØ1
  - senile HØ2.Ø39
    - left HØ2.Ø36
      - lower HØ2.Ø35
      - upper HØ2.Ø34
    - right HØ2.Ø33
      - lower HØ2.Ø32
      - upper HØ2.Ø31
  - spastic HØ2.Ø49
    - left HØ2.Ø46
      - lower HØ2.Ø45
      - upper HØ2.Ø44
    - right HØ2.Ø43
      - lower HØ2.Ø42
      - upper HØ2.Ø41
- **Enucleated eye** (traumatic, current) SØ5.7- ☑
- **Enuresis** R32
  - functional F98.Ø
  - habit disturbance F98.Ø
  - nocturnal N39.44
    - psychogenic F98.Ø
  - nonorganic origin F98.Ø
  - psychogenic F98.Ø
- **Eosinopenia** — *see* Agranulocytosis
- **Eosinophilia** (allergic) (idiopathic) (secondary) D72.1Ø
  - with
    - angiolymphoid hyperplasia (ALHE) D18.Ø1
  - familial D72.19
  - hereditary D72.19
  - in disease classified elsewhere D72.18
  - infiltrative — *see* Eosinophilia, pulmonary
  - Löffler's J82.89
  - peritoneal — *see* Peritonitis, eosinophilic
  - pulmonary NEC J82.89
    - acute J82.82
    - asthmatic J82.83
    - chronic J82.81
  - specified NEC D72.19
  - tropical (pulmonary) J82.89
- **Eosinophilia-myalgia syndrome** M35.89
- **Ependymitis** (acute) (cerebral) (chronic) (granular) — *see* Encephalomyelitis
- **Ependymoblastoma**
  - specified site — *see* Neoplasm, malignant, by site
  - unspecified site C71.9
- **Ependymoma** (epithelial) (malignant)
  - anaplastic
    - specified site — *see* Neoplasm, malignant, by site
    - unspecified site C71.9
  - benign
    - specified site — *see* Neoplasm, benign, by site
    - unspecified site D33.2
  - myxopapillary D43.2
    - specified site — *see* Neoplasm, uncertain behavior, by site
    - unspecified site D43.2
  - papillary D43.2
    - specified site — *see* Neoplasm, uncertain behavior, by site
    - unspecified site D43.2
  - specified site — *see* Neoplasm, malignant, by site
  - unspecified site C71.9
- **Ependymopathy** G93.89
- **Ephelis, ephelides** L81.2
- **Epiblepharon** (congenital) Q1Ø.3
- **Epicanthus, epicanthic fold** (eyelid) (congenital) Q1Ø.3
- **Epicondylitis** (elbow)
  - lateral M77.1- ☑
  - medial M77.Ø- ☑
- **Epicystitis** — *see* Cystitis
- **Epidemic** — *see* condition
- **Epidermalization, cervix** — *see* Dysplasia, cervix
- **Epidermis, epidermal** — *see* condition
- **Epidermodysplasia verruciformis** BØ7.8
- **Epidermolysis**
  - bullosa (congenital) Q81.9
    - acquired L12.3Ø
      - drug-induced L12.31
      - specified cause NEC L12.35
    - dystrophica Q81.2
    - letalis Q81.1
    - simplex Q81.Ø
    - specified NEC Q81.8
  - necroticans combustiformis L51.2
    - due to drug — *see* Table of Drugs and Chemicals, by drug
- **Epidermophytid** — *see* Dermatophytosis
- **Epidermophytosis** (infected) — *see* Dermatophytosis
- **Epididymis** — *see* condition
- **Epididymitis** (acute) (nonvenereal) (recurrent) (residual) N45.1
  - with orchitis N45.3
  - blennorrhagic (gonococcal) A54.23
  - caseous (tuberculous) A18.15
  - chlamydial A56.19
  - filarial — *see also* Infestation, filarial B74.9 *[N51]*
  - gonococcal A54.23
  - syphilitic A52.76
  - tuberculous A18.15
- **Epididymo-orchitis** — *see also* Epididymitis N45.3
- **Epidural** — *see* condition
- **Epigastrium, epigastric** — *see* condition
- **Epigastrocele** — *see* Hernia, ventral
- **Epiglottis** — *see* condition
- **Epiglottitis, epiglottiditis** (acute) JØ5.1Ø
  - with obstruction JØ5.11
  - chronic J37.Ø
- **Epignathus** Q89.4
- **Epilepsia partialis continua** — *see also* Kozhevnikof's epilepsy G4Ø.1- ☑
- **Epilepsy, epileptic, epilepsia** (attack) (cerebral) (convulsion) (fit) (seizure) G4Ø.9Ø9

Note: the following terms are to be considered equivalent to intractable: pharmacoresistant (pharmacologically resistant), treatment resistant, refractory (medically) and poorly controlled

- **Epilepsy, epileptic, epilepsia** (continued)
  - with
    - complex partial seizures — *see* Epilepsy, localization-related, symptomatic, with complex partial seizures
    - grand mal seizures on awakening — *see* Epilepsy, generalized, specified NEC
    - myoclonic absences — *see* Epilepsy, generalized, specified NEC
    - myoclonic-astatic seizures — *see* Epilepsy, generalized, specified NEC
    - simple partial seizures — *see* Epilepsy, localization-related, symptomatic, with simple partial seizures
  - akinetic — *see* Epilepsy, generalized, specified NEC
- **Epilepsy, epileptic, epilepsia** — *continued*
  - benign childhood with centrotemporal EEG spikes — *see* Epilepsy, localization-related, idiopathic
  - benign myoclonic in infancy G4Ø.8Ø- ☑
  - Bravais-jacksonian — *see* Epilepsy, localization-related, symptomatic, with simple partial seizures
  - childhood
    - with occipital EEG paroxysms — *see* Epilepsy, localization-related, idiopathic
    - absence G4Ø.AØ9 (*following* G4Ø.3)
      - intractable G4Ø.A19 (*following* G4Ø.3)
        - with status epilepticus G4Ø.A11 (*following* G4Ø.3)
        - without status epilepticus G4Ø.A19 (*following* G4Ø.3)
      - not intractable G4Ø.AØ9 (*following* G4Ø.3)
        - with status epilepticus G4Ø.AØ1 (*following* G4Ø.3)
        - without status epilepticus G4Ø.AØ9 (*following* G4Ø.3)
  - climacteric — *see* Epilepsy, specified NEC
  - cysticercosis B69.Ø
  - deterioration (mental) FØ6.8
  - due to syphilis A52.19
  - focal — *see* Epilepsy, localization-related, symptomatic, with simple partial seizures
  - generalized
    - idiopathic G4Ø.3Ø9
      - intractable G4Ø.319
        - with status epilepticus G4Ø.311
        - without status epilepticus G4Ø.319
      - not intractable G4Ø.3Ø9
        - with status epilepticus G4Ø.3Ø1
        - without status epilepticus G4Ø.3Ø9
    - specified NEC G4Ø.4Ø9
      - intractable G4Ø.419
        - with status epilepticus G4Ø.411
        - without status epilepticus G4Ø.419
      - not intractable G4Ø.4Ø9
        - with status epilepticus G4Ø.4Ø1
        - without status epilepticus G4Ø.4Ø9
  - impulsive petit mal — *see* Epilepsy, juvenile myoclonic
  - intractable G4Ø.919
    - with status epilepticus G4Ø.911
    - without status epilepticus G4Ø.919
  - juvenile absence G4Ø.AØ9 (*following* G4Ø.3)
    - intractable G4Ø.A19 (*following* G4Ø.3)
      - with status epilepticus G4Ø.A11 (*following* G4Ø.3)
      - without status epilepticus G4Ø.A19 (*following* G4Ø.3)
    - not intractable G4Ø.AØ9 (*following* G4Ø.3)
      - with status epilepticus G4Ø.AØ1 (*following* G4Ø.3)
      - without status epilepticus G4Ø.AØ9 (*following* G4Ø.3)
  - juvenile myoclonic G4Ø.BØ9 (*following* G4Ø.3)
    - intractable G4Ø.B19 (*following* G4Ø.3)
      - with status epilepticus G4Ø.B11 (*following* G4Ø.3)
      - without status epilepticus G4Ø.B19 (*following* G4Ø.3)
    - not intractable G4Ø.BØ9 (*following* G4Ø.3)
      - with status epilepticus G4Ø.BØ1 (*following* G4Ø.3)
      - without status epilepticus G4Ø.BØ9 (*following* G4Ø.3)
  - localization-related (focal) (partial)
    - idiopathic G4Ø.ØØ9
      - with seizures of localized onset G4Ø.ØØ9
        - intractable G4Ø.Ø19
          - with status epilepticus G4Ø.Ø11
          - without status epilepticus G4Ø.Ø19
        - not intractable G4Ø.ØØ9
          - with status epilepticus G4Ø.ØØ1
          - without status epilepticus G4Ø.ØØ9
    - symptomatic
      - with complex partial seizures G4Ø.2Ø9
        - intractable G4Ø.219
          - with status epilepticus G4Ø.211
          - without status epilepticus G4Ø.219
        - not intractable G4Ø.2Ø9
          - with status epilepticus G4Ø.2Ø1
          - without status epilepticus G4Ø.2Ø9
      - with simple partial seizures G4Ø.1Ø9
        - intractable G4Ø.119
          - with status epilepticus G4Ø.111
          - without status epilepticus G4Ø.119
        - not intractable G4Ø.1Ø9
          - with status epilepticus G4Ø.1Ø1
          - without status epilepticus G4Ø.1Ø9

Epilepsy, epileptic, epilepsia — *continued*
myoclonus, myoclonic — *see also* Epilepsy, generalized, specified NEC
progressive — *see* Epilepsy, generalized, idiopathic
severe, in infancy (SMEI) G4Ø.83- ☑
not intractable G4Ø.9Ø9
with status epilepticus G4Ø.9Ø1
without status epilepticus G4Ø.9Ø9
on awakening — *see* Epilepsy, generalized, specified NEC
parasitic NOS B71.9 *[G94]*
partialis continua — *see also* Kozhevnikof's epilepsy G4Ø.1- ☑
peripheral — *see* Epilepsy, specified NEC
polymorphic, in infancy (PMEI) G4Ø.83- ☑
procursiva — *see* Epilepsy, localization-related, symptomatic, with simple partial seizures
progressive (familial) myoclonic — *see* Epilepsy, generalized, idiopathic
reflex — *see* Epilepsy, specified NEC
related to
alcohol G4Ø.5Ø9
not intractable G4Ø.5Ø9
with status epilepticus G4Ø.5Ø1
without status epliepticus G4Ø.5Ø9
drugs G4Ø.5Ø9
not intractable G4Ø.5Ø9
with status epilepticus G4Ø.5Ø1
without status epliepticus G4Ø.5Ø9
external causes G4Ø.5Ø9
not intractable G4Ø.5Ø9
with status epilepticus G4Ø.5Ø1
without status epliepticus G4Ø.5Ø9
hormonal changes G4Ø.5Ø9
not intractable G4Ø.5Ø9
with status epilepticus G4Ø.5Ø1
without status epliepticus G4Ø.5Ø9
sleep deprivation G4Ø.5Ø9
not intractable G4Ø.5Ø9
with status epilepticus G4Ø.5Ø1
without status epliepticus G4Ø.5Ø9
stress G4Ø.5Ø9
not intractable G4Ø.5Ø9
with status epilepticus G4Ø.5Ø1
without status epliepticus G4Ø.5Ø9
somatomotor — *see* Epilepsy, localization-related, symptomatic, with simple partial seizures
somatosensory — *see* Epilepsy, localization-related, symptomatic, with simple partial seizures
spasms G4Ø.822
intractable G4Ø.824
with status epilepticus G4Ø.823
without status epilepticus G4Ø.824
not intractable G4Ø.822
with status epilepticus G4Ø.821
without status epilepticus G4Ø.822
specified NEC G4Ø.8Ø2
intractable G4Ø.8Ø4
with status epilepticus G4Ø.8Ø3
without status epilepticus G4Ø.8Ø4
not intractable G4Ø.8Ø2
with status epilepticus G4Ø.8Ø1
without status epilepticus G4Ø.8Ø2
syndromes
generalized
idiopathic G4Ø.3Ø9
intractable G4Ø.319
with status epilepticus G4Ø.311
without status epilepticus G4Ø.319
not intractable G4Ø.3Ø9
with status epilepticus G4Ø.3Ø1
without status epilepticus G4Ø.3Ø9
specified NEC G4Ø.4Ø9
intractable G4Ø.419
with status epilepticus G4Ø.411
without status epilepticus G4Ø.419
not intractable G4Ø.4Ø9
with status epilepticus G4Ø.4Ø1
without status epilepticus G4Ø.4Ø9
localization-related (focal) (partial)
idiopathic G4Ø.ØØ9
with seizures of localized onset G4Ø.ØØ9
intractable G4Ø.Ø19
with status epilepticus G4Ø.Ø11
without status epilepticus G4Ø.Ø19
not intractable G4Ø.ØØ9
with status epilepticus G4Ø.ØØ1
without status epilepticus G4Ø.ØØ9

Epilepsy, epileptic, epilepsia — *continued*
syndromes — *continued*
localization-related — *continued*
symptomatic
with complex partial seizures G4Ø.2Ø9
intractable G4Ø.219
with status epilepticus G4Ø.211
without status epilepticus G4Ø.219
not intractable G4Ø.2Ø9
with status epilepticus G4Ø.2Ø1
without status epilepticus G4Ø.2Ø9
with simple partial seizures G4Ø.1Ø9
intractable G4Ø.119
with status epilepticus G4Ø.111
without status epilepticus G4Ø.119
not intractable G4Ø.1Ø9
with status epilepticus G4Ø.1Ø1
without status epilepticus G4Ø.1Ø9
specified NEC G4Ø.8Ø2
intractable G4Ø.8Ø4
with status epilepticus G4Ø.8Ø3
without status epilepticus G4Ø.8Ø4
not intractable G4Ø.8Ø2
with status epilepticus G4Ø.8Ø1
without status epilepticus G4Ø.8Ø2
tonic (-clonic) — *see* Epilepsy, generalized, specified NEC
twilight FØ5
uncinate (gyrus) — *see* Epilepsy, localization-related, symptomatic, with complex partial seizures
Unverricht (-Lundborg) (familial myoclonic) — *see* Epilepsy, generalized, idiopathic
visceral — *see* Epilepsy, specified NEC
visual — *see* Epilepsy, specified NEC
Epiloia Q85.1
Epimenorrhea N92.Ø
Epipharyngitis — *see* Nasopharyngitis
Epiphora HØ4.2Ø- ☑
due to
excess lacrimation HØ4.21- ☑
insufficient drainage HØ4.22- ☑
Epiphyseal arrest — *see* Arrest, epiphyseal
Epiphyseolysis, epiphysiolysis — *see* Osteochondropathy
Epiphysitis — *see also* Osteochondropathy
juvenile M92.9
syphilitic (congenital) A5Ø.Ø2
Epiplocele — *see* Hernia, abdomen
Epiploitis — *see* Peritonitis
Epiplosarcomphalocele — *see* Hernia, umbilicus
Episcleritis (suppurative) H15.1Ø- ☑
in (due to)
syphilis A52.71
tuberculosis A18.51
nodular H15.12- ☑
periodica fugax H15.11- ☑
angioneurotic — *see* Edema, angioneurotic
syphilitic (late) A52.71
tuberculous A18.51
Episode
affective, mixed F39
depersonalization (in neurotic state) F48.1
depressive F32.A
major F32.9
mild F32.Ø
moderate F32.1
severe (without psychotic symptoms) F32.2
with psychotic symptoms F32.3
recurrent F33.9
brief F33.8
specified NEC F32.89
hypomanic F3Ø.8
manic F3Ø.9
with
psychotic symptoms F3Ø.2
remission (full) F3Ø.4
partial F3Ø.3
other specified F3Ø.8
recurrent F31.89
without psychotic symptoms F3Ø.1Ø
mild F3Ø.11
moderate F3Ø.12
severe (without psychotic symptoms) F3Ø.13
with psychotic symptoms F3Ø.2
psychotic F23
organic FØ6.8
schizophrenic (acute) NEC, brief F23
Epispadias (female) (male) Q64.Ø

Episplenitis D73.89
Epistaxis (multiple) RØ4.Ø
hereditary I78.Ø
vicarious menstruation N94.89
Epithelioma (malignant) — *see also* Neoplasm, malignant, by site
adenoides cysticum — *see* Neoplasm, skin, benign
basal cell — *see* Neoplasm, skin, malignant
benign — *see* Neoplasm, benign, by site
Bowen's — *see* Neoplasm, skin, in situ
calcifying, of Malherbe — *see* Neoplasm, skin, benign
external site — *see* Neoplasm, skin, malignant
intraepidermal, Jadassohn — *see* Neoplasm, skin, benign
squamous cell — *see* Neoplasm, malignant, by site
Epitheliomatosis pigmented Q82.1
Epitheliopathy, multifocal placoid pigment H3Ø.14- ☑
Epithelium, epithelial — *see* condition
Epituberculosis (with atelectasis) (allergic) A15.7
Eponychia Q84.6
Epstein's
nephrosis or syndrome — *see* Nephrosis
pearl KØ9.8
Epulis (gingiva) (fibrous) (giant cell) KØ6.8
Equinia A24.Ø
Equinovarus (congenital) (talipes) Q66.Ø- ☑
acquired — *see* Deformity, limb, clubfoot
Equivalent
convulsive (abdominal) — *see* Epilepsy, specified NEC
epileptic (psychic) — *see* Epilepsy, localization-related, symptomatic, with complex partial seizures
Erb (-Duchenne) **paralysis** (birth injury) (newborn) P14.Ø
Erb-Goldflam disease or syndrome G7Ø.ØØ
with exacerbation (acute) G7Ø.Ø1
in crisis G7Ø.Ø1
Erb's
disease G71.Ø2
palsy, paralysis (brachial) (birth) (newborn) P14.Ø
spinal (spastic) syphilitic A52.17
pseudohypertrophic muscular dystrophy G71.Ø2
Erdheim's syndrome (acromegalic macrospondylitis) E22.Ø
Erection, painful (persistent) — *see* Priapism
Ergosterol deficiency (vitamin D) E55.9
with
adult osteomalacia M83.8
rickets — *see* Rickets
Ergotism — *see also* Poisoning, food, noxious, plant
from ergot used as drug (migraine therapy) — *see* Table of Drugs and Chemicals
Erosio interdigitalis blastomycetica B37.2
Erosion
artery I77.2
without rupture I77.89
bone — *see* Disorder, bone, density and structure, specified NEC
bronchus J98.Ø9
cartilage (joint) — *see* Disorder, cartilage, specified type NEC
cervix (uteri) (acquired) (chronic) (congenital) N86
with cervicitis N72
cornea (nontraumatic) — *see* Ulcer, cornea
recurrent H18.83- ☑
traumatic — *see* Abrasion, cornea
dental (idiopathic) (occupational) (due to diet, drugs or vomiting) KØ3.2
duodenum, postpyloric — *see* Ulcer, duodenum
esophagus K22.1Ø
with bleeding K22.11
gastric — *see* Ulcer, stomach
gastrojejunal — *see* Ulcer, gastrojejunal
implanted mesh — *see* Complications, prosthetic device or implant, mesh
intestine K63.3
lymphatic vessel I89.8
pylorus, pyloric (ulcer) — *see* Ulcer, stomach
spine, aneurysmal A52.Ø9
stomach — *see* Ulcer, stomach
subcutaneous device pocket
nervous system prosthetic device, implant, or graft T85.89Ø ☑
other internal prosthetic device, implant, or graft T85.898 ☑
teeth (idiopathic) (occupational) (due to diet, drugs or vomiting) KØ3.2
urethra N36.8

- **Erosion** — *continued*
  - uterus N85.8
- **Erotomania** F52.8
- **Error**
  - metabolism, inborn — *see* Disorder, metabolism
  - refractive — *see* Disorder, refraction
- **Eructation** R14.2
  - nervous or psychogenic F45.8
- **Eruption**
  - creeping B76.9
  - drug (generalized) (taken internally) L27.Ø
    - fixed L27.1
    - in contact with skin — *see* Dermatitis, due to drugs
    - localized L27.1
  - Hutchinson, summer L56.4
  - Kaposi's varicelliform BØØ.Ø
  - napkin L22
  - polymorphous light (sun) L56.4
  - recalcitrant pustular L13.8
  - ringed R23.8
  - skin (nonspecific) R21
    - creeping (meaning hookworm) B76.9
    - due to inoculation/vaccination (generalized) — *see also* Dermatitis, due to, vaccine L27.Ø
      - localized L27.1
    - erysipeloid A26.Ø
    - feigned L98.1
    - Kaposi's varicelliform BØØ.Ø
    - lichenoid L28.Ø
    - meaning dermatitis — *see* Dermatitis
    - toxic NEC L53.Ø
  - tooth, teeth, abnormal (incomplete) (late) (premature) (sequence) KØØ.6
  - vesicular R23.8
- **Erysipelas** (gangrenous) (infantile) (newborn) (phlegmonous) (suppurative) A46
  - external ear A46 *[H62.4Ø]*
  - puerperal, postpartum O86.89
- **Erysipeloid** A26.9
  - cutaneous (Rosenbach's) A26.Ø
  - disseminated A26.8
  - sepsis A26.7
  - specified NEC A26.8
- **Erythema, erythematous** (infectional) (inflammation) L53.9
  - ab igne L59.Ø
  - annulare (centrifugum) (rheumaticum) L53.1
  - arthriticum epidemicum A25.1
  - brucellum — *see* Brucellosis
  - chronic figurate NEC L53.3
  - chronicum migrans (Borrelia burgdorferi) A69.2Ø
  - diaper L22
  - due to
    - chemical NEC L53.Ø
      - in contact with skin L24.5
    - drug (internal use) — *see* Dermatitis, due to, drugs
  - elevatum diutinum L95.1
  - endemic E52
  - epidemic, arthritic A25.1
  - figuratum perstans L53.3
  - gluteal L22
  - heat — *code by site under* Burn, first degree
  - ichthyosiforme congenitum bullous Q8Ø.3
  - in diseases classified elsewhere L54
  - induratum (nontuberculous) L52
    - tuberculous A18.4
  - infectiosum BØ8.3
  - intertrigo L3Ø.4
  - iris L51.9
  - marginatum L53.2
    - in (due to) acute rheumatic fever IØØ
  - medicamentosum — *see* Dermatitis, due to, drugs
  - migrans A26.Ø
    - chronicum A69.2Ø
    - tongue K14.1
  - multiforme (major) (minor) L51.9
    - bullous, bullosum L51.1
    - conjunctiva L51.1
    - nonbullous L51.Ø
    - pemphigoides L12.Ø
    - specified NEC L51.8
  - napkin L22
  - neonatorum P83.88
    - toxic P83.1
  - nodosum L52
    - tuberculous A18.4
  - palmar L53.8
  - pernio T69.1 ☑
- **Erythema, erythematous** — *continued*
  - rash, newborn P83.88
  - scarlatiniform (recurrent) (exfoliative) L53.8
  - solare L55.Ø
  - specified NEC L53.8
  - toxic, toxicum NEC L53.Ø
    - newborn P83.1
  - tuberculous (primary) A18.4
- **Erythematous, erythematosus** — *see* condition
- **Erythermalgia** (primary) I73.81
- **Erythralgia** I73.81
- **Erythrasma** LØ8.1
- **Erythredema** (polyneuropathy) — *see* Poisoning, mercury
- **Erythremia** (acute) C94.Ø- ☑
  - chronic D45
  - secondary D75.1
- **Erythroblastopenia** — *see also* Aplasia, red cell D6Ø.9
  - congenital D61.Ø1
- **Erythroblastophthisis** D61.Ø9
- **Erythroblastosis** (fetalis) (newborn) P55.9
  - due to
    - ABO (antibodies) (incompatibility) (isoimmunization) P55.1
    - Rh (antibodies) (incompatibility) (isoimmunization) P55.Ø
- **Erythrocyanosis** (crurum) I73.89
- **Erythrocythemia** — *see* Erythremia
- **Erythrocytosis** (megalosplenic) (secondary) D75.1
  - familial D75.Ø
  - oval, hereditary — *see* Elliptocytosis
  - secondary D75.1
  - stress D75.1
- **Erythroderma** (secondary) — *see also* Erythema L53.9
  - bullous ichthyosiform, congenital Q8Ø.3
  - desquamativum L21.1
  - ichthyosiform, congenital (bullous) Q8Ø.3
  - neonatorum P83.88
  - psoriaticum L4Ø.8
- **Erythrodysesthesia, palmar plantar** (PPE) L27.1
- **Erythrogenesis imperfecta** D61.Ø9
- **Erythroleukemia** C94.Ø- ☑
- **Erythromelalgia** I73.81
- **Erythrophagocytosis** D75.89
- **Erythrophobia** F4Ø.298
- **Erythroplakia, oral epithelium, and tongue** K13.29
- **Erythroplasia** (Queyrat) DØ7.4
  - specified site — *see* Neoplasm, skin, in situ
  - unspecified site DØ7.4
- **Escherichia coli** (E. coli), **as cause of disease classified elsewhere** B96.2Ø
  - non-O157 Shiga toxin-producing (with known O group) B96.22
  - non-Shiga toxin-producing B96.29
  - O157 B96.21
  - O157 with confirmation of Shiga toxin when H antigen is unknown, or is not H7 B96.21
  - O157:H- (nonmotile) with confirmation of Shiga toxin B96.21
  - O157:H7 with or without confirmation of Shiga toxin-production B96.21
  - specified NEC B96.22
  - Shiga toxin-producing (with unspecified O group) (STEC) B96.23
  - specified NEC B96.29
- **Esophagismus** K22.4
- **Esophagitis** (acute) (alkaline) (chemical) (chronic) (infectional) (necrotic) (peptic) (postoperative) (without bleeding) K2Ø.9Ø
  - with bleeding K2Ø.91
  - candidal B37.81
  - due to gastrointestinal reflux disease (without bleeding) K21.ØØ
    - with bleeding K21.Ø1
  - eosinophilic K2Ø.Ø
  - reflux K21.ØØ
  - specified NEC (without bleeding) K2Ø.8Ø
    - with bleeding K2Ø.81
  - tuberculous A18.83
  - ulcerative K22.1Ø
    - with bleeding K22.11
- **Esophagocele** K22.5
- **Esophagomalacia** K22.89
- **Esophagospasm** K22.4
- **Esophagostenosis** K22.2
- **Esophagostomiasis** B81.8
- **Esophagotracheal** — *see* condition
- **Esophagus** — *see* condition
- **Esophoria** H5Ø.51
  - convergence, excess H51.12
  - divergence, insufficiency H51.8
- **Esotropia** — *see* Strabismus, convergent concomitant
- **Espundia** B55.2
- **Essential** — *see* condition
- **Esthesioneuroblastoma** C3Ø.Ø
- **Esthesioneurocytoma** C3Ø.Ø
- **Esthesioneuroepithelioma** C3Ø.Ø
- **Esthiomene** A55
- **Estivo-autumnal malaria** (fever) B5Ø.9
- **Estrangement** (marital) Z63.5
  - parent-child NEC Z62.89Ø
- **Estriasis** — *see* Myiasis
- **Ethanolism** — *see* Alcoholism
- **Etherism** — *see* Dependence, drug, inhalant
- **Ethmoid, ethmoidal** — *see* condition
- **Ethmoiditis** (chronic) (nonpurulent) (purulent) — *see also* Sinusitis, ethmoidal
  - influenzal — *see* Influenza, with, respiratory manifestations NEC
  - Woakes' J33.1
- **Ethylism** — *see* Alcoholism
- **Eulenburg's disease** (congenital paramyotonia) G71.19
- **Eumycetoma** B47.Ø
- **Eunuchoidism** E29.1
  - hypogonadotropic E23.Ø
- **European blastomycosis** — *see* Cryptococcosis
- **Eustachian** — *see* condition
- **Evaluation** (for) (of)
  - development state
    - adolescent ZØØ.3
    - period of
      - delayed growth in childhood ZØØ.7Ø
        - with abnormal findings ZØØ.71
      - rapid growth in childhood ZØØ.2
    - puberty ZØØ.3
  - growth and developmental state (period of rapid growth) ZØØ.2
    - delayed growth ZØØ.7Ø
      - with abnormal findings ZØØ.71
  - mental health (status) ZØØ.8
    - requested by authority ZØ4.6
  - period of
    - delayed growth in childhood ZØØ.7Ø
      - with abnormal findings ZØØ.71
    - rapid growth in childhood ZØØ.2
  - suspected condition — *see* Observation
- **Evans syndrome** D69.41
- **Event**
  - apparent life threatening in newborn and infant (ALTE) R68.13
  - brief resolved unexplained event (BRUE) R68.13
- **Eventration** — *see also* Hernia, ventral
  - colon into chest — *see* Hernia, diaphragm
  - diaphragm (congenital) Q79.1
- **Eversion**
  - bladder N32.89
  - cervix (uteri) N86
    - with cervicitis N72
  - foot NEC — *see also* Deformity, valgus, ankle
    - congenital Q66.6
  - punctum lacrimale (postinfectional) (senile) HØ4.52- ☑
  - ureter (meatus) N28.89
  - urethra (meatus) N36.8
  - uterus N81.4
- **Evidence**
  - cytologic
    - of malignancy on anal smear R85.614
    - of malignancy on cervical smear R87.614
    - of malignancy on vaginal smear R87.624
- **Evisceration**
  - birth injury P15.8
  - traumatic NEC
    - eye — *see* Enucleated eye
- **Evulsion** — *see* Avulsion
- **Ewing's sarcoma or tumor** — *see* Neoplasm, bone, malignant
- **Examination** (for) (following) (general) (of) (routine) ZØØ.ØØ
  - with abnormal findings ZØØ.Ø1
  - abuse, physical (alleged), ruled out
    - adult ZØ4.71
    - child ZØ4.72
  - adolescent (development state) ZØØ.3
  - alleged rape or sexual assault (victim), ruled out
    - adult ZØ4.41
    - child ZØ4.42

- **Examination** — *continued*
  - allergy Z01.82
  - annual (adult) (periodic) (physical) Z00.00
    - with abnormal findings Z00.01
    - gynecological Z01.419
      - with abnormal findings Z01.411
  - antibody response Z01.84
  - blood — *see* Examination, laboratory
  - blood pressure Z01.30
    - with abnormal findings Z01.31
  - cancer staging — *see* Neoplasm, malignant, by site
  - cervical Papanicolaou smear Z12.4
    - as part of routine gynecological examination Z01.419
      - with abnormal findings Z01.411
  - child (over 28 days old) Z00.129
    - with abnormal findings Z00.121
    - under 28 days old — *see* Newborn, examination
  - clinical research control or normal comparison (control) (participant) Z00.6
  - contraceptive (drug) maintenance (routine) Z30.8
    - device (intrauterine) Z30.431
  - dental Z01.20
    - with abnormal findings Z01.21
  - developmental — *see* Examination, child
  - donor (potential) Z00.5
  - ear Z01.10
    - with abnormal findings NEC Z01.118
  - eye Z01.00
    - with abnormal findings Z01.01
    - following failed vision screening Z01.020
      - with abnormal findings Z01.021
  - follow-up (routine) (following) Z09
    - chemotherapy NEC Z09
      - malignant neoplasm Z08
    - fracture Z09
    - malignant neoplasm Z08
    - postpartum Z39.2
    - psychotherapy Z09
    - radiotherapy NEC Z09
      - malignant neoplasm Z08
    - surgery NEC Z09
      - malignant neoplasm Z08
  - following
    - accident NEC Z04.3
      - transport Z04.1
      - work Z04.2
    - assault, alleged, ruled out
      - adult Z04.71
      - child Z04.72
    - motor vehicle accident Z04.1
    - treatment (for) Z09
      - combined NEC Z09
        - fracture Z09
        - malignant neoplasm Z08
      - malignant neoplasm Z08
      - mental disorder Z09
      - specified condition NEC Z09
  - forced sexual exploitation Z04.81
  - forced labor exploitation Z04.82
  - gynecological Z01.419
    - with abnormal findings Z01.411
    - for contraceptive maintenance Z30.8
  - health — *see* Examination, medical
  - hearing Z01.10
    - with abnormal findings NEC Z01.118
    - following failed hearing screening Z01.110
    - infant or child (over 28 days old) Z00.129
      - with abnormal findings Z00.121
  - immunity status testing Z01.84
  - laboratory (as part of a general medical examination) Z00.00
    - with abnormal findings Z00.01
    - preprocedural Z01.812
  - lactating mother Z39.1
  - medical (adult) (for) (of) Z00.00
    - with abnormal findings Z00.01
    - administrative purpose only Z02.9
      - specified NEC Z02.89
    - admission to
      - armed forces Z02.3
      - old age home Z02.2
      - prison Z02.89
      - residential institution Z02.2
      - school Z02.0
        - following illness or medical treatment Z02.0
      - summer camp Z02.89
    - adoption Z02.82
    - blood alcohol or drug level Z02.83

- **Examination** — *continued*
  - medical — *continued*
    - camp (summer) Z02.89
    - clinical research, normal subject (control) (participant) Z00.6
    - control subject in clinical research (normal comparison) (participant) Z00.6
    - donor (potential) Z00.5
    - driving license Z02.4
    - general (adult) Z00.00
      - with abnormal findings Z00.01
    - immigration Z02.89
    - insurance purposes Z02.6
    - marriage Z02.89
    - medicolegal reasons NEC Z04.89
    - naturalization Z02.89
    - participation in sport Z02.5
    - paternity testing Z02.81
    - population survey Z00.8
    - pre-employment Z02.1
    - pre-operative — *see* Examination, pre-procedural
    - pre-procedural
      - cardiovascular Z01.810
      - respiratory Z01.811
      - specified NEC Z01.818
    - preschool children
      - for admission to school Z02.0
    - prisoners
      - for entrance into prison Z02.89
    - recruitment for armed forces Z02.3
    - specified NEC Z00.8
    - sport competition Z02.5
  - medicolegal reason NEC Z04.89
    - following
      - forced sexual exploitation Z04.81
      - forced labor exploitation Z04.82
  - newborn — *see* Newborn, examination
  - pelvic (annual) (periodic) Z01.419
    - with abnormal findings Z01.411
  - period of rapid growth in childhood Z00.2
  - periodic (adult) (annual) (routine) Z00.00
    - with abnormal findings Z00.01
  - physical (adult) — *see also* Examination, medical Z00.00
    - sports Z02.5
  - postpartum
    - immediately after delivery Z39.0
    - routine follow-up Z39.2
  - pre-chemotherapy (antineoplastic) Z01.818
  - prenatal (normal pregnancy) — *see also* Pregnancy, normal Z34.9- ☑
  - pre-procedural (pre-operative)
    - cardiovascular Z01.810
    - laboratory Z01.812
    - respiratory Z01.811
    - specified NEC Z01.818
  - prior to chemotherapy (antineoplastic) Z01.818
  - psychiatric NEC Z00.8
    - follow-up not needing further care Z09
    - requested by authority Z04.6
  - radiological (as part of a general medical examination) Z00.00
    - with abnormal findings Z00.01
  - repeat cervical smear to confirm findings of recent normal smear following initial abnormal smear Z01.42
  - skin (hypersensitivity) Z01.82
  - special — *see also* Examination, by type Z01.89
    - specified type NEC Z01.89
  - specified type or reason NEC Z04.89
  - teeth Z01.20
    - with abnormal findings Z01.21
  - urine — *see* Examination, laboratory
  - vision Z01.00
    - with abnormal findings Z01.01
    - following failed vision screening Z01.020
      - with abnormal findings Z01.021
    - infant or child (over 28 days old) Z00.129
      - with abnormal findings Z00.121
- **Exanthem, exanthema** — *see also* Rash
  - with enteroviral vesicular stomatitis B08.4
  - Boston A88.0
  - epidemic with meningitis A88.0 *[G02]*
  - subitum B08.20
    - due to human herpesvirus 6 B08.21
    - due to human herpesvirus 7 B08.22
  - viral, virus B09
    - specified type NEC B08.8

- **Excess, excessive, excessively**
  - alcohol level in blood R78.0
  - androgen (ovarian) E28.1
  - attrition, tooth, teeth K03.0
  - carotene, carotin (dietary) E67.1
  - cold, effects of T69.9 ☑
    - specified effect NEC T69.8 ☑
  - convergence H51.12
  - crying
    - in child, adolescent, or adult R45.83
    - in infant R68.11
  - development, breast N62
  - divergence H51.8
  - drinking (alcohol) NEC (without dependence) F10.10
    - habitual (continual) (without remission) F10.20
  - eating R63.2
  - estrogen E28.0
  - fat — *see also* Obesity
    - in heart — *see* Degeneration, myocardial
    - localized E65
  - foreskin N47.8
  - gas R14.0
  - glucagon E16.3
  - heat — *see* Heat
  - intermaxillary vertical dimension of fully erupted teeth M26.37
  - interocclusal distance of fully erupted teeth M26.37
  - kalium E87.5
  - large
    - colon K59.39
      - congenital Q43.8
    - infant P08.0
    - organ or site, congenital NEC — *see* Anomaly, by site
  - long
    - organ or site, congenital NEC — *see* Anomaly, by site
  - menstruation (with regular cycle) N92.0
    - with irregular cycle N92.1
  - napping Z72.821
  - natrium E87.0
  - number of teeth K00.1
  - nutrient (dietary) NEC R63.2
  - potassium (K) E87.5
  - salivation K11.7
  - secretion — *see also* Hypersecretion
    - milk O92.6
    - sputum R09.3
    - sweat R61
  - sexual drive F52.8
  - short
    - organ or site, congenital NEC — *see* Anomaly, by site
    - umbilical cord in labor or delivery O69.3 ☑
  - skin L98.7
    - and subcutaneous tissue L98.7
    - eyelid (acquired) — *see* Blepharochalasis
      - congenital Q10.3
  - sodium (Na) E87.0
  - spacing of fully erupted teeth M26.32
  - sputum R09.3
  - sweating R61
  - thirst R63.1
    - due to deprivation of water T73.1 ☑
  - transportation time Z59.82
  - tuberosity of jaw M26.07
  - vitamin
    - A (dietary) E67.0
      - administered as drug (prolonged intake) — *see* Table of Drugs and Chemicals, vitamins, adverse effect
      - overdose or wrong substance given or taken — *see* Table of Drugs and Chemicals, vitamins, poisoning
    - D (dietary) E67.3
      - administered as drug (prolonged intake) — *see* Table of Drugs and Chemicals, vitamins, adverse effect
      - overdose or wrong substance given or taken — *see* Table of Drugs and Chemicals, vitamins, poisoning
  - weight
    - gain R63.5
    - loss R63.4
- **Excitability, abnormal, under minor stress** (personality disorder) F60.3
- **Excitation**
  - anomalous atrioventricular I45.6

Excitation — *continued*
- psychogenic F30.8
- reactive (from emotional stress, psychological trauma) F30.8

Excitement
- hypomanic F30.8
- manic F30.9
- mental, reactive (from emotional stress, psychological trauma) F30.8
- state, reactive (from emotional stress, psychological trauma) F30.8

Excoriation (traumatic) — *see also* Abrasion
- neurotic L98.1
- skin picking disorder F42.4

Exfoliation
- due to erythematous conditions according to extent of body surface involved L49.0
  - 10-19 percent of body surface L49.1
  - 20-29 percent of body surface L49.2
  - 30-39 percent of body surface L49.3
  - 40-49 percent of body surface L49.4
  - 50-59 percent of body surface L49.5
  - 60-69 percent of body surface L49.6
  - 70-79 percent of body surface L49.7
  - 80-89 percent of body surface L49.8
  - 90-99 percent of body surface L49.9
  - less than 10 percent of body surface L49.0
- teeth, due to systemic causes K08.0

Exfoliative — *see* condition

Exhaustion, exhaustive (physical NEC) R53.83
- battle F43.0
- cardiac — *see* Failure, heart
- delirium F43.0
- due to
  - cold T69.8 ☑
  - excessive exertion T73.3 ☑
  - exposure T73.2 ☑
  - neurasthenia F48.8
- heart — *see* Failure, heart
- heat — *see also* Heat, exhaustion T67.5 ☑
  - due to
    - salt depletion T67.4 ☑
    - water depletion T67.3 ☑
- maternal, complicating delivery O75.81
- mental F48.8
- myocardium, myocardial — *see* Failure, heart
- nervous F48.8
- old age R54
- psychogenic F48.8
- psychosis F43.0
- senile R54
- vital NEC Z73.0

Exhibitionism F65.2

Exocervicitis — *see* Cervicitis

Exomphalos Q79.2
- meaning hernia — *see* Hernia, umbilicus

Exophoria H50.52
- convergence, insufficiency H51.11
- divergence, excess H51.8

Exophthalmos H05.2- ☑
- congenital Q15.8
- constant NEC H05.24- ☑
- displacement, globe — *see* Displacement, globe
- due to thyrotoxicosis (hyperthyroidism) — *see* Hyperthyroidism, with, goiter (diffuse)
- dysthyroid — *see* Hyperthyroidism, with, goiter (diffuse)
- goiter — *see* Hyperthyroidism, with, goiter (diffuse)
- intermittent NEC H05.25- ☑
- malignant — *see* Hyperthyroidism, with, goiter (diffuse)
- orbital
  - edema — *see* Edema, orbit
  - hemorrhage — *see* Hemorrhage, orbit
- pulsating NEC H05.26- ☑
- thyrotoxic, thyrotropic — *see* Hyperthyroidism, with, goiter (diffuse)

Exostosis — *see also* Disorder, bone
- cartilaginous — *see* Neoplasm, bone, benign
- congenital (multiple) Q78.6
- external ear canal H61.81- ☑
- gonococcal A54.49
- jaw (bone) M27.8
- multiple, congenital Q78.6
- orbit H05.35- ☑
- osteocartilaginous — *see* Neoplasm, bone, benign
- syphilitic A52.77

Exotropia — *see* Strabismus, divergent concomitant

Explanation of
- investigation finding Z71.2
- medication Z71.89

Exploitation
- labor
  - confirmed
    - adult forced T74.61 ☑
    - child forced T74.62 ☑
  - suspected
    - adult forced T76.61 ☑
    - child forced T76.62 ☑
- sexual
  - confirmed
    - adult forced T74.51 ☑
    - child T74.52 ☑
  - suspected
    - adult forced T76.51 ☑
    - child T76.52 ☑

Exposure (to) — *see also* Contact, with T75.89 ☑
- acariasis Z20.7
- AIDS virus Z20.6
- air pollution Z77.110
- algae and algae toxins Z77.121
- algae bloom Z77.121
- anthrax Z20.810
- aromatic amines Z77.020
- aromatic (hazardous) compounds NEC Z77.028
- aromatic dyes NOS Z77.028
- arsenic Z77.010
- asbestos Z77.090
- bacterial disease NEC Z20.818
- benzene Z77.021
- blue-green algae bloom Z77.121
- body fluids (potentially hazardous) Z77.21
- brown tide Z77.121
- chemicals (chiefly nonmedicinal) (hazardous) NEC Z77.098
- cholera Z20.09
- chromium compounds Z77.018
- cold, effects of T69.9 ☑
  - specified effect NEC T69.8 ☑
- communicable disease Z20.9
  - bacterial NEC Z20.818
  - specified NEC Z20.89
  - viral NEC Z20.828
  - Zika virus Z20.821
- coronavirus (disease) (novel) 2019 Z20.822
- COVID-19 Z20.822
- cyanobacteria bloom Z77.121
- disaster Z65.5
- discrimination Z60.5
- dyes Z77.098
- effects of T73.9 ☑
- environmental tobacco smoke (acute) (chronic) Z77.22
- Escherichia coli (E. coli) Z20.01
- exhaustion due to T73.2 ☑
- fiberglass — *see* Table of Drugs and Chemicals, fiberglass
- German measles Z20.4
- gonorrhea Z20.2
- hazardous metals NEC Z77.018
- hazardous substances NEC Z77.29
- hazards in the physical environment NEC Z77.128
- hazards to health NEC Z77.9
- human immunodeficiency virus (HIV) Z20.6
- human T-lymphotropic virus type-1 (HTLV-1) Z20.89
- implanted
  - mesh — *see* Complications, prosthetic device or implant, mesh
  - prosthetic materials NEC — *see* Complications, prosthetic materials NEC
- infestation (parasitic) NEC Z20.7
- intestinal infectious disease NEC Z20.09
  - Escherichia coli (E. coli) Z20.01
- lead Z77.011
- meningococcus Z20.811
- mold (toxic) Z77.120
- nickel dust Z77.018
- noise Z77.122
- occupational
  - air contaminants NEC Z57.39
  - dust Z57.2
  - environmental tobacco smoke Z57.31
  - extreme temperature Z57.6
  - noise Z57.0
  - radiation Z57.1
  - risk factors Z57.9
    - specified NEC Z57.8

Exposure — *continued*
- occupational — *continued*
  - toxic agents (gases) (liquids) (solids) (vapors) in agriculture Z57.4
  - toxic agents (gases) (liquids) (solids) (vapors) in industry NEC Z57.5
  - vibration Z57.7
- parasitic disease NEC Z20.7
- pediculosis Z20.7
- persecution Z60.5
- pfiesteria piscicida Z77.121
- poliomyelitis Z20.89
- pollution
  - air Z77.110
  - environmental NEC Z77.118
  - soil Z77.112
  - water Z77.111
- polycyclic aromatic hydrocarbons Z77.028
- prenatal (drugs) (toxic chemicals) — *see* Newborn, affected by, noxious substances transmitted via placenta or breast milk
- rabies Z20.3
- radiation, naturally occurring NEC Z77.123
- radon Z77.123
- red tide (Florida) Z77.121
- rubella Z20.4
- SARS-CoV-2 Z20.822
- second hand tobacco smoke (acute) (chronic) Z77.22
  - in the perinatal period P96.81
- sexually-transmitted disease Z20.2
- smallpox (laboratory) Z20.89
- syphilis Z20.2
- terrorism Z65.4
- torture Z65.4
- tuberculosis Z20.1
- uranium Z77.012
- varicella Z20.820
- venereal disease Z20.2
- viral disease NEC Z20.828
- war Z65.5
- water pollution Z77.111
- Zika virus Z20.821

Exsanguination — *see* Hemorrhage

Exstrophy
- abdominal contents Q45.8
- bladder Q64.10
  - cloacal Q64.12
  - specified type NEC Q64.19
  - supravesical fissure Q64.11

Extensive — *see* condition

Extra — *see also* Accessory
- marker chromosomes (normal individual) Q92.61
  - in abnormal individual Q92.62
- rib Q76.6
  - cervical Q76.5

Extrasystoles (supraventricular) I49.49
- atrial I49.1
- auricular I49.1
- junctional I49.2
- ventricular I49.3

Extrauterine gestation or pregnancy — *see* Pregnancy, by site

Extravasation
- blood R58
- chyle into mesentery I89.8
- pelvicalyceal N13.8
- pyelosinus N13.8
- urine (from ureter) R39.0
- vesicant agent
  - antineoplastic chemotherapy T80.810 ☑
  - other agent NEC T80.818 ☑

Extremity — *see* condition, limb

Extrophy — *see* Exstrophy

Extroversion
- bladder Q64.19
- uterus N81.4
  - complicating delivery O71.2
  - postpartal (old) N81.4

Extruded tooth (teeth) M26.34

Extrusion
- breast implant (prosthetic) T85.42 ☑
- eye implant (globe) (ball) T85.328 ☑
- intervertebral disc — *see* Displacement, intervertebral disc
- ocular lens implant (prosthetic) — *see* Complications, intraocular lens
- vitreous — *see* Prolapse, vitreous

Exudate
- pleural — *see* Effusion, pleura
- retina H35.89
- wound fluids L24.A9

Exudative — *see* condition
Eye, eyeball, eyelid — *see* condition
Eyestrain — *see* Disturbance, vision, subjective
Eyeworm disease of Africa B74.3

F

Faber's syndrome (achlorhydric anemia) D5Ø.9
Fabry (-Anderson) **disease** E75.21
Facet syndrome M47.89- ☑
Faciocephalalgia, autonomic — *see also* Neuropathy, peripheral, autonomic G9Ø.Ø9
Factor(s)
- psychic, associated with diseases classified elsewhere F54
- psychological
  - affecting physical conditions F54
  - or behavioral
    - affecting general medical condition F54
    - associated with disorders or diseases classified elsewhere F54

Fahr disease (of brain) G23.8
Fahr Volhard disease (of kidney) I12.- ☑
Failure, failed
- abortion — *see* Abortion, attempted
- aortic (valve) I35.8
  - rheumatic IØ6.8
- attempted abortion — *see* Abortion, attempted
- biventricular I5Ø.82
  - due to left heart failure I5Ø.814
- bone marrow — *see* Anemia, aplastic
- cardiac — *see* Failure, heart
- cardiorenal (chronic) — *see also* Failure, renal, and Failure, heart I5Ø.9
  - hypertensive I13.2
- cardiorespiratory — *see also* Failure, heart RØ9.2
- cardiovascular (chronic) — *see* Failure, heart
- cerebrovascular I67.9
- cervical dilatation in labor O62.Ø
- circulation, circulatory (peripheral) R57.9
  - newborn P29.89
- compensation — *see* Disease, heart
- compliance with medical treatment or regimen — *see* Noncompliance
- congestive — *see* Failure, heart, congestive
- dental implant (endosseous) M27.69
  - due to
    - failure of dental prosthesis M27.63
    - lack of attached gingiva M27.62
    - occlusal trauma (poor prosthetic design) M27.62
    - parafunctional habits M27.62
    - periodontal infection (peri-implantitis) M27.62
    - poor oral hygiene M27.62
  - osseointegration M27.61
    - due to
      - complications of systemic disease M27.61
      - poor bone quality M27.61
    - iatrogenic M27.61
  - post-osseointegration
    - biological M27.62
    - due to complications of systemic disease M27.62
    - iatrogenic M27.62
    - mechanical M27.63
  - pre-integration M27.61
  - pre-osseointegration M27.61
  - specified NEC M27.69
- descent of head (at term) of pregnancy (mother) O32.4 ☑
- endosseous dental implant — *see* Failure, dental implant
- engagement of head (term of pregnancy) (mother) O32.4 ☑
- erection (penile) — *see also* Dysfunction, sexual, male, erectile N52.9
  - nonorganic F52.21
- examination(s), anxiety concerning Z55.2
- expansion terminal respiratory units (newborn) (primary) P28.Ø
- forceps NOS (with subsequent cesarean delivery) O66.5
- gain weight (child over 28 days old) R62.51
  - adult R62.7
  - newborn P92.6
- genital response (male) F52.21
  - female F52.22

Failure, failed — *continued*
- heart (acute) (senile) (sudden) I5Ø.9
  - with
    - acute pulmonary edema — *see* Failure, ventricular, left
    - decompensation I5Ø.9
      - with
        - normal ejection fraction I5Ø.33
        - preserved ejection fraction I5Ø.33
        - reduced ejection fraction I5Ø.23
          - with diastolic dysfunction I5Ø.43
      - combined systolic and diastolic I5Ø.43
      - diastolic I5Ø.33
      - right I5Ø.813
      - systolic I5Ø.23
    - dilatation — *see* Disease, heart
    - hypertension — *see* Hypertension, heart
    - normal ejection fraction — *see* Failure, heart, diastolic
    - preserved ejection fraction — *see* Failure, heart, diastolic
    - reduced ejection fraction — *see* Failure, heart, systolic
  - arteriosclerotic I7Ø.9Ø
  - biventricular I5Ø.82
    - due to left heart failure I5Ø.814
  - combined left-right sided I5Ø.82
    - due to left heart failure I5Ø.814
  - compensated — *see also* Failure, heart, by type as diastolic or systolic, chronic I5Ø.9
  - complicating
    - anesthesia (general) (local) or other sedation
      - in labor and delivery O74.2
      - in pregnancy O29.12- ☑
      - postpartum, puerperal O89.1
    - delivery (cesarean) (instrumental) O75.4
  - congestive I5Ø.9
    - with rheumatic fever (conditions in IØØ)
      - active IØ1.8
      - inactive or quiescent (with chorea) IØ9.81
    - newborn P29.Ø
    - rheumatic (chronic) (inactive) (with chorea) IØ9.81
      - active or acute IØ1.8
        - with chorea IØ2.Ø
  - decompensated — *see also* Failure, heart, by type as diastolic or systolic, acute and chronic I5Ø.9
  - degenerative — *see* Degeneration, myocardial
  - diastolic (congestive) (left ventricular) I5Ø.3Ø
    - acute (congestive) I5Ø.31
      - and (on) chronic (congestive) I5Ø.33
    - chronic (congestive) I5Ø.32
      - and (on) acute (congestive) I5Ø.33
    - combined with systolic (congestive) I5Ø.4Ø
      - acute (congestive) I5Ø.41
        - and (on) chronic (congestive) I5Ø.43
      - chronic (congestive) I5Ø.42
        - and (on) acute (congestive) I5Ø.43
  - due to presence of cardiac prosthesis I97.13- ☑
  - end stage — *see also* Failure, heart, by type as diastolic or systolic, chronic I5Ø.84
  - following cardiac surgery I97.13- ☑
  - high output NOS I5Ø.83
  - hypertensive — *see* Hypertension, heart
  - left (ventricular) — *see also* Failure, ventricular, left
    - combined diastolic and systolic — *see* Failure, heart, diastolic, combined with systolic
    - diastolic — *see* Failure, heart, diastolic
    - systolic — *see* Failure, heart, systolic
  - low output (syndrome) NOS I5Ø.9
  - newborn P29.Ø
  - organic — *see* Disease, heart
  - peripartum O9Ø.3
  - postprocedural I97.13- ☑
  - rheumatic (chronic) (inactive) IØ9.9
  - right (isolated) (ventricular) I5Ø.81Ø
    - acute I5Ø.811
      - and (on) chronic I5Ø.813
    - chronic I5Ø.812
      - and acute I5Ø.813
    - secondary to left heart failure I5Ø.814
  - specified NEC I5Ø.89

Note: heart failure stages A, B, C, and D are based on the American College of Cardiology and American Heart Association stages of heart failure, which complement and should not be confused with the New York Heart Association Classification of Heart Failure, into Class I, Class II, Class III, and Class IV

Failure, failed — *continued*
- heart — *continued*
  - stage A Z91.89
  - stage B — *see also* Failure, heart, by type as diastolic or systolic I5Ø.9
  - stage C — *see also* Failure, heart, by type as diastolic or systolic I5Ø.9
  - stage D — *see also* Failure, heart, by type as diastolic or systolic, chronic I5Ø.84
  - systolic (congestive) (left ventricular) I5Ø.2Ø
    - acute (congestive) I5Ø.21
      - and (on) chronic (congestive) I5Ø.23
    - chronic (congestive) I5Ø.22
      - and (on) acute (congestive) I5Ø.23
    - combined with diastolic (congestive) I5Ø.4Ø
      - acute (congestive) I5Ø.41
        - and (on) chronic (congestive) I5Ø.43
      - chronic (congestive) I5Ø.42
        - and (on) acute (congestive) I5Ø.43
  - thyrotoxic — *see also* Thyrotoxicosis EØ5.9Ø *[I43]*
    - with
      - high output — *see also* Thyrotoxicosis I5Ø.83
      - thyroid storm EØ5.91 *[I43]*
        - high output — *see also* Thyrotoxicosis I5Ø.83
  - valvular — *see* Endocarditis
- hepatic K72.9Ø
  - with coma K72.91
  - acute or subacute K72.ØØ
    - with coma K72.Ø1
    - due to drugs K71.1Ø
      - with coma K71.11
  - alcoholic (acute) (chronic) (subacute) K7Ø.4Ø
    - with coma K7Ø.41
  - chronic K72.1Ø
    - with coma K72.11
    - due to drugs (acute) (subacute) (chronic) K71.1Ø
      - with coma K71.11
  - due to drugs (acute) (subacute) (chronic) K71.1Ø
    - with coma K71.11
  - postprocedural K91.82
- hepatorenal K76.7
- induction (of labor) O61.9
  - abortion — *see* Abortion, attempted
  - by
    - oxytocic drugs O61.Ø
    - prostaglandins O61.Ø
  - instrumental O61.1
  - mechanical O61.1
  - medical O61.Ø
  - specified NEC O61.8
  - surgical O61.1
- intubation during anesthesia T88.4 ☑
  - in pregnancy O29.6- ☑
  - labor and delivery O74.7
  - postpartum, puerperal O89.6
- involution, thymus (gland) E32.Ø
- kidney — *see also* Disease, kidney, chronic N19
  - acute — *see also* Failure, renal, acute N17.9
- lactation (complete) O92.3
  - partial O92.4
- Leydig's cell, adult E29.1
- liver — *see* Failure, hepatic
- menstruation at puberty N91.Ø
- mitral IØ5.8
- myocardial, myocardium — *see also* Failure, heart I5Ø.9
  - chronic — *see also* Failure, heart, congestive I5Ø.9
  - congestive — *see also* Failure, heart, congestive I5Ø.9
- newborn screening — *see* Abnormal, neonatal screening
  - neonatal congenital heart disease PØ9.5
- orgasm (female) (psychogenic) F52.31
  - male F52.32
- ovarian (primary) E28.39
  - iatrogenic E89.4Ø
    - asymptomatic E89.4Ø
    - symptomatic E89.41
  - postprocedural (postablative) (postirradiation) (postsurgical) E89.4Ø
    - asymptomatic E89.4Ø
    - symptomatic E89.41
- ovulation causing infertility N97.Ø
- polyglandular, autoimmune E31.Ø
- prosthetic joint implant — *see* Complications, joint prosthesis, mechanical, breakdown, by site
- renal N19

- **Failure, failed** — *continued*
  - renal — *continued*
    - with
      - tubular necrosis (acute) N17.Ø
    - acute N17.9
      - with
        - cortical necrosis N17.1
          - medullary necrosis N17.2
        - tubular necrosis N17.Ø
      - specified NEC N17.8
    - chronic N18.9
      - hypertensive — *see* Hypertension, kidney
    - congenital P96.Ø
    - end stage (chronic) N18.6
      - due to hypertension I12.Ø
    - following
      - abortion — *see* Abortion by type complicated by specified condition NEC
      - crushing T79.5 ☑
      - ectopic or molar pregnancy OØ8.4
      - labor and delivery (acute) O9Ø.4
    - hypertensive — *see* Hypertension, kidney
    - postprocedural N99.Ø
  - respiration, respiratory J96.9Ø
    - with
      - hypercapnia J96.92
      - hypercarbia J96.92
      - hypoxia J96.91
    - acute J96.ØØ
      - with
        - hypercapnia J96.Ø2
        - hypercarbia J96.Ø2
        - hypoxia J96.Ø1
    - center G93.89
    - acute and (on) chronic J96.2Ø
      - with
        - hypercapnia J96.22
        - hypercarbia J96.22
        - hypoxia J96.21
    - chronic J96.1Ø
      - with
        - hypercapnia J96.12
        - hypercarbia J96.12
        - hypoxia J96.11
    - newborn P28.5
    - postprocedural (acute) J95.821
      - acute and chronic J95.822
  - rotation
    - cecum Q43.3
    - colon Q43.3
    - intestine Q43.3
    - kidney Q63.2
  - sedation (conscious) (moderate) during procedure T88.52 ☑
    - history of Z92.83
  - segmentation — *see also* Fusion
    - fingers — *see* Syndactylism, complex, fingers
    - vertebra Q76.49
      - with scoliosis Q76.3
  - seminiferous tubule, adult E29.1
  - senile (general) R54
  - sexual arousal (male) F52.21
    - female F52.22
  - testicular endocrine function E29.1
  - to thrive (child over 28 days old) R62.51
    - adult R62.7
    - newborn P92.6
  - transplant T86.92
    - bone T86.831
      - marrow T86.Ø2
    - cornea T86.841- ☑
    - heart T86.22
      - with lung(s) T86.32
    - intestine T86.851
    - kidney T86.12
    - liver T86.42
    - lung(s) T86.811
      - with heart T86.32
    - pancreas T86.891
    - skin (allograft) (autograft) T86.821
    - specified organ or tissue NEC T86.891
    - stem cell (peripheral blood) (umbilical cord) T86.5
  - trial of labor (with subsequent cesarean delivery) O66.4Ø
    - following previous cesarean delivery O66.41
  - tubal ligation N99.89
  - urinary — *see* Disease, kidney, chronic
- **Failure, failed** — *continued*
  - vacuum extraction NOS (with subsequent cesarean delivery) O66.5
  - vasectomy N99.89
  - ventouse NOS (with subsequent cesarean delivery) O66.5
  - ventricular — *see also* Failure, heart I5Ø.9
    - left — *see also* Failure, heart, left I5Ø.1
      - with rheumatic fever (conditions in IØØ)
        - active IØ1.8
          - with chorea IØ2.Ø
        - inactive or quiescent (with chorea) IØ9.81
      - rheumatic (chronic) (inactive) (with chorea) IØ9.81
        - active or acute IØ1.8
          - with chorea IØ2.Ø
    - right — *see* Failure, heart, right
  - vital centers, newborn P91.88
- **Fainting** (fit) R55
- **Fallen arches** — *see* Deformity, limb, flat foot
- **Falling, falls** (repeated) R29.6
  - any organ or part — *see* Prolapse
- **Fallopian**
  - insufflation Z31.41
  - tube — *see* condition
- **Fallot's**
  - pentalogy Q21.8
  - tetrad or tetralogy Q21.3
  - triad or trilogy Q22.3
- **False** — *see also* condition
  - croup J38.5
  - joint — *see* Nonunion, fracture
  - labor (pains) O47.9
    - at or after 37 completed weeks of gestation O47.1
    - before 37 completed weeks of gestation O47.Ø- ☑
  - passage, urethra (prostatic) N36.5
  - pregnancy F45.8
- **Family, familial** — *see also* condition
  - disruption Z63.8
    - involving divorce or separation Z63.5
  - Li-Fraumeni (syndrome) Z15.Ø1
  - planning advice Z3Ø.Ø9
  - problem Z63.9
    - specified NEC Z63.8
  - retinoblastoma C69.2- ☑
- **Famine** (effects of) T73.Ø ☑
  - edema — *see* Malnutrition, severe
- **Fanconi** (-de Toni)(-Debré) **syndrome** E72.Ø9
  - with cystinosis E72.Ø4
- **Fanconi's anemia** (congenital pancytopenia) D61.Ø9
- **Farber's disease or syndrome** E75.29
- **Farcy** A24.Ø
- **Farmer's**
  - lung J67.Ø
  - skin L57.8
- **Farsightedness** — *see* Hypermetropia
- **Fascia** — *see* condition
- **Fasciculation** R25.3
- **Fasciitis** M72.9
  - diffuse (eosinophilic) M35.4
  - infective M72.8
    - necrotizing M72.6
  - necrotizing M72.6
  - nodular M72.4
  - perirenal (with ureteral obstruction) N13.5
    - with infection N13.6
  - plantar M72.2
  - specified NEC M72.8
  - traumatic (old) M72.8
    - current — *code by* site under Sprain
- **Fascioliasis** B66.3
- **Fasciolopsis, fasciolopsiasis** (intestinal) B66.5
- **Fascioscapulohumeral myopathy** G71.Ø2
- **Fast pulse** RØØ.Ø
- **Fat**
  - embolism — *see* Embolism, fat
  - excessive — *see also* Obesity
    - in heart — *see* Degeneration, myocardial
  - in stool R19.5
  - localized (pad) E65
    - heart — *see* Degeneration, myocardial
    - knee M79.4
    - retropatellar M79.4
  - necrosis
    - breast N64.1
    - mesentery K65.4
    - omentum K65.4
  - pad E65
- **Fat** — *continued*
  - pad — *continued*
    - knee M79.4
- **Fatigue** R53.83
  - auditory deafness — *see* Deafness
  - chronic R53.82
  - combat F43.Ø
  - general R53.83
    - psychogenic F48.8
  - heat (transient) T67.6 ☑
  - muscle M62.89
  - myocardium — *see* Failure, heart
  - neoplasm-related R53.Ø
  - nervous, neurosis F48.8
  - operational F48.8
  - psychogenic (general) F48.8
  - senile R54
  - voice R49.8
- **Fatness** — *see* Obesity
- **Fatty** — *see also* condition
  - apron E65
  - degeneration — *see* Degeneration, fatty
  - heart (enlarged) — *see* Degeneration, myocardial
  - liver NEC K76.Ø
    - alcoholic K7Ø.Ø
    - nonalcoholic K76.Ø
  - necrosis — *see* Degeneration, fatty
- **Fauces** — *see* condition
- **Fauchard's disease** (periodontitis) — *see* Periodontitis
- **Faucitis** JØ2.9
- **Favism** (anemia) D55.Ø
- **Favus** — *see* Dermatophytosis
- **Fazio-Londe disease or syndrome** G12.1
- **Fear complex or reaction** F4Ø.9
- **Fear of** — *see* Phobia
- **Feared complaint unfounded** Z71.1
- **Febris, febrile** — *see also* Fever
  - flava — *see also* Fever, yellow A95.9
  - melitensis A23.Ø
  - pestis — *see* Plague
  - recurrens — *see* Fever, relapsing
  - rubra A38.9
- **Fecal**
  - incontinence R15.9
  - smearing R15.1
  - soiling R15.1
  - urgency R15.2
- **Fecalith** (impaction) K56.41
  - appendix K38.1
  - congenital P76.8
- **Fede's disease** K14.Ø
- **Feeble rapid pulse due to shock following injury** T79.4 ☑
- **Feeble-minded** F7Ø
- **Feeding**
  - difficulties R63.3Ø
  - problem (elderly) (infant) R63.39
    - newborn P92.9
      - specified NEC P92.8
    - nonorganic (adult) — *see* Disorder, eating
- **Feeling** (of)
  - foreign body in throat RØ9.89
- **Feer's disease** — *see* Poisoning, mercury
- **Feet** — *see* condition
- **Feigned illness** Z76.5
- **Feil-Klippel syndrome** (brevicollis) Q76.1
- **Feinmesser's** (hidrotic) **ectodermal dysplasia** Q82.4
- **Felinophobia** F4Ø.218
- **Felon** — *see also* Cellulitis, digit
  - with lymphangitis — *see* Lymphangitis, acute, digit
- **Felty's syndrome** MØ5.ØØ
  - ankle MØ5.Ø7- ☑
  - elbow MØ5.Ø2- ☑
  - foot joint MØ5.Ø7- ☑
  - hand joint MØ5.Ø4- ☑
  - hip MØ5.Ø5- ☑
  - knee MØ5.Ø6- ☑
  - multiple site MØ5.Ø9
  - shoulder MØ5.Ø1- ☑
  - vertebra — *see* Spondylitis, ankylosing
  - wrist MØ5.Ø3- ☑
- **Female genital cutting status** — *see* Female genital mutilation status (FGM)
- **Female genital mutilation status** (FGM) N9Ø.81Ø
  - specified NEC N9Ø.818
  - type I (clitorectomy status) N9Ø.811

- **Female genital mutilation status** — *continued*
  - type II (clitorectomy with excision of labia minora status) N9Ø.812
  - type III (infibulation status) N9Ø.813
  - type IV N9Ø.818
- **Femur, femoral** — *see* condition
- **Fenestration, fenestrated** — *see also* Imperfect, closure
  - aortico-pulmonary Q21.4
  - atrial septum Q21.11
  - cusps, heart valve NEC Q24.8
    - pulmonary Q22.3
  - pulmonic cusps Q22.3
- **Fernell's disease** (aortic aneurysm) I71.9
- **Fertile eunuch syndrome** E23.Ø
- **Fetid**
  - breath R19.6
  - sweat L75.Ø
- **Fetishism** F65.Ø
  - transvestic F65.1
- **Fetus, fetal** — *see also* condition
  - alcohol syndrome (dysmorphic) Q86.Ø
  - compressus O31.Ø- ☑
  - hydantoin syndrome Q86.1
  - lung tissue P28.Ø
  - papyraceous O31.Ø- ☑
- **Fever** (inanition) (of unknown origin) (persistent) (with chills) (with rigor) R5Ø.9
  - abortus A23.1
  - Aden (dengue) A9Ø
  - African tick bite A77.8
  - African tick-borne A68.1
  - American
    - mountain (tick) A93.2
    - spotted A77.Ø
  - aphthous BØ8.8
  - arbovirus, arboviral A94
    - hemorrhagic A94
    - specified NEC A93.8
  - Argentinian hemorrhagic A96.Ø
  - Assam B55.Ø
  - Australian Q A78
  - Bangkok hemorrhagic A91
  - Barmah forest A92.8
  - Bartonella A44.Ø
  - bilious, hemoglobinuric B5Ø.8
  - blackwater B5Ø.8
  - blister BØØ.1
  - Bolivian hemorrhagic A96.1
  - Bonvale dam T73.3 ☑
  - boutonneuse A77.1
  - brain — *see* Encephalitis
  - Brazilian purpuric A48.4
  - breakbone A9Ø
  - Bullis A77.Ø
  - Bunyamwera A92.8
  - Burdwan B55.Ø
  - Bwamba A92.8
  - Cameroon — *see* Malaria
  - Canton A75.9
  - catarrhal (acute) JØØ
    - chronic J31.Ø
  - cat-scratch A28.1
  - Central Asian hemorrhagic A98.Ø
  - cerebral — *see* Encephalitis
  - cerebrospinal meningococcal A39.Ø
  - Chagres B5Ø.9
  - Chandipura A92.8
  - Changuinola A93.1
  - Charcot's (biliary) (hepatic) (intermittent) — *see* Calculus, bile duct
  - Chikungunya (viral) (hemorrhagic) A92.Ø
  - Chitral A93.1
  - Colombo — *see* Fever, paratyphoid
  - Colorado tick (virus) A93.2
  - congestive (remittent) — *see* Malaria
  - Congo virus A98.Ø
  - continued malarial B5Ø.9
  - Corsican — *see* Malaria
  - Crimean-Congo hemorrhagic A98.Ø
  - Cyprus — *see* Brucellosis
  - dandy A9Ø
  - deer fly — *see* Tularemia
  - dengue (virus) A9Ø
    - hemorrhagic A91
    - sandfly A93.1
  - desert B38.Ø
  - drug induced R5Ø.2
- **Fever** — *continued*
  - due to
    - conditions classified elsewhere R5Ø.81
    - heat T67.Ø1 ☑
  - enteric AØ1.ØØ
  - enteroviral exanthematous (Boston exanthem) A88.Ø
  - ephemeral (of unknown origin) R5Ø.9
  - epidemic hemorrhagic A98.5
  - erysipelatous — *see* Erysipelas
  - estivo-autumnal (malarial) B5Ø.9
  - famine A75.Ø
  - five day A79.Ø
  - following delivery O86.4
  - Fort Bragg A27.89
  - gastroenteric AØ1.ØØ
  - gastromalarial — *see* Malaria
  - Gibraltar — *see* Brucellosis
  - glandular — *see* Mononucleosis, infectious
  - Guama (viral) A92.8
  - Haverhill A25.1
  - hay (allergic) J3Ø.1
    - with asthma (bronchial) J45.9Ø9
      - with
        - exacerbation (acute) J45.9Ø1
        - status asthmaticus J45.9Ø2
    - due to
      - allergen other than pollen J3Ø.89
      - pollen, any plant or tree J3Ø.1
  - heat (effects) T67.Ø1 ☑
  - hematuric, bilious B5Ø.8
  - hemoglobinuric (malarial) (bilious) B5Ø.8
  - hemorrhagic (arthropod-borne) NOS A94
    - with renal syndrome A98.5
    - arenaviral A96.9
      - specified NEC A96.8
    - Argentinian A96.Ø
    - Bangkok A91
    - Bolivian A96.1
    - Central Asian A98.Ø
    - Chikungunya A92.Ø
    - Crimean-Congo A98.Ø
    - dengue (virus) A91
    - epidemic A98.5
    - Junin (virus) A96.Ø
    - Korean A98.5
    - Kyasanur forest A98.2
    - Machupo (virus) A96.1
    - mite-borne A93.8
    - mosquito-borne A92.8
    - Omsk A98.1
    - Philippine A91
    - Russian A98.5
    - Singapore A91
    - Southeast Asia A91
    - Thailand A91
    - tick-borne NEC A93.8
    - viral A99
      - specified NEC A98.8
  - hepatic — *see* Cholecystitis
  - herpetic — *see* Herpes
  - icterohemorrhagic A27.Ø
  - Indiana A93.8
  - infective B99.9
    - specified NEC B99.8
  - intermittent (bilious) — *see also* Malaria
    - of unknown origin R5Ø.9
    - pernicious B5Ø.9
  - iodide R5Ø.2
  - Japanese river A75.3
  - jungle — *see also* Malaria
    - yellow A95.Ø
  - Junin (virus) hemorrhagic A96.Ø
  - Katayama B65.2
  - kedani A75.3
  - Kenya (tick) A77.1
  - Kew Garden A79.1
  - Korean hemorrhagic A98.5
  - Lassa A96.2
  - Lone Star A77.Ø
  - Machupo (virus) hemorrhagic A96.1
  - malaria, malarial — *see* Malaria
  - Malta A23.9
  - Marseilles A77.1
  - marsh — *see* Malaria
  - Mayaro (viral) A92.8
  - Mediterranean — *see also* Brucellosis A23.9
    - familial MØ4.1
    - tick A77.1
- **Fever** — *continued*
  - meningeal — *see* Meningitis
  - Meuse A79.Ø
  - Mexican A75.2
  - mianeh A68.1
  - miasmatic — *see* Malaria
  - mosquito-borne (viral) A92.9
    - hemorrhagic A92.8
  - mountain — *see also* Brucellosis
    - meaning Rocky Mountain spotted fever A77.Ø
    - tick (American) (Colorado) (viral) A93.2
  - Mucambo (viral) A92.8
  - mud A27.9
  - Neapolitan — *see* Brucellosis
  - neutropenic D7Ø.9
  - newborn P81.9
    - environmental P81.Ø
  - Nine-Mile A78
  - non-exanthematous tick A93.2
  - North Asian tick-borne A77.2
  - Omsk hemorrhagic A98.1
  - O'nyong-nyong (viral) A92.1
  - Oropouche (viral) A93.Ø
  - Oroya A44.Ø
  - pacific coast tick A77.8
  - paludal — *see* Malaria
  - Panama (malarial) B5Ø.9
  - Pappataci A93.1
  - paratyphoid AØ1.4
    - A AØ1.1
    - B AØ1.2
    - C AØ1.3
  - parrot A7Ø
  - periodic (Mediterranean) MØ4.1
  - persistent (of unknown origin) R5Ø.9
  - petechial A39.Ø
  - pharyngoconjunctival B3Ø.2
  - Philippine hemorrhagic A91
  - phlebotomus A93.1
  - Piry (virus) A93.8
  - Pixuna (viral) A92.8
  - Plasmodium ovale B53.Ø
  - polioviral (nonparalytic) A8Ø.4
  - Pontiac A48.2
  - postimmunization R5Ø.83
  - postoperative R5Ø.82
    - due to infection T81.4Ø ☑
  - posttransfusion R5Ø.84
  - postvaccination R5Ø.83
  - presenting with conditions classified elsewhere R5Ø.81
  - pretibial A27.89
  - puerperal O86.4
  - Q A78
  - quadrilateral A78
  - quartan (malaria) B52.9
  - Queensland (coastal) (tick) A77.3
  - quintan A79.Ø
  - rabbit — *see* Tularemia
  - rat-bite A25.9
    - due to
      - Spirillum A25.Ø
      - Streptobacillus moniliformis A25.1
  - recurrent — *see* Fever, relapsing
  - relapsing (Borrelia) A68.9
    - Carter's (Asiatic) A68.1
    - Dutton's (West African) A68.1
    - Koch's A68.9
    - louse-borne A68.Ø
    - Novy's
      - louse-borne A68.Ø
      - tick-borne A68.1
    - Obermeyer's (European) A68.Ø
    - tick-borne A68.1
  - remittent (bilious) (congestive) (gastric) — *see* Malaria
  - rheumatic (active) (acute) (chronic) (subacute) IØØ
    - with central nervous system involvement IØ2.9
    - active with heart involvement — *see* category IØ1 ☑
    - inactive or quiescent with
      - cardiac hypertrophy IØ9.89
      - carditis IØ9.9
      - endocarditis IØ9.1
        - aortic (valve) IØ6.9
          - with mitral (valve) disease IØ8.Ø
        - mitral (valve) IØ5.9
          - with aortic (valve) disease IØ8.Ø
        - pulmonary (valve) IØ9.89
        - tricuspid (valve) IØ7.8
      - heart disease NEC IØ9.89

Fever — *continued*
rheumatic — *continued*
inactive or quiescent with — *continued*
heart failure (congestive) (conditions in category I5Ø.) IØ9.81
left ventricular failure (conditions in I5Ø.1-I5Ø.4-) IØ9.81
myocarditis, myocardial degeneration (conditions in I51.4) IØ9.Ø
pancarditis IØ9.9
pericarditis IØ9.2
Rift Valley (viral) A92.4
Rocky Mountain spotted A77.Ø
rose J3Ø.1
Ross River B33.1
Russian hemorrhagic A98.5
San Joaquin (Valley) B38.Ø
sandfly A93.1
Sao Paulo A77.Ø
scarlet A38.9
seven day (leptospirosis) (autumnal) (Japanese) A27.89
dengue A9Ø
shin-bone A79.Ø
Singapore hemorrhagic A91
solar A9Ø
Songo A98.5
sore BØØ.1
South African tick-bite A68.1
Southeast Asia hemorrhagic A91
spinal — *see* Meningitis
spirillary A25.Ø
splenic — *see* Anthrax
spotted A77.9
American A77.Ø
Brazilian A77.Ø
cerebrospinal meningitis A39.Ø
Colombian A77.Ø
due to Rickettsia
africae (African tick bite fever) A77.8
australis A77.3
conorii A77.1
parkeri A77.8
rickettsii A77.Ø
sibirica A77.2
specified type NEC A77.8
Ehrlichiosis A77.4Ø
due to
E. chafeensis A77.41
specified organism NEC A77.49
Rocky Mountain A77.Ø
steroid R5Ø.2
streptobacillary A25.1
subtertian B5Ø.9
Sumatran mite A75.3
sun A9Ø
swamp A27.9
swine AØ2.8
sylvatic, yellow A95.Ø
Tahyna B33.8
tertian — *see* Malaria, tertian
Thailand hemorrhagic A91
thermic T67.Ø1 ☑
three-day A93.1
tick
American mountain A93.2
Colorado A93.2
Kemerovo A93.8
Mediterranean A77.1
mountain A93.2
nonexanthematous A93.2
Quaranfil A93.8
tick-bite NEC A93.8
tick-borne (hemorrhagic) NEC A93.8
trench A79.Ø
tsutsugamushi A75.3
typhogastric AØ1.ØØ
typhoid (abortive) (hemorrhagic) (intermittent) (malignant) AØ1.ØØ
complicated by
arthritis AØ1.Ø4
heart involvement AØ1.Ø2
meningitis AØ1.Ø1
osteomyelitis AØ1.Ø5
pneumonia AØ1.Ø3
specified NEC AØ1.Ø9
typhomalarial — *see* Malaria
typhus — *see* Typhus (fever)
undulant — *see* Brucellosis

Fever — *continued*
unknown origin R5Ø.9
uveoparotid D86.89
valley B38.Ø
Venezuelan equine A92.2
vesicular stomatitis A93.8
viral hemorrhagic — *see* Fever, hemorrhagic, by type of virus
Volhynian A79.Ø
Wesselsbron (viral) A92.8
West
African B5Ø.8
Nile (viral) A92.3Ø
with
complications NEC A92.39
cranial nerve disorders A92.32
encephalitis A92.31
encephalomyelitis A92.31
neurologic manifestation NEC A92.32
optic neuritis A92.32
polyradiculitis A92.32
Whitmore's — *see* Melioidosis
Wolhynian A79.Ø
worm B83.9
yellow A95.9
jungle A95.Ø
sylvatic A95.Ø
urban A95.1
Zika virus A92.5
Fibrillation
atrial or auricular (established) I48.91
chronic I48.2Ø
persistent I48.19
paroxysmal I48.Ø
permanent I48.21
persistent (chronic) (NOS) (other) I48.19
longstanding I48.11
cardiac I49.8
heart I49.8
muscular M62.89
ventricular I49.Ø1
Fibrin
ball or bodies, pleural (sac) J94.1
chamber, anterior (eye) (gelatinous exudate) — *see* Iridocyclitis, acute
Fibrinogenolysis — *see* Fibrinolysis
Fibrinogenopenia D68.8
acquired D65
congenital D68.2
Fibrinolysis (hemorrhagic) (acquired) D65
antepartum hemorrhage — *see* Hemorrhage, antepartum, with coagulation defect
following
abortion — *see* Abortion by type complicated by hemorrhage
ectopic or molar pregnancy OØ8.1
intrapartum O67.Ø
newborn, transient P6Ø
postpartum O72.3
Fibrinopenia (hereditary) D68.2
acquired D68.4
Fibrinopurulent — *see* condition
Fibrinous — *see* condition
Fibroadenoma
cellular intracanalicular D24- ☑
giant D24- ☑
intracanalicular
cellular D24- ☑
giant D24- ☑
specified site — *see* Neoplasm, benign, by site
unspecified site D24- ☑
juvenile D24- ☑
pericanalicular
specified site — *see* Neoplasm, benign, by site
unspecified site D24- ☑
phyllodes D24- ☑
prostate D29.1
specified site NEC — *see* Neoplasm, benign, by site
unspecified site D24- ☑
Fibroadenosis, breast (chronic) (cystic) (diffuse) (periodic) (segmental) N6Ø.2- ☑
Fibroangioma — *see also* Neoplasm, benign, by site
juvenile
specified site — *see* Neoplasm, benign, by site
unspecified site D1Ø.6
Fibrochondrosarcoma — *see* Neoplasm, cartilage, malignant

Fibrocystic
disease — *see also* Fibrosis, cystic
breast — *see* Mastopathy, cystic
jaw M27.49
kidney (congenital) Q61.8
liver Q44.6
pancreas E84.9
kidney (congenital) Q61.8
Fibrodysplasia ossificans progressiva — *see* Myositis, ossificans, progressiva
Fibroelastosis (cordis) (endocardial) (endomyocardial) I42.4
Fibroid (tumor) — *see also* Neoplasm, connective tissue, benign
disease, lung (chronic) — *see* Fibrosis, lung
heart (disease) — *see* Myocarditis
in pregnancy or childbirth O34.1- ☑
causing obstructed labor O65.5
induration, lung (chronic) — *see* Fibrosis, lung
lung — *see* Fibrosis, lung
pneumonia (chronic) — *see* Fibrosis, lung
uterus — *see also* Leiomyoma, uterus D25.9
Fibrolipoma — *see* Lipoma
Fibroliposarcoma — *see* Neoplasm, connective tissue, malignant
Fibroma — *see also* Neoplasm, connective tissue, benign
ameloblastic — *see* Cyst, calcifying odontogenic
bone (nonossifying) — *see* Disorder, bone, specified type NEC
ossifying — *see* Neoplasm, bone, benign
cementifying — *see* Neoplasm, bone, benign
chondromyxoid — *see* Neoplasm, bone, benign
desmoplastic — *see* Neoplasm, connective tissue, uncertain behavior
durum — *see* Neoplasm, connective tissue, benign
fascial — *see* Neoplasm, connective tissue, benign
invasive — *see* Neoplasm, connective tissue, uncertain behavior
molle — *see* Lipoma
myxoid — *see* Neoplasm, connective tissue, benign
nasopharynx, nasopharyngeal (juvenile) D1Ø.6
nonosteogenic (nonossifying) — *see* Dysplasia, fibrous
odontogenic (central) — *see* Cyst, calcifying odontogenic
ossifying — *see* Neoplasm, bone, benign
periosteal — *see* Neoplasm, bone, benign
soft — *see* Lipoma
Fibromatosis M72.9
abdominal — *see* Neoplasm, connective tissue, uncertain behavior
aggressive — *see* Neoplasm, connective tissue, uncertain behavior
congenital generalized — *see* Neoplasm, connective tissue, uncertain behavior
Dupuytren's M72.Ø
gingival KØ6.1
palmar (fascial) M72.Ø
plantar (fascial) M72.2
pseudosarcomatous (proliferative) (subcutaneous) M72.4
retroperitoneal D48.3
specified NEC M72.8
Fibromyalgia M79.7
Fibromyoma — *see also* Neoplasm, connective tissue, benign
uterus (corpus) — *see also* Leiomyoma, uterus
in pregnancy or childbirth — *see* Fibroid, in pregnancy or childbirth
causing obstructed labor O65.5
Fibromyositis M79.7
Fibromyxolipoma D17.9
Fibromyxoma — *see* Neoplasm, connective tissue, benign
Fibromyxosarcoma — *see* Neoplasm, connective tissue, malignant
Fibro-odontoma, ameloblastic — *see* Cyst, calcifying odontogenic
Fibro-osteoma — *see* Neoplasm, bone, benign
Fibroplasia, retrolental H35.17- ☑
Fibropurulent — *see* condition
Fibrosarcoma — *see also* Neoplasm, connective tissue, malignant
ameloblastic C41.1
upper jaw (bone) C41.Ø
congenital — *see* Neoplasm, connective tissue, malignant
fascial — *see* Neoplasm, connective tissue, malignant

- **Fibrosarcoma** — *continued*
  - infantile — *see* Neoplasm, connective tissue, malignant
  - odontogenic C41.1
    - upper jaw (bone) C41.Ø
  - periosteal — *see* Neoplasm, bone, malignant
- **Fibrosclerosis**
  - breast N6Ø.3- ☑
  - multifocal M35.5
  - penis (corpora cavernosa) N48.6
- **Fibrosis, fibrotic**
  - adrenal (gland) E27.8
  - amnion O41.8X- ☑
  - anal papillae K62.89
  - arteriocapillary — *see* Arteriosclerosis
  - bladder N32.89
    - interstitial — *see* Cystitis, chronic, interstitial
    - localized submucosal — *see* Cystitis, chronic, interstitial
    - panmural — *see* Cystitis, chronic, interstitial
  - breast — *see* Fibrosclerosis, breast
  - capillary — *see also* Arteriosclerosis I7Ø.9Ø
    - lung (chronic) — *see* Fibrosis, lung
  - cardiac — *see* Myocarditis
  - cervix N88.8
  - chorion O41.8X- ☑
  - corpus cavernosum (sclerosing) N48.6
  - cystic (of pancreas) E84.9
    - with
      - distal intestinal obstruction syndrome E84.19
      - fecal impaction E84.19
      - intestinal manifestations NEC E84.19
      - pulmonary manifestations E84.Ø
      - specified manifestations NEC E84.8
  - due to device, implant or graft — *see also* Complications, by site and type, specified NEC T85.828 ☑
    - arterial graft NEC T82.828 ☑
    - breast (implant) T85.828 ☑
    - catheter NEC T85.828 ☑
      - dialysis (renal) T82.828 ☑
        - intraperitoneal T85.828 ☑
      - infusion NEC T82.828 ☑
        - spinal (epidural) (subdural) T85.82Ø ☑
      - urinary (indwelling) T83.82 ☑
    - electronic (electrode) (pulse generator) (stimulator)
      - bone T84.82 ☑
      - cardiac T82.827 ☑
      - nervous system (brain) (peripheral nerve) (spinal) T85.82Ø ☑
      - urinary T83.82 ☑
    - fixation, internal (orthopedic) NEC T84.82 ☑
    - gastrointestinal (bile duct) (esophagus) T85.828 ☑
    - genital NEC T83.82 ☑
    - heart NEC T82.827 ☑
    - joint prosthesis T84.82 ☑
    - ocular (corneal graft) (orbital implant) NEC T85.828 ☑
    - orthopedic NEC T84.82 ☑
    - specified NEC T85.828 ☑
    - urinary NEC T83.82 ☑
    - vascular NEC T82.828 ☑
    - ventricular intracranial shunt T85.82Ø ☑
  - ejaculatory duct N5Ø.89
  - endocardium — *see* Endocarditis
  - endomyocardial (tropical) I42.3
  - epididymis N5Ø.89
  - eye muscle — *see* Strabismus, mechanical
  - heart — *see* Myocarditis
  - hepatic — *see* Fibrosis, liver
  - hepatolienal (portal hypertension) K76.6
  - hepatosplenic (portal hypertension) K76.6
  - infrapatellar fat pad M79.4
  - intrascrotal N5Ø.89
  - kidney N26.9
  - liver K74.ØØ
    - with sclerosis K74.2
    - advanced K74.Ø2
    - alcoholic K7Ø.2
    - early K74.Ø1
    - stage
      - F1 or F2 K74.Ø1
      - F3 K74.Ø2
  - lung (atrophic) (chronic) (confluent) (massive) (perialveolar) (peribronchial) J84.1Ø
    - with
      - anthracosilicosis J6Ø
      - anthracosis J6Ø
      - asbestosis J61
- **Fibrosis, fibrotic** — *continued*
  - lung — *continued*
    - with — *continued*
      - bagassosis J67.1
      - bauxite J63.1
      - berylliosis J63.2
      - byssinosis J66.Ø
      - calcicosis J62.8
      - chalicosis J62.8
      - dust reticulation J64
      - farmer's lung J67.Ø
      - ganister disease J62.8
      - graphite J63.3
      - pneumoconiosis NOS J64
      - siderosis J63.4
      - silicosis J62.8
    - capillary J84.1Ø
    - congenital P27.8
    - diffuse (idiopathic) J84.1Ø
      - chemicals, gases, fumes or vapors (inhalation) J68.4
      - interstitial J84.1Ø
        - acute J84.114
      - talc J62.Ø
    - following radiation J7Ø.1
    - idiopathic J84.112
    - postinflammatory J84.1Ø
    - silicotic J62.8
    - tuberculous — *see* Tuberculosis, pulmonary
  - lymphatic gland I89.8
  - median bar — *see* Hyperplasia, prostate
  - mediastinum (idiopathic) J98.59
  - meninges G96.198
  - myocardium, myocardial — *see* Myocarditis
  - ovary N83.8
  - oviduct N83.8
  - pancreas K86.89
  - penis NEC N48.6
  - pericardium I31.Ø
  - perineum, in pregnancy or childbirth O34.7- ☑
    - causing obstructed labor O65.5
  - pleura J94.1
  - popliteal fat pad M79.4
  - prostate (chronic) — *see* Hyperplasia, prostate
  - pulmonary — *see also* Fibrosis, lung J84.1Ø
    - congenital P27.8
    - idiopathic J84.112
  - rectal sphincter K62.89
  - retroperitoneal, idiopathic (with ureteral obstruction) N13.5
    - with infection N13.6
  - sclerosing mesenteric (idiopathic) K65.4
  - scrotum N5Ø.89
  - seminal vesicle N5Ø.89
  - senile R54
  - skin L9Ø.5
  - spermatic cord N5Ø.89
  - spleen D73.89
    - in schistosomiasis (bilharziasis) B65.9 *[D77]*
  - subepidermal nodular — *see* Neoplasm, skin, benign
  - submucous (oral) (tongue) K13.5
  - testis N44.8
    - chronic, due to syphilis A52.76
  - thymus (gland) E32.8
  - tongue, submucous K13.5
  - tunica vaginalis N5Ø.89
  - uterus (non-neoplastic) N85.8
  - vagina N89.8
  - valve, heart — *see* Endocarditis
  - vas deferens N5Ø.89
  - vein I87.8
- **Fibrositis** (periarticular) M79.7
  - nodular, chronic (Jaccoud's) (rheumatoid) — *see* Arthropathy, postrheumatic, chronic
- **Fibrothorax** J94.1
- **Fibrotic** — *see* Fibrosis
- **Fibrous** — *see* condition
- **Fibroxanthoma** — *see also* Neoplasm, connective tissue, benign
  - atypical — *see* Neoplasm, connective tissue, uncertain behavior
  - malignant — *see* Neoplasm, connective tissue, malignant
- **Fibroxanthosarcoma** — *see* Neoplasm, connective tissue, malignant
- **Fiedler's**
  - disease (icterohemorrhagic leptospirosis) A27.Ø
  - myocarditis (acute) I4Ø.1
- **Fifth disease** BØ8.3
  - venereal A55
- **Filaria, filarial, filariasis** — *see* Infestation, filarial
- **Filatov's disease** — *see* Mononucleosis, infectious
- **File-cutter's disease** — *see* Poisoning, lead
- **Filling defect**
  - biliary tract R93.2
  - bladder R93.41
  - duodenum R93.3
  - gallbladder R93.2
  - gastrointestinal tract R93.3
  - intestine R93.3
  - kidney R93.42- ☑
  - stomach R93.3
  - ureter R93.41
  - urinary organs, specified NEC R93.49
- **Fimbrial cyst** Q5Ø.4
- **Financial problem affecting care NOS** Z59.9
  - bankruptcy Z59.89
  - foreclosure on loan Z59.89
    - home loan Z59.81- ☑
  - strain Z59.86
- **Findings, abnormal, inconclusive, without diagnosis** — *see also* Abnormal
  - 17-ketosteroids, elevated R82.5
  - acetonuria R82.4
  - alcohol in blood R78.Ø
  - anisocytosis R71.8
  - antenatal screening of mother O28.9
    - biochemical O28.1
    - chromosomal O28.5
    - cytological O28.2
    - genetic O28.5
    - hematological O28.Ø
    - radiological O28.4
    - specified NEC O28.8
    - ultrasonic O28.3
  - antibody titer, elevated R76.Ø
  - anticardiolipin antibody R76.Ø
  - antiphosphatidylglycerol antibody R76.Ø
  - antiphosphatidylinositol antibody R76.Ø
  - antiphosphatidylserine antibody R76.Ø
  - antiphospholipid antibody R76.Ø
  - bacteriuria R82.71
  - bicarbonate E87.8
  - bile in urine R82.2
  - blood sugar R73.Ø9
    - high R73.9
    - low (transient) E16.2
  - body fluid or substance, specified NEC R88.8
  - casts, urine R82.998
  - catecholamines R82.5
  - cells, urine R82.998
  - chloride E87.8
  - cholesterol E78.9
    - high E78.ØØ
      - with high triglycerides E78.2
  - chyluria R82.Ø
  - cloudy
    - dialysis effluent R88.Ø
    - urine R82.9Ø
  - creatinine clearance R94.4
  - crystals, urine R82.998
  - culture
    - blood R78.81
    - positive — *see* Positive, culture
  - echocardiogram R93.1
  - electrolyte level, urinary R82.998
  - function study NEC R94.8
    - bladder R94.8
    - endocrine NEC R94.7
      - thyroid R94.6
    - kidney R94.4
    - liver R94.5
    - pancreas R94.8
    - placenta R94.8
    - pulmonary R94.2
    - spleen R94.8
  - gallbladder, nonvisualization R93.2
  - glucose (tolerance test) (non-fasting) R73.Ø9
  - glycosuria R81
  - heart
    - shadow R93.1
    - sounds RØ1.2
  - hematinuria R82.3
  - hematocrit drop (precipitous) R71.Ø
  - hemoglobinuria R82.3

- **Findings, abnormal, inconclusive, without diagnosis** — *continued*
  - human papillomavirus (HPV) DNA test positive
    - cervix
      - high risk R87.81Ø
      - low risk R87.82Ø
    - vagina
      - high risk R87.811
      - low risk R87.821
  - in blood (of substance not normally found in blood) R78.9
    - addictive drug NEC R78.4
    - alcohol (excessive level) R78.Ø
    - cocaine R78.2
    - hallucinogen R78.3
    - heavy metals (abnormal level) R78.79
    - lead R78.71
    - lithium (abnormal level) R78.89
    - opiate drug R78.1
    - psychotropic drug R78.5
    - specified substance NEC R78.89
    - steroid agent R78.6
  - indoleacetic acid, elevated R82.5
  - ketonuria R82.4
  - lactic acid dehydrogenase (LDH) R74.Ø2
  - liver function test — *see also* Elevated, liver function, test R79.89
  - mammogram NEC R92.8
    - calcification (calculus) R92.1
    - inconclusive result (due to dense breasts) R92.2
    - microcalcification R92.Ø
  - mediastinal shift R93.89
  - melanin, urine R82.998
  - myoglobinuria R82.1
  - neonatal screening — *see* Abnormal, neonatal screening
  - newborn screens, state mandated — *see* Abnormal, neonatal screening
  - nonvisualization of gallbladder R93.2
  - odor of urine NOS R82.9Ø
  - Papanicolaou cervix R87.619
    - non-atypical endometrial cells R87.618
  - pneumoencephalogram R93.Ø
  - poikilocytosis R71.8
  - potassium (deficiency) E87.6
    - excess E87.5
  - PPD R76.11
  - radiologic (X-ray) R93.89
    - abdomen R93.5
    - biliary tract R93.2
    - breast R92.8
    - gastrointestinal tract R93.3
    - genitourinary organs R93.89
    - head R93.Ø
    - inconclusive due to excess body fat of patient R93.9
    - intrathoracic organs NEC R93.1
    - musculoskeletal
      - limbs R93.6
      - other than limb R93.7
    - placenta R93.89
    - retroperitoneum R93.5
    - skin R93.89
    - skull R93.Ø
    - subcutaneous tissue R93.89
    - testis R93.81- ☑
  - red blood cell (count) (morphology) (sickling) (volume) R71.8
  - scan NEC R94.8
    - bladder R94.8
    - bone R94.8
    - kidney R94.4
    - liver R93.2
    - lung R94.2
    - pancreas R94.8
    - placental R94.8
    - spleen R94.8
    - thyroid R94.6
  - sedimentation rate, elevated R7Ø.Ø
  - SGOT R74.Ø1
  - SGPT R74.Ø1
  - sodium (deficiency) E87.1
    - excess E87.Ø
  - specified body fluid NEC R88.8
  - stress test R94.39
  - testis R93.81- ☑
  - thyroid (function) (metabolic rate) (scan) (uptake) R94.6
  - transaminase (level) R74.Ø1
  - triglycerides E78.9
    - high E78.1
- **Findings, abnormal, inconclusive, without diagnosis** — *continued*
  - triglycerides — *continued*
    - high — *continued*
      - with high cholesterol E78.2
  - tuberculin skin test (without active tuberculosis) R76.11
  - urine R82.9Ø
    - acetone R82.4
    - bacteria R82.71
    - bile R82.2
    - casts or cells R82.998
    - chyle R82.Ø
    - culture positive R82.79
    - glucose R81
    - hemoglobin R82.3
    - ketone R82.4
    - sugar R81
  - vanillylmandelic acid (VMA), elevated R82.5
  - vectorcardiogram (VCG) R94.39
  - ventriculogram R93.Ø
  - white blood cell (count) (differential) (morphology) D72.9
  - xerography R92.8
- **Finger** — *see* condition
- **Fire, Saint Anthony's** — *see* Erysipelas
- **Fire-setting**
  - pathological (compulsive) F63.1
- **Fish hook stomach** K31.89
- **Fishmeal-worker's lung** J67.8
- **Fissure, fissured**
  - anus, anal K6Ø.2
    - acute K6Ø.Ø
    - chronic K6Ø.1
    - congenital Q43.8
  - ear, lobule, congenital Q17.8
  - epiglottis (congenital) Q31.8
  - larynx J38.7
    - congenital Q31.8
  - lip K13.Ø
    - congenital — *see* Cleft, lip
  - nipple N64.Ø
    - associated with
      - lactation O92.13
      - pregnancy O92.11- ☑
      - puerperium O92.12
  - nose Q3Ø.2
  - palate (congenital) — *see* Cleft, palate
  - skin R23.4
  - spine (congenital) — *see also* Spina bifida
    - with hydrocephalus — *see* Spina bifida, by site, with hydrocephalus
  - tongue (acquired) K14.5
    - congenital Q38.3
- **Fistula** (cutaneous) L98.8
  - abdomen (wall) K63.2
    - bladder N32.2
    - intestine NEC K63.2
    - ureter N28.89
    - uterus N82.5
  - abdominorectal K63.2
  - abdominosigmoidal K63.2
  - abdominothoracic J86.Ø
  - abdominouterine N82.5
    - congenital Q51.7
  - abdominovesical N32.2
  - accessory sinuses — *see* Sinusitis
  - actinomycotic — *see* Actinomycosis
  - alveolar antrum — *see* Sinusitis, maxillary
  - alveolar process KØ4.6
  - anorectal K6Ø.5
  - antrobuccal — *see* Sinusitis, maxillary
  - antrum — *see* Sinusitis, maxillary
  - anus, anal (recurrent) (infectional) K6Ø.3
    - congenital Q43.6
      - with absence, atresia and stenosis Q42.2
    - tuberculous A18.32
  - aorta-duodenal I77.2
  - appendix, appendicular K38.3
  - arteriovenous (acquired) (nonruptured) I77.Ø
    - brain I67.1
      - congenital Q28.2
        - ruptured — *see* Fistula, arteriovenous, brain, ruptured
      - ruptured I6Ø.8
        - intracerebral I61.8
        - intraparenchymal I61.8
        - intraventricular I61.5
        - subarachnoid I6Ø.8
- **Fistula** — *continued*
  - arteriovenous — *continued*
    - cerebral — *see* Fistula, arteriovenous, brain
    - congenital (peripheral) — *see also* Malformation, arteriovenous
      - brain Q28.2
        - ruptured — *see* Fistula, arteriovenous, brain, ruptured
      - coronary Q24.5
      - pulmonary Q25.72
    - coronary I25.41
      - congenital Q24.5
    - pulmonary I28.Ø
      - congenital Q25.72
    - surgically created (for dialysis) Z99.2
      - complication — *see* Complication, arteriovenous, fistula, surgically created
    - traumatic — *see* Injury, blood vessel
  - artery I77.2
  - aural (mastoid) — *see* Mastoiditis, chronic
  - auricle — *see also* Disorder, pinna, specified type NEC
    - congenital Q18.1
  - Bartholin's gland N82.8
  - bile duct (common) (hepatic) K83.3
    - with calculus, stones — *see also* Calculus, bile duct K83.3
  - biliary (tract) — *see* Fistula, bile duct
  - bladder (sphincter) NEC — *see also* Fistula, vesico- N32.2
    - into seminal vesicle N32.2
  - bone — *see also* Disorder, bone, specified type NEC
    - with osteomyelitis, chronic — *see* Osteomyelitis, chronic, with draining sinus
  - brain G93.89
    - arteriovenous (acquired) — *see also* Fistula, arteriovenous, brain I67.1
      - congenital Q28.2
  - branchial (cleft) Q18.Ø
  - branchiogenous Q18.Ø
  - breast N61.Ø
    - puerperal, postpartum or gestational, due to mastitis (purulent) — *see* Mastitis, obstetric, purulent
  - bronchial J86.Ø
  - bronchocutaneous, bronchomediastinal, bronchopleural, bronchopleuromediastinal (infective) J86.Ø
    - tuberculous NEC A15.5
  - bronchoesophageal J86.Ø
    - congenital Q39.2
      - with atresia of esophagus Q39.1
  - bronchovisceral J86.Ø
  - buccal cavity (infective) K12.2
  - cecosigmoidal K63.2
  - cecum K63.2
  - cerebrospinal (fluid) G96.Ø8
  - cervical, lateral Q18.1
  - cervicoaural Q18.1
  - cervicosigmoidal N82.4
  - cervicovesical N82.1
  - cervix N82.8
  - chest (wall) J86.Ø
  - cholecystenteric — *see* Fistula, gallbladder
  - cholecystocolic — *see* Fistula, gallbladder
  - cholecystocolonic — *see* Fistula, gallbladder
  - cholecystoduodenal — *see* Fistula, gallbladder
  - cholecystogastric — *see* Fistula, gallbladder
  - cholecystointestinal — *see* Fistula, gallbladder
  - choledochoduodenal — *see* Fistula, bile duct
  - cholocolic K82.3
  - coccyx — *see* Sinus, pilonidal
  - colon K63.2
  - colostomy K94.Ø9
  - colovesical N32.1
  - common duct — *see* Fistula, bile duct
  - congenital, site not listed — *see* Anomaly, by site
  - coronary, arteriovenous I25.41
    - congenital Q24.5
  - costal region J86.Ø
  - cul-de-sac, Douglas' N82.8
  - cystic duct — *see also* Fistula, gallbladder
    - congenital Q44.5
  - dental KØ4.6
  - diaphragm J86.Ø
  - duodenum K31.6
  - ear (external) (canal) — *see* Disorder, ear, external, specified type NEC
  - enterocolic K63.2
  - enterocutaneous K63.2
  - enterouterine N82.4

Fistula — *continued*
  enterouterine — *continued*
    congenital Q51.7
  enterovaginal N82.4
    congenital Q52.2
    large intestine N82.3
    small intestine N82.2
  enterovesical N32.1
  epididymis N5Ø.89
    tuberculous A18.15
  esophagobronchial J86.Ø
    congenital Q39.2
      with atresia of esophagus Q39.1
  esophagocutaneous K22.89
  esophagopleural-cutaneous J86.Ø
  esophagotracheal J86.Ø
    congenital Q39.2
      with atresia of esophagus Q39.1
  esophagus K22.89
    congenital Q39.2
      with atresia of esophagus Q39.1
  ethmoid — *see* Sinusitis, ethmoidal
  eyeball (cornea) (sclera) — *see* Disorder, globe, hypotony
  eyelid HØ1.8
  fallopian tube, external N82.5
  fecal K63.2
    congenital Q43.6
  from periapical abscess KØ4.6
  frontal sinus — *see* Sinusitis, frontal
  gallbladder K82.3
    with calculus, cholelithiasis, stones — *see* Calculus, gallbladder
  gastric K31.6
  gastrocolic K31.6
    congenital Q4Ø.2
    tuberculous A18.32
  gastroenterocolic K31.6
  gastroesophageal K31.6
  gastrojejunal K31.6
  gastrojejunocolic K31.6
  genital tract (female) N82.9
    specified NEC N82.8
    to intestine NEC N82.4
    to skin N82.5
  hepatic artery-portal vein, congenital Q26.6
  hepatopleural J86.Ø
  hepatopulmonary J86.Ø
  ileorectal or ileosigmoidal K63.2
  ileovaginal N82.2
  ileovesical N32.1
  ileum K63.2
  in ano K6Ø.3
    tuberculous A18.32
  inner ear (labyrinth) — *see* subcategory H83.1 ☑
  intestine NEC K63.2
  intestinocolonic (abdominal) K63.2
  intestinoureteral N28.89
  intestinouterine N82.4
  intestinovaginal N82.4
    large intestine N82.3
    small intestine N82.2
  intestinovesical N32.1
  ischiorectal (fossa) K61.39
  jejunum K63.2
  joint M25.1Ø
    ankle M25.17- ☑
    elbow M25.12- ☑
    foot joint M25.17- ☑
    hand joint M25.14- ☑
    hip M25.15- ☑
    knee M25.16- ☑
    shoulder M25.11- ☑
    specified joint NEC M25.18
    tuberculous — *see* Tuberculosis, joint
    vertebrae M25.18
    wrist M25.13- ☑
  kidney N28.89
  labium (majus) (minus) N82.8
  labyrinth — *see* subcategory H83.1 ☑
  lacrimal (gland) (sac) HØ4.61- ☑
  lacrimonasal duct — *see* Fistula, lacrimal
  laryngotracheal, congenital Q34.8
  larynx J38.7
  lip K13.Ø
    congenital Q38.Ø
  lumbar, tuberculous A18.Ø1
  lung J86.Ø

Fistula — *continued*
  lymphatic I89.8
  mammary (gland) N61.Ø
  mastoid (process) (region) — *see* Mastoiditis, chronic
  maxillary J32.Ø
  medial, face and neck Q18.8
  mediastinal J86.Ø
  mediastinobronchial J86.Ø
  mediastinocutaneous J86.Ø
  middle ear — *see* subcategory H74.8 ☑
  mouth K12.2
  nasal J34.89
    sinus — *see* Sinusitis
  nasopharynx J39.2
  nipple N64.Ø
  nose J34.89
  oral (cutaneous) K12.2
    maxillary J32.Ø
    nasal (with cleft palate) — *see* Cleft, palate
  orbit, orbital — *see* Disorder, orbit, specified type NEC
  oroantral J32.Ø
  oviduct, external N82.5
  palate (hard) M27.8
  pancreatic K86.89
  pancreaticoduodenal K86.89
  parotid (gland) K11.4
    region K12.2
  penis N48.89
  perianal K6Ø.3
  pericardium (pleura) (sac) — *see* Pericarditis
  pericecal K63.2
  perineorectal K6Ø.4
  perineosigmoidal K63.2
  perineum, perineal (with urethral involvement) NEC N36.Ø
    tuberculous A18.13
    ureter N28.89
  perirectal K6Ø.4
    tuberculous A18.32
  peritoneum K65.9
  pharyngoesophageal J39.2
  pharynx J39.2
    branchial cleft (congenital) Q18.Ø
  pilonidal (infected) (rectum) — *see* Sinus, pilonidal
  pleura, pleural, pleurocutaneous, pleuroperitoneal J86.Ø
    tuberculous NEC A15.6
  pleuropericardial I31.8
  portal vein-hepatic artery, congenital Q26.6
  postauricular H7Ø.81- ☑
  postoperative, persistent T81.83 ☑
    specified site — *see* Fistula, by site
  preauricular (congenital) Q18.1
  prostate N42.89
  pulmonary J86.Ø
    arteriovenous I28.Ø
      congenital Q25.72
    tuberculous — *see* Tuberculosis, pulmonary
  pulmonoperitoneal J86.Ø
  rectolabial N82.4
  rectosigmoid (intercommunicating) K63.2
  rectoureteral N28.89
  rectourethral N36.Ø
    congenital Q64.73
  rectouterine N82.4
    congenital Q51.7
  rectovaginal N82.3
    congenital Q52.2
    tuberculous A18.18
  rectovesical N32.1
    congenital Q64.79
  rectovesicovaginal N82.3
  rectovulval N82.4
    congenital Q52.79
  rectum (to skin) K6Ø.4
    congenital Q43.6
      with absence, atresia and stenosis Q42.Ø
    tuberculous A18.32
  renal N28.89
  retroauricular — *see* Fistula, postauricular
  salivary duct or gland (any) K11.4
    congenital Q38.4
  scrotum (urinary) N5Ø.89
    tuberculous A18.15
  semicircular canals — *see* subcategory H83.1 ☑
  sigmoid K63.2
    to bladder N32.1
  sinus — *see* Sinusitis

Fistula — *continued*
  skin L98.8
    to genital tract (female) N82.5
  splenocolic D73.89
  stercoral K63.2
  stomach K31.6
  sublingual gland K11.4
  submandibular gland K11.4
  submaxillary (gland) K11.4
    region K12.2
  thoracic J86.Ø
    duct I89.8
  thoracoabdominal J86.Ø
  thoracogastric J86.Ø
  thoracointestinal J86.Ø
  thorax J86.Ø
  thyroglossal duct Q89.2
  thyroid EØ7.89
  trachea, congenital (external) (internal) Q32.1
  tracheoesophageal J86.Ø
    congenital Q39.2
      with atresia of esophagus Q39.1
    following tracheostomy J95.Ø4
  traumatic arteriovenous — *see* Injury, blood vessel, by site
  tuberculous — *code by* site under Tuberculosis
  typhoid AØ1.Ø9
  umbilicourinary Q64.8
  urachus, congenital Q64.4
  ureter (persistent) N28.89
  ureteroabdominal N28.89
  ureterorectal N28.89
  ureterosigmoido-abdominal N28.89
  ureterovaginal N82.1
  ureterovesical N32.2
  urethra N36.Ø
    congenital Q64.79
    tuberculous A18.13
  urethroperineal N36.Ø
  urethroperineovesical N32.2
  urethrorectal N36.Ø
    congenital Q64.73
  urethroscrotal N5Ø.89
  urethrovaginal N82.1
  urethrovesical N32.2
  urinary (tract) (persistent) (recurrent) N36.Ø
  uteroabdominal N82.5
    congenital Q51.7
  uteroenteric, uterointestinal N82.4
    congenital Q51.7
  uterorectal N82.4
    congenital Q51.7
  uteroureteric N82.1
  uterourethral Q51.7
  uterovaginal N82.8
  uterovesical N82.1
    congenital Q51.7
  uterus N82.8
  vagina (postpartal) (wall) N82.8
  vaginocutaneous (postpartal) N82.5
  vaginointestinal NEC N82.4
    large intestine N82.3
    small intestine N82.2
  vaginoperineal N82.5
  vasocutaneous, congenital Q55.7
  vesical NEC N32.2
  vesicoabdominal N32.2
  vesicocervicovaginal N82.1
  vesicocolic N32.1
  vesicocutaneous N32.2
  vesicoenteric N32.1
  vesicointestinal N32.1
  vesicometrorectal N82.4
  vesicoperineal N32.2
  vesicorectal N32.1
    congenital Q64.79
  vesicosigmoidal N32.1
  vesicosigmoidovaginal N82.3
  vesicoureteral N32.2
  vesicoureterovaginal N82.1
  vesicourethral N32.2
  vesicourethrorectal N32.1
  vesicouterine N82.1
    congenital Q51.7
  vesicovaginal N82.Ø
  vulvorectal N82.4
    congenital Q52.79
Fit R56.9
  epileptic — *see* Epilepsy

- **Fit** — *continued*
  - fainting R55
  - hysterical F44.5
  - newborn P9Ø
- **Fitting** (and adjustment) (of)
  - artificial
    - arm — *see* Admission, adjustment, artificial, arm
    - breast Z44.3 ☑
    - eye Z44.2 ☑
    - leg — *see* Admission, adjustment, artificial, leg
  - automatic implantable cardiac defibrillator (with synchronous cardiac pacemaker) Z45.Ø2
  - brain neuropacemaker Z46.2
    - implanted Z45.42
  - cardiac defibrillator — *see* Fitting (and adjustment) (of), automatic implantable cardiac defibrillator
  - catheter, non-vascular Z46.82
  - colostomy belt Z46.89
  - contact lenses Z46.Ø
  - CRT-D (resynchronization therapy defibrillator) Z45.Ø2
  - CRT-P (cardiac resynchronization therapy pacemaker) Z45.Ø18
    - pulse generator Z45.Ø1Ø
  - cystostomy device Z46.6
  - defibrillator, cardiac — *see* Fitting (and adjustment) (of), automatic implantable cardiac defibrillator
  - dentures Z46.3
  - device NOS Z46.9
    - abdominal Z46.89
    - gastrointestinal NEC Z46.59
    - implanted NEC Z45.89
    - nervous system Z46.2
      - implanted — *see* Admission, adjustment, device, implanted, nervous system
    - orthodontic Z46.4
    - orthoptic Z46.Ø
    - orthotic Z46.89
    - prosthetic (external) Z44.9
      - breast Z44.3 ☑
      - dental Z46.3
      - eye Z44.2 ☑
      - specified NEC Z44.8
    - specified NEC Z46.89
    - substitution
      - auditory Z46.2
        - implanted — *see* Admission, adjustment, device, implanted, hearing device
      - nervous system Z46.2
        - implanted — *see* Admission, adjustment, device, implanted, nervous system
      - visual Z46.2
        - implanted Z45.31
    - urinary Z46.6
  - gastric lap band Z46.51
  - gastrointestinal appliance NEC Z46.59
  - glasses (reading) Z46.Ø
  - hearing aid Z46.1
  - ileostomy device Z46.89
  - insulin pump Z46.81
  - intestinal appliance NEC Z46.89
  - myringotomy device (stent) (tube) Z45.82
  - neuropacemaker Z46.2
    - implanted Z45.42
  - non-vascular catheter Z46.82
  - orthodontic device Z46.4
  - orthopedic device (brace) (cast) (corset) (shoes) Z46.89
  - pacemaker (cardiac) (cardiac resynchronization therapy (CRT-P)) Z45.Ø18
    - nervous system (brain) (peripheral nerve) (spinal cord) Z46.2
      - implanted Z45.42
    - pulse generator Z45.Ø1Ø
  - portacath (port-a-cath) Z45.2
  - prosthesis (external) Z44.9
    - arm — *see* Admission, adjustment, artificial, arm
    - breast Z44.3 ☑
    - dental Z46.3
    - eye Z44.2 ☑
    - leg — *see* Admission, adjustment, artificial, leg
    - specified NEC Z44.8
  - spectacles Z46.Ø
  - wheelchair Z46.89
- **Fitzhugh-Curtis syndrome**
  - due to
    - Chlamydia trachomatis A74.81
    - Neisseria gonorrhorea (gonococcal peritonitis) A54.85
- **Fitz's syndrome** (acute hemorrhagic pancreatitis) — *see also* Pancreatitis, acute K85.8Ø
- **Fixation**
  - joint — *see* Ankylosis
  - larynx J38.7
  - stapes — *see* Ankylosis, ear ossicles
    - deafness — *see* Deafness, conductive
  - uterus (acquired) — *see* Malposition, uterus
  - vocal cord J38.3
- **Flabby ridge** KØ6.8
- **Flaccid** — *see also* condition
  - palate, congenital Q38.5
- **Flail**
  - chest S22.5 ☑
    - associated with chest compression and cardiopulmonary resuscitation M96.A4
    - newborn (birth injury) P13.8
  - joint (paralytic) M25.2Ø
    - ankle M25.27- ☑
    - elbow M25.22- ☑
    - foot joint M25.27- ☑
    - hand joint M25.24- ☑
    - hip M25.25- ☑
    - knee M25.26- ☑
    - shoulder M25.21- ☑
    - specified joint NEC M25.28
    - wrist M25.23- ☑
- **Flajani's disease** — *see* Hyperthyroidism, with, goiter (diffuse)
- **Flap, liver** K71.3
- **Flashbacks** (residual to hallucinogen use) F16.283
- **Flat**
  - chamber (eye) — *see* Disorder, globe, hypotony, flat anterior chamber
  - chest, congenital Q67.8
  - foot (acquired) (fixed type) (painful) (postural) — *see also* Deformity, limb, flat foot
    - congenital (rigid) (spastic (everted)) Q66.5- ☑
    - rachitic sequelae (late effect) E64.3
  - organ or site, congenital NEC — *see* Anomaly, by site
  - pelvis M95.5
    - with disproportion (fetopelvic) O33.Ø
      - causing obstructed labor O65.Ø
    - congenital Q74.2
- **Flatau-Schilder disease** G37.Ø
- **Flatback syndrome** M4Ø.3Ø
  - lumbar region M4Ø.36
  - lumbosacral region M4Ø.37
  - thoracolumbar region M4Ø.35
- **Flattening**
  - head, femur M89.8X5
  - hip — *see* Coxa, plana
  - lip (congenital) Q18.8
  - nose (congenital) Q67.4
    - acquired M95.Ø
- **Flatulence** R14.3
  - psychogenic F45.8
- **Flatus** R14.3
  - vaginalis N89.8
- **Flax-dresser's disease** J66.1
- **Flea bite** — *see* Injury, bite, by site, superficial, insect
- **Flecks, glaucomatous** (subcapsular) — *see* Cataract, complicated
- **Fleischer (-Kayser) ring** (cornea) H18.Ø4- ☑
- **Fleshy mole** OØ2.Ø
- **Flexibilitas cerea** — *see* Catalepsy
- **Flexion**
  - amputation stump (surgical) T87.89
  - cervix — *see* Malposition, uterus
  - contracture, joint — *see* Contraction, joint
  - deformity, joint — *see also* Deformity, limb, flexion M21.2Ø
    - hip, congenital Q65.89
  - uterus — *see also* Malposition, uterus
    - lateral — *see* Lateroversion, uterus
- **Flexner-Boyd dysentery** AØ3.2
- **Flexner's dysentery** AØ3.1
- **Flexure** — *see* Flexion
- **Flint murmur** (aortic insufficiency) I35.1
- **Floater, vitreous** — *see* Opacity, vitreous
- **Floating**
  - cartilage (joint) — *see also* Loose, body, joint
    - knee — *see* Derangement, knee, loose body
  - gallbladder, congenital Q44.1
  - kidney N28.89
    - congenital Q63.8
  - spleen D73.89
- **Flooding** N92.Ø
- **Floor** — *see* condition
- **Floppy**
  - baby syndrome (nonspecific) P94.2
  - iris syndrome (intraoperative) (IFIS) H21.81
  - nonrheumatic mitral valve syndrome I34.1
- **Flu** — *see also* Influenza
  - avian — *see also* Influenza, due to, identified novel influenza A virus JØ9.X2
  - bird — *see also* Influenza, due to, identified novel influenza A virus JØ9.X2
  - intestinal NEC AØ8.4
  - swine (viruses that normally cause infections in pigs) — *see also* Influenza, due to, identified novel influenza A virus JØ9.X2
- **Fluctuating blood pressure** I99.8
- **Fluid**
  - abdomen R18.8
  - chest J94.8
  - heart — *see* Failure, heart, congestive
  - joint — *see* Effusion, joint
  - loss (acute) E86.9
  - lung — *see* Edema, lung
  - overload E87.7Ø
    - specified NEC E87.79
  - peritoneal cavity R18.8
  - pleural cavity J94.8
  - retention R6Ø.9
- **Flukes NEC** — *see also* Infestation, fluke
  - blood NEC — *see* Schistosomiasis
  - liver B66.3
- **Fluor** (vaginalis) N89.8
  - trichomonal or due to Trichomonas (vaginalis) A59.ØØ
- **Fluorosis**
  - dental KØØ.3
  - skeletal M85.1Ø
    - ankle M85.17- ☑
    - foot M85.17- ☑
    - forearm M85.13- ☑
    - hand M85.14- ☑
    - lower leg M85.16- ☑
    - multiple site M85.19
    - neck M85.18
    - rib M85.18
    - shoulder M85.11- ☑
    - skull M85.18
    - specified site NEC M85.18
    - thigh M85.15- ☑
    - toe M85.17- ☑
    - upper arm M85.12- ☑
    - vertebra M85.18
- **Flush syndrome** E34.Ø
- **Flushing** R23.2
  - menopausal N95.1
- **Flutter**
  - atrial or auricular I48.92
    - atypical I48.4
    - type I I48.3
    - type II I48.4
    - typical I48.3
  - heart I49.8
    - atrial or auricular I48.92
      - atypical I48.4
      - type I I48.3
      - type II I48.4
      - typical I48.3
    - ventricular I49.Ø2
  - ventricular I49.Ø2
- **FNHTR** (febrile nonhemolytic transfusion reaction) R5Ø.84
- **Fochier's abscess** — *code by* site under Abscess
- **Focus, Assmann's** — *see* Tuberculosis, pulmonary
- **Fogo selvagem** L1Ø.3
- **Foix-Alajouanine syndrome** G95.19
- **Fold, folds** (anomalous) — *see also* Anomaly, by site
  - Descemet's membrane — *see* Change, corneal membrane, Descemet's, fold
  - epicanthic Q1Ø.3
  - heart Q24.8
- **Folie à deux** F24
- **Follicle**
  - cervix (nabothian) (ruptured) N88.8
  - graafian, ruptured, with hemorrhage N83.Ø- ☑
  - nabothian N88.8
- **Follicular** — *see* condition
- **Folliculitis** (superficial) L73.9
  - abscedens et suffodiens L66.3
  - cyst N83.Ø- ☑

- **Folliculitis** — *continued*
  - decalvans L66.2
  - deep — *see* Furuncle, by site
  - gonococcal (acute) (chronic) A54.Ø1
  - keloid, keloidalis L73.Ø
  - pustular LØ1.Ø2
  - ulerythematosa reticulata L66.4
- **Folliculome lipidique**
  - specified site — *see* Neoplasm, benign, by site
  - unspecified site
    - female D27.9
    - male D29.2Ø
- **Følling's disease** E7Ø.Ø
- **Follow-up** — *see* Examination, follow-up
- **Fong's syndrome** (hereditary osteo-onychodysplasia) Q87.2
- **Food**
  - allergy L27.2
  - asphyxia (from aspiration or inhalation) — *see* Foreign body, by site
  - choked on — *see* Foreign body, by site
  - deprivation T73.Ø ☑
    - specified kind of food NEC E63.8
  - insecurity Z59.41
  - intoxication — *see* Poisoning, food
  - lack of T73.Ø ☑
  - poisoning — *see* Poisoning, food
  - rejection NEC — *see* Disorder, eating
  - strangulation or suffocation — *see* Foreign body, by site
  - toxemia — *see* Poisoning, food
- **Foot** — *see* condition
- **Foramen ovale** (nonclosure) (patent) (persistent) Q21.12
- **Forbes' glycogen storage disease** E74.Ø3
- **Fordyce-Fox disease** L75.2
- **Fordyce's disease** (mouth) Q38.6
- **Forearm** — *see* condition
- **Foreclosure on loan** Z59.89
- **Foreign body**
  - with
    - laceration — *see* Laceration, by site, with foreign body
    - puncture wound — *see* Puncture, by site, with foreign body
  - accidentally left following a procedure T81.5Ø9 ☑
    - aspiration T81.5Ø6 ☑
      - resulting in
        - adhesions T81.516 ☑
        - obstruction T81.526 ☑
        - perforation T81.536 ☑
        - specified complication NEC T81.596 ☑
    - cardiac catheterization T81.5Ø5 ☑
      - resulting in
        - acute reaction T81.6Ø ☑
          - aseptic peritonitis T81.61 ☑
          - specified NEC T81.69 ☑
        - adhesions T81.515 ☑
        - obstruction T81.525 ☑
        - perforation T81.535 ☑
        - specified complication NEC T81.595 ☑
    - causing
      - acute reaction T81.6Ø ☑
        - aseptic peritonitis T81.61 ☑
        - specified complication NEC T81.69 ☑
      - adhesions T81.519 ☑
      - aseptic peritonitis T81.61 ☑
      - obstruction T81.529 ☑
      - perforation T81.539 ☑
      - specified complication NEC T81.599 ☑
    - endoscopy T81.5Ø4 ☑
      - resulting in
        - adhesions T81.514 ☑
        - obstruction T81.524 ☑
        - perforation T81.534 ☑
        - specified complication NEC T81.594 ☑
    - immunization T81.5Ø3 ☑
      - resulting in
        - adhesions T81.513 ☑
        - obstruction T81.523 ☑
        - perforation T81.533 ☑
        - specified complication NEC T81.593 ☑
    - infusion T81.5Ø1 ☑
      - resulting in
        - adhesions T81.511 ☑
        - obstruction T81.521 ☑
        - perforation T81.531 ☑

- **Foreign body** — *continued*
  - accidentally left following a procedure — *continued*
    - infusion — *continued*
      - resulting in — *continued*
        - specified complication NEC T81.591 ☑
    - injection T81.5Ø3 ☑
      - resulting in
        - adhesions T81.513 ☑
        - obstruction T81.523 ☑
        - perforation T81.533 ☑
        - specified complication NEC T81.593 ☑
    - kidney dialysis T81.5Ø2 ☑
      - resulting in
        - adhesions T81.512 ☑
        - obstruction T81.522 ☑
        - perforation T81.532 ☑
        - specified complication NEC T81.592 ☑
    - packing removal T81.5Ø7 ☑
      - resulting in
        - acute reaction T81.6Ø ☑
          - aseptic peritonitis T81.61 ☑
          - specified NEC T81.69 ☑
        - adhesions T81.517 ☑
        - obstruction T81.527 ☑
        - perforation T81.537 ☑
        - specified complication NEC T81.597 ☑
    - puncture T81.5Ø6 ☑
      - resulting in
        - adhesions T81.516 ☑
        - obstruction T81.526 ☑
        - perforation T81.536 ☑
        - specified complication NEC T81.596 ☑
    - specified procedure NEC T81.5Ø8 ☑
      - resulting in
        - acute reaction T81.6Ø ☑
          - aseptic peritonitis T81.61 ☑
          - specified NEC T81.69 ☑
        - adhesions T81.518 ☑
        - obstruction T81.528 ☑
        - perforation T81.538 ☑
        - specified complication NEC T81.598 ☑
    - surgical operation T81.5ØØ ☑
      - resulting in
        - acute reaction T81.6Ø ☑
          - aseptic peritonitis T81.61 ☑
          - specified NEC T81.69 ☑
        - adhesions T81.51Ø ☑
        - obstruction T81.52Ø ☑
        - perforation T81.53Ø ☑
        - specified complication NEC T81.59Ø ☑
    - transfusion T81.5Ø1 ☑
      - resulting in
        - adhesions T81.511 ☑
        - obstruction T81.521 ☑
        - perforation T81.531 ☑
        - specified complication NEC T81.591 ☑
  - alimentary tract T18.9 ☑
    - anus T18.5 ☑
    - colon T18.4 ☑
    - esophagus — *see* Foreign body, esophagus
    - mouth T18.Ø ☑
    - multiple sites T18.8 ☑
    - rectosigmoid (junction) T18.5 ☑
    - rectum T18.5 ☑
    - small intestine T18.3 ☑
    - specified site NEC T18.8 ☑
    - stomach T18.2 ☑
  - anterior chamber (eye) SØ5.5- ☑
  - auditory canal — *see* Foreign body, entering through orifice, ear
  - bronchus T17.5Ø8 ☑
    - causing
      - asphyxiation T17.5ØØ ☑
        - food (bone) (seed) T17.52Ø ☑
        - gastric contents (vomitus) T17.51Ø ☑
        - specified type NEC T17.59Ø ☑
      - injury NEC T17.5Ø8 ☑
        - food (bone) (seed) T17.528 ☑
        - gastric contents (vomitus) T17.518 ☑
        - specified type NEC T17.598 ☑
  - canthus — *see* Foreign body, conjunctival sac
  - ciliary body (eye) SØ5.5- ☑
  - conjunctival sac T15.1- ☑
  - cornea T15.Ø- ☑
  - entering through orifice
    - accessory sinus T17.Ø ☑

- **Foreign body** — *continued*
  - entering through orifice — *continued*
    - alimentary canal T18.9 ☑
      - multiple parts T18.8 ☑
      - specified part NEC T18.8 ☑
    - alveolar process T18.Ø ☑
    - antrum (Highmore's) T17.Ø ☑
    - anus T18.5 ☑
    - appendix T18.4 ☑
    - auditory canal — *see* Foreign body, entering through orifice, ear
    - auricle — *see* Foreign body, entering through orifice, ear
    - bladder T19.1 ☑
    - bronchioles — *see* Foreign body, respiratory tract, specified site NEC
    - bronchus (main) — *see* Foreign body, bronchus
    - buccal cavity T18.Ø ☑
    - canthus (inner) — *see* Foreign body, conjunctival sac
    - cecum T18.4 ☑
    - cervix (canal) (uteri) T19.3 ☑
    - colon T18.4 ☑
    - conjunctival sac — *see* Foreign body, conjunctival sac
    - cornea — *see* Foreign body, cornea
    - digestive organ or tract NOS T18.9 ☑
      - multiple parts T18.8 ☑
      - specified part NEC T18.8 ☑
    - duodenum T18.3 ☑
    - ear (external) T16.- ☑
    - esophagus — *see* Foreign body, esophagus
    - eye (external) NOS T15.9- ☑
      - conjunctival sac — *see* Foreign body, conjunctival sac
      - cornea — *see* Foreign body, cornea
      - specified part NEC T15.8- ☑
    - eyeball — *see also* Foreign body, entering through orifice, eye, specified part NEC
      - with penetrating wound — *see* Puncture, eyeball
    - eyelid — *see also* Foreign body, conjunctival sac
      - with
        - laceration — *see* Laceration, eyelid, with foreign body
        - puncture — *see* Puncture, eyelid, with foreign body
        - superficial injury — *see* Foreign body, superficial, eyelid
    - gastrointestinal tract T18.9 ☑
      - multiple parts T18.8 ☑
      - specified part NEC T18.8 ☑
    - genitourinary tract T19.9 ☑
      - multiple parts T19.8 ☑
      - specified part NEC T19.8 ☑
    - globe — *see* Foreign body, entering through orifice, eyeball
    - gum T18.Ø ☑
    - Highmore's antrum T17.Ø ☑
    - hypopharynx — *see* Foreign body, pharynx
    - ileum T18.3 ☑
    - intestine (small) T18.3 ☑
      - large T18.4 ☑
    - lacrimal apparatus (punctum) — *see* Foreign body, entering through orifice, eye, specified part NEC
    - large intestine T18.4 ☑
    - larynx — *see* Foreign body, larynx
    - lung — *see* Foreign body, respiratory tract, specified site NEC
    - maxillary sinus T17.Ø ☑
    - mouth T18.Ø ☑
    - nasal sinus T17.Ø ☑
    - nasopharynx — *see* Foreign body, pharynx
    - nose (passage) T17.1 ☑
    - nostril T17.1 ☑
    - oral cavity T18.Ø ☑
    - palate T18.Ø ☑
    - penis T19.4 ☑
    - pharynx — *see* Foreign body, pharynx
    - piriform sinus — *see* Foreign body, pharynx
    - rectosigmoid (junction) T18.5 ☑
    - rectum T18.5 ☑
    - respiratory tract — *see* Foreign body, respiratory tract
    - sinus (accessory) (frontal) (maxillary) (nasal) T17.Ø ☑
      - piriform — *see* Foreign body, pharynx

Foreign body — *continued*
entering through orifice — *continued*
small intestine T18.3 ☑
stomach T18.2 ☑
suffocation by — *see* Foreign body, by site
tear ducts or glands — *see* Foreign body, entering through orifice, eye, specified part NEC
throat — *see* Foreign body, pharynx
tongue T18.0 ☑
tonsil, tonsillar (fossa) — *see* Foreign body, pharynx
trachea — *see* Foreign body, trachea
ureter T19.8 ☑
urethra T19.0 ☑
uterus (any part) T19.3 ☑
vagina T19.2 ☑
vulva T19.2 ☑
esophagus T18.108 ☑
causing
injury NEC T18.108 ☑
food (bone) (seed) T18.128 ☑
gastric contents (vomitus) T18.118 ☑
specified type NEC T18.198 ☑
tracheal compression T18.100 ☑
food (bone) (seed) T18.120 ☑
gastric contents (vomitus) T18.110 ☑
specified type NEC T18.190 ☑
feeling of, in throat R09.89
fragment — *see* Retained, foreign body fragments (type of)
genitourinary tract T19.9 ☑
bladder T19.1 ☑
multiple parts T19.8 ☑
penis T19.4 ☑
specified site NEC T19.8 ☑
urethra T19.0 ☑
uterus T19.3 ☑
IUD Z97.5
vagina T19.2 ☑
contraceptive device Z97.5
vulva T19.2 ☑
granuloma (old) (soft tissue) — *see also* Granuloma, foreign body
skin L92.3
in
laceration — *see* Laceration, by site, with foreign body
puncture wound — *see* Puncture, by site, with foreign body
soft tissue (residual) M79.5
inadvertently left in operation wound — *see* Foreign body, accidentally left during a procedure
ingestion, ingested NOS T18.9 ☑
inhalation or inspiration — *see* Foreign body, by site
internal organ, not entering through a natural orifice — code as specific injury with foreign body
intraocular S05.5- ☑
old, retained (nonmagnetic) H44.70- ☑
anterior chamber H44.71- ☑
ciliary body H44.72- ☑
iris H44.72- ☑
lens H44.73- ☑
magnetic H44.60- ☑
anterior chamber H44.61- ☑
ciliary body H44.62- ☑
iris H44.62- ☑
lens H44.63- ☑
posterior wall H44.64- ☑
specified site NEC H44.69- ☑
vitreous body H44.65- ☑
posterior wall H44.74- ☑
specified site NEC H44.79- ☑
vitreous body H44.75- ☑
iris — *see* Foreign body, intraocular
lacrimal punctum — *see* Foreign body, entering through orifice, eye, specified part NEC
larynx T17.308 ☑
causing
asphyxiation T17.300 ☑
food (bone) (seed) T17.320 ☑
gastric contents (vomitus) T17.310 ☑
specified type NEC T17.390 ☑
injury NEC T17.308 ☑
food (bone) (seed) T17.328 ☑
gastric contents (vomitus) T17.318 ☑
specified type NEC T17.398 ☑
lens — *see* Foreign body, intraocular

Foreign body — *continued*
ocular muscle S05.4- ☑
old, retained — *see* Foreign body, orbit, old
old or residual
soft tissue (residual) M79.5
operation wound, left accidentally — *see* Foreign body, accidentally left during a procedure
orbit S05.4- ☑
old, retained H05.5- ☑
pharynx T17.208 ☑
causing
asphyxiation T17.200 ☑
food (bone) (seed) T17.220 ☑
gastric contents (vomitus) T17.210 ☑
specified type NEC T17.290 ☑
injury NEC T17.208 ☑
food (bone) (seed) T17.228 ☑
gastric contents (vomitus) T17.218 ☑
specified type NEC T17.298 ☑
respiratory tract T17.908 ☑
bronchioles — *see* Foreign body, respiratory tract, specified site NEC
bronchus — *see* Foreign body, bronchus
causing
asphyxiation T17.900 ☑
food (bone) (seed) T17.920 ☑
gastric contents (vomitus) T17.910 ☑
specified type NEC T17.990 ☑
injury NEC T17.908 ☑
food (bone) (seed) T17.928 ☑
gastric contents (vomitus) T17.918 ☑
specified type NEC T17.998 ☑
larynx — *see* Foreign body, larynx
lung — *see* Foreign body, respiratory tract, specified site NEC
multiple parts — *see* Foreign body, respiratory tract, specified site NEC
nasal sinus T17.0 ☑
nasopharynx — *see* Foreign body, pharynx
nose T17.1 ☑
nostril T17.1 ☑
pharynx — *see* Foreign body, pharynx
specified site NEC T17.808 ☑
causing
asphyxiation T17.800 ☑
food (bone) (seed) T17.820 ☑
gastric contents (vomitus) T17.810 ☑
specified type NEC T17.890 ☑
injury NEC T17.808 ☑
food (bone) (seed) T17.828 ☑
gastric contents (vomitus) T17.818 ☑
specified type NEC T17.898 ☑
throat — *see* Foreign body, pharynx
trachea — *see* Foreign body, trachea
retained (old) (nonmagnetic) (in)
anterior chamber (eye) — *see* Foreign body, intraocular, old, retained, anterior chamber
magnetic — *see* Foreign body, intraocular, old, retained, magnetic, anterior chamber
ciliary body — *see* Foreign body, intraocular, old, retained, ciliary body
magnetic — *see* Foreign body, intraocular, old, retained, magnetic, ciliary body
eyelid H02.819
left H02.816
lower H02.815
upper H02.814
right H02.813
lower H02.812
upper H02.811
fragments — *see* Retained, foreign body fragments (type of)
globe — *see* Foreign body, intraocular, old, retained
magnetic — *see* Foreign body, intraocular, old, retained, magnetic
intraocular — *see* Foreign body, intraocular, old, retained
magnetic — *see* Foreign body, intraocular, old, retained, magnetic
iris — *see* Foreign body, intraocular, old, retained, iris
magnetic — *see* Foreign body, intraocular, old, retained, magnetic, iris
lens — *see* Foreign body, intraocular, old, retained, lens
magnetic — *see* Foreign body, intraocular, old, retained, magnetic, lens

Foreign body — *continued*
retained — *continued*
muscle — *see* Foreign body, retained, soft tissue
orbit — *see* Foreign body, orbit, old
posterior wall of globe — *see* Foreign body, intraocular, old, retained, posterior wall
magnetic — *see* Foreign body, intraocular, old, retained, magnetic, posterior wall
retrobulbar — *see* Foreign body, orbit, old, retrobulbar
soft tissue M79.5
vitreous — *see* Foreign body, intraocular, old, retained, vitreous body
magnetic — *see* Foreign body, intraocular, old, retained, magnetic, vitreous body
retina S05.5- ☑
superficial, without open wound
abdomen, abdominal (wall) S30.851 ☑
alveolar process S00.552 ☑
ankle S90.55- ☑
antecubital space — *see* Foreign body, superficial, forearm
anus S30.857 ☑
arm (upper) S40.85- ☑
auditory canal — *see* Foreign body, superficial, ear
auricle — *see* Foreign body, superficial, ear
axilla — *see* Foreign body, superficial, arm
back, lower S30.850 ☑
breast S20.15- ☑
brow S00.85 ☑
buttock S30.850 ☑
calf — *see* Foreign body, superficial, leg
canthus — *see* Foreign body, superficial, eyelid
cheek S00.85 ☑
internal S00.552 ☑
chest wall — *see* Foreign body, superficial, thorax
chin S00.85 ☑
clitoris S30.854 ☑
costal region — *see* Foreign body, superficial, thorax
digit(s)
foot — *see* Foreign body, superficial, toe
hand — *see* Foreign body, superficial, finger
ear S00.45- ☑
elbow S50.35- ☑
epididymis S30.853 ☑
epigastric region S30.851 ☑
epiglottis S10.15 ☑
esophagus, cervical S10.15 ☑
eyebrow — *see* Foreign body, superficial, eyelid
eyelid S00.25- ☑
face S00.85 ☑
finger(s) S60.459 ☑
index S60.45- ☑
little S60.45- ☑
middle S60.45- ☑
ring S60.45- ☑
flank S30.851 ☑
foot (except toe(s) alone) S90.85- ☑
toe — *see* Foreign body, superficial, toe
forearm S50.85- ☑
elbow only — *see* Foreign body, superficial, elbow
forehead S00.85 ☑
genital organs, external
female S30.856 ☑
male S30.855 ☑
groin S30.851 ☑
gum S00.552 ☑
hand S60.55- ☑
head S00.95 ☑
ear — *see* Foreign body, superficial, ear
eyelid — *see* Foreign body, superficial, eyelid
lip S00.551 ☑
nose S00.35 ☑
oral cavity S00.552 ☑
scalp S00.05 ☑
specified site NEC S00.85 ☑
heel — *see* Foreign body, superficial, foot
hip S70.25- ☑
inguinal region S30.851 ☑
interscapular region S20.459 ☑
jaw S00.85 ☑
knee S80.25- ☑
labium (majus) (minus) S30.854 ☑
larynx S10.15 ☑
leg (lower) S80.85- ☑

Foreign body — *continued*
  superficial, without open wound — *continued*
    leg — *continued*
      knee — *see* Foreign body, superficial, knee
      upper — *see* Foreign body, superficial, thigh
    lip S00.551 ☑
    lower back S30.850 ☑
    lumbar region S30.850 ☑
    malar region S00.85 ☑
    mammary — *see* Foreign body, superficial, breast
    mastoid region S00.85 ☑
    mouth S00.552 ☑
    nail
      finger — *see* Foreign body, superficial, finger
      toe — *see* Foreign body, superficial, toe
    nape S10.85 ☑
    nasal S00.35 ☑
    neck S10.95 ☑
      specified site NEC S10.85 ☑
      throat S10.15 ☑
    nose S00.35 ☑
    occipital region S00.05 ☑
    oral cavity S00.552 ☑
    orbital region — *see* Foreign body, superficial, eyelid
    palate S00.552 ☑
    palm — *see* Foreign body, superficial, hand
    parietal region S00.05 ☑
    pelvis S30.850 ☑
    penis S30.852 ☑
    perineum
      female S30.854 ☑
      male S30.850 ☑
    periocular area — *see* Foreign body, superficial, eyelid
    phalanges
      finger — *see* Foreign body, superficial, finger
      toe — *see* Foreign body, superficial, toe
    pharynx S10.15 ☑
    pinna — *see* Foreign body, superficial, ear
    popliteal space — *see* Foreign body, superficial, knee
    prepuce S30.852 ☑
    pubic region S30.850 ☑
    pudendum
      female S30.856 ☑
      male S30.855 ☑
    sacral region S30.850 ☑
    scalp S00.05 ☑
    scapular region — *see* Foreign body, superficial, shoulder
    scrotum S30.853 ☑
    shin — *see* Foreign body, superficial, leg
    shoulder S40.25- ☑
    sternal region S20.359 ☑
    submaxillary region S00.85 ☑
    submental region S00.85 ☑
    subungual
      finger(s) — *see* Foreign body, superficial, finger
      toe(s) — *see* Foreign body, superficial, toe
    supraclavicular fossa S10.85 ☑
    supraorbital S00.85 ☑
    temple S00.85 ☑
    temporal region S00.85 ☑
    testis S30.853 ☑
    thigh S70.35- ☑
    thorax, thoracic (wall) S20.95 ☑
      back S20.45- ☑
      front S20.35- ☑
    throat S10.15 ☑
    thumb S60.35- ☑
    toe(s) (lesser) S90.456 ☑
      great S90.45- ☑
    tongue S00.552 ☑
    trachea S10.15 ☑
    tunica vaginalis S30.853 ☑
    tympanum, tympanic membrane — *see* Foreign body, superficial, ear
    uvula S00.552 ☑
    vagina S30.854 ☑
    vocal cords S10.15 ☑
    vulva S30.854 ☑
    wrist S60.85- ☑
  swallowed T18.9 ☑
  trachea T17.408 ☑
    causing
      asphyxiation T17.400 ☑

Foreign body — *continued*
  trachea — *continued*
    causing — *continued*
      asphyxiation — *continued*
        food (bone) (seed) T17.420 ☑
        gastric contents (vomitus) T17.410 ☑
        specified type NEC T17.490 ☑
      injury NEC T17.408 ☑
        food (bone) (seed) T17.428 ☑
        gastric contents (vomitus) T17.418 ☑
        specified type NEC T17.498 ☑
  type of fragment — *see* Retained, foreign body fragments (type of)
  vitreous (humor) S05.5- ☑
Forestier's disease (rhizomelic pseudopolyarthritis) M35.3
  meaning ankylosing hyperostosis — *see* Hyperostosis, ankylosing
Formation
  hyalin in cornea — *see* Degeneration, cornea
  sequestrum in bone (due to infection) — *see* Osteomyelitis, chronic
  valve
    colon, congenital Q43.8
    ureter (congenital) Q62.39
Formication R20.2
Fort Bragg fever A27.89
Fossa — *see also* condition
  pyriform — *see* condition
Foster-Kennedy syndrome H47.14- ☑
Fothergill's
  disease (trigeminal neuralgia) — *see also* Neuralgia, trigeminal
  scarlatina anginosa A38.9
Foul breath R19.6
Foundling Z76.1
Fournier disease or gangrene N49.3
  female N76.82
  vagina and vulva N76.82
Fourth
  cranial nerve — *see* condition
  molar K00.1
Foville's (peduncular) **disease or syndrome** G46.3
Fox (-Fordyce) disease (apocrine miliaria) L75.2
FPIES (food protein-induced enterocolitis syndrome) K52.21
Fracture, burst — *see* Fracture, traumatic, by site
Fracture, chronic — *see* Fracture, pathological, by site
Fracture, insufficiency — *see* Fracture, pathological, by site
Fracture, nontraumatic, NEC
  atypical
    femur M84.750- ☑
      complete
        oblique M84.759 ☑
          left side M84.758 ☑
          right side M84.757 ☑
        transverse M84.756 ☑
          left side M84.755 ☑
          right side M84.754 ☑
      incomplete M84.753 ☑
        left side M84.752 ☑
        right side M84.751 ☑
Fracture, pathological (pathologic) — *see also* Fracture, traumatic M84.40 ☑
  ankle M84.47- ☑
  carpus M84.44- ☑
  clavicle M84.41- ☑
  compression (not due to trauma) — *see also* Collapse, vertebra M48.50- ☑
  dental implant M27.63
  dental restorative material K08.539
    with loss of material K08.531
    without loss of material K08.530
  due to
    neoplastic disease NEC — *see also* Neoplasm M84.50 ☑
      ankle M84.57- ☑
      carpus M84.54- ☑
      clavicle M84.51- ☑
      femur M84.55- ☑
      fibula M84.56- ☑
      finger M84.54- ☑
      hip M84.559 ☑
      humerus M84.52- ☑
      ilium M84.550 ☑

Fracture, pathological — *continued*
  due to — *continued*
    neoplastic disease — *see also* Neoplasm — *continued*
      ischium M84.550 ☑
      metacarpus M84.54- ☑
      metatarsus M84.57- ☑
      neck M84.58 ☑
      pelvis M84.550 ☑
      radius M84.53- ☑
      rib M84.58 ☑
      scapula M84.51- ☑
      skull M84.58 ☑
      specified site NEC M84.58 ☑
      tarsus M84.57- ☑
      tibia M84.56- ☑
      toe M84.57- ☑
      ulna M84.53- ☑
      vertebra M84.58 ☑
    osteoporosis M80.00 ☑
      disuse — *see* Osteoporosis, specified type NEC, with pathological fracture
      drug-induced — *see* Osteoporosis, drug induced, with pathological fracture
      idiopathic — *see* Osteoporosis, specified type NEC, with pathological fracture
      postmenopausal — *see* Osteoporosis, postmenopausal, with pathological fracture
      postoophorectomy — *see* Osteoporosis, postoophorectomy, with pathological fracture
      postsurgical malabsorption — *see* Osteoporosis, specified type NEC, with pathological fracture
      specified cause NEC — *see* Osteoporosis, specified type NEC, with pathological fracture
    specified disease NEC M84.60 ☑
      ankle M84.67- ☑
      carpus M84.64- ☑
      clavicle M84.61- ☑
      femur M84.65- ☑
      fibula M84.66- ☑
      finger M84.64- ☑
      hip M84.65- ☑
      humerus M84.62- ☑
      ilium M84.650 ☑
      ischium M84.650 ☑
      metacarpus M84.64- ☑
      metatarsus M84.67- ☑
      neck M84.68 ☑
      radius M84.63- ☑
      rib M84.68 ☑
      scapula M84.61- ☑
      skull M84.68 ☑
      tarsus M84.67- ☑
      tibia M84.66- ☑
      toe M84.67- ☑
      ulna M84.63- ☑
      vertebra M84.68 ☑
  femur M84.45- ☑
  fibula M84.46- ☑
  finger M84.44- ☑
  hip M84.459 ☑
  humerus M84.42- ☑
  ilium M84.454 ☑
  ischium M84.454 ☑
  joint prosthesis — *see* Complications, joint prosthesis, mechanical, breakdown, by site
    periprosthetic — *see* Fracture, pathological, periprosthetic
  metacarpus M84.44- ☑
  metatarsus M84.47- ☑
  neck M84.48 ☑
  pelvis M84.454 ☑
  periprosthetic M97.9 ☑
    ankle M97.2- ☑
    elbow M97.4- ☑
    finger M97.8 ☑
    hip M97.0- ☑
    knee M97.1- ☑
    other specified joint M97.8 ☑
    shoulder M97.3- ☑
    spinal joint M97.8 ☑
    toe joint M97.8 ☑
    wrist joint M97.8 ☑
  radius M84.43- ☑
  restorative material (dental) K08.539

- **Fracture, pathological** — *continued*
  - restorative material — *continued*
    - with loss of material KØ8.531
    - without loss of material KØ8.53Ø
  - rib M84.48 ☑
  - scapula M84.41- ☑
  - skull M84.48 ☑
  - tarsus M84.47- ☑
  - tibia M84.46- ☑
  - toe M84.47- ☑
  - ulna M84.43- ☑
  - vertebra M84.48 ☑
- **Fracture, traumatic** (abduction) (adduction) (separation) — *see also* Fracture, pathological T14.8 ☑
  - acetabulum S32.4Ø- ☑
    - column
      - anterior (displaced) (iliopubic) S32.43- ☑
        - nondisplaced S32.436 ☑
      - posterior (displaced) (ilioischial) S32.443 ☑
        - nondisplaced S32.44- ☑
    - dome (displaced) S32.48- ☑
      - nondisplaced S32.48 ☑
    - specified NEC S32.49- ☑
    - transverse (displaced) S32.45- ☑
      - with associated posterior wall fracture (displaced) S32.46- ☑
        - nondisplaced S32.46- ☑
      - nondisplaced S32.45- ☑
    - wall
      - anterior (displaced) S32.41- ☑
        - nondisplaced S32.41- ☑
      - medial (displaced) S32.47- ☑
        - nondisplaced S32.47- ☑
      - posterior (displaced) S32.42- ☑
        - with associated transverse fracture (displaced) S32.46- ☑
          - nondisplaced S32.46- ☑
        - nondisplaced S32.42- ☑
  - acromion — *see* Fracture, scapula, acromial process
  - ankle S82.899 ☑
    - bimalleolar (displaced) S82.84- ☑
      - nondisplaced S82.84- ☑
    - lateral malleolus only (displaced) S82.6- ☑
      - nondisplaced S82.6- ☑
    - medial malleolus (displaced) S82.5- ☑
      - associated with Maisonneuve's fracture — *see* Fracture, Maisonneuve's
      - nondisplaced S82.5- ☑
    - talus — *see* Fracture, tarsal, talus
    - trimalleolar (displaced) S82.85- ☑
      - nondisplaced S82.85- ☑
  - arm (upper) — *see also* Fracture, humerus, shaft
    - humerus — *see* Fracture, humerus
    - radius — *see* Fracture, radius
    - ulna — *see* Fracture, ulna
  - associated with chest compression and cardiopulmonary resuscitation M96.A9
  - astragalus — *see* Fracture, tarsal, talus
  - atlas — *see* Fracture, neck, cervical vertebra, first
  - axis — *see* Fracture, neck, cervical vertebra, second
  - back — *see* Fracture, vertebra
  - Barton's — *see* Barton's fracture
  - base of skull — *see* Fracture, skull, base
  - basicervical (basal) (femoral) S72.Ø ☑
  - Bennett's — *see* Bennett's fracture
  - bimalleolar — *see* Fracture, ankle, bimalleolar
  - blow-out SØ2.3- ☑
  - bone NEC T14.8 ☑
    - birth injury P13.9
    - following insertion of orthopedic implant, joint prosthesis or bone plate — *see* Fracture, following insertion of orthopedic implant, joint prosthesis or bone plate
    - in (due to) neoplastic disease NEC — *see* Fracture, pathological, due to, neoplastic disease
    - pathological (cause unknown) — *see* Fracture, pathological
  - breast bone — *see* Fracture, sternum
  - bucket handle (semilunar cartilage) — *see* Tear, meniscus
  - buckle — *see* Fracture, by site, torus
  - burst — *see* Fracture, traumatic, by site
  - calcaneus — *see* Fracture, tarsal, calcaneus
  - carpal bone(s) S62.1Ø- ☑
    - capitate (displaced) S62.13- ☑
      - nondisplaced S62.13- ☑

- **Fracture, traumatic** — *continued*
  - carpal bone(s) — *continued*
    - cuneiform — *see* Fracture, carpal bone, triquetrum
    - hamate (body) (displaced) S62.143 ☑
      - hook process (displaced) S62.15- ☑
        - nondisplaced S62.15- ☑
      - nondisplaced S62.14- ☑
    - larger multangular — *see* Fracture, carpal bones, trapezium
    - lunate (displaced) S62.12- ☑
      - nondisplaced S62.12- ☑
    - navicular S62.ØØ- ☑
      - distal pole (displaced) S62.Ø1- ☑
        - nondisplaced S62.Ø1- ☑
      - middle third (displaced) S62.Ø2- ☑
        - nondisplaced S62.Ø2- ☑
      - proximal third (displaced) S62.Ø3- ☑
        - nondisplaced S62.Ø3- ☑
      - volar tuberosity — *see* Fracture, carpal bones, navicular, distal pole
    - os magnum — *see* Fracture, carpal bones, capitate
    - pisiform (displaced) S62.16- ☑
      - nondisplaced S62.16- ☑
    - semilunar — *see* Fracture, carpal bones, lunate
    - smaller multangular — *see* Fracture, carpal bones, trapezoid
    - trapezium (displaced) S62.17- ☑
      - nondisplaced S62.17- ☑
    - trapezoid (displaced) S62.18- ☑
      - nondisplaced S62.18- ☑
    - triquetrum (displaced) S62.11- ☑
      - nondisplaced S62.11- ☑
    - unciform — *see* Fracture, carpal bones, hamate
  - cervical — *see* Fracture, vertebra, cervical
  - clavicle S42.ØØ- ☑
    - acromial end (displaced) S42.Ø3- ☑
      - nondisplaced S42.Ø3- ☑
    - birth injury P13.4
    - lateral end — *see* Fracture, clavicle, acromial end
    - shaft (displaced) S42.Ø2- ☑
      - nondisplaced S42.Ø2- ☑
    - sternal end (anterior) (displaced) S42.Ø1- ☑
      - nondisplaced S42.Ø1- ☑
      - posterior S42.Ø1- ☑
  - coccyx S32.2 ☑
  - collapsed — *see* Collapse, vertebra
  - collar bone — *see* Fracture, clavicle
  - Colles' — *see* Colles' fracture
  - coronoid process — *see* Fracture, ulna, upper end, coronoid process
  - corpus cavernosum penis S39.84Ø ☑
  - costochondral cartilage S23.41 ☑
  - costochondral, costosternal junction — *see* Fracture, rib
  - cranium — *see* Fracture, skull
  - cricoid cartilage S12.8 ☑
  - cuboid (ankle) — *see* Fracture, tarsal, cuboid
  - cuneiform
    - foot — *see* Fracture, tarsal, cuneiform
    - wrist — *see* Fracture, carpal, triquetrum
  - delayed union — *see* Delay, union, fracture
  - dental restorative material KØ8.539
    - with loss of material KØ8.531
    - without loss of material KØ8.53Ø
  - due to
    - birth injury — *see* Birth, injury, fracture
    - osteoporosis — *see* Osteoporosis, with fracture
  - Dupuytren's — *see* Fracture, ankle, lateral malleolus
  - elbow S42.4Ø- ☑
  - ethmoid (bone) (sinus) — *see* Fracture, skull, base
  - face bone SØ2.92 ☑
  - fatigue — *see also* Fracture, stress
    - vertebra M48.4Ø ☑
      - cervical region M48.42 ☑
      - cervicothoracic region M48.43 ☑
      - lumbar region M48.46 ☑
      - lumbosacral region M48.47 ☑
      - occipito-atlanto-axial region M48.41 ☑
      - sacrococcygeal region M48.48 ☑
      - thoracic region M48.44 ☑
      - thoracolumbar region M48.45 ☑
  - femur, femoral S72.9- ☑
    - basicervical (basal) S72.Ø ☑
    - birth injury P13.2
    - capital epiphyseal S79.Ø1- ☑

- **Fracture, traumatic** — *continued*
  - femur, femoral — *continued*
    - condyles, epicondyles — *see* Fracture, femur, lower end
    - distal end — *see* Fracture, femur, lower end
    - epiphysis
      - head — *see* Fracture, femur, upper end, epiphysis
      - lower — *see* Fracture, femur, lower end, epiphysis
      - upper — *see* Fracture, femur, upper end, epiphysis
    - following insertion of implant, prosthesis or plate M96.66- ☑
    - head — *see* Fracture, femur, upper end, head
    - intertrochanteric — *see* Fracture, femur, trochanteric
    - intratrochanteric — *see* Fracture, femur, trochanteric
    - lower end S72.4Ø- ☑
      - condyle (displaced) S72.41- ☑
        - lateral (displaced) S72.42- ☑
          - nondisplaced S72.42- ☑
        - medial (displaced) S72.43- ☑
          - nondisplaced S72.43- ☑
        - nondisplaced S72.41- ☑
      - epiphysis (displaced) S72.44- ☑
        - nondisplaced S72.44- ☑
      - physeal S79.1Ø- ☑
        - Salter-Harris
          - Type I S79.11- ☑
          - Type II S79.12- ☑
          - Type III S79.13- ☑
          - Type IV S79.14- ☑
        - specified NEC S79.19- ☑
      - specified NEC S72.49- ☑
      - supracondylar (displaced) S72.45- ☑
        - with intracondylar extension (displaced) S72.46- ☑
          - nondisplaced S72.46- ☑
        - nondisplaced S72.45- ☑
      - torus S72.47- ☑
    - neck — *see* Fracture, femur, upper end, neck
    - pertrochanteric — *see* Fracture, femur, trochanteric
    - shaft (lower third) (middle third) (upper third) S72.3Ø- ☑
      - comminuted (displaced) S72.35- ☑
        - nondisplaced S72.35- ☑
      - oblique (displaced) S72.33- ☑
        - nondisplaced S72.33- ☑
      - segmental (displaced) S72.36- ☑
        - nondisplaced S72.36- ☑
      - specified NEC S72.39- ☑
      - spiral (displaced) S72.34- ☑
        - nondisplaced S72.34- ☑
      - transverse (displaced) S72.32- ☑
        - nondisplaced S72.32- ☑
    - specified site NEC — *see* subcategory S72.8 ☑
    - subcapital (displaced) S72.Ø1- ☑
    - subtrochanteric (region) (section) (displaced) S72.2- ☑
    - nondisplaced S72.2- ☑
    - transcervical — *see* Fracture, femur, midcervical
    - transtrochanteric — *see* Fracture, femur, trochanteric
    - trochanteric S72.1Ø- ☑
      - apophyseal (displaced) S72.13- ☑
        - nondisplaced S72.13- ☑
      - greater trochanter (displaced) S72.11- ☑
        - nondisplaced S72.11- ☑
      - intertrochanteric (displaced) S72.14- ☑
        - nondisplaced S72.14- ☑
      - lesser trochanter (displaced) S72.12- ☑
        - nondisplaced S72.12- ☑
    - upper end S72.ØØ- ☑
      - apophyseal (displaced) S72.13- ☑
        - nondisplaced S72.13- ☑
      - cervicotrochanteric — *see* Fracture, femur, upper end, neck, base
      - epiphysis (displaced) S72.Ø2- ☑
        - nondisplaced S72.Ø2- ☑
      - head S72.Ø5- ☑
        - articular (displaced) S72.Ø6- ☑
          - nondisplaced S72.Ø6- ☑
        - specified NEC S72.Ø9- ☑
      - intertrochanteric (displaced) S72.14- ☑
        - nondisplaced S72.14- ☑

Fracture, traumatic — *continued*
femur, femoral — *continued*
upper end — *continued*
intracapsular S72.Ø1- ☑
midcervical (displaced) S72.Ø3- ☑
nondisplaced S72.Ø3- ☑
neck S72.ØØ- ☑
base (displaced) S72.Ø4- ☑
nondisplaced S72.Ø4- ☑
specified NEC S72.Ø9- ☑
pertrochanteric — *see* Fracture, femur, upper end, trochanteric
physeal S79.ØØ- ☑
Salter-Harris type I S79.Ø1- ☑
specified NEC S79.Ø9- ☑
subcapital (displaced) S72.Ø1- ☑
subtrochanteric (displaced) S72.2- ☑
nondisplaced S72.2- ☑
transcervical — *see* Fracture, femur, upper end, midcervical
trochanteric S72.1Ø- ☑
greater (displaced) S72.11- ☑
nondisplaced S72.11- ☑
lesser (displaced) S72.12- ☑
nondisplaced S72.12- ☑
fibula (shaft) (styloid) S82.4Ø- ☑
comminuted (displaced) S82.45- ☑
nondisplaced S82.45- ☑
following insertion of implant, prosthesis or plate M96.67- ☑
involving ankle or malleolus — *see* Fracture, fibula, lateral malleolus
lateral malleolus (displaced) S82.6- ☑
nondisplaced S82.6- ☑
lower end
physeal S89.3Ø- ☑
Salter-Harris
Type I S89.31- ☑
Type II S89.32- ☑
specified NEC S89.39- ☑
specified NEC S82.83- ☑
torus S82.82- ☑
oblique (displaced) S82.43- ☑
nondisplaced S82.43- ☑
segmental (displaced) S82.46- ☑
nondisplaced S82.46- ☑
specified NEC S82.49- ☑
spiral (displaced) S82.44- ☑
nondisplaced S82.44- ☑
transverse (displaced) S82.42- ☑
nondisplaced S82.42- ☑
upper end
physeal S89.2Ø- ☑
Salter-Harris
Type I S89.21- ☑
Type II S89.22- ☑
specified NEC S89.29- ☑
specified NEC S82.83- ☑
torus S82.81- ☑
finger (except thumb) S62.6Ø- ☑
distal phalanx (displaced) S62.63- ☑
nondisplaced S62.66- ☑
index S62.6Ø- ☑
distal phalanx (displaced) S62.63- ☑
nondisplaced S62.66- ☑
middle phalanx (displaced) S62.62- ☑
nondisplaced S62.65- ☑
proximal phalanx (displaced) S62.61- ☑
nondisplaced S62.64- ☑
little S62.6Ø- ☑
distal phalanx (displaced) S62.63- ☑
nondisplaced S62.66- ☑
middle phalanx (displaced) S62.62- ☑
nondisplaced S62.65- ☑
proximal phalanx (displaced) S62.61- ☑
nondisplaced S62.64- ☑
middle S62.6Ø- ☑
distal phalanx (displaced) S62.63- ☑
nondisplaced S62.66- ☑
middle phalanx (displaced) S62.62- ☑
nondisplaced S62.65- ☑
proximal phalanx (displaced) S62.61- ☑
nondisplaced S62.64- ☑
middle phalanx (displaced) S62.62- ☑
nondisplaced S62.65- ☑
proximal phalanx (displaced) S62.61- ☑

Fracture, traumatic — *continued*
finger — *continued*
proximal phalanx — *continued*
nondisplaced S62.64- ☑
ring S62.6Ø- ☑
distal phalanx (displaced) S62.63- ☑
nondisplaced S62.66- ☑
middle phalanx (displaced) S62.62- ☑
nondisplaced S62.65- ☑
proximal phalanx (displaced) S62.61- ☑
nondisplaced S62.64- ☑
thumb — *see* Fracture, thumb
following insertion (intraoperative) (postoperative) of orthopedic implant, joint prosthesis or bone plate M96.69
femur M96.66- ☑
fibula M96.67- ☑
humerus M96.62- ☑
pelvis M96.65
radius M96.63- ☑
specified bone NEC M96.69
tibia M96.67- ☑
ulna M96.63- ☑
foot S92.9Ø- ☑
astragalus — *see* Fracture, tarsal, talus
calcaneus — *see* Fracture, tarsal, calcaneus
cuboid — *see* Fracture, tarsal, cuboid
cuneiform — *see* Fracture, tarsal, cuneiform
metatarsal — *see* Fracture, metatarsal
navicular — *see* Fracture, tarsal, navicular
sesamoid S92.81- ☑
specified NEC S92.81- ☑
talus — *see* Fracture, tarsal, talus
tarsal — *see* Fracture, tarsal
toe — *see* Fracture, toe
forearm S52.9- ☑
radius — *see* Fracture, radius
ulna — *see* Fracture, ulna
fossa (anterior) (middle) (posterior) SØ2.19 ☑
fragility — *see* Fracture, pathological, due to osteoporosis
frontal (bone) (skull) SØ2.Ø ☑
sinus SØ2.19 ☑
glenoid (cavity) (scapula) — *see* Fracture, scapula, glenoid cavity
greenstick — *see* Fracture, by site
hallux — *see* Fracture, toe, great
hand S62.9- ☑
carpal — *see* Fracture, carpal bone
finger (except thumb) — *see* Fracture, finger
metacarpal — *see* Fracture, metacarpal
navicular (scaphoid) (hand) — *see* Fracture, carpal bone, navicular
thumb — *see* Fracture, thumb
healed or old
with complications — *code by* Nature of the complication
heel bone — *see* Fracture, tarsal, calcaneus
Hill-Sachs S42.29- ☑
hip — *see* Fracture, femur, neck
humerus S42.3Ø- ☑
anatomical neck — *see* Fracture, humerus, upper end
articular process — *see* Fracture, humerus, lower end
capitellum — *see* Fracture, humerus, lower end, condyle, lateral
distal end — *see* Fracture, humerus, lower end
epiphysis
lower — *see* Fracture, humerus, lower end, physeal
upper — *see* Fracture, humerus, upper end, physeal
external condyle — *see* Fracture, humerus, lower end, condyle, lateral
following insertion of implant, prosthesis or plate M96.62- ☑
great tuberosity — *see* Fracture, humerus, upper end, greater tuberosity
intercondylar — *see* Fracture, humerus, lower end
internal epicondyle — *see* Fracture, humerus, lower end, epicondyle, medial
lesser tuberosity — *see* Fracture, humerus, upper end, lesser tuberosity
lower end S42.4Ø- ☑
condyle
lateral (displaced) S42.45- ☑

Fracture, traumatic — *continued*
humerus — *continued*
lower end — *continued*
condyle — *continued*
lateral — *continued*
nondisplaced S42.45- ☑
medial (displaced) S42.46- ☑
nondisplaced S42.46- ☑
epicondyle
lateral (displaced) S42.43- ☑
nondisplaced S42.43- ☑
medial (displaced) S42.44- ☑
incarcerated S42.44- ☑
nondisplaced S42.44- ☑
physeal S49.1Ø- ☑
Salter-Harris
Type I S49.11- ☑
Type II S49.12- ☑
Type III S49.13- ☑
Type IV S49.14- ☑
specified NEC S49.19- ☑
specified NEC (displaced) S42.49- ☑
nondisplaced S42.49- ☑
supracondylar (simple) (displaced) S42.41- ☑
with intercondylar fracture — *see* Fracture, humerus, lower end
comminuted (displaced) S42.42- ☑
nondisplaced S42.42- ☑
nondisplaced S42.41- ☑
torus S42.48- ☑
transcondylar (displaced) S42.47- ☑
nondisplaced S42.47- ☑
proximal end — *see* Fracture, humerus, upper end
shaft S42.3Ø- ☑
comminuted (displaced) S42.35- ☑
nondisplaced S42.35- ☑
greenstick S42.31- ☑
oblique (displaced) S42.33- ☑
nondisplaced S42.33- ☑
segmental (displaced) S42.36- ☑
nondisplaced S42.36- ☑
specified NEC S42.39- ☑
spiral (displaced) S42.34- ☑
nondisplaced S42.34- ☑
transverse (displaced) S42.32- ☑
nondisplaced S42.32- ☑
supracondylar — *see* Fracture, humerus, lower end
surgical neck — *see* Fracture, humerus, upper end, surgical neck
trochlea — *see* Fracture, humerus, lower end, condyle, medial
tuberosity — *see* Fracture, humerus, upper end
upper end S42.2Ø- ☑
anatomical neck — *see* Fracture, humerus, upper end, specified NEC
articular head — *see* Fracture, humerus, upper end, specified NEC
epiphysis — *see* Fracture, humerus, upper end, physeal
greater tuberosity (displaced) S42.25- ☑
nondisplaced S42.25- ☑
lesser tuberosity (displaced) S42.26- ☑
nondisplaced S42.26- ☑
physeal S49.ØØ- ☑
Salter-Harris
Type I S49.Ø1- ☑
Type II S49.Ø2- ☑
Type III S49.Ø3- ☑
Type IV S49.Ø4- ☑
specified NEC S49.Ø9- ☑
specified NEC (displaced) S42.29- ☑
nondisplaced S42.29- ☑
surgical neck (displaced) S42.21- ☑
four-part S42.24- ☑
nondisplaced S42.21- ☑
three-part S42.23- ☑
two-part (displaced) S42.22- ☑
nondisplaced S42.22- ☑
torus S42.27- ☑
transepiphyseal — *see* Fracture, humerus, upper end, physeal
hyoid bone S12.8 ☑
ilium S32.3Ø- ☑
with disruption of pelvic ring — *see* Disruption, pelvic ring
avulsion (displaced) S32.31- ☑

- **Fracture, traumatic** — *continued*
  - ilium — *continued*
    - avulsion — *continued*
      - nondisplaced S32.31- ☑
    - specified NEC S32.39- ☑
  - impaction, impacted — *code as* Fracture, by site
  - innominate bone — *see* Fracture, ilium
  - instep — *see* Fracture, foot
  - ischium S32.60- ☑
    - with disruption of pelvic ring — *see* Disruption, pelvic ring
    - avulsion (displaced) S32.61- ☑
      - nondisplaced S32.61- ☑
    - specified NEC S32.69- ☑
  - jaw (bone) (lower) — *see* Fracture, mandible
    - upper — *see* Fracture, maxilla
  - joint prosthesis — *see* Complications, joint prosthesis, mechanical, breakdown, by site
    - periprosthetic — *see* Fracture, traumatic, periprosthetic
  - knee cap — *see* Fracture, patella
  - larynx S12.8 ☑
  - late effects — *see* Sequelae, fracture
  - leg (lower) S82.9- ☑
    - ankle — *see* Fracture, ankle
    - femur — *see* Fracture, femur
    - fibula — *see* Fracture, fibula
    - malleolus — *see* Fracture, ankle
    - patella — *see* Fracture, patella
    - specified site NEC S82.89- ☑
    - tibia — *see* Fracture, tibia
  - lumbar spine — *see* Fracture, vertebra, lumbar
  - lumbosacral spine S32.9 ☑
  - Maisonneuve's (displaced) S82.86- ☑
    - nondisplaced S82.86- ☑
  - malar bone — *see also* Fracture, maxilla S02.400 ☑
    - left side S02.40B ☑
    - right side S02.40A ☑
  - malleolus — *see* Fracture, ankle
  - malunion — *see* Fracture, by site
  - mandible (lower jaw (bone)) S02.609 ☑
    - alveolus S02.67- ☑
    - angle (of jaw) S02.65- ☑
    - body, unspecified S02.600 ☑
      - left side S02.602 ☑
      - right side S02.601 ☑
    - condylar process S02.61- ☑
    - coronoid process S02.63- ☑
    - ramus, unspecified S02.64- ☑
    - specified site NEC S02.69 ☑
    - subcondylar process S02.62- ☑
    - symphysis S02.66 ☑
  - manubrium (sterni) S22.21 ☑
    - dissociation from sternum S22.23 ☑
  - march — *see* Fracture, traumatic, stress, by site
  - maxilla, maxillary (bone) (sinus) (superior) (upper jaw) S02.401 ☑
    - alveolus S02.42 ☑
    - inferior — *see* Fracture, mandible
    - LeFort I S02.411 ☑
    - LeFort II S02.412 ☑
    - LeFort III S02.413 ☑
    - left side S02.40D ☑
    - right side S02.40C ☑
  - metacarpal S62.309 ☑
    - base (displaced) S62.319 ☑
      - nondisplaced S62.349 ☑
    - fifth S62.30- ☑
      - base (displaced) S62.31- ☑
        - nondisplaced S62.34- ☑
      - neck (displaced) S62.33- ☑
        - nondisplaced S62.36- ☑
      - shaft (displaced) S62.32- ☑
        - nondisplaced S62.35- ☑
      - specified NEC S62.398 ☑
    - first S62.20- ☑
      - base NEC (displaced) S62.23- ☑
        - nondisplaced S62.23- ☑
      - Bennett's — *see* Bennett's fracture
      - neck (displaced) S62.25- ☑
        - nondisplaced S62.25- ☑
      - shaft (displaced) S62.24- ☑
        - nondisplaced S62.24- ☑
      - specified NEC S62.29- ☑
    - fourth S62.30- ☑
      - base (displaced) S62.31- ☑

- **Fracture, traumatic** — *continued*
  - metacarpal — *continued*
    - fourth — *continued*
      - base — *continued*
        - nondisplaced S62.34- ☑
      - neck (displaced) S62.33- ☑
        - nondisplaced S62.36- ☑
      - shaft (displaced) S62.32- ☑
        - nondisplaced S62.35- ☑
      - specified NEC S62.39- ☑
    - neck (displaced) S62.33- ☑
      - nondisplaced S62.36- ☑
    - Rolando's — *see* Rolando's fracture
    - second S62.30- ☑
      - base (displaced) S62.31- ☑
        - nondisplaced S62.34- ☑
      - neck (displaced) S62.33- ☑
        - nondisplaced S62.36- ☑
      - shaft (displaced) S62.32- ☑
        - nondisplaced S62.35- ☑
      - specified NEC S62.39- ☑
    - shaft (displaced) S62.32- ☑
      - nondisplaced S62.35- ☑
    - specified NEC S62.399 ☑
    - third S62.30- ☑
      - base (displaced) S62.31- ☑
        - nondisplaced S62.34- ☑
      - neck (displaced) S62.33- ☑
        - nondisplaced S62.36- ☑
      - shaft (displaced) S62.32- ☑
        - nondisplaced S62.35- ☑
      - specified NEC S62.39- ☑
  - metaphyseal — *see* Fracture, traumatic, by site, shaft
  - metastatic — *see* Fracture, pathological, due to, neoplastic disease — *see also* Neoplasm
  - metatarsal bone S92.30- ☑
    - fifth (displaced) S92.35- ☑
      - nondisplaced S92.35- ☑
    - first (displaced) S92.31- ☑
      - nondisplaced S92.31- ☑
    - fourth (displaced) S92.34- ☑
      - nondisplaced S92.34- ☑
    - physeal S99.10- ☑
      - Salter-Harris
        - Type I S99.11- ☑
        - Type II S99.12- ☑
        - Type III S99.13- ☑
        - Type IV S99.14- ☑
      - specified NEC S99.19- ☑
    - second (displaced) S92.32- ☑
      - nondisplaced S92.32- ☑
    - third (displaced) S92.33- ☑
      - nondisplaced S92.33- ☑
  - Monteggia's — *see* Monteggia's fracture
  - multiple
    - hand (and wrist) NEC — *see* Fracture, by site
    - ribs — *see* Fracture, rib, multiple
  - nasal (bone(s)) S02.2 ☑
  - navicular (scaphoid) (foot) — *see also* Fracture, tarsal, navicular
    - hand — *see* Fracture, carpal, navicular
  - neck S12.9 ☑
    - cervical vertebra S12.9 ☑
      - fifth (displaced) S12.400 ☑
        - nondisplaced S12.401 ☑
        - specified type NEC (displaced) S12.490 ☑
          - nondisplaced S12.491 ☑
      - first (displaced) S12.000 ☑
        - burst (stable) S12.01 ☑
          - unstable S12.02 ☑
        - lateral mass (displaced) S12.040 ☑
          - nondisplaced S12.041 ☑
        - nondisplaced S12.001 ☑
        - posterior arch (displaced) S12.030 ☑
          - nondisplaced S12.031 ☑
        - specified type NEC (displaced) S12.090 ☑
          - nondisplaced S12.091 ☑
      - fourth (displaced) S12.300 ☑
        - nondisplaced S12.301 ☑
        - specified type NEC (displaced) S12.390 ☑
          - nondisplaced S12.391 ☑
      - second (displaced) S12.100 ☑
        - dens (anterior) (displaced) (type II) S12.110 ☑
          - nondisplaced S12.112 ☑
          - posterior S12.111 ☑
          - specified type NEC (displaced) S12.120 ☑

- **Fracture, traumatic** — *continued*
  - neck — *continued*
    - cervical vertebra — *continued*
      - second — *continued*
        - dens — *continued*
          - specified type — *continued*
            - nondisplaced S12.121 ☑
        - nondisplaced S12.101 ☑
        - specified type NEC (displaced) S12.190 ☑
          - nondisplaced S12.191 ☑
      - seventh (displaced) S12.600 ☑
        - nondisplaced S12.601 ☑
        - specified type NEC (displaced) S12.690 ☑
          - nondisplaced S12.691 ☑
      - sixth (displaced) S12.500 ☑
        - nondisplaced S12.501 ☑
        - specified type NEC (displaced) S12.590 ☑
          - nondisplaced S12.591 ☑
      - third (displaced) S12.200 ☑
        - nondisplaced S12.201 ☑
        - specified type NEC (displaced) S12.290 ☑
          - nondisplaced S12.291 ☑
    - hyoid bone S12.8 ☑
    - larynx S12.8 ☑
    - specified site NEC S12.8 ☑
    - thyroid cartilage S12.8 ☑
    - trachea S12.8 ☑
  - neoplastic NEC — *see* Fracture, pathological, due to, neoplastic disease
  - neural arch — *see* Fracture, vertebra
  - newborn — *see* Birth, injury, fracture
  - nontraumatic — *see* Fracture, pathological
  - nonunion — *see* Nonunion, fracture
  - nose, nasal (bone) (septum) S02.2 ☑
  - occiput — *see* Fracture, skull, base, occiput
  - odontoid process — *see* Fracture, neck, cervical vertebra, second
  - olecranon (process) (ulna) — *see* Fracture, ulna, upper end, olecranon process
  - orbit, orbital (bone) (region) S02.85 ☑
    - floor (blow-out) S02.3- ☑
    - roof S02.12- ☑
    - wall S02.85 ☑
      - lateral S02.84- ☑
      - medial S02.83- ☑
  - os
    - calcis — *see* Fracture, tarsal, calcaneus
    - magnum — *see* Fracture, carpal, capitate
    - pubis — *see* Fracture, pubis
  - palate S02.8- ☑
  - parietal bone (skull) S02.0 ☑
  - patella S82.00- ☑
    - comminuted (displaced) S82.04- ☑
      - nondisplaced S82.04- ☑
    - longitudinal (displaced) S82.02- ☑
      - nondisplaced S82.02- ☑
    - osteochondral (displaced) S82.01- ☑
      - nondisplaced S82.01- ☑
    - specified NEC S82.09- ☑
    - transverse (displaced) S82.03- ☑
      - nondisplaced S82.03- ☑
  - pedicle (of vertebral arch) — *see* Fracture, vertebra
  - pelvis, pelvic (bone) S32.9 ☑
    - acetabulum — *see* Fracture, acetabulum
    - circle — *see* Disruption, pelvic ring
    - following insertion of implant, prosthesis or plate M96.65
    - ilium — *see* Fracture, ilium
    - ischium — *see* Fracture, ischium
    - multiple
      - with disruption of pelvic ring (circle) — *see* Disruption, pelvic ring
      - without disruption of pelvic ring (circle) S32.82 ☑
    - pubis — *see* Fracture, pubis
    - sacrum — *see* Fracture, sacrum
    - specified site NEC S32.89 ☑
  - periprosthetic, around internal prosthetic joint M97.9 ☑
    - ankle M97.2- ☑
    - elbow M97.4- ☑
    - finger M97.8 ☑
    - hip M97.0- ☑
    - knee M97.1- ☑
    - shoulder M97.3- ☑
    - specified joint NEC M97.8 ☑

Fracture, traumatic — *continued*
periprosthetic, around internal prosthetic joint — *continued*
spine M97.8 ☑
toe M97.8 ☑
wrist M97.8 ☑
phalanx
foot — *see* Fracture, toe
hand — *see* Fracture, finger
pisiform — *see* Fracture, carpal, pisiform
pond — *see* Fracture, skull
prosthetic device, internal — *see* Complications, prosthetic device, by site, mechanical
pubis S32.5Ø- ☑
with disruption of pelvic ring — *see* Disruption, pelvic ring
specified site NEC S32.59- ☑
superior rim S32.51- ☑
radius S52.9- ☑
distal end — *see* Fracture, radius, lower end
following insertion of implant, prosthesis or plate M96.63- ☑
head — *see* Fracture, radius, upper end, head
lower end S52.5Ø- ☑
Barton's — *see* Barton's fracture
Colles' — *see* Colles' fracture
extraarticular NEC S52.55- ☑
intraarticular NEC S52.57- ☑
physeal S59.2Ø- ☑
Salter-Harris
Type I S59.21- ☑
Type II S59.22- ☑
Type III S59.23- ☑
Type IV S59.24- ☑
specified NEC S59.29- ☑
Smith's — *see* Smith's fracture
specified NEC S52.59- ☑
styloid process (displaced) S52.51- ☑
nondisplaced S52.51- ☑
torus S52.52- ☑
neck — *see* Fracture, radius, upper end
proximal end — *see* Fracture, radius, upper end
shaft S52.3Ø- ☑
bent bone S52.38- ☑
comminuted (displaced) S52.35- ☑
nondisplaced S52.35- ☑
Galeazzi's — *see* Galeazzi's fracture
greenstick S52.31- ☑
oblique (displaced) S52.33- ☑
nondisplaced S52.33- ☑
segmental (displaced) S52.36- ☑
nondisplaced S52.36- ☑
specified NEC S52.39- ☑
spiral (displaced) S52.34- ☑
nondisplaced S52.34- ☑
transverse (displaced) S52.32- ☑
nondisplaced S52.32- ☑
upper end S52.1Ø- ☑
head (displaced) S52.12- ☑
nondisplaced S52.12- ☑
neck (displaced) S52.13- ☑
nondisplaced S52.13- ☑
physeal S59.1Ø- ☑
Salter-Harris
Type I S59.11- ☑
Type II S59.12- ☑
Type III S59.13- ☑
Type IV S59.14- ☑
specified NEC S59.19- ☑
specified NEC S52.18- ☑
torus S52.11- ☑
ramus
inferior or superior, pubis — *see* Fracture, pubis
mandible — *see* Fracture, mandible
restorative material (dental) KØ8.539
with loss of material KØ8.531
without loss of material KØ8.53Ø
rib S22.3- ☑
with flail chest — *see* Flail, chest
associated with chest compression and cardiopulmonary resuscitation M96.A2
multiple S22.4- ☑
with flail chest — *see* Flail, chest
associated with chest compression and cardiopulmonary resuscitation M96.A3
root, tooth — *see* Fracture, tooth

Fracture, traumatic — *continued*
sacrum S32.1Ø ☑
specified NEC S32.19 ☑
Type
1 S32.14 ☑
2 S32.15 ☑
3 S32.16 ☑
4 S32.17 ☑
Zone
I S32.119 ☑
displaced (minimally) S32.111 ☑
severely S32.112 ☑
nondisplaced S32.11Ø ☑
II S32.129 ☑
displaced (minimally) S32.121 ☑
severely S32.122 ☑
nondisplaced S32.12Ø ☑
III S32.139 ☑
displaced (minimally) S32.131 ☑
severely S32.132 ☑
nondisplaced S32.13Ø ☑
scaphoid (hand) — *see also* Fracture, carpal, navicular
foot — *see* Fracture, tarsal, navicular
scapula S42.1Ø- ☑
acromial process (displaced) S42.12- ☑
nondisplaced S42.12- ☑
body (displaced) S42.11- ☑
nondisplaced S42.11- ☑
coracoid process (displaced) S42.13- ☑
nondisplaced S42.13- ☑
glenoid cavity (displaced) S42.14- ☑
nondisplaced S42.14- ☑
neck (displaced) S42.15- ☑
nondisplaced S42.15- ☑
specified NEC S42.19- ☑
semilunar bone, wrist — *see* Fracture, carpal, lunate
sequelae — *see* Sequelae, fracture
sesamoid bone
foot S92.81- ☑
hand — *see* Fracture, carpal
other — *see* Fracture, traumatic, by site
shepherd's — *see* Fracture, tarsal, talus
shoulder (girdle) S42.9- ☑
blade — *see* Fracture, scapula
sinus (ethmoid) (frontal) SØ2.19 ☑
skull SØ2.91 ☑
base SØ2.1Ø- ☑
occiput SØ2.119 ☑
condyle SØ2.113 ☑
specified NEC SØ2.118 ☑
left side SØ2.11H ☑
right side SØ2.11G ☑
type I SØ2.11Ø ☑
left side SØ2.11B ☑
right side SØ2.11A ☑
type II SØ2.111 ☑
left side SØ2.11D ☑
right side SØ2.11C ☑
type III SØ2.112 ☑
left side SØ2.11F ☑
right side SØ2.11E ☑
specified NEC SØ2.19 ☑
birth injury P13.Ø
frontal bone SØ2.Ø ☑
parietal bone SØ2.Ø ☑
specified site NEC SØ2.8- ☑
temporal bone SØ2.19 ☑
vault SØ2.Ø ☑
Smith's — *see* Smith's fracture
sphenoid (bone) (sinus) SØ2.19 ☑
spine — *see* Fracture, vertebra
spinous process — *see* Fracture, vertebra
spontaneous (cause unknown) — *see* Fracture, pathological
stave (of thumb) — *see* Fracture, metacarpal, first
sternum S22.2Ø ☑
with flail chest — *see* Flail, chest
associated with chest compression and cardiopulmonary resuscitation M96.A1
body S22.22 ☑
manubrium S22.21 ☑
xiphoid (process) S22.24 ☑
associated with chest compression and cardiopulmonary resuscitation M96.A1
stress M84.3Ø ☑
ankle M84.37- ☑

Fracture, traumatic — *continued*
stress — *continued*
carpus M84.34- ☑
clavicle M84.31- ☑
femoral neck M84.359 ☑
femur M84.35- ☑
fibula M84.36- ☑
finger M84.34- ☑
hip M84.359 ☑
humerus M84.32- ☑
ilium M84.35Ø ☑
ischium M84.35Ø ☑
metacarpus M84.34- ☑
metatarsus M84.37- ☑
neck — *see* Fracture, fatigue, vertebra
pelvis M84.35Ø ☑
radius M84.33- ☑
rib M84.38 ☑
scapula M84.31- ☑
skull M84.38 ☑
tarsus M84.37- ☑
tibia M84.36- ☑
toe M84.37- ☑
ulna M84.33- ☑
vertebra — *see* Fracture, fatigue, vertebra
supracondylar, elbow — *see* Fracture, humerus, lower end, supracondylar
symphysis pubis — *see* Fracture, pubis
talus (ankle bone) — *see* Fracture, tarsal, talus
tarsal bone(s) S92.2Ø- ☑
astragalus — *see* Fracture, tarsal, talus
calcaneus S92.ØØ- ☑
anterior process (displaced) S92.Ø2- ☑
nondisplaced S92.Ø2- ☑
body (displaced) S92.Ø1- ☑
nondisplaced S92.Ø1- ☑
extraarticular NEC (displaced) S92.Ø5- ☑
nondisplaced S92.Ø5- ☑
intraarticular (displaced) S92.Ø6- ☑
nondisplaced S92.Ø6- ☑
physeal S99.ØØ- ☑
Salter-Harris
Type I S99.Ø1- ☑
Type II S99.Ø2- ☑
Type III S99.Ø3- ☑
Type IV S99.Ø4- ☑
specified NEC S99.Ø9- ☑
tuberosity (displaced) S92.Ø4- ☑
avulsion (displaced) S92.Ø3- ☑
nondisplaced S92.Ø3- ☑
nondisplaced S92.Ø4- ☑
cuboid (displaced) S92.21- ☑
nondisplaced S92.21- ☑
cuneiform
intermediate (displaced) S92.23- ☑
nondisplaced S92.23- ☑
lateral (displaced) S92.22- ☑
nondisplaced S92.22- ☑
medial (displaced) S92.24- ☑
nondisplaced S92.24- ☑
navicular (displaced) S92.25- ☑
nondisplaced S92.25- ☑
scaphoid — *see* Fracture, tarsal, navicular
talus S92.1Ø- ☑
avulsion (displaced) S92.15- ☑
nondisplaced S92.15- ☑
body (displaced) S92.12- ☑
nondisplaced S92.12- ☑
dome (displaced) S92.14- ☑
nondisplaced S92.14- ☑
head (displaced) S92.12- ☑
nondisplaced S92.12- ☑
lateral process (displaced) S92.14- ☑
nondisplaced S92.14- ☑
neck (displaced) S92.11- ☑
nondisplaced S92.11- ☑
posterior process (displaced) S92.13- ☑
nondisplaced S92.13- ☑
specified NEC S92.19- ☑
temporal bone (styloid) SØ2.19 ☑
thorax (bony) S22.9 ☑
with flail chest — *see* Flail, chest
rib S22.3- ☑
multiple S22.4- ☑
with flail chest — *see* Flail, chest
sternum S22.2Ø ☑

Fracture, traumatic — *continued*
- thorax — *continued*
  - sternum — *continued*
    - body S22.22 ☑
    - manubrium S22.21 ☑
    - xiphoid process S22.24 ☑
      - associated with chest compression and cardiopulmonary resuscitation M96.A1
  - vertebra (displaced) S22.009 ☑
    - burst (stable) S22.001 ☑
      - unstable S22.002 ☑
    - eighth S22.069 ☑
      - burst (stable) S22.061 ☑
        - unstable S22.062 ☑
      - specified type NEC S22.068 ☑
      - wedge compression S22.060 ☑
    - eleventh S22.089 ☑
      - burst (stable) S22.081 ☑
        - unstable S22.082 ☑
      - specified type NEC S22.088 ☑
      - wedge compression S22.080 ☑
    - fifth S22.059 ☑
      - burst (stable) S22.051 ☑
        - unstable S22.052 ☑
      - specified type NEC S22.058 ☑
      - wedge compression S22.050 ☑
    - first S22.019 ☑
      - burst (stable) S22.011 ☑
        - unstable S22.012 ☑
      - specified type NEC S22.018 ☑
      - wedge compression S22.010 ☑
    - fourth S22.049 ☑
      - burst (stable) S22.041 ☑
        - unstable S22.042 ☑
      - specified type NEC S22.048 ☑
      - wedge compression S22.040 ☑
    - ninth S22.079 ☑
      - burst (stable) S22.071 ☑
        - unstable S22.072 ☑
      - specified type NEC S22.078 ☑
      - wedge compression S22.070 ☑
    - nondisplaced S22.001 ☑
    - second S22.029 ☑
      - burst (stable) S22.021 ☑
        - unstable S22.022 ☑
      - specified type NEC S22.028 ☑
      - wedge compression S22.020 ☑
    - seventh S22.069 ☑
      - burst (stable) S22.061 ☑
        - unstable S22.062 ☑
      - specified type NEC S22.068 ☑
      - wedge compression S22.060 ☑
    - sixth S22.059 ☑
      - burst (stable) S22.051 ☑
        - unstable S22.052 ☑
      - specified type NEC S22.058 ☑
      - wedge compression S22.050 ☑
    - specified type NEC S22.008 ☑
    - tenth S22.079 ☑
      - burst (stable) S22.071 ☑
        - unstable S22.072 ☑
      - specified type NEC S22.078 ☑
      - wedge compression S22.070 ☑
    - third S22.039 ☑
      - burst (stable) S22.031 ☑
        - unstable S22.032 ☑
      - specified type NEC S22.038 ☑
      - wedge compression S22.030 ☑
    - twelfth S22.089 ☑
      - burst (stable) S22.081 ☑
        - unstable S22.082 ☑
      - specified type NEC S22.088 ☑
      - wedge compression S22.080 ☑
    - wedge compression S22.000 ☑
- thumb S62.50- ☑
  - distal phalanx (displaced) S62.52- ☑
    - nondisplaced S62.52- ☑
  - proximal phalanx (displaced) S62.51- ☑
    - nondisplaced S62.51- ☑
- thyroid cartilage S12.8 ☑
- tibia (shaft) S82.20- ☑
  - comminuted (displaced) S82.25- ☑
    - nondisplaced S82.25- ☑
  - condyles — *see* Fracture, tibia, upper end
  - distal end — *see* Fracture, tibia, lower end

Fracture, traumatic — *continued*
- tibia — *continued*
  - epiphysis
    - lower — *see* Fracture, tibia, lower end
    - upper — *see* Fracture, tibia, upper end
  - following insertion of implant, prosthesis or plate M96.67- ☑
  - head (involving knee joint) — *see* Fracture, tibia, upper end
  - intercondyloid eminence — *see* Fracture, tibia, upper end
  - involving ankle or malleolus — *see* Fracture, ankle, medial malleolus
  - lower end S82.30- ☑
    - physeal S89.10- ☑
      - Salter-Harris
        - Type I S89.11- ☑
        - Type II S89.12- ☑
        - Type III S89.13- ☑
        - Type IV S89.14- ☑
      - specified NEC S89.19- ☑
    - pilon (displaced) S82.87- ☑
      - nondisplaced S82.87- ☑
    - specified NEC S82.39- ☑
    - torus S82.31- ☑
  - malleolus — *see* Fracture, ankle, medial malleolus
  - oblique (displaced) S82.23- ☑
    - nondisplaced S82.23- ☑
  - pilon — *see* Fracture, tibia, lower end, pilon
  - proximal end — *see* Fracture, tibia, upper end
  - segmental (displaced) S82.26- ☑
    - nondisplaced S82.26- ☑
  - specified NEC S82.29- ☑
  - spine — *see* Fracture, tibia, upper end, spine
  - spiral (displaced) S82.24- ☑
    - nondisplaced S82.24- ☑
  - transverse (displaced) S82.22- ☑
    - nondisplaced S82.22- ☑
  - tuberosity — *see* Fracture, tibia, upper end, tuberosity
  - upper end S82.10- ☑
    - bicondylar (displaced) S82.14- ☑
      - nondisplaced S82.14- ☑
    - lateral condyle (displaced) S82.12- ☑
      - nondisplaced S82.12- ☑
    - medial condyle (displaced) S82.13- ☑
      - nondisplaced S82.13- ☑
    - physeal S89.00- ☑
      - Salter-Harris
        - Type I S89.01- ☑
        - Type II S89.02- ☑
        - Type III S89.03- ☑
        - Type IV S89.04- ☑
      - specified NEC S89.09- ☑
    - plateau — *see* Fracture, tibia, upper end, bicondylar
    - specified NEC S82.19- ☑
    - spine (displaced) S82.11- ☑
      - nondisplaced S82.11- ☑
    - torus S82.16- ☑
    - tuberosity (displaced) S82.15- ☑
      - nondisplaced S82.15- ☑
- toe S92.91- ☑
  - great (displaced) S92.40- ☑
    - distal phalanx (displaced) S92.42- ☑
      - nondisplaced S92.42- ☑
    - nondisplaced S92.40- ☑
    - proximal phalanx (displaced) S92.41- ☑
      - nondisplaced S92.41- ☑
    - specified NEC S92.49- ☑
  - lesser (displaced) S92.50- ☑
    - distal phalanx (displaced) S92.53- ☑
      - nondisplaced S92.53- ☑
    - middle phalanx (displaced) S92.52- ☑
      - nondisplaced S92.52- ☑
    - nondisplaced S92.50- ☑
    - proximal phalanx (displaced) S92.51- ☑
      - nondisplaced S92.51- ☑
    - specified NEC S92.59- ☑
  - physeal
    - phalanx S99.20- ☑
      - Salter-Harris
        - Type I S99.21- ☑
        - Type II S99.22- ☑
        - Type III S99.23- ☑
        - Type IV S99.24- ☑

Fracture, traumatic — *continued*
- toe — *continued*
  - physeal — *continued*
    - phalanx — *continued*
      - specified NEC S99.29- ☑
- tooth (root) S02.5 ☑
- trachea (cartilage) S12.8 ☑
- transverse process — *see* Fracture, vertebra
- trapezium or trapezoid bone — *see* Fracture, carpal
- trimalleolar — *see* Fracture, ankle, trimalleolar
- triquetrum (cuneiform of carpus) — *see* Fracture, carpal, triquetrum
- trochanter — *see* Fracture, femur, trochanteric
- tuberosity (external) — *see* Fracture, traumatic, by site
- ulna (shaft) S52.20- ☑
  - bent bone S52.28- ☑
  - coronoid process — *see* Fracture, ulna, upper end, coronoid process
  - distal end — *see* Fracture, ulna, lower end
  - following insertion of implant, prosthesis or plate M96.63- ☑
  - head S52.60- ☑
  - lower end S52.60- ☑
    - physeal S59.00- ☑
      - Salter-Harris
        - Type I S59.01- ☑
        - Type II S59.02- ☑
        - Type III S59.03- ☑
        - Type IV S59.04- ☑
      - specified NEC S59.09- ☑
    - specified NEC S52.69- ☑
    - styloid process (displaced) S52.61- ☑
      - nondisplaced S52.61- ☑
    - torus S52.62- ☑
  - proximal end — *see* Fracture, ulna, upper end
  - shaft S52.20- ☑
    - comminuted (displaced) S52.25- ☑
      - nondisplaced S52.25- ☑
    - greenstick S52.21- ☑
    - Monteggia's — *see* Monteggia's fracture
    - oblique (displaced) S52.23- ☑
      - nondisplaced S52.23- ☑
    - segmental (displaced) S52.26- ☑
      - nondisplaced S52.26- ☑
    - specified NEC S52.29- ☑
    - spiral (displaced) S52.24- ☑
      - nondisplaced S52.24- ☑
    - transverse (displaced) S52.22- ☑
      - nondisplaced S52.22- ☑
  - upper end S52.00- ☑
    - coronoid process (displaced) S52.04- ☑
      - nondisplaced S52.04- ☑
    - olecranon process (displaced) S52.02- ☑
      - with intraarticular extension S52.03- ☑
      - nondisplaced S52.02- ☑
        - with intraarticular extension S52.03- ☑
    - specified NEC S52.09- ☑
    - torus S52.01- ☑
- unciform — *see* Fracture, carpal, hamate
- vault of skull S02.0 ☑
- vertebra, vertebral (arch) (body) (column) (neural arch) (pedicle) (spinous process) (transverse process)
  - atlas — *see* Fracture, neck, cervical vertebra, first
  - axis — *see* Fracture, neck, cervical vertebra, second
  - cervical (teardrop) S12.9 ☑
    - axis — *see* Fracture, neck, cervical vertebra, second
    - first (atlas) — *see* Fracture, neck, cervical vertebra, first
    - second (axis) — *see* Fracture, neck, cervical vertebra, second
  - chronic M84.48 ☑
  - coccyx S32.2 ☑
  - dorsal — *see* Fracture, thorax, vertebra
  - lumbar S32.009 ☑
    - burst (stable) S32.001 ☑
      - unstable S32.002 ☑
    - fifth S32.059 ☑
      - burst (stable) S32.051 ☑
        - unstable S32.052 ☑
      - specified type NEC S32.058 ☑
      - wedge compression S32.050 ☑
    - first S32.019 ☑
      - burst (stable) S32.011 ☑
        - unstable S32.012 ☑
      - specified type NEC S32.018 ☑

- **Fracture, traumatic** — *continued*
  - vertebra, vertebral — *continued*
    - lumbar — *continued*
      - first — *continued*
        - wedge compression S32.Ø1Ø ☑
      - fourth S32.Ø49 ☑
        - burst (stable) S32.Ø41 ☑
          - unstable S32.Ø42 ☑
        - specified type NEC S32.Ø48 ☑
        - wedge compression S32.Ø4Ø ☑
      - second S32.Ø29 ☑
        - burst (stable) S32.Ø21 ☑
          - unstable S32.Ø22 ☑
        - specified type NEC S32.Ø28 ☑
        - wedge compression S32.Ø2Ø ☑
      - specified type NEC S32.ØØ8 ☑
      - third S32.Ø39 ☑
        - burst (stable) S32.Ø31 ☑
          - unstable S32.Ø32 ☑
        - specified type NEC S32.Ø38 ☑
        - wedge compression S32.Ø3Ø ☑
      - wedge compression S32.ØØØ ☑
    - metastatic — *see* Collapse, vertebra, in, specified disease NEC — *see also* Neoplasm
    - newborn (birth injury) P11.5
    - sacrum S32.1Ø ☑
      - specified NEC S32.19 ☑
      - Type
        - 1 S32.14 ☑
        - 2 S32.15 ☑
        - 3 S32.16 ☑
        - 4 S32.17 ☑
      - Zone
        - I S32.119 ☑
          - displaced (minimally) S32.111 ☑
            - severely S32.112 ☑
          - nondisplaced S32.11Ø ☑
        - II S32.129 ☑
          - displaced (minimally) S32.121 ☑
            - severely S32.122 ☑
          - nondisplaced S32.12Ø ☑
        - III S32.139 ☑
          - displaced (minimally) S32.131 ☑
            - severely S32.132 ☑
          - nondisplaced S32.13Ø ☑
    - thoracic — *see* Fracture, thorax, vertebra
  - vertex SØ2.Ø ☑
  - vomer (bone) SØ2.2 ☑
  - wrist S62.1Ø- ☑
    - carpal — *see* Fracture, carpal bone
    - navicular (scaphoid) (hand) — *see* Fracture, carpal, navicular
  - xiphisternum, xiphoid (process) S22.24 ☑
    - associated with chest compression and cardiopulmonary resuscitation M96.A1
  - zygoma SØ2.4Ø2 ☑
    - left side SØ2.4ØF ☑
    - right side SØ2.4ØE ☑
- **Fragile, fragility**
  - autosomal site Q95.5
  - bone, congenital (with blue sclera) Q78.Ø
  - capillary (hereditary) D69.8
  - hair L67.8
  - nails L6Ø.3
  - non-sex chromosome site Q95.5
  - X chromosome Q99.2
- **Fragilitas**
  - crinium L67.8
  - ossium (with blue sclerae) (hereditary) Q78.Ø
  - unguium L6Ø.3
    - congenital Q84.6
- **Fragments, cataract** (lens), **following cataract surgery** H59.Ø2- ☑
  - retained foreign body — *see* Retained, foreign body fragments (type of)
- **Frailty** (frail) R54
  - mental R41.81
- **Frambesia, frambesial** (tropica) — *see also* Yaws
  - initial lesion or ulcer A66.Ø
  - primary A66.Ø
- **Frambeside**
  - gummatous A66.4
  - of early yaws A66.2
- **Frambesioma** A66.1
- **Franceschetti-Klein** (-Wildervanck) **disease or syndrome** Q75.4
- **Francis' disease** — *see* Tularemia
- **Franklin disease** C88.2
- **Frank's essential thrombocytopenia** D69.3
- **Fraser's syndrome** Q87.Ø
- **Freckle**(s) L81.2
  - malignant melanoma in — *see* Melanoma
  - melanotic (Hutchinson's) — *see* Melanoma, in situ
  - retinal D49.81
- **Frederickson's hyperlipoproteinemia, type**
  - I and V E78.3
  - IIA E78.ØØ
  - IIB and III E78.2
  - IV E78.1
- **Freeman Sheldon syndrome** Q87.Ø
- **Freezing** — *see also* Effect, adverse, cold T69.9 ☑
- **Freiberg's disease** (infraction of metatarsal head or osteochondrosis) — *see* Osteochondrosis, juvenile, metatarsus
- **Frei's disease** A55
- **Fremitus, friction, cardiac** RØ1.2
- **Frenum, frenulum**
  - external os Q51.828
  - tongue (shortening) (congenital) Q38.1
- **Frequency micturition** (nocturnal) R35.Ø
  - psychogenic F45.8
- **Frey's syndrome**
  - auriculotemporal G5Ø.8
  - hyperhidrosis L74.52
- **Friction**
  - burn — *see* Burn, by site
  - fremitus, cardiac RØ1.2
  - precordial RØ1.2
  - sounds, chest RØ9.89
- **Friderichsen-Waterhouse syndrome or disease** A39.1
- **Friedländer's B** (bacillus) **NEC** — *see also* condition A49.8
- **Friedreich's**
  - ataxia G11.11
  - combined systemic disease G11.11
  - facial hemihypertrophy Q67.4
  - sclerosis (cerebellum) (spinal cord) G11.11
- **Frigidity** F52.22
- **Fröhlich's syndrome** E23.6
- **Frontal** — *see also* condition
  - lobe syndrome FØ7.Ø
- **Frostbite** (superficial) T33.9Ø ☑
  - with
    - partial thickness skin loss — *see* Frostbite (superficial), by site
    - tissue necrosis T34.9Ø ☑
  - abdominal wall T33.3 ☑
    - with tissue necrosis T34.3 ☑
  - ankle T33.81- ☑
    - with tissue necrosis T34.81- ☑
  - arm T33.4- ☑
    - with tissue necrosis T34.4- ☑
    - finger(s) — *see* Frostbite, finger
    - hand — *see* Frostbite, hand
    - wrist — *see* Frostbite, wrist
  - ear T33.Ø1- ☑
    - with tissue necrosis T34.Ø1- ☑
  - face T33.Ø9 ☑
    - with tissue necrosis T34.Ø9 ☑
  - finger T33.53- ☑
    - with tissue necrosis T34.53- ☑
  - foot T33.82- ☑
    - with tissue necrosis T34.82- ☑
  - hand T33.52- ☑
    - with tissue necrosis T34.52- ☑
  - head T33.Ø9 ☑
    - with tissue necrosis T34.Ø9 ☑
    - ear — *see* Frostbite, ear
    - nose — *see* Frostbite, nose
  - hip (and thigh) T33.6- ☑
    - with tissue necrosis T34.6- ☑
  - knee T33.7- ☑
    - with tissue necrosis T34.7- ☑
  - leg T33.9- ☑
    - with tissue necrosis T34.9- ☑
    - ankle — *see* Frostbite, ankle
    - foot — *see* Frostbite, foot
    - knee — *see* Frostbite, knee
    - lower T33.7- ☑
      - with tissue necrosis T34.7- ☑
    - thigh — *see* Frostbite, hip
    - toe — *see* Frostbite, toe
  - limb
    - lower T33.99 ☑
- **Frostbite** — *continued*
  - limb — *continued*
    - lower — *continued*
      - with tissue necrosis T34.99 ☑
    - upper — *see* Frostbite, arm
  - neck T33.1 ☑
    - with tissue necrosis T34.1 ☑
  - nose T33.Ø2 ☑
    - with tissue necrosis T34.Ø2 ☑
  - pelvis T33.3 ☑
    - with tissue necrosis T34.3 ☑
  - specified site NEC T33.99 ☑
    - with tissue necrosis T34.99 ☑
  - thigh — *see* Frostbite, hip
  - thorax T33.2 ☑
    - with tissue necrosis T34.2 ☑
  - toes T33.83- ☑
    - with tissue necrosis T34.83- ☑
  - trunk T33.99 ☑
    - with tissue necrosis T34.99 ☑
  - wrist T33.51- ☑
    - with tissue necrosis T34.51- ☑
- **Frotteurism** F65.81
- **Frozen** — *see also* Effect, adverse, cold T69.9 ☑
  - pelvis (female) N94.89
    - male K66.8
  - shoulder — *see* Capsulitis, adhesive
- **Fructokinase deficiency** E74.11
- **Fructose 1,6 diphosphatase deficiency** E74.19
- **Fructosemia** (benign) (essential) E74.12
- **Fructosuria** (benign) (essential) E74.11
- **Fuchs'**
  - black spot (myopic) — *see also* Myopia, degenerative H44.2- ☑
  - dystrophy (corneal endothelium) H18.51- ☑
  - heterochromic cyclitis — *see* Cyclitis, Fuchs' heterochromic
- **Fucosidosis** E77.1
- **Fugue** R68.89
  - dissociative F44.1
  - hysterical (dissociative) F44.1
  - postictal in epilepsy — *see* Epilepsy
  - reaction to exceptional stress (transient) F43.Ø
- **Fulminant, fulminating** — *see* condition
- **Functional** — *see also* condition
  - bleeding (uterus) N93.8
- **Functioning, intellectual, borderline** R41.83
- **Fundus** — *see* condition
- **Fungemia NOS** B49
- **Fungus, fungous**
  - cerebral G93.89
  - disease NOS B49
  - infection — *see* Infection, fungus
- **Funiculitis** (acute) (chronic) (endemic) N49.1
  - gonococcal (acute) (chronic) A54.23
  - tuberculous A18.15
- **Funnel**
  - breast (acquired) M95.4
    - congenital Q67.6
    - sequelae (late effect) of rickets E64.3
  - chest (acquired) M95.4
    - congenital Q67.6
    - sequelae (late effect) of rickets E64.3
  - pelvis (acquired) M95.5
    - with disproportion (fetopelvic) O33.3 ☑
      - causing obstructed labor O65.3
    - congenital Q74.2
- **FUO** (fever of unknown origin) R5Ø.9
- **Furfur** L21.Ø
  - microsporon B36.Ø
- **Furrier's lung** J67.8
- **Furrowed** K14.5
  - nail(s) (transverse) L6Ø.4
    - congenital Q84.6
  - tongue K14.5
    - congenital Q38.3
- **Furuncle** LØ2.92
  - abdominal wall LØ2.221
  - ankle — *see* Furuncle, lower limb
  - antecubital space — *see* Furuncle, upper limb
  - anus K61.Ø
  - arm — *see* Furuncle, upper limb
  - auditory canal, external — *see* Abscess, ear, external
  - auricle (ear) — *see* Abscess, ear, external
  - axilla (region) LØ2.42- ☑
  - back (any part) LØ2.222
  - breast N61.1

Furuncle — *continued*
- buttock LØ2.32
- cheek (external) LØ2.Ø2
- chest wall LØ2.223
- chin LØ2.Ø2
- corpus cavernosum N48.21
- ear, external — *see* Abscess, ear, external
- external auditory canal — *see* Abscess, ear, external
- eyelid — *see* Abscess, eyelid
- face LØ2.Ø2
- femoral (region) — *see* Furuncle, lower limb
- finger — *see* Furuncle, hand
- flank LØ2.221
- foot LØ2.62- ☑
- forehead LØ2.Ø2
- gluteal (region) LØ2.32
- groin LØ2.224
- hand LØ2.52- ☑
- head LØ2.821
  - face LØ2.Ø2
- hip — *see* Furuncle, lower limb
- kidney — *see* Abscess, kidney
- knee — *see* Furuncle, lower limb
- labium (majus) (minus) N76.4
- lacrimal
  - gland — *see* Dacryoadenitis
  - passages (duct) (sac) — *see* Inflammation, lacrimal, passages, acute
- leg (any part) — *see* Furuncle, lower limb
- lower limb LØ2.42- ☑
- malignant A22.Ø
- mouth K12.2
- navel LØ2.226
- neck LØ2.12
- nose J34.Ø
- orbit, orbital — *see* Abscess, orbit
- palmar (space) — *see* Furuncle, hand
- partes posteriores LØ2.32
- pectoral region LØ2.223
- penis N48.21
- perineum LØ2.225
- pinna — *see* Abscess, ear, external
- popliteal — *see* Furuncle, lower limb
- prepatellar — *see* Furuncle, lower limb
- scalp LØ2.821
- seminal vesicle N49.Ø
- shoulder — *see* Furuncle, upper limb
- specified site NEC LØ2.828
- submandibular K12.2
- temple (region) LØ2.Ø2
- thumb — *see* Furuncle, hand
- toe — *see* Furuncle, foot
- trunk LØ2.229
  - abdominal wall LØ2.221
  - back LØ2.222
  - chest wall LØ2.223
  - groin LØ2.224
  - perineum LØ2.225
  - umbilicus LØ2.226
- umbilicus LØ2.226
- upper limb LØ2.42- ☑
- vulva N76.4

Furunculosis — *see* Furuncle

Fused — *see* Fusion, fused

Fusion, fused (congenital)
- astragaloscaphoid Q74.2
- atria Q21.19
- auditory canal Q16.1
- auricles, heart Q21.19
- binocular with defective stereopsis H53.32
- bone Q79.8
- cervical spine M43.22
- choanal Q3Ø.Ø
- commissure, mitral valve Q23.2
- cusps, heart valve NEC Q24.8
  - mitral Q23.2
  - pulmonary Q22.1
  - tricuspid Q22.4
- ear ossicles Q16.3
- fingers Q7Ø.Ø ☑
- hymen Q52.3
- joint (acquired) — *see also* Ankylosis
  - congenital Q74.8
- kidneys (incomplete) Q63.1
- labium (majus) (minus) Q52.5
- larynx and trachea Q34.8
- limb, congenital Q74.8
  - lower Q74.2
  - upper Q74.Ø
- lobes, lung Q33.8
- lumbosacral (acquired) M43.27
  - arthrodesis status Z98.1
  - congenital Q76.49
  - postprocedural status Z98.1
- nares, nose, nasal, nostril(s) Q3Ø.Ø
- organ or site not listed — *see* Anomaly, by site
- ossicles Q79.9
  - auditory Q16.3
- pulmonic cusps Q22.1
- ribs Q76.6
- sacroiliac (joint) (acquired) M43.28
  - arthrodesis status Z98.1
  - congenital Q74.2
  - postprocedural status Z98.1
- spine (acquired) NEC M43.2Ø
  - arthrodesis status Z98.1
  - cervical region M43.22
  - cervicothoracic region M43.23
  - congenital Q76.49
  - lumbar M43.26
  - lumbosacral region M43.27
  - occipito-atlanto-axial region M43.21
  - postoperative status Z98.1
  - sacrococcygeal region M43.28
  - thoracic region M43.24
  - thoracolumbar region M43.25
- sublingual duct with submaxillary duct at opening in mouth Q38.4
- testes Q55.1
- toes Q7Ø.2- ☑
- tooth, teeth KØØ.2
- trachea and esophagus Q39.8
- twins Q89.4
- vagina Q52.4
- ventricles, heart Q21.Ø
- vertebra (arch) — *see* Fusion, spine
- vulva Q52.5

Fusospirillosis (mouth) (tongue) (tonsil) A69.1

Fussy baby R68.12

G

Gain in weight (abnormal) (excessive) — *see also* Weight, gain
Gaisböck's disease (polycythemia hypertonica) D75.1
Gait abnormality R26.9
ataxic R26.Ø
falling R29.6
hysterical (ataxic) (staggering) F44.4
paralytic R26.1
spastic R26.1
specified type NEC R26.89
staggering R26.Ø
unsteadiness R26.81
walking difficulty NEC R26.2
Galactocele (breast) N64.89
puerperal, postpartum O92.79
Galactokinase deficiency E74.29
Galactophoritis N61.Ø
gestational, puerperal, postpartum O91.2- ☑
Galactorrhea O92.6
not associated with childbirth N64.3
Galactosemia (classic) (congenital) E74.21
Galactosuria E74.29
Galacturia R82.Ø
schistosomiasis (bilharziasis) B65.Ø
GALD (gestational alloimmune liver disease) P78.84
Galeazzi's fracture S52.37- ☑
Galen's vein — *see* condition
Galeophobia F4Ø.218
Gall duct — *see* condition
Gallbladder — *see also* condition
acute K81.Ø
Gallop rhythm RØØ.8
Gallstone (colic) (cystic duct) (gallbladder) (impacted) (multiple) — *see also* Calculus, gallbladder
with
cholecystitis — *see* Calculus, gallbladder, with cholecystitis
bile duct (common) (hepatic) — *see* Calculus, bile duct
causing intestinal obstruction K56.3
specified NEC K8Ø.8Ø
with obstruction K8Ø.81
Gambling Z72.6
pathological (compulsive) F63.Ø
Gammopathy (of undetermined significance [MGUS]) D47.2
associated with lymphoplasmacytic dyscrasia D47.2
monoclonal D47.2
polyclonal D89.Ø
Gamna's disease (siderotic splenomegaly) D73.1
Gamophobia F4Ø.298
Gampsodactylia (congenital) Q66.7- ☑
Gamstorp's disease (adynamia episodica hereditaria) G72.3
Gandy-Nanta disease (siderotic splenomegaly) D73.1
Gang
membership offenses Z72.81Ø
Gangliocytoma D36.1Ø
Ganglioglioma — *see* Neoplasm, uncertain behavior, by site
Ganglion (compound) (diffuse) (joint) (tendon (sheath)) M67.4Ø
ankle M67.47- ☑
foot M67.47- ☑
forearm M67.43- ☑
hand M67.44- ☑
lower leg M67.46- ☑
multiple sites M67.49
of yaws (early) (late) A66.6
pelvic region M67.45- ☑
periosteal — *see* Periostitis
shoulder region M67.41- ☑
specified site NEC M67.48
thigh region M67.45- ☑
tuberculous A18.Ø9
upper arm M67.42- ☑
wrist M67.43- ☑
Ganglioneuroblastoma — *see* Neoplasm, nerve, malignant
Ganglioneuroma D36.1Ø
malignant — *see* Neoplasm, nerve, malignant
Ganglioneuromatosis D36.1Ø
Ganglionitis
fifth nerve — *see* Neuralgia, trigeminal
gasserian (postherpetic) (postzoster) BØ2.21
Ganglionitis — *continued*
geniculate G51.1
newborn (birth injury) P11.3
postherpetic, postzoster BØ2.21
herpes zoster BØ2.21
postherpetic geniculate BØ2.21
Gangliosidosis E75.1Ø
GM1 E75.19
GM2 E75.ØØ
other specified E75.Ø9
Sandhoff disease E75.Ø1
Tay-Sachs disease E75.Ø2
GM3 E75.19
mucolipidosis IV E75.11
Gangosa A66.5
Gangrene, gangrenous (connective tissue) (dropsical) (dry) (moist) (skin) (ulcer) — *see also* Necrosis I96
with diabetes (mellitus) — *see* Diabetes, with, gangrene
abdomen (wall) I96
alveolar M27.3
appendix K35.8Ø
with
peritonitis, localized — *see also* Appendicitis K35.31
arteriosclerotic (general) (senile) — *see* Arteriosclerosis, extremities, with, gangrene
auricle I96
Bacillus welchii A48.Ø
bladder (infectious) — *see* Cystitis, specified type NEC
bowel, cecum, or colon — *see* Gangrene, intestine
Clostridium perfringens or welchii A48.Ø
cornea H18.89- ☑
corpora cavernosa N48.29
noninfective N48.89
cutaneous, spreading I96
decubital — *see* Ulcer, pressure, by site
diabetic (any site) — *see* Diabetes, with, gangrene
emphysematous — *see* Gangrene, gas
epidemic — *see* Poisoning, food, noxious, plant
epididymis (infectional) N45.1
erysipelas — *see* Erysipelas
extremity (lower) (upper) I96
Fournier N49.3
female N76.82
vagina and vulva N76.82
fusospirochetal A69.Ø
gallbladder — *see* Cholecystitis, acute
gas (bacillus) A48.Ø
following
abortion — *see* Abortion by type complicated by infection
ectopic or molar pregnancy OØ8.Ø
glossitis K14.Ø
hernia — *see* Hernia, by site, with gangrene
intestine, intestinal (hemorrhagic) (massive) — *see also* Infarct, intestine K55.Ø69
with
mesenteric embolism — *see also* Infarct, intestine K55.Ø69
obstruction — *see* Obstruction, intestine
laryngitis JØ4.Ø
limb (lower) (upper) I96
lung J85.Ø
spirochetal A69.8
lymphangitis I89.1
Meleney's (synergistic) — *see* Ulcer, skin
mesentery — *see also* Infarct, intestine K55.Ø69
with
embolism — *see also* Infarct, intestine K55.Ø69
intestinal obstruction — *see* Obstruction, intestine
mouth A69.Ø
ovary — *see* Oophoritis
pancreas — *see* Pancreatitis, acute
penis N48.29
noninfective N48.89
perineum I96
pharynx — *see also* Pharyngitis
Vincent's A69.1
presenile I73.1
progressive synergistic — *see* Ulcer, skin
pulmonary J85.Ø
pulpal (dental) KØ4.1
quinsy J36
Raynaud's (symmetric gangrene) I73.Ø1
retropharyngeal J39.2
scrotum N49.3
noninfective N5Ø.89
Gangrene, gangrenous — *continued*
senile (atherosclerotic) — *see* Arteriosclerosis, extremities, with, gangrene
spermatic cord N49.1
noninfective N5Ø.89
spine I96
spirochetal NEC A69.8
spreading cutaneous I96
stomatitis A69.Ø
symmetrical I73.Ø1
testis (infectional) N45.2
noninfective N44.8
throat — *see also* Pharyngitis
diphtheritic A36.Ø
Vincent's A69.1
thyroid (gland) EØ7.89
tooth (pulp) KØ4.1
tuberculous NEC — *see* Tuberculosis
tunica vaginalis N49.1
noninfective N5Ø.89
umbilicus I96
uterus — *see* Endometritis
uvulitis K12.2
vas deferens N49.1
noninfective N5Ø.89
vulva N76.82
Ganister disease J62.8
Ganser's syndrome (hysterical) F44.89
Gardner-Diamond syndrome (autoerythrocyte sensitization) D69.2
Gargoylism E76.Ø1
Garré's disease, osteitis (sclerosing), osteomyelitis — *see* Osteomyelitis, specified type NEC
Garrod's pad, knuckle M72.1
Gartner's duct
cyst Q52.4
persistent Q5Ø.6
Gas R14.3
asphyxiation, inhalation, poisoning, suffocation NEC — *see* Table of Drugs and Chemicals
excessive R14.Ø
gangrene A48.Ø
following
abortion — *see* Abortion by type complicated by infection
ectopic or molar pregnancy OØ8.Ø
on stomach R14.Ø
pains R14.1
Gastralgia — *see also* Pain, abdominal
Gastrectasis K31.Ø
psychogenic F45.8
Gastric — *see* condition
Gastrinoma
malignant
pancreas C25.4
specified site NEC — *see* Neoplasm, malignant, by site
unspecified site C25.4
specified site — *see* Neoplasm, uncertain behavior
unspecified site D37.9
Gastritis (simple) K29.7Ø
with bleeding K29.71
acute (erosive) K29.ØØ
with bleeding K29.Ø1
alcoholic K29.2Ø
with bleeding K29.21
allergic K29.6Ø
with bleeding K29.61
atrophic (chronic) K29.4Ø
with bleeding K29.41
chronic (antral) (fundal) K29.5Ø
with bleeding K29.51
atrophic K29.4Ø
with bleeding K29.41
superficial K29.3Ø
with bleeding K29.31
dietary counseling and surveillance Z71.3
due to diet deficiency E63.9
eosinophilic K52.81
giant hypertrophic K29.6Ø
with bleeding K29.61
granulomatous K29.6Ø
with bleeding K29.61
hypertrophic (mucosa) K29.6Ø
with bleeding K29.61
nervous F54
spastic K29.6Ø
with bleeding K29.61

- **Gastritis** — *continued*
  - specified NEC K29.6Ø
    - with bleeding K29.61
  - superficial chronic K29.3Ø
    - with bleeding K29.31
  - tuberculous A18.83
  - viral NEC AØ8.4
- **Gastrocarcinoma** — *see* Neoplasm, malignant, stomach
- **Gastrocolic** — *see* condition
- **Gastrodisciasis, gastrodiscoidiasis** B66.8
- **Gastroduodenitis** K29.9Ø
  - with bleeding K29.91
  - virus, viral AØ8.4
    - specified type NEC AØ8.39
- **Gastrodynia** — *see* Pain, abdominal
- **Gastroenteritis** (acute) (chronic) (noninfectious) — *see also* Enteritis K52.9
  - allergic K52.29
    - with
      - eosinophilic gastritis or gastroenteritis K52.81
      - food protein-induced enterocolitis syndrome K52.21
      - food protein-induced enteropathy K52.22
  - dietetic — *see also* Gastroenteritis, allergic K52.29
  - drug-induced K52.1
  - due to
    - Cryptosporidium AØ7.2
    - drugs K52.1
    - food poisoning — *see* Intoxication, foodborne
    - radiation K52.Ø
  - eosinophilic K52.81
  - epidemic (infectious) AØ9
  - food hypersensitivity — *see also* Gastroenteritis, allergic K52.29
  - infectious — *see* Enteritis, infectious
  - influenzal — *see* Influenza, with gastroenteritis
  - noninfectious K52.9
    - specified NEC K52.89
  - rotaviral AØ8.Ø
  - Salmonella AØ2.Ø
  - toxic K52.1
  - viral NEC AØ8.4
    - acute infectious AØ8.39
      - type Norwalk AØ8.11
    - infantile (acute) AØ8.39
    - Norwalk agent AØ8.11
    - rotaviral AØ8.Ø
    - severe of infants AØ8.39
    - specified type NEC AØ8.39
- **Gastroenteropathy** — *see also* Gastroenteritis K52.9
  - acute, due to Norovirus AØ8.11
  - acute, due to Norwalk agent AØ8.11
  - infectious AØ9
- **Gastroenteroptosis** K63.4
- **Gastroesophageal laceration- hemorrhage syndrome** K22.6
- **Gastrointestinal** — *see* condition
- **Gastrojejunal** — *see* condition
- **Gastrojejunitis** — *see also* Enteritis K52.9
- **Gastrojejunocolic** — *see* condition
- **Gastroliths** K31.89
- **Gastromalacia** K31.89
- **Gastroparalysis** K31.84
  - diabetic — *see* Diabetes, gastroparalysis
- **Gastroparesis** K31.84
  - diabetic — *see* Diabetes, by type, with gastroparesis
- **Gastropathy** K31.9
  - congestive portal — *see also* Hypertension, portal K31.89
  - erythematous K29.7Ø
  - exudative K9Ø.89
  - portal hypertensive — *see also* Hypertension, portal K31.89
- **Gastroptosis** K31.89
- **Gastrorrhagia** K92.2
  - psychogenic F45.8
- **Gastroschisis** (congenital) Q79.3
- **Gastrospasm** (neurogenic) (reflex) K31.89
  - neurotic F45.8
  - psychogenic F45.8
- **Gastrostaxis** — *see* Gastritis, with bleeding
- **Gastrostenosis** K31.89
- **Gastrostomy**
  - attention to Z43.1
  - status Z93.1
- **Gastrosuccorrhea** (continuous) (intermittent) K31.89
  - neurotic F45.8
  - psychogenic F45.8
- **Gatophobia** F4Ø.218
- **Gaucher's disease or splenomegaly** (adult) (infantile) E75.22
- **Gee** (-Herter)(-Thaysen) **disease** (nontropical sprue) K9Ø.Ø
- **Gélineau's syndrome** G47.419
  - with cataplexy G47.411
- **Gemination, tooth, teeth** KØØ.2
- **Gemistocytoma**
  - specified site — *see* Neoplasm, malignant, by site
  - unspecified site C71.9
- **General, generalized** — *see* condition
- **Genetic**
  - carrier (status)
    - cystic fibrosis Z14.1
    - hemophilia A (asymptomatic) Z14.Ø1
      - symptomatic Z14.Ø2
    - specified NEC Z14.8
  - susceptibility to disease NEC Z15.89
    - malignant neoplasm Z15.Ø9
      - breast Z15.Ø1
      - endometrium Z15.Ø4
      - ovary Z15.Ø2
      - prostate Z15.Ø3
      - specified NEC Z15.Ø9
    - multiple endocrine neoplasia Z15.81
- **Genital** — *see* condition
- **Genito-anorectal syndrome** A55
- **Genitourinary system** — *see* condition
- **Genu**
  - congenital Q74.1
  - extrorsum (acquired) — *see also* Deformity, varus, knee
    - congenital Q74.1
    - sequelae (late effect) of rickets E64.3
  - introrsum (acquired) — *see also* Deformity, valgus, knee
    - congenital Q74.1
    - sequelae (late effect) of rickets E64.3
  - rachitic (old) E64.3
  - recurvatum (acquired) — *see also* Deformity, limb, specified type NEC, lower leg
    - congenital Q68.2
    - sequelae (late effect) of rickets E64.3
  - valgum (acquired) (knock-knee) M21.Ø6- ☑
    - congenital Q74.1
    - sequelae (late effect) of rickets E64.3
  - varum (acquired) (bowleg) M21.16- ☑
    - congenital Q74.1
    - sequelae (late effect) of rickets E64.3
- **Geographic tongue** K14.1
- **Geophagia** — *see* Pica
- **Geotrichosis** B48.3
  - stomatitis B48.3
- **Gephyrophobia** F4Ø.242
- **Gerbode defect** Q21.Ø
- **GERD** (gastroesophageal reflux disease) K21.9
- **Gerhardt's**
  - disease (erythromelalgia) I73.81
  - syndrome (vocal cord paralysis) J38.ØØ
    - bilateral J38.Ø2
    - unilateral J38.Ø1
- **German measles** — *see also* Rubella
  - exposure to Z2Ø.4
- **Germinoblastoma** (diffuse) C85.9- ☑
  - follicular C82.9- ☑
- **Germinoma** — *see* Neoplasm, malignant, by site
- **Gerontoxon** — *see* Degeneration, cornea, senile
- **Gerstmann's syndrome** R48.8
  - developmental F81.2
- **Gerstmann-Sträussler-Scheinker syndrome** (GSS) A81.82
- **Gestation** (period) — *see also* Pregnancy
  - ectopic — *see* Pregnancy, by site
  - multiple O3Ø.9- ☑
    - greater than quadruplets — *see* Pregnancy, multiple (gestation), specified NEC
    - specified NEC — *see* Pregnancy, multiple (gestation), specified NEC
- **Gestational**
  - mammary abscess O91.11- ☑
  - purulent mastitis O91.11- ☑
  - subareolar abscess O91.11- ☑
- **Ghon tubercle, primary infection** A15.7
- **Ghost**
  - teeth KØØ.4
  - vessels (cornea) H16.41- ☑
- **Ghoul hand** A66.3
- **Gianotti-Crosti disease** L44.4
- **Giant**
  - cell
    - epulis KØ6.8
    - peripheral granuloma KØ6.8
  - esophagus, congenital Q39.5
  - kidney, congenital Q63.3
  - urticaria T78.3 ☑
    - hereditary D84.1
- **Giardiasis** AØ7.1
- **Gibert's disease or pityriasis** L42
- **Giddiness** R42
  - hysterical F44.89
  - psychogenic F45.8
- **Gierke's disease** (glycogenosis I) E74.Ø1
- **Gigantism** (cerebral) (hypophyseal) (pituitary) E22.Ø
  - constitutional E34.4
- **Gilbert's disease or syndrome** E8Ø.4
- **Gilchrist's disease** B4Ø.9
- **Gilford-Hutchinson disease** E34.8
- **Gilles de la Tourette's disease or syndrome** (motor-verbal tic) F95.2
- **Gingivitis** KØ5.1Ø
  - acute (catarrhal) KØ5.ØØ
    - necrotizing A69.1
    - nonplaque induced KØ5.Ø1
    - plaque induced KØ5.ØØ
  - chronic (desquamative) (hyperplastic) (simple marginal) (pregnancy associated) (ulcerative) KØ5.1Ø
    - nonplaque induced KØ5.11
    - plaque induced KØ5.1Ø
  - expulsiva — *see* Periodontitis
  - necrotizing ulcerative (acute) A69.1
  - pellagrous E52
    - acute necrotizing A69.1
  - Vincent's A69.1
- **Gingivoglossitis** K14.Ø
- **Gingivopericementitis** — *see* Periodontitis
- **Gingivosis** — *see* Gingivitis, chronic
- **Gingivostomatitis** KØ5.1Ø
  - herpesviral BØØ.2
  - necrotizing ulcerative (acute) A69.1
- **Gland, glandular** — *see* condition
- **Glanders** A24.Ø
- **Glanzmann** (-Naegeli) **disease or thrombasthenia** D69.1
- **Glasgow coma scale**
  - total score
    - 3-8 R4Ø.243 ☑
    - 9-12 R4Ø.242 ☑
    - 13-15 R4Ø.241 ☑
- **Glass-blower's disease** (cataract) — *see* Cataract, specified NEC
- **Glaucoma** H4Ø.9
  - with
    - increased episcleral venous pressure H4Ø.81- ☑
    - pseudoexfoliation of lens — *see* Glaucoma, open angle, primary, capsular
  - absolute H44.51- ☑
  - angle-closure (primary) H4Ø.2Ø- ☑
    - acute (attack) (crisis) H4Ø.21- ☑
    - chronic H4Ø.22- ☑
    - intermittent H4Ø.23- ☑
    - residual stage H4Ø.24- ☑
  - borderline H4Ø.ØØ- ☑
  - capsular (with pseudoexfoliation of lens) — *see* Glaucoma, open angle, primary, capsular
  - childhood Q15.Ø
  - closed angle — *see* Glaucoma, angle-closure
  - congenital Q15.Ø
  - corticosteroid-induced — *see* Glaucoma, secondary, drugs
  - hypersecretion H4Ø.82- ☑
  - in (due to)
    - amyloidosis E85.4 *[H42]*
    - aniridia Q13.1 *[H42]*
    - concussion of globe — *see* Glaucoma, secondary, trauma
    - dislocation of lens — *see* Glaucoma, secondary
    - disorder of lens NEC — *see* Glaucoma, secondary
    - drugs — *see* Glaucoma, secondary, drugs
    - endocrine disease NOS E34.9 *[H42]*
    - eye
      - inflammation — *see* Glaucoma, secondary, inflammation
      - trauma — *see* Glaucoma, secondary, trauma
    - hypermature cataract — *see* Glaucoma, secondary

- **Glaucoma** — *continued*
  - in — *continued*
    - iridocyclitis — *see* Glaucoma, secondary, inflammation
    - lens disorder — *see* Glaucoma, secondary
    - Lowe's syndrome E72.Ø3 *[H42]*
    - metabolic disease NOS E88.9 *[H42]*
    - ocular disorders NEC — *see* Glaucoma, secondary
    - onchocerciasis B73.Ø2
    - pupillary block — *see* Glaucoma, secondary
    - retinal vein occlusion — *see* Glaucoma, secondary
    - Rieger's anomaly Q13.81 *[H42]*
    - rubeosis of iris — *see* Glaucoma, secondary
    - tumor of globe — *see* Glaucoma, secondary
  - infantile Q15.Ø
  - low tension — *see* Glaucoma, open angle, primary, low-tension
  - malignant H4Ø.83- ☑
  - narrow angle — *see* Glaucoma, angle-closure
  - newborn Q15.Ø
  - noncongestive (chronic) — *see* Glaucoma, open angle
  - nonobstructive — *see* Glaucoma, open angle
  - obstructive — *see also* Glaucoma, angle-closure
    - due to lens changes — *see* Glaucoma, secondary
  - open angle H4Ø.1Ø- ☑
    - primary H4Ø.11- ☑
      - capsular (with pseudoexfoliation of lens) H4Ø.14- ☑
      - low-tension H4Ø.12- ☑
      - pigmentary H4Ø.13- ☑
      - residual stage H4Ø.15- ☑
  - phacolytic — *see* Glaucoma, secondary
  - pigmentary — *see* Glaucoma, open angle, primary, pigmentary
  - postinfectious — *see* Glaucoma, secondary, inflammation
  - secondary (to) H4Ø.5- ☑
    - drugs H4Ø.6- ☑
    - inflammation H4Ø.4- ☑
    - trauma H4Ø.3- ☑
  - simple (chronic) H4Ø.11- ☑
  - simplex H4Ø.11- ☑
  - specified type NEC H4Ø.89
  - suspect H4Ø.ØØ- ☑
  - syphilitic A52.71
  - traumatic — *see also* Glaucoma, secondary, trauma
    - newborn (birth injury) P15.3
  - tuberculous A18.59
- **Glaucomatous flecks** (subcapsular) — *see* Cataract, complicated
- **Glazed tongue** K14.4
- **Gleet** (gonococcal) A54.Ø1
- **Glénard's disease** K63.4
- **Glioblastoma** (multiforme)
  - with sarcomatous component
    - specified site — *see* Neoplasm, malignant, by site
    - unspecified site C71.9
  - giant cell
    - specified site — *see* Neoplasm, malignant, by site
    - unspecified site C71.9
  - specified site — *see* Neoplasm, malignant, by site
  - unspecified site C71.9
- **Glioma** (malignant)
  - astrocytic
    - specified site — *see* Neoplasm, malignant, by site
    - unspecified site C71.9
  - mixed
    - specified site — *see* Neoplasm, malignant, by site
    - unspecified site C71.9
  - nose Q3Ø.8
  - specified site NEC — *see* Neoplasm, malignant, by site
  - subependymal D43.2
    - specified site — *see* Neoplasm, uncertain behavior, by site
    - unspecified site D43.2
  - unspecified site C71.9
- **Gliomatosis cerebri** C71.Ø
- **Glioneuroma** — *see* Neoplasm, uncertain behavior, by site
- **Gliosarcoma**
  - specified site — *see* Neoplasm, malignant, by site
  - unspecified site C71.9
- **Gliosis** (cerebral) G93.89
  - spinal G95.89
- **Glisson's disease** — *see* Rickets
- **Globinuria** R82.3
- **Globus** (hystericus) F45.8
- **Glomangioma** D18.ØØ
  - intra-abdominal D18.Ø3
  - intracranial D18.Ø2
  - skin D18.Ø1
  - specified site NEC D18.Ø9
- **Glomangiomyoma** D18.ØØ
  - intra-abdominal D18.Ø3
  - intracranial D18.Ø2
  - skin D18.Ø1
  - specified site NEC D18.Ø9
- **Glomangiosarcoma** — *see* Neoplasm, connective tissue, malignant
- **Glomerular**
  - disease in syphilis A52.75
  - nephritis — *see* Glomerulonephritis
- **Glomerulitis** — *see* Glomerulonephritis
- **Glomerulonephritis** — *see also* Nephritis NØ5.9
  - with
    - C3
      - glomerulonephritis NØ5.A
      - glomerulopathy NØ5.A
        - with dense deposit disease NØ5.6
    - edema — *see* Nephrosis
    - minimal change NØ5.Ø
    - minor glomerular abnormality NØ5.Ø
  - acute NØØ.9
  - chronic NØ3.9
  - crescentic (diffuse) NEC — *see also* NØØ-NØ7 with fourth character .7 NØ5.7
  - dense deposit — *see also* NØØ-NØ7 with fourth character .6 NØ5.6
  - diffuse
    - crescentic — *see also* NØØ-NØ7 with fourth character .7 NØ5.7
    - endocapillary proliferative — *see also* NØØ-NØ7 with fourth character .4 NØ5.4
    - membranous — *see also* NØØ-NØ7 with fourth character .2 NØ5.2
    - mesangial proliferative — *see also* NØØ-NØ7 with fourth character .3 NØ5.3
    - mesangiocapillary — *see also* NØØ-NØ7 with fourth character .5 NØ5.5
    - sclerosing N18.9
  - endocapillary proliferative (diffuse) NEC — *see also* NØØ-NØ7 with fourth character .4 NØ5.4
  - extracapillary NEC — *see also* NØØ-NØ7 with fourth character .7 NØ5.7
  - focal (and segmental) — *see also* NØØ-NØ7 with fourth character .1 NØ5.1
  - hypocomplementemic — *see* Glomerulonephritis, membranoproliferative
  - IgA — *see* Nephropathy, IgA
  - immune complex (circulating) NEC NØ5.8
  - in (due to)
    - amyloidosis E85.4 *[NØ8]*
    - bilharziasis B65.9 *[NØ8]*
    - cryoglobulinemia D89.1 *[NØ8]*
    - defibrination syndrome D65 *[NØ8]*
    - diabetes mellitus — *see* Diabetes, glomerulosclerosis
    - disseminated intravascular coagulation D65 *[NØ8]*
    - Fabry (-Anderson) disease E75.21 *[NØ8]*
    - Goodpasture's syndrome M31.Ø
    - hemolytic-uremic syndrome — *see* Syndrome, hemolytic-uremic
    - Henoch (-Schönlein) purpura D69.Ø *[NØ8]*
    - lecithin cholesterol acyltransferase deficiency E78.6 *[NØ8]*
    - microscopic polyangiitis M31.7 *[NØ8]*
    - multiple myeloma C9Ø.Ø- ☑ *[NØ8]*
    - Plasmodium malariae B52.Ø
    - schistosomiasis B65.9 *[NØ8]*
    - sepsis A41.9 *[NØ8]*
      - streptococcal A4Ø- ☑ *[NØ8]*
    - sickle-cell disorders D57.- ☑ *[NØ8]*
    - strongyloidiasis B78.9 *[NØ8]*
    - subacute bacterial endocarditis I33.Ø *[NØ8]*
    - syphilis (late) congenital A5Ø.59 *[NØ8]*
    - systemic lupus erythematosus M32.14
    - thrombotic thrombocytopenic purpura M31.19 *[NØ8]*
    - typhoid fever AØ1.Ø9
    - Waldenström macroglobulinemia C88.Ø *[NØ8]*
    - Wegener's granulomatosis M31.31
  - latent or quiescent NØ3.9
  - lobular, lobulonodular — *see* Glomerulonephritis, membranoproliferative
- **Glomerulonephritis** — *continued*
  - membranoproliferative (diffuse)(type 1 or 3) — *see also* NØØ-NØ7 with fourth character .5 NØ5.5
    - dense deposit (type 2) NEC — *see also* NØØ-NØ7 with fourth character .6 NØ5.6
  - membranous (diffuse) NEC — *see also* NØØ-NØ7 with fourth character .2 NØ5.2
  - mesangial
    - IgA/IgG — *see* Nephropathy, IgA
    - proliferative (diffuse) NEC — *see also* NØØ-NØ7 with fourth character .3 NØ5.3
  - mesangiocapillary (diffuse) NEC — *see also* NØØ-NØ7 with fourth character .5 NØ5.5
  - necrotic, necrotizing NEC — *see also* NØØ- NØ7 with fourth character .8 NØ5.8
  - nodular — *see* Glomerulonephritis, membranoproliferative
  - poststreptococcal NEC NØ5.9
    - acute NØØ.9
    - chronic NØ3.9
    - rapidly progressive NØ1.9
  - proliferative NEC — *see also* NØØ-NØ7 with fourth character .8 NØ5.8
    - diffuse (lupus) M32.14
  - rapidly progressive NØ1.9
  - sclerosing, diffuse N18.9
  - specified pathology NEC — *see also* NØØ- NØ7 with fourth character .8 NØ5.8
  - subacute NØ1.9
- **Glomerulopathy** — *see* Glomerulonephritis
- **Glomerulosclerosis** — *see also* Sclerosis, renal
  - intercapillary (nodular) (with diabetes) — *see* Diabetes, glomerulosclerosis
  - intracapillary — *see* Diabetes, glomerulosclerosis
- **Glossagra** K14.6
- **Glossalgia** K14.6
- **Glossitis** (chronic superficial) (gangrenous) (Moeller's) K14.Ø
  - areata exfoliativa K14.1
  - atrophic K14.4
  - benign migratory K14.1
  - cortical superficial, sclerotic K14.Ø
  - Hunter's D51.Ø
  - interstitial, sclerous K14.Ø
  - median rhomboid K14.2
  - pellagrous E52
  - superficial, chronic K14.Ø
- **Glossocele** K14.8
- **Glossodynia** K14.6
  - exfoliativa K14.4
- **Glossoncus** K14.8
- **Glossopathy** K14.9
- **Glossophytia** K14.3
- **Glossoplegia** K14.8
- **Glossoptosis** K14.8
- **Glossopyrosis** K14.6
- **Glossotrichia** K14.3
- **Glossy skin** L9Ø.8
- **Glottis** — *see* condition
- **Glottitis** — *see also* Laryngitis JØ4.Ø
- **Glucagonoma**
  - pancreas
    - benign D13.7
    - malignant C25.4
    - uncertain behavior D37.8
  - specified site NEC
    - benign — *see* Neoplasm, benign, by site
    - malignant — *see* Neoplasm, malignant, by site
    - uncertain behavior — *see* Neoplasm, uncertain behavior, by site
  - unspecified site
    - benign D13.7
    - malignant C25.4
    - uncertain behavior D37.8
- **Glucoglycinuria** E72.51
- **Glucose-galactose malabsorption** E74.39
- **Glue**
  - ear — *see* Otitis, media, nonsuppurative, chronic, mucoid
  - sniffing (airplane) — *see* Abuse, drug, inhalant
    - dependence — *see* Dependence, drug, inhalant
- **GLUT1 deficiency syndrome 1, infantile onset** E74.81Ø
- **GLUT1 deficiency syndrome 2, childhood onset** E74.81Ø
- **Glutaric aciduria** E72.3
- **Glycinemia** E72.51
- **Glycinuria** (renal) (with ketosis) E72.Ø9

- **Glycogen**
  - infiltration — *see* Disease, glycogen storage
  - storage disease — *see* Disease, glycogen storage
- **Glycogenosis** (diffuse) (generalized) — *see also* Disease, glycogen storage
  - cardiac E74.02 *[I43]*
  - diabetic, secondary — *see* Diabetes, glycogenosis, secondary
  - pulmonary interstitial J84.842
- **Glycopenia** E16.2
- **Glycosuria** R81
  - renal E74.818
- **Gnathostoma spinigerum** (infection) (infestation), **gnathostomiasis** (wandering swelling) B83.1
- **Goiter** (plunging) (substernal) E04.9
  - with
    - hyperthyroidism (recurrent) — *see* Hyperthyroidism, with, goiter
    - thyrotoxicosis — *see* Hyperthyroidism, with, goiter
  - adenomatous — *see* Goiter, nodular
  - cancerous C73
  - congenital (nontoxic) E03.0
    - diffuse E03.0
    - parenchymatous E03.0
    - transitory, with normal functioning P72.0
  - cystic E04.2
    - due to iodine-deficiency E01.1
  - due to
    - enzyme defect in synthesis of thyroid hormone E07.1
    - iodine-deficiency (endemic) E01.2
  - dyshormonogenetic (familial) E07.1
  - endemic (iodine-deficiency) E01.2
    - diffuse E01.0
    - multinodular E01.1
  - exophthalmic — *see* Hyperthyroidism, with, goiter
  - iodine-deficiency (endemic) E01.2
    - diffuse E01.0
    - multinodular E01.1
    - nodular E01.1
  - lingual Q89.2
  - lymphadenoid E06.3
  - malignant C73
  - multinodular (cystic) (nontoxic) E04.2
    - toxic or with hyperthyroidism E05.20
      - with thyroid storm E05.21
  - neonatal NEC P72.0
  - nodular (nontoxic) (due to) E04.9
    - with
      - hyperthyroidism E05.20
        - with thyroid storm E05.21
      - thyrotoxicosis E05.20
        - with thyroid storm E05.21
    - endemic E01.1
    - iodine-deficiency E01.1
    - sporadic E04.9
    - toxic E05.20
      - with thyroid storm E05.21
  - nontoxic E04.9
    - diffuse (colloid) E04.0
    - multinodular E04.2
    - simple E04.0
    - specified NEC E04.8
    - uninodular E04.1
  - simple E04.0
  - toxic — *see* Hyperthyroidism, with, goiter
  - uninodular (nontoxic) E04.1
    - toxic or with hyperthyroidism E05.10
      - with thyroid storm E05.11
- **Goiter-deafness syndrome** E07.1
- **Goldberg syndrome** Q89.8
- **Goldberg-Maxwell syndrome** E34.51
- **Goldblatt's hypertension or kidney** I70.1
- **Goldenhar** (-Gorlin) **syndrome** Q87.0
- **Goldflam-Erb disease or syndrome** G70.00
  - with exacerbation (acute) G70.01
  - in crisis G70.01
- **Goldscheider's disease** Q81.8
- **Goldstein's disease** (familial hemorrhagic telangiectasia) I78.0
- **Golfer's elbow** — *see* Epicondylitis, medial
- **Gonadoblastoma**
  - specified site — *see* Neoplasm, uncertain behavior, by site
  - unspecified site
    - female D39.10
    - male D40.10
- **Gonecystitis** — *see* Vesiculitis
- **Gongylonemiasis** B83.8
- **Goniosynechiae** — *see* Adhesions, iris, goniosynechiae
- **Gonococcemia** A54.86
- **Gonococcus, gonococcal** (disease) (infection) — *see also* condition A54.9
  - anus A54.6
  - bursa, bursitis A54.49
  - conjunctiva, conjunctivitis (neonatorum) A54.31
  - endocardium A54.83
  - eye A54.30
    - conjunctivitis A54.31
    - iridocyclitis A54.32
    - keratitis A54.33
    - newborn A54.31
    - other specified A54.39
  - fallopian tubes (acute) (chronic) A54.24
  - genitourinary (organ) (system) (tract) (acute)
    - lower A54.00
      - with abscess (accessory gland) (periurethral) A54.1
    - upper — *see also* condition A54.29
  - heart A54.83
  - iridocyclitis A54.32
  - joint A54.42
  - lymphatic (gland) (node) A54.89
  - meninges, meningitis A54.81
  - musculoskeletal A54.40
    - arthritis A54.42
    - osteomyelitis A54.43
    - other specified A54.49
    - spondylopathy A54.41
  - pelviperitonitis A54.24
  - pelvis (acute) (chronic) A54.24
  - pharynx A54.5
  - proctitis A54.6
  - pyosalpinx (acute) (chronic) A54.24
  - rectum A54.6
  - skin A54.89
  - specified site NEC A54.89
  - tendon sheath A54.49
  - throat A54.5
  - urethra (acute) (chronic) A54.01
    - with abscess (accessory gland) (periurethral) A54.1
  - vulva (acute) (chronic) A54.02
- **Gonocytoma**
  - specified site — *see* Neoplasm, uncertain behavior, by site
  - unspecified site
    - female D39.10
    - male D40.10
- **Gonorrhea** (acute) (chronic) A54.9
  - Bartholin's gland (acute) (chronic) (purulent) A54.02
    - with abscess (accessory gland) (periurethral) A54.1
  - bladder A54.01
  - cervix A54.03
  - conjunctiva, conjunctivitis (neonatorum) A54.31
  - contact Z20.2
  - Cowper's gland (with abscess) A54.1
  - exposure to Z20.2
  - fallopian tube (acute) (chronic) A54.24
  - kidney (acute) (chronic) A54.21
  - lower genitourinary tract A54.00
    - with abscess (accessory gland) (periurethral) A54.1
  - ovary (acute) (chronic) A54.24
  - pelvis (acute) (chronic) A54.24
    - female pelvic inflammatory disease A54.24
  - penis A54.09
  - prostate (acute) (chronic) A54.22
  - seminal vesicle (acute) (chronic) A54.23
  - specified site not listed — *see also* Gonococcus A54.89
  - spermatic cord (acute) (chronic) A54.23
  - urethra A54.01
    - with abscess (accessory gland) (periurethral) A54.1
  - vagina A54.02
  - vas deferens (acute) (chronic) A54.23
  - vulva A54.02
- **Goodall's disease** A08.19
- **Goodpasture's syndrome** M31.0
- **Gopalan's syndrome** (burning feet) E53.0
- **Gorlin-Chaudry-Moss syndrome** Q87.0
- **Gottron's papules** L94.4
- **Gougerot-Blum syndrome** (pigmented purpuric lichenoid dermatitis) L81.7
- **Gougerot-Carteaud disease or syndrome** (confluent reticulate papillomatosis) L83
- **Gougerot's syndrome** (trisymptomatic) L81.7
- **Gouley's syndrome** (constrictive pericarditis) I31.1
- **Goundou** A66.6
- **Gout, chronic** — *see also* Gout, gouty M1A.9 ☑ *(following M08)*
  - drug-induced M1A.20 ☑ *(following M08)*
    - ankle M1A.27- ☑ *(following M08)*
    - elbow M1A.22- ☑ *(following M08)*
    - foot joint M1A.27- ☑ *(following M08)*
    - hand joint M1A.24- ☑ *(following M08)*
    - hip M1A.25- ☑ *(following M08)*
    - knee M1A.26- ☑ *(following M08)*
    - multiple site M1A.29- ☑ *(following M08)*
    - shoulder M1A.21- ☑ *(following M08)*
    - vertebrae M1A.28 ☑ *(following M08)*
    - wrist M1A.23- ☑ *(following M08)*
  - idiopathic M1A.00 ☑ *(following M08)*
    - ankle M1A.07- ☑ *(following M08)*
    - elbow M1A.02- ☑ *(following M08)*
    - foot joint M1A.07- ☑ *(following M08)*
    - hand joint M1A.04- ☑ *(following M08)*
    - hip M1A.05- ☑ *(following M08)*
    - knee M1A.06- ☑ *(following M08)*
    - multiple site M1A.09 ☑ *(following M08)*
    - shoulder M1A.01- ☑ *(following M08)*
    - vertebrae M1A.08 ☑ *(following M08)*
    - wrist M1A.03- ☑ *(following M08)*
  - in (due to) renal impairment M1A.30 ☑ *(following M08)*
    - ankle M1A.37- ☑ *(following M08)*
    - elbow M1A.32- ☑ *(following M08)*
    - foot joint M1A.37- ☑ *(following M08)*
    - hand joint M1A.34- ☑ *(following M08)*
    - hip M1A.35- ☑ *(following M08)*
    - knee M1A.36- ☑ *(following M08)*
    - multiple site M1A.39 ☑ *(following M08)*
    - shoulder M1A.31- ☑ *(following M08)*
    - vertebrae M1A.38 ☑ *(following M08)*
    - wrist M1A.33- ☑ *(following M08)*
  - lead-induced M1A.10 ☑ *(following M08)*
    - ankle M1A.17- ☑ *(following M08)*
    - elbow M1A.12- ☑ *(following M08)*
    - foot joint M1A.17- ☑ *(following M08)*
    - hand joint M1A.14- ☑ *(following M08)*
    - hip M1A.15- ☑ *(following M08)*
    - knee M1A.16- ☑ *(following M08)*
    - multiple site M1A.19 ☑ *(following M08)*
    - shoulder M1A.11- ☑ *(following M08)*
    - vertebrae M1A.18 ☑ *(following M08)*
    - wrist M1A.13- ☑ *(following M08)*
  - primary — *see* Gout, chronic, idiopathic
  - saturnine — *see* Gout, chronic, lead-induced
  - secondary NEC M1A.40 ☑ *(following M08)*
    - ankle M1A.47- ☑ *(following M08)*
    - elbow M1A.42- ☑ *(following M08)*
    - foot joint M1A.47- ☑ *(following M08)*
    - hand joint M1A.44- ☑ *(following M08)*
    - hip M1A.45- ☑ *(following M08)*
    - knee M1A.46- ☑ *(following M08)*
    - multiple site M1A.49 ☑ *(following M08)*
    - shoulder M1A.41- ☑ *(following M08)*
    - vertebrae M1A.48 ☑ *(following M08)*
    - wrist M1A.43- ☑ *(following M08)*
  - syphilitic — *see also* subcategory M14.8- A52.77
  - tophi M1A.9 ☑ *(following M08)*
- **Gout, gouty** (acute) (attack) (flare) — *see also* Gout, chronic M10.9
  - drug-induced M10.20
    - ankle M10.27- ☑
    - elbow M10.22- ☑
    - foot joint M10.27- ☑
    - hand joint M10.24- ☑
    - hip M10.25- ☑
    - knee M10.26- ☑
    - multiple site M10.29
    - shoulder M10.21- ☑
    - vertebrae M10.28
    - wrist M10.23- ☑
  - idiopathic M10.00
    - ankle M10.07- ☑
    - elbow M10.02- ☑
    - foot joint M10.07- ☑
    - hand joint M10.04- ☑
    - hip M10.05- ☑
    - knee M10.06- ☑
    - multiple site M10.09
    - shoulder M10.01- ☑
    - vertebrae M10.08
    - wrist M10.03- ☑
  - in (due to) renal impairment M10.30

- **Gout, gouty** — *continued*
  - in renal impairment — *continued*
    - ankle M1Ø.37- ☑
    - elbow M1Ø.32- ☑
    - foot joint M1Ø.37- ☑
    - hand joint M1Ø.34- ☑
    - hip M1Ø.35- ☑
    - knee M1Ø.36- ☑
    - multiple site M1Ø.39
    - shoulder M1Ø.31- ☑
    - vertebrae M1Ø.38
    - wrist M1Ø.33- ☑
  - lead-induced M1Ø.1Ø
    - ankle M1Ø.17- ☑
    - elbow M1Ø.12- ☑
    - foot joint M1Ø.17- ☑
    - hand joint M1Ø.14- ☑
    - hip M1Ø.15- ☑
    - knee M1Ø.16- ☑
    - multiple site M1Ø.19
    - shoulder M1Ø.11- ☑
    - vertebrae M1Ø.18
    - wrist M1Ø.13- ☑
  - primary — *see* Gout, idiopathic
  - saturnine — *see* Gout, lead-induced
  - secondary NEC M1Ø.4Ø
    - ankle M1Ø.47- ☑
    - elbow M1Ø.42- ☑
    - foot joint M1Ø.47- ☑
    - hand joint M1Ø.44- ☑
    - hip M1Ø.45- ☑
    - knee M1Ø.46- ☑
    - multiple site M1Ø.49
    - shoulder M1Ø.41- ☑
    - vertebrae M1Ø.48
    - wrist M1Ø.43- ☑
  - syphilitic — *see also* subcategory M14.8- A52.77
  - tophi — *see* Gout, chronic
- **Gower's**
  - muscular dystrophy G71.Ø1
  - syndrome (vasovagal attack) R55
- **Gradenigo's syndrome** — *see* Otitis, media, suppurative, acute
- **Graefe's disease** — *see* Strabismus, paralytic, ophthalmoplegia, progressive
- **Graft-versus-host disease** D89.813
  - acute D89.81Ø
  - acute on chronic D89.812
  - chronic D89.811
- **Grain mite** (itch) B88.Ø
- **Grainhandler's disease or lung** J67.8
- **Grand mal** — *see* Epilepsy, generalized, specified NEC
- **Grand multipara status only** (not pregnant) Z64.1
  - pregnant — *see* Pregnancy, complicated by, grand multiparity
- **Granite worker's lung** J62.8
- **Granular** — *see also* condition
  - inflammation, pharynx J31.2
  - kidney (contracting) — *see* Sclerosis, renal
  - liver K74.69
- **Granulation tissue** (abnormal) (excessive) L92.9
  - postmastoidectomy cavity — *see* Complications, postmastoidectomy, granulation
- **Granulocytopenia** (primary) (malignant) — *see* Agranulocytosis
- **Granuloma** L92.9
  - abdomen K66.8
    - from residual foreign body L92.3
    - pyogenicum L98.Ø
  - actinic L57.5
  - annulare (perforating) L92.Ø
  - apical KØ4.5
  - aural — *see* Otitis, externa, specified NEC
  - beryllium (skin) L92.3
  - bone
    - eosinophilic C96.6
    - from residual foreign body — *see* Osteomyelitis, specified type NEC
    - lung C96.6
  - brain (any site) GØ6.Ø
    - schistosomiasis B65.9 *[GØ7]*
  - canaliculus lacrimalis — *see* Granuloma, lacrimal
  - candidal (cutaneous) B37.2
  - cerebral (any site) GØ6.Ø
  - coccidioidal (primary) (progressive) B38.7
    - lung B38.1
    - meninges B38.4

- **Granuloma** — *continued*
  - colon K63.89
  - conjunctiva H11.22- ☑
  - dental KØ4.5
  - ear, middle — *see* Cholesteatoma
  - eosinophilic C96.6
    - bone C96.6
    - lung C96.6
    - oral mucosa K13.4
    - skin L92.2
  - eyelid HØ1.8
  - facial (e) L92.2
  - foreign body (in soft tissue) NEC M6Ø.2Ø
    - ankle M6Ø.27- ☑
    - foot M6Ø.27- ☑
    - forearm M6Ø.23- ☑
    - hand M6Ø.24- ☑
    - in operation wound — *see* Foreign body, accidentally left during a procedure
    - lower leg M6Ø.26- ☑
    - pelvic region M6Ø.25- ☑
    - shoulder region M6Ø.21- ☑
    - skin L92.3
    - specified site NEC M6Ø.28
    - subcutaneous tissue L92.3
    - thigh M6Ø.25- ☑
    - upper arm M6Ø.22- ☑
  - gangraenescens M31.2
  - genito-inguinale A58
  - giant cell (central) (reparative) (jaw) M27.1
    - gingiva (peripheral) KØ6.8
  - gland (lymph) I88.8
  - hepatic NEC K75.3
    - in (due to)
      - berylliosis J63.2 *[K77]*
      - sarcoidosis D86.89
  - Hodgkin C81.9 ☑
  - ileum K63.89
  - infectious B99.9
    - specified NEC B99.8
  - inguinale (Donovan) (venereal) A58
  - intestine NEC K63.89
  - intracranial (any site) GØ6.Ø
  - intraspinal (any part) GØ6.1
  - iridocyclitis — *see* Iridocyclitis, chronic
  - jaw (bone) (central) M27.1
    - reparative giant cell M27.1
  - kidney — *see also* Infection, kidney N15.8
  - lacrimal HØ4.81- ☑
  - larynx J38.7
  - lethal midline (faciale(e)) M31.2
  - liver NEC — *see* Granuloma, hepatic
  - lung (infectious) — *see also* Fibrosis, lung
    - coccidioidal B38.1
    - eosinophilic C96.6
  - Majocchi's B35.8
  - malignant (facial(e)) M31.2
  - mandible (central) M27.1
  - midline (lethal) M31.2
  - monilial (cutaneous) B37.2
  - nasal sinus — *see* Sinusitis
  - operation wound T81.89 ☑
    - foreign body — *see* Foreign body, accidentally left during a procedure
    - stitch T81.89 ☑
    - talc — *see* Foreign body, accidentally left during a procedure
  - oral mucosa K13.4
  - orbit, orbital HØ5.11- ☑
  - paracoccidioidal B41.8
  - penis, venereal A58
  - periapical KØ4.5
  - peritoneum K66.8
    - due to ova of helminths NOS — *see also* Helminthiasis B83.9 *[K67]*
  - postmastoidectomy cavity — *see* Complications, postmastoidectomy, recurrent cholesteatoma
  - prostate N42.89
  - pudendi (ulcerating) A58
  - pulp, internal (tooth) KØ3.3
  - pyogenic, pyogenicum (of) (skin) L98.Ø
    - gingiva KØ6.8
    - maxillary alveolar ridge KØ4.5
    - oral mucosa K13.4
  - rectum K62.89
  - reticulohistiocytic D76.3
  - rubrum nasi L74.8
  - Schistosoma — *see* Schistosomiasis

- **Granuloma** — *continued*
  - septic (skin) L98.Ø
  - silica (skin) L92.3
  - sinus (accessory) (infective) (nasal) — *see* Sinusitis
  - skin L92.9
    - from residual foreign body L92.3
    - pyogenicum L98.Ø
  - spine
    - syphilitic (epidural) A52.19
    - tuberculous A18.Ø1
  - stitch (postoperative) T81.89 ☑
  - suppurative (skin) L98.Ø
  - swimming pool A31.1
  - talc — *see also* Granuloma, foreign body
    - in operation wound — *see* Foreign body, accidentally left during a procedure
  - telangiectaticum (skin) L98.Ø
  - tracheostomy J95.Ø9
  - trichophyticum B35.8
  - tropicum A66.4
  - umbilical P83.81
  - umbilicus P83.81
  - urethra N36.8
  - uveitis — *see* Iridocyclitis, chronic
  - vagina A58
  - venereum A58
  - vocal cord J38.3
- **Granulomatosis** L92.9
  - with polyangiitis M31.3- ☑
  - eosinophilic, with polyangiitis [EGPA] M3Ø.1
  - lymphoid C83.8- ☑
  - miliary (listerial) A32.89
  - necrotizing, respiratory M31.3Ø
  - progressive septic D71
  - specified NEC L92.8
  - Wegener's M31.3Ø
    - with renal involvement M31.31
- **Granulomatous tissue** (abnormal) (excessive) L92.9
- **Granulosis rubra nasi** L74.8
- **Graphite fibrosis** (of lung) J63.3
- **Graphospasm** F48.8
  - organic G25.89
- **Grating scapula** M89.8X1
- **Gravel** (urinary) — *see* Calculus, urinary
- **Graves' disease** — *see* Hyperthyroidism, with, goiter
- **Gravis** — *see* condition
- **Grawitz tumor** C64.- ☑
- **Gray syndrome** (newborn) P93.Ø
- **Grayness, hair** (premature) L67.1
  - congenital Q84.2
- **Green sickness** D5Ø.8
- **Greenfield's disease**
  - meaning
    - concentric sclerosis (encephalitis periaxialis concentrica) G37.5
    - metachromatic leukodystrophy E75.25
- **Greenstick fracture** — *code as* Fracture, by site
- **Grey syndrome** (newborn) P93.Ø
- **Grief** F43.21
  - complicated F34.81
  - prolonged F43.29
  - reaction — *see also* Disorder, adjustment F43.2Ø
- **Griesinger's disease** B76.Ø
- **Grinder's lung or pneumoconiosis** J62.8
- **Grinding, teeth**
  - psychogenic F45.8
  - sleep related G47.63
- **Grip**
  - Dabney's B33.Ø
  - devil's B33.Ø
- **Grippe, grippal** — *see also* Influenza
  - Balkan A78
  - summer, of Italy A93.1
- **Grisel's disease** M43.6
- **Groin** — *see* condition
- **Grooved tongue** K14.5
- **Ground itch** B76.9
- **Grover's disease or syndrome** L11.1
- **Growing pains, children** R29.898
- **Growth** (fungoid) (neoplastic) (new) — *see also* Neoplasm
  - adenoid (vegetative) J35.8
  - benign — *see* Neoplasm, benign, by site
  - malignant — *see* Neoplasm, malignant, by site
  - rapid, childhood ZØØ.2
  - secondary — *see* Neoplasm, secondary, by site
- **Gruby's disease** B35.Ø
- **Gubler-Millard paralysis or syndrome** G46.3

- **Guerin-Stern syndrome** Q74.3
- **Guidance, insufficient anterior** (occlusal) M26.54
- **Guillain-Barré disease or syndrome** G61.Ø
  - sequelae G65.Ø
- **Guinea worms** (infection) (infestation) B72
- **Guinon's disease** (motor-verbal tic) F95.2
- **Gull's disease** EØ3.4
- **Gum** — *see* condition
- **Gumboil** KØ4.7
  - with sinus KØ4.6
- **Gumma** (syphilitic) A52.79
  - artery A52.Ø9
    - cerebral A52.Ø4
  - bone A52.77
    - of yaws (late) A66.6
  - brain A52.19
  - cauda equina A52.19
  - central nervous system A52.3
  - ciliary body A52.71
  - congenital A5Ø.59
  - eyelid A52.71
  - heart A52.Ø6
  - intracranial A52.19
  - iris A52.71
  - kidney A52.75
  - larynx A52.73
  - leptomeninges A52.19
  - liver A52.74
  - meninges A52.19
  - myocardium A52.Ø6
  - nasopharynx A52.73
  - neurosyphilitic A52.3
  - nose A52.73
  - orbit A52.71
  - palate (soft) A52.79
  - penis A52.76
  - pericardium A52.Ø6
  - pharynx A52.73
  - pituitary A52.79
  - scrofulous (tuberculous) A18.4
  - skin A52.79
  - specified site NEC A52.79
  - spinal cord A52.19
  - tongue A52.79
  - tonsil A52.73
  - trachea A52.73
  - tuberculous A18.4
  - ulcerative due to yaws A66.4
  - ureter A52.75
  - yaws A66.4
    - bone A66.6
- **Gunn's syndrome** QØ7.8
- **Gunshot wound** — *see also* Puncture, open
  - fracture — *code as* Fracture, by site
  - internal organs — *see* Injury, by site
- **Gynandrism** Q56.Ø
- **Gynandroblastoma**
  - specified site — *see* Neoplasm, uncertain behavior, by site
  - unspecified site
    - female D39.1Ø
    - male D4Ø.1Ø
- **Gynecological examination** (periodic) (routine) ZØ1.419
  - with abnormal findings ZØ1.411
- **Gynecomastia** N62
- **Gynephobia** F4Ø.291
- **Gyrate scalp** Q82.8

H

- H (Hartnup's) **disease** E72.Ø2
- **Haas' disease or osteochondrosis** (juvenile) (head of humerus) — *see* Osteochondrosis, juvenile, humerus
- **Habit, habituation**
  - bad sleep Z72.821
  - chorea F95.8
  - disturbance, child F98.9
  - drug — *see* Dependence, drug
  - irregular sleep Z72.821
  - laxative F55.2
  - spasm — *see* Tic
  - tic — *see* Tic
- **Haemophilus** (H.) **influenzae, as cause of disease classified elsewhere** B96.3
- **Haff disease** — *see* Poisoning, mercury
- **Hageman's factor defect, deficiency or disease** D68.2
- **Haglund's disease or osteochondrosis** (juvenile) (os tibiale externum) — *see* Osteochondrosis, juvenile, tarsus
- **Hailey-Hailey disease** Q82.8
- **Hair** — *see also* condition
  - plucking F63.3
    - in stereotyped movement disorder F98.4
  - tourniquet syndrome — *see also* Constriction, external, by site
    - finger S6Ø.44- ☑
    - penis S3Ø.842 ☑
    - thumb S6Ø.34- ☑
    - toe S9Ø.44- ☑
- **Hairball in stomach** T18.2 ☑
- **Hair-pulling, pathological** (compulsive) F63.3
- **Hairy black tongue** K14.3
- **Half vertebra** Q76.49
- **Halitosis** R19.6
- **Hallerman-Streiff syndrome** Q87.Ø
- **Hallervorden-Spatz disease** G23.Ø
- **Hallopeau's acrodermatitis or disease** L4Ø.2
- **Hallucination** R44.3
  - auditory R44.Ø
  - gustatory R44.2
  - olfactory R44.2
  - specified NEC R44.2
  - tactile R44.2
  - visual R44.1
- **Hallucinosis** (chronic) F28
  - alcoholic (acute) F1Ø.951
    - in
      - abuse F1Ø.151
      - dependence F1Ø.251
  - drug-induced F19.951
    - cannabis F12.951
    - cocaine F14.951
    - hallucinogen F16.151
    - in
      - abuse F19.151
        - cannabis F12.151
        - cocaine F14.151
        - hallucinogen F16.151
        - inhalant F18.151
        - opioid F11.151
        - sedative, anxiolytic or hypnotic F13.151
        - stimulant NEC F15.151
      - dependence F19.251
        - cannabis F12.251
        - cocaine F14.251
        - hallucinogen F16.251
        - inhalant F18.251
        - opioid F11.251
        - sedative, anxiolytic or hypnotic F13.251
        - stimulant NEC F15.251
    - inhalant F18.951
    - opioid F11.951
    - sedative, anxiolytic or hypnotic F13.951
    - stimulant NEC F15.951
  - organic FØ6.Ø
- **Hallux**
  - deformity (acquired) NEC M2Ø.5X- ☑
  - limitus M2Ø.5X- ☑
  - malleus (acquired) NEC M2Ø.3- ☑
  - rigidus (acquired) M2Ø.2- ☑
    - congenital Q74.2
    - sequelae (late effect) of rickets E64.3
  - valgus (acquired) M2Ø.1- ☑
    - congenital Q66.6
  - varus (acquired) M2Ø.3- ☑
    - congenital Q66.3- ☑
- **Halo, visual** H53.19
- **Hamartoma, hamartoblastoma** Q85.9
  - epithelial (gingival), odontogenic, central or peripheral — *see* Cyst, calcifying odontogenic
- **Hamartosis** Q85.9
- **Hamman-Rich syndrome** J84.114
- **Hammer toe** (acquired) NEC — *see also* Deformity, toe, hammer toe
  - congenital Q66.89
  - sequelae (late effect) of rickets E64.3
- **Hand** — *see* condition
- **Hand-foot syndrome** L27.1
- **Handicap, handicapped**
  - educational Z55.9
    - specified NEC Z55.8
- **Hand-Schüller-Christian disease or syndrome** C96.5
- **Hanging** (asphyxia) (strangulation) (suffocation) — *see* Asphyxia, traumatic, due to mechanical threat
- **Hangnail** — *see also* Cellulitis, digit
  - with lymphangitis — *see* Lymphangitis, acute, digit
- **Hangover** (alcohol) F1Ø.129
- **Hanhart's syndrome** Q87.Ø
- **Hanot-Chauffard** (-Troisier) **syndrome** E83.19
- **Hanot's cirrhosis or disease** K74.3
- **Hansen's disease** — *see* Leprosy
- **Hantaan virus disease** (Korean hemorrhagic fever) A98.5
- **Hantavirus disease** (with renal manifestations) (Dobrava) (Puumala) (Seoul) A98.5
  - with pulmonary manifestations (Andes) (Bayou) (Bermejo) (Black Creek Canal) (Choclo) (Juquitiba) (Laguna negra) (Lechiguanas) (New York) (Oran) (Sin nombre) B33.4
- **Happy puppet syndrome** Q93.51
- **Harada's disease or syndrome** H3Ø.81- ☑
- **Hardening**
  - artery — *see* Arteriosclerosis
  - brain G93.89
- **Hardship, material** Z59.87
- **Harelip** (complete) (incomplete) — *see* Cleft, lip
- **Harlequin** (newborn) Q8Ø.4
- **Harley's disease** D59.6
- **Harmful use** (of)
  - alcohol F1Ø.1Ø
  - anxiolytics — *see* Abuse, drug, sedative
  - cannabinoids — *see* Abuse, drug, cannabis
  - cocaine — *see* Abuse, drug, cocaine
  - drug — *see* Abuse, drug
  - hallucinogens — *see* Abuse, drug, hallucinogen
  - hypnotics — *see* Abuse, drug, sedative
  - opioids — *see* Abuse, drug, opioid
  - PCP (phencyclidine) — *see* Abuse, drug, hallucinogen
  - sedatives — *see* Abuse, drug, sedative
  - stimulants NEC — *see* Abuse, drug, stimulant
- **Harris' lines** — *see* Arrest, epiphyseal
- **Hartnup's disease** E72.Ø2
- **Harvester's lung** J67.Ø
- **Harvesting ovum for in vitro fertilization** Z31.83
- **Hashimoto's disease or thyroiditis** EØ6.3
- **Hashitoxicosis** (transient) EØ6.3
- **Hassal-Henle bodies or warts** (cornea) H18.49
- **Haut mal** — *see* Epilepsy, generalized, specified NEC
- **Haverhill fever** A25.1
- **Hay fever** — *see also* Fever, hay J3Ø.1
- **Hayem-Widal syndrome** D59.8
- **Haygarth's nodes** M15.8
- **Haymaker's lung** J67.Ø
- **Hb** (abnormal)
  - Bart's disease D56.Ø
  - disease — *see* Disease, hemoglobin
  - trait — *see* Trait
- **Head** — *see* condition
- **Headache** R51.9
  - with
    - orthostatic component NEC R51.Ø
    - positional component NEC R51.Ø
  - allergic NEC G44.89
  - associated with sexual activity G44.82
  - cervicogenic G44.86
  - chronic daily R51.9
  - cluster G44.ØØ9
    - chronic G44.Ø29
      - intractable G44.Ø21
      - not intractable G44.Ø29
    - episodic G44.Ø19
      - intractable G44.Ø11
      - not intractable G44.Ø19
    - intractable G44.ØØ1
    - not intractable G44.ØØ9
  - cough (primary) G44.83
  - daily chronic R51.9
  - drug-induced NEC G44.4Ø
    - intractable G44.41
    - not intractable G44.4Ø
  - exertional (primary) G44.84
  - histamine G44.ØØ9
    - intractable G44.ØØ1
    - not intractable G44.ØØ9
  - hypnic G44.81
  - lumbar puncture G97.1
  - medication overuse G44.4Ø
    - intractable G44.41
    - not intractable G44.4Ø
  - menstrual — *see* Migraine, menstrual

- **Headache** — *continued*
  - migraine (type) — *see also* Migraine G43.9Ø9
  - nasal septum R51.9
  - neuralgiform, short lasting unilateral, with conjunctival injection and tearing (SUNCT) G44.Ø59
    - intractable G44.Ø51
    - not intractable G44.Ø59
  - new daily persistent (NDPH) G44.52
  - orgasmic G44.82
  - periodic syndromes in adults and children G43.CØ (*following* G43.7)
    - with refractory migraine G43.C1 (*following* G43.7)
    - intractable G43.C1 (*following* G43.7)
    - not intractable G43.CØ (*following* G43.7)
    - without refractory migraine G43.CØ (*following* G43.7)
  - postspinal puncture G97.1
  - post-traumatic G44.3Ø9
    - acute G44.319
      - intractable G44.311
      - not intractable G44.319
    - chronic G44.329
      - intractable G44.321
      - not intractable G44.329
    - intractable G44.3Ø1
    - not intractable G44.3Ø9
  - pre-menstrual — *see* Migraine, menstrual
  - preorgasmic G44.82
  - primary
    - cough G44.83
    - exertional G44.84
    - stabbing G44.85
    - thunderclap G44.53
  - rebound G44.4Ø
    - intractable G44.41
    - not intractable G44.4Ø
  - short lasting unilateral neuralgiform, with conjunctival injection and tearing (SUNCT) G44.Ø59
    - intractable G44.Ø51
    - not intractable G44.Ø59
  - specified syndrome NEC G44.89
  - spinal and epidural anesthesia - induced T88.59 ☑
    - in labor and delivery O74.5
    - in pregnancy O29.4- ☑
    - postpartum, puerperal O89.4
  - spinal fluid loss (from puncture) G97.1
  - stabbing (primary) G44.85
  - tension (-type) G44.2Ø9
    - chronic G44.229
      - intractable G44.221
      - not intractable G44.229
    - episodic G44.219
      - intractable G44.211
      - not intractable G44.219
    - intractable G44.2Ø1
    - not intractable G44.2Ø9
  - thunderclap (primary) G44.53
  - vascular NEC G44.1
- **Healthy**
  - infant
    - accompanying sick mother Z76.3
    - receiving care Z76.2
  - person accompanying sick person Z76.3
- **Hearing examination** ZØ1.1Ø
  - with abnormal findings NEC ZØ1.118
  - following failed hearing screening ZØ1.11Ø
  - for hearing conservation and treatment ZØ1.12
  - infant or child (over 28 days old) ZØØ.129
    - with abnormal findings ZØØ.121
- **Heart** — *see* condition
- **Heart beat**
  - abnormality RØØ.9
    - specified NEC RØØ.8
  - awareness RØØ.2
  - rapid RØØ.Ø
  - slow RØØ.1
- **Heartburn** R12
  - psychogenic F45.8
- **Heartland virus disease** A93.8
- **Heat** (effects) T67.9 ☑
  - apoplexy T67.Ø1 ☑
  - burn — *see also* Burn L55.9
  - collapse T67.1 ☑
  - cramps T67.2 ☑
  - dermatitis or eczema L59.Ø
  - edema T67.7 ☑
  - erythema — *code by site under* Burn, first degree
  - excessive T67.9 ☑
    - specified effect NEC T67.8 ☑
- **Heat** — *continued*
  - exhaustion T67.5 ☑
    - anhydrotic T67.3 ☑
    - due to
      - salt (and water) depletion T67.4 ☑
      - water depletion T67.3 ☑
        - with salt depletion T67.4 ☑
  - fatigue (transient) T67.6 ☑
  - fever T67.Ø1 ☑
  - hyperpyrexia T67.Ø1 ☑
  - prickly L74.Ø
  - prostration — *see* Heat, exhaustion
  - pyrexia T67.Ø1 ☑
  - rash L74.Ø
  - specified effect NEC T67.8 ☑
  - stroke T67.Ø1 ☑
    - exertional T67.Ø2 ☑
    - specified NEC T67.Ø9 ☑
  - sunburn — *see* Sunburn
  - syncope T67.1 ☑
- **Heavy-for-dates NEC** (infant) (4ØØØg to 4499g) PØ8.1
  - exceptionally (45ØØg or more) PØ8.Ø
- **Hebephrenia, hebephrenic** (schizophrenia) F2Ø.1
- **Heberden's disease or nodes** (with arthropathy) M15.1
- **Hebra's**
  - pityriasis L26
  - prurigo L28.2
- **Heel** — *see* condition
- **Heerfordt's disease** D86.89
- **Hegglin's anomaly or syndrome** D72.Ø
- **Heilmeyer-Schoner disease** D45
- **Heine-Medin disease** A8Ø.9
- **Heinz body anemia, congenital** D58.2
- **Heliophobia** F4Ø.228
- **Heller's disease or syndrome** F84.3
- **HELLP syndrome** (hemolysis, elevated liver enzymes and low platelet count) O14.2- ☑
  - complicating
    - childbirth O14.24
    - puerperium O14.25
- **Helminthiasis** — *see also* Infestation, helminth
  - Ancylostoma B76.Ø
  - intestinal B82.Ø
    - mixed types (types classifiable to more than one of the titles B65.Ø-B81.3 and B81.8) B81.4
    - specified type NEC B81.8
  - mixed types (intestinal) (types classifiable to more than one of the titles B65.Ø-B81.3 and B81.8) B81.4
  - Necator (americanus) B76.1
  - specified type NEC B83.8
- **Heloma** L84
- **Hemangioblastoma** — *see* Neoplasm, connective tissue, uncertain behavior
  - malignant — *see* Neoplasm, connective tissue, malignant
- **Hemangioendothelioma** — *see also* Neoplasm, uncertain behavior, by site
  - benign D18.ØØ
    - intra-abdominal D18.Ø3
    - intracranial D18.Ø2
    - skin D18.Ø1
    - specified site NEC D18.Ø9
  - bone (diffuse) — *see* Neoplasm, bone, malignant
  - epithelioid — *see also* Neoplasm, uncertain behavior, by site
    - malignant — *see* Neoplasm, malignant, by site
  - malignant — *see* Neoplasm, connective tissue, malignant
- **Hemangiofibroma** — *see* Neoplasm, benign, by site
- **Hemangiolipoma** — *see* Lipoma
- **Hemangioma** D18.ØØ
  - arteriovenous D18.ØØ
    - intra-abdominal D18.Ø3
    - intracranial D18.Ø2
    - skin D18.Ø1
    - specified site NEC D18.Ø9
  - capillary I78.1
    - intra-abdominal D18.Ø3
    - intracranial D18.Ø2
    - skin D18.Ø1
    - specified site NEC D18.Ø9
  - cavernous D18.ØØ
    - intra-abdominal D18.Ø3
    - intracranial D18.Ø2
    - skin D18.Ø1
    - specified site NEC D18.Ø9
  - epithelioid D18.ØØ
- **Hemangioma** — *continued*
  - epithelioid — *continued*
    - intra-abdominal D18.Ø3
    - intracranial D18.Ø2
    - skin D18.Ø1
    - specified site NEC D18.Ø9
  - histiocytoid D18.ØØ
    - intra-abdominal D18.Ø3
    - intracranial D18.Ø2
    - skin D18.Ø1
    - specified site NEC D18.Ø9
  - infantile D18.ØØ
    - intra-abdominal D18.Ø3
    - intracranial D18.Ø2
    - skin D18.Ø1
    - specified site NEC D18.Ø9
  - intra-abdominal D18.Ø3
  - intracranial D18.Ø2
  - intramuscular D18.ØØ
    - intra-abdominal D18.Ø3
    - intracranial D18.Ø2
    - skin D18.Ø1
    - specified site NEC D18.Ø9
  - intrathoracic structures D18.Ø9
  - juvenile D18.ØØ
  - malignant — *see* Neoplasm,connective tissue, malignant
  - plexiform D18.ØØ
    - intra-abdominal D18.Ø3
    - intracranial D18.Ø2
    - skin D18.Ø1
    - specified site NEC D18.Ø9
  - racemose D18.ØØ
    - intra-abdominal D18.Ø3
    - intracranial D18.Ø2
    - skin D18.Ø1
    - specified site NEC D18.Ø9
  - sclerosing — *see* Neoplasm, skin, benign
  - simplex D18.ØØ
    - intra-abdominal D18.Ø3
    - intracranial D18.Ø2
    - skin D18.Ø1
    - specified site NEC D18.Ø9
  - skin D18.Ø1
  - specified site NEC D18.Ø9
  - venous D18.ØØ
    - intra-abdominal D18.Ø3
    - intracranial D18.Ø2
    - skin D18.Ø1
    - specified site NEC D18.Ø9
  - verrucous keratotic D18.ØØ
    - intra-abdominal D18.Ø3
    - intracranial D18.Ø2
    - skin D18.Ø1
    - specified site NEC D18.Ø9
- **Hemangiomatosis** (systemic) I78.8
  - involving single site — *see* Hemangioma
- **Hemangiopericytoma** — *see also* Neoplasm, connective tissue, uncertain behavior
  - benign — *see* Neoplasm, connective tissue, benign
  - malignant — *see* Neoplasm, connective tissue, malignant
- **Hemangiosarcoma** — *see* Neoplasm, connective tissue, malignant
- **Hemarthrosis** (nontraumatic) M25.ØØ
  - ankle M25.Ø7- ☑
  - elbow M25.Ø2- ☑
  - foot joint M25.Ø7- ☑
  - hand joint M25.Ø4- ☑
  - hip M25.Ø5- ☑
  - in hemophilic arthropathy — *see* Arthropathy, hemophilic
  - knee M25.Ø6- ☑
  - shoulder M25.Ø1- ☑
  - specified joint NEC M25.Ø8
  - traumatic — *see* Sprain, by site
  - vertebrae M25.Ø8
  - wrist M25.Ø3- ☑
- **Hematemesis** K92.Ø
  - with ulcer — *code by site under* Ulcer, with hemorrhage K27.4
  - newborn, neonatal P54.Ø
    - due to swallowed maternal blood P78.2
- **Hematidrosis** L74.8
- **Hematinuria** — *see also* Hemoglobinuria
  - malarial B5Ø.8
- **Hematobilia** K83.8

Hematocele
female NEC N94.89
with ectopic pregnancy O00.90
with intrauterine pregnancy O00.91
ovary N83.8
male N50.1
Hematochezia — *see also* Melena K92.1
Hematochyluria — *see also* Infestation, filarial
schistosomiasis (bilharziasis) B65.0
Hematocolpos (with hematometra or hematosalpinx) N89.7
Hematocornea — *see* Pigmentation, cornea, stromal
Hematogenous — *see* condition
Hematoma (traumatic) (skin surface intact) — *see also* Contusion
with
injury of internal organs — *see* Injury, by site
open wound — *see* Wound, open
amputation stump (surgical) (late) T87.89
aorta, dissecting I71.00
abdominal I71.02
thoracic — *see also* Dissection, aorta, thoracic I71.019
thoracoabdominal I71.03
aortic intramural — *see* Dissection, aorta
arterial (complicating trauma) — *see* Injury, blood vessel, by site
auricle — *see* Contusion, ear
nontraumatic — *see* Disorder, pinna, hematoma
birth injury NEC P15.8
brain (traumatic)
with
cerebral laceration or contusion (diffuse) — *see* Injury, intracranial, diffuse
focal — *see* Injury, intracranial, focal
cerebellar, traumatic S06.37- ☑
intracerebral, traumatic — *see* Injury, intracranial, intracerebral hemorrhage
newborn NEC P52.4
birth injury P10.1
nontraumatic — *see* Hemorrhage, intracranial
subarachnoid, arachnoid, traumatic — *see* Injury, intracranial, subarachnoid hemorrhage
subdural, traumatic — *see* Injury, intracranial, subdural hemorrhage
breast (nontraumatic) N64.89
broad ligament (nontraumatic) N83.7
traumatic S37.892 ☑
cerebellar, traumatic S06.37- ☑
cerebral — *see* Hematoma, brain
cerebrum S06.36- ☑
left S06.35- ☑
right S06.34- ☑
cesarean delivery wound O90.2
complicating delivery (perineal) (pelvic) (vagina) (vulva) O71.7
corpus cavernosum (nontraumatic) N48.89
epididymis (nontraumatic) N50.1
epidural (traumatic) — *see* Injury, intracranial, epidural hemorrhage
spinal — *see* Injury, spinal cord, by region
episiotomy O90.2
face, birth injury P15.4
genital organ NEC (nontraumatic)
female (nonobstetric) N94.89
traumatic S30.202 ☑
male N50.1
traumatic S30.201 ☑
internal organs — *see* Injury, by site
intracerebral, traumatic — *see* Injury, intracranial, intracerebral hemorrhage
intraoperative — *see* Complications, intraoperative, hemorrhage
labia (nontraumatic) (nonobstetric) N90.89
liver (subcapsular) (nontraumatic) K76.89
birth injury P15.0
mediastinum — *see* Injury, intrathoracic
mesosalpinx (nontraumatic) N83.7
traumatic S37.898 ☑
muscle — code by site under Contusion
nontraumatic
muscle M79.81
soft tissue M79.81
obstetrical surgical wound O90.2
orbit, orbital (nontraumatic) — *see also* Hemorrhage, orbit
traumatic — *see* Contusion, orbit

Hematoma — *continued*
pelvis (female) (nontraumatic) (nonobstetric) N94.89
obstetric O71.7
traumatic — *see* Injury, by site
penis (nontraumatic) N48.89
birth injury P15.5
perianal (nontraumatic) K64.5
perineal S30.23 ☑
complicating delivery O71.7
perirenal — *see* Injury, kidney
pinna — *see* Contusion, ear
nontraumatic — *see* Disorder, pinna, hematoma
placenta O43.89- ☑
postoperative (postprocedural) — *see* Complication, postprocedural, hematoma
retroperitoneal (nontraumatic) K66.1
traumatic S36.892 ☑
scrotum, superficial S30.22 ☑
birth injury P15.5
seminal vesicle (nontraumatic) N50.1
traumatic S37.892 ☑
spermatic cord (traumatic) S37.892 ☑
nontraumatic N50.1
spinal (cord) (meninges) — *see also* Injury, spinal cord, by region
newborn (birth injury) P11.5
spleen D73.5
intraoperative — *see* Complications, intraoperative, hemorrhage, spleen
postprocedural (postoperative) — *see* Complications, postprocedural, hemorrhage, spleen
sternocleidomastoid, birth injury P15.2
sternomastoid, birth injury P15.2
subarachnoid (traumatic) — *see* Injury, intracranial, subarachnoid hemorrhage
newborn (nontraumatic) P52.5
due to birth injury P10.3
nontraumatic — *see* Hemorrhage, intracranial, subarachnoid
subdural (traumatic) — *see* Injury, intracranial, subdural hemorrhage
newborn (localized) P52.8
birth injury P10.0
nontraumatic — *see* Hemorrhage, intracranial, subdural
superficial, newborn P54.5
testis (nontraumatic) N50.1
birth injury P15.5
tunica vaginalis (nontraumatic) N50.1
umbilical cord, complicating delivery O69.5 ☑
uterine ligament (broad) (nontraumatic) N83.7
traumatic S37.892 ☑
vagina (ruptured) (nontraumatic) N89.8
complicating delivery O71.7
vas deferens (nontraumatic) N50.1
traumatic S37.892 ☑
vitreous — *see* Hemorrhage, vitreous
vulva (nontraumatic) (nonobstetric) N90.89
complicating delivery O71.7
newborn (birth injury) P15.5
Hematometra N85.7
with hematocolpos N89.7
Hematomyelia (central) G95.19
newborn (birth injury) P11.5
traumatic T14.8 ☑
Hematomyelitis G04.90
Hematoperitoneum — *see* Hemoperitoneum
Hematophobia F40.230
Hematopneumothorax (see Hemothorax)
Hematopoiesis, cyclic D70.4
Hematoporphyria — *see* Porphyria
Hematorachis, hematorrhachis G95.19
newborn (birth injury) P11.5
Hematosalpinx N83.6
with
hematocolpos N89.7
hematometra N85.7
with hematocolpos N89.7
infectional — *see* Salpingitis
Hematospermia R36.1
Hematothorax (see Hemothorax)
Hematuria R31.9
benign (familial) (of childhood) — *see also* Hematuria, idiopathic
essential microscopic R31.1
due to sulphonamide, sulfonamide — *see* Table of Drugs and Chemicals, by drug

Hematuria — *continued*
endemic — *see also* Schistosomiasis B65.0
gross R31.0
idiopathic N02.9
with glomerular lesion
C3
glomerulonephritis N02.A
glomerulopathy N02.A
with dense deposit disease N02.6
crescentic (diffuse) glomerulonephritis N02.7
dense deposit disease N02.6
endocapillary proliferative glomerulonephritis N02.4
focal and segmental hyalinosis or sclerosis N02.1
membranoproliferative (diffuse) N02.5
membranous (diffuse) N02.2
mesangial proliferative (diffuse) N02.3
mesangiocapillary (diffuse) N02.5
minor abnormality N02.0
proliferative NEC N02.8
specified pathology NEC N02.8
intermittent — *see* Hematuria, idiopathic
malarial B50.8
microscopic NEC (with symptoms) R31.29
asymptomatic R31.21
benign essential R31.1
paroxysmal — *see also* Hematuria, idiopathic
nocturnal D59.5
persistent — *see* Hematuria, idiopathic
recurrent — *see* Hematuria, idiopathic
tropical — *see also* Schistosomiasis B65.0
tuberculous A18.13
Hemeralopia (day blindness) H53.11
vitamin A deficiency E50.5
Hemi-akinesia R41.4
Hemianalgesia R20.0
Hemianencephaly Q00.0
Hemianesthesia R20.0
Hemianopia, hemianopsia (heteronymous) H53.47
homonymous H53.46- ☑
syphilitic A52.71
Hemiathetosis R25.8
Hemiatrophy R68.89
cerebellar G31.9
face, facial, progressive (Romberg) G51.8
tongue K14.8
Hemiballism (us) G25.5
Hemicardia Q24.8
Hemicephalus, hemicephaly Q00.0
Hemichorea G25.5
Hemicolitis, left — *see* Colitis, left sided
Hemicrania
congenital malformation Q00.0
continua G44.51
meaning migraine — *see also* Migraine G43.909
paroxysmal G44.039
chronic G44.049
intractable G44.041
not intractable G44.049
episodic G44.039
intractable G44.031
not intractable G44.039
intractable G44.031
not intractable G44.039
Hemidystrophy — *see* Hemiatrophy
Hemiectromelia Q73.8
Hemihypalgesia R20.8
Hemihypesthesia R20.1
Hemi-inattention R41.4
Hemimelia Q73.8
lower limb — *see* Defect, reduction, lower limb, specified type NEC
upper limb — *see* Defect, reduction, upper limb, specified type NEC
Hemiparalysis — *see* Hemiplegia
Hemiparesis — *see* Hemiplegia
Hemiparesthesia R20.2
Hemiparkinsonism G20
Hemiplegia G81.9- ☑
alternans facialis G83.89
ascending NEC G81.90
spinal G95.89
congenital (cerebral) G80.8
spastic G80.2
embolic (current episode) I63.4- ☑
flaccid G81.0- ☑
following
cerebrovascular disease I69.959

- **Hemiplegia** — *continued*
  - following — *continued*
    - cerebrovascular disease — *continued*
      - cerebral infarction I69.35- ☑
      - intracerebral hemorrhage I69.15- ☑
      - nontraumatic intracranial hemorrhage NEC I69.25- ☑
      - specified disease NEC I69.85- ☑
      - stroke NOS I69.35- ☑
      - subarachnoid hemorrhage I69.Ø5- ☑
  - hysterical F44.4
  - newborn NEC P91.88
    - birth injury P11.9
  - spastic G81.1- ☑
    - congenital G8Ø.2
  - thrombotic (current episode) I63.3- ☑
- **Hemisection, spinal cord** — *see* Injury, spinal cord, by region
- **Hemispasm** (facial) R25.2
- **Hemisporosis** B48.8
- **Hemitremor** R25.1
- **Hemivertebra** Q76.49
  - failure of segmentation with scoliosis Q76.3
  - fusion with scoliosis Q76.3
- **Hemochromatosis** E83.119
  - with refractory anemia D46.1
  - due to repeated red blood cell transfusion E83.111
  - hereditary (primary) E83.11Ø
  - neonatal P78.84
  - primary E83.11Ø
  - specified NEC E83.118
- **Hemoglobin** — *see also* condition
  - abnormal (disease) — *see* Disease, hemoglobin
  - AS genotype D57.3
  - Constant Spring D58.2
  - E-beta thalassemia D56.5
  - fetal, hereditary persistence (HPFH) D56.4
  - H Constant Spring D56.Ø
  - low NOS D64.9
  - S (Hb S), heterozygous D57.3
- **Hemoglobinemia** D59.9
  - due to blood transfusion T8Ø.89 ☑
  - paroxysmal D59.6
    - nocturnal D59.5
- **Hemoglobinopathy** (mixed) D58.2
  - with thalassemia D56.8
  - sickle-cell D57.1
    - with thalassemia D57.4Ø
    - with
      - acute chest syndrome D57.411
      - cerebral vascular involvement D57.413
      - crisis (painful) D57.419
        - with specified complication NEC D57.418
      - splenic sequestration D57.412
      - vasoocclusive pain D57.419
    - without crisis D57.4Ø
- **Hemoglobinuria** R82.3
  - with anemia, hemolytic, acquired (chronic) NEC D59.6
  - cold (paroxysmal) (with Raynaud's syndrome) D59.6
    - agglutinin D59.12
  - due to exertion or hemolysis NEC D59.6
  - intermittent D59.6
  - malarial B5Ø.8
  - march D59.6
  - nocturnal (paroxysmal) D59.5
  - paroxysmal (cold) D59.6
    - nocturnal D59.5
- **Hemolymphangioma** D18.1
- **Hemolysis**
  - intravascular
    - with
      - abortion — *see* Abortion, by type, complicated by, hemorrhage
      - ectopic or molar pregnancy OØ8.1
      - hemorrhage
        - antepartum — *see* Hemorrhage, antepartum, with coagulation defect
        - intrapartum — *see also* Hemorrhage, complicating, delivery O67.Ø
    - postpartum O72.3
  - neonatal (excessive) P58.9
    - specified NEC P58.8
- **Hemolytic** — *see* condition
- **Hemopericardium** I31.2
  - following acute myocardial infarction (current complication) I23.Ø
  - newborn P54.8
  - traumatic — *see* Injury, heart, with hemopericardium
- **Hemoperitoneum** K66.1
  - infectional K65.9
  - traumatic S36.899 ☑
    - with open wound — *see* Wound, open, with penetration into peritoneal cavity
- **Hemophilia** (classical) (familial) (hereditary) D66
  - A D66
  - acquired D68.311
  - autoimmune D68.311
  - B D67
  - C D68.1
  - calcipriva — *see also* Defect, coagulation D68.4
  - nonfamilial — *see also* Defect, coagulation D68.4
  - secondary D68.311
  - vascular — *see* Disease, von Willebrand
- **Hemophthalmos** H44.81- ☑
- **Hemopneumothorax** — *see also* Hemothorax
  - traumatic S27.2 ☑
- **Hemoptysis** RØ4.2
  - newborn P26.9
  - tuberculous — *see* Tuberculosis, pulmonary
- **Hemorrhage, hemorrhagic** (concealed) R58
  - abdomen R58
  - accidental antepartum — *see* Hemorrhage, antepartum
  - acute idiopathic pulmonary, in infants RØ4.81
  - adenoid J35.8
  - adrenal (capsule) (gland) E27.49
    - medulla E27.8
    - newborn P54.4
  - after delivery — *see* Hemorrhage, postpartum
  - alveolar
    - lung, newborn P26.8
    - process KØ8.89
  - alveolus KØ8.89
  - amputation stump (surgical) T87.89
  - anemia (chronic) D5Ø.Ø
    - acute D62
  - antepartum (with) O46.9Ø
    - with coagulation defect O46.ØØ- ☑
      - afibrinogenemia O46.Ø1- ☑
      - disseminated intravascular coagulation O46.Ø2- ☑
      - hypofibrinogenemia O46.Ø1- ☑
      - specified defect NEC O46.Ø9- ☑
    - before 2Ø weeks gestation O2Ø.9
      - specified type NEC O2Ø.8
      - threatened abortion O2Ø.Ø
    - due to
      - abruptio placenta — *see also* Abruptio placentae O45.9- ☑
      - leiomyoma, uterus — *see* Hemorrhage, antepartum, specified cause NEC
      - placenta previa O44.1- ☑
    - specified cause NEC — *see* subcategory O46.8X- ☑
  - anus (sphincter) K62.5
  - apoplexy (stroke) — *see* Hemorrhage, intracranial, intracerebral
  - arachnoid — *see* Hemorrhage, intracranial, subarachnoid
  - artery R58
    - brain — *see* Hemorrhage, intracranial, intracerebral
  - basilar (ganglion) I61.Ø
  - bladder N32.89
  - bowel K92.2
    - newborn P54.3
  - brain (miliary) (nontraumatic) — *see* Hemorrhage, intracranial, intracerebral
    - due to
      - birth injury P1Ø.1
      - syphilis A52.Ø5
    - epidural or extradural (traumatic) — *see* Injury, intracranial, epidural hemorrhage
    - newborn P52.4
      - birth injury P1Ø.1
    - subarachnoid — *see* Hemorrhage, intracranial, subarachnoid
    - subdural — *see* Hemorrhage, intracranial, subdural
  - brainstem (nontraumatic) I61.3
    - traumatic SØ6.38- ☑
  - breast N64.59
  - bronchial tube — *see* Hemorrhage, lung
  - bronchopulmonary — *see* Hemorrhage, lung
  - bronchus — *see* Hemorrhage, lung
  - bulbar I61.5
  - capillary I78.8
    - primary D69.8
  - cecum K92.2
- **Hemorrhage, hemorrhagic** — *continued*
  - cerebellar, cerebellum (nontraumatic) I61.4
    - newborn P52.6
    - traumatic SØ6.37- ☑
  - cerebral, cerebrum — *see also* Hemorrhage, intracranial, intracerebral
    - lobe I61.1
    - newborn (anoxic) P52.4
      - birth injury P1Ø.1
  - cerebromeningeal I61.8
  - cerebrospinal — *see* Hemorrhage, intracranial, intracerebral
  - cervix (uteri) (stump) NEC N88.8
  - chamber, anterior (eye) — *see* Hyphema
  - childbirth — *see* Hemorrhage, complicating, delivery
  - choroid H31.3Ø- ☑
    - expulsive H31.31- ☑
  - ciliary body — *see* Hyphema
  - cochlea — *see* subcategory H83.8 ☑
  - colon K92.2
  - complicating
    - abortion — *see* Abortion, by type, complicated by, hemorrhage
    - delivery O67.9
      - associated with coagulation defect (afibrinogenemia) (DIC) (hyperfibrinolysis) O67.Ø
      - specified cause NEC O67.8
    - surgical procedure — *see* Hemorrhage, intraoperative
  - conjunctiva H11.3- ☑
    - newborn P54.8
  - cord, newborn (stump) P51.9
  - corpus luteum (ruptured) cyst N83.1- ☑
  - cortical (brain) I61.1
  - cranial — *see* Hemorrhage, intracranial
  - cutaneous R23.3
    - due to autosensitivity, erythrocyte D69.2
    - newborn P54.5
  - delayed
    - following ectopic or molar pregnancy OØ8.1
    - postpartum O72.2
  - diathesis (familial) D69.9
  - disease D69.9
    - newborn P53
    - specified type NEC D69.8
  - due to or associated with
    - afibrinogenemia or other coagulation defect (conditions in categories D65- D69)
      - antepartum — *see* Hemorrhage, antepartum, with coagulation defect
      - intrapartum O67.Ø
    - dental implant M27.61
    - device, implant or graft — *see also* Complications, by site and type, specified NEC T85.838 ☑
      - arterial graft NEC T82.838 ☑
      - breast T85.838 ☑
      - catheter NEC T85.838 ☑
        - dialysis (renal) T82.838 ☑
          - intraperitoneal T85.838 ☑
        - infusion NEC T82.838 ☑
          - spinal (epidural) (subdural) T85.83Ø ☑
        - urinary (indwelling) T83.83 ☑
      - electronic (electrode) (pulse generator) (stimulator)
        - bone T84.83 ☑
        - cardiac T82.837 ☑
        - nervous system (brain) (peripheral nerve) (spinal) T85.83Ø ☑
        - urinary T83.83 ☑
      - fixation, internal (orthopedic) NEC T84.83 ☑
      - gastrointestinal (bile duct) (esophagus) T85.838 ☑
      - genital NEC T83.83 ☑
      - heart NEC T82.837 ☑
      - joint prosthesis T84.83 ☑
      - ocular (corneal graft) (orbital implant) NEC T85.838 ☑
      - orthopedic NEC T84.83 ☑
        - bone graft T86.838
      - specified NEC T85.838 ☑
      - urinary NEC T83.83 ☑
      - vascular NEC T82.838 ☑
      - ventricular intracranial shunt T85.83Ø ☑
  - duodenum, duodenal K92.2
    - ulcer — *see* Ulcer, duodenum, with hemorrhage
  - dura mater — *see* Hemorrhage, intracranial, subdural
  - endotracheal — *see* Hemorrhage, lung

Hemorrhage, hemorrhagic — *continued*
- epicranial subaponeurotic (massive), birth injury P12.2
- epidural (traumatic) — *see also* Injury, intracranial, epidural hemorrhage
  - nontraumatic I62.1
- esophagus K22.89
  - varix I85.Ø1
    - secondary I85.11
- excessive, following ectopic gestation (subsequent episode) OØ8.1
- extradural (traumatic) — *see* Injury, intracranial, epidural hemorrhage
  - birth injury P1Ø.8
  - newborn (anoxic) (nontraumatic) P52.8
  - nontraumatic I62.1
- eye NEC H57.89
  - fundus — *see* Hemorrhage, retina
  - lid — *see* Disorder, eyelid, specified type NEC
- fallopian tube N83.6
- fibrinogenolysis — *see* Fibrinolysis
- fibrinolytic (acquired) — *see* Fibrinolysis
- from
  - ear (nontraumatic) — *see* Otorrhagia
  - tracheostomy stoma J95.Ø1
- fundus, eye — *see* Hemorrhage, retina
- funis — *see* Hemorrhage, umbilicus, cord
- gastric — *see* Hemorrhage, stomach
- gastroenteric K92.2
  - newborn P54.3
- gastrointestinal (tract) K92.2
  - newborn P54.3
- genital organ, male N5Ø.1
- genitourinary (tract) NOS R31.9
- gingiva KØ6.8
- globe (eye) — *see* Hemophthalmos
- graafian follicle cyst (ruptured) N83.Ø- ☑
- gum KØ6.8
- heart I51.89
- hypopharyngeal (throat) RØ4.1
- intermenstrual (regular) N92.3
  - irregular N92.1
- internal (organs) NEC R58
  - capsule I61.Ø
  - ear — *see* subcategory H83.8 ☑
  - newborn P54.8
- intestine K92.2
  - newborn P54.3
- intra-abdominal R58
- intra-alveolar (lung), newborn P26.8
- intracerebral (nontraumatic) — *see* Hemorrhage, intracranial, intracerebral
- intracranial (nontraumatic) I62.9
  - birth injury P1Ø.9
  - epidural, nontraumatic I62.1
  - extradural, nontraumatic I62.1
  - intracerebral (nontraumatic) (in) I61.9
    - brain stem I61.3
    - cerebellum I61.4
    - hemisphere I61.2
      - cortical (superficial) I61.1
      - subcortical (deep) I61.Ø
    - intraoperative
      - during a nervous system procedure G97.31
      - during other procedure G97.32
    - intraventricular I61.5
    - multiple localized I61.6
    - newborn P52.4
      - birth injury P1Ø.1
    - postprocedural
      - following a nervous system procedure G97.51
      - following other procedure G97.52
    - specified NEC I61.8
    - superficial I61.1
    - traumatic (diffuse) — *see* Injury, intracranial, diffuse
      - focal — *see* Injury, intracranial, focal
  - newborn P52.9
    - specified NEC P52.8
  - subarachnoid (nontraumatic) (from) I6Ø.9
    - intracranial (cerebral) artery I6Ø.7
      - anterior communicating I6Ø.2
      - basilar I6Ø.4
      - carotid siphon and bifurcation I6Ø.Ø- ☑
      - communicating I6Ø.7
        - anterior I6Ø.2
        - posterior I6Ø.3- ☑
      - middle cerebral I6Ø.1- ☑
      - posterior communicating I6Ø.3- ☑

Hemorrhage, hemorrhagic — *continued*
- intracranial — *continued*
  - subarachnoid — *continued*
    - intracranial artery — *continued*
      - specified artery NEC I6Ø.6
      - vertebral I6Ø.5- ☑
    - newborn P52.5
      - birth injury P1Ø.3
    - specified NEC I6Ø.8
    - traumatic SØ6.6X- ☑
  - subdural (nontraumatic) I62.ØØ
    - acute I62.Ø1
    - birth injury P1Ø.Ø
    - chronic I62.Ø3
    - newborn (anoxic) (hypoxic) P52.8
      - birth injury P1Ø.Ø
    - spinal G95.19
    - subacute I62.Ø2
    - traumatic — *see* Injury, intracranial, subdural hemorrhage
  - traumatic — *see* Injury, intracranial, focal brain injury
- intramedullary NEC G95.19
- intraocular — *see* Hemophthalmos
- intraoperative, intraprocedural — *see* Complication, hemorrhage (hematoma), intraoperative (intraprocedural), by site
- intrapartum — *see* Hemorrhage, complicating, delivery
- intrapelvic
  - female N94.89
  - male K66.1
- intraperitoneal K66.1
- intrapontine I61.3
- intraprocedural — *see* Complication, hemorrhage (hematoma), intraoperative (intraprocedural), by site
- intrauterine N85.7
  - complicating delivery — *see also* Hemorrhage, complicating, delivery O67.9
  - postpartum — *see* Hemorrhage, postpartum
- intraventricular I61.5
  - newborn (nontraumatic) — *see also* Newborn, affected by, hemorrhage P52.3
    - due to birth injury P1Ø.2
    - grade
      - 1 P52.Ø
      - 2 P52.1
      - 3 P52.21
      - 4 P52.22
- intravesical N32.89
- iris (postinfectional) (postinflammatory) (toxic) — *see* Hyphema
- joint (nontraumatic) — *see* Hemarthrosis
- kidney N28.89
- knee (joint) (nontraumatic) — *see* Hemarthrosis, knee
- labyrinth — *see* subcategory H83.8 ☑
- lenticular striate artery I61.Ø
- ligature, vessel — *see* Hemorrhage, postoperative
- liver K76.89
- lung RØ4.89
  - newborn P26.9
    - massive P26.1
    - specified NEC P26.8
  - tuberculous — *see* Tuberculosis, pulmonary
- massive umbilical, newborn P51.Ø
- mediastinum — *see* Hemorrhage, lung
- medulla I61.3
- membrane (brain) I6Ø.8
  - spinal cord — *see* Hemorrhage, spinal cord
- meninges, meningeal (brain) (middle) I6Ø.8
  - spinal cord — *see* Hemorrhage, spinal cord
- mesentery K66.1
- metritis — *see* Endometritis
- mouth K13.79
- mucous membrane NEC R58
  - newborn P54.8
- muscle M62.89
- nail (subungual) L6Ø.8
- nasal turbinate RØ4.Ø
  - newborn P54.8
- navel, newborn P51.9
- newborn P54.9
  - specified NEC P54.8
- nipple N64.59
- nose RØ4.Ø
  - newborn P54.8
- omentum K66.1
- optic nerve (sheath) H47.Ø2- ☑

Hemorrhage, hemorrhagic — *continued*
- orbit, orbital HØ5.23- ☑
- ovary NEC N83.8
- oviduct N83.6
- pancreas K86.89
- parathyroid (gland) (spontaneous) E21.4
- parturition — *see* Hemorrhage, complicating, delivery
- penis N48.89
- pericardium, pericarditis I31.2
- peritoneum, peritoneal K66.1
- peritonsillar tissue J35.8
  - due to infection J36
- petechial R23.3
  - due to autosensitivity, erythrocyte D69.2
- pituitary (gland) E23.6
- pleura — *see* Hemorrhage, lung
- polioencephalitis, superior E51.2
- polymyositis — *see* Polymyositis
- pons, pontine I61.3
- posterior fossa (nontraumatic) I61.8
  - newborn P52.6
- postmenopausal N95.Ø
- postnasal RØ4.Ø
- postoperative — *see* Complications, postprocedural, hemorrhage, by site
- postpartum NEC (following delivery of placenta) O72.1
  - delayed or secondary O72.2
  - retained placenta O72.Ø
  - third stage O72.Ø
- pregnancy — *see* Hemorrhage, antepartum
- preretinal — *see* Hemorrhage, retina
- prostate N42.1
- puerperal — *see* Hemorrhage, postpartum
  - delayed or secondary O72.2
- pulmonary RØ4.89
  - newborn P26.9
    - massive P26.1
    - specified NEC P26.8
  - tuberculous — *see* Tuberculosis, pulmonary
- purpura (primary) D69.3
- rectum (sphincter) K62.5
  - newborn P54.2
- recurring, following initial hemorrhage at time of injury T79.2 ☑
- renal N28.89
- respiratory passage or tract RØ4.9
  - specified NEC RØ4.89
- retina, retinal (vessels) H35.6- ☑
  - diabetic — *see* Microaneurysm, retinal, diabetic
- retroperitoneal R58
- scalp R58
- scrotum N5Ø.1
- secondary (nontraumatic) R58
  - following initial hemorrhage at time of injury T79.2 ☑
- seminal vesicle N5Ø.1
- skin R23.3
  - newborn P54.5
- slipped umbilical ligature P51.8
- spermatic cord N5Ø.1
- spinal (cord) G95.19
  - newborn (birth injury) P11.5
- spleen D73.5
  - intraoperative — *see* Complications, intraoperative, hemorrhage, spleen
  - postprocedural — *see* Complications, postprocedural, hemorrhage, spleen
- stomach K92.2
  - newborn P54.3
  - ulcer — *see* Ulcer, stomach, with hemorrhage
- subarachnoid (nontraumatic) — *see* Hemorrhage, intracranial, subarachnoid
- subconjunctival — *see also* Hemorrhage, conjunctiva
  - birth injury P15.3
- subcortical (brain) I61.Ø
- subcutaneous R23.3
- subdiaphragmatic R58
- subdural (acute) (nontraumatic) — *see* Hemorrhage, intracranial, subdural
- subependymal
  - newborn P52.Ø
    - with intraventricular extension P52.1
      - and intracerebral extension P52.22
- subgaleal P12.2
- subhyaloid — *see* Hemorrhage, retina
- subperiosteal — *see* Disorder, bone, specified type NEC
- subretinal — *see* Hemorrhage, retina
- subtentorial — *see* Hemorrhage, intracranial, subdural

Index

Hemorrhage, hemorrhagic — Hemorrhage, hemorrhagic

Hemorrhage, hemorrhagic — *continued*
- subungual L6Ø.8
- suprarenal (capsule) (gland) E27.49
  - newborn P54.4
- tentorium (traumatic) NEC — *see* Hemorrhage, brain
  - newborn (birth injury) P1Ø.4
- testis N5Ø.1
- third stage (postpartum) O72.Ø
- thorax — *see* Hemorrhage, lung
- throat RØ4.1
- thymus (gland) E32.8
- thyroid (cyst) (gland) EØ7.89
- tongue K14.8
- tonsil J35.8
- trachea — *see* Hemorrhage, lung
- tracheobronchial RØ4.89
  - newborn P26.Ø
- traumatic — *code to* specific injury
  - cerebellar — *see* Hemorrhage, brain
  - intracranial — *see* Hemorrhage, brain
  - recurring or secondary (following initial hemorrhage at time of injury) T79.2 ☑
- tuberculous NEC — *see also* Tuberculosis, pulmonary A15.Ø
- tunica vaginalis N5Ø.1
- ulcer — *code by* site under Ulcer, with hemorrhage K27.4
- umbilicus, umbilical
  - cord
    - after birth, newborn P51.9
    - complicating delivery O69.5 ☑
  - newborn P51.9
    - massive P51.Ø
    - slipped ligature P51.8
  - stump P51.9
- urethra (idiopathic) N36.8
- uterus, uterine (abnormal) N93.9
  - climacteric N92.4
  - complicating delivery — *see* Hemorrhage, complicating, delivery
  - dysfunctional or functional N93.8
  - intermenstrual (regular) N92.3
    - irregular N92.1
  - postmenopausal N95.Ø
  - postpartum — *see* Hemorrhage, postpartum
  - preclimacteric or premenopausal N92.4
  - prepubertal N93.8
  - pubertal N92.2
- vagina (abnormal) N93.9
  - newborn P54.6
- vas deferens N5Ø.1
- vasa previa O69.4 ☑
- ventricular I61.5
- vesical N32.89
- viscera NEC R58
  - newborn P54.8
- vitreous (humor) (intraocular) H43.1- ☑
- vulva N9Ø.89

Hemorrhoids (bleeding) (without mention of degree) K64.9
- 1st degree (grade/stage I) (without prolapse outside of anal canal) K64.Ø
- 2nd degree (grade/stage II) (that prolapse with straining but retract spontaneously) K64.1
- 3rd degree (grade/stage III) (that prolapse with straining and require manual replacement back inside anal canal) K64.2
- 4th degree (grade/stage IV) (with prolapsed tissue that cannot be manually replaced) K64.3
- complicating
  - pregnancy O22.4 ☑
  - puerperium O87.2
- external K64.4
  - with
    - thrombosis K64.5
- internal (without mention of degree) K64.8
- prolapsed K64.8
- skin tags
  - anus K64.4
  - residual K64.4
- specified NEC K64.8
- strangulated — *see also* Hemorrhoids, by degree K64.8
- thrombosed — *see also* Hemorrhoids, by degree K64.5
- ulcerated — *see also* Hemorrhoids, by degree K64.8

Hemosalpinx N83.6
- with
  - hematocolpos N89.7
  - hematometra N85.7

Hemosalpinx — *continued*
- with — *continued*
  - hematometra — *continued*
    - with hematocolpos N89.7

Hemosiderosis (dietary) E83.19
- pulmonary, idiopathic E83.1- ☑ *[J84.Ø3]*
- transfusion T8Ø.89 ☑

Hemothorax (bacterial) (nontuberculous) J94.2
- newborn P54.8
- traumatic S27.1 ☑
  - with pneumothorax S27.2 ☑
- tuberculous NEC A15.6

Henoch (-Schönlein) **disease or syndrome** (purpura) D69.Ø

Henpue, henpuye A66.6

Hepar lobatum (syphilitic) A52.74

Hepatalgia K76.89

Hepatitis K75.9
- acute B17.9
  - with coma K72.Ø1
  - with hepatic failure — *see* Failure, hepatic
  - alcoholic — *see* Hepatitis, alcoholic
  - infectious B17.9
  - non-viral K72.Ø ☑
  - viral B17.9
- alcoholic (acute) (chronic) K7Ø.1Ø
  - with ascites K7Ø.11
- amebic — *see* Abscess, liver, amebic
- anicteric, (viral) — *see* Hepatitis, viral
- antigen-associated (HAA) — *see* Hepatitis, B
- Australia-antigen (positive) — *see* Hepatitis, B
- autoimmune K75.4
- B B19.1Ø
  - with hepatic coma B19.11
  - acute B16.9
    - with
      - delta-agent (coinfection) (without hepatic coma) B16.1
        - with hepatic coma B16.Ø
      - hepatic coma (without delta-agent coinfection) B16.2
  - chronic B18.1
    - with delta-agent B18.Ø
- bacterial NEC K75.89
- C (viral) B19.2Ø
  - with hepatic coma B19.21
  - acute B17.1Ø
    - with hepatic coma B17.11
  - chronic B18.2
- catarrhal (acute) B15.9
  - with hepatic coma B15.Ø
- cholangiolitic K75.89
- cholestatic K75.89
- chronic K73.9
  - active NEC K73.2
  - lobular NEC K73.1
  - persistent NEC K73.Ø
  - specified NEC K73.8
- cytomegaloviral B25.1
- due to ethanol (acute) (chronic) — *see* Hepatitis, alcoholic
- epidemic B15.9
  - with hepatic coma B15.Ø
- fulminant NEC (viral) — *see* Hepatitis, viral
- granulomatous NEC K75.3
- herpesviral BØØ.81
- history of
  - B Z86.19
  - C Z86.19
- homologous serum — *see* Hepatitis, viral, type B
- in (due to)
  - mumps B26.81
  - toxoplasmosis (acquired) B58.1
    - congenital (active) P37.1 *[K77]*
- infectious, infective B15.9
  - acute (subacute) B17.9
  - chronic B18.9
- inoculation — *see* Hepatitis, viral, type B
- interstitial (chronic) K74.69
- ischemia, ischemic K72.ØØ
- lupoid NEC K75.4
- malignant NEC (with hepatic failure) K72.9Ø
  - with coma K72.91
- neonatal (idiopathic) (toxic) P59.29
- neonatal giant cell P59.29
- newborn P59.29
- non-viral K72.Ø ☑
- postimmunization — *see* Hepatitis, viral, type B

Hepatitis — *continued*
- post-transfusion — *see* Hepatitis, viral, type B
- reactive, nonspecific K75.2
- serum — *see* Hepatitis, viral, type B
- shock K72.ØØ
- specified type NEC
  - with hepatic failure — *see* Failure, hepatic
- syphilitic (late) A52.74
  - congenital (early) A5Ø.Ø8 *[K77]*
    - late A5Ø.59 *[K77]*
  - secondary A51.45
- toxic — *see also* Disease, liver, toxic K71.6
- tuberculous A18.83
- viral, virus B19.9
  - with hepatic coma B19.Ø
  - acute B17.9
  - chronic B18.9
    - specified NEC B18.8
    - type
      - B B18.1
        - with delta-agent B18.Ø
      - C B18.2
  - congenital P35.3
  - coxsackie B33.8 *[K77]*
  - cytomegalic inclusion B25.1
  - in remission, any type — *code to* Hepatitis, chronic, by type
  - non-A, non-B B17.8
  - specified type NEC (with or without coma) B17.8
  - type
    - A B15.9
      - with hepatic coma B15.Ø
    - B B19.1Ø
      - with hepatic coma B19.11
      - acute B16.9
        - with
          - delta-agent (coinfection) (without hepatic coma) B16.1
            - with hepatic coma B16.Ø
          - hepatic coma (without delta-agent coinfection) B16.2
      - chronic B18.1
        - with delta-agent B18.Ø
    - C B19.2Ø
      - with hepatic coma B19.21
      - acute B17.1Ø
        - with hepatic coma B17.11
      - chronic B18.2
    - E B17.2
    - non-A, non-B B17.8

Hepatization lung (acute) — *see* Pneumonia, lobar

Hepatoblastoma C22.2

Hepatocarcinoma C22.Ø

Hepatocholangiocarcinoma C22.Ø

Hepatocholangioma, benign D13.4

Hepatocholangitis K75.89

Hepatolenticular degeneration E83.Ø1

Hepatoma (malignant) C22.Ø
- benign D13.4
- embryonal C22.Ø

Hepatomegaly — *see also* Hypertrophy, liver
- with splenomegaly R16.2
- congenital Q44.7
- in mononucleosis
  - gammaherpesviral B27.Ø9
  - infectious specified NEC B27.89

Hepatoptosis K76.89

Hepatorenal syndrome following labor and delivery O9Ø.4

Hepatosis K76.89

Hepatosplenomegaly R16.2
- hyperlipemic (Bürger-Grütz type) E78.3 *[K77]*

Hereditary — *see* condition

Hereditary alpha tryptasemia (syndrome) D89.44

Heredodegeneration, macular — *see* Dystrophy, retina

Heredopathia atactica polyneuritiformis G6Ø.1

Heredosyphilis — *see* Syphilis, congenital

Herlitz' syndrome Q81.1

Hermansky-Pudlak syndrome E7Ø.331

Hermaphrodite, hermaphroditism (true) Q56.Ø
- 46,XX with streak gonads Q99.1
- 46,XX/46,XY Q99.Ø
- 46,XY with streak gonads Q99.1
- chimera 46,XX/46,XY Q99.Ø

Hernia, hernial (acquired) (recurrent) K46.9
- with
  - gangrene — *see* Hernia, by site, with, gangrene
  - incarceration — *see* Hernia, by site, with, obstruction

- **Hernia, hernial** — *continued*
  - with — *continued*
    - irreducible — *see* Hernia, by site, with, obstruction
    - obstruction — *see* Hernia, by site, with, obstruction
    - strangulation — *see* Hernia, by site, with, obstruction
  - abdomen, abdominal K46.9
    - with
      - gangrene (and obstruction) K46.1
      - obstruction K46.Ø
    - femoral — *see* Hernia, femoral
    - incisional — *see* Hernia, incisional
    - inguinal — *see* Hernia, inguinal
    - specified site NEC K45.8
      - with
        - gangrene (and obstruction) K45.1
        - obstruction K45.Ø
    - umbilical — *see* Hernia, umbilical
    - wall — *see* Hernia, ventral
  - appendix — *see* Hernia, abdomen
  - bladder (mucosa) (sphincter)
    - congenital (female) (male) Q79.51
    - female — *see* Cystocele
    - male N32.89
  - brain, congenital — *see* Encephalocele
  - cartilage, vertebra — *see* Displacement, intervertebral disc
  - cerebral, congenital — *see also* Encephalocele
    - endaural QØ1.8
  - ciliary body (traumatic) SØ5.2- ☑
  - colon — *see* Hernia, abdomen
  - Cooper's — *see* Hernia, abdomen, specified site NEC
  - crural — *see* Hernia, femoral
  - diaphragm, diaphragmatic K44.9
    - with
      - gangrene (and obstruction) K44.1
      - obstruction K44.Ø
    - congenital Q79.Ø
  - direct (inguinal) — *see* Hernia, inguinal
  - diverticulum, intestine — *see* Hernia, abdomen
  - double (inguinal) — *see* Hernia, inguinal, bilateral
  - due to adhesions (with obstruction) K56.5Ø
  - epigastric — *see also* Hernia, ventral K43.9
  - esophageal hiatus — *see* Hernia, hiatal
  - external (inguinal) — *see* Hernia, inguinal
  - fallopian tube N83.4- ☑
  - fascia M62.89
  - femoral K41.9Ø
    - with
      - gangrene (and obstruction) K41.4Ø
        - not specified as recurrent K41.4Ø
        - recurrent K41.41
      - obstruction K41.3Ø
        - not specified as recurrent K41.3Ø
        - recurrent K41.31
    - not specified as recurrent K41.9Ø
    - recurrent K41.91
    - bilateral K41.2Ø
      - with
        - gangrene (and obstruction) K41.1Ø
          - not specified as recurrent K41.1Ø
          - recurrent K41.11
        - obstruction K41.ØØ
          - not specified as recurrent K41.ØØ
          - recurrent K41.Ø1
      - not specified as recurrent K41.2Ø
      - recurrent K41.21
    - unilateral K41.9Ø
      - with
        - gangrene (and obstruction) K41.4Ø
          - not specified as recurrent K41.4Ø
          - recurrent K41.41
        - obstruction K41.3Ø
          - not specified as recurrent K41.3Ø
          - recurrent K41.31
      - not specified as recurrent K41.9Ø
      - recurrent K41.91
  - foramen magnum G93.5
    - congenital QØ1.8
  - funicular (umbilical) — *see also* Hernia, umbilicus
    - spermatic (cord) — *see* Hernia, inguinal
  - gastrointestinal tract — *see* Hernia, abdomen
  - Hesselbach's — *see* Hernia, femoral, specified site NEC
  - hiatal (esophageal) (sliding) K44.9
    - with
      - gangrene (and obstruction) K44.1
      - obstruction K44.Ø
    - congenital Q4Ø.1

- **Hernia, hernial** — *continued*
  - hypogastric — *see* Hernia, ventral
  - incarcerated — *see also* Hernia, by site, with obstruction
    - with gangrene — *see* Hernia, by site, with gangrene
  - incisional K43.2
    - with
      - gangrene (and obstruction) K43.1
      - obstruction K43.Ø
  - indirect (inguinal) — *see* Hernia, inguinal
  - inguinal (direct) (external) (funicular) (indirect) (internal) (oblique) (scrotal) (sliding) K4Ø.9Ø
    - with
      - gangrene (and obstruction) K4Ø.4Ø
        - not specified as recurrent K4Ø.4Ø
        - recurrent K4Ø.41
      - obstruction K4Ø.3Ø
        - not specified as recurrent K4Ø.3Ø
        - recurrent K4Ø.31
    - not specified as recurrent K4Ø.9Ø
    - recurrent K4Ø.91
    - bilateral K4Ø.2Ø
      - with
        - gangrene (and obstruction) K4Ø.1Ø
          - not specified as recurrent K4Ø.1Ø
          - recurrent K4Ø.11
        - obstruction K4Ø.ØØ
          - not specified as recurrent K4Ø.ØØ
          - recurrent K4Ø.Ø1
      - not specified as recurrent K4Ø.2Ø
      - recurrent K4Ø.21
    - unilateral K4Ø.9Ø
      - with
        - gangrene (and obstruction) K4Ø.4Ø
          - not specified as recurrent K4Ø.4Ø
          - recurrent K4Ø.41
        - obstruction K4Ø.3Ø
          - not specified as recurrent K4Ø.3Ø
          - recurrent K4Ø.31
      - not specified as recurrent K4Ø.9Ø
      - recurrent K4Ø.91
  - internal — *see also* Hernia, abdomen
    - inguinal — *see* Hernia, inguinal
  - interstitial — *see* Hernia, abdomen
  - intervertebral cartilage or disc — *see* Displacement, intervertebral disc
  - intestine, intestinal — *see* Hernia, by site
  - intra-abdominal — *see* Hernia, abdomen
  - iris (traumatic) SØ5.2- ☑
  - irreducible — *see also* Hernia, by site, with obstruction
    - with gangrene — *see* Hernia, by site, with gangrene
  - ischiatic — *see* Hernia, abdomen, specified site NEC
  - ischiorectal — *see* Hernia, abdomen, specified site NEC
  - lens (traumatic) SØ5.2- ☑
  - linea (alba) (semilunaris) — *see* Hernia, ventral
  - Littre's — *see* Hernia, abdomen
  - lumbar — *see* Hernia, abdomen, specified site NEC
  - lung (subcutaneous) J98.4
  - mediastinum J98.59
  - mesenteric (internal) — *see* Hernia, abdomen
  - midline — *see* Hernia, ventral
  - muscle (sheath) M62.89
  - nucleus pulposus — *see* Displacement, intervertebral disc
  - oblique (inguinal) — *see* Hernia, inguinal
  - obstructive — *see also* Hernia, by site, with obstruction
    - with gangrene — *see* Hernia, by site, with gangrene
  - obturator — *see* Hernia, abdomen, specified site NEC
  - omental — *see* Hernia, abdomen
  - ovary N83.4- ☑
  - oviduct N83.4- ☑
  - paraesophageal — *see also* Hernia, diaphragm
    - congenital Q4Ø.1
  - parastomal K43.5
    - with
      - gangrene (and obstruction) K43.4
      - obstruction K43.3
  - paraumbilical — *see* Hernia, umbilicus
  - perineal — *see* Hernia, abdomen, specified site NEC
  - Petit's — *see* Hernia, abdomen, specified site NEC
  - postoperative — *see* Hernia, incisional
  - pregnant uterus — *see* Abnormal, uterus in pregnancy or childbirth
  - prevesical N32.89
  - properitoneal — *see* Hernia, abdomen, specified site NEC
  - pudendal — *see* Hernia, abdomen, specified site NEC
  - rectovaginal N81.6

- **Hernia, hernial** — *continued*
  - retroperitoneal — *see* Hernia, abdomen, specified site NEC
  - Richter's — *see* Hernia, abdomen, with obstruction
  - Rieux's, Riex's — *see* Hernia, abdomen, specified site NEC
  - sac condition (adhesion) (dropsy) (inflammation) (laceration) (suppuration) — *code by site under* Hernia
  - sciatic — *see* Hernia, abdomen, specified site NEC
  - scrotum, scrotal — *see* Hernia, inguinal
  - sliding (inguinal) — *see also* Hernia, inguinal
    - hiatus — *see* Hernia, hiatal
  - spigelian — *see* Hernia, ventral
  - spinal — *see* Spina bifida
  - strangulated — *see also* Hernia, by site, with obstruction
    - with gangrene — *see* Hernia, by site, with gangrene
  - subxiphoid — *see* Hernia, ventral
  - supra-umbilicus — *see* Hernia, ventral
  - tendon — *see* Disorder, tendon, specified type NEC
  - Treitz's (fossa) — *see* Hernia, abdomen, specified site NEC
  - tunica vaginalis Q55.29
  - umbilicus, umbilical K42.9
    - with
      - gangrene (and obstruction) K42.1
      - obstruction K42.Ø
  - ureter N28.89
  - urethra, congenital Q64.79
  - urinary meatus, congenital Q64.79
  - uterus N81.4
    - pregnant — *see* Abnormal, uterus in pregnancy or childbirth
  - vaginal (anterior) (wall) — *see* Cystocele
  - Velpeau's — *see* Hernia, femoral
  - ventral K43.9
    - with
      - gangrene (and obstruction) K43.7
      - obstruction K43.6
    - incisional K43.2
      - with
        - gangrene (and obstruction) K43.1
        - obstruction K43.Ø
    - recurrent — *see* Hernia, incisional
    - specified NEC K43.9
      - with
        - gangrene (and obstruction) K43.7
        - obstruction K43.6
  - vesical
    - congenital (female) (male) Q79.51
    - female — *see* Cystocele
    - male N32.89
  - vitreous (into wound) SØ5.2- ☑
    - into anterior chamber — *see* Prolapse, vitreous
- **Herniation** — *see also* Hernia
  - brain (stem) G93.5
    - nontraumatic G93.5
    - traumatic SØ6.A1 ☑
      - cerebellar SØ6.A1 ☑
      - subfalcine (cingulate) SØ6.A1 ☑
      - tonsillar SØ6.A1 ☑
      - transtentorial (central) (upward cerebellar) SØ6.A1 ☑
      - uncal SØ6.A1 ☑
  - cerebral G93.5
    - nontraumatic G93.5
    - traumatic SØ6.A1 ☑
  - mediastinum J98.59
  - nucleus pulposus — *see* Displacement, intervertebral disc
- **Herpangina** BØ8.5
- **Herpes, herpesvirus, herpetic** BØØ.9
  - anogenital A6Ø.9
    - perianal skin A6Ø.1
    - rectum A6Ø.1
    - urogenital tract A6Ø.ØØ
      - cervix A6Ø.Ø3
      - male genital organ NEC A6Ø.Ø2
      - penis A6Ø.Ø1
      - specified site NEC A6Ø.Ø9
      - vagina A6Ø.Ø4
      - vulva A6Ø.Ø4
  - blepharitis (zoster) BØ2.39
    - simplex BØØ.59
  - circinatus B35.4
    - bullosus L12.Ø
  - conjunctivitis (simplex) BØØ.53

- **Herpes, herpesvirus, herpetic** — *continued*
  - conjunctivitis — *continued*
    - zoster B02.31
  - cornea B02.33
  - encephalitis B00.4
    - due to herpesvirus 6 B10.01
    - due to herpesvirus 7 B10.09
    - specified NEC B10.09
  - eye (zoster) B02.30
    - simplex B00.50
  - eyelid (zoster) B02.39
    - simplex B00.59
  - facialis B00.1
  - febrilis B00.1
  - geniculate ganglionitis B02.21
  - genital, genitalis A60.00
    - female A60.09
    - male A60.02
  - gestational, gestationis O26.4- ☑
  - gingivostomatitis B00.2
  - human B00.9
    - 1 — *see* Herpes, simplex
    - 2 — *see* Herpes, simplex
    - 3 — *see* Varicella
    - 4 — *see* Mononucleosis, Epstein-Barr (virus)
    - 5 — *see* Disease, cytomegalic inclusion (generalized)
    - 6
      - encephalitis B10.01
      - specified NEC B10.81
    - 7
      - encephalitis B10.09
      - specified NEC B10.82
    - 8 B10.89
  - infection NEC B10.89
    - Kaposi's sarcoma associated B10.89
  - iridocyclitis (simplex) B00.51
    - zoster B02.32
  - iris (vesicular erythema multiforme) L51.9
  - iritis (simplex) B00.51
  - Kaposi's sarcoma associated B10.89
  - keratitis (simplex) (dendritic) (disciform) (interstitial) B00.52
    - zoster (interstitial) B02.33
  - keratoconjunctivitis (simplex) B00.52
    - zoster B02.33
  - labialis B00.1
  - lip B00.1
  - meningitis (simplex) B00.3
    - zoster B02.1
  - ophthalmicus (zoster) NEC B02.30
    - simplex B00.50
  - penis A60.01
  - perianal skin A60.1
  - pharyngitis, pharyngotonsillitis B00.2
  - rectum A60.1
  - scrotum A60.02
  - sepsis B00.7
  - simplex B00.9
    - complicated NEC B00.89
    - congenital P35.2
    - conjunctivitis B00.53
    - external ear B00.1
    - eyelid B00.59
    - hepatitis B00.81
    - keratitis (interstitial) B00.52
    - myleitis B00.82
    - specified complication NEC B00.89
    - visceral B00.89
  - stomatitis B00.2
  - tonsurans B35.0
  - visceral B00.89
  - vulva A60.04
  - whitlow B00.89
  - zoster — *see also* condition B02.9
    - auricularis B02.21
    - complicated NEC B02.8
    - conjunctivitis B02.31
    - disseminated B02.7
    - encephalitis B02.0
    - eye (lid) B02.39
    - geniculate ganglionitis B02.21
    - keratitis (interstitial) B02.33
    - meningitis B02.1
    - myelitis B02.24
    - neuritis, neuralgia B02.29
    - ophthalmicus NEC B02.30
    - oticus B02.21
    - polyneuropathy B02.23
- **Herpes, herpesvirus, herpetic** — *continued*
  - zoster — *see also* condition — *continued*
    - specified complication NEC B02.8
    - trigeminal neuralgia B02.22
- **Herpesvirus** (human) — *see* Herpes
- **Herpetophobia** F40.218
- **Herrick's anemia** — *see* Disease, sickle-cell
- **Hers' disease** E74.09
- **Herter-Gee syndrome** K90.0
- **Herxheimer's reaction** R68.89
- **Hesitancy**
  - of micturition R39.11
  - urinary R39.11
- **Hesselbach's hernia** — *see* Hernia, femoral, specified site NEC
- **Heterochromia** (congenital) Q13.2
  - cataract — *see* Cataract, complicated
  - cyclitis (Fuchs) — *see* Cyclitis, Fuchs' heterochromic
  - hair L67.1
  - iritis — *see* Cyclitis, Fuchs' heterochromic
  - retained metallic foreign body (nonmagnetic) — *see* Foreign body, intraocular, old, retained
    - magnetic — *see* Foreign body, intraocular, old, retained, magnetic
  - uveitis — *see* Cyclitis, Fuchs' heterochromic
- **Heterophoria** — *see* Strabismus, heterophoria
- **Heterophyes, heterophyiasis** (small intestine) B66.8
- **Heterotopia, heterotopic** — *see also* Malposition, congenital
  - cerebralis Q04.8
- **Heterotropia** — *see* Strabismus
- **Heubner-Herter disease** K90.0
- **Hexadactylism** Q69.9
- **HGSIL** (cytology finding) (high grade squamous intraepithelial lesion on cytologic smear) (Pap smear finding)
  - anus R85.613
  - cervix R87.613
    - biopsy (histology) finding — *see* Neoplasia, intraepithelial, cervix, grade II or grade III
  - vagina R87.623
    - biopsy (histology) finding — *see* Neoplasia, intraepithelial, cervix, grade II or grade III
- **Hibernoma** — *see* Lipoma
- **Hiccup, hiccough** R06.6
  - epidemic B33.0
  - psychogenic F45.8
- **Hidden penis** (congenital) Q55.64
  - acquired N48.83
- **Hidradenitis** (axillaris) (suppurative) L73.2
- **Hidradenoma** (nodular) — *see also* Neoplasm, skin, benign
  - clear cell — *see* Neoplasm, skin, benign
  - papillary — *see* Neoplasm, skin, benign
- **Hidrocystoma** — *see* Neoplasm, skin, benign
- **High**
  - altitude effects T70.20 ☑
    - anoxia T70.29 ☑
    - on
      - ears T70.0 ☑
      - sinuses T70.1 ☑
    - polycythemia D75.1
  - arch
    - foot Q66.7- ☑
    - palate, congenital Q38.5
  - arterial tension — *see* Hypertension
  - basal metabolic rate R94.8
  - blood pressure — *see also* Hypertension
    - borderline R03.0
    - reading (incidental) (isolated) (nonspecific), without diagnosis of hypertension R03.0
  - cholesterol E78.00
    - with high triglycerides E78.2
  - diaphragm (congenital) Q79.1
  - expressed emotional level within family Z63.8
  - head at term O32.4 ☑
  - palate, congenital Q38.5
  - risk
    - infant NEC Z76.2
    - sexual behavior (heterosexual) Z72.51
      - bisexual Z72.53
      - homosexual Z72.52
  - scrotal testis, testes
    - bilateral Q53.23
    - unilateral Q53.13
  - temperature (of unknown origin) R50.9
  - thoracic rib Q76.6
- **High** — *continued*
  - triglycerides E78.1
    - with high cholesterol E78.2
- **Hildenbrand's disease** A75.0
- **Hilum** — *see* condition
- **Hip** — *see* condition
- **Hippel's disease** Q85.83
- **Hippophobia** F40.218
- **Hippus** H57.09
- **Hirschsprung's disease or megacolon** Q43.1
- **Hirsutism, hirsuties** L68.0
- **Hirudiniasis**
  - external B88.3
  - internal B83.4
- **Hiss-Russell dysentery** A03.1
- **Histidinemia, histidinuria** E70.41
- **Histiocytoma** — *see also* Neoplasm, skin, benign
  - fibrous — *see also* Neoplasm, skin, benign
    - atypical — *see* Neoplasm, connective tissue, uncertain behavior
    - malignant — *see* Neoplasm, connective tissue, malignant
- **Histiocytosis** D76.3
  - acute differentiated progressive C96.0
  - Langerhans' cell NEC C96.6
    - multifocal X
      - multisystemic (disseminated) C96.0
      - unisystemic C96.5
    - pulmonary, adult (adult PLCH) J84.82
    - unifocal (X) C96.6
  - lipid, lipoid D76.3
    - essential E75.29
  - malignant C96.A (*following* C96.6)
  - mononuclear phagocytes NEC D76.1
    - Langerhans' cells C96.6
  - non-Langerhans cell D76.3
  - polyostotic sclerosing D76.3
  - sinus, with massive lymphadenopathy D76.3
  - syndrome NEC D76.3
  - X NEC C96.6
    - acute (progressive) C96.0
    - chronic C96.6
    - multifocal C96.5
    - multisystemic C96.0
    - unifocal C96.6
- **Histoplasmosis** B39.9
  - with pneumonia NEC B39.2
  - African B39.5
  - American — *see* Histoplasmosis, capsulati
  - capsulati B39.4
    - disseminated B39.3
    - generalized B39.3
    - pulmonary B39.2
      - acute B39.0
      - chronic B39.1
  - Darling's B39.4
  - duboisii B39.5
  - lung NEC B39.2
- **History**
  - family (of) — *see also* History, personal (of)
    - alcohol abuse Z81.1
    - allergy NEC Z84.89
    - anemia Z83.2
    - arthritis Z82.61
    - asthma Z82.5
    - blindness Z82.1
    - cardiac death (sudden) Z82.41
    - carrier of genetic disease Z84.81
    - chromosomal anomaly Z82.79
    - chronic
      - disabling disease NEC Z82.8
      - lower respiratory disease Z82.5
    - colonic polyps Z83.71
    - congenital malformations and deformations Z82.79
      - polycystic kidney Z82.71
    - consanguinity Z84.3
    - deafness Z82.2
    - diabetes mellitus Z83.3
    - disability NEC Z82.8
    - disease or disorder (of)
      - allergic NEC Z84.89
      - behavioral NEC Z81.8
      - blood and blood-forming organs Z83.2
      - cardiovascular NEC Z82.49
      - chronic disabling NEC Z82.8
      - digestive Z83.79
      - ear NEC Z83.52
      - elevated lipoprotein (a) (Lp(a)) Z83.430

History — *continued*
- family — *see also* History, personal — *continued*
  - disease or disorder — *continued*
    - endocrine NEC Z83.49
    - eye NEC Z83.518
      - glaucoma Z83.511
    - familial hypercholesterolemia Z83.42
    - genitourinary NEC Z84.2
    - glaucoma Z83.511
    - hematological Z83.2
    - immune mechanism Z83.2
    - infectious NEC Z83.1
    - ischemic heart Z82.49
    - kidney Z84.1
    - lipoprotein metabolism Z83.438
    - mental NEC Z81.8
    - metabolic Z83.49
    - musculoskeletal NEC Z82.69
    - neurological NEC Z82.Ø
    - nutritional Z83.49
    - parasitic NEC Z83.1
    - psychiatric NEC Z81.8
    - respiratory NEC Z83.6
    - skin and subcutaneous tissue NEC Z84.Ø
    - specified NEC Z84.89
  - drug abuse NEC Z81.3
  - elevated lipoprotein (a) (Lp(a)) Z83.43Ø
  - epilepsy Z82.Ø
  - familial hypercholesterolemia Z83.42
  - genetic disease carrier Z84.81
  - glaucoma Z83.511
  - hearing loss Z82.2
  - human immunodeficiency virus (HIV) infection Z83.Ø
  - Huntington's chorea Z82.Ø
  - hyperlipidemia, familial combined Z83.438
  - intellectual disability Z81.Ø
  - leukemia Z8Ø.6
  - lipidemia NEC Z83.438
  - malignant neoplasm (of) NOS Z8Ø.9
    - bladder Z8Ø.52
    - breast Z8Ø.3
    - bronchus Z8Ø.1
    - digestive organ Z8Ø.Ø
    - gastrointestinal tract Z8Ø.Ø
    - genital organ Z8Ø.49
      - ovary Z8Ø.41
      - prostate Z8Ø.42
      - specified organ NEC Z8Ø.49
      - testis Z8Ø.43
    - hematopoietic NEC Z8Ø.7
    - intrathoracic organ NEC Z8Ø.2
    - kidney Z8Ø.51
    - lung Z8Ø.1
    - lymphatic NEC Z8Ø.7
    - ovary Z8Ø.41
    - prostate Z8Ø.42
    - respiratory organ NEC Z8Ø.2
    - specified site NEC Z8Ø.8
    - testis Z8Ø.43
    - trachea Z8Ø.1
    - urinary organ or tract Z8Ø.59
      - bladder Z8Ø.52
      - kidney Z8Ø.51
  - mental
    - disorder NEC Z81.8
  - multiple endocrine neoplasia (MEN) syndrome Z83.41
  - osteoporosis Z82.62
  - polycystic kidney Z82.71
  - polyps (colon) Z83.71
  - psychiatric disorder Z81.8
  - psychoactive substance abuse NEC Z81.3
  - respiratory condition NEC Z83.6
    - asthma and other lower respiratory conditions Z82.5
  - self-harmful behavior Z81.8
  - SIDS (sudden infant death syndrome) Z84.82
  - skin condition Z84.Ø
  - specified condition NEC Z84.89
  - stroke (cerebrovascular) Z82.3
  - substance abuse NEC Z81.4
    - alcohol Z81.1
    - drug NEC Z81.3
    - psychoactive NEC Z81.3
    - tobacco Z81.2
  - sudden
    - cardiac death Z82.41
    - infant death syndrome (SIDS) Z84.82
  - tobacco abuse Z81.2

History — *continued*
- family — *see also* History, personal — *continued*
  - violence, violent behavior Z81.8
  - visual loss Z82.1
- personal (of) — *see also* History, family (of)
  - abuse
    - adult Z91.419
      - forced labor or sexual exploitation Z91.42
      - physical and sexual Z91.41Ø
      - psychological Z91.411
    - childhood Z62.819
      - forced labor or sexual exploitation in childhood Z62.813
      - physical Z62.81Ø
      - psychological Z62.811
      - sexual Z62.81Ø
  - alcohol dependence F1Ø.21
  - allergy (to) Z88.9
    - analgesic agent NEC Z88.6
    - anesthetic Z88.4
    - antibiotic agent NEC Z88.1
    - anti-infective agent NEC Z88.3
    - contrast media Z91.Ø41
    - drugs, medicaments and biological substances Z88.9
      - specified NEC Z88.8
    - food Z91.Ø18
      - additives Z91.Ø2
      - beef Z91.Ø14
      - eggs Z91.Ø12
      - lamb Z91.Ø14
      - mammalian meats Z91.Ø14
      - milk products Z91.Ø11
      - peanuts Z91.Ø1Ø
      - pork Z91.Ø14
      - red meats Z91.Ø14
      - seafood Z91.Ø13
      - specified food NEC Z91.Ø18
    - insect Z91.Ø38
      - bee Z91.Ø3Ø
    - latex Z91.Ø4Ø
    - medicinal agents Z88.9
      - specified NEC Z88.8
    - narcotic agent NEC Z88.5
    - nonmedicinal agents Z91.Ø48
    - penicillin Z88.Ø
    - serum Z88.7
    - specified NEC Z91.Ø9
    - sulfonamides Z88.2
    - vaccine Z88.7
  - anaphylactic shock Z87.892
  - anaphylaxis Z87.892
  - behavioral disorders Z86.59
  - benign carcinoid tumor Z86.Ø12
  - benign neoplasm Z86.Ø18
    - brain Z86.Ø11
    - carcinoid Z86.Ø12
    - colonic polyps Z86.Ø1Ø
  - brain injury (traumatic) Z87.82Ø
  - breast implant removal Z98.86
  - calculi, renal Z87.442
  - cancer — *see* History, personal (of), malignant neoplasm (of)
  - cardiac arrest (death), successfully resuscitated Z86.74
  - CAR-T (Chimeric Antigen Receptor T-cell) therapy Z92.85Ø
  - cellular therapy Z92.859
    - specified NEC Z92.858
  - cerebral infarction without residual deficit Z86.73
  - certain (corrected) conditions arising in the perinatal period, specified NEC Z87.68
  - cervical dysplasia Z87.41Ø
  - chemotherapy for neoplastic condition Z92.21
  - childhood abuse — *see* History, personal (of), abuse
  - Chimeric Antigen Receptor T-cell (CAR-T) therapy Z92.85Ø
  - cleft lip (corrected) Z87.73Ø
  - cleft palate (corrected) Z87.73Ø
  - cloaca, persistent Z87.732
  - cloacal malformations Z87.732
  - collapsed vertebra (healed) Z87.311
    - due to osteoporosis Z87.31Ø
  - combat and operational stress reaction Z86.51
  - congenital malformation (corrected) Z87.798
    - circulatory system (corrected) Z87.74
    - diaphragmatic hernia Z87.76Ø
    - digestive system (corrected) NEC Z87.738
    - ear (corrected) Z87.721

History — *continued*
- personal — *see also* History, family — *continued*
  - congenital malformation — *continued*
    - eye (corrected) Z87.72Ø
    - face and neck (corrected) Z87.79Ø
    - gastroschisis Z87.761
    - genitourinary system (corrected) NEC Z87.718
    - heart (corrected) Z87.74
    - integument (corrected) Z87.768
    - limb(s) (corrected) Z87.768
    - malformations
      - abdominal wall Z87.763
      - diaphragm NEC Z87.76Ø
      - integument Z87.768
      - limbs Z87.768
      - musculoskeletal system Z87.768
      - prune belly Z87.762
    - musculoskeletal system (corrected) Z87.768
    - neck (corrected) Z87.79Ø
    - nervous system (corrected) NEC Z87.728
    - respiratory system (corrected) Z87.75
    - sense organs (corrected) NEC Z87.728
    - specified NEC Z87.798
  - contraception Z92.Ø
  - coronavirus (disease) (novel) 2Ø19 Z86.16
  - COVID-19 Z86.16
  - deployment (military) Z91.82
  - diabetic foot ulcer Z86.31
  - disease or disorder (of) Z87.898
    - anaphylaxis Z87.892
    - blood and blood-forming organs Z86.2
    - circulatory system Z86.79
      - specified condition NEC Z86.79
    - connective tissue Z87.39
    - digestive system Z87.19
      - colonic polyp Z86.Ø1Ø
      - peptic ulcer disease Z87.11
      - specified condition NEC Z87.19
    - ear Z86.69
    - endocrine Z86.39
      - diabetic foot ulcer Z86.31
      - gestational diabetes Z86.32
      - specified type NEC Z86.39
    - eye Z86.69
    - genital (track) system NEC
      - female Z87.42
      - male Z87.438
    - hematological Z86.2
    - Hodgkin Z85.71
    - immune mechanism Z86.2
    - infectious Z86.19
      - coronavirus (disease) (novel) 2Ø19 Z86.16
      - COVID-19 Z86.16
      - malaria Z86.13
      - Methicillin resistant Staphylococcus aureus (MRSA) Z86.14
      - poliomyelitis Z86.12
      - SARS-CoV-2 Z86.16
      - specified NEC Z86.19
      - tuberculosis Z86.11
    - mental NEC Z86.59
    - metabolic Z86.39
      - diabetic foot ulcer Z86.31
      - gestational diabetes Z86.32
      - specified type NEC Z86.39
    - musculoskeletal NEC Z87.39
    - nervous system Z86.69
    - nutritional Z86.39
    - parasitic Z86.19
    - respiratory system NEC Z87.Ø9
    - sense organs Z86.69
    - skin Z87.2
    - specified site or type NEC Z87.898
    - subcutaneous tissue Z87.2
    - trophoblastic Z87.59
    - urinary system NEC Z87.448
  - drug dependence — *see* Dependence, drug, by type, in remission
  - drug therapy
    - antineoplastic chemotherapy Z92.21
    - estrogen Z92.23
    - immunosuppression Z92.25
    - inhaled steroids Z92.24Ø
    - monoclonal drug Z92.22
    - specified NEC Z92.29
    - steroid Z92.241
    - systemic steroids Z92.241
  - dysplasia
    - cervical (mild) (moderate) Z87.41Ø

History — *continued*
personal — *see also* History, family — *continued*
dysplasia — *continued*
cervical — *continued*
severe (grade III) Z86.001
prostatic Z87.430
vaginal (mild) (moderate) Z87.411
severe (grade III) Z86.002
vulvar (mild) (moderate) Z87.412
severe (grade III) Z86.002
embolism (venous) Z86.718
pulmonary Z86.711
encephalitis Z86.61
estrogen therapy Z92.23
extracorporeal membrane oxygenation (ECMO) Z92.81
failed conscious sedation Z92.83
failed moderate sedation Z92.83
fall, falling Z91.81
forced labor or sexual exploitation Z91.42
in childhood Z62.813
fracture (healed)
fatigue Z87.312
fragility Z87.310
osteoporosis Z87.310
pathological NEC Z87.311
stress Z87.312
traumatic Z87.81
gene therapy Z92.86
gestational diabetes Z86.32
hepatitis
B Z86.19
C Z86.19
Hodgkin disease Z85.71
hyperthermia, malignant Z88.4
hypospadias (corrected) Z87.710
hysterectomy Z90.710
immunosuppression therapy Z92.25
in situ neoplasm
breast Z86.000
cervix uteri Z86.001
digestive organs, specified NEC Z86.004
esophagus Z86.003
genital organs, specified NEC Z86.002
melanoma Z86.006
middle ear Z86.005
oral cavity Z86.003
respiratory system Z86.005
skin Z86.007
specified NEC Z86.008
stomach Z86.003
in utero procedure during pregnancy Z98.870
in utero procedure while a fetus Z98.871
infection NEC Z86.19
central nervous system Z86.61
coronavirus (disease) (novel) 2019 Z86.16
COVID-19 Z86.16
latent tuberculosis Z86.15
Methicillin resistant Staphylococcus aureus (MRSA) Z86.14
SARS-CoV-2 Z86.16
urinary (recurrent) (tract) Z87.440
injury NEC Z87.828
irradiation Z92.3
kidney stones Z87.442
latent tuberculosis infection Z86.15
leukemia Z85.6
lymphoma (non-Hodgkin) Z85.72
malignant melanoma (skin) Z85.820
malignant neoplasm (of) Z85.9
accessory sinuses Z85.22
anus NEC Z85.048
carcinoid Z85.040
bladder Z85.51
bone Z85.830
brain Z85.841
breast Z85.3
bronchus NEC Z85.118
carcinoid Z85.110
carcinoid — *see* History, personal (of), malignant neoplasm, by site, carcinioid
cervix Z85.41
colon NEC Z85.038
carcinoid Z85.030
digestive organ Z85.00
specified NEC Z85.09
endocrine gland NEC Z85.858
epididymis Z85.48
esophagus Z85.01

History — *continued*
personal — *see also* History, family — *continued*
malignant neoplasm — *continued*
eye Z85.840
gastrointestinal tract — *see* History, malignant neoplasm, digestive organ
genital organ
female Z85.40
specified NEC Z85.44
male Z85.45
specified NEC Z85.49
hematopoietic NEC Z85.79
intrathoracic organ Z85.20
kidney NEC Z85.528
carcinoid Z85.520
large intestine NEC Z85.038
carcinoid Z85.030
larynx Z85.21
liver Z85.05
lung NEC Z85.118
carcinoid Z85.110
mediastinum Z85.29
Merkel cell Z85.821
middle ear Z85.22
nasal cavities Z85.22
nervous system NEC Z85.848
oral cavity Z85.819
specified site NEC Z85.818
ovary Z85.43
pancreas Z85.07
pelvis Z85.53
pharynx Z85.819
specified site NEC Z85.818
pleura Z85.29
prostate Z85.46
rectosigmoid junction NEC Z85.048
carcinoid Z85.040
rectum NEC Z85.048
carcinoid Z85.040
respiratory organ Z85.20
sinuses, accessory Z85.22
skin NEC Z85.828
melanoma Z85.820
Merkel cell Z85.821
small intestine NEC Z85.068
carcinoid Z85.060
soft tissue Z85.831
specified site NEC Z85.89
stomach NEC Z85.028
carcinoid Z85.020
testis Z85.47
thymus NEC Z85.238
carcinoid Z85.230
thyroid Z85.850
tongue Z85.810
trachea Z85.12
urinary organ or tract Z85.50
specified NEC Z85.59
uterus Z85.42
maltreatment Z91.89
medical treatment NEC Z92.89
melanoma Z85.820
in situ Z86.006
malignant (skin) Z85.820
meningitis Z86.61
mental disorder Z86.59
Merkel cell carcinoma (skin) Z85.821
Methicillin resistant Staphylococcus aureus (MRSA) Z86.14
military deployment Z91.82
military war, peacekeeping and humanitarian deployment (current or past conflict) Z91.82
myocardial infarction (old) I25.2
necrotizing enterocolitis of newborn (corrected) Z87.61
neglect (in)
adult Z91.412
childhood Z62.812
neoplasia
anal intraepithelial, III [AIN III] Z86.004
high-grade prostatic intraepithelial, III [HGPIN III] Z86.002
vaginal intraepithelial, III [VAIN III] Z86.002
vulvar intraepithelial, III [VIN III] Z86.002
neoplasm
benign Z86.018
brain Z86.011
colon polyp Z86.010

History — *continued*
personal — *see also* History, family — *continued*
neoplasm — *continued*
in situ
breast Z86.000
cervix uteri Z86.001
digestive organs, specified NEC Z86.004
esophagus Z86.003
genital organs, specified NEC Z86.002
melanoma Z86.006
middle ear Z86.005
oral cavity Z86.003
respiratory system Z86.005
skin Z86.007
specified NEC Z86.008
stomach Z86.003
malignant — *see* History of, malignant neoplasm
uncertain behavior Z86.03
nephrotic syndrome Z87.441
nicotine dependence Z87.891
noncompliance with medical treatment or regimen — *see* Noncompliance
nutritional deficiency Z86.39
obstetric complications Z87.59
childbirth Z87.59
pregnancy Z87.59
pre-term labor Z87.51
puerperium Z87.59
osteoporosis fractures Z87.31 ☑
parasuicide (attempt) Z91.51
physical trauma NEC Z87.828
self-harm or suicide attempt Z91.51
pneumonia (recurrent) Z87.01
poisoning NEC Z91.89
self-harm or suicide attempt Z91.51
poor personal hygiene Z91.89
preterm labor Z87.51
procedure during pregnancy Z98.870
procedure while a fetus Z98.871
prolonged reversible ischemic neurologic deficit (PRIND) Z86.73
prostatic dysplasia Z87.430
psychological
abuse
adult Z91.411
child Z62.811
trauma, specified NEC Z91.49
radiation therapy Z92.3
removal
implant
breast Z98.86
renal calculi Z87.442
respiratory condition NEC Z87.09
retained foreign body fully removed Z87.821
risk factors NEC Z91.89
SARS-CoV-2 infection Z86.16
self-harm
nonsuicidal Z91.52
suicidal Z91.51
self-inflicted injury without suicidal intent Z91.52
self-injury
nonsuicidal Z91.52
self-mutilation Z91.52
self-poisoning attempt Z91.51
sex reassignment Z87.890
sleep-wake cycle problem Z72.821
specified NEC Z87.898
steroid therapy (systemic) Z92.241
inhaled Z92.240
stroke without residual deficits Z86.73
substance abuse NEC F10-F19
sudden cardiac arrest Z86.74
sudden cardiac death successfully resuscitated Z86.74
suicidal behavior Z91.51
suicide attempt Z91.51
surgery NEC Z98.890
with uterine scar Z98.891
sex reassignment Z87.890
transplant — *see* Transplant
thrombophlebitis Z86.72
thrombosis (venous) Z86.718
pulmonary Z86.711
tobacco dependence Z87.891
tracheoesophageal
atresia Z87.731
fistula Z87.731
transient ischemic attack (TIA) without residual deficits Z86.73

- **History** — *continued*
  - personal — *see also* History, family — *continued*
    - trauma (physical) NEC Z87.828
      - psychological NEC Z91.49
      - self-harm Z91.51
    - traumatic brain injury Z87.82Ø
    - tuberculosis, latent infection Z86.15
    - unhealthy sleep-wake cycle Z72.821
    - unintended awareness under general anesthesia Z92.84
    - urinary calculi Z87.442
    - urinary (recurrent) (tract) infection(s) Z87.44Ø
    - uterine scar from previous surgery Z98.891
    - vaginal dysplasia Z87.411
    - venous thrombosis or embolism Z86.718
      - pulmonary Z86.711
    - vulvar dysplasia Z87.412
- **His-Werner disease** A79.Ø
- **HIV** — *see also* Human, immunodeficiency virus B2Ø
  - laboratory evidence (nonconclusive) R75
  - nonconclusive test (in infants) R75
  - positive, seropositive Z21
- **Hives** (bold) — *see* Urticaria
- **Hoarseness** R49.Ø
- **Hobo** Z59.ØØ
- **Hodgkin disease** — *see* Lymphoma, Hodgkin
- **Hodgson's** — *see also* Aneurysm, aorta, thorax I71.2Ø
  - ruptured — *see also* Aneurysm, aorta, thorax, ruptured I71.1Ø
- **Hoffa-Kastert disease** E88.89
- **Hoffa's disease** E88.89
- **Hoffmann-Bouveret syndrome** I47.9
- **Hoffmann's syndrome** EØ3.9 *[G73.7]*
- **Hole** (round)
  - macula H35.34- ☑
  - retina (without detachment) — *see* Break, retina, round hole
    - with detachment — *see* Detachment, retina, with retinal, break
- **Holiday relief care** Z75.5
- **Hollenhorst's plaque** — *see* Occlusion, artery, retina
- **Hollow foot** (congenital) Q66.7- ☑
  - acquired — *see* Deformity, limb, foot, specified NEC
- **Holoprosencephaly** QØ4.2
- **Holt-Oram syndrome** Q87.2
- **Homelessness** Z59.ØØ
  - sheltered Z59.Ø1
  - unsheltered Z59.Ø2
- **Homesickness** — *see* Disorder, adjustment
- **Homocysteinemia** R79.83
- **Homocystinemia, homocystinuria** E72.11
- **Homogentisate 1,2-dioxygenase deficiency** E7Ø.29
- **Homologous serum hepatitis** (prophylactic) (therapeutic) — *see* Hepatitis, viral, type B
- **Honeycomb lung** J98.4
  - congenital Q33.Ø
- **Hooded**
  - clitoris Q52.6
  - penis Q55.69
- **Hookworm** (disease) (infection) (infestation) B76.9
  - with anemia B76.9 *[D63.8]*
  - specified NEC B76.8
- **Hordeolum** (eyelid) (externum) (recurrent) HØØ.Ø19
  - internum HØØ.Ø29
    - left HØØ.Ø26
      - lower HØØ.Ø25
      - upper HØØ.Ø24
    - right HØØ.Ø23
      - lower HØØ.Ø22
      - upper HØØ.Ø21
  - left HØØ.Ø16
    - lower HØØ.Ø15
    - upper HØØ.Ø14
  - right HØØ.Ø13
    - lower HØØ.Ø12
    - upper HØØ.Ø11
- **Horn**
  - cutaneous L85.8
  - nail L6Ø.2
    - congenital Q84.6
- **Horner** (-Claude Bernard) **syndrome** G9Ø.2
  - traumatic — *see* Injury, nerve, cervical sympathetic
- **Horseshoe kidney** (congenital) Q63.1
- **Horton's headache or neuralgia** G44.Ø99
  - intractable G44.Ø91
  - not intractable G44.Ø99
- **Hospital hopper syndrome** — *see* Disorder, factitious
- **Hospitalism in children** — *see* Disorder, adjustment
- **Hostility** R45.5
  - towards child Z62.3
- **Hot flashes**
  - menopausal N95.1
- **Hourglass** (contracture) — *see also* Contraction, hourglass
  - stomach K31.89
    - congenital Q4Ø.2
    - stricture K31.2
- **Household, housing circumstance affecting care** Z59.9
  - specified NEC Z59.89
- **Housemaid's knee** — *see* Bursitis, prepatellar
- **HSCT-TMA** (hematopoietic stem cell transplantation-associated thrombotic microangiopathy) M31.11
- **Hudson** (-Stähli) **line** (cornea) — *see* Pigmentation, cornea, anterior
- **Human**
  - bite (open wound) — *see also* Bite
    - intact skin surface — *see* Bite, superficial
  - herpesvirus — *see* Herpes
  - immunodeficiency virus (HIV) disease (infection) B2Ø
    - asymptomatic status Z21
    - contact Z2Ø.6
    - counseling Z71.7
    - dementia — *see also* Dementia, in, diseases specified elsewhere B2Ø *[FØ2.8Ø]*
      - with behavioral disturbance — *see also* Dementia, in, diseases specified elsewhere B2Ø *[FØ2.81-]* ☑
    - exposure to Z2Ø.6
    - laboratory evidence R75
    - type-2 (HIV 2) as cause of disease classified elsewhere B97.35
  - papillomavirus (HPV)
    - DNA test positive
      - high risk
        - cervix R87.81Ø
        - vagina R87.811
      - low risk
        - cervix R87.82Ø
        - vagina R87.821
    - screening for Z11.51
  - T-cell lymphotropic virus
    - type-1 (HTLV-I) infection B33.3
      - as cause of disease classified elsewhere B97.33
      - carrier Z22.6
    - type-2 (HTLV-II) as cause of disease classified elsewhere B97.34
- **Humidifier lung or pneumonitis** J67.7
- **Humiliation** (experience) **in childhood** Z62.898
- **Humpback** (acquired) — *see* Kyphosis
- **Hunchback** (acquired) — *see* Kyphosis
- **Hunger** T73.Ø ☑
  - air, psychogenic F45.8
- **Hungry bone syndrome** E83.81
- **Hunner's ulcer** — *see* Cystitis, chronic, interstitial
- **Hunter's**
  - glossitis D51.Ø
  - syndrome E76.1
- **Huntington's disease or chorea** G1Ø
  - with dementia — *see also* Dementia, in, diseases specified elsewhere G1Ø *[FØ2.8Ø]*
    - with behavioral disturbance — *see also* Dementia, in, diseases specified elsewhere G1Ø *[FØ2.81-]* ☑
- **Hunt's**
  - disease or syndrome (herpetic geniculate ganglionitis) BØ2.21
    - dyssynergia cerebellaris myoclonica G11.19
  - neuralgia BØ2.21
- **Hurler** (-Scheie) **disease or syndrome** E76.Ø2
- **Hurst's disease** G36.1
- **Hurthle cell**
  - adenocarcinoma C73
  - adenoma D34
  - carcinoma C73
  - tumor D34
- **Hutchinson-Boeck disease or syndrome** — *see* Sarcoidosis
- **Hutchinson-Gilford disease or syndrome** E34.8
- **Hutchinson's**
  - disease, meaning
    - angioma serpiginosum L81.7
    - pompholyx (cheiropompholyx) L3Ø.1
    - prurigo estivalis L56.4
    - summer eruption or summer prurigo L56.4
- **Hutchinson's** — *continued*
  - melanotic freckle — *see* Melanoma, in situ
    - malignant melanoma in — *see* Melanoma
  - teeth or incisors (congenital syphilis) A5Ø.52
  - triad (congenital syphilis) A5Ø.53
- **Hyalin plaque, sclera, senile** H15.89
- **Hyaline membrane** (disease) (lung) (pulmonary) (newborn) P22.Ø
- **Hyalinosis**
  - cutis (et mucosae) E78.89
  - focal and segmental (glomerular) — *see also* NØØ-NØ7 with fourth character .1 NØ5.1
- **Hyalitis, hyalosis, asteroid** — *see also* Deposit, crystalline
  - syphilitic (late) A52.71
- **Hydatid**
  - cyst or tumor — *see* Echinococcus
  - mole — *see* Hydatidiform mole
  - Morgagni
    - female Q5Ø.5
    - male (epididymal) Q55.4
      - testicular Q55.29
- **Hydatidiform mole** (benign) (complicating pregnancy) (delivered) (undelivered) OØ1.9
  - classical OØ1.Ø
  - complete OØ1.Ø
  - incomplete OØ1.1
  - invasive D39.2
  - malignant D39.2
  - partial OØ1.1
- **Hydatidosis** — *see* Echinococcus
- **Hydradenitis** (axillaris) (suppurative) L73.2
- **Hydradenoma** — *see* Hidradenoma
- **Hydramnios** O4Ø.- ☑
- **Hydrancephaly, hydranencephaly** QØ4.3
  - with spina bifida — *see* Spina bifida, with hydrocephalus
- **Hydrargyrism NEC** — *see* Poisoning, mercury
- **Hydrarthrosis** — *see also* Effusion, joint
  - gonococcal A54.42
  - intermittent M12.4Ø
    - ankle M12.47- ☑
    - elbow M12.42- ☑
    - foot joint M12.47- ☑
    - hand joint M12.44- ☑
    - hip M12.45- ☑
    - knee M12.46- ☑
    - multiple site M12.49
    - shoulder M12.41- ☑
    - specified joint NEC M12.48
    - wrist M12.43- ☑
  - of yaws (early) (late) — *see also* subcategory M14.8- A66.6
  - syphilitic (late) A52.77
    - congenital A5Ø.55 *[M12.8Ø]*
- **Hydremia** D64.89
- **Hydrencephalocele** (congenital) — *see* Encephalocele
- **Hydrencephalomeningocele** (congenital) — *see* Encephalocele
- **Hydroa** R23.8
  - aestivale L56.4
  - vacciniforme L56.4
- **Hydroadenitis** (axillaris) (suppurative) L73.2
- **Hydrocalycosis** — *see* Hydronephrosis
- **Hydrocele** (spermatic cord) (testis) (tunica vaginalis) N43.3
  - canal of Nuck N94.89
  - communicating N43.2
    - congenital P83.5
  - congenital P83.5
  - encysted N43.Ø
  - female NEC N94.89
  - infected N43.1
  - newborn P83.5
  - round ligament N94.89
  - specified NEC N43.2
  - spinalis — *see* Spina bifida
  - vulva N9Ø.89
- **Hydrocephalus** (acquired) (external) (internal) (malignant) (recurrent) G91.9
  - aqueduct Sylvius stricture QØ3.Ø
  - causing disproportion O33.6 ☑
    - with obstructed labor O66.3
  - communicating G91.Ø
  - congenital (external) (internal) QØ3.9
    - with spina bifida QØ5.4
      - cervical QØ5.Ø

Hydrocephalus — *continued*
- congenital — *continued*
  - with spina bifida — *continued*
    - dorsal QØ5.1
    - lumbar QØ5.2
    - lumbosacral QØ5.2
    - sacral QØ5.3
    - thoracic QØ5.1
    - thoracolumbar QØ5.1
  - specified NEC QØ3.8
- due to toxoplasmosis (congenital) P37.1
- foramen Magendie block (acquired) G91.1
  - congenital — *see also* Hydrocephalus, congenital QØ3.1
- in (due to)
  - infectious disease NEC B89 *[G91.4]*
  - neoplastic disease NEC — *see also* Neoplasm G91.4
  - parasitic disease B89 *[G91.4]*
- newborn QØ3.9
  - with spina bifida — *see* Spina bifida, with hydrocephalus
- noncommunicating G91.1
- normal pressure G91.2
  - secondary G91.Ø
- obstructive G91.1
- otitic G93.2
- post-traumatic NEC G91.3
- secondary G91.4
  - post-traumatic G91.3
- specified NEC G91.8
- syphilitic, congenital A5Ø.49

Hydrocolpos (congenital) N89.8
Hydrocystoma — *see* Neoplasm, skin, benign
Hydroencephalocele (congenital) — *see* Encephalocele
Hydroencephalomeningocele (congenital) — *see* Encephalocele
Hydrohematopneumothorax — *see* Hemothorax
Hydromeningitis — *see* Meningitis
Hydromeningocele (spinal) — *see also* Spina bifida
- cranial — *see* Encephalocele

Hydrometra N85.8
Hydrometrocolpos N89.8
Hydromicrocephaly QØ2
Hydromphalos (since birth) Q45.8
Hydromyelia QØ6.4
Hydromyelocele — *see* Spina bifida
Hydronephrosis (atrophic) (early) (functionless) (intermittent) (primary) (secondary) NEC N13.3Ø
- with
  - infection N13.6
  - obstruction (by) (of)
    - renal calculus N13.2
      - with infection N13.6
    - ureteral NEC N13.1
      - with infection N13.6
      - calculus N13.2
        - with infection N13.6
    - ureteropelvic junction (congenital) Q62.11
      - acquired N13.Ø
        - with infection N13.6
  - ureteral stricture NEC N13.1
    - with infection N13.6
- congenital Q62.Ø
  - due to acquired occlusion of ureteropelvic junction N13.Ø
- specified type NEC N13.39
- tuberculous A18.11

Hydropericarditis — *see* Pericarditis
Hydropericardium — *see* Pericarditis
Hydroperitoneum R18.8
Hydrophobia — *see* Rabies
Hydrophthalmos Q15.Ø
Hydropneumohemothorax — *see* Hemothorax
Hydropneumopericarditis — *see* Pericarditis
Hydropneumopericardium — *see* Pericarditis
Hydropneumothorax J94.8
- traumatic — *see* Injury, intrathoracic, lung
- tuberculous NEC A15.6

Hydrops R6Ø.9
- abdominis R18.8
- articulorum intermittens — *see* Hydrarthrosis, intermittent
- cardiac — *see* Failure, heart, congestive
- causing obstructed labor (mother) O66.3
- endolymphatic H81.Ø- ☑
- fetal — *see* Pregnancy, complicated by, hydrops, fetalis
- fetalis P83.2

Hydrops — *continued*
- fetalis — *continued*
  - due to
    - ABO isoimmunization P56.Ø
    - alpha thalassemia D56.Ø
    - hemolytic disease P56.9Ø
      - specified NEC P56.99
    - isoimmunization (ABO) (Rh) P56.Ø
    - other specified nonhemolytic disease NEC P83.2
    - Rh incompatibility P56.Ø
  - during pregnancy — *see* Pregnancy, complicated by, hydrops, fetalis
- gallbladder K82.1
- joint — *see* Effusion, joint
- labyrinth H81.Ø- ☑
- newborn (idiopathic) P83.2
  - due to
    - ABO isoimmunization P56.Ø
    - alpha thalassemia D56.Ø
    - hemolytic disease P56.9Ø
      - specified NEC P56.99
    - isoimmunization (ABO) (Rh) P56.Ø
    - Rh incompatibility P56.Ø
- nutritional — *see* Malnutrition, severe
- pericardium — *see* Pericarditis
- pleura — *see* Hydrothorax
- spermatic cord — *see* Hydrocele

Hydropyonephrosis N13.6
Hydrorachis QØ6.4
Hydrorrhea (nasal) J34.89
- pregnancy — *see* Rupture, membranes, premature

Hydrosadenitis (axillaris) (suppurative) L73.2
Hydrosalpinx (fallopian tube) (follicularis) N7Ø.11
Hydrothorax (double) (pleura) J94.8
- chylous (nonfilarial) I89.8
  - filarial — *see also* Infestation, filarial B74.9 *[J91.8]*
- traumatic — *see* Injury, intrathoracic
- tuberculous NEC (non primary) A15.6

Hydroureter — *see also* Hydronephrosis N13.4
- with infection N13.6
- congenital Q62.39

Hydroureteronephrosis — *see* Hydronephrosis
Hydrourethra N36.8
Hydroxykynureninuria E7Ø.89
Hydroxylysinemia E72.3
Hydroxyprolinemia E72.59
Hygiene, sleep
- abuse Z72.821
- inadequate Z72.821
- poor Z72.821

Hygroma (congenital) (cystic) D18.1
- praepatellare, prepatellar — *see* Bursitis, prepatellar

Hymen — *see* condition
Hymenolepis, hymenolepiasis (diminuta) (infection) (infestation) (nana) B71.Ø
Hypalgesia R2Ø.8
Hyperacidity (gastric) K31.89
- psychogenic F45.8

Hyperactive, hyperactivity F9Ø.9
- basal cell, uterine cervix — *see* Dysplasia, cervix
- bowel sounds R19.12
- cervix epithelial (basal) — *see* Dysplasia, cervix
- child F9Ø.9
  - attention deficit — *see* Disorder, attention-deficit hyperactivity
- detrusor muscle N32.81
- gastrointestinal K31.89
  - psychogenic F45.8
- nasal mucous membrane J34.3
- stomach K31.89
- thyroid (gland) — *see* Hyperthyroidism

Hyperacusis H93.23- ☑
Hyperadrenalism E27.5
Hyperadrenocorticism E24.9
- congenital E25.Ø
- iatrogenic E24.2
  - correct substance properly administered — *see* Table of Drugs and Chemicals, by drug, adverse effect
  - overdose or wrong substance given or taken — *see* Table of Drugs and Chemicals, by drug, poisoning
- not associated with Cushing's syndrome E27.Ø
- pituitary-dependent E24.Ø

Hyperaldosteronism E26.9
- familial (type I) E26.Ø2
- glucocorticoid-remediable E26.Ø2

Hyperaldosteronism — *continued*
- primary (due to (bilateral) adrenal hyperplasia) E26.Ø9
- primary NEC E26.Ø9
- secondary E26.1
- specified NEC E26.89

Hyperalgesia R2Ø.8
Hyperalimentation R63.2
- carotene, carotin E67.1
- specified NEC E67.8
- vitamin
  - A E67.Ø
  - D E67.3

Hyperaminoaciduria
- arginine E72.21
- cystine E72.Ø1
- lysine E72.3
- ornithine E72.4

Hyperammonemia (congenital) E72.2Ø
Hyperazotemia — *see* Uremia
Hyperbetalipoproteinemia (familial) E78.ØØ
- with prebetalipoproteinemia E78.2

Hyperbicarbonatemia P74.41
Hyperbilirubinemia
- constitutional E8Ø.6
- familial conjugated E8Ø.6
- neonatal (transient) — *see* Jaundice, newborn

Hypercalcemia, hypocalciuric, familial E83.52
Hypercalciuria, idiopathic R82.994
Hypercapnia RØ6.89
- newborn P84

Hypercarotenemia (dietary) E67.1
Hypercementosis KØ3.4
Hyperchloremia E87.8
Hyperchlorhydria K31.89
- neurotic F45.8
- psychogenic F45.8

Hypercholesterinemia — *see* Hypercholesterolemia
Hypercholesterolemia (essential) (primary) (pure) E78.ØØ
- with hyperglyceridemia, endogenous E78.2
- dietary counseling and surveillance Z71.3
- familial E78.Ø1
- hereditary E78.Ø1

Hyperchylia gastrica, psychogenic F45.8
Hyperchylomicronemia (familial) (primary) E78.3
- with hyperbetalipoproteinemia E78.3

Hypercoagulable (state) D68.59
- activated protein C resistance D68.51
- antithrombin (III) deficiency D68.59
- factor V Leiden mutation D68.51
- primary NEC D68.59
- protein C deficiency D68.59
- protein S deficiency D68.59
- prothrombin gene mutation D68.52
- secondary D68.69
- specified NEC D68.69

Hypercoagulation (state) D68.59
Hypercorticalism, pituitary-dependent E24.Ø
Hypercorticosolism — *see* Cushing's, syndrome
Hypercorticosteronism E24.2
- correct substance properly administered — *see* Table of Drugs and Chemicals, by drug, adverse effect
- overdose or wrong substance given or taken — *see* Table of Drugs and Chemicals, by drug, poisoning

Hypercortisonism E24.2
- correct substance properly administered — *see* Table of Drugs and Chemicals, by drug, adverse effect
- overdose or wrong substance given or taken — *see* Table of Drugs and Chemicals, by drug, poisoning

Hyperekplexia Q89.8
Hyperelectrolytemia E87.8
Hyperemesis R11.1Ø
- with nausea R11.2
- gravidarum (mild) O21.Ø
  - with
    - carbohydrate depletion O21.1
    - dehydration O21.1
    - electrolyte imbalance O21.1
    - metabolic disturbance O21.1
  - severe (with metabolic disturbance) O21.1
- projectile R11.12
- psychogenic F45.8

Hyperemia (acute) (passive) R68.89
- anal mucosa K62.89
- bladder N32.89
- cerebral I67.89
- conjunctiva H11.43- ☑
- ear internal, acute — *see* subcategory H83.Ø ☑
- enteric K59.89

Hyperemia — *continued*
- eye — *see* Hyperemia, conjunctiva
- eyelid (active) (passive) — *see* Disorder, eyelid, specified type NEC
- intestine K59.89
- iris — *see* Disorder, iris, vascular
- kidney N28.89
- labyrinth — *see* subcategory H83.Ø ☑
- liver (active) K76.89
- lung (passive) — *see* Edema, lung
- pulmonary (passive) — *see* Edema, lung
- renal N28.89
- retina H35.89
- stomach K31.89

Hyperesthesia (body surface) R2Ø.3
- larynx (reflex) J38.7
  - hysterical F44.89
- pharynx (reflex) J39.2
  - hysterical F44.89

Hyperestrogenism (drug-induced) (iatrogenic) E28.Ø

Hyperexplexia Q89.8

Hyperfibrinolysis — *see* Fibrinolysis

Hyperfructosemia E74.19

Hyperfunction
- adrenal cortex, not associated with Cushing's syndrome E27.Ø
  - medulla E27.5
    - adrenomedullary E27.5
  - virilism E25.9
    - congenital E25.Ø
- ovarian E28.8
- pancreas K86.89
- parathyroid (gland) E21.3
- pituitary (gland) (anterior) E22.9
  - specified NEC E22.8
- polyglandular E31.1
- testicular E29.Ø

Hypergammaglobulinemia D89.2
- polyclonal D89.Ø
- Waldenström D89.Ø

Hypergastrinemia E16.4

Hyperglobulinemia R77.1

Hyperglycemia, hyperglycemic (transient) R73.9
- coma — *see* Diabetes, by type, with coma
- postpancreatectomy E89.1

Hyperglyceridemia (endogenous) (essential) (familial) (hereditary) (pure) E78.1
- mixed E78.3

Hyperglycinemia (non-ketotic) E72.51

Hypergonadism
- ovarian E28.8
- testicular (primary) (infantile) E29.Ø

Hyperheparinemia D68.32

Hyperhidrosis, hyperidrosis R61
- focal
  - primary L74.519
    - axilla L74.51Ø
    - face L74.511
    - palms L74.512
    - soles L74.513
  - secondary L74.52
- generalized R61
- localized
  - primary L74.519
    - axilla L74.51Ø
    - face L74.511
    - palms L74.512
    - soles L74.513
  - secondary L74.52
- psychogenic F45.8
- secondary R61
  - focal L74.52

Hyperhistidinemia E7Ø.41

Hyperhomocysteinemia E72.11

Hyperhydroxyprolinemia E72.59

Hyperinsulinism (functional) E16.1
- with
  - coma (hypoglycemic) E15
  - encephalopathy E16.1 *[G94]*
- ectopic E16.1
- therapeutic misadventure (from administration of insulin) — *see* subcategory T38.3 ☑

Hyperkalemia E87.5

Hyperkeratosis — *see also* Keratosis L85.9
- cervix N88.Ø
- due to yaws (early) (late) (palmar or plantar) A66.3
- follicularis Q82.8
  - penetrans (in cutem) L87.Ø

Hyperkeratosis — *continued*
- palmoplantaris climacterica L85.1
- pinta A67.1
- senile (with pruritus) L57.Ø
- universalis congenita Q8Ø.8
- vocal cord J38.3
- vulva N9Ø.4

Hyperkinesia, hyperkinetic (disease) (reaction) (syndrome) (childhood) (adolescence) — *see also* Disorder, attention-deficit hyperactivity
- heart I51.89

Hyperleucine-isoleucinemia E71.19

Hyperlipemia, hyperlipidemia E78.5
- combined E78.2
  - familial E78.49
- group
  - A E78.ØØ
  - B E78.1
  - C E78.2
  - D E78.3
- mixed E78.2
- specified NEC E78.49

Hyperlipidosis E75.6
- hereditary NEC E75.5

Hyperlipoproteinemia E78.5
- Fredrickson's type
  - I E78.3
  - IIa E78.ØØ
  - IIb E78.2
  - III E78.2
  - IV E78.1
  - V E78.3
- low-density-lipoprotein-type (LDL) E78.ØØ
- very-low-density-lipoprotein-type (VLDL) E78.1

Hyperlucent lung, unilateral J43.Ø

Hyperlysinemia E72.3

Hypermagnesemia E83.41
- neonatal P71.8

Hypermenorrhea N92.Ø

Hypermethioninemia E72.19

Hypermetropia (congenital) H52.Ø- ☑

Hypermobility, hypermotility
- cecum — *see* Syndrome, irritable bowel
- coccyx — *see* subcategory M53.2 ☑
- colon — *see* Syndrome, irritable bowel
  - psychogenic F45.8
- ileum K58.9
- intestine — *see also* Syndrome, irritable bowel K58.9
  - psychogenic F45.8
- meniscus (knee) — *see* Derangement, knee, meniscus
- scapula — *see* Instability, joint, shoulder
- stomach K31.89
  - psychogenic F45.8
- syndrome M35.7
- urethra N36.41
  - with intrinsic sphincter deficiency N36.43

Hypernasality R49.21

Hypernatremia E87.Ø

Hypernephroma C64.- ☑

Hyperopia — *see* Hypermetropia

Hyperorexia nervosa F5Ø.2

Hyperornithinemia E72.4

Hyperosmia R43.1

Hyperosmolality E87.Ø

Hyperostosis (monomelic) — *see also* Disorder, bone, density and structure, specified NEC
- ankylosing (spine) M48.1Ø
  - cervical region M48.12
  - cervicothoracic region M48.13
  - lumbar region M48.16
  - lumbosacral region M48.17
  - multiple sites M48.19
  - occipito-atlanto-axial region M48.11
  - sacrococcygeal region M48.18
  - thoracic region M48.14
  - thoracolumbar region M48.15
- cortical (skull) M85.2
  - infantile M89.8X- ☑
- frontal, internal of skull M85.2
- interna frontalis M85.2
- skeletal, diffuse idiopathic — *see* Hyperostosis, ankylosing
- skull M85.2
  - congenital Q75.8
- vertebral, ankylosing — *see* Hyperostosis, ankylosing

Hyperovarism E28.8

Hyperoxaluria R82.992
- primary E72.53

Hyperparathyroidism E21.3
- primary E21.Ø
- secondary (renal) N25.81
  - non-renal E21.1
- specified NEC E21.2
- tertiary E21.2

Hyperpathia R2Ø.8

Hyperperistalsis R19.2
- psychogenic F45.8

Hyperpermeability, capillary I78.8

Hyperphagia R63.2

Hyperphenylalaninemia NEC E7Ø.1

Hyperphoria (alternating) H5Ø.53

Hyperphosphatemia E83.39

Hyperpiesis, hyperpiesia — *see* Hypertension

Hyperpigmentation — *see also* Pigmentation
- melanin NEC L81.4
- postinflammatory L81.Ø

Hyperpinealism E34.8

Hyperpituitarism E22.9

Hyperplasia, hyperplastic
- adenoids J35.2
- adrenal (capsule) (cortex) (gland) E27.8
  - with
    - sexual precocity (male) E25.9
      - congenital E25.Ø
    - virilism, adrenal E25.9
      - congenital E25.Ø
    - virilization (female) E25.9
      - congenital E25.Ø
  - congenital E25.Ø
    - salt-losing E25.Ø
- adrenomedullary E27.5
- angiolymphoid, eosinophilia (ALHE) D18.Ø1
- appendix (lymphoid) K38.Ø
- artery, fibromuscular I77.3
- bone — *see also* Hypertrophy, bone
  - marrow D75.89
- breast — *see also* Hypertrophy, breast
  - atypical, atypia N6Ø.9- ☑
    - ductal N6Ø.9- ☑
    - lobular N6Ø.9- ☑
- C-cell, thyroid EØ7.Ø
- cementation (tooth) (teeth) KØ3.4
- cervical gland R59.Ø
- cervix (uteri) (basal cell) (endometrium) (polypoid) — *see also* Dysplasia, cervix
  - congenital Q51.828
- clitoris, congenital Q52.6
- denture KØ6.2
- endocervicitis N72
- endometrium, endometrial (adenomatous) (cystic) (glandular) (glandular-cystic) (polypoid) N85.ØØ
  - with atypia N85.Ø2
  - benign N85.Ø1
  - cervix — *see* Dysplasia, cervix
  - complex (without atypia) N85.Ø1
  - simple (without atypia) N85.Ø1
- epithelial L85.9
  - focal, oral, including tongue K13.29
  - nipple N62
  - skin L85.9
  - tongue K13.29
  - vaginal wall N89.3
- erythroid D75.89
- fibromuscular of artery (carotid) (renal) I77.3
- genital
  - female NEC N94.89
  - male N5Ø.89
- gingiva KØ6.1
- glandularis cystica uteri (interstitialis) — *see also* Hyperplasia, endometrial N85.ØØ
- gum KØ6.1
- hymen, congenital Q52.4
- irritative, edentulous (alveolar) KØ6.2
- jaw M26.Ø9
  - alveolar M26.79
  - lower M26.Ø3
    - alveolar M26.72
  - upper M26.Ø1
    - alveolar M26.71
- kidney (congenital) Q63.3
- labia N9Ø.69
  - epithelial N9Ø.3
- liver (congenital) Q44.7
  - nodular, focal K76.89
- lymph gland or node R59.9
- mandible, mandibular M26.Ø3

- **Hyperplasia, hyperplastic** — *continued*
  - mandible, mandibular — *continued*
    - alveolar M26.72
    - unilateral condylar M27.8
  - maxilla, maxillary M26.01
    - alveolar M26.71
  - myometrium, myometrial N85.2
  - neuroendocrine cell, of infancy J84.841
  - nose
    - lymphoid J34.89
    - polypoid J33.9
  - oral mucosa (irritative) K13.6
  - organ or site, congenital NEC — *see* Anomaly, by site
  - ovary N83.8
  - palate, papillary (irritative) K13.6
  - pancreatic islet cells E16.9
    - alpha E16.8
      - with excess
        - gastrin E16.4
        - glucagon E16.3
    - beta E16.1
  - parathyroid (gland) E21.0
  - pharynx (lymphoid) J39.2
  - prostate (adenofibromatous) (nodular) N40.0
    - with lower urinary tract symptoms (LUTS) N40.1
    - without lower urinary tract symtpoms (LUTS) N40.0
  - renal artery I77.89
  - reticulo-endothelial (cell) D75.89
  - salivary gland (any) K11.1
  - Schimmelbusch's — *see* Mastopathy, cystic
  - suprarenal capsule (gland) E27.8
  - thymus (gland) (persistent) E32.0
  - thyroid (gland) — *see* Goiter
  - tonsils (faucial) (infective) (lingual) (lymphoid) J35.1
    - with adenoids J35.3
  - unilateral condylar M27.8
  - uterus, uterine N85.2
    - endometrium (glandular) — *see also* Hyperplasia, endometrial N85.00
  - vulva N90.69
    - epithelial N90.3
- **Hyperpnea** — *see* Hyperventilation
- **Hyperpotassemia** E87.5
- **Hyperprebetalipoproteinemia** (familial) E78.1
- **Hyperprolactinemia** E22.1
- **Hyperprolinemia** (type I) (type II) E72.59
- **Hyperproteinemia** E88.09
- **Hyperprothrombinemia, causing coagulation factor deficiency** D68.4
- **Hyperpyrexia** R50.9
  - heat (effects) T67.01 ☑
  - malignant, due to anesthetic T88.3 ☑
  - rheumatic — *see* Fever, rheumatic
  - unknown origin R50.9
- **Hyper-reflexia** R29.2
- **Hypersalivation** K11.7
- **Hypersecretion**
  - ACTH (not associated with Cushing's syndrome) E27.0
    - pituitary E24.0
  - adrenaline E27.5
  - adrenomedullary E27.5
  - androgen (testicular) E29.0
    - ovarian (drug-induced) (iatrogenic) E28.1
  - calcitonin E07.0
  - catecholamine E27.5
  - corticoadrenal E24.9
  - cortisol E24.9
  - epinephrine E27.5
  - estrogen E28.0
  - gastric K31.89
    - psychogenic F45.8
  - gastrin E16.4
  - glucagon E16.3
  - hormone(s)
    - ACTH (not associated with Cushing's syndrome) E27.0
      - pituitary E24.0
    - antidiuretic E22.2
    - growth E22.0
    - intestinal NEC E34.1
    - ovarian androgen E28.1
    - pituitary E22.9
    - testicular E29.0
    - thyroid stimulating E05.80
      - with thyroid storm E05.81
  - insulin — *see* Hyperinsulinism
  - lacrimal glands — *see* Epiphora
  - medulloadrenal E27.5
- **Hypersecretion** — *continued*
  - milk O92.6
  - ovarian androgens E28.1
  - salivary gland (any) K11.7
  - thyrocalcitonin E07.0
  - upper respiratory J39.8
- **Hypersegmentation, leukocytic, hereditary** D72.0
- **Hypersensitive, hypersensitiveness, hypersensitivity** — *see also* Allergy
  - carotid sinus G90.01
  - colon — *see* Irritable, colon
  - drug T88.7 ☑
  - gastrointestinal K52.29
    - immediate K52.29
    - psychogenic F45.8
  - labyrinth — *see* subcategory H83.2 ☑
  - pain R20.8
  - pneumonitis — *see* Pneumonitis, allergic
  - reaction T78.40 ☑
    - upper respiratory tract NEC J39.3
- **Hypersomnia** (organic) G47.10
  - due to
    - alcohol
      - abuse F10.182
      - dependence F10.282
      - use F10.982
    - amphetamines
      - abuse F15.182
      - dependence F15.282
      - use F15.982
    - caffeine
      - abuse F15.182
      - dependence F15.282
      - use F15.982
    - cocaine
      - abuse F14.182
      - dependence F14.282
      - use F14.982
    - drug NEC
      - abuse F19.182
      - dependence F19.282
      - use F19.982
    - medical condition G47.14
    - mental disorder F51.13
    - opioid
      - abuse F11.182
      - dependence F11.282
      - use F11.982
    - psychoactive substance NEC
      - abuse F19.182
      - dependence F19.282
      - use F19.982
    - sedative, hypnotic, or anxiolytic
      - abuse F13.182
      - dependence F13.282
      - use F13.982
    - stimulant NEC
      - abuse F15.182
      - dependence F15.282
      - use F15.982
  - idiopathic G47.11
    - with long sleep time G47.11
    - without long sleep time G47.12
  - menstrual related G47.13
  - nonorganic origin F51.11
    - specified NEC F51.19
  - not due to a substance or known physiological condition F51.11
    - specified NEC F51.19
  - primary F51.11
  - recurrent G47.13
  - specified NEC G47.19
- **Hypersplenia, hypersplenism** D73.1
- **Hyperstimulation, ovaries** (associated with induced ovulation) N98.1
- **Hypersusceptibility** — *see* Allergy
- **Hypertelorism** (ocular) (orbital) Q75.2
- **Hypertension, hypertensive** (accelerated) (benign) (essential) (idiopathic) (malignant) (systemic) I10
  - with
    - heart failure (congestive) I11.0
    - heart involvement (conditions in I50.- or I51.4-I51.7, I51.89, I51.9, due to hypertension) — *see* Hypertension, heart
    - kidney involvement — *see* Hypertension, kidney
  - benign, intracranial G93.2
  - borderline R03.0
  - cardiorenal (disease) I13.10
- **Hypertension, hypertensive** — *continued*
  - cardiorenal — *continued*
    - with heart failure I13.0
      - with stage 1 through stage 4 chronic kidney disease I13.0
      - with stage 5 or end stage renal disease I13.2
    - without heart failure I13.10
      - with stage 1 through stage 4 chronic kidney disease I13.10
      - with stage 5 or end stage renal disease I13.11
  - cardiovascular
    - disease (arteriosclerotic) (sclerotic) — *see* Hypertension, heart
    - renal (disease) — *see* Hypertension, cardiorenal
  - chronic venous — *see* Hypertension, venous (chronic)
  - complicating
    - childbirth (labor) O16.4
      - pre-existing O10.92
        - with
          - heart disease O10.12
            - with renal disease O10.32
          - pre-eclampsia O11.4
          - renal disease O10.22
            - with heart disease O10.32
        - essential O10.02
        - secondary O10.42
    - pregnancy O16.- ☑
      - with edema — *see also* Pre-eclampsia O14.9- ☑
      - gestational (pregnancy induced) (without proteinuria) O13.- ☑
        - with proteinuria O14.9- ☑
          - mild pre-eclampsia O14.0- ☑
          - moderate pre-eclampsia O14.0- ☑
          - severe pre-eclampsia O14.1- ☑
            - with hemolysis, elevated liver enzymes and low platelet count (HELLP) O14.2- ☑
      - pre-existing O10.91- ☑
        - with
          - heart disease O10.11- ☑
            - with renal disease O10.31- ☑
          - pre-eclampsia — *see* category O11
          - renal disease O10.21- ☑
            - with heart disease O10.31- ☑
        - essential O10.01- ☑
        - secondary O10.41- ☑
      - transient O13- ☑
    - puerperium, pre-existing O16.5
      - pre-existing
        - with
          - heart disease O10.13
            - with renal disease O10.33
          - pre-eclampsia O11.5
          - renal disease O10.23
            - with heart disease O10.33
        - essential O10.03
      - pregnancy-induced O13.9
      - secondary O10.43
  - crisis I16.9
  - due to
    - endocrine disorders I15.2
    - pheochromocytoma I15.2
    - renal disorders NEC I15.1
      - arterial I15.0
    - renovascular disorders I15.0
    - specified disease NEC I15.8
  - emergency I16.1
  - encephalopathy I67.4
  - gestational (without significant proteinuria) (pregnancy-induced) (transient) O13.- ☑
    - with significant proteinuria — *see* Pre-eclampsia
    - complicating
      - delivery O13.4
      - puerperium O13.5
  - Goldblatt's I70.1
  - heart (disease) (conditions in I51.4-I51.9 due to hypertension) I11.9
    - with
      - heart failure (congestive) I11.0
      - kidney disease (chronic) — *see* Hypertension, cardiorenal
  - intracranial, benign G93.2
  - kidney I12.9
    - with
      - heart disease — *see* Hypertension, cardiorenal
      - stage 1 through stage 4 chronic kidney disease I12.9

- **Hypertension, hypertensive** — *continued*
  - kidney — *continued*
    - with — *continued*
      - stage 5 chronic kidney disease (CKD) or end stage renal disease (ESRD) I12.Ø
  - lesser circulation I27.Ø
  - maternal O16- ☑
  - newborn P29.2
    - pulmonary (persistent) P29.3Ø
  - ocular H4Ø.Ø5- ☑
  - pancreatic duct — *code to* underlying condition
    - with chronic pancreatitis K86.1
  - portal (due to chronic liver disease) (idiopathic) K76.6
    - gastropathy K31.89
    - in (due to) schistosomiasis (bilharziasis) B65.9 *[K77]*
  - postoperative I97.3
  - psychogenic F45.8
  - pulmonary I27.2Ø
    - with
      - cor pulmonale (chronic) I27.29
        - acute I26.Ø9
      - right heart ventricular strain/failure I27.29
        - acute I26.Ø9
      - right to left shunt related to congenital heart disease I27.83
      - unclear multifactorial mechanisms I27.29
    - arterial (associated) (drug-induced) (toxin-induced) I27.21
    - chronic thromboembolic I27.24
    - due to
      - hematologic disorders I27.29
      - kyphoscoliotic heart disease I27.1
      - left heart disease I27.22
      - lung diseases and hypoxia I27.23
      - metabolic disorders I27.29
      - specified systemic disorders I27.29
    - group 1 (associated) (drug-induced) (toxin-induced) I27.21
    - group 2 I27.22
    - group 3 I27.23
    - group 4 I27.24
    - group 5 I27.29
    - of newborn (persistent) P29.3Ø
    - primary (idiopathic) I27.Ø
    - secondary
      - arterial I27.21
      - specified NEC I27.29
  - renal — *see* Hypertension, kidney
  - renovascular I15.Ø
  - secondary NEC I15.9
    - due to
      - endocrine disorders I15.2
      - pheochromocytoma I15.2
      - renal disorders NEC I15.1
        - arterial I15.Ø
      - renovascular disorders I15.Ø
    - specified NEC I15.8
  - transient RØ3.Ø
    - of pregnancy O13.- ☑
  - urgency I16.Ø
  - venous (chronic)
    - due to
      - deep vein thrombosis — *see* Syndrome, post-thrombotic
    - idiopathic I87.3Ø9
      - with
        - inflammation I87.32- ☑
          - with ulcer I87.33- ☑
        - specified complication NEC I87.39- ☑
        - ulcer I87.31- ☑
          - with inflammation I87.33- ☑
      - asymptomatic I87.3Ø- ☑
- **Hypertensive urgency** — *see* Hypertension
- **Hyperthecosis ovary** E28.8
- **Hyperthermia** (of unknown origin) — *see also* Hyperpyrexia
  - malignant, due to anesthesia T88.3 ☑
  - newborn P81.9
    - environmental P81.Ø
- **Hyperthyroid** (recurrent) — *see* Hyperthyroidism
- **Hyperthyroidism** (latent) (pre-adult) (recurrent) EØ5.9Ø
  - with
    - goiter (diffuse) EØ5.ØØ
      - with thyroid storm EØ5.Ø1
      - nodular (multinodular) EØ5.2Ø
        - with thyroid storm EØ5.21
        - uninodular EØ5.1Ø
          - with thyroid storm EØ5.11
- **Hyperthyroidism** — *continued*
  - with — *continued*
    - storm EØ5.91
  - due to ectopic thyroid tissue EØ5.3Ø
    - with thyroid storm EØ5.31
  - neonatal, transitory P72.1
  - specified NEC EØ5.8Ø
    - with thyroid storm EØ5.81
- **Hypertony, hypertonia, hypertonicity**
  - bladder N31.8
  - congenital P94.1
  - stomach K31.89
    - psychogenic F45.8
  - uterus, uterine (contractions) (complicating delivery) O62.4
- **Hypertrichosis** L68.9
  - congenital Q84.2
  - eyelid HØ2.869
    - left HØ2.866
      - lower HØ2.865
      - upper HØ2.864
    - right HØ2.863
      - lower HØ2.862
      - upper HØ2.861
  - lanuginosa Q84.2
    - acquired L68.1
  - localized L68.2
  - specified NEC L68.8
- **Hypertriglyceridemia, essential** E78.1
- **Hypertrophy, hypertrophic**
  - adenofibromatous, prostate — *see* Enlargement, enlarged, prostate
  - adenoids (infective) J35.2
    - with tonsils J35.3
  - adrenal cortex E27.8
  - alveolar process or ridge — *see* Anomaly, alveolar
  - anal papillae K62.89
  - artery I77.89
    - congenital NEC Q27.8
      - digestive system Q27.8
      - lower limb Q27.8
      - specified site NEC Q27.8
      - upper limb Q27.8
  - auricular — *see* Hypertrophy, cardiac
  - Bartholin's gland N75.8
  - bile duct (common) (hepatic) K83.8
  - bladder (sphincter) (trigone) N32.89
  - bone M89.3Ø
    - carpus M89.34- ☑
    - clavicle M89.31- ☑
    - femur M89.35- ☑
    - fibula M89.36- ☑
    - finger M89.34- ☑
    - humerus M89.32- ☑
    - ilium M89.359
    - ischium M89.359
    - metacarpus M89.34- ☑
    - metatarsus M89.37- ☑
    - multiple sites M89.39
    - neck M89.38
    - radius M89.33- ☑
    - rib M89.38
    - scapula M89.31- ☑
    - skull M89.38
    - tarsus M89.37- ☑
    - tibia M89.36- ☑
    - toe M89.37- ☑
    - ulna M89.33- ☑
    - vertebra M89.38
  - brain G93.89
  - breast N62
    - cystic — *see* Mastopathy, cystic
    - newborn P83.4
    - pubertal, massive N62
    - puerperal, postpartum — *see* Disorder, breast, specified type NEC
    - senile (parenchymatous) N62
  - cardiac (chronic) (idiopathic) I51.7
    - with rheumatic fever (conditions in IØØ)
      - active IØ1.8
      - inactive or quiescent (with chorea) IØ9.89
    - congenital NEC Q24.8
    - fatty — *see* Degeneration, myocardial
    - hypertensive — *see* Hypertension, heart
    - rheumatic (with chorea) IØ9.89
      - active or acute IØ1.8
        - with chorea IØ2.Ø
    - valve — *see* Endocarditis
- **Hypertrophy, hypertrophic** — *continued*
  - cartilage — *see* Disorder, cartilage, specified type NEC
  - cecum — *see* Megacolon
  - cervix (uteri) N88.8
    - congenital Q51.828
    - elongation N88.4
  - clitoris (cirrhotic) N9Ø.89
    - congenital Q52.6
  - colon — *see also* Megacolon
    - congenital Q43.2
  - conjunctiva, lymphoid H11.89
  - corpora cavernosa N48.89
  - cystic duct K82.8
  - duodenum K31.89
  - endometrium (glandular) — *see also* Hyperplasia, endometrial N85.ØØ
    - cervix N88.8
  - epididymis N5Ø.89
  - esophageal hiatus (congenital) Q79.1
    - with hernia — *see* Hernia, hiatal
  - eyelid — *see* Disorder, eyelid, specified type NEC
  - facet joint — *see also* Spondylosis M47.819
  - fat pad E65
    - knee (infrapatellar) (popliteal) (prepatellar) (retropatellar) M79.4
  - foot (congenital) Q74.2
  - frenulum, frenum (tongue) K14.8
    - lip K13.Ø
  - gallbladder K82.8
  - gastric mucosa K29.6Ø
    - with bleeding K29.61
  - gland, glandular R59.9
    - generalized R59.1
    - localized R59.Ø
  - gum (mucous membrane) KØ6.1
  - heart (idiopathic) — *see also* Hypertrophy, cardiac
    - valve — *see also* Endocarditis I38
  - hemifacial Q67.4
  - hepatic — *see* Hypertrophy, liver
  - hiatus (esophageal) Q79.1
  - hilus gland R59.Ø
  - hymen, congenital Q52.4
  - ileum K63.89
  - intestine NEC K63.89
  - jejunum K63.89
  - kidney (compensatory) N28.81
    - congenital Q63.3
  - labium (majus) (minus) N9Ø.6Ø
  - ligament — *see* Disorder, ligament
  - lingual tonsil (infective) J35.1
    - with adenoids J35.3
  - lip K13.Ø
    - congenital Q18.6
  - liver R16.Ø
    - acute K76.89
    - cirrhotic — *see* Cirrhosis, liver
    - congenital Q44.7
    - fatty — *see* Fatty, liver
  - lymph, lymphatic gland R59.9
    - generalized R59.1
    - localized R59.Ø
    - tuberculous — *see* Tuberculosis, lymph gland
  - mammary gland — *see* Hypertrophy, breast
  - Meckel's diverticulum (congenital) Q43.Ø
    - malignant — *see* Table of Neoplasms, small intestine, malignant
  - median bar — *see* Hyperplasia, prostate
  - meibomian gland — *see* Chalazion
  - meniscus, knee, congenital Q74.1
  - metatarsal head — *see* Hypertrophy, bone, metatarsus
  - metatarsus — *see* Hypertrophy, bone, metatarsus
  - mucous membrane
    - alveolar ridge KØ6.2
    - gum KØ6.1
    - nose (turbinate) J34.3
  - muscle M62.89
  - muscular coat, artery I77.89
  - myocardium — *see also* Hypertrophy, cardiac
    - idiopathic I42.2
  - myometrium N85.2
  - nail L6Ø.2
    - congenital Q84.5
  - nasal J34.89
    - alae J34.89
    - bone J34.89
    - cartilage J34.89
    - mucous membrane (septum) J34.3
    - sinus J34.89

Hypertrophy, hypertrophic — *continued*
- nasal — *continued*
  - turbinate J34.3
- nasopharynx, lymphoid (infectional) (tissue) (wall) J35.2
- nipple N62
- organ or site, congenital NEC — *see* Anomaly, by site
- ovary N83.8
- palate (hard) M27.8
  - soft K13.79
- pancreas, congenital Q45.3
- parathyroid (gland) E21.Ø
- parotid gland K11.1
- penis N48.89
- pharyngeal tonsil J35.2
- pharynx J39.2
  - lymphoid (infectional) (tissue) (wall) J35.2
- pituitary (anterior) (fossa) (gland) E23.6
- prepuce (congenital) N47.8
  - female N9Ø.89
- prostate — *see* Enlargement, enlarged, prostate
  - congenital Q55.4
- pseudomuscular — *see also* Dystrophy, muscular, by type, if applicable G71.Ø9
- pylorus (adult) (muscle) (sphincter) K31.1
  - congenital or infantile Q4Ø.Ø
- rectal, rectum (sphincter) K62.89
- rhinitis (turbinate) J31.Ø
- salivary gland (any) K11.1
  - congenital Q38.4
- scaphoid (tarsal) — *see* Hypertrophy, bone, tarsus
- scar L91.Ø
- scrotum N5Ø.89
- seminal vesicle N5Ø.89
- sigmoid — *see* Megacolon
- skin L91.9
  - specified NEC L91.8
- spermatic cord N5Ø.89
- spleen — *see* Splenomegaly
- spondylitis — *see* Spondylosis
- stomach K31.89
- sublingual gland K11.1
- submandibular gland K11.1
- suprarenal cortex (gland) E27.8
- synovial NEC M67.2Ø
  - acromioclavicular M67.21- ☑
  - ankle M67.27- ☑
  - elbow M67.22- ☑
  - foot M67.27- ☑
  - hand M67.24- ☑
  - hip M67.25- ☑
  - knee M67.26- ☑
  - multiple sites M67.29
  - specified site NEC M67.28
  - wrist M67.23- ☑
- tendon — *see* Disorder, tendon, specified type NEC
- testis N44.8
  - congenital Q55.29
- thymic, thymus (gland) (congenital) E32.Ø
- thyroid (gland) — *see* Goiter
- toe (congenital) Q74.2
  - acquired — *see also* Deformity, toe, specified NEC
- tongue K14.8
  - congenital Q38.2
  - papillae (foliate) K14.3
- tonsils (faucial) (infective) (lingual) (lymphoid) J35.1
  - with adenoids J35.3
- tunica vaginalis N5Ø.89
- ureter N28.89
- urethra N36.8
- uterus N85.2
  - neck (with elongation) N88.4
  - puerperal O9Ø.89
- uvula K13.79
- vagina N89.8
- vas deferens N5Ø.89
- vein I87.8
- ventricle, ventricular (heart) — *see also* Hypertrophy, cardiac
  - congenital Q24.8
  - in tetralogy of Fallot Q21.3
- verumontanum N36.8
- vocal cord J38.3
- vulva N9Ø.6Ø
  - stasis (nonfilarial) N9Ø.69

Hypertropia H5Ø.2- ☑
Hypertyrosinemia E7Ø.21
Hyperuricemia (asymptomatic) E79.Ø
Hyperuricosuria R82.993
Hypervalinemia E71.19
Hyperventilation (tetany) RØ6.4
- hysterical F45.8
- psychogenic F45.8
- syndrome F45.8

Hypervitaminosis (dietary) NEC E67.8
- A E67.Ø
  - administered as drug (prolonged intake) — *see* Table of Drugs and Chemicals, vitamins, adverse effect
  - overdose or wrong substance given or taken — *see* Table of Drugs and Chemicals, vitamins, poisoning
- B6 E67.2
- D E67.3
  - administered as drug (prolonged intake) — *see* Table of Drugs and Chemicals, vitamins, adverse effect
  - overdose or wrong substance given or taken — *see* Table of Drugs and Chemicals, vitamins, poisoning
- K E67.8
  - administered as drug (prolonged intake) — *see* Table of Drugs and Chemicals, vitamins, adverse effect
  - overdose or wrong substance given or taken — *see* Table of Drugs and Chemicals, vitamins, poisoning

Hypervolemia E87.7Ø
- specified NEC E87.79

Hypesthesia R2Ø.1
- cornea — *see* Anesthesia, cornea

Hyphema H21.Ø- ☑
- traumatic SØ5.1- ☑

Hypoacidity, gastric K31.89
- psychogenic F45.8

Hypoadrenalism, hypoadrenia E27.4Ø
- primary E27.1
- tuberculous A18.7

Hypoadrenocorticism E27.4Ø
- pituitary E23.Ø
- primary E27.1

Hypoalbuminemia E88.Ø9
Hypoaldosteronism E27.4Ø
Hypoalphalipoproteinemia E78.6
Hypobarism T7Ø.29 ☑
Hypobaropathy T7Ø.29 ☑
Hypobetalipoproteinemia (familial) E78.6
Hypocalcemia E83.51
- dietary E58
- neonatal P71.1
  - due to cow's milk P71.Ø
- phosphate-loading (newborn) P71.1

Hypochloremia E87.8
Hypochlorhydria K31.89
- neurotic F45.8
- psychogenic F45.8

Hypochondria, hypochondriac, hypochondriasis (reaction) F45.21
- sleep F51.Ø3

Hypochondrogenesis Q77.Ø
Hypochondroplasia Q77.4
Hypochromasia, blood cells D5Ø.8
Hypocitraturia R82.991
Hypodontia — *see* Anodontia
Hypoeosinophilia D72.89
Hypoesthesia R2Ø.1
Hypofibrinogenemia D68.8
- acquired D65
- congenital (hereditary) D68.2

Hypofunction
- adrenocortical E27.4Ø
  - drug-induced E27.3
  - postprocedural E89.6
  - primary E27.1
- adrenomedullary, postprocedural E89.6
- cerebral R29.818
- corticoadrenal NEC E27.4Ø
- intestinal K59.89
- labyrinth — *see* subcategory H83.2 ☑
- ovary E28.39
- pituitary (gland) (anterior) E23.Ø
- testicular E29.1
  - postprocedural (postsurgical) (postirradiation) (iatrogenic) E89.5

Hypogalactia O92.4
Hypogammaglobulinemia — *see also* Agammaglobulinemia D8Ø.1
- hereditary D8Ø.Ø
- nonfamilial D8Ø.1
- transient, of infancy D8Ø.7

Hypogenitalism (congenital) — *see* Hypogonadism
Hypoglossia Q38.3
Hypoglycemia (spontaneous) E16.2
- coma E15
  - diabetic — *see* Diabetes, by type, with hypoglycemia, with coma
- diabetic — *see* Diabetes, hypoglycemia
- dietary counseling and surveillance Z71.3
- drug-induced E16.Ø
  - with coma (nondiabetic) E15
- due to insulin E16.Ø
  - with coma (nondiabetic) E15
  - therapeutic misadventure — *see* subcategory T38.3 ☑
- functional, nonhyperinsulinemic E16.1
- iatrogenic E16.Ø
  - with coma (nondiabetic) E15
- in infant of diabetic mother P7Ø.1
  - gestational diabetes P7Ø.Ø
- infantile E16.1
- leucine-induced E71.19
- neonatal (transitory) P7Ø.4
  - iatrogenic P7Ø.3
- reactive (not drug-induced) E16.1
- transitory neonatal P7Ø.4

Hypogonadism
- female E28.39
- hypogonadotropic E23.Ø
- male E29.1
- ovarian (primary) E28.39
- pituitary E23.Ø
- testicular (primary) E29.1

Hypohidrosis, hypoidrosis L74.4
Hypoinsulinemia, postprocedural E89.1
Hypokalemia E87.6
Hypoleukocytosis — *see* Agranulocytosis
Hypolipoproteinemia (alpha) (beta) E78.6
Hypomagnesemia E83.42
- neonatal P71.2

Hypomania, hypomanic reaction F3Ø.8
Hypomenorrhea — *see* Oligomenorrhea
Hypometabolism R63.8
Hypomotility
- gastrointestinal (tract) K31.89
  - psychogenic F45.8
- intestine K59.89
  - psychogenic F45.8
- stomach K31.89
  - psychogenic F45.8

Hyponasality R49.22
Hyponatremia E87.1
Hypo-osmolality E87.1
Hypo-ovarianism, hypo-ovarism E28.39
Hypoparathyroidism E2Ø.9
- familial E2Ø.8
- idiopathic E2Ø.Ø
- neonatal, transitory P71.4
- postprocedural E89.2
- specified NEC E2Ø.8

Hypoperfusion (in)
- newborn P96.89

Hypopharyngitis — *see* Laryngopharyngitis
Hypophoria H5Ø.53
Hypophosphatemia, hypophosphatasia (acquired) (congenital) (renal) E83.39
- familial E83.31

Hypophyseal, hypophysis — *see also* condition
- dwarfism E23.Ø
- gigantism E22.Ø

Hypopiesis — *see* Hypotension
Hypopinealism E34.8
Hypopituitarism (juvenile) E23.Ø
- drug-induced E23.1
- due to
  - hypophysectomy E89.3
  - radiotherapy E89.3
- iatrogenic NEC E23.1
- postirradiation E89.3
- postpartum O99.285
- postprocedural E89.3

Hypoplasia, hypoplastic
- adrenal (gland), congenital Q89.1
- alimentary tract, congenital Q45.8

- **Hypoplasia, hypoplastic** — *continued*
  - alimentary tract, congenital — *continued*
    - upper Q4Ø.8
  - anus, anal (canal) Q42.3
    - with fistula Q42.2
  - aorta, aortic Q25.42
    - ascending, in hypoplastic left heart syndrome Q23.4
    - valve Q23.1
      - in hypoplastic left heart syndrome Q23.4
  - areola, congenital Q83.8
  - arm (congenital) — *see* Defect, reduction, upper limb
  - artery (peripheral) Q27.8
    - brain (congenital) Q28.3
    - coronary Q24.5
    - digestive system Q27.8
    - lower limb Q27.8
    - pulmonary Q25.79
      - functional, unilateral J43.Ø
    - retinal (congenital) Q14.1
    - specified site NEC Q27.8
    - umbilical Q27.Ø
    - upper limb Q27.8
  - auditory canal Q17.8
    - causing impairment of hearing Q16.9
  - biliary duct or passage Q44.5
  - bone NOS Q79.9
    - face Q75.8
    - marrow D61.9
      - megakaryocytic D69.49
    - skull — *see* Hypoplasia, skull
  - brain QØ2
    - gyri QØ4.3
    - part of QØ4.3
  - breast (areola) N64.82
  - bronchus Q32.4
  - cardiac Q24.8
  - carpus — *see* Defect, reduction, upper limb, specified type NEC
  - cartilage hair Q78.8
  - cecum Q42.8
  - cementum KØØ.4
  - cephalic QØ2
  - cerebellum QØ4.3
  - cervix (uteri), congenital Q51.821
  - clavicle (congenital) Q74.Ø
  - coccyx Q76.49
  - colon Q42.9
    - specified NEC Q42.8
  - corpus callosum QØ4.Ø
  - cricoid cartilage Q31.2
  - digestive organ(s) or tract NEC Q45.8
    - upper (congenital) Q4Ø.8
  - ear (auricle) (lobe) Q17.2
    - middle Q16.4
  - enamel of teeth (neonatal) (postnatal) (prenatal) KØØ.4
  - endocrine (gland) NEC Q89.2
  - endometrium N85.8
  - epididymis (congenital) Q55.4
  - epiglottis Q31.2
  - erythroid, congenital D61.Ø1
  - esophagus (congenital) Q39.8
  - eustachian tube Q17.8
  - eye Q11.2
  - eyelid (congenital) Q1Ø.3
  - face Q18.8
    - bone(s) Q75.8
  - femur (congenital) — *see* Defect, reduction, lower limb, specified type NEC
  - fibula (congenital) — *see* Defect, reduction, lower limb, specified type NEC
  - finger (congenital) — *see* Defect, reduction, upper limb, specified type NEC
  - focal dermal Q82.8
  - foot — *see* Defect, reduction, lower limb, specified type NEC
  - gallbladder Q44.Ø
  - genitalia, genital organ(s)
    - female, congenital Q52.8
      - external Q52.79
      - internal NEC Q52.8
    - in adiposogenital dystrophy E23.6
  - glottis Q31.2
  - hair Q84.2
  - hand (congenital) — *see* Defect, reduction, upper limb, specified type NEC
  - heart Q24.8
  - humerus (congenital) — *see* Defect, reduction, upper limb, specified type NEC
- **Hypoplasia, hypoplastic** — *continued*
  - intestine (small) Q41.9
    - large Q42.9
      - specified NEC Q42.8
  - jaw M26.Ø9
    - alveolar M26.79
    - lower M26.Ø4
      - alveolar M26.74
    - upper M26.Ø2
      - alveolar M26.73
  - kidney(s) Q6Ø.5
    - bilateral Q6Ø.4
    - unilateral Q6Ø.3
  - labium (majus) (minus), congenital Q52.79
  - larynx Q31.2
  - left heart syndrome Q23.4
  - leg (congenital) — *see* Defect, reduction, lower limb
  - limb Q73.8
    - lower (congenital) — *see* Defect, reduction, lower limb
    - upper (congenital) — *see* Defect, reduction, upper limb
  - liver Q44.7
  - lung (lobe) (not associated with short gestation) Q33.6
    - associated with immaturity, low birth weight, prematurity, or short gestation P28.Ø
  - mammary (areola), congenital Q83.8
  - mandible, mandibular M26.Ø4
    - alveolar M26.74
    - unilateral condylar M27.8
  - maxillary M26.Ø2
    - alveolar M26.73
  - medullary D61.9
  - megakaryocytic D69.49
  - metacarpus — *see* Defect, reduction, upper limb, specified type NEC
  - metatarsus — *see* Defect, reduction, lower limb, specified type NEC
  - muscle Q79.8
  - nail(s) Q84.6
  - nose, nasal Q3Ø.1
  - optic nerve H47.Ø3- ☑
  - osseous meatus (ear) Q17.8
  - ovary, congenital Q5Ø.39
  - pancreas Q45.Ø
  - parathyroid (gland) Q89.2
  - parotid gland Q38.4
  - patella Q74.1
  - pelvis, pelvic girdle Q74.2
  - penis (congenital) Q55.62
  - peripheral vascular system Q27.8
    - digestive system Q27.8
    - lower limb Q27.8
    - specified site NEC Q27.8
    - upper limb Q27.8
  - pituitary (gland) (congenital) Q89.2
  - pulmonary (not associated with short gestation) Q33.6
    - artery, functional J43.Ø
    - associated with short gestation P28.Ø
  - radioulnar — *see* Defect, reduction, upper limb, specified type NEC
  - radius — *see* Defect, reduction, upper limb
  - rectum Q42.1
    - with fistula Q42.Ø
  - respiratory system NEC Q34.8
  - rib Q76.6
  - right heart syndrome Q22.6
  - sacrum Q76.49
  - scapula Q74.Ø
  - scrotum Q55.1
  - shoulder girdle Q74.Ø
  - skin Q82.8
  - skull (bone) Q75.8
    - with
      - anencephaly QØØ.Ø
      - encephalocele — *see* Encephalocele
      - hydrocephalus QØ3.9
        - with spina bifida — *see* Spina bifida, by site, with hydrocephalus
      - microcephaly QØ2
  - spinal (cord) (ventral horn cell) QØ6.1
  - spine Q76.49
  - sternum Q76.7
  - tarsus — *see* Defect, reduction, lower limb, specified type NEC
  - testis Q55.1
  - thymic, with immunodeficiency D82.1
  - thymus (gland) Q89.2
- **Hypoplasia, hypoplastic** — *continued*
  - thymus — *continued*
    - with immunodeficiency D82.1
  - thyroid (gland) EØ3.1
    - cartilage Q31.2
  - tibiofibular (congenital) — *see* Defect, reduction, lower limb, specified type NEC
  - toe — *see* Defect, reduction, lower limb, specified type NEC
  - tongue Q38.3
  - Turner's KØØ.4
  - ulna (congenital) — *see* Defect, reduction, upper limb
  - umbilical artery Q27.Ø
  - unilateral condylar M27.8
  - ureter Q62.8
  - uterus, congenital Q51.811
  - vagina Q52.4
  - vascular NEC peripheral Q27.8
    - brain Q28.3
    - digestive system Q27.8
    - lower limb Q27.8
    - specified site NEC Q27.8
    - upper limb Q27.8
  - vein(s) (peripheral) Q27.8
    - brain Q28.3
    - digestive system Q27.8
    - great Q26.8
    - lower limb Q27.8
    - specified site NEC Q27.8
    - upper limb Q27.8
  - vena cava (inferior) (superior) Q26.8
  - vertebra Q76.49
  - vulva, congenital Q52.79
  - zonule (ciliary) Q12.8
- **Hypoplasminogenemia** E88.Ø2
- **Hypopnea, obstructive sleep apnea** G47.33
- **Hypopotassemia** E87.6
- **Hypoproconvertinemia, congenital** (hereditary) D68.2
- **Hypoproteinemia** E77.8
- **Hypoprothrombinemia** (congenital) (hereditary) (idiopathic) D68.2
  - acquired D68.4
  - newborn, transient P61.6
- **Hypoptyalism** K11.7
- **Hypopyon** (eye) (anterior chamber) — *see* Iridocyclitis, acute, hypopyon
- **Hypopyrexia** R68.Ø
- **Hyporeflexia** R29.2
- **Hyposecretion**
  - ACTH E23.Ø
  - antidiuretic hormone E23.2
  - ovary E28.39
  - salivary gland (any) K11.7
  - vasopressin E23.2
- **Hyposegmentation, leukocytic, hereditary** D72.Ø
- **Hyposiderinemia** D5Ø.9
- **Hypospadias** Q54.9
  - balanic Q54.Ø
  - coronal Q54.Ø
  - glandular Q54.Ø
  - penile Q54.1
  - penoscrotal Q54.2
  - perineal Q54.3
  - specified NEC Q54.8
- **Hypospermatogenesis** — *see* Oligospermia
- **Hyposplenism** D73.Ø
- **Hypostasis pulmonary, passive** — *see* Edema, lung
- **Hypostatic** — *see* condition
- **Hyposthenuria** N28.89
- **Hypotension** (arterial) (constitutional) I95.9
  - chronic I95.89
  - due to (of) hemodialysis I95.3
  - drug-induced I95.2
  - iatrogenic I95.89
  - idiopathic (permanent) I95.Ø
  - intracranial G96.81Ø
    - following
      - lumbar cerebrospinal fluid shunting G97.83
      - specified procedure NEC G97.84
      - ventricular shunting (ventriculostomy) G97.2
    - specified NEC G96.819
    - spontaneous G96.811
  - intra-dialytic I95.3
  - maternal, syndrome (following labor and delivery) O26.5- ☑
  - neurogenic, orthostatic G9Ø.3
  - orthostatic (chronic) I95.1
    - due to drugs I95.2

Hypotension — *continued*
orthostatic — *continued*
neurogenic G9Ø.3
postoperative I95.81
postural I95.1
specified NEC I95.89
Hypothermia (accidental) T68 ☑
due to anesthesia, anesthetic T88.51 ☑
low environmental temperature T68 ☑
neonatal P8Ø.9
environmental (mild) NEC P8Ø.8
mild P8Ø.8
severe (chronic) (cold injury syndrome) P8Ø.Ø
specified NEC P8Ø.8
not associated with low environmental temperature R68.Ø
Hypothyroidism (acquired) EØ3.9
autoimmune — *see* Thyroiditis, autoimmune
congenital (without goiter) EØ3.1
with goiter (diffuse) EØ3.Ø
due to
exogenous substance NEC EØ3.2
iodine-deficiency, acquired EØ1.8
subclinical EØ2
irradiation therapy E89.Ø
medicament NEC EØ3.2
P-aminosalicylic acid (PAS) EØ3.2
phenylbutazone EØ3.2
resorcinol EØ3.2
sulfonamide EØ3.2
surgery E89.Ø
thiourea group drugs EØ3.2
iatrogenic NEC EØ3.2
iodine-deficiency (acquired) EØ1.8
congenital — *see* Syndrome, iodine- deficiency, congenital
subclinical EØ2
neonatal, transitory P72.2
postinfectious EØ3.3
postirradiation E89.Ø
postprocedural E89.Ø
postsurgical E89.Ø
specified NEC EØ3.8
subclinical, iodine-deficiency related EØ2
Hypotonia, hypotonicity, hypotony
bladder N31.2
congenital (benign) P94.2
eye — *see* Disorder, globe, hypotony
Hypotrichosis — *see* Alopecia
Hypotropia H5Ø.2- ☑
Hypoventilation RØ6.89
congenital central alveolar G47.35
sleep related
idiopathic nonobstructive alveolar G47.34
in conditions classified elsewhere G47.36
Hypovitaminosis — *see* Deficiency, vitamin
Hypovolemia E86.1
surgical shock T81.19 ☑
traumatic (shock) T79.4 ☑
Hypoxemia RØ9.Ø2
newborn P84
sleep related, in conditions classified elsewhere G47.36
Hypoxia — *see also* Anoxia RØ9.Ø2
cerebral, during a procedure NEC G97.81
postprocedural NEC G97.82
intrauterine P84
myocardial — *see* Insufficiency, coronary
newborn P84
sleep-related G47.34
Hypsarhythmia — *see* Epilepsy, generalized, specified NEC
Hysteralgia, pregnant uterus O26.89- ☑
Hysteria, hysterical (conversion) (dissociative state) F44.9
anxiety F41.8
convulsions F44.5
psychosis, acute F44.9
Hysteroepilepsy F44.5

I

IBDU (colonic inflammatory bowel dissease unclassified) K52.3
ICANS (immune effector cell-associated neurotoxicity syndrome) — *see* Syndrome, immune effector cell-associated neurotoxicity
Ichthyoparasitism due to Vandellia cirrhosa B88.8
Ichthyosis (congenital) Q8Ø.9
Ichthyosis — *continued*
acquired L85.Ø
fetalis Q8Ø.4
hystrix Q8Ø.8
lamellar Q8Ø.2
lingual K13.29
palmaris and plantaris Q82.8
simplex Q8Ø.Ø
vera Q8Ø.8
vulgaris Q8Ø.Ø
X-linked Q8Ø.1
Ichthyotoxism — *see* Poisoning, fish
bacterial — *see* Intoxication, foodborne
Icteroanemia, hemolytic (acquired) D59.9
congenital — *see* Spherocytosis
Icterus — *see also* Jaundice
conjunctiva R17
gravis, newborn P55.Ø
hematogenous (acquired) D59.9
hemolytic (acquired) D59.9
congenital — *see* Spherocytosis
hemorrhagic (acute) (leptospiral) (spirochetal) A27.Ø
newborn P53
infectious B15.9
with hepatic coma B15.Ø
leptospiral A27.Ø
spirochetal A27.Ø
neonatorum — *see* Jaundice, newborn
newborn P59.9
spirochetal A27.Ø
Ictus solaris, solis T67.Ø1 ☑
Id reaction (due to bacteria) L3Ø.2
Ideation
homicidal R45.85Ø
suicidal R45.851
Identity disorder (child) F64.9
gender role F64.2
psychosexual F64.2
Idioglossia F8Ø.Ø
Idiopathic — *see* condition
Idiot, idiocy (congenital) F73
amaurotic (Bielschowsky(-Jansky)) (family) (infantile (late)) (juvenile (late)) (Vogt-Spielmeyer) E75.4
microcephalic QØ2
IgE asthma J45.9Ø9
IIAC (idiopathic infantile arterial calcification) Q28.8
Ileitis (chronic) (noninfectious) — *see also* Enteritis K52.9
backwash — *see* Pancolitis, ulcerative (chronic)
infectious AØ9
regional (ulcerative) — *see* Enteritis, regional, small intestine
segmental — *see* Enteritis, regional
terminal (ulcerative) — *see* Enteritis, regional, small intestine
Ileocolitis — *see also* Enteritis K52.9
infectious AØ9
regional — *see* Enteritis, regional
ulcerative K51.Ø- ☑
Ileostomy
attention to Z43.2
malfunctioning K94.13
status Z93.2
with complication — *see* Complications, enterostomy
Ileotyphus — *see* Typhoid
Ileum — *see* condition
Ileus (bowel) (colon) (inhibitory) (intestine) K56.7
adynamic K56.Ø
due to gallstone (in intestine) K56.3
duodenal (chronic) K31.5
gallstone K56.3
mechanical NEC — *see also* Obstruction, intestine, specified NEC K56.699
meconium P76.Ø
in cystic fibrosis E84.11
meaning meconium plug (without cystic fibrosis) P76.Ø
myxedema K59.89
neurogenic K56.Ø
Hirschsprung's disease or megacolon Q43.1
newborn
due to meconium P76.Ø
in cystic fibrosis E84.11
meaning meconium plug (without cystic fibrosis) P76.Ø
transitory P76.1
obstructive — *see also* Obstruction, intestine, specified NEC K56.699
Ileus — *continued*
paralytic K56.Ø
postoperative K91.89
Iliac — *see* condition
Iliotibial band syndrome M76.3- ☑
Illiteracy Z55.Ø
Illness — *see also* Disease R69
manic-depressive — *see* Disorder, bipolar
Imbalance R26.89
autonomic G9Ø.8
constituents of food intake E63.1
electrolyte E87.8
with
abortion — *see* Abortion by type, complicated by, electrolyte imbalance
molar pregnancy OØ8.5
due to hyperemesis gravidarum O21.1
following ectopic or molar pregnancy OØ8.5
neonatal, transitory NEC P74.49
potassium
hyperkalemia P74.31
hypokalemia P74.32
sodium
hypernatremia P74.21
hyponatremia P74.22
endocrine E34.9
eye muscle NOS H5Ø.9
hormone E34.9
hysterical F44.4
labyrinth — *see* subcategory H83.2 ☑
posture R29.3
protein-energy — *see* Malnutrition
sympathetic G9Ø.8
Imbecile, imbecility (I.Q. 35-49) F71
Imbedding, intrauterine device T83.39 ☑
Imbibition, cholesterol (gallbladder) K82.4
Imbrication, teeth,, fully erupted M26.3Ø
Imerslund (-Gräsbeck) **syndrome** D51.1
Immature — *see also* Immaturity
birth (less than 37 completed weeks) — *see* Preterm, newborn
extremely (less than 28 completed weeks) — *see* Immaturity, extreme
personality F6Ø.89
Immaturity (less than 37 completed weeks) — *see also* Preterm, newborn
extreme of newborn (less than 28 completed weeks of gestation) (less than 196 completed days of gestation) (unspecified weeks of gestation) PØ7.2Ø
gestational age
23 completed weeks (23 weeks, Ø days through 23 weeks, 6 days) PØ7.22
24 completed weeks (24 weeks, Ø days through 24 weeks, 6 days) PØ7.23
25 completed weeks (25 weeks, Ø days through 25 weeks, 6 days) PØ7.24
26 completed weeks (26 weeks, Ø days through 26 weeks, 6 days) PØ7.25
27 completed weeks (27 weeks, Ø days through 27 weeks, 6 days) PØ7.26
less than 23 completed weeks PØ7.21
fetus or infant light-for-dates — *see* Light-for-dates
lung, newborn P28.Ø
organ or site NEC — *see* Hypoplasia
pulmonary, newborn P28.Ø
reaction F6Ø.89
sexual (female) (male), after puberty E3Ø.Ø
Immersion T75.1 ☑
foot T69.Ø2- ☑
hand T69.Ø1- ☑
Immobile, immobility
complete, due to severe physical disability or frailty R53.2
intestine K59.89
syndrome (paraplegic) M62.3
Immune reconstitution (inflammatory) syndrome [IRIS] D89.3
Immunization — *see also* Vaccination
ABO — *see* Incompatibility, ABO
in newborn P55.1
appropriate for age
child (over 28 days old) ZØØ.129
with abnormal findings ZØØ.121
complication — *see* Complications, vaccination
encounter for Z23
not done (not carried out) — *see also* Underimmunization status Z28.9

Immunization — *continued*
- not done — *see also* Underimmunization status — *continued*
  - because (of)
    - acute illness of patient Z28.Ø1
    - allergy to vaccine (or component) Z28.Ø4
    - caregiver refusal Z28.82
    - chronic illness of patient Z28.Ø2
    - contraindication NEC Z28.Ø9
    - delay in delivery of vaccine Z28.83
    - group pressure Z28.1
    - guardian refusal Z28.82
    - immune compromised state of patient Z28.Ø3
    - lack of availability of vaccine Z28.83
    - manufacturer delay of vaccine Z28.83
    - parent refusal Z28.82
    - patient had disease being vaccinated against Z28.81
    - patient refusal Z28.21
    - patient's belief Z28.1
    - religious beliefs of patient Z28.1
    - specified reason NEC Z28.89
      - of patient Z28.29
    - unavailability of vaccine Z28.83
    - unspecified patient reason Z28.2Ø
- partial — *see also* Underimmunization status
  - for COVID-19 Z28.311
- Rh factor
  - affecting management of pregnancy NEC O36.Ø9- ☑
    - anti-D antibody O36.Ø1- ☑
  - from transfusion — *see* Complication(s), transfusion, incompatibility reaction, Rh (factor)

Immunocompromised NOS D84.9

Immunocytoma C83.Ø- ☑

Immunodeficiency D84.9
- with
  - adenosine-deaminase deficiency — *see also* Deficiency, adenosine deaminase D81.3Ø
  - antibody defects D8Ø.9
    - specified type NEC D8Ø.8
  - hyperimmunoglobulinemia D8Ø.6
  - increased immunoglobulin M (IgM) D8Ø.5
  - major defect D82.9
    - specified type NEC D82.8
  - partial albinism D82.8
  - short-limbed stature D82.2
  - thrombocytopenia and eczema D82.Ø
- antibody with
  - hyperimmunoglobulinemia D8Ø.6
  - near-normal immunoglobulins D8Ø.6
- autosomal recessive, Swiss type D8Ø.Ø
- combined D81.9
  - biotin-dependent carboxylase D81.819
    - biotinidase D81.81Ø
    - holocarboxylase synthetase D81.818
    - specified type NEC D81.818
  - severe (SCID) D81.9
    - with
      - low or normal B-cell numbers D81.2
      - low T- and B-cell numbers D81.1
      - reticular dysgenesis D81.Ø
  - specified type NEC D81.89
- common variable D83.9
  - with
    - abnormalities of B-cell numbers and function D83.Ø
    - autoantibodies to B- or T-cells D83.2
    - immunoregulatory T-cell disorders D83.1
  - specified type NEC D83.8
- due to
  - conditions classified elsewhere D84.81
  - drugs D84.821
  - external causes D84.822
  - medication (current or past) D84.821
- following hereditary defective response to Epstein-Barr virus (EBV) D82.3
- selective, immunoglobulin
  - A (IgA) D8Ø.2
  - G (IgG) (subclasses) D8Ø.3
  - M (IgM) D8Ø.4
- severe combined (SCID) D81.9
  - due to adenosine deaminase deficiency D81.31
- specified type NEC D84.89
- X-linked, with increased IgM D8Ø.5

Immunodeficient NOS D84.9

Immunosuppressed NOS D84.9

Immunotherapy (encounter for)
- antineoplastic Z51.12

Impaction, impacted
- bowel, colon, rectum — *see also* Impaction, fecal K56.49
  - by gallstone K56.3
- calculus — *see* Calculus
- cerumen (ear) (external) H61.2- ☑
- cuspid — *see* Impaction, tooth
- dental (same or adjacent tooth) KØ1.1
- fecal, feces K56.41
- fracture — *see* Fracture, by site
- gallbladder — *see* Calculus, gallbladder
- gallstone(s) — *see* Calculus, gallbladder
  - bile duct (common) (hepatic) — *see* Calculus, bile duct
  - cystic duct — *see* Calculus, gallbladder
  - in intestine, with obstruction (any part) K56.3
- intestine (calculous) NEC — *see also* Impaction, fecal K56.49
  - gallstone, with ileus K56.3
- intrauterine device (IUD) T83.39 ☑
- molar — *see* Impaction, tooth
- shoulder, causing obstructed labor O66.Ø
- tooth, teeth KØ1.1
- turbinate J34.89

Impaired, impairment (function)
- auditory discrimination — *see* Abnormal, auditory perception
- cognitive, mild, of uncertain or unknown etiology G31.84
- dual sensory Z73.82
- fasting glucose R73.Ø1
- glucose tolerance (oral) R73.Ø2
- hearing — *see* Deafness
- heart — *see* Disease, heart
- kidney N28.9
  - disorder resulting from N25.9
    - specified NEC N25.89
- liver K72.9Ø
  - with coma K72.91
- mastication KØ8.89
- mild cognitive G31.84
  - of uncertain or unknown etiology G31.84
- mild neurocognitive
  - due to known physiological condition (without behavioral disturbance) FØ6.7Ø
    - with behavioral disturbance FØ6.71
- mobility
  - ear ossicles — *see* Ankylosis, ear ossicles
  - requiring care provider Z74.Ø9
- myocardium, myocardial — *see* Insufficiency, myocardial
- rectal sphincter R19.8
- renal (acute) (chronic) N28.9
  - disorder resulting from N25.9
    - specified NEC N25.89
- vision NEC H54.7
  - both eyes H54.3

Impediment, speech — *see also* Disorder, speech R47.9
- psychogenic (childhood) F98.8
- slurring R47.81
- specified NEC R47.89

Impending
- coronary syndrome I2Ø.Ø
- delirium tremens F1Ø.239
- myocardial infarction I2Ø.Ø

Imperception auditory (acquired) — *see also* Deafness
- congenital H93.25

Imperfect
- aeration, lung (newborn) NEC — *see* Atelectasis
- closure (congenital)
  - alimentary tract NEC Q45.8
    - lower Q43.8
    - upper Q4Ø.8
  - atrioventricular ostium Q21.2Ø
  - atrium (secundum) Q21.11
  - branchial cleft NOS Q18.2
    - cyst Q18.Ø
    - fistula Q18.Ø
    - sinus Q18.Ø
  - choroid Q14.3
  - cricoid cartilage Q31.8
  - cusps, heart valve NEC Q24.8
    - pulmonary Q22.3
  - ductus
    - arteriosus Q25.Ø
    - Botalli Q25.Ø
  - ear drum (causing impairment of hearing) Q16.4

Imperfect — *continued*
- closure — *continued*
  - esophagus with communication to bronchus or trachea Q39.1
  - eyelid Q1Ø.3
  - foramen
    - botalli Q21.12
    - ovale Q21.12
  - genitalia, genital organ(s) or system
    - female Q52.8
      - external Q52.79
      - internal NEC Q52.8
    - male Q55.8
  - glottis Q31.8
  - interatrial ostium or septum Q21.19
  - interauricular ostium or septum Q21.19
  - interventricular ostium or septum Q21.Ø
  - larynx Q31.8
  - lip — *see* Cleft, lip
  - nasal septum Q3Ø.3
  - nose Q3Ø.2
  - omphalomesenteric duct Q43.Ø
  - optic nerve entry Q14.2
  - organ or site not listed — *see* Anomaly, by site
  - ostium
    - interatrial Q21.19
    - interauricular Q21.19
    - interventricular Q21.Ø
  - palate — *see* Cleft, palate
  - preauricular sinus Q18.1
  - retina Q14.1
  - roof of orbit Q75.8
  - sclera Q13.5
  - septum
    - aorticopulmonary Q21.4
    - atrial (secundum) Q21.19
    - between aorta and pulmonary artery Q21.4
    - heart Q21.9
    - interatrial (secundum) Q21.19
    - interauricular (secundum) Q21.19
    - interventricular Q21.Ø
      - in tetralogy of Fallot Q21.3
    - nasal Q3Ø.3
    - ventricular Q21.Ø
      - with pulmonary stenosis or atresia, dextraposition of aorta, and hypertrophy of right ventricle Q21.3
      - in tetralogy of Fallot Q21.3
  - skull Q75.Ø
    - with
      - anencephaly QØØ.Ø
      - encephalocele — *see* Encephalocele
      - hydrocephalus QØ3.9
        - with spina bifida — *see* Spina bifida, by site, with hydrocephalus
      - microcephaly QØ2
  - spine (with meningocele) — *see* Spina bifida
  - trachea Q32.1
  - tympanic membrane (causing impairment of hearing) Q16.4
  - uterus Q51.818
  - vitelline duct Q43.Ø
- erection — *see* Dysfunction, sexual, male, erectile
- fusion — *see* Imperfect, closure
- inflation, lung (newborn) — *see* Atelectasis
- posture R29.3
- rotation, intestine Q43.3
- septum, ventricular Q21.Ø

Imperfectly descended testis — *see* Cryptorchid

Imperforate (congenital) — *see also* Atresia
- anus Q42.3
  - with fistula Q42.2
- cervix (uteri) Q51.828
- esophagus Q39.Ø
  - with tracheoesophageal fistula Q39.1
- hymen Q52.3
- jejunum Q41.1
- pharynx Q38.8
- rectum Q42.1
  - with fistula Q42.Ø
- urethra Q64.39
- vagina Q52.4

Impervious (congenital) — *see also* Atresia
- anus Q42.3
  - with fistula Q42.2
- bile duct Q44.2
- esophagus Q39.Ø
  - with tracheoesophageal fistula Q39.1

- **Impervious** — *continued*
  - intestine (small) Q41.9
    - large Q42.9
      - specified NEC Q42.8
  - rectum Q42.1
    - with fistula Q42.Ø
  - ureter — *see* Atresia, ureter
  - urethra Q64.39
- **Impetiginization of dermatoses** LØ1.1
- **Impetigo** (any organism) (any site) (circinate) (contagiosa) (simplex) (vulgaris) LØ1.ØØ
  - Bockhart's LØ1.Ø2
  - bullous, bullosa LØ1.Ø3
  - external ear LØ1.ØØ *[H62.4Ø]*
  - follicularis LØ1.Ø2
  - furfuracea L3Ø.5
  - herpetiformis L4Ø.1
    - nonobstetrical L4Ø.1
  - neonatorum LØ1.Ø3
  - nonbullous LØ1.Ø1
  - specified type NEC LØ1.Ø9
  - ulcerative LØ1.Ø9
- **Impingement** (on teeth)
  - joint — *see* Disorder, joint, specified type NEC
  - soft tissue
    - anterior M26.81
    - posterior M26.82
- **Implant, endometrial** N8Ø.9
- **Implantation**
  - anomalous — *see* Anomaly, by site
    - ureter Q62.63
  - cyst
    - external area or site (skin) NEC L72.Ø
    - iris — *see* Cyst, iris, implantation
    - vagina N89.8
    - vulva N9Ø.7
  - dermoid (cyst) — *see* Implantation, cyst
- **Impotence** (sexual) N52.9
  - counseling Z7Ø.1
  - organic origin — *see also* Dysfunction, sexual, male, erectile N52.9
  - psychogenic F52.21
- **Impression, basilar** Q75.8
- **Imprisonment, anxiety concerning** Z65.1
- **Improper care** (child) (newborn) — *see* Maltreatment
- **Improperly tied umbilical cord** (causing hemorrhage) P51.8
- **Impulsiveness** (impulsive) R45.87
- **Inability to swallow** — *see* Aphagia
  - comply with dietary regimen Z91.118
  - swallow — *see* Aphagia
- **Inaccessible, inaccessibility**
  - health care NEC Z75.3
    - due to
      - waiting period Z75.2
        - for admission to facility elsewhere Z75.1
  - other helping agencies Z75.4
  - transportation Z59.82
- **Inactive** — *see* condition
- **Inadequate, inadequacy**
  - aesthetics of dental restoration KØ8.56
  - biologic, constitutional, functional, or social F6Ø.7
  - development
    - child R62.5Ø
    - genitalia
      - after puberty NEC E3Ø.Ø
      - congenital
        - female Q52.8
          - external Q52.79
          - internal Q52.8
        - male Q55.8
    - lungs Q33.6
      - associated with short gestation P28.Ø
    - organ or site not listed — *see* Anomaly, by site
  - diet (causing nutritional deficiency) E63.9
  - drinking-water supply Z58.6
  - eating habits Z72.4
  - environment, household Z59.1
  - family support Z63.8
  - food (supply) NEC Z59.48
    - hunger effects T73.Ø ☑
  - functional F6Ø.7
  - household care, due to
    - family member
      - handicapped or ill Z74.2
      - on vacation Z75.5
      - temporarily away from home Z74.2
    - technical defects in home Z59.1
- **Inadequate, inadequacy** — *continued*
  - household care, due to — *continued*
    - temporary absence from home of person rendering care Z74.2
  - housing (heating) (space) Z59.1
  - income (financial) Z59.6
  - intrafamilial communication Z63.8
  - material resources Z59.87
  - mental — *see* Disability, intellectual
  - parental supervision or control of child Z62.Ø
  - personality F6Ø.7
  - pulmonary
    - function RØ6.89
      - newborn P28.5
    - ventilation, newborn P28.5
  - sample of cytologic smear
    - anus R85.615
    - cervix R87.615
    - vagina R87.625
  - social F6Ø.7
    - insurance Z59.7
    - skills NEC Z73.4
  - supervision of child by parent Z62.Ø
  - teaching affecting education Z55.8
  - transportation Z59.82
  - welfare support Z59.7
- **Inanition** R64
  - with edema — *see* Malnutrition, severe
  - due to
    - deprivation of food T73.Ø ☑
    - malnutrition — *see* Malnutrition
  - fever R5Ø.9
- **Inappropriate**
  - change in quantitative human chorionic gonadotropin (hCG) in early pregnancy OØ2.81
  - diet or eating habits Z72.4
  - level of quantitative human chorionic gonadotropin (hCG) for gestational age in early pregnancy OØ2.81
  - secretion
    - antidiuretic hormone (ADH) (excessive) E22.2
      - deficiency E23.2
    - pituitary (posterior) E22.2
- **Inattention at or after birth** — *see* Neglect
- **Incarceration, incarcerated**
  - enterocele K46.Ø
    - gangrenous K46.1
  - epiplocele K46.Ø
    - gangrenous K46.1
  - exomphalos K42.Ø
    - gangrenous K42.1
  - hernia — *see also* Hernia, by site, with obstruction
    - with gangrene — *see* Hernia, by site, with gangrene
  - iris, in wound — *see* Injury, eye, laceration, with prolapse
  - lens, in wound — *see* Injury, eye, laceration, with prolapse
  - omphalocele K42.Ø
  - prison, anxiety concerning Z65.1
  - rupture — *see* Hernia, by site
  - sarcoepiplocele K46.Ø
    - gangrenous K46.1
  - sarcoepiplomphalocele K42.Ø
    - with gangrene K42.1
  - uterus N85.8
    - gravid O34.51- ☑
      - causing obstructed labor O65.5
- **Incised wound**
  - external — *see* Laceration
  - internal organs — *see* Injury, by site
- **Incision, incisional**
  - hernia K43.2
    - with
      - gangrene (and obstruction) K43.1
      - obstruction K43.Ø
  - surgical, complication — *see* Complications, surgical procedure
  - traumatic
    - external — *see* Laceration
    - internal organs — *see* Injury, by site
- **Inclusion**
  - azurophilic leukocytic D72.Ø
  - blennorrhea (neonatal) (newborn) P39.1
  - gallbladder in liver (congenital) Q44.1
- **Incompatibility**
  - ABO
    - affecting management of pregnancy O36.11- ☑
      - anti-A sensitization O36.11- ☑
- **Incompatibility** — *continued*
  - ABO — *continued*
    - affecting management of pregnancy — *continued*
      - anti-B sensitization O36.19- ☑
      - specified NEC O36.19- ☑
    - infusion or transfusion reaction — *see* Complication(s), transfusion, incompatibility reaction, ABO
    - newborn P55.1
  - blood (group) (Duffy) (K) (Kell) (Kidd) (Lewis) (M) (S) NEC
    - affecting management of pregnancy O36.11- ☑
      - anti-A sensitization O36.11- ☑
      - anti-B sensitization O36.19- ☑
    - infusion or transfusion reaction T8Ø.89 ☑
    - newborn P55.8
  - divorce or estrangement Z63.5
  - Rh (blood group) (factor) Z31.82
    - affecting management of pregnancy NEC O36.Ø9- ☑
      - anti-D antibody O36.Ø1- ☑
    - infusion or transfusion reaction — *see* Complication(s), transfusion, incompatibility reaction, Rh (factor)
    - newborn P55.Ø
  - rhesus — *see* Incompatibility, Rh
- **Incompetency, incompetent, incompetence**
  - annular
    - aortic (valve) — *see* Insufficiency, aortic
    - mitral (valve) I34.Ø
    - pulmonary valve (heart) I37.1
  - aortic (valve) — *see* Insufficiency, aortic
  - cardiac valve — *see* Endocarditis
  - cervix, cervical (os) N88.3
    - in pregnancy O34.3- ☑
  - chronotropic I45.89
    - with
      - autonomic dysfunction G9Ø.8
      - ischemic heart disease I25.89
      - left ventricular dysfunction I51.89
      - sinus node dysfunction I49.8
  - esophagogastric (junction) (sphincter) K22.Ø
  - mitral (valve) — *see* Insufficiency, mitral
  - pelvic fundus N81.89
  - pubocervical tissue N81.82
  - pulmonary valve (heart) I37.1
    - congenital Q22.3
  - rectovaginal tissue N81.83
  - tricuspid (annular) (valve) — *see* Insufficiency, tricuspid
  - valvular — *see* Endocarditis
    - congenital Q24.8
  - vein, venous (saphenous) (varicose) — *see* Varix, leg
- **Incomplete** — *see also* condition
  - atrioventricular
    - canal Q21.21
    - septal defect Q21.21
  - bladder, emptying R33.9
  - defecation R15.Ø
  - endocardial cushion defect Q21.21
  - expansion lungs (newborn) NEC — *see* Atelectasis
  - rotation, intestine Q43.3
- **Inconclusive**
  - diagnostic imaging due to excess body fat of patient R93.9
  - findings on diagnostic imaging of breast NEC R92.8
  - mammogram (due to dense breasts) R92.2
- **Incontinence** R32
  - anal sphincter R15.9
  - coital N39.491
  - feces R15.9
    - nonorganic origin F98.1
  - insensible (urinary) N39.42
  - overflow N39.49Ø
  - postural (urinary) N39.492
  - psychogenic F45.8
  - rectal R15.9
  - reflex N39.498
  - stress (female) (male) N39.3
    - and urge N39.46
  - urethral sphincter R32
  - urge N39.41
    - and stress (female) (male) N39.46
  - urine (urinary) R32
    - continuous N39.45
    - due to cognitive impairment, or severe physical disability or immobility R39.81
    - functional R39.81
    - insensible N39.42

- **Incontinence** — *continued*
  - urine — *continued*
    - mixed (stress and urge) N39.46
    - nocturnal N39.44
    - nonorganic origin F98.Ø
    - overflow N39.49Ø
    - post dribbling N39.43
    - postural N39.492
    - reflex N39.498
    - specified NEC N39.498
    - stress (female) (male) N39.3
      - and urge N39.46
    - total N39.498
    - unaware N39.42
    - urge N39.41
      - and stress (female) (male) N39.46
- **Incontinentia pigmenti** Q82.3
- **Incoordinate, incoordination**
  - esophageal-pharyngeal (newborn) — *see* Dysphagia
  - muscular R27.8
  - uterus (action) (contractions) (complicating delivery) O62.4
- **Increase, increased**
  - abnormal, in development R63.8
  - androgens (ovarian) E28.1
  - anticoagulants (antithrombin) (anti-VIIIa) (anti-IXa) (anti-Xa) (anti-XIa) — *see* Circulating anticoagulants
  - cold sense R2Ø.8
  - estrogen E28.Ø
  - function
    - adrenal
      - cortex — *see* Cushing's, syndrome
      - medulla E27.5
    - pituitary (gland) (anterior) (lobe) E22.9
      - posterior E22.2
  - heat sense R2Ø.8
  - intracranial pressure (benign) G93.2
  - permeability, capillaries I78.8
  - pressure, intracranial G93.2
  - secretion
    - gastrin E16.4
    - glucagon E16.3
    - pancreas, endocrine E16.9
      - growth hormone-releasing hormone E16.8
      - pancreatic polypeptide E16.8
      - somatostatin E16.8
      - vasoactive-intestinal polypeptide E16.8
  - sphericity, lens Q12.4
  - splenic activity D73.1
  - venous pressure I87.8
    - portal K76.6
- **Increta placenta** O43.22- ☑
- **Incrustation, cornea, foreign body** (lead)(zinc) — *see* Foreign body, cornea
- **Incyclophoria** H5Ø.54
- **Incyclotropia** — *see* Cyclotropia
- **Indeterminate sex** Q56.4
- **India rubber skin** Q82.8
- **Indigestion** (acid) (bilious) (functional) K3Ø
  - catarrhal K31.89
  - due to decomposed food NOS AØ5.9
  - nervous F45.8
  - psychogenic F45.8
- **Indirect** — *see* condition
- **Induratio penis plastica** N48.6
- **Induration, indurated**
  - brain G93.89
  - breast (fibrous) N64.51
    - puerperal, postpartum O92.29
  - broad ligament N83.8
  - chancre
    - anus A51.1
    - congenital A5Ø.Ø7
    - extragenital NEC A51.2
  - corpora cavernosa (penis) (plastic) N48.6
  - liver (chronic) K76.89
  - lung (black) (chronic) (fibroid) — *see also* Fibrosis, lung J84.1Ø
    - essential brown J84.Ø3
  - penile (plastic) N48.6
  - phlebitic — *see* Phlebitis
  - skin R23.4
- **Inebriety** (without dependence) — *see* Alcohol, intoxication
- **Inefficiency, kidney** N28.9
- **Inelasticity, skin** R23.4
- **Inequality, leg** (length) (acquired) — *see also* Deformity, limb, unequal length
  - congenital — *see* Defect, reduction, lower limb
  - lower leg — *see* Deformity, limb, unequal length
- **Inertia**
  - bladder (neurogenic) N31.2
  - stomach K31.89
    - psychogenic F45.8
  - uterus, uterine during labor O62.2
    - during latent phase of labor O62.Ø
    - primary O62.Ø
    - secondary O62.1
  - vesical (neurogenic) N31.2
- **Infancy, infantile, infantilism** — *see also* condition
  - celiac K9Ø.Ø
  - genitalia, genitals (after puberty) E3Ø.Ø
  - Herter's (nontropical sprue) K9Ø.Ø
  - intestinal K9Ø.Ø
  - Lorain E23.Ø
  - pancreatic K86.89
  - pelvis M95.5
    - with disproportion (fetopelvic) O33.1
      - causing obstructed labor O65.1
  - pituitary E23.Ø
  - renal N25.Ø
  - uterus — *see* Infantile, genitalia
- **Infant**(s) — *see also* Infancy
  - excessive crying R68.11
  - irritable child R68.12
  - lack of care — *see* Neglect
  - liveborn (singleton) Z38.2
    - born in hospital Z38.ØØ
      - by cesarean Z38.Ø1
    - born outside hospital Z38.1
    - multiple NEC Z38.8
      - born in hospital Z38.68
        - by cesarean Z38.69
      - born outside hospital Z38.7
    - quadruplet Z38.8
      - born in hospital Z38.63
        - by cesarean Z38.64
      - born outside hospital Z38.7
    - quintuplet Z38.8
      - born in hospital Z38.65
        - by cesarean Z38.66
      - born outside hospital Z38.7
    - triplet Z38.8
      - born in hospital Z38.61
        - by cesarean Z38.62
      - born outside hospital Z38.7
    - twin Z38.5
      - born in hospital Z38.3Ø
        - by cesarean Z38.31
      - born outside hospital Z38.4
  - of diabetic mother (syndrome of) P7Ø.1
    - gestational diabetes P7Ø.Ø
- **Infantile** — *see also* condition
  - genitalia, genitals E3Ø.Ø
  - os, uterine E3Ø.Ø
  - penis E3Ø.Ø
  - testis E29.1
  - uterus E3Ø.Ø
- **Infantilism** — *see* Infancy
- **Infarct, infarction**
  - adrenal (capsule) (gland) E27.49
  - appendices epiploicae — *see also* Infarct, intestine K55.Ø69
  - bowel — *see also* Infarct, intestine K55.Ø69
  - brain (stem) — *see* Infarct, cerebral
  - breast N64.89
  - brewer's (kidney) N28.Ø
  - cardiac — *see* Infarct, myocardium
  - cerebellar — *see* Infarct, cerebral
  - cerebral (acute) (chronic) — *see also* Occlusion, artery cerebral or precerebral, with infarction I63.9-
    - aborted I63.9
    - cortical I63.9
    - due to
      - cerebral venous thrombosis, nonpyogenic I63.6
      - embolism
        - cerebral arteries I63.4- ☑
        - precerebral arteries I63.1- ☑
      - occlusion NEC
        - cerebral arteries I63.5- ☑
        - precerebral arteries I63.2- ☑
        - small artery I63.81
      - stenosis NEC
        - cerebral arteries I63.5- ☑

- **Infarct, infarction** — *continued*
  - cerebral — *see also* Occlusion, artery cerebral or precerebral, with infarction — *continued*
    - due to — *continued*
      - stenosis — *continued*
        - precerebral arteries I63.2- ☑
        - small artery I63.81
      - thrombosis
        - cerebral artery I63.3- ☑
        - precerebral artery I63.Ø- ☑
    - intraoperative
      - during cardiac surgery I97.81Ø
      - during other surgery I97.811
    - neonatal P91.82- ☑
    - perinatal (arterial ischemic) P91.82- ☑
    - postprocedural
      - following cardiac surgery I97.82Ø
      - following other surgery I97.821
    - specified NEC I63.89
  - colon (acute) (agnogenic) (embolic) (hemorrhagic) (nonocclusive) (nonthrombotic) (occlusive) (segmental) (thrombotic) (with gangrene) — *see also* Infarct, intestine K55.Ø49
  - coronary artery — *see* Infarct, myocardium
  - embolic — *see* Embolism
  - fallopian tube N83.8
  - gallbladder K82.8
  - heart — *see* Infarct, myocardium
  - hepatic K76.3
  - hypophysis (anterior lobe) E23.6
  - impending (myocardium) I2Ø.Ø
  - intestine (acute) (agnogenic) (embolic) (hemorrhagic) (nonocclusive) (nonthrombotic) (occlusive) (thrombotic) (with gangrene) K55.Ø69
    - diffuse K55.Ø62
    - focal K55.Ø61
    - large K55.Ø49
      - diffuse K55.Ø42
      - focal K55.Ø41
    - small K55.Ø29
      - diffuse K55.Ø22
      - focal K55.Ø21
  - kidney N28.Ø
  - lacunar I63.81
  - liver K76.3
  - lung (embolic) (thrombotic) — *see* Embolism, pulmonary
  - lymph node I89.8
  - mesentery, mesenteric (embolic) (thrombotic) (with gangrene) — *see also* Infarct, intestine K55.Ø69
  - muscle (ischemic) M62.2Ø
    - ankle M62.27- ☑
    - foot M62.27- ☑
    - forearm M62.23- ☑
    - hand M62.24- ☑
    - lower leg M62.26- ☑
    - pelvic region M62.25- ☑
    - shoulder region M62.21- ☑
    - specified site NEC M62.28
    - thigh M62.25- ☑
    - upper arm M62.22- ☑
  - myocardium, myocardial (acute) (with stated duration of 4 weeks or less) I21.9
    - associated with revascularization procedure I21.A9
    - diagnosed on ECG, but presenting no symptoms I25.2
    - due to
      - demand ischemia I21.A1
      - ischemic imbalance I21.A1
    - healed or old I25.2
    - intraoperative — *see also* Infarct, myocardium, associated with revascularization procedure
      - during cardiac surgery I97.79Ø
      - during other surgery I97.791
    - non-Q wave I21.4
    - non-ST elevation (NSTEMI) I21.4
      - subsequent I22.2
    - nontransmural I21.4
    - past (diagnosed on ECG or other investigation, but currently presenting no symptoms) I25.2
    - postprocedural — *see also* Infarct, myocardium, associated with revascularization procedure
      - following cardiac surgery — *see also* Infarct, myocardium, type 4 or type 5 I97.19Ø
      - following other surgery I97.191
    - Q wave (*see also* Infarct, myocardium, by site) I21.3
    - secondary to
      - demand ischemia I21.A1

Infarct, infarction — *continued*
  myocardium, myocardial — *continued*
    secondary to — *continued*
      ischemic imbalance I21.A1
    ST elevation (STEMI) I21.3
      anterior (anteroapical) (anterolateral) (anteroseptal) (Q wave) (wall) I21.Ø9
        subsequent I22.Ø
      inferior (diaphragmatic) (inferolateral) (inferoposterior) (wall) NEC I21.19
        subsequent I22.1
      inferoposterior transmural (Q wave) I21.11
      involving
        coronary artery of anterior wall NEC I21.Ø9
        coronary artery of inferior wall NEC I21.19
        diagonal coronary artery I21.Ø2
        left anterior descending coronary artery I21.Ø2
        left circumflex coronary artery I21.21
        left main coronary artery I21.Ø1
        oblique marginal coronary artery I21.21
        right coronary artery I21.11
      lateral (apical-lateral) (basal-lateral) (high) I21.29
        subsequent I22.8
      posterior (posterobasal) (posterolateral) (posteroseptal) (true) I21.29
        subsequent I22.8
      septal I21.29
        subsequent I22.8
      specified NEC I21.29
        subsequent I22.8
      subsequent I22.9
    subsequent (recurrent) (reinfarction) I22.9
      anterior (anteroapical) (anterolateral) (anteroseptal) (wall) I22.Ø
      diaphragmatic (wall) I22.1
      inferior (diaphragmatic) (inferolateral) (inferoposterior) (wall) I22.1
      lateral (apical-lateral) (basal-lateral) (high) I22.8
      non-ST elevation (NSTEMI) I22.2
      posterior (posterobasal) (posterolateral) (posteroseptal) (true) I22.8
      septal I22.8
      specified NEC I22.8
      ST elevation I22.9
        anterior (anteroapical) (anterolateral) (anteroseptal) (wall) I22.Ø
        inferior (diaphragmatic) (inferolateral) (inferoposterior) (wall) I22.1
        specified NEC I22.8
      subendocardial I22.2
      transmural I22.9
        anterior (anteroapical) (anterolateral) (anteroseptal) (wall) I22.Ø
        diaphragmatic (wall) I22.1
        inferior (diaphragmatic) (inferolateral) (inferoposterior) (wall) I22.1
        lateral (apical-lateral) (basal-lateral) (high) I22.8
        posterior (posterobasal) (posterolateral) (posteroseptal) (true) I22.8
        specified NEC I22.8
      type 1 — *see also* Infarction, myocardial, subsequent, by site, or by ST elevation or non-ST elevation I22.9
      type 2 I21.A1
      type 3 I21.A9
      type 4 I21.A9
      type 5 I21.A9
    syphilitic A52.Ø6
    transmural I21.9
      anterior (anteroapical) (anterolateral) (anteroseptal) (Q wave) (wall) NEC I21.Ø9
      inferior (diaphragmatic) (inferolateral) (inferoposterior) (Q wave) (wall) NEC I21.19
      inferoposterior (Q wave) I21.11
      lateral (apical-lateral) (basal-lateral) (high) NEC I21.29
      posterior (posterobasal) (posterolateral) (posteroseptal) (true) NEC I21.29
      septal NEC I21.29
      specified NEC I21.29
    type 1 — *see also* Infarction, myocardial, by site, or by ST elevation or non-ST elevation I21.9
    type 2 I21.A1
    type 3 I21.A9
    type 4 (a) (b) (c) I21.A9
    type 5 I21.A9
  nontransmural I21.4
  omentum — *see also* Infarct, intestine K55.Ø69

Infarct, infarction — *continued*
  ovary N83.8
  pancreas K86.89
  papillary muscle — *see* Infarct, myocardium
  parathyroid gland E21.4
  pituitary (gland) E23.6
  placenta O43.81- ☑
  prostate N42.89
  pulmonary (artery) (vein) (hemorrhagic) — *see* Embolism, pulmonary
  renal (embolic) (thrombotic) N28.Ø
  retina, retinal (artery) — *see* Occlusion, artery, retina
  spinal (cord) (acute) (embolic) (nonembolic) G95.11
  spleen D73.5
    embolic or thrombotic I74.8
  subendocardial (acute) (nontransmural) I21.4
  suprarenal (capsule) (gland) E27.49
  testis N5Ø.1
  thrombotic — *see also* Thrombosis
    artery, arterial — *see* Embolism
  thyroid (gland) EØ7.89
  ventricle (heart) — *see* Infarct, myocardium
Infecting — *see* condition
Infection, infected, infective (opportunistic) B99.9
  with
    drug resistant organism — *see* Resistance (to), drug — *see also* specific organism
    lymphangitis — *see* Lymphangitis
    organ dysfunction (acute) R65.2Ø
      with septic shock R65.21
  abscess (skin) — *code by* site under Abscess
  Absidia — *see* Mucormycosis
  Acanthamoeba — *see* Acanthamebiasis
  Acanthocheilonema (perstans) (streptocerca) B74.4
  accessory sinus (chronic) — *see* Sinusitis
  achorion — *see* Dermatophytosis
  Acremonium falciforme B47.Ø
  acromioclavicular MØØ.9
  Actinobacillus (actinomycetem-comitans) A28.8
    mallei A24.Ø
    muris A25.1
  Actinomadura B47.1
  Actinomyces (israelii) — *see also* Actinomycosis A42.9
  Actinomycetales — *see* Actinomycosis
  actinomycotic NOS — *see* Actinomycosis
  adenoid (and tonsil) JØ3.9Ø
    chronic J35.Ø2
  adenovirus NEC
    as cause of disease classified elsewhere B97.Ø
    unspecified nature or site B34.Ø
  aerogenes capsulatus A48.Ø
  aertrycke — *see* Infection, salmonella
  alimentary canal NOS — *see* Enteritis, infectious
  Allescheria boydii B48.2
  Alternaria B48.8
  alveolus, alveolar (process) KØ4.7
  Ameba, amebic (histolytica) — *see* Amebiasis
  amniotic fluid, sac or cavity O41.1Ø- ☑
    chorioamnionitis O41.12- ☑
    placentitis O41.14- ☑
  amputation stump (surgical) — *see* Complication, amputation stump, infection
  Ancylostoma (duodenalis) B76.Ø
  Anisakiasis, Anisakis larvae B81.Ø
  anthrax — *see* Anthrax
  antrum (chronic) — *see* Sinusitis, maxillary
  anus, anal (papillae) (sphincter) K62.89
  arbovirus (arbor virus) A94
    specified type NEC A93.8
  artificial insemination N98.Ø
  Ascaris lumbricoides — *see* Ascariasis
  Ascomycetes B47.Ø
  Aspergillus (flavus) (fumigatus) (terreus) — *see* Aspergillosis
  atypical
    acid-fast (bacilli) — *see* Mycobacterium, atypical
    mycobacteria — *see* Mycobacterium, atypical
    virus A81.9
      specified type NEC A81.89
  auditory meatus (external) — *see* Otitis, externa, infective
  auricle (ear) — *see* Otitis, externa, infective
  axillary gland (lymph) LØ4.2
  Bacillus A49.9
    abortus A23.1
    anthracis — *see* Anthrax
    Ducrey's (any location) A57
    Flexner's AØ3.1

Infection, infected, infective — *continued*
  Bacillus — *continued*
    Friedländer's NEC A49.8
    gas (gangrene) A48.Ø
    mallei A24.Ø
    melitensis A23.Ø
    paratyphoid, paratyphosus AØ1.4
      A AØ1.1
      B AØ1.2
      C AØ1.3
    Shiga (-Kruse) AØ3.Ø
    suipestifer — *see* Infection, salmonella
    swimming pool A31.1
    typhosa AØ1.ØØ
    welchii — *see* Gangrene, gas
  bacterial NOS A49.9
    as cause of disease classified elsewhere B96.89
      Bacteroides fragilis [B. fragilis] B96.6
      Clostridium perfringens [C. perfringens] B96.7
      Enterobacter sakazakii B96.89
      Enterococcus B95.2
      Escherichia coli [E. coli] — *see also* Escherichia coli B96.2Ø
      Helicobacter pylori [H.pylori] B96.81
      Hemophilus influenzae [H. influenzae] B96.3
      Klebsiella pneumoniae [K. pneumoniae] B96.1
      Mycoplasma pneumoniae [M. pneumoniae] B96.Ø
      Proteus (mirabilis) (morganii) B96.4
      Pseudomonas (aeruginosa) (mallei) (pseudomallei) B96.5
      Staphylococcus B95.8
        aureus (methicillin susceptible) (MSSA) B95.61
          methicillin resistant (MRSA) B95.62
        specified NEC B95.7
      Streptococcus B95.5
        group A B95.Ø
        group B B95.1
        pneumoniae B95.3
        specified NEC B95.4
      Vibrio vulnificus B96.82
    specified NEC A48.8
  Bacterium
    paratyphosum AØ1.4
      A AØ1.1
      B AØ1.2
      C AØ1.3
    typhosum AØ1.ØØ
  Bacteroides NEC A49.8
    fragilis, as cause of disease classified elsewhere B96.6
  Balantidium coli AØ7.Ø
  Bartholin's gland N75.8
  Basidiobolus B46.8
  bile duct (common) (hepatic) — *see* Cholangitis
  bladder — *see* Cystitis
  Blastomyces, blastomycotic — *see also* Blastomycosis
    brasiliensis — *see* Paracoccidioidomycosis
    dermatitidis — *see* Blastomycosis
    European — *see* Cryptococcosis
    Loboi B48.Ø
    North American B4Ø.9
    South American — *see* Paracoccidioidomycosis
  bleb, postprocedure — *see* Blebitis
  bone — *see* Osteomyelitis
  Bordetella — *see* Whooping cough
  Borrelia bergdorfi A69.2Ø
  brain — *see also* Encephalitis GØ4.9Ø
    membranes — *see* Meningitis
    septic GØ6.Ø
      meninges — *see* Meningitis, bacterial
  branchial cyst Q18.Ø
  breast — *see* Mastitis
  bronchus — *see* Bronchitis
  Brucella A23.9
    abortus A23.1
    canis A23.3
    melitensis A23.Ø
    mixed A23.8
    specified NEC A23.8
    suis A23.2
  Brugia (malayi) B74.1
    timori B74.2
  bursa — *see* Bursitis, infective
  buttocks (skin) LØ8.9
  Campylobacter, intestinal AØ4.5
    as cause of disease classified elsewhere B96.81
  Candida (albicans) (tropicalis) — *see* Candidiasis

Infection, infected, infective — *continued*

- candiru B88.8
- Capillaria (intestinal) B81.1
  - hepatica B83.8
  - philippinensis B81.1
- cartilage — *see* Disorder, cartilage, specified type NEC
- cat liver fluke B66.0
- catheter-related bloodstream (CRBSI) T80.211 ☑
- cellulitis — *code by* site under Cellulitis
- central line-associated T80.219 ☑
  - bloodstream (CLABSI) T80.211 ☑
  - specified NEC T80.218 ☑
- Cephalosporium falciforme B47.0
- cerebrospinal — *see* Meningitis
- cervical gland (lymph) L04.0
- cervix — *see* Cervicitis
- cesarean delivery wound (puerperal) O86.00
- cestodes — *see* Infestation, cestodes
- chest J22
- Chilomastix (intestinal) A07.8
- Chlamydia, chlamydial A74.9
  - anus A56.3
  - genitourinary tract A56.2
    - lower A56.00
    - specified NEC A56.19
  - lymphogranuloma A55
  - pharynx A56.4
  - psittaci A70
  - rectum A56.3
  - sexually transmitted NEC A56.8
- cholera — *see* Cholera
- Cladosporium
  - bantianum (brain abscess) B43.1
  - carrionii B43.0
  - castellanii B36.1
  - trichoides (brain abscess) B43.1
  - werneckii B36.1
- Clonorchis (sinensis) (liver) B66.1
- Clostridium NEC
  - bifermentans A48.0
  - botulinum (food poisoning) A05.1
    - infant A48.51
    - wound A48.52
  - difficile
    - as cause of disease classified elsewhere B96.89
    - foodborne (disease)
      - not specified as recurrent A04.72
      - recurrent A04.71
    - gas gangrene A48.0
    - necrotizing enterocolitis
      - not specified as recurrent A04.72
      - recurrent A04.71
    - sepsis A41.4
  - gas-forming NEC A48.0
  - histolyticum A48.0
  - novyi, causing gas gangrene A48.0
  - oedematiens A48.0
  - perfringens
    - as cause of disease classified elsewhere B96.7
    - due to food A05.2
    - foodborne (disease) A05.2
    - gas gangrene A48.0
    - sepsis A41.4
  - septicum, causing gas gangrene A48.0
  - sordellii, causing gas gangrene A48.0
  - welchii
    - as cause of disease classified elsewhere B96.7
    - foodborne (disease) A05.2
    - gas gangrene A48.0
    - necrotizing enteritis A05.2
    - sepsis A41.4
- Coccidioides (immitis) — *see* Coccidioidomycosis
- colon — *see* Enteritis, infectious
- colostomy K94.02
- common duct — *see* Cholangitis
- congenital P39.9
  - Candida (albicans) P37.5
  - cytomegalovirus P35.1
  - hepatitis, viral P35.3
  - herpes simplex P35.2
  - infectious or parasitic disease P37.9
    - specified NEC P37.8
  - listeriosis (disseminated) P37.2
  - malaria NEC P37.4
    - falciparum P37.3
  - Plasmodium falciparum P37.3
  - poliomyelitis P35.8
  - rubella P35.0

Infection, infected, infective — *continued*

- congenital — *continued*
  - skin P39.4
  - toxoplasmosis (acute) (subacute) (chronic) P37.1
  - tuberculosis P37.0
  - urinary (tract) P39.3
  - vaccinia P35.8
  - virus P35.9
    - specified type NEC P35.8
- Conidiobolus B46.8
- coronavirus-2019 U07.1
- coronavirus NEC B34.2
  - as cause of disease classified elsewhere B97.29
  - severe acute respiratory syndrome (SARS associated) B97.21
- corpus luteum — *see* Salpingo-oophoritis
- Corynebacterium diphtheriae — *see* Diphtheria
- cotia virus B08.8
- COVID-19 — *see also* COVID-19 U07.1
- Coxiella burnetii A78
- coxsackie — *see* Coxsackie
- Cryptococcus neoformans — *see* Cryptococcosis
- Cryptosporidium A07.2
- Cunninghamella — *see* Mucormycosis
- cyst — *see* Cyst
- cystic duct — *see also* Cholecystitis K81.9
- Cysticercus cellulosae — *see* Cysticercosis
- cytomegalovirus, cytomegaloviral B25.9
  - congenital P35.1
  - maternal, maternal care for (suspected) damage to fetus O35.3 ☑
  - mononucleosis B27.10
    - with
      - complication NEC B27.19
      - meningitis B27.12
      - polyneuropathy B27.11
- delta-agent (acute), in hepatitis B carrier B17.0
- dental (pulpal origin) K04.7
- Deuteromycetes B47.0
- Dicrocoelium dendriticum B66.2
- Dipetalonema (perstans) (streptocerca) B74.4
- diphtherial — *see* Diphtheria
- Diphyllobothrium (adult) (latum) (pacificum) B70.0
  - larval B70.1
- Diplogonoporus (grandis) B71.8
- Dipylidium caninum B67.4
- Dirofilaria B74.8
- Dracunculus medinensis B72
- Drechslera (hawaiiensis) B43.8
- Ducrey Haemophilus (any location) A57
- due to or resulting from
  - artificial insemination N98.0
  - Babesia
    - divergens (-like) strain B60.03
    - duncani (-type) species B60.02
    - microti B60.01
    - species
      - specified NEC B60.09
  - central venous catheter T80.219 ☑
    - bloodstream T80.211 ☑
    - exit or insertion site T80.212 ☑
    - localized T80.212 ☑
    - port or reservoir T80.212 ☑
    - specified NEC T80.218 ☑
    - tunnel T80.212 ☑
  - device, implant or graft — *see also* Complications, by site and type, infection or inflammation T85.79 ☑
    - arterial graft NEC T82.7 ☑
    - breast (implant) T85.79 ☑
    - catheter NEC T85.79 ☑
      - dialysis (renal) T82.7 ☑
        - central line T80.211 ☑
        - intraperitoneal T85.71 ☑
      - infusion NEC T82.7 ☑
        - cranial T85.735 ☑
        - intrathecal T85.735 ☑
        - spinal (epidural) (subdural) T85.735 ☑
        - subarachnoid T85.735 ☑
      - urinary T83.518 ☑
        - cystostomy T83.510 ☑
        - Hopkins T83.518 ☑
        - ileostomy T83.518 ☑
        - nephrostomy T83.512 ☑
        - specified NEC T83.518 ☑
        - urethral indwelling T83.511 ☑
        - urostomy T83.518 ☑

Infection, infected, infective — *continued*

- due to or resulting from — *continued*
  - device, implant or graft — *see also* Complications, by site and type, infection or inflammation — *continued*
    - electronic (electrode) (pulse generator) (stimulator)
      - bone T84.7 ☑
      - cardiac T82.7 ☑
      - nervous system T85.738 ☑
        - brain T85.731 ☑
        - cranial nerve T85.732 ☑
        - gastric nerve T85.732 ☑
        - generator pocket T85.734 ☑
        - neurostimulator generator T85.734 ☑
        - peripheral nerve T85.732 ☑
        - sacral nerve T85.732 ☑
        - spinal cord T85.733 ☑
        - vagal nerve T85.732 ☑
      - urinary (indwelling) T83.51 ☑
    - fixation, internal (orthopedic) NEC — *see* Complication, fixation device, infection
    - gastrointestinal (bile duct) (esophagus) T85.79 ☑
      - neurostimulator electrode (lead) T85.732 ☑
    - genital NEC T83.69 ☑
    - heart NEC T82.7 ☑
      - valve (prosthesis) T82.6 ☑
        - graft T82.7 ☑
    - joint prosthesis — *see* Complication, joint prosthesis, infection
    - ocular (corneal graft) (orbital implant) NEC T85.79 ☑
    - orthopedic NEC T84.7 ☑
    - penile (cylinder) (pump) (resevoir) T83.61 ☑
    - specified NEC T85.79 ☑
    - testicular T83.62 ☑
    - urinary NEC T83.598 ☑
      - ileal conduit stent T83.593 ☑
      - implanted neurostimulation T83.590 ☑
      - implanted sphincter T83.591 ☑
      - indwelling ureteral stent T83.592 ☑
      - nephroureteral stent T83.593 ☑
      - specified stent NEC T83.593 ☑
    - vascular NEC T82.7 ☑
    - ventricular intracranial (communicating) shunt T85.730 ☑
  - Hickman catheter T80.219 ☑
    - bloodstream T80.211 ☑
    - localized T80.212 ☑
    - specified NEC T80.218 ☑
  - immunization or vaccination T88.0 ☑
  - infusion, injection or transfusion NEC T80.29 ☑
  - injury NEC — *code by* site under Wound, open
  - peripherally inserted central catheter (PICC) T80.219 ☑
    - bloodstream T80.211 ☑
    - localized T80.212 ☑
    - specified NEC T80.218 ☑
  - portacath (port-a-cath) T80.219 ☑
    - bloodstream T80.211 ☑
    - localized T80.212 ☑
    - specified NEC T80.218 ☑
  - protozoa of the order Piroplasmida NEC B60.09
  - pulmonary artery catheter — *see* Infection, due to or resulting from, central venous catheter
  - surgery T81.40 ☑
  - Swan Ganz catheter — *see* Infection, due to or resulting from, central venous catheter
  - triple lumen catheter T80.219 ☑
    - bloodstream T80.211 ☑
    - localized T80.212 ☑
    - specified NEC T80.218 ☑
  - umbilical venous catheter T80.219 ☑
    - bloodstream T80.211 ☑
    - localized T80.212 ☑
    - specified NEC T80.218 ☑
- during labor NEC O75.3
- ear (middle) — *see also* Otitis media
  - external — *see* Otitis, externa, infective
  - inner — *see* subcategory H83.0 ☑
- Eberthella typhosa A01.00
- Echinococcus — *see* Echinococcus
- echovirus
  - as cause of disease classified elsewhere B97.12
  - unspecified nature or site B34.1
- endocardium I33.0

- **Infection, infected, infective** — *continued*
  - endocervix — *see* Cervicitis
  - Entamoeba — *see* Amebiasis
  - enteric — *see* Enteritis, infectious
  - Enterobacter sakazakii B96.89
  - Enterobius vermicularis B8Ø
  - enterostomy K94.12
  - enterovirus B34.1
    - as cause of disease classified elsewhere B97.1Ø
      - coxsackievirus B97.11
      - echovirus B97.12
      - specified NEC B97.19
  - Entomophthora B46.8
  - Epidermophyton — *see* Dermatophytosis
  - epididymis — *see* Epididymitis
  - episiotomy (puerperal) O86.Ø9
  - Erysipelothrix (insidiosa) (rhusiopathiae) — *see* Erysipeloid
  - erythema infectiosum BØ8.3
  - Escherichia (E.) coli NEC A49.8
    - as cause of disease classified elsewhere — *see also* Escherichia coli B96.2Ø
    - congenital P39.8
      - sepsis P36.4
    - generalized A41.51
    - intestinal — *see* Enteritis, infectious, due to, Escherichia coli
  - ethmoidal (chronic) (sinus) — *see* Sinusitis, ethmoidal
  - eustachian tube (ear) — *see* Salpingitis, eustachian
  - external auditory canal (meatus) NEC — *see* Otitis, externa, infective
  - eye (purulent) — *see* Endophthalmitis, purulent
  - eyelid — *see* Inflammation, eyelid
  - fallopian tube — *see* Salpingo-oophoritis
  - Fasciola (gigantica) (hepatica) (indica) B66.3
  - Fasciolopsis (buski) B66.5
  - filarial — *see* Infestation, filarial
  - finger (skin) LØ8.9
    - nail LØ3.Ø1- ☑
      - fungus B35.1
  - fish tapeworm B7Ø.Ø
    - larval B7Ø.1
  - flagellate, intestinal AØ7.9
  - fluke — *see* Infestation, fluke
  - focal
    - teeth (pulpal origin) KØ4.7
    - tonsils J35.Ø1
  - Fonsecaea (compactum) (pedrosoi) B43.Ø
  - food — *see* Intoxication, foodborne
  - foot (skin) LØ8.9
    - dermatophytic fungus B35.3
  - Francisella tularensis — *see* Tularemia
  - frontal (sinus) (chronic) — *see* Sinusitis, frontal
  - fungus NOS B49
    - beard B35.Ø
    - dermatophytic — *see* Dermatophytosis
    - foot B35.3
    - groin B35.6
    - hand B35.2
    - nail B35.1
    - pathogenic to compromised host only B48.8
    - perianal (area) B35.6
    - scalp B35.Ø
    - skin B36.9
      - foot B35.3
      - hand B35.2
      - toenails B35.1
  - Fusarium B48.8
  - gallbladder — *see* Cholecystitis
  - gas bacillus — *see* Gangrene, gas
  - gastrointestinal — *see* Enteritis, infectious
  - generalized NEC — *see* Sepsis
  - generator pocket, implanted electronic neurostimulator T85.734 ☑
  - genital organ or tract
    - female — *see* Disease, pelvis, inflammatory
    - male N49.9
      - multiple sites N49.8
      - specified NEC N49.8
  - Ghon tubercle, primary A15.7
  - Giardia lamblia AØ7.1
  - gingiva (chronic) KØ5.1Ø
    - acute KØ5.ØØ
      - nonplaque induced KØ5.Ø1
      - plaque induced KØ5.ØØ
    - nonplaque induced KØ5.11
    - plaque induced KØ5.1Ø
  - glanders A24.Ø

- **Infection, infected, infective** — *continued*
  - glenosporopsis B48.Ø
  - Gnathostoma (spinigerum) B83.1
  - Gongylonema B83.8
  - gonococcal — *see* Gonococcus
  - gram-negative bacilli NOS A49.9
  - guinea worm B72
  - gum (chronic) KØ5.1Ø
    - acute KØ5.ØØ
      - nonplaque induced KØ5.Ø1
      - plaque induced KØ5.ØØ
    - nonplaque induced KØ5.11
    - plaque induced KØ5.1Ø
  - Haemophilus — *see* Infection, Hemophilus
  - heart — *see* Carditis
  - Helicobacter pylori AØ4.8
    - as cause of disease classified elsewhere B96.81
  - helminths B83.9
    - intestinal B82.Ø
      - mixed (types classifiable to more than one of the titles B65.Ø-B81.3 and B81.8) B81.4
      - specified type NEC B81.8
    - specified type NEC B83.8
  - Hemophilus
    - aegyptius, systemic A48.4
    - ducrey (any location) A57
    - generalized A41.3
    - influenzae NEC A49.2
      - as cause of disease classified elsewhere B96.3
  - herpes (simplex) — *see also* Herpes
    - congenital P35.2
    - disseminated BØØ.7
    - zoster BØ2.9
  - herpesvirus, herpesviral — *see* Herpes
  - Heterophyes (heterophyes) B66.8
  - hip (joint) NEC MØØ.9
    - due to internal joint prosthesis
      - left T84.52 ☑
      - right T84.51 ☑
    - skin NEC LØ8.9
  - Histoplasma — *see* Histoplasmosis
    - American B39.4
    - capsulatum B39.4
  - hookworm B76.9
  - human
    - papilloma virus A63.Ø
    - T-cell lymphotropic virus type-1 (HTLV-1) B33.3
  - hydrocele N43.Ø
  - Hymenolepis B71.Ø
  - hypopharynx — *see* Pharyngitis
  - inguinal (lymph) glands LØ4.1
    - due to soft chancre A57
  - intervertebral disc, pyogenic M46.3Ø
    - cervical region M46.32
    - cervicothoracic region M46.33
    - lumbar region M46.36
    - lumbosacral region M46.37
    - multiple sites M46.39
    - occipito-atlanto-axial region M46.31
    - sacrococcygeal region M46.38
    - thoracic region M46.34
    - thoracolumbar region M46.35
  - intestine, intestinal — *see* Enteritis, infectious
    - specified NEC AØ8.8
  - intra-amniotic affecting newborn NEC P39.2
  - intrauterine inflammation O41.12- ☑
  - Isospora belli or hominis AØ7.3
  - Japanese B encephalitis A83.Ø
  - jaw (bone) (lower) (upper) M27.2
  - joint NEC MØØ.9
    - due to internal joint prosthesis T84.5Ø ☑
  - kidney (cortex) (hematogenous) N15.9
    - with calculus N2Ø.Ø
      - with hydronephrosis N13.6
    - following ectopic gestation OØ8.83
    - pelvis and ureter (cystic) N28.85
    - puerperal (postpartum) O86.21
    - specified NEC N15.8
  - Klebsiella (K.) pneumoniae NEC A49.8
    - as cause of disease classified elsewhere B96.1
  - knee (joint) NEC MØØ.9
    - joint MØØ.9
    - due to internal joint prosthesis
      - left T84.54 ☑
      - right T84.53 ☑
    - skin LØ8.9
  - Koch's — *see* Tuberculosis
  - labia (majora) (minora) (acute) — *see* Vulvitis

- **Infection, infected, infective** — *continued*
  - lacrimal
    - gland — *see* Dacryoadenitis
    - passages (duct) (sac) — *see* Inflammation, lacrimal, passages
  - lancet fluke B66.2
  - larynx NEC J38.7
  - leg (skin) NOS LØ8.9
  - Legionella pneumophila A48.1
    - nonpneumonic A48.2
  - Leishmania — *see also* Leishmaniasis
    - aethiopica B55.1
    - braziliensis B55.2
    - chagasi B55.Ø
    - donovani B55.Ø
    - infantum B55.Ø
    - major B55.1
    - mexicana B55.1
    - tropica B55.1
  - lentivirus, as cause of disease classified elsewhere B97.31
  - Leptosphaeria senegalensis B47.Ø
  - Leptospira interrogans A27.9
    - autumnalis A27.89
    - canicola A27.89
    - hebdomadis A27.89
    - icterohaemorrhagiae A27.Ø
    - pomona A27.89
    - specified type NEC A27.89
  - leptospirochetal NEC — *see* Leptospirosis
  - Listeria monocytogenes — *see also* Listeriosis
    - congenital P37.2
  - Loa loa B74.3
    - with conjunctival infestation B74.3
    - eyelid B74.3
  - Loboa loboi B48.Ø
  - local, skin (staphylococcal) (streptococcal) LØ8.9
    - abscess — *code by* site under Abscess
    - cellulitis — *code by* site under Cellulitis
    - specified NEC LØ8.89
    - ulcer — *see* Ulcer, skin
  - Loefflerella mallei A24.Ø
  - lung — *see also* Pneumonia J18.9
    - atypical Mycobacterium A31.Ø
    - spirochetal A69.8
    - tuberculous — *see* Tuberculosis, pulmonary
    - virus — *see* Pneumonia, viral
  - lymph gland — *see also* Lymphadenitis, acute
    - mesenteric I88.Ø
  - lymphoid tissue, base of tongue or posterior pharynx, NEC (chronic) J35.Ø3
  - Madurella (grisea) (mycetomii) B47.Ø
  - major
    - following ectopic or molar pregnancy OØ8.Ø
    - puerperal, postpartum, childbirth O85
  - Malassezia furfur B36.Ø
  - Malleomyces
    - mallei A24.Ø
    - pseudomallei (whitmori) — *see* Melioidosis
  - mammary gland N61.Ø
  - Mansonella (ozzardi) (perstans) (streptocerca) B74.4
  - mastoid — *see* Mastoiditis
  - maxilla, maxillary M27.2
    - sinus (chronic) — *see* Sinusitis, maxillary
  - mediastinum J98.51
  - Medina (worm) B72
  - meibomian cyst or gland — *see* Hordeolum
  - meninges — *see* Meningitis, bacterial
  - meningococcal — *see also* condition A39.9
    - adrenals A39.1
    - brain A39.81
    - cerebrospinal A39.Ø
    - conjunctiva A39.89
    - endocardium A39.51
    - heart A39.5Ø
      - endocardium A39.51
      - myocardium A39.52
      - pericardium A39.53
    - joint A39.83
    - meninges A39.Ø
    - meningococcemia A39.4
      - acute A39.2
      - chronic A39.3
    - myocardium A39.52
    - pericardium A39.53
    - retrobulbar neuritis A39.82
    - specified site NEC A39.89
  - mesenteric lymph nodes or glands NEC I88.Ø

Infection, infected, infective — *continued*

- Metagonimus B66.8
- metatarsophalangeal MØØ.9
- methicillin
  - resistant Staphylococcus aureus (MRSA) A49.Ø2
  - susceptible Staphylococcus aureus (MSSA) A49.Ø1
- Microsporum, microsporic — *see* Dermatophytosis
- mixed flora (bacterial) NEC A49.8
- Monilia — *see* Candidiasis
- Monosporium apiospermum B48.2
- mouth, parasitic B37.Ø
- Mucor — *see* Mucormycosis
- muscle NEC — *see* Myositis, infective
- mycelium NOS B49
- mycetoma B47.9
  - actinomycotic NEC B47.1
  - mycotic NEC B47.Ø
- Mycobacterium, mycobacterial — *see* Mycobacterium
- Mycoplasma NEC A49.3
  - pneumoniae, as cause of disease classified elsewhere B96.Ø
- mycotic NOS B49
  - pathogenic to compromised host only B48.8
  - skin NOS B36.9
- myocardium NEC I4Ø.Ø
- nail (chronic)
  - with lymphangitis — *see* Lymphangitis, acute, digit
  - finger LØ3.Ø1- ☑
    - fungus B35.1
  - ingrowing L6Ø.Ø
  - toe LØ3.Ø3- ☑
    - fungus B35.1
- nasal sinus (chronic) — *see* Sinusitis
- nasopharynx — *see* Nasopharyngitis
- navel LØ8.82
- Necator americanus B76.1
- Neisseria — *see* Gonococcus
- Neotestudina rosatii B47.Ø
- newborn P39.9
  - intra-amniotic NEC P39.2
  - skin P39.4
  - specified type NEC P39.8
- nipple N61.Ø
  - associated with
    - lactation O91.Ø3
    - pregnancy O91.Ø1- ☑
    - puerperium O91.Ø2
- Nocardia — *see* Nocardiosis
- obstetrical surgical wound (puerperal) O86.ØØ
  - incisional site
    - deep O86.Ø2
    - superficial O86.Ø1
  - organ and space site O86.Ø3
  - surgical site specified NEC O86.Ø9
- Oesophagostomum (apiostomum) B81.8
- Oestrus ovis — *see* Myiasis
- Oidium albicans B37.9
- Onchocerca (volvulus) — *see* Onchocerciasis
- oncovirus, as cause of disease classified elsewhere B97.32
- operation wound T81.49 ☑
- Opisthorchis (felineus) (viverrini) B66.Ø
- orbit, orbital — *see* Inflammation, orbit
- orthopoxvirus NEC BØ8.Ø9
- ovary — *see* Salpingo-oophoritis
- Oxyuris vermicularis B8Ø
- pancreas (acute) — *see* Pancreatitis, acute
  - abscess — *see* Pancreatitis, acute
  - specified NEC — *see also* Pancreatitis, acute K85.8Ø
- papillomavirus, as cause of disease classified elsewhere B97.7
- papovavirus NEC B34.4
- Paracoccidioides brasiliensis — *see* Paracoccidioidomycosis
- Paragonimus (westermani) B66.4
- parainfluenza virus B34.8
- parameningococcus NOS A39.9
- parapoxvirus BØ8.6Ø
  - specified NEC BØ8.69
- parasitic B89
- Parastrongylus
  - cantonensis B83.2
  - costaricensis B81.3
  - paratyphoid AØ1.4
    - Type A AØ1.1
    - Type B AØ1.2
    - Type C AØ1.3
- paraurethral ducts N34.2

Infection, infected, infective — *continued*

- parotid gland — *see* Sialoadenitis
- parvovirus NEC B34.3
  - as cause of disease classified elsewhere B97.6
- Pasteurella NEC A28.Ø
  - multocida A28.Ø
  - pestis — *see* Plague
  - pseudotuberculosis A28.Ø
  - septica (cat bite) (dog bite) A28.Ø
  - tularensis — *see* Tularemia
- pelvic, female — *see* Disease, pelvis, inflammatory
- Penicillium (marneffei) B48.4
- penis (glans) (retention) NEC N48.29
- periapical KØ4.5
- peridental, periodontal KØ5.2Ø
  - generalized — *see* Periodontitis, aggressive, generalized
  - localized — *see* Periodontitis, aggressive, localized
- perinatal period P39.9
  - specified type NEC P39.8
- perineal repair (puerperal) O86.Ø9
- periorbital — *see* Inflammation, orbit
- perirectal K62.89
- perirenal — *see* Infection, kidney
- peritoneal — *see* Peritonitis
- periureteral N28.89
- Petriellidium boydii B48.2
- pharynx — *see also* Pharyngitis
  - coxsackievirus BØ8.5
  - posterior, lymphoid (chronic) J35.Ø3
- Phialophora
  - gougerotii (subcutaneous abscess or cyst) B43.2
  - jeanselmei (subcutaneous abscess or cyst) B43.2
  - verrucosa (skin) B43.Ø
- Piedraia hortae B36.3
- pinta A67.9
  - intermediate A67.1
  - late A67.2
  - mixed A67.3
  - primary A67.Ø
- pinworm B8Ø
- pityrosporum furfur B36.Ø
- pleuro-pneumonia-like organism (PPLO) NEC A49.3
  - as cause of disease classified elsewhere B96.Ø
- pneumococcus, pneumococcal NEC A49.1
  - as cause of disease classified elsewhere B95.3
  - generalized (purulent) A4Ø.3
    - with pneumonia J13
- Pneumocystis carinii (pneumonia) B59
- Pneumocystis jiroveci (pneumonia) B59
- port or reservoir T8Ø.212 ☑
- postoperative T81.4Ø ☑
- postoperative wound T81.49 ☑
  - surgical site
    - deep incisional T81.42 ☑
    - organ and space T81.43 ☑
    - specified NEC T81.49 ☑
    - superficial incisional T81.41 ☑
- postprocedural T81.4Ø ☑
- postvaccinal T88.Ø ☑
- prepuce NEC N47.7
  - with penile inflammation N47.6
- prion — *see* Disease, prion, central nervous system
- prostate (capsule) — *see* Prostatitis
- Proteus (mirabilis) (morganii) (vulgaris) NEC A49.8
  - as cause of disease classified elsewhere B96.4
- protozoal NEC B64
  - intestinal AØ7.9
    - specified NEC AØ7.8
  - specified NEC B6Ø.8
- Pseudoallescheria boydii B48.2
- Pseudomonas NEC A49.8
  - as cause of disease classified elsewhere B96.5
  - mallei A24.Ø
  - pneumonia J15.1
  - pseudomallei — *see* Melioidosis
- puerperal O86.4
  - genitourinary tract NEC O86.89
  - major or generalized O85
  - minor O86.4
  - specified NEC O86.89
- pulmonary — *see* Infection, lung
- purulent — *see* Abscess
- Pyrenochaeta romeroi B47.Ø
- Q fever A78
- rectum (sphincter) K62.89
- renal — *see also* Infection, kidney
  - pelvis and ureter (cystic) N28.85

Infection, infected, infective — *continued*

- reovirus, as cause of disease classified elsewhere B97.5
- respiratory (tract) NEC J98.8
  - acute J22
  - chronic J98.8
  - influenzal (upper) (acute) — *see* Influenza, with, respiratory manifestations NEC
  - lower (acute) J22
    - chronic — *see* Bronchitis, chronic
  - rhinovirus JØØ
  - syncytial virus (RSV) — *see* Infection, virus, respiratory syncytial (RSV)
  - upper (acute) NOS JØ6.9
    - chronic J39.8
    - streptococcal JØ6.9
    - viral NOS JØ6.9
      - due to respiratory syncytial virus (RSV) JØ6.9 *[B97.4]*
- resulting from
  - presence of internal prosthesis, implant, graft — *see* Complications, by site and type, infection
- retortamoniasis AØ7.8
- retroperitoneal NEC K68.9
- retrovirus B33.3
  - as cause of disease classified elsewhere B97.3Ø
    - human
      - immunodeficiency, type 2 (HIV 2) B97.35
      - T-cell lymphotropic
        - type I (HTLV-I) B97.33
        - type II (HTLV-II) B97.34
    - lentivirus B97.31
    - oncovirus B97.32
    - specified NEC B97.39
- Rhinosporidium (seeberi) B48.1
- rhinovirus
  - as cause of disease classified elsewhere B97.89
  - unspecified nature or site B34.8
- Rhizopus — *see* Mucormycosis
- rickettsial NOS A79.9
- roundworm (large) NEC B82.Ø
  - Ascariasis — *see also* Ascariasis B77.9
- rubella — *see* Rubella
- Saccharomyces — *see* Candidiasis
- salivary duct or gland (any) — *see* Sialoadenitis
- Salmonella (aertrycke) (arizonae) (callinarum) (choleraesuis) (enteritidis) (suipestifer) (typhimurium) AØ2.9
  - with
    - (gastro)enteritis AØ2.Ø
    - sepsis AØ2.1
    - specified manifestation NEC AØ2.8
  - due to food (poisoning) AØ2.9
  - hirschfeldii AØ1.3
  - localized AØ2.2Ø
    - arthritis AØ2.23
    - meningitis AØ2.21
    - osteomyelitis AØ2.24
    - pneumonia AØ2.22
    - pyelonephritis AØ2.25
    - specified NEC AØ2.29
  - paratyphi AØ1.4
    - A AØ1.1
    - B AØ1.2
    - C AØ1.3
  - schottmuelleri AØ1.2
  - typhi, typhosa — *see* Typhoid
- Sarcocystis AØ7.8
- SARS-CoV-2 — *see* Infection, COVID-19
- scabies B86
- Schistosoma — *see* Infestation, Schistosoma
- scrotum (acute) NEC N49.2
- seminal vesicle — *see* Vesiculitis
- septic
  - localized, skin — *see* Abscess
- sheep liver fluke B66.3
- Shigella AØ3.9
  - boydii AØ3.2
  - dysenteriae AØ3.Ø
  - flexneri AØ3.1
  - group
    - A AØ3.Ø
    - B AØ3.1
    - C AØ3.2
    - D AØ3.3
  - Schmitz (-Stutzer) AØ3.Ø
  - schmitzii AØ3.Ø
  - shigae AØ3.Ø
  - sonnei AØ3.3

- **Infection, infected, infective** — *continued*
  - Shigella — *continued*
    - specified NEC A03.8
  - shoulder (joint) NEC M00.9
    - due to internal joint prosthesis T84.59 ☑
    - skin NEC L08.9
  - sinus (accessory) (chronic) (nasal) — *see also* Sinusitis
    - pilonidal — *see* Sinus, pilonidal
    - skin NEC L08.89
  - Skene's duct or gland — *see* Urethritis
  - skin (local) (staphylococcal) (streptococcal) L08.9
    - abscess — *code by* site under Abscess
    - cellulitis — *code by* site under Cellulitis
    - due to fungus B36.9
      - specified type NEC B36.8
    - mycotic B36.9
      - specified type NEC B36.8
    - newborn P39.4
    - ulcer — *see* Ulcer, skin
  - slow virus A81.9
    - specified NEC A81.89
  - Sparganum (mansoni) (proliferum) (baxteri) B70.1
  - specific — *see also* Syphilis
    - to perinatal period — *see* Infection, congenital
  - specified NEC B99.8
  - spermatic cord NEC N49.1
  - sphenoidal (sinus) — *see* Sinusitis, sphenoidal
  - spinal cord NOS — *see also* Myelitis G04.91
    - abscess G06.1
    - meninges — *see* Meningitis
    - streptococcal G04.89
  - Spirillum A25.0
  - spirochetal NOS A69.9
    - lung A69.8
    - specified NEC A69.8
  - Spirometra larvae B70.1
  - spleen D73.89
  - Sporotrichum, Sporothrix (schenckii) — *see* Sporotrichosis
  - staphylococcal, unspecified site
    - as cause of disease classified elsewhere B95.8
      - aureus (methicillin susceptible) (MSSA) B95.61
        - methicillin resistant (MRSA) B95.62
      - specified NEC B95.7
    - aureus (methicillin susceptible) (MSSA) A49.01
      - methicillin resistant (MRSA) A49.02
    - food poisoning A05.0
    - generalized (purulent) A41.2
    - pneumonia — *see* Pneumonia, staphylococcal
  - Stellantchasmus falcatus B66.8
  - streptobacillus moniliformis A25.1
  - streptococcal NEC A49.1
    - as cause of disease classified elsewhere B95.5
    - B genitourinary complicating
      - childbirth O98.82
      - pregnancy O98.81- ☑
      - puerperium O98.83
    - congenital
      - sepsis P36.10
        - group B P36.0
        - specified NEC P36.19
    - generalized (purulent) A40.9
  - Streptomyces B47.1
  - Strongyloides (stercoralis) — *see* Strongyloidiasis
  - stump (amputation) (surgical) — *see* Complication, amputation stump, infection
  - subcutaneous tissue, local L08.9
  - suipestifer — *see* Infection, salmonella
  - swimming pool bacillus A31.1
  - Taenia — *see* Infestation, Taenia
  - Taeniarhynchus saginatus B68.1
  - tapeworm — *see* Infestation, tapeworm
  - tendon (sheath) — *see* Tenosynovitis, infective NEC
  - Ternidens diminutus B81.8
  - testis — *see* Orchitis
  - threadworm B80
  - throat — *see* Pharyngitis
  - thyroglossal duct K14.8
  - toe (skin) L08.9
    - cellulitis L03.03- ☑
      - fungus B35.1
    - nail L03.03- ☑
      - fungus B35.1
  - tongue NEC K14.0
    - parasitic B37.0
  - tonsil (and adenoid) (faucial) (lingual) (pharyngeal) — *see* Tonsillitis
  - tooth, teeth K04.7

- **Infection, infected, infective** — *continued*
  - tooth, teeth — *continued*
    - periapical K04.7
    - peridental, periodontal K05.20
      - generalized — *see* Periodontitis, aggressive, generalized
      - localized — *see* Periodontitis, aggressive, localized
    - pulp K04.01
      - irreversible K04.02
      - reversible K04.01
    - socket M27.3
  - TORCH — *see* Infection, congenital
    - without active infection P00.2
  - Torula histolytica — *see* Cryptococcosis
  - Toxocara (canis) (cati) (felis) B83.0
  - Toxoplasma gondii — *see* Toxoplasma
  - trachea, chronic J42
  - trematode NEC — *see* Infestation, fluke
  - trench fever A79.0
  - Treponema pallidum — *see* Syphilis
  - Trichinella (spiralis) B75
  - Trichomonas A59.9
    - cervix A59.09
    - intestine A07.8
    - prostate A59.02
    - specified site NEC A59.8
    - urethra A59.03
    - urogenitalis A59.00
    - vagina A59.01
    - vulva A59.01
  - Trichophyton, trichophytic — *see* Dermatophytosis
  - Trichosporon (beigelii) cutaneum B36.2
  - Trichostrongylus B81.2
  - Trichuris (trichiura) B79
  - Trombicula (irritans) B88.0
  - Trypanosoma
    - brucei
      - gambiense B56.0
      - rhodesiense B56.1
    - cruzi — *see* Chagas' disease
  - tubal — *see* Salpingo-oophoritis
  - tuberculous
    - latent (LTBI) Z22.7
    - NEC — *see* Tuberculosis
  - tubo-ovarian — *see* Salpingo-oophoritis
  - tunica vaginalis N49.1
  - tunnel T80.212 ☑
  - tympanic membrane NEC — *see* Myringitis
  - typhoid (abortive) (ambulant) (bacillus) — *see* Typhoid
  - typhus A75.9
    - flea-borne A75.2
    - mite-borne A75.3
    - recrudescent A75.1
    - tick-borne A77.9
      - African A77.1
      - North Asian A77.2
  - umbilicus L08.82
  - ureter — *see* Ureteritis
  - urethra — *see* Urethritis
  - urinary (tract) N39.0
    - bladder — *see* Cystitis
    - complicating
      - pregnancy O23.4- ☑
        - specified type NEC O23.3- ☑
    - kidney — *see* Infection, kidney
    - newborn P39.3
    - puerperal (postpartum) O86.20
    - tuberculous A18.13
    - urethra — *see* Urethritis
  - uterus, uterine — *see* Endometritis
  - vaccination T88.0 ☑
  - vaccinia not from vaccination B08.011
  - vagina (acute) — *see* Vaginitis
  - varicella B01.9
  - varicose veins — *see* Varix
  - vas deferens NEC N49.1
  - vesical — *see* Cystitis
  - Vibrio
    - cholerae A00.0
      - El Tor A00.1
    - parahaemolyticus (food poisoning) A05.3
    - vulnificus
      - as cause of disease classified elsewhere B96.82
      - foodborne intoxication A05.5
  - Vincent's (gum) (mouth) (tonsil) A69.1
  - virus, viral NOS B34.9

- **Infection, infected, infective** — *continued*
  - virus, viral — *continued*
    - adenovirus
      - as cause of disease classified elsewhere B97.0
      - unspecified nature or site B34.0
    - arborvirus, arbovirus arthropod-borne A94
    - as cause of disease classified elsewhere B97.89
      - adenovirus B97.0
      - coronavirus B97.29
        - SARS-associated B97.21
      - coxsackievirus B97.11
      - echovirus B97.12
      - enterovirus B97.10
        - coxsackievirus B97.11
        - echovirus B97.12
        - specified NEC B97.19
      - human
        - immunodeficiency, type 2 (HIV 2) B97.35
        - metapneumovirus B97.81
        - T-cell lymphotropic,
          - type I (HTLV-I) B97.33
          - type II (HTLV-II) B97.34
      - papillomavirus B97.7
      - parvovirus B97.6
      - reovirus B97.5
      - respiratory syncytial (RSV) — *see* Infection, virus, respiratory syncytial (RSV)
      - retrovirus B97.30
        - human
          - immunodeficiency, type 2 (HIV 2) B97.35
          - T-cell lymphotropic,
            - type I (HTLV-I) B97.33
            - type II (HTLV-II) B97.34
        - lentivirus B97.31
        - oncovirus B97.32
        - specified NEC B97.39
      - specified NEC B97.89
    - central nervous system A89
      - atypical A81.9
        - specified NEC A81.89
      - enterovirus NEC A88.8
        - meningitis A87.0
      - slow virus A81.9
        - specified NEC A81.89
      - specified NEC A88.8
    - chest J98.8
    - cotia B08.8
    - COVID-19 U07.1
    - coxsackie — *see also* Infection, coxsackie B34.1
      - as cause of disease classified elsewhere B97.11
    - ECHO
      - as cause of disease classified elsewhere B97.12
      - unspecified nature or site B34.1
    - encephalitis, tick-borne A84.9
    - enterovirus, as cause of disease classified elsewhere B97.10
      - coxsackievirus B97.11
      - echovirus B97.12
      - specified NEC B97.19
    - exanthem NOS B09
    - human metapneumovirus as cause of disease classified elsewhere B97.81
    - human papilloma as cause of disease classified elsewhere B97.7
    - intestine — *see* Enteritis, viral
    - respiratory syncytial (RSV)
      - as cause of disease classified elsewhere B97.4
      - bronchiolitis J21.0
      - bronchitis J20.5
      - bronchopneumonia J12.1
      - otitis media H65- ☑ *[B97.4]*
      - pneumonia J12.1
      - upper respiratory infection J06.9 *[B97.4]*
    - rhinovirus
      - as cause of disease classified elsewhere B97.89
      - unspecified nature or site B34.8
    - slow A81.9
      - specified NEC A81.89
    - specified type NEC B33.8
      - as cause of disease classified elsewhere B97.89
      - unspecified nature or site B34.8
    - unspecified nature or site B34.9
    - West Nile — *see* Virus, West Nile
  - vulva (acute) — *see* Vulvitis
  - West Nile — *see* Virus, West Nile
  - whipworm B79
  - worms B83.9
    - specified type NEC B83.8

Infection, infected, infective — *continued*
Wuchereria (bancrofti) B74.Ø
malayi B74.1
yatapoxvirus BØ8.7Ø
specified NEC BØ8.79
yeast — *see also* Candidiasis B37.9
yellow fever — *see* Fever, yellow
Yersinia
enterocolitica (intestinal) AØ4.6
pestis — *see* Plague
pseudotuberculosis A28.2
Zeis' gland — *see* Hordeolum
Zika virus A92.5
congenital P35.4
zoonotic bacterial NOS A28.9
Zopfia senegalensis B47.Ø
Infective, infectious — *see* condition
Infertility
female N97.9
age-related N97.8
associated with
anovulation N97.Ø
cervical (mucus) disease or anomaly N88.3
congenital anomaly
cervix N88.3
fallopian tube N97.1
uterus N97.2
vagina N97.8
dysmucorrhea N88.3
fallopian tube disease or anomaly N97.1
pituitary-hypothalamic origin E23.Ø
specified origin NEC N97.8
Stein-Leventhal syndrome E28.2
uterine disease or anomaly N97.2
vaginal disease or anomaly N97.8
due to
cervical anomaly N88.3
fallopian tube anomaly N97.1
ovarian failure E28.39
Stein-Leventhal syndrome E28.2
uterine anomaly N97.2
vaginal anomaly N97.8
nonimplantation N97.2
origin
cervical N88.3
tubal (block) (occlusion) (stenosis) N97.1
uterine N97.2
vaginal N97.8
male N46.9
azoospermia N46.Ø1
extratesticular cause N46.Ø29
drug therapy N46.Ø21
efferent duct obstruction N46.Ø23
infection N46.Ø22
radiation N46.Ø24
specified cause NEC N46.Ø29
systemic disease N46.Ø25
oligospermia N46.11
extratesticular cause N46.129
drug therapy N46.121
efferent duct obstruction N46.123
infection N46.122
radiation N46.124
specified cause NEC N46.129
systemic disease N46.125
specified type NEC N46.8
Infestation B88.9
Acanthocheilonema (perstans) (streptocerca) B74.4
Acariasis B88.Ø
demodex folliculorum B88.Ø
sarcoptes scabiei B86
trombiculae B88.Ø
Agamofilaria streptocerca B74.4
Ancylostoma, ankylostoma (braziliense) (caninum) (ceylanicum) (duodenale) B76.Ø
americanum B76.1
new world B76.1
Anisakis larvae, anisakiasis B81.Ø
arthropod NEC B88.2
Ascaris lumbricoides — *see* Ascariasis
Balantidium coli AØ7.Ø
beef tapeworm B68.1
Bothriocephalus (latus) B7Ø.Ø
larval B7Ø.1
broad tapeworm B7Ø.Ø
larval B7Ø.1
Brugia (malayi) B74.1
timori B74.2

Infestation — *continued*
candiru B88.8
Capillaria
hepatica B83.8
philippinensis B81.1
cat liver fluke B66.Ø
cestodes B71.9
diphyllobothrium — *see* Infestation, diphyllobothrium
dipylidiasis B71.1
hymenolepiasis B71.Ø
specified type NEC B71.8
chigger B88.Ø
chigo, chigoe B88.1
Clonorchis (sinensis) (liver) B66.1
coccidial AØ7.3
crab-lice B85.3
Cysticercus cellulosae — *see* Cysticercosis
Demodex (folliculorum) B88.Ø
Dermanyssus gallinae B88.Ø
Dermatobia (hominis) — *see* Myiasis
Dibothriocephalus (latus) B7Ø.Ø
larval B7Ø.1
Dicrocoelium dendriticum B66.2
Diphyllobothrium (adult) (latum) (intestinal) (pacificum) B7Ø.Ø
larval B7Ø.1
Diplogonoporus (grandis) B71.8
Dipylidium caninum B67.4
Distoma hepaticum B66.3
dog tapeworm B67.4
Dracunculus medinensis B72
dragon worm B72
dwarf tapeworm B71.Ø
Echinococcus — *see* Echinococcus
Echinostomum ilocanum B66.8
Entamoeba (histolytica) — *see* Infection, Ameba
Enterobius vermicularis B8Ø
eyelid
in (due to)
leishmaniasis B55.1
loiasis B74.3
onchocerciasis B73.Ø9
phthiriasis B85.3
parasitic NOS B89
eyeworm B74.3
Fasciola (gigantica) (hepatica) (indica) B66.3
Fasciolopsis (buski) (intestine) B66.5
filarial B74.9
bancroftian B74.Ø
conjunctiva B74.9
due to
Acanthocheilonema (perstans) (streptocerca) B74.4
Brugia (malayi) B74.1
timori B74.2
Dracunculus medinensis B72
guinea worm B72
loa loa B74.3
Mansonella (ozzardi) (perstans) (streptocerca) B74.4
Onchocerca volvulus B73.ØØ
eye B73.ØØ
eyelid B73.Ø9
Wuchereria (bancrofti) B74.Ø
Malayan B74.1
ozzardi B74.4
specified type NEC B74.8
fish tapeworm B7Ø.Ø
larval B7Ø.1
fluke B66.9
blood NOS — *see* Schistosomiasis
cat liver B66.Ø
intestinal B66.5
lancet B66.2
liver (sheep) B66.3
cat B66.Ø
Chinese B66.1
due to clonorchiasis B66.1
oriental B66.1
lung (oriental) B66.4
sheep liver B66.3
specified type NEC B66.8
fly larvae — *see* Myiasis
Gasterophilus (intestinalis) — *see* Myiasis
Gastrodiscoides hominis B66.8
Giardia lamblia AØ7.1
Gnathostoma (spinigerum) B83.1

Infestation — *continued*
Gongylonema B83.8
guinea worm B72
helminth B83.9
angiostrongyliasis B83.2
intestinal B81.3
gnathostomiasis B83.1
hirudiniasis, internal B83.4
intestinal B82.Ø
angiostrongyliasis B81.3
anisakiasis B81.Ø
ascariasis — *see* Ascariasis
capillariasis B81.1
cysticercosis — *see* Cysticercosis
diphyllobothriasis — *see* Infestation, diphyllobothriasis
dracunculiasis B72
echinococcus — *see* Echinococcosis
enterobiasis B8Ø
filariasis — *see* Infestation, filarial
fluke — *see* Infestation, fluke
hookworm — *see* Infestation, hookworm
mixed (types classifiable to more than one of the titles B65.Ø-B81.3 and B81.8) B81.4
onchocerciasis — *see* Onchocerciasis
schistosomiasis — *see* Infestation, schistosoma
specified
cestode NEC — *see* Infestation, cestode
type NEC B81.8
strongyloidiasis — *see* Strongyloidiasis
taenia — *see* Infestation, taenia
trichinellosis B75
trichostrongyliasis B81.2
trichuriasis B79
specified type NEC B83.8
syngamiasis B83.3
visceral larva migrans B83.Ø
Heterophyes (heterophyes) B66.8
hookworm B76.9
ancylostomiasis B76.Ø
necatoriasis B76.1
specified type NEC B76.8
Hymenolepis (diminuta) (nana) B71.Ø
intestinal NEC B82.9
leeches (aquatic) (land) — *see* Hirudiniasis
Leishmania — *see* Leishmaniasis
lice, louse — *see* Infestation, Pediculus
Linguatula B88.8
Liponyssoides sanguineus B88.Ø
Loa loa B74.3
conjunctival B74.3
eyelid B74.3
louse — *see* Infestation, Pediculus
maggots — *see* Myiasis
Mansonella (ozzardi) (perstans) (streptocerca) B74.4
Medina (worm) B72
Metagonimus (yokogawai) B66.8
microfilaria streptocerca — *see* Onchocerciasis
eye B73.ØØ
eyelid B73.Ø9
mites B88.9
scabic B86
Monilia (albicans) — *see* Candidiasis
mouth B37.Ø
Necator americanus B76.1
nematode NEC (intestinal) B82.Ø
Ancylostoma B76.Ø
conjunctiva NEC B83.9
Enterobius vermicularis B8Ø
Gnathostoma spinigerum B83.1
physaloptera B8Ø
specified NEC B81.8
trichostrongylus B81.2
trichuris (trichuria) B79
Oesophagostomum (apiostomum) B81.8
Oestrus ovis — *see also* Myiasis B87.9
Onchocerca (volvulus) — *see* Onchocerciasis
Opisthorchis (felineus) (viverrini) B66.Ø
orbit, parasitic NOS B89
Oxyuris vermicularis B8Ø
Paragonimus (westermani) B66.4
parasite, parasitic B89
eyelid B89
intestinal NOS B82.9
mouth B37.Ø
skin B88.9
tongue B37.Ø

- **Infestation** — *continued*
  - Parastrongylus
    - cantonensis B83.2
    - costaricensis B81.3
  - Pediculus B85.2
    - body B85.1
    - capitis (humanus) (any site) B85.0
    - corporis (humanus) (any site) B85.1
    - head B85.0
    - mixed (classifiable to more than one of the titles B85.0 - B85.3) B85.4
    - pubis (any site) B85.3
  - Pentastoma B88.8
  - Phthirus (pubis) (any site) B85.3
    - with any infestation classifiable to B85.0 - B85.2 B85.4
  - pinworm B80
  - pork tapeworm (adult) B68.0
  - protozoal NEC B64
    - intestinal A07.9
      - specified NEC A07.8
    - specified NEC B60.8
  - pubic, louse B85.3
  - rat tapeworm B71.0
  - red bug B88.0
  - roundworm (large) NEC B82.0
    - Ascariasis — *see also* Ascariasis B77.9
  - sandflea B88.1
  - Sarcoptes scabiei B86
  - scabies B86
  - Schistosoma B65.9
    - bovis B65.8
    - cercariae B65.3
    - haematobium B65.0
    - intercalatum B65.8
    - japonicum B65.2
    - mansoni B65.1
    - mattheei B65.8
    - mekongi B65.8
    - specified type NEC B65.8
    - spindale B65.8
  - screw worms — *see* Myiasis
  - skin NOS B88.9
  - Sparganum (mansoni) (proliferum) (baxteri) B70.1
    - larval B70.1
  - specified type NEC B88.8
  - Spirometra larvae B70.1
  - Stellantchasmus falcatus B66.8
  - Strongyloides stercoralis — *see* Strongyloidiasis
  - Taenia B68.9
    - diminuta B71.0
    - echinococcus — *see* Echinococcus
    - mediocanellata B68.1
    - nana B71.0
    - saginata B68.1
    - solium (intestinal form) B68.0
      - larval form — *see* Cysticercosis
  - Taeniarhynchus saginatus B68.1
  - tapeworm B71.9
    - beef B68.1
    - broad B70.0
      - larval B70.1
    - dog B67.4
    - dwarf B71.0
    - fish B70.0
      - larval B70.1
    - pork B68.0
    - rat B71.0
  - Ternidens diminutus B81.8
  - Tetranychus molestissimus B88.0
  - threadworm B80
  - tongue B37.0
  - Toxocara (canis) (cati) (felis) B83.0
  - trematode(s) NEC — *see* Infestation, fluke
  - Trichinella (spiralis) B75
  - Trichocephalus B79
  - Trichomonas — *see* Trichomoniasis
  - Trichostrongylus B81.2
  - Trichuris (trichiura) B79
  - Trombicula (irritans) B88.0
  - Tunga penetrans B88.1
  - Uncinaria americana B76.1
  - Vandellia cirrhosa B88.8
  - whipworm B79
  - worms B83.9
    - intestinal B82.0
  - Wuchereria (bancrofti) B74.0
- **Infiltrate, infiltration**
  - amyloid (generalized) (localized) — *see* Amyloidosis
  - calcareous NEC R89.7
    - localized — *see* Degeneration, by site
  - calcium salt R89.7
  - cardiac
    - fatty — *see* Degeneration, myocardial
    - glycogenic E74.02 *[I43]*
  - corneal — *see* Edema, cornea
  - eyelid — *see* Inflammation, eyelid
  - glycogen, glycogenic — *see* Disease, glycogen storage
  - heart, cardiac
    - fatty — *see* Degeneration, myocardial
    - glycogenic E74.02 *[I43]*
  - inflammatory in vitreous H43.89
  - kidney N28.89
  - leukemic — *see* Leukemia
  - liver K76.89
    - fatty — *see* Fatty, liver NEC
    - glycogen — *see also* Disease, glycogen storage E74.03 *[K77]*
  - lung R91.8
    - eosinophilic — *see* Eosinophilia, pulmonary
  - lymphatic — *see also* Leukemia, lymphatic C91.9- ☑
    - gland I88.9
  - muscle, fatty M62.89
  - myocardium, myocardial
    - fatty — *see* Degeneration, myocardial
    - glycogenic E74.02 *[I43]*
  - on chest x-ray R91.8
  - pulmonary R91.8
    - with eosinophilia — *see* Eosinophilia, pulmonary
  - skin (lymphocytic) L98.6
  - thymus (gland) (fatty) E32.8
  - urine R39.0
  - vesicant agent
    - antineoplastic chemotherapy T80.810 ☑
    - other agent NEC T80.818 ☑
  - vitreous body H43.89
- **Infirmity** R68.89
  - senile R54
- **Inflammation, inflamed, inflammatory** (with exudation)
  - abducent (nerve) — *see* Strabismus, paralytic, sixth nerve
  - accessory sinus (chronic) — *see* Sinusitis
  - adrenal (gland) E27.8
  - alveoli, teeth M27.3
    - scorbutic E54
  - anal canal, anus K62.89
  - antrum (chronic) — *see* Sinusitis, maxillary
  - appendix — *see* Appendicitis
  - arachnoid — *see* Meningitis
  - areola N61.0
    - puerperal, postpartum or gestational — *see* Infection, nipple
  - areolar tissue NOS L08.9
  - artery — *see* Arteritis
  - auditory meatus (external) — *see* Otitis, externa
  - Bartholin's gland N75.8
  - bile duct (common) (hepatic) or passage — *see* Cholangitis
  - bladder — *see* Cystitis
  - bone — *see* Osteomyelitis
  - brain — *see also* Encephalitis
    - membrane — *see* Meningitis
  - breast N61.0
    - puerperal, postpartum, gestational — *see* Mastitis, obstetric
  - broad ligament — *see* Disease, pelvis, inflammatory
  - bronchi — *see* Bronchitis
  - catarrhal J00
  - cecum — *see* Appendicitis
  - cerebral — *see also* Encephalitis
    - membrane — *see* Meningitis
  - cerebrospinal
    - meningococcal A39.0
  - cervix (uteri) — *see* Cervicitis
  - chest J98.8
  - chorioretinal H30.9- ☑
    - cyclitis — *see* Cyclitis
    - disseminated H30.10- ☑
      - generalized H30.13- ☑
      - peripheral H30.12- ☑
      - posterior pole H30.11- ☑
    - epitheliopathy — *see* Epitheliopathy
    - focal H30.00- ☑
- **Inflammation, inflamed, inflammatory** — *continued*
  - chorioretinal — *continued*
    - focal — *continued*
      - juxtapapillary H30.01- ☑
      - macular H30.04- ☑
      - paramacular — *see* Inflammation, chorioretinal, focal, macular
      - peripheral H30.03- ☑
      - posterior pole H30.02- ☑
    - specified type NEC H30.89- ☑
  - choroid — *see* Inflammation, chorioretinal
  - chronic, postmastoidectomy cavity — *see* Complications, postmastoidectomy, inflammation
  - colon — *see* Enteritis
  - connective tissue (diffuse) NEC — *see* Disorder, soft tissue, specified type NEC
  - cornea — *see* Keratitis
  - corpora cavernosa N48.29
  - cranial nerve — *see* Disorder, nerve, cranial
  - Douglas' cul-de-sac or pouch (chronic) N73.0
  - due to device, implant or graft — *see also* Complications, by site and type, infection or inflammation
    - arterial graft T82.7 ☑
    - breast (implant) T85.79 ☑
    - catheter T85.79 ☑
      - dialysis (renal) T82.7 ☑
        - intraperitoneal T85.71 ☑
      - infusion T82.7 ☑
        - cranial T85.735 ☑
        - intrathecal T85.735 ☑
        - spinal (epidural) (subdural) T85.735 ☑
        - subarachnoid T85.735 ☑
      - urinary T83.518 ☑
        - cystostomy T83.510 ☑
        - Hopkins T83.518 ☑
        - ileostomy T83.518 ☑
        - nephrostomy T83.512 ☑
        - specified NEC T83.518 ☑
        - urethral indwelling T83.511 ☑
        - urostomy T83.518 ☑
    - electronic (electrode) (pulse generator) (stimulator)
      - bone T84.7 ☑
      - cardiac T82.7 ☑
      - nervous system T85.738 ☑
        - brain T85.731 ☑
        - cranial nerve T85.732 ☑
        - gastric nerve T85.732 ☑
        - neurostimulator generator T85.734 ☑
        - peripheral nerve T85.732 ☑
        - sacral nerve T85.732 ☑
        - spinal cord T85.733 ☑
        - vagal nerve T85.732 ☑
      - urinary T83.590 ☑
    - fixation, internal (orthopedic) NEC — *see* Complication, fixation device, infection
    - gastrointestinal (bile duct) (esophagus) T85.79 ☑
      - neurostimulator electrode (lead) T85.732 ☑
    - genital NEC T83.69 ☑
    - heart NEC T82.7 ☑
      - valve (prosthesis) T82.6 ☑
        - graft T82.7 ☑
    - joint prosthesis — *see* Complication, joint prosthesis, infection
    - ocular (corneal graft) (orbital implant) NEC T85.79 ☑
    - orthopedic NEC T84.7 ☑
    - penile (cylinder) (pump) (resevoir) T83.61 ☑
    - specified NEC T85.79 ☑
    - testicular T83.62 ☑
    - urinary NEC T83.598 ☑
      - ileal conduit stent T83.593 ☑
      - implanted neurostimulation T83.590 ☑
      - implanted sphincter T83.591 ☑
      - indwelling ureteral stent T83.592 ☑
      - nephroureteral stent T83.593 ☑
      - specified stent NEC T83.593 ☑
    - vascular NEC T82.7 ☑
    - ventricular intracranial (communicating) shunt T85.730 ☑
  - duodenum K29.80
    - with bleeding K29.81
  - dura mater — *see* Meningitis
  - ear (middle) — *see also* Otitis, media
    - external — *see* Otitis, externa
    - inner — *see* subcategory H83.0 ☑
  - epididymis — *see* Epididymitis

- **Inflammation, inflamed, inflammatory** — *continued*
  - esophagus — *see* Esophagitis
  - ethmoidal (sinus) (chronic) — *see* Sinusitis, ethmoidal
  - eustachian tube (catarrhal) — *see* Salpingitis, eustachian
  - eyelid HØ1.9
    - abscess — *see* Abscess, eyelid
    - blepharitis — *see* Blepharitis
    - chalazion — *see* Chalazion
    - dermatosis (noninfectious) — *see* Dermatosis, eyelid
    - hordeolum — *see* Hordeolum
    - specified NEC HØ1.8
  - fallopian tube — *see* Salpingo-oophoritis
  - fascia — *see* Myositis
  - follicular, pharynx J31.2
  - frontal (sinus) (chronic) — *see* Sinusitis, frontal
  - gallbladder — *see* Cholecystitis
  - gastric — *see* Gastritis
  - gastrointestinal — *see* Enteritis
  - genital organ (internal) (diffuse)
    - female — *see* Disease, pelvis, inflammatory
    - male N49.9
      - multiple sites N49.8
      - specified NEC N49.8
  - gland (lymph) — *see* Lymphadenitis
  - glottis — *see* Laryngitis
  - granular, pharynx J31.2
  - gum KØ5.1Ø
    - nonplaque induced KØ5.11
    - plaque induced KØ5.1Ø
  - heart — *see* Carditis
  - hepatic duct — *see* Cholangitis
  - ileoanal (internal) pouch K91.85Ø
  - ileum — *see also* Enteritis
    - regional or terminal — *see* Enteritis, regional
  - intestinal pouch K91.85Ø
  - intestine (any part) — *see* Enteritis
  - jaw (acute) (bone) (chronic) (lower) (suppurative) (upper) M27.2
  - joint NEC — *see* Arthritis
    - sacroiliac M46.1
  - kidney — *see* Nephritis
  - knee (joint) M13.169
    - tuberculous A18.Ø2
  - labium (majus) (minus) — *see* Vulvitis
  - lacrimal
    - gland — *see* Dacryoadenitis
    - passages (duct) (sac) — *see also* Dacryocystitis
      - canaliculitis — *see* Canaliculitis, lacrimal
  - larynx — *see* Laryngitis
  - leg NOS LØ8.9
  - lip K13.Ø
  - liver (capsule) — *see also* Hepatitis
    - chronic K73.9
    - suppurative K75.Ø
  - lung (acute) — *see also* Pneumonia
    - chronic J98.4
  - lymph gland or node — *see* Lymphadenitis
  - lymphatic vessel — *see* Lymphangitis
  - maxilla, maxillary M27.2
    - sinus (chronic) — *see* Sinusitis, maxillary
  - membranes of brain or spinal cord — *see* Meningitis
  - meninges — *see* Meningitis
  - mouth K12.1
  - muscle — *see* Myositis
  - myocardium — *see* Myocarditis
  - nasal sinus (chronic) — *see* Sinusitis
  - nasopharynx — *see* Nasopharyngitis
  - navel LØ8.82
  - nerve NEC — *see* Neuritis
  - nipple N61.Ø
    - puerperal, postpartum or gestational — *see* Infection, nipple
  - nose — *see* Rhinitis
  - oculomotor (nerve) — *see* Strabismus, paralytic, third nerve
  - optic nerve — *see* Neuritis, optic
  - orbit (chronic) HØ5.1Ø
    - acute HØ5.ØØ
      - abscess — *see* Abscess, orbit
      - cellulitis — *see* Cellulitis, orbit
      - osteomyelitis — *see* Osteomyelitis, orbit
      - periostitis — *see* Periostitis, orbital
      - tenonitis — *see* Tenonitis, eye
    - granuloma — *see* Granuloma, orbit
    - myositis — *see* Myositis, orbital

- **Inflammation, inflamed, inflammatory** — *continued*
  - ovary — *see* Salpingo-oophoritis
  - oviduct — *see* Salpingo-oophoritis
  - pancreas (acute) — *see* Pancreatitis
  - parametrium N73.Ø
  - parotid region LØ8.9
  - pelvis, female — *see* Disease, pelvis, inflammatory
  - penis (corpora cavernosa) N48.29
  - perianal K62.89
  - pericardium — *see* Pericarditis
  - perineum (female) (male) LØ8.9
  - perirectal K62.89
  - peritoneum — *see* Peritonitis
  - periuterine — *see* Disease, pelvis, inflammatory
  - perivesical — *see* Cystitis
  - petrous bone (acute) (chronic) — *see* Petrositis
  - pharynx (acute) — *see* Pharyngitis
  - pia mater — *see* Meningitis
  - pleura — *see* Pleurisy
  - polyp, colon — *see also* Polyp, colon, inflammatory K51.4Ø
  - prostate — *see also* Prostatitis
    - specified type NEC N41.8
  - rectosigmoid — *see* Rectosigmoiditis
  - rectum — *see also* Proctitis K62.89
  - respiratory, upper — *see also* Infection, respiratory, upper JØ6.9
    - acute, due to radiation J7Ø.Ø
    - chronic, due to external agent — *see* condition, respiratory, chronic, due to
    - due to
      - chemicals, gases, fumes or vapors (inhalation) J68.2
      - radiation J7Ø.1
  - retina — *see* Chorioretinitis
  - retrocecal — *see* Appendicitis
  - retroperitoneal — *see* Peritonitis
  - salivary duct or gland (any) (suppurative) — *see* Sialoadenitis
  - scorbutic, alveoli, teeth E54
  - scrotum N49.2
  - seminal vesicle — *see* Vesiculitis
  - sigmoid — *see* Enteritis
  - sinus — *see* Sinusitis
  - Skene's duct or gland — *see* Urethritis
  - skin LØ8.9
  - spermatic cord N49.1
  - sphenoidal (sinus) — *see* Sinusitis, sphenoidal
  - spinal
    - cord — *see* Encephalitis
    - membrane — *see* Meningitis
    - nerve — *see* Disorder, nerve
  - spine — *see* Spondylopathy, inflammatory
  - spleen (capsule) D73.89
  - stomach — *see* Gastritis
  - subcutaneous tissue LØ8.9
  - suprarenal (gland) E27.8
  - synovial — *see* Tenosynovitis
  - tendon (sheath) NEC — *see* Tenosynovitis
  - testis — *see* Orchitis
  - throat (acute) — *see* Pharyngitis
  - thymus (gland) E32.8
  - thyroid (gland) — *see* Thyroiditis
  - tongue K14.Ø
  - tonsil — *see* Tonsillitis
  - trachea — *see* Tracheitis
  - trochlear (nerve) — *see* Strabismus, paralytic, fourth nerve
  - tubal — *see* Salpingo-oophoritis
  - tuberculous NEC — *see* Tuberculosis
  - tubo-ovarian — *see* Salpingo-oophoritis
  - tunica vaginalis N49.1
  - tympanic membrane — *see* Tympanitis
  - umbilicus, umbilical LØ8.82
  - uterine ligament — *see* Disease, pelvis, inflammatory
  - uterus (catarrhal) — *see* Endometritis
  - uveal tract (anterior) NOS — *see also* Iridocyclitis
    - posterior — *see* Chorioretinitis
  - vagina — *see* Vaginitis
  - vas deferens N49.1
  - vein — *see also* Phlebitis
    - intracranial or intraspinal (septic) GØ8
    - thrombotic I8Ø.9
      - leg — *see* Phlebitis, leg
      - lower extremity — *see* Phlebitis, leg
  - vocal cord J38.3

- **Inflammation, inflamed, inflammatory** — *continued*
  - vulva — *see* Vulvitis
  - Wharton's duct (suppurative) — *see* Sialoadenitis
- **Inflation, lung, imperfect** (newborn) — *see* Atelectasis
- **Influenza** (bronchial) (epidemic) (respiratory (upper)) (unidentified influenza virus) J11.1
  - with
    - digestive manifestations J11.2
    - encephalopathy J11.81
    - enteritis J11.2
    - gastroenteritis J11.2
    - gastrointestinal manifestations J11.2
    - laryngitis J11.1
    - myocarditis J11.82
    - otitis media J11.83
    - pharyngitis J11.1
    - pneumonia J11.ØØ
      - specified type J11.Ø8
    - respiratory manifestations NEC J11.1
    - specified manifestation NEC J11.89
  - A (non-novel) J1Ø- ☑
  - A/H5N1 — *see also* Influenza, due to, identified novel influenza A virus JØ9.X2
  - avian — *see also* Influenza, due to, identified novel influenza A virus JØ9.X2
  - B J1Ø- ☑
  - bird — *see also* Influenza, due to, identified novel influenza A virus JØ9.X2
  - C J1Ø- ☑
  - due to
    - avian — *see also* Influenza, due to, identified novel influenza A virus JØ9.X2
    - identified influenza virus NEC J1Ø.1
      - with
        - digestive manifestations J1Ø.2
        - encephalopathy J1Ø.81
        - enteritis J1Ø.2
        - gastroenteritis J1Ø.2
        - gastrointestinal manifestations J1Ø.2
        - laryngitis J1Ø.1
        - myocarditis J1Ø.82
        - otitis media J1Ø.83
        - pharyngitis J1Ø.1
        - pneumonia (unspecified type) J1Ø.ØØ
          - with same identified influenza virus J1Ø.Ø1
          - specified type NEC J1Ø.Ø8
        - respiratory manifestations NEC J1Ø.1
        - specified manifestation NEC J1Ø.89
    - identified novel influenza A virus JØ9.X2
      - with
        - digestive manifestations JØ9.X3
        - encephalopathy JØ9.X9
        - enteritis JØ9.X3
        - gastroenteritis JØ9.X3
        - gastrointestinal manifestations JØ9.X3
        - laryngitis JØ9.X2
        - myocarditis JØ9.X9
        - otitis media JØ9.X9
        - pharyngitis JØ9.X2
        - pneumonia JØ9.X1
        - respiratory manifestations NEC JØ9.X2
        - specified manifestation NEC JØ9.X9
        - upper respiratory symptoms JØ9.X2
  - novel (2ØØ9) H1N1 influenza — *see also* Influenza, due to, identified influenza virus NEC J1Ø.1
  - novel influenza A/H1N1 — *see also* Influenza, due to, identified influenza virus NEC J1Ø.1
  - of other animal origin, not bird or swine — *see also* Influenza, due to, identified novel influenza A virus JØ9.X2
  - swine (viruses that normally cause infections in pigs) — *see also* Influenza, due to, identified novel influenza A virus JØ9.X2
- **Influenzal** — *see* Influenza
- **Influenza-like disease** — *see* Influenza
- **Infraction, Freiberg's** (metatarsal head) — *see* Osteochondrosis, juvenile, metatarsus
- **Infraeruption of tooth** (teeth) M26.34
- **Infusion complication, misadventure, or reaction** — *see* Complications, infusion
- **Ingestion**
  - chemical — *see* Table of Drugs and Chemicals, by substance, poisoning

Index Inflammation, inflamed, inflammatory — Ingestion

- **Ingestion** — *continued*
  - drug or medicament
    - correct substance properly administered — *see* Table of Drugs and Chemicals, by drug, adverse effect
    - overdose or wrong substance given or taken — *see* Table of Drugs and Chemicals, by drug, poisoning
  - foreign body — *see* Foreign body, alimentary tract
  - multiple drug — *see* Table of Drugs and Chemicals, multiple
  - tularemia A21.3
- **Ingrowing**
  - hair (beard) L73.1
  - nail (finger) (toe) L6Ø.Ø
- **Inguinal** — *see also* condition
  - testicle Q53.9
    - bilateral Q53.212
    - unilateral Q53.112
- **Inhalant-induced**
  - anxiety disorder F18.98Ø
  - depressive disorder F18.94
  - major neurocognitive disorder F18.97
  - mild neurocognitive disorder F18.988
  - psychotic disorder F18.959
- **Inhalation**
  - anthrax A22.1
  - flame T27.3 ☑
  - food or foreign body — *see* Foreign body, by site
  - gases, fumes, or vapors T59.9- ☑
    - specified agent NEC — *see* Table of Drugs and Chemicals, by substance T59.89- ☑
  - liquid or vomitus — *see* Asphyxia
  - meconium (newborn) P24.ØØ
    - with
      - with respiratory symptoms P24.Ø1
      - pneumonia (pneumonitis) P24.Ø1
  - mucus — *see* Asphyxia, mucus
  - oil or gasoline (causing suffocation) — *see* Foreign body, by site
  - smoke T59.81- ☑
    - with respiratory conditions J7Ø.5
      - due to chemicals, gases, fumes and vapors J68.9
  - steam — *see also* Burn, respiratory tract T59.9- ☑
  - stomach contents or secretions — *see* Foreign body, by site
    - due to anesthesia (general) (local) or other sedation T88.59
      - in labor and delivery O74.Ø
      - in pregnancy O29.Ø1- ☑
      - postpartum, puerperal O89.Ø1
- **Inhibition, orgasm**
  - female F52.31
  - male F52.32
- **Inhibitor, systemic lupus erythematosus** (presence of) D68.62
- **Iniencephalus, iniencephaly** QØØ.2
- **Injection, traumatic jet** (air) (industrial) (water) (paint or dye) T7Ø.4 ☑
- **Injury** — *see also* specified injury type T14.9Ø ☑
  - abdomen, abdominal S39.91 ☑
    - blood vessel — *see* Injury, blood vessel, abdomen
    - cavity — *see* Injury, intra-abdominal
    - contusion S3Ø.1 ☑
    - internal — *see* Injury, intra-abdominal
    - intra-abdominal organ — *see* Injury, intra-abdominal
    - nerve — *see* Injury, nerve, abdomen
    - open — *see* Wound, open, abdomen
    - specified NEC S39.81 ☑
    - superficial — *see* Injury, superficial, abdomen
  - Achilles tendon S86.ØØ- ☑
    - laceration S86.Ø2- ☑
    - specified type NEC S86.Ø9- ☑
    - strain S86.Ø1- ☑
  - acoustic, resulting in deafness — *see* Injury, nerve, acoustic
  - adrenal (gland) S37.819 ☑
    - contusion S37.812 ☑
    - laceration S37.813 ☑
    - specified type NEC S37.818 ☑
  - alveolar (process) SØ9.93 ☑
  - ankle S99.91- ☑
    - contusion — *see* Contusion, ankle
    - dislocation — *see* Dislocation, ankle
    - fracture — *see* Fracture, ankle
    - nerve — *see* Injury, nerve, ankle

- **Injury** — *continued*
  - ankle — *continued*
    - open — *see* Wound, open, ankle
    - specified type NEC S99.81- ☑
    - sprain — *see* Sprain, ankle
    - superficial — *see* Injury, superficial, ankle
  - anterior chamber, eye — *see* Injury, eye, specified site NEC
  - anus — *see* Injury, abdomen
  - aorta (thoracic) S25.ØØ ☑
    - abdominal S35.ØØ ☑
      - laceration (minor) (superficial) S35.Ø1 ☑
        - major S35.Ø2 ☑
      - specified type NEC S35.Ø9 ☑
    - laceration (minor) (superficial) S25.Ø1 ☑
      - major S25.Ø2 ☑
    - specified type NEC S25.Ø9 ☑
  - arm (upper) S49.9- ☑
    - blood vessel — *see* Injury, blood vessel, arm
    - contusion — *see* Contusion, arm, upper
    - fracture — *see* Fracture, humerus
    - lower — *see* Injury, forearm
    - muscle — *see* Injury, muscle, shoulder
    - nerve — *see* Injury, nerve, arm
    - open — *see* Wound, open, arm
    - specified type NEC S49.8- ☑
    - superficial — *see* Injury, superficial, arm
  - artery (complicating trauma) — *see also* Injury, blood vessel, by site
    - cerebral or meningeal — *see* Injury, intracranial
  - auditory canal (external) (meatus) SØ9.91 ☑
  - auricle, auris, ear SØ9.91 ☑
  - axilla — *see* Injury, shoulder
  - back — *see* Injury, back, lower
  - bile duct S36.13 ☑
  - birth — *see also* Birth, injury P15.9
  - bladder (sphincter) S37.2Ø ☑
    - at delivery O71.5
    - contusion S37.22 ☑
    - laceration S37.23 ☑
    - obstetrical trauma O71.5
    - specified type NEC S37.29 ☑
  - blast (air) (hydraulic) (immersion) (underwater) NEC T14.8 ☑
    - acoustic nerve trauma — *see* Injury, nerve, acoustic
    - bladder — *see* Injury, bladder
    - brain — *see* Concussion
      - primary, specified NEC SØ6.8A- ☑
    - colon — *see* Injury, intestine, large
    - ear (primary) SØ9.31- ☑
      - secondary SØ9.39- ☑
    - generalized T7Ø.8 ☑
    - lung — *see* Injury, intrathoracic, lung
    - multiple body organs T7Ø.8 ☑
    - peritoneum S36.81 ☑
    - rectum S36.61 ☑
    - retroperitoneum S36.898 ☑
    - small intestine S36.419 ☑
      - duodenum S36.41Ø ☑
      - specified site NEC S36.418 ☑
    - specified
      - intra-abdominal organ NEC S36.898 ☑
      - pelvic organ NEC S37.899 ☑
  - blood vessel NEC T14.8 ☑
    - abdomen S35.9 ☑
      - aorta — *see* Injury, aorta, abdominal
      - celiac artery — *see* Injury, blood vessel, celiac artery
      - iliac vessel — *see* Injury, blood vessel, iliac
      - laceration S35.91 ☑
      - mesenteric vessel — *see* Injury, mesenteric
      - portal vein — *see* Injury, blood vessel, portal vein
      - renal vessel — *see* Injury, blood vessel, renal
      - specified vessel NEC S35.8X- ☑
      - splenic vessel — *see* Injury, blood vessel, splenic
      - vena cava — *see* Injury, vena cava, inferior
    - ankle — *see* Injury, blood vessel, foot
    - aorta (abdominal) (thoracic) — *see* Injury, aorta
    - arm (upper) NEC S45.9Ø- ☑
      - forearm — *see* Injury, blood vessel, forearm
      - laceration S45.91- ☑
      - specified
        - site NEC S45.8Ø- ☑
          - laceration S45.81- ☑
          - specified type NEC S45.89- ☑
        - type NEC S45.99- ☑

- **Injury** — *continued*
  - blood vessel — *continued*
    - arm — *continued*
      - superficial vein S45.3Ø- ☑
        - laceration S45.31- ☑
        - specified type NEC S45.39- ☑
    - axillary
      - artery S45.ØØ- ☑
        - laceration S45.Ø1- ☑
        - specified type NEC S45.Ø9- ☑
      - vein S45.2Ø- ☑
        - laceration S45.21- ☑
        - specified type NEC S45.29- ☑
    - azygos vein — *see* Injury, blood vessel, thoracic, specified site NEC
    - brachial
      - artery S45.1Ø- ☑
        - laceration S45.11- ☑
        - specified type NEC S45.19- ☑
      - vein S45.2Ø- ☑
        - laceration S45.219 ☑
        - specified type NEC S45.29- ☑
    - carotid artery (common) (external) (internal, extracranial) S15.ØØ- ☑
      - internal, intracranial SØ6.8- ☑
      - laceration (minor) (superficial) S15.Ø1- ☑
        - major S15.Ø2- ☑
      - specified type NEC S15.Ø9- ☑
    - celiac artery S35.219 ☑
      - branch S35.299 ☑
        - laceration (minor) (superficial) S35.291 ☑
          - major S35.292 ☑
        - specified NEC S35.298 ☑
      - laceration (minor) (superficial) S35.211 ☑
        - major S35.212 ☑
      - specified type NEC S35.218 ☑
    - cerebral — *see* Injury, intracranial
    - deep plantar — *see* Injury, blood vessel, plantar artery
    - digital (hand) — *see* Injury, blood vessel, finger
    - dorsal
      - artery (foot) S95.ØØ- ☑
        - laceration S95.Ø1- ☑
        - specified type NEC S95.Ø9- ☑
      - vein (foot) S95.2Ø- ☑
        - laceration S95.21- ☑
        - specified type NEC S95.29- ☑
    - due to accidental laceration during procedure — *see* Laceration, accidental complicating surgery
    - extremity — *see* Injury, blood vessel, limb
    - femoral
      - artery (common) (superficial) S75.ØØ- ☑
        - laceration (minor) (superficial) S75.Ø1- ☑
          - major S75.Ø2- ☑
        - specified type NEC S75.Ø9- ☑
      - vein (hip level) (thigh level) S75.1Ø- ☑
        - laceration (minor) (superficial) S75.11- ☑
          - major S75.12- ☑
        - specified type NEC S75.19- ☑
    - finger S65.5Ø- ☑
      - index S65.5Ø- ☑
        - laceration S65.51- ☑
        - specified type NEC S65.59- ☑
      - laceration S65.51- ☑
      - little S65.5Ø- ☑
        - laceration S65.51- ☑
        - specified type NEC S65.59- ☑
      - middle S65.5Ø- ☑
        - laceration S65.51- ☑
        - specified type NEC S65.59- ☑
      - specified type NEC S65.59- ☑
      - thumb — *see* Injury, blood vessel, thumb
    - foot S95.9Ø- ☑
      - dorsal
        - artery — *see* Injury, blood vessel, dorsal, artery
        - vein — *see* Injury, blood vessel, dorsal, vein
      - laceration S95.91- ☑
      - plantar artery — *see* Injury, blood vessel, plantar artery
      - specified
        - site NEC S95.8Ø- ☑
          - laceration S95.81- ☑
          - specified type NEC S95.89- ☑
        - specified type NEC S95.99- ☑

Injury — *continued*
blood vessel — *continued*
forearm S55.9Ø- ☑
laceration S55.91- ☑
radial artery — *see* Injury, blood vessel, radial artery
specified
site NEC S55.8Ø- ☑
laceration S55.81- ☑
specified type NEC S55.89- ☑
type NEC S55.99- ☑
ulnar artery — *see* Injury, blood vessel, ulnar artery
vein S55.2Ø- ☑
laceration S55.21- ☑
specified type NEC S55.29- ☑
gastric
artery — *see* Injury, mesenteric, artery, branch
vein — *see* Injury, blood vessel, abdomen
gastroduodenal artery — *see* Injury, mesenteric, artery, branch
greater saphenous vein (lower leg level) S85.3Ø- ☑
hip (and thigh) level S75.2Ø- ☑
laceration (minor) (superficial) S75.21- ☑
major S75.22- ☑
specified type NEC S75.29- ☑
laceration S85.31- ☑
specified type NEC S85.39- ☑
hand (level) S65.9Ø- ☑
finger — *see* Injury, blood vessel, finger
laceration S65.91- ☑
palmar arch — *see* Injury, blood vessel, palmar arch
radial artery — *see* Injury, blood vessel, radial artery, hand
specified
site NEC S65.8Ø- ☑
laceration S65.81- ☑
specified type NEC S65.89- ☑
type NEC S65.99- ☑
thumb — *see* Injury, blood vessel, thumb
ulnar artery — *see* Injury, blood vessel, ulnar artery, hand
head S09.0 ☑
intracranial — *see* Injury, intracranial
multiple S09.0 ☑
hepatic
artery — *see* Injury, mesenteric, artery
vein — *see* Injury, vena cava, inferior
hip S75.9Ø- ☑
femoral artery — *see* Injury, blood vessel, femoral, artery
femoral vein — *see* Injury, blood vessel, femoral, vein
greater saphenous vein — *see* Injury, blood vessel, greater saphenous, hip level
laceration S75.91- ☑
specified
site NEC S75.8Ø- ☑
laceration S75.81- ☑
specified type NEC S75.89- ☑
type NEC S75.99- ☑
hypogastric (artery) (vein) — *see* Injury, blood vessel, iliac
iliac S35.5- ☑
artery S35.51- ☑
specified vessel NEC S35.5- ☑
uterine vessel — *see* Injury, blood vessel, uterine
vein S35.51- ☑
innominate — *see* Injury, blood vessel, thoracic, innominate
intercostal (artery) (vein) — *see* Injury, blood vessel, thoracic, intercostal
jugular vein (external) S15.2Ø- ☑
internal S15.3Ø- ☑
laceration (minor) (superficial) S15.31- ☑
major S15.32- ☑
specified type NEC S15.39- ☑
laceration (minor) (superficial) S15.21- ☑
major S15.22- ☑
specified type NEC S15.29- ☑
leg (level) (lower) S85.9Ø- ☑
greater saphenous — *see* Injury, blood vessel, greater saphenous
laceration S85.91- ☑

Injury — *continued*
blood vessel — *continued*
leg — *continued*
lesser saphenous — *see* Injury, blood vessel, lesser saphenous
peroneal artery — *see* Injury, blood vessel, peroneal artery
popliteal
artery — *see* Injury, blood vessel, popliteal, artery
vein — *see* Injury, blood vessel, popliteal, vein
specified
site NEC S85.8Ø- ☑
laceration S85.81- ☑
specified type NEC S85.89- ☑
type NEC S85.99- ☑
thigh — *see* Injury, blood vessel, hip
tibial artery — *see* Injury, blood vessel, tibial artery
lesser saphenous vein (lower leg level) S85.4Ø- ☑
laceration S85.41- ☑
specified type NEC S85.49- ☑
limb
lower — *see* Injury, blood vessel, leg
upper — *see* Injury, blood vessel, arm
lower back — *see* Injury, blood vessel, abdomen
specified NEC — *see* Injury, blood vessel, abdomen, specified, site NEC
mammary (artery) (vein) — *see* Injury, blood vessel, thoracic, specified site NEC
mesenteric (inferior) (superior)
artery — *see* Injury, mesenteric, artery
vein — *see* Injury, blood vessel, mesenteric, vein
neck S15.9 ☑
specified site NEC S15.8 ☑
ovarian (artery) (vein) — *see* subcategory S35.8 ☑
palmar arch (superficial) S65.2Ø- ☑
deep S65.3Ø- ☑
laceration S65.31- ☑
specified type NEC S65.39- ☑
laceration S65.21- ☑
specified type NEC S65.29- ☑
pelvis — *see* Injury, blood vessel, abdomen
specified NEC — *see* Injury, blood vessel, abdomen, specified, site NEC
peroneal artery S85.2Ø- ☑
laceration S85.21- ☑
specified type NEC S85.29- ☑
plantar artery (deep) (foot) S95.1Ø- ☑
laceration S95.11- ☑
specified type NEC S95.19- ☑
popliteal
artery S85.ØØ- ☑
laceration S85.Ø1- ☑
specified type NEC S85.Ø9- ☑
vein S85.5Ø- ☑
laceration S85.51- ☑
specified type NEC S85.59- ☑
portal vein S35.319 ☑
laceration S35.311 ☑
specified type NEC S35.318 ☑
precerebral — *see* Injury, blood vessel, neck
pulmonary (artery) (vein) — *see* Injury, blood vessel, thoracic, pulmonary
radial artery (forearm level) S55.1Ø- ☑
hand and wrist (level) S65.1Ø- ☑
laceration S65.11- ☑
specified type NEC S65.19- ☑
laceration S55.11- ☑
specified type NEC S55.19- ☑
renal
artery S35.4Ø- ☑
laceration S35.41- ☑
specified NEC S35.49- ☑
vein S35.4Ø- ☑
laceration S35.41- ☑
specified NEC S35.49- ☑
saphenous vein (greater) (lower leg level) — *see* Injury, blood vessel, greater saphenous
hip and thigh level — *see* Injury, blood vessel, greater saphenous, hip level
lesser — *see* Injury, blood vessel, lesser saphenous
shoulder
specified NEC — *see* Injury, blood vessel, arm, specified site NEC

Injury — *continued*
blood vessel — *continued*
shoulder — *continued*
superficial vein — *see* Injury, blood vessel, arm, superficial vein
specified NEC T14.8 ☑
splenic
artery — *see* Injury, blood vessel, celiac artery, branch
vein S35.329 ☑
laceration S35.321 ☑
specified NEC S35.328 ☑
subclavian — *see* Injury, blood vessel, thoracic, innominate
thigh — *see* Injury, blood vessel, hip
thoracic S25.9Ø ☑
aorta S25.ØØ ☑
laceration (minor) (superficial) S25.Ø1 ☑
major S25.Ø2 ☑
specified type NEC S25.Ø9 ☑
azygos vein — *see* Injury, blood vessel, thoracic, specified, site NEC
innominate
artery S25.1Ø- ☑
laceration (minor) (superficial) S25.11- ☑
major S25.12- ☑
specified type NEC S25.19- ☑
vein S25.3Ø- ☑
laceration (minor) (superficial) S25.31- ☑
major S25.32- ☑
specified type NEC S25.39- ☑
intercostal S25.5Ø- ☑
laceration S25.51- ☑
specified type NEC S25.59- ☑
laceration S25.91 ☑
mammary vessel — *see* Injury, blood vessel, thoracic, specified, site NEC
pulmonary S25.4Ø- ☑
laceration (minor) (superficial) S25.41- ☑
major S25.42- ☑
specified type NEC S25.49- ☑
specified
site NEC S25.8Ø- ☑
laceration S25.81 ☑
specified type NEC S25.89 ☑
type NEC S25.99 ☑
subclavian — *see* Injury, blood vessel, thoracic, innominate
vena cava (superior) S25.2Ø ☑
laceration (minor) (superficial) S25.21 ☑
major S25.22 ☑
specified type NEC S25.29 ☑
thumb S65.4Ø- ☑
laceration S65.41- ☑
specified type NEC S65.49- ☑
tibial artery S85.1Ø- ☑
anterior S85.13- ☑
laceration S85.14- ☑
specified injury NEC S85.15- ☑
laceration S85.11 ☑
posterior S85.16- ☑
laceration S85.17- ☑
specified injury NEC S85.18- ☑
specified injury NEC S85.12- ☑
ulnar artery (forearm level) S55.ØØ- ☑
hand and wrist (level) S65.ØØ- ☑
laceration S65.Ø1- ☑
specified type NEC S65.Ø9- ☑
laceration S55.Ø1- ☑
specified type NEC S55.Ø9- ☑
upper arm (level) — *see* Injury, blood vessel, arm
superficial vein — *see* Injury, blood vessel, arm, superficial vein
uterine S35.5- ☑
artery S35.53- ☑
vein S35.53- ☑
vena cava — *see* Injury, vena cava
vertebral artery S15.1Ø- ☑
laceration (minor) (superficial) S15.11- ☑
major S15.12- ☑
specified type NEC S15.19- ☑
wrist (level) — *see* Injury, blood vessel, hand
brachial plexus S14.3 ☑
newborn P14.3
brain (traumatic) SØ6.9- ☑
diffuse (axonal) SØ6.2X- ☑

- **Injury** — *continued*
  - brain — *continued*
    - focal SØ6.3Ø- ☑
  - brainstem SØ6.38- ☑
  - breast NOS S29.9 ☑
  - broad ligament — *see* Injury, pelvic organ, specified site NEC
  - bronchus, bronchi — *see* Injury, intrathoracic, bronchus
  - brow SØ9.9Ø ☑
  - buttock S39.92 ☑
  - canthus, eye SØ5.9Ø ☑
  - cardiac plexus — *see* Injury, nerve, thorax, sympathetic
  - cauda equina S34.3 ☑
  - cavernous sinus — *see* Injury, intracranial
  - cecum — *see* Injury, colon
  - celiac ganglion or plexus — *see* Injury, nerve, lumbosacral, sympathetic
  - cerebellum — *see* Injury, intracranial
  - cerebral — *see* Injury, intracranial
  - cervix (uteri) — *see* Injury, uterus
  - cheek (wall) SØ9.93 ☑
  - chest — *see* Injury, thorax
  - childbirth (newborn) — *see also* Birth, injury
    - maternal NEC O71.9
  - chin SØ9.93 ☑
  - choroid (eye) — *see* Injury, eye, specified site NEC
  - clitoris S39.94 ☑
  - coccyx — *see also* Injury, back, lower
    - complicating delivery O71.6
  - colon — *see* Injury, intestine, large
  - common bile duct — *see* Injury, liver
  - conjunctiva (superficial) — *see* Injury, eye, conjunctiva
  - conus medullaris — *see* Injury, spinal, sacral
  - cord
    - spermatic (pelvic region) S37.898 ☑
      - scrotal region S39.848 ☑
    - spinal — *see* Injury, spinal cord, by region
  - cornea — *see* Injury, eye, specified site NEC
    - abrasion — *see* Injury, eye, cornea, abrasion
  - cortex (cerebral) — *see also* Injury, intracranial
    - visual — *see* Injury, nerve, optic
  - costal region NEC S29.9 ☑
  - costochondral NEC S29.9 ☑
  - cranial
    - cavity — *see* Injury, intracranial
    - nerve — *see* Injury, nerve, cranial
  - crushing — *see* Crush
  - cutaneous sensory nerve
  - cystic duct — *see* Injury, liver
  - deep tissue — *see* Contusion, by site
    - meaning pressure ulcer — *see* Ulcer, pressure L89 with final character .6
  - delivery (newborn) P15.9
    - maternal NEC O71.9
  - Descemet's membrane — *see* Injury, eyeball, penetrating
  - diaphragm — *see* Injury, intrathoracic, diaphragm
  - duodenum — *see* Injury, intestine, small, duodenum
  - ear (auricle) (external) (canal) SØ9.91 ☑
    - abrasion — *see* Abrasion, ear
    - bite — *see* Bite, ear
    - blister — *see* Blister, ear
    - bruise — *see* Contusion, ear
    - contusion — *see* Contusion, ear
    - external constriction — *see* Constriction, external, ear
    - hematoma — *see* Hematoma, ear
    - inner — *see* Injury, ear, middle
    - laceration — *see* Laceration, ear
    - middle SØ9.3Ø- ☑
      - blast — *see* Injury, blast, ear
      - specified NEC SØ9.39- ☑
    - puncture — *see* Puncture, ear
    - superficial — *see* Injury, superficial, ear
  - eighth cranial nerve (acoustic or auditory) — *see* Injury, nerve, acoustic
  - elbow S59.9Ø- ☑
    - contusion — *see* Contusion, elbow
    - dislocation — *see* Dislocation, elbow
    - fracture — *see* Fracture, ulna, upper end
    - open — *see* Wound, open, elbow
    - specified NEC S59.8Ø- ☑
    - sprain — *see* Sprain, elbow
    - superficial — *see* Injury, superficial, elbow
  - eleventh cranial nerve (accessory) — *see* Injury, nerve, accessory

- **Injury** — *continued*
  - epididymis S39.94 ☑
  - epigastric region S39.91 ☑
  - epiglottis NEC S19.89 ☑
  - esophageal plexus — *see* Injury, nerve, thorax, sympathetic
  - esophagus (thoracic part) — *see also* Injury, intrathoracic, esophagus
    - cervical NEC S19.85 ☑
  - eustachian tube SØ9.3Ø ☑
  - eye SØ5.9- ☑
    - avulsion SØ5.7- ☑
    - ball — *see* Injury, eyeball
    - conjunctiva SØ5.Ø- ☑
    - cornea
      - abrasion SØ5.Ø- ☑
    - laceration SØ5.3- ☑
      - with prolapse SØ5.2- ☑
    - lacrimal apparatus SØ5.8X- ☑
    - orbit penetration SØ5.4- ☑
    - specified site NEC SØ5.8X- ☑
  - eyeball SØ5.8X- ☑
    - contusion SØ5.1- ☑
    - penetrating SØ5.6- ☑
      - with
        - foreign body SØ5.5- ☑
        - prolapse or loss of intraocular tissue SØ5.2- ☑
      - without prolapse or loss of intraocular tissue SØ5.3- ☑
    - specified type NEC SØ5.8- ☑
  - eyebrow SØ9.93 ☑
  - eyelid SØ9.93 ☑
    - abrasion — *see* Abrasion, eyelid
    - contusion — *see* Contusion, eyelid
    - open — *see* Wound, open, eyelid
  - face SØ9.93 ☑
  - fallopian tube S37.5Ø9 ☑
    - bilateral S37.5Ø2 ☑
      - blast injury S37.512 ☑
      - contusion S37.522 ☑
      - laceration S37.532 ☑
      - specified type NEC S37.592 ☑
    - blast injury (primary) S37.519 ☑
      - bilateral S37.512 ☑
      - secondary — *see* Injury, fallopian tube, specified type NEC
      - unilateral S37.511 ☑
    - contusion S37.529 ☑
      - bilateral S37.522 ☑
      - unilateral S37.521 ☑
    - laceration S37.539 ☑
      - bilateral S37.532 ☑
      - unilateral S37.531 ☑
    - specified type NEC S37.599 ☑
      - bilateral S37.592 ☑
      - unilateral S37.591 ☑
    - unilateral S37.5Ø1 ☑
      - blast injury S37.511 ☑
      - contusion S37.521 ☑
      - laceration S37.531 ☑
      - specified type NEC S37.591 ☑
  - fascia — *see* Injury, muscle
  - fifth cranial nerve (trigeminal) — *see* Injury, nerve, trigeminal
  - finger (nail) S69.9- ☑
    - blood vessel — *see* Injury, blood vessel, finger
    - contusion — *see* Contusion, finger
    - dislocation — *see* Dislocation, finger
    - fracture — *see* Fracture, finger
    - muscle — *see* Injury, muscle, finger
    - nerve — *see* Injury, nerve, digital, finger
    - open — *see* Wound, open, finger
    - specified NEC S69.8- ☑
    - sprain — *see* Sprain, finger
    - superficial — *see* Injury, superficial, finger
  - first cranial nerve (olfactory) — *see* Injury, nerve, olfactory
  - flank — *see* Injury, abdomen
  - foot S99.92- ☑
    - blood vessel — *see* Injury, blood vessel, foot
    - contusion — *see* Contusion, foot
    - dislocation — *see* Dislocation, foot
    - fracture — *see* Fracture, foot
    - muscle — *see* Injury, muscle, foot
    - open — *see* Wound, open, foot
    - specified type NEC S99.82- ☑

- **Injury** — *continued*
  - foot — *continued*
    - sprain — *see* Sprain, foot
    - superficial — *see* Injury, superficial, foot
  - forceps NOS P15.9
  - forearm S59.91- ☑
    - blood vessel — *see* Injury, blood vessel, forearm
    - contusion — *see* Contusion, forearm
    - fracture — *see* Fracture, forearm
    - muscle — *see* Injury, muscle, forearm
    - nerve — *see* Injury, nerve, forearm
    - open — *see* Wound, open, forearm
    - specified NEC S59.81- ☑
    - superficial — *see* Injury, superficial, forearm
  - forehead SØ9.9Ø ☑
  - fourth cranial nerve (trochlear) — *see* Injury, nerve, trochlear
  - gallbladder S36.129 ☑
    - contusion S36.122 ☑
    - laceration S36.123 ☑
    - specified NEC S36.128 ☑
  - ganglion
    - celiac, coeliac — *see* Injury, nerve, lumbosacral, sympathetic
    - gasserian — *see* Injury, nerve, trigeminal
    - stellate — *see* Injury, nerve, thorax, sympathetic
    - thoracic sympathetic — *see* Injury, nerve, thorax, sympathetic
  - gasserian ganglion — *see* Injury, nerve, trigeminal
  - gastric artery — *see* Injury, blood vessel, celiac artery, branch
  - gastroduodenal artery — *see* Injury, blood vessel, celiac artery, branch
  - gastrointestinal tract — *see* Injury, intra-abdominal
    - with open wound into abdominal cavity — *see* Wound, open, with penetration into peritoneal cavity
    - colon — *see* Injury, intestine, large
    - rectum — *see* Injury, intestine, large, rectum
      - with open wound into abdominal cavity S36.61 ☑
    - small intestine — *see* Injury, intestine, small
    - specified site NEC — *see* Injury, intra-abdominal, specified, site NEC
    - stomach — *see* Injury, stomach
  - genital organ(s)
    - external S39.94 ☑
      - specified NEC S39.848 ☑
    - internal S37.9Ø ☑
      - fallopian tube — *see* Injury, fallopian tube
      - ovary — *see* Injury, ovary
      - prostate — *see* Injury, prostate
      - seminal vesicle — *see* Injury, pelvis, organ, specified site NEC
      - uterus — *see* Injury, uterus
      - vas deferens — *see* Injury, pelvis, organ, specified site NEC
    - obstetrical trauma O71.9
  - gland
    - lacrimal laceration — *see* Injury, eye, specified site NEC
    - salivary SØ9.93 ☑
    - thyroid NEC S19.84 ☑
  - globe (eye) SØ5.9Ø ☑
    - specified NEC SØ5.8X- ☑
  - groin — *see* Injury, abdomen
  - gum SØ9.9Ø ☑
  - hand S69.9- ☑
    - blood vessel — *see* Injury, blood vessel, hand
    - contusion — *see* Contusion, hand
    - fracture — *see* Fracture, hand
    - muscle — *see* Injury, muscle, hand
    - nerve — *see* Injury, nerve, hand
    - open — *see* Wound, open, hand
    - specified NEC S69.8- ☑
    - sprain — *see* Sprain, hand
    - superficial — *see* Injury, superficial, hand
  - head SØ9.9Ø ☑
    - with loss of consciousness SØ6.9- ☑
    - specified NEC SØ9.8 ☑
  - heart (traumatic) S26.9Ø ☑
    - with hemopericardium S26.ØØ ☑
      - contusion S26.Ø1 ☑
      - laceration (mild) S26.Ø2Ø ☑
        - major S26.Ø22 ☑
        - moderate S26.Ø21 ☑

- **Injury** — *continued*
  - heart — *continued*
    - with hemopericardium — *continued*
      - specified type NEC S26.09 ☑
    - contusion S26.91 ☑
    - laceration S26.92 ☑
    - non-traumatic (acute) (chronic) (non-ischemic) I5A
    - specified type NEC S26.99 ☑
    - without hemopericardium S26.10 ☑
      - contusion S26.11 ☑
      - laceration S26.12 ☑
      - specified type NEC S26.19 ☑
  - heel — *see* Injury, foot
  - hepatic
    - artery — *see* Injury, blood vessel, celiac artery, branch
    - duct — *see* Injury, liver
    - vein — *see* Injury, vena cava, inferior
  - hip S79.91- ☑
    - blood vessel — *see* Injury, blood vessel, hip
    - contusion — *see* Contusion, hip
    - dislocation — *see* Dislocation, hip
    - fracture — *see* Fracture, femur, neck
    - muscle — *see* Injury, muscle, hip
    - nerve — *see* Injury, nerve, hip
    - open — *see* Wound, open, hip
    - specified NEC S79.81- ☑
    - sprain — *see* Sprain, hip
    - superficial — *see* Injury, superficial, hip
  - hymen S39.94 ☑
  - hypogastric
    - blood vessel — *see* Injury, blood vessel, iliac
    - plexus — *see* Injury, nerve, lumbosacral, sympathetic
  - ileum — *see* Injury, intestine, small
  - iliac region S39.91 ☑
  - instrumental (during surgery) — *see* Laceration, accidental complicating surgery
    - birth injury — *see* Birth, injury
    - nonsurgical — *see* Injury, by site
    - obstetrical O71.9
      - bladder O71.5
      - cervix O71.3
      - high vaginal O71.4
      - perineal NOS O70.9
      - urethra O71.5
      - uterus O71.5
        - with rupture or perforation O71.1
  - internal T14.8 ☑
    - aorta — *see* Injury, aorta
    - bladder (sphincter) — *see* Injury, bladder
      - with
        - ectopic or molar pregnancy O08.6
        - following ectopic or molar pregnancy O08.6
        - obstetrical trauma O71.5
    - bronchus, bronchi — *see* Injury, intrathoracic, bronchus
    - cecum — *see* Injury, intestine, large
    - cervix (uteri) — *see also* Injury, uterus
      - with ectopic or molar pregnancy O08.6
      - following ectopic or molar pregnancy O08.6
      - obstetrical trauma O71.3
    - chest — *see* Injury, intrathoracic
    - gastrointestinal tract — *see* Injury, intra-abdominal
    - heart — *see* Injury, heart
    - intestine NEC — *see* Injury, intestine
    - intrauterine — *see* Injury, uterus
    - mesentery — *see* Injury, intra-abdominal, specified, site NEC
    - pelvis, pelvic (organ) S37.90 ☑
      - following ectopic or molar pregnancy (subsequent episode) O08.6
      - obstetrical trauma NEC O71.5
        - rupture or perforation O71.1
      - specified NEC S39.83 ☑
    - rectum — *see* Injury, intestine, large, rectum
    - stomach — *see* Injury, stomach
    - ureter — *see* Injury, ureter
    - urethra (sphincter) following ectopic or molar pregnancy O08.6
    - uterus — *see* Injury, uterus
  - interscapular area — *see* Injury, thorax
  - intestine
    - large S36.509 ☑
      - ascending (right) S36.500 ☑
        - blast injury (primary) S36.510 ☑
          - secondary S36.590 ☑

- **Injury** — *continued*
  - intestine — *continued*
    - large — *continued*
      - ascending — *continued*
        - contusion S36.520 ☑
        - laceration S36.530 ☑
        - specified type NEC S36.590 ☑
      - blast injury (primary) S36.519 ☑
        - ascending (right) S36.510 ☑
        - descending (left) S36.512 ☑
        - rectum S36.61 ☑
        - sigmoid S36.513 ☑
        - specified site NEC S36.518 ☑
        - transverse S36.511 ☑
      - contusion S36.529 ☑
        - ascending (right) S36.520 ☑
        - descending (left) S36.522 ☑
        - rectum S36.62 ☑
        - sigmoid S36.523 ☑
        - specified site NEC S36.528 ☑
        - transverse S36.521 ☑
      - descending (left) S36.502 ☑
        - blast injury (primary) S36.512 ☑
          - secondary S36.592 ☑
        - contusion S36.522 ☑
        - laceration S36.532 ☑
        - specified type NEC S36.592 ☑
      - laceration S36.539 ☑
        - ascending (right) S36.530 ☑
        - descending (left) S36.532 ☑
        - rectum S36.63 ☑
        - sigmoid S36.533 ☑
        - specified site NEC S36.538 ☑
        - transverse S36.531 ☑
      - rectum S36.60 ☑
        - blast injury (primary) S36.61 ☑
          - secondary S36.69 ☑
        - contusion S36.62 ☑
        - laceration S36.63 ☑
        - specified type NEC S36.69 ☑
      - sigmoid S36.503 ☑
        - blast injury (primary) S36.513 ☑
          - secondary S36.593 ☑
        - contusion S36.523 ☑
        - laceration S36.533 ☑
        - specified type NEC S36.593 ☑
      - specified
        - site NEC S36.508 ☑
          - blast injury (primary) S36.518 ☑
            - secondary S36.598 ☑
          - contusion S36.528 ☑
          - laceration S36.538 ☑
          - specified type NEC S36.598 ☑
        - type NEC S36.599 ☑
          - ascending (right) S36.590 ☑
          - descending (left) S36.592 ☑
          - rectum S36.69 ☑
          - sigmoid S36.593 ☑
          - specified site NEC S36.598 ☑
          - transverse S36.591 ☑
      - transverse S36.501 ☑
        - blast injury (primary) S36.511 ☑
          - secondary S36.591 ☑
        - contusion S36.521 ☑
        - laceration S36.531 ☑
        - specified type NEC S36.591 ☑
    - small S36.409 ☑
      - blast injury (primary) S36.419 ☑
        - duodenum S36.410 ☑
        - secondary S36.499 ☑
          - duodenum S36.490 ☑
          - specified site NEC S36.498 ☑
        - specified site NEC S36.418 ☑
      - contusion S36.429 ☑
        - duodenum S36.420 ☑
        - specified site NEC S36.428 ☑
      - duodenum S36.400 ☑
        - blast injury (primary) S36.410 ☑
          - secondary S36.490 ☑
        - contusion S36.420 ☑
        - laceration S36.430 ☑
        - specified NEC S36.490 ☑
      - laceration S36.439 ☑
        - duodenum S36.430 ☑
        - specified site NEC S36.438 ☑

- **Injury** — *continued*
  - intestine — *continued*
    - small — *continued*
      - specified
        - site NEC S36.408 ☑
        - type NEC S36.499 ☑
          - duodenum S36.490 ☑
          - specified site NEC S36.498 ☑
  - intra-abdominal S36.90 ☑
    - adrenal gland — *see* Injury, adrenal gland
    - bladder — *see* Injury, bladder
    - colon — *see* Injury, intestine, large
    - contusion S36.92 ☑
    - fallopian tube — *see* Injury, fallopian tube
    - gallbladder — *see* Injury, gallbladder
    - intestine — *see* Injury, intestine
    - kidney — *see* Injury, kidney
    - laceration S36.93 ☑
    - liver — *see* Injury, liver
    - ovary — *see* Injury, ovary
    - pancreas — *see* Injury, pancreas
    - pelvic NOS S37.90 ☑
    - peritoneum — *see* Injury, intra-abdominal, specified, site NEC
    - prostate — *see* Injury, prostate
    - rectum — *see* Injury, intestine, large, rectum
    - retroperitoneum — *see* Injury, intra-abdominal, specified, site NEC
    - seminal vesicle — *see* Injury, pelvis, organ, specified site NEC
    - small intestine — *see* Injury, intestine, small
    - specified
      - pelvic S37.90 ☑
        - specified
          - site NEC S37.899 ☑
            - specified type NEC S37.898 ☑
          - type NEC S37.99 ☑
      - site NEC S36.899 ☑
        - contusion S36.892 ☑
        - laceration S36.893 ☑
        - specified type NEC S36.898 ☑
      - type NEC S36.99 ☑
    - spleen — *see* Injury, spleen
    - stomach — *see* Injury, stomach
    - ureter — *see* Injury, ureter
    - urethra — *see* Injury, urethra
    - uterus — *see* Injury, uterus
    - vas deferens — *see* Injury, pelvis, organ, specified site NEC
  - intracranial (traumatic) — *see also* if applicable, Compression, brain, traumatic S06.9- ☑
    - cerebellar hemorrhage, traumatic — *see* Injury, intracranial, focal
    - cerebral edema, traumatic S06.1X- ☑
      - diffuse S06.1X- ☑
      - focal S06.1X- ☑
    - diffuse (axonal) S06.2X- ☑
    - epidural hemorrhage (traumatic) S06.4X- ☑
    - focal brain injury S06.30- ☑
      - contusion — *see* Contusion, cerebral
      - laceration — *see* Laceration, cerebral
    - intracerebral hemorrhage, traumatic S06.36- ☑
      - left side S06.35- ☑
      - right side S06.34- ☑
    - specified NEC S06.89- ☑
    - subarachnoid hemorrhage, traumatic S06.6X- ☑
    - subdural hemorrhage, traumatic S06.5X- ☑
  - intraocular — *see* Injury, eyeball, penetrating
  - intrathoracic S27.9 ☑
    - bronchus S27.409 ☑
      - bilateral S27.402 ☑
      - blast injury (primary) S27.419 ☑
        - bilateral S27.412 ☑
        - secondary — *see* Injury, intrathoracic, bronchus, specified type NEC
        - unilateral S27.411 ☑
      - contusion S27.429 ☑
        - bilateral S27.422 ☑
        - unilateral S27.421 ☑
      - laceration S27.439 ☑
        - bilateral S27.432 ☑
        - unilateral S27.431 ☑
      - specified type NEC S27.499 ☑
        - bilateral S27.492 ☑
        - unilateral S27.491 ☑
      - unilateral S27.401 ☑

- **Injury** — *continued*
  - intrathoracic — *continued*
    - diaphragm S27.8Ø9 ☑
      - contusion S27.8Ø2 ☑
      - laceration S27.8Ø3 ☑
      - specified type NEC S27.8Ø8 ☑
    - esophagus (thoracic) S27.819 ☑
      - contusion S27.812 ☑
      - laceration S27.813 ☑
      - specified type NEC S27.818 ☑
    - heart — *see* Injury, heart
    - hemopneumothorax S27.2 ☑
    - hemothorax S27.1 ☑
    - lung S27.3Ø9 ☑
      - aspiration J69.Ø
      - bilateral S27.3Ø2 ☑
      - blast injury (primary) S27.319 ☑
        - bilateral S27.312 ☑
        - secondary — *see* Injury, intrathoracic, lung, specified type NEC
        - unilateral S27.311 ☑
      - contusion S27.329 ☑
        - bilateral S27.322 ☑
        - unilateral S27.321 ☑
      - laceration S27.339 ☑
        - bilateral S27.332 ☑
        - unilateral S27.331 ☑
      - specified type NEC S27.399 ☑
        - bilateral S27.392 ☑
        - unilateral S27.391 ☑
      - unilateral S27.3Ø1 ☑
    - pleura S27.6Ø ☑
      - laceration S27.63 ☑
      - specified type NEC S27.69 ☑
    - pneumothorax S27.Ø ☑
    - specified organ NEC S27.899 ☑
      - contusion S27.892 ☑
      - laceration S27.893 ☑
      - specified type NEC S27.898 ☑
    - thoracic duct — *see* Injury, intrathoracic, specified organ NEC
    - thymus gland — *see* Injury, intrathoracic, specified organ NEC
    - trachea, thoracic S27.5Ø ☑
      - blast (primary) S27.51 ☑
      - contusion S27.52 ☑
      - laceration S27.53 ☑
      - specified type NEC S27.59 ☑
  - iris — *see* Injury, eye, specified site NEC
    - penetrating — *see* Injury, eyeball, penetrating
  - jaw SØ9.93 ☑
  - jejunum — *see* Injury, intestine, small
  - joint NOS T14.8 ☑
    - old or residual — *see* Disorder, joint, specified type NEC
  - kidney S37.ØØ- ☑
    - acute (nontraumatic) N17.9
    - contusion — *see* Contusion, kidney
    - laceration — *see* Laceration, kidney
    - specified NEC S37.Ø9- ☑
  - knee S89.9- ☑
    - contusion — *see* Contusion, knee
    - dislocation — *see* Dislocation, knee
    - meniscus (lateral) (medial) — *see* Sprain, knee, specified site NEC
    - old injury or tear — *see* Derangement, knee, meniscus, due to old injury
    - open — *see* Wound, open, knee
    - specified NEC S89.8- ☑
    - sprain — *see* Sprain, knee
    - superficial — *see* Injury, superficial, knee
  - labium (majus) (minus) S39.94 ☑
  - labyrinth, ear SØ9.3Ø- ☑
  - lacrimal apparatus, duct, gland, or sac — *see* Injury, eye, specified site NEC
  - larynx NEC S19.81 ☑
  - leg (lower) S89.9- ☑
    - blood vessel — *see* Injury, blood vessel, leg
    - contusion — *see* Contusion, leg
    - fracture — *see* Fracture, leg
    - muscle — *see* Injury, muscle, leg
    - nerve — *see* Injury, nerve, leg
    - open — *see* Wound, open, leg
    - specified NEC S89.8- ☑
    - superficial — *see* Injury, superficial, leg
  - lens, eye — *see* Injury, eye, specified site NEC

- **Injury** — *continued*
  - lens, eye — *see* Injury, eye, specified site — *continued*
    - penetrating — *see* Injury, eyeball, penetrating
  - limb NEC T14.8 ☑
  - lip SØ9.93 ☑
  - liver S36.119 ☑
    - contusion S36.112 ☑
    - laceration S36.113 ☑
      - major (stellate) S36.116 ☑
      - minor S36.114 ☑
      - moderate S36.115 ☑
    - specified NEC S36.118 ☑
  - lower back S39.92 ☑
    - specified NEC S39.82 ☑
  - lumbar, lumbosacral (region) S39.92 ☑
    - plexus — *see* Injury, lumbosacral plexus
  - lumbosacral plexus S34.4 ☑
  - lung — *see also* Injury, intrathoracic, lung
    - aspiration J69.Ø
    - dabbing (related) UØ7.Ø
    - electronic cigarette (related) UØ7.Ø
    - EVALI - [e-cigarette, or vaping, product use associated] UØ7.Ø
    - transfusion-related (TRALI) J95.84
    - vaping (associated) (device) (product) (use) UØ7.Ø
  - lymphatic thoracic duct — *see* Injury, intrathoracic, specified organ NEC
  - malar region SØ9.93 ☑
  - mastoid region SØ9.9Ø ☑
  - maxilla SØ9.93 ☑
  - mediastinum — *see* Injury, intrathoracic, specified organ NEC
  - membrane, brain — *see* Injury, intracranial
  - meningeal artery — *see* Injury, intracranial, subdural hemorrhage
  - meninges (cerebral) — *see* Injury, intracranial
  - mesenteric
    - artery
      - branch S35.299 ☑
        - laceration (minor) (superficial) S35.291 ☑
          - major S35.292 ☑
        - specified NEC S35.298 ☑
      - inferior S35.239 ☑
        - laceration (minor) (superficial) S35.231 ☑
          - major S35.232 ☑
        - specified NEC S35.238 ☑
      - superior S35.229 ☑
        - laceration (minor) (superficial) S35.221 ☑
          - major S35.222 ☑
        - specified NEC S35.228 ☑
    - plexus (inferior) (superior) — *see* Injury, nerve, lumbosacral, sympathetic
    - vein
      - inferior S35.349 ☑
        - laceration S35.341 ☑
        - specified NEC S35.348 ☑
      - superior S35.339 ☑
        - laceration S35.331 ☑
        - specified NEC S35.338 ☑
  - mesentery — *see* Injury, intra-abdominal, specified site NEC
  - mesosalpinx — *see* Injury, pelvic organ, specified site NEC
  - middle ear SØ9.3Ø- ☑
  - midthoracic region NOS S29.9 ☑
  - mouth SØ9.93 ☑
  - multiple NOS TØ7 ☑
  - muscle (and fascia) (and tendon)
    - abdomen S39.ØØ1 ☑
      - laceration S39.Ø21 ☑
      - specified type NEC S39.Ø91 ☑
      - strain S39.Ø11 ☑
    - abductor
      - thumb, forearm level — *see* Injury, muscle, thumb, abductor
    - adductor
      - thigh S76.2Ø- ☑
        - laceration S76.22- ☑
        - specified type NEC S76.29- ☑
        - strain S76.21- ☑
    - ankle — *see* Injury, muscle, foot
    - anterior muscle group, at leg level (lower) S86.2Ø- ☑
      - laceration S86.22- ☑
      - specified type NEC S86.29- ☑
      - strain S86.21- ☑

- **Injury** — *continued*
  - muscle — *continued*
    - arm (upper) — *see* Injury, muscle, shoulder
    - biceps (parts NEC) S46.2Ø- ☑
      - laceration S46.22- ☑
      - long head S46.1Ø- ☑
        - laceration S46.12- ☑
        - specified type NEC S46.19- ☑
        - strain S46.11- ☑
      - specified type NEC S46.29- ☑
      - strain S46.21- ☑
    - extensor
      - finger(s) (other than thumb) — *see* Injury, muscle, finger by site, extensor
      - forearm level, specified NEC — *see* Injury, muscle, forearm, extensor
      - thumb — *see* Injury, muscle, thumb, extensor
      - toe (large) (ankle level) (foot level) — *see* Injury, muscle, toe, extensor
    - finger
      - extensor (forearm level) S56.4Ø- ☑
        - hand level S66.3Ø9 ☑
          - laceration S66.329 ☑
          - specified type NEC S66.399 ☑
          - strain S66.319 ☑
        - laceration S56.429 ☑
        - specified type NEC S56.499 ☑
        - strain S56.419 ☑
      - flexor (forearm level) S56.1Ø- ☑
        - hand level S66.1Ø9 ☑
          - laceration S66.129 ☑
          - specified type NEC S66.199 ☑
          - strain S66.119 ☑
        - laceration S56.129 ☑
        - specified type NEC S56.199 ☑
        - strain S56.119 ☑
      - index
        - extensor (forearm level)
          - hand level S66.3Ø8 ☑
            - laceration S66.32- ☑
            - specified type NEC S66.39- ☑
            - strain S66.31- ☑
          - specified type NEC S56.492- ☑
        - flexor (forearm level)
          - hand level S66.1Ø8 ☑
            - laceration S66.12- ☑
            - specified type NEC S66.19- ☑
            - strain S66.11- ☑
          - specified type NEC S56.19- ☑
          - strain S56.11- ☑
        - intrinsic S66.5Ø- ☑
          - laceration S66.52- ☑
          - specified type NEC S66.59- ☑
          - strain S66.51- ☑
      - intrinsic S66.5Ø9 ☑
        - laceration S66.529 ☑
        - specified type NEC S66.599 ☑
        - strain S66.519 ☑
      - little
        - extensor (forearm level)
          - hand level S66.3Ø- ☑
            - laceration S66.32- ☑
            - specified type NEC S66.39- ☑
            - strain S66.31- ☑
          - laceration S56.42- ☑
          - specified type NEC S56.49- ☑
          - strain S56.41- ☑
        - flexor (forearm level)
          - hand level S66.1Ø- ☑
            - laceration S66.12- ☑
            - specified type NEC S66.19- ☑
            - strain S66.11- ☑
          - laceration S56.12- ☑
          - specified type NEC S56.19- ☑
          - strain S56.11- ☑
        - intrinsic S66.5Ø- ☑
          - laceration S66.52- ☑
          - specified type NEC S66.59- ☑
          - strain S66.51- ☑
      - middle
        - extensor (forearm level)
          - hand level S66.3Ø- ☑
            - laceration S66.32- ☑
            - specified type NEC S66.39- ☑
            - strain S66.31- ☑
          - laceration S56.42- ☑

- **Injury** — *continued*
  - muscle — *continued*
    - finger — *continued*
      - middle — *continued*
        - extensor — *continued*
          - specified type NEC S56.49- ☑
          - strain S56.41- ☑
        - flexor (forearm level)
          - hand level S66.1Ø- ☑
            - laceration S66.12- ☑
            - specified type NEC S66.19- ☑
            - strain S66.11- ☑
          - laceration S56.12- ☑
          - specified type NEC S56.19- ☑
          - strain S56.11- ☑
        - intrinsic S66.5Ø- ☑
          - laceration S66.52- ☑
          - specified type NEC S66.59- ☑
          - strain S66.51- ☑
      - ring
        - extensor (forearm level)
          - hand level S66.3Ø- ☑
            - laceration S66.32- ☑
            - specified type NEC S66.39- ☑
            - strain S66.31- ☑
          - laceration S56.42- ☑
          - specified type NEC S56.49- ☑
          - strain S56.41- ☑
        - flexor (forearm level)
          - hand level S66.1Ø- ☑
            - laceration S66.12- ☑
            - specified type NEC S66.19- ☑
            - strain S66.11- ☑
          - laceration S56.12- ☑
          - specified type NEC S56.19- ☑
          - strain S56.11- ☑
        - intrinsic S66.5Ø- ☑
          - laceration S66.52- ☑
          - specified type NEC S66.59- ☑
          - strain S66.51- ☑
    - flexor
      - finger(s) (other than thumb) — *see* Injury, muscle, finger
      - forearm level, specified NEC — *see* Injury, muscle, forearm, flexor
      - thumb — *see* Injury, muscle, thumb, flexor
      - toe (long) (ankle level) (foot level) — *see* Injury, muscle, toe, flexor
    - foot S96.9Ø- ☑
      - intrinsic S96.2Ø- ☑
        - laceration S96.22- ☑
        - specified type NEC S96.29- ☑
        - strain S96.21- ☑
      - laceration S96.92- ☑
      - long extensor, toe — *see* Injury, muscle, toe, extensor
      - long flexor, toe — *see* Injury, muscle, toe, flexor
      - specified
        - site NEC S96.8Ø- ☑
          - laceration S96.82- ☑
          - specified type NEC S96.89- ☑
          - strain S96.81- ☑
        - type NEC S96.99- ☑
      - strain S96.91- ☑
    - forearm (level) S56.9Ø- ☑
      - extensor S56.5Ø- ☑
        - laceration S56.52- ☑
        - specified type NEC S56.59- ☑
        - strain S56.51- ☑
      - flexor S56.2Ø- ☑
        - laceration S56.22- ☑
        - specified type NEC S56.29- ☑
        - strain S56.21- ☑
      - laceration S56.92- ☑
      - specified S56.99- ☑
        - site NEC S56.8Ø- ☑
          - laceration S56.82- ☑
          - strain S56.81- ☑
        - type NEC S56.89- ☑
      - strain S56.91- ☑
    - hand (level) S66.9Ø- ☑
      - laceration S66.92- ☑
      - specified
        - site NEC S66.8Ø- ☑
          - laceration S66.82- ☑
          - specified type NEC S66.89- ☑

- **Injury** — *continued*
  - muscle — *continued*
    - hand — *continued*
      - specified — *continued*
        - site — *continued*
          - strain S66.81- ☑
        - type NEC S66.99- ☑
      - strain S66.91- ☑
    - head SØ9.1Ø ☑
      - laceration SØ9.12 ☑
      - specified type NEC SØ9.19 ☑
      - strain SØ9.11 ☑
    - hip NEC S76.ØØ- ☑
      - laceration S76.Ø2- ☑
      - specified type NEC S76.Ø9- ☑
      - strain S76.Ø1- ☑
    - intrinsic
      - ankle and foot level — *see* Injury, muscle, foot, intrinsic
      - finger (other than thumb) — *see* Injury, muscle, finger by site, intrinsic
      - foot (level) — *see* Injury, muscle, foot, intrinsic
      - thumb — *see* Injury, muscle, thumb, intrinsic
    - leg (level) (lower) S86.9Ø- ☑
      - Achilles tendon — *see* Injury, Achilles tendon
      - anterior muscle group — *see* Injury, muscle, anterior muscle group
      - laceration S86.92- ☑
      - peroneal muscle group — *see* Injury, muscle, peroneal muscle group
      - posterior muscle group — *see* Injury, muscle, posterior muscle group, leg level
      - specified
        - site NEC S86.8Ø- ☑
          - laceration S86.82- ☑
          - specified type NEC S86.89- ☑
          - strain S86.81- ☑
        - type NEC S86.99- ☑
      - strain S86.91- ☑
    - long
      - extensor toe, at ankle and foot level — *see* Injury, muscle, toe, extensor
      - flexor, toe, at ankle and foot level — *see* Injury, muscle, toe, flexor
      - head, biceps — *see* Injury, muscle, biceps, long head
    - lower back S39.ØØ2 ☑
      - laceration S39.Ø22 ☑
      - specified type NEC S39.Ø92 ☑
      - strain S39.Ø12 ☑
    - neck (level) S16.9 ☑
      - laceration S16.2 ☑
      - specified type NEC S16.8 ☑
      - strain S16.1 ☑
    - pelvis S39.ØØ3 ☑
      - laceration S39.Ø23 ☑
      - specified type NEC S39.Ø93 ☑
      - strain S39.Ø13 ☑
    - peroneal muscle group, at leg level (lower) S86.3Ø- ☑
      - laceration S86.32- ☑
      - specified type NEC S86.39- ☑
      - strain S86.31- ☑
    - posterior muscle (group)
      - leg level (lower) S86.1Ø- ☑
        - laceration S86.12- ☑
        - specified type NEC S86.19- ☑
        - strain S86.11- ☑
      - thigh level S76.3Ø- ☑
        - laceration S76.32- ☑
        - specified type NEC S76.39- ☑
        - strain S76.31- ☑
    - quadriceps (thigh) S76.1Ø- ☑
      - laceration S76.12- ☑
      - specified type NEC S76.19- ☑
      - strain S76.11- ☑
    - shoulder S46.9Ø- ☑
      - laceration S46.92- ☑
      - rotator cuff — *see* Injury, rotator cuff
      - specified site NEC S46.8Ø- ☑
        - laceration S46.82- ☑
        - specified type NEC S46.89- ☑
        - strain S46.81- ☑
      - specified type NEC S46.99- ☑
      - strain S46.91- ☑
    - thigh NEC (level) S76.9Ø- ☑

- **Injury** — *continued*
  - muscle — *continued*
    - thigh — *continued*
      - adductor — *see* Injury, muscle, adductor, thigh
      - laceration S76.92- ☑
      - posterior muscle (group) — *see* Injury, muscle, posterior muscle, thigh level
      - quadriceps — *see* Injury, muscle, quadriceps
      - specified
        - site NEC S76.8Ø- ☑
          - laceration S76.82- ☑
          - specified type NEC S76.89- ☑
          - strain S76.81- ☑
        - type NEC S76.99- ☑
      - strain S76.91- ☑
    - thorax (level) S29.ØØ9 ☑
      - back wall S29.ØØ2 ☑
      - front wall S29.ØØ1 ☑
      - laceration S29.Ø29 ☑
        - back wall S29.Ø22 ☑
        - front wall S29.Ø21 ☑
      - specified type NEC S29.Ø99 ☑
        - back wall S29.Ø92 ☑
        - front wall S29.Ø91 ☑
      - strain S29.Ø19 ☑
        - back wall S29.Ø12 ☑
        - front wall S29.Ø11 ☑
    - thumb
      - abductor (forearm level) S56.3Ø- ☑
        - laceration S56.32- ☑
        - specified type NEC S56.39- ☑
        - strain S56.31- ☑
      - extensor (forearm level) S56.3Ø- ☑
        - hand level S66.2Ø- ☑
          - laceration S66.22- ☑
          - specified type NEC S66.29- ☑
          - strain S66.21- ☑
        - laceration S56.32- ☑
        - specified type NEC S56.39- ☑
        - strain S56.31- ☑
      - flexor (forearm level) S56.ØØ- ☑
        - hand level S66.ØØ- ☑
          - laceration S66.Ø2- ☑
          - specified type NEC S66.Ø9- ☑
          - strain S66.Ø1- ☑
        - laceration S56.Ø2- ☑
        - specified type NEC S56.Ø9- ☑
        - strain S56.Ø1- ☑
        - wrist level — *see* Injury, muscle, thumb, flexor, hand level
      - intrinsic S66.4Ø- ☑
        - laceration S66.42- ☑
        - specified type NEC S66.49- ☑
        - strain S66.41- ☑
    - toe — *see also* Injury, muscle, foot
      - extensor, long S96.1Ø- ☑
        - laceration S96.12- ☑
        - specified type NEC S96.19- ☑
        - strain S96.11- ☑
      - flexor, long S96.ØØ- ☑
        - laceration S96.Ø2- ☑
        - specified type NEC S96.Ø9- ☑
        - strain S96.Ø1- ☑
    - triceps S46.3Ø- ☑
      - laceration S46.32- ☑
      - specified type NEC S46.39- ☑
      - strain S46.31- ☑
    - wrist (and hand) level — *see* Injury, muscle, hand
  - musculocutaneous nerve — *see* Injury, nerve, musculocutaneous
  - myocardial (acute) (chronic) (non-ischemic) (non-traumatic) I5A
    - traumatic — *see* Injury, heart
  - myocardium — *see also* Injury, heart
    - non-traumatic — *see* Injury, myocardial
  - nape — *see* Injury, neck
  - nasal (septum) (sinus) SØ9.92 ☑
  - nasopharynx SØ9.92 ☑
  - neck S19.9 ☑
    - specified NEC S19.8Ø ☑
      - specified site NEC S19.89 ☑
  - nerve NEC T14.8 ☑
    - abdomen S34.9 ☑
      - peripheral S34.6 ☑
      - specified site NEC S34.8 ☑
    - abducens SØ4.4- ☑

- **Injury** — *continued*
  - nerve — *continued*
    - abducens — *continued*
      - contusion SØ4.4- ☑
      - laceration SØ4.4- ☑
      - specified type NEC SØ4.4- ☑
    - abducent — *see* Injury, nerve, abducens
    - accessory SØ4.7- ☑
      - contusion SØ4.7- ☑
      - laceration SØ4.7- ☑
      - specified type NEC SØ4.7- ☑
    - acoustic SØ4.6- ☑
      - contusion SØ4.6- ☑
      - laceration SØ4.6- ☑
      - specified type NEC SØ4.6- ☑
    - ankle S94.9- ☑
      - cutaneous sensory S94.3- ☑
      - specified site NEC — *see* subcategory S94.8 ☑
    - anterior crural, femoral — *see* Injury, nerve, femoral
    - arm (upper) S44.9- ☑
      - axillary — *see* Injury, nerve, axillary
      - cutaneous — *see* Injury, nerve, cutaneous, arm
      - median — *see* Injury, nerve, median, upper arm
      - musculocutaneous — *see* Injury, nerve, musculocutaneous
      - radial — *see* Injury, nerve, radial, upper arm
      - specified site NEC — *see* subcategory S44.8 ☑
      - ulnar — *see* Injury, nerve, ulnar, arm
    - auditory — *see* Injury, nerve, acoustic
    - axillary S44.3- ☑
    - brachial plexus — *see* Injury, brachial plexus
    - cervical sympathetic S14.5 ☑
    - cranial SØ4.9 ☑
      - contusion SØ4.9 ☑
      - eighth (acoustic or auditory) — *see* Injury, nerve, acoustic
      - eleventh (accessory) — *see* Injury, nerve, accessory
      - fifth (trigeminal) — *see* Injury, nerve, trigeminal
      - first (olfactory) — *see* Injury, nerve, olfactory
      - fourth (trochlear) — *see* Injury, nerve, trochlear
      - laceration SØ4.9 ☑
      - ninth (glossopharyngeal) — *see* Injury, nerve, glossopharyngeal
      - second (optic) — *see* Injury, nerve, optic
      - seventh (facial) — *see* Injury, nerve, facial
      - sixth (abducent) — *see* Injury, nerve, abducens
      - specified
        - nerve NEC SØ4.89- ☑
          - contusion SØ4.89- ☑
          - laceration SØ4.89- ☑
          - specified type NEC SØ4.89- ☑
        - type NEC SØ4.9 ☑
      - tenth (pneumogastric or vagus) — *see* Injury, nerve, vagus
      - third (oculomotor) — *see* Injury, nerve, oculomotor
      - twelfth (hypoglossal) — *see* Injury, nerve, hypoglossal
    - cutaneous sensory
      - ankle (level) S94.3- ☑
      - arm (upper) (level) S44.5- ☑
      - foot (level) — *see* Injury, nerve, cutaneous sensory, ankle
      - forearm (level) S54.3- ☑
      - hip (level) S74.2- ☑
      - leg (lower level) S84.2- ☑
      - shoulder (level) — *see* Injury, nerve, cutaneous sensory, arm
      - thigh (level) — *see* Injury, nerve, cutaneous sensory, hip
    - deep peroneal — *see* Injury, nerve, peroneal, foot
    - digital
      - finger S64.4- ☑
        - index S64.49- ☑
        - little S64.49- ☑
        - middle S64.49- ☑
        - ring S64.49- ☑
      - thumb S64.3- ☑
      - toe — *see* Injury, nerve, ankle, specified site NEC
    - eighth cranial (acoustic or auditory) — *see* Injury, nerve, acoustic
    - eleventh cranial (accessory) — *see* Injury, nerve, accessory
    - facial SØ4.5- ☑
      - contusion SØ4.5- ☑

- **Injury** — *continued*
  - nerve — *continued*
    - facial — *continued*
      - laceration SØ4.5- ☑
      - newborn P11.3
      - specified type NEC SØ4.5- ☑
    - femoral (hip level) (thigh level) S74.1- ☑
    - fifth cranial (trigeminal) — *see* Injury, nerve, trigeminal
    - finger (digital) — *see* Injury, nerve, digital, finger
    - first cranial (olfactory) — *see* Injury, nerve, olfactory
    - foot S94.9- ☑
      - cutaneous sensory S94.3- ☑
      - deep peroneal S94.2- ☑
      - lateral plantar S94.Ø- ☑
      - medial plantar S94.1- ☑
      - specified site NEC — *see* subcategory S94.8 ☑
    - forearm (level) S54.9- ☑
      - cutaneous sensory — *see* Injury, nerve, cutaneous sensory, forearm
      - median — *see* Injury, nerve, median
      - radial — *see* Injury, nerve, radial
      - specified site NEC — *see* subcategory S54.8 ☑
      - ulnar — *see* Injury, nerve, ulnar
    - fourth cranial (trochlear) — *see* Injury, nerve, trochlear
    - glossopharyngeal SØ4.89- ☑
      - specified type NEC SØ4.89- ☑
    - hand S64.9- ☑
      - median — *see* Injury, nerve, median, hand
      - radial — *see* Injury, nerve, radial, hand
      - specified NEC — *see* subcategory S64.8 ☑
      - ulnar — *see* Injury, nerve, ulnar, hand
    - hip (level) S74.9- ☑
      - cutaneous sensory — *see* Injury, nerve, cutaneous sensory, hip
      - femoral — *see* Injury, nerve, femoral
      - sciatic — *see* Injury, nerve, sciatic
      - specified site NEC — *see* subcategory S74.8 ☑
    - hypoglossal SØ4.89- ☑
      - specified type NEC SØ4.89- ☑
    - lateral plantar S94.Ø- ☑
    - leg (lower) S84.9- ☑
      - cutaneous sensory — *see* Injury, nerve, cutaneous sensory, leg
      - peroneal — *see* Injury, nerve, peroneal
      - specified site NEC — *see* subcategory S84.8 ☑
      - tibial — *see* Injury, nerve, tibial
      - upper — *see* Injury, nerve, thigh
    - lower
      - back — *see* Injury, nerve, abdomen, specified site NEC
        - peripheral — *see* Injury, nerve, abdomen, peripheral
      - limb — *see* Injury, nerve, leg
    - lumbar plexus — *see* Injury, nerve, lumbosacral, sympathetic
    - lumbar spinal — *see* Injury, spinal, lumbar
      - peripheral S34.6 ☑
      - root S34.21 ☑
      - sympathetic S34.5 ☑
    - lumbosacral
      - plexus — *see* Injury, nerve, lumbosacral, sympathetic
      - sympathetic S34.5 ☑
    - medial plantar S94.1- ☑
    - median (forearm level) S54.1- ☑
      - hand (level) S64.1- ☑
      - upper arm (level) S44.1- ☑
      - wrist (level) — *see* Injury, nerve, median, hand
    - musculocutaneous S44.4- ☑
    - musculospiral (upper arm level) — *see* Injury, nerve, radial, upper arm
    - neck S14.9 ☑
      - peripheral S14.4 ☑
      - specified site NEC S14.8 ☑
      - sympathetic S14.5 ☑
    - ninth cranial (glossopharyngeal) — *see* Injury, nerve, glossopharyngeal
    - oculomotor SØ4.1- ☑
      - contusion SØ4.1- ☑
      - laceration SØ4.1- ☑
      - specified type NEC SØ4.1- ☑
    - olfactory SØ4.81- ☑
      - specified type NEC SØ4.81- ☑
    - optic SØ4.Ø1- ☑

- **Injury** — *continued*
  - nerve — *continued*
    - optic — *continued*
      - contusion SØ4.Ø1- ☑
      - laceration SØ4.Ø1- ☑
      - specified type NEC SØ4.Ø1- ☑
    - pelvic girdle — *see* Injury, nerve, hip
    - pelvis — *see* Injury, nerve, abdomen, specified site NEC
      - peripheral — *see* Injury, nerve, abdomen, peripheral
    - peripheral NEC T14.8 ☑
      - abdomen — *see* Injury, nerve, abdomen, peripheral
      - lower back — *see* Injury, nerve, abdomen, peripheral
      - neck — *see* Injury, nerve, neck, peripheral
      - pelvis — *see* Injury, nerve, abdomen, peripheral
      - specified NEC T14.8 ☑
    - peroneal (lower leg level) S84.1- ☑
      - foot S94.2- ☑
    - plexus
      - brachial — *see* Injury, brachial plexus
      - celiac, coeliac — *see* Injury, nerve, lumbosacral, sympathetic
      - mesenteric, inferior — *see* Injury, nerve, lumbosacral, sympathetic
      - sacral — *see* Injury, lumbosacral plexus
      - spinal
        - brachial — *see* Injury, brachial plexus
        - lumbosacral — *see* Injury, lumbosacral plexus
    - pneumogastric — *see* Injury, nerve, vagus
    - radial (forearm level) S54.2- ☑
      - hand (level) S64.2- ☑
      - upper arm (level) S44.2- ☑
      - wrist (level) — *see* Injury, nerve, radial, hand
    - root — *see* Injury, nerve, spinal, root
    - sacral plexus — *see* Injury, lumbosacral plexus
    - sacral spinal — *see* Injury, spinal, sacral
      - peripheral S34.6 ☑
      - root S34.22 ☑
      - sympathetic S34.5 ☑
    - sciatic (hip level) (thigh level) S74.Ø- ☑
    - second cranial (optic) — *see* Injury, nerve, optic
    - seventh cranial (facial) — *see* Injury, nerve, facial
    - shoulder — *see* Injury, nerve, arm
    - sixth cranial (abducent) — *see* Injury, nerve, abducens
    - spinal
      - plexus — *see* Injury, nerve, plexus, spinal
      - root
        - cervical S14.2 ☑
        - dorsal S24.2 ☑
        - lumbar S34.21 ☑
        - sacral S34.22 ☑
        - thoracic — *see* Injury, nerve, spinal, root, dorsal
    - splanchnic — *see* Injury, nerve, lumbosacral, sympathetic
    - sympathetic NEC — *see* Injury, nerve, lumbosacral, sympathetic
      - cervical — *see* Injury, nerve, cervical sympathetic
    - tenth cranial (pneumogastric or vagus) — *see* Injury, nerve, vagus
    - thigh (level) — *see* Injury, nerve, hip
      - cutaneous sensory — *see* Injury, nerve, cutaneous sensory, hip
      - femoral — *see* Injury, nerve, femoral
      - sciatic — *see* Injury, nerve, sciatic
      - specified NEC — *see* Injury, nerve, hip
    - third cranial (oculomotor) — *see* Injury, nerve, oculomotor
    - thorax S24.9 ☑
      - peripheral S24.3 ☑
      - specified site NEC S24.8 ☑
      - sympathetic S24.4 ☑
    - thumb, digital — *see* Injury, nerve, digital, thumb
    - tibial (lower leg level) (posterior) S84.Ø- ☑
    - toe — *see* Injury, nerve, ankle
    - trigeminal SØ4.3- ☑
      - contusion SØ4.3- ☑
      - laceration SØ4.3- ☑
      - specified type NEC SØ4.3- ☑
    - trochlear SØ4.2- ☑
      - contusion SØ4.2- ☑
      - laceration SØ4.2- ☑

Injury — *continued*
nerve — *continued*
trochlear — *continued*
specified type NEC S04.2- ☑
twelfth cranial (hypoglossal) — *see* Injury, nerve, hypoglossal
ulnar (forearm level) S54.0- ☑
arm (upper) (level) S44.0- ☑
hand (level) S64.0- ☑
wrist (level) — *see* Injury, nerve, ulnar, hand
vagus S04.89- ☑
specified type NEC S04.89- ☑
wrist (level) — *see* Injury, nerve, hand
ninth cranial nerve (glossopharyngeal) — *see* Injury, nerve, glossopharyngeal
nose (septum) S09.92 ☑
obstetrical O71.9
specified NEC O71.89
occipital (region) (scalp) S09.90 ☑
lobe — *see* Injury, intracranial
optic chiasm S04.02 ☑
optic radiation S04.03- ☑
optic tract and pathways S04.03- ☑
orbit, orbital (region) — *see* Injury, eye
penetrating (with foreign body) — *see* Injury, eye, orbit, penetrating
specified NEC — *see* Injury, eye, specified site NEC
ovary, ovarian S37.409 ☑
bilateral S37.402 ☑
contusion S37.422 ☑
laceration S37.432 ☑
specified type NEC S37.492 ☑
blood vessel — *see* Injury, blood vessel, ovarian
contusion S37.429 ☑
bilateral S37.422 ☑
unilateral S37.421 ☑
laceration S37.439 ☑
bilateral S37.432 ☑
unilateral S37.431 ☑
specified type NEC S37.499 ☑
bilateral S37.492 ☑
unilateral S37.491 ☑
unilateral S37.401 ☑
contusion S37.421 ☑
laceration S37.431 ☑
specified type NEC S37.491 ☑
palate (hard) (soft) S09.93 ☑
pancreas S36.209 ☑
body S36.201 ☑
contusion S36.221 ☑
laceration S36.231 ☑
major S36.261 ☑
minor S36.241 ☑
moderate S36.251 ☑
specified type NEC S36.291 ☑
contusion S36.229 ☑
head S36.200 ☑
contusion S36.220 ☑
laceration S36.230 ☑
major S36.260 ☑
minor S36.240 ☑
moderate S36.250 ☑
specified type NEC S36.290 ☑
laceration S36.239 ☑
major S36.269 ☑
minor S36.249 ☑
moderate S36.259 ☑
specified type NEC S36.299 ☑
tail S36.202 ☑
contusion S36.222 ☑
laceration S36.232 ☑
major S36.262 ☑
minor S36.242 ☑
moderate S36.252 ☑
specified type NEC S36.292 ☑
parietal (region) (scalp) S09.90 ☑
lobe — *see* Injury, intracranial
patellar ligament (tendon) S76.10- ☑
laceration S76.12- ☑
specified NEC S76.19- ☑
strain S76.11- ☑
pelvis, pelvic (floor) S39.93 ☑
complicating delivery O70.1
joint or ligament, complicating delivery O71.6
organ S37.90 ☑
with ectopic or molar pregnancy O08.6

Injury — *continued*
pelvis, pelvic — *continued*
organ — *continued*
complication of abortion — *see* Abortion
contusion S37.92 ☑
following ectopic or molar pregnancy O08.6
laceration S37.93 ☑
obstetrical trauma NEC O71.5
specified
site NEC S37.899 ☑
contusion S37.892 ☑
laceration S37.893 ☑
specified type NEC S37.898 ☑
type NEC S37.99 ☑
specified NEC S39.83 ☑
penis S39.94 ☑
perineum S39.94 ☑
peritoneum S36.81 ☑
laceration S36.893 ☑
periurethral tissue — *see* Injury, urethra
complicating delivery O71.82
phalanges
foot — *see* Injury, foot
hand — *see* Injury, hand
pharynx NEC S19.85 ☑
pleura — *see* Injury, intrathoracic, pleura
plexus
brachial — *see* Injury, brachial plexus
cardiac — *see* Injury, nerve, thorax, sympathetic
celiac, coeliac — *see* Injury, nerve, lumbosacral, sympathetic
esophageal — *see* Injury, nerve, thorax, sympathetic
hypogastric — *see* Injury, nerve, lumbosacral, sympathetic
lumbar, lumbosacral — *see* Injury, lumbosacral plexus
mesenteric — *see* Injury, nerve, lumbosacral, sympathetic
pulmonary — *see* Injury, nerve, thorax, sympathetic
postcardiac surgery (syndrome) I97.0
prepuce S39.94 ☑
pressure
injury — *see* Ulcer, pressure, by site
prostate S37.829 ☑
contusion S37.822 ☑
laceration S37.823 ☑
specified type NEC S37.828 ☑
pubic region S39.94 ☑
pudendum S39.94 ☑
pulmonary plexus — *see* Injury, nerve, thorax, sympathetic
rectovaginal septum NEC S39.83 ☑
rectum — *see* Injury, intestine, large, rectum
retina — *see* Injury, eye, specified site NEC
penetrating — *see* Injury, eyeball, penetrating
retroperitoneal — *see* Injury, intra-abdominal, specified site NEC
rotator cuff (muscle(s)) (tendon(s)) S46.00- ☑
laceration S46.02- ☑
specified type NEC S46.09- ☑
strain S46.01- ☑
round ligament — *see* Injury, pelvic organ, specified site NEC
sacral plexus — *see* Injury, lumbosacral plexus
salivary duct or gland S09.93 ☑
scalp S09.90 ☑
newborn (birth injury) P12.9
due to monitoring (electrode) (sampling incision) P12.4
specified NEC P12.89
caput succedaneum P12.81
scapular region — *see* Injury, shoulder
sclera — *see* Injury, eye, specified site NEC
penetrating — *see* Injury, eyeball, penetrating
scrotum S39.94 ☑
second cranial nerve (optic) — *see* Injury, nerve, optic
self-inflicted, without suicidal intent R45.88
seminal vesicle — *see* Injury, pelvic organ, specified site NEC
seventh cranial nerve (facial) — *see* Injury, nerve, facial
shoulder S49.9- ☑
blood vessel — *see* Injury, blood vessel, arm
contusion — *see* Contusion, shoulder
dislocation — *see* Dislocation, shoulder
fracture — *see* Fracture, shoulder
muscle — *see* Injury, muscle, shoulder
nerve — *see* Injury, nerve, shoulder

Injury — *continued*
shoulder — *continued*
open — *see* Wound, open, shoulder
specified type NEC S49.8- ☑
sprain — *see* Sprain, shoulder girdle
superficial — *see* Injury, superficial, shoulder
sinus
cavernous — *see* Injury, intracranial
nasal S09.92 ☑
sixth cranial nerve (abducent) — *see* Injury, nerve, abducens
skeleton, birth injury P13.9
specified part NEC P13.8
skin NEC T14.8 ☑
surface intact — *see* Injury, superficial
skull NEC S09.90 ☑
specified NEC T14.8 ☑
spermatic cord (pelvic region) S37.898 ☑
scrotal region S39.848 ☑
spinal (cord)
cervical (neck) S14.109 ☑
anterior cord syndrome S14.139 ☑
C1 level S14.131 ☑
C2 level S14.132 ☑
C3 level S14.133 ☑
C4 level S14.134 ☑
C5 level S14.135 ☑
C6 level S14.136 ☑
C7 level S14.137 ☑
C8 level S14.138 ☑
Brown-Séquard syndrome S14.149 ☑
C1 level S14.141 ☑
C2 level S14.142 ☑
C3 level S14.143 ☑
C4 level S14.144 ☑
C5 level S14.145 ☑
C6 level S14.146 ☑
C7 level S14.147 ☑
C8 level S14.148 ☑
C1 level S14.101 ☑
C2 level S14.102 ☑
C3 level S14.103 ☑
C4 level S14.104 ☑
C5 level S14.105 ☑
C6 level S14.106 ☑
C7 level S14.107 ☑
C8 level S14.108 ☑
central cord syndrome S14.129 ☑
C1 level S14.121 ☑
C2 level S14.122 ☑
C3 level S14.123 ☑
C4 level S14.124 ☑
C5 level S14.125 ☑
C6 level S14.126 ☑
C7 level S14.127 ☑
C8 level S14.128 ☑
complete lesion S14.119 ☑
C1 level S14.111 ☑
C2 level S14.112 ☑
C3 level S14.113 ☑
C4 level S14.114 ☑
C5 level S14.115 ☑
C6 level S14.116 ☑
C7 level S14.117 ☑
C8 level S14.118 ☑
concussion S14.0 ☑
edema S14.0 ☑
incomplete lesion specified NEC S14.159 ☑
C1 level S14.151 ☑
C2 level S14.152 ☑
C3 level S14.153 ☑
C4 level S14.154 ☑
C5 level S14.155 ☑
C6 level S14.156 ☑
C7 level S14.157 ☑
C8 level S14.158 ☑
posterior cord syndrome S14.159 ☑
C1 level S14.151 ☑
C2 level S14.152 ☑
C3 level S14.153 ☑
C4 level S14.154 ☑
C5 level S14.155 ☑
C6 level S14.156 ☑
C7 level S14.157 ☑
C8 level S14.158 ☑
dorsal — *see* Injury, spinal, thoracic

- **Injury** — *continued*
  - spinal — *continued*
    - lumbar S34.109 ☑
      - complete lesion S34.119 ☑
        - L1 level S34.111 ☑
        - L2 level S34.112 ☑
        - L3 level S34.113 ☑
        - L4 level S34.114 ☑
        - L5 level S34.115 ☑
      - concussion S34.01 ☑
      - edema S34.01 ☑
      - incomplete lesion S34.129 ☑
        - L1 level S34.121 ☑
        - L2 level S34.122 ☑
        - L3 level S34.123 ☑
        - L4 level S34.124 ☑
        - L5 level S34.125 ☑
      - L1 level S34.101 ☑
      - L2 level S34.102 ☑
      - L3 level S34.103 ☑
      - L4 level S34.104 ☑
      - L5 level S34.105 ☑
    - nerve root NEC
      - cervical — *see* Injury, nerve, spinal, root, cervical
      - dorsal — *see* Injury, nerve, spinal, root, dorsal
      - lumbar S34.21 ☑
      - sacral S34.22 ☑
      - thoracic — *see* Injury, nerve, spinal, root, dorsal
    - plexus
      - brachial — *see* Injury, brachial plexus
      - lumbosacral — *see* Injury, lumbosacral plexus
    - sacral S34.139 ☑
      - complete lesion S34.131 ☑
      - incomplete lesion S34.132 ☑
    - thoracic S24.109 ☑
      - anterior cord syndrome S24.139 ☑
        - T1 level S24.131 ☑
        - T2-T6 level S24.132 ☑
        - T7-T10 level S24.133 ☑
        - T11-T12 level S24.134 ☑
      - Brown-Séquard syndrome S24.149 ☑
        - T1 level S24.141 ☑
        - T2-T6 level S24.142 ☑
        - T7-T10 level S24.143 ☑
        - T11-T12 level S24.144 ☑
      - complete lesion S24.119 ☑
        - T1 level S24.111 ☑
        - T2-T6 level S24.112 ☑
        - T7-T10 level S24.113 ☑
        - T11-T12 level S24.114 ☑
      - concussion S24.0 ☑
      - edema S24.0 ☑
      - incomplete lesion specified NEC S24.159 ☑
        - T1 level S24.151 ☑
        - T2-T6 level S24.152 ☑
        - T7-T10 level S24.153 ☑
        - T11-T12 level S24.154 ☑
      - posterior cord syndrome S24.159 ☑
        - T1 level S24.151 ☑
        - T2-T6 level S24.152 ☑
        - T7-T10 level S24.153 ☑
        - T11-T12 level S24.154 ☑
      - T1 level S24.101 ☑
      - T2-T6 level S24.102 ☑
      - T7-T10 level S24.103 ☑
      - T11-T12 level S24.104 ☑
  - splanchnic nerve — *see* Injury, nerve, lumbosacral, sympathetic
  - spleen S36.00 ☑
    - contusion S36.029 ☑
      - major S36.021 ☑
      - minor S36.020 ☑
    - laceration S36.039 ☑
      - major (massive) (stellate) S36.032 ☑
      - moderate S36.031 ☑
      - superficial (capsular) (minor) S36.030 ☑
    - specified type NEC S36.09 ☑
  - splenic artery — *see* Injury, blood vessel, celiac artery, branch
  - stellate ganglion — *see* Injury, nerve, thorax, sympathetic
  - sternal region S29.9 ☑
  - stomach S36.30 ☑
    - contusion S36.32 ☑
    - laceration S36.33 ☑
    - specified type NEC S36.39 ☑
- **Injury** — *continued*
  - subconjunctival — *see* Injury, eye, conjunctiva
  - subcutaneous NEC T14.8 ☑
  - submaxillary region S09.93 ☑
  - submental region S09.93 ☑
  - subungual
    - fingers — *see* Injury, hand
    - toes — *see* Injury, foot
  - superficial NEC T14.8 ☑
    - abdomen, abdominal (wall) S30.92 ☑
      - abrasion S30.811 ☑
      - bite S30.871 ☑
        - insect S30.861 ☑
      - contusion S30.1 ☑
      - external constriction S30.841 ☑
      - foreign body S30.851 ☑
    - abrasion — *see* Abrasion, by site
    - adnexa, eye NEC — *see* Injury, eye, specified site NEC
    - alveolar process — *see* Injury, superficial, oral cavity
    - ankle S90.91- ☑
      - abrasion — *see* Abrasion, ankle
      - bite — *see* Bite, ankle
      - blister — *see* Blister, ankle
      - contusion — *see* Contusion, ankle
      - external constriction — *see* Constriction, external, ankle
      - foreign body — *see* Foreign body, superficial, ankle
    - anus S30.98 ☑
    - arm (upper) S40.92- ☑
      - abrasion — *see* Abrasion, arm
      - bite — *see* Bite, superficial, arm
      - blister — *see* Blister, arm (upper)
      - contusion — *see* Contusion, arm
      - external constriction — *see* Constriction, external, arm
      - foreign body — *see* Foreign body, superficial, arm
    - auditory canal (external) (meatus) — *see* Injury, superficial, ear
    - auricle — *see* Injury, superficial, ear
    - axilla — *see* Injury, superficial, arm
    - back — *see also* Injury, superficial, thorax, back
      - lower S30.91 ☑
        - abrasion S30.810 ☑
        - contusion S30.0 ☑
        - external constriction S30.840 ☑
        - superficial
          - bite NEC S30.870 ☑
            - insect S30.860 ☑
          - foreign body S30.850 ☑
    - bite NEC — *see* Bite, superficial NEC, by site
    - blister — *see* Blister, by site
    - breast S20.10- ☑
      - abrasion — *see* Abrasion, breast
      - bite — *see* Bite, superficial, breast
      - contusion — *see* Contusion, breast
      - external constriction — *see* Constriction, external, breast
      - foreign body — *see* Foreign body, superficial, breast
    - brow — *see* Injury, superficial, head, specified NEC
    - buttock S30.91 ☑
    - calf — *see* Injury, superficial, leg
    - canthus, eye — *see* Injury, superficial, periocular area
    - cheek (external) — *see* Injury, superficial, head, specified NEC
      - internal — *see* Injury, superficial, oral cavity
    - chest wall — *see* Injury, superficial, thorax
    - chin — *see* Injury, superficial, head NEC
    - clitoris S30.95 ☑
    - conjunctiva — *see* Injury, eye, conjunctiva
      - with foreign body (in conjunctival sac) — *see* Foreign body, conjunctival sac
    - contusion — *see* Contusion, by site
    - costal region — *see* Injury, superficial, thorax
    - digit(s)
      - hand — *see* Injury, superficial, finger
    - ear (auricle) (canal) (external) S00.40- ☑
      - abrasion — *see* Abrasion, ear
      - bite — *see* Bite, superficial, ear
      - contusion — *see* Contusion, ear
      - external constriction — *see* Constriction, external, ear
- **Injury** — *continued*
  - superficial — *continued*
    - ear — *continued*
      - foreign body — *see* Foreign body, superficial, ear
    - elbow S50.90- ☑
      - abrasion — *see* Abrasion, elbow
      - bite — *see* Bite, superficial, elbow
      - blister — *see* Blister, elbow
      - contusion — *see* Contusion, elbow
      - external constriction — *see* Constriction, external, elbow
      - foreign body — *see* Foreign body, superficial, elbow
    - epididymis S30.94 ☑
    - epigastric region S30.92 ☑
    - epiglottis — *see* Injury, superficial, throat
    - esophagus
      - cervical — *see* Injury, superficial, throat
    - external constriction — *see* Constriction, external, by site
    - extremity NEC T14.8 ☑
    - eyeball NEC — *see* Injury, eye, specified site NEC
    - eyebrow — *see* Injury, superficial, periocular area
    - eyelid S00.20- ☑
      - abrasion — *see* Abrasion, eyelid
      - bite — *see* Bite, superficial, eyelid
      - contusion — *see* Contusion, eyelid
      - external constriction — *see* Constriction, external, eyelid
      - foreign body — *see* Foreign body, superficial, eyelid
    - face NEC — *see* Injury, superficial, head, specified NEC
    - finger(s) S60.949 ☑
      - abrasion — *see* Abrasion, finger
      - bite — *see* Bite, superficial, finger
      - blister — *see* Blister, finger
      - contusion — *see* Contusion, finger
      - external constriction — *see* Constriction, external, finger
      - foreign body — *see* Foreign body, superficial, finger
      - index S60.94- ☑
      - insect bite — *see* Bite, by site, superficial, insect
      - little S60.94- ☑
      - middle S60.94- ☑
      - ring S60.94- ☑
    - flank S30.92 ☑
    - foot S90.92- ☑
      - abrasion — *see* Abrasion, foot
      - bite — *see* Bite, foot
      - blister — *see* Blister, foot
      - contusion — *see* Contusion, foot
      - external constriction — *see* Constriction, external, foot
      - foreign body — *see* Foreign body, superficial, foot
    - forearm S50.91- ☑
      - abrasion — *see* Abrasion, forearm
      - bite — *see* Bite, forearm, superficial
      - blister — *see* Blister, forearm
      - contusion — *see* Contusion, forearm
      - elbow only — *see* Injury, superficial, elbow
      - external constriction — *see* Constriction, external, forearm
      - foreign body — *see* Foreign body, superficial, forearm
    - forehead — *see* Injury, superficial, head NEC
    - foreign body — *see* Foreign body, superficial
    - genital organs, external
      - female S30.97 ☑
      - male S30.96 ☑
    - globe (eye) — *see* Injury, eye, specified site NEC
    - groin S30.92 ☑
    - gum — *see* Injury, superficial, oral cavity
    - hand S60.92- ☑
      - abrasion — *see* Abrasion, hand
      - bite — *see* Bite, superficial, hand
      - contusion — *see* Contusion, hand
      - external constriction — *see* Constriction, external, hand
      - foreign body — *see* Foreign body, superficial, hand
    - head S00.90 ☑
      - ear — *see* Injury, superficial, ear

Injury — *continued*
  superficial — *continued*
    head — *continued*
      eyelid — *see* Injury, superficial, eyelid
      nose S00.30 ☑
      oral cavity S00.502 ☑
      scalp S00.00 ☑
      specified site NEC S00.80 ☑
    heel — *see* Injury, superficial, foot
    hip S70.91- ☑
      abrasion — *see* Abrasion, hip
      bite — *see* Bite, superficial, hip
      blister — *see* Blister, hip
      contusion — *see* Contusion, hip
      external constriction — *see* Constriction, external, hip
      foreign body — *see* Foreign body, superficial, hip
    iliac region — *see* Injury, superficial, abdomen
    inguinal region — *see* Injury, superficial, abdomen
    insect bite — *see* Bite, by site, superficial, insect
    interscapular region — *see* Injury, superficial, thorax, back
    jaw — *see* Injury, superficial, head, specified NEC
    knee S80.91- ☑
      abrasion — *see* Abrasion, knee
      bite — *see* Bite, superficial, knee
      blister — *see* Blister, knee
      contusion — *see* Contusion, knee
      external constriction — *see* Constriction, external, knee
      foreign body — *see* Foreign body, superficial, knee
    labium (majus) (minus) S30.95 ☑
    lacrimal (apparatus) (gland) (sac) — *see* Injury, eye, specified site NEC
    larynx — *see* Injury, superficial, throat
    leg (lower) S80.92- ☑
      abrasion — *see* Abrasion, leg
      bite — *see* Bite, superficial, leg
      contusion — *see* Contusion, leg
      external constriction — *see* Constriction, external, leg
      foreign body — *see* Foreign body, superficial, leg
      knee — *see* Injury, superficial, knee
    limb NEC T14.8 ☑
    lip S00.501 ☑
    lower back S30.91 ☑
    lumbar region S30.91 ☑
    malar region — *see* Injury, superficial, head, specified NEC
    mammary — *see* Injury, superficial, breast
    mastoid region — *see* Injury, superficial, head, specified NEC
    mouth — *see* Injury, superficial, oral cavity
    muscle NEC T14.8 ☑
    nail NEC T14.8 ☑
      finger — *see* Injury, superficial, finger
      toe — *see* Injury, superficial, toe
    nasal (septum) — *see* Injury, superficial, nose
    neck S10.90 ☑
      specified site NEC S10.80 ☑
    nose (septum) S00.30 ☑
    occipital region — *see* Injury, superficial, scalp
    oral cavity S00.502 ☑
    orbital region — *see* Injury, superficial, periocular area
    palate — *see* Injury, superficial, oral cavity
    palm — *see* Injury, superficial, hand
    parietal region — *see* Injury, superficial, scalp
    pelvis S30.91 ☑
      girdle — *see* Injury, superficial, hip
    penis S30.93 ☑
    perineum
      female S30.95 ☑
      male S30.91 ☑
    periocular area S00.20- ☑
      abrasion — *see* Abrasion, eyelid
      bite — *see* Bite, superficial, eyelid
      contusion — *see* Contusion, eyelid
      external constriction — *see* Constriction, external, eyelid
      foreign body — *see* Foreign body, superficial, eyelid

Injury — *continued*
  superficial — *continued*
    phalanges
      finger — *see* Injury, superficial, finger
      toe — *see* Injury, superficial, toe
    pharynx — *see* Injury, superficial, throat
    pinna — *see* Injury, superficial, ear
    popliteal space — *see* Injury, superficial, knee
    prepuce S30.93 ☑
    pubic region S30.91 ☑
    pudendum
      female S30.97 ☑
      male S30.96 ☑
    sacral region S30.91 ☑
    scalp S00.00 ☑
    scapular region — *see* Injury, superficial, shoulder
    sclera — *see* Injury, eye, specified site NEC
    scrotum S30.94 ☑
    shin — *see* Injury, superficial, leg
    shoulder S40.91- ☑
      abrasion — *see* Abrasion, shoulder
      bite — *see* Bite, superficial, shoulder
      blister — *see* Blister, shoulder
      contusion — *see* Contusion, shoulder
      external constriction — *see* Constriction, external, shoulder
      foreign body — *see* Foreign body, superficial, shoulder
    skin NEC T14.8 ☑
    sternal region — *see* Injury, superficial, thorax, front
    subconjunctival — *see* Injury, eye, specified site NEC
    subcutaneous NEC T14.8 ☑
    submaxillary region — *see* Injury, superficial, head, specified NEC
    submental region — *see* Injury, superficial, head, specified NEC
    subungual
      finger(s) — *see* Injury, superficial, finger
      toe(s) — *see* Injury, superficial, toe
    supraclavicular fossa — *see* Injury, superficial, neck
    supraorbital — *see* Injury, superficial, head, specified NEC
    temple — *see* Injury, superficial, head, specified NEC
    temporal region — *see* Injury, superficial, head, specified NEC
    testis S30.94 ☑
    thigh S70.92- ☑
      abrasion — *see* Abrasion, thigh
      bite — *see* Bite, superficial, thigh
      blister — *see* Blister, thigh
      contusion — *see* Contusion, thigh
      external constriction — *see* Constriction, external, thigh
      foreign body — *see* Foreign body, superficial, thigh
    thorax, thoracic (wall) S20.90 ☑
      abrasion — *see* Abrasion, thorax
      back S20.40- ☑
      bite — *see* Bite, thorax, superficial
      blister — *see* Blister, thorax
      contusion — *see* Contusion, thorax
      external constriction — *see* Constriction, external, thorax
      foreign body — *see* Foreign body, superficial, thorax
      front S20.30- ☑
    throat S10.10 ☑
      abrasion S10.11 ☑
      bite S10.17 ☑
        insect S10.16 ☑
      blister S10.12 ☑
      contusion S10.0 ☑
      external constriction S10.14 ☑
      foreign body S10.15 ☑
    thumb S60.93- ☑
      abrasion — *see* Abrasion, thumb
      bite — *see* Bite, superficial, thumb
      blister — *see* Blister, thumb
      contusion — *see* Contusion, thumb
      external constriction — *see* Constriction, external, thumb
      foreign body — *see* Foreign body, superficial, thumb
      insect bite — *see* Bite, by site, superficial, insect
      specified type NEC S60.39 ☑
    toe(s) S90.93- ☑

Injury — *continued*
  superficial — *continued*
    toe(s) — *continued*
      abrasion — *see* Abrasion, toe
      bite — *see* Bite, toe
      blister — *see* Blister, toe
      contusion — *see* Contusion, toe
      external constriction — *see* Constriction, external, toe
      foreign body — *see* Foreign body, superficial, toe
      great S90.93- ☑
    tongue — *see* Injury, superficial, oral cavity
    tooth, teeth — *see* Injury, superficial, oral cavity
    trachea S10.10 ☑
    tunica vaginalis S30.94 ☑
    tympanum, tympanic membrane — *see* Injury, superficial, ear
    uvula — *see* Injury, superficial, oral cavity
    vagina S30.95 ☑
    vocal cords — *see* Injury, superficial, throat
    vulva S30.95 ☑
    wrist S60.91- ☑
  supraclavicular region — *see* Injury, neck
  supraorbital S09.93 ☑
  suprarenal gland (multiple) — *see* Injury, adrenal
  surgical complication (external or internal site) — *see* Laceration, accidental complicating surgery
  temple S09.90 ☑
  temporal region S09.90 ☑
  tendon — *see also* Injury, muscle, by site
    abdomen — *see* Injury, muscle, abdomen
    Achilles — *see* Injury, Achilles tendon
    lower back — *see* Injury, muscle, lower back
    pelvic organs — *see* Injury, muscle, pelvis
  tenth cranial nerve (pneumogastric or vagus) — *see* Injury, nerve, vagus
  testis S39.94 ☑
  thigh S79.92- ☑
    blood vessel — *see* Injury, blood vessel, hip
    contusion — *see* Contusion, thigh
    fracture — *see* Fracture, femur
    muscle — *see* Injury, muscle, thigh
    nerve — *see* Injury, nerve, thigh
    open — *see* Wound, open, thigh
    specified NEC S79.82- ☑
    superficial — *see* Injury, superficial, thigh
  third cranial nerve (oculomotor) — *see* Injury, nerve, oculomotor
  thorax, thoracic S29.9 ☑
    blood vessel — *see* Injury, blood vessel, thorax
    cavity — *see* Injury, intrathoracic
    dislocation — *see* Dislocation, thorax
    external (wall) S29.9 ☑
      contusion — *see* Contusion, thorax
      nerve — *see* Injury, nerve, thorax
      open — *see* Wound, open, thorax
      specified NEC S29.8 ☑
      sprain — *see* Sprain, thorax
      superficial — *see* Injury, superficial, thorax
    fracture — *see* Fracture, thorax
    internal — *see* Injury, intrathoracic
    intrathoracic organ — *see* Injury, intrathoracic
    sympathetic ganglion — *see* Injury, nerve, thorax, sympathetic
  throat — *see also* Injury, neck S19.9 ☑
  thumb S69.9- ☑
    blood vessel — *see* Injury, blood vessel, thumb
    contusion — *see* Contusion, thumb
    dislocation — *see* Dislocation, thumb
    fracture — *see* Fracture, thumb
    muscle — *see* Injury, muscle, thumb
    nerve — *see* Injury, nerve, digital, thumb
    open — *see* Wound, open, thumb
    specified NEC S69.8- ☑
    sprain — *see* Sprain, thumb
    superficial — *see* Injury, superficial, thumb
  thymus (gland) — *see* Injury, intrathoracic, specified organ NEC
  thyroid (gland) NEC S19.84 ☑
  toe S99.92- ☑
    contusion — *see* Contusion, toe
    dislocation — *see* Dislocation, toe
    fracture — *see* Fracture, toe
    muscle — *see* Injury, muscle, toe
    open — *see* Wound, open, toe

Injury — *continued*
- toe — *continued*
  - specified type NEC S99.82- ☑
  - sprain — *see* Sprain, toe
  - superficial — *see* Injury, superficial, toe
- tongue SØ9.93 ☑
- tonsil SØ9.93 ☑
- tooth SØ9.93 ☑
- trachea (cervical) NEC S19.82 ☑
  - thoracic — *see* Injury, intrathoracic, trachea, thoracic
- transfusion-related acute lung (TRALI) J95.84
- tunica vaginalis S39.94 ☑
- twelfth cranial nerve (hypoglossal) — *see* Injury, nerve, hypoglossal
- ureter S37.1Ø ☑
  - contusion S37.12 ☑
  - laceration S37.13 ☑
  - specified type NEC S37.19 ☑
- urethra (sphincter) S37.3Ø ☑
  - at delivery O71.5
  - contusion S37.32 ☑
  - laceration S37.33 ☑
  - specified type NEC S37.39 ☑
- urinary organ S37.9Ø ☑
  - contusion S37.92 ☑
  - laceration S37.93 ☑
  - specified
    - site NEC S37.899 ☑
      - contusion S37.892 ☑
      - laceration S37.893 ☑
      - specified type NEC S37.898 ☑
    - type NEC S37.99 ☑
- uterus, uterine S37.6Ø ☑
  - with ectopic or molar pregnancy OØ8.6
  - blood vessel — *see* Injury, blood vessel, iliac
  - contusion S37.62 ☑
  - laceration S37.63 ☑
    - cervix at delivery O71.3
  - rupture associated with obstetrics — *see* Rupture, uterus
  - specified type NEC S37.69 ☑
- uvula SØ9.93 ☑
- vagina S39.93 ☑
  - abrasion S3Ø.814 ☑
  - bite S31.45 ☑
    - insect S3Ø.864 ☑
    - superficial NEC S3Ø.874 ☑
  - contusion S3Ø.23 ☑
  - crush S38.Ø3 ☑
  - during delivery — *see* Laceration, vagina, during delivery
  - external constriction S3Ø.844 ☑
  - insect bite S3Ø.864 ☑
  - laceration S31.41 ☑
    - with foreign body S31.42 ☑
  - open wound S31.4Ø ☑
  - puncture S31.43 ☑
    - with foreign body S31.44 ☑
  - superficial S3Ø.95 ☑
    - foreign body S3Ø.854 ☑
- vas deferens — *see* Injury, pelvic organ, specified site NEC
- vascular NEC T14.8
- vein — *see* Injury, blood vessel
- vena cava (superior) S25.2Ø ☑
  - inferior S35.1Ø ☑
    - laceration (minor) (superficial) S35.11 ☑
      - major S35.12 ☑
    - specified type NEC S35.19 ☑
  - laceration (minor) (superficial) S25.21 ☑
    - major S25.22 ☑
  - specified type NEC S25.29 ☑
- vesical (sphincter) — *see* Injury, bladder
- visual cortex SØ4.Ø4- ☑
- vitreous (humor) SØ5.9Ø ☑
  - specified NEC SØ5.8X- ☑
- vocal cord NEC S19.83 ☑
- vulva S39.94 ☑
  - abrasion S3Ø.814 ☑
  - bite S31.45 ☑
    - insect S3Ø.864 ☑
    - superficial NEC S3Ø.874 ☑
  - contusion S3Ø.23 ☑
  - crush S38.Ø3 ☑
  - during delivery — *see* Laceration, perineum, female, during delivery

Injury — *continued*
- vulva — *continued*
  - external constriction S3Ø.844 ☑
  - insect bite S3Ø.864 ☑
  - laceration S31.41 ☑
    - with foreign body S31.42 ☑
  - open wound S31.4Ø ☑
  - puncture S31.43 ☑
    - with foreign body S31.44 ☑
  - superficial S3Ø.95 ☑
    - foreign body S3Ø.854 ☑
- whiplash (cervical spine) S13.4 ☑
- wrist S69.9- ☑
  - blood vessel — *see* Injury, blood vessel, hand
  - contusion — *see* Contusion, wrist
  - dislocation — *see* Dislocation, wrist
  - fracture — *see* Fracture, wrist
  - muscle — *see* Injury, muscle, hand
  - nerve — *see* Injury, nerve, hand
  - open — *see* Wound, open, wrist
  - specified NEC S69.8- ☑
  - sprain — *see* Sprain, wrist
  - superficial — *see* Injury, superficial, wrist

Inoculation — *see also* Vaccination
- complication or reaction — *see* Complications, vaccination

Insanity, insane — *see also* Psychosis
- adolescent — *see* Schizophrenia
- confusional F28
  - acute or subacute FØ5
- delusional F22
- senile FØ3 ☑

Insect
- bite — *see* Bite, by site, superficial, insect
- venomous, poisoning NEC (by) — *see* Venom, arthropod

Insecurity
- financial Z59.86
- food Z59.41
- transportation Z59.82

Insensitivity
- adrenocorticotropin hormone (ACTH) E27.49
- androgen E34.5Ø
  - complete E34.51
  - partial E34.52

Insertion
- cord (umbilical) lateral or velamentous O43.12- ☑
- intrauterine contraceptive device (encounter for) — *see* Intrauterine contraceptive device

Insolation (sunstroke) T67.Ø1 ☑

Insomnia (organic) G47.ØØ
- adjustment F51.Ø2
- adjustment disorder F51.Ø2
- behavioral, of childhood Z73.819
  - combined type Z73.812
  - limit setting type Z73.811
  - sleep-onset association type Z73.81Ø
- childhood Z73.819
- chronic F51.Ø4
  - somatized tension F51.Ø4
- conditioned F51.Ø4
- due to
  - alcohol
    - abuse F1Ø.182
    - dependence F1Ø.282
    - use F1Ø.982
  - amphetamines
    - abuse F15.182
    - dependence F15.282
    - use F15.982
  - anxiety disorder F51.Ø5
  - caffeine
    - abuse F15.182
    - dependence F15.282
    - use F15.982
  - cocaine
    - abuse F14.182
    - dependence F14.282
    - use F14.982
  - depression F51.Ø5
  - drug NEC
    - abuse F19.182
    - dependence F19.282
    - use F19.982
  - medical condition G47.Ø1
  - mental disorder NEC F51.Ø5

Insomnia — *continued*
- due to — *continued*
  - opioid
    - abuse F11.182
    - dependence F11.282
    - use F11.982
  - psychoactive substance NEC
    - abuse F19.182
    - dependence F19.182
    - use F19.982
  - sedative, hypnotic, or anxiolytic
    - abuse F13.182
    - dependence F13.282
    - use F13.982
  - stimulant NEC
    - abuse F15.182
    - dependence F15.282
    - use F15.982
- fatal familial (FFI) A81.83
- idiopathic F51.Ø1
- learned F51.3
- nonorganic origin F51.Ø1
- not due to a substance or known physiological condition F51.Ø1
  - specified NEC F51.Ø9
- paradoxical F51.Ø3
- primary F51.Ø1
- psychiatric F51.Ø5
- psychophysiologic F51.Ø4
- related to psychopathology F51.Ø5
- short-term F51.Ø2
- specified NEC G47.Ø9
- stress-related F51.Ø2
- transient F51.Ø2
- without objective findings F51.Ø2

Inspiration
- food or foreign body — *see* Foreign body, by site
- mucus — *see* Asphyxia, mucus

Inspissated bile syndrome (newborn) P59.1

Instability
- emotional (excessive) F6Ø.3
- housing
  - housed Z59.819
    - with risk of homelessness Z59.811
    - homelessness in past 12 months Z59.812
- joint (post-traumatic) M25.3Ø
  - ankle M25.37- ☑
  - due to old ligament injury — *see* Disorder, ligament
  - elbow M25.32- ☑
  - flail — *see* Flail, joint
  - foot M25.37- ☑
  - hand M25.34- ☑
  - hip M25.35- ☑
  - knee M25.36- ☑
  - lumbosacral — *see* subcategory M53.2 ☑
  - prosthesis — *see* Complications, joint prosthesis, mechanical, displacement, by site
  - sacroiliac — *see* subcategory M53.2 ☑
  - secondary to
    - old ligament injury — *see* Disorder, ligament
    - removal of joint prosthesis M96.89
  - shoulder (region) M25.31- ☑
  - specified site NEC M25.39
  - spine — *see* subcategory M53.2 ☑
  - wrist M25.33- ☑
- knee (chronic) M23.5- ☑
- lumbosacral — *see* subcategory M53.2 ☑
- nervous F48.8
- personality (emotional) F6Ø.3
- spine — *see* Instability, joint, spine
- vasomotor R55

Institutional syndrome (childhood) F94.2

Institutionalization, affecting child Z62.22
- disinhibited attachment F94.2

Insufficiency, insufficient
- accommodation, old age H52.4
- adrenal (gland) E27.4Ø
  - primary E27.1
- adrenocortical E27.4Ø
  - drug-induced E27.3
  - iatrogenic E27.3
  - primary E27.1
- anatomic crown height KØ8.89
- anterior (occlusal) guidance M26.54
- anus K62.89
- aortic (valve) I35.1
  - with
    - mitral (valve) disease IØ8.Ø

Insufficiency, insufficient — *continued*
- aortic — *continued*
  - with — *continued*
    - mitral disease — *continued*
      - with tricuspid (valve) disease I08.3
    - stenosis I35.2
    - tricuspid (valve) disease I08.2
      - with mitral (valve) disease I08.3
  - congenital Q23.1
  - rheumatic I06.1
    - with
      - mitral (valve) disease I08.0
        - with tricuspid (valve) disease I08.3
      - stenosis I06.2
        - with mitral (valve) disease I08.0
          - with tricuspid (valve) disease I08.3
      - tricuspid (valve) disease I08.2
        - with mitral (valve) disease I08.3
  - specified cause NEC I35.1
  - syphilitic A52.03
- arterial I77.1
  - basilar G45.0
  - carotid (hemispheric) G45.1
  - cerebral I67.81
  - coronary (acute or subacute) I24.8
  - mesenteric K55.1
  - peripheral I73.9
  - precerebral (multiple) (bilateral) G45.2
  - vertebral G45.0
- arteriovenous I99.8
- biliary K83.8
- cardiac — *see also* Insufficiency, myocardial
  - due to presence of (cardiac) prosthesis I97.11- ☑
  - postprocedural I97.11- ☑
- cardiorenal, hypertensive I13.2
- cardiovascular — *see* Disease, cardiovascular
- cerebrovascular (acute) I67.81
  - with transient focal neurological signs and symptoms G45.8
- circulatory NEC I99.8
  - newborn P29.89
- clinical crown length K08.89
- convergence H51.11
- coronary (acute or subacute) I24.8
  - chronic or with a stated duration of over 4 weeks I25.89
- corticoadrenal E27.40
  - primary E27.1
- dietary E63.9
- divergence H51.8
- food T73.0 ☑
- gastroesophageal K22.89
- gonadal
  - ovary E28.39
  - testis E29.1
- heart — *see also* Insufficiency, myocardial
  - newborn P29.0
  - valve — *see* Endocarditis
- hepatic — *see* Failure, hepatic
- idiopathic autonomic G90.09
- interocclusal distance of fully erupted teeth (ridge) M26.36
- kidney N28.9
  - acute N28.9
  - chronic N18.9
- lacrimal (secretion) H04.12- ☑
  - passages — *see* Stenosis, lacrimal
- liver — *see* Failure, hepatic
- lung — *see* Insufficiency, pulmonary
- mental (congenital) — *see* Disability, intellectual
- mesenteric K55.1
- mitral (valve) I34.0
  - with
    - aortic valve disease I08.0
      - with tricuspid (valve) disease I08.3
    - obstruction or stenosis I05.2
      - with aortic valve disease I08.0
    - tricuspid (valve) disease I08.1
      - with aortic (valve) disease I08.3
  - congenital Q23.3
  - rheumatic I05.1
    - with
      - aortic valve disease I08.0
        - with tricuspid (valve) disease I08.3
      - obstruction or stenosis I05.2
        - with aortic valve disease I08.0
          - with tricuspid (valve) disease I08.3
      - tricuspid (valve) disease I08.1

Insufficiency, insufficient — *continued*
- mitral — *continued*
  - rheumatic — *continued*
    - with — *continued*
      - tricuspid disease — *continued*
        - with aortic (valve) disease I08.3
    - active or acute I01.1
      - with chorea, rheumatic (Sydenham's) I02.0
  - specified cause, except rheumatic I34.0
- muscle — *see also* Disease, muscle
  - heart — *see* Insufficiency, myocardial
  - ocular NEC H50.9
- myocardial, myocardium (with arteriosclerosis) — *see also* Failure, heart I50.9
  - with
    - rheumatic fever (conditions in I00) I09.0
      - active, acute or subacute I01.2
        - with chorea I02.0
      - inactive or quiescent (with chorea) I09.0
  - congenital Q24.8
  - hypertensive — *see* Hypertension, heart
  - newborn P29.0
  - rheumatic I09.0
    - active, acute, or subacute I01.2
  - syphilitic A52.06
- nourishment — *see also* Nutrition deficient T73.0 ☑
- pancreatic K86.89
  - exocrine K86.81
- parathyroid (gland) E20.9
- peripheral vascular (arterial) I73.9
- pituitary E23.0
- placental (mother) O36.51- ☑
- platelets D69.6
- prenatal care affecting management of pregnancy O09.3- ☑
- progressive pluriglandular E31.0
- pulmonary J98.4
  - acute, following surgery (nonthoracic) J95.2
    - thoracic J95.1
  - chronic, following surgery J95.3
  - following
    - shock J98.4
    - trauma J98.4
  - newborn P28.89
  - valve I37.1
    - with stenosis I37.2
    - congenital Q22.2
    - rheumatic I09.89
      - with aortic, mitral or tricuspid (valve) disease I08.8
- pyloric K31.89
- renal (acute) N28.9
  - chronic N18.9
- respiratory R06.89
  - newborn P28.5
- rotation — *see* Malrotation
- sleep syndrome F51.12
- social insurance Z59.7
- suprarenal E27.40
  - primary E27.1
- tarso-orbital fascia, congenital Q10.3
- testis E29.1
- thyroid (gland) (acquired) E03.9
  - congenital E03.1
- tricuspid (valve) (rheumatic) I07.1
  - with
    - aortic (valve) disease I08.2
      - with mitral (valve) disease I08.3
    - mitral (valve) disease I08.1
      - with aortic (valve) disease I08.3
    - obstruction or stenosis I07.2
      - with aortic (valve) disease I08.2
        - with mitral (valve) disease I08.3
  - congenital Q22.8
  - nonrheumatic I36.1
    - with stenosis I36.2
- urethral sphincter R32
- valve, valvular (heart) I38
  - aortic — *see* Insufficiency, aortic (valve)
  - congenital Q24.8
  - mitral — *see* Insufficiency, mitral (valve)
  - pulmonary — *see* Insufficiency, pulmonary, valve
  - tricuspid — *see* Insufficiency, tricuspid (valve)
- vascular I99.8
  - intestine K55.9
    - acute — *see also* Ischemia, intestine, acute K55.059
  - mesenteric K55.1

Insufficiency, insufficient — *continued*
- vascular — *continued*
  - peripheral I73.9
  - renal — *see* Hypertension, kidney
- velopharyngeal
  - acquired K13.79
  - congenital Q38.8
- venous (chronic) (peripheral) I87.2
- ventricular — *see* Insufficiency, myocardial
- welfare support Z59.7

Insufflation, fallopian Z31.41

Insular — *see* condition

Insulinoma
- pancreas
  - benign D13.7
  - malignant C25.4
  - uncertain behavior D37.8
- specified site
  - benign — *see* Neoplasm, by site, benign
  - malignant — *see* Neoplasm, by site, malignant
  - uncertain behavior — *see* Neoplasm, by site, uncertain behavior
- unspecified site
  - benign D13.7
  - malignant C25.4
  - uncertain behavior D37.8

Insuloma — *see* Insulinoma

Interference
- balancing side M26.56
- non-working side M26.56

Intermenstrual — *see* condition

Intermittent — *see* condition

Internal — *see* condition

Interrogation
- cardiac defibrillator (automatic) (implantable) Z45.02
- cardiac pacemaker Z45.018
- cardiac (event) (loop) recorder Z45.09
- infusion pump (implanted) (intrathecal) Z45.1
- neurostimulator Z46.2

Interruption
- aortic arch Q25.21
- bundle of His I44.30
- phase-shift, sleep cycle — *see* Disorder, sleep, circadian rhythm
- sleep phase-shift, or 24 hour sleep-wake cycle — *see* Disorder, sleep, circadian rhythm

Interstitial — *see* condition

Intertrigo L30.4
- labialis K13.0

Intervertebral disc — *see* condition

Intestine, intestinal — *see* condition

Intolerance
- carbohydrate K90.49
- disaccharide, hereditary E73.0
- fat NEC K90.49
  - pancreatic K90.3
- food K90.49
  - dietary counseling and surveillance Z71.3
- fructose E74.10
  - hereditary E74.12
- glucose (-galactose) E74.39
- gluten K90.41
- lactose E73.9
  - specified NEC E73.8
- lysine E72.3
- milk NEC K90.49
  - lactose E73.9
  - orthostatic, chronic G90.A
- protein K90.49
- starch NEC K90.49
- sucrose (-isomaltose) E74.31

Intoxicated NEC (without dependence) — *see* Alcohol, intoxication

Intoxication
- acid — *see also* Acidosis E87.29
- alcoholic (acute) (without dependence) — *see* Alcohol, intoxication
- alimentary canal K52.1
- amphetamine (without dependence) — *see also* Abuse, drug, stimulant, with intoxication
  - with dependence — *see* Dependence, drug, stimulant, with intoxication
  - stimulant NEC F15.10
    - with
      - anxiety disorder F15.180
      - intoxication F15.129
        - with
          - delirium F15.121

Intoxication — *continued*
amphetamine — *see also* Abuse, drug, stimulant, with intoxication — *continued*
stimulant — *continued*
with — *continued*
intoxication — *continued*
with — *continued*
perceptual disturbance F15.122
anxiolytic (acute) (without dependence) — *see* Abuse, drug, sedative, with intoxication
with dependence — *see* Dependence, drug, sedative, with intoxication
caffeine F15.929
with dependence — *see* Dependence, drug, stimulant, with intoxication
cannabinoids (acute) (without dependence) — *see* Use, cannabis, with intoxication
with
abuse — *see* Abuse, drug, cannabis, with intoxication
dependence — *see* Dependence, drug, cannabis, with intoxication
chemical — *see* Table of Drugs and Chemicals
via placenta or breast milk — *see* - Absorption, chemical, through placenta
cocaine (acute) (without dependence) — *see* Abuse, drug, cocaine, with intoxication
with dependence — *see* Dependence, drug, cocaine, with intoxication
drug
acute (without dependence) — *see* Abuse, drug, by type with intoxication
with dependence — *see* Dependence, drug, by type with intoxication
addictive
via placenta or breast milk — *see* Absorption, drug, addictive, through placenta
newborn P93.8
gray baby syndrome P93.Ø
overdose or wrong substance given or taken — *see* Table of Drugs and Chemicals, by drug, poisoning
enteric K52.1
foodborne AØ5.9
bacterial AØ5.9
classical (Clostridium botulinum) AØ5.1
due to
Bacillus cereus AØ5.4
bacterium AØ5.9
specified NEC AØ5.8
Clostridium
botulinum AØ5.1
perfringens AØ5.2
welchii AØ5.2
Salmonella AØ2.9
with
(gastro)enteritis AØ2.Ø
localized infection(s) AØ2.2Ø
arthritis AØ2.23
meningitis AØ2.21
osteomyelitis AØ2.24
pneumonia AØ2.22
pyelonephritis AØ2.25
specified NEC AØ2.29
sepsis AØ2.1
specified manifestation NEC AØ2.8
Staphylococcus AØ5.Ø
Vibrio
parahaemolyticus AØ5.3
vulnificus AØ5.5
enterotoxin, staphylococcal AØ5.Ø
noxious — *see* Poisoning, food, noxious
gastrointestinal K52.1
hallucinogenic (without dependence) — *see* Abuse, drug, hallucinogen, with intoxication
with dependence — *see* Dependence, drug, hallucinogen, with intoxication
hepatocerebral intoxication K76.82
hypnotic (acute) (without dependence) — *see* Abuse, drug, sedative, with intoxication
with dependence — *see* Dependence, drug, sedative, with intoxication
inhalant (acute) (without dependence) — *see* Abuse, drug, inhalant, with intoxication
with dependence — *see* Dependence, drug, inhalant, with intoxication
meaning
inebriation — *see* category F1Ø ☑

Intoxication — *continued*
meaning — *continued*
poisoning — *see* Table of Drugs and Chemicals
methyl alcohol (acute) (without dependence) — *see* Alcohol, intoxication
opioid (acute) (without dependence) — *see* Abuse, drug, opioid, with intoxication
with dependence — *see* Dependence, drug, opioid, with intoxication
pathologic NEC (without dependence) — *see* Alcohol, intoxication
phencyclidine (without dependence) — *see* Abuse, drug, hallucinogen, with intoxication
with dependence — *see* Dependence, drug, hallucinogen, with intoxication
potassium (K) E87.5
psychoactive substance NEC (without dependence) — *see* Abuse, drug, psychoactive NEC, with intoxication
with dependence — *see* Dependence, drug, psychoactive NEC, with intoxication
sedative (acute) (without dependence) — *see* Abuse, drug, sedative, with intoxication
with dependence — *see* Dependence, drug, sedative, with intoxication
serum — *see also* Reaction, serum T8Ø.69 ☑
uremic — *see* Uremia
volatile solvents (acute) (without dependence) — *see* Abuse, drug, inhalant, with intoxication
with dependence — *see* Dependence, drug, inhalant, with intoxication
water E87.79
Intraabdominal testis, testes
bilateral Q53.211
unilateral Q53.111
Intracranial — *see* condition
Intrahepatic gallbladder Q44.1
Intraligamentous — *see* condition
Intrathoracic — *see also* condition
kidney Q63.2
Intrauterine contraceptive device
checking Z3Ø.431
in situ Z97.5
insertion Z3Ø.43Ø
immediately following removal Z3Ø.433
management Z3Ø.431
reinsertion Z3Ø.433
removal Z3Ø.432
replacement Z3Ø.433
retention in pregnancy O26.3- ☑
Intraventricular — *see* condition
Intrinsic deformity — *see* Deformity
Intubation, difficult or failed T88.4 ☑
Intumescence, lens (eye) (cataract) — *see* Cataract
Intussusception (bowel) (colon) (enteric) (ileocecal) (ileocolic) (intestine) (rectum) K56.1
appendix K38.8
congenital Q43.8
ureter (with obstruction) N13.5
Invagination (bowel, colon, intestine or rectum) K56.1
Inversion
albumin-globulin (A-G) ratio E88.Ø9
bladder N32.89
cecum — *see* Intussusception
cervix N88.8
chromosome in normal individual Q95.1
circadian rhythm — *see* Disorder, sleep, circadian rhythm
nipple N64.59
congenital Q83.8
gestational — *see* Retraction, nipple
puerperal, postpartum — *see* Retraction, nipple
nyctohemeral rhythm — *see* Disorder, sleep, circadian rhythm
optic papilla Q14.2
organ or site, congenital NEC — *see* Anomaly, by site
sleep rhythm — *see* Disorder, sleep, circadian rhythm
testis (congenital) Q55.29
uterus (chronic) (postinfectional) (postpartal, old) N85.5
postpartum O71.2
vagina (posthysterectomy) N99.3
ventricular Q2Ø.5
Investigation — *see also* Examination ZØ4.9
clinical research subject (control) (normal comparison) (participant) ZØØ.6
Involuntary movement, abnormal R25.9
Involution, involutional — *see also* condition

Involution, involutional — *continued*
breast, cystic — *see* Dysplasia, mammary, specified type NEC
depression (single episode) F32.89
recurrent episode F33.9
melancholia (single episode) F32.89
recurrent episode F33.8
ovary, senile — *see* Atrophy, ovary
thymus failure E32.8
I.Q.
2Ø-34 F72
35-49 F71
5Ø-69 F7Ø
under 2Ø F73
IRDS (type I) P22.Ø
type II P22.1
Irideremia Q13.1
Iridis rubeosis — *see* Disorder, iris, vascular
Iridochoroiditis (panuveitis) — *see* Panuveitis
Iridocyclitis H2Ø.9
acute H2Ø.Ø- ☑
hypopyon H2Ø.Ø5- ☑
primary H2Ø.Ø1- ☑
recurrent H2Ø.Ø2- ☑
secondary (noninfectious) H2Ø.Ø4- ☑
infectious H2Ø.Ø3- ☑
chronic H2Ø.1- ☑
due to allergy — *see* Iridocyclitis, acute, secondary
endogenous — *see* Iridocyclitis, acute, primary
Fuchs' — *see* Cyclitis, Fuchs' heterochromic
gonococcal A54.32
granulomatous — *see* Iridocyclitis, chronic
herpes, herpetic (simplex) BØØ.51
zoster BØ2.32
hypopyon — *see* Iridocyclitis, acute, hypopyon
in (due to)
ankylosing spondylitis M45.9
gonococcal infection A54.32
herpes (simplex) virus BØØ.51
zoster BØ2.32
infectious disease NOS B99 ☑
parasitic disease NOS B89 *[H22]*
sarcoidosis D86.83
syphilis A51.43
tuberculosis A18.54
zoster BØ2.32
lens-induced H2Ø.2- ☑
nongranulomatous — *see* Iridocyclitis, acute
recurrent — *see* Iridocyclitis, acute, recurrent
rheumatic — *see* Iridocyclitis, chronic
subacute — *see* Iridocyclitis, acute
sympathetic — *see* Uveitis, sympathetic
syphilitic (secondary) A51.43
tuberculous (chronic) A18.54
Vogt-Koyanagi H2Ø.82- ☑
Iridocyclochoroiditis (panuveitis) — *see* Panuveitis
Iridodialysis H21.53- ☑
Iridodonesis H21.89
Iridoplegia (complete) (partial) (reflex) H57.Ø9
Iridoschisis H21.25- ☑
Iris — *see also* condition
bombé — *see* Membrane, pupillary
Iritis — *see also* Iridocyclitis
chronic — *see* Iridocyclitis, chronic
diabetic — *see* EØ8-E13 with .39
due to
herpes simplex BØØ.51
leprosy A3Ø.9 *[H22]*
gonococcal A54.32
gouty — *see also* Gout, by type M1Ø.9 *[H22]*
granulomatous — *see* Iridocyclitis, chronic
lens induced — *see* Iridocyclitis, lens-induced
papulosa (syphilitic) A52.71
rheumatic — *see* Iridocyclitis, chronic
syphilitic (secondary) A51.43
congenital (early) A5Ø.Ø1
late A52.71
tuberculous A18.54
Iron — *see* condition
Iron-miner's lung J63.4
Irradiated enamel (tooth, teeth) KØ3.89
Irradiation effects, adverse T66 ☑
Irreducible, irreducibility — *see* condition
Irregular, irregularity
action, heart I49.9
alveolar process KØ8.89
bleeding N92.6

- **Irregular, irregularity** — *continued*
  - breathing RØ6.89
  - contour of cornea (acquired) — *see* Deformity, cornea
    - congenital Q13.4
  - contour, reconstructed breast N65.Ø
  - dentin (in pulp) KØ4.3
  - eye movements H55.89
    - deficient
      - saccadic H55.81
      - smooth H55.82
    - nystagmus — *see* Nystagmus
  - labor O62.2
  - menstruation (cause unknown) N92.6
  - periods N92.6
  - prostate N42.9
  - pupil — *see* Abnormality, pupillary
  - reconstructed breast N65.Ø
  - respiratory RØ6.89
  - septum (nasal) J34.2
  - shape, organ or site, congenital NEC — *see* Distortion
  - sleep-wake pattern (rhythm) G47.23
- **Irritable, irritability** R45.4
  - bladder N32.89
  - bowel (syndrome) K58.9
    - with
      - constipation K58.1
      - diarrhea K58.Ø
    - mixed K58.2
    - psychogenic F45.8
    - specified NEC K58.8
  - bronchial — *see* Bronchitis
  - cerebral, in newborn P91.3
  - colon — *see also* Irritable, bowel K58.9
    - with diarrhea K58.Ø
    - psychogenic F45.8
  - duodenum K59.89
  - heart (psychogenic) F45.8
  - hip — *see* Derangement, joint, specified type NEC, hip
  - ileum K59.89
  - infant R68.12
  - jejunum K59.89
  - rectum K59.89
  - stomach K31.89
    - psychogenic F45.8
  - sympathetic G9Ø.8
  - urethra N36.8
- **Irritation**
  - anus K62.89
  - axillary nerve G54.Ø
  - bladder N32.89
  - brachial plexus G54.Ø
  - bronchial — *see* Bronchitis
  - cervical plexus G54.2
  - cervix — *see* Cervicitis
  - choroid, sympathetic — *see* Endophthalmitis
  - cranial nerve — *see* Disorder, nerve, cranial
  - gastric K31.89
    - psychogenic F45.8
  - globe, sympathetic — *see* Uveitis, sympathetic
  - labyrinth — *see* subcategory H83.2 ☑
  - lumbosacral plexus G54.1
  - meninges (traumatic) — *see* Injury, intracranial
    - nontraumatic — *see* Meningismus
  - nerve — *see* Disorder, nerve
  - nervous R45.Ø
  - penis N48.89
  - perineum NEC L29.3
  - peripheral autonomic nervous system G9Ø.8
  - peritoneum — *see* Peritonitis
  - pharynx J39.2
  - plantar nerve — *see* Lesion, nerve, plantar
  - spinal (cord) (traumatic) — *see also* Injury, spinal cord, by region
    - nerve G58.9
      - root NEC — *see* Radiculopathy
    - nontraumatic — *see* Myelopathy
  - stomach K31.89
    - psychogenic F45.8
  - sympathetic nerve NEC G9Ø.8
  - ulnar nerve — *see* Lesion, nerve, ulnar
  - vagina N89.8
- **Ischemia, ischemic** I99.8
  - bowel (transient)
    - acute — *see also* Ischemia, intestine, acute K55.Ø59
    - chronic K55.1
    - due to mesenteric artery insufficiency K55.1
  - brain — *see* Ischemia, cerebral
  - cardiac (see Disease, heart, ischemic)
- **Ischemia, ischemic** — *continued*
  - cardiomyopathy I25.5
  - cerebral (chronic) (generalized) I67.82
    - arteriosclerotic I67.2
    - intermittent G45.9
    - newborn P91.Ø
    - recurrent focal G45.8
    - transient G45.9
  - colon chronic (due to mesenteric artery insufficiency) K55.1
  - coronary — *see* Disease, heart, ischemic
  - demand (coronary) — *see also* Angina I24.8
    - with myocardial infarction I21.A1
    - resulting in myocardial infarction I21.A1
  - heart (chronic or with a stated duration of over 4 weeks) I25.9
    - acute or with a stated duration of 4 weeks or less I24.9
    - subacute I24.9
  - infarction, muscle — *see* Infarct, muscle
  - intestine (large) (small) (transient) K55.9
    - acute K55.Ø59
      - diffuse K55.Ø52
      - focal K55.Ø51
      - large K55.Ø39
        - diffuse K55.Ø32
        - focal K55.Ø31
      - small K55.Ø19
        - diffuse K55.Ø12
        - focal K55.Ø11
    - chronic K55.1
    - due to mesenteric artery insufficiency K55.1
  - kidney N28.Ø
  - limb, critical — *see* Arteriosclerosis, with critical limb ischemia
  - limb-threatening, chronic — *see* Arteriosclerosis, with critical limb ischemia
  - mesenteric, acute — *see also* Ischemia, intestine, acute K55.Ø59
  - muscle, traumatic T79.6 ☑
  - myocardium, myocardial (chronic or with a stated duration of over 4 weeks) I25.9
    - acute, without myocardial infarction I51.3
    - silent (asymptomatic) I25.6
    - transient of newborn P29.4
  - renal N28.Ø
  - retina, retinal — *see* Occlusion, artery, retina
  - small bowel
    - acute K55.Ø19
      - diffuse K55.Ø12
      - focal K55.Ø11
    - chronic K55.1
    - due to mesenteric artery insufficiency K55.1
  - spinal cord G95.11
  - subendocardial — *see* Insufficiency, coronary
  - supply (coronary) — *see also* Angina I25.9
    - due to vasospasm I2Ø.1
- **Ischial spine** — *see* condition
- **Ischialgia** — *see* Sciatica
- **Ischiopagus** Q89.4
- **Ischium, ischial** — *see* condition
- **Ischuria** R34
- **Iselin's disease or osteochondrosis** — *see* Osteochondrosis, juvenile, metatarsus
- **Islands of**
  - parotid tissue in
    - lymph nodes Q38.6
    - neck structures Q38.6
  - submaxillary glands in
    - fascia Q38.6
    - lymph nodes Q38.6
    - neck muscles Q38.6
- **Islet cell tumor, pancreas** D13.7
- **Isoimmunization NEC** — *see also* Incompatibility
  - affecting management of pregnancy (ABO) (with hydrops fetalis) O36.11- ☑
    - anti-A sensitization O36.11- ☑
    - anti-B sensitization O36.19- ☑
    - anti-c sensitization O36.Ø9- ☑
    - anti-C sensitization O36.Ø9- ☑
    - anti-e sensitization O36.Ø9- ☑
    - anti-E sensitization O36.Ø9- ☑
    - Rh NEC O36.Ø9- ☑
      - anti-D antibody O36.Ø1- ☑
    - specified NEC O36.19- ☑
  - newborn P55.9
    - with
      - hydrops fetalis P56.Ø
- **Isoimmunization** — *continued*
  - newborn — *continued*
    - with — *continued*
      - kernicterus P57.Ø
    - ABO (blood groups) P55.1
    - Rhesus (Rh) factor P55.Ø
    - specified type NEC P55.8
- **Isolation, isolated**
  - dwelling Z59.89
  - family Z63.79
  - social Z6Ø.4
- **Isoleucinosis** E71.19
- **Isomerism atrial appendages** (with asplenia or polysplenia) Q2Ø.6
- **Isosporiasis, isosporosis** AØ7.3
- **Isovaleric acidemia** E71.11Ø
- **Issue of**
  - medical certificate ZØ2.79
    - for disability determination ZØ2.71
  - repeat prescription (appliance) (glasses) (medicinal substance, medicament, medicine) Z76.Ø
    - contraception — *see* Contraception
- **Itch, itching** — *see also* Pruritus
  - baker's L23.6
  - barber's B35.Ø
  - bricklayer's L24.5
  - cheese B88.Ø
  - clam digger's B65.3
  - coolie B76.9
  - copra B88.Ø
  - dew B76.9
  - dhobi B35.6
  - filarial — *see* Infestation, filarial
  - grain B88.Ø
  - grocer's B88.Ø
  - ground B76.9
  - harvest B88.Ø
  - jock B35.6
  - Malabar B35.5
    - beard B35.Ø
    - foot B35.3
    - scalp B35.Ø
  - meaning scabies B86
  - Norwegian B86
  - perianal L29.Ø
  - poultrymen's B88.Ø
  - sarcoptic B86
  - scabies B86
  - scrub B88.Ø
  - straw B88.Ø
  - swimmer's B65.3
  - water B76.9
  - winter L29.8
- **Ivemark's syndrome** (asplenia with congenital heart disease) Q89.Ø1
- **Ivory bones** Q78.2
- **Ixodiasis NEC** B88.8

J

- **Jaccoud's syndrome** — *see* Arthropathy, postrheumatic, chronic
- **Jackson's**
  - membrane Q43.3
  - paralysis or syndrome G83.89
  - veil Q43.3
- **Jacquet's dermatitis** (diaper dermatitis) L22
- **Jadassohn-Pellizari's disease or anetoderma** L9Ø.2
- **Jadassohn's**
  - blue nevus — *see* Nevus
  - intraepidermal epithelioma — *see* Neoplasm, skin, benign
- **Jaffe-Lichtenstein (-Uehlinger) syndrome** — *see* Dysplasia, fibrous, bone NEC
- **Jakob-Creutzfeldt disease or syndrome** — *see* Creutzfeldt-Jakob disease or syndrome
- **Jaksch-Luzet disease** D64.89
- **Jamaican**
  - neuropathy G92.8
  - paraplegic tropical ataxic-spastic syndrome G92.8
- **Janet's disease** F48.8
- **Janiceps** Q89.4
- **Jansky-Bielschowsky amaurotic idiocy** E75.4
- **Japanese**
  - B-type encephalitis A83.Ø
  - river fever A75.3
- **Jaundice** (yellow) R17

Jaundice — *continued*
  acholuric (familial) (splenomegalic) — *see also* Spherocytosis
    acquired D59.8
  breast-milk (inhibitor) P59.3
  catarrhal (acute) B15.9
    with hepatic coma B15.0
  cholestatic (benign) R17
  due to or associated with
    delayed conjugation P59.8
      associated with (due to) preterm delivery P59.0
    preterm delivery P59.0
  epidemic (catarrhal) B15.9
    with hepatic coma B15.0
    leptospiral A27.0
    spirochetal A27.0
  familial nonhemolytic (congenital) (Gilbert) E80.4
    Crigler-Najjar E80.5
  febrile (acute) B15.9
    with hepatic coma B15.0
    leptospiral A27.0
    spirochetal A27.0
  hematogenous D59.9
  hemolytic (acquired) D59.9
    congenital — *see* Spherocytosis
  hemorrhagic (acute) (leptospiral) (spirochetal) A27.0
  infectious (acute) (subacute) B15.9
    with hepatic coma B15.0
    leptospiral A27.0
    spirochetal A27.0
  leptospiral (hemorrhagic) A27.0
  malignant (without coma) K72.90
    with coma K72.91
  neonatal — *see* Jaundice, newborn
  newborn P59.9
    due to or associated with
      ABO
        antibodies P55.1
        incompatibility, maternal/fetal P55.1
        isoimmunization P55.1
      absence or deficiency of enzyme system for bilirubin conjugation (congenital) P59.8
      bleeding P58.1
      breast milk inhibitors to conjugation P59.3
        associated with preterm delivery P59.0
      bruising P58.0
      Crigler-Najjar syndrome E80.5
      delayed conjugation P59.8
        associated with preterm delivery P59.0
      drugs or toxins
        given to newborn P58.42
        transmitted from mother P58.41
      excessive hemolysis P58.9
        due to
          bleeding P58.1
          bruising P58.0
          drugs or toxins
            given to newborn P58.42
            transmitted from mother P58.41
          infection P58.2
          polycythemia P58.3
          swallowed maternal blood P58.5
        specified type NEC P58.8
      galactosemia E74.21
      Gilbert syndrome E80.4
      hemolytic disease P55.9
        ABO isoimmunization P55.1
        Rh isoimmunization P55.0
        specified NEC P55.8
      hepatocellular damage P59.20
        specified NEC P59.29
      hereditary hemolytic anemia P58.8
      hypothyroidism, congenital E03.1
      incompatibility, maternal/fetal NOS P55.9
      infection P58.2
      inspissated bile syndrome P59.1
      isoimmunization NOS P55.9
      mucoviscidosis E84.9
      polycythemia P58.3
      preterm delivery P59.0
      Rh
        antibodies P55.0
        incompatibility, maternal/fetal P55.0
        isoimmunization P55.0
      specified cause NEC P59.8
      swallowed maternal blood P58.5
    spherocytosis (congenital) D58.0
  nonhemolytic congenital familial (Gilbert) E80.4

Jaundice — *continued*
  nuclear, newborn — *see also* Kernicterus of newborn P57.9
  obstructive — *see also* Obstruction, bile duct K83.1
  post-immunization — *see* Hepatitis, viral, type, B
  post-transfusion — *see* Hepatitis, viral, type, B
  regurgitation — *see also* Obstruction, bile duct K83.1
  serum (homologous) (prophylactic) (therapeutic) — *see* Hepatitis, viral, type, B
  spirochetal (hemorrhagic) A27.0
  symptomatic R17
    newborn P59.9
Jaw — *see* condition
Jaw-winking phenomenon or syndrome Q07.8
Jealousy
  alcoholic F10.988
  childhood F93.8
  sibling F93.8
Jejunitis — *see* Enteritis
Jejunostomy status Z93.4
Jejunum, jejunal — *see* condition
Jensen's disease — *see* Inflammation, chorioretinal, focal, juxtapapillary
Jerks, myoclonic G25.3
Jervell-Lange-Nielsen syndrome I45.81
Jeune's disease Q77.2
Jigger disease B88.1
Job's syndrome (chronic granulomatous disease) D71
Joint — *see also* condition
  mice — *see* Loose, body, joint
    knee M23.4- ☑
Jordan's anomaly or syndrome D72.0
Joseph-Diamond-Blackfan anemia (congenital hypoplastic) D61.01
Jungle yellow fever A95.0
Jüngling's disease — *see* Sarcoidosis
Juvenile — *see* condition

K

Kahler's disease C90.0- ☑
Kakke E51.11
Kala-azar B55.0
Kallmann's syndrome E23.0
Kanner's syndrome (autism) — *see* Psychosis, childhood
Kaposi's
  dermatosis (xeroderma pigmentosum) Q82.1
  lichen ruber L44.0
    acuminatus L44.0
  sarcoma
    colon C46.4
    connective tissue C46.1
    gastrointestinal organ C46.4
    lung C46.5- ☑
    lymph node (multiple) C46.3
    palate (hard) (soft) C46.2
    rectum C46.4
    skin (multiple sites) C46.0
    specified site NEC C46.7
    stomach C46.4
    unspecified site C46.9
  varicelliform eruption B00.0
    vaccinia T88.1 ☑
Kartagener's syndrome or triad (sinusitis, bronchiectasis, situs inversus) Q89.3
Karyotype
  with abnormality except iso (Xq) Q96.2
  45,X Q96.0
  46,X
    iso (Xq) Q96.1
  46,XX Q98.3
    with streak gonads Q50.32
    hermaphrodite (true) Q99.1
    male Q98.3
  46,XY
    with streak gonads Q56.1
    female Q97.3
    hermaphrodite (true) Q99.1
  47,XXX Q97.0
  47,XXY Q98.0
  47,XYY Q98.5
Kaschin-Beck disease — *see* Disease, Kaschin-Beck
Katayama's disease or fever B65.2
Kawasaki's syndrome M30.3
Kayser-Fleischer ring (cornea) (pseudosclerosis) H18.04- ☑

Kaznelson's syndrome (congenital hypoplastic anemia) D61.01
Kearns-Sayre syndrome H49.81- ☑
Kedani fever A75.3
Kelis L91.0
Kelly (-Patterson) syndrome (sideropenic dysphagia) D50.1
Keloid, cheloid L91.0
  acne L73.0
  Addison's L94.0
  cornea — *see* Opacity, cornea
  Hawkin's L91.0
  scar L91.0
Keloma L91.0
Kenya fever A77.1
Keratectasia — *see also* Ectasia, cornea
  congenital Q13.4
Keratinization of alveolar ridge mucosa
  excessive K13.23
  minimal K13.22
Keratinized residual ridge mucosa
  excessive K13.23
  minimal K13.22
Keratitis (nodular) (nonulcerative) (simple) (zonular) H16.9
  with ulceration (central) (marginal) (perforated) (ring) — *see* Ulcer, cornea
  actinic — *see* Photokeratitis
  arborescens (herpes simplex) B00.52
  areolar H16.11- ☑
  bullosa H16.8
  deep H16.309
    specified type NEC H16.399
  dendritic (a) (herpes simplex) B00.52
  disciform (is) (herpes simplex) B00.52
    varicella B01.81
  filamentary H16.12- ☑
  gonococcal (congenital or prenatal) A54.33
  herpes, herpetic (simplex) B00.52
    zoster B02.33
  in (due to)
    acanthamebiasis B60.13
    adenovirus B30.0
    exanthema — *see also* Exanthem B09
    herpes (simplex) virus B00.52
    measles B05.81
    syphilis A50.31
    tuberculosis A18.52
    zoster B02.33
  interstitial (nonsyphilitic) H16.30- ☑
    diffuse H16.32- ☑
    herpes, herpetic (simplex) B00.52
      zoster B02.33
    sclerosing H16.33- ☑
    specified type NEC H16.39- ☑
    syphilitic (congenital) (late) A50.31
    tuberculous A18.52
  macular H16.11- ☑
  nummular H16.11- ☑
  oyster shuckers' H16.8
  parenchymatous — *see* Keratitis, interstitial
  petrificans H16.8
  postmeasles B05.81
  punctata
    leprosa A30.9 *[H16.14-]* ☑
    syphilitic (profunda) A50.31
  punctate H16.14- ☑
  purulent H16.8
  rosacea L71.8
  sclerosing H16.33- ☑
  specified type NEC H16.8
  stellate H16.11- ☑
  striate H16.11- ☑
  superficial H16.10- ☑
    with conjunctivitis — *see* Keratoconjunctivitis
    due to light — *see* Photokeratitis
  suppurative H16.8
  syphilitic (congenital) (prenatal) A50.31
  trachomatous A71.1
    sequelae B94.0
  tuberculous A18.52
  vesicular H16.8
  xerotic — *see also* Keratomalacia H16.8
    vitamin A deficiency E50.4
Keratoacanthoma L85.8
Keratocele — *see* Descemetocele
Keratoconjunctivitis H16.20- ☑

Keratoconjunctivitis — *continued*
Acanthamoeba B6Ø.13
adenoviral B3Ø.Ø
epidemic B3Ø.Ø
exposure H16.21- ☑
herpes, herpetic (simplex) BØØ.52
zoster BØ2.33
in exanthema — *see also* Exanthem BØ9
infectious B3Ø.Ø
lagophthalmic — *see* Keratoconjunctivitis, specified type NEC
neurotrophic H16.23- ☑
phlyctenular H16.25- ☑
postmeasles BØ5.81
shipyard B3Ø.Ø
sicca (Sjogren's) M35.Ø- ☑
not Sjogren's H16.22- ☑
specified type NEC H16.29- ☑
tuberculous (phlyctenular) A18.52
vernal H16.26- ☑
Keratoconus H18.6Ø- ☑
congenital Q13.4
stable H18.61- ☑
unstable H18.62- ☑
Keratocyst (dental) (odontogenic) — *see* Cyst, calcifying odontogenic
Keratoderma, keratodermia (congenital) (palmaris et plantaris) (symmetrical) Q82.8
acquired L85.1
in diseases classified elsewhere L86
climactericum L85.1
gonococcal A54.89
gonorrheal A54.89
punctata L85.2
Reiter's — *see* Reiter's disease
Keratodermatocele — *see* Descemetocele
Keratoglobus H18.79 ☑
congenital Q15.8
with glaucoma Q15.Ø
Keratohemia — *see* Pigmentation, cornea, stromal
Keratoiritis — *see also* Iridocyclitis
syphilitic A5Ø.39
tuberculous A18.54
Keratoma L57.Ø
palmaris and plantaris hereditarium Q82.8
senile L57.Ø
Keratomalacia H18.44- ☑
vitamin A deficiency E5Ø.4
Keratomegaly Q13.4
Keratomycosis B49
nigrans, nigricans (palmaris) B36.1
Keratopathy H18.9
band H18.42- ☑
bullous (aphakic), following cataract surgery H59.Ø1- ☑
bullous H18.1- ☑
Keratoscleritis, tuberculous A18.52
Keratosis L57.Ø
actinic L57.Ø
arsenical L85.8
congenital, specified NEC Q8Ø.8
female genital NEC N94.89
follicularis Q82.8
acquired L11.Ø
congenita Q82.8
et parafollicularis in cutem penetrans L87.Ø
spinulosa (decalvans) Q82.8
vitamin A deficiency E5Ø.8
gonococcal A54.89
male genital (external) N5Ø.89
nigricans L83
obturans, external ear (canal) — *see* Cholesteatoma, external ear
palmaris et plantaris (inherited) (symmetrical) Q82.8
acquired L85.1
penile N48.89
pharynx J39.2
pilaris, acquired L85.8
punctata (palmaris et plantaris) L85.2
scrotal N5Ø.89
seborrheic L82.1
inflamed L82.Ø
senile L57.Ø
solar L57.Ø
tonsillaris J35.8
vagina N89.4
vegetans Q82.8
vitamin A deficiency E5Ø.8
vocal cord J38.3
Kerato-uveitis — *see* Iridocyclitis
Kerion (celsi) B35.Ø
Kernicterus of newborn (not due to isoimmunization) P57.9
due to isoimmunization (conditions in P55.Ø-P55.9) P57.Ø
specified type NEC P57.8
Kerunoparalysis T75.Ø9 ☑
Keshan disease E59
Ketoacidosis E87.29
diabetic — *see* Diabetes, by type, with ketoacidosis
Ketonuria R82.4
Ketosis NEC E88.89
diabetic — *see* Diabetes, by type, with ketoacidosis
Kew Garden fever A79.1
Kidney — *see* condition
Kienböck's disease — *see also* Osteochondrosis, juvenile, hand, carpal lunate
adult M93.1
Kimmelstiel (-Wilson) **disease** — *see* Diabetes, Kimmelstiel (-Wilson) disease
Kink, kinking
artery I77.1
hair (acquired) L67.8
ileum or intestine — *see* Obstruction, intestine
Lane's — *see* Obstruction, intestine
organ or site, congenital NEC — *see* Anomaly, by site
ureter (pelvic junction) N13.5
with
hydronephrosis N13.1
with infection N13.6
pyelonephritis (chronic) N11.1
congenital Q62.39
vein(s) I87.8
caval I87.1
peripheral I87.1
Kinnier Wilson's disease (hepatolenticular degeneration) E83.Ø1
Kissing spine M48.2Ø
cervical region M48.22
cervicothoracic region M48.23
lumbar region M48.26
lumbosacral region M48.27
occipito-atlanto-axial region M48.21
thoracic region M48.24
thoracolumbar region M48.25
Klatskin's tumor C22.1
Klauder's disease A26.8
Klebs' disease — *see also* Glomerulonephritis NØ5- ☑
Klebsiella (K.) **pneumoniae, as cause of disease classified elsewhere** B96.1
Klein (e)**-Levin syndrome** G47.13
Kleptomania F63.2
Klinefelter's syndrome Q98.4
karyotype 47,XXY Q98.Ø
male with more than two X chromosomes Q98.1
Klippel-Feil deficiency, disease, or syndrome (brevicollis) Q76.1
Klippel's disease I67.2
Klippel-Trenaunay (-Weber) **syndrome** Q87.2
Klumpke (-Déjerine) **palsy, paralysis** (birth) (newborn) P14.1
Knee — *see* condition
Knock knee (acquired) M21.Ø6- ☑
congenital Q74.1
Knot(s)
intestinal, syndrome (volvulus) K56.2
surfer S89.8- ☑
umbilical cord (true) O69.2 ☑
Knotting (of)
hair L67.8
intestine K56.2
Knuckle pad (Garrod's) M72.1
Koch's
infection — *see* Tuberculosis
relapsing fever A68.9
Koch-Weeks' conjunctivitis — *see* Conjunctivitis, acute, mucopurulent
Köebner's syndrome Q81.8
Köenig's disease (osteochondritis dissecans) — *see* Osteochondritis, dissecans
Köhler-Pellegrini-Steida disease or syndrome (calcification, knee joint) — *see* Bursitis, tibial collateral
Köhler's disease
patellar — *see* Osteochondrosis, juvenile, patella
tarsal navicular — *see* Osteochondrosis, juvenile, tarsus
Koilonychia L6Ø.3
Koilonychia — *continued*
congenital Q84.6
Kojevnikov's, epilepsy — *see* Kozhevnikof's epilepsy
Koplik's spots BØ5.9
Kopp's asthma E32.8
Korsakoff's (Wernicke) **disease, psychosis or syndrome** (alcoholic) F1Ø.96
with dependence F1Ø.26
drug-induced
due to drug abuse — *see* Abuse, drug, by type, with amnestic disorder
due to drug dependence — *see* Dependence, drug, by type, with amnestic disorder
nonalcoholic FØ4
Korsakov's disease, psychosis or syndrome — *see* Korsakoff's disease
Korsakow's disease, psychosis or syndrome — *see* Korsakoff's disease
Kostmann's disease or syndrome (infantile genetic agranulocytosis) — *see* Agranulocytosis
Kozhevnikof's epilepsy G4Ø.1Ø9
intractable G4Ø.119
with status epilepticus G4Ø.111
without status epilepticus G4Ø.119
not intractable G4Ø.1Ø9
with status epilepticus G4Ø.1Ø1
without status epilepticus G4Ø.1Ø9
Krabbe's
disease E75.23
syndrome, congenital muscle hypoplasia Q79.8
Kraepelin-Morel disease — *see* Schizophrenia
Kraft-Weber-Dimitri disease Q85.89
Kraurosis
ani K62.89
penis N48.Ø
vagina N89.8
vulva N9Ø.4
Kreotoxism AØ5.9
Krukenberg's
spindle — *see* Pigmentation, cornea, posterior
tumor C79.6- ☑
Kufs' disease E75.4
Kugelberg-Welander disease G12.1
Kuhnt-Junius degeneration — *see also* Degeneration, macula H35.32- ☑
Kümmell's disease or spondylitis — *see* Spondylopathy, traumatic
Kupffer cell sarcoma C22.3
Kuru A81.81
Kussmaul's
disease M3Ø.Ø
respiration E87.29
in diabetic acidosis — *see* Diabetes, by type, with ketoacidosis
Kwashiorkor E4Ø
marasmic, marasmus type E42
Kyasanur Forest disease A98.2
Kyphoscoliosis, kyphoscoliotic (acquired) — *see also* Scoliosis M41.9
congenital Q67.5
heart (disease) I27.1
sequelae of rickets E64.3
tuberculous A18.Ø1
Kyphosis, kyphotic (acquired) M4Ø.2Ø9
cervical region M4Ø.2Ø2
cervicothoracic region M4Ø.2Ø3
congenital Q76.419
cervical region Q76.412
cervicothoracic region Q76.413
occipito-atlanto-axial region Q76.411
thoracic region Q76.414
thoracolumbar region Q76.415
Morquio-Brailsford type (spinal) — *see also* subcategory M49.8 E76.219
postlaminectomy M96.3
postradiation therapy M96.2
postural (adolescent) M4Ø.ØØ
cervicothoracic region M4Ø.Ø3
thoracic region M4Ø.Ø4
thoracolumbar region M4Ø.Ø5
secondary NEC M4Ø.1Ø
cervical region M4Ø.12
cervicothoracic region M4Ø.13
thoracic region M4Ø.14
thoracolumbar region M4Ø.15
sequelae of rickets E64.3
specified type NEC M4Ø.299
cervical region M4Ø.292

- **Kyphosis, kyphotic** — *continued*
  - specified type — *continued*
    - cervicothoracic region M4Ø.293
    - thoracic region M4Ø.294
    - thoracolumbar region M4Ø.295
  - syphilitic, congenital A5Ø.56
  - thoracic region M4Ø.2Ø4
  - thoracolumbar region M4Ø.2Ø5
  - tuberculous A18.Ø1
- **Kyrle disease** L87.Ø

L

- **Labia, labium** — *see* condition
- **Labile**
  - blood pressure RØ9.89
  - vasomotor system I73.9
- **Labioglossal paralysis** G12.29
- **Labium leporinum** — *see* Cleft, lip
- **Labor** — *see* Delivery
- **Labored breathing** — *see* Hyperventilation
- **Labyrinthitis** (circumscribed) (destructive) (diffuse) (inner ear) (latent) (purulent) (suppurative) — *see also* subcategory H83.Ø ☑
  - syphilitic A52.79
- **Laceration**
  - with abortion — *see* Abortion, by type, complicated by laceration of pelvic organs
  - abdomen, abdominal
    - wall S31.119 ☑
      - with
        - foreign body S31.129 ☑
        - penetration into peritoneal cavity S31.619 ☑
          - with foreign body S31.629 ☑
      - epigastric region S31.112 ☑
        - with
          - foreign body S31.122 ☑
          - penetration into peritoneal cavity S31.612 ☑
            - with foreign body S31.622 ☑
      - left
        - lower quadrant S31.114 ☑
          - with
            - foreign body S31.124 ☑
            - penetration into peritoneal cavity S31.614 ☑
              - with foreign body S31.624 ☑
        - upper quadrant S31.111 ☑
          - with
            - foreign body S31.121 ☑
            - penetration into peritoneal cavity S31.611 ☑
              - with foreign body S31.621 ☑
      - periumbilic region S31.115 ☑
        - with
          - foreign body S31.125 ☑
          - penetration into peritoneal cavity S31.615 ☑
            - with foreign body S31.625 ☑
      - right
        - lower quadrant S31.113 ☑
          - with
            - foreign body S31.123 ☑
            - penetration into peritoneal cavity S31.613 ☑
              - with foreign body S31.623 ☑
        - upper quadrant S31.11Ø ☑
          - with
            - foreign body S31.12Ø ☑
            - penetration into peritoneal cavity S31.61Ø ☑
              - with foreign body S31.62Ø ☑
  - accidental, complicating surgery — *see* Complications, surgical, accidental puncture or laceration
  - Achilles tendon S86.Ø2- ☑
  - adrenal gland S37.813 ☑
  - alveolar (process) — *see* Laceration, oral cavity
  - ankle S91.Ø1- ☑
    - with
      - foreign body S91.Ø2- ☑
  - antecubital space — *see* Laceration, elbow
  - anus (sphincter) S31.831 ☑
    - with
      - ectopic or molar pregnancy OØ8.6
      - foreign body S31.832 ☑
    - complicating delivery — *see* Delivery, complicated, by, laceration, anus (sphincter)

- **Laceration** — *continued*
  - anus — *continued*
    - following ectopic or molar pregnancy OØ8.6
    - nontraumatic, nonpuerperal — *see* Fissure, anus
  - arm (upper) S41.11- ☑
    - with foreign body S41.12- ☑
    - lower — *see* Laceration, forearm
  - auditory canal (external) (meatus) — *see* Laceration, ear
  - auricle, ear — *see* Laceration, ear
  - axilla — *see* Laceration, arm
  - back — *see also* Laceration, thorax, back
    - lower S31.Ø1Ø ☑
      - with
        - foreign body S31.Ø2Ø ☑
          - with penetration into retroperitoneal space S31.Ø21 ☑
        - penetration into retroperitoneal space S31.Ø11 ☑
  - bile duct S36.13 ☑
  - bladder S37.23 ☑
    - with ectopic or molar pregnancy OØ8.6
    - following ectopic or molar pregnancy OØ8.6
    - obstetrical trauma O71.5
  - blood vessel — *see* Injury, blood vessel
  - bowel — *see also* Laceration, intestine
    - with ectopic or molar pregnancy OØ8.6
    - complicating abortion — *see* Abortion, by type, complicated by, specified condition NEC
    - following ectopic or molar pregnancy OØ8.6
    - obstetrical trauma O71.5
  - brain (any part) (cortex) (diffuse) (membrane) — *see also* Injury, intracranial, diffuse
    - during birth P1Ø.8
      - with hemorrhage P1Ø.1
    - focal — *see* Injury, intracranial, focal brain injury
  - brainstem SØ6.38- ☑
  - breast S21.Ø1- ☑
    - with foreign body S21.Ø2- ☑
  - broad ligament S37.893 ☑
    - with ectopic or molar pregnancy OØ8.6
    - following ectopic or molar pregnancy OØ8.6
    - laceration syndrome N83.8
    - obstetrical trauma O71.6
    - syndrome (laceration) N83.8
  - buttock S31.8Ø1 ☑
    - with foreign body S31.8Ø2 ☑
    - left S31.821 ☑
      - with foreign body S31.822 ☑
    - right S31.811 ☑
      - with foreign body S31.812 ☑
  - calf — *see* Laceration, leg
  - canaliculus lacrimalis — *see* Laceration, eyelid
  - canthus, eye — *see* Laceration, eyelid
  - capsule, joint — *see* Sprain
  - causing eversion of cervix uteri (old) N86
  - central (perineal), complicating delivery O7Ø.9
  - cerebellum, traumatic SØ6.37- ☑
  - cerebral SØ6.33- ☑
    - during birth P1Ø.8
      - with hemorrhage P1Ø.1
    - left side SØ6.32- ☑
    - right side SØ6.31- ☑
  - cervix (uteri)
    - with ectopic or molar pregnancy OØ8.6
    - following ectopic or molar pregnancy OØ8.6
    - nonpuerperal, nontraumatic N88.1
    - obstetrical trauma (current) O71.3
    - old (postpartal) N88.1
    - traumatic S37.63 ☑
  - cheek (external) SØ1.41- ☑
    - with foreign body SØ1.42- ☑
    - internal — *see* Laceration, oral cavity
  - chest wall — *see* Laceration, thorax
  - chin — *see* Laceration, head, specified site NEC
  - chordae tendinae NEC I51.1
    - concurrent with acute myocardial infarction — *see* Infarct, myocardium
    - following acute myocardial infarction (current complication) I23.4
  - clitoris — *see* Laceration, vulva
  - colon — *see* Laceration, intestine, large, colon
  - common bile duct S36.13 ☑
  - cortex (cerebral) — *see* Injury, intracranial, diffuse
  - costal region — *see* Laceration, thorax
  - cystic duct S36.13 ☑
  - diaphragm S27.8Ø3 ☑

- **Laceration** — *continued*
  - digit(s)
    - foot — *see* Laceration, toe
    - hand — *see* Laceration, finger
  - duodenum S36.43Ø ☑
  - ear (canal) (external) SØ1.31- ☑
    - with foreign body SØ1.32- ☑
    - drum SØ9.2- ☑
  - elbow S51.Ø1- ☑
    - with
      - foreign body S51.Ø2- ☑
  - epididymis — *see* Laceration, testis
  - epigastric region — *see* Laceration, abdomen, wall, epigastric region
  - esophagus K22.89
    - traumatic
      - cervical S11.21 ☑
        - with foreign body S11.22 ☑
      - thoracic S27.813 ☑
  - eye (ball) SØ5.3- ☑
    - with prolapse or loss of intraocular tissue SØ5.2- ☑
    - penetrating SØ5.6- ☑
  - eyebrow — *see* Laceration, eyelid
  - eyelid SØ1.11- ☑
    - with foreign body SØ1.12- ☑
  - face NEC — *see* Laceration, head, specified site NEC
  - fallopian tube S37.539 ☑
    - bilateral S37.532 ☑
    - unilateral S37.531 ☑
  - finger(s) S61.219 ☑
    - with
      - damage to nail S61.319 ☑
        - with
          - foreign body S61.329 ☑
      - foreign body S61.229 ☑
    - index S61.218 ☑
      - with
        - damage to nail S61.318 ☑
          - with
            - foreign body S61.328 ☑
        - foreign body S61.228 ☑
      - left S61.211 ☑
        - with
          - damage to nail S61.311 ☑
            - with
              - foreign body S61.321 ☑
          - foreign body S61.221 ☑
      - right S61.21Ø ☑
        - with
          - damage to nail S61.31Ø ☑
            - with
              - foreign body S61.32Ø ☑
          - foreign body S61.22Ø ☑
    - little S61.218 ☑
      - with
        - damage to nail S61.318 ☑
          - with
            - foreign body S61.328 ☑
        - foreign body S61.228 ☑
      - left S61.217 ☑
        - with
          - damage to nail S61.317 ☑
            - with
              - foreign body S61.327 ☑
          - foreign body S61.227 ☑
      - right S61.216 ☑
        - with
          - damage to nail S61.316 ☑
            - with
              - foreign body S61.326 ☑
          - foreign body S61.226 ☑
    - middle S61.218 ☑
      - with
        - damage to nail S61.318 ☑
          - with
            - foreign body S61.328 ☑
        - foreign body S61.228 ☑
      - left S61.213 ☑
        - with
          - damage to nail S61.313 ☑
            - with
              - foreign body S61.323 ☑
          - foreign body S61.223 ☑
      - right S61.212 ☑
        - with
          - damage to nail S61.312 ☑

Laceration — *continued*
finger(s) — *continued*
middle — *continued*
right — *continued*
with — *continued*
damage to nail — *continued*
with
foreign body S61.322 ☑
foreign body S61.222 ☑
ring S61.218 ☑
with
damage to nail S61.318 ☑
with
foreign body S61.328 ☑
foreign body S61.228 ☑
left S61.215 ☑
with
damage to nail S61.315 ☑
with
foreign body S61.325 ☑
foreign body S61.225 ☑
right S61.214 ☑
with
damage to nail S61.314 ☑
with
foreign body S61.324 ☑
foreign body S61.224 ☑
flank S31.119 ☑
with foreign body S31.129 ☑
foot (except toe(s) alone) S91.319 ☑
with foreign body S91.329 ☑
left S91.312 ☑
with foreign body S91.322 ☑
right S91.311 ☑
with foreign body S91.321 ☑
toe — *see* Laceration, toe
forearm S51.819 ☑
with
foreign body S51.829 ☑
elbow only — *see* Laceration, elbow
left S51.812 ☑
with
foreign body S51.822 ☑
right S51.811 ☑
with
foreign body S51.821 ☑
forehead S01.81 ☑
with foreign body S01.82 ☑
fourchette O70.0
with ectopic or molar pregnancy O08.6
complicating delivery O70.0
following ectopic or molar pregnancy O08.6
gallbladder S36.123 ☑
genital organs, external
female S31.512 ☑
with foreign body S31.522 ☑
vagina — *see* Laceration, vagina
vulva — *see* Laceration, vulva
male S31.511 ☑
with foreign body S31.521 ☑
penis — *see* Laceration, penis
scrotum — *see* Laceration, scrotum
testis — *see* Laceration, testis
groin — *see* Laceration, abdomen, wall
gum — *see* Laceration, oral cavity
hand S61.419 ☑
with
foreign body S61.429 ☑
finger — *see* Laceration, finger
left S61.412 ☑
with
foreign body S61.422 ☑
right S61.411 ☑
with
foreign body S61.421 ☑
thumb — *see* Laceration, thumb
head S01.91 ☑
with foreign body S01.92 ☑
cheek — *see* Laceration, cheek
ear — *see* Laceration, ear
eyelid — *see* Laceration, eyelid
lip — *see* Laceration, lip
nose — *see* Laceration, nose
oral cavity — *see* Laceration, oral cavity
scalp S01.01 ☑
with foreign body S01.02 ☑

Laceration — *continued*
head — *continued*
specified site NEC S01.81 ☑
with foreign body S01.82 ☑
temporomandibular area — *see* Laceration, cheek
heart — *see* Injury, heart, laceration
heel — *see* Laceration, foot
hepatic duct S36.13 ☑
hip S71.019 ☑
with foreign body S71.029 ☑
left S71.012 ☑
with foreign body S71.022 ☑
right S71.011 ☑
with foreign body S71.021 ☑
hymen — *see* Laceration, vagina
hypochondrium — *see* Laceration, abdomen, wall
hypogastric region — *see* Laceration, abdomen, wall
ileum S36.438 ☑
inguinal region — *see* Laceration, abdomen, wall
instep — *see* Laceration, foot
internal organ — *see* Injury, by site
interscapular region — *see* Laceration, thorax, back
intestine
large
colon S36.539 ☑
ascending S36.530 ☑
descending S36.532 ☑
sigmoid S36.533 ☑
specified site NEC S36.538 ☑
rectum S36.63 ☑
transverse S36.531 ☑
small S36.439 ☑
duodenum S36.430 ☑
specified site NEC S36.438 ☑
intra-abdominal organ S36.93 ☑
intestine — *see* Laceration, intestine
liver — *see* Laceration, liver
pancreas — *see* Laceration, pancreas
peritoneum S36.81 ☑
specified site NEC S36.893 ☑
spleen — *see* Laceration, spleen
stomach — *see* Laceration, stomach
intracranial NEC — *see also* Injury, intracranial, diffuse
birth injury P10.9
jaw — *see* Laceration, head, specified site NEC
jejunum S36.438 ☑
joint capsule — *see* Sprain, by site
kidney S37.03- ☑
major (greater than 3 cm) (massive) (stellate) S37.06- ☑
minor (less than 1 cm) S37.04- ☑
moderate (1 to 3 cm) S37.05- ☑
multiple S37.06- ☑
knee S81.01- ☑
with foreign body S81.02- ☑
labium (majus) (minus) — *see* Laceration, vulva
lacrimal duct — *see* Laceration, eyelid
large intestine — *see* Laceration, intestine, large
larynx S11.011 ☑
with foreign body S11.012 ☑
leg (lower) S81.819 ☑
with foreign body S81.829 ☑
foot — *see* Laceration, foot
knee — *see* Laceration, knee
left S81.812 ☑
with foreign body S81.822 ☑
right S81.811 ☑
with foreign body S81.821 ☑
upper — *see* Laceration, thigh
ligament — *see* Sprain
lip S01.511 ☑
with foreign body S01.521 ☑
liver S36.113 ☑
major (stellate) S36.116 ☑
minor S36.114 ☑
moderate S36.115 ☑
loin — *see* Laceration, abdomen, wall
lower back — *see* Laceration, back, lower
lumbar region — *see* Laceration, back, lower
lung S27.339 ☑
bilateral S27.332 ☑
unilateral S27.331 ☑
malar region — *see* Laceration, head, specified site NEC
mammary — *see* Laceration, breast
mastoid region — *see* Laceration, head, specified site NEC

Laceration — *continued*
meninges — *see* Injury, intracranial, diffuse
meniscus — *see* Tear, meniscus
mesentery S36.893 ☑
mesosalpinx S37.893 ☑
mouth — *see* Laceration, oral cavity
muscle — *see* Injury, muscle, by site, laceration
nail
finger — *see* Laceration, finger, with damage to nail
toe — *see* Laceration, toe, with damage to nail
nasal (septum) (sinus) — *see* Laceration, nose
nasopharynx — *see* Laceration, head, specified site NEC
neck S11.91 ☑
with foreign body S11.92 ☑
involving
cervical esophagus S11.21 ☑
with foreign body S11.22 ☑
larynx — *see* Laceration, larynx
pharynx — *see* Laceration, pharynx
thyroid gland — *see* Laceration, thyroid gland
trachea — *see* Laceration, trachea
specified site NEC S11.81 ☑
with foreign body S11.82 ☑
nerve — *see* Injury, nerve
nose (septum) (sinus) S01.21 ☑
with foreign body S01.22 ☑
ocular NOS S05.3- ☑
adnexa NOS S01.11- ☑
oral cavity S01.512 ☑
with foreign body S01.522 ☑
orbit (eye) — *see* Wound, open, ocular, orbit
ovary S37.439 ☑
bilateral S37.432 ☑
unilateral S37.431 ☑
palate — *see* Laceration, oral cavity
palm — *see* Laceration, hand
pancreas S36.239 ☑
pelvic S31.010 ☑
with
foreign body S31.020 ☑
penetration into retroperitoneal cavity S31.021 ☑
penetration into retroperitoneal cavity S31.011 ☑
floor — *see also* Laceration, back, lower
with ectopic or molar pregnancy O08.6
complicating delivery O70.1
following ectopic or molar pregnancy O08.6
old (postpartal) N81.89
organ S37.93 ☑
penis S31.21 ☑
with foreign body S31.22 ☑
perineum
female S31.41 ☑
with
ectopic or molar pregnancy O08.6
foreign body S31.42 ☑
during delivery O70.9
first degree O70.0
fourth degree O70.3
second degree O70.1
third degree — *see also* Delivery, complicated, by, laceration, perineum, third degree O70.20
old (postpartal) N81.89
postpartal N81.89
secondary (postpartal) O90.1
male S31.119 ☑
with foreign body S31.129 ☑
periocular area (with or without lacrimal passages) — *see* Laceration, eyelid
peritoneum S36.893 ☑
periumbilic region — *see* Laceration, abdomen, wall, periumbilic
periurethral tissue — *see* Laceration, urethra
phalanges
finger — *see* Laceration, finger
toe — *see* Laceration, toe
pharynx S11.21 ☑
with foreign body S11.22 ☑
pinna — *see* Laceration, ear
popliteal space — *see* Laceration, knee
prepuce — *see* Laceration, penis
prostate S37.823 ☑
pubic region S31.119 ☑
with foreign body S31.129 ☑

Laceration — *continued*
pudendum — *see* Laceration, genital organs, external
rectovaginal septum — *see* Laceration, vagina
rectum S36.63 ☑
retroperitoneum S36.893 ☑
round ligament S37.893 ☑
sacral region — *see* Laceration, back, lower
sacroiliac region — *see* Laceration, back, lower
salivary gland — *see* Laceration, oral cavity
scalp S01.01 ☑
with foreign body S01.02 ☑
scapular region — *see* Laceration, shoulder
scrotum S31.31 ☑
with foreign body S31.32 ☑
seminal vesicle S37.893 ☑
shin — *see* Laceration, leg
shoulder S41.019 ☑
with foreign body S41.029 ☑
left S41.012 ☑
with foreign body S41.022 ☑
right S41.011 ☑
with foreign body S41.021 ☑
small intestine — *see* Laceration, intestine, small
spermatic cord — *see* Laceration, testis
spinal cord (meninges) — *see also* Injury, spinal cord, by region
due to injury at birth P11.5
newborn (birth injury) P11.5
spleen S36.039 ☑
major (massive) (stellate) S36.032 ☑
moderate S36.031 ☑
superficial (minor) S36.030 ☑
sternal region — *see* Laceration, thorax, front
stomach S36.33 ☑
submaxillary region — *see* Laceration, head, specified site NEC
submental region — *see* Laceration, head, specified site NEC
subungual
finger(s) — *see* Laceration, finger, with damage to nail
toe(s) — *see* Laceration, toe, with damage to nail
suprarenal gland — *see* Laceration, adrenal gland
temple, temporal region — *see* Laceration, head, specified site NEC
temporomandibular area — *see* Laceration, cheek
tendon — *see* Injury, muscle, by site, laceration
Achilles S86.02- ☑
tentorium cerebelli — *see* Injury, intracranial, diffuse
testis S31.31 ☑
with foreign body S31.32 ☑
thigh S71.11- ☑
with foreign body S71.12- ☑
thorax, thoracic (wall) S21.91 ☑
with foreign body S21.92 ☑
back S21.22- ☑
with penetration into thoracic cavity S21.42- ☑
front S21.12- ☑
with penetration into thoracic cavity S21.32- ☑
back S21.21- ☑
with
foreign body S21.22- ☑
with penetration into thoracic cavity S21.42- ☑
penetration into thoracic cavity S21.41- ☑
breast — *see* Laceration, breast
front S21.11- ☑
with
foreign body S21.12- ☑
with penetration into thoracic cavity S21.32- ☑
penetration into thoracic cavity S21.31- ☑
thumb S61.019 ☑
with
damage to nail S61.119 ☑
with
foreign body S61.129 ☑
foreign body S61.029 ☑
left S61.012 ☑
with
damage to nail S61.112 ☑
with
foreign body S61.122 ☑
foreign body S61.022 ☑

Laceration — *continued*
thumb — *continued*
right S61.011 ☑
with
damage to nail S61.111 ☑
with
foreign body S61.121 ☑
foreign body S61.021 ☑
thyroid gland S11.11 ☑
with foreign body S11.12 ☑
toe(s) S91.119 ☑
with
damage to nail S91.219 ☑
with
foreign body S91.229 ☑
foreign body S91.129 ☑
great S91.113 ☑
with
damage to nail S91.213 ☑
with
foreign body S91.223 ☑
foreign body S91.123 ☑
left S91.112 ☑
with
damage to nail S91.212 ☑
with
foreign body S91.222 ☑
foreign body S91.122 ☑
right S91.111 ☑
with
damage to nail S91.211 ☑
with
foreign body S91.221 ☑
foreign body S91.121 ☑
lesser S91.116 ☑
with
damage to nail S91.216 ☑
with
foreign body S91.226 ☑
foreign body S91.126 ☑
left S91.115 ☑
with
damage to nail S91.215 ☑
with
foreign body S91.225 ☑
foreign body S91.125 ☑
right S91.114 ☑
with
damage to nail S91.214 ☑
with
foreign body S91.224 ☑
foreign body S91.124 ☑
tongue — *see* Laceration, oral cavity
trachea S11.021 ☑
with foreign body S11.022 ☑
tunica vaginalis — *see* Laceration, testis
tympanum, tympanic membrane — *see* Laceration, ear, drum
umbilical region S31.115 ☑
with foreign body S31.125 ☑
ureter S37.13 ☑
urethra S37.33 ☑
with or following ectopic or molar pregnancy O08.6
obstetrical trauma O71.5
urinary organ NEC S37.893 ☑
uterus S37.63 ☑
with ectopic or molar pregnancy O08.6
following ectopic or molar pregnancy O08.6
nonpuerperal, nontraumatic N85.8
obstetrical trauma NEC O71.81
old (postpartal) N85.8
uvula — *see* Laceration, oral cavity
vagina S31.41 ☑
with
ectopic or molar pregnancy O08.6
foreign body S31.42 ☑
during delivery O71.4
with perineal laceration — *see* Laceration, perineum, female, during delivery
following ectopic or molar pregnancy O08.6
nonpuerperal, nontraumatic N89.8
old (postpartal) N89.8
vas deferens S37.893 ☑
vesical — *see* Laceration, bladder
vocal cords S11.031 ☑
with foreign body S11.032 ☑
vulva S31.41 ☑

Laceration — *continued*
vulva — *continued*
with
ectopic or molar pregnancy O08.6
foreign body S31.42 ☑
complicating delivery O70.0
following ectopic or molar pregnancy O08.6
nonpuerperal, nontraumatic N90.89
old (postpartal) N90.89
wrist S61.519 ☑
with
foreign body S61.529 ☑
left S61.512 ☑
with
foreign body S61.522 ☑
right S61.511 ☑
with
foreign body S61.521 ☑
Lack of
achievement in school Z55.3
adequate
food Z59.48
intermaxillary vertical dimension of fully erupted teeth M26.36
sleep Z72.820
appetite (see Anorexia) R63.0
awareness R41.9
care
in home Z74.2
of infant (at or after birth) T76.02 ☑
confirmed T74.02 ☑
cognitive functions R41.9
coordination R27.9
ataxia R27.0
specified type NEC R27.8
development (physiological) R62.50
failure to thrive (child over 28 days old) R62.51
adult R62.7
newborn P92.6
short stature R62.52
specified type NEC R62.59
energy R53.83
financial resources Z59.6
food Z59.48
growth R62.52
heating Z59.1
housing (permanent) (temporary) Z59.00
adequate Z59.1
learning experiences in childhood Z62.898
leisure time (affecting life-style) Z73.2
material resources Z59.87
memory — *see also* Amnesia
mild, following organic brain damage F06.8
ovulation N97.0
parental supervision or control of child Z62.0
person able to render necessary care Z74.2
physical exercise Z72.3
play experience in childhood Z62.898
posterior occlusal support M26.57
relaxation (affecting life-style) Z73.2
safe drinking water Z58.6
sexual
desire F52.0
enjoyment F52.1
shelter Z59.02
sleep (adequate) Z72.820
supervision of child by parent Z62.0
support, posterior occlusal M26.57
transportation Z59.82
water T73.1 ☑
safe drinking Z58.6
Lacrimal — *see* condition
Lacrimation, abnormal — *see* Epiphora
Lacrimonasal duct — *see* condition
Lactation, lactating (breast) (puerperal, postpartum)
associated
cracked nipple O92.13
retracted nipple O92.03
defective O92.4
disorder NEC O92.79
excessive O92.6
failed (complete) O92.3
partial O92.4
mastitis NEC — *see* Mastitis, obstetric
mother (care and/or examination) Z39.1
nonpuerperal N64.3
Lacticemia, excessive — *see also* Acidosis E87.20
Lacunar skull Q75.8

Laennec's cirrhosis K70.30
  with ascites K70.31
  nonalcoholic K74.69
Lafora's disease — *see* Epilepsy, generalized, idiopathic
Lag, lid (nervous) — *see* Retraction, lid
Lagophthalmos (eyelid) (nervous) H02.209
  bilateral, upper and lower eyelids H02.20C
  cicatricial H02.219
    bilateral, upper and lower eyelids H02.21C
    left H02.216
      lower H02.215
      upper H02.214
      upper and lower eyelids H02.21B
    right H02.213
      lower H02.212
      upper H02.211
      upper and lower eyelids H02.21A
  keratoconjunctivitis — *see* Keratoconjunctivitis
  left H02.206
    lower H02.205
    upper H02.204
    upper and lower eyelids H02.20B
  mechanical H02.229
    bilateral, upper and lower eyelids H02.22C
    left H02.226
      lower H02.225
      upper H02.224
      upper and lower eyelids H02.22B
    right H02.223
      lower H02.222
      upper H02.221
      upper and lower eyelids H02.22A
  paralytic H02.239
    bilateral, upper and lower eyelids H02.23C
    left H02.236
      lower H02.235
      upper H02.234
      upper and lower eyelids H02.23B
    right H02.233
      lower H02.232
      upper H02.231
      upper and lower eyelids H02.23A
  right H02.203
    lower H02.202
    upper H02.201
    upper and lower eyelids H02.20A
Laki-Lorand factor deficiency — *see* Defect, coagulation, specified type NEC
Lalling F80.0
Lambert-Eaton syndrome — *see* Syndrome, Lambert-Eaton
Lambliasis, lambliosis A07.1
Landau-Kleffner syndrome — *see* Epilepsy, specified NEC
Landouzy-Déjérine dystrophy or facioscapulohumeral atrophy G71.02
Landouzy's disease (icterohemorrhagic leptospirosis) A27.0
Landry-Guillain-Barré, syndrome or paralysis G61.0
Landry's disease or paralysis G61.0
Lane's
  band Q43.3
  kink — *see* Obstruction, intestine
  syndrome K90.2
Langdon Down syndrome — *see* Trisomy, 21
Lapsed immunization schedule status Z28.39
Large
  baby (regardless of gestational age) (4000g to 4499g) P08.1
  ear, congenital Q17.1
  physiological cup Q14.2
  stature R68.89
Large-for-dates NEC (infant) (4000g to 4499g) P08.1
  affecting management of pregnancy O36.6- ☑
  exceptionally (4500g or more) P08.0
Larsen-Johansson disease orosteochondrosis — *see* Osteochondrosis, juvenile, patella
Larsen's syndrome (flattened facies and multiple congenital dislocations) Q74.8
Larva migrans
  cutaneous B76.9
    Ancylostoma B76.0
  visceral B83.0
Laryngeal — *see* condition
Laryngismus (stridulus) J38.5
  congenital P28.89
  diphtheritic A36.2
Laryngitis (acute) (edematous) (fibrinous) (infective) (infiltrative) (malignant) (membranous) (phlegmonous) (pneumococcal) (pseudomembranous) (septic) (subglottic) (suppurative) (ulcerative) J04.0
  with
    influenza, flu, or grippe — *see* Influenza, with, laryngitis
    tracheitis (acute) — *see* Laryngotracheitis
  atrophic J37.0
  catarrhal J37.0
  chronic J37.0
    with tracheitis (chronic) J37.1
  diphtheritic A36.2
  due to external agent — *see* Inflammation, respiratory, upper, due to
  H. influenzae J04.0
  Hemophilus influenzae J04.0
  hypertrophic J37.0
  influenzal — *see* Influenza, with, respiratory manifestations NEC
  obstructive J05.0
  sicca J37.0
  spasmodic J05.0
    acute J04.0
  streptococcal J04.0
  stridulous J05.0
  syphilitic (late) A52.73
    congenital A50.59 *[J99]*
      early A50.03 *[J99]*
  tuberculous A15.5
  Vincent's A69.1
Laryngocele (congenital) (ventricular) Q31.3
Laryngofissure J38.7
  congenital Q31.8
Laryngomalacia (congenital) Q31.5
Laryngopharyngitis (acute) J06.0
  chronic J37.0
  due to external agent — *see* Inflammation, respiratory, upper, due to
Laryngoplegia J38.00
  bilateral J38.02
  unilateral J38.01
Laryngoptosis J38.7
Laryngospasm J38.5
Laryngostenosis J38.6
Laryngotracheitis (acute) (Infectional) (infective) (viral) J04.2
  atrophic J37.1
  catarrhal J37.1
  chronic J37.1
  diphtheritic A36.2
  due to external agent — *see* Inflammation, respiratory, upper, due to
  Hemophilus influenzae J04.2
  hypertrophic J37.1
  influenzal — *see* Influenza, with, respiratory manifestations NEC
  pachydermic J38.7
  sicca J37.1
  spasmodic J38.5
    acute J05.0
  streptococcal J04.2
  stridulous J38.5
  syphilitic (late) A52.73
    congenital A50.59 *[J99]*
      early A50.03 *[J99]*
  tuberculous A15.5
  Vincent's A69.1
Laryngotracheobronchitis — *see* Bronchitis
Larynx, laryngeal — *see* condition
Lassa fever A96.2
Lassitude — *see* Weakness
Late
  talker R62.0
  walker R62.0
Late effect(s) — *see* Sequelae
Latent — *see* condition
Laterocession — *see* Lateroversion
Lateroflexion — *see* Lateroversion
Lateroversion
  cervix — *see* Lateroversion, uterus
  uterus, uterine (cervix) (postinfectional) (postpartal, old) N85.4
    congenital Q51.818
    in pregnancy or childbirth O34.59- ☑
Lathyrism — *see* Poisoning, food, noxious, plant
Launois' syndrome (pituitary gigantism) E22.0
Launois-Bensaude adenolipomatosis E88.89
Laurence-Moon (-Bardet)-**Biedl syndrome** Q87.89
Lax, laxity — *see also* Relaxation
  ligament (ous) — *see also* Disorder, ligament
    familial M35.7
    knee — *see* Derangement, knee
  skin (acquired) L57.4
    congenital Q82.8
Laxative habit F55.2
Lazy leukocyte syndrome D70.8
Lead miner's lung J63.6
Leak, leakage
  air NEC J93.82
    postprocedural J95.812
  amniotic fluid — *see* Rupture, membranes, premature
  blood (microscopic), fetal, into maternal circulation
    affecting management of pregnancy — *see* Pregnancy, complicated by
  cerebrospinal fluid G96.00
    cranial
      postoperative G96.08
      specified NEC G96.08
      spontaneous G96.01
      traumatic G96.08
    from spinal (lumbar) puncture G97.0
    spinal
      postoperative G96.09
      post-traumatic G96.09
      specified NEC G96.09
      spontaneous G96.02
    spontaneous
      from
        skull base G96.01
        spine G96.02
  CSF — *see* Leak, cerebrospinal fluid
  device, implant or graft — *see also* Complications, by site and type, mechanical
    arterial graft NEC — *see* Complication vascular, graft, mechanical, leakage T82.838 ☑
    breast (implant) T85.43 ☑
    catheter NEC T85.638 ☑
      dialysis (renal) T82.43 ☑
        intraperitoneal T85.631 ☑
      infusion NEC T82.534 ☑
        spinal (epidural) (subdural) T85.630 ☑
      urinary T83.038 ☑
        cystostomy T83.030 ☑
        Hopkins T83.038 ☑
        ileostomy T83.038 ☑
        indwelling T83.031 ☑
        nephrostomy T83.032 ☑
        specified T83.038 ☑
        urostomy T83.038 ☑
    gastrointestinal — *see* Complications, prosthetic device, mechanical, gastrointestinal device
    genital NEC T83.498 ☑
      penile prosthesis (cylinder) (implanted) (pump) (reservoir) T83.490 ☑
      testicular prosthesis T83.491 ☑
    heart NEC — *see* Complication, cardiovascular device, mechanical
    joint prosthesis — *see* Complications, joint prosthesis, mechanical, specified NEC, by site
    ocular NEC — *see* Complications, prosthetic device, mechanical, ocular device
    orthopedic NEC — *see* Complication, orthopedic, device, mechanical
    persistent air J93.82
    specified NEC T85.638 ☑
    urinary NEC — *see also* Complication, genitourinary, device, urinary, mechanical
      graft T83.23 ☑
    vascular NEC — *see* Complication, cardiovascular device, mechanical
    ventricular intracranial shunt T85.03 ☑
  urine — *see* Incontinence
Leaky heart — *see* Endocarditis
Learning defect (specific) F81.9
Leather bottle stomach C16.9
Leber's
  congenital amaurosis H35.50
  optic atrophy (hereditary) H47.22
Lederer's anemia D59.19
Leeches (external) — *see* Hirudiniasis
Leg — *see* condition
Legg (-Calvé)-**Perthes disease, syndrome or osteochondrosis** M91.1- ☑
Legionellosis A48.1

- **Legionellosis** — *continued*
  - nonpneumonic A48.2
- **Legionnaires'**
  - disease A48.1
    - nonpneumonic A48.2
  - pneumonia A48.1
- **Leigh's disease** G31.82
- **Leiner's disease** L21.1
- **Leiofibromyoma** — *see* Leiomyoma
- **Leiomyoblastoma** — *see* Neoplasm, connective tissue, benign
- **Leiomyofibroma** — *see also* Neoplasm, connective tissue, benign
  - uterus (cervix) (corpus) D25.9
- **Leiomyoma** — *see also* Neoplasm, connective tissue, benign
  - bizarre — *see* Neoplasm, connective tissue, benign
  - cellular — *see* Neoplasm, connective tissue, benign
  - epithelioid — *see* Neoplasm, connective tissue, benign
  - uterus (cervix) (corpus) D25.9
    - intramural D25.1
    - submucous D25.Ø
    - subserosal D25.2
  - vascular — *see* Neoplasm, connective tissue, benign
- **Leiomyoma, leiomyomatosis** (intravascular) — *see* Neoplasm, connective tissue, uncertain behavior
- **Leiomyosarcoma** — *see also* Neoplasm, connective tissue, malignant
  - epithelioid — *see* Neoplasm, connective tissue, malignant
  - myxoid — *see* Neoplasm, connective tissue, malignant
- **Leishmaniasis** B55.9
  - American (mucocutaneous) B55.2
    - cutaneous B55.1
  - Asian Desert B55.1
  - Brazilian B55.2
  - cutaneous (any type) B55.1
  - dermal — *see also* Leishmaniasis, cutaneous
    - post-kala-azar B55.Ø
  - eyelid B55.1
  - infantile B55.Ø
  - Mediterranean B55.Ø
  - mucocutaneous (American) (New World) B55.2
  - naso-oral B55.2
  - nasopharyngeal B55.2
  - old world B55.1
  - tegumentaria diffusa B55.1
  - visceral B55.Ø
- **Leishmanoid, dermal** — *see also* Leishmaniasis, cutaneous
  - post-kala-azar B55.Ø
- **Lenegre's disease** I44.2
- **Lengthening, leg** — *see* Deformity, limb, unequal length
- **Lennert's lymphoma** — *see* Lymphoma, Lennert's
- **Lennox-Gastaut syndrome** G4Ø.812
  - intractable G4Ø.814
    - with status epilepticus G4Ø.813
    - without status epilepticus G4Ø.814
  - not intractable G4Ø.812
    - with status epilepticus G4Ø.811
    - without status epilepticus G4Ø.812
- **Lens** — *see* condition
- **Lenticonus** (anterior) (posterior) (congenital) Q12.8
- **Lenticular degeneration, progressive** E83.Ø1
- **Lentiglobus** (posterior) (congenital) Q12.8
- **Lentigo** (congenital) L81.4
  - maligna — *see also* Melanoma, in situ
    - melanoma — *see* Melanoma
- **Lentivirus, as cause of disease classified elsewhere** B97.31
- **Leontiasis**
  - ossium M85.2
  - syphilitic (late) A52.78
    - congenital A5Ø.59
- **Lepothrix** A48.8
- **Lepra** — *see* Leprosy
- **Leprechaunism** E34.8
- **Leprosy** A3Ø.- ☑
  - with muscle disorder A3Ø.9 *[M63.8Ø]*
    - ankle A3Ø.9 *[M63.87-]* ☑
    - foot A3Ø.9 *[M63.87-]* ☑
    - forearm A3Ø.9 *[M63.83-]* ☑
    - hand A3Ø.9 *[M63.84-]* ☑
    - lower leg A3Ø.9 *[M63.86-]* ☑
    - multiple sites A3Ø.9 *[M63.89]*
    - pelvic region A3Ø.9 *[M63.85-]* ☑
    - shoulder region A3Ø.9 *[M63.81-]* ☑
- **Leprosy** — *continued*
  - with muscle disorder — *continued*
    - specified site NEC A3Ø.9 *[M63.88]*
    - thigh A3Ø.9 *[M63.85-]* ☑
    - upper arm A3Ø.9 *[M63.82-]* ☑
  - anesthetic A3Ø.9
  - BB A3Ø.3
  - BL A3Ø.4
  - borderline (infiltrated) (neuritic) A3Ø.3
    - lepromatous A3Ø.4
    - tuberculoid A3Ø.2
  - BT A3Ø.2
  - dimorphous (infiltrated) (neuritic) A3Ø.3
  - I A3Ø.Ø
  - indeterminate (macular) (neuritic) A3Ø.Ø
  - lepromatous (diffuse) (infiltrated) (macular) (neuritic) (nodular) A3Ø.5
  - LL A3Ø.5
  - macular (early) (neuritic) (simple) A3Ø.9
  - maculoanesthetic A3Ø.9
  - mixed A3Ø.3
  - neural A3Ø.9
  - nodular A3Ø.5
  - primary neuritic A3Ø.3
  - specified type NEC A3Ø.8
  - TT A3Ø.1
  - tuberculoid (major) (minor) A3Ø.1
- **Leptocytosis, hereditary** D56.9
- **Leptomeningitis** (chronic) (circumscribed) (hemorrhagic) (nonsuppurative) — *see* Meningitis
- **Leptomeningopathy** G96.198
- **Leptospiral** — *see* condition
- **Leptospirochetal** — *see* condition
- **Leptospirosis** A27.9
  - canicola A27.89
  - due to Leptospira interrogans serovar icterohaemorrhagiae A27.Ø
  - icterohemorrhagica A27.Ø
  - pomona A27.89
  - Weil's disease A27.Ø
- **Leptus dermatitis** B88.Ø
- **Leriche's syndrome** (aortic bifurcation occlusion) I74.Ø9
- **Leri's pleonosteosis** Q78.8
- **Leri-Weill syndrome** Q77.8
- **Lermoyez' syndrome** — *see* Vertigo, peripheral NEC
- **Lesch-Nyhan syndrome** E79.1
- **Leser-Trélat disease** L82.1
  - inflamed L82.Ø
- **Lesion**(s) (nontraumatic)
  - abducens nerve — *see* Strabismus, paralytic, sixth nerve
  - alveolar process KØ8.9
  - angiocentric immunoproliferative D47.Z9 (*following* D47.4)
  - anorectal K62.9
  - aortic (valve) I35.9
  - auditory nerve — *see* subcategory H93.3 ☑
  - basal ganglion G25.9
  - bile duct — *see* Disease, bile duct
  - biomechanical M99.9
    - specified type NEC M99.89
      - abdomen M99.89
      - acromioclavicular M99.87
      - cervical region M99.81
      - cervicothoracic M99.81
      - costochondral M99.88
      - costovertebral M99.88
      - head region M99.8Ø
      - hip M99.85
      - lower extremity M99.86
      - lumbar region M99.83
      - lumbosacral M99.83
      - occipitocervical M99.8Ø
      - pelvic region M99.85
      - pubic M99.85
      - rib cage M99.88
      - sacral region M99.84
      - sacrococcygeal M99.84
      - sacroiliac M99.84
      - specified NEC M99.89
      - sternochondral M99.88
      - sternoclavicular M99.87
      - thoracic region M99.82
      - thoracolumbar M99.82
      - upper extremity M99.87
  - bladder N32.9
  - bone — *see* Disorder, bone
  - brachial plexus G54.Ø
  - brain G93.9
- **Lesion**(s) — *continued*
  - brain — *continued*
    - congenital QØ4.9
    - vascular I67.9
      - degenerative I67.9
      - hypertensive I67.4
  - buccal cavity K13.79
  - calcified — *see* Calcification
  - canthus — *see* Disorder, eyelid
  - carate — *see* Pinta, lesions
  - cardia K31.9
  - cardiac — *see also* Disease, heart I51.9
    - congenital Q24.9
    - valvular — *see* Endocarditis
  - cauda equina G83.4
  - cecum K63.9
  - cerebral — *see* Lesion, brain
  - cerebrovascular I67.9
    - degenerative I67.9
    - hypertensive I67.4
  - cervical (nerve) root NEC G54.2
  - chiasmal — *see* Disorder, optic, chiasm
  - chorda tympani G51.8
  - coin, lung R91.1
  - colon K63.9
  - combined periodontic - endodontic KØ5.5
  - congenital — *see* Anomaly, by site
  - conjunctiva H11.9
  - conus medullaris — *see* Injury, conus medullaris
  - coronary artery — *see* Ischemia, heart
  - cranial nerve G52.9
    - eighth — *see* Disorder, ear
    - eleventh G52.9
    - fifth G5Ø.9
    - first G52.Ø
    - fourth — *see* Strabismus, paralytic, fourth nerve
    - seventh G51.9
    - sixth — *see* Strabismus, paralytic, sixth nerve
    - tenth G52.2
    - twelfth G52.3
  - cystic — *see* Cyst
  - degenerative — *see* Degeneration
  - duodenum K31.9
  - edentulous (alveolar) ridge, associated with trauma, due to traumatic occlusion KØ6.2
  - en coup de sabre L94.1
  - eyelid — *see* Disorder, eyelid
  - gasserian ganglion G5Ø.8
  - gastric K31.9
  - gastroduodenal K31.9
  - gastrointestinal K63.9
  - gingiva, associated with trauma KØ6.2
  - glomerular
    - focal and segmental — *see also* NØØ-NØ7 with fourth character .1 NØ5.1
    - minimal change — *see also* NØØ-NØ7 with fourth character .Ø NØ5.Ø
  - heart (organic) — *see* Disease, heart
  - hyperchromic, due to pinta (carate) A67.1
  - hyperkeratotic — *see* Hyperkeratosis
  - hypothalamic E23.7
  - ileocecal K63.9
  - ileum K63.9
  - iliohypogastric nerve G57.8- ☑
  - inflammatory — *see* Inflammation
  - intestine K63.9
  - intracerebral — *see* Lesion, brain
  - intrachiasmal (optic) — *see* Disorder, optic, chiasm
  - intracranial, space-occupying R9Ø.Ø
  - joint — *see* Disorder, joint
    - sacroiliac (old) M53.3
  - keratotic — *see* Keratosis
  - kidney — *see* Disease, renal
  - laryngeal nerve (recurrent) G52.2
  - lip K13.Ø
  - liver K76.9
  - lumbosacral
    - plexus G54.1
    - root (nerve) NEC G54.4
  - lung (coin) R91.1
  - maxillary sinus J32.Ø
  - mitral IØ5.9
  - Morel-Lavallée — *see* Hematoma, by site
  - motor cortex NEC G93.89
  - mouth K13.79
  - nerve G58.9
    - femoral G57.2- ☑
    - median G56.1- ☑

- **Lesion**(s) — *continued*
  - nerve — *continued*
    - median — *continued*
      - carpal tunnel syndrome — *see* Syndrome, carpal tunnel
    - plantar G57.6- ☑
    - popliteal (lateral) G57.3- ☑
      - medial G57.4- ☑
    - radial G56.3- ☑
    - sciatic G57.Ø- ☑
    - spinal — *see* Injury, nerve, spinal
    - ulnar G56.2- ☑
  - nervous system, congenital QØ7.9
  - nonallopathic — *see* Lesion, biomechanical
  - nose (internal) J34.89
  - obstructive — *see* Obstruction
  - obturator nerve G57.8- ☑
  - oral mucosa K13.7Ø
  - organ or site NEC — *see* Disease, by site
  - osteolytic — *see* Osteolysis
  - peptic K27.9
  - periodontal, due to traumatic occlusion KØ5.5
  - pharynx J39.2
  - pigment, pigmented (skin) L81.9
  - pinta — *see* Pinta, lesions
  - polypoid — *see* Polyp
  - prechiasmal (optic) — *see* Disorder, optic, chiasm
  - primary — *see also* Syphilis, primary A51.Ø
    - carate A67.Ø
    - pinta A67.Ø
    - yaws A66.Ø
  - pulmonary J98.4
    - valve I37.9
  - pylorus K31.9
  - rectosigmoid K63.9
  - retina, retinal H35.9
  - sacroiliac (joint) (old) M53.3
  - salivary gland K11.9
    - benign lymphoepithelial K11.8
  - saphenous nerve G57.8- ☑
  - sciatic nerve G57.Ø- ☑
  - secondary — *see* Syphilis, secondary
  - shoulder (region) M75.9- ☑
    - specified NEC M75.8- ☑
  - sigmoid K63.9
  - sinus (accessory) (nasal) J34.89
  - skin L98.9
    - suppurative LØ8.Ø
  - SLAP S43.43- ☑
  - spinal cord G95.9
    - congenital QØ6.9
  - spleen D73.89
  - stomach K31.9
  - superior glenoid labrum S43.43- ☑
  - syphilitic — *see* Syphilis
  - tertiary — *see* Syphilis, tertiary
  - thoracic root (nerve) NEC G54.3
  - tonsillar fossa J35.9
  - tooth, teeth KØ8.9
    - white spot
      - chewing surface KØ2.51
      - pit and fissure surface KØ2.51
      - smooth surface KØ2.61
  - traumatic — *see* specific type of injury by site
  - tricuspid (valve) IØ7.9
    - nonrheumatic I36.9
  - trigeminal nerve G5Ø.9
  - ulcerated or ulcerative — *see* Ulcer, skin
  - uterus N85.9
  - vagina N89.8
  - vagus nerve G52.2
  - valvular — *see* Endocarditis
  - vascular I99.9
    - affecting central nervous system I67.9
    - following trauma NEC T14.8 ☑
    - umbilical cord, complicating delivery O69.5 ☑
  - vulva N9Ø.89
  - warty — *see* Verruca
  - white spot (tooth)
    - chewing surface KØ2.51
    - pit and fissure surface KØ2.51
    - smooth surface KØ2.61
- **Less than a high school diploma** Z55.5
- **Lethargic** — *see* condition
- **Lethargy** R53.83
- **Letterer-Siwe's disease** C96.Ø
- **Leukemia, leukemic** C95.9- ☑
- **Leukemia, leukemic** — *continued*
  - acute basophilic C94.8- ☑
  - acute bilineal C95.Ø- ☑
  - acute erythroid C94.Ø- ☑
  - acute lymphoblastic C91.Ø- ☑
  - acute megakaryoblastic C94.2- ☑
  - acute megakaryocytic C94.2- ☑
  - acute mixed lineage C95.Ø- ☑
  - acute monoblastic (monoblastic/monocytic) C93.Ø- ☑
  - acute monocytic (monoblastic/monocytic) C93.Ø- ☑
  - acute myeloblastic (minimal differentiation) (with maturation) C92.Ø- ☑
  - acute myeloid, NOS C92.Ø- ☑
    - with
      - 11q23-abnormality C92.6- ☑
      - dysplasia of remaining hematopoesis and/or myelodysplastic disease in its history C92.A- ☑ (*following* C92.6)
      - multilineage dysplasia C92.A- ☑ (*following* C92.6)
      - variation of MLL-gene C92.6- ☑
    - M6 (a)(b) C94.Ø- ☑
    - M7 C94.2- ☑
  - acute myelomonocytic C92.5- ☑
  - acute promyelocytic C92.4- ☑
  - adult T-cell (HTLV-1-associated) (acute variant) (chronic variant) (lymphomatoid variant) (smouldering variant) C91.5- ☑
  - aggressive NK-cell C94.8- ☑
  - AML (1/ETO) (MØ) (M1) (M2) (without a FAB classification) C92.Ø- ☑
  - AML M3 C92.4- ☑
  - AML M4 (Eo with inv(16) or t(16;16)) C92.5- ☑
  - AML M5 C93.Ø- ☑
  - AML M5a C93.Ø- ☑
  - AML M5b C93.Ø- ☑
  - AML Me with t (15;17) and variants C92.4- ☑
  - atypical chronic myeloid, BCR/ABL-negative C92.2- ☑
  - biphenotypic acute C95.Ø- ☑
  - blast cell C95.Ø- ☑
  - Burkitt-type, mature B-cell C91.A- ☑ (*following* C91.6)
  - chronic eosinophilic — *see also* Syndrome, hypereosinophilic, myeloid C94.8- ☑
  - chronic lymphocytic, of B-cell type C91.1- ☑
  - chronic monocytic C93.1- ☑
  - chronic myelogenous (Philadelphia chromosome (Ph1) positive) (t(9;22)) (q34;q11) (with crisis of blast cells) C92.1- ☑
  - chronic myeloid, BCR/ABL-positive C92.1- ☑
    - atypical, BCR/ABL-negative C92.2- ☑
  - chronic myelomonocytic C93.1- ☑
  - chronic neutrophilic D47.1
  - CMML (-1) (-2) (with eosinophilia) C93.1- ☑
  - granulocytic — *see also* Category C92 C92.9- ☑
  - hairy cell C91.4- ☑
  - juvenile myelomonocytic C93.3- ☑
  - lymphoid C91.9- ☑
    - specified NEC C91.Z- ☑ (*following* C91.6)
  - mast cell C94.3- ☑
  - mature B-cell, Burkitt-type C91.A- ☑ (*following* C91.6)
  - monocytic (subacute) C93.9- ☑
    - specified NEC C93.Z- ☑ (*following* C93.3)
  - myelogenous — *see also* Category C92 C92.9- ☑
  - myeloid C92.9- ☑
    - specified NEC C92.Z- ☑ (*following* C92.6)
  - plasma cell C9Ø.1- ☑
  - plasmacytic C9Ø.1- ☑
  - prolymphocytic
    - of B-cell type C91.3- ☑
    - of T-cell type C91.6- ☑
  - specified NEC C94.8- ☑
  - stem cell, of unclear lineage C95.Ø- ☑
  - subacute lymphocytic C91.9- ☑
  - T-cell large granular lymphocytic C91.Z- ☑ (*following* C91.6)
  - unspecified cell type C95.9- ☑
    - acute C95.Ø- ☑
    - chronic C95.1- ☑
- **Leukemoid reaction** — *see also* Reaction, leukemoid D72.823
- **Leukoaraiosis** (hypertensive) I67.81
- **Leukoariosis** — *see* Leukoaraiosis
- **Leukocoria** — *see* Disorder, globe, degenerated condition, leucocoria
- **Leukocytopenia** D72.819
- **Leukocytosis** D72.829
- **Leukocytosis** — *continued*
  - eosinophilic D72.19
- **Leukoderma, leukodermia NEC** L81.5
  - syphilitic A51.39
    - late A52.79
- **Leukodystrophy** E75.29
- **Leukoedema, oral epithelium** K13.29
- **Leukoencephalitis** GØ4.81
  - acute (subacute) hemorrhagic G36.1
    - postimmunization or postvaccinal GØ4.Ø2
  - postinfectious GØ4.Ø1
  - subacute sclerosing A81.1
  - van Bogaert's (sclerosing) A81.1
- **Leukoencephalopathy** — *see also* Encephalopathy G93.49
  - Binswanger's I67.3
  - heroin vapor G92.8
  - metachromatic E75.25
  - multifocal (progressive) A81.2
  - postimmunization and postvaccinal GØ4.Ø2
  - progressive multifocal A81.2
  - reversible, posterior G93.6
  - van Bogaert's (sclerosing) A81.1
  - vascular, progressive I67.3
- **Leukoerythroblastosis** D75.9
- **Leukokeratosis** — *see also* Leukoplakia
  - mouth K13.21
  - nicotina palati K13.24
  - oral mucosa K13.21
  - tongue K13.21
  - vocal cord J38.3
- **Leukokraurosis vulva** (e) N9Ø.4
- **Leukoma** (cornea) — *see also* Opacity, cornea
  - adherent H17.Ø- ☑
  - interfering with central vision — *see* Opacity, cornea, central
- **Leukomalacia, cerebral, newborn** P91.2
  - periventricular P91.2
- **Leukomelanopathy, hereditary** D72.Ø
- **Leukonychia** (punctata) (striata) L6Ø.8
  - congenital Q84.4
- **Leukopathia unguium** L6Ø.8
  - congenital Q84.4
- **Leukopenia** D72.819
  - basophilic D72.818
  - chemotherapy (cancer) induced D7Ø.1
  - congenital D7Ø.Ø
  - cyclic D7Ø.Ø
  - drug induced NEC D7Ø.2
    - due to cytoreductive cancer chemotherapy D7Ø.1
  - eosinophilic D72.818
  - familial D7Ø.Ø
  - infantile genetic D7Ø.Ø
  - malignant D7Ø.9
  - periodic D7Ø.Ø
  - transitory neonatal P61.5
- **Leukopenic** — *see* condition
- **Leukoplakia**
  - anus K62.89
  - bladder (postinfectional) N32.89
  - buccal K13.21
  - cervix (uteri) N88.Ø
  - esophagus K22.89
  - gingiva K13.21
  - hairy (oral mucosa) (tongue) K13.3
  - kidney (pelvis) N28.89
  - larynx J38.7
  - lip K13.21
  - mouth K13.21
  - oral epithelium, including tongue (mucosa) K13.21
  - palate K13.21
  - pelvis (kidney) N28.89
  - penis (infectional) N48.Ø
  - rectum K62.89
  - syphilitic (late) A52.79
  - tongue K13.21
  - ureter (postinfectional) N28.89
  - urethra (postinfectional) N36.8
  - uterus N85.8
  - vagina N89.4
  - vocal cord J38.3
  - vulva N9Ø.4
- **Leukorrhea** N89.8
  - due to Trichomonas (vaginalis) A59.ØØ
  - trichomonal A59.ØØ
- **Leukosarcoma** C85.9- ☑
- **Levocardia** (isolated) Q24.1
  - with situs inversus Q89.3

Levotransposition Q2Ø.5
Lev's disease or syndrome (acquired complete heart block) I44.2
Levulosuria — *see* Fructosuria
Levurid L3Ø.2
Lewy body (ies) (disease) G31.83
Leyden-Möbius dystrophy — *see* Dystrophy, Leyden-Möbius
Leydig cell
- carcinoma
  - specified site — *see* Neoplasm, malignant, by site
  - unspecified site
    - female C56.9
    - male C62.9- ☑
- tumor
  - benign
    - specified site — *see* Neoplasm, benign, by site
    - unspecified site
      - female D27.- ☑
      - male D29.2- ☑
  - malignant
    - specified site — *see* Neoplasm, malignant, by site
    - unspecified site
      - female C56.- ☑
      - male C62.9- ☑
  - specified site — *see* Neoplasm, uncertain behavior, by site
  - unspecified site
    - female D39.1- ☑
    - male D4Ø.1- ☑

Leydig-Sertoli cell tumor
- specified site — *see* Neoplasm, benign, by site
- unspecified site
  - female D27.- ☑
  - male D29.2- ☑

LGMD — *see* Dystrophy, muscular, limb-girdle
LGSIL (Low grade squamous intraepithelial lesion on cytologic smear of)
- anus R85.612
- cervix R87.612
- vagina R87.622

Liar, pathologic F6Ø.2
Libido
- decreased R68.82

Libman-Sacks disease M32.11
Lice (infestation) B85.2
- body (Pediculus corporis) B85.1
- crab B85.3
- head (Pediculus capitis) B85.Ø
- mixed (classifiable to more than one of the titles B85.Ø-B85.3) B85.4
- pubic (Phthirus pubis) B85.3

Lichen L28.Ø
- albus L9Ø.Ø
  - penis N48.Ø
  - vulva N9Ø.4
- amyloidosis E85.4 *[L99]*
- atrophicus L9Ø.Ø
  - penis N48.Ø
  - vulva N9Ø.4
- congenital Q82.8
- myxedematosus L98.5
- nitidus L44.1
- pilaris Q82.8
  - acquired L85.8
- planopilaris L66.1
- planus (chronicus) L43.9
  - annularis L43.8
  - bullous L43.1
  - follicular L66.1
  - hypertrophic L43.Ø
  - moniliformis L44.3
  - of Wilson L43.9
  - specified NEC L43.8
  - subacute (active) L43.3
  - tropicus L43.3
- ruber
  - acuminatus L44.Ø
  - moniliformis L44.3
  - planus L43.9
- sclerosus (et atrophicus) L9Ø.Ø
  - penis N48.Ø
  - vulva N9Ø.4
- scrofulosus (primary) (tuberculous) A18.4
- simplex (chronicus) (circumscriptus) L28.Ø
- striatus L44.2
- urticatus L28.2

Lichenification L28.Ø
Lichenoides tuberculosis (primary) A18.4
Lichtheim's disease or syndrome D51.Ø
Lien migrans D73.89
Ligament — *see* condition
Light
- for gestational age — *see* Light for dates
- headedness R42

Light-for-dates (infant) PØ5.ØØ
- with weight of
  - 499 grams or less PØ5.Ø1
  - 5ØØ-749 grams PØ5.Ø2
  - 75Ø-999 grams PØ5.Ø3
  - 1ØØØ-1249 grams PØ5.Ø4
  - 125Ø-1499 grams PØ5.Ø5
  - 15ØØ-1749 grams PØ5.Ø6
  - 175Ø-1999 grams PØ5.Ø7
  - 2ØØØ-2499 grams PØ5.Ø8
  - 25ØØ grams and over PØ5.Ø9
- affecting management of pregnancy O36.59- ☑
- and small-for-dates — *see* Small for dates
- specified NEC PØ5.Ø9

Lightning (effects) (stroke) (struck by) T75.ØØ ☑
- burn — *see* Burn
- foot E53.8
- shock T75.Ø1 ☑
- specified effect NEC T75.Ø9 ☑

Lightwood-Albright syndrome N25.89
Lightwood's disease or syndrome (renal tubular acidosis) N25.89
Lignac (-de Toni) (-Fanconi) (-Debré) **disease or syndrome** E72.Ø9
- with cystinosis E72.Ø4

Ligneous thyroiditis EØ6.5
Likoff's syndrome I2Ø.8
Limb — *see* condition
Limbic epilepsy personality syndrome FØ7.Ø
Limitation, limited
- activities due to disability Z73.6
- cardiac reserve — *see* Disease, heart
- eye muscle duction, traumatic — *see* Strabismus, mechanical
- mandibular range of motion M26.52

Lindau (-von Hippel) **disease** Q85.83
Line(s)
- Beau's L6Ø.4
- Harris' — *see* Arrest, epiphyseal
- Hudson's (cornea) — *see* Pigmentation, cornea, anterior
- Stähli's (cornea) — *see* Pigmentation, cornea, anterior

Linea corneae senilis — *see* Change, cornea, senile
Lingua
- geographica K14.1
- nigra (villosa) K14.3
- plicata K14.5
- tylosis K13.29

Lingual — *see* condition
Linguatulosis B88.8
Linitis (gastric) **plastica** C16.9
Lip — *see* condition
Lipedema — *see* Edema
Lipemia — *see also* Hyperlipidemia
- retina, retinalis E78.3

Lipidosis E75.6
- cerebral (infantile) (juvenile) (late) E75.4
- cerebroretinal E75.4
- cerebroside E75.22
- cholesterol (cerebral) E75.5
- glycolipid E75.21
- hepatosplenomegalic E78.3
- sphingomyelin — *see* Niemann-Pick disease or syndrome
- sulfatide E75.29

Lipoadenoma — *see* Neoplasm, benign, by site
Lipoblastoma — *see* Lipoma
Lipoblastomatosis — *see* Lipoma
Lipochondrodystrophy E76.Ø1
Lipochrome histiocytosis (familial) D71
Lipodermatosclerosis — *see* Varix, leg, with, inflammation
- ulcerated — *see* Varix, leg, with, ulcer, with inflammation by site

Lipodystrophia progressiva E88.1
Lipodystrophy (progressive) E88.1
- insulin E88.1
- intestinal K9Ø.81
- mesenteric K65.4

Lipofibroma — *see* Lipoma
Lipofuscinosis, neuronal (with ceroidosis) E75.4
Lipogranuloma, sclerosing L92.8
Lipogranulomatosis E78.89
Lipoid — *see also* condition
- histiocytosis D76.3
  - essential E75.29
- nephrosis NØ4.9
- proteinosis of Urbach E78.89

Lipoidemia — *see* Hyperlipidemia
Lipoidosis — *see* Lipidosis
Lipoma D17.9
- fetal D17.9
  - fat cell D17.9
- infiltrating D17.9
- intramuscular D17.9
- pleomorphic D17.9
- site classification
  - arms (skin) (subcutaneous) D17.2- ☑
  - connective tissue D17.3Ø
    - intra-abdominal D17.5
    - intrathoracic D17.4
    - peritoneum D17.79
    - retroperitoneum D17.79
    - specified site NEC D17.39
    - spermatic cord D17.6
  - face (skin) (subcutaneous) D17.Ø
  - genitourinary organ NEC D17.72
  - head (skin) (subcutaneous) D17.Ø
  - intra-abdominal D17.5
  - intrathoracic D17.4
  - kidney D17.71
  - legs (skin) (subcutaneous) D17.2- ☑
  - neck (skin) (subcutaneous) D17.Ø
  - peritoneum D17.79
  - retroperitoneum D17.79
  - skin D17.3Ø
    - specified site NEC D17.39
  - specified site NEC D17.79
  - spermatic cord D17.6
  - subcutaneous D17.3Ø
    - specified site NEC D17.39
  - trunk (skin) (subcutaneous) D17.1
  - unspecified D17.9
- spindle cell D17.9

Lipomatosis E88.2
- dolorosa (Dercum) E88.2
- fetal — *see* Lipoma
- Launois-Bensaude E88.89

Lipomyoma — *see* Lipoma
Lipomyxoma — *see* Lipoma
Lipomyxosarcoma — *see* Neoplasm, connective tissue, malignant
Lipoprotein metabolism disorder E78.9
Lipoproteinemia E78.5
- broad-beta E78.2
- floating-beta E78.2
- hyper-pre-beta E78.1

Liposarcoma — *see also* Neoplasm, connective tissue, malignant
- dedifferentiated — *see* Neoplasm, connective tissue, malignant
- differentiated type — *see* Neoplasm, connective tissue, malignant
- embryonal — *see* Neoplasm, connective tissue, malignant
- mixed type — *see* Neoplasm, connective tissue, malignant
- myxoid — *see* Neoplasm, connective tissue, malignant
- pleomorphic — *see* Neoplasm, connective tissue, malignant
- round cell — *see* Neoplasm, connective tissue, malignant
- well differentiated type — *see* Neoplasm, connective tissue, malignant

Liposynovitis prepatellaris E88.89
Lipping, cervix N86
Lipschütz disease or ulcer N76.6
Lipuria R82.Ø
- schistosomiasis (bilharziasis) B65.Ø

Lisping F8Ø.Ø
Lissauer's paralysis A52.17
Lissencephalia, lissencephaly QØ4.3
Listeriosis, listerellosis A32.9
- congenital (disseminated) P37.2
- cutaneous A32.Ø
- neonatal, newborn (disseminated) P37.2
- oculoglandular A32.81
- specified NEC A32.89

- **Lithemia** E79.Ø
- **Lithiasis** — *see* Calculus
- **Lithosis** J62.8
- **Lithuria** R82.998
- **Litigation, anxiety concerning** Z65.3
- **Little leaguer's elbow** — *see* Epicondylitis, medial
- **Little's disease** G8Ø.9
- **Littre's**
  - gland — *see* condition
  - hernia — *see* Hernia, abdomen
- **Littritis** — *see* Urethritis
- **Livedo** (annularis) (racemosa) (reticularis) R23.1
- **Liver** — *see* condition
- **Living alone** (problems with) Z6Ø.2
  - with handicapped person Z74.2
- **Living in a shelter** (motel) (scattered site housing) (temporary or transitional living situation) Z59.Ø1
- **Lloyd's syndrome** — *see* Adenomatosis, endocrine
- **Loa loa, loaiasis, loasis** B74.3
- **Lobar** — *see* condition
- **Lobomycosis** B48.Ø
- **Lobo's disease** B48.Ø
- **Lobotomy syndrome** FØ7.Ø
- **Lobstein** (-Ekman) **disease or syndrome** Q78.Ø
- **Lobster-claw hand** Q71.6- ☑
- **Lobulation** (congenital) — *see also* Anomaly, by site
  - kidney, Q63.1
  - liver, abnormal Q44.7
  - spleen Q89.Ø9
- **Lobule, lobular** — *see* condition
- **Local, localized** — *see* condition
- **Locked twins causing obstructed labor** O66.1
- **Locked-in state** G83.5
- **Locking**
  - joint — *see* Derangement, joint, specified type NEC
    - knee — *see* Derangement, knee
- **Lockjaw** — *see* Tetanus
- **Löffler's**
  - endocarditis I42.3
  - eosinophilia J82.89
  - pneumonia J82.89
  - syndrome (eosinophilic pneumonitis) J82.89
- **Loiasis** (with conjunctival infestation) (eyelid) B74.3
- **Lone Star fever** A77.Ø
- **Long**
  - COVID (-19) — *see also* COVID-19 UØ9.9
  - labor O63.9
    - first stage O63.Ø
    - second stage O63.1
  - QT syndrome I45.81
- **Longitudinal stripes or grooves, nails** L6Ø.8
  - congenital Q84.6
- **Long-term** (current) (prophylactic) **drug therapy** (use of)
  - 5-fluorouracil Z79.631
  - 6-mercaptopurine Z79.631
  - adalimumab Z79.62Ø
  - agents affecting estrogen receptors and estrogen levels NEC Z79.818
  - alkylating agent Z79.63Ø
  - anastrozole (Arimidex) Z79.811
  - antibiotics Z79.2
    - short-term use — *omit code*
  - anticoagulants Z79.Ø1
  - antidiabetic drugs, injectable, non-insulin Z79.85
  - anti-inflammatory, non-steroidal (NSAID) Z79.1
  - antimetabolite agent Z79.631
  - antiplatelet Z79.Ø2
  - antithrombotics Z79.Ø2
  - antitumor antibiotic Z79.632
  - apremilast Z79.61
  - aromatase inhibitors Z79.811
  - aspirin Z79.82
  - azathioprine Z79.624
  - birth control pill or patch Z79.3
  - bisphosphonates Z79.83
  - bleomycin Z79.632
  - calcineurin inhibitor Z79.621
  - chlorambucil Z79.63Ø
  - cisplatin Z79.63Ø
  - contraceptive, oral Z79.3
  - cyclophosphamide Z79.63Ø
  - cyclosporine Z79.621
  - cytarabine Z79.631
  - doxorubicin Z79.632
  - drug, specified NEC Z79.899
  - estrogen receptor downregulators Z79.818

- **Long-term** (current) (prophylactic) **drug therapy** — *continued*
  - etanercept Z79.62Ø
  - etoposide Z79.634
  - Evista Z79.81Ø
  - exemestane (Aromasin) Z79.811
  - Fareston Z79.81Ø
  - fulvestrant (Faslodex) Z79.818
  - gonadotropin-releasing hormone (GnRH) agonist Z79.818
  - goserelin acetate (Zoladex) Z79.818
  - hormone replacement Z79.89Ø
  - hydroxyurea Z79.64
  - immunomodulators, unspecified Z79.6Ø
    - specified NEC Z79.69
  - immunomodulatory imide drug Z79.61
  - immunosuppressants, unspecified Z79.6Ø
    - specified NEC Z79.69
  - immunosuppressive biologic Z79.62Ø
  - infliximab Z79.62Ø
  - inhibitors of nucleotide synthesis Z79.624
  - insulin Z79.4
  - irinotecan Z79.634
  - Janus kinase inhibitor Z79.622
  - lenalidomide Z79.61
  - letrozole (Femara) Z79.811
  - leuprolide acetate (leuprorelin) (Lupron) Z79.818
  - mammalian target of rapamycin (mTOR) inhibitor Z79.623
  - megestrol acetate (Megace) Z79.818
  - methadone for pain management Z79.891
  - mitomycin C Z79.632
  - mitotic inhibitor Z79.633
  - monoclonal antibodies Z79.62Ø
  - myelosuppressive agent Z79.64
  - Nolvadex Z79.81Ø
  - non-insulin antidiabetic drug, injectable Z79.899
  - non-steroidal anti-inflammatories (NSAID) Z79.1
  - omycophenolate Z79.624
  - opiate analgesic Z79.891
  - oral
    - antidiabetic Z79.84
    - contraceptive Z79.3
    - hypoglycemic Z79.84
  - paclitaxel Z79.633
  - plant alkaloids Z79.633
  - pomalidomide Z79.61
  - purine synthesis (IMDH) inhibitors Z79.624
  - raloxifene (Evista) Z79.81Ø
  - selective estrogen receptor modulators (SERMs) Z79.81Ø
  - sirolimus Z79.623
  - steroids
    - inhaled Z79.51
    - systemic Z79.52
  - tacrolimus Z79.621
  - tamoxifen (Nolvadex) Z79.81Ø
  - tofacitinib Z79.622
  - topoisomerase inhibitor Z79.634
  - topotecan Z79.634
  - toremifene (Fareston) Z79.81Ø
  - vinblastine Z79.633
  - vincristine Z79.633
- **Loop**
  - intestine — *see* Volvulus
  - vascular on papilla (optic) Q14.2
- **Loose** — *see also* condition
  - body
    - joint M24.ØØ
      - ankle M24.Ø7- ☑
      - elbow M24.Ø2- ☑
      - hand M24.Ø4- ☑
      - hip M24.Ø5- ☑
      - knee M23.4- ☑
      - shoulder (region) M24.Ø1- ☑
      - specified site NEC M24.Ø8
      - toe M24.Ø7- ☑
      - vertebra M24.Ø8
      - wrist M24.Ø3- ☑
    - knee M23.4- ☑
    - sheath, tendon — *see* Disorder, tendon, specified type NEC
  - cartilage — *see* Loose, body, joint
  - skin and subcutaneous tissue (following bariatric surgery weight loss) (following dietary weight loss) L98.7
  - tooth, teeth KØ8.89

- **Loosening**
  - aseptic
    - joint prosthesis — *see* Complications, joint prosthesis, mechanical, loosening, by site
  - epiphysis — *see* Osteochondropathy
  - mechanical
    - joint prosthesis — *see* Complications, joint prosthesis, mechanical, loosening, by site
- **Looser-Milkman** (-Debray) **syndrome** M83.8
- **Lop ear** (deformity) Q17.3
- **Lorain** (-Levi) **short stature syndrome** E23.Ø
- **Lordosis** M4Ø.5Ø
  - acquired — *see* Lordosis, specified type NEC
  - congenital Q76.429
    - lumbar region Q76.426
    - lumbosacral region Q76.427
    - sacral region Q76.428
    - sacrococcygeal region Q76.428
    - thoracolumbar region Q76.425
  - lumbar region M4Ø.56
  - lumbosacral region M4Ø.57
  - postsurgical M96.4
  - postural — *see* Lordosis, specified type NEC
  - rachitic (late effect) (sequelae) E64.3
  - sequelae of rickets E64.3
  - specified type NEC M4Ø.4Ø
    - lumbar region M4Ø.46
    - lumbosacral region M4Ø.47
    - thoracolumbar region M4Ø.45
  - thoracolumbar region M4Ø.55
  - tuberculous A18.Ø1
- **Loss** (of)
  - appetite — *see also* Anorexia R63.Ø
    - hysterical F5Ø.89
    - nonorganic origin F5Ø.89
    - psychogenic F5Ø.89
  - blood — *see* Hemorrhage
  - bone —*see* Loss, substance of, bone
  - consciousness, transient R55
    - traumatic — *see* Injury, intracranial
  - control, sphincter, rectum R15.9
    - nonorganic origin F98.1
  - elasticity, skin R23.4
  - family (member) in childhood Z62.898
  - fluid (acute) E86.9
  - function of labyrinth — *see* subcategory H83.2 ☑
  - hair, nonscarring — *see* Alopecia
  - hearing — *see also* Deafness
    - central NOS H9Ø.5
    - conductive H9Ø.2
      - bilateral H9Ø.Ø
      - unilateral
        - with
          - restricted hearing on the contralateral side H9Ø.A1- ☑
          - unrestricted hearing on the contralateral side H9Ø.1- ☑
    - mixed conductive and sensorineural hearing loss H9Ø.8
      - bilateral H9Ø.6
      - unilateral
        - with
          - restricted hearing on the contralateral side H9Ø.A3- ☑
          - unrestricted hearing on the contralateral side H9Ø.7- ☑
    - neural NOS H9Ø.5
    - perceptive NOS H9Ø.5
    - sensorineural NOS H9Ø.5
      - bilateral H9Ø.3
      - unilateral
        - with
          - restricted hearing onthe contralateral side H9Ø.A2- ☑
          - unrestricted hearing on the contralateral side H9Ø.4- ☑
    - sensory NOS H9Ø.5
  - height R29.89Ø
  - limb or member, traumatic, current — *see* Amputation, traumatic
  - love relationship in childhood Z62.898
  - memory — *see also* Amnesia
    - mild, following organic brain damage FØ6.8
  - mind — *see* Psychosis
  - occlusal vertical dimension of fully erupted teeth M26.37
  - organ or part — *see* Absence, by site, acquired
  - ossicles, ear (partial) H74.32- ☑

Index

Lithemia — Loss

- **Loss** — *continued*
  - parent in childhood Z63.4
  - pregnancy, recurrent N96
    - care in current pregnancy O26.2- ☑
    - without current pregnancy N96
  - recurrent pregnancy — *see* Loss, pregnancy, recurrent
  - self-esteem, in childhood Z62.898
  - sense of
    - smell — *see* Disturbance, sensation, smell
    - taste — *see* Disturbance, sensation, taste
    - touch R2Ø.8
  - sensory R44.9
    - dissociative F44.6
  - sexual desire F52.Ø
  - sight (acquired) (complete) (congenital) — *see* Blindness
  - substance of
    - bone — *see* Disorder, bone, density and structure, specified NEC
      - horizontal alveolar KØ6.3
    - cartilage — *see* Disorder, cartilage, specified type NEC
      - auricle (ear) — *see* Disorder, pinna, specified type NEC
    - vitreous (humor) H15.89
  - tooth, teeth — *see* Absence, teeth, acquired
  - vision, visual H54.7
    - both eyes H54.3
    - one eye H54.6Ø
      - left (normal vision on right) H54.62
      - right (normal vision on left) H54.61
    - specified as blindness — *see* Blindness
    - subjective
      - sudden H53.13- ☑
      - transient H53.12- ☑
  - vitreous — *see* Prolapse, vitreous
  - voice — *see* Aphonia
  - weight (abnormal) (cause unknown) R63.4
- **Louis-Bar syndrome** (ataxia-telangiectasia) G11.3
- **Louping ill** (encephalitis) A84.89
- **Louse, lousiness** — *see* Lice
- **Low**
  - achiever, school Z55.3
  - back syndrome M54.5Ø
  - basal metabolic rate R94.8
  - birthweight (2499 grams or less) PØ7.1Ø
    - with weight of
      - 1ØØØ-1249 grams PØ7.14
      - 125Ø-1499 grams PØ7.15
      - 15ØØ-1749 grams PØ7.16
      - 175Ø-1999 grams PØ7.17
      - 2ØØØ-2499 grams PØ7.18
    - extreme (999 grams or less) PØ7.ØØ
    - with weight of
      - 499 grams or less PØ7.Ø1
      - 5ØØ-749 grams PØ7.Ø2
      - 75Ø-999 grams PØ7.Ø3
    - for gestational age — *see* Light for dates
  - blood pressure — *see also* Hypotension
    - reading (incidental) (isolated) (nonspecific) RØ3.1
  - cardiac reserve — *see* Disease, heart
  - function — *see also* Hypofunction
    - kidney N28.9
  - hematocrit D64.9
  - hemoglobin D64.9
  - income Z59.6
  - level of literacy Z55.Ø
  - lying
    - kidney N28.89
    - organ or site, congenital — *see* Malposition, congenital
  - output syndrome (cardiac) — *see* Failure, heart
  - platelets (blood) — *see* Thrombocytopenia
  - reserve, kidney N28.89
  - salt syndrome E87.1
  - self esteem R45.81
  - set ears Q17.4
  - vision H54.2X- ☑
    - one eye (other eye normal) H54.5Ø
      - left (normal vision on right) H54.52A- ☑
      - other eye blind — *see* Blindness
      - right (normal vision on left) H54.511- ☑
  - von Willebrand factor R79.1
- **Low-density-lipoprotein-type** (LDL) **hyperlipoproteinemia** E78.ØØ
- **Lowe's syndrome** E72.Ø3
- **Lown-Ganong-Levine syndrome** I45.6
- **LSD reaction** (acute) (without dependence) F16.9Ø
- **LSD reaction** — *continued*
  - with dependence F16.2Ø
- **L-shaped kidney** Q63.8
- **LTBI** (latent tuberculosis infection) Z22.7
- **Ludwig's angina or disease** K12.2
- **Lues** (venerea), **luetic** — *see* Syphilis
- **Luetscher's syndrome** (dehydration) E86.Ø
- **Lumbago, lumbalgia** M54.5Ø
  - with sciatica M54.4- ☑
    - due to intervertebral disc disorder M51.17
  - due to displacement, intervertebral disc M51.27
    - with sciatica M51.17
- **Lumbar** — *see* condition
- **Lumbarization, vertebra, congenital** Q76.49
- **Lumbermen's itch** B88.Ø
- **Lump** — *see also* Mass
  - breast N63.Ø
    - axillary tail
      - left N63.32
      - right N63.31
    - left
      - lower inner quadrant N63.24
      - lower outer quadrant N63.23
      - overlapping quadrants N63.25
      - unspecified quadrant N63.2Ø
      - upper inner quadrant N63.22
      - upper outer quadrant N63.21
    - right
      - lower inner quadrant N63.14
      - lower outer quadrant N63.13
      - overlapping quadrants N63.15
      - unspecified quadrant N63.1Ø
      - upper inner quadrant N63.12
      - upper outer quadrant N63.11
    - subareolar
      - left N63.42
      - right N63.41
- **Lunacy** — *see* Psychosis
- **Lung** — *see* condition
- **Lupoid** (miliary) **of Boeck** D86.3
- **Lupus**
  - anticoagulant D68.62
    - with
      - hemorrhagic disorder D68.312
      - hypercoagulable state D68.62
    - finding without diagnosis R76.Ø
  - discoid (local) L93.Ø
  - erythematosus (discoid) (local) L93.Ø
    - disseminated — *see* Lupus, erythematosus, systemic
    - eyelid HØ1.129
      - left HØ1.126
        - lower HØ1.125
        - upper HØ1.124
      - right HØ1.123
        - lower HØ1.122
        - upper HØ1.121
    - profundus L93.2
    - specified NEC L93.2
    - subacute cutaneous L93.1
    - systemic M32.9
      - with organ or system involvement M32.1Ø
        - endocarditis M32.11
        - lung M32.13
        - pericarditis M32.12
        - renal (glomerular) M32.14
          - tubulo-interstitial M32.15
        - specified organ or system NEC M32.19
      - drug-induced M32.Ø
      - inhibitor (presence of) D68.62
        - with
          - hemorrhagic disorder D68.312
          - hypercoagulable state D68.62
        - finding without diagnosis R76.Ø
      - specified NEC M32.8
  - exedens A18.4
  - hydralazine M32.Ø
    - correct substance properly administered — *see* Table of Drugs and Chemicals, by drug, adverse effect
    - overdose or wrong substance given or taken — *see* Table of Drugs and Chemicals, by drug, poisoning
  - nephritis (chronic) M32.14
  - nontuberculous, not disseminated L93.Ø
  - panniculitis L93.2
  - pernio (Besnier) D86.3
  - systemic — *see* Lupus, erythematosus, systemic
  - tuberculous A18.4
- **Lupus** — *continued*
  - tuberculous — *continued*
    - eyelid A18.4
  - vulgaris A18.4
    - eyelid A18.4
- **Luteinoma** D27.- ☑
- **Lutembacher's disease or syndrome** (atrial septal defect with mitral stenosis) Q21.19
- **Luteoma** D27.- ☑
- **Lutz** (-Splendore-de Almeida) **disease** — *see* Paracoccidioidomycosis
- **Luxation** — *see also* Dislocation
  - eyeball (nontraumatic) — *see* Luxation, globe
    - birth injury P15.3
  - globe, nontraumatic H44.82- ☑
  - lacrimal gland — *see* Dislocation, lacrimal gland
  - lens (old) (partial) (spontaneous)
    - congenital Q12.1
      - syphilitic A5Ø.39
- **Lycanthropy** F22
- **Lyell's syndrome** L51.2
  - due to drug L51.2
    - correct substance properly administered — *see* Table of Drugs and Chemicals, by drug, adverse effect
    - overdose or wrong substance given or taken — *see* Table of Drugs and Chemicals, by drug, poisoning
- **Lyme disease** A69.2Ø
- **Lymph**
  - gland or node — *see* condition
  - scrotum — *see* Infestation, filarial
- **Lymphadenitis** I88.9
  - with ectopic or molar pregnancy OØ8.Ø
  - acute LØ4.9
    - axilla LØ4.2
    - face LØ4.Ø
    - head LØ4.Ø
    - hip LØ4.3
    - limb
      - lower LØ4.3
      - upper LØ4.2
    - neck LØ4.Ø
    - shoulder LØ4.2
    - specified site NEC LØ4.8
    - trunk LØ4.1
  - anthracosis (occupational) J6Ø
  - any site, except mesenteric I88.9
    - chronic I88.1
    - subacute I88.1
  - breast
    - gestational — *see* Mastitis, obstetric
    - puerperal, postpartum (nonpurulent) O91.22
  - chancroidal (congenital) A57
  - chronic I88.1
    - mesenteric I88.Ø
  - due to
    - Brugia (malayi) B74.1
      - timori B74.2
    - chlamydial lymphogranuloma A55
    - diphtheria (toxin) A36.89
    - lymphogranuloma venereum A55
    - Wuchereria bancrofti B74.Ø
  - following ectopic or molar pregnancy OØ8.Ø
  - gonorrheal A54.89
  - infective — *see* Lymphadenitis, acute
  - mesenteric (acute) (chronic) (nonspecific) (subacute) I88.Ø
    - due to Salmonella typhi AØ1.Ø9
    - tuberculous A18.39
  - mycobacterial A31.8
  - purulent — *see* Lymphadenitis, acute
  - pyogenic — *see* Lymphadenitis, acute
  - regional, nonbacterial I88.8
  - septic — *see* Lymphadenitis, acute
  - subacute, unspecified site I88.1
  - suppurative — *see* Lymphadenitis, acute
  - syphilitic (early) (secondary) A51.49
    - late A52.79
  - tuberculous — *see* Tuberculosis, lymph gland
  - venereal (chlamydial) A55
- **Lymphadenoid goiter** EØ6.3
- **Lymphadenopathy** (generalized) R59.1
  - angioimmunoblastic, with dysproteinemia (AILD) C86.5
  - due to toxoplasmosis (acquired) B58.89
    - congenital (acute) (subacute) (chronic) P37.1
  - localized R59.Ø
  - syphilitic (early) (secondary) A51.49

Lymphadenosis R59.1
Lymphangiectasis I89.0
- conjunctiva H11.89
- postinfectional I89.0
- scrotum I89.0

Lymphangiectatic elephantiasis, nonfilarial I89.0
Lymphangioendothelioma D18.1
- malignant — *see* Neoplasm, connective tissue, malignant

Lymphangioleiomyomatosis J84.81
Lymphangioma D18.1
- capillary D18.1
- cavernous D18.1
- cystic D18.1
- malignant — *see* Neoplasm, connective tissue, malignant

Lymphangiomyoma D18.1
Lymphangiomyomatosis J84.81
Lymphangiosarcoma — *see* Neoplasm, connective tissue, malignant
Lymphangitis I89.1
- with
  - abscess — *code by* site under Abscess
  - cellulitis — *code by* site under Cellulitis
  - ectopic or molar pregnancy O08.0
- acute L03.91
  - abdominal wall L03.321
  - ankle — *see* Lymphangitis, acute, lower limb
  - arm — *see* Lymphangitis, acute, upper limb
  - auricle (ear) — *see* Lymphangitis, acute, ear
  - axilla L03.12- ☑
  - back (any part) L03.322
  - buttock L03.327
  - cervical (meaning neck) L03.222
  - cheek (external) L03.212
  - chest wall L03.323
  - digit
    - finger — *see* Lymphangitis, acute, finger
    - toe — *see* Lymphangitis, acute, toe
  - ear (external) H60.1- ☑
  - external auditory canal — *see* Lymphangitis, acute, ear
  - eyelid — *see* Abscess, eyelid
  - face NEC L03.212
  - finger (intrathecal) (periosteal) (subcutaneous) (subcuticular) L03.02- ☑
  - foot — *see* Lymphangitis, acute, lower limb
  - gluteal (region) L03.327
  - groin L03.324
  - hand — *see* Lymphangitis, acute, upper limb
  - head NEC L03.891
    - face (any part, except ear, eye and nose) L03.212
  - heel — *see* Lymphangitis, acute, lower limb
  - hip — *see* Lymphangitis, acute, lower limb
  - jaw (region) L03.212
  - knee — *see* Lymphangitis, acute, lower limb
  - leg — *see* Lymphangitis, acute, lower limb
  - lower limb L03.12- ☑
    - toe — *see* Lymphangitis, acute, toe
  - navel L03.326
  - neck (region) L03.222
  - orbit, orbital — *see* Cellulitis, orbit
  - pectoral (region) L03.323
  - perineal, perineum L03.325
  - scalp (any part) L03.891
  - shoulder — *see* Lymphangitis, acute, upper limb
  - specified site NEC L03.898
  - thigh — *see* Lymphangitis, acute, lower limb
  - thumb (intrathecal) (periosteal) (subcutaneous) (subcuticular) — *see* Lymphangitis, acute, finger
  - toe (intrathecal) (periosteal) (subcutaneous) (subcuticular) L03.04- ☑
  - trunk L03.329
    - abdominal wall L03.321
    - back (any part) L03.322
    - buttock L03.327
    - chest wall L03.323
    - groin L03.324
    - perineal, perineum L03.325
    - umbilicus L03.326
  - umbilicus L03.326
  - upper limb L03.12- ☑
    - axilla — *see* Lymphangitis, acute, axilla
    - finger — *see* Lymphangitis, acute, finger
    - thumb — *see* Lymphangitis, acute, finger
  - wrist — *see* Lymphangitis, acute, upper limb

Lymphangitis — *continued*
- breast
  - gestational — *see* Mastitis, obstetric
- chancroidal A57
- chronic (any site) I89.1
- due to
  - Brugia (malayi) B74.1
    - timori B74.2
  - Wuchereria bancrofti B74.0
- following ectopic or molar pregnancy O08.89
- penis
  - acute N48.29
  - gonococcal (acute) (chronic) A54.09
- puerperal, postpartum, childbirth O86.89
- strumous, tuberculous A18.2
- subacute (any site) I89.1
- tuberculous — *see* Tuberculosis, lymph gland

Lymphatic (vessel) — *see* condition
Lymphatism E32.8
Lymphectasia I89.0
Lymphedema (acquired) — *see also* Elephantiasis
- congenital Q82.0
- hereditary (chronic) (idiopathic) Q82.0
- postmastectomy I97.2
- praecox I89.0
- secondary I89.0
- surgical NEC I97.89
  - postmastectomy (syndrome) I97.2

Lymphoblastic — *see* condition
Lymphoblastoma (diffuse) — *see* Lymphoma, lymphoblastic (diffuse)
- giant follicular — *see* Lymphoma, lymphoblastic (diffuse)
- macrofollicular — *see* Lymphoma, lymphoblastic (diffuse)

Lymphocele I89.8
Lymphocytic
- chorioencephalitis (acute) (serous) A87.2
- choriomeningitis (acute) (serous) A87.2
- meningoencephalitis A87.2

Lymphocytoma, benign cutis L98.8
Lymphocytopenia D72.810
Lymphocytosis (symptomatic) D72.820
- infectious (acute) B33.8

Lymphoepithelioma — *see* Neoplasm, malignant, by site
Lymphogranuloma (malignant) — *see also* Lymphoma, Hodgkin
- chlamydial A55
- inguinale A55
- venereum (any site) (chlamydial) (with stricture of rectum) A55

Lymphogranulomatosis (malignant) — *see also* Lymphoma, Hodgkin
- benign (Boeck's sarcoid) (Schaumann's) D86.1

Lymphohistiocytosis, hemophagocytic (familial) D76.1
Lymphoid — *see* condition
Lymphoma (of) (malignant) C85.90
- adult T-cell (HTLV-1-associated) (acute variant) (chronic variant) (lymphomatoid variant) (smouldering variant) C91.5 ☑
- anaplastic large cell
  - ALK-negative C84.7- ☑
  - ALK-positive C84.6- ☑
  - breast implant associated (BIA-ALCL) C84.7A
  - CD30-positive C84.6- ☑
  - primary cutaneous C86.6
- angioimmunoblastic T-cell C86.5
- BALT C88.4
- B-cell C85.1- ☑
- blastic NK-cell C86.4
- blastic plasmacytoid dendritic cell neoplasm (BPDCN) C86.4
- B-precursor C83.5- ☑
- bronchial-associated lymphoid tissue [BALT-lymphoma] C88.4
- Burkitt (atypical) C83.7- ☑
- Burkitt-like C83.7- ☑
- centrocytic C83.1- ☑
- cutaneous follicle center C82.6- ☑
- cutaneous T-cell C84.A- ☑ (*following* C84.7)
- diffuse follicle center C82.5- ☑
- diffuse large cell C83.3- ☑
  - anaplastic C83.3- ☑
  - B-cell C83.3- ☑
  - CD30-positive C83.3- ☑
  - centroblastic C83.3- ☑

Lymphoma — *continued*
- diffuse large cell — *continued*
  - immunoblastic C83.3- ☑
  - plasmablastic C83.3- ☑
  - subtype not specified C83.3- ☑
  - T-cell rich C83.3- ☑
- enteropathy-type (associated) (intestinal) T-cell C86.2
- extranodal marginal zone B-cell lymphoma of mucosa-associated lymphoid tissue [MALT-lymphoma] C88.4
- extranodal NK/T-cell, nasal type C86.0
- follicular C82.9- ☑
  - grade
    - I C82.0- ☑
    - II C82.1- ☑
    - III C82.2- ☑
    - IIIa C82.3- ☑
    - IIIb C82.4- ☑
  - specified NEC C82.8- ☑
- hepatosplenic T-cell (alpha-beta) (gamma-delta) C86.1
- histiocytic C85.9- ☑
  - true C96.A (*following* C96.6)
- Hodgkin C81.9 ☑
  - lymphocyte depleted (classical) C81.3- ☑
  - lymphocyte-rich (classical) C81.4- ☑
  - mixed cellularity (classical) C81.2- ☑
  - nodular
    - lymphocyte predominant C81.0- ☑
    - sclerosis (classical) C81.1- ☑
  - nodular sclerosis (classical) C81.1- ☑
  - specified NEC (classical) C81.7- ☑
- intravascular large B-cell C83.8- ☑
- Lennert's C84.4- ☑
- lymphoblastic (diffuse) C83.5- ☑
- lymphoblastic B-cell C83.5- ☑
- lymphoblastic T-cell C83.5- ☑
- lymphoepithelioid C84.4- ☑
- lymphoplasmacytic C83.0- ☑
  - with IgM-production C88.0
- MALT C88.4
- mantle cell C83.1- ☑
- mature T-cell NEC C84.4- ☑
- mature T/NK-cell C84.9- ☑
  - specified NEC C84.Z- ☑ (*following* C84.7)
- mediastinal (thymic) large B-cell C85.2- ☑
- Mediterranean C88.3
- mucosa-associated lymphoid tissue [MALT-lymphoma] C88.4
- NK/T cell C84.9- ☑
- nodal marginal zone C83.0- ☑
- non-follicular (diffuse) C83.9- ☑
  - specified NEC C83.8- ☑
- non-Hodgkin — *see also* Lymphoma, by type C85.9- ☑
  - specified NEC C85.8- ☑
- non-leukemic variant of B-CLL C83.0- ☑
- peripheral T-cell NEC C84.4- ☑
- primary cutaneous
  - anaplastic large cell C86.6
  - CD30-positive large T-cell C86.6
- primary effusion B-cell C83.8- ☑
- SALT C88.4
- skin-associated lymphoid tissue [SALT-lymphoma] C88.4
- small cell B-cell C83.0- ☑
- splenic marginal zone C83.0- ☑
- subcutaneous panniculitis-like T-cell C86.3
- T-precursor C83.5- ☑
- true histiocytic C96.A (*following* C96.6)

Lymphomatosis — *see* Lymphoma
Lymphopathia venereum, veneris A55
Lymphopenia D72.810
Lymphoplasmacytic leukemia — *see* Leukemia, chronic lymphocytic, B-cell type
Lymphoproliferation, X-linked disease D82.3
Lymphoreticulosis, benign (of inoculation) A28.1
Lymphorrhea I89.8
Lymphosarcoma (diffuse) — *see also* Lymphoma C85.9- ☑
Lymphostasis I89.8
Lypemania — *see* Melancholia
Lysine and hydroxylysine metabolism disorder E72.3
Lyssa — *see* Rabies

M

Macacus ear Q17.3

Index

Lymphadenosis — Macacus ear

- **Maceration, wet feet, tropical** (syndrome) T69.Ø2- ☑
- **MacLeod's syndrome** J43.Ø
- **Macrocephalia, macrocephaly** Q75.3
- **Macrocheilia, macrochilia** (congenital) Q18.6
- **Macrocolon** — *see also* Megacolon Q43.1
- **Macrocornea** Q15.8
  - with glaucoma Q15.Ø
- **Macrocytic** — *see* condition
- **Macrocytosis** D75.89
- **Macrodactylia, macrodactylism** (fingers) (thumbs) Q74.Ø
  - toes Q74.2
- **Macrodontia** KØØ.2
- **Macrogenia** M26.Ø5
- **Macrogenitosomia** (adrenal) (male) (praecox) E25.9
  - congenital E25.Ø
- **Macroglobulinemia** (idiopathic) (primary) C88.Ø
  - monoclonal (essential) D47.2
  - Waldenström C88.Ø
- **Macroglossia** (congenital) Q38.2
  - acquired K14.8
- **Macrognathia, macrognathism** (congenital) (mandibular) (maxillary) M26.Ø9
- **Macrogyria** (congenital) QØ4.8
- **Macrohydrocephalus** — *see* Hydrocephalus
- **Macromastia** — *see* Hypertrophy, breast
- **Macrophthalmos** Q11.3
  - in congenital glaucoma Q15.Ø
- **Macropsia** H53.15
- **Macrosigmoid** K59.39
  - congenital Q43.2
- **Macrospondylitis , acromegalic** E22.Ø
- **Macrostomia** (congenital) Q18.4
- **Macrotia** (external ear) (congenital) Q17.1
- **Macula**
  - cornea, corneal — *see* Opacity, cornea
  - degeneration (atrophic) (exudative) (senile) — *see also* Degeneration, macula
    - hereditary — *see* Dystrophy, retina
- **Maculae ceruleae** B85.1
- **Maculopathy, toxic** — *see* Degeneration, macula, toxic
- **Madarosis** (eyelid) HØ2.729
  - left HØ2.726
    - lower HØ2.725
    - upper HØ2.724
  - right HØ2.723
    - lower HØ2.722
    - upper HØ2.721
- **Madelung's**
  - deformity (radius) Q74.Ø
  - disease
    - radial deformity Q74.Ø
    - symmetrical lipomas, neck E88.89
- **Madness** — *see* Psychosis
- **Madura**
  - foot B47.9
    - actinomycotic B47.1
    - mycotic B47.Ø
- **Maduromycosis** B47.Ø
- **Maffucci's syndrome** Q78.4
- **Magnesium metabolism disorder** — *see* Disorder, metabolism, magnesium
- **Main en griffe** (acquired) — *see also* Deformity, limb, clawhand
  - congenital Q68.1
- **Maintenance** (encounter for)
  - antineoplastic chemotherapy Z51.11
  - antineoplastic radiation therapy Z51.Ø
  - methadone F11.2Ø
- **Majocchi's**
  - disease L81.7
  - granuloma B35.8
- **Major** — *see* condition
- **Mal de los pintos** — *see* Pinta
- **Mal de mer** T75.3 ☑
- **Malabar itch** (any site) B35.5
- **Malabsorption** K9Ø.9
  - calcium K9Ø.89
  - carbohydrate K9Ø.49
  - disaccharide E73.9
  - fat K9Ø.49
  - galactose E74.2Ø
  - glucose (-galactose) E74.39
  - intestinal K9Ø.9
    - specified NEC K9Ø.89
  - isomaltose E74.31
  - lactose E73.9

Malabsorption — *continued*

  - methionine E72.19
  - monosaccharide E74.39
  - postgastrectomy K91.2
  - postsurgical K91.2
  - protein K9Ø.49
  - starch K9Ø.49
  - sucrose E74.39
  - syndrome K9Ø.9
    - postsurgical K91.2
- **Malacia, bone** (adult) M83.9
  - juvenile — *see* Rickets
- **Malacoplakia**
  - bladder N32.89
  - pelvis (kidney) N28.89
  - ureter N28.89
  - urethra N36.8
- **Malacosteon, juvenile** — *see* Rickets
- **Maladaptation** — *see* Maladjustment
- **Maladie de Roger** Q21.Ø
- **Maladjustment**
  - conjugal Z63.Ø
    - involving divorce or estrangement Z63.5
  - educational Z55.4
  - family Z63.9
  - marital Z63.Ø
    - involving divorce or estrangement Z63.5
  - occupational NEC Z56.89
  - simple, adult — *see* Disorder, adjustment
  - situational — *see* Disorder, adjustment
  - social Z6Ø.9
    - due to
      - acculturation difficulty Z6Ø.3
      - discrimination and persecution (perceived) Z6Ø.5
      - exclusion and isolation Z6Ø.4
      - life-cycle (phase of life) transition Z6Ø.Ø
      - rejection Z6Ø.4
      - specified reason NEC Z6Ø.8
- **Malaise** R53.81
- **Malakoplakia** — *see* Malacoplakia
- **Malaria, malarial** (fever) B54
  - with
    - blackwater fever B5Ø.8
      - hemoglobinuric (bilious) B5Ø.8
    - hemoglobinuria B5Ø.8
  - accidentally induced (therapeutically) — *code by* type under Malaria
  - algid B5Ø.9
  - cerebral B5Ø.Ø *[G94]*
  - clinically diagnosed (without parasitological confirmation) B54
  - congenital NEC P37.4
    - falciparum P37.3
  - congestion, congestive B54
  - continued (fever) B5Ø.9
  - estivo-autumnal B5Ø.9
  - falciparum B5Ø.9
    - with complications NEC B5Ø.8
      - cerebral B5Ø.Ø *[G94]*
    - severe B5Ø.8
  - hemorrhagic B54
  - malariae B52.9
    - with
      - complications NEC B52.8
      - glomerular disorder B52.Ø
  - malignant (tertian) — *see* Malaria, falciparum
  - mixed infections — *code to* first listed type in B5Ø-B53
  - ovale B53.Ø
  - parasitologically confirmed NEC B53.8
  - pernicious, acute — *see* Malaria, falciparum
  - Plasmodium (P.)
    - falciparum NEC — *see* Malaria, falciparum
    - malariae NEC B52.9
      - with Plasmodium
        - falciparum (and or vivax) — *see* Malaria, falciparum
        - vivax — *see also* Malaria, vivax
          - and falciparum — *see* Malaria, falciparum
    - ovale B53.Ø
      - with Plasmodium malariae — *see also* Malaria, malariae
        - and vivax — *see also* Malaria, vivax
          - and falciparum — *see* Malaria, falciparum
    - simian B53.1
      - with Plasmodium malariae — *see also* Malaria, malariae
        - and vivax — *see also* Malaria, vivax
          - and falciparum — *see* Malaria, falciparum

Malaria, malarial — *continued*

  - Plasmodium — *continued*
    - vivax NEC B51.9
      - with Plasmodium falciparum — *see* Malaria, falciparum
  - quartan — *see* Malaria, malariae
  - quotidian — *see* Malaria, falciparum
  - recurrent B54
  - remittent B54
  - specified type NEC (parasitologically confirmed) B53.8
  - spleen B54
  - subtertian (fever) — *see* Malaria, falciparum
  - tertian (benign) — *see also* Malaria, vivax
    - malignant B5Ø.9
  - tropical B5Ø.9
  - typhoid B54
  - vivax B51.9
    - with
      - complications NEC B51.8
      - ruptured spleen B51.Ø
- **Malassez's disease** (cystic) N5Ø.89
- **Malassimilation** K9Ø.9
- **Maldescent, testis** Q53.9
  - bilateral Q53.2Ø
    - abdominal Q53.211
    - perineal Q53.22
  - unilateral Q53.1Ø
    - abdominal Q53.111
    - perineal Q53.12
- **Maldevelopment** — *see also* Anomaly
  - brain QØ7.9
  - colon Q43.9
  - hip Q74.2
    - congenital dislocation Q65.2
      - bilateral Q65.1
      - unilateral Q65.Ø- ☑
  - mastoid process Q75.8
  - middle ear Q16.4
    - except ossicles Q16.4
    - ossicles Q16.3
  - ossicles Q16.3
  - spine Q76.49
  - toe Q74.2
- **Male type pelvis** Q74.2
  - with disproportion (fetopelvic) O33.3 ☑
    - causing obstructed labor O65.3
- **Malformation** (congenital) — *see also* Anomaly
  - adrenal gland Q89.1
  - affecting multiple systems with skeletal changes NEC Q87.5
  - alimentary tract Q45.9
    - specified type NEC Q45.8
    - upper Q4Ø.9
      - specified type NEC Q4Ø.8
  - aorta Q25.4Ø
    - absence Q25.41
    - aneurysm, congenital Q25.43
    - aplasia Q25.41
    - atresia Q25.29
      - aortic arch Q25.21
    - coarctation (preductal) (postductal) Q25.1
    - dilatation, congenital Q25.44
    - hypoplasia Q25.42
    - patent ductus arteriosus Q25.Ø
    - specified type NEC Q25.49
    - stenosis Q25.1
      - supravalvular Q25.3
  - aortic valve Q23.9
    - specified NEC Q23.8
  - arteriovenous, aneurysmatic (congenital) Q27.3Ø
    - brain Q28.2
      - ruptured I6Ø.8
        - intracerebral I61.8
        - intraparenchymal I61.8
        - intraventricular I61.5
        - subarachnoid I6Ø.8
    - cerebral — *see also* Malformation, arteriovenous, brain Q28.2
    - peripheral Q27.3Ø
      - digestive system — *see* Angiodysplasia
        - congenital Q27.33
      - lower limb Q27.32
      - other specified site Q27.39
      - renal vessel Q27.34
      - upper limb Q27.31
    - precerebral vessels (nonruptured) Q28.Ø
  - auricle
    - ear (congenital) Q17.3

Malformation — *continued*
- auricle — *continued*
  - ear — *continued*
    - acquired H61.119
      - left H61.112
        - with right H61.113
      - right H61.111
        - with left H61.113
- bile duct Q44.5
- bladder Q64.79
  - aplasia Q64.5
  - diverticulum Q64.6
  - exstrophy — *see* Exstrophy, bladder
  - neck obstruction Q64.31
- bone Q79.9
  - face Q75.9
    - specified type NEC Q75.8
  - skull Q75.9
    - specified type NEC Q75.8
- brain (multiple) Q04.9
  - arteriovenous Q28.2
  - specified type NEC Q04.8
- branchial cleft Q18.2
- breast Q83.9
  - specified type NEC Q83.8
- broad ligament Q50.6
- bronchus Q32.4
- bursa Q79.9
- cardiac
  - chambers Q20.9
    - specified type NEC Q20.8
  - septum Q21.9
    - specified type NEC Q21.8
- cerebral Q04.9
  - vessels Q28.3
- cervix uteri Q51.9
  - specified type NEC Q51.828
- Chiari
  - Type I G93.5
  - Type II Q07.01
- choroid (congenital) Q14.3
  - plexus Q07.8
- circulatory system Q28.9
- cochlea Q16.5
- cornea Q13.4
- coronary vessels Q24.5
- corpus callosum (congenital) Q04.0
- diaphragm Q79.1
- digestive system NEC, specified type NEC Q45.8
- dura Q07.9
  - brain Q04.9
  - spinal Q06.9
- ear Q17.9
  - causing impairment of hearing Q16.9
  - external Q17.9
    - accessory auricle Q17.0
    - causing impairment of hearing Q16.9
      - absence of
        - auditory canal Q16.1
        - auricle Q16.0
    - macrotia Q17.1
    - microtia Q17.2
    - misplacement Q17.4
    - misshapen NEC Q17.3
    - prominence Q17.5
    - specified type NEC Q17.8
  - inner Q16.5
  - middle Q16.4
    - absence of eustachian tube Q16.2
    - ossicles (fusion) Q16.3
  - ossicles Q16.3
  - specified type NEC Q17.8
- epididymis Q55.4
- esophagus Q39.9
  - specified type NEC Q39.8
- eye Q15.9
  - lid Q10.3
  - specified NEC Q15.8
- fallopian tube Q50.6
- genital organ — *see* Anomaly, genitalia
- great
  - artery Q25.9
    - aorta — *see* Malformation, aorta
    - pulmonary artery — *see* Malformation, pulmonary, artery
    - specified type NEC Q25.8
  - vein Q26.9
    - anomalous
      - portal venous connection Q26.5

Malformation — *continued*
- great — *continued*
  - vein — *continued*
    - anomalous — *continued*
      - pulmonary venous connection Q26.4
        - partial Q26.3
        - total Q26.2
    - persistent left superior vena cava Q26.1
    - portal vein-hepatic artery fistula Q26.6
    - specified type NEC Q26.8
    - vena cava stenosis, congenital Q26.0
- gum Q38.6
- hair Q84.2
- heart Q24.9
  - specified type NEC Q24.8
- integument Q84.9
  - specified type NEC Q84.8
- internal ear Q16.5
- intestine Q43.9
  - specified type NEC Q43.8
- iris Q13.2
- joint Q74.9
  - ankle Q74.2
  - lumbosacral Q76.49
  - sacroiliac Q74.2
  - specified type NEC Q74.8
- kidney Q63.9
  - accessory Q63.0
  - giant Q63.3
  - horseshoe Q63.1
  - hydronephrosis Q62.0
  - malposition Q63.2
  - specified type NEC Q63.8
- lacrimal apparatus Q10.6
- lingual Q38.3
- lip Q38.0
- liver Q44.7
- lung Q33.9
- meninges or membrane (congenital) Q07.9
  - cerebral Q04.8
  - spinal (cord) Q06.9
- middle ear Q16.4
  - ossicles Q16.3
- mitral valve Q23.9
  - specified NEC Q23.8
- Mondini's (congenital) (malformation, cochlea) Q16.5
- mouth (congenital) Q38.6
- multiple types NEC Q89.7
- musculoskeletal system Q79.9
- myocardium Q24.8
- nail Q84.6
- nervous system (central) Q07.9
- nose Q30.9
  - specified type NEC Q30.8
- optic disc Q14.2
- orbit Q10.7
- ovary Q50.39
- palate Q38.5
- parathyroid gland Q89.2
- pelvic organs or tissues NEC
  - in pregnancy or childbirth O34.8- ☑
    - causing obstructed labor O65.5
- penis Q55.69
  - aplasia Q55.5
  - curvature (lateral) Q55.61
  - hypoplasia Q55.62
- pericardium Q24.8
- peripheral vascular system Q27.9
  - specified type NEC Q27.8
- pharynx Q38.8
- precerebral vessels Q28.1
- prostate Q55.4
- pulmonary
  - arteriovenous Q25.72
  - artery Q25.9
    - atresia Q25.5
    - specified type NEC Q25.79
    - stenosis Q25.6
  - valve Q22.3
- renal artery Q27.2
- respiratory system Q34.9
- retina Q14.1
- scrotum — *see* Malformation, testis and scrotum
- seminal vesicles Q55.4
- sense organs NEC Q07.9
- skin Q82.9
- specified NEC Q89.8
- spinal
  - cord Q06.9

Malformation — *continued*
- spinal — *continued*
  - nerve root Q07.8
- spine Q76.49
  - kyphosis — *see* Kyphosis, congenital
  - lordosis — *see* Lordosis, congenital
- spleen Q89.09
- stomach Q40.3
  - specified type NEC Q40.2
- teeth, tooth K00.9
- tendon Q79.9
- testis and scrotum Q55.20
  - aplasia Q55.0
  - hypoplasia Q55.1
  - polyorchism Q55.21
  - retractile testis Q55.22
  - scrotal transposition Q55.23
  - specified NEC Q55.29
- thorax, bony Q76.9
- throat Q38.8
- thyroid gland Q89.2
- tongue (congenital) Q38.3
  - hypertrophy Q38.2
  - tie Q38.1
- trachea Q32.1
- tricuspid valve Q22.9
  - specified type NEC Q22.8
- umbilical cord NEC (complicating delivery) O69.89 ☑
- umbilicus Q89.9
- ureter Q62.8
  - agenesis Q62.4
  - duplication Q62.5
  - malposition — *see* Malposition, congenital, ureter
  - obstructive defect — *see* Defect, obstructive, ureter
  - vesico-uretero-renal reflux Q62.7
- urethra Q64.79
  - aplasia Q64.5
  - duplication Q64.74
  - posterior valves Q64.2
  - prolapse Q64.71
  - stricture Q64.32
- urinary system Q64.9
- uterus Q51.9
  - specified type NEC Q51.818
- vagina Q52.4
- vas deferens Q55.4
  - atresia Q55.3
- vascular system, peripheral Q27.9
- venous — *see* Anomaly, vein(s)
- vulva Q52.70

Malfunction — *see also* Dysfunction
- cardiac electronic device T82.119 ☑
  - electrode T82.110 ☑
  - pulse generator T82.111 ☑
  - specified type NEC T82.118 ☑
- catheter device NEC T85.618 ☑
  - cystostomy T83.010 ☑
  - dialysis (renal) (vascular) T82.41 ☑
    - intraperitoneal T85.611 ☑
  - infusion NEC T82.514 ☑
    - cranial T85.610 ☑
    - epidural T85.610 ☑
    - intrathecal T85.610 ☑
    - spinal T85.610 ☑
    - subarachnoid T85.610 ☑
    - subdural T85.610 ☑
  - urinary — *see also* Breakdown, device, catheter T83.018 ☑
- colostomy K94.03
  - valve K94.03
- cystostomy (stoma) N99.512
  - catheter T83.010 ☑
- enteric stoma K94.13
- enterostomy K94.13
- esophagostomy K94.33
- gastroenteric K31.89
- gastrostomy K94.23
- ileostomy K94.13
  - valve K94.13
- intrathecal infusion pump T85.615 ☑
- jejunostomy K94.13
- nervous system device, implant or graft, specified NEC T85.615 ☑
- pacemaker — *see* Malfunction, cardiac electronic device
- prosthetic device, internal — *see* Complications, prosthetic device, by site, mechanical
- tracheostomy J95.03

Malfunction — *continued*
urinary device NEC — *see* Complication, genitourinary, device, urinary, mechanical
valve
colostomy K94.Ø3
heart T82.Ø9 ☑
ileostomy K94.13
vascular graft or shunt NEC — *see* Complication, cardiovascular device, mechanical, vascular
ventricular (communicating shunt) T85.Ø1 ☑
Malherbe's tumor — *see* Neoplasm, skin, benign
Malibu disease L98.8
Malignancy — *see also* Neoplasm, malignant, by site
unspecified site (primary) C8Ø.1
Malignant — *see* condition
Malingerer, malingering Z76.5
Mallet finger (acquired) — *see* Deformity, finger, mallet finger
congenital Q74.Ø
sequelae of rickets E64.3
Malleus A24.Ø
Mallory's bodies R89.7
Mallory-Weiss syndrome K22.6
Malnutrition E46
degree
first E44.1
mild (protein) E44.1
moderate (protein) E44.Ø
second E44.Ø
severe (protein-energy) E43
intermediate form E42
with
kwashiorkor E42
marasmus E41
third E43
following gastrointestinal surgery K91.2
intrauterine
light-for-dates — *see* Light for dates
small-for-dates — *see* Small for dates
lack of care, or neglect (child) (infant) T76.Ø2 ☑
confirmed T74.Ø2 ☑
malignant E4Ø
protein E46
calorie E46
mild E44.1
moderate E44.Ø
severe E43
intermediate form E42
with
kwashiorkor (and marasmus) E42
marasmus E41
energy E46
mild E44.1
moderate E44.Ø
severe E43
intermediate form E42
with
kwashiorkor (and marasmus) E42
marasmus E41
severe (protein-energy) E43
with
kwashiorkor (and marasmus) E42
marasmus E41
Malocclusion (teeth) M26.4
Angle's M26.219
class I M26.211
class II M26.212
class III M26.213
due to
abnormal swallowing M26.59
mouth breathing M26.59
tongue, lip or finger habits M26.59
temporomandibular (joint) M26.69
Malposition
cervix — *see* Malposition, uterus
congenital
adrenal (gland) Q89.1
alimentary tract Q45.8
lower Q43.8
upper Q4Ø.8
aorta Q25.49
appendix Q43.8
arterial trunk Q2Ø.Ø
artery (peripheral) Q27.8
coronary Q24.5
digestive system Q27.8
lower limb Q27.8
pulmonary Q25.79

Malposition — *continued*
congenital — *continued*
artery — *continued*
specified site NEC Q27.8
upper limb Q27.8
auditory canal Q17.8
causing impairment of hearing Q16.9
auricle (ear) Q17.4
causing impairment of hearing Q16.9
cervical Q18.2
biliary duct or passage Q44.5
bladder (mucosa) — *see* Exstrophy, bladder
brachial plexus QØ7.8
brain tissue QØ4.8
breast Q83.8
bronchus Q32.4
cecum Q43.8
clavicle Q74.Ø
colon Q43.8
digestive organ or tract NEC Q45.8
lower Q43.8
upper Q4Ø.8
ear (auricle) (external) Q17.4
ossicles Q16.3
endocrine (gland) NEC Q89.2
epiglottis Q31.8
eustachian tube Q17.8
eye Q15.8
facial features Q18.8
fallopian tube Q5Ø.6
finger(s) Q68.1
supernumerary Q69.Ø
foot Q66.9- ☑
gallbladder Q44.1
gastrointestinal tract Q45.8
genitalia, genital organ(s) or tract
female Q52.8
external Q52.79
internal NEC Q52.8
male Q55.8
glottis Q31.8
hand Q68.1
heart Q24.8
dextrocardia Q24.Ø
with complete transposition of viscera Q89.3
hepatic duct Q44.5
hip (joint) Q65.89
intestine (large) (small) Q43.8
with anomalous adhesions, fixation or malrotation Q43.3
joint NEC Q68.8
kidney Q63.2
larynx Q31.8
limb Q68.8
lower Q68.8
upper Q68.8
liver Q44.7
lung (lobe) Q33.8
nail(s) Q84.6
nerve QØ7.8
nervous system NEC QØ7.8
nose, nasal (septum) Q3Ø.8
organ or site not listed — *see* Anomaly, by site
ovary Q5Ø.39
pancreas Q45.3
parathyroid (gland) Q89.2
patella Q74.1
peripheral vascular system Q27.8
pituitary (gland) Q89.2
respiratory organ or system NEC Q34.8
rib (cage) Q76.6
supernumerary in cervical region Q76.5
scapula Q74.Ø
shoulder Q74.Ø
spinal cord QØ6.8
spleen Q89.Ø9
sternum NEC Q76.7
stomach Q4Ø.2
symphysis pubis Q74.2
thymus (gland) Q89.2
thyroid (gland) (tissue) Q89.2
cartilage Q31.8
toe(s) Q66.9- ☑
supernumerary Q69.2
tongue Q38.3
trachea Q32.1
ureter Q62.6Ø
deviation Q62.61
displacement Q62.62

Malposition — *continued*
congenital — *continued*
ureter — *continued*
ectopia Q62.63
specified type NEC Q62.69
uterus Q51.818
vein(s) (peripheral) Q27.8
great Q26.8
vena cava (inferior) (superior) Q26.8
device, implant or graft — *see also* Complications, by site and type, mechanical T85.628 ☑
arterial graft NEC — *see* Complication, cardiovascular device, mechanical, vascular
breast (implant) T85.42 ☑
catheter NEC T85.628 ☑
cystostomy T83.Ø2Ø ☑
dialysis (renal) T82.42 ☑
intraperitoneal T85.621 ☑
infusion NEC T82.524 ☑
spinal (epidural) (subdural) T85.62Ø ☑
urinary — *see* also Displacement, device, catheter, urinary T83.Ø28 ☑
electronic (electrode) (pulse generator) (stimulator)
bone T84.32Ø ☑
cardiac T82.129 ☑
electrode T82.12Ø ☑
pulse generator T82.121 ☑
specified type NEC T82.128 ☑
nervous system — *see* Complication, prosthetic device, mechanical, electronic nervous system stimulator
urinary — *see* Complication, genitourinary, device, urinary, mechanical
fixation, internal (orthopedic) NEC — *see* Complication, fixation device, mechanical
gastrointestinal — *see* Complications, prosthetic device, mechanical, gastrointestinal device
genital NEC T83.428 ☑
intrauterine contraceptive device (string) T83.32 ☑
penile prosthesis (cylinder) (implanted) (pump) (reservoir) T83.42Ø ☑
testicular prosthesis T83.421 ☑
heart NEC — *see* Complication, cardiovascular device, mechanical
joint prosthesis — *see* Complication, joint prosthesis, mechanical
ocular NEC — *see* Complications, prosthetic device, mechanical, ocular device
orthopedic NEC — *see* Complication, orthopedic, device, mechanical
specified NEC T85.628 ☑
urinary NEC — *see also* Complication, genitourinary, device, urinary, mechanical
graft T83.22 ☑
vascular NEC — *see* Complication, cardiovascular device, mechanical
ventricular intracranial shunt T85.Ø2 ☑
fetus — *see* Pregnancy, complicated by (management affected by), presentation, fetal
gallbladder K82.8
gastrointestinal tract, congenital Q45.8
heart, congenital NEC Q24.8
joint prosthesis — *see* Complications, joint prosthesis, mechanical, displacement, by site
stomach K31.89
congenital Q4Ø.2
tooth, teeth, fully erupted M26.3Ø
uterus (acute) (acquired) (adherent) (asymptomatic) (postinfectional) (postpartal, old) N85.4
anteflexion or anteversion N85.4
congenital Q51.818
flexion N85.4
lateral — *see* Lateroversion, uterus
inversion N85.5
lateral (flexion) (version) — *see* Lateroversion, uterus
in pregnancy or childbirth — *see* subcategory O34.5 ☑
retroflexion or retroversion — *see* Retroversion, uterus
Malposture R29.3
Malrotation
cecum Q43.3
colon Q43.3
intestine Q43.3
kidney Q63.2
Malta fever — *see* Brucellosis

Maltreatment
adult
abandonment
confirmed T74.Ø1 ☑
suspected T76.Ø1 ☑
bullying
confirmed T74.31 ☑
suspected T76.31 ☑
confirmed T74.91 ☑
history of Z91.419
intimidation (through social media)
confirmed T74.31 ☑
suspected T76.31 ☑
neglect
confirmed T74.Ø1 ☑
suspected T76.Ø1 ☑
physical abuse
confirmed T74.11 ☑
suspected T76.11 ☑
psychological abuse
confirmed T74.31 ☑
history of Z91.411
suspected T76.31 ☑
sexual abuse
confirmed T74.21 ☑
suspected T76.21 ☑
suspected T76.91 ☑
child
abandonment
confirmed T74.Ø2 ☑
suspected T76.Ø2 ☑
bullying
confirmed T74.32 ☑
suspected T76.32 ☑
confirmed T74.92 ☑
history of — *see* History, personal (of), abuse
intimidation (through social media)
confirmed T74.32 ☑
suspected T76.32 ☑
neglect
confirmed T74.Ø2 ☑
history of — *see* History, personal (of), abuse
suspected T76.Ø2 ☑
physical abuse
confirmed T74.12 ☑
history of — *see* History, personal (of), abuse
suspected T76.12 ☑
psychological abuse
confirmed T74.32 ☑
history of — *see* History, personal (of), abuse
suspected T76.32 ☑
sexual abuse
confirmed T74.22 ☑
history of — *see* History, personal (of), abuse
suspected T76.22 ☑
suspected T76.92 ☑
personal history of Z91.89
Maltworker's lung J67.4
Malunion, fracture — *see* Fracture, by site
Mammillitis N61.Ø
puerperal, postpartum O91.Ø2
Mammitis — *see* Mastitis
Mammogram (examination) Z12.39
routine Z12.31
Mammoplasia N62
Management (of)
bone conduction hearing device (implanted) Z45.32Ø
cardiac pacemaker NEC Z45.Ø18
cerebrospinal fluid drainage device Z45.41
cochlear device (implanted) Z45.321
contraceptive Z3Ø.9
specified NEC Z3Ø.8
implanted device Z45.9
specified NEC Z45.89
infusion pump Z45.1
procreative Z31.9
male factor infertility in female Z31.81
specified NEC Z31.89
prosthesis (external) — *see also* Fitting Z44.9
implanted Z45.9
specified NEC Z45.89
renal dialysis catheter Z49.Ø1
vascular access device Z45.2
Mangled — *see* specified injury by site
Mania (monopolar) — *see also* Disorder, mood, manic episode
with psychotic symptoms F3Ø.2
Mania — *continued*
without psychotic symptoms F3Ø.1Ø
mild F3Ø.11
moderate F3Ø.12
severe F3Ø.13
Bell's F3Ø.8
chronic (recurrent) F31.89
hysterical F44.89
puerperal F3Ø.8
recurrent F31.89
Manic depression F31.9
Manic-depressive insanity, psychosis, or syndrome — *see* Disorder, bipolar
Mannosidosis E77.1
Mansonelliasis, mansonellosis B74.4
Manson's
disease B65.1
schistosomiasis B65.1
Manual — *see* condition
Maple-bark-stripper's lung (disease) J67.6
Maple-syrup-urine disease E71.Ø
Marable's syndrome (celiac artery compression) I77.4
Marasmus E41
due to malnutrition E41
intestinal E41
nutritional E41
senile R54
tuberculous NEC — *see* Tuberculosis
Marble
bones Q78.2
skin R23.8
Marburg virus disease A98.3
March
fracture — *see* Fracture, traumatic, stress, by site
hemoglobinuria D59.6
Marchesani (-Weill) **syndrome** Q87.Ø
Marchiafava (-Bignami) **syndrome or disease** G37.1
Marchiafava-Micheli syndrome D59.5
Marcus Gunn's syndrome QØ7.8
Marfan's syndrome — *see* Syndrome, Marfan's
Marie-Bamberger disease — *see* Osteoarthropathy, hypertrophic, specified NEC
Marie-Charcot-Tooth neuropathic muscular atrophy G6Ø.Ø
Marie's
cerebellar ataxia (late-onset) G11.2
disease or syndrome (acromegaly) E22.Ø
Marie-Strümpell arthritis, disease or spondylitis — *see* Spondylitis, ankylosing
Marion's disease (bladder neck obstruction) N32.Ø
Marital conflict Z63.Ø
Mark
port wine Q82.5
raspberry Q82.5
strawberry Q82.5
stretch L9Ø.6
tattoo L81.8
Marker heterochromatin — *see* Extra, marker chromosomes
Maroteaux-Lamy syndrome (mild) (severe) E76.29
Marrow (bone)
arrest D61.9
poor function D75.89
Marseilles fever A77.1
Marsh fever — *see* Malaria
Marshall's (hidrotic) **ectodermal dysplasia** Q82.4
Marsh's disease (exophthalmic goiter) EØ5.ØØ
with storm EØ5.Ø1
Masculinization (female) **with adrenal hyperplasia** E25.9
congenital E25.Ø
Masculinovoblastoma D27.- ☑
Masochism (sexual) F65.51
Mason's lung J62.8
Mass
abdominal R19.ØØ
epigastric R19.Ø6
generalized R19.Ø7
left lower quadrant R19.Ø4
left upper quadrant R19.Ø2
periumbilic R19.Ø5
right lower quadrant R19.Ø3
right upper quadrant R19.Ø1
specified site NEC R19.Ø9
breast — *see also* Lump, breast N63.Ø
chest R22.2
cystic — *see* Cyst
Mass — *continued*
ear H93.8- ☑
head R22.Ø
intra-abdominal (diffuse) (generalized) — *see* Mass, abdominal
kidney N28.89
liver R16.Ø
localized (skin) R22.9
chest R22.2
head R22.Ø
limb
lower R22.4- ☑
upper R22.3- ☑
neck R22.1
trunk R22.2
lung R91.8
malignant — *see* Neoplasm, malignant, by site
neck R22.1
pelvic (diffuse) (generalized) — *see* Mass, abdominal
specified organ NEC — *see* Disease, by site
splenic R16.1
substernal thyroid — *see* Goiter
superficial (localized) R22.9
umbilical (diffuse) (generalized) R19.Ø9
Massive — *see* condition
Mast cell
disease, systemic tissue D47.Ø2
leukemia C94.3- ☑
neoplasm
malignant C96.2Ø
specified type NEC C96.29
of uncertain behavior NEC D47.Ø9
sarcoma C96.22
tumor D47.Ø9
Mastalgia N64.4
Masters-Allen syndrome N83.8
Mastitis (acute) (diffuse) (nonpuerperal) (subacute) N61.Ø
with abscess N61.1
chronic (cystic) — *see* Mastopathy, cystic
cystic (Schimmelbusch's type) — *see* Mastopathy, cystic
fibrocystic — *see* Mastopathy, cystic
granulomatous N61.2- ☑
infective N61.Ø
newborn P39.Ø
interstitial, gestational or puerperal — *see* Mastitis, obstetric
neonatal (noninfective) P83.4
infective P39.Ø
obstetric (interstitial) (nonpurulent)
associated with
lactation O91.23
pregnancy O91.21- ☑
puerperium O91.22
purulent
associated with
lactation O91.13
pregnancy O91.11- ☑
puerperium O91.12
periductal — *see* Ectasia, mammary duct
phlegmonous — *see* Mastopathy, cystic
plasma cell — *see* Ectasia, mammary duct
without abscess N61.Ø
Mastocytoma (extracutaneous) D47.Ø9
malignant C96.29
solitary D47.Ø1
Mastocytosis D47.Ø9
aggressive systemic C96.21
cutaneous (diffuse) (maculopapular) D47.Ø1
congenital Q82.2
of neonatal onset Q82.2
of newborn onset Q82.2
indolent systemic D47.Ø2
isolated bone marrow D47.Ø2
malignant C96.29
systemic (indolent) (smoldering)
with an associated hematological non-mast cell lineage disease (SM-AHNMD) D47.Ø2
Mastodynia N64.4
Mastoid — *see* condition
Mastoidalgia — *see* subcategory H92.Ø ☑
Mastoiditis (coalescent) (hemorrhagic) (suppurative) H7Ø.9- ☑
acute, subacute H7Ø.ØØ- ☑
complicated NEC H7Ø.Ø9- ☑
subperiosteal H7Ø.Ø1- ☑
chronic (necrotic) (recurrent) H7Ø.1- ☑

Mastoiditis — *continued*
- in (due to)
  - infectious disease NEC B99 ☑ *[H75.Ø-]* ☑
  - parasitic disease NEC B89 *[H75.Ø-]* ☑
  - tuberculosis A18.Ø3
- petrositis — *see* Petrositis
- postauricular fistula — *see* Fistula, postauricular
- specified NEC H7Ø.89- ☑
- tuberculous A18.Ø3

Mastopathy, mastopathia N64.9
- chronica cystica — *see* Mastopathy, cystic
- cystic (chronic) (diffuse) N6Ø.1- ☑
  - with epithelial proliferation N6Ø.3- ☑
- diffuse cystic — *see* Mastopathy, cystic
- estrogenic, oestrogenica N64.89
- ovarian origin N64.89

Mastoplasia, mastoplastia N62
Masturbation (excessive) F98.8
Maternal care (for) — *see* Pregnancy (complicated by) (management affected by)
Matheiu's disease (leptospiral jaundice) A27.Ø
Mauclaire's disease or osteochondrosis — *see* Osteochondrosis, juvenile, hand, metacarpal
Maxcy's disease A75.2
Maxilla, maxillary — *see* condition
May (-Hegglin) **anomaly or syndrome** D72.Ø
McArdle (-Schmid)(-Pearson) **disease** (glycogen storage) E74.Ø4
McCune-Albright syndrome Q78.1
McQuarrie's syndrome (idiopathic familial hypoglycemia) E16.2
Meadow's syndrome Q86.1
Measles (black) (hemorrhagic) (suppressed) BØ5.9
- with
  - complications NEC BØ5.89
  - encephalitis BØ5.Ø
  - intestinal complications BØ5.4
  - keratitis (keratoconjunctivitis) BØ5.81
  - meningitis BØ5.1
  - otitis media BØ5.3
  - pneumonia BØ5.2
- French — *see* Rubella
- German — *see* Rubella
- Liberty — *see* Rubella

Meatitis, urethral — *see* Urethritis
Meatus, meatal — *see* condition
Meat-wrappers' asthma J68.9
ME/CFS (myalgic encephalomyelitis/chronic fatigue syndrome) G93.32
Meckel-Gruber syndrome Q61.9
Meckel's diverticulitis, diverticulum (displaced) (hypertrophic) Q43.Ø
- malignant — *see* Table of Neoplasms, small intestine, malignant

Meconium
- ileus, newborn P76.Ø
  - in cystic fibrosis E84.11
  - meaning meconium plug (without cystic fibrosis) P76.Ø
- obstruction, newborn P76.Ø
  - due to fecaliths P76.Ø
  - in mucoviscidosis E84.11
- peritonitis P78.Ø
- plug syndrome (newborn) NEC P76.Ø

Median — *see also* condition
- arcuate ligament syndrome I77.4
- bar (prostate) (vesical orifice) — *see* Hyperplasia, prostate
- rhomboid glossitis K14.2

Mediastinal shift R93.89
Mediastinitis (acute) (chronic) J98.51
- syphilitic A52.73
- tuberculous A15.8

Mediastinopericarditis — *see also* Pericarditis
- acute I3Ø.9
- adhesive I31.Ø
- chronic I31.8
  - rheumatic IØ9.2

Mediastinum, mediastinal — *see* condition
Medicine poisoning — *see* Table of Drugs and Chemicals, by drug, poisoning
Mediterranean
- fever — *see* Brucellosis
  - familial MØ4.1
  - tick A77.1
- kala-azar B55.Ø
- leishmaniasis B55.Ø

Mediterranean — *continued*
- tick fever A77.1

Medulla — *see* condition
Medullary cystic kidney Q61.5
Medullated fibers
- optic (nerve) Q14.8
- retina Q14.1

Medulloblastoma
- desmoplastic C71.6
- specified site — *see* Neoplasm, malignant, by site
- unspecified site C71.6

Medulloepithelioma — *see also* Neoplasm, malignant, by site
- teratoid — *see* Neoplasm, malignant, by site

Medullomyoblastoma
- specified site — *see* Neoplasm, malignant, by site
- unspecified site C71.6

Meekeren-Ehlers-Danlos syndrome — *see also* Syndrome, Ehlers-Danlos Q79.69
Megacolon (acquired) (functional) (not Hirschsprung's disease) (in) K59.39
- Chagas' disease B57.32
- congenital, congenitum (aganglionic) Q43.1
- Hirschsprung's (disease) Q43.1
- toxic NEC K59.31
  - due to Clostridium difficile
    - not specified as recurrent AØ4.72
    - recurrent AØ4.71

Megaesophagus (functional) K22.Ø
- congenital Q39.5
- in (due to) Chagas' disease B57.31

Megalencephaly QØ4.5
Megalerythema (epidemic) BØ8.3
Megaloappendix Q43.8
Megalocephalus, megalocephaly NEC Q75.3
Megalocornea Q15.8
- with glaucoma Q15.Ø

Megalocytic anemia D53.1
Megalodactylia (fingers) (thumbs) (congenital) Q74.Ø
- toes Q74.2

Megaloduodenum Q43.8
Megaloesophagus (functional) K22.Ø
- congenital Q39.5

Megalogastria (acquired) K31.89
- congenital Q4Ø.2

Megalophthalmos Q11.3
Megalopsia H53.15
Megalosplenia — *see* Splenomegaly
Megaloureter N28.82
- congenital Q62.2

Megarectum K62.89
Megasigmoid K59.39
- congenital Q43.2

Megaureter N28.82
- congenital Q62.2

Megavitamin-B6 syndrome E67.2
Megrim — *see* Migraine
Meibomian
- cyst, infected — *see* Hordeolum
- gland — *see* condition
- sty, stye — *see* Hordeolum

Meibomitis — *see* Hordeolum
Meige-Milroy disease (chronic hereditary edema) Q82.Ø
Meige's syndrome Q82.Ø
Melalgia, nutritional E53.8
Melancholia F32.A
- climacteric (single episode) F32.89
  - recurrent episode F33.8
- hypochondriac F45.29
- intermittent (single episode) F32.89
  - recurrent episode F33.8
- involutional (single episode) F32.89
  - recurrent episode F33.8
- menopausal (single episode) F32.89
  - recurrent episode F33.8
- puerperal F32.89
- reactive (emotional stress or trauma) F32.3
- recurrent F33.9
- senile FØ3 ☑
- stuporous (single episode) F32.89
  - recurrent episode F33.8

Melanemia R79.89
Melanoameloblastoma — *see* Neoplasm, bone, benign
Melanoblastoma — *see* Melanoma
Melanocarcinoma — *see* Melanoma
Melanocytoma, eyeball D31.9- ☑
Melanocytosis, neurocutaneous Q82.8

Melanoderma, melanodermia L81.4
Melanodontia, infantile KØ3.89
Melanodontoclasia KØ3.89
Melanoepithelioma — *see* Melanoma
Melanoma (malignant) C43.9
- acral lentiginous, malignant — *see* Melanoma, skin, by site
- amelanotic — *see* Melanoma, skin, by site
- balloon cell — *see* Melanoma, skin, by site
- benign — *see* Nevus
- desmoplastic, malignant — *see* Melanoma, skin, by site
- epithelioid cell — *see* Melanoma, skin, by site
  - with spindle cell, mixed — *see* Melanoma, skin, by site
- in
  - giant pigmented nevus — *see* Melanoma, skin, by site
  - Hutchinson's melanotic freckle — *see* Melanoma, skin, by site
  - junctional nevus — *see* Melanoma, skin, by site
  - precancerous melanosis — *see* Melanoma, skin, by site
- in situ DØ3.9
  - abdominal wall DØ3.59
  - ala nasi DØ3.39
  - ankle DØ3.7- ☑
  - anus, anal (margin) (skin) DØ3.51
  - arm DØ3.6- ☑
  - auditory canal DØ3.2- ☑
  - auricle (ear) DØ3.2- ☑
  - auricular canal (external) DØ3.2- ☑
  - axilla, axillary fold DØ3.59
  - back DØ3.59
  - breast DØ3.52
  - brow DØ3.39
  - buttock DØ3.59
  - canthus (eye) DØ3.1- ☑
  - cheek (external) DØ3.39
  - chest wall DØ3.59
  - chin DØ3.39
  - choroid DØ3.8
  - conjunctiva DØ3.8
  - ear (external) DØ3.2- ☑
  - external meatus (ear) DØ3.2- ☑
  - eye DØ3.8
  - eyebrow DØ3.39
  - eyelid (lower) (upper) DØ3.1- ☑
  - face DØ3.3Ø
    - specified NEC DØ3.39
  - female genital organ (external) NEC DØ3.8
  - finger DØ3.6- ☑
  - flank DØ3.59
  - foot DØ3.7- ☑
  - forearm DØ3.6- ☑
  - forehead DØ3.39
  - foreskin DØ3.8
  - gluteal region DØ3.59
  - groin DØ3.59
  - hand DØ3.6- ☑
  - heel DØ3.7- ☑
  - helix DØ3.2- ☑
  - hip DØ3.7- ☑
  - interscapular region DØ3.59
  - iris DØ3.8
  - jaw DØ3.39
  - knee DØ3.7- ☑
  - labium (majus) (minus) DØ3.8
  - lacrimal gland DØ3.8
  - leg DØ3.7- ☑
  - lip (lower) (upper) DØ3.Ø
  - lower limb NEC DØ3.7- ☑
  - male genital organ (external) NEC DØ3.8
  - nail DØ3.9
    - finger DØ3.6- ☑
    - toe DØ3.7- ☑
  - neck DØ3.4
  - nose (external) DØ3.39
  - orbit DØ3.8
  - penis DØ3.8
  - perianal skin DØ3.51
  - perineum DØ3.51
  - pinna DØ3.2- ☑
  - popliteal fossa or space DØ3.7- ☑
  - prepuce DØ3.8
  - pudendum DØ3.8
  - retina DØ3.8

- **Melanoma** — *continued*
  - in situ — *continued*
    - retrobulbar DØ3.8
    - scalp DØ3.4
    - scrotum DØ3.8
    - shoulder DØ3.6- ☑
    - specified site NEC DØ3.8
    - submammary fold DØ3.52
    - temple DØ3.39
    - thigh DØ3.7- ☑
    - toe DØ3.7- ☑
    - trunk NEC DØ3.59
    - umbilicus DØ3.59
    - upper limb NEC DØ3.6- ☑
    - vulva DØ3.8
  - juvenile — *see* Nevus
  - malignant, of soft parts except skin — *see* Neoplasm, connective tissue, malignant
  - metastatic
    - breast C79.81
    - genital organ C79.82
    - specified site NEC C79.89
  - neurotropic, malignant — *see* Melanoma, skin, by site
  - nodular — *see* Melanoma, skin, by site
  - regressing, malignant — *see* Melanoma, skin, by site
  - skin C43.9
    - abdominal wall C43.59
    - ala nasi C43.31
    - ankle C43.7- ☑
    - anus, anal (skin) C43.51
    - arm C43.6- ☑
    - auditory canal (external) C43.2- ☑
    - auricle (ear) C43.2- ☑
    - auricular canal (external) C43.2- ☑
    - axilla, axillary fold C43.59
    - back C43.59
    - breast (female) (male) C43.52
    - brow C43.39
    - buttock C43.59
    - canthus (eye) C43.1- ☑
    - cheek (external) C43.39
    - chest wall C43.59
    - chin C43.39
    - ear (external) C43.2- ☑
    - elbow C43.6- ☑
    - external meatus (ear) C43.2- ☑
    - eyebrow C43.39
    - eyelid (lower) (upper) C43.1- ☑
    - face C43.3Ø
      - specified NEC C43.39
    - female genital organ (external) NEC C51.9
    - finger C43.6- ☑
    - flank C43.59
    - foot C43.7- ☑
    - forearm C43.6- ☑
    - forehead C43.39
    - foreskin C6Ø.Ø
    - glabella C43.39
    - gluteal region C43.59
    - groin C43.59
    - hand C43.6- ☑
    - heel C43.7- ☑
    - helix C43.2- ☑
    - hip C43.7- ☑
    - interscapular region C43.59
    - jaw (external) C43.39
    - knee C43.7- ☑
    - labium C51.9
      - majus C51.Ø
      - minus C51.1
    - leg C43.7- ☑
    - lip (lower) (upper) C43.Ø
    - lower limb NEC C43.7- ☑
    - male genital organ (external) NEC C63.9
    - nail
      - finger C43.6- ☑
      - toe C43.7- ☑
    - nasolabial groove C43.39
    - nates C43.59
    - neck C43.4
    - nose (external) C43.31
    - overlapping site C43.8
    - palpebra C43.1- ☑
    - penis C6Ø.9
    - perianal skin C43.51
    - perineum C43.51
    - pinna C43.2- ☑
- **Melanoma** — *continued*
  - skin — *continued*
    - popliteal fossa or space C43.7- ☑
    - prepuce C6Ø.Ø
    - pudendum C51.9
    - scalp C43.4
    - scrotum C63.2
    - shoulder C43.6- ☑
    - skin NEC C43.9
    - submammary fold C43.52
    - temple C43.39
    - thigh C43.7- ☑
    - toe C43.7- ☑
    - trunk NEC C43.59
    - umbilicus C43.59
    - upper limb NEC C43.6- ☑
    - vulva C51.9
      - overlapping sites C51.8
  - spindle cell
    - with epithelioid, mixed — *see* Melanoma, skin, by site
    - type A C69.4- ☑
    - type B C69.4- ☑
  - superficial spreading — *see* Melanoma, skin, by site
- **Melanosarcoma** — *see also* Melanoma
  - epithelioid cell — *see* Melanoma
- **Melanosis** L81.4
  - addisonian E27.1
    - tuberculous A18.7
  - adrenal E27.1
  - colon K63.89
  - conjunctiva — *see* Pigmentation, conjunctiva
    - congenital Q13.89
  - cornea (presenile) (senile) — *see also* Pigmentation, cornea
    - congenital Q13.4
  - eye NEC H57.89
    - congenital Q15.8
  - lenticularis progressiva Q82.1
  - liver K76.89
  - precancerous — *see also* Melanoma, in situ
    - malignant melanoma in — *see* Melanoma
  - Riehl's L81.4
  - sclera H15.89
    - congenital Q13.89
  - suprarenal E27.1
  - tar L81.4
  - toxic L81.4
- **Melanuria** R82.998
- **MELAS syndrome** E88.41
- **Melasma** L81.1
  - adrenal (gland) E27.1
  - suprarenal (gland) E27.1
- **Melena** K92.1
  - with ulcer — *code by* site under Ulcer, with hemorrhage K27.4
  - due to swallowed maternal blood P78.2
  - newborn, neonatal P54.1
    - due to swallowed maternal blood P78.2
- **Meleney's**
  - gangrene (cutaneous) — *see* Ulcer, skin
  - ulcer (chronic undermining) — *see* Ulcer, skin
- **Melioidosis** A24.9
  - acute A24.1
  - chronic A24.2
  - fulminating A24.1
  - pneumonia A24.1
  - pulmonary (chronic) A24.2
    - acute A24.1
    - subacute A24.2
  - sepsis A24.1
  - specified NEC A24.3
  - subacute A24.2
- **Melitensis, febris** A23.Ø
- **Melkersson** (-Rosenthal) **syndrome** G51.2
- **Mellitus, diabetes** — *see* Diabetes
- **Melorheostosis** (bone) — *see* Disorder, bone, density and structure, specified NEC
- **Meloschisis** Q18.4
- **Melotia** Q17.4
- **Membrana**
  - capsularis lentis posterior Q13.89
  - epipapillaris Q14.2
- **Membranacea placenta** O43.19- ☑
- **Membranaceous uterus** N85.8
- **Membrane**(s), membranous — *see also* condition
  - cyclitic — *see* Membrane, pupillary
- **Membrane(s), membranous** — *continued*
  - folds, congenital — *see* Web
  - Jackson's Q43.3
  - over face of newborn P28.9
  - premature rupture — *see* Rupture, membranes, premature
  - pupillary H21.4- ☑
    - persistent Q13.89
  - retained (with hemorrhage) (complicating delivery) O72.2
    - without hemorrhage O73.1
  - secondary cataract — *see* Cataract, secondary
  - unruptured (causing asphyxia) — *see* Asphyxia, newborn
  - vitreous — *see* Opacity, vitreous, membranes and strands
- **Membranitis** — *see* Chorioamnionitis
- **Memory disturbance, lack or loss** — *see also* Amnesia
  - mild, following organic brain damage FØ6.8
- **Menadione deficiency** E56.1
- **Menarche**
  - delayed E3Ø.Ø
  - precocious E3Ø.1
- **Mendacity, pathologic** F6Ø.2
- **Mendelson's syndrome** (due to anesthesia) J95.4
  - in labor and delivery O74.Ø
  - in pregnancy O29.Ø1- ☑
  - obstetric O74.Ø
  - postpartum, puerperal O89.Ø1
- **Ménétrier's disease or syndrome** K29.6Ø
  - with bleeding K29.61
- **Ménière's disease, syndrome or vertigo** H81.Ø- ☑
- **Meninges, meningeal** — *see* condition
- **Meningioma** — *see also* Neoplasm, meninges, benign
  - angioblastic — *see* Neoplasm, meninges, benign
  - angiomatous — *see* Neoplasm, meninges, benign
  - atypical — *see* Neoplasm, meninges, uncertain behavior
  - endotheliomatous — *see* Neoplasm, meninges, benign
  - fibroblastic — *see* Neoplasm, meninges, benign
  - fibrous — *see* Neoplasm, meninges, benign
  - hemangioblastic — *see* Neoplasm, meninges, benign
  - hemangiopericytic — *see* Neoplasm, meninges, benign
  - malignant — *see* Neoplasm, meninges, malignant
  - meningiothelial — *see* Neoplasm, meninges, benign
  - meningotheliomatous — *see* Neoplasm, meninges, benign
  - mixed — *see* Neoplasm, meninges, benign
  - multiple — *see* Neoplasm, meninges, uncertain behavior
  - papillary — *see* Neoplasm, meninges, uncertain behavior
  - psammomatous — *see* Neoplasm, meninges, benign
  - syncytial — *see* Neoplasm, meninges, benign
  - transitional — *see* Neoplasm, meninges, benign
- **Meningiomatosis** (diffuse) — *see* Neoplasm, meninges, uncertain behavior
- **Meningism** — *see* Meningismus
- **Meningismus** (infectional) (pneumococcal) R29.1
  - due to serum or vaccine R29.1
  - influenzal — *see* Influenza, with, manifestations NEC
- **Meningitis** (basal) (basic) (brain) (cerebral) (cervical) (congestive) (diffuse) (hemorrhagic) (infantile) (membranous) (metastatic) (nonspecific) (pontine) (progressive) (simple) (spinal) (subacute) (sympathetic) (toxic) GØ3.9
  - abacterial GØ3.Ø
  - actinomycotic A42.81
  - adenoviral A87.1
  - arbovirus A87.8
  - aseptic (acute) GØ3.Ø
  - bacterial GØØ.9
    - Escherichia coli (E. coli) GØØ.8
    - Friedländer (bacillus) GØØ.8
    - gram-negative GØØ.9
    - H. influenzae GØØ.Ø
    - Klebsiella GØØ.8
    - pneumococcal GØØ.1
    - specified organism NEC GØØ.8
    - staphylococcal GØØ.3
    - streptococcal (acute) GØØ.2
  - benign recurrent (Mollaret) GØ3.2
  - candidal B37.5
  - caseous (tuberculous) A17.Ø
  - cerebrospinal A39.Ø
  - chronic NEC GØ3.1
  - clear cerebrospinal fluid NEC GØ3.Ø

- **Meningitis** — *continued*
  - coxsackievirus A87.Ø
  - cryptococcal B45.1
  - diplococcal (gram positive) A39.Ø
  - echovirus A87.Ø
  - enteroviral A87.Ø
  - eosinophilic B83.2
  - epidemic NEC A39.Ø
  - Escherichia coli (E. coli) GØØ.8
  - fibrinopurulent GØØ.9
    - specified organism NEC GØØ.8
  - Friedländer (bacillus) GØØ.8
  - gonococcal A54.81
  - gram-negative cocci GØØ.9
  - gram-positive cocci GØØ.9
  - H. influenzae GØØ.Ø
  - Haemophilus (influenzae) GØØ.Ø
  - in (due to)
    - adenovirus A87.1
    - African trypanosomiasis B56.9 *[GØ2]*
    - anthrax A22.8
    - bacterial disease NEC A48.8 *[GØ1]*
    - Chagas' disease (chronic) B57.41
    - chickenpox BØ1.Ø
    - coccidioidomycosis B38.4
    - Diplococcus pneumoniae GØØ.1
    - enterovirus A87.Ø
    - herpes (simplex) virus BØØ.3
      - zoster BØ2.1
    - infectious mononucleosis B27.92
    - leptospirosis A27.81
    - Listeria monocytogenes A32.11
    - Lyme disease A69.21
    - measles BØ5.1
    - mumps (virus) B26.1
    - neurosyphilis (late) A52.13
    - parasitic disease NEC B89 *[GØ2]*
    - poliovirus A8Ø.9 *[GØ2]*
    - preventive immunization, inoculation or vaccination GØ3.8
    - rubella BØ6.Ø2
    - Salmonella infection AØ2.21
    - specified cause NEC GØ3.8
    - Streptococcal pneumoniae GØØ.1
    - typhoid fever AØ1.Ø1
    - varicella BØ1.Ø
    - viral disease NEC A87.8
    - whooping cough A37.9Ø
    - zoster BØ2.1
  - infectious GØØ.9
  - influenzal (H. influenzae) GØØ.Ø
  - Klebsiella GØØ.8
  - leptospiral (aseptic) A27.81
  - lymphocytic (acute) (benign) (serous) A87.2
  - meningococcal A39.Ø
  - Mima polymorpha GØØ.8
  - Mollaret (benign recurrent) GØ3.2
  - monilial B37.5
  - mycotic NEC B49 *[GØ2]*
  - Neisseria A39.Ø
  - nonbacterial GØ3.Ø
  - nonpyogenic NEC GØ3.Ø
  - ossificans G96.198
  - pneumococcal streptococcus pneumoniae GØØ.1
  - poliovirus A8Ø.9 *[GØ2]*
  - postmeasles BØ5.1
  - purulent GØØ.9
    - specified organism NEC GØØ.8
  - pyogenic GØØ.9
    - specified organism NEC GØØ.8
  - Salmonella (arizonae) (Cholerae-Suis) (enteritidis) (typhimurium) AØ2.21
  - septic GØØ.9
    - specified organism NEC GØØ.8
  - serosa circumscripta NEC GØ3.Ø
  - serous NEC G93.2
  - specified organism NEC GØØ.8
  - sporotrichosis B42.81
  - staphylococcal GØØ.3
  - sterile GØ3.Ø
  - Streptococcal (acute) GØØ.2
    - pneumoniae GØØ.1
  - suppurative GØØ.9
    - specified organism NEC GØØ.8
  - syphilitic (late) (tertiary) A52.13
    - acute A51.41
    - congenital A5Ø.41
    - secondary A51.41
  - Torula histolytica (cryptococcal) B45.1

- **Meningitis** — *continued*
  - traumatic (complication of injury) T79.8 ☑
  - tuberculous A17.Ø
  - typhoid AØ1.Ø1
  - viral NEC A87.9
  - Yersinia pestis A2Ø.3
- **Meningocele** (spinal) — *see also* Spina bifida
  - with hydrocephalus — *see* Spina bifida, by site, with hydrocephalus
  - acquired (traumatic) G96.198
  - cerebral — *see* Encephalocele
- **Meningocerebritis** — *see* Meningoencephalitis
- **Meningococcemia** A39.4
  - acute A39.2
  - chronic A39.3
- **Meningococcus, meningococcal** — *see also* condition A39.9
  - adrenalitis, hemorrhagic A39.1
  - carrier (suspected) of Z22.31
  - meningitis (cerebrospinal) A39.Ø
- **Meningoencephalitis** — *see also* Encephalitis GØ4.9Ø
  - acute NEC — *see also* Encephalitis, viral A86
  - bacterial NEC GØ4.2
  - California A83.5
  - diphasic A84.1
  - eosinophilic B83.2
  - epidemic A39.81
  - herpesviral, herpetic BØØ.4
    - due to herpesvirus 6 B1Ø.Ø1
    - due to herpesvirus 7 B1Ø.Ø9
    - specified NEC B1Ø.Ø9
  - in (due to)
    - blastomycosis NEC B4Ø.81
    - diseases classified elsewhere GØ5.3
    - free-living amebae B6Ø.2
    - H. influenzae GØØ.Ø
    - Hemophilus influenzae (H .influenzae) GØØ.Ø
    - herpes BØØ.4
      - due to herpesvirus 6 B1Ø.Ø1
      - due to herpesvirus 7 B1Ø.Ø9
      - specified NEC B1Ø.Ø9
    - Lyme disease A69.22
    - mercury — *see* subcategory T56.1 ☑
    - mumps B26.2
    - Naegleria (amebae) (organisms) (fowleri) B6Ø.2
    - Parastrongylus cantonensis B83.2
    - toxoplasmosis (acquired) B58.2
      - congenital P37.1
  - infectious (acute) (viral) A86
  - influenzal (H. influenzae) GØØ.Ø
  - Listeria monocytogenes A32.12
  - lymphocytic (serous) A87.2
  - mumps B26.2
  - parasitic NEC B89 *[GØ5.3]*
  - pneumococcal GØ4.2
  - primary amebic B6Ø.2
  - specific (syphilitic) A52.14
  - specified organism NEC GØ4.81
  - staphylococcal GØ4.2
  - streptococcal GØ4.2
  - syphilitic A52.14
  - toxic NEC G92.8
    - due to mercury — *see* subcategory T56.1 ☑
  - tuberculous A17.82
  - virus NEC A86
- **Meningoencephalocele** — *see also* Encephalocele
  - syphilitic A52.19
    - congenital A5Ø.49
- **Meningoencephalomyelitis** — *see also* Meningoencephalitis
  - acute NEC (viral) A86
    - disseminated GØ4.ØØ
      - postimmunization or postvaccination GØ4.Ø2
      - postinfectious GØ4.Ø1
  - due to
    - actinomycosis A42.82
    - Torula B45.1
    - Toxoplasma or toxoplasmosis (acquired) B58.2
      - congenital P37.1
  - postimmunization or postvaccination GØ4.Ø2
- **Meningoencephalomyelopathy** G96.9
- **Meningoencephalopathy** G96.9
- **Meningomyelitis** — *see also* Meningoencephalitis
  - bacterial NEC GØ4.2
  - blastomycotic NEC B4Ø.81
  - cryptococcal B45.1
  - in diseases classified elsewhere GØ5.4
  - meningococcal A39.81

- **Meningomyelitis** — *continued*
  - syphilitic A52.14
  - tuberculous A17.82
- **Meningomyelocele** — *see also* Spina bifida
  - syphilitic A52.19
- **Meningomyeloneuritis** — *see* Meningoencephalitis
- **Meningoradiculitis** — *see* Meningitis
- **Meningovascular** — *see* condition
- **Menkes' disease or syndrome** E83.Ø9
  - meaning maple-syrup-urine disease E71.Ø
- **Menometrorrhagia** N92.1
- **Menopause, menopausal** (asymptomatic) (state) Z78.Ø
  - arthritis (any site) NEC — *see* Arthritis, specified form NEC
  - bleeding N92.4
  - depression (single episode) F32.89
    - agitated (single episode) F32.2
      - recurrent episode F33.9
    - psychotic (single episode) F32.89
      - recurrent episode F33.9
    - recurrent episode F33.8
  - melancholia (single episode) F32.89
    - recurrent episode F33.8
  - paranoid state F22
  - postirradiation (postprocedural)
    - asymptomatic E89.4Ø
    - symptomatic E89.41
  - premature E28.319
    - asymptomatic E28.319
      - postirradiation E89.4Ø
      - postsurgical E89.4Ø
    - symptomatic E28.31Ø
      - postirradiation E89.41
      - postsurgical E89.41
  - psychosis NEC F28
  - symptomatic N95.1
  - toxic polyarthritis NEC — *see* Arthritis, specified form NEC
- **Menorrhagia** (primary) N92.Ø
  - climacteric N92.4
    - menopausal N92.4
  - menopausal N92.4
  - perimenopausal N92.4
  - postclimacteric N95.Ø
  - postmenopausal N95.Ø
  - preclimacteric or premenopausal N92.4
  - pubertal (menses retained) N92.2
- **Menostaxis** N92.Ø
- **Menses, retention** N94.89
- **Menstrual** — *see* Menstruation
- **Menstruation**
  - absent — *see* Amenorrhea
  - anovulatory N97.Ø
  - cycle, irregular N92.6
  - delayed N91.Ø
  - disorder N93.9
    - psychogenic F45.8
  - during pregnancy O2Ø.8
  - excessive (with regular cycle) N92.Ø
    - with irregular cycle N92.1
    - at puberty N92.2
  - frequent N92.Ø
  - infrequent — *see* Oligomenorrhea
  - irregular N92.6
    - specified NEC N92.5
  - latent N92.5
  - membranous N92.5
  - painful — *see also* Dysmenorrhea N94.6
    - primary N94.4
    - psychogenic F45.8
    - secondary N94.5
  - passage of clots N92.Ø
  - precocious E3Ø.1
  - protracted N92.5
  - rare — *see* Oligomenorrhea
  - retained N94.89
  - retrograde N92.5
  - scanty — *see* Oligomenorrhea
  - suppression N94.89
  - vicarious (nasal) N94.89
- **Mental** — *see also* condition
  - deficiency — *see* Disability, intellectual
  - deterioration — *see* Psychosis
  - disorder — *see* Disorder, mental
  - exhaustion F48.8
  - insufficiency (congenital) — *see* Disability, intellectual
  - observation without need for further medical care ZØ3.89

- **Mental** — *continued*
  - retardation — *see* Disability, intellectual
  - subnormality — *see* Disability, intellectuall
  - upset — *see* Disorder, mental
- **Meralgia paresthetica** G57.1- ☑
- **Mercurial** — *see* condition
- **Mercurialism** — *see* subcategory T56.1 ☑
- **Merkel cell tumor** — *see* Carcinoma, Merkel cell
- **Merocele** — *see* Hernia, femoral
- **Meromelia**
  - lower limb — *see* Defect, reduction, lower limb
    - intercalary
      - femur — *see* Defect, reduction, lower limb, specified type NEC
      - tibiofibular (complete) (incomplete) — *see* Defect, reduction, lower limb
  - upper limb — *see* Defect, reduction, upper limb
    - intercalary, humeral, radioulnar — *see* Agenesis, arm, with hand present
- **MERRF syndrome** (myoclonic epilepsy associated with ragged-red fiber) E88.42
- **Merzbacher-Pelizaeus disease** E75.29
- **Mesaortitis** — *see* Aortitis
- **Mesarteritis** — *see* Arteritis
- **Mesencephalitis** — *see* Encephalitis
- **Mesenchymoma** — *see also* Neoplasm, connective tissue, uncertain behavior
  - benign — *see* Neoplasm, connective tissue, benign
  - malignant — *see* Neoplasm, connective tissue, malignant
- **Mesenteritis**
  - retractile K65.4
  - sclerosing K65.4
- **Mesentery, mesenteric** — *see* condition
- **Mesiodens, mesiodentes** KØØ.1
- **Mesio-occlusion** M26.213
- **Mesocolon** — *see* condition
- **Mesonephroma** (malignant) — *see* Neoplasm, malignant, by site
  - benign — *see* Neoplasm, benign, by site
- **Mesophlebitis** — *see* Phlebitis
- **Mesostromal dysgenesia** Q13.89
- **Mesothelioma** (malignant) C45.9
  - benign
    - mesentery D19.1
    - mesocolon D19.1
    - omentum D19.1
    - peritoneum D19.1
    - pleura D19.Ø
    - specified site NEC D19.7
    - unspecified site D19.9
  - biphasic C45.9
    - benign
      - mesentery D19.1
      - mesocolon D19.1
      - omentum D19.1
      - peritoneum D19.1
      - pleura D19.Ø
      - specified site NEC D19.7
      - unspecified site D19.9
  - cystic D48.4
  - epithelioid C45.9
    - benign
      - mesentery D19.1
      - mesocolon D19.1
      - omentum D19.1
      - peritoneum D19.1
      - pleura D19.Ø
      - specified site NEC D19.7
      - unspecified site D19.9
  - fibrous C45.9
    - benign
      - mesentery D19.1
      - mesocolon D19.1
      - omentum D19.1
      - peritoneum D19.1
      - pleura D19.Ø
      - specified site NEC D19.7
      - unspecified site D19.9
  - site classification
    - liver C45.7
    - lung C45.7
    - mediastinum C45.7
    - mesentery C45.1
    - mesocolon C45.1
    - omentum C45.1
    - pericardium C45.2
    - peritoneum C45.1
- **Mesothelioma** — *continued*
  - site classification — *continued*
    - pleura C45.Ø
      - parietal C45.Ø
    - retroperitoneum C45.7
    - specified site NEC C45.7
    - unspecified C45.9
- **Metabolic syndrome** E88.81
- **Metagonimiasis** B66.8
- **Metagonimus infestation** (intestine) B66.8
- **Metal**
  - pigmentation L81.8
  - polisher's disease J62.8
- **Metamorphopsia** H53.15
- **Metaplasia**
  - apocrine (breast) — *see* Dysplasia, mammary, specified type NEC
  - cervix (squamous) — *see* Dysplasia, cervix
  - endometrium (squamous) (uterus) N85.8
  - esophagus K22.7- ☑
  - gastric intestinal K31.AØ
    - with dysplasia K31.A29
      - high grade K31.A22
      - low grade K31.A21
    - indefinite for dysplasia K31.AØ
    - without dysplasia K31.A19
      - involving
        - antrum K31.A11
        - body (corpus) K31.A12
        - cardia K31.A14
        - fundus K31.A13
        - multiple sites K31.A15
  - kidney (pelvis) (squamous) N28.89
  - myelogenous D73.1
  - myeloid (agnogenic) (megakaryocytic) D73.1
  - spleen D73.1
  - squamous cell, bladder N32.89
- **Metastasis, metastatic**
  - abscess — *see* Abscess
  - calcification E83.59
  - cancer
    - from specified site — *see* Neoplasm, malignant, by site
    - to specified site — *see* Neoplasm, secondary, by site
  - deposits (in) — *see* Neoplasm, secondary, by site
  - disease — *see also* Neoplasm, secondary, by site C79.9
  - spread (to) — *see* Neoplasm, secondary, by site
- **Metastrongyliasis** B83.8
- **Metatarsalgia** M77.4- ☑
  - anterior G57.6- ☑
  - Morton's G57.6- ☑
- **Metatarsus, metatarsal** — *see also* condition
  - adductus, congenital Q66.22- ☑
  - valgus (abductus), congenital Q66.6
  - varus (congenital) Q66.22- ☑
    - primus Q66.21- ☑
- **Methadone use** — *see* Use, opioid
- **Methemoglobinemia** D74.9
  - acquired (with sulfhemoglobinemia) D74.8
  - congenital D74.Ø
  - enzymatic (congenital) D74.Ø
  - Hb M disease D74.Ø
  - hereditary D74.Ø
  - toxic D74.8
- **Methemoglobinuria** — *see* Hemoglobinuria
- **Methioninemia** E72.19
- **Methylmalonic acidemia** E71.12Ø
- **Metritis** (catarrhal) (hemorrhagic) (septic) (suppurative) — *see also* Endometritis
  - cervical — *see* Cervicitis
- **Metropathia hemorrhagica** N93.8
- **Metroperitonitis** — *see* Peritonitis, pelvic, female
- **Metrorrhagia** N92.1
  - climacteric N92.4
  - menopausal N92.4
  - perimenopausal N92.4
  - postpartum NEC (atonic) (following delivery of placenta) O72.1
    - delayed or secondary O72.2
  - preclimacteric or premenopausal N92.4
  - psychogenic F45.8
- **Metrorrhexis** — *see* Rupture, uterus
- **Metrosalpingitis** N7Ø.91
- **Metrostaxis** N93.8
- **Metrovaginitis** — *see* Endometritis
- **Meyer-Schwickerath and Weyers syndrome** Q87.Ø
- **Meynert's amentia** (nonalcoholic) FØ4
- **Meynert's amentia** — *continued*
  - alcoholic F1Ø.96
    - with dependence F1Ø.26
- **Mibelli's disease** (porokeratosis) Q82.8
- **Mice, joint** — *see* Loose, body, joint
  - knee M23.4- ☑
- **Micrencephalon, micrencephaly** QØ2
- **Microalbuminuria** R8Ø.9
- **Microaneurysm, retinal** — *see also* Disorder, retina, microaneurysms
  - diabetic — *see* EØ8-E13 with .31
- **Microangiopathy** (peripheral) I73.9
  - thrombotic M31.1Ø
    - hematopoietic stem cell transplantation-associated [HSCT-TMA] M31.1Ø
- **Microcalcifications, breast** R92.Ø
- **Microcephalus, microcephalic, microcephaly** QØ2
  - due to toxoplasmosis (congenital) P37.1
- **Microcheilia** Q18.7
- **Microcolon** (congenital) Q43.8
- **Microcornea** (congenital) Q13.4
- **Microcytic** — *see* condition
- **Microdeletions NEC** Q93.88
- **Microdontia** KØØ.2
- **Microdrepanocytosis** D57.4Ø
  - with
    - acute chest syndrome D57.411
    - cerebral vascular involvement D57.413
    - crisis (painful) D57.419
      - with specified complication NEC D57.418
    - splenic sequestration D57.412
    - vasoocclusive pain D57.419
- **Microembolism**
  - atherothrombotic — *see* Atheroembolism
  - retinal — *see* Occlusion, artery, retina
- **Microencephalon** QØ2
- **Microfilaria streptocerca infestation** — *see* Onchocerciasis
- **Microgastria** (congenital) Q4Ø.2
- **Microgenia** M26.Ø6
- **Microgenitalia, congenital**
  - female Q52.8
  - male Q55.8
- **Microglioma** — *see* Lymphoma, non-Hodgkin, specified NEC
- **Microglossia** (congenital) Q38.3
- **Micrognathia, micrognathism** (congenital) (mandibular) (maxillary) M26.Ø9
- **Microgyria** (congenital) QØ4.3
- **Microinfarct of heart** — *see* Insufficiency, coronary
- **Microlentia** (congenital) Q12.8
- **Microlithiasis, alveolar, pulmonary** J84.Ø2
- **Micromastia** N64.82
- **Micromyelia** (congenital) QØ6.8
- **Micropenis** Q55.62
- **Microphakia** (congenital) Q12.8
- **Microphthalmos, microphthalmia** (congenital) Q11.2
  - due to toxoplasmosis P37.1
- **Micropsia** H53.15
- **Microscopic polyangiitis** (polyarteritis) M31.7
- **Microsporidiosis** B6Ø.8
  - intestinal AØ7.8
- **Microsporon furfur infestation** B36.Ø
- **Microsporosis** — *see also* Dermatophytosis
  - nigra B36.1
- **Microstomia** (congenital) Q18.5
- **Microtia** (congenital) (external ear) Q17.2
- **Microtropia** H5Ø.4Ø
- **Microvillus inclusion disease** (MVD) (MVID) Q43.8
- **Micturition**
  - disorder NEC — *see also* Difficulty, micturition R39.198
    - psychogenic F45.8
  - frequency R35.Ø
    - psychogenic F45.8
  - hesitancy R39.11
  - incomplete emptying R39.14
  - nocturnal R35.1
  - painful R3Ø.9
    - dysuria R3Ø.Ø
    - psychogenic F45.8
    - tenesmus R3Ø.1
  - poor stream R39.12
  - position dependent R39.192
  - split stream R39.13
  - straining R39.16
  - urgency R39.15
- **Mid plane** — *see* condition

Middle
ear — *see* condition
lobe (right) syndrome J98.19
Miescher's elastoma L87.2
Mietens' syndrome Q87.2
Migraine (idiopathic) G43.909
with refractory migraine G43.919
with status migrainosus G43.911
without status migrainosus G43.919
with aura (acute-onset) (prolonged) (typical) (without headache) G43.109
with refractory migraine G43.119
with status migrainosus G43.111
without status migrainosus G43.119
intractable G43.119
with status migrainosus G43.111
without status migrainosus G43.119
not intractable G43.109
with status migrainosus G43.101
without status migrainosus G43.109
persistent G43.509
with cerebral infarction G43.609
with refractory migraine G43.619
with status migrainosus G43.611
without status migrainosus G43.619
intractable G43.619
with status migrainosus G43.611
without status migrainosus G43.619
not intractable G43.609
with status migrainosus G43.601
without status migrainosus G43.609
without refractory migraine G43.609
with status migrainosus G43.601
without status migrainosus G43.609
without cerebral infarction G43.509
with refractory migraine G43.519
with status migrainosus G43.511
without status migrainosus G43.519
intractable G43.519
with status migrainosus G43.511
without status migrainosus G43.519
not intractable G43.509
with status migrainosus G43.501
without status migrainosus G43.509
without refractory migraine G43.509
with status migrainosus G43.501
without status migrainosus G43.509
without mention of refractory migraine G43.109
with status migrainosus G43.101
without status migrainosus G43.109
abdominal G43.D0 (*following* G43.7)
with refractory migraine G43.D1 (*following* G43.7)
intractable G43.D1 (*following* G43.7)
not intractable G43.D0 (*following* G43.7)
without refractory migraine G43.D0 (*following* G43.7)
basilar — *see* Migraine, with aura
classical — *see* Migraine, with aura
common — *see* Migraine, without aura
complicated G43.109
equivalents — *see* Migraine, with aura
familiar — *see* Migraine, hemiplegic
hemiplegic G43.409
with refractory migraine G43.419
with status migrainosus G43.411
without status migrainosus G43.419
intractable G43.419
with status migrainosus G43.411
without status migrainosus G43.419
not intractable G43.409
with status migrainosus G43.401
without status migrainosus G43.409
without refractory migraine G43.409
with status migrainosus G43.401
without status migrainosus G43.409
intractable G43.919
with status migrainosus G43.911
without status migrainosus G43.919
menstrual G43.829
with refractory migraine G43.839
with status migrainosus G43.831
without status migrainosus G43.839
intractable G43.839
with status migrainosus G43.831
without status migrainosus G43.839
not intractable G43.829
with status migrainosus G43.821
without status migrainosus G43.829
without refractory migraine G43.829

Migraine — *continued*
menstrual — *continued*
without refractory migraine — *continued*
with status migrainosus G43.821
without status migrainosus G43.829
menstrually related — *see* Migraine, menstrual
not intractable G43.909
with status migrainosus G43.901
without status migrainosus G43.919
ophthalmoplegic G43.B0 (*following* G43.7)
with refractory migraine G43.B1 (*following* G43.7)
intractable G43.B1 (*following* G43.7)
not intractable G43.B0 (*following* G43.7)
without refractory migraine G43.B0 (*following* G43.7)
persistent aura (with, without) cerebral infarction — *see* Migraine, with aura, persistent
preceded or accompanied by transient focal neurological phenomena — *see* Migraine, with aura
pre-menstrual — *see* Migraine, menstrual
pure menstrual — *see* Migraine, menstrual
retinal — *see* Migraine, with aura
specified NEC G43.809
intractable G43.819
with status migrainosus G43.811
without status migrainosus G43.819
not intractable G43.809
with status migrainosus G43.801
without status migrainosus G43.809
sporadic — *see* Migraine, hemiplegic
transformed — *see* Migraine, without aura, chronic
triggered seizures — *see* Migraine, with aura
without aura G43.009
with refractory migraine G43.019
with status migrainosus G43.011
without status migrainosus G43.019
chronic G43.709
with refractory migraine G43.719
with status migrainosus G43.711
without status migrainosus G43.719
intractable
with status migrainosus G43.711
without status migrainosus G43.719
not intractable
with status migrainosus G43.701
without status migrainosus G43.709
without refractory migraine G43.709
with status migrainosus G43.701
without status migrainosus G43.709
intractable
with status migrainosus G43.011
without status migrainosus G43.019
not intractable
with status migrainosus G43.001
without status migrainosus G43.009
without mention of refractory migraine G43.009
with status migrainosus G43.001
without status migrainosus G43.009
without refractory migraine G43.909
with status migrainosus G43.901
without status migrainosus G43.909
Migrant, social Z59.00
Migration, anxiety concerning Z60.3
Migratory, migrating — *see also* condition
person Z59.00
testis Q55.29
Mikity-Wilson disease or syndrome P27.0
Mikulicz' disease or syndrome K11.8
Miliaria L74.3
alba L74.1
apocrine L75.2
crystallina L74.1
profunda L74.2
rubra L74.0
tropicalis L74.2
Miliary — *see* condition
Milium L72.0
colloid L57.8
Milk
crust L21.0
excessive secretion O92.6
poisoning — *see* Poisoning, food, noxious
retention O92.79
sickness — *see* Poisoning, food, noxious
spots I31.0
Milk-alkali disease or syndrome E83.52
Milk-leg (deep vessels) (nonpuerperal) — *see* Embolism, vein, lower extremity
complicating pregnancy O22.3- ☑

Milk-leg — *continued*
puerperal, postpartum, childbirth O87.1
Milkman's disease or syndrome M83.8
Milky urine — *see* Chyluria
Millard-Gubler (-Foville) **paralysis or syndrome** G46.3
Millar's asthma J38.5
Miller Fisher syndrome G61.0
Mills' disease — *see* Hemiplegia
Millstone maker's pneumoconiosis J62.8
Milroy's disease (chronic hereditary edema) Q82.0
Minamata disease T56.1 ☑
Miners' asthma or lung J60
Minkowski-Chauffard syndrome — *see* Spherocytosis
Minor — *see* condition
Minor's disease (hematomyelia) G95.19
Minot's disease (hemorrhagic disease), newborn P53
Minot-von Willebrand-Jurgens disease or syndrome (angiohemophilia) — *see* Disease, von Willebrand
Minus (and plus) **hand** (intrinsic) — *see* Deformity, limb, specified type NEC, forearm
Miosis (pupil) H57.03
Mirizzi's syndrome (hepatic duct stenosis) K83.1
Mirror writing F81.0
MIS-A M35.81
Misadventure (of) (prophylactic) (therapeutic) — *see also* Complications T88.9 ☑
administration of insulin (by accident) — *see* subcategory T38.3 ☑
infusion — *see* Complications, infusion
local applications (of fomentations, plasters, etc.) T88.9 ☑
burn or scald — *see* Burn
specified NEC T88.8 ☑
medical care (early) (late) T88.9 ☑
adverse effect of drugs or chemicals — *see* Table of Drugs and Chemicals
burn or scald — *see* Burn
specified NEC T88.8 ☑
specified NEC T88.8 ☑
surgical procedure (early) (late) — *see* Complications, surgical procedure
transfusion — *see* Complications, transfusion
vaccination or other immunological procedure — *see* Complications, vaccination
MIS-C M35.81
Miscarriage O03.9
Misdirection, aqueous H40.83- ☑
Misperception, sleep state F51.02
Misplaced, misplacement
ear Q17.4
kidney (acquired) N28.89
congenital Q63.2
organ or site, congenital NEC — *see* Malposition, congenital
Missed
abortion O02.1
delivery O36.4 ☑
Missing — *see also* Absence
string of intrauterine contraceptive device T83.32- ☑
Misuse of drugs F19.99
Mitchell's disease (erythromelalgia) I73.81
Mite(s) (infestation) B88.9
diarrhea B88.0
grain (itch) B88.0
hair follicle (itch) B88.0
in sputum B88.0
Mitral — *see* condition
Mittelschmerz N94.0
Mixed — *see* condition
MMN (multifocal motor neuropathy) G61.82
MNGIE (Mitochondrial Neurogastrointestinal Encephalopathy) **syndrome** E88.49
Mobile, mobility
cecum Q43.3
excessive — *see* Hypermobility
gallbladder, congenital Q44.1
kidney N28.89
organ or site, congenital NEC — *see* Malposition, congenital
Mobitz heart block (atrioventricular) I44.1
Moebius, Möbius
disease (ophthalmoplegic migraine) — *see* Migraine, ophthalmoplegic
syndrome Q87.0
congenital oculofacial paralysis (with other anomalies) Q87.0

Moebius, Möbius — *continued*
syndrome — *continued*
ophthalmoplegic migraine — *see* Migraine, ophthalmoplegic
Moeller's glossitis K14.0
Mohr's syndrome (Types I and II) Q87.0
Mola destruens D39.2
Molar pregnancy O02.0
Molarization of premolars K00.2
Molding, head (during birth) — *omit code*
Mole (pigmented) — *see also* Nevus
blood O02.0
Breus' O02.0
cancerous — *see* Melanoma
carneous O02.0
destructive D39.2
fleshy O02.0
hydatid, hydatidiform (benign) (complicating pregnancy) (delivered) (undelivered) O01.9
classical O01.0
complete O01.0
incomplete O01.1
invasive D39.2
malignant D39.2
partial O01.1
intrauterine O02.0
invasive (hydatidiform) D39.2
malignant
meaning
malignant hydatidiform mole D39.2
melanoma — *see* Melanoma
nonhydatidiform O02.0
nonpigmented — *see* Nevus
pregnancy NEC O02.0
skin — *see* Nevus
tubal O00.10- ☑
with intrauterine pregnancy O00.11- ☑
vesicular — *see* Mole, hydatidiform
Molimen, molimina (menstrual) N94.3
Molluscum contagiosum (epitheliale) B08.1
Mönckeberg's arteriosclerosis, disease, or sclerosis — *see* Arteriosclerosis, extremities
Mondini's malformation (cochlea) Q16.5
Mondor's disease I80.8
Monge's disease T70.29 ☑
Monilethrix (congenital) Q84.1
Moniliasis — *see also* Candidiasis B37.9
neonatal P37.5
Monitoring (encounter for)
therapeutic drug level Z51.81
Monkey malaria B53.1
Monkeypox B04
Monoarthritis M13.10
ankle M13.17- ☑
elbow M13.12- ☑
foot joint M13.17- ☑
hand joint M13.14- ☑
hip M13.15- ☑
knee M13.16- ☑
shoulder M13.11- ☑
wrist M13.13- ☑
Monoblastic — *see* condition
Monochromat (ism), monochromatopsia (acquired) (congenital) H53.51
Monocytic — *see* condition
Monocytopenia D72.818
Monocytosis (symptomatic) D72.821
Monomania — *see* Psychosis
Mononeuritis G58.9
cranial nerve — *see* Disorder, nerve, cranial
femoral nerve G57.2- ☑
lateral
cutaneous nerve of thigh G57.1- ☑
popliteal nerve G57.3- ☑
lower limb G57.9- ☑
specified nerve NEC G57.8- ☑
medial popliteal nerve G57.4- ☑
median nerve G56.1- ☑
multiplex G58.7
plantar nerve G57.6- ☑
posterior tibial nerve G57.5- ☑
radial nerve G56.3- ☑
sciatic nerve G57.0- ☑
specified NEC G58.8
tibial nerve G57.4- ☑
ulnar nerve G56.2- ☑
upper limb G56.9- ☑

Mononeuritis — *continued*
upper limb — *continued*
specified nerve NEC G56.8- ☑
vestibular — *see* subcategory H93.3 ☑
Mononeuropathy G58.9
carpal tunnel syndrome — *see* Syndrome, carpal tunnel
diabetic NEC — *see* E08-E13 with .41
femoral nerve — *see* Lesion, nerve, femoral
ilioinguinal nerve G57.8- ☑
in diseases classified elsewhere — *see* category G59
intercostal G58.0
lower limb G57.9- ☑
causalgia — *see* Causalgia, lower limb
femoral nerve — *see* Lesion, nerve, femoral
meralgia paresthetica G57.1- ☑
plantar nerve — *see* Lesion, nerve, plantar
popliteal nerve — *see* Lesion, nerve, popliteal
sciatic nerve — *see* Lesion, nerve, sciatic
specified NEC G57.8- ☑
tarsal tunnel syndrome — *see* Syndrome, tarsal tunnel
median nerve — *see* Lesion, nerve, median
multiplex G58.7
obturator nerve G57.8- ☑
popliteal nerve — *see* Lesion, nerve, popliteal
radial nerve — *see* Lesion, nerve, radial
saphenous nerve G57.8- ☑
specified NEC G58.8
tarsal tunnel syndrome — *see* Syndrome, tarsal tunnel
tuberculous A17.83
ulnar nerve — *see* Lesion, nerve, ulnar
upper limb G56.9- ☑
carpal tunnel syndrome — *see* Syndrome, carpal tunnel
causalgia — *see* Causalgia
median nerve — *see* Lesion, nerve, median
radial nerve — *see* Lesion, nerve, radial
specified site NEC G56.8- ☑
ulnar nerve — *see* Lesion, nerve, ulnar
Mononucleosis, infectious B27.90
with
complication NEC B27.99
meningitis B27.92
polyneuropathy B27.91
cytomegaloviral B27.10
with
complication NEC B27.19
meningitis B27.12
polyneuropathy B27.11
Epstein-Barr (virus) B27.00
with
complication NEC B27.09
meningitis B27.02
polyneuropathy B27.01
gammaherpesviral B27.00
with
complication NEC B27.09
meningitis B27.02
polyneuropathy B27.01
specified NEC B27.80
with
complication NEC B27.89
meningitis B27.82
polyneuropathy B27.81
Monoplegia G83.3- ☑
congenital (cerebral) G80.8
spastic G80.1
embolic (current episode) I63.4- ☑
following
cerebrovascular disease
cerebral infarction
lower limb I69.34- ☑
upper limb I69.33- ☑
intracerebral hemorrhage
lower limb I69.14- ☑
upper limb I69.13- ☑
lower limb I69.94- ☑
nontraumatic intracranial hemorrhage NEC
lower limb I69.24- ☑
upper limb I69.23- ☑
specified disease NEC
lower limb I69.84- ☑
upper limb I69.83- ☑
stroke NOS
lower limb I69.34- ☑
upper limb I69.33- ☑

Monoplegia — *continued*
following — *continued*
cerebrovascular disease — *continued*
subarachnoid hemorrhage
lower limb I69.04- ☑
upper limb I69.03- ☑
upper limb I69.93- ☑
hysterical (transient) F44.4
lower limb G83.1- ☑
psychogenic (conversion reaction) F44.4
thrombotic (current episode) I63.3- ☑
transient R29.818
upper limb G83.2- ☑
Monorchism, monorchidism Q55.0
Monosomy — *see also* Deletion, chromosome Q93.9
specified NEC Q93.89
whole chromosome
meiotic nondisjunction Q93.0
mitotic nondisjunction Q93.1
mosaicism Q93.1
X Q96.9
Monster, monstrosity (single) Q89.7
acephalic Q00.0
twin Q89.4
Monteggia's fracture (-dislocation) S52.27- ☑
Mooren's ulcer (cornea) — *see* Ulcer, cornea, Mooren's
Moore's syndrome — *see* Epilepsy, specified NEC
Mooser-Neill reaction A75.2
Mooser's bodies A75.2
Morbidity not stated or unknown R69
Morbilli — *see* Measles
Morbus — *see also* Disease
angelicus, anglorum E55.0
Beigel B36.2
caducus — *see* Epilepsy
celiacus K90.0
comitialis — *see* Epilepsy
cordis — *see also* Disease, heart I51.9
valvulorum — *see* Endocarditis
coxae senilis M16.9
tuberculous A18.02
hemorrhagicus neonatorum P53
maculosus neonatorum P54.5
Morel (-Stewart)(-Morgagni) **syndrome** M85.2
Morel-Kraepelin disease — *see* Schizophrenia
Morel-Moore syndrome M85.2
Morgagni's
cyst, organ, hydatid, or appendage
female Q50.5
male (epididymal) Q55.4
testicular Q55.29
syndrome M85.2
Morgagni-Stewart-Morel syndrome M85.2
Morgagni-Stokes-Adams syndrome I45.9
Morgagni-Turner (-Albright) **syndrome** Q96.9
Moria F07.0
Moron (I.Q. 50-69) F70
Morphea L94.0
Morphinism (without remission) F11.20
with remission F11.21
Morphinomania (without remission) F11.20
with remission F11.21
Morquio (-Ullrich)(-Brailsford) **disease or syndrome** — *see* Mucopolysaccharidosis
Mortification (dry) (moist) — *see* Gangrene
Morton's metatarsalgia (neuralgia) (neuroma) (syndrome) G57.6- ☑
Morvan's disease or syndrome G60.8
Mosaicism, mosaic (autosomal) (chromosomal)
45,X/46,XX Q96.3
45,X/other cell lines NEC with abnormal sex chromosome Q96.4
sex chromosome
female Q97.8
lines with various numbers of X chromosomes Q97.2
male Q98.7
XY Q96.3
Moschowitz' disease M31.19
Mother yaw A66.0
Motion sickness (from travel, any vehicle) (from roundabouts or swings) T75.3 ☑
Mottled, mottling, teeth (enamel) (endemic) (nonendemic) K00.3
Mounier-Kuhn syndrome Q32.4
with bronchiectasis J47.9
exacerbation (acute) J47.1
lower respiratory infection J47.0

Mounier-Kuhn syndrome — *continued*
acquired J98.09
with bronchiectasis J47.9
with
exacerbation (acute) J47.1
lower respiratory infection J47.0
Mountain
sickness T70.29 ☑
with polycythemia , acquired (acute) D75.1
tick fever A93.2
Mouse, joint — *see* Loose, body, joint
knee M23.4- ☑
Mouth — *see* condition
Movable
coccyx — *see* subcategory M53.2 ☑
kidney N28.89
congenital Q63.8
spleen D73.89
Movements, dystonic R25.8
Moyamoya disease I67.5
MRSA (Methicillin resistant Staphylococcus aureus)
infection A49.02
as the cause of diseases classified elsewhere B95.62
sepsis A41.02
MSD (multiple sulfatase deficiency) E75.26
MSSA (Methicillin susceptible Staphylococcus aureus)
infection A49.01
as the cause of diseases classified elsewhere B95.61
sepsis A41.01
Mucha-Habermann disease L41.0
Mucinosis (cutaneous) (focal) (papular) (skin) L98.5
oral K13.79
Mucocele
appendix K38.8
buccal cavity K13.79
gallbladder K82.1
lacrimal sac, chronic H04.43- ☑
nasal sinus J34.1
nose J34.1
salivary gland (any) K11.6
sinus (accessory) (nasal) J34.1
turbinate (bone) (middle) (nasal) J34.1
uterus N85.8
Mucolipidosis
I E77.1
II, III E77.0
IV E75.11
Mucopolysaccharidosis E76.3
beta-gluduronidase deficiency E76.29
cardiopathy E76.3 *[I52]*
Hunter's syndrome E76.1
Hurler's syndrome E76.01
Hurler-Scheie syndrome E76.02
Maroteaux-Lamy syndrome E76.29
Morquio syndrome E76.219
A E76.210
B E76.211
classic E76.210
Sanfilippo syndrome E76.22
Scheie's syndrome E76.03
specified NEC E76.29
type
I
Hurler's syndrome E76.01
Hurler-Scheie syndrome E76.02
Scheie's syndrome E76.03
II E76.1
III E76.22
IV E76.219
IVA E76.210
IVB E76.211
VI E76.29
VII E76.29
Mucormycosis B46.5
cutaneous B46.3
disseminated B46.4
gastrointestinal B46.2
generalized B46.4
pulmonary B46.0
rhinocerebral B46.1
skin B46.3
subcutaneous B46.3
Mucositis (ulcerative) K12.30
due to drugs NEC K12.32
gastrointestinal K92.81
mouth (oral) (oropharyngeal) K12.30
due to antineoplastic therapy K12.31
due to drugs NEC K12.32

Mucositis — *continued*
mouth — *continued*
due to radiation K12.33
specified NEC K12.39
viral K12.39
nasal J34.81
oral cavity — *see* Mucositis, mouth
oral soft tissues — *see* Mucositis, mouth
vagina and vulva N76.81
Mucositis necroticans agranulocytica — *see* Agranulocytosis
Mucous — *see also* condition
patches (syphilitic) A51.39
congenital A50.07
Mucoviscidosis E84.9
with meconium obstruction E84.11
Mucus
asphyxia or suffocation — *see* Asphyxia, mucus
in stool R19.5
plug — *see* Asphyxia, mucus
Muguet B37.0
Mulberry molars (congenital syphilis) A50.52
Müllerian mixed tumor
specified site — *see* Neoplasm, malignant, by site
unspecified site C54.9
Multicystic kidney (development) Q61.4
Multiparity (grand) Z64.1
affecting management of pregnancy, labor and delivery (supervision only) O09.4- ☑
requiring contraceptive management — *see* Contraception
Multipartita placenta O43.19- ☑
Multiple, multiplex — *see also* condition
digits (congenital) Q69.9
endocrine neoplasia — *see* Neoplasia, endocrine, multiple (MEN)
personality F44.81
Multisystem inflammatory syndrome (in adult) (in children) M35.81
Mumps B26.9
arthritis B26.85
complication NEC B26.89
encephalitis B26.2
hepatitis B26.81
meningitis (aseptic) B26.1
meningoencephalitis B26.2
myocarditis B26.82
oophoritis B26.89
orchitis B26.0
pancreatitis B26.3
polyneuropathy B26.84
Mumu — *see also* Infestation, filarial B74.9 *[N51]*
Münchhausen's syndrome — *see* Disorder, factitious
Münchmeyer's syndrome — *see* Myositis, ossificans, progressiva
Mural — *see* condition
Murmur (cardiac) (heart) (organic) R01.1
abdominal R19.15
aortic (valve) — *see* Endocarditis, aortic
benign R01.0
diastolic — *see* Endocarditis
Flint I35.1
functional R01.0
Graham Steell I37.1
innocent R01.0
mitral (valve) — *see* Insufficiency, mitral
nonorganic R01.0
presystolic, mitral — *see* Insufficiency, mitral
pulmonic (valve) I37.8
systolic R01.1
tricuspid (valve) I07.9
valvular — *see* Endocarditis
Murri's disease (intermittent hemoglobinuria) D59.6
Muscle, muscular — *see also* condition
carnitine (palmityltransferase) deficiency E71.314
Musculoneuralgia — *see* Neuralgia
Mushrooming hip — *see* Derangement, joint, specified NEC, hip
Mushroom-workers' (pickers') **disease or lung** J67.5
Mutation(s)
factor V Leiden D68.51
prothrombin gene D68.52
surfactant, of lung J84.83
Mutism — *see also* Aphasia
deaf (acquired) (congenital) NEC H91.3
elective (adjustment reaction) (childhood) F94.0
hysterical F44.4

Mutism — *continued*
selective (childhood) F94.0
MVD (microvillus inclusion disease) Q43.8
MVID (microvillus inclusion disease) Q43.8
Myalgia M79.10
auxiliary muscles, head and neck M79.12
epidemic (cervical) B33.0
mastication muscle M79.11
site specified NEC M79.18
traumatic NEC T14.8 ☑
Myasthenia G70.9
congenital G70.2
cordis — *see* Failure, heart
developmental G70.2
gravis G70.00
with exacerbation (acute) G70.01
in crisis G70.01
neonatal, transient P94.0
pseudoparalytica G70.00
with exacerbation (acute) G70.01
in crisis G70.01
stomach, psychogenic F45.8
syndrome
in
diabetes mellitus — *see* E08-E13 with .44
neoplastic disease — *see also* Neoplasm D49.9 *[G73.3]*
pernicious anemia D51.0 *[G73.3]*
thyrotoxicosis E05.90 *[G73.3]*
with thyroid storm E05.91 *[G73.3]*
Myasthenic M62.81
Mycelium infection B49
Mycetismus — *see* Poisoning, food, noxious, mushroom
Mycetoma B47.9
actinomycotic B47.1
bone (mycotic) B47.9 *[M90.80]*
eumycotic B47.0
foot B47.9
actinomycotic B47.1
mycotic B47.0
madurae NEC B47.9
mycotic B47.0
maduromycotic B47.0
mycotic B47.0
nocardial B47.1
Mycobacteriosis — *see* Mycobacterium
Mycobacterium, mycobacterial (infection) A31.9
anonymous A31.9
atypical A31.9
cutaneous A31.1
pulmonary A31.0
tuberculous — *see* Tuberculosis, pulmonary
specified site NEC A31.8
avium (intracellulare complex) A31.0
balnei A31.1
Battey A31.0
chelonei A31.8
cutaneous A31.1
extrapulmonary systemic A31.8
fortuitum A31.8
intracellulare (Battey bacillus) A31.0
kakaferifu A31.8
kansasii (yellow bacillus) A31.0
kasongo A31.8
leprae — *see also* Leprosy A30.9
luciflavum A31.1
marinum (M. balnei) A31.1
nonspecific — *see* Mycobacterium, atypical
pulmonary (atypical) A31.0
tuberculous — *see* Tuberculosis, pulmonary
scrofulaceum A31.8
simiae A31.8
systemic, extrapulmonary A31.8
szulgai A31.8
terrae A31.8
triviale A31.8
tuberculosis (human, bovine) — *see* Tuberculosis
ulcerans A31.1
xenopi A31.8
Mycoplasma (M.) **pneumoniae, as cause of disease classified elsewhere** B96.0
Mycosis, mycotic B49
cutaneous NEC B36.9
ear B36.9
in
aspergillosis B44.89
candidiasis B37.84
moniliasis B37.84

Mycosis, mycotic — *continued*
  fungoides (extranodal) (solid organ) C84.Ø- ☑
  mouth B37.Ø
  nails B35.1
  opportunistic B48.8
  skin NEC B36.9
  specified NEC B48.8
  stomatitis B37.Ø
  vagina, vaginitis (candidal) (acute) B37.31
    chronic (recurrent) B37.32
Mydriasis (pupil) H57.Ø4
Myelatelia QØ6.1
Myelinolysis, pontine, central G37.2
Myelitis (acute) (ascending) (childhood) (chronic) (descending) (diffuse) (disseminated) (idiopathic) (pressure) (progressive) (spinal cord) (subacute) — *see also* Encephalitis GØ4.91
  flaccid GØ4.82
  herpes simplex BØØ.82
  herpes zoster BØ2.24
  in diseases classified elsewhere GØ5.4
  necrotizing, subacute G37.4
  optic neuritis in G36.Ø
  postchickenpox BØ1.12
  postherpetic BØ2.24
  postimmunization GØ4.Ø2
  postinfectious NEC GØ4.89
  postvaccinal GØ4.Ø2
  specified NEC GØ4.89
  syphilitic (transverse) A52.14
  toxic G92.9
  transverse (in demyelinating diseases of central nervous system) G37.3
  tuberculous A17.82
  varicella BØ1.12
Myeloblastic — *see* condition
Myeloblastoma
  granular cell — *see also* Neoplasm, connective tissue
    malignant — *see* Neoplasm, connective tissue, malignant
    tongue D1Ø.1
Myelocele — *see* Spina bifida
Myelocystocele — *see* Spina bifida
Myelocytic — *see* condition
Myelodysplasia D46.9
  specified NEC D46.Z (*following* D46.4)
  spinal cord (congenital) QØ6.1
Myelodysplastic syndrome — *see also* Syndrome, myelodysplastic D46.9
  with
    5q deletion D46.C (*following* D46.2)
    isolated del (5q) chromosomal abnormality D46.C (*following* D46.2)
  specified NEC D46.Z (*following* D46.4)
Myeloencephalitis — *see* Encephalitis
Myelofibrosis D75.81
  with myeloid metaplasia D47.4
  acute C94.4- ☑
  idiopathic (chronic) D47.4
  primary D47.1
  secondary D75.81
    in myeloproliferative disease D47.4
Myelogenous — *see* condition
Myeloid — *see* condition
Myelokathexis D7Ø.9
Myeloleukodystrophy E75.29
Myelolipoma — *see* Lipoma
Myeloma (multiple) C9Ø.Ø- ☑
  monostotic C9Ø.3 ☑
    plasma cell C9Ø.Ø- ☑
  plasma cell C9Ø.Ø- ☑
  solitary — *see also* Plasmacytoma, solitary C9Ø.3- ☑
Myelomalacia G95.89
Myelomatosis C9Ø.Ø- ☑
Myelomeningitis — *see* Meningoencephalitis
Myelomeningocele (spinal cord) — *see* Spina bifida
Myelo-osteo-musculodysplasia hereditaria Q79.8
Myelopathic
  anemia D64.89
  muscle atrophy — *see* Atrophy, muscle, spinal
  pain syndrome G89.Ø
Myelopathy (spinal cord) G95.9
  drug-induced G95.89
  in (due to)
    degeneration or displacement, intervertebral disc NEC — *see* Disorder, disc, with, myelopathy
    infection — *see* Encephalitis

Myelopathy — *continued*
  in — *continued*
    intervertebral disc disorder — *see also* Disorder, disc, with, myelopathy
    mercury — *see* subcategory T56.1 ☑
    neoplastic disease — *see also* Neoplasm D49.9 *[G99.2]*
    pernicious anemia D51.Ø *[G99.2]*
    spondylosis — *see* Spondylosis, with myelopathy NEC
  necrotic (subacute) (vascular) G95.19
  radiation-induced G95.89
  spondylogenic NEC — *see* Spondylosis, with myelopathy NEC
  toxic G95.89
  transverse, acute G37.3
  vascular G95.19
  vitamin B12 E53.8 *[G32.Ø]*
Myelophthisis D61.82
Myeloradiculitis GØ4.91
Myeloradiculodysplasia (spinal) QØ6.1
Myelosarcoma C92.3- ☑
Myelosclerosis D75.89
  with myeloid metaplasia D47.4
  disseminated, of nervous system G35
  megakaryocytic D47.4
    with myeloid metaplasia D47.4
Myelosis
  acute C92.Ø- ☑
  aleukemic C92.9- ☑
  chronic D47.1
  erythremic (acute) C94.Ø- ☑
  megakaryocytic C94.2- ☑
  nonleukemic D72.828
  subacute C92.9- ☑
Myiasis (cavernous) B87.9
  aural B87.4
  creeping B87.Ø
  cutaneous B87.Ø
  dermal B87.Ø
  ear (external) (middle) B87.4
  eye B87.2
  genitourinary B87.81
  intestinal B87.82
  laryngeal B87.3
  nasopharyngeal B87.3
  ocular B87.2
  orbit B87.2
  skin B87.Ø
  specified site NEC B87.89
  traumatic B87.1
  wound B87.1
Myoadenoma, prostate — *see* Hyperplasia, prostate
Myoblastoma
  granular cell — *see also* Neoplasm, connective tissue, benign
    malignant — *see* Neoplasm, connective tissue, malignant
  tongue D1Ø.1
Myocardial — *see* condition
Myocardiopathy (congestive) (constrictive) (familial) (hypertrophic nonobstructive) (idiopathic) (infiltrative) (obstructive) (primary) (restrictive) (sporadic) — *see also* Cardiomyopathy I42.9
  alcoholic I42.6
  cobalt-beer I42.6
  glycogen storage E74.Ø2 *[I43]*
  hypertrophic obstructive I42.1
  in (due to)
    beriberi E51.12
    cardiac glycogenosis E74.Ø2 *[I43]*
    Friedreich's ataxia G11.11 *[I43]*
    myotonia atrophica G71.11 *[I43]*
    progressive muscular dystrophy — *see also* Dystrophy, muscular, by type G71.Ø9 *[I43]*
  obscure (African) I42.8
  secondary I42.9
  thyrotoxic EØ5.9Ø *[I43]*
    with storm EØ5.91 *[I43]*
  toxic NEC I42.7
Myocarditis (with arteriosclerosis) (chronic) (fibroid) (interstitial) (old) (progressive) (senile) I51.4
  with
    rheumatic fever (conditions in IØØ) IØ9.Ø
      active — *see* Myocarditis, acute, rheumatic
      inactive or quiescent (with chorea) IØ9.Ø
  active I4Ø.9

Myocarditis — *continued*
  active — *continued*
    rheumatic IØ1.2
      with chorea (acute) (rheumatic) (Sydenham's) IØ2.Ø
  acute or subacute (interstitial) I4Ø.9
    due to
      streptococcus (beta-hemolytic) IØ1.2
    idiopathic I4Ø.1
    rheumatic IØ1.2
      with chorea (acute) (rheumatic) (Sydenham's) IØ2.Ø
    specified NEC I4Ø.8
  aseptic of newborn B33.22
  bacterial (acute) I4Ø.Ø
  Coxsackie (virus) B33.22
  diphtheritic A36.81
  eosinophilic I4Ø.1
  epidemic of newborn (Coxsackie) B33.22
  Fiedler's (acute) (isolated) I4Ø.1
  giant cell (acute) (subacute) I4Ø.1
  gonococcal A54.83
  granulomatous (idiopathic) (isolated) (nonspecific) I4Ø.1
  hypertensive — *see* Hypertension, heart
  idiopathic (granulomatous) I4Ø.1
  in (due to)
    diphtheria A36.81
    epidemic louse-borne typhus A75.Ø *[I41]*
    Lyme disease A69.29
    sarcoidosis D86.85
    scarlet fever A38.1
    toxoplasmosis (acquired) B58.81
    typhoid AØ1.Ø2
    typhus NEC A75.9 *[I41]*
  infective I4Ø.Ø
  influenzal — *see* Influenza, with, myocarditis
  isolated (acute) I4Ø.1
  meningococcal A39.52
  mumps B26.82
  nonrheumatic, active I4Ø.9
  parenchymatous I4Ø.9
  pneumococcal I4Ø.Ø
  rheumatic (chronic) (inactive) (with chorea) IØ9.Ø
    active or acute IØ1.2
      with chorea (acute) (rheumatic) (Sydenham's) IØ2.Ø
  rheumatoid — *see* Rheumatoid, carditis
  septic I4Ø.Ø
  staphylococcal I4Ø.Ø
  suppurative I4Ø.Ø
  syphilitic (chronic) A52.Ø6
  toxic I4Ø.8
    rheumatic — *see* Myocarditis, acute, rheumatic
  tuberculous A18.84
  typhoid AØ1.Ø2
  valvular — *see* Endocarditis
  virus, viral I4Ø.Ø
    of newborn (Coxsackie) B33.22
Myocardium, myocardial — *see* condition
Myocardosis — *see* Cardiomyopathy
Myoclonus, myoclonic, myoclonia (familial) (essential) (multifocal) (simplex) G25.3
  drug-induced G25.3
  epilepsy — *see also* Epilepsy, generalized, specified NEC G4Ø.4- ☑
    familial (progressive) G25.3
  epileptica G4Ø.4Ø9
    with status epilepticus G4Ø.4Ø1
  facial G51.3- ☑
  familial progressive G25.3
  Friedreich's G25.3
  jerks G25.3
  massive G25.3
  palatal G25.3
  pharyngeal G25.3
Myocytolysis I51.5
Myodiastasis — *see* Diastasis, muscle
Myoendocarditis — *see* Endocarditis
Myoepithelioma — *see* Neoplasm, benign, by site
Myofasciitis (acute) — *see* Myositis
Myofibroma — *see also* Neoplasm, connective tissue, benign
  uterus (cervix) (corpus) — *see* Leiomyoma
Myofibromatosis D48.1
  infantile Q89.8
Myofibrosis M62.89
  heart — *see* Myocarditis
  scapulohumeral — *see* Lesion, shoulder, specified NEC

- **Myofibrositis** M79.7
  - scapulohumeral — *see* Lesion, shoulder, specified NEC
- **Myoglobulinuria, myoglobinuria** (primary) R82.1
- **Myokymia, facial** G51.4
- **Myolipoma** — *see* Lipoma
- **Myoma** — *see also* Neoplasm, connective tissue, benign
  - malignant — *see* Neoplasm, connective tissue, malignant
  - prostate D29.1
  - uterus (cervix) (corpus) — *see* Leiomyoma
- **Myomalacia** M62.89
- **Myometritis** — *see* Endometritis
- **Myometrium** — *see* condition
- **Myonecrosis, clostridial** A48.0
- **Myopathy** G72.9
  - acute
    - necrotizing G72.81
    - quadriplegic G72.81
  - alcoholic G72.1
  - benign congenital G71.20
  - central core G71.29
  - centronuclear G71.228
    - autosomal (dominant) (recessive) G71.228
    - other specified NEC G71.228
  - congenital (benign) G71.20
  - critical illness G72.81
  - distal G71.09
  - drug-induced G72.0
  - endocrine NEC E34.9 *[G73.7]*
  - extraocular muscles H05.82- ☑
  - facioscapulohumeral G71.02
  - hereditary G71.9
    - specified NEC G71.8
  - hyaline body G71.29
  - immune NEC G72.49
  - in (due to)
    - Addison's disease E27.1 *[G73.7]*
    - alcohol G72.1
    - amyloidosis E85.0 *[G73.7]*
    - cretinism E00.9 *[G73.7]*
    - Cushing's syndrome E24.9 *[G73.7]*
    - drugs G72.0
    - endocrine disease NEC E34.9 *[G73.7]*
    - giant cell arteritis M31.6 *[G73.7]*
    - glycogen storage disease E74.00 *[G73.7]*
    - hyperadrenocorticism E24.9 *[G73.7]*
    - hyperparathyroidism NEC E21.3 *[G73.7]*
    - hypoparathyroidism E20.9 *[G73.7]*
    - hypopituitarism E23.0 *[G73.7]*
    - hypothyroidism E03.9 *[G73.7]*
    - infectious disease NEC B99 ☑ *[G73.7]*
    - lipid storage disease E75.6 *[G73.7]*
    - metabolic disease NEC E88.9 *[G73.7]*
    - myxedema E03.9 *[G73.7]*
    - parasitic disease NEC B89 *[G73.7]*
    - polyarteritis nodosa M30.0 *[G73.7]*
    - rheumatoid arthritis — *see* Rheumatoid, myopathy
    - sarcoidosis D86.87
    - scleroderma M34.82
    - sicca syndrome M35.03
    - Sjögren's syndrome M35.03
    - systemic lupus erythematosus M32.19
    - thyrotoxicosis (hyperthyroidism) E05.90 *[G73.7]*
      - with thyroid storm E05.91 *[G73.7]*
    - toxic agent NEC G72.2
  - inflammatory NEC G72.49
  - intensive care (ICU) G72.81
  - limb-girdle — *see* Dystrophy, muscular, limb-girdle
  - mitochondrial NEC
  - Miyoshi, type 3 G71.035
  - myosin storage G71.29
  - myotubular (centronuclear) G71.220
    - X-linked G71.220
  - mytonic, proximal (PROMM) G71.11
  - nemaline G71.21
  - ocular G71.09
  - oculopharyngeal G71.09
  - of critical illness G72.81
  - primary G71.9
    - specified NEC G71.8
  - progressive NEC G72.89
  - proximal myotonic (PROMM) G71.11
  - rod (body) G71.21
  - scapulohumeral G71.02
  - specified NEC G72.89
  - toxic G72.2
- **Myopericarditis** — *see also* Pericarditis
  - chronic rheumatic I09.2
- **Myopia** (axial) (congenital) H52.1- ☑
  - degenerative (malignant) H44.20
    - with
      - choroidal neovascularization H44.2A- ☑
      - foveoschisis H44.2D- ☑
      - macular hole H44.2B- ☑
      - retinal detachment H44.2C- ☑
      - specified maculopathy NEC H44.2E- ☑
    - bilateral H44.23
    - left eye H44.22
    - right eye H44.21
  - malignant — *see also* Myopia, degenerative H44.2- ☑
  - pernicious — *see also* Myopia, degenerative H44.2- ☑
  - progressive high (degenerative) — *see also* Myopia, degenerative H44.2- ☑
- **Myosarcoma** — *see* Neoplasm, connective tissue, malignant
- **Myosis** (pupil) H57.03
  - stromal (endolymphatic) D39.0
- **Myositis** M60.9
  - clostridial A48.0
  - due to posture — *see* Myositis, specified type NEC
  - epidemic B33.0
  - fibrosa or fibrous (chronic), Volkmann's T79.6 ☑
  - foreign body granuloma — *see* Granuloma, foreign body
  - in (due to)
    - bilharziasis B65.9 *[M63.8-]* ☑
    - cysticercosis B69.81
    - leprosy A30.9 *[M63.8-]* ☑
    - mycosis B49 *[M63.8-]* ☑
    - sarcoidosis D86.87
    - schistosomiasis B65.9 *[M63.8-]* ☑
    - syphilis
      - late A52.78
      - secondary A51.49
    - toxoplasmosis (acquired) B58.82
    - trichinellosis B75 *[M63.8-]* ☑
    - tuberculosis A18.09
  - inclusion body [IBM] G72.41
  - infective M60.009
    - arm M60.002
      - left M60.001
      - right M60.000
    - leg M60.005
      - left M60.004
      - right M60.003
    - lower limb M60.005
      - ankle M60.07- ☑
      - foot M60.07- ☑
      - lower leg M60.06- ☑
      - thigh M60.05- ☑
      - toe M60.07- ☑
    - multiple sites M60.09
    - specified site NEC M60.08
    - upper limb M60.002
      - finger M60.04- ☑
      - forearm M60.03- ☑
      - hand M60.04- ☑
      - shoulder region M60.01- ☑
      - upper arm M60.02- ☑
  - interstitial M60.10
    - ankle M60.17- ☑
    - foot M60.17- ☑
    - forearm M60.13- ☑
    - hand M60.14- ☑
    - lower leg M60.16- ☑
    - multiple sites M60.19
    - shoulder region M60.11- ☑
    - specified site NEC M60.18
    - thigh M60.15- ☑
    - upper arm M60.12- ☑
  - mycotic B49 *[M63.8-]* ☑
  - orbital, chronic H05.12- ☑
  - ossificans or ossifying (circumscripta) — *see also* Ossification, muscle, specified NEC
    - in (due to)
      - burns M61.30
        - ankle M61.37- ☑
        - foot M61.37- ☑
        - forearm M61.33- ☑
        - hand M61.34- ☑
        - lower leg M61.36- ☑
        - multiple sites M61.39
        - pelvic region M61.35- ☑
        - shoulder region M61.31- ☑
        - specified site NEC M61.38
- **Myositis** — *continued*
  - ossificans or ossifying — *see also* Ossification, muscle, specified — *continued*
    - in — *continued*
      - burns — *continued*
        - thigh M61.35- ☑
        - upper arm M61.32- ☑
      - quadriplegia or paraplegia M61.20
        - ankle M61.27- ☑
        - foot M61.27- ☑
        - forearm M61.23- ☑
        - hand M61.24- ☑
        - lower leg M61.26- ☑
        - multiple sites M61.29
        - pelvic region M61.25- ☑
        - shoulder region M61.21- ☑
        - specified site NEC M61.28
        - thigh M61.25- ☑
        - upper arm M61.22- ☑
    - progressiva M61.10
      - ankle M61.17- ☑
      - finger M61.14- ☑
      - foot M61.17- ☑
      - forearm M61.13- ☑
      - hand M61.14- ☑
      - lower leg M61.16- ☑
      - multiple sites M61.19
      - pelvic region M61.15- ☑
      - shoulder region M61.11- ☑
      - specified site NEC M61.18
      - thigh M61.15- ☑
      - toe M61.17- ☑
      - upper arm M61.12- ☑
    - traumatica M61.00
      - ankle M61.07- ☑
      - foot M61.07- ☑
      - forearm M61.03- ☑
      - hand M61.04- ☑
      - lower leg M61.06- ☑
      - multiple sites M61.09
      - pelvic region M61.05- ☑
      - shoulder region M61.01- ☑
      - specified site NEC M61.08
      - thigh M61.05- ☑
      - upper arm M61.02- ☑
  - purulent — *see* Myositis, infective
  - specified type NEC M60.80
    - ankle M60.87- ☑
    - foot M60.87- ☑
    - forearm M60.83- ☑
    - hand M60.84- ☑
    - lower leg M60.86- ☑
    - multiple sites M60.89
    - pelvic region M60.85- ☑
    - shoulder region M60.81- ☑
    - specified site NEC M60.88
    - thigh M60.85- ☑
    - upper arm M60.82- ☑
  - suppurative — *see* Myositis, infective
  - traumatic (old) — *see* Myositis, specified type NEC
- **Myospasia impulsiva** F95.2
- **Myotonia** (acquisita) (intermittens) M62.89
  - atrophica G71.11
  - chondrodystrophic G71.13
  - congenita (acetazolamide responsive) (dominant) (recessive) G71.12
  - drug-induced G71.14
  - dystrophica G71.11
  - fluctuans G71.19
  - levior G71.12
  - permanens G71.19
  - symptomatic G71.19
- **Myotonic pupil** — *see* Anomaly, pupil, function, tonic pupil
- **Myriapodiasis** B88.2
- **Myringitis** H73.2- ☑
  - with otitis media — *see* Otitis, media
  - acute H73.00- ☑
    - bullous H73.01- ☑
    - specified NEC H73.09- ☑
  - bullous — *see* Myringitis, acute, bullous
  - chronic H73.1- ☑
- **Mysophobia** F40.228
- **Mytilotoxism** — *see* Poisoning, fish
- **Myxadenitis labialis** K13.0

Myxedema (adult) (idiocy) (infantile) (juvenile) — *see also* Hypothyroidism EØ3.9
- circumscribed EØ5.9Ø
  - with storm EØ5.91
- coma EØ3.5
- congenital EØØ.1
- cutis L98.5
- localized (pretibial) EØ5.9Ø
  - with storm EØ5.91

Myxedema — *continued*
- papular L98.5

Myxochondrosarcoma — *see* Neoplasm, cartilage, malignant

Myxofibroma — *see* Neoplasm, connective tissue, benign
- odontogenic — *see* Cyst, calcifying odontogenic

Myxofibrosarcoma — *see* Neoplasm, connective tissue, malignant

Myxolipoma D17.9

Myxoliposarcoma — *see* Neoplasm, connective tissue, malignant

Myxoma — *see also* Neoplasm, connective tissue, benign
- nerve sheath — *see* Neoplasm, nerve, benign
- odontogenic — *see* Cyst, calcifying odontogenic

Myxosarcoma — *see* Neoplasm, connective tissue, malignant

Index

Myxedema — Myxosarcoma

N

- **Naegeli's**
  - disease Q82.8
  - leukemia, monocytic C93.1- ☑
- **Naegleriasis** (with meningoencephalitis) B6Ø.2
- **Naffziger's syndrome** G54.Ø
- **Naga sore** — *see* Ulcer, skin
- **Nägele's pelvis** M95.5
  - with disproportion (fetopelvic) O33.Ø
    - causing obstructed labor O65.Ø
- **Nail** — *see also* condition
  - biting F98.8
  - patella syndrome Q87.2
- **Nanism, nanosomia** — *see* Dwarfism
- **Nanophyetiasis** B66.8
- **Nanukayami** A27.89
- **Napkin rash** L22
- **Narcolepsy** G47.419
  - with cataplexy G47.411
  - in conditions classified elsewhere G47.429
    - with cataplexy G47.421
- **Narcosis** RØ6.89
- **Narcotism** — *see* Dependence
- **NARP** (Neuropathy, Ataxia and Retinitis pigmentosa) syndrome E88.49
- **Narrow**
  - anterior chamber angle H4Ø.Ø3- ☑
  - gingival width (of periodontal soft tissue) KØ5.5
  - pelvis — *see* Contraction, pelvis
- **Narrowing** — *see also* Stenosis
  - artery I77.1
    - auditory, internal I65.8
    - basilar — *see* Occlusion, artery, basilar
    - carotid — *see* Occlusion, artery, carotid
    - cerebellar — *see* Occlusion, artery, cerebellar
    - cerebral — *see* Occlusion artery, cerebral
    - choroidal — *see* Occlusion, artery, precerebral, specified NEC
    - communicating posterior — *see* Occlusion, artery, precerebral, specified NEC
    - coronary — *see also* Disease, heart, ischemic, atherosclerotic
      - congenital Q24.5
        - syphilitic A5Ø.54 *[I52]*
      - due to syphilis NEC A52.Ø6
    - hypophyseal — *see* Occlusion, artery, precerebral, specified NEC
    - pontine — *see* Occlusion, artery, precerebral, specified NEC
    - precerebral — *see* Occlusion, artery, precerebral
    - vertebral — *see* Occlusion, artery, vertebral
  - auditory canal (external) — *see* Stenosis, external ear canal
  - eustachian tube — *see* Obstruction, eustachian tube
  - eyelid — *see* Disorder, eyelid function
  - larynx J38.6
  - mesenteric artery — *see also* Ischemia, intestine, acute K55.Ø59
  - palate M26.89
  - palpebral fissure — *see* Disorder, eyelid function
  - ureter N13.5
    - with infection N13.6
  - urethra — *see* Stricture, urethra
- **Narrowness, abnormal, eyelid** Q1Ø.3
- **Nasal** — *see* condition
- **Nasolachrymal, nasolacrimal** — *see* condition
- **Nasopharyngeal** — *see also* condition
  - pituitary gland Q89.2
  - torticollis M43.6
- **Nasopharyngitis** (acute) (infective) (streptococcal) (subacute) JØØ
  - chronic (suppurative) (ulcerative) J31.1
- **Nasopharynx, nasopharyngeal** — *see* condition
- **Natal tooth, teeth** KØØ.6
- **Nausea** (without vomiting) R11.Ø
  - with vomiting R11.2
  - gravidarum — *see* Hyperemesis, gravidarum
  - marina T75.3 ☑
  - navalis T75.3 ☑
- **Navel** — *see* condition
- **Neapolitan fever** — *see* Brucellosis
- **Near drowning** T75.1 ☑
- **Nearsightedness** — *see* Myopia
- **Near-syncope** R55
- **Nebula, cornea** — *see* Opacity, cornea
- **Necator americanus infestation** B76.1
- **Necatoriasis** B76.1
- **Neck** — *see* condition
- **Necrobiosis** R68.89
  - lipoidica NEC L92.1
    - with diabetes — *see* EØ8-E13 with .62Ø
- **Necrolysis, toxic epidermal** L51.2
  - due to drug
    - correct substance properly administered — *see* Table of Drugs and Chemicals, by drug, adverse effect
    - overdose or wrong substance given or taken — *see* Table of Drugs and Chemicals, by drug, poisoning
- **Necrophilia** F65.89
- **Necrosis, necrotic** (ischemic) — *see also* Gangrene
  - adrenal (capsule) (gland) E27.49
  - amputation stump (surgical) (late) T87.5Ø
    - arm T87.5- ☑
    - leg T87.5- ☑
  - antrum J32.Ø
  - aorta (hyaline) — *see also* Aneurysm, aorta
    - cystic medial — *see* Dissection, aorta
  - artery I77.5
  - bladder (aseptic) (sphincter) N32.89
  - bone — *see also* Osteonecrosis M87.9
    - aseptic or avascular — *see* Osteonecrosis
      - idiopathic M87.ØØ
    - ethmoid J32.2
    - jaw M27.2
    - tuberculous — *see* Tuberculosis, bone
  - brain I67.89
  - breast (aseptic) (fat) (segmental) N64.1
  - bronchus J98.Ø9
  - central nervous system NEC I67.89
  - cerebellar I67.89
  - cerebral I67.89
  - colon — *see also* Infarct, intestine K55.Ø49
  - cornea H18.89- ☑
  - cortical (acute) (renal) N17.1
  - cystic medial (aorta) — *see* Dissection, aorta
  - dental pulp KØ4.1
  - esophagus K22.89
  - ethmoid (bone) J32.2
  - eyelid — *see* Disorder, eyelid, degenerative
  - fat, fatty (generalized) — *see also* Disorder, soft tissue, specified type NEC)
    - abdominal wall K65.4
    - breast (aseptic) (segmental) N64.1
    - localized — *see* Degeneration, by site, fatty
    - mesentery K65.4
    - omentum K65.4
    - pancreas K86.89
    - peritoneum K65.4
    - skin (subcutaneous), newborn P83.Ø
    - subcutaneous, due to birth injury P15.6
  - gallbladder — *see* Cholecystitis, acute
  - heart — *see* Infarct, myocardium
  - hip, aseptic or avascular — *see* Osteonecrosis, by type, femur
  - intestine (acute) (hemorrhagic) (massive) — *see also* Infarct, intestine K55.Ø69
  - jaw M27.2
  - kidney (bilateral) N28.Ø
    - acute N17.9
    - cortical (acute) (bilateral) N17.1
      - with ectopic or molar pregnancy OØ8.4
    - medullary (bilateral) (in acute renal failure) (papillary) N17.2
    - papillary (bilateral) (in acute renal failure) N17.2
    - tubular N17.Ø
      - with ectopic or molar pregnancy OØ8.4
      - complicating
        - abortion — *see* Abortion, by type, complicated by, tubular necrosis
        - ectopic or molar pregnancy OØ8.4
        - pregnancy — *see* Pregnancy, complicated by, diseases of, specified type or system NEC
      - following ectopic or molar pregnancy OØ8.4
      - traumatic T79.5 ☑
  - larynx J38.7
  - liver (with hepatic failure) (cell) — *see* Failure, hepatic
    - hemorrhagic, central K76.2
  - lung J85.Ø
  - lymphatic gland — *see* Lymphadenitis, acute
  - mammary gland (fat) (segmental) N64.1
  - mastoid (chronic) — *see* Mastoiditis, chronic

Necrosis, necrotic — *continued*

  - medullary (acute) (renal) N17.2
  - mesentery — *see also* Infarct, intestine K55.Ø69
    - fat K65.4
  - mitral valve — *see* Insufficiency, mitral
  - myocardium, myocardial — *see* Infarct, myocardium
  - nose J34.Ø
  - omentum (with mesenteric infarction) — *see also* Infarct, intestine K55.Ø69
    - fat K65.4
  - orbit, orbital — *see* Osteomyelitis, orbit
  - ossicles, ear — *see* Abnormal, ear ossicles
  - ovary N7Ø.92
  - pancreas (aseptic) (duct) (fat) K86.89
    - acute (infective) — *see* Pancreatitis, acute
    - infective — *see* Pancreatitis, acute
  - papillary (acute) (renal) N17.2
  - perineum N9Ø.89
  - peritoneum (with mesenteric infarction) — *see also* Infarct, intestine K55.Ø69
    - fat K65.4
  - pharynx JØ2.9
    - in granulocytopenia — *see* Neutropenia
    - Vincent's A69.1
  - phosphorus — *see* subcategory T54.2 ☑
  - pituitary (gland) E23.Ø
    - postpartum O99.285
    - Sheehan O99.285
  - pressure — *see* Ulcer, pressure, by site
  - pulmonary J85.Ø
  - pulp (dental) KØ4.1
  - radiation — *see* Necrosis, by site
  - radium — *see* Necrosis, by site
  - renal — *see* Necrosis, kidney
  - sclera H15.89
  - scrotum N5Ø.89
  - skin or subcutaneous tissue NEC I96
  - spine, spinal (column) — *see also* Osteonecrosis, by type, vertebra
    - cord G95.19
  - spleen D73.5
  - stomach K31.89
  - stomatitis (ulcerative) A69.Ø
  - subcutaneous fat, newborn P83.88
  - subendocardial (acute) I21.4
    - chronic I25.89
  - suprarenal (capsule) (gland) E27.49
  - testis N5Ø.89
  - thymus (gland) E32.8
  - tonsil J35.8
  - trachea J39.8
  - tuberculous NEC — *see* Tuberculosis
  - tubular (acute) (anoxic) (renal) (toxic) N17.Ø
    - postprocedural N99.Ø
  - vagina N89.8
  - vertebra — *see also* Osteonecrosis, by type, vertebra
    - tuberculous A18.Ø1
  - vulva N9Ø.89
  - X-ray — *see* Necrosis, by site
- **Necrospermia** — *see* Infertility, male
- **Need** (for)
  - care provider because (of)
    - assistance with personal care Z74.1
    - continuous supervision required Z74.3
    - impaired mobility Z74.Ø9
    - no other household member able to render care Z74.2
    - specified reason NEC Z74.8
  - immunization — *see* Vaccination
  - vaccination — *see* Vaccination
- **Neglect**
  - adult
    - confirmed T74.Ø1 ☑
    - history of Z91.412
    - suspected T76.Ø1 ☑
  - child (childhood)
    - confirmed T74.Ø2 ☑
    - history of Z62.812
    - suspected T76.Ø2 ☑
  - emotional, in childhood Z62.898
  - hemispatial R41.4
  - left-sided R41.4
  - sensory R41.4
  - visuospatial R41.4
- **Neisserian infection NEC** — *see* Gonococcus
- **Nelaton's syndrome** G6Ø.8
- **Nelson's syndrome** E24.1
- **Nematodiasis** (intestinal) B82.Ø

- **Nematodiasis** — *continued*
  - Ancylostoma B76.Ø
- **Neonatal** — *see also* Newborn
  - acne L7Ø.4
  - bradycardia P29.12
  - screening, abnormal findings on — *see* Abnormal, neonatal screening
  - tachycardia P29.11
  - tooth, teeth KØØ.6
- **Neonatorum** — *see* condition
- **Neoplasia**
  - endocrine, multiple (MEN) E31.2Ø
    - type I E31.21
    - type IIA E31.22
    - type IIB E31.23
  - intraepithelial (histologically confirmed)
    - anal (AIN) (histologically confirmed) K62.82
      - grade I K62.82
      - grade II K62.82
      - severe DØ1.3
    - cervical glandular (histologically confirmed) DØ6.9
    - cervix (uteri) (CIN) (histologically confirmed) N87.9
      - glandular DØ6.9
      - grade I N87.Ø
      - grade II N87.1
      - grade III (severe dysplasia) — *see also* Carcinoma, cervix uteri, in situ DØ6.9
    - prostate (histologically confirmed) (PIN) N42.31
      - grade I N42.31
      - grade II N42.31
      - grade III (severe dysplasia) DØ7.5
    - vagina (histologically confirmed) (VAIN) N89.3
      - grade I N89.Ø
      - grade II N89.1
      - grade III (severe dysplasia) DØ7.2
    - vulva (histologically confirmed) (VIN) N9Ø.3
      - grade I N9Ø.Ø
      - grade II N9Ø.1
      - grade III (severe dysplasia) DØ7.1
- **Neoplasm, neoplastic** — *see also* Table of Neoplasms
  - lipomatous, benign — *see* Lipoma
  - malignant mast cell C96.2Ø
    - specified type NEC C96.29
  - mast cell, of uncertain behavior NEC D47.Ø9
  - myelodysplastic/myeloproliferative, unclassifiable C94.6
- **Neovascularization**
  - ciliary body — *see* Disorder, iris, vascular
  - cornea H16.4Ø- ☑
    - deep H16.44- ☑
    - ghost vessels — *see* Ghost, vessels
    - localized H16.43- ☑
    - pannus — *see* Pannus
  - iris — *see* Disorder, iris, vascular
  - retina H35.Ø5- ☑
- **Nephralgia** N23
- **Nephritis, nephritic** (albuminuric) (azotemic) (congenital) (disseminated) (epithelial) (familial) (focal) (granulomatous) (hemorrhagic) (infantile) (nonsuppurative, excretory) (uremic) NØ5.9
  - with
    - C3
      - glomerulonephritis NØ5.A
      - glomerulopathy NØ5.A
        - with dense deposit disease NØ5.6
    - dense deposit disease NØ5.6
    - diffuse
      - crescentic glomerulonephritis NØ5.7
      - endocapillary proliferative glomerulonephritis NØ5.4
      - membranous glomerulonephritis NØ5.2
      - mesangial proliferative glomerulonephritis NØ5.3
      - mesangiocapillary glomerulonephritis NØ5.5
    - edema — *see* Nephrosis
    - focal and segmental glomerular lesions NØ5.1
    - foot process disease NØ4.9
    - glomerular lesion
      - diffuse sclerosing NØ5.8
      - hypocomplementemic — *see* Nephritis, membranoproliferative
      - IgA — *see* Nephropathy, IgA
      - lobular, lobulonodular — *see* Nephritis, membranoproliferative
      - nodular — *see* Nephritis, membranoproliferative
    - lesion of
      - glomerulonephritis, proliferative NØ5.8
      - renal necrosis NØ5.9
    - minor glomerular abnormality NØ5.Ø

- **Nephritis, nephritic** — *continued*
  - with — *continued*
    - specified morphological changes NEC NØ5.8
  - acute NØØ.9
    - with
      - C3
        - glomerulonephritis NØØ.A
        - glomerulopathy NØØ.A
          - with dense deposit disease NØØ.6
      - dense deposit disease NØØ.6
      - diffuse
        - crescentic glomerulonephritis NØØ.7
        - endocapillary proliferative glomerulonephritis NØØ.4
        - membranous glomerulonephritis NØØ.2
        - mesangial proliferative glomerulonephritis NØØ.3
        - mesangiocapillary glomerulonephritis NØØ.5
      - focal and segmental glomerular lesions NØØ.1
      - minor glomerular abnormality NØØ.Ø
      - specified morphological changes NEC NØØ.8
  - amyloid E85.4 *[NØ8]*
  - antiglomerular basement membrane (anti-GBM) antibody NEC
    - in Goodpasture's syndrome M31.Ø
  - antitubular basement membrane (tubulo-interstitial) NEC N12
    - toxic — *see* Nephropathy, toxic
  - arteriolar — *see* Hypertension, kidney
  - arteriosclerotic — *see* Hypertension, kidney
  - ascending — *see* Nephritis, tubulo-interstitial
  - atrophic NØ3.9
  - Balkan (endemic) N15.Ø
  - calculous, calculus — *see* Calculus, kidney
  - cardiac — *see* Hypertension, kidney
  - cardiovascular — *see* Hypertension, kidney
  - chronic NØ3.9
    - with
      - C3
        - glomerulonephritis NØ3.A
        - glomerulopathy NØ3.A
          - with dense deposit disease NØ3.6
      - dense deposit disease NØ3.6
      - diffuse
        - crescentic glomerulonephritis NØ3.7
        - endocapillary proliferative glomerulonephritis NØ3.4
        - membranous glomerulonephritis NØ3.2
        - mesangial proliferative glomerulonephritis NØ3.3
        - mesangiocapillary glomerulonephritis NØ3.5
      - focal and segmental glomerular lesions NØ3.1
      - minor glomerular abnormality NØ3.Ø
      - specified morphological changes NEC NØ3.8
    - arteriosclerotic — *see* Hypertension, kidney
  - cirrhotic N26.9
  - complicating pregnancy O26.83- ☑
  - croupous NØØ.9
  - degenerative — *see* Nephrosis
  - diffuse sclerosing NØ5.8
  - due to
    - diabetes mellitus — *see* EØ8-E13 with .21
    - subacute bacterial endocarditis I33.Ø
    - systemic lupus erythematosus (chronic) M32.14
    - typhoid fever AØ1.Ø9
  - gonococcal (acute) (chronic) A54.21
  - hypocomplementemic — *see* Nephritis, membranoproliferative
  - IgA — *see* Nephropathy, IgA
  - immune complex (circulating) NEC NØ5.8
  - infective — *see* Nephritis, tubulo-interstitial
  - interstitial — *see* Nephritis, tubulo-interstitial
  - lead N14.3
  - membranoproliferative (diffuse) (type 1 or 3) — *see also* NØØ-NØ7 with fourth character .5 NØ5.5
    - type 2 — *see also* NØØ-NØ7 with fourth character .6 NØ5.6
  - minimal change NØ5.Ø
  - necrotic, necrotizing NEC — *see also* NØØ-NØ7 with fourth character .8 NØ5.8
  - nephrotic — *see* Nephrosis
  - nodular — *see* Nephritis, membranoproliferative
  - polycystic Q61.3
    - adult type Q61.2
    - autosomal
      - dominant Q61.2
      - recessive NEC Q61.19
    - childhood type NEC Q61.19

- **Nephritis, nephritic** — *continued*
  - polycystic — *continued*
    - infantile type NEC Q61.19
  - poststreptococcal NØ5.9
    - acute NØØ.9
    - chronic NØ3.9
    - rapidly progressive NØ1.9
  - proliferative NEC — *see also* NØØ-NØ7 with fourth character .8 NØ5.8
  - purulent — *see* Nephritis, tubulo-interstitial
  - rapidly progressive NØ1.9
    - with
      - C3
        - glomerulonephritis NØ1.A
        - glomerulopathy NØ1.A
          - with dense deposit disease NØ1.6
      - dense deposit disease NØ1.6
      - diffuse
        - crescentic glomerulonephritis NØ1.7
        - endocapillary proliferative glomerulonephritis NØ1.4
        - membranous glomerulonephritis NØ1.2
        - mesangial proliferative glomerulonephritis NØ1.3
        - mesangiocapillary glomerulonephritis NØ1.5
      - focal and segmental glomerular lesions NØ1.1
      - minor glomerular abnormality NØ1.Ø
      - specified morphological changes NEC NØ1.8
  - salt losing or wasting NEC N28.89
  - saturnine N14.3
  - sclerosing, diffuse NØ5.8
  - septic — *see* Nephritis, tubulo-interstitial
  - specified pathology NEC — *see also* NØØ-NØ7 with fourth character .8 NØ5.8
  - subacute NØ1.9
  - suppurative — *see* Nephritis, tubulo-interstitial
  - syphilitic (late) A52.75
    - congenital A5Ø.59 *[NØ8]*
    - early (secondary) A51.44
  - toxic — *see* Nephropathy, toxic
  - tubal, tubular — *see* Nephritis, tubulo-interstitial
  - tuberculous A18.11
  - tubulo-interstitial (in) N12
    - acute (infectious) N1Ø
    - chronic (infectious) N11.9
      - nonobstructive N11.8
        - reflux-associated N11.Ø
      - obstructive N11.1
      - specified NEC N11.8
    - due to
      - brucellosis A23.9 *[N16]*
      - cryoglobulinemia D89.1 *[N16]*
      - glycogen storage disease E74.ØØ *[N16]*
    - Sjögren's syndrome M35.Ø4
  - vascular — *see* Hypertension, kidney
  - war NØØ.9
- **Nephroblastoma** (epithelial) (mesenchymal) C64- ☑
- **Nephrocalcinosis** E83.59 *[N29]*
- **Nephrocystitis, pustular** — *see* Nephritis, tubulo-interstitial
- **Nephrolithiasis** (congenital) (pelvis) (recurrent) — *see also* Calculus, kidney
- **Nephroma** C64- ☑
  - mesoblastic D41.Ø- ☑
- **Nephronephritis** — *see* Nephrosis
- **Nephronophthisis** Q61.5
- **Nephropathia epidemica** A98.5
- **Nephropathy** — *see also* Nephritis N28.9
  - with
    - edema — *see* Nephrosis
    - glomerular lesion — *see* Glomerulonephritis
  - amyloid, hereditary E85.Ø
  - analgesic N14.Ø
    - with medullary necrosis, acute N17.2
  - Balkan (endemic) N15.Ø
  - chemical — *see* Nephropathy, toxic
  - contrast medium, radiography N14.11
  - contrast-induced N14.11
  - diabetic — *see* EØ8-E13 with .21
  - drug-induced N14.2
    - contrast-induced N14.11
    - specified NEC N14.19
  - focal and segmental hyalinosis or sclerosis NØ2.1
  - heavy metal-induced N14.3
  - hereditary NEC NØ7.9
    - with
      - C3
        - glomerulonephritis NØ7.A

- **Nephropathy** — *continued*
  - hereditary — *continued*
    - with — *continued*
      - C3 — *continued*
        - glomerulopathy NØ7.A
          - with dense deposit disease NØ7.6
        - dense deposit disease NØ7.6
      - diffuse
        - crescentic glomerulonephritis NØ7.7
        - endocapillary proliferative glomerulonephritis NØ7.4
        - membranous glomerulonephritis NØ7.2
        - mesangial proliferative glomerulonephritis NØ7.3
        - mesangiocapillary glomerulonephritis NØ7.5
      - focal and segmental glomerular lesions NØ7.1
      - minor glomerular abnormality NØ7.Ø
      - specified morphological changes NEC NØ7.8
  - hypercalcemic N25.89
  - hypertensive — *see* Hypertension, kidney
  - hypokalemic (vacuolar) N25.89
  - IgA NØ2.8
    - with glomerular lesion NØ2.9
      - focal and segmental hyalinosis or sclerosis NØ2.1
      - membranoproliferative (diffuse) NØ2.5
      - membranous (diffuse) NØ2.2
      - mesangial proliferative (diffuse) NØ2.3
      - mesangiocapillary (diffuse) NØ2.5
      - proliferative NEC NØ2.8
      - specified pathology NEC NØ2.8
  - lead N14.3
  - membranoproliferative (diffuse) NØ2.5
  - membranous (diffuse) NØ2.2
  - mesangial (IgA/IgG) — *see* Nephropathy, IgA
    - proliferative (diffuse) NØ2.3
  - mesangiocapillary (diffuse) NØ2.5
  - obstructive N13.8
  - phenacetin N17.2
  - phosphate-losing N25.Ø
  - potassium depletion N25.89
  - pregnancy-related O26.83- ☑
  - proliferative NEC — *see also* NØØ-NØ7 with fourth character .8 NØ5.8
  - protein-losing N25.89
  - saturnine N14.3
  - sickle-cell D57.- ☑ *[NØ8]*
  - toxic NEC N14.4
    - due to
      - drugs N14.2
        - analgesic N14.Ø
        - specified NEC N14.19
      - heavy metals N14.3
  - vasomotor N17.Ø
  - water-losing N25.89
- **Nephroptosis** N28.83
- **Nephropyosis** — *see* Abscess, kidney
- **Nephrorrhagia** N28.89
- **Nephrosclerosis** (arteriolar) (arteriosclerotic) (chronic) (hyaline) — *see also* Hypertension, kidney
  - hyperplastic — *see* Hypertension, kidney
  - senile N26.9
- **Nephrosis, nephrotic** (Epstein's) (syndrome) (congenital) NØ4.9
  - with
    - foot process disease NØ4.9
    - glomerular lesion NØ4.1
    - hypocomplementemic NØ4.5
  - acute NØ4.9
  - anoxic — *see* Nephrosis, tubular
  - chemical — *see* Nephrosis, tubular
  - cholemic K76.7
  - diabetic — *see* EØ8-E13 with .21
  - Finnish type (congenital) Q89.8
  - hemoglobin N1Ø
  - hemoglobinuric — *see* Nephrosis, tubular
  - in
    - amyloidosis E85.4 *[NØ8]*
    - diabetes mellitus — *see* EØ8-E13 with .21
    - epidemic hemorrhagic fever A98.5
    - malaria (malariae) B52.Ø
  - ischemic — *see* Nephrosis, tubular
  - lipoid NØ4.9
  - lower nephron — *see* Nephrosis, tubular
  - malarial (malariae) B52.Ø
  - minimal change NØ4.Ø
  - myoglobin N1Ø
  - necrotizing — *see* Nephrosis, tubular
  - osmotic (sucrose) N25.89
- **Nephrosis, nephrotic** — *continued*
  - radiation NØ4.9
  - syphilitic (late) A52.75
  - toxic — *see* Nephrosis, tubular
  - tubular (acute) N17.Ø
    - postprocedural N99.Ø
    - radiation NØ4.9
- **Nephrosonephritis, hemorrhagic** (endemic) A98.5
- **Nephrostomy**
  - attention to Z43.6
  - status Z93.6
- **Nerve** — *see also* condition
  - injury — *see* Injury, nerve, by body site
- **Nerves** R45.Ø
- **Nervous** — *see also* condition R45.Ø
  - heart F45.8
  - stomach F45.8
  - tension R45.Ø
- **Nervousness** R45.Ø
- **Nesidioblastoma**
  - pancreas D13.7
  - specified site NEC — *see* Neoplasm, benign, by site
  - unspecified site D13.7
- **Nettleship's syndrome** — *see* Urticaria pigmentosa
- **Neumann's disease or syndrome** L1Ø.1
- **Neuralgia, neuralgic** (acute) M79.2
  - accessory (nerve) G52.8
  - acoustic (nerve) — *see* subcategory H93.3 ☑
  - auditory (nerve) — *see* subcategory H93.3 ☑
  - ciliary G44.ØØ9
    - intractable G44.ØØ1
    - not intractable G44.ØØ9
  - cranial
    - nerve — *see also* Disorder, nerve, cranial
      - fifth or trigeminal — *see* Neuralgia, trigeminal
    - postherpetic, postzoster BØ2.29
  - ear — *see* subcategory H92.Ø ☑
  - facialis vera G51.1
  - Fothergill's — *see* Neuralgia, trigeminal
  - glossopharyngeal (nerve) G52.1
  - Horton's G44.Ø99
    - intractable G44.Ø91
    - not intractable G44.Ø99
  - Hunt's BØ2.21
  - hypoglossal (nerve) G52.3
  - infraorbital — *see* Neuralgia, trigeminal
  - malarial — *see* Malaria
  - migrainous G44.ØØ9
    - intractable G44.ØØ1
    - not intractable G44.ØØ9
  - Morton's G57.6- ☑
  - nerve, cranial — *see* Disorder, nerve, cranial
  - nose G52.Ø
  - occipital M54.81
  - olfactory G52.Ø
  - penis N48.9
  - perineum R1Ø.2
  - postherpetic NEC BØ2.29
    - trigeminal BØ2.22
  - pubic region R1Ø.2
  - scrotum R1Ø.2
  - Sluder's G44.89
  - specified nerve NEC G58.8
  - spermatic cord R1Ø.2
  - sphenopalatine (ganglion) G9Ø.Ø9
  - trifacial — *see* Neuralgia, trigeminal
  - trigeminal G5Ø.Ø
    - postherpetic, postzoster BØ2.22
  - vagus (nerve) G52.2
  - writer's F48.8
    - organic G25.89
- **Neurapraxia** — *see* Injury, nerve
- **Neurasthenia** F48.8
  - cardiac F45.8
  - gastric F45.8
  - heart F45.8
- **Neurilemmoma** — *see also* Neoplasm, nerve, benign
  - acoustic (nerve) D33.3
  - malignant — *see also* Neoplasm, nerve, malignant
    - acoustic (nerve) C72.4- ☑
- **Neurilemmosarcoma** — *see* Neoplasm, nerve, malignant
- **Neurinoma** — *see* Neoplasm, nerve, benign
- **Neurinomatosis** — *see* Neoplasm, nerve, uncertain behavior
- **Neuritis** (rheumatoid) M79.2
  - abducens (nerve) — *see* Strabismus, paralytic, sixth nerve
  - accessory (nerve) G52.8
- **Neuritis** — *continued*
  - acoustic (nerve) — *see also* subcategory H93.3 ☑
    - in (due to)
      - infectious disease NEC B99 ☑ *[H94.Ø-]* ☑
      - parasitic disease NEC B89 *[H94.Ø-]* ☑
    - syphilitic A52.15
  - alcoholic G62.1
    - with psychosis — *see* Psychosis, alcoholic
  - amyloid, any site E85.4 *[G63]*
  - auditory (nerve) — *see* subcategory H93.3 ☑
  - brachial — *see* Radiculopathy
    - due to displacement, intervertebral disc — *see* Disorder, disc, cervical, with neuritis
  - cranial nerve
    - due to Lyme disease A69.22
    - eighth or acoustic or auditory — *see* subcategory H93.3 ☑
    - eleventh or accessory G52.8
    - fifth or trigeminal G5Ø.- ☑
    - first or olfactory G52.Ø
    - fourth or trochlear — *see* Strabismus, paralytic, fourth nerve
    - second or optic — *see* Neuritis, optic
    - seventh or facial G51.8
      - newborn (birth injury) P11.3
    - sixth or abducent — *see* Strabismus, paralytic, sixth nerve
    - tenth or vagus G52.2
    - third or oculomotor — *see* Strabismus, paralytic, third nerve
    - twelfth or hypoglossal G52.3
  - Déjérine-Sottas G6Ø.Ø
  - diabetic (mononeuropathy) — *see* EØ8-E13 with .41
    - polyneuropathy — *see* EØ8-E13 with .42
  - due to
    - beriberi E51.11
    - displacement, prolapse or rupture, intervertebral disc — *see* Disorder, disc, with, radiculopathy
    - herniation, nucleus pulposus M51.9 *[G55]*
  - endemic E51.11
  - facial G51.8
    - newborn (birth injury) P11.3
  - general — *see* Polyneuropathy
  - geniculate ganglion G51.1
    - due to herpes (zoster) BØ2.21
  - gouty — *see also* Gout, by type M1Ø.9 *[G63]*
  - hypoglossal (nerve) G52.3
  - ilioinguinal (nerve) G57.9- ☑
  - infectious (multiple) NEC G61.Ø
  - interstitial hypertrophic progressive G6Ø.Ø
  - lumbar M54.16
  - lumbosacral M54.17
  - multiple — *see also* Polyneuropathy
    - endemic E51.11
    - infective, acute G61.Ø
  - multiplex endemica E51.11
  - nerve root — *see* Radiculopathy
  - oculomotor (nerve) — *see* Strabismus, paralytic, third nerve
  - olfactory nerve G52.Ø
  - optic (nerve) (hereditary) (sympathetic) H46.9
    - with demyelination G36.Ø
    - in myelitis G36.Ø
    - nutritional H46.2
    - papillitis — *see* Papillitis, optic
    - retrobulbar H46.1- ☑
    - specified type NEC H46.8
    - toxic H46.3
  - peripheral (nerve) G62.9
    - multiple — *see* Polyneuropathy
    - single — *see* Mononeuritis
  - pneumogastric (nerve) G52.2
  - postherpetic, postzoster BØ2.29
  - progressive hypertrophic interstitial G6Ø.Ø
  - retrobulbar — *see also* Neuritis, optic, retrobulbar
    - in (due to)
      - late syphilis A52.15
      - meningococcal infection A39.82
    - meningococcal A39.82
    - syphilitic A52.15
  - sciatic (nerve) — *see also* Sciatica
    - due to displacement of intervertebral disc — *see* Disorder, disc, with, radiculopathy
  - serum — *see also* Reaction, serum T8Ø.69 ☑
  - shoulder-girdle G54.5
  - specified nerve NEC G58.8
  - spinal (nerve) root — *see* Radiculopathy
  - syphilitic A52.15

Neuritis — *continued*
- thenar (median) G56.1- ☑
- thoracic M54.14
- toxic NEC G62.2
- trochlear (nerve) — *see* Strabismus, paralytic, fourth nerve
- vagus (nerve) G52.2

Neuroastrocytoma — *see* Neoplasm, uncertain behavior, by site
Neuroavitaminosis E56.9 *[G99.8]*
Neuroblastoma
- olfactory C3Ø.Ø
- specified site — *see* Neoplasm, malignant, by site
- unspecified site C74.9Ø

Neurochorioretinitis — *see* Chorioretinitis
Neurocirculatory asthenia F45.8
Neurocysticercosis B69.Ø
Neurocytoma — *see* Neoplasm, benign, by site
Neurodermatitis (circumscribed) (circumscripta) (local) L28.Ø
- atopic L2Ø.81
- diffuse (Brocq) L2Ø.81
- disseminated L2Ø.81

Neuroencephalomyelopathy, optic G36.Ø
Neuroepithelioma — *see also* Neoplasm, malignant, by site
- olfactory C3Ø.Ø

Neurofibroma — *see also* Neoplasm, nerve, benign
- melanotic — *see* Neoplasm, nerve, benign
- multiple — *see* Neurofibromatosis
- plexiform — *see* Neoplasm, nerve, benign

Neurofibromatosis (multiple) (nonmalignant) Q85.ØØ
- acoustic Q85.Ø2
- malignant — *see* Neoplasm, nerve, malignant
- specified NEC Q85.Ø9
- type 1 (von Recklinghausen) Q85.Ø1
- type 2 Q85.Ø2

Neurofibrosarcoma — *see* Neoplasm, nerve, malignant
Neurogenic — *see also* condition
- bladder — *see also* Dysfunction, bladder, neuromuscular N31.9
  - cauda equina syndrome G83.4
- bowel NEC K59.2
- heart F45.8

Neuroglioma — *see* Neoplasm, uncertain behavior, by site
Neurolabyrinthitis (of Dix and Hallpike) — *see* Neuronitis, vestibular
Neurolathyrism — *see* Poisoning, food, noxious, plant
Neuroleprosy A3Ø.9
Neuroma — *see also* Neoplasm, nerve, benign
- acoustic (nerve) D33.3
- amputation (stump) (traumatic) (surgical complication) (late) T87.3- ☑
  - arm T87.3- ☑
  - leg T87.3- ☑
- digital (toe) G57.6- ☑
- interdigital G58.8
  - lower limb (toe) G57.8- ☑
  - upper limb G56.8- ☑
- intermetatarsal G57.8- ☑
- Morton's G57.6- ☑
- nonneoplastic
  - arm G56.9- ☑
  - leg G57.9- ☑
  - lower extremity G57.9- ☑
  - upper extremity G56.9- ☑
- optic (nerve) D33.3
- plantar G57.6- ☑
- plexiform — *see* Neoplasm, nerve, benign
- surgical (nonneoplastic)
  - arm G56.9- ☑
  - leg G57.9- ☑
  - lower extremity G57.9- ☑
  - upper extremity G56.9- ☑

Neuromyalgia — *see* Neuralgia
Neuromyasthenia (epidemic) (postinfectious) G93.39
Neuromyelitis G36.9
- ascending G61.Ø
- optica G36.Ø

Neuromyopathy G7Ø.9
- paraneoplastic D49.9 *[G13.Ø]*

Neuromyotonia (Isaacs) G71.19
Neuronevus — *see* Nevus
Neuronitis G58.9
- ascending (acute) G57.2- ☑
- vestibular H81.2- ☑

Neuroparalytic — *see* condition
Neuropathy, neuropathic G62.9
- acute motor G62.81
- alcoholic G62.1
  - with psychosis — *see* Psychosis, alcoholic
- arm G56.9- ☑
- autonomic, peripheral — *see* Neuropathy, peripheral, autonomic
- axillary G56.9- ☑
- bladder N31.9
  - atonic (motor) (sensory) N31.2
  - autonomous N31.2
  - flaccid N31.2
  - nonreflex N31.2
  - reflex N31.1
  - uninhibited N31.Ø
- brachial plexus G54.Ø
- cervical plexus G54.2
- chronic
  - progressive segmentally demyelinating G62.89
  - relapsing demyelinating G62.89
- Déjérine-Sottas G6Ø.Ø
- diabetic — *see* EØ8-E13 with .4Ø
  - mononeuropathy — *see* EØ8-E13 with .41
  - polyneuropathy — *see* EØ8-E13 with .42
- entrapment G58.9
  - iliohypogastric nerve G57.8- ☑
  - ilioinguinal nerve G57.8- ☑
  - lateral cutaneous nerve of thigh G57.1- ☑
  - median nerve G56.Ø- ☑
  - obturator nerve G57.8- ☑
  - peroneal nerve G57.3- ☑
  - posterior tibial nerve G57.5- ☑
  - saphenous nerve G57.8- ☑
  - ulnar nerve G56.2- ☑
- facial nerve G51.9
- hereditary G6Ø.9
  - motor and sensory (types I-IV) G6Ø.Ø
  - sensory G6Ø.8
  - specified NEC G6Ø.8
- hypertrophic G6Ø.Ø
  - Charcot-Marie-Tooth G6Ø.Ø
  - Déjérine-Sottas G6Ø.Ø
  - interstitial progressive G6Ø.Ø
  - of infancy G6Ø.Ø
  - Refsum G6Ø.1
- idiopathic G6Ø.9
  - progressive G6Ø.3
  - specified NEC G6Ø.8
- in association with hereditary ataxia G6Ø.2
- intercostal G58.Ø
- ischemic — *see* Disorder, nerve
- Jamaica (ginger) G62.2
- leg NEC G57.9- ☑
- lower extremity G57.9- ☑
- lumbar plexus G54.1
- median nerve G56.1- ☑
- motor and sensory — *see also* Polyneuropathy
  - hereditary (types I-IV) G6Ø.Ø
- multifocal motor (MMN) G61.82
- multiple (acute) (chronic) — *see* Polyneuropathy
- optic (nerve) — *see also* Neuritis, optic
  - ischemic H47.Ø1- ☑
- paraneoplastic (sensorial) (Denny Brown) D49.9 *[G13.Ø]*
- peripheral (nerve) — *see also* Polyneuropathy G62.9
  - autonomic G9Ø.9
    - idiopathic G9Ø.Ø9
    - in (due to)
      - amyloidosis E85.4 *[G99.Ø]*
      - diabetes mellitus — *see* EØ8-E13 with .43
      - endocrine disease NEC E34.9 *[G99.Ø]*
      - gout M1Ø.ØØ *[G99.Ø]*
      - hyperthyroidism EØ5.9Ø *[G99.Ø]*
        - with thyroid storm EØ5.91 *[G99.Ø]*
      - metabolic disease NEC E88.9 *[G99.Ø]*
  - idiopathic G6Ø.9
    - progressive G6Ø.3
  - in (due to)
    - antitetanus serum G62.Ø
    - arsenic G62.2
    - drugs NEC G62.Ø
    - lead G62.2
    - organophosphate compounds G62.2
    - toxic agent NEC G62.2
- plantar nerves G57.6- ☑
- progressive
  - hypertrophic interstitial G6Ø.Ø

Neuropathy, neuropathic — *continued*
- progressive — *continued*
  - inflammatory G62.81
- radicular NEC — *see* Radiculopathy
- sacral plexus G54.1
- sciatic G57.Ø- ☑
- serum G61.1
- toxic NEC G62.2
- trigeminal sensory G5Ø.8
- ulnar nerve G56.2- ☑
- uremic N18.9 *[G63]*
- vitamin B12 E53.8 *[G63]*
  - with anemia (pernicious) D51.Ø *[G63]*
    - due to dietary deficiency D51.3 *[G63]*

Neurophthisis — *see also* Disorder, nerve
- peripheral, diabetic — *see* EØ8-E13 with .42

Neuroretinitis — *see* Chorioretinitis
Neuroretinopathy, hereditary optic H47.22
Neurosarcoma — *see* Neoplasm, nerve, malignant
Neurosclerosis — *see* Disorder, nerve
Neurosis, neurotic F48.9
- anankastic F42.8
- anxiety (state) F41.1
  - panic type F41.Ø
- asthenic F48.8
- bladder F45.8
- cardiac (reflex) F45.8
- cardiovascular F45.8
- character F6Ø.9
- colon F45.8
- compensation F68.1Ø
- compulsive, compulsion F42.8
- conversion F44.9
- craft F48.8
- cutaneous F45.8
- depersonalization F48.1
- depressive (reaction) (type) F34.1
- environmental F48.8
- excoriation L98.1
- fatigue F48.8
- functional — *see* Disorder, somatoform
- gastric F45.8
- gastrointestinal F45.8
- heart F45.8
- hypochondriacal F45.21
- hysterical F44.9
- incoordination F45.8
  - larynx F45.8
  - vocal cord F45.8
- intestine F45.8
- larynx (sensory) F45.8
  - hysterical F44.4
- mixed NEC F48.8
- musculoskeletal F45.8
- obsessional F42.8
- obsessive-compulsive F42.8
- occupational F48.8
- ocular NEC F45.8
- organ — *see* Disorder, somatoform
- pharynx F45.8
- phobic F4Ø.9
- posttraumatic (situational) F43.1Ø
  - acute F43.11
  - chronic F43.12
- psychasthenic (type) F48.8
- railroad F48.8
- rectum F45.8
- respiratory F45.8
- rumination F45.8
- sexual F65.9
- situational F48.8
- social F4Ø.1Ø
  - generalized F4Ø.11
- specified type NEC F48.8
- state F48.9
  - with depersonalization episode F48.1
- stomach F45.8
- traumatic F43.1Ø
  - acute F43.11
  - chronic F43.12
- vasomotor F45.8
- visceral F45.8
- war F48.8

Neurospongioblastosis diffusa Q85.1
Neurosyphilis (arrested) (early) (gumma) (late) (latent) (recurrent) (relapse) A52.3
- with ataxia (cerebellar) (locomotor) (spastic) (spinal) A52.19

Neurosyphilis — *continued*
  aneurysm (cerebral) A52.Ø5
  arachnoid (adhesive) A52.13
  arteritis (any artery) (cerebral) A52.Ø4
  asymptomatic A52.2
  congenital A5Ø.4Ø
  dura (mater) A52.13
  general paresis A52.17
  hemorrhagic A52.Ø5
  juvenile (asymptomatic) (meningeal) A5Ø.4Ø
  leptomeninges (aseptic) A52.13
  meningeal, meninges (adhesive) A52.13
  meningitis A52.13
  meningovascular (diffuse) A52.13
  optic atrophy A52.15
  parenchymatous (degenerative) A52.19
  paresis, paretic A52.17
    juvenile A5Ø.45
  remission in (sustained) A52.3
  serological (without symptoms) A52.2
  specified nature or site NEC A52.19
  tabes, tabetic (dorsalis) A52.11
    juvenile A5Ø.45
  taboparesis A52.17
    juvenile A5Ø.45
  thrombosis (cerebral) A52.Ø5
  vascular (cerebral) NEC A52.Ø5
Neurothekeoma — *see* Neoplasm, nerve, benign
Neurotic — *see* Neurosis
Neurotoxemia — *see* Toxemia
Neutroclusion M26.211
Neutropenia, neutropenic (chronic) (genetic) (idiopathic) (immune) (infantile) (malignant) (pernicious) (splenic) D7Ø.9
  congenital (primary) D7Ø.Ø
  cyclic D7Ø.4
  cytoreductive cancer chemotherapy sequela D7Ø.1
  drug-induced D7Ø.2
    due to cytoreductive cancer chemotherapy D7Ø.1
  due to infection D7Ø.3
  fever D7Ø.9
  neonatal, transitory (isoimmune) (maternal transfer) P61.5
  periodic D7Ø.4
  secondary (cyclic) (periodic) (splenic) D7Ø.4
    drug-induced D7Ø.2
      due to cytoreductive cancer chemotherapy D7Ø.1
  toxic D7Ø.8
Neutrophilia, hereditary giant D72.Ø
Nevocarcinoma — *see* Melanoma
Nevus D22.9
  achromic — *see* Neoplasm, skin, benign
  amelanotic — *see* Neoplasm, skin, benign
  angiomatous D18.ØØ
    intra-abdominal D18.Ø3
    intracranial D18.Ø2
    skin D18.Ø1
    specified site NEC D18.Ø9
  araneus I78.1
  balloon cell — *see* Neoplasm, skin, benign
  bathing trunk D48.5
  blue — *see* Neoplasm, skin, benign
    cellular — *see* Neoplasm, skin, benign
    giant — *see* Neoplasm, skin, benign
    Jadassohn's — *see* Neoplasm, skin, benign
    malignant — *see* Melanoma
  capillary D18.ØØ
    intra-abdominal D18.Ø3
    intracranial D18.Ø2
    skin D18.Ø1
    specified site NEC D18.Ø9
  cavernous D18.ØØ
    intra-abdominal D18.Ø3
    intracranial D18.Ø2
    skin D18.Ø1
    specified site NEC D18.Ø9
  cellular — *see* Neoplasm, skin, benign
    blue — *see* Neoplasm, skin, benign
  choroid D31.3- ☑
  comedonicus Q82.5
  conjunctiva D31.Ø- ☑
  dermal — *see* Neoplasm, skin, benign
    with epidermal nevus — *see* Neoplasm, skin, benign
  dysplastic — *see* Neoplasm, skin, benign
  eye D31.9- ☑
  flammeus Q82.5
  hemangiomatous D18.ØØ
    intra-abdominal D18.Ø3
Nevus — *continued*
  hemangiomatous — *continued*
    intracranial D18.Ø2
    skin D18.Ø1
    specified site NEC D18.Ø9
  iris D31.4- ☑
  lacrimal gland D31.5- ☑
  lymphatic D18.1
  magnocellular
    specified site — *see* Neoplasm, benign, by site
    unspecified site D31.4Ø
  malignant — *see* Melanoma
  meaning hemangioma D18.ØØ
    intra-abdominal D18.Ø3
    intracranial D18.Ø2
    skin D18.Ø1
    specified site NEC D18.Ø9
  mouth (mucosa) D1Ø.3Ø
    specified site NEC D1Ø.39
    white sponge Q38.6
  multiplex Q85.1
  non-neoplastic I78.1
  oral mucosa D1Ø.3Ø
    specified site NEC D1Ø.39
    white sponge Q38.6
  orbit D31.6- ☑
  pigmented
    giant — *see also* Neoplasm, skin, uncertain behavior D48.5
      malignant melanoma in — *see* Melanoma
  portwine Q82.5
  retina D31.2- ☑
  retrobulbar D31.6- ☑
  sanguineous Q82.5
  senile I78.1
  skin D22.9
    abdominal wall D22.5
    ala nasi D22.39
    ankle D22.7- ☑
    anus, anal D22.5
    arm D22.6- ☑
    auditory canal (external) D22.2- ☑
    auricle (ear) D22.2- ☑
    auricular canal (external) D22.2- ☑
    axilla, axillary fold D22.5
    back D22.5
    breast D22.5
    brow D22.39
    buttock D22.5
    canthus (eye) D22.1- ☑
    cheek (external) D22.39
    chest wall D22.5
    chin D22.39
    ear (external) D22.2- ☑
    external meatus (ear) D22.2- ☑
    eyebrow D22.39
    eyelid (lower) (upper) D22.1- ☑
    face D22.3Ø
      specified NEC D22.39
    female genital organ (external) NEC D28.Ø
    finger D22.6- ☑
    flank D22.5
    foot D22.7- ☑
    forearm D22.6- ☑
    forehead D22.39
    foreskin D29.Ø
    genital organ (external) NEC
      female D28.Ø
      male D29.9
    gluteal region D22.5
    groin D22.5
    hand D22.6- ☑
    heel D22.7- ☑
    helix D22.2- ☑
    hip D22.7- ☑
    interscapular region D22.5
    jaw D22.39
    knee D22.7- ☑
    labium (majus) (minus) D28.Ø
    leg D22.7- ☑
    lip (lower) (upper) D22.Ø
    lower limb D22.7- ☑
    male genital organ (external) D29.9
    nail D22.9
      finger D22.6- ☑
      toe D22.7- ☑
    nasolabial groove D22.39
    nates D22.5
Nevus — *continued*
  skin — *continued*
    neck D22.4
    nose (external) D22.39
    palpebra D22.1- ☑
    penis D29.Ø
    perianal skin D22.5
    perineum D22.5
    pinna D22.2- ☑
    popliteal fossa or space D22.7- ☑
    prepuce D29.Ø
    pudendum D28.Ø
    scalp D22.4
    scrotum D29.4
    shoulder D22.6- ☑
    submammary fold D22.5
    temple D22.39
    thigh D22.7- ☑
    toe D22.7- ☑
    trunk NEC D22.5
    umbilicus D22.5
    upper limb D22.6- ☑
    vulva D28.Ø
  specified site NEC — *see* Neoplasm, by site, benign
  spider I78.1
  stellar I78.1
  strawberry Q82.5
  Sutton's benign D22.9
  unius lateris Q82.5
  Unna's Q82.5
  vascular Q82.5
  verrucous Q82.5
Newborn (infant) (liveborn) (singleton) Z38.2
  abstinence syndrome P96.1
  acne L7Ø.4
  affected by
    abnormalities of membranes PØ2.9
      specified NEC PØ2.8
    abruptio placenta PØ2.1
    amino-acid metabolic disorder, transitory P74.8
    amniocentesis (while in utero) PØØ.6
    amnionitis PØ2.78
    apparent life threatening event (ALTE) R68.13
    bleeding (into)
      cerebral cortex P52.22
      germinal matrix P52.Ø
      ventricles P52.1
    breech delivery PØ3.Ø
    cardiac arrest P29.81
    cardiomyopathy I42.8
      congenital I42.4
    cerebral ischemia P91.Ø
    Cesarean delivery PØ3.4
    chemotherapy agents PØ4.11
    chorioamnionitis PØ2.78
    cocaine (crack) PØ4.41
    complications of labor and delivery PØ3.9
      specified NEC PØ3.89
    compression of umbilical cord NEC PØ2.5
    contracted pelvis PØ3.1
    cyanosis P28.2
    delivery PØ3.9
      Cesarean PØ3.4
      forceps PØ3.2
      vacuum extractor PØ3.3
    drugs of addiction PØ4.4Ø
      cocaine PØ4.41
      hallucinogens PØ4.42
      specified drug NEC PØ4.49
    entanglement (knot) in umbilical cord PØ2.5
    environmental chemicals PØ4.6
    fetal (intrauterine)
      growth retardation PØ5.9
      inflammatory response syndrome (FIRS) PØ2.7Ø
      malnutrition not light or small for gestational age PØ5.2
    FIRS (fetal inflammatory response syndrome) PØ2.7Ø
    forceps delivery PØ3.2
    heart rate abnormalities
      bradycardia P29.12
      intrauterine PØ3.819
        before onset of labor PØ3.81Ø
        during labor PØ3.811
      tachycardia P29.11
    hemorrhage (antepartum) PØ2.1
      cerebellar (nontraumatic) P52.6
      intracerebral (nontraumatic) P52.4
      intracranial (nontraumatic) P52.9

- **Newborn** — *continued*
  - affected by — *continued*
    - hemorrhage — *continued*
      - intracranial — *continued*
        - specified NEC P52.8
      - intraventricular (nontraumatic) P52.3
        - grade 1 P52.Ø
        - grade 2 P52.1
        - grade 3 P52.21
        - grade 4 P52.22
      - posterior fossa (nontraumatic) P52.6
      - subarachnoid (nontraumatic) P52.5
      - subependymal P52.Ø
        - with intracerebral extension P52.22
        - with intraventricular extension P52.1
          - with enlargment of ventricles P52.21
        - without intraventricular extension P52.Ø
    - hypoxic ischemic encephalopathy [HIE] P91.6Ø
      - mild P91.61
      - moderate P91.62
      - severe P91.63
    - induction of labor PØ3.89
    - intestinal perforation P78.Ø
    - intrauterine (fetal) blood loss P5Ø.9
      - due to (from)
        - cut end of co-twin cord P5Ø.5
        - hemorrhage into
          - co-twin P5Ø.3
          - maternal circulation P5Ø.4
        - placenta P5Ø.2
        - ruptured cord blood P5Ø.1
        - vasa previa P5Ø.Ø
      - specified NEC P5Ø.8
    - intrauterine (fetal) hemorrhage P5Ø.9
    - intrauterine (in utero) procedure P96.5
    - malpresentation (malposition) NEC PØ3.1
    - maternal (complication of) (use of)
      - alcohol PØ4.3
      - amphetamines PØ4.16
      - analgesia (maternal) PØ4.Ø
      - anesthesia (maternal) PØ4.Ø
      - anticonvulsants PØ4.13
      - antidepressants PØ4.15
      - antineoplastic chemotherapy PØ4.11
      - anxiolytics PØ4.1A
      - blood loss PØ2.1
      - cannabis PØ4.81
      - circulatory disease PØØ.3
      - condition PØØ.9
        - specified NEC PØØ.89
      - cytotoxic drugs PØ4.12
      - delivery PØ3.9
        - Cesarean PØ3.4
        - forceps PØ3.2
        - vacuum extractor PØ3.3
      - diabetes mellitus (pre-existing) P7Ø.1
      - disorder PØØ.9
        - specified NEC PØØ.89
      - drugs (addictive) (illegal) NEC PØ4.49
      - ectopic pregnancy PØ1.4
      - gestational diabetes P7Ø.Ø
      - group B streptococcus (GBS) colonization (positive) PØØ.82
      - hemorrhage PØ2.1
      - hypertensive disorder PØØ.Ø
      - incompetent cervix PØ1.Ø
      - infectious disease PØØ.2
      - injury PØØ.5
      - labor and delivery PØ3.9
      - malpresentation before labor PØ1.7
      - maternal death PØ1.6
      - medical procedure PØØ.7
      - medication PØ4.19
        - specified type NEC PØ4.18
      - multiple pregnancy PØ1.5
      - nutritional disorder PØØ.4
      - oligohydramnios PØ1.2
      - opiates PØ4.14
        - administered for procedures during pregnancy or labor and delivery PØ4.Ø
      - parasitic disease PØØ.2
      - periodontal disease PØØ.81
      - placenta previa PØ2.Ø
      - polyhydramnios PØ1.3
      - precipitate delivery PØ3.5
      - pregnancy PØ1.9
        - specified PØ1.8
      - premature rupture of membranes PØ1.1
      - renal disease PØØ.1
      - respiratory disease PØØ.3
      - sedative-hypnotics PØ4.17
      - surgical procedure PØØ.6
      - tranquilizers administered for procedures during pregnancy or labor and delivery PØ4.Ø
      - urinary tract disease PØØ.1
      - uterine contraction (abnormal) PØ3.6
    - meconium peritonitis P78.Ø
    - medication (legal) (maternal use) (prescribed) PØ4.19
    - membrane abnormalities PØ2.9
      - specified NEC PØ2.8
    - membranitis PØ2.78
    - methamphetamine(s) PØ4.49
    - mixed metabolic and respiratory acidosis P84
    - neonatal abstinence syndrome P96.1
    - noxious substances transmitted via placenta or breast milk PØ4.9
      - cannabis PØ4.81
      - specified NEC PØ4.89
    - nutritional supplements PØ4.5
    - placenta previa PØ2.Ø
    - placental
      - abnormality (functional) (morphological) PØ2.2Ø
        - specified NEC PØ2.29
      - dysfunction PØ2.29
      - infarction PØ2.29
      - insufficiency PØ2.29
      - separation NEC PØ2.1
      - transfusion syndromes PØ2.3
    - placentitis PØ2.78
    - precipitate delivery PØ3.5
    - prolapsed cord PØ2.4
    - respiratory arrest P28.81
    - slow intrauterine growth PØ5.9
    - tobacco PØ4.2
    - twin to twin transplacental transfusion PØ2.3
    - umbilical cord (tightly) around neck PØ2.5
    - umbilical cord condition PØ2.6Ø
      - short cord PØ2.69
      - specified NEC PØ2.69
    - uterine contractions (abnormal) PØ3.6
    - vasa previa PØ2.69
      - from intrauterine blood loss P5Ø.Ø
  - apnea — *see also* Apnea, newborn P28.4Ø
    - obstructive P28.42
    - primary — *see also* Apnea, newborn, sleep, primary P28.3Ø
    - sleep (central) (obstructive) (primary) — *see also* Apnea, newborn, sleep, primary P28.3Ø
  - born in hospital Z38.ØØ
    - by cesarean Z38.Ø1
  - born outside hospital Z38.1
  - breast buds P96.89
  - breast engorgement P83.4
  - check-up — *see* Newborn, examination
  - convulsion P9Ø
  - dehydration P74.1
  - examination
    - 8 to 28 days old ZØØ.111
    - under 8 days old ZØØ.11Ø
  - fever P81.9
    - environmentally-induced P81.Ø
  - hyperbilirubinemia P59.9
    - of prematurity P59.Ø
  - hypernatremia P74.21
  - hyponatremia P74.22
  - infection P39.9
    - candidal P37.5
    - specified NEC P39.8
    - urinary tract P39.3
  - jaundice P59.9
    - due to
      - breast milk inhibitor P59.3
      - hepatocellular damage P59.2Ø
        - specified NEC P59.29
      - preterm delivery P59.Ø
    - of prematurity P59.Ø
    - specified NEC P59.8
  - late metabolic acidosis P74.Ø
  - mastitis P39.Ø
    - infective P39.Ø
    - noninfective P83.4
  - multiple born NEC Z38.8
    - born in hospital Z38.68
      - by cesarean Z38.69
    - born outside hospital Z38.7
  - omphalitis P38.9
    - with mild hemorrhage P38.1
    - without hemorrhage P38.9
  - post-term PØ8.21
  - prolonged gestation (over 42 completed weeks) PØ8.22
  - quadruplet Z38.8
    - born in hospital Z38.63
      - by cesarean Z38.64
    - born outside hospital Z38.7
  - quintuplet Z38.8
    - born in hospital Z38.65
      - by cesarean Z38.66
    - born outside hospital Z38.7
  - seizure P9Ø
  - sepsis (congenital) P36.9
    - due to
      - anaerobes NEC P36.5
      - Escherichia coli P36.4
      - Staphylococcus P36.3Ø
        - aureus P36.2
        - specified NEC P36.39
      - Streptococcus P36.1Ø
        - group B P36.Ø
        - specified NEC P36.19
    - specified NEC P36.8
  - triplet Z38.8
    - born in hospital Z38.61
      - by cesarean Z38.62
    - born outside hospital Z38.7
  - twin Z38.5
    - born in hospital Z38.3Ø
      - by cesarean Z38.31
    - born outside hospital Z38.4
  - vomiting P92.Ø9
    - bilious P92.Ø1
  - weight check ZØØ.111
- **Newcastle conjunctivitis or disease** B3Ø.8
- **Nezelof's syndrome** (pure alymphocytosis) D81.4
- **Niacin** (amide) **deficiency** E52
- **Nicolas** (-Durand)**-Favre disease** A55
- **Nicotine** — *see* Tobacco
- **Nicotinic acid deficiency** E52
- **Niemann-Pick disease or syndrome** E75.249
  - specified NEC E75.248
  - type
    - A E75.24Ø
    - A/B E75.244
    - B E75.241
    - C E75.242
    - D E75.243
- **Night**
  - blindness — *see* Blindness, night
  - sweats R61
  - terrors (child) F51.4
- **Nightmares** (REM sleep type) F51.5
- **NIHSS** (National Institutes of Health Stroke Scale) **score** R29.7- ☑
- **Nipple** — *see* condition
- **Nisbet's chancre** A57
- **Nishimoto** (-Takeuchi) **disease** I67.5
- **Nitritoid crisis or reaction** — *see* Crisis, nitritoid
- **Nitrosohemoglobinemia** D74.8
- **Njovera** A65
- **No general equivalence degree** (GED) Z55.5
- **Nocardiosis, nocardiasis** A43.9
  - cutaneous A43.1
  - lung A43.Ø
  - pneumonia A43.Ø
  - pulmonary A43.Ø
  - specified site NEC A43.8
- **Nocturia** R35.1
  - psychogenic F45.8
- **Nocturnal** — *see* condition
- **Nodal rhythm** I49.8
- **Node**(s) — *see also* Nodule
  - Bouchard's (with arthropathy) M15.2
  - Haygarth's M15.8
  - Heberden's (with arthropathy) M15.1
  - larynx J38.7
  - lymph — *see* condition
  - milker's BØ8.Ø3
  - Osler's I33.Ø
  - Schmorl's — *see* Schmorl's disease
  - singer's J38.2
  - teacher's J38.2

- **Node(s)** — *continued*
  - tuberculous — *see* Tuberculosis, lymph gland
  - vocal cord J38.2
- **Nodule**(s), **nodular**
  - actinomycotic — *see* Actinomycosis
  - breast NEC — *see also* Lump, breast N63.Ø
  - colloid (cystic), thyroid EØ4.1
  - cutaneous — *see* Swelling, localized
  - endometrial (stromal) D26.1
  - Haygarth's M15.8
  - inflammatory — *see* Inflammation
  - juxta-articular
    - syphilitic A52.77
    - yaws A66.7
  - larynx J38.7
  - lung, solitary (subsegmental branch of the bronchial tree) R91.1
    - multiple R91.8
  - milker's BØ8.Ø3
  - prostate N4Ø.2
    - with lower urinary tract symptoms (LUTS) N4Ø.3
    - without lower urinary tract symtpoms (LUTS) N4Ø.2
  - pulmonary, solitary (subsegmental branch of the bronchial tree) R91.1
  - retrocardiac RØ9.89
  - rheumatoid MØ6.3Ø
    - ankle MØ6.37- ☑
    - elbow MØ6.32- ☑
    - foot joint MØ6.37- ☑
    - hand joint MØ6.34- ☑
    - hip MØ6.35- ☑
    - knee MØ6.36- ☑
    - multiple site MØ6.39
    - shoulder MØ6.31- ☑
    - vertebra MØ6.38
    - wrist MØ6.33- ☑
  - scrotum (inflammatory) N49.2
  - singer's J38.2
  - solitary, lung (subsegmental branch of the bronchial tree) R91.1
    - multiple R91.8
  - subcutaneous — *see* Swelling, localized
  - teacher's J38.2
  - thyroid (cold) (gland) (nontoxic) EØ4.1
    - with thyrotoxicosis EØ5.2Ø
      - with thyroid storm EØ5.21
    - toxic or with hyperthyroidism EØ5.2Ø
      - with thyroid storm EØ5.21
  - vocal cord J38.2
- **Noma** (gangrenous) (hospital) (infective) A69.Ø
  - auricle I96
  - mouth A69.Ø
  - pudendi N76.89
  - vulvae N76.89
- **Nomad, nomadism** Z59.ØØ
- **NOMID** (neonatal onset multisystemic inflammatory disorder) MØ4.2
- **Nonadherence to medical treatment, specified NEC** Z91.199
  - due to
    - financial hardship Z91.19Ø
    - specified reason NEC Z91.198
- **Nonautoimmune hemolytic anemia** D59.4
  - drug-induced D59.2
- **Nonclosure** — *see also* Imperfect, closure
  - ductus arteriosus (Botallo's) Q25.Ø
  - foramen
    - botalli Q21.12
    - ovale Q21.12
- **Noncompliance** Z91.199
  - with
    - dialysis Z91.15
    - dietary regimen Z91.119
      - due to
        - financial hardship Z91.11Ø
        - specified reason NEC Z91.118
    - medical treatment, specified NEC Z91.199
      - due to
        - financial hardship Z91.19Ø
        - specified reason NEC Z91.198
    - medication regimen NEC Z91.14
      - underdosing — *see also* Table of Drugs and Chemicals, categories T36-T5Ø, with final character 6 Z91.14
        - intentional NEC Z91.128
          - by caregiver Z91.A4
            - due to
              - financial hardship Z91.A2Ø
- **Noncompliance** — *continued*
  - with — *continued*
    - medication regimen — *continued*
      - underdosing — *see also* Table of Drugs and Chemicals, categories T36-T5Ø, with final character 6 — *continued*
        - intentional — *continued*
          - by caregiver — *continued*
            - due to — *continued*
              - specified reason NEC Z91.A28
          - due to financial hardship of patient Z91.12Ø
        - unintentional NEC Z91.138
          - by caregiver Z91.A3
          - due to patient's age related debility Z91.13Ø
    - renal dialysis Z91.15
  - caregiver
    - with patient's
      - dietary regimen
        - due to
          - financial hardship Z91.A1Ø
          - specified reason NEC Z91.A18
      - medical treatment and regimen Z91.A9
      - medication regimen, specified NEC Z91.A4
      - renal dialysis Z91.A5
- **Nondescent** (congenital) — *see also* Malposition, congenital
  - cecum Q43.3
  - colon Q43.3
  - testicle Q53.9
    - bilateral Q53.2Ø
      - abdominal Q53.211
      - perineal Q53.22
    - unilateral Q53.1Ø
      - abdominal Q53.111
      - perineal Q53.12
- **Nondevelopment**
  - brain QØ2
    - part of QØ4.3
  - heart Q24.8
  - organ or site, congenital NEC — *see* Hypoplasia
- **Nonengagement**
  - head NEC O32.4 ☑
    - in labor, causing obstructed labor O64.8 ☑
- **Nonexanthematous tick fever** A93.2
- **Nonexpansion, lung** (newborn) P28.Ø
- **Nonfunctioning**
  - cystic duct — *see also* Disease, gallbladder K82.8
  - gallbladder — *see also* Disease, gallbladder K82.8
  - kidney N28.9
  - labyrinth — *see* subcategory H83.2 ☑
- **Non-Hodgkin lymphoma NEC** — *see* Lymphoma, non-Hodgkin
- **Nonimplantation, ovum** N97.2
- **Noninsufflation, fallopian tube** N97.1
- **Non-ketotic hyperglycinemia** E72.51
- **Nonne-Milroy syndrome** Q82.Ø
- **Nonovulation** N97.Ø
- **Non-palpable testicle**(s)
  - bilateral R39.84
  - unilateral R39.83
- **Nonpatent fallopian tube** N97.1
- **Nonpneumatization, lung NEC** P28.Ø
- **Nonrotation** — *see* Malrotation
- **Nonsecretion, urine** — *see* Anuria
- **Nonunion**
  - fracture — *see* Fracture, by site
  - joint, following fusion or arthrodesis M96.Ø
  - organ or site, congenital NEC — *see* Imperfect, closure
  - symphysis pubis, congenital Q74.2
- **Nonvisualization, gallbladder** R93.2
- **Nonvital, nonvitalized tooth** KØ4.99
- **Non-working side interference** M26.56
- **Noonan's syndrome** Q87.19
- **Normocytic anemia** (infectional) due to blood loss (chronic) D5Ø.Ø
  - acute D62
- **Norrie's disease** (congenital) Q15.8
- **North American blastomycosis** B4Ø.9
- **Norwegian itch** B86
- **Nose, nasal** — *see* condition
- **Nosebleed** RØ4.Ø
- **Nose-picking** F98.8
- **Nosomania** F45.21
- **Nosophobia** F45.22
- **Nostalgia** F43.2Ø
- **Notch of iris** Q13.2
- **Notching nose, congenital** (tip) Q3Ø.2
- **Nothnagel's**
  - syndrome — *see* Strabismus, paralytic, third nerve
  - vasomotor acroparesthesia I73.89
- **Novy's relapsing fever** A68.9
  - louse-borne A68.Ø
  - tick-borne A68.1
- **Noxious**
  - foodstuffs, poisoning by — *see* Poisoning, food, noxious, plant
  - substances transmitted through placenta or breast milk PØ4.9
- **Nucleus pulposus** — *see* condition
- **Numbness** R2Ø.Ø
- **Nuns' knee** — *see* Bursitis, prepatellar
- **Nursemaid's elbow** S53.Ø3- ☑
- **Nutcracker esophagus** K22.4
- **Nutmeg liver** K76.1
- **Nutrient element deficiency** E61.9
  - specified NEC E61.8
- **Nutrition deficient or insufficient** — *see also* Malnutrition E63.9
  - due to
    - insufficient food T73.Ø ☑
    - lack of
      - care (child) T76.Ø2 ☑
        - adult T76.Ø1 ☑
      - food T73.Ø ☑
  - specific element deficiency — *see* Nutrient element deficiency, or by element
  - sequelae — *see* Sequalae, nutritional deficiency
  - specified NEC E63.8
- **Nutritional stunting** E45
- **Nyctalopia** (night blindness) — *see* Blindness, night
- **Nycturia** R35.1
  - psychogenic F45.8
- **Nymphomania** F52.8
- **Nystagmus** H55.ØØ
  - benign paroxysmal — *see* Vertigo, benign paroxysmal
  - central positional H81.4
  - congenital H55.Ø1
  - dissociated H55.Ø4
  - latent H55.Ø2
  - miners' H55.Ø9
  - positional
    - benign paroxysmal H81.4
    - central H81.4
  - specified form NEC H55.Ø9
  - visual deprivation H55.Ø3

O

- **Obermeyer's relapsing fever** (European) A68.Ø
- **Obesity** E66.9
  - with alveolar hypoventilation E66.2
  - adrenal E27.8
  - complicating
    - childbirth O99.214
    - pregnancy O99.21- ☑
    - puerperium O99.215
  - constitutional E66.8
  - dietary counseling and surveillance Z71.3
  - drug-induced E66.1
  - due to
    - drug E66.1
    - excess calories E66.Ø9
      - morbid E66.Ø1
      - severe E66.Ø1
  - endocrine E66.8
  - endogenous E66.8
  - exogenous E66.Ø9
  - familial E66.8
  - glandular E66.8
  - hypothyroid — *see* Hypothyroidism
  - hypoventilation syndrome (OHS) E66.2
  - morbid E66.Ø1
    - with
      - alveolar hypoventilation E66.2
      - obesity hypoventilation syndrome (OHS) E66.2
    - due to excess calories E66.Ø1
  - nutritional E66.Ø9
  - pituitary E23.6
  - severe E66.Ø1
  - specified type NEC E66.8
- **Oblique** — *see* condition

- **Obliteration**
  - appendix (lumen) K38.8
  - artery I77.1
  - bile duct (noncalculous) K83.1
  - common duct (noncalculous) K83.1
  - cystic duct — *see* Obstruction, gallbladder
  - disease, arteriolar I77.1
  - endometrium N85.8
  - eye, anterior chamber — *see* Disorder, globe, hypotony
  - fallopian tube N97.1
  - lymphatic vessel I89.Ø
    - due to mastectomy I97.2
  - organ or site, congenital NEC — *see* Atresia, by site
  - ureter N13.5
    - with infection N13.6
  - urethra — *see* Stricture, urethra
  - vein I87.8
  - vestibule (oral) KØ8.89
- **Observation** (following) (for) (without need for further medical care) ZØ4.9
  - accident NEC ZØ4.3
    - at work ZØ4.2
    - transport ZØ4.1
  - adverse effect of drug ZØ3.6
  - alleged rape or sexual assault (victim), ruled out
    - adult ZØ4.41
    - child ZØ4.42
  - criminal assault ZØ4.89
  - development state
    - adolescent ZØØ.3
    - period of rapid growth in childhood ZØØ.2
    - puberty ZØØ.3
  - disease, specified NEC ZØ3.89
  - following work accident ZØ4.2
  - forced sexual exploitation ZØ4.81
  - forced labor exploitation ZØ4.82
  - growth and development state — *see* Observation, development state
  - injuries (accidental) NEC — *see also* Observation, accident
  - newborn (for)
    - suspected condition, related to exposure from the mother or birth process — *see* Newborn, affected by, maternal
      - ruled out ZØ5.9
        - cardiac ZØ5.Ø
        - connective tissue ZØ5.73
        - gastrointestinal ZØ5.5
        - genetic ZØ5.41
        - genitourinary ZØ5.6
        - immunologic ZØ5.43
        - infectious ZØ5.1
        - metabolic ZØ5.42
        - musculoskeletal ZØ5.72
        - neurological ZØ5.2
        - respiratory ZØ5.3
        - skin and subcutaneous tissue ZØ5.71
        - specified condition NEC ZØ5.8
  - postpartum
    - immediately after delivery Z39.Ø
    - routine follow-up Z39.2
  - pregnancy (normal) (without complication) Z34.9- ☑
    - high risk OØ9.9- ☑
  - suicide attempt, alleged NEC ZØ3.89
    - self-poisoning ZØ3.6
  - suspected, ruled out — *see also* Suspected condition, ruled out
    - abuse, physical
      - adult ZØ4.71
      - child ZØ4.72
    - accident at work ZØ4.2
    - adult battering victim ZØ4.71
    - child battering victim ZØ4.72
    - condition NEC ZØ3.89
      - newborn — *see also* Observation, newborn (for), suspected condition, ruled out ZØ5.9
    - drug poisoning or adverse effect ZØ3.6
    - exposure (to)
      - anthrax ZØ3.81Ø
      - biological agent NEC ZØ3.818
    - foreign body
      - aspirated (inhaled) ZØ3.822
      - ingested ZØ3.821
      - inserted (injected), in (eye) (orifice) (skin) ZØ3.823
    - inflicted injury NEC ZØ4.89
    - suicide attempt, alleged ZØ3.89
      - self-poisoning ZØ3.6

- **Observation** — *continued*
  - suspected, ruled out — *see also* Suspected condition, ruled out — *continued*
    - toxic effects from ingested substance (drug) (poison) ZØ3.6
  - toxic effects from ingested substance (drug) (poison) ZØ3.6
- **Obsession, obsessional state** F42.8
  - mixed thoughts and acts F42.2
- **Obsessive-compulsive neurosis or reaction** F42.8
- **Obstetric embolism, septic** — *see* Embolism, obstetric, septic
- **Obstetrical trauma** (complicating delivery) O71.9
  - with or following ectopic or molar pregnancy OØ8.6
  - specified type NEC O71.89
- **Obstipation** — *see* Constipation
- **Obstruction, obstructed, obstructive**
  - airway J98.8
    - with
      - allergic alveolitis J67.9
      - asthma J45.9Ø9
        - with
          - exacerbation (acute) J45.9Ø1
          - status asthmaticus J45.9Ø2
      - bronchiectasis J47.9
        - with
          - exacerbation (acute) J47.1
          - lower respiratory infection J47.Ø
      - bronchitis (chronic) J44.9
      - emphysema J43.9
    - chronic J44.9
      - with
        - allergic alveolitis — *see* Pneumonitis, hypersensitivity
        - bronchiectasis J47.9
          - with
            - exacerbation (acute) J47.1
            - lower respiratory infection J47.Ø
    - due to
      - foreign body — *see* Foreign body, by site, causing asphyxia
      - inhalation of fumes or vapors J68.9
      - laryngospasm J38.5
  - ampulla of Vater K83.1
  - aortic (heart) (valve) — *see* Stenosis, aortic
  - aortoiliac I74.Ø9
  - aqueduct of Sylvius G91.1
    - congenital QØ3.Ø
      - with spina bifida — *see* Spina bifida, by site, with hydrocephalus
  - Arnold-Chiari — *see* Arnold-Chiari disease
  - artery — *see also* Atherosclerosis, artery I7Ø.9 ☑
    - basilar (complete) (partial) — *see* Occlusion, artery, basilar
    - carotid (complete) (partial) — *see* Occlusion, artery, carotid
    - cerebellar — *see* Occlusion, artery, cerebellar
    - cerebral (anterior) (middle) (posterior) — *see* Occlusion, artery, cerebral
    - precerebral — *see* Occlusion, artery, precerebral
    - renal N28.Ø
    - retinal NEC — *see* Occlusion, artery, retina
    - stent — *see* Restenosis, stent
    - vertebral (complete) (partial) — *see* Occlusion, artery, vertebral
  - band (intestinal) — *see also* Obstruction, intestine, specified NEC K56.699
  - bile duct or passage (common) (hepatic) (noncalculous) K83.1
    - with calculus K8Ø.51
    - congenital (causing jaundice) Q44.3
  - biliary (duct) (tract) K83.1
    - gallbladder K82.Ø
  - bladder-neck (acquired) N32.Ø
    - congenital Q64.31
    - due to hyperplasia (hypertrophy) of prostate — *see* Hyperplasia, prostate
  - bowel — *see* Obstruction, intestine
  - bronchus J98.Ø9
  - canal, ear — *see* Stenosis, external ear canal
  - cardia K22.2
  - caval veins (inferior) (superior) I87.1
  - cecum — *see* Obstruction, intestine
  - circulatory I99.8
  - colon — *see* Obstruction, intestine
  - common duct (noncalculous) K83.1
  - coronary (artery) — *see* Occlusion, coronary
  - cystic duct — *see also* Obstruction, gallbladder

- **Obstruction, obstructed, obstructive** — *continued*
  - cystic duct — *see also* Obstruction, gallbladder — *continued*
    - with calculus K8Ø.21
  - device, implant or graft — *see also* Complications, by site and type, mechanical T85.698 ☑
    - arterial graft NEC — *see* Complication, cardiovascular device, mechanical, vascular
    - catheter NEC T85.628 ☑
      - cystostomy T83.Ø9Ø ☑
      - dialysis (renal) T82.49 ☑
        - intraperitoneal T85.691 ☑
      - Hopkins T83.Ø98 ☑
      - ileostomy T83.Ø98 ☑
      - infusion NEC T82.594 ☑
        - spinal (epidural) (subdural) T85.69Ø ☑
      - nephrostomy T83.Ø92 ☑
      - urethral indwelling T83.Ø91 ☑
      - urinary T83.Ø98 ☑
      - urostomy T83.Ø98 ☑
    - due to infection T85.79 ☑
    - gastrointestinal — *see* Complications, prosthetic device, mechanical, gastrointestinal device
    - genital NEC T83.498 ☑
      - intrauterine contraceptive device T83.39 ☑
      - penile prosthesis (cylinder) (implanted) (pump) (resevoir) T83.49Ø ☑
      - testicular prosthesis T83.491 ☑
    - heart NEC — *see* Complication, cardiovascular device, mechanical
    - joint prosthesis — *see* Complications, joint prosthesis, mechanical, specified NEC, by site
    - orthopedic NEC — *see* Complication, orthopedic, device, mechanical
    - specified NEC T85.628 ☑
    - urinary NEC — *see also* Complication, genitourinary, device, urinary, mechanical
      - graft T83.29 ☑
    - vascular NEC — *see* Complication, cardiovascular device, mechanical
    - ventricular intracranial shunt T85.Ø9 ☑
  - due to foreign body accidentally left in operative wound T81.529 ☑
  - duodenum K31.5
  - ejaculatory duct N5Ø.89
  - esophagus K22.2
  - eustachian tube (complete) (partial) H68.1Ø- ☑
    - cartilagenous (extrinsic) H68.13- ☑
      - intrinsic H68.12- ☑
    - osseous H68.11- ☑
  - fallopian tube (bilateral) N97.1
  - fecal K56.41
    - with hernia — *see* Hernia, by site, with obstruction
  - foramen of Monro (congenital) QØ3.8
    - with spina bifida — *see* Spina bifida, by site, with hydrocephalus
  - foreign body — *see* Foreign body
  - gallbladder K82.Ø
    - with calculus, stones K8Ø.21
    - congenital Q44.1
  - gastric outlet K31.1
  - gastrointestinal — *see* Obstruction, intestine
  - hepatic K76.89
    - duct (noncalculous) K83.1
  - ileum — *see* Obstruction, intestine
  - iliofemoral (artery) I74.5
  - intestine K56.6Ø9
    - with
      - adhesions (intestinal) (peritoneal) K56.5Ø
        - complete K56.52
        - incomplete K56.51
        - partial K56.51
    - adynamic K56.Ø
    - by gallstone K56.3
    - complete K56.6Ø1
    - congenital (small) Q41.9
      - large Q42.9
        - specified part NEC Q42.8
    - incomplete K56.6ØØ
    - neurogenic K56.Ø
      - Hirschsprung's disease or megacolon Q43.1
    - newborn P76.9
      - due to
        - fecaliths P76.8
        - inspissated milk P76.2
        - meconium (plug) P76.Ø
          - in mucoviscidosis E84.11

Obstruction, obstructed, obstructive — *continued*
- intestine — *continued*
  - newborn — *continued*
    - specified NEC P76.8
  - partial K56.6ØØ
  - postoperative K91.3Ø
    - complete K91.32
    - incomplete K91.31
    - partial K91.31
  - reflex K56.Ø
  - specified NEC K56.699
    - complete K56.691
    - incomplete K56.69Ø
    - partial K56.69Ø
  - volvulus K56.2
- intracardiac ball valve prosthesis T82.Ø9 ☑
- jejunum — *see* Obstruction, intestine
- joint prosthesis — *see* Complications, joint prosthesis, mechanical, specified NEC, by site
- kidney (calices) — *see also* Hydronephrosis N28.89
- labor — *see* Delivery
- lacrimal (passages) (duct)
  - by
    - dacryolith — *see* Dacryolith
    - stenosis — *see* Stenosis, lacrimal
  - congenital Q1Ø.5
  - neonatal HØ4.53- ☑
- lacrimonasal duct — *see* Obstruction, lacrimal
- lacteal, with steatorrhea K9Ø.2
- laryngitis — *see* Laryngitis
- larynx NEC J38.6
  - congenital Q31.8
- lung J98.4
  - disease, chronic J44.9
- lymphatic I89.Ø
- meconium (plug)
  - newborn P76.Ø
    - due to fecaliths P76.Ø
    - in mucoviscidosis E84.11
- mitral — *see* Stenosis, mitral
- nasal J34.89
- nasolacrimal duct — *see also* Obstruction, lacrimal
  - congenital Q1Ø.5
- nasopharynx J39.2
- nose J34.89
- organ or site, congenital NEC — *see* Atresia, by site
- pancreatic duct K86.89
- parotid duct or gland K11.8
- pelviureteral junction N13.5
  - with hydronephrosis N13.Ø
  - congenital Q62.39
- pharynx J39.2
- portal (circulation) (vein) I81
- prostate — *see also* Hyperplasia, prostate
  - valve (urinary) N32.Ø
- pulmonary valve (heart) I37.Ø
- pyelonephritis (chronic) N11.1
- pylorus
  - adult K31.1
  - congenital or infantile Q4Ø.Ø
- rectosigmoid — *see* Obstruction, intestine
- rectum K62.4
- renal — *see also* Hydronephrosis N28.89
  - outflow N13.8
  - pelvis, congenital Q62.39
- respiratory J98.8
  - chronic J44.9
- retinal (vessels) H34.9
- salivary duct (any) K11.8
  - with calculus K11.5
- sigmoid — *see* Obstruction, intestine
- sinus (accessory) (nasal) J34.89
- Stensen's duct K11.8
- stomach NEC K31.89
  - acute K31.Ø
  - congenital Q4Ø.2
  - due to pylorospasm K31.3
- submandibular duct K11.8
- submaxillary gland K11.8
  - with calculus K11.5
- thoracic duct I89.Ø
- thrombotic — *see* Thrombosis
- trachea J39.8
- tracheostomy airway J95.Ø3
- tricuspid (valve) — *see* Stenosis, tricuspid
- upper respiratory, congenital Q34.8
- ureter (functional) (pelvic junction) NEC N13.5

Obstruction, obstructed, obstructive — *continued*
- ureter — *continued*
  - with
    - hydronephrosis N13.1
      - with infection N13.6
    - congenital Q62.39
    - pyelonephritis (chronic) N11.1
  - congenital Q62.39
  - due to calculus — *see* Calculus, ureter
- urethra NEC N36.8
  - congenital Q64.39
- urinary (moderate) N13.9
  - due to hyperplasia (hypertrophy) of prostate — *see* Hyperplasia, prostate
  - organ or tract (lower) N13.9
  - prostatic valve N32.Ø
  - specified NEC N13.8
- uropathy N13.9
- uterus N85.8
- vagina N89.5
- valvular — *see* Endocarditis
- vein, venous I87.1
  - caval (inferior) (superior) I87.1
  - thrombotic — *see* Thrombosis
- vena cava (inferior) (superior) I87.1
- vesical NEC N32.Ø
- vesicourethral orifice N32.Ø
  - congenital Q64.31
- vessel NEC I99.8
  - stent — *see* Restenosis, stent

Obturator — *see* condition

Occlusal wear, teeth KØ3.Ø

Occlusio pupillae — *see* Membrane, pupillary

Occlusion, occluded
- anus K62.4
  - congenital Q42.3
    - with fistula Q42.2
- aortoiliac (chronic) I74.Ø9
- aqueduct of Sylvius G91.1
  - congenital QØ3.Ø
    - with spina bifida — *see* Spina bifida, by site, with hydrocephalus
- artery — *see also* Atherosclerosis, artery I7Ø.9 ☑
  - auditory, internal I65.8
  - basilar I65.1
    - with
      - infarction I63.22
        - due to
          - embolism I63.12
          - thrombosis I63.Ø2
  - brain or cerebral I66.9
    - with infarction (due to) I63.5- ☑
      - embolism I63.4- ☑
      - thrombosis I63.3- ☑
  - carotid I65.2- ☑
    - with
      - infarction I63.23- ☑
        - due to
          - embolism I63.13- ☑
          - thrombosis I63.Ø3- ☑
  - cerebellar (anterior inferior) (posterior inferior) (superior) I66.3
    - with infarction I63.54- ☑
      - due to
        - embolism I63.44- ☑
        - thrombosis I63.34- ☑
  - cerebral I66.9
    - with infarction I63.5Ø
      - due to
        - embolism I63.4Ø
          - specified NEC I63.49
        - thrombosis I63.3Ø
          - specified NEC I63.39
    - anterior I66.1- ☑
      - with infarction I63.52- ☑
        - due to
          - embolism I63.42- ☑
          - thrombosis I63.32- ☑
    - middle I66.Ø- ☑
      - with infarction I63.51- ☑
        - due to
          - embolism I63.41- ☑
          - thrombosis I63.31- ☑
    - posterior I66.2- ☑
      - with infarction I63.53- ☑
        - due to
          - embolism I63.43- ☑

Occlusion, occluded — *continued*
- artery — *see also* Atherosclerosis, artery — *continued*
  - cerebral — *continued*
    - posterior — *continued*
      - with infarction — *continued*
        - due to — *continued*
          - thrombosis I63.33- ☑
    - specified NEC I66.8
      - with infarction I63.59
        - due to
          - embolism I63.4- ☑
          - thrombosis I63.3- ☑
  - choroidal (anterior) — *see* Occlusion, artery, precerebral, specified NEC
  - communicating posterior — *see* Occlusion, artery, precerebral, specified NEC
  - complete
    - coronary I25.82
    - extremities I7Ø.92
  - coronary (acute) (thrombotic) (without myocardial infarction) I24.Ø
    - with myocardial infarction — *see* Infarction, myocardium
    - chronic total I25.82
    - complete I25.82
    - healed or old I25.2
    - total (chronic) I25.82
  - hypophyseal — *see* Occlusion, artery, precerebral, specified NEC
  - iliac I74.5
  - lower extremities due to stenosis or stricture I77.1
  - mesenteric (embolic) (thrombotic) — *see also* Infarct, intestine K55.Ø69
  - perforating — *see* Occlusion, artery, cerebral, specified NEC
  - peripheral I77.9
    - thrombotic or embolic I74.4
  - pontine — *see* Occlusion, artery, precerebral, specified NEC
  - precerebral I65.9
    - with infarction I63.2Ø
      - specified NEC I63.29
      - due to
        - embolism I63.1Ø
          - specified NEC I63.19
        - thrombosis I63.ØØ
          - specified NEC I63.Ø9
    - basilar — *see* Occlusion, artery, basilar
    - carotid — *see* Occlusion, artery, carotid
    - puerperal O88.23
    - specified NEC I65.8
      - with infarction I63.29
        - due to
          - embolism I63.19
          - thrombosis I63.Ø9
    - vertebral — *see* Occlusion, artery, vertebral
  - renal N28.Ø
  - retinal
    - branch H34.23- ☑
    - central H34.1- ☑
    - partial H34.21- ☑
    - transient H34.Ø- ☑
  - spinal — *see* Occlusion, artery, precerebral, vertebral
  - total (chronic)
    - coronary I25.82
    - extremities I7Ø.92
  - vertebral I65.Ø- ☑
    - with
      - infarction I63.21- ☑
        - due to
          - embolism I63.11- ☑
          - thrombosis I63.Ø1- ☑
- basilar artery — *see* Occlusion, artery, basilar
- bile duct (common) (hepatic) (noncalculous) K83.1
- bowel — *see* Obstruction, intestine
- carotid (artery) (common) (internal) — *see* Occlusion, artery, carotid
- centric (of teeth) M26.59
  - maximum intercuspation discrepancy M26.55
- cerebellar (artery) — *see* Occlusion, artery, cerebellar
- cerebral (artery) — *see* Occlusion, artery, cerebral
- cerebrovascular — *see also* Occlusion, artery, cerebral
  - with infarction I63.5- ☑
- cervical canal — *see* Stricture, cervix
- cervix (uteri) — *see* Stricture, cervix
- choanal Q3Ø.Ø

Occlusion, occluded — *continued*
- choroidal (artery) — *see* Occlusion, artery, precerebral, specified NEC
- colon — *see* Obstruction, intestine
- communicating posterior artery — *see* Occlusion, artery, precerebral, specified NEC
- coronary (artery) (vein) (thrombotic) — *see also* Infarct, myocardium
  - chronic total I25.82
  - healed or old I25.2
  - not resulting in infarction I24.Ø
  - total (chronic) I25.82
- cystic duct — *see* Obstruction, gallbladder
- embolic — *see* Embolism
- fallopian tube N97.1
  - congenital Q5Ø.6
- gallbladder — *see also* Obstruction, gallbladder
  - congenital (causing jaundice) Q44.1
- gingiva, traumatic KØ6.2
- hymen N89.6
  - congenital Q52.3
- hypophyseal (artery) — *see* Occlusion, artery, precerebral, specified NEC
- iliac artery I74.5
- intestine — *see* Obstruction, intestine
- lacrimal passages — *see* Obstruction, lacrimal
- lung J98.4
- lymph or lymphatic channel I89.Ø
- mammary duct N64.89
- mesenteric artery (embolic) (thrombotic) — *see also* Infarct, intestine K55.Ø69
- nose J34.89
  - congenital Q3Ø.Ø
- organ or site, congenital NEC — *see* Atresia, by site
- oviduct N97.1
  - congenital Q5Ø.6
- peripheral arteries
  - due to stricture or stenosis I77.1
  - upper extremity I74.2
- pontine (artery) — *see* Occlusion, artery, precerebral, specified NEC
- posterior lingual, of mandibular teeth M26.29
- precerebral artery — *see* Occlusion, artery, precerebral
- punctum lacrimale — *see* Obstruction, lacrimal
- pupil — *see* Membrane, pupillary
- pylorus, adult — *see also* Stricture, pylorus K31.1
- renal artery N28.Ø
- retina, retinal
  - artery — *see* Occlusion, artery, retinal
  - vein (central) H34.81- ☑
    - engorgement H34.82- ☑
    - tributary H34.83- ☑
  - vessels H34.9
- spinal artery — *see* Occlusion, artery, precerebral, vertebral
- teeth (mandibular) (posterior lingual) M26.29
- thoracic duct I89.Ø
- thrombotic — *see* Thrombosis, artery
- traumatic
  - edentulous (alveolar) ridge KØ6.2
  - gingiva KØ6.2
  - periodontal KØ5.5
- tubal N97.1
- ureter (complete) (partial) N13.5
  - congenital Q62.1Ø
- ureteropelvic junction N13.5
  - congenital Q62.11
- ureterovesical orifice N13.5
  - congenital Q62.12
- urethra — *see* Stricture, urethra
- uterus N85.8
- vagina N89.5
- vascular NEC I99.8
- vein — *see* Thrombosis
  - retinal — *see* Occlusion, retinal, vein
- vena cava (inferior) (superior) — *see* Embolism, vena cava
- ventricle (brain) NEC G91.1
- vertebral (artery) — *see* Occlusion, artery, vertebral
- vessel (blood) I99.8
- vulva N9Ø.5

Occult
- blood in feces (stools) R19.5

Occupational
- problems NEC Z56.89

Ochlophobia — *see* Agoraphobia

Ochronosis (endogenous) E7Ø.29

Ocular muscle — *see* condition

Oculogyric crisis or disturbance H51.8
- psychogenic F45.8

Oculomotor syndrome H51.9

Oculopathy
- syphilitic NEC A52.71
  - congenital
    - early A5Ø.Ø1
    - late A5Ø.3Ø
  - early (secondary) A51.43
  - late A52.71

Oddi's sphincter spasm K83.4

Odontalgia KØ8.89

Odontoameloblastoma — *see* Cyst, calcifying odontogenic

Odontoclasia KØ3.89

Odontodysplasia, regional KØØ.4

Odontogenesis imperfecta KØØ.5

Odontoma (ameloblastic) (complex) (compound) (fibroameloblastic) — *see* Cyst, calcifying odontogenic

Odontomyelitis (closed) (open) KØ4.Ø1
- irreversible KØ4.Ø2
- reversible KØ4.Ø1

Odontorrhagia KØ8.89

Odontosarcoma, ameloblastic C41.1
- upper jaw (bone) C41.Ø

Oestriasis — *see* Myiasis

Oguchi's disease H53.63

Ohara's disease — *see* Tularemia

OHS (obesity hypoventilation syndrome) E66.2

Oidiomycosis — *see* Candidiasis

Oidium albicans infection — *see* Candidiasis

Old age (without mention of debility) R54
- dementia FØ3 ☑

Old (previous) **myocardial infarction** I25.2

Olfactory — *see* condition

Oligemia — *see* Anemia

Oligoastrocytoma
- specified site — *see* Neoplasm, malignant, by site
- unspecified site C71.9

Oligocythemia D64.9

Oligodendroblastoma
- specified site — *see* Neoplasm, malignant
- unspecified site C71.9

Oligodendroglioma
- anaplastic type
  - specified site — *see* Neoplasm, malignant, by site
  - unspecified site C71.9
- specified site — *see* Neoplasm, malignant, by site
- unspecified site C71.9

Oligodontia — *see* Anodontia

Oligoencephalon QØ2

Oligohidrosis L74.4

Oligohydramnios O41.Ø- ☑

Oligohydrosis L74.4

Oligomenorrhea N91.5
- primary N91.3
- secondary N91.4

Oligophrenia — *see also* Disability, intellectual
- phenylpyruvic E7Ø.Ø

Oligospermia N46.11
- due to
  - drug therapy N46.121
  - efferent duct obstruction N46.123
  - infection N46.122
  - radiation N46.124
  - specified cause NEC N46.129
  - systemic disease N46.125

Oligotrichia — *see* Alopecia

Oliguria R34
- with, complicating or following ectopic or molar pregnancy OØ8.4
- postprocedural N99.Ø

Ollier's disease Q78.4

Omenotocele — *see* Hernia, abdomen, specified site NEC

Omentitis — *see* Peritonitis

Omentum, omental — *see* condition

Omphalitis (congenital) (newborn) P38.9
- with mild hemorrhage P38.1
- without hemorrhage P38.9
- not of newborn LØ8.82
- tetanus A33

Omphalocele Q79.2

Omphalomesenteric duct, persistent Q43.Ø

Omphalorrhagia, newborn P51.9

Omsk hemorrhagic fever A98.1

Onanism (excessive) F98.8

Onchocerciasis, onchocercosis B73.1

Onchocerciasis, onchocercosis — *continued*
- with
  - eye disease B73.ØØ
    - endophthalmitis B73.Ø1
    - eyelid B73.Ø9
    - glaucoma B73.Ø2
    - specified NEC B73.Ø9
- eyelid B73.Ø9
- eye NEC B73.ØØ

Oncocytoma — *see* Neoplasm, benign, by site

Oncovirus, as cause of disease classified elsewhere B97.32

Ondine's curse — *see* Apnea, sleep

Oneirophrenia F23

Onychauxis L6Ø.2
- congenital Q84.5

Onychia — *see also* Cellulitis, digit
- with lymphangitis — *see* Lymphangitis, acute, digit
- candidal B37.2
- dermatophytic B35.1

Onychitis — *see also* Cellulitis, digit
- with lymphangitis — *see* Lymphangitis, acute, digit

Onychocryptosis L6Ø.Ø

Onychodystrophy L6Ø.3
- congenital Q84.6

Onychogryphosis, onychogryposis L6Ø.2

Onycholysis L6Ø.1

Onychomadesis L6Ø.8

Onychomalacia L6Ø.3

Onychomycosis (finger) (toe) B35.1

Onycho-osteodysplasia Q87.2

Onychophagia F98.8

Onychophosis L6Ø.8

Onychoptosis L6Ø.8

Onychorrhexis L6Ø.3
- congenital Q84.6

Onychoschizia L6Ø.3

Onyxis (finger) (toe) L6Ø.Ø

Onyxitis — *see also* Cellulitis, digit
- with lymphangitis — *see* Lymphangitis, acute, digit

Oophoritis (cystic) (infectional) (interstitial) N7Ø.92
- with salpingitis N7Ø.93
- acute N7Ø.Ø2
  - with salpingitis N7Ø.Ø3
- chronic N7Ø.12
  - with salpingitis N7Ø.13
- complicating abortion — *see* Abortion, by type, complicated by, oophoritis

Oophorocele N83.4- ☑

Opacity, opacities
- cornea H17.- ☑
  - central H17.1- ☑
  - congenital Q13.3
  - degenerative — *see* Degeneration, cornea
  - hereditary — *see* Dystrophy, cornea
  - inflammatory — *see* Keratitis
  - minor H17.81- ☑
  - peripheral H17.82- ☑
  - sequelae of trachoma (healed) B94.Ø
  - specified NEC H17.89
- enamel (teeth) (fluoride) (nonfluoride) KØØ.3
- lens — *see* Cataract
- snowball — *see* Deposit, crystalline
- vitreous (humor) NEC H43.39- ☑
  - congenital Q14.Ø
  - membranes and strands H43.31- ☑

Opalescent dentin (hereditary) KØØ.5

Open, opening
- abnormal, organ or site, congenital — *see* Imperfect, closure
- angle with
  - borderline
    - findings
      - high risk H4Ø.Ø2- ☑
      - low risk H4Ø.Ø1- ☑
    - intraocular pressure H4Ø.ØØ- ☑
  - cupping of discs H4Ø.Ø1- ☑
  - glaucoma (primary) — *see* Glaucoma, open angle
- bite
  - anterior M26.22Ø
  - posterior M26.221
- false — *see* Imperfect, closure
- margin on tooth restoration KØ8.51
- restoration margins of tooth KØ8.51
- wound — *see* Wound, open

Operational fatigue F48.8

Operative — *see* condition

- **Operculitis** — *see* Periodontitis
- **Operculum** — *see* Break, retina
- **Ophiasis** L63.2
- **Ophthalmia** — *see also* Conjunctivitis H1Ø.9
  - actinic rays — *see* Photokeratitis
  - allergic (acute) — *see* Conjunctivitis, acute, atopic
  - blennorrhagic (gonococcal) (neonatorum) A54.31
  - diphtheritic A36.86
  - Egyptian A71.1
  - electrica — *see* Photokeratitis
  - gonococcal (neonatorum) A54.31
  - metastatic — *see* Endophthalmitis, purulent
  - migraine — *see* Migraine, ophthalmoplegic
  - neonatorum, newborn P39.1
    - gonococcal A54.31
  - nodosa H16.24- ☑
  - purulent — *see* Conjunctivitis, acute, mucopurulent
  - spring — *see* Conjunctivitis, acute, atopic
  - sympathetic — *see* Uveitis, sympathetic
- **Ophthalmitis** — *see* Ophthalmia
- **Ophthalmocele** (congenital) Q15.8
- **Ophthalmoneuromyelitis** G36.Ø
- **Ophthalmoplegia** — *see also* Strabismus, paralytic
  - anterior internuclear — *see* Ophthalmoplegia, internuclear
  - ataxia-areflexia G61.Ø
  - diabetic — *see* EØ8-E13 with .39
  - exophthalmic EØ5.ØØ
    - with thyroid storm EØ5.Ø1
  - external H49.88- ☑
    - progressive H49.4- ☑
      - with pigmentary retinopathy — *see* Kearns-Sayre syndrome
    - total H49.3- ☑
  - internal (complete) (total) H52.51- ☑
  - internuclear H51.2- ☑
  - migraine — *see* Migraine, ophthalmoplegic
  - Parinaud's H49.88- ☑
  - progressive external — *see* Ophthalmoplegia, external, progressive
  - supranuclear, progressive G23.1
  - total (external) — *see* Ophthalmoplegia, external, total
- **Opioid**(s)
  - abuse — *see* Abuse, drug, opioids
  - dependence — *see* Dependence, drug, opioids
  - induced, without use disorder
    - anxiety disorder F11.988
    - delirium F11.921
    - depressive disorder F11.94
    - sexual dysfunction F11.981
    - sleep disorder F11.982
- **Opisthognathism** M26.Ø9
- **Opisthorchiasis** (felineus) (viverrini) B66.Ø
- **Opitz' disease** D73.2
- **Opiumism** — *see* Dependence, drug, opioid
- **Oppenheim's disease** G7Ø.2
- **Oppenheim-Urbach disease** (necrobiosis lipoidica diabeticorum) — *see* EØ8-E13 with .62Ø
- **Optic nerve** — *see* condition
- **Orbit** — *see* condition
- **Orchioblastoma** C62.9- ☑
- **Orchitis** (gangrenous) (nonspecific) (septic) (suppurative) N45.2
  - blennorrhagic (gonococcal) (acute) (chronic) A54.23
  - chlamydial A56.19
  - filarial — *see also* Infestation, filarial B74.9 *[N51]*
  - gonococcal (acute) (chronic) A54.23
  - mumps B26.Ø
  - syphilitic A52.76
  - tuberculous A18.15
- **Orf** (virus disease) BØ8.Ø2
- **Organic** — *see also* condition
  - brain syndrome FØ9
  - heart — *see* Disease, heart
  - mental disorder FØ9
  - psychosis FØ9
- **Orgasm**
  - anejaculatory N53.13
- **Oriental**
  - bilharziasis B65.2
  - schistosomiasis B65.2
- **Orifice** — *see* condition
- **Origin of both great vessels from right ventricle** Q2Ø.1
- **Ormond's disease** (with ureteral obstruction) N13.5
  - with infection N13.6
- **Ornithine metabolism disorder** E72.4
- **Ornithinemia** (Type I) (Type II) E72.4
- **Ornithosis** A7Ø
- **Orotaciduria, oroticaciduria** (congenital) (hereditary) (pyrimidine deficiency) E79.8
  - anemia D53.Ø
- **Orthodontics**
  - adjustment Z46.4
  - fitting Z46.4
- **Orthopnea** RØ6.Ø1
- **Orthopoxvirus** BØ8.Ø9
- **Os, uterus** — *see* condition
- **Osgood-Schlatter disease or osteochondrosis** M92.52- ☑
- **Osler** (-Weber)-**Rendu disease** I78.Ø
- **Osler's nodes** I33.Ø
- **Osmidrosis** L75.Ø
- **Osseous** — *see* condition
- **Ossification**
  - artery — *see* Arteriosclerosis
  - auricle (ear) — *see* Disorder, pinna, specified type NEC
  - bronchial J98.Ø9
  - cardiac — *see* Degeneration, myocardial
  - cartilage (senile) — *see* Disorder, cartilage, specified type NEC
  - coronary (artery) — *see* Disease, heart, ischemic, atherosclerotic
  - diaphragm J98.6
  - ear, middle — *see* Otosclerosis
  - falx cerebri G96.198
  - fontanel, premature Q75.Ø
  - heart — *see also* Degeneration, myocardial
    - valve — *see* Endocarditis
  - larynx J38.7
  - ligament — *see* Disorder, tendon, specified type NEC
    - posterior longitudinal — *see* Spondylopathy, specified NEC
  - meninges (cerebral) (spinal) G96.198
  - multiple, eccentric centers — *see* Disorder, bone, development or growth
  - muscle — *see also* Calcification, muscle
    - due to burns — *see* Myositis, ossificans, in, burns
    - paralytic — *see* Myositis, ossificans, in, quadriplegia
    - progressive — *see* Myositis, ossificans, progressiva
    - specified NEC M61.5Ø
      - ankle M61.57- ☑
      - foot M61.57- ☑
      - forearm M61.53- ☑
      - hand M61.54- ☑
      - lower leg M61.56- ☑
      - multiple sites M61.59
      - pelvic region M61.55- ☑
      - shoulder region M61.51- ☑
      - specified site NEC M61.58
      - thigh M61.55- ☑
      - upper arm M61.52- ☑
    - traumatic — *see* Myositis, ossificans, traumatica
  - myocardium, myocardial — *see* Degeneration, myocardial
  - penis N48.89
  - periarticular — *see* Disorder, joint, specified type NEC
  - pinna — *see* Disorder, pinna, specified type NEC
  - rider's bone — *see* Ossification, muscle, specified NEC
  - sclera H15.89
  - subperiosteal, post-traumatic M89.8X- ☑
  - tendon — *see* Disorder, tendon, specified type NEC
  - trachea J39.8
  - tympanic membrane — *see* Disorder, tympanic membrane, specified NEC
  - vitreous (humor) — *see* Deposit, crystalline
- **Osteitis** — *see also* Osteomyelitis
  - alveolar M27.3
  - condensans M85.3Ø
    - ankle M85.37- ☑
    - foot M85.37- ☑
    - forearm M85.33- ☑
    - hand M85.34- ☑
    - lower leg M85.36- ☑
    - multiple site M85.39
    - neck M85.38
    - rib M85.38
    - shoulder M85.31- ☑
    - skull M85.38
    - specified site NEC M85.38
    - thigh M85.35- ☑
    - toe M85.37- ☑
    - upper arm M85.32- ☑
    - vertebra M85.38
- **Osteitis** — *continued*
  - deformans M88.9
    - in (due to)
      - malignant neoplasm of bone C41.9 *[M9Ø.6Ø]*
      - neoplastic disease — *see also* Neoplasm D49.9 *[M9Ø.6Ø]*
        - carpus D49.9 *[M9Ø.64-]* ☑
        - clavicle D49.9 *[M9Ø.61-]* ☑
        - femur D49.9 *[M9Ø.65-]* ☑
        - fibula D49.9 *[M9Ø.66-]* ☑
        - finger D49.9 *[M9Ø.64-]* ☑
        - humerus D49.9 *[M9Ø.62-]* ☑
        - ilium D49.9 *[M9Ø.65-]* ☑
        - ischium D49.9 *[M9Ø.65-]* ☑
        - metacarpus D49.9 *[M9Ø.64-]* ☑
        - metatarsus D49.9 *[M9Ø.67-]* ☑
        - multiple sites D49.9 *[M9Ø.69]*
        - neck D49.9 *[M9Ø.68]*
        - radius D49.9 *[M9Ø.63-]* ☑
        - rib D49.9 *[M9Ø.68]*
        - scapula D49.9 *[M9Ø.61-]* ☑
        - skull D49.9 *[M9Ø.68]*
        - tarsus D49.9 *[M9Ø.67-]* ☑
        - tibia D49.9 *[M9Ø.66-]* ☑
        - toe D49.9 *[M9Ø.67-]* ☑
        - ulna D49.9 *[M9Ø.63-]* ☑
        - vertebra D49.9 *[M9Ø.68]*
    - skull M88.Ø
    - specified NEC — *see* Paget's disease, bone, by site
    - vertebra M88.1
  - due to yaws A66.6
  - fibrosa NEC — *see* Cyst, bone, by site
    - circumscripta — *see* Dysplasia, fibrous, bone NEC
    - cystica (generalisata) E21.Ø
    - disseminata Q78.1
    - osteoplastica E21.Ø
  - fragilitans Q78.Ø
  - Garr's (sclerosing) — *see* Osteomyelitis, specified type NEC
  - jaw (acute) (chronic) (lower) (suppurative) (upper) M27.2
  - parathyroid E21.Ø
  - petrous bone (acute) (chronic) — *see* Petrositis
  - sclerotic, nonsuppurative — *see* Osteomyelitis, specified type NEC
  - tuberculosa A18.Ø9
    - cystica D86.89
    - multiplex cystoides D86.89
- **Osteoarthritis** M19.9Ø
  - ankle M19.Ø7- ☑
    - post-traumatic M19.17- ☑
    - primary M19.Ø7- ☑
    - secondary M19.27- ☑
  - elbow M19.Ø2- ☑
    - post-traumatic M19.12- ☑
    - primary M19.Ø2- ☑
    - secondary M19.22- ☑
  - foot joint M19.Ø7- ☑
    - post-traumatic M19.17- ☑
    - primary M19.Ø7- ☑
    - secondary M19.27- ☑
  - generalized (multiple joints) M15.9
    - erosive M15.4
    - primary M15.Ø
    - specified NEC M15.8
  - hand joint M19.Ø4- ☑
    - first carpometacarpal joint M18.9
      - post-traumatic — *see* Osteoarthritis, post-traumatic NEC, hand joint, first carpometacarpal joint
      - primary — *see* Osteoarthritis, primary, hand joint, first carpometacarpal joint
      - secondary — *see* Osteoarthritis, secondary, hand joint, first carpometacarpal joint
    - post-traumatic M19.14- ☑
    - primary M19.Ø4- ☑
    - secondary M19.24- ☑
  - hip M16.9
    - bilateral M16.Ø
      - due to hip dysplasia M16.2
      - post-traumatic M16.4
      - secondary M16.6
    - due to hip dysplasia (unilateral) M16.3- ☑
      - bilateral M16.2
    - post-traumatic — *see* Osteoarthritis, post-traumatic, hip
    - primary M16.1- ☑

Index

Operculitis — Osteoarthritis

- **Osteoarthritis** — *continued*
  - hip — *continued*
    - secondary — *see* Osteoarthritis, secondary, hip
    - unilateral M16.1- ☑
      - due to hip dysplasia M16.3- ☑
      - post-traumatic M16.5- ☑
      - primary M16.1- ☑
      - secondary NEC M16.7
  - interphalangeal
    - distal (Heberden) M15.1
    - proximal (Bouchard) M15.2
  - knee M17.9
    - bilateral M17.Ø
      - post-traumatic M17.2
      - secondary M17.4
    - post-traumatic — *see* Osteoarthritis, post-traumatic, knee
    - primary M17.1- ☑
      - bilateral M17.Ø
    - secondary — *see* Osteoarthritis, secondary, knee
    - unilateral M17.1- ☑
      - post-traumatic M17.3- ☑
      - primary M17.1- ☑
      - secondary NEC M17.5
  - post-traumatic NEC M19.92
    - ankle M19.17- ☑
    - elbow M19.12- ☑
    - foot joint M19.17- ☑
    - hand joint M19.14- ☑
      - first carpometacarpal joint M18.3- ☑
        - bilateral M18.2
    - hip M16.5- ☑
      - bilateral M16.4
    - knee M17.3- ☑
      - bilateral M17.2
    - shoulder M19.11- ☑
    - specified site NEC M19.19
    - wrist M19.13- ☑
  - primary M19.91
    - ankle M19.Ø7- ☑
    - elbow M19.Ø2- ☑
    - foot joint M19.Ø7- ☑
    - hand joint M19.Ø4- ☑
      - first carpometacarpal joint M18.1- ☑
        - bilateral M18.Ø
    - hip M16.1- ☑
      - bilateral M16.Ø
    - knee M17.1- ☑
      - bilateral M17.Ø
    - multiple sites M15.9
    - shoulder M19.Ø1- ☑
    - specified site NEC M19.Ø9
    - spine — *see* Spondylosis
    - wrist M19.Ø3- ☑
  - secondary M19.93
    - ankle M19.27- ☑
    - elbow M19.22- ☑
    - foot joint M19.27- ☑
    - hand joint M19.24- ☑
      - first carpometacarpal joint M18.5- ☑
        - bilateral M18.4
    - hip M16.7-
      - bilateral M16.6
    - knee M17.5-
      - bilateral M17.4
    - multiple M15.3
    - shoulder M19.21- ☑
    - specified site NEC M19.29
    - spine — *see* Spondylosis
    - wrist M19.23- ☑
  - shoulder M19.Ø1- ☑
    - post-traumatic M19.11- ☑
    - primary M19.Ø1- ☑
    - secondary M19.21- ☑
  - specified site NEC M19.Ø9
  - spine — *see* Spondylosis
  - wrist M19.Ø3- ☑
    - first carpometacarpal joint — *see* Osteoarthritis, hand joint, first carpometacarpal joint
    - post-traumatic M19.13- ☑
    - primary M19.Ø3- ☑
    - secondary M19.23 ☑
- **Osteoarthropathy** (hypertrophic) M19.9Ø
  - ankle — *see* Osteoarthritis, primary, ankle
  - elbow — *see* Osteoarthritis, primary, elbow
  - foot joint — *see* Osteoarthritis, primary, foot
  - hand joint — *see* Osteoarthritis, primary, hand joint
- **Osteoarthropathy** — *continued*
  - knee joint — *see* Osteoarthritis, primary, knee
  - multiple site — *see* Osteoarthritis, primary, multiple joint
  - pulmonary — *see also* Osteoarthropathy, specified type NEC
    - hypertrophic — *see* Osteoarthropathy, hypertrophic, specified type NEC
  - secondary — *see* Osteoarthropathy, specified type NEC
  - secondary hypertrophic — *see* Osteoarthropathy, specified type NEC
  - shoulder — *see* Osteoarthritis, primary, shoulder
  - specified joint NEC — *see* Osteoarthritis, primary, specified joint NEC
  - specified type NEC M89.4Ø
    - carpus M89.44- ☑
    - clavicle M89.41- ☑
    - femur M89.45- ☑
    - fibula M89.46- ☑
    - finger M89.44- ☑
    - humerus M89.42- ☑
    - ilium M89.459
    - ischium M89.459
    - metacarpus M89.44- ☑
    - metatarsus M89.47- ☑
    - multiple sites M89.49
    - neck M89.48
    - radius M89.43- ☑
    - rib M89.48
    - scapula M89.41- ☑
    - skull M89.48
    - tarsus M89.47- ☑
    - tibia M89.46- ☑
    - toe M89.47- ☑
    - ulna M89.43- ☑
    - vertebra M89.48
  - spine — *see* Spondylosis
  - wrist — *see* Osteoarthritis, primary, wrist
- **Osteoarthrosis** (degenerative) (hypertrophic) (joint) — *see also* Osteoarthritis
  - deformans alkaptonurica E7Ø.29 *[M36.8]*
  - erosive M15.4
  - generalized M15.9
    - primary M15.Ø
  - polyarticular M15.9
  - spine — *see* Spondylosis
- **Osteoblastoma** — *see* Neoplasm, bone, benign
  - aggressive — *see* Neoplasm, bone, uncertain behavior
- **Osteochondritis** — *see also* Osteochondropathy, by site
  - Brailsford's — *see* Osteochondrosis, juvenile, radius
  - dissecans M93.2Ø
    - ankle M93.27- ☑
    - elbow M93.22- ☑
    - foot M93.27- ☑
    - hand M93.24- ☑
    - hip M93.25- ☑
    - knee M93.26- ☑
    - multiple sites M93.29
    - shoulder joint M93.21- ☑
    - specified site NEC M93.28
    - wrist M93.23- ☑
  - juvenile M92.9
    - patellar — *see* Osteochondrosis, juvenile, patella
  - syphilitic (congenital) (early) A5Ø.Ø2 *[M9Ø.8Ø]*
    - ankle A5Ø.Ø2 *[M9Ø.87-]* ☑
    - elbow A5Ø.Ø2 *[M9Ø.82-]* ☑
    - foot A5Ø.Ø2 *[M9Ø.87-]* ☑
    - forearm A5Ø.Ø2 *[M9Ø.83-]* ☑
    - hand A5Ø.Ø2 *[M9Ø.84-]* ☑
    - hip A5Ø.Ø2 *[M9Ø.85-]* ☑
    - knee A5Ø.Ø2 *[M9Ø.86-]* ☑
    - multiple sites A5Ø.Ø2 *[M9Ø.89]*
    - shoulder joint A5Ø.Ø2 *[M9Ø.81-]* ☑
    - specified site NEC A5Ø.Ø2 *[M9Ø.88]*
- **Osteochondroarthrosis deformans endemica** — *see* Disease, Kaschin-Beck
- **Osteochondrodysplasia** Q78.9
  - with defects of growth of tubular bones and spine Q77.9
    - specified NEC Q77.8
  - specified NEC Q78.8
- **Osteochondrodystrophy** E78.9
- **Osteochondrolysis** — *see* Osteochondritis, dissecans
- **Osteochondroma** — *see* Neoplasm, bone, benign
- **Osteochondromatosis** D16.9
  - syndrome Q78.4
- **Osteochondromyxosarcoma** — *see* Neoplasm, bone, malignant
- **Osteochondropathy** M93.9Ø
  - ankle M93.97- ☑
  - elbow M93.92- ☑
  - foot M93.97- ☑
  - hand M93.94- ☑
  - hip M93.95- ☑
  - Kienböck's disease of adults M93.1
  - knee M93.96- ☑
  - multiple joints M93.99
  - osteochondritis dissecans — *see* Osteochondritis, dissecans
  - osteochondrosis — *see* Osteochondrosis
  - shoulder region M93.91- ☑
  - slipped upper femoral epiphysis — *see* Slipped, epiphysis, upper femoral
  - specified joint NEC M93.98
  - specified type NEC M93.8Ø
    - ankle M93.87- ☑
    - elbow M93.82- ☑
    - foot M93.87- ☑
    - hand M93.84- ☑
    - hip M93.85- ☑
    - knee M93.86- ☑
    - multiple joints M93.89
    - shoulder region M93.81- ☑
    - specified joint NEC M93.88
    - wrist M93.83- ☑
  - syphilitic, congenital
    - early A5Ø.Ø2 *[M9Ø.8Ø]*
    - late A5Ø.56 *[M9Ø.8Ø]*
  - wrist M93.93- ☑
- **Osteochondrosarcoma** — *see* Neoplasm, bone, malignant
- **Osteochondrosis** — *see also* Osteochondropathy, by site
  - acetabulum (juvenile) M91.Ø
  - adult — *see* Osteochondropathy, specified type NEC, by site
  - astragalus (juvenile) — *see* Osteochondrosis, juvenile, tarsus
  - Blount M92.51- ☑
  - Buchanan's M91.Ø
  - Burns' — *see* Osteochondrosis, juvenile, ulna
  - calcaneus (juvenile) — *see* Osteochondrosis, juvenile, tarsus
  - capitular epiphysis (femur) (juvenile) — *see* Legg-Calvé-Perthes disease
  - carpal (juvenile) (lunate) (scaphoid) — *see* Osteochondrosis, juvenile, hand, carpal lunate
    - adult M93.1
  - coxae juvenilis — *see* Legg-Calvé-Perthes disease
  - deformans juvenilis, coxae — *see* Legg-Calvé-Perthes disease
  - Diaz's — *see* Osteochondrosis, juvenile, tarsus
  - dissecans (knee) (shoulder) — *see* Osteochondritis, dissecans
  - femoral capital epiphysis (juvenile) — *see* Legg-Calvé-Perthes disease
  - femur (head), juvenile — *see* Legg-Calvé-Perthes disease
  - fibula (juvenile) — *see* Osteochondrosis, juvenile, fibula
  - foot NEC (juvenile) M92.8
  - Freiberg's — *see* Osteochondrosis, juvenile, metatarsus
  - Haas' (juvenile) — *see* Osteochondrosis, juvenile, humerus
  - Haglund's — *see* Osteochondrosis, juvenile, tarsus
  - hip (juvenile) — *see* Legg-Calvé-Perthes disease
  - humerus (capitulum) (head) (juvenile) — *see* Osteochondrosis, juvenile, humerus
  - ilium, iliac crest (juvenile) M91.Ø
  - ischiopubic synchondrosis M91.Ø
  - Iselin's — *see* Osteochondrosis, juvenile, metatarsus
  - juvenile, juvenilis M92.9
    - after congenital dislocation of hip reduction — *see* Osteochondrosis, juvenile, hip, specified NEC
    - arm — *see* Osteochondrosis, juvenile, upper limb NEC
    - capitular epiphysis (femur) — *see* Legg-Calvé-Perthes disease
    - clavicle, sternal epiphysis — *see* Osteochondrosis, juvenile, upper limb NEC
    - coxae — *see* Legg-Calvé-Perthes disease
    - deformans M92.9
    - fibula M92.5Ø- ☑

Index

Osteoarthritis — Osteochondrosis

- **Osteochondrosis** — *continued*
  - juvenile, juvenilis — *continued*
    - foot NEC M92.8
    - hand M92.2Ø- ☑
      - carpal lunate M92.21- ☑
      - metacarpal head M92.22- ☑
      - specified site NEC M92.29- ☑
    - head of femur — *see* Legg-Calvé-Perthes disease
    - hip and pelvis M91.9- ☑
      - coxa plana — *see* Coxa, plana
      - femoral head — *see* Legg-Calvé-Perthes disease
      - pelvis M91.Ø
      - pseudocoxalgia — *see* Pseudocoxalgia
      - specified NEC M91.8- ☑
    - humerus M92.Ø- ☑
    - limb
      - lower NEC M92.8
      - upper NEC — *see* Osteochondrosis, juvenile, upper limb NEC
    - medial cuneiform bone — *see* Osteochondrosis, juvenile, tarsus
    - metatarsus M92.7- ☑
    - patella M92.4- ☑
    - radius M92.1- ☑
    - specified
      - site NEC M92.8
      - type NEC M92.8
        - tibia and fibula M92.59- ☑
    - spine M42.ØØ
      - cervical region M42.Ø2
      - cervicothoracic region M42.Ø3
      - lumbar region M42.Ø6
      - lumbosacral region M42.Ø7
      - multiple sites M42.Ø9
      - occipito-atlanto-axial region M42.Ø1
      - sacrococcygeal region M42.Ø8
      - thoracic region M42.Ø4
      - thoracolumbar region M42.Ø5
    - tarsus M92.6- ☑
    - tibia M92.5Ø- ☑
      - proximal M92.51- ☑
      - tubercle M92.52- ☑
    - ulna M92.1- ☑
    - upper limb NEC M92.3- ☑
    - vertebra (body) (epiphyseal plates) (Calvé's) (Scheuermann's) — *see* Osteochondrosis, juvenile, spine
  - Kienböck's — *see* Osteochondrosis, juvenile, hand, carpal lunate
    - adult M93.1
  - Köhler's
    - patellar — *see* Osteochondrosis, juvenile, patella
    - tarsal navicular — *see* Osteochondrosis, juvenile, tarsus
  - Legg-Perthes (-Calvé) (-Waldenström) — *see* Legg-Calvé-Perthes disease
  - limb
    - lower NEC (juvenile) M92.8
      - tibia and fibula M92.59- ☑
    - upper NEC (juvenile) — *see* Osteochondrosis, juvenile, upper limb NEC
  - lunate bone (carpal) (juvenile) — *see also* Osteochondrosis, juvenile, hand, carpal lunate
    - adult M93.1
  - Mauclaire's — *see* Osteochondrosis, juvenile, hand, metacarpal
  - metacarpal (head) (juvenile) — *see* Osteochondrosis, juvenile, hand, metacarpal
  - metatarsus (fifth) (head) (juvenile) (second) — *see* Osteochondrosis, juvenile, metatarsus
  - navicular (juvenile) — *see* Osteochondrosis, juvenile, tarsus
  - os
    - calcis (juvenile) — *see* Osteochondrosis, juvenile, tarsus
    - tibiale externum (juvenile) — *see* Osteochondrosis, juvenile, tarsus
  - Osgood-Schlatter M92.52- ☑
  - Panner's — *see* Osteochondrosis, juvenile, humerus
  - patellar center (juvenile) (primary) (secondary) — *see* Osteochondrosis, juvenile, patella
  - pelvis (juvenile) M91.Ø
  - Pierson's M91.Ø
  - radius (head) (juvenile) — *see* Osteochondrosis, juvenile, radius
  - Scheuermann's — *see* Osteochondrosis, juvenile, spine
  - Sever's — *see* Osteochondrosis, juvenile, tarsus
- **Osteochondrosis** — *continued*
  - Sinding-Larsen — *see* Osteochondrosis, juvenile, patella
  - spine M42.9
    - adult M42.1Ø
      - cervical region M42.12
      - cervicothoracic region M42.13
      - lumbar region M42.16
      - lumbosacral region M42.17
      - multiple sites M42.19
      - occipito-atlanto-axial region M42.11
      - sacrococcygeal region M42.18
      - thoracic region M42.14
      - thoracolumbar region M42.15
    - juvenile — *see* Osteochondrosis, juvenile, spine
  - symphysis pubis (juvenile) M91.Ø
  - syphilitic (congenital) A5Ø.Ø2
  - talus (juvenile) — *see* Osteochondrosis, juvenile, tarsus
  - tarsus (navicular) (juvenile) — *see* Osteochondrosis, juvenile, tarsus
  - tibia (proximal) (tubercle) (juvenile) — *see* Osteochondrosis, juvenile, tibia
  - tuberculous — *see* Tuberculosis, bone
  - ulna (lower) (juvenile) — *see* Osteochondrosis, juvenile, ulna
  - van Neck's M91.Ø
  - vertebral — *see* Osteochondrosis, spine
- **Osteoclastoma** D48.Ø
  - malignant — *see* Neoplasm, bone, malignant
- **Osteodynia** — *see* Disorder, bone, specified type NEC
- **Osteodystrophy** Q78.9
  - azotemic N25.Ø
  - congenital Q78.9
  - parathyroid, secondary E21.1
  - renal N25.Ø
- **Osteofibroma** — *see* Neoplasm, bone, benign
- **Osteofibrosarcoma** — *see* Neoplasm, bone, malignant
- **Osteogenesis imperfecta** Q78.Ø
- **Osteogenic** — *see* condition
- **Osteolysis** M89.5Ø
  - carpus M89.54- ☑
  - clavicle M89.51- ☑
  - femur M89.55- ☑
  - fibula M89.56- ☑
  - finger M89.54- ☑
  - humerus M89.52- ☑
  - ilium M89.559
  - ischium M89.559
  - joint prosthesis (periprosthetic) — *see* Complications, joint prosthesis, mechanical, periprosthetic, osteolysis, by site
  - metacarpus M89.54- ☑
  - metatarsus M89.57- ☑
  - multiple sites M89.59
  - neck M89.58
  - periprosthetic — *see* Complications, joint prosthesis, mechanical, periprosthetic, osteolysis, by site
  - radius M89.53- ☑
  - rib M89.58
  - scapula M89.51- ☑
  - skull M89.58
  - tarsus M89.57- ☑
  - tibia M89.56- ☑
  - toe M89.57- ☑
  - ulna M89.53- ☑
  - vertebra M89.58
- **Osteoma** — *see also* Neoplasm, bone, benign
  - osteoid — *see also* Neoplasm, bone, benign
    - giant — *see* Neoplasm, bone, benign
- **Osteomalacia** M83.9
  - adult M83.9
    - drug-induced NEC M83.5
    - due to
      - malabsorption (postsurgical) M83.2
      - malnutrition M83.3
    - specified NEC M83.8
  - aluminium-induced M83.4
  - infantile — *see* Rickets
  - juvenile — *see* Rickets
  - oncogenic E83.89
  - pelvis M83.8
  - puerperal M83.Ø
  - senile M83.1
  - vitamin-D-resistant in adults E83.31 *[M9Ø.8-]* ☑
    - carpus E83.31 *[M9Ø.84-]* ☑
    - clavicle E83.31 *[M9Ø.81-]* ☑
    - femur E83.31 *[M9Ø.85-]* ☑
- **Osteomalacia** — *continued*
  - vitamin-D-resistant in adults — *continued*
    - fibula E83.31 *[M9Ø.86-]* ☑
    - finger E83.31 *[M9Ø.84-]* ☑
    - humerus E83.31 *[M9Ø.82-]* ☑
    - ilium E83.31 *[M9Ø.859]*
    - ischium E83.31 *[M9Ø.859]*
    - metacarpus E83.31 *[M9Ø.84-]* ☑
    - metatarsus E83.31 *[M9Ø.87-]* ☑
    - multiple sites E83.31 *[M9Ø.89]*
    - neck E83.31 *[M9Ø.88]*
    - radius E83.31 *[M9Ø.83-]* ☑
    - rib E83.31 *[M9Ø.88]*
    - scapula E83.31 *[M9Ø.819]*
    - skull E83.31 *[M9Ø.88]*
    - tarsus E83.31 *[M9Ø.879]*
    - tibia E83.31 *[M9Ø.869]*
    - toe E83.31 *[M9Ø.879]*
    - ulna E83.31 *[M9Ø.839]*
    - vertebra E83.31 *[M9Ø.88]*
- **Osteomyelitis** (general) (infective) (localized) (neonatal) (purulent) (septic) (staphylococcal) (streptococcal) (suppurative) (with periostitis) M86.9
  - acute M86.1Ø
    - carpus M86.14- ☑
    - clavicle M86.11- ☑
    - femur M86.15- ☑
    - fibula M86.16- ☑
    - finger M86.14- ☑
    - hematogenous M86.ØØ
      - carpus M86.Ø4- ☑
      - clavicle M86.Ø1- ☑
      - femur M86.Ø5- ☑
      - fibula M86.Ø6- ☑
      - finger M86.Ø4- ☑
      - humerus M86.Ø2- ☑
      - ilium M86.Ø8
      - ischium M86.Ø8
      - mandible M27.2
      - metacarpus M86.Ø4- ☑
      - metatarsus M86.Ø7- ☑
      - multiple sites M86.Ø9
      - neck M86.Ø8
      - orbit HØ5.Ø2- ☑
      - petrous bone — *see* Petrositis
      - radius M86.Ø3- ☑
      - rib M86.Ø8
      - scapula M86.Ø1- ☑
      - skull M86.Ø8
      - tarsus M86.Ø7- ☑
      - tibia M86.Ø6- ☑
      - toe M86.Ø7- ☑
      - ulna M86.Ø3- ☑
      - vertebra — *see* Osteomyelitis, vertebra
    - humerus M86.12- ☑
    - ilium M86.18
    - ischium M86.18
    - mandible M27.2
    - metacarpus M86.14- ☑
    - metatarsus M86.17- ☑
    - multiple sites M86.19
    - neck M86.18
    - orbit HØ5.Ø2- ☑
    - petrous bone — *see* Petrositis
    - radius M86.13- ☑
    - rib M86.18
    - scapula M86.11- ☑
    - skull M86.18
    - tarsus M86.17- ☑
    - tibia M86.16- ☑
    - toe M86.17- ☑
    - ulna M86.13- ☑
    - vertebra — *see* Osteomyelitis, vertebra
  - chronic (or old) M86.6Ø
    - with draining sinus M86.4Ø
      - carpus M86.44- ☑
      - clavicle M86.41- ☑
      - femur M86.45- ☑
      - fibula M86.46- ☑
      - finger M86.44- ☑
      - humerus M86.42- ☑
      - ilium M86.459
      - ischium M86.459
      - mandible M27.2
      - metacarpus M86.44- ☑
      - metatarsus M86.47- ☑

Osteomyelitis — *continued*
chronic — *continued*
with draining sinus — *continued*
multiple sites M86.49
neck M86.48
orbit HØ5.Ø2- ☑
petrous bone — *see* Petrositis
radius M86.43- ☑
rib M86.48
scapula M86.41- ☑
skull M86.48
tarsus M86.47- ☑
tibia M86.46- ☑
toe M86.47- ☑
ulna M86.43- ☑
vertebra — *see* Osteomyelitis, vertebra
carpus M86.64- ☑
clavicle M86.61- ☑
femur M86.65- ☑
fibula M86.66- ☑
finger M86.64- ☑
hematogenous NEC M86.5Ø
carpus M86.54- ☑
clavicle M86.51- ☑
femur M86.55- ☑
fibula M86.56- ☑
finger M86.54- ☑
humerus M86.52- ☑
ilium M86.559
ischium M86.559
mandible M27.2
metacarpus M86.54- ☑
metatarsus M86.57- ☑
multifocal M86.3Ø
carpus M86.34- ☑
clavicle M86.31- ☑
femur M86.35- ☑
fibula M86.36- ☑
finger M86.34- ☑
humerus M86.32- ☑
ilium M86.359
ischium M86.359
metacarpus M86.34- ☑
metatarsus M86.37- ☑
multiple sites M86.39
neck M86.38
radius M86.33- ☑
rib M86.38
scapula M86.31- ☑
skull M86.38
tarsus M86.37- ☑
tibia M86.36- ☑
toe M86.37- ☑
ulna M86.33- ☑
vertebra — *see* Osteomyelitis, vertebra
multiple sites M86.59
neck M86.58
orbit HØ5.Ø2- ☑
petrous bone — *see* Petrositis
radius M86.53- ☑
rib M86.58
scapula M86.51- ☑
skull M86.58
tarsus M86.57- ☑
tibia M86.56- ☑
toe M86.57- ☑
ulna M86.53- ☑
vertebra — *see* Osteomyelitis, vertebra
humerus M86.62- ☑
ilium M86.659
ischium M86.659
mandible M27.2
metacarpus M86.64- ☑
metatarsus M86.67- ☑
multifocal — *see* Osteomyelitis, chronic, hematogenous, multifocal
multiple sites M86.69
neck M86.68
orbit HØ5.Ø2- ☑
petrous bone — *see* Petrositis
radius M86.63- ☑
rib M86.68
scapula M86.61- ☑
skull M86.68
tarsus M86.67- ☑
tibia M86.66- ☑
toe M86.67- ☑

Osteomyelitis — *continued*
chronic — *continued*
ulna M86.63- ☑
vertebra — *see* Osteomyelitis, vertebra
echinococcal B67.2
Garr's — *see* Osteomyelitis, specified type NEC
in diabetes mellitus — *see* EØ8-E13 with .69
jaw (acute) (chronic) (lower) (neonatal) (suppurative) (upper) M27.2
nonsuppurating — *see* Osteomyelitis, specified type NEC
orbit HØ5.Ø2- ☑
petrous bone — *see* Petrositis
Salmonella (arizonae) (cholerae-suis) (enteritidis) (typhimurium) AØ2.24
sclerosing, nonsuppurative — *see* Osteomyelitis, specified type NEC
specified type NEC — *see also* subcategory M86.8X- ☑
mandible M27.2
orbit HØ5.Ø2- ☑
petrous bone — *see* Petrositis
vertebra — *see* Osteomyelitis, vertebra
subacute M86.2Ø
carpus M86.24- ☑
clavicle M86.21- ☑
femur M86.25- ☑
fibula M86.26- ☑
finger M86.24- ☑
humerus M86.22- ☑
mandible M27.2
metacarpus M86.24- ☑
metatarsus M86.27- ☑
multiple sites M86.29
neck M86.28
orbit HØ5.Ø2- ☑
petrous bone — *see* Petrositis
radius M86.23- ☑
rib M86.28
scapula M86.21- ☑
skull M86.28
tarsus M86.27- ☑
tibia M86.26- ☑
toe M86.27- ☑
ulna M86.23- ☑
vertebra — *see* Osteomyelitis, vertebra
syphilitic A52.77
congenital (early) A5Ø.Ø2 *[M9Ø.8Ø]*
tuberculous — *see* Tuberculosis, bone
typhoid AØ1.Ø5
vertebra M46.2Ø
cervical region M46.22
cervicothoracic region M46.23
lumbar region M46.26
lumbosacral region M46.27
occipito-atlanto-axial region M46.21
sacrococcygeal region M46.28
thoracic region M46.24
thoracolumbar region M46.25
Osteomyelofibrosis D47.4
Osteomyelosclerosis D75.89
Osteonecrosis M87.9
due to
drugs — *see* Osteonecrosis, secondary, due to, drugs
trauma — *see* Osteonecrosis, secondary, due to, trauma
idiopathic aseptic M87.ØØ
ankle M87.Ø7- ☑
carpus M87.Ø3- ☑
clavicle M87.Ø1- ☑
femur M87.Ø5- ☑
fibula M87.Ø6- ☑
finger M87.Ø4- ☑
humerus M87.Ø2- ☑
ilium M87.Ø5Ø
ischium M87.Ø5Ø
metacarpus M87.Ø4- ☑
metatarsus M87.Ø7- ☑
multiple sites M87.Ø9
neck M87.Ø8
pelvis M87.Ø5Ø
radius M87.Ø3- ☑
rib M87.Ø8
scapula M87.Ø1- ☑
skull M87.Ø8
tarsus M87.Ø7- ☑
tibia M87.Ø6- ☑
toe M87.Ø7- ☑

Osteonecrosis — *continued*
idiopathic aseptic — *continued*
ulna M87.Ø3- ☑
vertebra M87.Ø8
secondary NEC M87.3Ø
carpus M87.33- ☑
clavicle M87.31- ☑
due to
drugs M87.1Ø
carpus M87.13- ☑
clavicle M87.11- ☑
femur M87.15- ☑
fibula M87.16- ☑
finger M87.14- ☑
humerus M87.12- ☑
ilium M87.159
ischium M87.159
jaw M87.18Ø
metacarpus M87.14- ☑
metatarsus M87.17- ☑
multiple sites M87.19
neck M87.18 ☑
radius M87.13- ☑
rib M87.18 ☑
scapula M87.11- ☑
skull M87.18 ☑
tarsus M87.17- ☑
tibia M87.16- ☑
toe M87.17- ☑
ulna M87.13- ☑
vertebra M87.18 ☑
hemoglobinopathy NEC D58.2 *[M9Ø.5Ø]*
carpus D58.2 *[M9Ø.54-]* ☑
clavicle D58.2 *[M9Ø.51-]* ☑
femur D58.2 *[M9Ø.55-]* ☑
fibula D58.2 *[M9Ø.56-]* ☑
finger D58.2 *[M9Ø.54-]* ☑
humerus D58.2 *[M9Ø.52-]* ☑
ilium D58.2 *[M9Ø.55-]* ☑
ischium D58.2 *[M9Ø.55-]* ☑
metacarpus D58.2 *[M9Ø.54-]* ☑
metatarsus D58.2 *[M9Ø.57-]* ☑
multiple sites D58.2 *[M9Ø.58]*
neck D58.2 *[M9Ø.58]*
radius D58.2 *[M9Ø.53-]* ☑
rib D58.2 *[M9Ø.58]*
scapula D58.2 *[M9Ø.51-]* ☑
skull D58.2 *[M9Ø.58]*
tarsus D58.2 *[M9Ø.57-]* ☑
tibia D58.2 *[M9Ø.56-]* ☑
toe D58.2 *[M9Ø.57-]* ☑
ulna D58.2 *[M9Ø.53-]* ☑
vertebra D58.2 *[M9Ø.58]*
trauma (previous) M87.2Ø
carpus M87.23- ☑
clavicle M87.21- ☑
femur M87.25- ☑
fibula M87.26- ☑
finger M87.24- ☑
humerus M87.22 ☑
ilium M87.25- ☑
ischium M87.25- ☑
metacarpus M87.24- ☑
metatarsus M87.27- ☑
multiple sites M87.29
neck M87.28
radius M87.23- ☑
rib M87.28
scapula M87.21- ☑
skull M87.28
tarsus M87.27- ☑
tibia M87.26- ☑
toe M87.27- ☑
ulna M87.23- ☑
vertebra M87.28
femur M87.35- ☑
fibula M87.36- ☑
finger M87.34- ☑
humerus M87.32- ☑
ilium M87.35Ø
in
caisson disease T7Ø.3 ☑ *[M9Ø.5Ø]*
carpus T7Ø.3 ☑ *[M9Ø.54-]* ☑
clavicle T7Ø.3 ☑ *[M9Ø.51-]* ☑
femur T7Ø.3 ☑ *[M9Ø.55-]* ☑
fibula T7Ø.3 ☑ *[M9Ø.56-]* ☑

- **Osteonecrosis** — *continued*
  - secondary — *continued*
    - in — *continued*
      - caisson disease — *continued*
        - finger T7Ø.3 ☑ *[M9Ø.54-]* ☑
        - humerus T7Ø.3 ☑ *[M9Ø.52-]* ☑
        - ilium T7Ø.3 ☑ *[M9Ø.55-]* ☑
        - ischium T7Ø.3 ☑ *[M9Ø.55-]* ☑
        - metacarpus T7Ø.3 ☑ *[M9Ø.54-]* ☑
        - metatarsus T7Ø.3 ☑ *[M9Ø.57-]* ☑
        - multiple sites T7Ø.3 ☑ *[M9Ø.59]*
        - neck T7Ø.3 ☑ *[M9Ø.58]*
        - radius T7Ø.3 ☑ *[M9Ø.53-]* ☑
        - rib T7Ø.3 ☑ *[M9Ø.58]*
        - scapula T7Ø.3 ☑ *[M9Ø.51-]* ☑
        - skull T7Ø.3 ☑ *[M9Ø.58]*
        - tarsus T7Ø.3 ☑ *[M9Ø.57-]* ☑
        - tibia T7Ø.3 ☑ *[M9Ø.56-]* ☑
        - toe T7Ø.3 ☑ *[M9Ø.57-]* ☑
        - ulna T7Ø.3 ☑ *[M9Ø.53-]* ☑
        - vertebra T7Ø.3 ☑ *[M9Ø.58]*
    - ischium M87.35Ø
    - metacarpus M87.34- ☑
    - metatarsus M87.37- ☑
    - multiple site M87.39
    - neck M87.38
    - radius M87.33- ☑
    - rib M87.38
    - scapula M87.319
    - skull M87.38
    - tarsus M87.379
    - tibia M87.366
    - toe M87.379
    - ulna M87.33- ☑
    - vertebra M87.38
  - specified type NEC M87.8Ø
    - carpus M87.83- ☑
    - clavicle M87.81- ☑
    - femur M87.85- ☑
    - fibula M87.86- ☑
    - finger M87.84- ☑
    - humerus M87.82- ☑
    - ilium M87.85- ☑
    - ischium M87.85- ☑
    - metacarpus M87.84- ☑
    - metatarsus M87.87- ☑
    - multiple sites M87.89
    - neck M87.88
    - radius M87.83- ☑
    - rib M87.88
    - scapula M87.81- ☑
    - skull M87.88
    - tarsus M87.87- ☑
    - tibia M87.86- ☑
    - toe M87.87- ☑
    - ulna M87.83- ☑
    - vertebra M87.88
- **Osteo-onycho-arthro-dysplasia** Q87.2
- **Osteo-onychodysplasia, hereditary** Q87.2
- **Osteopathia condensans disseminata** Q78.8
- **Osteopathy** — *see also* Osteomyelitis, Osteonecrosis, Osteoporosis
  - after poliomyelitis M89.6Ø
    - carpus M89.64- ☑
    - clavicle M89.61- ☑
    - femur M89.65- ☑
    - fibula M89.66- ☑
    - finger M89.64- ☑
    - humerus M89.62- ☑
    - ilium M89.659
    - ischium M89.659
    - metacarpus M89.64- ☑
    - metatarsus M89.67- ☑
    - multiple sites M89.69
    - neck M89.68
    - radius M89.63- ☑
    - rib M89.68
    - scapula M89.61- ☑
    - skull M89.68
    - tarsus M89.67- ☑
    - tibia M89.66- ☑
    - toe M89.67- ☑
    - ulna M89.63- ☑
    - vertebra M89.68
  - in (due to)
    - renal osteodystrophy N25.Ø

- **Osteopathy** — *continued*
  - in — *continued*
    - specified diseases classified elsewhere — *see* subcategory M9Ø.8 ☑
- **Osteopenia** M85.8- ☑
  - borderline M85.8- ☑
- **Osteoperiostitis** — *see* Osteomyelitis, specified type NEC
- **Osteopetrosis** (familial) Q78.2
- **Osteophyte** M25.7Ø
  - ankle M25.77- ☑
  - elbow M25.72- ☑
  - foot joint M25.77- ☑
  - hand joint M25.74- ☑
  - hip M25.75- ☑
  - knee M25.76- ☑
  - shoulder M25.71- ☑
  - spine M25.78
  - vertebrae M25.78
  - wrist M25.73- ☑
- **Osteopoikilosis** Q78.8
- **Osteoporosis** (female) (male) M81.Ø
  - with current pathological fracture M8Ø.ØØ ☑
  - age-related M81.Ø
    - with current pathologic fracture M8Ø.ØØ ☑
      - carpus M8Ø.Ø4- ☑
      - clavicle M8Ø.Ø1- ☑
      - fibula M8Ø.Ø6- ☑
      - finger M8Ø.Ø4- ☑
      - humerus M8Ø.Ø2- ☑
      - ilium M8Ø.Ø5- ☑
      - ischium M8Ø.Ø5- ☑
      - metacarpus M8Ø.Ø4- ☑
      - metatarsus M8Ø.Ø7- ☑
      - pelvis M8Ø.Ø5- ☑
      - radius M8Ø.Ø3- ☑
      - rib(s) — *see* Osteoporosis, specified site NEC
      - scapula M8Ø.Ø1- ☑
      - site specified NEC M8Ø.ØA ☑
      - specified site NEC M8Ø.ØA ☑
      - tarsus M8Ø.Ø7- ☑
      - tibia M8Ø.Ø6- ☑
      - toe M8Ø.Ø7- ☑
      - ulna M8Ø.Ø3- ☑
      - vertebra M8Ø.Ø8 ☑
  - disuse M81.8
    - with current pathological fracture M8Ø.8Ø ☑
      - carpus M8Ø.84- ☑
      - clavicle M8Ø.81- ☑
      - fibula M8Ø.86- ☑
      - finger M8Ø.84- ☑
      - humerus M8Ø.82- ☑
      - ilium M8Ø.85- ☑
      - ischium M8Ø.85- ☑
      - metacarpus M8Ø.84- ☑
      - metatarsus M8Ø.87- ☑
      - pelvis M8Ø.85- ☑
      - radius M8Ø.83- ☑
      - scapula M8Ø.81- ☑
      - site specified NEC M8Ø.8A ☑
      - tarsus M8Ø.87- ☑
      - tibia M8Ø.86- ☑
      - toe M8Ø.87- ☑
      - ulna M8Ø.83- ☑
      - vertebra M8Ø.88 ☑
  - drug-induced — *see* Osteoporosis, specified type NEC
  - idiopathic — *see* Osteoporosis, specified type NEC
  - involutional — *see* Osteoporosis, age-related
  - Lequesne M81.6
  - localized M81.6
  - postmenopausal M81.Ø
    - with pathological fracture M8Ø.ØØ ☑
      - carpus M8Ø.Ø4- ☑
      - clavicle M8Ø.Ø1- ☑
      - fibula M8Ø.Ø6- ☑
      - finger M8Ø.Ø4- ☑
      - humerus M8Ø.Ø2- ☑
      - ilium M8Ø.Ø5- ☑
      - ischium M8Ø.Ø5- ☑
      - metacarpus M8Ø.Ø4- ☑
      - metatarsus M8Ø.Ø7- ☑
      - pelvis M8Ø.Ø5- ☑
      - radius M8Ø.Ø3- ☑
      - scapula M8Ø.Ø1- ☑
      - site specified NEC M8Ø.ØA ☑
      - tarsus M8Ø.Ø7- ☑

- **Osteoporosis** — *continued*
  - postmenopausal — *continued*
    - with pathological fracture — *continued*
      - tibia M8Ø.Ø6- ☑
      - toe M8Ø.Ø7- ☑
      - ulna M8Ø.Ø3- ☑
      - vertebra M8Ø.Ø8 ☑
  - postoophorectomy — *see* Osteoporosis, specified type NEC
  - postsurgical malabsorption — *see* Osteoporosis, specified type NEC
  - post-traumatic — *see* Osteoporosis, specified type NEC
  - senile — *see* Osteoporosis, age-related
  - specified type NEC M81.8
    - with pathological fracture M8Ø.8Ø ☑
      - carpus M8Ø.84- ☑
      - clavicle M8Ø.81- ☑
      - fibula M8Ø.86- ☑
      - finger M8Ø.84- ☑
      - humerus M8Ø.82- ☑
      - ilium M8Ø.85- ☑
      - ischium M8Ø.85- ☑
      - metacarpus M8Ø.84- ☑
      - metatarsus M8Ø.87- ☑
      - pelvis M8Ø.85- ☑
      - radius M8Ø.83- ☑
      - scapula M8Ø.81- ☑
      - site specified NEC M8Ø.8A ☑
      - tarsus M8Ø.87- ☑
      - tibia M8Ø.86- ☑
      - toe M8Ø.87- ☑
      - ulna M8Ø.83- ☑
      - vertebra M8Ø.88 ☑
- **Osteopsathyrosis** (idiopathica) Q78.Ø
- **Osteoradionecrosis, jaw** (acute) (chronic) (lower) (suppurative) (upper) M27.2
- **Osteosarcoma** (any form) — *see* Neoplasm, bone, malignant
- **Osteosclerosis** Q78.2
  - acquired M85.8- ☑
  - congenita Q77.4
  - fragilitas (generalisata) Q78.2
  - myelofibrosis D75.81
- **Osteosclerotic anemia** D64.89
- **Osteosis**
  - cutis L94.2
  - renal fibrocystic N25.Ø
- **Österreicher-Turner syndrome** Q87.2
- **Ostium**
  - atrioventriculare commune Q21.23
  - primum (arteriosum) (defect) (persistent) Q21.2Ø
  - secundum (arteriosum) (defect) (patent) (persistent) Q21.11
- **Ostrum-Furst syndrome** Q75.8
- **Otalgia** H92.Ø ☑
- **Otitis** (acute) H66.9Ø
  - with effusion — *see also* Otitis, media, nonsuppurative
    - purulent — *see* Otitis, media, suppurative
  - adhesive — *see* subcategory H74.1 ☑
  - chronic — *see also* Otitis, media, chronic
    - with effusion — *see also* Otitis, media, nonsuppurative, chronic
  - externa H6Ø.9- ☑
    - abscess — *see* Abscess, ear, external
    - acute (noninfective) H6Ø.5Ø- ☑
      - actinic H6Ø.51- ☑
      - chemical H6Ø.52- ☑
      - contact H6Ø.53- ☑
      - eczematoid H6Ø.54- ☑
      - infective — *see* Otitis, externa, infective
      - reactive H6Ø.55- ☑
      - specified NEC H6Ø.59- ☑
    - cellulitis — *see* Cellulitis, ear
    - chronic H6Ø.6- ☑
    - diffuse — *see* Otitis, externa, infective, diffuse
    - hemorrhagic — *see* Otitis, externa, infective, hemorrhagic
    - in (due to)
      - aspergillosis B44.89
      - candidiasis B37.84
      - erysipelas A46 *[H62.4Ø]*
      - herpes (simplex) virus infection BØØ.1
        - zoster BØ2.8
      - impetigo LØ1.ØØ *[H62.4Ø]*
      - infectious disease NEC B99 ☑ *[H62.4-]* ☑
      - mycosis NEC B36.9 *[H62.4Ø]*

Otitis — *continued*
  externa — *continued*
    in — *continued*
      parasitic disease NEC B89 *[H62.4Ø]*
      viral disease NEC B34.9 *[H62.4Ø]*
      zoster BØ2.8
    infective NEC H6Ø.39- ☑
      abscess — *see* Abscess, ear, external
      cellulitis — *see* Cellulitis, ear
      diffuse H6Ø.31- ☑
      hemorrhagic H6Ø.32- ☑
      swimmer's ear — *see* Swimmer's, ear
    malignant H6Ø.2- ☑
    mycotic NEC B36.9 *[H62.4Ø]*
      in
        aspergillosis B44.89
        candidiasis B37.84
        moniliasis B37.84
    necrotizing — *see* Otitis, externa, malignant
    Pseudomonas aeruginosa — *see* Otitis, externa, malignant
    reactive — *see* Otitis, externa, acute, reactive
    specified NEC — *see* subcategory H6Ø.8 ☑
    tropical NEC B36.9 *[H62.4Ø]*
      in
        aspergillosis B44.89
        candidiasis B37.84
        moniliasis B37.84
  insidiosa — *see* Otosclerosis
  interna H83.Ø ☑
  media (hemorrhagic) (staphylococcal) (streptococcal) H66.9- ☑
    with effusion (nonpurulent) — *see* Otitis, media, nonsuppurative
    acute, subacute H66.9Ø
      allergic — *see* Otitis, media, nonsuppurative, acute, allergic
      exudative — *see* Otitis, media, suppurative, acute
      mucoid — *see* Otitis, media, nonsuppurative, acute
      necrotizing — *see also* Otitis, media, suppurative, acute
        in
          measles BØ5.3
          scarlet fever A38.Ø
      nonsuppurative NEC — *see* Otitis, media, nonsuppurative, acute
      purulent — *see* Otitis, media, suppurative, acute
      sanguinous — *see* Otitis, media, nonsuppurative, acute
      secretory — *see* Otitis, media, nonsuppurative, acute, serous
      seromucinous — *see* Otitis, media, nonsuppurative, acute
      serous — *see* Otitis, media, nonsuppurative, acute, serous
      suppurative — *see* Otitis, media, suppurative, acute
    allergic — *see* Otitis, media, nonsuppurative
    catarrhal — *see* Otitis, media, nonsuppurative
    chronic H66.9Ø
      with effusion (nonpurulent) — *see* Otitis, media, nonsuppurative, chronic
      allergic — *see* Otitis, media, nonsuppurative, chronic, allergic
      benign suppurative — *see* Otitis, media, suppurative, chronic, tubotympanic
      catarrhal — *see* Otitis, media, nonsuppurative, chronic, serous
      exudative — *see* Otitis, media, nonsuppurative, chronic
      mucinous — *see* Otitis, media, nonsuppurative, chronic, mucoid
      mucoid — *see* Otitis, media, nonsuppurative, chronic, mucoid
      nonsuppurative NEC — *see* Otitis, media, nonsuppurative, chronic
      purulent — *see* Otitis, media, suppurative, chronic
      secretory — *see* Otitis, media, nonsuppurative, chronic, mucoid
      seromucinous — *see* Otitis, media, nonsuppurative, chronic
      serous — *see* Otitis, media, nonsuppurative, chronic, serous
      suppurative — *see* Otitis, media, suppurative, chronic

Otitis — *continued*
  media — *continued*
    chronic — *continued*
      transudative — *see* Otitis, media, nonsuppurative, chronic, mucoid
    exudative — *see* Otitis, media, suppurative
    in (due to) (with)
      influenza — *see* Influenza, with, otitis media
      measles BØ5.3
      scarlet fever A38.Ø
      tuberculosis A18.6
      viral disease NEC B34.- ☑ *[H67.-]* ☑
    mucoid — *see* Otitis, media, nonsuppurative
    nonsuppurative H65.9- ☑
      acute or subacute NEC H65.19- ☑
        allergic H65.11- ☑
          recurrent H65.11- ☑
        recurrent H65.19- ☑
        secretory — *see* Otitis, media, nonsuppurative, serous
        serous H65.Ø- ☑
          recurrent H65.Ø- ☑
      chronic H65.49- ☑
        allergic H65.41- ☑
        mucoid H65.3- ☑
        serous H65.2- ☑
    postmeasles BØ5.3
    purulent — *see* Otitis, media, suppurative
    secretory — *see* Otitis, media, nonsuppurative
    seromucinous — *see* Otitis, media, nonsuppurative
    serous — *see* Otitis, media, nonsuppurative
    suppurative H66.4- ☑
      acute H66.ØØ- ☑
        with rupture of ear drum H66.Ø1- ☑
        recurrent H66.ØØ- ☑
          with rupture of ear drum H66.Ø1- ☑
      chronic — *see also* subcategory H66.3 ☑
        atticoantral H66.2- ☑
        benign — *see* Otitis, media, suppurative, chronic, tubotympanic
        tubotympanic H66.1- ☑
    transudative — *see* Otitis, media, nonsuppurative
    tuberculous A18.6
Otocephaly Q18.2
Otolith syndrome — *see* subcategory H81.8 ☑
Otomycosis (diffuse) **NEC** B36.9 *[H62.4Ø]*
  in
    aspergillosis B44.89
    candidiasis B37.84
    moniliasis B37.84
Otoporosis — *see* Otosclerosis
Otorrhagia (nontraumatic) H92.2- ☑
  traumatic — *code by* Type of injury
Otorrhea H92.1- ☑
  cerebrospinal (fluid) G96.Ø1
    postoperative G96.Ø8
    specified NEC G96.Ø8
    spontaneous G96.Ø1
    traumatic G96.Ø8
Otosclerosis (general) H8Ø.9- ☑
  cochlear (endosteal) H8Ø.2- ☑
  involving
    otic capsule — *see* Otosclerosis, cochlear
    oval window
      nonobliterative H8Ø.Ø- ☑
      obliterative H8Ø.1- ☑
    round window — *see* Otosclerosis, cochlear
  nonobliterative — *see* Otosclerosis, involving, oval window, nonobliterative
  obliterative — *see* Otosclerosis, involving, oval window, obliterative
  specified NEC H8Ø.8- ☑
Otospongiosis — *see* Otosclerosis
Otto's disease or pelvis M24.7
Outcome of delivery Z37.9
  multiple births Z37.9
    all liveborn Z37.5Ø
      quadruplets Z37.52
      quintuplets Z37.53
      sextuplets Z37.54
      specified number NEC Z37.59
      triplets Z37.51
    all stillborn Z37.7
    some liveborn Z37.6Ø
      quadruplets Z37.62
      quintuplets Z37.63
      sextuplets Z37.64

Outcome of delivery — *continued*
  multiple births — *continued*
    some liveborn — *continued*
      specified number NEC Z37.69
      triplets Z37.61
  single NEC Z37.9
    liveborn Z37.Ø
    stillborn Z37.1
  twins NEC Z37.9
    both liveborn Z37.2
    both stillborn Z37.4
    one liveborn, one stillborn Z37.3
Outlet — *see* condition
Ovalocytosis (congenital) (hereditary) — *see* Elliptocytosis
Ovarian — *see* Condition
Ovariocele N83.4- ☑
Ovaritis (cystic) — *see* Oophoritis
Ovary, ovarian — *see also* condition
  resistant syndrome E28.39
  vein syndrome N13.8
Overactive — *see also* Hyperfunction
  adrenal cortex NEC E27.Ø
  bladder N32.81
  hypothalamus E23.3
  thyroid — *see* Hyperthyroidism
Overactivity R46.3
  child — *see* Disorder, attention-deficit hyperactivity
Overbite (deep) (excessive) (horizontal) (vertical) M26.29
Overbreathing — *see* Hyperventilation
Overconscientious personality F6Ø.5
Overdevelopment — *see* Hypertrophy
Overdistension — *see* Distension
Overdose, overdosage (drug) — *see* Table of Drugs and Chemicals, by drug, poisoning
Overeating R63.2
  nonorganic origin F5Ø.89
  psychogenic F5Ø.89
Overexertion (effects) (exhaustion) T73.3 ☑
Overexposure (effects) T73.9 ☑
  exhaustion T73.2 ☑
Overfeeding — *see* Overeating
  newborn P92.4
Overfill, endodontic M27.52
Overgrowth, bone — *see* Hypertrophy, bone
Overhanging of dental restorative material (unrepairable) KØ8.52
Overheated (places) (effects) — *see* Heat
Overjet (excessive horizontal) M26.23
Overlaid, overlying (suffocation) — *see* Asphyxia, traumatic, due to mechanical threat
Overlap, excessive horizontal (teeth) M26.23
Overlapping toe (acquired) — *see also* Deformity, toe, specified NEC
  congenital (fifth toe) Q66.89
Overload
  circulatory, due to transfusion (blood) (blood components) (TACO) E87.71
  fluid E87.7Ø
    due to transfusion (blood) (blood components) E87.71
    specified NEC E87.79
  iron, due to repeated red blood cell transfusions E83.111
  potassium (K) E87.5
  sodium (Na) E87.Ø
Overnutrition — *see* Hyperalimentation
Overproduction — *see also* Hypersecretion
  ACTH E27.Ø
  catecholamine E27.5
  growth hormone E22.Ø
Overprotection, child by parent Z62.1
Overriding
  aorta Q25.49
  finger (acquired) — *see* Deformity, finger
    congenital Q68.1
  toe (acquired) — *see also* Deformity, toe, specified NEC
    congenital Q66.89
Overstrained R53.83
  heart — *see* Hypertrophy, cardiac
Overuse, muscle NEC M7Ø.8- ☑
Overweight E66.3
Overworked R53.83
Oviduct — *see* condition
Ovotestis Q56.Ø
Ovulation (cycle)
  failure or lack of N97.Ø

Ovulation — *continued*
- pain N94.Ø

Ovum — *see* condition
Owren's disease or syndrome (parahemophilia) D68.2
Ox heart — *see* Hypertrophy, cardiac
Oxalosis E72.53
Oxaluria E72.53
Oxycephaly, oxycephalic Q75.Ø
- syphilitic, congenital A5Ø.Ø2

Oxyuriasis B8Ø
Oxyuris vermicularis (infestation) B8Ø
Ozena J31.Ø

P

Pachyderma, pachydermia L85.9
- larynx (verrucosa) J38.7

Pachydermatocele (congenital) Q82.8
Pachydermoperiostosis — *see also* Osteoarthropathy, hypertrophic, specified type NEC
- clubbed nail M89.4Ø *[L62]*

Pachygyria QØ4.3
Pachymeningitis (adhesive) (basal) (brain) (cervical) (chronic) (circumscribed) (external) (fibrous) (hemorrhagic) (hypertrophic) (internal) (purulent) (spinal) (suppurative) — *see* Meningitis
Pachyonychia (congenital) Q84.5
Pacinian tumor — *see* Neoplasm, skin, benign
Pad, knuckle or Garrod's M72.1
Paget's disease
- with infiltrating duct carcinoma — *see* Neoplasm, breast, malignant
- bone M88.9
  - carpus M88.84- ☑
  - clavicle M88.81- ☑
  - femur M88.85- ☑
  - fibula M88.86- ☑
  - finger M88.84- ☑
  - humerus M88.82- ☑
  - ilium M88.85- ☑
  - in neoplastic disease — *see* Osteitis, deformans, in neoplastic disease
  - ischium M88.85- ☑
  - metacarpus M88.84- ☑
  - metatarsus M88.87- ☑
  - multiple sites M88.89
  - neck M88.88
  - radius M88.83- ☑
  - rib M88.88
  - scapula M88.81- ☑
  - skull M88.Ø
  - specified NEC M88.88
  - tarsus M88.87- ☑
  - tibia M88.86- ☑
  - toe M88.87- ☑
  - ulna M88.83- ☑
  - vertebra M88.1
- breast (female) C5Ø.Ø1- ☑
  - male C5Ø.Ø2- ☑
- extramammary — *see also* Neoplasm, skin, malignant
  - anus C21.Ø
    - margin C44.59Ø
    - skin C44.59Ø
- intraductal carcinoma — *see* Neoplasm, breast, malignant
- malignant — *see* Neoplasm, skin, malignant
  - breast (female) C5Ø.Ø1- ☑
    - male C5Ø.Ø2- ☑
  - unspecified site (female) C5Ø.Ø1- ☑
    - male C5Ø.Ø2- ☑
- mammary — *see* Paget's disease, breast
- nipple — *see* Paget's disease, breast
- osteitis deformans — *see* Paget's disease, bone

Paget-Schroetter syndrome I82.89Ø
Pain(s) — *see also* Painful R52
- abdominal R1Ø.9
  - colic R1Ø.83
  - generalized R1Ø.84
    - with acute abdomen R1Ø.Ø
  - lower R1Ø.3Ø
    - left quadrant R1Ø.32
    - pelvic or perineal R1Ø.2
    - periumbilical R1Ø.33
    - right quadrant R1Ø.31
  - rebound — *see* Tenderness, abdominal, rebound
  - severe with abdominal rigidity R1Ø.Ø
  - tenderness — *see* Tenderness, abdominal
  - upper R1Ø.1Ø
    - epigastric R1Ø.13
    - left quadrant R1Ø.12
    - right quadrant R1Ø.11
- acute R52
  - due to trauma G89.11
  - neoplasm related G89.3
  - postprocedural NEC G89.18
  - post-thoracotomy G89.12
  - specified by site — *code to* Pain, by site
- adnexa (uteri) R1Ø.2
- anginoid — *see* Pain, precordial
- anus K62.89
- arm — *see* Pain, limb, upper
- axillary (axilla) M79.62- ☑
- back (postural) M54.9
- bladder R39.89
  - associated with micturition — *see* Micturition, painful
  - chronic R39.82
- bone — *see* Disorder, bone, specified type NEC
- breast N64.4
- broad ligament R1Ø.2
- cancer associated (acute) (chronic) G89.3
- cecum — *see* Pain, abdominal
- cervicobrachial M53.1
- chest (central) RØ7.9
  - anterior wall RØ7.89
  - atypical RØ7.89
  - ischemic I2Ø.9
  - musculoskeletal RØ7.89
  - non-cardiac RØ7.89
  - on breathing RØ7.1
  - pleurodynia RØ7.81
  - precordial RØ7.2
  - wall (anterior) RØ7.89
- chronic G89.29
  - associated with significant psychosocial dysfunction G89.4
  - due to trauma G89.21
  - neoplasm related G89.3
  - postoperative NEC G89.28
  - postprocedural NEC G89.28
  - post-thoracotomy G89.22
  - specified NEC G89.29
- coccyx M53.3
- colon — *see* Pain, abdominal
- coronary — *see* Angina
- costochondral RØ7.1
- diaphragm RØ7.1
- due to cancer G89.3
- due to device, implant or graft — *see also* Complications, by site and type, specified NEC T85.848 ☑
  - arterial graft NEC T82.848 ☑
  - breast (implant) T85.848 ☑
  - catheter NEC T85.848 ☑
    - dialysis (renal) T82.848 ☑
      - intraperitoneal T85.848 ☑
    - infusion NEC T82.848 ☑
      - spinal (epidural) (subdural) T85.84Ø ☑
    - urinary (indwelling) T83.84 ☑
  - electronic (electrode) (pulse generator) (stimulator)
    - bone T85.84Ø ☑
    - cardiac T82.847 ☑
    - nervous system (brain) (peripheral nerve) (spinal) T85.84 ☑
    - urinary T83.84 ☑
  - fixation, internal (orthopedic) NEC T84.84 ☑
  - gastrointestinal (bile duct) (esophagus) T85.848 ☑
  - genital NEC T83.84 ☑
  - heart NEC T82.847 ☑
  - infusion NEC T85.848 ☑
  - joint prosthesis T84.84 ☑
  - ocular (corneal graft) (orbital implant) NEC T85.848 ☑
  - orthopedic NEC T84.84 ☑
  - specified NEC T85.848 ☑
  - urinary NEC T83.84 ☑
  - vascular NEC T82.848 ☑
  - ventricular intracranial shunt T85.84Ø ☑
- due to malignancy (primary) (secondary) G89.3
- ear — *see* subcategory H92.Ø ☑
- epigastric, epigastrium R1Ø.13
- eye — *see* Pain, ocular
- face, facial R51.9
  - atypical G5Ø.1
- female genital organs NEC N94.89
- finger — *see* Pain, limb, upper
- flank — *see* Pain, abdominal
- foot — *see* Pain, limb, lower
- gallbladder K82.9
- gas (intestinal) R14.1
- gastric — *see* Pain, abdominal
- generalized NOS R52
- genital organ
  - female N94.89
  - male N5Ø.89
- groin — *see* Pain, abdominal, lower
- hand — *see* Pain, limb, upper
- head — *see* Headache
- heart — *see* Pain, precordial
- infra-orbital — *see* Neuralgia, trigeminal
- intercostal RØ7.82
- intermenstrual N94.Ø
- jaw R68.84
- joint M25.5Ø
  - ankle M25.57- ☑
  - elbow M25.52- ☑
  - finger M25.54- ☑
  - foot M25.57- ☑
  - hand M25.54- ☑
  - hip M25.55- ☑
  - knee M25.56- ☑
  - shoulder M25.51- ☑
  - specified site NEC M25.59
  - toe M25.57- ☑
  - wrist M25.53- ☑
- kidney N23
- laryngeal RØ7.Ø
- leg — *see* Pain, limb, lower
- limb M79.6Ø9
  - lower M79.6Ø- ☑
    - foot M79.67- ☑
    - lower leg M79.66- ☑
    - thigh M79.65- ☑
    - toe M79.67- ☑
  - upper M79.6Ø- ☑
    - axilla M79.62- ☑
    - finger M79.64- ☑
    - forearm M79.63- ☑
    - hand M79.64- ☑
    - upper arm M79.62- ☑
- loin M54.5Ø
- low back M54.5Ø
  - specified NEC M54.59
  - vertebral end plate M54.51
  - vertebrogenic M54.51
- lumbar region M54.5Ø
  - vertebral end plate M54.51
  - vertebrogenic M54.51
- mandibular R68.84
- mastoid — *see* subcategory H92.Ø ☑
- maxilla R68.84
- menstrual — *see also* Dysmenorrhea N94.6
- metacarpophalangeal (joint) — *see* Pain, joint, hand
- metatarsophalangeal (joint) — *see* Pain, joint, foot
- mouth K13.79
- muscle — *see* Myalgia
- musculoskeletal — *see also* Pain, by site M79.18
- myofascial M79.18
- nasal J34.89
- nasopharynx J39.2
- neck NEC M54.2
- nerve NEC — *see* Neuralgia
- neuromuscular — *see* Neuralgia
- nose J34.89
- ocular H57.1- ☑
- ophthalmic — *see* Pain, ocular
- orbital region — *see* Pain, ocular
- ovary N94.89
- over heart — *see* Pain, precordial
- ovulation N94.Ø
- pelvic (female) R1Ø.2
- penis N48.89
- pericardial — *see* Pain, precordial
- perineal, perineum R1Ø.2
- pharynx J39.2
- pleura, pleural, pleuritic RØ7.81
- postoperative NOS G89.18
- postprocedural NOS G89.18

☑ **Additional Character Required — Refer to the Tabular List for Character Selection**

Pain(s) — *continued*
- post-thoracotomy G89.12
- precordial (region) RØ7.2
- premenstrual N94.3
- psychogenic (persistent) (any site) F45.41
- radicular (spinal) — *see* Radiculopathy
- rectum K62.89
- respiration RØ7.1
- retrosternal RØ7.2
- rheumatoid, muscular — *see* Myalgia
- rib RØ7.81
- root (spinal) — *see* Radiculopathy
- round ligament (stretch) R1Ø.2
- sacroiliac M53.3
- sciatic — *see* Sciatica
- scrotum N5Ø.82
- seminal vesicle N5Ø.89
- shoulder M25.51- ☑
- spermatic cord N5Ø.89
- spinal root — *see* Radiculopathy
- spine M54.9
  - cervical M54.2
  - low back M54.5Ø
    - with sciatica M54.4- ☑
  - thoracic M54.6
- stomach — *see* Pain, abdominal
- substernal RØ7.2
- temporomandibular (joint) M26.62- ☑
- testis N5Ø.81- ☑
- thoracic spine M54.6
  - with radicular and visceral pain M54.14
- throat RØ7.Ø
- tibia — *see* Pain, limb, lower
- toe — *see* Pain, limb, lower
- tongue K14.6
- tooth KØ8.89
- trigeminal — *see* Neuralgia, trigeminal
- tumor associated G89.3
- ureter N23
- urinary (organ) (system) N23
- uterus NEC N94.89
- vagina R1Ø.2
- vertebral end plate — *see* Pain, vertebrogenic
- vertebrogenic M54.89
  - low back M54.51
  - lumbar M54.51
  - syndrome M54.89
- vesical R39.89
  - associated with micturition — *see* Micturition, painful
- vulva R1Ø.2

Painful — *see also* Pain
- coitus
  - female N94.1Ø
  - male N53.12
  - psychogenic F52.6
- ejaculation (semen) N53.12
  - psychogenic F52.6
- erection — *see* Priapism
- feet syndrome E53.8
- joint replacement (hip) (knee) T84.84 ☑
- menstruation — *see* Dysmenorrhea
  - psychogenic F45.8
- micturition — *see* Micturition, painful
- respiration RØ7.1
- scar NEC L9Ø.5
- wire sutures T81.89 ☑

Painter's colic — *see* subcategory T56.Ø ☑

Palate — *see* condition

Palatoplegia K13.79

Palatoschisis — *see* Cleft, palate

Palilalia R48.8

Palliative care Z51.5

Pallor R23.1
- optic disc, temporal — *see* Atrophy, optic

Palmar — *see also* condition
- fascia — *see* condition

Palpable
- cecum K63.89
- kidney N28.89
- ovary N83.8
- prostate N42.9
- spleen — *see* Splenomegaly

Palpitations (heart) RØØ.2
- psychogenic F45.8

Palsy — *see also* Paralysis G83.9
- atrophic diffuse (progressive) G12.22
- Bell's — *see also* Palsy, facial

Palsy — *continued*
- Bell's — *see also* Palsy, facial — *continued*
  - newborn P11.3
- brachial plexus NEC G54.Ø
  - newborn (birth injury) P14.3
- brain — *see* Palsy, cerebral
- bulbar (progressive) (chronic) G12.22
  - of childhood (Fazio-Londe) G12.1
  - pseudo NEC G12.29
  - supranuclear (progressive) G23.1
- cerebral (congenital) G8Ø.9
  - ataxic G8Ø.4
  - athetoid G8Ø.3
  - choreathetoid G8Ø.3
  - diplegic G8Ø.8
    - spastic G8Ø.1
  - dyskinetic G8Ø.3
    - athetoid G8Ø.3
    - choreathetoid G8Ø.3
    - distonic G8Ø.3
  - dystonic G8Ø.3
  - hemiplegic G8Ø.8
    - spastic G8Ø.2
  - mixed G8Ø.8
  - monoplegic G8Ø.8
    - spastic G8Ø.1
  - paraplegic G8Ø.8
    - spastic G8Ø.1
  - quadriplegic G8Ø.8
    - spastic G8Ø.Ø
  - spastic G8Ø.1
    - diplegic G8Ø.1
    - hemiplegic G8Ø.2
    - monoplegic G8Ø.1
    - quadriplegic G8Ø.Ø
    - specified NEC G8Ø.1
    - tetrapelgic G8Ø.Ø
  - specified NEC G8Ø.8
  - syphilitic A52.12
    - congenital A5Ø.49
  - tetraplegic G8Ø.8
    - spastic G8Ø.Ø
- cranial nerve — *see also* Disorder, nerve, cranial
  - multiple G52.7
    - in
      - infectious disease B99 ☑ *[G53]*
      - neoplastic disease — *see also* Neoplasm D49.9 *[G53]*
      - parasitic disease B89 *[G53]*
      - sarcoidosis D86.82
- creeping G12.22
- diver's T7Ø.3 ☑
- Erb's P14.Ø
- facial G51.Ø
  - newborn (birth injury) P11.3
- glossopharyngeal G52.1
- Klumpke (-Déjérine) P14.1
- lead — *see* subcategory T56.Ø ☑
- median nerve (tardy) G56.1- ☑
- nerve G58.9
  - specified NEC G58.8
- peroneal nerve (acute) (tardy) G57.3- ☑
- progressive supranuclear G23.1
- pseudobulbar NEC G12.29
- radial nerve (acute) G56.3- ☑
- seventh nerve — *see also* Palsy, facial
  - newborn P11.3
- shaking — *see* Parkinsonism
- spastic (cerebral) (spinal) G8Ø.1
- ulnar nerve (tardy) G56.2- ☑
- wasting G12.29

Paludism — *see* Malaria

Panangiitis M3Ø.Ø

Panaris, panaritium — *see also* Cellulitis, digit
- with lymphangitis — *see* Lymphangitis, acute, digit

Panarteritis nodosa M3Ø.Ø
- brain or cerebral I67.7

Pancake heart R93.1
- with cor pulmonale (chronic) I27.81

Pancarditis (acute) (chronic) I51.89
- rheumatic IØ9.89
  - active or acute IØ1.8

Pancoast's syndrome or tumor C34.1- ☑

Pancolitis, ulcerative (chronic) K51.ØØ
- with
  - abscess K51.Ø14
  - complication K51.Ø19
  - fistula K51.Ø13

Pancolitis, ulcerative — *continued*
- with — *continued*
  - obstruction K51.Ø12
  - rectal bleeding K51.Ø11
  - specified complication NEC K51.Ø18

Pancreas, pancreatic — *see* condition

Pancreatitis (annular) (apoplectic) (calcareous) (edematous) (hemorrhagic) (malignant) (subacute) (suppurative) K85.9Ø
- with necrosis (uninfected) K85.91
  - infected K85.92
- acute (without necrosis or infection) K85.9Ø
  - with necrosis (uninfected) K85.91
    - infected K85.92
  - alcohol induced (without necrosis or infection) K85.2Ø
    - with necrosis (uninfected) K85.21
      - infected K85.22
  - biliary (without necrosis or infection) K85.1Ø
    - with necrosis (uninfected) K85.11
      - infected K85.12
  - drug induced (without necrosis or infection) K85.3Ø
    - with necrosis (uninfected) K85.31
      - infected K85.32
  - gallstone (without necrosis or infection) K85.1Ø
    - with necrosis (uninfected) K85.11
      - infected K85.12
  - idiopathic (without necrosis or infection) K85.ØØ
    - with necrosis (uninfected) K85.Ø1
      - infected K85.Ø2
  - specified NEC (without necrosis or infection) K85.8Ø
    - with necrosis (uninfected) K85.81
      - infected K85.82
- chronic (infectious) K86.1
  - alcohol-induced K86.Ø
  - recurrent K86.1
  - relapsing K86.1
- cystic (chronic) K86.1
- cytomegaloviral B25.2
- fibrous (chronic) K86.1
- gallstone (without necrosis or infection) K85.1Ø
  - with necrosis (uninfected) K85.11
    - infected K85.12
- gangrenous — *see* Pancreatitis, acute
- interstitial (chronic) K86.1
  - acute — *see also* Pancreatitis, acute K85.8Ø
- mumps B26.3
- recurrent
  - acute — *see* Pancreatitis, acute by type
  - chronic K86.1
- relapsing, chronic K86.1
- syphilitic A52.74

Pancreatoblastoma — *see* Neoplasm, pancreas, malignant

Pancreolithiasis K86.89

Pancytolysis D75.89

Pancytopenia (acquired) D61.818
- with
  - malformations D61.Ø9
  - myelodysplastic syndrome — *see* Syndrome, myelodysplastic
- antineoplastic chemotherapy induced D61.81Ø
- congenital D61.Ø9
- drug-induced NEC D61.811

PANDAS (pediatric autoimmune neuropsychiatric disorders associated with streptococcal infections syndrome) D89.89

Panencephalitis, subacute, sclerosing A81.1

Panhematopenia D61.9
- congenital D61.Ø9
- constitutional D61.Ø9
- splenic, primary D73.1

Panhemocytopenia D61.9
- congenital D61.Ø9
- constitutional D61.Ø9

Panhypogonadism E29.1

Panhypopituitarism E23.Ø
- prepubertal E23.Ø

Panic (attack) (state) F41.Ø
- reaction to exceptional stress (transient) F43.Ø

Panmyelopathy, familial, constitutional D61.Ø9

Panmyelophthisis D61.82
- congenital D61.Ø9

Panmyelosis (acute) (with myelofibrosis) C94.4- ☑

Panner's disease — *see* Osteochondrosis, juvenile, humerus

Panneuritis endemica E51.11

Panniculitis (nodular) (nonsuppurative) M79.3

Panniculitis — *continued*
back M54.ØØ
cervical region M54.Ø2
cervicothoracic region M54.Ø3
lumbar region M54.Ø6
lumbosacral region M54.Ø7
multiple sites M54.Ø9
occipito-atlanto-axial region M54.Ø1
sacrococcygeal region M54.Ø8
thoracic region M54.Ø4
thoracolumbar region M54.Ø5
lupus L93.2
mesenteric K65.4
neck M54.Ø2
cervicothoracic region M54.Ø3
occipito-atlanto-axial region M54.Ø1
relapsing M35.6
Panniculus adiposus (abdominal) E65
Pannus (allergic) (cornea) (degenerativus) (keratic) H16.42- ☑
abdominal (symptomatic) E65
trachomatosus, trachomatous (active) A71.1
Panophthalmitis H44.Ø1- ☑
Pansinusitis (chronic) (hyperplastic) (nonpurulent) (purulent) J32.4
acute JØ1.4Ø
recurrent JØ1.41
tuberculous A15.8
Panuveitis (sympathetic) H44.11- ☑
Panvalvular disease IØ8.9
specified NEC IØ8.8
PAPA (pyogenic arthritis, pyoderma gangrenosum, and acne syndrome) MØ4.8
Papanicolaou smear, cervix Z12.4
as part of routine gynecological examination ZØ1.419
with abnormal findings ZØ1.411
for suspected neoplasm Z12.4
nonspecific abnormal finding R87.619
routine ZØ1.419
with abnormal findings ZØ1.411
Papilledema (choked disc) H47.1Ø
associated with
decreased ocular pressure H47.12
increased intracranial pressure H47.11
retinal disorder H47.13
Foster-Kennedy syndrome H47.14- ☑
Papillitis H46.ØØ
anus K62.89
chronic lingual K14.4
necrotizing, kidney N17.2
optic H46.Ø- ☑
rectum K62.89
renal, necrotizing N17.2
tongue K14.Ø
Papilloma — *see also* Neoplasm, benign, by site
acuminatum (female) (male) (anogenital) A63.Ø
basal cell L82.1
inflamed L82.Ø
benign pinta (primary) A67.Ø
bladder (urinary) (transitional cell) D41.4
choroid plexus (lateral ventricle) (third ventricle) D33.Ø
anaplastic C71.5
fourth ventricle D33.1
malignant C71.5
renal pelvis (transitional cell) D41.1- ☑
benign D3Ø.1- ☑
Schneiderian
specified site — *see* Neoplasm, benign, by site
unspecified site D14.Ø
serous surface
borderline malignancy
specified site — *see* Neoplasm, uncertain behavior, by site
unspecified site D39.1Ø
specified site — *see* Neoplasm, benign, by site
unspecified site D27.9
transitional (cell)
bladder (urinary) D41.4
inverted type — *see* Neoplasm, uncertain behavior, by site
renal pelvis D41.1- ☑
ureter D41.2- ☑
ureter (transitional cell) D41.2- ☑
benign D3Ø.2- ☑
urothelial — *see* Neoplasm, uncertain behavior, by site
villous — *see* Neoplasm, uncertain behavior, by site
adenocarcinoma in — *see* Neoplasm, malignant, by site
Papilloma — *continued*
villous — *see* Neoplasm, uncertain behavior, by site — *continued*
adenocarcinoma in — *see* Neoplasm, malignant, by site — *continued*
in situ — *see* Neoplasm, in situ
yaws, plantar or palmar A66.1
Papillomata, multiple, of yaws A66.1
Papillomatosis — *see also* Neoplasm, benign, by site
confluent and reticulated L83
cystic, breast — *see* Mastopathy, cystic
ductal, breast — *see* Mastopathy, cystic
intraductal (diffuse) — *see* Neoplasm, benign, by site
subareolar duct D24- ☑
Papillomavirus, as cause of disease classified elsewhere B97.7
Papillon-Léage and Psaume syndrome Q87.Ø
Papule(s) R23.8
carate (primary) A67.Ø
fibrous, of nose D22.39
Gottron's L94.4
pinta (primary) A67.Ø
Papulosis
lymphomatoid C86.6
malignant I77.89
Papyraceous fetus O31.Ø- ☑
Para-albuminemia E88.Ø9
Paracephalus Q89.7
Parachute mitral valve Q23.2
Paracoccidioidomycosis B41.9
disseminated B41.7
generalized B41.7
mucocutaneous-lymphangitic B41.8
pulmonary B41.Ø
specified NEC B41.8
visceral B41.8
Paradentosis KØ5.4
Paraffinoma T88.8 ☑
Paraganglioma D44.7
adrenal D35.Ø- ☑
malignant C74.1- ☑
aortic body D44.7
malignant C75.5
carotid body D44.6
malignant C75.4
chromaffin — *see also* Neoplasm, benign, by site
malignant — *see* Neoplasm, malignant, by site
extra-adrenal D44.7
malignant C75.5
specified site — *see* Neoplasm, malignant, by site
unspecified site C75.5
specified site — *see* Neoplasm, uncertain behavior, by site
unspecified site D44.7
gangliocytic D13.2
specified site — *see* Neoplasm, benign, by site
unspecified site D13.2
glomus jugulare D44.7
malignant C75.5
jugular D44.7
malignant C75.5
specified site — *see* Neoplasm, malignant, by site
unspecified site C75.5
nonchromaffin D44.7
malignant C75.5
specified site — *see* Neoplasm, malignant, by site
unspecified site C75.5
specified site — *see* Neoplasm, uncertain behavior, by site
unspecified site D44.7
parasympathetic D44.7
specified site — *see* Neoplasm, uncertain behavior, by site
unspecified site D44.7
specified site — *see* Neoplasm, uncertain behavior, by site
sympathetic D44.7
specified site — *see* Neoplasm, uncertain behavior, by site
unspecified site D44.7
unspecified site D44.7
Parageusia R43.2
psychogenic F45.8
Paragonimiasis B66.4
Paragranuloma, Hodgkin — *see* Lymphoma, Hodgkin, specified NEC
Parahemophilia — *see also* Defect, coagulation D68.2
Parakeratosis R23.4
variegata L41.Ø
Paralysis, paralytic (complete) (incomplete) G83.9
with
syphilis A52.17
abducens, abducent (nerve) — *see* Strabismus, paralytic, sixth nerve
abductor, lower extremity G57.9- ☑
accessory nerve G52.8
accommodation — *see also* Paresis, of accommodation
hysterical F44.89
acoustic nerve (except Deafness) H93.3 ☑
agitans — *see also* Parkinsonism G2Ø
arteriosclerotic G21.4
alternating (oculomotor) G83.89
amyotrophic G12.21
ankle G57.9- ☑
anus (sphincter) K62.89
arm — *see* Monoplegia, upper limb
ascending (spinal), acute G61.Ø
association G12.29
asthenic bulbar G7Ø.ØØ
with exacerbation (acute) G7Ø.Ø1
in crisis G7Ø.Ø1
ataxic (hereditary) G11.9
general (syphilitic) A52.17
atrophic G58.9
infantile, acute — *see* Poliomyelitis, paralytic
progressive G12.22
spinal (acute) — *see* Poliomyelitis, paralytic
axillary G54.Ø
Babinski-Nageotte's G83.89
Bell's G51.Ø
newborn P11.3
Benedikt's G46.3
birth injury P14.9
spinal cord P11.5
bladder (neurogenic) (sphincter) N31.2
bowel, colon or intestine K56.Ø
brachial plexus G54.Ø
birth injury P14.3
newborn (birth injury) P14.3
brain G83.9
diplegia G83.Ø
triplegia G83.89
bronchial J98.Ø9
Brown-Séquard G83.81
bulbar (chronic) (progressive) G12.22
infantile — *see* Poliomyelitis, paralytic
poliomyelitic — *see* Poliomyelitis, paralytic
pseudo G12.29
bulbospinal G7Ø.ØØ
with exacerbation (acute) G7Ø.Ø1
in crisis G7Ø.Ø1
cardiac — *see also* Failure, heart I5Ø.9
cerebrocerebellar, diplegic G8Ø.1
cervical
plexus G54.2
sympathetic G9Ø.Ø9
Céstan-Chenais G46.3
Charcot-Marie-Tooth type G6Ø.Ø
Clark's G8Ø.9
colon K56.Ø
compressed air T7Ø.3 ☑
compression
arm G56.9- ☑
leg G57.9- ☑
lower extremity G57.9- ☑
upper extremity G56.9- ☑
congenital (cerebral) — *see* Palsy, cerebral
conjugate movement (gaze) (of eye) H51.Ø
cortical (nuclear) (supranuclear) H51.Ø
cordis — *see* Failure, heart
cranial or cerebral nerve G52.9
creeping G12.22
crossed leg G83.89
crutch — *see* Injury, brachial plexus
deglutition R13.Ø
hysterical F44.4
dementia A52.17
descending (spinal) NEC G12.29
diaphragm (flaccid) J98.6
due to accidental dissection of phrenic nerve during procedure — *see* Puncture, accidental complicating surgery

Paralysis, paralytic — *continued*
- digestive organs NEC K59.89
- diplegic — *see* Diplegia
- divergence (nuclear) H51.8
- diver's T7Ø.3 ☑
- Duchenne's
  - birth injury P14.Ø
  - due to or associated with
    - motor neuron disease G12.22
    - muscular dystrophy G71.Ø1
- due to intracranial or spinal birth injury — *see* Palsy, cerebral
- embolic (current episode) I63.4- ☑
- Erb (-Duchenne) (birth) (newborn) P14.Ø
- Erb's syphilitic spastic spinal A52.17
- esophagus K22.89
- eye muscle (extrinsic) H49.9
  - intrinsic — *see also* Paresis, of accommodation
- facial (nerve) G51.Ø
  - birth injury P11.3
  - congenital P11.3
  - following operation NEC — *see* Puncture, accidental complicating surgery
  - newborn (birth injury) P11.3
- familial (recurrent) (periodic) G72.3
  - spastic G11.4
- fauces J39.2
- finger G56.9- ☑
- gait R26.1
- gastric nerve (nondiabetic) G52.2
- gaze, conjugate H51.Ø
- general (progressive) (syphilitic) A52.17
  - juvenile A5Ø.45
- glottis J38.ØØ
  - bilateral J38.Ø2
  - unilateral J38.Ø1
- gluteal G54.1
- Gubler (-Millard) G46.3
- hand — *see* Monoplegia, upper limb
- heart — *see* Arrest, cardiac
- hemiplegic — *see* Hemiplegia
- hyperkalemic periodic (familial) G72.3
- hypoglossal (nerve) G52.3
- hypokalemic periodic G72.3
- hysterical F44.4
- ileus K56.Ø
- infantile — *see also* Poliomyelitis, paralytic A8Ø.3Ø
  - bulbar — *see* Poliomyelitis, paralytic
  - cerebral — *see* Palsy, cerebral
  - spastic — *see* Palsy, cerebral, spastic
- infective — *see* Poliomyelitis, paralytic
- inferior nuclear G83.9
- internuclear — *see* Ophthalmoplegia, internuclear
- intestine K56.Ø
- iris H57.Ø9
  - due to diphtheria (toxin) A36.89
- ischemic, Volkmann's (complicating trauma) T79.6 ☑
- Jackson's G83.89
- jake — *see* Poisoning, food, noxious, plant
- Jamaica ginger (jake) G62.2
- juvenile general A5Ø.45
- Klumpke (-Déjérine) (birth) (newborn) P14.1
- labioglossal (laryngeal) (pharyngeal) G12.29
- Landry's G61.Ø
- laryngeal nerve (recurrent) (superior) (unilateral) J38.ØØ
  - bilateral J38.Ø2
  - unilateral J38.Ø1
- larynx J38.ØØ
  - bilateral J38.Ø2
  - due to diphtheria (toxin) A36.2
  - unilateral J38.Ø1
- lateral G12.23
- lead T56.Ø ☑
- left side — *see* Hemiplegia
- leg G83.1- ☑
  - both — *see* Paraplegia
  - crossed G83.89
  - hysterical F44.4
  - psychogenic F44.4
  - transient or transitory R29.818
    - traumatic NEC — *see* Injury, nerve, leg
- levator palpebrae superioris — *see* Blepharoptosis, paralytic
- limb — *see* Monoplegia
- lip K13.Ø
- Lissauer's A52.17
- lower limb — *see* Monoplegia, lower limb
  - both — *see* Paraplegia

Paralysis, paralytic — *continued*
- lung J98.4
- median nerve G56.1- ☑
- medullary (tegmental) G83.89
- mesencephalic NEC G83.89
  - tegmental G83.89
- middle alternating G83.89
- Millard-Gubler-Foville G46.3
- monoplegic — *see* Monoplegia
- motor G83.9
- muscle, muscular NEC G72.89
  - due to nerve lesion G58.9
  - eye (extrinsic) H49.9
    - intrinsic — *see* Paresis, of accommodation
    - oblique — *see* Strabismus, paralytic, fourth nerve
  - iris sphincter H21.9
  - ischemic (Volkmann's) (complicating trauma) T79.6 ☑
  - progressive G12.21
  - progressive, spinal G12.25
  - pseudohypertrophic G71.Ø2
  - spinal progressive G12.25
- musculocutaneous nerve G56.9- ☑
- musculospiral G56.9- ☑
- nerve — *see also* Disorder, nerve
  - abducent — *see* Strabismus, paralytic, sixth nerve
  - accessory G52.8
  - auditory (except Deafness) H93.3 ☑
  - birth injury P14.9
  - cranial or cerebral G52.9
  - facial G51.Ø
    - birth injury P11.3
    - congenital P11.3
    - newborn (birth injury) P11.3
  - fourth or trochlear — *see* Strabismus, paralytic, fourth nerve
  - newborn (birth injury) P14.9
  - oculomotor — *see* Strabismus, paralytic, third nerve
  - phrenic (birth injury) P14.2
  - radial G56.3- ☑
  - seventh or facial G51.Ø
    - newborn (birth injury) P11.3
  - sixth or abducent — *see* Strabismus, paralytic, sixth nerve
  - syphilitic A52.15
  - third or oculomotor — *see* Strabismus, paralytic, third nerve
  - trigeminal G5Ø.9
  - trochlear — *see* Strabismus, paralytic, fourth nerve
  - ulnar G56.2- ☑
- normokalemic periodic G72.3
- ocular H49.9
  - alternating G83.89
- oculofacial, congenital (Moebius) Q87.Ø
- oculomotor (external bilateral) (nerve) — *see* Strabismus, paralytic, third nerve
- palate (soft) K13.79
- paratrigeminal G5Ø.9
- periodic (familial) (hyperkalemic) (hypokalemic) (myotonic) (normokalemic) (potassium sensitive) (secondary) G72.3
- peripheral autonomic nervous system — *see* Neuropathy, peripheral, autonomic
- peroneal (nerve) G57.3- ☑
- pharynx J39.2
- phrenic nerve G56.8- ☑
- plantar nerve(s) G57.6- ☑
- pneumogastric nerve G52.2
- poliomyelitis (current) — *see* Poliomyelitis, paralytic
- popliteal nerve G57.3- ☑
- postepileptic transitory G83.84
- progressive (atrophic) (bulbar) (spinal) G12.22
  - general A52.17
  - infantile acute — *see* Poliomyelitis, paralytic
  - supranuclear G23.1
- pseudobulbar G12.29
- pseudohypertrophic (muscle) — *see also* Dystrophy, muscular, by type, if applicable G71.Ø9
- psychogenic F44.4
- quadriceps G57.9- ☑
- quadriplegic — *see* Tetraplegia
- radial nerve G56.3- ☑
- rectus muscle (eye) H49.9
- recurrent isolated sleep G47.53
- respiratory (muscle) (system) (tract) RØ6.81
  - center NEC G93.89
  - congenital P28.89
  - newborn P28.89

Paralysis, paralytic — *continued*
- right side — *see* Hemiplegia
- saturnine T56.Ø ☑
- sciatic nerve G57.Ø- ☑
- senile G83.9
- shaking — *see* Parkinsonism
- shoulder G56.9- ☑
- sleep, recurrent isolated G47.53
- spastic G83.9
  - cerebral — *see* Palsy, cerebral, spastic
  - congenital (cerebral) — *see* Palsy, cerebral, spastic
  - familial G11.4
  - hereditary G11.4
  - quadriplegic G8Ø.Ø
  - syphilitic (spinal) A52.17
- sphincter, bladder — *see* Paralysis, bladder
- spinal (cord) G83.9
  - accessory nerve G52.8
  - acute — *see* Poliomyelitis, paralytic
  - ascending acute G61.Ø
  - atrophic (acute) — *see also* Poliomyelitis, paralytic
    - spastic, syphilitic A52.17
  - congenital NEC — *see* Palsy, cerebral
  - hereditary G95.89
  - infantile — *see* Poliomyelitis, paralytic
  - progressive G12.21
    - muscle G12.25
  - sequelae NEC G83.89
- sternomastoid G52.8
- stomach K31.84
  - diabetic — *see* Diabetes, by type, with gastroparesis
  - nerve G52.2
    - diabetic — *see* Diabetes, by type, with gastroparesis
- stroke — *see* Infarct, brain
- subcapsularis G56.8- ☑
- supranuclear (progressive) G23.1
- sympathetic G9Ø.8
  - cervical G9Ø.Ø9
  - nervous system — *see* Neuropathy, peripheral, autonomic
- syndrome G83.9
  - specified NEC G83.89
- syphilitic spastic spinal (Erb's) A52.17
- thigh G57.9- ☑
- throat J39.2
  - diphtheritic A36.Ø
  - muscle J39.2
- thrombotic (current episode) I63.3- ☑
- thumb G56.9- ☑
- tick — *see* Toxicity, venom, arthropod, specified NEC
- Todd's (postepileptic transitory paralysis) G83.84
- toe G57.6- ☑
- tongue K14.8
- transient R29.5
  - arm or leg NEC R29.818
  - traumatic NEC — *see* Injury, nerve
- trapezius G52.8
- traumatic, transient NEC — *see* Injury, nerve
- trembling — *see* Parkinsonism
- triceps brachii G56.9 ☑
- trigeminal nerve G5Ø.9
- trochlear (nerve) — *see* Strabismus, paralytic, fourth nerve
- ulnar nerve G56.2- ☑
- upper limb — *see* Monoplegia, upper limb
- uremic N18.9 *[G99.8]*
- uveoparotitic D86.89
- uvula K13.79
  - postdiphtheritic A36.Ø
- vagus nerve G52.2
- vasomotor NEC G9Ø.8
- velum palati K13.79
- vesical — *see* Paralysis, bladder
- vestibular nerve (except Vertigo) H93.3 ☑
- vocal cords J38.ØØ
  - bilateral J38.Ø2
  - unilateral J38.Ø1
- Volkmann's (complicating trauma) T79.6 ☑
- wasting G12.29
- Weber's G46.3
- wrist G56.9- ☑

Paramedial urethrovesical orifice Q64.79

Paramenia N92.6

Parametritis — *see also* Disease, pelvis, inflammatory N73.2
- acute N73.Ø

Parametritis — *continued*
complicating abortion — *see* Abortion, by type, complicated by, parametritis
Parametrium, parametric — *see* condition
Paramnesia — *see* Amnesia
Paramolar K00.1
Paramyloidosis E85.89
Paramyoclonus multiplex G25.3
Paramyotonia (congenita) G71.19
Parangi — *see* Yaws
Paranoia (querulans) F22
senile F03 ☑
Paranoid
dementia (senile) F03 ☑
praecox — *see* Schizophrenia
personality F60.0
psychosis (climacteric) (involutional) (menopausal) F22
psychogenic (acute) F23
senile F03 ☑
reaction (acute) F23
chronic F22
schizophrenia F20.0
state (climacteric) (involutional) (menopausal) (simple) F22
senile F03 ☑
tendencies F60.0
traits F60.0
trends F60.0
type, psychopathic personality F60.0
Paraparesis — *see* Paraplegia
Paraphasia R47.02
Paraphilia F65.9
Paraphimosis (congenital) N47.2
chancroidal A57
Paraphrenia, paraphrenic (late) F22
schizophrenia F20.0
Paraplegia (lower) G82.20
ataxic — *see* Degeneration, combined, spinal cord
complete G82.21
congenital (cerebral) G80.8
spastic G80.1
familial spastic G11.4
functional (hysterical) F44.4
hereditary, spastic G11.4
hysterical F44.4
incomplete G82.22
Pott's A18.01
psychogenic F44.4
spastic
Erb's spinal, syphilitic A52.17
hereditary G11.4
tropical G04.1
syphilitic (spastic) A52.17
traumatic
current injury — code to injury with seventh character A
sequela of previous injury — code to injury with seventh character S
tropical spastic G04.1
Parapoxvirus B08.60
specified NEC B08.69
Paraproteinemia D89.2
benign (familial) D89.2
monoclonal D47.2
secondary to malignant disease D47.2
Parapsoriasis L41.9
en plaques L41.4
guttata L41.1
large plaque L41.4
retiform, retiformis L41.5
small plaque L41.3
specified NEC L41.8
varioliformis (acuta) L41.0
Parasitic — *see also* condition
disease NEC B89
stomatitis B37.0
sycosis (beard) (scalp) B35.0
twin Q89.4
Parasitism B89
intestinal B82.9
skin B88.9
specified — *see* Infestation
Parasitophobia F40.218
Parasomnia G47.50
due to
alcohol
abuse F10.182
dependence F10.282

Parasomnia — *continued*
due to — *continued*
alcohol — *continued*
use F10.982
amphetamines
abuse F15.182
dependence F15.282
use F15.982
caffeine
abuse F15.182
dependence F15.282
use F15.982
cocaine
abuse F14.182
dependence F14.282
use F14.982
drug NEC
abuse F19.182
dependence F19.282
use F19.982
opioid
abuse F11.182
dependence F11.282
use F11.982
psychoactive substance NEC
abuse F19.182
dependence F19.282
use F19.982
sedative, hypnotic, or anxiolytic
abuse F13.182
dependence F13.282
use F13.982
stimulant NEC
abuse F15.182
dependence F15.282
use F15.982
in conditions classified elsewhere G47.54
nonorganic origin F51.8
organic G47.50
specified NEC G47.59
Paraspadias Q54.9
Paraspasmus facialis G51.8
Parasuicide (attempt)
history of (personal) Z91.51
in family Z81.8
Parathyroid gland — *see* condition
Parathyroid tetany E20.9
Paratrachoma A74.0
Paratyphilitis — *see* Appendicitis
Paratyphoid (fever) — *see* Fever, paratyphoid
Paratyphus — *see* Fever, paratyphoid
Paraurethral duct Q64.79
Paraurethritis — *see also* Urethritis
gonococcal (acute) (chronic) (with abscess) A54.1
Paravaccinia NEC B08.04
Paravaginitis — *see* Vaginitis
Parencephalitis — *see also* Encephalitis
sequelae G09
Parent-child conflict — *see* Conflict, parent-child
estrangement NEC Z62.890
Paresis — *see also* Paralysis
accommodation — *see* Paresis, of accommodation
Bernhardt's G57.1- ☑
bladder (sphincter) — *see also* Paralysis, bladder
tabetic A52.17
bowel, colon or intestine K56.0
extrinsic muscle, eye H49.9
general (progressive) (syphilitic) A52.17
juvenile A50.45
heart — *see* Failure, heart
insane (syphilitic) A52.17
juvenile (general) A50.45
of accommodation H52.52- ☑
peripheral progressive (idiopathic) G60.3
pseudohypertrophic — *see also* Dystrophy, muscular, by type, if applicable G71.09
senile G83.9
syphilitic (general) A52.17
congenital A50.45
vesical NEC N31.2
Paresthesia — *see also* Disturbance, sensation, skin R20.2
Bernhardt G57.1- ☑
Paretic — *see* condition
Parinaud's
conjunctivitis H10.89
oculoglandular syndrome H10.89
ophthalmoplegia H49.88- ☑
Parkinsonism (idiopathic) (primary) G20

Parkinsonism — *continued*
with neurogenic orthostatic hypotension (symptomatic) G90.3
arteriosclerotic G21.4
dementia — *see also* Dementia, in, diseases specified elsewhere G20 *[F02.80]*
with behavioral disturbance — *see also* Dementia, in, diseases specified elsewhere G20 *[F02.81-]* ☑
due to
drugs NEC G21.19
neuroleptic G21.11
medication-induced NEC G21.19
neuroleptic induced G21.11
postencephalitic G21.3
secondary G21.9
due to
arteriosclerosis G21.4
drugs NEC G21.19
neuroleptic G21.11
encephalitis G21.3
external agents NEC G21.2
syphilis A52.19
specified NEC G21.8
syphilitic A52.19
treatment-induced NEC G21.19
vascular G21.4
Parkinson's disease, syndrome or tremor — *see* Parkinsonism
Parodontitis — *see* Periodontitis
Parodontosis K05.4
Paronychia — *see also* Cellulitis, digit
with lymphangitis — *see* Lymphangitis, acute, digit
candidal (chronic) B37.2
tuberculous (primary) A18.4
Parorexia (psychogenic) F50.89
Parosmia R43.1
psychogenic F45.8
Parotid gland — *see* condition
Parotitis, parotiditis (allergic) (nonspecific toxic) (purulent) (septic) (suppurative) — *see also* Sialoadenitis
epidemic — *see* Mumps
infectious — *see* Mumps
postoperative K91.89
surgical K91.89
Parrot fever A70
Parrot's disease (early congenital syphilitic pseudoparalysis) A50.02
Parry-Romberg syndrome G51.8
Parry's disease or syndrome E05.00
with thyroid storm E05.01
Pars planitis — *see* Cyclitis
Parsonage (-Aldren)-**Turner syndrome** G54.5
Parson's disease (exophthalmic goiter) E05.00
with thyroid storm E05.01
Particolored infant Q82.8
Parturition — *see* Delivery
Parulis K04.7
with sinus K04.6
Parvovirus, as cause of disease classified elsewhere B97.6
Pasini and Pierini's atrophoderma L90.3
Passage
false, urethra N36.5
meconium (newborn) during delivery P03.82
of sounds or bougies — *see* Attention to, artificial, opening
Passive — *see* condition
smoking Z77.22
Past due on rent or mortgage Z59.81- ☑
Pasteurella septica A28.0
Pasteurellosis — *see* Infection, Pasteurella
PAT (paroxysmal atrial tachycardia) I47.1
Patau's syndrome — *see* Trisomy, 13
Patches
mucous (syphilitic) A51.39
congenital A50.07
smokers' (mouth) K13.24
Patellar — *see* condition
Patent — *see also* Imperfect, closure
canal of Nuck Q52.4
cervix N88.3
ductus arteriosus or Botallo's Q25.0
foramen
botalli Q21.12
ovale Q21.12
interauricular septum Q21.19

Patent — *continued*
- interventricular septum Q21.Ø
- omphalomesenteric duct Q43.Ø
- os (uteri) — *see* Patent, cervix
- ostium secundum (type II) Q21.11
- urachus Q64.4
- vitelline duct Q43.Ø

Paterson (-Brown) (-Kelly) **syndrome or web** D5Ø.1

Pathologic, pathological — *see also* condition
- asphyxia R09.Ø1
- fire-setting F63.1
- gambling F63.Ø
- ovum OØ2.Ø
- resorption, tooth KØ3.3
- stealing F63.2

Pathology (of) — *see* Disease
- periradicular, associated with previous endodontic treatment NEC M27.59

Pattern, sleep-wake, irregular G47.23

Patulous — *see also* Imperfect, closure (congenital)
- alimentary tract Q45.8
  - lower Q43.8
  - upper Q4Ø.8
- eustachian tube H69.Ø- ☑

Pause, sinoatrial I49.5

Paxton's disease B36.2

Pearl(s)
- enamel KØØ.2
- Epstein's KØ9.8

Pearl-worker's disease — *see* Osteomyelitis, specified type NEC

Pectenosis K62.4

Pectoral — *see* condition

Pectus
- carinatum (congenital) Q67.7
  - acquired M95.4
  - rachitic sequelae (late effect) E64.3
- excavatum (congenital) Q67.6
  - acquired M95.4
  - rachitic sequelae (late effect) E64.3
- recurvatum (congenital) Q67.6

Pedatrophia E41

Pederosis F65.4

Pediatric inflammatory multisystem syndrome M35.81

Pediculosis (infestation) B85.2
- capitis (head-louse) (any site) B85.Ø
- corporis (body-louse) (any site) B85.1
- eyelid B85.Ø
- mixed (classifiable to more than one of the titles B85.Ø-B85.3) B85.4
- pubis (pubic louse) (any site) B85.3
- vestimenti B85.1
- vulvae B85.3

Pediculus (infestation) — *see* Pediculosis

Pedophilia F65.4

Peg-shaped teeth KØØ.2

Pelade — *see* Alopecia, areata

Pelger-Huët anomaly or syndrome D72.Ø

Peliosis (rheumatica) D69.Ø
- hepatis K76.4
  - with toxic liver disease K71.8

Pelizaeus-Merzbacher disease E75.29

Pellagra (alcoholic) (with polyneuropathy) E52

Pellagra-cerebellar-ataxia-renal aminoaciduria syndrome E72.Ø2

Pellegrini (-Stieda) **disease or syndrome** — *see* Bursitis, tibial collateral

Pellizzi's syndrome E34.8

Pel's crisis A52.11

Pelvic — *see also* condition
- examination (periodic) (routine) ZØ1.419
  - with abnormal findings ZØ1.411
- kidney, congenital Q63.2

Pelviolithiasis — *see* Calculus, kidney

Pelviperitonitis — *see also* Peritonitis, pelvic
- gonococcal A54.24
- puerperal O85

Pelvis — *see* condition or type

Pemphigoid L12.9
- benign, mucous membrane L12.1
- bullous L12.Ø
- cicatricial L12.1
- juvenile L12.2
- ocular L12.1
- specified NEC L12.8

Pemphigus L1Ø.9
- benign familial (chronic) Q82.8

Pemphigus — *continued*
- Brazilian L1Ø.3
- circinatus L13.Ø
- conjunctiva L12.1
- drug-induced L1Ø.5
- erythematosus L1Ø.4
- foliaceous L1Ø.2
- gangrenous — *see* Gangrene
- neonatorum LØ1.Ø3
- ocular L12.1
- paraneoplastic L1Ø.81
- specified NEC L1Ø.89
- syphilitic (congenital) A5Ø.Ø6
- vegetans L1Ø.1
- vulgaris L1Ø.Ø
- wildfire L1Ø.3

Pendred's syndrome EØ7.1

Pendulous
- abdomen, in pregnancy — *see* Pregnancy, complicated by, abnormal, pelvic organs or tissues NEC
- breast N64.89

Penetrating wound — *see also* Puncture
- with internal injury — *see* Injury, by site
- eyeball — *see* Puncture, eyeball
- orbit (with or without foreign body) — *see* Puncture, orbit
- uterus by instrument with or following ectopic or molar pregnancy OØ8.6

Penicillosis B48.4

Penis — *see* condition

Penitis N48.29

Pentalogy of Fallot Q21.8

Pentasomy X syndrome Q97.1

Pentosuria (essential) E74.89

Percreta placenta - O43.23 ☑

Peregrinating patient — *see* Disorder, factitious

Perforation, perforated (nontraumatic) (of)
- accidental during procedure (blood vessel) (nerve) (organ) — *see* Complication, accidental puncture or laceration
- antrum — *see* Sinusitis, maxillary
- appendix K35.32
  - with localized peritonitis K35.32
- atrial septum, multiple Q21.19
- attic, ear — *see* Perforation, tympanum, attic
- bile duct (common) (hepatic) K83.2
  - cystic K82.2
- bladder (urinary)
  - with or following ectopic or molar pregnancy OØ8.6
  - obstetrical trauma O71.5
  - traumatic S37.29 ☑
    - at delivery O71.5
- bowel K63.1
  - with or following ectopic or molar pregnancy OØ8.6
  - newborn P78.Ø
  - obstetrical trauma O71.5
  - traumatic — *see* Laceration, intestine
- broad ligament N83.8
  - with or following ectopic or molar pregnancy OØ8.6
  - obstetrical trauma O71.6
- by
  - device, implant or graft — *see also* Complications, by site and type, mechanical T85.628 ☑
    - arterial graft NEC — *see* Complication, cardiovascular device, mechanical, vascular
    - breast (implant) T85.49 ☑
    - catheter NEC T85.698 ☑
      - cystostomy T83.Ø9Ø ☑
      - dialysis (renal) T82.49 ☑
        - intraperitoneal T85.691 ☑
      - infusion NEC T82.594 ☑
        - spinal (epidural) (subdural) T85.69Ø ☑
      - urinary — *see also* Complications, catheter, urinary T83.Ø98 ☑
    - electronic (electrode) (pulse generator) (stimulator)
      - bone T84.39Ø ☑
      - cardiac T82.199 ☑
        - electrode T82.19Ø ☑
        - pulse generator T82.191 ☑
        - specified type NEC T82.198 ☑
      - nervous system — *see* Complication, prosthetic device, mechanical, electronic nervous system stimulator
      - urinary — *see* Complication, genitourinary, device, urinary, mechanical

Perforation, perforated — *continued*
- by — *continued*
  - device, implant or graft — *see also* Complications, by site and type, mechanical — *continued*
    - fixation, internal (orthopedic) NEC — *see* Complication, fixation device, mechanical
    - gastrointestinal — *see* Complications, prosthetic device, mechanical, gastrointestinal device
    - genital NEC T83.498 ☑
      - intrauterine contraceptive device T83.39 ☑
      - penile prosthesis T83.49Ø ☑
    - heart NEC — *see* Complication, cardiovascular device, mechanical
    - joint prosthesis — *see* Complications, joint prosthesis, mechanical, specified NEC, by site
    - ocular NEC — *see* Complications, prosthetic device, mechanical, ocular device
    - orthopedic NEC — *see* Complication, orthopedic, device, mechanical
    - specified NEC T85.628 ☑
    - urinary NEC — *see also* Complication, genitourinary, device, urinary, mechanical
      - graft T83.29 ☑
    - vascular NEC — *see* Complication, cardiovascular device, mechanical
    - ventricular intracranial shunt T85.Ø9 ☑
  - foreign body left accidentally in operative wound T81.539 ☑
  - instrument (any) during a procedure, accidental — *see* Puncture, accidental complicating surgery
- cecum K35.32
  - with localized peritonitis K35.32
- cervix (uteri) N88.8
  - with or following ectopic or molar pregnancy OØ8.6
  - obstetrical trauma O71.3
- colon K63.1
  - newborn P78.Ø
  - obstetrical trauma O71.5
  - traumatic — *see* Laceration, intestine, large
- common duct (bile) K83.2
- cornea (due to ulceration) — *see* Ulcer, cornea, perforated
- cystic duct K82.2
- diverticulum (intestine) K57.8Ø
  - with bleeding K57.81
  - large intestine K57.2Ø
    - with
      - bleeding K57.21
      - small intestine K57.4Ø
        - with bleeding K57.41
  - small intestine K57.ØØ
    - with
      - bleeding K57.Ø1
      - large intestine K57.4Ø
        - with bleeding K57.41
- ear drum — *see* Perforation, tympanum
- esophagus K22.3
- ethmoidal sinus — *see* Sinusitis, ethmoidal
- frontal sinus — *see* Sinusitis, frontal
- gallbladder K82.2
- heart valve — *see* Endocarditis
- ileum K63.1
  - newborn P78.Ø
  - obstetrical trauma O71.5
  - traumatic — *see* Laceration, intestine, small
- instrumental, surgical (accidental) (blood vessel) (nerve) (organ) — *see* Puncture, accidental complicating surgery
- intestine NEC K63.1
  - with ectopic or molar pregnancy OØ8.6
  - newborn P78.Ø
  - obstetrical trauma O71.5
  - traumatic — *see* Laceration, intestine
  - ulcerative NEC K63.1
    - newborn P78.Ø
- jejunum, jejunal K63.1
  - obstetrical trauma O71.5
  - traumatic — *see* Laceration, intestine, small
  - ulcer — *see* Ulcer, gastrojejunal, with perforation
- joint prosthesis — *see* Complications, joint prosthesis, mechanical, specified NEC, by site
- mastoid (antrum) (cell) — *see* Disorder, mastoid, specified NEC
- maxillary sinus — *see* Sinusitis, maxillary
- membrana tympani — *see* Perforation, tympanum
- nasal
  - septum J34.89

- **Perforation, perforated** — *continued*
  - nasal — *continued*
    - septum — *continued*
      - congenital Q3Ø.3
      - syphilitic A52.73
    - sinus J34.89
      - congenital Q3Ø.8
      - due to sinusitis — *see* Sinusitis
  - palate — *see also* Cleft, palate Q35.9
    - syphilitic A52.79
  - palatine vault — *see also* Cleft, palate, hard Q35.1
    - syphilitic A52.79
      - congenital A5Ø.59
  - pars flaccida (ear drum) — *see* Perforation, tympanum, attic
  - pelvic
    - floor S31.03Ø ☑
      - with
        - ectopic or molar pregnancy OØ8.6
        - penetration into retroperitoneal space S31.Ø31 ☑
        - retained foreign body S31.Ø4Ø ☑
          - with penetration into retroperitoneal space S31.Ø41 ☑
      - following ectopic or molar pregnancy OØ8.6
      - obstetrical trauma O7Ø.1
    - organ S37.99 ☑
      - adrenal gland S37.818 ☑
      - bladder — *see* Perforation, bladder
      - fallopian tube S37.599 ☑
        - bilateral S37.592 ☑
        - unilateral S37.591 ☑
      - kidney S37.Ø9- ☑
      - obstetrical trauma O71.5
      - ovary S37.499 ☑
        - bilateral S37.492 ☑
        - unilateral S37.491 ☑
      - prostate S37.828 ☑
      - specified organ NEC S37.898 ☑
      - ureter — *see* Perforation, ureter
      - urethra — *see* Perforation, urethra
      - uterus — *see* Perforation, uterus
  - perineum — *see* Laceration, perineum
  - pharynx J39.2
  - rectum K63.1
    - newborn P78.Ø
    - obstetrical trauma O71.5
    - traumatic S36.63 ☑
  - root canal space due to endodontic treatment M27.51
  - sigmoid K63.1
    - newborn P78.Ø
    - obstetrical trauma O71.5
    - traumatic S36.533 ☑
  - sinus (accessory) (chronic) (nasal) J34.89
  - sphenoidal sinus — *see* Sinusitis, sphenoidal
  - surgical (accidental) (by instrument) (blood vessel) (nerve) (organ) — *see* Puncture, accidental complicating surgery
  - traumatic
    - external — *see* Puncture
    - eye — *see* Puncture, eyeball
    - internal organ — *see* Injury, by site
  - tympanum, tympanic (membrane) (persistent post-traumatic) (postinflammatory) H72.9- ☑
    - attic H72.1- ☑
      - multiple — *see* Perforation, tympanum, multiple
      - total — *see* Perforation, tympanum, total
    - central H72.Ø- ☑
      - multiple — *see* Perforation, tympanum, multiple
      - total — *see* Perforation, tympanum, total
    - marginal NEC — *see* subcategory H72.2 ☑
    - multiple H72.81- ☑
    - pars flaccida — *see* Perforation, tympanum, attic
    - total H72.82- ☑
    - traumatic, current episode SØ9.2- ☑
  - typhoid, gastrointestinal — *see* Typhoid
  - ulcer — *see* Ulcer, by site, with perforation
  - ureter N28.89
    - traumatic S37.19 ☑
  - urethra N36.8
    - with ectopic or molar pregnancy OØ8.6
    - following ectopic or molar pregnancy OØ8.6
    - obstetrical trauma O71.5
    - traumatic S37.39 ☑
      - at delivery O71.5
  - uterus
    - with ectopic or molar pregnancy OØ8.6
    - by intrauterine contraceptive device T83.39 ☑
    - following ectopic or molar pregnancy OØ8.6
    - obstetrical trauma O71.1
    - traumatic S37.69 ☑
      - obstetric O71.1
  - uvula K13.79
    - syphilitic A52.79
  - vagina O71.4
    - obstetrical trauma O71.4
    - other trauma — *see* Puncture, vagina
- **Periadenitis mucosa necrotica recurrens** K12.Ø
- **Periappendicitis** (acute) — *see* Appendicitis
- **Periarteritis nodosa** (disseminated) (infectious) (necrotizing) M3Ø.Ø
- **Periarthritis** (joint) — *see also* Enthesopathy
  - Duplay's M75.Ø- ☑
  - gonococcal A54.42
  - humeroscapularis — *see* Capsulitis, adhesive
  - scapulohumeral — *see* Capsulitis, adhesive
  - shoulder — *see* Capsulitis, adhesive
  - wrist M77.2- ☑
- **Periarthrosis** (angioneural) — *see* Enthesopathy
- **Pericapsulitis, adhesive** (shoulder) — *see* Capsulitis, adhesive
- **Pericarditis** (with decompensation) (with effusion) I31.9
  - with rheumatic fever (conditions in IØØ)
    - active — *see* Pericarditis, rheumatic
    - inactive or quiescent IØ9.2
  - acute (hemorrhagic) (nonrheumatic) (Sicca) I3Ø.9
    - with chorea (acute) (rheumatic) (Sydenham's) IØ2.Ø
    - benign I3Ø.8
    - nonspecific I3Ø.Ø
    - rheumatic IØ1.Ø
      - with chorea (acute) (Sydenham's) IØ2.Ø
  - adhesive or adherent (chronic) (external) (internal) I31.Ø
    - acute — *see* Pericarditis, acute
    - rheumatic IØ9.2
  - bacterial (acute) (subacute) (with serous or seropurulent effusion) I3Ø.1
  - calcareous I31.1
  - cholesterol (chronic) I31.8
    - acute I3Ø.9
  - chronic (nonrheumatic) I31.9
    - rheumatic IØ9.2
  - constrictive (chronic) I31.1
  - coxsackie B33.23
  - fibrinocaseous (tuberculous) A18.84
  - fibrinopurulent I3Ø.1
  - fibrinous I3Ø.8
  - fibrous I31.Ø
  - gonococcal A54.83
  - idiopathic I3Ø.Ø
  - in systemic lupus erythematosus M32.12
  - infective I3Ø.1
  - meningococcal A39.53
  - neoplastic (chronic) I31.8
    - acute I3Ø.9
  - obliterans, obliterating I31.Ø
  - plastic I31.Ø
  - pneumococcal I3Ø.1
  - postinfarction I24.1
  - purulent I3Ø.1
  - rheumatic (active) (acute) (with effusion) (with pneumonia) IØ1.Ø
    - with chorea (acute) (rheumatic) (Sydenham's) IØ2.Ø
    - chronic or inactive (with chorea) IØ9.2
  - rheumatoid — *see* Rheumatoid, carditis
  - septic I3Ø.1
  - serofibrinous I3Ø.8
  - staphylococcal I3Ø.1
  - streptococcal I3Ø.1
  - suppurative I3Ø.1
  - syphilitic A52.Ø6
  - tuberculous A18.84
  - uremic N18.9 *[I32]*
  - viral I3Ø.1
- **Pericardium, pericardial** — *see* condition
- **Pericellulitis** — *see* Cellulitis
- **Pericementitis** (chronic) (suppurative) — *see also* Periodontitis
  - acute KØ5.2Ø
    - generalized — *see* Periodontitis, aggressive, generalized
    - localized — *see* Periodontitis, aggressive, localized
- **Perichondritis**
  - auricle — *see* Perichondritis, ear
- **Perichondritis** — *continued*
  - bronchus J98.Ø9
  - ear (external) H61.ØØ- ☑
    - acute H61.Ø1- ☑
    - chronic H61.Ø2- ☑
  - external auditory canal — *see* Perichondritis, ear
  - larynx J38.7
    - syphilitic A52.73
    - typhoid AØ1.Ø9
  - nose J34.89
  - pinna — *see* Perichondritis, ear
  - trachea J39.8
- **Periclasia** KØ5.4
- **Pericoronitis** — *see* Periodontitis
- **Pericystitis** N3Ø.9Ø
  - with hematuria N3Ø.91
- **Peridiverticulitis** (intestine) K57.92
  - cecum — *see* Diverticulitis, intestine, large
  - colon — *see* Diverticulitis, intestine, large
  - duodenum — *see* Diverticulitis, intestine, small
  - intestine — *see* Diverticulitis, intestine
  - jejunum — *see* Diverticulitis, intestine, small
  - rectosigmoid — *see* Diverticulitis, intestine, large
  - rectum — *see* Diverticulitis, intestine, large
  - sigmoid — *see* Diverticulitis, intestine, large
- **Periendocarditis** — *see* Endocarditis
- **Periepididymitis** N45.1
- **Perifolliculitis** LØ1.Ø2
  - abscedens, caput, scalp L66.3
  - capitis, abscedens (et suffodiens) L66.3
  - superficial pustular LØ1.Ø2
- **Perihepatitis** K65.8
- **Perilabyrinthitis** (acute) — *see* subcategory H83.Ø ☑
- **Perimeningitis** — *see* Meningitis
- **Perimetritis** — *see* Endometritis
- **Perimetrosalpingitis** — *see* Salpingo-oophoritis
- **Perineocele** N81.81
- **Perinephric, perinephritic** — *see* condition
- **Perinephritis** — *see also* Infection, kidney
  - purulent — *see* Abscess, kidney
- **Perineum, perineal** — *see* condition
- **Perineuritis NEC** — *see* Neuralgia
- **Periodic** — *see* condition
- **Periodontitis** (chronic) (complex) (compound) (local) (simplex) KØ5.3Ø
  - acute KØ5.2Ø
    - generalized KØ5.229
      - moderate KØ5.222
      - severe KØ5.223
      - slight KØ5.221
    - localized KØ5.219
      - moderate KØ5.212
      - severe KØ5.213
      - slight KØ5.211
  - aggressive KØ5.2Ø
    - generalized KØ5.229
      - moderate KØ5.222
      - severe KØ5.223
      - slight KØ5.221
    - localized KØ5.219
      - moderate KØ5.212
      - severe KØ5.213
      - slight KØ5.211
  - apical KØ4.5
    - acute (pulpal origin) KØ4.4
  - generalized KØ5.329
    - moderate KØ5.322
    - severe KØ5.323
    - slight KØ5.321
  - localized KØ5.319
    - moderate KØ5.312
    - severe KØ5.313
    - slight KØ5.311
- **Periodontoclasia** KØ5.4
- **Periodontosis** (juvenile) KØ5.4
- **Periods** — *see also* Menstruation
  - heavy N92.Ø
  - irregular N92.6
  - shortened intervals (irregular) N92.1
- **Perionychia** — *see also* Cellulitis, digit
  - with lymphangitis — *see* Lymphangitis, acute, digit
- **Perioophoritis** — *see* Salpingo-oophoritis
- **Periorchitis** N45.2
- **Periosteum, periosteal** — *see* condition
- **Periostitis** (albuminosa) (circumscribed) (diffuse) (infective) (monomelic) — *see also* Osteomyelitis
  - alveolar M27.3

- **Periostitis** — *continued*
  - alveolodental M27.3
  - dental M27.3
  - gonorrheal A54.43
  - jaw (lower) (upper) M27.2
  - orbit HØ5.Ø3- ☑
  - syphilitic A52.77
    - congenital (early) A5Ø.Ø2 *[M9Ø.8Ø]*
    - secondary A51.46
  - tuberculous — *see* Tuberculosis, bone
  - yaws (hypertrophic) (early) (late) A66.6 *[M9Ø.8Ø]*
- **Periostosis** (hyperplastic) — *see also* Disorder, bone, specified type NEC
  - with osteomyelitis — *see* Osteomyelitis, specified type NEC
- **Peripartum**
  - cardiomyopathy O9Ø.3
- **Periphlebitis** — *see* Phlebitis
- **Periproctitis** K62.89
- **Periprostatitis** — *see* Prostatitis
- **Perirectal** — *see* condition
- **Perirenal** — *see* condition
- **Perisalpingitis** — *see* Salpingo-oophoritis
- **Perisplenitis** (infectional) D73.89
- **Peristalsis, visible or reversed** R19.2
- **Peritendinitis** — *see* Enthesopathy
- **Peritoneum, peritoneal** — *see* condition
- **Peritonitis** (adhesive) (bacterial) (fibrinous) (hemorrhagic) (idiopathic) (localized) (perforative) (primary) (with adhesions) (with effusion) K65.9
  - with or following
    - abscess K65.1
    - appendicitis
      - with perforation or rupture K35.32
      - generalized — *see also* Appendicitis K35.2Ø
      - localized — *see also* Appendicitis K35.3Ø
    - diverticular disease (intestine) K57.8Ø
      - with bleeding K57.81
      - ectopic or molar pregnancy OØ8.Ø
      - large intestine K57.2Ø
        - with
          - bleeding K57.21
          - small intestine K57.4Ø
            - with bleeding K57.41
      - small intestine K57.ØØ
        - with
          - bleeding K57.Ø1
          - large intestine K57.4Ø
            - with bleeding K57.41
  - acute (generalized) K65.Ø
  - aseptic T81.61 ☑
  - bile, biliary K65.3
  - chemical T81.61 ☑
  - chlamydial A74.81
  - chronic proliferative K65.8
  - complicating abortion — *see* Abortion, by type, complicated by, pelvic peritonitis
  - congenital P78.1
  - diaphragmatic K65.Ø
  - diffuse K65.Ø
  - diphtheritic A36.89
  - disseminated K65.Ø
  - due to
    - bile K65.3
    - foreign
      - body or object accidentally left during a procedure (instrument) (sponge) (swab) T81.599 ☑
      - substance accidentally left during a procedure (chemical) (powder) (talc) T81.61 ☑
    - talc T81.61 ☑
    - urine K65.8
  - eosinophilic K65.8
    - acute K65.Ø
  - fibrocaseous (tuberculous) A18.31
  - fibropurulent K65.Ø
  - following ectopic or molar pregnancy OØ8.Ø
  - general (ized) K65.Ø
  - gonococcal A54.85
  - meconium (newborn) P78.Ø
  - neonatal P78.1
    - meconium P78.Ø
  - pancreatic K65.Ø
  - paroxysmal, familial E85.Ø
    - benign E85.Ø
  - pelvic
    - female N73.5
      - acute N73.3
- **Peritonitis** — *continued*
  - pelvic — *continued*
    - female — *continued*
      - chronic N73.4
        - with adhesions N73.6
    - male K65.Ø
  - periodic, familial E85.Ø
  - proliferative, chronic K65.8
  - puerperal, postpartum, childbirth O85
  - purulent K65.Ø
  - septic K65.Ø
  - specified NEC K65.8
  - spontaneous bacterial K65.2
  - subdiaphragmatic K65.Ø
  - subphrenic K65.Ø
  - suppurative K65.Ø
  - syphilitic A52.74
    - congenital (early) A5Ø.Ø8 *[K67]*
  - talc T81.61 ☑
  - tuberculous A18.31
  - urine K65.8
- **Peritonsillar** — *see* condition
- **Peritonsillitis** J36
- **Perityphlitis** — *see also* Cecitis K37
- **Periureteritis** N28.89
- **Periurethral** — *see* condition
- **Periurethritis** (gangrenous) — *see* Urethritis
- **Periuterine** — *see* condition
- **Perivaginitis** — *see* Vaginitis
- **Perivasculitis, retinal** H35.Ø6- ☑
- **Perivasitis** (chronic) N49.1
- **Perivesiculitis** (seminal) — *see* Vesiculitis
- **Perlèche NEC** K13.Ø
  - due to
    - candidiasis B37.83
    - moniliasis B37.83
    - riboflavin deficiency E53.Ø
    - vitamin B2 (riboflavin) deficiency E53.Ø
- **Pernicious** — *see* condition
- **Pernio, perniosis** T69.1 ☑
- **Perpetrator** (of abuse) — *see* Index to External Causes of Injury, Perpetrator
- **Persecution**
  - delusion F22
  - social Z6Ø.5
- **Perseveration** (tonic) R48.8
- **Persistence, persistent** (congenital)
  - anal membrane Q42.3
    - with fistula Q42.2
  - arteria stapedia Q16.3
  - atrioventricular canal Q21.2Ø
  - branchial cleft NOS Q18.2
    - cyst Q18.Ø
    - fistula Q18.Ø
    - sinus Q18.Ø
  - bulbus cordis in left ventricle Q21.8
  - canal of Cloquet Q14.Ø
  - capsule (opaque) Q12.8
  - cilioretinal artery or vein Q14.8
  - cloaca Q43.7
  - communication — *see* Fistula, congenital
  - convolutions
    - aortic arch Q25.46
    - fallopian tube Q5Ø.6
    - oviduct Q5Ø.6
    - uterine tube Q5Ø.6
  - double aortic arch Q25.45
  - ductus arteriosus (Botalli) Q25.Ø
  - fetal
    - circulation P29.38
    - form of cervix (uteri) Q51.828
    - hemoglobin, hereditary (HPFH) D56.4
  - foramen
    - Botalli Q21.12
    - ovale Q21.12
  - Gartner's duct Q52.4
  - hemoglobin, fetal (hereditary) (HPFH) D56.4
  - hyaloid
    - artery (generally incomplete) Q14.Ø
    - system Q14.8
  - hymen, in pregnancy or childbirth — *see* Pregnancy, complicated by, abnormal, vulva
  - lanugo Q84.2
  - left
    - posterior cardinal vein Q26.8
    - root with right arch of aorta Q25.49
    - superior vena cava Q26.1
  - Meckel's diverticulum Q43.Ø
- **Persistence, persistent** — *continued*
  - Meckel's diverticulum — *continued*
    - malignant — *see* Table of Neoplasms, small intestine, malignant
  - mucosal disease (middle ear) — *see* Otitis, media, suppurative, chronic, tubotympanic
  - nail(s), anomalous Q84.6
  - omphalomesenteric duct Q43.Ø
  - organ or site not listed — *see* Anomaly, by site
  - ostium
    - atrioventriculare commune Q21.23
    - primum Q21.2Ø
    - secundum Q21.11
  - ovarian rests in fallopian tube Q5Ø.6
  - pancreatic tissue in intestinal tract Q43.8
  - primary (deciduous)
    - teeth KØØ.6
    - vitreous hyperplasia Q14.Ø
  - pupillary membrane Q13.89
  - rhesus (Rh) titer — *see* Complication(s), transfusion, incompatibility reaction, Rh (factor)
  - right aortic arch Q25.47
  - sinus
    - urogenitalis
      - female Q52.8
      - male Q55.8
    - venosus with imperfect incorporation in right auricle Q26.8
  - thymus (gland) (hyperplasia) E32.Ø
  - thyroglossal duct Q89.2
  - thyrolingual duct Q89.2
  - truncus arteriosus or communis Q2Ø.Ø
  - tunica vasculosa lentis Q12.2
  - umbilical sinus Q64.4
  - urachus Q64.4
  - vitelline duct Q43.Ø
- **Person** (with)
  - admitted for clinical research, as a control subject (normal comparison) (participant) ZØØ.6
  - awaiting admission to adequate facility elsewhere Z75.1
  - concern (normal) about sick person in family Z63.6
  - consulting on behalf of another Z71.Ø
  - feigning illness Z76.5
  - living (in)
    - alone Z6Ø.2
    - boarding school Z59.3
    - residential institution Z59.3
    - without
      - adequate housing (heating) (space) Z59.1
      - housing (permanent) (temporary) Z59.ØØ
      - person able to render necessary care Z74.2
      - shelter Z59.Ø2
  - on waiting list Z75.1
  - sick or handicapped in family Z63.6
- **Personality** (disorder) F6Ø.9
  - accentuation of traits (type A pattern) Z73.1
  - affective F34.Ø
  - aggressive F6Ø.3
  - amoral F6Ø.2
  - anacastic, anankastic F6Ø.5
  - antisocial F6Ø.2
  - anxious F6Ø.6
  - asocial F6Ø.2
  - asthenic F6Ø.7
  - avoidant F6Ø.6
  - borderline F6Ø.3
  - change due to organic condition (enduring) FØ7.Ø
  - compulsive F6Ø.5
  - cycloid F34.Ø
  - cyclothymic F34.Ø
  - dependent F6Ø.7
  - depressive F34.1
  - dissocial F6Ø.2
  - dual F44.81
  - eccentric F6Ø.89
  - emotionally unstable F6Ø.3
  - expansive paranoid F6Ø.Ø
  - explosive F6Ø.3
  - fanatic F6Ø.Ø
  - haltlose type F6Ø.89
  - histrionic F6Ø.4
  - hyperthymic F34.Ø
  - hypothymic F34.1
  - hysterical F6Ø.4
  - immature F6Ø.89
  - inadequate F6Ø.7
  - labile (emotional) F6Ø.3
  - mixed (nonspecific) F6Ø.89

Personality — *continued*
- morally defective F6Ø.2
- multiple F44.81
- narcissistic F6Ø.81
- obsessional F6Ø.5
- obsessive (-compulsive) F6Ø.5
- organic FØ7.Ø
- overconscientious F6Ø.5
- paranoid F6Ø.Ø
- passive (-dependent) F6Ø.7
- passive-aggressive F6Ø.89
- pathologic F6Ø.9
- pattern defect or disturbance F6Ø.9
- pseudopsychopathic (organic) FØ7.Ø
- pseudoretarded (organic) FØ7.Ø
- psychoinfantile F6Ø.4
- psychoneurotic NEC F6Ø.89
- psychopathic F6Ø.2
- querulant F6Ø.Ø
- sadistic F6Ø.89
- schizoid F6Ø.1
- self-defeating F6Ø.89
- sensitive paranoid F6Ø.Ø
- sociopathic (amoral) (antisocial) (asocial) (dissocial) F6Ø.2
- specified NEC F6Ø.89
- type A Z73.1
- unstable (emotional) F6Ø.3

Perthes' disease — *see* Legg-Calvé-Perthes disease

Pertussis — *see also* Whooping cough A37.9Ø

Perversion, perverted
- appetite F5Ø.89
  - psychogenic F5Ø.89
- function
  - pituitary gland E23.2
    - posterior lobe E22.2
  - sense of smell and taste R43.8
    - psychogenic F45.8
- sexual — *see* Deviation, sexual

Pervious, congenital — *see also* Imperfect, closure
- ductus arteriosus Q25.Ø

Pes (congenital) — *see also* Talipes
- acquired — *see also* Deformity, limb, foot, specified NEC
  - planus — *see* Deformity, limb, flat foot
- adductus Q66.89
- cavus Q66.7- ☑
- deformity NEC, acquired — *see* Deformity, limb, foot, specified NEC
- planus (acquired) (any degree) — *see also* Deformity, limb, flat foot
  - rachitic sequelae (late effect) E64.3
- valgus Q66.6

Pest, pestis — *see* Plague

Petechia, petechiae R23.3
- newborn P54.5

Petechial typhus A75.9

Peter's anomaly Q13.4

Petit mal seizure — *see* Epilepsy, childhood, absence

Petit's hernia — *see* Hernia, abdomen, specified site NEC

Petrellidosis B48.2

Petrositis H7Ø.2Ø- ☑
- acute H7Ø.21- ☑
- chronic H7Ø.22- ☑

Peutz-Jeghers disease or syndrome Q85.89

Peyronie's disease N48.6

PFAPA (periodic fever, aphthous stomatitis, pharyngitis, and adenopathy syndrome) MØ4.8

Pfeiffer's disease — *see* Mononucleosis, infectious

Phagedena (dry) (moist) (sloughing) — *see also* Gangrene
- geometric L88
- penis N48.29
- tropical — *see* Ulcer, skin
- vulva N76.6

Phagedenic — *see* condition

Phakoma H35.89

Phakomatosis — *see also* specific eponymous syndromes Q85.9
- Bourneville's Q85.1
- specified NEC Q85.89

Phantom limb syndrome (without pain) G54.7
- with pain G54.6

Pharyngeal pouch syndrome D82.1

Pharyngitis (acute) (catarrhal) (gangrenous) (infective) (malignant) (membranous) (phlegmonous) (pseudomembranous) (simple) (subacute) (suppurative) (ulcerative) (viral) JØ2.9

Pharyngitis — *continued*
- with influenza, flu, or grippe — *see* Influenza, with, pharyngitis
- aphthous BØ8.5
- atrophic J31.2
- chlamydial A56.4
- chronic (atrophic) (granular) (hypertrophic) J31.2
- coxsackievirus BØ8.5
- diphtheritic A36.Ø
- enteroviral vesicular BØ8.5
- follicular (chronic) J31.2
- fusospirochetal A69.1
- gonococcal A54.5
- granular (chronic) J31.2
- herpesviral BØØ.2
- hypertrophic J31.2
- infectional, chronic J31.2
- influenzal — *see* Influenza, with, respiratory manifestations NEC
- lymphonodular, acute (enteroviral) BØ8.8
- pneumococcal JØ2.8
- purulent JØ2.9
- putrid JØ2.9
- septic JØ2.Ø
- sicca J31.2
- specified organism NEC JØ2.8
- staphylococcal JØ2.8
- streptococcal JØ2.Ø
- syphilitic, congenital (early) A5Ø.Ø3
- tuberculous A15.8
- vesicular, enteroviral BØ8.5
- viral NEC JØ2.8

Pharyngoconjunctivitis, viral B3Ø.2

Pharyngolaryngitis (acute) JØ6.Ø
- chronic J37.Ø

Pharyngoplegia J39.2

Pharyngotonsillitis, herpesviral BØØ.2

Pharyngotracheitis, chronic J42

Pharynx, pharyngeal — *see* condition

Phencyclidine-induced
- anxiety disorder F16.98Ø
- bipolar and related disorder F16.94
- depressive disorder F16.94
- psychotic disorder F16.959

Phenomenon
- Arthus' — *see* Arthus' phenomenon
- jaw-winking QØ7.8
- lupus erythematosus (LE) cell M32.9
- Raynaud's (secondary) I73.ØØ
  - with gangrene I73.Ø1
- vasomotor R55
- vasospastic I73.9
- vasovagal R55
- Wenckebach's I44.1

Phenylketonuria E7Ø.1
- classical E7Ø.Ø
- maternal E7Ø.1

Pheochromoblastoma
- specified site — *see* Neoplasm, malignant, by site
- unspecified site C74.1Ø

Pheochromocytoma
- malignant
  - specified site — *see* Neoplasm, malignant, by site
  - unspecified site C74.1Ø
- specified site — *see* Neoplasm, benign, by site
- unspecified site D35.ØØ

Pheohyphomycosis — *see* Chromomycosis

Pheomycosis — *see* Chromomycosis

Phimosis (congenital) (due to infection) N47.1
- chancroidal A57

Phlebectasia — *see also* Varix
- congenital Q27.4

Phlebitis (infective) (pyemic) (septic) (suppurative) I8Ø.9
- antepartum — *see* Thrombophlebitis, antepartum
- blue — *see* Phlebitis, leg, deep
- breast, superficial I8Ø.8
- calf muscular vein (NOS) I8Ø.25- ☑
- cavernous (venous) sinus — *see* Phlebitis, intracranial (venous) sinus
- cerebral (venous) sinus — *see* Phlebitis, intracranial (venous) sinus
- chest wall, superficial I8Ø.8
- cranial (venous) sinus — *see* Phlebitis, intracranial (venous) sinus
- deep (vessels) — *see* Phlebitis, leg, deep
- due to implanted device — *see* Complications, by site and type, specified NEC
- during or resulting from a procedure T81.72 ☑

Phlebitis — *continued*
- femoral vein (superficial) I8Ø.1- ☑
- femoropopliteal vein I8Ø.Ø- ☑
- gastrocnemial vein I8Ø.25- ☑
- gestational — *see* Phlebopathy, gestational
- hepatic veins I8Ø.8
- iliac vein (common) (external) (internal) I8Ø.21- ☑
- iliofemoral — *see* Phlebitis, femoral vein
- intracranial (venous) sinus (any) GØ8
  - nonpyogenic I67.6
- intraspinal venous sinuses and veins GØ8
  - nonpyogenic G95.19
- lateral (venous) sinus — *see* Phlebitis, intracranial (venous) sinus
- leg I8Ø.3
  - antepartum — *see* Thrombophlebitis, antepartum
  - deep (vessels) NEC I8Ø.2Ø- ☑
    - iliac I8Ø.21- ☑
    - popliteal vein I8Ø.22- ☑
    - specified vessel NEC I8Ø.29- ☑
    - tibial vein (anterior) (posterior) I8Ø.23- ☑
  - femoral vein (superficial) I8Ø.1- ☑
  - superficial (vessels) I8Ø.Ø- ☑
- longitudinal sinus — *see* Phlebitis, intracranial (venous) sinus
- lower limb — *see* Phlebitis, leg
- migrans, migrating (superficial) I82.1
- pelvic
  - with ectopic or molar pregnancy OØ8.Ø
  - following ectopic or molar pregnancy OØ8.Ø
  - puerperal, postpartum O87.1
- peroneal vein I8Ø.24- ☑
- popliteal vein — *see* Phlebitis, leg, deep, popliteal
- portal (vein) K75.1
- postoperative T81.72 ☑
- pregnancy — *see* Thrombophlebitis, antepartum
- puerperal, postpartum, childbirth O87.Ø
  - deep O87.1
  - pelvic O87.1
  - superficial O87.Ø
- retina — *see* Vasculitis, retina
- saphenous (accessory) (great) (long) (small) — *see* Phlebitis, leg, superficial
- sinus (meninges) — *see* Phlebitis, intracranial (venous) sinus
- soleal vein I8Ø.25- ☑
- specified site NEC I8Ø.8
- syphilitic A52.Ø9
- tibial vein — *see* Phlebitis, leg, deep, tibial
- ulcerative I8Ø.9
  - leg — *see* Phlebitis, leg
- umbilicus I8Ø.8
- uterus (septic) — *see* Endometritis
- varicose (leg) (lower limb) — *see* Varix, leg, with, inflammation

Phlebofibrosis I87.8

Phleboliths I87.8

Phlebopathy,
- gestational O22.9- ☑
- puerperal O87.9

Phlebosclerosis I87.8

Phlebothrombosis — *see also* Thrombosis
- antepartum — *see* Thrombophlebitis, antepartum
- pregnancy — *see* Thrombophlebitis, antepartum
- puerperal — *see* Thrombophlebitis, puerperal

Phlebotomus fever A93.1

Phlegmasia
- alba dolens O87.1
  - nonpuerperal — *see* Phlebitis, femoral vein
- cerulea dolens — *see* Phlebitis, leg, deep

Phlegmon — *see* Abscess

Phlegmonous — *see* condition

Phlyctenulosis (allergic) (keratoconjunctivitis) (nontuberculous) — *see also* Keratoconjunctivitis
- cornea — *see* Keratoconjunctivitis
- tuberculous A18.52

Phobia, phobic F4Ø.9
- animal F4Ø.218
  - spiders F4Ø.21Ø
- examination F4Ø.298
- reaction F4Ø.9
- simple F4Ø.298
- social F4Ø.1Ø
  - generalized F4Ø.11
- specific (isolated) F4Ø.298
  - animal F4Ø.218
    - spiders F4Ø.21Ø

Phobia, phobic — *continued*
specific — *continued*
blood F40.230
injection F40.231
injury F40.233
men F40.290
natural environment F40.228
thunderstorms F40.220
situational F40.248
bridges F40.242
closed in spaces F40.240
flying F40.243
heights F40.241
specified focus NEC F40.298
transfusion F40.231
women F40.291
specified NEC F40.8
medical care NEC F40.232
state F40.9
Phocas' disease — *see* Mastopathy, cystic
Phocomelia Q73.1
lower limb — *see* Agenesis, leg, with foot present
upper limb — *see* Agenesis, arm, with hand present
Phoria H50.50
Phosphate-losing tubular disorder N25.0
Phosphatemia E83.39
Phosphaturia E83.39
Photodermatitis (sun) L56.8
chronic L57.8
due to drug L56.8
light other than sun L59.8
Photokeratitis H16.13- ☑
Photophobia H53.14- ☑
Photophthalmia — *see* Photokeratitis
Photopsia H53.19
Photoretinitis — *see* Retinopathy, solar
Photosensitivity, photosensitization (sun) skin L56.8
light other than sun L59.8
Phrenitis — *see* Encephalitis
Phrynoderma (vitamin A deficiency) E50.8
Phthiriasis (pubis) B85.3
with any infestation classifiable to B85.0-B85.2 B85.4
Phthirus infestation — *see* Phthiriasis
Phthisis — *see also* Tuberculosis
bulbi (infectional) — *see* Disorder, globe, degenerated condition, atrophy
eyeball (due to infection) — *see* Disorder, globe, degenerated condition, atrophy
PHTS Q85.81
Phycomycosis — *see* Zygomycosis
Physalopteriasis B81.8
Physical restraint status Z78.1
Phytobezoar T18.9 ☑
intestine T18.3 ☑
stomach T18.2 ☑
Pian — *see* Yaws
Pianoma A66.1
Pica F50.89
in adults F50.89
infant or child F98.3
Picking, nose F98.8
Pick-Niemann disease — *see* Niemann-Pick disease or syndrome
Pick's
cerebral atrophy — *see also* Dementia, in, diseases specified elsewhere G31.01 *[F02.80]*
with behavioral disturbance — *see also* Dementia, in, diseases specified elsewhere G31.01 *[F02.81-]* ☑
disease or syndrome (brain) — *see also* Dementia, in, diseases specified elsewhere G31.01 *[F02.80]*
with behavioral disturbance — *see also* Dementia, in, diseases specified elsewhere G31.01 *[F02.81-]* ☑
brain — *see also* Dementia, in, diseases specified elsewhere G31.01 *[F02.80]*
with behavioral disturbance — *see also* Dementia, in, diseases specified elsewhere G31.01 *[F02.81-]* ☑
pericardium (pericardial pseudocirrhosis of liver) I31.1
syndrome
brain — *see also* Dementia, in, diseases specified elsewhere G31.01 *[F02.80]*
with behavioral disturbance — *see also* Dementia, in, diseases specified elsewhere G31.01 *[F02.81-]* ☑

Pick's — *continued*
syndrome — *continued*
of heart (pericardial pseudocirrhosis of liver) I31.1
Pickwickian syndrome E66.2
Piebaldism E70.39
Piedra (beard) (scalp) B36.8
black B36.3
white B36.2
Pierre Robin deformity or syndrome Q87.0
Pierson's disease or osteochondrosis M91.0
Pig-bel A05.2
Pigeon
breast or chest (acquired) M95.4
congenital Q67.7
rachitic sequelae (late effect) E64.3
breeder's disease or lung J67.2
fancier's disease or lung J67.2
toe — *see* Deformity, toe, specified NEC
Pigmentation (abnormal) (anomaly) L81.9
conjunctiva H11.13- ☑
cornea (anterior) H18.01- ☑
posterior H18.05- ☑
stromal H18.06- ☑
diminished melanin formation NEC L81.6
iron L81.8
lids, congenital Q82.8
limbus corneae — *see* Pigmentation, cornea
metals L81.8
optic papilla, congenital Q14.2
retina, congenital (grouped) (nevoid) Q14.1
scrotum, congenital Q82.8
tattoo L81.8
Piles — *see also* Hemorrhoids K64.9
Pili
annulati or torti (congenital) Q84.1
incarnati L73.1
Pill roller hand (intrinsic) — *see* Parkinsonism
Pilomatrixoma — *see* Neoplasm, skin, benign
malignant — *see* Neoplasm, skin, malignant
Pilonidal — *see* condition
Pimple R23.8
PIMS M35.81
PIN — *see* Neoplasia, intraepithelial, prostate
Pinched nerve — *see* Neuropathy, entrapment
Pindborg tumor — *see* Cyst, calcifying odontogenic
Pineal body or gland — *see* condition
Pinealoblastoma C75.3
Pinealoma D44.5
malignant C75.3
Pineoblastoma C75.3
Pineocytoma D44.5
Pinguecula H11.15- ☑
Pingueculitis H10.81- ☑
Pinhole meatus — *see also* Stricture, urethra N35.919
Pink
disease — *see* subcategory T56.1 ☑
eye — *see* Conjunctivitis, acute, mucopurulent
Pinkus' disease (lichen nitidus) L44.1
Pinpoint
meatus — *see* Stricture, urethra
os (uteri) — *see* Stricture, cervix
Pins and needles R20.2
Pinta A67.9
cardiovascular lesions A67.2
chancre (primary) A67.0
erythematous plaques A67.1
hyperchromic lesions A67.1
hyperkeratosis A67.1
lesions A67.9
cardiovascular A67.2
hyperchromic A67.1
intermediate A67.1
late A67.2
mixed A67.3
primary A67.0
skin (achromic) (cicatricial) (dyschromic) A67.2
hyperchromic A67.1
mixed (achromic and hyperchromic) A67.3
papule (primary) A67.0
skin lesions (achromic) (cicatricial) (dyschromic) A67.2
hyperchromic A67.1
mixed (achromic and hyperchromic) A67.3
vitiligo A67.2
Pintids A67.1
Pinworm (disease) (infection) (infestation) B80
Piroplasmosis — *see also* Babesiosis B60.00
specified NEC B60.09

Pistol wound — *see* Gunshot wound
Pitchers' elbow — *see* Derangement, joint, specified type NEC, elbow
Pithecoid pelvis Q74.2
with disproportion (fetopelvic) O33.0
causing obstructed labor O65.0
Pithiatism F48.8
Pitted — *see* Pitting
Pitting — *see also* Edema R60.9
lip R60.0
nail L60.8
teeth K00.4
Pituitary gland — *see* condition
Pituitary-snuff-taker's disease J67.8
Pityriasis (capitis) L21.0
alba L30.5
circinata (et maculata) L42
furfuracea L21.0
Hebra's L26
lichenoides L41.0
chronica L41.1
et varioliformis (acuta) L41.0
maculata (et circinata) L30.5
nigra B36.1
pilaris, Hebra's L44.0
rosea L42
rotunda L44.8
rubra (Hebra) pilaris L44.0
simplex L30.5
specified type NEC L30.5
streptogenes L30.5
versicolor (scrotal) B36.0
Placenta, placental — *see* Pregnancy, complicated by (care of) (management affected by), specified condition
Placentitis O41.14- ☑
Plagiocephaly Q67.3
Plague A20.9
abortive A20.8
ambulatory A20.8
asymptomatic A20.8
bubonic A20.0
cellulocutaneous A20.1
cutaneobubonic A20.1
lymphatic gland A20.0
meningitis A20.3
pharyngeal A20.8
pneumonic (primary) (secondary) A20.2
pulmonary, pulmonic A20.2
septicemic A20.7
tonsillar A20.8
septicemic A20.7
Planning, family
contraception Z30.9
procreation Z31.69
Plaque(s)
artery, arterial — *see* Arteriosclerosis
calcareous — *see* Calcification
coronary, lipid rich I25.83
epicardial I31.8
erythematous, of pinta A67.1
Hollenhorst's — *see* Occlusion, artery, retina
lipid rich, coronary I25.83
pleural (without asbestos) J92.9
with asbestos J92.0
tongue K13.29
Plasmacytoma C90.3- ☑
extramedullary C90.2- ☑
medullary C90.0- ☑
solitary C90.3- ☑
Plasmacytopenia D72.818
Plasmacytosis D72.822
Plaster ulcer — *see* Ulcer, pressure, by site
Plateau iris syndrome (post-iridectomy) (postprocedural) (without glaucoma) H21.82
with glaucoma H40.22- ☑
Platybasia Q75.8
Platyonychia (congenital) Q84.6
acquired L60.8
Platypelloid pelvis M95.5
with disproportion (fetopelvic) O33.0
causing obstructed labor O65.0
congenital Q74.2
Platyspondylisis Q76.49
Plaut (-Vincent) disease — *see also* Vincent's A69.1
Plethora R23.2
newborn P61.1
Pleura, pleural — *see* condition

Pleuralgia RØ7.81
Pleurisy (acute) (adhesive) (chronic) (costal) (diaphragmatic) (double) (dry) (fibrinous) (fibrous) (interlobar) (latent) (plastic) (primary) (residual) (sicca) (sterile) (subacute) (unresolved) RØ9.1
with
adherent pleura J86.Ø
effusion J9Ø
chylous, chyliform J94.Ø
tuberculous (non primary) A15.6
primary (progressive) A15.7
tuberculosis — *see* Pleurisy, tuberculous (non primary)
encysted — *see* Pleurisy, with effusion
exudative — *see* Pleurisy, with effusion
fibrinopurulent, fibropurulent — *see* Pyothorax
hemorrhagic — *see* Hemothorax
pneumococcal J9Ø
purulent — *see* Pyothorax
septic — *see* Pyothorax
serofibrinous — *see* Pleurisy, with effusion
seropurulent — *see* Pyothorax
serous — *see* Pleurisy, with effusion
staphylococcal J86.9
streptococcal J9Ø
suppurative — *see* Pyothorax
traumatic (post) (current) — *see* Injury, intrathoracic, pleura
tuberculous (with effusion) (non primary) A15.6
primary (progressive) A15.7
Pleuritis sicca — *see* Pleurisy
Pleurobronchopneumonia — *see* Pneumonia, broncho-
Pleurodynia RØ7.81
epidemic B33.Ø
viral B33.Ø
Pleuropericarditis — *see also* Pericarditis
acute I3Ø.9
Pleuropneumonia (acute) (bilateral) (double) (septic) — *see also* Pneumonia J18.8
chronic — *see* Fibrosis, lung
Pleuro-pneumonia-like-organism (PPLO), as cause of disease classified elsewhere B96.Ø
Pleurorrhea — *see* Pleurisy, with effusion
Plexitis, brachial G54.Ø
Plica
polonica B85.Ø
syndrome, knee M67.5- ☑
tonsil J35.8
Plicated tongue K14.5
Plug
bronchus NEC J98.Ø9
meconium (newborn) NEC syndrome P76.Ø
mucus — *see* Asphyxia, mucus
Plumbism — *see* subcategory T56.Ø ☑
Plummer's disease EØ5.2Ø
with thyroid storm EØ5.21
Plummer-Vinson syndrome D5Ø.1
Pluricarential syndrome of infancy E4Ø
Plus (and minus) **hand** (intrinsic) — *see* Deformity, limb, specified type NEC, forearm
PMEI (polymorphic epilepsy in infancy) G4Ø.83- ☑
Pneumathemia — *see* Air, embolism
Pneumatic hammer (drill) syndrome T75.21 ☑
Pneumatocele (lung) J98.4
intracranial G93.89
tension J44.9
Pneumatosis
cystoides intestinalis K63.89
intestinalis K63.89
peritonei K66.8
Pneumaturia R39.89
Pneumoblastoma — *see* Neoplasm, lung, malignant
Pneumocephalus G93.89
Pneumococcemia A4Ø.3
Pneumococcus, pneumococcal — *see* condition
Pneumoconiosis (due to) (inhalation of) J64
with tuberculosis (any type in A15) J65
aluminum J63.Ø
asbestos J61
bagasse, bagassosis J67.1
bauxite J63.1
beryllium J63.2
coal miners' (simple) J6Ø
coalworkers' (simple) J6Ø
collier's J6Ø
cotton dust J66.Ø
diatomite (diatomaceous earth) J62.8
Pneumoconiosis — *continued*
dust
inorganic NEC J63.6
lime J62.8
marble J62.8
organic NEC J66.8
fumes or vapors (from silo) J68.9
graphite J63.3
grinder's J62.8
kaolin J62.8
mica J62.8
millstone maker's J62.8
mineral fibers NEC J61
miner's J6Ø
moldy hay J67.Ø
potter's J62.8
rheumatoid — *see* Rheumatoid, lung
sandblaster's J62.8
silica, silicate NEC J62.8
with carbon J6Ø
stonemason's J62.8
talc (dust) J62.Ø
Pneumocystis carinii pneumonia B59
Pneumocystis jiroveci (pneumonia) B59
Pneumocystosis (with pneumonia) B59
Pneumohemopericardium I31.2
Pneumohemothorax J94.2
traumatic S27.2 ☑
Pneumohydropericardium — *see* Pericarditis
Pneumohydrothorax — *see* Hydrothorax
Pneumomediastinum J98.2
congenital or perinatal P25.2
Pneumomycosis B49 *[J99]*
Pneumonia (acute) (double) (migratory) (purulent) (septic) (unresolved) J18.9
with
influenza — *see* Influenza, with, pneumonia
lung abscess J85.1
due to specified organism — *see* Pneumonia, in (due to)
2Ø19 (novel) coronavirus J12.82
adenoviral J12.Ø
adynamic J18.2
alba A5Ø.Ø4
allergic — *see also* Pneumonitis, hypersensitivity J82.89
alveolar — *see* Pneumonia, lobar
anaerobes J15.8
anthrax A22.1
apex, apical — *see* Pneumonia, lobar
Ascaris B77.81
aspiration J69.Ø
due to
aspiration of microorganisms
bacterial J15.9
viral J12.9
food (regurgitated) J69.Ø
gastric secretions J69.Ø
milk (regurgitated) J69.Ø
oils, essences J69.1
solids, liquids NEC J69.8
vomitus J69.Ø
newborn P24.81
amniotic fluid (clear) P24.11
blood P24.21
food (regurgitated) P24.31
liquor (amnii) P24.11
meconium P24.Ø1
milk P24.31
mucus P24.11
specified NEC P24.81
stomach contents P24.31
postprocedural J95.4
atypical NEC J18.9
bacillus J15.9
specified NEC J15.8
bacterial J15.9
specified NEC J15.8
Bacteroides (fragilis) (oralis) (melaninogenicus) J15.8
basal, basic, basilar — *see* Pneumonia, by type
bronchiolitis obliterans organized (BOOP) J84.89
broncho-, bronchial (confluent) (croupous) (diffuse) (disseminated) (hemorrhagic) (involving lobes) (lobar) (terminal) J18.Ø
allergic — *see also* Pneumonitis, hypersensitivity J82.89
aspiration — *see* Pneumonia, aspiration
bacterial J15.9
specified NEC J15.8
Pneumonia — *continued*
broncho-, bronchial — *continued*
chronic — *see* Fibrosis, lung
diplococcal J13
Eaton's agent J15.7
Escherichia coli (E. coli) J15.5
Friedländer's bacillus J15.Ø
Hemophilus influenzae J14
hypostatic J18.2
inhalation — *see also* Pneumonia, aspiration
due to fumes or vapors (chemical) J68.Ø
of oils or essences J69.1
Klebsiella (pneumoniae) J15.Ø
lipid, lipoid J69.1
endogenous J84.89
Mycoplasma (pneumoniae) J15.7
pleuro-pneumonia-like-organisms (PPLO) J15.7
pneumococcal J13
Proteus J15.6
Pseudomonas J15.1
Serratia marcescens J15.6
specified organism NEC J16.8
staphylococcal — *see* Pneumonia, staphylococcal
streptococcal NEC J15.4
group B J15.3
pneumoniae J13
viral, virus — *see* Pneumonia, viral
Butyrivibrio (fibriosolvens) J15.8
Candida B37.1
caseous — *see* Tuberculosis, pulmonary
catarrhal — *see* Pneumonia, broncho
chlamydial J16.Ø
congenital P23.1
cholesterol J84.89
cirrhotic (chronic) — *see* Fibrosis, lung
Clostridium (haemolyticum) (novyi) J15.8
confluent — *see* Pneumonia, broncho
congenital (infective) P23.9
due to
bacterium NEC P23.6
Chlamydia P23.1
Escherichia coli P23.4
Haemophilus influenzae P23.6
infective organism NEC P23.8
Klebsiella pneumoniae P23.6
Mycoplasma P23.6
Pseudomonas P23.5
Staphylococcus P23.2
Streptococcus (except group B) P23.6
group B P23.3
viral agent P23.Ø
specified NEC P23.8
coronavirus (novel) (disease) 2Ø19 J12.82
COVID-19 J12.82
croupous — *see* Pneumonia, lobar
cryptogenic organizing J84.116
cytomegalic inclusion B25.Ø
cytomegaloviral B25.Ø
deglutition — *see* Pneumonia, aspiration
desquamative interstitial J84.117
diffuse — *see* Pneumonia, broncho
diplococcal, diplococcus (broncho-) (lobar) J13
disseminated (focal) — *see* Pneumonia, broncho
Eaton's agent J15.7
embolic, embolism — *see* Embolism, pulmonary
Enterobacter J15.6
eosinophilic J82.81
acute J82.82
chronic J82.81
Escherichia coli (E. coli) J15.5
Eubacterium J15.8
fibrinous — *see* Pneumonia, lobar
fibroid, fibrous (chronic) — *see* Fibrosis, lung
Friedländer's bacillus J15.Ø
Fusobacterium (nucleatum) J15.8
gangrenous J85.Ø
giant cell (measles) BØ5.2
gonococcal A54.84
gram-negative bacteria NEC J15.6
anaerobic J15.8
Hemophilus influenzae (broncho) (lobar) J14
human metapneumovirus J12.3
hypostatic (broncho) (lobar) J18.2
in (due to)
actinomycosis A42.Ø
adenovirus J12.Ø
anthrax A22.1
ascariasis B77.81

- **Pneumonia** — *continued*
  - in — *continued*
    - aspergillosis B44.9
    - Bacillus anthracis A22.1
    - Bacterium anitratum J15.6
    - candidiasis B37.1
    - chickenpox BØ1.2
    - Chlamydia J16.Ø
      - neonatal P23.1
    - coccidioidomycosis B38.2
      - acute B38.Ø
      - chronic B38.1
    - cytomegalovirus disease B25.Ø
    - Diplococcus (pneumoniae) J13
    - Eaton's agent J15.7
    - Enterobacter J15.6
    - Escherichia coli (E. coli) J15.5
    - Friedländer's bacillus J15.Ø
    - fumes and vapors (chemical) (inhalation) J68.Ø
    - gonorrhea A54.84
    - Hemophilus influenzae (H. influenzae) J14
    - Herellea J15.6
    - histoplasmosis B39.2
      - acute B39.Ø
      - chronic B39.1
    - human metapneumovirus J12.3
    - Klebsiella (pneumoniae) J15.Ø
    - measles BØ5.2
    - Mycoplasma (pneumoniae) J15.7
    - nocardiosis, nocardiasis A43.Ø
    - ornithosis A7Ø
    - parainfluenza virus J12.2
    - pleuro-pneumonia-like-organism (PPLO) J15.7
    - pneumococcus J13
    - pneumocystosis (Pneumocystis carinii) (Pneumocystis jiroveci) B59
    - Proteus J15.6
    - Pseudomonas NEC J15.1
      - pseudomallei A24.1
    - psittacosis A7Ø
    - Q fever A78
    - respiratory syncytial virus (RSV) J12.1
    - rheumatic fever IØØ *[J17]*
    - rubella BØ6.81
    - Salmonella (infection) AØ2.22
      - typhi AØ1.Ø3
    - schistosomiasis B65.9 *[J17]*
    - Serratia marcescens J15.6
    - specified
      - bacterium NEC J15.8
      - organism NEC J16.8
    - spirochetal NEC A69.8
    - Staphylococcus J15.2Ø
      - aureus (methicillin susceptible) (MSSA) J15.211
        - methicillin resistant (MRSA) J15.212
      - specified NEC J15.29
    - Streptococcus J15.4
      - group B J15.3
      - pneumoniae J13
      - specified NEC J15.4
    - toxoplasmosis B58.3
    - tularemia A21.2
    - typhoid (fever) AØ1.Ø3
    - varicella BØ1.2
    - virus — *see* Pneumonia, viral
    - whooping cough A37.91
      - due to
        - Bordetella parapertussis A37.11
        - Bordetella pertussis A37.Ø1
        - specified NEC A37.81
    - Yersinia pestis A2Ø.2
  - inhalation of food or vomit — *see* Pneumonia, aspiration
  - interstitial J84.9
    - chronic J84.111
    - desquamative J84.117
    - due to
      - collagen vascular disease J84.178
      - known underlying cause J84.178
    - idiopathic NOS J84.111
    - in disease classified elsewhere J84.178
    - lymphocytic (due to collagen vascular disease) (in diseases classified elsewhere) J84.178
    - lymphoid J84.2
    - non-specific J84.89
      - due to
        - collagen vascular disease J84.178
        - known underlying cause J84.178
      - idiopathic J84.113

- **Pneumonia** — *continued*
  - interstitial — *continued*
    - non-specific — *continued*
      - in diseases classified elsewhere J84.178
    - plasma cell B59
    - pseudomonas J15.1
    - usual J84.112
      - due to collagen vascular disease J84.178
      - idiopathic J84.112
      - in diseases classified elsewhere J84.178
  - Klebsiella (pneumoniae) J15.Ø
  - lipid, lipoid (exogenous) J69.1
    - endogenous J84.89
  - lobar (disseminated) (double) (interstitial) J18.1
    - bacterial J15.9
      - specified NEC J15.8
    - chronic — *see* Fibrosis, lung
    - Escherichia coli (E. coli) J15.5
    - Friedländer's bacillus J15.Ø
    - Hemophilus influenzae J14
    - hypostatic J18.2
    - Klebsiella (pneumoniae) J15.Ø
    - pneumococcal J13
    - Proteus J15.6
    - Pseudomonas J15.1
    - specified organism NEC J16.8
    - staphylococcal — *see* Pneumonia, staphylococcal
    - streptococcal NEC J15.4
    - Streptococcus pneumoniae J13
    - viral, virus — *see* Pneumonia, viral
  - lobular — *see* Pneumonia, broncho
  - Löffler's J82.89
  - lymphoid interstitial J84.2
  - massive — *see* Pneumonia, lobar
  - meconium P24.Ø1
  - MRSA (methicillin resistant Staphylococcus aureus) J15.212
  - MSSA (methicillin susceptible Staphylococcus aureus) J15.211
  - multilobar — *see* Pneumonia, by type
  - Mycoplasma (pneumoniae) J15.7
  - necrotic J85.Ø
  - neonatal P23.9
    - aspiration — *see* Aspiration, by substance, with pneumonia
  - nitrogen dioxide J68.Ø
  - organizing J84.89
    - due to
      - collagen vascular disease J84.178
      - known underlying cause J84.178
    - in diseases classified elsewhere J84.178
  - orthostatic J18.2
  - parainfluenza virus J12.2
  - parenchymatous — *see* Fibrosis, lung
  - passive J18.2
  - patchy — *see* Pneumonia, broncho
  - Peptococcus J15.8
  - Peptostreptococcus J15.8
  - plasma cell (of infants) B59
  - pleurolobar — *see* Pneumonia, lobar
  - pleuro-pneumonia-like organism (PPLO) J15.7
  - pneumococcal (broncho) (lobar) J13
  - Pneumocystis (carinii) (jiroveci) B59
  - postinfectional NEC B99 ☑ *[J17]*
  - postmeasles BØ5.2
  - Proteus J15.6
  - Pseudomonas J15.1
  - psittacosis A7Ø
  - radiation J7Ø.Ø
  - respiratory syncytial virus (RSV) J12.1
  - resulting from a procedure J95.89
  - rheumatic IØØ *[J17]*
  - Salmonella (arizonae) (cholerae-suis) (enteritidis) (typhimurium) AØ2.22
    - typhi AØ1.Ø3
    - typhoid fever AØ1.Ø3
  - SARS-associated coronavirus J12.81
  - SARS-CoV-2 J12.82
  - segmented, segmental — *see* Pneumonia, broncho-
  - Serratia marcescens J15.6
  - specified NEC J18.8
    - bacterium NEC J15.8
    - organism NEC J16.8
    - virus NEC J12.89
  - spirochetal NEC A69.8
  - staphylococcal (broncho) (lobar) J15.2Ø
    - aureus (methicillin susceptible) (MSSA) J15.211
      - methicillin resistant (MRSA) J15.212

- **Pneumonia** — *continued*
  - staphylococcal — *continued*
    - specified NEC J15.29
  - static, stasis J18.2
  - streptococcal NEC (broncho) (lobar) J15.4
    - group
      - A J15.4
      - B J15.3
    - specified NEC J15.4
  - Streptococcus pneumoniae J13
  - syphilitic, congenital (early) A5Ø.Ø4
  - traumatic (complication) (early) (secondary) T79.8 ☑
  - tuberculous (any) — *see* Tuberculosis, pulmonary
  - tularemic A21.2
  - varicella BØ1.2
  - Veillonella J15.8
  - ventilator associated J95.851
  - viral, virus (broncho) (interstitial) (lobar) J12.9
    - adenoviral J12.Ø
    - congenital P23.Ø
    - human metapneumovirus J12.3
    - parainfluenza J12.2
    - respiratory syncytial (RSV) J12.1
    - SARS-associated coronavirus J12.81
    - specified NEC J12.89
  - white (congenital) A5Ø.Ø4
- **Pneumonic** — *see* condition
- **Pneumonitis** (acute) (primary) — *see also* Pneumonia
  - air-conditioner J67.7
  - allergic (due to) J67.9
    - organic dust NEC J67.8
    - red cedar dust J67.8
    - sequoiosis J67.8
    - wood dust J67.8
  - aspiration J69.Ø
    - due to
      - anesthesia J95.4
        - during
          - labor and delivery O74.Ø
          - pregnancy O29.Ø1- ☑
          - puerperium O89.Ø1
      - fumes or gases J68.Ø
    - obstetric O74.Ø
  - chemical (due to gases, fumes or vapors) (inhalation) J68.Ø
    - due to anesthesia J95.4
  - cholesterol J84.89
  - chronic — *see* Fibrosis, lung
  - congenital rubella P35.Ø
  - crack (cocaine) J68.Ø
  - due to
    - beryllium J68.Ø
    - cadmium J68.Ø
    - crack (cocaine) J68.Ø
    - detergent J69.8
    - fluorocarbon-polymer J68.Ø
    - food, vomit (aspiration) J69.Ø
    - fumes or vapors J68.Ø
    - gases, fumes or vapors (inhalation) J68.Ø
    - inhalation
      - blood J69.8
      - essences J69.1
      - food (regurgitated), milk, vomit J69.Ø
      - oils, essences J69.1
      - saliva J69.Ø
      - solids, liquids NEC J69.8
    - manganese J68.Ø
    - nitrogen dioxide J68.Ø
    - oils, essences J69.1
    - solids, liquids NEC J69.8
    - toxoplasmosis (acquired) B58.3
      - congenital P37.1
    - vanadium J68.Ø
    - ventilator J95.851
  - eosinophilic J82.81
    - acute J82.82
    - chronic J82.81
  - hypersensitivity J67.9
    - air conditioner lung J67.7
    - bagassosis J67.1
    - bird fancier's lung J67.2
    - farmer's lung J67.Ø
    - maltworker's lung J67.4
    - maple bark-stripper's lung J67.6
    - mushroom worker's lung J67.5
    - specified organic dust NEC J67.8
    - suberosis J67.3
  - interstitial (chronic) J84.89

- **Pneumonitis** — *continued*
  - interstitial — *continued*
    - acute J84.114
    - lymphoid J84.2
    - non-specific J84.89
      - idiopathic J84.113
  - lymphoid, interstitial J84.2
  - meconium P24.Ø1
  - postanesthetic J95.4
    - correct substance properly administered — *see* Table of Drugs and Chemicals, by drug, adverse effect
    - in labor and delivery O74.Ø
    - in pregnancy O29.Ø1- ☑
    - obstetric O74.Ø
    - overdose or wrong substance given or taken (by accident) — *see* Table of Drugs and Chemicals, by drug, poisoning
    - postpartum, puerperal O89.Ø1
  - postoperative J95.4
    - obstetric O74.Ø
  - radiation J7Ø.Ø
  - rubella, congenital P35.Ø
  - ventilation (air-conditioning) J67.7
  - ventilator associated J95.851
  - wood-dust J67.8
- **Pneumonoconiosis** — *see* Pneumoconiosis
- **Pneumoparotid** K11.8
- **Pneumopathy NEC** J98.4
  - alveolar J84.Ø9
  - due to organic dust NEC J66.8
  - parietoalveolar J84.Ø9
- **Pneumopericarditis** — *see also* Pericarditis
  - acute I3Ø.9
- **Pneumopericardium** — *see also* Pericarditis
  - congenital P25.3
  - newborn P25.3
  - traumatic (post) — *see* Injury, heart
- **Pneumophagia** (psychogenic) F45.8
- **Pneumopleurisy, pneumopleuritis** — *see also* Pneumonia J18.8
- **Pneumopyopericardium** I3Ø.1
- **Pneumopyothorax** — *see* Pyopneumothorax
  - with fistula J86.Ø
- **Pneumorrhagia** — *see also* Hemorrhage, lung
  - tuberculous — *see* Tuberculosis, pulmonary
- **Pneumothorax NOS** J93.9
  - acute J93.83
  - chronic J93.81
  - congenital P25.1
  - perinatal period P25.1
  - postprocedural J95.811
  - specified NEC J93.83
  - spontaneous NOS J93.83
    - newborn P25.1
    - primary J93.11
    - secondary J93.12
    - tension J93.Ø
  - tense valvular, infectional J93.Ø
  - tension (spontaneous) J93.Ø
  - traumatic S27.Ø ☑
    - with hemothorax S27.2 ☑
  - tuberculous — *see* Tuberculosis, pulmonary
- **Podagra** — *see also* Gout M1Ø.9
- **Podencephalus** QØ1.9
- **Poikilocytosis** R71.8
- **Poikiloderma** L81.6
  - Civatte's L57.3
  - congenital Q82.8
  - vasculare atrophicans L94.5
- **Poikilodermatomyositis** M33.1Ø
  - with
    - myopathy M33.12
    - respiratory involvement M33.11
    - specified organ involvement NEC M33.19
  - amyopathic M33.13
  - without myopathy M33.13
- **Pointed ear** (congenital) Q17.3
- **Poison ivy, oak, sumac or other plant dermatitis** (allergic) (contact) L23.7
- **Poisoning** (acute) — *see also* Table of Drugs and Chemicals
  - algae and toxins T65.82- ☑
  - Bacillus B (aertrycke) (cholerae (suis)) (paratyphosus) (suipestifer) AØ2.9
    - botulinus AØ5.1
  - bacterial toxins AØ5.9
  - berries, noxious — *see* Poisoning, food, noxious, berries
- **Poisoning** — *continued*
  - botulism AØ5.1
  - ciguatera fish T61.Ø- ☑
  - Clostridium botulinum AØ5.1
  - death-cap (Amanita phalloides) (Amanita verna) — *see* Poisoning, food, noxious, mushrooms
  - drug — *see* Table of Drugs and Chemicals, by drug, poisoning
  - epidemic, fish (noxious) — *see* Poisoning, seafood
    - bacterial AØ5.9
  - fava bean D55.Ø
  - fish (noxious) T61.9- ☑
    - bacterial — *see* Intoxication, foodborne, by agent
    - ciguatera fish — *see* Poisoning, ciguatera fish
    - scombroid fish — *see* Poisoning, scombroid fish
    - specified type NEC T61.77- ☑
  - food NEC AØ5.9
    - bacterial — *see* Intoxication, foodborne, by agent
    - due to
      - Bacillus (aertrycke) (choleraesuis) (paratyphosus) (suipestifer) AØ2.9
        - botulinus AØ5.1
      - Clostridium (perfringens) (Welchii) AØ5.2
      - salmonella (aertrycke) (callinarum) (choleraesuis) (enteritidis) (paratyphi) (suipestifer) AØ2.9
        - with
          - gastroenteritis AØ2.Ø
          - sepsis AØ2.1
      - staphylococcus AØ5.Ø
      - Vibrio
        - parahaemolyticus AØ5.3
        - vulnificus AØ5.5
    - noxious or naturally toxic T62.9- ☑
      - berries — *see* subcategory T62.1 ☑
      - fish — *see* Poisoning, seafood
      - mushrooms — *see* subcategory T62.ØX ☑
      - plants NEC — *see* subcategory T62.2X ☑
      - seafood — *see* Poisoning, seafood
      - specified NEC — *see* subcategory T62.8X ☑
  - ichthyotoxism — *see* Poisoning, seafood
  - kreotoxism, food AØ5.9
  - latex T65.81- ☑
  - lead T56.Ø- ☑
  - mushroom — *see* Poisoning, food, noxious, mushroom
  - mussels — *see also* Poisoning, shellfish
    - bacterial — *see* Intoxication, foodborne, by agent
  - nicotine (tobacco) T65.2- ☑
  - noxious foodstuffs — *see* Poisoning, food, noxious
  - plants, noxious — *see* Poisoning, food, noxious, plants NEC
  - ptomaine — *see* Poisoning, food
  - radiation J7Ø.Ø
  - Salmonella (arizonae) (cholerae-suis) (enteritidis) (typhimurium) AØ2.9
  - scombroid fish T61.1- ☑
  - seafood (noxious) T61.9- ☑
    - bacterial — *see* Intoxication, foodborne, by agent
    - fish — *see* Poisoning, fish
    - shellfish — *see* Poisoning, shellfish
    - specified NEC — *see* subcategory T61.8X ☑
  - shellfish (amnesic) (azaspiracid) (diarrheic) (neurotoxic) (noxious) (paralytic) T61.78- ☑
    - bacterial — *see* Intoxication, foodborne, by agent
    - ciguatera mollusk — *see* Poisoning, ciguatera fish
  - specified substance NEC T65.891 ☑
  - Staphylococcus, food AØ5.Ø
  - tobacco (nicotine) T65.2- ☑
  - water E87.79
- **Poker spine** — *see* Spondylitis, ankylosing
- **Poland syndrome** Q79.8
- **Polioencephalitis** (acute) (bulbar) A8Ø.9
  - inferior G12.22
  - influenzal — *see* Influenza, with, encephalopathy
  - superior hemorrhagic (acute) (Wernicke's) E51.2
  - Wernicke's E51.2
- **Polioencephalomyelitis** (acute) (anterior) A8Ø.9
  - with beriberi E51.2
- **Polioencephalopathy, superior hemorrhagic** E51.2
  - with
    - beriberi E51.11
    - pellagra E52
- **Poliomeningoencephalitis** — *see* Meningoencephalitis
- **Poliomyelitis** (acute) (anterior) (epidemic) A8Ø.9
  - with paralysis (bulbar) — *see* Poliomyelitis, paralytic
  - abortive A8Ø.4
  - ascending (progressive) — *see* Poliomyelitis, paralytic
  - bulbar (paralytic) — *see* Poliomyelitis, paralytic
- **Poliomyelitis** — *continued*
  - congenital P35.8
  - nonepidemic A8Ø.9
  - nonparalytic A8Ø.4
  - paralytic A8Ø.3Ø
    - specified NEC A8Ø.39
    - vaccine-associated A8Ø.Ø
    - wild virus
      - imported A8Ø.1
      - indigenous A8Ø.2
  - spinal, acute A8Ø.9
- **Poliosis** (eyebrow) (eyelashes) L67.1
  - circumscripta, acquired L67.1
- **Pollakiuria** R35.Ø
  - psychogenic F45.8
- **Pollinosis** J3Ø.1
- **Pollitzer's disease** L73.2
- **Polyadenitis** — *see also* Lymphadenitis
  - malignant A2Ø.Ø
- **Polyalgia** M79.89
- **Polyangiitis** M3Ø.Ø
  - microscopic M31.7
  - overlap syndrome M3Ø.8
- **Polyarteritis**
  - microscopic M31.7
  - nodosa M3Ø.Ø
    - with lung involvement M3Ø.1
    - juvenile M3Ø.2
    - related condition NEC M3Ø.8
- **Polyarthralgia** — *see* Pain, joint
- **Polyarthritis, polyarthropathy** — *see also* Arthritis M13.Ø
  - due to or associated with other specified conditions — *see* Arthritis
  - epidemic (Australian) (with exanthema) B33.1
  - infective — *see* Arthritis, pyogenic or pyemic
  - inflammatory MØ6.4
  - juvenile (chronic) (seronegative) MØ8.3
  - migratory M13.8- ☑
  - rheumatic, acute — *see* Fever, rheumatic
- **Polyarthrosis** M15.9
  - post-traumatic M15.3
  - primary M15.Ø
  - specified NEC M15.8
- **Polycarential syndrome of infancy** E4Ø
- **Polychondritis** (atrophic) (chronic) — *see also* Disorder, cartilage, specified type NEC
  - relapsing M94.1
- **Polycoria** Q13.2
- **Polycystic** (disease)
  - degeneration, kidney Q61.3
    - autosomal dominant (adult type) Q61.2
    - autosomal recessive (infantile type) NEC Q61.19
  - kidney Q61.3
    - autosomal
      - dominant Q61.2
      - recessive NEC Q61.19
    - autosomal dominant (adult type) Q61.2
    - autosomal recessive (childhood type) NEC Q61.19
    - infantile type NEC Q61.19
  - liver Q44.6
  - lung J98.4
    - congenital Q33.Ø
  - ovary, ovaries E28.2
  - spleen Q89.Ø9
- **Polycythemia** (secondary) D75.1
  - acquired D75.1
  - benign (familial) D75.Ø
  - due to
    - donor twin P61.1
    - erythropoietin D75.1
    - fall in plasma volume D75.1
    - high altitude D75.1
    - maternal-fetal transfusion P61.1
    - stress D75.1
  - emotional D75.1
  - erythropoietin D75.1
  - familial (benign) D75.Ø
  - Gaisböck's (hypertonica) D75.1
  - high altitude D75.1
  - hypertonica D75.1
  - hypoxemic D75.1
  - neonatorum P61.1
  - nephrogenous D75.1
  - relative D75.1
  - secondary D75.1
  - spurious D75.1
  - stress D75.1

- **Polycythemia** — *continued*
  - vera D45
- **Polycytosis cryptogenica** D75.1
- **Polydactylism, polydactyly** Q69.9
  - toes Q69.2
- **Polydipsia** R63.1
- **Polydystrophy, pseudo-Hurler** E77.Ø
- **Polyembryoma** — *see* Neoplasm, malignant, by site
- **Polyglandular**
  - deficiency E31.Ø
  - dyscrasia E31.9
  - dysfunction E31.9
  - syndrome E31.8
- **Polyhydramnios** O4Ø.- ☑
- **Polymastia** Q83.1
- **Polymenorrhea** N92.Ø
- **Polymyalgia** M35.3
  - arteritica, giant cell M31.5
  - rheumatica M35.3
    - with giant cell arteritis M31.5
- **Polymyositis** (acute) (chronic) (hemorrhagic) M33.2Ø
  - with
    - myopathy M33.22
    - respiratory involvement M33.21
    - skin involvement — *see* Dermatopolymyositis
    - specified organ involvement NEC M33.29
  - ossificans (generalisata) (progressiva) — *see* Myositis, ossificans, progressiva
- **Polyneuritis, polyneuritic** — *see also* Polyneuropathy
  - acute (post-)infective G61.Ø
  - alcoholic G62.1
  - cranialis G52.7
  - demyelinating, chronic inflammatory (CIDP) G61.81
  - diabetic — *see* Diabetes, polyneuropathy
  - diphtheritic A36.83
  - due to lack of vitamin NEC E56.9 *[G63]*
  - endemic E51.11
  - erythredema — *see* subcategory T56.1 ☑
  - febrile, acute G61.Ø
  - hereditary ataxic G6Ø.1
  - idiopathic, acute G61.Ø
  - infective (acute) G61.Ø
  - inflammatory, chronic demyelinating (CIDP) G61.81
  - nutritional E63.9 *[G63]*
  - postinfective (acute) G61.Ø
  - specified NEC G62.89
- **Polyneuropathy** (peripheral) G62.9
  - alcoholic G62.1
  - amyloid (Portuguese) E85.1 *[G63]*
    - transthyretin-related (ATTR) familial E85.1 *[G63]*
  - arsenical G62.2
  - critical illness G62.81
  - demyelinating, chronic inflammatory (CIDP) G61.81
  - diabetic — *see* Diabetes, polyneuropathy
  - drug-induced G62.Ø
  - hereditary G6Ø.9
    - specified NEC G6Ø.8
  - idiopathic G6Ø.9
    - progressive G6Ø.3
  - in (due to)
    - alcohol G62.1
      - sequelae G65.2
    - amyloidosis, familial (Portuguese) E85.1 *[G63]*
    - antitetanus serum G61.1
    - arsenic G62.2
      - sequelae G65.2
    - avitaminosis NEC E56.9 *[G63]*
    - beriberi E51.11
    - collagen vascular disease NEC M35.9 *[G63]*
    - deficiency (of)
      - B (-complex) vitamins E53.9 *[G63]*
      - vitamin B6 E53.1 *[G63]*
    - diabetes — *see* Diabetes, polyneuropathy
    - diphtheria A36.83
    - drug or medicament G62.Ø
      - correct substance properly administered — *see* Table of Drugs and Chemicals, by drug, adverse effect
      - overdose or wrong substance given or taken — *see* Table of Drugs and Chemicals, by drug, poisoning
    - endocrine disease NEC E34.9 *[G63]*
    - herpes zoster BØ2.23
    - hypoglycemia E16.2 *[G63]*
    - infectious
      - disease NEC B99 ☑ *[G63]*
      - mononucleosis B27.91
    - lack of vitamin NEC E56.9 *[G63]*

- **Polyneuropathy** — *continued*
  - in — *continued*
    - lead G62.2
      - sequelae G65.2
    - leprosy A3Ø.9 *[G63]*
    - Lyme disease A69.22
    - metabolic disease NEC E88.9 *[G63]*
    - microscopic polyangiitis M31.7 *[G63]*
    - mumps B26.84
    - neoplastic disease — *see also* Neoplasm D49.9 *[G63]*
    - nutritional deficiency NEC E63.9 *[G63]*
    - organophosphate compounds G62.2
      - sequelae G65.2
    - parasitic disease NEC B89 *[G63]*
    - pellagra E52 *[G63]*
    - polyarteritis nodosa M3Ø.Ø
    - porphyria E8Ø.2Ø *[G63]*
    - radiation G62.82
    - rheumatoid arthritis — *see* Rheumatoid, polyneuropathy
    - sarcoidosis D86.89
    - serum G61.1
    - syphilis (late) A52.15
      - congenital A5Ø.43
    - systemic
      - connective tissue disorder M35.9 *[G63]*
      - lupus erythematosus M32.19
    - toxic agent NEC G62.2
      - sequelae G65.2
    - transthyretin-related (ATTR) familial amyloid E85.1
    - triorthocresyl phosphate G62.2
      - sequelae G65.2
    - tuberculosis A17.89
    - uremia N18.9 *[G63]*
    - vitamin B12 deficiency E53.8 *[G63]*
      - with anemia (pernicious) D51.Ø *[G63]*
        - due to dietary deficiency D51.3, G63
    - zoster BØ2.23
  - inflammatory G61.9
    - chronic demyelinating (CIDP) G61.81
    - sequelae G65.1
    - specified NEC G61.89
  - lead G62.2
    - sequelae G65.2
  - nutritional NEC E63.9 *[G63]*
  - postherpetic (zoster) BØ2.23
  - progressive G6Ø.3
  - radiation-induced G62.82
  - sensory (hereditary) (idiopathic) G6Ø.8
  - specified NEC G62.89
  - syphilitic (late) A52.15
    - congenital A5Ø.43
- **Polyopia** H53.8
- **Polyorchism, polyorchidism** Q55.21
- **Polyosteoarthritis** — *see also* Osteoarthritis, generalized M15.9
  - post-traumatic M15.3
  - specified NEC M15.8
- **Polyostotic fibrous dysplasia** Q78.1
- **Polyotia** Q17.Ø
- **Polyp, polypus**
  - accessory sinus J33.8
  - adenocarcinoma in — *see* Neoplasm, malignant, by site
  - adenocarcinoma in situ in — *see* Neoplasm, in situ, by site
  - adenoid tissue J33.Ø
  - adenomatous — *see also* Neoplasm, benign, by site
    - adenocarcinoma in — *see* Neoplasm, malignant, by site
    - adenocarcinoma in situ in — *see* Neoplasm, in situ, by site
    - carcinoma in — *see* Neoplasm, malignant, by site
    - carcinoma in situ in — *see* Neoplasm, in situ, by site
    - multiple — *see* Neoplasm, benign
      - adenocarcinoma in — *see* Neoplasm, malignant, by site
      - adenocarcinoma in situ in — *see* Neoplasm, in situ, by site
  - antrum J33.8
  - anus, anal (canal) K62.Ø
  - Bartholin's gland N84.3
  - bladder D41.4
  - carcinoma in — *see* Neoplasm, malignant, by site
  - carcinoma in situ in — *see* Neoplasm, in situ, by site
  - cecum D12.Ø
  - cervix (uteri) N84.1

- **Polyp, polypus** — *continued*
  - cervix — *continued*
    - in pregnancy or childbirth — *see* Pregnancy, complicated by, abnormal, cervix
    - mucous N84.1
    - nonneoplastic N84.1
  - choanal J33.Ø
  - cholesterol K82.4
  - clitoris N84.3
  - colon K63.5
    - adenomatous D12.6
      - ascending D12.2
      - cecum D12.Ø
      - descending D12.4
      - sigmoid D12.5
      - transverse D12.3
    - ascending K63.5
    - cecum K63.5
    - descending K63.5
    - hyperplastic, (any site) K63.5
    - inflammatory K51.4Ø
      - with
        - abscess K51.414
        - complication K51.419
          - specified NEC K51.418
        - fistula K51.413
        - intestinal obstruction K51.412
        - rectal bleeding K51.411
    - sigmoid K63.5
    - transverse K63.5
  - corpus uteri N84.Ø
  - dental KØ4.Ø1
    - irreversible KØ4.Ø2
    - reversible KØ4.Ø1
  - duodenum K31.7
  - ear (middle) H74.4- ☑
  - endometrium N84.Ø
  - esophageal K22.81
  - esophagogastric junction K22.82
  - ethmoidal (sinus) J33.8
  - fallopian tube N84.8
  - female genital tract N84.9
    - specified NEC N84.8
  - frontal (sinus) J33.8
  - gallbladder K82.4
  - gingiva, gum KØ6.8
  - labia, labium (majus) (minus) N84.3
  - larynx (mucous) J38.1
    - adenomatous D14.1
  - malignant — *see* Neoplasm, malignant, by site
  - maxillary (sinus) J33.8
  - middle ear — *see* Polyp, ear (middle)
  - myometrium N84.Ø
  - nares
    - anterior J33.9
    - posterior J33.Ø
  - nasal (mucous) J33.9
    - cavity J33.Ø
    - septum J33.Ø
  - nasopharyngeal J33.Ø
  - nose (mucous) J33.9
  - oviduct N84.8
  - pharynx J39.2
  - placenta O9Ø.89
  - prostate — *see* Enlargement, enlarged, prostate
  - pudenda, pudendum N84.3
  - pulpal (dental) KØ4.Ø1
    - irreversible KØ4.Ø2
    - reversible KØ4.Ø1
  - rectum (nonadenomatous) K62.1
    - adenomatous — *see* Polyp, adenomatous
  - septum (nasal) J33.Ø
  - sinus (accessory) (ethmoidal) (frontal) (maxillary) (sphenoidal) J33.8
  - sphenoidal (sinus) J33.8
  - stomach K31.7
    - adenomatous D13.1
  - tube, fallopian N84.8
  - turbinate, mucous membrane J33.8
  - umbilical, newborn P83.6
  - ureter N28.89
  - urethra N36.2
  - uterus (body) (corpus) (mucous) N84.Ø
    - cervix N84.1
    - in pregnancy or childbirth — *see* Pregnancy, complicated by, tumor, uterus
  - vagina N84.2
  - vocal cord (mucous) J38.1

- **Polyp, polypus** — *continued*
  - vulva N84.3
- **Polyphagia** R63.2
- **Polyploidy** Q92.7
- **Polypoid** — *see* condition
- **Polyposis** — *see also* Polyp
  - coli (adenomatous) D12.6
    - adenocarcinoma in C18.9
    - adenocarcinoma in situ in — *see* Neoplasm, in situ, by site
    - carcinoma in C18.9
  - colon (adenomatous) D12.6
  - familial D12.6
    - adenocarcinoma in situ in — *see* Neoplasm, in situ, by site
  - intestinal (adenomatous) D12.6
  - malignant lymphomatous C83.1- ☑
  - multiple, adenomatous — *see also* Neoplasm, benign D36.9
- **Polyradiculitis** — *see* Polyneuropathy
- **Polyradiculoneuropathy** (acute) (postinfective) (segmentally demyelinating) G61.Ø
- **Polyserositis**
  - due to pericarditis I31.1
  - pericardial I31.1
  - periodic, familial E85.Ø
  - tuberculous A19.9
    - acute A19.1
    - chronic A19.8
- **Polysplenia syndrome** Q89.Ø9
- **Polysyndactyly** — *see also* Syndactylism, syndactyly Q7Ø.4
- **Polytrichia** L68.3
- **Polyunguia** Q84.6
- **Polyuria** R35.89
  - nocturnal R35.81
  - psychogenic F45.8
  - specified NEC R35.89
- **Pompe's disease** (glycogen storage) E74.Ø2
- **Pompholyx** L3Ø.1
- **Poncet's disease** (tuberculous rheumatism) A18.Ø9
- **Pond fracture** — *see* Fracture, skull
- **Ponos** B55.Ø
- **Pons, pontine** — *see* condition
- **Poor**
  - aesthetic of existing restoration of tooth KØ8.56
  - contractions, labor O62.2
  - gingival margin to tooth restoration KØ8.51
  - personal hygiene R46.Ø
  - prenatal care, affecting management of pregnancy — *see* Pregnancy, complicated by, insufficient, prenatal care
  - sucking reflex (newborn) R29.2
  - urinary stream R39.12
  - vision NEC H54.7
- **Poradenitis, nostras inguinalis or venerea** A55
- **Porencephaly** (congenital) (developmental) (true) QØ4.6
  - acquired G93.Ø
  - nondevelopmental G93.Ø
  - traumatic (post) FØ7.89
- **Porocephaliasis** B88.8
- **Porokeratosis** Q82.8
- **Poroma, eccrine** — *see* Neoplasm, skin, benign
- **Porphyria** (South African) E8Ø.2Ø
  - acquired E8Ø.2Ø
  - acute intermittent (hepatic) (Swedish) E8Ø.21
  - cutanea tarda (hereditary) (symptomatic) E8Ø.1
  - due to drugs E8Ø.2Ø
    - correct substance properly administered — *see* Table of Drugs and Chemicals, by drug, adverse effect
    - overdose or wrong substance given or taken — *see* Table of Drugs and Chemicals, by drug, poisoning
  - erythropoietic (congenital) (hereditary) E8Ø.Ø
  - hepatocutaneous type E8Ø.1
  - secondary E8Ø.2Ø
  - toxic NEC E8Ø.2Ø
  - variegata E8Ø.2Ø
- **Porphyrinuria** — *see* Porphyria
- **Porphyruria** — *see* Porphyria
- **Port wine nevus, mark, or stain** Q82.5
- **Portal** — *see* condition
- **Posadas-Wernicke disease** B38.9
- **Positive**
  - culture (nonspecific)
    - blood R78.81
    - bronchial washings R84.5
- **Positive** — *continued*
  - culture — *continued*
    - cerebrospinal fluid R83.5
    - cervix uteri R87.5
    - nasal secretions R84.5
    - nipple discharge R89.5
    - nose R84.5
      - staphylococcus (Methicillin susceptible) Z22.321
        - Methicillin resistant Z22.322
    - peritoneal fluid R85.5
    - pleural fluid R84.5
    - prostatic secretions R86.5
    - saliva R85.5
    - seminal fluid R86.5
    - sputum R84.5
    - synovial fluid R89.5
    - throat scrapings R84.5
    - urine R82.79
    - vagina R87.5
    - vulva R87.5
    - wound secretions R89.5
  - PPD (skin test) R76.11
  - serology for syphilis A53.Ø
    - false R76.8
    - with signs or symptoms — *code as* Syphilis, by site and stage
  - skin test, tuberculin (without active tuberculosis) R76.11
  - test, human immunodeficiency virus (HIV) R75
  - VDRL A53.Ø
    - with signs or symptoms — *code by* site and stage under Syphilis A53.9
  - Wassermann reaction A53.Ø
- **Post COVID-19 condition, unspecified** UØ9.9
- **Postcardiotomy syndrome** I97.Ø
- **Postcaval ureter** Q62.62
- **Postcholecystectomy syndrome** K91.5
- **Postclimacteric bleeding** N95.Ø
- **Postcommissurotomy syndrome** I97.Ø
- **Postconcussional syndrome** FØ7.81
- **Postcontusional syndrome** FØ7.81
- **Postcricoid region** — *see* condition
- **Post-dates** (4Ø-42 weeks) (pregnancy) (mother) O48.Ø
  - more than 42 weeks gestation O48.1
- **Postencephalitic syndrome** FØ7.89
- **Posterior** — *see* condition
- **Posterolateral sclerosis** (spinal cord) — *see* Degeneration, combined
- **Postexanthematous** — *see* condition
- **Postfebrile** — *see* condition
- **Postgastrectomy dumping syndrome** K91.1
- **Posthemiplegic chorea** — *see* Monoplegia
- **Posthemorrhagic anemia** (chronic) D5Ø.Ø
  - acute D62
  - newborn P61.3
- **Postherpetic neuralgia** (zoster) BØ2.29
  - trigeminal BØ2.22
- **Posthitis** N47.7
- **Postimmunization complication or reaction** — *see* Complications, vaccination
- **Postinfectious** — *see* condition
- **Postlaminectomy syndrome NEC** M96.1
- **Postleukotomy syndrome** FØ7.Ø
- **Postmastectomy lymphedema** (syndrome) I97.2
- **Postmaturity, postmature** (over 42 weeks)
  - maternal (over 42 weeks gestation) O48.1
  - newborn PØ8.22
- **Postmeasles complication NEC** — *see also* condition BØ5.89
- **Postmenopausal**
  - endometrium (atrophic) N95.8
    - suppurative — *see also* Endometritis N71.9
  - osteoporosis — *see* Osteoporosis, postmenopausal
- **Postnasal drip** RØ9.82
  - due to
    - allergic rhinitis — *see* Rhinitis, allergic
    - common cold JØØ
    - gastroesophageal reflux — *see* Reflux, gastroesophageal
    - nasopharyngitis — *see* Nasopharyngitis
    - other known condition — *code to* condition
    - sinusitis — *see* Sinusitis
- **Postnatal** — *see* condition
- **Postoperative** (postprocedural) — *see* Complication, postoperative
  - pneumothorax, therapeutic Z98.3
  - state NEC Z98.89Ø
- **Postpancreatectomy hyperglycemia** E89.1
- **Postpartum** — *see* Puerperal
- **Postphlebitic syndrome** — *see* Syndrome, postthrombotic
- **Postpolio** (myelitic) **syndrome** G14
- **Postpoliomyelitic** — *see also* condition
  - osteopathy — *see* Osteopathy, after poliomyelitis
- **Postprocedural** — *see also* Postoperative
  - hypoinsulinemia E89.1
- **Postschizophrenic depression** F32.89
- **Postsurgery status** — *see also* Status (post)
  - pneumothorax, therapeutic Z98.3
- **Post-term** (4Ø-42 weeks) (pregnancy) (mother) O48.Ø
  - infant PØ8.21
  - more than 42 weeks gestation (mother) O48.1
- **Post-traumatic brain syndrome, nonpsychotic** FØ7.81
- **Post-typhoid abscess** AØ1.Ø9
- **Postures, hysterical** F44.2
- **Postvaccinal reaction or complication** — *see* Complications, vaccination
- **Postvalvulotomy syndrome** I97.Ø
- **Potain's**
  - disease (pulmonary edema) — *see* Edema, lung
  - syndrome (gastrectasis with dyspepsia) K31.Ø
- **POTS** (postural orthostatic tachycardia syndrome) G9Ø.A
- **Potter's**
  - asthma J62.8
  - facies Q6Ø.6
  - lung J62.8
  - syndrome (with renal agenesis) Q6Ø.6
- **Pott's**
  - curvature (spinal) A18.Ø1
  - disease or paraplegia A18.Ø1
  - spinal curvature A18.Ø1
  - tumor, puffy — *see* Osteomyelitis, specified type NEC
- **Pouch**
  - bronchus Q32.4
  - Douglas' — *see* condition
  - esophagus, esophageal, congenital Q39.6
    - acquired K22.5
  - gastric K31.4
  - Hartmann's K82.8
  - pharynx, pharyngeal (congenital) Q38.7
- **Pouchitis** K91.85Ø
- **Poultrymen's itch** B88.Ø
- **Poverty NEC** Z59.6
  - extreme Z59.5
- **Poxvirus NEC** BØ8.8
- **Prader-Willi syndrome** Q87.11
- **Prader-Willi-like syndrome** Q87.19
- **Preauricular appendage or tag** Q17.Ø
- **Prebetalipoproteinemia** (acquired) (essential) (familial) (hereditary) (primary) (secondary) E78.1
  - with chylomicronemia E78.3
- **Precipitate labor or delivery** O62.3
- **Preclimacteric bleeding** (menorrhagia) N92.4
- **Precocious**
  - adrenarche E3Ø.1
  - menarche E3Ø.1
  - menstruation E3Ø.1
  - pubarche E3Ø.1
  - puberty E3Ø.1
    - central E22.8
  - sexual development NEC E3Ø.1
  - thelarche E3Ø.8
- **Precocity, sexual** (constitutional) (cryptogenic) (female) (idiopathic) (male) E3Ø.1
  - with adrenal hyperplasia E25.9
    - congenital E25.Ø
- **Precordial pain** RØ7.2
- **Predeciduous teeth** KØØ.2
- **Prediabetes, prediabetic** R73.Ø3
  - complicating
    - pregnancy — *see* Pregnancy, complicated by, diseases of, specified type or system NEC
    - puerperium O99.893
- **Predislocation status of hip at birth** Q65.6
- **Pre-eclampsia** O14.9- ☑
  - with pre-existing hypertension — *see* Hypertension, complicating pregnancy, pre-existing, with, pre-eclampsia
  - complicating
    - childbirth O14.94
    - puerperium O14.95
  - mild O14.Ø- ☑
    - complicating
      - childbirth O14.Ø4
      - puerperium O14.Ø5

Pre-eclampsia — *continued*
moderate O14.Ø- ☑
complicating
childbirth O14.Ø4
puerperium O14.Ø5
severe O14.1- ☑
with hemolysis, elevated liver enzymes and low platelet count (HELLP) O14.2- ☑
complicating
childbirth O14.24
puerperium O14.25
complicating
childbirth O14.14
puerperium O14.15
Pre-eruptive color change, teeth, tooth KØØ.8
Pre-excitation atrioventricular conduction I45.6
Preglaucoma H4Ø.ØØ- ☑
Pregnancy (single) (uterine) — *see also* Delivery and Puerperal Z33.1

Note: The Tabular must be reviewed for assignment of appropriate seventh character for multiple gestation codes in Chapter 15

Note: The Tabular must be reviewed for assignment of the appropriate character indicating the trimester of the pregnancy

abdominal (ectopic) OØØ.ØØ
with intrauterine pregnancy OØØ.Ø1
with viable fetus O36.7- ☑
ampullar OØØ.1Ø- ☑
with intrauterine pregnancy OØØ.11- ☑
biochemical OØ2.81
broad ligament OØØ.8Ø
with intrauterine pregnancy OØØ.81
cervical OØØ.8
with intrauterine pregnancy OØØ.81
chemical OØ2.81
complicated by (care of) (management affected by)
abnormal, abnormality
cervix O34.4- ☑
causing obstructed labor O65.5
cord (umbilical) O69.9 ☑
fetal heart rate or rhythm O36.83- ☑
findings on antenatal screening of mother O28.9
biochemical O28.1
chromosomal O28.5
cytological O28.2
genetic O28.5
hematological O28.Ø
radiological O28.4
specified NEC O28.8
ultrasonic O28.3
glucose (tolerance) NEC O99.81Ø
pelvic organs O34.9- ☑
specified NEC O34.8- ☑
causing obstructed labor O65.5
pelvis (bony) (major) NEC O33.Ø
perineum O34.7- ☑
position
placenta O44.Ø- ☑
with hemorrhage O44.1- ☑
uterus O34.59- ☑
uterus O34.59- ☑
causing obstructed labor O65.5
congenital O34.Ø- ☑
vagina O34.6- ☑
causing obstructed labor O65.5
vulva O34.7- ☑
causing obstructed labor O65.5
abruptio placentae — *see* Abruptio placentae
abscess or cellulitis
bladder O23.1- ☑
breast O91.11- ☑
genital organ or tract O23.9- ☑
abuse
physical O9A.31 ☑ (*following* O99)
psychological O9A.51 ☑ (*following* O99)
sexual O9A.41 ☑ (*following* O99)
adverse effect anesthesia O29.9- ☑
aspiration pneumonitis O29.Ø1- ☑
cardiac arrest O29.11- ☑
cardiac complication NEC O29.19- ☑
cardiac failure O29.12- ☑
central nervous system complication NEC O29.29- ☑
cerebral anoxia O29.21- ☑

Pregnancy — *continued*
complicated by — *continued*
adverse effect anesthesia — *continued*
failed or difficult intubation O29.6- ☑
inhalation of stomach contents or secretions NOS O29.Ø1- ☑
local, toxic reaction O29.3X ☑
Mendelson's syndrome O29.Ø1- ☑
pressure collapse of lung O29.Ø2- ☑
pulmonary complications NEC O29.Ø9- ☑
specified NEC O29.8X- ☑
spinal and epidural type NEC O29.5X ☑
induced headache O29.4- ☑
albuminuria — *see also* Proteinuria, gestational O12.1- ☑
alcohol use O99.31- ☑
amnionitis O41.12- ☑
anaphylactoid syndrome of pregnancy O88.Ø1- ☑
anemia (conditions in D5Ø-D64) (pre-existing) O99.Ø1- ☑
complicating the puerperium O99.Ø3
antepartum hemorrhage O46.9- ☑
with coagulation defect — *see* Hemorrhage, antepartum, with coagulation defect
specified NEC O46.8X- ☑
appendicitis O99.61- ☑
atrophy (yellow) (acute) liver (subacute) O26.61- ☑
bariatric surgery status O99.84- ☑
bicornis or bicornuate uterus O34.Ø- ☑
biliary tract problems O26.61- ☑
breech presentation O32.1 ☑
cardiovascular diseases (conditions in IØØ-IØ9, I2Ø-I52, I7Ø-I99) O99.41- ☑
cerebrovascular disorders (conditions in I6Ø-I69) O99.41- ☑
cervical shortening O26.87- ☑
cervicitis O23.51- ☑
cesarean scar defect (isthmocele) O34.22
chloasma (gravidarum) O26.89- ☑
cholecystitis O99.61- ☑
cholestasis (intrahepatic) O26.61- ☑
chorioamnionitis O41.12- ☑
circulatory system disorder (conditions in IØØ-IØ9, I2Ø-I99, O99.41-)
compound presentation O32.6 ☑
conjoined twins O3Ø.Ø2- ☑
connective system disorders (conditions in MØØ-M99) O99.891
contracted pelvis (general) O33.1
inlet O33.2
outlet O33.3 ☑
convulsions (eclamptic) (uremic) — *see also* Eclampsia O15.9
cracked nipple O92.11- ☑
cystitis O23.1- ☑
cystocele O34.8- ☑
death of fetus (near term) O36.4 ☑
early pregnancy OØ2.1
of one fetus or more in multiple gestation O31.2- ☑
deciduitis O41.14- ☑
decreased fetal movement O36.81- ☑
dental problems O99.61- ☑
diabetes (mellitus) O24.91- ☑
gestational (pregnancy induced) — *see* Diabetes, gestational
pre-existing O24.31- ☑
specified NEC O24.81- ☑
type 1 O24.Ø1- ☑
type 2 O24.11- ☑
digestive system disorders (conditions in KØØ-K93) O99.61- ☑
diseases of — *see* Pregnancy, complicated by, specified body system disease
biliary tract O26.61- ☑
blood NEC (conditions in D65-D77) O99.11- ☑
liver O26.61- ☑
specified NEC O99.891
disorders of — *see* Pregnancy, complicated by, specified body system disorder
amniotic fluid and membranes O41.9- ☑
specified NEC O41.8X- ☑
biliary tract O26.61- ☑
ear and mastoid process (conditions in H6Ø-H95) O99.891
eye and adnexa (conditions in HØØ-H59) O99.891

Pregnancy — *continued*
complicated by — *continued*
disorders of — *see* Pregnancy, complicated by, specified body system disorder — *continued*
liver O26.61- ☑
skin (conditions in LØØ-L99) O99.71- ☑
specified NEC O99.891
displacement, uterus NEC O34.59- ☑
causing obstructed labor O65.5
disproportion (due to) O33.9
fetal (ascites) (hydrops) (meningomyelocele) (sacral teratoma) (tumor) deformities NEC O33.7 ☑
generally contracted pelvis O33.1
hydrocephalic fetus O33.6 ☑
inlet contraction of pelvis O33.2
mixed maternal and fetal origin O33.4 ☑
specified NEC O33.8
double uterus O34.Ø- ☑
causing obstructed labor O65.5
drug use (conditions in F11-F19) O99.32- ☑
eclampsia, eclamptic (coma) (convulsions) (delirium) (nephritis) (uremia) — *see also* Eclampsia O15.- ☑
ectopic pregnancy — *see* Pregnancy, ectopic
edema O12.Ø- ☑
with
gestational hypertension, mild — *see also* Pre-eclampsia O14.Ø- ☑
proteinuria O12.2- ☑
effusion, amniotic fluid — *see* Pregnancy, complicated by, premature rupture of membranes
elderly
multigravida OØ9.52- ☑
primigravida OØ9.51- ☑
embolism — *see also* Embolism, obstetric, pregnancy O88.- ☑
endocrine diseases NEC O99.28- ☑
endometritis O86.12
excessive weight gain O26.Ø- ☑
exhaustion O26.81- ☑
during labor and delivery O75.81
face presentation O32.3 ☑
failed induction of labor O61.9
instrumental O61.1
mechanical O61.1
medical O61.Ø
specified NEC O61.8
surgical O61.1
failed or difficult intubation for anesthesia O29.6- ☑
false labor (pains) O47.9
at or after 37 completed weeks of pregnancy O47.1
before 37 completed weeks of pregnancy O47.Ø- ☑
fatigue O26.81- ☑
during labor and delivery O75.81
fatty metamorphosis of liver O26.61- ☑
female genital mutilation O34.8- ☑ *[N9Ø.81-]* ☑
fetal (maternal care for)
abnormality or damage O35.9 ☑
acid-base balance O68
specified type NEC O35.8 ☑
acidemia O68
acidosis O68
agenesis of corpus callosum O35.Ø1 ☑
alkalosis O68
anemia and thrombocytopenia O36.82- ☑
anencephaly O35.Ø2 ☑
bradycardia O36.83- ☑
cardiac anomalies O35.B ☑
central nervous system malformation or damage O35.ØØ ☑
specified type NEC O35.Ø9 ☑
choroid plexus cysts O35.Ø3 ☑
chromosomal abnormality (conditions in Q9Ø-Q99) O35.1Ø ☑
sex chromosome O35.15 ☑
specified NEC O35.19 ☑
Trisomy 13 O35.11 ☑
Trisomy 18 O35.12 ☑
Trisomy 21 O35.13 ☑
Turner Syndrome O35.14 ☑
conjoined twins O3Ø.Ø2- ☑
damage from
amniocentesis O35.7 ☑

- **Pregnancy** — *continued*
  - complicated by — *continued*
    - fetal — *continued*
      - damage from — *continued*
        - biopsy procedures O35.7 ☑
        - drug addiction O35.5 ☑
        - hematological investigation O35.7 ☑
        - intrauterine contraceptive device O35.7 ☑
        - maternal
          - alcohol addiction O35.4 ☑
          - cytomegalovirus infection O35.3 ☑
          - disease NEC O35.8 ☑
          - drug addiction O35.5 ☑
          - listeriosis O35.8 ☑
          - rubella O35.3 ☑
          - toxoplasmosis O35.8 ☑
          - viral infection O35.3 ☑
        - medical procedure NEC O35.7 ☑
        - radiation O35.6 ☑
      - death (near term) O36.4 ☑
        - early pregnancy O02.1
      - decreased movement O36.81- ☑
      - depressed heart rate tones O36.83- ☑
      - disproportion due to deformity (fetal) O33.7 ☑
      - encephalocele O35.Ø4 ☑
      - excessive growth (large for dates) O36.6- ☑
      - facial anomalies O35.A ☑
      - gastrointestinal anomalies O35.D ☑
      - genitourinary anomalies O35.E ☑
      - growth retardation O36.59- ☑
        - light for dates O36.59- ☑
        - small for dates O36.59- ☑
      - heart rate irregularity (abnormal variability) (bradycardia) (decelerations) (tachycardia) O36.83- ☑
      - hereditary disease O35.2 ☑
      - holoprosencephaly O35.Ø5 ☑
      - hydrocephalus O35.Ø6 ☑
      - hydrocephaly O35.Ø6 ☑
      - intrauterine death O36.4 ☑
      - microcephaly O35.Ø7 ☑
      - musculoskeletal anomalies
        - lower extremities O35.H ☑
        - trunk O35.F ☑
        - upper extremities O35.G ☑
      - non-reassuring heart rate or rhythm O36.83- ☑
      - poor growth O36.59- ☑
        - light for dates O36.59- ☑
        - small for dates O36.59- ☑
      - problem O36.9- ☑
        - specified NEC O36.89- ☑
      - pulmonary anomalies O35.C ☑
      - reduction (elective) O31.3- ☑
      - selective termination O31.3- ☑
      - spina bifida O35.Ø8 ☑
      - thrombocytopenia O36.82- ☑
    - fibroid (tumor) (uterus) O34.1- ☑
    - fissure of nipple O92.11- ☑
    - gallstones O99.61- ☑
    - gastric banding status O99.84- ☑
    - gastric bypass status O99.84- ☑
    - genital herpes (asymptomatic) (history of) (inactive) O98.3- ☑
    - genital tract infection O23.9- ☑
    - glomerular diseases (conditions in NØØ-NØ7) O26.83- ☑
      - with hypertension, pre-existing — *see* Hypertension, complicating, pregnancy, pre-existing, with, renal disease
    - gonorrhea O98.21- ☑
    - grand multiparity OØ9.4 ☑
    - habitual aborter — *see* Pregnancy, complicated by, recurrent pregnancy loss
    - HELLP syndrome (hemolysis, elevated liver enzymes and low platelet count) O14.2- ☑
    - hemorrhage
      - antepartum — *see* Hemorrhage, antepartum
      - before 2Ø completed weeks gestation O2Ø.9
        - specified NEC O2Ø.8
      - due to premature separation, placenta — *see also* Abruptio placentae O45.9- ☑
      - early O2Ø.9
        - specified NEC O2Ø.8
      - threatened abortion O2Ø.Ø
    - hemorrhoids O22.4- ☑
    - hepatitis (viral) O98.41- ☑

- **Pregnancy** — *continued*
  - complicated by — *continued*
    - herniation of uterus O34.59- ☑
    - high
      - head at term O32.4 ☑
      - risk — *see* Supervision (of) (for), high-risk
    - history of in utero procedure during previous pregnancy OØ9.82- ☑
    - HIV O98.71- ☑
    - human immunodeficiency virus (HIV) disease O98.71- ☑
    - hydatidiform mole — *see also* Mole, hydatidiform OØ1.9
    - hydramnios O4Ø.- ☑
    - hydrocephalic fetus (disproportion) O33.6 ☑
    - hydrops
      - amnii O4Ø.- ☑
      - fetalis O36.2- ☑
        - associated with isoimmunization — *see also* Pregnancy, complicated by, isoimmunization O36.11- ☑
    - hydrorrhea O42.9Ø
    - hyperemesis (gravidarum) (mild) — *see also* Hyperemesis, gravidarum O21.Ø
    - hypertension — *see* Hypertension, complicating pregnancy
    - hypertensive
      - heart and renal disease, pre-existing — *see* Hypertension, complicating, pregnancy, pre-existing, with, heart disease, with renal disease
      - heart disease, pre-existing — *see* Hypertension, complicating, pregnancy, pre-existing, with, heart disease
      - renal disease, pre-existing — *see* Hypertension, complicating, pregnancy, pre-existing, with, renal disease
    - hypotension O26.5- ☑
    - immune disorders NEC (conditions in D8Ø-D89) O99.11- ☑
    - incarceration, uterus O34.51- ☑
    - incompetent cervix O34.3- ☑
    - inconclusive fetal viability O36.8Ø ☑
    - infection(s) O98.91- ☑
      - amniotic fluid or sac O41.1Ø- ☑
      - bladder O23.1- ☑
      - carrier state NEC O99.83Ø
        - streptococcus B O99.82Ø
      - genital organ or tract O23.9- ☑
        - specified NEC O23.59- ☑
      - genitourinary tract O23.9- ☑
      - gonorrhea O98.21- ☑
      - hepatitis (viral) O98.41- ☑
      - HIV O98.71- ☑
      - human immunodeficiency virus (HIV) O98.71- ☑
      - intrauterine O41.12 ☑
      - kidney O23.Ø- ☑
      - nipple O91.Ø1- ☑
      - parasitic disease O98.91- ☑
        - specified NEC O98.81- ☑
      - protozoal disease O98.61- ☑
      - sexually transmitted NEC O98.31- ☑
      - specified type NEC O98.81- ☑
      - syphilis O98.11- ☑
      - tuberculosis O98.Ø1- ☑
      - urethra O23.2- ☑
      - urinary (tract) O23.4- ☑
        - specified NEC O23.3- ☑
      - viral disease O98.51- ☑
    - inflammation
      - intrauterine O41.12 ☑
    - injury or poisoning (conditions in SØØ-T88) O9A.21- ☑ (*following* O99)
      - due to abuse
        - physical O9A.31- ☑ (*following* O99)
        - psychological O9A.51- ☑ (*following* O99)
        - sexual O9A.41- ☑ (*following* O99)
    - insufficient
      - prenatal care OØ9.3- ☑
      - weight gain O26.1- ☑
    - insulin resistance O26.89 ☑
    - intrauterine fetal death (near term) O36.4 ☑
      - early pregnancy OØ2.1
      - multiple gestation (one fetus or more) O31.2- ☑
    - isoimmunization O36.11- ☑
      - anti-A sensitization O36.11- ☑

- **Pregnancy** — *continued*
  - complicated by — *continued*
    - isoimmunization — *continued*
      - anti-B sensitization O36.19- ☑
      - Rh O36.Ø9- ☑
        - anti-D antibody O36.Ø1- ☑
      - specified NEC O36.19- ☑
    - laceration of uterus NEC O71.81
    - malformation
      - central nervous system O35.ØØ ☑
        - specified type NEC O35.Ø9 ☑
      - placenta, placental (vessel) O43.1Ø- ☑
        - specified NEC O43.19- ☑
      - uterus (congenital) O34.Ø- ☑
    - malnutrition (conditions in E4Ø-E46) O25.1- ☑
    - maternal hypotension syndrome O26.5- ☑
    - mental disorders (conditions in FØ1-FØ9, F2Ø-F52 and F54-F99) O99.34- ☑
      - alcohol use O99.31- ☑
      - drug use O99.32- ☑
      - smoking O99.33- ☑
    - mentum presentation O32.3 ☑
    - metabolic disorders O99.28- ☑
    - missed
      - abortion OØ2.1
      - delivery O36.4 ☑
    - multiple gestations O3Ø.9- ☑
      - conjoined twins O3Ø.Ø2- ☑
      - quadruplet — *see* Pregnancy, quadruplet
      - specified complication NEC O31.8X- ☑
      - specified number of multiples NEC — *see* Pregnancy, multiple (gestation), specified NEC
      - triplet — *see* Pregnancy, triplet
      - twin — *see* Pregnancy, twin
    - musculoskeletal condition (conditions is MØØ-M99) O99.891
    - necrosis, liver (conditions in K72) O26.61- ☑
    - neoplasm
      - benign
        - cervix O34.4- ☑
        - corpus uteri O34.1- ☑
        - uterus O34.1- ☑
      - malignant O9A.11- ☑ (*following* O99)
    - nephropathy NEC O26.83- ☑
    - nervous system condition (conditions in GØØ-G99) O99.35- ☑
    - nutritional diseases NEC O99.28- ☑
    - obesity (pre-existing) O99.21- ☑
    - obesity surgery status O99.84- ☑
    - oblique lie or presentation O32.2 ☑
    - older mother — *see* Pregnancy, complicated by, elderly
    - oligohydramnios O41.Ø- ☑
      - with premature rupture of membranes — *see also* Pregnancy, complicated by, premature rupture of membranes O42.- ☑
    - onset (spontaneous) of labor after 37 completed weeks of gestation but before 39 completed weeks gestation, with delivery by (planned) cesarean section O75.82
    - oophoritis O23.52- ☑
    - overdose, drug — *see also* Table of Drugs and Chemicals, by drug, poisoning O9A.21- ☑ (*following* O99)
    - oversize fetus O33.5 ☑
    - papyraceous fetus O31.Ø- ☑
    - pelvic inflammatory disease O99.891
    - periodontal disease O99.61- ☑
    - peripheral neuritis O26.82- ☑
    - peritoneal (pelvic) adhesions O99.891
    - phlebitis O22.9- ☑
    - phlebopathy O22.9- ☑
    - phlebothrombosis (superficial) O22.2- ☑
      - deep O22.3- ☑
    - placenta accreta O43.21- ☑
    - placenta increta O43.22- ☑
    - placenta percreta O43.23- ☑
    - placenta previa O44.Ø- ☑
      - complete O44.Ø- ☑
        - with hemorrhage O44.1- ☑
      - marginal O44.2- ☑
        - with hemorrhage O44.3- ☑
      - partial O44.2- ☑
        - with hemorrhage O44.3- ☑
    - placental disorder O43.9- ☑
      - specified NEC O43.89- ☑

- **Pregnancy** — *continued*
  - complicated by — *continued*
    - placental dysfunction O43.89- ☑
    - placental infarction O43.81- ☑
    - placental insufficiency O36.51- ☑
    - placental transfusion syndromes
      - fetomaternal O43.Ø1- ☑
      - fetus to fetus O43.Ø2- ☑
      - maternofetal O43.Ø1- ☑
    - placentitis O41.14- ☑
    - pneumonia O99.51- ☑
    - poisoning — *see also* Table of Drugs and Chemicals O9A.21 ☑ (*following* O99)
    - polyhydramnios O4Ø- ☑
    - polymorphic eruption of pregnancy O26.86
    - poor obstetric history NEC O09.29- ☑
    - postmaturity (post-term) (4Ø to 42 weeks) O48.Ø
      - more than 42 completed weeks gestation (prolonged) O48.1
    - pre-eclampsia O14.9- ☑
      - mild O14.Ø- ☑
      - moderate O14.Ø- ☑
      - severe O14.1- ☑
        - with hemolysis, elevated liver enzymes and low platelet count (HELLP) O14.2- ☑
    - premature labor — *see* Pregnancy, complicated by, preterm labor
    - premature rupture of membranes O42.9Ø
      - with onset of labor
        - within 24 hours O42.ØØ
          - at or after 37 weeks gestation, onset of labor within 24 hours of rupture O42.Ø2
          - pre-term (before 37 completed weeks of gestation) O42.Ø1- ☑
        - after 24 hours O42.1Ø
          - at or after 37 weeks gestation, onset of labor more than 24 hours following rupture O42.12
          - pre-term (before 37 completed weeks of gestation) O42.11- ☑
      - at or after 37 weeks gestation, unspecified as to length of time between rupture and onset of labor O42.92
      - full-term, unspecified as to length of time between rupture and onset of labor O42.92
      - pre-term (before 37 completed weeks of gestation) O42.91- ☑
    - premature separation of placenta — *see also* Abruptio placentae O45.9- ☑
    - presentation, fetal — *see* Delivery, complicated by, malposition
    - preterm delivery O6Ø.1Ø ☑
    - preterm labor
      - with delivery O6Ø.1Ø ☑
        - preterm O6Ø.1Ø ☑
        - term O6Ø.2Ø ☑
      - second trimester
        - with term delivery O6Ø.22 ☑
        - without delivery O6Ø.Ø2
        - with preterm delivery
          - second trimester O6Ø.12 ☑
          - third trimester O6Ø.13 ☑
      - third trimester
        - with term delivery O6Ø.23 ☑
        - without delivery O6Ø.Ø3
        - with third trimester preterm delivery O6Ø.14 ☑
      - without delivery O6Ø.ØØ
        - second trimester O6Ø.Ø2
        - third trimester O6Ø.Ø3
    - previous history of — *see* Pregnancy, supervision of, high-risk
    - prolapse, uterus O34.52- ☑
    - proteinuria (gestational) — *see also* Proteinuria, gestational O12.1- ☑
      - with edema O12.2- ☑
    - pruritic urticarial papules and plaques of pregnancy (PUPPP) O26.86
    - pruritus (neurogenic) O26.89- ☑
    - psychosis or psychoneurosis (puerperal) F53.1
    - ptyalism O26.89- ☑
    - PUPPP (pruritic urticarial papules and plaques of pregnancy) O26.86
    - pyelitis O23.Ø- ☑
    - recurrent pregnancy loss O26.2- ☑
    - renal disease or failure NEC O26.83- ☑
      - with secondary hypertension, pre-existing — *see* Hypertension, complicating, pregnancy, pre-existing, secondary
      - hypertensive, pre-existing — *see* Hypertension, complicating, pregnancy, pre-existing, with, renal disease
    - respiratory condition (conditions in JØØ-J99) O99.51- ☑
    - retained, retention
      - dead ovum O02.Ø
      - intrauterine contraceptive device O26.3- ☑
    - retroversion, uterus O34.53- ☑
    - Rh immunization, incompatibility or sensitization NEC O36.Ø9- ☑
      - anti-D antibody O36.Ø1- ☑
    - rupture
      - amnion (premature) — *see also* Pregnancy, complicated by, premature rupture of membranes O42- ☑
      - membranes (premature) — *see also* Pregnancy, complicated by, premature rupture of membranes O42- ☑
      - uterus (during labor) O71.1
        - before onset of labor O71.Ø- ☑
    - salivation (excessive) O26.89- ☑
    - salpingitis O23.52- ☑
    - salpingo-oophoritis O23.52- ☑
    - sepsis (conditions in A4Ø, A41) O98.81- ☑
    - size date discrepancy (uterine) O26.84- ☑
    - skin condition (conditions in LØØ-L99) O99.71- ☑
    - smoking (tobacco) O99.33- ☑
    - social problem O09.7- ☑
    - specified condition NEC O26.89- ☑
    - spotting O26.85- ☑
    - streptococcus group B (GBS) carrier state O99.82Ø
    - subluxation of symphysis (pubis) O26.71- ☑
    - syphilis (conditions in A5Ø-A53) O98.11- ☑
    - threatened
      - abortion O2Ø.Ø
      - labor O47.9
        - at or after 37 completed weeks of gestation O47.1
        - before 37 completed weeks of gestation O47.Ø- ☑
    - thrombophlebitis (superficial) O22.2- ☑
    - thrombosis O22.9- ☑
      - cerebral venous O22.5- ☑
      - cerebrovenous sinus O22.5- ☑
      - deep O22.3- ☑
    - tobacco use disorder (smoking) O99.33- ☑
    - torsion of uterus O34.59- ☑
    - toxemia O14.9- ☑
    - transverse lie or presentation O32.2 ☑
    - tuberculosis (conditions in A15-A19) O98.Ø1- ☑
    - tumor (benign)
      - cervix O34.4- ☑
      - malignant O9A.11- ☑ (*following* O99)
      - uterus O34.1- ☑
    - unstable lie O32.Ø ☑
    - upper respiratory infection O99.51- ☑
    - urethritis O23.2- ☑
    - uterine size date discrepancy O26.84- ☑
    - vaginitis or vulvitis O23.59- ☑
    - varicose veins (lower extremities) O22.Ø- ☑
      - genitals O22.1- ☑
      - legs O22.Ø- ☑
      - perineal O22.1- ☑
      - vaginal or vulval O22.1- ☑
    - venereal disease NEC (conditions in A63.8) O98.31- ☑
    - venous disorders O22.9- ☑
      - specified NEC O22.8X- ☑
    - very young mother — *see* Pregnancy, complicated by, young mother
    - viral diseases (conditions in A8Ø-BØ9, B25-B34) O98.51- ☑
    - vomiting O21.9
      - due to diseases classified elsewhere O21.8
      - hyperemesis gravidarum (mild) — *see also* Hyperemesis, gravidarum O21.Ø
      - late (occurring after 2Ø weeks of gestation) O21.2
    - young mother
      - multigravida O09.62- ☑
      - primigravida O09.61- ☑
  - complicated NOS O26.9- ☑
  - concealed O09.3- ☑
  - continuing following
    - elective fetal reduction of one or more fetus O31.3- ☑
    - intrauterine death of one or more fetus O31.2- ☑
    - spontaneous abortion of one or more fetus O31.1- ☑
  - cornual OØØ.8Ø
    - with intrauterine pregnancy OØØ.81
  - ectopic (ruptured) OØØ.9Ø
    - with intrauterine pregnancy OØØ.91
    - abdominal OØØ.ØØ
      - with
        - intrauterine pregnancy OØØ.Ø1
        - viable fetus O36.7- ☑
    - cervical OØØ.8Ø
      - with intrauterine pregnancy OØØ.81
    - complicated (by) OØ8.9
      - afibrinogenemia OØ8.1
      - cardiac arrest OØ8.81
      - chemical damage of pelvic organ(s) OØ8.6
      - circulatory collapse OØ8.3
      - defibrination syndrome OØ8.1
      - electrolyte imbalance OØ8.5
      - embolism (amniotic fluid) (blood clot) (pulmonary) (septic) OØ8.2
      - endometritis OØ8.Ø
      - genital tract and pelvic infection OØ8.Ø
      - hemorrhage (delayed) (excessive) OØ8.1
      - infection
        - genital tract or pelvic OØ8.Ø
        - kidney OØ8.83
        - urinary tract OØ8.83
      - intravascular coagulation OØ8.1
      - laceration of pelvic organ(s) OØ8.6
      - metabolic disorder OØ8.5
      - oliguria OØ8.4
      - oophoritis OØ8.Ø
      - parametritis OØ8.Ø
      - pelvic peritonitis OØ8.Ø
      - perforation of pelvic organ(s) OØ8.6
      - renal failure or shutdown OØ8.4
      - salpingitis or salpingo-oophoritis OØ8.Ø
      - sepsis OØ8.82
      - shock OØ8.83
        - septic OØ8.82
      - specified condition NEC OØ8.89
      - tubular necrosis (renal) OØ8.4
      - uremia OØ8.4
      - urinary infection OØ8.83
      - venous complication NEC OØ8.7
        - embolism OØ8.2
    - cornual OØØ.8Ø
      - with intrauterine pregnancy OØØ.81
    - intraligamentous OØØ.8Ø
      - with intrauterine pregnancy OØØ.81
    - mural OØØ.8Ø
      - with intrauterine pregnancy OØØ.81
    - ovarian OØØ.2Ø- ☑
      - with intrauterine pregnancy OØØ.21- ☑
    - specified site NEC OØØ.8Ø
      - with intrauterine pregnancy OØØ.81
    - tubal (ruptured) OØØ.1Ø- ☑
      - with intrauterine pregnancy OØØ.11- ☑
  - examination (normal) Z34.9- ☑
    - first Z34.Ø- ☑
    - high-risk — *see* Pregnancy, supervision of, high-risk
    - specified Z34.8- ☑
  - extrauterine — *see* Pregnancy, ectopic
  - fallopian OØØ.1Ø- ☑
    - with intrauterine pregnancy OØØ.11- ☑
  - false F45.8
  - gestational carrier Z33.3
  - heptachorionic, hepta-amniotic (septuplets) O3Ø.83- ☑
  - hexachorionic, hexa-amniotic (sextuplets) O3Ø.83- ☑
  - hidden O09.3- ☑
  - high-risk — *see* Pregnancy, supervision of, high-risk
  - incidental finding Z33.1
  - interstitial OØØ.8Ø
    - with intrauterine pregnancy OØØ.81
  - intraligamentous OØØ.8Ø
    - with intrauterine pregnancy OØØ.81
  - intramural OØØ.8Ø
    - with intrauterine pregnancy OØØ.81
  - intraperitoneal OØØ.ØØ
    - with intrauterine pregnancy OØØ.Ø1

Pregnancy — *continued*
  isthmian OØØ.1Ø- ☑
    with intrauterine pregnancy OØØ.11- ☑
  mesometric (mural) OØØ.8Ø
    with intrauterine pregnancy OØØ.81
  molar NEC OØ2.Ø
    complicated (by) OØ8.9
      afibrinogenemia OØ8.1
      cardiac arrest OØ8.81
      chemical damage of pelvic organ(s) OØ8.6
      circulatory collapse OØ8.3
      defibrination syndrome OØ8.1
      electrolyte imbalance OØ8.5
      embolism (amniotic fluid) (blood clot) (pulmonary) (septic) OØ8.2
      endometritis OØ8.Ø
      genital tract and pelvic infection OØ8.Ø
      hemorrhage (delayed) (excessive) OØ8.1
      infection
        genital tract or pelvic OØ8.Ø
        kidney OØ8.83
        urinary tract OØ8.83
      intravascular coagulation OØ8.1
      laceration of pelvic organ(s) OØ8.6
      metabolic disorder OØ8.5
      oliguria OØ8.4
      oophoritis OØ8.Ø
      parametritis OØ8.Ø
      pelvic peritonitis OØ8.Ø
      perforation of pelvic organ(s) OØ8.6
      renal failure or shutdown OØ8.4
      salpingitis or salpingo-oophoritis OØ8.Ø
      sepsis OØ8.82
      shock OØ8.3
        septic OØ8.82
      specified condition NEC OØ8.89
      tubular necrosis (renal) OØ8.4
      uremia OØ8.4
      urinary infection OØ8.83
      venous complication NEC OØ8.7
        embolism OØ8.2
    hydatidiform — *see also* Mole, hydatidiform OØ1.9
  multiple (gestation) O3Ø.9- ☑
    greater than quadruplets — *see* Pregnancy, multiple (gestation), specified NEC
    specified NEC O3Ø.8Ø- ☑
      with
        two or more monoamniotic fetuses O3Ø.82- ☑
        two or more monochorionic fetuses O3Ø.81- ☑
      number of chorions and amnions are both equal to the number of fetuses O3Ø.83- ☑
      two or more monoamniotic fetuses O3Ø.82- ☑
      two or more monochorionic fetuses O3Ø.81- ☑
      unable to determine number of placenta and number of amniotic sacs O3Ø.89- ☑
      unspecified number of placenta and unspecified number of amniotic sacs O3Ø.8Ø- ☑
  mural OØØ.8Ø
    with intrauterine pregnancy OØØ.81
  normal (supervision of) Z34.9- ☑
    first Z34.Ø- ☑
    high-risk — *see* Pregnancy, supervision of, high-risk
    specified Z34.8- ☑
  ovarian OØØ.2Ø- ☑
    with intrauterine pregnancy OØØ.21- ☑
  pentachorionic, penta-amniotic (quintuplets) O3Ø.83- ☑
  postmature (4Ø to 42 weeks) O48.Ø
    more than 42 weeks gestation O48.1
  post-term (4Ø to 42 weeks) O48.Ø
  prenatal care only Z34.9- ☑
    first Z34.Ø- ☑
    high-risk — *see* Pregnancy, supervision of, high-risk
    specified Z34.8- ☑
  prolonged (more than 42 weeks gestation) O48.1
  quadruplet O3Ø.2Ø- ☑
    with
      two or more monoamniotic fetuses O3Ø.22- ☑
      two or more monochorionic fetuses O3Ø.21- ☑
    quadrachorionic/quadra-amniotic O3Ø.23- ☑
    two or more monoamniotic fetuses O3Ø.22- ☑
    two or more monochorionic fetuses O3Ø.21- ☑
    unable to determine number of placenta and number of amniotic sacs O3Ø.29- ☑
    unspecified number of placenta and unspecified number of amniotic sacs O3Ø.2Ø- ☑

Pregnancy — *continued*
  quintuplet — *see* Pregnancy, multiple (gestation), specified NEC
  sextuplet — *see* Pregnancy, multiple (gestation), specified NEC
  supervision of
    concealed pregnancy OØ9.3- ☑
    elderly mother
      multigravida OØ9.52- ☑
      primigravida OØ9.51- ☑
    hidden pregnancy OØ9.3- ☑
    high-risk OØ9.9- ☑
      due to (history of)
        ectopic pregnancy OØ9.1- ☑
        elderly — *see* Pregnancy, supervision, elderly mother
        grand multiparity OØ9.4 ☑
        in utero procedure during previous pregnancy OØ9.82- ☑
        in vitro fertilization OØ9.81- ☑
        infertility OØ9.Ø- ☑
        insufficient prenatal care OØ9.3- ☑
        molar pregnancy OØ9.A- ☑
        multiple previous pregnancies OØ9.4- ☑
        older mother — *see* Pregnancy, supervision of, elderly mother
        poor reproductive or obstetric history NEC OØ9.29- ☑
        pre-term labor OØ9.21- ☑
        previous
          neonatal death OØ9.29- ☑
        social problems OØ9.7- ☑
        specified NEC OØ9.89- ☑
        very young mother — *see* Pregnancy, supervision, young mother
      resulting from in vitro fertilization OØ9.81- ☑
    normal Z34.9- ☑
      first Z34.Ø- ☑
      specified NEC Z34.8- ☑
    young mother
      multigravida OØ9.62- ☑
      primigravida OØ9.61- ☑
  triplet O3Ø.1Ø- ☑
    with
      two or more monoamniotic fetuses O3Ø.12- ☑
      two or more monochorionic fetuses O3Ø.11- ☑
    trichorionic/triamniotic O3Ø.13- ☑
    two or more monoamniotic fetuses O3Ø.12- ☑
    two or more monochorionic fetuses O3Ø.11- ☑
    unable to determine number of placenta and number of amniotic sacs O3Ø.19- ☑
    unspecified number of placenta and unspecified number of amniotic sacs O3Ø.1Ø- ☑
  tubal (with abortion) (with rupture) OØØ.1Ø- ☑
    with intrauterine pregnancy OØØ.11- ☑
  twin O3Ø.ØØ- ☑
    conjoined O3Ø.Ø2- ☑
    dichorionic/diamniotic (two placenta, two amniotic sacs) O3Ø.Ø4- ☑
    monochorionic/diamniotic (one placenta, two amniotic sacs) O3Ø.Ø3- ☑
    monochorionic/monoamniotic (one placenta, one amniotic sac) O3Ø.Ø1- ☑
    unable to determine number of placenta and number of amniotic sacs O3Ø.Ø9- ☑
    unspecified number of placenta and unspecified number of amniotic sacs O3Ø.ØØ- ☑
  unwanted Z64.Ø
  weeks of gestation
    8 weeks Z3A.Ø8 (*following* Z36)
    9 weeks Z3A.Ø9 (*following* Z36)
    1Ø weeks Z3A.1Ø (*following* Z36)
    11 weeks Z3A.11 (*following* Z36)
    12 weeks Z3A.12 (*following* Z36)
    13 weeks Z3A.13 (*following* Z36)
    14 weeks Z3A.14 (*following* Z36)
    15 weeks Z3A.15 (*following* Z36)
    16 weeks Z3A.16 (*following* Z36)
    17 weeks Z3A.17 (*following* Z36)
    18 weeks Z3A.18 (*following* Z36)
    19 weeks Z3A.19 (*following* Z36)
    2Ø weeks Z3A.2Ø (*following* Z36)
    21 weeks Z3A.21 (*following* Z36)
    22 weeks Z3A.22 (*following* Z36)
    23 weeks Z3A.23 (*following* Z36)
    24 weeks Z3A.24 (*following* Z36)
    25 weeks Z3A.25 (*following* Z36)

Pregnancy — *continued*
  weeks of gestation — *continued*
    26 weeks Z3A.26 (*following* Z36)
    27 weeks Z3A.27 (*following* Z36)
    28 weeks Z3A.28 (*following* Z36)
    29 weeks Z3A.29 (*following* Z36)
    3Ø weeks Z3A.3Ø (*following* Z36)
    31 weeks Z3A.31 (*following* Z36)
    32 weeks Z3A.32 (*following* Z36)
    33 weeks Z3A.33 (*following* Z36)
    34 weeks Z3A.34 (*following* Z36)
    35 weeks Z3A.35 (*following* Z36)
    36 weeks Z3A.36 (*following* Z36)
    37 weeks Z3A.37 (*following* Z36)
    38 weeks Z3A.38 (*following* Z36)
    39 weeks Z3A.39 (*following* Z36)
    4Ø weeks Z3A.4Ø (*following* Z36)
    41 weeks Z3A.41 (*following* Z36)
    42 weeks Z3A.42 (*following* Z36)
    greater than 42 weeks Z3A.49 (*following* Z36)
    less than 8 weeks Z3A.Ø1 (*following* Z36)
    not specified Z3A.ØØ (*following* Z36)
Preiser's disease — *see* Osteonecrosis, secondary, due to, trauma, metacarpus
Pre-kwashiorkor — *see* Malnutrition, severe
Preleukemia (syndrome) D46.9
Preluxation, hip, congenital Q65.6
Premature — *see also* condition
  adrenarche E27.Ø
  aging E34.8
  beats I49.4Ø
    atrial I49.1
    auricular I49.1
    supraventricular I49.1
  birth NEC — *see* Preterm, newborn
  closure, foramen ovale Q21.8
  contraction
    atrial I49.1
    atrioventricular I49.2
    auricular I49.1
    auriculoventricular I49.49
    heart (extrasystole) I49.49
    junctional I49.2
    ventricular I49.3
  delivery — *see also* Pregnancy, complicated by, preterm labor O6Ø.1Ø ☑
  ejaculation F52.4
  infant NEC — *see* Preterm, newborn
    light-for-dates — *see* Light for dates
  labor — *see* Pregnancy, complicated by, preterm labor
  lungs P28.Ø
  menopause E28.319
    asymptomatic E28.319
    symptomatic E28.31Ø
  newborn
    extreme (less than 28 completed weeks) — *see* Immaturity, extreme
    less than 37 completed weeks — *see* Preterm, newborn
  puberty E3Ø.1
  rupture membranes or amnion — *see* Pregnancy, complicated by, premature rupture of membranes
  senility E34.8
  thelarche E3Ø.8
  ventricular systole I49.3
Prematurity NEC (less than 37 completed weeks) — *see* Preterm, newborn
  extreme (less than 28 completed weeks) — *see* Immaturity, extreme
Premenstrual
  dysphoric disorder (PMDD) F32.81
  tension (syndrome) N94.3
Premolarization, cuspids KØØ.2
Prenatal
  care, normal pregnancy — *see* Pregnancy, normal
  screening of mother — *see also* Encounter, antenatal screening Z36.9
  teeth KØØ.6
Preparatory care for subsequent treatment NEC
  for dialysis Z49.Ø1
    peritoneal Z49.Ø2
Prepartum — *see* condition
Preponderance, left or right ventricular I51.7
Prepuce — *see* condition
PRES (posterior reversible encephalopathy syndrome) I67.83
Presbycardia R54

- **Presbycusis, presbyacusia** H91.1- ☑
- **Presbyesophagus** K22.89
- **Presbyophrenia** FØ3 ☑
- **Presbyopia** H52.4
- **Prescription of contraceptives** (initial) Z3Ø.Ø19
  - barrier Z3Ø.Ø18
  - diaphragm Z3Ø.Ø18
  - emergency (postcoital) Z3Ø.Ø12
  - implantable subdermal Z3Ø.Ø17
  - injectable Z3Ø.Ø13
  - intrauterine contraceptive device Z3Ø.Ø14
  - pills Z3Ø.Ø11
  - postcoital (emergency) Z3Ø.Ø12
  - repeat Z3Ø.4Ø
    - barrier Z3Ø.49
    - diaphragm Z3Ø.49
    - implantable subdermal Z3Ø.46
    - injectable Z3Ø.42
    - pills Z3Ø.41
    - specified type NEC Z3Ø.49
    - transdermal patch hormonal Z3Ø.45
    - vaginal ring hormonal Z3Ø.44
  - specified type NEC Z3Ø.Ø18
    - transdermal patch hormonal Z3Ø.Ø16
    - vaginal ring hormonal Z3Ø.Ø15
- **Presence** (of)
  - ankle-joint implant (functional) (prosthesis) Z96.66- ☑
  - aortocoronary (bypass) graft Z95.1
  - arterial-venous shunt (dialysis) Z99.2
  - artificial
    - eye (globe) Z97.Ø
    - heart (fully implantable) (mechanical) Z95.812
      - valve Z95.2
    - larynx Z96.3
    - lens (intraocular) Z96.1
    - limb (complete) (partial) Z97.1- ☑
      - arm Z97.1- ☑
        - bilateral Z97.15
      - leg Z97.1- ☑
        - bilateral Z97.16
  - audiological implant (functional) Z96.29
  - bladder implant (functional) Z96.Ø
  - bone
    - conduction hearing device Z96.29
    - implant (functional) NEC Z96.7
    - joint (prosthesis) — *see* Presence, joint implant
  - cardiac
    - defibrillator (functional) (with synchronous cardiac pacemaker) Z95.81Ø
    - implant or graft Z95.9
      - specified type NEC Z95.818
    - pacemaker Z95.Ø
    - resynchronization therapy
      - defibrillator Z95.81Ø
      - pacemaker Z95.Ø
  - cardioverter-defibrillator (ICD) Z95.81Ø
  - cerebrospinal fluid drainage device Z98.2
  - cochlear implant (functional) Z96.21
  - contact lens (es) Z97.3
  - coronary artery graft or prosthesis Z95.5
  - CRT-D (cardiac resynchronization therapy defibrillator) Z95.81Ø
  - CRT-P (cardiac resynchronization therapy pacemaker) Z95.Ø
  - CSF shunt Z98.2
  - dental prosthesis device Z97.2
  - dentures Z97.2
  - device (external) NEC Z97.8
    - cardiac NEC Z95.818
    - heart assist Z95.811
    - implanted (functional) Z96.9
      - specified NEC Z96.89
    - prosthetic Z97.8
  - ear implant Z96.2Ø
    - cochlear implant Z96.21
    - myringotomy tube Z96.22
    - specified type NEC Z96.29
  - elbow-joint implant (functional) (prosthesis) Z96.62- ☑
  - endocrine implant (functional) NEC Z96.49
  - eustachian tube stent or device (functional) Z96.29
  - external hearing-aid or device Z97.4
  - finger-joint implant (functional) (prosthetic) Z96.69- ☑
  - functional implant Z96.9
    - specified NEC Z96.89
  - graft
    - cardiac NEC Z95.818
    - vascular NEC Z95.828
  - hearing-aid or device (external) Z97.4

- **Presence** — *continued*
  - hearing-aid or device — *continued*
    - implant (bone) (cochlear) (functional) Z96.21
  - heart assist device Z95.811
  - heart valve implant (functional) Z95.2
    - prosthetic Z95.2
    - specified type NEC Z95.4
    - xenogenic Z95.3
  - hip-joint implant (functional) (prosthesis) Z96.64- ☑
  - ICD (cardioverter-defibrillator) Z95.81Ø
  - implanted device (artificial) (functional) (prosthetic) Z96.9
    - automatic cardiac defibrillator (with synchronous cardiac pacemaker) Z95.81Ø
    - cardiac pacemaker Z95.Ø
    - cochlear Z96.21
    - dental Z96.5
    - heart Z95.812
    - heart valve Z95.2
      - prosthetic Z95.2
      - specified NEC Z95.4
      - xenogenic Z95.3
    - insulin pump Z96.41
    - intraocular lens Z96.1
    - joint Z96.6Ø
      - ankle Z96.66- ☑
      - elbow Z96.62- ☑
      - finger Z96.69- ☑
      - hip Z96.64- ☑
      - knee Z96.65- ☑
      - shoulder Z96.61- ☑
      - specified NEC Z96.698
      - wrist Z96.63- ☑
    - larynx Z96.3
    - myringotomy tube Z96.22
    - otological Z96.2Ø
      - cochlear Z96.21
      - eustachian stent Z96.29
      - myringotomy Z96.22
      - specified NEC Z96.29
      - stapes Z96.29
    - skin Z96.81
    - skull plate Z96.7
    - specified NEC Z96.89
    - urogenital Z96.Ø
  - insulin pump (functional) Z96.41
  - intestinal bypass or anastomosis Z98.Ø
  - intraocular lens (functional) Z96.1
  - intrauterine contraceptive device (IUD) Z97.5
  - intravascular implant (functional) (prosthetic) NEC Z95.9
    - coronary artery Z95.5
    - defibrillator (with synchronous cardiac pacemaker) Z95.81Ø
    - peripheral vessel (with angioplasty) Z95.82Ø
  - joint implant (prosthetic) (any) Z96.6Ø
    - ankle — *see* Presence, ankle joint implant
    - elbow — *see* Presence, elbow joint implant
    - finger — *see* Presence, finger joint implant
    - hip — *see* Presence, hip joint implant
    - knee — *see* Presence, knee joint implant
    - shoulder — *see* Presence, shoulder joint implant
    - specified joint NEC Z96.698
    - wrist — *see* Presence, wrist joint implant
  - knee-joint implant (functional) (prosthesis) Z96.65- ☑
  - laryngeal implant (functional) Z96.3
  - mandibular implant (dental) Z96.5
  - myringotomy tube(s) Z96.22
  - neurostimulator (brain) (gastric) (peripheral nerve) (sacral nerve) (spinal cord) (vagus nerve) Z96.82
  - orthopedic-joint implant (prosthetic) (any) — *see* Presence, joint implant
  - otological implant (functional) Z96.29
  - shoulder-joint implant (functional) (prosthesis) Z96.61- ☑
  - skull-plate implant Z96.7
  - spectacles Z97.3
  - stapes implant (functional) Z96.29
  - systemic lupus erythematosus [SLE] inhibitor D68.62
  - tendon implant (functional) (graft) Z96.7
  - tooth root(s) implant Z96.5
  - ureteral stent Z96.Ø
  - urethral stent Z96.Ø
  - urogenital implant (functional) Z96.Ø
  - vascular implant or device Z95.9
    - access port device Z95.828
    - specified type NEC Z95.828
  - wrist-joint implant (functional) (prosthesis) Z96.63- ☑

- **Presenile** — *see also* condition
  - dementia FØ3 ☑
  - premature aging E34.8
- **Presentation, fetal** — *see* Delivery, complicated by, malposition
- **Prespondylolisthesis** (congenital) Q76.2
- **Pressure**
  - area, skin — *see* Ulcer, pressure, by site
  - brachial plexus G54.Ø
  - brain G93.5
    - injury at birth NEC P11.1
  - cerebral — *see* Pressure, brain
  - chest RØ7.89
  - cone, tentorial G93.5
  - hyposystolic — *see also* Hypotension
    - incidental reading, without diagnosis of hypotension RØ3.1
  - increased
    - intracranial benign G93.2
      - injury at birth P11.Ø
    - intraocular H4Ø.Ø5- ☑
  - injury — *see* Ulcer, pressure, by site
  - lumbosacral plexus G54.1
  - mediastinum J98.59
  - necrosis (chronic) — *see* Ulcer, pressure, by site
  - parental, inappropriate (excessive) Z62.6
  - sore (chronic) — *see* Ulcer, pressure, by site
  - spinal cord G95.2Ø
  - ulcer (chronic) — *see* Ulcer, pressure, by site
  - venous, increased I87.8
- **Pre-syncope** R55
- **Preterm**
  - delivery — *see also* Pregnancy, complicated by, preterm labor O6Ø.1Ø ☑
  - labor — *see* Pregnancy, complicated by, preterm labor
  - newborn (infant) PØ7.3Ø
    - gestational age
      - 28 completed weeks (28 weeks, Ø days through 28 weeks, 6 days) PØ7.31
      - 29 completed weeks (29 weeks, Ø days through 29 weeks, 6 days) PØ7.32
      - 3Ø completed weeks (3Ø weeks, Ø days through 3Ø weeks, 6 days) PØ7.33
      - 31 completed weeks (31 weeks, Ø days through 31 weeks, 6 days) PØ7.34
      - 32 completed weeks (32 weeks, Ø days through 32 weeks, 6 days) PØ7.35
      - 33 completed weeks (33 weeks, Ø days through 33 weeks, 6 days) PØ7.36
      - 34 completed weeks (34 weeks, Ø days through 34 weeks, 6 days) PØ7.37
      - 35 completed weeks (35 weeks, Ø days through 35 weeks, 6 days) PØ7.38
      - 36 completed weeks (36 weeks, Ø days through 36 weeks, 6 days) PØ7.39
- **Previa**
  - placenta (total) (without hemorrhage) O44.Ø- ☑
    - with hemorrhage O44.1- ☑
    - complete O44.Ø- ☑
      - with hemorrhage O44.1- ☑
    - low — *see also* Delivery, complicated, by, placenta, low O44.4- ☑
      - with hemorrhage O44.5- ☑
    - marginal O44.2- ☑
      - with hemorrhage O44.3- ☑
    - partial O44.2- ☑
      - with hemorrhage O44.3- ☑
  - vasa O69.4 ☑
- **Priapism** N48.3Ø
  - due to
    - disease classified elsewhere N48.32
    - drug N48.33
    - specified cause NEC N48.39
    - trauma N48.31
- **Prickling sensation** (skin) R2Ø.2
- **Prickly heat** L74.Ø
- **Primary** — *see* condition
- **Primigravida**
  - elderly, affecting management of pregnancy, labor and delivery (supervision only) — *see* Pregnancy, complicated by, elderly, primigravida
  - older, affecting management of pregnancy, labor and delivery (supervision only) — *see* Pregnancy, complicated by, elderly, primigravida
  - very young, affecting management of pregnancy, labor and delivery (supervision only) — *see* Pregnancy, complicated by, young mother, primigravida

- **Primipara**
  - elderly, affecting management of pregnancy, labor and delivery (supervision only) — *see* Pregnancy, complicated by, elderly, primigravida
  - older, affecting management of pregnancy, labor and delivery (supervision only) — *see* Pregnancy, complicated by, elderly, primigravida
  - very young, affecting management of pregnancy, labor and delivery (supervision only) — *see* Pregnancy, complicated by, young mother, primigravida
- **Primus varus** Q66.21- ☑
- **PRIND** (Prolonged reversible ischemic neurologic deficit) I63.9
- **Pringle's disease** (tuberous sclerosis) Q85.1
- **Prinzmetal angina** I2Ø.1
- **Prizefighter ear** — *see* Cauliflower ear
- **Problem** (with) (related to)
  - academic Z55.8
  - acculturation Z6Ø.3
  - adjustment (to)
    - change of job Z56.1
    - life-cycle transition Z6Ø.Ø
    - pension Z6Ø.Ø
    - retirement Z6Ø.Ø
  - adopted child Z62.821
  - alcoholism in family Z63.72
  - atypical parenting situation Z62.9
  - bankruptcy Z59.89
  - behavioral (adult) F69
    - drug seeking Z76.5
  - birth of sibling affecting child Z62.898
  - care (of)
    - provider dependency Z74.9
      - specified NEC Z74.8
    - sick or handicapped person in family or household Z63.6
  - child
    - abuse (affecting the child) — *see* Maltreatment, child
    - custody or support proceedings Z65.3
    - in care of non-parental family member Z62.21
    - in foster care Z62.21
    - in welfare custody Z62.21
    - living in orphanage or group home Z62.22
  - child-rearing Z62.9
    - specified NEC Z62.898
  - communication (developmental) F8Ø.9
  - conflict or discord (with)
    - boss Z56.4
    - classmates Z55.4
    - counselor Z64.4
    - employer Z56.4
    - family Z63.9
      - specified NEC Z63.8
    - probation officer Z64.4
    - social worker Z64.4
    - teachers Z55.4
    - workmates Z56.4
  - conviction in legal proceedings Z65.Ø
    - with imprisonment Z65.1
  - counselor Z64.4
  - creditors Z59.89
  - digestive K92.9
  - drug addict in family Z63.72
  - ear — *see* Disorder, ear
  - economic Z59.9
    - affecting care Z59.9
    - specified NEC Z59.89
    - strain Z59.86
  - education Z55.9
    - specified NEC Z55.8
  - employment Z56.9
    - change of job Z56.1
    - discord Z56.4
    - environment Z56.5
    - sexual harassment Z56.81
    - specified NEC Z56.89
    - stressful schedule Z56.3
    - stress NEC Z56.6
    - threat of job loss Z56.2
    - unemployment Z56.Ø
  - enuresis, child F98.Ø
  - eye H57.9
  - failed examinations (school) Z55.2
  - falling Z91.81
  - family — *see also* Disruption, family Z63.9
    - specified NEC Z63.8
  - feeding (elderly) (infant) R63.39

- **Problem** — *continued*
  - feeding — *continued*
    - newborn P92.9
      - breast P92.5
      - overfeeding P92.4
      - slow P92.2
      - specified NEC P92.8
      - underfeeding P92.3
    - nonorganic F5Ø.89
  - finance Z59.9
    - specified NEC Z59.89
  - foreclosure on loan Z59.89
  - foster child Z62.822
  - frightening experience(s) in childhood Z62.898
  - genital NEC
    - female N94.9
    - male N5Ø.9
  - health care Z75.9
    - specified NEC Z75.8
  - hearing — *see* Deafness
  - homelessness Z59.ØØ
  - housing Z59.9
    - inadequate Z59.1
    - isolated Z59.89
    - specified NEC Z59.89
  - identity (of childhood) F93.8
  - illegitimate pregnancy (unwanted) Z64.Ø
  - illiteracy Z55.Ø
  - impaired mobility Z74.Ø9
  - imprisonment or incarceration Z65.1
  - inadequate teaching affecting education Z55.8
  - inappropriate (excessive) parental pressure Z62.6
  - influencing health status NEC Z78.9
  - in-law Z63.1
  - institutionalization, affecting child Z62.22
  - intrafamilial communication Z63.8
  - jealousy, child F93.8
  - landlord Z59.2
  - language (developmental) F8Ø.9
  - learning (developmental) F81.9
  - legal Z65.3
    - conviction without imprisonment Z65.Ø
    - imprisonment Z65.1
    - release from prison Z65.2
  - life-management Z73.9
    - specified NEC Z73.89
  - life-style Z72.9
    - gambling Z72.6
    - high-risk sexual behavior (heterosexual) Z72.51
      - bisexual Z72.53
      - homosexual Z72.52
    - inappropriate eating habits Z72.4
    - self-damaging behavior NEC Z72.89
    - specified NEC Z72.89
    - tobacco use Z72.Ø
  - literacy Z55.9
    - low level Z55.Ø
    - specified NEC Z55.8
  - living alone Z6Ø.2
  - lodgers Z59.2
  - loss of love relationship in childhood Z62.898
  - marital Z63.Ø
    - involving
      - divorce Z63.5
      - estrangement Z63.5
      - gender identity F66
  - mastication KØ8.89
  - medical
    - care, within family Z63.6
    - facilities Z75.9
      - specified NEC Z75.8
  - mental F48.9
  - money Z59.86
  - multiparity Z64.1
  - negative life events in childhood Z62.9
    - altered pattern of family relationships Z62.898
    - frightening experience Z62.898
    - loss of
      - love relationship Z62.898
      - self-esteem Z62.898
    - physical abuse (alleged) — *see* Maltreatment, child
    - removal from home Z62.29
    - specified event NEC Z62.898
  - neighbor Z59.2
  - neurological NEC R29.818
  - new step-parent affecting child Z62.898
  - none (feared complaint unfounded) Z71.1
  - occupational NEC Z56.89
  - parent-child — *see* Conflict, parent-child

- **Problem** — *continued*
  - personal hygiene Z91.89
  - personality F69
  - phase-of-life transition, adjustment Z6Ø.Ø
  - presence of sick or disabled person in family or household Z63.79
    - needing care Z63.6
  - primary support group (family) Z63.9
    - specified NEC Z63.8
  - probation officer Z64.4
  - psychiatric F99
  - psychosexual (development) F66
  - psychosocial Z65.9
    - religious or spiritual Z65.8
    - specified NEC Z65.8
  - relationship Z63.9
    - childhood F93.8
  - release from prison Z65.2
    - religious or spiritual Z65.8
  - removal from home affecting child Z62.29
  - seeking and accepting known hazardous and harmful
    - behavioral or psychological interventions Z65.8
    - chemical, nutritional or physical interventions Z65.8
  - sexual function (nonorganic) F52.9
  - sight H54.7
  - sleep disorder, child F51.9
  - smell — *see* Disturbance, sensation, smell
  - social
    - environment Z6Ø.9
      - specified NEC Z6Ø.8
    - exclusion and rejection Z6Ø.4
    - worker Z64.4
  - speech R47.9
    - developmental F8Ø.9
    - specified NEC R47.89
  - swallowing — *see* Dysphagia
  - taste — *see* Disturbance, sensation, taste
  - tic, child F95.Ø
  - underachievement in school Z55.3
  - unemployment Z56.Ø
    - threatened Z56.2
  - unwanted pregnancy Z64.Ø
  - upbringing Z62.9
    - specified NEC Z62.898
  - urinary N39.9
  - voice production R47.89
  - work schedule (stressful) Z56.3
- **Procedure** (surgical)
  - converted
    - arthroscopic to open Z53.33
    - laparoscopic to open Z53.31
    - specified procedure NEC to open Z53.39
    - thoracoscopic to open Z53.32
  - for purpose other than remedying health state Z41.9
    - specified NEC Z41.8
  - not done Z53.9
    - because of
      - administrative reasons Z53.8
      - contraindication Z53.Ø9
        - smoking Z53.Ø1
      - patient's decision Z53.2Ø
        - for reasons of belief or group pressure Z53.1
        - left against medical advice (AMA) Z53.29
        - left without being seen Z53.21
        - specified reason NEC Z53.29
      - specified reason NEC Z53.8
- **Procidentia** (uteri) N81.3
- **Proctalgia** K62.89
  - fugax K59.4
  - spasmodic K59.4
- **Proctitis** K62.89
  - amebic (acute) AØ6.Ø
  - chlamydial A56.3
  - gonococcal A54.6
  - granulomatous — *see* Enteritis, regional, large intestine
  - herpetic A6Ø.1
  - radiation K62.7
  - tuberculous A18.32
  - ulcerative (chronic) K51.2Ø
    - with
      - complication K51.219
        - abscess K51.214
        - fistula K51.213
        - obstruction K51.212
        - rectal bleeding K51.211
        - specified NEC K51.218
- **Proctocele**
  - female (without uterine prolapse) N81.6

- **Proctocele** — *continued*
  - female — *continued*
    - with uterine prolapse N81.2
      - complete N81.3
  - male K62.3
- **Proctocolitis**
  - allergic K52.29
  - food protein-induced K52.29
  - food-induced eosinophilic K52.29
  - milk protein-induced K52.29
  - mucosal — *see* Rectosigmoiditis, ulcerative
- **Proctoptosis** K62.3
- **Proctorrhagia** K62.5
- **Proctosigmoiditis** K63.89
  - ulcerative (chronic) — *see* Rectosigmoiditis, ulcerative
- **Proctospasm** K59.4
  - psychogenic F45.8
- **Profichet's disease** — *see* Disorder, soft tissue, specified type NEC
- **Progeria** E34.8
- **Prognathism** (mandibular) (maxillary) M26.19
- **Progonoma** (melanotic) — *see* Neoplasm, benign, by site
- **Progressive** — *see* condition
- **Prolactinoma**
  - specified site — *see* Neoplasm, benign, by site
  - unspecified site D35.2
- **Prolapse, prolapsed**
  - anus, anal (canal) (sphincter) K62.2
  - arm or hand O32.2 ☑
    - causing obstructed labor O64.4 ☑
  - bladder (mucosa) (sphincter) (acquired)
    - congenital Q79.4
    - female — *see* Cystocele
    - male N32.89
  - breast implant (prosthetic) T85.49 ☑
  - cecostomy K94.Ø9
  - cecum K63.4
  - cervix, cervical (hypertrophied) N81.2
    - anterior lip, obstructing labor O65.5
    - congenital Q51.828
    - postpartal, old N81.2
    - stump N81.85
  - ciliary body (traumatic) — *see* Laceration, eye(ball), with prolapse or loss of interocular tissue
  - colon (pedunculated) K63.4
  - colostomy K94.Ø9
  - disc (intervertebral) — *see* Displacement, intervertebral disc
  - eye implant (orbital) T85.398 ☑
    - lens (ocular) — *see* Complications, intraocular lens
  - fallopian tube N83.4- ☑
  - gastric (mucosa) K31.89
  - genital, female N81.9
    - specified NEC N81.89
  - globe, nontraumatic — *see* Luxation, globe
  - ileostomy bud K94.19
  - intervertebral disc — *see* Displacement, intervertebral disc
  - intestine (small) K63.4
  - iris (traumatic) — *see* Laceration, eye(ball), with prolapse or loss of interocular tissue
    - nontraumatic H21.89
  - kidney N28.83
    - congenital Q63.2
  - laryngeal muscles or ventricle J38.7
  - liver K76.89
  - meatus urinarius N36.8
  - mitral (valve) I34.1
  - ocular lens implant — *see* Complications, intraocular lens
  - organ or site, congenital NEC — *see* Malposition, congenital
  - ovary N83.4- ☑
  - pelvic floor, female N81.89
  - perineum, female N81.89
  - rectum (mucosa) (sphincter) K62.3
    - due to trichuris trichuria B79
  - spleen D73.89
  - stomach K31.89
  - umbilical cord
    - complicating delivery O69.Ø ☑
  - urachus, congenital Q64.4
  - ureter N28.89
    - with obstruction N13.5
      - with infection N13.6
  - ureterovesical orifice N28.89
  - urethra (acquired) (infected) (mucosa) N36.8
- **Prolapse, prolapsed** — *continued*
  - urethra — *continued*
    - congenital Q64.71
  - urinary meatus N36.8
    - congenital Q64.72
  - uterovaginal N81.4
    - complete N81.3
    - incomplete N81.2
  - uterus (with prolapse of vagina) N81.4
    - complete N81.3
    - congenital Q51.818
    - first degree N81.2
    - in pregnancy or childbirth — *see* Pregnancy, complicated by, abnormal, uterus
    - incomplete N81.2
    - postpartal (old) N81.4
    - second degree N81.2
    - third degree N81.3
  - uveal (traumatic) — *see* Laceration, eye(ball), with prolapse or loss of interocular tissue
  - vagina (anterior) (wall) — *see* Cystocele
    - with prolapse of uterus N81.4
      - complete N81.3
      - incomplete N81.2
    - posterior wall N81.6
    - posthysterectomy N99.3
  - vitreous (humor) H43.Ø- ☑
    - in wound — *see* Laceration, eye(ball), with prolapse or loss of interocular tissue
  - womb — *see* Prolapse, uterus
- **Prolapsus, female** N81.9
  - specified NEC N81.89
- **Proliferation(s)**
  - primary cutaneous CD3Ø-positive large T-cell C86.6
  - prostate, atypical small acinar N42.32
- **Proliferative** — *see* condition
- **Prolonged, prolongation** (of)
  - bleeding (time) (idiopathic) R79.1
  - coagulation (time) R79.1
  - gestation (over 42 completed weeks)
    - mother O48.1
    - newborn PØ8.22
  - interval I44.Ø
  - labor O63.9
    - first stage O63.Ø
    - second stage O63.1
  - partial thromboplastin time (PTT) R79.1
  - pregnancy (more than 42 weeks gestation) O48.1
  - prothrombin time R79.1
  - QT interval R94.31
  - uterine contractions in labor O62.4
- **Prominence, prominent**
  - auricle (congenital) (ear) Q17.5
  - ischial spine or sacral promontory with disproportion (fetopelvic) O33.Ø
    - causing obstructed labor O65.Ø
  - nose (congenital) acquired M95.Ø
- **Promiscuity** — *see* High, risk, sexual behavior
- **Pronation**
  - ankle — *see* Deformity, limb, foot, specified NEC
  - foot — *see also* Deformity, limb, foot, specified NEC
    - congenital Q74.2
- **Prophylactic**
  - administration of
    - antibiotics, long-term Z79.2
      - short-term use — *omit code*
    - drug — *see also* Long-term (current) drug therapy (use of) Z79.899
  - medication Z79.899
  - organ removal (for neoplasia management) Z4Ø.ØØ
    - breast Z4Ø.Ø1
    - fallopian tube(s) Z4Ø.Ø3
      - with ovary(s) Z4Ø.Ø2
    - ovary(s) Z4Ø.Ø2
    - specified site NEC Z4Ø.Ø9
  - surgery Z4Ø.9
    - for risk factors related to malignant neoplasm — *see* Prophylactic, organ removal
    - specified NEC Z4Ø.8
  - vaccination Z23
- **Propionic acidemia** E71.121
- **Proptosis** (ocular) — *see also* Exophthalmos
  - thyroid — *see* Hyperthyroidism, with goiter
- **Prosecution, anxiety concerning** Z65.3
- **Prosopagnosia** R48.3
- **Prostadynia** N42.81
- **Prostate, prostatic** — *see* condition
- **Prostatism** — *see* Hyperplasia, prostate
- **Prostatitis** (congestive) (suppurative) (with cystitis) N41.9
  - acute N41.Ø
  - cavitary N41.8
  - chronic N41.1
  - diverticular N41.8
  - due to Trichomonas (vaginalis) A59.Ø2
  - fibrous N41.1
  - gonococcal (acute) (chronic) A54.22
  - granulomatous N41.4
  - hypertrophic N41.1
  - subacute N41.1
  - trichomonal A59.Ø2
  - tuberculous A18.14
- **Prostatocystitis** N41.3
- **Prostatorrhea** N42.89
- **Prostatosis** N42.82
- **Prostration** R53.83
  - heat — *see also* Heat, exhaustion
    - anhydrotic T67.3 ☑
    - due to
      - salt (and water) depletion T67.4 ☑
      - water depletion T67.3 ☑
  - nervous F48.8
  - senile R54
- **Protanomaly** (anomalous trichromat) H53.54
- **Protanopia** (complete) (incomplete) H53.54
- **Protection** (against) (from) — *see* Prophylactic
- **Protein**
  - deficiency NEC — *see* Malnutrition
  - malnutrition — *see* Malnutrition
  - sickness — *see also* Reaction, serum T8Ø.69 ☑
- **Proteinemia** R77.9
- **Proteinosis**
  - alveolar (pulmonary) J84.Ø1
  - lipid or lipoid (of Urbach) E78.89
- **Proteinuria** R8Ø.9
  - Bence Jones R8Ø.3
  - complicating pregnancy — *see* Proteinuria, gestational
  - gestational
    - complicating
      - childbirth O12.14
      - pregnancy O12.1- ☑
        - with edema O12.2- ☑
      - puerperium O12.15
  - idiopathic R8Ø.Ø
  - isolated R8Ø.Ø
    - with glomerular lesion NØ6.9
      - C3
        - glomerulonephritis NØ6.A
        - glomerulopathy NØ6.A
          - with dense deposit disease NØ6.6
      - dense deposit disease NØ6.6
      - diffuse
        - crescentic glomerulonephritis NØ6.7
        - endocapillary proliferative glomerulonephritis NØ6.4
        - mesangiocapillary glomerulonephritis NØ6.5
      - focal and segmental hyalinosis or sclerosis NØ6.1
      - membranous (diffuse) NØ6.2
      - mesangial proliferative (diffuse) NØ6.3
      - minimal change NØ6.Ø
      - specified pathology NEC NØ6.8
  - orthostatic R8Ø.2
    - with glomerular lesion — *see* Proteinuria, isolated, with glomerular lesion
  - persistent R8Ø.1
    - with glomerular lesion — *see* Proteinuria, isolated, with glomerular lesion
  - postural R8Ø.2
    - with glomerular lesion — *see* Proteinuria, isolated, with glomerular lesion
  - pre-eclamptic — *see* Pre-eclampsia
  - puerperal O12.15
  - specified type NEC R8Ø.8
- **Proteolysis, pathologic** D65
- **Proteus** (mirabilis) (morganii), **as cause of disease classified elsewhere** B96.4
- **Prothrombin gene mutation** D68.52
- **Protoporphyria, erythropoietic** E8Ø.Ø
- **Protozoal** — *see also* condition
  - disease B64
    - specified NEC B6Ø.8
- **Protrusion, protrusio**
  - acetabuli M24.7
  - acetabulum (into pelvis) M24.7
  - device, implant or graft — *see also* Complications, by site and type, mechanical T85.698 ☑

Protrusion, protrusio — *continued*
device, implant or graft — *see also* Complications, by site and type, mechanical — *continued*
arterial graft NEC — *see* Complication, cardiovascular device, mechanical, vascular
breast (implant) T85.49 ☑
catheter NEC T85.698 ☑
cystostomy T83.090 ☑
dialysis (renal) T82.49 ☑
intraperitoneal T85.691 ☑
infusion NEC T82.594 ☑
spinal (epidural) (subdural) T85.690 ☑
urinary — *see also* Complications, catheter, urinary T83.098 ☑
electronic (electrode) (pulse generator) (stimulator) bone T84.390 ☑
nervous system — *see* Complication, prosthetic device, mechanical, electronic nervous system stimulator
fixation, internal (orthopedic) NEC — *see* Complication, fixation device, mechanical
gastrointestinal — *see* Complications, prosthetic device, mechanical, gastrointestinal device
genital NEC T83.498 ☑
intrauterine contraceptive device T83.39 ☑
penile prosthesis (cylinder) (implanted) (pump) (resevoir) T83.490 ☑
testicular prosthesis T83.491 ☑
heart NEC — *see* Complication, cardiovascular device, mechanical
joint prosthesis — *see* Complications, joint prosthesis, mechanical, specified NEC, by site
ocular NEC — *see* Complications, prosthetic device, mechanical, ocular device
orthopedic NEC — *see* Complication, orthopedic, device, mechanical
specified NEC T85.628 ☑
urinary NEC — *see also* Complication, genitourinary, device, urinary, mechanical
graft T83.29 ☑
vascular NEC — *see* Complication, cardiovascular device, mechanical
ventricular intracranial shunt T85.09 ☑
intervertebral disc — *see* Displacement, intervertebral disc
joint prosthesis — *see* Complications, joint prosthesis, mechanical, specified NEC, by site
nucleus pulposus — *see* Displacement, intervertebral disc
Prune belly (syndrome) Q79.4
Prurigo (ferox) (gravis) (Hebrae) (Hebra's) (mitis) (simplex) L28.2
Besnier's L20.0
estivalis L56.4
nodularis L28.1
psychogenic F45.8
Pruritus, pruritic (essential) L29.9
ani, anus L29.0
psychogenic F45.8
anogenital L29.3
psychogenic F45.8
due to onchocerca volvulus B73.1
gravidarum — *see* Pregnancy, complicated by, specified pregnancy-related condition NEC
hiemalis L29.8
neurogenic (any site) F45.8
perianal L29.0
psychogenic (any site) F45.8
scroti, scrotum L29.1
psychogenic F45.8
senile, senilis L29.8
specified NEC L29.8
psychogenic F45.8
Trichomonas A59.9
vulva, vulvae L29.2
psychogenic F45.8
Pseudarthrosis, pseudoarthrosis (bone) — *see* Nonunion, fracture
clavicle, congenital Q74.0
joint, following fusion or arthrodesis M96.0
Pseudoaneurysm — *see* Aneurysm
Pseudoangina (pectoris) — *see* Angina
Pseudoangioma I81
Pseudoarteriosus Q28.8
Pseudoarthrosis — *see* Pseudarthrosis
Pseudobulbar affect (PBA) F48.2
Pseudochromhidrosis L67.8
Pseudocirrhosis, liver, pericardial I31.1
Pseudocowpox B08.03
Pseudocoxalgia M91.3- ☑
Pseudocroup J38.5
Pseudo-Cushing's syndrome, alcohol-induced E24.4
Pseudocyesis F45.8
Pseudocyst
lung J98.4
pancreas K86.3
retina — *see* Cyst, retina
Pseudoelephantiasis neuroarthritica Q82.0
Pseudoexfoliation, capsule (lens) — *see* Cataract, specified NEC
Pseudofolliculitis barbae L73.1
Pseudoglioma H44.89
Pseudohemophilia (Bernuth's) (hereditary) (type B) — *see* Disease, von Willebrand
Type A D69.8
vascular D69.8
Pseudohermaphroditism Q56.3
adrenal E25.8
female — *see also* Disorder, adrenogenital Q56.2
with adrenocortical disorder E25.8
without adrenocortical disorder Q56.2
adrenal (congenital) E25.0
male — *see also* Disorder, adrenogenital Q56.1
with
5-alpha-reductase deficiency E29.1
adrenocortical disorder E25.8
androgen resistance E34.51
cleft scrotum Q56.1
feminizing testis E34.51
without gonadal disorder Q56.1
adrenal E25.8
Pseudo-Hurler's polydystrophy E77.0
Pseudohydrocephalus G93.2
Pseudohypertrophic muscular dystrophy (Erb's) G71.02
Pseudohypertrophy, muscle — *see also* Dystrophy, muscular, by type, if applicable G71.09
Pseudohypoparathyroidism E20.1
Pseudoinsomnia F51.03
Pseudoleukemia, infantile D64.89
Pseudomembranous — *see* condition
Pseudomeningocele (cerebral) (infective) (post-traumatic) G96.198
postprocedural (spinal) G97.82
Pseudomenses (newborn) P54.6
Pseudomenstruation (newborn) P54.6
Pseudomonas
aeruginosa, as cause of disease classified elsewhere B96.5
mallei infection A24.0
as cause of disease classified elsewhere B96.5
pseudomallei, as cause of disease classified elsewhere B96.5
Pseudomyotonia G71.19
Pseudomyxoma peritonei C78.6
Pseudoneuritis, optic (nerve) (disc) (papilla), **congenital** Q14.2
Pseudo-obstruction intestine (acute) (chronic) (idiopathic) (intermittent secondary) (primary) K59.89
colonic K59.81
Pseudopapilledema H47.33- ☑
congenital Q14.2
Pseudoparalysis
arm or leg R29.818
atonic, congenital P94.2
Pseudopelade L66.0
Pseudophakia Z96.1
Pseudopolyarthritis, rhizomelic M35.3
Pseudopolycythemia D75.1
Pseudopseudohypoparathyroidism E20.1
Pseudopterygium H11.81- ☑
Pseudoptosis (eyelid) — *see* Blepharochalasis
Pseudopuberty, precocious
female heterosexual E25.8
male isosexual E25.8
Pseudorickets (renal) N25.0
Pseudorubella B08.20
Pseudosclerema, newborn P83.88
Pseudosclerosis (brain)
Jakob's — *see* Creutzfeldt-Jakob disease or syndrome
of Westphal (Strümpell) E83.01
spastic — *see* Creutzfeldt-Jakob disease or syndrome
Pseudotetanus — *see* Convulsions
Pseudotetany R29.0
Pseudotetany — *continued*
hysterical F44.5
Pseudotruncus arteriosus Q25.49
Pseudotuberculosis A28.2
enterocolitis A04.8
pasteurella (infection) A28.0
Pseudotumor G93.2
cerebri G93.2
orbital H05.11 ☑
Pseudoxanthoma elasticum Q82.8
Psilosis (sprue) (tropical) K90.1
nontropical K90.0
Psittacosis A70
Psoitis M60.88
Psoriasis L40.9
arthropathic L40.50
arthritis mutilans L40.52
distal interphalangeal L40.51
juvenile L40.54
other specified L40.59
spondylitis L40.53
buccal K13.29
flexural L40.8
guttate L40.4
mouth K13.29
nummular L40.0
plaque L40.0
psychogenic F54
pustular (generalized) L40.1
palmaris et plantaris L40.3
specified NEC L40.8
vulgaris L40.0
Psychasthenia F48.8
Psychiatric disorder or problem F99
Psychogenic — *see also* condition
factors associated with physical conditions F54
Psychological and behavioral factors affecting medical condition F59
Psychoneurosis, psychoneurotic — *see also* Neurosis
anxiety (state) F41.1
depersonalization F48.1
hypochondriacal F45.21
hysteria F44.9
neurasthenic F48.8
personality NEC F60.89
Psychopathy, psychopathic
affectionless F94.2
autistic F84.5
constitution, post-traumatic F07.81
personality — *see* Disorder, personality
sexual — *see* Deviation, sexual
state F60.2
Psychosexual identity disorder of childhood F64.2
Psychosis, psychotic F29
acute (transient) F23
hysterical F44.9
affective — *see* Disorder, mood
alcoholic F10.959
with
abuse F10.159
anxiety disorder F10.980
with
abuse F10.180
dependence F10.280
delirium tremens F10.231
delusions F10.950
with
abuse F10.150
dependence F10.250
dementia F10.97
with dependence F10.27
dependence F10.259
hallucinosis F10.951
with
abuse F10.151
dependence F10.251
mood disorder F10.94
with
abuse F10.14
dependence F10.24
paranoia F10.950
with
abuse F10.150
dependence F10.250
persisting amnesia F10.96
with dependence F10.26
amnestic confabulatory F10.96
with dependence F10.26

Psychosis, psychotic — *continued*
- alcoholic — *continued*
  - delirium tremens F1Ø.231
  - Korsakoff's, Korsakov's, Korsakow's F1Ø.26
  - paranoid type F1Ø.95Ø
  - with
    - abuse F1Ø.15Ø
    - dependence F1Ø.25Ø
- anergastic — *see* Psychosis, organic
- arteriosclerotic (simple type) (uncomplicated) — *see also* Dementia, vascular FØ1.5Ø
  - with behavioral disturbance — *see* Dementia, vascular
- childhood F84.Ø
  - atypical F84.8
- climacteric — *see* Psychosis, involutional
- confusional F29
  - acute or subacute FØ5
  - reactive F23
- cycloid F23
- depressive — *see* Disorder, depressive
- disintegrative (childhood) F84.3
- drug-induced — *see* F11-F19 with .X59
  - paranoid and hallucinatory states — *see* F11-F19 with .X5Ø or .X51
- due to or associated with
  - addiction, drug — *see* F11-F19 with .X59
  - dependence
    - alcohol F1Ø.259
    - drug — *see* F11-F19 with .X59
  - epilepsy FØ6.8
  - Huntington's chorea FØ6.8
  - ischemia, cerebrovascular (generalized) FØ6.8
  - multiple sclerosis FØ6.8
  - physical disease FØ6.8
  - presenile dementia FØ3 ☑
  - senile dementia FØ3 ☑
  - vascular disease (arteriosclerotic) (cerebral) — *see also* Dementia, vascular FØ1.5Ø
    - with behavioral disturbance — *see* Dementia, vascular
- epileptic FØ6.8
- episode F23
  - due to or associated with physical condition FØ6.8
- exhaustive F43.Ø
- hallucinatory, chronic F28
- hypomanic F3Ø.8
- hysterical (acute) F44.9
- induced F24
- infantile F84.Ø
  - atypical F84.8
- infective (acute) (subacute) FØ5
- involutional F28
  - depressive — *see* Disorder, depressive
  - melancholic — *see* Disorder, depressive
  - paranoid (state) F22
- Korsakoff's, Korsakov's, Korsakow's (nonalcoholic) FØ4
  - alcoholic F1Ø.96
    - in dependence F1Ø.26
  - induced by other psychoactive substance — *see* categories F11-F19 with .X5X
- mania, manic (single episode) F3Ø.2
  - recurrent type F31.89
- manic-depressive — *see* Disorder, bipolar
- menopausal — *see* Psychosis, involutional
- mixed schizophrenic and affective F25.8
- multi-infarct (cerebrovascular) — *see also* Dementia, vascular FØ1.5Ø
  - with behavioral disturbance — *see* Dementia, vascular
- nonorganic F29
  - specified NEC F28
- organic FØ9
  - due to or associated with
    - arteriosclerosis (cerebral) — *see* Psychosis, arteriosclerotic
    - cerebrovascular disease, arteriosclerotic — *see* Psychosis, arteriosclerotic
    - childbirth — *see* Psychosis, puerperal
    - Creutzfeldt-Jakob disease or syndrome — *see* Creutzfeldt-Jakob disease or syndrome
    - dependence, alcohol F1Ø.259
    - disease
      - alcoholic liver F1Ø.259
      - brain, arteriosclerotic — *see* Psychosis, arteriosclerotic
      - cerebrovascular — *see also* Dementia, vascular FØ1.5Ø

Psychosis, psychotic — *continued*
- organic — *continued*
  - due to or associated with — *continued*
    - disease — *continued*
      - cerebrovascular — *see also* Dementia, vascular — *continued*
        - with behavioral disturbance — *see* Dementia, vascular
      - Creutzfeldt-Jakob — *see* Creutzfeldt-Jakob disease or syndrome
      - endocrine or metabolic FØ6.8
        - acute or subacute FØ5
      - liver, alcoholic F1Ø.259
    - epilepsy transient (acute) FØ5
    - infection
      - brain (intracranial) FØ6.8
        - acute or subacute FØ5
    - intoxication
      - alcoholic (acute) F1Ø.259
      - drug F11-F19 with .x59
    - ischemia, cerebrovascular (generalized) — *see* Psychosis, arteriosclerotic
    - puerperium — *see* Psychosis, puerperal
    - trauma, brain (birth) (from electric current) (surgical) FØ6.8
      - acute or subacute FØ5
  - infective FØ6.8
    - acute or subacute FØ5
  - post-traumatic FØ6.8
    - acute or subacute FØ5
- paranoiac F22
- paranoid (climacteric) (involutional) (menopausal) F22
  - psychogenic (acute) F23
  - schizophrenic F2Ø.Ø
  - senile FØ3 ☑
- postpartum (NOS) F53.1
- presbyophrenic (type) FØ3 ☑
- presenile FØ3 ☑
- psychogenic (paranoid) F23
  - depressive F32.3
- puerperal (NOS) F53.1
  - specified type — *see* Psychosis, by type
- reactive (brief) (transient) (emotional stress) (psychological trauma) F23
  - depressive F32.3
    - recurrent F33.3
  - excitative type F3Ø.8
- schizoaffective F25.9
  - depressive type F25.1
  - manic type F25.Ø
- schizophrenia, schizophrenic — *see* Schizophrenia
- schizophrenia-like, in epilepsy FØ6.2
- schizophreniform F2Ø.81
  - affective type F25.9
  - brief F23
  - confusional type F23
  - mixed type F25.Ø
- senile NEC FØ3 ☑
  - depressed or paranoid type FØ3 ☑
  - simple deterioration FØ3 ☑
  - specified type — *code to* condition
- shared F24
- situational (reactive) F23
- symbiotic (childhood) F84.3
- symptomatic FØ9

Psychosomatic — *see* Disorder, psychosomatic

Psychosyndrome, organic FØ7.9

Psychotic episode due to or associated with physical condition FØ6.8

Pterygium (eye) H11.ØØ- ☑
- amyloid H11.Ø1- ☑
- central H11.Ø2- ☑
- colli Q18.3
- double H11.Ø3- ☑
- peripheral
  - progressive H11.Ø5- ☑
  - stationary H11.Ø4- ☑
- recurrent H11.Ø6- ☑

Ptilosis (eyelid) — *see* Madarosis

Ptomaine (poisoning) — *see* Poisoning, food

Ptosis — *see also* Blepharoptosis
- adiposa (false) — *see* Blepharoptosis
- breast N64.81-
- brow H57.81- ☑
- cecum K63.4
- colon K63.4
- congenital (eyelid) Q1Ø.Ø
  - specified site NEC — *see* Anomaly, by site

Ptosis — *continued*
- eyebrow H57.81- ☑
- eyelid — *see* Blepharoptosis
  - congenital Q1Ø.Ø
- gastric K31.89
- intestine K63.4
- kidney N28.83
- liver K76.89
- renal N28.83
- splanchnic K63.4
- spleen D73.89
- stomach K31.89
- viscera K63.4

PTP D69.51

Ptyalism (periodic) K11.7
- hysterical F45.8
- pregnancy — *see* Pregnancy, complicated by, specified pregnancy-related condition NEC
- psychogenic F45.8

Ptyalolithiasis K11.5

Pubarche, precocious E3Ø.1

Pubertas praecox E3Ø.1

Puberty (development state) ZØØ.3
- bleeding (excessive) N92.2
- delayed E3Ø.Ø
- precocious (constitutional) (cryptogenic) (idiopathic) E3Ø.1
  - central E22.8
  - due to
    - ovarian hyperfunction E28.1
      - estrogen E28.Ø
    - testicular hyperfunction E29.Ø
- premature E3Ø.1
  - due to
    - adrenal cortical hyperfunction E25.8
    - pineal tumor E34.8
    - pituitary (anterior) hyperfunction E22.8

Puckering, macula — *see* Degeneration, macula, puckering

Pudenda, pudendum — *see* condition

Puente's disease (simple glandular cheilitis) K13.Ø

Puerperal, puerperium (complicated by, complications)
- abnormal glucose (tolerance test) O99.815
- abscess
  - areola O91.Ø2
    - associated with lactation O91.Ø3
  - Bartholin's gland O86.19
  - breast O91.12
    - associated with lactation O91.13
  - cervix (uteri) O86.11
  - genital organ NEC O86.19
  - kidney O86.21
  - mammary O91.12
    - associated with lactation O91.13
  - nipple O91.Ø2
    - associated with lactation O91.Ø3
  - peritoneum O85
  - subareolar O91.12
    - associated with lactation O91.13
  - urinary tract — *see* Puerperal, infection, urinary
  - uterus O86.12
  - vagina (wall) O86.13
  - vaginorectal O86.13
  - vulvovaginal gland O86.13
- adnexitis O86.19
- afibrinogenemia, or other coagulation defect O72.3
- albuminuria (acute) (subacute) — *see* Proteinuria, gestational
- alcohol use O99.315
- anemia O9Ø.81
  - pre-existing (pre-pregnancy) O99.Ø3
- anesthetic death O89.8
- apoplexy O99.43
- bariatric surgery status O99.845
- blood disorder NEC O99.13
- blood dyscrasia O72.3
- cardiomyopathy O9Ø.3
- cerebrovascular disorder (conditions in I6Ø-I69) O99.43
- cervicitis O86.11
- circulatory system disorder O99.43
- coagulopathy (any) O99.13
  - with hemorrhage O72.3
- complications O9Ø.9
  - specified NEC O9Ø.89
- convulsions — *see* Eclampsia
- cystitis O86.22
- cystopyelitis O86.29
- delirium NEC FØ5

Puerperal, puerperium — *continued*
- diabetes O24.93
  - gestational — *see* Puerperal, gestational diabetes
  - pre-existing O24.33
    - specified NEC O24.83
    - type 1 O24.Ø3
    - type 2 O24.13
- digestive system disorder O99.63
- disease O9Ø.9
  - breast NEC O92.29
  - cerebrovascular (acute) O99.43
  - nonobstetric NEC O99.893
  - tubo-ovarian O86.19
  - Valsuani's O99.Ø3
- disorder O9Ø.9
  - biliary tract O26.63
  - lactation O92.7Ø
  - liver O26.63
  - nonobstetric NEC O99.893
- disruption
  - cesarean wound O9Ø.Ø
  - episiotomy wound O9Ø.1
  - perineal laceration wound O9Ø.1
- drug use O99.325
- eclampsia (with pre-existing hypertension) O15.2
- embolism (pulmonary) (blood clot) — *see* Embolism, obstetric, puerperal
- endocrine, nutritional or metabolic disease NEC O99.285
- endophlebitis — *see* Puerperal, phlebitis
- endotrachelitis O86.11
- failure
  - lactation (complete) O92.3
    - partial O92.4
  - renal, acute O9Ø.4
- fever (of unknown origin) O86.4
  - septic O85
- fissure, nipple O92.12
  - associated with lactation O92.13
- fistula
  - breast (due to mastitis) O91.12
    - associated with lactation O91.13
  - nipple O91.Ø2
    - associated with lactation O91.Ø3
- galactophoritis O91.22
  - associated with lactation O91.23
- galactorrhea O92.6
- gastric banding status O99.845
- gastric bypass status O99.845
- gastrointestinal disease NEC O99.63
- gestational
  - diabetes O24.439
    - diet controlled O24.43Ø
    - insulin (and diet) controlled O24.434
    - oral drug controlled (antidiabetic) (hypoglycemic) O24.435
  - edema O12.Ø5
    - with proteinuria O12.25
  - proteinuria O12.15
- gonorrhea O98.23
- hematoma, subdural O99.43
- hemiplegia, cerebral O99.355
  - due to cerbrovascular disorder O99.43
- hemorrhage O72.1
  - brain O99.43
  - bulbar O99.43
  - cerebellar O99.43
  - cerebral O99.43
  - cortical O99.43
  - delayed or secondary O72.2
  - extradural O99.43
  - internal capsule O99.43
  - intracranial O99.43
  - intrapontine O99.43
  - meningeal O99.43
  - pontine O99.43
  - retained placenta O72.Ø
  - subarachnoid O99.43
  - subcortical O99.43
  - subdural O99.43
  - third stage O72.Ø
  - uterine, delayed O72.2
  - ventricular O99.43
- hemorrhoids O87.2
- hepatorenal syndrome O9Ø.4
- hypertension — *see* Hypertension, complicating, puerperium
- hypertrophy, breast O92.29
- induration breast (fibrous) O92.29

Puerperal, puerperium — *continued*
- infection O86.4
  - cervix O86.11
  - generalized O85
  - genital tract NEC O86.19
    - obstetric surgical wound O86.Ø9
  - kidney (bacillus coli) O86.21
  - maternal O98.93
    - carrier state NEC O99.835
    - gonorrhea O98.23
    - human immunodeficiency virus (HIV) O98.73
    - protozoal O98.63
    - sexually transmitted NEC O98.33
    - specified NEC O98.83
    - streptococcus group B (GBS) carrier state O99.825
    - syphilis O98.13
    - tuberculosis O98.Ø3
    - viral hepatitis O98.43
    - viral NEC O98.53
  - nipple O91.Ø2
    - associated with lactation O91.Ø3
  - peritoneum O85
  - renal O86.21
  - specified NEC O86.89
  - urinary (asymptomatic) (tract) NEC O86.2Ø
    - bladder O86.22
    - kidney O86.21
    - specified site NEC O86.29
    - urethra O86.22
  - vagina O86.13
  - vein — *see* Puerperal, phlebitis
- ischemia, cerebral O99.43
- lymphangitis O86.89
  - breast O91.22
    - associated with lactation O91.23
- malignancy O9A.13 (*following* O99)
- malnutrition O25.3
- mammillitis O91.Ø2
  - associated with lactation O91.Ø3
- mammitis O91.22
  - associated with lactation O91.23
- mania F3Ø.8
- mastitis O91.22
  - associated with lactation O91.23
  - purulent O91.12
    - associated with lactation O91.13
- melancholia — *see* Disorder, depressive
- mental disorder NEC O99.345
- metroperitonitis O85
- metrorrhagia — *see* Hemorrhage, postpartum
- metrosalpingitis O86.19
- metrovaginitis O86.13
- milk leg O87.1
- monoplegia, cerebral O99.43
- mood disturbance O9Ø.6
- necrosis, liver (acute) (subacute) (conditions in subcategory K72.Ø) O26.63
  - with renal failure O9Ø.4
- nervous system disorder O99.355
- obesity (pre-existing prior to pregnancy) O99.215
- obesity surgery status O99.845
- occlusion, precerebral artery O99.43
- paralysis
  - bladder (sphincter) O9Ø.89
  - cerebral O99.43
- paralytic stroke O99.43
- parametritis O85
- paravaginitis O86.13
- pelviperitonitis O85
- perimetritis O86.12
- perimetrosalpingitis O86.19
- perinephritis O86.21
- periphlebitis — *see* Puerperal phlebitis
- peritoneal infection O85
- peritonitis (pelvic) O85
- perivaginitis O86.13
- phlebitis O87.Ø
  - deep O87.1
  - pelvic O87.1
  - superficial O87.Ø
- phlebothrombosis, deep O87.1
- phlegmasia alba dolens O87.1
- placental polyp O9Ø.89
- pneumonia, embolic — *see* Embolism, obstetric, puerperal
- pre-eclampsia — *see* Pre-eclampsia
- psychosis (NOS) F53.1
- pyelitis O86.21
- pyelocystitis O86.29

Puerperal, puerperium — *continued*
- pyelonephritis O86.21
- pyelonephrosis O86.21
- pyemia O85
- pyocystitis O86.29
- pyohemia O85
- pyometra O86.12
- pyonephritis O86.21
- pyosalpingitis O86.19
- pyrexia (of unknown origin) O86.4
- renal
  - disease NEC O9Ø.89
  - failure O9Ø.4
- respiratory disease NEC O99.53
- retention
  - decidua — *see* Retention, decidua
  - placenta O72.Ø
  - secundines — *see* Retention, secundines
- retrated nipple O92.Ø2
- salpingo-ovaritis O86.19
- salpingoperitonitis O85
- secondary perineal tear O9Ø.1
- sepsis (pelvic) O85
- sepsis O85
- septic thrombophlebitis O86.81
- skin disorder NEC O99.73
- specified condition NEC O99.893
- stroke O99.43
- subinvolution (uterus) O9Ø.89
- subluxation of symphysis (pubis) O26.73
- suppuration — *see* Puerperal, abscess
- tetanus A34
- thelitis O91.Ø2
  - associated with lactation O91.Ø3
- thrombocytopenia O72.3
- thrombophlebitis (superficial) O87.Ø
  - deep O87.1
  - pelvic O87.1
  - septic O86.81
- thrombosis (venous) — *see* Thrombosis, puerperal
- thyroiditis O9Ø.5
- toxemia (eclamptic) (pre-eclamptic) (with convulsions) O15.2
- trauma, non-obstetric O9A.23 (*following* O99)
  - caused by abuse (physical) (suspected) O9A.33 (*following* O99)
    - confirmed O9A.33 (*following* O99)
    - psychological (suspected) O9A.53 (*following* O99)
      - confirmed O9A.53 (*following* O99)
    - sexual (suspected) O9A.43 (*following* O99)
      - confirmed O9A.43 (*following* O99)
- uremia (due to renal failure) O9Ø.4
- urethritis O86.22
- vaginitis O86.13
- varicose veins (legs) O87.4
  - vulva or perineum O87.8
- venous O87.9
- vulvitis O86.19
- vulvovaginitis O86.13
- white leg O87.1

Puerperium — *see* Puerperal

Pulmolithiasis J98.4

Pulmonary — *see* condition

Pulpitis (acute) (anachoretic) (chronic) (hyperplastic) (putrescent) (suppurative) (ulcerative) KØ4.Ø1
- irreversible KØ4.Ø2
- reversible KØ4.Ø1

Pulpless tooth KØ4.99

Pulse
- alternating RØØ.8
- bigeminal RØØ.8
- fast RØØ.Ø
- feeble, rapid due to shock following injury T79.4 ☑
- rapid RØØ.Ø
- weak RØ9.89

Pulsus alternans or trigeminus RØØ.8

Punch drunk FØ7.81

Punctum lacrimale occlusion — *see* Obstruction, lacrimal

Puncture
- abdomen, abdominal
  - wall S31.139 ☑
    - with
      - foreign body S31.149 ☑
      - penetration into peritoneal cavity S31.639 ☑
        - with foreign body S31.649 ☑
    - epigastric region S31.132 ☑

Puncture — *continued*
abdomen, abdominal — *continued*
wall — *continued*
epigastric region — *continued*
with
foreign body S31.142 ☑
penetration into peritoneal cavity S31.632 ☑
with foreign body S31.642 ☑
left
lower quadrant S31.134 ☑
with
foreign body S31.144 ☑
penetration into peritoneal cavity S31.634 ☑
with foreign body S31.644 ☑
upper quadrant S31.131 ☑
with
foreign body S31.141 ☑
penetration into peritoneal cavity S31.631 ☑
with foreign body S31.641 ☑
periumbilic region S31.135 ☑
with
foreign body S31.145 ☑
penetration into peritoneal cavity S31.635 ☑
with foreign body S31.645 ☑
right
lower quadrant S31.133 ☑
with
foreign body S31.143 ☑
penetration into peritoneal cavity S31.633 ☑
with foreign body S31.643 ☑
upper quadrant S31.130 ☑
with
foreign body S31.140 ☑
penetration into peritoneal cavity S31.630 ☑
with foreign body S31.640 ☑
accidental, complicating surgery — *see* Complication, accidental puncture or laceration
alveolar (process) — *see* Puncture, oral cavity
ankle S91.039 ☑
with
foreign body S91.049 ☑
left S91.032 ☑
with
foreign body S91.042 ☑
right S91.031 ☑
with
foreign body S91.041 ☑
anus S31.833 ☑
with foreign body S31.834 ☑
arm (upper) S41.139 ☑
with foreign body S41.149 ☑
left S41.132 ☑
with foreign body S41.142 ☑
lower — *see* Puncture, forearm
right S41.131 ☑
with foreign body S41.141 ☑
auditory canal (external) (meatus) — *see* Puncture, ear
auricle, ear — *see* Puncture, ear
axilla — *see* Puncture, arm
back — *see also* Puncture, thorax, back
lower S31.030 ☑
with
foreign body S31.040 ☑
with penetration into retroperitoneal space S31.041 ☑
penetration into retroperitoneal space S31.031 ☑
bladder (traumatic) S37.29 ☑
nontraumatic N32.89
breast S21.039 ☑
with foreign body S21.049 ☑
left S21.032 ☑
with foreign body S21.042 ☑
right S21.031 ☑
with foreign body S21.041 ☑
buttock S31.803 ☑
with foreign body S31.804 ☑
left S31.823 ☑
with foreign body S31.824 ☑
right S31.813 ☑

Puncture — *continued*
buttock — *continued*
right — *continued*
with foreign body S31.814 ☑
by
device, implant or graft — *see* Complications, by site and type, mechanical
foreign body left accidentally in operative wound T81.539 ☑
instrument (any) during a procedure, accidental — *see* Puncture, accidental complicating surgery
calf — *see* Puncture, leg
canaliculus lacrimalis — *see* Puncture, eyelid
canthus, eye — *see* Puncture, eyelid
cervical esophagus S11.23 ☑
with foreign body S11.24 ☑
cheek (external) S01.439 ☑
with foreign body S01.449 ☑
internal — *see* Puncture, oral cavity
left S01.432 ☑
with foreign body S01.442 ☑
right S01.431 ☑
with foreign body S01.441 ☑
chest wall — *see* Puncture, thorax
chin — *see* Puncture, head, specified site NEC
clitoris — *see* Puncture, vulva
costal region — *see* Puncture, thorax
digit(s)
foot — *see* Puncture, toe
hand — *see* Puncture, finger
ear (canal) (external) S01.339 ☑
with foreign body S01.349 ☑
drum S09.2- ☑
left S01.332 ☑
with foreign body S01.342 ☑
right S01.331 ☑
with foreign body S01.341 ☑
elbow S51.039 ☑
with
foreign body S51.049 ☑
left S51.032 ☑
with
foreign body S51.042 ☑
right S51.031 ☑
with
foreign body S51.041 ☑
epididymis — *see* Puncture, testis
epigastric region — *see* Puncture, abdomen, wall, epigastric
epiglottis S11.83 ☑
with foreign body S11.84 ☑
esophagus
cervical S11.23 ☑
with foreign body S11.24 ☑
thoracic S27.818 ☑
eyeball S05.6- ☑
with foreign body S05.5- ☑
eyebrow — *see* Puncture, eyelid
eyelid S01.13- ☑
with foreign body S01.14- ☑
left S01.132 ☑
with foreign body S01.142 ☑
right S01.131 ☑
with foreign body S01.141 ☑
face NEC — *see* Puncture, head, specified site NEC
finger(s) S61.239 ☑
with
damage to nail S61.339 ☑
with
foreign body S61.349 ☑
foreign body S61.249 ☑
index S61.238 ☑
with
damage to nail S61.338 ☑
with
foreign body S61.348 ☑
foreign body S61.248 ☑
left S61.231 ☑
with
damage to nail S61.331 ☑
with
foreign body S61.341 ☑
foreign body S61.241 ☑
right S61.230 ☑
with
damage to nail S61.330 ☑

Puncture — *continued*
finger(s) — *continued*
index — *continued*
right — *continued*
with — *continued*
damage to nail — *continued*
with
foreign body S61.340 ☑
foreign body S61.240 ☑
little S61.238 ☑
with
damage to nail S61.338 ☑
with
foreign body S61.348 ☑
foreign body S61.248 ☑
left S61.237 ☑
with
damage to nail S61.337 ☑
with
foreign body S61.347 ☑
foreign body S61.247 ☑
right S61.236 ☑
with
damage to nail S61.336 ☑
with
foreign body S61.346 ☑
foreign body S61.246 ☑
middle S61.238 ☑
with
damage to nail S61.338 ☑
with
foreign body S61.348 ☑
foreign body S61.248 ☑
left S61.233 ☑
with
damage to nail S61.333 ☑
with
foreign body S61.343 ☑
foreign body S61.243 ☑
right S61.232 ☑
with
damage to nail S61.332 ☑
with
foreign body S61.342 ☑
foreign body S61.242 ☑
ring S61.238 ☑
with
damage to nail S61.338 ☑
with
foreign body S61.348 ☑
foreign body S61.248 ☑
left S61.235 ☑
with
damage to nail S61.335 ☑
with
foreign body S61.345 ☑
foreign body S61.245 ☑
right S61.234 ☑
with
damage to nail S61.334 ☑
with
foreign body S61.344 ☑
foreign body S61.244 ☑
flank S31.139 ☑
with foreign body S31.149 ☑
foot (except toe(s) alone) S91.339 ☑
with foreign body S91.349 ☑
left S91.332 ☑
with foreign body S91.342 ☑
right S91.331 ☑
with foreign body S91.341 ☑
toe — *see* Puncture, toe
forearm S51.839 ☑
with
foreign body S51.849 ☑
elbow only — *see* Puncture, elbow
left S51.832 ☑
with
foreign body S51.842 ☑
right S51.831 ☑
with
foreign body S51.841 ☑
forehead — *see* Puncture, head, specified site NEC
genital organs, external
female S31.532 ☑
with foreign body S31.542 ☑

Puncture — *continued*
genital organs, external — *continued*
female — *continued*
vagina — *see* Puncture, vagina
vulva — *see* Puncture, vulva
male S31.531 ☑
with foreign body S31.541 ☑
penis — *see* Puncture, penis
scrotum — *see* Puncture, scrotum
testis — *see* Puncture, testis
groin — *see* Puncture, abdomen, wall
gum — *see* Puncture, oral cavity
hand S61.439 ☑
with
foreign body S61.449 ☑
finger — *see* Puncture, finger
left S61.432 ☑
with
foreign body S61.442 ☑
right S61.431 ☑
with
foreign body S61.441 ☑
thumb — *see* Puncture, thumb
head SØ1.93 ☑
with foreign body SØ1.94 ☑
cheek — *see* Puncture, cheek
ear — *see* Puncture, ear
eyelid — *see* Puncture, eyelid
lip — *see* Puncture, oral cavity
nose — *see* Puncture, nose
oral cavity — *see* Puncture, oral cavity
scalp SØ1.Ø3 ☑
with foreign body SØ1.Ø4 ☑
specified site NEC SØ1.83 ☑
with foreign body SØ1.84 ☑
temporomandibular area — *see* Puncture, cheek
heart S26.99 ☑
with hemopericardium S26.Ø9 ☑
without hemopericardium S26.19 ☑
heel — *see* Puncture, foot
hip S71.Ø39 ☑
with foreign body S71.Ø49 ☑
left S71.Ø32 ☑
with foreign body S71.Ø42 ☑
right S71.Ø31 ☑
with foreign body S71.Ø41 ☑
hymen — *see* Puncture, vagina
hypochondrium — *see* Puncture, abdomen, wall
hypogastric region — *see* Puncture, abdomen, wall
inguinal region — *see* Puncture, abdomen, wall
instep — *see* Puncture, foot
internal organs — *see* Injury, by site
interscapular region — *see* Puncture, thorax, back
intestine
large
colon S36.599 ☑
ascending S36.59Ø ☑
descending S36.592 ☑
sigmoid S36.593 ☑
specified site NEC S36.598 ☑
transverse S36.591 ☑
rectum S36.69 ☑
small S36.499 ☑
duodenum S36.49Ø ☑
specified site NEC S36.498 ☑
intra-abdominal organ S36.99 ☑
gallbladder S36.128 ☑
intestine — *see* Puncture, intestine
liver S36.118 ☑
pancreas — *see* Puncture, pancreas
peritoneum S36.81 ☑
specified site NEC S36.898 ☑
spleen S36.Ø9 ☑
stomach S36.39 ☑
jaw — *see* Puncture, head, specified site NEC
knee S81.Ø39 ☑
with foreign body S81.Ø49 ☑
left S81.Ø32 ☑
with foreign body S81.Ø42 ☑
right S81.Ø31 ☑
with foreign body S81.Ø41 ☑
labium (majus) (minus) — *see* Puncture, vulva
lacrimal duct — *see* Puncture, eyelid
larynx S11.Ø13 ☑
with foreign body S11.Ø14 ☑
leg (lower) S81.839 ☑

Puncture — *continued*
leg — *continued*
with foreign body S81.849 ☑
foot — *see* Puncture, foot
knee — *see* Puncture, knee
left S81.832 ☑
with foreign body S81.842 ☑
right S81.831 ☑
with foreign body S81.841 ☑
upper — *see* Puncture, thigh
lip SØ1.531 ☑
with foreign body SØ1.541 ☑
loin — *see* Puncture, abdomen, wall
lower back — *see* Puncture, back, lower
lumbar region — *see* Puncture, back, lower
malar region — *see* Puncture, head, specified site NEC
mammary — *see* Puncture, breast
mastoid region — *see* Puncture, head, specified site NEC
mouth — *see* Puncture, oral cavity
nail
finger — *see* Puncture, finger, with damage to nail
toe — *see* Puncture, toe, with damage to nail
nasal (septum) (sinus) — *see* Puncture, nose
nasopharynx — *see* Puncture, head, specified site NEC
neck S11.93 ☑
with foreign body S11.94 ☑
involving
cervical esophagus — *see* Puncture, cervical esophagus
larynx — *see* Puncture, larynx
pharynx — *see* Puncture, pharynx
thyroid gland — *see* Puncture, thyroid gland
trachea — *see* Puncture, trachea
specified site NEC S11.83 ☑
with foreign body S11.84 ☑
nose (septum) (sinus) SØ1.23 ☑
with foreign body SØ1.24 ☑
ocular — *see* Puncture, eyeball
oral cavity SØ1.532 ☑
with foreign body SØ1.542 ☑
orbit SØ5.4- ☑
palate — *see* Puncture, oral cavity
palm — *see* Puncture, hand
pancreas S36.299 ☑
body S36.291 ☑
head S36.29Ø ☑
tail S36.292 ☑
pelvis — *see* Puncture, back, lower
penis S31.23 ☑
with foreign body S31.24 ☑
perineum
female S31.43 ☑
with foreign body S31.44 ☑
male S31.139 ☑
with foreign body S31.149 ☑
periocular area (with or without lacrimal passages) — *see* Puncture, eyelid
phalanges
finger — *see* Puncture, finger
toe — *see* Puncture, toe
pharynx S11.23 ☑
with foreign body S11.24 ☑
pinna — *see* Puncture, ear
popliteal space — *see* Puncture, knee
prepuce — *see* Puncture, penis
pubic region S31.139 ☑
with foreign body S31.149 ☑
pudendum — *see* Puncture, genital organs, external
rectovaginal septum — *see* Puncture, vagina
sacral region — *see* Puncture, back, lower
sacroiliac region — *see* Puncture, back, lower
salivary gland — *see* Puncture, oral cavity
scalp SØ1.Ø3 ☑
with foreign body SØ1.Ø4 ☑
scapular region — *see* Puncture, shoulder
scrotum S31.33 ☑
with foreign body S31.34 ☑
shin — *see* Puncture, leg
shoulder S41.Ø39 ☑
with foreign body S41.Ø49 ☑
left S41.Ø32 ☑
with foreign body S41.Ø42 ☑
right S41.Ø31 ☑
with foreign body S41.Ø41 ☑
spermatic cord — *see* Puncture, testis

Puncture — *continued*
sternal region — *see* Puncture, thorax, front
submaxillary region — *see* Puncture, head, specified site NEC
submental region — *see* Puncture, head, specified site NEC
subungual
finger(s) — *see* Puncture, finger, with damage to nail
toe — *see* Puncture, toe, with damage to nail
supraclavicular fossa — *see* Puncture, neck, specified site NEC
temple, temporal region — *see* Puncture, head, specified site NEC
temporomandibular area — *see* Puncture, cheek
testis S31.33 ☑
with foreign body S31.34 ☑
thigh S71.139 ☑
with foreign body S71.149 ☑
left S71.132 ☑
with foreign body S71.142 ☑
right S71.131 ☑
with foreign body S71.141 ☑
thorax, thoracic (wall) S21.93 ☑
with foreign body S21.94 ☑
back S21.23- ☑
with
foreign body S21.24- ☑
with penetration S21.44 ☑
penetration S21.43 ☑
breast — *see* Puncture, breast
front S21.13- ☑
with
foreign body S21.14- ☑
with penetration S21.34 ☑
penetration S21.33 ☑
throat — *see* Puncture, neck
thumb S61.Ø39 ☑
with
damage to nail S61.139 ☑
with
foreign body S61.149 ☑
foreign body S61.Ø49 ☑
left S61.Ø32 ☑
with
damage to nail S61.132 ☑
with
foreign body S61.142 ☑
foreign body S61.Ø42 ☑
right S61.Ø31 ☑
with
damage to nail S61.131 ☑
with
foreign body S61.141 ☑
foreign body S61.Ø41 ☑
thyroid gland S11.13 ☑
with foreign body S11.14 ☑
toe(s) S91.139 ☑
with
damage to nail S91.239 ☑
with
foreign body S91.249 ☑
foreign body S91.149 ☑
great S91.133 ☑
with
damage to nail S91.233 ☑
with
foreign body S91.243 ☑
foreign body S91.143 ☑
left S91.132 ☑
with
damage to nail S91.232 ☑
with
foreign body S91.242 ☑
foreign body S91.142 ☑
right S91.131 ☑
with
damage to nail S91.231 ☑
with
foreign body S91.241 ☑
foreign body S91.141 ☑
lesser S91.136 ☑
with
damage to nail S91.236 ☑
with
foreign body S91.246 ☑

- **Puncture** — *continued*
  - toe(s) — *continued*
    - lesser — *continued*
      - with — *continued*
        - foreign body S91.146 ☑
    - left S91.135 ☑
      - with
        - damage to nail S91.235 ☑
          - with
            - foreign body S91.245 ☑
        - foreign body S91.145 ☑
    - right S91.134 ☑
      - with
        - damage to nail S91.234 ☑
          - with
            - foreign body S91.244 ☑
        - foreign body S91.144 ☑
  - tongue — *see* Puncture, oral cavity
  - trachea S11.Ø23 ☑
    - with foreign body S11.Ø24 ☑
  - tunica vaginalis — *see* Puncture, testis
  - tympanum, tympanic membrane SØ9.2- ☑
  - umbilical region S31.135 ☑
    - with foreign body S31.145 ☑
  - uvula — *see* Puncture, oral cavity
  - vagina S31.43 ☑
    - with foreign body S31.44 ☑
  - vocal cords S11.Ø33 ☑
    - with foreign body S11.Ø34 ☑
  - vulva S31.43 ☑
    - with foreign body S31.44 ☑
  - wrist S61.539 ☑
    - with
      - foreign body S61.549 ☑
    - left S61.532 ☑
      - with
        - foreign body S61.542 ☑
    - right S61.531 ☑
      - with
        - foreign body S61.541 ☑
- **PUO** (pyrexia of unknown origin) R5Ø.9
- **Pupillary membrane** (persistent) Q13.89
- **Pupillotonia** — *see* Anomaly, pupil, function, tonic pupil
- **Purpura** D69.2
  - abdominal D69.Ø
  - allergic D69.Ø
  - anaphylactoid D69.Ø
  - annularis telangiectodes L81.7
  - arthritic D69.Ø
  - autoerythrocyte sensitization D69.2
  - autoimmune D69.Ø
  - bacterial D69.Ø
  - Bateman's (senile) D69.2
  - capillary fragility (hereditary) (idiopathic) D69.8
  - cryoglobulinemic D89.1
  - Devil's pinches D69.2
  - fibrinolytic — *see* Fibrinolysis
  - fulminans, fulminous D65
  - gangrenous D65
  - hemorrhagic, hemorrhagica D69.3
    - not due to thrombocytopenia D69.Ø
  - Henoch (-Schönlein) (allergic) D69.Ø
  - hypergammaglobulinemic (benign) (Waldenström) D89.Ø
  - idiopathic (thrombocytopenic) D69.3
    - nonthrombocytopenic D69.Ø
  - immune thrombocytopenic D69.3
  - infectious D69.Ø
  - malignant D69.Ø
  - neonatorum P54.5
  - nervosa D69.Ø
  - newborn P54.5
  - nonthrombocytopenic D69.2
    - hemorrhagic D69.Ø
    - idiopathic D69.Ø
  - nonthrombopenic D69.2
  - peliosis rheumatica D69.Ø
  - posttransfusion (post-transfusion) (from (fresh) whole blood or blood products) D69.51
  - primary D69.49
  - red cell membrane sensitivity D69.2
  - rheumatica D69.Ø
  - Schönlein (-Henoch) (allergic) D69.Ø
  - scorbutic E54 *[D77]*
  - senile D69.2
  - simplex D69.2
  - symptomatica D69.Ø
- **Purpura** — *continued*
  - telangiectasia annularis L81.7
  - thrombocytopenic D69.49
    - congenital D69.42
    - hemorrhagic D69.3
    - hereditary D69.42
    - idiopathic D69.3
    - immune D69.3
    - neonatal, transitory P61.Ø
    - thrombotic M31.19
  - thrombohemolytic — *see* Fibrinolysis
  - thrombolytic — *see* Fibrinolysis
  - thrombopenic D69.49
  - thrombotic, thrombocytopenic M31.19
  - toxic D69.Ø
  - vascular D69.Ø
  - visceral symptoms D69.Ø
- **Purpuric spots** R23.3
- **Purulent** — *see* condition
- **Pus**
  - in
    - stool R19.5
    - urine N39.Ø
  - tube (rupture) — *see* Salpingo-oophoritis
- **Pustular rash** LØ8.Ø
- **Pustule** (nonmalignant) LØ8.9
  - malignant A22.Ø
- **Pustulosis palmaris et plantaris** L4Ø.3
- **Putnam** (-Dana) **disease or syndrome** — *see* Degeneration, combined
- **Putrescent pulp** (dental) KØ4.1
- **Pyarthritis, pyarthrosis** — *see* Arthritis, pyogenic or pyemic
  - tuberculous — *see* Tuberculosis, joint
- **Pyelectasis** — *see* Hydronephrosis
- **Pyelitis** (congenital) (uremic) — *see also* Pyelonephritis
  - with
    - calculus — *see* category N2Ø ☑
      - with hydronephrosis N13.6
    - contracted kidney N11.9
  - acute N1Ø
  - chronic N11.9
    - with calculus — *see* category N2Ø ☑
      - with hydronephrosis N13.6
  - cystica N28.84
  - puerperal (postpartum) O86.21
  - tuberculous A18.11
- **Pyelocystitis** — *see* Pyelonephritis
- **Pyelonephritis** — *see also* Nephritis, tubulo-interstitial
  - with
    - calculus — *see* category N2Ø ☑
      - with hydronephrosis N13.6
    - contracted kidney N11.9
  - acute N1Ø
  - calculous — *see* category N2Ø ☑
    - with hydronephrosis N13.6
  - chronic N11.9
    - with calculus — *see* category N2Ø ☑
      - with hydronephrosis N13.6
    - associated with ureteral obstruction or stricture N11.1
    - nonobstructive N11.8
      - with reflux (vesicoureteral) N11.Ø
    - obstructive N11.1
    - specified NEC N11.8
  - in (due to)
    - brucellosis A23.9 *[N16]*
    - cryoglobulinemia (mixed) D89.1 *[N16]*
    - cystinosis E72.Ø4
    - diphtheria A36.84
    - glycogen storage disease E74.Ø9 *[N16]*
    - leukemia NEC C95.9- ☑ *[N16]*
    - lymphoma NEC C85.9Ø *[N16]*
    - multiple myeloma C9Ø.Ø- ☑ *[N16]*
    - obstruction N11.1
    - Salmonella infection AØ2.25
    - sarcoidosis D86.84
    - sepsis A41.9 *[N16]*
    - Sjögren's disease M35.Ø4
    - toxoplasmosis B58.83
    - transplant rejection T86.91 *[N16]*
    - Wilson's disease E83.Ø1 *[N16]*
  - nonobstructive N12
    - with reflux (vesicoureteral) N11.Ø
    - chronic N11.8
  - syphilitic A52.75
- **Pyelonephrosis** (obstructive) N11.1
  - chronic N11.9
- **Pyelophlebitis** I8Ø.8
- **Pyeloureteritis cystica** N28.85
- **Pyemia, pyemic** (fever) (infection) (purulent) — *see also* Sepsis
  - joint — *see* Arthritis, pyogenic or pyemic
  - liver K75.1
  - pneumococcal A4Ø.3
  - portal K75.1
  - postvaccinal T88.Ø ☑
  - puerperal, postpartum, childbirth O85
  - specified organism NEC A41.89
  - tuberculous — *see* Tuberculosis, miliary
- **Pygopagus** Q89.4
- **Pyknoepilepsy** (idiopathic) — *see* Pyknolepsy
- **Pyknolepsy** G4Ø.AØ9 *(following G4Ø.3)*
  - intractable G4Ø.A19 *(following G4Ø.3)*
    - with status epilepticus G4Ø.A11 *(following G4Ø.3)*
    - without status epilepticus G4Ø.A19 *(following G4Ø.3)*
  - not intractable G4Ø.AØ9 *(following G4Ø.3)*
    - with status epilepticus G4Ø.AØ1 *(following G4Ø.3)*
    - without status epilepticus G4Ø.AØ9 *(following G4Ø.3)*
- **Pylephlebitis** K75.1
- **Pyle's syndrome** Q78.5
- **Pylethrombophlebitis** K75.1
- **Pylethrombosis** K75.1
- **Pyloritis** K29.9Ø
  - with bleeding K29.91
- **Pylorospasm** (reflex) **NEC** K31.3
  - congenital or infantile Q4Ø.Ø
  - neurotic F45.8
  - newborn Q4Ø.Ø
  - psychogenic F45.8
- **Pylorus, pyloric** — *see* condition
- **Pyoarthrosis** — *see* Arthritis, pyogenic or pyemic
- **Pyocele**
  - mastoid — *see* Mastoiditis, acute
  - sinus (accessory) — *see* Sinusitis
  - turbinate (bone) J32.9
  - urethra — *see also* Urethritis N34.Ø
- **Pyocolpos** — *see* Vaginitis
- **Pyocystitis** N3Ø.8Ø
  - with hematuria N3Ø.81
- **Pyoderma, pyodermia** LØ8.Ø
  - gangrenosum L88
  - newborn P39.4
  - phagedenic L88
  - vegetans LØ8.81
- **Pyodermatitis** LØ8.Ø
  - vegetans LØ8.81
- **Pyogenic** — *see* condition
- **Pyohydronephrosis** N13.6
- **Pyometra, pyometrium, pyometritis** — *see* Endometritis
- **Pyomyositis** (tropical) — *see* Myositis, infective
- **Pyonephritis** N12
- **Pyonephrosis** N13.6
  - tuberculous A18.11
- **Pyo-oophoritis** — *see* Salpingo-oophoritis
- **Pyo-ovarium** — *see* Salpingo-oophoritis
- **Pyopericarditis, pyopericardium** I3Ø.1
- **Pyophlebitis** — *see* Phlebitis
- **Pyopneumopericardium** I3Ø.1
- **Pyopneumothorax** (infective) J86.9
  - with fistula J86.Ø
  - tuberculous NEC A15.6
- **Pyosalpinx, pyosalpingitis** — *see also* Salpingo-oophoritis
- **Pyothorax** J86.9
  - with fistula J86.Ø
  - tuberculous NEC A15.6
- **Pyoureter** N28.89
  - tuberculous A18.11
- **Pyramidopallidonigral syndrome** G2Ø
- **Pyrexia** (of unknown origin) R5Ø.9
  - atmospheric T67.Ø1 ☑
  - during labor NEC O75.2
  - heat T67.Ø1 ☑
  - newborn P81.9
    - environmentally-induced P81.Ø
  - persistent R5Ø.9
  - puerperal O86.4
- **Pyroglobulinemia NEC** E88.Ø9
- **Pyromania** F63.1
- **Pyrosis** R12
- **Pyuria** (bacterial) (sterile) R82.81

Q

Q fever A78
- with pneumonia A78

Quadricuspid aortic valve Q23.8
Quadrilateral fever A78
Quadriparesis — *see* Quadriplegia
- meaning muscle weakness M62.81

Quadriplegia G82.5Ø
- complete
  - C1-C4 level G82.51
  - C5-C7 level G82.53
- congenital (cerebral) (spinal) G8Ø.8
  - spastic G8Ø.Ø
- embolic (current episode) I63.4- ☑
- functional R53.2
- incomplete
  - C1-C4 level G82.52
  - C5-C7 level G82.54
- thrombotic (current episode) I63.3- ☑
- traumatic — *code to* injury with seventh character S
  - current episode — *see* Injury, spinal (cord), cervical

Quadruplet, pregnancy — *see* Pregnancy, quadruplet
Quarrelsomeness F6Ø.3
Queensland fever A77.3
Quervain's disease M65.4
- thyroid EØ6.1

Queyrat's erythroplasia DØ7.4
- penis DØ7.4
- specified site — *see* Neoplasm, skin, in situ
- unspecified site DØ7.4

Quincke's disease or edema T78.3 ☑
- hereditary D84.1

Quinsy (gangrenous) J36
Quintan fever A79.Ø
Quintuplet, pregnancy — *see* Pregnancy, quintuplet

R

Rabbit fever — *see* Tularemia
Rabies A82.9
- contact Z2Ø.3
- exposure to Z2Ø.3
- inoculation reaction — *see* Complications, vaccination
- sylvatic A82.Ø
- urban A82.1

Rachischisis — *see* Spina bifida
Rachitic — *see also* condition
- deformities of spine (late effect) (sequelae) E64.3
- pelvis (late effect) (sequelae) E64.3
  - with disproportion (fetopelvic) O33.Ø
    - causing obstructed labor O65.Ø

Rachitis, rachitism (acute) (tarda) — *see also* Rickets
- renalis N25.Ø
- sequelae E64.3

Radial nerve — *see* condition
Radiation
- burn — *see* Burn
- effects NOS T66 ☑
- sickness NOS T66 ☑
- therapy, encounter for Z51.Ø

Radiculitis (pressure) (vertebrogenic) — *see* Radiculopathy
Radiculomyelitis — *see also* Encephalitis
- toxic, due to
  - Clostridium tetani A35
  - Corynebacterium diphtheriae A36.82

Radiculopathy M54.1Ø
- cervical region M54.12
- cervicothoracic region M54.13
- due to
  - disc disorder
    - C3 M5Ø.11
    - C4 M5Ø.11
    - C5 M5Ø.121
    - C6 M5Ø.122
    - C7 M5Ø.123
  - displacement of intervertebral disc — *see* Disorder, disc, with, radiculopathy
- leg M54.1- ☑
- lumbar region M54.16
- lumbosacral region M54.17
- occipito-atlanto-axial region M54.11
- postherpetic BØ2.29
- sacrococcygeal region M54.18
- syphilitic A52.11

Radiculopathy — *continued*
- thoracic region (with visceral pain) M54.14
- thoracolumbar region M54.15

Radiodermal burns (acute, chronic, or occupational) — *see* Burn
Radiodermatitis L58.9
- acute L58.Ø
- chronic L58.1

Radiotherapy session Z51.Ø
RAEB (refractory anemia with excess blasts) D46.2- ☑
Rage, meaning rabies — *see* Rabies
Ragpicker's disease A22.1
Ragsorter's disease A22.1
Raillietiniasis B71.8
Railroad neurosis F48.8
Railway spine F48.8
Raised — *see also* Elevated
- antibody titer R76.Ø

Rake teeth, tooth M26.39
Rales RØ9.89
Ramifying renal pelvis Q63.8
Ramsay-Hunt disease or syndrome — *see also* Hunt's disease BØ2.21
- meaning dyssynergia cerebellaris myoclonica G11.19

Ranula K11.6
- congenital Q38.4

Rape
- adult
  - confirmed T74.21 ☑
  - suspected T76.21 ☑
- alleged, observation or examination, ruled out
  - adult ZØ4.41
  - child ZØ4.42
- child
  - confirmed T74.22 ☑
  - suspected T76.22 ☑

Rapid
- feeble pulse, due to shock, following injury T79.4 ☑
- heart (beat) RØØ.Ø
  - psychogenic F45.8
- second stage (delivery) O62.3
- time-zone change syndrome G47.25

Rarefaction, bone — *see* Disorder, bone, density and structure, specified NEC
Rash (toxic) R21
- canker A38.9
- diaper L22
- drug (internal use) L27.Ø
  - contact — *see also* Dermatitis, due to, drugs, external L25.1
- following immunization T88.1 ☑
- food — *see* Dermatitis, due to, food
- heat L74.Ø
- napkin (psoriasiform) L22
- nettle — *see* Urticaria
- pustular LØ8.Ø
- rose R21
  - epidemic BØ6.9
- scarlet A38.9
- serum — *see also* Reaction, serum T8Ø.69 ☑
- wandering tongue K14.1

Rasmussen aneurysm — *see* Tuberculosis, pulmonary
Rasmussen encephalitis GØ4.81
Rat-bite fever A25.9
- due to Streptobacillus moniliformis A25.1
- spirochetal (morsus muris) A25.Ø

Rathke's pouch tumor D44.3
Raymond (-Céstan) **syndrome** I65.8
Raynaud's disease, phenomenon or syndrome (secondary) I73.ØØ
- with gangrene (symmetric) I73.Ø1

RDS (newborn) (type I) P22.Ø
- type II P22.1

Reaction — *see also* Disorder
- withdrawing, child or adolescent F93.8
- adaptation — *see* Disorder, adjustment
- adjustment (anxiety) (conduct disorder) (depressiveness) (distress) — *see* Disorder, adjustment
  - with
    - mutism, elective (child) (adolescent) F94.Ø
- adverse
  - food (any) (ingested) NEC T78.1 ☑
    - anaphylactic — *see* Shock, anaphylactic, due to food
- affective — *see* Disorder, mood
- allergic — *see* Allergy
- anaphylactic — *see* Shock, anaphylactic

Reaction — *continued*
- anaphylactoid — *see* Shock, anaphylactic
- anesthesia — *see* Anesthesia, complication
- antitoxin (prophylactic) (therapeutic) — *see* Complications, vaccination
- anxiety F41.1
- Arthus — *see* Arthus' phenomenon
- asthenic F48.8
- combat and operational stress F43.Ø
- compulsive F42.8
- conversion F44.9
- crisis, acute F43.Ø
- deoxyribonuclease (DNA) (DNase) hypersensitivity D69.2
- depressive (single episode) F32.9
  - affective (single episode) F31.4
    - recurrent episode F33.9
  - neurotic F34.1
  - psychoneurotic F34.1
  - psychotic F32.3
  - recurrent — *see* Disorder, depressive, recurrent
- dissociative F44.9
- drug NEC T88.7 ☑
  - addictive — *see* Dependence, drug
    - transmitted via placenta or breast milk — *see* Absorption, drug, addictive, through placenta
  - allergic — *see* Allergy, drug
  - lichenoid L43.2
  - newborn P93.8
    - gray baby syndrome P93.Ø
  - overdose or poisoning (by accident) — *see* Table of Drugs and Chemicals, by drug, poisoning
  - photoallergic L56.1
  - phototoxic L56.Ø
  - withdrawal — *see* Dependence, by drug, with, withdrawal
    - infant of dependent mother P96.1
    - newborn P96.1
  - wrong substance given or taken (by accident) — *see* Table of Drugs and Chemicals, by drug, poisoning
- fear F4Ø.9
  - child (abnormal) F93.8
- febrile nonhemolytic transfusion (FNHTR) R5Ø.84
- fluid loss, cerebrospinal G97.1
- foreign
  - body NEC — *see* Granuloma, foreign body
    - in operative wound (inadvertently left) — *see* Foreign body, accidentally left during a procedure
  - substance accidentally left during a procedure (chemical) (powder) (talc) T81.6Ø ☑
    - aseptic peritonitis T81.61 ☑
    - body or object (instrument) (sponge) (swab) — *see* Foreign body, accidentally left during a procedure
    - specified reaction NEC T81.69 ☑
- grief — *see* Disorder, adjustment
- Herxheimer's R68.89
- hyperkinetic — *see* Hyperkinesia
- hypochondriacal F45.2Ø
- hypoglycemic, due to insulin E16.Ø
  - with coma (diabetic) — *see* Diabetes, coma
    - nondiabetic E15
  - therapeutic misadventure — *see* subcategory T38.3 ☑
- hypomanic F3Ø.8
- hysterical F44.9
- immunization — *see* Complications, vaccination
- incompatibility
  - ABO blood group (infusion) (transfusion) — *see* Complication(s), transfusion, incompatibility reaction, ABO
    - delayed serologic T8Ø.39 ☑
  - minor blood group (Duffy) (E) (K) (Kell) (Kidd) (Lewis) (M) (N) (P) (S) T8Ø.89 ☑
  - Rh (factor) (infusion) (transfusion) — *see* Complication(s), transfusion, incompatibility reaction, Rh (factor)
- inflammatory — *see* Infection
- infusion — *see* Complications, infusion
- inoculation (immune serum) — *see* Complications, vaccination
- insulin T38.3- ☑
- involutional psychotic — *see* Disorder, depressive
- leukemoid D72.823
  - basophilic D72.823

- **Reaction** — *continued*
  - leukemoid — *continued*
    - lymphocytic D72.823
    - monocytic D72.823
    - myelocytic D72.823
    - neutrophilic D72.823
  - LSD (acute)
    - due to drug abuse — *see* Abuse, drug, hallucinogen
    - due to drug dependence — *see* Dependence, drug, hallucinogen
  - lumbar puncture G97.1
  - manic-depressive — *see* Disorder, bipolar
  - neurasthenic F48.8
  - neurogenic — *see* Neurosis
  - neurotic F48.9
  - neurotic-depressive F34.1
  - nitritoid — *see* Crisis, nitritoid
  - nonspecific
    - to
      - cell mediated immunity measurement of gamma interferon antigen response without active tuberculosis R76.12
      - QuantiFERON-TB test (QFT) without active tuberculosis R76.12
      - tuberculin test — *see also* Reaction, tuberculin skin test R76.11
  - obsessive-compulsive F42.8
  - organic, acute or subacute — *see* Delirium
  - paranoid (acute) F23
    - chronic F22
    - senile F03 ☑
  - passive dependency F60.7
  - phobic F40.9
  - post-traumatic stress, uncomplicated Z73.3
  - psychogenic F99
  - psychoneurotic — *see also* Neurosis
    - compulsive F42.8
    - depersonalization F48.1
    - depressive F34.1
    - hypochondriacal F45.20
    - neurasthenic F48.8
    - obsessive F42.8
  - psychophysiologic — *see* Disorder, somatoform
  - psychosomatic — *see* Disorder, somatoform
  - psychotic — *see* Psychosis
  - scarlet fever toxin — *see* Complications, vaccination
  - schizophrenic F23
    - acute (brief) (undifferentiated) F23
    - latent F21
    - undifferentiated (acute) (brief) F23
  - serological for syphilis — *see* Serology for syphilis
  - serum T80.69 ☑
    - anaphylactic (immediate) — *see also* Shock, anaphylactic T80.59 ☑
    - specified reaction NEC
      - due to
        - administration of blood and blood products T80.61 ☑
        - immunization T80.62 ☑
        - serum specified NEC T80.69 ☑
        - vaccination T80.62 ☑
  - situational — *see* Disorder, adjustment
  - somatization — *see* Disorder, somatoform
  - spinal puncture G97.1
    - dural G97.1
  - stress (severe) F43.9
    - acute (agitation) ("daze") (disorientation) (disturbance of consciousness) (flight reaction) (fugue) F43.0
    - specified NEC F43.89
  - surgical procedure — *see* Complications, surgical procedure
  - tetanus antitoxin — *see* Complications, vaccination
  - toxic, to local anesthesia T88.59 ☑
    - in labor and delivery O74.4
    - in pregnancy O29.3X- ☑
    - postpartum, puerperal O89.3
  - toxin-antitoxin — *see* Complications, vaccination
  - transfusion (blood) (bone marrow) (lymphocytes) (allergic) — *see* Complications, transfusion
  - tuberculin skin test, abnormal R76.11
  - vaccination (any) — *see* Complications, vaccination
- **Reactive airway disease** — *see* Asthma
- **Reactive depression** — *see* Reaction, depressive
- **Rearrangement**
  - chromosomal
    - balanced (in) Q95.9
      - abnormal individual (autosomal) Q95.2
- **Rearrangement** — *continued*
  - chromosomal — *continued*
    - balanced — *continued*
      - abnormal individual — *continued*
        - non-sex (autosomal) chromosomes Q95.2
        - sex/non-sex chromosomes Q95.3
      - specified NEC Q95.8
- **Recalcitrant patient** — *see* Noncompliance
- **Recanalization, thrombus** — *see* Thrombosis
- **Recession, receding**
  - chamber angle (eye) H21.55- ☑
  - chin M26.09
  - gingival (postinfective) (postoperative)
    - generalized K06.020
      - minimal K06.021
      - moderate K06.022
      - severe K06.023
    - localized K06.010
      - minimal K06.011
      - moderate K06.012
      - severe K06.013
- **Recklinghausen disease** Q85.01
  - bones E21.0
- **Reclus' disease** (cystic) — *see* Mastopathy, cystic
- **Recrudescent typhus** (fever) A75.1
- **Recruitment, auditory** H93.21- ☑
- **Rectalgia** K62.89
- **Rectitis** K62.89
- **Rectocele**
  - female (without uterine prolapse) N81.6
    - with uterine prolapse N81.4
      - incomplete N81.2
  - in pregnancy — *see* Pregnancy, complicated by, abnormal, pelvic organs or tissues NEC
  - male K62.3
- **Rectosigmoid junction** — *see* condition
- **Rectosigmoiditis** K63.89
  - ulcerative (chronic) K51.30
    - with
      - complication K51.319
        - abscess K51.314
        - fistula K51.313
        - obstruction K51.312
        - rectal bleeding K51.311
        - specified NEC K51.318
- **Rectourethral** — *see* condition
- **Rectovaginal** — *see* condition
- **Rectovesical** — *see* condition
- **Rectum, rectal** — *see* condition
- **Recurrent** — *see* condition
  - pregnancy loss — *see* Loss (of), pregnancy, recurrent
- **Red bugs** B88.0
- **Red tide** — *see also* Table of Drugs and Chemicals T65.82- ☑
- **Red-cedar lung or pneumonitis** J67.8
- **Reduced**
  - mobility Z74.09
  - ventilatory or vital capacity R94.2
- **Redundant, redundancy**
  - anus (congenital) Q43.8
  - clitoris N90.89
  - colon (congenital) Q43.8
  - foreskin (congenital) N47.8
  - intestine (congenital) Q43.8
  - labia N90.69
  - organ or site, congenital NEC — *see* Accessory
  - panniculus (abdominal) E65
  - prepuce (congenital) N47.8
  - pylorus K31.89
  - rectum (congenital) Q43.8
  - scrotum N50.89
  - sigmoid (congenital) Q43.8
  - skin L98.7
    - and subcutaneous tissue L98.7
      - of face L57.4
        - eyelids — *see* Blepharochalasis
  - stomach K31.89
- **Reduplication** — *see* Duplication
- **Reflex** R29.2
  - hyperactive gag J39.2
  - pupillary, abnormal — *see* Anomaly, pupil, function
  - vasoconstriction I73.9
  - vasovagal R55
- **Reflux** K21.9
  - acid K21.9
  - esophageal K21.9
    - with esophagitis (without bleeding) K21.00
      - with bleeding K21.01
- **Reflux** — *continued*
  - esophageal — *continued*
    - newborn P78.83
  - gastroesophageal K21.9
    - with esophagitis (without bleeding) K21.00
      - with bleeding K21.01
  - mitral — *see* Insufficiency, mitral
  - ureteral — *see* Reflux, vesicoureteral
  - vesicoureteral (with scarring) N13.70
    - with
      - nephropathy N13.729
        - with hydroureter N13.739
          - bilateral N13.732
          - unilateral N13.731
        - bilateral N13.722
        - unilateral N13.721
        - without hydroureter N13.729
          - bilateral N13.722
          - unilateral N13.721
      - pyelonephritis (chronic) N11.0
    - congenital Q62.7
    - without nephropathy N13.71
- **Reforming, artificial openings** — *see* Attention to, artificial, opening
- **Refractive error** — *see* Disorder, refraction
- **Refsum's disease or syndrome** G60.1
- **Refusal of**
  - food, psychogenic F50.89
  - treatment (because of) Z53.20
    - left against medical advice (AMA) Z53.29
    - left without being seen Z53.21
    - patient's decision NEC Z53.29
    - reasons of belief or group pressure Z53.1
- **Regional** — *see* condition
- **Regurgitation** R11.10
  - aortic (valve) — *see* Insufficiency, aortic
  - food — *see also* Vomiting
    - with reswallowing — *see* Rumination
    - newborn P92.1
  - gastric contents — *see* Vomiting
  - heart — *see* Endocarditis
  - mitral (valve) — *see* Insufficiency, mitral
    - congenital Q23.3
  - myocardial — *see* Endocarditis
  - pulmonary (valve) (heart) I37.1
    - congenital Q22.2
    - syphilitic A52.03
  - tricuspid — *see* Insufficiency, tricuspid
  - valve, valvular — *see* Endocarditis
    - congenital Q24.8
  - vesicoureteral — *see* Reflux, vesicoureteral
- **Reichmann's disease or syndrome** K31.89
- **Reifenstein syndrome** E34.52
- **Reinsertion**
  - implantable subdermal contraceptive Z30.46
  - intrauterine contraceptive device Z30.433
- **Reiter's disease, syndrome, or urethritis** M02.30
  - ankle M02.37- ☑
  - elbow M02.32- ☑
  - foot joint M02.37- ☑
  - hand joint M02.34- ☑
  - hip M02.35- ☑
  - knee M02.36- ☑
  - multiple site M02.39
  - shoulder M02.31- ☑
  - vertebra M02.38
  - wrist M02.33- ☑
- **Rejection**
  - food, psychogenic F50.89
  - transplant T86.91
    - bone T86.830
      - marrow T86.01
    - cornea T86.840- ☑
    - heart T86.21
      - with lung(s) T86.31
    - intestine T86.850
    - kidney T86.11
    - liver T86.41
    - lung(s) T86.810
      - with heart T86.31
    - organ (immune or nonimmune cause) T86.91
    - pancreas T86.890
    - skin (allograft) (autograft) T86.820
    - specified NEC T86.890
    - stem cell (peripheral blood) (umbilical cord) T86.5
- **Relapsing fever** A68.9
  - Carter's (Asiatic) A68.1
  - Dutton's (West African) A68.1

- **Relapsing fever** — *continued*
  - Koch's A68.9
  - louse-borne (epidemic) A68.Ø
  - Novy's (American) A68.1
  - Obermeyers's (European) A68.Ø
  - Spirillum A68.9
  - tick-borne (endemic) A68.1
- **Relationship**
  - occlusal
    - open anterior M26.22Ø
    - open posterior M26.221
- **Relaxation**
  - anus (sphincter) K62.89
    - psychogenic F45.8
  - arch (foot) — *see also* Deformity, limb, flat foot
  - back ligaments — *see* Instability, joint, spine
  - bladder (sphincter) N31.2
  - cardioesophageal K21.9
  - cervix — *see* Incompetency, cervix
  - diaphragm J98.6
  - joint (capsule) (ligament) (paralytic) — *see* Flail, joint
    - congenital NEC Q74.8
  - lumbosacral (joint) — *see* subcategory M53.2 ☑
  - pelvic floor N81.89
  - perineum N81.89
  - posture R29.3
  - rectum (sphincter) K62.89
  - sacroiliac (joint) — *see* subcategory M53.2 ☑
  - scrotum N5Ø.89
  - urethra (sphincter) N36.44
  - vesical N31.2
- **Release from prison, anxiety concerning** Z65.2
- **Remains**
  - canal of Cloquet Q14.Ø
  - capsule (opaque) Q14.8
- **Remittent fever** (malarial) B54
- **Remnant**
  - canal of Cloquet Q14.Ø
  - capsule (opaque) Q14.8
  - cervix, cervical stump (acquired) (postoperative) N88.8
  - cystic duct, postcholecystectomy K91.5
  - fingernail L6Ø.8
    - congenital Q84.6
  - meniscus, knee — *see* Derangement, knee, meniscus, specified NEC
  - thyroglossal duct Q89.2
  - tonsil J35.8
    - infected (chronic) J35.Ø1
  - urachus Q64.4
- **Removal** (from) (of)
  - artificial
    - arm Z44.ØØ- ☑
      - complete Z44.Ø1- ☑
      - partial Z44.Ø2- ☑
    - eye Z44.2- ☑
    - leg Z44.1Ø- ☑
      - complete Z44.11- ☑
      - partial Z44.12- ☑
  - breast implant Z45.81 ☑
  - cardiac pulse generator (battery) (end-of-life) Z45.Ø1Ø
  - catheter (urinary) (indwelling) Z46.6
    - from artificial opening — *see* Attention to, artificial, opening
    - non-vascular Z46.82
    - vascular NEC Z45.2
  - device Z46.9
    - contraceptive Z3Ø.432
      - implantable subdermal Z3Ø.46
    - implanted NEC Z45.89
    - specified NEC Z46.89
  - drains Z48.Ø3
  - dressing (nonsurgical) Z48.ØØ
    - surgical Z48.Ø1
  - external
    - fixation device — *code to* fracture with seventh character D
    - prosthesis, prosthetic device Z44.9
      - breast Z44.3- ☑
      - specified NEC Z44.8
  - home in childhood (to foster home or institution) Z62.29
  - ileostomy Z43.2
  - insulin pump Z46.81
  - myringotomy device (stent) (tube) Z45.82
  - nervous system device NEC Z46.2
    - brain neuropacemaker Z46.2
    - visual substitution device Z46.2
      - implanted Z45.31
- **Removal** — *continued*
  - non-vascular catheter Z46.82
  - organ, prophylactic (for neoplasia management) — *see* Prophylactic, organ removal
  - orthodontic device Z46.4
  - staples Z48.Ø2
  - stent
    - ureteral Z46.6
  - suture Z48.Ø2
  - urinary device Z46.6
  - vascular access device or catheter Z45.2
- **Ren**
  - arcuatus Q63.1
  - mobile, mobilis N28.89
    - congenital Q63.8
  - unguliformis Q63.1
- **Renal** — *see* condition
- **Rendu-Osler-Weber disease or syndrome** I78.Ø
- **Reninoma** D41.Ø- ☑
- **Renon-Delille syndrome** E23.3
- **Reovirus, as cause of disease classified elsewhere** B97.5
- **Repeated falls NEC** R29.6
- **Replaced chromosome by dicentric ring** Q93.2
- **Replacement by artificial or mechanical device or prosthesis of**
  - bladder Z96.Ø
  - blood vessel NEC Z95.828
  - bone NEC Z96.7
  - cochlea Z96.21
  - coronary artery Z95.5
  - eustachian tube Z96.29
  - eye globe Z97.Ø
  - heart Z95.812
    - valve Z95.2
      - prosthetic Z95.2
      - specified NEC Z95.4
      - xenogenic Z95.3
  - intestine Z96.89
  - joint Z96.6Ø
    - hip — *see* Presence, hip joint implant
    - knee — *see* Presence, knee joint implant
    - specified site NEC Z96.698
  - larynx Z96.3
  - lens Z96.1
  - limb(s) — *see* Presence, artificial, limb
  - mandible NEC (for tooth root implant(s)) Z96.5
  - organ NEC Z96.89
  - peripheral vessel NEC Z95.828
  - stapes Z96.29
  - teeth Z97.2
  - tendon Z96.7
  - tissue NEC Z96.89
  - tooth root(s) Z96.5
  - vessel NEC Z95.828
    - coronary (artery) Z95.5
- **Request for expert evidence** ZØ4.89
- **Reserve, decreased or low**
  - cardiac — *see* Disease, heart
  - kidney N28.89
- **Residing**
  - in place not meant for human habitation (abandoned building) (car) (park) (sidewalk) Z59.Ø2
  - on the street Z59.Ø2
- **Residual** — *see also* condition
  - ovary syndrome N99.83
  - state, schizophrenic F2Ø.5
  - urine R39.198
- **Resistance, resistant** (to)
  - activated protein C D68.51
  - complicating pregnancy O26.89 ☑
  - insulin E88.81
  - organism(s)
    - to
      - drug Z16.3Ø
        - aminoglycosides Z16.29
        - amoxicillin Z16.11
        - ampicillin Z16.11
        - antibiotic(s) Z16.2Ø
          - multiple Z16.24
          - specified NEC Z16.29
        - antifungal Z16.32
        - antimicrobial (single) Z16.3Ø
          - multiple Z16.35
          - specified NEC Z16.39
        - antimycobacterial (single) Z16.341
          - multiple Z16.342
        - antiparasitic Z16.31
- **Resistance, resistant** — *continued*
  - organism(s) — *continued*
    - to — *continued*
      - drug — *continued*
        - antiviral Z16.33
        - beta lactam antibiotics Z16.1Ø
          - specified NEC Z16.19
        - cephalosporins Z16.19
        - extended beta lactamase (ESBL) Z16.12
        - fluoroquinolones Z16.23
        - macrolides Z16.29
        - methicillin — *see* MRSA
        - multiple drugs (MDRO)
          - antibiotics Z16.24
          - antimicrobial Z16.35
          - antimycobacterials Z16.342
        - penicillins Z16.11
        - quinine (and related compounds) Z16.31
        - quinolones Z16.23
        - sulfonamides Z16.29
        - tetracyclines Z16.29
        - tuberculostatics (single) Z16.341
          - multiple Z16.342
        - vancomycin Z16.21
          - related antibiotics Z16.22
  - thyroid hormone EØ7.89
- **Resorption**
  - dental (roots) KØ3.3
    - alveoli M26.79
  - teeth (external) (internal) (pathological) (roots) KØ3.3
- **Respiration**
  - Cheyne-Stokes RØ6.3
  - decreased due to shock, following injury T79.4 ☑
  - disorder of, psychogenic F45.8
  - insufficient, or poor RØ6.89
    - newborn P28.5
  - painful RØ7.1
  - sighing, psychogenic F45.8
- **Respiratory** — *see also* condition
  - distress syndrome (newborn) (type I) P22.Ø
    - type II P22.1
  - syncytial virus, as cause of disease classified elsewhere — *see also* Virus, respiratory syncytial (RSV) B97.4
- **Respite care** Z75.5
- **Response** (drug)
  - photoallergic L56.1
  - phototoxic L56.Ø
- **Restenosis**
  - stent
    - vascular
      - end stent
        - adjacent to stent — *see* Arteriosclerosis
        - within the stent
          - coronary T82.855 ☑
          - peripheral T82.856 ☑
      - in stent
        - coronary vessel T82.855 ☑
        - peripheral vessel T82.856 ☑
- **Restless legs** (syndrome) G25.81
- **Restlessness** R45.1
- **Restoration** (of)
  - dental
    - aesthetically inadequate or displeasing KØ8.56
    - defective KØ8.5Ø
      - specified NEC KØ8.59
    - failure of marginal integrity KØ8.51
    - failure of periodontal anatomical intergrity KØ8.54
  - organ continuity from previous sterilization (tuboplasty) (vasoplasty) Z31.Ø
    - aftercare Z31.42
  - tooth (existing)
    - contours biologically incompatible with oral health KØ8.54
    - open margins KØ8.51
    - overhanging KØ8.52
    - poor aesthetic KØ8.56
    - poor gingival margins KØ8.51
  - unsatisfactory, of tooth KØ8.5Ø
    - specified NEC KØ8.59
- **Restorative material** (dental)
  - allergy to KØ8.55
  - fractured KØ8.539
    - with loss of material KØ8.531
    - without loss of material KØ8.53Ø
  - unrepairable overhanging of KØ8.52
- **Restriction of housing space** Z59.1
- **Rests, ovarian, in fallopian tube** Q5Ø.6
- **Restzustand** (schizophrenic) F2Ø.5

- **Retained** — *see also* Retention
  - cholelithiasis following cholecystectomy K91.86
  - foreign body fragments (type of) Z18.9
    - acrylics Z18.2
    - animal quill(s) or spines Z18.31
    - cement Z18.83
    - concrete Z18.83
    - crystalline Z18.83
    - depleted isotope Z18.Ø9
    - depleted uranium Z18.Ø1
    - diethylhexyl phthalates Z18.2
    - glass Z18.81
    - isocyanate Z18.2
    - magnetic metal Z18.11
    - metal Z18.1Ø
    - nonmagnectic metal Z18.12
    - nontherapeutic radioactive Z18.Ø9
    - organic NEC Z18.39
    - plastic Z18.2
    - quill(s) (animal) Z18.31
    - radioactive (nontherapeutic) NEC Z18.Ø9
    - specified NEC Z18.89
    - spine(s) (animal) Z18.31
    - stone Z18.83
    - tooth (teeth) Z18.32
    - wood Z18.33
  - fragments (type of) Z18.9
    - acrylics Z18.2
    - animal quill(s) or spines Z18.31
    - cement Z18.83
    - concrete Z18.83
    - crystalline Z18.83
    - depleted isotope Z18.Ø9
    - depleted uranium Z18.Ø1
    - diethylhexyl phthalates Z18.2
    - glass Z18.81
    - isocyanate Z18.2
    - magnetic metal Z18.11
    - metal Z18.1Ø
    - nonmagnectic metal Z18.12
    - nontherapeutic radioactive Z18.Ø9
    - organic NEC Z18.39
    - plastic Z18.2
    - quill(s) (animal) Z18.31
    - radioactive (nontherapeutic) NEC Z18.Ø9
    - specified NEC Z18.89
    - spine(s) (animal) Z18.31
    - stone Z18.83
    - tooth (teeth) Z18.32
    - wood Z18.33
  - gallstones, following cholecystectomy K91.86
- **Retardation**
  - development, developmental, specific — *see* Disorder, developmental
  - endochondral bone growth — *see* Disorder, bone, development or growth
  - growth R62.5Ø
    - due to malnutrition E45
  - mental — *see* Disability, intellectual
  - motor function, specific F82
  - physical (child) R62.52
    - due to malnutrition E45
  - reading (specific) F81.Ø
  - spelling (specific) (without reading disorder) F81.81
- **Retching** — *see* Vomiting
- **Retention** — *see also* Retained
  - bladder — *see* Retention, urine
  - carbon dioxide E87.29
  - cholelithiasis following cholecystectomy K91.86
  - cyst — *see* Cyst
  - dead
    - fetus (at or near term) (mother) O36.4 ☑
      - early fetal death OØ2.1
    - ovum OØ2.Ø
  - decidua (fragments) (following delivery) (with hemorrhage) O72.2
    - without hemorrhage O73.1
  - deciduous tooth KØØ.6
  - dental root KØ8.3
  - fecal — *see* Constipation
  - fetus
    - dead O36.4 ☑
      - early OØ2.1
  - fluid R6Ø.9
  - foreign body — *see also* Foreign body, retained
    - current trauma — *code as* Foreign body, by site or type
  - gallstones, following cholecystectomy K91.86

- **Retention** — *continued*
  - gastric K31.89
  - intrauterine contraceptive device, in pregnancy — *see* Pregnancy, complicated by, retention, intrauterine device
  - membranes (complicating delivery) (with hemorrhage) O72.2
    - with abortion — *see* Abortion, by type
    - without hemorrhage O73.1
  - meniscus — *see* Derangement, meniscus
  - menses N94.89
  - milk (puerperal, postpartum) O92.79
  - nitrogen, extrarenal R39.2
  - ovary syndrome N99.83
  - placenta (total) (with hemorrhage) O72.Ø
    - without hemorrhage O73.Ø
    - portions or fragments (with hemorrhage) O72.2
      - without hemorrhage O73.1
  - products of conception
    - early pregnancy (dead fetus) OØ2.1
    - following
      - delivery (with hemorrhage) O72.2
        - without hemorrhage O73.1
  - secundines (following delivery) (with hemorrhage) O72.Ø
    - without hemorrhage O73.Ø
    - complicating puerperium (delayed hemorrhage) O72.2
    - partial O72.2
      - without hemorrhage O73.1
  - smegma, clitoris N9Ø.89
  - urine R33.9
    - due to hyperplasia (hypertrophy) of prostate — *see* Hyperplasia, prostate
    - drug-induced R33.Ø
    - organic R33.8
      - drug-induced R33.Ø
    - psychogenic F45.8
    - specified NEC R33.8
  - water (in tissues) — *see* Edema
- **Reticulation, dust** — *see* Pneumoconiosis
- **Reticulocytosis** R7Ø.1
- **Reticuloendotheliosis**
  - acute infantile C96.Ø
  - leukemic C91.4- ☑
  - nonlipid C96.Ø
- **Reticulohistiocytoma** (giant-cell) D76.3
- **Reticuloid, actinic** L57.1
- **Reticulosis** (skin)
  - acute of infancy C96.Ø
  - hemophagocytic, familial D76.1
  - histiocytic medullary C96.A (*following* C96.6)
  - lipomelanotic I89.8
  - malignant (midline) C86.Ø
  - polymorphic C83.8- ☑
  - Sézary — *see* Sézary disease
- **Retina, retinal** — *see also* condition
  - dark area D49.81
- **Retinitis** — *see also* Inflammation, chorioretinal
  - albuminurica N18.9 *[H32]*
  - diabetic — *see* Diabetes, retinitis
  - disciformis — *see* Degeneration, macula
  - focal — *see* Inflammation, chorioretinal, focal
  - gravidarum — *see* Pregnancy, complicated by, specified pregnancy-related condition NEC
  - juxtapapillaris — *see* Inflammation, chorioretinal, focal, juxtapapillary
  - luetic — *see* Retinitis, syphilitic
  - pigmentosa H35.52
  - proliferans — *see* Disorder, globe, degenerative, specified type NEC
  - proliferating — *see* Disorder, globe, degenerative, specified type NEC
  - renal N18.9 *[H32]*
  - syphilitic (early) (secondary) A51.43
    - central, recurrent A52.71
    - congenital (early) A5Ø.Ø1 *[H32]*
    - late A52.71
  - tuberculous A18.53
- **Retinoblastoma** C69.2- ☑
  - differentiated C69.2- ☑
  - undifferentiated C69.2- ☑
- **Retinochoroiditis** — *see also* Inflammation, chorioretinal
  - disseminated — *see* Inflammation, chorioretinal, disseminated
    - syphilitic A52.71
  - focal — *see* Inflammation, chorioretinal

- **Retinochoroiditis** — *continued*
  - juxtapapillaris — *see* Inflammation, chorioretinal, focal, juxtapapillary
- **Retinopathy** (background) H35.ØØ
  - arteriosclerotic I7Ø.8 *[H35.Ø-]* ☑
  - atherosclerotic I7Ø.8 *[H35.Ø-]* ☑
  - central serous — *see* Chorioretinopathy, central serous
  - Coats H35.Ø2- ☑
  - diabetic — *see* Diabetes, retinopathy
  - exudative H35.Ø2- ☑
  - hypertensive H35.Ø3- ☑
  - in (due to)
    - diabetes — *see* Diabetes, retinopathy
    - sickle-cell disorders D57.- ☑ *[H36]*
  - of prematurity H35.1Ø- ☑
    - stage Ø H35.11- ☑
    - stage 1 H35.12- ☑
    - stage 2 H35.13- ☑
    - stage 3 H35.14- ☑
    - stage 4 H35.15- ☑
    - stage 5 H35.16- ☑
  - pigmentary, congenital — *see* Dystrophy, retina
  - proliferative NEC H35.2- ☑
    - diabetic — *see* Diabetes, retinopathy, proliferative
    - sickle-cell D57.- ☑ *[H36]*
  - solar H31.Ø2- ☑
- **Retinoschisis** H33.1Ø- ☑
  - congenital Q14.1
  - specified type NEC H33.19- ☑
- **Retortamoniasis** AØ7.8
- **Retractile testis** Q55.22
- **Retraction**
  - cervix — *see* Retroversion, uterus
  - drum (membrane) — *see* Disorder, tympanic membrane, specified NEC
  - finger — *see* Deformity, finger
  - lid HØ2.539
    - left HØ2.536
      - lower HØ2.535
      - upper HØ2.534
    - right HØ2.533
      - lower HØ2.532
      - upper HØ2.531
  - lung J98.4
  - mediastinum J98.59
  - nipple N64.53
    - associated with
      - lactation O92.Ø3
      - pregnancy O92.Ø1- ☑
      - puerperium O92.Ø2
    - congenital Q83.8
  - palmar fascia M72.Ø
  - pleura — *see* Pleurisy
  - ring, uterus (Bandl's) (pathological) O62.4
  - sternum (congenital) Q76.7
    - acquired M95.4
  - uterus — *see* Retroversion, uterus
  - valve (heart) — *see* Endocarditis
- **Retrobulbar** — *see* condition
- **Retrocecal** — *see* condition
- **Retrocession** — *see* Retroversion
- **Retrodisplacement** — *see* Retroversion
- **Retroflection, retroflexion** — *see* Retroversion
- **Retrognathia, retrognathism** (mandibular) (maxillary) M26.19
- **Retrograde menstruation** N92.5
- **Retroperineal** — *see* condition
- **Retroperitoneal** — *see* condition
- **Retroperitonitis** K68.9
- **Retropharyngeal** — *see* condition
- **Retroplacental** — *see* condition
- **Retroposition** — *see* Retroversion
- **Retroprosthetic membrane** T85.398 ☑
- **Retrosternal thyroid** (congenital) Q89.2
- **Retroversion, retroverted**
  - cervix — *see* Retroversion, uterus
  - female NEC — *see* Retroversion, uterus
  - iris H21.89
  - testis (congenital) Q55.29
  - uterus (acquired) (acute) (any degree) (asymptomatic) (cervix) (postinfectional) (postpartal, old) N85.4
    - congenital Q51.818
    - in pregnancy O34.53- ☑
- **Retrovirus, as cause of disease classified elsewhere** B97.3Ø
  - human
    - immunodeficiency, type 2 (HIV 2) B97.35

- **Retrovirus, as cause of disease classified elsewhere** — *continued*
  - human — *continued*
    - T-cell lymphotropic
      - type I (HTLV-I) B97.33
      - type II (HTLV-II) B97.34
  - lentivirus B97.31
  - oncovirus B97.32
  - specified NEC B97.39
- **Retrusion, premaxilla** (developmental) M26.Ø9
- **Rett's disease or syndrome** F84.2
- **Reverse peristalsis** R19.2
- **Reye's syndrome** G93.7
- **Rh** (factor)
  - hemolytic disease (newborn) P55.Ø
  - incompatibility, immunization or sensitization
    - affecting management of pregnancy NEC O36.Ø9- ☑
      - anti-D antibody O36.Ø1- ☑
    - newborn P55.Ø
    - transfusion reaction — *see* Complication(s), transfusion, incompatibility reaction, Rh (factor)
  - negative mother affecting newborn P55.Ø
  - titer elevated — *see* Complication(s), transfusion, incompatibility reaction, Rh (factor)
  - transfusion reaction — *see* Complication(s), transfusion, incompatibility reaction, Rh (factor)
- **Rhabdomyolysis** (idiopathic) NEC M62.82
  - traumatic T79.6 ☑
- **Rhabdomyoma** — *see also* Neoplasm, connective tissue, benign
  - adult — *see* Neoplasm, connective tissue, benign
  - fetal — *see* Neoplasm, connective tissue, benign
  - glycogenic — *see* Neoplasm, connective tissue, benign
- **Rhabdomyosarcoma** (any type) — *see* Neoplasm, connective tissue, malignant
- **Rhabdosarcoma** — *see* Rhabdomyosarcoma
- **Rhesus** (factor) **incompatibility** — *see* Rh, incompatibility
- **Rheumatic** (acute) (subacute)
  - adherent pericardium IØ9.2
  - chronic IØ9.89
  - coronary arteritis IØ1.8
  - degeneration, myocardium IØ9.Ø
  - fever (acute) — *see* Fever, rheumatic
  - heart — *see* Disease, heart, rheumatic
  - myocardial degeneration — *see* Degeneration, myocardium
  - myocarditis (chronic) (inactive) (with chorea) IØ9.Ø
    - active or acute IØ1.2
      - with chorea (acute) (rheumatic) (Sydenham's) IØ2.Ø
  - pancarditis, acute IØ1.8
    - with chorea (acute (rheumatic) Sydenham's) IØ2.Ø
  - pericarditis (active) (acute) (with effusion) (with pneumonia) IØ1.Ø
    - with chorea (acute) (rheumatic) (Sydenham's) IØ2.Ø
    - chronic or inactive IØ9.2
  - pneumonia IØØ *[J17]*
  - torticollis M43.6
  - typhoid fever AØ1.Ø9
- **Rheumatism** (articular) (neuralgic) (nonarticular) M79.Ø
  - gout — *see* Arthritis, rheumatoid
  - intercostal, meaning Tietze's disease M94.Ø
  - palindromic (any site) M12.3Ø
    - ankle M12.37- ☑
    - elbow M12.32- ☑
    - foot joint M12.37- ☑
    - hand joint M12.34- ☑
    - hip M12.35- ☑
    - knee M12.36- ☑
    - multiple site M12.39
    - shoulder M12.31- ☑
    - specified joint NEC M12.38
    - vertebrae M12.38
    - wrist M12.33- ☑
  - sciatic M54.4- ☑
- **Rheumatoid** — *see also* condition
  - arthritis — *see also* Arthritis, rheumatoid
    - with involvement of organs NEC MØ5.6Ø
      - ankle MØ5.67- ☑
      - elbow MØ5.62- ☑
      - foot joint MØ5.67- ☑
      - hand joint MØ5.64- ☑
      - hip MØ5.65- ☑
      - knee MØ5.66- ☑
      - multiple site MØ5.69
      - shoulder MØ5.61- ☑
      - vertebra — *see* Spondylitis, ankylosing
- **Rheumatoid** — *continued*
  - arthritis — *see also* Arthritis, rheumatoid — *continued*
    - with involvement of organs — *continued*
      - wrist MØ5.63- ☑
    - seronegative — *see* Arthritis, rheumatoid, seronegative
    - seropositive — *see* Arthritis, rheumatoid, seropositive
  - carditis MØ5.3Ø
    - ankle MØ5.37- ☑
    - elbow MØ5.32- ☑
    - foot joint MØ5.37- ☑
    - hand joint MØ5.34- ☑
    - hip MØ5.35- ☑
    - knee MØ5.36- ☑
    - multiple site MØ5.39
    - shoulder MØ5.31- ☑
    - vertebra — *see* Spondylitis, ankylosing
    - wrist MØ5.33- ☑
  - endocarditis — *see* Rheumatoid, carditis
  - lung (disease) MØ5.1Ø
    - ankle MØ5.17- ☑
    - elbow MØ5.12- ☑
    - foot joint MØ5.17- ☑
    - hand joint MØ5.14- ☑
    - hip MØ5.15- ☑
    - knee MØ5.16- ☑
    - multiple site MØ5.19
    - shoulder MØ5.11- ☑
    - vertebra — *see* Spondylitis, ankylosing
    - wrist MØ5.13- ☑
  - myocarditis — *see* Rheumatoid, carditis
  - myopathy MØ5.4Ø
    - ankle MØ5.47- ☑
    - elbow MØ5.42- ☑
    - foot joint MØ5.47- ☑
    - hand joint MØ5.44- ☑
    - hip MØ5.45- ☑
    - knee MØ5.46- ☑
    - multiple site MØ5.49
    - shoulder MØ5.41- ☑
    - vertebra — *see* Spondylitis, ankylosing
    - wrist MØ5.43- ☑
  - pericarditis — *see* Rheumatoid, carditis
  - polyarthritis — *see* Arthritis, rheumatoid
  - polyneuropathy MØ5.5Ø
    - ankle MØ5.57- ☑
    - elbow MØ5.52- ☑
    - foot joint MØ5.57- ☑
    - hand joint MØ5.54- ☑
    - hip MØ5.55- ☑
    - knee MØ5.56- ☑
    - multiple site MØ5.59
    - shoulder MØ5.51- ☑
    - vertebra — *see* Spondylitis, ankylosing
    - wrist MØ5.53- ☑
  - vasculitis MØ5.2Ø
    - ankle MØ5.27- ☑
    - elbow MØ5.22- ☑
    - foot joint MØ5.27- ☑
    - hand joint MØ5.24- ☑
    - hip MØ5.25- ☑
    - knee MØ5.26- ☑
    - multiple site MØ5.29
    - shoulder MØ5.21- ☑
    - vertebra — *see* Spondylitis, ankylosing
    - wrist MØ5.23- ☑
- **Rhinitis** (atrophic) (catarrhal) (chronic) (croupous) (fibrinous) (granulomatous) (hyperplastic) (hypertrophic) (membranous) (obstructive) (purulent) (suppurative) (ulcerative) J31.Ø
  - with
    - sore throat — *see* Nasopharyngitis
  - acute JØØ
  - allergic J3Ø.9
    - with asthma J45.9Ø9
      - with
        - exacerbation (acute) J45.9Ø1
        - status asthmaticus J45.9Ø2
    - due to
      - food J3Ø.5
      - pollen J3Ø.1
    - nonseasonal J3Ø.89
    - perennial J3Ø.89
    - seasonal NEC J3Ø.2
    - specified NEC J3Ø.89
- **Rhinitis** — *continued*
  - infective JØØ
  - pneumococcal JØØ
  - syphilitic A52.73
    - congenital A5Ø.Ø5 *[J99]*
  - tuberculous A15.8
  - vasomotor J3Ø.Ø
- **Rhinoantritis** (chronic) — *see* Sinusitis, maxillary
- **Rhinodacryolith** — *see* Dacryolith
- **Rhinolith** (nasal sinus) J34.89
- **Rhinomegaly** J34.89
- **Rhinopharyngitis** (acute) (subacute) — *see also* Nasopharyngitis
  - chronic J31.1
  - destructive ulcerating A66.5
  - mutilans A66.5
- **Rhinophyma** L71.1
- **Rhinorrhea** J34.89
  - cerebrospinal (fluid) G96.Ø1
    - postoperative G96.Ø8
    - specified NEC G96.Ø8
    - spontaneous G96.Ø1
    - traumatic G96.Ø8
  - paroxysmal — *see* Rhinitis, allergic
  - spasmodic — *see* Rhinitis, allergic
- **Rhinosalpingitis** — *see* Salpingitis, eustachian
- **Rhinoscleroma** A48.8
- **Rhinosporidiosis** B48.1
- **Rhinovirus infection NEC** B34.8
- **Rhizomelic chondrodysplasia punctata** E71.54Ø
- **Rhythm**
  - atrioventricular nodal I49.8
  - disorder I49.9
    - coronary sinus I49.8
    - ectopic I49.8
    - nodal I49.8
  - escape I49.9
  - heart, abnormal I49.9
  - idioventricular I44.2
  - nodal I49.8
  - sleep, inversion G47.2- ☑
    - nonorganic origin — *see* Disorder, sleep, circadian rhythm, psychogenic
- **Rhytidosis facialis** L98.8
- **Rib** — *see also* condition
  - cervical Q76.5
- **Riboflavin deficiency** E53.Ø
- **Rice bodies** — *see also* Loose, body, joint
  - knee M23.4- ☑
- **Richter syndrome** — *see* Leukemia, chronic lymphocytic, B-cell type
- **Richter's hernia** — *see* Hernia, abdomen, with obstruction
- **Ricinism** — *see* Poisoning, food, noxious, plant
- **Rickets** (active) (acute) (adolescent) (chest wall) (congenital) (current) (infantile) (intestinal) E55.Ø
  - adult — *see* Osteomalacia
  - celiac K9Ø.Ø
  - hypophosphatemic with nephrotic-glycosuric dwarfism E72.Ø9
  - inactive E64.3
  - kidney N25.Ø
  - renal N25.Ø
  - sequelae, any E64.3
  - vitamin-D-resistant E83.31 *[M9Ø.8Ø]*
- **Rickettsia 364D/R. philipii** (Pacific Coast tick fever) A77.8
- **Rickettsial disease** A79.9
  - specified type NEC A79.89
- **Rickettsialpox** (Rickettsia akari) A79.1
- **Rickettsiosis** A79.9
  - due to
    - Ehrlichia sennetsu A79.81
    - Neorickettsia sennetsu A79.81
    - Rickettsia akari (rickettsialpox) A79.1
  - specified type NEC A79.89
  - tick-borne A77.9
  - vesicular A79.1
- **Rider's bone** — *see* Ossification, muscle, specified NEC
- **Ridge, alveolus** — *see also* condition
  - flabby KØ6.8
- **Ridged ear, congenital** Q17.3
- **Riedel's**
  - lobe, liver Q44.7
  - struma, thyroiditis or disease EØ6.5
- **Rieger's anomaly or syndrome** Q13.81
- **Riehl's melanosis** L81.4

Rietti-Greppi-Micheli anemia D56.9
Rieux's hernia — *see* Hernia, abdomen, specified site NEC
Riga (-Fede) **disease** K14.Ø
Riggs' disease — *see* Periodontitis
Right aortic arch Q25.47
Right middle lobe syndrome J98.11
Rigid, rigidity — *see also* condition
abdominal R19.3Ø
with severe abdominal pain R1Ø.Ø
epigastric R19.36
generalized R19.37
left lower quadrant R19.34
left upper quadrant R19.32
periumbilic R19.35
right lower quadrant R19.33
right upper quadrant R19.31
articular, multiple, congenital Q68.8
cervix (uteri) in pregnancy — *see* Pregnancy, complicated by, abnormal, cervix
hymen (acquired) (congenital) N89.6
nuchal R29.1
pelvic floor in pregnancy — *see* Pregnancy, complicated by, abnormal, pelvic organs or tissues NEC
perineum or vulva in pregnancy — *see* Pregnancy, complicated by, abnormal, vulva
spine — *see* Dorsopathy, specified NEC
vagina in pregnancy — *see* Pregnancy, complicated by, abnormal, vagina
Rigors R68.89
with fever R5Ø.9
Riley-Day syndrome G9Ø.1
RIND (reversible ischemic neurologic deficit) I63.9
Ring(s)
aorta (vascular) Q25.45
Bandl's O62.4
contraction, complicating delivery O62.4
esophageal, lower (muscular) K22.2
Fleischer's (cornea) H18.Ø4- ☑
hymenal, tight (acquired) (congenital) N89.6
Kayser-Fleischer (cornea) H18.Ø4- ☑
retraction, uterus, pathological O62.4
Schatzki's (esophagus) (lower) K22.2
congenital Q39.3
Soemmerring's — *see* Cataract, secondary
vascular (congenital) Q25.8
aorta Q25.45
Ringed hair (congenital) Q84.1
Ringworm B35.9
beard B35.Ø
black dot B35.Ø
body B35.4
Burmese B35.5
corporeal B35.4
foot B35.3
groin B35.6
hand B35.2
honeycomb B35.Ø
nails B35.1
perianal (area) B35.6
scalp B35.Ø
specified NEC B35.8
Tokelau B35.5
Rise, venous pressure I87.8
Rising, PSA following treatment for malignant neoplasm of prostate R97.21
Risk
for
dental caries Z91.849
high Z91.843
low Z91.841
moderate Z91.842
homelessness, imminent Z59.811
suffocation (smothering) under another while sleeping Z72.823
suicidal
meaning personal history of attempted suicide Z91.51
meaning suicidal ideation — *see* Ideation, suicidal
Ritter's disease LØØ
Rivalry, sibling Z62.891
Rivalta's disease A42.2
River blindness B73.Ø1
Robert's pelvis Q74.2
with disproportion (fetopelvic) O33.Ø
causing obstructed labor O65.Ø
Robin (-Pierre) **syndrome** Q87.Ø
Robinow-Silvermann-Smith syndrome Q87.19
Robinson's (hidrotic) **ectodermal dysplasia or syndrome** Q82.4
Robles' disease B73.Ø1
Rocky Mountain (spotted) **fever** A77.Ø
Roetheln — *see* Rubella
Roger's disease Q21.Ø
Rokitansky-Aschoff sinuses (gallbladder) K82.8
Rolando's fracture (displaced) S62.22- ☑
nondisplaced S62.22- ☑
Romano-Ward (prolonged QT interval) **syndrome** I45.81
Romberg's disease or syndrome G51.8
Roof, mouth — *see* condition
Rosacea L71.9
acne L71.9
keratitis L71.8
specified NEC L71.8
Rosary, rachitic E55.Ø
Rose
cold J3Ø.1
fever J3Ø.1
rash R21
epidemic BØ6.9
Rosenbach's erysipeloid A26.Ø
Rosenthal's disease or syndrome D68.1
Roseola BØ9
infantum BØ8.2Ø
due to human herpesvirus 6 BØ8.21
due to human herpesvirus 7 BØ8.22
Ross River disease or fever B33.1
Rossbach's disease K31.89
psychogenic F45.8
Rostan's asthma (cardiac) — *see* Failure, ventricular, left
Rotation
anomalous, incomplete or insufficient, intestine Q43.3
cecum (congenital) Q43.3
colon (congenital) Q43.3
spine, incomplete or insufficient — *see* Dorsopathy, deforming, specified NEC
tooth, teeth, fully erupted M26.35
vertebra, incomplete or insufficient — *see* Dorsopathy, deforming, specified NEC
Rotes Quérol disease or syndrome — *see* Hyperostosis, ankylosing
Roth (-Bernhardt) **disease or syndrome** — *see* Meralgia paraesthetica
Rothmund (-Thomson) **syndrome** Q82.8
Rotor's disease or syndrome E8Ø.6
Round
back (with wedging of vertebrae) — *see* Kyphosis
sequelae (late effect) of rickets E64.3
worms (large) (infestation) NEC B82.Ø
Ascariasis — *see also* Ascariasis B77.9
Roussy-Lévy syndrome G6Ø.Ø
Rubella (German measles) BØ6.9
complication NEC BØ6.Ø9
neurological BØ6.ØØ
congenital P35.Ø
contact Z2Ø.4
exposure to Z2Ø.4
maternal
care for (suspected) damage to fetus O35.3 ☑
manifest rubella in infant P35.Ø
suspected damage to fetus affecting management of pregnancy O35.3 ☑
specified complications NEC BØ6.89
Rubeola (meaning measles) — *see* Measles
meaning rubella — *see* Rubella
Rubeosis, iris — *see* Disorder, iris, vascular
Rubinstein-Taybi syndrome Q87.2
Rudimentary (congenital) — *see also* Agenesis
arm — *see* Defect, reduction, upper limb
bone Q79.9
cervix uteri Q51.828
eye Q11.2
lobule of ear Q17.3
patella Q74.1
respiratory organs in thoracopagus Q89.4
tracheal bronchus Q32.4
uterus Q51.818
in male Q56.1
vagina Q52.Ø
Ruled out condition — *see* Observation, suspected
Rumination R11.1Ø
with nausea R11.2
disorder of infancy F98.21
neurotic F42.8
newborn P92.1
Rumination — *continued*
obsessional F42.8
psychogenic F42.8
Runeberg's disease D51.Ø
Running out of money Z59.86
Runny nose RØ9.89
Rupia (syphilitic) A51.39
congenital A5Ø.Ø6
tertiary A52.79
Rupture, ruptured
abscess (spontaneous) — *code by* site under Abscess
aneurysm — *see* Aneurysm
anus (sphincter) — *see* Laceration, anus
aorta, aortic I71.8
abdominal I71.3Ø
infrarenal I71.33
juxtarenal I71.32
pararenal I71.31
arch I71.12
ascending I71.11
descending I71.8
abdominal I71.3Ø
thoracic I71.13
syphilitic A52.Ø1
thoracoabdominal I71.5Ø
paravisceral I71.52
supraceliac I71.51
thorax, thoracic I71.1Ø
transverse I71.12
traumatic — *see* Injury, aorta, laceration, major
valve or cusp — *see also* Endocarditis, aortic I35.8
appendix (with peritonitis) — *see also* Appendicitis K35.32
with localized peritonitis — *see also* Appendicitis K35.32
arteriovenous fistula, brain — *see* Fistula, arteriovenous, brain, ruptured
artery I77.2
brain — *see* Hemorrhage, intracranial, intracerebral
coronary — *see* Infarct, myocardium
heart — *see* Infarct, myocardium
pulmonary I28.8
traumatic (complication) — *see* Injury, blood vessel
bile duct (common) (hepatic) K83.2
cystic K82.2
bladder (sphincter) (nontraumatic) (spontaneous) N32.89
following ectopic or molar pregnancy OØ8.6
obstetrical trauma O71.5
traumatic S37.29 ☑
blood vessel — *see also* Hemorrhage
brain — *see* Hemorrhage, intracranial, intracerebral
heart — *see* Infarct, myocardium
traumatic (complication) — *see* Injury, blood vessel, laceration, major, by site
bone — *see* Fracture
bowel (nontraumatic) K63.1
brain
aneurysm (congenital) — *see also* Hemorrhage, intracranial, subarachnoid
syphilitic A52.Ø5
hemorrhagic — *see* Hemorrhage, intracranial, intracerebral
capillaries I78.8
cardiac (auricle) (ventricle) (wall) I23.3
with hemopericardium I23.Ø
infectional I4Ø.9
traumatic — *see* Injury, heart
cartilage (articular) (current) — *see also* Sprain
knee S83.3- ☑
semilunar — *see* Tear, meniscus
cecum (with peritonitis) K65.Ø
with peritoneal abscess K35.33
traumatic S36.598 ☑
celiac artery, traumatic — *see* Injury, blood vessel, celiac artery, laceration, major
cerebral aneurysm (congenital) (see Hemorrhage, intracranial, subarachnoid)
cervix (uteri)
with ectopic or molar pregnancy OØ8.6
following ectopic or molar pregnancy OØ8.6
obstetrical trauma O71.3
traumatic S37.69 ☑
chordae tendineae NEC I51.1
concurrent with acute myocardial infarction — *see* Infarct, myocardium
following acute myocardial infarction (current complication) I23.4

Rupture, ruptured — *continued*
- choroid (direct) (indirect) (traumatic) H31.32- ☑
- circle of Willis I6Ø.6
- colon (nontraumatic) K63.1
  - traumatic — *see* Injury, intestine, large
- cornea (traumatic) — *see* Injury, eye, laceration
- coronary (artery) (thrombotic) — *see* Infarct, myocardium
- corpus luteum (infected) (ovary) N83.1- ☑
- cyst — *see* Cyst
- cystic duct K82.2
- Descemet's membrane — *see* Change, corneal membrane, Descemet's, rupture
  - traumatic — *see* Injury, eye, laceration
- diaphragm, traumatic — *see* Injury, intrathoracic, diaphragm
- disc — *see* Rupture, intervertebral disc
- diverticulum (intestine) K57.8Ø
  - with bleeding K57.81
  - bladder N32.3
  - large intestine K57.2Ø
    - with
      - bleeding K57.21
      - small intestine K57.4Ø
        - with bleeding K57.41
  - small intestine K57.ØØ
    - with
      - bleeding K57.Ø1
      - large intestine K57.4Ø
        - with bleeding K57.41
- duodenal stump K31.89
- ear drum (nontraumatic) — *see also* Perforation, tympanum
  - traumatic SØ9.2- ☑
    - due to blast injury — *see* Injury, blast, ear
- esophagus K22.3
- eye (without prolapse or loss of intraocular tissue) — *see* Injury, eye, laceration
- fallopian tube NEC (nonobstetric) (nontraumatic) N83.8
  - due to pregnancy OØØ.1Ø- ☑
    - with intrauterine pregnancy OØØ.11- ☑
- fontanel P13.1
- gallbladder K82.2
  - traumatic S36.128 ☑
- gastric — *see also* Rupture, stomach
  - vessel K92.2
- globe (eye) (traumatic) — *see* Injury, eye, laceration
- graafian follicle (hematoma) N83.Ø- ☑
- heart — *see* Rupture, cardiac
- hymen (nontraumatic) (nonintentional) N89.8
- internal organ, traumatic — *see* Injury, by site
- intervertebral disc — *see* Displacement, intervertebral disc
  - traumatic — *see* Rupture, traumatic, intervertebral disc
- intestine NEC (nontraumatic) K63.1
  - traumatic — *see* Injury, intestine
- iris — *see also* Abnormality, pupillary
  - traumatic — *see* Injury, eye, laceration
- joint capsule, traumatic — *see* Sprain
- kidney (traumatic) S37.Ø6- ☑
  - birth injury P15.8
  - nontraumatic N28.89
- lacrimal duct (traumatic) — *see* Injury, eye, specified site NEC
- lens (cataract) (traumatic) — *see* Cataract, traumatic
- ligament, traumatic — *see* Rupture, traumatic, ligament, by site
- liver S36.116 ☑
  - birth injury P15.Ø
- lymphatic vessel I89.8
- marginal sinus (placental) (with hemorrhage) — *see* Hemorrhage, antepartum, specified cause NEC
- membrana tympani (nontraumatic) — *see* Perforation, tympanum
- membranes (spontaneous)
  - artificial
    - delayed delivery following O75.5
  - delayed delivery following — *see* Pregnancy, complicated by, premature rupture of membranes
- meningeal artery I6Ø.8
- meniscus (knee) — *see also* Tear, meniscus
  - old — *see* Derangement, meniscus
  - site other than knee — *code as* Sprain
- mesenteric artery, traumatic — *see* Injury, mesenteric, artery, laceration, major
- mesentery (nontraumatic) K66.8

Rupture, ruptured — *continued*
- mesentery — *continued*
  - traumatic — *see* Injury, intra-abdominal, specified, site NEC
- mitral (valve) I34.89
- muscle (traumatic) — *see also* Strain
  - diastasis — *see* Diastasis, muscle
  - nontraumatic M62.1Ø
    - ankle M62.17- ☑
    - foot M62.17- ☑
    - forearm M62.13- ☑
    - hand M62.14- ☑
    - lower leg M62.16- ☑
    - pelvic region M62.15- ☑
    - shoulder region M62.11- ☑
    - specified site NEC M62.18
    - thigh M62.15- ☑
    - upper arm M62.12- ☑
  - traumatic — *see* Strain, by site
- musculotendinous junction NEC, nontraumatic — *see* Rupture, tendon, spontaneous
- mycotic aneurysm causing cerebral hemorrhage — *see* Hemorrhage, intracranial, subarachnoid
- myocardium, myocardial — *see* Rupture, cardiac
  - traumatic — *see* Injury, heart
- nontraumatic, meaning hernia — *see* Hernia
- obstructed — *see* Hernia, by site, obstructed
- operation wound — *see* Disruption, wound, operation
- ovary, ovarian N83.8
  - corpus luteum cyst N83.1- ☑
  - follicle (graafian) N83.Ø- ☑
- oviduct (nonobstetric) (nontraumatic) N83.8
  - due to pregnancy OØØ.1Ø- ☑
    - with intrauterine pregnancy OØØ.11- ☑
- pancreas (nontraumatic) K86.89
  - traumatic S36.299 ☑
- papillary muscle NEC I51.2
  - following acute myocardial infarction (current complication) I23.5
- pelvic
  - floor, complicating delivery O7Ø.1
  - organ NEC, obstetrical trauma O71.5
- perineum (nonobstetric) (nontraumatic) N9Ø.89
  - complicating delivery — *see* Delivery, complicated, by, laceration, anus (sphincter)
- postoperative wound — *see* Disruption, wound, operation
- prostate (traumatic) S37.828 ☑
- pulmonary
  - artery I28.8
  - valve (heart) I37.8
  - vein I28.8
  - vessel I28.8
- pus tube — *see* Salpingitis
- pyosalpinx — *see* Salpingitis
- rectum (nontraumatic) K63.1
  - traumatic S36.69 ☑
- retina, retinal (traumatic) (without detachment) — *see also* Break, retina
  - with detachment — *see* Detachment, retina, with retinal, break
- rotator cuff (nontraumatic) M75.1Ø- ☑
  - complete M75.12- ☑
  - incomplete M75.11- ☑
- sclera — *see* Injury, eye, laceration
- sigmoid (nontraumatic) K63.1
  - traumatic S36.593 ☑
- spinal cord — *see also* Injury, spinal cord, by region
  - due to injury at birth P11.5
  - newborn (birth injury) P11.5
- spleen (traumatic) S36.Ø9 ☑
  - birth injury P15.1
  - congenital (birth injury) P15.1
  - due to P. vivax malaria B51.Ø
  - nontraumatic D73.5
  - spontaneous D73.5
- splenic vein R58
  - traumatic — *see* Injury, blood vessel, splenic vein
- stomach (nontraumatic) (spontaneous) K31.89
  - traumatic S36.39 ☑
- supraspinatus (complete) (incomplete) (nontraumatic) — *see* Tear, rotator cuff
- symphysis pubis
  - obstetric O71.6
  - traumatic S33.4 ☑
- synovium (cyst) M66.1Ø
  - ankle M66.17- ☑

Rupture, ruptured — *continued*
- synovium — *continued*
  - elbow M66.12- ☑
  - finger M66.14- ☑
  - foot M66.17- ☑
  - forearm M66.13- ☑
  - hand M66.14- ☑
  - pelvic region M66.15- ☑
  - shoulder region M66.11- ☑
  - specified site NEC M66.18
  - thigh M66.15- ☑
  - toe M66.17- ☑
  - upper arm M66.12- ☑
  - wrist M66.13- ☑
- tendon (traumatic) — *see* Strain
  - nontraumatic (spontaneous) M66.9
    - ankle M66.87- ☑
    - extensor M66.2Ø
      - ankle M66.27- ☑
      - foot M66.27- ☑
      - forearm M66.23- ☑
      - hand M66.24- ☑
      - lower leg M66.26- ☑
      - multiple sites M66.29
      - pelvic region M66.25- ☑
      - shoulder region M66.21- ☑
      - specified site NEC M66.28
      - thigh M66.25- ☑
      - upper arm M66.22- ☑
    - flexor M66.3Ø
      - ankle M66.37- ☑
      - foot M66.37- ☑
      - forearm M66.33- ☑
      - hand M66.34- ☑
      - lower leg M66.36- ☑
      - multiple sites M66.39
      - pelvic region M66.35- ☑
      - shoulder region M66.31- ☑
      - specified site NEC M66.38
      - thigh M66.35- ☑
      - upper arm M66.32- ☑
    - foot M66.87- ☑
    - forearm M66.83- ☑
    - hand M66.84- ☑
    - lower leg M66.86- ☑
    - multiple sites M66.89
    - pelvic region M66.85- ☑
    - shoulder region M66.81- ☑
    - specified
      - site NEC M66.88
      - tendon M66.8Ø
    - thigh M66.85- ☑
    - upper arm M66.82- ☑
- thoracic duct I89.8
- tonsil J35.8
- traumatic
  - aorta — *see* Injury, aorta, laceration, major
  - diaphragm — *see* Injury, intrathoracic, diaphragm
  - external site — *see* Wound, open, by site
  - eye — *see* Injury, eye, laceration
  - internal organ — *see* Injury, by site
  - intervertebral disc
    - cervical S13.Ø ☑
    - lumbar S33.Ø ☑
    - thoracic S23.Ø ☑
  - kidney S37.Ø6- ☑
  - ligament — *see also* Sprain
    - ankle — *see* Sprain, ankle
    - carpus — *see* Rupture, traumatic, ligament, wrist
    - collateral (hand) — *see* Rupture, traumatic, ligament, finger, collateral
    - finger (metacarpophalangeal) (interphalangeal) S63.4Ø- ☑
      - collateral S63.41- ☑
        - index S63.41- ☑
        - little S63.41- ☑
        - middle S63.41- ☑
        - ring S63.41- ☑
      - index S63.4Ø- ☑
      - little S63.4Ø- ☑
      - middle S63.4Ø- ☑
      - palmar S63.42- ☑
        - index S63.42- ☑
        - little S63.42- ☑
        - middle S63.42- ☑
        - ring S63.42- ☑

Rupture, ruptured — *continued*
traumatic — *continued*
ligament — *see also* Sprain — *continued*
finger — *continued*
ring S63.40- ☑
specified site NEC S63.499 ☑
index S63.49- ☑
little S63.49- ☑
middle S63.49- ☑
ring S63.49- ☑
volar plate S63.43- ☑
index S63.43- ☑
little S63.43- ☑
middle S63.43- ☑
ring S63.43- ☑
foot — *see* Sprain, foot
radial collateral S53.2- ☑
radiocarpal — *see* Rupture, traumatic, ligament, wrist, radiocarpal
ulnar collateral S53.3- ☑
ulnocarpal — *see* Rupture, traumatic, ligament, wrist, ulnocarpal
wrist S63.30- ☑
collateral S63.31- ☑
radiocarpal S63.32- ☑
specified site NEC S63.39- ☑
ulnocarpal (palmar) S63.33- ☑
liver S36.116 ☑
membrana tympani — *see* Rupture, ear drum, traumatic
muscle or tendon — *see* Strain
myocardium — *see* Injury, heart
pancreas S36.299 ☑
rectum S36.69 ☑
sigmoid S36.593 ☑
spleen S36.09 ☑
stomach S36.39 ☑
symphysis pubis S33.4 ☑
tympanum, tympanic (membrane) — *see* Rupture, ear drum, traumatic
ureter S37.19 ☑
uterus S37.69 ☑
vagina — *see* Injury, vagina
vena cava — *see* Injury, vena cava, laceration, major
tricuspid (heart) (valve) I07.8
tube, tubal (nonobstetric) (nontraumatic) N83.8
abscess — *see* Salpingitis
due to pregnancy O00.10- ☑
with intrauterine pregnancy O00.11- ☑
tympanum, tympanic (membrane) (nontraumatic) — *see also* Perforation, tympanic membrane H72.9- ☑
traumatic — *see* Rupture, ear drum, traumatic
umbilical cord, complicating delivery O69.89 ☑
ureter (traumatic) S37.19 ☑
nontraumatic N28.89
urethra (nontraumatic) N36.8
with ectopic or molar pregnancy O08.6
following ectopic or molar pregnancy O08.6
obstetrical trauma O71.5
traumatic S37.39 ☑
uterosacral ligament (nonobstetric) (nontraumatic) N83.8
uterus (traumatic) S37.69 ☑
before labor O71.0- ☑
during or after labor O71.1
nonpuerperal, nontraumatic N85.8
pregnant (during labor) O71.1
before labor O71.0- ☑
vagina — *see* Injury, vagina
valve, valvular (heart) — *see* Endocarditis
varicose vein — *see* Varix
varix — *see* Varix
vena cava R58
traumatic — *see* Injury, vena cava, laceration, major
vesical (urinary) N32.89
vessel (blood) R58
pulmonary I28.8
traumatic — *see* Injury, blood vessel
viscus R19.8
vulva complicating delivery O70.0
Russell-Silver syndrome Q87.19
Russian spring-summer type encephalitis A84.0
Rust's disease (tuberculous cervical spondylitis) A18.01
Ruvalcaba-Myhre-Smith syndrome E71.440
Rytand-Lipsitch syndrome I44.2

S

Saber, sabre shin or tibia (syphilitic) A50.56 *[M90.8-]* ☑
Sac lacrimal — *see* condition
Saccharomyces infection B37.9
Saccharopinuria E72.3
Saccular — *see* condition
Sacculation
aorta (nonsyphilitic) — *see* Aneurysm, aorta
bladder N32.3
intralaryngeal (congenital) (ventricular) Q31.3
larynx (congenital) (ventricular) Q31.3
organ or site, congenital — *see* Distortion
pregnant uterus — *see* Pregnancy, complicated by, abnormal, uterus
ureter N28.89
urethra N36.1
vesical N32.3
Sachs' amaurotic familial idiocy or disease E75.02
Sachs-Tay disease E75.02
Sacks-Libman disease M32.11
Sacralgia M53.3
Sacralization Q76.49
Sacrodynia M53.3
Sacroiliac joint — *see* condition
Sacroiliitis NEC M46.1
Sacrum — *see* condition
Saddle
back — *see* Lordosis
embolus
abdominal aorta I74.01
pulmonary artery I26.92
with acute cor pulmonale I26.02
injury — *code to* condition
nose M95.0
due to syphilis A50.57
Sadism (sexual) F65.52
Sadness, postpartal O90.6
Sadomasochism F65.50
Saemisch's ulcer (cornea) — *see* Ulcer, cornea, central
Sagging
skin and subcutaneous tissue (following bariatric surgery weight loss) (following dietary weight loss) L98.7
Sahib disease B55.0
Sailors' skin L57.8
Saint
Anthony's fire — *see* Erysipelas
triad — *see* Hernia, diaphragm
Vitus' dance — *see* Chorea, Sydenham's
Salaam
attack(s) — *see* Epilepsy, spasms
tic R25.8
Salicylism
abuse F55.8
overdose or wrong substance given — *see* Table of Drugs and Chemicals, by drug, poisoning
Salivary duct or gland — *see* condition
Salivation, excessive K11.7
Salmonella — *see* Infection, Salmonella
Salmonellosis A02.0
Salpingitis (catarrhal) (fallopian tube) (nodular) (pseudofollicular) (purulent) (septic) N70.91
with oophoritis N70.93
acute N70.01
with oophoritis N70.03
chlamydial A56.11
chronic N70.11
with oophoritis N70.13
complicating abortion — *see* Abortion, by type, complicated by, salpingitis
ear — *see* Salpingitis, eustachian
eustachian (tube) H68.00- ☑
acute H68.01- ☑
chronic H68.02- ☑
follicularis N70.11
with oophoritis N70.13
gonococcal (acute) (chronic) A54.24
interstitial, chronic N70.11
with oophoritis N70.13
isthmica nodosa N70.11
with oophoritis N70.13
specific (gonococcal) (acute) (chronic) A54.24
tuberculous (acute) (chronic) A18.17
venereal (gonococcal) (acute) (chronic) A54.24
Salpingocele N83.4- ☑
Salpingo-oophoritis (catarrhal) (purulent) (ruptured) (septic) (suppurative) N70.93
acute N70.03
with ectopic or molar pregnancy O08.0
following ectopic or molar pregnancy O08.0
gonococcal A54.24
chronic N70.13
following ectopic or molar pregnancy O08.0
gonococcal (acute) (chronic) A54.24
puerperal O86.19
specific (gonococcal) (acute) (chronic) A54.24
subacute N70.03
tuberculous (acute) (chronic) A18.17
venereal (gonococcal) (acute) (chronic) A54.24
Salpingo-ovaritis — *see* Salpingo-oophoritis
Salpingoperitonitis — *see* Salpingo-oophoritis
Salzmann's nodular dystrophy — *see* Degeneration, cornea, nodular
Sampson's cyst or tumor N80.10- ☑
San Joaquin (Valley) **fever** B38.0
Sandblaster's asthma, lung or pneumoconiosis J62.8
Sander's disease (paranoia) F22
Sandfly fever A93.1
Sandhoff's disease E75.01
Sanfilippo (Type B) (Type C) (Type D) **syndrome** E76.22
Sanger-Brown ataxia G11.2
Sao Paulo fever or typhus A77.0
Saponification, mesenteric K65.8
Sarcocele (benign)
syphilitic A52.76
congenital A50.59
Sarcocystosis A07.8
Sarcoepiplocele — *see* Hernia
Sarcoepiplomphalocele Q79.2
Sarcoglycanopathy G71.0340
alpha G71.0341
beta G71.0342
delta G71.0349
gamma G71.0349
Sarcoid — *see also* Sarcoidosis
arthropathy D86.86
Boeck's D86.9
Darier-Roussy D86.3
iridocyclitis D86.83
meningitis D86.81
myocarditis D86.85
myositis D86.87
pyelonephritis D86.84
Spiegler-Fendt L08.89
Sarcoidosis D86.9
with
cranial nerve palsies D86.82
hepatic granuloma D86.89
polyarthritis D86.86
tubulo-interstitial nephropathy D86.84
combined sites NEC D86.89
lung D86.0
and lymph nodes D86.2
lymph nodes D86.1
and lung D86.2
meninges D86.81
skin D86.3
specified type NEC D86.89
Sarcoma (of) — *see also* Neoplasm, connective tissue, malignant
alveolar soft part — *see* Neoplasm, connective tissue, malignant
ameloblastic C41.1
upper jaw (bone) C41.0
botryoid — *see* Neoplasm, connective tissue, malignant
botryoides — *see* Neoplasm, connective tissue, malignant
cerebellar C71.6
circumscribed (arachnoidal) C71.6
circumscribed (arachnoidal) cerebellar C71.6
clear cell — *see also* Neoplasm, connective tissue, malignant
kidney C64.- ☑
dendritic cells (accessory cells) C96.4
embryonal — *see* Neoplasm, connective tissue, malignant
endometrial (stromal) C54.1
isthmus C54.0
epithelioid (cell) — *see* Neoplasm, connective tissue, malignant
Ewing's — *see* Neoplasm, bone, malignant
follicular dendritic cell C96.4

Sarcoma — *continued*
  germinoblastic (diffuse) — *see* Lymphoma, diffuse large cell
    follicular — *see* Lymphoma, follicular, specified NEC
  giant cell (except of bone) — *see also* Neoplasm, connective tissue, malignant
    bone — *see* Neoplasm, bone, malignant
  glomoid — *see* Neoplasm, connective tissue, malignant
  granulocytic C92.3- ☑
  hemangioendothelial — *see* Neoplasm, connective tissue, malignant
  hemorrhagic, multiple — *see* Sarcoma, Kaposi's
  histiocytic C96.A (*following* C96.6)
  Hodgkin — *see* Lymphoma, Hodgkin
  immunoblastic (diffuse) — *see* Lymphoma, diffuse large cell
  interdigitating dendritic cell C96.4
  Kaposi's
    colon C46.4
    connective tissue C46.1
    gastrointestinal organ C46.4
    lung C46.5- ☑
    lymph node(s) C46.3
    palate (hard) (soft) C46.2
    rectum C46.4
    skin C46.Ø
    specified site NEC C46.7
    stomach C46.4
    unspecified site C46.9
  Kupffer cell C22.3
  Langerhans cell C96.4
  leptomeningeal — *see* Neoplasm, meninges, malignant
  liver NEC C22.4
  lymphangioendothelial — *see* Neoplasm, connective tissue, malignant
  lymphoblastic — *see* Lymphoma, lymphoblastic (diffuse)
  lymphocytic — *see* Lymphoma, small cell B-cell
  mast cell C96.22
  melanotic — *see* Melanoma
  meningeal — *see* Neoplasm, meninges, malignant
  meningothelial — *see* Neoplasm, meninges, malignant
  mesenchymal — *see also* Neoplasm, connective tissue, malignant
    mixed — *see* Neoplasm, connective tissue, malignant
  mesothelial — *see* Mesothelioma
  monstrocellular
    specified site — *see* Neoplasm, malignant, by site
    unspecified site C71.9
  myeloid C92.3- ☑
  neurogenic — *see* Neoplasm, nerve, malignant
  odontogenic C41.1
    upper jaw (bone) C41.Ø
  osteoblastic — *see* Neoplasm, bone, malignant
  osteogenic — *see also* Neoplasm, bone, malignant
    juxtacortical — *see* Neoplasm, bone, malignant
    periosteal — *see* Neoplasm, bone, malignant
  periosteal — *see also* Neoplasm, bone, malignant
    osteogenic — *see* Neoplasm, bone, malignant
  pleomorphic cell — *see* Neoplasm, connective tissue, malignant
  reticulum cell (diffuse) — *see* Lymphoma, diffuse large cell
    nodular — *see* Lymphoma, follicular
    pleomorphic cell type — *see* Lymphoma, diffuse large cell
  rhabdoid — *see* Neoplasm, malignant, by site
  round cell — *see* Neoplasm, connective tissue, malignant
  small cell — *see* Neoplasm, connective tissue, malignant
  soft tissue — *see* Neoplasm, connective tissue, malignant
  spindle cell — *see* Neoplasm, connective tissue, malignant
  stromal (endometrial) C54.1
    isthmus C54.Ø
  synovial — *see also* Neoplasm, connective tissue, malignant
    biphasic — *see* Neoplasm, connective tissue, malignant
    epithelioid cell — *see* Neoplasm, connective tissue, malignant
    spindle cell — *see* Neoplasm, connective tissue, malignant

Sarcomatosis
  meningeal — *see* Neoplasm, meninges, malignant
  specified site NEC — *see* Neoplasm, connective tissue, malignant
  unspecified site C8Ø.1
Sarcopenia (age-related) M62.84
Sarcosinemia E72.59
Sarcosporidiosis (intestinal) AØ7.8
SARS-CoV-2 — *see also* COVID-19
  sequelae (post acute) UØ9.9
Satiety, early R68.81
Saturnine — *see* condition
Saturnism
  overdose or wrong substance given or taken — *see* Table of Drugs and Chemicals, by drug, poisoning
Satyriasis F52.8
Sauriasis — *see* Ichthyosis
SBE (subacute bacterial endocarditis) I33.Ø
Scabies (any site) B86
Scabs R23.4
Scaglietti-Dagnini syndrome E22.Ø
Scald — *see* Burn
Scalenus anticus (anterior) **syndrome** G54.Ø
Scales R23.4
Scaling, skin R23.4
Scalp — *see* condition
Scapegoating affecting child Z62.3
Scaphocephaly Q75.Ø
Scapulalgia M89.8X1
Scapulohumeral myopathy G71.Ø2
Scar, scarring — *see also* Cicatrix L9Ø.5
  adherent L9Ø.5
  atrophic L9Ø.5
  cervix
    in pregnancy or childbirth — *see* Pregnancy, complicated by, abnormal cervix
  cheloid L91.Ø
  chorioretinal H31.ØØ- ☑
    posterior pole macula H31.Ø1- ☑
    postsurgical H59.81- ☑
    solar retinopathy H31.Ø2- ☑
    specified type NEC H31.Ø9- ☑
  choroid — *see* Scar, chorioretinal
  conjunctiva H11.24- ☑
  cornea H17.9
    xerophthalmic — *see also* Opacity, cornea
      vitamin A deficiency E5Ø.6
  defect (isthmocele) O34.22
  duodenum, obstructive K31.5
  hypertrophic L91.Ø
  keloid L91.Ø
  labia N9Ø.89
  lung (base) J98.4
  macula — *see* Scar, chorioretinal, posterior pole
  muscle M62.89
  myocardium, myocardial I25.2
  painful L9Ø.5
  posterior pole (eye) — *see* Scar, chorioretinal, posterior pole
  retina — *see* Scar, chorioretinal
  trachea J39.8
  transmural uterine, in pregnancy O34.29
  uterus N85.8
    in pregnancy O34.29
  vagina N89.8
    postoperative N99.2
  vulva N9Ø.89
Scarabiasis B88.2
Scarlatina (anginosa) (maligna) A38.9
  myocarditis (acute) A38.1
    old — *see* Myocarditis
  otitis media A38.Ø
  ulcerosa A38.8
Scarlet fever (albuminuria) (angina) A38.9
Schamberg's disease (progressive pigmentary dermatosis) L81.7
Schatzki's ring (acquired) (esophagus) (lower) K22.2
  congenital Q39.3
Schaufenster krankheit I2Ø.8
Schaumann's
  benign lymphogranulomatosis D86.1
  disease or syndrome — *see* Sarcoidosis
Scheie's syndrome E76.Ø3
Schenck's disease B42.1
Scheuermann's disease or osteochondrosis — *see* Osteochondrosis, juvenile, spine
Schilder (-Flatau) **disease** G37.Ø

Schilling-type monocytic leukemia C93.Ø- ☑
Schimmelbusch's disease, cystic mastitis, or hyperplasia — *see* Mastopathy, cystic
Schistosoma infestation — *see* Infestation, Schistosoma
Schistosomiasis B65.9
  with muscle disorder B65.9 *[M63.8Ø]*
    ankle B65.9 *[M63.87-]* ☑
    foot B65.9 *[M63.87-]* ☑
    forearm B65.9 *[M63.83-]* ☑
    hand B65.9 *[M63.84-]* ☑
    lower leg B65.9 *[M63.86-]* ☑
    multiple sites B65.9 *[M63.89]*
    pelvic region B65.9 *[M63.85-]* ☑
    shoulder region B65.9 *[M63.81-]* ☑
    specified site NEC B65.9 *[M63.88]*
    thigh B65.9 *[M63.85-]* ☑
    upper arm B65.9 *[M63.82-]* ☑
  Asiatic B65.2
  bladder B65.Ø
  chestermani B65.8
  colon B65.1
  cutaneous B65.3
  due to
    S. haematobium B65.Ø
    S. japonicum B65.2
    S. mansoni B65.1
    S. mattheii B65.8
  Eastern B65.2
  genitourinary tract B65.Ø
  intestinal B65.1
  lung NEC B65.9 *[J99]*
    pneumonia B65.9 *[J17]*
  Manson's (intestinal) B65.1
  oriental B65.2
  pulmonary NEC B65.9 *[J99]*
    pneumonia B65.9
  Schistosoma
    haematobium B65.Ø
    japonicum B65.2
    mansoni B65.1
  specified type NEC B65.8
  urinary B65.Ø
  vesical B65.Ø
Schizencephaly QØ4.6
Schizoaffective psychosis F25.9
Schizodontia KØØ.2
Schizoid personality F6Ø.1
Schizophrenia, schizophrenic F2Ø.9
  acute (brief) (undifferentiated) F23
  atypical (form) F2Ø.3
  borderline F21
  catalepsy F2Ø.2
  catatonic (type) (excited) (withdrawn) F2Ø.2
  cenesthopathic, cenesthesiopathic F2Ø.89
  childhood type F84.5
  chronic undifferentiated F2Ø.9
  cyclic F25.Ø
  disorganized (type) F2Ø.1
  flexibilitas cerea F2Ø.2
  hebephrenic (type) F2Ø.1
  incipient F21
  latent F21
  negative type F2Ø.5
  paranoid (type) F2Ø.Ø
  paraphrenic F2Ø.Ø
  post-psychotic depression F32.89
  prepsychotic F21
  prodromal F21
  pseudoneurotic F21
  pseudopsychopathic F21
  reaction F23
  residual (state) (type) F2Ø.5
  restzustand F2Ø.5
  schizoaffective (type) — *see* Psychosis, schizoaffective
  simple (type) F2Ø.89
  simplex F2Ø.89
  specified type NEC F2Ø.89
  spectrum and other psychotic disorder F29
    specified NEC F28
  stupor F2Ø.2
  syndrome of childhood F84.5
  undifferentiated (type) F2Ø.3
    chronic F2Ø.9
Schizothymia (persistent) F6Ø.1
Schlatter-Osgood disease or osteochondrosis M92.52- ☑
Schlatter's tibia — *see* Osteochondrosis, juvenile, tibia
Schmidt's syndrome (polyglandular, autoimmune) E31.Ø

Schmincke's carcinoma or tumor — *see* Neoplasm, nasopharynx, malignant
Schmitz (-Stutzer) **dysentery** A03.0
Schmorl's disease or nodes
lumbar region M51.46
lumbosacral region M51.47
sacrococcygeal region M53.3
thoracic region M51.44
thoracolumbar region M51.45
Schneiderian
papilloma — *see* Neoplasm, nasopharynx, benign
specified site — *see* Neoplasm, benign, by site
unspecified site D14.0
specified site — *see* Neoplasm, malignant, by site
unspecified site C30.0
Scholte's syndrome (malignant carcinoid) E34.0
Scholz (-Bielchowsky-Henneberg) **disease or syndrome** E75.25
Schönlein (-Henoch) disease or purpura (primary) (rheumatic) D69.0
Schottmuller's disease A01.4
Schroeder's syndrome (endocrine hypertensive) E27.0
Schüller-Christian disease or syndrome C96.5
Schultze's type acroparesthesia, simple I73.89
Schultz's disease or syndrome — *see* Agranulocytosis
Schwalbe-Ziehen-Oppenheim disease G24.1
Schwannoma — *see also* Neoplasm, nerve, benign
malignant — *see also* Neoplasm, nerve, malignant
with rhabdomyoblastic differentiation — *see* Neoplasm, nerve, malignant
melanocytic — *see* Neoplasm, nerve, benign
pigmented — *see* Neoplasm, nerve, benign
Schwannomatosis Q85.03
Schwartz (-Jampel) **syndrome** G71.13
Schwartz-Bartter syndrome E22.2
Schweniger-Buzzi anetoderma L90.1
Sciatic — *see* condition
Sciatica (infective) M54.3 ☑
with lumbago M54.4- ☑
due to intervertebral disc disorder — *see* Disorder, disc, with, radiculopathy
due to displacement of intervertebral disc (with lumbago) — *see* Disorder, disc, with, radiculopathy
wallet M54.3- ☑
Scimitar syndrome Q26.8
Sclera — *see* condition
Sclerectasia H15.84- ☑
Scleredema
adultorum — *see* Sclerosis, systemic
Buschke's — *see* Sclerosis, systemic
newborn P83.0
Sclerema (adiposum) (edematosum) (neonatorum) (newborn) P83.0
adultorum — *see* Sclerosis, systemic
Scleriasis — *see* Scleroderma
Scleritis H15.00- ☑
with corneal involvement H15.04- ☑
anterior H15.01- ☑
brawny H15.02- ☑
in (due to) zoster B02.34
posterior H15.03- ☑
specified type NEC H15.09- ☑
syphilitic A52.71
tuberculous (nodular) A18.51
Sclerochoroiditis H31.8
Scleroconjunctivitis — *see* Scleritis
Sclerocystic ovary syndrome E28.2
Sclerodactyly, sclerodactylia L94.3
Scleroderma, sclerodermia (acrosclerotic) (diffuse) (generalized) (progressive) (pulmonary) — *see also* Sclerosis, systemic M34.9
circumscribed L94.0
linear L94.1
localized L94.0
newborn P83.88
systemic M34.9
Sclerokeratitis H16.8
tuberculous A18.52
Scleroma nasi A48.8
Scleromalacia (perforans) H15.05- ☑
Scleromyxedema L98.5
Sclérose en plaques G35
Sclerosis, sclerotic
adrenal (gland) E27.8
Alzheimer's — *see* Disease, Alzheimer's
amyotrophic (lateral) G12.21
aorta, aortic I70.0
Sclerosis, sclerotic — *continued*
aorta, aortic — *continued*
valve — *see* Endocarditis, aortic
artery, arterial, arteriolar, arteriovascular — *see* Arteriosclerosis
ascending multiple G35
brain (generalized) (lobular) G37.9
artery, arterial I67.2
diffuse G37.0
disseminated G35
insular G35
Krabbe's E75.23
miliary G35
multiple G35
presenile (Alzheimer's) — *see* Disease, Alzheimer's, early onset
senile (arteriosclerotic) I67.2
stem, multiple G35
tuberous Q85.1
bulbar, multiple G35
bundle of His I44.39
cardiac — *see* Disease, heart, ischemic, atherosclerotic
cardiorenal — *see* Hypertension, cardiorenal
cardiovascular — *see also* Disease, cardiovascular
renal — *see* Hypertension, cardiorenal
cerebellar — *see* Sclerosis, brain
cerebral — *see* Sclerosis, brain
cerebrospinal (disseminated) (multiple) G35
cerebrovascular I67.2
choroid — *see* Degeneration, choroid
combined (spinal cord) — *see also* Degeneration, combined
multiple G35
concentric (Balo) G37.5
cornea — *see* Opacity, cornea
coronary (artery) I25.10
with angina pectoris — *see* Arteriosclerosis, coronary (artery),
corpus cavernosum
female N90.89
male N48.6
diffuse (brain) (spinal cord) G37.0
disseminated G35
dorsal G35
dorsolateral (spinal cord) — *see* Degeneration, combined
endometrium N85.5
extrapyramidal G25.9
eye, nuclear (senile) — *see* Cataract, senile, nuclear
focal and segmental (glomerular) — *see also* N00-N07 with fourth character .1 N05.1
Friedreich's (spinal cord) G11.11
funicular (spermatic cord) N50.89
general (vascular) — *see* Arteriosclerosis
gland (lymphatic) I89.8
hepatic K74.1
alcoholic K70.2
hereditary
cerebellar G11.9
spinal (Friedreich's ataxia) G11.11
hippocampal G93.81
insular G35
kidney — *see* Sclerosis, renal
larynx J38.7
lateral (amyotrophic) (descending) (spinal) G12.21
primary G12.23
lens, senile nuclear — *see* Cataract, senile, nuclear
liver K74.1
with fibrosis K74.2
alcoholic K70.2
alcoholic K70.2
cardiac K76.1
lung — *see* Fibrosis, lung
mastoid — *see* Mastoiditis, chronic
mesial temporal G93.81
mitral I05.8
Mönckeberg's (medial) — *see* Arteriosclerosis, extremities
multiple (brain stem) (cerebral) (generalized) (spinal cord) G35
myocardium, myocardial — *see* Disease, heart, ischemic, atherosclerotic
nuclear (senile), eye — *see* Cataract, senile, nuclear
ovary N83.8
pancreas K86.89
penis N48.6
peripheral arteries — *see* Arteriosclerosis, extremities
plaques G35
Sclerosis, sclerotic — *continued*
pluriglandular E31.8
polyglandular E31.8
posterolateral (spinal cord) — *see* Degeneration, combined
presenile (Alzheimer's) — *see* Disease, Alzheimer's, early onset
primary, lateral G12.23
progressive, systemic M34.0
pulmonary — *see* Fibrosis, lung
artery I27.0
valve (heart) — *see* Endocarditis, pulmonary
renal N26.9
with
cystine storage disease E72.09
hypertensive heart disease (conditions in I11) — *see* Hypertension, cardiorenal
arteriolar (hyaline) (hyperplastic) — *see* Hypertension, kidney
retina (senile) (vascular) H35.00
senile (vascular) — *see* Arteriosclerosis
spinal (cord) (progressive) G95.89
ascending G61.0
combined — *see also* Degeneration, combined
multiple G35
syphilitic A52.11
disseminated G35
dorsolateral — *see* Degeneration, combined
hereditary (Friedreich's) (mixed form) G11.11
lateral (amyotrophic) G12.21
progressive G12.23
multiple G35
posterior (syphilitic) A52.11
stomach K31.89
subendocardial, congenital I42.4
systemic M34.9
with
lung involvement M34.81
myopathy M34.82
polyneuropathy M34.83
drug-induced M34.2
due to chemicals NEC M34.2
progressive M34.0
specified NEC M34.89
temporal (mesial) G93.81
tricuspid (heart) (valve) I07.8
tuberous (brain) Q85.1
tympanic membrane — *see* Disorder, tympanic membrane, specified NEC
valve, valvular (heart) — *see* Endocarditis
vascular — *see* Arteriosclerosis
vein I87.8
Scoliosis (acquired) (postural) M41.9
adolescent (idiopathic) — *see* Scoliosis, idiopathic, adolescent
congenital Q67.5
due to bony malformation Q76.3
failure of segmentation (hemivertebra) Q76.3
hemivertebra fusion Q76.3
postural Q67.5
degenerative M41.5- ☑
idiopathic M41.20
adolescent M41.129
cervical region M41.122
cervicothoracic region M41.123
lumbar region M41.126
lumbosacral region M41.127
thoracic region M41.124
thoracolumbar region M41.125
cervical region M41.22
cervicothoracic region M41.23
infantile M41.00
cervical region M41.02
cervicothoracic region M41.03
lumbar region M41.06
lumbosacral region M41.07
sacrococcygeal region M41.08
thoracic region M41.04
thoracolumbar region M41.05
juvenile M41.119
cervical region M41.112
cervicothoracic region M41.113
lumbar region M41.116
lumbosacral region M41.117
thoracic region M41.114
thoracolumbar region M41.115
lumbar region M41.26
lumbosacral region M41.27

- **Scoliosis** — *continued*
  - idiopathic — *continued*
    - thoracic region M41.24
    - thoracolumbar region M41.25
  - infantile — *see* Scoliosis, idiopathic, infantile
  - neuromuscular M41.40
    - cervical region M41.42
    - cervicothoracic region M41.43
    - lumbar region M41.46
    - lumbosacral region M41.47
    - occipito-atlanto-axial region M41.41
    - thoracic region M41.44
    - thoracolumbar region M41.45
  - paralytic — *see* Scoliosis, neuromuscular
  - postradiation therapy M96.5
  - rachitic (late effect or sequelae) E64.3 *[M49.80]*
    - cervical region E64.3 *[M49.82]*
    - cervicothoracic region E64.3 *[M49.83]*
    - lumbar region E64.3 *[M49.86]*
    - lumbosacral region E64.3 *[M49.87]*
    - multiple sites E64.3 *[M49.89]*
    - occipito-atlanto-axial region E64.3 *[M49.81]*
    - sacrococcygeal region E64.3 *[M49.88]*
    - thoracic region E64.3 *[M49.84]*
    - thoracolumbar region E64.3 *[M49.85]*
  - sciatic M54.4- ☑
  - secondary (to) NEC M41.50
    - cerebral palsy, Friedreich's ataxia, poliomyelitis, neuromuscular disorders — *see* Scoliosis, neuromuscular
    - cervical region M41.52
    - cervicothoracic region M41.53
    - lumbar region M41.56
    - lumbosacral region M41.57
    - thoracic region M41.54
    - thoracolumbar region M41.55
  - specified form NEC M41.80
    - cervical region M41.82
    - cervicothoracic region M41.83
    - lumbar region M41.86
    - lumbosacral region M41.87
    - thoracic region M41.84
    - thoracolumbar region M41.85
  - thoracogenic M41.30
    - thoracic region M41.34
    - thoracolumbar region M41.35
  - tuberculous A18.01
- **Scoliotic pelvis**
  - with disproportion (fetopelvic) O33.0
    - causing obstructed labor O65.0
- **Scorbutus, scorbutic** — *see also* Scurvy
  - anemia D53.2
- **Score, NIHSS** (National Institutes of Health Stroke Scale) R29.7- ☑
- **Scotoma** (arcuate) (Bjerrum) (central) (ring) — *see also* Defect, visual field, localized, scotoma
  - scintillating H53.12- ☑
- **Scratch** — *see* Abrasion
- **Scratchy throat** R09.89
- **Screening** (for) Z13.9
  - alcoholism Z13.39
  - anemia Z13.0
  - anomaly, congenital Z13.89
  - antenatal, of mother — *see also* Encounter, antenatal screening Z36.9
  - arterial hypertension Z13.6
  - arthropod-borne viral disease NEC Z11.59
  - autism Z13.41
  - bacteriuria, asymptomatic Z13.89
  - behavioral disorder Z13.30
    - specified NEC Z13.39
  - brain injury, traumatic Z13.850
  - bronchitis, chronic Z13.83
  - brucellosis Z11.2
  - cardiovascular disorder Z13.6
  - cataract Z13.5
  - chlamydial diseases Z11.8
  - cholera Z11.0
  - chromosomal abnormalities (nonprocreative) NEC Z13.79
  - colonoscopy Z12.11
  - congenital
    - dislocation of hip Z13.89
    - eye disorder Z13.5
    - malformation or deformation Z13.89
  - contamination NEC Z13.88
  - coronavirus (disease) (novel) 2019 Z11.52
  - COVID-19 Z11.52
- **Screening** — *continued*
  - cystic fibrosis Z13.228
  - dengue fever Z11.59
  - dental disorder Z13.84
  - depression (adult) (adolescent) (child) Z13.31
    - maternal Z13.32
    - perinatal Z13.32
  - developmental
    - delays Z13.40
      - global (milestones) Z13.42
      - specified NEC Z13.49
    - handicap Z13.42
      - in early childhood Z13.42
  - diabetes mellitus Z13.1
  - diphtheria Z11.2
  - disability, intellectual Z13.39
  - disease or disorder Z13.9
    - bacterial NEC Z11.2
      - intestinal infectious Z11.0
      - respiratory tuberculosis Z11.1
    - behavioral Z13.30
      - specified NEC Z13.39
    - blood or blood-forming organ Z13.0
    - cardiovascular Z13.6
    - Chagas' Z11.6
    - chlamydial Z11.8
    - coronavirus (novel) 2019 Z11.52
    - COVID-19 Z11.52
    - dental Z13.89
    - developmental delays Z13.40
      - global (milestones) Z13.42
      - specified NEC Z13.49
    - digestive tract NEC Z13.818
      - lower GI Z13.811
      - upper GI Z13.810
    - ear Z13.5
    - endocrine Z13.29
    - eye Z13.5
    - genitourinary Z13.89
    - heart Z13.6
    - human immunodeficiency virus (HIV) infection Z11.4
    - immunity Z13.0
    - infection
      - intestinal Z11.0
        - specified NEC Z11.6
    - infectious Z11.9
    - mental health and behavioral Z13.30
      - specified NEC Z13.39
    - metabolic Z13.228
    - neurological Z13.89
    - nutritional Z13.21
      - metabolic Z13.228
        - lipoid disorders Z13.220
    - protozoal Z11.6
      - intestinal Z11.0
    - respiratory Z13.83
    - rheumatic Z13.828
    - rickettsial Z11.8
    - sexually-transmitted NEC Z11.3
      - human immunodeficiency virus (HIV) Z11.4
    - sickle-cell (trait) Z13.0
    - skin Z13.89
    - specified NEC Z13.89
    - spirochetal Z11.8
    - thyroid Z13.29
    - vascular Z13.6
    - venereal Z11.3
    - viral NEC Z11.59
      - coronavirus (novel) 2019 Z11.52
      - COVID-19 Z11.52
      - human immunodeficiency virus (HIV) Z11.4
      - intestinal Z11.0
      - SARS-CoV-2 Z11.52
  - elevated titer Z13.89
  - emphysema Z13.83
  - encephalitis, viral (mosquito- or tick-borne) Z11.59
  - exposure to contaminants (toxic) Z13.88
  - fever
    - dengue Z11.59
    - hemorrhagic Z11.59
    - yellow Z11.59
  - filariasis Z11.6
  - galactosemia Z13.228
  - gastrointestinal condition Z13.818
  - genetic (nonprocreative) - for procreative management — *see* Testing, genetic, for procreative management
    - disease carrier status (nonprocreative) Z13.71
    - specified NEC (nonprocreative) Z13.79
- **Screening** — *continued*
  - genitourinary condition Z13.89
  - glaucoma Z13.5
  - gonorrhea Z11.3
  - gout Z13.89
  - helminthiasis (intestinal) Z11.6
  - hematopoietic malignancy Z12.89
  - hemoglobinopathies NEC Z13.0
  - hemorrhagic fever Z11.59
  - Hodgkin disease Z12.89
  - human immunodeficiency virus (HIV) Z11.4
  - human papillomavirus Z11.51
  - hypertension Z13.6
  - immunity disorders Z13.0
  - infant or child (over 28 days old) Z00.129
    - with abnormal findings Z00.121
  - infection
    - mycotic Z11.8
    - parasitic Z11.8
  - ingestion of radioactive substance Z13.88
  - intellectual disability Z13.39
  - intestinal
    - helminthiasis Z11.6
    - infectious disease Z11.0
  - leishmaniasis Z11.6
  - leprosy Z11.2
  - leptospirosis Z11.8
  - leukemia Z12.89
  - lymphoma Z12.89
  - malaria Z11.6
  - malnutrition Z13.29
    - metabolic Z13.228
    - nutritional Z13.21
  - measles Z11.59
  - mental health disorder Z13.30
    - specified NEC Z13.39
  - metabolic errors, inborn Z13.228
  - multiphasic Z13.89
  - musculoskeletal disorder Z13.828
    - osteoporosis Z13.820
  - mycoses Z11.8
  - myocardial infarction (acute) Z13.6
  - neoplasm (malignant) (of) Z12.9
    - bladder Z12.6
    - blood Z12.89
    - breast Z12.39
      - routine mammogram Z12.31
    - cervix Z12.4
    - colon Z12.11
    - genitourinary organs NEC Z12.79
      - bladder Z12.6
      - cervix Z12.4
      - ovary Z12.73
      - prostate Z12.5
      - testis Z12.71
      - vagina Z12.72
    - hematopoietic system Z12.89
    - intestinal tract Z12.10
      - colon Z12.11
      - rectum Z12.12
      - small intestine Z12.13
    - lung Z12.2
    - lymph (glands) Z12.89
    - nervous system Z12.82
    - oral cavity Z12.81
    - prostate Z12.5
    - rectum Z12.12
    - respiratory organs Z12.2
    - skin Z12.83
    - small intestine Z12.13
    - specified site NEC Z12.89
    - stomach Z12.0
  - nephropathy Z13.89
  - nervous system disorders NEC Z13.858
  - neurological condition Z13.89
  - osteoporosis Z13.820
  - parasitic infestation Z11.9
    - specified NEC Z11.8
  - phenylketonuria Z13.228
  - plague Z11.2
  - poisoning (chemical) (heavy metal) Z13.88
  - poliomyelitis Z11.59
  - postnatal, chromosomal abnormalities Z13.89
  - prenatal, of mother — *see also* Encounter, antenatal screening Z36.9
  - protozoal disease Z11.6
    - intestinal Z11.0
  - pulmonary tuberculosis Z11.1
  - radiation exposure Z13.88

Screening — *continued*
- respiratory condition Z13.83
- respiratory tuberculosis Z11.1
- rheumatoid arthritis Z13.828
- rubella Z11.59
- SARS-CoV-2 Z11.52
- schistosomiasis Z11.6
- sexually-transmitted disease NEC Z11.3
  - human immunodeficiency virus (HIV) Z11.4
- sickle-cell disease or trait Z13.Ø
- skin condition Z13.89
- sleeping sickness Z11.6
- special Z13.9
  - specified NEC Z13.89
- syphilis Z11.3
- tetanus Z11.2
- trachoma Z11.8
- traumatic brain injury Z13.85Ø
- trypanosomiasis Z11.6
- tuberculosis, respiratory Z11.1
  - active Z11.1
  - latent Z11.7
- venereal disease Z11.3
- viral encephalitis (mosquito- or tick-borne) Z11.59
- whooping cough Z11.2
- worms, intestinal Z11.6
- yaws Z11.8
- yellow fever Z11.59

Scrofula, scrofulosis (tuberculosis of cervical lymph glands) A18.2
Scrofulide (primary) (tuberculous) A18.4
Scrofuloderma, scrofulodermia (any site) (primary) A18.4
Scrofulosus lichen (primary) (tuberculous) A18.4
Scrofulous — *see* condition
Scrotal tongue K14.5
Scrotum — *see* condition
Scurvy, scorbutic E54
- anemia D53.2
- gum E54
- infantile E54
- rickets E55.Ø *[M9Ø.8Ø]*

Sealpox BØ8.62
Seasickness T75.3 ☑
Seatworm (infection) (infestation) B8Ø
Sebaceous — *see also* condition
- cyst — *see* Cyst, sebaceous

Seborrhea, seborrheic L21.9
- capillitii R23.8
- capitis L21.Ø
- dermatitis L21.9
  - infantile L21.1
- eczema L21.9
  - infantile L21.1
- sicca L21.Ø

Seckel's syndrome Q87.19
Seclusion, pupil — *see* Membrane, pupillary
Second hand tobacco smoke exposure (acute) (chronic) Z77.22
- in the perinatal period P96.81

Secondary
- dentin (in pulp) KØ4.3
- neoplasm, secondaries — *see* Table of Neoplasms, secondary

Secretion
- antidiuretic hormone, inappropriate E22.2
- catecholamine, by pheochromocytoma E27.5
- hormone
  - antidiuretic, inappropriate (syndrome) E22.2
  - by
    - carcinoid tumor E34.Ø
    - pheochromocytoma E27.5
  - ectopic NEC E34.2
- urinary
  - excessive R35.89
  - suppression R34

Section
- nerve, traumatic — *see* Injury, nerve

Sedative, hypnotic, or anxiolytic-induced
- anxiety disorder F13.98Ø
- bipolar and related disorder F13.94
- delirium F13.921
- depressive disorder F13.94
- major neurocognitive disorder F13.97
- mild neurocognitive disorder F13.988
- psychotic disorder F13.959
- sexual dysfunction F13.981
- sleep disorder F13.982

Segmentation, incomplete (congenital) — *see also* Fusion
- bone NEC Q78.8
- lumbosacral (joint) (vertebra) Q76.49

SEID (systemic exertion intolerance disease) G93.32
Seitelberger's syndrome (infantile neuraxonal dystrophy) G31.89
Seizure(s) — *see also* Convulsions R56.9
- absence G4Ø.A- ☑ (*following* G4Ø.3)
- akinetic — *see* Epilepsy, generalized, specified NEC
- atonic — *see* Epilepsy, generalized, specified NEC
- autonomic (hysterical) F44.5
- convulsive — *see* Convulsions
- cortical (focal) (motor) — *see* Epilepsy, localization-related, symptomatic, with simple partial seizures
- disorder — *see also* Epilepsy G4Ø.9Ø9
- due to stroke — *see* Sequelae (of), disease, cerebrovascular, by type, specified NEC
- epileptic — *see* Epilepsy
- febrile (simple) R56.ØØ
  - with status epilepticus G4Ø.9Ø1
  - complex (atypical) (complicated) R56.Ø1
    - with status epilepticus G4Ø.9Ø1
- grand mal G4Ø.4Ø9
  - intractable G4Ø.419
    - with status epilepticus G4Ø.411
    - without status epilepticus G4Ø.419
  - not intractable G4Ø.4Ø9
    - with status epilepticus G4Ø.4Ø1
    - without status epilepticus G4Ø.4Ø9
- heart — *see* Disease, heart
- hysterical F44.5
- intractable G4Ø.919
  - with status epilepticus G4Ø.911
- Jacksonian (focal) (motor type) (sensory type) — *see* Epilepsy, localization-related, symptomatic, with simple partial seizures
- newborn P9Ø
- nonspecific epileptic
  - atonic — *see* Epilepsy, generalized, specified NEC
  - clonic — *see* Epilepsy, generalized, specified NEC
  - myoclonic — *see* Epilepsy, generalized, specified NEC
  - tonic — *see* Epilepsy, generalized, specified NEC
  - tonic-clonic — *see* Epilepsy, generalized, specified NEC
- partial, developing into secondarily generalized seizures
  - complex — *see* Epilepsy, localization-related, symptomatic, with complex partial seizures
  - simple — *see* Epilepsy, localization-related, symptomatic, with simple partial seizures
- petit mal G4Ø.A- ☑ (*following* G4Ø.3)
  - intractable G4Ø.A1- ☑ (*following* G4Ø.3)
    - with status epilepticus G4Ø.A11 (*following* G4Ø.3)
    - without status epilepticus G4Ø.A19 (*following* G4Ø.3)
  - not intractable G4Ø.AØ- ☑ (*following* G4Ø.3)
    - with status epilepticus G4Ø.AØ1 (*following* G4Ø.3)
    - without status epilepticus G4Ø.AØ9 (*following* G4Ø.3)
- post traumatic R56.1
- recurrent G4Ø.9Ø9
- specified NEC G4Ø.89
- uncinate — *see* Epilepsy, localization-related, symptomatic, with complex partial seizures

Selenium deficiency, dietary E59
Self-damaging behavior (life-style) Z72.89
Self-harm (attempted)
- history (personal)
  - in family Z81.8
  - nonsuicidal Z91.52
  - suicidal Z91.51
- nonsuicidal R45.88

Self-injury, nonsuicidal R45.88
- personal history Z91.52

Self-mutilation (attempted)
- history (personal)
  - in family Z81.8
  - nonsuicidal Z91.52
  - suicidal Z91.51
- nonsuicidal R45.88

Self-poisoning
- history (personal) Z91.51
  - in family Z81.8
- observation following (alleged) attempt ZØ3.6

Semicoma R4Ø.1
Seminal vesiculitis N49.Ø
Seminoma C62.9- ☑
- specified site — *see* Neoplasm, malignant, by site

Senear-Usher disease or syndrome L1Ø.4
Senectus R54
Senescence (without mention of psychosis) R54
Senile, senility — *see also* condition R41.81
- with
  - acute confusional state FØ5
  - mental changes NOS FØ3 ☑
  - psychosis NEC — *see* Psychosis, senile
- asthenia R54
- cervix (atrophic) N88.8
- debility R54
- endometrium (atrophic) N85.8
- fallopian tube (atrophic) — *see* Atrophy, fallopian tube
- heart (failure) R54
- ovary (atrophic) — *see* Atrophy, ovary
- premature E34.8
- vagina, vaginitis (atrophic) N95.2
- wart L82.1

Sensation
- burning (skin) R2Ø.8
  - tongue K14.6
- loss of R2Ø.8
- prickling (skin) R2Ø.2
- tingling (skin) R2Ø.2

Sense loss
- smell — *see* Disturbance, sensation, smell
- taste — *see* Disturbance, sensation, taste
- touch R2Ø.8

Sensibility disturbance (cortical) (deep) (vibratory) R2Ø.9
Sensitive, sensitivity — *see also* Allergy
- carotid sinus G9Ø.Ø1
- child (excessive) F93.8
- cold, autoimmune D59.12
- dentin KØ3.89
- gluten (non-celiac) K9Ø.41
- latex Z91.Ø4Ø
- methemoglobin D74.8
- tuberculin, without clinical or radiological symptoms R76.11
- visual
  - glare H53.71
  - impaired contrast H53.72

Sensitiver Beziehungswahn F22
Sensitization, auto-erythrocytic D69.2
Separation
- anxiety, abnormal (of childhood) F93.Ø
- apophysis, traumatic — *code as* Fracture, by site
- choroid — *see* Detachment, choroid
- epiphysis, epiphyseal
  - nontraumatic — *see also* Osteochondropathy, specified type NEC
    - upper femoral — *see* Slipped, epiphysis, upper femoral
  - traumatic — *code as* Fracture, by site
- fracture — *see* Fracture
- infundibulum cardiac from right ventricle by a partition Q24.3
- joint (traumatic) (current) — *code by* site under Dislocation
- muscle (nontraumatic) — *see* Diastasis, muscle
- pubic bone, obstetrical trauma O71.6
- retina, retinal — *see* Detachment, retina
- symphysis pubis, obstetrical trauma O71.6
- tracheal ring, incomplete, congenital Q32.1

Sepsis (generalized) (unspecified organism) A41.9
- with
  - organ dysfunction (acute) (multiple) R65.2Ø
    - with septic shock R65.21
- actinomycotic A42.7
- adrenal hemorrhage syndrome (meningococcal) A39.1
- anaerobic A41.4
- Bacillus anthracis A22.7
- Brucella — *see also* Brucellosis A23.9
- candidal B37.7
- cryptogenic A41.9
- due to device, implant or graft T85.79 ☑
  - arterial graft NEC T82.7 ☑
  - breast (implant) T85.79 ☑
  - catheter NEC T85.79 ☑
    - dialysis (renal) T82.7 ☑
      - intraperitoneal T85.71 ☑
    - infusion NEC T82.7 ☑
      - spinal (cranial) (epidural) (intrathecal) (spinal) (subarachnoid) (subdural) T85.735 ☑
    - urethral indwelling T83.511 ☑

Sepsis — *continued*
due to device, implant or graft — *continued*
catheter — *continued*
urinary T83.518 ☑
ectopic or molar pregnancy O08.82
electronic (electrode) (pulse generator) (stimulator)
bone T84.7 ☑
cardiac T82.7 ☑
nervous system T85.738 ☑
brain T85.731 ☑
neurostimulator generator T85.734 ☑
peripheral nerve T85.732 ☑
spinal cord T85.733 ☑
urinary T83.590 ☑
fixation, internal (orthopedic) — *see* Complication, fixation device, infection
gastrointestinal (bile duct) (esophagus) T85.79 ☑
neurostimulator electrode (lead) T85.732 ☑
genital T83.69 ☑
heart NEC T82.7 ☑
valve (prosthesis) T82.6 ☑
graft T82.7 ☑
joint prosthesis — *see* Complication, joint prosthesis, infection
ocular (corneal graft) (orbital implant) T85.79 ☑
orthopedic NEC T84.7 ☑
fixation device, internal — *see* Complication, fixation device, infection
specified NEC T85.79 ☑
vascular T82.7 ☑
ventricular intracranial (communicating) shunt T85.730 ☑
during labor O75.3
Enterococcus A41.81
Erysipelothrix (rhusiopathiae) (erysipeloid) A26.7
Escherichia coli (E. coli) A41.5 ☑
extraintestinal yersiniosis A28.2
following
abortion (subsequent episode) O08.0
current episode — *see* Abortion
ectopic or molar pregnancy O08.82
immunization T88.0 ☑
infusion, therapeutic injection or transfusion NEC T80.29 ☑
obstetrical procedure O86.04
gangrenous A41.9
gonococcal A54.86
Gram-negative (organism) A41.5 ☑
anaerobic A41.4
Haemophilus influenzae A41.3
herpesviral B00.7
intra-abdominal K65.1
intraocular — *see* Endophthalmitis, purulent
Listeria monocytogenes A32.7
localized — *code to* specific localized infection
in operation wound T81.49 ☑
skin — *see* Abscess
malleus A24.0
melioidosis A24.1
meningeal — *see* Meningitis
meningococcal A39.4
acute A39.2
chronic A39.3
MSSA (Methicillin susceptible Staphylococcus aureus) A41.01
newborn P36.9
due to
anaerobes NEC P36.5
Escherichia coli P36.4
Staphylococcus P36.30
aureus P36.2
specified NEC P36.39
Streptococcus P36.10
group B P36.0
specified NEC P36.19
specified NEC P36.8
Pasteurella multocida A28.0
pelvic, puerperal, postpartum, childbirth O85
pneumococcal A40.3
postprocedural T81.44 ☑
puerperal, postpartum, childbirth (pelvic) O85
Salmonella (arizonae) (cholerae-suis) (enteritidis) (typhimurium) A02.1
severe R65.20
with septic shock R65.21
Shigella — *see also* Dysentery, bacillary A03.9
skin, localized — *see* Abscess

Sepsis — *continued*
specified organism NEC A41.89
Staphylococcus, staphylococcal A41.2
aureus (methicillin susceptible) (MSSA) A41.01
methicillin resistant (MRSA) A41.02
coagulase-negative A41.1
specified NEC A41.1
Streptococcus, streptococcal A40.9
agalactiae A40.1
group
A A40.0
B A40.1
D A41.81
neonatal P36.10
group B P36.0
specified NEC P36.19
pneumoniae A40.3
pyogenes A40.0
specified NEC A40.8
tracheostomy stoma J95.02
tularemic A21.7
umbilical, umbilical cord (newborn) — *see* Sepsis, newborn
Yersinia pestis A20.7
Septate — *see* Septum
Septic — *see* condition
arm — *see* Cellulitis, upper limb
with lymphangitis — *see* Lymphangitis, acute, upper limb
embolus — *see* Embolism
finger — *see* Cellulitis, digit
with lymphangitis — *see* Lymphangitis, acute, digit
foot — *see* Cellulitis, lower limb
with lymphangitis — *see* Lymphangitis, acute, lower limb
gallbladder (acute) K81.0
hand — *see* Cellulitis, upper limb
with lymphangitis — *see* Lymphangitis, acute, upper limb
joint — *see* Arthritis, pyogenic or pyemic
leg — *see* Cellulitis, lower limb
with lymphangitis — *see* Lymphangitis, acute, lower limb
nail — *see also* Cellulitis, digit
with lymphangitis — *see* Lymphangitis, acute, digit
sore — *see also* Abscess
throat J02.0
streptococcal J02.0
spleen (acute) D73.89
teeth, tooth (pulpal origin) K04.4
throat — *see* Pharyngitis
thrombus — *see* Thrombosis
toe — *see* Cellulitis, digit
with lymphangitis — *see* Lymphangitis, acute, digit
tonsils, chronic J35.01
with adenoiditis J35.03
uterus — *see* Endometritis
Septicemia A41.9
meaning sepsis — *see* Sepsis
Septum, septate (congenital) — *see also* Anomaly, by site
anal Q42.3
with fistula Q42.2
aqueduct of Sylvius Q03.0
with spina bifida — *see* Spina bifida, by site, with hydrocephalus
uterus Q51.28
complete Q51.21
partial Q51.22
specified NEC Q51.28
vagina Q52.10
in pregnancy — *see* Pregnancy, complicated by, abnormal vagina
causing obstructed labor O65.5
longitudinal Q52.129
microperforate
left side Q52.124
right side Q52.123
nonobstruction Q52.120
obstructing Q52.129
left side Q52.122
right side Q52.121
transverse Q52.11
Sequelae (of) — *see also* condition
abscess, intracranial or intraspinal (conditions in G06) G09

Sequelae — *continued*
amputation — *code to* injury with seventh character S
burn and corrosion — *code to* injury with seventh character S
calcium deficiency E64.8
cerebrovascular disease — *see* Sequelae, disease, cerebrovascular
childbirth O94
contusion — *code to* injury with seventh character S
corrosion — *see* Sequelae, burn and corrosion
COVID-19 (post acute) U09.9
crushing injury — *code to* injury with seventh character S
disease
cerebrovascular I69.90
alteration of sensation I69.998
aphasia I69.920
apraxia I69.990
ataxia I69.993
cognitive deficits I69.91 ☑
disturbance of vision I69.998
dysarthria I69.922
dysphagia I69.991
dysphasia I69.921
facial droop I69.992
facial weakness I69.992
fluency disorder I69.923
hemiplegia I69.95- ☑
hemorrhage
intracerebral — *see* Sequelae, hemorrhage, intracerebral
intracranial, nontraumatic NEC — *see* Sequelae, hemorrhage, intracranial, nontraumatic
subarachnoid — *see* Sequelae, hemorrhage, subarachnoid
language deficit I69.928
monoplegia
lower limb I69.94- ☑
upper limb I69.93- ☑
paralytic syndrome I69.96- ☑
specified effect NEC I69.998
specified type NEC I69.80
alteration of sensation I69.898
aphasia I69.820
apraxia I69.890
ataxia I69.893
cognitive deficits I69.81 ☑
disturbance of vision I69.898
dysarthria I69.822
dysphagia I69.891
dysphasia I69.821
facial droop I69.892
facial weakness I69.892
fluency disorder I69.823
hemiplegia I69.85- ☑
language deficit I69.828
monoplegia
lower limb I69.84- ☑
upper limb I69.83- ☑
paralytic syndrome I69.86- ☑
specified effect NEC I69.898
speech deficit I69.928
speech deficit I69.828
stroke NOS — *see* Sequelae, stroke NOS
dislocation — *code to* injury with seventh character S
encephalitis or encephalomyelitis (conditions in G04) G09
in infectious disease NEC B94.8
viral B94.1
external cause — *code to* injury with seventh character S
foreign body entering natural orifice — *code to* injury with seventh character S
fracture — *code to* injury with seventh character S
frostbite — *code to* injury with seventh character S
Hansen's disease B92
hemorrhage
intracerebral I69.10
alteration of sensation I69.198
aphasia I69.120
apraxia I69.190
ataxia I69.193
cognitive deficits I69.11 ☑
disturbance of vision I69.198
dysarthria I69.122
dysphagia I69.191

Sequelae — *continued*
- hemorrhage — *continued*
  - intracerebral — *continued*
    - dysphasia I69.121
    - facial droop I69.192
    - facial weakness I69.192
    - fluency disorder I69.123
    - hemiplegia I69.15- ☑
    - language deficit NEC I69.128
    - monoplegia
      - lower limb I69.14- ☑
      - upper limb I69.13- ☑
    - paralytic syndrome I69.16- ☑
    - specified effect NEC I69.198
    - speech deficit NEC I69.128
  - intracranial, nontraumatic NEC I69.2Ø
    - alteration of sensation I69.298
    - aphasia I69.22Ø
    - apraxia I69.29Ø
    - ataxia I69.293
    - cognitive deficits I69.21 ☑
    - disturbance of vision I69.298
    - dysarthria I69.222
    - dysphagia I69.291
    - dysphasia I69.221
    - facial droop I69.292
    - facial weakness I69.292
    - fluency disorder I69.223
    - hemiplegia I69.25- ☑
    - language deficit NEC I69.228
    - monoplegia
      - lower limb I69.24- ☑
      - upper limb I69.23- ☑
    - paralytic syndrome I69.26- ☑
    - specified effect NEC I69.298
    - speech deficit NEC I69.228
  - subarachnoid I69.ØØ
    - alteration of sensation I69.Ø98
    - aphasia I69.Ø2Ø
    - apraxia I69.Ø9Ø
    - ataxia I69.Ø93
    - cognitive deficits — *see* subcategory I69.Ø1- ☑
    - disturbance of vision I69.Ø98
    - dysarthria I69.Ø22
    - dysphagia I69.Ø91
    - dysphasia I69.Ø21
    - facial droop I69.Ø92
    - facial weakness I69.Ø92
    - fluency disorder I69.Ø23
    - hemiplegia I69.Ø5- ☑
    - language deficit NEC I69.Ø28
    - monoplegia
      - lower limb I69.Ø4- ☑
      - upper limb I69.Ø3- ☑
    - paralytic syndrome I69.Ø6- ☑
    - specified effect NEC I69.Ø98
    - speech deficit NEC I69.Ø28
- hepatitis, viral B94.2
- hyperalimentation E68
- infarction
  - cerebral I69.3Ø
    - alteration of sensation I69.398
    - aphasia I69.32Ø
    - apraxia I69.39Ø
    - ataxia I69.393
    - cognitive deficits I69.31 ☑
    - disturbance of vision I69.398
    - dysarthria I69.322
    - dysphagia I69.391
    - dysphasia I69.321
    - facial droop I69.392
    - facial weakness I69.392
    - fluency disorder I69.323
    - hemiplegia I69.35- ☑
    - language deficit NEC I69.328
    - monoplegia
      - lower limb I69.34- ☑
      - upper limb I69.33- ☑
    - paralytic syndrome I69.36- ☑
    - specified effect NEC I69.398
    - speech deficit NEC I69.328
- infection, pyogenic, intracranial or intraspinal GØ9
- infectious disease B94.9
  - specified NEC B94.8
- injury — *code to* injury with seventh character S
- leprosy B92
- meningitis
  - bacterial (conditions in GØØ) GØ9

Sequelae — *continued*
- meningitis — *continued*
  - other or unspecified cause (conditions in GØ3) GØ9
- muscle (and tendon) injury — *code to* injury with seventh character S
- myelitis — *see* Sequelae, encephalitis
- niacin deficiency E64.8
- nutritional deficiency E64.9
  - specified NEC E64.8
- obstetrical condition O94
- parasitic disease B94.9
- phlebitis or thrombophlebitis of intracranial or intraspinal venous sinuses and veins (conditions in GØ8) GØ9
- poisoning — *code to* poisoning with seventh character S
  - nonmedicinal substance — *see* Sequelae, toxic effect, nonmedicinal substance
- poliomyelitis (acute) B91
- pregnancy O94
- protein-energy malnutrition E64.Ø
- puerperium O94
- rickets E64.3
- SARS-CoV-2 (post acute) UØ9.9
- selenium deficiency E64.8
- sprain and strain — *code to* injury with seventh character S
- stroke NOS I69.3Ø
  - alteration in sensation I69.398
  - aphasia I69.32Ø
  - apraxia I69.39Ø
  - ataxia I69.393
  - cognitive deficits I69.31 ☑
  - disturbance of vision I69.398
  - dysarthria I69.322
  - dysphagia I69.391
  - dysphasia I69.321
  - facial droop I69.392
  - facial weakness I69.392
  - hemiplegia I69.35- ☑
  - language deficit NEC I69.328
  - monoplegia
    - lower limb I69.34- ☑
    - upper limb I69.33- ☑
  - paralytic syndrome I69.36- ☑
  - specified effect NEC I69.398
  - speech deficit NEC I69.328
- tendon and muscle injury — *code to* injury with seventh character S
- thiamine deficiency E64.8
- trachoma B94.Ø
- tuberculosis B9Ø.9
  - bones and joints B9Ø.2
  - central nervous system B9Ø.Ø
  - genitourinary B9Ø.1
  - pulmonary (respiratory) B9Ø.9
  - specified organs NEC B9Ø.8
- viral
  - encephalitis B94.1
  - hepatitis B94.2
- vitamin deficiency NEC E64.8
  - A E64.1
  - B E64.8
  - C E64.2
- wound, open — *code to* injury with seventh character S

Sequestration — *see also* Sequestrum
- disc — *see* Displacement, intervertebral disc
- lung, congenital Q33.2

Sequestrum
- bone — *see* Osteomyelitis, chronic
- dental M27.2
- jaw bone M27.2
- orbit — *see* Osteomyelitis, orbit
- sinus (accessory) (nasal) — *see* Sinusitis

Sequoiosis lung or pneumonitis J67.8

Serology for syphilis
- doubtful
  - with signs or symptoms — *code by* site and stage under Syphilis
  - follow-up of latent syphilis — *see* Syphilis, latent
- negative, with signs or symptoms — *code by* site and stage under Syphilis
- positive A53.Ø
  - with signs or symptoms — *code by* site and stage under Syphilis
- reactivated A53.Ø

Seroma — *see also* Hematoma

Seroma — *continued*
- postprocedural — *see* Complication, postprocedural, seroma
- traumatic, secondary and recurrent T79.2 ☑

Seropurulent — *see* condition

Serositis, multiple K65.8
- pericardial I31.1
- peritoneal K65.8

Serous — *see* condition

Sertoli cell
- adenoma
  - specified site — *see* Neoplasm, benign, by site
  - unspecified site
    - female D27.9
    - male D29.2Ø
- carcinoma
  - specified site — *see* Neoplasm, malignant, by site
  - unspecified site (male) C62.9- ☑
    - female C56.9
- tumor
  - with lipid storage
    - specified site — *see* Neoplasm, benign, by site
    - unspecified site
      - female D27.9
      - male D29.2Ø
  - specified site — *see* Neoplasm, benign, by site
  - unspecified site
    - female D27.9
    - male D29.2Ø

Sertoli-Leydig cell tumor — *see* Neoplasm, benign, by site
- specified site — *see* Neoplasm, benign, by site
- unspecified site
  - female D27.9
  - male D29.2Ø

Serum
- allergy, allergic reaction — *see also* Reaction, serum T8Ø.69 ☑
  - shock — *see also* Shock, anaphylactic T8Ø.59 ☑
- arthritis — *see also* Reaction, serum T8Ø.69 ☑
- complication or reaction NEC — *see also* Reaction, serum T8Ø.69 ☑
- disease NEC — *see also* Reaction, serum T8Ø.69 ☑
- hepatitis — *see also* Hepatitis, viral, type B
  - carrier (suspected) of B18.1
- intoxication — *see also* Reaction, serum T8Ø.69 ☑
- neuritis — *see also* Reaction, serum T8Ø.69 ☑
- neuropathy G61.1
- poisoning NEC — *see also* Reaction, serum T8Ø.69 ☑
- rash NEC — *see also* Reaction, serum T8Ø.69 ☑
- reaction NEC — *see also* Reaction, serum T8Ø.69 ☑
- sickness NEC — *see also* Reaction, serum T8Ø.69 ☑
- urticaria — *see also* Reaction, serum T8Ø.69 ☑

Sesamoiditis M25.8- ☑

Severe sepsis R65.2Ø
- with septic shock R65.21

Sever's disease or osteochondrosis — *see* Osteochondrosis, juvenile, tarsus

Sex
- chromosome mosaics Q97.8
  - lines with various numbers of X chromosomes Q97.2
- education Z7Ø.8
- reassignment surgery status Z87.89Ø

Sextuplet pregnancy — *see* Pregnancy, sextuplet

Sexual
- function, disorder of (psychogenic) F52.9
- immaturity (female) (male) E3Ø.Ø
- impotence (psychogenic) organic origin NEC — *see* Dysfunction, sexual, male
- precocity (constitutional) (cryptogenic) (female) (idiopathic) (male) E3Ø.1

Sexuality, pathologic — *see* Deviation, sexual

Sézary disease C84.1- ☑

Shadow, lung R91.8

Shaking palsy or paralysis — *see* Parkinsonism

Shallowness, acetabulum — *see* Derangement, joint, specified type NEC, hip

Shaver's disease J63.1

Sheath (tendon) — *see* condition

Sheathing, retinal vessels H35.Ø1- ☑

Shedding
- nail L6Ø.8
- premature, primary (deciduous) teeth KØØ.6

Sheehan's disease or syndrome E23.Ø

Shelf, rectal K62.89

Shell teeth KØØ.5

Shellshock (current) F43.Ø

Shellshock — *continued*
- lasting state — *see* Disorder, post-traumatic stress

Shield kidney Q63.1
Shift
- auditory threshold (temporary) H93.24- ☑
- mediastinal R93.89

Shifting sleep-work schedule (affecting sleep) G47.26
Shiga (-Kruse) **dysentery** AØ3.Ø
Shiga's bacillus AØ3.Ø
Shigella (dysentery) — *see* Dysentery, bacillary
Shigellosis AØ3.9
- Group A AØ3.Ø
- Group B AØ3.1
- Group C AØ3.2
- Group D AØ3.3

Shin splints S86.89- ☑
Shingles — *see* Herpes, zoster
Shipyard disease or eye B3Ø.Ø
Shirodkar suture, in pregnancy — *see* Pregnancy, complicated by, incompetent cervix
Shock R57.9
- with ectopic or molar pregnancy OØ8.3
- adrenal (cortical) (Addisonian) E27.2
- adverse food reaction (anaphylactic) — *see* Shock, anaphylactic, due to food
- allergic — *see* Shock, anaphylactic
- anaphylactic T78.2 ☑
  - chemical — *see* Table of Drugs and Chemicals
  - due to drug or medicinal substance
    - correct substance properly administered T88.6 ☑
    - overdose or wrong substance given or taken (by accident) — *see* Table of Drugs and Chemicals, by drug, poisoning
  - due to food (nonpoisonous) T78.ØØ ☑
    - additives T78.Ø6 ☑
    - dairy products T78.Ø7 ☑
    - eggs T78.Ø8 ☑
    - fish T78.Ø3 ☑
      - shellfish T78.Ø2 ☑
    - fruit T78.Ø4 ☑
    - milk T78.Ø7 ☑
    - nuts T78.Ø5 ☑
      - multiple types T78.Ø5 ☑
      - peanuts T78.Ø1 ☑
    - peanuts T78.Ø1 ☑
    - seeds T78.Ø5 ☑
    - specified type NEC T78.Ø9 ☑
    - vegetable T78.Ø4 ☑
  - following sting(s) — *see* Venom
  - immunization T8Ø.52 ☑
  - serum T8Ø.59 ☑
    - blood and blood products T8Ø.51 ☑
    - immunization T8Ø.52 ☑
    - specified NEC T8Ø.59 ☑
    - vaccination T8Ø.52 ☑
- anaphylactoid — *see* Shock, anaphylactic
- anesthetic
  - correct substance properly administered T88.2 ☑
  - overdose or wrong substance given or taken — *see* Table of Drugs and Chemicals, by drug, poisoning
    - specified anesthetic — *see* Table of Drugs and Chemicals, by drug, poisoning
- cardiogenic R57.Ø
- chemical substance — *see* Table of Drugs and Chemicals
- complicating ectopic or molar pregnancy OØ8.3
- culture — *see* Disorder, adjustment
- drug
  - due to correct substance properly administered T88.6 ☑
  - overdose or wrong substance given or taken (by accident) — *see* Table of Drugs and Chemicals, by drug, poisoning
- during or after labor and delivery O75.1
- electric T75.4 ☑
  - (taser) T75.4 ☑
- endotoxic R65.21
  - postprocedural (resulting from a procedure, not elsewhere classified) T81.12 ☑
- following
  - ectopic or molar pregnancy OØ8.3
  - injury (immediate) (delayed) T79.4 ☑
  - labor and delivery O75.1
- food (anaphylactic) — *see* Shock, anaphylactic, due to food
- from electroshock gun (taser) T75.4 ☑

Shock — *continued*
- gram-negative R65.21
  - postprocedural (resulting from a procedure, not elsewhere classified) T81.12 ☑
- hematologic R57.8
- hemorrhagic R57.8
  - surgery (intraoperative) (postoperative) T81.19 ☑
  - trauma T79.4 ☑
- hypovolemic R57.1
  - surgical T81.19 ☑
  - traumatic T79.4 ☑
- insulin E15
  - therapeutic misadventure — *see* subcategory T38.3 ☑
- kidney N17.Ø
  - traumatic (following crushing) T79.5 ☑
- lightning T75.Ø1 ☑
- liver K72.ØØ
- lung J8Ø
- obstetric O75.1
  - with ectopic or molar pregnancy OØ8.3
  - following ectopic or molar pregnancy OØ8.3
- pleural (surgical) T81.19 ☑
  - due to trauma T79.4 ☑
- postprocedural (postoperative) T81.1Ø ☑
  - with ectopic or molar pregnancy OØ8.3
  - cardiogenic T81.11 ☑
  - endotoxic T81.12 ☑
  - following ectopic or molar pregnancy OØ8.3
  - gram-negative T81.12 ☑
  - hypovolemic T81.19 ☑
  - septic T81.12 ☑
  - specified type NEC T81.19 ☑
- psychic F43.Ø
- septic (due to severe sepsis) R65.21
- specified NEC R57.8
- surgical T81.1Ø ☑
- taser gun (taser) T75.4 ☑
- therapeutic misadventure NEC T81.1Ø ☑
- thyroxin
  - overdose or wrong substance given or taken — *see* Table of Drugs and Chemicals, by drug, poisoning
- toxic, syndrome A48.3
- transfusion — *see* Complications, transfusion
- traumatic (immediate) (delayed) T79.4 ☑

Shoemaker's chest M95.4
Short, shortening, shortness
- arm (acquired) — *see also* Deformity, limb, unequal length
  - congenital Q71.81- ☑
  - forearm — *see* Deformity, limb, unequal length
- bowel syndrome K91.2
- breath RØ6.Ø2
- cervical (complicating pregnancy) O26.87- ☑
  - non-gravid uterus N88.3
- common bile duct, congenital Q44.5
- cord (umbilical), complicating delivery O69.3 ☑
- cystic duct, congenital Q44.5
- esophagus (congenital) Q39.8
- femur (acquired) — *see* Deformity, limb, unequal length, femur
  - congenital — *see* Defect, reduction, lower limb, longitudinal, femur
- frenum, frenulum, linguae (congenital) Q38.1
- hip (acquired) — *see also* Deformity, limb, unequal length
  - congenital Q65.89
- leg (acquired) — *see also* Deformity, limb, unequal length
  - congenital Q72.81- ☑
  - lower leg — *see also* Deformity, limb, unequal length
- limbed stature, with immunodeficiency D82.2
- lower limb (acquired) — *see also* Deformity, limb, unequal length
  - congenital Q72.81- ☑
- organ or site, congenital NEC — *see* Distortion
- palate, congenital Q38.5
- radius (acquired) — *see also* Deformity, limb, unequal length
  - congenital — *see* Defect, reduction, upper limb, longitudinal, radius
- rib syndrome Q77.2
- stature (child) (hereditary) (idiopathic) NEC R62.52
  - constitutional E34.31

Short, shortening, shortness — *continued*
- stature — *continued*
  - due to
    - endocrine disorder E34.3Ø
      - specified type NEC, due to endocrine dosorder E34.39
    - genetic causes E34.329
      - ACAN gene variant E34.328
      - acid-labile subunit gene (IGFALS) defect E34.321
      - aggrecan deficiency E34.328
      - genetic syndrome with resistance to insulin-like growth factor-1 E34.322
      - growth hormone gene 1 (GH1) defect with growth hormone neutralizing antibodies E34.321
      - growth hormone insensitivity syndrome (GHIS) E34.321
      - insulin-like growth factor 1 gene (IGF1) defect E34.321
      - insulin-like growth factor-1 receptor (IGF-1R) defect E34.322
      - insulin-like growth factor-1 (IGF-1) resistance E34.322
      - NPR-2 gene variant E34.328
      - post-insulin-like growth factor-1 receptor signaling defect E34.322
      - primary insulin-like growth factor-1 (IGF-1) deficiency E34.321
      - severe primary insulin-like growth factor-1 deficiency (SPIGFD) E34.321
      - signal transducer and activator of transcription 5B gene (STAT5b) defect E34.321
      - specified genetic cause NEC E34.328
  - Laron-type E34.321
- tendon — *see also* Contraction, tendon
  - with contracture of joint — *see* Contraction, joint
  - Achilles (acquired) M67.Ø- ☑
    - congenital Q66.89
  - congenital Q79.8
- thigh (acquired) — *see also* Deformity, limb, unequal length, femur
  - congenital — *see* Defect, reduction, lower limb, longitudinal, femur
- tibialis anterior (tendon) — *see* Contraction, tendon
- umbilical cord
  - complicating delivery O69.3 ☑
- upper limb, congenital — *see* Defect, reduction, upper limb, specified type NEC
- urethra N36.8
- uvula, congenital Q38.5
- vagina (congenital) Q52.4

Shortsightedness — *see* Myopia
Shoshin (acute fulminating beriberi) E51.11
Shoulder — *see* condition
Shovel-shaped incisors KØØ.2
Shower, thromboembolic — *see* Embolism
Shunt
- arterial-venous (dialysis) Z99.2
- arteriovenous, pulmonary (acquired) I28.Ø
  - congenital Q25.72
- cerebral ventricle (communicating) in situ Z98.2
- surgical, prosthetic, with complications — *see* Complications, cardiovascular, device or implant

Shutdown, renal N28.9
Shy-Drager syndrome G9Ø.3
Sialadenitis, sialadenosis (any gland) (chronic) (periodic) (suppurative) — *see* Sialoadenitis
Sialectasia K11.8
Sialidosis E77.1
Sialitis, silitis (any gland) (chronic) (suppurative) — *see* Sialoadenitis
Sialoadenitis (any gland) (periodic) (suppurative) K11.2Ø
- acute K11.21
  - recurrent K11.22
- chronic K11.23

Sialoadenopathy K11.9
Sialoangitis — *see* Sialoadenitis
Sialodochitis (fibrinosa) — *see* Sialoadenitis
Sialodocholithiasis K11.5
Sialolithiasis K11.5
Sialometaplasia, necrotizing K11.8
Sialorrhea — *see also* Ptyalism
- periodic — *see* Sialoadenitis

Sialosis K11.7
Siamese twin Q89.4
Sibling rivalry Z62.891
Sicard's syndrome G52.7

Sicca syndrome — *see* Syndrome, Sjögren
Sick R69
  or handicapped person in family Z63.79
    needing care at home Z63.6
  sinus (syndrome) I49.5
Sick-euthyroid syndrome EØ7.81
Sickle-cell
  anemia — *see* Disease, sickle-cell
  beta plus — *see* Disease, sickle-cell, thalassemia, beta plus
  beta zero — *see* Disease, sickle-cell, thalassemia, beta zero
  trait D57.3
Sicklemia — *see also* Disease, sickle-cell
  trait D57.3
Sickness
  air (travel) T75.3 ☑
  airplane T75.3 ☑
  alpine T7Ø.29 ☑
  altitude T7Ø.2Ø ☑
  Andes T7Ø.29 ☑
  aviator's T7Ø.29 ☑
  balloon T7Ø.29 ☑
  car T75.3 ☑
  compressed air T7Ø.3 ☑
  decompression T7Ø.3 ☑
  green D5Ø.8
  milk — *see* Poisoning, food, noxious
  motion T75.3 ☑
  mountain T7Ø.29 ☑
    acute D75.1
  protein — *see also* Reaction, serum T8Ø.69 ☑
  radiation T66 ☑
  roundabout (motion) T75.3 ☑
  sea T75.3 ☑
  serum NEC — *see also* Reaction, serum T8Ø.69 ☑
  sleeping (African) B56.9
    by Trypanosoma B56.9
      brucei
        gambiense B56.Ø
        rhodesiense B56.1
    East African B56.1
    Gambian B56.Ø
    Rhodesian B56.1
    West African B56.Ø
  swing (motion) T75.3 ☑
  train (railway) (travel) T75.3 ☑
  travel (any vehicle) T75.3 ☑
Sideropenia — *see* Anemia, iron deficiency
Siderosilicosis J62.8
Siderosis (lung) J63.4
  brain G93.89
  eye (globe) — *see* Disorder, globe, degenerative, siderosis
Siemens' syndrome (ectodermal dysplasia) Q82.8
Sighing RØ6.89
  psychogenic F45.8
Sigmoid — *see also* condition
  flexure — *see* condition
  kidney Q63.1
Sigmoiditis — *see also* Enteritis K52.9
  infectious AØ9
  noninfectious K52.9
Silfverskïöld's syndrome Q78.9
Silicosiderosis J62.8
Silicosis, silicotic (simple) (complicated) J62.8
  with tuberculosis J65
Silicotuberculosis J65
Silo-fillers' disease J68.8
  bronchitis J68.Ø
  pneumonitis J68.Ø
  pulmonary edema J68.1
Silver's syndrome Q87.19
Simian malaria B53.1
Simmonds' cachexia or disease E23.Ø
Simons' disease or syndrome (progressive lipodystrophy) E88.1
Simple, simplex — *see* condition
Simulation, conscious (of illness) Z76.5
Simultagnosia (asimultagnosia) R48.3
Sin Nombre virus disease (Hantavirus) (cardio)-pulmonary syndrome) B33.4
Sinding-Larsen disease or osteochondrosis — *see* Osteochondrosis, juvenile, patella
Singapore hemorrhagic fever A91
Singer's node or nodule J38.2
Single
  atrium Q21.2Ø
  coronary artery Q24.5
  umbilical artery Q27.Ø
  ventricle Q2Ø.4
Singultus RØ6.6
  epidemicus B33.Ø
Sinus — *see also* Fistula
  abdominal K63.89
  arrest I45.5
  arrhythmia I49.8
  bradycardia RØØ.1
  branchial cleft (internal) (external) Q18.Ø
  coccygeal — *see* Sinus, pilonidal
  dental KØ4.6
  dermal (congenital) QØ6.8
    with abscess QØ6.8
    coccygeal, pilonidal — *see* Sinus, coccygeal
  infected, skin NEC LØ8.89
  marginal, ruptured or bleeding — *see* Hemorrhage, antepartum, specified cause NEC
  medial, face and neck Q18.8
  pause I45.5
  pericranii QØ1.9
  pilonidal (infected) (rectum) LØ5.92
    with abscess LØ5.02
  preauricular Q18.1
  rectovaginal N82.3
  Rokitansky-Aschoff (gallbladder) K82.8
  sacrococcygeal (dermoid) (infected) — *see* Sinus, pilonidal
  tachycardia RØØ.Ø
    paroxysmal I47.1
  tarsi syndrome M25.57- ☑
  testis N5Ø.89
  tract (postinfective) — *see* Fistula
  urachus Q64.4
Sinusitis (accessory) (chronic) (hyperplastic) (nasal) (nonpurulent) (purulent) J32.9
  acute JØ1.9Ø
    ethmoidal JØ1.2Ø
      recurrent JØ1.21
    frontal JØ1.1Ø
      recurrent JØ1.11
    involving more than one sinus, other than pansinusitis JØ1.8Ø
      recurrent JØ1.81
    maxillary JØ1.ØØ
      recurrent JØ1.Ø1
    pansinusitis JØ1.4Ø
      recurrent JØ1.41
    recurrent JØ1.91
    specified NEC JØ1.8Ø
      recurrent JØ1.81
    sphenoidal JØ1.3Ø
      recurrent JØ1.31
  allergic — *see* Rhinitis, allergic
  due to high altitude T7Ø.1 ☑
  ethmoidal J32.2
    acute JØ1.2Ø
      recurrent JØ1.21
  frontal J32.1
    acute JØ1.1Ø
      recurrent JØ1.11
  influenzal — *see* Influenza, with, respiratory manifestations NEC
  involving more than one sinus but not pansinusitis J32.8
    acute JØ1.8Ø
      recurrent JØ1.81
  maxillary J32.Ø
    acute JØ1.ØØ
      recurrent JØ1.Ø1
  sphenoidal J32.3
    acute JØ1.3Ø
      recurrent JØ1.31
  tuberculous, any sinus A15.8
Sinusitis-bronchiectasis-situs inversus (syndrome) (triad) Q89.3
Sipple's syndrome E31.22
Sirenomelia (syndrome) Q87.2
Siriasis T67.Ø1 ☑
Sirkari's disease B55.Ø
Siti A65
Situation, psychiatric F99
Situational
  disturbance (transient) — *see* Disorder, adjustment
    acute F43.Ø
Situational — *continued*
  maladjustment — *see* Disorder, adjustment
  reaction — *see* Disorder, adjustment
    acute F43.Ø
Situs inversus or transversus (abdominalis) (thoracis) Q89.3
Sixth disease BØ8.2Ø
  due to human herpesvirus 6 BØ8.21
  due to human herpesvirus 7 BØ8.22
Sjögren-Larsson syndrome Q87.19
Sjögren's syndrome or disease — *see* Syndrome, Sjögren
Skeletal — *see* condition
Skene's gland — *see* condition
Skenitis — *see* Urethritis
Skerljevo A65
Skevas-Zerfus disease — *see* Toxicity, venom, marine animal, sea anemone
Skin — *see also* condition
  clammy R23.1
  donor — *see* Donor, skin
  dry L85.3
  hidebound M35.9
Slate-dressers' or slate-miners' lung J62.8
Sleep
  apnea — *see* Apnea, sleep
  deprivation Z72.82Ø
  disorder or disturbance G47.9
    child F51.9
    nonorganic origin F51.9
    specified NEC G47.8
  disturbance G47.9
    nonorganic origin F51.9
  drunkenness F51.9
  rhythm inversion G47.2- ☑
  terrors F51.4
  walking F51.3
    hysterical F44.89
Sleep hygiene
  abuse Z72.821
  inadequate Z72.821
  poor Z72.821
Sleeping sickness — *see* Sickness, sleeping
Sleeplessness — *see* Insomnia
  menopausal N95.1
Sleep-wake schedule disorder G47.2Ø
Slim disease (in HIV infection) B2Ø
Slipped, slipping
  epiphysis (traumatic) — *see also* Osteochondropathy, specified type NEC
    capital femoral (traumatic) [SCFE]
      acute (on chronic) S79.Ø1- ☑
      nontraumatic M93.ØØ- ☑
    current traumatic — *code as* Fracture, by site
    upper femoral (nontraumatic) [SUFE] M93.ØØ- ☑
      acute M93.Ø1- ☑
        on chronic M93.Ø3- ☑
      chronic M93.Ø2- ☑
  intervertebral disc — *see* Displacement, intervertebral disc
  ligature, umbilical P51.8
  patella — *see* Disorder, patella, derangement NEC
  rib M89.8X8
  sacroiliac joint — *see* subcategory M53.2 ☑
  tendon — *see* Disorder, tendon
  ulnar nerve, nontraumatic — *see* Lesion, nerve, ulnar
  vertebra NEC — *see* Spondylolisthesis
Slocumb's syndrome E27.Ø
Sloughing (multiple) (phagedena) (skin) — *see also* Gangrene
  abscess — *see* Abscess
  appendix K38.8
  fascia — *see* Disorder, soft tissue, specified type NEC
  scrotum N5Ø.89
  tendon — *see* Disorder, tendon
  transplanted organ — *see* Rejection, transplant
  ulcer — *see* Ulcer, skin
Slow
  feeding, newborn P92.2
  flow syndrome, coronary I2Ø.8
  heart (beat) RØØ.1
Slowing, urinary stream R39.198
Sluder's neuralgia (syndrome) G44.89
Slurred, slurring speech R47.81
Small (ness)
  for gestational age — *see* Small for dates
  introitus, vagina N89.6

- **Small** — *continued*
  - kidney (unknown cause) N27.9
    - bilateral N27.1
    - unilateral N27.Ø
  - ovary (congenital) Q5Ø.39
  - pelvis
    - with disproportion (fetopelvic) O33.1
      - causing obstructed labor O65.1
  - uterus N85.8
  - white kidney NØ3.9
- **Small-and-light-for-dates** — *see* Small for dates
- **Small-for-dates** (infant) PØ5.1Ø
  - with weight of
    - 499 grams or less PØ5.11
    - 5ØØ-749 grams PØ5.12
    - 75Ø-999 grams PØ5.13
    - 1ØØØ-1249 grams PØ5.14
    - 125Ø-1499 grams PØ5.15
    - 15ØØ-1749 grams PØ5.16
    - 175Ø-1999 grams PØ5.17
    - 2ØØØ-2499 grams PØ5.18
    - 25ØØ grams and over PØ5.19
  - specified NEC PØ5.19
- **Smallpox** BØ3
- **Smearing, fecal** R15.1
- **SMEI** (severe myoclonic epilepsy in infancy) G4Ø.83- ☑
- **Smith-Lemli-Opitz syndrome** E78.72
- **Smith's fracture** S52.54- ☑
- **Smoker** — *see* Dependence, drug, nicotine
- **Smoker's**
  - bronchitis J41.Ø
  - cough J41.Ø
  - palate K13.24
  - throat J31.2
  - tongue K13.24
- **Smoking**
  - passive Z77.22
- **Smothering spells** RØ6.81
- **Snaggle teeth, tooth** M26.39
- **Snapping**
  - finger — *see* Trigger finger
  - hip — *see* Derangement, joint, specified type NEC, hip
    - involving the iliotiblial band M76.3- ☑
  - knee — *see* Derangement, knee
    - involving the iliotiblial band M76.3- ☑
- **Sneddon-Wilkinson disease or syndrome** (sub-corneal pustular dermatosis) L13.1
- **Sneezing** (intractable) RØ6.7
- **Sniffing**
  - cocaine
    - abuse — *see* Abuse, drug, cocaine
    - dependence — *see* Dependence, drug, cocaine
  - gasoline
    - abuse — *see* Abuse, drug, inhalant
    - dependence — *see* Dependence, drug, inhalant
  - glue (airplane)
    - abuse — *see* Abuse, drug, inhalant
    - drug dependence — *see* Dependence, drug, inhalant
- **Sniffles**
  - newborn P28.89
- **Snoring** RØ6.83
- **Snow blindness** — *see* Photokeratitis
- **Snuffles** (non-syphilitic) RØ6.5
  - newborn P28.89
  - syphilitic (infant) A5Ø.Ø5 *[J99]*
- **Social**
  - exclusion Z6Ø.4
    - due to discrimination or persecution (perceived) Z6Ø.5
  - migrant Z59.ØØ
    - acculturation difficulty Z6Ø.3
  - rejection Z6Ø.4
    - due to discrimination or persecution Z6Ø.5
  - role conflict NEC Z73.5
  - skills inadequacy NEC Z73.4
  - transplantation Z6Ø.3
- **Sodoku** A25.Ø
- **Soemmerring's ring** — *see* Cataract, secondary
- **Soft** — *see also* condition
  - nails L6Ø.3
- **Softening**
  - bone — *see* Osteomalacia
  - brain (necrotic) (progressive) G93.89
    - congenital QØ4.8
    - embolic I63.4- ☑
- **Softening** — *continued*
  - brain — *continued*
    - hemorrhagic — *see* Hemorrhage, intracranial, intracerebral
    - occlusive I63.5- ☑
    - thrombotic I63.3- ☑
  - cartilage M94.2- ☑
    - patella M22.4- ☑
  - cerebellar — *see* Softening, brain
  - cerebral — *see* Softening, brain
  - cerebrospinal — *see* Softening, brain
  - myocardial, heart — *see* Degeneration, myocardial
  - spinal cord G95.89
  - stomach K31.89
- **Soldier's**
  - heart F45.8
  - patches I31.Ø
- **Solitary**
  - cyst, kidney N28.1
  - kidney, congenital Q6Ø.Ø
- **Solvent abuse** — *see* Abuse, drug, inhalant
  - dependence — *see* Dependence, drug, inhalant
- **Somatization reaction, somatic reaction** — *see* Disorder, somatoform
- **Somnambulism** F51.3
  - hysterical F44.89
- **Somnolence** R4Ø.Ø
  - nonorganic origin F51.11
- **Sonne dysentery** AØ3.3
- **Soor** B37.Ø
- **Sore**
  - bed — *see* Ulcer, pressure, by site
  - chiclero B55.1
  - Delhi B55.1
  - desert — *see* Ulcer, skin
  - eye H57.1- ☑
  - Lahore B55.1
  - mouth K13.79
    - canker K12.Ø
  - muscle M79.1Ø
  - Naga — *see* Ulcer, skin
  - of skin — *see* Ulcer, skin
  - oriental B55.1
  - pressure — *see* Ulcer, pressure, by site
  - skin L98.9
  - soft A57
  - throat (acute) — *see also* Pharyngitis
    - with influenza, flu, or grippe — *see* Influenza, with, respiratory manifestations NEC
    - chronic J31.2
    - coxsackie (virus) BØ8.5
    - diphtheritic A36.Ø
    - herpesviral BØØ.2
    - influenzal — *see* Influenza, with, respiratory manifestations NEC
    - septic JØ2.Ø
    - streptococcal (ulcerative) JØ2.Ø
    - viral NEC JØ2.8
      - coxsackie BØ8.5
  - tropical — *see* Ulcer, skin
  - veldt — *see* Ulcer, skin
- **Soto's syndrome** (cerebral gigantism) Q87.3
- **South African cardiomyopathy syndrome** I42.8
- **Southeast Asian hemorrhagic fever** A91
- **Spacing**
  - abnormal, tooth, teeth, fully erupted M26.3Ø
  - excessive, tooth, fully erupted M26.32
- **Spade-like hand** (congenital) Q68.1
- **Spading nail** L6Ø.8
  - congenital Q84.6
- **Spanish collar** N47.1
- **Sparganosis** B7Ø.1
- **Spasm**(s), **spastic, spasticity** — *see also* condition R25.2
  - accommodation — *see* Spasm, of accommodation
  - ampulla of Vater K83.4
  - anus, ani (sphincter) (reflex) K59.4
    - psychogenic F45.8
  - artery I73.9
    - cerebral G45.9
  - Bell's G51.3- ☑
  - bladder (sphincter, external or internal) N32.89
    - psychogenic F45.8
  - bronchus, bronchiole J98.Ø1
  - cardia K22.Ø
  - cardiac I2Ø.1
  - carpopedal — *see* Tetany
  - cerebral (arteries) (vascular) G45.9
- **Spasm(s), spastic, spasticity** — *continued*
  - cervix, complicating delivery O62.4
  - ciliary body (of accommodation) — *see* Spasm, of accommodation
  - colon — *see also* Irritable, bowel K58.9
    - with diarrhea K58.Ø
    - psychogenic F45.8
  - common duct K83.8
  - compulsive — *see* Tic
  - conjugate H51.8
  - coronary (artery) I2Ø.1
  - diaphragm (reflex) RØ6.6
    - epidemic B33.Ø
    - psychogenic F45.8
  - duodenum K59.89
  - epidemic diaphragmatic (transient) B33.Ø
  - esophagus (diffuse) K22.4
    - psychogenic F45.8
  - facial G51.3- ☑
  - fallopian tube N83.8
  - gastrointestinal (tract) K31.89
    - psychogenic F45.8
  - glottis J38.5
    - hysterical F44.4
    - psychogenic F45.8
      - conversion reaction F44.4
    - reflex through recurrent laryngeal nerve J38.5
  - habit — *see* Tic
  - heart I2Ø.1
  - hemifacial (clonic) G51.3- ☑
  - hourglass — *see* Contraction, hourglass
  - hysterical F44.4
  - infantile — *see* Epilepsy, spasms
  - inferior oblique, eye H51.8
  - intestinal — *see also* Syndrome, irritable bowel K58.9
    - psychogenic F45.8
  - larynx, laryngeal J38.5
    - hysterical F44.4
    - psychogenic F45.8
      - conversion reaction F44.4
  - levator palpebrae superioris — *see* Disorder, eyelid function
  - muscle NEC M62.838
    - back M62.83Ø
  - nerve, trigeminal G51.Ø
  - nervous F45.8
  - nodding F98.4
  - occupational F48.8
  - oculogyric H51.8
    - psychogenic F45.8
  - of accommodation H52.53- ☑
  - ophthalmic artery — *see* Occlusion, artery, retina
  - perineal, female N94.89
  - peroneo-extensor — *see also* Deformity, limb, flat foot
  - pharynx (reflex) J39.2
    - hysterical F45.8
    - psychogenic F45.8
  - psychogenic F45.8
  - pylorus NEC K31.3
    - adult hypertrophic K31.89
    - congenital or infantile Q4Ø.Ø
    - psychogenic F45.8
  - rectum (sphincter) K59.4
    - psychogenic F45.8
  - retinal (artery) — *see* Occlusion, artery, retina
  - sigmoid — *see also* Syndrome, irritable bowel K58.9
    - psychogenic F45.8
  - sphincter of Oddi K83.4
  - stomach K31.89
    - neurotic F45.8
  - throat J39.2
    - hysterical F45.8
    - psychogenic F45.8
  - tic F95.9
    - chronic F95.1
    - transient of childhood F95.Ø
  - tongue K14.8
  - torsion (progressive) G24.1
  - trigeminal nerve — *see* Neuralgia, trigeminal
  - ureter N13.5
  - urethra (sphincter) N35.919
  - uterus N85.8
    - complicating labor O62.4
  - vagina N94.2
    - psychogenic F52.5
  - vascular I73.9
  - vasomotor I73.9
  - vein NEC I87.8

- **Spasm(s), spastic, spasticity** — *continued*
  - viscera — *see* Pain, abdominal
- **Spasmodic** — *see* condition
- **Spasmophilia** — *see* Tetany
- **Spasmus nutans** F98.4
- **Spastic, spasticity** — *see also* Spasm
  - child (cerebral) (congenital) (paralysis) G8Ø.1
- **Speaker's throat** R49.8
- **Specific, specified** — *see* condition
- **Speech**
  - defect, disorder, disturbance, impediment — *see* Disorder, speech R47.9
    - psychogenic, in childhood and adolescence F98.8
    - slurring R47.81
    - specified NEC R47.89
- **Spells, transient oxygen desaturation of newborn** — *see also* Apnea, newborn P28.4Ø
  - during sleep — *see also* Apnea, newborn, sleep, primary P28.3Ø
- **Spencer's disease** AØ8.19
- **Spens' syndrome** (syncope with heart block) I45.9
- **Sperm counts** (fertility testing) Z31.41
  - postvasectomy Z3Ø.8
    - reversal Z31.42
- **Spermatic cord** — *see* condition
- **Spermatocele** N43.4Ø
  - congenital Q55.4
  - multiple N43.42
  - single N43.41
- **Spermatocystitis** N49.Ø
- **Spermatocytoma** C62.9- ☑
  - specified site — *see* Neoplasm, malignant, by site
- **Spermatorrhea** N5Ø.89
- **Sphacelus** — *see* Gangrene
- **Sphenoidal** — *see* condition
- **Sphenoiditis** (chronic) — *see* Sinusitis, sphenoidal
- **Sphenopalatine ganglion neuralgia** G9Ø.Ø9
- **Sphericity, increased, lens** (congenital) Q12.4
- **Spherocytosis** (congenital) (familial) (hereditary) D58.Ø
  - hemoglobin disease D58.Ø
  - sickle-cell (disease) D57.8- ☑
- **Spherophakia** Q12.4
- **Sphincter** — *see* condition
- **Sphincteritis, sphincter of Oddi** — *see* Cholangitis
- **Sphingolipidosis** E75.3
  - specified NEC E75.29
- **Sphingomyelinosis** E75.3
- **Spicule tooth** KØØ.2
- **Spider**
  - bite — *see* Toxicity, venom, spider
    - nonvenomous — *see* Bite, by site, superficial, insect
  - fingers — *see* Syndrome, Marfan's
  - nevus I78.1
  - toes — *see* Syndrome, Marfan's
  - vascular I78.1
- **Spiegler-Fendt**
  - benign lymphocytoma L98.8
  - sarcoid LØ8.89
- **Spielmeyer-Vogt disease** E75.4
- **Spina bifida** (aperta) QØ5.9
  - with hydrocephalus NEC QØ5.4
  - cervical QØ5.5
    - with hydrocephalus QØ5.Ø
  - dorsal QØ5.6
    - with hydrocephalus QØ5.1
  - lumbar QØ5.7
    - with hydrocephalus QØ5.2
  - lumbosacral QØ5.7
    - with hydrocephalus QØ5.2
  - occulta Q76.Ø
  - sacral QØ5.8
    - with hydrocephalus QØ5.3
  - thoracic QØ5.6
    - with hydrocephalus QØ5.1
  - thoracolumbar QØ5.6
    - with hydrocephalus QØ5.1
- **Spindle, Krukenberg's** — *see* Pigmentation, cornea, posterior
- **Spine, spinal** — *see* condition
- **Spiradenoma** (eccrine) — *see* Neoplasm, skin, benign
- **Spirillosis** A25.Ø
- **Spirillum**
  - minus A25.Ø
  - obermeieri infection A68.Ø
- **Spirochetal** — *see* condition
- **Spirochetosis** A69.9
  - arthritic, arthritica A69.9
- **Spirochetosis** — *continued*
  - bronchopulmonary A69.8
  - icterohemorrhagic A27.Ø
  - lung A69.8
- **Spirometrosis** B7Ø.1
- **Spitting blood** — *see* Hemoptysis
- **Splanchnoptosis** K63.4
- **Spleen, splenic** — *see* condition
- **Splenectasis** — *see* Splenomegaly
- **Splenitis** (interstitial) (malignant) (nonspecific) D73.89
  - malarial — *see also* Malaria B54 *[D77]*
  - tuberculous A18.85
- **Splenocele** D73.89
- **Splenomegaly, splenomegalia** (Bengal) (cryptogenic) (idiopathic) (tropical) R16.1
  - with hepatomegaly R16.2
  - cirrhotic D73.2
  - congenital Q89.Ø9
  - congestive, chronic D73.2
  - Egyptian B65.1
  - Gaucher's E75.22
  - malarial — *see also* Malaria B54 *[D77]*
  - neutropenic D73.81
  - Niemann-Pick — *see* Niemann-Pick disease or syndrome
  - siderotic D73.2
  - syphilitic A52.79
    - congenital (early) A5Ø.Ø8 *[D77]*
- **Splenopathy** D73.9
- **Splenoptosis** D73.89
- **Splenosis** D73.89
- **Splinter** — *see* Foreign body, superficial, by site
- **Split, splitting**
  - foot Q72.7- ☑
  - hand Q71.6 ☑
  - heart sounds RØ1.2
  - lip, congenital — *see* Cleft, lip
  - nails L6Ø.3
  - urinary stream R39.13
- **Spondylarthrosis** — *see* Spondylosis
- **Spondylitis** (chronic) — *see also* Spondylopathy, inflammatory
  - ankylopoietica — *see* Spondylitis, ankylosing
  - ankylosing (chronic) M45.9
    - with lung involvement M45.9 *[J99]*
    - cervical region M45.2
    - cervicothoracic region M45.3
    - juvenile MØ8.1
    - lumbar region M45.6
    - lumbosacral region M45.7
    - multiple sites M45.Ø
    - occipito-atlanto-axial region M45.1
    - sacrococcygeal region M45.8
    - thoracic region M45.4
    - thoracolumbar region M45.5
  - atrophic (ligamentous) — *see* Spondylitis, ankylosing
  - deformans (chronic) — *see* Spondylosis
  - gonococcal A54.41
  - gouty — *see also* Gout, by type, vertebrae M1Ø.Ø8
  - in (due to)
    - brucellosis A23.9 *[M49.8Ø]*
      - cervical region A23.9 *[M49.82]*
      - cervicothoracic region A23.9 *[M49.83]*
      - lumbar region A23.9 *[M49.86]*
      - lumbosacral region A23.9 *[M49.87]*
      - multiple sites A23.9 *[M49.89]*
      - occipito-atlanto-axial region A23.9 *[M49.81]*
      - sacrococcygeal region A23.9 *[M49.88]*
      - thoracic region A23.9 *[M49.84]*
      - thoracolumbar region A23.9 *[M49.85]*
    - enterobacteria — *see also* subcategory M49.8 AØ4.9
    - tuberculosis A18.Ø1
  - infectious NEC — *see* Spondylopathy, infective
  - juvenile ankylosing (chronic) MØ8.1
  - Kümmell's — *see* Spondylopathy, traumatic
  - Marie-Strümpell — *see* Spondylitis, ankylosing
  - muscularis — *see* Spondylopathy, specified NEC
  - psoriatic L4Ø.53
  - rheumatoid — *see* Spondylitis, ankylosing
  - rhizomelica — *see* Spondylitis, ankylosing
  - sacroiliac NEC M46.1
  - senescent, senile — *see* Spondylosis
  - traumatic (chronic) or post-traumatic — *see* Spondylopathy, traumatic
  - tuberculous A18.Ø1
  - typhosa AØ1.Ø5
- **Spondyloarthritis**
  - axial — *see also* Spondlyitis, ankylosing
    - non-radiographic M45.AØ
      - cervical M45.A2
      - cervicothoracic M45.A3
      - lumbar M45.A6
      - lumbosacral M45.A7
      - multiple sites M45.AB
      - occipito-atlanto-axial region M45.A1
      - sacral and sacrococcygeal M45.A8
      - thoracic M45.A4
      - thoracolumbar M45.A5
- **Spondylolisthesis** (acquired) (degenerative) M43.1Ø
  - with disproportion (fetopelvic) O33.Ø
    - causing obstructed labor O65.Ø
  - cervical region M43.12
  - cervicothoracic region M43.13
  - congenital Q76.2
  - lumbar region M43.16
  - lumbosacral region M43.17
  - multiple sites M43.19
  - occipito-atlanto-axial region M43.11
  - sacrococcygeal region M43.18
  - thoracic region M43.14
  - thoracolumbar region M43.15
  - traumatic (old) M43.1Ø
    - acute
      - fifth cervical (displaced) S12.43Ø ☑
        - nondisplaced S12.431 ☑
        - specified type NEC (displaced) S12.45Ø ☑
          - nondisplaced S12.451 ☑
        - type III S12.44 ☑
      - fourth cervical (displaced) S12.33Ø ☑
        - nondisplaced S12.331 ☑
        - specified type NEC (displaced) S12.35Ø ☑
          - nondisplaced S12.351 ☑
        - type III S12.34 ☑
      - second cervical (displaced) S12.13Ø ☑
        - nondisplaced S12.131 ☑
        - specified type NEC (displaced) S12.15Ø ☑
          - nondisplaced S12.151 ☑
        - type III S12.14 ☑
      - seventh cervical (displaced) S12.63Ø ☑
        - nondisplaced S12.631 ☑
        - specified type NEC (displaced) S12.65Ø ☑
          - nondisplaced S12.651 ☑
        - type III S12.64 ☑
      - sixth cervical (displaced) S12.53Ø ☑
        - nondisplaced S12.531 ☑
        - specified type NEC (displaced) S12.55Ø ☑
          - nondisplaced S12.551 ☑
        - type III S12.54 ☑
      - third cervical (displaced) S12.23Ø ☑
        - nondisplaced S12.231 ☑
        - specified type NEC (displaced) S12.25Ø ☑
          - nondisplaced S12.251 ☑
        - type III S12.24 ☑
- **Spondylolysis** (acquired) M43.ØØ
  - cervical region M43.Ø2
  - cervicothoracic region M43.Ø3
  - congenital Q76.2
  - lumbar region M43.Ø6
  - lumbosacral region M43.Ø7
    - with disproportion (fetopelvic) O33.Ø
      - causing obstructed labor O65.8
  - multiple sites M43.Ø9
  - occipito-atlanto-axial region M43.Ø1
  - sacrococcygeal region M43.Ø8
  - thoracic region M43.Ø4
  - thoracolumbar region M43.Ø5
- **Spondylopathy** M48.9
  - infective NEC M46.5Ø
    - cervical region M46.52
    - cervicothoracic region M46.53
    - lumbar region M46.56
    - lumbosacral region M46.57
    - multiple sites M46.59
    - occipito-atlanto-axial region M46.51
    - sacrococcygeal region M46.58
    - thoracic region M46.54
    - thoracolumbar region M46.55
  - inflammatory M46.9Ø
    - cervical region M46.92
    - cervicothoracic region M46.93
    - lumbar region M46.96
    - lumbosacral region M46.97
    - multiple sites M46.99

Spondylopathy — *continued*
- inflammatory — *continued*
  - occipito-atlanto-axial region M46.91
  - sacrococcygeal region M46.98
  - specified type NEC M46.8Ø
    - cervical region M46.82
    - cervicothoracic region M46.83
    - lumbar region M46.86
    - lumbosacral region M46.87
    - multiple sites M46.89
    - occipito-atlanto-axial region M46.81
    - sacrococcygeal region M46.88
    - thoracic region M46.84
    - thoracolumbar region M46.85
  - thoracic region M46.94
  - thoracolumbar region M46.95
- neuropathic, in
  - syringomyelia and syringobulbia G95.Ø
  - tabes dorsalis A52.11
- specified NEC — *see* subcategory M48.8 ☑
- traumatic M48.3Ø
  - cervical region M48.32
  - cervicothoracic region M48.33
  - lumbar region M48.36
  - lumbosacral region M48.37
  - occipito-atlanto-axial region M48.31
  - sacrococcygeal region M48.38
  - thoracic region M48.34
  - thoracolumbar region M48.35

Spondylosis M47.9
- with
  - disproportion (fetopelvic) O33.Ø
    - causing obstructed labor O65.Ø
  - myelopathy NEC M47.1Ø
    - cervical region M47.12
    - cervicothoracic region M47.13
    - lumbar region M47.16
    - occipito-atlanto-axial region M47.11
    - thoracic region M47.14
    - thoracolumbar region M47.15
  - radiculopathy M47.2Ø
    - cervical region M47.22
    - cervicothoracic region M47.23
    - lumbar region M47.26
    - lumbosacral region M47.27
    - occipito-atlanto-axial region M47.21
    - sacrococcygeal region M47.28
    - thoracic region M47.24
    - thoracolumbar region M47.25
- specified NEC M47.899
  - cervical region M47.892
  - cervicothoracic region M47.893
  - facet joint — *see also* Spondylosis M47.819
  - lumbar region M47.896
  - lumbosacral region M47.897
  - occipito-atlanto-axial region M47.891
  - sacrococcygeal region M47.898
  - thoracic region M47.894
  - thoracolumbar region M47.895
- traumatic — *see* Spondylopathy, traumatic
- without myelopathy or radiculopathy M47.819
  - cervical region M47.812
  - cervicothoracic region M47.813
  - lumbar region M47.816
  - lumbosacral region M47.817
  - occipito-atlanto-axial region M47.811
  - sacrococcygeal region M47.818
  - thoracic region M47.814
  - thoracolumbar region M47.815

Sponge
- inadvertently left in operation wound — *see* Foreign body, accidentally left during a procedure
- kidney (medullary) Q61.5

Sponge-diver's disease — *see* Toxicity, venom, marine animal, sea anemone

Spongioblastoma (any type) — *see* Neoplasm, malignant, by site
- specified site — *see* Neoplasm, malignant, by site
- unspecified site C71.9

Spongioneuroblastoma — *see* Neoplasm, malignant, by site

Spontaneous — *see also* condition
- fracture (cause unknown) — *see* Fracture, pathological

Spoon nail L6Ø.3
- congenital Q84.6

Sporadic — *see* condition

Sporothrix schenckii infection — *see* Sporotrichosis

Sporotrichosis B42.9

Sporotrichosis — *continued*
- arthritis B42.82
- disseminated B42.7
- generalized B42.7
- lymphocutaneous (fixed) (progressive) B42.1
- pulmonary B42.Ø
- specified NEC B42.89

Spots, spotting (in) (of)
- Bitot's — *see also* Pigmentation, conjunctiva
  - in the young child E5Ø.1
  - vitamin A deficiency E5Ø.1
- café, au lait L81.3
- Cayenne pepper I78.1
- cotton wool, retina — *see* Occlusion, artery, retina
- de Morgan's (senile angiomas) I78.1
- Fuchs' black (myopic) — *see also* Myopia, degenerative H44.2- ☑
- intermenstrual (regular) N92.Ø
  - irregular N92.1
- Koplik's BØ5.9
- liver L81.4
- pregnancy O26.85- ☑
- purpuric R23.3
- ruby I78.1

Spotted fever — *see* Fever, spotted A77.9

Sprain (joint) (ligament)
- acromioclavicular joint or ligament S43.5- ☑
- ankle S93.4Ø- ☑
  - calcaneofibular ligament S93.41- ☑
  - deltoid ligament S93.42- ☑
  - internal collateral ligament — *see* Sprain, ankle, specified ligament NEC
  - specified ligament NEC S93.49- ☑
  - talofibular ligament — *see* Sprain, ankle, specified ligament NEC
  - tibiofibular ligament S93.43- ☑
- anterior longitudinal, cervical S13.4 ☑
- atlas, atlanto-axial, atlanto-occipital S13.4 ☑
- breast bone — *see* Sprain, sternum
- calcaneofibular — *see* Sprain, ankle
- carpal — *see* Sprain, wrist
- carpometacarpal — *see* Sprain, hand, specified site NEC
- cartilage
  - costal S23.41 ☑
  - semilunar (knee) — *see* Sprain, knee, specified site NEC
    - with current tear — *see* Tear, meniscus
  - thyroid region S13.5 ☑
  - xiphoid — *see* Sprain, sternum
- cervical, cervicodorsal, cervicothoracic S13.4 ☑
- chondrosternal S23.421 ☑
- coracoclavicular S43.8- ☑
- coracohumeral S43.41- ☑
- coronary, knee — *see* Sprain, knee, specified site NEC
- costal cartilage S23.41 ☑
- cricoarytenoid articulation or ligament S13.5 ☑
- cricothyroid articulation S13.5 ☑
- cruciate, knee — *see* Sprain, knee, cruciate
- deltoid, ankle — *see* Sprain, ankle
- dorsal (spine) S23.3 ☑
- elbow S53.4Ø- ☑
  - radial collateral ligament S53.43- ☑
  - radiohumeral S53.41- ☑
  - rupture
    - radial collateral ligament — *see* Rupture, traumatic, ligament, radial collateral
    - ulnar collateral ligament — *see* Rupture, traumatic, ligament, ulnar collateral
  - specified type NEC S53.49- ☑
  - ulnar collateral ligament S53.44- ☑
  - ulnohumeral S53.42- ☑
- femur, head — *see* Sprain, hip
- fibular collateral, knee — *see* Sprain, knee, collateral
- fibulocalcaneal — *see* Sprain, ankle
- finger(s) S63.61- ☑
  - index S63.61- ☑
  - interphalangeal (joint) S63.63- ☑
    - index S63.63- ☑
    - little S63.63- ☑
    - middle S63.63- ☑
    - ring S63.63- ☑
  - little S63.61- ☑
  - metacarpophalangeal (joint) S63.65- ☑
  - middle S63.61- ☑
  - ring S63.61- ☑

Sprain — *continued*
- finger(s) — *continued*
  - specified site NEC S63.69- ☑
    - index S63.69- ☑
    - little S63.69- ☑
    - middle S63.69- ☑
    - ring S63.69- ☑
- foot S93.6Ø- ☑
  - specified ligament NEC S93.69- ☑
  - tarsal ligament S93.61- ☑
  - tarsometatarsal ligament S93.62- ☑
  - toe — *see* Sprain, toe
- hand S63.9- ☑
  - finger — *see* Sprain, finger
  - specified site NEC — *see* subcategory S63.8 ☑
  - thumb — *see* Sprain, thumb
- head SØ3.9 ☑
- hip S73.1Ø- ☑
  - iliofemoral ligament S73.11- ☑
  - ischiocapsular (ligament) S73.12- ☑
  - specified NEC S73.19- ☑
- iliofemoral — *see* Sprain, hip
- innominate
  - acetabulum — *see* Sprain, hip
  - sacral junction S33.6 ☑
- internal
  - collateral, ankle — *see* Sprain, ankle
  - semilunar cartilage — *see* Sprain, knee, specified site NEC
- interphalangeal
  - finger — *see* Sprain, finger, interphalangeal (joint)
  - toe — *see* Sprain, toe, interphalangeal joint
- ischiocapsular — *see* Sprain, hip
- ischiofemoral — *see* Sprain, hip
- jaw (articular disc) (cartilage) (meniscus) SØ3.4- ☑
  - old M26.69
- knee S83.9- ☑
  - collateral ligament S83.4Ø- ☑
    - lateral (fibular) S83.42- ☑
    - medial (tibial) S83.41- ☑
  - cruciate ligament S83.5Ø- ☑
    - anterior S83.51- ☑
    - posterior S83.52- ☑
  - lateral (fibular) collateral ligament S83.42- ☑
  - medial (tibial) collateral ligament S83.41- ☑
  - patellar ligament S76.11- ☑
  - specified site NEC S83.8X- ☑
  - superior tibiofibular joint (ligament) S83.6- ☑
- lateral collateral, knee — *see* Sprain, knee, collateral
- lumbar (spine) S33.5 ☑
- lumbosacral S33.9 ☑
- mandible (articular disc) SØ3.4- ☑
  - old M26.69
- medial collateral, knee — *see* Sprain, knee, collateral
- meniscus
  - jaw SØ3.4- ☑
    - old M26.69
  - knee — *see* Sprain, knee, specified site NEC
    - with current tear — *see* Tear, meniscus
      - old — *see* Derangement, knee, meniscus, due to old tear
  - mandible SØ3.4- ☑
    - old M26.69
- metacarpal (distal) (proximal) — *see* Sprain, hand, specified site NEC
- metacarpophalangeal — *see* Sprain, finger, metacarpophalangeal (joint)
- metatarsophalangeal — *see* Sprain, toe, metatarsophalangeal joint
- midcarpal — *see* Sprain, hand, specified site NEC
- midtarsal — *see* Sprain, foot, specified site NEC
- neck S13.9 ☑
  - anterior longitudinal cervical ligament S13.4 ☑
  - atlanto-axial joint S13.4 ☑
  - atlanto-occipital joint S13.4 ☑
  - cervical spine S13.4 ☑
  - cricoarytenoid ligament S13.5 ☑
  - cricothyroid ligament S13.5 ☑
  - specified site NEC S13.8 ☑
  - thyroid region (cartilage) S13.5 ☑
- nose SØ3.8 ☑
- orbicular, hip — *see* Sprain, hip
- patella — *see* Sprain, knee, specified site NEC
- patellar ligament S76.11- ☑
- pelvis NEC S33.8 ☑

- **Sprain** — *continued*
  - phalanx
    - finger — *see* Sprain, finger
    - toe — *see* Sprain, toe
  - pubofemoral — *see* Sprain, hip
  - radiocarpal — *see* Sprain, wrist
  - radiohumeral — *see* Sprain, elbow
  - radius, collateral — *see* Rupture, traumatic, ligament, radial collateral
  - rib (cage) S23.41 ☑
  - rotator cuff (capsule) S43.42- ☑
  - sacroiliac (region)
    - chronic or old — *see* subcategory M53.2 ☑
    - joint S33.6 ☑
  - scaphoid (hand) — *see* Sprain, hand, specified site NEC
  - scapula (r) — *see* Sprain, shoulder girdle, specified site NEC
  - semilunar cartilage (knee) — *see* Sprain, knee, specified site NEC
    - with current tear — *see* Tear, meniscus
      - old — *see* Derangement, knee, meniscus, due to old tear
  - shoulder joint S43.40- ☑
    - acromioclavicular joint (ligament) — *see* Sprain, acromioclavicular joint
    - blade — *see* Sprain, shoulder, girdle, specified site NEC
    - coracoclavicular joint (ligament) — *see* Sprain, coracoclavicular joint
    - coracohumeral ligament — *see* Sprain, coracohumeral joint
    - girdle S43.9- ☑
      - specified site NEC S43.8- ☑
    - rotator cuff — *see* Sprain, rotator cuff
    - specified site NEC S43.49- ☑
    - sternoclavicular joint (ligament) — *see* Sprain, sternoclavicular joint
  - spine
    - cervical S13.4 ☑
    - lumbar S33.5 ☑
    - thoracic S23.3 ☑
  - sternoclavicular joint S43.6- ☑
  - sternum S23.429 ☑
    - chondrosternal joint S23.421 ☑
    - specified site NEC S23.428 ☑
    - sternoclavicular (joint) (ligament) S23.420 ☑
  - symphysis
    - jaw S03.4- ☑
      - old M26.69
    - mandibular S03.4- ☑
      - old M26.69
  - talofibular — *see* Sprain, ankle
  - tarsal — *see* Sprain, foot, specified site NEC
  - tarsometatarsal — *see* Sprain, foot, specified site NEC
  - temporomandibular S03.4- ☑
    - old M26.69
  - thorax S23.9 ☑
    - ribs S23.41 ☑
    - specified site NEC S23.8 ☑
    - spine S23.3 ☑
    - sternum — *see* Sprain, sternum
  - thumb S63.60- ☑
    - interphalangeal (joint) S63.62- ☑
    - metacarpophalangeal (joint) S63.64- ☑
    - specified site NEC S63.68- ☑
  - thyroid cartilage or region S13.5 ☑
  - tibia (proximal end) — *see* Sprain, knee, specified site NEC
  - tibial collateral, knee — *see* Sprain, knee, collateral
  - tibiofibular
    - distal — *see* Sprain, ankle
    - superior — *see* Sprain, knee, specified site NEC
  - toe(s) S93.50- ☑
    - great S93.50- ☑
    - interphalangeal joint S93.51- ☑
      - great S93.51- ☑
      - lesser S93.51- ☑
    - lesser S93.50- ☑
    - metatarsophalangeal joint S93.52- ☑
      - great S93.52- ☑
      - lesser S93.52- ☑
  - ulna, collateral — *see* Rupture, traumatic, ligament, ulnar collateral
  - ulnohumeral — *see* Sprain, elbow
  - wrist S63.50- ☑
    - carpal S63.51- ☑

- **Sprain** — *continued*
  - wrist — *continued*
    - radiocarpal S63.52- ☑
    - specified site NEC S63.59- ☑
  - xiphoid cartilage — *see* Sprain, sternum
- **Sprengel's deformity** (congenital) Q74.0
- **Sprue** (tropical) K90.1
  - celiac K90.0
  - idiopathic K90.49
  - meaning thrush B37.0
  - nontropical K90.0
- **Spur, bone** — *see also* Enthesopathy
  - calcaneal M77.3- ☑
  - iliac crest M76.2- ☑
  - nose (septum) J34.89
- **Spurway's syndrome** Q78.0
- **Sputum**
  - abnormal (amount) (color) (odor) (purulent) R09.3
  - blood-stained R04.2
  - excessive (cause unknown) R09.3
- **Squamous** — *see also* condition
  - epithelium in
    - cervical canal (congenital) Q51.828
    - uterine mucosa (congenital) Q51.818
- **Squashed nose** M95.0
  - congenital Q67.4
- **Squeeze, diver's** T70.3 ☑
- **Squint** — *see also* Strabismus
  - accommodative — *see* Strabismus, convergent concomitant
- **SSADHD** (succinic semialdehyde dehydrogenase deficiency) E72.81
- **St. Hubert's disease** A82.9
- **Stab** — *see also* Laceration
  - internal organs — *see* Injury, by site
- **Stafne's cyst or cavity** M27.0
- **Staggering gait** R26.0
  - hysterical F44.4
- **Staghorn calculus** — *see* Calculus, kidney
- **Stähli's line** (cornea) (pigment) — *see* Pigmentation, cornea, anterior
- **Stain, staining**
  - meconium (newborn) P96.83
  - port wine Q82.5
  - tooth, teeth (hard tissues) (extrinsic) K03.6
    - due to
      - accretions K03.6
      - deposits (betel) (black) (green) (materia alba) (orange) (soft) (tobacco) K03.6
      - metals (copper) (silver) K03.7
      - nicotine K03.6
      - pulpal bleeding K03.7
      - tobacco K03.6
    - intrinsic K00.8
- **Stammering** — *see also* Disorder, fluency F80.81
- **Standstill**
  - auricular I45.5
  - cardiac — *see* Arrest, cardiac
  - sinoatrial I45.5
  - ventricular — *see* Arrest, cardiac
- **Stannosis** J63.5
- **Stanton's disease** — *see* Melioidosis
- **Staphylitis** (acute) (catarrhal) (chronic) (gangrenous) (membranous) (suppurative) (ulcerative) K12.2
- **Staphylococcal scalded skin syndrome** L00
- **Staphylococcemia** A41.2
- **Staphylococcus, staphylococcal** — *see also* condition
  - as cause of disease classified elsewhere B95.8
    - aureus (methicillin susceptible) (MSSA) B95.61
      - methicillin resistant (MRSA) B95.62
  - specified NEC, as cause of disease classified elsewhere B95.7
- **Staphyloma** (sclera)
  - cornea H18.72- ☑
  - equatorial H15.81- ☑
  - localized (anterior) H15.82- ☑
  - posticum H15.83- ☑
  - ring H15.85- ☑
- **Stargardt's disease** — *see* Dystrophy, retina
- **Starvation** (inanition) (due to lack of food) T73.0 ☑
  - edema — *see* Malnutrition, severe
- **Stasis**
  - bile (noncalculous) K83.1
  - bronchus J98.09
    - with infection — *see* Bronchitis
  - cardiac — *see* Failure, heart, congestive
  - cecum K59.89

- **Stasis** — *continued*
  - colon K59.89
  - dermatitis I87.2
    - with
      - varicose ulcer — *see* Varix, leg, with ulcer, with inflammation
      - varicose veins — *see* Varix, leg, with, inflammation
    - due to postthrombotic syndrome — *see* Syndrome, postthrombotic
  - duodenal K31.5
  - eczema — *see* Varix, leg, with, inflammation
  - edema — *see* Hypertension, venous (chronic), idiopathic
  - foot T69.0- ☑
  - ileocecal coil K59.89
  - ileum K59.89
  - intestinal K59.89
  - jejunum K59.89
  - kidney N19
  - liver (cirrhotic) K76.1
  - lymphatic I89.8
  - pneumonia J18.2
  - pulmonary — *see* Edema, lung
  - rectal K59.89
  - renal N19
    - tubular N17.0
  - ulcer — *see* Varix, leg, with, ulcer
    - without varicose veins I87.2
  - urine — *see* Retention, urine
  - venous I87.8
- **State** (of)
  - affective and paranoid, mixed, organic psychotic F06.8
  - agitated R45.1
    - acute reaction to stress F43.0
  - anxiety (neurotic) F41.1
  - apprehension F41.1
  - burn-out Z73.0
  - climacteric, female Z78.0
    - symptomatic N95.1
  - compulsive F42.8
    - mixed with obsessional thoughts F42.2
  - confusional (psychogenic) F44.89
    - acute — *see also* Delirium
      - with
        - arteriosclerotic dementia — *see also* Dementia, vascular F01.50
          - with behavioral disturbance — *see* Dementia, vascular
        - senility or dementia F05
      - alcoholic F10.231
    - epileptic F05
    - reactive (from emotional stress, psychological trauma) F44.89
    - subacute — *see* Delirium
  - convulsive — *see* Convulsions
  - crisis F43.0
  - depressive F32.A
    - neurotic F34.1
  - dissociative F44.9
  - emotional shock (stress) R45.7
  - hypercoagulation — *see* Hypercoagulable
  - locked-in G83.5
  - menopausal Z78.0
    - symptomatic N95.1
  - neurotic F48.9
    - with depersonalization F48.1
  - obsessional F42.8
  - oneiroid (schizophrenia-like) F23
  - organic
    - hallucinatory (nonalcoholic) F06.0
    - paranoid (-hallucinatory) F06.2
  - panic F41.0
  - paranoid F22
    - climacteric F22
    - involutional F22
    - menopausal F22
    - organic F06.2
    - senile F03 ☑
    - simple F22
  - persistent vegetative R40.3
  - phobic F40.9
  - postleukotomy F07.0
  - pregnant
    - gestational carrier Z33.3
    - incidental Z33.1
  - psychogenic, twilight F44.89
  - psychopathic (constitutional) F60.2

State — *continued*
- psychotic, organic — *see also* Psychosis, organic
  - mixed paranoid and affective F06.8
  - senile or presenile F03 ☑
  - transient NEC F06.8
    - with
      - depression F06.31
      - hallucinations F06.0
- residual schizophrenic F20.5
- restlessness R45.1
- stress (emotional) R45.7
- tension (mental) F48.9
  - specified NEC F48.8
- transient organic psychotic NEC F06.8
  - depressive type F06.31
  - hallucinatory type F06.0
- twilight
  - epileptic F05
  - psychogenic F44.89
- vegetative, persistent R40.3
- vital exhaustion Z73.0
- withdrawal, — *see* Withdrawal, state

Status (post) — *see also* Presence (of)
- absence, epileptic — *see* Epilepsy, by type, with status epilepticus
- administration of tPA (rtPA) in a different facility within the last 24 hours prior to admission to current facility Z92.82
- adrenalectomy (unilateral) (bilateral) E89.6
- anastomosis Z98.0
- anginosus I20.9
- angioplasty (peripheral) Z98.62
  - with implant Z95.820
  - coronary artery Z98.61
    - with implant Z95.5
- aortocoronary bypass Z95.1
- arthrodesis Z98.1
- artificial opening (of) Z93.9
  - gastrointestinal tract Z93.4
  - specified NEC Z93.8
  - urinary tract Z93.6
  - vagina Z93.8
- asthmaticus — *see* Asthma, by type, with status asthmaticus
- awaiting organ transplant Z76.82
- bariatric surgery Z98.84
- bed confinement Z74.01
- bleb, filtering (vitreous), after glaucoma surgery Z98.83
- breast implant Z98.82
  - removal Z98.86
- cataract extraction Z98.4- ☑
- cholecystectomy Z90.49
- clitorectomy N90.811
  - with excision of labia minora N90.812
- colectomy (complete) (partial) Z90.49
- colonization — *see* Carrier (suspected) of
- colostomy Z93.3
- convulsivus idiopathicus — *see* Epilepsy, by type, with status epilepticus
- coronary artery angioplasty — *see* Status, angioplasty, coronary artery
- coronary artery bypass graft Z95.1
- cystectomy (urinary bladder) Z90.6
- cystostomy Z93.50
  - appendico-vesicostomy Z93.52
  - cutaneous Z93.51
  - specified NEC Z93.59
- delinquent immunization Z28.39
  - COVID-19 Z28.31- ☑
- dental Z98.818
  - crown Z98.811
  - fillings Z98.811
  - restoration Z98.811
  - sealant Z98.810
  - specified NEC Z98.818
- deployment (current) (military) Z56.82
- dialysis (hemodialysis) (peritoneal) Z99.2
- do not resuscitate (DNR) Z66
- donor — *see* Donor
- embedded fragments — *see* Retained, foreign body fragments (type of)
- embedded splinter — *see* Retained, foreign body fragments (type of)
- enterostomy Z93.4
- epileptic, epilepticus — *see also* Epilepsy, by type, with status epilepticus G40.901
- estrogen receptor
  - negative Z17.1

Status — *continued*
- estrogen receptor — *continued*
  - positive Z17.0
- female genital cutting — *see* Female genital mutilation status
- female genital mutilation — *see* Female genital mutilation status
- filtering (vitreous) bleb after glaucoma surgery Z98.83
- gastrectomy (complete) (partial) Z90.3
- gastric banding Z98.84
- gastric bypass for obesity Z98.84
- gastrostomy Z93.1
- human immunodeficiency virus (HIV) infection, asymptomatic Z21
- hysterectomy (complete) (total) Z90.710
  - partial (with remaining cervial stump) Z90.711
- ileostomy Z93.2
- implant
  - breast Z98.82
- infibulation N90.813
- intestinal bypass Z98.0
- jejunostomy Z93.4
- lapsed immunization schedule Z28.39
- laryngectomy Z90.02
- lymphaticus E32.8
- malignancy
  - castrate resistant prostate Z19.2
  - hormone resistant Z19.2
  - hormone sensitive Z19.1
- marmoratus G80.3
- mastectomy (unilateral) (bilateral) Z90.1- ☑
- military deployment status (current) Z56.82
  - in theater or in support of military war, peacekeeping and humanitarian operations Z56.82
- nephrectomy (unilateral) (bilateral) Z90.5
- nephrostomy Z93.6
- obesity surgery Z98.84
- oophorectomy
  - bilateral Z90.722
  - unilateral Z90.721
- organ replacement
  - by artificial or mechanical device or prosthesis of
    - artery Z95.828
    - bladder Z96.0
    - blood vessel Z95.828
    - breast Z97.8
    - eye globe Z97.0
    - heart Z95.812
      - valve Z95.2
    - intestine Z97.8
    - joint Z96.60
      - hip — *see* Presence, hip joint implant
      - knee — *see* Presence, knee joint implant
      - specified site NEC Z96.698
    - kidney Z97.8
    - larynx Z96.3
    - lens Z96.1
    - limbs — *see* Presence, artificial, limb
    - liver Z97.8
    - lung Z97.8
    - pancreas Z97.8
  - by organ transplant (heterologous) (homologous) — *see* Transplant
- pacemaker
  - brain Z96.89
  - cardiac Z95.0
  - specified NEC Z96.89
- pancreatectomy Z90.410
  - complete Z90.410
  - partial Z90.411
  - total Z90.410
- physical restraint Z78.1
- pneumonectomy (complete) (partial) Z90.2
- pneumothorax, therapeutic Z98.3
- postcommotio cerebri F07.81
- postoperative (postprocedural) NEC Z98.890
  - breast implant Z98.82
  - dental Z98.818
    - crown Z98.811
    - fillings Z98.811
    - restoration Z98.811
    - sealant Z98.810
    - specified NEC Z98.818
  - pneumothorax, therapeutic Z98.3
  - uterine scar Z98.891
- postpartum (routine follow-up) Z39.2
  - care immediately after delivery Z39.0
- postsurgical (postprocedural) NEC Z98.890
  - pneumothorax, therapeutic Z98.3

Status — *continued*
- pregnancy, incidental Z33.1
- prosthesis coronary angioplasty Z95.5
- pseudophakia Z96.1
- renal dialysis (hemodialysis) (peritoneal) Z99.2
- retained foreign body — *see* Retained, foreign body fragments (type of)
- reversed jejunal transposition (for bypass) Z98.0
- salpingo-oophorectomy
  - bilateral Z90.722
  - unilateral Z90.721
- sex reassignment surgery status Z87.890
- shunt
  - arteriovenous (for dialysis) Z99.2
  - cerebrospinal fluid Z98.2
  - ventricular (communicating) (for drainage) Z98.2
- splenectomy Z90.81
- thymicolymphaticus E32.8
- thymicus E32.8
- thymolymphaticus E32.8
- thyroidectomy (hypothyroidism) E89.0
- tooth (teeth) extraction — *see also* Absence, teeth, acquired K08.409
- tPA (rtPA) administration in a different facility within the last 24 hours prior to admission to current facility Z92.82
- tracheostomy Z93.0
- transplant — *see* Transplant
  - organ removed Z98.85
- tubal ligation Z98.51
- underimmunization Z28.39
  - COVID-19 Z28.31- ☑
    - partially vaccinated (for) Z28.311
    - unvaccinated (for) Z28.310
- ureterostomy Z93.6
- urethrostomy Z93.6
- vagina, artificial Z93.8
- vasectomy Z98.52
- wheelchair confinement Z99.3

Stealing
- child problem F91.8
  - in company with others Z72.810
- pathological (compulsive) F63.2

Steam burn — *see* Burn

Steatocystoma multiplex L72.2

Steatohepatitis (nonalcoholic) (NASH) K75.81

Steatoma L72.3
- eyelid (cystic) — *see* Dermatosis, eyelid
  - infected — *see* Hordeolum

Steatorrhea (chronic) K90.9
- with lacteal obstruction K90.2
- idiopathic (adult) (infantile) K90.9
- pancreatic K90.3
- primary K90.0
- tropical K90.1

Steatosis E88.89
- heart — *see* Degeneration, myocardial
- kidney N28.89
- liver NEC K76.0

Steele-Richardson-Olszewski disease or syndrome G23.1

Steinbrocker's syndrome G90.8

Steinert's disease G71.11

Stein-Leventhal syndrome E28.2

Stein's syndrome E28.2

STEMI — *see also* Infarct, myocardium, ST elevation I21.3

Stenocardia I20.8

Stenocephaly Q75.8

Stenosis, stenotic (cicatricial) — *see also* Stricture
- ampulla of Vater K83.1
- anus, anal (canal) (sphincter) K62.4
  - and rectum K62.4
  - congenital Q42.3
    - with fistula Q42.2
- aorta (ascending) (supraventricular) (congenital) Q25.1
  - arteriosclerotic I70.0
  - calcified I70.0
  - supravalvular Q25.3
- aortic (valve) I35.0
  - with insufficiency I35.2
  - congenital Q23.0
  - rheumatic I06.0
    - with
      - incompetency, insufficiency or regurgitation I06.2
        - with mitral (valve) disease I08.0
          - with tricuspid (valve) disease I08.3
      - mitral (valve) disease I08.0

Stenosis, stenotic — *continued*
- aortic — *continued*
  - rheumatic — *continued*
    - with — *continued*
      - mitral disease — *continued*
        - with tricuspid (valve) disease I08.3
      - tricuspid (valve) disease I08.2
        - with mitral (valve) disease I08.3
  - specified cause NEC I35.Ø
  - syphilitic A52.Ø3
- aqueduct of Sylvius (congenital) QØ3.Ø
  - with spina bifida — *see* Spina bifida, by site, with hydrocephalus
  - acquired G91.1
- artery NEC — *see also* Arteriosclerosis I77.1
  - celiac I77.4
  - cerebral — *see* Occlusion, artery, cerebral
  - extremities — *see* Arteriosclerosis, extremities
  - precerebral — *see* Occlusion, artery, precerebral
  - pulmonary (congenital) Q25.6
    - acquired I28.8
  - renal I7Ø.1
  - stent
    - coronary T82.855 ☑
    - peripheral T82.856 ☑
- bile duct (common) (hepatic) K83.1
  - congenital Q44.3
- bladder-neck (acquired) N32.Ø
  - congenital Q64.31
- brain G93.89
- bronchus J98.Ø9
  - congenital Q32.3
  - syphilitic A52.72
- cardia (stomach) K22.2
  - congenital Q39.3
- cardiovascular — *see* Disease, cardiovascular
- caudal M48.Ø8
- cervix, cervical (canal) N88.2
  - congenital Q51.828
  - in pregnancy or childbirth — *see* Pregnancy, complicated by, abnormal cervix
- colon — *see also* Obstruction, intestine
  - congenital Q42.9
    - specified NEC Q42.8
- colostomy K94.Ø3
- common (bile) duct K83.1
  - congenital Q44.3
- coronary (artery) — *see* Disease, heart, ischemic, atherosclerotic
- cystic duct — *see* Obstruction, gallbladder
- due to presence of device, implant or graft — *see also* Complications, by site and type, specified NEC T85.858 ☑
  - arterial graft NEC T82.858 ☑
  - breast (implant) T85.858 ☑
  - catheter T85.858 ☑
    - dialysis (renal) T82.858 ☑
      - intraperitoneal T85.858 ☑
    - infusion NEC T82.858 ☑
      - spinal (epidural) (subdural) T85.85Ø ☑
    - urinary (indwelling) T83.85 ☑
  - fixation, internal (orthopedic) NEC T84.85 ☑
  - gastrointestinal (bile duct) (esophagus) T85.858 ☑
  - genital NEC T83.85 ☑
  - heart NEC T82.857 ☑
  - joint prosthesis T84.85 ☑
  - ocular (corneal graft) (orbital implant) NEC T85.858 ☑
  - orthopedic NEC T84.85 ☑
  - specified NEC T85.858 ☑
  - urinary NEC T83.85 ☑
  - vascular NEC T82.858 ☑
  - ventricular intracranial shunt T85.85Ø ☑
- duodenum K31.5
  - congenital Q41.Ø
- ejaculatory duct NEC N5Ø.89
  - stent
    - vascular
      - end stent
        - adjacent to stent — *see* Arteriosclerosis
        - within the stent
          - coronary T82.855 ☑
          - peripheral T82.856 ☑
      - in stent
        - coronary vessel T82.855 ☑
        - peripheral vessel T82.856 ☑
- endocervical os — *see* Stenosis, cervix

Stenosis, stenotic — *continued*
- enterostomy K94.13
- esophagus K22.2
  - congenital Q39.3
  - syphilitic A52.79
    - congenital A5Ø.59 *[K23]*
- eustachian tube — *see* Obstruction, eustachian tube
- external ear canal (acquired) H61.3Ø- ☑
  - congenital Q16.1
  - due to
    - inflammation H61.32- ☑
    - trauma H61.31- ☑
  - postprocedural H95.81- ☑
  - specified cause NEC H61.39- ☑
- gallbladder — *see* Obstruction, gallbladder
- glottis J38.6
- heart valve — *see also* Endocarditis I38
  - aortic — *see* Stenosis, aortic
  - congenital Q24.8
  - mitral — *see* Stenosis, mitral
  - pulmonary — *see* Stenosis, pulmonary valve
  - tricuspid — *see* Stenosis, tricuspid
- hepatic duct K83.1
- hymen N89.6
- hypertrophic subaortic (idiopathic) I42.1
- ileum — *see also* Obstruction, intestine, specified NEC K56.699
  - congenital Q41.2
- infundibulum cardia Q24.3
- intervertebral foramina — *see also* Lesion, biomechanical, specified NEC
  - connective tissue M99.79
    - abdomen M99.79
    - cervical region M99.71
    - cervicothoracic M99.71
    - head region M99.7Ø
    - lumbar region M99.73
    - lumbosacral M99.73
    - occipitocervical M99.7Ø
    - sacral region M99.74
    - sacrococcygeal M99.74
    - sacroiliac M99.74
    - specified NEC M99.79
    - thoracic region M99.72
    - thoracolumbar M99.72
  - disc M99.79
    - abdomen M99.79
    - cervical region M99.71
    - cervicothoracic M99.71
    - head region M99.7Ø
    - lower extremity M99.76
    - lumbar region M99.73
    - lumbosacral M99.73
    - occipitocervical M99.7Ø
    - pelvic M99.75
    - rib cage M99.78
    - sacral region M99.74
    - sacrococcygeal M99.74
    - sacroiliac M99.74
    - specified NEC M99.79
    - thoracic region M99.72
    - thoracolumbar M99.72
    - upper extremity M99.77
  - osseous M99.69
    - abdomen M99.69
    - cervical region M99.61
    - cervicothoracic M99.61
    - head region M99.6Ø
    - lower extremity M99.66
    - lumbar region M99.63
    - lumbosacral M99.63
    - occipitocervical M99.6Ø
    - pelvic M99.65
    - rib cage M99.68
    - sacral region M99.64
    - sacrococcygeal M99.64
    - sacroiliac M99.64
    - specified NEC M99.69
    - thoracic region M99.62
    - thoracolumbar M99.62
    - upper extremity M99.67
  - subluxation — *see* Stenosis, intervertebral foramina, osseous
- intestine — *see also* Obstruction, intestine
  - congenital (small) Q41.9
    - large Q42.9
      - specified NEC Q42.8
    - specified NEC Q41.8

Stenosis, stenotic — *continued*
- jejunum — *see also* Obstruction, intestine, specified NEC K56.699
  - congenital Q41.1
- lacrimal (passage)
  - canaliculi HØ4.54- ☑
  - congenital Q1Ø.5
  - duct HØ4.55- ☑
  - punctum HØ4.56- ☑
  - sac HØ4.57- ☑
- lacrimonasal duct — *see* Stenosis, lacrimal, duct
  - congenital Q1Ø.5
- larynx J38.6
  - congenital NEC Q31.8
    - subglottic Q31.1
  - syphilitic A52.73
    - congenital A5Ø.59 *[J99]*
- mitral (chronic) (inactive) (valve) IØ5.Ø
  - with
    - aortic valve disease IØ8.Ø
    - incompetency, insufficiency or regurgitation IØ5.2
  - active or acute IØ1.1
    - with rheumatic or Sydenham's chorea IØ2.Ø
  - congenital Q23.2
  - specified cause, except rheumatic I34.2
  - syphilitic A52.Ø3
- myocardium, myocardial — *see also* Degeneration, myocardial
  - hypertrophic subaortic (idiopathic) I42.1
- nares (anterior) (posterior) J34.89
  - congenital Q3Ø.Ø
- nasal duct — *see also* Stenosis, lacrimal, duct
  - congenital Q1Ø.5
- nasolacrimal duct — *see also* Stenosis, lacrimal, duct
  - congenital Q1Ø.5
- neural canal — *see also* Lesion, biomechanical, specified NEC
  - connective tissue M99.49
    - abdomen M99.49
    - cervical region M99.41
    - cervicothoracic M99.41
    - head region M99.4Ø
    - lower extremity M99.46
    - lumbar region M99.43
    - lumbosacral M99.43
    - occipitocervical M99.4Ø
    - pelvic M99.45
    - rib cage M99.48
    - sacral region M99.44
    - sacrococcygeal M99.44
    - sacroiliac M99.44
    - specified NEC M99.49
    - thoracic region M99.42
    - thoracolumbar M99.42
    - upper extremity M99.47
  - intervertebral disc M99.59
    - abdomen M99.59
    - cervical region M99.51
    - cervicothoracic M99.51
    - head region M99.5Ø
    - lower extremity M99.56
    - lumbar region M99.53
    - lumbosacral M99.53
    - occipitocervical M99.5Ø
    - pelvic M99.55
    - rib cage M99.58
    - sacral region M99.54
    - sacrococcygeal M99.54
    - sacroiliac M99.54
    - specified NEC M99.59
    - thoracic region M99.52
    - thoracolumbar M99.52
    - upper extremity M99.57
  - osseous M99.39
    - abdomen M99.39
    - cervical region M99.31
    - cervicothoracic M99.31
    - head region M99.3Ø
    - lower extremity M99.36
    - lumbar region M99.33
    - lumbosacral M99.33
    - occipitocervical M99.3Ø
    - pelvic M99.35
    - rib cage M99.38
    - sacral region M99.34
    - sacrococcygeal M99.34
    - sacroiliac M99.34

Stenosis, stenotic — *continued*
  neural canal — *see also* Lesion, biomechanical, specified — *continued*
    osseous — *continued*
      specified NEC M99.39
      thoracic region M99.32
      thoracolumbar M99.32
      upper extremity M99.37
    subluxation M99.29
      cervical region M99.21
      cervicothoracic M99.21
      head region M99.2Ø
      lower extremity M99.26
      lumbar region M99.23
      lumbosacral M99.23
      occipitocervical M99.2Ø
      pelvic M99.25
      rib cage M99.28
      sacral region M99.24
      sacrococcygeal M99.24
      sacroiliac M99.24
      specified NEC M99.29
      thoracic region M99.22
      thoracolumbar M99.22
      upper extremity M99.27
  organ or site, congenital NEC — *see* Atresia, by site
  papilla of Vater K83.1
  pulmonary (artery) (congenital) Q25.6
    with ventricular septal defect, transposition of aorta, and hypertrophy of right ventricle Q21.3
    acquired I28.8
    in tetralogy of Fallot Q21.3
    infundibular Q24.3
    subvalvular Q24.3
    supravalvular Q25.6
    valve I37.Ø
      with insufficiency I37.2
      congenital Q22.1
      rheumatic IØ9.89
        with aortic, mitral or tricuspid (valve) disease IØ8.8
    vein, acquired I28.8
    vessel NEC I28.8
  pulmonic (congenital) Q22.1
    infundibular Q24.3
    subvalvular Q24.3
  pylorus (hypertrophic) (acquired) K31.1
    adult K31.1
    congenital Q4Ø.Ø
    infantile Q4Ø.Ø
  rectum (sphincter) — *see* Stricture, rectum
  renal artery I7Ø.1
    congenital Q27.1
  salivary duct (any) K11.8
  sphincter of Oddi K83.1
  spinal M48.ØØ
    cervical region M48.Ø2
    cervicothoracic region M48.Ø3
    lumbar region (NOS) (without neurogenic claudication) M48.Ø61
      with neurogenic claudication M48.Ø62
    lumbosacral region M48.Ø7
    occipito-atlanto-axial region M48.Ø1
    sacrococcygeal region M48.Ø8
    thoracic region M48.Ø4
    thoracolumbar region M48.Ø5
  stomach, hourglass K31.2
  subaortic (congenital) Q24.4
    hypertrophic (idiopathic) I42.1
  subglottic J38.6
    congenital Q31.1
    postprocedural J95.5
  trachea J39.8
    congenital Q32.1
    syphilitic A52.73
    tuberculous NEC A15.5
  tracheostomy J95.Ø3
  tricuspid (valve) IØ7.Ø
    with
      aortic (valve) disease IØ8.2
      incompetency, insufficiency or regurgitation IØ7.2
        with aortic (valve) disease IØ8.2
          with mitral (valve) disease IØ8.3
      mitral (valve) disease IØ8.1
        with aortic (valve) disease IØ8.3
    congenital Q22.4
    nonrheumatic I36.Ø
      with insufficiency I36.2

Stenosis, stenotic — *continued*
  tubal N97.1
  ureter — *see* Atresia, ureter
  ureteropelvic junction, congenital Q62.11
  ureterovesical orifice, congenital Q62.12
  urethra (valve) *see also* Stricture, urethra
    congenital Q64.32
  urinary meatus, congenital Q64.33
  vagina N89.5
    congenital Q52.4
    in pregnancy — *see* Pregnancy, complicated by, abnormal vagina
      causing obstructed labor O65.5
  valve (cardiac) (heart) — *see also* Endocarditis I38
    congenital Q24.8
      aortic Q23.Ø
      mitral Q23.2
      pulmonary Q22.1
      tricuspid Q22.4
  vena cava (inferior) (superior) I87.1
    congenital Q26.Ø
  vesicourethral orifice Q64.31
  vulva N9Ø.5
Stent jail T82.897 ☑
Stercolith (impaction) K56.41
  appendix K38.1
Stercoraceous, stercoral ulcer K63.3
  anus or rectum K62.6
Stereotypies NEC F98.4
Sterility — *see* Infertility
Sterilization — *see* Encounter (for), sterilization
Sternalgia — *see* Angina
Sternopagus Q89.4
Sternum bifidum Q76.7
Steroid
  effects (adverse) (adrenocortical) (iatrogenic)
    cushingoid E24.2
      correct substance properly administered — *see* Table of Drugs and Chemicals, by drug, adverse effect
      overdose or wrong substance given or taken — *see* Table of Drugs and Chemicals, by drug, poisoning
    diabetes — *see* subcategory EØ9 ☑
      correct substance properly administered — *see* Table of Drugs and Chemicals, by drug, adverse effect
      overdose or wrong substance given or taken — *see* Table of Drugs and Chemicals, by drug, poisoning
    fever R5Ø.2
    insufficiency E27.3
      correct substance properly administered — *see* Table of Drugs and Chemicals, by drug, adverse effect
      overdose or wrong substance given or taken — *see* Table of Drugs and Chemicals, by drug, poisoning
  responder H4Ø.Ø4- ☑
Stevens-Johnson disease or syndrome L51.1
  toxic epidermal necrolysis overlap L51.3
Stewart-Morel syndrome M85.2
Sticker's disease BØ8.3
Sticky eye — *see* Conjunctivitis, acute, mucopurulent
Stieda's disease — *see* Bursitis, tibial collateral
Stiff neck — *see* Torticollis
Stiff-man syndrome G25.82
Stiffness, joint NEC M25.6Ø
  ankle M25.67- ☑
  ankylosis — *see* Ankylosis, joint
  contracture — *see* Contraction, joint
  elbow M25.62- ☑
  foot M25.67- ☑
  hand M25.64- ☑
  hip M25.65- ☑
  knee M25.66- ☑
  shoulder M25.61- ☑
  specified site NEC M25.69
  wrist M25.63- ☑
Stigmata congenital syphilis A5Ø.59
Stillbirth P95
Still-Felty syndrome — *see* Felty's syndrome
Still's disease or syndrome (juvenile) MØ8.2Ø
  adult-onset MØ6.1
  ankle MØ8.27- ☑
  elbow MØ8.22- ☑
  foot joint MØ8.27- ☑

Still's disease or syndrome — *continued*
  hand joint MØ8.24- ☑
  hip MØ8.25- ☑
  knee MØ8.26- ☑
  multiple site MØ8.29
  shoulder MØ8.21- ☑
  specified site NEC MØ8.2A
  vertebra MØ8.28
  wrist MØ8.23- ☑
Stimulation, ovary E28.1
Sting (venomous) (with allergic or anaphylactic shock) — *see* Table of Drugs and Chemicals, by animal or substance, poisoning
Stippled epiphyses Q78.8
Stitch
  abscess T81.41 ☑
  burst (in operation wound) — *see* Disruption, wound, operation
Stokes' disease EØ5.ØØ
  with thyroid storm EØ5.Ø1
Stokes-Adams disease or syndrome I45.9
Stokvis (-Talma) **disease** D74.8
Stoma malfunction
  colostomy K94.Ø3
  enterostomy K94.13
  gastrostomy K94.23
  ileostomy K94.13
  tracheostomy J95.Ø3
Stomach — *see* condition
Stomatitis (denture) (ulcerative) K12.1
  angular K13.Ø
    due to dietary or vitamin deficiency E53.Ø
  aphthous K12.Ø
  bovine BØ8.61
  candidal B37.Ø
  catarrhal K12.1
  diphtheritic A36.89
  due to
    dietary deficiency E53.Ø
    thrush B37.Ø
    vitamin deficiency
      B group NEC E53.9
      B2 (riboflavin) E53.Ø
  epidemic BØ8.8
  epizootic BØ8.8
  follicular K12.1
  gangrenous A69.Ø
  Geotrichum B48.3
  herpesviral, herpetic BØØ.2
  herpetiformis K12.Ø
  malignant K12.1
  membranous acute K12.1
  monilial B37.Ø
  mycotic B37.Ø
  necrotizing ulcerative A69.Ø
  parasitic B37.Ø
  septic K12.1
  spirochetal A69.1
  suppurative (acute) K12.2
  ulceromembranous A69.1
  vesicular K12.1
    with exanthem (enteroviral) BØ8.4
    virus disease A93.8
  Vincent's A69.1
Stomatocytosis D58.8
Stomatomycosis B37.Ø
Stomatorrhagia K13.79
Stone(s) — *see also* Calculus
  bladder (diverticulum) N21.Ø
  cystine E72.Ø9
  heart syndrome I5Ø.1
  kidney N2Ø.Ø
  prostate N42.Ø
  pulpal (dental) KØ4.2
  renal N2Ø.Ø
  salivary gland or duct (any) K11.5
  urethra (impacted) N21.1
  urinary (duct) (impacted) (passage) N2Ø.9
    bladder (diverticulum) N21.Ø
    lower tract N21.9
    specified NEC N21.8
  xanthine E79.8 *[N22]*
Stonecutter's lung J62.8
Stonemason's asthma, disease, lung or pneumoconiosis J62.8
Stoppage
  heart — *see* Arrest, cardiac
  urine — *see* Retention, urine

Storm, thyroid — *see* Thyrotoxicosis
Strabismus (congenital) (nonparalytic) H5Ø.9
- concomitant H5Ø.4Ø
  - convergent — *see* Strabismus, convergent concomitant
  - divergent — *see* Strabismus, divergent concomitant
- convergent concomitant H5Ø.ØØ
  - accommodative component H5Ø.43
  - alternating H5Ø.Ø5
    - with
      - A pattern H5Ø.Ø6
      - specified nonconcomitances NEC H5Ø.Ø8
      - V pattern H5Ø.Ø7
  - monocular H5Ø.Ø1- ☑
    - with
      - A pattern H5Ø.Ø2- ☑
      - specified nonconcomitances NEC H5Ø.Ø4- ☑
      - V pattern H5Ø.Ø3- ☑
  - intermittent H5Ø.31- ☑
    - alternating H5Ø.32
- cyclotropia H5Ø.41 ☑
- divergent concomitant H5Ø.1Ø
  - alternating H5Ø.15
    - with
      - A pattern H5Ø.16
      - specified noncomitances NEC H5Ø.18
      - V pattern H5Ø.17
  - monocular H5Ø.11- ☑
    - with
      - A pattern H5Ø.12- ☑
      - specified noncomitances NEC H5Ø.14- ☑
      - V pattern H5Ø.13- ☑
  - intermittent H5Ø.33 ☑
    - alternating H5Ø.34
- Duane's syndrome H5Ø.81- ☑
- due to adhesions, scars H5Ø.69
- heterophoria H5Ø.5Ø
  - alternating H5Ø.55
  - cyclophoria H5Ø.54
  - esophoria H5Ø.51
  - exophoria H5Ø.52
  - vertical H5Ø.53
- heterotropia H5Ø.4Ø
  - intermittent H5Ø.3Ø
- hypertropia H5Ø.2- ☑
- hypotropia — *see* Hypertropia
- latent H5Ø.5Ø
- mechanical H5Ø.6Ø
  - Brown's sheath syndrome H5Ø.61- ☑
  - specified type NEC H5Ø.69
- monofixation syndrome H5Ø.42
- paralytic H49.9
  - abducens nerve H49.2- ☑
  - fourth nerve H49.1- ☑
  - Kearns-Sayre syndrome H49.81- ☑
  - ophthalmoplegia (external)
    - progressive H49.4- ☑
      - with pigmentary retinopathy H49.81- ☑
    - total H49.3- ☑
  - sixth nerve H49.2- ☑
  - specified type NEC H49.88- ☑
  - third nerve H49.Ø- ☑
  - trochlear nerve H49.1- ☑
- specified type NEC H5Ø.89
- vertical H5Ø.2- ☑

Strain
- back S39.Ø12 ☑
- cervical S16.1 ☑
- eye NEC — *see* Disturbance, vision, subjective
- heart — *see* Disease, heart
- low back S39.Ø12 ☑
- mental NOS Z73.3
  - work-related Z56.6
- muscle (tendon) — *see* Injury, muscle, by site, strain
- neck S16.1 ☑
- physical NOS Z73.3
  - work-related Z56.6
- postural — *see also* Disorder, soft tissue, due to use
- psychological NEC Z73.3
- tendon — *see* Injury, muscle, by site, strain

Straining, on urination R39.16
Strand, vitreous — *see* Opacity, vitreous, membranes and strands
Strangulation, strangulated — *see also* Asphyxia, traumatic
- appendix K38.8
- bladder-neck N32.Ø

Strangulation, strangulated — *continued*
- bowel or colon K56.2
- food or foreign body — *see* Foreign body, by site
- hemorrhoids — *see* Hemorrhoids, with complication
- hernia — *see also* Hernia, by site, with obstruction
  - with gangrene — *see* Hernia, by site, with gangrene
- intestine (large) (small) K56.2
  - with hernia — *see also* Hernia, by site, with obstruction
    - with gangrene — *see* Hernia, by site, with gangrene
- mesentery K56.2
- mucus — *see* Asphyxia, mucus
- omentum K56.2
- organ or site, congenital NEC — *see* Atresia, by site
- ovary — *see* Torsion, ovary
- penis N48.89
  - foreign body T19.4 ☑
- rupture — *see* Hernia, by site, with obstruction
- stomach due to hernia — *see also* Hernia, by site, with obstruction
  - with gangrene — *see* Hernia, by site, with gangrene
- vesicourethral orifice N32.Ø

Strangury R3Ø.Ø
Straw itch B88.Ø
Strawberry
- gallbladder K82.4
- mark Q82.5
- tongue (red) (white) K14.3

Streak(s)
- macula, angioid H35.33
- ovarian Q5Ø.32

Strephosymbolia F81.Ø
- secondary to organic lesion R48.8

Streptobacillary fever A25.1
Streptobacillosis A25.1
Streptobacillus moniliformis A25.1
Streptococcus, streptococcal — *see also* condition
- as cause of disease classified elsewhere B95.5
- group
  - A, as cause of disease classified elsewhere B95.Ø
  - B, as cause of disease classified elsewhere B95.1
  - D, as cause of disease classified elsewhere B95.2
- pneumoniae, as cause of disease classified elsewhere B95.3
- specified NEC, as cause of disease classified elsewhere B95.4

Streptomycosis B47.1
Streptotrichosis A48.8
Stress F43.9
- family — *see* Disruption, family
- fetal P84
  - complicating pregnancy O77.9
    - due to drug administration O77.1
- mental NEC Z73.3
  - work-related Z56.6
- physical NEC Z73.3
  - work-related Z56.6
- polycythemia D75.1
- reaction — *see also* Reaction, stress F43.9
- work schedule Z56.3

Stretching, nerve — *see* Injury, nerve
Striae albicantes, atrophicae or distensae (cutis) L9Ø.6
Stricture — *see also* Stenosis
- ampulla of Vater K83.1
- anus (sphincter) K62.4
  - congenital Q42.3
    - with fistula Q42.2
  - infantile Q42.3
    - with fistula Q42.2
- aorta (ascending) (congenital) Q25.1
  - arteriosclerotic I7Ø.Ø
  - calcified I7Ø.Ø
  - supravalvular, congenital Q25.3
- aortic (valve) — *see* Stenosis, aortic
- aqueduct of Sylvius (congenital) QØ3.Ø
  - with spina bifida — *see* Spina bifida, by site, with hydrocephalus
  - acquired G91.1
- artery I77.1
  - basilar — *see* Occlusion, artery, basilar
  - carotid — *see* Occlusion, artery, carotid
  - celiac I77.4
  - congenital (peripheral) Q27.8
    - cerebral Q28.3
    - coronary Q24.5
    - digestive system Q27.8
    - lower limb Q27.8

Stricture — *continued*
- artery — *continued*
  - congenital — *continued*
    - retinal Q14.1
    - specified site NEC Q27.8
    - umbilical Q27.Ø
    - upper limb Q27.8
  - coronary — *see* Disease, heart, ischemic, atherosclerotic
    - congenital Q24.5
  - precerebral — *see* Occlusion, artery, precerebral
  - pulmonary (congenital) Q25.6
    - acquired I28.8
  - renal I7Ø.1
  - vertebral — *see* Occlusion, artery, vertebral
- auditory canal (external) (congenital)
  - acquired — *see* Stenosis, external ear canal
- bile duct (common) (hepatic) K83.1
  - congenital Q44.3
  - postoperative K91.89
- bladder N32.89
  - neck N32.Ø
- bowel — *see* Obstruction, intestine
- brain G93.89
- bronchus J98.Ø9
  - congenital Q32.3
  - syphilitic A52.72
- cardia (stomach) K22.2
  - congenital Q39.3
- cardiac — *see also* Disease, heart
  - orifice (stomach) K22.2
- cecum — *see* Obstruction, intestine
- cervix, cervical (canal) N88.2
  - congenital Q51.828
  - in pregnancy — *see* Pregnancy, complicated by, abnormal cervix
    - causing obstructed labor O65.5
- colon — *see also* Obstruction, intestine
  - congenital Q42.9
    - specified NEC Q42.8
- colostomy K94.Ø3
- common (bile) duct K83.1
- coronary (artery) — *see* Disease, heart, ischemic, atherosclerotic
- cystic duct — *see* Obstruction, gallbladder
- digestive organs NEC, congenital Q45.8
- duodenum K31.5
  - congenital Q41.Ø
- ear canal (external) (congenital) Q16.1
  - acquired — *see* Stricture, auditory canal, acquired
- ejaculatory duct N5Ø.89
- enterostomy K94.13
- esophagus K22.2
  - congenital Q39.3
  - syphilitic A52.79
    - congenital A5Ø.59 *[K23]*
- eustachian tube — *see also* Obstruction, eustachian tube
  - congenital Q17.8
- fallopian tube N97.1
  - gonococcal A54.24
  - tuberculous A18.17
- gallbladder — *see* Obstruction, gallbladder
- glottis J38.6
- heart — *see also* Disease, heart
  - valve — *see also* Endocarditis I38
    - aortic Q23.Ø
    - mitral Q23.2
    - pulmonary Q22.1
    - tricuspid Q22.4
- hepatic duct K83.1
- hourglass, of stomach K31.2
- hymen N89.6
- hypopharynx J39.2
- ileum — *see also* Obstruction, intestine, specified NEC K56.699
  - congenital Q41.2
- intestine — *see also* Obstruction, intestine
  - congenital (small) Q41.9
    - large Q42.9
      - specified NEC Q42.8
    - specified NEC Q41.8
  - ischemic K55.1
- jejunum — *see also* Obstruction, intestine, specified NEC K56.699
  - congenital Q41.1
- lacrimal passages — *see also* Stenosis, lacrimal
  - congenital Q1Ø.5

Stricture — *continued*
  larynx J38.6
    congenital NEC Q31.8
      subglottic Q31.1
    syphilitic A52.73
      congenital A5Ø.59 *[J99]*
  meatus
    ear (congenital) Q16.1
      acquired — *see* Stricture, auditory canal, acquired
    osseous (ear) (congenital) Q16.1
      acquired — *see* Stricture, auditory canal, acquired
    urinarius — *see also* Stricture, urethra
      congenital Q64.33
  mitral (valve) — *see* Stenosis, mitral
  myocardium, myocardial I51.5
    hypertrophic subaortic (idiopathic) I42.1
  nares (anterior) (posterior) J34.89
    congenital Q3Ø.Ø
  nasal duct — *see also* Stenosis, lacrimal, duct
    congenital Q1Ø.5
  nasolacrimal duct — *see also* Stenosis, lacrimal, duct
    congenital Q1Ø.5
  nasopharynx J39.2
    syphilitic A52.73
  nose J34.89
    congenital Q3Ø.Ø
  nostril (anterior) (posterior) J34.89
    congenital Q3Ø.Ø
    syphilitic A52.73
      congenital A5Ø.59 *[J99]*
  organ or site, congenital NEC — *see* Atresia, by site
  os uteri — *see* Stricture, cervix
  osseous meatus (ear) (congenital) Q16.1
    acquired — *see* Stricture, auditory canal, acquired
  oviduct — *see* Stricture, fallopian tube
  pelviureteric junction (congenital) Q62.11
    acquired, with hydronephrosis N13.Ø
  penis, by foreign body T19.4 ☑
  pharynx J39.2
  prostate N42.89
  pulmonary, pulmonic
    artery (congenital) Q25.6
      acquired I28.8
      noncongenital I28.8
    infundibulum (congenital) Q24.3
    valve I37.Ø
      congenital Q22.1
    vein, acquired I28.8
    vessel NEC I28.8
  punctum lacrimale — *see also* Stenosis, lacrimal, punctum
    congenital Q1Ø.5
  pylorus (hypertrophic) K31.1
    adult K31.1
    congenital Q4Ø.Ø
    infantile Q4Ø.Ø
  rectosigmoid — *see also* Obstruction, intestine, specified NEC K56.699
  rectum (sphincter) K62.4
    congenital Q42.1
      with fistula Q42.Ø
    due to
      chlamydial lymphogranuloma A55
      irradiation K91.89
      lymphogranuloma venereum A55
    gonococcal A54.6
    inflammatory (chlamydial) A55
    syphilitic A52.74
    tuberculous A18.32
  renal artery I7Ø.1
    congenital Q27.1
  salivary duct or gland (any) K11.8
  sigmoid (flexure) — *see* Obstruction, intestine
  spermatic cord N5Ø.89
  stoma (following) (of)
    colostomy K94.Ø3
    enterostomy K94.13
    gastrostomy K94.23
    ileostomy K94.13
    tracheostomy J95.Ø3
  stomach K31.89
    congenital Q4Ø.2
    hourglass K31.2
  subaortic Q24.4
    hypertrophic (acquired) (idiopathic) I42.1
  subglottic J38.6

Stricture — *continued*
  syphilitic NEC A52.79
  trachea J39.8
    congenital Q32.1
    syphilitic A52.73
    tuberculous NEC A15.5
  tracheostomy J95.Ø3
  tricuspid (valve) — *see* Stenosis, tricuspid
  tunica vaginalis N5Ø.89
  ureter (postoperative) N13.5
    with
      hydronephrosis N13.1
        with infection N13.6
      pyelonephritis (chronic) N11.1
    congenital — *see* Atresia, ureter
    tuberculous A18.11
  ureteropelvic junction (congenital) Q62.11
    acquired, with hydronephrosis N13.Ø
  ureterovesical orifice N13.5
    with infection N13.6
  urethra (organic) (spasmodic) — *see also* Stricture, urethra, male N35.919
    associated with schistosomiasis B65.Ø *[N37]*
    congenital Q64.39
      valvular (posterior) Q64.2
    due to
      infection — *see* Stricture, urethra, postinfective
      trauma — *see* Stricture, urethra, post-traumatic
    female N35.92
    gonococcal, gonorrheal A54.Ø1
    infective NEC — *see* Stricture, urethra, postinfective
    late effect (sequelae) of injury — *see* Stricture, urethra, post-traumatic
    male N35.919
      anterior urethra N35.914
      bulbous urethra N35.912
      meatal N35.911
      membranous urethra N35.913
      overlapping sites N35.916
    postcatheterization — *see* Stricture, urethra, postprocedural
    postinfective NEC
      female N35.12
      male N35.119
        anterior urethra N35.114
        bulbous urethra N35.112
        meatal N35.111
        membranous urethra N35.113
        overlapping sites N35.116
    postobstetric N35.Ø21
    postoperative — *see* Stricture, urethra, postprocedural
    postprocedural
      female N99.12
      male N99.114
        anterior bulbous urethra N99.113
        bulbous urethra N99.111
        fossa navicularis N99.115
        meatal N99.11Ø
        membranous urethra N99.112
        overlapping sites N99.116
    post-traumatic
      female N35.Ø28
        due to childbirth N35.Ø21
      male N35.Ø14
        anterior urethra N35.Ø13
        bulbous urethra N35.Ø11
        meatal N35.Ø1Ø
        membranous urethra N35.Ø12
        overlapping sites N35.Ø16
    sequela (late effect) of
      childbirth N35.Ø21
      injury — *see* Stricture, urethra, post-traumatic
    specified cause NEC
      female N35.82
      male N35.819
        anterior urethra N35.814
        bulbous urethra N35.812
        meatal N35.811
        membranous urethra N35.813
        overlapping sites N35.816
    syphilitic A52.76
    traumatic — *see* Stricture, urethra, post-traumatic
    valvular (posterior), congenital Q64.2
  urinary meatus — *see* Stricture, urethra
  uterus, uterine (synechiae) N85.6
    os (external) (internal) — *see* Stricture, cervix
  vagina (outlet) — *see* Stenosis, vagina

Stricture — *continued*
  valve (cardiac) (heart) — *see also* Endocarditis
    congenital
      aortic Q23.Ø
      mitral Q23.2
      pulmonary Q22.1
      tricuspid Q22.4
  vas deferens N5Ø.89
    congenital Q55.4
  vein I87.1
  vena cava (inferior) (superior) NEC I87.1
    congenital Q26.Ø
  vesicourethral orifice N32.Ø
    congenital Q64.31
  vulva (acquired) N9Ø.5
Stridor RØ6.1
  congenital (larynx) P28.89
Stridulous — *see* condition
Stroke (apoplectic) (brain) (embolic) (ischemic) (paralytic) (thrombotic) I63.9
  cerebral, perinatal P91.82- ☑
  cryptogenic — *see also* infarction, cerebral I63.9
  epileptic — *see* Epilepsy
  heat T67.Ø1 ☑
    exertional T67.Ø2 ☑
    specified NEC T67.Ø9 ☑
  in evolution I63.9
  intraoperative
    during cardiac surgery I97.81Ø
    during other surgery I97.811
  ischemic, perinatal arterial P91.82- ☑
  lightning — *see* Lightning
  meaning
    cerebral hemorrhage — *code to* Hemorrhage, intracranial
    cerebral infarction *code to* Infarction, cerebral
  neonatal P91.82- ☑
  postprocedural
    following cardiac surgery I97.82Ø
    following other surgery I97.821
  sun T67.Ø1 ☑
    specified NEC T67.Ø9 ☑
  unspecified (NOS) I63.9
Stromatosis, endometrial D39.Ø
Strongyloidiasis, strongyloidosis B78.9
  cutaneous B78.1
  disseminated B78.7
  intestinal B78.Ø
Strophulus pruriginosus L28.2
Struck by lightning — *see* Lightning
Struma — *see also* Goiter
  Hashimoto EØ6.3
  lymphomatosa EØ6.3
  nodosa (simplex) EØ4.9
    endemic EØ1.2
      multinodular EØ1.1
    multinodular EØ4.2
      iodine-deficiency related EØ1.1
    toxic or with hyperthyroidism EØ5.2Ø
      with thyroid storm EØ5.21
      multinodular EØ5.2Ø
        with thyroid storm EØ5.21
      uninodular EØ5.1Ø
        with thyroid storm EØ5.11
    toxicosa EØ5.2Ø
      with thyroid storm EØ5.21
      multinodular EØ5.2Ø
        with thyroid storm EØ5.21
      uninodular EØ5.1Ø
        with thyroid storm EØ5.11
    uninodular EØ4.1
  ovarii D27.- ☑
  Riedel's EØ6.5
Strumipriva cachexia EØ3.4
Strümpell-Marie spine — *see* Spondylitis, ankylosing
Strümpell-Westphal pseudosclerosis E83.Ø1
Stuart deficiency disease (factor X) D68.2
Stuart-Prower factor deficiency (factor X) D68.2
Student's elbow — *see* Bursitis, elbow, olecranon
Stump — *see* Amputation
Stunting, nutritional E45
Stupor (catatonic) R4Ø.1
  depressive (single episode) F32.89
    recurrent episode F33.8
  dissociative F44.2
  manic F3Ø.2
  manic-depressive F31.89
  psychogenic (anergic) F44.2

Stupor — *continued*
- reaction to exceptional stress (transient) F43.Ø

Sturge (-Weber) (-Dimitri) (-Kalischer) **disease or syndrome** Q85.89
Stuttering F8Ø.81
- adult onset F98.5
- childhood onset F8Ø.81
- following cerebrovascular disease — *see* Disorder, fluency, following cerebrovascular disease
- in conditions classified elsewhere R47.82

Sty, stye (external) (internal) (meibomian) (zeisian) — *see* Hordeolum
Subacidity, gastric K31.89
- psychogenic F45.8

Subacute — *see* condition
Subarachnoid — *see* condition
Subcortical — *see* condition
Subcostal syndrome, nerve compression — *see* Mononeuropathy, upper limb, specified site NEC
Subcutaneous, subcuticular — *see* condition
Subdural — *see* condition
Subendocardium — *see* condition
Subependymoma
- specified site — *see* Neoplasm, uncertain behavior, by site
- unspecified site D43.2

Suberosis J67.3
Subglossitis — *see* Glossitis
Subhemophilia D66
Subinvolution
- breast (postlactational) (postpuerperal) N64.89
- puerperal O9Ø.89
- uterus (chronic) (nonpuerperal) N85.3
  - puerperal O9Ø.89

Sublingual — *see* condition
Sublinguitis — *see* Sialoadenitis
Subluxatable hip Q65.6
Subluxation — *see also* Dislocation
- acromioclavicular S43.11- ☑
- ankle S93.Ø- ☑
- atlantoaxial, recurrent M43.4
  - with myelopathy M43.3
- carpometacarpal (joint) NEC S63.Ø5- ☑
  - thumb S63.Ø4- ☑
- complex, vertebral — *see* Complex, subluxation
- congenital — *see also* Malposition, congenital
  - hip — *see* Dislocation, hip, congenital, partial
  - joint (excluding hip)
    - lower limb Q68.8
    - shoulder Q68.8
    - upper limb Q68.8
- elbow (traumatic) S53.1Ø- ☑
  - anterior S53.11- ☑
  - lateral S53.14- ☑
  - medial S53.13- ☑
  - posterior S53.12- ☑
  - specified type NEC S53.19- ☑
- finger S63.2Ø- ☑
  - index S63.2Ø- ☑
  - interphalangeal S63.22- ☑
    - distal S63.24- ☑
      - index S63.24- ☑
      - little S63.24- ☑
      - middle S63.24- ☑
      - ring S63.24- ☑
    - index S63.22- ☑
    - little S63.22- ☑
    - middle S63.22- ☑
    - proximal S63.23- ☑
      - index S63.23- ☑
      - little S63.23- ☑
      - middle S63.23- ☑
      - ring S63.23- ☑
    - ring S63.22- ☑
  - little S63.2Ø- ☑
  - metacarpophalangeal S63.21- ☑
    - index S63.21- ☑
    - little S63.21- ☑
    - middle S63.21- ☑
    - ring S63.21- ☑
  - middle S63.2Ø- ☑
  - ring S63.2Ø- ☑
- foot S93.3Ø- ☑
  - specified site NEC S93.33- ☑
  - tarsal joint S93.31- ☑
  - tarsometatarsal joint S93.32- ☑

Subluxation — *continued*
- foot — *continued*
  - toe — *see* Subluxation, toe
- hip S73.ØØ- ☑
  - anterior S73.Ø3- ☑
    - obturator S73.Ø2- ☑
  - central S73.Ø4- ☑
  - posterior S73.Ø1- ☑
- interphalangeal (joint)
  - finger S63.22- ☑
    - distal joint S63.24- ☑
      - index S63.24- ☑
      - little S63.24- ☑
      - middle S63.24- ☑
      - ring S63.24- ☑
    - index S63.22- ☑
    - little S63.22- ☑
    - middle S63.22- ☑
    - proximal joint S63.23- ☑
      - index S63.23- ☑
      - little S63.23- ☑
      - middle S63.23- ☑
      - ring S63.23- ☑
    - ring S63.22- ☑
  - thumb S63.12- ☑
  - toe S93.13- ☑
    - great S93.13- ☑
    - lesser S93.13- ☑
- joint prosthesis — *see* Complications, joint prosthesis, mechanical, displacement, by site
- knee S83.1Ø- ☑
  - cap — *see* Subluxation, patella
  - patella — *see* Subluxation, patella
  - proximal tibia
    - anteriorly S83.11- ☑
    - laterally S83.14- ☑
    - medially S83.13- ☑
    - posteriorly S83.12- ☑
  - specified type NEC S83.19- ☑
- lens — *see* Dislocation, lens, partial
- ligament, traumatic — *see* Sprain, by site
- metacarpal (bone)
  - proximal end S63.Ø6- ☑
- metacarpophalangeal (joint)
  - finger S63.21- ☑
    - index S63.21- ☑
    - little S63.21- ☑
    - middle S63.21- ☑
    - ring S63.21- ☑
  - thumb S63.11- ☑
- metatarsophalangeal joint S93.14- ☑
  - great toe S93.14- ☑
  - lesser toe S93.14- ☑
- midcarpal (joint) S63.Ø3- ☑
- patella S83.ØØ- ☑
  - lateral S83.Ø1- ☑
  - recurrent (nontraumatic) — *see* Dislocation, patella, recurrent, incomplete
  - specified type NEC S83.Ø9- ☑
- pathological — *see* Dislocation, pathological
- radial head S53.ØØ- ☑
  - anterior S53.Ø1- ☑
  - nursemaid's elbow S53.Ø3- ☑
  - posterior S53.Ø2- ☑
  - specified type NEC S53.Ø9- ☑
- radiocarpal (joint) S63.Ø2- ☑
- radioulnar (joint)
  - distal S63.Ø1- ☑
  - proximal — *see* Subluxation, elbow
- shoulder
  - congenital Q68.8
  - girdle S43.3Ø- ☑
    - scapula S43.31- ☑
    - specified site NEC S43.39- ☑
  - traumatic S43.ØØ- ☑
    - anterior S43.Ø1- ☑
    - inferior S43.Ø3- ☑
    - posterior S43.Ø2- ☑
    - specified type NEC S43.Ø8- ☑
- sternoclavicular (joint) S43.2Ø- ☑
  - anterior S43.21- ☑
  - posterior S43.22- ☑
- symphysis (pubis) — *see also* Dislocation, symphysis pubis
- thumb S63.1Ø3 ☑

Subluxation — *continued*
- thumb — *continued*
  - interphalangeal joint — *see* Subluxation, interphalangeal (joint), thumb
  - metacarpophalangeal joint — *see* Subluxation, metacarpophalangeal (joint), thumb
- toe(s) S93.1Ø- ☑
  - great S93.1Ø- ☑
    - interphalangeal joint S93.13- ☑
    - metatarsophalangeal joint S93.14- ☑
  - interphalangeal joint S93.13- ☑
  - lesser S93.1Ø- ☑
    - interphalangeal joint S93.13- ☑
    - metatarsophalangeal joint S93.14- ☑
  - metatarsophalangeal joint S93.149 ☑
- ulna
  - distal end S63.Ø7- ☑
  - proximal end — *see* Subluxation, elbow
- ulnohumeral joint — *see* Subluxation, elbow
- vertebral
  - recurrent NEC — *see* subcategory M43.5 ☑
  - traumatic
    - cervical S13.1ØØ ☑
      - atlantoaxial joint S13.12Ø ☑
      - atlantooccipital joint S13.11Ø ☑
      - atloidooccipital joint S13.11Ø ☑
      - joint between
        - CØ and C1 S13.11Ø ☑
        - C1 and C2 S13.12Ø ☑
        - C2 and C3 S13.13Ø ☑
        - C3 and C4 S13.14Ø ☑
        - C4 and C5 S13.15Ø ☑
        - C5 and C6 S13.16Ø ☑
        - C6 and C7 S13.17Ø ☑
        - C7 and T1 S13.18Ø ☑
      - occipitoatloid joint S13.11Ø ☑
    - lumbar S33.1ØØ ☑
      - joint between
        - L1 and L2 S33.11Ø ☑
        - L2 and L3 S33.12Ø ☑
        - L3 and L4 S33.13Ø ☑
        - L4 and L5 S33.14Ø ☑
    - thoracic S23.1ØØ ☑
      - joint between
        - T1 and T2 S23.11Ø ☑
        - T2 and T3 S23.12Ø ☑
        - T3 and T4 S23.122 ☑
        - T4 and T5 S23.13Ø ☑
        - T5 and T6 S23.132 ☑
        - T6 and T7 S23.14Ø ☑
        - T7 and T8 S23.142 ☑
        - T8 and T9 S23.15Ø ☑
        - T9 and T1Ø S23.152 ☑
        - T1Ø and T11 S23.16Ø ☑
        - T11 and T12 S23.162 ☑
        - T12 and L1 S23.17Ø ☑
- wrist (carpal bone) S63.ØØ- ☑
  - carpometacarpal joint — *see* Subluxation, carpometacarpal (joint)
  - distal radioulnar joint — *see* Subluxation, radioulnar (joint), distal
  - metacarpal bone, proximal — *see* Subluxation, metacarpal (bone), proximal end
  - midcarpal — *see* Subluxation, midcarpal (joint)
  - radiocarpal joint — *see* Subluxation, radiocarpal (joint)
  - recurrent — *see* Dislocation, recurrent, wrist
  - specified site NEC S63.Ø9- ☑
  - ulna — *see* Subluxation, ulna, distal end

Submaxillary — *see* condition
Submersion (fatal) (nonfatal) T75.1 ☑
Submucous — *see* condition
Subnormal, subnormality
- accommodation (old age) H52.4
- mental — *see* Disability, intellectual
- temperature (accidental) T68

Subphrenic — *see* condition
Subscapular nerve — *see* condition
Subseptus uterus Q51.28
Subsiding appendicitis K36
Substance (other psychoactive) **-induced**
- anxiety disorder F19.98Ø
- bipolar and related disorder F19.94
- delirium F19.921
- depressive disorder F19.94
- major neurocognitive disorder F19.97

- **Substance** (other psychoactive) **-induced** — *continued*
  - mild neurocognitive disorder F19.988
  - obsessive-compulsive and related disorder F19.988
  - psychotic disorder F19.959
  - sexual dysfunction F19.981
  - sleep disorder F19.982
- **Substernal thyroid** EØ4.9
  - congenital Q89.2
- **Substitution disorder** F44.9
- **Subtentorial** — *see* condition
- **Subthyroidism** (acquired) — *see also* Hypothyroidism
  - congenital EØ3.1
- **Succenturiate placenta** O43.19- ☑
- **Sucking thumb, child** (excessive) F98.8
- **Sudamen, sudamina** L74.1
- **Sudanese kala-azar** B55.Ø
- **Sudden**
  - hearing loss — *see* Deafness, sudden
  - heart failure — *see* Failure, heart
- **Sudeck's atrophy, disease, or syndrome** — *see* Algoneurodystrophy
- **Suffocation** — *see* Asphyxia, traumatic
- **Sugar**
  - blood
    - high (transient) R73.9
    - low (transient) E16.2
  - in urine R81
- **Suicide, suicidal** (attempted) T14.91 ☑
  - by poisoning — *see* Table of Drugs and Chemicals
  - history of (personal) Z91.51
    - in family Z81.8
  - ideation — *see* Ideation, suicidal
  - risk
    - meaning personal history of attempted suicide Z91.51
    - meaning suicidal ideation — *see* Ideation, suicidal
  - tendencies
    - meaning personal history of attempted suicide Z91.51
    - meaning suicidal ideation — *see* Ideation, suicidal
  - trauma — *see* nature of injury by site
- **Suipestifer infection** — *see* Infection, salmonella
- **Sulfhemoglobinemia, sulphemoglobinemia** (acquired) (with methemoglobinemia) D74.8
- **Sumatran mite fever** A75.3
- **Summer** — *see* condition
- **Sunburn** L55.9
  - due to
    - tanning bed (acute) L56.8
      - chronic L57.8
    - ultraviolet radiation (acute) L56.8
      - chronic L57.8
  - first degree L55.Ø
  - second degree L55.1
  - third degree L55.2
- **SUNCT** (short lasting unilateral neuralgiform headache with conjunctival injection and tearing) G44.Ø59
  - intractable G44.Ø51
  - not intractable G44.Ø59
- **Sundowning** FØ5
- **Sunken acetabulum** — *see* Derangement, joint, specified type NEC, hip
- **Sunstroke** T67.Ø1 ☑
  - specified NEC T67.Ø9 ☑
- **Superfecundation** — *see* Pregnancy, multiple
- **Superfetation** — *see* Pregnancy, multiple
- **Superinvolution** (uterus) N85.8
- **Supernumerary** (congenital)
  - aortic cusps Q23.8
  - auditory ossicles Q16.3
  - bone Q79.8
  - breast Q83.1
  - carpal bones Q74.Ø
  - cusps, heart valve NEC Q24.8
    - aortic Q23.8
    - mitral Q23.2
    - pulmonary Q22.3
  - digit(s) Q69.9
  - ear (lobule) Q17.Ø
  - fallopian tube Q5Ø.6
  - finger Q69.Ø
  - hymen Q52.4
  - kidney Q63.Ø
  - lacrimonasal duct Q1Ø.6
  - lobule (ear) Q17.Ø
  - mitral cusps Q23.2
  - muscle Q79.8
- **Supernumerary** — *continued*
  - nipple(s) Q83.3
  - organ or site not listed — *see* Accessory
  - ossicles, auditory Q16.3
  - ovary Q5Ø.31
  - oviduct Q5Ø.6
  - pulmonary, pulmonic cusps Q22.3
  - rib Q76.6
    - cervical or first (syndrome) Q76.5
  - roots (of teeth) KØØ.2
  - spleen Q89.Ø9
  - tarsal bones Q74.2
  - teeth KØØ.1
  - testis Q55.29
  - thumb Q69.1
  - toe Q69.2
  - uterus Q51.28
  - vagina Q52.1 ☑
  - vertebra Q76.49
- **Supervision** (of)
  - contraceptive — *see* Prescription, contraceptives
  - dietary (for) Z71.3
    - allergy (food) Z71.3
    - colitis Z71.3
    - diabetes mellitus Z71.3
    - food allergy or intolerance Z71.3
    - gastritis Z71.3
    - hypercholesterolemia Z71.3
    - hypoglycemia Z71.3
    - intolerance (food) Z71.3
    - obesity Z71.3
    - specified NEC Z71.3
  - healthy infant or child Z76.2
    - foundling Z76.1
  - high-risk pregnancy — *see* Pregnancy, supervision of, high-risk
  - lactation Z39.1
  - pregnancy — *see* Pregnancy, supervision of
- **Supplemental teeth** KØØ.1
- **Suppression**
  - binocular vision H53.34
  - lactation O92.5
  - menstruation N94.89
  - ovarian secretion E28.39
  - renal N28.9
  - urine, urinary secretion R34
- **Suppuration, suppurative** — *see also* condition
  - accessory sinus (chronic) — *see* Sinusitis
  - adrenal gland
  - antrum (chronic) — *see* Sinusitis, maxillary
  - bladder — *see* Cystitis
  - brain GØ6.Ø
    - sequelae GØ9
  - breast N61.1
    - puerperal, postpartum or gestational — *see* Mastitis, obstetric, purulent
  - dental periosteum M27.3
  - ear (middle) — *see also* Otitis, media
    - external NEC — *see* Otitis, externa, infective
    - internal — *see* subcategory H83.Ø ☑
  - ethmoidal (chronic) (sinus) — *see* Sinusitis, ethmoidal
  - fallopian tube — *see* Salpingo-oophoritis
  - frontal (chronic) (sinus) — *see* Sinusitis, frontal
  - gallbladder (acute) K81.Ø
  - gum KØ5.2Ø
    - generalized — *see* Periodontitis, aggressive, generalized
    - localized — *see* Periodontitis, aggressive, localized
  - intracranial GØ6.Ø
  - joint — *see* Arthritis, pyogenic or pyemic
  - labyrinthine — *see* subcategory H83.Ø ☑
  - lung — *see* Abscess, lung
  - mammary gland N61.1
    - puerperal, postpartum O91.12
      - associated with lactation O91.13
  - maxilla, maxillary M27.2
    - sinus (chronic) — *see* Sinusitis, maxillary
  - muscle — *see* Myositis, infective
  - nasal sinus (chronic) — *see* Sinusitis
  - pancreas, acute — *see also* Pancreatitis, acute K85.8Ø
  - parotid gland — *see* Sialoadenitis
  - pelvis, pelvic
    - female — *see* Disease, pelvis, inflammatory
    - male K65.Ø
  - pericranial — *see* Osteomyelitis
  - salivary duct or gland (any) — *see* Sialoadenitis
  - sinus (accessory) (chronic) (nasal) — *see* Sinusitis
  - sphenoidal sinus (chronic) — *see* Sinusitis, sphenoidal
- **Suppuration, suppurative** — *continued*
  - thymus (gland) E32.1
  - thyroid (gland) EØ6.Ø
  - tonsil — *see* Tonsillitis
  - uterus — *see* Endometritis
- **Supraeruption of tooth** (teeth) M26.34
- **Supraglottitis** JØ4.3Ø
  - with obstruction JØ4.31
- **Suprarenal** (gland) — *see* condition
- **Suprascapular nerve** — *see* condition
- **Suprasellar** — *see* condition
- **Surfer's knots or nodules** S89.8- ☑
- **Surgical**
  - emphysema T81.82 ☑
  - procedures, complication or misadventure — *see* Complications, surgical procedures
  - shock T81.1Ø ☑
- **Surveillance** (of) (for) — *see also* Observation
  - alcohol abuse Z71.41
  - contraceptive — *see* Prescription, contraceptives
  - dietary Z71.3
  - drug abuse Z71.51
- **Susceptibility to disease, genetic** Z15.89
  - malignant neoplasm Z15.Ø9
    - breast Z15.Ø1
    - endometrium Z15.Ø4
    - ovary Z15.Ø2
    - prostate Z15.Ø3
    - specified NEC Z15.Ø9
  - multiple endocrine neoplasia Z15.81
- **Suspected condition, ruled out** — *see also* Observation, suspected
  - amniotic cavity and membrane ZØ3.71
  - cervical shortening ZØ3.75
  - fetal anomaly ZØ3.73
  - fetal growth ZØ3.74
  - maternal and fetal conditions NEC ZØ3.79
  - newborn — *see also* Observation, newborn, suspected condition ruled out ZØ5.9
  - oligohydramnios ZØ3.71
  - placental problem ZØ3.72
  - polyhydramnios ZØ3.71
- **Suspended uterus**
  - in pregnancy or childbirth — *see* Pregnancy, complicated by, abnormal uterus
- **Sutton's nevus** D22.9
- **Suture**
  - burst (in operation wound) T81.31 ☑
    - external operation wound T81.31 ☑
    - internal operation wound T81.32 ☑
  - inadvertently left in operation wound — *see* Foreign body, accidentally left during a procedure
  - removal Z48.Ø2
- **Swab inadvertently left in operation wound** — *see* Foreign body, accidentally left during a procedure
- **Swallowed, swallowing**
  - difficulty — *see* Dysphagia
  - foreign body — *see* Foreign body, alimentary tract
- **Swan-neck deformity** (finger) — *see* Deformity, finger, swan-neck
- **Swearing, compulsive** F42.8
  - in Gilles de la Tourette's syndrome F95.2
- **Sweat, sweats**
  - fetid L75.Ø
  - night R61
- **Sweating, excessive** R61
- **Sweeley-Klionsky disease** E75.21
- **Sweet's disease or dermatosis** L98.2
- **Swelling** (of) R6Ø.9
  - abdomen, abdominal (not referable to any particular organ) — *see* Mass, abdominal
  - ankle — *see* Effusion, joint, ankle
  - arm M79.89
    - forearm M79.89
  - breast — *see also* Lump, breast N63.Ø
  - Calabar B74.3
  - cervical gland R59.Ø
  - chest, localized R22.2
  - ear H93.8- ☑
  - extremity (lower) (upper) — *see* Disorder, soft tissue, specified type NEC
  - finger M79.89
  - foot M79.89
  - glands R59.9
    - generalized R59.1
    - localized R59.Ø
  - hand M79.89

Swelling — *continued*
head (localized) R22.Ø
inflammatory — *see* Inflammation
intra-abdominal — *see* Mass, abdominal
joint — *see* Effusion, joint
leg M79.89
lower M79.89
limb — *see* Disorder, soft tissue, specified type NEC
localized (skin) R22.9
chest R22.2
head R22.Ø
limb
lower — *see* Mass, localized, limb, lower
upper — *see* Mass, localized, limb, upper
neck R22.1
trunk R22.2
neck (localized) R22.1
pelvic — *see* Mass, abdominal
scrotum N5Ø.89
splenic — *see* Splenomegaly
testis N5Ø.89
toe M79.89
umbilical R19.Ø9
wandering, due to Gnathostoma (spinigerum) B83.1
white — *see* Tuberculosis, arthritis
Swift (-Feer) disease
overdose or wrong substance given or taken — *see* Table of Drugs and Chemicals, by drug, poisoning
Swimmer's
cramp T75.1 ☑
ear H6Ø.33- ☑
itch B65.3
Swimming in the head R42
Swollen — *see* Swelling
Swyer syndrome Q99.1
Sycosis L73.8
barbae (not parasitic) L73.8
contagiosa (mycotic) B35.Ø
lupoides L73.8
mycotic B35.Ø
parasitic B35.Ø
vulgaris L73.8
Sydenham's chorea — *see* Chorea, Sydenham's
Sylvatic yellow fever A95.Ø
Sylvest's disease B33.Ø
Symblepharon H11.23- ☑
congenital Q1Ø.3
Symond's syndrome G93.2
Sympathetic — *see* condition
Sympatheticotonia G9Ø.8
Sympathicoblastoma
specified site — *see* Neoplasm, malignant, by site
unspecified site C74.9Ø
Sympathogonioma — *see* Sympathicoblastoma
Symphalangy (fingers) (toes) Q7Ø.9
Symptoms NEC R68.89
breast NEC N64.59
cold JØØ
development NEC R63.8
factitious, self-induced — *see* Disorder, factitious
genital organs, female R1Ø.2
involving
abdomen NEC R19.8
appearance NEC R46.89
awareness R41.9
altered mental status R41.82
amnesia — *see* Amnesia
borderline intellectual functioning R41.83
coma — *see* Coma
disorientation R41.Ø
neurologic neglect syndrome R41.4
senile cognitive decline R41.81
specified symptom NEC R41.89
behavior NEC R46.89
cardiovascular system NEC RØ9.89
chest NEC RØ9.89
circulatory system NEC RØ9.89
cognitive functions R41.9
altered mental status R41.82
amnesia — *see* Amnesia
borderline intellectual functioning R41.83
coma — *see* Coma
disorientation R41.Ø
neurologic neglect syndrome R41.4
senile cognitive decline R41.81
specified symptom NEC R41.89
development NEC R62.5Ø
digestive system NEC R19.8
Symptoms — *continued*
involving — *continued*
emotional state NEC R45.89
emotional lability R45.86
food and fluid intake R63.8
general perceptions and sensations R44.9
specified NEC R44.8
musculoskeletal system R29.91
specified NEC R29.898
nervous system R29.9Ø
specified NEC R29.818
pelvis NEC R19.8
respiratory system NEC RØ9.89
skin and integument R23.9
urinary system R39.9
menopausal N95.1
metabolism NEC R63.8
neurotic F48.8
of infancy R68.19
pelvis NEC, female R1Ø.2
skin and integument NEC R23.9
subcutaneous tissue NEC R23.9
viral cold JØØ
Sympus Q74.2
Syncephalus Q89.4
Synchondrosis
abnormal (congenital) Q78.8
ischiopubic M91.Ø
Synchysis (scintillans) (senile) (vitreous body) H43.89
Syncope (near) (pre-) R55
anginosa I2Ø.8
bradycardia RØØ.1
cardiac R55
carotid sinus G9Ø.Ø1
due to spinal (lumbar) puncture G97.1
heart R55
heat T67.1 ☑
laryngeal RØ5.4
psychogenic F48.8
tussive RØ5.8
vasoconstriction R55
vasodepressor R55
vasomotor R55
vasovagal R55
Syndactylism, syndactyly Q7Ø.9
complex (with synostosis)
fingers Q7Ø.Ø- ☑
toes Q7Ø.2- ☑
simple (without synostosis)
fingers Q7Ø.1- ☑
toes Q7Ø.3- ☑
Syndrome — *see also* Disease
5q minus NOS D46.C (*following* D46.2)
48,XXXX Q97.1
49,XXXXX Q97.1
abdominal
acute R1Ø.Ø
muscle deficiency Q79.4
abnormal innervation HØ2.519
left HØ2.516
lower HØ2.515
upper HØ2.514
right HØ2.513
lower HØ2.512
upper HØ2.511
abstinence, neonatal P96.1
acid pulmonary aspiration, obstetric O74.Ø
acquired immunodeficiency — *see* Human, immunodeficiency virus (HIV) disease
activated phosphoinositide 3-kinase delta syndrome [APDS] D81.82
acute abdominal R1Ø.Ø
acute respiratory distress (adult) (child) J8Ø
idiopathic J84.114
Adair-Dighton Q78.Ø
Adams-Stokes (-Morgagni) I45.9
adiposogenital E23.6
adrenal
hemorrhage (meningococcal) A39.1
meningococcic A39.1
adrenocortical — *see* Cushing's, syndrome
adrenogenital E25.9
congenital, associated with enzyme deficiency E25.Ø
afferent loop NEC K91.89
Alagille's Q44.7
alcohol withdrawal (without convulsions) — *see* Dependence, alcohol, with, withdrawal
Alder's D72.Ø
Syndrome — *continued*
Aldrich (-Wiskott) D82.Ø
alien hand R41.4
Alport Q87.81
alveolar hypoventilation E66.2
alveolocapillary block J84.1Ø
amnesic, amnestic (confabulatory) (due to) — *see* Disorder, amnesic
amyostatic (Wilson's disease) E83.Ø1
androgen insensitivity E34.5Ø
complete E34.51
partial E34.52
androgen resistance — *see also* Syndrome, androgen insensitivity E34.5Ø
Angelman Q93.51
anginal — *see* Angina
ankyloglossia superior Q38.1
anterior
chest wall RØ7.89
cord G83.82
spinal artery G95.19
compression M47.Ø19
cervical region M47.Ø12
cervicothoracic region M47.Ø13
lumbar region M47.Ø16
occipito-atlanto-axial region M47.Ø11
thoracic region M47.Ø14
thoracolumbar region M47.Ø15
tibial M76.81- ☑
antibody deficiency D8Ø.9
agammaglobulinemic D8Ø.1
hereditary D8Ø.Ø
congenital D8Ø.Ø
hypogammaglobulinemic D8Ø.1
hereditary D8Ø.Ø
anticardiolipin (-antibody) D68.61
antidepressant discontinuation T43.2Ø5 ☑
antiphospholipid (-antibody) D68.61
aortic
arch M31.4
bifurcation I74.Ø9
aortomesenteric duodenum occlusion K31.5
apical ballooning (transient left ventricular) I51.81
arcuate ligament I77.4
argentaffin, argintaffinoma E34.Ø
Arnold-Chiari — *see* Arnold-Chiari disease
Arrillaga-Ayerza I27.Ø
arterial tortuosity Q87.82
arteriovenous steal T82.898- ☑
Asherman's N85.6
aspiration, of newborn — *see* Aspiration, by substance, with pneumonia
meconium P24.Ø1
ataxia-telangiectasia G11.3
auriculotemporal G5Ø.8
autoerythrocyte sensitization (Gardner-Diamond) D69.2
autoimmune lymphoproliferative [ALPS] D89.82
autoimmune polyglandular E31.Ø
autoinflammatory MØ4.9
specified type NEC MØ4.8
autosomal — *see* Abnormal, autosomes
Avellis' G46.8
Ayerza (-Arrillaga) I27.Ø
Babinski-Nageotte G83.89
Bakwin-Krida Q78.5
bare lymphocyte D81.6
Barré-Guillain G61.Ø
Barré-Liéou M53.Ø
Barrett's — *see* Barrett's, esophagus
Barsony-Polgar K22.4
Bársony-Teschendorf K22.4
Barth E78.71
Bartter's E26.81
basal cell nevus Q87.89
Basedow's EØ5.ØØ
with thyroid storm EØ5.Ø1
basilar artery G45.Ø
Batten-Steinert G71.11
battered
baby or child — *see* Maltreatment, child, physical abuse
spouse — *see* Maltreatment, adult, physical abuse
Beals Q87.4Ø
Beau's I51.5
Beck's I65.8
Benedikt's G46.3
Béquez César (-Steinbrinck-Chédiak-Higashi) E7Ø.33Ø
Bernhardt-Roth — *see* Meralgia paresthetica

- **Syndrome** — *continued*
  - Bernheim's — *see* Failure, heart, right
  - big spleen D73.1
  - bilateral polycystic ovarian E28.2
  - Bing-Horton's — *see* Horton's headache
  - Birt-Hogg-Dube syndrome Q87.89
  - Björck (-Thorsen) E34.Ø
  - black
    - lung J6Ø
    - widow spider bite — *see* Toxicity, venom, spider, black widow
  - Blackfan-Diamond D61.Ø1
  - Blau MØ4.8
  - blind loop K9Ø.2
    - congenital Q43.8
    - postsurgical K91.2
  - blue sclera Q78.Ø
  - blue toe I75.Ø2- ☑
  - Boder-Sedgewick G11.3
  - Boerhaave's K22.3
  - Borjeson Forssman Lehmann Q89.8
  - Bouillaud's IØ1.9
  - Bourneville (-Pringle) Q85.1
  - Bouveret (-Hoffman) I47.9
  - brachial plexus G54.Ø
  - bradycardia-tachycardia I49.5
  - brain (nonpsychotic) FØ9
    - with psychosis, psychotic reaction FØ9
    - acute or subacute — *see* Delirium
    - congenital — *see* Disability, intellectual
    - organic FØ9
      - post-traumatic (nonpsychotic) FØ7.81
        - psychotic FØ9
    - personality change FØ7.Ø
    - postcontusional FØ7.81
    - post-traumatic, nonpsychotic FØ7.81
    - psycho-organic FØ9
    - psychotic FØ6.8
  - brain stem stroke G46.3
  - Brandt's (acrodermatitis enteropathica) E83.2
  - broad ligament laceration N83.8
  - Brock's J98.11
  - bronze baby P83.88
  - Brown-Sequard G83.81
  - Brugada I49.8
  - bubbly lung P27.Ø
  - Buchem's M85.2
  - Budd-Chiari I82.Ø
  - bulbar (progressive) G12.22
  - Bürger-Grütz E78.3
  - Burke's K86.89
  - Burnett's (milk-alkali) E83.52
  - burning feet E53.9
  - Bywaters' T79.5 ☑
  - Call-Fleming I67.841
  - carbohydrate-deficient glycoprotein (CDGS) E77.8
  - carcinogenic thrombophlebitis I82.1
  - carcinoid E34.Ø
  - cardiac asthma I5Ø.1
  - cardiacos negros I27.Ø
  - cardiofaciocutaneous Q87.89
  - cardiopulmonary-obesity E66.2
  - cardiorenal — *see* Hypertension, cardiorenal
  - cardiorespiratory distress (idiopathic), newborn P22.Ø
  - cardiovascular renal — *see* Hypertension, cardiorenal
  - carotid
    - artery (hemispheric) (internal) G45.1
    - body G9Ø.Ø1
    - sinus G9Ø.Ø1
  - carpal tunnel G56.Ø- ☑
  - Cassidy (-Scholte) E34.Ø
  - cat cry Q93.4
  - cat eye Q92.8
  - cauda equina G83.4
  - causalgia — *see* Causalgia
  - celiac K9Ø.Ø
    - artery compression I77.4
    - axis I77.4
  - central pain G89.Ø
  - cerebellar
    - hereditary G11.9
    - stroke G46.4
  - cerebellomedullary malformation — *see* Spina bifida
  - cerebral
    - artery
      - anterior G46.1
      - middle G46.Ø
      - posterior G46.2
- **Syndrome** — *continued*
  - cerebral — *continued*
    - gigantism E22.Ø
  - cervical (root) M53.1
    - disc — *see* Disorder, disc, cervical, with neuritis
    - fusion Q76.1
    - posterior, sympathicus M53.Ø
    - rib Q76.5
    - sympathetic paralysis G9Ø.2
  - cervicobrachial (diffuse) M53.1
  - cervicocranial M53.Ø
  - cervicodorsal outlet G54.2
  - cervicothoracic outlet G54.Ø
  - Céstan (-Raymond) I65.8
  - Charcot's (angina cruris) (intermittent claudication) I73.9
  - Charcot-Weiss-Baker G9Ø.Ø9
  - CHARGE Q89.8
  - Chédiak-Higashi (-Steinbrinck) E7Ø.33Ø
  - chest wall RØ7.1
  - Chiari's (hepatic vein thrombosis) I82.Ø
  - Chilaiditi's Q43.3
  - child maltreatment — *see* Maltreatment, child
  - chondrocostal junction M94.Ø
  - chondroectodermal dysplasia Q77.6
  - chromosome 4 short arm deletion Q93.3
  - chromosome 5 short arm deletion Q93.4
  - chronic
    - infantile neurological, cutaneous and articular (CINCA) MØ4.2
    - pain G89.4
      - personality F68.8
  - Churg-Strauss M3Ø.1
  - Clarke-Hadfield K86.89
  - Clerambault's automatism G93.89
  - Clouston's (hidrotic ectodermal dysplasia) Q82.4
  - clumsiness, clumsy child F82
  - cluster headache G44.ØØ9
    - intractable G44.ØØ1
    - not intractable G44.ØØ9
  - Coffin-Lowry Q89.8
  - cold injury (newborn) P8Ø.Ø
  - combined immunity deficiency D81.9
  - compartment (deep) (posterior) (traumatic) T79.AØ ☑ (*following* T79.7)
    - abdomen T79.A3 ☑ (*following* T79.7)
    - lower extremity (hip, buttock, thigh, leg, foot, toes) T79.A2 ☑ (*following* T79.7)
    - nontraumatic
      - abdomen M79.A3 (*following* M79.7)
      - lower extremity (hip, buttock, thigh, leg, foot, toes) M79.A2- ☑ (*following* M79.7)
      - specified site NEC M79.A9 (*following* M79.7)
      - upper extremity (shoulder, arm, forearm, wrist, hand, fingers) M79.A1- ☑ (*following* M79.7)
    - postprocedural — *see* Syndrome, compartment, nontraumatic
    - specified site NEC T79.A9 ☑ (*following* T79.7)
    - upper extremity (shoulder, arm, forearm, wrist, hand, fingers) T79.A1 ☑ (*following* T79.7)
  - complex regional pain — *see* Syndrome, pain, complex regional
  - compression T79.5 ☑
    - anterior spinal — *see* Syndrome, anterior, spinal artery, compression
    - cauda equina G83.4
    - celiac artery I77.4
    - vertebral artery M47.Ø29
      - cervical region M47.Ø22
      - occipito-atlanto-axial region M47.Ø21
  - concussion FØ7.81
  - congenital
    - affecting multiple systems NEC Q87.89
    - central alveolar hypoventilation G47.35
    - facial diplegia Q87.Ø
    - muscular hypertrophy-cerebral Q87.89
    - oculo-auriculovertebral Q87.Ø
    - oculofacial diplegia (Moebius) Q87.Ø
    - rubella (manifest) P35.Ø
  - congestion-fibrosis (pelvic), female N94.89
  - congestive dysmenorrhea N94.6
  - connective tissue M35.9
    - overlap NEC M35.1
  - Conn's E26.Ø1
  - conus medullaris G95.81
  - cord
    - anterior G83.82
- **Syndrome** — *continued*
  - cord — *continued*
    - posterior G83.83
  - coronary
    - acute NEC I24.9
    - insufficiency or intermediate I2Ø.Ø
    - slow flow I2Ø.8
  - Costen's (complex) M26.69
  - costochondral junction M94.Ø
  - costoclavicular G54.Ø
  - costovertebral E22.Ø
  - Cowden
    - PTEN related Q85.81
    - specified NEC Q85.82
  - craniovertebral M53.Ø
  - Creutzfeldt-Jakob — *see* Creutzfeldt-Jakob disease or syndrome
  - crib death R99
  - cricopharyngeal — *see* Dysphagia
  - cri-du-chat Q93.4
  - croup JØ5.Ø
  - CRPS I — *see* Syndrome, pain, complex regional I
  - crush T79.5 ☑
  - cryopyrin-associated perodic MØ4.2
  - cryptophthalmos Q87.Ø
  - cubital tunnel — *see* Lesion, nerve, ulnar
  - Curschmann (-Batten) (-Steinert) G71.11
  - Cushing's E24.9
    - alcohol-induced E24.4
    - due to
      - alcohol
      - drugs E24.2
      - ectopic ACTH E24.3
      - overproduction of pituitary ACTH E24.Ø
    - drug-induced E24.2
    - overdose or wrong substance given or taken — *see* Table of Drugs and Chemicals, by drug, poisoning
    - pituitary-dependent E24.Ø
    - specified type NEC E24.8
  - cystic duct stump K91.5
  - cytokine release D89.839
    - grade 1 D89.831
    - grade 2 D89.832
    - grade 3 D89.833
    - grade 4 D89.834
    - grade 5 D89.835
  - Dana-Putnam D51.Ø
  - Danbolt (-Cross) (acrodermatitis enteropathica) E83.2
  - Dandy-Walker QØ3.1
    - with spina bifida QØ7.Ø1
  - Danlos' — *see also* Syndrome, Ehlers-Danlos Q79.6Ø
  - De Quervain E34.51
  - de Toni-Fanconi (-Debré) E72.Ø9
    - with cystinosis E72.Ø4
  - de Vivo syndrome E74.81Ø
  - defibrination — *see also* Fibrinolysis
    - with
      - antepartum hemorrhage — *see* Hemorrhage, antepartum, with coagulation defect
      - intrapartum hemorrhage — *see* Hemorrhage, complicating, delivery
    - newborn P6Ø
    - postpartum O72.3
  - Degos' I77.89
  - Déjérine-Roussy G89.Ø
  - delayed sleep phase G47.21
  - demyelinating G37.9
  - dependence — *see* F1Ø-F19 with fourth character .2
  - depersonalization (-derealization) F48.1
  - di George's D82.1
  - diabetes mellitus in newborn infant P7Ø.2
  - diabetes mellitus-hypertension-nephrosis — *see* Diabetes, nephrosis
  - diabetes-nephrosis — *see* Diabetes, nephrosis
  - diabetic amyotrophy — *see* Diabetes, amyotrophy
  - dialysis associated steal T82.898- ☑
  - Diamond-Blackfan D61.Ø1
  - Diamond-Gardener D69.2
  - DIC (diffuse or disseminated intravascular coagulopathy) D65
  - Dighton's Q78.Ø
  - disequilibrium E87.8
  - Döhle body-panmyelopathic D72.Ø
  - dorsolateral medullary G46.4
  - double athetosis G8Ø.3
  - Down — *see also* Down syndrome Q9Ø.9
  - Dravet (intractable) G4Ø.834

- **Syndrome** — *continued*
  - Dravet — *continued*
    - with status epilepticus G4Ø.833
    - without status epilepticus G4Ø.834
  - Dresbach's (elliptocytosis) D58.1
  - DRESS (drug rash with eosinophilia and systemic symptoms) D72.12
  - Dressler's (postmyocardial infarction) I24.1
    - postcardiotomy I97.Ø
  - drug rash with eosinophilia and systemic symptoms (DRESS) D72.12
  - drug withdrawal, infant of dependent mother P96.1
  - dry eye HØ4.12- ☑
  - due to abnormality
    - chromosomal Q99.9
      - sex
        - female phenotype Q97.9
        - male phenotype Q98.9
      - specified NEC Q99.8
  - dumping (postgastrectomy) K91.1
    - nonsurgical K31.89
  - Dupré's (meningism) R29.1
  - dysmetabolic X E88.81
  - dyspraxia, developmental F82
  - Eagle-Barrett Q79.4
  - Eaton-Lambert — *see* Syndrome, Lambert-Eaton
  - Ebstein's Q22.5
  - ectopic ACTH E24.3
  - eczema-thrombocytopenia D82.Ø
  - Eddowes' Q78.Ø
  - effort (psychogenic) F45.8
  - Ehlers-Danlos Q79.6Ø
    - classical (cEDS) (classical EDS) Q79.61
    - hypermobile (hEDS) (hypermobile EDS) Q79.62
    - specified NEC Q79.69
    - vascular (vascular EDS) (vEDS) Q79.63
  - Eisenmenger's I27.83
  - Ekman's Q78.Ø
  - electric feet E53.8
  - Ellis-van Creveld Q77.6
  - empty nest Z6Ø.Ø
  - endocrine-hypertensive E27.Ø
  - entrapment — *see* Neuropathy, entrapment
  - eosinophilia-myalgia M35.89
  - epileptic — *see also* Epilepsy, by type
    - absence G4Ø.AØ9 (*following* G4Ø.3)
      - intractable G4Ø.A19 (*following* G4Ø.3)
        - with status epilepticus G4Ø.A11 (*following* G4Ø.3)
        - without status epilepticus G4Ø.A19 (*following* G4Ø.3)
      - not intractable G4Ø.AØ9 (*following* G4Ø.3)
        - with status epilepticus G4Ø.AØ1 (*following* G4Ø.3)
        - without status epilepticus G4Ø.AØ9 (*following* G4Ø.3)
  - Erdheim-Chester (ECD) E88.89
  - Erdheim's E22.Ø
  - erythrocyte fragmentation D59.4
  - Evans D69.41
  - exhaustion F48.8
  - extrapyramidal G25.9
    - specified NEC G25.89
  - eye retraction — *see* Strabismus
  - eyelid-malar-mandible Q87.Ø
  - Faber's D5Ø.9
  - facet M47.89- ☑
  - facet joint — *see also* Spondylosis M47.819
  - facial pain, paroxysmal G5Ø.Ø
  - Fallot's Q21.3
  - familial cold autoinflammatory MØ4.2
  - familial eczema-thrombocytopenia (Wiskott-Aldrich) D82.Ø
  - Fanconi (-de Toni) (-Debré) E72.Ø9
    - with cystinosis E72.Ø4
  - Fanconi's (anemia) (congenital pancytopenia) D61.Ø9
  - fatigue
    - chronic G93.32
    - postviral G93.31
    - psychogenic F48.8
  - faulty bowel habit K59.39
  - Feil-Klippel (brevicollis) Q76.1
  - Felty's — *see* Felty's syndrome
  - fertile eunuch E23.Ø
  - fetal
    - alcohol (dysmorphic) Q86.Ø
    - hydantoin Q86.1
  - Fiedler's I4Ø.1

- **Syndrome** — *continued*
  - first arch Q87.Ø
  - fish odor E72.89
  - Fisher's G61.Ø
  - Fitzhugh-Curtis
    - due to
      - Chlamydia trachomatis A74.81
      - Neisseria gonorrhorea (gonococcal peritonitis) A54.85
  - Fitz's — *see also* Pancreatitis, acute K85.8Ø
  - Flajani (-Basedow) EØ5.ØØ
    - with thyroid storm EØ5.Ø1
  - flatback — *see* Flatback syndrome
  - floppy
    - baby P94.2
    - iris (intraoeprative) (IFIS) H21.81
    - mitral valve I34.1
  - flush E34.Ø
  - Foix-Alajouanine G95.19
  - Fong's Q87.2
  - food protein-induced enterocolitis (FPIES) K52.21
  - foramen magnum G93.5
  - Foster-Kennedy H47.14- ☑
  - Foville's (peduncular) G46.3
  - fragile X Q99.2
  - Franceschetti Q75.4
  - Frey's
    - auriculotemporal G5Ø.8
    - hyperhidrosis L74.52
  - Friderichsen-Waterhouse A39.1
  - Froin's G95.89
  - frontal lobe FØ7.Ø
  - Fukuhara E88.49
  - functional
    - bowel K59.9
    - prepubertal castrate E29.1
  - Gaisböck's D75.1
  - ganglion (basal ganglia brain) G25.9
    - geniculi G51.1
  - Gardner-Diamond D69.2
  - gastroesophageal
    - junction K22.Ø
    - laceration-hemorrhage K22.6
  - gastrojejunal loop obstruction K91.89
  - Gee-Herter-Heubner K9Ø.Ø
  - Gelineau's G47.419
    - with cataplexy G47.411
  - genito-anorectal A55
  - Gerstmann-Sträussler-Scheinker (GSS) A81.82
  - Gianotti-Crosti L44.4
  - giant platelet (Bernard-Soulier) D69.1
  - Gilles de la Tourette's F95.2
  - Glass Q87.89
  - Gleich's D72.118
  - goiter-deafness EØ7.1
  - Goldberg Q89.8
  - Goldberg-Maxwell E34.51
  - Good's D83.8
  - Gopalan' (burning feet) E53.8
  - Gorlin's Q87.89
  - Gougerot-Blum L81.7
  - Gouley's I31.1
  - Gower's R55
  - gray or grey (newborn) P93.Ø
    - platelet D69.1
  - Gubler-Millard G46.3
  - Guillain-Barré (-Strohl) G61.Ø
  - gustatory sweating G5Ø.8
  - Hadfield-Clarke K86.89
  - hair tourniquet — *see* Constriction, external, by site
  - Hamman's J98.19
  - hand-foot L27.1
  - hand-shoulder G9Ø.8
  - hantavirus (cardio)-pulmonary (HPS) (HCPS) B33.4
  - happy puppet Q93.51
  - Harada's H3Ø.81- ☑
  - Hayem-Faber D5Ø.9
  - headache NEC G44.89
    - complicated NEC G44.59
  - Heberden's I2Ø.8
  - Hedinger's E34.Ø
  - Hegglin's D72.Ø
  - HELLP (hemolysis, elevated liver enzymes and low platelet count) O14.2- ☑
    - complicating
      - childbirth O14.24
      - puerperium O14.25
  - hemolytic-uremic D59.3Ø
    - atypical D59.39

- **Syndrome** — *continued*
  - hemolytic-uremic — *continued*
    - atypical — *continued*
      - genetic D59.32
      - hereditary D59.32
      - infection-associated D59.31
      - secondary D59.39
      - specified NEC D59.39
    - due to genetic disorder D59.32
    - familial D59.32
    - hereditary D59.32
    - infection-associated D59.31
    - secondary D59.39
    - Shiga toxin-producing E. coli [STEC] related D59.31
    - specified NEC D59.39
    - typical D59.31
  - hemophagocytic, infection-associated D76.2
  - Henoch-Schönlein D69.Ø
  - hepatic flexure K59.89
  - hepatopulmonary K76.81
  - hepatorenal K76.7
    - following delivery O9Ø.4
    - postoperative or postprocedural K91.83
    - postpartum, puerperal O9Ø.4
  - hepatourologic K76.7
  - hereditary alpha tryptasemia D89.44
  - Herter (-Gee) (nontropical sprue) K9Ø.Ø
  - Heubner-Herter K9Ø.Ø
  - Heyd's K76.7
  - Hilger's G9Ø.Ø9
  - histamine-like (fish poisoning) — *see* Poisoning, fish
  - histiocytic D76.3
  - histiocytosis NEC D76.3
  - HIV infection, acute B2Ø
  - Hoffmann-Werdnig G12.Ø
  - Hollander-Simons E88.1
  - Hoppe-Goldflam G7Ø.ØØ
    - with exacerbation (acute) G7Ø.Ø1
    - in crisis G7Ø.Ø1
  - Horner's G9Ø.2
  - hungry bone E83.81
  - hunterian glossitis D51.Ø
  - Hutchinson's triad A5Ø.53
  - hyperabduction G54.Ø
  - hyperammonemia-hyperornithinemia-homocitrullinemia E72.4
  - hypereosinophilic (HES) D72.119
    - idiopathic (IHES) D72.11Ø
    - lymphocytic variant (LHES) D72.111
    - myeloid D72.118
    - specified NEC D72.118
  - hyperimmunoglobulin D MØ4.1
  - hyperimmunoglobulin E (IgE) D82.4
  - hyperkalemic E87.5
  - hyperkinetic — *see* Hyperkinesia
  - hypermobility M35.7
  - hypernatremia E87.Ø
  - hyperosmolarity E87.Ø
  - hyperperfusion G97.82
  - hypersplenic D73.1
  - hypertransfusion, newborn P61.1
  - hyperventilation F45.8
  - hyperviscosity (of serum)
    - polycythemic D75.1
    - sclerothymic D58.8
  - hypoglycemic (familial) (neonatal) E16.2
  - hypokalemic E87.6
  - hyponatremic E87.1
  - hypopituitarism E23.Ø
  - hypoplastic left-heart Q23.4
  - hypopotassemia E87.6
  - hyposmolality E87.1
  - hypotension, maternal O26.5- ☑
  - hypothenar hammer I73.89
  - hypoventilation, obesity (OHS) E66.2
  - ICF (intravascular coagulation-fibrinolysis) D65
  - idiopathic
    - cardiorespiratory distress, newborn P22.Ø
    - nephrotic (infantile) NØ4.9
  - iliotibial band M76.3- ☑
  - immobility, immobilization (paraplegic) M62.3
  - immune effector cell-associated neurotoxicity (ICANS) G92.ØØ
    - grade
      - 1 G92.Ø1
      - 2 G92.Ø2
      - 3 G92.Ø3
      - 4 G92.Ø4
      - 5 G92.Ø5

- **Syndrome** — *continued*
  - immune effector cell-associated neurotoxicity — *continued*
    - grade — *continued*
      - unspecified G92.ØØ
  - immune reconstitution D89.3
  - immune reconstitution inflammatory [IRIS] D89.3
  - immunity deficiency, combined D81.9
  - immunodeficiency
    - acquired — *see* Human, immunodeficiency virus (HIV) disease
    - combined D81.9
  - impending coronary I2Ø.Ø
  - impingement, shoulder M75.4- ☑
  - inappropriate secretion of antidiuretic hormone E22.2
  - infant
    - gestational diabetes P7Ø.Ø
    - of diabetic mother P7Ø.1
  - infantilism (pituitary) E23.Ø
  - inferior vena cava I87.1
  - inspissated bile (newborn) P59.1
  - institutional (childhood) F94.2
  - insufficient sleep F51.12
  - intermediate coronary (artery) I2Ø.Ø
  - interspinous ligament — *see* Spondylopathy, specified NEC
  - intestinal
    - carcinoid E34.Ø
    - knot K56.2
  - intravascular coagulation-fibrinolysis (ICF) D65
  - iodine-deficiency, congenital EØØ.9
    - type
      - mixed EØØ.2
      - myxedematous EØØ.1
      - neurological EØØ.Ø
  - IRDS (idiopathic respiratory distress, newborn) P22.Ø
  - irritable
    - bowel K58.9
      - with
        - constipation K58.1
        - diarrhea K58.Ø
      - mixed K58.2
      - psychogenic F45.8
      - specified NEC K58.8
    - heart (psychogenic) F45.8
    - weakness F48.8
  - ischemic
    - bowel (transient) K55.9
      - chronic K55.1
      - due to mesenteric artery insufficiency K55.1
    - steal T82.898 ☑
  - IVC (intravascular coagulopathy) D65
  - Ivemark's Q89.Ø1
  - Jaccoud's — *see* Arthropathy, postrheumatic, chronic
  - Jackson's G83.89
  - Jakob-Creutzfeldt — *see* Creutzfeldt-Jakob disease or syndrome
  - jaw-winking QØ7.8
  - Jervell-Lange-Nielsen I45.81
  - jet lag G47.25
  - Job's D71
  - Joseph-Diamond-Blackfan D61.Ø1
  - jugular foramen G52.7
  - Kabuki Q89.8
  - Kanner's (autism) F84.Ø
  - Kartagener's Q89.3
  - Kelly's D5Ø.1
  - Kimmelstiel-Wilson — *see* Diabetes, specified type, with Kimmelstiel-Wilson disease
  - Klein (e)-Levine G47.13
  - Klippel-Feil (brevicollis) Q76.1
  - Köhler-Pellegrini-Steida — *see* Bursitis, tibial collateral
  - König's K59.89
  - Korsakoff (-Wernicke) (nonalcoholic) FØ4
    - alcoholic F1Ø.26
  - Kostmann's D7Ø.Ø
  - Krabbe's congenital muscle hypoplasia Q79.8
  - labyrinthine — *see* subcategory H83.2 ☑
  - lacunar NEC G46.7
  - Lambert-Eaton G7Ø.8Ø
    - in
      - neoplastic disease G73.1
      - specified disease NEC G7Ø.81
  - Landau-Kleffner — *see* Epilepsy, specified NEC
  - Larsen's Q74.8
  - lateral
    - cutaneous nerve of thigh G57.1- ☑
    - medullary G46.4
  - Launois' E22.Ø
  - lazy
    - leukocyte D7Ø.8
    - posture M62.3
  - Lemiere I8Ø.8
  - Lennox-Gastaut G4Ø.812
    - intractable G4Ø.814
      - with status epilepticus G4Ø.813
      - without status epilepticus G4Ø.814
    - not intractable G4Ø.812
      - with status epilepticus G4Ø.811
      - without status epilepticus G4Ø.812
  - lenticular, progressive E83.Ø1
  - Leopold-Levi's EØ5.9Ø
  - Lev's I44.2
  - Lichtheim's D51.Ø
  - Li-Fraumeni Z15.Ø1
  - Lightwood's N25.89
  - Lignac (de Toni) (-Fanconi) (-Debré) E72.Ø9
    - with cystinosis E72.Ø4
  - Likoff's I2Ø.8
  - limbic epilepsy personality FØ7.Ø
  - liver-kidney K76.7
  - lobotomy FØ7.Ø
  - Löffler's J82.89
  - long arm 18 or 21 deletion Q93.89
  - long QT I45.81
  - Louis-Barré G11.3
  - low
    - atmospheric pressure T7Ø.29 ☑
    - back M54.5Ø
    - output (cardiac) I5Ø.9
  - lower radicular, newborn (birth injury) P14.8
  - Luetscher's (dehydration) E86.Ø
  - Lupus anticoagulant D68.62
  - Lutembacher's Q21.19
  - macrophage activation D76.1
    - due to infection D76.2
  - magnesium-deficiency R29.Ø
  - Majeed MØ4.8
  - Mal de Debarquement R42
  - malabsorption K9Ø.9
    - postsurgical K91.2
  - malformation, congenital, due to
    - alcohol Q86.Ø
    - exogenous cause NEC Q86.8
    - hydantoin Q86.1
    - warfarin Q86.2
  - malignant
    - carcinoid E34.Ø
    - neuroleptic G21.Ø
  - Mallory-Weiss K22.6
  - mandibulofacial dysostosis Q75.4
  - manic-depressive — *see* Disorder, bipolar
  - maple-syrup-urine E71.Ø
  - Marable's I77.4
  - Marfan's Q87.4Ø
    - with
      - cardiovascular manifestations Q87.418
        - aortic dilation Q87.41Ø
      - ocular manifestations Q87.42
      - skeletal manifestations Q87.43
  - Marie's (acromegaly) E22.Ø
  - mast cell activation — *see* Activation, mast cell
  - maternal hypotension — *see* Syndrome, hypotension, maternal
  - May (-Hegglin) D72.Ø
  - McArdle (-Schmidt) (-Pearson) E74.Ø4
  - McQuarrie's E16.2
  - meconium plug (newborn) P76.Ø
  - median arcuate ligament I77.4
  - Meekeren-Ehlers-Danlos Q79.6 ☑
  - megavitamin-B6 E67.2
  - Meige G24.4
  - MELAS E88.41
  - Mendelson's O74.Ø
  - MERRF (myoclonic epilepsy associated with ragged-red fibers) E88.42
  - mesenteric
    - artery (superior) K55.1
    - vascular insufficiency K55.1
  - metabolic E88.81
  - metastatic carcinoid E34.Ø
  - micrognathia-glossoptosis Q87.Ø
  - midbrain NEC G93.89
  - middle lobe (lung) J98.19
  - middle radicular G54.Ø
  - migraine — *see also* Migraine G43.9Ø9
  - Mikulicz' K11.8
  - milk-alkali E83.52
  - Millard-Gubler G46.3
  - Miller-Dieker Q93.88
  - Miller-Fisher G61.Ø
  - Minkowski-Chauffard D58.Ø
  - Mirizzi's K83.1
  - MNGIE (Mitochondrial Neurogastrointestinal Encephalopathy) E88.49
  - Möbius, ophthalmoplegic migraine — *see* Migraine, ophthalmoplegic
  - monofixation H5Ø.42
  - Morel-Moore M85.2
  - Morel-Morgagni M85.2
  - Morgagni (-Morel) (-Stewart) M85.2
  - Morgagni-Adams-Stokes I45.9
  - Mounier-Kuhn Q32.4
    - with bronchiectasis J47.9
      - with
        - exacerbation (acute) J47.1
        - lower respiratory infection J47.Ø
    - acquired J98.Ø9
      - with bronchiectasis J47.9
        - with
          - exacerbation (acute) J47.1
          - lower respiratory infection J47.Ø
  - Muckle-Wells MØ4.2
  - mucocutaneous lymph node (acute febrile) (MCLS) M3Ø.3
  - multiple endocrine neoplasia (MEN) — *see* Neoplasia, endocrine, multiple (MEN)
  - multiple operations — *see* Disorder, factitious
  - multisystem inflammatory (in adults) (in children) M35.81
  - myasthenic G7Ø.9
    - in
      - diabetes mellitus — *see* Diabetes, amyotrophy
      - endocrine disease NEC E34.9 *[G73.3]*
      - neoplastic disease — *see also* Neoplasm D49.9 *[G73.3]*
      - thyrotoxicosis (hyperthyroidism) EØ5.9Ø *[G73.3]*
        - with thyroid storm EØ5.91 *[G73.3]*
  - myelodysplastic D46.9
    - with
      - 5q deletion D46.C (*following* D46.2)
      - isolated del (5q) chromosomal abnormality D46.C (*following* D46.2)
      - multilineage dysplasia D46.A (*following* D46.2)
        - with ringed sideroblasts D46.B (*following* D46.2)
    - lesions, low grade D46.2Ø
    - specified NEC D46.Z (*following* D46.4)
  - myeloid hypereosinophilic D72.118
  - myelopathic pain G89.Ø
  - myeloproliferative (chronic) D47.1
  - myofascial pain M79.18
  - Naffziger's G54.Ø
  - nail patella Q87.2
  - NARP (Neuropathy, Ataxia and Retinitis pigmentosa) E88.49
  - neonatal abstinence P96.1
  - nephritic — *see also* Nephritis
    - with edema — *see* Nephrosis
    - acute NØØ.9
    - chronic NØ3.9
    - rapidly progressive NØ1.9
  - nephrotic (congenital) — *see also* Nephrosis NØ4.9
    - with
      - C3
        - glomerulonephritis NØ4.A
        - glomerulopathy NØ4.A
          - with dense deposit disease NØ4.6
      - dense deposit disease NØ4.6
      - diffuse
        - crescentic glomerulonephritis NØ4.7
        - endocapillary proliferative glomerulonephritis NØ4.4
        - membranous glomerulonephritis NØ4.2
        - mesangial proliferative glomerulonephritis NØ4.3
        - mesangiocapillary glomerulonephritis NØ4.5
      - focal and segmental glomerular lesions NØ4.1
      - minor glomerular abnormality NØ4.Ø
      - specified morphological changes NEC NØ4.8
    - diabetic — *see* Diabetes, nephrosis
  - neurologic neglect R41.4
  - Nezelof's D81.4

- **Syndrome** — *continued*
  - Nonne-Milroy-Meige Q82.Ø
  - Nothnagel's vasomotor acroparesthesia I73.89
  - obesity hypoventilation (OHS) E66.2
  - oculomotor H51.9
  - Ogilvie K59.81
  - ophthalmoplegia-cerebellar ataxia — *see* Strabismus, paralytic, third nerve
  - oral allergy T78.1 ☑
  - oral-facial-digital Q87.Ø
  - organic
    - affective FØ6.3Ø
    - amnesic (not alcohol- or drug-induced) FØ4
    - brain FØ9
    - depressive FØ6.31
    - hallucinosis FØ6.Ø
    - personality FØ7.Ø
  - Ormond's N13.5
  - oro-facial-digital Q87.Ø
  - os trigonum Q68.8
  - Osler-Weber-Rendu I78.Ø
  - osteoporosis-osteomalacia M83.8
  - Osterreicher-Turner Q87.2
  - otolith — *see* subcategory H81.8 ☑
  - oto-palatal-digital Q87.Ø
  - outlet (thoracic) G54.Ø
  - ovary
    - polycystic E28.2
    - resistant E28.39
    - sclerocystic E28.2
  - Owren's D68.2
  - Paget-Schroetter I82.89Ø
  - pain — *see also* Pain
    - complex regional I G9Ø.5Ø
      - lower limb G9Ø.52- ☑
      - specified site NEC G9Ø.59
      - upper limb G9Ø.51- ☑
    - complex regional II — *see* Causalgia
  - painful
    - bruising D69.2
    - feet E53.8
    - prostate N42.81
  - paralysis agitans — *see* Parkinsonism
  - paralytic G83.9
    - specified NEC G83.89
  - Parinaud's H51.Ø
  - parkinsonian — *see* Parkinsonism
  - Parkinson's — *see* Parkinsonism
  - paroxysmal facial pain G5Ø.Ø
  - Parry's EØ5.ØØ
    - with thyroid storm EØ5.Ø1
  - Parsonage (-Aldren)-Turner G54.5
  - patella clunk M25.86- ☑
  - Paterson (-Brown) (-Kelly) D5Ø.1
  - pectoral girdle I77.89
  - pectoralis minor I77.89
  - pediatric autoimmune neuropsychiatric disorders associated with streptococcal infections (PANDAS) D89.89
  - pediatric inflammatory multisystem M35.81
  - Pelger Huet D72.Ø
  - pellagra-cerebellar ataxia-renal aminoaciduria E72.Ø2
  - pellagroid E52
  - Pellegrini-Stieda — *see* Bursitis, tibial collateral
  - pelvic congestion-fibrosis, female N94.89
  - penta X Q97.1
  - peptic ulcer — *see* Ulcer, peptic
  - perabduction I77.89
  - periodic fever MØ4.1
  - periodic fever, aphthous stomatitis, pharyngitis, and adenopathy [PFAPA] MØ4.8
  - periodic headache, in adults and children — *see* Headache, periodic syndromes in adults and children
  - periurethral fibrosis N13.5
  - Peutz-Jeghers Q85.89
  - phantom limb (without pain) G54.7
    - with pain G54.6
  - pharyngeal pouch D82.1
  - Pick's — *see* Disease, Pick's
  - Pickwickian E66.2
  - PIE (pulmonary infiltration with eosinophilia) — *see also* Eosinophilia, pulmonary J82.89
  - pigmentary pallidal degeneration (progressive) G23.Ø
  - pineal E34.8
  - pituitary E22.Ø
  - placental transfusion — *see* Pregnancy, complicated by, placental transfusion syndromes

- **Syndrome** — *continued*
  - plantar fascia M72.2
  - plateau iris (post-iridectomy) (postprocedural) H21.82
  - Plummer-Vinson D5Ø.1
  - pluricarential of infancy E4Ø
  - plurideficiency E4Ø
  - pluriglandular (compensatory) E31.8
    - autoimmune E31.Ø
  - pneumatic hammer T75.21 ☑
  - polyangiitis overlap M3Ø.8
  - polycarential of infancy E4Ø
  - polyglandular E31.8
    - autoimmune E31.Ø
  - polysplenia Q89.Ø9
  - pontine NEC G93.89
  - popliteal
    - artery entrapment I77.89
    - web Q87.89
  - post chemoembolization — *code to* associated conditions
  - post endometrial ablation N99.85
  - postbacterial fatigue G93.39
  - postcardiac injury
    - postcardiotomy I97.Ø
    - postmyocardial infarction I24.1
  - postcardiotomy I97.Ø
  - postcholecystectomy K91.5
  - postcommissurotomy I97.Ø
  - postconcussional FØ7.81
  - postcontusional FØ7.81
  - post-COVID (-19) UØ9.9
  - postencephalitic FØ7.89
  - posterior
    - cervical sympathetic M53.Ø
    - cord G83.83
    - fossa compression G93.5
    - reversible encephalopathy (PRES) I67.83
  - postgastrectomy (dumping) K91.1
  - postgastric surgery K91.1
  - postinfarction I24.1
  - postinfectious fatigue G93.39
  - postlaminectomy NEC M96.1
  - postleukotomy FØ7.Ø
  - postmastectomy lymphedema I97.2
  - postmyocardial infarction I24.1
  - postoperative NEC T81.9 ☑
    - blind loop K9Ø.2
  - postpartum panhypopituitary (Sheehan) E23.Ø
  - postpolio (myelitic) G14
  - postthrombotic I87.ØØ9
    - with
      - inflammation I87.Ø2- ☑
        - with ulcer I87.Ø3- ☑
      - specified complication NEC I87.Ø9- ☑
      - ulcer I87.Ø1- ☑
        - with inflammation I87.Ø3- ☑
    - asymptomatic I87.ØØ- ☑
  - postural
    - orthostatic tachycardia [POTS] G9Ø.A
    - tachycardia G9Ø.A
  - postvagotomy K91.1
  - postvalvulotomy I97.Ø
  - postviral NEC G93.31
    - fatigue G93.31
  - Potain's K31.Ø
  - potassium intoxication E87.5
  - Prader-Willi Q87.11
  - Prader-Willi-like Q87.19
  - precerebral artery (multiple) (bilateral) G45.2
  - preinfarction I2Ø.Ø
  - preleukemic D46.9
  - premature senility E34.8
  - premenstrual dysphoric F32.81
  - premenstrual tension N94.3
  - Prinzmetal-Massumi RØ7.1
  - prune belly Q79.4
  - pseudo -Turner's Q87.19
  - pseudocarpal tunnel (sublimis) — *see* Syndrome, carpal tunnel
  - pseudoparalytica G7Ø.ØØ
    - with exacerbation (acute) G7Ø.Ø1
    - in crisis G7Ø.Ø1
  - psycho-organic (nonpsychotic severity) FØ7.9
    - acute or subacute FØ5
    - depressive type FØ6.31
    - hallucinatory type FØ6.Ø
    - nonpsychotic severity FØ7.Ø
    - specified NEC FØ7.89

- **Syndrome** — *continued*
  - PTEN (hamartoma) tumor Q85.81
  - pulmonary
    - arteriosclerosis I27.Ø
    - dysmaturity (Wilson-Mikity) P27.Ø
    - hypoperfusion (idiopathic) P22.Ø
    - renal (hemorrhagic) (Goodpasture's) M31.Ø
  - pure
    - motor lacunar G46.5
    - sensory lacunar G46.6
  - Putnam-Dana D51.Ø
  - pyogenic arthritis, pyoderma gangrenosum, and acne [PAPA] MØ4.8
  - pyramidopallidonigral G2Ø
  - pyriformis — *see* Lesion, nerve, sciatic
  - QT interval prolongation I45.81
  - radicular NEC — *see* Radiculopathy
    - upper limbs, newborn (birth injury) P14.3
  - rapid time-zone change G47.25
  - Rasmussen GØ4.81
  - Raymond (-Céstan) I65.8
  - Raynaud's I73.ØØ
    - with gangrene I73.Ø1
  - RDS (respiratory distress syndrome, newborn) P22.Ø
  - reactive airways dysfunction J68.3
  - Refsum's G6Ø.1
  - Reifenstein E34.52
  - renal glomerulohyalinosis-diabetic — *see* Diabetes, nephrosis
  - Rendu-Osler-Weber I78.Ø
  - residual ovary N99.83
  - resistant ovary E28.39
  - respiratory
    - distress
      - acute J8Ø
        - adult J8Ø
        - child J8Ø
        - idiopathic J84.114
      - newborn (idiopathic) (type I) P22.Ø
        - type II P22.1
  - restless legs G25.81
  - retinoblastoma (familial) C69.2 ☑
  - retroperitoneal fibrosis N13.5
  - retroviral seroconversion (acute) Z21
  - Reye's G93.7
  - Richter — *see* Leukemia, chronic lymphocytic, B-cell type
  - Ridley's I5Ø.1
  - right
    - heart, hypoplastic Q22.6
    - ventricular obstruction — *see* Failure, heart, right
  - Romano-Ward (prolonged QT interval) I45.81
  - rotator cuff, shoulder — *see also* Tear, rotator cuff M75.1Ø- ☑
  - Rotes Quérol — *see* Hyperostosis, ankylosing
  - Roth — *see* Meralgia paresthetica
  - rubella (congenital) P35.Ø
  - Ruvalcaba-Myhre-Smith E71.44Ø
  - Rytand-Lipsitch I44.2
  - salt
    - depletion E87.1
      - due to heat NEC T67.8 ☑
        - causing heat exhaustion or prostration T67.4 ☑
    - low E87.1
  - salt-losing N28.89
  - SATB2-associated Q87.89
  - Scaglietti-Dagnini E22.Ø
  - scalenus anticus (anterior) G54.Ø
  - scapulocostal — *see* Mononeuropathy, upper limb, specified site NEC
  - scapuloperoneal G71.Ø9
  - schizophrenic, of childhood NEC F84.5
  - Schnitzler D47.2
  - Scholte's E34.Ø
  - Schroeder's E27.Ø
  - Schüller-Christian C96.5
  - Schwachman's — *see* Syndrome, Shwachman's
  - Schwartz (-Jampel) G71.13
  - Schwartz-Bartter E22.2
  - scimitar Q26.8
  - sclerocystic ovary E28.2
  - Seitelberger's G31.89
  - septicemic adrenal hemorrhage A39.1
  - seroconversion, retroviral (acute) Z21
  - serous meningitis G93.2
  - severe acute respiratory (SARS) J12.81
    - coronavirus 2 (*see also* COVID-19) UØ7.1

- **Syndrome** — *continued*
  - severe acute respiratory — *continued*
    - coronavirus 2 (*see also* COVID-19) — *continued*
      - pneumonia J12.82
  - shaken infant T74.4 ☑
  - shock (traumatic) T79.4 ☑
    - kidney N17.Ø
      - following crush injury T79.5 ☑
    - toxic A48.3
  - shock-lung J8Ø
  - Shone's — *code to* specific anomalies
  - short
    - bowel K91.2
    - rib Q77.2
  - shoulder-hand — *see* Algoneurodystrophy
  - Shwachman's D7Ø.4
  - sicca — *see* Syndrome, Sjögren
  - sick
    - cell E87.1
    - sinus I49.5
  - sick-euthyroid EØ7.81
  - sideropenic D5Ø.1
  - Siemens' ectodermal dysplasia Q82.4
  - Silfverskiöld's Q78.9
  - Simons' E88.1
  - sinus tarsi M25.57- ☑
  - sinusitis-bronchiectasis-situs inversus Q89.3
  - Sipple's E31.22
  - sirenomelia Q87.2
  - Sjögren M35.ØØ
    - with
      - central nervous system involvement M35.Ø7
      - dental involvement M35.ØC
      - gastrointestinal involvement M35.Ø8
      - glomerular disease M35.ØA
      - inflammatory arthritis M35.Ø5
      - keratoconjunctivitis M35.Ø1
      - lung involvement M35.Ø2
      - myopathy M35.Ø3
      - peripheral nervous system involvement M35.Ø6
      - renal tubular acidosis M35.Ø4
      - specified organ involvement, NEC M35.Ø9
      - tubulo-interstitial nephropathy M35.Ø4
      - vasculitis M35.ØB
  - Slocumb's E27.Ø
  - slow flow, coronary I2Ø.8
  - Sluder's G44.89
  - Smith-Magenis Q93.88
  - Sneddon-Wilkinson L13.1
  - Sotos' Q87.3
  - South African cardiomyopathy I42.8
  - spasmodic
    - upward movement, eyes H51.8
    - winking F95.8
  - Spen's I45.9
  - splenic
    - agenesis Q89.Ø1
    - flexure K59.89
    - neutropenia D73.81
  - Spurway's Q78.Ø
  - staphylococcal scalded skin LØØ
  - steal
    - arteriovenous T82.898- ☑
    - ischemic T82.898- ☑
    - subclavian G45.8
  - Stein-Leventhal E28.2
  - Stein's E28.2
  - Stevens-Johnson syndrome L51.1
    - toxic epidermal necrolysis overlap L51.3
  - Stewart-Morel M85.2
  - Stickler Q89.8
  - stiff baby Q89.8
  - stiff man G25.82
  - Still-Felty — *see* Felty's syndrome
  - Stokes (-Adams) I45.9
  - stone heart I5Ø.1
  - straight back, congenital Q76.49
  - Sturge-Weber (-Dimitri) Q85.89
  - subclavian steal G45.8
  - subcoracoid-pectoralis minor G54.Ø
  - subcostal nerve compression I77.89
  - subphrenic interposition Q43.3
  - superior
    - cerebellar artery I63.89
    - mesenteric artery K55.1
    - semi-circular canal dehiscence H83.8X- ☑
    - vena cava I87.1
- **Syndrome** — *continued*
  - supine hypotensive (maternal) — *see* Syndrome, hypotension, maternal
  - suprarenal cortical E27.Ø
  - supraspinatus — *see also* Tear, rotator cuff M75.1Ø- ☑
  - Susac G93.49
  - swallowed blood P78.2
  - sweat retention L74.Ø
  - Swyer Q99.1
  - Symond's G93.2
  - sympathetic
    - cervical paralysis G9Ø.2
    - pelvic, female N94.89
  - systemic inflammatory response (SIRS), of non-infectious origin (without organ dysfunction) R65.1Ø
    - with acute organ dysfunction R65.11
  - tachycardia-bradycardia I49.5
  - takotsubo I51.81
  - TAR (thrombocytopenia with absent radius) Q87.2
  - tarsal tunnel G57.5- ☑
  - teething KØØ.7
  - tegmental G93.89
  - telangiectasic-pigmentation-cataract Q82.8
  - temporal pyramidal apex — *see* Otitis, media, suppurative, acute
  - temporomandibular joint-pain-dysfunction M26.62- ☑
  - Terry's — *see also* Myopia, degenerative H44.2- ☑
  - testicular feminization — *see also* Syndrome, androgen insensitivity E34.51
  - thalamic pain (hyperesthetic) G89.Ø
  - thoracic outlet (compression) G54.Ø
  - Thorson-Björck E34.Ø
  - thrombocytopenia with absent radius (TAR) Q87.2
  - thrombosis with thrombocytopenia D75.84
  - thyroid-adrenocortical insufficiency E31.Ø
  - tibial
    - anterior M76.81- ☑
    - posterior M76.82- ☑
  - Tietze's M94.Ø
  - time-zone (rapid) G47.25
  - Toni-Fanconi E72.Ø9
    - with cystinosis E72.Ø4
  - Touraine's Q79.8
  - tourniquet — *see* Constriction, external, by site
  - toxic shock A48.3
  - transient left ventricular apical ballooning I51.81
  - traumatic vasospastic T75.22 ☑
  - Treacher Collins Q75.4
  - triple X, female Q97.Ø
  - trisomy Q92.9
    - 13 Q91.7
      - meiotic nondisjunction Q91.4
      - mitotic nondisjunction Q91.5
      - mosaicism Q91.5
      - translocation Q91.6
    - 18 Q91.3
      - meiotic nondisjunction Q91.Ø
      - mitotic nondisjunction Q91.1
      - mosaicism Q91.1
      - translocation Q91.2
    - 2Ø (q)(p) Q92.8
    - 21 Q9Ø.9
      - meiotic nondisjunction Q9Ø.Ø
      - mitotic nondisjunction Q9Ø.1
      - mosaicism Q9Ø.1
      - translocation Q9Ø.2
    - 22 Q92.8
  - tropical wet feet T69.Ø- ☑
  - Trousseau's I82.1
  - tumor lysis (following antineoplastic chemotherapy) (spontaneous) NEC E88.3
  - tumor necrosis factor receptor associated periodic (TRAPS) MØ4.1
  - Twiddler's (due to)
    - automatic implantable defibrillator T82.198 ☑
    - cardiac pacemaker T82.198 ☑
  - Unverricht (-Lundborg) — *see* Epilepsy, generalized, idiopathic
  - upward gaze H51.8
  - uremia, chronic — *see also* Disease, kidney, chronic N18.9
  - urethral N34.3
  - urethro-oculo-articular — *see* Reiter's disease
  - urohepatic K76.7
  - vago-hypoglossal G52.7
  - van Buchem's M85.2
  - van der Hoeve's Q78.Ø
  - vascular NEC in cerebrovascular disease G46.8
- **Syndrome** — *continued*
  - vasoconstriction, reversible cerebrovascular I67.841
  - vasomotor I73.9
  - vasospastic (traumatic) T75.22 ☑
  - vasovagal R55
  - VATER Q87.2
  - velo-cardio-facial Q93.81
  - vena cava (inferior) (superior) (obstruction) I87.1
  - vertebral
    - artery G45.Ø
      - compression — *see* Syndrome, anterior, spinal artery, compression
    - steal G45.Ø
  - vertebro-basilar artery G45.Ø
  - vertebrogenic (pain) — *see also* Pain, vertebrogenic M54.89
  - vertiginous — *see* Disorder, vestibular function
  - Vinson-Plummer D5Ø.1
  - virus B34.9
  - visceral larva migrans B83.Ø
  - visual disorientation H53.8
  - vitamin B6 deficiency E53.1
  - vitreal corneal H59.Ø1- ☑
  - vitreous (touch) H59.Ø1- ☑
  - Vogt-Koyanagi H2Ø.82- ☑
  - Volkmann's T79.6 ☑
  - von Hippel-Lindau Q85.83
  - von Schroetter's I82.89Ø
  - von Willebrand (-Jürgen) — *see* Disease, von Willebrand
    - acquired — *see also* Disease, von Willebrand D68.Ø4
  - Waldenström-Kjellberg D5Ø.1
  - Wallenberg's G46.3
  - water retention E87.79
  - Waterhouse (-Friderichsen) A39.1
  - Weber-Gubler G46.3
  - Weber-Leyden G46.3
  - Weber's G46.3
  - Wegener's M31.3Ø
    - with
      - kidney involvement M31.31
      - lung involvement M31.3Ø
        - with kidney involvement M31.31
  - Weingarten's (tropical eosinophilia) J82.89
  - Weiss-Baker G9Ø.Ø9
  - Werdnig-Hoffman G12.Ø
  - Wermer's E31.21
  - Werner's E34.8
  - Wernicke-Korsakoff (nonalcoholic) FØ4
    - alcoholic F1Ø.26
  - Westphal-Strümpell E83.Ø1
  - West's — *see* Epilepsy, spasms
  - wet
    - feet (maceration) (tropical) T69.Ø- ☑
    - lung, newborn P22.1
  - whiplash S13.4 ☑
  - whistling face Q87.Ø
  - Wilkie's K55.1
  - Wilkinson-Sneddon L13.1
  - Willebrand (-Jürgens) — *see* Disease, von Willebrand
  - Williams Q93.82
  - Wilson's (hepatolenticular degeneration) E83.Ø1
  - Wiskott-Aldrich D82.Ø
  - withdrawal — *see* Withdrawal, state
    - drug
      - infant of dependent mother P96.1
      - therapeutic use, newborn P96.2
  - Woakes' (ethmoiditis) J33.1
  - Wright's (hyperabduction) G54.Ø
  - X I2Ø.9
  - XXXX Q97.1
  - XXXXX Q97.1
  - XXXXY Q98.1
  - XXY Q98.Ø
  - Yao MØ4.8
  - yellow nail L6Ø.5
  - Zahorsky's BØ8.5
  - Zellweger syndrome E71.51Ø
  - Zellweger-like syndrome E71.541
- **Synechia** (anterior) (iris) (posterior) (pupil) — *see also* Adhesions, iris
  - intra-uterine (traumatic) N85.6
- **Synesthesia** R2Ø.8
- **Syngamiasis, syngamosis** B83.3
- **Synodontia** KØØ.2
- **Synorchidism, synorchism** Q55.1
- **Synostosis** (congenital) Q78.8
  - astragalo-scaphoid Q74.2

Synostosis — *continued*
radioulnar Q74.0
Synovial sarcoma — *see* Neoplasm, connective tissue, malignant
Synovioma (malignant) — *see also* Neoplasm, connective tissue, malignant
benign — *see* Neoplasm, connective tissue, benign
Synoviosarcoma — *see* Neoplasm, connective tissue, malignant
Synovitis — *see also* Tenosynovitis M65.9
crepitant
hand M70.0- ☑
wrist M70.03- ☑
gonococcal A54.49
gouty — *see* Gout
in (due to)
crystals M65.8- ☑
gonorrhea A54.49
syphilis (late) A52.78
use, overuse, pressure — *see* Disorder, soft tissue, due to use
infective NEC — *see* Tenosynovitis, infective NEC
specified NEC — *see* Tenosynovitis, specified type NEC
syphilitic A52.78
congenital (early) A50.02
toxic — *see* Synovitis, transient
transient M67.3- ☑
ankle M67.37- ☑
elbow M67.32- ☑
foot joint M67.37- ☑
hand joint M67.34- ☑
hip M67.35- ☑
knee M67.36- ☑
multiple site M67.39
pelvic region M67.35- ☑
shoulder M67.31- ☑
specified joint NEC M67.38
wrist M67.33- ☑
traumatic, current — *see* Sprain
tuberculous — *see* Tuberculosis, synovitis
villonodular (pigmented) M12.2- ☑
ankle M12.27- ☑
elbow M12.22- ☑
foot joint M12.27- ☑
hand joint M12.24- ☑
hip M12.25- ☑
knee M12.26- ☑
multiple site M12.29
pelvic region M12.25- ☑
shoulder M12.21- ☑
specified joint NEC M12.28
vertebrae M12.28
wrist M12.23- ☑
Syphilid A51.39
congenital A50.06
newborn A50.06
tubercular (late) A52.79
Syphilis, syphilitic (acquired) A53.9
abdomen (late) A52.79
acoustic nerve A52.15
adenopathy (secondary) A51.49
adrenal (gland) (with cortical hypofunction) A52.79
age under 2 years NOS — *see also* Syphilis, congenital, early
acquired A51.9
alopecia (secondary) A51.32
anemia (late) A52.79 *[D63.8]*
aneurysm (aorta) (ruptured) A52.01
central nervous system A52.05
congenital A50.54 *[I79.0]*
anus (late) A52.74
primary A51.1
secondary A51.39
aorta (arch) (abdominal) (thoracic) A52.02
aneurysm A52.01
aortic (insufficiency) (regurgitation) (stenosis) A52.03
aneurysm A52.01
arachnoid (adhesive) (cerebral) (spinal) A52.13
asymptomatic — *see* Syphilis, latent
ataxia (locomotor) A52.11
atrophoderma maculatum A51.39
auricular fibrillation A52.06
bladder (late) A52.76
bone A52.77
secondary A51.46
brain A52.17
breast (late) A52.79

Syphilis, syphilitic — *continued*
bronchus (late) A52.72
bubo (primary) A51.0
bulbar palsy A52.19
bursa (late) A52.78
cardiac decompensation A52.06
cardiovascular A52.00
central nervous system (late) (recurrent) (relapse) (tertiary) A52.3
with
ataxia A52.11
general paralysis A52.17
juvenile A50.45
paresis (general) A52.17
juvenile A50.45
tabes (dorsalis) A52.11
juvenile A50.45
taboparesis A52.17
juvenile A50.45
aneurysm A52.05
congenital A50.40
juvenile A50.40
remission in (sustained) A52.3
serology doubtful, negative, or positive A52.3
specified nature or site NEC A52.19
vascular A52.05
cerebral A52.17
meningovascular A52.13
nerves (multiple palsies) A52.15
sclerosis A52.17
thrombosis A52.05
cerebrospinal (tabetic type) A52.12
cerebrovascular A52.05
cervix (late) A52.76
chancre (multiple) A51.0
extragenital A51.2
Rollet's A51.0
Charcot's joint A52.16
chorioretinitis A51.43
congenital A50.01
late A52.71
prenatal A50.01
choroiditis — *see* Syphilitic chorioretinitis
choroidoretinitis — *see* Syphilitic chorioretinitis
ciliary body (secondary) A51.43
late A52.71
colon (late) A52.74
combined spinal sclerosis A52.11
condyloma (latum) A51.31
congenital A50.9
with
paresis (general) A50.45
tabes (dorsalis) A50.45
taboparesis A50.45
chorioretinitis, choroiditis A50.01 *[H32]*
early, or less than 2 years after birth NEC A50.2
with manifestations — *see* Syphilis, congenital, early, symptomatic
latent (without manifestations) A50.1
negative spinal fluid test A50.1
serology positive A50.1
symptomatic A50.09
cutaneous A50.06
mucocutaneous A50.07
oculopathy A50.01
osteochondropathy A50.02
pharyngitis A50.03
pneumonia A50.04
rhinitis A50.05
visceral A50.08
interstitial keratitis A50.31
juvenile neurosyphilis A50.45
late, or 2 years or more after birth NEC A50.7
chorioretinitis, choroiditis A50.32
interstitial keratitis A50.31
juvenile neurosyphilis A50.45
latent (without manifestations) A50.6
negative spinal fluid test A50.6
serology positive A50.6
symptomatic or with manifestations NEC A50.59
arthropathy A50.55
cardiovascular A50.54
Clutton's joints A50.51
Hutchinson's teeth A50.52
Hutchinson's triad A50.53
osteochondropathy A50.56
saddle nose A50.57
conjugal A53.9
tabes A52.11

Syphilis, syphilitic — *continued*
conjunctiva (late) A52.71
contact Z20.2
cord bladder A52.19
cornea, late A52.71
coronary (artery) (sclerosis) A52.06
coryza, congenital A50.05
cranial nerve A52.15
multiple palsies A52.15
cutaneous — *see* Syphilis, skin
dacryocystitis (late) A52.71
degeneration, spinal cord A52.12
dementia paralytica A52.17
juvenilis A50.45
destruction of bone A52.77
dilatation, aorta A52.01
due to blood transfusion A53.9
dura mater A52.13
ear A52.79
inner A52.79
nerve (eighth) A52.15
neurorecurrence A52.15
early A51.9
cardiovascular A52.00
central nervous system A52.3
latent (without manifestations) (less than 2 years after infection) A51.5
negative spinal fluid test A51.5
serological relapse after treatment A51.5
serology positive A51.5
relapse (treated, untreated) A51.9
skin A51.39
symptomatic A51.9
extragenital chancre A51.2
primary, except extragenital chancre A51.0
secondary — *see also* Syphilis, secondary A51.39
relapse (treated, untreated) A51.49
ulcer A51.39
eighth nerve (neuritis) A52.15
endemic A65
endocarditis A52.03
aortic A52.03
pulmonary A52.03
epididymis (late) A52.76
epiglottis (late) A52.73
epiphysitis (congenital) (early) A50.02
episcleritis (late) A52.71
esophagus A52.79
eustachian tube A52.73
exposure to Z20.2
eye A52.71
eyelid (late) (with gumma) A52.71
fallopian tube (late) A52.76
fracture A52.77
gallbladder (late) A52.74
gastric (polyposis) (late) A52.74
general A53.9
paralysis A52.17
juvenile A50.45
genital (primary) A51.0
glaucoma A52.71
gumma NEC A52.79
cardiovascular system A52.00
central nervous system A52.3
congenital A50.59
heart (block) (decompensation) (disease) (failure) A52.06 *[I52]*
valve NEC A52.03
hemianesthesia A52.19
hemianopsia A52.71
hemiparesis A52.17
hemiplegia A52.17
hepatic artery A52.09
hepatis A52.74
hepatomegaly, congenital A50.08
hereditaria tarda — *see* Syphilis, congenital, late
hereditary — *see* Syphilis, congenital
Hutchinson's teeth A50.52
hyalitis A52.71
inactive — *see* Syphilis, latent
infantum — *see* Syphilis, congenital
inherited — *see* Syphilis, congenital
internal ear A52.79
intestine (late) A52.74
iris, iritis (secondary) A51.43
late A52.71
joint (late) A52.77
keratitis (congenital) (interstitial) (late) A50.31

Index

Synostosis — Syphilis, syphilitic

Syphilis, syphilitic — *continued*
- kidney (late) A52.75
- lacrimal passages (late) A52.71
- larynx (late) A52.73
- late A52.9
  - cardiovascular A52.ØØ
  - central nervous system A52.3
  - kidney A52.75
  - latent or 2 years or more after infection (without manifestations) A52.8
  - negative spinal fluid test A52.8
  - serology positive A52.8
  - paresis A52.17
  - specified site NEC A52.79
  - symptomatic or with manifestations A52.79
  - tabes A52.11
- latent A53.Ø
  - with signs or symptoms — *code by* site and stage under Syphilis
  - central nervous system A52.2
  - date of infection unspecified A53.Ø
  - early, or less than 2 years after infection A51.5
  - follow-up of latent syphilis A53.Ø
    - date of infection unspecified A53.Ø
    - late, or 2 years or more after infection A52.8
  - late, or 2 years or more after infection A52.8
  - positive serology (only finding) A53.Ø
    - date of infection unspecified A53.Ø
    - early, or less than 2 years after infection A51.5
    - late, or 2 years or more after infection A52.8
- lens (late) A52.71
- leukoderma A51.39
  - late A52.79
- lienitis A52.79
- lip A51.39
  - chancre (primary) A51.2
  - late A52.79
- Lissauer's paralysis A52.17
- liver A52.74
- locomotor ataxia A52.11
- lung A52.72
- lymph gland (early) (secondary) A51.49
  - late A52.79
- lymphadenitis (secondary) A51.49
- macular atrophy of skin A51.39
  - striated A52.79
- mediastinum (late) A52.73
- meninges (adhesive) (brain) (spinal cord) A52.13
- meningitis A52.13
  - acute (secondary) A51.41
  - congenital A5Ø.41
- meningoencephalitis A52.14
- meningovascular A52.13
  - congenital A5Ø.41
- mesarteritis A52.Ø9
  - brain A52.Ø4
- middle ear A52.77
- mitral stenosis A52.Ø3
- monoplegia A52.17
- mouth (secondary) A51.39
  - late A52.79
- mucocutaneous (secondary) A51.39
  - late A52.79
- mucous
  - membrane (secondary) A51.39
    - late A52.79
  - patches A51.39
    - congenital A5Ø.Ø7
- mulberry molars A5Ø.52
- muscle A52.78
- myocardium A52.Ø6
- nasal sinus (late) A52.73
- neonatorum — *see* Syphilis, congenital
- nephrotic syndrome (secondary) A51.44
- nerve palsy (any cranial nerve) A52.15
  - multiple A52.15
- nervous system, central A52.3
- neuritis A52.15
  - acoustic A52.15
- neurorecidive of retina A52.19
- neuroretinitis A52.19
- newborn — *see* Syphilis, congenital
- nodular superficial (late) A52.79
- nonvenereal A65
- nose (late) A52.73
  - saddle back deformity A5Ø.57
- occlusive arterial disease A52.Ø9
- oculopathy A52.71
- ophthalmic (late) A52.71

Syphilis, syphilitic — *continued*
- optic nerve (atrophy) (neuritis) (papilla) A52.15
- orbit (late) A52.71
- organic A53.9
- osseous (late) A52.77
- osteochondritis (congenital) (early) A5Ø.Ø2 *[M9Ø.8Ø]*
- osteoporosis A52.77
- ovary (late) A52.76
- oviduct (late) A52.76
- palate (late) A52.79
- pancreas (late) A52.74
- paralysis A52.17
  - general A52.17
    - juvenile A5Ø.45
- paresis (general) A52.17
  - juvenile A5Ø.45
- paresthesia A52.19
- Parkinson's disease or syndrome A52.19
- paroxysmal tachycardia A52.Ø6
- pemphigus (congenital) A5Ø.Ø6
- penis (chancre) A51.Ø
  - late A52.76
- pericardium A52.Ø6
- perichondritis, larynx (late) A52.73
- periosteum (late) A52.77
  - congenital (early) A5Ø.Ø2 *[M9Ø.8Ø]*
  - early (secondary) A51.46
- peripheral nerve A52.79
- petrous bone (late) A52.77
- pharynx (late) A52.73
  - secondary A51.39
- pituitary (gland) A52.79
- pleura (late) A52.73
- pneumonia, white A5Ø.Ø4
- pontine lesion A52.17
- portal vein A52.Ø9
- primary A51.Ø
  - anal A51.1
  - and secondary — *see* Syphilis, secondary
  - central nervous system A52.3
  - extragenital chancre NEC A51.2
  - fingers A51.2
  - genital A51.Ø
  - lip A51.2
  - specified site NEC A51.2
  - tonsils A51.2
- prostate (late) A52.76
- ptosis (eyelid) A52.71
- pulmonary (late) A52.72
  - artery A52.Ø9
- pyelonephritis (late) A52.75
- recently acquired, symptomatic A51.9
- rectum (late) A52.74
- respiratory tract (late) A52.73
- retina, late A52.71
- retrobulbar neuritis A52.15
- salpingitis A52.76
- sclera (late) A52.71
- sclerosis
  - cerebral A52.17
  - coronary A52.Ø6
  - multiple A52.11
- scotoma (central) A52.71
- scrotum (late) A52.76
- secondary (and primary) A51.49
  - adenopathy A51.49
  - anus A51.39
  - bone A51.46
  - chorioretinitis, choroiditis A51.43
  - hepatitis A51.45
  - liver A51.45
  - lymphadenitis A51.49
  - meningitis (acute) A51.41
  - mouth A51.39
  - mucous membranes A51.39
  - periosteum, periostitis A51.46
  - pharynx A51.39
  - relapse (treated, untreated) A51.49
  - skin A51.39
  - specified form NEC A51.49
  - tonsil A51.39
  - ulcer A51.39
  - viscera NEC A51.49
  - vulva A51.39
- seminal vesicle (late) A52.76

Syphilis, syphilitic — *continued*
- seronegative with signs or symptoms — *code by* site and stage under Syphilis
- seropositive
  - with signs or symptoms — *code by* site and stage under Syphilis
  - follow-up of latent syphilis — *see* Syphilis, latent
  - only finding — *see* Syphilis, latent
- seventh nerve (paralysis) A52.15
- sinus, sinusitis (late) A52.73
- skeletal system A52.77
- skin (with ulceration) (early) (secondary) A51.39
  - late or tertiary A52.79
- small intestine A52.74
- spastic spinal paralysis A52.17
- spermatic cord (late) A52.76
- spinal (cord) A52.12
- spleen A52.79
- splenomegaly A52.79
- spondylitis A52.77
- staphyloma A52.71
- stigmata (congenital) A5Ø.59
- stomach A52.74
- synovium A52.78
- tabes dorsalis (late) A52.11
  - juvenile A5Ø.45
- tabetic type A52.11
  - juvenile A5Ø.45
- taboparesis A52.17
  - juvenile A5Ø.45
- tachycardia A52.Ø6
- tendon (late) A52.78
- tertiary A52.9
  - with symptoms NEC A52.79
  - cardiovascular A52.ØØ
  - central nervous system A52.3
  - multiple NEC A52.79
  - specified site NEC A52.79
- testis A52.76
- thorax A52.73
- throat A52.73
- thymus (gland) (late) A52.79
- thyroid (late) A52.79
- tongue (late) A52.79
- tonsil (lingual) (late) A52.73
  - primary A51.2
  - secondary A51.39
- trachea (late) A52.73
- tunica vaginalis (late) A52.76
- ulcer (any site) (early) (secondary) A51.39
  - late A52.79
  - perforating A52.79
    - foot A52.11
- urethra (late) A52.76
- urogenital (late) A52.76
- uterus (late) A52.76
- uveal tract (secondary) A51.43
  - late A52.71
- uveitis (secondary) A51.43
  - late A52.71
- uvula (late) (perforated) A52.79
- vagina A51.Ø
  - late A52.76
- valvulitis NEC A52.Ø3
- vascular A52.ØØ
  - brain (cerebral) A52.Ø5
- ventriculi A52.74
- vesicae urinariae (late) A52.76
- viscera (abdominal) (late) A52.74
  - secondary A51.49
- vitreous (opacities) (late) A52.71
  - hemorrhage A52.71
- vulva A51.Ø
  - late A52.76
  - secondary A51.39

Syphiloma A52.79
- cardiovascular system A52.ØØ
- central nervous system A52.3
- circulatory system A52.ØØ
- congenital A5Ø.59

Syphilophobia F45.29

Syringadenoma — *see also* Neoplasm, skin, benign
- papillary — *see* Neoplasm, skin, benign

Syringobulbia G95.Ø

Syringocystadenoma — *see* Neoplasm, skin, benign
- papillary — *see* Neoplasm, skin, benign

Syringoma — *see also* Neoplasm, skin, benign
- chondroid — *see* Neoplasm, skin, benign

Syringomyelia G95.Ø
Syringomyelitis — *see* Encephalitis
Syringomyelocele — *see* Spina bifida
Syringopontia G95.Ø
System, systemic — *see also* condition
disease, combined — *see* Degeneration, combined
inflammatory response syndrome (SIRS) of non-infectious origin (without organ dysfunction) R65.1Ø
with acute organ dysfunction R65.11
System, systemic — *continued*
lupus erythematosus M32.9
inhibitor present D68.62
Systemic exertion intolerance disease [SEID] G93.32

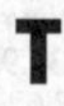

- **Tabacism, tabacosis, tabagism** — *see also* Poisoning, tobacco
  - meaning dependence (without remission) F17.2ØØ
    - with
      - disorder F17.299
        - in remission F17.211
        - specified disorder NEC F17.298
        - withdrawal F17.2Ø3
- **Tabardillo** A75.9
  - flea-borne A75.2
  - louse-borne A75.Ø
- **Tabes, tabetic** A52.1Ø
  - with
    - central nervous system syphilis A52.1Ø
    - Charcot's joint A52.16
    - cord bladder A52.19
    - crisis, viscera (any) A52.19
    - paralysis, general A52.17
    - paresis (general) A52.17
    - perforating ulcer (foot) A52.19
  - arthropathy (Charcot) A52.16
  - bladder A52.19
  - bone A52.11
  - cerebrospinal A52.12
  - congenital A5Ø.45
  - conjugal A52.1Ø
  - dorsalis A52.11
    - juvenile A5Ø.49
  - juvenile A5Ø.49
  - latent A52.19
  - mesenterica A18.39
  - paralysis, insane, general A52.17
  - spasmodic A52.17
  - syphilis (cerebrospinal) A52.12
- **Taboparalysis** A52.17
- **Taboparesis** (remission) A52.17
  - juvenile A5Ø.45
- **TAC** (trigeminal autonomic cephalgia) **NEC** G44.Ø99
  - intractable G44.Ø91
  - not intractable G44.Ø99
- **Tache noir** S6Ø.22- ☑
- **Tachyalimentation** K91.2
- **Tachyarrhythmia, tachyrhythmia** — *see* Tachycardia
- **Tachycardia** RØØ.Ø
  - atrial (paroxysmal) I47.1
  - auricular I47.1
  - AV nodal re-entry (re-entrant) I47.1
  - junctional (paroxysmal) I47.1
  - newborn P29.11
  - nodal (paroxysmal) I47.1
  - non-paroxysmal AV nodal I45.89
  - paroxysmal (sustained) (nonsustained) I47.9
    - with sinus bradycardia I49.5
    - atrial (PAT) I47.1
    - atrioventricular (AV) (re-entrant) I47.1
      - psychogenic F54
    - junctional I47.1
      - ectopic I47.1
    - nodal I47.1
    - psychogenic (atrial) (supraventricular) (ventricular) F54
    - supraventricular (sustained) I47.1
      - psychogenic F54
    - ventricular I47.2Ø
      - psychogenic F54
      - specified type NEC I47.29
  - psychogenic F45.8
  - sick sinus I49.5
  - sinoauricular NOS RØØ.Ø
    - paroxysmal I47.1
  - sinus [sinusal] NOS RØØ.Ø
    - paroxysmal I47.1
  - supraventricular I47.1
  - ventricular (paroxysmal) (sustained) I47.2Ø
    - psychogenic F54
    - specified NEC I47.29
- **Tachygastria** K31.89
- **Tachypnea** RØ6.82
  - hysterical F45.8
  - newborn (idiopathic) (transitory) P22.1
  - psychogenic F45.8
  - transitory, of newborn P22.1
- **TACO** (transfusion associated circulatory overload) E87.71
- **TAD** (transfusion-associated dyspnea) J95.87
- **Taenia** (infection) (infestation) B68.9
- **Taenia** — *continued*
  - diminuta B71.Ø
  - echinococcal infestation B67.9Ø
  - mediocanellata B68.1
  - nana B71.Ø
  - saginata B68.1
  - solium (intestinal form) B68.Ø
    - larval form — *see* Cysticercosis
- **Taeniasis** (intestine) — *see* Taenia
- **Tag** (hypertrophied skin) (infected) L91.8
  - adenoid J35.8
  - anus K64.4
  - hemorrhoidal K64.4
  - hymen N89.8
  - perineal N9Ø.89
  - preauricular Q17.Ø
  - sentinel K64.4
  - skin L91.8
    - accessory (congenital) Q82.8
    - anus K64.4
    - congenital Q82.8
    - preauricular Q17.Ø
  - tonsil J35.8
  - urethra, urethral N36.8
  - vulva N9Ø.89
- **Tahyna fever** B33.8
- **Takahara's disease** E8Ø.3
- **Takayasu's disease or syndrome** M31.4
- **Talaromycosis** B48.4
- **Talcosis** (pulmonary) J62.Ø
- **Talipes** (congenital) Q66.89
  - acquired, planus — *see* Deformity, limb, flat foot
  - asymmetric Q66.89
  - calcaneovalgus Q66.4- ☑
  - calcaneovarus Q66.1- ☑
  - calcaneus Q66.89
  - cavus Q66.7- ☑
  - equinovalgus Q66.6
  - equinovarus Q66.Ø- ☑
  - equinus Q66.89
  - percavus Q66.7- ☑
  - planovalgus Q66.6
  - planus (acquired) (any degree) — *see also* Deformity, limb, flat foot
    - congenital Q66.5- ☑
    - due to rickets (sequelae) E64.3
  - valgus Q66.6
  - varus Q66.3- ☑
- **Tall stature, constitutional** E34.4
- **Talma's disease** M62.89
- **Talon noir** S9Ø.3- ☑
  - hand S6Ø.22- ☑
  - heel S9Ø.3- ☑
  - toe S9Ø.1- ☑
- **Tamponade, heart** I31.4
- **Tanapox** (virus disease) BØ8.71
- **Tangier disease** E78.6
- **Tantrum, child problem** F91.8
- **Tapeworm** (infection) (infestation) — *see* Infestation, tapeworm
- **Tapia's syndrome** G52.7
- **TAR** (thrombocytopenia with absent radius) **syndrome** Q87.2
- **Tarral-Besnier disease** L44.Ø
- **Tarsal tunnel syndrome** — *see* Syndrome, tarsal tunnel
- **Tarsalgia** — *see* Pain, limb, lower
- **Tarsitis** (eyelid) HØ1.8
  - syphilitic A52.71
  - tuberculous A18.4
- **Tartar** (teeth) (dental calculus) KØ3.6
- **Tattoo** (mark) L81.8
- **Tauri's disease** E74.Ø9
- **Taurodontism** KØØ.2
- **Taussig-Bing syndrome** Q2Ø.1
- **Taybi's syndrome** Q87.2
- **Tay-Sachs amaurotic familial idiocy or disease** E75.Ø2
- **TBI** (traumatic brain injury) SØ6.9 ☑
- **Teacher's node or nodule** J38.2
- **Tear, torn** (traumatic) — *see also* Laceration
  - with abortion — *see* Abortion
  - annular fibrosis M51.35
  - anus, anal (sphincter) S31.831 ☑
    - complicating delivery
      - with third degree perineal laceration — *see also* Delivery, complicated, by, laceration, perineum, third degree O7Ø.2Ø
        - with mucosa O7Ø.3
- **Tear, torn** — *continued*
  - anus, anal — *continued*
    - complicating delivery — *continued*
      - without third degree perineal laceration O7Ø.4
    - nontraumatic (healed) (old) K62.81
  - articular cartilage, old — *see* Derangement, joint, articular cartilage, by site
  - bladder
    - with ectopic or molar pregnancy OØ8.6
    - following ectopic or molar pregnancy OØ8.6
    - obstetrical O71.5
    - traumatic — *see* Injury, bladder
  - bowel
    - with ectopic or molar pregnancy OØ8.6
    - following ectopic or molar pregnancy OØ8.6
    - obstetrical trauma O71.5
  - broad ligament
    - with ectopic or molar pregnancy OØ8.6
    - following ectopic or molar pregnancy OØ8.6
    - obstetrical trauma O71.6
  - bucket handle (knee) (meniscus) — *see* Tear, meniscus
  - capsule, joint — *see* Sprain
  - cartilage — *see also* Sprain
    - articular, old — *see* Derangement, joint, articular cartilage, by site
  - cervix
    - with ectopic or molar pregnancy OØ8.6
    - following ectopic or molar pregnancy OØ8.6
    - obstetrical trauma (current) O71.3
    - old N88.1
    - traumatic — *see* Injury, uterus
  - dural G97.41
    - nontraumatic G96.11
  - internal organ — *see* Injury, by site
  - knee cartilage
    - articular (current) S83.3- ☑
    - old — *see* Derangement, knee, meniscus, due to old tear
  - ligament — *see* Sprain
  - meniscus (knee) (current injury) S83.2Ø9 ☑
    - bucket-handle S83.2Ø- ☑
    - lateral
      - bucket-handle S83.25- ☑
      - complex S83.27- ☑
      - peripheral S83.26- ☑
      - specified type NEC S83.28- ☑
    - medial
      - bucket-handle S83.21- ☑
      - complex S83.23- ☑
      - peripheral S83.22- ☑
      - specified type NEC S83.24- ☑
    - old — *see* Derangement, knee, meniscus, due to old tear
    - site other than knee — *code as* Sprain
    - specified type NEC S83.2Ø- ☑
  - muscle — *see* Strain
  - pelvic
    - floor, complicating delivery O7Ø.1
    - organ NEC, obstetrical trauma O71.5
      - with ectopic or molar pregnancy OØ8.6
      - following ectopic or molar pregnancy OØ8.6
  - perineal, secondary O9Ø.1
  - periurethral tissue, obstetrical trauma O71.82
    - with ectopic or molar pregnancy OØ8.6
    - following ectopic or molar pregnancy OØ8.6
  - rectovaginal septum — *see* Laceration, vagina
  - retina, retinal (without detachment) (horseshoe) — *see also* Break, retina, horseshoe
    - with detachment — *see* Detachment, retina, with retinal, break
  - rotator cuff (nontraumatic) M75.1Ø- ☑
    - complete M75.12- ☑
    - incomplete M75.11- ☑
    - traumatic S46.Ø1- ☑
      - capsule S43.42- ☑
  - semilunar cartilage, knee — *see* Tear, meniscus
  - supraspinatus (complete) (incomplete) (nontraumatic) — *see also* Tear, rotator cuff M75.1Ø- ☑
  - tendon — *see* Strain
  - tentorial, at birth P1Ø.4
  - umbilical cord
    - complicating delivery O69.89 ☑
  - urethra
    - with ectopic or molar pregnancy OØ8.6
    - following ectopic or molar pregnancy OØ8.6
    - obstetrical trauma O71.5
  - uterus — *see* Injury, uterus

- **Tear, torn** — *continued*
  - vagina — *see* Laceration, vagina
  - vessel, from catheter — *see* Puncture, accidental complicating surgery
  - vulva, complicating delivery O7Ø.Ø
- **Tear-stone** — *see* Dacryolith
- **Teeth** — *see also* condition
  - grinding
    - psychogenic F45.8
    - sleep related G47.63
- **Teething** (syndrome) KØØ.7
- **Telangiectasia, telangiectasis** (verrucous) I78.1
  - ataxic (cerebellar) (Louis-Bar) G11.3
  - familial I78.Ø
  - hemorrhagic, hereditary (congenital) (senile) I78.Ø
  - hereditary, hemorrhagic (congenital) (senile) I78.Ø
  - juxtafoveal H35.Ø7- ☑
  - macular H35.Ø7- ☑
  - macularis eruptiva perstans D47.Ø1
  - parafoveal H35.Ø7- ☑
  - retinal (idiopathic) (juxtafoveal) (macular) (parafoveal) H35.Ø7- ☑
  - spider I78.1
- **Telephone scatologia** F65.89
- **Telescoped bowel or intestine** K56.1
  - congenital Q43.8
- **Temperature**
  - body, high (of unknown origin) R5Ø.9
  - cold, trauma from T69.9 ☑
    - newborn P8Ø.Ø
    - specified effect NEC T69.8 ☑
- **Temple** — *see* condition
- **Temporal** — *see* condition
- **Temporomandibular joint pain-dysfunction syndrome** M26.62- ☑
- **Temporosphenoidal** — *see* condition
- **Tendency**
  - bleeding — *see* Defect, coagulation
  - suicide
    - meaning personal history of attempted suicide Z91.51
    - meaning suicidal ideation — *see* Ideation, suicidal
  - to fall R29.6
- **Tenderness, abdominal** R1Ø.819
  - epigastric R1Ø.816
  - generalized R1Ø.817
  - left lower quadrant R1Ø.814
  - left upper quadrant R1Ø.812
  - periumbilic R1Ø.815
  - rebound R1Ø.829
    - epigastric R1Ø.826
    - generalized R1Ø.827
    - left lower quadrant R1Ø.824
    - left upper quadrant R1Ø.822
    - periumbilic R1Ø.825
    - right lower quadrant R1Ø.823
    - right upper quadrant R1Ø.821
  - right lower quadrant R1Ø.813
  - right upper quadrant R1Ø.811
- **Tendinitis, tendonitis** — *see also* Enthesopathy
  - Achilles M76.6- ☑
  - adhesive — *see* Tenosynovitis, specified type NEC
    - shoulder — *see* Capsulitis, adhesive
  - bicipital M75.2- ☑
  - calcific M65.2- ☑
    - ankle M65.27- ☑
    - foot M65.27- ☑
    - forearm M65.23- ☑
    - hand M65.24- ☑
    - lower leg M65.26- ☑
    - multiple sites M65.29
    - pelvic region M65.25- ☑
    - shoulder M75.3- ☑
    - specified site NEC M65.28
    - thigh M65.25- ☑
    - upper arm M65.22- ☑
  - due to use, overuse, pressure — *see also* Disorder, soft tissue, due to use
    - specified NEC — *see* Disorder, soft tissue, due to use, specified NEC
  - gluteal M76.Ø- ☑
  - patellar M76.5- ☑
  - peroneal M76.7- ☑
  - psoas M76.1- ☑
  - tibial (posterior) M76.82- ☑
    - anterior M76.81- ☑
  - trochanteric — *see* Bursitis, hip, trochanteric
- **Tendon** — *see* condition
- **Tendosynovitis** — *see* Tenosynovitis
- **Tenesmus** (rectal) R19.8
  - vesical R3Ø.1
- **Tennis elbow** — *see* Epicondylitis, lateral
- **Tenonitis** — *see also* Tenosynovitis
  - eye (capsule) HØ5.Ø4- ☑
- **Tenontosynovitis** — *see* Tenosynovitis
- **Tenontothecitis** — *see* Tenosynovitis
- **Tenophyte** — *see* Disorder, synovium, specified type NEC
- **Tenosynovitis** — *see also* Synovitis M65.9
  - adhesive — *see* Tenosynovitis, specified type NEC
    - shoulder — *see* Capsulitis, adhesive
  - bicipital (calcifying) — *see* Tendinitis, bicipital
  - gonococcal A54.49
  - in (due to)
    - crystals M65.8- ☑
    - gonorrhea A54.49
    - syphilis (late) A52.78
    - use, overuse, pressure — *see also* Disorder, soft tissue, due to use
      - specified NEC — *see* Disorder, soft tissue, due to use, specified NEC
  - infective NEC M65.1- ☑
    - ankle M65.17- ☑
    - foot M65.17- ☑
    - forearm M65.13- ☑
    - hand M65.14- ☑
    - lower leg M65.16- ☑
    - multiple sites M65.19
    - pelvic region M65.15- ☑
    - shoulder region M65.11- ☑
    - specified site NEC M65.18
    - thigh M65.15- ☑
    - upper arm M65.12- ☑
  - radial styloid M65.4
  - shoulder region M65.81- ☑
    - adhesive — *see* Capsulitis, adhesive
  - specified type NEC M65.88
    - ankle M65.87- ☑
    - foot M65.87- ☑
    - forearm M65.83- ☑
    - hand M65.84- ☑
    - lower leg M65.86- ☑
    - multiple sites M65.89
    - pelvic region M65.85- ☑
    - shoulder region M65.81- ☑
    - specified site NEC M65.88
    - thigh M65.85- ☑
    - upper arm M65.82- ☑
  - tuberculous — *see* Tuberculosis, tenosynovitis
- **Tenovaginitis** — *see* Tenosynovitis
- **Tension**
  - arterial, high — *see also* Hypertension
    - without diagnosis of hypertension RØ3.Ø
  - headache G44.2Ø9
    - intractable G44.2Ø1
    - not intractable G44.2Ø9
  - nervous R45.Ø
  - pneumothorax J93.Ø
  - premenstrual N94.3
  - state (mental) F48.9
- **Tentorium** — *see* condition
- **Teratencephalus** Q89.8
- **Teratism** Q89.7
- **Teratoblastoma** (malignant) — *see* Neoplasm, malignant, by site
- **Teratocarcinoma** — *see also* Neoplasm, malignant, by site
  - liver C22.7
- **Teratoma** (solid) — *see also* Neoplasm, uncertain behavior, by site
  - with embryonal carcinoma, mixed — *see* Neoplasm, malignant, by site
  - with malignant transformation — *see* Neoplasm, malignant, by site
  - adult (cystic) — *see* Neoplasm, benign, by site
  - benign — *see* Neoplasm, benign, by site
  - combined with choriocarcinoma — *see* Neoplasm, malignant, by site
  - cystic (adult) — *see* Neoplasm, benign, by site
  - differentiated — *see* Neoplasm, benign, by site
  - embryonal — *see also* Neoplasm, malignant, by site
    - liver C22.7
  - immature — *see* Neoplasm, malignant, by site
  - liver C22.7
- **Teratoma** — *continued*
  - liver — *continued*
    - adult, benign, cystic, differentiated type or mature D13.4
  - malignant — *see also* Neoplasm, malignant, by site
    - anaplastic — *see* Neoplasm, malignant, by site
    - intermediate — *see* Neoplasm, malignant, by site
      - specified site — *see* Neoplasm, malignant, by site
      - unspecified site C62.9Ø
    - undifferentiated — *see* Neoplasm, malignant, by site
  - mature — *see* Neoplasm, uncertain behavior, by site
    - malignant — *see* Neoplasm, by site, malignant, by site
  - ovary D27.- ☑
    - embryonal, immature or malignant C56- ☑
  - solid — *see* Neoplasm, uncertain behavior, by site
  - testis C62.9- ☑
    - adult, benign, cystic, differentiated type or mature D29.2- ☑
    - scrotal C62.1- ☑
    - undescended C62.Ø- ☑
- **Termination**
  - anomalous — *see also* Malposition, congenital
    - right pulmonary vein Q26.3
  - pregnancy, elective Z33.2
- **Ternidens diminutus infestation** B81.8
- **Ternidensiasis** B81.8
- **Terror(s) night** (child) F51.4
- **Terrorism, victim of** Z65.4
- **Terry's syndrome** — *see also* Myopia, degenerative H44.2- ☑
- **Tertiary** — *see* condition
- **Test, tests, testing** (for)
  - adequacy (for dialysis)
    - hemodialysis Z49.31
    - peritoneal Z49.32
  - blood pressure ZØ1.3Ø
    - abnormal reading — *see* Blood, pressure
  - blood typing ZØ1.83
    - Rh typing ZØ1.83
  - blood-alcohol ZØ2.83
    - positive — *see* Findings, abnormal, in blood
  - blood-drug ZØ2.83
    - positive — *see* Findings, abnormal, in blood
  - cardiac pulse generator (battery) Z45.Ø1Ø
  - fertility Z31.41
  - genetic
    - disease carrier status for procreative management
      - female Z31.43Ø
      - male Z31.44Ø
    - male partner of patient with recurrent pregnancy loss Z31.441
    - procreative management NEC
      - female Z31.438
      - male Z31.448
  - hearing ZØ1.1Ø
    - with abnormal findings NEC ZØ1.118
    - infant or child (over 28 days old) ZØØ.129
      - with abnormal findings ZØØ.121
  - HIV (human immunodeficiency virus)
    - nonconclusive (in infants) R75
    - positive Z21
    - seropositive Z21
  - immunity status ZØ1.84
  - intelligence NEC ZØ1.89
  - laboratory (as part of a general medical examination) ZØØ.ØØ
    - with abnormal finding ZØØ.Ø1
    - for medicolegal reason NEC ZØ4.89
  - male partner of patient with recurrent pregnancy loss Z31.441
  - Mantoux (for tuberculosis) Z11.1
    - abnormal result R76.11
  - pregnancy, positive first pregnancy — *see* Pregnancy, normal, first
  - procreative Z31.49
    - fertility Z31.41
  - skin, diagnostic
    - allergy ZØ1.82
      - special screening examination — *see* Screening, by name of disease
    - Mantoux Z11.1
    - tuberculin Z11.1
  - specified NEC ZØ1.89
  - tuberculin Z11.1
    - abnormal result R76.11

- **Test, tests, testing** — *continued*
  - vision Z01.00
    - with abnormal findings Z01.01
    - following failed vision screening Z01.020
      - with abnormal findings Z01.021
    - infant or child (over 28 days old) Z00.129
      - with abnormal findings Z00.121
  - Wassermann Z11.3
    - positive — *see* Serology for syphilis, positive
- **Testicle, testicular, testis** — *see also* condition
  - feminization syndrome — *see also* Syndrome, androgen insensitivity E34.51
  - migrans Q55.29
- **Tetanus, tetanic** (cephalic) (convulsions) A35
  - with
    - abortion A34
    - ectopic or molar pregnancy O08.0
  - following ectopic or molar pregnancy O08.0
  - inoculation reaction (due to serum) — *see* Complications, vaccination
  - neonatorum A33
  - obstetrical A34
  - puerperal, postpartum, childbirth A34
- **Tetany** (due to) R29.0
  - alkalosis E87.3
  - associated with rickets E55.0
  - convulsions R29.0
    - hysterical F44.5
  - functional (hysterical) F44.5
  - hyperkinetic R29.0
    - hysterical F44.5
  - hyperpnea R06.4
    - hysterical F44.5
    - psychogenic F45.8
  - hyperventilation — *see also* Hyperventilation R06.4
    - hysterical F44.5
  - neonatal (without calcium or magnesium deficiency) P71.3
  - parathyroid (gland) E20.9
  - parathyroprival E89.2
  - post- (para)thyroidectomy E89.2
  - postoperative E89.2
  - pseudotetany R29.0
  - psychogenic (conversion reaction) F44.5
- **Tetralogy of Fallot** Q21.3
- **Tetraplegia** (chronic) — *see also* Quadriplegia G82.50
- **Thailand hemorrhagic fever** A91
- **Thalassanemia** — *see* Thalassemia
- **Thalassemia** (anemia) (disease) D56.9
  - with other hemoglobinopathy D56.8
  - alpha (major) (severe) (triple gene defect) D56.0
    - minor D56.3
    - silent carrier D56.3
    - trait D56.3
  - beta (severe) D56.1
    - homozygous D56.1
    - major D56.1
    - minor D56.3
    - trait D56.3
  - delta-beta (homozygous) D56.2
    - minor D56.3
    - trait D56.3
  - dominant D56.8
  - hemoglobin
    - C D56.8
    - E-beta D56.5
  - intermedia D56.1
  - major D56.1
  - minor D56.3
  - mixed D56.8
  - sickle-cell — *see* Disease, sickle-cell, thalassemia
  - specified type NEC D56.8
  - trait D56.3
  - variants D56.8
- **Thanatophoric dwarfism or short stature** Q77.1
- **Thaysen-Gee disease** (nontropical sprue) K90.0
- **Thaysen's disease** K90.0
- **Thecoma** D27- ☑
  - luteinized D27- ☑
  - malignant C56- ☑
- **Thelarche, premature** E30.8
- **Thelaziasis** B83.8
- **Thelitis** N61.0
  - puerperal, postpartum or gestational — *see* Infection, nipple
- **Therapeutic** — *see* condition
- **Therapy**
  - drug, long-term (current) (prophylactic)
    - agents affecting estrogen receptors and estrogen levels NEC Z79.818
    - anastrozole (Arimidex) Z79.811
    - antibiotics Z79.2
      - short-term use — *omit code*
    - anticoagulants Z79.01
    - anti-inflammatory Z79.1
    - antiplatelet Z79.02
    - antithrombotics Z79.02
    - aromatase inhibitors Z79.811
    - aspirin Z79.82
    - birth control pill or patch Z79.3
    - bisphosphonates Z79.83
    - contraceptive, oral Z79.3
    - drug, specified NEC Z79.899
    - estrogen receptor downregulators Z79.818
    - Evista Z79.810
    - exemestane (Aromasin) Z79.811
    - Fareston Z79.810
    - fulvestrant (Faslodex) Z79.818
    - gonadotropin-releasing hormone (GnRH) agonist Z79.818
    - goserelin acetate (Zoladex) Z79.818
    - hormone replacement Z79.890
    - insulin Z79.4
    - letrozole (Femara) Z79.811
    - leuprolide acetate (leuprorelin) (Lupron) Z79.818
    - megestrol acetate (Megace) Z79.818
    - methadone
      - for pain management Z79.891
      - maintenance therapy F11.20
    - Nolvadex Z79.810
    - opiate analgesic Z79.891
    - oral contraceptive Z79.3
    - raloxifene (Evista) Z79.810
    - selective estrogen receptor modulators (SERMs) Z79.810
    - short term — *omit code*
    - steroids
      - inhaled Z79.51
      - systemic Z79.52
    - tamoxifen (Nolvadex) Z79.810
    - toremifene (Fareston) Z79.810
- **Thermic** — *see* condition
- **Thermography** (abnormal) — *see also* Abnormal, diagnostic imaging R93.89
  - breast R92.8
- **Thermoplegia** T67.01 ☑
- **Thesaurismosis, glycogen** — *see* Disease, glycogen storage
- **Thiamin deficiency** E51.9
  - specified NEC E51.8
- **Thiaminic deficiency with beriberi** E51.11
- **Thibierge-Weissenbach syndrome** — *see* Sclerosis, systemic
- **Thickening**
  - bone — *see* Hypertrophy, bone
  - breast N64.59
  - endometrium R93.89
  - epidermal L85.9
    - specified NEC L85.8
  - hymen N89.6
  - larynx J38.7
  - nail L60.2
    - congenital Q84.5
  - periosteal — *see* Hypertrophy, bone
  - pleura J92.9
    - with asbestos J92.0
  - skin R23.4
  - subepiglottic J38.7
  - tongue K14.8
  - valve, heart — *see* Endocarditis
- **Thigh** — *see* condition
- **Thinning vertebra** — *see* Spondylopathy, specified NEC
- **Thirst, excessive** R63.1
  - due to deprivation of water T73.1 ☑
- **Thomsen disease** G71.12
- **Thoracic** — *see also* condition
  - kidney Q63.2
  - outlet syndrome G54.0
- **Thoracogastroschisis** (congenital) Q79.8
- **Thoracopagus** Q89.4
- **Thorax** — *see* condition
- **Thorn's syndrome** N28.89
- **Thorson-Björck syndrome** E34.0
- **Threadworm** (infection) (infestation) B80
- **Threatened**
  - abortion O20.0
    - with subsequent abortion O03.9
  - job loss, anxiety concerning Z56.2
  - labor (without delivery) O47.9
    - at or after 37 completed weeks of gestation O47.1
    - before 37 completed weeks of gestation O47.0- ☑
  - loss of job, anxiety concerning Z56.2
  - miscarriage O20.0
  - unemployment, anxiety concerning Z56.2
- **Three-day fever** A93.1
- **Threshers' lung** J67.0
- **Thrix annulata** (congenital) Q84.1
- **Throat** — *see* condition
- **Thrombasthenia** (Glanzmann) (hemorrhagic) (hereditary) D69.1
- **Thromboangiitis** I73.1
  - obliterans (general) I73.1
    - cerebral I67.89
    - vessels
      - brain I67.89
      - spinal cord I67.89
- **Thromboarteritis** — *see* Arteritis
- **Thromboasthenia** (Glanzmann) (hemorrhagic) (hereditary) D69.1
- **Thrombocytasthenia** (Glanzmann) D69.1
- **Thrombocythemia** (hemorrhagic) *see also* Thrombocytosis D75.839
  - essential D47.3
  - idiopathic D47.3
  - primary D47.3
- **Thrombocytopathy** (dystrophic) (granulopenic) D69.1
- **Thrombocytopenia, thrombocytopenic** D69.6
  - with absent radius (TAR) Q87.2
  - congenital D69.42
  - dilutional D69.59
  - due to
    - (massive) blood transfusion D69.59
    - drugs D69.59
    - extracorporeal circulation of blood D69.59
    - platelet alloimmunization D69.59
  - essential D69.3
  - heparin induced (HIT) D75.829
    - delayed-onset D75.828
    - immune-mediated D75.822
    - non-immune D75.821
    - persisting D75.828
    - syndrome
      - autoimmune D75.828
      - specified NEC D75.828
      - spontaneous (without heparin exposure) D75.84
    - type 1 D75.821
    - type 2 D75.822
  - heparin-associated D75.821
  - hereditary D69.42
  - idiopathic D69.3
  - neonatal, transitory P61.0
    - due to
      - exchange transfusion P61.0
      - idiopathic maternal thrombocytopenia P61.0
      - isoimmunization P61.0
  - primary NEC D69.49
    - idiopathic D69.3
  - puerperal, postpartum O72.3
  - secondary D69.59
  - transient neonatal P61.0
  - vaccine-induced thrombotic D75.84
- **Thrombocytosis** D75.839
  - essential D47.3
  - idiopathic D47.3
  - primary D47.3
  - reactive D75.838
  - secondary D75.838
  - specified NEC D75.838
- **Thromboembolism** — *see* Embolism
- **Thrombopathy** (Bernard-Soulier) D69.1
  - constitutional — *see* Disease, von Willebrand
  - Willebrand-Jurgens — *see* Disease, von Willebrand
- **Thrombopenia** — *see* Thrombocytopenia
- **Thrombophilia** D68.59
  - primary NEC D68.59
  - secondary NEC D68.69
  - specified NEC D68.69
- **Thrombophlebitis** I80.9
  - antepartum O22.2- ☑
    - deep O22.3- ☑
    - superficial O22.2- ☑
  - calf muscular vein (NOS) I80.25- ☑

Thrombophlebitis — *continued*
  cavernous (venous) sinus GØ8
    complicating pregnancy O22.5- ☑
    nonpyogenic I67.6
  cerebral (sinus) (vein) GØ8
    nonpyogenic I67.6
    sequelae GØ9
  due to implanted device — *see* Complications, by site and type, specified NEC
  during or resulting from a procedure NEC T81.72 ☑
  femoral vein (superficial) I8Ø.1- ☑
  femoropopliteal vein I8Ø.Ø- ☑
  gastrocnemial vein I8Ø.25- ☑
  hepatic (vein) I8Ø.8
  idiopathic, recurrent I82.1
  iliac vein (common) (external) (internal) I8Ø.21- ☑
  iliofemoral I8Ø.1- ☑
  intracranial venous sinus (any) GØ8
    nonpyogenic I67.6
    sequelae GØ9
  intraspinal venous sinuses and veins GØ8
    nonpyogenic G95.19
  lateral (venous) sinus GØ8
    nonpyogenic I67.6
  leg I8Ø.3
    superficial I8Ø.Ø- ☑
  longitudinal (venous) sinus GØ8
    nonpyogenic I67.6
  lower extremity I8Ø.299
  migrans, migrating I82.1
  pelvic
    with ectopic or molar pregnancy OØ8.Ø
    following ectopic or molar pregnancy OØ8.Ø
    puerperal O87.1
  peroneal vein I8Ø.24- ☑
  popliteal vein — *see* Phlebitis, leg, deep, popliteal
  portal (vein) K75.1
  postoperative T81.72 ☑
  pregnancy — *see* Thrombophlebitis, antepartum
  puerperal, postpartum, childbirth O87.Ø
    deep O87.1
    pelvic O87.1
    septic O86.81
    superficial O87.Ø
  saphenous (greater) (lesser) I8Ø.Ø- ☑
  sinus (intracranial) GØ8
    nonpyogenic I67.6
  soleal vein I8Ø.25- ☑
  specified site NEC I8Ø.8
  tibial vein (anterior) (posterior) I8Ø.23- ☑

Thrombosis, thrombotic (bland) (multiple) (progressive) (silent) (vessel) I82.9Ø
  anal K64.5
  antepartum — *see* Thrombophlebitis, antepartum
  aorta, aortic I74.1Ø
    abdominal I74.Ø9
      saddle I74.Ø1
    bifurcation I74.Ø9
    saddle I74.Ø1
    specified site NEC I74.19
    terminal I74.Ø9
    thoracic I74.11
    valve — *see* Endocarditis, aortic
  apoplexy I63.3- ☑
  artery, arteries (postinfectional) I74.9
    auditory, internal — *see* Occlusion, artery, precerebral, specified NEC
    basilar — *see* Occlusion, artery, basilar
    carotid (common) (internal) — *see* Occlusion, artery, carotid
    cerebellar (anterior inferior) (posterior inferior) (superior) — *see* Occlusion, artery, cerebellar
    cerebral — *see* Occlusion, artery, cerebral
    choroidal (anterior) — *see* Occlusion, artery, precerebral, specified NEC
    communicating, posterior — *see* Occlusion, artery, precerebral, specified NEC
    coronary — *see also* Infarct, myocardium
      not resulting in infarction I24.Ø
    hepatic I74.8
    hypophyseal — *see* Occlusion, artery, precerebral, specified NEC
    iliac I74.5
    limb I74.4
      lower I74.3
      upper I74.2
    meningeal, anterior or posterior — *see* Occlusion, artery, cerebral, specified NEC

Thrombosis, thrombotic — *continued*
  artery, arteries — *continued*
    mesenteric (with gangrene) — *see also* Infarct, intestine K55.Ø69
    ophthalmic — *see* Occlusion, artery, retina
    pontine — *see* Occlusion, artery, precerebral, specified NEC
    precerebral — *see* Occlusion, artery, precerebral
    pulmonary (iatrogenic) — *see* Embolism, pulmonary
    renal N28.Ø
    retinal — *see* Occlusion, artery, retina
    spinal, anterior or posterior G95.11
    traumatic NEC T14.8 ☑
    vertebral — *see* Occlusion, artery, vertebral
  atrium, auricular — *see also* Infarct, myocardium
    following acute myocardial infarction (current complication) I23.6
    not resulting in infarction I51.3
    old I51.3
  basilar (artery) — *see* Occlusion, artery, basilar
  brain (artery) (stem) — *see also* Occlusion, artery, cerebral
    due to syphilis A52.Ø5
    puerperal O99.43
    sinus — *see* Thrombosis, intracranial venous sinus
  capillary I78.8
  cardiac — *see also* Infarct, myocardium
    not resulting in infarction I51.3
    old I51.3
    valve — *see* Endocarditis
  carotid (artery) (common) (internal) — *see* Occlusion, artery, carotid
  cavernous (venous) sinus — *see* Thrombosis, intracranial venous sinus
  cerebellar artery (anterior inferior) (posterior inferior) (superior) I66.3
  cerebral (artery) — *see* Occlusion, artery, cerebral
  cerebrovenous sinus — *see also* Thrombosis, intracranial venous sinus
    puerperium O87.3
  chronic I82.91
  coronary (artery) (vein) — *see also* Infarct, myocardium
    not resulting in infarction I24.Ø
  corpus cavernosum N48.89
  cortical I66.9
  deep — *see* Embolism, vein, lower extremity
  due to device, implant or graft — *see also* Complications, by site and type, specified NEC T85.868 ☑
    arterial graft NEC T82.868 ☑
    breast (implant) T85.868 ☑
    catheter NEC T85.868 ☑
      dialysis (renal) T82.868 ☑
        intraperitoneal T85.868 ☑
      infusion NEC T82.868 ☑
        spinal (epidural) (subdural) T85.86Ø ☑
      urinary (indwelling) T83.86 ☑
    electronic (electrode) (pulse generator) (stimulator)
      bone T84.86 ☑
      cardiac T82.867 ☑
      nervous system (brain) (peripheral nerve) (spinal) T85.86Ø ☑
      urinary T83.86 ☑
    fixation, internal (orthopedic) NEC T84.86 ☑
    gastrointestinal (bile duct) (esophagus) T85.868 ☑
    genital NEC T83.86 ☑
    heart T82.867 ☑
    joint prosthesis T84.86 ☑
    ocular (corneal graft) (orbital implant) NEC T85.868 ☑
    orthopedic NEC T84.86 ☑
    specified NEC T85.868 ☑
    urinary NEC T83.86 ☑
    vascular NEC T82.868 ☑
    ventricular intracranial shunt T85.86Ø ☑
  during the puerperium — *see* Thrombosis, puerperal
  endocardial — *see also* Infarct, myocardium
    not resulting in infarction I51.3
  eye — *see* Occlusion, retina
  genital organ
    female NEC N94.89
      pregnancy — *see* Thrombophlebitis, antepartum
    male N5Ø.1
  gestational — *see* Phlebopathy, gestational
  heart (chamber) — *see also* Infarct, myocardium
    not resulting in infarction I51.3
    old I51.3
  hepatic (vein) I82.Ø

Thrombosis, thrombotic — *continued*
  hepatic — *continued*
    artery I74.8
  history (of) Z86.718
  intestine (with gangrene) — *see also* Infarct, intestine K55.Ø69
  intracardiac NEC (apical) (atrial) (auricular) (ventricular) (old) I51.3
  intracranial (arterial) I66.9
    venous sinus (any) GØ8
      nonpyogenic origin I67.6
      puerperium O87.3
  intramural — *see also* Infarct, myocardium
    not resulting in infarction I51.3
    old I51.3
  intraspinal venous sinuses and veins GØ8
    nonpyogenic G95.19
  kidney (artery) N28.Ø
  lateral (venous) sinus — *see* Thrombosis, intracranial venous sinus
  leg — *see* Thrombosis, vein, lower extremity
    arterial I74.3
  liver (venous) I82.Ø
    artery I74.8
    portal vein I81
  longitudinal (venous) sinus — *see* Thrombosis, intracranial venous sinus
  lower limb — *see* Thrombosis, vein, lower extremity
  lung (iatrogenic) (postoperative) — *see* Embolism, pulmonary
  meninges (brain) (arterial) I66.8
  mesenteric (artery) (with gangrene) — *see also* Infarct, intestine K55.Ø69
    vein (inferior) (superior) K55.Ø- ☑
  mitral I34.89
  mural — *see also* Infarct, myocardium
    due to syphilis A52.Ø6
    not resulting in infarction I51.3
    old I51.3
  omentum (with gangrene) — *see also* Infarct, intestine K55.Ø69
  ophthalmic — *see* Occlusion, retina
  pampiniform plexus (male) N5Ø.1
  parietal — *see also* Infarct, myocardium
    not resulting in infarction I24.Ø
  penis, superficial vein N48.81
  perianal venous K64.5
  peripheral arteries I74.4
    upper I74.2
  personal history (of) Z86.718
  portal I81
    due to syphilis A52.Ø9
  precerebral artery — *see* Occlusion, artery, precerebral
  puerperal, postpartum O87.Ø
    brain (artery) O99.43
      venous (sinus) O87.3
    cardiac O99.43
    cerebral (artery) O99.43
      venous (sinus) O87.3
    superficial O87.Ø
  pulmonary (artery) (iatrogenic) (postoperative) (vein) — *see* Embolism, pulmonary
  renal (artery) N28.Ø
    vein I82.3
  resulting from presence of device, implant or graft — *see* Complications, by site and type, specified NEC
  retina, retinal — *see* Occlusion, retina
  scrotum N5Ø.1
  seminal vesicle N5Ø.1
  sigmoid (venous) sinus — *see* Thrombosis, intracranial venous sinus
  sinus, intracranial (any) — *see* Thrombosis, intracranial venous sinus
  specified site NEC I82.89Ø
    chronic I82.891
  spermatic cord N5Ø.1
  spinal cord (arterial) G95.11
    due to syphilis A52.Ø9
    pyogenic origin GØ6.1
  spleen, splenic D73.5
    artery I74.8
  testis N5Ø.1
  traumatic NEC T14.8 ☑
  tricuspid IØ7.8
  tumor — *see* Neoplasm, unspecified behavior, by site
  tunica vaginalis N5Ø.1
  umbilical cord (vessels), complicating delivery O69.5 ☑

- **Thrombosis, thrombotic** — *continued*
  - vas deferens N5Ø.1
  - vein (acute) I82.9Ø
    - antecubital I82.61- ☑
      - chronic I82.71- ☑
    - axillary I82.A1- ☑ (*following* I82.7)
      - chronic I82.A2- ☑ (*following* I82.7)
    - basilic I82.61- ☑
      - chronic I82.71- ☑
    - brachial I82.62- ☑
      - chronic I82.72- ☑
    - brachiocephalic (innominate) I82.29Ø
      - chronic I82.291
    - cephalic I82.61- ☑
      - chronic I82.71- ☑
    - cerebral, nonpyogenic I67.6
    - chronic I82.91
    - deep (DVT) I82.4Ø- ☑
      - calf I82.4Z- ☑
        - chronic I82.5Z- ☑
      - lower leg I82.4Z- ☑
        - chronic I82.5Z- ☑
      - thigh I82.4Y- ☑
        - chronic I82.5Y- ☑
      - upper leg I82.4Y- ☑
        - chronic I82.5Y- ☑
    - femoral I82.41- ☑
      - chronic I82.51- ☑
    - iliac (iliofemoral) I82.42- ☑
      - chronic I82.52- ☑
    - innominate I82.29Ø
      - chronic I82.291
    - internal jugular I82.C1- ☑ (*following* I82.7)
      - chronic I82.C2- ☑ (*following* I82.7)
    - lower extremity
      - deep I82.4Ø- ☑
        - chronic I82.5Ø- ☑
        - specified NEC I82.49- ☑
          - chronic NEC I82.59- ☑
      - distal
        - deep I82.4Z- ☑
      - proximal
        - deep I82.4Y- ☑
          - chronic I82.5Y- ☑
      - superficial I82.81- ☑
    - perianal K64.5
    - popliteal I82.43- ☑
      - chronic I82.53- ☑
    - radial I82.62- ☑
      - chronic I82.72- ☑
    - renal I82.3
    - saphenous (greater) (lesser) I82.81- ☑
    - specified NEC I82.89Ø
      - chronic NEC I82.891
    - subclavian I82.B1- ☑ (*following* I82.7)
      - chronic I82.B2- ☑ (*following* I82.7)
    - thoracic NEC I82.29Ø
      - chronic I82.291
    - tibial I82.44- ☑
      - chronic I82.54- ☑
    - ulnar I82.62- ☑
      - chronic I82.72- ☑
    - upper extremity I82.6Ø- ☑
      - chronic I82.7Ø- ☑
      - deep I82.62- ☑
        - chronic I82.72- ☑
      - superficial I82.61- ☑
        - chronic I82.71- ☑
  - vena cava
    - inferior I82.22Ø
      - chronic I82.221
    - superior I82.21Ø
      - chronic I82.211
  - venous, perianal K64.5
  - ventricle — *see also* Infarct, myocardium
    - following acute myocardial infarction (current complication) I23.6
    - not resulting in infarction I24.Ø
    - old I51.3
- **Thrombus** — *see* Thrombosis
- **Thrush** — *see also* Candidiasis
  - newborn P37.5
  - oral B37.Ø
  - vaginal (acute) B37.31
    - chronic (recurrent) B37.32
- **Thumb** — *see also* condition
  - sucking (child problem) F98.8
- **Thymitis** E32.8
- **Thymoma** — *see also* Neoplasm, thymus, by type
  - malignant C37
  - metaplastic C37
  - microscopic D15.Ø
  - sclerosing C37
  - type A C37
  - type AB C37
  - type B1 C37
  - type B2 C37
  - type B3 C37
- **Thymus, thymic** (gland) — *see* condition
- **Thyrocele** — *see* Goiter
- **Thyroglossal** — *see also* condition
  - cyst Q89.2
  - duct, persistent Q89.2
- **Thyroid** (gland) (body) — *see also* condition
  - hormone resistance EØ7.89
  - lingual Q89.2
  - nodule (cystic) (nontoxic) (single) EØ4.1
- **Thyroiditis** EØ6.9
  - acute (nonsuppurative) (pyogenic) (suppurative) EØ6.Ø
  - autoimmune EØ6.3
  - chronic (nonspecific) (sclerosing) EØ6.5
    - with thyrotoxicosis, transient EØ6.2
    - fibrous EØ6.5
    - lymphadenoid EØ6.3
    - lymphocytic EØ6.3
    - lymphoid EØ6.3
  - de Quervain's EØ6.1
  - drug-induced EØ6.4
  - fibrous (chronic) EØ6.5
  - giant-cell (follicular) EØ6.1
  - granulomatous (de Quervain) (subacute) EØ6.1
  - Hashimoto's (struma lymphomatosa) EØ6.3
  - iatrogenic EØ6.4
  - ligneous EØ6.5
  - lymphocytic (chronic) EØ6.3
  - lymphoid EØ6.3
  - lymphomatous EØ6.3
  - nonsuppurative EØ6.1
  - postpartum, puerperal O9Ø.5
  - pseudotuberculous EØ6.1
  - pyogenic EØ6.Ø
  - radiation EØ6.4
  - Riedel's EØ6.5
  - subacute (granulomatous) EØ6.1
  - suppurative EØ6.Ø
  - tuberculous A18.81
  - viral EØ6.1
  - woody EØ6.5
- **Thyrolingual duct, persistent** Q89.2
- **Thyromegaly** EØ1.Ø
- **Thyrotoxic**
  - crisis — *see* Thyrotoxicosis
  - heart disease or failure — *see also* Thyrotoxicosis EØ5.9Ø *[I43]*
    - with thyroid storm EØ5.91 *[I43]*
  - storm — *see* Thyrotoxicosis
- **Thyrotoxicosis** (recurrent) EØ5.9Ø
  - with
    - goiter (diffuse) EØ5.ØØ
      - with thyroid storm EØ5.Ø1
      - adenomatous uninodular EØ5.1Ø
        - with thyroid storm EØ5.11
      - multinodular EØ5.2Ø
        - with thyroid storm EØ5.21
      - nodular EØ5.2Ø
        - with thyroid storm EØ5.21
      - uninodular EØ5.1Ø
        - with thyroid storm EØ5.11
    - infiltrative
      - dermopathy EØ5.ØØ
        - with thyroid storm EØ5.Ø1
      - ophthalmopathy EØ5.ØØ
        - with thyroid storm EØ5.Ø1
    - single thyroid nodule EØ5.1Ø
      - with thyroid storm EØ5.11
    - thyroid storm EØ5.91
  - due to
    - ectopic thyroid nodule or tissue EØ5.3Ø
      - with thyroid storm EØ5.31
    - ingestion of (excessive) thyroid material EØ5.4Ø
      - with thyroid storm EØ5.41
    - overproduction of thyroid-stimulating hormone EØ5.8Ø
      - with thyroid storm EØ5.81
    - specified cause NEC EØ5.8Ø
- **Thyrotoxicosis** — *continued*
  - due to — *continued*
    - specified cause — *continued*
      - with thyroid storm EØ5.81
  - factitia EØ5.4Ø
    - with thyroid storm EØ5.41
  - heart — *see also* Failure, heart, high-output EØ5.9Ø *[I43]*
    - with thyroid storm — *see also* Failure, heart, high-output EØ5.91 *[I43]*
    - failure — *see also* Failure, heart, high-output EØ5.9Ø *[I43]*
  - neonatal (transient) P72.1
  - transient with chronic thyroiditis EØ6.2
- **Tibia vara** M92.51- ☑
- **Tic** (disorder) F95.9
  - breathing F95.8
  - child problem F95.Ø
  - compulsive F95.1
  - de la Tourette F95.2
  - degenerative (generalized) (localized) G25.69
    - facial G25.69
  - disorder
    - chronic
      - motor F95.1
      - vocal F95.1
    - combined vocal and multiple motor F95.2
    - transient F95.Ø
  - douloureux G5Ø.Ø
    - atypical G5Ø.1
    - postherpetic, postzoster BØ2.22
  - drug-induced G25.61
  - eyelid F95.8
  - habit F95.9
    - chronic F95.1
    - transient of childhood F95.Ø
  - lid, transient of childhood F95.Ø
  - motor-verbal F95.2
  - occupational F48.8
  - orbicularis F95.8
    - transient of childhood F95.Ø
  - organic origin G25.69
  - postchoreic G25.69
  - provisional F95.Ø
  - psychogenic, compulsive F95.1
  - salaam R25.8
  - spasm (motor or vocal) F95.9
    - chronic F95.1
    - transient of childhood F95.Ø
  - specified NEC F95.8
- **Tick-borne** — *see* condition
- **Tietze's disease or syndrome** M94.Ø
- **Tight, tightness**
  - anus K62.89
  - chest RØ7.89
  - fascia (lata) M62.89
  - foreskin (congenital) N47.1
  - hymen, hymenal ring N89.6
  - introitus (acquired) (congenital) N89.6
  - rectal sphincter K62.89
  - tendon — *see* Short, tendon
  - urethral sphincter N35.919
- **Tilting vertebra** — *see* Dorsopathy, deforming, specified NEC
- **Timidity, child** F93.8
- **Tinea** (intersecta) (tarsi) B35.9
  - amiantacea L44.8
  - asbestina B35.Ø
  - barbae B35.Ø
  - beard B35.Ø
  - black dot B35.Ø
  - blanca B36.2
  - capitis B35.Ø
  - corporis B35.4
  - cruris B35.6
  - flava B36.Ø
  - foot B35.3
  - furfuracea B36.Ø
  - imbricata (Tokelau) B35.5
  - kerion B35.Ø
  - manuum B35.2
  - microsporic — *see* Dermatophytosis
  - nigra B36.1
  - nodosa — *see* Piedra
  - pedis B35.3
  - scalp B35.Ø
  - specified NEC B35.8
  - sycosis B35.Ø
  - tonsurans B35.Ø

Tinea — *continued*
trichophytic — *see* Dermatophytosis
unguium B35.1
versicolor B36.Ø
Tingling sensation (skin) R2Ø.2
Tin-miner's lung J63.5
Tinnitus NOS H93.1- ☑
audible H93.1- ☑
aurium H93.1- ☑
pulsatile H93.A- ☑
subjective H93.1- ☑
Tipped tooth (teeth) M26.33
Tipping
pelvis M95.5
with disproportion (fetopelvic) O33.Ø
causing obstructed labor O65.Ø
tooth (teeth), fully erupted M26.33
Tiredness R53.83
Tissue — *see* condition
Tobacco (nicotine)
abuse — *see* Tobacco, use
dependence — *see* Dependence, drug, nicotine
harmful use Z72.Ø
heart — *see* Tobacco, toxic effect
maternal use, affecting newborn PØ4.2
toxic effect — *see* Table of Drugs and Chemicals, by substance, poisoning
chewing tobacco — *see* Table of Drugs and Chemicals, by substance, poisoning
cigarettes — *see* Table of Drugs and Chemicals, by substance, poisoning
use Z72.Ø
complicating
childbirth O99.334
pregnancy O99.33- ☑
puerperium O99.335
counseling and surveillance Z71.6
history Z87.891
withdrawal state — *see also* Dependence, drug, nicotine F17.2Ø3
Tocopherol deficiency E56.Ø
Todd's
cirrhosis K74.3
paralysis (postepileptic) (transitory) G83.84
Toe — *see* condition
Toilet, artificial opening — *see* Attention to, artificial, opening
Tokelau (ringworm) B35.5
Tollwut — *see* Rabies
Tommaselli's disease R31.9
correct substance properly administered — *see* Table of Drugs and Chemicals, by drug, adverse effect
overdose or wrong substance given or taken — *see* Table of Drugs and Chemicals, by drug, poisoning
Tongue — *see also* condition
tie Q38.1
Tonic pupil — *see* Anomaly, pupil, function, tonic pupil
Toni-Fanconi syndrome (cystinosis) E72.Ø9
with cystinosis E72.Ø4
Tonsil — *see* condition
Tonsillitis (acute) (catarrhal) (croupous) (follicular) (gangrenous) (infective) (lacunar) (lingual) (malignant) (membranous) (parenchymatous) (phlegmonous) (pseudomembranous) (purulent) (septic) (subacute) (suppurative) (toxic) (ulcerative) (vesicular) (viral) JØ3.9Ø
chronic J35.Ø1
with adenoiditis J35.Ø3
diphtheritic A36.Ø
hypertrophic J35.Ø1
with adenoiditis J35.Ø3
recurrent JØ3.91
specified organism NEC JØ3.8Ø
recurrent JØ3.81
staphylococcal JØ3.8Ø
recurrent JØ3.81
streptococcal JØ3.ØØ
recurrent JØ3.Ø1
tuberculous A15.8
Vincent's A69.1
Tooth, teeth — *see* condition
Toothache KØ8.89
Topagnosis R2Ø.8
Tophi — *see* Gout, chronic
TORCH infection — *see* Infection, congenital
without active infection PØØ.2
Torn — *see* Tear
Tornwaldt's cyst or disease J39.2
Torsades de pointes I47.21
Torsion
accessory tube — *see* Torsion, fallopian tube
adnexa (female) — *see* Torsion, fallopian tube
aorta, acquired I77.1
appendix epididymis N44.Ø4
appendix testis N44.Ø3
bile duct (common) (hepatic) K83.8
congenital Q44.5
bowel, colon or intestine K56.2
cervix — *see* Malposition, uterus
cystic duct K82.8
dystonia — *see* Dystonia, torsion
epididymis (appendix) N44.Ø4
fallopian tube N83.52- ☑
with ovary N83.53
gallbladder K82.8
congenital Q44.1
hydatid of Morgagni
female N83.52- ☑
male N44.Ø3
kidney (pedicle) (leading to infarction) N28.Ø
Meckel's diverticulum (congenital) Q43.Ø
malignant — *see* Table of Neoplasms, small intestine, malignant
mesentery K56.2
omentum K56.2
organ or site, congenital NEC — *see* Anomaly, by site
ovary (pedicle) N83.51- ☑
with fallopian tube N83.53
congenital Q5Ø.2
oviduct — *see* Torsion, fallopian tube
penis (acquired) N48.82
congenital Q55.63
spasm — *see* Dystonia, torsion
spermatic cord N44.Ø2
extravaginal N44.Ø1
intravaginal N44.Ø2
spleen D73.5
testis, testicle N44.ØØ
appendix N44.Ø3
tibia — *see* Deformity, limb, specified type NEC, lower leg
uterus — *see* Malposition, uterus
Torticollis (intermittent) (spastic) M43.6
congenital (sternomastoid) Q68.Ø
due to birth injury P15.8
hysterical F44.4
ocular R29.891
psychogenic F45.8
conversion reaction F44.4
rheumatic M43.6
rheumatoid MØ6.88
spasmodic G24.3
traumatic, current S13.4 ☑
Tortipelvis G24.1
Tortuous
aortic arch Q25.46
artery I77.1
organ or site, congenital NEC — *see* Distortion
retinal vessel, congenital Q14.1
ureter N13.8
urethra N36.8
vein — *see* Varix
Torture, victim of Z65.4
Torula, torular (histolytica) (infection) — *see* Cryptococcosis
Torulosis — *see* Cryptococcosis
Torus (mandibularis) (palatinus) M27.Ø
fracture — *see* Fracture, by site, torus
Touraine's syndrome Q79.8
Tourette's syndrome F95.2
Tourniquet syndrome — *see* Constriction, external, by site
Tower skull Q75.Ø
with exophthalmos Q87.Ø
Toxemia R68.89
bacterial — *see* Sepsis
burn — *see* Burn
eclamptic (with pre-existing hypertension) — *see* Eclampsia
erysipelatous — *see* Erysipelas
fatigue R68.89
food — *see* Poisoning, food
gastrointestinal K52.1
intestinal K52.1
kidney — *see* Uremia
Toxemia — *continued*
malarial — *see* Malaria
myocardial — *see* Myocarditis, toxic
of pregnancy — *see* Pre-eclampsia
pre-eclamptic — *see* Pre-eclampsia
small intestine K52.1
staphylococcal, due to food AØ5.Ø
stasis R68.89
uremic — *see* Uremia
urinary — *see* Uremia
Toxemica cerebropathia psychica (nonalcoholic) FØ4
alcoholic — *see* Alcohol, amnestic disorder
Toxic (poisoning) — *see also* condition T65.91 ☑
effect — *see* Table of Drugs and Chemicals, by substance, poisoning
shock syndrome A48.3
thyroid (gland) — *see* Thyrotoxicosis
Toxicemia — *see* Toxemia
Toxicity — *see* Table of Drugs and Chemicals, by substance, poisoning
fava bean D55.Ø
food, noxious — *see* Poisoning, food
from drug or nonmedicinal substance — *see* Table of Drugs and Chemicals, by drug
Toxicosis — *see also* Toxemia
capillary, hemorrhagic D69.Ø
Toxinfection, gastrointestinal K52.1
Toxocariasis B83.Ø
Toxoplasma, toxoplasmosis (acquired) B58.9
with
hepatitis B58.1
meningoencephalitis B58.2
ocular involvement B58.ØØ
other organ involvement B58.89
pneumonia, pneumonitis B58.3
congenital (acute) (subacute) (chronic) P37.1
maternal, manifest toxoplasmosis in infant (acute) (subacute) (chronic) P37.1
tPA (rtPA) **administation in a different facility within the last 24 hours prior to admission to current facility** Z92.82
Trabeculation, bladder N32.89
Trachea — *see* condition
Tracheitis (catarrhal) (infantile) (membranous) (plastic) (septal) (suppurative) (viral) JØ4.1Ø
with
bronchitis (15 years of age and above) J4Ø
acute or subacute — *see* Bronchitis, acute
chronic J42
tuberculous NEC A15.5
under 15 years of age J2Ø.9
laryngitis (acute) JØ4.2
chronic J37.1
tuberculous NEC A15.5
acute JØ4.1Ø
with obstruction JØ4.11
chronic J42
with
bronchitis (chronic) J42
laryngitis (chronic) J37.1
diphtheritic (membranous) A36.89
due to external agent — *see* Inflammation, respiratory, upper, due to
syphilitic A52.73
tuberculous A15.5
Trachelitis (nonvenereal) — *see* Cervicitis
Tracheobronchial — *see* condition
Tracheobronchitis (15 years of age and above) — *see also* Bronchitis
due to
Bordetella bronchiseptica A37.8Ø
with pneumonia A37.81
Francisella tularensis A21.8
Tracheobronchomegaly Q32.4
with bronchiectasis J47.9
with
exacerbation (acute) J47.1
lower respiratory infection J47.Ø
acquired J98.Ø9
with bronchiectasis J47.9
with
exacerbation (acute) J47.1
lower respiratory infection J47.Ø
Tracheobronchopneumonitis — *see* Pneumonia, broncho-
Tracheocele (external) (internal) J39.8
congenital Q32.1
Tracheomalacia J39.8

- **Tracheomalacia** — *continued*
  - congenital Q32.Ø
- **Tracheopharyngitis** (acute) J06.9
  - chronic J42
  - due to external agent — *see* Inflammation, respiratory, upper, due to
- **Tracheostenosis** J39.8
- **Tracheostomy**
  - complication — *see* Complication, tracheostomy
  - status Z93.Ø
    - attention to Z43.Ø
    - malfunctioning J95.Ø3
- **Trachoma, trachomatous** A71.9
  - active (stage) A71.1
  - contraction of conjunctiva A71.1
  - dubium A71.Ø
  - healed or sequelae B94.Ø
  - initial (stage) A71.Ø
  - pannus A71.1
  - Türck's J37.Ø
- **Traction, vitreomacular** H43.82- ☑
- **Train sickness** T75.3 ☑
- **Trait**(s)
  - Hb-S D57.3
  - hemoglobin
    - abnormal NEC D58.2
      - with thalassemia D56.3
    - C — *see* Disease, hemoglobin C
    - S (Hb-S) D57.3
  - Lepore D56.3
  - personality, accentuated Z73.1
  - sickle-cell D57.3
    - with elliptocytosis or spherocytosis D57.3
  - type A personality Z73.1
- **Tramp** Z59.ØØ
- **Trance** R41.89
  - hysterical F44.89
- **Transaminasemia** R74.Ø1
- **Transection**
  - abdomen (partial) S38.3 ☑
  - aorta (incomplete) — *see also* Injury, aorta
    - complete — *see* Injury, aorta, laceration, major
  - carotid artery (incomplete) — *see also* Injury, blood vessel, carotid, laceration
    - complete — *see* Injury, blood vessel, carotid, laceration, major
  - celiac artery (incomplete) S35.211 ☑
    - branch (incomplete) S35.291 ☑
      - complete S35.292 ☑
    - complete S35.212 ☑
  - innominate
    - artery (incomplete) — *see also* Injury, blood vessel, thoracic, innominate, artery, laceration
      - complete — *see* Injury, blood vessel, thoracic, innominate, artery, laceration, major
    - vein (incomplete) — *see also* Injury, blood vessel, thoracic, innominate, vein, laceration
      - complete — *see* Injury, blood vessel, thoracic, innominate, vein, laceration, major
  - jugular vein (external) (incomplete) — *see also* Injury, blood vessel, jugular vein, laceration
    - complete — *see* Injury, blood vessel, jugular vein, laceration, major
    - internal (incomplete) — *see also* Injury, blood vessel, jugular vein, internal, laceration
      - complete — *see* Injury, blood vessel, jugular vein, internal, laceration, major
  - mesenteric artery (incomplete) — *see also* Injury, mesenteric, artery, laceration
    - complete — *see* Injury, mesenteric artery, laceration, major
  - pulmonary vessel (incomplete) — *see also* Injury, blood vessel, thoracic, pulmonary, laceration
    - complete — *see* Injury, blood vessel, thoracic, pulmonary, laceration, major
  - subclavian — *see* Transection, innominate
  - vena cava (incomplete) — *see also* Injury, vena cava
    - complete — *see* Injury, vena cava, laceration, major
  - vertebral artery (incomplete) — *see also* Injury, blood vessel, vertebral, laceration
    - complete — *see* Injury, blood vessel, vertebral, laceration, major
- **Transfusion**
  - associated (red blood cell) hemochromatosis E83.111
  - blood
    - ABO incompatible — *see* Complication(s), transfusion, incompatibility reaction, ABO
- **Transfusion** — *continued*
  - blood — *continued*
    - minor blood group (Duffy) (E) (K) (Kell) (Kidd) (Lewis) (M) (N) (P) (S) T8Ø.89 ☑
    - reaction or complication — *see* Complications, transfusion
  - fetomaternal (mother) — *see* Pregnancy, complicated by, placenta, transfusion syndrome
  - maternofetal (mother) — *see* Pregnancy, complicated by, placenta, transfusion syndrome
  - placental (syndrome) (mother) — *see* Pregnancy, complicated by, placenta, transfusion syndrome
  - reaction (adverse) — *see* Complications, transfusion
  - related acute lung injury (TRALI) J95.84
  - twin-to-twin — *see* Pregnancy, complicated by, placenta, transfusion syndrome, fetus to fetus
- **Transient** (meaning homeless) — *see also* condition Z59.ØØ
- **Translocation**
  - balanced autosomal Q95.9
    - in normal individual Q95.Ø
  - chromosomes NEC Q99.8
    - balanced and insertion in normal individual Q95.Ø
  - Down syndrome Q9Ø.2
  - trisomy
    - 13 Q91.6
    - 18 Q91.2
    - 21 Q9Ø.2
- **Translucency, iris** — *see* Degeneration, iris
- **Transmission of chemical substances through the placenta** — *see* Absorption, chemical, through placenta
- **Transparency, lung, unilateral** J43.Ø
- **Transplant** (ed) (status) Z94.9
  - awaiting organ Z76.82
  - bone Z94.6
    - marrow Z94.81
  - candidate Z76.82
  - complication — *see* Complication, transplant
  - cornea Z94.7
  - heart Z94.1
    - and lung(s) Z94.3
    - valve Z95.2
      - prosthetic Z95.2
      - specified NEC Z95.4
      - xenogenic Z95.3
  - intestine Z94.82
  - kidney Z94.Ø
  - liver Z94.4
  - lung(s) Z94.2
    - and heart Z94.3
  - organ (failure) (infection) (rejection) Z94.9
    - removal status Z98.85
  - pancreas Z94.83
  - skin Z94.5
  - social Z6Ø.3
  - specified organ or tissue NEC Z94.89
  - stem cells Z94.84
  - tissue Z94.9
- **Transplants, ovarian, endometrial** N8Ø.1Ø- ☑
- **Transposed** — *see* Transposition
- **Transposition** (congenital) — *see also* Malposition, congenital
  - abdominal viscera Q89.3
  - aorta (dextra) Q2Ø.3
  - appendix Q43.8
  - colon Q43.8
  - corrected Q2Ø.5
  - great vessels (complete) (partial) Q2Ø.3
  - heart Q24.Ø
    - with complete transposition of viscera Q89.3
  - intestine (large) (small) Q43.8
  - reversed jejunal (for bypass) (status) Z98.Ø
  - scrotum Q55.23
  - stomach Q4Ø.2
    - with general transposition of viscera Q89.3
  - tooth, teeth, fully erupted M26.3Ø
  - vessels, great (complete) (partial) Q2Ø.3
  - viscera (abdominal) (thoracic) Q89.3
- **Transsexualism** F64.Ø
- **Transverse** — *see also* condition
  - arrest (deep), in labor O64.Ø ☑
  - lie (mother) O32.2 ☑
    - causing obstructed labor O64.8 ☑
- **Transvestism, transvestitism** (dual-role) F64.1
  - fetishistic F65.1
- **Trapped placenta** (with hemorrhage) O72.Ø
  - without hemorrhage O73.Ø
- **TRAPS** (tumor necrosis factor receptor associated periodic syndrome) MØ4.1
- **Trauma, traumatism** — *see also* Injury
  - acoustic — *see* subcategory H83.3 ☑
  - birth — *see* Birth, injury
  - complicating ectopic or molar pregnancy OØ8.6
  - during delivery O71.9
  - following ectopic or molar pregnancy OØ8.6
  - obstetric O71.9
    - specified NEC O71.89
  - occusal
    - primary KØ8.81
    - secondary KØ8.82
- **Traumatic** — *see also* condition
  - brain injury SØ6.9 ☑
- **Treacher Collins syndrome** Q75.4
- **Treitz's hernia** — *see* Hernia, abdomen, specified site NEC
- **Trematode infestation** — *see* Infestation, fluke
- **Trematodiasis** — *see* Infestation, fluke
- **Trembling paralysis** — *see* Parkinsonism
- **Tremor(s)** R25.1
  - drug induced G25.1
  - essential (benign) G25.Ø
  - familial G25.Ø
  - hereditary G25.Ø
  - hysterical F44.4
  - intention G25.2
  - medication induced postural G25.1
  - mercurial — *see* subcategory T56.1 ☑
  - Parkinson's — *see* Parkinsonism
  - psychogenic (conversion reaction) F44.4
  - senilis R54
  - specified type NEC G25.2
- **Trench**
  - fever A79.Ø
  - foot — *see* Immersion, foot
  - mouth A69.1
- **Treponema pallidum infection** — *see* Syphilis
- **Treponematosis**
  - due to
    - T. pallidum — *see* Syphilis
    - T. pertenue — *see* Yaws
- **Triad**
  - Hutchinson's (congenital syphilis) A5Ø.53
  - Kartagener's Q89.3
  - Saint's — *see* Hernia, diaphragm
- **Trichiasis** (eyelid) HØ2.Ø59
  - with entropion — *see* Entropion
  - left HØ2.Ø56
    - lower HØ2.Ø55
    - upper HØ2.Ø54
  - right HØ2.Ø53
    - lower HØ2.Ø52
    - upper HØ2.Ø51
- **Trichinella spiralis** (infection) (infestation) B75
- **Trichinellosis, trichiniasis, trichinelliasis, trichinosis** B75
  - with muscle disorder B75 *[M63.8Ø]*
    - ankle B75 *[M63.87-]* ☑
    - foot B75 *[M63.87-]* ☑
    - forearm B75 *[M63.83-]* ☑
    - hand B75 *[M63.84-]* ☑
    - lower leg B75 *[M63.86-]* ☑
    - multiple sites B75 *[M63.89]*
    - pelvic region B75 *[M63.85-]* ☑
    - shoulder region B75 *[M63.81-]* ☑
    - specified site NEC B75 *[M63.88]*
    - thigh B75 *[M63.85-]* ☑
    - upper arm B75 *[M63.82-]* ☑
- **Trichobezoar** T18.9 ☑
  - intestine T18.3 ☑
  - stomach T18.2 ☑
- **Trichocephaliasis, trichocephalosis** B79
- **Trichocephalus infestation** B79
- **Trichoclasis** L67.8
- **Trichoepithelioma** — *see also* Neoplasm, skin, benign
  - malignant — *see* Neoplasm, skin, malignant
- **Trichofolliculoma** — *see* Neoplasm, skin, benign
- **Tricholemmoma** — *see* Neoplasm, skin, benign
- **Trichomoniasis** A59.9
  - bladder A59.Ø3
  - cervix A59.Ø9
  - intestinal AØ7.8
  - prostate A59.Ø2
  - seminal vesicles A59.Ø9
  - specified site NEC A59.8

Trichomoniasis — *continued*
urethra A59.03
urogenitalis A59.00
vagina A59.01
vulva A59.01
Trichomycosis
axillaris A48.8
nodosa, nodularis B36.8
Trichonodosis L67.8
Trichophytid, trichophyton infection — *see* Dermatophytosis
Trichophytobezoar T18.9 ☑
intestine T18.3 ☑
stomach T18.2 ☑
Trichophytosis — *see* Dermatophytosis
Trichoptilosis L67.8
Trichorrhexis (nodosa) (invaginata) L67.0
Trichosis axillaris A48.8
Trichosporosis nodosa B36.2
Trichostasis spinulosa (congenital) Q84.1
Trichostrongyliasis, trichostrongylosis (small intestine) B81.2
Trichostrongylus infection B81.2
Trichotillomania F63.3
Trichromat, trichromatopsia, anomalous (congenital) H53.55
Trichuriasis B79
Trichuris trichiura (infection) (infestation) (any site) B79
Tricuspid (valve) — *see* condition
Trifid — *see also* Accessory
kidney (pelvis) Q63.8
tongue Q38.3
Trigeminal neuralgia — *see* Neuralgia, trigeminal
Trigeminy R00.8
Trigger finger (acquired) M65.30
congenital Q74.0
index finger M65.32- ☑
little finger M65.35- ☑
middle finger M65.33- ☑
ring finger M65.34- ☑
thumb M65.31- ☑
Trigonitis (bladder) (chronic) (pseudomembranous) N30.30
with hematuria N30.31
Trigonocephaly Q75.0
Trilocular heart — *see* Cor triloculare
Trimethylaminuria E72.52
Tripartite placenta O43.19- ☑
Triphalangeal thumb Q74.0
Triple — *see also* Accessory
kidneys Q63.0
uteri Q51.818
X, female Q97.0
Triple I O41.12- ☑
Triplegia G83.89
congenital G80.8
Triplet (newborn) — *see also* Newborn, triplet
complicating pregnancy — *see* Pregnancy, triplet
Triplication — *see* Accessory
Triploidy Q92.7
Trismus R25.2
neonatorum A33
newborn A33
Trisomy (syndrome) Q92.9
13 (partial) Q91.7
meiotic nondisjunction Q91.4
mitotic nondisjunction Q91.5
mosaicism Q91.5
translocation Q91.6
18 (partial) Q91.3
meiotic nondisjunction Q91.0
mitotic nondisjunction Q91.1
mosaicism Q91.1
translocation Q91.2
20 Q92.8
21 (partial) Q90.9
meiotic nondisjunction Q90.0
mitotic nondisjunction Q90.1
mosaicism Q90.1
translocation Q90.2
22 Q92.8
autosomes Q92.9
chromosome specified NEC Q92.8
partial Q92.2
due to unbalanced translocation Q92.5
specified NEC Q92.8
Trisomy — *continued*
chromosome specified — *continued*
whole (nonsex chromosome)
meiotic nondisjunction Q92.0
mitotic nondisjunction Q92.1
mosaicism Q92.1
due to
dicentrics — *see* Extra, marker chromosomes
extra rings — *see* Extra, marker chromosomes
isochromosomes — *see* Extra, marker chromosomes
specified NEC Q92.8
whole chromosome Q92.9
meiotic nondisjunction Q92.0
mitotic nondisjunction Q92.1
mosaicism Q92.1
partial Q92.9
specified NEC Q92.8
Tritanomaly, tritanopia H53.55
Trombiculosis, trombiculiasis, trombidiosis B88.0
Trophedema (congenital) (hereditary) Q82.0
Trophoblastic disease — *see also* Mole, hydatidiform O01.9
Tropholymphedema Q82.0
Trophoneurosis NEC G96.89
disseminated M34.9
Tropical — *see* condition
Trouble — *see also* Disease
heart — *see* Disease, heart
kidney — *see* Disease, renal
nervous R45.0
sinus — *see* Sinusitis
Trousseau's syndrome (thrombophlebitis migrans) I82.1
Truancy, childhood
from school Z72.810
Truncus
arteriosus (persistent) Q20.0
communis Q20.0
Trunk — *see* condition
Trypanosomiasis
African B56.9
by Trypanosoma brucei
gambiense B56.0
rhodesiense B56.1
American — *see* Chagas' disease
Brazilian — *see* Chagas' disease
by Trypanosoma
brucei gambiense B56.0
brucei rhodesiense B56.1
cruzi — *see* Chagas' disease
gambiensis, Gambian B56.0
rhodesiensis, Rhodesian B56.1
South American — *see* Chagas' disease
where
African trypanosomiasis is prevalent B56.9
Chagas' disease is prevalent B57.2
Tryptasemia, hereditary alpha D89.44
T-shaped incisors K00.2
Tsutsugamushi (disease) (fever) A75.3
Tube, tubal, tubular — *see* condition
Tubercle — *see also* Tuberculosis
brain, solitary A17.81
Darwin's Q17.8
Ghon, primary infection A15.7
Tuberculid, tuberculide (indurating, subcutaneous) (lichenoid) (miliary) (papulonecrotic) (primary) (skin) A18.4
Tuberculoma — *see also* Tuberculosis
brain A17.81
meninges (cerebral) (spinal) A17.1
spinal cord A17.81
Tuberculosis, tubercular, tuberculous (calcification) (calcified) (caseous) (chromogenic acid-fast bacilli) (degeneration) (fibrocaseous) (fistula) (interstitial) (isolated circumscribed lesions) (necrosis) (parenchymatous) (ulcerative) A15.9
with pneumoconiosis (any condition in J60-J64) J65
abdomen (lymph gland) A18.39
abscess (respiratory) A15.9
bone A18.03
hip A18.02
knee A18.02
sacrum A18.01
specified site NEC A18.03
spinal A18.01
vertebra A18.01
brain A17.81
breast A18.89
Cowper's gland A18.15
Tuberculosis, tubercular, tuberculous — *continued*
abscess — *continued*
dura (mater) (cerebral) (spinal) A17.81
epidural (cerebral) (spinal) A17.81
female pelvis A18.17
frontal sinus A15.8
genital organs NEC A18.10
genitourinary A18.10
gland (lymphatic) — *see* Tuberculosis, lymph gland
hip A18.02
intestine A18.32
ischiorectal A18.32
joint NEC A18.02
hip A18.02
knee A18.02
specified NEC A18.02
vertebral A18.01
kidney A18.11
knee A18.02
latent Z22.7
lumbar (spine) A18.01
lung — *see* Tuberculosis, pulmonary
meninges (cerebral) (spinal) A17.0
muscle A18.09
perianal (fistula) A18.32
perinephritic A18.11
perirectal A18.32
rectum A18.32
retropharyngeal A15.8
sacrum A18.01
scrofulous A18.2
scrotum A18.15
skin (primary) A18.4
spinal cord A17.81
spine or vertebra (column) A18.01
subdiaphragmatic A18.31
testis A18.15
urinary A18.13
uterus A18.17
accessory sinus — *see* Tuberculosis, sinus
Addison's disease A18.7
adenitis — *see* Tuberculosis, lymph gland
adenoids A15.8
adenopathy — *see* Tuberculosis, lymph gland
adherent pericardium A18.84
adnexa (uteri) A18.17
adrenal (capsule) (gland) A18.7
alimentary canal A18.32
anemia A18.89
ankle (joint) (bone) A18.02
anus A18.32
apex, apical — *see* Tuberculosis, pulmonary
appendicitis, appendix A18.32
arachnoid A17.0
artery, arteritis A18.89
cerebral A18.89
arthritis (chronic) (synovial) A18.02
spine or vertebra (column) A18.01
articular — *see* Tuberculosis, joint
ascites A18.31
asthma — *see* Tuberculosis, pulmonary
axilla, axillary (gland) A18.2
bladder A18.12
bone A18.03
hip A18.02
knee A18.02
limb NEC A18.03
sacrum A18.01
spine or vertebral column A18.01
bowel (miliary) A18.32
brain A17.81
breast A18.89
broad ligament A18.17
bronchi, bronchial, bronchus A15.5
ectasia, ectasis (bronchiectasis) — *see* Tuberculosis, pulmonary
fistula A15.5
primary (progressive) A15.7
gland or node A15.4
primary (progressive) A15.7
lymph gland or node A15.4
primary (progressive) A15.7
bronchiectasis — *see* Tuberculosis, pulmonary
bronchitis A15.5
bronchopleural A15.6
bronchopneumonia, bronchopneumonic — *see* Tuberculosis, pulmonary
bronchorrhagia A15.5

Tuberculosis, tubercular, tuberculous — *continued*
bronchotracheal A15.5
bronze disease A18.7
buccal cavity A18.83
bulbourethral gland A18.15
bursa A18.Ø9
cachexia A15.9
cardiomyopathy A18.84
caries — *see* Tuberculosis, bone
cartilage A18.Ø2
intervertebral A18.Ø1
catarrhal — *see* Tuberculosis, respiratory
cecum A18.32
cellulitis (primary) A18.4
cerebellum A17.81
cerebral, cerebrum A17.81
cerebrospinal A17.81
meninges A17.Ø
cervical (lymph gland or node) A18.2
cervicitis, cervix (uteri) A18.16
chest — *see* Tuberculosis, respiratory
chorioretinitis A18.53
choroid, choroiditis A18.53
ciliary body A18.54
colitis A18.32
collier's J65
colliquativa (primary) A18.4
colon A18.32
complex, primary A15.7
congenital P37.Ø
conjunctiva A18.59
connective tissue (systemic) A18.89
contact Z2Ø.1
cornea (ulcer) A18.52
Cowper's gland A18.15
coxae A18.Ø2
coxalgia A18.Ø2
cul-de-sac of Douglas A18.17
curvature, spine A18.Ø1
cutis (colliquativa) (primary) A18.4
cyst, ovary A18.18
cystitis A18.12
dactylitis A18.Ø3
diarrhea A18.32
diffuse — *see* Tuberculosis, miliary
digestive tract A18.32
disseminated — *see* Tuberculosis, miliary
duodenum A18.32
dura (mater) (cerebral) (spinal) A17.Ø
abscess (cerebral) (spinal) A17.81
dysentery A18.32
ear (inner) (middle) A18.6
bone A18.Ø3
external (primary) A18.4
skin (primary) A18.4
elbow A18.Ø2
emphysema — *see* Tuberculosis, pulmonary
empyema A15.6
encephalitis A17.82
endarteritis A18.89
endocarditis A18.84
aortic A18.84
mitral A18.84
pulmonary A18.84
tricuspid A18.84
endocrine glands NEC A18.82
endometrium A18.17
enteric, enterica, enteritis A18.32
enterocolitis A18.32
epididymis, epididymitis A18.15
epidural abscess (cerebral) (spinal) A17.81
epiglottis A15.5
episcleritis A18.51
erythema (induratum) (nodosum) (primary) A18.4
esophagus A18.83
eustachian tube A18.6
exposure (to) Z2Ø.1
exudative — *see* Tuberculosis, pulmonary
eye A18.5Ø
eyelid (primary) (lupus) A18.4
fallopian tube (acute) (chronic) A18.17
fascia A18.Ø9
fauces A15.8
female pelvic inflammatory disease A18.17
finger A18.Ø3
first infection A15.7
gallbladder A18.83
ganglion A18.Ø9

Tuberculosis, tubercular, tuberculous — *continued*
gastritis A18.83
gastrocolic fistula A18.32
gastroenteritis A18.32
gastrointestinal tract A18.32
general, generalized — *see* Tuberculosis, miliary
genital organs A18.1Ø
genitourinary A18.1Ø
genu A18.Ø2
glandula suprarenalis A18.7
glandular, general A18.2
glottis A15.5
grinder's J65
gum A18.83
hand A18.Ø3
heart A18.84
hematogenous — *see* Tuberculosis, miliary
hemoptysis — *see* Tuberculosis, pulmonary
hemorrhage NEC — *see* Tuberculosis, pulmonary
hemothorax A15.6
hepatitis A18.83
hilar lymph nodes A15.4
primary (progressive) A15.7
hip (joint) (disease) (bone) A18.Ø2
hydropneumothorax A15.6
hydrothorax A15.6
hypoadrenalism A18.7
hypopharynx A15.8
ileocecal (hyperplastic) A18.32
ileocolitis A18.32
ileum A18.32
iliac spine (superior) A18.Ø3
immunological findings only A15.7
indurativa (primary) A18.4
infantile A15.7
infection A15.9
without clinical manifestations A15.7
infraclavicular gland A18.2
inguinal gland A18.2
inguinalis A18.2
intestine (any part) A18.32
iridocyclitis A18.54
iris, iritis A18.54
ischiorectal A18.32
jaw A18.Ø3
jejunum A18.32
joint A18.Ø2
vertebral A18.Ø1
keratitis (interstitial) A18.52
keratoconjunctivitis A18.52
kidney A18.11
knee (joint) A18.Ø2
kyphosis, kyphoscoliosis A18.Ø1
laryngitis A15.5
larynx A15.5
latent Z22.7
leptomeninges, leptomeningitis (cerebral) (spinal) A17.Ø
lichenoides (primary) A18.4
linguae A18.83
lip A18.83
liver A18.83
lordosis A18.Ø1
lung — *see* Tuberculosis, pulmonary
lupus vulgaris A18.4
lymph gland or node (peripheral) A18.2
abdomen A18.39
bronchial A15.4
primary (progressive) A15.7
cervical A18.2
hilar A15.4
primary (progressive) A15.7
intrathoracic A15.4
primary (progressive) A15.7
mediastinal A15.4
primary (progressive) A15.7
mesenteric A18.39
retroperitoneal A18.39
tracheobronchial A15.4
primary (progressive) A15.7
lymphadenitis — *see* Tuberculosis, lymph gland
lymphangitis — *see* Tuberculosis, lymph gland
lymphatic (gland) (vessel) — *see* Tuberculosis, lymph gland
mammary gland A18.89
marasmus A15.9
mastoiditis A18.Ø3
mediastinal lymph gland or node A15.4

Tuberculosis, tubercular, tuberculous — *continued*
mediastinal lymph gland or node — *continued*
primary (progressive) A15.7
mediastinitis A15.8
primary (progressive) A15.7
mediastinum A15.8
primary (progressive) A15.7
medulla A17.81
melanosis, Addisonian A18.7
meninges, meningitis (basilar) (cerebral) (cerebrospinal) (spinal) A17.Ø
meningoencephalitis A17.82
mesentery, mesenteric (gland or node) A18.39
miliary A19.9
acute A19.2
multiple sites A19.1
single specified site A19.Ø
chronic A19.8
specified NEC A19.8
millstone makers' J65
miner's J65
molder's J65
mouth A18.83
multiple A19.9
acute A19.1
chronic A19.8
muscle A18.Ø9
myelitis A17.82
myocardium, myocarditis A18.84
nasal (passage) (sinus) A15.8
nasopharynx A15.8
neck gland A18.2
nephritis A18.11
nerve (mononeuropathy) A17.83
nervous system A17.9
nose (septum) A15.8
ocular A18.5Ø
omentum A18.31
oophoritis (acute) (chronic) A18.17
optic (nerve trunk) (papilla) A18.59
orbit A18.59
orchitis A18.15
organ, specified NEC A18.89
osseous — *see* Tuberculosis, bone
osteitis — *see* Tuberculosis, bone
osteomyelitis — *see* Tuberculosis, bone
otitis media A18.6
ovary, ovaritis (acute) (chronic) A18.17
oviduct (acute) (chronic) A18.17
pachymeningitis A17.Ø
palate (soft) A18.83
pancreas A18.83
papulonecrotic (a) (primary) A18.4
parathyroid glands A18.82
paronychia (primary) A18.4
parotid gland or region A18.83
pelvis (bony) A18.Ø3
penis A18.15
peribronchitis A15.5
pericardium, pericarditis A18.84
perichondritis, larynx A15.5
periostitis — *see* Tuberculosis, bone
perirectal fistula A18.32
peritoneum NEC A18.31
peritonitis A18.31
pharynx, pharyngitis A15.8
phlyctenulosis (keratoconjunctivitis) A18.52
phthisis NEC — *see* Tuberculosis, pulmonary
pituitary gland A18.82
pleura, pleural, pleurisy, pleuritis (fibrinous) (obliterative) (purulent) (simple plastic) (with effusion) A15.6
primary (progressive) A15.7
pneumonia, pneumonic — *see* Tuberculosis, pulmonary
pneumothorax (spontaneous) (tense valvular) — *see* Tuberculosis, pulmonary
polyneuropathy A17.89
polyserositis A19.9
acute A19.1
chronic A19.8
potter's J65
prepuce A18.15
primary (complex) A15.7
proctitis A18.32
prostate, prostatitis A18.14
pulmonalis — *see* Tuberculosis, pulmonary

Tuberculosis, tubercular, tuberculous — *continued*
pulmonary (cavitated) (fibrotic) (infiltrative) (nodular) A15.Ø
childhood type or first infection A15.7
primary (complex) A15.7
pyelitis A18.11
pyelonephritis A18.11
pyemia — *see* Tuberculosis, miliary
pyonephrosis A18.11
pyopneumothorax A15.6
pyothorax A15.6
rectum (fistula) (with abscess) A18.32
reinfection stage — *see* Tuberculosis, pulmonary
renal A18.11
renis A18.11
respiratory A15.9
primary A15.7
specified site NEC A15.8
retina, retinitis A18.53
retroperitoneal (lymph gland or node) A18.39
rheumatism NEC A18.Ø9
rhinitis A15.8
sacroiliac (joint) A18.Ø1
sacrum A18.Ø1
salivary gland A18.83
salpingitis (acute) (chronic) A18.17
sandblaster's J65
sclera A18.51
scoliosis A18.Ø1
scrofulous A18.2
scrotum A18.15
seminal tract or vesicle A18.15
senile A15.9
septic — *see* Tuberculosis, miliary
shoulder (joint) A18.Ø2
blade A18.Ø3
sigmoid A18.32
sinus (any nasal) A15.8
bone A18.Ø3
epididymis A18.15
skeletal NEC A18.Ø3
skin (any site) (primary) A18.4
small intestine A18.32
soft palate A18.83
spermatic cord A18.15
spine, spinal (column) A18.Ø1
cord A17.81
medulla A17.81
membrane A17.Ø
meninges A17.Ø
spleen, splenitis A18.85
spondylitis A18.Ø1
sternoclavicular joint A18.Ø2
stomach A18.83
stonemason's J65
subcutaneous tissue (cellular) (primary) A18.4
subcutis (primary) A18.4
subdeltoid bursa A18.83
submaxillary (region) A18.83
supraclavicular gland A18.2
suprarenal (capsule) (gland) A18.7
swelling, joint (*see also* category MØ1) — *see also* Tuberculosis, joint A18.Ø2
symphysis pubis A18.Ø2
synovitis A18.Ø9
articular A18.Ø2
spine or vertebra A18.Ø1
systemic — *see* Tuberculosis, miliary
tarsitis A18.4
tendon (sheath) — *see* Tuberculosis, tenosynovitis
tenosynovitis A18.Ø9
spine or vertebra A18.Ø1
testis A18.15
throat A15.8
thymus gland A18.82
thyroid gland A18.81
tongue A18.83
tonsil, tonsillitis A15.8
trachea, tracheal A15.5
lymph gland or node A15.4
primary (progressive) A15.7
tracheobronchial A15.5
lymph gland or node A15.4
primary (progressive) A15.7
tubal (acute) (chronic) A18.17
tunica vaginalis A18.15
ulcer (skin) (primary) A18.4
bowel or intestine A18.32

Tuberculosis, tubercular, tuberculous — *continued*
ulcer — *continued*
specified NEC — *see* Tuberculosis, by site
unspecified site A15.9
ureter A18.11
urethra, urethral (gland) A18.13
urinary organ or tract A18.13
uterus A18.17
uveal tract A18.54
uvula A18.83
vagina A18.18
vas deferens A18.15
verruca, verrucosa (cutis) (primary) A18.4
vertebra (column) A18.Ø1
vesiculitis A18.15
vulva A18.18
wrist (joint) A18.Ø2
Tuberculum
Carabelli — *see* Excludes Note at KØØ.2
occlusal — *see* Excludes Note at KØØ.2
paramolare KØØ.2
Tuberosity, enitre maxillary M26.Ø7
Tuberous sclerosis (brain) Q85.1
Tubo-ovarian — *see* condition
Tuboplasty, after previous sterilization Z31.Ø
aftercare Z31.42
Tubotympanitis, catarrhal (chronic) — *see* Otitis, media, nonsuppurative, chronic, serous
Tularemia A21.9
with
conjunctivitis A21.1
pneumonia A21.2
abdominal A21.3
bronchopneumonic A21.2
conjunctivitis A21.1
cryptogenic A21.3
enteric A21.3
gastrointestinal A21.3
generalized A21.7
ingestion A21.3
intestinal A21.3
oculoglandular A21.1
ophthalmic A21.1
pneumonia (any), pneumonic A21.2
pulmonary A21.2
sepsis A21.7
specified NEC A21.8
typhoidal A21.7
ulceroglandular A21.Ø
Tularensis conjunctivitis A21.1
Tumefaction — *see also* Swelling
liver — *see* Hypertrophy, liver
Tumor — *see also* Neoplasm, unspecified behavior, by site
acinar cell — *see* Neoplasm, uncertain behavior, by site
acinic cell — *see* Neoplasm, uncertain behavior, by site
adenocarcinoid — *see* Neoplasm, malignant, by site
adenomatoid — *see also* Neoplasm, benign, by site
odontogenic — *see* Cyst, calcifying odontogenic
adnexal (skin) — *see* Neoplasm, skin, benign, by site
adrenal
cortical (benign) D35.Ø- ☑
malignant C74.Ø- ☑
rest — *see* Neoplasm, benign, by site
alpha-cell
malignant
pancreas C25.4
specified site NEC — *see* Neoplasm, malignant, by site
unspecified site C25.4
pancreas D13.7
specified site NEC — *see* Neoplasm, benign, by site
unspecified site D13.7
aneurysmal — *see* Aneurysm
aortic body D44.7
malignant C75.5
Askin's — *see* Neoplasm, connective tissue, malignant
basal cell — *see also* Neoplasm, skin, uncertain behavior D48.5
Bednar — *see* Neoplasm, skin, malignant
benign (unclassified) — *see* Neoplasm, benign, by site
beta-cell
malignant
pancreas C25.4
specified site NEC — *see* Neoplasm, malignant, by site
unspecified site C25.4
pancreas D13.7

Tumor — *continued*
beta-cell — *continued*
specified site NEC — *see* Neoplasm, benign, by site
unspecified site D13.7
Brenner D27.9
borderline malignancy D39.1- ☑
malignant C56- ☑
proliferating D39.1- ☑
bronchial alveolar, intravascular D38.1
Brooke's — *see* Neoplasm, skin, benign
brown fat — *see* Lipoma
Burkitt — *see* Lymphoma, Burkitt
calcifying epithelial odontogenic — *see* Cyst, calcifying odontogenic
carcinoid D3A.ØØ (*following* D36)
benign D3A.ØØ (*following* D36)
appendix D3A.Ø2Ø (*following* D36)
ascending colon D3A.Ø22 (*following* D36)
bronchus (lung) D3A.Ø9Ø (*following* D36)
cecum D3A.Ø21 (*following* D36)
colon D3A.Ø29 (*following* D36)
descending colon D3A.Ø24 (*following* D36)
duodenum D3A.Ø1Ø (*following* D36)
foregut NOS D3A.Ø94 (*following* D36)
hindgut NOS D3A.Ø96 (*following* D36)
ileum D3A.Ø12 (*following* D36)
jejunum D3A.Ø11 (*following* D36)
kidney D3A.Ø93 (*following* D36)
large intestine D3A.Ø29 (*following* D36)
lung (bronchus) D3A.Ø9Ø (*following* D36)
midgut NOS D3A.Ø95 (*following* D36)
rectum D3A.Ø26 (*following* D36)
sigmoid colon D3A.Ø25 (*following* D36)
small intestine D3A.Ø19 (*following* D36)
specified NEC D3A.Ø98 (*following* D36)
stomach D3A.Ø92 (*following* D36)
thymus D3A.Ø91 (*following* D36)
transverse colon D3A.Ø23 (*following* D36)
malignant C7A.ØØ (*following* C75)
appendix C7A.Ø2Ø (*following* C75)
ascending colon C7A.Ø22 (*following* C75)
bronchus (lung) C7A.Ø9Ø (*following* C75)
cecum C7A.Ø21 (*following* C75)
colon C7A.Ø29 (*following* C75)
descending colon C7A.Ø24 (*following* C75)
duodenum C7A.Ø1Ø (*following* C75)
foregut NOS C7A.Ø94 (*following* C75)
hindgut NOS C7A.Ø96 (*following* C75)
ileum C7A.Ø12 (*following* C75)
jejunum C7A.Ø11 (*following* C75)
kidney C7A.Ø93 (*following* C75)
large intestine C7A.Ø29 (*following* C75)
lung (bronchus) C7A.Ø9Ø (*following* C75)
midgut NOS C7A.Ø95 (*following* C75)
rectum C7A.Ø26 (*following* C75)
sigmoid colon C7A.Ø25 (*following* C75)
small intestine C7A.Ø19 (*following* C75)
specified NEC C7A.Ø98 (*following* C75)
stomach C7A.Ø92 (*following* C75)
thymus C7A.Ø91 (*following* C75)
transverse colon C7A.Ø23 (*following* C75)
mesentary metastasis C7B.Ø4 (*following* C75)
secondary C7B.ØØ (*following* C75)
bone C7B.Ø3 (*following* C75)
distant lymph nodes C7B.Ø1 (*following* C75)
liver C7B.Ø2 (*following* C75)
peritoneum C7B.Ø4 (*following* C75)
specified NEC C7B.Ø9 (*following* C75)
carotid body D44.6
malignant C75.4
cells — *see also* Neoplasm, unspecified behavior, by site
benign — *see* Neoplasm, benign, by site
malignant — *see* Neoplasm, malignant, by site
uncertain whether benign or malignant — *see* Neoplasm, uncertain behavior, by site
cervix, in pregnancy or childbirth — *see* Pregnancy, complicated by, tumor, cervix
chondromatous giant cell — *see* Neoplasm, bone, benign
chromaffin — *see also* Neoplasm, benign, by site
malignant — *see* Neoplasm, malignant, by site
Cock's peculiar L72.3
Codman's — *see* Neoplasm, bone, benign
dentigerous, mixed — *see* Cyst, calcifying odontogenic
dermoid — *see* Neoplasm, benign, by site
with malignant transformation C56- ☑

Tumor — *continued*
- desmoid (extra-abdominal) — *see also* Neoplasm, connective tissue, uncertain behavior
  - abdominal — *see* Neoplasm, connective tissue, uncertain behavior
- embolus — *see* Neoplasm, secondary, by site
- embryonal (mixed) — *see also* Neoplasm, uncertain behavior, by site
  - liver C22.7
- endodermal sinus
  - specified site — *see* Neoplasm, malignant, by site
  - unspecified site
    - female C56.- ☑
    - male C62.9Ø
- epithelial
  - benign — *see* Neoplasm, benign, by site
  - malignant — *see* Neoplasm, malignant, by site
- Ewing's — *see* Neoplasm, bone, malignant, by site
- fatty — *see* Lipoma
- fibroid — *see* Leiomyoma
- G cell
  - malignant
    - pancreas C25.4
    - specified site NEC — *see* Neoplasm, malignant, by site
    - unspecified site C25.4
  - specified site — *see* Neoplasm, uncertain behavior, by site
  - unspecified site D37.8
- germ cell — *see also* Neoplasm, malignant, by site
  - mixed — *see* Neoplasm, malignant, by site
- ghost cell, odontogenic — *see* Cyst, calcifying odontogenic
- giant cell — *see also* Neoplasm, uncertain behavior, by site
  - bone D48.Ø
    - malignant — *see* Neoplasm, bone, malignant
  - chondromatous — *see* Neoplasm, bone, benign
  - malignant — *see* Neoplasm, malignant, by site
  - soft parts — *see* Neoplasm, connective tissue, uncertain behavior
    - malignant — *see* Neoplasm, connective tissue, malignant
- glomus D18.ØØ
  - intra-abdominal D18.Ø3
  - intracranial D18.Ø2
  - jugulare D44.7
    - malignant C75.5
  - skin D18.Ø1
  - specified site NEC D18.Ø9
- gonadal stromal — *see* Neoplasm, uncertain behavior, by site
- granular cell — *see also* Neoplasm, connective tissue, benign
  - malignant — *see* Neoplasm, connective tissue, malignant
- granulosa cell D39.1- ☑
  - juvenile D39.1- ☑
  - malignant C56- ☑
- granulosa cell-theca cell D39.1- ☑
  - malignant C56- ☑
- Grawitz's C64- ☑
- hemorrhoidal — *see* Hemorrhoids
- hilar cell D27- ☑
- hilus cell D27- ☑
- Hurthle cell (benign) D34
  - malignant C73
- hydatid — *see* Echinococcus
- hypernephroid — *see also* Neoplasm, uncertain behavior, by site
- interstitial cell — *see also* Neoplasm, uncertain behavior, by site
  - benign — *see* Neoplasm, benign, by site
  - malignant — *see* Neoplasm, malignant, by site
- intravascular bronchial alveolar D38.1
- islet cell — *see* Neoplasm, benign, by site
  - malignant — *see* Neoplasm, malignant, by site
    - pancreas C25.4
    - specified site NEC — *see* Neoplasm, malignant, by site
    - unspecified site C25.4
  - pancreas D13.7
  - specified site NEC — *see* Neoplasm, benign, by site
  - unspecified site D13.7
- juxtaglomerular D41.Ø- ☑
- Klatskin's C22.1
- Krukenberg's C79.6- ☑

Tumor — *continued*
- Leydig cell — *see* Neoplasm, uncertain behavior, by site
  - benign — *see* Neoplasm, benign, by site
    - specified site — *see* Neoplasm, benign, by site
    - unspecified site
      - female D27.9
      - male D29.2Ø
  - malignant — *see* Neoplasm, malignant, by site
    - specified site — *see* Neoplasm, malignant, by site
    - unspecified site
      - female C56.9
      - male C62.9Ø
  - specified site — *see* Neoplasm, uncertain behavior, by site
  - unspecified site
    - female D39.1Ø
    - male D4Ø.1Ø
- lipid cell, ovary D27- ☑
- lipoid cell, ovary D27- ☑
- malignant — *see also* Neoplasm, malignant, by site C8Ø.1
  - fusiform cell (type) C8Ø.1
  - giant cell (type) C8Ø.1
  - localized, plasma cell — *see* Plasmacytoma, solitary
  - mixed NEC C8Ø.1
  - small cell (type) C8Ø.1
  - spindle cell (type) C8Ø.1
  - unclassified C8Ø.1
- mast cell D47.Ø9
- melanotic, neuroectodermal — *see* Neoplasm, benign, by site
- Merkel cell — *see* Carcinoma, Merkel cell
- mesenchymal
  - malignant — *see* Neoplasm, connective tissue, malignant
  - mixed — *see* Neoplasm, connective tissue, uncertain behavior
- mesodermal, mixed — *see also* Neoplasm, malignant, by site
  - liver C22.4
- mesonephric — *see also* Neoplasm, uncertain behavior, by site
  - malignant — *see* Neoplasm, malignant, by site
- metastatic
  - from specified site — *see* Neoplasm, malignant, by site
  - of specified site — *see* Neoplasm, malignant, by site
  - to specified site — *see* Neoplasm, secondary, by site
- mixed NEC — *see also* Neoplasm, benign, by site
  - malignant — *see* Neoplasm, malignant, by site
- mucinous of low malignant potential
  - specified site — *see* Neoplasm, malignant, by site
  - unspecified site C56.9
- mucocarcinoid
  - specified site — *see* Neoplasm, malignant, by site
  - unspecified site C18.1
- mucoepidermoid — *see* Neoplasm, uncertain behavior, by site
- Müllerian, mixed
  - specified site — *see* Neoplasm, malignant, by site
  - unspecified site C54.9
- myoepithelial — *see* Neoplasm, benign, by site
- neuroectodermal (peripheral) — *see* Neoplasm, malignant, by site
  - primitive
    - specified site — *see* Neoplasm, malignant, by site
    - unspecified site C71.9
- neuroendocrine D3A.8 (*following* D36)
  - malignant poorly differentiated C7A.1 (*following* C75)
  - secondary NEC C7B.8 (*following* C75)
  - specified NEC C7A.8 (*following* C75)
- neurogenic olfactory C3Ø.Ø
- nonencapsulated sclerosing C73
- odontogenic (adenomatoid) (benign) (calcifying epithelial) (keratocystic) (squamous) — *see* Cyst, calcifying odontogenic
  - malignant C41.1
    - upper jaw (bone) C41.Ø
- ovarian stromal D39.1- ☑
- ovary, in pregnancy — *see* Pregnancy, complicated by
- pacinian — *see* Neoplasm, skin, benign
- Pancoast's — *see* Pancoast's syndrome
- papillary — *see also* Papilloma
  - cystic D37.9

Tumor — *continued*
- papillary — *see also* Papilloma — *continued*
  - mucinous of low malignant potential C56- ☑
    - specified site — *see* Neoplasm, malignant, by site
    - unspecified site C56.9
  - serous of low malignant potential
    - specified site — *see* Neoplasm, malignant, by site
    - unspecified site C56.9
- pelvic, in pregnancy or childbirth — *see* Pregnancy, complicated by
- phantom F45.8
- phyllodes D48.6- ☑
  - benign D24- ☑
  - malignant — *see* Neoplasm, breast, malignant
- Pindborg — *see* Cyst, calcifying odontogenic
- placental site trophoblastic D39.2
- plasma cell (malignant) (localized) — *see* Plasmacytoma, solitary
- polyvesicular vitelline
  - specified site — *see* Neoplasm, malignant, by site
  - unspecified site
    - female C56.9
    - male C62.9Ø
- Pott's puffy — *see* Osteomyelitis, specified NEC
- Rathke's pouch D44.3
- retinal anlage — *see* Neoplasm, benign, by site
- salivary gland type, mixed — *see* Neoplasm, salivary gland, benign
  - malignant — *see* Neoplasm, salivary gland, malignant
- Sampson's N8Ø.1Ø- ☑
- Schmincke's — *see* Neoplasm, nasopharynx, malignant
- sclerosing stromal D27- ☑
- sebaceous — *see* Cyst, sebaceous
- secondary — *see* Neoplasm, secondary, by site
  - carcinoid C7B.ØØ (*following* C75)
    - bone C7B.Ø3 (*following* C75)
    - distant lymph nodes C7B.Ø1 (*following* C75)
    - liver C7B.Ø2 (*following* C75)
    - peritoneum C7B.Ø4 (*following* C75)
    - specified NEC C7B.Ø9 (*following* C75)
  - neuroendocrine NEC C7B.8 (*following* C75)
- serous of low malignant potential
  - specified site — *see* Neoplasm, malignant, by site
  - unspecified site C56.9
- Sertoli cell — *see* Neoplasm, benign, by site
  - with lipid storage
    - specified site — *see* Neoplasm, benign, by site
    - unspecified site
      - female D27.9
      - male D29.2Ø
  - specified site — *see* Neoplasm, benign, by site
  - unspecified site
    - female D27.9
    - male D29.2Ø
- Sertoli-Leydig cell — *see* Neoplasm, benign, by site
  - specified site — *see* Neoplasm, benign, by site
  - unspecified site
    - female D27.9
    - male D29.2Ø
- sex cord (-stromal) — *see* Neoplasm, uncertain behavior, by site
  - with annular tubules D39.1- ☑
- skin appendage — *see* Neoplasm, skin, benign
- smooth muscle — *see* Neoplasm, connective tissue, uncertain behavior
- soft tissue
  - benign — *see* Neoplasm, connective tissue, benign
  - malignant — *see* Neoplasm, connective tissue, malignant
- sternomastoid (congenital) Q68.Ø
- stromal
  - endometrial D39.Ø
  - gastric D48.1
    - benign D21.4
    - malignant C16.9
    - uncertain behavior D48.1
  - gastrointestinal C49.A- ☑
    - benign D21.4
    - esophagus C49.A1
    - malignant C49.AØ
      - colon C49.A4
      - duodenum C49.A3
      - esophagus C49.A1
      - ileum C49.A3
      - jejunum C49.A3

- **Tumor** — *continued*
  - stromal — *continued*
    - gastrointestinal — *continued*
      - malignant — *continued*
        - large intestine C49.A4
        - Meckel diverticulum C49.A3
        - omentum C49.A9
        - peritoneum C49.A9
        - rectum C49.A5
        - small intestine C49.A3
        - specified site NEC C49.A9
        - stomach C49.A2
      - rectum C49.A5
      - small intestine C49.A3
      - specified site NEC C49.A9
      - stomach C49.A2
      - uncertain behavior D48.1
    - intestine
      - benign D21.4
      - malignant
        - large C49.A4
        - small C49.A3
      - uncertain behavior D48.1
    - ovarian D39.1- ☑
    - stomach C49.A2
      - benign D21.4
      - malignant C49.A2
      - uncertain behavior D48.1
  - sweat gland — *see also* Neoplasm, skin, uncertain behavior
    - benign — *see* Neoplasm, skin, benign
    - malignant — *see* Neoplasm, skin, malignant
  - syphilitic, brain A52.17
  - testicular D40.10
  - testicular stromal D40.1- ☑
  - theca cell D27.- ☑
  - theca cell-granulosa cell D39.1- ☑
  - Triton, malignant — *see* Neoplasm, nerve, malignant
  - trophoblastic, placental site D39.2
  - turban D23.4
  - uterus (body), in pregnancy or childbirth — *see* Pregnancy, complicated by, tumor, uterus
  - vagina, in pregnancy or childbirth — *see* Pregnancy, complicated by
  - varicose — *see* Varix
  - von Recklinghausen's — *see* Neurofibromatosis
  - vulva or perineum, in pregnancy or childbirth — *see* Pregnancy, complicated by
    - causing obstructed labor O65.5
  - Warthin's — *see* Neoplasm, salivary gland, benign
  - Wilms' C64- ☑
  - yolk sac — *see* Neoplasm, malignant, by site
    - specified site — *see* Neoplasm, malignant, by site
    - unspecified site
      - female C56.9
      - male C62.90
- **Tumor lysis syndrome** (following antineoplastic chemotherapy) (spontaneous) NEC E88.3
- **Tumorlet** — *see* Neoplasm, uncertain behavior, by site
- **Tungiasis** B88.1
- **Tunica vasculosa lentis** Q12.2
- **Turban tumor** D23.4
- **Türck's trachoma** J37.0
- **Turner-Kieser syndrome** Q87.2
- **Turner-like syndrome** Q87.19
- **Turner's**
  - hypoplasia (tooth) K00.4
  - syndrome Q96.9
    - specified NEC Q96.8
  - tooth K00.4
- **Turner-Ullrich syndrome** Q96.9
- **Tussis convulsiva** — *see* Whooping cough
- **Twiddler's syndrome** (due to)
  - automatic implantable defibrillatorT82.198
  - cardiac pacemaker T82.198 ☑
- **Twilight state**
  - epileptic F05
  - psychogenic F44.89
- **Twin** (newborn) — *see also* Newborn, twin
  - conjoined Q89.4
  - pregnancy — *see* Pregnancy, twin
- **Twinning, teeth** K00.2
- **Twist, twisted**
  - bowel, colon or intestine K56.2
  - hair (congenital) Q84.1
  - mesentery K56.2
  - omentum K56.2
  - organ or site, congenital NEC — *see* Anomaly, by site
- **Twist, twisted** — *continued*
  - ovarian pedicle — *see* Torsion, ovary
- **Twitching** R25.3
- **Tylosis** (acquired) L84
  - buccalis K13.29
  - linguae K13.29
  - palmaris et plantaris (congenital) (inherited) Q82.8
    - acquired L85.1
- **Tympanism** R14.0
- **Tympanites** (abdominal) (intestinal) R14.0
- **Tympanitis** — *see* Myringitis
- **Tympanosclerosis** H74.0 ☑
- **Tympanum** — *see* condition
- **Tympany**
  - abdomen R14.0
  - chest R09.89
- **Type A behavior pattern** Z73.1
- **Typhlitis** — *see* Cecitis
- **Typhoenteritis** — *see* Typhoid
- **Typhoid** (abortive) (ambulant) (any site) (clinical) (fever) (hemorrhagic) (infection) (intermittent) (malignant) (rheumatic) (Widal negative) A01.00
  - with pneumonia A01.03
  - abdominal A01.09
  - arthritis A01.04
  - carrier (suspected) of Z22.0
  - cholecystitis (current) A01.09
  - endocarditis A01.02
  - heart involvement A01.02
  - inoculation reaction — *see* Complications, vaccination
  - meningitis A01.01
  - mesenteric lymph nodes A01.09
  - myocarditis A01.02
  - osteomyelitis A01.05
  - perichondritis, larynx A01.09
  - pneumonia A01.03
  - specified NEC A01.09
  - spine A01.05
  - ulcer (perforating) A01.09
- **Typhomalaria** (fever) — *see* Malaria
- **Typhomania** A01.00
- **Typhoperitonitis** A01.09
- **Typhus** (fever) A75.9
  - abdominal, abdominalis — *see* Typhoid
  - African tick A77.1
  - amarillic A95.9
  - brain A75.9 *[G94]*
  - cerebral A75.9 *[G94]*
  - classical A75.0
  - due to Rickettsia
    - prowazekii A75.0
      - recrudescent A75.1
    - tsutsugamushi A75.3
    - typhi A75.2
  - endemic (flea-borne) A75.2
  - epidemic (louse-borne) A75.0
  - exanthematicus SAI A75.0
    - brillii SAI A75.1
    - mexicanus SAI A75.2
    - typhus murinus A75.2
  - exanthematic NEC A75.0
  - flea-borne A75.2
  - India tick A77.1
  - Kenya (tick) A77.1
  - louse-borne A75.0
  - Mexican A75.2
  - mite-borne A75.3
  - murine A75.2
  - North Asian tick-borne A77.2
  - Orientia Tsutsugamushi (scrub typhus) A75.3
  - petechial A75.9
  - Queensland tick A77.3
  - rat A75.2
  - recrudescent A75.1
  - recurrens — *see* Fever, relapsing
  - Sao Paulo A77.0
  - scrub (China) (India) (Malaysia) (New Guinea) A75.3
  - shop (of Malaysia) A75.2
  - Siberian tick A77.2
  - tick-borne A77.9
  - tropical (mite-borne) A75.3
- **Tyrosinemia** E70.21
  - newborn, transitory P74.5
- **Tyrosinosis** E70.21
- **Tyrosinuria** E70.29

U

- **Uhl's anomaly or disease** Q24.8
- **Ulcer, ulcerated, ulcerating, ulceration, ulcerative**
  - alveolar process M27.3
  - amebic (intestine) A06.1
    - skin A06.7
  - anastomotic — *see* Ulcer, gastrojejunal
  - anorectal K62.6
  - antral — *see* Ulcer, stomach
  - anus (sphincter) (solitary) K62.6
  - aorta — *see* Aneurysm
  - aphthous (oral) (recurrent) K12.0
    - genital organ(s)
      - female N76.6
      - male N50.89
  - artery I77.2
  - atrophic — *see* Ulcer, skin
    - decubitus — *see* Ulcer, pressure, by site
  - back L98.429
    - with
      - bone involvement without evidence of necrosis L98.426
      - bone necrosis L98.424
      - exposed fat layer L98.422
      - muscle involvement without evidence of necrosis L98.425
      - muscle necrosis L98.423
      - skin breakdown only L98.421
      - specified severity NEC L98.428
  - Barrett's (esophagus) K22.10
    - with bleeding K22.11
  - bile duct (common) (hepatic) K83.8
  - bladder (solitary) (sphincter) NEC N32.89
    - bilharzial B65.9 *[N33]*
    - in schistosomiasis (bilharzial) B65.9 *[N33]*
    - submucosal — *see* Cystitis, interstitial
    - tuberculous A18.12
  - bleeding K27.4
  - bone — *see* Osteomyelitis, specified type NEC
  - bowel — *see* Ulcer, intestine
  - breast N61.1
  - bronchus J98.09
  - buccal (cavity) (traumatic) K12.1
  - Buruli A31.1
  - buttock L98.419
    - with
      - bone involvement without evidence of necrosis L98.416
      - bone necrosis L98.414
      - exposed fat layer L98.412
      - muscle involvement without evidence of necrosis L98.415
      - muscle necrosis L98.413
      - skin breakdown only L98.411
      - specified severity NEC L98.418
  - cancerous — *see* Neoplasm, malignant, by site
  - cardia K22.10
    - with bleeding K22.11
  - cardioesophageal (peptic) K22.10
    - with bleeding K22.11
  - cecum — *see* Ulcer, intestine
  - cervix (uteri) (decubitus) (trophic) N86
    - with cervicitis N72
  - chancroidal A57
  - chiclero B55.1
  - chronic (cause unknown) — *see* Ulcer, skin
  - Cochin-China B55.1
  - colon — *see* Ulcer, intestine
  - conjunctiva H10.89
  - cornea H16.00- ☑
    - with hypopyon H16.03- ☑
    - central H16.01- ☑
    - dendritic (herpes simplex) B00.52
    - marginal H16.04- ☑
    - Mooren's H16.05- ☑
    - mycotic H16.06- ☑
    - perforated H16.07- ☑
    - ring H16.02- ☑
    - tuberculous (phlyctenular) A18.52
  - corpus cavernosum (chronic) N48.5
  - crural — *see* Ulcer, lower limb
  - Curling's — *see* Ulcer, peptic, acute
  - Cushing's — *see* Ulcer, peptic, acute
  - cystic duct K82.8
  - cystitis (interstitial) — *see* Cystitis, interstitial
  - decubitus — *see* Ulcer, pressure, by site

Ulcer, ulcerated, ulcerating, ulceration, ulcerative — *continued*
dendritic, cornea (herpes simplex) BØØ.52
diabetes, diabetic — *see* Diabetes, ulcer
Dieulafoy's K25.Ø
due to
infection NEC — *see* Ulcer, skin
radiation NEC L59.8
trophic disturbance (any region) — *see* Ulcer, skin
X-ray L58.1
duodenum, duodenal (eroded) (peptic) K26.9
with
hemorrhage K26.4
and perforation K26.6
perforation K26.5
acute K26.3
with
hemorrhage K26.Ø
and perforation K26.2
perforation K26.1
chronic K26.7
with
hemorrhage K26.4
and perforation K26.6
perforation K26.5
dysenteric AØ9
elusive — *see* Cystitis, interstitial
endocarditis (acute) (chronic) (subacute) I28.8
epiglottis J38.7
esophagus (peptic) K22.1Ø
with bleeding K22.11
due to
aspirin K22.1Ø
with bleeding K22.11
gastrointestinal reflux disease (without bleeding) K21.ØØ
with bleeding K21.Ø1
ingestion of chemical or medicament K22.1Ø
with bleeding K22.11
fungal K22.1Ø
with bleeding K22.11
infective K22.1Ø
with bleeding K22.11
varicose — *see* Varix, esophagus
eyelid (region) HØ1.8
fauces J39.2
Fenwick (-Hunner) (solitary) — *see* Cystitis, interstitial
fistulous — *see* Ulcer, skin
foot (indolent) (trophic) — *see* Ulcer, lower limb
frambesial, initial A66.Ø
frenum (tongue) K14.Ø
gallbladder or duct K82.8
gangrenous — *see* Gangrene
gastric — *see* Ulcer, stomach
gastrocolic — *see* Ulcer, gastrojejunal
gastroduodenal — *see* Ulcer, peptic
gastroesophageal — *see* Ulcer, stomach
gastrointestinal — *see* Ulcer, gastrojejunal
gastrojejunal (peptic) K28.9
with
hemorrhage K28.4
and perforation K28.6
perforation K28.5
acute K28.3
with
hemorrhage K28.Ø
and perforation K28.2
perforation K28.1
chronic K28.7
with
hemorrhage K28.4
and perforation K28.6
perforation K28.5
gastrojejunocolic — *see* Ulcer, gastrojejunal
gingiva KØ6.8
gingivitis KØ5.1Ø
nonplaque induced KØ5.11
plaque induced KØ5.1Ø
glottis J38.7
granuloma of pudenda A58
gum KØ6.8
gumma, due to yaws A66.4
heel — *see* Ulcer, lower limb
hemorrhoid — *see also* Hemorrhoids, by degree K64.8
Hunner's — *see* Cystitis, interstitial
hypopharynx J39.2
hypopyon (chronic) (subacute) — *see* Ulcer, cornea, with hypopyon

Ulcer, ulcerated, ulcerating, ulceration, ulcerative — *continued*
hypostaticum — *see* Ulcer, varicose
ileum — *see* Ulcer, intestine
intestine, intestinal K63.3
with perforation K63.1
amebic AØ6.1
duodenal — *see* Ulcer, duodenum
granulocytopenic (with hemorrhage) — *see* Neutropenia
marginal — *see* Ulcer, gastrojejunal
perforating K63.1
newborn P78.Ø
primary, small intestine K63.3
rectum K62.6
stercoraceous, stercoral K63.3
tuberculous A18.32
typhoid (fever) — *see* Typhoid
varicose I86.8
jejunum, jejunal — *see* Ulcer, gastrojejunal
keratitis — *see* Ulcer, cornea
knee — *see* Ulcer, lower limb
labium (majus) (minus) N76.6
laryngitis — *see* Laryngitis
larynx (aphthous) (contact) J38.7
diphtheritic A36.2
leg — *see* Ulcer, lower limb
lip K13.Ø
Lipschütz's N76.6
lower limb (atrophic) (chronic) (neurogenic) (perforating) (pyogenic) (trophic) (tropical) L97.9Ø9
with
bone involvement without evidence of necrosis L97.9Ø6
bone necrosis L97.9Ø4
exposed fat layer L97.9Ø2
muscle involvement without evidence of necrosis L97.9Ø5
muscle necrosis L97.9Ø3
skin breakdown only L97.9Ø1
specified severity NEC L97.9Ø8
ankle L97.3Ø9
with
bone involvement without evidence of necrosis L97.3Ø6
bone necrosis L97.3Ø4
exposed fat layer L97.3Ø2
muscle involvement without evidence of necrosis L97.3Ø5
muscle necrosis L97.3Ø3
skin breakdown only L97.3Ø1
specified severity NEC L97.3Ø8
left L97.329
with
bone involvement without evidence of necrosis L97.326
bone necrosis L97.324
exposed fat layer L97.322
muscle involvement without evidence of necrosis L97.325
muscle necrosis L97.323
skin breakdown only L97.321
specified severity NEC L97.328
right L97.319
with
bone involvement without evidence of necrosis L97.316
bone necrosis L97.314
exposed fat layer L97.312
muscle involvement without evidence of necrosis L97.315
muscle necrosis L97.313
skin breakdown only L97.311
specified severity NEC L97.318
calf L97.2Ø9
with
bone involvement without evidence of necrosis L97.2Ø6
bone necrosis L97.2Ø4
exposed fat layer L97.2Ø2
muscle involvement without evidence of necrosis L97.2Ø5
muscle necrosis L97.2Ø3
skin breakdown only L97.2Ø1
specified severity NEC L97.2Ø8
left L97.229

Ulcer, ulcerated, ulcerating, ulceration, ulcerative — *continued*
lower limb — *continued*
calf — *continued*
left — *continued*
with
bone involvement without evidence of necrosis L97.226
bone necrosis L97.224
exposed fat layer L97.222
muscle involvement without evidence of necrosis L97.225
muscle necrosis L97.223
skin breakdown only L97.221
specified severity NEC L97.228
right L97.219
with
bone involvement without evidence of necrosis L97.216
bone necrosis L97.214
exposed fat layer L97.212
muscle involvement without evidence of necrosis L97.215
muscle necrosis L97.213
skin breakdown only L97.211
specified severity NEC L97.218
decubitus — *see* Ulcer, pressure, by site
foot specified NEC L97.5Ø9
with
bone involvement without evidence of necrosis L97.5Ø6
bone necrosis L97.5Ø4
exposed fat layer L97.5Ø2
muscle involvement without evidence of necrosis L97.5Ø5
muscle necrosis L97.5Ø3
skin breakdown only L97.5Ø1
specified severity NEC L97.5Ø8
left L97.529
with
bone involvement without evidence of necrosis L97.526
bone necrosis L97.524
exposed fat layer L97.522
muscle involvement without evidence of necrosis L97.525
muscle necrosis L97.523
skin breakdown only L97.521
specified severity NEC L97.528
right L97.519
with
bone involvement without evidence of necrosis L97.516
bone necrosis L97.514
exposed fat layer L97.512
muscle involvement without evidence of necrosis L97.515
muscle necrosis L97.513
skin breakdown only L97.511
specified severity NEC L97.518
heel L97.4Ø9
with
bone involvement without evidence of necrosis L97.4Ø6
bone necrosis L97.4Ø4
exposed fat layer L97.4Ø2
muscle involvement without evidence of necrosis L97.4Ø5
muscle necrosis L97.4Ø3
skin breakdown only L97.4Ø1
specified severity NEC L97.4Ø8
left L97.429
with
bone involvement without evidence of necrosis L97.426
bone necrosis L97.424
exposed fat layer L97.422
muscle involvement without evidence of necrosis L97.425
muscle necrosis L97.423
skin breakdown only L97.421
specified severity NEC L97.428
right L97.419
with
bone involvement without evidence of necrosis L97.416
bone necrosis L97.414
exposed fat layer L97.412

Ulcer, ulcerated, ulcerating, ulceration, ulcerative *— continued*
- lower limb *— continued*
  - heel *— continued*
    - right *— continued*
      - with *— continued*
        - muscle involvement without evidence of necrosis L97.415
        - muscle necrosis L97.413
        - skin breakdown only L97.411
        - specified severity NEC L97.418
  - left L97.929
    - with
      - bone involvement without evidence of necrosis L97.926
      - bone necrosis L97.924
      - exposed fat layer L97.922
      - muscle involvement without evidence of necrosis L97.925
      - muscle necrosis L97.923
      - skin breakdown only L97.921
      - specified severity NEC L97.928
  - leprous A30.1
  - lower leg NOS L97.909
    - with
      - bone involvement without evidence of necrosis L97.906
      - bone necrosis L97.904
      - exposed fat layer L97.902
      - muscle involvement without evidence of necrosis L97.905
      - muscle necrosis L97.903
      - skin breakdown only L97.901
      - specified severity NEC L97.908
    - left L97.929
      - with
        - bone involvement without evidence of necrosis L97.926
        - bone necrosis L97.924
        - exposed fat layer L97.922
        - muscle involvement without evidence of necrosis L97.925
        - muscle necrosis L97.923
        - skin breakdown only L97.921
        - specified severity NEC L97.928
    - right L97.919
      - with
        - bone involvement without evidence of necrosis L97.916
        - bone necrosis L97.914
        - exposed fat layer L97.912
        - muscle involvement without evidence of necrosis L97.915
        - muscle necrosis L97.913
        - skin breakdown only L97.911
        - specified severity NEC L97.918
    - specified site NEC L97.809
      - with
        - bone involvement without evidence of necrosis L97.806
        - bone necrosis L97.804
        - exposed fat layer L97.802
        - muscle involvement without evidence of necrosis L97.805
        - muscle necrosis L97.803
        - skin breakdown only L97.801
        - specified severity NEC L97.808
      - left L97.829
        - with
          - bone involvement without evidence of necrosis L97.826
          - bone necrosis L97.824
          - exposed fat layer L97.822
          - muscle involvement without evidence of necrosis L97.825
          - muscle necrosis L97.823
          - skin breakdown only L97.821
          - specified severity NEC L97.828
      - right L97.819
        - with
          - bone involvement without evidence of necrosis L97.816
          - bone necrosis L97.814
          - exposed fat layer L97.812
          - muscle involvement without evidence of necrosis L97.815
          - muscle necrosis L97.813
          - skin breakdown only L97.811
          - specified severity NEC L97.818

Ulcer, ulcerated, ulcerating, ulceration, ulcerative *— continued*
- lower limb *— continued*
  - midfoot L97.409
    - with
      - bone involvement without evidence of necrosis L97.406
      - bone necrosis L97.404
      - exposed fat layer L97.402
      - muscle involvement without evidence of necrosis L97.405
      - muscle necrosis L97.403
      - skin breakdown only L97.401
      - specified severity NEC L97.408
    - left L97.429
      - with
        - bone involvement without evidence of necrosis L97.426
        - bone necrosis L97.424
        - exposed fat layer L97.422
        - muscle involvement without evidence of necrosis L97.425
        - muscle necrosis L97.423
        - skin breakdown only L97.421
        - specified severity NEC L97.428
    - right L97.419
      - with
        - bone involvement without evidence of necrosis L97.416
        - bone necrosis L97.414
        - exposed fat layer L97.412
        - muscle involvement without evidence of necrosis L97.415
        - muscle necrosis L97.413
        - skin breakdown only L97.411
        - specified severity NEC L97.418
  - right L97.919
    - with
      - bone involvement without evidence of necrosis L97.916
      - bone necrosis L97.914
      - exposed fat layer L97.912
      - muscle involvement without evidence of necrosis L97.915
      - muscle necrosis L97.913
      - skin breakdown only L97.911
      - specified severity NEC L97.918
  - syphilitic A52.19
  - thigh L97.109
    - with
      - bone involvement without evidence of necrosis L97.106
      - bone necrosis L97.104
      - exposed fat layer L97.102
      - muscle involvement without evidence of necrosis L97.105
      - muscle necrosis L97.103
      - skin breakdown only L97.101
      - specified severity NEC L97.108
    - left L97.129
      - with
        - bone involvement without evidence of necrosis L97.126
        - bone necrosis L97.124
        - exposed fat layer L97.122
        - muscle involvement without evidence of necrosis L97.125
        - muscle necrosis L97.123
        - skin breakdown only L97.121
        - specified severity NEC L97.128
    - right L97.119
      - with
        - bone involvement without evidence of necrosis L97.116
        - bone necrosis L97.114
        - exposed fat layer L97.112
        - muscle involvement without evidence of necrosis L97.115
        - muscle necrosis L97.113
        - skin breakdown only L97.111
        - specified severity NEC L97.118
  - toe L97.509
    - with
      - bone involvement without evidence of necrosis L97.506
      - bone necrosis L97.504
      - exposed fat layer L97.502
      - muscle involvement without evidence of necrosis L97.505

Ulcer, ulcerated, ulcerating, ulceration, ulcerative *— continued*
- lower limb *— continued*
  - toe *— continued*
    - with *— continued*
      - muscle necrosis L97.503
      - skin breakdown only L97.501
      - specified severity NEC L97.508
    - left L97.529
      - with
        - bone involvement without evidence of necrosis L97.526
        - bone necrosis L97.524
        - exposed fat layer L97.522
        - muscle involvement without evidence of necrosis L97.525
        - muscle necrosis L97.523
        - skin breakdown only L97.521
        - specified severity NEC L97.528
    - right L97.519
      - with
        - bone involvement without evidence of necrosis L97.516
        - bone necrosis L97.514
        - exposed fat layer L97.512
        - muscle involvement without evidence of necrosis L97.515
        - muscle necrosis L97.513
        - skin breakdown only L97.511
        - specified severity NEC L97.518
  - varicose *— see* Varix, leg, with, ulcer
- luetic *— see* Ulcer, syphilitic
- lung J98.4
  - tuberculous *— see* Tuberculosis, pulmonary
- malignant *— see* Neoplasm, malignant, by site
- marginal NEC *— see* Ulcer, gastrojejunal
- meatus (urinarius) N34.2
- Meckel's diverticulum Q43.0
  - malignant *— see* Table of Neoplasms, small intestine, malignant
- Meleney's (chronic undermining) *— see* Ulcer, skin
- Mooren's (cornea) *— see* Ulcer, cornea, Mooren's
- mycobacterial (skin) A31.1
- nasopharynx J39.2
- neck, uterus N86
- neurogenic NEC *— see* Ulcer, skin
- nose, nasal (passage) (infective) (septum) J34.0
  - skin *— see* Ulcer, skin
  - spirochetal A69.8
  - varicose (bleeding) I86.8
- oral mucosa (traumatic) K12.1
- palate (soft) K12.1
- penis (chronic) N48.5
- peptic (site unspecified) K27.9
  - with
    - hemorrhage K27.4
      - and perforation K27.6
    - perforation K27.5
  - acute K27.3
    - with
      - hemorrhage K27.0
        - and perforation K27.2
      - perforation K27.1
  - chronic K27.7
    - with
      - hemorrhage K27.4
        - and perforation K27.6
      - perforation K27.5
  - esophagus K22.10
    - with bleeding K22.11
  - newborn P78.82
- perforating K27.5
  - skin *— see* Ulcer, skin
- peritonsillar J35.8
- phagedenic (tropical) *— see* Ulcer, skin
- pharynx J39.2
- phlebitis *— see* Phlebitis
- plaster *— see* Ulcer, pressure, by site
- popliteal space *— see* Ulcer, lower limb
- postpyloric *— see* Ulcer, duodenum
- prepuce N47.7
- prepyloric *— see* Ulcer, stomach
- pressure (pressure area) L89.9- ☑
  - ankle L89.5- ☑
  - back L89.1- ☑
  - buttock L89.3- ☑
  - coccyx L89.15- ☑
  - contiguous site of back, buttock, hip L89.4- ☑

Ulcer, ulcerated, ulcerating, ulceration, ulcerative *— continued*
- pressure *— continued*
  - elbow L89.Ø- ☑
  - face L89.81- ☑
  - head L89.81- ☑
  - heel L89.6- ☑
  - hip L89.2- ☑
  - sacral region (tailbone) L89.15- ☑
  - specified site NEC L89.89- ☑
  - stage 1 (healing) (pre-ulcer skin changes limited to persistent focal edema)
    - ankle L89.5- ☑
    - back L89.1- ☑
    - buttock L89.3- ☑
    - coccyx L89.15- ☑
    - contiguous site of back, buttock, hip L89.4- ☑
    - elbow L89.Ø- ☑
    - face L89.81- ☑
    - head L89.81- ☑
    - heel L89.6- ☑
    - hip L89.2- ☑
    - sacral region (tailbone) L89.15- ☑
    - specified site NEC L89.89- ☑
  - stage 2 (healing) (abrasion, blister, partial thickness skin loss involving epidermis and/or dermis)
    - ankle L89.5- ☑
    - back L89.1- ☑
    - buttock L89.3- ☑
    - coccyx L89.15- ☑
    - contiguous site of back, buttock, hip L89.4- ☑
    - elbow L89.Ø- ☑
    - face L89.81- ☑
    - head L89.81- ☑
    - heel L89.6- ☑
    - hip L89.2- ☑
    - sacral region (tailbone) L89.15- ☑
    - specified site NEC L89.89- ☑
  - stage 3 (healing) (full thickness skin loss involving damage or necrosis of subcutaneous tissue)
    - ankle L89.5- ☑
    - back L89.1- ☑
    - buttock L89.3- ☑
    - coccyx L89.15- ☑
    - contiguous site of back, buttock, hip L89.4- ☑
    - elbow L89.Ø- ☑
    - face L89.81- ☑
    - head L89.81- ☑
    - heel L89.6- ☑
    - hip L89.2- ☑
    - sacral region (tailbone) L89.15- ☑
    - specified site NEC L89.89- ☑
  - stage 4 (healing) (necrosis of soft tissues through to underlying muscle, tendon, or bone)
    - ankle L89.5- ☑
    - back L89.1- ☑
    - buttock L89.3- ☑
    - coccyx L89.15- ☑
    - contiguous site of back, buttock, hip L89.4- ☑
    - elbow L89.Ø- ☑
    - face L89.81- ☑
    - head L89.81- ☑
    - heel L89.6- ☑
    - hip L89.2- ☑
    - sacral region (tailbone) L89.15- ☑
    - specified site NEC L89.89- ☑
  - unspecified stage
    - ankle L89.5- ☑
    - back L89.1- ☑
    - buttock L89.3- ☑
    - coccyx L89.15- ☑
    - contiguous site of back, buttock, hip L89.4- ☑
    - elbow L89.Ø- ☑
    - face L89.81- ☑
    - head L89.81- ☑
    - heel L89.6- ☑
    - hip L89.2- ☑
    - sacral region (tailbone) L89.15- ☑
    - specified site NEC L89.89- ☑
  - unstageable
    - ankle L89.5- ☑
    - back L89.1- ☑
    - buttock L89.3- ☑
    - coccyx L89.15- ☑
    - contiguous site of back, buttock, hip L89.4- ☑
    - elbow L89.Ø- ☑

Ulcer, ulcerated, ulcerating, ulceration, ulcerative *— continued*
- pressure *— continued*
  - unstageable *— continued*
    - face L89.81- ☑
    - head L89.81- ☑
    - heel L89.6- ☑
    - hip L89.2- ☑
    - sacral region (tailbone) L89.15- ☑
    - specified site NEC L89.89- ☑
- primary of intestine K63.3
  - with perforation K63.1
- prostate N41.9
- pyloric *— see* Ulcer, stomach
- rectosigmoid K63.3
  - with perforation K63.1
- rectum (sphincter) (solitary) K62.6
  - stercoraceous, stercoral K62.6
- retina *— see* Inflammation, chorioretinal
- rodent *— see also* Neoplasm, skin, malignant
- sclera *— see* Scleritis
- scrofulous (tuberculous) A18.2
- scrotum N5Ø.89
  - tuberculous A18.15
  - varicose I86.1
- seminal vesicle N5Ø.89
- sigmoid *— see* Ulcer, intestine
- skin (atrophic) (chronic) (neurogenic) (non-healing) (perforating) (pyogenic) (trophic) (tropical) L98.499
  - with gangrene *— see* Gangrene
  - amebic AØ6.7
  - back *— see* Ulcer, back
  - buttock *— see* Ulcer, buttock
  - decubitus *— see* Ulcer, pressure
  - lower limb *— see* Ulcer, lower limb
  - mycobacterial A31.1
  - specified site NEC L98.499
    - with
      - bone involvement without evidence of necrosis L98.496
      - bone necrosis L98.494
      - exposed fat layer L98.492
      - muscle involvement without evidence of necrosis L98.495
      - muscle necrosis L98.493
      - skin breakdown only L98.491
      - specified severity NEC L98.498
  - tuberculous (primary) A18.4
  - varicose *— see* Ulcer, varicose
- sloughing *— see* Ulcer, skin
- solitary, anus or rectum (sphincter) K62.6
- sore throat JØ2.9
  - streptococcal JØ2.Ø
- spermatic cord N5Ø.89
- spine (tuberculous) A18.Ø1
- stasis (venous) *— see* Varix, leg, with, ulcer
  - without varicose veins I87.2
- stercoraceous, stercoral K63.3
  - with perforation K63.1
  - anus or rectum K62.6
- stoma, stomal *— see* Ulcer, gastrojejunal
- stomach (eroded) (peptic) (round) K25.9
  - with
    - hemorrhage K25.4
      - and perforation K25.6
    - perforation K25.5
  - acute K25.3
    - with
      - hemorrhage K25.Ø
        - and perforation K25.2
      - perforation K25.1
  - chronic K25.7
    - with
      - hemorrhage K25.4
        - and perforation K25.6
      - perforation K25.5
- stomal *— see* Ulcer, gastrojejunal
- stomatitis K12.1
- stress *— see* Ulcer, peptic
- strumous (tuberculous) A18.2
- submucosal, bladder *— see* Cystitis, interstitial
- syphilitic (any site) (early) (secondary) A51.39
  - late A52.79
  - perforating A52.79
    - foot A52.11
- testis N5Ø.89
- thigh *— see* Ulcer, lower limb

Ulcer, ulcerated, ulcerating, ulceration, ulcerative *— continued*
- throat J39.2
  - diphtheritic A36.Ø
- toe *— see* Ulcer, lower limb
- tongue (traumatic) K14.Ø
- tonsil J35.8
  - diphtheritic A36.Ø
- trachea J39.8
- trophic *— see* Ulcer, skin
- tropical *— see* Ulcer, skin
- tuberculous *— see* Tuberculosis, ulcer
- tunica vaginalis N5Ø.89
- turbinate J34.89
- typhoid (perforating) *— see* Typhoid
- unspecified site *— see* Ulcer, skin
- urethra (meatus) *— see* Urethritis
- uterus N85.8
  - cervix N86
    - with cervicitis N72
  - neck N86
    - with cervicitis N72
- vagina N76.5
  - in Behçet's disease M35.2 *[N77.Ø]*
  - pessary N89.8
- valve, heart I33.Ø
- varicose (lower limb, any part) *— see also* Varix, leg, with, ulcer
  - broad ligament I86.2
  - esophagus *— see* Varix, esophagus
  - inflamed or infected *— see* Varix, leg, with ulcer, with inflammation
  - nasal septum I86.8
  - perineum I86.3
  - scrotum I86.1
  - specified site NEC I86.8
  - sublingual I86.Ø
  - vulva I86.3
- vas deferens N5Ø.89
- vulva (acute) (infectional) N76.6
  - in (due to)
    - Behçet's disease M35.2 *[N77.Ø]*
    - herpesviral (herpes simplex) infection A6Ø.Ø4
    - tuberculosis A18.18
- vulvobuccal, recurring N76.6
- X-ray L58.1
- yaws A66.4

Ulcerosa scarlatina A38.8

Ulcus *— see also* Ulcer
- cutis tuberculosum A18.4
- duodeni *— see* Ulcer, duodenum
- durum (syphilitic) A51.Ø
  - extragenital A51.2
- gastrojejunale *— see* Ulcer, gastrojejunal
- hypostaticum *— see* Ulcer, varicose
- molle (cutis) (skin) A57
- serpens corneae *— see* Ulcer, cornea, central
- ventriculi *— see* Ulcer, stomach

Ulegyria QØ4.8

Ulerythema
- ophryogenes, congenital Q84.2
- sycosiforme L73.8

Ullrich (-Bonnevie) (-Turner) syndrome *— see also* Turner's syndrome Q87.19

Ullrich-Feichtiger syndrome Q87.Ø

Ulnar *— see* condition

Ulorrhagia, ulorrhea KØ6.8

Umbilicus, umbilical *— see* condition

Unable to
- make ends meet Z59.86
- obtain
  - adequate
    - childcare Z59.87
    - clothing Z59.87
    - utilities Z59.87
  - basic needs Z59.87

Unacceptable
- contours of tooth KØ8.54
- morphology of tooth KØ8.54

Unaffordable transportation Z59.82

Unavailability (of)
- bed at medical facility Z75.1
- health service-related agencies Z75.4
- medical facilities (at) Z75.3
  - due to
    - investigation by social service agency Z75.2
    - lack of services at home Z75.Ø
    - remoteness from facility Z75.3

- **Unavailability** — *continued*
  - medical facilities — *continued*
    - due to — *continued*
      - waiting list Z75.1
    - home Z75.Ø
    - outpatient clinic Z75.3
  - schooling Z55.1
  - social service agencies Z75.4
- **Uncinaria americana infestation** B76.1
- **Uncinariasis** B76.9
- **Uncongenial work** Z56.5
- **Unconscious** (ness) — *see* Coma
- **Under observation** — *see* Observation
- **Underachievement in school** Z55.3
- **Underdevelopment** — *see also* Undeveloped
  - nose Q3Ø.1
  - sexual E3Ø.Ø
- **Underdosing** — *see also* Table of Drugs and Chemicals, categories T36-T5Ø, with final character 6 Z91.14
  - intentional NEC Z91.128
    - due to financial hardship of patient Z91.12Ø
  - unintentional NEC Z91.138
    - due to patient's age related debility Z91.13Ø
- **Underfeeding, newborn** P92.3
- **Underfill, endodontic** M27.53
- **Underimmunization status** Z28.39
  - COVID-19 Z28.31- ☑
    - partially vaccinated (for) Z28.311
    - unvaccinated (for) Z28.31Ø
- **Undernourishment** — *see* Malnutrition
- **Undernutrition** — *see* Malnutrition
- **Underweight** R63.6
  - for gestational age — *see* Light for dates
- **Underwood's disease** P83.Ø
- **Undescended** — *see also* Malposition, congenital
  - cecum Q43.3
  - colon Q43.3
  - testicle — *see* Cryptorchid
- **Undeveloped, undevelopment** — *see also* Hypoplasia
  - brain (congenital) QØ2
  - cerebral (congenital) QØ2
  - heart Q24.8
  - lung Q33.6
  - testis E29.1
  - uterus E3Ø.Ø
- **Undiagnosed** (disease) R69
- **Undulant fever** — *see* Brucellosis
- **Unemployment, anxiety concerning** Z56.Ø
  - threatened Z56.2
- **Unequal length** (acquired) (limb) — *see also* Deformity, limb, unequal length
  - leg — *see also* Deformity, limb, unequal length
    - congenital Q72.9- ☑
- **Unextracted dental root** KØ8.3
- **Unguis incarnatus** L6Ø.Ø
- **Unhappiness** R45.2
- **Unicornate uterus** Q51.4
  - in pregnancy or childbirth O34.ØØ
- **Unilateral** — *see also* condition
  - development, breast N64.89
  - organ or site, congenital NEC — *see* Agenesis, by site
- **Unilocular heart** Q2Ø.8
- **Unimmunized** — *see also* Underimmunization status for COVID-19 Z28.31Ø
- **Union, abnormal** — *see also* Fusion
  - larynx and trachea Q34.8
- **Universal mesentery** Q43.3
- **Unreliable transportation** Z59.82
- **Unrepairable overhanging of dental restorative materials** KØ8.52
- **Unroofed coronary sinus** Q21.13
- **Unsafe transportation** Z59.82
- **Unsatisfactory**
  - restoration of tooth KØ8.5Ø
    - specified NEC KØ8.59
  - sample of cytologic smear
    - anus R85.615
    - cervix R87.615
    - vagina R87.625
  - surroundings Z59.1
    - work Z56.5
- **Unsoundness of mind** — *see* Psychosis
- **Unstable**
  - back NEC — *see* Instability, joint, spine
  - hip (congenital) Q65.6
    - acquired — *see* Derangement, joint, specified type NEC, hip
- **Unstable** — *continued*
  - joint — *see* Instability, joint
    - secondary to removal of joint prosthesis M96.89
  - lie (mother) O32.Ø ☑
  - lumbosacral joint (congenital) — *see* subcategory M53.2
  - sacroiliac — *see* subcategory M53.2 ☑
  - spine NEC — *see* Instability, joint, spine
- **Unsteadiness on feet** R26.81
- **Untruthfulness, child problem** F91.8
- **Unvaccinated** — *see also* Underimmunization status for COVID-19 Z28.31Ø
- **Unverricht** (-Lundborg) **disease or epilepsy** — *see* Epilepsy, generalized, idiopathic
- **Unwanted**
  - multiple moves in the last 12 months Z59.81- ☑
  - pregnancy Z64.Ø
- **Upbringing, institutional** Z62.22
  - away from parents NEC Z62.29
  - in care of non-parental family member Z62.21
  - in foster care Z62.21
  - in orphanage or group home Z62.22
  - in welfare custody Z62.21
- **Upper respiratory** — *see* condition
- **Upset**
  - gastric K3Ø
  - gastrointestinal K3Ø
    - psychogenic F45.8
  - intestinal (large) (small) K59.9
    - psychogenic F45.8
  - menstruation N93.9
  - mental F48.9
  - stomach K3Ø
    - psychogenic F45.8
- **Urachus** — *see also* condition
  - patent or persistent Q64.4
- **Urbach-Oppenheim disease** (necrobiosis lipoidica diabeticorum) — *see* EØ8-E13 with .62Ø
- **Urbach's lipoid proteinosis** E78.89
- **Urbach-Wiethe disease** E78.89
- **Urban yellow fever** A95.1
- **Urea**
  - blood, high — *see* Uremia
  - cycle metabolism disorder — *see* Disorder, urea cycle metabolism
- **Uremia, uremic** N19
  - with
    - ectopic or molar pregnancy OØ8.4
    - polyneuropathy N18.9 *[G63]*
  - chronic NOS — *see also* Disease, kidney, chronic N18.9
    - due to hypertension — *see* Hypertensive, kidney
  - complicating
    - ectopic or molar pregnancy OØ8.4
  - congenital P96.Ø
  - extrarenal R39.2
  - following ectopic or molar pregnancy OØ8.4
  - newborn P96.Ø
  - prerenal R39.2
- **Ureter, ureteral** — *see* condition
- **Ureteralgia** N23
- **Ureterectasis** — *see* Hydroureter
- **Ureteritis** N28.89
  - cystica N28.86
  - due to calculus N2Ø.1
    - with calculus, kidney N2Ø.2
      - with hydronephrosis N13.2
  - gonococcal (acute) (chronic) A54.21
  - nonspecific N28.89
- **Ureterocele** N28.89
  - congenital (orthotopic) Q62.31
    - ectopic Q62.32
- **Ureterolith, ureterolithiasis** — *see* Calculus, ureter
- **Ureterostomy**
  - attention to Z43.6
  - status Z93.6
- **Urethra, urethral** — *see* condition
- **Urethralgia** R39.89
- **Urethritis** (anterior) (posterior) N34.2
  - calculous N21.1
  - candidal B37.41
  - chlamydial A56.Ø1
  - diplococcal (gonococcal) A54.Ø1
    - with abscess (accessory gland) (periurethral) A54.1
  - gonococcal A54.Ø1
    - with abscess (accessory gland) (periurethral) A54.1
  - nongonococcal N34.1
    - Reiter's — *see* Reiter's disease
- **Urethritis** — *continued*
  - nonspecific N34.1
  - nonvenereal N34.1
  - postmenopausal N34.2
  - puerperal O86.22
  - Reiter's — *see* Reiter's disease
  - specified NEC N34.2
  - trichomonal or due to Trichomonas (vaginalis) A59.Ø3
- **Urethrocele** N81.Ø
  - with
    - cystocele — *see* Cystocele
    - prolapse of uterus — *see* Prolapse, uterus
- **Urethrolithiasis** (with colic or infection) N21.1
- **Urethrorectal** — *see* condition
- **Urethrorrhagia** N36.8
- **Urethrorrhea** R36.9
- **Urethrostomy**
  - attention to Z43.6
  - status Z93.6
- **Urethrotrigonitis** — *see* Trigonitis
- **Urethrovaginal** — *see* condition
- **Urgency**
  - fecal R15.2
  - hypertensive — *see* Hypertension
  - urinary R39.15
- **Urhidrosis, uridrosis** L74.8
- **Uric acid in blood** (increased) E79.Ø
- **Uricacidemia** (asymptomatic) E79.Ø
- **Uricemia** (asymptomatic) E79.Ø
- **Uricosuria** R82.998
- **Urinary** — *see* condition
- **Urination**
  - frequent R35.Ø
  - painful R3Ø.9
- **Urine**
  - blood in — *see* Hematuria
  - discharge, excessive R35.89
  - enuresis, nonorganic origin F98.Ø
  - extravasation R39.Ø
  - frequency R35.Ø
  - incontinence R32
    - nonorganic origin F98.Ø
  - intermittent stream R39.198
  - pus in N39.Ø
  - retention or stasis R33.9
    - organic R33.8
      - drug-induced R33.Ø
    - psychogenic F45.8
  - secretion
    - deficient R34
    - excessive R35.89
    - frequency R35.Ø
  - stream
    - intermittent R39.198
    - slowing R39.198
    - splitting R39.13
    - weak R39.12
- **Urinemia** — *see* Uremia
- **Urinoma, urethra** N36.8
- **Uroarthritis, infectious** (Reiter's) — *see* Reiter's disease
- **Urodialysis** R34
- **Urolithiasis** — *see* Calculus, urinary
- **Uronephrosis** — *see* Hydronephrosis
- **Uropathy** N39.9
  - obstructive N13.9
    - specified NEC N13.8
  - reflux N13.9
    - specified NEC N13.8
  - vesicoureteral reflux-associated — *see* Reflux, vesicoureteral
- **Urosepsis** — *code to* condition
- **Urticaria** L5Ø.9
  - with angioneurotic edema T78.3 ☑
    - hereditary D84.1
  - allergic L5Ø.Ø
  - cholinergic L5Ø.5
  - chronic L5Ø.8
  - cold, familial L5Ø.2
  - contact L5Ø.6
  - dermatographic L5Ø.3
  - due to
    - cold or heat L5Ø.2
    - drugs L5Ø.Ø
    - food L5Ø.Ø
    - inhalants L5Ø.Ø
    - plants L5Ø.6
    - serum — *see also* Reaction, serum T8Ø.69 ☑
  - factitial L5Ø.3

- **Urticaria** — *continued*
  - familial cold M04.2
  - giant T78.3 ☑
    - hereditary D84.1
  - gigantea T78.3 ☑
  - idiopathic L50.1
  - larynx T78.3 ☑
    - hereditary D84.1
  - neonatorum P83.88
  - nonallergic L50.1
  - papulosa (Hebra) L28.2
  - pigmentosa D47.01
    - congenital Q82.2
    - of neonatal onset Q82.2
    - of newborn onset Q82.2
  - recurrent periodic L50.8
  - serum — *see also* Reaction, serum T80.69 ☑
  - solar L56.3
  - specified type NEC L50.8
  - thermal (cold) (heat) L50.2
  - vibratory L50.4
  - xanthelasmoidea — *see* Urticaria pigmentosa
- **Use** (of)
  - alcohol F10.90
    - with
      - intoxication F10.929
      - sleep disorder F10.982
      - withdrawal F10.939
        - with
          - perceptual disturbance F10.932
        - delirium F10.931
        - uncomplicated F10.930
    - harmful — *see* Abuse, alcohol
    - in remission F10.91
  - amphetamines — *see* Use, stimulant NEC
  - caffeine — *see* Use, stimulant NEC
  - cannabis F12.90
    - with
      - anxiety disorder F12.980
      - intoxication F12.929
        - with
          - delirium F12.921
          - perceptual disturbance F12.922
        - uncomplicated F12.920
      - other specified disorder F12.988
      - psychosis F12.959
        - delusions F12.950
        - hallucinations F12.951
      - unspecified disorder F12.99
      - withdrawal F12.93
    - in remission F12.91
  - cocaine F14.90
    - with
      - anxiety disorder F14.980
      - intoxication F14.929
        - with
          - delirium F14.921
          - perceptual disturbance F14.922
        - uncomplicated F14.920
      - other specified disorder F14.988
      - psychosis F14.959
        - delusions F14.950
        - hallucinations F14.951
      - sexual dysfunction F14.981
      - sleep disorder F14.982
      - unspecified disorder F14.99
      - withdrawal F14.93
    - harmful — *see* Abuse, drug, cocaine
    - in remission F14.91
  - drug(s) NEC F19.90
    - with sleep disorder F19.982
    - harmful — *see* Abuse, drug, by type
  - hallucinogen NEC F16.90
    - with
      - anxiety disorder F16.980
      - intoxication F16.929
        - with
          - delirium F16.921
        - uncomplicated F16.920
      - mood disorder F16.94
      - other specified disorder F16.988
      - perception disorder (flashbacks) F16.983
      - psychosis F16.959
        - delusions F16.950
        - hallucinations F16.951
      - unspecified disorder F16.99
    - harmful — *see* Abuse, drug, hallucinogen NEC
    - in remission F16.91
- **Use** — *continued*
  - inhalants F18.90
    - with
      - anxiety disorder F18.980
      - intoxication F18.929
        - with delirium F18.921
        - uncomplicated F18.920
      - mood disorder F18.94
      - other specified disorder F18.988
      - persisting dementia F18.97
      - psychosis F18.959
        - delusions F18.950
        - hallucinations F18.951
      - unspecified disorder F18.99
    - harmful — *see* Abuse, drug, inhalant
    - in remission F18.91
  - methadone — *see* Use, opioid
  - nonprescribed drugs F19.90
    - harmful — *see* Abuse, non-psychoactive substance
  - opioid F11.90
    - with
      - disorder F11.99
        - mood F11.94
        - sleep F11.982
        - specified type NEC F11.988
      - intoxication F11.929
        - with
          - delirium F11.921
          - perceptual disturbance F11.922
        - uncomplicated F11.920
      - withdrawal F11.93
    - harmful — *see* Abuse, drug, opioid
    - in remission F11.91
  - patent medicines F19.90
    - harmful — *see* Abuse, non-psychoactive substance
  - psychoactive drug NEC F19.90
    - with
      - anxiety disorder F19.980
      - intoxication F19.929
        - with
          - delirium F19.921
          - perceptual disturbance F19.922
        - uncomplicated F19.920
      - mood disorder F19.94
      - other specified disorder F19.988
      - persisting
        - amnestic disorder F19.96
        - dementia F19.97
      - psychosis F19.959
        - delusions F19.950
        - hallucinations F19.951
      - sexual dysfunction F19.981
      - sleep disorder F19.982
      - unspecified disorder F19.99
      - withdrawal F19.939
        - with
          - delirium F19.931
          - perceptual disturbance F19.932
        - uncomplicated F19.930
    - harmful — *see* Abuse, drug NEC, psychoactive NEC
    - in remission F19.91
  - sedative, hypnotic, or anxiolytic F13.90
    - with
      - anxiety disorder F13.980
      - intoxication F13.929
        - with
          - delirium F13.921
        - uncomplicated F13.920
      - other specified disorder F13.988
      - persisting
        - amnestic disorder F13.96
        - dementia F13.97
      - psychosis F13.959
        - delusions F13.950
        - hallucinations F13.951
      - sexual dysfunction F13.981
      - sleep disorder F13.982
      - unspecified disorder F13.99
    - harmful — *see* Abuse, drug, sedative, hypnotic, or anxiolytic
    - in remission F13.91
  - stimulant NEC F15.90
    - with
      - anxiety disorder F15.980
      - intoxication F15.929
        - with
          - delirium F15.921
          - perceptual disturbance F15.922
- **Use** — *continued*
  - stimulant — *continued*
    - with — *continued*
      - intoxication — *continued*
        - uncomplicated F15.920
      - mood disorder F15.94
      - other specified disorder F15.988
      - psychosis F15.959
        - delusions F15.950
        - hallucinations F15.951
      - sexual dysfunction F15.981
      - sleep disorder F15.982
      - unspecified disorder F15.99
      - withdrawal F15.93
    - harmful — *see* Abuse, drug, stimulant NEC
    - in remission F15.91
  - tobacco Z72.0
    - with dependence — *see* Dependence, drug, nicotine
  - volatile solvents — *see also* Use, inhalant F18.90
    - harmful — *see* Abuse, drug, inhalant
- **Usher-Senear disease or syndrome** L10.4
- **Uta** B55.1
- **Uteromegaly** N85.2
- **Uterovaginal** — *see* condition
- **Uterovesical** — *see* condition
- **Uveal** — *see* condition
- **Uveitis** (anterior) — *see also* Iridocyclitis
  - acute — *see* Iridocyclitis, acute
  - chronic — *see* Iridocyclitis, chronic
  - due to toxoplasmosis (acquired) B58.09
    - congenital P37.1
  - granulomatous — *see* Iridocyclitis, chronic
  - heterochromic — *see* Cyclitis, Fuchs' heterochromic
  - lens-induced — *see* Iridocyclitis, lens-induced
  - posterior — *see* Chorioretinitis
  - sympathetic H44.13- ☑
  - syphilitic (secondary) A51.43
    - congenital (early) A50.01
    - late A52.71
  - tuberculous A18.54
- **Uveoencephalitis** — *see* Inflammation, chorioretinal
- **Uveokeratitis** — *see* Iridocyclitis
- **Uveoparotitis** D86.89
- **Uvula** — *see* condition
- **Uvulitis** (acute) (catarrhal) (chronic) (membranous) (suppurative) (ulcerative) K12.2

V

- **Vaccination** (prophylactic)
  - complication or reaction — *see* Complications, vaccination
  - delayed Z28.9
  - encounter for Z23
  - not done — *see* Immunization, not done
  - partial — *see also* Underimmunization status
    - for COVID-19 Z28.311
- **Vaccinia** (generalized) (localized) T88.1 ☑
  - congenital P35.8
  - without vaccination B08.011
- **Vacuum, in sinus** (accessory) (nasal) J34.89
- **Vagabond, vagabondage** Z59.00
- **Vagabond's disease** B85.1
- **Vagina, vaginal** — *see* condition
- **Vaginalitis** (tunica) (testis) N49.1
- **Vaginismus** (reflex) N94.2
  - functional F52.5
  - nonorganic F52.5
  - psychogenic F52.5
  - secondary N94.2
- **Vaginitis** (acute) (circumscribed) (diffuse) (emphysematous) (nonvenereal) (ulcerative) N76.0
  - with ectopic or molar pregnancy O08.0
  - amebic A06.82
  - atrophic, postmenopausal N95.2
  - bacterial N76.0
  - blennorrhagic (gonococcal) A54.02
  - candidal (acute) B37.31
    - chronic (recurrent) B37.32
  - chlamydial A56.02
  - chronic N76.1
  - due to Trichomonas (vaginalis) A59.01
  - following ectopic or molar pregnancy O08.0
  - gonococcal A54.02
    - with abscess (accessory gland) (periurethral) A54.1
  - granuloma A58

Vaginitis — *continued*
  in (due to)
    candidiasis (acute) B37.31
      chronic (recurrent) B37.32
    herpesviral (herpes simplex) infection A6Ø.Ø4
    pinworm infection B8Ø *[N77.1]*
  monilial (acute) B37.31
    chronic (recurrent) B37.32
  mycotic (candidal) (acute) B37.31
    chronic (recurrent) B37.32
  postmenopausal atrophic N95.2
  puerperal (postpartum) O86.13
  senile (atrophic) N95.2
  subacute or chronic N76.1
  syphilitic (early) A51.Ø
    late A52.76
  trichomonal A59.Ø1
  tuberculous A18.18
Vaginosis — *see* Vaginitis
Vagotonia G52.2
Vagrancy Z59.ØØ
VAIN — *see* Neoplasia, intraepithelial, vagina
Vallecula — *see* condition
Valley fever B38.Ø
Valsuani's disease — *see* Anemia, obstetric
Valve, valvular (formation) — *see also* condition
  cerebral ventricle (communicating) in situ Z98.2
  cervix, internal os Q51.828
  congenital NEC — *see* Atresia, by site
  ureter (pelvic junction) (vesical orifice) Q62.39
  urethra (congenital) (posterior) Q64.2
Valvulitis (chronic) — *see* Endocarditis
Valvulopathy — *see* Endocarditis
Van Bogaert's leukoencephalopathy (sclerosing) (subacute) A81.1
Van Bogaert-Scherer-Epstein disease or syndrome E75.5
Van Buchem's syndrome M85.2
Van Creveld-von Gierke disease E74.Ø1
Van der Hoeve (-de Kleyn) **syndrome** Q78.Ø
Van der Woude's syndrome Q38.Ø
Van Neck's disease or osteochondrosis M91.Ø
Vanishing lung J44.9
Vapor asphyxia or suffocation T59.9 ☑
  specified agent — *see* Table of Drugs and Chemicals
Variance, lethal ball, prosthetic heart valve T82.Ø9 ☑
Variants, thalassemic D56.8
Variations in hair color L67.1
Varicella BØ1.9
  with
    complications NEC BØ1.89
    encephalitis BØ1.11
    encephalomyelitis BØ1.11
    meningitis BØ1.Ø
    myelitis BØ1.12
    pneumonia BØ1.2
  congenital P35.8
Varices — *see* Varix
Varicocele (scrotum) (thrombosed) I86.1
  ovary I86.2
  perineum I86.3
  spermatic cord (ulcerated) I86.1
Varicose
  aneurysm (ruptured) I77.Ø
  dermatitis — *see* Varix, leg, with, inflammation
  eczema — *see* Varix, leg, with, inflammation
  phlebitis — *see* Varix, with, inflammation
  tumor — *see* Varix
  ulcer (lower limb, any part) — *see also* Varix, leg, with, ulcer
    anus — *see also* Hemorrhoids K64.8
    esophagus — *see* Varix, esophagus
    inflamed or infected — *see* Varix, leg, with ulcer, with inflammation
    nasal septum I86.8
    perineum I86.3
    scrotum I86.1
    specified site NEC I86.8
  vein — *see* Varix
  vessel — *see* Varix, leg
Varicosis, varicosities, varicosity — *see* Varix
Variola (major) (minor) BØ3
Varioloid BØ3
Varix (lower limb) I83.9Ø
  with
    bleeding I83.899
    edema I83.899

Varix — *continued*
  with — *continued*
    inflammation I83.1Ø
      with ulcer (venous) I83.2Ø9
    pain I83.819
    rupture I83.899
    specified complication NEC I83.899
    stasis dermatitis I83.1Ø
      with ulcer (venous) I83.2Ø9
    swelling I83.899
    ulcer I83.ØØ9
      with inflammation I83.2Ø9
  aneurysmal I77.Ø
  asymptomatic I83.9- ☑
  bladder I86.2
  broad ligament I86.2
  complicating
    childbirth (lower extremity) O87.4
      anus or rectum O87.2
      genital (vagina, vulva or perineum) O87.8
    pregnancy (lower extremity) O22.Ø- ☑
      anus or rectum O22.4- ☑
      genital (vagina, vulva or perineum) O22.1- ☑
    puerperium (lower extremity) O87.4
      anus or rectum O87.2
      genital (vagina, vulva, perineum) O87.8
  congenital (any site) Q27.8
  esophagus (idiopathic) (primary) (ulcerated) I85.ØØ
    bleeding I85.Ø1
    congenital Q27.8
    in (due to)
      alcoholic liver disease I85.1Ø
        bleeding I85.11
      cirrhosis of liver I85.1Ø
        bleeding I85.11
      portal hypertension I85.1Ø
        bleeding I85.11
      schistosomiasis I85.1Ø
        bleeding I85.11
      toxic liver disease I85.1Ø
        bleeding I85.11
    secondary I85.1Ø
      bleeding I85.11
  gastric I86.4
  inflamed or infected I83.1Ø
    ulcerated I83.2Ø9
  labia (majora) I86.3
  leg (asymptomatic) I83.9- ☑
    with
      edema I83.899
      inflammation I83.1Ø
        with ulcer — *see* Varix, leg, with, ulcer, with inflammation by site
      pain I83.819
      specified complication NEC I83.899
      swelling I83.899
      ulcer I83.Ø- ☑
        with inflammation I83.2- ☑
        ankle I83.ØØ3
          with inflammation I83.2Ø3
        calf I83.ØØ2
          with inflammation I83.2Ø2
        foot NEC I83.ØØ5
          with inflammation I83.2Ø5
        heel I83.ØØ4
          with inflammation I83.2Ø4
        lower leg NEC I83.ØØ8
          with inflammation I83.2Ø8
        midfoot I83.ØØ4
          with inflammation I83.2Ø4
        thigh I83.ØØ1
          with inflammation I83.2Ø1
    bilateral (asymptomatic) I83.93
      with
        edema I83.893
        pain I83.813
        specified complication NEC I83.893
        swelling I83.893
        ulcer I83.Ø- ☑
          with inflammation I83.2Ø9
    left (asymptomatic) I83.92
      with
        edema I83.892
        inflammation I83.12
          with ulcer — *see* Varix, leg, with, ulcer, with inflammation by site
        pain I83.812
        specified complication NEC I83.892

Varix — *continued*
  leg — *continued*
    left — *continued*
      with — *continued*
        swelling I83.892
        ulcer I83.Ø29
          with inflammation I83.229
          ankle I83.Ø23
            with inflammation I83.223
          calf I83.Ø22
            with inflammation I83.222
          foot NEC I83.Ø25
            with inflammation I83.225
          heel I83.Ø24
            with inflammation I83.224
          lower leg NEC I83.Ø28
            with inflammation I83.228
          midfoot I83.Ø24
            with inflammation I83.224
          thigh I83.Ø21
            with inflammation I83.221
    right (asymptomatic) I83.91
      with
        edema I83.891
        inflammation I83.11
          with ulcer — *see* Varix, leg, with, ulcer, with inflammation by site
        pain I83.811
        specified complication NEC I83.891
        swelling I83.891
        ulcer I83.Ø19
          with inflammation I83.219
          ankle I83.Ø13
            with inflammation I83.213
          calf I83.Ø12
            with inflammation I83.212
          foot NEC I83.Ø15
            with inflammation I83.215
          heel I83.Ø14
            with inflammation I83.214
          lower leg NEC I83.Ø18
            with inflammation I83.218
          midfoot I83.Ø14
            with inflammation I83.214
          thigh I83.Ø11
            with inflammation I83.211
  nasal septum I86.8
  orbit I86.8
    congenital Q27.8
  ovary I86.2
  papillary I78.1
  pelvis I86.2
  perineum I86.3
  pharynx I86.8
  placenta O43.89- ☑
  renal papilla I86.8
  retina H35.Ø9
  scrotum (ulcerated) I86.1
  sigmoid colon I86.8
  specified site NEC I86.8
  spinal (cord) (vessels) I86.8
  spleen, splenic (vein) (with phlebolith) I86.8
  stomach I86.4
  sublingual I86.Ø
  ulcerated I83.ØØ9
    inflamed or infected I83.2Ø9
  uterine ligament I86.2
  vagina I86.8
  vocal cord I86.8
  vulva I86.3
Vas deferens — *see* condition
Vas deferentitis N49.1
Vasa previa O69.4 ☑
  hemorrhage from, affecting newborn P5Ø.Ø
Vascular — *see also* condition
  loop on optic papilla Q14.2
  spasm I73.9
  spider I78.1
Vascularization, cornea — *see* Neovascularization, cornea
Vasculitis I77.6
  allergic D69.Ø
  ANCA (antineutrophilic cytoplasmic antibody) associated I77.82
  ANCA (antineutrophilic cytoplasmic antibody) positive I77.82
  antineutrophilic cytoplasmic antibody [ANCA] I77.82
  cryoglobulinemic D89.1

- **Vasculitis** — *continued*
  - disseminated I77.6
  - hypocomplementemic M31.8
  - kidney I77.89
  - leukocytoclastic M31.Ø
  - livedoid L95.Ø
  - nodular L95.8
  - retina H35.Ø6- ☑
  - rheumatic — *see* Fever, rheumatic
  - rheumatoid — *see* Rheumatoid, vasculitis
  - skin (limited to) L95.9
    - specified NEC L95.8
  - systemic M31.8
- **Vasculopathy, necrotizing** M31.9
  - cardiac allograft T86.29Ø
  - specified NEC M31.8
- **Vasitis** (nodosa) N49.1
  - tuberculous A18.15
- **Vasodilation** I73.9
- **Vasomotor** — *see* condition
- **Vasoplasty, after previous sterilization** Z31.Ø
  - aftercare Z31.42
- **Vasospasm** (vasoconstriction) I73.9
  - cerebral (cerebrovascular) (artery) I67.848
    - reversible I67.841
  - coronary I2Ø.1
  - nerve
    - arm — *see* Mononeuropathy, upper limb
    - brachial plexus G54.Ø
    - cervical plexus G54.2
    - leg — *see* Mononeuropathy, lower limb
  - peripheral NOS I73.9
  - retina (artery) — *see* Occlusion, artery, retina
- **Vasospastic** — *see* condition
- **Vasovagal attack** (paroxysmal) R55
  - psychogenic F45.8
- **VATER syndrome** Q87.2
- **Vater's ampulla** — *see* condition
- **Vegetation, vegetative**
  - adenoid (nasal fossa) J35.8
  - endocarditis (acute) (any valve) (subacute) I33.Ø
  - heart (mycotic) (valve) I33.Ø
- **Veil**
  - Jackson's Q43.3
- **Vein, venous** — *see* condition
- **Veldt sore** — *see* Ulcer, skin
- **Velpeau's hernia** — *see* Hernia, femoral
- **Venereal**
  - bubo A55
  - disease A64
  - granuloma inguinale A58
  - lymphogranuloma (Durand-Nicolas-Favre) A55
- **Venofibrosis** I87.8
- **Venom, venomous** — *see* Table of Drugs and Chemicals, by animal or substance, poisoning
- **Venous** — *see* condition
- **Ventilator lung, newborn** P27.8
- **Ventral** — *see* condition
- **Ventricle, ventricular** — *see also* condition
  - escape I49.3
  - inversion Q2Ø.5
- **Ventriculitis** (cerebral) — *see also* Encephalitis GØ4.9Ø
- **Ventriculostomy status** Z98.2
- **Vernet's syndrome** G52.7
- **Verneuil's disease** (syphilitic bursitis) A52.78
- **Verruca** (due to HPV) (filiformis) (simplex) (viral) (vulgaris) BØ7.9
  - acuminata A63.Ø
  - necrogenica (primary) (tuberculosa) A18.4
  - plana BØ7.8
  - plantaris BØ7.Ø
  - seborrheica L82.1
    - inflamed L82.Ø
  - senile (seborrheic) L82.1
    - inflamed L82.Ø
  - tuberculosa (primary) A18.4
  - venerea A63.Ø
- **Verrucosities** — *see* Verruca
- **Verruga peruana, peruviana** A44.1
- **Version**
  - cervix — *see* Malposition, uterus
  - uterus (postinfectional) (postpartal, old) — *see* Malposition, uterus
- **Vertebra, vertebral** — *see* condition
- **Vertical talus** (congenital) Q66.8Ø
  - left foot Q66.82
  - right foot Q66.81
- **Vertigo** R42
  - auditory — *see* Vertigo, aural
  - aural H81.31- ☑
  - benign paroxysmal (positional) H81.1- ☑
  - central (origin) H81.4
  - cerebral H81.4
  - Dix and Hallpike (epidemic) — *see* Neuronitis, vestibular
  - due to infrasound T75.23 ☑
  - epidemic A88.1
    - Dix and Hallpike — *see* Neuronitis, vestibular
    - Pedersen's — *see* Neuronitis, vestibular
    - vestibular neuronitis — *see* Neuronitis, vestibular
  - hysterical F44.89
  - infrasound T75.23 ☑
  - labyrinthine — *see* subcategory H81.Ø ☑
  - laryngeal RØ5.4
  - malignant positional H81.4
  - Ménière's — *see* subcategory H81.Ø ☑
  - menopausal N95.1
  - otogenic — *see* Vertigo, aural
  - paroxysmal positional, benign — *see* Vertigo, benign paroxysmal
  - Pedersen's (epidemic) — *see* Neuronitis, vestibular
  - peripheral NEC H81.39- ☑
  - positional
    - benign paroxysmal — *see* Vertigo, benign paroxysmal
    - malignant H81.4
- **Very-low-density-lipoprotein-type** (VLDL) **hyperlipoproteinemia** E78.1
- **Vesania** — *see* Psychosis
- **Vesical** — *see* condition
- **Vesicle**
  - cutaneous R23.8
  - seminal — *see* condition
  - skin R23.8
- **Vesicocolic** — *see* condition
- **Vesicoperineal** — *see* condition
- **Vesicorectal** — *see* condition
- **Vesicourethrorectal** — *see* condition
- **Vesicovaginal** — *see* condition
- **Vesicular** — *see* condition
- **Vesiculitis** (seminal) N49.Ø
  - amebic AØ6.82
  - gonorrheal (acute) (chronic) A54.23
  - trichomonal A59.Ø9
  - tuberculous A18.15
- **Vestibulitis** (ear) — *see also* subcategory H83.Ø ☑
  - nose (external) J34.89
  - vulvar N94.81Ø
- **Vestibulopathy , acute peripheral** (recurrent) — *see* Neuronitis, vestibular
- **Vestige, vestigial** — *see also* Persistence
  - branchial Q18.Ø
  - structures in vitreous Q14.Ø
- **Vibration**
  - adverse effects T75.2Ø ☑
    - pneumatic hammer syndrome T75.21 ☑
    - specified effect NEC T75.29 ☑
    - vasospastic syndrome T75.22 ☑
    - vertigo from infrasound T75.23 ☑
  - exposure (occupational) Z57.7
  - vertigo T75.23 ☑
- **Vibriosis** A28.9
- **Victim** (of)
  - crime Z65.4
  - disaster Z65.5
  - terrorism Z65.4
  - torture Z65.4
  - war Z65.5
- **Vidal's disease** L28.Ø
- **Villaret's syndrome** G52.7
- **Villous** — *see* condition
- **VIN** — *see* Neoplasia, intraepithelial, vulva
- **Vincent's infection** (angina) (gingivitis) A69.1
  - stomatitis NEC A69.1
- **Vinson-Plummer syndrome** D5Ø.1
- **Violence, physical** R45.6
- **Viosterol deficiency** — *see* Deficiency, calciferol
- **Vipoma** — *see* Neoplasm, malignant, by site
- **Viremia** B34.9
- **Virilism** (adrenal) E25.9
  - congenital E25.Ø
- **Virilization** (female) (suprarenal) E25.9
  - congenital E25.Ø
  - isosexual E28.2
- **Virulent bubo** A57
- **Virus, viral** — *see also* condition
  - as cause of disease classified elsewhere B97.89
    - respiratory syncytial virus (RSV) — *see* Virus, respiratory syncytial (RSV)
  - cytomegalovirus B25.9
  - human immunodeficiency (HIV) — *see* Human, immunodeficiency virus (HIV) disease
  - infection — *see* Infection, virus
  - respiratory syncytial (RSV)
    - as cause of disease classified elsewhere B97.4
    - bronchiolitis J21.Ø
    - bronchitis J2Ø.5
    - bronchopneumonia J12.1
    - otitis media H65.- ☑ *[B97.4]*
    - pneumonia J12.1
    - upper respiratory infection JØ6.9 *[B97.4]*
  - specified NEC B34.8
  - swine influenza (viruses that normally cause infections in pigs) — *see also* Influenza, due to, identified novel influenza A virus JØ9.X2
  - West Nile (fever) A92.3Ø
    - with
      - complications NEC A92.39
      - cranial nerve disorders A92.32
      - encephalitis A92.31
      - encephalomyelitis A92.31
      - neurologic manifestation NEC A92.32
      - optic neuritis A92.32
      - polyradiculitis A92.32
- **Viscera, visceral** — *see* condition
- **Visceroptosis** K63.4
- **Visible peristalsis** R19.2
- **Vision, visual**
  - binocular, suppression H53.34
  - blurred, blurring H53.8
    - hysterical F44.6
  - defect, defective NEC H54.7
  - disorientation (syndrome) H53.8
  - disturbance H53.9
    - hysterical F44.6
  - double H53.2
  - examination ZØ1.ØØ
    - with abnormal findings ZØ1.Ø1
    - following failed vision screening ZØ1.Ø2Ø
      - with abnormal findings ZØ1.Ø21
  - field, limitation (defect) — *see* Defect, visual field
  - hallucinations R44.1
  - halos H53.19
  - loss — *see* Loss, vision
    - sudden — *see* Disturbance, vision, subjective, loss, sudden
  - low (both eyes) — *see* Low, vision
  - perception, simultaneous without fusion H53.33
- **Vitality, lack or want of** R53.83
  - newborn P96.89
- **Vitamin deficiency** — *see* Deficiency, vitamin
- **Vitelline duct, persistent** Q43.Ø
- **Vitiligo** L8Ø
  - eyelid HØ2.739
    - left HØ2.736
      - lower HØ2.735
      - upper HØ2.734
    - right HØ2.733
      - lower HØ2.732
      - upper HØ2.731
  - pinta A67.2
  - vulva N9Ø.89
- **Vitreal corneal syndrome** H59.Ø1- ☑
- **Vitreoretinopathy, proliferative** — *see also* Retinopathy, proliferative
  - with retinal detachment — *see* Detachment, retina, traction
- **Vitreous** — *see also* condition
  - touch syndrome — *see* Complication, postprocedural, following cataract surgery
- **Vocal cord** — *see* condition
- **Vogt-Koyanagi syndrome** H2Ø.82- ☑
- **Vogt's disease or syndrome** G8Ø.3
- **Vogt-Spielmeyer amaurotic idiocy or disease** E75.4
- **Voice**
  - change R49.9
    - specified NEC R49.8
  - loss — *see* Aphonia
- **Volhynian fever** A79.Ø
- **Volkmann's ischemic contracture or paralysis** (complicating trauma) T79.6 ☑
- **Volvulus** (bowel) (colon) (intestine) K56.2

- **Volvulus** — *continued*
  - with perforation K56.2
  - congenital Q43.8
  - duodenum K31.5
  - fallopian tube — *see* Torsion, fallopian tube
  - oviduct — *see* Torsion, fallopian tube
  - stomach (due to absence of gastrocolic ligament) K31.89
- **Vomiting** R11.1Ø
  - with nausea R11.2
  - asphyxia — *see* Foreign body, by site, causing asphyxia, gastric contents
  - bilious (cause unknown) R11.14
    - following gastro-intestinal surgery K91.Ø
    - in newborn P92.Ø1
  - blood — *see* Hematemesis
  - causing asphyxia, choking, or suffocation — *see* Foreign body, by site
  - cyclical, in migraine G43.AØ (*following* G43.7)
    - with refractory migraine G43.A1 (*following* G43.7)
    - intractable G43.A1 (*following* G43.7)
    - not intractable G43.AØ (*following* G43.7)
    - psychogenic F5Ø.89
    - without refractory migraine G43.AØ (*following* G43.7)
  - cyclical syndrome NOS (unrelated to migraine) R11.15
  - fecal mater R11.13
  - following gastrointestinal surgery K91.Ø
    - psychogenic F5Ø.89
  - functional K31.89
  - hysterical F5Ø.89
  - nervous F5Ø.89
  - neurotic F5Ø.89
  - newborn NEC P92.Ø9
    - bilious P92.Ø1
  - periodic R11.1Ø
    - psychogenic F5Ø.89
  - persistent R11.15
  - projectile R11.12
  - psychogenic F5Ø.89
  - uremic — *see* Uremia
  - without nausea R11.11
- **Vomito negro** — *see* Fever, yellow
- **Von Bezold's abscess** — *see* Mastoiditis, acute
- **Von Economo-Cruchet disease** A85.8
- **Von Eulenburg's disease** G71.19
- **Von Gierke's disease** E74.Ø1
- **Von Hippel** (-Lindau) **disease or syndrome** Q85.83
- **Von Jaksch's anemia or disease** D64.89
- **Von Recklinghausen**
  - disease (neurofibromatosis) Q85.Ø1
    - bones E21.Ø
- **Von Schroetter's syndrome** I82.89Ø
- **Von Willebrand** (-Jurgens) (-Minot) **disease or syndrome** — *see* Disease, von Willebrand
- **Von Zumbusch's disease** L4Ø.1
- **Voyeurism** F65.3
- **Vrolik's disease** Q78.Ø
- **Vulva** — *see* condition
- **Vulvismus** N94.2
- **Vulvitis** (acute) (allergic) (atrophic) (hypertrophic) (intertriginous) (senile) N76.2
  - with ectopic or molar pregnancy OØ8.Ø
  - adhesive, congenital Q52.79
  - blennorrhagic (gonococcal) A54.Ø2
  - candidal (acute) B37.31
    - chronic (recurrent) B37.32
  - chlamydial A56.Ø2
  - due to Haemophilus ducreyi A57
  - following ectopic or molar pregnancy OØ8.Ø
  - gonococcal A54.Ø2
    - with abscess (accessory gland) (periurethral) A54.1
  - herpesviral A6Ø.Ø4
  - leukoplakic N9Ø.4
  - monilial (acute) B37.31
    - chronic (recurrent) B37.32
  - puerperal (postpartum) O86.19
  - subacute or chronic N76.3
  - syphilitic (early) A51.Ø
    - late A52.76
  - trichomonal A59.Ø1
  - tuberculous A18.18
- **Vulvodynia** N94.819
  - specified NEC N94.818
- **Vulvorectal** — *see* condition
- **Vulvovaginitis** (acute) — *see* Vaginitis

W

- **Waiting list, person on** Z75.1
  - for organ transplant Z76.82
  - undergoing social agency investigation Z75.2
- **Waldenström**
  - hypergammaglobulinemia D89.Ø
  - syndrome or macroglobulinemia C88.Ø
- **Waldenström-Kjellberg syndrome** D5Ø.1
- **Walking**
  - difficulty R26.2
    - psychogenic F44.4
  - sleep F51.3
    - hysterical F44.89
- **Wall, abdominal** — *see* condition
- **Wallenberg's disease or syndrome** G46.3
- **Wallgren's disease** I87.8
- **Wandering**
  - gallbladder, congenital Q44.1
  - in diseases classified elsewhere Z91.83
  - kidney, congenital Q63.8
  - organ or site, congenital NEC — *see* Malposition, congenital, by site
  - pacemaker (heart) I49.8
  - spleen D73.89
- **War neurosis** F48.8
- **Wart** (due to HPV) (filiform) (infectious) (viral) BØ7.9
  - anogenital region (venereal) A63.Ø
  - common BØ7.8
  - external genital organs (venereal) A63.Ø
  - flat BØ7.8
  - Hassal-Henle's (of cornea) H18.49
  - Peruvian A44.1
  - plantar BØ7.Ø
  - prosector (tuberculous) A18.4
  - seborrheic L82.1
    - inflamed L82.Ø
  - senile (seborrheic) L82.1
    - inflamed L82.Ø
  - tuberculous A18.4
  - venereal A63.Ø
- **Warthin's tumor** — *see* Neoplasm, salivary gland, benign
- **Wassilieff's disease** A27.Ø
- **Wasting**
  - disease R64
    - due to malnutrition E43
      - with marasmus E41
  - extreme (due to malnutrition) E43
    - with marasmus E41
  - muscle NEC — *see* Atrophy, muscle
- **Water**
  - clefts (senile cataract) — *see* Cataract, senile, incipient
  - deprivation of T73.1 ☑
  - intoxication E87.79
  - itch B76.9
  - lack of T73.1 ☑
    - safe drinking Z58.6
  - loading E87.7Ø
  - on
    - brain — *see* Hydrocephalus
    - chest J94.8
  - poisoning E87.79
- **Waterbrash** R12
- **Waterhouse** (-Friderichsen) **syndrome or disease** (meningococcal) A39.1
- **Water-losing nephritis** N25.89
- **Watermelon stomach** K31.819
  - with hemorrhage K31.811
  - without hemorrhage K31.819
- **Watsoniasis** B66.8
- **Wax in ear** — *see* Impaction, cerumen
- **Weak, weakening, weakness** (generalized) R53.1
  - arches (acquired) — *see also* Deformity, limb, flat foot
  - bladder (sphincter) R32
  - facial R29.81Ø
    - following
      - cerebrovascular disease I69.992
        - cerebral infarction I69.392
        - intracerebral hemorrhage I69.192
        - nontraumatic intracranial hemorrhage NEC I69.292
        - specified disease NEC I69.892
        - stroke I69.392
        - subarachnoid hemorrhage I69.Ø92
  - foot (double) — *see also* Weak, arches
  - heart, cardiac — *see* Failure, heart
  - mind F7Ø
- **Weak, weakening, weakness** — *continued*
  - muscle M62.81
  - myocardium — *see* Failure, heart
  - newborn P96.89
  - pelvic fundus N81.89
  - pubocervical tissue N81.82
  - rectovaginal tissue N81.83
  - senile R54
  - urinary stream R39.12
  - valvular — *see* Endocarditis
- **Wear, worn** (with normal or routine use)
  - articular bearing surface of internal joint prosthesis — *see* Complications, joint prosthesis, mechanical, wear of articular bearing surfaces, by site
  - device, implant or graft — *see* Complications, by site, mechanical complication
  - tooth, teeth (approximal) (hard tissues) (interproximal) (occlusal) KØ3.Ø
- **Weather, weathered**
  - effects of
    - cold T69.9 ☑
      - specified effect NEC T69.8 ☑
    - hot — *see* Heat
  - skin L57.8
- **Weaver's syndrome** Q87.3
- **Web, webbed** (congenital)
  - duodenal Q43.8
  - esophagus Q39.4
  - fingers Q7Ø.1- ☑
  - larynx (glottic) (subglottic) Q31.Ø
  - neck (pterygium colli) Q18.3
  - Paterson-Kelly D5Ø.1
  - popliteal syndrome Q87.89
  - toes Q7Ø.3- ☑
- **Weber-Christian disease** M35.6
- **Weber-Cockayne syndrome** (epidermolysis bullosa) Q81.8
- **Weber-Gubler syndrome** G46.3
- **Weber-Leyden syndrome** G46.3
- **Weber-Osler syndrome** I78.Ø
- **Weber's paralysis or syndrome** G46.3
- **Wedge-shaped or wedging vertebra** — *see* Collapse, vertebra NEC
- **Wegener's granulomatosis or syndrome** M31.3Ø
  - with
    - kidney involvement M31.31
    - lung involvement M31.3Ø
      - with kidney involvement M31.31
- **Wegner's disease** A5Ø.Ø2
- **Weight**
  - 1ØØØ-2499 grams at birth (low) — *see* Low, birthweight
  - 999 grams or less at birth (extremely low) — *see* Low, birthweight, extreme
  - and length below 1Øth percentile for gestational age PØ5.1- ☑
  - below but length above 1Øth percentile for gestational age PØ5.Ø- ☑
  - gain (abnormal) (excessive) R63.5
    - in pregnancy — *see* Pregnancy, complicated by, excessive weight gain
    - low — *see* Pregnancy, complicated by, insufficient, weight gain
  - loss (abnormal) (cause unknown) R63.4
- **Weightlessness** (effect of) T75.82 ☑
- **Weil (l)-Marchesani syndrome** Q87.19
- **Weil's disease** A27.Ø
- **Weingarten's syndrome** J82.89
- **Weir Mitchell's disease** I73.81
- **Weiss-Baker syndrome** G9Ø.Ø9
- **Wells' disease** L98.3
- **Wen** — *see* Cyst, sebaceous
- **Wenckebach's block or phenomenon** I44.1
- **Werdnig-Hoffmann syndrome** (muscular atrophy) G12.Ø
- **Werlhof's disease** D69.3
- **Wermer's disease or syndrome** E31.21
- **Werner-His disease** A79.Ø
- **Werner's disease or syndrome** E34.8
- **Wernicke-Korsakoff's syndrome or psychosis** (alcoholic) F1Ø.96
  - with dependence F1Ø.26
  - drug-induced
    - due to drug abuse — *see* Abuse, drug, by type, with amnestic disorder
    - due to drug dependence — *see* Dependence, drug, by type, with amnestic disorder
  - nonalcoholic FØ4

Wernicke-Posadas disease B38.9
Wernicke's
  developmental aphasia F8Ø.2
  disease or syndrome E51.2
  encephalopathy E51.2
  polioencephalitis, superior E51.2
West African fever B5Ø.8
Westphal-Strümpell syndrome E83.Ø1
West's syndrome — *see* Epilepsy, spasms
Wet
  feet, tropical (maceration) (syndrome) — *see* Immersion, foot
  lung (syndrome), newborn P22.1
Wharton's duct — *see* condition
Wheal — *see* Urticaria
Wheezing RØ6.2
Whiplash injury S13.4 ☑
Whipple's disease — *see also* subcategory M14.8- K9Ø.81
Whipworm (disease) (infection) (infestation) B79
Whistling face Q87.Ø
White — *see also* condition
  kidney, small NØ3.9
  leg, puerperal, postpartum, childbirth O87.1
  mouth B37.Ø
  patches of mouth K13.29
  spot lesions, teeth
    chewing surface KØ2.51
    pit and fissure surface KØ2.51
    smooth surface KØ2.61
Whitehead L7Ø.Ø
Whitlow — *see also* Cellulitis, digit
  with lymphangitis — *see* Lymphangitis, acute, digit
  herpesviral BØØ.89
Whitmore's disease or fever — *see* Melioidosis
Whooping cough A37.9Ø
  with pneumonia A37.91
    due to Bordetella
      bronchiseptica A37.81
      parapertussis A37.11
      pertussis A37.Ø1
    specified organism NEC A37.81
  due to
    Bordetella
      bronchiseptica A37.8Ø
        with pneumonia A37.81
      parapertussis A37.1Ø
        with pneumonia A37.11
      pertussis A37.ØØ
        with pneumonia A37.Ø1
    specified NEC A37.8Ø
      with pneumonia A37.81
Wichman's asthma J38.5
Wide cranial sutures, newborn P96.3
Widening aorta — *see* Ectasia, aorta
  with aneurysm — *see* Aneurysm, aorta
Wilkie's disease or syndrome K55.1
Wilkinson-Sneddon disease or syndrome L13.1
Willebrand (-Jürgens) **thrombopathy** — *see* Disease, von Willebrand
Williams syndrome Q93.82
Willige-Hunt disease or syndrome G23.1
Wilms' tumor C64- ☑
Wilson-Mikity syndrome P27.Ø
Wilson's
  disease or syndrome E83.Ø1
  hepatolenticular degeneration E83.Ø1
  lichen ruber L43.9
Window — *see also* Imperfect, closure
  aorticopulmonary Q21.4
Winter — *see* condition
Wiskott-Aldrich syndrome D82.Ø
Withdrawal state — *see also* Dependence, drug by type, with withdrawal
  alcohol
    with perceptual disturbances F1Ø.232
      due to alcohol abuse F1Ø.132
      due to alcohol use F1Ø.932
    abuse — *see* Abuse, alcohol, with, withdrawal
    dependence — *see* Dependence, alcohol, with, withdrawal
    use — *see* Use, alcohol, with, withdrawal
    without perceptual disturbances F1Ø.239
      due to alcohol abuse F1Ø.139
      due to alcohol use F1Ø.939
  caffeine F15.93
  cannabis F12.23

Withdrawal state — *continued*
  newborn
    correct therapeutic substance properly administered P96.2
    infant of dependent mother P96.1
  therapeutic substance, neonatal P96.2
Witts' anemia D5Ø.8
Witzelsucht FØ7.Ø
Woakes' ethmoiditis or syndrome J33.1
Wolff-Hirschorn syndrome Q93.3
Wolff-Parkinson-White syndrome I45.6
Wolhynian fever A79.Ø
Wolman's disease E75.5
Wood lung or pneumonitis J67.8
Woolly, wooly hair (congenital) (nevus) Q84.1
Woolsorter's disease A22.1
Word
  blindness (congenital) (developmental) F81.Ø
  deafness (congenital) (developmental) H93.25
Worm(s) (infection) (infestation) — *see also* Infestation, helminth
  guinea B72
  in intestine NEC B82.Ø
Worm-eaten soles A66.3
Worn out — *see* Exhaustion
  cardiac
    defibrillator (with synchronous cardiac pacemaker) Z45.Ø2
    pacemaker
      battery Z45.Ø1Ø
      lead Z45.Ø18
  device, implant or graft — *see* Complications, by site, mechanical
Worried well Z71.1
Worries R45.82
Wound check Z48.Ø- ☑
  due to injury — *code to* Injury, by site, using appropriate seventh character for subsequent encounter
Wound, open T14.8- ☑
  abdomen, abdominal
    wall S31.1Ø9 ☑
      with penetration into peritoneal cavity S31.6Ø9 ☑
      bite — *see* Bite, abdomen, wall
      epigastric region S31.1Ø2 ☑
        with penetration into peritoneal cavity S31.6Ø2 ☑
        bite — *see* Bite, abdomen, wall, epigastric region
        laceration — *see* Laceration, abdomen, wall, epigastric region
        puncture — *see* Puncture, abdomen, wall, epigastric region
      laceration — *see* Laceration, abdomen, wall
      left
        lower quadrant S31.1Ø4 ☑
          with penetration into peritoneal cavity S31.6Ø4 ☑
          bite — *see* Bite, abdomen, wall, left, lower quadrant
          laceration — *see* Laceration, abdomen, wall, left, lower quadrant
          puncture — *see* Puncture, abdomen, wall, left, lower quadrant
        upper quadrant S31.1Ø1 ☑
          with penetration into peritoneal cavity S31.6Ø1 ☑
          bite — *see* Bite, abdomen, wall, left, upper quadrant
          laceration — *see* Laceration, abdomen, wall, left, upper quadrant
          puncture — *see* Puncture, abdomen, wall, left, upper quadrant
      periumbilic region S31.1Ø5 ☑
        with penetration into peritoneal cavity S31.6Ø5 ☑
        bite — *see* Bite, abdomen, wall, periumbilic region
        laceration — *see* Laceration, abdomen, wall, periumbilic region
        puncture — *see* Puncture, abdomen, wall, periumbilic region
      puncture — *see* Puncture, abdomen, wall
      right
        lower quadrant S31.1Ø3 ☑
          with penetration into peritoneal cavity S31.6Ø3 ☑

Wound, open — *continued*
  abdomen, abdominal — *continued*
    wall — *continued*
      right — *continued*
        lower quadrant — *continued*
          bite — *see* Bite, abdomen, wall, right, lower quadrant
          laceration — *see* Laceration, abdomen, wall, right, lower quadrant
          puncture — *see* Puncture, abdomen, wall, right, lower quadrant
        upper quadrant S31.1ØØ ☑
          with penetration into peritoneal cavity S31.6ØØ ☑
          bite — *see* Bite, abdomen, wall, right, upper quadrant
          laceration — *see* Laceration, abdomen, wall, right, upper quadrant
          puncture — *see* Puncture, abdomen, wall, right, upper quadrant
  alveolar (process) — *see* Wound, open, oral cavity
  ankle S91.ØØ- ☑
    bite — *see* Bite, ankle
    laceration — *see* Laceration, ankle
    puncture — *see* Puncture, ankle
  antecubital space — *see* Wound, open, elbow
  anterior chamber, eye — *see* Wound, open, ocular
  anus S31.839 ☑
    bite S31.835 ☑
    laceration — *see* Laceration, anus
    puncture — *see* Puncture, anus
  arm (upper) S41.1Ø- ☑
    with amputation — *see* Amputation, traumatic, arm
    bite — *see* Bite, arm
    forearm — *see* Wound, open, forearm
    laceration — *see* Laceration, arm
    puncture — *see* Puncture, arm
  auditory canal (external) (meatus) — *see* Wound, open, ear
  auricle, ear — *see* Wound, open, ear
  axilla — *see* Wound, open, arm
  back — *see also* Wound, open, thorax, back
    lower S31.ØØØ ☑
      with penetration into retroperitoneal space S31.ØØ1 ☑
      bite — *see* Bite, back, lower
      laceration — *see* Laceration, back, lower
      puncture — *see* Puncture, back, lower
  bite — *see* Bite
  blood vessel — *see* Injury, blood vessel
  breast S21.ØØ- ☑
    with amputation — *see* Amputation, traumatic, breast
    bite — *see* Bite, breast
    laceration — *see* Laceration, breast
    puncture — *see* Puncture, breast
  buttock S31.8Ø9 ☑
    bite — *see* Bite, buttock
    laceration — *see* Laceration, buttock
    left S31.829 ☑
    puncture — *see* Puncture, buttock
    right S31.819 ☑
  calf — *see* Wound, open, leg
  canaliculus lacrimalis — *see* Wound, open, eyelid
  canthus, eye — *see* Wound, open, eyelid
  cervical esophagus S11.2Ø ☑
    bite S11.25 ☑
    laceration — *see* Laceration, esophagus, traumatic, cervical
    puncture — *see* Puncture, cervical esophagus
  cheek (external) SØ1.4Ø- ☑
    bite — *see* Bite, cheek
    internal — *see* Wound, open, oral cavity
    laceration — *see* Laceration, cheek
    puncture — *see* Puncture, cheek
  chest wall — *see* Wound, open, thorax
  chin — *see* Wound, open, head, specified site NEC
  choroid — *see* Wound, open, ocular
  ciliary body (eye) — *see* Wound, open, ocular
  clitoris S31.4Ø ☑
    with amputation — *see* Amputation, traumatic, clitoris
    bite S31.45 ☑
    laceration — *see* Laceration, vulva
    puncture — *see* Puncture, vulva
  conjunctiva — *see* Wound, open, ocular

Wound, open — *continued*
- cornea — *see* Wound, open, ocular
- costal region — *see* Wound, open, thorax
- Descemet's membrane — *see* Wound, open, ocular
- digit(s)
  - foot — *see* Wound, open, toe
  - hand — *see* Wound, open, finger
- ear (canal) (external) S01.30- ☑
  - with amputation — *see* Amputation, traumatic, ear
  - bite — *see* Bite, ear
  - drum S09.2- ☑
  - laceration — *see* Laceration, ear
  - puncture — *see* Puncture, ear
- elbow S51.00- ☑
  - bite — *see* Bite, elbow
  - laceration — *see* Laceration, elbow
  - puncture — *see* Puncture, elbow
- epididymis — *see* Wound, open, testis
- epigastric region S31.102 ☑
  - with penetration into peritoneal cavity S31.602 ☑
  - bite — *see* Bite, abdomen, wall, epigastric region
  - laceration — *see* Laceration, abdomen, wall, epigastric region
  - puncture — *see* Puncture, abdomen, wall, epigastric region
- epiglottis — *see* Wound, open, neck, specified site NEC
- esophagus (thoracic) S27.819 ☑
  - cervical — *see* Wound, open, cervical esophagus
  - laceration S27.813 ☑
  - specified type NEC S27.818 ☑
- eye — *see* Wound, open, ocular
- eyeball — *see* Wound, open, ocular
- eyebrow — *see* Wound, open, eyelid
- eyelid S01.10- ☑
  - bite — *see* Bite, eyelid
  - laceration — *see* Laceration, eyelid
  - puncture — *see* Puncture, eyelid
- face NEC — *see* Wound, open, head, specified site NEC
- finger(s) S61.209 ☑
  - with
    - amputation — *see* Amputation, traumatic, finger
    - damage to nail S61.309 ☑
  - bite — *see* Bite, finger
  - index S61.208 ☑
    - with
      - damage to nail S61.308 ☑
    - left S61.201 ☑
      - with
        - damage to nail S61.301 ☑
    - right S61.200 ☑
      - with
        - damage to nail S61.300 ☑
  - laceration — *see* Laceration, finger
  - little S61.208 ☑
    - with
      - damage to nail S61.308 ☑
    - left S61.207 ☑
      - with damage to nail S61.307 ☑
    - right S61.206 ☑
      - with damage to nail S61.306 ☑
  - middle S61.208 ☑
    - with
      - damage to nail S61.308 ☑
    - left S61.203 ☑
      - with damage to nail S61.303 ☑
    - right S61.202 ☑
      - with damage to nail S61.302 ☑
  - puncture — *see* Puncture, finger
  - ring S61.208 ☑
    - with
      - damage to nail S61.308 ☑
    - left S61.205 ☑
      - with damage to nail S61.305 ☑
    - right S61.204 ☑
      - with damage to nail S61.304 ☑
- flank — *see* Wound, open, abdomen, wall
- foot (except toe(s) alone) S91.30- ☑
  - with amputation — *see* Amputation, traumatic, foot
  - bite — *see* Bite, foot
  - laceration — *see* Laceration, foot
  - puncture — *see* Puncture, foot
  - toe — *see* Wound, open, toe
- forearm S51.80- ☑
  - with
    - amputation — *see* Amputation, traumatic, forearm

Wound, open — *continued*
- forearm — *continued*
  - bite — *see* Bite, forearm
  - elbow only — *see* Wound, open, elbow
  - laceration — *see* Laceration, forearm
  - puncture — *see* Puncture, forearm
- forehead — *see* Wound, open, head, specified site NEC
- genital organs, external
  - with amputation — *see* Amputation, traumatic, genital organs
  - bite — *see* Bite, genital organ
  - female S31.502 ☑
    - vagina S31.40 ☑
    - vulva S31.40 ☑
  - laceration — *see* Laceration, genital organ
  - male S31.501 ☑
    - penis S31.20 ☑
    - scrotum S31.30 ☑
    - testes S31.30 ☑
  - puncture — *see* Puncture, genital organ
- globe (eye) — *see* Wound, open, ocular
- groin — *see* Wound, open, abdomen, wall
- gum — *see* Wound, open, oral cavity
- hand S61.40- ☑
  - with
    - amputation — *see* Amputation, traumatic, hand
  - bite — *see* Bite, hand
  - finger(s) — *see* Wound, open, finger
  - laceration — *see* Laceration, hand
  - puncture — *see* Puncture, hand
  - thumb — *see* Wound, open, thumb
- head S01.90 ☑
  - bite — *see* Bite, head
  - cheek — *see* Wound, open, cheek
  - ear — *see* Wound, open, ear
  - eyelid — *see* Wound, open, eyelid
  - laceration — *see* Laceration, head
  - lip — *see* Wound, open, lip
  - nose S01.20 ☑
  - oral cavity — *see* Wound, open, oral cavity
  - puncture — *see* Puncture, head
  - scalp — *see* Wound, open, scalp
  - specified site NEC S01.80 ☑
  - temporomandibular area — *see* Wound, open, cheek
- heel — *see* Wound, open, foot
- hip S71.00- ☑
  - with amputation — *see* Amputation, traumatic, hip
  - bite — *see* Bite, hip
  - laceration — *see* Laceration, hip
  - puncture — *see* Puncture, hip
- hymen S31.40 ☑
  - bite — *see* Bite, vulva
  - laceration — *see* Laceration, vagina
  - puncture — *see* Puncture, vagina
- hypochondrium S31.109 ☑
  - bite — *see* Bite, hypochondrium
  - laceration — *see* Laceration, hypochondrium
  - puncture — *see* Puncture, hypochondrium
- hypogastric region S31.109 ☑
  - bite — *see* Bite, hypogastric region
  - laceration — *see* Laceration, hypogastric region
  - puncture — *see* Puncture, hypogastric region
- iliac (region) — *see* Wound, open, inguinal region
- inguinal region S31.109 ☑
  - bite — *see* Bite, abdomen, wall, lower quadrant
  - laceration — *see* Laceration, inguinal region
  - puncture — *see* Puncture, inguinal region
- instep — *see* Wound, open, foot
- interscapular region — *see* Wound, open, thorax, back
- intraocular — *see* Wound, open, ocular
- iris — *see* Wound, open, ocular
- jaw — *see* Wound, open, head, specified site NEC
- knee S81.00- ☑
  - bite — *see* Bite, knee
  - laceration — *see* Laceration, knee
  - puncture — *see* Puncture, knee
- labium (majus) (minus) — *see* Wound, open, vulva
- laceration — *see* Laceration, by site
- lacrimal duct — *see* Wound, open, eyelid
- larynx S11.019 ☑
  - bite — *see* Bite, larynx
  - laceration — *see* Laceration, larynx
  - puncture — *see* Puncture, larynx
- left
  - lower quadrant S31.104 ☑

Wound, open — *continued*
- left — *continued*
  - lower quadrant — *continued*
    - with penetration into peritoneal cavity S31.604 ☑
    - bite — *see* Bite, abdomen, wall, left, lower quadrant
    - laceration — *see* Laceration, abdomen, wall, left, lower quadrant
    - puncture — *see* Puncture, abdomen, wall, left, lower quadrant
  - upper quadrant S31.101 ☑
    - with penetration into peritoneal cavity S31.601 ☑
    - bite — *see* Bite, abdomen, wall, left, upper quadrant
    - laceration — *see* Laceration, abdomen, wall, left, upper quadrant
    - puncture — *see* Puncture, abdomen, wall, left, upper quadrant
- leg (lower) S81.80- ☑
  - with amputation — *see* Amputation, traumatic, leg
  - ankle — *see* Wound, open, ankle
  - bite — *see* Bite, leg
  - foot — *see* Wound, open, foot
  - knee — *see* Wound, open, knee
  - laceration — *see* Laceration, leg
  - puncture — *see* Puncture, leg
  - toe — *see* Wound, open, toe
  - upper — *see* Wound, open, thigh
- lip S01.501 ☑
  - bite — *see* Bite, lip
  - laceration — *see* Laceration, lip
  - puncture — *see* Puncture, lip
- loin S31.109 ☑
  - bite — *see* Bite, abdomen, wall
  - laceration — *see* Laceration, loin
  - puncture — *see* Puncture, loin
- lower back — *see* Wound, open, back, lower
- lumbar region — *see* Wound, open, back, lower
- malar region — *see* Wound, open, head, specified site NEC
- mammary — *see* Wound, open, breast
- mastoid region — *see* Wound, open, head, specified site NEC
- mouth — *see* Wound, open, oral cavity
- nail
  - finger — *see* Wound, open, finger, with damage to nail
  - toe — *see* Wound, open, toe, with damage to nail
- nape (neck) — *see* Wound, open, neck
- nasal (septum) (sinus) — *see* Wound, open, nose
- nasopharynx — *see* Wound, open, head, specified site NEC
- neck S11.90 ☑
  - bite — *see* Bite, neck
  - involving
    - cervical esophagus S11.20 ☑
    - larynx — *see* Wound, open, larynx
    - pharynx S11.20 ☑
    - thyroid S11.10 ☑
    - trachea (cervical) S11.029 ☑
      - bite — *see* Bite, trachea
      - laceration S11.021 ☑
        - with foreign body S11.022 ☑
      - puncture S11.023 ☑
        - with foreign body S11.024 ☑
  - laceration — *see* Laceration, neck
  - puncture — *see* Puncture, neck
  - specified site NEC S11.80 ☑
    - specified type NEC S11.89 ☑
- nose (septum) (sinus) S01.20 ☑
  - with amputation — *see* Amputation, traumatic, nose
  - bite — *see* Bite, nose
  - laceration — *see* Laceration, nose
  - puncture — *see* Puncture, nose
- ocular S05.90 ☑
  - avulsion (traumatic enucleation) S05.7- ☑
  - eyeball S05.6- ☑
    - with foreign body S05.5- ☑
  - eyelid — *see* Wound, open, eyelid
  - laceration and rupture S05.3- ☑
    - with prolapse or loss of intraocular tissue S05.2- ☑

Wound, open — *continued*
ocular — *continued*
orbit (penetrating) (with or without foreign body) S05.4- ☑
periocular area — *see* Wound, open, eyelid
specified NEC S05.8X- ☑
oral cavity S01.502 ☑
bite S01.552 ☑
laceration — *see* Laceration, oral cavity
puncture — *see* Puncture, oral cavity
orbit — *see* Wound, open, ocular, orbit
palate — *see* Wound, open, oral cavity
palm — *see* Wound, open, hand
pelvis, pelvic — *see also* Wound, open, back, lower
girdle — *see* Wound, open, hip
penetrating — *see* Puncture, by site
penis S31.20 ☑
with amputation — *see* Amputation, traumatic, penis
bite S31.25 ☑
laceration — *see* Laceration, penis
puncture — *see* Puncture, penis
perineum
bite — *see* Bite, perineum
female S31.502 ☑
laceration — *see* Laceration, perineum
male S31.501 ☑
puncture — *see* Puncture, perineum
periocular area (with or without lacrimal passages) — *see* Wound, open, eyelid
periumbilic region S31.105 ☑
with penetration into peritoneal cavity S31.605 ☑
bite — *see* Bite, abdomen, wall, periumbilic region
laceration — *see* Laceration, abdomen, wall, periumbilic region
puncture — *see* Puncture, abdomen, wall, periumbilic region
phalanges
finger — *see* Wound, open, finger
toe — *see* Wound, open, toe
pharynx S11.20 ☑
pinna — *see* Wound, open, ear
popliteal space — *see* Wound, open, knee
prepuce — *see* Wound, open, penis
pubic region — *see* Wound, open, back, lower
pudendum — *see* Wound, open, genital organs, external
puncture wound — *see* Puncture
rectovaginal septum — *see* Wound, open, vagina
right
lower quadrant S31.103 ☑
with penetration into peritoneal cavity S31.603 ☑
bite — *see* Bite, abdomen, wall, right, lower quadrant
laceration — *see* Laceration, abdomen, wall, right, lower quadrant
puncture — *see* Puncture, abdomen, wall, right, lower quadrant
upper quadrant S31.100 ☑
with penetration into peritoneal cavity S31.600 ☑
bite — *see* Bite, abdomen, wall, right, upper quadrant
laceration — *see* Laceration, abdomen, wall, right, upper quadrant
puncture — *see* Puncture, abdomen, wall, right, upper quadrant
sacral region — *see* Wound, open, back, lower
sacroiliac region — *see* Wound, open, back, lower
salivary gland — *see* Wound, open, oral cavity
scalp S01.00 ☑
bite S01.05 ☑
laceration — *see* Laceration, scalp
puncture — *see* Puncture, scalp
scalpel, newborn (birth injury) P15.8
scapular region — *see* Wound, open, shoulder
sclera — *see* Wound, open, ocular
scrotum S31.30 ☑
with amputation — *see* Amputation, traumatic, scrotum
bite S31.35 ☑
laceration — *see* Laceration, scrotum
puncture — *see* Puncture, scrotum
shin — *see* Wound, open, leg
shoulder S41.00- ☑

Wound, open — *continued*
shoulder — *continued*
with amputation — *see* Amputation, traumatic, arm
bite — *see* Bite, shoulder
laceration — *see* Laceration, shoulder
puncture — *see* Puncture, shoulder
skin NOS T14.8 ☑
spermatic cord — *see* Wound, open, testis
sternal region — *see* Wound, open, thorax, front wall
submaxillary region — *see* Wound, open, head, specified site NEC
submental region — *see* Wound, open, head, specified site NEC
subungual
finger(s) — *see* Wound, open, finger
toe(s) — *see* Wound, open, toe
supraclavicular region — *see* Wound, open, neck, specified site NEC
temple, temporal region — *see* Wound, open, head, specified site NEC
temporomandibular area — *see* Wound, open, cheek
testis S31.30 ☑
with amputation — *see* Amputation, traumatic, testes
bite S31.35 ☑
laceration — *see* Laceration, testis
puncture — *see* Puncture, testis
thigh S71.10- ☑
with amputation — *see* Amputation, traumatic, hip
bite — *see* Bite, thigh
laceration — *see* Laceration, thigh
puncture — *see* Puncture, thigh
thorax, thoracic (wall) S21.90 ☑
back S21.20- ☑
with penetration S21.40 ☑
bite — *see* Bite, thorax
breast — *see* Wound, open, breast
front S21.10- ☑
with penetration S21.30 ☑
laceration — *see* Laceration, thorax
puncture — *see* Puncture, thorax
throat — *see* Wound, open, neck
thumb S61.009 ☑
with
amputation — *see* Amputation, traumatic, thumb
damage to nail S61.109 ☑
bite — *see* Bite, thumb
laceration — *see* Laceration, thumb
left S61.002 ☑
with
damage to nail S61.102 ☑
puncture — *see* Puncture, thumb
right S61.001 ☑
with
damage to nail S61.101 ☑
thyroid (gland) — *see* Wound, open, neck, thyroid
toe(s) S91.109 ☑
with
amputation — *see* Amputation, traumatic, toe
damage to nail S91.209 ☑
bite — *see* Bite, toe
great S91.103 ☑
with
damage to nail S91.203 ☑
left S91.102 ☑
with
damage to nail S91.202 ☑
right S91.101 ☑
with
damage to nail S91.201 ☑
laceration — *see* Laceration, toe
lesser S91.106 ☑
with
damage to nail S91.206 ☑
left S91.105 ☑
with
damage to nail S91.205 ☑
right S91.104 ☑
with
damage to nail S91.204 ☑
puncture — *see* Puncture, toe
tongue — *see* Wound, open, oral cavity
trachea (cervical region) — *see* Wound, open, neck, trachea
tunica vaginalis — *see* Wound, open, testis

Wound, open — *continued*
tympanum, tympanic membrane S09.2- ☑
laceration — *see* Laceration, ear, drum
puncture — *see* Puncture, tympanum
umbilical region — *see* Wound, open, abdomen, wall, periumbilic region
uvula — *see* Wound, open, oral cavity
vagina S31.40 ☑
bite S31.45 ☑
laceration — *see* Laceration, vagina
puncture — *see* Puncture, vagina
vitreous (humor) — *see* Wound, open, ocular
vocal cord S11.039 ☑
bite — *see* Bite, vocal cord
laceration S11.031 ☑
with foreign body S11.032 ☑
puncture S11.033 ☑
with foreign body S11.034 ☑
vulva S31.40 ☑
with amputation — *see* Amputation, traumatic, vulva
bite S31.45 ☑
laceration — *see* Laceration, vulva
puncture — *see* Puncture, vulva
wrist S61.50- ☑
bite — *see* Bite, wrist
laceration — *see* Laceration, wrist
puncture — *see* Puncture, wrist
Wound, superficial — *see* Injury — *see also* specified injury type
Wright's syndrome G54.0
Wrist — *see* condition
Wrong drug (by accident) (given in error) — *see* Table of Drugs and Chemicals, by drug, poisoning
Wry neck — *see* Torticollis
Wuchereria (bancrofti) **infestation** B74.0
Wuchereriasis B74.0
Wucherende Struma Langhans C73

X

Xanthelasma (eyelid) (palpebrarum) H02.60
left H02.66
lower H02.65
upper H02.64
right H02.63
lower H02.62
upper H02.61
Xanthelasmatosis (essential) E78.2
Xanthinuria, hereditary E79.8
Xanthoastrocytoma
specified site — *see* Neoplasm, malignant, by site
unspecified site C71.9
Xanthofibroma — *see* Neoplasm, connective tissue, benign
Xanthogranuloma D76.3
Xanthoma(s), xanthomatosis (primary) (familial) (hereditary) E75.5
with
hyperlipoproteinemia
Type I E78.3
Type III E78.2
Type IV E78.1
Type V E78.3
bone (generalisata) C96.5
cerebrotendinous E75.5
cutaneotendinous E75.5
disseminatum (skin) E78.2
eruptive E78.2
hypercholesterinemic E78.00
hypercholesterolemic E78.00
hyperlipidemic E78.5
joint E75.5
multiple (skin) E78.2
tendon (sheath) E75.5
tuberosum E78.2
tuberous E78.2
tubo-eruptive E78.2
verrucous, oral mucosa K13.4
Xanthosis R23.8
Xenophobia F40.10
Xeroderma — *see also* Ichthyosis
acquired L85.0
eyelid H01.149
left H01.146
lower H01.145
upper H01.144

Xeroderma — *continued*
- acquired — *continued*
  - eyelid — *continued*
    - right H01.143
      - lower H01.142
      - upper H01.141
- pigmentosum Q82.1
- vitamin A deficiency E50.8

Xerophthalmia (vitamin A deficiency) E50.7
- unrelated to vitamin A deficiency — *see* Keratoconjunctivitis

Xerosis
- conjunctiva H11.14- ☑
  - with Bitot's spots — *see also* Pigmentation, conjunctiva
    - vitamin A deficiency E50.1
  - vitamin A deficiency E50.0
- cornea H18.89- ☑
  - with ulceration — *see* Ulcer, cornea
    - vitamin A deficiency E50.3
  - vitamin A deficiency E50.2
- cutis (dry skin) L85.3
- skin L85.3

Xerostomia K11.7

Xiphopagus Q89.4

XO syndrome Q96.9

X-ray (of)
- abnormal findings — *see* Abnormal, diagnostic imaging
- breast (mammogram) (routine) Z12.31
- chest
  - routine (as part of a general medical examination) Z00.00
    - with abnormal findings Z00.01
- routine (as part of a general medical examination) Z00.00
  - with abnormal findings Z00.01

XXXXY syndrome Q98.1

XXY syndrome Q98.0

Y

Yaba pox (virus disease) B08.72

Yatapoxvirus B08.70
- specified NEC B08.79

Yawning R06.89
- psychogenic F45.8

Yaws A66.9
- bone lesions A66.6
- butter A66.1
- chancre A66.0
- cutaneous, less than five years after infection A66.2
- early (cutaneous) (macular) (maculopapular) (micropapular) (papular) A66.2
  - frambeside A66.2
  - skin lesions NEC A66.2
- eyelid A66.2
- ganglion A66.6
- gangosis, gangosa A66.5
- gumma, gummata A66.4
  - bone A66.6
- gummatous
  - frambeside A66.4
  - osteitis A66.6
  - periostitis A66.6
- hydrarthrosis — *see also* subcategory M14.8- A66.6
- hyperkeratosis (early) (late) A66.3
- initial lesions A66.0
- joint lesions — *see also* subcategory M14.8- A66.6
- juxta-articular nodules A66.7
- late nodular (ulcerated) A66.4
- latent (without clinical manifestations) (with positive serology) A66.8
- mother A66.0
- mucosal A66.7
- multiple papillomata A66.1
- nodular, late (ulcerated) A66.4
- osteitis A66.6
- papilloma, plantar or palmar A66.1
- periostitis (hypertrophic) A66.6
- specified NEC A66.7
- ulcers A66.4
- wet crab A66.1

Yeast infection — *see also* Candidiasis B37.9

Yellow
- atrophy (liver) — *see* Failure, hepatic
- fever — *see* Fever, yellow
- jack — *see* Fever, yellow
- jaundice — *see* Jaundice
- nail syndrome L60.5

Yersiniosis — *see also* Infection, Yersinia
- extraintestinal A28.2
- intestinal A04.6

Z

Zahorsky's syndrome (herpangina) B08.5

Zellweger's syndrome E71.510

Zenker's diverticulum (esophagus) K22.5

Ziehen-Oppenheim disease G24.1

Zieve's syndrome K70.0

Zika NOS A92.5
- congenital P35.4

Zinc
- deficiency, dietary E60
- metabolism disorder E83.2

Zollinger-Ellison syndrome E16.4

Zona — *see* Herpes, zoster

Zoophobia F40.218

Zoster (herpes) — *see* Herpes, zoster

Zygomycosis B46.9
- specified NEC B46.8

Zymotic — *see* condition

Note: The list below gives the code number for neoplasms by anatomical site. For each site there are six possible code numbers according to whether the neoplasm in question is malignant, benign, in situ, of uncertain behavior, or of unspecified nature. The description of the neoplasm will often indicate which of the six columns is appropriate; e.g., malignant melanoma of skin, benign fibroadenoma of breast, carcinoma in situ of cervix uteri. Where such descriptors are not present, the remainder of the Index should be consulted where guidance is given to the appropriate column for each morphological (histological) variety listed; e.g., Mesonephroma – see Neoplasm, malignant; Embryoma — see also Neoplasm, uncertain behavior; Disease, Bowen's – see Neoplasm, skin, in situ. However, the guidance in the Index can be overridden if one of the descriptors mentioned above is present; e.g., malignant adenoma of colon is coded to C18.9 and not to D12.6 as the adjective "malignant" overrides the Index entry "Adenoma — *see also* Neoplasm, benign, by site." Codes listed with a dash -, following the code have a required additional character for laterality. The tabular list must be reviewed for the complete code.

	Malignant Primary	Malignant Secondary	Ca in situ	Benign	Uncertain Behavior	Unspecified Behavior
Neoplasm, neoplastic	C80.1	C79.9	D09.9	D36.9	D48.9	D49.9
abdomen, abdominal	C76.2	C79.8-☑	D09.8	D36.7	D48.7	D49.89
cavity	C76.2	C79.8-☑	D09.8	D36.7	D48.7	D49.89
organ	C76.2	C79.8-☑	D09.8	D36.7	D48.7	D49.89
viscera	C76.2	C79.8-☑	D09.8	D36.7	D48.7	D49.89
wall — *see also* Neoplasm, abdomen, wall, skin	C44.509	C79.2	D04.5	D23.5	D48.5	D49.2
connective tissue	C49.4	C79.8-☑	—	D21.4	D48.1	D49.2
skin	C44.509	—	—	—	—	—
basal cell carcinoma	C44.519	—	—	—	—	—
specified type NEC	C44.599	—	—	—	—	—
squamous cell carcinoma	C44.529	—	—	—	—	—
abdominopelvic	C76.8	C79.8-☑	—	D36.7	D48.7	D49.89
accessory sinus — *see* Neoplasm, sinus						
acoustic nerve	C72.4-☑	C79.49	—	D33.3	D43.3	D49.7
adenoid (pharynx) (tissue)	C11.1	C79.89	D00.08	D10.6	D37.05	D49.0
adipose tissue — *see also* Neoplasm, connective tissue	C49.4	C79.89	—	D21.9	D48.1	D49.2
adnexa (uterine)	C57.4	C79.89	D07.39	D28.7	D39.8	D49.59
adrenal	C74.9-☑	C79.7-☑	D09.3	D35.0-☑	D44.1-☑	D49.7
capsule	C74.9-☑	C79.7-☑	D09.3	D35.0-☑	D44.1-☑	D49.7
cortex	C74.0-☑	C79.7-☑	D09.3	D35.0-☑	D44.1-☑	D49.7
gland	C74.9-☑	C79.7-☑	D09.3	D35.0-☑	D44.1-☑	D49.7
medulla	C74.1-☑	C79.7-☑	D09.3	D35.0-☑	D44.1-☑	D49.7
ala nasi (external) — *see also* Neoplasm, skin, nose	C44.301	C79.2	D04.39	D23.39	D48.5	D49.2
alimentary canal or tract NEC	C26.9	C78.80	D01.9	D13.9	D37.9	D49.0
alveolar	C03.9	C79.89	D00.03	D10.39	D37.09	D49.0
mucosa	C03.9	C79.89	D00.03	D10.39	D37.09	D49.0
lower	C03.1	C79.89	D00.03	D10.39	D37.09	D49.0
upper	C03.0	C79.89	D00.03	D10.39	D37.09	D49.0
ridge or process	C41.1	C79.51	—	D16.5	D48.0	D49.2
carcinoma	C03.9	C79.8-☑	—	—	—	—
lower	C03.1	C79.8-☑	—	—	—	—
upper	C03.0	C79.8-☑	—	—	—	—
lower	C41.1	C79.51	—	D16.5	D48.0	D49.2
mucosa	C03.9	C79.89	D00.03	D10.39	D37.09	D49.0
lower	C03.1	C79.89	D00.03	D10.39	D37.09	D49.0
upper	C03.0	C79.89	D00.03	D10.39	D37.09	D49.0
upper	C41.0	C79.51	—	D16.4	D48.0	D49.2
sulcus	C06.1	C79.89	D00.02	D10.39	D37.09	D49.0
alveolus	C03.9	C79.89	D00.03	D10.39	D37.09	D49.0
lower	C03.1	C79.89	D00.03	D10.39	D37.09	D49.0
upper	C03.0	C79.89	D00.03	D10.39	D37.09	D49.0
ampulla of Vater	C24.1	C78.89	D01.5	D13.5	D37.6	D49.0
ankle NEC	C76.5-☑	C79.89	D04.7-☑	D36.7	D48.7	D49.89
anorectum, anorectal (junction)	C21.8	C78.5	D01.3	D12.9	D37.8	D49.0
antecubital fossa or space	C76.4-☑	C79.89	D04.6-☑	D36.7	D48.7	D49.89
Neoplasm, neoplastic — *continued*						
antrum (Highmore) (maxillary)	C31.0	C78.39	D02.3	D14.0	D38.5	D49.1
pyloric	C16.3	C78.89	D00.2	D13.1	D37.1	D49.0
tympanicum	C30.1	C78.39	D02.3	D14.0	D38.5	D49.1
anus, anal	C21.0	C78.5	D01.3	D12.9	D37.8	D49.0
canal	C21.1	C78.5	D01.3	D12.9	D37.8	D49.0
cloacogenic zone	C21.2	C78.5	D01.3	D12.9	D37.8	D49.0
margin — *see also* Neoplasm, anus, skin	C44.500	C79.2	D04.5	D23.5	D48.5	D49.2
overlapping lesion with rectosigmoid junction or rectum	C21.8	—	—	—	—	—
skin	C44.500	C79.2	D04.5	D23.5	D48.5	D49.2
basal cell carcinoma	C44.510	—	—	—	—	—
specified type NEC	C44.590	—	—	—	—	—
squamous cell carcinoma	C44.520	—	—	—	—	—
sphincter	C21.1	C78.5	D01.3	D12.9	D37.8	D49.0
aorta (thoracic)	C49.3	C79.89	—	D21.3	D48.1	D49.2
abdominal	C49.4	C79.89	—	D21.4	D48.1	D49.2
aortic body	C75.5	C79.89	—	D35.6	D44.7	D49.7
aponeurosis	C49.9	C79.89	—	D21.9	D48.1	D49.2
palmar	C49.1-☑	C79.89	—	D21.1-☑	D48.1	D49.2
plantar	C49.2-☑	C79.89	—	D21.2-☑	D48.1	D49.2
appendix	C18.1	C78.5	D01.0	D12.1	D37.3	D49.0
arachnoid	C70.9	C79.49	—	D32.9	D42.9	D49.7
cerebral	C70.0	C79.32	—	D32.0	D42.0	D49.7
spinal	C70.1	C79.49	—	D32.1	D42.1	D49.7
areola	C50.0-☑	C79.81	D05-☑	D24-☑	D48.6-☑	D49.3
arm NEC	C76.4-☑	C79.89	D04.6-☑	D36.7	D48.7	D49.89
artery — *see* Neoplasm, connective tissue						
aryepiglottic fold	C13.1	C79.89	D00.08	D10.7	D37.05	D49.0
hypopharyngeal aspect	C13.1	C79.89	D00.08	D10.7	D37.05	D49.0
laryngeal aspect	C32.1	C78.39	D02.0	D14.1	D38.0	D49.1
marginal zone	C13.1	C79.89	D00.08	D10.7	D37.05	D49.0
arytenoid (cartilage)	C32.3	C78.39	D02.0	D14.1	D38.0	D49.1
fold — *see* Neoplasm, aryepiglottic						
associated with transplanted organ	C80.2	—	—	—	—	—
atlas	C41.2	C79.51	—	D16.6	D48.0	D49.2
atrium, cardiac	C38.0	C79.89	—	D15.1	D48.7	D49.89
auditory						
canal (external) (skin)	C44.20-☑	C79.2	D04.2-☑	D23.2-☑	D48.5	D49.2
internal	C30.1	C78.39	D02.3	D14.0	D38.5	D49.1
nerve	C72.4-☑	C79.49	—	D33.3	D43.3	D49.7
tube	C30.1	C78.39	D02.3	D14.0	D38.5	D49.1
opening	C11.2	C79.89	D00.08	D10.6	D37.05	D49.0
auricle, ear — *see also* Neoplasm, skin, ear	C44.20-☑	C79.2	D04.2-☑	D23.2-☑	D48.5	D49.2
auricular canal (external) — *see also* Neoplasm, skin, ear	C44.20-☑	C79.2	D04.2-☑	D23.2-☑	D48.5	D49.2
internal	C30.1	C78.39	D02.3	D14.0	D38.5	D49.2
autonomic nerve or nervous system NEC (see Neoplasm, nerve, peripheral)						
axilla, axillary	C76.1	C79.89	D09.8	D36.7	D48.7	D49.89
fold — *see also* Neoplasm, skin, trunk	C44.509	C79.2	D04.5	D23.5	D48.5	D49.2
back NEC	C76.8	C79.89	D04.5	D36.7	D48.7	D49.89
Bartholin's gland	C51.0	C79.82	D07.1	D28.0	D39.8	D49.59
basal ganglia	C71.0	C79.31	—	D33.0	D43.0	D49.6
basis pedunculi	C71.7	C79.31	—	D33.1	D43.1	D49.6
bile or biliary (tract)	C24.9	C78.89	D01.5	D13.5	D37.6	D49.0

	Malignant Primary	Malignant Secondary	Ca in situ	Benign	Uncertain Behavior	Unspecified Behavior
Neoplasm, neoplastic — *continued*						
bile or biliary — *continued*						
canaliculi (biliferi) (intrahepatic)	C22.1	C78.7	DØ1.5	D13.4	D37.6	D49.Ø
canals, interlobular	C22.1	C78.89	DØ1.5	D13.4	D37.6	D49.Ø
duct or passage (common) (cystic) (extrahepatic)	C24.Ø	C78.89	DØ1.5	D13.5	D37.6	D49.Ø
interlobular	C22.1	C78.89	DØ1.5	D13.4	D37.6	D49.Ø
intrahepatic	C22.1	C78.7	DØ1.5	D13.4	D37.6	D49.Ø
and extrahepatic	C24.8	C78.89	DØ1.5	D13.5	D37.6	D49.Ø
bladder (urinary)	C67.9	C79.11	DØ9.Ø	D3Ø.3	D41.4	D49.4
dome	C67.1	C79.11	DØ9.Ø	D3Ø.3	D41.4	D49.4
neck	C67.5	C79.11	DØ9.Ø	D3Ø.3	D41.4	D49.4
orifice	C67.9	C79.11	DØ9.Ø	D3Ø.3	D41.4	D49.4
ureteric	C67.6	C79.11	DØ9.Ø	D3Ø.3	D41.4	D49.4
urethral	C67.5	C79.11	DØ9.Ø	D3Ø.3	D41.4	D49.4
overlapping lesion	C67.8	—	—	—	—	—
sphincter	C67.8	C79.11	DØ9.Ø	D3Ø.3	D41.4	D49.4
trigone	C67.Ø	C79.11	DØ9.Ø	D3Ø.3	D41.4	D49.4
urachus	C67.7	C79.11	DØ9.Ø	D3Ø.3	D41.4	D49.4
wall	C67.9	C79.11	DØ9.Ø	D3Ø.3	D41.4	D49.4
anterior	C67.3	C79.11	DØ9.Ø	D3Ø.3	D41.4	D49.4
lateral	C67.2	C79.11	DØ9.Ø	D3Ø.3	D41.4	D49.4
posterior	C67.4	C79.11	DØ9.Ø	D3Ø.3	D41.4	D49.4
blood vessel — *see* Neoplasm, connective tissue						
bone (periosteum)	C41.9	C79.51	—	D16.9-	D48.Ø	D49.2
acetabulum						
ankle	C4Ø.3-☑	C79.51	—	D16.3-☑	—	—
arm NEC	C4Ø.Ø-☑	C79.51	—	D16.Ø-☑	—	—
astragalus	C4Ø.3-☑	C79.51	—	D16.3-☑	—	—
atlas	C41.2	C79.51	—	D16.6	D48.Ø	D49.2
axis	C41.2	C79.51	—	D16.6	D48.Ø	D49.2
back NEC	C41.2	C79.51	—	D16.6	D48.Ø	D49.2
calcaneus	C4Ø.3-☑	C79.51	—	D16.3-☑	—	—
calvarium	C41.Ø	C79.51	—	D16.4	D48.Ø	D49.2
carpus (any)	C4Ø.1-☑	C79.51	—	D16.1-☑	—	—
cartilage NEC	C41.9	C79.51	—	D16.9	D48.Ø	D49.2
clavicle	C41.3	C79.51	—	D16.7	D48.Ø	D49.2
clivus	C41.Ø	C79.51	—	D16.4	D48.Ø	D49.2
coccygeal vertebra	C41.4	C79.51	—	D16.8	D48.Ø	D49.2
coccyx	C41.4	C79.51	—	D16.8	D48.Ø	D49.2
costal cartilage	C41.3	C79.51	—	D16.7	D48.Ø	D49.2
costovertebral joint	C41.3	C79.51	—	D16.7	D48.Ø	D49.2
cranial	C41.Ø	C79.51	—	D16.4	D48.Ø	D49.2
cuboid	C4Ø.3-☑	C79.51	—	D16.3-☑	—	—
cuneiform	C41.9	C79.51	—	D16.9	D48.Ø	D49.2
elbow	C4Ø.Ø-☑	C79.51	—	D16.Ø-☑	—	—
ethmoid (labyrinth)	C41.Ø	C79.51	—	D16.4	D48.Ø	D49.2
face	C41.Ø	C79.51	—	D16.4	D48.Ø	D49.2
femur (any part)	C4Ø.2-☑	C79.51	—	D16.2-☑	—	—
fibula (any part)	C4Ø.2-☑	C79.51	—	D16.2-☑	—	—
finger (any)	C4Ø.1-☑	C79.51	—	D16.1-☑	—	—
foot	C4Ø.3-☑	C79.51	—	D16.3-☑	—	—
forearm	C4Ø.Ø-☑	C79.51	—	D16.Ø-☑	—	—
frontal	C41.Ø	C79.51	—	D16.4	D48.Ø	D49.2
hand	C4Ø.1-☑	C79.51	—	D16.1-☑	—	—
heel	C4Ø.3-☑	C79.51	—	D16.3-☑	—	—
hip	C41.4	C79.51	—	D16.8	D48.Ø	D49.2
humerus (any part)	C4Ø.Ø-☑	C79.51	—	D16.Ø-☑	—	—
hyoid	C41.Ø	C79.51	—	D16.4	D48.Ø	D49.2
ilium	C41.4	C79.51	—	D16.8	D48.Ø	D49.2
innominate	C41.4	C79.51	—	D16.8	D48.Ø	D49.2
intervertebral cartilage or disc	C41.2	C79.51	—	D16.6	D48.Ø	D49.2
ischium	C41.4	C79.51	—	D16.8	D48.Ø	D49.2
jaw (lower)	C41.1	C79.51	—	D16.5	D48.Ø	D49.2
knee	C4Ø.2-☑	C79.51	—	D16.2-☑	—	—
leg NEC	C4Ø.2-☑	C79.51	—	D16.2-☑	—	—
limb NEC	C4Ø.9-☑	C79.51	—	D16.9	—	—
Neoplasm, neoplastic — *continued*						
bone — *continued*						
limb — *continued*						
lower (long bones)	C4Ø.2-☑	C79.51	—	D16.2-☑	—	—
short bones	C4Ø.3-☑	C79.51	—	D16.3-☑	—	—
upper (long bones)	C4Ø.Ø-☑	C79.51	—	D16.Ø-☑	—	—
short bones	C4Ø.1-☑	C79.51	—	D16.1-☑	—	—
malar	C41.Ø	C79.51	—	D16.4	D48.Ø	D49.2
mandible	C41.1	C79.51	—	D16.5	D48.Ø	D49.2
marrow NEC (any bone)	C96.9	C79.52	—	—	D47.9	D49.89
mastoid	C41.Ø	C79.51	—	D16.4	D48.Ø	D49.2
maxilla, maxillary (superior)	C41.Ø	C79.51	—	D16.4	D48.Ø	D49.2
inferior	C41.1	C79.51	—	D16.5	D48.Ø	D49.2
metacarpus (any)	C4Ø.1-☑	C79.51	—	D16.1-☑	—	—
metatarsus (any)	C4Ø.3-☑	C79.51	—	D16.3-☑	—	—
navicular						
ankle	C4Ø.3-☑	C79.51	—	—	—	—
hand	C4Ø.1-☑	C79.51	—	—	—	—
nose, nasal	C41.Ø	C79.51	—	D16.4	D48.Ø	D49.2
occipital	C41.Ø	C79.51	—	D16.4	D48.Ø	D49.2
orbit	C41.Ø	C79.51	—	D16.4	D48.Ø	D49.2
overlapping sites	C4Ø.8-☑	—	—	—	—	—
parietal	C41.Ø	C79.51	—	D16.4	D48.Ø	D49.2
patella	C4Ø.2-☑	C79.51	—	—	—	—
pelvic	C41.4	C79.51	—	D16.8	D48.Ø	D49.2
phalanges						
foot	C4Ø.3-☑	C79.51	—	—	—	—
hand	C4Ø.1-☑	C79.51	—	—	—	—
pubic	C41.4	C79.51	—	D16.8	D48.Ø	D49.2
radius (any part)	C4Ø.Ø-☑	C79.51	—	D16.Ø-☑	—	—
rib	C41.3	C79.51	—	D16.7	D48.Ø	D49.2
sacral vertebra	C41.4	C79.51	—	D16.8	D48.Ø	D49.2
sacrum	C41.4	C79.51	—	D16.8	D48.Ø	D49.2
scaphoid						
of ankle	C4Ø.3-☑	C79.51	—	—	—	—
of hand	C4Ø.1-☑	C79.51	—	—	—	—
scapula (any part)	C4Ø.Ø-☑	C79.51	—	D16.Ø-☑	—	—
sella turcica	C41.Ø	C79.51	—	D16.4	D48.Ø	D49.2
shoulder	C4Ø.Ø-☑	C79.51	—	D16.Ø-☑	—	—
skull	C41.Ø	C79.51	—	D16.4	D48.Ø	D49.2
sphenoid	C41.Ø	C79.51	—	D16.4	D48.Ø	D49.2
spine, spinal (column)	C41.2	C79.51	—	D16.6	D48.Ø	D49.2
coccyx	C41.4	C79.51	—	D16.8	D48.Ø	D49.2
sacrum	C41.4	C79.51	—	D16.8	D48.Ø	D49.2
sternum	C41.3	C79.51	—	D16.7	D48.Ø	D49.2
tarsus (any)	C4Ø.3-☑	C79.51	—	—	—	—
temporal	C41.Ø	C79.51	—	D16.4	D48.Ø	D49.2
thumb	C4Ø.1-☑	C79.51	—	—	—	—
tibia (any part)	C4Ø.2-☑	C79.51	—	—	—	—
toe (any)	C4Ø.3-☑	C79.51	—	—	—	—
trapezium	C4Ø.1-☑	C79.51	—	—	—	—
trapezoid	C4Ø.1-☑	C79.51	—	—	—	—
turbinate	C41.Ø	C79.51	—	D16.4	D48.Ø	D49.2
ulna (any part)	C4Ø.Ø-☑	C79.51	—	D16.Ø-☑	—	—
unciform	C4Ø.1-☑	C79.51	—	—	—	—
vertebra (column)	C41.2	C79.51	—	D16.6	D48.Ø	D49.2
coccyx	C41.4	C79.51	—	D16.8	D48.Ø	D49.2
sacrum	C41.4	C79.51	—	D16.8	D48.Ø	D49.2
vomer	C41.Ø	C79.51	—	D16.4	D48.Ø	D49.2
wrist	C4Ø.1-☑	C79.51	—	—	—	—
xiphoid process	C41.3	C79.51	—	D16.7	D48.Ø	D49.2
zygomatic	C41.Ø	C79.51	—	D16.4	D48.Ø	D49.2
book-leaf (mouth) — *ventral surface of tongue and floor of mouth*	CØ6.89	C79.89	DØØ.ØØ	D1Ø.39	D37.Ø9	D49.Ø
bowel — *see* Neoplasm, intestine						
brachial plexus	C47.1-☑	C79.89	—	D36.12	D48.2	D49.2
brain NEC	C71.9	C79.31	—	D33.2	D43.2	D49.6

	Malignant Primary	Malignant Secondary	Ca in situ	Benign	Uncertain Behavior	Unspecified Behavior
Neoplasm, neoplastic — *continued*						
brain — *continued*						
basal ganglia	C71.Ø	C79.31	—	D33.Ø	D43.Ø	D49.6
cerebellopontine angle	C71.6	C79.31	—	D33.1	D43.1	D49.6
cerebellum NOS	C71.6	C79.31	—	D33.1	D43.1	D49.6
cerebrum	C71.Ø	C79.31	—	D33.Ø	D43.Ø	D49.6
choroid plexus	C71.7	C79.31	—	D33.1	D43.1	D49.6
corpus callosum	C71.8	C79.31	—	D33.2	D43.2	D49.6
corpus striatum	C71.Ø	C79.31	—	D33.Ø	D43.Ø	D49.6
cortex (cerebral)	C71.Ø	C79.31	—	D33.Ø	D43.Ø	D49.6
frontal lobe	C71.1	C79.31	—	D33.Ø	D43.Ø	D49.6
globus pallidus	C71.Ø	C79.31	—	D33.Ø	D43.Ø	D49.6
hippocampus	C71.2	C79.31	—	D33.Ø	D43.Ø	D49.6
hypothalamus	C71.Ø	C79.31	—	D33.Ø	D43.Ø	D49.6
internal capsule	C71.Ø	C79.31	—	D33.Ø	D43.Ø	D49.6
medulla oblongata	C71.7	C79.31	—	D33.1	D43.1	D49.6
meninges	C7Ø.Ø	C79.32	—	D32.Ø	D42.Ø	D49.7
midbrain	C71.7	C79.31	—	D33.1	D43.1	D49.6
occipital lobe	C71.4	C79.31	—	D33.Ø	D43.Ø	D49.6
overlapping lesion	C71.8	C79.31	—	—	—	—
parietal lobe	C71.3	C79.31	—	D33.Ø	D43.Ø	D49.6
peduncle	C71.7	C79.31	—	D33.1	D43.1	D49.6
pons	C71.7	C79.31	—	D33.1	D43.1	D49.6
stem	C71.7	C79.31	—	D33.1	D43.1	D49.6
tapetum	C71.8	C79.31	—	D33.2	D43.2	D49.6
temporal lobe	C71.2	C79.31	—	D33.Ø	D43.Ø	D49.6
thalamus	C71.Ø	C79.31	—	D33.Ø	D43.Ø	D49.6
uncus	C71.2	C79.31	—	D33.Ø	D43.Ø	D49.6
ventricle (floor)	C71.5	C79.31	—	D33.Ø	D43.Ø	D49.6
fourth	C71.7	C79.31	—	D33.1	D43.1	D49.6
branchial (cleft) (cyst) (vestiges)	C1Ø.4	C79.89	DØØ.Ø8	D1Ø.5	D37.Ø5	D49.Ø
breast (connective tissue) (glandular tissue) (soft parts)	C5Ø.9-☑	C79.81	DØ5.-☑	D24.-☑	D48.6-☑	D49.3
areola	C5Ø.Ø-☑	C79.81	DØ5.-☑	D24.-☑	D48.6-☑	D49.3
axillary tail	C5Ø.6-☑	C79.81	DØ5.-☑	D24.-☑	D48.6-☑	D49.3
central portion	C5Ø.1-☑	C79.81	DØ5.-☑	D24.-☑	D48.6-☑	D49.3
inner	C5Ø.8-☑	C79.81	DØ5.-☑	D24.-☑	D48.6-☑	D49.3
lower	C5Ø.8-☑	C79.81	DØ5.-☑	D24.-☑	D48.6-☑	D49.3
lower-inner quadrant	C5Ø.3-☑	C79.81	DØ5.-☑	D24.-☑	D48.6-☑	D49.3
lower-outer quadrant	C5Ø.5-☑	C79.81	DØ5.-☑	D24.-☑	D48.6-☑	D49.3
mastectomy site (skin) — *see also* Neoplasm, breast, skin	C44.5Ø1	C79.2	—	—	—	—
specified as breast tissue	C5Ø.8-☑	C79.81	—	—	—	—
midline	C5Ø.8-☑	C79.81	DØ5.-☑	D24.-☑	D48.6-☑	D49.3
nipple	C5Ø.Ø-☑	C79.81	DØ5.-☑	D24.-☑	D48.6-☑	D49.3
outer	C5Ø.8-☑	C79.81	DØ5.-☑	D24.-☑	D48.6-☑	D49.3
overlapping lesion	C5Ø.8-☑	—	—	—	—	—
skin	C44.5Ø1	C79.2	DØ4.5	D23.5	D48.5	D49.2
basal cell carcinoma	C44.511	—	—	—	—	—
specified type NEC	C44.591	—	—	—	—	—
squamous cell carcinoma	C44.521	—	—	—	—	—
tail (axillary)	C5Ø.6-☑	C79.81	DØ5.-☑	D24.-☑	D48.6-☑	D49.3
upper	C5Ø.8-☑	C79.81	DØ5.-☑	D24.-☑	D48.6-☑	D49.3
upper-inner quadrant	C5Ø.2-☑	C79.81	DØ5.-☑	D24.-☑	D48.6-☑	D49.3
upper-outer quadrant	C5Ø.4-☑	C79.81	DØ5.-☑	D24.-☑	D48.6-☑	D49.3
broad ligament	C57.1-☑	C79.82	DØ7.39	D28.2	D39.8	D49.59
bronchiogenic, bronchogenic (lung)	C34.9-☑	C78.Ø-☑	DØ2.2-☑	D14.3-☑	D38.1	D49.1
bronchiole	C34.9-☑	C78.Ø-☑	DØ2.2-☑	D14.3-☑	D38.1	D49.1
bronchus	C34.9-☑	C78.Ø-☑	DØ2.2-☑	D14.3-☑	D38.1	D49.1
carina	C34.Ø-☑	C78.Ø-☑	DØ2.2-☑	D14.3-☑	D38.1	D49.1
lower lobe of lung	C34.3-☑	C78.Ø-☑	DØ2.2-☑	D14.3-☑	D38.1	D49.1
Neoplasm, neoplastic — *continued*						
bronchus — *continued*						
main	C34.Ø-☑	C78.Ø-☑	DØ2.2-☑	D14.3-☑	D38.1	D49.1
middle lobe of lung	C34.2	C78.Ø-☑	DØ2.21	D14.31	D38.1	D49.1
overlapping lesion	C34.8-☑	—	—	—	—	—
upper lobe of lung	C34.1-☑	C78.Ø-☑	DØ2.2-☑	D14.3-☑	D38.1	D49.1
brow	C44.3Ø9	C79.2	DØ4.39	D23.39	D48.5	D49.2
basal cell carcinoma	C44.319	—	—	—	—	—
specified type NEC	C44.399	—	—	—	—	—
squamous cell carcinoma	C44.329	—	—	—	—	—
buccal (cavity)	CØ6.9	C79.89	DØØ.ØØ	D1Ø.39	D37.Ø9	D49.Ø
commissure	CØ6.Ø	C79.89	DØØ.Ø2	D1Ø.39	D37.Ø9	D49.Ø
groove (lower) (upper)	CØ6.1	C79.89	DØØ.Ø2	D1Ø.39	D37.Ø9	D49.Ø
mucosa	CØ6.Ø	C79.89	DØØ.Ø2	D1Ø.39	D37.Ø9	D49.Ø
sulcus (lower) (upper)	CØ6.1	C79.89	DØØ.Ø2	D1Ø.39	D37.Ø9	D49.Ø
bulbourethral gland	C68.Ø	C79.19	DØ9.19	D3Ø.4	D41.3	D49.59
bursa — *see* Neoplasm, connective tissue						
buttock NEC	C76.3	C79.89	DØ4.5	D36.7	D48.7	D49.89
calf	C76.5-☑	C79.89	DØ4.7-☑	D36.7	D48.7	D49.89
calvarium	C41.Ø	C79.51	—	D16.4	D48.Ø	D49.2
calyx, renal	C65.-☑	C79.Ø-☑	DØ9.19	D3Ø.1-☑	D41.1-☑	D49.51-☑
canal						
anal	C21.1	C78.5	DØ1.3	D12.9	D37.8	D49.Ø
auditory (external) — *see also* Neoplasm, skin, ear	C44.2Ø-☑	C79.2	DØ4.2-☑	D23.2-☑	D48.5	D49.2
auricular (external) — *see also* Neoplasm, skin, ear	C44.2Ø-☑	C79.2	DØ4.2-☑	D23.2-☑	D48.5	D49.2
canaliculi, biliary (biliferi) (intrahepatic)	C22.1	C78.7	DØ1.5	D13.4	D37.6	D49.Ø
canthus (eye) (inner) (outer)	C44.1Ø-☑	C79.2	DØ4.1-☑	D23.1-☑	D48.5	D49.2
basal cell carcinoma	C44.11-☑	—	—	—	—	—
sebaceous cell	C44.13-☑	—	—	—	—	—
specified type NEC	C44.19-☑	—	—	—	—	—
squamous cell carcinoma	C44.12-☑	—	—	—	—	—
capillary — *see* Neoplasm, connective tissue						
caput coli	C18.Ø	C78.5	DØ1.Ø	D12.Ø	D37.4	D49.Ø
carcinoid — *see* Tumor, carcinoid						
cardia (gastric)	C16.Ø	C78.89	DØØ.2	D13.1	D37.1	D49.Ø
cardiac orifice (stomach)	C16.Ø	C78.89	DØØ.2	D13.1	D37.1	D49.Ø
cardio-esophageal junction	C16.Ø	C78.89	DØØ.2	D13.1	D37.1	D49.Ø
cardio-esophagus	C16.Ø	C78.89	DØØ.2	D13.1	D37.1	D49.Ø
carina (bronchus)	C34.Ø-☑	C78.Ø-☑	DØ2.2-☑	D14.3-☑	D38.1	D49.1
carotid (artery)	C49.Ø	C79.89	—	D21.Ø	D48.1	D49.2
body	C75.4	C79.89	—	D35.5	D44.6	D49.7
carpus (any bone)	C4Ø.1-☑	C79.51	—	D16.1-☑	—	—
cartilage (articular) (joint) NEC — *see also* Neoplasm, bone	C41.9	C79.51	—	D16.9	D48.Ø	D49.2
arytenoid	C32.3	C78.39	DØ2.Ø	D14.1	D38.Ø	D49.1
auricular	C49.Ø	C79.89	—	D21.Ø	D48.1	D49.2
bronchi	C34.Ø-☑	C78.39	—	D14.3-☑	D38.1	D49.1
costal	C41.3	C79.51	—	D16.7	D48.Ø	D49.2
cricoid	C32.3	C78.39	DØ2.Ø	D14.1	D38.Ø	D49.1
cuneiform	C32.3	C78.39	DØ2.Ø	D14.1	D38.Ø	D49.1
ear (external)	C49.Ø	C79.89	—	D21.Ø	D48.1	D49.2
ensiform	C41.3	C79.51	—	D16.7	D48.Ø	D49.2
epiglottis	C32.1	C78.39	DØ2.Ø	D14.1	D38.Ø	D49.1

	Malignant Primary	Malignant Secondary	Ca in situ	Benign	Uncertain Behavior	Unspecified Behavior
Neoplasm, neoplastic — *continued*						
cartilage — *see also* Neoplasm, bone — *continued*						
epiglottis — *continued*						
anterior surface	C10.1	C79.89	D00.08	D10.5	D37.05	D49.0
eyelid	C49.0	C79.89	—	D21.0	D48.1	D49.2
intervertebral	C41.2	C79.51	—	D16.6	D48.0	D49.2
larynx, laryngeal	C32.3	C78.39	D02.0	D14.1	D38.0	D49.1
nose, nasal	C30.0	C78.39	D02.3	D14.0	D38.5	D49.1
pinna	C49.0	C79.89	—	D21.0	D48.1	D49.2
rib	C41.3	C79.51	—	D16.7	D48.0	D49.2
semilunar (knee)	C40.2-☑	C79.51	—	D16.2-☑	D48.0	D49.2
thyroid	C32.3	C78.39	D02.0	D14.1	D38.0	D49.1
trachea	C33	C78.39	D02.1	D14.2	D38.1	D49.1
cauda equina	C72.1	C79.49	—	D33.4	D43.4	D49.7
cavity						
buccal	C06.9	C79.89	D00.00	D10.30	D37.09	D49.0
nasal	C30.0	C78.39	D02.3	D14.0	D38.5	D49.1
oral	C06.9	C79.89	D00.00	D10.30	D37.09	D49.0
peritoneal	C48.2	C78.6	—	D20.1	D48.4	D49.0
tympanic	C30.1	C78.39	D02.3	D14.0	D38.5	D49.1
cecum	C18.0	C78.5	D01.0	D12.0	D37.4	D49.0
central nervous system	C72.9	C79.40	—	—	—	—
cerebellopontine (angle)	C71.6	C79.31	—	D33.1	D43.1	D49.6
cerebellum, cerebellar	C71.6	C79.31	—	D33.1	D43.1	D49.6
cerebrum, cerebra (cortex) (hemisphere) (white matter)	C71.0	C79.31	—	D33.0	D43.0	D49.6
meninges	C70.0	C79.32	—	D32.0	D42.0	D49.7
peduncle	C71.7	C79.31	—	D33.1	D43.1	D49.6
ventricle	C71.5	C79.31	—	D33.0	D43.0	D49.6
fourth	C71.7	C79.31	—	D33.1	D43.1	D49.6
cervical region	C76.0	C79.89	D09.8	D36.7	D48.7	D49.89
cervix (cervical) (uteri) (uterus)	C53.9	C79.82	D06.9	D26.0	D39.0	D49.59
canal	C53.0	C79.82	D06.0	D26.0	D39.0	D49.59
endocervix (canal) (gland)	C53.0	C79.82	D06.0	D26.0	D39.0	D49.59
exocervix	C53.1	C79.82	D06.1	D26.0	D39.0	D49.59
external os	C53.1	C79.82	D06.1	D26.0	D39.0	D49.59
internal os	C53.0	C79.82	D06.0	D26.0	D39.0	D49.59
nabothian gland	C53.0	C79.82	D06.0	D26.0	D39.0	D49.59
overlapping lesion	C53.8	—	—	—	—	—
squamocolumnar junction	C53.8	C79.82	D06.7	D26.0	D39.0	D49.59
stump	C53.8	C79.82	D06.7	D26.0	D39.0	D49.59
cheek	C76.0	C79.89	D09.8	D36.7	D48.7	D49.89
external	C44.309	C79.2	D04.39	D23.39	D48.5	D49.2
basal cell carcinoma	C44.319	—	—	—	—	—
specified type NEC	C44.399	—	—	—	—	—
squamous cell carcinoma	C44.329	—	—	—	—	—
inner aspect	C06.0	C79.89	D00.02	D10.39	D37.09	D49.0
internal	C06.0	C79.89	D00.02	D10.39	D37.09	D49.0
mucosa	C06.0	C79.89	D00.02	D10.39	D37.09	D49.0
chest (wall) NEC	C76.1	C79.89	D09.8	D36.7	D48.7	D49.89
chiasma opticum	C72.3-☑	C79.49	—	D33.3	D43.3	D49.7
chin	C44.309	C79.2	D04.39	D23.39	D48.5	D49.2
basal cell carcinoma	C44.319	—	—	—	—	—
specified type NEC	C44.399	—	—	—	—	—
squamous cell carcinoma	C44.329	—	—	—	—	—
choana	C11.3	C79.89	D00.08	D10.6	D37.05	D49.0
cholangiole	C22.1	C78.89	D01.5	D13.4	D37.6	D49.0
choledochal duct	C24.0	C78.89	D01.5	D13.5	D37.6	D49.0
choroid	C69.3-☑	C79.49	D09.2-☑	D31.3-☑	D48.7	D49.81
plexus	C71.5	C79.31	—	D33.0	D43.0	D49.6
ciliary body	C69.4-☑	C79.49	D09.2-☑	D31.4-☑	D48.7	D49.89
clavicle	C41.3	C79.51	—	D16.7	D48.0	D49.2
Neoplasm, neoplastic — *continued*						
clitoris	C51.2	C79.82	D07.1	D28.0	D39.8	D49.59
clivus	C41.0	C79.51	—	D16.4	D48.0	D49.2
cloacogenic zone	C21.2	C78.5	D01.3	D12.9	D37.8	D49.0
coccygeal						
body or glomus	C49.5	C79.89	—	D21.5	D48.1	D49.2
vertebra	C41.4	C79.51	—	D16.8	D48.0	D49.2
coccyx	C41.4	C79.51	—	D16.8	D48.0	D49.2
colon — *see also* Neoplasm, intestine, large	C18.9	C78.5	—	—	—	—
with rectum	C19	C78.5	D01.1	D12.7	D37.5	D49.0
columnella — *see also* Neoplasm, skin, face	C44.390	C79.2	D04.39	D23.39	D48.5	D49.2
column, spinal — *see* Neoplasm, spine						
commissure						
labial, lip	C00.6	C79.89	D00.01	D10.39	D37.01	D49.0
laryngeal	C32.0	C78.39	D02.0	D14.1	D38.0	D49.1
common (bile) duct	C24.0	C78.89	D01.5	D13.5	D37.6	D49.0
concha — *see also* Neoplasm, skin, ear	C44.20-☑	C79.2	D04.2-☑	D23.2-☑	D48.5	D49.2
nose	C30.0	C78.39	D02.3	D14.0	D38.5	D49.1
conjunctiva	C69.0-☑	C79.49	D09.2-☑	D31.0-☑	D48.7	D49.89
connective tissue NEC	C49.9	C79.89	—	D21.9	D48.1	D49.2

Note: For neoplasms of connective tissue (blood vessel, bursa, fascia, ligament, muscle, peripheral nerves, sympathetic and parasympathetic nerves and ganglia, synovia, tendon, etc.) or of morphological types that indicate connective tissue, code according to the list under "Neoplasm, connective tissue". For sites that do not appear in this list, code to neoplasm of that site; e.g., fibrosarcoma, pancreas (C25.9)

Note: Morphological types that indicate connective tissue appear in their proper place in the alphabetic index with the instruction "see Neoplasm, connective tissue ...."

	Malignant Primary	Malignant Secondary	Ca in situ	Benign	Uncertain Behavior	Unspecified Behavior
abdomen	C49.4	C79.89	—	D21.4	D48.1	D49.2
abdominal wall	C49.4	C79.89	—	D21.4	D48.1	D49.2
ankle	C49.2-☑	C79.89	—	D21.2-☑	D48.1	D49.2
antecubital fossa or space	C49.1-☑	C79.89	—	D21.1-☑	D48.1	D49.2
arm	C49.1-☑	C79.89	—	D21.1-☑	D48.1	D49.2
auricle (ear)	C49.0	C79.89	—	D21.0	D48.1	D49.2
axilla	C49.3	C79.89	—	D21.3	D48.1	D49.2
back	C49.6	C79.89	—	D21.6	D48.1	D49.2
breast — *see* Neoplasm, breast						
buttock	C49.5	C79.89	—	D21.5	D48.1	D49.2
calf	C49.2-☑	C79.89	—	D21.2-☑	D48.1	D49.2
cervical region	C49.0	C79.89	—	D21.0	D48.1	D49.2
cheek	C49.0	C79.89	—	D21.0	D48.1	D49.2
chest (wall)	C49.3	C79.89	—	D21.3	D48.1	D49.2
chin	C49.0	C79.89	—	D21.0	D48.1	D49.2
diaphragm	C49.3	C79.89	—	D21.3	D48.1	D49.2
ear (external)	C49.0	C79.89	—	D21.0	D48.1	D49.2
elbow	C49.1-☑	C79.89	—	D21.1-☑	D48.1	D49.2
extrarectal	C49.5	C79.89	—	D21.5	D48.1	D49.2
extremity	C49.9	C79.89	—	D21.9	D48.1	D49.2
lower	C49.2-☑	C79.89	—	D21.2-☑	D48.1	D49.2
upper	C49.1-☑	C79.89	—	D21.1-☑	D48.1	D49.2
eyelid	C49.0	C79.89	—	D21.0	D48.1	D49.2
face	C49.0	C79.89	—	D21.0	D48.1	D49.2
finger	C49.1-☑	C79.89	—	D21.1-☑	D48.1	D49.2
flank	C49.6	C79.89	—	D21.6	D48.1	D49.2
foot	C49.2-☑	C79.89	—	D21.2-☑	D48.1	D49.2
forearm	C49.1-☑	C79.89	—	D21.1-☑	D48.1	D49.2
forehead	C49.0	C79.89	—	D21.0	D48.1	D49.2
gastric	C49.4	C79.89	—	D21.4	D48.1	D49.2
gastrointestinal	C49.4	C79.89	—	D21.4	D48.1	D49.2
gluteal region	C49.5	C79.89	—	D21.5	D48.1	D49.2
great vessels NEC	C49.3	C79.89	—	D21.3	D48.1	D49.2
groin	C49.5	C79.89	—	D21.5	D48.1	D49.2
hand	C49.1-☑	C79.89	—	D21.1-☑	D48.1	D49.2
head	C49.0	C79.89	—	D21.0	D48.1	D49.2

	Malignant Primary	Malignant Secondary	Ca in situ	Benign	Uncertain Behavior	Unspecified Behavior
Neoplasm, neoplastic — *continued*						
connective tissue — *continued*						
heel	C49.2-☑	C79.89	—	D21.2-☑	D48.1	D49.2
hip	C49.2-☑	C79.89	—	D21.2-☑	D48.1	D49.2
hypochondrium	C49.4	C79.89	—	D21.4	D48.1	D49.2
iliopsoas muscle	C49.5	C79.89	—	D21.5	D48.1	D49.2
infraclavicular region	C49.3	C79.89	—	D21.3	D48.1	D49.2
inguinal (canal) (region)	C49.5	C79.89	—	D21.5	D48.1	D49.2
intestinal	C49.4	C79.89	—	D21.4	D48.1	D49.2
intrathoracic	C49.3	C79.89	—	D21.3	D48.1	D49.2
ischiorectal fossa	C49.5	C79.89	—	D21.5	D48.1	D49.2
jaw	C03.9	C79.89	D00.03	D10.39	D48.1	D49.0
knee	C49.2-☑	C79.89	—	D21.2-☑	D48.1	D49.2
leg	C49.2-☑	C79.89	—	D21.2-☑	D48.1	D49.2
limb NEC	C49.9	C79.89	—	D21.9	D48.1	D49.2
lower	C49.2-☑	C79.89	—	D21.2-☑	D48.1	D49.2
upper	C49.1-☑	C79.89	—	D21.1-☑	D48.1	D49.2
nates	C49.5	C79.89	—	D21.5	D48.1	D49.2
neck	C49.0	C79.89	—	D21.0	D48.1	D49.2
orbit	C69.6-☑	C79.49	D09.2-☑	D31.6-☑	D48.1	D49.89
overlapping lesion	C49.8	—	—	—	—	—
pararectal	C49.5	C79.89	—	D21.5	D48.1	D49.2
para-urethral	C49.5	C79.89	—	D21.5	D48.1	D49.2
paravaginal	C49.5	C79.89	—	D21.5	D48.1	D49.2
pelvis (floor)	C49.5	C79.89	—	D21.5	D48.1	D49.2
pelvo-abdominal	C49.8	C79.89	—	D21.6	D48.1	D49.2
perineum	C49.5	C79.89	—	D21.5	D48.1	D49.2
perirectal (tissue)	C49.5	C79.89	—	D21.5	D48.1	D49.2
periurethral (tissue)	C49.5	C79.89	—	D21.5	D48.1	D49.2
popliteal fossa or space	C49.2-☑	C79.89	—	D21.2-☑	D48.1	D49.2
presacral	C49.5	C79.89	—	D21.5	D48.1	D49.2
psoas muscle	C49.4	C79.89	—	D21.4	D48.1	D49.2
pterygoid fossa	C49.0	C79.89	—	D21.0	D48.1	D49.2
rectovaginal septum or wall	C49.5	C79.89	—	D21.5	D48.1	D49.2
rectovesical	C49.5	C79.89	—	D21.5	D48.1	D49.2
retroperitoneum	C48.0	C78.6	—	D20.0	D48.3	D49.0
sacrococcygeal region	C49.5	C79.89	—	D21.5	D48.1	D49.2
scalp	C49.0	C79.89	—	D21.0	D48.1	D49.2
scapular region	C49.3	C79.89	—	D21.3	D48.1	D49.2
shoulder	C49.1-☑	C79.89	—	D21.1-☑	D48.1	D49.2
skin (dermis) NEC — *see also* Neoplasm, skin, by site	C44.90	C79.2	D04.9	D23.9	D48.5	D49.2
stomach	C49.4	C79.89	—	D21.4	D48.1	D49.2
submental	C49.0	C79.89	—	D21.0	D48.1	D49.2
supraclavicular region	C49.0	C79.89	—	D21.0	D48.1	D49.2
temple	C49.0	C79.89	—	D21.0	D48.1	D49.2
temporal region	C49.0	C79.89	—	D21.0	D48.1	D49.2
thigh	C49.2-☑	C79.89	—	D21.2-☑	D48.1	D49.2
thoracic (duct) (wall)	C49.3	C79.89	—	D21.3	D48.1	D49.2
thorax	C49.3	C79.89	—	D21.3	D48.1	D49.2
thumb	C49.1-☑	C79.89	—	D21.1-☑	D48.1	D49.2
toe	C49.2-☑	C79.89	—	D21.2-☑	D48.1	D49.2
trunk	C49.6	C79.89	—	D21.6	D48.1	D49.2
umbilicus	C49.4	C79.89	—	D21.4	D48.1	D49.2
vesicorectal	C49.5	C79.89	—	D21.5	D48.1	D49.2
wrist	C49.1-☑	C79.89	—	D21.1-☑	D48.1	D49.2
conus medullaris	C72.0	C79.49	—	D33.4	D43.4	D49.7
cord (true) (vocal)	C32.0	C78.39	D02.0	D14.1	D38.0	D49.1
false	C32.1	C78.39	D02.0	D14.1	D38.0	D49.1
spermatic	C63.1-☑	C79.82	D07.69	D29.8	D40.8	D49.59
spinal (cervical) (lumbar) (thoracic)	C72.0	C79.49	—	D33.4	D43.4	D49.7
cornea (limbus)	C69.1-☑	C79.49	D09.2-☑	D31.1-☑	D48.7	D49.89
corpus						
albicans	C56.-☑	C79.6-☑	D07.39	D27.-☑	D39.1-☑	D49.59
callosum, brain	C71.0	C79.31	—	D33.2	D43.2	D49.6
Neoplasm, neoplastic — *continued*						
corpus — *continued*						
cavernosum	C60.2	C79.82	D07.4	D29.0	D40.8	D49.59
gastric	C16.2	C78.89	D00.2	D13.1	D37.1	D49.0
overlapping sites	C54.8	—	—	—	—	—
penis	C60.2	C79.82	D07.4	D29.0	D40.8	D49.59
striatum, cerebrum	C71.0	C79.31	—	D33.0	D43.0	D49.6
uteri	C54.9	C79.82	D07.0	D26.1	D39.0	D49.59
isthmus	C54.0	C79.82	D07.0	D26.1	D39.0	D49.59
cortex						
adrenal	C74.0-☑	C79.7-☑	D09.3	D35.0-☑	D44.1-☑	D49.7
cerebral	C71.0	C79.31	—	D33.0	D43.0	D49.6
costal cartilage	C41.3	C79.51	—	D16.7	D48.0	D49.2
costovertebral joint	C41.3	C79.51	—	D16.7	D48.0	D49.2
Cowper's gland	C68.0	C79.19	D09.19	D30.4	D41.3	D49.59
cranial (fossa, any)	C71.9	C79.31	—	D33.2	D43.2	D49.6
meninges	C70.0	C79.32	—	D32.0	D42.0	D49.7
nerve	C72.50	C79.49	—	D33.3	D43.3	D49.7
specified NEC	C72.59	C79.49	—	D33.3	D43.3	D49.7
craniobuccal pouch	C75.2	C79.89	D09.3	D35.2	D44.3	D49.7
craniopharyngeal (duct) (pouch)	C75.2	C79.89	D09.3	D35.3	D44.4	D49.7
cricoid	C13.0	C79.89	D00.08	D10.7	D37.05	D49.0
cartilage	C32.3	C78.39	D02.0	D14.1	D38.0	D49.1
cricopharynx	C13.0	C79.89	D00.08	D10.7	D37.05	D49.0
crypt of Morgagni	C21.8	C78.5	D01.3	D12.9	D37.8	D49.0
crystalline lens	C69.4-☑	C79.49	D09.2-☑	D31.4-☑	D48.7	D49.89
cul-de-sac (Douglas')	C48.1	C78.6	—	D20.1	D48.4	D49.0
cuneiform cartilage	C32.3	C78.39	D02.0	D14.1	D38.0	D49.1
cutaneous — *see* Neoplasm, skin						
cutis — *see* Neoplasm, skin						
cystic (bile) duct (common)	C24.0	C78.89	D01.5	D13.5	D37.6	D49.0
dermis — *see* Neoplasm, skin						
diaphragm	C49.3	C79.89	—	D21.3	D48.1	D49.2
digestive organs, system, tube, or tract NEC	C26.9	C78.89	D01.9	D13.9	D37.9	D49.0
disc, intervertebral	C41.2	C79.51	—	D16.6	D48.0	D49.2
disease, generalized	C80.0	—	—	—	—	—
disseminated	C80.0	—	—	—	—	—
Douglas' cul-de-sac or pouch	C48.1	C78.6	—	D20.1	D48.4	D49.0
duodenojejunal junction	C17.8	C78.4	D01.49	D13.39	D37.2	D49.0
duodenum	C17.0	C78.4	D01.49	D13.2	D37.2	D49.0
dura (cranial) (mater)	C70.9	C79.49	—	D32.9	D42.9	D49.7
cerebral	C70.0	C79.32	—	D32.0	D42.0	D49.7
spinal	C70.1	C79.49	—	D32.1	D42.1	D49.7
ear (external) — *see also* Neoplasm, skin, ear	C44.20-☑	C79.2	D04.2-☑	D23.2-☑	D48.5	D49.2
auricle or auris — *see also* Neoplasm, skin, ear	C44.20-☑	C79.2	D04.2-☑	D23.2-☑	D48.5	D49.2
canal, external — *see also* Neoplasm, skin, ear	C44.20-☑	C79.2	D04.2-☑	D23.2-☑	D48.5	D49.2
cartilage	C49.0	C79.89	—	D21.0	D48.1	D49.2
external meatus — *see also* Neoplasm, skin, ear	C44.20-☑	C79.2	D04.2-☑	D23.2-☑	D48.5	D49.2
inner	C30.1	C78.39	D02.3	D14.0	D38.5	D49.1
lobule — *see also* Neoplasm, skin, ear	C44.20-☑	C79.2	D04.2-☑	D23.2-☑	D48.5	D49.2
middle	C30.1	C78.39	D02.3	D14.0	D38.5	D49.1
overlapping lesion with accessory sinuses	C31.8	—	—	—	—	—

	Malignant Primary	Malignant Secondary	Ca in situ	Benign	Uncertain Behavior	Unspecified Behavior
Neoplasm, neoplastic *— continued*						
ear *— see also* Neoplasm, skin, ear *— continued*						
skin	C44.20-☑	C79.2	D04.2-☑	D23.2-☑	D48.5	D49.2
basal cell carcinoma	C44.21-☑	—	—	—	—	—
specified type NEC	C44.29-☑	—	—	—	—	—
squamous cell carcinoma	C44.22-☑	—	—	—	—	—
earlobe	C44.20-☑	C79.2	D04.2-☑	D23.2-☑	D48.5	D49.2
basal cell carcinoma	C44.21-☑	—	—	—	—	—
specified type NEC	C44.29-☑	—	—	—	—	—
squamous cell carcinoma	C44.22-☑	—	—	—	—	—
ejaculatory duct	C63.7	C79.82	D07.69	D29.8	D40.8	D49.59
elbow NEC	C76.4-☑	C79.89	D04.6-☑	D36.7	D48.7	D49.89
endocardium	C38.0	C79.89	—	D15.1	D48.7	D49.89
endocervix (canal) (gland)	C53.0	C79.82	D06.0	D26.0	D39.0	D49.59
endocrine gland NEC	C75.9	C79.89	D09.3	D35.9	D44.9	D49.7
pluriglandular	C75.8	C79.89	D09.3	D35.7	D44.9	D49.7
endometrium (gland) (stroma)	C54.1	C79.82	D07.0	D26.1	D39.0	D49.59
ensiform cartilage	C41.3	C79.51	—	D16.7	D48.0	D49.2
enteric *— see* Neoplasm, intestine						
ependyma (brain)	C71.5	C79.31	—	D33.0	D43.0	D49.6
fourth ventricle	C71.7	C79.31	—	D33.1	D43.1	D49.6
epicardium	C38.0	C79.89	—	D15.1	D48.7	D49.89
epididymis	C63.0-☑	C79.82	D07.69	D29.3-☑	D40.8	D49.59
epidural	C72.9	C79.49	—	D33.9	D43.9	D49.7
epiglottis	C32.1	C78.39	D02.0	D14.1	D38.0	D49.1
anterior aspect or surface	C10.1	C79.89	D00.08	D10.5	D37.05	D49.0
cartilage	C32.3	C78.39	D02.0	D14.1	D38.0	D49.1
free border (margin)	C10.1	C79.89	D00.08	D10.5	D37.05	D49.0
junctional region	C10.8	C79.89	D00.08	D10.5	D37.05	D49.0
posterior (laryngeal) surface	C32.1	C78.39	D02.0	D14.1	D38.0	D49.1
suprahyoid portion	C32.1	C78.39	D02.0	D14.1	D38.0	D49.1
esophagogastric junction	C16.0	C78.89	D00.2	D13.1	D37.1	D49.0
esophagus	C15.9	C78.89	D00.1	D13.0	D37.8	D49.0
abdominal	C15.5	C78.89	D00.1	D13.0	D37.8	D49.0
cervical	C15.3	C78.89	D00.1	D13.0	D37.8	D49.0
distal (third)	C15.5	C78.89	D00.1	D13.0	D37.8	D49.0
lower (third)	C15.5	C78.89	D00.1	D13.0	D37.8	D49.0
middle (third)	C15.4	C78.89	D00.1	D13.0	D37.8	D49.0
overlapping lesion	C15.8	—	—	—	—	—
proximal (third)	C15.3	C78.89	D00.1	D13.0	D37.8	D49.0
thoracic	C15.4	C78.89	D00.1	D13.0	D37.8	D49.0
upper (third)	C15.3	C78.89	D00.1	D13.0	D37.8	D49.0
ethmoid (sinus)	C31.1	C78.39	D02.3	D14.0	D38.5	D49.1
bone or labyrinth	C41.0	C79.51	—	D16.4	D48.0	D49.2
eustachian tube	C30.1	C78.39	D02.3	D14.0	D38.5	D49.1
exocervix	C53.1	C79.82	D06.1	D26.0	D39.0	D49.59
external						
meatus (ear) *— see also* Neoplasm, skin, ear	C44.20-☑	C79.2	D04.2-☑	D23.2-☑	D48.5	D49.2
os, cervix uteri	C53.1	C79.82	D06.1	D26.0	D39.0	D49.59
extradural	C72.9	C79.49	—	D33.9	D43.9	D49.7
extrahepatic (bile) duct	C24.0	C78.89	D01.5	D13.5	D37.6	D49.0
overlapping lesion with gallbladder	C24.8	—	—	—	—	—
extraocular muscle	C69.6-☑	C79.49	D09.2-☑	D31.6-☑	D48.7	D49.89
extrarectal	C76.3	C79.89	D09.8	D36.7	D48.7	D49.89
extremity	C76.8	C79.89	D04.8	D36.7	D48.7	D49.89
Neoplasm, neoplastic *— continued*						
extremity *— continued*						
lower	C76.5-☑	C79.89	D04.7-☑	D36.7	D48.7	D49.89
upper	C76.4-☑	C79.89	D04.6-☑	D36.7	D48.7	D49.89
eyeball	C69.9-☑	C79.49	D09.2-☑	D31.9-☑	D48.7	D49.89
eyebrow	C44.309	C79.2	D04.39	D23.39	D48.5	D49.2
basal cell carcinoma	C44.319	—	—	—	—	—
specified type NEC	C44.399	—	—	—	—	—
squamous cell carcinoma	C44.329	—	—	—	—	—
eyelid (lower) (skin) (upper)	C44.10-☑	—	—	—	—	—
basal cell carcinoma	C44.11-☑	—	—	—	—	—
cartilage	C49.0	C79.89	—	D21.0	D48.1	D49.2
sebaceous cell	C44.13-☑	—	—	—	—	—
specified type NEC	C44.19-☑	—	—	—	—	—
squamous cell carcinoma	C44.12-☑	—	—	—	—	—
eye NEC	C69.9-☑	C79.49	D09.2-☑	D31.9-☑	D48.7	D49.89
overlapping sites	C69.8-☑	—	—	—	—	—
face NEC	C76.0	C79.89	D04.39	D36.7	D48.7	D49.89
fallopian tube (accessory)	C57.0-☑	C79.82	D07.39	D28.2	D39.8	D49.59
falx (cerebella) (cerebri)	C70.0	C79.32	—	D32.0	D42.0	D49.7
fascia *— see also* Neoplasm, connective tissue						
palmar	C49.1-☑	C79.89	—	D21.1-☑	D48.1	D49.2
plantar	C49.2-☑	C79.89	—	D21.2-☑	D48.1	D49.2
fatty tissue *— see* Neoplasm, connective tissue						
fauces, faucial NEC	C10.9	C79.89	D00.08	D10.5	D37.05	D49.0
pillars	C09.1	C79.89	D00.08	D10.5	D37.05	D49.0
tonsil	C09.9	C79.89	D00.08	D10.4	D37.05	D49.0
femur (any part)	C40.2-☑	—	—	D16.2-☑	—	—
fetal membrane	C58	C79.82	D07.0	D26.7	D39.2	D49.59
fibrous tissue *— see* Neoplasm, connective tissue						
fibula (any part)	C40.2-☑	C79.51	—	D16.2-☑	—	—
filum terminale	C72.0	C79.49	—	D33.4	D43.4	D49.7
finger NEC	C76.4-☑	C79.89	D04.6-☑	D36.7	D48.7	D49.89
flank NEC	C76.8	C79.89	D04.5	D36.7	D48.7	D49.89
follicle, nabothian	C53.0	C79.82	D06.0	D26.0	D39.0	D49.59
foot NEC	C76.5-☑	C79.89	D04.7-☑	D36.7	D48.7	D49.89
forearm NEC	C76.4-☑	C79.89	D04.6-☑	D36.7	D48.7	D49.89
forehead (skin)	C44.309	C79.2	D04.39	D23.39	D48.5	D49.2
basal cell carcinoma	C44.319	—	—	—	—	—
specified type NEC	C44.399	—	—	—	—	—
squamous cell carcinoma	C44.329	—	—	—	—	—
foreskin	C60.0	C79.82	D07.4	D29.0	D40.8	D49.59
fornix						
pharyngeal	C11.3	C79.89	D00.08	D10.6	D37.05	D49.0
vagina	C52	C79.82	D07.2	D28.1	D39.8	D49.59
fossa (of)						
anterior (cranial)	C71.9	C79.31	—	D33.2	D43.2	D49.6
cranial	C71.9	C79.31	—	D33.2	D43.2	D49.6
ischiorectal	C76.3	C79.89	D09.8	D36.7	D48.7	D49.89
middle (cranial)	C71.9	C79.31	—	D33.2	D43.2	D49.6
piriform	C12	C79.89	D00.08	D10.7	D37.05	D49.0
pituitary	C75.1	C79.89	D09.3	D35.2	D44.3	D49.7
posterior (cranial)	C71.9	C79.31	—	D33.2	D43.2	D49.6
pterygoid	C49.0	C79.89	—	D21.0	D48.1	D49.2
pyriform	C12	C79.89	D00.08	D10.7	D37.05	D49.0
Rosenmuller	C11.2	C79.89	D00.08	D10.6	D37.05	D49.0
tonsillar	C09.0	C79.89	D00.08	D10.5	D37.05	D49.0
fourchette	C51.9	C79.82	D07.1	D28.0	D39.8	D49.59
frenulum						
labii *— see* Neoplasm, lip, internal						

	Malignant Primary	Malignant Secondary	Ca in situ	Benign	Uncertain Behavior	Unspecified Behavior
Neoplasm, neoplastic — *continued*						
frenulum — *continued*						
linguae	CØ2.2	C79.89	DØØ.Ø7	D1Ø.1	D37.Ø2	D49.Ø
frontal						
bone	C41.Ø	C79.51	—	D16.4	D48.Ø	D49.2
lobe, brain	C71.1	C79.31	—	D33.Ø	D43.Ø	D49.6
pole	C71.1	C79.31	—	D33.Ø	D43.Ø	D49.6
sinus	C31.2	C78.39	DØ2.3	D14.Ø	D38.5	D49.1
fundus						
stomach	C16.1	C78.89	DØØ.2	D13.1	D37.1	D49.Ø
uterus	C54.3	C79.82	DØ7.Ø	D26.1	D39.Ø	D49.59
gallbladder	C23	C78.89	DØ1.5	D13.5	D37.6	D49.Ø
overlapping lesion with extrahepatic bile ducts	C24.8	—	—	—	—	
gall duct (extrahepatic)	C24.Ø	C78.89	DØ1.5	D13.5	D37.6	D49.Ø
intrahepatic	C22.1	C78.7	DØ1.5	D13.4	D37.6	D49.Ø
ganglia — *see also* Neoplasm, nerve, peripheral	C47.9	C79.89	—	D36.1Ø	D48.2	D49.2
basal	C71.Ø	C79.31	—	D33.Ø	D43.Ø	D49.6
cranial nerve	C72.5Ø	C79.49	—	D33.3	D43.3	D49.7
Gartner's duct	C52	C79.82	DØ7.2	D28.1	D39.8	D49.59
gastric — *see* Neoplasm, stomach						
gastrocolic	C26.9	C78.89	DØ1.9	D13.9	D37.9	D49.Ø
gastroesophageal junction	C16.Ø	C78.89	DØØ.2	D13.1	D37.1	D49.Ø
gastrointestinal (tract) NEC	C26.9	C78.89	DØ1.9	D13.9	D37.9	D49.Ø
generalized	C8Ø.Ø	—	—	—	—	—
genital organ or tract						
female NEC	C57.9	C79.82	DØ7.3Ø	D28.9	D39.9	D49.59
overlapping lesion	C57.8	—	—	—	—	—
specified site NEC	C57.7	C79.82	DØ7.39	D28.7	D39.8	D49.59
male NEC	C63.9	C79.82	DØ7.6Ø	D29.9	D4Ø.9	D49.59
overlapping lesion	C63.8	—	—	—	—	—
specified site NEC	C63.7	C79.82	DØ7.69	D29.8	D4Ø.8	D49.59
genitourinary tract						
female	C57.9	C79.82	DØ7.3Ø	D28.9	D39.9	D49.59
male	C63.9	C79.82	DØ7.6Ø	D29.9	D4Ø.9	D49.59
gingiva (alveolar) (marginal)	CØ3.9	C79.89	DØØ.Ø3	D1Ø.39	D37.Ø9	D49.Ø
lower	CØ3.1	C79.89	DØØ.Ø3	D1Ø.39	D37.Ø9	D49.Ø
mandibular	CØ3.1	C79.89	DØØ.Ø3	D1Ø.39	D37.Ø9	D49.Ø
maxillary	CØ3.Ø	C79.89	DØØ.Ø3	D1Ø.39	D37.Ø9	D49.Ø
upper	CØ3.Ø	C79.89	DØØ.Ø3	D1Ø.39	D37.Ø9	D49.Ø
gland, glandular (lymphatic) (system) — *see also* Neoplasm, lymph gland						
endocrine NEC	C75.9	C79.89	DØ9.3	D35.9	D44.9	D49.7
salivary — *see* Neoplasm, salivary gland						
glans penis	C6Ø.1	C79.82	DØ7.4	D29.Ø	D4Ø.8	D49.59
globus pallidus	C71.Ø	C79.31	—	D33.Ø	D43.Ø	D49.6
glomus						
coccygeal	C49.5	C79.89	—	D21.5	D48.1	D49.2
jugularis	C75.5	C79.89	—	D35.6	D44.7	D49.7
glosso-epiglottic fold(s)	C1Ø.1	C79.89	DØØ.Ø8	D1Ø.5	D37.Ø5	D49.Ø
glossopalatine fold	CØ9.1	C79.89	DØØ.Ø8	D1Ø.5	D37.Ø5	D49.Ø
glossopharyngeal sulcus	CØ9.Ø	C79.89	DØØ.Ø8	D1Ø.5	D37.Ø5	D49.Ø
glottis	C32.Ø	C78.39	DØ2.Ø	D14.1	D38.Ø	D49.1
gluteal region	C76.3	C79.89	DØ4.5	D36.7	D48.7	D49.89
great vessels NEC	C49.3	C79.89	—	D21.3	D48.1	D49.2
groin NEC	C76.3	C79.89	DØ4.5	D36.7	D48.7	D49.89
gum	CØ3.9	C79.89	DØØ.Ø3	D1Ø.39	D37.Ø9	D49.Ø
lower	CØ3.1	C79.89	DØØ.Ø3	D1Ø.39	D37.Ø9	D49.Ø
upper	CØ3.Ø	C79.89	DØØ.Ø3	D1Ø.39	D37.Ø9	D49.Ø
hand NEC	C76.4-☑	C79.89	DØ4.6-☑	D36.7	D48.7	D49.89
head NEC	C76.Ø	C79.89	DØ4.4	D36.7	D48.7	D49.89
heart	C38.Ø	C79.89	—	D15.1	D48.7	D49.89

	Malignant Primary	Malignant Secondary	Ca in situ	Benign	Uncertain Behavior	Unspecified Behavior
Neoplasm, neoplastic — *continued*						
heel NEC	C76.5-☑	C79.89	DØ4.7-☑	D36.7	D48.7	D49.89
helix — *see also* Neoplasm, skin, ear	C44.2Ø-☑	C79.2	DØ4.2-☑	D23.2-☑	D48.5	D49.2
hematopoietic, hemopoietic tissue NEC	C96.9	—	—	—	—	—
specified NEC	C96.Z	—	—	—	—	—
hemisphere, cerebral	C71.Ø	C79.31	—	D33.Ø	D43.Ø	D49.6
hemorrhoidal zone	C21.1	C78.5	DØ1.3	D12.9	D37.8	D49.Ø
hepatic — *see also* Index to disease, by histology	C22.9	C78.7	DØ1.5	D13.4	D37.6	D49.Ø
duct (bile)	C24.Ø	C78.89	DØ1.5	D13.5	D37.6	D49.Ø
flexure (colon)	C18.3	C78.5	DØ1.Ø	D12.3	D37.4	D49.Ø
primary	C22.8	C78.7	DØ1.5	D13.4	D37.6	D49.Ø
hepatobiliary	C24.9	C78.89	DØ1.5	D13.5	D37.6	D49.Ø
hepatoblastoma	C22.2	C78.7	DØ1.5	D13.4	D37.6	D49.Ø
hepatoma	C22.Ø	C78.7	DØ1.5	D13.4	D37.6	D49.Ø
hilus of lung	C34.Ø-☑	C78.Ø-☑	DØ2.2-☑	D14.3-☑	D38.1	D49.1
hippocampus, brain	C71.2	C79.31	—	D33.Ø	D43.Ø	D49.6
hip NEC	C76.5-☑	C79.89	DØ4.7-☑	D36.7	D48.7	D49.89
humerus (any part)	C4Ø.Ø-☑	C79.51	—	D16.Ø-☑	—	—
hymen	C52	C79.82	DØ7.2	D28.1	D39.8	D49.59
hypopharynx, hypopharyngeal NEC	C13.9	C79.89	DØØ.Ø8	D1Ø.7	D37.Ø5	D49.Ø
overlapping lesion	C13.8	—	—	—	—	—
postcricoid region	C13.Ø	C79.89	DØØ.Ø8	D1Ø.7	D37.Ø5	D49.Ø
posterior wall	C13.2	C79.89	DØØ.Ø8	D1Ø.7	D37.Ø5	D49.Ø
pyriform fossa (sinus)	C12	C79.89	DØØ.Ø8	D1Ø.7	D37.Ø5	D49.Ø
hypophysis	C75.1	C79.89	DØ9.3	D35.2	D44.3	D49.7
hypothalamus	C71.Ø	C79.31	—	D33.Ø	D43.Ø	D49.6
ileocecum, ileocecal (coil) (junction) (valve)	C18.Ø	C78.5	DØ1.Ø	D12.Ø	D37.4	D49.Ø
ileum	C17.2	C78.4	DØ1.49	D13.39	D37.2	D49.Ø
ilium	C41.4	C79.51	—	D16.8	D48.Ø	D49.2
immunoproliferative NEC	C88.9	—	—	—	—	—
infraclavicular (region)	C76.1	C79.89	DØ4.5	D36.7	D48.7	D49.89
inguinal (region)	C76.3	C79.89	DØ4.5	D36.7	D48.7	D49.89
insula	C71.Ø	C79.31	—	D33.Ø	D43.Ø	D49.6
insular tissue (pancreas)	C25.4	C78.89	DØ1.7	D13.7	D37.8	D49.Ø
brain	C71.Ø	C79.31	—	D33.Ø	D43.Ø	D49.6
interarytenoid fold	C13.1	C78.39	DØØ.Ø8	D1Ø.7	D37.Ø5	D49.Ø
hypopharyngeal aspect	C13.1	C79.89	DØØ.Ø8	D1Ø.7	D37.Ø5	D49.Ø
laryngeal aspect	C32.1	C78.39	DØ2.Ø	D14.1	D38.Ø	D49.1
marginal zone	C13.1	C79.89	DØØ.Ø8	D1Ø.7	D37.Ø5	D49.Ø
interdental papillae	CØ3.9	C79.89	DØØ.Ø3	D1Ø.39	D37.Ø9	D49.Ø
lower	CØ3.1	C79.89	DØØ.Ø3	D1Ø.39	D37.Ø9	D49.Ø
upper	CØ3.Ø	C79.89	DØØ.Ø3	D1Ø.39	D37.Ø9	D49.Ø
internal						
capsule	C71.Ø	C79.31	—	D33.Ø	D43.Ø	D49.6
os (cervix)	C53.Ø	C79.82	DØ6.Ø	D26.Ø	D39.Ø	D49.59
intervertebral cartilage or disc	C41.2	C79.51	—	D16.6	D48.Ø	D49.2
intestine, intestinal	C26.Ø	C78.8Ø	DØ1.4Ø	D13.9	D37.8	D49.Ø
large	C18.9	C78.5	DØ1.Ø	D12.6	D37.4	D49.Ø
appendix	C18.1	C78.5	DØ1.Ø	D12.1	D37.3	D49.Ø
caput coli	C18.Ø	C78.5	DØ1.Ø	D12.Ø	D37.4	D49.Ø
cecum	C18.Ø	C78.5	DØ1.Ø	D12.Ø	D37.4	D49.Ø
colon	C18.9	C78.5	DØ1.Ø	D12.6	D37.4	D49.Ø
and rectum	C19	C78.5	DØ1.1	D12.7	D37.5	D49.Ø
ascending	C18.2	C78.5	DØ1.Ø	D12.2	D37.4	D49.Ø
caput	C18.Ø	C78.5	DØ1.Ø	D12.Ø	D37.4	D49.Ø
descending	C18.6	C78.5	DØ1.Ø	D12.4	D37.4	D49.Ø
distal	C18.6	C78.5	DØ1.Ø	D12.4	D37.4	D49.Ø

	Malignant Primary	Malignant Secondary	Ca in situ	Benign	Uncertain Behavior	Unspecified Behavior
Neoplasm, neoplastic — *continued*						
intestine, intestinal — *continued*						
large — *continued*						
colon — *continued*						
left	C18.6	C78.5	DØ1.Ø	D12.4	D37.4	D49.Ø
overlapping lesion	C18.8	—	—	—	—	—
pelvic	C18.7	C78.5	DØ1.Ø	D12.5	D37.4	D49.Ø
right	C18.2	C78.5	DØ1.Ø	D12.2	D37.4	D49.Ø
sigmoid (flexure)	C18.7	C78.5	DØ1.Ø	D12.5	D37.4	D49.Ø
transverse	C18.4	C78.5	DØ1.Ø	D12.3	D37.4	D49.Ø
hepatic flexure	C18.3	C78.5	DØ1.Ø	D12.3	D37.4	D49.Ø
ileocecum, ileocecal (coil) (valve)	C18.Ø	C78.5	DØ1.Ø	D12.Ø	D37.4	D49.Ø
overlapping lesion	C18.8	—	—	—	—	—
sigmoid flexure (lower) (upper)	C18.7	C78.5	DØ1.Ø	D12.5	D37.4	D49.Ø
splenic flexure	C18.5	C78.5	DØ1.Ø	D12.3	D37.4	D49.Ø
small	C17.9	C78.4	DØ1.4Ø	D13.3Ø	D37.2	D49.Ø
duodenum	C17.Ø	C78.4	DØ1.49	D13.2	D37.2	D49.Ø
ileum	C17.2	C78.4	DØ1.49	D13.39	D37.2	D49.Ø
jejunum	C17.1	C78.4	DØ1.49	D13.39	D37.2	D49.Ø
overlapping lesion	C17.8	—	—	—	—	—
tract NEC	C26.Ø	C78.89	DØ1.4Ø	D13.9	D37.8	D49.Ø
intra-abdominal	C76.2	C79.89	DØ9.8	D36.7	D48.7	D49.89
intracranial NEC	C71.9	C79.31	—	D33.2	D43.2	D49.6
intrahepatic (bile) duct	C22.1	C78.7	DØ1.5	D13.4	D37.6	D49.Ø
intraocular	C69.9-☑	C79.49	DØ9.2-☑	D31.9-☑	D48.7	D49.89
intraorbital	C69.6-☑	C79.49	DØ9.2-☑	D31.6-☑	D48.7	D49.89
intrasellar	C75.1	C79.89	DØ9.3	D35.2	D44.3	D49.7
intrathoracic (cavity) (organs)	C76.1	C79.89	DØ9.8	D15.9	D48.7	D49.89
specified NEC	C76.1	C79.89	DØ9.8	D15.7	—	—
iris	C69.4-☑	C79.49	DØ9.2-☑	D31.4-☑	D48.7	D49.89
ischiorectal (fossa)	C76.3	C79.89	DØ9.8	D36.7	D48.7	D49.89
ischium	C41.4	C79.51	—	D16.8	D48.Ø	D49.2
island of Reil	C71.Ø	C79.31	—	D33.Ø	D43.Ø	D49.6
islands or islets of Langerhans	C25.4	C78.89	DØ1.7	D13.7	D37.8	D49.Ø
isthmus uteri	C54.Ø	C79.82	DØ7.Ø	D26.1	D39.Ø	D49.59
jaw	C76.Ø	C79.89	DØ9.8	D36.7	D48.7	D49.89
bone	C41.1	C79.51	—	D16.5	D48.Ø	D49.2
lower	C41.1	C79.51	—	D16.5	—	—
upper	C41.Ø	C79.51	—	D16.4	—	—
carcinoma (any type) (lower) (upper)	C76.Ø	C79.89	—	—	—	—
skin — *see also* Neoplasm, skin, face	C44.3Ø9	C79.2	DØ4.39	D23.39	D48.5	D49.2
soft tissues	CØ3.9	C79.89	DØØ.Ø3	D1Ø.39	D37.Ø9	D49.Ø
lower	CØ3.1	C79.89	DØØ.Ø3	D1Ø.39	D37.Ø9	D49.Ø
upper	CØ3.Ø	C79.89	DØØ.Ø3	D1Ø.39	D37.Ø9	D49.Ø
jejunum	C17.1	C78.4	DØ1.49	D13.39	D37.2	D49.Ø
joint NEC — *see also* Neoplasm, bone	C41.9	C79.51	—	D16.9	D48.Ø	D49.2
acromioclavicular	C4Ø.Ø-☑	C79.51	—	D16.Ø-☑	—	—
bursa or synovial membrane — *see* Neoplasm, connective tissue						
costovertebral	C41.3	C79.51	—	D16.7	D48.Ø	D49.2
sternocostal	C41.3	C79.51	—	D16.7	D48.Ø	D49.2
temporomandibular	C41.1	C79.51	—	D16.5	D48.Ø	D49.2
junction						
anorectal	C21.8	C78.5	DØ1.3	D12.9	D37.8	D49.Ø
cardioesophageal	C16.Ø	C78.89	DØØ.2	D13.1	D37.1	D49.Ø
esophagogastric	C16.Ø	C78.89	DØØ.2	D13.1	D37.1	D49.Ø
gastroesophageal	C16.Ø	C78.89	DØØ.2	D13.1	D37.1	D49.Ø
hard and soft palate	CØ5.9	C79.89	DØØ.ØØ	D1Ø.39	D37.Ø9	D49.Ø
ileocecal	C18.Ø	C78.5	DØ1.Ø	D12.Ø	D37.4	D49.Ø
Neoplasm, neoplastic — *continued*						
junction — *continued*						
pelvirectal	C19	C78.5	DØ1.1	D12.7	D37.5	D49.Ø
pelviureteric	C65.-☑	C79.Ø-☑	DØ9.19	D3Ø.1-☑	D41.1-☑	D49.59
rectosigmoid	C19	C78.5	DØ1.1	D12.7	D37.5	D49.Ø
squamocolumnar, of cervix	C53.8	C79.82	DØ6.7	D26.Ø	D39.Ø	D49.59
Kaposi's sarcoma — *see* Kaposi's, sarcoma						
kidney (parenchymal)	C64.-☑	C79.Ø-☑	DØ9.19	D3Ø.Ø-☑	D41.Ø-☑	D49.51-☑
calyx	C65.-☑	C79.Ø-☑	DØ9.19	D3Ø.1-☑	D41.1-☑	D49.51-☑
hilus	C65.-☑	C79.Ø-☑	DØ9.19	D3Ø.1-☑	D41.1-☑	D49.51-☑
pelvis	C65.-☑	C79.Ø-☑	DØ9.19	D3Ø.1-☑	D41.1-☑	D49.51-☑
knee NEC	C76.5-☑	C79.89	DØ4.7-☑	D36.7	D48.7	D49.89
labia (skin)	C51.9	C79.82	DØ7.1	D28.Ø	D39.8	D49.59
majora	C51.Ø	C79.82	DØ7.1	D28.Ø	D39.8	D49.59
minora	C51.1	C79.82	DØ7.1	D28.Ø	D39.8	D49.59
labial — *see also* Neoplasm, lip	CØØ.9	C79.89	DØØ.Ø1	D1Ø.Ø	D37.Ø1	D49.Ø
sulcus (lower) (upper)	CØ6.1	C79.89	DØØ.Ø2	D1Ø.39	D37.Ø9	D49.Ø
labium (skin)	C51.9	C79.82	DØ7.1	D28.Ø	D39.8	D49.59
majus	C51.Ø	C79.82	DØ7.1	D28.Ø	D39.8	D49.59
minus	C51.1	C79.82	DØ7.1	D28.Ø	D39.8	D49.59
lacrimal						
canaliculi	C69.5-☑	C79.49	DØ9.2-☑	D31.5-☑	D48.7	D49.89
duct (nasal)	C69.5-☑	C79.49	DØ9.2-☑	D31.5-☑	D48.7	D49.89
gland	C69.5-☑	C79.49	DØ9.2-☑	D31.5-☑	D48.7	D49.89
punctum	C69.5-☑	C79.49	DØ9.2-☑	D31.5-☑	D48.7	D49.89
sac	C69.5-☑	C79.49	DØ9.2-☑	D31.5-☑	D48.7	D49.89
Langerhans, islands or islets	C25.4	C78.89	DØ1.7	D13.7	D37.8	D49.Ø
laryngopharynx	C13.9	C79.89	DØØ.Ø8	D1Ø.7	D37.Ø5	D49.Ø
larynx, laryngeal NEC	C32.9	C78.39	DØ2.Ø	D14.1	D38.Ø	D49.1
aryepiglottic fold	C32.1	C78.39	DØ2.Ø	D14.1	D38.Ø	D49.1
cartilage (arytenoid) (cricoid) (cuneiform) (thyroid)	C32.3	C78.39	DØ2.Ø	D14.1	D38.Ø	D49.1
commissure (anterior) (posterior)	C32.Ø	C78.39	DØ2.Ø	D14.1	D38.Ø	D49.1
extrinsic NEC	C32.1	C78.39	DØ2.Ø	D14.1	D38.Ø	D49.1
meaning hypopharynx	C13.9	C79.89	DØØ.Ø8	D1Ø.7	D37.Ø5	D49.Ø
interarytenoid fold	C32.1	C78.39	DØ2.Ø	D14.1	D38.Ø	D49.1
intrinsic	C32.Ø	C78.39	DØ2.Ø	D14.1	D38.Ø	D49.1
overlapping lesion	C32.8	—	—	—	—	—
ventricular band	C32.1	C78.39	DØ2.Ø	D14.1	D38.Ø	D49.1
leg NEC	C76.5-☑	C79.89	DØ4.7-☑	D36.7	D48.7	D49.89
lens, crystalline	C69.4-☑	C79.49	DØ9.2-☑	D31.4-☑	D48.7	D49.89
lid (lower) (upper)	C44.1Ø-☑	C79.2	DØ4.1-☑	D23.1-☑	D48.5	D49.2
basal cell carcinoma	C44.11-☑	—	—	—	—	—
sebaceous cell	C44.13-☑	—	—	—	—	—
specified type NEC	C44.19-☑	—	—	—	—	—
squamous cell carcinoma	C44.12-☑	—	—	—	—	—
ligament — *see also* Neoplasm, connective tissue						
broad	C57.1-☑	C79.82	DØ7.39	D28.2	D39.8	D49.59
Mackenrodt's	C57.7	C79.82	DØ7.39	D28.7	D39.8	D49.59
non-uterine — *see* Neoplasm, connective tissue						
round	C57.2-☑	C79.82	—	D28.2	D39.8	D49.59
sacro-uterine	C57.3	C79.82	—	D28.2	D39.8	D49.59
uterine	C57.3	C79.82	—	D28.2	D39.8	D49.59
utero-ovarian	C57.7	C79.82	DØ7.39	D28.2	D39.8	D49.59
uterosacral	C57.3	C79.82	—	D28.2	D39.8	D49.59
limb	C76.8	C79.89	DØ4.8	D36.7	D48.7	D49.89
lower	C76.5-☑	C79.89	DØ4.7-☑	D36.7	D48.7	D49.89
upper	C76.4-☑	C79.89	DØ4.6-☑	D36.7	D48.7	D49.89
limbus of cornea	C69.1-☑	C79.49	DØ9.2-☑	D31.1-☑	D48.7	D49.89

	Malignant Primary	Malignant Secondary	Ca in situ	Benign	Uncertain Behavior	Unspecified Behavior
Neoplasm, neoplastic *— continued*						
lingual NEC — *see also* Neoplasm, tongue	C02.9	C79.89	D00.07	D10.1	D37.02	D49.0
lingula, lung	C34.1-☑	C78.0-☑	D02.2-☑	D14.3-☑	D38.1	D49.1
lip	C00.9	C79.89	D00.01	D10.0	D37.01	D49.0
buccal aspect — *see* Neoplasm, lip, internal						
commissure	C00.6	C79.89	D00.01	D10.0	D37.01	D49.0
external	C00.2	C79.89	D00.01	D10.0	D37.01	D49.0
lower	C00.1	C79.89	D00.01	D10.0	D37.01	D49.0
upper	C00.0	C79.89	D00.01	D10.0	D37.01	D49.0
frenulum — *see* Neoplasm, lip, internal						
inner aspect — *see* Neoplasm, lip, internal						
internal	C00.5	C79.89	D00.01	D10.0	D37.01	D49.0
lower	C00.4	C79.89	D00.01	D10.0	D37.01	D49.0
upper	C00.3	C79.89	D00.01	D10.0	D37.01	D49.0
lipstick area	C00.2	C79.89	D00.01	D10.0	D37.01	D49.0
lower	C00.1	C79.89	D00.01	D10.0	D37.01	D49.0
upper	C00.0	C79.89	D00.01	D10.0	D37.01	D49.0
lower	C00.1	C79.89	D00.01	D10.0	D37.01	D49.0
internal	C00.4	C79.89	D00.01	D10.0	D37.01	D49.0
mucosa — *see* Neoplasm, lip, internal						
oral aspect — *see* Neoplasm, lip, internal						
overlapping lesion	C00.8	—	—	—	—	—
with oral cavity or pharynx	C14.8	—	—	—	—	—
skin (commissure) (lower) (upper)	C44.00	C79.2	D04.0	D23.0	D48.5	D49.2
basal cell carcinoma	C44.01	—	—	—	—	—
specified type NEC	C44.09	—	—	—	—	—
squamous cell carcinoma	C44.02	—	—	—	—	—
upper	C00.0	C79.89	D00.01	D10.0	D37.01	D49.0
internal	C00.3	C79.89	D00.01	D10.0	D37.01	D49.0
vermilion border	C00.2	C79.89	D00.01	D10.0	D37.01	D49.0
lower	C00.1	C79.89	D00.01	D10.0	D37.01	D49.0
upper	C00.0	C79.89	D00.01	D10.0	D37.01	D49.0
lipomatous — *see* Lipoma, by site						
liver — *see also* Index to disease, by histology	C22.9	C78.7	D01.5	D13.4	D37.6	D49.0
primary	C22.8	C78.7	D01.5	D13.4	D37.6	D49.0
lumbosacral plexus	C47.5	C79.89	—	D36.16	D48.2	D49.2
lung	C34.9-☑	C78.0-☑	D02.2-☑	D14.3-☑	D38.1	D49.1
azygos lobe	C34.1-☑	C78.0-☑	D02.2-☑	D14.3-☑	D38.1	D49.1
carina	C34.0-☑	C78.0-☑	D02.2-☑	D14.3-☑	D38.1	D49.1
hilus	C34.0-☑	C78.0-☑	D02.2-☑	D14.3-☑	D38.1	D49.1
linqula	C34.1-☑	C78.0-☑	D02.2-☑	D14.3-☑	D38.1	D49.1
lobe NEC	C34.9-☑	C78.0-☑	D02.2-☑	D14.3-☑	D38.1	D49.1
lower lobe	C34.3-☑	C78.0-☑	D02.2-☑	D14.3-☑	D38.1	D49.1
main bronchus	C34.0-☑	C78.0-☑	D02.2-☑	D14.3-☑	D38.1	D49.1
mesothelioma — *see* Mesothelioma						
middle lobe	C34.2	C78.0-☑	D02.21	D14.31	D38.1	D49.1
overlapping lesion	C34.8-☑	—	—	—	—	—
upper lobe	C34.1-☑	C78.0-☑	D02.2-☑	D14.3-☑	D38.1	D49.1
lymph, lymphatic channel NEC	C49.9	C79.89	—	D21.9	D48.1	D49.2
gland (secondary)	—	C77.9	—	D36.0	D48.7	D49.89
abdominal	—	C77.2	—	D36.0	D48.7	D49.89
aortic	—	C77.2	—	D36.0	D48.7	D49.89
arm	—	C77.3	—	D36.0	D48.7	D49.89

	Malignant Primary	Malignant Secondary	Ca in situ	Benign	Uncertain Behavior	Unspecified Behavior
Neoplasm, neoplastic *— continued*						
lymph, lymphatic channel — *continued*						
gland — *continued*						
auricular (anterior) (posterior)	—	C77.0	—	D36.0	D48.7	D49.89
axilla, axillary	—	C77.3	—	D36.0	D48.7	D49.89
brachial	—	C77.3	—	D36.0	D48.7	D49.89
bronchial	—	C77.1	—	D36.0	D48.7	D49.89
bronchopulmonary	—	C77.1	—	D36.0	D48.7	D49.89
celiac	—	C77.2	—	D36.0	D48.7	D49.89
cervical	—	C77.0	—	D36.0	D48.7	D49.89
cervicofacial	—	C77.0	—	D36.0	D48.7	D49.89
Cloquet	—	C77.4	—	D36.0	D48.7	D49.89
colic	—	C77.2	—	D36.0	D48.7	D49.89
common duct	—	C77.2	—	D36.0	D48.7	D49.89
cubital	—	C77.3	—	D36.0	D48.7	D49.89
diaphragmatic	—	C77.1	—	D36.0	D48.7	D49.89
epigastric, inferior	—	C77.1	—	D36.0	D48.7	D49.89
epitrochlear	—	C77.3	—	D36.0	D48.7	D49.89
esophageal	—	C77.1	—	D36.0	D48.7	D49.89
face	—	C77.0	—	D36.0	D48.7	D49.89
femoral	—	C77.4	—	D36.0	D48.7	D49.89
gastric	—	C77.2	—	D36.0	D48.7	D49.89
groin	—	C77.4	—	D36.0	D48.7	D49.89
head	—	C77.0	—	D36.0	D48.7	D49.89
hepatic	—	C77.2	—	D36.0	D48.7	D49.89
hilar (pulmonary)	—	C77.1	—	D36.0	D48.7	D49.89
splenic	—	C77.2	—	D36.0	D48.7	D49.89
hypogastric	—	C77.5	—	D36.0	D48.7	D49.89
ileocolic	—	C77.2	—	D36.0	D48.7	D49.89
iliac	—	C77.5	—	D36.0	D48.7	D49.89
infraclavicular	—	C77.3	—	D36.0	D48.7	D49.89
inguina, inguinal	—	C77.4	—	D36.0	D48.7	D49.89
innominate	—	C77.1	—	D36.0	D48.7	D49.89
intercostal	—	C77.1	—	D36.0	D48.7	D49.89
intestinal	—	C77.2	—	D36.0	D48.7	D49.89
intrabdominal	—	C77.2	—	D36.0	D48.7	D49.89
intrapelvic	—	C77.5	—	D36.0	D48.7	D49.89
intrathoracic	—	C77.1	—	D36.0	D48.7	D49.89
jugular	—	C77.0	—	D36.0	D48.7	D49.89
leg	—	C77.4	—	D36.0	D48.7	D49.89
limb						
lower	—	C77.4	—	D36.0	D48.7	D49.89
upper	—	C77.3	—	D36.0	D48.7	D49.89
lower limb	—	C77.4	—	D36.0	D48.7	D49.89
lumbar	—	C77.2	—	D36.0	D48.7	D49.89
mandibular	—	C77.0	—	D36.0	D48.7	D49.89
mediastinal	—	C77.1	—	D36.0	D48.7	D49.89
mesenteric (inferior) (superior)	—	C77.2	—	D36.0	D48.7	D49.89
midcolic	—	C77.2	—	D36.0	D48.7	D49.89
multiple sites in categories C77.0 - C77.5	—	C77.8	—	D36.0	D48.7	D49.89
neck	—	C77.0	—	D36.0	D48.7	D49.89
obturator	—	C77.5	—	D36.0	D48.7	D49.89
occipital	—	C77.0	—	D36.0	D48.7	D49.89
pancreatic	—	C77.2	—	D36.0	D48.7	D49.89
para-aortic	—	C77.2	—	D36.0	D48.7	D49.89
paracervical	—	C77.5	—	D36.0	D48.7	D49.89
parametrial	—	C77.5	—	D36.0	D48.7	D49.89
parasternal	—	C77.1	—	D36.0	D48.7	D49.89
parotid	—	C77.0	—	D36.0	D48.7	D49.89
pectoral	—	C77.3	—	D36.0	D48.7	D49.89
pelvic	—	C77.5	—	D36.0	D48.7	D49.89
peri-aortic	—	C77.2	—	D36.0	D48.7	D49.89
peripancreatic	—	C77.2	—	D36.0	D48.7	D49.89
popliteal	—	C77.4	—	D36.0	D48.7	D49.89
porta hepatis	—	C77.2	—	D36.0	D48.7	D49.89
portal	—	C77.2	—	D36.0	D48.7	D49.89
preauricular	—	C77.0	—	D36.0	D48.7	D49.89
prelaryngeal	—	C77.0	—	D36.0	D48.7	D49.89
presymphysial	—	C77.5	—	D36.0	D48.7	D49.89
pretracheal	—	C77.0	—	D36.0	D48.7	D49.89
primary (any site) NEC	C96.9	—	—	—	—	—

	Malignant Primary	Malignant Secondary	Ca in situ	Benign	Uncertain Behavior	Unspecified Behavior
Neoplasm, neoplastic — *continued*						
lymph, lymphatic channel — *continued*						
gland — *continued*						
pulmonary (hiler)	—	C77.1	—	D36.0	D48.7	D49.89
pyloric	—	C77.2	—	D36.0	D48.7	D49.89
retroperitoneal	—	C77.2	—	D36.0	D48.7	D49.89
retropharyngeal	—	C77.0	—	D36.0	D48.7	D49.89
Rosenmuller's	—	C77.4	—	D36.0	D48.7	D49.89
sacral	—	C77.5	—	D36.0	D48.7	D49.89
scalene	—	C77.0	—	D36.0	D48.7	D49.89
site NEC	—	C77.9	—	D36.0	D48.7	D49.89
splenic (hilar)	—	C77.2	—	D36.0	D48.7	D49.89
subclavicular	—	C77.3	—	D36.0	D48.7	D49.89
subinguinal	—	C77.4	—	D36.0	D48.7	D49.89
sublingual	—	C77.0	—	D36.0	D48.7	D49.89
submandibular	—	C77.0	—	D36.0	D48.7	D49.89
submaxillary	—	C77.0	—	D36.0	D48.7	D49.89
submental	—	C77.0	—	D36.0	D48.7	D49.89
subscapular	—	C77.3	—	D36.0	D48.7	D49.89
supraclavicular	—	C77.0	—	D36.0	D48.7	D49.89
thoracic	—	C77.1	—	D36.0	D48.7	D49.89
tibial	—	C77.4	—	D36.0	D48.7	D49.89
tracheal	—	C77.1	—	D36.0	D48.7	D49.89
tracheobronchial	—	C77.1	—	D36.0	D48.7	D49.89
upper limb	—	C77.3	—	D36.0	D48.7	D49.89
Virchow's	—	C77.0	—	D36.0	D48.7	D49.89
node — *see also* Neoplasm, lymph gland						
primary NEC	C96.9	—	—	—	—	—
vessel — *see also* Neoplasm, connective tissue	C49.9	C79.89	—	D21.9	D48.1	D49.2
Mackenrodt's ligament	C57.7	C79.82	D07.39	D28.7	D39.8	D49.59
malar	C41.0	C79.51	—	D16.4	D48.0	D49.2
region — *see* Neoplasm, cheek						
mammary gland — *see* Neoplasm, breast						
mandible	C41.1	C79.51	—	D16.5	D48.0	D49.2
alveolar						
mucosa (carcinoma)	C03.1	C79.89	D00.03	D10.39	D37.09	D49.0
ridge or process	C41.1	C79.51	—	D16.5	D48.0	D49.2
marrow (bone)						
NEC	C96.9	C79.52	—	—	D47.9	D49.89
mastectomy site (skin) — *see also* Neoplasm, breast, skin	C44.501	C79.2	—	—	—	—
specified as breast tissue	C50.8-☑	C79.81	—	—	—	—
mastoid (air cells) (antrum) (cavity)	C30.1	C78.39	D02.3	D14.0	D38.5	D49.1
bone or process	C41.0	C79.51	—	D16.4	D48.0	D49.2
maxilla, maxillary (superior)	C41.0	C79.51	—	D16.4	D48.0	D49.2
alveolar						
mucosa	C03.0	C79.89	D00.03	D10.39	D37.09	D49.0
ridge or process (carcinoma)	C41.0	C79.51	—	D16.4	D48.0	D49.2
antrum	C31.0	C78.39	D02.3	D14.0	D38.5	D49.1
carcinoma	C03.0	C79.51	—	—	—	—
inferior — *see* Neoplasm, mandible						
sinus	C31.0	C78.39	D02.3	D14.0	D38.5	D49.1
meatus external (ear) — *see also* Neoplasm, skin, ear	C44.20-☑	C79.2	D04.2-☑	D23.2-☑	D48.5	D49.2
Meckel diverticulum, malignant	C17.3	C78.4	D01.49	D13.39	D37.2	D49.0
mediastinum, mediastinal	C38.3	C78.1	—	D15.2	D38.3	D49.89
anterior	C38.1	C78.1	—	D15.2	D38.3	D49.89
Neoplasm, neoplastic — *continued*						
mediastinum, mediastinal — *continued*						
posterior	C38.2	C78.1	—	D15.2	D38.3	D49.89
medulla						
adrenal	C74.1-☑	C79.7-☑	D09.3	D35.0-☑	D44.1-☑	D49.7
oblongata	C71.7	C79.31	—	D33.1	D43.1	D49.6
meibomian gland	C44.10-☑	C79.2	D04.1-☑	D23.1-☑	D48.5	D49.2
basal cell carcinoma	C44.11-☑	—	—	—	—	—
sebaceous cell	C44.13-☑	—	—	—	—	—
specified type NEC	C44.19-☑	—	—	—	—	—
squamous cell carcinoma	C44.12-☑	—	—	—	—	—
melanoma — *see* Melanoma						
meninges	C70.9	C79.49	—	D32.9	D42.9	D49.7
brain	C70.0	C79.32	—	D32.0	D42.0	D49.7
cerebral	C70.0	C79.32	—	D32.0	D42.0	D49.7
crainial	C70.0	C79.32	—	D32.0	D42.0	D49.7
intracranial	C70.0	C79.32	—	D32.0	D42.0	D49.7
spinal (cord)	C70.1	C79.49	—	D32.1	D42.1	D49.7
meniscus, knee joint (lateral) (medial)	C40.2-☑	C79.51	—	D16.2-☑	D48.0	D49.2
Merkel cell — *see* Carcinoma, Merkel cell						
mesentery, mesenteric	C48.1	C78.6	—	D20.1	D48.4	D49.0
mesoappendix	C48.1	C78.6	—	D20.1	D48.4	D49.0
mesocolon	C48.1	C78.6	—	D20.1	D48.4	D49.0
mesopharynx — *see* Neoplasm, oropharynx						
mesosalpinx	C57.1-☑	C79.82	D07.39	D28.2	D39.8	D49.59
mesothelial tissue — *see* Mesothelioma						
mesothelioma — *see* Mesothelioma						
mesovarium	C57.1-☑	C79.82	D07.39	D28.2	D39.8	D49.59
metacarpus (any bone)	C40.1-☑	C79.51	—	D16.1-☑	—	—
metastatic NEC — *see also* Neoplasm, by site, secondary	—	C79.9	—	—	—	—
metatarsus (any bone)	C40.3-☑	C79.51	—	D16.3-☑	—	—
midbrain	C71.7	C79.31	—	D33.1	D43.1	D49.6
milk duct — *see* Neoplasm, breast						
mons						
pubis	C51.9	C79.82	D07.1	D28.0	D39.8	D49.59
veneris	C51.9	C79.82	D07.1	D28.0	D39.8	D49.59
motor tract	C72.9	C79.49	—	D33.9	D43.9	D49.7
brain	C71.9	C79.31	—	D33.2	D43.2	D49.6
cauda equina	C72.1	C79.49	—	D33.4	D43.4	D49.7
spinal	C72.0	C79.49	—	D33.4	D43.4	D49.7
mouth	C06.9	C79.89	D00.00	D10.30	D37.09	D49.0
book-leaf	C06.89	C79.89	—	—	—	—
floor	C04.9	C79.89	D00.06	D10.2	D37.09	D49.0
anterior portion	C04.0	C79.89	D00.06	D10.2	D37.09	D49.0
lateral portion	C04.1	C79.89	D00.06	D10.2	D37.09	D49.0
overlapping lesion	C04.8	—	—	—	—	—
overlapping NEC	C06.80	—	—	—	—	—
roof	C05.9	C79.89	D00.00	D10.39	D37.09	D49.0
specified part NEC	C06.89	C79.89	D00.00	D10.39	D37.09	D49.0
vestibule	C06.1	C79.89	D00.00	D10.39	D37.09	D49.0
mucosa						
alveolar (ridge or process)	C03.9	C79.89	D00.03	D10.39	D37.09	D49.0
lower	C03.1	C79.89	D00.03	D10.39	D37.09	D49.0
upper	C03.0	C79.89	D00.03	D10.39	D37.09	D49.0
buccal	C06.0	C79.89	D00.02	D10.39	D37.09	D49.0
cheek	C06.0	C79.89	D00.02	D10.39	D37.09	D49.0

	Malignant Primary	Malignant Secondary	Ca in situ	Benign	Uncertain Behavior	Unspecified Behavior
Neoplasm, neoplastic — *continued*						
mucosa — *continued*						
lip — *see* Neoplasm, lip, internal						
nasal	C3Ø.Ø	C78.39	DØ2.3	D14.Ø	D38.5	D49.1
oral	CØ6.Ø	C79.89	DØØ.Ø2	D1Ø.39	D37.Ø9	D49.Ø
Mullerian duct						
female	C57.7	C79.82	DØ7.39	D28.7	D39.8	D49.59
male	C63.7	C79.82	DØ7.69	D29.8	D4Ø.8	D49.59
muscle — *see also* Neoplasm, connective tissue						
extraocular	C69.6-☑	C79.49	DØ9.2-☑	D31.6-☑	D48.7	D49.89
myocardium	C38.Ø	C79.89	—	D15.1	D48.7	D49.89
myometrium	C54.2	C79.82	DØ7.Ø	D26.1	D39.Ø	D49.59
myopericardium	C38.Ø	C79.89	—	D15.1	D48.7	D49.89
nabothian gland (follicle)	C53.Ø	C79.82	DØ6.Ø	D26.Ø	D39.Ø	D49.59
nail — *see also* Neoplasm, skin, limb	C44.9Ø	C79.2	DØ4.9	D23.9	D48.5	D49.2
finger — *see also* Neoplasm, skin, limb, upper	C44.6Ø-☑	C79.2	DØ4.6-☑	D23.6-☑	D48.5	D49.2
toe — *see also* Neoplasm, skin, limb, lower	C44.7Ø-☑	C79.2	DØ4.7-☑	D23.7-☑	D48.5	D49.2
nares, naris (anterior) (posterior)	C3Ø.Ø	C78.39	DØ2.3	D14.Ø	D38.5	D49.1
nasal — *see* Neoplasm, nose						
nasolabial groove — *see also* Neoplasm, skin, face	C44.3Ø9	C79.2	DØ4.39	D23.39	D48.5	D49.2
nasolacrimal duct	C69.5-☑	C79.49	DØ9.2-☑	D31.5-☑	D48.7	D49.89
nasopharynx, nasopharyngeal	C11.9	C79.89	DØØ.Ø8	D1Ø.6	D37.Ø5	D49.Ø
floor	C11.3	C79.89	DØØ.Ø8	D1Ø.6	D37.Ø5	D49.Ø
overlapping lesion	C11.8	—	—	—	—	—
roof	C11.Ø	C79.89	DØØ.Ø8	D1Ø.6	D37.Ø5	D49.Ø
wall	C11.9	C79.89	DØØ.Ø8	D1Ø.6	D37.Ø5	D49.Ø
anterior	C11.3	C79.89	DØØ.Ø8	D1Ø.6	D37.Ø5	D49.Ø
lateral	C11.2	C79.89	DØØ.Ø8	D1Ø.6	D37.Ø5	D49.Ø
posterior	C11.1	C79.89	DØØ.Ø8	D1Ø.6	D37.Ø5	D49.Ø
superior	C11.Ø	C79.89	DØØ.Ø8	D1Ø.6	D37.Ø5	D49.Ø
nates — *see also* Neoplasm, skin, trunk	C44.5Ø9	C79.2	DØ4.5	D23.5	D48.5	D49.2
neck NEC	C76.Ø	C79.89	DØ9.8	D36.7	D48.7	D49.89
skin	C44.4Ø	—	—	—	—	—
basal cell carcinoma	C44.41	—	—	—	—	—
specified type NEC	C44.49	—	—	—	—	—
squamous cell carcinoma	C44.42	—	—	—	—	—
nerve (ganglion)	C47.9	C79.89	—	D36.1Ø	D48.2	D49.2
abducens	C72.59	C79.49	—	D33.3	D43.3	D49.7
accessory (spinal)	C72.59	C79.49	—	D33.3	D43.3	D49.7
acoustic	C72.4-☑	C79.49	—	D33.3	D43.3	D49.7
auditory	C72.4-☑	C79.49	—	D33.3	D43.3	D49.7
autonomic NEC — *see also* Neoplasm, nerve, peripheral	C47.9	C79.89	—	D36.1Ø	D48.2	D49.2
brachial	C47.1-☑	C79.89	—	D36.12	D48.2	D49.2
cranial	C72.5Ø	C79.49	—	D33.3	D43.3	D49.7
specified NEC	C72.59	C79.49	—	D33.3	D43.3	D49.7
facial	C72.59	C79.49	—	D33.3	D43.3	D49.7
femoral	C47.2-☑	C79.89	—	D36.13	D48.2	D49.2
ganglion NEC — *see also* Neoplasm, nerve, peripheral	C47.9	C79.89	—	D36.1Ø	D48.2	D49.2
glossopharyngeal	C72.59	C79.49	—	D33.3	D43.3	D49.7
hypoglossal	C72.59	C79.49	—	D33.3	D43.3	D49.7
intercostal	C47.3	C79.89	—	D36.14	D48.2	D49.2
lumbar	C47.6	C79.89	—	D36.17	D48.2	D49.2
median	C47.1-☑	C79.89	—	D36.12	D48.2	D49.2
obturator	C47.2-☑	C79.89	—	D36.13	D48.2	D49.2

	Malignant Primary	Malignant Secondary	Ca in situ	Benign	Uncertain Behavior	Unspecified Behavior
Neoplasm, neoplastic — *continued*						
nerve — *continued*						
oculomotor	C72.59	C79.49	—	D33.3	D43.3	D49.7
olfactory	C47.2-☑	C79.49	—	D33.3	D43.3	D49.7
optic	C72.3-☑	C79.49	—	D33.3	D43.3	D49.7
parasympathetic NEC	C47.9	C79.89	—	D36.1Ø	D48.2	D49.2
peripheral NEC	C47.9	C79.89	—	D36.1Ø	D48.2	D49.2
abdomen	C47.4	C79.89	—	D36.15	D48.2	D49.2
abdominal wall	C47.4	C79.89	—	D36.15	D48.2	D49.2
ankle	C47.2-☑	C79.89	—	D36.13	D48.2	D49.2
antecubital fossa or space	C47.1-☑	C79.89	—	D36.12	D48.2	D49.2
arm	C47.1-☑	C79.89	—	D36.12	D48.2	D49.2
auricle (ear)	C47.Ø	C79.89	—	D36.11	D48.2	D49.2
axilla	C47.3	C79.89	—	D36.12	D48.2	D49.2
back	C47.6	C79.89	—	D36.17	D48.2	D49.2
buttock	C47.5	C79.89	—	D36.16	D48.2	D49.2
calf	C47.2-☑	C79.89	—	D36.13	D48.2	D49.2
cervical region	C47.Ø	C79.89	—	D36.11	D48.2	D49.2
cheek	C47.Ø	C79.89	—	D36.11	D48.2	D49.2
chest (wall)	C47.3	C79.89	—	D36.14	D48.2	D49.2
chin	C47.Ø	C79.89	—	D36.11	D48.2	D49.2
ear (external)	C47.Ø	C79.89	—	D36.11	D48.2	D49.2
elbow	C47.1-☑	C79.89	—	D36.12	D48.2	D49.2
extrarectal	C47.5	C79.89	—	D36.16	D48.2	D49.2
extremity	C47.9	C79.89	—	D36.1Ø	D48.2	D49.2
lower	C47.2-☑	C79.89	—	D36.13	D48.2	D49.2
upper	C47.1-☑	C79.89	—	D36.12	D48.2	D49.2
eyelid	C47.Ø	C79.89	—	D36.11	D48.2	D49.2
face	C47.Ø	C79.89	—	D36.11	D48.2	D49.2
finger	C47.1-☑	C79.89	—	D36.12	D48.2	D49.2
flank	C47.6	C79.89	—	D36.17	D48.2	D49.2
foot	C47.2-☑	C79.89	—	D36.13	D48.2	D49.2
forearm	C47.1-☑	C79.89	—	D36.12	D48.2	D49.2
forehead	C47.Ø	C79.89	—	D36.11	D48.2	D49.2
gluteal region	C47.5	C79.89	—	D36.16	D48.2	D49.2
groin	C47.5	C79.89	—	D36.16	D48.2	D49.2
hand	C47.1-☑	C79.89	—	D36.12	D48.2	D49.2
head	C47.Ø	C79.89	—	D36.11	D48.2	D49.2
heel	C47.2-☑	C79.89	—	D36.13	D48.2	D49.2
hip	C47.2-☑	C79.89	—	D36.13	D48.2	D49.2
infraclavicular region	C47.3	C79.89	—	D36.14	D48.2	D49.2
inguinal (canal) (region)	C47.5	C79.89	—	D36.16	D48.2	D49.2
intrathoracic	C47.3	C79.89	—	D36.14	D48.2	D49.2
ischiorectal fossa	C47.5	C79.89	—	D36.16	D48.2	D49.2
knee	C47.2-☑	C79.89	—	D36.13	D48.2	D49.2
leg	C47.2-☑	C79.89	—	D36.13	D48.2	D49.2
limb NEC	C47.9	C79.89	—	D36.1Ø	D48.2	D49.2
lower	C47.2-☑	C79.89	—	D36.13	D48.2	D49.2
upper	C47.1-☑	C79.89	—	D36.12	D48.2	D49.2
nates	C47.5	C79.89	—	D36.16	D48.2	D49.2
neck	C47.Ø	C79.89	—	D36.11	D48.2	D49.2
orbit	C69.6-☑	C79.49	—	D31.6-☑	D48.7	D49.2
pararectal	C47.5	C79.89	—	D36.16	D48.2	D49.2
paraurethral	C47.5	C79.89	—	D36.16	D48.2	D49.2
paravaginal	C47.5	C79.89	—	D36.16	D48.2	D49.2
pelvis (floor)	C47.5	C79.89	—	D36.16	D48.2	D49.2
pelvoabdominal	C47.8	C79.89	—	D36.17	D48.2	D49.2
perineum	C47.5	C79.89	—	D36.16	D48.2	D49.2
perirectal (tissue)	C47.5	C79.89	—	D36.16	D48.2	D49.2
periurethral (tissue)	C47.5	C79.89	—	D36.16	D48.2	D49.2
popliteal fossa or space	C47.2-☑	C79.89	—	D36.13	D48.2	D49.2
presacral	C47.5	C79.89	—	D36.16	D48.2	D49.2
pterygoid fossa	C47.Ø	C79.89	—	D36.11	D48.2	D49.2
rectovaginal septum or wall	C47.5	C79.89	—	D36.16	D48.2	D49.2
rectovesical	C47.5	C79.89	—	D36.16	D48.2	D49.2
sacrococcygeal region	C47.5	C79.89	—	D36.16	D48.2	D49.2
scalp	C47.Ø	C79.89	—	D36.11	D48.2	D49.2

☑ **Additional Character Required — Refer to the Tabular List for Character Selection**

	Malignant Primary	Malignant Secondary	Ca in situ	Benign	Uncertain Behavior	Unspecified Behavior
Neoplasm, neoplastic — *continued*						
nerve — *continued*						
peripheral — *continued*						
scapular region	C47.3	C79.89	—	D36.14	D48.2	D49.2
shoulder	C47.1-☑	C79.89	—	D36.12	D48.2	D49.2
submental	C47.Ø	C79.89	—	D36.11	D48.2	D49.2
supraclavicular region	C47.Ø	C79.89	—	D36.11	D48.2	D49.2
temple	C47.Ø	C79.89	—	D36.11	D48.2	D49.2
temporal region	C47.Ø	C79.89	—	D36.11	D48.2	D49.2
thigh	C47.2-☑	C79.89	—	D36.13	D48.2	D49.2
thoracic (duct) (wall)	C47.3	C79.89	—	D36.14	D48.2	D49.2
thorax	C47.3	C79.89	—	D36.14	D48.2	D49.2
thumb	C47.1-☑	C79.89	—	D36.12	D48.2	D49.2
toe	C47.2-☑	C79.89	—	D36.13	D48.2	D49.2
trunk	C47.6	C79.89	—	D36.17	D48.2	D49.2
umbilicus	C47.4	C79.89	—	D36.15	D48.2	D49.2
vesicorectal	C47.5	C79.89	—	D36.16	D48.2	D49.2
wrist	C47.1-☑	C79.89	—	D36.12	D48.2	D49.2
radial	C47.1-☑	C79.89	—	D36.12	D48.2	D49.2
sacral	C47.5	C79.89	—	D36.16	D48.2	D49.2
sciatic	C47.2-☑	C79.89	—	D36.13	D48.2	D49.2
spinal NEC	C47.9	C79.89	—	D36.1Ø	D48.2	D49.2
accessory	C72.59	C79.49	—	D33.3	D43.3	D49.7
sympathetic NEC — *see also* Neoplasm, nerve, peripheral	C47.9	C79.89	—	D36.1Ø	D48.2	D49.2
trigeminal	C72.59	C79.49	—	D33.3	D43.3	D49.7
trochlear	C72.59	C79.49	—	D33.3	D43.3	D49.7
ulnar	C47.1-☑	C79.89	—	D36.12	D48.2	D49.2
vagus	C72.59	C79.49	—	D33.3	D43.3	D49.7
nervous system (central)	C72.9	C79.4Ø	—	D33.9	D43.9	D49.7
autonomic — *see* Neoplasm, nerve, peripheral						
parasympathetic — *see* Neoplasm, nerve, peripheral						
specified site NEC	—	C79.49	—	D33.7	D43.8	—
sympathetic — *see* Neoplasm, nerve, peripheral						
nevus — *see* Nevus						
nipple	C5Ø.Ø-☑	C79.81	DØ5.-☑	D24.-☑	—	—
nose, nasal	C76.Ø	C79.89	DØ9.8	D36.7	D48.7	D49.89
ala (external) (nasi) — *see also* Neoplasm, nose, skin	C44.3Ø1	C79.2	DØ4.39	D23.39	D48.5	D49.2
bone	C41.Ø	C79.51	—	D16.4	D48.Ø	D49.2
cartilage	C3Ø.Ø	C78.39	DØ2.3	D14.Ø	D38.5	D49.1
cavity	C3Ø.Ø	C78.39	DØ2.3	D14.Ø	D38.5	D49.1
choana	C11.3	C79.89	DØØ.Ø8	D1Ø.6	D37.Ø5	D49.Ø
external (skin) — *see also* Neoplasm, nose, skin	C44.3Ø1	C79.2	DØ4.39	D23.39	D48.5	D49.2
fossa	C3Ø.Ø	C78.39	DØ2.3	D14.Ø	D38.5	D49.1
internal	C3Ø.Ø	C78.39	DØ2.3	D14.Ø	D38.5	D49.1
mucosa	C3Ø.Ø	C78.39	DØ2.3	D14.Ø	D38.5	D49.1
septum	C3Ø.Ø	C78.39	DØ2.3	D14.Ø	D38.5	D49.1
posterior margin	C11.3	C79.89	DØØ.Ø8	D1Ø.6	D37.Ø5	D49.Ø
sinus — *see* Neoplasm, sinus						
skin	C44.3Ø1	C79.2	DØ4.39	D23.39	D48.5	D49.2
basal cell carcinoma	C44.311	—	—	—	—	—
specified type NEC	C44.391	—	—	—	—	—
squamous cell carcinoma	C44.321	—	—	—	—	—
turbinate (mucosa)	C3Ø.Ø	C78.39	DØ2.3	D14.Ø	D38.5	D49.1
bone	C41.Ø	C79.51	—	D16.4	D48.Ø	D49.2
vestibule	C3Ø.Ø	C78.39	DØ2.3	D14.Ø	D38.5	D49.1
Neoplasm, neoplastic — *continued*						
nostril	C3Ø.Ø	C78.39	DØ2.3	D14.Ø	D38.5	D49.1
nucleus pulposus	C41.2	C79.51	—	D16.6	D48.Ø	D49.2
occipital						
bone	C41.Ø	C79.51	—	D16.4	D48.Ø	D49.2
lobe or pole, brain	C71.4	C79.31	—	D33.Ø	D43.Ø	D49.6
odontogenic — *see* Neoplasm, jaw bone						
olfactory nerve or bulb	C72.2-☑	C79.49	—	D33.3	D43.3	D49.7
olive (brain)	C71.7	C79.31	—	D33.1	D43.1	D49.6
omentum	C48.1	C78.6	—	D2Ø.1	D48.4	D49.Ø
operculum (brain)	C71.Ø	C79.31	—	D33.Ø	D43.Ø	D49.6
optic nerve, chiasm, or tract	C72.3-☑	C79.49	—	D33.3	D43.3	D49.7
oral (cavity)	CØ6.9	C79.89	DØØ.ØØ	D1Ø.3Ø	D37.Ø9	D49.Ø
ill-defined	C14.8	C79.89	DØØ.ØØ	D1Ø.3Ø	D37.Ø9	D49.Ø
mucosa	CØ6.Ø	C79.89	DØØ.Ø2	D1Ø.39	D37.Ø9	D49.Ø
orbit	C69.6-☑	C79.49	DØ9.2-☑	D31.6-☑	D48.7	D49.89
autonomic nerve	C69.6-☑	C79.49	—	D31.6-☑	D48.7	D49.2
bone	C41.Ø	C79.51	—	D16.4	D48.Ø	D49.2
eye	C69.6-☑	C79.49	DØ9.2-☑	D31.6-☑	D48.7	D49.89
peripheral nerves	C69.6-☑	C79.49	—	D31.6-☑	D48.7	D49.2
soft parts	C69.6-☑	C79.49	DØ9.2-☑	D31.6-☑	D48.7	D49.89
organ of Zuckerkandl	C75.5	C79.89	—	D35.6	D44.7	D49.7
oropharynx	C1Ø.9	C79.89	DØØ.Ø8	D1Ø.5	D37.Ø5	D49.Ø
branchial cleft (vestige)	C1Ø.4	C79.89	DØØ.Ø8	D1Ø.5	D37.Ø5	D49.Ø
junctional region	C1Ø.8	C79.89	DØØ.Ø8	D1Ø.5	D37.Ø5	D49.Ø
lateral wall	C1Ø.2	C79.89	DØØ.Ø8	D1Ø.5	D37.Ø5	D49.Ø
overlapping lesion	C1Ø.8	—	—	—	—	—
pillars or fauces	CØ9.1	C79.89	DØØ.Ø8	D1Ø.5	D37.Ø5	D49.Ø
posterior wall	C1Ø.3	C79.89	DØØ.Ø8	D1Ø.5	D37.Ø5	D49.Ø
vallecula	C1Ø.Ø	C79.89	DØØ.Ø8	D1Ø.5	D37.Ø5	D49.Ø
os						
external	C53.1	C79.82	DØ6.1	D26.Ø	D39.Ø	D49.59
internal	C53.Ø	C79.82	DØ6.Ø	D26.Ø	D39.Ø	D49.59
ovary	C56.-☑	C79.6-☑	DØ7.39	D27.-☑	D39.1-☑	D49.59
oviduct	C57.Ø-☑	C79.82	DØ7.39	D28.2	D39.8	D49.59
palate	CØ5.9	C79.89	DØØ.ØØ	D1Ø.39	D37.Ø9	D49.Ø
hard	CØ5.Ø	C79.89	DØØ.Ø5	D1Ø.39	D37.Ø9	D49.Ø
junction of hard and soft palate	CØ5.9	C79.89	DØØ.ØØ	D1Ø.39	D37.Ø9	D49.Ø
overlapping lesions	CØ5.8	—	—	—	—	—
soft	CØ5.1	C79.89	DØØ.Ø4	D1Ø.39	D37.Ø9	D49.Ø
nasopharyngeal surface	C11.3	C79.89	DØØ.Ø8	D1Ø.6	D37.Ø5	D49.Ø
posterior surface	C11.3	C79.89	DØØ.Ø8	D1Ø.6	D37.Ø5	D49.Ø
superior surface	C11.3	C79.89	DØØ.Ø8	D1Ø.6	D37.Ø5	D49.Ø
palatoglossal arch	CØ9.1	C79.89	DØØ.ØØ	D1Ø.5	D37.Ø9	D49.Ø
palatopharyngeal arch	CØ9.1	C79.89	DØØ.ØØ	D1Ø.5	D37.Ø9	D49.Ø
pallium	C71.Ø	C79.31	—	D33.Ø	D43.Ø	D49.6
palpebra	C44.1Ø-☑	C79.2	DØ4.1-☑	D23.1-☑	D48.5	D49.2
basal cell carcinoma	C44.11-☑	—	—	—	—	—
sebaceous cell	C44.13-☑	—	—	—	—	—
specified type NEC	C44.19-☑	—	—	—	—	—
squamous cell carcinoma	C44.12-☑	—	—	—	—	—
pancreas	C25.9	C78.89	DØ1.7	D13.6	D37.8	D49.Ø
body	C25.1	C78.89	DØ1.7	D13.6	D37.8	D49.Ø
duct (of Santorini) (of Wirsung)	C25.3	C78.89	DØ1.7	D13.6	D37.8	D49.Ø
ectopic tissue	C25.7	C78.89	—	D13.6	D37.8	D49.Ø
head	C25.Ø	C78.89	DØ1.7	D13.6	D37.8	D49.Ø
islet cells	C25.4	C78.89	DØ1.7	D13.7	D37.8	D49.Ø
neck	C25.7	C78.89	DØ1.7	D13.6	D37.8	D49.Ø
overlapping lesion	C25.8	—	—	—	—	—
tail	C25.2	C78.89	DØ1.7	D13.6	D37.8	D49.Ø

Neoplasm, neoplastic — *continued*	Malignant Primary	Malignant Secondary	Ca in situ	Benign	Uncertain Behavior	Unspecified Behavior
para-aortic body	C75.5	C79.89	—	D35.6	D44.7	D49.7
paraganglion NEC	C75.5	C79.89	—	D35.6	D44.7	D49.7
parametrium	C57.3	C79.82	—	D28.2	D39.8	D49.59
paranephric	C48.Ø	C78.6	—	D2Ø.Ø	D48.3	D49.Ø
pararectal	C76.3	C79.89	—	D36.7	D48.7	D49.89
parasagittal (region)	C76.Ø	C79.89	DØ9.8	D36.7	D48.7	D49.89
parasellar	C72.9	C79.49	—	D33.9	D43.8	D49.7
parathyroid (gland)	C75.Ø	C79.89	DØ9.3	D35.1	D44.2	D49.7
paraurethral	C76.3	C79.89	—	D36.7	D48.7	D49.89
gland	C68.1	C79.19	DØ9.19	D3Ø.8	D41.8	D49.59
paravaginal	C76.3	C79.89	—	D36.7	D48.7	D49.89
parenchyma, kidney	C64.-☑	C79.Ø-☑	DØ9.19	D3Ø.Ø-☑	D41.Ø-☑	D49.51-☑
parietal						
bone	C41.Ø	C79.51	—	D16.4	D48.Ø	D49.2
lobe, brain	C71.3	C79.31	—	D33.Ø	D43.Ø	D49.6
paroophoron	C57.1-☑	C79.82	DØ7.39	D28.2	D39.8	D49.59
parotid (duct) (gland)	CØ7	C79.89	DØØ.ØØ	D11.Ø	D37.Ø3Ø	D49.Ø
parovarium	C57.1-☑	C79.82	DØ7.39	D28.2	D39.8	D49.59
patella	C4Ø.2Ø	C79.51	—	—	—	—
peduncle, cerebral	C71.7	C79.31	—	D33.1	D43.1	D49.6
pelvirectal junction	C19	C78.5	DØ1.1	D12.7	D37.5	D49.Ø
pelvis, pelvic	C76.3	C79.89	DØ9.8	D36.7	D48.7	D49.89
bone	C41.4	C79.51	—	D16.8	D48.Ø	D49.2
floor	C76.3	C79.89	DØ9.8	D36.7	D48.7	D49.89
renal	C65.-☑	C79.Ø-☑	DØ9.19	D3Ø.1-☑	D41.1-☑	D49.51-☑
viscera	C76.3	C79.89	DØ9.8	D36.7	D48.7	D49.89
wall	C76.3	C79.89	DØ9.8	D36.7	D48.7	D49.89
pelvo-abdominal	C76.8	C79.89	DØ9.8	D36.7	D48.7	D49.89
penis	C6Ø.9	C79.82	DØ7.4	D29.Ø	D4Ø.8	D49.59
body	C6Ø.2	C79.82	DØ7.4	D29.Ø	D4Ø.8	D49.59
corpus (cavernosum)	C6Ø.2	C79.82	DØ7.4	D29.Ø	D4Ø.8	D49.59
glans	C6Ø.1	C79.82	DØ7.4	D29.Ø	D4Ø.8	D49.59
overlapping sites	C6Ø.8	—	—	—	—	—
skin NEC	C6Ø.9	C79.82	DØ7.4	D29.Ø	D4Ø.8	D49.59
periadrenal (tissue)	C48.Ø	C78.6	—	D2Ø.Ø	D48.3	D49.Ø
perianal (skin) — *see also* Neoplasm, anus, skin	C44.5ØØ	C79.2	DØ4.5	D23.5	D48.5	D49.2
pericardium	C38.Ø	C79.89	—	D15.1	D48.7	D49.89
perinephric	C48.Ø	C78.6	—	D2Ø.Ø	D48.3	D49.Ø
perineum	C76.3	C79.89	DØ9.8	D36.7	D48.7	D49.89
periodontal tissue NEC	CØ3.9	C79.89	DØØ.Ø3	D1Ø.39	D37.Ø9	D49.Ø
periosteum — *see* Neoplasm, bone						
peripancreatic	C48.Ø	C78.6	—	D2Ø.Ø	D48.3	D49.Ø
peripheral nerve NEC	C47.9	C79.89	—	D36.1Ø	D48.2	D49.2
perirectal (tissue)	C76.3	C79.89	—	D36.7	D48.7	D49.89
perirenal (tissue)	C48.Ø	C78.6	—	D2Ø.Ø	D48.3	D49.Ø
peritoneum, peritoneal (cavity)	C48.2	C78.6	—	D2Ø.1	D48.4	D49.Ø
benign mesothelial tissue — *see* Mesothelioma, benign						
overlapping lesion	C48.8	—	—	—	—	—
with digestive organs	C26.9	—	—	—	—	—
parietal	C48.1	C78.6	—	D2Ø.1	D48.4	D49.Ø
pelvic	C48.1	C78.6	—	D2Ø.1	D48.4	D49.Ø
specified part NEC	C48.1	C78.6	—	D2Ø.1	D48.4	D49.Ø
peritonsillar (tissue)	C76.Ø	C79.89	DØ9.8	D36.7	D48.7	D49.89
periurethral tissue	C76.3	C79.89	—	D36.7	D48.7	D49.89
phalanges						
foot	C4Ø.3-☑	C79.51	—	D16.3-☑	—	—
hand	C4Ø.1-☑	C79.51	—	D16.1-☑	—	—
pharynx, pharyngeal	C14.Ø	C79.89	DØØ.Ø8	D1Ø.9	D37.Ø5	D49.Ø
bursa	C11.1	C79.89	DØØ.Ø8	D1Ø.6	D37.Ø5	D49.Ø

Neoplasm, neoplastic — *continued*	Malignant Primary	Malignant Secondary	Ca in situ	Benign	Uncertain Behavior	Unspecified Behavior
pharynx, pharyngeal — *continued*						
fornix	C11.3	C79.89	DØØ.Ø8	D1Ø.6	D37.Ø5	D49.Ø
recess	C11.2	C79.89	DØØ.Ø8	D1Ø.6	D37.Ø5	D49.Ø
region	C14.Ø	C79.89	DØØ.Ø8	D1Ø.9	D37.Ø5	D49.Ø
tonsil	C11.1	C79.89	DØØ.Ø8	D1Ø.6	D37.Ø5	D49.Ø
wall (lateral) (posterior)	C14.Ø	C79.89	DØØ.Ø8	D1Ø.9	D37.Ø5	D49.Ø
pia mater	C7Ø.9	C79.4Ø	—	D32.9	D42.9	D49.7
cerebral	C7Ø.Ø	C79.32	—	D32.Ø	D42.Ø	D49.7
cranial	C7Ø.Ø	C79.32	—	D32.Ø	D42.Ø	D49.7
spinal	C7Ø.1	C79.49	—	D32.1	D42.1	D49.7
pillars of fauces	CØ9.1	C79.89	DØØ.Ø8	D1Ø.5	D37.Ø5	D49.Ø
pineal (body) (gland)	C75.3	C79.89	DØ9.3	D35.4	D44.5	D49.7
pinna (ear) NEC — *see also* Neoplasm, skin, ear	C44.2Ø-☑	C79.2	DØ4.2-☑	D23.2-☑	D48.5	D49.2
piriform fossa or sinus	C12	C79.89	DØØ.Ø8	D1Ø.7	D37.Ø5	D49.Ø
pituitary (body) (fossa) (gland) (lobe)	C75.1	C79.89	DØ9.3	D35.2	D44.3	D49.7
placenta	C58	C79.82	DØ7.Ø	D26.7	D39.2	D49.59
pleura, pleural (cavity)	C38.4	C78.2	—	D19.Ø	D38.2	D49.1
overlapping lesion with heart or mediastinum	C38.8	—	—	—	—	—
parietal	C38.4	C78.2	—	D19.Ø	D38.2	D49.1
visceral	C38.4	C78.2	—	D19.Ø	D38.2	D49.1
plexus						
brachial	C47.1-☑	C79.89	—	D36.12	D48.2	D49.2
cervical	C47.Ø	C79.89	—	D36.11	D48.2	D49.2
choroid	C71.5	C79.31	—	D33.Ø	D43.Ø	D49.6
lumbosacral	C47.5	C79.89	—	D36.16	D48.2	D49.2
sacral	C47.5	C79.89	—	D36.16	D48.2	D49.2
pluriendocrine	C75.8	C79.89	DØ9.3	D35.7	D44.9	D49.7
pole						
frontal	C71.1	C79.31	—	D33.Ø	D43.Ø	D49.6
occipital	C71.4	C79.31	—	D33.Ø	D43.Ø	D49.6
pons (varolii)	C71.7	C79.31	—	D33.1	D43.1	D49.6
popliteal fossa or space	C76.5-☑	C79.89	DØ4.7-☑	D36.7	D48.7	D49.89
postcricoid (region)	C13.Ø	C79.89	DØØ.Ø8	D1Ø.7	D37.Ø5	D49.Ø
posterior fossa (cranial)	C71.9	C79.31	—	D33.2	D43.2	D49.6
postnasal space	C11.9	C79.89	DØØ.Ø8	D1Ø.6	D37.Ø5	D49.Ø
prepuce	C6Ø.Ø	C79.82	DØ7.4	D29.Ø	D4Ø.8	D49.59
prepylorus	C16.4	C78.89	DØØ.2	D13.1	D37.1	D49.Ø
presacral (region)	C76.3	C79.89	—	D36.7	D48.7	D49.89
prostate (gland)	C61	C79.82	DØ7.5	D29.1	D4Ø.Ø	D49.59
utricle	C68.Ø	C79.19	DØ9.19	D3Ø.4	D41.3	D49.59
pterygoid fossa	C49.Ø	C79.89	—	D21.Ø	D48.1	D49.2
pubic bone	C41.4	C79.51	—	D16.8	D48.Ø	D49.2
pudenda, pudendum (femaie)	C51.9	C79.82	DØ7.1	D28.Ø	D39.8	D49.59
pulmonary — *see also* Neoplasm, lung	C34.9-☑	C78.Ø-☑	DØ2.2-☑	D14.3-☑	D38.1	D49.1
putamen	C71.Ø	C79.31	—	D33.Ø	D43.Ø	D49.6
pyloric						
antrum	C16.3	C78.89	DØØ.2	D13.1	D37.1	D49.Ø
canal	C16.4	C78.89	DØØ.2	D13.1	D37.1	D49.Ø
pylorus	C16.4	C78.89	DØØ.2	D13.1	D37.1	D49.Ø
pyramid (brain)	C71.7	C79.31	—	D33.1	D43.1	D49.6
pyriform fossa or sinus	C12	C79.89	DØØ.Ø8	D1Ø.7	D37.Ø5	D49.Ø
radius (any part)	C4Ø.Ø-☑	C79.51	—	D16.Ø-☑	—	—
Rathke's pouch	C75.1	C79.89	DØ9.3	D35.2	D44.3	D49.7
rectosigmoid (junction)	C19	C78.5	DØ1.1	D12.7	D37.5	D49.Ø
overlapping lesion with anus or rectum	C21.8	—	—	—	—	—
rectouterine pouch	C48.1	C78.6	—	D2Ø.1	D48.4	D49.Ø
rectovaginal septum or wall	C76.3	C79.89	DØ9.8	D36.7	D48.7	D49.89
rectovesical septum	C76.3	C79.89	DØ9.8	D36.7	D48.7	D49.89
rectum (ampulla)	C2Ø	C78.5	DØ1.2	D12.8	D37.5	D49.Ø

☑ **Additional Character Required — Refer to the Tabular List for Character Selection**

	Malignant Primary	Malignant Secondary	Ca in situ	Benign	Uncertain Behavior	Unspecified Behavior
Neoplasm, neoplastic — *continued*						
rectum — *continued*						
and colon	C19	C78.5	DØ1.1	D12.7	D37.5	D49.Ø
overlapping lesion with anus or rectosigmoid junction	C21.8	—	—	—	—	—
renal	C64.-☑	C79.Ø-☑	DØ9.19	D3Ø.Ø-☑	D41.Ø-☑	D49.51-☑
calyx	C65.-☑	C79.Ø-☑	DØ9.19	D3Ø.1-☑	D41.1-☑	D49.51-☑
hilus	C65.-☑	C79.Ø-☑	DØ9.19	D3Ø.1-☑	D41.1-☑	D49.51-☑
parenchyma	C64.-☑	C79.Ø-☑	DØ9.19	D3Ø.Ø-☑	D41.Ø-☑	D49.51-☑
pelvis	C65.-☑	C79.Ø-☑	DØ9.19	D3Ø.1-☑	D41.1-☑	D49.51-☑
respiratory						
organs or system NEC	C39.9	C78.3Ø	DØ2.4	D14.4	D38.6	D49.1
tract NEC	C39.9	C78.3Ø	DØ2.4	D14.4	D38.5	D49.1
upper	C39.Ø	C78.3Ø	DØ2.4	D14.4	D38.5	D49.1
retina	C69.2-☑	C79.49	DØ9.2-☑	D31.2-☑	D48.7	D49.81
retrobulbar	C69.6-☑	C79.49	—	D31.6-☑	D48.7	D49.89
retrocecal	C48.Ø	C78.6	—	D2Ø.Ø	D48.3	D49.Ø
retromolar (area) (triangle) (trigone)	CØ6.2	C79.89	DØØ.ØØ	D1Ø.39	D37.Ø9	D49.Ø
retro-orbital	C76.Ø	C79.89	DØ9.8	D36.7	D48.7	D49.89
retroperitoneal (space) (tissue)	C48.Ø	C78.6	—	D2Ø.Ø	D48.3	D49.Ø
retroperitoneum	C48.Ø	C78.6	—	D2Ø.Ø	D48.3	D49.Ø
retropharyngeal	C14.Ø	C79.89	DØØ.Ø8	D1Ø.9	D37.Ø5	D49.Ø
retrovesical (septum)	C76.3	C79.89	DØ9.8	D36.7	D48.7	D49.89
rhinencephalon	C71.Ø	C79.31	—	D33.Ø	D43.Ø	D49.6
rib	C41.3	C79.51	—	D16.7	D48.Ø	D49.2
Rosenmuller's fossa	C11.2	C79.89	DØØ.Ø8	D1Ø.6	D37.Ø5	D49.Ø
round ligament	C57.2-☑	C79.82	—	D28.2	D39.8	D49.59
sacrococcyx, sacrococcygeal	C41.4	C79.51	—	D16.8	D48.Ø	D49.2
region	C76.3	C79.89	DØ9.8	D36.7	D48.7	D49.89
sacrouterine ligament	C57.3	C79.82	—	D28.2	D39.8	D49.59
sacrum, sacral (vertebra)	C41.4	C79.51	—	D16.8	D48.Ø	D49.2
salivary gland or duct (major)	CØ8.9	C79.89	DØØ.ØØ	D11.9	D37.Ø39	D49.Ø
minor NEC	CØ6.9	C79.89	DØØ.ØØ	D1Ø.39	D37.Ø4	D49.Ø
overlapping lesion	CØ8.9	—	—	—	—	—
parotid	CØ7	C79.89	DØØ.ØØ	D11.Ø	D37.Ø3Ø	D49.Ø
pluriglandular	CØ8.9	C79.89	DØØ.ØØ	D11.9	D37.Ø39	D49.Ø
sublingual	CØ8.1	C79.89	DØØ.ØØ	D11.7	D37.Ø31	D49.Ø
submandibular	CØ8.Ø	C79.89	DØØ.ØØ	D11.7	D37.Ø32	D49.Ø
submaxillary	CØ8.Ø	C79.89	DØØ.ØØ	D11.7	D37.Ø32	D49.Ø
salpinx (uterine)	C57.Ø-☑	C79.82	DØ7.39	D28.2	D39.8	D49.59
Santorini's duct	C25.3	C78.89	DØ1.7	D13.6	D37.8	D49.Ø
scalp	C44.4Ø	C79.2	DØ4.4	D23.4	D48.5	D49.2
basal cell carcinoma	C44.41	—	—	—	—	—
specified type NEC	C44.49	—	—	—	—	—
squamous cell carcinoma	C44.42	—	—	—	—	—
scapula (any part)	C4Ø.Ø-☑	C79.51	—	D16.Ø-☑	—	—
scapular region	C76.1	C79.89	DØ9.8	D36.7	D48.7	D49.89
scar NEC — *see also* Neoplasm, skin, by site	C44.9Ø	C79.2	DØ4.9	D23.9	D48.5	D49.2
sciatic nerve	C47.2-☑	C79.89	—	D36.13	D48.2	D49.2
sclera	C69.4-☑	C79.49	DØ9.2-☑	D31.4-☑	D48.7	D49.89
scrotum (skin)	C63.2	C79.82	DØ7.61	D29.4	D4Ø.8	D49.59
sebaceous gland — *see* Neoplasm, skin						
sella turcica	C75.1	C79.89	DØ9.3	D35.2	D44.3	D49.7
bone	C41.Ø	C79.51	—	D16.4	D48.Ø	D49.2
semilunar cartilage (knee)	C4Ø.2-☑	C79.51	—	D16.2-☑	D48.Ø	D49.2
seminal vesicle	C63.7	C79.82	DØ7.69	D29.8	D4Ø.8	D49.59
septum						
nasal	C3Ø.Ø	C78.39	DØ2.3	D14.Ø	D38.5	D49.1
posterior margin	C11.3	C79.89	DØØ.Ø8	D1Ø.6	D37.Ø5	D49.Ø
rectovaginal	C76.3	C79.89	DØ9.8	D36.7	D48.7	D49.89
rectovesical	C76.3	C79.89	DØ9.8	D36.7	D48.7	D49.89

	Malignant Primary	Malignant Secondary	Ca in situ	Benign	Uncertain Behavior	Unspecified Behavior
Neoplasm, neoplastic — *continued*						
septum — *continued*						
urethrovaginal	C57.9	C79.82	DØ7.3Ø	D28.9	D39.9	D49.59
vesicovaginal	C57.9	C79.82	DØ7.3Ø	D28.9	D39.9	D49.59
shoulder NEC	C76.4-☑	C79.89	DØ4.6-☑	D36.7	D48.7	D49.89
sigmoid flexure (lower) (upper)	C18.7	C78.5	DØ1.Ø	D12.5	D37.4	D49.Ø
sinus (accessory)	C31.9	C78.39	DØ2.3	D14.Ø	D38.5	D49.1
bone (any)	C41.Ø	C79.51	—	D16.4	D48.Ø	D49.2
ethmoidal	C31.1	C78.39	DØ2.3	D14.Ø	D38.5	D49.1
frontal	C31.2	C78.39	DØ2.3	D14.Ø	D38.5	D49.1
maxillary	C31.Ø	C78.39	DØ2.3	D14.Ø	D38.5	D49.1
nasal, paranasal NEC	C31.9	C78.39	DØ2.3	D14.Ø	D38.5	D49.1
overlapping lesion	C31.8	—	—	—	—	—
pyriform	C12	C79.89	DØØ.Ø8	D1Ø.7	D37.Ø5	D49.Ø
sphenoid	C31.3	C78.39	DØ2.3	D14.Ø	D38.5	D49.1
skeleton, skeletal NEC	C41.9	C79.51	—	D16.9	D48.Ø	D49.2
Skene's gland	C68.1	C79.19	DØ9.19	D3Ø.8	D41.8	D49.59
skin NOS	C44.9Ø	C79.2	DØ4.9	D23.9	D48.5	D49.2
abdominal wall	C44.5Ø9	C79.2	DØ4.5	D23.5	D48.5	D49.2
basal cell carcinoma	C44.519	—	—	—	—	—
specified type NEC	C44.599	—	—	—	—	—
squamous cell carcinoma	C44.529	—	—	—	—	—
ala nasi — *see also* Neoplasm, nose, skin	C44.3Ø1	C79.2	DØ4.39	D23.39	D48.5	D49.2
ankle — *see also* Neoplasm, skin, limb, lower	C44.7Ø-☑	C79.2	DØ4.7-☑	D23.7-☑	D48.5	D49.2
antecubital space — *see also* Neoplasm, skin, limb, upper	C44.6Ø-☑	C79.2	DØ4.6-☑	D23.6-☑	D48.5	D49.2
anus	C44.5ØØ	C79.2	DØ4.5	D23.5	D48.5	D49.2
basal cell carcinoma	C44.51Ø	—	—	—	—	—
specified type NEC	C44.59Ø	—	—	—	—	—
squamous cell carcinoma	C44.52Ø	—	—	—	—	—
arm — *see also* Neoplasm, skin, limb, upper	C44.6Ø-☑	C79.2	DØ4.6-☑	D23.6-☑	D48.5	D49.2
auditory canal (external) — *see also* Neoplasm, skin, ear	C44.2Ø-☑	C79.2	DØ4.2-☑	D23.2-☑	D48.5	D49.2
auricle (ear) — *see also* Neoplasm, skin, ear	C44.2Ø-☑	C79.2	DØ4.2-☑	D23.2-☑	D48.5	D49.2
auricular canal (external) — *see also* Neoplasm, skin, ear	C44.2Ø-☑	C79.2	DØ4.2-☑	D23.2-☑	D48.5	D49.2
axilla, axillary fold — *see also* Neoplasm, skin, trunk	C44.5Ø9	C79.2	DØ4.5	D23.5	D48.5	D49.2
back — *see also* Neoplasm, skin, trunk	C44.5Ø9	C79.2	DØ4.5	D23.5	D48.5	D49.2
basal cell carcinoma	C44.91	—	—	—	—	—
breast	C44.5Ø1	C79.2	DØ4.5	D23.5	D48.5	D49.2
basal cell carcinoma	C44.511	—	—	—	—	—
specified type NEC	C44.591	—	—	—	—	—
squamous cell carcinoma	C44.521	—	—	—	—	—
brow — *see also* Neoplasm, skin, face	C44.3Ø9	C79.2	DØ4.39	D23.39	D48.5	D49.2
buttock — *see also* Neoplasm, skin, trunk	C44.5Ø9	C79.2	DØ4.5	D23.5	D48.5	D49.2

Neoplasm, neoplastic	Malignant Primary	Malignant Secondary	Ca in situ	Benign	Uncertain Behavior	Unspecified Behavior
Neoplasm, neoplastic — *continued*						
skin — *continued*						
calf — *see also* Neoplasm, skin, limb, lower	C44.7Ø-☑	C79.2	DØ4.7-☑	D23.7-☑	D48.5	D49.2
canthus (eye) (inner) (outer)	C44.1Ø-☑	C79.2	DØ4.1-☑	D23.1-☑	D48.5	D49.2
basal cell carcinoma	C44.11-☑	—	—	—	—	—
sebaceous cell	C44.13-☑	—	—	—	—	—
specified type NEC	C44.19-☑	—	—	—	—	—
squamous cell carcinoma	C44.12-☑	—	—	—	—	—
cervical region — *see also* Neoplasm, skin, neck	C44.4Ø	C79.2	DØ4.4	D23.4	D48.5	D49.2
cheek (external) — *see also* Neoplasm, skin, face	C44.3Ø9	C79.2	DØ4.39	D23.39	D48.5	D49.2
chest (wall) — *see also* Neoplasm, skin, trunk	C44.5Ø9	C79.2	DØ4.5	D23.5	D48.5	D49.2
chin — *see also* Neoplasm, skin, face	C44.3Ø9	C79.2	DØ4.39	D23.39	D48.5	D49.2
clavicular area — *see also* Neoplasm, skin, trunk	C44.5Ø9	C79.2	DØ4.5	D23.5	D48.5	D49.2
clitoris	C51.2	C79.82	DØ7.1	D28.Ø	D39.8	D49.59
columnella — *see also* Neoplasm, skin, face	C44.3Ø9	C79.2	DØ4.39	D23.39	D48.5	D49.2
concha — *see also* Neoplasm, skin, ear	C44.2Ø-☑	C79.2	DØ4.2-☑	D23.2-☑	D48.5	D49.2
ear (external)	C44.2Ø-☑	C79.2	DØ4.2-☑	D23.2-☑	D48.5	D49.2
basal cell carcinoma	C44.21-☑	—	—	—	—	—
specified type NEC	C44.29-☑	—	—	—	—	—
squamous cell carcinoma	C44.22-☑	—	—	—	—	—
elbow — *see also* Neoplasm, skin, limb, upper	C44.6Ø-☑	C79.2	DØ4.6-☑	D23.6-☑	D48.5	D49.2
eyebrow — *see also* Neoplasm, skin, face	C44.3Ø9	C79.2	DØ4.39	D23.39	D48.5	D49.2
eyelid	C44.1Ø-☑	C79.2	DØ4.1-☑	D23.1-☑	D48.5	D49.2
basal cell carcinoma	C44.11-☑	—	—	—	—	—
sebaceous cell	C44.13-☑	—	—	—	—	—
specified type NEC	C44.19-☑	—	—	—	—	—
squamous cell carcinoma	C44.12-☑	—	—	—	—	—
face NOS	C44.3ØØ	C79.2	DØ4.3Ø	D23.3Ø	D48.5	D49.2
basal cell carcinoma	C44.31Ø	—	—	—	—	—
specified type NEC	C44.39Ø	—	—	—	—	—
squamous cell carcinoma	C44.32Ø	—	—	—	—	—
female genital organs (external)	C51.9	C79.82	DØ7.1	D28.Ø	D39.8	D49.59
clitoris	C51.2	C79.82	DØ7.1	D28.Ø	D39.8	D49.59
labium NEC	C51.9	C79.82	DØ7.1	D28.Ø	D39.8	D49.59
majus	C51.Ø	C79.82	DØ7.1	D28.Ø	D39.8	D49.59
minus	C51.1	C79.82	DØ7.1	D28.Ø	D39.8	D49.59
pudendum	C51.9	C79.82	DØ7.1	D28.Ø	D39.8	D49.59
vulva	C51.9	C79.82	DØ7.1	D28.Ø	D39.8	D49.59
finger — *see also* Neoplasm, skin, limb, upper	C44.6Ø-☑	C79.2	DØ4.6-☑	D23.6-☑	D48.5	D49.2
flank — *see also* Neoplasm, skin, trunk	C44.5Ø9	C79.2	DØ4.5	D23.5	D48.5	D49.2
foot — *see also* Neoplasm, skin, limb, lower	C44.7Ø-☑	C79.2	DØ4.7-☑	D23.7-☑	D48.5	D49.2
Neoplasm, neoplastic — *continued*						
skin — *continued*						
forearm — *see also* Neoplasm, skin, limb, upper	C44.6Ø-☑	C79.2	DØ4.6-☑	D23.6-☑	D48.5	D49.2
forehead — *see also* Neoplasm, skin, face	C44.3Ø9	C79.2	DØ4.39	D23.39	D48.5	D49.2
glabella — *see also* Neoplasm, skin, face	C44.3Ø9	C79.2	DØ4.39	D23.39	D48.5	D49.2
gluteal region — *see also* Neoplasm, skin, trunk	C44.5Ø9	C79.2	DØ4.5	D23.5	D48.5	D49.2
groin — *see also* Neoplasm, skin, trunk	C44.5Ø9	C79.2	DØ4.5	D23.5	D48.5	D49.2
hand — *see also* Neoplasm, skin, limb, upper	C44.6Ø-☑	C79.2	DØ4.6-☑	D23.6-☑	D48.5	D49.2
head NEC — *see also* Neoplasm, skin, scalp	C44.4Ø	C79.2	DØ4.4	D23.4	D48.5	D49.2
heel — *see also* Neoplasm, skin, limb, lower	C44.7Ø-☑	C79.2	DØ4.7-☑	D23.7-☑	D48.5	D49.2
helix — *see also* Neoplasm, skin, ear	C44.2Ø-☑	C79.2	DØ4.2-☑	D23.2-☑	D48.5	D49.2
hip — *see also* Neoplasm, skin, limb, lower	C44.7Ø-☑	C79.2	DØ4.7-☑	D23.7-☑	D48.5	D49.2
infraclavicular region — *see also* Neoplasm, skin, trunk	C44.5Ø9	C79.2	DØ4.5	D23.5	D48.5	D49.2
inguinal region — *see also* Neoplasm, skin, trunk	C44.5Ø9	C79.2	DØ4.5	D23.5	D48.5	D49.2
jaw — *see also* Neoplasm, skin, face	C44.3Ø9	C79.2	DØ4.39	D23.39	D48.5	D49.2
Kaposi's sarcoma — *see* Kaposi's, sarcoma, skin						
knee — *see also* Neoplasm, skin, limb, lower	C44.7Ø-☑	C79.2	DØ4.7-☑	D23.7-☑	D48.5	D49.2
labia						
majora	C51.Ø	C79.82	DØ7.1	D28.Ø	D39.8	D49.59
minora	C51.1	C79.82	DØ7.1	D28.Ø	D39.8	D49.59
leg — *see also* Neoplasm, skin, limb, lower	C44.7Ø-☑	C79.2	DØ4.7-☑	D23.7-☑	D48.5	D49.2
lid (lower) (upper)	C44.1Ø-☑	C79.2	DØ4.1-☑	D23.1-☑	D48.5	D49.2
basal cell carcinoma	C44.11-☑	—	—	—	—	—
sebaceous cell	C44.13-☑	—	—	—	—	—
specified type NEC	C44.19-☑	—	—	—	—	—
squamous cell carcinoma	C44.12-☑	—	—	—	—	—
limb NEC	C44.9Ø	C79.2	DØ4.9	D23.9	D48.5	D49.2
basal cell carcinoma	C44.91	—	—	—	—	—
lower	C44.7Ø-☑	C79.2	DØ4.7-☑	D23.7-☑	D48.5	D49.2
basal cell carcinoma	C44.71-☑	—	—	—	—	—
specified type NEC	C44.79-☑	—	—	—	—	—
squamous cell carcinoma	C44.72-☑	—	—	—	—	—
upper	C44.6Ø-☑	C79.2	DØ4.6-☑	D23.6-☑	D48.5	D49.2
basal cell carcinoma	C44.61-☑	—	—	—	—	—
specified type NEC	C44.69-☑	—	—	—	—	—
squamous cell carcinoma	C44.62-☑	—	—	—	—	—
lip (lower) (upper)	C44.ØØ	C79.2	DØ4.Ø	D23.Ø	D48.5	D49.2

	Malignant Primary	Malignant Secondary	Ca in situ	Benign	Uncertain Behavior	Unspecified Behavior
Neoplasm, neoplastic — *continued*						
skin — *continued*						
lip — *continued*						
basal cell carcinoma	C44.01	—	—	—	—	—
specified type NEC	C44.09	—	—	—	—	—
squamous cell carcinoma	C44.02	—	—	—	—	—
male genital organs	C63.9	C79.82	D07.60	D29.9	D40.8	D49.59
penis	C60.9	C79.82	D07.4	D29.0	D40.8	D49.59
prepuce	C60.0	C79.82	D07.4	D29.0	D40.8	D49.59
scrotum	C63.2	C79.82	D07.61	D29.4	D40.8	D49.59
mastectomy site (skin) — *see also* Neoplasm, skin, breast	C44.501	C79.2	—	—	—	—
specified as breast tissue	C50.8-☑	C79.81	—	—	—	—
meatus, acoustic (external) — *see also* Neoplasm, skin, ear	C44.20-☑	C79.2	D04.2-☑	D23.2-☑	D48.5	D49.2
melanotic — *see* Melanoma						
Merkel cell — *see* Carcinoma, Merkel cell						
nates — *see also* Neoplasm, skin, trunk	C44.509	C79.2	D04.5	D23.5	D48.5	D49.2
neck	C44.40	C79.2	D04.4	D23.4	D48.5	D49.2
basal cell carcinoma	C44.41	—	—	—	—	—
specified type NEC	C44.49	—	—	—	—	—
squamous cell carcinoma	C44.42	—	—	—	—	—
nevus — *see* Nevus, skin						
nose (external) — *see also* Neoplasm, nose, skin	C44.301	C79.2	D04.39	D23.39	D48.5	D49.2
overlapping lesion	C44.80	—	—	—	—	—
basal cell carcinoma	C44.81	—	—	—	—	—
specified type NEC	C44.89	—	—	—	—	—
squamous cell carcinoma	C44.82	—	—	—	—	—
palm — *see also* Neoplasm, skin, limb, upper	C44.60-☑	C79.2	D04.6-☑	D23.6-☑	D48.5	D49.2
palpebra	C44.10-☑	C79.2	D04.1-☑	D23.1-☑	D48.5	D49.2
basal cell carcinoma	C44.11-☑	—	—	—	—	—
sebaceous cell	C44.13-☑	—	—	—	—	—
specified type NEC	C44.19-☑	—	—	—	—	—
squamous cell carcinoma	C44.12-☑	—	—	—	—	—
penis NEC	C60.9	C79.82	D07.4	D29.0	D40.8	D49.59
perianal — *see also* Neoplasm, skin, anus	C44.500	C79.2	D04.5	D23.5	D48.5	D49.2
perineum — *see also* Neoplasm, skin, anus	C44.500	C79.2	D04.5	D23.5	D48.5	D49.2
pinna — *see also* Neoplasm, skin, ear	C44.20-☑	C79.2	D04.2-☑	D23.2-☑	D48.5	D49.2
plantar — *see also* Neoplasm, skin, limb, lower	C44.70-☑	C79.2	D04.7-☑	D23.7-☑	D48.5	D49.2
popliteal fossa or space — *see also* Neoplasm, skin, limb, lower	C44.70-☑	C79.2	D04.7-☑	D23.7-☑	D48.5	D49.2
prepuce	C60.0	C79.82	D07.4	D29.0	D40.8	D49.59
Neoplasm, neoplastic — *continued*						
skin — *continued*						
pubes — *see also* Neoplasm, skin, trunk	C44.509	C79.2	D04.5	D23.5	D48.5	D49.2
sacrococcygeal region — *see also* Neoplasm, skin, trunk	C44.509	C79.2	D04.5	D23.5	D48.5	D49.2
scalp	C44.40	C79.2	D04.4	D23.4	D48.5	D49.2
basal cell carcinoma	C44.41	—	—	—	—	—
specified type NEC	C44.49	—	—	—	—	—
squamous cell carcinoma	C44.42	—	—	—	—	—
scapular region — *see also* Neoplasm, skin, trunk	C44.509	C79.2	D04.5	D23.5	D48.5	D49.2
scrotum	C63.2	C79.82	D07.61	D29.4	D40.8	D49.59
shoulder — *see also* Neoplasm, skin, limb, upper	C44.60-☑	C79.2	D04.6-☑	D23.6-☑	D48.5	D49.2
sole (foot) — *see also* Neoplasm, skin, limb, lower	C44.70-☑	C79.2	D04.7-☑	D23.7-☑	D48.5	D49.2
specified sites NEC	C44.80	C79.2	D04.8	D23.9	D48.5	D49.2
basal cell carcinoma	C44.81	—	—	—	—	—
specified type NEC	C44.89	—	—	—	—	—
squamous cell carcinoma	C44.82	—	—	—	—	—
specified type NEC	C44.99	—	—	—	—	—
squamous cell carcinoma	C44.92	—	—	—	—	—
submammary fold — *see also* Neoplasm, skin, trunk	C44.509	C79.2	D04.5	D23.5	D48.5	D49.2
supraclavicular region — *see also* Neoplasm, skin, neck	C44.40	C79.2	D04.4	D23.4	D48.5	D49.2
temple — *see also* Neoplasm, skin, face	C44.309	C79.2	D04.39	D23.39	D48.5	D49.2
thigh — *see also* Neoplasm, skin, limb, lower	C44.70-☑	C79.2	D04.7-☑	D23.7-☑	D48.5	D49.2
thoracic wall — *see also* Neoplasm, skin, trunk	C44.509	C79.2	D04.5	D23.5	D48.5	D49.2
thumb — *see also* Neoplasm, skin, limb, upper	C44.60-☑	C79.2	D04.6-☑	D23.6-☑	D48.5	D49.2
toe — *see also* Neoplasm, skin, limb, lower	C44.70-☑	C79.2	D04.7-☑	D23.7-☑	D48.5	D49.2
tragus — *see also* Neoplasm, skin, ear	C44.20-☑	C79.2	D04.2-☑	D23.2-☑	D48.5	D49.2
trunk	C44.509	C79.2	D04.5	D23.5	D48.5	D49.2
basal cell carcinoma	C44.519	—	—	—	—	—
specified type NEC	C44.599	—	—	—	—	—
squamous cell carcinoma	C44.529	—	—	—	—	—
umbilicus — *see also* Neoplasm, skin, trunk	C44.509	C79.2	D04.5	D23.5	D48.5	D49.2
vulva	C51.9	C79.82	D07.1	D28.0	D39.8	D49.59
overlapping lesion	C51.8	—	—	—	—	—
wrist — *see also* Neoplasm, skin, limb, upper	C44.60-☑	C79.2	D04.6-☑	D23.6-☑	D48.5	D49.2
skull	C41.0	C79.51	—	D16.4	D48.0	D49.2

	Malignant Primary	Malignant Secondary	Ca in situ	Benign	Uncertain Behavior	Unspecified Behavior
Neoplasm, neoplastic — *continued*						
soft parts or tissues — *see* Neoplasm, connective tissue						
specified site NEC	C76.8	C79.89	DØ9.8	D36.7	D48.7	D49.89
spermatic cord	C63.1-☑	C79.82	DØ7.69	D29.8	D4Ø.8	D49.59
sphenoid	C31.3	C78.39	DØ2.3	D14.Ø	D38.5	D49.1
bone	C41.Ø	C79.51	—	D16.4	D48.Ø	D49.2
sinus	C31.3	C78.39	DØ2.3	D14.Ø	D38.5	D49.1
sphincter						
anal	C21.1	C78.5	DØ1.3	D12.9	D37.8	D49.Ø
of Oddi	C24.Ø	C78.89	DØ1.5	D13.5	D37.6	D49.Ø
spine, spinal (column)	C41.2	C79.51	—	D16.6	D48.Ø	D49.2
bulb	C71.7	C79.31	—	D33.1	D43.1	D49.6
coccyx	C41.4	C79.51	—	D16.8	D48.Ø	D49.2
cord (cervical) (lumbar) (sacral) (thoracic)	C72.Ø	C79.49	—	D33.4	D43.4	D49.7
dura mater	C7Ø.1	C79.49	—	D32.1	D42.1	D49.7
lumbosacral	C41.2	C79.51	—	D16.6	D48.Ø	D49.2
marrow NEC	C96.9	C79.52	—	—	D47.9	D49.89
membrane	C7Ø.1	C79.49	—	D32.1	D42.1	D49.7
meninges	C7Ø.1	C79.49	—	D32.1	D42.1	D49.7
nerve (root)	C47.9	C79.89	—	D36.1Ø	D48.2	D49.2
pia mater	C7Ø.1	C79.49	—	D32.1	D42.1	D49.7
root	C47.9	C79.89	—	D36.1Ø	D48.2	D49.2
sacrum	C41.4	C79.51	—	D16.8	D48.Ø	D49.2
spleen, splenic						
NEC	C26.1	C78.89	DØ1.7	D13.9	D37.8	D49.Ø
flexure (colon)	C18.5	C78.5	DØ1.Ø	D12.3	D37.4	D49.Ø
stem, brain	C71.7	C79.31	—	D33.1	D43.1	D49.6
Stensen's duct	CØ7	C79.89	DØØ.ØØ	D11.Ø	D37.Ø3Ø	D49.Ø
sternum	C41.3	C79.51	—	D16.7	D48.Ø	D49.2
stomach	C16.9	C78.89	DØØ.2	D13.1	D37.1	D49.Ø
antrum (pyloric)	C16.3	C78.89	DØØ.2	D13.1	D37.1	D49.Ø
body	C16.2	C78.89	DØØ.2	D13.1	D37.1	D49.Ø
cardia	C16.Ø	C78.89	DØØ.2	D13.1	D37.1	D49.Ø
cardiac orifice	C16.Ø	C78.89	DØØ.2	D13.1	D37.1	D49.Ø
corpus	C16.2	C78.89	DØØ.2	D13.1	D37.1	D49.Ø
fundus	C16.1	C78.89	DØØ.2	D13.1	D37.1	D49.Ø
greater curvature NEC	C16.6	C78.89	DØØ.2	D13.1	D37.1	D49.Ø
lesser curvature NEC	C16.5	C78.89	DØØ.2	D13.1	D37.1	D49.Ø
overlapping lesion	C16.8	—	—	—	—	—
prepylorus	C16.4	C78.89	DØØ.2	D13.1	D37.1	D49.Ø
pylorus	C16.4	C78.89	DØØ.2	D13.1	D37.1	D49.Ø
wall NEC	C16.9	C78.89	DØØ.2	D13.1	D37.1	D49.Ø
anterior NEC	C16.8	C78.89	DØØ.2	D13.1	D37.1	D49.Ø
posterior NEC	C16.8	C78.89	DØØ.2	D13.1	D37.1	D49.Ø
stroma, endometrial	C54.1	C79.82	DØ7.Ø	D26.1	D39.Ø	D49.59
stump, cervical	C53.8	C79.82	DØ6.7	D26.Ø	D39.Ø	D49.59
subcutaneous (nodule) (tissue) NEC — *see* Neoplasm, connective tissue						
subdural	C7Ø.9	C79.32	—	D32.9	D42.9	D49.7
subglottis, subglottic	C32.2	C78.39	DØ2.Ø	D14.1	D38.Ø	D49.1
sublingual	CØ4.9	C79.89	DØØ.Ø6	D1Ø.2	D37.Ø9	D49.Ø
gland or duct	CØ8.1	C79.89	DØØ.ØØ	D11.7	D37.Ø31	D49.Ø
submandibular gland	CØ8.Ø	C79.89	DØØ.ØØ	D11.7	D37.Ø32	D49.Ø
submaxillary gland or duct	CØ8.Ø	C79.89	DØØ.ØØ	D11.7	D37.Ø32	D49.Ø
submental	C76.Ø	C79.89	DØ9.8	D36.7	D48.7	D49.89
subpleural	C34.9-☑	C78.Ø-☑	DØ2.2-☑	D14.3-☑	D38.1	D49.1
substernal	C38.1	C78.1	—	D15.2	D38.3	D49.89
sudoriferous, sudoriparous gland, site						
unspecified	C44.9Ø	C79.2	DØ4.9	D23.9	D48.5	D49.2
specified site — *see* Neoplasm, skin						
supraclavicular region	C76.Ø	C79.89	DØ9.8	D36.7	D48.7	D49.89
supraglottis	C32.1	C78.39	DØ2.Ø	D14.1	D38.Ø	D49.1
suprarenal	C74.9-☑	C79.7-☑	DØ9.3	D35.Ø-☑	D44.1-☑	D49.7
capsule	C74.9-☑	C79.7-☑	DØ9.3	D35.Ø-☑	D44.1-☑	D49.7

	Malignant Primary	Malignant Secondary	Ca in situ	Benign	Uncertain Behavior	Unspecified Behavior
Neoplasm, neoplastic — *continued*						
suprarenal — *continued*						
cortex	C74.Ø-☑	C79.7-☑	DØ9.3	D35.Ø-☑	D44.1-☑	D49.7
gland	C74.9-☑	C79.7-☑	DØ9.3	D35.Ø-☑	D44.1-☑	D49.7
medulla	C74.1-☑	C79.7-☑	DØ9.3	D35.Ø-☑	D44.1-☑	D49.7
suprasellar (region)	C71.9	C79.31	—	D33.2	D43.2	D49.6
supratentorial (brain) NEC	C71.Ø	C79.31	—	D33.Ø	D43.Ø	D49.6
sweat gland (apocrine) (eccrine), site						
unspecified	C44.9Ø	C79.2	DØ4.9	D23.9	D48.5	D49.2
specified site — *see* Neoplasm, skin						
sympathetic nerve or nervous system NEC	C47.9	C79.89	—	D36.1Ø	D48.2	D49.2
symphysis pubis	C41.4	C79.51	—	D16.8	D48.Ø	D49.2
synovial membrane — *see* Neoplasm, connective tissue						
tapetum, brain	C71.8	C79.31	—	D33.2	D43.2	D49.6
tarsus (any bone)	C4Ø.3-☑	C79.51	—	D16.3-☑	—	—
temple (skin) — *see also* Neoplasm, skin, face	C44.3Ø9	C79.2	DØ4.39	D23.39	D48.5	D49.2
temporal						
bone	C41.Ø	C79.51	—	D16.4	D48.Ø	D49.2
lobe or pole	C71.2	C79.31	—	D33.Ø	D43.Ø	D49.6
region	C76.Ø	C79.89	DØ9.8	D36.7	D48.7	D49.89
skin — *see also* Neoplasm, skin, face	C44.3Ø9	C79.2	DØ4.39	D23.39	D48.5	D49.2
tendon (sheath) — *see* Neoplasm, connective tissue						
tentorium (cerebelli)	C7Ø.Ø	C79.32	—	D32.Ø	D42.Ø	D49.7
testis, testes	C62.9-☑	C79.82	DØ7.69	D29.2-☑	D4Ø.1-☑	D49.59
descended	C62.1-☑	C79.82	DØ7.69	D29.2-☑	D4Ø.1-☑	D49.59
ectopic	C62.Ø-☑	C79.82	DØ7.69	D29.2-☑	D4Ø.1-☑	D49.59
retained	C62.Ø-☑	C79.82	DØ7.69	D29.2-☑	D4Ø.1-☑	D49.59
scrotal	C62.1-☑	C79.82	DØ7.69	D29.2-☑	D4Ø.1-☑	D49.59
undescended	C62.Ø-☑	C79.82	DØ7.69	D29.2-☑	D4Ø.1-☑	D49.59
unspecified whether descended or undescended	C62.9-☑	C79.82	DØ7.69	D29.2-☑	D4Ø.1-☑	D49.59
thalamus	C71.Ø	C79.31	—	D33.Ø	D43.Ø	D49.6
thigh NEC	C76.5-☑	C79.89	DØ4.7-☑	D36.7	D48.7	D49.89
thorax, thoracic (cavity) (organs NEC)	C76.1	C79.89	DØ9.8	D36.7	D48.7	D49.89
duct	C49.3	C79.89	—	D21.3	D48.1	D49.2
wall NEC	C76.1	C79.89	DØ9.8	D36.7	D48.7	D49.89
throat	C14.Ø	C79.89	DØØ.Ø8	D1Ø.9	D37.Ø5	D49.Ø
thumb NEC	C76.4-☑	C79.89	DØ4.6-☑	D36.7	D48.7	D49.89
thymus (gland)	C37	C79.89	DØ9.3	D15.Ø	D38.4	D49.89
thyroglossal duct	C73	C79.89	DØ9.3	D34	D44.Ø	D49.7
thyroid (gland)	C73	C79.89	DØ9.3	D34	D44.Ø	D49.7
cartilage	C32.3	C78.39	DØ2.Ø	D14.1	D38.Ø	D49.1
tibia (any part)	C4Ø.2-☑	C79.51	—	D16.2-☑	—	—
toe NEC	C76.5-☑	C79.89	DØ4.7-☑	D36.7	D48.7	D49.89
tongue	CØ2.9	C79.89	DØØ.Ø7	D1Ø.1	D37.Ø2	D49.Ø
anterior (two-thirds) NEC	CØ2.3	C79.89	DØØ.Ø7	D1Ø.1	D37.Ø2	D49.Ø
dorsal surface	CØ2.Ø	C79.89	DØØ.Ø7	D1Ø.1	D37.Ø2	D49.Ø
ventral surface	CØ2.2	C79.89	DØØ.Ø7	D1Ø.1	D37.Ø2	D49.Ø
base (dorsal surface)	CØ1	C79.89	DØØ.Ø7	D1Ø.1	D37.Ø2	D49.Ø
border (lateral)	CØ2.1	C79.89	DØØ.Ø7	D1Ø.1	D37.Ø2	D49.Ø
dorsal surface NEC	CØ2.Ø	C79.89	DØØ.Ø7	D1Ø.1	D37.Ø2	D49.Ø
fixed part NEC	CØ1	C79.89	DØØ.Ø7	D1Ø.1	D37.Ø2	D49.Ø
foreamen cecum	CØ2.Ø	C79.89	DØØ.Ø7	D1Ø.1	D37.Ø2	D49.Ø
frenulum linguae	CØ2.2	C79.89	DØØ.Ø7	D1Ø.1	D37.Ø2	D49.Ø
junctional zone	CØ2.8	C79.89	DØØ.Ø7	D1Ø.1	D37.Ø2	D49.Ø
margin (lateral)	CØ2.1	C79.89	DØØ.Ø7	D1Ø.1	D37.Ø2	D49.Ø
midline NEC	CØ2.Ø	C79.89	DØØ.Ø7	D1Ø.1	D37.Ø2	D49.Ø
mobile part NEC	CØ2.3	C79.89	DØØ.Ø7	D1Ø.1	D37.Ø2	D49.Ø

	Malignant Primary	Malignant Secondary	Ca in situ	Benign	Uncertain Behavior	Unspecified Behavior
Neoplasm, neoplastic — *continued*						
tongue — *continued*						
overlapping lesion	CØ2.8	—	—	—	—	—
posterior (third)	CØ1	C79.89	DØØ.Ø7	D1Ø.1	D37.Ø2	D49.Ø
root	CØ1	C79.89	DØØ.Ø7	D1Ø.1	D37.Ø2	D49.Ø
surface (dorsal)	CØ2.Ø	C79.89	DØØ.Ø7	D1Ø.1	D37.Ø2	D49.Ø
base	CØ1	C79.89	DØØ.Ø7	D1Ø.1	D37.Ø2	D49.Ø
ventral	CØ2.2	C79.89	DØØ.Ø7	D1Ø.1	D37.Ø2	D49.Ø
tip	CØ2.1	C79.89	DØØ.Ø7	D1Ø.1	D37.Ø2	D49.Ø
tonsil	CØ2.4	C79.89	DØØ.Ø7	D1Ø.1	D37.Ø2	D49.Ø
tonsil	CØ9.9	C79.89	DØØ.Ø8	D1Ø.4	D37.Ø5	D49.Ø
fauces, faucial	CØ9.9	C79.89	DØØ.Ø8	D1Ø.4	D37.Ø5	D49.Ø
lingual	CØ2.4	C79.89	DØØ.Ø7	D1Ø.1	D37.Ø2	D49.Ø
overlapping sites	CØ9.8	—	—	—	—	—
palatine	CØ9.9	C79.89	DØØ.Ø8	D1Ø.4	D37.Ø5	D49.Ø
pharyngeal	C11.1	C79.89	DØØ.Ø8	D1Ø.6	D37.Ø5	D49.Ø
pillar (anterior) (posterior)	CØ9.1	C79.89	DØØ.Ø8	D1Ø.5	D37.Ø5	D49.Ø
tonsillar fossa	CØ9.Ø	C79.89	DØØ.Ø8	D1Ø.5	D37.Ø5	D49.Ø
tooth socket NEC	CØ3.9	C79.89	DØØ.Ø3	D1Ø.39	D37.Ø9	D49.Ø
trachea (cartilage) (mucosa)	C33	C78.39	DØ2.1	D14.2	D38.1	D49.1
overlapping lesion with bronchus or lung	C34.8-☑	—	—	—	—	—
tracheobronchial	C34.8-☑	C78.39	DØ2.1	D14.2	D38.1	D49.1
overlapping lesion with lung	C34.8-☑	—	—	—	—	—
tragus — *see also* Neoplasm, skin, ear	C44.2Ø-☑	C79.2	DØ4.2-☑	D23.2-☑	D48.5	D49.2
trunk NEC	C76.8	C79.89	DØ4.5	D36.7	D48.7	D49.89
tubo-ovarian	C57.8	C79.82	DØ7.39	D28.7	D39.8	D49.59
tunica vaginalis	C63.7	C79.82	DØ7.69	D29.8	D4Ø.8	D49.59
turbinate (bone)	C41.Ø	C79.51	—	D16.4	D48.Ø	D49.2
nasal	C3Ø.Ø	C78.39	DØ2.3	D14.Ø	D38.5	D49.1
tympanic cavity	C3Ø.1	C78.39	DØ2.3	D14.Ø	D38.5	D49.1
ulna (any part)	C4Ø.Ø-☑	C79.51	—	D16.Ø-☑	—	—
umbilicus, umbilical — *see also* Neoplasm, skin, trunk	C44.5Ø9	C79.2	DØ4.5	D23.5	D48.5	D49.2
uncus, brain	C71.2	C79.31	—	D33.Ø	D43.Ø	D49.6
unknown site or unspecified	C8Ø.1	C79.9	DØ9.9	D36.9	D48.9	D49.9
urachus	C67.7	C79.11	DØ9.Ø	D3Ø.3	D41.4	D49.4
ureter-bladder (junction)	C67.6	C79.11	DØ9.Ø	D3Ø.3	D41.4	D49.4
ureter, ureteral	C66.-☑	C79.19	DØ9.19	D3Ø.2-☑	D41.2-☑	D49.59
orifice (bladder)	C67.6	C79.11	DØ9.Ø	D3Ø.3	D41.4	D49.4
urethra, urethral (gland)	C68.Ø	C79.19	DØ9.19	D3Ø.4	D41.3	D49.59
orifice, internal	C67.5	C79.11	DØ9.Ø	D3Ø.3	D41.4	D49.4
urethrovaginal (septum)	C57.9	C79.82	DØ7.3Ø	D28.9	D39.8	D49.59
urinary organ or system	C68.9	C79.1Ø	DØ9.1Ø	D3Ø.9	D41.9	D49.59
bladder — *see* Neoplasm, bladder						
overlapping lesion	C68.8	—	—	—	—	—
specified sites NEC	C68.8	C79.19	DØ9.19	D3Ø.8	D41.8	D49.59
utero-ovarian	C57.8	C79.82	DØ7.39	D28.7	D39.8	D49.59
ligament	C57.1-☑	C79.82	DØ7.39	D28.2	D39.8	D49.59
uterosacral ligament	C57.3	C79.82	—	D28.2	D39.8	D49.59
uterus, uteri, uterine	C55	C79.82	DØ7.Ø	D26.9	D39.Ø	D49.59
adnexa NEC	C57.4	C79.82	DØ7.39	D28.7	D39.8	D49.59
body	C54.9	C79.82	DØ7.Ø	D26.1	D39.Ø	D49.59
cervix	C53.9	C79.82	DØ6.9	D26.Ø	D39.Ø	D49.59
cornu	C54.9	C79.82	DØ7.Ø	D26.1	D39.Ø	D49.59
corpus	C54.9	C79.82	DØ7.Ø	D26.1	D39.Ø	D49.59
endocervix (canal) (gland)	C53.Ø	C79.82	DØ6.Ø	D26.Ø	D39.Ø	D49.59
endometrium	C54.1	C79.82	DØ7.Ø	D26.1	D39.Ø	D49.59
exocervix	C53.1	C79.82	DØ6.1	D26.Ø	D39.Ø	D49.59
external os	C53.1	C79.82	DØ6.1	D26.Ø	D39.Ø	D49.59
fundus	C54.3	C79.82	DØ7.Ø	D26.1	D39.Ø	D49.59
Neoplasm, neoplastic — *continued*						
uterus, uteri, uterine — *continued*						
internal os	C53.Ø	C79.82	DØ6.Ø	D26.Ø	D39.Ø	D49.59
isthmus	C54.Ø	C79.82	DØ7.Ø	D26.1	D39.Ø	D49.59
ligament	C57.3	C79.82	—	D28.2	D39.8	D49.59
broad	C57.1-☑	C79.82	DØ7.39	D28.2	D39.8	D49.59
round	C57.2-☑	C79.82	—	D28.2	D39.8	D49.59
lower segment	C54.Ø	C79.82	DØ7.Ø	D26.1	D39.Ø	D49.59
myometrium	C54.2	C79.82	DØ7.Ø	D26.1	D39.Ø	D49.59
overlapping sites	C54.8	—	—	—	—	—
squamocolumnar junction	C53.8	C79.82	DØ6.7	D26.Ø	D39.Ø	D49.59
tube	C57.Ø-☑	C79.82	DØ7.39	D28.2	D39.8	D49.59
utricle, prostatic	C68.Ø	C79.19	DØ9.19	D3Ø.4	D41.3	D49.59
uveal tract	C69.4-☑	C79.49	DØ9.2-☑	D31.4-☑	D48.7	D49.89
uvula	CØ5.2	C79.89	DØØ.Ø4	D1Ø.39	D37.Ø9	D49.Ø
vagina, vaginal (fornix) (vault) (wall)	C52	C79.82	DØ7.2	D28.1	D39.8	D49.59
vaginovesical	C57.9	C79.82	DØ7.3Ø	D28.9	D39.9	D49.59
septum	C57.9	C79.82	DØ7.3Ø	D28.9	D39.9	D49.59
vallecula (epiglottis)	C1Ø.Ø	C79.89	DØØ.Ø8	D1Ø.5	D37.Ø5	D49.Ø
vascular — *see* Neoplasm, connective tissue						
vas deferens	C63.1-☑	C79.82	DØ7.69	D29.8	D4Ø.8	D49.59
Vater's ampulla	C24.1	C78.89	DØ1.5	D13.5	D37.6	D49.Ø
vein, venous — *see* Neoplasm, connective tissue						
vena cava (abdominal) (inferior)	C49.4	C79.89	—	D21.4	D48.1	D49.2
superior	C49.3	C79.89	—	D21.3	D48.1	D49.2
ventricle (cerebral) (floor) (lateral) (third)	C71.5	C79.31	—	D33.Ø	D43.Ø	D49.6
cardiac (left) (right)	C38.Ø	C79.89	—	D15.1	D48.7	D49.89
fourth	C71.7	C79.31	—	D33.1	D43.1	D49.6
ventricular band of larynx	C32.1	C78.39	DØ2.Ø	D14.1	D38.Ø	D49.1
ventriculus — *see* Neoplasm, stomach						
vermillion border — *see* Neoplasm, lip						
vermis, cerebellum	C71.6	C79.31	—	D33.1	D43.1	D49.6
vertebra (column)	C41.2	C79.51	—	D16.6	D48.Ø	D49.2
coccyx	C41.4	C79.51	—	D16.8	D48.Ø	D49.2
marrow NEC	C96.9	C79.52	—	—	D47.9	D49.89
sacrum	C41.4	C79.51	—	D16.8	D48.Ø	D49.2
vesical — *see* Neoplasm, bladder						
vesicle, seminal	C63.7	C79.82	DØ7.69	D29.8	D4Ø.8	D49.59
vesicocervical tissue	C57.9	C79.82	DØ7.3Ø	D28.9	D39.9	D49.59
vesicorectal	C76.3	C79.82	DØ9.8	D36.7	D48.7	D49.89
vesicovaginal	C57.9	C79.82	DØ7.3Ø	D28.9	D39.9	D49.59
septum	C57.9	C79.82	DØ7.3Ø	D28.9	D39.8	D49.59
vessel (blood) — *see* Neoplasm, connective tissue						
vestibular gland, greater	C51.Ø	C79.82	DØ7.1	D28.Ø	D39.8	D49.59
vestibule						
mouth	CØ6.1	C79.89	DØØ.ØØ	D1Ø.39	D37.Ø9	D49.Ø
nose	C3Ø.Ø	C78.39	DØ2.3	D14.Ø	D38.5	D49.1
Virchow's gland	C77.Ø	C77.Ø	—	D36.Ø	D48.7	D49.89
viscera NEC	C76.8	C79.89	DØ9.8	D36.7	D48.7	D49.89
vocal cords (true)	C32.Ø	C78.39	DØ2.Ø	D14.1	D38.Ø	D49.1
false	C32.1	C78.39	DØ2.Ø	D14.1	D38.Ø	D49.1
vomer	C41.Ø	C79.51	—	D16.4	D48.Ø	D49.2
vulva	C51.9	C79.82	DØ7.1	D28.Ø	D39.8	D49.59
vulvovaginal gland	C51.Ø	C79.82	DØ7.1	D28.Ø	D39.8	D49.59
Waldeyer's ring	C14.2	C79.89	DØØ.Ø8	D1Ø.9	D37.Ø5	D49.Ø
Wharton's duct	CØ8.Ø	C79.89	DØØ.ØØ	D11.7	D37.Ø32	D49.Ø
white matter (central) (cerebral)	C71.Ø	C79.31	—	D33.Ø	D43.Ø	D49.6

Neoplasm Table

	Malignant Primary	Malignant Secondary	Ca in situ	Benign	Uncertain Behavior	Unspecified Behavior
Neoplasm, neoplastic						
— *continued*						
windpipe	C33	C78.39	DØ2.1	D14.2	D38.1	D49.1
Wirsung's duct	C25.3	C78.89	DØ1.7	D13.6	D37.8	D49.Ø
wolffian (body) (duct)						
female	C57.7	C79.82	DØ7.39	D28.7	D39.8	D49.59
male	C63.7	C79.82	DØ7.69	D29.8	D4Ø.8	D49.59
womb — *see* Neoplasm, uterus						
wrist NEC	C76.4-☑	C79.89	DØ4.6-☑	D36.7	D48.7	D49.89
xiphoid process	C41.3	C79.51	—	D16.7	D48.Ø	D49.2
Zuckerkandl organ	C75.5	C79.89	—	D35.6	D44.7	D49.7

Neoplasm, windpipe — Neoplasm, Zuckerkandl organ

Substance	Poisoning, Accidental (unintentional)	Poisoning, Intentional Self-harm	Poisoning, Assault	Poisoning, Undetermined	Adverse Effect	Under-dosing
14-hydroxydihydro-morphinone	T40.2X1	T40.2X2	T40.2X3	T40.2X4	T40.2X5	T40.2X6
1-Propanol	T51.3X1	T51.3X2	T51.3X3	T51.3X4	—	—
2,3,7,8-Tetrachlorodibenzo-p-dioxin	T53.7X1	T53.7X2	T53.7X3	T53.7X4	—	—
2,4,5-T (trichloro-phenoxyacetic acid)	T60.1X1	T60.1X2	T60.1X3	T60.1X4	—	—
2,4,5-Trichlorophen-oxyacetic acid	T60.3X1	T60.3X2	T60.3X3	T60.3X4	—	—
2,4-D (dichlorophen-oxyacetic acid)	T60.3X1	T60.3X2	T60.3X3	T60.3X4	—	—
2,4-Toluene diisocyanate	T65.0X1	T65.0X2	T65.0X3	T65.0X4	—	—
2-Deoxy-5-fluorouridine	T45.1X1	T45.1X2	T45.1X3	T45.1X4	T45.1X5	T45.1X6
2-Ethoxyethanol	T52.3X1	T52.3X2	T52.3X3	T52.3X4	—	—
2-Methoxyethanol	T52.3X1	T52.3X2	T52.3X3	T52.3X4	—	—
2-Propanol	T51.2X1	T51.2X2	T51.2X3	T51.2X4	—	—
3,4-methylenedioxymeth-amphetamine	T43.641	T43.642	T43.643	T43.644	—	—
4-Aminobutyric acid	T43.8X1	T43.8X2	T43.8X3	T43.8X4	T43.8X5	T43.8X6
4-Aminophenol derivatives	T39.1X1	T39.1X2	T39.1X3	T39.1X4	T39.1X5	T39.1X6
5-Deoxy-5-fluorouridine	T45.1X1	T45.1X2	T45.1X3	T45.1X4	T45.1X5	T45.1X6
5-Methoxypsoralen (5-MOP)	T50.991	T50.992	T50.993	T50.994	T50.995	T50.996
8-Aminoquinoline drugs	T37.2X1	T37.2X2	T37.2X3	T37.2X4	T37.2X5	T37.2X6
8-Methoxypsoralen (8-MOP)	T50.991	T50.992	T50.993	T50.994	T50.995	T50.996
9-hydoxyrisperidone*	T43.591	T43.592	T43.593	T43.594	T43.595	T43.596
ABOB	T37.5X1	T37.5X2	T37.5X3	T37.5X4	T37.5X5	T37.5X6
Abrine	T62.2X1	T62.2X2	T62.2X3	T62.2X4	—	—
Abrus (seed)	T62.2X1	T62.2X2	T62.2X3	T62.2X4	—	—
Absinthe	T51.0X1	T51.0X2	T51.0X3	T51.0X4	—	—
beverage	T51.0X1	T51.0X2	T51.0X3	T51.0X4	—	—
Acaricide	T60.8X1	T60.8X2	T60.8X3	T60.8X4	—	—
Acebutolol	T44.7X1	T44.7X2	T44.7X3	T44.7X4	T44.7X5	T44.7X6
Acecarbromal	T42.6X1	T42.6X2	T42.6X3	T42.6X4	T42.6X5	T42.6X6
Aceclidine	T44.1X1	T44.1X2	T44.1X3	T44.1X4	T44.1X5	T44.1X6
Acedapsone	T37.0X1	T37.0X2	T37.0X3	T37.0X4	T37.0X5	T37.0X6
Acefylline piperazine	T48.6X1	T48.6X2	T48.6X3	T48.6X4	T48.6X5	T48.6X6
Acemorphan	T40.2X1	T40.2X2	T40.2X3	T40.2X4	T40.2X5	T40.2X6
Acenocoumarin	T45.511	T45.512	T45.513	T45.514	T45.515	T45.516
Acenocoumarol	T45.511	T45.512	T45.513	T45.514	T45.515	T45.516
Aceon*	T46.4X1	T46.4X2	T46.4X3	T46.4X4	T46.4X5	T46.4X6
Acepifylline	T48.6X1	T48.6X2	T48.6X3	T48.6X4	T48.6X5	T48.6X6
Acepromazine	T43.3X1	T43.3X2	T43.3X3	T43.3X4	T43.3X5	T43.3X6
Acesulfamethoxypyridazine	T37.0X1	T37.0X2	T37.0X3	T37.0X4	T37.0X5	T37.0X6
Acetal	T52.8X1	T52.8X2	T52.8X3	T52.8X4	—	—
Acetaldehyde (vapor)	T52.8X1	T52.8X2	T52.8X3	T52.8X4	—	—
liquid	T65.891	T65.892	T65.893	T65.894	—	—
Acetaminophen	T39.1X1	T39.1X2	T39.1X3	T39.1X4	T39.1X5	T39.1X6
Acetaminosalol	T39.1X1	T39.1X2	T39.1X3	T39.1X4	T39.1X5	T39.1X6
Acetanilide	T39.1X1	T39.1X2	T39.1X3	T39.1X4	T39.1X5	T39.1X6
Acetarsol	T37.3X1	T37.3X2	T37.3X3	T37.3X4	T37.3X5	T37.3X6
Acetazolamide	T50.2X1	T50.2X2	T50.2X3	T50.2X4	T50.2X5	T50.2X6
Acetiamine	T45.2X1	T45.2X2	T45.2X3	T45.2X4	T45.2X5	T45.2X6
Acetic						
acid	T54.2X1	T54.2X2	T54.2X3	T54.2X4	—	—
with sodium acetate (ointment)	T49.3X1	T49.3X2	T49.3X3	T49.3X4	T49.3X5	T49.3X6
ester (solvent)(vapor)	T52.8X1	T52.8X2	T52.8X3	T52.8X4	—	—
irrigating solution	T50.3X1	T50.3X2	T50.3X3	T50.3X4	T50.3X5	T50.3X6
medicinal (lotion)	T49.2X1	T49.2X2	T49.2X3	T49.2X4	T49.2X5	T49.2X6
anhydride	T65.891	T65.892	T65.893	T65.894	—	—
ether (vapor)	T52.8X1	T52.8X2	T52.8X3	T52.8X4	—	—
Acetohexamide	T38.3X1	T38.3X2	T38.3X3	T38.3X4	T38.3X5	T38.3X6
Acetohydroxamic acid	T50.991	T50.992	T50.993	T50.994	T50.995	T50.996
Acetomenaphthone	T45.7X1	T45.7X2	T45.7X3	T45.7X4	T45.7X5	T45.7X6
Acetomorphine	T40.1X1	T40.1X2	T40.1X3	T40.1X4	—	—
Acetone (oils)	T52.4X1	T52.4X2	T52.4X3	T52.4X4	—	—
chlorinated	T52.4X1	T52.4X2	T52.4X3	T52.4X4	—	—
vapor	T52.4X1	T52.4X2	T52.4X3	T52.4X4	—	—
Acetonitrile	T52.8X1	T52.8X2	T52.8X3	T52.8X4	—	—
Acetophenazine	T43.3X1	T43.3X2	T43.3X3	T43.3X4	T43.3X5	T43.3X6
Acetophenetedin	T39.1X1	T39.1X2	T39.1X3	T39.1X4	T39.1X5	T39.1X6
Acetophenone	T52.4X1	T52.4X2	T52.4X3	T52.4X4	—	—
Acetorphine	T40.2X1	T40.2X2	T40.2X3	T40.2X4	—	—
Acetosulfone (sodium)	T37.1X1	T37.1X2	T37.1X3	T37.1X4	T37.1X5	T37.1X6
Acetrizoate (sodium)	T50.8X1	T50.8X2	T50.8X3	T50.8X4	T50.8X5	T50.8X6
Acetrizoic acid	T50.8X1	T50.8X2	T50.8X3	T50.8X4	T50.8X5	T50.8X6
Acetyl						
bromide	T53.6X1	T53.6X2	T53.6X3	T53.6X4	—	—
chloride	T53.6X1	T53.6X2	T53.6X3	T53.6X4	—	—
Acetylcarbromal	T42.6X1	T42.6X2	T42.6X3	T42.6X4	T42.6X5	T42.6X6
Acetylcholine						

Substance	Poisoning, Accidental (unintentional)	Poisoning, Intentional Self-harm	Poisoning, Assault	Poisoning, Undetermined	Adverse Effect	Under-dosing
Acetylcholine — *continued*						
chloride	T44.1X1	T44.1X2	T44.1X3	T44.1X4	T44.1X5	T44.1X6
derivative	T44.1X1	T44.1X2	T44.1X3	T44.1X4	T44.1X5	T44.1X6
Acetylcysteine	T48.4X1	T48.4X2	T48.4X3	T48.4X4	T48.4X5	T48.4X6
Acetyldigitoxin	T46.0X1	T46.0X2	T46.0X3	T46.0X4	T46.0X5	T46.0X6
Acetyldigoxin	T46.0X1	T46.0X2	T46.0X3	T46.0X4	T46.0X5	T46.0X6
Acetyldihydrocodeine	T40.2X1	T40.2X2	T40.2X3	T40.2X4	—	—
Acetyldihydrocodeinone	T40.2X1	T40.2X2	T40.2X3	T40.2X4	—	—
Acetylene (gas)	T59.891	T59.892	T59.893	T59.894	—	—
dichloride	T53.6X1	T53.6X2	T53.6X3	T53.6X4	—	—
incomplete combustion of	T58.11	T58.12	T58.13	T58.14	—	—
industrial	T59.891	T59.892	T59.893	T59.894	—	—
tetrachloride	T53.6X1	T53.6X2	T53.6X3	T53.6X4	—	—
vapor	T53.6X1	T53.6X2	T53.6X3	T53.6X4	—	—
Acetylpheneturide	T42.6X1	T42.6X2	T42.6X3	T42.6X4	T42.6X5	T42.6X6
Acetylphenylhydrazine	T39.8X1	T39.8X2	T39.8X3	T39.8X4	T39.8X5	T39.8X6
Acetylsalicylic acid (salts)	T39.011	T39.012	T39.013	T39.014	T39.015	T39.016
enteric coated	T39.011	T39.012	T39.013	T39.014	T39.015	T39.016
Acetylsulfamethoxypyridazine	T37.0X1	T37.0X2	T37.0X3	T37.0X4	T37.0X5	T37.0X6
Achromycin	T36.4X1	T36.4X2	T36.4X3	T36.4X4	T36.4X5	T36.4X6
ophthalmic preparation	T49.5X1	T49.5X2	T49.5X3	T49.5X4	T49.5X5	T49.5X6
topical NEC	T49.0X1	T49.0X2	T49.0X3	T49.0X4	T49.0X5	T49.0X6
Aciclovir	T37.5X1	T37.5X2	T37.5X3	T37.5X4	T37.5X5	T37.5X6
Acidifying agent NEC	T50.901	T50.902	T50.903	T50.904	T50.905	T50.906
Acid (corrosive) **NEC**	T54.2X1	T54.2X2	T54.2X3	T54.2X4	—	—
AcipHex*	T47.1X1	T47.1X2	T47.1X3	T47.1X4	T47.1X5	T47.1X6
Acipimox	T46.6X1	T46.6X2	T46.6X3	T46.6X4	T46.6X5	T46.6X6
Acitretin	T50.991	T50.992	T50.993	T50.994	T50.995	T50.996
Aclarubicin	T45.1X1	T45.1X2	T45.1X3	T45.1X4	T45.1X5	T45.1X6
Aclatonium napadisilate	T48.1X1	T48.1X2	T48.1X3	T48.1X4	T48.1X5	T48.1X6
Aconite (wild)	T46.991	T46.992	T46.993	T46.994	T46.995	T46.996
Aconitine	T46.991	T46.992	T46.993	T46.994	T46.995	T46.996
Aconitum ferox	T46.991	T46.992	T46.993	T46.994	T46.995	T46.996
Acridine	T65.6X1	T65.6X2	T65.6X3	T65.6X4	—	—
vapor	T59.891	T59.892	T59.893	T59.894	—	—
Acriflavine	T37.91	T37.92	T37.93	T37.94	T37.95	T37.96
Acriflavinium chloride	T49.0X1	T49.0X2	T49.0X3	T49.0X4	T49.0X5	T49.0X6
Acrinol	T49.0X1	T49.0X2	T49.0X3	T49.0X4	T49.0X5	T49.0X6
Acrisorcin	T49.0X1	T49.0X2	T49.0X3	T49.0X4	T49.0X5	T49.0X6
Acrivastine	T45.0X1	T45.0X2	T45.0X3	T45.0X4	T45.0X5	T45.0X6
Acrolein (gas)	T59.891	T59.892	T59.893	T59.894	—	—
liquid	T54.1X1	T54.1X2	T54.1X3	T54.1X4	—	—
Acrylamide	T65.891	T65.892	T65.893	T65.894	—	—
Acrylic resin	T49.3X1	T49.3X2	T49.3X3	T49.3X4	T49.3X5	T49.3X6
Acrylonitrile	T65.891	T65.892	T65.893	T65.894	—	—
Actaea spicata	T62.2X1	T62.2X2	T62.2X3	T62.2X4	—	—
berry	T62.1X1	T62.1X2	T62.1X3	T62.1X4	—	—
Acterol	T37.3X1	T37.3X2	T37.3X3	T37.3X4	T37.3X5	T37.3X6
ACTH	T38.811	T38.812	T38.813	T38.814	T38.815	T38.816
Actinomycin C	T45.1X1	T45.1X2	T45.1X3	T45.1X4	T45.1X5	T45.1X6
Actinomycin D	T45.1X1	T45.1X2	T45.1X3	T45.1X4	T45.1X5	T45.1X6
Activated charcoal — *see also* Charcoal, medicinal	T47.6X1	T47.6X2	T47.6X3	T47.6X4	T47.6X5	T47.6X6
Activella*	T38.5X1	T38.5X2	T38.5X3	T38.5X4	T38.5X5	T38.5X6
Acyclovir	T37.5X1	T37.5X2	T37.5X3	T37.5X4	T37.5X5	T37.5X6
Adenine	T45.2X1	T45.2X2	T45.2X3	T45.2X4	T45.2X5	T45.2X6
arabinoside	T37.5X1	T37.5X2	T37.5X3	T37.5X4	T37.5X5	T37.5X6
Adenosine (phosphate)	T46.2X1	T46.2X2	T46.2X3	T46.2X4	T46.2X5	T46.2X6
ADH	T38.891	T38.892	T38.893	T38.894	T38.895	T38.896
Adhesive NEC	T65.891	T65.892	T65.893	T65.894	—	—
Adicillin	T36.0X1	T36.0X2	T36.0X3	T36.0X4	T36.0X5	T36.0X6
Adiphenine	T44.3X1	T44.3X2	T44.3X3	T44.3X4	T44.3X5	T44.3X6
Adipiodone	T50.8X1	T50.8X2	T50.8X3	T50.8X4	T50.8X5	T50.8X6
Adjunct, pharmaceutical	T50.901	T50.902	T50.903	T50.904	T50.905	T50.906
Adrenal (extract, cortex or medulla) (glucocorticoids) (hormones) (mineralocorticoids)	T38.0X1	T38.0X2	T38.0X3	T38.0X4	T38.0X5	T38.0X6
ENT agent	T49.6X1	T49.6X2	T49.6X3	T49.6X4	T49.6X5	T49.6X6
ophthalmic preparation	T49.5X1	T49.5X2	T49.5X3	T49.5X4	T49.5X5	T49.5X6
topical NEC	T49.0X1	T49.0X2	T49.0X3	T49.0X4	T49.0X5	T49.0X6
Adrenalin — *see* Adrenaline						
Adrenaline	T44.5X1	T44.5X2	T44.5X3	T44.5X4	T44.5X5	T44.5X6
Adrenergic NEC	T44.901	T44.902	T44.903	T44.904	T44.905	T44.906
blocking agent NEC	T44.8X1	T44.8X2	T44.8X3	T44.8X4	T44.8X5	T44.8X6
beta, heart	T44.7X1	T44.7X2	T44.7X3	T44.7X4	T44.7X5	T44.7X6
specified NEC	T44.991	T44.992	T44.993	T44.994	T44.995	T44.996
Adrenochrome						
derivative	T46.991	T46.992	T46.993	T46.994	T46.995	T46.996
(mono) semicarbazone	T46.991	T46.992	T46.993	T46.994	T46.995	T46.996
Adrenocorticotrophic hormone	T38.811	T38.812	T38.813	T38.814	T38.815	T38.816
Adrenocorticotrophin	T38.811	T38.812	T38.813	T38.814	T38.815	T38.816

Substance	Poisoning, Accidental (unintentional)	Poisoning, Intentional Self-harm	Poisoning, Assault	Poisoning, Undetermined	Adverse Effect	Under-dosing
Adriamycin	T45.1X1	T45.1X2	T45.1X3	T45.1X4	T45.1X5	T45.1X6
Adrucil*	T45.1X1	T45.1X2	T45.1X3	T45.1X4	T45.1X5	T45.1X6
Aerosol spray NEC	T65.91	T65.92	T65.93	T65.94	—	—
Aerosporin	T36.8X1	T36.8X2	T36.8X3	T36.8X4	T36.8X5	T36.8X6
ENT agent	T49.6X1	T49.6X2	T49.6X3	T49.6X4	T49.6X5	T49.6X6
ophthalmic preparation	T49.5X1	T49.5X2	T49.5X3	T49.5X4	T49.5X5	T49.5X6
topical NEC	T49.ØX1	T49.ØX2	T49.ØX3	T49.ØX4	T49.ØX5	T49.ØX6
Aethusa cynapium	T62.2X1	T62.2X2	T62.2X3	T62.2X4	—	—
Afghanistan black	T4Ø.711	T4Ø.712	T4Ø.713	T4Ø.714	T4Ø.715	T4Ø.716
Aflatoxin	T64.Ø1	T64.Ø2	T64.Ø3	T64.Ø4	—	—
Afloqualone	T42.8X1	T42.8X2	T42.8X3	T42.8X4	T42.8X5	T42.8X6
African boxwood	T62.2X1	T62.2X2	T62.2X3	T62.2X4	—	—
Agar	T47.4X1	T47.4X2	T47.4X3	T47.4X4	T47.4X5	T47.4X6
Agonist						
predominantly						
alpha-adrenoreceptor	T44.4X1	T44.4X2	T44.4X3	T44.4X4	T44.4X5	T44.4X6
beta-adrenoreceptor	T44.5X1	T44.5X2	T44.5X3	T44.5X4	T44.5X5	T44.5X6
Agricultural agent NEC	T65.91	T65.92	T65.93	T65.94	—	—
Agrypnal	T42.3X1	T42.3X2	T42.3X3	T42.3X4	T42.3X5	T42.3X6
AHLG	T5Ø.Z11	T5Ø.Z12	T5Ø.Z13	T5Ø.Z14	T5Ø.Z15	T5Ø.Z16
Air contaminant(s), source/type NOS	T65.91	T65.92	T65.93	T65.94	—	—
Ajmaline	T46.2X1	T46.2X2	T46.2X3	T46.2X4	T46.2X5	T46.2X6
Akee	T62.1X1	T62.1X2	T62.1X3	T62.1X4	—	—
Akne-Mycin*	T49.ØX1	T49.ØX2	T49.ØX3	T49.ØX4	T49.ØX5	T49.ØX6
Akrinol	T49.ØX1	T49.ØX2	T49.ØX3	T49.ØX4	T49.ØX5	T49.ØX6
Akritoin	T37.8X1	T37.8X2	T37.8X3	T37.8X4	T37.8X5	T37.8X6
Alacepril	T46.4X1	T46.4X2	T46.4X3	T46.4X4	T46.4X5	T46.4X6
Alantolactone	T37.4X1	T37.4X2	T37.4X3	T37.4X4	T37.4X5	T37.4X6
Albamycin	T36.8X1	T36.8X2	T36.8X3	T36.8X4	T36.8X5	T36.8X6
Albendazole	T37.4X1	T37.4X2	T37.4X3	T37.4X4	T37.4X5	T37.4X6
Albigutide*	T38.3X1	T38.3X2	T38.3X3	T38.3X4	T38.3X5	T38.3X6
Albumin						
bovine	T45.8X1	T45.8X2	T45.8X3	T45.8X4	T45.8X5	T45.8X6
human serum	T45.8X1	T45.8X2	T45.8X3	T45.8X4	T45.8X5	T45.8X6
salt-poor	T45.8X1	T45.8X2	T45.8X3	T45.8X4	T45.8X5	T45.8X6
normal human serum	T45.8X1	T45.8X2	T45.8X3	T45.8X4	T45.8X5	T45.8X6
Albuterol	T48.6X1	T48.6X2	T48.6X3	T48.6X4	T48.6X5	T48.6X6
Albutoin	T42.ØX1	T42.ØX2	T42.ØX3	T42.ØX4	T42.ØX5	T42.ØX6
Alclometasone	T49.ØX1	T49.ØX2	T49.ØX3	T49.ØX4	T49.ØX5	T49.ØX6
Alcohol	T51.91	T51.92	T51.93	T51.94	—	—
absolute	T51.ØX1	T51.ØX2	T51.ØX3	T51.ØX4	—	—
beverage	T51.ØX1	T51.ØX2	T51.ØX3	T51.ØX4	—	—
allyl	T51.8X1	T51.8X2	T51.8X3	T51.8X4	—	—
amyl	T51.3X1	T51.3X2	T51.3X3	T51.3X4	—	—
antifreeze	T51.1X1	T51.1X2	T51.1X3	T51.1X4	—	—
beverage	T51.ØX1	T51.ØX2	T51.ØX3	T51.ØX4	—	—
butyl	T51.3X1	T51.3X2	T51.3X3	T51.3X4	—	—
dehydrated	T51.ØX1	T51.ØX2	T51.ØX3	T51.ØX4	—	—
beverage	T51.ØX1	T51.ØX2	T51.ØX3	T51.ØX4	—	—
denatured	T51.ØX1	T51.ØX2	T51.ØX3	T51.ØX4	—	—
deterrent NEC	T5Ø.6X1	T5Ø.6X2	T5Ø.6X3	T5Ø.6X4	T5Ø.6X5	T5Ø.6X6
diagnostic (gastric function)	T5Ø.8X1	T5Ø.8X2	T5Ø.8X3	T5Ø.8X4	T5Ø.8X5	T5Ø.8X6
ethyl	T51.ØX1	T51.ØX2	T51.ØX3	T51.ØX4	—	—
beverage	T51.ØX1	T51.ØX2	T51.ØX3	T51.ØX4	—	—
grain	T51.ØX1	T51.ØX2	T51.ØX3	T51.ØX4	—	—
beverage	T51.ØX1	T51.ØX2	T51.ØX3	T51.ØX4	—	—
industrial	T51.ØX1	T51.ØX2	T51.ØX3	T51.ØX4	—	—
isopropyl	T51.2X1	T51.2X2	T51.2X3	T51.2X4	—	—
methyl	T51.1X1	T51.1X2	T51.1X3	T51.1X4	—	—
preparation for consumption	T51.ØX1	T51.ØX2	T51.ØX3	T51.ØX4	—	—
propyl	T51.3X1	T51.3X2	T51.3X3	T51.3X4	—	—
secondary	T51.2X1	T51.2X2	T51.2X3	T51.2X4	—	—
radiator	T51.1X1	T51.1X2	T51.1X3	T51.1X4	—	—
rubbing	T51.2X1	T51.2X2	T51.2X3	T51.2X4	—	—
specified type NEC	T51.8X1	T51.8X2	T51.8X3	T51.8X4	—	—
surgical	T51.ØX1	T51.ØX2	T51.ØX3	T51.ØX4	—	—
vapor (from any type of Alcohol)	T59.891	T59.892	T59.893	T59.894	—	—
wood	T51.1X1	T51.1X2	T51.1X3	T51.1X4	—	—
Alcuronium (chloride)	T48.1X1	T48.1X2	T48.1X3	T48.1X4	T48.1X5	T48.1X6
Aldactone	T5Ø.ØX1	T5Ø.ØX2	T5Ø.ØX3	T5Ø.ØX4	T5Ø.ØX5	T5Ø.ØX6
Aldesulfone sodium	T37.1X1	T37.1X2	T37.1X3	T37.1X4	T37.1X5	T37.1X6
Aldicarb	T6Ø.ØX1	T6Ø.ØX2	T6Ø.ØX3	T6Ø.ØX4	—	—
Aldomet	T46.5X1	T46.5X2	T46.5X3	T46.5X4	T46.5X5	T46.5X6
Aldosterone	T5Ø.ØX1	T5Ø.ØX2	T5Ø.ØX3	T5Ø.ØX4	T5Ø.ØX5	T5Ø.ØX6
Aldrin (dust)	T6Ø.1X1	T6Ø.1X2	T6Ø.1X3	T6Ø.1X4	—	—
Aleve — *see* Naproxen						
Alexitol sodium	T47.1X1	T47.1X2	T47.1X3	T47.1X4	T47.1X5	T47.1X6
Alfacalcidol	T45.2X1	T45.2X2	T45.2X3	T45.2X4	T45.2X5	T45.2X6
Alfadolone	T41.1X1	T41.1X2	T41.1X3	T41.1X4	T41.1X5	T41.1X6

Substance	Poisoning, Accidental (unintentional)	Poisoning, Intentional Self-harm	Poisoning, Assault	Poisoning, Undetermined	Adverse Effect	Under-dosing
Alfaxalone	T41.1X1	T41.1X2	T41.1X3	T41.1X4	T41.1X5	T41.1X6
Alfentanil	T4Ø.411	T4Ø.412	T4Ø.413	T4Ø.414	T4Ø.415	T4Ø.416
Alfuzosin (hydrochloride)	T44.8X1	T44.8X2	T44.8X3	T44.8X4	T44.8X5	T44.8X6
Algae (harmful) (toxin)	T65.821	T65.822	T65.823	T65.824	—	—
Algeldrate	T47.1X1	T47.1X2	T47.1X3	T47.1X4	T47.1X5	T47.1X6
Algin	T47.8X1	T47.8X2	T47.8X3	T47.8X4	T47.8X5	T47.8X6
Alglucerase	T45.3X1	T45.3X2	T45.3X3	T45.3X4	T45.3X5	T45.3X6
Alidase	T45.3X1	T45.3X2	T45.3X3	T45.3X4	T45.3X5	T45.3X6
Alimemazine	T43.3X1	T43.3X2	T43.3X3	T43.3X4	T43.3X5	T43.3X6
Aliphatic thiocyanates	T65.ØX1	T65.ØX2	T65.ØX3	T65.ØX4	—	—
Alitretinoin*	T49.ØX1	T49.ØX2	T49.ØX3	T49.ØX4	T49.ØX5	T49.ØX6
Alizapride	T45.ØX1	T45.ØX2	T45.ØX3	T45.ØX4	T45.ØX5	T45.ØX6
Alkali (caustic)	T54.3X1	T54.3X2	T54.3X3	T54.3X4	—	—
Alkaline antiseptic solution (aromatic)	T49.6X1	T49.6X2	T49.6X3	T49.6X4	T49.6X5	T49.6X6
Alkalinizing agents (medicinal)	T5Ø.9Ø1	T5Ø.9Ø2	T5Ø.9Ø3	T5Ø.9Ø4	T5Ø.9Ø5	T5Ø.9Ø6
Alkalizing agent NEC	T5Ø.9Ø1	T5Ø.9Ø2	T5Ø.9Ø3	T5Ø.9Ø4	T5Ø.9Ø5	T5Ø.9Ø6
Alka-seltzer	T39.Ø11	T39.Ø12	T39.Ø13	T39.Ø14	T39.Ø15	T39.Ø16
Alkavervir	T46.5X1	T46.5X2	T46.5X3	T46.5X4	T46.5X5	T46.5X6
Alkeran*	T45.1X1	T45.1X2	T45.1X3	T45.1X4	T45.1X5	T45.1X6
Alkonium (bromide)	T49.ØX1	T49.ØX2	T49.ØX3	T49.ØX4	T49.ØX5	T49.ØX6
Alkylating drug NEC	T45.1X1	T45.1X2	T45.1X3	T45.1X4	T45.1X5	T45.1X6
antimyeloproliferative	T45.1X1	T45.1X2	T45.1X3	T45.1X4	T45.1X5	T45.1X6
lymphatic	T45.1X1	T45.1X2	T45.1X3	T45.1X4	T45.1X5	T45.1X6
Alkylisocyanate	T65.ØX1	T65.ØX2	T65.ØX3	T65.ØX4	—	—
Allantoin	T49.4X1	T49.4X2	T49.4X3	T49.4X4	T49.4X5	T49.4X6
Allegron	T43.Ø11	T43.Ø12	T43.Ø13	T43.Ø14	T43.Ø15	T43.Ø16
Allethrin	T49.ØX1	T49.ØX2	T49.ØX3	T49.ØX4	T49.ØX5	T49.ØX6
Allobarbital	T42.3X1	T42.3X2	T42.3X3	T42.3X4	T42.3X5	T42.3X6
Allopurinol	T5Ø.4X1	T5Ø.4X2	T5Ø.4X3	T5Ø.4X4	T5Ø.4X5	T5Ø.4X6
Allyl						
alcohol	T51.8X1	T51.8X2	T51.8X3	T51.8X4	—	—
disulfide	T46.6X1	T46.6X2	T46.6X3	T46.6X4	T46.6X5	T46.6X6
Allylestrenol	T38.5X1	T38.5X2	T38.5X3	T38.5X4	T38.5X5	T38.5X6
Allylisopropylacetylurea	T42.6X1	T42.6X2	T42.6X3	T42.6X4	T42.6X5	T42.6X6
Allylisopropylmalonylurea	T42.3X1	T42.3X2	T42.3X3	T42.3X4	T42.3X5	T42.3X6
Allylthiourea	T49.3X1	T49.3X2	T49.3X3	T49.3X4	T49.3X5	T49.3X6
Allyltribromide	T42.6X1	T42.6X2	T42.6X3	T42.6X4	T42.6X5	T42.6X6
Allypropymal	T42.3X1	T42.3X2	T42.3X3	T42.3X4	T42.3X5	T42.3X6
Almagate	T47.1X1	T47.1X2	T47.1X3	T47.1X4	T47.1X5	T47.1X6
Almasilate	T47.1X1	T47.1X2	T47.1X3	T47.1X4	T47.1X5	T47.1X6
Almitrine	T5Ø.7X1	T5Ø.7X2	T5Ø.7X3	T5Ø.7X4	T5Ø.7X5	T5Ø.7X6
Aloes	T47.2X1	T47.2X2	T47.2X3	T47.2X4	T47.2X5	T47.2X6
Aloglutamol	T47.1X1	T47.1X2	T47.1X3	T47.1X4	T47.1X5	T47.1X6
Aloin	T47.2X1	T47.2X2	T47.2X3	T47.2X4	T47.2X5	T47.2X6
Aloxidone	T42.2X1	T42.2X2	T42.2X3	T42.2X4	T42.2X5	T42.2X6
Alpha						
acetyldigoxin	T46.ØX1	T46.ØX2	T46.ØX3	T46.ØX4	T46.ØX5	T46.ØX6
adrenergic blocking drug	T44.6X1	T44.6X2	T44.6X3	T44.6X4	T44.6X5	T44.6X6
amylase	T45.3X1	T45.3X2	T45.3X3	T45.3X4	T45.3X5	T45.3X6
tocoferol (acetate)	T45.2X1	T45.2X2	T45.2X3	T45.2X4	T45.2X5	T45.2X6
tocopherol	T45.2X1	T45.2X2	T45.2X3	T45.2X4	T45.2X5	T45.2X6
Alphadolone	T41.1X1	T41.1X2	T41.1X3	T41.1X4	T41.1X5	T41.1X6
Alphaprodine	T4Ø.491	T4Ø.492	T4Ø.493	T4Ø.494	T4Ø.495	T4Ø.496
Alphaxalone	T41.1X1	T41.1X2	T41.1X3	T41.1X4	T41.1X5	T41.1X6
Alprazolam	T42.4X1	T42.4X2	T42.4X3	T42.4X4	T42.4X5	T42.4X6
Alprenolol	T44.7X1	T44.7X2	T44.7X3	T44.7X4	T44.7X5	T44.7X6
Alprostadil	T46.7X1	T46.7X2	T46.7X3	T46.7X4	T46.7X5	T46.7X6
Alsactide	T38.811	T38.812	T38.813	T38.814	T38.815	T38.816
Alseroxylon	T46.5X1	T46.5X2	T46.5X3	T46.5X4	T46.5X5	T46.5X6
Alteplase	T45.611	T45.612	T45.613	T45.614	T45.615	T45.616
Altizide	T5Ø.2X1	T5Ø.2X2	T5Ø.2X3	T5Ø.2X4	T5Ø.2X5	T5Ø.2X6
Altoprev*	T46.6X1	T46.6X2	T46.6X3	T46.6X4	T46.6X5	T46.6X6
Altretamine	T45.1X1	T45.1X2	T45.1X3	T45.1X4	T45.1X5	T45.1X6
Alum (medicinal)	T49.4X1	T49.4X2	T49.4X3	T49.4X4	T49.4X5	T49.4X6
nonmedicinal (ammonium) (potassium)	T56.891	T56.892	T56.893	T56.894	—	—
Aluminium, aluminum						
acetate	T49.2X1	T49.2X2	T49.2X3	T49.2X4	T49.2X5	T49.2X6
solution	T49.ØX1	T49.ØX2	T49.ØX3	T49.ØX4	T49.ØX5	T49.ØX6
aspirin	T39.Ø11	T39.Ø12	T39.Ø13	T39.Ø14	T39.Ø15	T39.Ø16
bis (acetylsalicylate)	T39.Ø11	T39.Ø12	T39.Ø13	T39.Ø14	T39.Ø15	T39.Ø16
carbonate (gel, basic)	T47.1X1	T47.1X2	T47.1X3	T47.1X4	T47.1X5	T47.1X6
chlorhydroxide-complex	T47.1X1	T47.1X2	T47.1X3	T47.1X4	T47.1X5	T47.1X6
chloride	T49.2X1	T49.2X2	T49.2X3	T49.2X4	T49.2X5	T49.2X6
clofibrate	T46.6X1	T46.6X2	T46.6X3	T46.6X4	T46.6X5	T46.6X6
diacetate	T49.2X1	T49.2X2	T49.2X3	T49.2X4	T49.2X5	T49.2X6
glycinate	T47.1X1	T47.1X2	T47.1X3	T47.1X4	T47.1X5	T47.1X6
hydroxide (gel)	T47.1X1	T47.1X2	T47.1X3	T47.1X4	T47.1X5	T47.1X6
hydroxide-magnesium carb. gel	T47.1X1	T47.1X2	T47.1X3	T47.1X4	T47.1X5	T47.1X6
magnesium silicate	T47.1X1	T47.1X2	T47.1X3	T47.1X4	T47.1X5	T47.1X6

Substance	Poisoning, Accidental (unintentional)	Poisoning, Intentional Self-harm	Poisoning, Assault	Poisoning, Undetermined	Adverse Effect	Under-dosing
Aluminium, aluminum — *continued*						
nicotinate	T46.7X1	T46.7X2	T46.7X3	T46.7X4	T46.7X5	T46.7X6
ointment (surgical) (topical)	T49.3X1	T49.3X2	T49.3X3	T49.3X4	T49.3X5	T49.3X6
phosphate	T47.1X1	T47.1X2	T47.1X3	T47.1X4	T47.1X5	T47.1X6
salicylate	T39.Ø91	T39.Ø92	T39.Ø93	T39.Ø94	T39.Ø95	T39.Ø96
silicate	T47.1X1	T47.1X2	T47.1X3	T47.1X4	T47.1X5	T47.1X6
sodium silicate	T47.1X1	T47.1X2	T47.1X3	T47.1X4	T47.1X5	T47.1X6
subacetate	T49.2X1	T49.2X2	T49.2X3	T49.2X4	T49.2X5	T49.2X6
sulfate	T49.ØX1	T49.ØX2	T49.ØX3	T49.ØX4	T49.ØX5	T49.ØX6
tannate	T47.6X1	T47.6X2	T47.6X3	T47.6X4	T47.6X5	T47.6X6
topical NEC	T49.3X1	T49.3X2	T49.3X3	T49.3X4	T49.3X5	T49.3X6
Alurate	T42.3X1	T42.3X2	T42.3X3	T42.3X4	T42.3X5	T42.3X6
Alverine	T44.3X1	T44.3X2	T44.3X3	T44.3X4	T44.3X5	T44.3X6
Alvodine	T4Ø.2X1	T4Ø.2X2	T4Ø.2X3	T4Ø.2X4	T4Ø.2X5	T4Ø.2X6
Amanita phalloides	T62.ØX1	T62.ØX2	T62.ØX3	T62.ØX4	—	—
Amanitine	T62.ØX1	T62.ØX2	T62.ØX3	T62.ØX4	—	—
Amantadine	T42.8X1	T42.8X2	T42.8X3	T42.8X4	T42.8X5	T42.8X6
Ambazone	T49.6X1	T49.6X2	T49.6X3	T49.6X4	T49.6X5	T49.6X6
Ambenonium (chloride)	T44.ØX1	T44.ØX2	T44.ØX3	T44.ØX4	T44.ØX5	T44.ØX6
Ambroxol	T48.4X1	T48.4X2	T48.4X3	T48.4X4	T48.4X5	T48.4X6
Ambuphylline	T48.6X1	T48.6X2	T48.6X3	T48.6X4	T48.6X5	T48.6X6
Ambutonium bromide	T44.3X1	T44.3X2	T44.3X3	T44.3X4	T44.3X5	T44.3X6
Amcinonide	T49.ØX1	T49.ØX2	T49.ØX3	T49.ØX4	T49.ØX5	T49.ØX6
Amdinocilline	T36.ØX1	T36.ØX2	T36.ØX3	T36.ØX4	T36.ØX5	T36.ØX6
Americaine*	T41.3X1	T41.3X2	T41.3X3	T41.3X4	T41.3X5	T41.3X6
Ametazole	T5Ø.8X1	T5Ø.8X2	T5Ø.8X3	T5Ø.8X4	T5Ø.8X5	T5Ø.8X6
Amethocaine	T41.3X1	T41.3X2	T41.3X3	T41.3X4	T41.3X5	T41.3X6
regional	T41.3X1	T41.3X2	T41.3X3	T41.3X4	T41.3X5	T41.3X6
spinal	T41.3X1	T41.3X2	T41.3X3	T41.3X4	T41.3X5	T41.3X6
Amethopterin	T45.1X1	T45.1X2	T45.1X3	T45.1X4	T45.1X5	T45.1X6
Amezinium metilsulfate	T44.991	T44.992	T44.993	T44.994	T44.995	T44.996
Amfebutamone	T43.291	T43.292	T43.293	T43.294	T43.295	T43.296
Amfepramone	T5Ø.5X1	T5Ø.5X2	T5Ø.5X3	T5Ø.5X4	T5Ø.5X5	T5Ø.5X6
Amfetamine	T43.621	T43.622	T43.623	T43.624	T43.625	T43.626
Amfetaminil	T43.621	T43.622	T43.623	T43.624	T43.625	T43.626
Amfomycin	T36.8X1	T36.8X2	T36.8X3	T36.8X4	T36.8X5	T36.8X6
Amidefrine mesilate	T48.5X1	T48.5X2	T48.5X3	T48.5X4	T48.5X5	T48.5X6
Amidone	T4Ø.3X1	T4Ø.3X2	T4Ø.3X3	T4Ø.3X4	T4Ø.3X5	T4Ø.3X6
Amidopyrine	T39.2X1	T39.2X2	T39.2X3	T39.2X4	T39.2X5	T39.2X6
Amidotrizoate	T5Ø.8X1	T5Ø.8X2	T5Ø.8X3	T5Ø.8X4	T5Ø.8X5	T5Ø.8X6
Amiflamine	T43.1X1	T43.1X2	T43.1X3	T43.1X4	T43.1X5	T43.1X6
Amikacin	T36.5X1	T36.5X2	T36.5X3	T36.5X4	T36.5X5	T36.5X6
Amikhelline	T46.3X1	T46.3X2	T46.3X3	T46.3X4	T46.3X5	T46.3X6
Amiloride	T5Ø.2X1	T5Ø.2X2	T5Ø.2X3	T5Ø.2X4	T5Ø.2X5	T5Ø.2X6
Aminacrine	T49.ØX1	T49.ØX2	T49.ØX3	T49.ØX4	T49.ØX5	T49.ØX6
Amineptine	T43.Ø11	T43.Ø12	T43.Ø13	T43.Ø14	T43.Ø15	T43.Ø16
Aminitrozole	T37.3X1	T37.3X2	T37.3X3	T37.3X4	T37.3X5	T37.3X6
Aminoacetic acid (derivatives)	T5Ø.3X1	T5Ø.3X2	T5Ø.3X3	T5Ø.3X4	T5Ø.3X5	T5Ø.3X6
Amino acids	T5Ø.3X1	T5Ø.3X2	T5Ø.3X3	T5Ø.3X4	T5Ø.3X5	T5Ø.3X6
Aminoacridine	T49.ØX1	T49.ØX2	T49.ØX3	T49.ØX4	T49.ØX5	T49.ØX6
Aminobenzoic acid (-p)	T49.3X1	T49.3X2	T49.3X3	T49.3X4	T49.3X5	T49.3X6
Aminocaproic acid	T45.621	T45.622	T45.623	T45.624	T45.625	T45.626
Aminoethylisothiourium	T45.8X1	T45.8X2	T45.8X3	T45.8X4	T45.8X5	T45.8X6
Aminofenazone	T39.2X1	T39.2X2	T39.2X3	T39.2X4	T39.2X5	T39.2X6
Aminoglutethimide	T45.1X1	T45.1X2	T45.1X3	T45.1X4	T45.1X5	T45.1X6
Aminoglycosides*	T36.5X1	T36.5X2	T36.5X3	T36.5X4	T36.5X5	T36.5X6
Aminohippuric acid	T5Ø.8X1	T5Ø.8X2	T5Ø.8X3	T5Ø.8X4	T5Ø.8X5	T5Ø.8X6
Aminomethylbenzoic acid	T45.691	T45.692	T45.693	T45.694	T45.695	T45.696
Aminometradine	T5Ø.2X1	T5Ø.2X2	T5Ø.2X3	T5Ø.2X4	T5Ø.2X5	T5Ø.2X6
Aminopentamide	T44.3X1	T44.3X2	T44.3X3	T44.3X4	T44.3X5	T44.3X6
Aminophenazone	T39.2X1	T39.2X2	T39.2X3	T39.2X4	T39.2X5	T39.2X6
Aminophenol	T54.ØX1	T54.ØX2	T54.ØX3	T54.ØX4	—	—
Aminophenylpyridone	T43.591	T43.592	T43.593	T43.594	T43.595	T43.596
Aminophylline	T48.6X1	T48.6X2	T48.6X3	T48.6X4	T48.6X5	T48.6X6
Aminopterin sodium	T45.1X1	T45.1X2	T45.1X3	T45.1X4	T45.1X5	T45.1X6
Aminopyrine	T39.2X1	T39.2X2	T39.2X3	T39.2X4	T39.2X5	T39.2X6
Aminorex	T5Ø.5X1	T5Ø.5X2	T5Ø.5X3	T5Ø.5X4	T5Ø.5X5	T5Ø.5X6
Aminosalicylic acid	T37.1X1	T37.1X2	T37.1X3	T37.1X4	T37.1X5	T37.1X6
Aminosalylum	T37.1X1	T37.1X2	T37.1X3	T37.1X4	T37.1X5	T37.1X6
Amiodarone	T46.2X1	T46.2X2	T46.2X3	T46.2X4	T46.2X5	T46.2X6
Amiphenazole	T5Ø.7X1	T5Ø.7X2	T5Ø.7X3	T5Ø.7X4	T5Ø.7X5	T5Ø.7X6
Amiquinsin	T46.5X1	T46.5X2	T46.5X3	T46.5X4	T46.5X5	T46.5X6
Amisometradine	T5Ø.2X1	T5Ø.2X2	T5Ø.2X3	T5Ø.2X4	T5Ø.2X5	T5Ø.2X6
Amisulpride	T43.591	T43.592	T43.593	T43.594	T43.595	T43.596
Amitriptyline	T43.Ø11	T43.Ø12	T43.Ø13	T43.Ø14	T43.Ø15	T43.Ø16
Amitriptylinoxide	T43.Ø11	T43.Ø12	T43.Ø13	T43.Ø14	T43.Ø15	T43.Ø16
Amlexanox	T48.6X1	T48.6X2	T48.6X3	T48.6X4	T48.6X5	T48.6X6
Ammonia (fumes) (gas) (vapor)	T59.891	T59.892	T59.893	T59.894	—	—
aromatic spirit	T48.991	T48.992	T48.993	T48.994	T48.995	T48.996
Ammonia — *continued*						
liquid (household)	T54.3X1	T54.3X2	T54.3X3	T54.3X4	—	—
Ammoniated mercury	T49.ØX1	T49.ØX2	T49.ØX3	T49.ØX4	T49.ØX5	T49.ØX6
Ammonium						
acid tartrate	T49.5X1	T49.5X2	T49.5X3	T49.5X4	T49.5X5	T49.5X6
bromide	T42.6X1	T42.6X2	T42.6X3	T42.6X4	T42.6X5	T42.6X6
carbonate	T54.3X1	T54.3X2	T54.3X3	T54.3X4	—	—
chloride	T5Ø.991	T5Ø.992	T5Ø.993	T5Ø.994	T5Ø.995	T5Ø.996
expectorant	T48.4X1	T48.4X2	T48.4X3	T48.4X4	T48.4X5	T48.4X6
compounds (household)	T54.3X1	T54.3X2	T54.3X3	T54.3X4	—	—
NEC						
fumes (any usage)	T59.891	T59.892	T59.893	T59.894	—	—
industrial	T54.3X1	T54.3X2	T54.3X3	T54.3X4	—	—
ichthyosulronate	T49.4X1	T49.4X2	T49.4X3	T49.4X4	T49.4X5	T49.4X6
mandelate	T37.91	T37.92	T37.93	T37.94	T37.95	T37.96
sulfamate	T6Ø.3X1	T6Ø.3X2	T6Ø.3X3	T6Ø.3X4	—	—
sulfonate resin	T47.8X1	T47.8X2	T47.8X3	T47.8X4	T47.8X5	T47.8X6
Amobarbital (sodium)	T42.3X1	T42.3X2	T42.3X3	T42.3X4	T42.3X5	T42.3X6
Amodiaquine	T37.2X1	T37.2X2	T37.2X3	T37.2X4	T37.2X5	T37.2X6
Amopyroquin (e)	T37.2X1	T37.2X2	T37.2X3	T37.2X4	T37.2X5	T37.2X6
Amoxapine	T43.Ø11	T43.Ø12	T43.Ø13	T43.Ø14	T43.Ø15	T43.Ø16
Amoxicillin	T36.ØX1	T36.ØX2	T36.ØX3	T36.ØX4	T36.ØX5	T36.ØX6
Amperozide	T43.591	T43.592	T43.593	T43.594	T43.595	T43.596
Amphenidone	T43.591	T43.592	T43.593	T43.594	T43.595	T43.596
Amphetamine NEC	T43.621	T43.622	T43.623	T43.624	T43.625	T43.626
Amphogel*	T47.1X1	T47.1X2	T47.1X3	T47.1X4	T47.1X5	T47.1X6
Amphomycin	T36.8X1	T36.8X2	T36.8X3	T36.8X4	T36.8X5	T36.8X6
Amphotalide	T37.4X1	T37.4X2	T37.4X3	T37.4X4	T37.4X5	T37.4X6
Amphotericin B	T36.7X1	T36.7X2	T36.7X3	T36.7X4	T36.7X5	T36.7X6
topical	T49.ØX1	T49.ØX2	T49.ØX3	T49.ØX4	T49.ØX5	T49.ØX6
Ampicillin	T36.ØX1	T36.ØX2	T36.ØX3	T36.ØX4	T36.ØX5	T36.ØX6
Amprotropine	T44.3X1	T44.3X2	T44.3X3	T44.3X4	T44.3X5	T44.3X6
Amsacrine	T45.1X1	T45.1X2	T45.1X3	T45.1X4	T45.1X5	T45.1X6
Amygdaline	T62.2X1	T62.2X2	T62.2X3	T62.2X4	—	—
Amyl						
acetate	T52.8X1	T52.8X2	T52.8X3	T52.8X4	—	—
vapor	T59.891	T59.892	T59.893	T59.894	—	—
alcohol	T51.3X1	T51.3X2	T51.3X3	T51.3X4	—	—
chloride	T53.6X1	T53.6X2	T53.6X3	T53.6X4	—	—
formate	T52.8X1	T52.8X2	T52.8X3	T52.8X4	—	—
nitrite	T46.3X1	T46.3X2	T46.3X3	T46.3X4	T46.3X5	T46.3X6
propionate	T65.891	T65.892	T65.893	T65.894	—	—
Amylase	T47.5X1	T47.5X2	T47.5X3	T47.5X4	T47.5X5	T47.5X6
Amyleine, regional	T41.3X1	T41.3X2	T41.3X3	T41.3X4	T41.3X5	T41.3X6
Amylene						
dichloride	T53.6X1	T53.6X2	T53.6X3	T53.6X4	—	—
hydrate	T51.3X1	T51.3X2	T51.3X3	T51.3X4	—	—
Amylmetacresol	T49.6X1	T49.6X2	T49.6X3	T49.6X4	T49.6X5	T49.6X6
Amylobarbitone	T42.3X1	T42.3X2	T42.3X3	T42.3X4	T42.3X5	T42.3X6
Amylocaine, regional	T41.3X1	T41.3X2	T41.3X3	T41.3X4	T41.3X5	T41.3X6
infiltration (subcutaneous)	T41.3X1	T41.3X2	T41.3X3	T41.3X4	T41.3X5	T41.3X6
nerve block (peripheral) (plexus)	T41.3X1	T41.3X2	T41.3X3	T41.3X4	T41.3X5	T41.3X6
spinal	T41.3X1	T41.3X2	T41.3X3	T41.3X4	T41.3X5	T41.3X6
topical (surface)	T41.3X1	T41.3X2	T41.3X3	T41.3X4	T41.3X5	T41.3X6
Amylopectin	T47.6X1	T47.6X2	T47.6X3	T47.6X4	T47.6X5	T47.6X6
Amytal (sodium)	T42.3X1	T42.3X2	T42.3X3	T42.3X4	T42.3X5	T42.3X6
Anabolic steroid	T38.7X1	T38.7X2	T38.7X3	T38.7X4	T38.7X5	T38.7X6
Anacaine*	T41.3X1	T41.3X2	T41.3X3	T41.3X4	T41.3X5	T41.3X6
Analeptic NEC	T5Ø.7X1	T5Ø.7X2	T5Ø.7X3	T5Ø.7X4	T5Ø.7X5	T5Ø.7X6
Analgesic	T39.91	T39.92	T39.93	T39.94	T39.95	T39.96
anti-inflammatory NEC	T39.91	T39.92	T39.93	T39.94	T39.95	T39.96
propionic acid derivative	T39.311	T39.312	T39.313	T39.314	T39.315	T39.316
antirheumatic NEC	T39.4X1	T39.4X2	T39.4X3	T39.4X4	T39.4X5	T39.4X6
aromatic NEC	T39.1X1	T39.1X2	T39.1X3	T39.1X4	T39.1X5	T39.1X6
narcotic NEC	T4Ø.6Ø1	T4Ø.6Ø2	T4Ø.6Ø3	T4Ø.6Ø4	T4Ø.6Ø5	T4Ø.6Ø6
combination	T4Ø.6Ø1	T4Ø.6Ø2	T4Ø.6Ø3	T4Ø.6Ø4	T4Ø.6Ø5	T4Ø.6Ø6
obstetric	T4Ø.6Ø1	T4Ø.6Ø2	T4Ø.6Ø3	T4Ø.6Ø4	T4Ø.6Ø5	T4Ø.6Ø6
non-narcotic NEC	T39.91	T39.92	T39.93	T39.94	T39.95	T39.96
combination	T39.91	T39.92	T39.93	T39.94	T39.95	T39.96
pyrazole	T39.2X1	T39.2X2	T39.2X3	T39.2X4	T39.2X5	T39.2X6
specified NEC	T39.8X1	T39.8X2	T39.8X3	T39.8X4	T39.8X5	T39.8X6
Analgin	T39.2X1	T39.2X2	T39.2X3	T39.2X4	T39.2X5	T39.2X6
Anamirta cocculus	T62.1X1	T62.1X2	T62.1X3	T62.1X4	—	—
Ancillin	T36.ØX1	T36.ØX2	T36.ØX3	T36.ØX4	T36.ØX5	T36.ØX6
Ancrod	T45.691	T45.692	T45.693	T45.694	T45.695	T45.696
Androgen	T38.7X1	T38.7X2	T38.7X3	T38.7X4	T38.7X5	T38.7X6
Androgen-estrogen mixture	T38.7X1	T38.7X2	T38.7X3	T38.7X4	T38.7X5	T38.7X6
Androstalone	T38.7X1	T38.7X2	T38.7X3	T38.7X4	T38.7X5	T38.7X6
Androstanolone	T38.7X1	T38.7X2	T38.7X3	T38.7X4	T38.7X5	T38.7X6
Androsterone	T38.7X1	T38.7X2	T38.7X3	T38.7X4	T38.7X5	T38.7X6
Anemone pulsatilla	T62.2X1	T62.2X2	T62.2X3	T62.2X4	—	—

Substance	Poisoning, Accidental (unintentional)	Poisoning, Intentional Self-harm	Poisoning, Assault	Poisoning, Undetermined	Adverse Effect	Under-dosing
Anesthesia						
caudal	T41.3X1	T41.3X2	T41.3X3	T41.3X4	T41.3X5	T41.3X6
endotracheal	T41.ØX1	T41.ØX2	T41.ØX3	T41.ØX4	T41.ØX5	T41.ØX6
epidural	T41.3X1	T41.3X2	T41.3X3	T41.3X4	T41.3X5	T41.3X6
inhalation	T41.ØX1	T41.ØX2	T41.ØX3	T41.ØX4	T41.ØX5	T41.ØX6
local	T41.3X1	T41.3X2	T41.3X3	T41.3X4	T41.3X5	T41.3X6
mucosal	T41.3X1	T41.3X2	T41.3X3	T41.3X4	T41.3X5	T41.3X6
muscle relaxation	T48.1X1	T48.1X2	T48.1X3	T48.1X4	T48.1X5	T48.1X6
nerve blocking	T41.3X1	T41.3X2	T41.3X3	T41.3X4	T41.3X5	T41.3X6
plexus blocking	T41.3X1	T41.3X2	T41.3X3	T41.3X4	T41.3X5	T41.3X6
potentiated	T41.201	T41.202	T41.203	T41.204	T41.205	T41.206
rectal	T41.201	T41.202	T41.203	T41.204	T41.205	T41.206
— general	T41.201	T41.202	T41.203	T41.204	T41.205	T41.206
— local	T41.3X1	T41.3X2	T41.3X3	T41.3X4	T41.3X5	T41.3X6
regional	T41.3X1	T41.3X2	T41.3X3	T41.3X4	T41.3X5	T41.3X6
surface	T41.3X1	T41.3X2	T41.3X3	T41.3X4	T41.3X5	T41.3X6
Anesthetic NEC — *see also* Anesthesia	T41.41	T41.42	T41.43	T41.44	T41.45	T41.46
with muscle relaxant	T41.201	T41.202	T41.203	T41.204	T41.205	T41.206
— general	T41.201	T41.202	T41.203	T41.204	T41.205	T41.206
— local	T41.3X1	T41.3X2	T41.3X3	T41.3X4	T41.3X5	T41.3X6
gaseous NEC	T41.ØX1	T41.ØX2	T41.ØX3	T41.ØX4	T41.ØX5	T41.ØX6
general NEC	T41.201	T41.202	T41.203	T41.204	T41.205	T41.206
halogenated hydrocarbon derivatives NEC	T41.ØX1	T41.ØX2	T41.ØX3	T41.ØX4	T41.ØX5	T41.ØX6
infiltration NEC	T41.3X1	T41.3X2	T41.3X3	T41.3X4	T41.3X5	T41.3X6
intravenous NEC	T41.1X1	T41.1X2	T41.1X3	T41.1X4	T41.1X5	T41.1X6
local NEC	T41.3X1	T41.3X2	T41.3X3	T41.3X4	T41.3X5	T41.3X6
rectal	T41.201	T41.202	T41.203	T41.204	T41.205	T41.206
— general	T41.201	T41.202	T41.203	T41.204	T41.205	T41.206
— local	T41.3X1	T41.3X2	T41.3X3	T41.3X4	T41.3X5	T41.3X6
regional NEC	T41.3X1	T41.3X2	T41.3X3	T41.3X4	T41.3X5	T41.3X6
spinal NEC	T41.3X1	T41.3X2	T41.3X3	T41.3X4	T41.3X5	T41.3X6
thiobarbiturate	T41.1X1	T41.1X2	T41.1X3	T41.1X4	T41.1X5	T41.1X6
topical	T41.3X1	T41.3X2	T41.3X3	T41.3X4	T41.3X5	T41.3X6
Aneurine	T45.2X1	T45.2X2	T45.2X3	T45.2X4	T45.2X5	T45.2X6
Angeliq*	T38.5X1	T38.5X2	T38.5X3	T38.5X4	T38.5X5	T38.5X6
Angio-Conray	T5Ø.8X1	T5Ø.8X2	T5Ø.8X3	T5Ø.8X4	T5Ø.8X5	T5Ø.8X6
Angiotensin	T44.5X1	T44.5X2	T44.5X3	T44.5X4	T44.5X5	T44.5X6
Angiotensinamide	T44.991	T44.992	T44.993	T44.994	T44.995	T44.996
Anhydrohydroxy-progesterone	T38.5X1	T38.5X2	T38.5X3	T38.5X4	T38.5X5	T38.5X6
Anhydron	T5Ø.2X1	T5Ø.2X2	T5Ø.2X3	T5Ø.2X4	T5Ø.2X5	T5Ø.2X6
Anileridine	T4Ø.491	T4Ø.492	T4Ø.493	T4Ø.494	T4Ø.495	T4Ø.496
Aniline (dye) (liquid)	T65.3X1	T65.3X2	T65.3X3	T65.3X4		
analgesic	T39.1X1	T39.1X2	T39.1X3	T39.1X4	T39.1X5	T39.1X6
derivatives, therapeutic NEC	T39.1X1	T39.1X2	T39.1X3	T39.1X4	T39.1X5	T39.1X6
vapor	T65.3X1	T65.3X2	T65.3X3	T65.3X4	—	—
Aniscoropine	T44.3X1	T44.3X2	T44.3X3	T44.3X4	T44.3X5	T44.3X6
Anise oil	T47.5X1	T47.5X2	T47.5X3	T47.5X4	T47.5X5	T47.5X6
Anisidine	T65.3X1	T65.3X2	T65.3X3	T65.3X4	—	—
Anisindione	T45.511	T45.512	T45.513	T45.514	T45.515	T45.516
Anisotropine methyl-bromide	T44.3X1	T44.3X2	T44.3X3	T44.3X4	T44.3X5	T44.3X6
Anistreplase	T45.611	T45.612	T45.613	T45.614	T45.615	T45.616
Anorexiant (central)	T5Ø.5X1	T5Ø.5X2	T5Ø.5X3	T5Ø.5X4	T5Ø.5X5	T5Ø.5X6
Anorexic agents	T5Ø.5X1	T5Ø.5X2	T5Ø.5X3	T5Ø.5X4	T5Ø.5X5	T5Ø.5X6
Ansaid*	T39.311	T39.312	T39.313	T39.314	T39.315	T39.316
Ansamycin	T36.6X1	T36.6X2	T36.6X3	T36.6X4	T36.6X5	T36.6X6
Ant (bite) (sting)	T63.421	T63.422	T63.423	T63.424	—	—
Antabuse	T5Ø.6X1	T5Ø.6X2	T5Ø.6X3	T5Ø.6X4	T5Ø.6X5	T5Ø.6X6
Antacid NEC	T47.1X1	T47.1X2	T47.1X3	T47.1X4	T47.1X5	T47.1X6
Antagonist						
Aldosterone	T5Ø.ØX1	T5Ø.ØX2	T5Ø.ØX3	T5Ø.ØX4	T5Ø.ØX5	T5Ø.ØX6
alpha-adrenoreceptor	T44.6X1	T44.6X2	T44.6X3	T44.6X4	T44.6X5	T44.6X6
anticoagulant	T45.7X1	T45.7X2	T45.7X3	T45.7X4	T45.7X5	T45.7X6
beta-adrenoreceptor	T44.7X1	T44.7X2	T44.7X3	T44.7X4	T44.7X5	T44.7X6
extrapyramidal NEC	T44.3X1	T44.3X2	T44.3X3	T44.3X4	T44.3X5	T44.3X6
folic acid	T45.1X1	T45.1X2	T45.1X3	T45.1X4	T45.1X5	T45.1X6
H2 receptor	T47.ØX1	T47.ØX2	T47.ØX3	T47.ØX4	T47.ØX5	T47.ØX6
heavy metal	T45.8X1	T45.8X2	T45.8X3	T45.8X4	T45.8X5	T45.8X6
narcotic analgesic	T5Ø.7X1	T5Ø.7X2	T5Ø.7X3	T5Ø.7X4	T5Ø.7X5	T5Ø.7X6
opiate	T5Ø.7X1	T5Ø.7X2	T5Ø.7X3	T5Ø.7X4	T5Ø.7X5	T5Ø.7X6
pyrimidine	T45.1X1	T45.1X2	T45.1X3	T45.1X4	T45.1X5	T45.1X6
serotonin	T46.5X1	T46.5X2	T46.5X3	T46.5X4	T46.5X5	T46.5X6
Antazolin (e)	T45.ØX1	T45.ØX2	T45.ØX3	T45.ØX4	T45.ØX5	T45.ØX6
Anterior pituitary hormone NEC	T38.811	T38.812	T38.813	T38.814	T38.815	T38.816
Anthelmintic NEC	T37.4X1	T37.4X2	T37.4X3	T37.4X4	T37.4X5	T37.4X6
Anthiolimine	T37.4X1	T37.4X2	T37.4X3	T37.4X4	T37.4X5	T37.4X6
Anthralin	T49.4X1	T49.4X2	T49.4X3	T49.4X4	T49.4X5	T49.4X6
Anthramycin	T45.1X1	T45.1X2	T45.1X3	T45.1X4	T45.1X5	T45.1X6
Antiadrenergic NEC	T44.8X1	T44.8X2	T44.8X3	T44.8X4	T44.8X5	T44.8X6
Antiallergic NEC	T45.ØX1	T45.ØX2	T45.ØX3	T45.ØX4	T45.ØX5	T45.ØX6
Antiandrogen NEC	T38.6X1	T38.6X2	T38.6X3	T38.6X4	T38.6X5	T38.6X6
Anti-anemic (drug) (preparation)	T45.8X1	T45.8X2	T45.8X3	T45.8X4	T45.8X5	T45.8X6
Antianxiety drug NEC	T43.5Ø1	T43.5Ø2	T43.5Ø3	T43.5Ø4	T43.5Ø5	T43.5Ø6
Antiaris toxicaria	T65.891	T65.892	T65.893	T65.894	—	—
Antiarteriosclerotic drug	T46.6X1	T46.6X2	T46.6X3	T46.6X4	T46.6X5	T46.6X6
Antiasthmatic drug NEC	T48.6X1	T48.6X2	T48.6X3	T48.6X4	T48.6X5	T48.6X6
Antibiotic Otic Suspension (Solution)*	T49.6X1	T49.6X2	T49.6X3	T49.6X4	T49.6X5	T49.6X6
Antibiotic NEC	T36.91	T36.92	T36.93	T36.94	T36.95	T36.96
aminoglycoside	T36.5X1	T36.5X2	T36.5X3	T36.5X4	T36.5X5	T36.5X6
anticancer	T45.1X1	T45.1X2	T45.1X3	T45.1X4	T45.1X5	T45.1X6
antifungal	T36.7X1	T36.7X2	T36.7X3	T36.7X4	T36.7X5	T36.7X6
antimycobacterial	T36.5X1	T36.5X2	T36.5X3	T36.5X4	T36.5X5	T36.5X6
antineoplastic	T45.1X1	T45.1X2	T45.1X3	T45.1X4	T45.1X5	T45.1X6
b-lactam NEC	T36.1X1	T36.1X2	T36.1X3	T36.1X4	T36.1X5	T36.1X6
cephalosporin (group)	T36.1X1	T36.1X2	T36.1X3	T36.1X4	T36.1X5	T36.1X6
chloramphenicol (group)	T36.2X1	T36.2X2	T36.2X3	T36.2X4	T36.2X5	T36.2X6
ENT	T49.6X1	T49.6X2	T49.6X3	T49.6X4	T49.6X5	T49.6X6
eye	T49.5X1	T49.5X2	T49.5X3	T49.5X4	T49.5X5	T49.5X6
fungicidal (local)	T49.ØX1	T49.ØX2	T49.ØX3	T49.ØX4	T49.ØX5	T49.ØX6
intestinal	T36.8X1	T36.8X2	T36.8X3	T36.8X4	T36.8X5	T36.8X6
local	T49.ØX1	T49.ØX2	T49.ØX3	T49.ØX4	T49.ØX5	T49.ØX6
macrolides	T36.3X1	T36.3X2	T36.3X3	T36.3X4	T36.3X5	T36.3X6
polypeptide	T36.8X1	T36.8X2	T36.8X3	T36.8X4	T36.8X5	T36.8X6
specified NEC	T36.8X1	T36.8X2	T36.8X3	T36.8X4	T36.8X5	T36.8X6
tetracycline (group)	T36.4X1	T36.4X2	T36.4X3	T36.4X4	T36.4X5	T36.4X6
throat	T49.6X1	T49.6X2	T49.6X3	T49.6X4	T49.6X5	T49.6X6
Anticancer agents NEC	T45.1X1	T45.1X2	T45.1X3	T45.1X4	T45.1X5	T45.1X6
Anticholesterolemic drug NEC	T46.6X1	T46.6X2	T46.6X3	T46.6X4	T46.6X5	T46.6X6
Anticholinergic NEC	T44.3X1	T44.3X2	T44.3X3	T44.3X4	T44.3X5	T44.3X6
Anticholinesterase	T44.ØX1	T44.ØX2	T44.ØX3	T44.ØX4	T44.ØX5	T44.ØX6
organophosphorus	T44.ØX1	T44.ØX2	T44.ØX3	T44.ØX4	T44.ØX5	T44.ØX6
insecticide	T6Ø.ØX1	T6Ø.ØX2	T6Ø.ØX3	T6Ø.ØX4	—	—
nerve gas	T59.891	T59.892	T59.893	T59.894	—	—
reversible	T44.ØX1	T44.ØX2	T44.ØX3	T44.ØX4	T44.ØX5	T44.ØX6
ophthalmological	T49.5X1	T49.5X2	T49.5X3	T49.5X4	T49.5X5	T49.5X6
Anticoagulant NEC	T45.511	T45.512	T45.513	T45.514	T45.515	T45.516
Antagonist	T45.7X1	T45.7X2	T45.7X3	T45.7X4	T45.7X5	T45.7X6
Anti-common-cold drug NEC	T48.5X1	T48.5X2	T48.5X3	T48.5X4	T48.5X5	T48.5X6
Anticonvulsant	T42.71	T42.72	T42.73	T42.74	T42.75	T42.76
barbiturate	T42.3X1	T42.3X2	T42.3X3	T42.3X4	T42.3X5	T42.3X6
combination (with barbiturate)	T42.3X1	T42.3X2	T42.3X3	T42.3X4	T42.3X5	T42.3X6
hydantoin	T42.ØX1	T42.ØX2	T42.ØX3	T42.ØX4	T42.ØX5	T42.ØX6
hypnotic NEC	T42.6X1	T42.6X2	T42.6X3	T42.6X4	T42.6X5	T42.6X6
oxazolidinedione	T42.2X1	T42.2X2	T42.2X3	T42.2X4	T42.2X5	T42.2X6
pyrimidinedione	T42.6X1	T42.6X2	T42.6X3	T42.6X4	T42.6X5	T42.6X6
specified NEC	T42.6X1	T42.6X2	T42.6X3	T42.6X4	T42.6X5	T42.6X6
succinimide	T42.2X1	T42.2X2	T42.2X3	T42.2X4	T42.2X5	T42.2X6
Antidepressant	T43.2Ø1	T43.2Ø2	T43.2Ø3	T43.2Ø4	T43.2Ø5	T43.2Ø6
monoamine oxidase inhibitor	T43.1X1	T43.1X2	T43.1X3	T43.1X4	T43.1X5	T43.1X6
selective serotonin norepinephrine reuptake inhibitor	T43.211	T43.212	T43.213	T43.214	T43.215	T43.216
selective serotonin reuptake inhibitor	T43.221	T43.222	T43.223	T43.224	T43.225	T43.226
specified NEC	T43.291	T43.292	T43.293	T43.294	T43.295	T43.296
tetracyclic	T43.Ø21	T43.Ø22	T43.Ø23	T43.Ø24	T43.Ø25	T43.Ø26
triazolopyridine	T43.211	T43.212	T43.213	T43.214	T43.215	T43.216
tricyclic	T43.Ø11	T43.Ø12	T43.Ø13	T43.Ø14	T43.Ø15	T43.Ø16
Antidiabetic NEC	T38.3X1	T38.3X2	T38.3X3	T38.3X4	T38.3X5	T38.3X6
biguanide	T38.3X1	T38.3X2	T38.3X3	T38.3X4	T38.3X5	T38.3X6
and sulfonyl combined	T38.3X1	T38.3X2	T38.3X3	T38.3X4	T38.3X5	T38.3X6
combined	T38.3X1	T38.3X2	T38.3X3	T38.3X4	T38.3X5	T38.3X6
sulfonylurea	T38.3X1	T38.3X2	T38.3X3	T38.3X4	T38.3X5	T38.3X6
Antidiarrheal drug NEC	T47.6X1	T47.6X2	T47.6X3	T47.6X4	T47.6X5	T47.6X6
absorbent	T47.6X1	T47.6X2	T47.6X3	T47.6X4	T47.6X5	T47.6X6
Anti-D immunoglobulin (human)	T5Ø.Z11	T5Ø.Z12	T5Ø.Z13	T5Ø.Z14	T5Ø.Z15	T5Ø.Z16
Antidiphtheria serum	T5Ø.Z11	T5Ø.Z12	T5Ø.Z13	T5Ø.Z14	T5Ø.Z15	T5Ø.Z16
Antidiuretic hormone	T38.891	T38.892	T38.893	T38.894	T38.895	T38.896
Antidote NEC	T5Ø.6X1	T5Ø.6X2	T5Ø.6X3	T5Ø.6X4	T5Ø.6X5	T5Ø.6X6
heavy metal	T45.8X1	T45.8X2	T45.8X3	T45.8X4	T45.8X5	T45.8X6
Antidysrhythmic NEC	T46.2X1	T46.2X2	T46.2X3	T46.2X4	T46.2X5	T46.2X6
Antiemetic drug	T45.ØX1	T45.ØX2	T45.ØX3	T45.ØX4	T45.ØX5	T45.ØX6
Antiepilepsy agent	T42.71	T42.72	T42.73	T42.74	T42.75	T42.76
combination	T42.5X1	T42.5X2	T42.5X3	T42.5X4	T42.5X5	T42.5X6
mixed	T42.5X1	T42.5X2	T42.5X3	T42.5X4	T42.5X5	T42.5X6

Substance	Poisoning, Accidental (unintentional)	Poisoning, Intentional Self-harm	Poisoning, Assault	Poisoning, Undetermined	Adverse Effect	Under-dosing
Antiepilepsy agent — *continued*						
specified, NEC	T42.6X1	T42.6X2	T42.6X3	T42.6X4	T42.6X5	T42.6X6
Antiestrogen NEC	T38.6X1	T38.6X2	T38.6X3	T38.6X4	T38.6X5	T38.6X6
Antifertility pill	T38.4X1	T38.4X2	T38.4X3	T38.4X4	T38.4X5	T38.4X6
Antifibrinolytic drug	T45.621	T45.622	T45.623	T45.624	T45.625	T45.626
Antifilarial drug	T37.4X1	T37.4X2	T37.4X3	T37.4X4	T37.4X5	T37.4X6
Antiflatulent	T47.5X1	T47.5X2	T47.5X3	T47.5X4	T47.5X5	T47.5X6
Antifreeze	T65.91	T65.92	T65.93	T65.94	—	—
alcohol	T51.1X1	T51.1X2	T51.1X3	T51.1X4	—	—
ethylene glycol	T51.8X1	T51.8X2	T51.8X3	T51.8X4		
Antifungal						
antibiotic (systemic)	T36.7X1	T36.7X2	T36.7X3	T36.7X4	T36.7X5	T36.7X6
anti-infective NEC	T37.91	T37.92	T37.93	T37.94	T37.95	T37.96
disinfectant, local	T49.ØX1	T49.ØX2	T49.ØX3	T49.ØX4	T49.ØX5	T49.ØX6
nonmedicinal (spray)	T6Ø.3X1	T6Ø.3X2	T6Ø.3X3	T6Ø.3X4		
topical	T49.ØX1	T49.ØX2	T49.ØX3	T49.ØX4	T49.ØX5	T49.ØX6
Anti-gastric-secretion drug NEC	T47.1X1	T47.1X2	T47.1X3	T47.1X4	T47.1X5	T47.1X6
Antigonadotrophin NEC	T38.6X1	T38.6X2	T38.6X3	T38.6X4	T38.6X5	T38.6X6
Antihallucinogen	T43.5Ø1	T43.5Ø2	T43.5Ø3	T43.5Ø4	T43.5Ø5	T43.5Ø6
Antihelmintics	T37.4X1	T37.4X2	T37.4X3	T37.4X4	T37.4X5	T37.4X6
Antihemophilic						
factor	T45.8X1	T45.8X2	T45.8X3	T45.8X4	T45.8X5	T45.8X6
fraction	T45.8X1	T45.8X2	T45.8X3	T45.8X4	T45.8X5	T45.8X6
globulin concentrate	T45.7X1	T45.7X2	T45.7X3	T45.7X4	T45.7X5	T45.7X6
human plasma	T45.8X1	T45.8X2	T45.8X3	T45.8X4	T45.8X5	T45.8X6
plasma, dried	T45.7X1	T45.7X2	T45.7X3	T45.7X4	T45.7X5	T45.7X6
Antihemorrhoidal preparation	T49.2X1	T49.2X2	T49.2X3	T49.2X4	T49.2X5	T49.2X6
Antiheparin drug	T45.7X1	T45.7X2	T45.7X3	T45.7X4	T45.7X5	T45.7X6
Antihistamine	T45.ØX1	T45.ØX2	T45.ØX3	T45.ØX4	T45.ØX5	T45.ØX6
Antihookworm drug	T37.4X1	T37.4X2	T37.4X3	T37.4X4	T37.4X5	T37.4X6
Anti-human lymphocytic globulin	T5Ø.Z11	T5Ø.Z12	T5Ø.Z13	T5Ø.Z14	T5Ø.Z15	T5Ø.Z16
Antihyperlipidemic drug	T46.6X1	T46.6X2	T46.6X3	T46.6X4	T46.6X5	T46.6X6
Antihypertensive drug NEC	T46.5X1	T46.5X2	T46.5X3	T46.5X4	T46.5X5	T46.5X6
Anti-infective NEC	T37.91	T37.92	T37.93	T37.94	T37.95	T37.96
anthelmintic	T37.4X1	T37.4X2	T37.4X3	T37.4X4	T37.4X5	T37.4X6
antibiotics	T36.91	T36.92	T36.93	T36.94	T36.95	T36.96
specified NEC	T36.8X1	T36.8X2	T36.8X3	T36.8X4	T36.8X5	T36.8X6
antimalarial	T37.2X1	T37.2X2	T37.2X3	T37.2X4	T37.2X5	T37.2X6
antimycobacterial NEC	T37.1X1	T37.1X2	T37.1X3	T37.1X4	T37.1X5	T37.1X6
antibiotics	T36.5X1	T36.5X2	T36.5X3	T36.5X4	T36.5X5	T36.5X6
antiprotozoal NEC	T37.3X1	T37.3X2	T37.3X3	T37.3X4	T37.3X5	T37.3X6
blood	T37.2X1	T37.2X2	T37.2X3	T37.2X4	T37.2X5	T37.2X6
antiviral	T37.5X1	T37.5X2	T37.5X3	T37.5X4	T37.5X5	T37.5X6
arsenical	T37.8X1	T37.8X2	T37.8X3	T37.8X4	T37.8X5	T37.8X6
bismuth, local	T49.ØX1	T49.ØX2	T49.ØX3	T49.ØX4	T49.ØX5	T49.ØX6
ENT	T49.6X1	T49.6X2	T49.6X3	T49.6X4	T49.6X5	T49.6X6
eye NEC	T49.5X1	T49.5X2	T49.5X3	T49.5X4	T49.5X5	T49.5X6
heavy metals NEC	T37.8X1	T37.8X2	T37.8X3	T37.8X4	T37.8X5	T37.8X6
local NEC	T49.ØX1	T49.ØX2	T49.ØX3	T49.ØX4	T49.ØX5	T49.ØX6
specified NEC	T49.ØX1	T49.ØX2	T49.ØX3	T49.ØX4	T49.ØX5	T49.ØX6
mixed	T37.91	T37.92	T37.93	T37.94	T37.95	T37.96
ophthalmic preparation	T49.5X1	T49.5X2	T49.5X3	T49.5X4	T49.5X5	T49.5X6
topical NEC	T49.ØX1	T49.ØX2	T49.ØX3	T49.ØX4	T49.ØX5	T49.ØX6
Anti-inflammatory drug NEC	T39.391	T39.392	T39.393	T39.394	T39.395	T39.396
local	T49.ØX1	T49.ØX2	T49.ØX3	T49.ØX4	T49.ØX5	T49.ØX6
nonsteroidal NEC	T39.391	T39.392	T39.393	T39.394	T39.395	T39.396
propionic acid derivative	T39.311	T39.312	T39.313	T39.314	T39.315	T39.316
specified NEC	T39.391	T39.392	T39.393	T39.394	T39.395	T39.396
Antikaluretic	T5Ø.3X1	T5Ø.3X2	T5Ø.3X3	T5Ø.3X4	T5Ø.3X5	T5Ø.3X6
Antiknock (tetraethyl lead)	T56.ØX1	T56.ØX2	T56.ØX3	T56.ØX4	—	—
Antilipemic drug NEC	T46.6X1	T46.6X2	T46.6X3	T46.6X4	T46.6X5	T46.6X6
Antilysin*	T45.621	T45.622	T45.623	T45.624	T45.625	T45.626
Antimalarial	T37.2X1	T37.2X2	T37.2X3	T37.2X4	T37.2X5	T37.2X6
prophylactic NEC	T37.2X1	T37.2X2	T37.2X3	T37.2X4	T37.2X5	T37.2X6
pyrimidine derivative	T37.2X1	T37.2X2	T37.2X3	T37.2X4	T37.2X5	T37.2X6
Antimetabolite	T45.1X1	T45.1X2	T45.1X3	T45.1X4	T45.1X5	T45.1X6
Antimitotic agent	T45.1X1	T45.1X2	T45.1X3	T45.1X4	T45.1X5	T45.1X6
Antimony (compounds) (vapor) **NEC**	T56.891	T56.892	T56.893	T56.894	—	—
anti-infectives	T37.8X1	T37.8X2	T37.8X3	T37.8X4	T37.8X5	T37.8X6
dimercaptosuccinate	T37.3X1	T37.3X2	T37.3X3	T37.3X4	T37.3X5	T37.3X6
hydride	T56.891	T56.892	T56.893	T56.894	—	—
pesticide (vapor)	T6Ø.8X1	T6Ø.8X2	T6Ø.8X3	T6Ø.8X4	—	—
potassium (sodium)	T37.8X1	T37.8X2	T37.8X3	T37.8X4	T37.8X5	T37.8X6
tartrate						
sodium dimercaptosuccinate	T37.3X1	T37.3X2	T37.3X3	T37.3X4	T37.3X5	T37.3X6
tartrated	T37.8X1	T37.8X2	T37.8X3	T37.8X4	T37.8X5	T37.8X6

Substance	Poisoning, Accidental (unintentional)	Poisoning, Intentional Self-harm	Poisoning, Assault	Poisoning, Undetermined	Adverse Effect	Under-dosing
Antimuscarinic NEC	T44.3X1	T44.3X2	T44.3X3	T44.3X4	T44.3X5	T44.3X6
Antimycobacterial drug NEC	T37.1X1	T37.1X2	T37.1X3	T37.1X4	T37.1X5	T37.1X6
antibiotics	T36.5X1	T36.5X2	T36.5X3	T36.5X4	T36.5X5	T36.5X6
combination	T37.1X1	T37.1X2	T37.1X3	T37.1X4	T37.1X5	T37.1X6
Antinausea drug	T45.ØX1	T45.ØX2	T45.ØX3	T45.ØX4	T45.ØX5	T45.ØX6
Antinematode drug	T37.4X1	T37.4X2	T37.4X3	T37.4X4	T37.4X5	T37.4X6
Antineoplastic NEC	T45.1X1	T45.1X2	T45.1X3	T45.1X4	T45.1X5	T45.1X6
alkaloidal	T45.1X1	T45.1X2	T45.1X3	T45.1X4	T45.1X5	T45.1X6
antibiotics	T45.1X1	T45.1X2	T45.1X3	T45.1X4	T45.1X5	T45.1X6
combination	T45.1X1	T45.1X2	T45.1X3	T45.1X4	T45.1X5	T45.1X6
estrogen	T38.5X1	T38.5X2	T38.5X3	T38.5X4	T38.5X5	T38.5X6
steroid	T38.7X1	T38.7X2	T38.7X3	T38.7X4	T38.7X5	T38.7X6
Antiparasitic drug (systemic)	T37.91	T37.92	T37.93	T37.94	T37.95	T37.96
local	T49.ØX1	T49.ØX2	T49.ØX3	T49.ØX4	T49.ØX5	T49.ØX6
specified NEC	T37.8X1	T37.8X2	T37.8X3	T37.8X4	T37.8X5	T37.8X6
Antiparkinsonism drug NEC	T42.8X1	T42.8X2	T42.8X3	T42.8X4	T42.8X5	T42.8X6
Antiperspirant NEC	T49.2X1	T49.2X2	T49.2X3	T49.2X4	T49.2X5	T49.2X6
Antiphlogistic NEC	T39.4X1	T39.4X2	T39.4X3	T39.4X4	T39.4X5	T39.4X6
Antiplatyhelmintic drug	T37.4X1	T37.4X2	T37.4X3	T37.4X4	T37.4X5	T37.4X6
Antiprotozoal drug NEC	T37.3X1	T37.3X2	T37.3X3	T37.3X4	T37.3X5	T37.3X6
blood	T37.2X1	T37.2X2	T37.2X3	T37.2X4	T37.2X5	T37.2X6
local	T49.ØX1	T49.ØX2	T49.ØX3	T49.ØX4	T49.ØX5	T49.ØX6
Antipruritic drug NEC	T49.1X1	T49.1X2	T49.1X3	T49.1X4	T49.1X5	T49.1X6
Antipsychotic drug	T43.5Ø1	T43.5Ø2	T43.5Ø3	T43.5Ø4	T43.5Ø5	T43.5Ø6
specified NEC	T43.591	T43.592	T43.593	T43.594	T43.595	T43.596
Antipyretic	T39.91	T39.92	T39.93	T39.94	T39.95	T39.96
specified NEC	T39.8X1	T39.8X2	T39.8X3	T39.8X4	T39.8X5	T39.8X6
Antipyrine	T39.2X1	T39.2X2	T39.2X3	T39.2X4	T39.2X5	T39.2X6
Antirabies hyperimmune serum	T5Ø.Z11	T5Ø.Z12	T5Ø.Z13	T5Ø.Z14	T5Ø.Z15	T5Ø.Z16
Antirheumatic NEC	T39.4X1	T39.4X2	T39.4X3	T39.4X4	T39.4X5	T39.4X6
Antirigidity drug NEC	T42.8X1	T42.8X2	T42.8X3	T42.8X4	T42.8X5	T42.8X6
Antischistosomal drug	T37.4X1	T37.4X2	T37.4X3	T37.4X4	T37.4X5	T37.4X6
Antiscorpion sera	T5Ø.Z11	T5Ø.Z12	T5Ø.Z13	T5Ø.Z14	T5Ø.Z15	T5Ø.Z16
Antiseborrheics	T49.4X1	T49.4X2	T49.4X3	T49.4X4	T49.4X5	T49.4X6
Antiseptics (external) (medicinal)	T49.ØX1	T49.ØX2	T49.ØX3	T49.ØX4	T49.ØX5	T49.ØX6
Antistine	T45.ØX1	T45.ØX2	T45.ØX3	T45.ØX4	T45.ØX5	T45.ØX6
Antitapeworm drug	T37.4X1	T37.4X2	T37.4X3	T37.4X4	T37.4X5	T37.4X6
Antitetanus immunoglobulin	T5Ø.Z11	T5Ø.Z12	T5Ø.Z13	T5Ø.Z14	T5Ø.Z15	T5Ø.Z16
Antithrombin III*	T45.511	T45.512	T45.513	T45.514	T45.515	T45.516
Antithrombotic	T45.521	T45.522	T45.523	T45.524	T45.525	T45.526
Antithyroid drug NEC	T38.2X1	T38.2X2	T38.2X3	T38.2X4	T38.2X5	T38.2X6
Antitoxin	T5Ø.Z11	T5Ø.Z12	T5Ø.Z13	T5Ø.Z14	T5Ø.Z15	T5Ø.Z16
diphtheria	T5Ø.Z11	T5Ø.Z12	T5Ø.Z13	T5Ø.Z14	T5Ø.Z15	T5Ø.Z16
gas gangrene	T5Ø.Z11	T5Ø.Z12	T5Ø.Z13	T5Ø.Z14	T5Ø.Z15	T5Ø.Z16
tetanus	T5Ø.Z11	T5Ø.Z12	T5Ø.Z13	T5Ø.Z14	T5Ø.Z15	T5Ø.Z16
Antitrichomonal drug	T37.3X1	T37.3X2	T37.3X3	T37.3X4	T37.3X5	T37.3X6
Antituberculars	T37.1X1	T37.1X2	T37.1X3	T37.1X4	T37.1X5	T37.1X6
antibiotics	T36.5X1	T36.5X2	T36.5X3	T36.5X4	T36.5X5	T36.5X6
Antitussive NEC	T48.3X1	T48.3X2	T48.3X3	T48.3X4	T48.3X5	T48.3X6
codeine mixture	T4Ø.2X1	T4Ø.2X2	T4Ø.2X3	T4Ø.2X4	T4Ø.2X5	T4Ø.2X6
opiate	T4Ø.2X1	T4Ø.2X2	T4Ø.2X3	T4Ø.2X4	T4Ø.2X5	T4Ø.2X6
Antivaricose drug	T46.8X1	T46.8X2	T46.8X3	T46.8X4	T46.8X5	T46.8X6
Antivenin, antivenom (sera)	T5Ø.Z11	T5Ø.Z12	T5Ø.Z13	T5Ø.Z14	T5Ø.Z15	T5Ø.Z16
crotaline	T5Ø.Z11	T5Ø.Z12	T5Ø.Z13	T5Ø.Z14	T5Ø.Z15	T5Ø.Z16
spider bite	T5Ø.Z11	T5Ø.Z12	T5Ø.Z13	T5Ø.Z14	T5Ø.Z15	T5Ø.Z16
Antivert*	T45.ØX1	T45.ØX2	T45.ØX3	T45.ØX4	T45.ØX5	T45.ØX6
Antivertigo drug	T45.ØX1	T45.ØX2	T45.ØX3	T45.ØX4	T45.ØX5	T45.ØX6
Antiviral drug NEC	T37.5X1	T37.5X2	T37.5X3	T37.5X4	T37.5X5	T37.5X6
eye	T49.5X1	T49.5X2	T49.5X3	T49.5X4	T49.5X5	T49.5X6
Antiwhipworm drug	T37.4X1	T37.4X2	T37.4X3	T37.4X4	T37.4X5	T37.4X6
Ant poison — *see* Insecticide						
Antrol — *see also* by specific chemical substance	T6Ø.91	T6Ø.92	T6Ø.93	T6Ø.94	—	—
fungicide	T6Ø.91	T6Ø.92	T6Ø.93	T6Ø.94	—	—
ANTU (alpha naphthylthiourea)	T6Ø.4X1	T6Ø.4X2	T6Ø.4X3	T6Ø.4X4	—	—
Apalcillin	T36.ØX1	T36.ØX2	T36.ØX3	T36.ØX4	T36.ØX5	T36.ØX6
APC	T48.5X1	T48.5X2	T48.5X3	T48.5X4	T48.5X5	T48.5X6
Aplonidine	T44.4X1	T44.4X2	T44.4X3	T44.4X4	T44.4X5	T44.4X6
Apomorphine	T47.7X1	T47.7X2	T47.7X3	T47.7X4	T47.7X5	T47.7X6
Appetite depressants, central	T5Ø.5X1	T5Ø.5X2	T5Ø.5X3	T5Ø.5X4	T5Ø.5X5	T5Ø.5X6
Apraclonidine (hydrochloride)	T44.4X1	T44.4X2	T44.4X3	T44.4X4	T44.4X5	T44.4X6
Apresoline	T46.5X1	T46.5X2	T46.5X3	T46.5X4	T46.5X5	T46.5X6
Apri*	T38.4X1	T38.4X2	T38.4X3	T38.4X4	T38.4X5	T38.4X6

Substance	Poisoning, Accidental (unintentional)	Poisoning, Intentional Self-harm	Poisoning, Assault	Poisoning, Undetermined	Adverse Effect	Under-dosing
Aprindine	T46.2X1	T46.2X2	T46.2X3	T46.2X4	T46.2X5	T46.2X6
Aprobarbital	T42.3X1	T42.3X2	T42.3X3	T42.3X4	T42.3X5	T42.3X6
Apronalide	T42.6X1	T42.6X2	T42.6X3	T42.6X4	T42.6X5	T42.6X6
Aprotinin	T45.621	T45.622	T45.623	T45.624	T45.625	T45.626
Aptocaine	T41.3X1	T41.3X2	T41.3X3	T41.3X4	T41.3X5	T41.3X6
Aqua fortis	T54.2X1	T54.2X2	T54.2X3	T54.2X4	—	—
Ara-A	T37.5X1	T37.5X2	T37.5X3	T37.5X4	T37.5X5	T37.5X6
Ara-C	T45.1X1	T45.1X2	T45.1X3	T45.1X4	T45.1X5	T45.1X6
Arachis oil	T49.3X1	T49.3X2	T49.3X3	T49.3X4	T49.3X5	T49.3X6
cathartic	T47.4X1	T47.4X2	T47.4X3	T47.4X4	T47.4X5	T47.4X6
Aralen	T37.2X1	T37.2X2	T37.2X3	T37.2X4	T37.2X5	T37.2X6
Arecoline	T44.1X1	T44.1X2	T44.1X3	T44.1X4	T44.1X5	T44.1X6
Arginine	T5Ø.991	T5Ø.992	T5Ø.993	T5Ø.994	T5Ø.995	T5Ø.996
glutamate	T5Ø.991	T5Ø.992	T5Ø.993	T5Ø.994	T5Ø.995	T5Ø.996
Argyrol	T49.ØX1	T49.ØX2	T49.ØX3	T49.ØX4	T49.ØX5	T49.ØX6
ENT agent	T49.6X1	T49.6X2	T49.6X3	T49.6X4	T49.6X5	T49.6X6
ophthalmic preparation	T49.5X1	T49.5X2	T49.5X3	T49.5X4	T49.5X5	T49.5X6
Aristocort	T38.ØX1	T38.ØX2	T38.ØX3	T38.ØX4	T38.ØX5	T38.ØX6
ENT agent	T49.6X1	T49.6X2	T49.6X3	T49.6X4	T49.6X5	T49.6X6
ophthalmic preparation	T49.5X1	T49.5X2	T49.5X3	T49.5X4	T49.5X5	T49.5X6
topical NEC	T49.ØX1	T49.ØX2	T49.ØX3	T49.ØX4	T49.ØX5	T49.ØX6
Aromatics, corrosive	T54.1X1	T54.1X2	T54.1X3	T54.1X4	—	—
disinfectants	T54.1X1	T54.1X2	T54.1X3	T54.1X4	—	—
Arsenate of lead	T57.ØX1	T57.ØX2	T57.ØX3	T57.ØX4	—	—
herbicide	T57.ØX1	T57.ØX2	T57.ØX3	T57.ØX4	—	—
Arsenic, arsenicals (compounds) (dust) (vapor) **NEC**	T57.ØX1	T57.ØX2	T57.ØX3	T57.ØX4	—	—
anti-infectives	T37.8X1	T37.8X2	T37.8X3	T37.8X4	T37.8X5	T37.8X6
pesticide (dust) (fumes)	T57.ØX1	T57.ØX2	T57.ØX3	T57.ØX4	—	—
Arsine (gas)	T57.ØX1	T57.ØX2	T57.ØX3	T57.ØX4	—	—
Arsobal*	T37.3X1	T37.3X2	T37.3X3	T37.3X4	T37.3X5	T37.3X6
Arsphenamine (silver)	T37.8X1	T37.8X2	T37.8X3	T37.8X4	T37.8X5	T37.8X6
Arsthinol	T37.3X1	T37.3X2	T37.3X3	T37.3X4	T37.3X5	T37.3X6
Artane	T44.3X1	T44.3X2	T44.3X3	T44.3X4	T44.3X5	T44.3X6
Arthropod (venomous) **NEC**	T63.481	T63.482	T63.483	T63.484	—	—
Articaine	T41.3X1	T41.3X2	T41.3X3	T41.3X4	T41.3X5	T41.3X6
Asbestos	T57.8X1	T57.8X2	T57.8X3	T57.8X4	—	—
Ascaridole	T37.4X1	T37.4X2	T37.4X3	T37.4X4	T37.4X5	T37.4X6
Ascorbic acid	T45.2X1	T45.2X2	T45.2X3	T45.2X4	T45.2X5	T45.2X6
Asiaticoside	T49.ØX1	T49.ØX2	T49.ØX3	T49.ØX4	T49.ØX5	T49.ØX6
Asparaginase	T45.1X1	T45.1X2	T45.1X3	T45.1X4	T45.1X5	T45.1X6
Aspidium (oleoresin)	T37.4X1	T37.4X2	T37.4X3	T37.4X4	T37.4X5	T37.4X6
Aspirin (aluminum) (soluble)	T39.Ø11	T39.Ø12	T39.Ø13	T39.Ø14	T39.Ø15	T39.Ø16
Aspoxicillin	T36.ØX1	T36.ØX2	T36.ØX3	T36.ØX4	T36.ØX5	T36.ØX6
Astemizole	T45.ØX1	T45.ØX2	T45.ØX3	T45.ØX4	T45.ØX5	T45.ØX6
Astringent (local)	T49.2X1	T49.2X2	T49.2X3	T49.2X4	T49.2X5	T49.2X6
specified NEC	T49.2X1	T49.2X2	T49.2X3	T49.2X4	T49.2X5	T49.2X6
Astromicin	T36.5X1	T36.5X2	T36.5X3	T36.5X4	T36.5X5	T36.5X6
Ataractic drug NEC	T43.5Ø1	T43.5Ø2	T43.5Ø3	T43.5Ø4	T43.5Ø5	T43.5Ø6
Atenolol	T44.7X1	T44.7X2	T44.7X3	T44.7X4	T44.7X5	T44.7X6
Atonia drug, intestinal	T47.4X1	T47.4X2	T47.4X3	T47.4X4	T47.4X5	T47.4X6
Atophan	T5Ø.4X1	T5Ø.4X2	T5Ø.4X3	T5Ø.4X4	T5Ø.4X5	T5Ø.4X6
Atracurium besilate	T48.1X1	T48.1X2	T48.1X3	T48.1X4	T48.1X5	T48.1X6
Atropine	T44.3X1	T44.3X2	T44.3X3	T44.3X4	T44.3X5	T44.3X6
derivative	T44.3X1	T44.3X2	T44.3X3	T44.3X4	T44.3X5	T44.3X6
methonitrate	T44.3X1	T44.3X2	T44.3X3	T44.3X4	T44.3X5	T44.3X6
Atrovent*	T48.6X1	T48.6X2	T48.6X3	T48.6X4	T48.6X5	T48.6X6
Attapulgite	T47.6X1	T47.6X2	T47.6X3	T47.6X4	T47.6X5	T47.6X6
Auramine	T65.891	T65.892	T65.893	T65.894	—	—
dye	T65.6X1	T65.6X2	T65.6X3	T65.6X4	—	—
fungicide	T6Ø.3X1	T6Ø.3X2	T6Ø.3X3	T6Ø.3X4	—	—
Auranofin	T39.4X1	T39.4X2	T39.4X3	T39.4X4	T39.4X5	T39.4X6
Aurantiin	T46.991	T46.992	T46.993	T46.994	T46.995	T46.996
Aureomycin	T36.4X1	T36.4X2	T36.4X3	T36.4X4	T36.4X5	T36.4X6
ophthalmic preparation	T49.5X1	T49.5X2	T49.5X3	T49.5X4	T49.5X5	T49.5X6
topical NEC	T49.ØX1	T49.ØX2	T49.ØX3	T49.ØX4	T49.ØX5	T49.ØX6
Aurothioglucose	T39.4X1	T39.4X2	T39.4X3	T39.4X4	T39.4X5	T39.4X6
Aurothioglycanide	T39.4X1	T39.4X2	T39.4X3	T39.4X4	T39.4X5	T39.4X6
Aurothiomalate sodium	T39.4X1	T39.4X2	T39.4X3	T39.4X4	T39.4X5	T39.4X6
Aurotioprol	T39.4X1	T39.4X2	T39.4X3	T39.4X4	T39.4X5	T39.4X6
Automobile fuel	T52.ØX1	T52.ØX2	T52.ØX3	T52.ØX4	—	—
Autonomic nervous system agent NEC	T44.9Ø1	T44.9Ø2	T44.9Ø3	T44.9Ø4	T44.9Ø5	T44.9Ø6
Avelox*	T36.8X1	T36.8X2	T36.8X3	T36.8X4	T36.8X5	T36.8X6
Avlosulfon	T37.1X1	T37.1X2	T37.1X3	T37.1X4	T37.1X5	T37.1X6
Avomine	T42.6X1	T42.6X2	T42.6X3	T42.6X4	T42.6X5	T42.6X6
Axerophthol	T45.2X1	T45.2X2	T45.2X3	T45.2X4	T45.2X5	T45.2X6
Azacitidine	T45.1X1	T45.1X2	T45.1X3	T45.1X4	T45.1X5	T45.1X6
Azacyclonol	T43.591	T43.592	T43.593	T43.594	T43.595	T43.596
Azadirachta	T6Ø.2X1	T6Ø.2X2	T6Ø.2X3	T6Ø.2X4	—	—
Azanidazole	T37.3X1	T37.3X2	T37.3X3	T37.3X4	T37.3X5	T37.3X6
Azapetine	T46.7X1	T46.7X2	T46.7X3	T46.7X4	T46.7X5	T46.7X6
Azapropazone	T39.2X1	T39.2X2	T39.2X3	T39.2X4	T39.2X5	T39.2X6
Azaribine	T45.1X1	T45.1X2	T45.1X3	T45.1X4	T45.1X5	T45.1X6
Azaserine	T45.1X1	T45.1X2	T45.1X3	T45.1X4	T45.1X5	T45.1X6
Azatadine	T45.ØX1	T45.ØX2	T45.ØX3	T45.ØX4	T45.ØX5	T45.ØX6
Azatepa	T45.1X1	T45.1X2	T45.1X3	T45.1X4	T45.1X5	T45.1X6
Azathioprine	T45.1X1	T45.1X2	T45.1X3	T45.1X4	T45.1X5	T45.1X6
Azelaic acid	T49.ØX1	T49.ØX2	T49.ØX3	T49.ØX4	T49.ØX5	T49.ØX6
Azelastine	T45.ØX1	T45.ØX2	T45.ØX3	T45.ØX4	T45.ØX5	T45.ØX6
Azidocillin	T36.ØX1	T36.ØX2	T36.ØX3	T36.ØX4	T36.ØX5	T36.ØX6
Azidothymidine	T37.5X1	T37.5X2	T37.5X3	T37.5X4	T37.5X5	T37.5X6
Azinphos (ethyl) (methyl)	T6Ø.ØX1	T6Ø.ØX2	T6Ø.ØX3	T6Ø.ØX4	—	—
Aziridine (chelating)	T54.1X1	T54.1X2	T54.1X3	T54.1X4	—	—
Azithromycin	T36.3X1	T36.3X2	T36.3X3	T36.3X4	T36.3X5	T36.3X6
Azlocillin	T36.ØX1	T36.ØX2	T36.ØX3	T36.ØX4	T36.ØX5	T36.ØX6
Azobenzene smoke	T65.3X1	T65.3X2	T65.3X3	T65.3X4	—	—
acaricide	T6Ø.8X1	T6Ø.8X2	T6Ø.8X3	T6Ø.8X4	—	—
Azo-Standard*	T49.ØX1	T49.ØX2	T49.ØX3	T49.ØX4	T49.ØX5	T49.ØX6
Azosulfamide	T37.ØX1	T37.ØX2	T37.ØX3	T37.ØX4	T37.ØX5	T37.ØX6
AZT	T37.5X1	T37.5X2	T37.5X3	T37.5X4	T37.5X5	T37.5X6
Aztreonam	T36.1X1	T36.1X2	T36.1X3	T36.1X4	T36.1X5	T36.1X6
Azulfidine	T37.ØX1	T37.ØX2	T37.ØX3	T37.ØX4	T37.ØX5	T37.ØX6
Azuresin	T5Ø.8X1	T5Ø.8X2	T5Ø.8X3	T5Ø.8X4	T5Ø.8X5	T5Ø.8X6
b-acetyldigoxin	T46.ØX1	T46.ØX2	T46.ØX3	T46.ØX4	T46.ØX5	T46.ØX6
P-Acetamidophenol	T39.1X1	T39.1X2	T39.1X3	T39.1X4	T39.1X5	T39.1X6
Bacampicillin	T36.ØX1	T36.ØX2	T36.ØX3	T36.ØX4	T36.ØX5	T36.ØX6
Bacillus						
lactobacillus	T47.8X1	T47.8X2	T47.8X3	T47.8X4	T47.8X5	T47.8X6
subtilis	T47.6X1	T47.6X2	T47.6X3	T47.6X4	T47.6X5	T47.6X6
Bacimycin	T49.ØX1	T49.ØX2	T49.ØX3	T49.ØX4	T49.ØX5	T49.ØX6
ophthalmic preparation	T49.5X1	T49.5X2	T49.5X3	T49.5X4	T49.5X5	T49.5X6
Bacitracin zinc	T49.ØX1	T49.ØX2	T49.ØX3	T49.ØX4	T49.ØX5	T49.ØX6
with neomycin	T49.ØX1	T49.ØX2	T49.ØX3	T49.ØX4	T49.ØX5	T49.ØX6
ENT agent	T49.6X1	T49.6X2	T49.6X3	T49.6X4	T49.6X5	T49.6X6
ophthalmic preparation	T49.5X1	T49.5X2	T49.5X3	T49.5X4	T49.5X5	T49.5X6
topical NEC	T49.ØX1	T49.ØX2	T49.ØX3	T49.ØX4	T49.ØX5	T49.ØX6
Baclofen	T42.8X1	T42.8X2	T42.8X3	T42.8X4	T42.8X5	T42.8X6
Baking soda	T5Ø.991	T5Ø.992	T5Ø.993	T5Ø.994	T5Ø.995	T5Ø.996
BAL	T45.8X1	T45.8X2	T45.8X3	T45.8X4	T45.8X5	T45.8X6
Bambuterol	T48.6X1	T48.6X2	T48.6X3	T48.6X4	T48.6X5	T48.6X6
Bamethan (sulfate)	T46.7X1	T46.7X2	T46.7X3	T46.7X4	T46.7X5	T46.7X6
Bamifylline	T48.6X1	T48.6X2	T48.6X3	T48.6X4	T48.6X5	T48.6X6
Bamipine	T45.ØX1	T45.ØX2	T45.ØX3	T45.ØX4	T45.ØX5	T45.ØX6
Baneberry — *see* Actaea spicata						
Banewort — *see* Belladonna						
Barbenyl	T42.3X1	T42.3X2	T42.3X3	T42.3X4	T42.3X5	T42.3X6
Barbexaclone	T42.6X1	T42.6X2	T42.6X3	T42.6X4	T42.6X5	T42.6X6
Barbital	T42.3X1	T42.3X2	T42.3X3	T42.3X4	T42.3X5	T42.3X6
sodium	T42.3X1	T42.3X2	T42.3X3	T42.3X4	T42.3X5	T42.3X6
Barbitone	T42.3X1	T42.3X2	T42.3X3	T42.3X4	T42.3X5	T42.3X6
Barbiturate NEC	T42.3X1	T42.3X2	T42.3X3	T42.3X4	T42.3X5	T42.3X6
with tranquilizer	T42.3X1	T42.3X2	T42.3X3	T42.3X4	T42.3X5	T42.3X6
anesthetic (intravenous)	T41.1X1	T41.1X2	T41.1X3	T41.1X4	T41.1X5	T41.1X6
Barium (carbonate) (chloride) (sulfite)	T57.8X1	T57.8X2	T57.8X3	T57.8X4	—	—
diagnostic agent	T5Ø.8X1	T5Ø.8X2	T5Ø.8X3	T5Ø.8X4	T5Ø.8X5	T5Ø.8X6
pesticide	T6Ø.4X1	T6Ø.4X2	T6Ø.4X3	T6Ø.4X4	—	—
rodenticide	T6Ø.4X1	T6Ø.4X2	T6Ø.4X3	T6Ø.4X4	—	—
sulfate (medicinal)	T5Ø.8X1	T5Ø.8X2	T5Ø.8X3	T5Ø.8X4	T5Ø.8X5	T5Ø.8X6
Barrier cream	T49.3X1	T49.3X2	T49.3X3	T49.3X4	T49.3X5	T49.3X6
Basic fuchsin	T49.ØX1	T49.ØX2	T49.ØX3	T49.ØX4	T49.ØX5	T49.ØX6
Basiliximab*	T45.1X1	T45.1X2	T45.1X3	T45.1X4	T45.1X5	T45.1X6
Battery acid or fluid	T54.2X1	T54.2X2	T54.2X3	T54.2X4	—	—
Bay rum	T51.8X1	T51.8X2	T51.8X3	T51.8X4	—	—
b-benzalbutyramide	T46.6X1	T46.6X2	T46.6X3	T46.6X4	T46.6X5	T46.6X6
BCG (vaccine)	T5Ø.A91	T5Ø.A92	T5Ø.A93	T5Ø.A94	T5Ø.A95	T5Ø.A96
BCNU	T45.1X1	T45.1X2	T45.1X3	T45.1X4	T45.1X5	T45.1X6
Bearsfoot	T62.2X1	T62.2X2	T62.2X3	T62.2X4	—	—
Beclamide	T42.6X1	T42.6X2	T42.6X3	T42.6X4	T42.6X5	T42.6X6
Beclomethasone	T44.5X1	T44.5X2	T44.5X3	T44.5X4	T44.5X5	T44.5X6
Bee (sting) (venom)	T63.441	T63.442	T63.443	T63.444	—	—
Befunolol	T49.5X1	T49.5X2	T49.5X3	T49.5X4	T49.5X5	T49.5X6
Bekanamycin	T36.5X1	T36.5X2	T36.5X3	T36.5X4	T36.5X5	T36.5X6
Belladonna — *see also* Nightshade						
alkaloids	T44.3X1	T44.3X2	T44.3X3	T44.3X4	T44.3X5	T44.3X6
extract	T44.3X1	T44.3X2	T44.3X3	T44.3X4	T44.3X5	T44.3X6
herb	T44.3X1	T44.3X2	T44.3X3	T44.3X4	T44.3X5	T44.3X6
Belviq*	T5Ø.5X1	T5Ø.5X2	T5Ø.5X3	T5Ø.5X4	T5Ø.5X5	T5Ø.5X6
Bemegride	T5Ø.7X1	T5Ø.7X2	T5Ø.7X3	T5Ø.7X4	T5Ø.7X5	T5Ø.7X6
Benactyzine	T44.3X1	T44.3X2	T44.3X3	T44.3X4	T44.3X5	T44.3X6
Benadryl	T45.ØX1	T45.ØX2	T45.ØX3	T45.ØX4	T45.ØX5	T45.ØX6
Benaprizine	T44.3X1	T44.3X2	T44.3X3	T44.3X4	T44.3X5	T44.3X6
Benazepril	T46.4X1	T46.4X2	T46.4X3	T46.4X4	T46.4X5	T46.4X6

Substance	Poisoning, Accidental (unintentional)	Poisoning, Intentional Self-harm	Poisoning, Assault	Poisoning, Undetermined	Adverse Effect	Under-dosing
Bencyclane	T46.7X1	T46.7X2	T46.7X3	T46.7X4	T46.7X5	T46.7X6
Bendazol	T46.3X1	T46.3X2	T46.3X3	T46.3X4	T46.3X5	T46.3X6
Bendrofluazide	T5Ø.2X1	T5Ø.2X2	T5Ø.2X3	T5Ø.2X4	T5Ø.2X5	T5Ø.2X6
Bendroflumethiazide	T5Ø.2X1	T5Ø.2X2	T5Ø.2X3	T5Ø.2X4	T5Ø.2X5	T5Ø.2X6
Benemid	T5Ø.4X1	T5Ø.4X2	T5Ø.4X3	T5Ø.4X4	T5Ø.4X5	T5Ø.4X6
Benethamine penicillin	T36.ØX1	T36.ØX2	T36.ØX3	T36.ØX4	T36.ØX5	T36.ØX6
Benexate	T47.1X1	T47.1X2	T47.1X3	T47.1X4	T47.1X5	T47.1X6
Benfluorex	T46.6X1	T46.6X2	T46.6X3	T46.6X4	T46.6X5	T46.6X6
Benfotiamine	T45.2X1	T45.2X2	T45.2X3	T45.2X4	T45.2X5	T45.2X6
Benisone	T49.ØX1	T49.ØX2	T49.ØX3	T49.ØX4	T49.ØX5	T49.ØX6
Benomyl	T6Ø.ØX1	T6Ø.ØX2	T6Ø.ØX3	T6Ø.ØX4	—	—
Benoquin	T49.8X1	T49.8X2	T49.8X3	T49.8X4	T49.8X5	T49.8X6
Benoxinate	T41.3X1	T41.3X2	T41.3X3	T41.3X4	T41.3X5	T41.3X6
Benperidol	T43.4X1	T43.4X2	T43.4X3	T43.4X4	T43.4X5	T43.4X6
Benproperine	T48.3X1	T48.3X2	T48.3X3	T48.3X4	T48.3X5	T48.3X6
Benserazide	T42.8X1	T42.8X2	T42.8X3	T42.8X4	T42.8X5	T42.8X6
Bentazepam	T42.4X1	T42.4X2	T42.4X3	T42.4X4	T42.4X5	T42.4X6
Bentiromide	T5Ø.8X1	T5Ø.8X2	T5Ø.8X3	T5Ø.8X4	T5Ø.8X5	T5Ø.8X6
Bentonite	T49.3X1	T49.3X2	T49.3X3	T49.3X4	T49.3X5	T49.3X6
Benzalbutyramide	T46.6X1	T46.6X2	T46.6X3	T46.6X4	T46.6X5	T46.6X6
Benzalkonium (chloride)	T49.ØX1	T49.ØX2	T49.ØX3	T49.ØX4	T49.ØX5	T49.ØX6
ophthalmic preparation	T49.5X1	T49.5X2	T49.5X3	T49.5X4	T49.5X5	T49.5X6
Benzamidosalicylate (calcium)	T37.1X1	T37.1X2	T37.1X3	T37.1X4	T37.1X5	T37.1X6
Benzamine	T41.3X1	T41.3X2	T41.3X3	T41.3X4	T41.3X5	T41.3X6
lactate	T49.1X1	T49.1X2	T49.1X3	T49.1X4	T49.1X5	T49.1X6
Benzamphetamine	T5Ø.5X1	T5Ø.5X2	T5Ø.5X3	T5Ø.5X4	T5Ø.5X5	T5Ø.5X6
Benzapril hydrochloride	T46.5X1	T46.5X2	T46.5X3	T46.5X4	T46.5X5	T46.5X6
Benzathine benzylpenicillin	T36.ØX1	T36.ØX2	T36.ØX3	T36.ØX4	T36.ØX5	T36.ØX6
Benzathine penicillin	T36.ØX1	T36.ØX2	T36.ØX3	T36.ØX4	T36.ØX5	T36.ØX6
Benzatropine	T42.8X1	T42.8X2	T42.8X3	T42.8X4	T42.8X5	T42.8X6
Benzbromarone	T5Ø.4X1	T5Ø.4X2	T5Ø.4X3	T5Ø.4X4	T5Ø.4X5	T5Ø.4X6
Benzcarbimine	T45.1X1	T45.1X2	T45.1X3	T45.1X4	T45.1X5	T45.1X6
Benzedrex	T44.991	T44.992	T44.993	T44.994	T44.995	T44.996
Benzedrine (amphetamine)	T43.621	T43.622	T43.623	T43.624	T43.625	T43.626
Benzenamine	T65.3X1	T65.3X2	T65.3X3	T65.3X4	—	—
Benzene	T52.1X1	T52.1X2	T52.1X3	T52.1X4	—	—
homologues (acetyl) (dimethyl) (methyl) (solvent)	T52.2X1	T52.2X2	T52.2X3	T52.2X4	—	—
Benzethonium (chloride)	T49.ØX1	T49.ØX2	T49.ØX3	T49.ØX4	T49.ØX5	T49.ØX6
Benzfetamine	T5Ø.5X1	T5Ø.5X2	T5Ø.5X3	T5Ø.5X4	T5Ø.5X5	T5Ø.5X6
Benzhexol	T44.3X1	T44.3X2	T44.3X3	T44.3X4	T44.3X5	T44.3X6
Benzhydramine (chloride)	T45.ØX1	T45.ØX2	T45.ØX3	T45.ØX4	T45.ØX5	T45.ØX6
Benzidine	T65.891	T65.892	T65.893	T65.894	—	—
Benzilonium bromide	T44.3X1	T44.3X2	T44.3X3	T44.3X4	T44.3X5	T44.3X6
Benzimidazole	T6Ø.3X1	T6Ø.3X2	T6Ø.3X3	T6Ø.3X4	—	—
Benzin (e) — *see* Ligroin						
Benziodarone	T46.3X1	T46.3X2	T46.3X3	T46.3X4	T46.3X5	T46.3X6
Benznidazole	T37.3X1	T37.3X2	T37.3X3	T37.3X4	T37.3X5	T37.3X6
Benzocaine	T41.3X1	T41.3X2	T41.3X3	T41.3X4	T41.3X5	T41.3X6
Benzocol*	T41.3X1	T41.3X2	T41.3X3	T41.3X4	T41.3X5	T41.3X6
Benzodiapin	T42.4X1	T42.4X2	T42.4X3	T42.4X4	T42.4X5	T42.4X6
Benzodiazepine NEC	T42.4X1	T42.4X2	T42.4X3	T42.4X4	T42.4X5	T42.4X6
Benzoic acid	T49.ØX1	T49.ØX2	T49.ØX3	T49.ØX4	T49.ØX5	T49.ØX6
with salicylic acid	T49.ØX1	T49.ØX2	T49.ØX3	T49.ØX4	T49.ØX5	T49.ØX6
Benzoin (tincture)	T48.5X1	T48.5X2	T48.5X3	T48.5X4	T48.5X5	T48.5X6
Benzol (benzene)	T52.1X1	T52.1X2	T52.1X3	T52.1X4	—	—
vapor	T52.ØX1	T52.ØX2	T52.ØX3	T52.ØX4	—	—
Benzomorphan	T4Ø.2X1	T4Ø.2X2	T4Ø.2X3	T4Ø.2X4	T4Ø.2X5	T4Ø.2X6
Benzonatate	T48.3X1	T48.3X2	T48.3X3	T48.3X4	T48.3X5	T48.3X6
Benzophenones	T49.3X1	T49.3X2	T49.3X3	T49.3X4	T49.3X5	T49.3X6
Benzopyrone	T46.991	T46.992	T46.993	T46.994	T46.995	T46.996
Benzothiadiazides	T5Ø.2X1	T5Ø.2X2	T5Ø.2X3	T5Ø.2X4	T5Ø.2X5	T5Ø.2X6
Benzoxonium chloride	T49.ØX1	T49.ØX2	T49.ØX3	T49.ØX4	T49.ØX5	T49.ØX6
Benzoylpas calcium	T37.1X1	T37.1X2	T37.1X3	T37.1X4	T37.1X5	T37.1X6
Benzoyl peroxide	T49.ØX1	T49.ØX2	T49.ØX3	T49.ØX4	T49.ØX5	T49.ØX6
Benzperidin	T43.591	T43.592	T43.593	T43.594	T43.595	T43.596
Benzperidol	T43.591	T43.592	T43.593	T43.594	T43.595	T43.596
Benzphetamine	T5Ø.5X1	T5Ø.5X2	T5Ø.5X3	T5Ø.5X4	T5Ø.5X5	T5Ø.5X6
Benzpyrinium bromide	T44.1X1	T44.1X2	T44.1X3	T44.1X4	T44.1X5	T44.1X6
Benzquinamide	T45.ØX1	T45.ØX2	T45.ØX3	T45.ØX4	T45.ØX5	T45.ØX6
Benzthiazide	T5Ø.2X1	T5Ø.2X2	T5Ø.2X3	T5Ø.2X4	T5Ø.2X5	T5Ø.2X6
Benztropine						
anticholinergic	T44.3X1	T44.3X2	T44.3X3	T44.3X4	T44.3X5	T44.3X6
antiparkinson	T42.8X1	T42.8X2	T42.8X3	T42.8X4	T42.8X5	T42.8X6
Benzydamine	T49.ØX1	T49.ØX2	T49.ØX3	T49.ØX4	T49.ØX5	T49.ØX6
Benzyl						
acetate	T52.8X1	T52.8X2	T52.8X3	T52.8X4	—	—
alcohol	T49.ØX1	T49.ØX2	T49.ØX3	T49.ØX4	T49.ØX5	T49.ØX6
benzoate	T49.ØX1	T49.ØX2	T49.ØX3	T49.ØX4	T49.ØX5	T49.ØX6
Benzoic acid	T49.ØX1	T49.ØX2	T49.ØX3	T49.ØX4	T49.ØX5	T49.ØX6
hydroquinone*	T49.4X1	T49.4X2	T49.4X3	T49.4X4	T49.4X5	T49.4X6
Benzyl — *continued*						
morphine	T4Ø.2X1	T4Ø.2X2	T4Ø.2X3	T4Ø.2X4	—	—
nicotinate	T46.6X1	T46.6X2	T46.6X3	T46.6X4	T46.6X5	T46.6X6
penicillin	T36.ØX1	T36.ØX2	T36.ØX3	T36.ØX4	T36.ØX5	T36.ØX6
Benzylhydrochlorthiazide	T5Ø.2X1	T5Ø.2X2	T5Ø.2X3	T5Ø.2X4	T5Ø.2X5	T5Ø.2X6
Benzylpenicillin	T36.ØX1	T36.ØX2	T36.ØX3	T36.ØX4	T36.ØX5	T36.ØX6
Benzylthiouracil	T38.2X1	T38.2X2	T38.2X3	T38.2X4	T38.2X5	T38.2X6
Bephenium hydroxynaphthoate	T37.4X1	T37.4X2	T37.4X3	T37.4X4	T37.4X5	T37.4X6
Bepridil	T46.1X1	T46.1X2	T46.1X3	T46.1X4	T46.1X5	T46.1X6
Bergamot oil	T65.891	T65.892	T65.893	T65.894	—	—
Bergapten	T5Ø.991	T5Ø.992	T5Ø.993	T5Ø.994	T5Ø.995	T5Ø.996
Berries, poisonous	T62.1X1	T62.1X2	T62.1X3	T62.1X4	—	—
Beryllium (compounds)	T56.7X1	T56.7X2	T56.7X3	T56.7X4	—	—
beta adrenergic blocking agent, heart	T44.7X1	T44.7X2	T44.7X3	T44.7X4	T44.7X5	T44.7X6
Betacarotene	T45.2X1	T45.2X2	T45.2X3	T45.2X4	T45.2X5	T45.2X6
Beta-Chlor	T42.6X1	T42.6X2	T42.6X3	T42.6X4	T42.6X5	T42.6X6
Betahistine	T46.7X1	T46.7X2	T46.7X3	T46.7X4	T46.7X5	T46.7X6
Betaine	T47.5X1	T47.5X2	T47.5X3	T47.5X4	T47.5X5	T47.5X6
Betamethasone	T49.ØX1	T49.ØX2	T49.ØX3	T49.ØX4	T49.ØX5	T49.ØX6
topical	T49.ØX1	T49.ØX2	T49.ØX3	T49.ØX4	T49.ØX5	T49.ØX6
Betamicin	T36.8X1	T36.8X2	T36.8X3	T36.8X4	T36.8X5	T36.8X6
Betanidine	T46.5X1	T46.5X2	T46.5X3	T46.5X4	T46.5X5	T46.5X6
Betaxolol	T44.7X1	T44.7X2	T44.7X3	T44.7X4	T44.7X5	T44.7X6
Betazole	T5Ø.8X1	T5Ø.8X2	T5Ø.8X3	T5Ø.8X4	T5Ø.8X5	T5Ø.8X6
Bethanechol	T44.1X1	T44.1X2	T44.1X3	T44.1X4	T44.1X5	T44.1X6
chloride	T44.1X1	T44.1X2	T44.1X3	T44.1X4	T44.1X5	T44.1X6
Bethanidine	T46.5X1	T46.5X2	T46.5X3	T46.5X4	T46.5X5	T46.5X6
Betoxycaine	T41.3X1	T41.3X2	T41.3X3	T41.3X4	T41.3X5	T41.3X6
Betula oil	T49.3X1	T49.3X2	T49.3X3	T49.3X4	T49.3X5	T49.3X6
Bevantolol	T44.7X1	T44.7X2	T44.7X3	T44.7X4	T44.7X5	T44.7X6
Bevonium metilsulfate	T44.3X1	T44.3X2	T44.3X3	T44.3X4	T44.3X5	T44.3X6
Bezafibrate	T46.6X1	T46.6X2	T46.6X3	T46.6X4	T46.6X5	T46.6X6
Bezitramide	T4Ø.491	T4Ø.492	T4Ø.493	T4Ø.494	T4Ø.495	T4Ø.496
BHA	T5Ø.991	T5Ø.992	T5Ø.993	T5Ø.994	T5Ø.995	T5Ø.996
Bhang	T4Ø.711	T4Ø.712	T4Ø.713	T4Ø.714	T4Ø.715	T4Ø.716
BHC (medicinal)	T49.ØX1	T49.ØX2	T49.ØX3	T49.ØX4	T49.ØX5	T49.ØX6
nonmedicinal (vapor)	T53.6X1	T53.6X2	T53.6X3	T53.6X4	—	—
Bialamicol	T37.3X1	T37.3X2	T37.3X3	T37.3X4	T37.3X5	T37.3X6
Bibenzonium bromide	T48.3X1	T48.3X2	T48.3X3	T48.3X4	T48.3X5	T48.3X6
Bibrocathol	T49.5X1	T49.5X2	T49.5X3	T49.5X4	T49.5X5	T49.5X6
Bichloride of mercury — *see* Mercury, chloride						
Bichromates (calcium) (potassium)(sodium) (crystals)	T57.8X1	T57.8X2	T57.8X3	T57.8X4	—	—
fumes	T56.2X1	T56.2X2	T56.2X3	T56.2X4	—	—
Biclotymol	T49.6X1	T49.6X2	T49.6X3	T49.6X4	T49.6X5	T49.6X6
BiCNU*	T45.1X1	T45.1X2	T45.1X3	T45.1X4	T45.1X5	T45.1X6
Bicuculline	T5Ø.7X1	T5Ø.7X2	T5Ø.7X3	T5Ø.7X4	T5Ø.7X5	T5Ø.7X6
Bifemelane	T43.291	T43.292	T43.293	T43.294	T43.295	T43.296
Biguanide derivatives, oral	T38.3X1	T38.3X2	T38.3X3	T38.3X4	T38.3X5	T38.3X6
Bile salts	T47.5X1	T47.5X2	T47.5X3	T47.5X4	T47.5X5	T47.5X6
Biligrafin	T5Ø.8X1	T5Ø.8X2	T5Ø.8X3	T5Ø.8X4	T5Ø.8X5	T5Ø.8X6
Bilopaque	T5Ø.8X1	T5Ø.8X2	T5Ø.8X3	T5Ø.8X4	T5Ø.8X5	T5Ø.8X6
Binifibrate	T46.6X1	T46.6X2	T46.6X3	T46.6X4	T46.6X5	T46.6X6
Binitrobenzol	T65.3X1	T65.3X2	T65.3X3	T65.3X4	—	—
Bioflavonoid(s)	T46.991	T46.992	T46.993	T46.994	T46.995	T46.996
Biological substance NEC	T5Ø.9Ø1	T5Ø.9Ø2	T5Ø.9Ø3	T5Ø.9Ø4	T5Ø.9Ø5	T5Ø.9Ø6
Biotin	T45.2X1	T45.2X2	T45.2X3	T45.2X4	T45.2X5	T45.2X6
Biperiden	T44.3X1	T44.3X2	T44.3X3	T44.3X4	T44.3X5	T44.3X6
Bisacodyl	T47.2X1	T47.2X2	T47.2X3	T47.2X4	T47.2X5	T47.2X6
Bisbentiamine	T45.2X1	T45.2X2	T45.2X3	T45.2X4	T45.2X5	T45.2X6
Bisbutiamine	T45.2X1	T45.2X2	T45.2X3	T45.2X4	T45.2X5	T45.2X6
Bisdequalinium (salts) (diacetate)	T49.6X1	T49.6X2	T49.6X3	T49.6X4	T49.6X5	T49.6X6
Bishydroxycoumarin	T45.511	T45.512	T45.513	T45.514	T45.515	T45.516
Bismarsen	T37.8X1	T37.8X2	T37.8X3	T37.8X4	T37.8X5	T37.8X6
Bismuth salts	T47.6X1	T47.6X2	T47.6X3	T47.6X4	T47.6X5	T47.6X6
aluminate	T47.1X1	T47.1X2	T47.1X3	T47.1X4	T47.1X5	T47.1X6
anti-infectives	T37.8X1	T37.8X2	T37.8X3	T37.8X4	T37.8X5	T37.8X6
formic iodide	T49.ØX1	T49.ØX2	T49.ØX3	T49.ØX4	T49.ØX5	T49.ØX6
glycolylarsenate	T49.ØX1	T49.ØX2	T49.ØX3	T49.ØX4	T49.ØX5	T49.ØX6
nonmedicinal (compounds)	T65.91	T65.92	T65.93	T65.94	—	—
NEC						
subcarbonate	T47.6X1	T47.6X2	T47.6X3	T47.6X4	T47.6X5	T47.6X6
subsalicylate	T37.8X1	T37.8X2	T37.8X3	T37.8X4	T37.8X5	T37.8X6
sulfarsphenamine	T37.8X1	T37.8X2	T37.8X3	T37.8X4	T37.8X5	T37.8X6
Bisoprolol	T44.7X1	T44.7X2	T44.7X3	T44.7X4	T44.7X5	T44.7X6
Bisoxatin	T47.2X1	T47.2X2	T47.2X3	T47.2X4	T47.2X5	T47.2X6
Bisulepin (hydrochloride)	T45.ØX1	T45.ØX2	T45.ØX3	T45.ØX4	T45.ØX5	T45.ØX6

Substance	Poisoning, Accidental (unintentional)	Poisoning, Intentional Self-harm	Poisoning, Assault	Poisoning, Undetermined	Adverse Effect	Under-dosing
Bithionol	T37.8X1	T37.8X2	T37.8X3	T37.8X4	T37.8X5	T37.8X6
anthelminthic	T37.4X1	T37.4X2	T37.4X3	T37.4X4	T37.4X5	T37.4X6
Bitolterol	T48.6X1	T48.6X2	T48.6X3	T48.6X4	T48.6X5	T48.6X6
Bitoscanate	T37.4X1	T37.4X2	T37.4X3	T37.4X4	T37.4X5	T37.4X6
Bitter almond oil	T62.8X1	T62.8X2	T62.8X3	T62.8X4	—	—
Bittersweet	T62.2X1	T62.2X2	T62.2X3	T62.2X4	—	—
Bivalirudin*	T45.511	T45.512	T45.513	T45.514	T45.515	T45.516
Black						
flag	T6Ø.91	T6Ø.92	T6Ø.93	T6Ø.94	—	—
henbane	T62.2X1	T62.2X2	T62.2X3	T62.2X4	—	—
leaf (40)	T6Ø.91	T6Ø.92	T6Ø.93	T6Ø.94	—	—
widow spider (bite)	T63.311	T63.312	T63.313	T63.314	—	—
antivenin	T5Ø.Z11	T5Ø.Z12	T5Ø.Z13	T5Ø.Z14	T5Ø.Z15	T5Ø.Z16
Blast furnace gas (carbon monoxide from)	T58.8X1	T58.8X2	T58.8X3	T58.8X4	—	—
Bleach	T54.91	T54.92	T54.93	T54.94	—	—
Bleaching agent (medicinal)	T49.4X1	T49.4X2	T49.4X3	T49.4X4	T49.4X5	T49.4X6
Bleomycin	T45.1X1	T45.1X2	T45.1X3	T45.1X4	T45.1X5	T45.1X6
Blockain	T41.3X1	T41.3X2	T41.3X3	T41.3X4	T41.3X5	T41.3X6
infiltration (subcutaneous)	T41.3X1	T41.3X2	T41.3X3	T41.3X4	T41.3X5	T41.3X6
nerve block (peripheral) (plexus)	T41.3X1	T41.3X2	T41.3X3	T41.3X4	T41.3X5	T41.3X6
topical (surface)	T41.3X1	T41.3X2	T41.3X3	T41.3X4	T41.3X5	T41.3X6
Blockers, calcium channel	T46.1X1	T46.1X2	T46.1X3	T46.1X4	T46.1X5	T46.1X6
Blood (derivatives) (natural) (plasma) (whole)	T45.8X1	T45.8X2	T45.8X3	T45.8X4	T45.8X5	T45.8X6
dried	T45.8X1	T45.8X2	T45.8X3	T45.8X4	T45.8X5	T45.8X6
drug affecting NEC	T45.91	T45.92	T45.93	T45.94	T45.95	T45.96
expander NEC	T45.8X1	T45.8X2	T45.8X3	T45.8X4	T45.8X5	T45.8X6
fraction NEC	T45.8X1	T45.8X2	T45.8X3	T45.8X4	T45.8X5	T45.8X6
substitute (macromolecular)	T45.8X1	T45.8X2	T45.8X3	T45.8X4	T45.8X5	T45.8X6
Blue velvet	T4Ø.2X1	T4Ø.2X2	T4Ø.2X3	T4Ø.2X4	—	—
Bone meal	T62.8X1	T62.8X2	T62.8X3	T62.8X4	—	—
Bonine	T45.ØX1	T45.ØX2	T45.ØX3	T45.ØX4	T45.ØX5	T45.ØX6
Bontril*	T5Ø.5X1	T5Ø.5X2	T5Ø.5X3	T5Ø.5X4	T5Ø.5X5	T5Ø.5X6
Bopindolol	T44.7X1	T44.7X2	T44.7X3	T44.7X4	T44.7X5	T44.7X6
Boracic acid	T49.ØX1	T49.ØX2	T49.ØX3	T49.ØX4	T49.ØX5	T49.ØX6
ENT agent	T49.6X1	T49.6X2	T49.6X3	T49.6X4	T49.6X5	T49.6X6
ophthalmic preparation	T49.5X1	T49.5X2	T49.5X3	T49.5X4	T49.5X5	T49.5X6
Borane complex	T57.8X1	T57.8X2	T57.8X3	T57.8X4	—	—
Borate(s)	T57.8X1	T57.8X2	T57.8X3	T57.8X4	—	—
buffer	T5Ø.991	T5Ø.992	T5Ø.993	T5Ø.994	T5Ø.995	T5Ø.996
cleanser	T54.91	T54.92	T54.93	T54.94	—	—
sodium	T57.8X1	T57.8X2	T57.8X3	T57.8X4	—	—
Borax (cleanser)	T54.91	T54.92	T54.93	T54.94	—	—
Bordeaux mixture	T6Ø.3X1	T6Ø.3X2	T6Ø.3X3	T6Ø.3X4	—	—
Boric acid	T49.ØX1	T49.ØX2	T49.ØX3	T49.ØX4	T49.ØX5	T49.ØX6
ENT agent	T49.6X1	T49.6X2	T49.6X3	T49.6X4	T49.6X5	T49.6X6
ophthalmic preparation	T49.5X1	T49.5X2	T49.5X3	T49.5X4	T49.5X5	T49.5X6
Bornaprine	T44.3X1	T44.3X2	T44.3X3	T44.3X4	T44.3X5	T44.3X6
Boron	T57.8X1	T57.8X2	T57.8X3	T57.8X4	—	—
hydride NEC	T57.8X1	T57.8X2	T57.8X3	T57.8X4	—	—
fumes or gas	T57.8X1	T57.8X2	T57.8X3	T57.8X4	—	—
trifluoride	T59.891	T59.892	T59.893	T59.894	—	—
Botox	T48.291	T48.292	T48.293	T48.294	T48.295	T48.296
Botulinus anti-toxin (type A, B)	T5Ø.Z11	T5Ø.Z12	T5Ø.Z13	T5Ø.Z14	T5Ø.Z15	T5Ø.Z16
Brake fluid vapor	T59.891	T59.892	T59.893	T59.894	—	—
Brallobarbital	T42.3X1	T42.3X2	T42.3X3	T42.3X4	T42.3X5	T42.3X6
Bran (wheat)	T47.4X1	T47.4X2	T47.4X3	T47.4X4	T47.4X5	T47.4X6
Brass (fumes)	T56.891	T56.892	T56.893	T56.894	—	—
Brasso	T52.ØX1	T52.ØX2	T52.ØX3	T52.ØX4	—	—
Bretylium tosilate	T46.2X1	T46.2X2	T46.2X3	T46.2X4	T46.2X5	T46.2X6
Brevital (sodium)	T41.1X1	T41.1X2	T41.1X3	T41.1X4	T41.1X5	T41.1X6
Brinase	T45.3X1	T45.3X2	T45.3X3	T45.3X4	T45.3X5	T45.3X6
British antilewisite	T45.8X1	T45.8X2	T45.8X3	T45.8X4	T45.8X5	T45.8X6
Brodalumab*	T5Ø.991	T5Ø.992	T5Ø.993	T5Ø.994	T5Ø.995	T5Ø.996
Brodifacoum	T6Ø.4X1	T6Ø.4X2	T6Ø.4X3	T6Ø.4X4	—	—
Bromal (hydrate)	T42.6X1	T42.6X2	T42.6X3	T42.6X4	T42.6X5	T42.6X6
Bromazepam	T42.4X1	T42.4X2	T42.4X3	T42.4X4	T42.4X5	T42.4X6
Bromazine	T45.ØX1	T45.ØX2	T45.ØX3	T45.ØX4	T45.ØX5	T45.ØX6
Brombenzylcyanide	T59.3X1	T59.3X2	T59.3X3	T59.3X4	—	—
Bromelains	T45.3X1	T45.3X2	T45.3X3	T45.3X4	T45.3X5	T45.3X6
Bromethalin	T6Ø.4X1	T6Ø.4X2	T6Ø.4X3	T6Ø.4X4	—	—
Bromhexine	T48.4X1	T48.4X2	T48.4X3	T48.4X4	T48.4X5	T48.4X6
Bromide salts	T42.6X1	T42.6X2	T42.6X3	T42.6X4	T42.6X5	T42.6X6
Bromindione	T45.511	T45.512	T45.513	T45.514	T45.515	T45.516
Bromine						
compounds (medicinal)	T42.6X1	T42.6X2	T42.6X3	T42.6X4	T42.6X5	T42.6X6
sedative	T42.6X1	T42.6X2	T42.6X3	T42.6X4	T42.6X5	T42.6X6
vapor	T59.891	T59.892	T59.893	T59.894	—	—
Bromisoval	T42.6X1	T42.6X2	T42.6X3	T42.6X4	T42.6X5	T42.6X6
Bromisovalum	T42.6X1	T42.6X2	T42.6X3	T42.6X4	T42.6X5	T42.6X6
Bromobenzylcyanide	T59.3X1	T59.3X2	T59.3X3	T59.3X4	—	—
Bromochlorosalicylani-lide	T49.ØX1	T49.ØX2	T49.ØX3	T49.ØX4	T49.ØX5	T49.ØX6
Bromocriptine	T42.8X1	T42.8X2	T42.8X3	T42.8X4	T42.8X5	T42.8X6
Bromodiphenhydramine	T45.ØX1	T45.ØX2	T45.ØX3	T45.ØX4	T45.ØX5	T45.ØX6
Bromoform	T42.6X1	T42.6X2	T42.6X3	T42.6X4	T42.6X5	T42.6X6
Bromophenol blue reagent	T5Ø.991	T5Ø.992	T5Ø.993	T5Ø.994	T5Ø.995	T5Ø.996
Bromopride	T47.8X1	T47.8X2	T47.8X3	T47.8X4	T47.8X5	T47.8X6
Bromosalicylchloranitide	T49.ØX1	T49.ØX2	T49.ØX3	T49.ØX4	T49.ØX5	T49.ØX6
Bromosalicylhydroxamic acid	T37.1X1	T37.1X2	T37.1X3	T37.1X4	T37.1X5	T37.1X6
Bromo-seltzer	T39.1X1	T39.1X2	T39.1X3	T39.1X4	T39.1X5	T39.1X6
Bromoxynil	T6Ø.3X1	T6Ø.3X2	T6Ø.3X3	T6Ø.3X4	—	—
Bromperidol	T43.4X1	T43.4X2	T43.4X3	T43.4X4	T43.4X5	T43.4X6
Brompheniramine	T45.ØX1	T45.ØX2	T45.ØX3	T45.ØX4	T45.ØX5	T45.ØX6
Bromsulfophthalein	T5Ø.8X1	T5Ø.8X2	T5Ø.8X3	T5Ø.8X4	T5Ø.8X5	T5Ø.8X6
Bromural	T42.6X1	T42.6X2	T42.6X3	T42.6X4	T42.6X5	T42.6X6
Bromvaletone	T42.6X1	T42.6X2	T42.6X3	T42.6X4	T42.6X5	T42.6X6
Bronchodilator NEC	T48.6X1	T48.6X2	T48.6X3	T48.6X4	T48.6X5	T48.6X6
Brotizolam	T42.4X1	T42.4X2	T42.4X3	T42.4X4	T42.4X5	T42.4X6
Brovincamine	T46.7X1	T46.7X2	T46.7X3	T46.7X4	T46.7X5	T46.7X6
Brown recluse spider (bite) (venom)	T63.331	T63.332	T63.333	T63.334	—	—
Brown spider (bite) (venom)	T63.391	T63.392	T63.393	T63.394	—	—
Broxaterol	T48.6X1	T48.6X2	T48.6X3	T48.6X4	T48.6X5	T48.6X6
Broxuridine	T45.1X1	T45.1X2	T45.1X3	T45.1X4	T45.1X5	T45.1X6
Broxyquinoline	T37.8X1	T37.8X2	T37.8X3	T37.8X4	T37.8X5	T37.8X6
Bruceine	T48.291	T48.292	T48.293	T48.294	T48.295	T48.296
Brucia	T62.2X1	T62.2X2	T62.2X3	T62.2X4	—	—
Brucine	T65.1X1	T65.1X2	T65.1X3	T65.1X4	—	—
Brunswick green — *see* Copper						
Bruten — *see* Ibuprofen						
Bryonia	T47.2X1	T47.2X2	T47.2X3	T47.2X4	T47.2X5	T47.2X6
Buclizine	T45.ØX1	T45.ØX2	T45.ØX3	T45.ØX4	T45.ØX5	T45.ØX6
Buclosamide	T49.ØX1	T49.ØX2	T49.ØX3	T49.ØX4	T49.ØX5	T49.ØX6
Budesonide	T44.5X1	T44.5X2	T44.5X3	T44.5X4	T44.5X5	T44.5X6
Budralazine	T46.5X1	T46.5X2	T46.5X3	T46.5X4	T46.5X5	T46.5X6
Bufferin	T39.Ø11	T39.Ø12	T39.Ø13	T39.Ø14	T39.Ø15	T39.Ø16
Buflomedil	T46.7X1	T46.7X2	T46.7X3	T46.7X4	T46.7X5	T46.7X6
Buformin	T38.3X1	T38.3X2	T38.3X3	T38.3X4	T38.3X5	T38.3X6
Bufotenine	T4Ø.991	T4Ø.992	T4Ø.993	T4Ø.994	—	—
Bufrolin	T48.6X1	T48.6X2	T48.6X3	T48.6X4	T48.6X5	T48.6X6
Bufylline	T48.6X1	T48.6X2	T48.6X3	T48.6X4	T48.6X5	T48.6X6
Bulgaricum IB*	T47.6X1	T47.6X2	T47.6X3	T47.6X4	T47.6X5	T47.6X6
Bulk filler	T5Ø.5X1	T5Ø.5X2	T5Ø.5X3	T5Ø.5X4	T5Ø.5X5	T5Ø.5X6
cathartic	T47.4X1	T47.4X2	T47.4X3	T47.4X4	T47.4X5	T47.4X6
Bumetanide	T5Ø.1X1	T5Ø.1X2	T5Ø.1X3	T5Ø.1X4	T5Ø.1X5	T5Ø.1X6
Bunaftine	T46.2X1	T46.2X2	T46.2X3	T46.2X4	T46.2X5	T46.2X6
Bunamiodyl	T5Ø.8X1	T5Ø.8X2	T5Ø.8X3	T5Ø.8X4	T5Ø.8X5	T5Ø.8X6
Bunazosin	T44.6X1	T44.6X2	T44.6X3	T44.6X4	T44.6X5	T44.6X6
Bunitrolol	T44.7X1	T44.7X2	T44.7X3	T44.7X4	T44.7X5	T44.7X6
Buphenine	T46.7X1	T46.7X2	T46.7X3	T46.7X4	T46.7X5	T46.7X6
Bupivacaine	T41.3X1	T41.3X2	T41.3X3	T41.3X4	T41.3X5	T41.3X6
infiltration (subcutaneous)	T41.3X1	T41.3X2	T41.3X3	T41.3X4	T41.3X5	T41.3X6
nerve block (peripheral) (plexus)	T41.3X1	T41.3X2	T41.3X3	T41.3X4	T41.3X5	T41.3X6
spinal	T41.3X1	T41.3X2	T41.3X3	T41.3X4	T41.3X5	T41.3X6
Bupranolol	T44.7X1	T44.7X2	T44.7X3	T44.7X4	T44.7X5	T44.7X6
Buprenorphine	T4Ø.491	T4Ø.492	T4Ø.493	T4Ø.494	T4Ø.495	T4Ø.496
Bupropion	T43.291	T43.292	T43.293	T43.294	T43.295	T43.296
Burimamide	T47.1X1	T47.1X2	T47.1X3	T47.1X4	T47.1X5	T47.1X6
Buserelin	T38.891	T38.892	T38.893	T38.894	T38.895	T38.896
Buspirone	T43.591	T43.592	T43.593	T43.594	T43.595	T43.596
Busulfan, busulphan	T45.1X1	T45.1X2	T45.1X3	T45.1X4	T45.1X5	T45.1X6
Busulfex*	T45.1X1	T45.1X2	T45.1X3	T45.1X4	T45.1X5	T45.1X6
Butabarbital (sodium)	T42.3X1	T42.3X2	T42.3X3	T42.3X4	T42.3X5	T42.3X6
Butabarbitone	T42.3X1	T42.3X2	T42.3X3	T42.3X4	T42.3X5	T42.3X6
Butabarpal	T42.3X1	T42.3X2	T42.3X3	T42.3X4	T42.3X5	T42.3X6
Butacaine	T41.3X1	T41.3X2	T41.3X3	T41.3X4	T41.3X5	T41.3X6
Butalamine	T46.7X1	T46.7X2	T46.7X3	T46.7X4	T46.7X5	T46.7X6
Butalbital	T42.3X1	T42.3X2	T42.3X3	T42.3X4	T42.3X5	T42.3X6
Butallylonal	T42.3X1	T42.3X2	T42.3X3	T42.3X4	T42.3X5	T42.3X6
Butamben	T41.3X1	T41.3X2	T41.3X3	T41.3X4	T41.3X5	T41.3X6
Butamirate	T48.3X1	T48.3X2	T48.3X3	T48.3X4	T48.3X5	T48.3X6
Butane (distributed in mobile container)	T59.891	T59.892	T59.893	T59.894	—	—
distributed through pipes	T59.891	T59.892	T59.893	T59.894	—	—
incomplete combustion	T58.11	T58.12	T58.13	T58.14	—	—
Butanilicaine	T41.3X1	T41.3X2	T41.3X3	T41.3X4	T41.3X5	T41.3X6
Butanol	T51.3X1	T51.3X2	T51.3X3	T51.3X4	—	—

Substance	Poisoning, Accidental (unintentional)	Poisoning, Intentional Self-harm	Poisoning, Assault	Poisoning, Undetermined	Adverse Effect	Under-dosing
Butanone, 2-butanone	T52.4X1	T52.4X2	T52.4X3	T52.4X4	—	—
Butantrone	T49.4X1	T49.4X2	T49.4X3	T49.4X4	T49.4X5	T49.4X6
Butaperazine	T43.3X1	T43.3X2	T43.3X3	T43.3X4	T43.3X5	T43.3X6
Butazolidin	T39.2X1	T39.2X2	T39.2X3	T39.2X4	T39.2X5	T39.2X6
Butetamate	T48.6X1	T48.6X2	T48.6X3	T48.6X4	T48.6X5	T48.6X6
Butethal	T42.3X1	T42.3X2	T42.3X3	T42.3X4	T42.3X5	T42.3X6
Butethamate	T44.3X1	T44.3X2	T44.3X3	T44.3X4	T44.3X5	T44.3X6
Buthalitone (sodium)	T41.1X1	T41.1X2	T41.1X3	T41.1X4	T41.1X5	T41.1X6
Butisol (sodium)	T42.3X1	T42.3X2	T42.3X3	T42.3X4	T42.3X5	T42.3X6
Butizide	T50.2X1	T50.2X2	T50.2X3	T50.2X4	T50.2X5	T50.2X6
Butobarbital	T42.3X1	T42.3X2	T42.3X3	T42.3X4	T42.3X5	T42.3X6
sodium	T42.3X1	T42.3X2	T42.3X3	T42.3X4	T42.3X5	T42.3X6
Butobarbitone	T42.3X1	T42.3X2	T42.3X3	T42.3X4	T42.3X5	T42.3X6
Butoconazole (nitrate)	T49.ØX1	T49.ØX2	T49.ØX3	T49.ØX4	T49.ØX5	T49.ØX6
Butorphanol	T40.491	T40.492	T40.493	T40.494	T40.495	T40.496
Butriptyline	T43.Ø11	T43.Ø12	T43.Ø13	T43.Ø14	T43.Ø15	T43.Ø16
Butropium bromide	T44.3X1	T44.3X2	T44.3X3	T44.3X4	T44.3X5	T44.3X6
Buttercups	T62.2X1	T62.2X2	T62.2X3	T62.2X4	—	—
Butter of antimony — *see* Antimony						
Butyl						
acetate (secondary)	T52.8X1	T52.8X2	T52.8X3	T52.8X4	—	—
alcohol	T51.3X1	T51.3X2	T51.3X3	T51.3X4	—	—
aminobenzoate	T41.3X1	T41.3X2	T41.3X3	T41.3X4	T41.3X5	T41.3X6
butyrate	T52.8X1	T52.8X2	T52.8X3	T52.8X4	—	—
carbinol	T51.3X1	T51.3X2	T51.3X3	T51.3X4	—	—
carbitol	T52.3X1	T52.3X2	T52.3X3	T52.3X4	—	—
cellosolve	T52.3X1	T52.3X2	T52.3X3	T52.3X4	—	—
chloral (hydrate)	T42.6X1	T42.6X2	T42.6X3	T42.6X4	T42.6X5	T42.6X6
formate	T52.8X1	T52.8X2	T52.8X3	T52.8X4	—	—
lactate	T52.8X1	T52.8X2	T52.8X3	T52.8X4	—	—
propionate	T52.8X1	T52.8X2	T52.8X3	T52.8X4	—	—
scopolamine bromide	T44.3X1	T44.3X2	T44.3X3	T44.3X4	T44.3X5	T44.3X6
thiobarbital sodium	T41.1X1	T41.1X2	T41.1X3	T41.1X4	T41.1X5	T41.1X6
Butylated hydroxyanisole	T50.991	T50.992	T50.993	T50.994	T50.995	T50.996
Butylchloral hydrate	T42.6X1	T42.6X2	T42.6X3	T42.6X4	T42.6X5	T42.6X6
Butyltoluene	T52.2X1	T52.2X2	T52.2X3	T52.2X4	—	—
Butyn	T41.3X1	T41.3X2	T41.3X3	T41.3X4	T41.3X5	T41.3X6
Butyrophenone (-based tranquilizers)	T43.4X1	T43.4X2	T43.4X3	T43.4X4	T43.4X5	T43.4X6
Cabazitaxel*	T45.1X1	T45.1X2	T45.1X3	T45.1X4	T45.1X5	T45.1X6
Cabergoline	T42.8X1	T42.8X2	T42.8X3	T42.8X4	T42.8X5	T42.8X6
Cacodyl, cacodylic acid	T57.ØX1	T57.ØX2	T57.ØX3	T57.ØX4	—	—
Cactinomycin	T45.1X1	T45.1X2	T45.1X3	T45.1X4	T45.1X5	T45.1X6
Cade oil	T49.4X1	T49.4X2	T49.4X3	T49.4X4	T49.4X5	T49.4X6
Cadexomer iodine	T49.ØX1	T49.ØX2	T49.ØX3	T49.ØX4	T49.ØX5	T49.ØX6
Cadmium (chloride) (fumes) (oxide)	T56.3X1	T56.3X2	T56.3X3	T56.3X4	—	—
sulfide (medicinal) NEC	T49.4X1	T49.4X2	T49.4X3	T49.4X4	T49.4X5	T49.4X6
Cadralazine	T46.5X1	T46.5X2	T46.5X3	T46.5X4	T46.5X5	T46.5X6
Caffeine	T43.611	T43.612	T43.613	T43.614	T43.615	T43.616
Calabar bean	T62.2X1	T62.2X2	T62.2X3	T62.2X4	—	—
Caladium seguinum	T62.2X1	T62.2X2	T62.2X3	T62.2X4	—	—
Calamine (lotion)	T49.3X1	T49.3X2	T49.3X3	T49.3X4	T49.3X5	T49.3X6
Calcifediol	T45.2X1	T45.2X2	T45.2X3	T45.2X4	T45.2X5	T45.2X6
Calciferol	T45.2X1	T45.2X2	T45.2X3	T45.2X4	T45.2X5	T45.2X6
Calcijex*	T45.2X1	T45.2X2	T45.2X3	T45.2X4	T45.2X5	T45.2X6
Calcitonin	T50.991	T50.992	T50.993	T50.994	T50.995	T50.996
Calcitriol	T45.2X1	T45.2X2	T45.2X3	T45.2X4	T45.2X5	T45.2X6
Calcium	T50.3X1	T50.3X2	T50.3X3	T50.3X4	T50.3X5	T50.3X6
actylsalicylate	T39.Ø11	T39.Ø12	T39.Ø13	T39.Ø14	T39.Ø15	T39.Ø16
benzamidosalicylate	T37.1X1	T37.1X2	T37.1X3	T37.1X4	T37.1X5	T37.1X6
bromide	T42.6X1	T42.6X2	T42.6X3	T42.6X4	T42.6X5	T42.6X6
bromolactobionate	T42.6X1	T42.6X2	T42.6X3	T42.6X4	T42.6X5	T42.6X6
carbaspirin	T39.Ø11	T39.Ø12	T39.Ø13	T39.Ø14	T39.Ø15	T39.Ø16
carbimide	T50.6X1	T50.6X2	T50.6X3	T50.6X4	T50.6X5	T50.6X6
carbonate	T47.1X1	T47.1X2	T47.1X3	T47.1X4	T47.1X5	T47.1X6
chloride	T50.991	T50.992	T50.993	T50.994	T50.995	T50.996
anhydrous	T50.991	T50.992	T50.993	T50.994	T50.995	T50.996
cyanide	T57.8X1	T57.8X2	T57.8X3	T57.8X4	—	—
dioctyl sulfosuccinate	T47.4X1	T47.4X2	T47.4X3	T47.4X4	T47.4X5	T47.4X6
disodium edathamil	T45.8X1	T45.8X2	T45.8X3	T45.8X4	T45.8X5	T45.8X6
disodium edetate	T45.8X1	T45.8X2	T45.8X3	T45.8X4	T45.8X5	T45.8X6
dobesilate	T46.991	T46.992	T46.993	T46.994	T46.995	T46.996
EDTA	T45.8X1	T45.8X2	T45.8X3	T45.8X4	T45.8X5	T45.8X6
ferrous citrate	T45.4X1	T45.4X2	T45.4X3	T45.4X4	T45.4X5	T45.4X6
folinate	T45.8X1	T45.8X2	T45.8X3	T45.8X4	T45.8X5	T45.8X6
glubionate	T50.3X1	T50.3X2	T50.3X3	T50.3X4	T50.3X5	T50.3X6
gluconate	T50.3X1	T50.3X2	T50.3X3	T50.3X4	T50.3X5	T50.3X6
gluconogalactogluconate	T50.3X1	T50.3X2	T50.3X3	T50.3X4	T50.3X5	T50.3X6
hydrate, hydroxide	T54.3X1	T54.3X2	T54.3X3	T54.3X4	—	—
hypochlorite	T54.3X1	T54.3X2	T54.3X3	T54.3X4	—	—
iodide	T48.4X1	T48.4X2	T48.4X3	T48.4X4	T48.4X5	T48.4X6

Substance	Poisoning, Accidental (unintentional)	Poisoning, Intentional Self-harm	Poisoning, Assault	Poisoning, Undetermined	Adverse Effect	Under-dosing
Calcium — *continued*						
ipodate	T50.8X1	T50.8X2	T50.8X3	T50.8X4	T50.8X5	T50.8X6
lactate	T50.3X1	T50.3X2	T50.3X3	T50.3X4	T50.3X5	T50.3X6
leucovorin	T45.8X1	T45.8X2	T45.8X3	T45.8X4	T45.8X5	T45.8X6
mandelate	T37.91	T37.92	T37.93	T37.94	T37.95	T37.96
oxide	T54.3X1	T54.3X2	T54.3X3	T54.3X4	—	—
pantothenate	T45.2X1	T45.2X2	T45.2X3	T45.2X4	T45.2X5	T45.2X6
phosphate	T50.3X1	T50.3X2	T50.3X3	T50.3X4	T50.3X5	T50.3X6
salicylate	T39.Ø91	T39.Ø92	T39.Ø93	T39.Ø94	T39.Ø95	T39.Ø96
salts	T50.3X1	T50.3X2	T50.3X3	T50.3X4	T50.3X5	T50.3X6
Calculus-dissolving drug	T50.991	T50.992	T50.993	T50.994	T50.995	T50.996
Calomel	T49.ØX1	T49.ØX2	T49.ØX3	T49.ØX4	T49.ØX5	T49.ØX6
Caloric agent	T50.3X1	T50.3X2	T50.3X3	T50.3X4	T50.3X5	T50.3X6
Calusterone	T38.7X1	T38.7X2	T38.7X3	T38.7X4	T38.7X5	T38.7X6
Camazepam	T42.4X1	T42.4X2	T42.4X3	T42.4X4	T42.4X5	T42.4X6
Camomile	T49.ØX1	T49.ØX2	T49.ØX3	T49.ØX4	T49.ØX5	T49.ØX6
Camoquin	T37.2X1	T37.2X2	T37.2X3	T37.2X4	T37.2X5	T37.2X6
Camphor						
insecticide	T60.2X1	T60.2X2	T60.2X3	T60.2X4	—	—
medicinal	T49.8X1	T49.8X2	T49.8X3	T49.8X4	T49.8X5	T49.8X6
Camylofin	T44.3X1	T44.3X2	T44.3X3	T44.3X4	T44.3X5	T44.3X6
Cancer chemotherapy drug regimen	T45.1X1	T45.1X2	T45.1X3	T45.1X4	T45.1X5	T45.1X6
Candeptin	T49.ØX1	T49.ØX2	T49.ØX3	T49.ØX4	T49.ØX5	T49.ØX6
Candicidin	T49.ØX1	T49.ØX2	T49.ØX3	T49.ØX4	T49.ØX5	T49.ØX6
Cankaid*	T49.6X1	T49.6X2	T49.6X3	T49.6X4	T49.6X5	T49.6X6
Cannabinoids, synthetic	T40.721	T40.722	T40.723	T40.724	T40.725	T40.726
Cannabinol	T40.711	T40.712	T40.713	T40.714	T40.715	T40.716
Cannabis (derivatives)	T40.711	T40.712	T40.713	T40.714	T40.715	T40.716
Canned heat	T51.1X1	T51.1X2	T51.1X3	T51.1X4	—	—
Canrenoic acid	T50.ØX1	T50.ØX2	T50.ØX3	T50.ØX4	T50.ØX5	T50.ØX6
Canrenone	T50.ØX1	T50.ØX2	T50.ØX3	T50.ØX4	T50.ØX5	T50.ØX6
Cantharides, cantharidin, cantharis	T49.8X1	T49.8X2	T49.8X3	T49.8X4	T49.8X5	T49.8X6
Canthaxanthin	T50.991	T50.992	T50.993	T50.994	T50.995	T50.996
Capillary-active drug NEC	T46.9Ø1	T46.9Ø2	T46.9Ø3	T46.9Ø4	T46.9Ø5	T46.9Ø6
Capreomycin	T36.8X1	T36.8X2	T36.8X3	T36.8X4	T36.8X5	T36.8X6
Capresla*	T45.1X1	T45.1X2	T45.1X3	T45.1X4	T45.1X5	T45.1X6
Capsicum	T49.4X1	T49.4X2	T49.4X3	T49.4X4	T49.4X5	T49.4X6
Captafol	T60.3X1	T60.3X2	T60.3X3	T60.3X4	—	—
Captan	T60.3X1	T60.3X2	T60.3X3	T60.3X4	—	—
Captodiame, captodiamine	T43.591	T43.592	T43.593	T43.594	T43.595	T43.596
Captopril	T46.4X1	T46.4X2	T46.4X3	T46.4X4	T46.4X5	T46.4X6
Caramiphen	T44.3X1	T44.3X2	T44.3X3	T44.3X4	T44.3X5	T44.3X6
Carazolol	T44.7X1	T44.7X2	T44.7X3	T44.7X4	T44.7X5	T44.7X6
Carbachol	T44.1X1	T44.1X2	T44.1X3	T44.1X4	T44.1X5	T44.1X6
Carbacrylamine (resin)	T50.3X1	T50.3X2	T50.3X3	T50.3X4	T50.3X5	T50.3X6
Carbamate (insecticide)	T60.ØX1	T60.ØX2	T60.ØX3	T60.ØX4	—	—
Carbamate (sedative)	T42.6X1	T42.6X2	T42.6X3	T42.6X4	T42.6X5	T42.6X6
herbicide	T60.ØX1	T60.ØX2	T60.ØX3	T60.ØX4	—	—
insecticide	T60.ØX1	T60.ØX2	T60.ØX3	T60.ØX4	—	—
Carbamazepine	T42.1X1	T42.1X2	T42.1X3	T42.1X4	T42.1X5	T42.1X6
Carbamide	T47.3X1	T47.3X2	T47.3X3	T47.3X4	T47.3X5	T47.3X6
peroxide	T49.ØX1	T49.ØX2	T49.ØX3	T49.ØX4	T49.ØX5	T49.ØX6
topical	T49.8X1	T49.8X2	T49.8X3	T49.8X4	T49.8X5	T49.8X6
Carbamylcholine chloride	T44.1X1	T44.1X2	T44.1X3	T44.1X4	T44.1X5	T44.1X6
Carbaril	T60.ØX1	T60.ØX2	T60.ØX3	T60.ØX4	—	—
Carbarsone	T37.3X1	T37.3X2	T37.3X3	T37.3X4	T37.3X5	T37.3X6
Carbaryl	T60.ØX1	T60.ØX2	T60.ØX3	T60.ØX4	—	—
Carbaspirin	T39.Ø11	T39.Ø12	T39.Ø13	T39.Ø14	T39.Ø15	T39.Ø16
Carbastat*	T49.5X1	T49.5X2	T49.5X3	T49.5X4	T49.5X5	T49.5X6
Carbazochrome (salicylate) (sodium sulfonate)	T49.4X1	T49.4X2	T49.4X3	T49.4X4	T49.4X5	T49.4X6
Carbenicillin	T36.ØX1	T36.ØX2	T36.ØX3	T36.ØX4	T36.ØX5	T36.ØX6
Carbenoxolone	T47.1X1	T47.1X2	T47.1X3	T47.1X4	T47.1X5	T47.1X6
Carbetapentane	T48.3X1	T48.3X2	T48.3X3	T48.3X4	T48.3X5	T48.3X6
Carbethyl salicylate	T39.Ø91	T39.Ø92	T39.Ø93	T39.Ø94	T39.Ø95	T39.Ø96
Carbidopa (with levodopa)	T42.8X1	T42.8X2	T42.8X3	T42.8X4	T42.8X5	T42.8X6
Carbimazole	T38.2X1	T38.2X2	T38.2X3	T38.2X4	T38.2X5	T38.2X6
Carbinol	T51.1X1	T51.1X2	T51.1X3	T51.1X4	—	—
Carbinoxamine	T45.ØX1	T45.ØX2	T45.ØX3	T45.ØX4	T45.ØX5	T45.ØX6
Carbiphene	T39.8X1	T39.8X2	T39.8X3	T39.8X4	T39.8X5	T39.8X6
Carbitol	T52.3X1	T52.3X2	T52.3X3	T52.3X4	—	—
Carbocaine	T41.3X1	T41.3X2	T41.3X3	T41.3X4	T41.3X5	T41.3X6
infiltration (subcutaneous)	T41.3X1	T41.3X2	T41.3X3	T41.3X4	T41.3X5	T41.3X6
nerve block (peripheral) (plexus)	T41.3X1	T41.3X2	T41.3X3	T41.3X4	T41.3X5	T41.3X6
topical (surface)	T41.3X1	T41.3X2	T41.3X3	T41.3X4	T41.3X5	T41.3X6
Carbocisteine	T48.4X1	T48.4X2	T48.4X3	T48.4X4	T48.4X5	T48.4X6
Carbocromen	T46.3X1	T46.3X2	T46.3X3	T46.3X4	T46.3X5	T46.3X6
Carbol fuchsin	T49.ØX1	T49.ØX2	T49.ØX3	T49.ØX4	T49.ØX5	T49.ØX6

Substance	Poisoning, Accidental (unintentional)	Poisoning, Intentional Self-harm	Poisoning, Assault	Poisoning, Undetermined	Adverse Effect	Under-dosing
Carbolic acid — *see also* Phenol	T54.ØX1	T54.ØX2	T54.ØX3	T54.ØX4	—	—
Carbolonium (bromide)	T48.1X1	T48.1X2	T48.1X3	T48.1X4	T48.1X5	T48.1X6
Carbo medicinalis	T47.6X1	T47.6X2	T47.6X3	T47.6X4	T47.6X5	T47.6X6
Carbomycin	T36.8X1	T36.8X2	T36.8X3	T36.8X4	T36.8X5	T36.8X6
Carbon						
bisulfide (liquid)	T65.4X1	T65.4X2	T65.4X3	T65.4X4	—	—
vapor	T65.4X1	T65.4X2	T65.4X3	T65.4X4	—	—
dioxide (gas)	T59.7X1	T59.7X2	T59.7X3	T59.7X4	—	—
medicinal	T41.5X1	T41.5X2	T41.5X3	T41.5X4	T41.5X5	T41.5X6
nonmedicinal	T59.7X1	T59.7X2	T59.7X3	T59.7X4	—	—
snow	T49.4X1	T49.4X2	T49.4X3	T49.4X4	T49.4X5	T49.4X6
disulfide (liquid)	T65.4X1	T65.4X2	T65.4X3	T65.4X4	—	—
vapor	T65.4X1	T65.4X2	T65.4X3	T65.4X4	—	—
monoxide (from incomplete combustion)	T58.91	T58.92	T58.93	T58.94	—	—
blast furnace gas	T58.8X1	T58.8X2	T58.8X3	T58.8X4	—	—
butane (distributed in mobile container)	T58.11	T58.12	T58.13	T58.14	—	—
distributed through pipes	T58.11	T58.12	T58.13	T58.14	—	—
charcoal fumes	T58.2X1	T58.2X2	T58.2X3	T58.2X4	—	—
coal	T58.2X1	T58.2X2	T58.2X3	T58.2X4	—	—
coke (in domestic stoves, fireplaces)	T58.2X1	T58.2X2	T58.2X3	T58.2X4	—	—
exhaust gas (motor) not in transit	T58.Ø1	T58.Ø2	T58.Ø3	T58.Ø4	—	—
combustion engine, any not in watercraft	T58.Ø1	T58.Ø2	T58.Ø3	T58.Ø4	—	—
farm tractor, not in transit	T58.Ø1	T58.Ø2	T58.Ø3	T58.Ø4	—	—
gas engine	T58.Ø1	T58.Ø2	T58.Ø3	T58.Ø4	—	—
motor pump	T58.Ø1	T58.Ø2	T58.Ø3	T58.Ø4	—	—
motor vehicle, not in transit	T58.Ø1	T58.Ø2	T58.Ø3	T58.Ø4	—	—
fuel (in domestic use)	T58.2X1	T58.2X2	T58.2X3	T58.2X4	—	—
gas (piped)	T58.11	T58.12	T58.13	T58.14	—	—
in mobile container	T58.11	T58.12	T58.13	T58.14	—	—
piped (natural)	T58.11	T58.12	T58.13	T58.14	—	—
utility	T58.11	T58.12	T58.13	T58.14	—	—
in mobile container	T58.11	T58.12	T58.13	T58.14	—	—
gas (piped)	T58.11	T58.12	T58.13	T58.14	—	—
illuminating gas	T58.11	T58.12	T58.13	T58.14	—	—
industrial fuels or gases, any	T58.8X1	T58.8X2	T58.8X3	T58.8X4	—	—
kerosene (in domestic stoves, fireplaces)	T58.2X1	T58.2X2	T58.2X3	T58.2X4	—	—
kiln gas or vapor	T58.8X1	T58.8X2	T58.8X3	T58.8X4	—	—
motor exhaust gas, not in transit	T58.Ø1	T58.Ø2	T58.Ø3	T58.Ø4	—	—
piped gas (manufactured) (natural)	T58.11	T58.12	T58.13	T58.14	—	—
producer gas	T58.8X1	T58.8X2	T58.8X3	T58.8X4	—	—
propane (distributed in mobile container)	T58.11	T58.12	T58.13	T58.14	—	—
distributed through pipes	T58.11	T58.12	T58.13	T58.14	—	—
solid (in domestic stoves, fireplaces)	T58.2X1	T58.2X2	T58.2X3	T58.2X4	—	—
specified source NEC	T58.8X1	T58.8X2	T58.8X3	T58.8X4	—	—
stove gas	T58.11	T58.12	T58.13	T58.14	—	—
piped	T58.11	T58.12	T58.13	T58.14	—	—
utility gas	T58.11	T58.12	T58.13	T58.14	—	—
piped	T58.11	T58.12	T58.13	T58.14	—	—
water gas	T58.11	T58.12	T58.13	T58.14	—	—
wood (in domestic stoves, fireplaces)	T58.2X1	T58.2X2	T58.2X3	T58.2X4	—	—
tetrachloride (vapor) NEC	T53.ØX1	T53.ØX2	T53.ØX3	T53.ØX4	—	—
liquid (cleansing agent) NEC	T53.ØX1	T53.ØX2	T53.ØX3	T53.ØX4	—	—
solvent	T53.ØX1	T53.ØX2	T53.ØX3	T53.ØX4	—	—
Carbonic acid gas	T59.7X1	T59.7X2	T59.7X3	T59.7X4	—	—
anhydrase inhibitor NEC	T5Ø.2X1	T5Ø.2X2	T5Ø.2X3	T5Ø.2X4	T5Ø.2X5	T5Ø.2X6
Carbophenothion	T6Ø.ØX1	T6Ø.ØX2	T6Ø.ØX3	T6Ø.ØX4	—	—
Carboplatin	T45.1X1	T45.1X2	T45.1X3	T45.1X4	T45.1X5	T45.1X6
Carboprost	T48.ØX1	T48.ØX2	T48.ØX3	T48.ØX4	T48.ØX5	T48.ØX6
Carboquone	T45.1X1	T45.1X2	T45.1X3	T45.1X4	T45.1X5	T45.1X6
Carbowax	T49.3X1	T49.3X2	T49.3X3	T49.3X4	T49.3X5	T49.3X6
Carboxymethylcellulose	T47.4X1	T47.4X2	T47.4X3	T47.4X4	T47.4X5	T47.4X6
Carbrital	T42.3X1	T42.3X2	T42.3X3	T42.3X4	T42.3X5	T42.3X6
Carbromal	T42.6X1	T42.6X2	T42.6X3	T42.6X4	T42.6X5	T42.6X6
Carbutamide	T38.3X1	T38.3X2	T38.3X3	T38.3X4	T38.3X5	T38.3X6
Carbuterol	T48.6X1	T48.6X2	T48.6X3	T48.6X4	T48.6X5	T48.6X6
Cardiac						
depressants	T46.2X1	T46.2X2	T46.2X3	T46.2X4	T46.2X5	T46.2X6
rhythm regulator	T46.2X1	T46.2X2	T46.2X3	T46.2X4	T46.2X5	T46.2X6
specified NEC	T46.2X1	T46.2X2	T46.2X3	T46.2X4	T46.2X5	T46.2X6
Cardiografin	T5Ø.8X1	T5Ø.8X2	T5Ø.8X3	T5Ø.8X4	T5Ø.8X5	T5Ø.8X6
Cardiogreen	T5Ø.8X1	T5Ø.8X2	T5Ø.8X3	T5Ø.8X4	T5Ø.8X5	T5Ø.8X6
Cardiotonic (glycoside) **NEC**	T46.ØX1	T46.ØX2	T46.ØX3	T46.ØX4	T46.ØX5	T46.ØX6
Cardiovascular drug NEC	T46.9Ø1	T46.9Ø2	T46.9Ø3	T46.9Ø4	T46.9Ø5	T46.9Ø6
Cardizem*	T46.1X1	T46.1X2	T46.1X3	T46.1X4	T46.1X5	T46.1X6
Cardrase	T5Ø.2X1	T5Ø.2X2	T5Ø.2X3	T5Ø.2X4	T5Ø.2X5	T5Ø.2X6
Carfecillin	T36.ØX1	T36.ØX2	T36.ØX3	T36.ØX4	T36.ØX5	T36.ØX6
Carfenazine	T43.3X1	T43.3X2	T43.3X3	T43.3X4	T43.3X5	T43.3X6
Carfusin	T49.ØX1	T49.ØX2	T49.ØX3	T49.ØX4	T49.ØX5	T49.ØX6
Carindacillin	T36.ØX1	T36.ØX2	T36.ØX3	T36.ØX4	T36.ØX5	T36.ØX6
Carisoprodol	T42.8X1	T42.8X2	T42.8X3	T42.8X4	T42.8X5	T42.8X6
Carmellose	T47.4X1	T47.4X2	T47.4X3	T47.4X4	T47.4X5	T47.4X6
Carminative	T47.5X1	T47.5X2	T47.5X3	T47.5X4	T47.5X5	T47.5X6
Carmofur	T45.1X1	T45.1X2	T45.1X3	T45.1X4	T45.1X5	T45.1X6
Carmustine	T45.1X1	T45.1X2	T45.1X3	T45.1X4	T45.1X5	T45.1X6
Carotene	T45.2X1	T45.2X2	T45.2X3	T45.2X4	T45.2X5	T45.2X6
Carphenazine	T43.3X1	T43.3X2	T43.3X3	T43.3X4	T43.3X5	T43.3X6
Carpipramine	T42.4X1	T42.4X2	T42.4X3	T42.4X4	T42.4X5	T42.4X6
Carprofen	T39.311	T39.312	T39.313	T39.314	T39.315	T39.316
Carpronium chloride	T44.3X1	T44.3X2	T44.3X3	T44.3X4	T44.3X5	T44.3X6
Carrageenan	T47.8X1	T47.8X2	T47.8X3	T47.8X4	T47.8X5	T47.8X6
Carteolol	T44.7X1	T44.7X2	T44.7X3	T44.7X4	T44.7X5	T44.7X6
Carter's Little Pills	T47.2X1	T47.2X2	T47.2X3	T47.2X4	T47.2X5	T47.2X6
Cartia*	T46.1X1	T46.1X2	T46.1X3	T46.1X4	T46.1X5	T46.1X6
Cascara (sagrada)	T47.2X1	T47.2X2	T47.2X3	T47.2X4	T47.2X5	T47.2X6
Cassava	T62.2X1	T62.2X2	T62.2X3	T62.2X4	—	—
Castellani's paint	T49.ØX1	T49.ØX2	T49.ØX3	T49.ØX4	T49.ØX5	T49.ØX6
Castor						
bean	T62.2X1	T62.2X2	T62.2X3	T62.2X4	—	—
oil	T47.2X1	T47.2X2	T47.2X3	T47.2X4	T47.2X5	T47.2X6
Catalase	T45.3X1	T45.3X2	T45.3X3	T45.3X4	T45.3X5	T45.3X6
Caterpillar (sting)	T63.431	T63.432	T63.433	T63.434	—	—
Catha (edulis) (tea)	T43.691	T43.692	T43.693	T43.694	—	—
Cathartic NEC	T47.4X1	T47.4X2	T47.4X3	T47.4X4	T47.4X5	T47.4X6
anthacene derivative	T47.2X1	T47.2X2	T47.2X3	T47.2X4	T47.2X5	T47.2X6
bulk	T47.4X1	T47.4X2	T47.4X3	T47.4X4	T47.4X5	T47.4X6
contact	T47.2X1	T47.2X2	T47.2X3	T47.2X4	T47.2X5	T47.2X6
emollient NEC	T47.4X1	T47.4X2	T47.4X3	T47.4X4	T47.4X5	T47.4X6
irritant NEC	T47.2X1	T47.2X2	T47.2X3	T47.2X4	T47.2X5	T47.2X6
mucilage	T47.4X1	T47.4X2	T47.4X3	T47.4X4	T47.4X5	T47.4X6
saline	T47.3X1	T47.3X2	T47.3X3	T47.3X4	T47.3X5	T47.3X6
vegetable	T47.2X1	T47.2X2	T47.2X3	T47.2X4	T47.2X5	T47.2X6
Cathine	T5Ø.5X1	T5Ø.5X2	T5Ø.5X3	T5Ø.5X4	T5Ø.5X5	T5Ø.5X6
Cathomycin	T36.8X1	T36.8X2	T36.8X3	T36.8X4	T36.8X5	T36.8X6
Cation exchange resin	T5Ø.3X1	T5Ø.3X2	T5Ø.3X3	T5Ø.3X4	T5Ø.3X5	T5Ø.3X6
Caustic(s) **NEC**	T54.91	T54.92	T54.93	T54.94	—	—
alkali	T54.3X1	T54.3X2	T54.3X3	T54.3X4	—	—
hydroxide	T54.3X1	T54.3X2	T54.3X3	T54.3X4	—	—
potash	T54.3X1	T54.3X2	T54.3X3	T54.3X4	—	—
soda	T54.3X1	T54.3X2	T54.3X3	T54.3X4	—	—
specified NEC	T54.91	T54.92	T54.93	T54.94	—	—
Ceepryn	T49.ØX1	T49.ØX2	T49.ØX3	T49.ØX4	T49.ØX5	T49.ØX6
ENT agent	T49.6X1	T49.6X2	T49.6X3	T49.6X4	T49.6X5	T49.6X6
lozenges	T49.6X1	T49.6X2	T49.6X3	T49.6X4	T49.6X5	T49.6X6
Cefacetrile	T36.1X1	T36.1X2	T36.1X3	T36.1X4	T36.1X5	T36.1X6
Cefaclor	T36.1X1	T36.1X2	T36.1X3	T36.1X4	T36.1X5	T36.1X6
Cefadroxil	T36.1X1	T36.1X2	T36.1X3	T36.1X4	T36.1X5	T36.1X6
Cefalexin	T36.1X1	T36.1X2	T36.1X3	T36.1X4	T36.1X5	T36.1X6
Cefaloglycin	T36.1X1	T36.1X2	T36.1X3	T36.1X4	T36.1X5	T36.1X6
Cefaloridine	T36.1X1	T36.1X2	T36.1X3	T36.1X4	T36.1X5	T36.1X6
Cefalosporins	T36.1X1	T36.1X2	T36.1X3	T36.1X4	T36.1X5	T36.1X6
Cefalotin	T36.1X1	T36.1X2	T36.1X3	T36.1X4	T36.1X5	T36.1X6
Cefamandole	T36.1X1	T36.1X2	T36.1X3	T36.1X4	T36.1X5	T36.1X6
Cefamycin antibiotic	T36.1X1	T36.1X2	T36.1X3	T36.1X4	T36.1X5	T36.1X6
Cefapirin	T36.1X1	T36.1X2	T36.1X3	T36.1X4	T36.1X5	T36.1X6
Cefatrizine	T36.1X1	T36.1X2	T36.1X3	T36.1X4	T36.1X5	T36.1X6
Cefazedone	T36.1X1	T36.1X2	T36.1X3	T36.1X4	T36.1X5	T36.1X6
Cefazolin	T36.1X1	T36.1X2	T36.1X3	T36.1X4	T36.1X5	T36.1X6
Cefbuperazone	T36.1X1	T36.1X2	T36.1X3	T36.1X4	T36.1X5	T36.1X6
Cefetamet	T36.1X1	T36.1X2	T36.1X3	T36.1X4	T36.1X5	T36.1X6
Cefixime	T36.1X1	T36.1X2	T36.1X3	T36.1X4	T36.1X5	T36.1X6
Cefmenoxime	T36.1X1	T36.1X2	T36.1X3	T36.1X4	T36.1X5	T36.1X6
Cefmetazole	T36.1X1	T36.1X2	T36.1X3	T36.1X4	T36.1X5	T36.1X6
Cefminox	T36.1X1	T36.1X2	T36.1X3	T36.1X4	T36.1X5	T36.1X6
Cefonicid	T36.1X1	T36.1X2	T36.1X3	T36.1X4	T36.1X5	T36.1X6
Cefoperazone	T36.1X1	T36.1X2	T36.1X3	T36.1X4	T36.1X5	T36.1X6
Ceforanide	T36.1X1	T36.1X2	T36.1X3	T36.1X4	T36.1X5	T36.1X6
Cefotaxime	T36.1X1	T36.1X2	T36.1X3	T36.1X4	T36.1X5	T36.1X6
Cefotetan	T36.1X1	T36.1X2	T36.1X3	T36.1X4	T36.1X5	T36.1X6

Substance	Poisoning, Accidental (unintentional)	Poisoning, Intentional Self-harm	Poisoning, Assault	Poisoning, Undetermined	Adverse Effect	Under-dosing
Cefotiam	T36.1X1	T36.1X2	T36.1X3	T36.1X4	T36.1X5	T36.1X6
Cefoxitin	T36.1X1	T36.1X2	T36.1X3	T36.1X4	T36.1X5	T36.1X6
Cefpimizole	T36.1X1	T36.1X2	T36.1X3	T36.1X4	T36.1X5	T36.1X6
Cefpiramide	T36.1X1	T36.1X2	T36.1X3	T36.1X4	T36.1X5	T36.1X6
Cefradine	T36.1X1	T36.1X2	T36.1X3	T36.1X4	T36.1X5	T36.1X6
Cefroxadine	T36.1X1	T36.1X2	T36.1X3	T36.1X4	T36.1X5	T36.1X6
Cefsulodin	T36.1X1	T36.1X2	T36.1X3	T36.1X4	T36.1X5	T36.1X6
Ceftazidime	T36.1X1	T36.1X2	T36.1X3	T36.1X4	T36.1X5	T36.1X6
Cefteram	T36.1X1	T36.1X2	T36.1X3	T36.1X4	T36.1X5	T36.1X6
Ceftezole	T36.1X1	T36.1X2	T36.1X3	T36.1X4	T36.1X5	T36.1X6
Ceftin*	T36.1X1	T36.1X2	T36.1X3	T36.1X4	T36.1X5	T36.1X6
Ceftizoxime	T36.1X1	T36.1X2	T36.1X3	T36.1X4	T36.1X5	T36.1X6
Ceftriaxone	T36.1X1	T36.1X2	T36.1X3	T36.1X4	T36.1X5	T36.1X6
Cefuroxime	T36.1X1	T36.1X2	T36.1X3	T36.1X4	T36.1X5	T36.1X6
Cefuzonam	T36.1X1	T36.1X2	T36.1X3	T36.1X4	T36.1X5	T36.1X6
Celestone	T38.ØX1	T38.ØX2	T38.ØX3	T38.ØX4	T38.ØX5	T38.ØX6
topical	T49.ØX1	T49.ØX2	T49.ØX3	T49.ØX4	T49.ØX5	T49.ØX6
Celiprolol	T44.7X1	T44.7X2	T44.7X3	T44.7X4	T44.7X5	T44.7X6
Cellosolve	T52.91	T52.92	T52.93	T52.94	—	—
Cell stimulants and proliferants	T49.8X1	T49.8X2	T49.8X3	T49.8X4	T49.8X5	T49.8X6
Cellulose						
cathartic	T47.4X1	T47.4X2	T47.4X3	T47.4X4	T47.4X5	T47.4X6
hydroxyethyl	T47.4X1	T47.4X2	T47.4X3	T47.4X4	T47.4X5	T47.4X6
nitrates (topical)	T49.3X1	T49.3X2	T49.3X3	T49.3X4	T49.3X5	T49.3X6
oxidized	T49.4X1	T49.4X2	T49.4X3	T49.4X4	T49.4X5	T49.4X6
Centipede (bite)	T63.411	T63.412	T63.413	T63.414	—	—
Central nervous system						
depressants	T42.71	T42.72	T42.73	T42.74	T42.75	T42.76
anesthetic (general) NEC	T41.2Ø1	T41.2Ø2	T41.2Ø3	T41.2Ø4	T41.2Ø5	T41.2Ø6
gases NEC	T41.ØX1	T41.ØX2	T41.ØX3	T41.ØX4	T41.ØX5	T41.ØX6
intravenous	T41.1X1	T41.1X2	T41.1X3	T41.1X4	T41.1X5	T41.1X6
barbiturates	T42.3X1	T42.3X2	T42.3X3	T42.3X4	T42.3X5	T42.3X6
benzodiazepines	T42.4X1	T42.4X2	T42.4X3	T42.4X4	T42.4X5	T42.4X6
bromides	T42.6X1	T42.6X2	T42.6X3	T42.6X4	T42.6X5	T42.6X6
cannabis sativa	T4Ø.711	T4Ø.712	T4Ø.713	T4Ø.714	T4Ø.715	T4Ø.716
chloral hydrate	T42.6X1	T42.6X2	T42.6X3	T42.6X4	T42.6X5	T42.6X6
ethanol	T51.ØX1	T51.ØX2	T51.ØX3	T51.ØX4	—	—
hallucinogenics	T4Ø.9Ø1	T4Ø.9Ø2	T4Ø.9Ø3	T4Ø.9Ø4	T4Ø.9Ø5	T4Ø.9Ø6
hypnotics	T42.71	T42.72	T42.73	T42.74	T42.75	T42.76
specified NEC	T42.6X1	T42.6X2	T42.6X3	T42.6X4	T42.6X5	T42.6X6
muscle relaxants	T42.8X1	T42.8X2	T42.8X3	T42.8X4	T42.8X5	T42.8X6
paraldehyde	T42.6X1	T42.6X2	T42.6X3	T42.6X4	T42.6X5	T42.6X6
sedatives;	T42.71	T42.72	T42.73	T42.74	T42.75	T42.76
sedative-hypnotics						
mixed NEC	T42.6X1	T42.6X2	T42.6X3	T42.6X4	T42.6X5	T42.6X6
specified NEC	T42.8X1	T42.8X2	T42.8X3	T42.8X4	T42.8X5	T42.8X6
muscle-tone depressants	T42.8X1	T42.8X2	T42.8X3	T42.8X4	T42.8X5	T42.8X6
stimulants	T43.6Ø1	T43.6Ø2	T43.6Ø3	T43.6Ø4	T43.6Ø5	T43.6Ø6
amphetamines	T43.621	T43.622	T43.623	T43.624	T43.625	T43.626
analeptics	T5Ø.7X1	T5Ø.7X2	T5Ø.7X3	T5Ø.7X4	T5Ø.7X5	T5Ø.7X6
antidepressants	T43.2Ø1	T43.2Ø2	T43.2Ø3	T43.2Ø4	T43.2Ø5	T43.2Ø6
opiate antagonists	T5Ø.7X1	T5Ø.7X2	T5Ø.7X3	T5Ø.7X4	T5Ø.7X5	T5Ø.7X6
specified NEC	T43.691	T43.692	T43.693	T43.694	T43.695	T43.696
Cepacol*	T41.3X1	T41.3X2	T41.3X3	T41.3X4	T41.3X5	T41.3X6
Cephalexin	T36.1X1	T36.1X2	T36.1X3	T36.1X4	T36.1X5	T36.1X6
Cephaloglycin	T36.1X1	T36.1X2	T36.1X3	T36.1X4	T36.1X5	T36.1X6
Cephaloridine	T36.1X1	T36.1X2	T36.1X3	T36.1X4	T36.1X5	T36.1X6
Cephalosporins	T36.1X1	T36.1X2	T36.1X3	T36.1X4	T36.1X5	T36.1X6
N (adicillin)	T36.ØX1	T36.ØX2	T36.ØX3	T36.ØX4	T36.ØX5	T36.ØX6
Cephalothin	T36.1X1	T36.1X2	T36.1X3	T36.1X4	T36.1X5	T36.1X6
Cephalotin	T36.1X1	T36.1X2	T36.1X3	T36.1X4	T36.1X5	T36.1X6
Cephradine	T36.1X1	T36.1X2	T36.1X3	T36.1X4	T36.1X5	T36.1X6
Cerbera (odallam)	T62.2X1	T62.2X2	T62.2X3	T62.2X4	—	—
Cerberin	T46.ØX1	T46.ØX2	T46.ØX3	T46.ØX4	T46.ØX5	T46.ØX6
Cerebral stimulants	T43.6Ø1	T43.6Ø2	T43.6Ø3	T43.6Ø4	T43.6Ø5	T43.6Ø6
psychotherapeutic	T43.6Ø1	T43.6Ø2	T43.6Ø3	T43.6Ø4	T43.6Ø5	T43.6Ø6
specified NEC	T43.691	T43.692	T43.693	T43.694	T43.695	T43.696
Cerium oxalate	T45.ØX1	T45.ØX2	T45.ØX3	T45.ØX4	T45.ØX5	T45.ØX6
Cerous oxalate	T45.ØX1	T45.ØX2	T45.ØX3	T45.ØX4	T45.ØX5	T45.ØX6
Ceruletide	T5Ø.8X1	T5Ø.8X2	T5Ø.8X3	T5Ø.8X4	T5Ø.8X5	T5Ø.8X6
Cetacort*	T49.ØX1	T49.ØX2	T49.ØX3	T49.ØX4	T49.ØX5	T49.ØX6
Cetalkonium (chloride)	T49.ØX1	T49.ØX2	T49.ØX3	T49.ØX4	T49.ØX5	T49.ØX6
Cethexonium chloride	T49.ØX1	T49.ØX2	T49.ØX3	T49.ØX4	T49.ØX5	T49.ØX6
Cetiedil	T46.7X1	T46.7X2	T46.7X3	T46.7X4	T46.7X5	T46.7X6
Cetirizine	T45.ØX1	T45.ØX2	T45.ØX3	T45.ØX4	T45.ØX5	T45.ØX6
Cetomacrogol	T5Ø.991	T5Ø.992	T5Ø.993	T5Ø.994	T5Ø.995	T5Ø.996
Cetotiamine	T45.2X1	T45.2X2	T45.2X3	T45.2X4	T45.2X5	T45.2X6
Cetoxime	T45.ØX1	T45.ØX2	T45.ØX3	T45.ØX4	T45.ØX5	T45.ØX6
Cetraxate	T47.1X1	T47.1X2	T47.1X3	T47.1X4	T47.1X5	T47.1X6
Cetrimide	T49.ØX1	T49.ØX2	T49.ØX3	T49.ØX4	T49.ØX5	T49.ØX6
Cetrimonium (bromide)	T49.ØX1	T49.ØX2	T49.ØX3	T49.ØX4	T49.ØX5	T49.ØX6
Cetylpyridinium chloride	T49.ØX1	T49.ØX2	T49.ØX3	T49.ØX4	T49.ØX5	T49.ØX6

Substance	Poisoning, Accidental (unintentional)	Poisoning, Intentional Self-harm	Poisoning, Assault	Poisoning, Undetermined	Adverse Effect	Under-dosing
Cetylpyridinium chloride — *continued*						
ENT agent	T49.6X1	T49.6X2	T49.6X3	T49.6X4	T49.6X5	T49.6X6
lozenges	T49.6X1	T49.6X2	T49.6X3	T49.6X4	T49.6X5	T49.6X6
Cevadilla — *see* Sabadilla						
Cevitamic acid	T45.2X1	T45.2X2	T45.2X3	T45.2X4	T45.2X5	T45.2X6
Chalk, precipitated	T47.1X1	T47.1X2	T47.1X3	T47.1X4	T47.1X5	T47.1X6
Chamomile	T49.ØX1	T49.ØX2	T49.ØX3	T49.ØX4	T49.ØX5	T49.ØX6
Ch'an su	T46.ØX1	T46.ØX2	T46.ØX3	T46.ØX4	T46.ØX5	T46.ØX6
Charcoal	T47.6X1	T47.6X2	T47.6X3	T47.6X4	T47.6X5	T47.6X6
activated — *see also* Charcoal, medicinal	T47.6X1	T47.6X2	T47.6X3	T47.6X4	T47.6X5	T47.6X6
fumes (Carbon monoxide)	T58.2X1	T58.2X2	T58.2X3	T58.2X4	—	—
industrial	T58.8X1	T58.8X2	T58.8X3	T58.8X4	—	—
medicinal (activated)	T47.6X1	T47.6X2	T47.6X3	T47.6X4	T47.6X5	T47.6X6
antidiarrheal	T47.6X1	T47.6X2	T47.6X3	T47.6X4	T47.6X5	T47.6X6
poison control	T47.8X1	T47.8X2	T47.8X3	T47.8X4	T47.8X5	T47.8X6
specified use other than for diarrhea	T47.8X1	T47.8X2	T47.8X3	T47.8X4	T47.8X5	T47.8X6
topical	T49.8X1	T49.8X2	T49.8X3	T49.8X4	T49.8X5	T49.8X6
Chaulmosulfone	T37.1X1	T37.1X2	T37.1X3	T37.1X4	T37.1X5	T37.1X6
Chelating agent NEC	T5Ø.6X1	T5Ø.6X2	T5Ø.6X3	T5Ø.6X4	T5Ø.6X5	T5Ø.6X6
Chelidonium majus	T62.2X1	T62.2X2	T62.2X3	T62.2X4	—	—
Chemical substance NEC	T65.91	T65.92	T65.93	T65.94	—	—
Chenodeoxycholic acid	T47.5X1	T47.5X2	T47.5X3	T47.5X4	T47.5X5	T47.5X6
Chenodiol	T47.5X1	T47.5X2	T47.5X3	T47.5X4	T47.5X5	T47.5X6
Chenopodium	T37.4X1	T37.4X2	T37.4X3	T37.4X4	T37.4X5	T37.4X6
Cherry laurel	T62.2X1	T62.2X2	T62.2X3	T62.2X4	—	—
Chiggertox*	T41.3X1	T41.3X2	T41.3X3	T41.3X4	T41.3X5	T41.3X6
Chinidin (e)	T46.2X1	T46.2X2	T46.2X3	T46.2X4	T46.2X5	T46.2X6
Chiniofon	T37.8X1	T37.8X2	T37.8X3	T37.8X4	T37.8X5	T37.8X6
Chlophedianol	T48.3X1	T48.3X2	T48.3X3	T48.3X4	T48.3X5	T48.3X6
Chloral	T42.6X1	T42.6X2	T42.6X3	T42.6X4	T42.6X5	T42.6X6
derivative	T42.6X1	T42.6X2	T42.6X3	T42.6X4	T42.6X5	T42.6X6
hydrate	T42.6X1	T42.6X2	T42.6X3	T42.6X4	T42.6X5	T42.6X6
Chloralamide	T42.6X1	T42.6X2	T42.6X3	T42.6X4	T42.6X5	T42.6X6
Chloralodol	T42.6X1	T42.6X2	T42.6X3	T42.6X4	T42.6X5	T42.6X6
Chloralose	T6Ø.4X1	T6Ø.4X2	T6Ø.4X3	T6Ø.4X4	—	—
Chlorambucil	T45.1X1	T45.1X2	T45.1X3	T45.1X4	T45.1X5	T45.1X6
Chloramine	T57.8X1	T57.8X2	T57.8X3	T57.8X4	—	—
T	T49.ØX1	T49.ØX2	T49.ØX3	T49.ØX4	T49.ØX5	T49.ØX6
topical	T49.ØX1	T49.ØX2	T49.ØX3	T49.ØX4	T49.ØX5	T49.ØX6
Chloramphenicol	T36.2X1	T36.2X2	T36.2X3	T36.2X4	T36.2X5	T36.2X6
ENT agent	T49.6X1	T49.6X2	T49.6X3	T49.6X4	T49.6X5	T49.6X6
ophthalmic preparation	T49.5X1	T49.5X2	T49.5X3	T49.5X4	T49.5X5	T49.5X6
topical NEC	T49.ØX1	T49.ØX2	T49.ØX3	T49.ØX4	T49.ØX5	T49.ØX6
Chlorate (potassium) (sodium) **NEC**	T6Ø.3X1	T6Ø.3X2	T6Ø.3X3	T6Ø.3X4	—	—
herbicide	T6Ø.3X1	T6Ø.3X2	T6Ø.3X3	T6Ø.3X4	—	—
Chlorazanil	T5Ø.2X1	T5Ø.2X2	T5Ø.2X3	T5Ø.2X4	T5Ø.2X5	T5Ø.2X6
Chlorbenzene, chlorbenzol	T53.7X1	T53.7X2	T53.7X3	T53.7X4	—	—
Chlorbenzoxamine	T44.3X1	T44.3X2	T44.3X3	T44.3X4	T44.3X5	T44.3X6
Chlorbutol	T42.6X1	T42.6X2	T42.6X3	T42.6X4	T42.6X5	T42.6X6
Chlorcyclizine	T45.ØX1	T45.ØX2	T45.ØX3	T45.ØX4	T45.ØX5	T45.ØX6
Chlordan (e) (dust)	T6Ø.1X1	T6Ø.1X2	T6Ø.1X3	T6Ø.1X4	—	—
Chlordantoin	T49.ØX1	T49.ØX2	T49.ØX3	T49.ØX4	T49.ØX5	T49.ØX6
Chlordiazepoxide	T42.4X1	T42.4X2	T42.4X3	T42.4X4	T42.4X5	T42.4X6
Chlordiethyl benzamide	T49.3X1	T49.3X2	T49.3X3	T49.3X4	T49.3X5	T49.3X6
Chloresium	T49.8X1	T49.8X2	T49.8X3	T49.8X4	T49.8X5	T49.8X6
Chlorethiazol	T42.6X1	T42.6X2	T42.6X3	T42.6X4	T42.6X5	T42.6X6
Chlorethyl — *see* Ethyl, chloride						
Chloretone	T42.6X1	T42.6X2	T42.6X3	T42.6X4	T42.6X5	T42.6X6
Chlorex	T53.6X1	T53.6X2	T53.6X3	T53.6X4	—	—
insecticide	T6Ø.1X1	T6Ø.1X2	T6Ø.1X3	T6Ø.1X4	—	—
Chlorfenvinphos	T6Ø.ØX1	T6Ø.ØX2	T6Ø.ØX3	T6Ø.ØX4	—	—
Chlorhexadol	T42.6X1	T42.6X2	T42.6X3	T42.6X4	T42.6X5	T42.6X6
Chlorhexamide	T45.1X1	T45.1X2	T45.1X3	T45.1X4	T45.1X5	T45.1X6
Chlorhexidine	T49.ØX1	T49.ØX2	T49.ØX3	T49.ØX4	T49.ØX5	T49.ØX6
Chlorhexidine Gluconate Oral Rinse*	T49.6X1	T49.6X2	T49.6X3	T49.6X4	T49.6X5	T49.6X6
Chlorhydroxyquinolin	T49.ØX1	T49.ØX2	T49.ØX3	T49.ØX4	T49.ØX5	T49.ØX6
Chloride of lime (bleach)	T54.3X1	T54.3X2	T54.3X3	T54.3X4	—	—
Chlorimipramine	T43.Ø11	T43.Ø12	T43.Ø13	T43.Ø14	T43.Ø15	T43.Ø16
Chlorinated						
camphene	T53.6X1	T53.6X2	T53.6X3	T53.6X4	—	—
diphenyl	T53.7X1	T53.7X2	T53.7X3	T53.7X4	—	—
hydrocarbons NEC	T53.91	T53.92	T53.93	T53.94	—	—
solvents	T53.91	T53.92	T53.93	T53.94	—	—
lime (bleach)	T54.3X1	T54.3X2	T54.3X3	T54.3X4	—	—
and boric acid solution	T49.ØX1	T49.ØX2	T49.ØX3	T49.ØX4	T49.ØX5	T49.ØX6
naphthalene (insecticide)	T6Ø.1X1	T6Ø.1X2	T6Ø.1X3	T6Ø.1X4	—	—

Substance	Poisoning, Accidental (unintentional)	Poisoning, Intentional Self-harm	Poisoning, Assault	Poisoning, Undetermined	Adverse Effect	Under-dosing
Chlorinated — *continued*						
naphthalene — *continued*						
industrial (non-pesticide)	T53.7X1	T53.7X2	T53.7X3	T53.7X4	—	—
pesticide NEC	T6Ø.8X1	T6Ø.8X2	T6Ø.8X3	T6Ø.8X4	—	—
soda — *see also* sodium hypochlorite						
solution	T49.ØX1	T49.ØX2	T49.ØX3	T49.ØX4	T49.ØX5	T49.ØX6
Chlorine (fumes) (gas)	T59.4X1	T59.4X2	T59.4X3	T59.4X4	—	—
bleach	T54.3X1	T54.3X2	T54.3X3	T54.3X4	—	—
compound gas NEC	T59.4X1	T59.4X2	T59.4X3	T59.4X4	—	—
disinfectant	T59.4X1	T59.4X2	T59.4X3	T59.4X4	—	—
releasing agents NEC	T59.4X1	T59.4X2	T59.4X3	T59.4X4	—	—
Chlorisondamine chloride	T46.991	T46.992	T46.993	T46.994	T46.995	T46.996
Chlormadinone	T38.5X1	T38.5X2	T38.5X3	T38.5X4	T38.5X5	T38.5X6
Chlormephos	T6Ø.ØX1	T6Ø.ØX2	T6Ø.ØX3	T6Ø.ØX4	—	—
Chlormerodrin	T5Ø.2X1	T5Ø.2X2	T5Ø.2X3	T5Ø.2X4	T5Ø.2X5	T5Ø.2X6
Chlormethiazole	T42.6X1	T42.6X2	T42.6X3	T42.6X4	T42.6X5	T42.6X6
Chlormethine	T45.1X1	T45.1X2	T45.1X3	T45.1X4	T45.1X5	T45.1X6
Chlormethylenecycline	T36.4X1	T36.4X2	T36.4X3	T36.4X4	T36.4X5	T36.4X6
Chlormezanone	T42.6X1	T42.6X2	T42.6X3	T42.6X4	T42.6X5	T42.6X6
Chloroacetic acid	T6Ø.3X1	T6Ø.3X2	T6Ø.3X3	T6Ø.3X4	—	—
Chloroacetone	T59.3X1	T59.3X2	T59.3X3	T59.3X4	—	—
Chloroacetophenone	T59.3X1	T59.3X2	T59.3X3	T59.3X4	—	—
Chloroaniline	T53.7X1	T53.7X2	T53.7X3	T53.7X4	—	—
Chlorobenzene, chlorobenzol	T53.7X1	T53.7X2	T53.7X3	T53.7X4	—	—
Chlorobromomethane (fire extinguisher)	T53.6X1	T53.6X2	T53.6X3	T53.6X4	—	—
Chlorobutanol	T49.ØX1	T49.ØX2	T49.ØX3	T49.ØX4	T49.ØX5	T49.ØX6
Chlorocresol	T49.ØX1	T49.ØX2	T49.ØX3	T49.ØX4	T49.ØX5	T49.ØX6
Chlorodehydromethyltestosterone	T38.7X1	T38.7X2	T38.7X3	T38.7X4	T38.7X5	T38.7X6
Chlorodeoxyadenosine*	T45.1X1	T45.1X2	T45.1X3	T45.1X4	T45.1X5	T45.1X6
Chlorodinitrobenzene	T53.7X1	T53.7X2	T53.7X3	T53.7X4	—	—
dust or vapor	T53.7X1	T53.7X2	T53.7X3	T53.7X4	—	—
Chlorodiphenyl	T53.7X1	T53.7X2	T53.7X3	T53.7X4	—	—
Chloroethane — *see* Ethyl, chloride						
Chloroethylene	T53.6X1	T53.6X2	T53.6X3	T53.6X4	—	—
Chlorofluorocarbons	T53.5X1	T53.5X2	T53.5X3	T53.5X4	—	—
Chloroform (fumes) (vapor)	T53.1X1	T53.1X2	T53.1X3	T53.1X4	—	—
anesthetic	T41.ØX1	T41.ØX2	T41.ØX3	T41.ØX4	T41.ØX5	T41.ØX6
solvent	T53.1X1	T53.1X2	T53.1X3	T53.1X4	—	—
water, concentrated	T41.ØX1	T41.ØX2	T41.ØX3	T41.ØX4	T41.ØX5	T41.ØX6
Chloroguanide	T37.2X1	T37.2X2	T37.2X3	T37.2X4	T37.2X5	T37.2X6
Chloromycetin	T36.2X1	T36.2X2	T36.2X3	T36.2X4	T36.2X5	T36.2X6
ENT agent	T49.6X1	T49.6X2	T49.6X3	T49.6X4	T49.6X5	T49.6X6
ophthalmic preparation	T49.5X1	T49.5X2	T49.5X3	T49.5X4	T49.5X5	T49.5X6
otic solution	T49.6X1	T49.6X2	T49.6X3	T49.6X4	T49.6X5	T49.6X6
topical NEC	T49.ØX1	T49.ØX2	T49.ØX3	T49.ØX4	T49.ØX5	T49.ØX6
Chloronitrobenzene	T53.7X1	T53.7X2	T53.7X3	T53.7X4	—	—
dust or vapor	T53.7X1	T53.7X2	T53.7X3	T53.7X4	—	—
Chlorophacinone	T6Ø.4X1	T6Ø.4X2	T6Ø.4X3	T6Ø.4X4	—	—
Chlorophenol	T53.7X1	T53.7X2	T53.7X3	T53.7X4	—	—
Chlorophenothane	T6Ø.1X1	T6Ø.1X2	T6Ø.1X3	T6Ø.1X4	—	—
Chlorophyll	T5Ø.991	T5Ø.992	T5Ø.993	T5Ø.994	T5Ø.995	T5Ø.996
Chloropicrin (fumes)	T53.6X1	T53.6X2	T53.6X3	T53.6X4	—	—
fumigant	T6Ø.8X1	T6Ø.8X2	T6Ø.8X3	T6Ø.8X4	—	—
fungicide	T6Ø.3X1	T6Ø.3X2	T6Ø.3X3	T6Ø.3X4	—	—
pesticide	T6Ø.8X1	T6Ø.8X2	T6Ø.8X3	T6Ø.8X4	—	—
Chloroprocaine	T41.3X1	T41.3X2	T41.3X3	T41.3X4	T41.3X5	T41.3X6
infiltration (subcutaneous)	T41.3X1	T41.3X2	T41.3X3	T41.3X4	T41.3X5	T41.3X6
nerve block (peripheral) (plexus)	T41.3X1	T41.3X2	T41.3X3	T41.3X4	T41.3X5	T41.3X6
spinal	T41.3X1	T41.3X2	T41.3X3	T41.3X4	T41.3X5	T41.3X6
Chloroptic	T49.5X1	T49.5X2	T49.5X3	T49.5X4	T49.5X5	T49.5X6
Chloropurine	T45.1X1	T45.1X2	T45.1X3	T45.1X4	T45.1X5	T45.1X6
Chloropyramine	T45.ØX1	T45.ØX2	T45.ØX3	T45.ØX4	T45.ØX5	T45.ØX6
Chloropyrifos	T6Ø.ØX1	T6Ø.ØX2	T6Ø.ØX3	T6Ø.ØX4	—	—
Chloropyrilene	T45.ØX1	T45.ØX2	T45.ØX3	T45.ØX4	T45.ØX5	T45.ØX6
Chloroquine	T37.2X1	T37.2X2	T37.2X3	T37.2X4	T37.2X5	T37.2X6
Chlorostat*	T49.ØX1	T49.ØX2	T49.ØX3	T49.ØX4	T49.ØX5	T49.ØX6
Chlorothalonil	T6Ø.3X1	T6Ø.3X2	T6Ø.3X3	T6Ø.3X4	—	—
Chlorothen	T45.ØX1	T45.ØX2	T45.ØX3	T45.ØX4	T45.ØX5	T45.ØX6
Chlorothiazide	T5Ø.2X1	T5Ø.2X2	T5Ø.2X3	T5Ø.2X4	T5Ø.2X5	T5Ø.2X6
Chlorothymol	T49.4X1	T49.4X2	T49.4X3	T49.4X4	T49.4X5	T49.4X6
Chlorotrianisene	T38.5X1	T38.5X2	T38.5X3	T38.5X4	T38.5X5	T38.5X6
Chlorovinyldichloroarsine, not in war	T57.ØX1	T57.ØX2	T57.ØX3	T57.ØX4	—	—
Chloroxine	T49.4X1	T49.4X2	T49.4X3	T49.4X4	T49.4X5	T49.4X6
Chloroxylenol	T49.ØX1	T49.ØX2	T49.ØX3	T49.ØX4	T49.ØX5	T49.ØX6
Chlorphenamine	T45.ØX1	T45.ØX2	T45.ØX3	T45.ØX4	T45.ØX5	T45.ØX6

Substance	Poisoning, Accidental (unintentional)	Poisoning, Intentional Self-harm	Poisoning, Assault	Poisoning, Undetermined	Adverse Effect	Under-dosing
Chlorphenesin	T42.8X1	T42.8X2	T42.8X3	T42.8X4	T42.8X5	T42.8X6
topical (antifungal)	T49.ØX1	T49.ØX2	T49.ØX3	T49.ØX4	T49.ØX5	T49.ØX6
Chlorpheniramine	T45.ØX1	T45.ØX2	T45.ØX3	T45.ØX4	T45.ØX5	T45.ØX6
Chlorphenoxamine	T45.ØX1	T45.ØX2	T45.ØX3	T45.ØX4	T45.ØX5	T45.ØX6
Chlorphentermine	T5Ø.5X1	T5Ø.5X2	T5Ø.5X3	T5Ø.5X4	T5Ø.5X5	T5Ø.5X6
Chlorprocaine — *see* Chloroprocaine						
Chlorproguanil	T37.2X1	T37.2X2	T37.2X3	T37.2X4	T37.2X5	T37.2X6
Chlorpromazine	T43.3X1	T43.3X2	T43.3X3	T43.3X4	T43.3X5	T43.3X6
Chlorpropamide	T38.3X1	T38.3X2	T38.3X3	T38.3X4	T38.3X5	T38.3X6
Chlorprothixene	T43.4X1	T43.4X2	T43.4X3	T43.4X4	T43.4X5	T43.4X6
Chlorquinaldol	T49.ØX1	T49.ØX2	T49.ØX3	T49.ØX4	T49.ØX5	T49.ØX6
Chlorquinol	T49.ØX1	T49.ØX2	T49.ØX3	T49.ØX4	T49.ØX5	T49.ØX6
Chlortalidone	T5Ø.2X1	T5Ø.2X2	T5Ø.2X3	T5Ø.2X4	T5Ø.2X5	T5Ø.2X6
Chlortetracycline	T36.4X1	T36.4X2	T36.4X3	T36.4X4	T36.4X5	T36.4X6
Chlorthalidone	T5Ø.2X1	T5Ø.2X2	T5Ø.2X3	T5Ø.2X4	T5Ø.2X5	T5Ø.2X6
Chlorthion	T6Ø.ØX1	T6Ø.ØX2	T6Ø.ØX3	T6Ø.ØX4	—	—
Chlorthiophos	T6Ø.ØX1	T6Ø.ØX2	T6Ø.ØX3	T6Ø.ØX4	—	—
Chlortrianisene	T38.5X1	T38.5X2	T38.5X3	T38.5X4	T38.5X5	T38.5X6
Chlor-Trimeton	T45.ØX1	T45.ØX2	T45.ØX3	T45.ØX4	T45.ØX5	T45.ØX6
Chlorzoxazone	T42.8X1	T42.8X2	T42.8X3	T42.8X4	T42.8X5	T42.8X6
Choke damp	T59.7X1	T59.7X2	T59.7X3	T59.7X4	—	—
Cholagogues	T47.5X1	T47.5X2	T47.5X3	T47.5X4	T47.5X5	T47.5X6
Cholebrine	T5Ø.8X1	T5Ø.8X2	T5Ø.8X3	T5Ø.8X4	T5Ø.8X5	T5Ø.8X6
Cholecalciferol	T45.2X1	T45.2X2	T45.2X3	T45.2X4	T45.2X5	T45.2X6
Cholecystokinin	T5Ø.8X1	T5Ø.8X2	T5Ø.8X3	T5Ø.8X4	T5Ø.8X5	T5Ø.8X6
Cholera vaccine	T5Ø.A91	T5Ø.A92	T5Ø.A93	T5Ø.A94	T5Ø.A95	T5Ø.A96
Choleretic	T47.5X1	T47.5X2	T47.5X3	T47.5X4	T47.5X5	T47.5X6
Cholesterol-lowering agents	T46.6X1	T46.6X2	T46.6X3	T46.6X4	T46.6X5	T46.6X6
Cholestyramine (resin)	T46.6X1	T46.6X2	T46.6X3	T46.6X4	T46.6X5	T46.6X6
Cholic acid	T47.5X1	T47.5X2	T47.5X3	T47.5X4	T47.5X5	T47.5X6
Choline	T48.6X1	T48.6X2	T48.6X3	T48.6X4	T48.6X5	T48.6X6
chloride	T5Ø.991	T5Ø.992	T5Ø.993	T5Ø.994	T5Ø.995	T5Ø.996
dihydrogen citrate	T5Ø.991	T5Ø.992	T5Ø.993	T5Ø.994	T5Ø.995	T5Ø.996
salicylate	T39.Ø91	T39.Ø92	T39.Ø93	T39.Ø94	T39.Ø95	T39.Ø96
theophyllinate	T48.6X1	T48.6X2	T48.6X3	T48.6X4	T48.6X5	T48.6X6
Cholinergic (drug) **NEC**	T44.1X1	T44.1X2	T44.1X3	T44.1X4	T44.1X5	T44.1X6
muscle tone enhancer	T44.1X1	T44.1X2	T44.1X3	T44.1X4	T44.1X5	T44.1X6
organophosphorus	T44.ØX1	T44.ØX2	T44.ØX3	T44.ØX4	T44.ØX5	T44.ØX6
insecticide	T6Ø.ØX1	T6Ø.ØX2	T6Ø.ØX3	T6Ø.ØX4	—	—
nerve gas	T59.891	T59.892	T59.893	T59.894	—	—
trimethyl ammonium propanediol	T44.1X1	T44.1X2	T44.1X3	T44.1X4	T44.1X5	T44.1X6
Cholinesterase reactivator	T5Ø.6X1	T5Ø.6X2	T5Ø.6X3	T5Ø.6X4	T5Ø.6X5	T5Ø.6X6
Cholografin	T5Ø.8X1	T5Ø.8X2	T5Ø.8X3	T5Ø.8X4	T5Ø.8X5	T5Ø.8X6
Chorionic gonadotropin	T38.891	T38.892	T38.893	T38.894	T38.895	T38.896
Chromate	T56.2X1	T56.2X2	T56.2X3	T56.2X4	—	—
dust or mist	T56.2X1	T56.2X2	T56.2X3	T56.2X4	—	—
lead — *see also* lead paint	T56.ØX1	T56.ØX2	T56.ØX3	T56.ØX4	—	—
Chromelin*	T49.3X1	T49.3X2	T49.3X3	T49.3X4	T49.3X5	T49.3X6
Chromic						
acid	T56.2X1	T56.2X2	T56.2X3	T56.2X4	—	—
dust or mist	T56.2X1	T56.2X2	T56.2X3	T56.2X4	—	—
phosphate 32P	T45.1X1	T45.1X2	T45.1X3	T45.1X4	T45.1X5	T45.1X6
Chromium	T56.2X1	T56.2X2	T56.2X3	T56.2X4	—	—
compounds — *see* Chromate						
sesquioxide	T5Ø.8X1	T5Ø.8X2	T5Ø.8X3	T5Ø.8X4	T5Ø.8X5	T5Ø.8X6
Chromomycin A3	T45.1X1	T45.1X2	T45.1X3	T45.1X4	T45.1X5	T45.1X6
Chromonar	T46.3X1	T46.3X2	T46.3X3	T46.3X4	T46.3X5	T46.3X6
Chromyl chloride	T56.2X1	T56.2X2	T56.2X3	T56.2X4	—	—
Chrysarobin	T49.4X1	T49.4X2	T49.4X3	T49.4X4	T49.4X5	T49.4X6
Chrysazin	T47.2X1	T47.2X2	T47.2X3	T47.2X4	T47.2X5	T47.2X6
Chymar	T45.3X1	T45.3X2	T45.3X3	T45.3X4	T45.3X5	T45.3X6
ophthalmic preparation	T49.5X1	T49.5X2	T49.5X3	T49.5X4	T49.5X5	T49.5X6
Chymopapain	T45.3X1	T45.3X2	T45.3X3	T45.3X4	T45.3X5	T45.3X6
Chymotrypsin	T45.3X1	T45.3X2	T45.3X3	T45.3X4	T45.3X5	T45.3X6
ophthalmic preparation	T49.5X1	T49.5X2	T49.5X3	T49.5X4	T49.5X5	T49.5X6
Cianidanol	T5Ø.991	T5Ø.992	T5Ø.993	T5Ø.994	T5Ø.995	T5Ø.996
Cianopramine	T43.Ø11	T43.Ø12	T43.Ø13	T43.Ø14	T43.Ø15	T43.Ø16
Cibenzoline	T46.2X1	T46.2X2	T46.2X3	T46.2X4	T46.2X5	T46.2X6
Ciclacillin	T36.ØX1	T36.ØX2	T36.ØX3	T36.ØX4	T36.ØX5	T36.ØX6
Ciclobarbital — *see* Hexobarbital						
Ciclonicate	T46.7X1	T46.7X2	T46.7X3	T46.7X4	T46.7X5	T46.7X6
Ciclopirox (olamine)	T49.ØX1	T49.ØX2	T49.ØX3	T49.ØX4	T49.ØX5	T49.ØX6
Ciclosporin	T45.1X1	T45.1X2	T45.1X3	T45.1X4	T45.1X5	T45.1X6
Cicuta maculata or virosa	T62.2X1	T62.2X2	T62.2X3	T62.2X4	—	—
Cicutoxin	T62.2X1	T62.2X2	T62.2X3	T62.2X4	—	—
Cigarette lighter fluid	T52.ØX1	T52.ØX2	T52.ØX3	T52.ØX4	—	—
Cigarettes (tobacco)	T65.221	T65.222	T65.223	T65.224	—	—
Ciguatoxin	T61.Ø1	T61.Ø2	T61.Ø3	T61.Ø4	—	—

Substance	Poisoning, Accidental (unintentional)	Poisoning, Intentional Self-harm	Poisoning, Assault	Poisoning, Undetermined	Adverse Effect	Under-dosing
Cilazapril	T46.4X1	T46.4X2	T46.4X3	T46.4X4	T46.4X5	T46.4X6
Cimetidine	T47.ØX1	T47.ØX2	T47.ØX3	T47.ØX4	T47.ØX5	T47.ØX6
Cimetropium bromide	T44.3X1	T44.3X2	T44.3X3	T44.3X4	T44.3X5	T44.3X6
Cinchocaine	T41.3X1	T41.3X2	T41.3X3	T41.3X4	T41.3X5	T41.3X6
topical (surface)	T41.3X1	T41.3X2	T41.3X3	T41.3X4	T41.3X5	T41.3X6
Cinchona	T37.2X1	T37.2X2	T37.2X3	T37.2X4	T37.2X5	T37.2X6
Cinchonine alkaloids	T37.2X1	T37.2X2	T37.2X3	T37.2X4	T37.2X5	T37.2X6
Cinchophen	T5Ø.4X1	T5Ø.4X2	T5Ø.4X3	T5Ø.4X4	T5Ø.4X5	T5Ø.4X6
Cinepazide	T46.7X1	T46.7X2	T46.7X3	T46.7X4	T46.7X5	T46.7X6
Cinnamedrine	T48.5X1	T48.5X2	T48.5X3	T48.5X4	T48.5X5	T48.5X6
Cinnarizine	T45.ØX1	T45.ØX2	T45.ØX3	T45.ØX4	T45.ØX5	T45.ØX6
Cinoxacin	T37.8X1	T37.8X2	T37.8X3	T37.8X4	T37.8X5	T37.8X6
Ciprofibrate	T46.6X1	T46.6X2	T46.6X3	T46.6X4	T46.6X5	T46.6X6
Ciprofloxacin	T36.8X1	T36.8X2	T36.8X3	T36.8X4	T36.8X5	T36.8X6
Cisapride	T47.8X1	T47.8X2	T47.8X3	T47.8X4	T47.8X5	T47.8X6
Cisplatin	T45.1X1	T45.1X2	T45.1X3	T45.1X4	T45.1X5	T45.1X6
Citalopram	T43.221	T43.222	T43.223	T43.224	T43.225	T43.226
Citanest	T41.3X1	T41.3X2	T41.3X3	T41.3X4	T41.3X5	T41.3X6
infiltration (subcutaneous)	T41.3X1	T41.3X2	T41.3X3	T41.3X4	T41.3X5	T41.3X6
nerve block (peripheral) (plexus)	T41.3X1	T41.3X2	T41.3X3	T41.3X4	T41.3X5	T41.3X6
Citracel*	T5Ø.3X1	T5Ø.3X2	T5Ø.3X3	T5Ø.3X4	T5Ø.3X5	T5Ø.3X6
Citric acid	T47.5X1	T47.5X2	T47.5X3	T47.5X4	T47.5X5	T47.5X6
Citrovorum (factor)	T45.8X1	T45.8X2	T45.8X3	T45.8X4	T45.8X5	T45.8X6
Claviceps purpurea	T62.2X1	T62.2X2	T62.2X3	T62.2X4	—	—
Clavulanic acid	T36.1X1	T36.1X2	T36.1X3	T36.1X4	T36.1X5	T36.1X6
Cleaner, cleansing agent, type not specified	T65.891	T65.892	T65.893	T65.894	—	—
of paint or varnish	T52.91	T52.92	T52.93	T52.94	—	—
specified type NEC	T65.891	T65.892	T65.893	T65.894	—	—
Clebopride	T47.8X1	T47.8X2	T47.8X3	T47.8X4	T47.8X5	T47.8X6
Clefamide	T37.3X1	T37.3X2	T37.3X3	T37.3X4	T37.3X5	T37.3X6
Clemastine	T45.ØX1	T45.ØX2	T45.ØX3	T45.ØX4	T45.ØX5	T45.ØX6
Clematis vitalba	T62.2X1	T62.2X2	T62.2X3	T62.2X4	—	—
Clemizole	T45.ØX1	T45.ØX2	T45.ØX3	T45.ØX4	T45.ØX5	T45.ØX6
penicillin	T36.ØX1	T36.ØX2	T36.ØX3	T36.ØX4	T36.ØX5	T36.ØX6
Clenbuterol	T48.6X1	T48.6X2	T48.6X3	T48.6X4	T48.6X5	T48.6X6
Clidinium bromide	T44.3X1	T44.3X2	T44.3X3	T44.3X4	T44.3X5	T44.3X6
Clinda-Derm*	T49.ØX1	T49.ØX2	T49.ØX3	T49.ØX4	T49.ØX5	T49.ØX6
Clindamycin	T36.8X1	T36.8X2	T36.8X3	T36.8X4	T36.8X5	T36.8X6
Clinofibrate	T46.6X1	T46.6X2	T46.6X3	T46.6X4	T46.6X5	T46.6X6
Clioquinol	T37.8X1	T37.8X2	T37.8X3	T37.8X4	T37.8X5	T37.8X6
Cliradon	T4Ø.2X1	T4Ø.2X2	T4Ø.2X3	T4Ø.2X4	—	—
Clobazam	T42.4X1	T42.4X2	T42.4X3	T42.4X4	T42.4X5	T42.4X6
Clobenzorex	T5Ø.5X1	T5Ø.5X2	T5Ø.5X3	T5Ø.5X4	T5Ø.5X5	T5Ø.5X6
Clobetasol	T49.ØX1	T49.ØX2	T49.ØX3	T49.ØX4	T49.ØX5	T49.ØX6
Clobetasone	T49.ØX1	T49.ØX2	T49.ØX3	T49.ØX4	T49.ØX5	T49.ØX6
Clobutinol	T48.3X1	T48.3X2	T48.3X3	T48.3X4	T48.3X5	T48.3X6
Clocortolone	T38.ØX1	T38.ØX2	T38.ØX3	T38.ØX4	T38.ØX5	T38.ØX6
Clodantoin	T49.ØX1	T49.ØX2	T49.ØX3	T49.ØX4	T49.ØX5	T49.ØX6
Clodronic acid	T5Ø.991	T5Ø.992	T5Ø.993	T5Ø.994	T5Ø.995	T5Ø.996
Clofazimine	T37.1X1	T37.1X2	T37.1X3	T37.1X4	T37.1X5	T37.1X6
Clofedanol	T48.3X1	T48.3X2	T48.3X3	T48.3X4	T48.3X5	T48.3X6
Clofenamide	T5Ø.2X1	T5Ø.2X2	T5Ø.2X3	T5Ø.2X4	T5Ø.2X5	T5Ø.2X6
Clofenotane	T49.ØX1	T49.ØX2	T49.ØX3	T49.ØX4	T49.ØX5	T49.ØX6
Clofezone	T39.2X1	T39.2X2	T39.2X3	T39.2X4	T39.2X5	T39.2X6
Clofibrate	T46.6X1	T46.6X2	T46.6X3	T46.6X4	T46.6X5	T46.6X6
Clofibride	T46.6X1	T46.6X2	T46.6X3	T46.6X4	T46.6X5	T46.6X6
Cloforex	T5Ø.5X1	T5Ø.5X2	T5Ø.5X3	T5Ø.5X4	T5Ø.5X5	T5Ø.5X6
Clomethiazole	T42.6X1	T42.6X2	T42.6X3	T42.6X4	T42.6X5	T42.6X6
Clometocillin	T36.ØX1	T36.ØX2	T36.ØX3	T36.ØX4	T36.ØX5	T36.ØX6
Clomifene	T38.5X1	T38.5X2	T38.5X3	T38.5X4	T38.5X5	T38.5X6
Clomiphene	T38.5X1	T38.5X2	T38.5X3	T38.5X4	T38.5X5	T38.5X6
Clomipramine	T43.Ø11	T43.Ø12	T43.Ø13	T43.Ø14	T43.Ø15	T43.Ø16
Clomocycline	T36.4X1	T36.4X2	T36.4X3	T36.4X4	T36.4X5	T36.4X6
Clonazepam	T42.4X1	T42.4X2	T42.4X3	T42.4X4	T42.4X5	T42.4X6
Clonidine	T46.5X1	T46.5X2	T46.5X3	T46.5X4	T46.5X5	T46.5X6
Clonixin	T39.8X1	T39.8X2	T39.8X3	T39.8X4	T39.8X5	T39.8X6
Clopamide	T5Ø.2X1	T5Ø.2X2	T5Ø.2X3	T5Ø.2X4	T5Ø.2X5	T5Ø.2X6
Clopenthixol	T43.4X1	T43.4X2	T43.4X3	T43.4X4	T43.4X5	T43.4X6
Cloperastine	T48.3X1	T48.3X2	T48.3X3	T48.3X4	T48.3X5	T48.3X6
Clophedianol	T48.3X1	T48.3X2	T48.3X3	T48.3X4	T48.3X5	T48.3X6
Cloponone	T36.2X1	T36.2X2	T36.2X3	T36.2X4	T36.2X5	T36.2X6
Cloprednol	T38.ØX1	T38.ØX2	T38.ØX3	T38.ØX4	T38.ØX5	T38.ØX6
Cloral betaine	T42.6X1	T42.6X2	T42.6X3	T42.6X4	T42.6X5	T42.6X6
Cloramfenicol	T36.2X1	T36.2X2	T36.2X3	T36.2X4	T36.2X5	T36.2X6
Clorazepate (dipotassium)	T42.4X1	T42.4X2	T42.4X3	T42.4X4	T42.4X5	T42.4X6
Clorexolone	T5Ø.2X1	T5Ø.2X2	T5Ø.2X3	T5Ø.2X4	T5Ø.2X5	T5Ø.2X6
Clorfenamine	T45.ØX1	T45.ØX2	T45.ØX3	T45.ØX4	T45.ØX5	T45.ØX6
Clorgiline	T43.1X1	T43.1X2	T43.1X3	T43.1X4	T43.1X5	T43.1X6
Clorotepine	T44.3X1	T44.3X2	T44.3X3	T44.3X4	T44.3X5	T44.3X6
Clorox (bleach)	T54.91	T54.92	T54.93	T54.94	—	—
Clorprenaline	T48.6X1	T48.6X2	T48.6X3	T48.6X4	T48.6X5	T48.6X6

Substance	Poisoning, Accidental (unintentional)	Poisoning, Intentional Self-harm	Poisoning, Assault	Poisoning, Undetermined	Adverse Effect	Under-dosing
Clortermine	T5Ø.5X1	T5Ø.5X2	T5Ø.5X3	T5Ø.5X4	T5Ø.5X5	T5Ø.5X6
Clotiapine	T43.591	T43.592	T43.593	T43.594	T43.595	T43.596
Clotiazepam	T42.4X1	T42.4X2	T42.4X3	T42.4X4	T42.4X5	T42.4X6
Clotibric acid	T46.6X1	T46.6X2	T46.6X3	T46.6X4	T46.6X5	T46.6X6
Clotrimazole	T49.ØX1	T49.ØX2	T49.ØX3	T49.ØX4	T49.ØX5	T49.ØX6
Cloxacillin	T36.ØX1	T36.ØX2	T36.ØX3	T36.ØX4	T36.ØX5	T36.ØX6
Cloxazolam	T42.4X1	T42.4X2	T42.4X3	T42.4X4	T42.4X5	T42.4X6
Cloxiquine	T49.ØX1	T49.ØX2	T49.ØX3	T49.ØX4	T49.ØX5	T49.ØX6
Clozapine	T42.4X1	T42.4X2	T42.4X3	T42.4X4	T42.4X5	T42.4X6
Coagulant NEC	T45.7X1	T45.7X2	T45.7X3	T45.7X4	T45.7X5	T45.7X6
Coal (carbon monoxide from) — *see also* Carbon, monoxide, coal	T58.2X1	T58.2X2	T58.2X3	T58.2X4	—	—
oil — *see* Kerosene						
tar	T49.1X1	T49.1X2	T49.1X3	T49.1X4	T49.1X5	T49.1X6
fumes	T59.891	T59.892	T59.893	T59.894	—	—
medicinal (ointment)	T49.4X1	T49.4X2	T49.4X3	T49.4X4	T49.4X5	T49.4X6
analgesics NEC	T39.2X1	T39.2X2	T39.2X3	T39.2X4	T39.2X5	T39.2X6
naphtha (solvent)	T52.ØX1	T52.ØX2	T52.ØX3	T52.ØX4	—	—
Coartem*	T37.2X1	T37.2X2	T37.2X3	T37.2X4	T37.2X5	T37.2X6
Cobalamine	T45.2X1	T45.2X2	T45.2X3	T45.2X4	T45.2X5	T45.2X6
Cobalt (nonmedicinal) (fumes) (industrial)	T56.891	T56.892	T56.893	T56.894	—	—
medicinal (trace) (chloride)	T45.8X1	T45.8X2	T45.8X3	T45.8X4	T45.8X5	T45.8X6
Cobra (venom)	T63.Ø41	T63.Ø42	T63.Ø43	T63.Ø44	—	—
Coca (leaf)	T4Ø.5X1	T4Ø.5X2	T4Ø.5X3	T4Ø.5X4	T4Ø.5X5	T4Ø.5X6
Cocaine	T4Ø.5X1	T4Ø.5X2	T4Ø.5X3	T4Ø.5X4	T4Ø.5X5	T4Ø.5X6
topical anesthetic	T41.3X1	T41.3X2	T41.3X3	T41.3X4	T41.3X5	T41.3X6
Cocarboxylase	T45.3X1	T45.3X2	T45.3X3	T45.3X4	T45.3X5	T45.3X6
Coccidioidin	T5Ø.8X1	T5Ø.8X2	T5Ø.8X3	T5Ø.8X4	T5Ø.8X5	T5Ø.8X6
Cocculus indicus	T62.1X1	T62.1X2	T62.1X3	T62.1X4	—	—
Cochineal	T65.6X1	T65.6X2	T65.6X3	T65.6X4	—	—
medicinal products	T5Ø.991	T5Ø.992	T5Ø.993	T5Ø.994	T5Ø.995	T5Ø.996
Codeine	T4Ø.2X1	T4Ø.2X2	T4Ø.2X3	T4Ø.2X4	T4Ø.2X5	T4Ø.2X6
Cod-liver oil	T45.2X1	T45.2X2	T45.2X3	T45.2X4	T45.2X5	T45.2X6
Coenzyme A	T5Ø.991	T5Ø.992	T5Ø.993	T5Ø.994	T5Ø.995	T5Ø.996
Coffee	T62.8X1	T62.8X2	T62.8X3	T62.8X4	—	—
Cogalactoisomerase	T5Ø.991	T5Ø.992	T5Ø.993	T5Ø.994	T5Ø.995	T5Ø.996
Cogentin	T44.3X1	T44.3X2	T44.3X3	T44.3X4	T44.3X5	T44.3X6
Coke fumes or gas (carbon monoxide)	T58.2X1	T58.2X2	T58.2X3	T58.2X4	—	—
industrial use	T58.8X1	T58.8X2	T58.8X3	T58.8X4	—	—
Colace	T47.4X1	T47.4X2	T47.4X3	T47.4X4	T47.4X5	T47.4X6
Colaspase	T45.1X1	T45.1X2	T45.1X3	T45.1X4	T45.1X5	T45.1X6
Colazal*	T47.8X1	T47.8X2	T47.8X3	T47.8X4	T47.8X5	T47.8X6
Colchicine	T5Ø.4X1	T5Ø.4X2	T5Ø.4X3	T5Ø.4X4	T5Ø.4X5	T5Ø.4X6
Colchicum	T62.2X1	T62.2X2	T62.2X3	T62.2X4	—	—
Cold cream	T49.3X1	T49.3X2	T49.3X3	T49.3X4	T49.3X5	T49.3X6
Colecalciferol	T45.2X1	T45.2X2	T45.2X3	T45.2X4	T45.2X5	T45.2X6
Colestipol	T46.6X1	T46.6X2	T46.6X3	T46.6X4	T46.6X5	T46.6X6
Colestyramine	T46.6X1	T46.6X2	T46.6X3	T46.6X4	T46.6X5	T46.6X6
Colimycin	T36.8X1	T36.8X2	T36.8X3	T36.8X4	T36.8X5	T36.8X6
Colistimethate	T36.8X1	T36.8X2	T36.8X3	T36.8X4	T36.8X5	T36.8X6
Colistin	T36.8X1	T36.8X2	T36.8X3	T36.8X4	T36.8X5	T36.8X6
sulfate (eye preparation)	T49.5X1	T49.5X2	T49.5X3	T49.5X4	T49.5X5	T49.5X6
Collagen	T5Ø.991	T5Ø.992	T5Ø.993	T5Ø.994	T5Ø.995	T5Ø.996
Collagenase	T49.4X1	T49.4X2	T49.4X3	T49.4X4	T49.4X5	T49.4X6
Collodion	T49.3X1	T49.3X2	T49.3X3	T49.3X4	T49.3X5	T49.3X6
Colocynth	T47.2X1	T47.2X2	T47.2X3	T47.2X4	T47.2X5	T47.2X6
Colophony adhesive	T49.3X1	T49.3X2	T49.3X3	T49.3X4	T49.3X5	T49.3X6
Colorant — *see also* Dye	T5Ø.991	T5Ø.992	T5Ø.993	T5Ø.994	T5Ø.995	T5Ø.996
Coloring matter — *see* Dye(s)						
Combustion gas (after combustion) — *see* Carbon, monoxide						
prior to combustion	T59.891	T59.892	T59.893	T59.894	—	—
Cometriq*	T45.1X1	T45.1X2	T45.1X3	T45.1X4	T45.1X5	T45.1X6
Compazine	T43.3X1	T43.3X2	T43.3X3	T43.3X4	T43.3X5	T43.3X6
Compound						
1080 (sodium fluoroacetate)	T6Ø.4X1	T6Ø.4X2	T6Ø.4X3	T6Ø.4X4	—	—
269 (endrin)	T6Ø.1X1	T6Ø.1X2	T6Ø.1X3	T6Ø.1X4	—	—
3422 (parathion)	T6Ø.ØX1	T6Ø.ØX2	T6Ø.ØX3	T6Ø.ØX4	—	—
3911 (phorate)	T6Ø.ØX1	T6Ø.ØX2	T6Ø.ØX3	T6Ø.ØX4	—	—
3956 (toxaphene)	T6Ø.1X1	T6Ø.1X2	T6Ø.1X3	T6Ø.1X4	—	—
4049 (malathion)	T6Ø.ØX1	T6Ø.ØX2	T6Ø.ØX3	T6Ø.ØX4	—	—
4069 (malathion)	T6Ø.ØX1	T6Ø.ØX2	T6Ø.ØX3	T6Ø.ØX4	—	—
4124 (dicapthon)	T6Ø.ØX1	T6Ø.ØX2	T6Ø.ØX3	T6Ø.ØX4	—	—
42 (warfarin)	T6Ø.4X1	T6Ø.4X2	T6Ø.4X3	T6Ø.4X4	—	—
497 (dieldrin)	T6Ø.1X1	T6Ø.1X2	T6Ø.1X3	T6Ø.1X4	—	—
E (cortisone)	T38.ØX1	T38.ØX2	T38.ØX3	T38.ØX4	T38.ØX5	T38.ØX6
F (hydrocortisone)	T38.ØX1	T38.ØX2	T38.ØX3	T38.ØX4	T38.ØX5	T38.ØX6
Comvax*	T5Ø.A21	T5Ø.A22	T5Ø.A23	T5Ø.A24	T5Ø.A25	T5Ø.A26

Substance	Poisoning, Accidental (unintentional)	Poisoning, Intentional Self-harm	Poisoning, Assault	Poisoning, Undetermined	Adverse Effect	Under-dosing
Congener, anabolic	T38.7X1	T38.7X2	T38.7X3	T38.7X4	T38.7X5	T38.7X6
Congo red	T5Ø.8X1	T5Ø.8X2	T5Ø.8X3	T5Ø.8X4	T5Ø.8X5	T5Ø.8X6
Coniine, conine	T62.2X1	T62.2X2	T62.2X3	T62.2X4	—	—
Conium (maculatum)	T62.2X1	T62.2X2	T62.2X3	T62.2X4	—	—
Conjugated estrogenic substances	T38.5X1	T38.5X2	T38.5X3	T38.5X4	T38.5X5	T38.5X6
Contac	T48.5X1	T48.5X2	T48.5X3	T48.5X4	T48.5X5	T48.5X6
Contact lens solution	T49.5X1	T49.5X2	T49.5X3	T49.5X4	T49.5X5	T49.5X6
Contraceptive (oral)	T38.4X1	T38.4X2	T38.4X3	T38.4X4	T38.4X5	T38.4X6
vaginal	T49.8X1	T49.8X2	T49.8X3	T49.8X4	T49.8X5	T49.8X6
Contrast medium, radiography	T5Ø.8X1	T5Ø.8X2	T5Ø.8X3	T5Ø.8X4	T5Ø.8X5	T5Ø.8X6
Convallaria glycosides	T46.ØX1	T46.ØX2	T46.ØX3	T46.ØX4	T46.ØX5	T46.ØX6
Convallaria majalis	T62.2X1	T62.2X2	T62.2X3	T62.2X4	—	—
berry	T62.1X1	T62.1X2	T62.1X3	T62.1X4	—	—
Copperhead snake (bite) (venom)	T63.Ø61	T63.Ø62	T63.Ø63	T63.Ø64	—	—
Copper (dust) (fumes) (nonmedicinal) **NEC**	T56.4X1	T56.4X2	T56.4X3	T56.4X4	—	—
arsenate, arsenite	T57.ØX1	T57.ØX2	T57.ØX3	T57.ØX4	—	—
insecticide	T6Ø.2X1	T6Ø.2X2	T6Ø.2X3	T6Ø.2X4	—	—
emetic	T47.7X1	T47.7X2	T47.7X3	T47.7X4	T47.7X5	T47.7X6
fungicide	T6Ø.3X1	T6Ø.3X2	T6Ø.3X3	T6Ø.3X4	—	—
gluconate	T49.ØX1	T49.ØX2	T49.ØX3	T49.ØX4	T49.ØX5	T49.ØX6
insecticide	T6Ø.2X1	T6Ø.2X2	T6Ø.2X3	T6Ø.2X4	—	—
medicinal (trace)	T45.8X1	T45.8X2	T45.8X3	T45.8X4	T45.8X5	T45.8X6
oleate	T49.ØX1	T49.ØX2	T49.ØX3	T49.ØX4	T49.ØX5	T49.ØX6
sulfate	T56.4X1	T56.4X2	T56.4X3	T56.4X4	—	—
cupric	T56.4X1	T56.4X2	T56.4X3	T56.4X4	—	—
fungicide	T6Ø.3X1	T6Ø.3X2	T6Ø.3X3	T6Ø.3X4	—	—
medicinal						
ear	T49.6X1	T49.6X2	T49.6X3	T49.6X4	T49.6X5	T49.6X6
emetic	T47.7X1	T47.7X2	T47.7X3	T47.7X4	T47.7X5	T47.7X6
eye	T49.5X1	T49.5X2	T49.5X3	T49.5X4	T49.5X5	T49.5X6
cuprous	T56.4X1	T56.4X2	T56.4X3	T56.4X4	—	—
fungicide	T6Ø.3X1	T6Ø.3X2	T6Ø.3X3	T6Ø.3X4	—	—
medicinal						
ear	T49.6X1	T49.6X2	T49.6X3	T49.6X4	T49.6X5	T49.6X6
emetic	T47.7X1	T47.7X2	T47.7X3	T47.7X4	T47.7X5	T47.7X6
eye	T49.5X1	T49.5X2	T49.5X3	T49.5X4	T49.5X5	T49.5X6
Coral (sting)	T63.691	T63.692	T63.693	T63.694	—	—
snake (bite) (venom)	T63.Ø21	T63.Ø22	T63.Ø23	T63.Ø24	—	—
Corbadrine	T49.6X1	T49.6X2	T49.6X3	T49.6X4	T49.6X5	T49.6X6
Cordite	T65.891	T65.892	T65.893	T65.894	—	—
vapor	T59.891	T59.892	T59.893	T59.894	—	—
Cordran	T49.ØX1	T49.ØX2	T49.ØX3	T49.ØX4	T49.ØX5	T49.ØX6
Cormax*	T49.ØX1	T49.ØX2	T49.ØX3	T49.ØX4	T49.ØX5	T49.ØX6
Corn cures	T49.4X1	T49.4X2	T49.4X3	T49.4X4	T49.4X5	T49.4X6
Cornhusker's lotion	T49.3X1	T49.3X2	T49.3X3	T49.3X4	T49.3X5	T49.3X6
Corn starch	T49.3X1	T49.3X2	T49.3X3	T49.3X4	T49.3X5	T49.3X6
Coronary vasodilator NEC	T46.3X1	T46.3X2	T46.3X3	T46.3X4	T46.3X5	T46.3X6
Corrosive NEC	T54.91	T54.92	T54.93	T54.94	—	—
acid NEC	T54.2X1	T54.2X2	T54.2X3	T54.2X4	—	—
aromatics	T54.1X1	T54.1X2	T54.1X3	T54.1X4	—	—
disinfectant	T54.1X1	T54.1X2	T54.1X3	T54.1X4	—	—
fumes NEC	T54.91	T54.92	T54.93	T54.94	—	—
specified NEC	T54.91	T54.92	T54.93	T54.94	—	—
sublimate	T56.1X1	T56.1X2	T56.1X3	T56.1X4	—	—
Cortate	T38.ØX1	T38.ØX2	T38.ØX3	T38.ØX4	T38.ØX5	T38.ØX6
Cort-Dome	T38.ØX1	T38.ØX2	T38.ØX3	T38.ØX4	T38.ØX5	T38.ØX6
ENT agent	T49.6X1	T49.6X2	T49.6X3	T49.6X4	T49.6X5	T49.6X6
ophthalmic preparation	T49.5X1	T49.5X2	T49.5X3	T49.5X4	T49.5X5	T49.5X6
topical NEC	T49.ØX1	T49.ØX2	T49.ØX3	T49.ØX4	T49.ØX5	T49.ØX6
Cortef	T38.ØX1	T38.ØX2	T38.ØX3	T38.ØX4	T38.ØX5	T38.ØX6
ENT agent	T49.6X1	T49.6X2	T49.6X3	T49.6X4	T49.6X5	T49.6X6
ophthalmic preparation	T49.5X1	T49.5X2	T49.5X3	T49.5X4	T49.5X5	T49.5X6
topical NEC	T49.ØX1	T49.ØX2	T49.ØX3	T49.ØX4	T49.ØX5	T49.ØX6
Corticosteroid	T38.ØX1	T38.ØX2	T38.ØX3	T38.ØX4	T38.ØX5	T38.ØX6
ENT agent	T49.6X1	T49.6X2	T49.6X3	T49.6X4	T49.6X5	T49.6X6
mineral	T5Ø.ØX1	T5Ø.ØX2	T5Ø.ØX3	T5Ø.ØX4	T5Ø.ØX5	T5Ø.ØX6
ophthalmic	T49.5X1	T49.5X2	T49.5X3	T49.5X4	T49.5X5	T49.5X6
topical NEC	T49.ØX1	T49.ØX2	T49.ØX3	T49.ØX4	T49.ØX5	T49.ØX6
Corticotropin	T38.811	T38.812	T38.813	T38.814	T38.815	T38.816
Cortisol	T49.ØX1	T49.ØX2	T49.ØX3	T49.ØX4	T49.ØX5	T49.ØX6
ENT agent	T49.6X1	T49.6X2	T49.6X3	T49.6X4	T49.6X5	T49.6X6
ophthalmic preparation	T49.5X1	T49.5X2	T49.5X3	T49.5X4	T49.5X5	T49.5X6
topical NEC	T49.ØX1	T49.ØX2	T49.ØX3	T49.ØX4	T49.ØX5	T49.ØX6
Cortisone (acetate)	T38.ØX1	T38.ØX2	T38.ØX3	T38.ØX4	T38.ØX5	T38.ØX6
ENT agent	T49.6X1	T49.6X2	T49.6X3	T49.6X4	T49.6X5	T49.6X6
ophthalmic preparation	T49.5X1	T49.5X2	T49.5X3	T49.5X4	T49.5X5	T49.5X6
topical NEC	T49.ØX1	T49.ØX2	T49.ØX3	T49.ØX4	T49.ØX5	T49.ØX6
Cortisporin*	T49.ØX1	T49.ØX2	T49.ØX3	T49.ØX4	T49.ØX5	T49.ØX6
Cortivazol	T38.ØX1	T38.ØX2	T38.ØX3	T38.ØX4	T38.ØX5	T38.ØX6
Cortogen	T38.ØX1	T38.ØX2	T38.ØX3	T38.ØX4	T38.ØX5	T38.ØX6
ENT agent	T49.6X1	T49.6X2	T49.6X3	T49.6X4	T49.6X5	T49.6X6
ophthalmic preparation	T49.5X1	T49.5X2	T49.5X3	T49.5X4	T49.5X5	T49.5X6
Cortone	T38.ØX1	T38.ØX2	T38.ØX3	T38.ØX4	T38.ØX5	T38.ØX6
ENT agent	T49.6X1	T49.6X2	T49.6X3	T49.6X4	T49.6X5	T49.6X6
ophthalmic preparation	T49.5X1	T49.5X2	T49.5X3	T49.5X4	T49.5X5	T49.5X6
Cortril	T38.ØX1	T38.ØX2	T38.ØX3	T38.ØX4	T38.ØX5	T38.ØX6
ENT agent	T49.6X1	T49.6X2	T49.6X3	T49.6X4	T49.6X5	T49.6X6
ophthalmic preparation	T49.5X1	T49.5X2	T49.5X3	T49.5X4	T49.5X5	T49.5X6
topical NEC	T49.ØX1	T49.ØX2	T49.ØX3	T49.ØX4	T49.ØX5	T49.ØX6
Corynebacterium parvum	T45.1X1	T45.1X2	T45.1X3	T45.1X4	T45.1X5	T45.1X6
Cosmetic preparation	T49.8X1	T49.8X2	T49.8X3	T49.8X4	T49.8X5	T49.8X6
Cosmetics	T49.8X1	T49.8X2	T49.8X3	T49.8X4	T49.8X5	T49.8X6
Cosyntropin	T38.811	T38.812	T38.813	T38.814	T38.815	T38.816
Cotarnine	T45.7X1	T45.7X2	T45.7X3	T45.7X4	T45.7X5	T45.7X6
Co-trimoxazole	T36.8X1	T36.8X2	T36.8X3	T36.8X4	T36.8X5	T36.8X6
Cottonseed oil	T49.3X1	T49.3X2	T49.3X3	T49.3X4	T49.3X5	T49.3X6
Cough mixture (syrup)	T48.4X1	T48.4X2	T48.4X3	T48.4X4	T48.4X5	T48.4X6
containing opiates	T4Ø.2X1	T4Ø.2X2	T4Ø.2X3	T4Ø.2X4	T4Ø.2X5	T4Ø.2X6
expectorants	T48.4X1	T48.4X2	T48.4X3	T48.4X4	T48.4X5	T48.4X6
Coumadin	T45.511	T45.512	T45.513	T45.514	T45.515	T45.516
rodenticide	T6Ø.4X1	T6Ø.4X2	T6Ø.4X3	T6Ø.4X4	—	—
Coumaphos	T6Ø.ØX1	T6Ø.ØX2	T6Ø.ØX3	T6Ø.ØX4	—	—
Coumarin	T45.511	T45.512	T45.513	T45.514	T45.515	T45.516
Coumetarol	T45.511	T45.512	T45.513	T45.514	T45.515	T45.516
Cowbane	T62.2X1	T62.2X2	T62.2X3	T62.2X4	—	—
Cozyme	T45.2X1	T45.2X2	T45.2X3	T45.2X4	T45.2X5	T45.2X6
Crack	T4Ø.5X1	T4Ø.5X2	T4Ø.5X3	T4Ø.5X4	—	—
Crataegus extract	T46.ØX1	T46.ØX2	T46.ØX3	T46.ØX4	T46.ØX5	T46.ØX6
Creolin	T54.1X1	T54.1X2	T54.1X3	T54.1X4	—	—
disinfectant	T54.1X1	T54.1X2	T54.1X3	T54.1X4	—	—
Creosol (compound)	T49.ØX1	T49.ØX2	T49.ØX3	T49.ØX4	T49.ØX5	T49.ØX6
Creosote (coal tar) (beechwood)	T49.ØX1	T49.ØX2	T49.ØX3	T49.ØX4	T49.ØX5	T49.ØX6
medicinal (expectorant)	T48.4X1	T48.4X2	T48.4X3	T48.4X4	T48.4X5	T48.4X6
syrup	T48.4X1	T48.4X2	T48.4X3	T48.4X4	T48.4X5	T48.4X6
Cresol(s)	T49.ØX1	T49.ØX2	T49.ØX3	T49.ØX4	T49.ØX5	T49.ØX6
and soap solution	T49.ØX1	T49.ØX2	T49.ØX3	T49.ØX4	T49.ØX5	T49.ØX6
Crestor*	T46.6X1	T46.6X2	T46.6X3	T46.6X4	T46.6X5	T46.6X6
Cresyl acetate	T49.ØX1	T49.ØX2	T49.ØX3	T49.ØX4	T49.ØX5	T49.ØX6
Cresylic acid	T49.ØX1	T49.ØX2	T49.ØX3	T49.ØX4	T49.ØX5	T49.ØX6
Crimidine	T6Ø.4X1	T6Ø.4X2	T6Ø.4X3	T6Ø.4X4	—	—
Croconazole	T37.8X1	T37.8X2	T37.8X3	T37.8X4	T37.8X5	T37.8X6
Cromoglicic acid	T48.6X1	T48.6X2	T48.6X3	T48.6X4	T48.6X5	T48.6X6
Cromolyn	T48.6X1	T48.6X2	T48.6X3	T48.6X4	T48.6X5	T48.6X6
Cromonar	T46.3X1	T46.3X2	T46.3X3	T46.3X4	T46.3X5	T46.3X6
Cropropamide	T39.8X1	T39.8X2	T39.8X3	T39.8X4	T39.8X5	T39.8X6
with crotethamide	T5Ø.7X1	T5Ø.7X2	T5Ø.7X3	T5Ø.7X4	T5Ø.7X5	T5Ø.7X6
Crotamiton	T49.ØX1	T49.ØX2	T49.ØX3	T49.ØX4	T49.ØX5	T49.ØX6
Crotethamide	T39.8X1	T39.8X2	T39.8X3	T39.8X4	T39.8X5	T39.8X6
with cropropamide	T5Ø.7X1	T5Ø.7X2	T5Ø.7X3	T5Ø.7X4	T5Ø.7X5	T5Ø.7X6
Croton (oil)	T47.2X1	T47.2X2	T47.2X3	T47.2X4	T47.2X5	T47.2X6
chloral	T42.6X1	T42.6X2	T42.6X3	T42.6X4	T42.6X5	T42.6X6
Crude oil	T52.ØX1	T52.ØX2	T52.ØX3	T52.ØX4	—	—
Cryogenine	T39.8X1	T39.8X2	T39.8X3	T39.8X4	T39.8X5	T39.8X6
Cryolite (vapor)	T6Ø.1X1	T6Ø.1X2	T6Ø.1X3	T6Ø.1X4	—	—
insecticide	T6Ø.1X1	T6Ø.1X2	T6Ø.1X3	T6Ø.1X4	—	—
Cryptenamine (tannates)	T46.5X1	T46.5X2	T46.5X3	T46.5X4	T46.5X5	T46.5X6
Crystal violet	T49.ØX1	T49.ØX2	T49.ØX3	T49.ØX4	T49.ØX5	T49.ØX6
Cuckoopint	T62.2X1	T62.2X2	T62.2X3	T62.2X4	—	—
Cumetharol	T45.511	T45.512	T45.513	T45.514	T45.515	T45.516
Cupric						
acetate	T6Ø.3X1	T6Ø.3X2	T6Ø.3X3	T6Ø.3X4	—	—
acetoarsenite	T57.ØX1	T57.ØX2	T57.ØX3	T57.ØX4	—	—
arsenate	T57.ØX1	T57.ØX2	T57.ØX3	T57.ØX4	—	—
gluconate	T49.ØX1	T49.ØX2	T49.ØX3	T49.ØX4	T49.ØX5	T49.ØX6
oleate	T49.ØX1	T49.ØX2	T49.ØX3	T49.ØX4	T49.ØX5	T49.ØX6
sulfate	T56.4X1	T56.4X2	T56.4X3	T56.4X4	—	—
Cuprimine*	T5Ø.6X1	T5Ø.6X2	T5Ø.6X3	T5Ø.6X4	T5Ø.6X5	T5Ø.6X6
Cuprous sulfate — *see also* Copper, sulfate	T56.4X1	T56.4X2	T56.4X3	T56.4X4	—	—
Curare, curarine	T48.1X1	T48.1X2	T48.1X3	T48.1X4	T48.1X5	T48.1X6
Cyamemazine	T43.3X1	T43.3X2	T43.3X3	T43.3X4	T43.3X5	T43.3X6
Cyamopsis tetragonoloba	T46.6X1	T46.6X2	T46.6X3	T46.6X4	T46.6X5	T46.6X6
Cyanacetyl hydrazide	T37.1X1	T37.1X2	T37.1X3	T37.1X4	T37.1X5	T37.1X6
Cyanic acid (gas)	T59.891	T59.892	T59.893	T59.894	—	—
Cyanide(s) (compounds) (potassium) (sodium) **NEC**	T65.ØX1	T65.ØX2	T65.ØX3	T65.ØX4	—	—
dust or gas (inhalation) NEC	T57.3X1	T57.3X2	T57.3X3	T57.3X4	—	—
fumigant	T65.ØX1	T65.ØX2	T65.ØX3	T65.ØX4	—	—
hydrogen	T57.3X1	T57.3X2	T57.3X3	T57.3X4	—	—

Substance	Poisoning, Accidental (unintentional)	Poisoning, Intentional Self-harm	Poisoning, Assault	Poisoning, Undetermined	Adverse Effect	Under-dosing
Cyanide(s) (compounds) (potassium) (sodium) **NEC** — *continued*						
mercuric — *see* Mercury						
pesticide (dust) (fumes)	T65.0X1	T65.0X2	T65.0X3	T65.0X4	—	—
Cyanoacrylate adhesive	T49.3X1	T49.3X2	T49.3X3	T49.3X4	T49.3X5	T49.3X6
Cyanocobalamin	T45.8X1	T45.8X2	T45.8X3	T45.8X4	T45.8X5	T45.8X6
Cyanogen (chloride) (gas) **NEC**	T59.891	T59.892	T59.893	T59.894	—	—
Cyclacillin	T36.0X1	T36.0X2	T36.0X3	T36.0X4	T36.0X5	T36.0X6
Cyclaine	T41.3X1	T41.3X2	T41.3X3	T41.3X4	T41.3X5	T41.3X6
Cyclamate	T50.991	T50.992	T50.993	T50.994	T50.995	T50.996
Cyclamen europaeum	T62.2X1	T62.2X2	T62.2X3	T62.2X4	—	—
Cyclandelate	T46.7X1	T46.7X2	T46.7X3	T46.7X4	T46.7X5	T46.7X6
Cyclazocine	T50.7X1	T50.7X2	T50.7X3	T50.7X4	T50.7X5	T50.7X6
Cyclizine	T45.0X1	T45.0X2	T45.0X3	T45.0X4	T45.0X5	T45.0X6
Cyclobarbital	T42.3X1	T42.3X2	T42.3X3	T42.3X4	T42.3X5	T42.3X6
Cyclobarbitone	T42.3X1	T42.3X2	T42.3X3	T42.3X4	T42.3X5	T42.3X6
Cyclobenzaprine	T48.1X1	T48.1X2	T48.1X3	T48.1X4	T48.1X5	T48.1X6
Cyclodrine	T44.3X1	T44.3X2	T44.3X3	T44.3X4	T44.3X5	T44.3X6
Cycloguanil embonate	T37.2X1	T37.2X2	T37.2X3	T37.2X4	T37.2X5	T37.2X6
Cyclohexane	T52.8X1	T52.8X2	T52.8X3	T52.8X4	—	—
Cyclohexanol	T51.8X1	T51.8X2	T51.8X3	T51.8X4	—	—
Cyclohexanone	T52.4X1	T52.4X2	T52.4X3	T52.4X4	—	—
Cycloheximide	T60.3X1	T60.3X2	T60.3X3	T60.3X4	—	—
Cyclohexyl acetate	T52.8X1	T52.8X2	T52.8X3	T52.8X4	—	—
Cycloleucin	T45.1X1	T45.1X2	T45.1X3	T45.1X4	T45.1X5	T45.1X6
Cyclomethycaine	T41.3X1	T41.3X2	T41.3X3	T41.3X4	T41.3X5	T41.3X6
Cyclopentamine	T44.4X1	T44.4X2	T44.4X3	T44.4X4	T44.4X5	T44.4X6
Cyclopenthiazide	T50.2X1	T50.2X2	T50.2X3	T50.2X4	T50.2X5	T50.2X6
Cyclopentolate	T44.3X1	T44.3X2	T44.3X3	T44.3X4	T44.3X5	T44.3X6
Cyclophosphamide	T45.1X1	T45.1X2	T45.1X3	T45.1X4	T45.1X5	T45.1X6
Cycloplegic drug	T49.5X1	T49.5X2	T49.5X3	T49.5X4	T49.5X5	T49.5X6
Cyclopropane	T41.291	T41.292	T41.293	T41.294	T41.295	T41.296
Cyclopyrabital	T39.8X1	T39.8X2	T39.8X3	T39.8X4	T39.8X5	T39.8X6
Cycloserine	T37.1X1	T37.1X2	T37.1X3	T37.1X4	T37.1X5	T37.1X6
Cyclosporin	T45.1X1	T45.1X2	T45.1X3	T45.1X4	T45.1X5	T45.1X6
Cyclothiazide	T50.2X1	T50.2X2	T50.2X3	T50.2X4	T50.2X5	T50.2X6
Cycrimine	T44.3X1	T44.3X2	T44.3X3	T44.3X4	T44.3X5	T44.3X6
Cyhalothrin	T60.1X1	T60.1X2	T60.1X3	T60.1X4	—	—
Cymarin	T46.0X1	T46.0X2	T46.0X3	T46.0X4	T46.0X5	T46.0X6
Cypermethrin	T60.1X1	T60.1X2	T60.1X3	T60.1X4	—	—
Cyphenothrin	T60.2X1	T60.2X2	T60.2X3	T60.2X4	—	—
Cyproheptadine	T45.0X1	T45.0X2	T45.0X3	T45.0X4	T45.0X5	T45.0X6
Cyproterone	T38.6X1	T38.6X2	T38.6X3	T38.6X4	T38.6X5	T38.6X6
Cystaran*	T49.5X1	T49.5X2	T49.5X3	T49.5X4	T49.5X5	T49.5X6
Cysteamine	T50.6X1	T50.6X2	T50.6X3	T50.6X4	T50.6X5	T50.6X6
Cytarabine	T45.1X1	T45.1X2	T45.1X3	T45.1X4	T45.1X5	T45.1X6
Cytisus						
laburnum	T62.2X1	T62.2X2	T62.2X3	T62.2X4	—	—
scoparius	T62.2X1	T62.2X2	T62.2X3	T62.2X4	—	—
Cytochrome C	T47.5X1	T47.5X2	T47.5X3	T47.5X4	T47.5X5	T47.5X6
Cytomel	T38.1X1	T38.1X2	T38.1X3	T38.1X4	T38.1X5	T38.1X6
Cytosine arabinoside	T45.1X1	T45.1X2	T45.1X3	T45.1X4	T45.1X5	T45.1X6
Cytoxan	T45.1X1	T45.1X2	T45.1X3	T45.1X4	T45.1X5	T45.1X6
Cytozyme	T45.7X1	T45.7X2	T45.7X3	T45.7X4	T45.7X5	T45.7X6
S-Carboxymethylcysteine	T48.4X1	T48.4X2	T48.4X3	T48.4X4	T48.4X5	T48.4X6
Dabigatran*	T45.511	T45.512	T45.513	T45.514	T45.515	T45.516
Dacarbazine	T45.1X1	T45.1X2	T45.1X3	T45.1X4	T45.1X5	T45.1X6
Dactinomycin	T45.1X1	T45.1X2	T45.1X3	T45.1X4	T45.1X5	T45.1X6
DADPS	T37.1X1	T37.1X2	T37.1X3	T37.1X4	T37.1X5	T37.1X6
Dakin's solution	T49.0X1	T49.0X2	T49.0X3	T49.0X4	T49.0X5	T49.0X6
Dalapon (sodium)	T60.3X1	T60.3X2	T60.3X3	T60.3X4	—	—
Dalmane	T42.4X1	T42.4X2	T42.4X3	T42.4X4	T42.4X5	T42.4X6
Danazol	T38.6X1	T38.6X2	T38.6X3	T38.6X4	T38.6X5	T38.6X6
Danilone	T45.511	T45.512	T45.513	T45.514	T45.515	T45.516
Danthron	T47.2X1	T47.2X2	T47.2X3	T47.2X4	T47.2X5	T47.2X6
Dantrolene	T42.8X1	T42.8X2	T42.8X3	T42.8X4	T42.8X5	T42.8X6
Dantron	T47.2X1	T47.2X2	T47.2X3	T47.2X4	T47.2X5	T47.2X6
Daphne (gnidium) (mezereum)	T62.2X1	T62.2X2	T62.2X3	T62.2X4	—	—
berry	T62.1X1	T62.1X2	T62.1X3	T62.1X4	—	—
Dapsone	T37.1X1	T37.1X2	T37.1X3	T37.1X4	T37.1X5	T37.1X6
Daraprim	T37.2X1	T37.2X2	T37.2X3	T37.2X4	T37.2X5	T37.2X6
Darnel	T62.2X1	T62.2X2	T62.2X3	T62.2X4	—	—
Darvon	T39.8X1	T39.8X2	T39.8X3	T39.8X4	T39.8X5	T39.8X6
Daunomycin	T45.1X1	T45.1X2	T45.1X3	T45.1X4	T45.1X5	T45.1X6
Daunorubicin	T45.1X1	T45.1X2	T45.1X3	T45.1X4	T45.1X5	T45.1X6
DBI	T38.3X1	T38.3X2	T38.3X3	T38.3X4	T38.3X5	T38.3X6
D-Con	T60.91	T60.92	T60.93	T60.94	—	—
insecticide	T60.2X1	T60.2X2	T60.2X3	T60.2X4	—	—
rodenticide	T60.4X1	T60.4X2	T60.4X3	T60.4X4	—	—
DDAVP	T38.891	T38.892	T38.893	T38.894	T38.895	T38.896

Substance	Poisoning, Accidental (unintentional)	Poisoning, Intentional Self-harm	Poisoning, Assault	Poisoning, Undetermined	Adverse Effect	Under-dosing
DDE (bis(chlorophenyl)-dichloroethylene)	T60.2X1	T60.2X2	T60.2X3	T60.2X4	—	—
DDS	T37.1X1	T37.1X2	T37.1X3	T37.1X4	T37.1X5	T37.1X6
DDT (dust)	T60.1X1	T60.1X2	T60.1X3	T60.1X4	—	—
Deadly nightshade — *see also* Belladonna	T62.2X1	T62.2X2	T62.2X3	T62.2X4	—	—
berry	T62.1X1	T62.1X2	T62.1X3	T62.1X4	—	—
Deamino-D-arginine vasopressin	T38.891	T38.892	T38.893	T38.894	T38.895	T38.896
Deanol (aceglumate)	T50.991	T50.992	T50.993	T50.994	T50.995	T50.996
Debrisoquine	T46.5X1	T46.5X2	T46.5X3	T46.5X4	T46.5X5	T46.5X6
Decaborane	T57.8X1	T57.8X2	T57.8X3	T57.8X4	—	—
fumes	T59.891	T59.892	T59.893	T59.894	—	—
Decadron	T38.0X1	T38.0X2	T38.0X3	T38.0X4	T38.0X5	T38.0X6
ENT agent	T49.6X1	T49.6X2	T49.6X3	T49.6X4	T49.6X5	T49.6X6
ophthalmic preparation	T49.5X1	T49.5X2	T49.5X3	T49.5X4	T49.5X5	T49.5X6
topical NEC	T49.0X1	T49.0X2	T49.0X3	T49.0X4	T49.0X5	T49.0X6
Decahydronaphthalene	T52.8X1	T52.8X2	T52.8X3	T52.8X4	—	—
Decalin	T52.8X1	T52.8X2	T52.8X3	T52.8X4	—	—
Decamethonium (bromide)	T48.1X1	T48.1X2	T48.1X3	T48.1X4	T48.1X5	T48.1X6
Decholin	T47.5X1	T47.5X2	T47.5X3	T47.5X4	T47.5X5	T47.5X6
Declomycin	T36.4X1	T36.4X2	T36.4X3	T36.4X4	T36.4X5	T36.4X6
Decongestant, nasal (mucosa)	T48.5X1	T48.5X2	T48.5X3	T48.5X4	T48.5X5	T48.5X6
combination	T48.5X1	T48.5X2	T48.5X3	T48.5X4	T48.5X5	T48.5X6
Deet	T60.8X1	T60.8X2	T60.8X3	T60.8X4	—	—
Deferoxamine	T45.8X1	T45.8X2	T45.8X3	T45.8X4	T45.8X5	T45.8X6
Deflazacort	T38.0X1	T38.0X2	T38.0X3	T38.0X4	T38.0X5	T38.0X6
Deglycyrrhizinized extract of licorice	T48.4X1	T48.4X2	T48.4X3	T48.4X4	T48.4X5	T48.4X6
Dehydrocholic acid	T47.5X1	T47.5X2	T47.5X3	T47.5X4	T47.5X5	T47.5X6
Dehydroemetine	T37.3X1	T37.3X2	T37.3X3	T37.3X4	T37.3X5	T37.3X6
Dekalin	T52.8X1	T52.8X2	T52.8X3	T52.8X4	—	—
Delafloxacin*	T36.8X1	T36.8X2	T36.8X3	T36.8X4	T36.8X5	T36.8X6
Delalutin	T38.5X1	T38.5X2	T38.5X3	T38.5X4	T38.5X5	T38.5X6
Delorazepam	T42.4X1	T42.4X2	T42.4X3	T42.4X4	T42.4X5	T42.4X6
Delphinium	T62.2X1	T62.2X2	T62.2X3	T62.2X4	—	—
Deltacortisone*	T38.0X1	T38.0X2	T38.0X3	T38.0X4	T38.0X5	T38.0X6
Deltamethrin	T60.1X1	T60.1X2	T60.1X3	T60.1X4	—	—
Deltasone	T38.0X1	T38.0X2	T38.0X3	T38.0X4	T38.0X5	T38.0X6
Deltra	T38.0X1	T38.0X2	T38.0X3	T38.0X4	T38.0X5	T38.0X6
Delvinal	T42.3X1	T42.3X2	T42.3X3	T42.3X4	T42.3X5	T42.3X6
Demecarium (bromide)	T49.5X1	T49.5X2	T49.5X3	T49.5X4	T49.5X5	T49.5X6
Demeclocycline	T36.4X1	T36.4X2	T36.4X3	T36.4X4	T36.4X5	T36.4X6
Demecolcine	T45.1X1	T45.1X2	T45.1X3	T45.1X4	T45.1X5	T45.1X6
Demegestone	T38.5X1	T38.5X2	T38.5X3	T38.5X4	T38.5X5	T38.5X6
Demelanizing agents	T49.8X1	T49.8X2	T49.8X3	T49.8X4	T49.8X5	T49.8X6
Demephion -O and -S	T60.0X1	T60.0X2	T60.0X3	T60.0X4	—	—
Demerol	T40.2X1	T40.2X2	T40.2X3	T40.2X4	T40.2X5	T40.2X6
Demethylchlortetracycline	T36.4X1	T36.4X2	T36.4X3	T36.4X4	T36.4X5	T36.4X6
Demethyltetracycline	T36.4X1	T36.4X2	T36.4X3	T36.4X4	T36.4X5	T36.4X6
Demeton -O and -S	T60.0X1	T60.0X2	T60.0X3	T60.0X4	—	—
Demulcent (external)	T49.3X1	T49.3X2	T49.3X3	T49.3X4	T49.3X5	T49.3X6
specified NEC	T49.3X1	T49.3X2	T49.3X3	T49.3X4	T49.3X5	T49.3X6
Demulen	T38.4X1	T38.4X2	T38.4X3	T38.4X4	T38.4X5	T38.4X6
Denatured alcohol	T51.0X1	T51.0X2	T51.0X3	T51.0X4	—	—
Dendrid	T49.5X1	T49.5X2	T49.5X3	T49.5X4	T49.5X5	T49.5X6
Dental drug, topical application NEC	T49.7X1	T49.7X2	T49.7X3	T49.7X4	T49.7X5	T49.7X6
Dentifrice	T49.7X1	T49.7X2	T49.7X3	T49.7X4	T49.7X5	T49.7X6
Deodorant spray (feminine hygiene)	T49.8X1	T49.8X2	T49.8X3	T49.8X4	T49.8X5	T49.8X6
Deoxycortone	T50.0X1	T50.0X2	T50.0X3	T50.0X4	T50.0X5	T50.0X6
Deoxyribonuclease (pancreatic)	T45.3X1	T45.3X2	T45.3X3	T45.3X4	T45.3X5	T45.3X6
Depilatory	T49.4X1	T49.4X2	T49.4X3	T49.4X4	T49.4X5	T49.4X6
Deprenalin	T42.8X1	T42.8X2	T42.8X3	T42.8X4	T42.8X5	T42.8X6
Deprenyl	T42.8X1	T42.8X2	T42.8X3	T42.8X4	T42.8X5	T42.8X6
Depressant						
appetite (central)	T50.5X1	T50.5X2	T50.5X3	T50.5X4	T50.5X5	T50.5X6
cardiac	T46.2X1	T46.2X2	T46.2X3	T46.2X4	T46.2X5	T46.2X6
central nervous system (anesthetic) — *see also* Central nervous system, depressants	T42.71	T42.72	T42.73	T42.74	T42.75	T42.76
general anesthetic	T41.201	T41.202	T41.203	T41.204	T41.205	T41.206
muscle tone	T42.8X1	T42.8X2	T42.8X3	T42.8X4	T42.8X5	T42.8X6
muscle tone, central	T42.8X1	T42.8X2	T42.8X3	T42.8X4	T42.8X5	T42.8X6
psychotherapeutic	T43.501	T43.502	T43.503	T43.504	T43.505	T43.506
Depressant, appetite	T50.5X1	T50.5X2	T50.5X3	T50.5X4	T50.5X5	T50.5X6
Deptropine	T45.0X1	T45.0X2	T45.0X3	T45.0X4	T45.0X5	T45.0X6
Dequalinium (chloride)	T49.0X1	T49.0X2	T49.0X3	T49.0X4	T49.0X5	T49.0X6
Derris root	T60.2X1	T60.2X2	T60.2X3	T60.2X4	—	—

Substance	Poisoning, Accidental (unintentional)	Poisoning, Intentional Self-harm	Poisoning, Assault	Poisoning, Undetermined	Adverse Effect	Under-dosing
Deserpidine	T46.5X1	T46.5X2	T46.5X3	T46.5X4	T46.5X5	T46.5X6
Desferrioxamine	T45.8X1	T45.8X2	T45.8X3	T45.8X4	T45.8X5	T45.8X6
Desipramine	T43.Ø11	T43.Ø12	T43.Ø13	T43.Ø14	T43.Ø15	T43.Ø16
Deslanoside	T46.ØX1	T46.ØX2	T46.ØX3	T46.ØX4	T46.ØX5	T46.ØX6
Desloughing agent	T49.4X1	T49.4X2	T49.4X3	T49.4X4	T49.4X5	T49.4X6
Desmethylimipramine	T43.Ø11	T43.Ø12	T43.Ø13	T43.Ø14	T43.Ø15	T43.Ø16
Desmopressin	T38.891	T38.892	T38.893	T38.894	T38.895	T38.896
Desocodeine	T4Ø.2X1	T4Ø.2X2	T4Ø.2X3	T4Ø.2X4	T4Ø.2X5	T4Ø.2X6
Desogestrel	T38.5X1	T38.5X2	T38.5X3	T38.5X4	T38.5X5	T38.5X6
Desomorphine	T4Ø.2X1	T4Ø.2X2	T4Ø.2X3	T4Ø.2X4	—	—
Desonide	T49.ØX1	T49.ØX2	T49.ØX3	T49.ØX4	T49.ØX5	T49.ØX6
Desoximetasone	T49.ØX1	T49.ØX2	T49.ØX3	T49.ØX4	T49.ØX5	T49.ØX6
Desoxycorticosteroid	T5Ø.ØX1	T5Ø.ØX2	T5Ø.ØX3	T5Ø.ØX4	T5Ø.ØX5	T5Ø.ØX6
Desoxycortone	T5Ø.ØX1	T5Ø.ØX2	T5Ø.ØX3	T5Ø.ØX4	T5Ø.ØX5	T5Ø.ØX6
Desoxyephedrine	T43.651	T43.652	T43.652	T43.654	T43.655	T43.656
Detaxtran	T46.6X1	T46.6X2	T46.6X3	T46.6X4	T46.6X5	T46.6X6
Detergent	T49.2X1	T49.2X2	T49.2X3	T49.2X4	T49.2X5	T49.2X6
external medication	T49.2X1	T49.2X2	T49.2X3	T49.2X4	T49.2X5	T49.2X6
local	T49.2X1	T49.2X2	T49.2X3	T49.2X4	T49.2X5	T49.2X6
medicinal	T49.2X1	T49.2X2	T49.2X3	T49.2X4	T49.2X5	T49.2X6
nonmedicinal	T55.1X1	T55.1X2	T55.1X3	T55.1X4	—	—
specified NEC	T55.1X1	T55.1X2	T55.1X3	T55.1X4	—	—
Deterrent, alcohol	T5Ø.6X1	T5Ø.6X2	T5Ø.6X3	T5Ø.6X4	T5Ø.6X5	T5Ø.6X6
Detoxifying agent	T5Ø.6X1	T5Ø.6X2	T5Ø.6X3	T5Ø.6X4	T5Ø.6X5	T5Ø.6X6
Detrothyronine	T38.1X1	T38.1X2	T38.1X3	T38.1X4	T38.1X5	T38.1X6
Dettol (external medication)	T49.ØX1	T49.ØX2	T49.ØX3	T49.ØX4	T49.ØX5	T49.ØX6
Dexamethasone	T38.ØX1	T38.ØX2	T38.ØX3	T38.ØX4	T38.ØX5	T38.ØX6
ENT agent	T49.6X1	T49.6X2	T49.6X3	T49.6X4	T49.6X5	T49.6X6
ophthalmic preparation	T49.5X1	T49.5X2	T49.5X3	T49.5X4	T49.5X5	T49.5X6
topical NEC	T49.ØX1	T49.ØX2	T49.ØX3	T49.ØX4	T49.ØX5	T49.ØX6
Dexamfetamine	T43.621	T43.622	T43.623	T43.624	T43.625	T43.626
Dexamphetamine	T43.621	T43.622	T43.623	T43.624	T43.625	T43.626
Dexbrompheniramine	T45.ØX1	T45.ØX2	T45.ØX3	T45.ØX4	T45.ØX5	T45.ØX6
Dexchlorpheniramine	T45.ØX1	T45.ØX2	T45.ØX3	T45.ØX4	T45.ØX5	T45.ØX6
Dexedrine	T43.621	T43.622	T43.623	T43.624	T43.625	T43.626
Dexetimide	T44.3X1	T44.3X2	T44.3X3	T44.3X4	T44.3X5	T44.3X6
Dexfenfluramine	T5Ø.5X1	T5Ø.5X2	T5Ø.5X3	T5Ø.5X4	T5Ø.5X5	T5Ø.5X6
Dexpanthenol	T45.2X1	T45.2X2	T45.2X3	T45.2X4	T45.2X5	T45.2X6
Dextran (40) (70) (150)	T45.8X1	T45.8X2	T45.8X3	T45.8X4	T45.8X5	T45.8X6
Dextriferron	T45.4X1	T45.4X2	T45.4X3	T45.4X4	T45.4X5	T45.4X6
Dextroamphetamine	T43.621	T43.622	T43.623	T43.624	T43.625	T43.626
Dextro calcium pantothenate	T45.2X1	T45.2X2	T45.2X3	T45.2X4	T45.2X5	T45.2X6
Dextromethorphan	T48.3X1	T48.3X2	T48.3X3	T48.3X4	T48.3X5	T48.3X6
Dextromoramide	T4Ø.491	T4Ø.492	T4Ø.493	T4Ø.494	—	—
topical	T49.8X1	T49.8X2	T49.8X3	T49.8X4	T49.8X5	T49.8X6
Dextro pantothenyl alcohol	T45.2X1	T45.2X2	T45.2X3	T45.2X4	T45.2X5	T45.2X6
Dextropropoxyphene	T4Ø.491	T4Ø.492	T4Ø.493	T4Ø.494	T4Ø.495	T4Ø.496
Dextrorphan	T4Ø.2X1	T4Ø.2X2	T4Ø.2X3	T4Ø.2X4	T4Ø.2X5	T4Ø.2X6
Dextrose	T5Ø.3X1	T5Ø.3X2	T5Ø.3X3	T5Ø.3X4	T5Ø.3X5	T5Ø.3X6
concentrated solution, intravenous	T46.8X1	T46.8X2	T46.8X3	T46.8X4	T46.8X5	T46.8X6
Dextrothyroxin	T38.1X1	T38.1X2	T38.1X3	T38.1X4	T38.1X5	T38.1X6
Dextrothyroxine sodium	T38.1X1	T38.1X2	T38.1X3	T38.1X4	T38.1X5	T38.1X6
DFP	T44.ØX1	T44.ØX2	T44.ØX3	T44.ØX4	T44.ØX5	T44.ØX6
DHE	T37.3X1	T37.3X2	T37.3X3	T37.3X4	T37.3X5	T37.3X6
45	T46.5X1	T46.5X2	T46.5X3	T46.5X4	T46.5X5	T46.5X6
DiaBeta*	T38.3X1	T38.3X2	T38.3X3	T38.3X4	T38.3X5	T38.3X6
Diabinese	T38.3X1	T38.3X2	T38.3X3	T38.3X4	T38.3X5	T38.3X6
Diacetone alcohol	T52.4X1	T52.4X2	T52.4X3	T52.4X4	—	—
Diacetyl monoxime	T5Ø.991	T5Ø.992	T5Ø.993	T5Ø.994	—	—
Diacetylmorphine	T4Ø.1X1	T4Ø.1X2	T4Ø.1X3	T4Ø.1X4	—	—
Diachylon plaster	T49.4X1	T49.4X2	T49.4X3	T49.4X4	T49.4X5	T49.4X6
Diaethylstilboestrolum	T38.5X1	T38.5X2	T38.5X3	T38.5X4	T38.5X5	T38.5X6
Diagnostic agent NEC	T5Ø.8X1	T5Ø.8X2	T5Ø.8X3	T5Ø.8X4	T5Ø.8X5	T5Ø.8X6
Dial (soap)	T49.2X1	T49.2X2	T49.2X3	T49.2X4	T49.2X5	T49.2X6
sedative	T42.3X1	T42.3X2	T42.3X3	T42.3X4	T42.3X5	T42.3X6
Dialkyl carbonate	T52.91	T52.92	T52.93	T52.94	—	—
Diallylbarbituric acid	T42.3X1	T42.3X2	T42.3X3	T42.3X4	T42.3X5	T42.3X6
Diallymal	T42.3X1	T42.3X2	T42.3X3	T42.3X4	T42.3X5	T42.3X6
Dialysis solution (intraperitoneal)	T5Ø.3X1	T5Ø.3X2	T5Ø.3X3	T5Ø.3X4	T5Ø.3X5	T5Ø.3X6
Diaminodiphenylsulfone	T37.1X1	T37.1X2	T37.1X3	T37.1X4	T37.1X5	T37.1X6
Diamorphine	T4Ø.1X1	T4Ø.1X2	T4Ø.1X3	T4Ø.1X4	—	—
Diamox	T5Ø.2X1	T5Ø.2X2	T5Ø.2X3	T5Ø.2X4	T5Ø.2X5	T5Ø.2X6
Diamthazole	T49.ØX1	T49.ØX2	T49.ØX3	T49.ØX4	T49.ØX5	T49.ØX6
Dianthone	T47.2X1	T47.2X2	T47.2X3	T47.2X4	T47.2X5	T47.2X6
Diaphenylsulfone	T37.ØX1	T37.ØX2	T37.ØX3	T37.ØX4	T37.ØX5	T37.ØX6
Diasone (sodium)	T37.1X1	T37.1X2	T37.1X3	T37.1X4	T37.1X5	T37.1X6
Diastase	T47.5X1	T47.5X2	T47.5X3	T47.5X4	T47.5X5	T47.5X6
Diastat*	T42.4X1	T42.4X2	T42.4X3	T42.4X4	T42.4X5	T42.4X6
Diatrizoate	T5Ø.8X1	T5Ø.8X2	T5Ø.8X3	T5Ø.8X4	T5Ø.8X5	T5Ø.8X6
Diazepam	T42.4X1	T42.4X2	T42.4X3	T42.4X4	T42.4X5	T42.4X6
Diazinon	T6Ø.ØX1	T6Ø.ØX2	T6Ø.ØX3	T6Ø.ØX4	—	—
Diazomethane (gas)	T59.891	T59.892	T59.893	T59.894	—	—
Diazoxide	T46.5X1	T46.5X2	T46.5X3	T46.5X4	T46.5X5	T46.5X6
Dibekacin	T36.5X1	T36.5X2	T36.5X3	T36.5X4	T36.5X5	T36.5X6
Dibenamine	T44.6X1	T44.6X2	T44.6X3	T44.6X4	T44.6X5	T44.6X6
Dibenzepin	T43.Ø11	T43.Ø12	T43.Ø13	T43.Ø14	T43.Ø15	T43.Ø16
Dibenzheptropine	T45.ØX1	T45.ØX2	T45.ØX3	T45.ØX4	T45.ØX5	T45.ØX6
Dibenzyline	T44.6X1	T44.6X2	T44.6X3	T44.6X4	T44.6X5	T44.6X6
Diborane (gas)	T59.891	T59.892	T59.893	T59.894	—	—
Dibromochloropropane	T6Ø.8X1	T6Ø.8X2	T6Ø.8X3	T6Ø.8X4	—	—
Dibromodulcitol	T45.1X1	T45.1X2	T45.1X3	T45.1X4	T45.1X5	T45.1X6
Dibromoethane	T53.6X1	T53.6X2	T53.6X3	T53.6X4	—	—
Dibromomannitol	T45.1X1	T45.1X2	T45.1X3	T45.1X4	T45.1X5	T45.1X6
Dibromopropamidine isethionate	T49.ØX1	T49.ØX2	T49.ØX3	T49.ØX4	T49.ØX5	T49.ØX6
Dibrompropamidine	T49.ØX1	T49.ØX2	T49.ØX3	T49.ØX4	T49.ØX5	T49.ØX6
Dibucaine	T41.3X1	T41.3X2	T41.3X3	T41.3X4	T41.3X5	T41.3X6
topical (surface)	T41.3X1	T41.3X2	T41.3X3	T41.3X4	T41.3X5	T41.3X6
Dibunate sodium	T48.3X1	T48.3X2	T48.3X3	T48.3X4	T48.3X5	T48.3X6
Dibutoline sulfate	T44.3X1	T44.3X2	T44.3X3	T44.3X4	T44.3X5	T44.3X6
Dicamba	T6Ø.3X1	T6Ø.3X2	T6Ø.3X3	T6Ø.3X4	—	—
Dicapthon	T6Ø.ØX1	T6Ø.ØX2	T6Ø.ØX3	T6Ø.ØX4	—	—
Dichlobenil	T6Ø.3X1	T6Ø.3X2	T6Ø.3X3	T6Ø.3X4	—	—
Dichlone	T6Ø.3X1	T6Ø.3X2	T6Ø.3X3	T6Ø.3X4	—	—
Dichloralphenozone	T42.6X1	T42.6X2	T42.6X3	T42.6X4	T42.6X5	T42.6X6
Dichlorbenzidine	T65.3X1	T65.3X2	T65.3X3	T65.3X4	—	—
Dichlorhydrin	T52.8X1	T52.8X2	T52.8X3	T52.8X4	—	—
Dichlorhydroxyquinoline	T37.8X1	T37.8X2	T37.8X3	T37.8X4	T37.8X5	T37.8X6
Dichlorobenzene	T53.7X1	T53.7X2	T53.7X3	T53.7X4	—	—
Dichlorobenzyl alcohol	T49.6X1	T49.6X2	T49.6X3	T49.6X4	T49.6X5	T49.6X6
Dichlorodifluoromethane	T53.5X1	T53.5X2	T53.5X3	T53.5X4	—	—
Dichloroethane	T52.8X1	T52.8X2	T52.8X3	T52.8X4	—	—
Dichloroethylene	T53.6X1	T53.6X2	T53.6X3	T53.6X4	—	—
Dichloroethyl sulfide, not in war	T59.891	T59.892	T59.893	T59.894	—	—
Dichloroformoxine, not in war	T59.891	T59.892	T59.893	T59.894	—	—
Dichlorohydrin, alpha-dichlorohydrin	T52.8X1	T52.8X2	T52.8X3	T52.8X4	—	—
Dichloromethane (solvent)	T53.4X1	T53.4X2	T53.4X3	T53.4X4	—	—
vapor	T53.4X1	T53.4X2	T53.4X3	T53.4X4	—	—
Dichloronaphthoquinone	T6Ø.3X1	T6Ø.3X2	T6Ø.3X3	T6Ø.3X4	—	—
Dichlorophen	T37.4X1	T37.4X2	T37.4X3	T37.4X4	T37.4X5	T37.4X6
Dichloropropene	T6Ø.3X1	T6Ø.3X2	T6Ø.3X3	T6Ø.3X4	—	—
Dichloropropionic acid	T6Ø.3X1	T6Ø.3X2	T6Ø.3X3	T6Ø.3X4	—	—
Dichlorphenamide	T5Ø.2X1	T5Ø.2X2	T5Ø.2X3	T5Ø.2X4	T5Ø.2X5	T5Ø.2X6
Dichlorvos	T6Ø.ØX1	T6Ø.ØX2	T6Ø.ØX3	T6Ø.ØX4	—	—
Dichysterol*	T45.2X1	T45.2X2	T45.2X3	T45.2X4	T45.2X5	T45.2X6
Diclofenac	T39.391	T39.392	T39.393	T39.394	T39.395	T39.396
Diclofenamide	T5Ø.2X1	T5Ø.2X2	T5Ø.2X3	T5Ø.2X4	T5Ø.2X5	T5Ø.2X6
Diclofensine	T43.291	T43.292	T43.293	T43.294	T43.295	T43.296
Diclonixine	T39.8X1	T39.8X2	T39.8X3	T39.8X4	T39.8X5	T39.8X6
Dicloxacillin	T36.ØX1	T36.ØX2	T36.ØX3	T36.ØX4	T36.ØX5	T36.ØX6
Dicophane	T49.ØX1	T49.ØX2	T49.ØX3	T49.ØX4	T49.ØX5	T49.ØX6
Dicoumarol, dicoumarin, dicumarol	T45.511	T45.512	T45.513	T45.514	T45.515	T45.516
Dicrotophos	T6Ø.ØX1	T6Ø.ØX2	T6Ø.ØX3	T6Ø.ØX4	—	—
Dicyanogen (gas)	T65.ØX1	T65.ØX2	T65.ØX3	T65.ØX4	—	—
Dicyclomine	T44.3X1	T44.3X2	T44.3X3	T44.3X4	T44.3X5	T44.3X6
Dicycloverine	T44.3X1	T44.3X2	T44.3X3	T44.3X4	T44.3X5	T44.3X6
Didanosine*	T37.5X1	T37.5X2	T37.5X3	T37.5X4	T37.5X5	T37.5X6
Dideoxycytidine	T37.5X1	T37.5X2	T37.5X3	T37.5X4	T37.5X5	T37.5X6
Dideoxyinosine	T37.5X1	T37.5X2	T37.5X3	T37.5X4	T37.5X5	T37.5X6
Dieldrin (vapor)	T6Ø.1X1	T6Ø.1X2	T6Ø.1X3	T6Ø.1X4	—	—
Diemal	T42.3X1	T42.3X2	T42.3X3	T42.3X4	T42.3X5	T42.3X6
Dienestrol	T38.5X1	T38.5X2	T38.5X3	T38.5X4	T38.5X5	T38.5X6
Dienoestrol	T38.5X1	T38.5X2	T38.5X3	T38.5X4	T38.5X5	T38.5X6
Dietetic drug NEC	T5Ø.9Ø1	T5Ø.9Ø2	T5Ø.9Ø3	T5Ø.9Ø4	T5Ø.9Ø5	T5Ø.9Ø6
Diethazine	T42.8X1	T42.8X2	T42.8X3	T42.8X4	T42.8X5	T42.8X6
Diethyl						
barbituric acid	T42.3X1	T42.3X2	T42.3X3	T42.3X4	T42.3X5	T42.3X6
carbamazine	T37.4X1	T37.4X2	T37.4X3	T37.4X4	T37.4X5	T37.4X6
carbinol	T51.3X1	T51.3X2	T51.3X3	T51.3X4	—	—
carbonate	T52.8X1	T52.8X2	T52.8X3	T52.8X4	—	—
ether (vapor) — *see also* ether	T41.ØX1	T41.ØX2	T41.ØX3	T41.ØX4	T41.ØX5	T41.ØX6
oxide	T52.8X1	T52.8X2	T52.8X3	T52.8X4	—	—
propion	T5Ø.5X1	T5Ø.5X2	T5Ø.5X3	T5Ø.5X4	T5Ø.5X5	T5Ø.5X6
stilbestrol	T38.5X1	T38.5X2	T38.5X3	T38.5X4	T38.5X5	T38.5X6
toluamide (nonmedicinal)	T6Ø.8X1	T6Ø.8X2	T6Ø.8X3	T6Ø.8X4	—	—
medicinal	T49.3X1	T49.3X2	T49.3X3	T49.3X4	T49.3X5	T49.3X6
Diethylcarbamazine	T37.4X1	T37.4X2	T37.4X3	T37.4X4	T37.4X5	T37.4X6

Substance	Poisoning, Accidental (unintentional)	Poisoning, Intentional Self-harm	Poisoning, Assault	Poisoning, Undetermined	Adverse Effect	Under-dosing
Diethylene						
dioxide	T52.8X1	T52.8X2	T52.8X3	T52.8X4	—	—
glycol (monoacetate)	T52.3X1	T52.3X2	T52.3X3	T52.3X4	—	—
(monobutyl ether)						
(monoethyl ether)						
Diethylhexylphthalate	T65.891	T65.892	T65.893	T65.894	—	—
Diethylpropion	T5Ø.5X1	T5Ø.5X2	T5Ø.5X3	T5Ø.5X4	T5Ø.5X5	T5Ø.5X6
Diethylstilbestrol	T38.5X1	T38.5X2	T38.5X3	T38.5X4	T38.5X5	T38.5X6
Diethylstilboestrol	T38.5X1	T38.5X2	T38.5X3	T38.5X4	T38.5X5	T38.5X6
Diethylsulfone-diethylmethane	T42.6X1	T42.6X2	T42.6X3	T42.6X4	T42.6X5	T42.6X6
Diethyltoluamide	T49.ØX1	T49.ØX2	T49.ØX3	T49.ØX4	T49.ØX5	T49.ØX6
Diethyltryptamine (DET)	T4Ø.991	T4Ø.992	T4Ø.993	T4Ø.994	—	—
Difebarbamate	T42.3X1	T42.3X2	T42.3X3	T42.3X4	T42.3X5	T42.3X6
Difencloxazine	T4Ø.2X1	T4Ø.2X2	T4Ø.2X3	T4Ø.2X4	T4Ø.2X5	T4Ø.2X6
Difenidol	T45.ØX1	T45.ØX2	T45.ØX3	T45.ØX4	T45.ØX5	T45.ØX6
Difenoxin	T47.6X1	T47.6X2	T47.6X3	T47.6X4	T47.6X5	T47.6X6
Difetarsone	T37.3X1	T37.3X2	T37.3X3	T37.3X4	T37.3X5	T37.3X6
Diffusin	T45.3X1	T45.3X2	T45.3X3	T45.3X4	T45.3X5	T45.3X6
Diflorasone	T49.ØX1	T49.ØX2	T49.ØX3	T49.ØX4	T49.ØX5	T49.ØX6
Diflos	T44.ØX1	T44.ØX2	T44.ØX3	T44.ØX4	T44.ØX5	T44.ØX6
Diflubenzuron	T6Ø.1X1	T6Ø.1X2	T6Ø.1X3	T6Ø.1X4	—	—
Diflucortolone	T49.ØX1	T49.ØX2	T49.ØX3	T49.ØX4	T49.ØX5	T49.ØX6
Diflunisal	T39.Ø91	T39.Ø92	T39.Ø93	T39.Ø94	T39.Ø95	T39.Ø96
Difluoromethyldopa	T42.8X1	T42.8X2	T42.8X3	T42.8X4	T42.8X5	T42.8X6
Difluorophate	T44.ØX1	T44.ØX2	T44.ØX3	T44.ØX4	T44.ØX5	T44.ØX6
Digestant NEC	T47.5X1	T47.5X2	T47.5X3	T47.5X4	T47.5X5	T47.5X6
Digitalin (e)	T46.ØX1	T46.ØX2	T46.ØX3	T46.ØX4	T46.ØX5	T46.ØX6
Digitalis (leaf)(glycoside)	T46.ØX1	T46.ØX2	T46.ØX3	T46.ØX4	T46.ØX5	T46.ØX6
lanata	T46.ØX1	T46.ØX2	T46.ØX3	T46.ØX4	T46.ØX5	T46.ØX6
purpurea	T46.ØX1	T46.ØX2	T46.ØX3	T46.ØX4	T46.ØX5	T46.ØX6
Digitoxin	T46.ØX1	T46.ØX2	T46.ØX3	T46.ØX4	T46.ØX5	T46.ØX6
Digitoxose	T46.ØX1	T46.ØX2	T46.ØX3	T46.ØX4	T46.ØX5	T46.ØX6
Digoxin	T46.ØX1	T46.ØX2	T46.ØX3	T46.ØX4	T46.ØX5	T46.ØX6
Digoxine	T46.ØX1	T46.ØX2	T46.ØX3	T46.ØX4	T46.ØX5	T46.ØX6
Dihydralazine	T46.5X1	T46.5X2	T46.5X3	T46.5X4	T46.5X5	T46.5X6
Dihydrazine	T46.5X1	T46.5X2	T46.5X3	T46.5X4	T46.5X5	T46.5X6
Dihydrocodeine	T4Ø.2X1	T4Ø.2X2	T4Ø.2X3	T4Ø.2X4	T4Ø.2X5	T4Ø.2X6
Dihydrocodeinone	T4Ø.2X1	T4Ø.2X2	T4Ø.2X3	T4Ø.2X4	T4Ø.2X5	T4Ø.2X6
Dihydroergocornine	T46.7X1	T46.7X2	T46.7X3	T46.7X4	T46.7X5	T46.7X6
Dihydroergocristine (mesilate)	T46.7X1	T46.7X2	T46.7X3	T46.7X4	T46.7X5	T46.7X6
Dihydroergokryptine	T46.7X1	T46.7X2	T46.7X3	T46.7X4	T46.7X5	T46.7X6
Dihydroergotamine	T46.5X1	T46.5X2	T46.5X3	T46.5X4	T46.5X5	T46.5X6
Dihydroergotoxine	T46.7X1	T46.7X2	T46.7X3	T46.7X4	T46.7X5	T46.7X6
mesilate	T46.7X1	T46.7X2	T46.7X3	T46.7X4	T46.7X5	T46.7X6
Dihydrohydroxycodeinone	T4Ø.2X1	T4Ø.2X2	T4Ø.2X3	T4Ø.2X4	T4Ø.2X5	T4Ø.2X6
Dihydrohydroxymorphinone	T4Ø.2X1	T4Ø.2X2	T4Ø.2X3	T4Ø.2X4	T4Ø.2X5	T4Ø.2X6
Dihydroisocodeine	T4Ø.2X1	T4Ø.2X2	T4Ø.2X3	T4Ø.2X4	T4Ø.2X5	T4Ø.2X6
Dihydromorphine	T4Ø.2X1	T4Ø.2X2	T4Ø.2X3	T4Ø.2X4	—	
Dihydromorphinone	T4Ø.2X1	T4Ø.2X2	T4Ø.2X3	T4Ø.2X4	T4Ø.2X5	T4Ø.2X6
Dihydrostreptomycin	T36.5X1	T36.5X2	T36.5X3	T36.5X4	T36.5X5	T36.5X6
Dihydrotachysterol	T45.2X1	T45.2X2	T45.2X3	T45.2X4	T45.2X5	T45.2X6
Dihydroxyacetone*	T49.3X1	T49.3X2	T49.3X3	T49.3X4	T49.3X5	T49.3X6
Dihydroxyaluminum aminoacetate	T47.1X1	T47.1X2	T47.1X3	T47.1X4	T47.1X5	T47.1X6
Dihydroxyaluminum sodium carbonate	T47.1X1	T47.1X2	T47.1X3	T47.1X4	T47.1X5	T47.1X6
Dihydroxyanthraquinone	T47.2X1	T47.2X2	T47.2X3	T47.2X4	T47.2X5	T47.2X6
Dihydroxycodeinone	T4Ø.2X1	T4Ø.2X2	T4Ø.2X3	T4Ø.2X4	T4Ø.2X5	T4Ø.2X6
Dihydroxypropyl theophylline	T5Ø.2X1	T5Ø.2X2	T5Ø.2X3	T5Ø.2X4	T5Ø.2X5	T5Ø.2X6
Diiodohydroxyquin	T37.8X1	T37.8X2	T37.8X3	T37.8X4	T37.8X5	T37.8X6
topical	T49.ØX1	T49.ØX2	T49.ØX3	T49.ØX4	T49.ØX5	T49.ØX6
Diiodohydroxyquinoline	T37.8X1	T37.8X2	T37.8X3	T37.8X4	T37.8X5	T37.8X6
Diiodotyrosine	T38.2X1	T38.2X2	T38.2X3	T38.2X4	T38.2X5	T38.2X6
Diisopromine	T44.3X1	T44.3X2	T44.3X3	T44.3X4	T44.3X5	T44.3X6
Diisopropylamine	T46.3X1	T46.3X2	T46.3X3	T46.3X4	T46.3X5	T46.3X6
Diisopropylfluorophosphonate	T44.ØX1	T44.ØX2	T44.ØX3	T44.ØX4	T44.ØX5	T44.ØX6
Dilantin	T42.ØX1	T42.ØX2	T42.ØX3	T42.ØX4	T42.ØX5	T42.ØX6
Dilatrate*	T46.3X1	T46.3X2	T46.3X3	T46.3X4	T46.3X5	T46.3X6
Dilaudid	T4Ø.2X1	T4Ø.2X2	T4Ø.2X3	T4Ø.2X4	T4Ø.2X5	T4Ø.2X6
Dilazep	T46.3X1	T46.3X2	T46.3X3	T46.3X4	T46.3X5	T46.3X6
Dill	T47.5X1	T47.5X2	T47.5X3	T47.5X4	T47.5X5	T47.5X6
Diloxanide	T37.3X1	T37.3X2	T37.3X3	T37.3X4	T37.3X5	T37.3X6
Diltiazem	T46.1X1	T46.1X2	T46.1X3	T46.1X4	T46.1X5	T46.1X6
Dimazole	T49.ØX1	T49.ØX2	T49.ØX3	T49.ØX4	T49.ØX5	T49.ØX6
Dimefline	T5Ø.7X1	T5Ø.7X2	T5Ø.7X3	T5Ø.7X4	T5Ø.7X5	T5Ø.7X6
Dimefox	T6Ø.ØX1	T6Ø.ØX2	T6Ø.ØX3	T6Ø.ØX4	—	—
Dimemorfan	T48.3X1	T48.3X2	T48.3X3	T48.3X4	T48.3X5	T48.3X6
Dimenhydrinate	T45.ØX1	T45.ØX2	T45.ØX3	T45.ØX4	T45.ØX5	T45.ØX6

Substance	Poisoning, Accidental (unintentional)	Poisoning, Intentional Self-harm	Poisoning, Assault	Poisoning, Undetermined	Adverse Effect	Under-dosing
Dimercaprol (British anti-lewisite)	T45.8X1	T45.8X2	T45.8X3	T45.8X4	T45.8X5	T45.8X6
Dimercaptopropanol	T45.8X1	T45.8X2	T45.8X3	T45.8X4	T45.8X5	T45.8X6
Dimestrol	T38.5X1	T38.5X2	T38.5X3	T38.5X4	T38.5X5	T38.5X6
Dimetane	T45.ØX1	T45.ØX2	T45.ØX3	T45.ØX4	T45.ØX5	T45.ØX6
Dimethicone	T47.1X1	T47.1X2	T47.1X3	T47.1X4	T47.1X5	T47.1X6
Dimethindene	T45.ØX1	T45.ØX2	T45.ØX3	T45.ØX4	T45.ØX5	T45.ØX6
Dimethisoquin	T49.1X1	T49.1X2	T49.1X3	T49.1X4	T49.1X5	T49.1X6
Dimethisterone	T38.5X1	T38.5X2	T38.5X3	T38.5X4	T38.5X5	T38.5X6
Dimethoate	T6Ø.ØX1	T6Ø.ØX2	T6Ø.ØX3	T6Ø.ØX4	—	—
Dimethocaine	T41.3X1	T41.3X2	T41.3X3	T41.3X4	T41.3X5	T41.3X6
Dimethoxanate	T48.3X1	T48.3X2	T48.3X3	T48.3X4	T48.3X5	T48.3X6
Dimethyl						
arsine, arsinic acid	T57.ØX1	T57.ØX2	T57.ØX3	T57.ØX4	—	—
carbinol	T51.2X1	T51.2X2	T51.2X3	T51.2X4	—	—
carbonate	T52.8X1	T52.8X2	T52.8X3	T52.8X4	—	—
diguanide	T38.3X1	T38.3X2	T38.3X3	T38.3X4	T38.3X5	T38.3X6
ketone	T52.4X1	T52.4X2	T52.4X3	T52.4X4	—	—
vapor	T52.4X1	T52.4X2	T52.4X3	T52.4X4	—	—
meperidine	T4Ø.2X1	T4Ø.2X2	T4Ø.2X3	T4Ø.2X4	T4Ø.2X5	T4Ø.2X6
parathion	T6Ø.ØX1	T6Ø.ØX2	T6Ø.ØX3	T6Ø.ØX4	—	—
phthlate	T49.3X1	T49.3X2	T49.3X3	T49.3X4	T49.3X5	T49.3X6
polysiloxane	T47.8X1	T47.8X2	T47.8X3	T47.8X4	T47.8X5	T47.8X6
sulfate (fumes)	T59.891	T59.892	T59.893	T59.894	—	—
liquid	T65.891	T65.892	T65.893	T65.894	—	—
sulfoxide (nonmedicinal)	T52.8X1	T52.8X2	T52.8X3	T52.8X4	—	—
medicinal	T49.4X1	T49.4X2	T49.4X3	T49.4X4	T49.4X5	T49.4X6
tryptamine	T4Ø.991	T4Ø.992	T4Ø.993	T4Ø.994	—	—
tubocurarine	T48.1X1	T48.1X2	T48.1X3	T48.1X4	T48.1X5	T48.1X6
Dimethylamine sulfate	T49.4X1	T49.4X2	T49.4X3	T49.4X4	T49.4X5	T49.4X6
Dimethylcysteine*	T5Ø.6X1	T5Ø.6X2	T5Ø.6X3	T5Ø.6X4	T5Ø.6X5	T5Ø.6X6
Dimethylformamide	T52.8X1	T52.8X2	T52.8X3	T52.8X4	—	—
Dimethyltubocurarinium chloride	T48.1X1	T48.1X2	T48.1X3	T48.1X4	T48.1X5	T48.1X6
Dimeticone	T47.1X1	T47.1X2	T47.1X3	T47.1X4	T47.1X5	T47.1X6
Dimetilan	T6Ø.ØX1	T6Ø.ØX2	T6Ø.ØX3	T6Ø.ØX4	—	—
Dimetindene	T45.ØX1	T45.ØX2	T45.ØX3	T45.ØX4	T45.ØX5	T45.ØX6
Dimetotiazine	T43.3X1	T43.3X2	T43.3X3	T43.3X4	T43.3X5	T43.3X6
Dimorpholamine	T5Ø.7X1	T5Ø.7X2	T5Ø.7X3	T5Ø.7X4	T5Ø.7X5	T5Ø.7X6
Dimoxyline	T46.3X1	T46.3X2	T46.3X3	T46.3X4	T46.3X5	T46.3X6
Dinitrobenzene	T65.3X1	T65.3X2	T65.3X3	T65.3X4	—	—
vapor	T59.891	T59.892	T59.893	T59.894	—	—
Dinitrobenzol	T65.3X1	T65.3X2	T65.3X3	T65.3X4	—	—
vapor	T59.891	T59.892	T59.893	T59.894	—	—
Dinitrobutylphenol	T65.3X1	T65.3X2	T65.3X3	T65.3X4	—	—
Dinitro (-ortho-)cresol (pesticide) (spray)	T65.3X1	T65.3X2	T65.3X3	T65.3X4	—	—
Dinitrocyclohexylphenol	T65.3X1	T65.3X2	T65.3X3	T65.3X4	—	—
Dinitrophenol	T65.3X1	T65.3X2	T65.3X3	T65.3X4	—	—
Dinoprost	T48.ØX1	T48.ØX2	T48.ØX3	T48.ØX4	T48.ØX5	T48.ØX6
Dinoprostone	T48.ØX1	T48.ØX2	T48.ØX3	T48.ØX4	T48.ØX5	T48.ØX6
Dinoseb	T6Ø.3X1	T6Ø.3X2	T6Ø.3X3	T6Ø.3X4	—	—
Dioctyl sulfosuccinate (calcium) (sodium)	T47.4X1	T47.4X2	T47.4X3	T47.4X4	T47.4X5	T47.4X6
Diodone	T5Ø.8X1	T5Ø.8X2	T5Ø.8X3	T5Ø.8X4	T5Ø.8X5	T5Ø.8X6
Diodoquin	T37.8X1	T37.8X2	T37.8X3	T37.8X4	T37.8X5	T37.8X6
Dionin	T4Ø.2X1	T4Ø.2X2	T4Ø.2X3	T4Ø.2X4	T4Ø.2X5	T4Ø.2X6
Diosmin	T46.991	T46.992	T46.993	T46.994	T46.995	T46.996
Diovan*	T46.5X1	T46.5X2	T46.5X3	T46.5X4	T46.5X5	T46.5X6
Dioxane	T52.8X1	T52.8X2	T52.8X3	T52.8X4	—	—
Dioxathion	T6Ø.ØX1	T6Ø.ØX2	T6Ø.ØX3	T6Ø.ØX4	—	—
Dioxin	T53.7X1	T53.7X2	T53.7X3	T53.7X4	—	—
Dioxopromethazine	T43.3X1	T43.3X2	T43.3X3	T43.3X4	T43.3X5	T43.3X6
Dioxyline	T46.3X1	T46.3X2	T46.3X3	T46.3X4	T46.3X5	T46.3X6
Dipentene	T52.8X1	T52.8X2	T52.8X3	T52.8X4	—	—
Diperodon	T41.3X1	T41.3X2	T41.3X3	T41.3X4	T41.3X5	T41.3X6
Diphacinone	T6Ø.4X1	T6Ø.4X2	T6Ø.4X3	T6Ø.4X4	—	—
Diphemanil	T44.3X1	T44.3X2	T44.3X3	T44.3X4	T44.3X5	T44.3X6
metilsulfate	T44.3X1	T44.3X2	T44.3X3	T44.3X4	T44.3X5	T44.3X6
Diphenadione	T45.511	T45.512	T45.513	T45.514	T45.515	T45.516
rodenticide	T6Ø.4X1	T6Ø.4X2	T6Ø.4X3	T6Ø.4X4	—	—
Diphenhydramine	T45.ØX1	T45.ØX2	T45.ØX3	T45.ØX4	T45.ØX5	T45.ØX6
Diphenidol	T45.ØX1	T45.ØX2	T45.ØX3	T45.ØX4	T45.ØX5	T45.ØX6
Diphenoxylate	T47.6X1	T47.6X2	T47.6X3	T47.6X4	T47.6X5	T47.6X6
Diphenylamine	T65.3X1	T65.3X2	T65.3X3	T65.3X4	—	—
Diphenylbutazone	T39.2X1	T39.2X2	T39.2X3	T39.2X4	T39.2X5	T39.2X6
Diphenylchloroarsine, not in war	T57.ØX1	T57.ØX2	T57.ØX3	T57.ØX4	—	—
Diphenylhydantoin	T42.ØX1	T42.ØX2	T42.ØX3	T42.ØX4	T42.ØX5	T42.ØX6
Diphenylmethane dye	T52.1X1	T52.1X2	T52.1X3	T52.1X4	—	—
Diphenylpyraline	T45.ØX1	T45.ØX2	T45.ØX3	T45.ØX4	T45.ØX5	T45.ØX6
Diphtheria						
antitoxin	T5Ø.Z11	T5Ø.Z12	T5Ø.Z13	T5Ø.Z14	T5Ø.Z15	T5Ø.Z16

Substance	Poisoning, Accidental (unintentional)	Poisoning, Intentional Self-harm	Poisoning, Assault	Poisoning, Undetermined	Adverse Effect	Under-dosing
Diphtheria — *continued*						
toxoid	T50.A91	T50.A92	T50.A93	T50.A94	T50.A95	T50.A96
with tetanus toxoid	T50.A21	T50.A22	T50.A23	T50.A24	T50.A25	T50.A26
with pertussis component	T50.A11	T50.A12	T50.A13	T50.A14	T50.A15	T50.A16
vaccine	T50.A91	T50.A92	T50.A93	T50.A94	T50.A95	T50.A96
combination						
without pertussis	T50.A21	T50.A22	T50.A23	T50.A24	T50.A25	T50.A26
including pertussis	T50.A11	T50.A12	T50.A13	T50.A14	T50.A15	T50.A16
Diphylline	T50.2X1	T50.2X2	T50.2X3	T50.2X4	T50.2X5	T50.2X6
Dipipanone	T40.491	T40.492	T40.493	T40.494	—	—
Dipivefrine	T49.5X1	T49.5X2	T49.5X3	T49.5X4	T49.5X5	T49.5X6
Diplovax	T50.B91	T50.B92	T50.B93	T50.B94	T50.B95	T50.B96
Diprophylline	T50.2X1	T50.2X2	T50.2X3	T50.2X4	T50.2X5	T50.2X6
Dipropyline	T48.291	T48.292	T48.293	T48.294	T48.295	T48.296
Dipyridamole	T46.3X1	T46.3X2	T46.3X3	T46.3X4	T46.3X5	T46.3X6
Dipyrone	T39.2X1	T39.2X2	T39.2X3	T39.2X4	T39.2X5	T39.2X6
Diquat (dibromide)	T60.3X1	T60.3X2	T60.3X3	T60.3X4	—	—
Disinfectant	T65.891	T65.892	T65.893	T65.894	—	—
alkaline	T54.3X1	T54.3X2	T54.3X3	T54.3X4	—	—
aromatic	T54.1X1	T54.1X2	T54.1X3	T54.1X4	—	—
intestinal	T37.8X1	T37.8X2	T37.8X3	T37.8X4	T37.8X5	T37.8X6
Disipal	T42.8X1	T42.8X2	T42.8X3	T42.8X4	T42.8X5	T42.8X6
Disodium edetate	T50.6X1	T50.6X2	T50.6X3	T50.6X4	T50.6X5	T50.6X6
Disoprofol	T41.291	T41.292	T41.293	T41.294	T41.295	T41.296
Disopyramide*	T46.2X1	T46.2X2	T46.2X3	T46.2X4	T46.2X5	T46.2X6
Distigmine (bromide)	T44.0X1	T44.0X2	T44.0X3	T44.0X4	T44.0X5	T44.0X6
Disulfamide	T50.2X1	T50.2X2	T50.2X3	T50.2X4	T50.2X5	T50.2X6
Disulfanilamide	T37.0X1	T37.0X2	T37.0X3	T37.0X4	T37.0X5	T37.0X6
Disulfiram	T50.6X1	T50.6X2	T50.6X3	T50.6X4	T50.6X5	T50.6X6
Disulfoton	T60.0X1	T60.0X2	T60.0X3	T60.0X4	—	—
Dithiazanine iodide	T37.4X1	T37.4X2	T37.4X3	T37.4X4	T37.4X5	T37.4X6
Dithiocarbamate	T60.0X1	T60.0X2	T60.0X3	T60.0X4	—	—
Dithranol	T49.4X1	T49.4X2	T49.4X3	T49.4X4	T49.4X5	T49.4X6
Diucardin	T50.2X1	T50.2X2	T50.2X3	T50.2X4	T50.2X5	T50.2X6
Diupres	T50.2X1	T50.2X2	T50.2X3	T50.2X4	T50.2X5	T50.2X6
Diuretic NEC	T50.2X1	T50.2X2	T50.2X3	T50.2X4	T50.2X5	T50.2X6
benzothiadiazine	T50.2X1	T50.2X2	T50.2X3	T50.2X4	T50.2X5	T50.2X6
carbonic acid anhydrase inhibitors	T50.2X1	T50.2X2	T50.2X3	T50.2X4	T50.2X5	T50.2X6
furfuryl NEC	T50.2X1	T50.2X2	T50.2X3	T50.2X4	T50.2X5	T50.2X6
loop (high-ceiling)	T50.1X1	T50.1X2	T50.1X3	T50.1X4	T50.1X5	T50.1X6
mercurial NEC	T50.2X1	T50.2X2	T50.2X3	T50.2X4	T50.2X5	T50.2X6
osmotic	T50.2X1	T50.2X2	T50.2X3	T50.2X4	T50.2X5	T50.2X6
purine NEC	T50.2X1	T50.2X2	T50.2X3	T50.2X4	T50.2X5	T50.2X6
saluretic NEC	T50.2X1	T50.2X2	T50.2X3	T50.2X4	T50.2X5	T50.2X6
sulfonamide	T50.2X1	T50.2X2	T50.2X3	T50.2X4	T50.2X5	T50.2X6
thiazide NEC	T50.2X1	T50.2X2	T50.2X3	T50.2X4	T50.2X5	T50.2X6
xanthine	T50.2X1	T50.2X2	T50.2X3	T50.2X4	T50.2X5	T50.2X6
Diurgin	T50.2X1	T50.2X2	T50.2X3	T50.2X4	T50.2X5	T50.2X6
Diuril	T50.2X1	T50.2X2	T50.2X3	T50.2X4	T50.2X5	T50.2X6
Diuron	T60.3X1	T60.3X2	T60.3X3	T60.3X4	—	—
Divalproex	T42.6X1	T42.6X2	T42.6X3	T42.6X4	T42.6X5	T42.6X6
Divinyl ether	T41.0X1	T41.0X2	T41.0X3	T41.0X4	T41.0X5	T41.0X6
Dixanthogen	T49.0X1	T49.0X2	T49.0X3	T49.0X4	T49.0X5	T49.0X6
Dixyrazine	T43.3X1	T43.3X2	T43.3X3	T43.3X4	T43.3X5	T43.3X6
D-lysergic acid diethylamide	T40.8X1	T40.8X2	T40.8X3	T40.8X4	—	—
DMCT	T36.4X1	T36.4X2	T36.4X3	T36.4X4	T36.4X5	T36.4X6
DMSO — *see* Dimethyl, sulfoxide						
DNBP	T60.3X1	T60.3X2	T60.3X3	T60.3X4	—	—
DNOC	T65.3X1	T65.3X2	T65.3X3	T65.3X4	—	—
Dobutamine	T44.5X1	T44.5X2	T44.5X3	T44.5X4	T44.5X5	T44.5X6
DOCA	T38.0X1	T38.0X2	T38.0X3	T38.0X4	T38.0X5	T38.0X6
Docusate sodium	T47.4X1	T47.4X2	T47.4X3	T47.4X4	T47.4X5	T47.4X6
Dodicin	T49.0X1	T49.0X2	T49.0X3	T49.0X4	T49.0X5	T49.0X6
Dofamium chloride	T49.0X1	T49.0X2	T49.0X3	T49.0X4	T49.0X5	T49.0X6
Dolophine	T40.3X1	T40.3X2	T40.3X3	T40.3X4	T40.3X5	T40.3X6
Doloxene	T39.8X1	T39.8X2	T39.8X3	T39.8X4	T39.8X5	T39.8X6
Domestic gas (after combustion) — *see* Gas, utility						
prior to combustion	T59.891	T59.892	T59.893	T59.894	—	—
Domiodol	T48.4X1	T48.4X2	T48.4X3	T48.4X4	T48.4X5	T48.4X6
Domiphen (bromide)	T49.0X1	T49.0X2	T49.0X3	T49.0X4	T49.0X5	T49.0X6
Domperidone	T45.0X1	T45.0X2	T45.0X3	T45.0X4	T45.0X5	T45.0X6
Donepezil*	T44.0X1	T44.0X2	T44.0X3	T44.0X4	T44.0X5	T44.0X6
Dopa	T42.8X1	T42.8X2	T42.8X3	T42.8X4	T42.8X5	T42.8X6
Dopamine	T44.991	T44.992	T44.993	T44.994	T44.995	T44.996
Doriden	T42.6X1	T42.6X2	T42.6X3	T42.6X4	T42.6X5	T42.6X6
Dormiral	T42.3X1	T42.3X2	T42.3X3	T42.3X4	T42.3X5	T42.3X6
Dormison	T42.6X1	T42.6X2	T42.6X3	T42.6X4	T42.6X5	T42.6X6
Dornase	T48.4X1	T48.4X2	T48.4X3	T48.4X4	T48.4X5	T48.4X6
Dorsacaine	T41.3X1	T41.3X2	T41.3X3	T41.3X4	T41.3X5	T41.3X6
Dosulepin	T43.011	T43.012	T43.013	T43.014	T43.015	T43.016
Dothiepin	T43.011	T43.012	T43.013	T43.014	T43.015	T43.016
Doxantrazole	T48.6X1	T48.6X2	T48.6X3	T48.6X4	T48.6X5	T48.6X6
Doxapram	T50.7X1	T50.7X2	T50.7X3	T50.7X4	T50.7X5	T50.7X6
Doxazosin	T44.6X1	T44.6X2	T44.6X3	T44.6X4	T44.6X5	T44.6X6
Doxepin	T43.011	T43.012	T43.013	T43.014	T43.015	T43.016
Doxifluridine	T45.1X1	T45.1X2	T45.1X3	T45.1X4	T45.1X5	T45.1X6
Doxil*	T45.1X1	T45.1X2	T45.1X3	T45.1X4	T45.1X5	T45.1X6
Doxorubicin	T45.1X1	T45.1X2	T45.1X3	T45.1X4	T45.1X5	T45.1X6
Doxycycline	T36.4X1	T36.4X2	T36.4X3	T36.4X4	T36.4X5	T36.4X6
Doxylamine	T45.0X1	T45.0X2	T45.0X3	T45.0X4	T45.0X5	T45.0X6
Dramamine	T45.0X1	T45.0X2	T45.0X3	T45.0X4	T45.0X5	T45.0X6
Drano (drain cleaner)	T54.3X1	T54.3X2	T54.3X3	T54.3X4	—	—
Dressing, live pulp	T49.7X1	T49.7X2	T49.7X3	T49.7X4	T49.7X5	T49.7X6
Drocode	T40.2X1	T40.2X2	T40.2X3	T40.2X4	T40.2X5	T40.2X6
Dromoran	T40.2X1	T40.2X2	T40.2X3	T40.2X4	T40.2X5	T40.2X6
Dromostanolone	T38.7X1	T38.7X2	T38.7X3	T38.7X4	T38.7X5	T38.7X6
Dronabinol	T40.711	T40.712	T40.713	T40.714	T40.715	T40.716
Droperidol	T43.591	T43.592	T43.593	T43.594	T43.595	T43.596
Dropropizine	T48.3X1	T48.3X2	T48.3X3	T48.3X4	T48.3X5	T48.3X6
Drostanolone	T38.7X1	T38.7X2	T38.7X3	T38.7X4	T38.7X5	T38.7X6
Drotaverine	T44.3X1	T44.3X2	T44.3X3	T44.3X4	T44.3X5	T44.3X6
Drotrecogin alfa	T45.511	T45.512	T45.513	T45.514	T45.515	T45.516
Drug NEC	T50.901	T50.902	T50.903	T50.904	T50.905	T50.906
specified NEC	T50.991	T50.992	T50.993	T50.994	T50.995	T50.996
DTIC	T45.1X1	T45.1X2	T45.1X3	T45.1X4	T45.1X5	T45.1X6
Duboisine	T44.3X1	T44.3X2	T44.3X3	T44.3X4	T44.3X5	T44.3X6
Dulcolax	T47.2X1	T47.2X2	T47.2X3	T47.2X4	T47.2X5	T47.2X6
Duponol (C) (EP)	T49.2X1	T49.2X2	T49.2X3	T49.2X4	T49.2X5	T49.2X6
Durabolin	T38.7X1	T38.7X2	T38.7X3	T38.7X4	T38.7X5	T38.7X6
Durezol*	T49.5X1	T49.5X2	T49.5X3	T49.5X4	T49.5X5	T49.5X6
Dyclone	T41.3X1	T41.3X2	T41.3X3	T41.3X4	T41.3X5	T41.3X6
Dyclonine	T41.3X1	T41.3X2	T41.3X3	T41.3X4	T41.3X5	T41.3X6
Dydrogesterone	T38.5X1	T38.5X2	T38.5X3	T38.5X4	T38.5X5	T38.5X6
Dye NEC	T65.6X1	T65.6X2	T65.6X3	T65.6X4	—	—
antiseptic	T49.0X1	T49.0X2	T49.0X3	T49.0X4	T49.0X5	T49.0X6
diagnostic agents	T50.8X1	T50.8X2	T50.8X3	T50.8X4	T50.8X5	T50.8X6
pharmaceutical NEC	T50.901	T50.902	T50.903	T50.904	T50.905	T50.906
Dyflos	T44.0X1	T44.0X2	T44.0X3	T44.0X4	T44.0X5	T44.0X6
Dymelor	T38.3X1	T38.3X2	T38.3X3	T38.3X4	T38.3X5	T38.3X6
Dynamite	T65.3X1	T65.3X2	T65.3X3	T65.3X4	—	—
fumes	T59.891	T59.892	T59.893	T59.894	—	—
Dyphylline	T44.3X1	T44.3X2	T44.3X3	T44.3X4	T44.3X5	T44.3X6
b-eucaine	T49.1X1	T49.1X2	T49.1X3	T49.1X4	T49.1X5	T49.1X6
Ear drug NEC	T49.6X1	T49.6X2	T49.6X3	T49.6X4	T49.6X5	T49.6X6
Ear preparations	T49.6X1	T49.6X2	T49.6X3	T49.6X4	T49.6X5	T49.6X6
Echothiophate, echothiopate, ecothiopate	T49.5X1	T49.5X2	T49.5X3	T49.5X4	T49.5X5	T49.5X6
Econazole	T49.0X1	T49.0X2	T49.0X3	T49.0X4	T49.0X5	T49.0X6
Ecothiopate iodide	T49.5X1	T49.5X2	T49.5X3	T49.5X4	T49.5X5	T49.5X6
Ecstasy	T43.641	T43.642	T43.643	T43.644	—	—
Ectylurea	T42.6X1	T42.6X2	T42.6X3	T42.6X4	T42.6X5	T42.6X6
Edathamil disodium	T45.8X1	T45.8X2	T45.8X3	T45.8X4	T45.8X5	T45.8X6
Edecrin	T50.1X1	T50.1X2	T50.1X3	T50.1X4	T50.1X5	T50.1X6
Edetate, disodium (calcium)	T45.8X1	T45.8X2	T45.8X3	T45.8X4	T45.8X5	T45.8X6
Edoxudine	T49.5X1	T49.5X2	T49.5X3	T49.5X4	T49.5X5	T49.5X6
Edrophonium	T44.0X1	T44.0X2	T44.0X3	T44.0X4	T44.0X5	T44.0X6
chloride	T44.0X1	T44.0X2	T44.0X3	T44.0X4	T44.0X5	T44.0X6
EDTA	T50.6X1	T50.6X2	T50.6X3	T50.6X4	T50.6X5	T50.6X6
Eflornithine	T37.2X1	T37.2X2	T37.2X3	T37.2X4	T37.2X5	T37.2X6
Efloxate	T46.3X1	T46.3X2	T46.3X3	T46.3X4	T46.3X5	T46.3X6
Elase	T49.8X1	T49.8X2	T49.8X3	T49.8X4	T49.8X5	T49.8X6
Elastase	T47.5X1	T47.5X2	T47.5X3	T47.5X4	T47.5X5	T47.5X6
Elaterium	T47.2X1	T47.2X2	T47.2X3	T47.2X4	T47.2X5	T47.2X6
Elcatonin	T50.991	T50.992	T50.993	T50.994	T50.995	T50.996
Elder	T62.2X1	T62.2X2	T62.2X3	T62.2X4	—	—
berry, (unripe)	T62.1X1	T62.1X2	T62.1X3	T62.1X4	—	—
Electrolyte balance drug	T50.3X1	T50.3X2	T50.3X3	T50.3X4	T50.3X5	T50.3X6
Electrolytes NEC	T50.3X1	T50.3X2	T50.3X3	T50.3X4	T50.3X5	T50.3X6
Electrolytic agent NEC	T50.3X1	T50.3X2	T50.3X3	T50.3X4	T50.3X5	T50.3X6
Elemental diet	T50.901	T50.902	T50.903	T50.904	T50.905	T50.906
Elliptinium acetate	T45.1X1	T45.1X2	T45.1X3	T45.1X4	T45.1X5	T45.1X6
Elocon*	T49.0X1	T49.0X2	T49.0X3	T49.0X4	T49.0X5	T49.0X6
Embramine	T45.0X1	T45.0X2	T45.0X3	T45.0X4	T45.0X5	T45.0X6
Emepronium (salts)	T44.3X1	T44.3X2	T44.3X3	T44.3X4	T44.3X5	T44.3X6
bromide	T44.3X1	T44.3X2	T44.3X3	T44.3X4	T44.3X5	T44.3X6
Emetic NEC	T47.7X1	T47.7X2	T47.7X3	T47.7X4	T47.7X5	T47.7X6
Emetine	T37.3X1	T37.3X2	T37.3X3	T37.3X4	T37.3X5	T37.3X6
Emollient NEC	T49.3X1	T49.3X2	T49.3X3	T49.3X4	T49.3X5	T49.3X6
Emorfazone	T39.8X1	T39.8X2	T39.8X3	T39.8X4	T39.8X5	T39.8X6
Emylcamate	T43.591	T43.592	T43.593	T43.594	T43.595	T43.596
Enalapril	T46.4X1	T46.4X2	T46.4X3	T46.4X4	T46.4X5	T46.4X6

☑ **Additional Character May Be Required — Refer to the Tabular List for Character Selection**

***Optum Value-Add**

Substance	Poisoning, Accidental (unintentional)	Poisoning, Intentional Self-harm	Poisoning, Assault	Poisoning, Undetermined	Adverse Effect	Under-dosing
Enalaprilat	T46.4X1	T46.4X2	T46.4X3	T46.4X4	T46.4X5	T46.4X6
Enbrel*	T39.4X1	T39.4X2	T39.4X3	T39.4X4	T39.4X5	T39.4X6
Encainide	T46.2X1	T46.2X2	T46.2X3	T46.2X4	T46.2X5	T46.2X6
Endocaine	T41.3X1	T41.3X2	T41.3X3	T41.3X4	T41.3X5	T41.3X6
Endosulfan	T60.2X1	T60.2X2	T60.2X3	T60.2X4	—	—
Endothall	T60.3X1	T60.3X2	T60.3X3	T60.3X4	—	—
Endralazine	T46.5X1	T46.5X2	T46.5X3	T46.5X4	T46.5X5	T46.5X6
Endrin	T60.1X1	T60.1X2	T60.1X3	T60.1X4	—	—
Enflurane	T41.0X1	T41.0X2	T41.0X3	T41.0X4	T41.0X5	T41.0X6
Enfuvirtide*	T37.5X1	T37.5X2	T37.5X3	T37.5X4	T37.5X5	T37.5X6
Enhexymal	T42.3X1	T42.3X2	T42.3X3	T42.3X4	T42.3X5	T42.3X6
Enocitabine	T45.1X1	T45.1X2	T45.1X3	T45.1X4	T45.1X5	T45.1X6
Enovid	T38.4X1	T38.4X2	T38.4X3	T38.4X4	T38.4X5	T38.4X6
Enoxacin	T36.8X1	T36.8X2	T36.8X3	T36.8X4	T36.8X5	T36.8X6
Enoxaparin (sodium)	T45.511	T45.512	T45.513	T45.514	T45.515	T45.516
Enpiprazole	T43.591	T43.592	T43.593	T43.594	T43.595	T43.596
Enprofylline	T48.6X1	T48.6X2	T48.6X3	T48.6X4	T48.6X5	T48.6X6
Enprostil	T47.1X1	T47.1X2	T47.1X3	T47.1X4	T47.1X5	T47.1X6
Enterogastrone	T38.891	T38.892	T38.893	T38.894	T38.895	T38.896
ENT preparations (anti-infectives)	T49.6X1	T49.6X2	T49.6X3	T49.6X4	T49.6X5	T49.6X6
Enviomycin	T36.8X1	T36.8X2	T36.8X3	T36.8X4	T36.8X5	T36.8X6
Enzodase	T45.3X1	T45.3X2	T45.3X3	T45.3X4	T45.3X5	T45.3X6
Enzyme NEC	T45.3X1	T45.3X2	T45.3X3	T45.3X4	T45.3X5	T45.3X6
depolymerizing	T49.8X1	T49.8X2	T49.8X3	T49.8X4	T49.8X5	T49.8X6
fibrolytic	T45.3X1	T45.3X2	T45.3X3	T45.3X4	T45.3X5	T45.3X6
gastric	T47.5X1	T47.5X2	T47.5X3	T47.5X4	T47.5X5	T47.5X6
intestinal	T47.5X1	T47.5X2	T47.5X3	T47.5X4	T47.5X5	T47.5X6
local action	T49.4X1	T49.4X2	T49.4X3	T49.4X4	T49.4X5	T49.4X6
proteolytic	T49.4X1	T49.4X2	T49.4X3	T49.4X4	T49.4X5	T49.4X6
thrombolytic	T45.3X1	T45.3X2	T45.3X3	T45.3X4	T45.3X5	T45.3X6
EPAB	T41.3X1	T41.3X2	T41.3X3	T41.3X4	T41.3X5	T41.3X6
Epanutin	T42.0X1	T42.0X2	T42.0X3	T42.0X4	T42.0X5	T42.0X6
Ephedra	T44.991	T44.992	T44.993	T44.994	T44.995	T44.996
Ephedrine	T44.991	T44.992	T44.993	T44.994	T44.995	T44.996
Epichlorhydrin, epichlorohydrin	T52.8X1	T52.8X2	T52.8X3	T52.8X4	—	—
Epicillin	T36.0X1	T36.0X2	T36.0X3	T36.0X4	T36.0X5	T36.0X6
Epiestriol	T38.5X1	T38.5X2	T38.5X3	T38.5X4	T38.5X5	T38.5X6
Epilim — *see* Sodium, valproate						
Epimestrol	T38.5X1	T38.5X2	T38.5X3	T38.5X4	T38.5X5	T38.5X6
Epinephrine	T44.5X1	T44.5X2	T44.5X3	T44.5X4	T44.5X5	T44.5X6
EpiPen*	T44.5X1	T44.5X2	T44.5X3	T44.5X4	T44.5X5	T44.5X6
Epirubicin	T45.1X1	T45.1X2	T45.1X3	T45.1X4	T45.1X5	T45.1X6
Epitiostanol	T38.7X1	T38.7X2	T38.7X3	T38.7X4	T38.7X5	T38.7X6
Epitizide	T50.2X1	T50.2X2	T50.2X3	T50.2X4	T50.2X5	T50.2X6
EPN	T60.0X1	T60.0X2	T60.0X3	T60.0X4	—	—
EPO	T45.8X1	T45.8X2	T45.8X3	T45.8X4	T45.8X5	T45.8X6
Epoetin alpha	T45.8X1	T45.8X2	T45.8X3	T45.8X4	T45.8X5	T45.8X6
Epomediol	T50.991	T50.992	T50.993	T50.994	T50.995	T50.996
Epoprostenol	T45.521	T45.522	T45.523	T45.524	T45.525	T45.526
Epoxy resin	T65.891	T65.892	T65.893	T65.894	—	—
Eprazinone	T48.4X1	T48.4X2	T48.4X3	T48.4X4	T48.4X5	T48.4X6
Epsilon aminocaproic acid	T45.621	T45.622	T45.623	T45.624	T45.625	T45.626
Epsom salt	T47.3X1	T47.3X2	T47.3X3	T47.3X4	T47.3X5	T47.3X6
Eptazocine	T40.491	T40.492	T40.493	T40.494	T40.495	T40.496
Equanil	T43.591	T43.592	T43.593	T43.594	T43.595	T43.596
Equisetum	T62.2X1	T62.2X2	T62.2X3	T62.2X4	—	—
diuretic	T50.2X1	T50.2X2	T50.2X3	T50.2X4	T50.2X5	T50.2X6
Ergobasine	T48.0X1	T48.0X2	T48.0X3	T48.0X4	T48.0X5	T48.0X6
Ergocalciferol	T45.2X1	T45.2X2	T45.2X3	T45.2X4	T45.2X5	T45.2X6
Ergoloid mesylates	T46.7X1	T46.7X2	T46.7X3	T46.7X4	T46.7X5	T46.7X6
Ergometrine	T48.0X1	T48.0X2	T48.0X3	T48.0X4	T48.0X5	T48.0X6
Ergonovine	T48.0X1	T48.0X2	T48.0X3	T48.0X4	T48.0X5	T48.0X6
Ergotamine	T46.5X1	T46.5X2	T46.5X3	T46.5X4	T46.5X5	T46.5X6
Ergotocine	T48.0X1	T48.0X2	T48.0X3	T48.0X4	T48.0X5	T48.0X6
Ergotrate	T48.0X1	T48.0X2	T48.0X3	T48.0X4	T48.0X5	T48.0X6
Ergot NEC	T64.81	T64.82	T64.83	T64.84	—	—
derivative	T48.0X1	T48.0X2	T48.0X3	T48.0X4	T48.0X5	T48.0X6
medicinal (alkaloids)	T48.0X1	T48.0X2	T48.0X3	T48.0X4	T48.0X5	T48.0X6
prepared	T48.0X1	T48.0X2	T48.0X3	T48.0X4	T48.0X5	T48.0X6
Eritrityl tetranitrate	T46.3X1	T46.3X2	T46.3X3	T46.3X4	T46.3X5	T46.3X6
Erythrityl tetranitrate	T46.3X1	T46.3X2	T46.3X3	T46.3X4	T46.3X5	T46.3X6
Erythrol tetranitrate	T46.3X1	T46.3X2	T46.3X3	T46.3X4	T46.3X5	T46.3X6
Erythromycin (salts)	T36.3X1	T36.3X2	T36.3X3	T36.3X4	T36.3X5	T36.3X6
ophthalmic preparation	T49.5X1	T49.5X2	T49.5X3	T49.5X4	T49.5X5	T49.5X6
topical NEC	T49.0X1	T49.0X2	T49.0X3	T49.0X4	T49.0X5	T49.0X6
Erythropoietin	T45.8X1	T45.8X2	T45.8X3	T45.8X4	T45.8X5	T45.8X6
human	T45.8X1	T45.8X2	T45.8X3	T45.8X4	T45.8X5	T45.8X6
Esbriet*	T48.991	T48.992	T48.993	T48.994	T48.995	T48.996
Escin	T46.991	T46.992	T46.993	T46.994	T46.995	T46.996
Esculin	T45.2X1	T45.2X2	T45.2X3	T45.2X4	T45.2X5	T45.2X6
Esculoside	T45.2X1	T45.2X2	T45.2X3	T45.2X4	T45.2X5	T45.2X6
ESDT (ether-soluble tar distillate)	T49.1X1	T49.1X2	T49.1X3	T49.1X4	T49.1X5	T49.1X6
Eserine	T49.5X1	T49.5X2	T49.5X3	T49.5X4	T49.5X5	T49.5X6
Esflurbiprofen	T39.311	T39.312	T39.313	T39.314	T39.315	T39.316
Eskabarb	T42.3X1	T42.3X2	T42.3X3	T42.3X4	T42.3X5	T42.3X6
Eskalith	T43.8X1	T43.8X2	T43.8X3	T43.8X4	T43.8X5	T43.8X6
Esmolol	T44.7X1	T44.7X2	T44.7X3	T44.7X4	T44.7X5	T44.7X6
Estanozolol	T38.7X1	T38.7X2	T38.7X3	T38.7X4	T38.7X5	T38.7X6
Estazolam	T42.4X1	T42.4X2	T42.4X3	T42.4X4	T42.4X5	T42.4X6
Estradiol	T38.5X1	T38.5X2	T38.5X3	T38.5X4	T38.5X5	T38.5X6
with testosterone	T38.7X1	T38.7X2	T38.7X3	T38.7X4	T38.7X5	T38.7X6
benzoate	T38.5X1	T38.5X2	T38.5X3	T38.5X4	T38.5X5	T38.5X6
Estramustine	T45.1X1	T45.1X2	T45.1X3	T45.1X4	T45.1X5	T45.1X6
Estriol	T38.5X1	T38.5X2	T38.5X3	T38.5X4	T38.5X5	T38.5X6
Estrogen	T38.5X1	T38.5X2	T38.5X3	T38.5X4	T38.5X5	T38.5X6
with progesterone	T38.5X1	T38.5X2	T38.5X3	T38.5X4	T38.5X5	T38.5X6
conjugated	T38.5X1	T38.5X2	T38.5X3	T38.5X4	T38.5X5	T38.5X6
Estrone	T38.5X1	T38.5X2	T38.5X3	T38.5X4	T38.5X5	T38.5X6
Estropipate	T38.5X1	T38.5X2	T38.5X3	T38.5X4	T38.5X5	T38.5X6
Etacrynate sodium	T50.1X1	T50.1X2	T50.1X3	T50.1X4	T50.1X5	T50.1X6
Etacrynic acid	T50.1X1	T50.1X2	T50.1X3	T50.1X4	T50.1X5	T50.1X6
Etafedrine	T48.6X1	T48.6X2	T48.6X3	T48.6X4	T48.6X5	T48.6X6
Etafenone	T46.3X1	T46.3X2	T46.3X3	T46.3X4	T46.3X5	T46.3X6
Etambutol	T37.1X1	T37.1X2	T37.1X3	T37.1X4	T37.1X5	T37.1X6
Etamiphyllin	T48.6X1	T48.6X2	T48.6X3	T48.6X4	T48.6X5	T48.6X6
Etamivan	T50.7X1	T50.7X2	T50.7X3	T50.7X4	T50.7X5	T50.7X6
Etamsylate	T45.7X1	T45.7X2	T45.7X3	T45.7X4	T45.7X5	T45.7X6
Etebenecid	T50.4X1	T50.4X2	T50.4X3	T50.4X4	T50.4X5	T50.4X6
Ethacridine	T49.0X1	T49.0X2	T49.0X3	T49.0X4	T49.0X5	T49.0X6
Ethacrynate*	T50.1X1	T50.1X2	T50.1X3	T50.1X4	T50.1X5	T50.1X6
Ethacrynic acid	T50.1X1	T50.1X2	T50.1X3	T50.1X4	T50.1X5	T50.1X6
Ethadione	T42.2X1	T42.2X2	T42.2X3	T42.2X4	T42.2X5	T42.2X6
Ethambutol	T37.1X1	T37.1X2	T37.1X3	T37.1X4	T37.1X5	T37.1X6
Ethamide	T50.2X1	T50.2X2	T50.2X3	T50.2X4	T50.2X5	T50.2X6
Ethamivan	T50.7X1	T50.7X2	T50.7X3	T50.7X4	T50.7X5	T50.7X6
Ethamsylate	T45.7X1	T45.7X2	T45.7X3	T45.7X4	T45.7X5	T45.7X6
Ethanol	T51.0X1	T51.0X2	T51.0X3	T51.0X4	—	—
beverage	T51.0X1	T51.0X2	T51.0X3	T51.0X4	—	—
Ethanolamine oleate	T46.8X1	T46.8X2	T46.8X3	T46.8X4	T46.8X5	T46.8X6
Ethaverine	T44.3X1	T44.3X2	T44.3X3	T44.3X4	T44.3X5	T44.3X6
Ethchlorvynol	T42.6X1	T42.6X2	T42.6X3	T42.6X4	T42.6X5	T42.6X6
Ethebenecid	T50.4X1	T50.4X2	T50.4X3	T50.4X4	T50.4X5	T50.4X6
Ether (vapor)	T41.0X1	T41.0X2	T41.0X3	T41.0X4	T41.0X5	T41.0X6
anesthetic	T41.0X1	T41.0X2	T41.0X3	T41.0X4	T41.0X5	T41.0X6
divinyl	T41.0X1	T41.0X2	T41.0X3	T41.0X4	T41.0X5	T41.0X6
ethyl (medicinal)	T41.0X1	T41.0X2	T41.0X3	T41.0X4	T41.0X5	T41.0X6
nonmedicinal	T52.8X1	T52.8X2	T52.8X3	T52.8X4	—	—
petroleum — *see* Ligroin						
solvent	T52.8X1	T52.8X2	T52.8X3	T52.8X4	—	—
Ethiazide	T50.2X1	T50.2X2	T50.2X3	T50.2X4	T50.2X5	T50.2X6
Ethidium chloride (vapor)	T59.891	T59.892	T59.893	T59.894	—	—
Ethinamate	T42.6X1	T42.6X2	T42.6X3	T42.6X4	T42.6X5	T42.6X6
Ethinylestradiol, ethinyloestradiol	T38.5X1	T38.5X2	T38.5X3	T38.5X4	T38.5X5	T38.5X6
with						
levonorgestrel	T38.4X1	T38.4X2	T38.4X3	T38.4X4	T38.4X5	T38.4X6
norethisterone	T38.4X1	T38.4X2	T38.4X3	T38.4X4	T38.4X5	T38.4X6
Ethiodized oil (131 I)	T50.8X1	T50.8X2	T50.8X3	T50.8X4	T50.8X5	T50.8X6
Ethiofos*	T50.991	T50.992	T50.993	T50.994	T50.995	T50.996
Ethion	T60.0X1	T60.0X2	T60.0X3	T60.0X4	—	—
Ethionamide	T37.1X1	T37.1X2	T37.1X3	T37.1X4	T37.1X5	T37.1X6
Ethioniamide	T37.1X1	T37.1X2	T37.1X3	T37.1X4	T37.1X5	T37.1X6
Ethisterone	T38.5X1	T38.5X2	T38.5X3	T38.5X4	T38.5X5	T38.5X6
Ethobral	T42.3X1	T42.3X2	T42.3X3	T42.3X4	T42.3X5	T42.3X6
Ethocaine (infiltration) (topical)	T41.3X1	T41.3X2	T41.3X3	T41.3X4	T41.3X5	T41.3X6
nerve block (peripheral) (plexus)	T41.3X1	T41.3X2	T41.3X3	T41.3X4	T41.3X5	T41.3X6
spinal	T41.3X1	T41.3X2	T41.3X3	T41.3X4	T41.3X5	T41.3X6
Ethoheptazine	T40.491	T40.492	T40.493	T40.494	T40.495	T40.496
Ethopropazine	T44.3X1	T44.3X2	T44.3X3	T44.3X4	T44.3X5	T44.3X6
Ethosuximide	T42.2X1	T42.2X2	T42.2X3	T42.2X4	T42.2X5	T42.2X6
Ethotoin	T42.0X1	T42.0X2	T42.0X3	T42.0X4	T42.0X5	T42.0X6
Ethoxazene	T37.91	T37.92	T37.93	T37.94	T37.95	T37.96
Ethoxazorutoside	T46.991	T46.992	T46.993	T46.994	T46.995	T46.996
Ethoxzolamide	T50.2X1	T50.2X2	T50.2X3	T50.2X4	T50.2X5	T50.2X6
Ethyl						
acetate	T52.8X1	T52.8X2	T52.8X3	T52.8X4	—	—
alcohol	T51.0X1	T51.0X2	T51.0X3	T51.0X4	—	—
beverage	T51.0X1	T51.0X2	T51.0X3	T51.0X4	—	—
aldehyde (vapor)	T59.891	T59.892	T59.893	T59.894	—	—
liquid	T52.8X1	T52.8X2	T52.8X3	T52.8X4	—	—
aminobenzoate	T41.3X1	T41.3X2	T41.3X3	T41.3X4	T41.3X5	T41.3X6

Substance	Poisoning, Accidental (unintentional)	Poisoning, Intentional Self-harm	Poisoning, Assault	Poisoning, Undetermined	Adverse Effect	Under-dosing
Ethyl — *continued*						
aminophenothiazine	T43.3X1	T43.3X2	T43.3X3	T43.3X4	T43.3X5	T43.3X6
benzoate	T52.8X1	T52.8X2	T52.8X3	T52.8X4	—	—
biscoumacetate	T45.511	T45.512	T45.513	T45.514	T45.515	T45.516
bromide (anesthetic)	T41.0X1	T41.0X2	T41.0X3	T41.0X4	T41.0X5	T41.0X6
carbamate	T45.1X1	T45.1X2	T45.1X3	T45.1X4	T45.1X5	T45.1X6
carbinol	T51.3X1	T51.3X2	T51.3X3	T51.3X4	—	—
carbonate	T52.8X1	T52.8X2	T52.8X3	T52.8X4	—	—
chaulmoograte	T37.1X1	T37.1X2	T37.1X3	T37.1X4	T37.1X5	T37.1X6
chloride (anesthetic)	T41.0X1	T41.0X2	T41.0X3	T41.0X4	T41.0X5	T41.0X6
anesthetic (local)	T41.3X1	T41.3X2	T41.3X3	T41.3X4	T41.3X5	T41.3X6
inhaled	T41.0X1	T41.0X2	T41.0X3	T41.0X4	T41.0X5	T41.0X6
local	T49.4X1	T49.4X2	T49.4X3	T49.4X4	T49.4X5	T49.4X6
solvent	T53.6X1	T53.6X2	T53.6X3	T53.6X4	—	—
dibunate	T48.3X1	T48.3X2	T48.3X3	T48.3X4	T48.3X5	T48.3X6
dichloroarsine (vapor)	T57.0X1	T57.0X2	T57.0X3	T57.0X4	—	—
estranol	T38.7X1	T38.7X2	T38.7X3	T38.7X4	T38.7X5	T38.7X6
ether — *see also* ether	T52.8X1	T52.8X2	T52.8X3	T52.8X4	—	—
formate NEC (solvent)	T52.0X1	T52.0X2	T52.0X3	T52.0X4	—	—
fumarate	T49.4X1	T49.4X2	T49.4X3	T49.4X4	T49.4X5	T49.4X6
hydroxyisobutyrate NEC (solvent)	T52.8X1	T52.8X2	T52.8X3	T52.8X4	—	—
iodoacetate	T59.3X1	T59.3X2	T59.3X3	T59.3X4	—	—
lactate NEC (solvent)	T52.8X1	T52.8X2	T52.8X3	T52.8X4	—	—
loflazepate	T42.4X1	T42.4X2	T42.4X3	T42.4X4	T42.4X5	T42.4X6
mercuric chloride	T56.1X1	T56.1X2	T56.1X3	T56.1X4	—	—
methylcarbinol	T51.8X1	T51.8X2	T51.8X3	T51.8X4	—	—
morphine	T40.2X1	T40.2X2	T40.2X3	T40.2X4	T40.2X5	T40.2X6
noradrenaline	T48.6X1	T48.6X2	T48.6X3	T48.6X4	T48.6X5	T48.6X6
oxybutyrate NEC (solvent)	T52.8X1	T52.8X2	T52.8X3	T52.8X4	—	—
Ethylene (gas)	T59.891	T59.892	T59.893	T59.894	—	—
anesthetic (general)	T41.0X1	T41.0X2	T41.0X3	T41.0X4	T41.0X5	T41.0X6
chlorohydrin	T52.8X1	T52.8X2	T52.8X3	T52.8X4	—	—
vapor	T53.6X1	T53.6X2	T53.6X3	T53.6X4	—	—
dichloride	T52.8X1	T52.8X2	T52.8X3	T52.8X4	—	—
vapor	T53.6X1	T53.6X2	T53.6X3	T53.6X4	—	—
dinitrate	T52.3X1	T52.3X2	T52.3X3	T52.3X4	—	—
glycol(s)	T52.8X1	T52.8X2	T52.8X3	T52.8X4	—	—
dinitrate	T52.3X1	T52.3X2	T52.3X3	T52.3X4	—	—
monobutyl ether	T52.3X1	T52.3X2	T52.3X3	T52.3X4	—	—
imine	T54.1X1	T54.1X2	T54.1X3	T54.1X4	—	—
oxide (fumigant) (nonmedicinal)	T59.891	T59.892	T59.893	T59.894	—	—
medicinal	T49.0X1	T49.0X2	T49.0X3	T49.0X4	T49.0X5	T49.0X6
Ethylenediaminetetra-acetic acid	T50.6X1	T50.6X2	T50.6X3	T50.6X4	T50.6X5	T50.6X6
Ethylenediamine theophylline	T48.6X1	T48.6X2	T48.6X3	T48.6X4	T48.6X5	T48.6X6
Ethylenedinitrilotetra-acetate	T50.6X1	T50.6X2	T50.6X3	T50.6X4	T50.6X5	T50.6X6
Ethylestrenol	T38.7X1	T38.7X2	T38.7X3	T38.7X4	T38.7X5	T38.7X6
Ethylhydroxycellulose	T47.4X1	T47.4X2	T47.4X3	T47.4X4	T47.4X5	T47.4X6
Ethylidene						
chloride NEC	T53.6X1	T53.6X2	T53.6X3	T53.6X4	—	—
diacetate	T60.3X1	T60.3X2	T60.3X3	T60.3X4	—	—
dicoumarin	T45.511	T45.512	T45.513	T45.514	T45.515	T45.516
dicoumarol	T45.511	T45.512	T45.513	T45.514	T45.515	T45.516
diethyl ether	T52.0X1	T52.0X2	T52.0X3	T52.0X4	—	—
Ethylmorphine	T40.2X1	T40.2X2	T40.2X3	T40.2X4	T40.2X5	T40.2X6
Ethylnorepinephrine	T48.6X1	T48.6X2	T48.6X3	T48.6X4	T48.6X5	T48.6X6
Ethylparachlorophen-oxyisobutyrate	T46.6X1	T46.6X2	T46.6X3	T46.6X4	T46.6X5	T46.6X6
Ethynodiol	T38.4X1	T38.4X2	T38.4X3	T38.4X4	T38.4X5	T38.4X6
with mestranol diacetate	T38.4X1	T38.4X2	T38.4X3	T38.4X4	T38.4X5	T38.4X6
Ethyol*	T50.991	T50.992	T50.993	T50.994	T50.995	T50.996
Etidocaine	T41.3X1	T41.3X2	T41.3X3	T41.3X4	T41.3X5	T41.3X6
infiltration (subcutaneous)	T41.3X1	T41.3X2	T41.3X3	T41.3X4	T41.3X5	T41.3X6
nerve (peripheral) (plexus)	T41.3X1	T41.3X2	T41.3X3	T41.3X4	T41.3X5	T41.3X6
Etidronate	T50.991	T50.992	T50.993	T50.994	T50.995	T50.996
Etidronic acid (disodium salt)	T50.991	T50.992	T50.993	T50.994	T50.995	T50.996
Etifoxine	T42.6X1	T42.6X2	T42.6X3	T42.6X4	T42.6X5	T42.6X6
Etilefrine	T44.4X1	T44.4X2	T44.4X3	T44.4X4	T44.4X5	T44.4X6
Etilfen	T42.3X1	T42.3X2	T42.3X3	T42.3X4	T42.3X5	T42.3X6
Etinodiol	T38.4X1	T38.4X2	T38.4X3	T38.4X4	T38.4X5	T38.4X6
Etiroxate	T46.6X1	T46.6X2	T46.6X3	T46.6X4	T46.6X5	T46.6X6
Etizolam	T42.4X1	T42.4X2	T42.4X3	T42.4X4	T42.4X5	T42.4X6
Etodolac	T39.391	T39.392	T39.393	T39.394	T39.395	T39.396
Etofamide	T37.3X1	T37.3X2	T37.3X3	T37.3X4	T37.3X5	T37.3X6
Etofibrate	T46.6X1	T46.6X2	T46.6X3	T46.6X4	T46.6X5	T46.6X6
Etofylline	T46.7X1	T46.7X2	T46.7X3	T46.7X4	T46.7X5	T46.7X6
clofibrate	T46.6X1	T46.6X2	T46.6X3	T46.6X4	T46.6X5	T46.6X6
Etoglucid	T45.1X1	T45.1X2	T45.1X3	T45.1X4	T45.1X5	T45.1X6
Etomidate	T41.1X1	T41.1X2	T41.1X3	T41.1X4	T41.1X5	T41.1X6

Substance	Poisoning, Accidental (unintentional)	Poisoning, Intentional Self-harm	Poisoning, Assault	Poisoning, Undetermined	Adverse Effect	Under-dosing
Etomide	T39.8X1	T39.8X2	T39.8X3	T39.8X4	T39.8X5	T39.8X6
Etomidoline	T44.3X1	T44.3X2	T44.3X3	T44.3X4	T44.3X5	T44.3X6
Etoposide	T45.1X1	T45.1X2	T45.1X3	T45.1X4	T45.1X5	T45.1X6
Etorphine	T40.2X1	T40.2X2	T40.2X3	T40.2X4	T40.2X5	T40.2X6
Etoval	T42.3X1	T42.3X2	T42.3X3	T42.3X4	T42.3X5	T42.3X6
Etozolin	T50.1X1	T50.1X2	T50.1X3	T50.1X4	T50.1X5	T50.1X6
Etravirine*	T37.5X1	T37.5X2	T37.5X3	T37.5X4	T37.5X5	T37.5X6
Etretinate	T50.991	T50.992	T50.993	T50.994	T50.995	T50.996
Etryptamine	T43.691	T43.692	T43.693	T43.694	T43.695	T43.696
Etybenzatropine	T44.3X1	T44.3X2	T44.3X3	T44.3X4	T44.3X5	T44.3X6
Etynodiol	T38.4X1	T38.4X2	T38.4X3	T38.4X4	T38.4X5	T38.4X6
Eucaine	T41.3X1	T41.3X2	T41.3X3	T41.3X4	T41.3X5	T41.3X6
Eucalyptus oil	T49.7X1	T49.7X2	T49.7X3	T49.7X4	T49.7X5	T49.7X6
Eucatropine	T49.5X1	T49.5X2	T49.5X3	T49.5X4	T49.5X5	T49.5X6
Eucodal	T40.2X1	T40.2X2	T40.2X3	T40.2X4	T40.2X5	T40.2X6
Euneryl	T42.3X1	T42.3X2	T42.3X3	T42.3X4	T42.3X5	T42.3X6
Euphthalmine	T44.3X1	T44.3X2	T44.3X3	T44.3X4	T44.3X5	T44.3X6
Eurax	T49.0X1	T49.0X2	T49.0X3	T49.0X4	T49.0X5	T49.0X6
Euresol	T49.4X1	T49.4X2	T49.4X3	T49.4X4	T49.4X5	T49.4X6
Euthroid	T38.1X1	T38.1X2	T38.1X3	T38.1X4	T38.1X5	T38.1X6
Evans blue	T50.8X1	T50.8X2	T50.8X3	T50.8X4	T50.8X5	T50.8X6
Evipal	T42.3X1	T42.3X2	T42.3X3	T42.3X4	T42.3X5	T42.3X6
sodium	T41.1X1	T41.1X2	T41.1X3	T41.1X4	T41.1X5	T41.1X6
Evipan	T42.3X1	T42.3X2	T42.3X3	T42.3X4	T42.3X5	T42.3X6
sodium	T41.1X1	T41.1X2	T41.1X3	T41.1X4	T41.1X5	T41.1X6
Exalamide	T49.0X1	T49.0X2	T49.0X3	T49.0X4	T49.0X5	T49.0X6
Exalgin	T39.1X1	T39.1X2	T39.1X3	T39.1X4	T39.1X5	T39.1X6
Excipients, pharmaceutical	T50.901	T50.902	T50.903	T50.904	T50.905	T50.906
Exhaust gas (engine) (motor vehicle)	T58.01	T58.02	T58.03	T58.04	—	—
Ex-Lax (phenolphthalein)	T47.2X1	T47.2X2	T47.2X3	T47.2X4	T47.2X5	T47.2X6
Expectorant NEC	T48.4X1	T48.4X2	T48.4X3	T48.4X4	T48.4X5	T48.4X6
Extended insulin zinc suspension	T38.3X1	T38.3X2	T38.3X3	T38.3X4	T38.3X5	T38.3X6
External medications (skin) (mucous membrane)	T49.91	T49.92	T49.93	T49.94	T49.95	T49.96
dental agent	T49.7X1	T49.7X2	T49.7X3	T49.7X4	T49.7X5	T49.7X6
ENT agent	T49.6X1	T49.6X2	T49.6X3	T49.6X4	T49.6X5	T49.6X6
ophthalmic preparation	T49.5X1	T49.5X2	T49.5X3	T49.5X4	T49.5X5	T49.5X6
specified NEC	T49.8X1	T49.8X2	T49.8X3	T49.8X4	T49.8X5	T49.8X6
Extina*	T49.0X1	T49.0X2	T49.0X3	T49.0X4	T49.0X5	T49.0X6
Extrapyramidal antagonist NEC	T44.3X1	T44.3X2	T44.3X3	T44.3X4	T44.3X5	T44.3X6
Eye agents (anti-infective)	T49.5X1	T49.5X2	T49.5X3	T49.5X4	T49.5X5	T49.5X6
Eye drug NEC	T49.5X1	T49.5X2	T49.5X3	T49.5X4	T49.5X5	T49.5X6
FAC (fluorouracil + doxorubicin + cyclophosphamide)	T45.1X1	T45.1X2	T45.1X3	T45.1X4	T45.1X5	T45.1X6
Factor						
I (fibrinogen)	T45.8X1	T45.8X2	T45.8X3	T45.8X4	T45.8X5	T45.8X6
III (thromboplastin)	T45.8X1	T45.8X2	T45.8X3	T45.8X4	T45.8X5	T45.8X6
IX complex	T45.7X1	T45.7X2	T45.7X3	T45.7X4	T45.7X5	T45.7X6
human	T45.8X1	T45.8X2	T45.8X3	T45.8X4	T45.8X5	T45.8X6
VIII (antihemophilic Factor) (concentrate)	T45.8X1	T45.8X2	T45.8X3	T45.8X4	T45.8X5	T45.8X6
Famotidine	T47.0X1	T47.0X2	T47.0X3	T47.0X4	T47.0X5	T47.0X6
Fat suspension, intravenous	T50.991	T50.992	T50.993	T50.994	T50.995	T50.996
Fazadinium bromide	T48.1X1	T48.1X2	T48.1X3	T48.1X4	T48.1X5	T48.1X6
Febarbamate	T42.3X1	T42.3X2	T42.3X3	T42.3X4	T42.3X5	T42.3X6
Fecal softener	T47.4X1	T47.4X2	T47.4X3	T47.4X4	T47.4X5	T47.4X6
Fedrilate	T48.3X1	T48.3X2	T48.3X3	T48.3X4	T48.3X5	T48.3X6
Felodipine	T46.1X1	T46.1X2	T46.1X3	T46.1X4	T46.1X5	T46.1X6
Felypressin	T38.891	T38.892	T38.893	T38.894	T38.895	T38.896
Femizol*	T49.0X1	T49.0X2	T49.0X3	T49.0X4	T49.0X5	T49.0X6
Femoxetine	T43.221	T43.222	T43.223	T43.224	T43.225	T43.226
Fenalcomine	T46.3X1	T46.3X2	T46.3X3	T46.3X4	T46.3X5	T46.3X6
Fenamisal	T37.1X1	T37.1X2	T37.1X3	T37.1X4	T37.1X5	T37.1X6
Fenazone	T39.2X1	T39.2X2	T39.2X3	T39.2X4	T39.2X5	T39.2X6
Fenbendazole	T37.4X1	T37.4X2	T37.4X3	T37.4X4	T37.4X5	T37.4X6
Fenbutrazate	T50.5X1	T50.5X2	T50.5X3	T50.5X4	T50.5X5	T50.5X6
Fencamfamine	T43.691	T43.692	T43.693	T43.694	T43.695	T43.696
Fendiline	T46.1X1	T46.1X2	T46.1X3	T46.1X4	T46.1X5	T46.1X6
Fenetylline	T43.691	T43.692	T43.693	T43.694	T43.695	T43.696
Fenflumizole	T39.391	T39.392	T39.393	T39.394	T39.395	T39.396
Fenfluramine	T50.5X1	T50.5X2	T50.5X3	T50.5X4	T50.5X5	T50.5X6
Fenobarbital	T42.3X1	T42.3X2	T42.3X3	T42.3X4	T42.3X5	T42.3X6
Fenofibrate	T46.6X1	T46.6X2	T46.6X3	T46.6X4	T46.6X5	T46.6X6
Fenoprofen	T39.311	T39.312	T39.313	T39.314	T39.315	T39.316
Fenoterol	T48.6X1	T48.6X2	T48.6X3	T48.6X4	T48.6X5	T48.6X6
Fenoverine	T44.3X1	T44.3X2	T44.3X3	T44.3X4	T44.3X5	T44.3X6
Fenoxazoline	T48.5X1	T48.5X2	T48.5X3	T48.5X4	T48.5X5	T48.5X6
Fenproporex	T50.5X1	T50.5X2	T50.5X3	T50.5X4	T50.5X5	T50.5X6

Substance	Poisoning, Accidental (unintentional)	Poisoning, Intentional Self-harm	Poisoning, Assault	Poisoning, Undetermined	Adverse Effect	Under-dosing
Fenquizone	T5Ø.2X1	T5Ø.2X2	T5Ø.2X3	T5Ø.2X4	T5Ø.2X5	T5Ø.2X6
Fentanyl (analogs)	T4Ø.411	T4Ø.412	T4Ø.413	T4Ø.414	T4Ø.415	T4Ø.416
Fentazin	T43.3X1	T43.3X2	T43.3X3	T43.3X4	T43.3X5	T43.3X6
Fenthion	T6Ø.ØX1	T6Ø.ØX2	T6Ø.ØX3	T6Ø.ØX4	—	—
Fenticlor	T49.ØX1	T49.ØX2	T49.ØX3	T49.ØX4	T49.ØX5	T49.ØX6
Fenylbutazone	T39.2X1	T39.2X2	T39.2X3	T39.2X4	T39.2X5	T39.2X6
Feprazone	T39.2X1	T39.2X2	T39.2X3	T39.2X4	T39.2X5	T39.2X6
Fer de lance (bite) (venom)	T63.Ø61	T63.Ø62	T63.Ø63	T63.Ø64	—	—
Ferrex*	T45.4X1	T45.4X2	T45.4X3	T45.4X4	T45.4X5	T45.4X6
Ferric — *see also* Iron						
chloride	T45.4X1	T45.4X2	T45.4X3	T45.4X4	T45.4X5	T45.4X6
citrate	T45.4X1	T45.4X2	T45.4X3	T45.4X4	T45.4X5	T45.4X6
hydroxide						
colloidal	T45.4X1	T45.4X2	T45.4X3	T45.4X4	T45.4X5	T45.4X6
polymaltose	T45.4X1	T45.4X2	T45.4X3	T45.4X4	T45.4X5	T45.4X6
pyrophosphate	T45.4X1	T45.4X2	T45.4X3	T45.4X4	T45.4X5	T45.4X6
Ferritin	T45.4X1	T45.4X2	T45.4X3	T45.4X4	T45.4X5	T45.4X6
Ferrocholinate	T45.4X1	T45.4X2	T45.4X3	T45.4X4	T45.4X5	T45.4X6
Ferrodextrane	T45.4X1	T45.4X2	T45.4X3	T45.4X4	T45.4X5	T45.4X6
Ferropolimaler	T45.4X1	T45.4X2	T45.4X3	T45.4X4	T45.4X5	T45.4X6
Ferrous — *see also* Iron						
phosphate	T45.4X1	T45.4X2	T45.4X3	T45.4X4	T45.4X5	T45.4X6
salt	T45.4X1	T45.4X2	T45.4X3	T45.4X4	T45.4X5	T45.4X6
with folic acid	T45.4X1	T45.4X2	T45.4X3	T45.4X4	T45.4X5	T45.4X6
Ferrous fumerate, gluconate, lactate, salt NEC, sulfate (medicinal)	T45.4X1	T45.4X2	T45.4X3	T45.4X4	T45.4X5	T45.4X6
Ferrovanadium (fumes)	T59.891	T59.892	T59.893	T59.894	—	—
Ferrum — *see* Iron						
Fertilizers NEC	T65.891	T65.892	T65.893	T65.894	—	—
with herbicide mixture	T6Ø.3X1	T6Ø.3X2	T6Ø.3X3	T6Ø.3X4	—	—
Fetoxilate	T47.6X1	T47.6X2	T47.6X3	T47.6X4	T47.6X5	T47.6X6
Fiber, dietary	T47.4X1	T47.4X2	T47.4X3	T47.4X4	T47.4X5	T47.4X6
Fiberglass	T65.831	T65.832	T65.833	T65.834	—	—
Fibrinogen (human)	T45.8X1	T45.8X2	T45.8X3	T45.8X4	T45.8X5	T45.8X6
Fibrinolysin (human)	T45.691	T45.692	T45.693	T45.694	T45.695	T45.696
Fibrinolysis						
affecting drug	T45.6Ø1	T45.6Ø2	T45.6Ø3	T45.6Ø4	T45.6Ø5	T45.6Ø6
inhibitor NEC	T45.621	T45.622	T45.623	T45.624	T45.625	T45.626
Fibrinolytic drug	T45.611	T45.612	T45.613	T45.614	T45.615	T45.616
Filix mas	T37.4X1	T37.4X2	T37.4X3	T37.4X4	T37.4X5	T37.4X6
Filtering cream	T49.3X1	T49.3X2	T49.3X3	T49.3X4	T49.3X5	T49.3X6
Finacea*	T49.ØX1	T49.ØX2	T49.ØX3	T49.ØX4	T49.ØX5	T49.ØX6
Fiorinal	T39.Ø11	T39.Ø12	T39.Ø13	T39.Ø14	T39.Ø15	T39.Ø16
Firedamp	T59.891	T59.892	T59.893	T59.894	—	—
Fish, noxious, nonbacterial						
ciguatera	T61.Ø1	T61.Ø2	T61.Ø3	T61.Ø4	—	—
scombroid	T61.11	T61.12	T61.13	T61.14	—	—
shell	T61.781	T61.782	T61.783	T61.784	—	—
specified NEC	T61.771	T61.772	T61.773	T61.774	—	—
Flagyl	T37.3X1	T37.3X2	T37.3X3	T37.3X4	T37.3X5	T37.3X6
Flavine adenine dinucleotide	T45.2X1	T45.2X2	T45.2X3	T45.2X4	T45.2X5	T45.2X6
Flavodic acid	T46.991	T46.992	T46.993	T46.994	T46.995	T46.996
Flavoxate	T44.3X1	T44.3X2	T44.3X3	T44.3X4	T44.3X5	T44.3X6
Flaxedil	T48.1X1	T48.1X2	T48.1X3	T48.1X4	T48.1X5	T48.1X6
Flaxseed (medicinal)	T49.3X1	T49.3X2	T49.3X3	T49.3X4	T49.3X5	T49.3X6
Flecainide	T46.2X1	T46.2X2	T46.2X3	T46.2X4	T46.2X5	T46.2X6
Fleroxacin	T36.8X1	T36.8X2	T36.8X3	T36.8X4	T36.8X5	T36.8X6
Floctafenine	T39.8X1	T39.8X2	T39.8X3	T39.8X4	T39.8X5	T39.8X6
Flomax	T44.6X1	T44.6X2	T44.6X3	T44.6X4	T44.6X5	T44.6X6
Flomoxef	T36.1X1	T36.1X2	T36.1X3	T36.1X4	T36.1X5	T36.1X6
Flopropione	T44.3X1	T44.3X2	T44.3X3	T44.3X4	T44.3X5	T44.3X6
FLORAjen*	T47.6X1	T47.6X2	T47.6X3	T47.6X4	T47.6X5	T47.6X6
Florantyrone	T47.5X1	T47.5X2	T47.5X3	T47.5X4	T47.5X5	T47.5X6
Floraquin	T37.8X1	T37.8X2	T37.8X3	T37.8X4	T37.8X5	T37.8X6
Florinef	T38.ØX1	T38.ØX2	T38.ØX3	T38.ØX4	T38.ØX5	T38.ØX6
ENT agent	T49.6X1	T49.6X2	T49.6X3	T49.6X4	T49.6X5	T49.6X6
ophthalmic preparation	T49.5X1	T49.5X2	T49.5X3	T49.5X4	T49.5X5	T49.5X6
topical NEC	T49.ØX1	T49.ØX2	T49.ØX3	T49.ØX4	T49.ØX5	T49.ØX6
Flowers of sulfur	T49.4X1	T49.4X2	T49.4X3	T49.4X4	T49.4X5	T49.4X6
Floxuridine	T45.1X1	T45.1X2	T45.1X3	T45.1X4	T45.1X5	T45.1X6
Fluanisone	T43.4X1	T43.4X2	T43.4X3	T43.4X4	T43.4X5	T43.4X6
Flubendazole	T37.4X1	T37.4X2	T37.4X3	T37.4X4	T37.4X5	T37.4X6
Fluclorolone acetonide	T49.ØX1	T49.ØX2	T49.ØX3	T49.ØX4	T49.ØX5	T49.ØX6
Flucloxacillin	T36.ØX1	T36.ØX2	T36.ØX3	T36.ØX4	T36.ØX5	T36.ØX6
Fluconazole	T37.8X1	T37.8X2	T37.8X3	T37.8X4	T37.8X5	T37.8X6
Flucytosine	T37.8X1	T37.8X2	T37.8X3	T37.8X4	T37.8X5	T37.8X6
Fludeoxyglucose (18F)	T5Ø.8X1	T5Ø.8X2	T5Ø.8X3	T5Ø.8X4	T5Ø.8X5	T5Ø.8X6
Fludiazepam	T42.4X1	T42.4X2	T42.4X3	T42.4X4	T42.4X5	T42.4X6
Fludrocortisone	T5Ø.ØX1	T5Ø.ØX2	T5Ø.ØX3	T5Ø.ØX4	T5Ø.ØX5	T5Ø.ØX6
ENT agent	T49.6X1	T49.6X2	T49.6X3	T49.6X4	T49.6X5	T49.6X6
Fludrocortisone — *continued*						
ophthalmic preparation	T49.5X1	T49.5X2	T49.5X3	T49.5X4	T49.5X5	T49.5X6
topical NEC	T49.ØX1	T49.ØX2	T49.ØX3	T49.ØX4	T49.ØX5	T49.ØX6
Fludroxycortide	T49.ØX1	T49.ØX2	T49.ØX3	T49.ØX4	T49.ØX5	T49.ØX6
Flufenamic acid	T39.391	T39.392	T39.393	T39.394	T39.395	T39.396
Fluindione	T45.511	T45.512	T45.513	T45.514	T45.515	T45.516
Flumequine	T37.8X1	T37.8X2	T37.8X3	T37.8X4	T37.8X5	T37.8X6
Flumethasone	T49.ØX1	T49.ØX2	T49.ØX3	T49.ØX4	T49.ØX5	T49.ØX6
Flumethiazide	T5Ø.2X1	T5Ø.2X2	T5Ø.2X3	T5Ø.2X4	T5Ø.2X5	T5Ø.2X6
Flumidin	T37.5X1	T37.5X2	T37.5X3	T37.5X4	T37.5X5	T37.5X6
Flunarizine	T46.7X1	T46.7X2	T46.7X3	T46.7X4	T46.7X5	T46.7X6
Flunidazole	T37.8X1	T37.8X2	T37.8X3	T37.8X4	T37.8X5	T37.8X6
Flunisolide	T48.6X1	T48.6X2	T48.6X3	T48.6X4	T48.6X5	T48.6X6
Flunitrazepam	T42.4X1	T42.4X2	T42.4X3	T42.4X4	T42.4X5	T42.4X6
Fluocinolone (acetonide)	T49.ØX1	T49.ØX2	T49.ØX3	T49.ØX4	T49.ØX5	T49.ØX6
Fluocinonide	T49.ØX1	T49.ØX2	T49.ØX3	T49.ØX4	T49.ØX5	T49.ØX6
Fluocortin (butyl)	T49.ØX1	T49.ØX2	T49.ØX3	T49.ØX4	T49.ØX5	T49.ØX6
Fluocortolone	T49.ØX1	T49.ØX2	T49.ØX3	T49.ØX4	T49.ØX5	T49.ØX6
Fluohydrocortisone	T38.ØX1	T38.ØX2	T38.ØX3	T38.ØX4	T38.ØX5	T38.ØX6
ENT agent	T49.6X1	T49.6X2	T49.6X3	T49.6X4	T49.6X5	T49.6X6
ophthalmic preparation	T49.5X1	T49.5X2	T49.5X3	T49.5X4	T49.5X5	T49.5X6
topical NEC	T49.ØX1	T49.ØX2	T49.ØX3	T49.ØX4	T49.ØX5	T49.ØX6
Fluonid	T49.ØX1	T49.ØX2	T49.ØX3	T49.ØX4	T49.ØX5	T49.ØX6
Fluopromazine	T43.3X1	T43.3X2	T43.3X3	T43.3X4	T43.3X5	T43.3X6
Fluoracetate	T6Ø.8X1	T6Ø.8X2	T6Ø.8X3	T6Ø.8X4	—	—
Fluorescein	T5Ø.8X1	T5Ø.8X2	T5Ø.8X3	T5Ø.8X4	T5Ø.8X5	T5Ø.8X6
Fluorhydrocortisone	T5Ø.ØX1	T5Ø.ØX2	T5Ø.ØX3	T5Ø.ØX4	T5Ø.ØX5	T5Ø.ØX6
Fluoride (nonmedicinal) (pesticide) (sodium) **NEC**	T6Ø.8X1	T6Ø.8X2	T6Ø.8X3	T6Ø.8X4	—	—
hydrogen — *see* Hydrofluoric acid						
medicinal NEC	T5Ø.991	T5Ø.992	T5Ø.993	T5Ø.994	T5Ø.995	T5Ø.996
dental use	T49.7X1	T49.7X2	T49.7X3	T49.7X4	T49.7X5	T49.7X6
not pesticide NEC	T54.91	T54.92	T54.93	T54.94	—	—
stannous	T49.7X1	T49.7X2	T49.7X3	T49.7X4	T49.7X5	T49.7X6
Fluorigard*	T47.7X1	T47.7X2	T47.7X3	T47.7X4	T47.7X5	T47.7X6
Fluorinated corticosteroids	T38.ØX1	T38.ØX2	T38.ØX3	T38.ØX4	T38.ØX5	T38.ØX6
Fluorine (gas)	T59.5X1	T59.5X2	T59.5X3	T59.5X4	—	—
salt — *see* Fluoride(s)						
Fluoristan	T49.7X1	T49.7X2	T49.7X3	T49.7X4	T49.7X5	T49.7X6
Fluormetholone	T49.ØX1	T49.ØX2	T49.ØX3	T49.ØX4	T49.ØX5	T49.ØX6
Fluoroacetate	T6Ø.8X1	T6Ø.8X2	T6Ø.8X3	T6Ø.8X4	—	—
Fluorocarbon monomer	T53.6X1	T53.6X2	T53.6X3	T53.6X4	—	—
Fluorocytosine	T37.8X1	T37.8X2	T37.8X3	T37.8X4	T37.8X5	T37.8X6
Fluorodeoxyuridine	T45.1X1	T45.1X2	T45.1X3	T45.1X4	T45.1X5	T45.1X6
Fluorometholone	T49.ØX1	T49.ØX2	T49.ØX3	T49.ØX4	T49.ØX5	T49.ØX6
ophthalmic preparation	T49.5X1	T49.5X2	T49.5X3	T49.5X4	T49.5X5	T49.5X6
Fluorophosphate insecticide	T6Ø.ØX1	T6Ø.ØX2	T6Ø.ØX3	T6Ø.ØX4	—	—
Fluorosol	T46.3X1	T46.3X2	T46.3X3	T46.3X4	T46.3X5	T46.3X6
Fluorouracil	T45.1X1	T45.1X2	T45.1X3	T45.1X4	T45.1X5	T45.1X6
Fluorphenylalanine	T49.5X1	T49.5X2	T49.5X3	T49.5X4	T49.5X5	T49.5X6
Fluothane	T41.ØX1	T41.ØX2	T41.ØX3	T41.ØX4	T41.ØX5	T41.ØX6
Fluoxetine	T43.221	T43.222	T43.223	T43.224	T43.225	T43.226
Fluoxymesterone	T38.7X1	T38.7X2	T38.7X3	T38.7X4	T38.7X5	T38.7X6
Flupenthixol	T43.4X1	T43.4X2	T43.4X3	T43.4X4	T43.4X5	T43.4X6
Flupentixol	T43.4X1	T43.4X2	T43.4X3	T43.4X4	T43.4X5	T43.4X6
Fluphenazine	T43.3X1	T43.3X2	T43.3X3	T43.3X4	T43.3X5	T43.3X6
Fluprednidene	T49.ØX1	T49.ØX2	T49.ØX3	T49.ØX4	T49.ØX5	T49.ØX6
Fluprednisolone	T38.ØX1	T38.ØX2	T38.ØX3	T38.ØX4	T38.ØX5	T38.ØX6
Fluradoline	T39.8X1	T39.8X2	T39.8X3	T39.8X4	T39.8X5	T39.8X6
Flurandrenolide	T49.ØX1	T49.ØX2	T49.ØX3	T49.ØX4	T49.ØX5	T49.ØX6
Flurandrenolone	T49.ØX1	T49.ØX2	T49.ØX3	T49.ØX4	T49.ØX5	T49.ØX6
Flurazepam	T42.4X1	T42.4X2	T42.4X3	T42.4X4	T42.4X5	T42.4X6
Flurbiprofen	T39.311	T39.312	T39.313	T39.314	T39.315	T39.316
Flurobate	T49.ØX1	T49.ØX2	T49.ØX3	T49.ØX4	T49.ØX5	T49.ØX6
Fluroxene	T41.ØX1	T41.ØX2	T41.ØX3	T41.ØX4	T41.ØX5	T41.ØX6
Fluspirilene	T43.591	T43.592	T43.593	T43.594	T43.595	T43.596
Flutamide	T38.6X1	T38.6X2	T38.6X3	T38.6X4	T38.6X5	T38.6X6
Flutazolam	T38.ØX1	T38.ØX2	T38.ØX3	T38.ØX4	T38.ØX5	T38.ØX6
Fluticasone propionate	T38.ØX1	T38.ØX2	T38.ØX3	T38.ØX4	T38.ØX5	T38.ØX6
Flutoprazepam	T42.4X1	T42.4X2	T42.4X3	T42.4X4	T42.4X5	T42.4X6
Flutropium bromide	T48.6X1	T48.6X2	T48.6X3	T48.6X4	T48.6X5	T48.6X6
Fluvoxamine	T43.221	T43.222	T43.223	T43.224	T43.225	T43.226
Folacin	T45.8X1	T45.8X2	T45.8X3	T45.8X4	T45.8X5	T45.8X6
Folic acid	T45.8X1	T45.8X2	T45.8X3	T45.8X4	T45.8X5	T45.8X6
with ferrous salt	T45.2X1	T45.2X2	T45.2X3	T45.2X4	T45.2X5	T45.2X6
antagonist	T45.1X1	T45.1X2	T45.1X3	T45.1X4	T45.1X5	T45.1X6
Folinic acid	T45.8X1	T45.8X2	T45.8X3	T45.8X4	T45.8X5	T45.8X6
Folium stramoniae	T48.6X1	T48.6X2	T48.6X3	T48.6X4	T48.6X5	T48.6X6
Follicle-stimulating hormone, human	T38.811	T38.812	T38.813	T38.814	T38.815	T38.816

Substance	Poisoning, Accidental (unintentional)	Poisoning, Intentional Self-harm	Poisoning, Assault	Poisoning, Undetermined	Adverse Effect	Under-dosing
Folpet	T6Ø.3X1	T6Ø.3X2	T6Ø.3X3	T6Ø.3X4	—	—
Fomepizole*	T5Ø.6X1	T5Ø.6X2	T5Ø.6X3	T5Ø.6X4	T5Ø.6X5	T5Ø.6X6
Fominoben	T48.3X1	T48.3X2	T48.3X3	T48.3X4	T48.3X5	T48.3X6
Food, foodstuffs, noxious, nonbacterial, NEC	T62.91	T62.92	T62.93	T62.94	—	—
berries	T62.1X1	T62.1X2	T62.1X3	T62.1X4	—	—
fish — *see also* Fish	T61.91	T61.92	T61.93	T61.94	—	—
mushrooms	T62.ØX1	T62.ØX2	T62.ØX3	T62.ØX4	—	—
plants	T62.2X1	T62.2X2	T62.2X3	T62.2X4	—	—
seafood	T61.91	T61.92	T61.93	T61.94	—	—
specified NEC	T61.8X1	T61.8X2	T61.8X3	T61.8X4	—	—
seeds	T62.2X1	T62.2X2	T62.2X3	T62.2X4	—	—
shellfish	T61.781	T61.782	T61.783	T61.784	—	—
specified NEC	T62.8X1	T62.8X2	T62.8X3	T62.8X4	—	—
Fool's parsley	T62.2X1	T62.2X2	T62.2X3	T62.2X4	—	—
Formaldehyde (solution), gas or vapor	T59.2X1	T59.2X2	T59.2X3	T59.2X4	—	—
fungicide	T6Ø.3X1	T6Ø.3X2	T6Ø.3X3	T6Ø.3X4	—	—
Formalin	T59.2X1	T59.2X2	T59.2X3	T59.2X4	—	—
fungicide	T6Ø.3X1	T6Ø.3X2	T6Ø.3X3	T6Ø.3X4	—	—
vapor	T59.2X1	T59.2X2	T59.2X3	T59.2X4	—	—
Formic acid	T54.2X1	T54.2X2	T54.2X3	T54.2X4	—	—
vapor	T59.891	T59.892	T59.893	T59.894	—	—
Formoterol*	T48.6X1	T48.6X2	T48.6X3	T48.6X4	T48.6X5	T48.6X6
Fortaz*	T36.1X1	T36.1X2	T36.1X3	T36.1X4	T36.1X5	T36.1X6
Foscarnet sodium	T37.5X1	T37.5X2	T37.5X3	T37.5X4	T37.5X5	T37.5X6
Fosfestrol	T38.5X1	T38.5X2	T38.5X3	T38.5X4	T38.5X5	T38.5X6
Fosfomycin	T36.8X1	T36.8X2	T36.8X3	T36.8X4	T36.8X5	T36.8X6
Fosfonet sodium	T37.5X1	T37.5X2	T37.5X3	T37.5X4	T37.5X5	T37.5X6
Fosinopril	T46.4X1	T46.4X2	T46.4X3	T46.4X4	T46.4X5	T46.4X6
sodium	T46.4X1	T46.4X2	T46.4X3	T46.4X4	T46.4X5	T46.4X6
Fowler's solution	T57.ØX1	T57.ØX2	T57.ØX3	T57.ØX4	—	—
Foxglove	T62.2X1	T62.2X2	T62.2X3	T62.2X4	—	—
Framycetin	T36.5X1	T36.5X2	T36.5X3	T36.5X4	T36.5X5	T36.5X6
Frangula	T47.2X1	T47.2X2	T47.2X3	T47.2X4	T47.2X5	T47.2X6
extract	T47.2X1	T47.2X2	T47.2X3	T47.2X4	T47.2X5	T47.2X6
Frei antigen	T5Ø.8X1	T5Ø.8X2	T5Ø.8X3	T5Ø.8X4	T5Ø.8X5	T5Ø.8X6
Freon	T53.5X1	T53.5X2	T53.5X3	T53.5X4	—	—
Fructose	T5Ø.3X1	T5Ø.3X2	T5Ø.3X3	T5Ø.3X4	T5Ø.3X5	T5Ø.3X6
Frusemide	T5Ø.1X1	T5Ø.1X2	T5Ø.1X3	T5Ø.1X4	T5Ø.1X5	T5Ø.1X6
FSH	T38.811	T38.812	T38.813	T38.814	T38.815	T38.816
Ftorafur	T45.1X1	T45.1X2	T45.1X3	T45.1X4	T45.1X5	T45.1X6
Fuel						
automobile	T52.ØX1	T52.ØX2	T52.ØX3	T52.ØX4	—	—
exhaust gas, not in transit	T58.Ø1	T58.Ø2	T58.Ø3	T58.Ø4	—	—
vapor NEC	T52.ØX1	T52.ØX2	T52.ØX3	T52.ØX4	—	—
gas (domestic use) — *see also* Carbon, monoxide, fuel, utility	T59.891	T59.892	T59.893	T59.894	—	—
utility	T59.891	T59.892	T59.893	T59.894	—	—
incomplete combustion of — *see* Carbon, monoxide, fuel, utility						
in mobile container	T59.891	T59.892	T59.893	T59.894	—	—
piped (natural)	T59.891	T59.892	T59.893	T59.894	—	—
industrial, incomplete combustion	T58.8X1	T58.8X2	T58.8X3	T58.8X4	—	—
Fugillin	T36.8X1	T36.8X2	T36.8X3	T36.8X4	T36.8X5	T36.8X6
Fulminate of mercury	T56.1X1	T56.1X2	T56.1X3	T56.1X4	—	—
Fulvicin	T36.7X1	T36.7X2	T36.7X3	T36.7X4	T36.7X5	T36.7X6
Fumadil	T36.8X1	T36.8X2	T36.8X3	T36.8X4	T36.8X5	T36.8X6
Fumagillin	T36.8X1	T36.8X2	T36.8X3	T36.8X4	T36.8X5	T36.8X6
Fumaric acid	T49.4X1	T49.4X2	T49.4X3	T49.4X4	T49.4X5	T49.4X6
Fumes (from)	T59.91	T59.92	T59.93	T59.94	—	—
carbon monoxide — *see* Carbon, monoxide						
charcoal (domestic use) — *see* Charcoal, fumes						
chloroform — *see* Chloroform						
coke (in domestic stoves, fireplaces) — *see* Coke fumes						
corrosive NEC	T54.91	T54.92	T54.93	T54.94	—	—
ether — *see* ether						
freons	T53.5X1	T53.5X2	T53.5X3	T53.5X4	—	—
hydrocarbons	T59.891	T59.892	T59.893	T59.894	—	—
petroleum (liquefied)	T59.891	T59.892	T59.893	T59.894	—	—
distributed through pipes (pure or mixed with air)	T59.891	T59.892	T59.893	T59.894	—	—
lead — *see* lead						
Fumes — *continued*						
metal — *see* Metals, or the specified metal						
nitrogen dioxide	T59.ØX1	T59.ØX2	T59.ØX3	T59.ØX4	—	—
pesticides — *see* Pesticide						
petroleum (liquefied)	T59.891	T59.892	T59.893	T59.894	—	—
distributed through pipes (pure or mixed with air)	T59.891	T59.892	T59.893	T59.894	—	—
polyester	T59.891	T59.892	T59.893	T59.894	—	—
specified source NEC — *see also* substance specified	T59.891	T59.892	T59.893	T59.894	—	—
sulfur dioxide	T59.1X1	T59.1X2	T59.1X3	T59.1X4	—	—
Fumigant NEC	T6Ø.91	T6Ø.92	T6Ø.93	T6Ø.94	—	—
Fungicide NEC (nonmedicinal)	T6Ø.3X1	T6Ø.3X2	T6Ø.3X3	T6Ø.3X4	—	—
Fungi, noxious, used as food	T62.ØX1	T62.ØX2	T62.ØX3	T62.ØX4	—	—
Fungizone	T36.7X1	T36.7X2	T36.7X3	T36.7X4	T36.7X5	T36.7X6
topical	T49.ØX1	T49.ØX2	T49.ØX3	T49.ØX4	T49.ØX5	T49.ØX6
Fungoid*	T49.ØX1	T49.ØX2	T49.ØX3	T49.ØX4	T49.ØX5	T49.ØX6
Furacin	T49.ØX1	T49.ØX2	T49.ØX3	T49.ØX4	T49.ØX5	T49.ØX6
Furadantin	T37.91	T37.92	T37.93	T37.94	T37.95	T37.96
Furazolidone	T37.8X1	T37.8X2	T37.8X3	T37.8X4	T37.8X5	T37.8X6
Furazolium chloride	T49.ØX1	T49.ØX2	T49.ØX3	T49.ØX4	T49.ØX5	T49.ØX6
Furfural	T52.8X1	T52.8X2	T52.8X3	T52.8X4	—	—
Furnace (coal burning) (domestic), gas from industrial	T58.8X1	T58.8X2	T58.8X3	T58.8X4	—	—
Furniture polish	T65.891	T65.892	T65.893	T65.894	—	—
Furosemide	T5Ø.1X1	T5Ø.1X2	T5Ø.1X3	T5Ø.1X4	T5Ø.1X5	T5Ø.1X6
Furoxone	T37.91	T37.92	T37.93	T37.94	T37.95	T37.96
Fursultiamine	T45.2X1	T45.2X2	T45.2X3	T45.2X4	T45.2X5	T45.2X6
Fusafungine	T36.8X1	T36.8X2	T36.8X3	T36.8X4	T36.8X5	T36.8X6
Fusel oil (any) (amyl) (butyl) (propyl), vapor	T51.3X1	T51.3X2	T51.3X3	T51.3X4	—	—
Fusidate (ethanolamine) (sodium)	T36.8X1	T36.8X2	T36.8X3	T36.8X4	T36.8X5	T36.8X6
Fusidic acid	T36.8X1	T36.8X2	T36.8X3	T36.8X4	T36.8X5	T36.8X6
Fytic acid, nonasodium	T5Ø.6X1	T5Ø.6X2	T5Ø.6X3	T5Ø.6X4	T5Ø.6X5	T5Ø.6X6
b-Galactosidase	T47.5X1	T47.5X2	T47.5X3	T47.5X4	T47.5X5	T47.5X6
GABA	T43.8X1	T43.8X2	T43.8X3	T43.8X4	T43.8X5	T43.8X6
Gabitril*	T42.6X1	T42.6X2	T42.6X3	T42.6X4	T42.6X5	T42.6X6
Gadopentetic acid	T5Ø.8X1	T5Ø.8X2	T5Ø.8X3	T5Ø.8X4	T5Ø.8X5	T5Ø.8X6
Galactose	T5Ø.3X1	T5Ø.3X2	T5Ø.3X3	T5Ø.3X4	T5Ø.3X5	T5Ø.3X6
Galantamine	T44.ØX1	T44.ØX2	T44.ØX3	T44.ØX4	T44.ØX5	T44.ØX6
Gallamine (triethiodide)	T48.1X1	T48.1X2	T48.1X3	T48.1X4	T48.1X5	T48.1X6
Gallium citrate	T5Ø.991	T5Ø.992	T5Ø.993	T5Ø.994	T5Ø.995	T5Ø.996
Gallopamil	T46.1X1	T46.1X2	T46.1X3	T46.1X4	T46.1X5	T46.1X6
Gamboge	T47.2X1	T47.2X2	T47.2X3	T47.2X4	T47.2X5	T47.2X6
Gamimune	T5Ø.Z11	T5Ø.Z12	T5Ø.Z13	T5Ø.Z14	T5Ø.Z15	T5Ø.Z16
Gamma-aminobutyric acid	T43.8X1	T43.8X2	T43.8X3	T43.8X4	T43.8X5	T43.8X6
Gamma-benzene hexachloride (medicinal)	T49.ØX1	T49.ØX2	T49.ØX3	T49.ØX4	T49.ØX5	T49.ØX6
nonmedicinal, vapor	T53.6X1	T53.6X2	T53.6X3	T53.6X4	—	—
Gamma-BHC (medicinal) — *see also* Gamma-benzene hexachloride	T49.ØX1	T49.ØX2	T49.ØX3	T49.ØX4	T49.ØX5	T49.ØX6
Gamma globulin	T5Ø.Z11	T5Ø.Z12	T5Ø.Z13	T5Ø.Z14	T5Ø.Z15	T5Ø.Z16
Gamulin	T5Ø.Z11	T5Ø.Z12	T5Ø.Z13	T5Ø.Z14	T5Ø.Z15	T5Ø.Z16
Ganciclovir (sodium)	T37.5X1	T37.5X2	T37.5X3	T37.5X4	T37.5X5	T37.5X6
Ganglionic blocking drug NEC	T44.2X1	T44.2X2	T44.2X3	T44.2X4	T44.2X5	T44.2X6
specified NEC	T44.2X1	T44.2X2	T44.2X3	T44.2X4	T44.2X5	T44.2X6
Ganja	T4Ø.711	T4Ø.712	T4Ø.713	T4Ø.714	T4Ø.715	T4Ø.716
Garamycin	T36.5X1	T36.5X2	T36.5X3	T36.5X4	T36.5X5	T36.5X6
ophthalmic preparation	T49.5X1	T49.5X2	T49.5X3	T49.5X4	T49.5X5	T49.5X6
topical NEC	T49.ØX1	T49.ØX2	T49.ØX3	T49.ØX4	T49.ØX5	T49.ØX6
Gardenal	T42.3X1	T42.3X2	T42.3X3	T42.3X4	T42.3X5	T42.3X6
Gardepanyl	T42.3X1	T42.3X2	T42.3X3	T42.3X4	T42.3X5	T42.3X6
Gaseous substance — *see* Gas						
Gasoline	T52.ØX1	T52.ØX2	T52.ØX3	T52.ØX4	—	—
vapor	T52.ØX1	T52.ØX2	T52.ØX3	T52.ØX4	—	—
Gastric enzymes	T47.5X1	T47.5X2	T47.5X3	T47.5X4	T47.5X5	T47.5X6
Gastrografin	T5Ø.8X1	T5Ø.8X2	T5Ø.8X3	T5Ø.8X4	T5Ø.8X5	T5Ø.8X6
Gastrointestinal drug	T47.91	T47.92	T47.93	T47.94	T47.95	T47.96
biological	T47.8X1	T47.8X2	T47.8X3	T47.8X4	T47.8X5	T47.8X6
specified NEC	T47.8X1	T47.8X2	T47.8X3	T47.8X4	T47.8X5	T47.8X6
Gas NEC	T59.91	T59.92	T59.93	T59.94	—	—
acetylene	T59.891	T59.892	T59.893	T59.894	—	—
incomplete combustion of	T58.11	T58.12	T58.13	T58.14	—	—

Substance	Poisoning, Accidental (unintentional)	Poisoning, Intentional Self-harm	Poisoning, Assault	Poisoning, Undetermined	Adverse Effect	Under-dosing
Gas — *continued*						
air contaminants, source or type not specified	T59.91	T59.92	T59.93	T59.94	—	—
anesthetic	T41.ØX1	T41.ØX2	T41.ØX3	T41.ØX4	T41.ØX5	T41.ØX6
blast furnace	T58.8X1	T58.8X2	T58.8X3	T58.8X4	—	—
butane — *see* butane						
carbon monoxide — *see* Carbon, monoxide						
chlorine	T59.4X1	T59.4X2	T59.4X3	T59.4X4	—	—
coal	T58.2X1	T58.2X2	T58.2X3	T58.2X4	—	—
cyanide	T57.3X1	T57.3X2	T57.3X3	T57.3X4	—	—
dicyanogen	T65.ØX1	T65.ØX2	T65.ØX3	T65.ØX4	—	—
domestic — *see* Domestic gas						
exhaust	T58.Ø1	T58.Ø2	T58.Ø3	T58.Ø4	—	—
from utility (for cooking, heating, or lighting) (after combustion) — *see* Carbon, monoxide, fuel, utility						
prior to combustion	T59.891	T59.892	T59.893	T59.894	—	—
from wood- or coal-burning stove or fireplace	T58.2X1	T58.2X2	T58.2X3	T58.2X4	—	—
fuel (domestic use) (after combustion) — *see also* Carbon, monoxide, fuel						
industrial use	T58.8X1	T58.8X2	T58.8X3	T58.8X4	—	—
prior to combustion	T59.891	T59.892	T59.893	T59.894	—	—
utility	T59.891	T59.892	T59.893	T59.894	—	—
incomplete combustion of — *see* Carbon, monoxide, fuel, utility						
in mobile container	T59.891	T59.892	T59.893	T59.894	—	—
piped (natural)	T59.891	T59.892	T59.893	T59.894	—	—
garage	T58.Ø1	T58.Ø2	T58.Ø3	T58.Ø4	—	—
hydrocarbon NEC	T59.891	T59.892	T59.893	T59.894	—	—
incomplete combustion of — *see* Carbon, monoxide, fuel, utility						
liquefied — *see* butane						
piped	T59.891	T59.892	T59.893	T59.894	—	—
hydrocyanic acid	T65.ØX1	T65.ØX2	T65.ØX3	T65.ØX4	—	—
illuminating (after combustion)	T58.11	T58.12	T58.13	T58.14	—	—
prior to combustion	T59.891	T59.892	T59.893	T59.894	—	—
incomplete combustion, any — *see* Carbon, monoxide						
kiln	T58.8X1	T58.8X2	T58.8X3	T58.8X4	—	—
lacrimogenic	T59.3X1	T59.3X2	T59.3X3	T59.3X4	—	—
liquefied petroleum — *see* butane						
marsh	T59.891	T59.892	T59.893	T59.894	—	—
motor exhaust, not in transit	T58.Ø1	T58.Ø2	T58.Ø3	T58.Ø4	—	—
mustard, not in war	T59.891	T59.892	T59.893	T59.894	—	—
natural	T59.891	T59.892	T59.893	T59.894	—	—
nerve, not in war	T59.91	T59.92	T59.93	T59.94	—	—
oil	T52.ØX1	T52.ØX2	T52.ØX3	T52.ØX4	—	—
petroleum (liquefied) (distributed in mobile containers)	T59.891	T59.892	T59.893	T59.894	—	—
piped (pure or mixed with air)	T59.891	T59.892	T59.893	T59.894	—	—
piped (manufactured) (natural) NEC	T59.891	T59.892	T59.893	T59.894	—	—
producer	T58.8X1	T58.8X2	T58.8X3	T58.8X4	—	—
propane — *see* propane						
refrigerant (chlorofluoro-carbon)	T53.5X1	T53.5X2	T53.5X3	T53.5X4	—	—
not chlorofluoro-carbon	T59.891	T59.892	T59.893	T59.894	—	—
sewer	T59.91	T59.92	T59.93	T59.94	—	—
specified source NEC	T59.91	T59.92	T59.93	T59.94	—	—
stove (after combustion)	T58.11	T58.12	T58.13	T58.14	—	—
prior to combustion	T59.891	T59.892	T59.893	T59.894	—	—
tear	T59.3X1	T59.3X2	T59.3X3	T59.3X4	—	—
therapeutic	T41.5X1	T41.5X2	T41.5X3	T41.5X4	T41.5X5	T41.5X6
utility (for cooking, heating, or lighting) (piped) NEC	T59.891	T59.892	T59.893	T59.894	—	—
incomplete combustion of — *see* Carbon, monoxide, fuel, utility						
in mobile container	T59.891	T59.892	T59.893	T59.894	—	—
piped (natural)	T59.891	T59.892	T59.893	T59.894	—	—
water	T58.11	T58.12	T58.13	T58.14	—	—

Substance	Poisoning, Accidental (unintentional)	Poisoning, Intentional Self-harm	Poisoning, Assault	Poisoning, Undetermined	Adverse Effect	Under-dosing
Gas — *continued*						
water — *continued*						
incomplete combustion of — *see* Carbon, monoxide, fuel, utility						
Gaultheria procumbens	T62.2X1	T62.2X2	T62.2X3	T62.2X4	—	—
Gaviscon*	T47.1X1	T47.1X2	T47.1X3	T47.1X4	T47.1X5	T47.1X6
Gefarnate	T44.3X1	T44.3X2	T44.3X3	T44.3X4	T44.3X5	T44.3X6
Gelatin (intravenous)	T45.8X1	T45.8X2	T45.8X3	T45.8X4	T45.8X5	T45.8X6
absorbable (sponge)	T45.7X1	T45.7X2	T45.7X3	T45.7X4	T45.7X5	T45.7X6
Gelfilm	T49.8X1	T49.8X2	T49.8X3	T49.8X4	T49.8X5	T49.8X6
Gelfoam	T45.7X1	T45.7X2	T45.7X3	T45.7X4	T45.7X5	T45.7X6
Gelsemine	T5Ø.991	T5Ø.992	T5Ø.993	T5Ø.994	T5Ø.995	T5Ø.996
Gelsemium (sempervirens)	T62.2X1	T62.2X2	T62.2X3	T62.2X4	—	—
Gemeprost	T48.ØX1	T48.ØX2	T48.ØX3	T48.ØX4	T48.ØX5	T48.ØX6
Gemfibrozil	T46.6X1	T46.6X2	T46.6X3	T46.6X4	T46.6X5	T46.6X6
Gemonil	T42.3X1	T42.3X2	T42.3X3	T42.3X4	T42.3X5	T42.3X6
Gentamicin	T36.5X1	T36.5X2	T36.5X3	T36.5X4	T36.5X5	T36.5X6
ophthalmic preparation	T49.5X1	T49.5X2	T49.5X3	T49.5X4	T49.5X5	T49.5X6
topical NEC	T49.ØX1	T49.ØX2	T49.ØX3	T49.ØX4	T49.ØX5	T49.ØX6
Gentasol*	T49.5X1	T49.5X2	T49.5X3	T49.5X4	T49.5X5	T49.5X6
Gentian	T47.5X1	T47.5X2	T47.5X3	T47.5X4	T47.5X5	T47.5X6
violet	T49.ØX1	T49.ØX2	T49.ØX3	T49.ØX4	T49.ØX5	T49.ØX6
Gepefrine	T44.4X1	T44.4X2	T44.4X3	T44.4X4	T44.4X5	T44.4X6
Gestonorone caproate	T38.5X1	T38.5X2	T38.5X3	T38.5X4	T38.5X5	T38.5X6
Gexane	T49.ØX1	T49.ØX2	T49.ØX3	T49.ØX4	T49.ØX5	T49.ØX6
Gila monster (venom)	T63.111	T63.112	T63.113	T63.114	—	—
Ginger	T47.5X1	T47.5X2	T47.5X3	T47.5X4	T47.5X5	T47.5X6
Jamaica — *see* Jamaica, ginger						
Gitalin	T46.ØX1	T46.ØX2	T46.ØX3	T46.ØX4	T46.ØX5	T46.ØX6
amorphous	T46.ØX1	T46.ØX2	T46.ØX3	T46.ØX4	T46.ØX5	T46.ØX6
Gitaloxin	T46.ØX1	T46.ØX2	T46.ØX3	T46.ØX4	T46.ØX5	T46.ØX6
Gitoxin	T46.ØX1	T46.ØX2	T46.ØX3	T46.ØX4	T46.ØX5	T46.ØX6
Glafenine	T39.8X1	T39.8X2	T39.8X3	T39.8X4	T39.8X5	T39.8X6
Glandular extract (medicinal) NEC	T5Ø.Z91	T5Ø.Z92	T5Ø.Z93	T5Ø.Z94	T5Ø.Z95	T5Ø.Z96
Glaucarubin	T37.3X1	T37.3X2	T37.3X3	T37.3X4	T37.3X5	T37.3X6
Glibenclamide	T38.3X1	T38.3X2	T38.3X3	T38.3X4	T38.3X5	T38.3X6
Glibornuride	T38.3X1	T38.3X2	T38.3X3	T38.3X4	T38.3X5	T38.3X6
Gliclazide	T38.3X1	T38.3X2	T38.3X3	T38.3X4	T38.3X5	T38.3X6
Glimidine	T38.3X1	T38.3X2	T38.3X3	T38.3X4	T38.3X5	T38.3X6
Glipizide	T38.3X1	T38.3X2	T38.3X3	T38.3X4	T38.3X5	T38.3X6
Gliquidone	T38.3X1	T38.3X2	T38.3X3	T38.3X4	T38.3X5	T38.3X6
Glisolamide	T38.3X1	T38.3X2	T38.3X3	T38.3X4	T38.3X5	T38.3X6
Glisoxepide	T38.3X1	T38.3X2	T38.3X3	T38.3X4	T38.3X5	T38.3X6
Globin zinc insulin	T38.3X1	T38.3X2	T38.3X3	T38.3X4	T38.3X5	T38.3X6
Globulin						
antilymphocytic	T5Ø.Z11	T5Ø.Z12	T5Ø.Z13	T5Ø.Z14	T5Ø.Z15	T5Ø.Z16
antirhesus	T5Ø.Z11	T5Ø.Z12	T5Ø.Z13	T5Ø.Z14	T5Ø.Z15	T5Ø.Z16
antivenin	T5Ø.Z11	T5Ø.Z12	T5Ø.Z13	T5Ø.Z14	T5Ø.Z15	T5Ø.Z16
antiviral	T5Ø.Z11	T5Ø.Z12	T5Ø.Z13	T5Ø.Z14	T5Ø.Z15	T5Ø.Z16
Glucagon	T38.3X1	T38.3X2	T38.3X3	T38.3X4	T38.3X5	T38.3X6
Glucocorticoids	T38.ØX1	T38.ØX2	T38.ØX3	T38.ØX4	T38.ØX5	T38.ØX6
Glucocorticosteroid	T38.ØX1	T38.ØX2	T38.ØX3	T38.ØX4	T38.ØX5	T38.ØX6
Gluconic acid	T5Ø.991	T5Ø.992	T5Ø.993	T5Ø.994	T5Ø.995	T5Ø.996
Glucosamine sulfate	T39.4X1	T39.4X2	T39.4X3	T39.4X4	T39.4X5	T39.4X6
Glucose	T5Ø.3X1	T5Ø.3X2	T5Ø.3X3	T5Ø.3X4	T5Ø.3X5	T5Ø.3X6
with sodium chloride	T5Ø.3X1	T5Ø.3X2	T5Ø.3X3	T5Ø.3X4	T5Ø.3X5	T5Ø.3X6
Glucosulfone sodium	T37.1X1	T37.1X2	T37.1X3	T37.1X4	T37.1X5	T37.1X6
Glucotrol*	T38.3X1	T38.3X2	T38.3X3	T38.3X4	T38.3X5	T38.3X6
Glucurolactone	T47.8X1	T47.8X2	T47.8X3	T47.8X4	T47.8X5	T47.8X6
Glue NEC	T52.8X1	T52.8X2	T52.8X3	T52.8X4	—	—
Glutamic acid	T47.5X1	T47.5X2	T47.5X3	T47.5X4	T47.5X5	T47.5X6
Glutaral (medicinal)	T49.ØX1	T49.ØX2	T49.ØX3	T49.ØX4	T49.ØX5	T49.ØX6
nonmedicinal	T65.891	T65.892	T65.893	T65.894	—	—
Glutaraldehyde (nonmedicinal)	T65.891	T65.892	T65.893	T65.894	—	—
medicinal	T49.ØX1	T49.ØX2	T49.ØX3	T49.ØX4	T49.ØX5	T49.ØX6
Glutathione	T5Ø.6X1	T5Ø.6X2	T5Ø.6X3	T5Ø.6X4	T5Ø.6X5	T5Ø.6X6
Glutethimide	T42.6X1	T42.6X2	T42.6X3	T42.6X4	T42.6X5	T42.6X6
Glyburide	T38.3X1	T38.3X2	T38.3X3	T38.3X4	T38.3X5	T38.3X6
Glycerin	T47.4X1	T47.4X2	T47.4X3	T47.4X4	T47.4X5	T47.4X6
Glycerol	T47.4X1	T47.4X2	T47.4X3	T47.4X4	T47.4X5	T47.4X6
borax	T49.6X1	T49.6X2	T49.6X3	T49.6X4	T49.6X5	T49.6X6
intravenous	T5Ø.3X1	T5Ø.3X2	T5Ø.3X3	T5Ø.3X4	T5Ø.3X5	T5Ø.3X6
iodinated	T48.4X1	T48.4X2	T48.4X3	T48.4X4	T48.4X5	T48.4X6
Glycerophosphate	T5Ø.991	T5Ø.992	T5Ø.993	T5Ø.994	T5Ø.995	T5Ø.996
Glyceryl						
gualacolate	T48.4X1	T48.4X2	T48.4X3	T48.4X4	T48.4X5	T48.4X6
nitrate	T46.3X1	T46.3X2	T46.3X3	T46.3X4	T46.3X5	T46.3X6
triacetate (topical)	T49.ØX1	T49.ØX2	T49.ØX3	T49.ØX4	T49.ØX5	T49.ØX6
trinitrate	T46.3X1	T46.3X2	T46.3X3	T46.3X4	T46.3X5	T46.3X6
Glycine	T5Ø.3X1	T5Ø.3X2	T5Ø.3X3	T5Ø.3X4	T5Ø.3X5	T5Ø.3X6

Substance	Poisoning, Accidental (unintentional)	Poisoning, Intentional Self-harm	Poisoning, Assault	Poisoning, Undetermined	Adverse Effect	Under-dosing
Glyclopyramide	T38.3X1	T38.3X2	T38.3X3	T38.3X4	T38.3X5	T38.3X6
Glycobiarsol	T37.3X1	T37.3X2	T37.3X3	T37.3X4	T37.3X5	T37.3X6
Glycols (ether)	T52.3X1	T52.3X2	T52.3X3	T52.3X4	—	—
Glyconiazide	T37.1X1	T37.1X2	T37.1X3	T37.1X4	T37.1X5	T37.1X6
Glycopyrrolate	T44.3X1	T44.3X2	T44.3X3	T44.3X4	T44.3X5	T44.3X6
Glycopyrronium	T44.3X1	T44.3X2	T44.3X3	T44.3X4	T44.3X5	T44.3X6
bromide	T44.3X1	T44.3X2	T44.3X3	T44.3X4	T44.3X5	T44.3X6
Glycoside, cardiac (stimulant)	T46.ØX1	T46.ØX2	T46.ØX3	T46.ØX4	T46.ØX5	T46.ØX6
Glycyclamide	T38.3X1	T38.3X2	T38.3X3	T38.3X4	T38.3X5	T38.3X6
Glycyrrhiza extract	T48.4X1	T48.4X2	T48.4X3	T48.4X4	T48.4X5	T48.4X6
Glycyrrhizic acid	T48.4X1	T48.4X2	T48.4X3	T48.4X4	T48.4X5	T48.4X6
Glycyrrhizinate potassium	T48.4X1	T48.4X2	T48.4X3	T48.4X4	T48.4X5	T48.4X6
Glymidine sodium	T38.3X1	T38.3X2	T38.3X3	T38.3X4	T38.3X5	T38.3X6
Glyphosate	T6Ø.3X1	T6Ø.3X2	T6Ø.3X3	T6Ø.3X4	—	—
Glyphylline	T48.6X1	T48.6X2	T48.6X3	T48.6X4	T48.6X5	T48.6X6
Gold						
colloidal (198Au)	T45.1X1	T45.1X2	T45.1X3	T45.1X4	T45.1X5	T45.1X6
salts	T39.4X1	T39.4X2	T39.4X3	T39.4X4	T39.4X5	T39.4X6
Golden sulfide of antimony	T56.891	T56.892	T56.893	T56.894	—	—
Goldylocks	T62.2X1	T62.2X2	T62.2X3	T62.2X4	—	—
Gonadal tissue extract	T38.9Ø1	T38.9Ø2	T38.9Ø3	T38.9Ø4	T38.9Ø5	T38.9Ø6
female	T38.5X1	T38.5X2	T38.5X3	T38.5X4	T38.5X5	T38.5X6
male	T38.7X1	T38.7X2	T38.7X3	T38.7X4	T38.7X5	T38.7X6
Gonadorelin	T38.891	T38.892	T38.893	T38.894	T38.895	T38.896
Gonadotropin	T38.891	T38.892	T38.893	T38.894	T38.895	T38.896
chorionic	T38.891	T38.892	T38.893	T38.894	T38.895	T38.896
pituitary	T38.811	T38.812	T38.813	T38.814	T38.815	T38.816
Goserelin	T45.1X1	T45.1X2	T45.1X3	T45.1X4	T45.1X5	T45.1X6
Grain alcohol	T51.ØX1	T51.ØX2	T51.ØX3	T51.ØX4	—	—
Gralise*	T42.6X1	T42.6X2	T42.6X3	T42.6X4	T42.6X5	T42.6X6
Gramicidin	T49.ØX1	T49.ØX2	T49.ØX3	T49.ØX4	T49.ØX5	T49.ØX6
Granisetron	T45.ØX1	T45.ØX2	T45.ØX3	T45.ØX4	T45.ØX5	T45.ØX6
Gratiola officinalis	T62.2X1	T62.2X2	T62.2X3	T62.2X4	—	—
Grease	T65.891	T65.892	T65.893	T65.894	—	—
Green hellebore	T62.2X1	T62.2X2	T62.2X3	T62.2X4	—	—
Green soap	T49.2X1	T49.2X2	T49.2X3	T49.2X4	T49.2X5	T49.2X6
Grifulvin	T36.7X1	T36.7X2	T36.7X3	T36.7X4	T36.7X5	T36.7X6
Griseofulvin	T36.7X1	T36.7X2	T36.7X3	T36.7X4	T36.7X5	T36.7X6
Growth hormone	T38.811	T38.812	T38.813	T38.814	T38.815	T38.816
Guaiacol derivatives	T48.4X1	T48.4X2	T48.4X3	T48.4X4	T48.4X5	T48.4X6
Guaiac reagent	T5Ø.991	T5Ø.992	T5Ø.993	T5Ø.994	T5Ø.995	T5Ø.996
Guaifenesin	T48.4X1	T48.4X2	T48.4X3	T48.4X4	T48.4X5	T48.4X6
Guaimesal	T48.4X1	T48.4X2	T48.4X3	T48.4X4	T48.4X5	T48.4X6
Guaiphenesin	T48.4X1	T48.4X2	T48.4X3	T48.4X4	T48.4X5	T48.4X6
Guaituss*	T48.4X1	T48.4X2	T48.4X3	T48.4X4	T48.4X5	T48.4X6
Guamecycline	T36.4X1	T36.4X2	T36.4X3	T36.4X4	T36.4X5	T36.4X6
Guanabenz	T46.5X1	T46.5X2	T46.5X3	T46.5X4	T46.5X5	T46.5X6
Guanacline	T46.5X1	T46.5X2	T46.5X3	T46.5X4	T46.5X5	T46.5X6
Guanadrel	T46.5X1	T46.5X2	T46.5X3	T46.5X4	T46.5X5	T46.5X6
Guanatol	T37.2X1	T37.2X2	T37.2X3	T37.2X4	T37.2X5	T37.2X6
Guanethidine	T46.5X1	T46.5X2	T46.5X3	T46.5X4	T46.5X5	T46.5X6
Guanfacine	T46.5X1	T46.5X2	T46.5X3	T46.5X4	T46.5X5	T46.5X6
Guano	T65.891	T65.892	T65.893	T65.894	—	—
Guanochlor	T46.5X1	T46.5X2	T46.5X3	T46.5X4	T46.5X5	T46.5X6
Guanoclor	T46.5X1	T46.5X2	T46.5X3	T46.5X4	T46.5X5	T46.5X6
Guanoctine	T46.5X1	T46.5X2	T46.5X3	T46.5X4	T46.5X5	T46.5X6
Guanoxabenz	T46.5X1	T46.5X2	T46.5X3	T46.5X4	T46.5X5	T46.5X6
Guanoxan	T46.5X1	T46.5X2	T46.5X3	T46.5X4	T46.5X5	T46.5X6
Guar gum (medicinal)	T46.6X1	T46.6X2	T46.6X3	T46.6X4	T46.6X5	T46.6X6
Hachimycin	T36.7X1	T36.7X2	T36.7X3	T36.7X4	T36.7X5	T36.7X6
Hair						
dye	T49.4X1	T49.4X2	T49.4X3	T49.4X4	T49.4X5	T49.4X6
preparation NEC	T49.4X1	T49.4X2	T49.4X3	T49.4X4	T49.4X5	T49.4X6
Halazepam	T42.4X1	T42.4X2	T42.4X3	T42.4X4	T42.4X5	T42.4X6
Halcinolone	T49.ØX1	T49.ØX2	T49.ØX3	T49.ØX4	T49.ØX5	T49.ØX6
Halcinonide	T49.ØX1	T49.ØX2	T49.ØX3	T49.ØX4	T49.ØX5	T49.ØX6
Halethazole	T49.ØX1	T49.ØX2	T49.ØX3	T49.ØX4	T49.ØX5	T49.ØX6
Hallucinogen NOS	T4Ø.9Ø1	T4Ø.9Ø2	T4Ø.9Ø3	T4Ø.9Ø4	T4Ø.9Ø5	T4Ø.9Ø6
specified NEC	T4Ø.991	T4Ø.992	T4Ø.993	T4Ø.994	T4Ø.995	T4Ø.996
Halofantrine	T37.2X1	T37.2X2	T37.2X3	T37.2X4	T37.2X5	T37.2X6
Halofenate	T46.6X1	T46.6X2	T46.6X3	T46.6X4	T46.6X5	T46.6X6
Halometasone	T49.ØX1	T49.ØX2	T49.ØX3	T49.ØX4	T49.ØX5	T49.ØX6
Haloperidol	T43.4X1	T43.4X2	T43.4X3	T43.4X4	T43.4X5	T43.4X6
Haloprogin	T49.ØX1	T49.ØX2	T49.ØX3	T49.ØX4	T49.ØX5	T49.ØX6
Halotex	T49.ØX1	T49.ØX2	T49.ØX3	T49.ØX4	T49.ØX5	T49.ØX6
Halothane	T41.ØX1	T41.ØX2	T41.ØX3	T41.ØX4	T41.ØX5	T41.ØX6
Haloxazolam	T42.4X1	T42.4X2	T42.4X3	T42.4X4	T42.4X5	T42.4X6
Halquinols	T49.ØX1	T49.ØX2	T49.ØX3	T49.ØX4	T49.ØX5	T49.ØX6
Hamamelis	T49.2X1	T49.2X2	T49.2X3	T49.2X4	T49.2X5	T49.2X6
Haptendextran	T45.8X1	T45.8X2	T45.8X3	T45.8X4	T45.8X5	T45.8X6
Harmonyl	T46.5X1	T46.5X2	T46.5X3	T46.5X4	T46.5X5	T46.5X6

Substance	Poisoning, Accidental (unintentional)	Poisoning, Intentional Self-harm	Poisoning, Assault	Poisoning, Undetermined	Adverse Effect	Under-dosing
Hartmann's solution	T5Ø.3X1	T5Ø.3X2	T5Ø.3X3	T5Ø.3X4	T5Ø.3X5	T5Ø.3X6
Hashish	T4Ø.711	T4Ø.712	T4Ø.713	T4Ø.714	T4Ø.715	T4Ø.716
Havrix*	T5Ø.B91	T5Ø.B92	T5Ø.B93	T5Ø.B94	T5Ø.B95	T5Ø.B96
Hawaiian Woodrose seeds	T4Ø.991	T4Ø.992	T4Ø.993	T4Ø.994	—	—
HCB	T6Ø.3X1	T6Ø.3X2	T6Ø.3X3	T6Ø.3X4	—	—
HCH	T53.6X1	T53.6X2	T53.6X3	T53.6X4	—	—
medicinal	T49.ØX1	T49.ØX2	T49.ØX3	T49.ØX4	T49.ØX5	T49.ØX6
HCN	T57.3X1	T57.3X2	T57.3X3	T57.3X4	—	—
Headache cures, drugs, powders NEC	T5Ø.9Ø1	T5Ø.9Ø2	T5Ø.9Ø3	T5Ø.9Ø4	T5Ø.9Ø5	T5Ø.9Ø6
Heavenly Blue (morning glory)	T4Ø.991	T4Ø.992	T4Ø.993	T4Ø.994	—	—
Heavy metal antidote	T45.8X1	T45.8X2	T45.8X3	T45.8X4	T45.8X5	T45.8X6
Hedaquinium	T49.ØX1	T49.ØX2	T49.ØX3	T49.ØX4	T49.ØX5	T49.ØX6
Hedge hyssop	T62.2X1	T62.2X2	T62.2X3	T62.2X4	—	—
Heet	T49.8X1	T49.8X2	T49.8X3	T49.8X4	T49.8X5	T49.8X6
Helenin	T37.4X1	T37.4X2	T37.4X3	T37.4X4	T37.4X5	T37.4X6
Helium (nonmedicinal) **NEC**	T59.891	T59.892	T59.893	T59.894	—	—
medicinal	T48.991	T48.992	T48.993	T48.994	T48.995	T48.996
Hellebore (black) (green) (white)	T62.2X1	T62.2X2	T62.2X3	T62.2X4	—	—
Hematin	T45.8X1	T45.8X2	T45.8X3	T45.8X4	T45.8X5	T45.8X6
Hematinic preparation	T45.8X1	T45.8X2	T45.8X3	T45.8X4	T45.8X5	T45.8X6
Hematological agent	T45.91	T45.92	T45.93	T45.94	T45.95	T45.96
specified NEC	T45.8X1	T45.8X2	T45.8X3	T45.8X4	T45.8X5	T45.8X6
Hemlock	T62.2X1	T62.2X2	T62.2X3	T62.2X4	—	—
Hemostatic	T45.621	T45.622	T45.623	T45.624	T45.625	T45.626
drug, systemic	T45.621	T45.622	T45.623	T45.624	T45.625	T45.626
Hemostyptic	T49.4X1	T49.4X2	T49.4X3	T49.4X4	T49.4X5	T49.4X6
Henbane	T62.2X1	T62.2X2	T62.2X3	T62.2X4	—	—
Heparin (sodium)	T45.511	T45.512	T45.513	T45.514	T45.515	T45.516
action reverser	T45.7X1	T45.7X2	T45.7X3	T45.7X4	T45.7X5	T45.7X6
Heparin-fraction	T45.511	T45.512	T45.513	T45.514	T45.515	T45.516
Heparinoid (systemic)	T45.511	T45.512	T45.513	T45.514	T45.515	T45.516
Hepatic secretion stimulant	T47.8X1	T47.8X2	T47.8X3	T47.8X4	T47.8X5	T47.8X6
Hepatitis A vaccine*	T5Ø.B91	T5Ø.B92	T5Ø.B93	T5Ø.B94	T5Ø.B95	T5Ø.B96
Hepatitis B						
immune globulin	T5Ø.Z11	T5Ø.Z12	T5Ø.Z13	T5Ø.Z14	T5Ø.Z15	T5Ø.Z16
vaccine	T5Ø.B91	T5Ø.B92	T5Ø.B93	T5Ø.B94	T5Ø.B95	T5Ø.B96
Hepronicate	T46.7X1	T46.7X2	T46.7X3	T46.7X4	T46.7X5	T46.7X6
Heptabarb	T42.3X1	T42.3X2	T42.3X3	T42.3X4	T42.3X5	T42.3X6
Heptabarbital	T42.3X1	T42.3X2	T42.3X3	T42.3X4	T42.3X5	T42.3X6
Heptabarbitone	T42.3X1	T42.3X2	T42.3X3	T42.3X4	T42.3X5	T42.3X6
Heptachlor	T6Ø.1X1	T6Ø.1X2	T6Ø.1X3	T6Ø.1X4	—	—
Heptalgin	T4Ø.2X1	T4Ø.2X2	T4Ø.2X3	T4Ø.2X4	T4Ø.2X5	T4Ø.2X6
Heptaminol	T46.3X1	T46.3X2	T46.3X3	T46.3X4	T46.3X5	T46.3X6
Herbicide NEC	T6Ø.3X1	T6Ø.3X2	T6Ø.3X3	T6Ø.3X4	—	—
Heroin	T4Ø.1X1	T4Ø.1X2	T4Ø.1X3	T4Ø.1X4	—	—
Herplex	T49.5X1	T49.5X2	T49.5X3	T49.5X4	T49.5X5	T49.5X6
HES	T45.8X1	T45.8X2	T45.8X3	T45.8X4	T45.8X5	T45.8X6
Hesperidin	T46.991	T46.992	T46.993	T46.994	T46.995	T46.996
Hetacillin	T36.ØX1	T36.ØX2	T36.ØX3	T36.ØX4	T36.ØX5	T36.ØX6
Hetastarch	T45.8X1	T45.8X2	T45.8X3	T45.8X4	T45.8X5	T45.8X6
HETP	T6Ø.ØX1	T6Ø.ØX2	T6Ø.ØX3	T6Ø.ØX4	—	—
Hexachlorobenzene (vapor)	T6Ø.3X1	T6Ø.3X2	T6Ø.3X3	T6Ø.3X4	—	—
Hexachlorocyclohexane	T53.6X1	T53.6X2	T53.6X3	T53.6X4	—	—
Hexachlorophene	T49.ØX1	T49.ØX2	T49.ØX3	T49.ØX4	T49.ØX5	T49.ØX6
Hexadiline	T46.3X1	T46.3X2	T46.3X3	T46.3X4	T46.3X5	T46.3X6
Hexadimethrine (bromide)	T45.7X1	T45.7X2	T45.7X3	T45.7X4	T45.7X5	T45.7X6
Hexadylamine	T46.3X1	T46.3X2	T46.3X3	T46.3X4	T46.3X5	T46.3X6
Hexaethyl tetraphosphate	T6Ø.ØX1	T6Ø.ØX2	T6Ø.ØX3	T6Ø.ØX4	—	—
Hexafluorenium bromide	T48.1X1	T48.1X2	T48.1X3	T48.1X4	T48.1X5	T48.1X6
Hexafluronium (bromide)	T48.1X1	T48.1X2	T48.1X3	T48.1X4	T48.1X5	T48.1X6
Hexa-germ	T49.2X1	T49.2X2	T49.2X3	T49.2X4	T49.2X5	T49.2X6
Hexahydrobenzol	T52.8X1	T52.8X2	T52.8X3	T52.8X4	—	—
Hexahydrocresol(s)	T51.8X1	T51.8X2	T51.8X3	T51.8X4	—	—
arsenide	T57.ØX1	T57.ØX2	T57.ØX3	T57.ØX4	—	—
arseniurated	T57.ØX1	T57.ØX2	T57.ØX3	T57.ØX4	—	—
cyanide	T57.3X1	T57.3X2	T57.3X3	T57.3X4	—	—
gas	T59.891	T59.892	T59.893	T59.894	—	—
Fluoride (liquid)	T57.8X1	T57.8X2	T57.8X3	T57.8X4	—	—
vapor	T59.891	T59.892	T59.893	T59.894	—	—
phophorated	T6Ø.ØX1	T6Ø.ØX2	T6Ø.ØX3	T6Ø.ØX4	—	—
sulfate	T57.8X1	T57.8X2	T57.8X3	T57.8X4	—	—
sulfide (gas)	T59.6X1	T59.6X2	T59.6X3	T59.6X4	—	—
arseniurated	T57.ØX1	T57.ØX2	T57.ØX3	T57.ØX4	—	—
sulfurated	T57.8X1	T57.8X2	T57.8X3	T57.8X4	—	—
Hexahydrophenol	T51.8X1	T51.8X2	T51.8X3	T51.8X4	—	—
Hexalen	T51.8X1	T51.8X2	T51.8X3	T51.8X4	—	—
Hexamethonium bromide	T44.2X1	T44.2X2	T44.2X3	T44.2X4	T44.2X5	T44.2X6
Hexamethylene	T52.8X1	T52.8X2	T52.8X3	T52.8X4	—	—

Substance	Poisoning, Accidental (unintentional)	Poisoning, Intentional Self-harm	Poisoning, Assault	Poisoning, Undetermined	Adverse Effect	Under-dosing
Hexamethylmelamine	T45.1X1	T45.1X2	T45.1X3	T45.1X4	T45.1X5	T45.1X6
Hexamidine	T49.ØX1	T49.ØX2	T49.ØX3	T49.ØX4	T49.ØX5	T49.ØX6
Hexamine (mandelate)	T37.8X1	T37.8X2	T37.8X3	T37.8X4	T37.8X5	T37.8X6
Hexanone, 2-hexanone	T52.4X1	T52.4X2	T52.4X3	T52.4X4	—	—
Hexanuorenium	T48.1X1	T48.1X2	T48.1X3	T48.1X4	T48.1X5	T48.1X6
Hexapropymate	T42.6X1	T42.6X2	T42.6X3	T42.6X4	T42.6X5	T42.6X6
Hexasonium iodide	T44.3X1	T44.3X2	T44.3X3	T44.3X4	T44.3X5	T44.3X6
Hexcarbacholine bromide	T48.1X1	T48.1X2	T48.1X3	T48.1X4	T48.1X5	T48.1X6
Hexemal	T42.3X1	T42.3X2	T42.3X3	T42.3X4	T42.3X5	T42.3X6
Hexestrol	T38.5X1	T38.5X2	T38.5X3	T38.5X4	T38.5X5	T38.5X6
Hexethal (sodium)	T42.3X1	T42.3X2	T42.3X3	T42.3X4	T42.3X5	T42.3X6
Hexetidine	T37.8X1	T37.8X2	T37.8X3	T37.8X4	T37.8X5	T37.8X6
Hexobarbital	T42.3X1	T42.3X2	T42.3X3	T42.3X4	T42.3X5	T42.3X6
rectal	T41.291	T41.292	T41.293	T41.294	T41.295	T41.296
sodium	T41.1X1	T41.1X2	T41.1X3	T41.1X4	T41.1X5	T41.1X6
Hexobendine	T46.3X1	T46.3X2	T46.3X3	T46.3X4	T46.3X5	T46.3X6
Hexocyclium	T44.3X1	T44.3X2	T44.3X3	T44.3X4	T44.3X5	T44.3X6
metilsulfate	T44.3X1	T44.3X2	T44.3X3	T44.3X4	T44.3X5	T44.3X6
Hexoestrol	T38.5X1	T38.5X2	T38.5X3	T38.5X4	T38.5X5	T38.5X6
Hexone	T52.4X1	T52.4X2	T52.4X3	T52.4X4	—	—
Hexoprenaline	T48.6X1	T48.6X2	T48.6X3	T48.6X4	T48.6X5	T48.6X6
Hexylcaine	T41.3X1	T41.3X2	T41.3X3	T41.3X4	T41.3X5	T41.3X6
Hexylresorcinol	T52.2X1	T52.2X2	T52.2X3	T52.2X4	—	—
HGH (human growth hormone)	T38.811	T38.812	T38.813	T38.814	T38.815	T38.816
Hibistat*	T49.ØX1	T49.ØX2	T49.ØX3	T49.ØX4	T49.ØX5	T49.ØX6
Hinkle's pills	T47.2X1	T47.2X2	T47.2X3	T47.2X4	T47.2X5	T47.2X6
Histalog	T5Ø.8X1	T5Ø.8X2	T5Ø.8X3	T5Ø.8X4	T5Ø.8X5	T5Ø.8X6
Histamine (phosphate)	T5Ø.8X1	T5Ø.8X2	T5Ø.8X3	T5Ø.8X4	T5Ø.8X5	T5Ø.8X6
Histolyn*	T5Ø.8X1	T5Ø.8X2	T5Ø.8X3	T5Ø.8X4	T5Ø.8X5	T5Ø.8X6
Histoplasmin	T5Ø.8X1	T5Ø.8X2	T5Ø.8X3	T5Ø.8X4	T5Ø.8X5	T5Ø.8X6
Holly berries	T62.2X1	T62.2X2	T62.2X3	T62.2X4	—	—
Homatropine	T44.3X1	T44.3X2	T44.3X3	T44.3X4	T44.3X5	T44.3X6
methylbromide	T44.3X1	T44.3X2	T44.3X3	T44.3X4	T44.3X5	T44.3X6
Homochlorcyclizine	T45.ØX1	T45.ØX2	T45.ØX3	T45.ØX4	T45.ØX5	T45.ØX6
Homosalate	T49.3X1	T49.3X2	T49.3X3	T49.3X4	T49.3X5	T49.3X6
Homo-tet	T5Ø.Z11	T5Ø.Z12	T5Ø.Z13	T5Ø.Z14	T5Ø.Z15	T5Ø.Z16
Hormone	T38.8Ø1	T38.8Ø2	T38.8Ø3	T38.8Ø4	T38.8Ø5	T38.8Ø6
adrenal cortical steroids	T38.ØX1	T38.ØX2	T38.ØX3	T38.ØX4	T38.ØX5	T38.ØX6
androgenic	T38.7X1	T38.7X2	T38.7X3	T38.7X4	T38.7X5	T38.7X6
anterior pituitary NEC	T38.811	T38.812	T38.813	T38.814	T38.815	T38.816
antidiabetic agents	T38.3X1	T38.3X2	T38.3X3	T38.3X4	T38.3X5	T38.3X6
antidiuretic	T38.891	T38.892	T38.893	T38.894	T38.895	T38.896
cancer therapy	T45.1X1	T45.1X2	T45.1X3	T45.1X4	T45.1X5	T45.1X6
follicle stimulating	T38.811	T38.812	T38.813	T38.814	T38.815	T38.816
gonadotropic	T38.891	T38.892	T38.893	T38.894	T38.895	T38.896
pituitary	T38.811	T38.812	T38.813	T38.814	T38.815	T38.816
growth	T38.811	T38.812	T38.813	T38.814	T38.815	T38.816
luteinizing	T38.811	T38.812	T38.813	T38.814	T38.815	T38.816
ovarian	T38.5X1	T38.5X2	T38.5X3	T38.5X4	T38.5X5	T38.5X6
oxytocic	T48.ØX1	T48.ØX2	T48.ØX3	T48.ØX4	T48.ØX5	T48.ØX6
parathyroid (derivatives)	T5Ø.991	T5Ø.992	T5Ø.993	T5Ø.994	T5Ø.995	T5Ø.996
pituitary (posterior) NEC	T38.891	T38.892	T38.893	T38.894	T38.895	T38.896
anterior	T38.811	T38.812	T38.813	T38.814	T38.815	T38.816
specified, NEC	T38.891	T38.892	T38.893	T38.894	T38.895	T38.896
thyroid	T38.1X1	T38.1X2	T38.1X3	T38.1X4	T38.1X5	T38.1X6
Hornet (sting)	T63.451	T63.452	T63.453	T63.454	—	—
Horse anti-human lymphocytic serum	T5Ø.Z11	T5Ø.Z12	T5Ø.Z13	T5Ø.Z14	T5Ø.Z15	T5Ø.Z16
Horticulture agent NEC	T65.91	T65.92	T65.93	T65.94	—	—
with pesticide	T6Ø.91	T6Ø.92	T6Ø.93	T6Ø.94	—	—
Human						
albumin	T45.8X1	T45.8X2	T45.8X3	T45.8X4	T45.8X5	T45.8X6
growth hormone (HGH)	T38.811	T38.812	T38.813	T38.814	T38.815	T38.816
immune serum	T5Ø.Z11	T5Ø.Z12	T5Ø.Z13	T5Ø.Z14	T5Ø.Z15	T5Ø.Z16
Hyaluronidase	T45.3X1	T45.3X2	T45.3X3	T45.3X4	T45.3X5	T45.3X6
Hyazyme	T45.3X1	T45.3X2	T45.3X3	T45.3X4	T45.3X5	T45.3X6
Hycodan	T4Ø.2X1	T4Ø.2X2	T4Ø.2X3	T4Ø.2X4	T4Ø.2X5	T4Ø.2X6
Hydantoin derivative NEC	T42.ØX1	T42.ØX2	T42.ØX3	T42.ØX4	T42.ØX5	T42.ØX6
Hydeltra	T38.ØX1	T38.ØX2	T38.ØX3	T38.ØX4	T38.ØX5	T38.ØX6
Hydergine	T44.6X1	T44.6X2	T44.6X3	T44.6X4	T44.6X5	T44.6X6
Hydrabamine penicillin	T36.ØX1	T36.ØX2	T36.ØX3	T36.ØX4	T36.ØX5	T36.ØX6
Hydralazine	T46.5X1	T46.5X2	T46.5X3	T46.5X4	T46.5X5	T46.5X6
Hydrargaphen	T49.ØX1	T49.ØX2	T49.ØX3	T49.ØX4	T49.ØX5	T49.ØX6
Hydrargyri aminochloridum	T49.ØX1	T49.ØX2	T49.ØX3	T49.ØX4	T49.ØX5	T49.ØX6
Hydrastine	T48.291	T48.292	T48.293	T48.294	T48.295	T48.296
Hydrazine	T54.1X1	T54.1X2	T54.1X3	T54.1X4	—	—
monoamine oxidase inhibitors	T43.1X1	T43.1X2	T43.1X3	T43.1X4	T43.1X5	T43.1X6
Hydrazoic acid, azides	T54.2X1	T54.2X2	T54.2X3	T54.2X4	—	—
Hydriodic acid	T48.4X1	T48.4X2	T48.4X3	T48.4X4	T48.4X5	T48.4X6
Hydrisalic*	T49.4X1	T49.4X2	T49.4X3	T49.4X4	T49.4X5	T49.4X6

Substance	Poisoning, Accidental (unintentional)	Poisoning, Intentional Self-harm	Poisoning, Assault	Poisoning, Undetermined	Adverse Effect	Under-dosing
Hydrocarbon gas	T59.891	T59.892	T59.893	T59.894	—	—
incomplete combustion of — *see* Carbon, monoxide, fuel, utility						
liquefied (mobile container)	T59.891	T59.892	T59.893	T59.894	—	—
piped (natural)	T59.891	T59.892	T59.893	T59.894	—	—
Hydrochloric acid (liquid)	T54.2X1	T54.2X2	T54.2X3	T54.2X4	—	—
medicinal (digestant)	T47.5X1	T47.5X2	T47.5X3	T47.5X4	T47.5X5	T47.5X6
vapor	T59.891	T59.892	T59.893	T59.894	—	—
Hydrochlorothiazide	T5Ø.2X1	T5Ø.2X2	T5Ø.2X3	T5Ø.2X4	T5Ø.2X5	T5Ø.2X6
Hydrocodone	T4Ø.2X1	T4Ø.2X2	T4Ø.2X3	T4Ø.2X4	T4Ø.2X5	T4Ø.2X6
Hydrocortisone (derivatives)	T38.ØX1	T38.ØX2	T38.ØX3	T38.ØX4	T38.ØX5	T38.ØX6
aceponate	T49.ØX1	T49.ØX2	T49.ØX3	T49.ØX4	T49.ØX5	T49.ØX6
ENT agent	T49.6X1	T49.6X2	T49.6X3	T49.6X4	T49.6X5	T49.6X6
ophthalmic preparation	T49.5X1	T49.5X2	T49.5X3	T49.5X4	T49.5X5	T49.5X6
topical NEC	T49.ØX1	T49.ØX2	T49.ØX3	T49.ØX4	T49.ØX5	T49.ØX6
Hydrocortone	T38.ØX1	T38.ØX2	T38.ØX3	T38.ØX4	T38.ØX5	T38.ØX6
ENT agent	T49.6X1	T49.6X2	T49.6X3	T49.6X4	T49.6X5	T49.6X6
ophthalmic preparation	T49.5X1	T49.5X2	T49.5X3	T49.5X4	T49.5X5	T49.5X6
topical NEC	T49.ØX1	T49.ØX2	T49.ØX3	T49.ØX4	T49.ØX5	T49.ØX6
Hydrocyanic acid (liquid)	T57.3X1	T57.3X2	T57.3X3	T57.3X4	—	—
gas	T65.ØX1	T65.ØX2	T65.ØX3	T65.ØX4	—	—
Hydroflumethiazide	T5Ø.2X1	T5Ø.2X2	T5Ø.2X3	T5Ø.2X4	T5Ø.2X5	T5Ø.2X6
Hydrofluoric acid (liquid)	T54.2X1	T54.2X2	T54.2X3	T54.2X4	—	—
vapor	T59.891	T59.892	T59.893	T59.894	—	—
Hydrogen	T59.891	T59.892	T59.893	T59.894	—	—
arsenide	T57.ØX1	T57.ØX2	T57.ØX3	T57.ØX4	—	—
arseniureted	T57.ØX1	T57.ØX2	T57.ØX3	T57.ØX4	—	—
chloride	T57.8X1	T57.8X2	T57.8X3	T57.8X4	—	—
cyanide (salts)	T57.3X1	T57.3X2	T57.3X3	T57.3X4	—	—
gas	T57.3X1	T57.3X2	T57.3X3	T57.3X4	—	—
Fluoride	T59.5X1	T59.5X2	T59.5X3	T59.5X4	—	—
vapor	T59.5X1	T59.5X2	T59.5X3	T59.5X4	—	—
peroxide	T49.ØX1	T49.ØX2	T49.ØX3	T49.ØX4	T49.ØX5	T49.ØX6
phosphureted	T57.1X1	T57.1X2	T57.1X3	T57.1X4	—	—
sulfide	T59.6X1	T59.6X2	T59.6X3	T59.6X4	—	—
arseniureted	T57.ØX1	T57.ØX2	T57.ØX3	T57.ØX4	—	—
sulfureted	T59.6X1	T59.6X2	T59.6X3	T59.6X4	—	—
Hydromethylpyridine	T46.7X1	T46.7X2	T46.7X3	T46.7X4	T46.7X5	T46.7X6
Hydromorphinol	T4Ø.2X1	T4Ø.2X2	T4Ø.2X3	T4Ø.2X4	—	—
Hydromorphinone	T4Ø.2X1	T4Ø.2X2	T4Ø.2X3	T4Ø.2X4	T4Ø.2X5	T4Ø.2X6
Hydromorphone	T4Ø.2X1	T4Ø.2X2	T4Ø.2X3	T4Ø.2X4	T4Ø.2X5	T4Ø.2X6
Hydromox	T5Ø.2X1	T5Ø.2X2	T5Ø.2X3	T5Ø.2X4	T5Ø.2X5	T5Ø.2X6
Hydrophilic lotion	T49.3X1	T49.3X2	T49.3X3	T49.3X4	T49.3X5	T49.3X6
Hydroquinidine	T46.2X1	T46.2X2	T46.2X3	T46.2X4	T46.2X5	T46.2X6
Hydroquinone	T52.2X1	T52.2X2	T52.2X3	T52.2X4	—	—
vapor	T59.891	T59.892	T59.893	T59.894	—	—
Hydro-ride*	T5Ø.2X1	T5Ø.2X2	T5Ø.2X3	T5Ø.2X4	T5Ø.2X5	T5Ø.2X6
Hydrosulfuric acid (gas)	T59.6X1	T59.6X2	T59.6X3	T59.6X4	—	—
Hydrotalcite	T47.1X1	T47.1X2	T47.1X3	T47.1X4	T47.1X5	T47.1X6
Hydrous wool fat	T49.3X1	T49.3X2	T49.3X3	T49.3X4	T49.3X5	T49.3X6
Hydroxide, caustic	T54.3X1	T54.3X2	T54.3X3	T54.3X4	—	—
Hydroxocobalamin	T45.8X1	T45.8X2	T45.8X3	T45.8X4	T45.8X5	T45.8X6
Hydroxyamphetamine	T49.5X1	T49.5X2	T49.5X3	T49.5X4	T49.5X5	T49.5X6
Hydroxycarbamide	T45.1X1	T45.1X2	T45.1X3	T45.1X4	T45.1X5	T45.1X6
Hydroxychloroquine	T37.8X1	T37.8X2	T37.8X3	T37.8X4	T37.8X5	T37.8X6
Hydroxydaunorubicin*	T45.1X1	T45.1X2	T45.1X3	T45.1X4	T45.1X5	T45.1X6
Hydroxydihydrocodeinone	T4Ø.2X1	T4Ø.2X2	T4Ø.2X3	T4Ø.2X4	T4Ø.2X5	T4Ø.2X6
Hydroxyestrone	T38.5X1	T38.5X2	T38.5X3	T38.5X4	T38.5X5	T38.5X6
Hydroxyethyl starch	T45.8X1	T45.8X2	T45.8X3	T45.8X4	T45.8X5	T45.8X6
Hydroxymethylpentanone	T52.4X1	T52.4X2	T52.4X3	T52.4X4	—	—
Hydroxyphenamate	T43.591	T43.592	T43.593	T43.594	T43.595	T43.596
Hydroxyphenylbutazone	T39.2X1	T39.2X2	T39.2X3	T39.2X4	T39.2X5	T39.2X6
Hydroxyprogesterone	T38.5X1	T38.5X2	T38.5X3	T38.5X4	T38.5X5	T38.5X6
caproate	T38.5X1	T38.5X2	T38.5X3	T38.5X4	T38.5X5	T38.5X6
Hydroxyquinoline (derivatives) **NEC**	T37.8X1	T37.8X2	T37.8X3	T37.8X4	T37.8X5	T37.8X6
Hydroxystilbamidine	T37.3X1	T37.3X2	T37.3X3	T37.3X4	T37.3X5	T37.3X6
Hydroxytoluene (nonmedicinal)	T54.ØX1	T54.ØX2	T54.ØX3	T54.ØX4	—	—
medicinal	T49.ØX1	T49.ØX2	T49.ØX3	T49.ØX4	T49.ØX5	T49.ØX6
Hydroxyurea	T45.1X1	T45.1X2	T45.1X3	T45.1X4	T45.1X5	T45.1X6
Hydroxyzine	T43.591	T43.592	T43.593	T43.594	T43.595	T43.596
Hyoscine	T44.3X1	T44.3X2	T44.3X3	T44.3X4	T44.3X5	T44.3X6
Hyoscyamine	T44.3X1	T44.3X2	T44.3X3	T44.3X4	T44.3X5	T44.3X6
Hyoscyamus	T44.3X1	T44.3X2	T44.3X3	T44.3X4	T44.3X5	T44.3X6
dry extract	T44.3X1	T44.3X2	T44.3X3	T44.3X4	T44.3X5	T44.3X6
Hypaque	T5Ø.8X1	T5Ø.8X2	T5Ø.8X3	T5Ø.8X4	T5Ø.8X5	T5Ø.8X6
HyperRAB*	T5Ø.Z11	T5Ø.Z12	T5Ø.Z13	T5Ø.Z14	T5Ø.Z15	T5Ø.Z16
Hypertussis	T5Ø.Z11	T5Ø.Z12	T5Ø.Z13	T5Ø.Z14	T5Ø.Z15	T5Ø.Z16
Hypnotic	T42.71	T42.72	T42.73	T42.74	T42.75	T42.76

Substance	Poisoning, Accidental (unintentional)	Poisoning, Intentional Self-harm	Poisoning, Assault	Poisoning, Undetermined	Adverse Effect	Under-dosing
Hypnotic — *continued*						
anticonvulsant	T42.71	T42.72	T42.73	T42.74	T42.75	T42.76
specified NEC	T42.6X1	T42.6X2	T42.6X3	T42.6X4	T42.6X5	T42.6X6
Hypochlorite	T49.ØX1	T49.ØX2	T49.ØX3	T49.ØX4	T49.ØX5	T49.ØX6
Hypophysis, posterior	T38.891	T38.892	T38.893	T38.894	T38.895	T38.896
Hypotensive NEC	T46.5X1	T46.5X2	T46.5X3	T46.5X4	T46.5X5	T46.5X6
Hypromellose	T49.5X1	T49.5X2	T49.5X3	T49.5X4	T49.5X5	T49.5X6
Ibacitabine	T37.5X1	T37.5X2	T37.5X3	T37.5X4	T37.5X5	T37.5X6
Ibopamine	T44.991	T44.992	T44.993	T44.994	T44.995	T44.996
Ibufenac	T39.311	T39.312	T39.313	T39.314	T39.315	T39.316
Ibuprofen	T39.311	T39.312	T39.313	T39.314	T39.315	T39.316
Ibuproxam	T39.311	T39.312	T39.313	T39.314	T39.315	T39.316
Ibuterol	T48.6X1	T48.6X2	T48.6X3	T48.6X4	T48.6X5	T48.6X6
Ichthammol	T49.ØX1	T49.ØX2	T49.ØX3	T49.ØX4	T49.ØX5	T49.ØX6
Ichthyol	T49.4X1	T49.4X2	T49.4X3	T49.4X4	T49.4X5	T49.4X6
Idarubicin	T45.1X1	T45.1X2	T45.1X3	T45.1X4	T45.1X5	T45.1X6
Idrocilamide	T42.8X1	T42.8X2	T42.8X3	T42.8X4	T42.8X5	T42.8X6
Ifenprodil	T46.7X1	T46.7X2	T46.7X3	T46.7X4	T46.7X5	T46.7X6
Ifosfamide	T45.1X1	T45.1X2	T45.1X3	T45.1X4	T45.1X5	T45.1X6
Iletin	T38.3X1	T38.3X2	T38.3X3	T38.3X4	T38.3X5	T38.3X6
Ilex	T62.2X1	T62.2X2	T62.2X3	T62.2X4	—	—
Illuminating gas (after combustion)	T58.11	T58.12	T58.13	T58.14	—	—
prior to combustion	T59.891	T59.892	T59.893	T59.894	—	—
Ilopan	T45.2X1	T45.2X2	T45.2X3	T45.2X4	T45.2X5	T45.2X6
Iloprost	T46.7X1	T46.7X2	T46.7X3	T46.7X4	T46.7X5	T46.7X6
Ilotycin	T36.3X1	T36.3X2	T36.3X3	T36.3X4	T36.3X5	T36.3X6
ophthalmic preparation	T49.5X1	T49.5X2	T49.5X3	T49.5X4	T49.5X5	T49.5X6
topical NEC	T49.ØX1	T49.ØX2	T49.ØX3	T49.ØX4	T49.ØX5	T49.ØX6
Imdur*	T46.3X1	T46.3X2	T46.3X3	T46.3X4	T46.3X5	T46.3X6
Imidazole-4-carboxamide	T45.1X1	T45.1X2	T45.1X3	T45.1X4	T45.1X5	T45.1X6
Iminostilbene	T42.1X1	T42.1X2	T42.1X3	T42.1X4	T42.1X5	T42.1X6
Imipenem	T36.ØX1	T36.ØX2	T36.ØX3	T36.ØX4	T36.ØX5	T36.ØX6
Imipramine	T43.011	T43.012	T43.013	T43.014	T43.015	T43.016
Immu-G	T5Ø.Z11	T5Ø.Z12	T5Ø.Z13	T5Ø.Z14	T5Ø.Z15	T5Ø.Z16
Immuglobin	T5Ø.Z11	T5Ø.Z12	T5Ø.Z13	T5Ø.Z14	T5Ø.Z15	T5Ø.Z16
Immune						
globulin	T5Ø.Z11	T5Ø.Z12	T5Ø.Z13	T5Ø.Z14	T5Ø.Z15	T5Ø.Z16
serum globulin	T5Ø.Z11	T5Ø.Z12	T5Ø.Z13	T5Ø.Z14	T5Ø.Z15	T5Ø.Z16
Immunoglobin human (intravenous) (normal)	T5Ø.Z11	T5Ø.Z12	T5Ø.Z13	T5Ø.Z14	T5Ø.Z15	T5Ø.Z16
unmodified	T5Ø.Z11	T5Ø.Z12	T5Ø.Z13	T5Ø.Z14	T5Ø.Z15	T5Ø.Z16
Immunosuppressive drug	T45.1X1	T45.1X2	T45.1X3	T45.1X4	T45.1X5	T45.1X6
Immu-tetanus	T5Ø.Z11	T5Ø.Z12	T5Ø.Z13	T5Ø.Z14	T5Ø.Z15	T5Ø.Z16
Indalpine	T43.221	T43.222	T43.223	T43.224	T43.225	T43.226
Indanazoline	T48.5X1	T48.5X2	T48.5X3	T48.5X4	T48.5X5	T48.5X6
Indandione (derivatives)	T45.511	T45.512	T45.513	T45.514	T45.515	T45.516
Indapamide	T46.5X1	T46.5X2	T46.5X3	T46.5X4	T46.5X5	T46.5X6
Indendione (derivatives)	T45.511	T45.512	T45.513	T45.514	T45.515	T45.516
Indenolol	T44.7X1	T44.7X2	T44.7X3	T44.7X4	T44.7X5	T44.7X6
Inderal	T44.7X1	T44.7X2	T44.7X3	T44.7X4	T44.7X5	T44.7X6
Indian						
hemp	T4Ø.711	T4Ø.712	T4Ø.713	T4Ø.714	T4Ø.715	T4Ø.716
tobacco	T62.2X1	T62.2X2	T62.2X3	T62.2X4	—	—
Indigo carmine	T5Ø.8X1	T5Ø.8X2	T5Ø.8X3	T5Ø.8X4	T5Ø.8X5	T5Ø.8X6
Indobufen	T45.521	T45.522	T45.523	T45.524	T45.525	T45.526
Indocin	T39.2X1	T39.2X2	T39.2X3	T39.2X4	T39.2X5	T39.2X6
Indocyanine green	T5Ø.8X1	T5Ø.8X2	T5Ø.8X3	T5Ø.8X4	T5Ø.8X5	T5Ø.8X6
Indometacin	T39.391	T39.392	T39.393	T39.394	T39.395	T39.396
Indomethacin	T39.391	T39.392	T39.393	T39.394	T39.395	T39.396
farnesil	T39.4X1	T39.4X2	T39.4X3	T39.4X4	T39.4X5	T39.4X6
Indoramin	T44.6X1	T44.6X2	T44.6X3	T44.6X4	T44.6X5	T44.6X6
Industrial						
alcohol	T51.ØX1	T51.ØX2	T51.ØX3	T51.ØX4	—	—
fumes	T59.891	T59.892	T59.893	T59.894	—	—
solvents (fumes) (vapors)	T52.91	T52.92	T52.93	T52.94	—	—
Inflectra*	T39.4X1	T39.4X2	T39.4X3	T39.4X4	T39.4X5	T39.4X6
Influenza vaccine	T5Ø.B91	T5Ø.B92	T5Ø.B93	T5Ø.B94	T5Ø.B95	T5Ø.B96
Ingested substance NEC	T65.91	T65.92	T65.93	T65.94	—	—
INH	T37.1X1	T37.1X2	T37.1X3	T37.1X4	T37.1X5	T37.1X6
Inhalation, gas (noxious) — *see* Gas						
Inhibitor						
angiotensin-converting enzyme	T46.4X1	T46.4X2	T46.4X3	T46.4X4	T46.4X5	T46.4X6
carbonic anhydrase	T5Ø.2X1	T5Ø.2X2	T5Ø.2X3	T5Ø.2X4	T5Ø.2X5	T5Ø.2X6
fibrinolysis	T45.621	T45.622	T45.623	T45.624	T45.625	T45.626
monoamine oxidase NEC	T43.1X1	T43.1X2	T43.1X3	T43.1X4	T43.1X5	T43.1X6
hydrazine	T43.1X1	T43.1X2	T43.1X3	T43.1X4	T43.1X5	T43.1X6
postsynaptic	T43.8X1	T43.8X2	T43.8X3	T43.8X4	T43.8X5	T43.8X6
prothrombin synthesis	T45.511	T45.512	T45.513	T45.514	T45.515	T45.516
Ink	T65.891	T65.892	T65.893	T65.894	—	—
Innopran*	T44.7X1	T44.7X2	T44.7X3	T44.7X4	T44.7X5	T44.7X6
Inorganic substance NEC	T57.91	T57.92	T57.93	T57.94	—	—
Inosine pranobex	T37.5X1	T37.5X2	T37.5X3	T37.5X4	T37.5X5	T37.5X6
Inositol	T5Ø.991	T5Ø.992	T5Ø.993	T5Ø.994	T5Ø.995	T5Ø.996
nicotinate	T46.7X1	T46.7X2	T46.7X3	T46.7X4	T46.7X5	T46.7X6
Inproquone	T45.1X1	T45.1X2	T45.1X3	T45.1X4	T45.1X5	T45.1X6
Insecticide NEC	T6Ø.91	T6Ø.92	T6Ø.93	T6Ø.94	—	—
carbamate	T6Ø.ØX1	T6Ø.ØX2	T6Ø.ØX3	T6Ø.ØX4	—	—
chlorinated	T6Ø.1X1	T6Ø.1X2	T6Ø.1X3	T6Ø.1X4	—	—
mixed	T6Ø.91	T6Ø.92	T6Ø.93	T6Ø.94	—	—
organochlorine	T6Ø.1X1	T6Ø.1X2	T6Ø.1X3	T6Ø.1X4	—	—
organophosphorus	T6Ø.ØX1	T6Ø.ØX2	T6Ø.ØX3	T6Ø.ØX4	—	—
Insect (sting), venomous	T63.481	T63.482	T63.483	T63.484	—	—
ant	T63.421	T63.422	T63.423	T63.424	—	—
bee	T63.441	T63.442	T63.443	T63.444	—	—
caterpillar	T63.431	T63.432	T63.433	T63.434	—	—
hornet	T63.451	T63.452	T63.453	T63.454	—	—
wasp	T63.461	T63.462	T63.463	T63.464	—	—
Insular tissue extract	T38.3X1	T38.3X2	T38.3X3	T38.3X4	T38.3X5	T38.3X6
Insulin (amorphous) (globin) (isophane) (Lente) (NPH) (Semilente) (Ultralente)	T38.3X1	T38.3X2	T38.3X3	T38.3X4	T38.3X5	T38.3X6
defalan	T38.3X1	T38.3X2	T38.3X3	T38.3X4	T38.3X5	T38.3X6
human	T38.3X1	T38.3X2	T38.3X3	T38.3X4	T38.3X5	T38.3X6
injection, soluble	T38.3X1	T38.3X2	T38.3X3	T38.3X4	T38.3X5	T38.3X6
biphasic	T38.3X1	T38.3X2	T38.3X3	T38.3X4	T38.3X5	T38.3X6
intermediate acting	T38.3X1	T38.3X2	T38.3X3	T38.3X4	T38.3X5	T38.3X6
protamine zinc	T38.3X1	T38.3X2	T38.3X3	T38.3X4	T38.3X5	T38.3X6
slow acting	T38.3X1	T38.3X2	T38.3X3	T38.3X4	T38.3X5	T38.3X6
zinc						
protamine injection	T38.3X1	T38.3X2	T38.3X3	T38.3X4	T38.3X5	T38.3X6
suspension (amorphous) (crystalline)	T38.3X1	T38.3X2	T38.3X3	T38.3X4	T38.3X5	T38.3X6
Interferon (alpha) (beta) (gamma)	T37.5X1	T37.5X2	T37.5X3	T37.5X4	T37.5X5	T37.5X6
Intestinal motility control drug	T47.6X1	T47.6X2	T47.6X3	T47.6X4	T47.6X5	T47.6X6
biological	T47.8X1	T47.8X2	T47.8X3	T47.8X4	T47.8X5	T47.8X6
Intranarcon	T41.1X1	T41.1X2	T41.1X3	T41.1X4	T41.1X5	T41.1X6
Intravenous						
amino acids	T5Ø.991	T5Ø.992	T5Ø.993	T5Ø.994	T5Ø.995	T5Ø.996
fat suspension	T5Ø.991	T5Ø.992	T5Ø.993	T5Ø.994	T5Ø.995	T5Ø.996
Inulin	T5Ø.8X1	T5Ø.8X2	T5Ø.8X3	T5Ø.8X4	T5Ø.8X5	T5Ø.8X6
Invanz*	T36.1X1	T36.1X2	T36.1X3	T36.1X4	T36.1X5	T36.1X6
Invert sugar	T5Ø.3X1	T5Ø.3X2	T5Ø.3X3	T5Ø.3X4	T5Ø.3X5	T5Ø.3X6
Inza — *see* Naproxen						
Iobenzamic acid	T5Ø.8X1	T5Ø.8X2	T5Ø.8X3	T5Ø.8X4	T5Ø.8X5	T5Ø.8X6
Iocarmic acid	T5Ø.8X1	T5Ø.8X2	T5Ø.8X3	T5Ø.8X4	T5Ø.8X5	T5Ø.8X6
Iocetamic acid	T5Ø.8X1	T5Ø.8X2	T5Ø.8X3	T5Ø.8X4	T5Ø.8X5	T5Ø.8X6
Iodamide	T5Ø.8X1	T5Ø.8X2	T5Ø.8X3	T5Ø.8X4	T5Ø.8X5	T5Ø.8X6
Iodide NEC — *see also* Iodine	T49.ØX1	T49.ØX2	T49.ØX3	T49.ØX4	T49.ØX5	T49.ØX6
mercury (ointment)	T49.ØX1	T49.ØX2	T49.ØX3	T49.ØX4	T49.ØX5	T49.ØX6
methylate	T49.ØX1	T49.ØX2	T49.ØX3	T49.ØX4	T49.ØX5	T49.ØX6
potassium (expectorant) NEC	T48.4X1	T48.4X2	T48.4X3	T48.4X4	T48.4X5	T48.4X6
Iodinated						
contrast medium	T5Ø.8X1	T5Ø.8X2	T5Ø.8X3	T5Ø.8X4	T5Ø.8X5	T5Ø.8X6
glycerol	T48.4X1	T48.4X2	T48.4X3	T48.4X4	T48.4X5	T48.4X6
human serum albumin (131I)	T5Ø.8X1	T5Ø.8X2	T5Ø.8X3	T5Ø.8X4	T5Ø.8X5	T5Ø.8X6
Iodine (antiseptic, external) (tincture) **NEC**	T49.ØX1	T49.ØX2	T49.ØX3	T49.ØX4	T49.ØX5	T49.ØX6
125 — *see also* Radiation sickness, and Exposure to radioactive isotopes	T5Ø.8X1	T5Ø.8X2	T5Ø.8X3	T5Ø.8X4	T5Ø.8X5	T5Ø.8X6
therapeutic	T5Ø.991	T5Ø.992	T5Ø.993	T5Ø.994	T5Ø.995	T5Ø.996
131 — *see also* Radiation sickness, and Exposure to radioactive isotopes	T5Ø.8X1	T5Ø.8X2	T5Ø.8X3	T5Ø.8X4	T5Ø.8X5	T5Ø.8X6
therapeutic	T38.2X1	T38.2X2	T38.2X3	T38.2X4	T38.2X5	T38.2X6
diagnostic	T5Ø.8X1	T5Ø.8X2	T5Ø.8X3	T5Ø.8X4	T5Ø.8X5	T5Ø.8X6
for thyroid conditions (antithyroid)	T38.2X1	T38.2X2	T38.2X3	T38.2X4	T38.2X5	T38.2X6
solution	T49.ØX1	T49.ØX2	T49.ØX3	T49.ØX4	T49.ØX5	T49.ØX6
vapor	T59.891	T59.892	T59.893	T59.894	—	—
Iodipamide	T5Ø.8X1	T5Ø.8X2	T5Ø.8X3	T5Ø.8X4	T5Ø.8X5	T5Ø.8X6
Iodized (poppy seed) oil	T5Ø.8X1	T5Ø.8X2	T5Ø.8X3	T5Ø.8X4	T5Ø.8X5	T5Ø.8X6
Iodobismitol	T37.8X1	T37.8X2	T37.8X3	T37.8X4	T37.8X5	T37.8X6
Iodochlorhydroxyquin	T37.8X1	T37.8X2	T37.8X3	T37.8X4	T37.8X5	T37.8X6
topical	T49.ØX1	T49.ØX2	T49.ØX3	T49.ØX4	T49.ØX5	T49.ØX6
Iodochlorhydroxyquinoline	T37.8X1	T37.8X2	T37.8X3	T37.8X4	T37.8X5	T37.8X6
Iodocholesterol (131I)	T5Ø.8X1	T5Ø.8X2	T5Ø.8X3	T5Ø.8X4	T5Ø.8X5	T5Ø.8X6
Iodoform	T49.ØX1	T49.ØX2	T49.ØX3	T49.ØX4	T49.ØX5	T49.ØX6

Substance	Poisoning, Accidental (unintentional)	Poisoning, Intentional Self-harm	Poisoning, Assault	Poisoning, Undetermined	Adverse Effect	Under-dosing
Iodohippuric acid	T5Ø.8X1	T5Ø.8X2	T5Ø.8X3	T5Ø.8X4	T5Ø.8X5	T5Ø.8X6
Iodopanoic acid	T5Ø.8X1	T5Ø.8X2	T5Ø.8X3	T5Ø.8X4	T5Ø.8X5	T5Ø.8X6
Iodophthalein (sodium)	T5Ø.8X1	T5Ø.8X2	T5Ø.8X3	T5Ø.8X4	T5Ø.8X5	T5Ø.8X6
Iodopyracet	T5Ø.8X1	T5Ø.8X2	T5Ø.8X3	T5Ø.8X4	T5Ø.8X5	T5Ø.8X6
Iodoquinol	T37.8X1	T37.8X2	T37.8X3	T37.8X4	T37.8X5	T37.8X6
Iodoxamic acid	T5Ø.8X1	T5Ø.8X2	T5Ø.8X3	T5Ø.8X4	T5Ø.8X5	T5Ø.8X6
Iofendylate	T5Ø.8X1	T5Ø.8X2	T5Ø.8X3	T5Ø.8X4	T5Ø.8X5	T5Ø.8X6
Ioglycamic acid	T5Ø.8X1	T5Ø.8X2	T5Ø.8X3	T5Ø.8X4	T5Ø.8X5	T5Ø.8X6
Iohexol	T5Ø.8X1	T5Ø.8X2	T5Ø.8X3	T5Ø.8X4	T5Ø.8X5	T5Ø.8X6
Ion exchange resin						
anion	T47.8X1	T47.8X2	T47.8X3	T47.8X4	T47.8X5	T47.8X6
cation	T5Ø.3X1	T5Ø.3X2	T5Ø.3X3	T5Ø.3X4	T5Ø.3X5	T5Ø.3X6
cholestyramine	T46.6X1	T46.6X2	T46.6X3	T46.6X4	T46.6X5	T46.6X6
intestinal	T47.8X1	T47.8X2	T47.8X3	T47.8X4	T47.8X5	T47.8X6
Iopamidol	T5Ø.8X1	T5Ø.8X2	T5Ø.8X3	T5Ø.8X4	T5Ø.8X5	T5Ø.8X6
Iopanoic acid	T5Ø.8X1	T5Ø.8X2	T5Ø.8X3	T5Ø.8X4	T5Ø.8X5	T5Ø.8X6
Iophenoic acid	T5Ø.8X1	T5Ø.8X2	T5Ø.8X3	T5Ø.8X4	T5Ø.8X5	T5Ø.8X6
Iopodate, sodium	T5Ø.8X1	T5Ø.8X2	T5Ø.8X3	T5Ø.8X4	T5Ø.8X5	T5Ø.8X6
Iopodic acid	T5Ø.8X1	T5Ø.8X2	T5Ø.8X3	T5Ø.8X4	T5Ø.8X5	T5Ø.8X6
Iopromide	T5Ø.8X1	T5Ø.8X2	T5Ø.8X3	T5Ø.8X4	T5Ø.8X5	T5Ø.8X6
Iopydol	T5Ø.8X1	T5Ø.8X2	T5Ø.8X3	T5Ø.8X4	T5Ø.8X5	T5Ø.8X6
Iotalamic acid	T5Ø.8X1	T5Ø.8X2	T5Ø.8X3	T5Ø.8X4	T5Ø.8X5	T5Ø.8X6
Iothalamate	T5Ø.8X1	T5Ø.8X2	T5Ø.8X3	T5Ø.8X4	T5Ø.8X5	T5Ø.8X6
Iothiouracil	T38.2X1	T38.2X2	T38.2X3	T38.2X4	T38.2X5	T38.2X6
Iotrol	T5Ø.8X1	T5Ø.8X2	T5Ø.8X3	T5Ø.8X4	T5Ø.8X5	T5Ø.8X6
Iotrolan	T5Ø.8X1	T5Ø.8X2	T5Ø.8X3	T5Ø.8X4	T5Ø.8X5	T5Ø.8X6
Iotroxate	T5Ø.8X1	T5Ø.8X2	T5Ø.8X3	T5Ø.8X4	T5Ø.8X5	T5Ø.8X6
Iotroxic acid	T5Ø.8X1	T5Ø.8X2	T5Ø.8X3	T5Ø.8X4	T5Ø.8X5	T5Ø.8X6
Ioversol	T5Ø.8X1	T5Ø.8X2	T5Ø.8X3	T5Ø.8X4	T5Ø.8X5	T5Ø.8X6
Ioxaglate	T5Ø.8X1	T5Ø.8X2	T5Ø.8X3	T5Ø.8X4	T5Ø.8X5	T5Ø.8X6
Ioxaglic acid	T5Ø.8X1	T5Ø.8X2	T5Ø.8X3	T5Ø.8X4	T5Ø.8X5	T5Ø.8X6
Ioxitalamic acid	T5Ø.8X1	T5Ø.8X2	T5Ø.8X3	T5Ø.8X4	T5Ø.8X5	T5Ø.8X6
Ipecac	T47.7X1	T47.7X2	T47.7X3	T47.7X4	T47.7X5	T47.7X6
Ipecacuanha	T48.4X1	T48.4X2	T48.4X3	T48.4X4	T48.4X5	T48.4X6
Ipodate, calcium	T5Ø.8X1	T5Ø.8X2	T5Ø.8X3	T5Ø.8X4	T5Ø.8X5	T5Ø.8X6
IPOL*	T5Ø.B91	T5Ø.B92	T5Ø.B93	T5Ø.B94	T5Ø.B95	T5Ø.B96
Ipral	T42.3X1	T42.3X2	T42.3X3	T42.3X4	T42.3X5	T42.3X6
Ipratropium (bromide)	T48.6X1	T48.6X2	T48.6X3	T48.6X4	T48.6X5	T48.6X6
Ipriflavone	T46.3X1	T46.3X2	T46.3X3	T46.3X4	T46.3X5	T46.3X6
Iprindole	T43.Ø11	T43.Ø12	T43.Ø13	T43.Ø14	T43.Ø15	T43.Ø16
Iproclozide	T43.1X1	T43.1X2	T43.1X3	T43.1X4	T43.1X5	T43.1X6
Iprofenin	T5Ø.8X1	T5Ø.8X2	T5Ø.8X3	T5Ø.8X4	T5Ø.8X5	T5Ø.8X6
Iproheptine	T49.2X1	T49.2X2	T49.2X3	T49.2X4	T49.2X5	T49.2X6
Iproniazid	T43.1X1	T43.1X2	T43.1X3	T43.1X4	T43.1X5	T43.1X6
Iproplatin	T45.1X1	T45.1X2	T45.1X3	T45.1X4	T45.1X5	T45.1X6
Iproveratril	T46.1X1	T46.1X2	T46.1X3	T46.1X4	T46.1X5	T46.1X6
Irinotecan*	T45.1X1	T45.1X2	T45.1X3	T45.1X4	T45.1X5	T45.1X6
Iron (compounds) (medicinal) **NEC**	T45.4X1	T45.4X2	T45.4X3	T45.4X4	T45.4X5	T45.4X6
ammonium	T45.4X1	T45.4X2	T45.4X3	T45.4X4	T45.4X5	T45.4X6
dextran injection	T45.4X1	T45.4X2	T45.4X3	T45.4X4	T45.4X5	T45.4X6
nonmedicinal	T56.891	T56.892	T56.893	T56.894	—	—
salts	T45.4X1	T45.4X2	T45.4X3	T45.4X4	T45.4X5	T45.4X6
sorbitex	T45.4X1	T45.4X2	T45.4X3	T45.4X4	T45.4X5	T45.4X6
sorbitol citric acid complex	T45.4X1	T45.4X2	T45.4X3	T45.4X4	T45.4X5	T45.4X6
Irrigating fluid (vaginal)	T49.8X1	T49.8X2	T49.8X3	T49.8X4	T49.8X5	T49.8X6
eye	T49.5X1	T49.5X2	T49.5X3	T49.5X4	T49.5X5	T49.5X6
Isepamicin	T36.5X1	T36.5X2	T36.5X3	T36.5X4	T36.5X5	T36.5X6
Isoaminile (citrate)	T48.3X1	T48.3X2	T48.3X3	T48.3X4	T48.3X5	T48.3X6
Isoamyl nitrite	T46.3X1	T46.3X2	T46.3X3	T46.3X4	T46.3X5	T46.3X6
Isobenzan	T6Ø.1X1	T6Ø.1X2	T6Ø.1X3	T6Ø.1X4	—	—
Isobutyl acetate	T52.8X1	T52.8X2	T52.8X3	T52.8X4	—	—
Isocarboxazid	T43.1X1	T43.1X2	T43.1X3	T43.1X4	T43.1X5	T43.1X6
Isoconazole	T49.ØX1	T49.ØX2	T49.ØX3	T49.ØX4	T49.ØX5	T49.ØX6
Isocyanate	T65.ØX1	T65.ØX2	T65.ØX3	T65.ØX4	—	—
Isoephedrine	T44.991	T44.992	T44.993	T44.994	T44.995	T44.996
Isoetarine	T48.6X1	T48.6X2	T48.6X3	T48.6X4	T48.6X5	T48.6X6
Isoethadione	T42.2X1	T42.2X2	T42.2X3	T42.2X4	T42.2X5	T42.2X6
Isoetharine	T44.5X1	T44.5X2	T44.5X3	T44.5X4	T44.5X5	T44.5X6
Isoflurane	T41.ØX1	T41.ØX2	T41.ØX3	T41.ØX4	T41.ØX5	T41.ØX6
Isoflurophate	T44.ØX1	T44.ØX2	T44.ØX3	T44.ØX4	T44.ØX5	T44.ØX6
Isomaltose, ferric complex	T45.4X1	T45.4X2	T45.4X3	T45.4X4	T45.4X5	T45.4X6
Isometheptene	T44.3X1	T44.3X2	T44.3X3	T44.3X4	T44.3X5	T44.3X6
Isoniazid	T37.1X1	T37.1X2	T37.1X3	T37.1X4	T37.1X5	T37.1X6
with						
rifampicin	T36.6X1	T36.6X2	T36.6X3	T36.6X4	T36.6X5	T36.6X6
thioacetazone	T37.1X1	T37.1X2	T37.1X3	T37.1X4	T37.1X5	T37.1X6
Isonicotinic acid hydrazide	T37.1X1	T37.1X2	T37.1X3	T37.1X4	T37.1X5	T37.1X6
Isonipecaine	T4Ø.491	T4Ø.492	T4Ø.493	T4Ø.494	T4Ø.495	T4Ø.496
Isopentaquine	T37.2X1	T37.2X2	T37.2X3	T37.2X4	T37.2X5	T37.2X6
Isophane insulin	T38.3X1	T38.3X2	T38.3X3	T38.3X4	T38.3X5	T38.3X6
Isophorone	T65.891	T65.892	T65.893	T65.894	—	—
Isophosphamide	T45.1X1	T45.1X2	T45.1X3	T45.1X4	T45.1X5	T45.1X6

Substance	Poisoning, Accidental (unintentional)	Poisoning, Intentional Self-harm	Poisoning, Assault	Poisoning, Undetermined	Adverse Effect	Under-dosing
Isopregnenone	T38.5X1	T38.5X2	T38.5X3	T38.5X4	T38.5X5	T38.5X6
Isoprenaline	T48.6X1	T48.6X2	T48.6X3	T48.6X4	T48.6X5	T48.6X6
Isopromethazine	T43.3X1	T43.3X2	T43.3X3	T43.3X4	T43.3X5	T43.3X6
Isopropamide	T44.3X1	T44.3X2	T44.3X3	T44.3X4	T44.3X5	T44.3X6
iodide	T44.3X1	T44.3X2	T44.3X3	T44.3X4	T44.3X5	T44.3X6
Isopropanol	T51.2X1	T51.2X2	T51.2X3	T51.2X4	—	—
Isopropyl						
acetate	T52.8X1	T52.8X2	T52.8X3	T52.8X4	—	—
alcohol	T51.2X1	T51.2X2	T51.2X3	T51.2X4	—	—
medicinal	T49.4X1	T49.4X2	T49.4X3	T49.4X4	T49.4X5	T49.4X6
ether	T52.8X1	T52.8X2	T52.8X3	T52.8X4	—	—
Isopropylaminophenazone	T39.2X1	T39.2X2	T39.2X3	T39.2X4	T39.2X5	T39.2X6
Isoproterenol	T48.6X1	T48.6X2	T48.6X3	T48.6X4	T48.6X5	T48.6X6
Isosorbide dinitrate	T46.3X1	T46.3X2	T46.3X3	T46.3X4	T46.3X5	T46.3X6
Isothipendyl	T45.ØX1	T45.ØX2	T45.ØX3	T45.ØX4	T45.ØX5	T45.ØX6
Isotretinoin	T5Ø.991	T5Ø.992	T5Ø.993	T5Ø.994	T5Ø.995	T5Ø.996
Isoxazolyl penicillin	T36.ØX1	T36.ØX2	T36.ØX3	T36.ØX4	T36.ØX5	T36.ØX6
Isoxicam	T39.391	T39.392	T39.393	T39.394	T39.395	T39.396
Isoxsuprine	T46.7X1	T46.7X2	T46.7X3	T46.7X4	T46.7X5	T46.7X6
Ispagula	T47.4X1	T47.4X2	T47.4X3	T47.4X4	T47.4X5	T47.4X6
husk	T47.4X1	T47.4X2	T47.4X3	T47.4X4	T47.4X5	T47.4X6
Isradipine	T46.1X1	T46.1X2	T46.1X3	T46.1X4	T46.1X5	T46.1X6
I-thyroxine sodium	T38.1X1	T38.1X2	T38.1X3	T38.1X4	T38.1X5	T38.1X6
Itraconazole	T37.8X1	T37.8X2	T37.8X3	T37.8X4	T37.8X5	T37.8X6
Itramin tosilate	T46.3X1	T46.3X2	T46.3X3	T46.3X4	T46.3X5	T46.3X6
Ivarest*	T41.3X1	T41.3X2	T41.3X3	T41.3X4	T41.3X5	T41.3X6
Ivermectin	T37.4X1	T37.4X2	T37.4X3	T37.4X4	T37.4X5	T37.4X6
Izoniazid	T37.1X1	T37.1X2	T37.1X3	T37.1X4	T37.1X5	T37.1X6
with thioacetazone	T37.1X1	T37.1X2	T37.1X3	T37.1X4	T37.1X5	T37.1X6
Jalap	T47.2X1	T47.2X2	T47.2X3	T47.2X4	T47.2X5	T47.2X6
Jamaica						
dogwood (bark)	T39.8X1	T39.8X2	T39.8X3	T39.8X4	T39.8X5	T39.8X6
ginger	T65.891	T65.892	T65.893	T65.894	—	—
root	T62.2X1	T62.2X2	T62.2X3	T62.2X4	—	—
Jantoven*	T45.511	T45.512	T45.513	T45.514	T45.515	T45.516
Jatropha	T62.2X1	T62.2X2	T62.2X3	T62.2X4	—	—
curcas	T62.2X1	T62.2X2	T62.2X3	T62.2X4	—	—
Jectofer	T45.4X1	T45.4X2	T45.4X3	T45.4X4	T45.4X5	T45.4X6
Jellyfish (sting)	T63.621	T63.622	T63.623	T63.624	—	—
Jequirity (bean)	T62.2X1	T62.2X2	T62.2X3	T62.2X4	—	—
Jimson weed (stramonium)	T62.2X1	T62.2X2	T62.2X3	T62.2X4	—	—
seeds	T62.2X1	T62.2X2	T62.2X3	T62.2X4	—	—
Josamycin	T36.3X1	T36.3X2	T36.3X3	T36.3X4	T36.3X5	T36.3X6
Juniper tar	T49.1X1	T49.1X2	T49.1X3	T49.1X4	T49.1X5	T49.1X6
Kaletra*	T37.5X1	T37.5X2	T37.5X3	T37.5X4	T37.5X5	T37.5X6
Kallidinogenase	T46.7X1	T46.7X2	T46.7X3	T46.7X4	T46.7X5	T46.7X6
Kallikrein	T46.7X1	T46.7X2	T46.7X3	T46.7X4	T46.7X5	T46.7X6
Kanamycin	T36.5X1	T36.5X2	T36.5X3	T36.5X4	T36.5X5	T36.5X6
Kantrex	T36.5X1	T36.5X2	T36.5X3	T36.5X4	T36.5X5	T36.5X6
Kaolin	T47.6X1	T47.6X2	T47.6X3	T47.6X4	T47.6X5	T47.6X6
light	T47.6X1	T47.6X2	T47.6X3	T47.6X4	T47.6X5	T47.6X6
Karaya (gum)	T47.4X1	T47.4X2	T47.4X3	T47.4X4	T47.4X5	T47.4X6
Kebuzone	T39.2X1	T39.2X2	T39.2X3	T39.2X4	T39.2X5	T39.2X6
Kelevan	T6Ø.1X1	T6Ø.1X2	T6Ø.1X3	T6Ø.1X4	—	—
Kemithal	T41.1X1	T41.1X2	T41.1X3	T41.1X4	T41.1X5	T41.1X6
Kenacort	T38.ØX1	T38.ØX2	T38.ØX3	T38.ØX4	T38.ØX5	T38.ØX6
Keratolytic drug NEC	T49.4X1	T49.4X2	T49.4X3	T49.4X4	T49.4X5	T49.4X6
anthracene	T49.4X1	T49.4X2	T49.4X3	T49.4X4	T49.4X5	T49.4X6
Keratoplastic NEC	T49.4X1	T49.4X2	T49.4X3	T49.4X4	T49.4X5	T49.4X6
Kerosene, kerosine (fuel) (solvent) **NEC**	T52.ØX1	T52.ØX2	T52.ØX3	T52.ØX4	—	—
insecticide	T52.ØX1	T52.ØX2	T52.ØX3	T52.ØX4	—	—
vapor	T52.ØX1	T52.ØX2	T52.ØX3	T52.ØX4	—	—
Ketamine	T41.291	T41.292	T41.293	T41.294	T41.295	T41.296
Ketazolam	T42.4X1	T42.4X2	T42.4X3	T42.4X4	T42.4X5	T42.4X6
Ketazon	T39.2X1	T39.2X2	T39.2X3	T39.2X4	T39.2X5	T39.2X6
Ketobemidone	T4Ø.491	T4Ø.492	T4Ø.493	T4Ø.494	—	—
Ketoconazole	T49.ØX1	T49.ØX2	T49.ØX3	T49.ØX4	T49.ØX5	T49.ØX6
Ketols	T52.4X1	T52.4X2	T52.4X3	T52.4X4	—	—
Ketone oils	T52.4X1	T52.4X2	T52.4X3	T52.4X4	—	—
Ketoprofen	T39.311	T39.312	T39.313	T39.314	T39.315	T39.316
Ketorolac	T39.8X1	T39.8X2	T39.8X3	T39.8X4	T39.8X5	T39.8X6
Ketotifen	T45.ØX1	T45.ØX2	T45.ØX3	T45.ØX4	T45.ØX5	T45.ØX6
Keytruda*	T45.1X1	T45.1X2	T45.1X3	T45.1X4	T45.1X5	T45.1X6
Khat	T43.691	T43.692	T43.693	T43.694	—	—
Khellin	T46.3X1	T46.3X2	T46.3X3	T46.3X4	T46.3X5	T46.3X6
Khelloside	T46.3X1	T46.3X2	T46.3X3	T46.3X4	T46.3X5	T46.3X6
Kiln gas or vapor (carbon monoxide)	T58.8X1	T58.8X2	T58.8X3	T58.8X4	—	—
Kineret*	T39.4X1	T39.4X2	T39.4X3	T39.4X4	T39.4X5	T39.4X6
Kitasamycin	T36.3X1	T36.3X2	T36.3X3	T36.3X4	T36.3X5	T36.3X6
Komgiblyze*	T38.3X1	T38.3X2	T38.3X3	T38.3X4	T38.3X5	T38.3X6
Konsyl	T47.4X1	T47.4X2	T47.4X3	T47.4X4	T47.4X5	T47.4X6

Substance	Poisoning, Accidental (unintentional)	Poisoning, Intentional Self-harm	Poisoning, Assault	Poisoning, Undetermined	Adverse Effect	Under-dosing
Kosam seed	T62.2X1	T62.2X2	T62.2X3	T62.2X4	—	—
Krait (venom)	T63.Ø91	T63.Ø92	T63.Ø93	T63.Ø94	—	—
Kwell (insecticide)	T6Ø.1X1	T6Ø.1X2	T6Ø.1X3	T6Ø.1X4	—	—
anti-infective (topical)	T49.ØX1	T49.ØX2	T49.ØX3	T49.ØX4	T49.ØX5	T49.ØX6
Labetalol	T44.8X1	T44.8X2	T44.8X3	T44.8X4	T44.8X5	T44.8X6
Laburnum (seeds)	T62.2X1	T62.2X2	T62.2X3	T62.2X4	—	—
leaves	T62.2X1	T62.2X2	T62.2X3	T62.2X4	—	—
Lachesine	T49.5X1	T49.5X2	T49.5X3	T49.5X4	T49.5X5	T49.5X6
Lacidipine	T46.5X1	T46.5X2	T46.5X3	T46.5X4	T46.5X5	T46.5X6
Lacquer	T65.6X1	T65.6X2	T65.6X3	T65.6X4	—	—
Lacrimogenic gas	T59.3X1	T59.3X2	T59.3X3	T59.3X4	—	—
Lactated potassic saline	T5Ø.3X1	T5Ø.3X2	T5Ø.3X3	T5Ø.3X4	T5Ø.3X5	T5Ø.3X6
Lactic acid	T49.8X1	T49.8X2	T49.8X3	T49.8X4	T49.8X5	T49.8X6
Lactobacillus						
acidophilus	T47.6X1	T47.6X2	T47.6X3	T47.6X4	T47.6X5	T47.6X6
compound	T47.6X1	T47.6X2	T47.6X3	T47.6X4	T47.6X5	T47.6X6
bifidus, lyophilized	T47.6X1	T47.6X2	T47.6X3	T47.6X4	T47.6X5	T47.6X6
bulgaricus	T47.6X1	T47.6X2	T47.6X3	T47.6X4	T47.6X5	T47.6X6
sporogenes	T47.6X1	T47.6X2	T47.6X3	T47.6X4	T47.6X5	T47.6X6
Lactoflavin	T45.2X1	T45.2X2	T45.2X3	T45.2X4	T45.2X5	T45.2X6
Lactose (as excipient)	T5Ø.9Ø1	T5Ø.9Ø2	T5Ø.9Ø3	T5Ø.9Ø4	T5Ø.9Ø5	T5Ø.9Ø6
Lactuca (virosa) (extract)	T42.6X1	T42.6X2	T42.6X3	T42.6X4	T42.6X5	T42.6X6
Lactucarium	T42.6X1	T42.6X2	T42.6X3	T42.6X4	T42.6X5	T42.6X6
Lactulose	T47.3X1	T47.3X2	T47.3X3	T47.3X4	T47.3X5	T47.3X6
Laevo — *see* Levo-						
Lanatosides	T46.ØX1	T46.ØX2	T46.ØX3	T46.ØX4	T46.ØX5	T46.ØX6
Lanolin	T49.3X1	T49.3X2	T49.3X3	T49.3X4	T49.3X5	T49.3X6
Lanoxin*	T46.ØX1	T46.ØX2	T46.ØX3	T46.ØX4	T46.ØX5	T46.ØX6
Largactil	T43.3X1	T43.3X2	T43.3X3	T43.3X4	T43.3X5	T43.3X6
Larkspur	T62.2X1	T62.2X2	T62.2X3	T62.2X4	—	—
Laroxyl	T43.Ø11	T43.Ø12	T43.Ø13	T43.Ø14	T43.Ø15	T43.Ø16
Lasix	T5Ø.1X1	T5Ø.1X2	T5Ø.1X3	T5Ø.1X4	T5Ø.1X5	T5Ø.1X6
Lassar's paste	T49.4X1	T49.4X2	T49.4X3	T49.4X4	T49.4X5	T49.4X6
Latamoxef	T36.1X1	T36.1X2	T36.1X3	T36.1X4	T36.1X5	T36.1X6
Latex	T65.811	T65.812	T65.813	T65.814	—	—
Lathyrus (seed)	T62.2X1	T62.2X2	T62.2X3	T62.2X4	—	—
Laudanum	T4Ø.ØX1	T4Ø.ØX2	T4Ø.ØX3	T4Ø.ØX4	T4Ø.ØX5	T4Ø.ØX6
Laudexium	T48.1X1	T48.1X2	T48.1X3	T48.1X4	T48.1X5	T48.1X6
Laughing gas	T41.ØX1	T41.ØX2	T41.ØX3	T41.ØX4	T41.ØX5	T41.ØX6
Laurel, black or cherry	T62.2X1	T62.2X2	T62.2X3	T62.2X4	—	—
Laurolinium	T49.ØX1	T49.ØX2	T49.ØX3	T49.ØX4	T49.ØX5	T49.ØX6
Lauryl sulfoacetate	T49.2X1	T49.2X2	T49.2X3	T49.2X4	T49.2X5	T49.2X6
Laxative NEC	T47.4X1	T47.4X2	T47.4X3	T47.4X4	T47.4X5	T47.4X6
osmotic	T47.3X1	T47.3X2	T47.3X3	T47.3X4	T47.3X5	T47.3X6
saline	T47.3X1	T47.3X2	T47.3X3	T47.3X4	T47.3X5	T47.3X6
stimulant	T47.2X1	T47.2X2	T47.2X3	T47.2X4	T47.2X5	T47.2X6
L-dopa	T42.8X1	T42.8X2	T42.8X3	T42.8X4	T42.8X5	T42.8X6
Lead (dust) (fumes) (vapor) **NEC**	T56.ØX1	T56.ØX2	T56.ØX3	T56.ØX4	—	—
acetate	T49.2X1	T49.2X2	T49.2X3	T49.2X4	T49.2X5	T49.2X6
alkyl (fuel additive)	T56.ØX1	T56.ØX2	T56.ØX3	T56.ØX4	—	—
anti-infectives	T37.8X1	T37.8X2	T37.8X3	T37.8X4	T37.8X5	T37.8X6
antiknock compound (tetraethyl)	T56.ØX1	T56.ØX2	T56.ØX3	T56.ØX4	—	—
arsenate, arsenite (dust)(herbicide) (insecticide) (vapor)	T57.ØX1	T57.ØX2	T57.ØX3	T57.ØX4	—	—
carbonate	T56.ØX1	T56.ØX2	T56.ØX3	T56.ØX4	—	—
paint	T56.ØX1	T56.ØX2	T56.ØX3	T56.ØX4	—	—
chromate	T56.ØX1	T56.ØX2	T56.ØX3	T56.ØX4	—	—
paint	T56.ØX1	T56.ØX2	T56.ØX3	T56.ØX4	—	—
dioxide	T56.ØX1	T56.ØX2	T56.ØX3	T56.ØX4	—	—
inorganic	T56.ØX1	T56.ØX2	T56.ØX3	T56.ØX4	—	—
iodide	T56.ØX1	T56.ØX2	T56.ØX3	T56.ØX4	—	—
pigment (paint)	T56.ØX1	T56.ØX2	T56.ØX3	T56.ØX4	—	—
monoxide (dust)	T56.ØX1	T56.ØX2	T56.ØX3	T56.ØX4	—	—
paint	T56.ØX1	T56.ØX2	T56.ØX3	T56.ØX4	—	—
organic	T56.ØX1	T56.ØX2	T56.ØX3	T56.ØX4	—	—
oxide	T56.ØX1	T56.ØX2	T56.ØX3	T56.ØX4	—	—
paint	T56.ØX1	T56.ØX2	T56.ØX3	T56.ØX4	—	—
paint	T56.ØX1	T56.ØX2	T56.ØX3	T56.ØX4	—	—
salts	T56.ØX1	T56.ØX2	T56.ØX3	T56.ØX4	—	—
specified compound NEC	T56.ØX1	T56.ØX2	T56.ØX3	T56.ØX4	—	—
tetra-ethyl	T56.ØX1	T56.ØX2	T56.ØX3	T56.ØX4	—	—
Lebanese red	T4Ø.711	T4Ø.712	T4Ø.713	T4Ø.714	T4Ø.715	T4Ø.716
Lefetamine	T39.8X1	T39.8X2	T39.8X3	T39.8X4	T39.8X5	T39.8X6
Lenperone	T43.4X1	T43.4X2	T43.4X3	T43.4X4	T43.4X5	T43.4X6
Lente lietin (insulin)	T38.3X1	T38.3X2	T38.3X3	T38.3X4	T38.3X5	T38.3X6
Leptazol	T5Ø.7X1	T5Ø.7X2	T5Ø.7X3	T5Ø.7X4	T5Ø.7X5	T5Ø.7X6
Leptophos	T6Ø.ØX1	T6Ø.ØX2	T6Ø.ØX3	T6Ø.ØX4	—	—
Leritine	T4Ø.2X1	T4Ø.2X2	T4Ø.2X3	T4Ø.2X4	T4Ø.2X5	T4Ø.2X6
Lescol*	T46.6X1	T46.6X2	T46.6X3	T46.6X4	T46.6X5	T46.6X6
Letosteine	T48.4X1	T48.4X2	T48.4X3	T48.4X4	T48.4X5	T48.4X6

Substance	Poisoning, Accidental (unintentional)	Poisoning, Intentional Self-harm	Poisoning, Assault	Poisoning, Undetermined	Adverse Effect	Under-dosing
Letter	T38.1X1	T38.1X2	T38.1X3	T38.1X4	T38.1X5	T38.1X6
Lettuce opium	T42.6X1	T42.6X2	T42.6X3	T42.6X4	T42.6X5	T42.6X6
Leucinocaine	T41.3X1	T41.3X2	T41.3X3	T41.3X4	T41.3X5	T41.3X6
Leucocianidol	T46.991	T46.992	T46.993	T46.994	T46.995	T46.996
Leucovorin (factor)	T45.8X1	T45.8X2	T45.8X3	T45.8X4	T45.8X5	T45.8X6
Leukeran	T45.1X1	T45.1X2	T45.1X3	T45.1X4	T45.1X5	T45.1X6
Leuprolide	T38.891	T38.892	T38.893	T38.894	T38.895	T38.896
Levalbuterol	T48.6X1	T48.6X2	T48.6X3	T48.6X4	T48.6X5	T48.6X6
Levallorphan	T5Ø.7X1	T5Ø.7X2	T5Ø.7X3	T5Ø.7X4	T5Ø.7X5	T5Ø.7X6
Levamisole	T37.4X1	T37.4X2	T37.4X3	T37.4X4	T37.4X5	T37.4X6
Levanil	T42.6X1	T42.6X2	T42.6X3	T42.6X4	T42.6X5	T42.6X6
Levarterenol	T44.4X1	T44.4X2	T44.4X3	T44.4X4	T44.4X5	T44.4X6
Levdropropizine	T48.3X1	T48.3X2	T48.3X3	T48.3X4	T48.3X5	T48.3X6
Levobunolol	T49.5X1	T49.5X2	T49.5X3	T49.5X4	T49.5X5	T49.5X6
Levocabastine (hydrochloride)	T45.ØX1	T45.ØX2	T45.ØX3	T45.ØX4	T45.ØX5	T45.ØX6
Levocarnitine	T5Ø.991	T5Ø.992	T5Ø.993	T5Ø.994	T5Ø.995	T5Ø.996
Levodopa	T42.8X1	T42.8X2	T42.8X3	T42.8X4	T42.8X5	T42.8X6
with carbidopa	T42.8X1	T42.8X2	T42.8X3	T42.8X4	T42.8X5	T42.8X6
Levo-dromoran	T4Ø.2X1	T4Ø.2X2	T4Ø.2X3	T4Ø.2X4	T4Ø.2X5	T4Ø.2X6
Levoglutamide	T5Ø.991	T5Ø.992	T5Ø.993	T5Ø.994	T5Ø.995	T5Ø.996
Levoid	T38.1X1	T38.1X2	T38.1X3	T38.1X4	T38.1X5	T38.1X6
Levo-isomethadone	T4Ø.3X1	T4Ø.3X2	T4Ø.3X3	T4Ø.3X4	T4Ø.3X5	T4Ø.3X6
Levomepromazine	T43.3X1	T43.3X2	T43.3X3	T43.3X4	T43.3X5	T43.3X6
Levonordefrin	T49.6X1	T49.6X2	T49.6X3	T49.6X4	T49.6X5	T49.6X6
Levonorgestrel	T38.4X1	T38.4X2	T38.4X3	T38.4X4	T38.4X5	T38.4X6
with ethinylestradiol	T38.5X1	T38.5X2	T38.5X3	T38.5X4	T38.5X5	T38.5X6
Levopromazine	T43.3X1	T43.3X2	T43.3X3	T43.3X4	T43.3X5	T43.3X6
Levoprome	T42.6X1	T42.6X2	T42.6X3	T42.6X4	T42.6X5	T42.6X6
Levopropoxyphene	T4Ø.491	T4Ø.492	T4Ø.493	T4Ø.494	T4Ø.495	T4Ø.496
Levopropylhexedrine	T5Ø.5X1	T5Ø.5X2	T5Ø.5X3	T5Ø.5X4	T5Ø.5X5	T5Ø.5X6
Levoproxyphylline	T48.6X1	T48.6X2	T48.6X3	T48.6X4	T48.6X5	T48.6X6
Levorphanol	T4Ø.491	T4Ø.492	T4Ø.493	T4Ø.494	T4Ø.495	T4Ø.496
Levothroid*	T38.1X1	T38.1X2	T38.1X3	T38.1X4	T38.1X5	T38.1X6
Levothyroxine	T38.1X1	T38.1X2	T38.1X3	T38.1X4	T38.1X5	T38.1X6
sodium	T38.1X1	T38.1X2	T38.1X3	T38.1X4	T38.1X5	T38.1X6
Levsin	T44.3X1	T44.3X2	T44.3X3	T44.3X4	T44.3X5	T44.3X6
Levulose	T5Ø.3X1	T5Ø.3X2	T5Ø.3X3	T5Ø.3X4	T5Ø.3X5	T5Ø.3X6
Lewisite (gas), not in war	T57.ØX1	T57.ØX2	T57.ØX3	T57.ØX4	—	—
Librium	T42.4X1	T42.4X2	T42.4X3	T42.4X4	T42.4X5	T42.4X6
Lidex	T49.ØX1	T49.ØX2	T49.ØX3	T49.ØX4	T49.ØX5	T49.ØX6
Lidocaine	T41.3X1	T41.3X2	T41.3X3	T41.3X4	T41.3X5	T41.3X6
regional	T41.3X1	T41.3X2	T41.3X3	T41.3X4	T41.3X5	T41.3X6
spinal	T41.3X1	T41.3X2	T41.3X3	T41.3X4	T41.3X5	T41.3X6
Lidofenin	T5Ø.8X1	T5Ø.8X2	T5Ø.8X3	T5Ø.8X4	T5Ø.8X5	T5Ø.8X6
Lidoflazine	T46.1X1	T46.1X2	T46.1X3	T46.1X4	T46.1X5	T46.1X6
Lighter fluid	T52.ØX1	T52.ØX2	T52.ØX3	T52.ØX4	—	—
Lignin hemicellulose	T47.6X1	T47.6X2	T47.6X3	T47.6X4	T47.6X5	T47.6X6
Lignocaine	T41.3X1	T41.3X2	T41.3X3	T41.3X4	T41.3X5	T41.3X6
regional	T41.3X1	T41.3X2	T41.3X3	T41.3X4	T41.3X5	T41.3X6
spinal	T41.3X1	T41.3X2	T41.3X3	T41.3X4	T41.3X5	T41.3X6
Ligroin (e) (solvent)	T52.ØX1	T52.ØX2	T52.ØX3	T52.ØX4	—	—
vapor	T59.891	T59.892	T59.893	T59.894	—	—
Ligustrum vulgare	T62.2X1	T62.2X2	T62.2X3	T62.2X4	—	—
Lily of the valley	T62.2X1	T62.2X2	T62.2X3	T62.2X4	—	—
Lime (chloride)	T54.3X1	T54.3X2	T54.3X3	T54.3X4	—	—
Limonene	T52.8X1	T52.8X2	T52.8X3	T52.8X4	—	—
Lincomycin	T36.8X1	T36.8X2	T36.8X3	T36.8X4	T36.8X5	T36.8X6
Lindane (insecticide) (nonmedicinal) (vapor)	T53.6X1	T53.6X2	T53.6X3	T53.6X4	—	—
medicinal	T49.ØX1	T49.ØX2	T49.ØX3	T49.ØX4	T49.ØX5	T49.ØX6
Liniments NEC	T49.91	T49.92	T49.93	T49.94	T49.95	T49.96
Linoleic acid	T46.6X1	T46.6X2	T46.6X3	T46.6X4	T46.6X5	T46.6X6
Linolenic acid	T46.6X1	T46.6X2	T46.6X3	T46.6X4	T46.6X5	T46.6X6
Linseed	T47.4X1	T47.4X2	T47.4X3	T47.4X4	T47.4X5	T47.4X6
Liothyronine	T38.1X1	T38.1X2	T38.1X3	T38.1X4	T38.1X5	T38.1X6
Liotrix	T38.1X1	T38.1X2	T38.1X3	T38.1X4	T38.1X5	T38.1X6
Lipancreatin	T47.5X1	T47.5X2	T47.5X3	T47.5X4	T47.5X5	T47.5X6
Lipo-alprostadil	T46.7X1	T46.7X2	T46.7X3	T46.7X4	T46.7X5	T46.7X6
Lipo-Lutin	T38.5X1	T38.5X2	T38.5X3	T38.5X4	T38.5X5	T38.5X6
Lipotropic drug NEC	T5Ø.9Ø1	T5Ø.9Ø2	T5Ø.9Ø3	T5Ø.9Ø4	T5Ø.9Ø5	T5Ø.9Ø6
Liquefied petroleum gases	T59.891	T59.892	T59.893	T59.894	—	—
piped (pure or mixed with air)	T59.891	T59.892	T59.893	T59.894	—	—
Liquid						
paraffin	T47.4X1	T47.4X2	T47.4X3	T47.4X4	T47.4X5	T47.4X6
petrolatum	T47.4X1	T47.4X2	T47.4X3	T47.4X4	T47.4X5	T47.4X6
topical	T49.3X1	T49.3X2	T49.3X3	T49.3X4	T49.3X5	T49.3X6
specified NEC	T65.891	T65.892	T65.893	T65.894	—	—
substance	T65.91	T65.92	T65.93	T65.94	—	—
Liquor creosolis compositus	T65.891	T65.892	T65.893	T65.894	—	—
Liquorice	T48.4X1	T48.4X2	T48.4X3	T48.4X4	T48.4X5	T48.4X6

Substance	Poisoning, Accidental (unintentional)	Poisoning, Intentional Self-harm	Poisoning, Assault	Poisoning, Undetermined	Adverse Effect	Under-dosing
Liquorice — *continued*						
extract	T47.8X1	T47.8X2	T47.8X3	T47.8X4	T47.8X5	T47.8X6
Liraglutide*	T38.3X1	T38.3X2	T38.3X3	T38.3X4	T38.3X5	T38.3X6
Lisinopril	T46.4X1	T46.4X2	T46.4X3	T46.4X4	T46.4X5	T46.4X6
Lisuride	T42.8X1	T42.8X2	T42.8X3	T42.8X4	T42.8X5	T42.8X6
Lithane	T43.8X1	T43.8X2	T43.8X3	T43.8X4	T43.8X5	T43.8X6
Lithium	T56.891	T56.892	T56.893	T56.894	—	—
gluconate	T43.591	T43.592	T43.593	T43.594	T43.595	T43.596
salts (carbonate)	T43.591	T43.592	T43.593	T43.594	T43.595	T43.596
Lithonate	T43.8X1	T43.8X2	T43.8X3	T43.8X4	T43.8X5	T43.8X6
Liver						
extract	T45.8X1	T45.8X2	T45.8X3	T45.8X4	T45.8X5	T45.8X6
for parenteral use	T45.8X1	T45.8X2	T45.8X3	T45.8X4	T45.8X5	T45.8X6
fraction 1	T45.8X1	T45.8X2	T45.8X3	T45.8X4	T45.8X5	T45.8X6
hydrolysate	T45.8X1	T45.8X2	T45.8X3	T45.8X4	T45.8X5	T45.8X6
Lizard (bite) (venom)	T63.121	T63.122	T63.123	T63.124	—	—
LMD	T45.8X1	T45.8X2	T45.8X3	T45.8X4	T45.8X5	T45.8X6
Lobelia	T62.2X1	T62.2X2	T62.2X3	T62.2X4	—	—
Lobeline	T50.7X1	T50.7X2	T50.7X3	T50.7X4	T50.7X5	T50.7X6
Local action drug NEC	T49.8X1	T49.8X2	T49.8X3	T49.8X4	T49.8X5	T49.8X6
Locorten	T49.ØX1	T49.ØX2	T49.ØX3	T49.ØX4	T49.ØX5	T49.ØX6
Lofepramine	T43.Ø11	T43.Ø12	T43.Ø13	T43.Ø14	T43.Ø15	T43.Ø16
Lolium temulentum	T62.2X1	T62.2X2	T62.2X3	T62.2X4	—	—
Lomotil	T47.6X1	T47.6X2	T47.6X3	T47.6X4	T47.6X5	T47.6X6
Lomustine	T45.1X1	T45.1X2	T45.1X3	T45.1X4	T45.1X5	T45.1X6
Lonidamine	T45.1X1	T45.1X2	T45.1X3	T45.1X4	T45.1X5	T45.1X6
LoOvral*	T38.4X1	T38.4X2	T38.4X3	T38.4X4	T38.4X5	T38.4X6
Loperamide	T47.6X1	T47.6X2	T47.6X3	T47.6X4	T47.6X5	T47.6X6
Loprazolam	T42.4X1	T42.4X2	T42.4X3	T42.4X4	T42.4X5	T42.4X6
Lorajmine	T46.2X1	T46.2X2	T46.2X3	T46.2X4	T46.2X5	T46.2X6
Loratidine	T45.ØX1	T45.ØX2	T45.ØX3	T45.ØX4	T45.ØX5	T45.ØX6
Lorazepam	T42.4X1	T42.4X2	T42.4X3	T42.4X4	T42.4X5	T42.4X6
Lorcainide	T46.2X1	T46.2X2	T46.2X3	T46.2X4	T46.2X5	T46.2X6
Lormetazepam	T42.4X1	T42.4X2	T42.4X3	T42.4X4	T42.4X5	T42.4X6
Lotions NEC	T49.91	T49.92	T49.93	T49.94	T49.95	T49.96
Lotrimin*	T49.ØX1	T49.ØX2	T49.ØX3	T49.ØX4	T49.ØX5	T49.ØX6
Lotusate	T42.3X1	T42.3X2	T42.3X3	T42.3X4	T42.3X5	T42.3X6
Lovastatin	T46.6X1	T46.6X2	T46.6X3	T46.6X4	T46.6X5	T46.6X6
Lowila	T49.2X1	T49.2X2	T49.2X3	T49.2X4	T49.2X5	T49.2X6
Loxapine	T43.591	T43.592	T43.593	T43.594	T43.595	T43.596
Lozenges (throat)	T49.6X1	T49.6X2	T49.6X3	T49.6X4	T49.6X5	T49.6X6
LSD	T40.8X1	T40.8X2	T40.8X3	T40.8X4	—	—
L-Tryptophan — *see* amino acid						
Lubricant, eye	T49.5X1	T49.5X2	T49.5X3	T49.5X4	T49.5X5	T49.5X6
Lubricating oil NEC	T52.ØX1	T52.ØX2	T52.ØX3	T52.ØX4	—	—
Lucanthone	T37.4X1	T37.4X2	T37.4X3	T37.4X4	T37.4X5	T37.4X6
Luminal	T42.3X1	T42.3X2	T42.3X3	T42.3X4	T42.3X5	T42.3X6
Lung irritant (gas) **NEC**	T59.91	T59.92	T59.93	T59.94	—	—
Luteinizing hormone	T38.811	T38.812	T38.813	T38.814	T38.815	T38.816
Lutocylol	T38.5X1	T38.5X2	T38.5X3	T38.5X4	T38.5X5	T38.5X6
Lutromone	T38.5X1	T38.5X2	T38.5X3	T38.5X4	T38.5X5	T38.5X6
Lututrin	T48.291	T48.292	T48.293	T48.294	T48.295	T48.296
Luveris*	T38.891	T38.892	T38.893	T38.894	T38.895	T38.896
Lye (concentrated)	T54.3X1	T54.3X2	T54.3X3	T54.3X4	—	—
Lygranum (skin test)	T50.8X1	T50.8X2	T50.8X3	T50.8X4	T50.8X5	T50.8X6
Lymecycline	T36.4X1	T36.4X2	T36.4X3	T36.4X4	T36.4X5	T36.4X6
Lymphogranuloma venereum antigen	T50.8X1	T50.8X2	T50.8X3	T50.8X4	T50.8X5	T50.8X6
Lynestrenol	T38.4X1	T38.4X2	T38.4X3	T38.4X4	T38.4X5	T38.4X6
Lyovac Sodium Edecrin	T50.1X1	T50.1X2	T50.1X3	T50.1X4	T50.1X5	T50.1X6
Lypressin	T38.891	T38.892	T38.893	T38.894	T38.895	T38.896
Lysergic acid diethylamide	T40.8X1	T40.8X2	T40.8X3	T40.8X4	—	—
Lysergide	T40.8X1	T40.8X2	T40.8X3	T40.8X4	—	—
Lysine vasopressin	T38.891	T38.892	T38.893	T38.894	T38.895	T38.896
Lysol	T54.1X1	T54.1X2	T54.1X3	T54.1X4	—	—
Lysozyme	T49.ØX1	T49.ØX2	T49.ØX3	T49.ØX4	T49.ØX5	T49.ØX6
Lytta (vitatta)	T49.8X1	T49.8X2	T49.8X3	T49.8X4	T49.8X5	T49.8X6
Mace	T59.3X1	T59.3X2	T59.3X3	T59.3X4	—	—
Macrogol	T50.991	T50.992	T50.993	T50.994	T50.995	T50.996
Macrolide						
anabolic drug	T38.7X1	T38.7X2	T38.7X3	T38.7X4	T38.7X5	T38.7X6
antibiotic	T36.3X1	T36.3X2	T36.3X3	T36.3X4	T36.3X5	T36.3X6
Mafenide	T49.ØX1	T49.ØX2	T49.ØX3	T49.ØX4	T49.ØX5	T49.ØX6
Magaldrate	T47.1X1	T47.1X2	T47.1X3	T47.1X4	T47.1X5	T47.1X6
Magic mushroom	T40.991	T40.992	T40.993	T40.994	—	—
Magnamycin	T36.8X1	T36.8X2	T36.8X3	T36.8X4	T36.8X5	T36.8X6
Magnesia magma	T47.1X1	T47.1X2	T47.1X3	T47.1X4	T47.1X5	T47.1X6
Magnesium NEC	T56.891	T56.892	T56.893	T56.894	—	—
carbonate	T47.1X1	T47.1X2	T47.1X3	T47.1X4	T47.1X5	T47.1X6
citrate	T47.4X1	T47.4X2	T47.4X3	T47.4X4	T47.4X5	T47.4X6
hydroxide	T47.1X1	T47.1X2	T47.1X3	T47.1X4	T47.1X5	T47.1X6
oxide	T47.1X1	T47.1X2	T47.1X3	T47.1X4	T47.1X5	T47.1X6
peroxide	T49.ØX1	T49.ØX2	T49.ØX3	T49.ØX4	T49.ØX5	T49.ØX6
Magnesium — *continued*						
salicylate	T39.Ø91	T39.Ø92	T39.Ø93	T39.Ø94	T39.Ø95	T39.Ø96
silicofluoride	T50.3X1	T50.3X2	T50.3X3	T50.3X4	T50.3X5	T50.3X6
sulfate	T47.4X1	T47.4X2	T47.4X3	T47.4X4	T47.4X5	T47.4X6
thiosulfate	T45.ØX1	T45.ØX2	T45.ØX3	T45.ØX4	T45.ØX5	T45.ØX6
trisilicate	T47.1X1	T47.1X2	T47.1X3	T47.1X4	T47.1X5	T47.1X6
Malathion (medicinal)	T49.ØX1	T49.ØX2	T49.ØX3	T49.ØX4	T49.ØX5	T49.ØX6
insecticide	T6Ø.ØX1	T6Ø.ØX2	T6Ø.ØX3	T6Ø.ØX4	—	—
Male fern extract	T37.4X1	T37.4X2	T37.4X3	T37.4X4	T37.4X5	T37.4X6
M-AMSA	T45.1X1	T45.1X2	T45.1X3	T45.1X4	T45.1X5	T45.1X6
Mandelic acid	T37.8X1	T37.8X2	T37.8X3	T37.8X4	T37.8X5	T37.8X6
Manganese (dioxide) (salts)	T57.2X1	T57.2X2	T57.2X3	T57.2X4	—	—
medicinal	T50.991	T50.992	T50.993	T50.994	T50.995	T50.996
Mannitol	T47.3X1	T47.3X2	T47.3X3	T47.3X4	T47.3X5	T47.3X6
hexanitrate	T46.3X1	T46.3X2	T46.3X3	T46.3X4	T46.3X5	T46.3X6
Mannomustine	T45.1X1	T45.1X2	T45.1X3	T45.1X4	T45.1X5	T45.1X6
MAO inhibitors	T43.1X1	T43.1X2	T43.1X3	T43.1X4	T43.1X5	T43.1X6
Mapharsen	T37.8X1	T37.8X2	T37.8X3	T37.8X4	T37.8X5	T37.8X6
Maphenide	T49.ØX1	T49.ØX2	T49.ØX3	T49.ØX4	T49.ØX5	T49.ØX6
Maprotiline	T43.Ø21	T43.Ø22	T43.Ø23	T43.Ø24	T43.Ø25	T43.Ø26
Marcaine	T41.3X1	T41.3X2	T41.3X3	T41.3X4	T41.3X5	T41.3X6
infiltration (subcutaneous)	T41.3X1	T41.3X2	T41.3X3	T41.3X4	T41.3X5	T41.3X6
nerve block (peripheral) (plexus)	T41.3X1	T41.3X2	T41.3X3	T41.3X4	T41.3X5	T41.3X6
Marezine	T45.ØX1	T45.ØX2	T45.ØX3	T45.ØX4	T45.ØX5	T45.ØX6
Marihuana	T40.711	T40.712	T40.713	T40.714	T40.715	T40.716
Marijuana	T40.711	T40.712	T40.713	T40.714	T40.715	T40.716
Marine (sting)	T63.691	T63.692	T63.693	T63.694	—	—
animals (sting)	T63.691	T63.692	T63.693	T63.694	—	—
plants (sting)	T63.711	T63.712	T63.713	T63.714	—	—
Marplan	T43.1X1	T43.1X2	T43.1X3	T43.1X4	T43.1X5	T43.1X6
Marsh gas	T59.891	T59.892	T59.893	T59.894	—	—
Marsilid	T43.1X1	T43.1X2	T43.1X3	T43.1X4	T43.1X5	T43.1X6
Massengill*	T49.ØX1	T49.ØX2	T49.ØX3	T49.ØX4	T49.ØX5	T49.ØX6
Matulane	T45.1X1	T45.1X2	T45.1X3	T45.1X4	T45.1X5	T45.1X6
Mazindol	T50.5X1	T50.5X2	T50.5X3	T50.5X4	T50.5X5	T50.5X6
MCPA	T60.3X1	T60.3X2	T60.3X3	T60.3X4	—	—
MDMA	T43.641	T43.642	T43.643	T43.644	—	—
Meadow saffron	T62.2X1	T62.2X2	T62.2X3	T62.2X4	—	—
Measles virus vaccine (attenuated)	T50.B91	T50.B92	T50.B93	T50.B94	T50.B95	T50.B96
Meat, noxious	T62.8X1	T62.8X2	T62.8X3	T62.8X4	—	—
Meballymal	T42.3X1	T42.3X2	T42.3X3	T42.3X4	T42.3X5	T42.3X6
Mebanazine	T43.1X1	T43.1X2	T43.1X3	T43.1X4	T43.1X5	T43.1X6
Mebaral	T42.3X1	T42.3X2	T42.3X3	T42.3X4	T42.3X5	T42.3X6
Mebendazole	T37.4X1	T37.4X2	T37.4X3	T37.4X4	T37.4X5	T37.4X6
Mebeverine	T44.3X1	T44.3X2	T44.3X3	T44.3X4	T44.3X5	T44.3X6
Mebhydrolin	T45.ØX1	T45.ØX2	T45.ØX3	T45.ØX4	T45.ØX5	T45.ØX6
Mebumal	T42.3X1	T42.3X2	T42.3X3	T42.3X4	T42.3X5	T42.3X6
Mebutamate	T43.591	T43.592	T43.593	T43.594	T43.595	T43.596
Mecamylamine	T44.2X1	T44.2X2	T44.2X3	T44.2X4	T44.2X5	T44.2X6
Mechlorethamine	T45.1X1	T45.1X2	T45.1X3	T45.1X4	T45.1X5	T45.1X6
Mecillinam	T36.ØX1	T36.ØX2	T36.ØX3	T36.ØX4	T36.ØX5	T36.ØX6
Meclizine (hydrochloride)	T45.ØX1	T45.ØX2	T45.ØX3	T45.ØX4	T45.ØX5	T45.ØX6
Meclocycline	T36.4X1	T36.4X2	T36.4X3	T36.4X4	T36.4X5	T36.4X6
Meclofenamate	T39.391	T39.392	T39.393	T39.394	T39.395	T39.396
Meclofenamic acid	T39.391	T39.392	T39.393	T39.394	T39.395	T39.396
Meclofenoxate	T43.691	T43.692	T43.693	T43.694	T43.695	T43.696
Meclozine	T45.ØX1	T45.ØX2	T45.ØX3	T45.ØX4	T45.ØX5	T45.ØX6
Mecobalamin	T45.8X1	T45.8X2	T45.8X3	T45.8X4	T45.8X5	T45.8X6
Mecoprop	T60.3X1	T60.3X2	T60.3X3	T60.3X4	—	—
Mecrilate	T49.3X1	T49.3X2	T49.3X3	T49.3X4	T49.3X5	T49.3X6
Mecysteine	T48.4X1	T48.4X2	T48.4X3	T48.4X4	T48.4X5	T48.4X6
Medazepam	T42.4X1	T42.4X2	T42.4X3	T42.4X4	T42.4X5	T42.4X6
Medicament NEC	T50.901	T50.902	T50.903	T50.904	T50.905	T50.906
Medinal	T42.3X1	T42.3X2	T42.3X3	T42.3X4	T42.3X5	T42.3X6
Medomin	T42.3X1	T42.3X2	T42.3X3	T42.3X4	T42.3X5	T42.3X6
Medrogestone	T38.5X1	T38.5X2	T38.5X3	T38.5X4	T38.5X5	T38.5X6
Medroxalol	T44.8X1	T44.8X2	T44.8X3	T44.8X4	T44.8X5	T44.8X6
Medroxyprogesterone acetate (depot)	T38.5X1	T38.5X2	T38.5X3	T38.5X4	T38.5X5	T38.5X6
Medrysone	T49.ØX1	T49.ØX2	T49.ØX3	T49.ØX4	T49.ØX5	T49.ØX6
Mefenamic acid	T39.391	T39.392	T39.393	T39.394	T39.395	T39.396
Mefenorex	T50.5X1	T50.5X2	T50.5X3	T50.5X4	T50.5X5	T50.5X6
Mefloquine	T37.2X1	T37.2X2	T37.2X3	T37.2X4	T37.2X5	T37.2X6
Mefoxin*	T36.1X1	T36.1X2	T36.1X3	T36.1X4	T36.1X5	T36.1X6
Mefruside	T50.2X1	T50.2X2	T50.2X3	T50.2X4	T50.2X5	T50.2X6
Megahallucinogen	T40.901	T40.902	T40.903	T40.904	T40.905	T40.906
Megestrol	T38.5X1	T38.5X2	T38.5X3	T38.5X4	T38.5X5	T38.5X6
Meglumine						
antimoniate	T37.8X1	T37.8X2	T37.8X3	T37.8X4	T37.8X5	T37.8X6
diatrizoate	T50.8X1	T50.8X2	T50.8X3	T50.8X4	T50.8X5	T50.8X6
iodipamide	T50.8X1	T50.8X2	T50.8X3	T50.8X4	T50.8X5	T50.8X6

Substance	Poisoning, Accidental (unintentional)	Poisoning, Intentional Self-harm	Poisoning, Assault	Poisoning, Undetermined	Adverse Effect	Under-dosing
Meglumine — *continued*						
iotroxate	T50.8X1	T50.8X2	T50.8X3	T50.8X4	T50.8X5	T50.8X6
MEK (methyl ethyl ketone)	T52.4X1	T52.4X2	T52.4X3	T52.4X4	—	—
Meladinin	T49.3X1	T49.3X2	T49.3X3	T49.3X4	T49.3X5	T49.3X6
Meladrazine	T44.3X1	T44.3X2	T44.3X3	T44.3X4	T44.3X5	T44.3X6
Melaleuca alternifolia oil	T49.ØX1	T49.ØX2	T49.ØX3	T49.ØX4	T49.ØX5	T49.ØX6
Melanizing agents	T49.3X1	T49.3X2	T49.3X3	T49.3X4	T49.3X5	T49.3X6
Melanocyte-stimulating hormone	T38.891	T38.892	T38.893	T38.894	T38.895	T38.896
Melarsonyl potassium	T37.3X1	T37.3X2	T37.3X3	T37.3X4	T37.3X5	T37.3X6
Melarsoprol	T37.3X1	T37.3X2	T37.3X3	T37.3X4	T37.3X5	T37.3X6
Melia azedarach	T62.2X1	T62.2X2	T62.2X3	T62.2X4	—	—
Melitracen	T43.Ø11	T43.Ø12	T43.Ø13	T43.Ø14	T43.Ø15	T43.Ø16
Mellaril	T43.3X1	T43.3X2	T43.3X3	T43.3X4	T43.3X5	T43.3X6
Meloxicam*	T39.391	T39.392	T39.393	T39.394	T39.395	T39.396
Meloxine	T49.3X1	T49.3X2	T49.3X3	T49.3X4	T49.3X5	T49.3X6
Melperone	T43.4X1	T43.4X2	T43.4X3	T43.4X4	T43.4X5	T43.4X6
Melphalan	T45.1X1	T45.1X2	T45.1X3	T45.1X4	T45.1X5	T45.1X6
Memantine	T43.8X1	T43.8X2	T43.8X3	T43.8X4	T43.8X5	T43.8X6
Menadiol	T45.7X1	T45.7X2	T45.7X3	T45.7X4	T45.7X5	T45.7X6
sodium sulfate	T45.7X1	T45.7X2	T45.7X3	T45.7X4	T45.7X5	T45.7X6
Menadione	T45.7X1	T45.7X2	T45.7X3	T45.7X4	T45.7X5	T45.7X6
sodium bisulfite	T45.7X1	T45.7X2	T45.7X3	T45.7X4	T45.7X5	T45.7X6
Menaphthone	T45.7X1	T45.7X2	T45.7X3	T45.7X4	T45.7X5	T45.7X6
Menaquinone	T45.7X1	T45.7X2	T45.7X3	T45.7X4	T45.7X5	T45.7X6
Menatetrenone	T45.7X1	T45.7X2	T45.7X3	T45.7X4	T45.7X5	T45.7X6
Meningococcal vaccine	T5Ø.A91	T5Ø.A92	T5Ø.A93	T5Ø.A94	T5Ø.A95	T5Ø.A96
Menningovax (-AC) (-C)	T5Ø.A91	T5Ø.A92	T5Ø.A93	T5Ø.A94	T5Ø.A95	T5Ø.A96
Menotropins	T38.811	T38.812	T38.813	T38.814	T38.815	T38.816
Menthol	T48.5X1	T48.5X2	T48.5X3	T48.5X4	T48.5X5	T48.5X6
Mepacrine	T37.2X1	T37.2X2	T37.2X3	T37.2X4	T37.2X5	T37.2X6
Meparfynol	T42.6X1	T42.6X2	T42.6X3	T42.6X4	T42.6X5	T42.6X6
Mepartricin	T36.7X1	T36.7X2	T36.7X3	T36.7X4	T36.7X5	T36.7X6
Mepazine	T43.3X1	T43.3X2	T43.3X3	T43.3X4	T43.3X5	T43.3X6
Mepenzolate	T44.3X1	T44.3X2	T44.3X3	T44.3X4	T44.3X5	T44.3X6
bromide	T44.3X1	T44.3X2	T44.3X3	T44.3X4	T44.3X5	T44.3X6
Meperidine	T4Ø.491	T4Ø.492	T4Ø.493	T4Ø.494	T4Ø.495	T4Ø.496
Mephebarbital	T42.3X1	T42.3X2	T42.3X3	T42.3X4	T42.3X5	T42.3X6
Mephenamin (e)	T42.8X1	T42.8X2	T42.8X3	T42.8X4	T42.8X5	T42.8X6
Mephenesin	T42.8X1	T42.8X2	T42.8X3	T42.8X4	T42.8X5	T42.8X6
Mephenhydramine	T45.ØX1	T45.ØX2	T45.ØX3	T45.ØX4	T45.ØX5	T45.ØX6
Mephenoxalone	T42.8X1	T42.8X2	T42.8X3	T42.8X4	T42.8X5	T42.8X6
Mephentermine	T44.991	T44.992	T44.993	T44.994	T44.995	T44.996
Mephenytoin	T42.ØX1	T42.ØX2	T42.ØX3	T42.ØX4	T42.ØX5	T42.ØX6
with phenobarbital	T42.3X1	T42.3X2	T42.3X3	T42.3X4	T42.3X5	T42.3X6
Mephobarbital	T42.3X1	T42.3X2	T42.3X3	T42.3X4	T42.3X5	T42.3X6
Mephosfolan	T6Ø.ØX1	T6Ø.ØX2	T6Ø.ØX3	T6Ø.ØX4	—	—
Mepindolol	T44.7X1	T44.7X2	T44.7X3	T44.7X4	T44.7X5	T44.7X6
Mepiperphenidol	T44.3X1	T44.3X2	T44.3X3	T44.3X4	T44.3X5	T44.3X6
Mepitiostane	T38.7X1	T38.7X2	T38.7X3	T38.7X4	T38.7X5	T38.7X6
Mepivacaine	T41.3X1	T41.3X2	T41.3X3	T41.3X4	T41.3X5	T41.3X6
epidural	T41.3X1	T41.3X2	T41.3X3	T41.3X4	T41.3X5	T41.3X6
Meprednisone	T38.ØX1	T38.ØX2	T38.ØX3	T38.ØX4	T38.ØX5	T38.ØX6
Meprobam	T43.591	T43.592	T43.593	T43.594	T43.595	T43.596
Meprobamate	T43.591	T43.592	T43.593	T43.594	T43.595	T43.596
Meproscillarin	T46.ØX1	T46.ØX2	T46.ØX3	T46.ØX4	T46.ØX5	T46.ØX6
Meprylcaine	T41.3X1	T41.3X2	T41.3X3	T41.3X4	T41.3X5	T41.3X6
Meptazinol	T39.8X1	T39.8X2	T39.8X3	T39.8X4	T39.8X5	T39.8X6
Mepyramine	T45.ØX1	T45.ØX2	T45.ØX3	T45.ØX4	T45.ØX5	T45.ØX6
Mequinol*	T49.8X1	T49.8X2	T49.8X3	T49.8X4	T49.8X5	T49.8X6
Mequitazine	T43.3X1	T43.3X2	T43.3X3	T43.3X4	T43.3X5	T43.3X6
Meralluride	T5Ø.2X1	T5Ø.2X2	T5Ø.2X3	T5Ø.2X4	T5Ø.2X5	T5Ø.2X6
Merbaphen	T5Ø.2X1	T5Ø.2X2	T5Ø.2X3	T5Ø.2X4	T5Ø.2X5	T5Ø.2X6
Merbromin	T49.ØX1	T49.ØX2	T49.ØX3	T49.ØX4	T49.ØX5	T49.ØX6
Mercaptobenzothiazole salts	T49.ØX1	T49.ØX2	T49.ØX3	T49.ØX4	T49.ØX5	T49.ØX6
Mercaptomerin	T5Ø.2X1	T5Ø.2X2	T5Ø.2X3	T5Ø.2X4	T5Ø.2X5	T5Ø.2X6
Mercaptopurine	T45.1X1	T45.1X2	T45.1X3	T45.1X4	T45.1X5	T45.1X6
Mercumatilin	T5Ø.2X1	T5Ø.2X2	T5Ø.2X3	T5Ø.2X4	T5Ø.2X5	T5Ø.2X6
Mercuramide	T5Ø.2X1	T5Ø.2X2	T5Ø.2X3	T5Ø.2X4	T5Ø.2X5	T5Ø.2X6
Mercurochrome	T49.ØX1	T49.ØX2	T49.ØX3	T49.ØX4	T49.ØX5	T49.ØX6
Mercurophylline	T5Ø.2X1	T5Ø.2X2	T5Ø.2X3	T5Ø.2X4	T5Ø.2X5	T5Ø.2X6
Mercury, mercurial, mercuric, mercurous (compounds) (cyanide) (fumes) (nonmedicinal) (vapor) **NEC**	T56.1X1	T56.1X2	T56.1X3	T56.1X4	—	—
ammoniated	T49.ØX1	T49.ØX2	T49.ØX3	T49.ØX4	T49.ØX5	T49.ØX6
anti-infective						
local	T49.ØX1	T49.ØX2	T49.ØX3	T49.ØX4	T49.ØX5	T49.ØX6
systemic	T37.8X1	T37.8X2	T37.8X3	T37.8X4	T37.8X5	T37.8X6
topical	T49.ØX1	T49.ØX2	T49.ØX3	T49.ØX4	T49.ØX5	T49.ØX6
chloride (ammoniated)	T49.ØX1	T49.ØX2	T49.ØX3	T49.ØX4	T49.ØX5	T49.ØX6
Mercury, mercurial, mercuric, mercurous (compounds) (cyanide) (fumes) (nonmedicinal) (vapor) **NEC** — *continued*						
chloride — *continued*						
fungicide	T56.1X1	T56.1X2	T56.1X3	T56.1X4	—	—
diuretic NEC	T5Ø.2X1	T5Ø.2X2	T5Ø.2X3	T5Ø.2X4	T5Ø.2X5	T5Ø.2X6
fungicide	T56.1X1	T56.1X2	T56.1X3	T56.1X4	—	—
organic (fungicide)	T56.1X1	T56.1X2	T56.1X3	T56.1X4	—	—
oxide, yellow	T49.ØX1	T49.ØX2	T49.ØX3	T49.ØX4	T49.ØX5	T49.ØX6
Mersalyl	T5Ø.2X1	T5Ø.2X2	T5Ø.2X3	T5Ø.2X4	T5Ø.2X5	T5Ø.2X6
Merthiolate	T49.ØX1	T49.ØX2	T49.ØX3	T49.ØX4	T49.ØX5	T49.ØX6
ophthalmic preparation	T49.5X1	T49.5X2	T49.5X3	T49.5X4	T49.5X5	T49.5X6
Meruvax	T5Ø.B91	T5Ø.B92	T5Ø.B93	T5Ø.B94	T5Ø.B95	T5Ø.B96
Mesalazine	T47.8X1	T47.8X2	T47.8X3	T47.8X4	T47.8X5	T47.8X6
Mescal buttons	T4Ø.991	T4Ø.992	T4Ø.993	T4Ø.994	—	—
Mescaline	T4Ø.991	T4Ø.992	T4Ø.993	T4Ø.994	—	—
Mesna	T48.4X1	T48.4X2	T48.4X3	T48.4X4	T48.4X5	T48.4X6
Mesoglycan	T46.6X1	T46.6X2	T46.6X3	T46.6X4	T46.6X5	T46.6X6
Mesoridazine	T43.3X1	T43.3X2	T43.3X3	T43.3X4	T43.3X5	T43.3X6
Mestanolone	T38.7X1	T38.7X2	T38.7X3	T38.7X4	T38.7X5	T38.7X6
Mesterolone	T38.7X1	T38.7X2	T38.7X3	T38.7X4	T38.7X5	T38.7X6
Mestranol	T38.5X1	T38.5X2	T38.5X3	T38.5X4	T38.5X5	T38.5X6
Mesulergine	T42.8X1	T42.8X2	T42.8X3	T42.8X4	T42.8X5	T42.8X6
Mesulfen	T49.ØX1	T49.ØX2	T49.ØX3	T49.ØX4	T49.ØX5	T49.ØX6
Mesuximide	T42.2X1	T42.2X2	T42.2X3	T42.2X4	T42.2X5	T42.2X6
Metabutethamine	T41.3X1	T41.3X2	T41.3X3	T41.3X4	T41.3X5	T41.3X6
Metactesylacetate	T49.ØX1	T49.ØX2	T49.ØX3	T49.ØX4	T49.ØX5	T49.ØX6
Metacycline	T36.4X1	T36.4X2	T36.4X3	T36.4X4	T36.4X5	T36.4X6
Metaldehyde (snail killer) **NEC**	T6Ø.8X1	T6Ø.8X2	T6Ø.8X3	T6Ø.8X4	—	—
Metals (heavy) (nonmedicinal)	T56.91	T56.92	T56.93	T56.94	—	—
dust, fumes, or vapor NEC	T56.91	T56.92	T56.93	T56.94	—	—
light NEC	T56.91	T56.92	T56.93	T56.94	—	—
dust, fumes, or vapor NEC	T56.91	T56.92	T56.93	T56.94	—	—
specified NEC	T56.891	T56.892	T56.893	T56.894	—	—
thallium	T56.811	T56.812	T56.813	T56.814	—	—
Metamfetamine	T43.651	T43.652	T43.652	T43.654	T43.655	T43.656
Metamizole sodium	T39.2X1	T39.2X2	T39.2X3	T39.2X4	T39.2X5	T39.2X6
Metampicillin	T36.ØX1	T36.ØX2	T36.ØX3	T36.ØX4	T36.ØX5	T36.ØX6
Metamucil	T47.4X1	T47.4X2	T47.4X3	T47.4X4	T47.4X5	T47.4X6
Metandienone	T38.7X1	T38.7X2	T38.7X3	T38.7X4	T38.7X5	T38.7X6
Metandrostenolone	T38.7X1	T38.7X2	T38.7X3	T38.7X4	T38.7X5	T38.7X6
Metaphen	T49.ØX1	T49.ØX2	T49.ØX3	T49.ØX4	T49.ØX5	T49.ØX6
Metaphos	T6Ø.ØX1	T6Ø.ØX2	T6Ø.ØX3	T6Ø.ØX4	—	—
Metapramine	T43.Ø11	T43.Ø12	T43.Ø13	T43.Ø14	T43.Ø15	T43.Ø16
Metaproterenol	T48.291	T48.292	T48.293	T48.294	T48.295	T48.296
Metaraminol	T44.4X1	T44.4X2	T44.4X3	T44.4X4	T44.4X5	T44.4X6
Metaxalone	T42.8X1	T42.8X2	T42.8X3	T42.8X4	T42.8X5	T42.8X6
Meted*	T49.4X1	T49.4X2	T49.4X3	T49.4X4	T49.4X5	T49.4X6
Metenolone	T38.7X1	T38.7X2	T38.7X3	T38.7X4	T38.7X5	T38.7X6
Metergoline	T42.8X1	T42.8X2	T42.8X3	T42.8X4	T42.8X5	T42.8X6
Metescufylline	T46.991	T46.992	T46.993	T46.994	T46.995	T46.996
Metetoin	T42.ØX1	T42.ØX2	T42.ØX3	T42.ØX4	T42.ØX5	T42.ØX6
Metformin	T38.3X1	T38.3X2	T38.3X3	T38.3X4	T38.3X5	T38.3X6
Methacholine	T44.1X1	T44.1X2	T44.1X3	T44.1X4	T44.1X5	T44.1X6
Methacycline	T36.4X1	T36.4X2	T36.4X3	T36.4X4	T36.4X5	T36.4X6
Methadone	T4Ø.3X1	T4Ø.3X2	T4Ø.3X3	T4Ø.3X4	T4Ø.3X5	T4Ø.3X6
Methadose*	T4Ø.3X1	T4Ø.3X2	T4Ø.3X3	T4Ø.3X4	T4Ø.3X5	T4Ø.3X6
Methallenestril	T38.5X1	T38.5X2	T38.5X3	T38.5X4	T38.5X5	T38.5X6
Methallenoestril	T38.5X1	T38.5X2	T38.5X3	T38.5X4	T38.5X5	T38.5X6
Methamphetamine	T43.651	T43.652	T43.652	T43.654	T43.655	T43.656
Methampyrone	T39.2X1	T39.2X2	T39.2X3	T39.2X4	T39.2X5	T39.2X6
Methandienone	T38.7X1	T38.7X2	T38.7X3	T38.7X4	T38.7X5	T38.7X6
Methandriol	T38.7X1	T38.7X2	T38.7X3	T38.7X4	T38.7X5	T38.7X6
Methandrostenolone	T38.7X1	T38.7X2	T38.7X3	T38.7X4	T38.7X5	T38.7X6
Methane	T59.891	T59.892	T59.893	T59.894	—	—
Methanethiol	T59.891	T59.892	T59.893	T59.894	—	—
Methaniazide	T37.1X1	T37.1X2	T37.1X3	T37.1X4	T37.1X5	T37.1X6
Methanol (vapor)	T51.1X1	T51.1X2	T51.1X3	T51.1X4	—	—
Methantheline	T44.3X1	T44.3X2	T44.3X3	T44.3X4	T44.3X5	T44.3X6
Methanthelinium bromide	T44.3X1	T44.3X2	T44.3X3	T44.3X4	T44.3X5	T44.3X6
Methaphenilene	T45.ØX1	T45.ØX2	T45.ØX3	T45.ØX4	T45.ØX5	T45.ØX6
Methapyrilene	T45.ØX1	T45.ØX2	T45.ØX3	T45.ØX4	T45.ØX5	T45.ØX6
Methaqualone (compound)	T42.6X1	T42.6X2	T42.6X3	T42.6X4	T42.6X5	T42.6X6
Metharbital	T42.3X1	T42.3X2	T42.3X3	T42.3X4	T42.3X5	T42.3X6
Methazolamide	T5Ø.2X1	T5Ø.2X2	T5Ø.2X3	T5Ø.2X4	T5Ø.2X5	T5Ø.2X6
Methdilazine	T43.3X1	T43.3X2	T43.3X3	T43.3X4	T43.3X5	T43.3X6
Methedrine	T43.651	T43.652	T43.652	T43.654	T43.655	T43.656
Methenamine (mandelate)	T37.8X1	T37.8X2	T37.8X3	T37.8X4	T37.8X5	T37.8X6
Methenolone	T38.7X1	T38.7X2	T38.7X3	T38.7X4	T38.7X5	T38.7X6

Substance	Poisoning, Accidental (unintentional)	Poisoning, Intentional Self-harm	Poisoning, Assault	Poisoning, Undetermined	Adverse Effect	Under-dosing
Methergine	T48.ØX1	T48.ØX2	T48.ØX3	T48.ØX4	T48.ØX5	T48.ØX6
Methetoin	T42.ØX1	T42.ØX2	T42.ØX3	T42.ØX4	T42.ØX5	T42.ØX6
Methiacil	T38.2X1	T38.2X2	T38.2X3	T38.2X4	T38.2X5	T38.2X6
Methicillin	T36.ØX1	T36.ØX2	T36.ØX3	T36.ØX4	T36.ØX5	T36.ØX6
Methimazole	T38.2X1	T38.2X2	T38.2X3	T38.2X4	T38.2X5	T38.2X6
Methiodal sodium	T5Ø.8X1	T5Ø.8X2	T5Ø.8X3	T5Ø.8X4	T5Ø.8X5	T5Ø.8X6
Methionine	T5Ø.991	T5Ø.992	T5Ø.993	T5Ø.994	T5Ø.995	T5Ø.996
Methisazone	T37.5X1	T37.5X2	T37.5X3	T37.5X4	T37.5X5	T37.5X6
Methisoprinol	T37.5X1	T37.5X2	T37.5X3	T37.5X4	T37.5X5	T37.5X6
Methitural	T42.3X1	T42.3X2	T42.3X3	T42.3X4	T42.3X5	T42.3X6
Methixene	T44.3X1	T44.3X2	T44.3X3	T44.3X4	T44.3X5	T44.3X6
Methobarbital, methobarbitone	T42.3X1	T42.3X2	T42.3X3	T42.3X4	T42.3X5	T42.3X6
Methocarbamol	T42.8X1	T42.8X2	T42.8X3	T42.8X4	T42.8X5	T42.8X6
skeletal muscle relaxant	T48.1X1	T48.1X2	T48.1X3	T48.1X4	T48.1X5	T48.1X6
Methohexital	T41.1X1	T41.1X2	T41.1X3	T41.1X4	T41.1X5	T41.1X6
Methohexitone	T41.1X1	T41.1X2	T41.1X3	T41.1X4	T41.1X5	T41.1X6
Methoin	T42.ØX1	T42.ØX2	T42.ØX3	T42.ØX4	T42.ØX5	T42.ØX6
Methopholine	T39.8X1	T39.8X2	T39.8X3	T39.8X4	T39.8X5	T39.8X6
Methopromazine	T43.3X1	T43.3X2	T43.3X3	T43.3X4	T43.3X5	T43.3X6
Methorate	T48.3X1	T48.3X2	T48.3X3	T48.3X4	T48.3X5	T48.3X6
Methoserpidine	T46.5X1	T46.5X2	T46.5X3	T46.5X4	T46.5X5	T46.5X6
Methotrexate	T45.1X1	T45.1X2	T45.1X3	T45.1X4	T45.1X5	T45.1X6
Methotrimeprazine	T43.3X1	T43.3X2	T43.3X3	T43.3X4	T43.3X5	T43.3X6
Methoxa-Dome	T49.3X1	T49.3X2	T49.3X3	T49.3X4	T49.3X5	T49.3X6
Methoxamine	T44.4X1	T44.4X2	T44.4X3	T44.4X4	T44.4X5	T44.4X6
Methoxsalen	T5Ø.991	T5Ø.992	T5Ø.993	T5Ø.994	T5Ø.995	T5Ø.996
Methoxyaniline	T65.3X1	T65.3X2	T65.3X3	T65.3X4	—	—
Methoxybenzyl penicillin	T36.ØX1	T36.ØX2	T36.ØX3	T36.ØX4	T36.ØX5	T36.ØX6
Methoxychlor	T53.7X1	T53.7X2	T53.7X3	T53.7X4	—	—
Methoxy-DDT	T53.7X1	T53.7X2	T53.7X3	T53.7X4	—	—
Methoxyflurane	T41.ØX1	T41.ØX2	T41.ØX3	T41.ØX4	T41.ØX5	T41.ØX6
Methoxyphenamine	T48.6X1	T48.6X2	T48.6X3	T48.6X4	T48.6X5	T48.6X6
Methoxypromazine	T43.3X1	T43.3X2	T43.3X3	T43.3X4	T43.3X5	T43.3X6
Methscopolamine bromide	T44.3X1	T44.3X2	T44.3X3	T44.3X4	T44.3X5	T44.3X6
Methsuximide	T42.2X1	T42.2X2	T42.2X3	T42.2X4	T42.2X5	T42.2X6
Methyclothiazide	T5Ø.2X1	T5Ø.2X2	T5Ø.2X3	T5Ø.2X4	T5Ø.2X5	T5Ø.2X6
Methyl						
acetate	T52.4X1	T52.4X2	T52.4X3	T52.4X4	—	—
acetone	T52.4X1	T52.4X2	T52.4X3	T52.4X4	—	—
acrylate	T65.891	T65.892	T65.893	T65.894	—	—
alcohol	T51.1X1	T51.1X2	T51.1X3	T51.1X4	—	—
aminophenol	T65.3X1	T65.3X2	T65.3X3	T65.3X4	—	—
amphetamine	T43.651	T43.652	T43.652	T43.654	T43.655	T43.656
androstanolone	T38.7X1	T38.7X2	T38.7X3	T38.7X4	T38.7X5	T38.7X6
atropine	T44.3X1	T44.3X2	T44.3X3	T44.3X4	T44.3X5	T44.3X6
benzene	T52.2X1	T52.2X2	T52.2X3	T52.2X4	—	—
benzoate	T52.8X1	T52.8X2	T52.8X3	T52.8X4	—	—
benzol	T52.2X1	T52.2X2	T52.2X3	T52.2X4	—	—
bromide (gas)	T59.891	T59.892	T59.893	T59.894	—	—
fumigant	T6Ø.8X1	T6Ø.8X2	T6Ø.8X3	T6Ø.8X4	—	—
butanol	T51.3X1	T51.3X2	T51.3X3	T51.3X4	—	—
carbinol	T51.1X1	T51.1X2	T51.1X3	T51.1X4	—	—
carbonate	T52.8X1	T52.8X2	T52.8X3	T52.8X4	—	—
CCNU	T45.1X1	T45.1X2	T45.1X3	T45.1X4	T45.1X5	T45.1X6
cellosolve	T52.91	T52.92	T52.93	T52.94		
cellulose	T47.4X1	T47.4X2	T47.4X3	T47.4X4	T47.4X5	T47.4X6
chloride (gas)	T59.891	T59.892	T59.893	T59.894	—	—
chloroformate	T59.3X1	T59.3X2	T59.3X3	T59.3X4	—	—
cyclohexane	T52.8X1	T52.8X2	T52.8X3	T52.8X4	—	—
cyclohexanol	T51.8X1	T51.8X2	T51.8X3	T51.8X4	—	—
cyclohexanone	T52.8X1	T52.8X2	T52.8X3	T52.8X4	—	—
cyclohexyl acetate	T52.8X1	T52.8X2	T52.8X3	T52.8X4	—	—
demeton	T6Ø.ØX1	T6Ø.ØX2	T6Ø.ØX3	T6Ø.ØX4	—	—
dihydromorphinone	T4Ø.2X1	T4Ø.2X2	T4Ø.2X3	T4Ø.2X4	T4Ø.2X5	T4Ø.2X6
ergometrine	T48.ØX1	T48.ØX2	T48.ØX3	T48.ØX4	T48.ØX5	T48.ØX6
ergonovine	T48.ØX1	T48.ØX2	T48.ØX3	T48.ØX4	T48.ØX5	T48.ØX6
ethyl ketone	T52.4X1	T52.4X2	T52.4X3	T52.4X4	—	—
glucamine antimonate	T37.8X1	T37.8X2	T37.8X3	T37.8X4	T37.8X5	T37.8X6
hydrazine	T65.891	T65.892	T65.893	T65.894	—	—
iodide	T65.891	T65.892	T65.893	T65.894	—	—
isobutyl ketone	T52.4X1	T52.4X2	T52.4X3	T52.4X4	—	—
isothiocyanate	T6Ø.3X1	T6Ø.3X2	T6Ø.3X3	T6Ø.3X4	—	—
mercaptan	T59.891	T59.892	T59.893	T59.894	—	—
morphine NEC	T4Ø.2X1	T4Ø.2X2	T4Ø.2X3	T4Ø.2X4	T4Ø.2X5	T4Ø.2X6
nicotinate	T49.4X1	T49.4X2	T49.4X3	T49.4X4	T49.4X5	T49.4X6
paraben	T49.ØX1	T49.ØX2	T49.ØX3	T49.ØX4	T49.ØX5	T49.ØX6
parafynol	T42.6X1	T42.6X2	T42.6X3	T42.6X4	T42.6X5	T42.6X6
parathion	T6Ø.ØX1	T6Ø.ØX2	T6Ø.ØX3	T6Ø.ØX4	—	—
peridol	T43.4X1	T43.4X2	T43.4X3	T43.4X4	T43.4X5	T43.4X6
phenidate	T43.631	T43.632	T43.633	T43.634	T43.635	T43.636
prednisolone	T38.ØX1	T38.ØX2	T38.ØX3	T38.ØX4	T38.ØX5	T38.ØX6
Methyl — *continued*						
prednisolone — *continued*						
ENT agent	T49.6X1	T49.6X2	T49.6X3	T49.6X4	T49.6X5	T49.6X6
ophthalmic preparation	T49.5X1	T49.5X2	T49.5X3	T49.5X4	T49.5X5	T49.5X6
topical NEC	T49.ØX1	T49.ØX2	T49.ØX3	T49.ØX4	T49.ØX5	T49.ØX6
propylcarbinol	T51.3X1	T51.3X2	T51.3X3	T51.3X4	—	—
rosaniline NEC	T49.ØX1	T49.ØX2	T49.ØX3	T49.ØX4	T49.ØX5	T49.ØX6
salicylate	T49.2X1	T49.2X2	T49.2X3	T49.2X4	T49.2X5	T49.2X6
sulfate (fumes)	T59.891	T59.892	T59.893	T59.894	—	—
liquid	T52.8X1	T52.8X2	T52.8X3	T52.8X4	—	—
sulfonal	T42.6X1	T42.6X2	T42.6X3	T42.6X4	T42.6X5	T42.6X6
testosterone	T38.7X1	T38.7X2	T38.7X3	T38.7X4	T38.7X5	T38.7X6
thiouracil	T38.2X1	T38.2X2	T38.2X3	T38.2X4	T38.2X5	T38.2X6
Methylacetoxyprogesterone*	T38.5X1	T38.5X2	T38.5X3	T38.5X4	T38.5X5	T38.5X6
Methylamphetamine	T43.651	T43.652	T43.652	T43.654	T43.655	T43.656
Methylated spirit	T51.1X1	T51.1X2	T51.1X3	T51.1X4	—	—
Methylatropine nitrate	T44.3X1	T44.3X2	T44.3X3	T44.3X4	T44.3X5	T44.3X6
Methylbenactyzium bromide	T44.3X1	T44.3X2	T44.3X3	T44.3X4	T44.3X5	T44.3X6
Methylbenzethonium chloride	T49.ØX1	T49.ØX2	T49.ØX3	T49.ØX4	T49.ØX5	T49.ØX6
Methylcellulose	T47.4X1	T47.4X2	T47.4X3	T47.4X4	T47.4X5	T47.4X6
laxative	T47.4X1	T47.4X2	T47.4X3	T47.4X4	T47.4X5	T47.4X6
Methylchlorophenoxyacetic acid	T6Ø.3X1	T6Ø.3X2	T6Ø.3X3	T6Ø.3X4	—	—
Methyldopa	T46.5X1	T46.5X2	T46.5X3	T46.5X4	T46.5X5	T46.5X6
Methyldopate	T46.5X1	T46.5X2	T46.5X3	T46.5X4	T46.5X5	T46.5X6
Methylene						
blue	T5Ø.6X1	T5Ø.6X2	T5Ø.6X3	T5Ø.6X4	T5Ø.6X5	T5Ø.6X6
chloride or dichloride (solvent)	T53.4X1	T53.4X2	T53.4X3	T53.4X4	—	—
NEC						
Methylenedioxyamphetamine	T43.621	T43.622	T43.623	T43.624	T43.625	T43.626
Methylenedioxymethamphetamine	T43.641	T43.642	T43.643	T43.644	—	—
Methylergometrine	T48.ØX1	T48.ØX2	T48.ØX3	T48.ØX4	T48.ØX5	T48.ØX6
Methylergonovine	T48.ØX1	T48.ØX2	T48.ØX3	T48.ØX4	T48.ØX5	T48.ØX6
Methylestrenolone	T38.5X1	T38.5X2	T38.5X3	T38.5X4	T38.5X5	T38.5X6
Methylethyl cellulose	T5Ø.991	T5Ø.992	T5Ø.993	T5Ø.994	T5Ø.995	T5Ø.996
Methylhexabital	T42.3X1	T42.3X2	T42.3X3	T42.3X4	T42.3X5	T42.3X6
Methylmorphine	T4Ø.2X1	T4Ø.2X2	T4Ø.2X3	T4Ø.2X4	T4Ø.2X5	T4Ø.2X6
Methylparaben (ophthalmic)	T49.5X1	T49.5X2	T49.5X3	T49.5X4	T49.5X5	T49.5X6
Methylparafynol	T42.6X1	T42.6X2	T42.6X3	T42.6X4	T42.6X5	T42.6X6
Methylpentynol, methylpenthynol	T42.6X1	T42.6X2	T42.6X3	T42.6X4	T42.6X5	T42.6X6
Methylphenidate	T43.631	T43.632	T43.633	T43.634	T43.635	T43.636
Methylphenobarbital	T42.3X1	T42.3X2	T42.3X3	T42.3X4	T42.3X5	T42.3X6
Methylpolysiloxane	T47.1X1	T47.1X2	T47.1X3	T47.1X4	T47.1X5	T47.1X6
Methylprednisolone — *see* Methyl, prednisolone						
Methylrosaniline	T49.ØX1	T49.ØX2	T49.ØX3	T49.ØX4	T49.ØX5	T49.ØX6
Methylrosanilinium chloride	T49.ØX1	T49.ØX2	T49.ØX3	T49.ØX4	T49.ØX5	T49.ØX6
Methyltestosterone	T38.7X1	T38.7X2	T38.7X3	T38.7X4	T38.7X5	T38.7X6
Methylthionine chloride	T5Ø.6X1	T5Ø.6X2	T5Ø.6X3	T5Ø.6X4	T5Ø.6X5	T5Ø.6X6
Methylthioninium chloride	T5Ø.6X1	T5Ø.6X2	T5Ø.6X3	T5Ø.6X4	T5Ø.6X5	T5Ø.6X6
Methylthiouracil	T38.2X1	T38.2X2	T38.2X3	T38.2X4	T38.2X5	T38.2X6
Methyprylon	T42.6X1	T42.6X2	T42.6X3	T42.6X4	T42.6X5	T42.6X6
Methysergide	T46.5X1	T46.5X2	T46.5X3	T46.5X4	T46.5X5	T46.5X6
Metiamide	T47.1X1	T47.1X2	T47.1X3	T47.1X4	T47.1X5	T47.1X6
Meticillin	T36.ØX1	T36.ØX2	T36.ØX3	T36.ØX4	T36.ØX5	T36.ØX6
Meticrane	T5Ø.2X1	T5Ø.2X2	T5Ø.2X3	T5Ø.2X4	T5Ø.2X5	T5Ø.2X6
Metildigoxin	T46.ØX1	T46.ØX2	T46.ØX3	T46.ØX4	T46.ØX5	T46.ØX6
Metipranolol	T49.5X1	T49.5X2	T49.5X3	T49.5X4	T49.5X5	T49.5X6
Metirosine	T46.5X1	T46.5X2	T46.5X3	T46.5X4	T46.5X5	T46.5X6
Metisazone	T37.5X1	T37.5X2	T37.5X3	T37.5X4	T37.5X5	T37.5X6
Metixene	T44.3X1	T44.3X2	T44.3X3	T44.3X4	T44.3X5	T44.3X6
Metizoline	T48.5X1	T48.5X2	T48.5X3	T48.5X4	T48.5X5	T48.5X6
Metoclopramide	T45.ØX1	T45.ØX2	T45.ØX3	T45.ØX4	T45.ØX5	T45.ØX6
Metofenazate	T43.3X1	T43.3X2	T43.3X3	T43.3X4	T43.3X5	T43.3X6
Metofoline	T39.8X1	T39.8X2	T39.8X3	T39.8X4	T39.8X5	T39.8X6
Metolazone	T5Ø.2X1	T5Ø.2X2	T5Ø.2X3	T5Ø.2X4	T5Ø.2X5	T5Ø.2X6
Metopon	T4Ø.2X1	T4Ø.2X2	T4Ø.2X3	T4Ø.2X4	T4Ø.2X5	T4Ø.2X6
Metoprine	T45.1X1	T45.1X2	T45.1X3	T45.1X4	T45.1X5	T45.1X6
Metoprolol	T44.7X1	T44.7X2	T44.7X3	T44.7X4	T44.7X5	T44.7X6
Metrifonate	T6Ø.ØX1	T6Ø.ØX2	T6Ø.ØX3	T6Ø.ØX4	—	—
Metrizamide	T5Ø.8X1	T5Ø.8X2	T5Ø.8X3	T5Ø.8X4	T5Ø.8X5	T5Ø.8X6
Metrizoic acid	T5Ø.8X1	T5Ø.8X2	T5Ø.8X3	T5Ø.8X4	T5Ø.8X5	T5Ø.8X6
Metronidazole	T37.8X1	T37.8X2	T37.8X3	T37.8X4	T37.8X5	T37.8X6
Metycaine	T41.3X1	T41.3X2	T41.3X3	T41.3X4	T41.3X5	T41.3X6
infiltration (subcutaneous)	T41.3X1	T41.3X2	T41.3X3	T41.3X4	T41.3X5	T41.3X6

Table of Drugs and Chemicals

Substance	Poisoning, Accidental (unintentional)	Poisoning, Intentional Self-harm	Poisoning, Assault	Poisoning, Undetermined	Adverse Effect	Under-dosing
Metycaine — *continued*						
nerve block (peripheral) (plexus)	T41.3X1	T41.3X2	T41.3X3	T41.3X4	T41.3X5	T41.3X6
topical (surface)	T41.3X1	T41.3X2	T41.3X3	T41.3X4	T41.3X5	T41.3X6
Metyrapone	T5Ø.8X1	T5Ø.8X2	T5Ø.8X3	T5Ø.8X4	T5Ø.8X5	T5Ø.8X6
Mevacor*	T46.6X1	T46.6X2	T46.6X3	T46.6X4	T46.6X5	T46.6X6
Mevinphos	T6Ø.ØX1	T6Ø.ØX2	T6Ø.ØX3	T6Ø.ØX4	—	—
Mexazolam	T42.4X1	T42.4X2	T42.4X3	T42.4X4	T42.4X5	T42.4X6
Mexenone	T49.3X1	T49.3X2	T49.3X3	T49.3X4	T49.3X5	T49.3X6
Mexiletine	T46.2X1	T46.2X2	T46.2X3	T46.2X4	T46.2X5	T46.2X6
Mezereon	T62.2X1	T62.2X2	T62.2X3	T62.2X4	—	—
berries	T62.1X1	T62.1X2	T62.1X3	T62.1X4	—	—
Mezlocillin	T36.ØX1	T36.ØX2	T36.ØX3	T36.ØX4	T36.ØX5	T36.ØX6
Mianserin	T43.Ø21	T43.Ø22	T43.Ø23	T43.Ø24	T43.Ø25	T43.Ø26
Micatin	T49.ØX1	T49.ØX2	T49.ØX3	T49.ØX4	T49.ØX5	T49.ØX6
Miconazole	T49.ØX1	T49.ØX2	T49.ØX3	T49.ØX4	T49.ØX5	T49.ØX6
Micronomicin	T36.5X1	T36.5X2	T36.5X3	T36.5X4	T36.5X5	T36.5X6
Microzide*	T5Ø.2X1	T5Ø.2X2	T5Ø.2X3	T5Ø.2X4	T5Ø.2X5	T5Ø.2X6
Midazolam	T42.4X1	T42.4X2	T42.4X3	T42.4X4	T42.4X5	T42.4X6
Midecamycin	T36.3X1	T36.3X2	T36.3X3	T36.3X4	T36.3X5	T36.3X6
Mifepristone	T38.6X1	T38.6X2	T38.6X3	T38.6X4	T38.6X5	T38.6X6
Milk of magnesia	T47.1X1	T47.1X2	T47.1X3	T47.1X4	T47.1X5	T47.1X6
Millipede (tropical) (venomous)	T63.411	T63.412	T63.413	T63.414	—	—
Miltown	T43.591	T43.592	T43.593	T43.594	T43.595	T43.596
Milverine	T44.3X1	T44.3X2	T44.3X3	T44.3X4	T44.3X5	T44.3X6
Minaprine	T43.291	T43.292	T43.293	T43.294	T43.295	T43.296
Minaxolone	T41.291	T41.292	T41.293	T41.294	T41.295	T41.296
Mineral						
acids	T54.2X1	T54.2X2	T54.2X3	T54.2X4	—	—
oil (laxative)(medicinal)	T47.4X1	T47.4X2	T47.4X3	T47.4X4	T47.4X5	T47.4X6
emulsion	T47.2X1	T47.2X2	T47.2X3	T47.2X4	T47.2X5	T47.2X6
nonmedicinal	T52.ØX1	T52.ØX2	T52.ØX3	T52.ØX4	—	—
topical	T49.3X1	T49.3X2	T49.3X3	T49.3X4	T49.3X5	T49.3X6
salt NEC	T5Ø.3X1	T5Ø.3X2	T5Ø.3X3	T5Ø.3X4	T5Ø.3X5	T5Ø.3X6
spirits	T52.ØX1	T52.ØX2	T52.ØX3	T52.ØX4	—	—
Mineralocorticosteroid	T5Ø.ØX1	T5Ø.ØX2	T5Ø.ØX3	T5Ø.ØX4	T5Ø.ØX5	T5Ø.ØX6
Minocycline	T36.4X1	T36.4X2	T36.4X3	T36.4X4	T36.4X5	T36.4X6
Minoxidil	T46.7X1	T46.7X2	T46.7X3	T46.7X4	T46.7X5	T46.7X6
Miokamycin	T36.3X1	T36.3X2	T36.3X3	T36.3X4	T36.3X5	T36.3X6
Miotic drug	T49.5X1	T49.5X2	T49.5X3	T49.5X4	T49.5X5	T49.5X6
Mipafox	T6Ø.ØX1	T6Ø.ØX2	T6Ø.ØX3	T6Ø.ØX4	—	—
Mipomersen*	T46.6X1	T46.6X2	T46.6X3	T46.6X4	T46.6X5	T46.6X6
Mirex	T6Ø.1X1	T6Ø.1X2	T6Ø.1X3	T6Ø.1X4	—	—
Mirtazapine	T43.Ø21	T43.Ø22	T43.Ø23	T43.Ø24	T43.Ø25	T43.Ø26
Misonidazole	T37.3X1	T37.3X2	T37.3X3	T37.3X4	T37.3X5	T37.3X6
Misoprostol	T47.1X1	T47.1X2	T47.1X3	T47.1X4	T47.1X5	T47.1X6
Mithramycin	T45.1X1	T45.1X2	T45.1X3	T45.1X4	T45.1X5	T45.1X6
Mitobronitol	T45.1X1	T45.1X2	T45.1X3	T45.1X4	T45.1X5	T45.1X6
Mitoguazone	T45.1X1	T45.1X2	T45.1X3	T45.1X4	T45.1X5	T45.1X6
Mitolactol	T45.1X1	T45.1X2	T45.1X3	T45.1X4	T45.1X5	T45.1X6
Mitomycin	T45.1X1	T45.1X2	T45.1X3	T45.1X4	T45.1X5	T45.1X6
Mitopodozide	T45.1X1	T45.1X2	T45.1X3	T45.1X4	T45.1X5	T45.1X6
Mitotane	T45.1X1	T45.1X2	T45.1X3	T45.1X4	T45.1X5	T45.1X6
Mitoxantrone	T45.1X1	T45.1X2	T45.1X3	T45.1X4	T45.1X5	T45.1X6
Mivacurium chloride	T48.1X1	T48.1X2	T48.1X3	T48.1X4	T48.1X5	T48.1X6
Miyari bacteria	T47.6X1	T47.6X2	T47.6X3	T47.6X4	T47.6X5	T47.6X6
Moclobemide	T43.1X1	T43.1X2	T43.1X3	T43.1X4	T43.1X5	T43.1X6
Moderil	T46.5X1	T46.5X2	T46.5X3	T46.5X4	T46.5X5	T46.5X6
Mofebutazone	T39.2X1	T39.2X2	T39.2X3	T39.2X4	T39.2X5	T39.2X6
Mogadon — *see* Nitrazepam						
Molindone	T43.591	T43.592	T43.593	T43.594	T43.595	T43.596
Molsidomine	T46.3X1	T46.3X2	T46.3X3	T46.3X4	T46.3X5	T46.3X6
Mometasone	T49.ØX1	T49.ØX2	T49.ØX3	T49.ØX4	T49.ØX5	T49.ØX6
Monistat	T49.ØX1	T49.ØX2	T49.ØX3	T49.ØX4	T49.ØX5	T49.ØX6
Monkshood	T62.2X1	T62.2X2	T62.2X3	T62.2X4	—	—
Monoamine oxidase inhibitor NEC	T43.1X1	T43.1X2	T43.1X3	T43.1X4	T43.1X5	T43.1X6
hydrazine	T43.1X1	T43.1X2	T43.1X3	T43.1X4	T43.1X5	T43.1X6
Monobenzone	T49.4X1	T49.4X2	T49.4X3	T49.4X4	T49.4X5	T49.4X6
Monochloroacetic acid	T6Ø.3X1	T6Ø.3X2	T6Ø.3X3	T6Ø.3X4	—	—
Monochlorobenzene	T53.7X1	T53.7X2	T53.7X3	T53.7X4	—	—
Monoethanolamine	T46.8X1	T46.8X2	T46.8X3	T46.8X4	T46.8X5	T46.8X6
oleate	T46.8X1	T46.8X2	T46.8X3	T46.8X4	T46.8X5	T46.8X6
Monooctanoin	T5Ø.991	T5Ø.992	T5Ø.993	T5Ø.994	T5Ø.995	T5Ø.996
Monophenylbutazone	T39.2X1	T39.2X2	T39.2X3	T39.2X4	T39.2X5	T39.2X6
Monopril*	T46.4X1	T46.4X2	T46.4X3	T46.4X4	T46.4X5	T46.4X6
Monosodium glutamate	T65.891	T65.892	T65.893	T65.894	—	—
Monosulfiram	T49.ØX1	T49.ØX2	T49.ØX3	T49.ØX4	T49.ØX5	T49.ØX6
Monoxide, carbon — *see* Carbon, monoxide						
Monoxidine hydrochloride	T46.1X1	T46.1X2	T46.1X3	T46.1X4	T46.1X5	T46.1X6
Monuron	T6Ø.3X1	T6Ø.3X2	T6Ø.3X3	T6Ø.3X4	—	—
Moperone	T43.4X1	T43.4X2	T43.4X3	T43.4X4	T43.4X5	T43.4X6
Mopidamol	T45.1X1	T45.1X2	T45.1X3	T45.1X4	T45.1X5	T45.1X6
MOPP (mechloreth-amine + vincristine + prednisone + procarba-zine)	T45.1X1	T45.1X2	T45.1X3	T45.1X4	T45.1X5	T45.1X6
Morfin	T4Ø.2X1	T4Ø.2X2	T4Ø.2X3	T4Ø.2X4	T4Ø.2X5	T4Ø.2X6
Morinamide	T37.1X1	T37.1X2	T37.1X3	T37.1X4	T37.1X5	T37.1X6
Morning glory seeds	T4Ø.991	T4Ø.992	T4Ø.993	T4Ø.994	—	—
Moroxydine	T37.5X1	T37.5X2	T37.5X3	T37.5X4	T37.5X5	T37.5X6
Morphazinamide	T37.1X1	T37.1X2	T37.1X3	T37.1X4	T37.1X5	T37.1X6
Morphine	T4Ø.2X1	T4Ø.2X2	T4Ø.2X3	T4Ø.2X4	T4Ø.2X5	T4Ø.2X6
antagonist	T5Ø.7X1	T5Ø.7X2	T5Ø.7X3	T5Ø.7X4	T5Ø.7X5	T5Ø.7X6
Morpholinylethylmorphine	T4Ø.2X1	T4Ø.2X2	T4Ø.2X3	T4Ø.2X4	—	—
Morsuximide	T42.2X1	T42.2X2	T42.2X3	T42.2X4	T42.2X5	T42.2X6
Mosapramine	T43.591	T43.592	T43.593	T43.594	T43.595	T43.596
Moth balls — *see also* Pesticide	T6Ø.2X1	T6Ø.2X2	T6Ø.2X3	T6Ø.2X4	—	—
naphthalene	T6Ø.2X1	T6Ø.2X2	T6Ø.2X3	T6Ø.2X4	—	—
paradichlorobenzene	T6Ø.1X1	T6Ø.1X2	T6Ø.1X3	T6Ø.1X4	—	—
Motor exhaust gas	T58.Ø1	T58.Ø2	T58.Ø3	T58.Ø4	—	—
Motrin*	T39.311	T39.312	T39.313	T39.314	T39.315	T39.316
Mouthwash (antiseptic) (zinc chloride)	T49.6X1	T49.6X2	T49.6X3	T49.6X4	T49.6X5	T49.6X6
Moxastine	T45.ØX1	T45.ØX2	T45.ØX3	T45.ØX4	T45.ØX5	T45.ØX6
Moxaverine	T44.3X1	T44.3X2	T44.3X3	T44.3X4	T44.3X5	T44.3X6
Moxisylyte	T46.7X1	T46.7X2	T46.7X3	T46.7X4	T46.7X5	T46.7X6
Mucilage, plant	T47.4X1	T47.4X2	T47.4X3	T47.4X4	T47.4X5	T47.4X6
Mucolytic drug	T48.4X1	T48.4X2	T48.4X3	T48.4X4	T48.4X5	T48.4X6
Mucomyst	T48.4X1	T48.4X2	T48.4X3	T48.4X4	T48.4X5	T48.4X6
Mucous membrane agents (external)	T49.91	T49.92	T49.93	T49.94	T49.95	T49.96
specified NEC	T49.8X1	T49.8X2	T49.8X3	T49.8X4	T49.8X5	T49.8X6
Multaq*	T46.2X1	T46.2X2	T46.2X3	T46.2X4	T46.2X5	T46.2X6
Multiple unspecified drugs, medicaments and biological substances	T5Ø.911	T5Ø.912	T5Ø.913	T5Ø.914	T5Ø.915	T5Ø.916
Mumps						
immune globulin (human)	T5Ø.Z11	T5Ø.Z12	T5Ø.Z13	T5Ø.Z14	T5Ø.Z15	T5Ø.Z16
skin test antigen	T5Ø.8X1	T5Ø.8X2	T5Ø.8X3	T5Ø.8X4	T5Ø.8X5	T5Ø.8X6
vaccine	T5Ø.B91	T5Ø.B92	T5Ø.B93	T5Ø.B94	T5Ø.B95	T5Ø.B96
Mumpsvax	T5Ø.B91	T5Ø.B92	T5Ø.B93	T5Ø.B94	T5Ø.B95	T5Ø.B96
Mupirocin	T49.ØX1	T49.ØX2	T49.ØX3	T49.ØX4	T49.ØX5	T49.ØX6
Muriatic acid — *see* Hydrochloric acid						
Muromonab-CD3	T45.1X1	T45.1X2	T45.1X3	T45.1X4	T45.1X5	T45.1X6
Muscle-action drug NEC	T48.2Ø1	T48.2Ø2	T48.2Ø3	T48.2Ø4	T48.2Ø5	T48.2Ø6
Muscle affecting agents NEC	T48.2Ø1	T48.2Ø2	T48.2Ø3	T48.2Ø4	T48.2Ø5	T48.2Ø6
oxytocic	T48.ØX1	T48.ØX2	T48.ØX3	T48.ØX4	T48.ØX5	T48.ØX6
relaxants	T48.2Ø1	T48.2Ø2	T48.2Ø3	T48.2Ø4	T48.2Ø5	T48.2Ø6
central nervous system	T42.8X1	T42.8X2	T42.8X3	T42.8X4	T42.8X5	T42.8X6
skeletal	T48.1X1	T48.1X2	T48.1X3	T48.1X4	T48.1X5	T48.1X6
smooth	T44.3X1	T44.3X2	T44.3X3	T44.3X4	T44.3X5	T44.3X6
Muscle relaxant — *see* Relaxant, muscle						
Muscle-tone depressant, central NEC	T42.8X1	T42.8X2	T42.8X3	T42.8X4	T42.8X5	T42.8X6
specified NEC	T42.8X1	T42.8X2	T42.8X3	T42.8X4	T42.8X5	T42.8X6
Mushroom, noxious	T62.ØX1	T62.ØX2	T62.ØX3	T62.ØX4	—	—
Mussel, noxious	T61.781	T61.782	T61.783	T61.784	—	—
Mustard (emetic)	T47.7X1	T47.7X2	T47.7X3	T47.7X4	T47.7X5	T47.7X6
black	T47.7X1	T47.7X2	T47.7X3	T47.7X4	T47.7X5	T47.7X6
gas, not in war	T59.91	T59.92	T59.93	T59.94	—	—
nitrogen	T45.1X1	T45.1X2	T45.1X3	T45.1X4	T45.1X5	T45.1X6
Mustine	T45.1X1	T45.1X2	T45.1X3	T45.1X4	T45.1X5	T45.1X6
M-vac	T45.1X1	T45.1X2	T45.1X3	T45.1X4	T45.1X5	T45.1X6
Mycifradin	T36.5X1	T36.5X2	T36.5X3	T36.5X4	T36.5X5	T36.5X6
topical	T49.ØX1	T49.ØX2	T49.ØX3	T49.ØX4	T49.ØX5	T49.ØX6
Mycitracin	T36.8X1	T36.8X2	T36.8X3	T36.8X4	T36.8X5	T36.8X6
ophthalmic preparation	T49.5X1	T49.5X2	T49.5X3	T49.5X4	T49.5X5	T49.5X6
Mycostatin	T36.7X1	T36.7X2	T36.7X3	T36.7X4	T36.7X5	T36.7X6
topical	T49.ØX1	T49.ØX2	T49.ØX3	T49.ØX4	T49.ØX5	T49.ØX6
Mycotoxins	T64.81	T64.82	T64.83	T64.84	—	—
aflatoxin	T64.Ø1	T64.Ø2	T64.Ø3	T64.Ø4	—	—
specified NEC	T64.81	T64.82	T64.83	T64.84	—	—
Mydriacyl	T44.3X1	T44.3X2	T44.3X3	T44.3X4	T44.3X5	T44.3X6
Mydriatic drug	T49.5X1	T49.5X2	T49.5X3	T49.5X4	T49.5X5	T49.5X6
Myelobromal	T45.1X1	T45.1X2	T45.1X3	T45.1X4	T45.1X5	T45.1X6
Myleran	T45.1X1	T45.1X2	T45.1X3	T45.1X4	T45.1X5	T45.1X6
Myochrysin (e)	T39.2X1	T39.2X2	T39.2X3	T39.2X4	T39.2X5	T39.2X6
Myoneural blocking agents	T48.1X1	T48.1X2	T48.1X3	T48.1X4	T48.1X5	T48.1X6
Myrac*	T36.4X1	T36.4X2	T36.4X3	T36.4X4	T36.4X5	T36.4X6

Metycaine — Myrac*

Substance	Poisoning, Accidental (unintentional)	Poisoning, Intentional Self-harm	Poisoning, Assault	Poisoning, Undetermined	Adverse Effect	Under-dosing
Myralact	T49.ØX1	T49.ØX2	T49.ØX3	T49.ØX4	T49.ØX5	T49.ØX6
Myristica fragrans	T62.2X1	T62.2X2	T62.2X3	T62.2X4	—	—
Myristicin	T65.891	T65.892	T65.893	T65.894	—	—
Mysoline	T42.3X1	T42.3X2	T42.3X3	T42.3X4	T42.3X5	T42.3X6
Nabilone	T4Ø.711	T4Ø.712	T4Ø.713	T4Ø.714	T4Ø.715	T4Ø.716
Nabumetone	T39.391	T39.392	T39.393	T39.394	T39.395	T39.396
Nadolol	T44.7X1	T44.7X2	T44.7X3	T44.7X4	T44.7X5	T44.7X6
Nafcillin	T36.ØX1	T36.ØX2	T36.ØX3	T36.ØX4	T36.ØX5	T36.ØX6
Nafoxidine	T38.6X1	T38.6X2	T38.6X3	T38.6X4	T38.6X5	T38.6X6
Naftazone	T46.991	T46.992	T46.993	T46.994	T46.995	T46.996
Naftidrofuryl (oxalate)	T46.7X1	T46.7X2	T46.7X3	T46.7X4	T46.7X5	T46.7X6
Naftifine	T49.ØX1	T49.ØX2	T49.ØX3	T49.ØX4	T49.ØX5	T49.ØX6
Nail polish remover	T52.91	T52.92	T52.93	T52.94	—	—
Nalbuphine	T4Ø.491	T4Ø.492	T4Ø.493	T4Ø.494	T4Ø.495	T4Ø.496
Naled	T6Ø.ØX1	T6Ø.ØX2	T6Ø.ØX3	T6Ø.ØX4	—	—
Nalidixic acid	T37.8X1	T37.8X2	T37.8X3	T37.8X4	T37.8X5	T37.8X6
Nalorphine	T5Ø.7X1	T5Ø.7X2	T5Ø.7X3	T5Ø.7X4	T5Ø.7X5	T5Ø.7X6
Naloxone	T5Ø.7X1	T5Ø.7X2	T5Ø.7X3	T5Ø.7X4	T5Ø.7X5	T5Ø.7X6
Naltrexone	T5Ø.7X1	T5Ø.7X2	T5Ø.7X3	T5Ø.7X4	T5Ø.7X5	T5Ø.7X6
Namenda	T43.8X1	T43.8X2	T43.8X3	T43.8X4	T43.8X5	T43.8X6
Nandrolone	T38.7X1	T38.7X2	T38.7X3	T38.7X4	T38.7X5	T38.7X6
Naphazoline	T48.5X1	T48.5X2	T48.5X3	T48.5X4	T48.5X5	T48.5X6
Naphtha (painters') (petroleum)	T52.ØX1	T52.ØX2	T52.ØX3	T52.ØX4	—	—
solvent	T52.ØX1	T52.ØX2	T52.ØX3	T52.ØX4	—	—
vapor	T52.ØX1	T52.ØX2	T52.ØX3	T52.ØX4	—	—
Naphthalene (non-chlorinated)	T6Ø.2X1	T6Ø.2X2	T6Ø.2X3	T6Ø.2X4	—	—
chlorinated	T6Ø.1X1	T6Ø.1X2	T6Ø.1X3	T6Ø.1X4	—	—
vapor	T6Ø.1X1	T6Ø.1X2	T6Ø.1X3	T6Ø.1X4	—	—
insecticide or moth repellent	T6Ø.2X1	T6Ø.2X2	T6Ø.2X3	T6Ø.2X4	—	—
chlorinated	T6Ø.1X1	T6Ø.1X2	T6Ø.1X3	T6Ø.1X4	—	—
vapor	T6Ø.2X1	T6Ø.2X2	T6Ø.2X3	T6Ø.2X4	—	—
chlorinated	T6Ø.1X1	T6Ø.1X2	T6Ø.1X3	T6Ø.1X4	—	—
Naphthol	T65.891	T65.892	T65.893	T65.894	—	—
Naphthylamine	T65.891	T65.892	T65.893	T65.894	—	—
Naphthylthiourea (ANTU)	T6Ø.4X1	T6Ø.4X2	T6Ø.4X3	T6Ø.4X4	—	—
Naprosyn — *see* Naproxen						
Naproxen	T39.311	T39.312	T39.313	T39.314	T39.315	T39.316
Narcotic (drug)	T4Ø.6Ø1	T4Ø.6Ø2	T4Ø.6Ø3	T4Ø.6Ø4	T4Ø.6Ø5	T4Ø.6Ø6
analgesic NEC	T4Ø.6Ø1	T4Ø.6Ø2	T4Ø.6Ø3	T4Ø.6Ø4	T4Ø.6Ø5	T4Ø.6Ø6
antagonist	T5Ø.7X1	T5Ø.7X2	T5Ø.7X3	T5Ø.7X4	T5Ø.7X5	T5Ø.7X6
specified NEC	T4Ø.691	T4Ø.692	T4Ø.693	T4Ø.694	T4Ø.695	T4Ø.696
synthetic	T4Ø.491	T4Ø.492	T4Ø.493	T4Ø.494	T4Ø.495	T4Ø.496
Narcotine	T48.3X1	T48.3X2	T48.3X3	T48.3X4	T48.3X5	T48.3X6
Nardil	T43.1X1	T43.1X2	T43.1X3	T43.1X4	T43.1X5	T43.1X6
Nasacort*	T49.5X1	T49.5X2	T49.5X3	T49.5X4	T49.5X5	T49.5X6
Nasal drug NEC	T49.6X1	T49.6X2	T49.6X3	T49.6X4	T49.6X5	T49.6X6
Natamycin	T49.ØX1	T49.ØX2	T49.ØX3	T49.ØX4	T49.ØX5	T49.ØX6
Natrium cyanide — *see* Cyanide(s)						
Natural						
blood (product)	T45.8X1	T45.8X2	T45.8X3	T45.8X4	T45.8X5	T45.8X6
gas (piped)	T59.891	T59.892	T59.893	T59.894	—	—
incomplete combustion	T58.11	T58.12	T58.13	T58.14		
Nealbarbital	T42.3X1	T42.3X2	T42.3X3	T42.3X4	T42.3X5	T42.3X6
Nectadon	T48.3X1	T48.3X2	T48.3X3	T48.3X4	T48.3X5	T48.3X6
Nedocromil	T48.6X1	T48.6X2	T48.6X3	T48.6X4	T48.6X5	T48.6X6
Nefopam	T39.8X1	T39.8X2	T39.8X3	T39.8X4	T39.8X5	T39.8X6
Nematocyst (sting)	T63.691	T63.692	T63.693	T63.694	—	—
Nembutal	T42.3X1	T42.3X2	T42.3X3	T42.3X4	T42.3X5	T42.3X6
Nemonapride	T43.591	T43.592	T43.593	T43.594	T43.595	T43.596
Neoarsphenamine	T37.8X1	T37.8X2	T37.8X3	T37.8X4	T37.8X5	T37.8X6
Neocinchophen	T5Ø.4X1	T5Ø.4X2	T5Ø.4X3	T5Ø.4X4	T5Ø.4X5	T5Ø.4X6
Neomycin (derivatives)	T36.5X1	T36.5X2	T36.5X3	T36.5X4	T36.5X5	T36.5X6
with						
bacitracin	T49.ØX1	T49.ØX2	T49.ØX3	T49.ØX4	T49.ØX5	T49.ØX6
neostigmine	T44.ØX1	T44.ØX2	T44.ØX3	T44.ØX4	T44.ØX5	T44.ØX6
ENT agent	T49.6X1	T49.6X2	T49.6X3	T49.6X4	T49.6X5	T49.6X6
ophthalmic preparation	T49.5X1	T49.5X2	T49.5X3	T49.5X4	T49.5X5	T49.5X6
topical NEC	T49.ØX1	T49.ØX2	T49.ØX3	T49.ØX4	T49.ØX5	T49.ØX6
Neonal	T42.3X1	T42.3X2	T42.3X3	T42.3X4	T42.3X5	T42.3X6
Neopham*	T5Ø.3X1	T5Ø.3X2	T5Ø.3X3	T5Ø.3X4	T5Ø.3X5	T5Ø.3X6
Neoprontosil	T37.ØX1	T37.ØX2	T37.ØX3	T37.ØX4	T37.ØX5	T37.ØX6
Neosalvarsan	T37.8X1	T37.8X2	T37.8X3	T37.8X4	T37.8X5	T37.8X6
Neosilversalvarsan	T37.8X1	T37.8X2	T37.8X3	T37.8X4	T37.8X5	T37.8X6
Neosporin	T36.8X1	T36.8X2	T36.8X3	T36.8X4	T36.8X5	T36.8X6
ENT agent	T49.6X1	T49.6X2	T49.6X3	T49.6X4	T49.6X5	T49.6X6
opthalmic preparation	T49.5X1	T49.5X2	T49.5X3	T49.5X4	T49.5X5	T49.5X6
topical NEC	T49.ØX1	T49.ØX2	T49.ØX3	T49.ØX4	T49.ØX5	T49.ØX6
Neostigmine bromide	T44.ØX1	T44.ØX2	T44.ØX3	T44.ØX4	T44.ØX5	T44.ØX6
Neraval	T42.3X1	T42.3X2	T42.3X3	T42.3X4	T42.3X5	T42.3X6

Substance	Poisoning, Accidental (unintentional)	Poisoning, Intentional Self-harm	Poisoning, Assault	Poisoning, Undetermined	Adverse Effect	Under-dosing
Neravan	T42.3X1	T42.3X2	T42.3X3	T42.3X4	T42.3X5	T42.3X6
Nerium oleander	T62.2X1	T62.2X2	T62.2X3	T62.2X4	—	—
Nerlynx*	T45.1X1	T45.1X2	T45.1X3	T45.1X4	T45.1X5	T45.1X6
Nerve gas, not in war	T59.91	T59.92	T59.93	T59.94	—	—
Nesacaine	T41.3X1	T41.3X2	T41.3X3	T41.3X4	T41.3X5	T41.3X6
infiltration (subcutaneous)	T41.3X1	T41.3X2	T41.3X3	T41.3X4	T41.3X5	T41.3X6
nerve block (peripheral) (plexus)	T41.3X1	T41.3X2	T41.3X3	T41.3X4	T41.3X5	T41.3X6
Netilmicin	T36.5X1	T36.5X2	T36.5X3	T36.5X4	T36.5X5	T36.5X6
Neurobarb	T42.3X1	T42.3X2	T42.3X3	T42.3X4	T42.3X5	T42.3X6
Neuroleptic drug NEC	T43.5Ø1	T43.5Ø2	T43.5Ø3	T43.5Ø4	T43.5Ø5	T43.5Ø6
Neuromuscular blocking drug	T48.1X1	T48.1X2	T48.1X3	T48.1X4	T48.1X5	T48.1X6
Neutral insulin injection	T38.3X1	T38.3X2	T38.3X3	T38.3X4	T38.3X5	T38.3X6
Neutral spirits	T51.ØX1	T51.ØX2	T51.ØX3	T51.ØX4	—	—
beverage	T51.ØX1	T51.ØX2	T51.ØX3	T51.ØX4	—	—
Niacin	T46.7X1	T46.7X2	T46.7X3	T46.7X4	T46.7X5	T46.7X6
Niacinamide	T45.2X1	T45.2X2	T45.2X3	T45.2X4	T45.2X5	T45.2X6
Nialamide	T43.1X1	T43.1X2	T43.1X3	T43.1X4	T43.1X5	T43.1X6
Niaprazine	T42.6X1	T42.6X2	T42.6X3	T42.6X4	T42.6X5	T42.6X6
Nicametate	T46.7X1	T46.7X2	T46.7X3	T46.7X4	T46.7X5	T46.7X6
Nicardipine	T46.1X1	T46.1X2	T46.1X3	T46.1X4	T46.1X5	T46.1X6
Nicergoline	T46.7X1	T46.7X2	T46.7X3	T46.7X4	T46.7X5	T46.7X6
Nickel (carbonyl) (tetra-carbonyl) (fumes) (vapor)	T56.891	T56.892	T56.893	T56.894	—	—
Nickelocene	T56.891	T56.892	T56.893	T56.894	—	—
Niclosamide	T37.4X1	T37.4X2	T37.4X3	T37.4X4	T37.4X5	T37.4X6
Nicofuranose	T46.7X1	T46.7X2	T46.7X3	T46.7X4	T46.7X5	T46.7X6
Nicomorphine	T4Ø.2X1	T4Ø.2X2	T4Ø.2X3	T4Ø.2X4	—	—
Nicorandil	T46.3X1	T46.3X2	T46.3X3	T46.3X4	T46.3X5	T46.3X6
Nicotiana (plant)	T62.2X1	T62.2X2	T62.2X3	T62.2X4	—	—
Nicotinamide	T45.2X1	T45.2X2	T45.2X3	T45.2X4	T45.2X5	T45.2X6
Nicotine (insecticide) (spray) (sulfate) **NEC**	T6Ø.2X1	T6Ø.2X2	T6Ø.2X3	T6Ø.2X4	—	—
from tobacco	T65.291	T65.292	T65.293	T65.294	—	—
cigarettes	T65.221	T65.222	T65.223	T65.224	—	—
not insecticide	T65.291	T65.292	T65.293	T65.294	—	—
Nicotinic acid	T46.7X1	T46.7X2	T46.7X3	T46.7X4	T46.7X5	T46.7X6
Nicotinyl alcohol	T46.7X1	T46.7X2	T46.7X3	T46.7X4	T46.7X5	T46.7X6
Nicoumalone	T45.511	T45.512	T45.513	T45.514	T45.515	T45.516
Nifedipine	T46.1X1	T46.1X2	T46.1X3	T46.1X4	T46.1X5	T46.1X6
Nifenazone	T39.2X1	T39.2X2	T39.2X3	T39.2X4	T39.2X5	T39.2X6
Nifuraldezone	T37.91	T37.92	T37.93	T37.94	T37.95	T37.96
Nifuratel	T37.8X1	T37.8X2	T37.8X3	T37.8X4	T37.8X5	T37.8X6
Nifurtimox	T37.3X1	T37.3X2	T37.3X3	T37.3X4	T37.3X5	T37.3X6
Nifurtoinol	T37.8X1	T37.8X2	T37.8X3	T37.8X4	T37.8X5	T37.8X6
Nightshade, deadly (solanum) — *see also* Belladonna	T62.2X1	T62.2X2	T62.2X3	T62.2X4	—	—
berry	T62.1X1	T62.1X2	T62.1X3	T62.1X4	—	—
Nikethamide	T5Ø.7X1	T5Ø.7X2	T5Ø.7X3	T5Ø.7X4	T5Ø.7X5	T5Ø.7X6
Nilstat	T36.7X1	T36.7X2	T36.7X3	T36.7X4	T36.7X5	T36.7X6
topical	T49.ØX1	T49.ØX2	T49.ØX3	T49.ØX4	T49.ØX5	T49.ØX6
Nilutamide	T38.6X1	T38.6X2	T38.6X3	T38.6X4	T38.6X5	T38.6X6
Nimesulide	T39.391	T39.392	T39.393	T39.394	T39.395	T39.396
Nimetazepam	T42.4X1	T42.4X2	T42.4X3	T42.4X4	T42.4X5	T42.4X6
Nimodipine	T46.1X1	T46.1X2	T46.1X3	T46.1X4	T46.1X5	T46.1X6
Nimorazole	T37.3X1	T37.3X2	T37.3X3	T37.3X4	T37.3X5	T37.3X6
Nimustine	T45.1X1	T45.1X2	T45.1X3	T45.1X4	T45.1X5	T45.1X6
Nipent*	T45.1X1	T45.1X2	T45.1X3	T45.1X4	T45.1X5	T45.1X6
Niridazole	T37.4X1	T37.4X2	T37.4X3	T37.4X4	T37.4X5	T37.4X6
Nisentil	T4Ø.2X1	T4Ø.2X2	T4Ø.2X3	T4Ø.2X4	T4Ø.2X5	T4Ø.2X6
Nisoldipine	T46.1X1	T46.1X2	T46.1X3	T46.1X4	T46.1X5	T46.1X6
Nitramine	T65.3X1	T65.3X2	T65.3X3	T65.3X4	—	—
Nitrate, organic	T46.3X1	T46.3X2	T46.3X3	T46.3X4	T46.3X5	T46.3X6
Nitrazepam	T42.4X1	T42.4X2	T42.4X3	T42.4X4	T42.4X5	T42.4X6
Nitrefazole	T5Ø.6X1	T5Ø.6X2	T5Ø.6X3	T5Ø.6X4	T5Ø.6X5	T5Ø.6X6
Nitrendipine	T46.1X1	T46.1X2	T46.1X3	T46.1X4	T46.1X5	T46.1X6
Nitric						
acid (liquid)	T54.2X1	T54.2X2	T54.2X3	T54.2X4	—	—
vapor	T59.891	T59.892	T59.893	T59.894	—	—
oxide (gas)	T59.ØX1	T59.ØX2	T59.ØX3	T59.ØX4	—	—
Nitrimidazine	T37.3X1	T37.3X2	T37.3X3	T37.3X4	T37.3X5	T37.3X6
Nitrite, amyl (medicinal) (vapor)	T46.3X1	T46.3X2	T46.3X3	T46.3X4	T46.3X5	T46.3X6
Nitroaniline	T65.3X1	T65.3X2	T65.3X3	T65.3X4	—	—
vapor	T59.891	T59.892	T59.893	T59.894	—	—
Nitrobenzene, nitrobenzol	T65.3X1	T65.3X2	T65.3X3	T65.3X4	—	—
vapor	T65.3X1	T65.3X2	T65.3X3	T65.3X4	—	—
Nitrocellulose	T65.891	T65.892	T65.893	T65.894	—	—
lacquer	T65.891	T65.892	T65.893	T65.894	—	—
Nitrodiphenyl	T65.3X1	T65.3X2	T65.3X3	T65.3X4	—	—
Nitrofural	T49.ØX1	T49.ØX2	T49.ØX3	T49.ØX4	T49.ØX5	T49.ØX6
Nitrofurantoin	T37.8X1	T37.8X2	T37.8X3	T37.8X4	T37.8X5	T37.8X6

*Optum Value-Add

☑ **Additional Character May Be Required — Refer to the Tabular List for Character Selection**

Substance	Poisoning, Accidental (unintentional)	Poisoning, Intentional Self-harm	Poisoning, Assault	Poisoning, Undetermined	Adverse Effect	Under-dosing
Nitrofurazone	T49.ØX1	T49.ØX2	T49.ØX3	T49.ØX4	T49.ØX5	T49.ØX6
Nitrogen	T59.ØX1	T59.ØX2	T59.ØX3	T59.ØX4	—	—
mustard	T45.1X1	T45.1X2	T45.1X3	T45.1X4	T45.1X5	T45.1X6
Nitroglycerin, nitroglycerol (medicinal)	T46.3X1	T46.3X2	T46.3X3	T46.3X4	T46.3X5	T46.3X6
nonmedicinal	T65.5X1	T65.5X2	T65.5X3	T65.5X4	—	—
fumes	T65.5X1	T65.5X2	T65.5X3	T65.5X4	—	—
Nitroglycol	T52.3X1	T52.3X2	T52.3X3	T52.3X4	—	—
Nitrohydrochloric acid	T54.2X1	T54.2X2	T54.2X3	T54.2X4	—	—
Nitromersol	T49.ØX1	T49.ØX2	T49.ØX3	T49.ØX4	T49.ØX5	T49.ØX6
Nitronaphthalene	T65.891	T65.892	T65.893	T65.894	—	—
Nitrophenol	T54.ØX1	T54.ØX2	T54.ØX3	T54.ØX4	—	—
Nitropropane	T52.8X1	T52.8X2	T52.8X3	T52.8X4	—	—
Nitroprusside	T46.5X1	T46.5X2	T46.5X3	T46.5X4	T46.5X5	T46.5X6
Nitrosodimethylamine	T65.3X1	T65.3X2	T65.3X3	T65.3X4	—	—
Nitrothiazol	T37.4X1	T37.4X2	T37.4X3	T37.4X4	T37.4X5	T37.4X6
Nitrotoluene, nitrotoluol	T65.3X1	T65.3X2	T65.3X3	T65.3X4	—	—
vapor	T65.3X1	T65.3X2	T65.3X3	T65.3X4	—	—
Nitrous						
acid (liquid)	T54.2X1	T54.2X2	T54.2X3	T54.2X4	—	—
fumes	T59.891	T59.892	T59.893	T59.894	—	—
ether spirit	T46.3X1	T46.3X2	T46.3X3	T46.3X4	T46.3X5	T46.3X6
oxide	T41.ØX1	T41.ØX2	T41.ØX3	T41.ØX4	T41.ØX5	T41.ØX6
Nitroxoline	T37.8X1	T37.8X2	T37.8X3	T37.8X4	T37.8X5	T37.8X6
Nitrozone	T49.ØX1	T49.ØX2	T49.ØX3	T49.ØX4	T49.ØX5	T49.ØX6
Nizatidine	T47.ØX1	T47.ØX2	T47.ØX3	T47.ØX4	T47.ØX5	T47.ØX6
Nizofenone	T43.8X1	T43.8X2	T43.8X3	T43.8X4	T43.8X5	T43.8X6
Noctec	T42.6X1	T42.6X2	T42.6X3	T42.6X4	T42.6X5	T42.6X6
No Doz*	T43.611	T43.612	T43.613	T43.614	T43.615	T43.616
Noludar	T42.6X1	T42.6X2	T42.6X3	T42.6X4	T42.6X5	T42.6X6
Nomegestrol	T38.5X1	T38.5X2	T38.5X3	T38.5X4	T38.5X5	T38.5X6
Nomifensine	T43.291	T43.292	T43.293	T43.294	T43.295	T43.296
Nonoxinol	T49.8X1	T49.8X2	T49.8X3	T49.8X4	T49.8X5	T49.8X6
Nonylphenoxy (polyethoxyethanol)	T49.8X1	T49.8X2	T49.8X3	T49.8X4	T49.8X5	T49.8X6
Noptil	T42.3X1	T42.3X2	T42.3X3	T42.3X4	T42.3X5	T42.3X6
Noradrenaline	T44.4X1	T44.4X2	T44.4X3	T44.4X4	T44.4X5	T44.4X6
Noramidopyrine	T39.2X1	T39.2X2	T39.2X3	T39.2X4	T39.2X5	T39.2X6
methanesulfonate sodium	T39.2X1	T39.2X2	T39.2X3	T39.2X4	T39.2X5	T39.2X6
Norbormide	T6Ø.4X1	T6Ø.4X2	T6Ø.4X3	T6Ø.4X4	—	—
Nordazepam	T42.4X1	T42.4X2	T42.4X3	T42.4X4	T42.4X5	T42.4X6
Norepinephrine	T44.4X1	T44.4X2	T44.4X3	T44.4X4	T44.4X5	T44.4X6
Norethandrolone	T38.7X1	T38.7X2	T38.7X3	T38.7X4	T38.7X5	T38.7X6
Norethindrone	T38.4X1	T38.4X2	T38.4X3	T38.4X4	T38.4X5	T38.4X6
Norethisterone (acetate) (enantate)	T38.4X1	T38.4X2	T38.4X3	T38.4X4	T38.4X5	T38.4X6
with ethinylestradiol	T38.5X1	T38.5X2	T38.5X3	T38.5X4	T38.5X5	T38.5X6
Noretynodrel	T38.5X1	T38.5X2	T38.5X3	T38.5X4	T38.5X5	T38.5X6
Norfenefrine	T44.4X1	T44.4X2	T44.4X3	T44.4X4	T44.4X5	T44.4X6
Norfloxacin	T36.8X1	T36.8X2	T36.8X3	T36.8X4	T36.8X5	T36.8X6
Norgestrel	T38.4X1	T38.4X2	T38.4X3	T38.4X4	T38.4X5	T38.4X6
Norgestrienone	T38.4X1	T38.4X2	T38.4X3	T38.4X4	T38.4X5	T38.4X6
Norlestrin	T38.4X1	T38.4X2	T38.4X3	T38.4X4	T38.4X5	T38.4X6
Norlutin	T38.4X1	T38.4X2	T38.4X3	T38.4X4	T38.4X5	T38.4X6
Normal serum albumin (human), salt-poor	T45.8X1	T45.8X2	T45.8X3	T45.8X4	T45.8X5	T45.8X6
Normethandrone	T38.5X1	T38.5X2	T38.5X3	T38.5X4	T38.5X5	T38.5X6
Normison — *see* Benzodiazepines						
Normorphine	T4Ø.2X1	T4Ø.2X2	T4Ø.2X3	T4Ø.2X4	—	—
Norpseudoephedrine	T5Ø.5X1	T5Ø.5X2	T5Ø.5X3	T5Ø.5X4	T5Ø.5X5	T5Ø.5X6
Nortestosterone (furanpropionate)	T38.7X1	T38.7X2	T38.7X3	T38.7X4	T38.7X5	T38.7X6
Nortriptyline	T43.Ø11	T43.Ø12	T43.Ø13	T43.Ø14	T43.Ø15	T43.Ø16
Norvasc*	T46.1X1	T46.1X2	T46.1X3	T46.1X4	T46.1X5	T46.1X6
Noscapine	T48.3X1	T48.3X2	T48.3X3	T48.3X4	T48.3X5	T48.3X6
Nose preparations	T49.6X1	T49.6X2	T49.6X3	T49.6X4	T49.6X5	T49.6X6
Novobiocin	T36.5X1	T36.5X2	T36.5X3	T36.5X4	T36.5X5	T36.5X6
Novocain (infiltration) (topical)	T41.3X1	T41.3X2	T41.3X3	T41.3X4	T41.3X5	T41.3X6
nerve block (peripheral) (plexus)	T41.3X1	T41.3X2	T41.3X3	T41.3X4	T41.3X5	T41.3X6
spinal	T41.3X1	T41.3X2	T41.3X3	T41.3X4	T41.3X5	T41.3X6
Noxious foodstuff	T62.91	T62.92	T62.93	T62.94	—	—
specified NEC	T62.8X1	T62.8X2	T62.8X3	T62.8X4	—	—
Noxiptiline	T43.Ø11	T43.Ø12	T43.Ø13	T43.Ø14	T43.Ø15	T43.Ø16
Noxytiolin	T49.ØX1	T49.ØX2	T49.ØX3	T49.ØX4	T49.ØX5	T49.ØX6
NPH Iletin (insulin)	T38.3X1	T38.3X2	T38.3X3	T38.3X4	T38.3X5	T38.3X6
Numorphan	T4Ø.2X1	T4Ø.2X2	T4Ø.2X3	T4Ø.2X4	T4Ø.2X5	T4Ø.2X6
Nunol	T42.3X1	T42.3X2	T42.3X3	T42.3X4	T42.3X5	T42.3X6
Nupercaine (spinal anesthetic)	T41.3X1	T41.3X2	T41.3X3	T41.3X4	T41.3X5	T41.3X6
topical (surface)	T41.3X1	T41.3X2	T41.3X3	T41.3X4	T41.3X5	T41.3X6
Nutmeg oil (liniment)	T49.3X1	T49.3X2	T49.3X3	T49.3X4	T49.3X5	T49.3X6
Nutrilipid*	T5Ø.991	T5Ø.992	T5Ø.993	T5Ø.994	T5Ø.995	T5Ø.996
Nutritional supplement	T5Ø.9Ø1	T5Ø.9Ø2	T5Ø.9Ø3	T5Ø.9Ø4	T5Ø.9Ø5	T5Ø.9Ø6
Nux vomica	T65.1X1	T65.1X2	T65.1X3	T65.1X4	—	—
Nydrazid	T37.1X1	T37.1X2	T37.1X3	T37.1X4	T37.1X5	T37.1X6
Nylidrin	T46.7X1	T46.7X2	T46.7X3	T46.7X4	T46.7X5	T46.7X6
Nystatin	T36.7X1	T36.7X2	T36.7X3	T36.7X4	T36.7X5	T36.7X6
topical	T49.ØX1	T49.ØX2	T49.ØX3	T49.ØX4	T49.ØX5	T49.ØX6
Nytol	T45.ØX1	T45.ØX2	T45.ØX3	T45.ØX4	T45.ØX5	T45.ØX6
Obidoxime chloride	T5Ø.6X1	T5Ø.6X2	T5Ø.6X3	T5Ø.6X4	T5Ø.6X5	T5Ø.6X6
Octafonium (chloride)	T49.3X1	T49.3X2	T49.3X3	T49.3X4	T49.3X5	T49.3X6
Octamethyl pyrophosphoramide	T6Ø.ØX1	T6Ø.ØX2	T6Ø.ØX3	T6Ø.ØX4	—	—
Octanoin	T5Ø.991	T5Ø.992	T5Ø.993	T5Ø.994	T5Ø.995	T5Ø.996
Octatropine methylbromide	T44.3X1	T44.3X2	T44.3X3	T44.3X4	T44.3X5	T44.3X6
Octotiamine	T45.2X1	T45.2X2	T45.2X3	T45.2X4	T45.2X5	T45.2X6
Octoxinol (9)	T49.8X1	T49.8X2	T49.8X3	T49.8X4	T49.8X5	T49.8X6
Octreotide	T38.991	T38.992	T38.993	T38.994	T38.995	T38.996
Octyl nitrite	T46.3X1	T46.3X2	T46.3X3	T46.3X4	T46.3X5	T46.3X6
Oestradiol	T38.5X1	T38.5X2	T38.5X3	T38.5X4	T38.5X5	T38.5X6
Oestriol	T38.5X1	T38.5X2	T38.5X3	T38.5X4	T38.5X5	T38.5X6
Oestrogen	T38.5X1	T38.5X2	T38.5X3	T38.5X4	T38.5X5	T38.5X6
Oestrone	T38.5X1	T38.5X2	T38.5X3	T38.5X4	T38.5X5	T38.5X6
Ofloxacin	T36.8X1	T36.8X2	T36.8X3	T36.8X4	T36.8X5	T36.8X6
Oil (of)	T65.891	T65.892	T65.893	T65.894	—	—
bitter almond	T62.8X1	T62.8X2	T62.8X3	T62.8X4	—	—
cloves	T49.7X1	T49.7X2	T49.7X3	T49.7X4	T49.7X5	T49.7X6
colors	T65.6X1	T65.6X2	T65.6X3	T65.6X4	—	—
fumes	T59.891	T59.892	T59.893	T59.894	—	—
lubricating	T52.ØX1	T52.ØX2	T52.ØX3	T52.ØX4	—	—
Niobe	T52.8X1	T52.8X2	T52.8X3	T52.8X4	—	—
vitriol (liquid)	T54.2X1	T54.2X2	T54.2X3	T54.2X4	—	—
fumes	T54.2X1	T54.2X2	T54.2X3	T54.2X4	—	—
wintergreen (bitter) NEC	T49.3X1	T49.3X2	T49.3X3	T49.3X4	T49.3X5	T49.3X6
Oily preparation (for skin)	T49.3X1	T49.3X2	T49.3X3	T49.3X4	T49.3X5	T49.3X6
Ointment NEC	T49.3X1	T49.3X2	T49.3X3	T49.3X4	T49.3X5	T49.3X6
Olanzapine	T43.591	T43.592	T43.593	T43.594	T43.595	T43.596
Oleander	T62.2X1	T62.2X2	T62.2X3	T62.2X4	—	—
Oleandomycin	T36.3X1	T36.3X2	T36.3X3	T36.3X4	T36.3X5	T36.3X6
Oleandrin	T46.ØX1	T46.ØX2	T46.ØX3	T46.ØX4	T46.ØX5	T46.ØX6
Oleic acid	T46.6X1	T46.6X2	T46.6X3	T46.6X4	T46.6X5	T46.6X6
Oleovitamin A	T45.2X1	T45.2X2	T45.2X3	T45.2X4	T45.2X5	T45.2X6
Oleum ricini	T47.2X1	T47.2X2	T47.2X3	T47.2X4	T47.2X5	T47.2X6
Olive oil (medicinal) **NEC**	T47.4X1	T47.4X2	T47.4X3	T47.4X4	T47.4X5	T47.4X6
Olivomycin	T45.1X1	T45.1X2	T45.1X3	T45.1X4	T45.1X5	T45.1X6
Olodaterol*	T48.6X1	T48.6X2	T48.6X3	T48.6X4	T48.6X5	T48.6X6
Olsalazine	T47.8X1	T47.8X2	T47.8X3	T47.8X4	T47.8X5	T47.8X6
Omeprazole	T47.1X1	T47.1X2	T47.1X3	T47.1X4	T47.1X5	T47.1X6
OMPA	T6Ø.ØX1	T6Ø.ØX2	T6Ø.ØX3	T6Ø.ØX4	—	—
Oncovin	T45.1X1	T45.1X2	T45.1X3	T45.1X4	T45.1X5	T45.1X6
Ondansetron	T45.ØX1	T45.ØX2	T45.ØX3	T45.ØX4	T45.ØX5	T45.ØX6
Ophthaine	T41.3X1	T41.3X2	T41.3X3	T41.3X4	T41.3X5	T41.3X6
Ophthetic	T41.3X1	T41.3X2	T41.3X3	T41.3X4	T41.3X5	T41.3X6
Opiate NEC	T4Ø.6Ø1	T4Ø.6Ø2	T4Ø.6Ø3	T4Ø.6Ø4	T4Ø.6Ø5	T4Ø.6Ø6
antagonists	T5Ø.7X1	T5Ø.7X2	T5Ø.7X3	T5Ø.7X4	T5Ø.7X5	T5Ø.7X6
Opioid NEC	T4Ø.2X1	T4Ø.2X2	T4Ø.2X3	T4Ø.2X4	T4Ø.2X5	T4Ø.2X6
Opipramol	T43.Ø11	T43.Ø12	T43.Ø13	T43.Ø14	T43.Ø15	T43.Ø16
Opium alkaloids (total)	T4Ø.ØX1	T4Ø.ØX2	T4Ø.ØX3	T4Ø.ØX4	T4Ø.ØX5	T4Ø.ØX6
standardized powdered	T4Ø.ØX1	T4Ø.ØX2	T4Ø.ØX3	T4Ø.ØX4	T4Ø.ØX5	T4Ø.ØX6
tincture (camphorated)	T4Ø.ØX1	T4Ø.ØX2	T4Ø.ØX3	T4Ø.ØX4	T4Ø.ØX5	T4Ø.ØX6
Optivar*	T49.5X1	T49.5X2	T49.5X3	T49.5X4	T49.5X5	T49.5X6
Oracon	T38.4X1	T38.4X2	T38.4X3	T38.4X4	T38.4X5	T38.4X6
Oragrafin	T5Ø.8X1	T5Ø.8X2	T5Ø.8X3	T5Ø.8X4	T5Ø.8X5	T5Ø.8X6
Oral contraceptives	T38.4X1	T38.4X2	T38.4X3	T38.4X4	T38.4X5	T38.4X6
Oral rehydration salts	T5Ø.3X1	T5Ø.3X2	T5Ø.3X3	T5Ø.3X4	T5Ø.3X5	T5Ø.3X6
Orazamide	T5Ø.991	T5Ø.992	T5Ø.993	T5Ø.994	T5Ø.995	T5Ø.996
Orciprenaline	T48.291	T48.292	T48.293	T48.294	T48.295	T48.296
Organidin	T48.4X1	T48.4X2	T48.4X3	T48.4X4	T48.4X5	T48.4X6
Organonitrate NEC	T46.3X1	T46.3X2	T46.3X3	T46.3X4	T46.3X5	T46.3X6
Organophosphates	T6Ø.ØX1	T6Ø.ØX2	T6Ø.ØX3	T6Ø.ØX4	—	—
Orimune	T5Ø.B91	T5Ø.B92	T5Ø.B93	T5Ø.B94	T5Ø.B95	T5Ø.B96
Orinase	T38.3X1	T38.3X2	T38.3X3	T38.3X4	T38.3X5	T38.3X6
Ormeloxifene	T38.6X1	T38.6X2	T38.6X3	T38.6X4	T38.6X5	T38.6X6
Ornidazole	T37.3X1	T37.3X2	T37.3X3	T37.3X4	T37.3X5	T37.3X6
Ornithine aspartate	T5Ø.991	T5Ø.992	T5Ø.993	T5Ø.994	T5Ø.995	T5Ø.996
Ornoprostil	T47.1X1	T47.1X2	T47.1X3	T47.1X4	T47.1X5	T47.1X6
Orphenadrine (hydrochloride)	T42.8X1	T42.8X2	T42.8X3	T42.8X4	T42.8X5	T42.8X6
Ortal (sodium)	T42.3X1	T42.3X2	T42.3X3	T42.3X4	T42.3X5	T42.3X6
Orthoboric acid	T49.ØX1	T49.ØX2	T49.ØX3	T49.ØX4	T49.ØX5	T49.ØX6
ENT agent	T49.6X1	T49.6X2	T49.6X3	T49.6X4	T49.6X5	T49.6X6
ophthalmic preparation	T49.5X1	T49.5X2	T49.5X3	T49.5X4	T49.5X5	T49.5X6

Substance	Poisoning, Accidental (unintentional)	Poisoning, Intentional Self-harm	Poisoning, Assault	Poisoning, Undetermined	Adverse Effect	Under-dosing
Orthocaine	T41.3X1	T41.3X2	T41.3X3	T41.3X4	T41.3X5	T41.3X6
Orthodichlorobenzene	T53.7X1	T53.7X2	T53.7X3	T53.7X4	—	—
Ortho-Novum	T38.4X1	T38.4X2	T38.4X3	T38.4X4	T38.4X5	T38.4X6
Orthotolidine (reagent)	T54.2X1	T54.2X2	T54.2X3	T54.2X4	—	—
Osmic acid (liquid)	T54.2X1	T54.2X2	T54.2X3	T54.2X4	—	—
fumes	T54.2X1	T54.2X2	T54.2X3	T54.2X4	—	—
Osmotic diuretics	T5Ø.2X1	T5Ø.2X2	T5Ø.2X3	T5Ø.2X4	T5Ø.2X5	T5Ø.2X6
Otilonium bromide	T44.3X1	T44.3X2	T44.3X3	T44.3X4	T44.3X5	T44.3X6
Otorhinolaryngological drug NEC	T49.6X1	T49.6X2	T49.6X3	T49.6X4	T49.6X5	T49.6X6
Ouabain (e)	T46.ØX1	T46.ØX2	T46.ØX3	T46.ØX4	T46.ØX5	T46.ØX6
Ovarian						
hormone	T38.5X1	T38.5X2	T38.5X3	T38.5X4	T38.5X5	T38.5X6
stimulant	T38.5X1	T38.5X2	T38.5X3	T38.5X4	T38.5X5	T38.5X6
Ovide*	T49.ØX1	T49.ØX2	T49.ØX3	T49.ØX4	T49.ØX5	T49.ØX6
Ovral	T38.4X1	T38.4X2	T38.4X3	T38.4X4	T38.4X5	T38.4X6
Ovulen	T38.4X1	T38.4X2	T38.4X3	T38.4X4	T38.4X5	T38.4X6
Oxacillin	T36.ØX1	T36.ØX2	T36.ØX3	T36.ØX4	T36.ØX5	T36.ØX6
Oxalic acid	T54.2X1	T54.2X2	T54.2X3	T54.2X4	—	—
ammonium salt	T5Ø.991	T5Ø.992	T5Ø.993	T5Ø.994	T5Ø.995	T5Ø.996
Oxamniquine	T37.4X1	T37.4X2	T37.4X3	T37.4X4	T37.4X5	T37.4X6
Oxanamide	T43.591	T43.592	T43.593	T43.594	T43.595	T43.596
Oxandrolone	T38.7X1	T38.7X2	T38.7X3	T38.7X4	T38.7X5	T38.7X6
Oxantel	T37.4X1	T37.4X2	T37.4X3	T37.4X4	T37.4X5	T37.4X6
Oxapium iodide	T44.3X1	T44.3X2	T44.3X3	T44.3X4	T44.3X5	T44.3X6
Oxaprotiline	T43.Ø21	T43.Ø22	T43.Ø23	T43.Ø24	T43.Ø25	T43.Ø26
Oxaprozin	T39.311	T39.312	T39.313	T39.314	T39.315	T39.316
Oxatomide	T45.ØX1	T45.ØX2	T45.ØX3	T45.ØX4	T45.ØX5	T45.ØX6
Oxazepam	T42.4X1	T42.4X2	T42.4X3	T42.4X4	T42.4X5	T42.4X6
Oxazimedrine	T5Ø.5X1	T5Ø.5X2	T5Ø.5X3	T5Ø.5X4	T5Ø.5X5	T5Ø.5X6
Oxazolam	T42.4X1	T42.4X2	T42.4X3	T42.4X4	T42.4X5	T42.4X6
Oxazolidine derivatives	T42.2X1	T42.2X2	T42.2X3	T42.2X4	T42.2X5	T42.2X6
Oxazolidinedione (derivative)	T42.2X1	T42.2X2	T42.2X3	T42.2X4	T42.2X5	T42.2X6
Ox bile extract	T47.5X1	T47.5X2	T47.5X3	T47.5X4	T47.5X5	T47.5X6
Oxcarbazepine	T42.1X1	T42.1X2	T42.1X3	T42.1X4	T42.1X5	T42.1X6
Oxedrine	T44.4X1	T44.4X2	T44.4X3	T44.4X4	T44.4X5	T44.4X6
Oxeladin (citrate)	T48.3X1	T48.3X2	T48.3X3	T48.3X4	T48.3X5	T48.3X6
Oxendolone	T38.5X1	T38.5X2	T38.5X3	T38.5X4	T38.5X5	T38.5X6
Oxetacaine	T41.3X1	T41.3X2	T41.3X3	T41.3X4	T41.3X5	T41.3X6
Oxethazine	T41.3X1	T41.3X2	T41.3X3	T41.3X4	T41.3X5	T41.3X6
Oxetorone	T39.8X1	T39.8X2	T39.8X3	T39.8X4	T39.8X5	T39.8X6
Oxiconazole	T49.ØX1	T49.ØX2	T49.ØX3	T49.ØX4	T49.ØX5	T49.ØX6
Oxidizing agent NEC	T54.91	T54.92	T54.93	T54.94	—	—
Oxipurinol	T5Ø.4X1	T5Ø.4X2	T5Ø.4X3	T5Ø.4X4	T5Ø.4X5	T5Ø.4X6
Oxitriptan	T43.291	T43.292	T43.293	T43.294	T43.295	T43.296
Oxitropium bromide	T48.6X1	T48.6X2	T48.6X3	T48.6X4	T48.6X5	T48.6X6
Oxodipine	T46.1X1	T46.1X2	T46.1X3	T46.1X4	T46.1X5	T46.1X6
Oxolamine	T48.3X1	T48.3X2	T48.3X3	T48.3X4	T48.3X5	T48.3X6
Oxolinic acid	T37.8X1	T37.8X2	T37.8X3	T37.8X4	T37.8X5	T37.8X6
Oxomemazine	T43.3X1	T43.3X2	T43.3X3	T43.3X4	T43.3X5	T43.3X6
Oxophenarsine	T37.3X1	T37.3X2	T37.3X3	T37.3X4	T37.3X5	T37.3X6
Oxprenolol	T44.7X1	T44.7X2	T44.7X3	T44.7X4	T44.7X5	T44.7X6
Oxsoralen	T49.3X1	T49.3X2	T49.3X3	T49.3X4	T49.3X5	T49.3X6
Oxtriphylline	T48.6X1	T48.6X2	T48.6X3	T48.6X4	T48.6X5	T48.6X6
Oxybate sodium	T41.291	T41.292	T41.293	T41.294	T41.295	T41.296
Oxybuprocaine	T41.3X1	T41.3X2	T41.3X3	T41.3X4	T41.3X5	T41.3X6
Oxybutynin	T44.3X1	T44.3X2	T44.3X3	T44.3X4	T44.3X5	T44.3X6
Oxychlorosene	T49.ØX1	T49.ØX2	T49.ØX3	T49.ØX4	T49.ØX5	T49.ØX6
Oxycodone	T4Ø.2X1	T4Ø.2X2	T4Ø.2X3	T4Ø.2X4	T4Ø.2X5	T4Ø.2X6
OxyContin*	T4Ø.2X1	T4Ø.2X2	T4Ø.2X3	T4Ø.2X4	T4Ø.2X5	T4Ø.2X6
Oxyfedrine	T46.3X1	T46.3X2	T46.3X3	T46.3X4	T46.3X5	T46.3X6
Oxygen	T41.5X1	T41.5X2	T41.5X3	T41.5X4	T41.5X5	T41.5X6
Oxylone	T49.ØX1	T49.ØX2	T49.ØX3	T49.ØX4	T49.ØX5	T49.ØX6
ophthalmic preparation	T49.5X1	T49.5X2	T49.5X3	T49.5X4	T49.5X5	T49.5X6
Oxymesterone	T38.7X1	T38.7X2	T38.7X3	T38.7X4	T38.7X5	T38.7X6
Oxymetazoline	T48.5X1	T48.5X2	T48.5X3	T48.5X4	T48.5X5	T48.5X6
Oxymetholone	T38.7X1	T38.7X2	T38.7X3	T38.7X4	T38.7X5	T38.7X6
Oxymorphone	T4Ø.2X1	T4Ø.2X2	T4Ø.2X3	T4Ø.2X4	T4Ø.2X5	T4Ø.2X6
Oxypertine	T43.591	T43.592	T43.593	T43.594	T43.595	T43.596
Oxyphenbutazone	T39.2X1	T39.2X2	T39.2X3	T39.2X4	T39.2X5	T39.2X6
Oxyphencyclimine	T44.3X1	T44.3X2	T44.3X3	T44.3X4	T44.3X5	T44.3X6
Oxyphenisatine	T47.2X1	T47.2X2	T47.2X3	T47.2X4	T47.2X5	T47.2X6
Oxyphenonium bromide	T44.3X1	T44.3X2	T44.3X3	T44.3X4	T44.3X5	T44.3X6
Oxypolygelatin	T45.8X1	T45.8X2	T45.8X3	T45.8X4	T45.8X5	T45.8X6
Oxyquinoline (derivatives)	T37.8X1	T37.8X2	T37.8X3	T37.8X4	T37.8X5	T37.8X6
Oxytetracycline	T36.4X1	T36.4X2	T36.4X3	T36.4X4	T36.4X5	T36.4X6
Oxytocic drug NEC	T48.ØX1	T48.ØX2	T48.ØX3	T48.ØX4	T48.ØX5	T48.ØX6
Oxytocin (synthetic)	T48.ØX1	T48.ØX2	T48.ØX3	T48.ØX4	T48.ØX5	T48.ØX6
Oxytrol*	T44.3X1	T44.3X2	T44.3X3	T44.3X4	T44.3X5	T44.3X6
Ozone	T59.891	T59.892	T59.893	T59.894	—	—
PABA	T49.3X1	T49.3X2	T49.3X3	T49.3X4	T49.3X5	T49.3X6
Packed red cells	T45.8X1	T45.8X2	T45.8X3	T45.8X4	T45.8X5	T45.8X6

Substance	Poisoning, Accidental (unintentional)	Poisoning, Intentional Self-harm	Poisoning, Assault	Poisoning, Undetermined	Adverse Effect	Under-dosing
Padimate	T49.3X1	T49.3X2	T49.3X3	T49.3X4	T49.3X5	T49.3X6
Paint NEC	T65.6X1	T65.6X2	T65.6X3	T65.6X4	—	—
cleaner	T52.91	T52.92	T52.93	T52.94	—	—
fumes NEC	T59.891	T59.892	T59.893	T59.894	—	—
lead (fumes)	T56.ØX1	T56.ØX2	T56.ØX3	T56.ØX4	—	—
solvent NEC	T52.8X1	T52.8X2	T52.8X3	T52.8X4	—	—
stripper	T52.8X1	T52.8X2	T52.8X3	T52.8X4	—	—
Palfium	T4Ø.2X1	T4Ø.2X2	T4Ø.2X3	T4Ø.2X4	—	—
Palm kernel oil	T5Ø.991	T5Ø.992	T5Ø.993	T5Ø.994	T5Ø.995	T5Ø.996
Paludrine	T37.2X1	T37.2X2	T37.2X3	T37.2X4	T37.2X5	T37.2X6
PAM (pralidoxime)	T5Ø.6X1	T5Ø.6X2	T5Ø.6X3	T5Ø.6X4	T5Ø.6X5	T5Ø.6X6
Pamaquine (naphthoute)	T37.2X1	T37.2X2	T37.2X3	T37.2X4	T37.2X5	T37.2X6
Panadol	T39.1X1	T39.1X2	T39.1X3	T39.1X4	T39.1X5	T39.1X6
Pancreatic						
digestive secretion stimulant	T47.8X1	T47.8X2	T47.8X3	T47.8X4	T47.8X5	T47.8X6
dornase	T45.3X1	T45.3X2	T45.3X3	T45.3X4	T45.3X5	T45.3X6
Pancreatin	T47.5X1	T47.5X2	T47.5X3	T47.5X4	T47.5X5	T47.5X6
Pancrelipase	T47.5X1	T47.5X2	T47.5X3	T47.5X4	T47.5X5	T47.5X6
Pancuronium (bromide)	T48.1X1	T48.1X2	T48.1X3	T48.1X4	T48.1X5	T48.1X6
Pangamic acid	T45.2X1	T45.2X2	T45.2X3	T45.2X4	T45.2X5	T45.2X6
Panthenol	T45.2X1	T45.2X2	T45.2X3	T45.2X4	T45.2X5	T45.2X6
topical	T49.8X1	T49.8X2	T49.8X3	T49.8X4	T49.8X5	T49.8X6
Pantopon	T4Ø.ØX1	T4Ø.ØX2	T4Ø.ØX3	T4Ø.ØX4	T4Ø.ØX5	T4Ø.ØX6
Pantoprazole*	T47.1X1	T47.1X2	T47.1X3	T47.1X4	T47.1X5	T47.1X6
Pantothenic acid	T45.2X1	T45.2X2	T45.2X3	T45.2X4	T45.2X5	T45.2X6
Panwarfin	T45.511	T45.512	T45.513	T45.514	T45.515	T45.516
Papain	T47.5X1	T47.5X2	T47.5X3	T47.5X4	T47.5X5	T47.5X6
digestant	T47.5X1	T47.5X2	T47.5X3	T47.5X4	T47.5X5	T47.5X6
Papaveretum	T4Ø.ØX1	T4Ø.ØX2	T4Ø.ØX3	T4Ø.ØX4	T4Ø.ØX5	T4Ø.ØX6
Papaverine	T44.3X1	T44.3X2	T44.3X3	T44.3X4	T44.3X5	T44.3X6
Para-acetamidophenol	T39.1X1	T39.1X2	T39.1X3	T39.1X4	T39.1X5	T39.1X6
Para-aminobenzoic acid	T49.3X1	T49.3X2	T49.3X3	T49.3X4	T49.3X5	T49.3X6
Para-aminophenol derivatives	T39.1X1	T39.1X2	T39.1X3	T39.1X4	T39.1X5	T39.1X6
Para-aminosalicylic acid	T37.1X1	T37.1X2	T37.1X3	T37.1X4	T37.1X5	T37.1X6
Paracetaldehyde	T42.6X1	T42.6X2	T42.6X3	T42.6X4	T42.6X5	T42.6X6
Paracetamol	T39.1X1	T39.1X2	T39.1X3	T39.1X4	T39.1X5	T39.1X6
Parachlorophenol (camphorated)	T49.ØX1	T49.ØX2	T49.ØX3	T49.ØX4	T49.ØX5	T49.ØX6
Paracodin	T4Ø.2X1	T4Ø.2X2	T4Ø.2X3	T4Ø.2X4	T4Ø.2X5	T4Ø.2X6
Paradione	T42.2X1	T42.2X2	T42.2X3	T42.2X4	T42.2X5	T42.2X6
Paraffin(s) (wax)	T52.ØX1	T52.ØX2	T52.ØX3	T52.ØX4	—	—
liquid (medicinal)	T47.4X1	T47.4X2	T47.4X3	T47.4X4	T47.4X5	T47.4X6
nonmedicinal	T52.ØX1	T52.ØX2	T52.ØX3	T52.ØX4	—	—
Paraformaldehyde	T6Ø.3X1	T6Ø.3X2	T6Ø.3X3	T6Ø.3X4	—	—
Paraldehyde	T42.6X1	T42.6X2	T42.6X3	T42.6X4	T42.6X5	T42.6X6
Paramethadione	T42.2X1	T42.2X2	T42.2X3	T42.2X4	T42.2X5	T42.2X6
Paramethasone	T38.ØX1	T38.ØX2	T38.ØX3	T38.ØX4	T38.ØX5	T38.ØX6
acetate	T49.ØX1	T49.ØX2	T49.ØX3	T49.ØX4	T49.ØX5	T49.ØX6
Paraoxon	T6Ø.ØX1	T6Ø.ØX2	T6Ø.ØX3	T6Ø.ØX4	—	—
Paraquat	T6Ø.3X1	T6Ø.3X2	T6Ø.3X3	T6Ø.3X4	—	—
Parasympatholytic NEC	T44.3X1	T44.3X2	T44.3X3	T44.3X4	T44.3X5	T44.3X6
Parasympathomimetic drug NEC	T44.1X1	T44.1X2	T44.1X3	T44.1X4	T44.1X5	T44.1X6
Parathion	T6Ø.ØX1	T6Ø.ØX2	T6Ø.ØX3	T6Ø.ØX4	—	—
Parathormone	T5Ø.991	T5Ø.992	T5Ø.993	T5Ø.994	T5Ø.995	T5Ø.996
Parathyroid extract	T5Ø.991	T5Ø.992	T5Ø.993	T5Ø.994	T5Ø.995	T5Ø.996
Paratyphoid vaccine	T5Ø.A91	T5Ø.A92	T5Ø.A93	T5Ø.A94	T5Ø.A95	T5Ø.A96
Paredrine	T44.4X1	T44.4X2	T44.4X3	T44.4X4	T44.4X5	T44.4X6
Paregoric	T4Ø.ØX1	T4Ø.ØX2	T4Ø.ØX3	T4Ø.ØX4	T4Ø.ØX5	T4Ø.ØX6
Pargyline	T46.5X1	T46.5X2	T46.5X3	T46.5X4	T46.5X5	T46.5X6
Paris green	T57.ØX1	T57.ØX2	T57.ØX3	T57.ØX4	—	—
insecticide	T57.ØX1	T57.ØX2	T57.ØX3	T57.ØX4	—	—
Parnate	T43.1X1	T43.1X2	T43.1X3	T43.1X4	T43.1X5	T43.1X6
Paromomycin	T36.5X1	T36.5X2	T36.5X3	T36.5X4	T36.5X5	T36.5X6
Paroxypropione	T45.1X1	T45.1X2	T45.1X3	T45.1X4	T45.1X5	T45.1X6
Parsabiv*	T5Ø.991	T5Ø.992	T5Ø.993	T5Ø.994	T5Ø.995	T5Ø.996
Parzone	T4Ø.2X1	T4Ø.2X2	T4Ø.2X3	T4Ø.2X4	T4Ø.2X5	T4Ø.2X6
PAS	T37.1X1	T37.1X2	T37.1X3	T37.1X4	T37.1X5	T37.1X6
Pasiniazid	T37.1X1	T37.1X2	T37.1X3	T37.1X4	T37.1X5	T37.1X6
PBB (polybrominated biphenyls)	T65.891	T65.892	T65.893	T65.894	—	—
PCB	T65.891	T65.892	T65.893	T65.894	—	—
PCP						
meaning pentachlorophenol	T6Ø.1X1	T6Ø.1X2	T6Ø.1X3	T6Ø.1X4	—	—
fungicide	T6Ø.3X1	T6Ø.3X2	T6Ø.3X3	T6Ø.3X4	—	—
herbicide	T6Ø.3X1	T6Ø.3X2	T6Ø.3X3	T6Ø.3X4	—	—
insecticide	T6Ø.1X1	T6Ø.1X2	T6Ø.1X3	T6Ø.1X4	—	—
meaning phencyclidine	T4Ø.991	T4Ø.992	T4Ø.993	T4Ø.994	—	—
Peach kernel oil (emulsion)	T47.4X1	T47.4X2	T47.4X3	T47.4X4	T47.4X5	T47.4X6
Peanut oil (emulsion) **NEC**	T47.4X1	T47.4X2	T47.4X3	T47.4X4	T47.4X5	T47.4X6

Substance	Poisoning, Accidental (unintentional)	Poisoning, Intentional Self-harm	Poisoning, Assault	Poisoning, Undetermined	Adverse Effect	Under-dosing
Peanut oil (emulsion) **NEC** — *continued*						
topical	T49.3X1	T49.3X2	T49.3X3	T49.3X4	T49.3X5	T49.3X6
Pearly Gates (morning glory seeds)	T4Ø.991	T4Ø.992	T4Ø.993	T4Ø.994	—	—
Pecazine	T43.3X1	T43.3X2	T43.3X3	T43.3X4	T43.3X5	T43.3X6
Pectin	T47.6X1	T47.6X2	T47.6X3	T47.6X4	T47.6X5	T47.6X6
Pediaflor*	T49.7X1	T49.7X2	T49.7X3	T49.7X4	T49.7X5	T49.7X6
Pefloxacin	T37.8X1	T37.8X2	T37.8X3	T37.8X4	T37.8X5	T37.8X6
Pegademase, bovine	T5Ø.Z91	T5Ø.Z92	T5Ø.Z93	T5Ø.Z94	T5Ø.Z95	T5Ø.Z96
Pelletierine tannate	T37.4X1	T37.4X2	T37.4X3	T37.4X4	T37.4X5	T37.4X6
Pemirolast (potassium)	T48.6X1	T48.6X2	T48.6X3	T48.6X4	T48.6X5	T48.6X6
Pemoline	T5Ø.7X1	T5Ø.7X2	T5Ø.7X3	T5Ø.7X4	T5Ø.7X5	T5Ø.7X6
Pempidine	T44.2X1	T44.2X2	T44.2X3	T44.2X4	T44.2X5	T44.2X6
Penamecillin	T36.ØX1	T36.ØX2	T36.ØX3	T36.ØX4	T36.ØX5	T36.ØX6
Penbutolol	T44.7X1	T44.7X2	T44.7X3	T44.7X4	T44.7X5	T44.7X6
Penethamate	T36.ØX1	T36.ØX2	T36.ØX3	T36.ØX4	T36.ØX5	T36.ØX6
Penfluridol	T43.591	T43.592	T43.593	T43.594	T43.595	T43.596
Penflutizide	T5Ø.2X1	T5Ø.2X2	T5Ø.2X3	T5Ø.2X4	T5Ø.2X5	T5Ø.2X6
Pengitoxin	T46.ØX1	T46.ØX2	T46.ØX3	T46.ØX4	T46.ØX5	T46.ØX6
Penicillamine	T5Ø.6X1	T5Ø.6X2	T5Ø.6X3	T5Ø.6X4	T5Ø.6X5	T5Ø.6X6
Penicillin (any)	T36.ØX1	T36.ØX2	T36.ØX3	T36.ØX4	T36.ØX5	T36.ØX6
Penicillinase	T45.3X1	T45.3X2	T45.3X3	T45.3X4	T45.3X5	T45.3X6
Penicilloyl polylysine	T5Ø.8X1	T5Ø.8X2	T5Ø.8X3	T5Ø.8X4	T5Ø.8X5	T5Ø.8X6
Penimepicycline	T36.4X1	T36.4X2	T36.4X3	T36.4X4	T36.4X5	T36.4X6
Pentacel*	T5Ø.A11	T5Ø.A12	T5Ø.A13	T5Ø.A14	T5Ø.A15	T5Ø.A16
Pentachloroethane	T53.6X1	T53.6X2	T53.6X3	T53.6X4	—	—
Pentachloronaphthalene	T53.7X1	T53.7X2	T53.7X3	T53.7X4	—	—
Pentachlorophenol (pesticide)	T6Ø.1X1	T6Ø.1X2	T6Ø.1X3	T6Ø.1X4	—	—
fungicide	T6Ø.3X1	T6Ø.3X2	T6Ø.3X3	T6Ø.3X4	—	—
herbicide	T6Ø.3X1	T6Ø.3X2	T6Ø.3X3	T6Ø.3X4	—	—
insecticide	T6Ø.1X1	T6Ø.1X2	T6Ø.1X3	T6Ø.1X4	—	—
Pentaerythritol	T46.3X1	T46.3X2	T46.3X3	T46.3X4	T46.3X5	T46.3X6
chloral	T42.6X1	T42.6X2	T42.6X3	T42.6X4	T42.6X5	T42.6X6
tetranitrate NEC	T46.3X1	T46.3X2	T46.3X3	T46.3X4	T46.3X5	T46.3X6
Pentaerythrityl tetranitrate	T46.3X1	T46.3X2	T46.3X3	T46.3X4	T46.3X5	T46.3X6
Pentagastrin	T5Ø.8X1	T5Ø.8X2	T5Ø.8X3	T5Ø.8X4	T5Ø.8X5	T5Ø.8X6
Pentalin	T53.6X1	T53.6X2	T53.6X3	T53.6X4	—	—
Pentamethonium bromide	T44.2X1	T44.2X2	T44.2X3	T44.2X4	T44.2X5	T44.2X6
Pentamidine	T37.3X1	T37.3X2	T37.3X3	T37.3X4	T37.3X5	T37.3X6
Pentanol	T51.3X1	T51.3X2	T51.3X3	T51.3X4	—	—
Pentapyrrolinium (bitartrate)	T44.2X1	T44.2X2	T44.2X3	T44.2X4	T44.2X5	T44.2X6
Pentaquine	T37.2X1	T37.2X2	T37.2X3	T37.2X4	T37.2X5	T37.2X6
Pentazocine	T4Ø.491	T4Ø.492	T4Ø.493	T4Ø.494	T4Ø.495	T4Ø.496
Pentetrazole	T5Ø.7X1	T5Ø.7X2	T5Ø.7X3	T5Ø.7X4	T5Ø.7X5	T5Ø.7X6
Penthienate bromide	T44.3X1	T44.3X2	T44.3X3	T44.3X4	T44.3X5	T44.3X6
Pentifylline	T46.7X1	T46.7X2	T46.7X3	T46.7X4	T46.7X5	T46.7X6
Pentobarbital	T42.3X1	T42.3X2	T42.3X3	T42.3X4	T42.3X5	T42.3X6
sodium	T42.3X1	T42.3X2	T42.3X3	T42.3X4	T42.3X5	T42.3X6
Pentobarbitone	T42.3X1	T42.3X2	T42.3X3	T42.3X4	T42.3X5	T42.3X6
Pentolonium tartrate	T44.2X1	T44.2X2	T44.2X3	T44.2X4	T44.2X5	T44.2X6
Pentosan polysulfate (sodium)	T39.8X1	T39.8X2	T39.8X3	T39.8X4	T39.8X5	T39.8X6
Pentostatin	T45.1X1	T45.1X2	T45.1X3	T45.1X4	T45.1X5	T45.1X6
Pentothal	T41.1X1	T41.1X2	T41.1X3	T41.1X4	T41.1X5	T41.1X6
Pentoxifylline	T46.7X1	T46.7X2	T46.7X3	T46.7X4	T46.7X5	T46.7X6
Pentoxyverine	T48.3X1	T48.3X2	T48.3X3	T48.3X4	T48.3X5	T48.3X6
Pentrinat	T46.3X1	T46.3X2	T46.3X3	T46.3X4	T46.3X5	T46.3X6
Pentylenetetrazole	T5Ø.7X1	T5Ø.7X2	T5Ø.7X3	T5Ø.7X4	T5Ø.7X5	T5Ø.7X6
Pentylsalicylamide	T37.1X1	T37.1X2	T37.1X3	T37.1X4	T37.1X5	T37.1X6
Pentymal	T42.3X1	T42.3X2	T42.3X3	T42.3X4	T42.3X5	T42.3X6
Pepcid*	T47.ØX1	T47.ØX2	T47.ØX3	T47.ØX4	T47.ØX5	T47.ØX6
Peplomycin	T45.1X1	T45.1X2	T45.1X3	T45.1X4	T45.1X5	T45.1X6
Peppermint (oil)	T47.5X1	T47.5X2	T47.5X3	T47.5X4	T47.5X5	T47.5X6
Pepsin	T47.5X1	T47.5X2	T47.5X3	T47.5X4	T47.5X5	T47.5X6
digestant	T47.5X1	T47.5X2	T47.5X3	T47.5X4	T47.5X5	T47.5X6
Pepstatin	T47.1X1	T47.1X2	T47.1X3	T47.1X4	T47.1X5	T47.1X6
Peptavlon	T5Ø.8X1	T5Ø.8X2	T5Ø.8X3	T5Ø.8X4	T5Ø.8X5	T5Ø.8X6
Perazine	T43.3X1	T43.3X2	T43.3X3	T43.3X4	T43.3X5	T43.3X6
Percaine (spinal)	T41.3X1	T41.3X2	T41.3X3	T41.3X4	T41.3X5	T41.3X6
topical (surface)	T41.3X1	T41.3X2	T41.3X3	T41.3X4	T41.3X5	T41.3X6
Perchloroethylene	T53.3X1	T53.3X2	T53.3X3	T53.3X4	—	—
medicinal	T37.4X1	T37.4X2	T37.4X3	T37.4X4	T37.4X5	T37.4X6
vapor	T53.3X1	T53.3X2	T53.3X3	T53.3X4	—	—
Percodan	T4Ø.2X1	T4Ø.2X2	T4Ø.2X3	T4Ø.2X4	T4Ø.2X5	T4Ø.2X6
Percogesic — *see also* acetaminophen	T45.ØX1	T45.ØX2	T45.ØX3	T45.ØX4	T45.ØX5	T45.ØX6
Percorten	T38.ØX1	T38.ØX2	T38.ØX3	T38.ØX4	T38.ØX5	T38.ØX6
Pergolide	T42.8X1	T42.8X2	T42.8X3	T42.8X4	T42.8X5	T42.8X6
Pergonal	T38.811	T38.812	T38.813	T38.814	T38.815	T38.816
Perhexilene	T46.3X1	T46.3X2	T46.3X3	T46.3X4	T46.3X5	T46.3X6
Perhexiline (maleate)	T46.3X1	T46.3X2	T46.3X3	T46.3X4	T46.3X5	T46.3X6
Periactin	T45.ØX1	T45.ØX2	T45.ØX3	T45.ØX4	T45.ØX5	T45.ØX6
Periciazine	T43.3X1	T43.3X2	T43.3X3	T43.3X4	T43.3X5	T43.3X6
Periclor	T42.6X1	T42.6X2	T42.6X3	T42.6X4	T42.6X5	T42.6X6
Perindopril	T46.4X1	T46.4X2	T46.4X3	T46.4X4	T46.4X5	T46.4X6
Perisoxal	T39.8X1	T39.8X2	T39.8X3	T39.8X4	T39.8X5	T39.8X6
Peritoneal dialysis solution	T5Ø.3X1	T5Ø.3X2	T5Ø.3X3	T5Ø.3X4	T5Ø.3X5	T5Ø.3X6
Peritrate	T46.3X1	T46.3X2	T46.3X3	T46.3X4	T46.3X5	T46.3X6
Perlapine	T42.4X1	T42.4X2	T42.4X3	T42.4X4	T42.4X5	T42.4X6
Permanganate	T65.891	T65.892	T65.893	T65.894	—	—
Permapen*	T36.ØX1	T36.ØX2	T36.ØX3	T36.ØX4	T36.ØX5	T36.ØX6
Permethrin	T6Ø.1X1	T6Ø.1X2	T6Ø.1X3	T6Ø.1X4	—	—
Pernocton	T42.3X1	T42.3X2	T42.3X3	T42.3X4	T42.3X5	T42.3X6
Pernoston	T42.3X1	T42.3X2	T42.3X3	T42.3X4	T42.3X5	T42.3X6
Peronine	T4Ø.2X1	T4Ø.2X2	T4Ø.2X3	T4Ø.2X4	—	—
Perphenazine	T43.3X1	T43.3X2	T43.3X3	T43.3X4	T43.3X5	T43.3X6
Pertofrane	T43.Ø11	T43.Ø12	T43.Ø13	T43.Ø14	T43.Ø15	T43.Ø16
Pertussis						
immune serum (human)	T5Ø.Z11	T5Ø.Z12	T5Ø.Z13	T5Ø.Z14	T5Ø.Z15	T5Ø.Z16
vaccine (with diphtheria toxoid) (with tetanus toxoid)	T5Ø.A11	T5Ø.A12	T5Ø.A13	T5Ø.A14	T5Ø.A15	T5Ø.A16
Peruvian balsam	T49.ØX1	T49.ØX2	T49.ØX3	T49.ØX4	T49.ØX5	T49.ØX6
Peruvoside	T46.ØX1	T46.ØX2	T46.ØX3	T46.ØX4	T46.ØX5	T46.ØX6
Pesticide (dust) (fumes) (vapor) **NEC**	T6Ø.91	T6Ø.92	T6Ø.93	T6Ø.94	—	—
arsenic	T57.ØX1	T57.ØX2	T57.ØX3	T57.ØX4	—	—
chlorinated	T6Ø.1X1	T6Ø.1X2	T6Ø.1X3	T6Ø.1X4	—	—
cyanide	T65.ØX1	T65.ØX2	T65.ØX3	T65.ØX4	—	—
kerosene	T52.ØX1	T52.ØX2	T52.ØX3	T52.ØX4	—	—
mixture (of compounds)	T6Ø.91	T6Ø.92	T6Ø.93	T6Ø.94	—	—
naphthalene	T6Ø.2X1	T6Ø.2X2	T6Ø.2X3	T6Ø.2X4	—	—
organochlorine (compounds)	T6Ø.1X1	T6Ø.1X2	T6Ø.1X3	T6Ø.1X4	—	—
petroleum (distillate) (products) NEC	T6Ø.8X1	T6Ø.8X2	T6Ø.8X3	T6Ø.8X4	—	—
specified ingredient NEC	T6Ø.8X1	T6Ø.8X2	T6Ø.8X3	T6Ø.8X4	—	—
strychnine	T65.1X1	T65.1X2	T65.1X3	T65.1X4	—	—
thallium	T6Ø.4X1	T6Ø.4X2	T6Ø.4X3	T6Ø.4X4	—	—
Pethidine	T4Ø.491	T4Ø.492	T4Ø.493	T4Ø.494	T4Ø.495	T4Ø.496
Petrichloral	T42.6X1	T42.6X2	T42.6X3	T42.6X4	T42.6X5	T42.6X6
Petrol	T52.ØX1	T52.ØX2	T52.ØX3	T52.ØX4	—	—
vapor	T52.ØX1	T52.ØX2	T52.ØX3	T52.ØX4	—	—
Petrolatum	T49.3X1	T49.3X2	T49.3X3	T49.3X4	T49.3X5	T49.3X6
hydrophilic	T49.3X1	T49.3X2	T49.3X3	T49.3X4	T49.3X5	T49.3X6
liquid	T47.4X1	T47.4X2	T47.4X3	T47.4X4	T47.4X5	T47.4X6
topical	T49.3X1	T49.3X2	T49.3X3	T49.3X4	T49.3X5	T49.3X6
nonmedicinal	T52.ØX1	T52.ØX2	T52.ØX3	T52.ØX4	—	—
red veterinary	T49.3X1	T49.3X2	T49.3X3	T49.3X4	T49.3X5	T49.3X6
white	T49.3X1	T49.3X2	T49.3X3	T49.3X4	T49.3X5	T49.3X6
Petroleum (products) **NEC**	T52.ØX1	T52.ØX2	T52.ØX3	T52.ØX4	—	—
benzine(s) — *see* Ligroin						
ether — *see* Ligroin						
jelly — *see* Petrolatum						
naphtha — *see* Ligroin						
pesticide	T6Ø.8X1	T6Ø.8X2	T6Ø.8X3	T6Ø.8X4	—	—
solids	T52.ØX1	T52.ØX2	T52.ØX3	T52.ØX4	—	—
solvents	T52.ØX1	T52.ØX2	T52.ØX3	T52.ØX4	—	—
vapor	T52.ØX1	T52.ØX2	T52.ØX3	T52.ØX4	—	—
Peyote	T4Ø.991	T4Ø.992	T4Ø.993	T4Ø.994	—	—
Phanodorm, phanodorn	T42.3X1	T42.3X2	T42.3X3	T42.3X4	T42.3X5	T42.3X6
Phanquinone	T37.3X1	T37.3X2	T37.3X3	T37.3X4	T37.3X5	T37.3X6
Phanquone	T37.3X1	T37.3X2	T37.3X3	T37.3X4	T37.3X5	T37.3X6
Pharmaceutical						
adjunct NEC	T5Ø.9Ø1	T5Ø.9Ø2	T5Ø.9Ø3	T5Ø.9Ø4	T5Ø.9Ø5	T5Ø.9Ø6
excipient NEC	T5Ø.9Ø1	T5Ø.9Ø2	T5Ø.9Ø3	T5Ø.9Ø4	T5Ø.9Ø5	T5Ø.9Ø6
sweetener	T5Ø.9Ø1	T5Ø.9Ø2	T5Ø.9Ø3	T5Ø.9Ø4	T5Ø.9Ø5	T5Ø.9Ø6
viscous agent	T5Ø.9Ø1	T5Ø.9Ø2	T5Ø.9Ø3	T5Ø.9Ø4	T5Ø.9Ø5	T5Ø.9Ø6
Phazyme*	T47.1X1	T47.1X2	T47.1X3	T47.1X4	T47.1X5	T47.1X6
Phemitone	T42.3X1	T42.3X2	T42.3X3	T42.3X4	T42.3X5	T42.3X6
Phenacaine	T41.3X1	T41.3X2	T41.3X3	T41.3X4	T41.3X5	T41.3X6
Phenacemide	T42.6X1	T42.6X2	T42.6X3	T42.6X4	T42.6X5	T42.6X6
Phenacetin	T39.1X1	T39.1X2	T39.1X3	T39.1X4	T39.1X5	T39.1X6
Phenadoxone	T4Ø.2X1	T4Ø.2X2	T4Ø.2X3	T4Ø.2X4	—	—
Phenaglycodol	T43.591	T43.592	T43.593	T43.594	T43.595	T43.596
Phenantoin	T42.ØX1	T42.ØX2	T42.ØX3	T42.ØX4	T42.ØX5	T42.ØX6
Phenaphthazine reagent	T5Ø.991	T5Ø.992	T5Ø.993	T5Ø.994	T5Ø.995	T5Ø.996
Phenazocine	T4Ø.491	T4Ø.492	T4Ø.493	T4Ø.494	T4Ø.495	T4Ø.496
Phenazone	T39.2X1	T39.2X2	T39.2X3	T39.2X4	T39.2X5	T39.2X6
Phenazopyridine	T39.8X1	T39.8X2	T39.8X3	T39.8X4	T39.8X5	T39.8X6
Phenbenicillin	T36.ØX1	T36.ØX2	T36.ØX3	T36.ØX4	T36.ØX5	T36.ØX6
Phenbutrazate	T5Ø.5X1	T5Ø.5X2	T5Ø.5X3	T5Ø.5X4	T5Ø.5X5	T5Ø.5X6

Substance	Poisoning, Accidental (unintentional)	Poisoning, Intentional Self-harm	Poisoning, Assault	Poisoning, Undetermined	Adverse Effect	Under-dosing
Phencyclidine	T40.991	T40.992	T40.993	T40.994	T40.995	T40.996
Phendimetrazine	T50.5X1	T50.5X2	T50.5X3	T50.5X4	T50.5X5	T50.5X6
Phenelzine	T43.1X1	T43.1X2	T43.1X3	T43.1X4	T43.1X5	T43.1X6
Phenemal	T42.3X1	T42.3X2	T42.3X3	T42.3X4	T42.3X5	T42.3X6
Phenergan	T42.6X1	T42.6X2	T42.6X3	T42.6X4	T42.6X5	T42.6X6
Pheneticillin	T36.0X1	T36.0X2	T36.0X3	T36.0X4	T36.0X5	T36.0X6
Pheneturide	T42.6X1	T42.6X2	T42.6X3	T42.6X4	T42.6X5	T42.6X6
Phenformin	T38.3X1	T38.3X2	T38.3X3	T38.3X4	T38.3X5	T38.3X6
Phenglutarimide	T44.3X1	T44.3X2	T44.3X3	T44.3X4	T44.3X5	T44.3X6
Phenicarbazide	T39.8X1	T39.8X2	T39.8X3	T39.8X4	T39.8X5	T39.8X6
Phenindamine	T45.0X1	T45.0X2	T45.0X3	T45.0X4	T45.0X5	T45.0X6
Phenindione	T45.511	T45.512	T45.513	T45.514	T45.515	T45.516
Pheniprazine	T43.1X1	T43.1X2	T43.1X3	T43.1X4	T43.1X5	T43.1X6
Pheniramine	T45.0X1	T45.0X2	T45.0X3	T45.0X4	T45.0X5	T45.0X6
Phenisatin	T47.2X1	T47.2X2	T47.2X3	T47.2X4	T47.2X5	T47.2X6
Phenmetrazine	T50.5X1	T50.5X2	T50.5X3	T50.5X4	T50.5X5	T50.5X6
Phenobal	T42.3X1	T42.3X2	T42.3X3	T42.3X4	T42.3X5	T42.3X6
Phenobarbital	T42.3X1	T42.3X2	T42.3X3	T42.3X4	T42.3X5	T42.3X6
with						
mephenytoin	T42.3X1	T42.3X2	T42.3X3	T42.3X4	T42.3X5	T42.3X6
phenytoin	T42.3X1	T42.3X2	T42.3X3	T42.3X4	T42.3X5	T42.3X6
sodium	T42.3X1	T42.3X2	T42.3X3	T42.3X4	T42.3X5	T42.3X6
Phenobarbitone	T42.3X1	T42.3X2	T42.3X3	T42.3X4	T42.3X5	T42.3X6
Phenobutiodil	T50.8X1	T50.8X2	T50.8X3	T50.8X4	T50.8X5	T50.8X6
Phenoctide	T49.0X1	T49.0X2	T49.0X3	T49.0X4	T49.0X5	T49.0X6
Phenol	T49.0X1	T49.0X2	T49.0X3	T49.0X4	T49.0X5	T49.0X6
disinfectant	T54.0X1	T54.0X2	T54.0X3	T54.0X4	—	—
in oil injection	T46.8X1	T46.8X2	T46.8X3	T46.8X4	T46.8X5	T46.8X6
medicinal	T49.1X1	T49.1X2	T49.1X3	T49.1X4	T49.1X5	T49.1X6
nonmedicinal NEC	T54.0X1	T54.0X2	T54.0X3	T54.0X4	—	—
pesticide	T60.8X1	T60.8X2	T60.8X3	T60.8X4	—	—
red	T50.8X1	T50.8X2	T50.8X3	T50.8X4	T50.8X5	T50.8X6
Phenolic preparation	T49.1X1	T49.1X2	T49.1X3	T49.1X4	T49.1X5	T49.1X6
Phenolphthalein	T47.2X1	T47.2X2	T47.2X3	T47.2X4	T47.2X5	T47.2X6
Phenolsulfonphthalein	T50.8X1	T50.8X2	T50.8X3	T50.8X4	T50.8X5	T50.8X6
Phenomorphan	T40.2X1	T40.2X2	T40.2X3	T40.2X4	—	—
Phenonyl	T42.3X1	T42.3X2	T42.3X3	T42.3X4	T42.3X5	T42.3X6
Phenoperidine	T40.491	T40.492	T40.493	T40.494	—	—
Phenopyrazone	T46.991	T46.992	T46.993	T46.994	T46.995	T46.996
Phenoquin	T50.4X1	T50.4X2	T50.4X3	T50.4X4	T50.4X5	T50.4X6
Phenothiazine (psychotropic) NEC	T43.3X1	T43.3X2	T43.3X3	T43.3X4	T43.3X5	T43.3X6
insecticide	T60.2X1	T60.2X2	T60.2X3	T60.2X4	—	—
Phenothrin	T49.0X1	T49.0X2	T49.0X3	T49.0X4	T49.0X5	T49.0X6
Phenoxybenzamine	T46.7X1	T46.7X2	T46.7X3	T46.7X4	T46.7X5	T46.7X6
Phenoxyethanol	T49.0X1	T49.0X2	T49.0X3	T49.0X4	T49.0X5	T49.0X6
Phenoxymethyl penicillin	T36.0X1	T36.0X2	T36.0X3	T36.0X4	T36.0X5	T36.0X6
Phenprobamate	T42.8X1	T42.8X2	T42.8X3	T42.8X4	T42.8X5	T42.8X6
Phenprocoumon	T45.511	T45.512	T45.513	T45.514	T45.515	T45.516
Phensuximide	T42.2X1	T42.2X2	T42.2X3	T42.2X4	T42.2X5	T42.2X6
Phentermine	T50.5X1	T50.5X2	T50.5X3	T50.5X4	T50.5X5	T50.5X6
Phenthicillin	T36.0X1	T36.0X2	T36.0X3	T36.0X4	T36.0X5	T36.0X6
Phentolamine	T46.7X1	T46.7X2	T46.7X3	T46.7X4	T46.7X5	T46.7X6
Phenyl						
butazone	T39.2X1	T39.2X2	T39.2X3	T39.2X4	T39.2X5	T39.2X6
enediamine	T65.3X1	T65.3X2	T65.3X3	T65.3X4	—	—
hydrazine	T65.3X1	T65.3X2	T65.3X3	T65.3X4	—	—
antineoplastic	T45.1X1	T45.1X2	T45.1X3	T45.1X4	T45.1X5	T45.1X6
mercuric compounds — *see* Mercury						
salicylate	T49.3X1	T49.3X2	T49.3X3	T49.3X4	T49.3X5	T49.3X6
Phenylalanine mustard	T45.1X1	T45.1X2	T45.1X3	T45.1X4	T45.1X5	T45.1X6
Phenylbutazone	T39.2X1	T39.2X2	T39.2X3	T39.2X4	T39.2X5	T39.2X6
Phenylenediamine	T65.3X1	T65.3X2	T65.3X3	T65.3X4	—	—
Phenylephrine	T44.4X1	T44.4X2	T44.4X3	T44.4X4	T44.4X5	T44.4X6
Phenylethylbiguanide	T38.3X1	T38.3X2	T38.3X3	T38.3X4	T38.3X5	T38.3X6
Phenylmercuric						
acetate	T49.0X1	T49.0X2	T49.0X3	T49.0X4	T49.0X5	T49.0X6
borate	T49.0X1	T49.0X2	T49.0X3	T49.0X4	T49.0X5	T49.0X6
nitrate	T49.0X1	T49.0X2	T49.0X3	T49.0X4	T49.0X5	T49.0X6
Phenylmethylbarbitone	T42.3X1	T42.3X2	T42.3X3	T42.3X4	T42.3X5	T42.3X6
Phenylpropanol	T47.5X1	T47.5X2	T47.5X3	T47.5X4	T47.5X5	T47.5X6
Phenylpropanolamine	T44.991	T44.992	T44.993	T44.994	T44.995	T44.996
Phenylsulfthion	T60.0X1	T60.0X2	T60.0X3	T60.0X4	—	—
Phenyltoloxamine	T45.0X1	T45.0X2	T45.0X3	T45.0X4	T45.0X5	T45.0X6
Phenyramidol, phenyramidon	T39.8X1	T39.8X2	T39.8X3	T39.8X4	T39.8X5	T39.8X6
Phenytek*	T42.0X1	T42.0X2	T42.0X3	T42.0X4	T42.0X5	T42.0X6
Phenytoin	T42.0X1	T42.0X2	T42.0X3	T42.0X4	T42.0X5	T42.0X6
with Phenobarbital	T42.3X1	T42.3X2	T42.3X3	T42.3X4	T42.3X5	T42.3X6
pHisoHex	T49.2X1	T49.2X2	T49.2X3	T49.2X4	T49.2X5	T49.2X6
Pholcodine	T48.3X1	T48.3X2	T48.3X3	T48.3X4	T48.3X5	T48.3X6
Pholedrine	T46.991	T46.992	T46.993	T46.994	T46.995	T46.996
Phorate	T60.0X1	T60.0X2	T60.0X3	T60.0X4	—	—
Phosdrin	T60.0X1	T60.0X2	T60.0X3	T60.0X4	—	—
Phosfolan	T60.0X1	T60.0X2	T60.0X3	T60.0X4	—	—
Phosgene (gas)	T59.891	T59.892	T59.893	T59.894	—	—
Phosphamidon	T60.0X1	T60.0X2	T60.0X3	T60.0X4	—	—
Phosphate	T65.891	T65.892	T65.893	T65.894	—	—
laxative	T47.4X1	T47.4X2	T47.4X3	T47.4X4	T47.4X5	T47.4X6
organic	T60.0X1	T60.0X2	T60.0X3	T60.0X4	—	—
solvent	T52.91	T52.92	T52.93	T52.94	—	—
tricresyl	T65.891	T65.892	T65.893	T65.894	—	—
Phosphine	T57.1X1	T57.1X2	T57.1X3	T57.1X4	—	—
fumigant	T57.1X1	T57.1X2	T57.1X3	T57.1X4	—	—
Phospholine	T49.5X1	T49.5X2	T49.5X3	T49.5X4	T49.5X5	T49.5X6
Phosphoric acid	T54.2X1	T54.2X2	T54.2X3	T54.2X4	—	—
Phosphorus (compound) **NEC**	T57.1X1	T57.1X2	T57.1X3	T57.1X4	—	—
pesticide	T60.0X1	T60.0X2	T60.0X3	T60.0X4	—	—
Photrexa*	T49.5X1	T49.5X2	T49.5X3	T49.5X4	T49.5X5	T49.5X6
Phthalates	T65.891	T65.892	T65.893	T65.894	—	—
Phthalic anhydride	T65.891	T65.892	T65.893	T65.894	—	—
Phthalimidoglutarimide	T42.6X1	T42.6X2	T42.6X3	T42.6X4	T42.6X5	T42.6X6
Phthalylsulfathiazole	T37.0X1	T37.0X2	T37.0X3	T37.0X4	T37.0X5	T37.0X6
Phylloquinone	T45.7X1	T45.7X2	T45.7X3	T45.7X4	T45.7X5	T45.7X6
Physeptone	T40.3X1	T40.3X2	T40.3X3	T40.3X4	T40.3X5	T40.3X6
Physostigma venenosum	T62.2X1	T62.2X2	T62.2X3	T62.2X4	—	—
Physostigmine	T49.5X1	T49.5X2	T49.5X3	T49.5X4	T49.5X5	T49.5X6
Phytolacca decandra	T62.2X1	T62.2X2	T62.2X3	T62.2X4	—	—
berries	T62.1X1	T62.1X2	T62.1X3	T62.1X4	—	—
Phytomenadione	T45.7X1	T45.7X2	T45.7X3	T45.7X4	T45.7X5	T45.7X6
Phytonadione	T45.7X1	T45.7X2	T45.7X3	T45.7X4	T45.7X5	T45.7X6
Picoperine	T48.3X1	T48.3X2	T48.3X3	T48.3X4	T48.3X5	T48.3X6
Picosulfate (sodium)	T47.2X1	T47.2X2	T47.2X3	T47.2X4	T47.2X5	T47.2X6
Picric (acid)	T54.2X1	T54.2X2	T54.2X3	T54.2X4	—	—
Picrotoxin	T50.7X1	T50.7X2	T50.7X3	T50.7X4	T50.7X5	T50.7X6
Piketoprofen	T49.0X1	T49.0X2	T49.0X3	T49.0X4	T49.0X5	T49.0X6
Pilocarpine	T44.1X1	T44.1X2	T44.1X3	T44.1X4	T44.1X5	T44.1X6
Pilocarpus (jaborandi) extract	T44.1X1	T44.1X2	T44.1X3	T44.1X4	T44.1X5	T44.1X6
Pilsicainide (hydrochloride)	T46.2X1	T46.2X2	T46.2X3	T46.2X4	T46.2X5	T46.2X6
Pimaricin	T36.7X1	T36.7X2	T36.7X3	T36.7X4	T36.7X5	T36.7X6
Pimeclone	T50.7X1	T50.7X2	T50.7X3	T50.7X4	T50.7X5	T50.7X6
Pimelic ketone	T52.8X1	T52.8X2	T52.8X3	T52.8X4	—	—
Pimethixene	T45.0X1	T45.0X2	T45.0X3	T45.0X4	T45.0X5	T45.0X6
Piminodine	T40.2X1	T40.2X2	T40.2X3	T40.2X4	T40.2X5	T40.2X6
Pimozide	T43.591	T43.592	T43.593	T43.594	T43.595	T43.596
Pinacidil	T46.5X1	T46.5X2	T46.5X3	T46.5X4	T46.5X5	T46.5X6
Pinaverium bromide	T44.3X1	T44.3X2	T44.3X3	T44.3X4	T44.3X5	T44.3X6
Pinazepam	T42.4X1	T42.4X2	T42.4X3	T42.4X4	T42.4X5	T42.4X6
Pindolol	T44.7X1	T44.7X2	T44.7X3	T44.7X4	T44.7X5	T44.7X6
Pindone	T60.4X1	T60.4X2	T60.4X3	T60.4X4	—	—
Pine oil (disinfectant)	T65.891	T65.892	T65.893	T65.894	—	—
Pinkroot	T37.4X1	T37.4X2	T37.4X3	T37.4X4	T37.4X5	T37.4X6
Pipadone	T40.2X1	T40.2X2	T40.2X3	T40.2X4	—	—
Pipamazine	T45.0X1	T45.0X2	T45.0X3	T45.0X4	T45.0X5	T45.0X6
Pipamperone	T43.4X1	T43.4X2	T43.4X3	T43.4X4	T43.4X5	T43.4X6
Pipazetate	T48.3X1	T48.3X2	T48.3X3	T48.3X4	T48.3X5	T48.3X6
Pipemidic acid	T37.8X1	T37.8X2	T37.8X3	T37.8X4	T37.8X5	T37.8X6
Pipenzolate bromide	T44.3X1	T44.3X2	T44.3X3	T44.3X4	T44.3X5	T44.3X6
Piperacetazine	T43.3X1	T43.3X2	T43.3X3	T43.3X4	T43.3X5	T43.3X6
Piperacillin	T36.0X1	T36.0X2	T36.0X3	T36.0X4	T36.0X5	T36.0X6
Piperazine	T37.4X1	T37.4X2	T37.4X3	T37.4X4	T37.4X5	T37.4X6
estrone sulfate	T38.5X1	T38.5X2	T38.5X3	T38.5X4	T38.5X5	T38.5X6
Piper cubeba	T62.2X1	T62.2X2	T62.2X3	T62.2X4	—	—
Piperidione	T48.3X1	T48.3X2	T48.3X3	T48.3X4	T48.3X5	T48.3X6
Piperidolate	T44.3X1	T44.3X2	T44.3X3	T44.3X4	T44.3X5	T44.3X6
Piperocaine	T41.3X1	T41.3X2	T41.3X3	T41.3X4	T41.3X5	T41.3X6
infiltration (subcutaneous)	T41.3X1	T41.3X2	T41.3X3	T41.3X4	T41.3X5	T41.3X6
nerve block (peripheral) (plexus)	T41.3X1	T41.3X2	T41.3X3	T41.3X4	T41.3X5	T41.3X6
topical (surface)	T41.3X1	T41.3X2	T41.3X3	T41.3X4	T41.3X5	T41.3X6
Piperonyl butoxide	T60.8X1	T60.8X2	T60.8X3	T60.8X4	—	—
Pipethanate	T44.3X1	T44.3X2	T44.3X3	T44.3X4	T44.3X5	T44.3X6
Pipobroman	T45.1X1	T45.1X2	T45.1X3	T45.1X4	T45.1X5	T45.1X6
Pipotiazine	T43.3X1	T43.3X2	T43.3X3	T43.3X4	T43.3X5	T43.3X6
Pipoxizine	T45.0X1	T45.0X2	T45.0X3	T45.0X4	T45.0X5	T45.0X6
Pipradrol	T43.691	T43.692	T43.693	T43.694	T43.695	T43.696
Piprinhydrinate	T45.0X1	T45.0X2	T45.0X3	T45.0X4	T45.0X5	T45.0X6
Pirarubicin	T45.1X1	T45.1X2	T45.1X3	T45.1X4	T45.1X5	T45.1X6
Pirazinamide	T37.1X1	T37.1X2	T37.1X3	T37.1X4	T37.1X5	T37.1X6
Pirbuterol	T48.6X1	T48.6X2	T48.6X3	T48.6X4	T48.6X5	T48.6X6
Pirenzepine	T47.1X1	T47.1X2	T47.1X3	T47.1X4	T47.1X5	T47.1X6
Piretanide	T50.1X1	T50.1X2	T50.1X3	T50.1X4	T50.1X5	T50.1X6
Pirfenidone*	T48.991	T48.992	T48.993	T48.994	T48.995	T48.996

Substance	Poisoning, Accidental (unintentional)	Poisoning, Intentional Self-harm	Poisoning, Assault	Poisoning, Undetermined	Adverse Effect	Under-dosing
Piribedil	T42.8X1	T42.8X2	T42.8X3	T42.8X4	T42.8X5	T42.8X6
Piridoxilate	T46.3X1	T46.3X2	T46.3X3	T46.3X4	T46.3X5	T46.3X6
Piritramide	T40.491	T40.492	T40.493	T40.494	—	—
Piromidic acid	T37.8X1	T37.8X2	T37.8X3	T37.8X4	T37.8X5	T37.8X6
Piroxicam	T39.391	T39.392	T39.393	T39.394	T39.395	T39.396
beta-cyclodextrin complex	T39.8X1	T39.8X2	T39.8X3	T39.8X4	T39.8X5	T39.8X6
Pirozadil	T46.6X1	T46.6X2	T46.6X3	T46.6X4	T46.6X5	T46.6X6
Piscidia (bark) (erythrina)	T39.8X1	T39.8X2	T39.8X3	T39.8X4	T39.8X5	T39.8X6
Pitch	T65.891	T65.892	T65.893	T65.894	—	—
Pitkin's solution	T41.3X1	T41.3X2	T41.3X3	T41.3X4	T41.3X5	T41.3X6
Pitocin	T48.ØX1	T48.ØX2	T48.ØX3	T48.ØX4	T48.ØX5	T48.ØX6
Pitressin (tannate)	T38.891	T38.892	T38.893	T38.894	T38.895	T38.896
Pituitary extracts (posterior)	T38.891	T38.892	T38.893	T38.894	T38.895	T38.896
anterior	T38.811	T38.812	T38.813	T38.814	T38.815	T38.816
Pituitrin	T38.891	T38.892	T38.893	T38.894	T38.895	T38.896
Pivampicillin	T36.ØX1	T36.ØX2	T36.ØX3	T36.ØX4	T36.ØX5	T36.ØX6
Pivmecillinam	T36.ØX1	T36.ØX2	T36.ØX3	T36.ØX4	T36.ØX5	T36.ØX6
Placental hormone	T38.891	T38.892	T38.893	T38.894	T38.895	T38.896
Placidyl	T42.6X1	T42.6X2	T42.6X3	T42.6X4	T42.6X5	T42.6X6
Plague vaccine	T5Ø.A91	T5Ø.A92	T5Ø.A93	T5Ø.A94	T5Ø.A95	T5Ø.A96
Plant						
food or fertilizer NEC	T65.891	T65.892	T65.893	T65.894	—	—
containing herbicide	T6Ø.3X1	T6Ø.3X2	T6Ø.3X3	T6Ø.3X4	—	—
noxious, used as food	T62.2X1	T62.2X2	T62.2X3	T62.2X4	—	—
berries	T62.1X1	T62.1X2	T62.1X3	T62.1X4	—	—
seeds	T62.2X1	T62.2X2	T62.2X3	T62.2X4	—	—
specified type NEC	T62.2X1	T62.2X2	T62.2X3	T62.2X4	—	—
Plasma	T45.8X1	T45.8X2	T45.8X3	T45.8X4	T45.8X5	T45.8X6
expander NEC	T45.8X1	T45.8X2	T45.8X3	T45.8X4	T45.8X5	T45.8X6
protein fraction (human)	T45.8X1	T45.8X2	T45.8X3	T45.8X4	T45.8X5	T45.8X6
Plasmanate	T45.8X1	T45.8X2	T45.8X3	T45.8X4	T45.8X5	T45.8X6
Plasminogen (tissue) activator	T45.611	T45.612	T45.613	T45.614	T45.615	T45.616
Plaster dressing	T49.3X1	T49.3X2	T49.3X3	T49.3X4	T49.3X5	T49.3X6
Plastic dressing	T49.3X1	T49.3X2	T49.3X3	T49.3X4	T49.3X5	T49.3X6
Plavix*	T45.521	T45.522	T45.523	T45.524	T45.525	T45.526
Plegicil	T43.3X1	T43.3X2	T43.3X3	T43.3X4	T43.3X5	T43.3X6
Plicamycin	T45.1X1	T45.1X2	T45.1X3	T45.1X4	T45.1X5	T45.1X6
Podophyllotoxin	T49.8X1	T49.8X2	T49.8X3	T49.8X4	T49.8X5	T49.8X6
Podophyllum (resin)	T49.4X1	T49.4X2	T49.4X3	T49.4X4	T49.4X5	T49.4X6
Poisonous berries	T62.1X1	T62.1X2	T62.1X3	T62.1X4	—	—
Poison NEC	T65.91	T65.92	T65.93	T65.94	—	—
Pokeweed (any part)	T62.2X1	T62.2X2	T62.2X3	T62.2X4	—	—
Poldine metilsulfate	T44.3X1	T44.3X2	T44.3X3	T44.3X4	T44.3X5	T44.3X6
Polidexide (sulfate)	T46.6X1	T46.6X2	T46.6X3	T46.6X4	T46.6X5	T46.6X6
Polidocanol	T46.8X1	T46.8X2	T46.8X3	T46.8X4	T46.8X5	T46.8X6
Poliomyelitis vaccine	T5Ø.B91	T5Ø.B92	T5Ø.B93	T5Ø.B94	T5Ø.B95	T5Ø.B96
Polish (car) (floor) (furniture) (metal) (porcelain) (silver)	T65.891	T65.892	T65.893	T65.894	—	—
abrasive	T65.891	T65.892	T65.893	T65.894	—	—
porcelain	T65.891	T65.892	T65.893	T65.894	—	—
Poloxalkol	T47.4X1	T47.4X2	T47.4X3	T47.4X4	T47.4X5	T47.4X6
Poloxamer	T47.4X1	T47.4X2	T47.4X3	T47.4X4	T47.4X5	T47.4X6
Polyaminostyrene resins	T5Ø.3X1	T5Ø.3X2	T5Ø.3X3	T5Ø.3X4	T5Ø.3X5	T5Ø.3X6
Polycarbophil	T47.4X1	T47.4X2	T47.4X3	T47.4X4	T47.4X5	T47.4X6
Polychlorinated biphenyl	T65.891	T65.892	T65.893	T65.894	—	—
Polycycline	T36.4X1	T36.4X2	T36.4X3	T36.4X4	T36.4X5	T36.4X6
Polyester fumes	T59.891	T59.892	T59.893	T59.894	—	—
Polyester resin hardener	T52.91	T52.92	T52.93	T52.94	—	—
fumes	T59.891	T59.892	T59.893	T59.894	—	—
Polyestradiol phosphate	T38.5X1	T38.5X2	T38.5X3	T38.5X4	T38.5X5	T38.5X6
Polyethanolamine alkyl sulfate	T49.2X1	T49.2X2	T49.2X3	T49.2X4	T49.2X5	T49.2X6
Polyethylene adhesive	T49.3X1	T49.3X2	T49.3X3	T49.3X4	T49.3X5	T49.3X6
Polyferose	T45.4X1	T45.4X2	T45.4X3	T45.4X4	T45.4X5	T45.4X6
Polygeline	T45.8X1	T45.8X2	T45.8X3	T45.8X4	T45.8X5	T45.8X6
Polymyxin	T36.8X1	T36.8X2	T36.8X3	T36.8X4	T36.8X5	T36.8X6
B	T36.8X1	T36.8X2	T36.8X3	T36.8X4	T36.8X5	T36.8X6
ENT agent	T49.6X1	T49.6X2	T49.6X3	T49.6X4	T49.6X5	T49.6X6
ophthalmic preparation	T49.5X1	T49.5X2	T49.5X3	T49.5X4	T49.5X5	T49.5X6
topical NEC	T49.ØX1	T49.ØX2	T49.ØX3	T49.ØX4	T49.ØX5	T49.ØX6
E sulfate (eye preparation)	T49.5X1	T49.5X2	T49.5X3	T49.5X4	T49.5X5	T49.5X6
Polynoxylin	T49.ØX1	T49.ØX2	T49.ØX3	T49.ØX4	T49.ØX5	T49.ØX6
Polyoestradiol phosphate	T38.5X1	T38.5X2	T38.5X3	T38.5X4	T38.5X5	T38.5X6
Polyoxymethyleneurea	T49.ØX1	T49.ØX2	T49.ØX3	T49.ØX4	T49.ØX5	T49.ØX6
Poly-Pred*	T49.5X1	T49.5X2	T49.5X3	T49.5X4	T49.5X5	T49.5X6
Polysilane	T47.8X1	T47.8X2	T47.8X3	T47.8X4	T47.8X5	T47.8X6
Polytetrafluoroethylene (inhaled)	T59.891	T59.892	T59.893	T59.894	—	—
Polythiazide	T5Ø.2X1	T5Ø.2X2	T5Ø.2X3	T5Ø.2X4	T5Ø.2X5	T5Ø.2X6
Polyvidone	T45.8X1	T45.8X2	T45.8X3	T45.8X4	T45.8X5	T45.8X6
Polyvinylpyrrolidone	T45.8X1	T45.8X2	T45.8X3	T45.8X4	T45.8X5	T45.8X6
Pontocaine (hydrochloride) (infiltration) (topical)	T41.3X1	T41.3X2	T41.3X3	T41.3X4	T41.3X5	T41.3X6
nerve block (peripheral) (plexus)	T41.3X1	T41.3X2	T41.3X3	T41.3X4	T41.3X5	T41.3X6
spinal	T41.3X1	T41.3X2	T41.3X3	T41.3X4	T41.3X5	T41.3X6
Porfiromycin	T45.1X1	T45.1X2	T45.1X3	T45.1X4	T45.1X5	T45.1X6
Portactant alfa*	T48.991	T48.992	T48.993	T48.994	T48.995	T48.996
Posterior pituitary hormone NEC	T38.891	T38.892	T38.893	T38.894	T38.895	T38.896
Pot	T4Ø.711	T4Ø.712	T4Ø.713	T4Ø.714	T4Ø.715	T4Ø.716
Potash (caustic)	T54.3X1	T54.3X2	T54.3X3	T54.3X4	—	—
Potassic saline injection (lactated)	T5Ø.3X1	T5Ø.3X2	T5Ø.3X3	T5Ø.3X4	T5Ø.3X5	T5Ø.3X6
Potassium (salts) **NEC**	T5Ø.3X1	T5Ø.3X2	T5Ø.3X3	T5Ø.3X4	T5Ø.3X5	T5Ø.3X6
aminobenzoate	T45.8X1	T45.8X2	T45.8X3	T45.8X4	T45.8X5	T45.8X6
aminosalicylate	T37.1X1	T37.1X2	T37.1X3	T37.1X4	T37.1X5	T37.1X6
antimony 'tartrate'	T37.8X1	T37.8X2	T37.8X3	T37.8X4	T37.8X5	T37.8X6
arsenite (solution)	T57.ØX1	T57.ØX2	T57.ØX3	T57.ØX4	—	—
bichromate	T56.2X1	T56.2X2	T56.2X3	T56.2X4	—	—
bisulfate	T47.3X1	T47.3X2	T47.3X3	T47.3X4	T47.3X5	T47.3X6
bromide	T42.6X1	T42.6X2	T42.6X3	T42.6X4	T42.6X5	T42.6X6
canrenoate	T5Ø.ØX1	T5Ø.ØX2	T5Ø.ØX3	T5Ø.ØX4	T5Ø.ØX5	T5Ø.ØX6
carbonate	T54.3X1	T54.3X2	T54.3X3	T54.3X4	—	—
chlorate NEC	T65.891	T65.892	T65.893	T65.894	—	—
chloride	T5Ø.3X1	T5Ø.3X2	T5Ø.3X3	T5Ø.3X4	T5Ø.3X5	T5Ø.3X6
citrate	T5Ø.991	T5Ø.992	T5Ø.993	T5Ø.994	T5Ø.995	T5Ø.996
cyanide	T65.ØX1	T65.ØX2	T65.ØX3	T65.ØX4	—	—
ferric hexacyanoferrate (medicinal)	T5Ø.6X1	T5Ø.6X2	T5Ø.6X3	T5Ø.6X4	T5Ø.6X5	T5Ø.6X6
nonmedicinal	T65.891	T65.892	T65.893	T65.894	—	—
Fluoride	T57.8X1	T57.8X2	T57.8X3	T57.8X4	—	—
glucaldrate	T47.1X1	T47.1X2	T47.1X3	T47.1X4	T47.1X5	T47.1X6
hydroxide	T54.3X1	T54.3X2	T54.3X3	T54.3X4	—	—
iodate	T49.ØX1	T49.ØX2	T49.ØX3	T49.ØX4	T49.ØX5	T49.ØX6
iodide	T48.4X1	T48.4X2	T48.4X3	T48.4X4	T48.4X5	T48.4X6
nitrate	T57.8X1	T57.8X2	T57.8X3	T57.8X4	—	—
oxalate	T65.891	T65.892	T65.893	T65.894	—	—
perchlorate (nonmedicinal) NEC	T65.891	T65.892	T65.893	T65.894	—	—
antithyroid	T38.2X1	T38.2X2	T38.2X3	T38.2X4	T38.2X5	T38.2X6
medicinal	T38.2X1	T38.2X2	T38.2X3	T38.2X4	T38.2X5	T38.2X6
Permanganate (nonmedicinal)	T65.891	T65.892	T65.893	T65.894	—	—
medicinal	T49.ØX1	T49.ØX2	T49.ØX3	T49.ØX4	T49.ØX5	T49.ØX6
sulfate	T47.2X1	T47.2X2	T47.2X3	T47.2X4	T47.2X5	T47.2X6
Potassium-removing resin	T5Ø.3X1	T5Ø.3X2	T5Ø.3X3	T5Ø.3X4	T5Ø.3X5	T5Ø.3X6
Potassium-retaining drug	T5Ø.3X1	T5Ø.3X2	T5Ø.3X3	T5Ø.3X4	T5Ø.3X5	T5Ø.3X6
Povidone	T45.8X1	T45.8X2	T45.8X3	T45.8X4	T45.8X5	T45.8X6
iodine	T49.ØX1	T49.ØX2	T49.ØX3	T49.ØX4	T49.ØX5	T49.ØX6
Practolol	T44.7X1	T44.7X2	T44.7X3	T44.7X4	T44.7X5	T44.7X6
Prajmalium bitartrate	T46.2X1	T46.2X2	T46.2X3	T46.2X4	T46.2X5	T46.2X6
Pralidoxime (iodide)	T5Ø.6X1	T5Ø.6X2	T5Ø.6X3	T5Ø.6X4	T5Ø.6X5	T5Ø.6X6
chloride	T5Ø.6X1	T5Ø.6X2	T5Ø.6X3	T5Ø.6X4	T5Ø.6X5	T5Ø.6X6
Pramiverine	T44.3X1	T44.3X2	T44.3X3	T44.3X4	T44.3X5	T44.3X6
Pramlintide*	T38.3X1	T38.3X2	T38.3X3	T38.3X4	T38.3X5	T38.3X6
Pramocaine	T49.1X1	T49.1X2	T49.1X3	T49.1X4	T49.1X5	T49.1X6
Pramoxine	T49.1X1	T49.1X2	T49.1X3	T49.1X4	T49.1X5	T49.1X6
Prasterone	T38.7X1	T38.7X2	T38.7X3	T38.7X4	T38.7X5	T38.7X6
Pravastatin	T46.6X1	T46.6X2	T46.6X3	T46.6X4	T46.6X5	T46.6X6
Prazepam	T42.4X1	T42.4X2	T42.4X3	T42.4X4	T42.4X5	T42.4X6
Praziquantel	T37.4X1	T37.4X2	T37.4X3	T37.4X4	T37.4X5	T37.4X6
Prazitone	T43.291	T43.292	T43.293	T43.294	T43.295	T43.296
Prazosin	T44.6X1	T44.6X2	T44.6X3	T44.6X4	T44.6X5	T44.6X6
Prednicarbate	T49.ØX1	T49.ØX2	T49.ØX3	T49.ØX4	T49.ØX5	T49.ØX6
Prednimustine	T45.1X1	T45.1X2	T45.1X3	T45.1X4	T45.1X5	T45.1X6
Prednisolone	T38.ØX1	T38.ØX2	T38.ØX3	T38.ØX4	T38.ØX5	T38.ØX6
ENT agent	T49.6X1	T49.6X2	T49.6X3	T49.6X4	T49.6X5	T49.6X6
ophthalmic preparation	T49.5X1	T49.5X2	T49.5X3	T49.5X4	T49.5X5	T49.5X6
steaglate	T49.ØX1	T49.ØX2	T49.ØX3	T49.ØX4	T49.ØX5	T49.ØX6
topical NEC	T49.ØX1	T49.ØX2	T49.ØX3	T49.ØX4	T49.ØX5	T49.ØX6
Prednisone	T38.ØX1	T38.ØX2	T38.ØX3	T38.ØX4	T38.ØX5	T38.ØX6
Prednylidene	T38.ØX1	T38.ØX2	T38.ØX3	T38.ØX4	T38.ØX5	T38.ØX6
Pregnandiol	T38.5X1	T38.5X2	T38.5X3	T38.5X4	T38.5X5	T38.5X6
Pregneninolone	T38.5X1	T38.5X2	T38.5X3	T38.5X4	T38.5X5	T38.5X6
Preludin	T43.691	T43.692	T43.693	T43.694	T43.695	T43.696
Premarin	T38.5X1	T38.5X2	T38.5X3	T38.5X4	T38.5X5	T38.5X6
Premedication anesthetic	T41.2Ø1	T41.2Ø2	T41.2Ø3	T41.2Ø4	T41.2Ø5	T41.2Ø6
Prenalterol	T44.5X1	T44.5X2	T44.5X3	T44.5X4	T44.5X5	T44.5X6
Prenoxdiazine	T48.3X1	T48.3X2	T48.3X3	T48.3X4	T48.3X5	T48.3X6
Prenylamine	T46.3X1	T46.3X2	T46.3X3	T46.3X4	T46.3X5	T46.3X6
Preparation H	T49.8X1	T49.8X2	T49.8X3	T49.8X4	T49.8X5	T49.8X6
Preparation, local	T49.4X1	T49.4X2	T49.4X3	T49.4X4	T49.4X5	T49.4X6

Substance	Poisoning, Accidental (unintentional)	Poisoning, Intentional Self-harm	Poisoning, Assault	Poisoning, Undetermined	Adverse Effect	Under-dosing
Preservative (nonmedicinal)	T65.891	T65.892	T65.893	T65.894	—	—
medicinal	T50.901	T50.902	T50.903	T50.904	T50.905	T50.906
wood	T60.91	T60.92	T60.93	T60.94	—	—
Prethcamide	T50.7X1	T50.7X2	T50.7X3	T50.7X4	T50.7X5	T50.7X6
Prevacid*	T47.1X1	T47.1X2	T47.1X3	T47.1X4	T47.1X5	T47.1X6
Pride of China	T62.2X1	T62.2X2	T62.2X3	T62.2X4	—	—
Pridinol	T44.3X1	T44.3X2	T44.3X3	T44.3X4	T44.3X5	T44.3X6
Prifinium bromide	T44.3X1	T44.3X2	T44.3X3	T44.3X4	T44.3X5	T44.3X6
Prilocaine	T41.3X1	T41.3X2	T41.3X3	T41.3X4	T41.3X5	T41.3X6
infiltration (subcutaneous)	T41.3X1	T41.3X2	T41.3X3	T41.3X4	T41.3X5	T41.3X6
nerve block (peripheral) (plexus)	T41.3X1	T41.3X2	T41.3X3	T41.3X4	T41.3X5	T41.3X6
regional	T41.3X1	T41.3X2	T41.3X3	T41.3X4	T41.3X5	T41.3X6
Primaquine	T37.2X1	T37.2X2	T37.2X3	T37.2X4	T37.2X5	T37.2X6
Primidone	T42.6X1	T42.6X2	T42.6X3	T42.6X4	T42.6X5	T42.6X6
Primula (veris)	T62.2X1	T62.2X2	T62.2X3	T62.2X4	—	—
Prinadol	T40.2X1	T40.2X2	T40.2X3	T40.2X4	T40.2X5	T40.2X6
Priscol, Priscoline	T44.6X1	T44.6X2	T44.6X3	T44.6X4	T44.6X5	T44.6X6
Pristinamycin	T36.3X1	T36.3X2	T36.3X3	T36.3X4	T36.3X5	T36.3X6
Pristiq*	T43.211	T43.212	T43.213	T43.214	T43.215	T43.216
Privet	T62.2X1	T62.2X2	T62.2X3	T62.2X4	—	—
berries	T62.1X1	T62.1X2	T62.1X3	T62.1X4	—	—
Privine	T44.4X1	T44.4X2	T44.4X3	T44.4X4	T44.4X5	T44.4X6
Pro-Banthine	T44.3X1	T44.3X2	T44.3X3	T44.3X4	T44.3X5	T44.3X6
Probarbital	T42.3X1	T42.3X2	T42.3X3	T42.3X4	T42.3X5	T42.3X6
Probenecid	T50.4X1	T50.4X2	T50.4X3	T50.4X4	T50.4X5	T50.4X6
Probucol	T46.6X1	T46.6X2	T46.6X3	T46.6X4	T46.6X5	T46.6X6
Procainamide	T46.2X1	T46.2X2	T46.2X3	T46.2X4	T46.2X5	T46.2X6
Procaine	T41.3X1	T41.3X2	T41.3X3	T41.3X4	T41.3X5	T41.3X6
benzylpenicillin	T36.0X1	T36.0X2	T36.0X3	T36.0X4	T36.0X5	T36.0X6
nerve block (periphreal) (plexus)	T41.3X1	T41.3X2	T41.3X3	T41.3X4	T41.3X5	T41.3X6
penicillin G	T36.0X1	T36.0X2	T36.0X3	T36.0X4	T36.0X5	T36.0X6
regional	T41.3X1	T41.3X2	T41.3X3	T41.3X4	T41.3X5	T41.3X6
spinal	T41.3X1	T41.3X2	T41.3X3	T41.3X4	T41.3X5	T41.3X6
Procalmidol	T43.591	T43.592	T43.593	T43.594	T43.595	T43.596
Procarbazine	T45.1X1	T45.1X2	T45.1X3	T45.1X4	T45.1X5	T45.1X6
Procaterol	T44.5X1	T44.5X2	T44.5X3	T44.5X4	T44.5X5	T44.5X6
Prochlorperazine	T43.3X1	T43.3X2	T43.3X3	T43.3X4	T43.3X5	T43.3X6
Procyclidine	T44.3X1	T44.3X2	T44.3X3	T44.3X4	T44.3X5	T44.3X6
Producer gas	T58.8X1	T58.8X2	T58.8X3	T58.8X4	—	—
Profadol	T40.491	T40.492	T40.493	T40.494	T40.495	T40.496
Profenamine	T44.3X1	T44.3X2	T44.3X3	T44.3X4	T44.3X5	T44.3X6
Profenil	T44.3X1	T44.3X2	T44.3X3	T44.3X4	T44.3X5	T44.3X6
Proflavine	T49.0X1	T49.0X2	T49.0X3	T49.0X4	T49.0X5	T49.0X6
Progabide	T42.6X1	T42.6X2	T42.6X3	T42.6X4	T42.6X5	T42.6X6
Progesterone	T38.5X1	T38.5X2	T38.5X3	T38.5X4	T38.5X5	T38.5X6
Progestin	T38.5X1	T38.5X2	T38.5X3	T38.5X4	T38.5X5	T38.5X6
oral contraceptive	T38.4X1	T38.4X2	T38.4X3	T38.4X4	T38.4X5	T38.4X6
Progestogen NEC	T38.5X1	T38.5X2	T38.5X3	T38.5X4	T38.5X5	T38.5X6
Progestone	T38.5X1	T38.5X2	T38.5X3	T38.5X4	T38.5X5	T38.5X6
Proglumide	T47.1X1	T47.1X2	T47.1X3	T47.1X4	T47.1X5	T47.1X6
Prograf*	T45.1X1	T45.1X2	T45.1X3	T45.1X4	T45.1X5	T45.1X6
Proguanil	T37.2X1	T37.2X2	T37.2X3	T37.2X4	T37.2X5	T37.2X6
Prolactin	T38.811	T38.812	T38.813	T38.814	T38.815	T38.816
Prolintane	T43.691	T43.692	T43.693	T43.694	T43.695	T43.696
Proloid	T38.1X1	T38.1X2	T38.1X3	T38.1X4	T38.1X5	T38.1X6
Proluton	T38.5X1	T38.5X2	T38.5X3	T38.5X4	T38.5X5	T38.5X6
Promacetin	T37.1X1	T37.1X2	T37.1X3	T37.1X4	T37.1X5	T37.1X6
Promazine	T43.3X1	T43.3X2	T43.3X3	T43.3X4	T43.3X5	T43.3X6
Promedol	T40.2X1	T40.2X2	T40.2X3	T40.2X4	—	—
Promegestone	T38.5X1	T38.5X2	T38.5X3	T38.5X4	T38.5X5	T38.5X6
Promethazine (teoclate)	T43.3X1	T43.3X2	T43.3X3	T43.3X4	T43.3X5	T43.3X6
Promin	T37.1X1	T37.1X2	T37.1X3	T37.1X4	T37.1X5	T37.1X6
Pronase	T45.3X1	T45.3X2	T45.3X3	T45.3X4	T45.3X5	T45.3X6
Pronestyl (hydrochloride)	T46.2X1	T46.2X2	T46.2X3	T46.2X4	T46.2X5	T46.2X6
Pronetalol	T44.7X1	T44.7X2	T44.7X3	T44.7X4	T44.7X5	T44.7X6
Prontosil	T37.0X1	T37.0X2	T37.0X3	T37.0X4	T37.0X5	T37.0X6
Propachlor	T60.3X1	T60.3X2	T60.3X3	T60.3X4	—	—
Propafenone	T46.2X1	T46.2X2	T46.2X3	T46.2X4	T46.2X5	T46.2X6
Propallylonal	T42.3X1	T42.3X2	T42.3X3	T42.3X4	T42.3X5	T42.3X6
Propamidine	T49.0X1	T49.0X2	T49.0X3	T49.0X4	T49.0X5	T49.0X6
Propane (distributed in mobile container)	T59.891	T59.892	T59.893	T59.894	—	—
distributed through pipes	T59.891	T59.892	T59.893	T59.894	—	—
incomplete combustion	T58.11	T58.12	T58.13	T58.14	—	—
Propanidid	T41.291	T41.292	T41.293	T41.294	T41.295	T41.296
Propanil	T60.3X1	T60.3X2	T60.3X3	T60.3X4	—	—
Propantheline	T44.3X1	T44.3X2	T44.3X3	T44.3X4	T44.3X5	T44.3X6
bromide	T44.3X1	T44.3X2	T44.3X3	T44.3X4	T44.3X5	T44.3X6
Proparacaine	T41.3X1	T41.3X2	T41.3X3	T41.3X4	T41.3X5	T41.3X6
Propatylnitrate	T46.3X1	T46.3X2	T46.3X3	T46.3X4	T46.3X5	T46.3X6

Substance	Poisoning, Accidental (unintentional)	Poisoning, Intentional Self-harm	Poisoning, Assault	Poisoning, Undetermined	Adverse Effect	Under-dosing
Propicillin	T36.0X1	T36.0X2	T36.0X3	T36.0X4	T36.0X5	T36.0X6
Propine*	T49.5X1	T49.5X2	T49.5X3	T49.5X4	T49.5X5	T49.5X6
Propiolactone	T49.0X1	T49.0X2	T49.0X3	T49.0X4	T49.0X5	T49.0X6
Propiomazine	T45.0X1	T45.0X2	T45.0X3	T45.0X4	T45.0X5	T45.0X6
Propionaldehyde (medicinal)	T42.6X1	T42.6X2	T42.6X3	T42.6X4	T42.6X5	T42.6X6
Propionate (calcium) (sodium)	T49.0X1	T49.0X2	T49.0X3	T49.0X4	T49.0X5	T49.0X6
Propion gel	T49.0X1	T49.0X2	T49.0X3	T49.0X4	T49.0X5	T49.0X6
Propitocaine	T41.3X1	T41.3X2	T41.3X3	T41.3X4	T41.3X5	T41.3X6
infiltration (subcutaneous)	T41.3X1	T41.3X2	T41.3X3	T41.3X4	T41.3X5	T41.3X6
nerve block (peripheral) (plexus)	T41.3X1	T41.3X2	T41.3X3	T41.3X4	T41.3X5	T41.3X6
Propofol	T41.291	T41.292	T41.293	T41.294	T41.295	T41.296
Propoxur	T60.0X1	T60.0X2	T60.0X3	T60.0X4	—	—
Propoxycaine	T41.3X1	T41.3X2	T41.3X3	T41.3X4	T41.3X5	T41.3X6
infiltration (subcutaneous)	T41.3X1	T41.3X2	T41.3X3	T41.3X4	T41.3X5	T41.3X6
nerve block (peripheral) (plexus)	T41.3X1	T41.3X2	T41.3X3	T41.3X4	T41.3X5	T41.3X6
topical (surface)	T41.3X1	T41.3X2	T41.3X3	T41.3X4	T41.3X5	T41.3X6
Propoxyphene	T40.491	T40.492	T40.493	T40.494	T40.495	T40.496
Propranolol	T44.7X1	T44.7X2	T44.7X3	T44.7X4	T44.7X5	T44.7X6
Propyl						
alcohol	T51.3X1	T51.3X2	T51.3X3	T51.3X4	—	—
carbinol	T51.3X1	T51.3X2	T51.3X3	T51.3X4	—	—
hexadrine	T44.4X1	T44.4X2	T44.4X3	T44.4X4	T44.4X5	T44.4X6
iodone	T50.8X1	T50.8X2	T50.8X3	T50.8X4	T50.8X5	T50.8X6
thiouracil	T38.2X1	T38.2X2	T38.2X3	T38.2X4	T38.2X5	T38.2X6
Propylaminophenothiazine	T43.3X1	T43.3X2	T43.3X3	T43.3X4	T43.3X5	T43.3X6
Propylene	T59.891	T59.892	T59.893	T59.894	—	—
Propylhexedrine	T48.5X1	T48.5X2	T48.5X3	T48.5X4	T48.5X5	T48.5X6
Propyliodone	T50.8X1	T50.8X2	T50.8X3	T50.8X4	T50.8X5	T50.8X6
Propylparaben (ophthalmic)	T49.5X1	T49.5X2	T49.5X3	T49.5X4	T49.5X5	T49.5X6
Propylthiouracil	T38.2X1	T38.2X2	T38.2X3	T38.2X4	T38.2X5	T38.2X6
Propyphenazone	T39.2X1	T39.2X2	T39.2X3	T39.2X4	T39.2X5	T39.2X6
Proquazone	T39.391	T39.392	T39.393	T39.394	T39.395	T39.396
Proscar*	T38.6X1	T38.6X2	T38.6X3	T38.6X4	T38.6X5	T38.6X6
Proscillaridin	T46.0X1	T46.0X2	T46.0X3	T46.0X4	T46.0X5	T46.0X6
Prostacyclin	T45.521	T45.522	T45.523	T45.524	T45.525	T45.526
Prostaglandin (I2)	T45.521	T45.522	T45.523	T45.524	T45.525	T45.526
E1	T46.7X1	T46.7X2	T46.7X3	T46.7X4	T46.7X5	T46.7X6
E2	T48.0X1	T48.0X2	T48.0X3	T48.0X4	T48.0X5	T48.0X6
F2 alpha	T48.0X1	T48.0X2	T48.0X3	T48.0X4	T48.0X5	T48.0X6
Prostigmin	T44.0X1	T44.0X2	T44.0X3	T44.0X4	T44.0X5	T44.0X6
Prosultiamine	T45.2X1	T45.2X2	T45.2X3	T45.2X4	T45.2X5	T45.2X6
Protamine sulfate	T45.7X1	T45.7X2	T45.7X3	T45.7X4	T45.7X5	T45.7X6
zinc insulin	T38.3X1	T38.3X2	T38.3X3	T38.3X4	T38.3X5	T38.3X6
Protease	T47.5X1	T47.5X2	T47.5X3	T47.5X4	T47.5X5	T47.5X6
Protectant, skin NEC	T49.3X1	T49.3X2	T49.3X3	T49.3X4	T49.3X5	T49.3X6
Protein hydrolysate	T50.991	T50.992	T50.993	T50.994	T50.995	T50.996
Prothiaden — *see* Dothiepin hydrochloride						
Prothionamide	T37.1X1	T37.1X2	T37.1X3	T37.1X4	T37.1X5	T37.1X6
Prothipendyl	T43.591	T43.592	T43.593	T43.594	T43.595	T43.596
Prothoate	T60.0X1	T60.0X2	T60.0X3	T60.0X4	—	—
Prothrombin						
activator	T45.7X1	T45.7X2	T45.7X3	T45.7X4	T45.7X5	T45.7X6
synthesis inhibitor	T45.511	T45.512	T45.513	T45.514	T45.515	T45.516
Protionamide	T37.1X1	T37.1X2	T37.1X3	T37.1X4	T37.1X5	T37.1X6
Protirelin	T38.891	T38.892	T38.893	T38.894	T38.895	T38.896
Protokylol	T48.6X1	T48.6X2	T48.6X3	T48.6X4	T48.6X5	T48.6X6
Protopam	T50.6X1	T50.6X2	T50.6X3	T50.6X4	T50.6X5	T50.6X6
Protoveratrine(s) (A) (B)	T46.5X1	T46.5X2	T46.5X3	T46.5X4	T46.5X5	T46.5X6
Protriptyline	T43.011	T43.012	T43.013	T43.014	T43.015	T43.016
Proventil*	T48.6X1	T48.6X2	T48.6X3	T48.6X4	T48.6X5	T48.6X6
Provera	T38.5X1	T38.5X2	T38.5X3	T38.5X4	T38.5X5	T38.5X6
Provitamin A	T45.2X1	T45.2X2	T45.2X3	T45.2X4	T45.2X5	T45.2X6
Proxibarbal	T42.3X1	T42.3X2	T42.3X3	T42.3X4	T42.3X5	T42.3X6
Proxymetacaine	T41.3X1	T41.3X2	T41.3X3	T41.3X4	T41.3X5	T41.3X6
Proxyphylline	T48.6X1	T48.6X2	T48.6X3	T48.6X4	T48.6X5	T48.6X6
Prozac — *see* Fluoxetine hydrochloride						
Prunus						
laurocerasus	T62.2X1	T62.2X2	T62.2X3	T62.2X4	—	—
virginiana	T62.2X1	T62.2X2	T62.2X3	T62.2X4	—	—
Prussian blue						
commercial	T65.891	T65.892	T65.893	T65.894	—	—
therapeutic	T50.6X1	T50.6X2	T50.6X3	T50.6X4	T50.6X5	T50.6X6
Prussic acid	T65.0X1	T65.0X2	T65.0X3	T65.0X4	—	—
vapor	T57.3X1	T57.3X2	T57.3X3	T57.3X4	—	—
Pseudoephedrine	T44.991	T44.992	T44.993	T44.994	T44.995	T44.996
Psilocin	T40.991	T40.992	T40.993	T40.994	—	—

Substance	Poisoning, Accidental (unintentional)	Poisoning, Intentional Self-harm	Poisoning, Assault	Poisoning, Undetermined	Adverse Effect	Under-dosing
Psilocybin	T4Ø.991	T4Ø.992	T4Ø.993	T4Ø.994	—	—
Psilocybine	T4Ø.991	T4Ø.992	T4Ø.993	T4Ø.994	—	—
Psoralene (nonmedicinal)	T65.891	T65.892	T65.893	T65.894	—	—
Psoralens (medicinal)	T5Ø.991	T5Ø.992	T5Ø.993	T5Ø.994	T5Ø.995	T5Ø.996
PSP (phenolsulfonphthalein)	T5Ø.8X1	T5Ø.8X2	T5Ø.8X3	T5Ø.8X4	T5Ø.8X5	T5Ø.8X6
Psychodysleptic drug NOS	T4Ø.9Ø1	T4Ø.9Ø2	T4Ø.9Ø3	T4Ø.9Ø4	T4Ø.9Ø5	T4Ø.9Ø6
specified NEC	T4Ø.991	T4Ø.992	T4Ø.993	T4Ø.994	T4Ø.995	T4Ø.996
Psychostimulant	T43.6Ø1	T43.6Ø2	T43.6Ø3	T43.6Ø4	T43.6Ø5	T43.6Ø6
amphetamine	T43.621	T43.622	T43.623	T43.624	T43.625	T43.626
caffeine	T43.611	T43.612	T43.613	T43.614	T43.615	T43.616
methylphenidate	T43.631	T43.632	T43.633	T43.634	T43.635	T43.636
specified NEC	T43.691	T43.692	T43.693	T43.694	T43.695	T43.696
Psychotherapeutic drug NEC	T43.91	T43.92	T43.93	T43.94	T43.95	T43.96
antidepressants — *see also* Antidepressant	T43.2Ø1	T43.2Ø2	T43.2Ø3	T43.2Ø4	T43.2Ø5	T43.2Ø6
specified NEC	T43.8X1	T43.8X2	T43.8X3	T43.8X4	T43.8X5	T43.8X6
tranquilizers NEC	T43.5Ø1	T43.5Ø2	T43.5Ø3	T43.5Ø4	T43.5Ø5	T43.5Ø6
Psychotomimetic agents	T4Ø.9Ø1	T4Ø.9Ø2	T4Ø.9Ø3	T4Ø.9Ø4	T4Ø.9Ø5	T4Ø.9Ø6
Psychotropic drug NEC	T43.91	T43.92	T43.93	T43.94	T43.95	T43.96
specified NEC	T43.8X1	T43.8X2	T43.8X3	T43.8X4	T43.8X5	T43.8X6
Psyllium hydrophilic mucilloid	T47.4X1	T47.4X2	T47.4X3	T47.4X4	T47.4X5	T47.4X6
Pteroylglutamic acid	T45.8X1	T45.8X2	T45.8X3	T45.8X4	T45.8X5	T45.8X6
Pteroyltriglutamate	T45.1X1	T45.1X2	T45.1X3	T45.1X4	T45.1X5	T45.1X6
PTFE — *see* Polytetrafluoroethylene						
Pulmicort*	T44.5X1	T44.5X2	T44.5X3	T44.5X4	T44.5X5	T44.5X6
Pulp						
devitalizing paste	T49.7X1	T49.7X2	T49.7X3	T49.7X4	T49.7X5	T49.7X6
dressing	T49.7X1	T49.7X2	T49.7X3	T49.7X4	T49.7X5	T49.7X6
Pulsatilla	T62.2X1	T62.2X2	T62.2X3	T62.2X4	—	—
Pumpkin seed extract	T37.4X1	T37.4X2	T37.4X3	T37.4X4	T37.4X5	T37.4X6
Purex (bleach)	T54.91	T54.92	T54.93	T54.94	—	—
Purgative NEC — *see also* Cathartic	T47.4X1	T47.4X2	T47.4X3	T47.4X4	T47.4X5	T47.4X6
Purine analogue (antineoplastic)	T45.1X1	T45.1X2	T45.1X3	T45.1X4	T45.1X5	T45.1X6
Purine diuretics	T5Ø.2X1	T5Ø.2X2	T5Ø.2X3	T5Ø.2X4	T5Ø.2X5	T5Ø.2X6
Purinethol	T45.1X1	T45.1X2	T45.1X3	T45.1X4	T45.1X5	T45.1X6
PVP	T45.8X1	T45.8X2	T45.8X3	T45.8X4	T45.8X5	T45.8X6
Pyrabital	T39.8X1	T39.8X2	T39.8X3	T39.8X4	T39.8X5	T39.8X6
Pyramidon	T39.2X1	T39.2X2	T39.2X3	T39.2X4	T39.2X5	T39.2X6
Pyrantel	T37.4X1	T37.4X2	T37.4X3	T37.4X4	T37.4X5	T37.4X6
Pyrathiazine	T45.ØX1	T45.ØX2	T45.ØX3	T45.ØX4	T45.ØX5	T45.ØX6
Pyrazinamide	T37.1X1	T37.1X2	T37.1X3	T37.1X4	T37.1X5	T37.1X6
Pyrazinoic acid (amide)	T37.1X1	T37.1X2	T37.1X3	T37.1X4	T37.1X5	T37.1X6
Pyrazole (derivatives)	T39.2X1	T39.2X2	T39.2X3	T39.2X4	T39.2X5	T39.2X6
Pyrazolone analgesic NEC	T39.2X1	T39.2X2	T39.2X3	T39.2X4	T39.2X5	T39.2X6
Pyrethrin, pyrethrum (nonmedicinal)	T6Ø.2X1	T6Ø.2X2	T6Ø.2X3	T6Ø.2X4	—	—
Pyrethrum extract	T49.ØX1	T49.ØX2	T49.ØX3	T49.ØX4	T49.ØX5	T49.ØX6
Pyribenzamine	T45.ØX1	T45.ØX2	T45.ØX3	T45.ØX4	T45.ØX5	T45.ØX6
Pyridine	T52.8X1	T52.8X2	T52.8X3	T52.8X4	—	—
aldoxime methiodide	T5Ø.6X1	T5Ø.6X2	T5Ø.6X3	T5Ø.6X4	T5Ø.6X5	T5Ø.6X6
aldoxime methyl chloride	T5Ø.6X1	T5Ø.6X2	T5Ø.6X3	T5Ø.6X4	T5Ø.6X5	T5Ø.6X6
vapor	T59.891	T59.892	T59.893	T59.894	—	—
Pyridium	T39.8X1	T39.8X2	T39.8X3	T39.8X4	T39.8X5	T39.8X6
Pyridostigmine bromide	T44.ØX1	T44.ØX2	T44.ØX3	T44.ØX4	T44.ØX5	T44.ØX6
Pyridoxal phosphate	T45.2X1	T45.2X2	T45.2X3	T45.2X4	T45.2X5	T45.2X6
Pyridoxine	T45.2X1	T45.2X2	T45.2X3	T45.2X4	T45.2X5	T45.2X6
Pyrilamine	T45.ØX1	T45.ØX2	T45.ØX3	T45.ØX4	T45.ØX5	T45.ØX6
Pyrimethamine	T37.2X1	T37.2X2	T37.2X3	T37.2X4	T37.2X5	T37.2X6
with sulfadoxine	T37.2X1	T37.2X2	T37.2X3	T37.2X4	T37.2X5	T37.2X6
Pyrimidine antagonist	T45.1X1	T45.1X2	T45.1X3	T45.1X4	T45.1X5	T45.1X6
Pyriminil	T6Ø.4X1	T6Ø.4X2	T6Ø.4X3	T6Ø.4X4	—	—
Pyrithione zinc	T49.4X1	T49.4X2	T49.4X3	T49.4X4	T49.4X5	T49.4X6
Pyrithyldione	T42.6X1	T42.6X2	T42.6X3	T42.6X4	T42.6X5	T42.6X6
Pyrogallic acid	T49.ØX1	T49.ØX2	T49.ØX3	T49.ØX4	T49.ØX5	T49.ØX6
Pyrogallol	T49.ØX1	T49.ØX2	T49.ØX3	T49.ØX4	T49.ØX5	T49.ØX6
Pyroxylin	T49.3X1	T49.3X2	T49.3X3	T49.3X4	T49.3X5	T49.3X6
Pyrrobutamine	T45.ØX1	T45.ØX2	T45.ØX3	T45.ØX4	T45.ØX5	T45.ØX6
Pyrrolizidine alkaloids	T62.8X1	T62.8X2	T62.8X3	T62.8X4	—	—
Pyrvinium chloride	T37.4X1	T37.4X2	T37.4X3	T37.4X4	T37.4X5	T37.4X6
PZI	T38.3X1	T38.3X2	T38.3X3	T38.3X4	T38.3X5	T38.3X6
Qbrelis*	T46.4X1	T46.4X2	T46.4X3	T46.4X4	T46.4X5	T46.4X6
Quaalude	T42.6X1	T42.6X2	T42.6X3	T42.6X4	T42.6X5	T42.6X6
Quarternary ammonium						
anti-infective	T49.ØX1	T49.ØX2	T49.ØX3	T49.ØX4	T49.ØX5	T49.ØX6
ganglion blocking	T44.2X1	T44.2X2	T44.2X3	T44.2X4	T44.2X5	T44.2X6
parasympatholytic	T44.3X1	T44.3X2	T44.3X3	T44.3X4	T44.3X5	T44.3X6
Quazepam	T42.4X1	T42.4X2	T42.4X3	T42.4X4	T42.4X5	T42.4X6

Substance	Poisoning, Accidental (unintentional)	Poisoning, Intentional Self-harm	Poisoning, Assault	Poisoning, Undetermined	Adverse Effect	Under-dosing
Quicklime	T54.3X1	T54.3X2	T54.3X3	T54.3X4	—	—
Quilbron-T*	T48.6X1	T48.6X2	T48.6X3	T48.6X4	T48.6X5	T48.6X6
Quillaja extract	T48.4X1	T48.4X2	T48.4X3	T48.4X4	T48.4X5	T48.4X6
Quinacrine	T37.2X1	T37.2X2	T37.2X3	T37.2X4	T37.2X5	T37.2X6
Quinaglute	T46.2X1	T46.2X2	T46.2X3	T46.2X4	T46.2X5	T46.2X6
Quinalbarbital	T42.3X1	T42.3X2	T42.3X3	T42.3X4	T42.3X5	T42.3X6
Quinalbarbitone sodium	T42.3X1	T42.3X2	T42.3X3	T42.3X4	T42.3X5	T42.3X6
Quinalphos	T6Ø.ØX1	T6Ø.ØX2	T6Ø.ØX3	T6Ø.ØX4	—	—
Quinapril	T46.4X1	T46.4X2	T46.4X3	T46.4X4	T46.4X5	T46.4X6
Quinestradiol	T38.5X1	T38.5X2	T38.5X3	T38.5X4	T38.5X5	T38.5X6
Quinestradol	T38.5X1	T38.5X2	T38.5X3	T38.5X4	T38.5X5	T38.5X6
Quinestrol	T38.5X1	T38.5X2	T38.5X3	T38.5X4	T38.5X5	T38.5X6
Quinethazone	T5Ø.2X1	T5Ø.2X2	T5Ø.2X3	T5Ø.2X4	T5Ø.2X5	T5Ø.2X6
Quingestanol	T38.4X1	T38.4X2	T38.4X3	T38.4X4	T38.4X5	T38.4X6
Quinidine	T46.2X1	T46.2X2	T46.2X3	T46.2X4	T46.2X5	T46.2X6
Quinine	T37.2X1	T37.2X2	T37.2X3	T37.2X4	T37.2X5	T37.2X6
Quiniobine	T37.8X1	T37.8X2	T37.8X3	T37.8X4	T37.8X5	T37.8X6
Quinisocaine	T49.1X1	T49.1X2	T49.1X3	T49.1X4	T49.1X5	T49.1X6
Quinocide	T37.2X1	T37.2X2	T37.2X3	T37.2X4	T37.2X5	T37.2X6
Quinoline (derivatives) **NEC**	T37.8X1	T37.8X2	T37.8X3	T37.8X4	T37.8X5	T37.8X6
Quinupramine	T43.Ø11	T43.Ø12	T43.Ø13	T43.Ø14	T43.Ø15	T43.Ø16
Quixin*	T49.5X1	T49.5X2	T49.5X3	T49.5X4	T49.5X5	T49.5X6
Quotane	T41.3X1	T41.3X2	T41.3X3	T41.3X4	T41.3X5	T41.3X6
Rabies						
immune globulin (human)	T5Ø.Z11	T5Ø.Z12	T5Ø.Z13	T5Ø.Z14	T5Ø.Z15	T5Ø.Z16
vaccine	T5Ø.B91	T5Ø.B92	T5Ø.B93	T5Ø.B94	T5Ø.B95	T5Ø.B96
Racemoramide	T4Ø.2X1	T4Ø.2X2	T4Ø.2X3	T4Ø.2X4	—	—
Racemorphan	T4Ø.2X1	T4Ø.2X2	T4Ø.2X3	T4Ø.2X4	T4Ø.2X5	T4Ø.2X6
Racepinefrin	T44.5X1	T44.5X2	T44.5X3	T44.5X4	T44.5X5	T44.5X6
Raclopride	T43.591	T43.592	T43.593	T43.594	T43.595	T43.596
Radiator alcohol	T51.1X1	T51.1X2	T51.1X3	T51.1X4	—	—
Radioactive drug NEC	T5Ø.8X1	T5Ø.8X2	T5Ø.8X3	T5Ø.8X4	T5Ø.8X5	T5Ø.8X6
Radio-opaque (drugs) (materials)	T5Ø.8X1	T5Ø.8X2	T5Ø.8X3	T5Ø.8X4	T5Ø.8X5	T5Ø.8X6
Ramifenazone	T39.2X1	T39.2X2	T39.2X3	T39.2X4	T39.2X5	T39.2X6
Ramipril	T46.4X1	T46.4X2	T46.4X3	T46.4X4	T46.4X5	T46.4X6
Ranitidine	T47.ØX1	T47.ØX2	T47.ØX3	T47.ØX4	T47.ØX5	T47.ØX6
Ranunculus	T62.2X1	T62.2X2	T62.2X3	T62.2X4	—	—
Rat poison NEC	T6Ø.4X1	T6Ø.4X2	T6Ø.4X3	T6Ø.4X4	—	—
Rattlesnake (venom)	T63.Ø11	T63.Ø12	T63.Ø13	T63.Ø14	—	—
Raubasine	T46.7X1	T46.7X2	T46.7X3	T46.7X4	T46.7X5	T46.7X6
Raudixin	T46.5X1	T46.5X2	T46.5X3	T46.5X4	T46.5X5	T46.5X6
Rautensin	T46.5X1	T46.5X2	T46.5X3	T46.5X4	T46.5X5	T46.5X6
Rautina	T46.5X1	T46.5X2	T46.5X3	T46.5X4	T46.5X5	T46.5X6
Rautotal	T46.5X1	T46.5X2	T46.5X3	T46.5X4	T46.5X5	T46.5X6
Rauwiloid	T46.5X1	T46.5X2	T46.5X3	T46.5X4	T46.5X5	T46.5X6
Rauwoldin	T46.5X1	T46.5X2	T46.5X3	T46.5X4	T46.5X5	T46.5X6
Rauwolfia (alkaloids)	T46.5X1	T46.5X2	T46.5X3	T46.5X4	T46.5X5	T46.5X6
Razadyne*	T44.ØX1	T44.ØX2	T44.ØX3	T44.ØX4	T44.ØX5	T44.ØX6
Razoxane	T45.1X1	T45.1X2	T45.1X3	T45.1X4	T45.1X5	T45.1X6
Realgar	T57.ØX1	T57.ØX2	T57.ØX3	T57.ØX4	—	—
Recombinant (R) — *see* specific protein						
Red blood cells, packed	T45.8X1	T45.8X2	T45.8X3	T45.8X4	T45.8X5	T45.8X6
Red squill (scilliroside)	T6Ø.4X1	T6Ø.4X2	T6Ø.4X3	T6Ø.4X4	—	—
Reducing agent, industrial NEC	T65.891	T65.892	T65.893	T65.894	—	—
Refrigerant gas (chlorofluorocarbon)	T53.5X1	T53.5X2	T53.5X3	T53.5X4	—	—
not chlorofluorocarbon	T59.891	T59.892	T59.893	T59.894	—	—
Regroton	T5Ø.2X1	T5Ø.2X2	T5Ø.2X3	T5Ø.2X4	T5Ø.2X5	T5Ø.2X6
Rehydration salts (oral)	T5Ø.3X1	T5Ø.3X2	T5Ø.3X3	T5Ø.3X4	T5Ø.3X5	T5Ø.3X6
Rela	T42.8X1	T42.8X2	T42.8X3	T42.8X4	T42.8X5	T42.8X6
Relaxant, muscle						
anesthetic	T48.1X1	T48.1X2	T48.1X3	T48.1X4	T48.1X5	T48.1X6
central nervous system	T42.8X1	T42.8X2	T42.8X3	T42.8X4	T42.8X5	T42.8X6
skeletal NEC	T48.1X1	T48.1X2	T48.1X3	T48.1X4	T48.1X5	T48.1X6
smooth NEC	T44.3X1	T44.3X2	T44.3X3	T44.3X4	T44.3X5	T44.3X6
Remoxipride	T43.591	T43.592	T43.593	T43.594	T43.595	T43.596
Renese	T5Ø.2X1	T5Ø.2X2	T5Ø.2X3	T5Ø.2X4	T5Ø.2X5	T5Ø.2X6
Renografin	T5Ø.8X1	T5Ø.8X2	T5Ø.8X3	T5Ø.8X4	T5Ø.8X5	T5Ø.8X6
Replacement solution	T5Ø.3X1	T5Ø.3X2	T5Ø.3X3	T5Ø.3X4	T5Ø.3X5	T5Ø.3X6
Reproterol	T48.6X1	T48.6X2	T48.6X3	T48.6X4	T48.6X5	T48.6X6
Rescinnamine	T46.5X1	T46.5X2	T46.5X3	T46.5X4	T46.5X5	T46.5X6
Reserpin (e)	T46.5X1	T46.5X2	T46.5X3	T46.5X4	T46.5X5	T46.5X6
Resorcin, resorcinol (nonmedicinal)	T65.891	T65.892	T65.893	T65.894	—	—
medicinal	T49.4X1	T49.4X2	T49.4X3	T49.4X4	T49.4X5	T49.4X6
Respaire	T48.4X1	T48.4X2	T48.4X3	T48.4X4	T48.4X5	T48.4X6
Respiratory drug NEC	T48.9Ø1	T48.9Ø2	T48.9Ø3	T48.9Ø4	T48.9Ø5	T48.9Ø6
antiasthmatic NEC	T48.6X1	T48.6X2	T48.6X3	T48.6X4	T48.6X5	T48.6X6
anti-common-cold NEC	T48.5X1	T48.5X2	T48.5X3	T48.5X4	T48.5X5	T48.5X6
expectorant NEC	T48.4X1	T48.4X2	T48.4X3	T48.4X4	T48.4X5	T48.4X6

Substance	Poisoning, Accidental (unintentional)	Poisoning, Intentional Self-harm	Poisoning, Assault	Poisoning, Undetermined	Adverse Effect	Under-dosing
Respiratory drug — *continued*						
stimulant	T48.901	T48.902	T48.903	T48.904	T48.905	T48.906
Restoril*	T42.4X1	T42.4X2	T42.4X3	T42.4X4	T42.4X5	T42.4X6
Retinoic acid	T49.0X1	T49.0X2	T49.0X3	T49.0X4	T49.0X5	T49.0X6
Retinol	T45.2X1	T45.2X2	T45.2X3	T45.2X4	T45.2X5	T45.2X6
Rh (D) immune globulin (human)	T50.Z11	T50.Z12	T50.Z13	T50.Z14	T50.Z15	T50.Z16
Rhodine	T39.011	T39.012	T39.013	T39.014	T39.015	T39.016
RhoGAM	T50.Z11	T50.Z12	T50.Z13	T50.Z14	T50.Z15	T50.Z16
Rhubarb						
dry extract	T47.2X1	T47.2X2	T47.2X3	T47.2X4	T47.2X5	T47.2X6
tincture, compound	T47.2X1	T47.2X2	T47.2X3	T47.2X4	T47.2X5	T47.2X6
Ribavirin	T37.5X1	T37.5X2	T37.5X3	T37.5X4	T37.5X5	T37.5X6
Riboflavin	T45.2X1	T45.2X2	T45.2X3	T45.2X4	T45.2X5	T45.2X6
Ribostamycin	T36.5X1	T36.5X2	T36.5X3	T36.5X4	T36.5X5	T36.5X6
Ricin	T62.2X1	T62.2X2	T62.2X3	T62.2X4	—	—
Ricinus communis	T62.2X1	T62.2X2	T62.2X3	T62.2X4	—	—
Rickettsial vaccine NEC	T50.A91	T50.A92	T50.A93	T50.A94	T50.A95	T50.A96
Rifabutin	T36.6X1	T36.6X2	T36.6X3	T36.6X4	T36.6X5	T36.6X6
Rifamide	T36.6X1	T36.6X2	T36.6X3	T36.6X4	T36.6X5	T36.6X6
Rifampicin	T36.6X1	T36.6X2	T36.6X3	T36.6X4	T36.6X5	T36.6X6
with isoniazid	T37.1X1	T37.1X2	T37.1X3	T37.1X4	T37.1X5	T37.1X6
Rifampin	T36.6X1	T36.6X2	T36.6X3	T36.6X4	T36.6X5	T36.6X6
Rifamycin	T36.6X1	T36.6X2	T36.6X3	T36.6X4	T36.6X5	T36.6X6
Rifaximin	T36.6X1	T36.6X2	T36.6X3	T36.6X4	T36.6X5	T36.6X6
Rimantadine	T37.5X1	T37.5X2	T37.5X3	T37.5X4	T37.5X5	T37.5X6
Rimazolium metilsulfate	T39.8X1	T39.8X2	T39.8X3	T39.8X4	T39.8X5	T39.8X6
Rimifon	T37.1X1	T37.1X2	T37.1X3	T37.1X4	T37.1X5	T37.1X6
Rimiterol	T48.6X1	T48.6X2	T48.6X3	T48.6X4	T48.6X5	T48.6X6
Ringer (lactate) **solution**	T50.3X1	T50.3X2	T50.3X3	T50.3X4	T50.3X5	T50.3X6
Risperdal*	T43.591	T43.592	T43.593	T43.594	T43.595	T43.596
Ristocetin	T36.8X1	T36.8X2	T36.8X3	T36.8X4	T36.8X5	T36.8X6
Ritalin	T43.631	T43.632	T43.633	T43.634	T43.635	T43.636
Ritodrine	T44.5X1	T44.5X2	T44.5X3	T44.5X4	T44.5X5	T44.5X6
Roach killer — *see* Insecticide						
Robitussin*	T48.3X1	T48.3X2	T48.3X3	T48.3X4	T48.3X5	T48.3X6
Rociverine	T44.3X1	T44.3X2	T44.3X3	T44.3X4	T44.3X5	T44.3X6
Rocky Mountain spotted fever vaccine	T50.A91	T50.A92	T50.A93	T50.A94	T50.A95	T50.A96
Rodenticide NEC	T60.4X1	T60.4X2	T60.4X3	T60.4X4	—	—
Rohypnol	T42.4X1	T42.4X2	T42.4X3	T42.4X4	T42.4X5	T42.4X6
Rokitamycin	T36.3X1	T36.3X2	T36.3X3	T36.3X4	T36.3X5	T36.3X6
Rolaids	T47.1X1	T47.1X2	T47.1X3	T47.1X4	T47.1X5	T47.1X6
Rolitetracycline	T36.4X1	T36.4X2	T36.4X3	T36.4X4	T36.4X5	T36.4X6
Romilar	T48.3X1	T48.3X2	T48.3X3	T48.3X4	T48.3X5	T48.3X6
Ronifibrate	T46.6X1	T46.6X2	T46.6X3	T46.6X4	T46.6X5	T46.6X6
Rosaprostol	T47.1X1	T47.1X2	T47.1X3	T47.1X4	T47.1X5	T47.1X6
Rose bengal sodium (131I)	T50.8X1	T50.8X2	T50.8X3	T50.8X4	T50.8X5	T50.8X6
Rose water ointment	T49.3X1	T49.3X2	T49.3X3	T49.3X4	T49.3X5	T49.3X6
Rosoxacin	T37.8X1	T37.8X2	T37.8X3	T37.8X4	T37.8X5	T37.8X6
Rotenone	T60.2X1	T60.2X2	T60.2X3	T60.2X4	—	—
Rotoxamine	T45.0X1	T45.0X2	T45.0X3	T45.0X4	T45.0X5	T45.0X6
Rough-on-rats	T60.4X1	T60.4X2	T60.4X3	T60.4X4	—	—
Roxatidine	T47.0X1	T47.0X2	T47.0X3	T47.0X4	T47.0X5	T47.0X6
Roxithromycin	T36.3X1	T36.3X2	T36.3X3	T36.3X4	T36.3X5	T36.3X6
Rt-PA	T45.611	T45.612	T45.613	T45.614	T45.615	T45.616
Rubbing alcohol	T51.2X1	T51.2X2	T51.2X3	T51.2X4	—	—
Rubefacient	T49.4X1	T49.4X2	T49.4X3	T49.4X4	T49.4X5	T49.4X6
Rubella vaccine	T50.B91	T50.B92	T50.B93	T50.B94	T50.B95	T50.B96
Rubeola vaccine	T50.B91	T50.B92	T50.B93	T50.B94	T50.B95	T50.B96
Rubidium chloride Rb82	T50.8X1	T50.8X2	T50.8X3	T50.8X4	T50.8X5	T50.8X6
Rubidomycin	T45.1X1	T45.1X2	T45.1X3	T45.1X4	T45.1X5	T45.1X6
Rue	T62.2X1	T62.2X2	T62.2X3	T62.2X4	—	—
Rufocromomycin	T45.1X1	T45.1X2	T45.1X3	T45.1X4	T45.1X5	T45.1X6
Russel's viper venin	T45.7X1	T45.7X2	T45.7X3	T45.7X4	T45.7X5	T45.7X6
Ruta (graveolens)	T62.2X1	T62.2X2	T62.2X3	T62.2X4	—	—
Rutinum	T46.991	T46.992	T46.993	T46.994	T46.995	T46.996
Rutoside	T46.991	T46.992	T46.993	T46.994	T46.995	T46.996
b-sitosterol(s)	T46.6X1	T46.6X2	T46.6X3	T46.6X4	T46.6X5	T46.6X6
Sabadilla (plant)	T62.2X1	T62.2X2	T62.2X3	T62.2X4	—	—
pesticide	T60.2X1	T60.2X2	T60.2X3	T60.2X4	—	—
Sabril*	T42.6X1	T42.6X2	T42.6X3	T42.6X4	T42.6X5	T42.6X6
Saccharated iron oxide	T45.8X1	T45.8X2	T45.8X3	T45.8X4	T45.8X5	T45.8X6
Saccharin	T50.901	T50.902	T50.903	T50.904	T50.905	T50.906
Saccharomyces boulardii	T47.6X1	T47.6X2	T47.6X3	T47.6X4	T47.6X5	T47.6X6
Safflower oil	T46.6X1	T46.6X2	T46.6X3	T46.6X4	T46.6X5	T46.6X6
Safrazine	T43.1X1	T43.1X2	T43.1X3	T43.1X4	T43.1X5	T43.1X6
Salazosulfapyridine	T37.0X1	T37.0X2	T37.0X3	T37.0X4	T37.0X5	T37.0X6
Salbutamol	T48.6X1	T48.6X2	T48.6X3	T48.6X4	T48.6X5	T48.6X6
Salicylamide	T39.091	T39.092	T39.093	T39.094	T39.095	T39.096
Salicylate NEC	T39.091	T39.092	T39.093	T39.094	T39.095	T39.096
methyl	T49.3X1	T49.3X2	T49.3X3	T49.3X4	T49.3X5	T49.3X6
theobromine calcium	T50.2X1	T50.2X2	T50.2X3	T50.2X4	T50.2X5	T50.2X6

Substance	Poisoning, Accidental (unintentional)	Poisoning, Intentional Self-harm	Poisoning, Assault	Poisoning, Undetermined	Adverse Effect	Under-dosing
Salicylazosulfapyridine	T37.0X1	T37.0X2	T37.0X3	T37.0X4	T37.0X5	T37.0X6
Salicylhydroxamic acid	T49.0X1	T49.0X2	T49.0X3	T49.0X4	T49.0X5	T49.0X6
Salicylic acid	T49.4X1	T49.4X2	T49.4X3	T49.4X4	T49.4X5	T49.4X6
with benzoic acid	T49.4X1	T49.4X2	T49.4X3	T49.4X4	T49.4X5	T49.4X6
congeners	T39.091	T39.092	T39.093	T39.094	T39.095	T39.096
derivative	T39.091	T39.092	T39.093	T39.094	T39.095	T39.096
salts	T39.091	T39.092	T39.093	T39.094	T39.095	T39.096
Salinazid	T37.1X1	T37.1X2	T37.1X3	T37.1X4	T37.1X5	T37.1X6
Salmeterol	T48.6X1	T48.6X2	T48.6X3	T48.6X4	T48.6X5	T48.6X6
Salol	T49.3X1	T49.3X2	T49.3X3	T49.3X4	T49.3X5	T49.3X6
Salsalate	T39.091	T39.092	T39.093	T39.094	T39.095	T39.096
Salt-replacing drug	T50.901	T50.902	T50.903	T50.904	T50.905	T50.906
Salt-retaining mineralocorticoid	T50.0X1	T50.0X2	T50.0X3	T50.0X4	T50.0X5	T50.0X6
Salt substitute	T50.901	T50.902	T50.903	T50.904	T50.905	T50.906
Saluretic NEC	T50.2X1	T50.2X2	T50.2X3	T50.2X4	T50.2X5	T50.2X6
Saluron	T50.2X1	T50.2X2	T50.2X3	T50.2X4	T50.2X5	T50.2X6
Salvarsan 606 (neosilver) (silver)	T37.8X1	T37.8X2	T37.8X3	T37.8X4	T37.8X5	T37.8X6
Sambucus canadensis	T62.2X1	T62.2X2	T62.2X3	T62.2X4	—	—
berry	T62.1X1	T62.1X2	T62.1X3	T62.1X4	—	—
Sandril	T46.5X1	T46.5X2	T46.5X3	T46.5X4	T46.5X5	T46.5X6
Sanguinaria canadensis	T62.2X1	T62.2X2	T62.2X3	T62.2X4	—	—
Saniflush (cleaner)	T54.2X1	T54.2X2	T54.2X3	T54.2X4	—	—
Santonin	T37.4X1	T37.4X2	T37.4X3	T37.4X4	T37.4X5	T37.4X6
Santyl	T49.8X1	T49.8X2	T49.8X3	T49.8X4	T49.8X5	T49.8X6
Saralasin	T46.5X1	T46.5X2	T46.5X3	T46.5X4	T46.5X5	T46.5X6
Sarcolysin	T45.1X1	T45.1X2	T45.1X3	T45.1X4	T45.1X5	T45.1X6
Sarilumab*	T39.4X1	T39.4X2	T39.4X3	T39.4X4	T39.4X5	T39.4X6
Sarkomycin	T45.1X1	T45.1X2	T45.1X3	T45.1X4	T45.1X5	T45.1X6
Saroten	T43.011	T43.012	T43.013	T43.014	T43.015	T43.016
Saturnine — *see* Lead						
Savin (oil)	T49.4X1	T49.4X2	T49.4X3	T49.4X4	T49.4X5	T49.4X6
Scammony	T47.2X1	T47.2X2	T47.2X3	T47.2X4	T47.2X5	T47.2X6
Scarlet red	T49.8X1	T49.8X2	T49.8X3	T49.8X4	T49.8X5	T49.8X6
Scheele's green	T57.0X1	T57.0X2	T57.0X3	T57.0X4	—	—
insecticide	T57.0X1	T57.0X2	T57.0X3	T57.0X4	—	—
Schizontozide (blood) (tissue)	T37.2X1	T37.2X2	T37.2X3	T37.2X4	T37.2X5	T37.2X6
Schradan	T60.0X1	T60.0X2	T60.0X3	T60.0X4	—	—
Schweinfurth green	T57.0X1	T57.0X2	T57.0X3	T57.0X4	—	—
insecticide	T57.0X1	T57.0X2	T57.0X3	T57.0X4	—	—
Scilla, rat poison	T60.4X1	T60.4X2	T60.4X3	T60.4X4	—	—
Scillaren	T60.4X1	T60.4X2	T60.4X3	T60.4X4	—	—
Sclerosing agent	T46.8X1	T46.8X2	T46.8X3	T46.8X4	T46.8X5	T46.8X6
Scombrotoxin	T61.11	T61.12	T61.13	T61.14	—	—
Scopolamine	T44.3X1	T44.3X2	T44.3X3	T44.3X4	T44.3X5	T44.3X6
Scopolia extract	T44.3X1	T44.3X2	T44.3X3	T44.3X4	T44.3X5	T44.3X6
Scouring powder	T65.891	T65.892	T65.893	T65.894	—	—
Sea						
anemone (sting)	T63.631	T63.632	T63.633	T63.634	—	—
cucumber (sting)	T63.691	T63.692	T63.693	T63.694	—	—
snake (bite) (venom)	T63.091	T63.092	T63.093	T63.094	—	—
urchin spine (puncture)	T63.691	T63.692	T63.693	T63.694	—	—
Seafood	T61.91	T61.92	T61.93	T61.94	—	—
specified NEC	T61.8X1	T61.8X2	T61.8X3	T61.8X4	—	—
Secbutabarbital	T42.3X1	T42.3X2	T42.3X3	T42.3X4	T42.3X5	T42.3X6
Secbutabarbitone	T42.3X1	T42.3X2	T42.3X3	T42.3X4	T42.3X5	T42.3X6
Secnidazole	T37.3X1	T37.3X2	T37.3X3	T37.3X4	T37.3X5	T37.3X6
Secobarbital	T42.3X1	T42.3X2	T42.3X3	T42.3X4	T42.3X5	T42.3X6
Seconal	T42.3X1	T42.3X2	T42.3X3	T42.3X4	T42.3X5	T42.3X6
Secretin	T50.8X1	T50.8X2	T50.8X3	T50.8X4	T50.8X5	T50.8X6
Sectral*	T44.7X1	T44.7X2	T44.7X3	T44.7X4	T44.7X5	T44.7X6
Sedative NEC	T42.71	T42.72	T42.73	T42.74	T42.75	T42.76
mixed NEC	T42.6X1	T42.6X2	T42.6X3	T42.6X4	T42.6X5	T42.6X6
Sedormid	T42.6X1	T42.6X2	T42.6X3	T42.6X4	T42.6X5	T42.6X6
Seed disinfectant or dressing	T60.8X1	T60.8X2	T60.8X3	T60.8X4	—	—
Seeds (poisonous)	T62.2X1	T62.2X2	T62.2X3	T62.2X4	—	—
Selegiline	T42.8X1	T42.8X2	T42.8X3	T42.8X4	T42.8X5	T42.8X6
Selenium NEC	T56.891	T56.892	T56.893	T56.894	—	—
disulfide or sulfide	T49.4X1	T49.4X2	T49.4X3	T49.4X4	T49.4X5	T49.4X6
fumes	T59.891	T59.892	T59.893	T59.894	—	—
sulfide	T49.4X1	T49.4X2	T49.4X3	T49.4X4	T49.4X5	T49.4X6
Selenomethionine (75Se)	T50.8X1	T50.8X2	T50.8X3	T50.8X4	T50.8X5	T50.8X6
Selsun	T49.4X1	T49.4X2	T49.4X3	T49.4X4	T49.4X5	T49.4X6
Semustine	T45.1X1	T45.1X2	T45.1X3	T45.1X4	T45.1X5	T45.1X6
Senega syrup	T48.4X1	T48.4X2	T48.4X3	T48.4X4	T48.4X5	T48.4X6
Senna	T47.2X1	T47.2X2	T47.2X3	T47.2X4	T47.2X5	T47.2X6
Sennoside A+B	T47.2X1	T47.2X2	T47.2X3	T47.2X4	T47.2X5	T47.2X6
Septisol	T49.2X1	T49.2X2	T49.2X3	T49.2X4	T49.2X5	T49.2X6
Seractide	T38.811	T38.812	T38.813	T38.814	T38.815	T38.816
Serax	T42.4X1	T42.4X2	T42.4X3	T42.4X4	T42.4X5	T42.4X6

*Optum Value-Add

☑ Additional Character May Be Required — Refer to the Tabular List for Character Selection

Substance	Poisoning, Accidental (unintentional)	Poisoning, Intentional Self-harm	Poisoning, Assault	Poisoning, Undetermined	Adverse Effect	Under-dosing
Serenesil	T42.6X1	T42.6X2	T42.6X3	T42.6X4	T42.6X5	T42.6X6
Serenium (hydrochloride)	T37.91	T37.92	T37.93	T37.94	T37.95	T37.96
Serepax — *see* Oxazepam						
Serevent*	T48.6X1	T48.6X2	T48.6X3	T48.6X4	T48.6X5	T48.6X6
Sermorelin	T38.891	T38.892	T38.893	T38.894	T38.895	T38.896
Sernyl	T41.1X1	T41.1X2	T41.1X3	T41.1X4	T41.1X5	T41.1X6
Serotonin	T5Ø.991	T5Ø.992	T5Ø.993	T5Ø.994	T5Ø.995	T5Ø.996
Serpasil	T46.5X1	T46.5X2	T46.5X3	T46.5X4	T46.5X5	T46.5X6
Serrapeptase	T45.3X1	T45.3X2	T45.3X3	T45.3X4	T45.3X5	T45.3X6
Serum						
antibotulinus	T5Ø.Z11	T5Ø.Z12	T5Ø.Z13	T5Ø.Z14	T5Ø.Z15	T5Ø.Z16
anticytotoxic	T5Ø.Z11	T5Ø.Z12	T5Ø.Z13	T5Ø.Z14	T5Ø.Z15	T5Ø.Z16
antidiphtheria	T5Ø.Z11	T5Ø.Z12	T5Ø.Z13	T5Ø.Z14	T5Ø.Z15	T5Ø.Z16
antimeningococcus	T5Ø.Z11	T5Ø.Z12	T5Ø.Z13	T5Ø.Z14	T5Ø.Z15	T5Ø.Z16
anti-Rh	T5Ø.Z11	T5Ø.Z12	T5Ø.Z13	T5Ø.Z14	T5Ø.Z15	T5Ø.Z16
anti-snake-bite	T5Ø.Z11	T5Ø.Z12	T5Ø.Z13	T5Ø.Z14	T5Ø.Z15	T5Ø.Z16
antitetanic	T5Ø.Z11	T5Ø.Z12	T5Ø.Z13	T5Ø.Z14	T5Ø.Z15	T5Ø.Z16
antitoxic	T5Ø.Z11	T5Ø.Z12	T5Ø.Z13	T5Ø.Z14	T5Ø.Z15	T5Ø.Z16
complement (inhibitor)	T45.8X1	T45.8X2	T45.8X3	T45.8X4	T45.8X5	T45.8X6
convalescent	T5Ø.Z11	T5Ø.Z12	T5Ø.Z13	T5Ø.Z14	T5Ø.Z15	T5Ø.Z16
hemolytic complement	T45.8X1	T45.8X2	T45.8X3	T45.8X4	T45.8X5	T45.8X6
immune (human)	T5Ø.Z11	T5Ø.Z12	T5Ø.Z13	T5Ø.Z14	T5Ø.Z15	T5Ø.Z16
protective NEC	T5Ø.Z11	T5Ø.Z12	T5Ø.Z13	T5Ø.Z14	T5Ø.Z15	T5Ø.Z16
Setastine	T45.ØX1	T45.ØX2	T45.ØX3	T45.ØX4	T45.ØX5	T45.ØX6
Setoperone	T43.591	T43.592	T43.593	T43.594	T43.595	T43.596
Sewer gas	T59.91	T59.92	T59.93	T59.94	—	—
Shampoo	T55.ØX1	T55.ØX2	T55.ØX3	T55.ØX4	—	—
Shellfish, noxious, nonbacterial	T61.781	T61.782	T61.783	T61.784	—	—
Sildenafil	T46.7X1	T46.7X2	T46.7X3	T46.7X4	T46.7X5	T46.7X6
Silibinin	T5Ø.991	T5Ø.992	T5Ø.993	T5Ø.994	T5Ø.995	T5Ø.996
Silicone NEC	T65.891	T65.892	T65.893	T65.894	—	—
medicinal	T49.3X1	T49.3X2	T49.3X3	T49.3X4	T49.3X5	T49.3X6
Silvadene	T49.ØX1	T49.ØX2	T49.ØX3	T49.ØX4	T49.ØX5	T49.ØX6
Silver	T49.ØX1	T49.ØX2	T49.ØX3	T49.ØX4	T49.ØX5	T49.ØX6
anti-infectives	T49.ØX1	T49.ØX2	T49.ØX3	T49.ØX4	T49.ØX5	T49.ØX6
arsphenamine	T37.8X1	T37.8X2	T37.8X3	T37.8X4	T37.8X5	T37.8X6
colloidal	T49.ØX1	T49.ØX2	T49.ØX3	T49.ØX4	T49.ØX5	T49.ØX6
nitrate	T49.ØX1	T49.ØX2	T49.ØX3	T49.ØX4	T49.ØX5	T49.ØX6
ophthalmic preparation	T49.5X1	T49.5X2	T49.5X3	T49.5X4	T49.5X5	T49.5X6
toughened (keratolytic)	T49.4X1	T49.4X2	T49.4X3	T49.4X4	T49.4X5	T49.4X6
nonmedicinal (dust)	T56.891	T56.892	T56.893	T56.894	—	—
protein	T49.5X1	T49.5X2	T49.5X3	T49.5X4	T49.5X5	T49.5X6
salvarsan	T37.8X1	T37.8X2	T37.8X3	T37.8X4	T37.8X5	T37.8X6
sulfadiazine	T49.4X1	T49.4X2	T49.4X3	T49.4X4	T49.4X5	T49.4X6
Silymarin	T5Ø.991	T5Ø.992	T5Ø.993	T5Ø.994	T5Ø.995	T5Ø.996
Simaldrate	T47.1X1	T47.1X2	T47.1X3	T47.1X4	T47.1X5	T47.1X6
Simazine	T6Ø.3X1	T6Ø.3X2	T6Ø.3X3	T6Ø.3X4	—	—
Simethicone	T47.1X1	T47.1X2	T47.1X3	T47.1X4	T47.1X5	T47.1X6
Simfibrate	T46.6X1	T46.6X2	T46.6X3	T46.6X4	T46.6X5	T46.6X6
Simvastatin	T46.6X1	T46.6X2	T46.6X3	T46.6X4	T46.6X5	T46.6X6
Sincalide	T5Ø.8X1	T5Ø.8X2	T5Ø.8X3	T5Ø.8X4	T5Ø.8X5	T5Ø.8X6
Sinequan	T43.Ø11	T43.Ø12	T43.Ø13	T43.Ø14	T43.Ø15	T43.Ø16
Singoserp	T46.5X1	T46.5X2	T46.5X3	T46.5X4	T46.5X5	T46.5X6
Singulair*	T48.6X1	T48.6X2	T48.6X3	T48.6X4	T48.6X5	T48.6X6
Sintrom	T45.511	T45.512	T45.513	T45.514	T45.515	T45.516
Sisomicin	T36.5X1	T36.5X2	T36.5X3	T36.5X4	T36.5X5	T36.5X6
Sitosterols	T46.6X1	T46.6X2	T46.6X3	T46.6X4	T46.6X5	T46.6X6
Skeletal muscle relaxants	T48.1X1	T48.1X2	T48.1X3	T48.1X4	T48.1X5	T48.1X6
Skin						
agents (external)	T49.91	T49.92	T49.93	T49.94	T49.95	T49.96
specified NEC	T49.8X1	T49.8X2	T49.8X3	T49.8X4	T49.8X5	T49.8X6
test antigen	T5Ø.8X1	T5Ø.8X2	T5Ø.8X3	T5Ø.8X4	T5Ø.8X5	T5Ø.8X6
Sleep-eze	T45.ØX1	T45.ØX2	T45.ØX3	T45.ØX4	T45.ØX5	T45.ØX6
Sleeping draught, pill	T42.71	T42.72	T42.73	T42.74	T42.75	T42.76
Smallpox vaccine	T5Ø.B11	T5Ø.B12	T5Ø.B13	T5Ø.B14	T5Ø.B15	T5Ø.B16
Smelter fumes NEC	T56.91	T56.92	T56.93	T56.94	—	—
Smog	T59.1X1	T59.1X2	T59.1X3	T59.1X4	—	—
Smoke NEC	T59.811	T59.812	T59.813	T59.814	—	—
Smooth muscle relaxant	T44.3X1	T44.3X2	T44.3X3	T44.3X4	T44.3X5	T44.3X6
Snail killer NEC	T6Ø.8X1	T6Ø.8X2	T6Ø.8X3	T6Ø.8X4	—	—
Snake venom or bite	T63.ØØ1	T63.ØØ2	T63.ØØ3	T63.ØØ4	—	—
hemocoagulase	T45.7X1	T45.7X2	T45.7X3	T45.7X4	T45.7X5	T45.7X6
Snuff	T65.211	T65.212	T65.213	T65.214	—	—
Soap (powder) (product)	T55.ØX1	T55.ØX2	T55.ØX3	T55.ØX4	—	—
enema	T47.4X1	T47.4X2	T47.4X3	T47.4X4	T47.4X5	T47.4X6
medicinal, soft	T49.2X1	T49.2X2	T49.2X3	T49.2X4	T49.2X5	T49.2X6
superfatted	T49.2X1	T49.2X2	T49.2X3	T49.2X4	T49.2X5	T49.2X6
Sobrerol	T48.4X1	T48.4X2	T48.4X3	T48.4X4	T48.4X5	T48.4X6
Soda (caustic)	T54.3X1	T54.3X2	T54.3X3	T54.3X4	—	—
bicarb	T47.1X1	T47.1X2	T47.1X3	T47.1X4	T47.1X5	T47.1X6
chlorinated — *see* Sodium, hypochlorite						

Substance	Poisoning, Accidental (unintentional)	Poisoning, Intentional Self-harm	Poisoning, Assault	Poisoning, Undetermined	Adverse Effect	Under-dosing
Sodium						
acetosulfone	T37.1X1	T37.1X2	T37.1X3	T37.1X4	T37.1X5	T37.1X6
acetrizoate	T5Ø.8X1	T5Ø.8X2	T5Ø.8X3	T5Ø.8X4	T5Ø.8X5	T5Ø.8X6
acid phosphate	T5Ø.3X1	T5Ø.3X2	T5Ø.3X3	T5Ø.3X4	T5Ø.3X5	T5Ø.3X6
alginate	T47.8X1	T47.8X2	T47.8X3	T47.8X4	T47.8X5	T47.8X6
amidotrizoate	T5Ø.8X1	T5Ø.8X2	T5Ø.8X3	T5Ø.8X4	T5Ø.8X5	T5Ø.8X6
aminohippurate*	T5Ø.8X1	T5Ø.8X2	T5Ø.8X3	T5Ø.8X4	T5Ø.8X5	T5Ø.8X6
aminopterin	T45.1X1	T45.1X2	T45.1X3	T45.1X4	T45.1X5	T45.1X6
amylosulfate	T47.8X1	T47.8X2	T47.8X3	T47.8X4	T47.8X5	T47.8X6
amytal	T42.3X1	T42.3X2	T42.3X3	T42.3X4	T42.3X5	T42.3X6
antimony gluconate	T37.3X1	T37.3X2	T37.3X3	T37.3X4	T37.3X5	T37.3X6
arsenate	T57.ØX1	T57.ØX2	T57.ØX3	T57.ØX4	—	—
aurothiomalate	T39.4X1	T39.4X2	T39.4X3	T39.4X4	T39.4X5	T39.4X6
aurothiosulfate	T39.4X1	T39.4X2	T39.4X3	T39.4X4	T39.4X5	T39.4X6
barbiturate	T42.3X1	T42.3X2	T42.3X3	T42.3X4	T42.3X5	T42.3X6
basic phosphate	T47.4X1	T47.4X2	T47.4X3	T47.4X4	T47.4X5	T47.4X6
bicarbonate	T47.1X1	T47.1X2	T47.1X3	T47.1X4	T47.1X5	T47.1X6
bichromate	T57.8X1	T57.8X2	T57.8X3	T57.8X4	—	—
biphosphate	T5Ø.3X1	T5Ø.3X2	T5Ø.3X3	T5Ø.3X4	T5Ø.3X5	T5Ø.3X6
bisulfate	T65.891	T65.892	T65.893	T65.894	—	—
borate						
cleanser	T57.8X1	T57.8X2	T57.8X3	T57.8X4	—	—
eye	T49.5X1	T49.5X2	T49.5X3	T49.5X4	T49.5X5	T49.5X6
therapeutic	T49.8X1	T49.8X2	T49.8X3	T49.8X4	T49.8X5	T49.8X6
bromide	T42.6X1	T42.6X2	T42.6X3	T42.6X4	T42.6X5	T42.6X6
cacodylate (nonmedicinal) NEC	T5Ø.8X1	T5Ø.8X2	T5Ø.8X3	T5Ø.8X4	T5Ø.8X5	T5Ø.8X6
anti-infective	T37.8X1	T37.8X2	T37.8X3	T37.8X4	T37.8X5	T37.8X6
herbicide	T6Ø.3X1	T6Ø.3X2	T6Ø.3X3	T6Ø.3X4	—	—
calcium edetate	T45.8X1	T45.8X2	T45.8X3	T45.8X4	T45.8X5	T45.8X6
carbonate NEC	T54.3X1	T54.3X2	T54.3X3	T54.3X4	—	—
chlorate NEC	T65.891	T65.892	T65.893	T65.894	—	—
herbicide	T54.91	T54.92	T54.93	T54.94	—	—
chloride	T5Ø.3X1	T5Ø.3X2	T5Ø.3X3	T5Ø.3X4	T5Ø.3X5	T5Ø.3X6
with glucose	T5Ø.3X1	T5Ø.3X2	T5Ø.3X3	T5Ø.3X4	T5Ø.3X5	T5Ø.3X6
chromate	T65.891	T65.892	T65.893	T65.894	—	—
citrate	T5Ø.991	T5Ø.992	T5Ø.993	T5Ø.994	T5Ø.995	T5Ø.996
cromoglicate	T48.6X1	T48.6X2	T48.6X3	T48.6X4	T48.6X5	T48.6X6
cyanide	T65.ØX1	T65.ØX2	T65.ØX3	T65.ØX4	—	—
cyclamate	T5Ø.3X1	T5Ø.3X2	T5Ø.3X3	T5Ø.3X4	T5Ø.3X5	T5Ø.3X6
dehydrocholate	T45.8X1	T45.8X2	T45.8X3	T45.8X4	T45.8X5	T45.8X6
diatrizoate	T5Ø.8X1	T5Ø.8X2	T5Ø.8X3	T5Ø.8X4	T5Ø.8X5	T5Ø.8X6
dibunate	T48.4X1	T48.4X2	T48.4X3	T48.4X4	T48.4X5	T48.4X6
dioctyl sulfosuccinate	T47.4X1	T47.4X2	T47.4X3	T47.4X4	T47.4X5	T47.4X6
dipantoyl ferrate	T45.8X1	T45.8X2	T45.8X3	T45.8X4	T45.8X5	T45.8X6
edetate	T45.8X1	T45.8X2	T45.8X3	T45.8X4	T45.8X5	T45.8X6
ethacrynate	T5Ø.1X1	T5Ø.1X2	T5Ø.1X3	T5Ø.1X4	T5Ø.1X5	T5Ø.1X6
etidronate*	T5Ø.991	T5Ø.992	T5Ø.993	T5Ø.994	T5Ø.995	T5Ø.996
feredetate	T45.8X1	T45.8X2	T45.8X3	T45.8X4	T45.8X5	T45.8X6
Fluoride — *see* Fluoride						
fluoroacetate (dust) (pesticide)	T6Ø.4X1	T6Ø.4X2	T6Ø.4X3	T6Ø.4X4	—	—
free salt	T5Ø.3X1	T5Ø.3X2	T5Ø.3X3	T5Ø.3X4	T5Ø.3X5	T5Ø.3X6
fusidate	T36.8X1	T36.8X2	T36.8X3	T36.8X4	T36.8X5	T36.8X6
glucaldrate	T47.1X1	T47.1X2	T47.1X3	T47.1X4	T47.1X5	T47.1X6
glucosulfone	T37.1X1	T37.1X2	T37.1X3	T37.1X4	T37.1X5	T37.1X6
glutamate	T45.8X1	T45.8X2	T45.8X3	T45.8X4	T45.8X5	T45.8X6
hydrogen carbonate	T5Ø.3X1	T5Ø.3X2	T5Ø.3X3	T5Ø.3X4	T5Ø.3X5	T5Ø.3X6
hydroxide	T54.3X1	T54.3X2	T54.3X3	T54.3X4	—	—
hypochlorite (bleach) NEC	T54.3X1	T54.3X2	T54.3X3	T54.3X4	—	—
disinfectant	T54.3X1	T54.3X2	T54.3X3	T54.3X4	—	—
medicinal (anti-infective) (external)	T49.ØX1	T49.ØX2	T49.ØX3	T49.ØX4	T49.ØX5	T49.ØX6
vapor	T54.3X1	T54.3X2	T54.3X3	T54.3X4	—	—
hyposulfite	T49.ØX1	T49.ØX2	T49.ØX3	T49.ØX4	T49.ØX5	T49.ØX6
indigotin disulfonate	T5Ø.8X1	T5Ø.8X2	T5Ø.8X3	T5Ø.8X4	T5Ø.8X5	T5Ø.8X6
iodide	T5Ø.991	T5Ø.992	T5Ø.993	T5Ø.994	T5Ø.995	T5Ø.996
I-131	T5Ø.8X1	T5Ø.8X2	T5Ø.8X3	T5Ø.8X4	T5Ø.8X5	T5Ø.8X6
therapeutic	T38.2X1	T38.2X2	T38.2X3	T38.2X4	T38.2X5	T38.2X6
iodohippurate (131I)	T5Ø.8X1	T5Ø.8X2	T5Ø.8X3	T5Ø.8X4	T5Ø.8X5	T5Ø.8X6
iopodate	T5Ø.8X1	T5Ø.8X2	T5Ø.8X3	T5Ø.8X4	T5Ø.8X5	T5Ø.8X6
iothalamate	T5Ø.8X1	T5Ø.8X2	T5Ø.8X3	T5Ø.8X4	T5Ø.8X5	T5Ø.8X6
iron edetate	T45.4X1	T45.4X2	T45.4X3	T45.4X4	T45.4X5	T45.4X6
lactate (compound solution)	T45.8X1	T45.8X2	T45.8X3	T45.8X4	T45.8X5	T45.8X6
lauryl (sulfate)	T49.2X1	T49.2X2	T49.2X3	T49.2X4	T49.2X5	T49.2X6
L-triiodothyronine	T38.1X1	T38.1X2	T38.1X3	T38.1X4	T38.1X5	T38.1X6
magnesium citrate	T5Ø.991	T5Ø.992	T5Ø.993	T5Ø.994	T5Ø.995	T5Ø.996
mersalate	T5Ø.2X1	T5Ø.2X2	T5Ø.2X3	T5Ø.2X4	T5Ø.2X5	T5Ø.2X6
metasilicate	T65.891	T65.892	T65.893	T65.894	—	—
metrizoate	T5Ø.8X1	T5Ø.8X2	T5Ø.8X3	T5Ø.8X4	T5Ø.8X5	T5Ø.8X6
monofluoroacetate (pesticide)	T6Ø.1X1	T6Ø.1X2	T6Ø.1X3	T6Ø.1X4	—	—

Substance	Poisoning, Accidental (unintentional)	Poisoning, Intentional Self-harm	Poisoning, Assault	Poisoning, Undetermined	Adverse Effect	Under-dosing
Sodium — *continued*						
morrhuate	T46.8X1	T46.8X2	T46.8X3	T46.8X4	T46.8X5	T46.8X6
nafcillin	T36.ØX1	T36.ØX2	T36.ØX3	T36.ØX4	T36.ØX5	T36.ØX6
nitrate (oxidizing agent)	T65.891	T65.892	T65.893	T65.894	—	—
nitrite	T5Ø.6X1	T5Ø.6X2	T5Ø.6X3	T5Ø.6X4	T5Ø.6X5	T5Ø.6X6
nitroferricyanide	T46.5X1	T46.5X2	T46.5X3	T46.5X4	T46.5X5	T46.5X6
nitroprusside	T46.5X1	T46.5X2	T46.5X3	T46.5X4	T46.5X5	T46.5X6
oxalate	T65.891	T65.892	T65.893	T65.894	—	—
oxide/peroxide	T65.891	T65.892	T65.893	T65.894	—	—
oxybate	T41.291	T41.292	T41.293	T41.294	T41.295	T41.296
para-aminohippurate	T5Ø.8X1	T5Ø.8X2	T5Ø.8X3	T5Ø.8X4	T5Ø.8X5	T5Ø.8X6
perborate (nonmedicinal) NEC	T65.891	T65.892	T65.893	T65.894	—	—
medicinal	T49.ØX1	T49.ØX2	T49.ØX3	T49.ØX4	T49.ØX5	T49.ØX6
soap	T55.ØX1	T55.ØX2	T55.ØX3	T55.ØX4	—	—
percarbonate — *see* Sodium, perborate						
pertechnetate Tc99m	T5Ø.8X1	T5Ø.8X2	T5Ø.8X3	T5Ø.8X4	T5Ø.8X5	T5Ø.8X6
phosphate						
cellulose	T45.8X1	T45.8X2	T45.8X3	T45.8X4	T45.8X5	T45.8X6
dibasic	T47.2X1	T47.2X2	T47.2X3	T47.2X4	T47.2X5	T47.2X6
monobasic	T47.2X1	T47.2X2	T47.2X3	T47.2X4	T47.2X5	T47.2X6
phytate	T5Ø.6X1	T5Ø.6X2	T5Ø.6X3	T5Ø.6X4	T5Ø.6X5	T5Ø.6X6
picosulfate	T47.2X1	T47.2X2	T47.2X3	T47.2X4	T47.2X5	T47.2X6
polyhydroxyaluminium monocarbonate	T47.1X1	T47.1X2	T47.1X3	T47.1X4	T47.1X5	T47.1X6
polystyrene sulfonate	T5Ø.3X1	T5Ø.3X2	T5Ø.3X3	T5Ø.3X4	T5Ø.3X5	T5Ø.3X6
propionate	T49.ØX1	T49.ØX2	T49.ØX3	T49.ØX4	T49.ØX5	T49.ØX6
propyl hydroxybenzoate	T5Ø.991	T5Ø.992	T5Ø.993	T5Ø.994	T5Ø.995	T5Ø.996
psylliate	T46.8X1	T46.8X2	T46.8X3	T46.8X4	T46.8X5	T46.8X6
removing resins	T5Ø.3X1	T5Ø.3X2	T5Ø.3X3	T5Ø.3X4	T5Ø.3X5	T5Ø.3X6
salicylate	T39.Ø91	T39.Ø92	T39.Ø93	T39.Ø94	T39.Ø95	T39.Ø96
salt NEC	T5Ø.3X1	T5Ø.3X2	T5Ø.3X3	T5Ø.3X4	T5Ø.3X5	T5Ø.3X6
selenate	T6Ø.2X1	T6Ø.2X2	T6Ø.2X3	T6Ø.2X4	—	—
stibogluconate	T37.3X1	T37.3X2	T37.3X3	T37.3X4	T37.3X5	T37.3X6
sulfate	T47.4X1	T47.4X2	T47.4X3	T47.4X4	T47.4X5	T47.4X6
sulfoxone	T37.1X1	T37.1X2	T37.1X3	T37.1X4	T37.1X5	T37.1X6
tetradecyl sulfate	T46.8X1	T46.8X2	T46.8X3	T46.8X4	T46.8X5	T46.8X6
thiopental	T41.1X1	T41.1X2	T41.1X3	T41.1X4	T41.1X5	T41.1X6
thiosalicylate	T39.Ø91	T39.Ø92	T39.Ø93	T39.Ø94	T39.Ø95	T39.Ø96
thiosulfate	T5Ø.6X1	T5Ø.6X2	T5Ø.6X3	T5Ø.6X4	T5Ø.6X5	T5Ø.6X6
tolbutamide	T38.3X1	T38.3X2	T38.3X3	T38.3X4	T38.3X5	T38.3X6
(L)-triiodothyronine	T38.1X1	T38.1X2	T38.1X3	T38.1X4	T38.1X5	T38.1X6
tyropanoate	T5Ø.8X1	T5Ø.8X2	T5Ø.8X3	T5Ø.8X4	T5Ø.8X5	T5Ø.8X6
valproate	T42.6X1	T42.6X2	T42.6X3	T42.6X4	T42.6X5	T42.6X6
versenate	T5Ø.6X1	T5Ø.6X2	T5Ø.6X3	T5Ø.6X4	T5Ø.6X5	T5Ø.6X6
Sodium-free salt	T5Ø.9Ø1	T5Ø.9Ø2	T5Ø.9Ø3	T5Ø.9Ø4	T5Ø.9Ø5	T5Ø.9Ø6
Sodium-removing resin	T5Ø.3X1	T5Ø.3X2	T5Ø.3X3	T5Ø.3X4	T5Ø.3X5	T5Ø.3X6
Soft soap	T55.ØX1	T55.ØX2	T55.ØX3	T55.ØX4	—	—
Solanine	T62.2X1	T62.2X2	T62.2X3	T62.2X4	—	—
berries	T62.1X1	T62.1X2	T62.1X3	T62.1X4	—	—
Solanum dulcamara	T62.2X1	T62.2X2	T62.2X3	T62.2X4	—	—
berries	T62.1X1	T62.1X2	T62.1X3	T62.1X4	—	—
Solapsone	T37.1X1	T37.1X2	T37.1X3	T37.1X4	T37.1X5	T37.1X6
Solaquin*	T49.8X1	T49.8X2	T49.8X3	T49.8X4	T49.8X5	T49.8X6
Solar lotion	T49.3X1	T49.3X2	T49.3X3	T49.3X4	T49.3X5	T49.3X6
Solasulfone	T37.1X1	T37.1X2	T37.1X3	T37.1X4	T37.1X5	T37.1X6
Soldering fluid	T65.891	T65.892	T65.893	T65.894	—	—
Solid substance	T65.91	T65.92	T65.93	T65.94	—	—
specified NEC	T65.891	T65.892	T65.893	T65.894	—	—
Solvent, industrial NEC	T52.91	T52.92	T52.93	T52.94	—	—
naphtha	T52.ØX1	T52.ØX2	T52.ØX3	T52.ØX4	—	—
petroleum	T52.ØX1	T52.ØX2	T52.ØX3	T52.ØX4	—	—
specified NEC	T52.8X1	T52.8X2	T52.8X3	T52.8X4	—	—
Soma	T42.8X1	T42.8X2	T42.8X3	T42.8X4	T42.8X5	T42.8X6
Somatorelin	T38.891	T38.892	T38.893	T38.894	T38.895	T38.896
Somatostatin	T38.991	T38.992	T38.993	T38.994	T38.995	T38.996
Somatotropin	T38.811	T38.812	T38.813	T38.814	T38.815	T38.816
Somatrem	T38.811	T38.812	T38.813	T38.814	T38.815	T38.816
Somatropin	T38.811	T38.812	T38.813	T38.814	T38.815	T38.816
Sominex	T45.ØX1	T45.ØX2	T45.ØX3	T45.ØX4	T45.ØX5	T45.ØX6
Somnos	T42.6X1	T42.6X2	T42.6X3	T42.6X4	T42.6X5	T42.6X6
Somonal	T42.3X1	T42.3X2	T42.3X3	T42.3X4	T42.3X5	T42.3X6
Soneryl	T42.3X1	T42.3X2	T42.3X3	T42.3X4	T42.3X5	T42.3X6
Soothing syrup	T5Ø.9Ø1	T5Ø.9Ø2	T5Ø.9Ø3	T5Ø.9Ø4	T5Ø.9Ø5	T5Ø.9Ø6
Sopor	T42.6X1	T42.6X2	T42.6X3	T42.6X4	T42.6X5	T42.6X6
Soporific	T42.71	T42.72	T42.73	T42.74	T42.75	T42.76
Soporific drug	T42.71	T42.72	T42.73	T42.74	T42.75	T42.76
specified type NEC	T42.6X1	T42.6X2	T42.6X3	T42.6X4	T42.6X5	T42.6X6
Sorbide nitrate	T46.3X1	T46.3X2	T46.3X3	T46.3X4	T46.3X5	T46.3X6
Sorbitol	T47.4X1	T47.4X2	T47.4X3	T47.4X4	T47.4X5	T47.4X6
Sotalol	T44.7X1	T44.7X2	T44.7X3	T44.7X4	T44.7X5	T44.7X6
Sotradecol	T46.8X1	T46.8X2	T46.8X3	T46.8X4	T46.8X5	T46.8X6

Substance	Poisoning, Accidental (unintentional)	Poisoning, Intentional Self-harm	Poisoning, Assault	Poisoning, Undetermined	Adverse Effect	Under-dosing
Soysterol	T46.6X1	T46.6X2	T46.6X3	T46.6X4	T46.6X5	T46.6X6
Spacoline	T44.3X1	T44.3X2	T44.3X3	T44.3X4	T44.3X5	T44.3X6
Spanish fly	T49.8X1	T49.8X2	T49.8X3	T49.8X4	T49.8X5	T49.8X6
Sparine	T43.3X1	T43.3X2	T43.3X3	T43.3X4	T43.3X5	T43.3X6
Sparteine	T48.ØX1	T48.ØX2	T48.ØX3	T48.ØX4	T48.ØX5	T48.ØX6
Spasmolytic						
anticholinergics	T44.3X1	T44.3X2	T44.3X3	T44.3X4	T44.3X5	T44.3X6
autonomic	T44.3X1	T44.3X2	T44.3X3	T44.3X4	T44.3X5	T44.3X6
bronchial NEC	T48.6X1	T48.6X2	T48.6X3	T48.6X4	T48.6X5	T48.6X6
quaternary ammonium	T44.3X1	T44.3X2	T44.3X3	T44.3X4	T44.3X5	T44.3X6
skeletal muscle NEC	T48.1X1	T48.1X2	T48.1X3	T48.1X4	T48.1X5	T48.1X6
Spectinomycin	T36.5X1	T36.5X2	T36.5X3	T36.5X4	T36.5X5	T36.5X6
Spectracef*	T36.1X1	T36.1X2	T36.1X3	T36.1X4	T36.1X5	T36.1X6
Speed	T43.651	T43.652	T43.652	T43.654	T43.655	T43.656
Spermicide	T49.8X1	T49.8X2	T49.8X3	T49.8X4	T49.8X5	T49.8X6
Spider (bite) (venom)	T63.391	T63.392	T63.393	T63.394	—	—
antivenin	T5Ø.Z11	T5Ø.Z12	T5Ø.Z13	T5Ø.Z14	T5Ø.Z15	T5Ø.Z16
Spigelia (root)	T37.4X1	T37.4X2	T37.4X3	T37.4X4	T37.4X5	T37.4X6
Spindle inactivator	T5Ø.4X1	T5Ø.4X2	T5Ø.4X3	T5Ø.4X4	T5Ø.4X5	T5Ø.4X6
Spiperone	T43.4X1	T43.4X2	T43.4X3	T43.4X4	T43.4X5	T43.4X6
Spiramycin	T36.3X1	T36.3X2	T36.3X3	T36.3X4	T36.3X5	T36.3X6
Spirapril	T46.4X1	T46.4X2	T46.4X3	T46.4X4	T46.4X5	T46.4X6
Spirilene	T43.591	T43.592	T43.593	T43.594	T43.595	T43.596
Spirit(s) (neutral) **NEC**	T51.ØX1	T51.ØX2	T51.ØX3	T51.ØX4	—	—
beverage	T51.ØX1	T51.ØX2	T51.ØX3	T51.ØX4	—	—
industrial	T51.ØX1	T51.ØX2	T51.ØX3	T51.ØX4	—	—
mineral	T52.ØX1	T52.ØX2	T52.ØX3	T52.ØX4	—	—
of salt — *see* Hydrochloric acid						
surgical	T51.ØX1	T51.ØX2	T51.ØX3	T51.ØX4	—	—
Spiriva*	T44.3X1	T44.3X2	T44.3X3	T44.3X4	T44.3X5	T44.3X6
Spironolactone	T5Ø.ØX1	T5Ø.ØX2	T5Ø.ØX3	T5Ø.ØX4	T5Ø.ØX5	T5Ø.ØX6
Spiroperidol	T43.4X1	T43.4X2	T43.4X3	T43.4X4	T43.4X5	T43.4X6
Sponge, absorbable (gelatin)	T45.7X1	T45.7X2	T45.7X3	T45.7X4	T45.7X5	T45.7X6
Sporostacin	T49.ØX1	T49.ØX2	T49.ØX3	T49.ØX4	T49.ØX5	T49.ØX6
Spray (aerosol)	T65.91	T65.92	T65.93	T65.94	—	—
cosmetic	T65.891	T65.892	T65.893	T65.894	—	—
medicinal NEC	T5Ø.9Ø1	T5Ø.9Ø2	T5Ø.9Ø3	T5Ø.9Ø4	T5Ø.9Ø5	T5Ø.9Ø6
pesticides — *see* Pesticide						
specified content — *see* specific substance						
Spurge flax	T62.2X1	T62.2X2	T62.2X3	T62.2X4	—	—
Spurges	T62.2X1	T62.2X2	T62.2X3	T62.2X4	—	—
Sputum viscosity-lowering drug	T48.4X1	T48.4X2	T48.4X3	T48.4X4	T48.4X5	T48.4X6
Squill	T46.ØX1	T46.ØX2	T46.ØX3	T46.ØX4	T46.ØX5	T46.ØX6
rat poison	T6Ø.4X1	T6Ø.4X2	T6Ø.4X3	T6Ø.4X4	—	—
Squirting cucumber (cathartic)	T47.2X1	T47.2X2	T47.2X3	T47.2X4	T47.2X5	T47.2X6
Stains	T65.6X1	T65.6X2	T65.6X3	T65.6X4	—	—
Stannous fluoride	T49.7X1	T49.7X2	T49.7X3	T49.7X4	T49.7X5	T49.7X6
Stanolone	T38.7X1	T38.7X2	T38.7X3	T38.7X4	T38.7X5	T38.7X6
Stanozolol	T38.7X1	T38.7X2	T38.7X3	T38.7X4	T38.7X5	T38.7X6
Staphisagria or stavesacre (pediculicide)	T49.ØX1	T49.ØX2	T49.ØX3	T49.ØX4	T49.ØX5	T49.ØX6
Starch	T5Ø.9Ø1	T5Ø.9Ø2	T5Ø.9Ø3	T5Ø.9Ø4	T5Ø.9Ø5	T5Ø.9Ø6
Stavzor*	T42.6X1	T42.6X2	T42.6X3	T42.6X4	T42.6X5	T42.6X6
Stelazine	T43.3X1	T43.3X2	T43.3X3	T43.3X4	T43.3X5	T43.3X6
Stemetil	T43.3X1	T43.3X2	T43.3X3	T43.3X4	T43.3X5	T43.3X6
Stepronin	T48.4X1	T48.4X2	T48.4X3	T48.4X4	T48.4X5	T48.4X6
Sterculia	T47.4X1	T47.4X2	T47.4X3	T47.4X4	T47.4X5	T47.4X6
Sternutator gas	T59.891	T59.892	T59.893	T59.894	—	—
Steroid	T38.ØX1	T38.ØX2	T38.ØX3	T38.ØX4	T38.ØX5	T38.ØX6
anabolic	T38.7X1	T38.7X2	T38.7X3	T38.7X4	T38.7X5	T38.7X6
androgenic	T38.7X1	T38.7X2	T38.7X3	T38.7X4	T38.7X5	T38.7X6
antineoplastic, hormone	T38.7X1	T38.7X2	T38.7X3	T38.7X4	T38.7X5	T38.7X6
estrogen	T38.5X1	T38.5X2	T38.5X3	T38.5X4	T38.5X5	T38.5X6
ENT agent	T49.6X1	T49.6X2	T49.6X3	T49.6X4	T49.6X5	T49.6X6
ophthalmic preparation	T49.5X1	T49.5X2	T49.5X3	T49.5X4	T49.5X5	T49.5X6
topical NEC	T49.ØX1	T49.ØX2	T49.ØX3	T49.ØX4	T49.ØX5	T49.ØX6
Stibine	T56.891	T56.892	T56.893	T56.894	—	—
Stibogluconate	T37.3X1	T37.3X2	T37.3X3	T37.3X4	T37.3X5	T37.3X6
Stibophen	T37.4X1	T37.4X2	T37.4X3	T37.4X4	T37.4X5	T37.4X6
Stilbamidine (isetionate)	T37.3X1	T37.3X2	T37.3X3	T37.3X4	T37.3X5	T37.3X6
Stilbestrol	T38.5X1	T38.5X2	T38.5X3	T38.5X4	T38.5X5	T38.5X6
Stilboestrol	T38.5X1	T38.5X2	T38.5X3	T38.5X4	T38.5X5	T38.5X6
Stimulant						
central nervous system — *see also* Psychostimulant	T43.6Ø1	T43.6Ø2	T43.6Ø3	T43.6Ø4	T43.6Ø5	T43.6Ø6
analeptics	T5Ø.7X1	T5Ø.7X2	T5Ø.7X3	T5Ø.7X4	T5Ø.7X5	T5Ø.7X6
opiate antagonist	T5Ø.7X1	T5Ø.7X2	T5Ø.7X3	T5Ø.7X4	T5Ø.7X5	T5Ø.7X6

*Optum Value-Add

☑ Additional Character May Be Required — Refer to the Tabular List for Character Selection

Substance	Poisoning, Accidental (unintentional)	Poisoning, Intentional Self-harm	Poisoning, Assault	Poisoning, Undetermined	Adverse Effect	Under-dosing
Stimulant — *continued*						
central nervous system — *see also* Psychostimulant — *continued*						
psychotherapeutic NEC — *see also* Psychotherapeutic drug	T43.6Ø1	T43.6Ø2	T43.6Ø3	T43.6Ø4	T43.6Ø5	T43.6Ø6
specified NEC	T43.691	T43.692	T43.693	T43.694	T43.695	T43.696
respiratory	T48.9Ø1	T48.9Ø2	T48.9Ø3	T48.9Ø4	T48.9Ø5	T48.9Ø6
Stone-dissolving drug	T5Ø.9Ø1	T5Ø.9Ø2	T5Ø.9Ø3	T5Ø.9Ø4	T5Ø.9Ø5	T5Ø.9Ø6
Storage battery (cells) (acid)	T54.2X1	T54.2X2	T54.2X3	T54.2X4	—	—
Stovaine	T41.3X1	T41.3X2	T41.3X3	T41.3X4	T41.3X5	T41.3X6
infiltration (subcutaneous)	T41.3X1	T41.3X2	T41.3X3	T41.3X4	T41.3X5	T41.3X6
nerve block (peripheral) (plexus)	T41.3X1	T41.3X2	T41.3X3	T41.3X4	T41.3X5	T41.3X6
spinal	T41.3X1	T41.3X2	T41.3X3	T41.3X4	T41.3X5	T41.3X6
topical (surface)	T41.3X1	T41.3X2	T41.3X3	T41.3X4	T41.3X5	T41.3X6
Stovarsal	T37.8X1	T37.8X2	T37.8X3	T37.8X4	T37.8X5	T37.8X6
Stove gas — *see* Gas, stove						
Stoxil	T49.5X1	T49.5X2	T49.5X3	T49.5X4	T49.5X5	T49.5X6
Stramonium	T48.6X1	T48.6X2	T48.6X3	T48.6X4	T48.6X5	T48.6X6
natural state	T62.2X1	T62.2X2	T62.2X3	T62.2X4	—	—
Streptodornase	T45.3X1	T45.3X2	T45.3X3	T45.3X4	T45.3X5	T45.3X6
Streptoduocin	T36.5X1	T36.5X2	T36.5X3	T36.5X4	T36.5X5	T36.5X6
Streptokinase	T45.611	T45.612	T45.613	T45.614	T45.615	T45.616
Streptomycin (derivative)	T36.5X1	T36.5X2	T36.5X3	T36.5X4	T36.5X5	T36.5X6
Streptonivicin	T36.5X1	T36.5X2	T36.5X3	T36.5X4	T36.5X5	T36.5X6
Streptovarycin	T36.5X1	T36.5X2	T36.5X3	T36.5X4	T36.5X5	T36.5X6
Streptozocin	T45.1X1	T45.1X2	T45.1X3	T45.1X4	T45.1X5	T45.1X6
Streptozotocin	T45.1X1	T45.1X2	T45.1X3	T45.1X4	T45.1X5	T45.1X6
Stripper (paint) (solvent)	T52.8X1	T52.8X2	T52.8X3	T52.8X4	—	—
Strobane	T6Ø.1X1	T6Ø.1X2	T6Ø.1X3	T6Ø.1X4	—	—
Strofantina	T46.ØX1	T46.ØX2	T46.ØX3	T46.ØX4	T46.ØX5	T46.ØX6
Stromectol*	T37.4X1	T37.4X2	T37.4X3	T37.4X4	T37.4X5	T37.4X6
Strophanthin (g) (k)	T46.ØX1	T46.ØX2	T46.ØX3	T46.ØX4	T46.ØX5	T46.ØX6
Strophanthus	T46.ØX1	T46.ØX2	T46.ØX3	T46.ØX4	T46.ØX5	T46.ØX6
Strophantin	T46.ØX1	T46.ØX2	T46.ØX3	T46.ØX4	T46.ØX5	T46.ØX6
Strophantin-g	T46.ØX1	T46.ØX2	T46.ØX3	T46.ØX4	T46.ØX5	T46.ØX6
Strychnine (nonmedicinal) (pesticide) (salts)	T65.1X1	T65.1X2	T65.1X3	T65.1X4	—	—
medicinal	T48.291	T48.292	T48.293	T48.294	T48.295	T48.296
Strychnos (ignatii) — *see* Strychnine						
Styramate	T42.8X1	T42.8X2	T42.8X3	T42.8X4	T42.8X5	T42.8X6
Styrene	T65.891	T65.892	T65.893	T65.894	—	—
Succinimide, antiepileptic or anticonvulsant	T42.2X1	T42.2X2	T42.2X3	T42.2X4	T42.2X5	T42.2X6
mercuric — *see* Mercury						
Succinylcholine	T48.1X1	T48.1X2	T48.1X3	T48.1X4	T48.1X5	T48.1X6
Succinylsulfathiazole	T37.ØX1	T37.ØX2	T37.ØX3	T37.ØX4	T37.ØX5	T37.ØX6
Sucralfate	T47.1X1	T47.1X2	T47.1X3	T47.1X4	T47.1X5	T47.1X6
Sucrose	T5Ø.3X1	T5Ø.3X2	T5Ø.3X3	T5Ø.3X4	T5Ø.3X5	T5Ø.3X6
Sufentanil	T4Ø.411	T4Ø.412	T4Ø.413	T4Ø.414	T4Ø.415	T4Ø.416
Sulbactam	T36.ØX1	T36.ØX2	T36.ØX3	T36.ØX4	T36.ØX5	T36.ØX6
Sulbenicillin	T36.ØX1	T36.ØX2	T36.ØX3	T36.ØX4	T36.ØX5	T36.ØX6
Sulbentine	T49.ØX1	T49.ØX2	T49.ØX3	T49.ØX4	T49.ØX5	T49.ØX6
Sulconazole*	T49.ØX1	T49.ØX2	T49.ØX3	T49.ØX4	T49.ØX5	T49.ØX6
Sulfacetamide	T49.ØX1	T49.ØX2	T49.ØX3	T49.ØX4	T49.ØX5	T49.ØX6
ophthalmic preparation	T49.5X1	T49.5X2	T49.5X3	T49.5X4	T49.5X5	T49.5X6
Sulfachlorpyridazine	T37.ØX1	T37.ØX2	T37.ØX3	T37.ØX4	T37.ØX5	T37.ØX6
Sulfacitine	T37.ØX1	T37.ØX2	T37.ØX3	T37.ØX4	T37.ØX5	T37.ØX6
Sulfadiasulfone sodium	T37.ØX1	T37.ØX2	T37.ØX3	T37.ØX4	T37.ØX5	T37.ØX6
Sulfadiazine	T37.ØX1	T37.ØX2	T37.ØX3	T37.ØX4	T37.ØX5	T37.ØX6
silver (topical)	T49.ØX1	T49.ØX2	T49.ØX3	T49.ØX4	T49.ØX5	T49.ØX6
Sulfadimethoxine	T37.ØX1	T37.ØX2	T37.ØX3	T37.ØX4	T37.ØX5	T37.ØX6
Sulfadimidine	T37.ØX1	T37.ØX2	T37.ØX3	T37.ØX4	T37.ØX5	T37.ØX6
Sulfadoxine	T37.ØX1	T37.ØX2	T37.ØX3	T37.ØX4	T37.ØX5	T37.ØX6
with pyrimethamine	T37.2X1	T37.2X2	T37.2X3	T37.2X4	T37.2X5	T37.2X6
Sulfaethidole	T37.ØX1	T37.ØX2	T37.ØX3	T37.ØX4	T37.ØX5	T37.ØX6
Sulfafurazole	T37.ØX1	T37.ØX2	T37.ØX3	T37.ØX4	T37.ØX5	T37.ØX6
Sulfaguanidine	T37.ØX1	T37.ØX2	T37.ØX3	T37.ØX4	T37.ØX5	T37.ØX6
Sulfalene	T37.ØX1	T37.ØX2	T37.ØX3	T37.ØX4	T37.ØX5	T37.ØX6
Sulfaloxate	T37.ØX1	T37.ØX2	T37.ØX3	T37.ØX4	T37.ØX5	T37.ØX6
Sulfaloxic acid	T37.ØX1	T37.ØX2	T37.ØX3	T37.ØX4	T37.ØX5	T37.ØX6
Sulfamazone	T39.2X1	T39.2X2	T39.2X3	T39.2X4	T39.2X5	T39.2X6
Sulfamerazine	T37.ØX1	T37.ØX2	T37.ØX3	T37.ØX4	T37.ØX5	T37.ØX6
Sulfameter	T37.ØX1	T37.ØX2	T37.ØX3	T37.ØX4	T37.ØX5	T37.ØX6
Sulfamethazine	T37.ØX1	T37.ØX2	T37.ØX3	T37.ØX4	T37.ØX5	T37.ØX6
Sulfamethizole	T37.ØX1	T37.ØX2	T37.ØX3	T37.ØX4	T37.ØX5	T37.ØX6
Sulfamethoxazole	T37.ØX1	T37.ØX2	T37.ØX3	T37.ØX4	T37.ØX5	T37.ØX6
with trimethoprim	T36.8X1	T36.8X2	T36.8X3	T36.8X4	T36.8X5	T36.8X6
Sulfamethoxydiazine	T37.ØX1	T37.ØX2	T37.ØX3	T37.ØX4	T37.ØX5	T37.ØX6
Sulfamethoxypyridazine	T37.ØX1	T37.ØX2	T37.ØX3	T37.ØX4	T37.ØX5	T37.ØX6
Sulfamethylthiazole	T37.ØX1	T37.ØX2	T37.ØX3	T37.ØX4	T37.ØX5	T37.ØX6
Sulfametoxydiazine	T37.ØX1	T37.ØX2	T37.ØX3	T37.ØX4	T37.ØX5	T37.ØX6
Sulfamidopyrine	T39.2X1	T39.2X2	T39.2X3	T39.2X4	T39.2X5	T39.2X6
Sulfamonomethoxine	T37.ØX1	T37.ØX2	T37.ØX3	T37.ØX4	T37.ØX5	T37.ØX6
Sulfamoxole	T37.ØX1	T37.ØX2	T37.ØX3	T37.ØX4	T37.ØX5	T37.ØX6
Sulfamylon	T49.ØX1	T49.ØX2	T49.ØX3	T49.ØX4	T49.ØX5	T49.ØX6
Sulfan blue (diagnostic dye)	T5Ø.8X1	T5Ø.8X2	T5Ø.8X3	T5Ø.8X4	T5Ø.8X5	T5Ø.8X6
Sulfanilamide	T37.ØX1	T37.ØX2	T37.ØX3	T37.ØX4	T37.ØX5	T37.ØX6
Sulfanilylguanidine	T37.ØX1	T37.ØX2	T37.ØX3	T37.ØX4	T37.ØX5	T37.ØX6
Sulfaperin	T37.ØX1	T37.ØX2	T37.ØX3	T37.ØX4	T37.ØX5	T37.ØX6
Sulfaphenazole	T37.ØX1	T37.ØX2	T37.ØX3	T37.ØX4	T37.ØX5	T37.ØX6
Sulfaphenylthiazole	T37.ØX1	T37.ØX2	T37.ØX3	T37.ØX4	T37.ØX5	T37.ØX6
Sulfaproxyline	T37.ØX1	T37.ØX2	T37.ØX3	T37.ØX4	T37.ØX5	T37.ØX6
Sulfapyridine	T37.ØX1	T37.ØX2	T37.ØX3	T37.ØX4	T37.ØX5	T37.ØX6
Sulfapyrimidine	T37.ØX1	T37.ØX2	T37.ØX3	T37.ØX4	T37.ØX5	T37.ØX6
Sulfarsphenamine	T37.8X1	T37.8X2	T37.8X3	T37.8X4	T37.8X5	T37.8X6
Sulfasalazine	T37.ØX1	T37.ØX2	T37.ØX3	T37.ØX4	T37.ØX5	T37.ØX6
Sulfasuxidine	T37.ØX1	T37.ØX2	T37.ØX3	T37.ØX4	T37.ØX5	T37.ØX6
Sulfasymazine	T37.ØX1	T37.ØX2	T37.ØX3	T37.ØX4	T37.ØX5	T37.ØX6
Sulfated amylopectin	T47.8X1	T47.8X2	T47.8X3	T47.8X4	T47.8X5	T47.8X6
Sulfathiazole	T37.ØX1	T37.ØX2	T37.ØX3	T37.ØX4	T37.ØX5	T37.ØX6
Sulfatostearate	T49.2X1	T49.2X2	T49.2X3	T49.2X4	T49.2X5	T49.2X6
Sulfatrim*	T36.8X1	T36.8X2	T36.8X3	T36.8X4	T36.8X5	T36.8X6
Sulfinpyrazone	T5Ø.4X1	T5Ø.4X2	T5Ø.4X3	T5Ø.4X4	T5Ø.4X5	T5Ø.4X6
Sulfiram	T49.ØX1	T49.ØX2	T49.ØX3	T49.ØX4	T49.ØX5	T49.ØX6
Sulfisomidine	T37.ØX1	T37.ØX2	T37.ØX3	T37.ØX4	T37.ØX5	T37.ØX6
Sulfisoxazole	T37.ØX1	T37.ØX2	T37.ØX3	T37.ØX4	T37.ØX5	T37.ØX6
ophthalmic preparation	T49.5X1	T49.5X2	T49.5X3	T49.5X4	T49.5X5	T49.5X6
Sulfobromophthalein (sodium)	T5Ø.8X1	T5Ø.8X2	T5Ø.8X3	T5Ø.8X4	T5Ø.8X5	T5Ø.8X6
Sulfobromphthalein	T5Ø.8X1	T5Ø.8X2	T5Ø.8X3	T5Ø.8X4	T5Ø.8X5	T5Ø.8X6
Sulfogaiacol	T48.4X1	T48.4X2	T48.4X3	T48.4X4	T48.4X5	T48.4X6
Sulfomyxin	T36.8X1	T36.8X2	T36.8X3	T36.8X4	T36.8X5	T36.8X6
Sulfonal	T42.6X1	T42.6X2	T42.6X3	T42.6X4	T42.6X5	T42.6X6
Sulfonamide NEC	T37.ØX1	T37.ØX2	T37.ØX3	T37.ØX4	T37.ØX5	T37.ØX6
eye	T49.5X1	T49.5X2	T49.5X3	T49.5X4	T49.5X5	T49.5X6
Sulfonazide	T37.1X1	T37.1X2	T37.1X3	T37.1X4	T37.1X5	T37.1X6
Sulfones	T37.1X1	T37.1X2	T37.1X3	T37.1X4	T37.1X5	T37.1X6
Sulfonethylmethane	T42.6X1	T42.6X2	T42.6X3	T42.6X4	T42.6X5	T42.6X6
Sulfonmethane	T42.6X1	T42.6X2	T42.6X3	T42.6X4	T42.6X5	T42.6X6
Sulfonphthal, sulfonphthol	T5Ø.8X1	T5Ø.8X2	T5Ø.8X3	T5Ø.8X4	T5Ø.8X5	T5Ø.8X6
Sulfonylurea derivatives, oral	T38.3X1	T38.3X2	T38.3X3	T38.3X4	T38.3X5	T38.3X6
Sulforidazine	T43.3X1	T43.3X2	T43.3X3	T43.3X4	T43.3X5	T43.3X6
Sulfoxone	T37.1X1	T37.1X2	T37.1X3	T37.1X4	T37.1X5	T37.1X6
Sulfuric acid	T54.2X1	T54.2X2	T54.2X3	T54.2X4	—	—
Sulfur, sulfurated, sulfuric, sulfurous, sulfuryl (compounds NEC) (medicinal)	T49.4X1	T49.4X2	T49.4X3	T49.4X4	T49.4X5	T49.4X6
acid	T54.2X1	T54.2X2	T54.2X3	T54.2X4	—	—
dioxide (gas)	T59.1X1	T59.1X2	T59.1X3	T59.1X4	—	—
ether — *see* Ether(s)						
hydrogen	T59.6X1	T59.6X2	T59.6X3	T59.6X4	—	—
medicinal (keratolytic) (ointment) NEC	T49.4X1	T49.4X2	T49.4X3	T49.4X4	T49.4X5	T49.4X6
ointment	T49.ØX1	T49.ØX2	T49.ØX3	T49.ØX4	T49.ØX5	T49.ØX6
pesticide (vapor)	T6Ø.91	T6Ø.92	T6Ø.93	T6Ø.94	—	—
vapor NEC	T59.891	T59.892	T59.893	T59.894	—	—
Sulglicotide	T47.1X1	T47.1X2	T47.1X3	T47.1X4	T47.1X5	T47.1X6
Sulindac	T39.391	T39.392	T39.393	T39.394	T39.395	T39.396
Sulisatin	T47.2X1	T47.2X2	T47.2X3	T47.2X4	T47.2X5	T47.2X6
Sulisobenzone	T49.3X1	T49.3X2	T49.3X3	T49.3X4	T49.3X5	T49.3X6
Sulkowitch's reagent	T5Ø.8X1	T5Ø.8X2	T5Ø.8X3	T5Ø.8X4	T5Ø.8X5	T5Ø.8X6
Sulmetozine	T44.3X1	T44.3X2	T44.3X3	T44.3X4	T44.3X5	T44.3X6
Suloctidil	T46.7X1	T46.7X2	T46.7X3	T46.7X4	T46.7X5	T46.7X6
Sulph- — *see also* Sulf-						
Sulphadiazine	T37.ØX1	T37.ØX2	T37.ØX3	T37.ØX4	T37.ØX5	T37.ØX6
Sulphadimethoxine	T37.ØX1	T37.ØX2	T37.ØX3	T37.ØX4	T37.ØX5	T37.ØX6
Sulphadimidine	T37.ØX1	T37.ØX2	T37.ØX3	T37.ØX4	T37.ØX5	T37.ØX6
Sulphadione	T37.1X1	T37.1X2	T37.1X3	T37.1X4	T37.1X5	T37.1X6
Sulphafurazole	T37.ØX1	T37.ØX2	T37.ØX3	T37.ØX4	T37.ØX5	T37.ØX6
Sulphamethizole	T37.ØX1	T37.ØX2	T37.ØX3	T37.ØX4	T37.ØX5	T37.ØX6
Sulphamethoxazole	T37.ØX1	T37.ØX2	T37.ØX3	T37.ØX4	T37.ØX5	T37.ØX6
Sulphan blue	T5Ø.8X1	T5Ø.8X2	T5Ø.8X3	T5Ø.8X4	T5Ø.8X5	T5Ø.8X6
Sulphaphenazole	T37.ØX1	T37.ØX2	T37.ØX3	T37.ØX4	T37.ØX5	T37.ØX6
Sulphapyridine	T37.ØX1	T37.ØX2	T37.ØX3	T37.ØX4	T37.ØX5	T37.ØX6
Sulphasalazine	T37.ØX1	T37.ØX2	T37.ØX3	T37.ØX4	T37.ØX5	T37.ØX6
Sulphinpyrazone	T5Ø.4X1	T5Ø.4X2	T5Ø.4X3	T5Ø.4X4	T5Ø.4X5	T5Ø.4X6
Sulpiride	T43.591	T43.592	T43.593	T43.594	T43.595	T43.596
Sulprostone	T48.ØX1	T48.ØX2	T48.ØX3	T48.ØX4	T48.ØX5	T48.ØX6

Substance	Poisoning, Accidental (unintentional)	Poisoning, Intentional Self-harm	Poisoning, Assault	Poisoning, Undetermined	Adverse Effect	Under-dosing
Sulpyrine	T39.2X1	T39.2X2	T39.2X3	T39.2X4	T39.2X5	T39.2X6
Sultamicillin	T36.ØX1	T36.ØX2	T36.ØX3	T36.ØX4	T36.ØX5	T36.ØX6
Sulthiame	T42.6X1	T42.6X2	T42.6X3	T42.6X4	T42.6X5	T42.6X6
Sultiame	T42.6X1	T42.6X2	T42.6X3	T42.6X4	T42.6X5	T42.6X6
Sultopride	T43.591	T43.592	T43.593	T43.594	T43.595	T43.596
Sumatriptan	T39.8X1	T39.8X2	T39.8X3	T39.8X4	T39.8X5	T39.8X6
Sumavel*	T39.8X1	T39.8X2	T39.8X3	T39.8X4	T39.8X5	T39.8X6
Sunflower seed oil	T46.6X1	T46.6X2	T46.6X3	T46.6X4	T46.6X5	T46.6X6
Superinone	T48.4X1	T48.4X2	T48.4X3	T48.4X4	T48.4X5	T48.4X6
Suprofen	T39.311	T39.312	T39.313	T39.314	T39.315	T39.316
Suramin (sodium)	T37.4X1	T37.4X2	T37.4X3	T37.4X4	T37.4X5	T37.4X6
Surfacaine	T41.3X1	T41.3X2	T41.3X3	T41.3X4	T41.3X5	T41.3X6
Surital	T41.1X1	T41.1X2	T41.1X3	T41.1X4	T41.1X5	T41.1X6
Sutilains	T45.3X1	T45.3X2	T45.3X3	T45.3X4	T45.3X5	T45.3X6
Suxamethonium (chloride)	T48.1X1	T48.1X2	T48.1X3	T48.1X4	T48.1X5	T48.1X6
Suxethonium (chloride)	T48.1X1	T48.1X2	T48.1X3	T48.1X4	T48.1X5	T48.1X6
Suxibuzone	T39.2X1	T39.2X2	T39.2X3	T39.2X4	T39.2X5	T39.2X6
Sweetener	T50.901	T50.902	T50.903	T50.904	T50.905	T50.906
Sweet niter spirit	T46.3X1	T46.3X2	T46.3X3	T46.3X4	T46.3X5	T46.3X6
Sweet oil (birch)	T49.3X1	T49.3X2	T49.3X3	T49.3X4	T49.3X5	T49.3X6
Sylvant*	T45.1X1	T45.1X2	T45.1X3	T45.1X4	T45.1X5	T45.1X6
Sym-dichloroethyl ether	T53.6X1	T53.6X2	T53.6X3	T53.6X4	—	—
Sympatholytic NEC	T44.8X1	T44.8X2	T44.8X3	T44.8X4	T44.8X5	T44.8X6
haloalkylamine	T44.8X1	T44.8X2	T44.8X3	T44.8X4	T44.8X5	T44.8X6
Sympathomimetic NEC	T44.901	T44.902	T44.903	T44.904	T44.905	T44.906
anti-common-cold	T48.5X1	T48.5X2	T48.5X3	T48.5X4	T48.5X5	T48.5X6
bronchodilator	T48.6X1	T48.6X2	T48.6X3	T48.6X4	T48.6X5	T48.6X6
specified NEC	T44.991	T44.992	T44.993	T44.994	T44.995	T44.996
Synagis	T50.B91	T50.B92	T50.B93	T50.B94	T50.B95	T50.B96
Synalar	T49.ØX1	T49.ØX2	T49.ØX3	T49.ØX4	T49.ØX5	T49.ØX6
Synthetic cannabinoids	T40.721	T40.722	T40.723	T40.724	T40.725	T40.726
Synthroid	T38.1X1	T38.1X2	T38.1X3	T38.1X4	T38.1X5	T38.1X6
Syntocinon	T48.ØX1	T48.ØX2	T48.ØX3	T48.ØX4	T48.ØX5	T48.ØX6
Syrosingopine	T46.5X1	T46.5X2	T46.5X3	T46.5X4	T46.5X5	T46.5X6
Systemic drug	T45.91	T45.92	T45.93	T45.94	T45.95	T45.96
specified NEC	T45.8X1	T45.8X2	T45.8X3	T45.8X4	T45.8X5	T45.8X6
Tablets — *see also* specified substance	T50.901	T50.902	T50.903	T50.904	T50.905	T50.906
Tace	T38.5X1	T38.5X2	T38.5X3	T38.5X4	T38.5X5	T38.5X6
Tacrine	T44.ØX1	T44.ØX2	T44.ØX3	T44.ØX4	T44.ØX5	T44.ØX6
Tadalafil	T46.7X1	T46.7X2	T46.7X3	T46.7X4	T46.7X5	T46.7X6
Talampicillin	T36.ØX1	T36.ØX2	T36.ØX3	T36.ØX4	T36.ØX5	T36.ØX6
Talbutal	T42.3X1	T42.3X2	T42.3X3	T42.3X4	T42.3X5	T42.3X6
Talc powder	T49.3X1	T49.3X2	T49.3X3	T49.3X4	T49.3X5	T49.3X6
Talcum	T49.3X1	T49.3X2	T49.3X3	T49.3X4	T49.3X5	T49.3X6
Taleranol	T38.6X1	T38.6X2	T38.6X3	T38.6X4	T38.6X5	T38.6X6
Taltz*	T39.391	T39.392	T39.393	T39.394	T39.395	T39.396
Tamoxifen	T38.6X1	T38.6X2	T38.6X3	T38.6X4	T38.6X5	T38.6X6
Tamsulosin	T44.6X1	T44.6X2	T44.6X3	T44.6X4	T44.6X5	T44.6X6
Tandearil, tanderil	T39.2X1	T39.2X2	T39.2X3	T39.2X4	T39.2X5	T39.2X6
Tannic acid	T49.2X1	T49.2X2	T49.2X3	T49.2X4	T49.2X5	T49.2X6
medicinal (astringent)	T49.2X1	T49.2X2	T49.2X3	T49.2X4	T49.2X5	T49.2X6
Tannin — *see* Tannic acid						
Tansy	T62.2X1	T62.2X2	T62.2X3	T62.2X4	—	—
TAO	T36.3X1	T36.3X2	T36.3X3	T36.3X4	T36.3X5	T36.3X6
Tapazole	T38.2X1	T38.2X2	T38.2X3	T38.2X4	T38.2X5	T38.2X6
Taractan	T43.591	T43.592	T43.593	T43.594	T43.595	T43.596
Tarantula (venomous)	T63.321	T63.322	T63.323	T63.324	—	—
Tartar emetic	T37.8X1	T37.8X2	T37.8X3	T37.8X4	T37.8X5	T37.8X6
Tartaric acid	T65.891	T65.892	T65.893	T65.894	—	—
Tartrated antimony (anti-infective)	T37.8X1	T37.8X2	T37.8X3	T37.8X4	T37.8X5	T37.8X6
Tartrate, laxative	T47.4X1	T47.4X2	T47.4X3	T47.4X4	T47.4X5	T47.4X6
Tar NEC	T52.ØX1	T52.ØX2	T52.ØX3	T52.ØX4	—	—
camphor	T60.1X1	T60.1X2	T60.1X3	T60.1X4	—	—
distillate	T49.1X1	T49.1X2	T49.1X3	T49.1X4	T49.1X5	T49.1X6
fumes	T59.891	T59.892	T59.893	T59.894	—	—
medicinal	T49.1X1	T49.1X2	T49.1X3	T49.1X4	T49.1X5	T49.1X6
ointment	T49.1X1	T49.1X2	T49.1X3	T49.1X4	T49.1X5	T49.1X6
Tauromustine	T45.1X1	T45.1X2	T45.1X3	T45.1X4	T45.1X5	T45.1X6
TCA — *see* Trichloroacetic acid						
TCDD	T53.7X1	T53.7X2	T53.7X3	T53.7X4	—	—
TDI (vapor)	T65.ØX1	T65.ØX2	T65.ØX3	T65.ØX4	—	—
Tear						
gas	T59.3X1	T59.3X2	T59.3X3	T59.3X4	—	—
solution	T49.5X1	T49.5X2	T49.5X3	T49.5X4	T49.5X5	T49.5X6
Tecentriq*	T45.1X1	T45.1X2	T45.1X3	T45.1X4	T45.1X5	T45.1X6
Teclothiazide	T50.2X1	T50.2X2	T50.2X3	T50.2X4	T50.2X5	T50.2X6
Teclozan	T37.3X1	T37.3X2	T37.3X3	T37.3X4	T37.3X5	T37.3X6
Tegafur	T45.1X1	T45.1X2	T45.1X3	T45.1X4	T45.1X5	T45.1X6
Tegretol	T42.1X1	T42.1X2	T42.1X3	T42.1X4	T42.1X5	T42.1X6
Teicoplanin	T36.8X1	T36.8X2	T36.8X3	T36.8X4	T36.8X5	T36.8X6
Telepaque	T50.8X1	T50.8X2	T50.8X3	T50.8X4	T50.8X5	T50.8X6

Substance	Poisoning, Accidental (unintentional)	Poisoning, Intentional Self-harm	Poisoning, Assault	Poisoning, Undetermined	Adverse Effect	Under-dosing
Tellurium	T56.891	T56.892	T56.893	T56.894	—	—
fumes	T56.891	T56.892	T56.893	T56.894	—	—
TEM	T45.1X1	T45.1X2	T45.1X3	T45.1X4	T45.1X5	T45.1X6
Temazepam	T42.4X1	T42.4X2	T42.4X3	T42.4X4	T42.4X5	T42.4X6
Temocillin	T36.ØX1	T36.ØX2	T36.ØX3	T36.ØX4	T36.ØX5	T36.ØX6
Tenamfetamine	T43.621	T43.622	T43.623	T43.624	T43.625	T43.626
Tenecteplase*	T45.611	T45.612	T45.613	T45.614	T45.615	T45.616
Teniposide	T45.1X1	T45.1X2	T45.1X3	T45.1X4	T45.1X5	T45.1X6
Tenitramine	T46.3X1	T46.3X2	T46.3X3	T46.3X4	T46.3X5	T46.3X6
Tenoglicin	T48.4X1	T48.4X2	T48.4X3	T48.4X4	T48.4X5	T48.4X6
Tenonitrozole	T37.3X1	T37.3X2	T37.3X3	T37.3X4	T37.3X5	T37.3X6
Tenoxicam	T39.391	T39.392	T39.393	T39.394	T39.395	T39.396
TEPA	T45.1X1	T45.1X2	T45.1X3	T45.1X4	T45.1X5	T45.1X6
TEPP	T60.ØX1	T60.ØX2	T60.ØX3	T60.ØX4	—	—
Teprotide	T46.5X1	T46.5X2	T46.5X3	T46.5X4	T46.5X5	T46.5X6
Terazosin	T44.6X1	T44.6X2	T44.6X3	T44.6X4	T44.6X5	T44.6X6
Terbufos	T60.ØX1	T60.ØX2	T60.ØX3	T60.ØX4	—	—
Terbutaline	T48.6X1	T48.6X2	T48.6X3	T48.6X4	T48.6X5	T48.6X6
Terconazole	T49.ØX1	T49.ØX2	T49.ØX3	T49.ØX4	T49.ØX5	T49.ØX6
Terfenadine	T45.ØX1	T45.ØX2	T45.ØX3	T45.ØX4	T45.ØX5	T45.ØX6
Teriparatide (acetate)	T50.991	T50.992	T50.993	T50.994	T50.995	T50.996
Terizidone	T37.1X1	T37.1X2	T37.1X3	T37.1X4	T37.1X5	T37.1X6
Terlipressin	T38.891	T38.892	T38.893	T38.894	T38.895	T38.896
Terodiline	T46.3X1	T46.3X2	T46.3X3	T46.3X4	T46.3X5	T46.3X6
Teroxalene	T37.4X1	T37.4X2	T37.4X3	T37.4X4	T37.4X5	T37.4X6
Terpin (cis) hydrate	T48.4X1	T48.4X2	T48.4X3	T48.4X4	T48.4X5	T48.4X6
Terramycin	T36.4X1	T36.4X2	T36.4X3	T36.4X4	T36.4X5	T36.4X6
Tertatolol	T44.7X1	T44.7X2	T44.7X3	T44.7X4	T44.7X5	T44.7X6
Tessalon	T48.3X1	T48.3X2	T48.3X3	T48.3X4	T48.3X5	T48.3X6
Testolactone	T38.7X1	T38.7X2	T38.7X3	T38.7X4	T38.7X5	T38.7X6
Testosterone	T38.7X1	T38.7X2	T38.7X3	T38.7X4	T38.7X5	T38.7X6
Tetanus toxoid or vaccine	T50.A91	T50.A92	T50.A93	T50.A94	T50.A95	T50.A96
antitoxin	T50.Z11	T50.Z12	T50.Z13	T50.Z14	T50.Z15	T50.Z16
immune globulin (human)	T50.Z11	T50.Z12	T50.Z13	T50.Z14	T50.Z15	T50.Z16
toxoid	T50.A91	T50.A92	T50.A93	T50.A94	T50.A95	T50.A96
with diphtheria toxoid	T50.A21	T50.A22	T50.A23	T50.A24	T50.A25	T50.A26
with pertussis	T50.A11	T50.A12	T50.A13	T50.A14	T50.A15	T50.A16
Tetrabenazine	T43.591	T43.592	T43.593	T43.594	T43.595	T43.596
Tetracaine	T41.3X1	T41.3X2	T41.3X3	T41.3X4	T41.3X5	T41.3X6
nerve block (peripheral) (plexus)	T41.3X1	T41.3X2	T41.3X3	T41.3X4	T41.3X5	T41.3X6
regional	T41.3X1	T41.3X2	T41.3X3	T41.3X4	T41.3X5	T41.3X6
spinal	T41.3X1	T41.3X2	T41.3X3	T41.3X4	T41.3X5	T41.3X6
Tetrachlorethylene — *see* Tetrachloroethylene						
Tetrachlormethiazide	T50.2X1	T50.2X2	T50.2X3	T50.2X4	T50.2X5	T50.2X6
Tetrachloroethane	T53.6X1	T53.6X2	T53.6X3	T53.6X4	—	—
vapor	T53.6X1	T53.6X2	T53.6X3	T53.6X4	—	—
paint or varnish	T53.6X1	T53.6X2	T53.6X3	T53.6X4	—	—
Tetrachloroethylene (liquid)	T53.3X1	T53.3X2	T53.3X3	T53.3X4	—	—
medicinal	T37.4X1	T37.4X2	T37.4X3	T37.4X4	T37.4X5	T37.4X6
vapor	T53.3X1	T53.3X2	T53.3X3	T53.3X4	—	—
Tetrachloromethane — *see* Carbon tetrachloride						
Tetracosactide	T38.811	T38.812	T38.813	T38.814	T38.815	T38.816
Tetracosactrin	T38.811	T38.812	T38.813	T38.814	T38.815	T38.816
Tetracycline	T36.4X1	T36.4X2	T36.4X3	T36.4X4	T36.4X5	T36.4X6
ophthalmic preparation	T49.5X1	T49.5X2	T49.5X3	T49.5X4	T49.5X5	T49.5X6
topical NEC	T49.ØX1	T49.ØX2	T49.ØX3	T49.ØX4	T49.ØX5	T49.ØX6
Tetradifon	T60.8X1	T60.8X2	T60.8X3	T60.8X4	—	—
Tetradotoxin	T61.771	T61.772	T61.773	T61.774	—	—
Tetraethyl						
lead	T56.ØX1	T56.ØX2	T56.ØX3	T56.ØX4	—	—
pyrophosphate	T60.ØX1	T60.ØX2	T60.ØX3	T60.ØX4	—	—
Tetraethylammonium chloride	T44.2X1	T44.2X2	T44.2X3	T44.2X4	T44.2X5	T44.2X6
Tetraethylthiuram disulfide	T50.6X1	T50.6X2	T50.6X3	T50.6X4	T50.6X5	T50.6X6
Tetrahydroaminoacridine	T44.ØX1	T44.ØX2	T44.ØX3	T44.ØX4	T44.ØX5	T44.ØX6
Tetrahydrocannabinol	T40.711	T40.712	T40.713	T40.714	T40.715	T40.716
Tetrahydrofuran	T52.8X1	T52.8X2	T52.8X3	T52.8X4	—	—
Tetrahydrolipstatin*	T47.8X1	T47.8X2	T47.8X3	T47.8X4	T47.8X5	T47.8X6
Tetrahydronaphthalene	T52.8X1	T52.8X2	T52.8X3	T52.8X4	—	—
Tetrahydrozoline	T49.5X1	T49.5X2	T49.5X3	T49.5X4	T49.5X5	T49.5X6
Tetralin	T52.8X1	T52.8X2	T52.8X3	T52.8X4	—	—
Tetramethrin	T60.2X1	T60.2X2	T60.2X3	T60.2X4	—	—
Tetramethylthiuram (disulfide) NEC	T60.3X1	T60.3X2	T60.3X3	T60.3X4	—	—
medicinal	T49.ØX1	T49.ØX2	T49.ØX3	T49.ØX4	T49.ØX5	T49.ØX6
Tetramisole	T37.4X1	T37.4X2	T37.4X3	T37.4X4	T37.4X5	T37.4X6
Tetranicotinoyl fructose	T46.7X1	T46.7X2	T46.7X3	T46.7X4	T46.7X5	T46.7X6
Tetrazepam	T42.4X1	T42.4X2	T42.4X3	T42.4X4	T42.4X5	T42.4X6

Substance	Poisoning, Accidental (unintentional)	Poisoning, Intentional Self-harm	Poisoning, Assault	Poisoning, Undetermined	Adverse Effect	Under-dosing
Tetronal	T42.6X1	T42.6X2	T42.6X3	T42.6X4	T42.6X5	T42.6X6
Tetryl	T65.3X1	T65.3X2	T65.3X3	T65.3X4	—	—
Tetrylammonium chloride	T44.2X1	T44.2X2	T44.2X3	T44.2X4	T44.2X5	T44.2X6
Tetryzoline	T49.5X1	T49.5X2	T49.5X3	T49.5X4	T49.5X5	T49.5X6
Thalidomide	T45.1X1	T45.1X2	T45.1X3	T45.1X4	T45.1X5	T45.1X6
Thallium (compounds) (dust)	T56.811	T56.812	T56.813	T56.814	—	—
NEC						
pesticide	T6Ø.4X1	T6Ø.4X2	T6Ø.4X3	T6Ø.4X4	—	—
THC	T4Ø.711	T4Ø.712	T4Ø.713	T4Ø.714	T4Ø.715	T4Ø.716
Thebacon	T48.3X1	T48.3X2	T48.3X3	T48.3X4	T48.3X5	T48.3X6
Thebaine	T4Ø.2X1	T4Ø.2X2	T4Ø.2X3	T4Ø.2X4	T4Ø.2X5	T4Ø.2X6
Thenoic acid	T49.6X1	T49.6X2	T49.6X3	T49.6X4	T49.6X5	T49.6X6
Thenyldiamine	T45.ØX1	T45.ØX2	T45.ØX3	T45.ØX4	T45.ØX5	T45.ØX6
Theobromine (calcium salicylate)	T48.6X1	T48.6X2	T48.6X3	T48.6X4	T48.6X5	T48.6X6
sodium salicylate	T48.6X1	T48.6X2	T48.6X3	T48.6X4	T48.6X5	T48.6X6
Theolair*	T48.6X1	T48.6X2	T48.6X3	T48.6X4	T48.6X5	T48.6X6
Theophyllamine	T48.6X1	T48.6X2	T48.6X3	T48.6X4	T48.6X5	T48.6X6
Theophylline	T48.6X1	T48.6X2	T48.6X3	T48.6X4	T48.6X5	T48.6X6
aminobenzoic acid	T48.6X1	T48.6X2	T48.6X3	T48.6X4	T48.6X5	T48.6X6
ethylenediamine	T48.6X1	T48.6X2	T48.6X3	T48.6X4	T48.6X5	T48.6X6
piperazine p-amino-benzoate	T48.6X1	T48.6X2	T48.6X3	T48.6X4	T48.6X5	T48.6X6
Therevac*	T47.4X1	T47.4X2	T47.4X3	T47.4X4	T47.4X5	T47.4X6
Thiabendazole	T37.4X1	T37.4X2	T37.4X3	T37.4X4	T37.4X5	T37.4X6
Thialbarbital	T41.1X1	T41.1X2	T41.1X3	T41.1X4	T41.1X5	T41.1X6
Thiamazole	T38.2X1	T38.2X2	T38.2X3	T38.2X4	T38.2X5	T38.2X6
Thiambutosine	T37.1X1	T37.1X2	T37.1X3	T37.1X4	T37.1X5	T37.1X6
Thiamine	T45.2X1	T45.2X2	T45.2X3	T45.2X4	T45.2X5	T45.2X6
Thiamphenicol	T36.2X1	T36.2X2	T36.2X3	T36.2X4	T36.2X5	T36.2X6
Thiamylal	T41.1X1	T41.1X2	T41.1X3	T41.1X4	T41.1X5	T41.1X6
sodium	T41.1X1	T41.1X2	T41.1X3	T41.1X4	T41.1X5	T41.1X6
Thiazesim	T43.291	T43.292	T43.293	T43.294	T43.295	T43.296
Thiazides (diuretics)	T5Ø.2X1	T5Ø.2X2	T5Ø.2X3	T5Ø.2X4	T5Ø.2X5	T5Ø.2X6
Thiazinamium metilsulfate	T43.3X1	T43.3X2	T43.3X3	T43.3X4	T43.3X5	T43.3X6
Thiethylperazine	T43.3X1	T43.3X2	T43.3X3	T43.3X4	T43.3X5	T43.3X6
Thimerosal	T49.ØX1	T49.ØX2	T49.ØX3	T49.ØX4	T49.ØX5	T49.ØX6
ophthalmic preparation	T49.5X1	T49.5X2	T49.5X3	T49.5X4	T49.5X5	T49.5X6
Thioacetazone	T37.1X1	T37.1X2	T37.1X3	T37.1X4	T37.1X5	T37.1X6
with isoniazid	T37.1X1	T37.1X2	T37.1X3	T37.1X4	T37.1X5	T37.1X6
Thiobarbital sodium	T41.1X1	T41.1X2	T41.1X3	T41.1X4	T41.1X5	T41.1X6
Thiobarbiturate anesthetic	T41.1X1	T41.1X2	T41.1X3	T41.1X4	T41.1X5	T41.1X6
Thiobismol	T37.8X1	T37.8X2	T37.8X3	T37.8X4	T37.8X5	T37.8X6
Thiobutabarbital sodium	T41.1X1	T41.1X2	T41.1X3	T41.1X4	T41.1X5	T41.1X6
Thiocarbamate (insecticide)	T6Ø.ØX1	T6Ø.ØX2	T6Ø.ØX3	T6Ø.ØX4	—	—
Thiocarbamide	T38.2X1	T38.2X2	T38.2X3	T38.2X4	T38.2X5	T38.2X6
Thiocarbarsone	T37.8X1	T37.8X2	T37.8X3	T37.8X4	T37.8X5	T37.8X6
Thiocarlide	T37.1X1	T37.1X2	T37.1X3	T37.1X4	T37.1X5	T37.1X6
Thioctamide	T5Ø.991	T5Ø.992	T5Ø.993	T5Ø.994	T5Ø.995	T5Ø.996
Thioctic acid	T5Ø.991	T5Ø.992	T5Ø.993	T5Ø.994	T5Ø.995	T5Ø.996
Thiofos	T6Ø.ØX1	T6Ø.ØX2	T6Ø.ØX3	T6Ø.ØX4		
Thioglycolate	T49.4X1	T49.4X2	T49.4X3	T49.4X4	T49.4X5	T49.4X6
Thioglycolic acid	T65.891	T65.892	T65.893	T65.894	—	—
Thioguanine	T45.1X1	T45.1X2	T45.1X3	T45.1X4	T45.1X5	T45.1X6
Thiomercaptomerin	T5Ø.2X1	T5Ø.2X2	T5Ø.2X3	T5Ø.2X4	T5Ø.2X5	T5Ø.2X6
Thiomerin	T5Ø.2X1	T5Ø.2X2	T5Ø.2X3	T5Ø.2X4	T5Ø.2X5	T5Ø.2X6
Thiomersal	T49.ØX1	T49.ØX2	T49.ØX3	T49.ØX4	T49.ØX5	T49.ØX6
Thionazin	T6Ø.ØX1	T6Ø.ØX2	T6Ø.ØX3	T6Ø.ØX4	—	—
Thiopental (sodium)	T41.1X1	T41.1X2	T41.1X3	T41.1X4	T41.1X5	T41.1X6
Thiopentone (sodium)	T41.1X1	T41.1X2	T41.1X3	T41.1X4	T41.1X5	T41.1X6
Thiopropazate	T43.3X1	T43.3X2	T43.3X3	T43.3X4	T43.3X5	T43.3X6
Thioproperazine	T43.3X1	T43.3X2	T43.3X3	T43.3X4	T43.3X5	T43.3X6
Thioridazine	T43.3X1	T43.3X2	T43.3X3	T43.3X4	T43.3X5	T43.3X6
Thiosinamine	T49.3X1	T49.3X2	T49.3X3	T49.3X4	T49.3X5	T49.3X6
Thiotepa	T45.1X1	T45.1X2	T45.1X3	T45.1X4	T45.1X5	T45.1X6
Thiothixene	T43.4X1	T43.4X2	T43.4X3	T43.4X4	T43.4X5	T43.4X6
Thiouracil (benzyl) (methyl) (propyl)	T38.2X1	T38.2X2	T38.2X3	T38.2X4	T38.2X5	T38.2X6
Thiourea	T38.2X1	T38.2X2	T38.2X3	T38.2X4	T38.2X5	T38.2X6
Thiphenamil	T44.3X1	T44.3X2	T44.3X3	T44.3X4	T44.3X5	T44.3X6
Thiram	T6Ø.3X1	T6Ø.3X2	T6Ø.3X3	T6Ø.3X4	—	—
medicinal	T49.2X1	T49.2X2	T49.2X3	T49.2X4	T49.2X5	T49.2X6
Thonzylamine (systemic)	T45.ØX1	T45.ØX2	T45.ØX3	T45.ØX4	T45.ØX5	T45.ØX6
mucosal decongestant	T48.5X1	T48.5X2	T48.5X3	T48.5X4	T48.5X5	T48.5X6
Thorazine	T43.3X1	T43.3X2	T43.3X3	T43.3X4	T43.3X5	T43.3X6
Thorium dioxide suspension	T5Ø.8X1	T5Ø.8X2	T5Ø.8X3	T5Ø.8X4	T5Ø.8X5	T5Ø.8X6
Thornapple	T62.2X1	T62.2X2	T62.2X3	T62.2X4	—	—
Throat drug NEC	T49.6X1	T49.6X2	T49.6X3	T49.6X4	T49.6X5	T49.6X6
Thrombate 111*	T45.511	T45.512	T45.513	T45.514	T45.515	T45.516

Substance	Poisoning, Accidental (unintentional)	Poisoning, Intentional Self-harm	Poisoning, Assault	Poisoning, Undetermined	Adverse Effect	Under-dosing
Thrombin	T45.7X1	T45.7X2	T45.7X3	T45.7X4	T45.7X5	T45.7X6
Thrombolysin	T45.611	T45.612	T45.613	T45.614	T45.615	T45.616
Thromboplastin	T45.7X1	T45.7X2	T45.7X3	T45.7X4	T45.7X5	T45.7X6
Thurfyl nicotinate	T46.7X1	T46.7X2	T46.7X3	T46.7X4	T46.7X5	T46.7X6
Thymol	T49.ØX1	T49.ØX2	T49.ØX3	T49.ØX4	T49.ØX5	T49.ØX6
Thymopentin	T37.5X1	T37.5X2	T37.5X3	T37.5X4	T37.5X5	T37.5X6
Thymoxamine	T46.7X1	T46.7X2	T46.7X3	T46.7X4	T46.7X5	T46.7X6
Thymus extract	T38.891	T38.892	T38.893	T38.894	T38.895	T38.896
Thyreotrophic hormone	T38.811	T38.812	T38.813	T38.814	T38.815	T38.816
Thyroglobulin	T38.1X1	T38.1X2	T38.1X3	T38.1X4	T38.1X5	T38.1X6
Thyroid (hormone)	T38.1X1	T38.1X2	T38.1X3	T38.1X4	T38.1X5	T38.1X6
Thyrolar	T38.1X1	T38.1X2	T38.1X3	T38.1X4	T38.1X5	T38.1X6
Thyrotrophin	T38.811	T38.812	T38.813	T38.814	T38.815	T38.816
Thyrotropic hormone	T38.811	T38.812	T38.813	T38.814	T38.815	T38.816
Thyroxine	T38.1X1	T38.1X2	T38.1X3	T38.1X4	T38.1X5	T38.1X6
Tiabendazole	T37.4X1	T37.4X2	T37.4X3	T37.4X4	T37.4X5	T37.4X6
Tiamizide	T5Ø.2X1	T5Ø.2X2	T5Ø.2X3	T5Ø.2X4	T5Ø.2X5	T5Ø.2X6
Tianeptine	T43.291	T43.292	T43.293	T43.294	T43.295	T43.296
Tiapamil	T46.1X1	T46.1X2	T46.1X3	T46.1X4	T46.1X5	T46.1X6
Tiapride	T43.591	T43.592	T43.593	T43.594	T43.595	T43.596
Tiaprofenic acid	T39.311	T39.312	T39.313	T39.314	T39.315	T39.316
Tiaramide	T39.8X1	T39.8X2	T39.8X3	T39.8X4	T39.8X5	T39.8X6
Ticagrelor*	T45.521	T45.522	T45.523	T45.524	T45.525	T45.526
Ticarcillin	T36.ØX1	T36.ØX2	T36.ØX3	T36.ØX4	T36.ØX5	T36.ØX6
Ticlatone	T49.ØX1	T49.ØX2	T49.ØX3	T49.ØX4	T49.ØX5	T49.ØX6
Ticlopidine	T45.521	T45.522	T45.523	T45.524	T45.525	T45.526
Ticrynafen	T5Ø.1X1	T5Ø.1X2	T5Ø.1X3	T5Ø.1X4	T5Ø.1X5	T5Ø.1X6
Tidiacic	T5Ø.991	T5Ø.992	T5Ø.993	T5Ø.994	T5Ø.995	T5Ø.996
Tiemonium	T44.3X1	T44.3X2	T44.3X3	T44.3X4	T44.3X5	T44.3X6
iodide	T44.3X1	T44.3X2	T44.3X3	T44.3X4	T44.3X5	T44.3X6
Tienilic acid	T5Ø.1X1	T5Ø.1X2	T5Ø.1X3	T5Ø.1X4	T5Ø.1X5	T5Ø.1X6
Tifenamil	T44.3X1	T44.3X2	T44.3X3	T44.3X4	T44.3X5	T44.3X6
Tigan	T45.ØX1	T45.ØX2	T45.ØX3	T45.ØX4	T45.ØX5	T45.ØX6
Tigloidine	T44.3X1	T44.3X2	T44.3X3	T44.3X4	T44.3X5	T44.3X6
Tilactase	T47.5X1	T47.5X2	T47.5X3	T47.5X4	T47.5X5	T47.5X6
Tiletamine	T41.291	T41.292	T41.293	T41.294	T41.295	T41.296
Tilidine	T4Ø.491	T4Ø.492	T4Ø.493	T4Ø.494	—	—
Timepidium bromide	T44.3X1	T44.3X2	T44.3X3	T44.3X4	T44.3X5	T44.3X6
Timiperone	T43.4X1	T43.4X2	T43.4X3	T43.4X4	T43.4X5	T43.4X6
Timolol	T44.7X1	T44.7X2	T44.7X3	T44.7X4	T44.7X5	T44.7X6
Tincture, iodine — *see* Iodine						
Tindal	T43.3X1	T43.3X2	T43.3X3	T43.3X4	T43.3X5	T43.3X6
Tinidazole	T37.3X1	T37.3X2	T37.3X3	T37.3X4	T37.3X5	T37.3X6
Tin (chloride) (dust) (oxide)	T56.6X1	T56.6X2	T56.6X3	T56.6X4	—	—
NEC						
anti-infectives	T37.8X1	T37.8X2	T37.8X3	T37.8X4	T37.8X5	T37.8X6
Tinoridine	T39.8X1	T39.8X2	T39.8X3	T39.8X4	T39.8X5	T39.8X6
Tiocarlide	T37.1X1	T37.1X2	T37.1X3	T37.1X4	T37.1X5	T37.1X6
Tioclomarol	T45.511	T45.512	T45.513	T45.514	T45.515	T45.516
Tioconazole	T49.ØX1	T49.ØX2	T49.ØX3	T49.ØX4	T49.ØX5	T49.ØX6
Tioguanine	T45.1X1	T45.1X2	T45.1X3	T45.1X4	T45.1X5	T45.1X6
Tiopronin	T5Ø.991	T5Ø.992	T5Ø.993	T5Ø.994	T5Ø.995	T5Ø.996
Tiotixene	T43.4X1	T43.4X2	T43.4X3	T43.4X4	T43.4X5	T43.4X6
Tioxolone	T49.4X1	T49.4X2	T49.4X3	T49.4X4	T49.4X5	T49.4X6
Tipepidine	T48.3X1	T48.3X2	T48.3X3	T48.3X4	T48.3X5	T48.3X6
Tiquizium bromide	T44.3X1	T44.3X2	T44.3X3	T44.3X4	T44.3X5	T44.3X6
Tiratricol	T38.1X1	T38.1X2	T38.1X3	T38.1X4	T38.1X5	T38.1X6
Tisopurine	T5Ø.4X1	T5Ø.4X2	T5Ø.4X3	T5Ø.4X4	T5Ø.4X5	T5Ø.4X6
Titanium (compounds) (vapor)	T56.891	T56.892	T56.893	T56.894	—	—
dioxide	T49.3X1	T49.3X2	T49.3X3	T49.3X4	T49.3X5	T49.3X6
ointment	T49.3X1	T49.3X2	T49.3X3	T49.3X4	T49.3X5	T49.3X6
oxide	T49.3X1	T49.3X2	T49.3X3	T49.3X4	T49.3X5	T49.3X6
tetrachloride	T56.891	T56.892	T56.893	T56.894	—	—
Titanocene	T56.891	T56.892	T56.893	T56.894	—	—
Titroid	T38.1X1	T38.1X2	T38.1X3	T38.1X4	T38.1X5	T38.1X6
Tizanidine	T42.8X1	T42.8X2	T42.8X3	T42.8X4	T42.8X5	T42.8X6
TMTD	T6Ø.3X1	T6Ø.3X2	T6Ø.3X3	T6Ø.3X4	—	—
TNT (fumes)	T65.3X1	T65.3X2	T65.3X3	T65.3X4	—	—
Toadstool	T62.ØX1	T62.ØX2	T62.ØX3	T62.ØX4	—	—
Tobacco NEC	T65.291	T65.292	T65.293	T65.294	—	—
cigarettes	T65.221	T65.222	T65.223	T65.224	—	—
Indian	T62.2X1	T62.2X2	T62.2X3	T62.2X4	—	—
smoke, second-hand	T65.221	T65.222	T65.223	T65.224	—	—
Tobraflex*	T49.5X1	T49.5X2	T49.5X3	T49.5X4	T49.5X5	T49.5X6
Tobramycin	T36.5X1	T36.5X2	T36.5X3	T36.5X4	T36.5X5	T36.5X6
Tocainide	T46.2X1	T46.2X2	T46.2X3	T46.2X4	T46.2X5	T46.2X6
Tocoferol	T45.2X1	T45.2X2	T45.2X3	T45.2X4	T45.2X5	T45.2X6
Tocopherol	T45.2X1	T45.2X2	T45.2X3	T45.2X4	T45.2X5	T45.2X6
acetate	T45.2X1	T45.2X2	T45.2X3	T45.2X4	T45.2X5	T45.2X6
Tocosamine	T48.ØX1	T48.ØX2	T48.ØX3	T48.ØX4	T48.ØX5	T48.ØX6
Todralazine	T46.5X1	T46.5X2	T46.5X3	T46.5X4	T46.5X5	T46.5X6
Tofisopam	T42.4X1	T42.4X2	T42.4X3	T42.4X4	T42.4X5	T42.4X6

Substance	Poisoning, Accidental (unintentional)	Poisoning, Intentional Self-harm	Poisoning, Assault	Poisoning, Undetermined	Adverse Effect	Under-dosing
Tofranil	T43.Ø11	T43.Ø12	T43.Ø13	T43.Ø14	T43.Ø15	T43.Ø16
Toilet deodorizer	T65.891	T65.892	T65.893	T65.894	—	—
Tolamolol	T44.7X1	T44.7X2	T44.7X3	T44.7X4	T44.7X5	T44.7X6
Tolazamide	T38.3X1	T38.3X2	T38.3X3	T38.3X4	T38.3X5	T38.3X6
Tolazoline	T46.7X1	T46.7X2	T46.7X3	T46.7X4	T46.7X5	T46.7X6
Tolbutamide (sodium)	T38.3X1	T38.3X2	T38.3X3	T38.3X4	T38.3X5	T38.3X6
Tolciclate	T49.ØX1	T49.ØX2	T49.ØX3	T49.ØX4	T49.ØX5	T49.ØX6
Tolmetin	T39.391	T39.392	T39.393	T39.394	T39.395	T39.396
Tolnaftate	T49.ØX1	T49.ØX2	T49.ØX3	T49.ØX4	T49.ØX5	T49.ØX6
Tolonidine	T46.5X1	T46.5X2	T46.5X3	T46.5X4	T46.5X5	T46.5X6
Toloxatone	T42.6X1	T42.6X2	T42.6X3	T42.6X4	T42.6X5	T42.6X6
Tolperisone	T44.3X1	T44.3X2	T44.3X3	T44.3X4	T44.3X5	T44.3X6
Tolserol	T42.8X1	T42.8X2	T42.8X3	T42.8X4	T42.8X5	T42.8X6
Toluene (liquid)	T52.2X1	T52.2X2	T52.2X3	T52.2X4	—	—
diisocyanate	T65.ØX1	T65.ØX2	T65.ØX3	T65.ØX4	—	—
Toluidine	T65.891	T65.892	T65.893	T65.894	—	—
vapor	T59.891	T59.892	T59.893	T59.894	—	—
Toluol (liquid)	T52.2X1	T52.2X2	T52.2X3	T52.2X4	—	—
vapor	T52.2X1	T52.2X2	T52.2X3	T52.2X4	—	—
Toluylenediamine	T65.3X1	T65.3X2	T65.3X3	T65.3X4	—	—
Tolylene-2,4-diisocyanate	T65.ØX1	T65.ØX2	T65.ØX3	T65.ØX4	—	—
Tonic NEC	T5Ø.9Ø1	T5Ø.9Ø2	T5Ø.9Ø3	T5Ø.9Ø4	T5Ø.9Ø5	T5Ø.9Ø6
Topical action drug NEC	T49.91	T49.92	T49.93	T49.94	T49.95	T49.96
ear, nose or throat	T49.6X1	T49.6X2	T49.6X3	T49.6X4	T49.6X5	T49.6X6
eye	T49.5X1	T49.5X2	T49.5X3	T49.5X4	T49.5X5	T49.5X6
skin	T49.91	T49.92	T49.93	T49.94	T49.95	T49.96
specified NEC	T49.8X1	T49.8X2	T49.8X3	T49.8X4	T49.8X5	T49.8X6
Toprol*	T44.7X1	T44.7X2	T44.7X3	T44.7X4	T44.7X5	T44.7X6
Toquizine	T44.3X1	T44.3X2	T44.3X3	T44.3X4	T44.3X5	T44.3X6
Toremifene	T38.6X1	T38.6X2	T38.6X3	T38.6X4	T38.6X5	T38.6X6
Tosylchloramide sodium	T49.8X1	T49.8X2	T49.8X3	T49.8X4	T49.8X5	T49.8X6
Toxaphene (dust) (spray)	T6Ø.1X1	T6Ø.1X2	T6Ø.1X3	T6Ø.1X4	—	—
Toxin, diphtheria (Schick Test)	T5Ø.8X1	T5Ø.8X2	T5Ø.8X3	T5Ø.8X4	T5Ø.8X5	T5Ø.8X6
Toxoid						
combined	T5Ø.A21	T5Ø.A22	T5Ø.A23	T5Ø.A24	T5Ø.A25	T5Ø.A26
diphtheria	T5Ø.A91	T5Ø.A92	T5Ø.A93	T5Ø.A94	T5Ø.A95	T5Ø.A96
tetanus	T5Ø.A91	T5Ø.A92	T5Ø.A93	T5Ø.A94	T5Ø.A95	T5Ø.A96
Trace element NEC	T45.8X1	T45.8X2	T45.8X3	T45.8X4	T45.8X5	T45.8X6
Tractor fuel NEC	T52.ØX1	T52.ØX2	T52.ØX3	T52.ØX4	—	—
Tragacanth	T5Ø.991	T5Ø.992	T5Ø.993	T5Ø.994	T5Ø.995	T5Ø.996
Tramadol	T4Ø.421	T4Ø.422	T4Ø.423	T4Ø.424	T4Ø.425	T4Ø.426
Tramazoline	T48.5X1	T48.5X2	T48.5X3	T48.5X4	T48.5X5	T48.5X6
Tranexamic acid	T45.621	T45.622	T45.623	T45.624	T45.625	T45.626
Tranilast	T45.ØX1	T45.ØX2	T45.ØX3	T45.ØX4	T45.ØX5	T45.ØX6
Tranquilizer NEC	T43.5Ø1	T43.5Ø2	T43.5Ø3	T43.5Ø4	T43.5Ø5	T43.5Ø6
with hypnotic or sedative	T42.6X1	T42.6X2	T42.6X3	T42.6X4	T42.6X5	T42.6X6
benzodiazepine NEC	T42.4X1	T42.4X2	T42.4X3	T42.4X4	T42.4X5	T42.4X6
butyrophenone NEC	T43.4X1	T43.4X2	T43.4X3	T43.4X4	T43.4X5	T43.4X6
carbamate	T43.591	T43.592	T43.593	T43.594	T43.595	T43.596
dimethylamine	T43.3X1	T43.3X2	T43.3X3	T43.3X4	T43.3X5	T43.3X6
ethylamine	T43.3X1	T43.3X2	T43.3X3	T43.3X4	T43.3X5	T43.3X6
hydroxyzine	T43.591	T43.592	T43.593	T43.594	T43.595	T43.596
major NEC	T43.5Ø1	T43.5Ø2	T43.5Ø3	T43.5Ø4	T43.5Ø5	T43.5Ø6
penothiazine NEC	T43.3X1	T43.3X2	T43.3X3	T43.3X4	T43.3X5	T43.3X6
phenothiazine-based	T43.3X1	T43.3X2	T43.3X3	T43.3X4	T43.3X5	T43.3X6
piperazine NEC	T43.3X1	T43.3X2	T43.3X3	T43.3X4	T43.3X5	T43.3X6
piperidine	T43.3X1	T43.3X2	T43.3X3	T43.3X4	T43.3X5	T43.3X6
propylamine	T43.3X1	T43.3X2	T43.3X3	T43.3X4	T43.3X5	T43.3X6
specified NEC	T43.591	T43.592	T43.593	T43.594	T43.595	T43.596
thioxanthene NEC	T43.591	T43.592	T43.593	T43.594	T43.595	T43.596
Tranxene	T42.4X1	T42.4X2	T42.4X3	T42.4X4	T42.4X5	T42.4X6
Tranylcypromine	T43.1X1	T43.1X2	T43.1X3	T43.1X4	T43.1X5	T43.1X6
Trapidil	T46.3X1	T46.3X2	T46.3X3	T46.3X4	T46.3X5	T46.3X6
Trasentine	T44.3X1	T44.3X2	T44.3X3	T44.3X4	T44.3X5	T44.3X6
Travert	T5Ø.3X1	T5Ø.3X2	T5Ø.3X3	T5Ø.3X4	T5Ø.3X5	T5Ø.3X6
Trazodone	T43.211	T43.212	T43.213	T43.214	T43.215	T43.216
Treanda*	T45.1X1	T45.1X2	T45.1X3	T45.1X4	T45.1X5	T45.1X6
Trecator	T37.1X1	T37.1X2	T37.1X3	T37.1X4	T37.1X5	T37.1X6
Treosulfan	T45.1X1	T45.1X2	T45.1X3	T45.1X4	T45.1X5	T45.1X6
Tretamine	T45.1X1	T45.1X2	T45.1X3	T45.1X4	T45.1X5	T45.1X6
Tretinoin	T49.ØX1	T49.ØX2	T49.ØX3	T49.ØX4	T49.ØX5	T49.ØX6
Tretoquinol	T48.6X1	T48.6X2	T48.6X3	T48.6X4	T48.6X5	T48.6X6
Triacetin	T49.ØX1	T49.ØX2	T49.ØX3	T49.ØX4	T49.ØX5	T49.ØX6
Triacetoxyanthracene	T49.4X1	T49.4X2	T49.4X3	T49.4X4	T49.4X5	T49.4X6
Triacetyloleandomycin	T36.3X1	T36.3X2	T36.3X3	T36.3X4	T36.3X5	T36.3X6
Triamcinolone	T38.ØX1	T38.ØX2	T38.ØX3	T38.ØX4	T38.ØX5	T38.ØX6
ENT agent	T49.6X1	T49.6X2	T49.6X3	T49.6X4	T49.6X5	T49.6X6
hexacetonide	T49.ØX1	T49.ØX2	T49.ØX3	T49.ØX4	T49.ØX5	T49.ØX6
ophthalmic preparation	T49.5X1	T49.5X2	T49.5X3	T49.5X4	T49.5X5	T49.5X6
topical NEC	T49.ØX1	T49.ØX2	T49.ØX3	T49.ØX4	T49.ØX5	T49.ØX6
Triampyzine	T44.3X1	T44.3X2	T44.3X3	T44.3X4	T44.3X5	T44.3X6
Triamterene	T5Ø.2X1	T5Ø.2X2	T5Ø.2X3	T5Ø.2X4	T5Ø.2X5	T5Ø.2X6
Triazine (herbicide)	T6Ø.3X1	T6Ø.3X2	T6Ø.3X3	T6Ø.3X4	—	—
Triaziquone	T45.1X1	T45.1X2	T45.1X3	T45.1X4	T45.1X5	T45.1X6
Triazolam	T42.4X1	T42.4X2	T42.4X3	T42.4X4	T42.4X5	T42.4X6
Triazole (herbicide)	T6Ø.3X1	T6Ø.3X2	T6Ø.3X3	T6Ø.3X4	—	—
Tribavirin*	T37.5X1	T37.5X2	T37.5X3	T37.5X4	T37.5X5	T37.5X6
Tribenoside	T46.991	T46.992	T46.993	T46.994	T46.995	T46.996
Tribromacetaldehyde	T42.6X1	T42.6X2	T42.6X3	T42.6X4	T42.6X5	T42.6X6
Tribromoethanol, rectal	T41.291	T41.292	T41.293	T41.294	T41.295	T41.296
Tribromomethane	T42.6X1	T42.6X2	T42.6X3	T42.6X4	T42.6X5	T42.6X6
Trichlorethane	T53.2X1	T53.2X2	T53.2X3	T53.2X4	—	—
Trichlorethylene	T53.2X1	T53.2X2	T53.2X3	T53.2X4	—	—
Trichlorfon	T6Ø.ØX1	T6Ø.ØX2	T6Ø.ØX3	T6Ø.ØX4	—	—
Trichlormethiazide	T5Ø.2X1	T5Ø.2X2	T5Ø.2X3	T5Ø.2X4	T5Ø.2X5	T5Ø.2X6
Trichlormethine	T45.1X1	T45.1X2	T45.1X3	T45.1X4	T45.1X5	T45.1X6
Trichloroacetic acid, Trichloracetic acid	T54.2X1	T54.2X2	T54.2X3	T54.2X4	—	—
medicinal	T49.4X1	T49.4X2	T49.4X3	T49.4X4	T49.4X5	T49.4X6
Trichloroethane	T53.2X1	T53.2X2	T53.2X3	T53.2X4	—	—
Trichloroethanol	T42.6X1	T42.6X2	T42.6X3	T42.6X4	T42.6X5	T42.6X6
Trichloroethylene (liquid) (vapor)	T53.2X1	T53.2X2	T53.2X3	T53.2X4	—	—
anesthetic (gas)	T41.ØX1	T41.ØX2	T41.ØX3	T41.ØX4	T41.ØX5	T41.ØX6
vapor NEC	T53.2X1	T53.2X2	T53.2X3	T53.2X4	—	—
Trichloroethyl phosphate	T42.6X1	T42.6X2	T42.6X3	T42.6X4	T42.6X5	T42.6X6
Trichlorofluoromethane NEC	T53.5X1	T53.5X2	T53.5X3	T53.5X4	—	—
Trichloronate	T6Ø.ØX1	T6Ø.ØX2	T6Ø.ØX3	T6Ø.ØX4	—	—
Trichloropropane	T53.6X1	T53.6X2	T53.6X3	T53.6X4	—	—
Trichlorotriethylamine	T45.1X1	T45.1X2	T45.1X3	T45.1X4	T45.1X5	T45.1X6
Trichomonacides NEC	T37.3X1	T37.3X2	T37.3X3	T37.3X4	T37.3X5	T37.3X6
Trichomycin	T36.7X1	T36.7X2	T36.7X3	T36.7X4	T36.7X5	T36.7X6
Triclobisonium chloride	T49.ØX1	T49.ØX2	T49.ØX3	T49.ØX4	T49.ØX5	T49.ØX6
Triclocarban	T49.ØX1	T49.ØX2	T49.ØX3	T49.ØX4	T49.ØX5	T49.ØX6
Triclofos	T42.6X1	T42.6X2	T42.6X3	T42.6X4	T42.6X5	T42.6X6
Triclosan	T49.ØX1	T49.ØX2	T49.ØX3	T49.ØX4	T49.ØX5	T49.ØX6
Tricosal*	T39.Ø91	T39.Ø92	T39.Ø93	T39.Ø94	T39.Ø95	T39.Ø96
Tricresyl phosphate	T65.891	T65.892	T65.893	T65.894	—	—
solvent	T52.91	T52.92	T52.93	T52.94	—	—
Tricyclamol chloride	T44.3X1	T44.3X2	T44.3X3	T44.3X4	T44.3X5	T44.3X6
Tridesilon	T49.ØX1	T49.ØX2	T49.ØX3	T49.ØX4	T49.ØX5	T49.ØX6
Tridihexethyl iodide	T44.3X1	T44.3X2	T44.3X3	T44.3X4	T44.3X5	T44.3X6
Tridione	T42.2X1	T42.2X2	T42.2X3	T42.2X4	T42.2X5	T42.2X6
Trientine	T45.8X1	T45.8X2	T45.8X3	T45.8X4	T45.8X5	T45.8X6
Triethanolamine NEC	T54.3X1	T54.3X2	T54.3X3	T54.3X4	—	—
detergent	T54.3X1	T54.3X2	T54.3X3	T54.3X4	—	—
trinitrate (biphosphate)	T46.3X1	T46.3X2	T46.3X3	T46.3X4	T46.3X5	T46.3X6
Triethanomelamine	T45.1X1	T45.1X2	T45.1X3	T45.1X4	T45.1X5	T45.1X6
Triethylenemelamine	T45.1X1	T45.1X2	T45.1X3	T45.1X4	T45.1X5	T45.1X6
Triethylenephosphoramide	T45.1X1	T45.1X2	T45.1X3	T45.1X4	T45.1X5	T45.1X6
Triethylenethiophosphoramide	T45.1X1	T45.1X2	T45.1X3	T45.1X4	T45.1X5	T45.1X6
Trifluoperazine	T43.3X1	T43.3X2	T43.3X3	T43.3X4	T43.3X5	T43.3X6
Trifluoroethyl vinyl ether	T41.ØX1	T41.ØX2	T41.ØX3	T41.ØX4	T41.ØX5	T41.ØX6
Trifluperidol	T43.4X1	T43.4X2	T43.4X3	T43.4X4	T43.4X5	T43.4X6
Triflupromazine	T43.3X1	T43.3X2	T43.3X3	T43.3X4	T43.3X5	T43.3X6
Trifluridine	T37.5X1	T37.5X2	T37.5X3	T37.5X4	T37.5X5	T37.5X6
Triflusal	T45.521	T45.522	T45.523	T45.524	T45.525	T45.526
Trihexyphenidyl	T44.3X1	T44.3X2	T44.3X3	T44.3X4	T44.3X5	T44.3X6
Triiodothyronine	T38.1X1	T38.1X2	T38.1X3	T38.1X4	T38.1X5	T38.1X6
Trilene	T41.ØX1	T41.ØX2	T41.ØX3	T41.ØX4	T41.ØX5	T41.ØX6
Trilostane	T38.991	T38.992	T38.993	T38.994	T38.995	T38.996
Trimebutine	T44.3X1	T44.3X2	T44.3X3	T44.3X4	T44.3X5	T44.3X6
Trimecaine	T41.3X1	T41.3X2	T41.3X3	T41.3X4	T41.3X5	T41.3X6
Trimeprazine (tartrate)	T44.3X1	T44.3X2	T44.3X3	T44.3X4	T44.3X5	T44.3X6
Trimetaphan camsilate	T44.2X1	T44.2X2	T44.2X3	T44.2X4	T44.2X5	T44.2X6
Trimetazidine	T46.7X1	T46.7X2	T46.7X3	T46.7X4	T46.7X5	T46.7X6
Trimethadione	T42.2X1	T42.2X2	T42.2X3	T42.2X4	T42.2X5	T42.2X6
Trimethaphan	T44.2X1	T44.2X2	T44.2X3	T44.2X4	T44.2X5	T44.2X6
Trimethidinium	T44.2X1	T44.2X2	T44.2X3	T44.2X4	T44.2X5	T44.2X6
Trimethobenzamide	T45.ØX1	T45.ØX2	T45.ØX3	T45.ØX4	T45.ØX5	T45.ØX6
Trimethoprim	T37.8X1	T37.8X2	T37.8X3	T37.8X4	T37.8X5	T37.8X6
with sulfamethoxazole	T36.8X1	T36.8X2	T36.8X3	T36.8X4	T36.8X5	T36.8X6
Trimethylcarbinol	T51.3X1	T51.3X2	T51.3X3	T51.3X4	—	—
Trimethylpsoralen	T49.3X1	T49.3X2	T49.3X3	T49.3X4	T49.3X5	T49.3X6
Trimeton	T45.ØX1	T45.ØX2	T45.ØX3	T45.ØX4	T45.ØX5	T45.ØX6
Trimetrexate	T45.1X1	T45.1X2	T45.1X3	T45.1X4	T45.1X5	T45.1X6
Trimipramine	T43.Ø11	T43.Ø12	T43.Ø13	T43.Ø14	T43.Ø15	T43.Ø16
Trimox*	T36.ØX1	T36.ØX2	T36.ØX3	T36.ØX4	T36.ØX5	T36.ØX6
Trimustine	T45.1X1	T45.1X2	T45.1X3	T45.1X4	T45.1X5	T45.1X6
Trinitrine	T46.3X1	T46.3X2	T46.3X3	T46.3X4	T46.3X5	T46.3X6
Trinitrobenzol	T65.3X1	T65.3X2	T65.3X3	T65.3X4	—	—
Trinitrophenol	T65.3X1	T65.3X2	T65.3X3	T65.3X4	—	—
Trinitrotoluene (fumes)	T65.3X1	T65.3X2	T65.3X3	T65.3X4	—	—

Substance	Poisoning, Accidental (unintentional)	Poisoning, Intentional Self-harm	Poisoning, Assault	Poisoning, Undetermined	Adverse Effect	Under-dosing
Trional	T42.6X1	T42.6X2	T42.6X3	T42.6X4	T42.6X5	T42.6X6
Triorthocresyl phosphate	T65.891	T65.892	T65.893	T65.894	—	—
Trioxide of arsenic	T57.ØX1	T57.ØX2	T57.ØX3	T57.ØX4	—	—
Trioxysalen	T49.4X1	T49.4X2	T49.4X3	T49.4X4	T49.4X5	T49.4X6
Tripamide	T5Ø.2X1	T5Ø.2X2	T5Ø.2X3	T5Ø.2X4	T5Ø.2X5	T5Ø.2X6
Triparanol	T46.6X1	T46.6X2	T46.6X3	T46.6X4	T46.6X5	T46.6X6
Tripelennamine	T45.ØX1	T45.ØX2	T45.ØX3	T45.ØX4	T45.ØX5	T45.ØX6
Triperiden	T44.3X1	T44.3X2	T44.3X3	T44.3X4	T44.3X5	T44.3X6
Triperidol	T43.4X1	T43.4X2	T43.4X3	T43.4X4	T43.4X5	T43.4X6
Triphenylphosphate	T65.891	T65.892	T65.893	T65.894	—	—
Triple						
bromides	T42.6X1	T42.6X2	T42.6X3	T42.6X4	T42.6X5	T42.6X6
carbonate	T47.1X1	T47.1X2	T47.1X3	T47.1X4	T47.1X5	T47.1X6
vaccine						
DPT	T5Ø.A11	T5Ø.A12	T5Ø.A13	T5Ø.A14	T5Ø.A15	T5Ø.A16
including pertussis	T5Ø.A11	T5Ø.A12	T5Ø.A13	T5Ø.A14	T5Ø.A15	T5Ø.A16
MMR	T5Ø.B91	T5Ø.B92	T5Ø.B93	T5Ø.B94	T5Ø.B95	T5Ø.B96
Triprolidine	T45.ØX1	T45.ØX2	T45.ØX3	T45.ØX4	T45.ØX5	T45.ØX6
Trisodium hydrogen edetate	T5Ø.6X1	T5Ø.6X2	T5Ø.6X3	T5Ø.6X4	T5Ø.6X5	T5Ø.6X6
Trisoralen	T49.3X1	T49.3X2	T49.3X3	T49.3X4	T49.3X5	T49.3X6
Trisulfapyrimidines	T37.ØX1	T37.ØX2	T37.ØX3	T37.ØX4	T37.ØX5	T37.ØX6
Trithiozine	T44.3X1	T44.3X2	T44.3X3	T44.3X4	T44.3X5	T44.3X6
Tritiozine	T44.3X1	T44.3X2	T44.3X3	T44.3X4	T44.3X5	T44.3X6
Tritoqualine	T45.ØX1	T45.ØX2	T45.ØX3	T45.ØX4	T45.ØX5	T45.ØX6
Trizivir*	T37.5X1	T37.5X2	T37.5X3	T37.5X4	T37.5X5	T37.5X6
Trofosfamide	T45.1X1	T45.1X2	T45.1X3	T45.1X4	T45.1X5	T45.1X6
Troleandomycin	T36.3X1	T36.3X2	T36.3X3	T36.3X4	T36.3X5	T36.3X6
Trolnitrate (phosphate)	T46.3X1	T46.3X2	T46.3X3	T46.3X4	T46.3X5	T46.3X6
Tromantadine	T37.5X1	T37.5X2	T37.5X3	T37.5X4	T37.5X5	T37.5X6
Trometamol	T5Ø.2X1	T5Ø.2X2	T5Ø.2X3	T5Ø.2X4	T5Ø.2X5	T5Ø.2X6
Tromethamine	T5Ø.2X1	T5Ø.2X2	T5Ø.2X3	T5Ø.2X4	T5Ø.2X5	T5Ø.2X6
Tronothane	T41.3X1	T41.3X2	T41.3X3	T41.3X4	T41.3X5	T41.3X6
Tropacine	T44.3X1	T44.3X2	T44.3X3	T44.3X4	T44.3X5	T44.3X6
Tropatepine	T44.3X1	T44.3X2	T44.3X3	T44.3X4	T44.3X5	T44.3X6
Tropicamide	T44.3X1	T44.3X2	T44.3X3	T44.3X4	T44.3X5	T44.3X6
Trospium chloride	T44.3X1	T44.3X2	T44.3X3	T44.3X4	T44.3X5	T44.3X6
Troxerutin	T46.991	T46.992	T46.993	T46.994	T46.995	T46.996
Troxidone	T42.2X1	T42.2X2	T42.2X3	T42.2X4	T42.2X5	T42.2X6
Tryparsamide	T37.3X1	T37.3X2	T37.3X3	T37.3X4	T37.3X5	T37.3X6
Trypsin	T45.3X1	T45.3X2	T45.3X3	T45.3X4	T45.3X5	T45.3X6
Tryptizol	T43.Ø11	T43.Ø12	T43.Ø13	T43.Ø14	T43.Ø15	T43.Ø16
TSH	T38.811	T38.812	T38.813	T38.814	T38.815	T38.816
Tuaminoheptane	T48.5X1	T48.5X2	T48.5X3	T48.5X4	T48.5X5	T48.5X6
Tuberculin, purified protein derivative (PPD)	T5Ø.8X1	T5Ø.8X2	T5Ø.8X3	T5Ø.8X4	T5Ø.8X5	T5Ø.8X6
Tubocurare	T48.1X1	T48.1X2	T48.1X3	T48.1X4	T48.1X5	T48.1X6
Tubocurarine (chloride)	T48.1X1	T48.1X2	T48.1X3	T48.1X4	T48.1X5	T48.1X6
Tulobuterol	T48.6X1	T48.6X2	T48.6X3	T48.6X4	T48.6X5	T48.6X6
Turpentine (spirits of)	T52.8X1	T52.8X2	T52.8X3	T52.8X4	—	—
vapor	T52.8X1	T52.8X2	T52.8X3	T52.8X4	—	—
Twinrix*	T5Ø.B91	T5Ø.B92	T5Ø.B93	T5Ø.B94	T5Ø.B95	T5Ø.B96
Tybamate	T43.591	T43.592	T43.593	T43.594	T43.595	T43.596
Tygacil*	T36.4X1	T36.4X2	T36.4X3	T36.4X4	T36.4X5	T36.4X6
Tyloxapol	T48.4X1	T48.4X2	T48.4X3	T48.4X4	T48.4X5	T48.4X6
Tymazoline	T48.5X1	T48.5X2	T48.5X3	T48.5X4	T48.5X5	T48.5X6
Tymlos*	T5Ø.991	T5Ø.992	T5Ø.993	T5Ø.994	T5Ø.995	T5Ø.996
Typhoid-paratyphoid vaccine	T5Ø.A91	T5Ø.A92	T5Ø.A93	T5Ø.A94	T5Ø.A95	T5Ø.A96
Typhus vaccine	T5Ø.A91	T5Ø.A92	T5Ø.A93	T5Ø.A94	T5Ø.A95	T5Ø.A96
Tyropanoate	T5Ø.8X1	T5Ø.8X2	T5Ø.8X3	T5Ø.8X4	T5Ø.8X5	T5Ø.8X6
Tyrothricin	T49.6X1	T49.6X2	T49.6X3	T49.6X4	T49.6X5	T49.6X6
ENT agent	T49.6X1	T49.6X2	T49.6X3	T49.6X4	T49.6X5	T49.6X6
ophthalmic preparation	T49.5X1	T49.5X2	T49.5X3	T49.5X4	T49.5X5	T49.5X6
Ufenamate	T39.391	T39.392	T39.393	T39.394	T39.395	T39.396
Ultraviolet light protectant	T49.3X1	T49.3X2	T49.3X3	T49.3X4	T49.3X5	T49.3X6
Unasyn*	T36.ØX1	T36.ØX2	T36.ØX3	T36.ØX4	T36.ØX5	T36.ØX6
Undecenoic acid	T49.ØX1	T49.ØX2	T49.ØX3	T49.ØX4	T49.ØX5	T49.ØX6
Undecoylium	T49.ØX1	T49.ØX2	T49.ØX3	T49.ØX4	T49.ØX5	T49.ØX6
Undecylenic acid (derivatives)	T49.ØX1	T49.ØX2	T49.ØX3	T49.ØX4	T49.ØX5	T49.ØX6
Unna's boot	T49.3X1	T49.3X2	T49.3X3	T49.3X4	T49.3X5	T49.3X6
Unsaturated fatty acid	T46.6X1	T46.6X2	T46.6X3	T46.6X4	T46.6X5	T46.6X6
Uracil mustard	T45.1X1	T45.1X2	T45.1X3	T45.1X4	T45.1X5	T45.1X6
Uramustine	T45.1X1	T45.1X2	T45.1X3	T45.1X4	T45.1X5	T45.1X6
Urapidil	T46.5X1	T46.5X2	T46.5X3	T46.5X4	T46.5X5	T46.5X6
Urari	T48.1X1	T48.1X2	T48.1X3	T48.1X4	T48.1X5	T48.1X6
Urate oxidase	T5Ø.4X1	T5Ø.4X2	T5Ø.4X3	T5Ø.4X4	T5Ø.4X5	T5Ø.4X6
Urea	T47.3X1	T47.3X2	T47.3X3	T47.3X4	T47.3X5	T47.3X6
peroxide	T49.ØX1	T49.ØX2	T49.ØX3	T49.ØX4	T49.ØX5	T49.ØX6
stibamine	T37.4X1	T37.4X2	T37.4X3	T37.4X4	T37.4X5	T37.4X6
topical	T49.8X1	T49.8X2	T49.8X3	T49.8X4	T49.8X5	T49.8X6

Substance	Poisoning, Accidental (unintentional)	Poisoning, Intentional Self-harm	Poisoning, Assault	Poisoning, Undetermined	Adverse Effect	Under-dosing
Ureaphil*	T48.ØX1	T48.ØX2	T48.ØX3	T48.ØX4	T48.ØX5	T48.ØX6
Urethane	T45.1X1	T45.1X2	T45.1X3	T45.1X4	T45.1X5	T45.1X6
Urginea (maritima) (scilla) — *see* Squill						
Uric acid metabolism drug NEC	T5Ø.4X1	T5Ø.4X2	T5Ø.4X3	T5Ø.4X4	T5Ø.4X5	T5Ø.4X6
Uricosuric agent	T5Ø.4X1	T5Ø.4X2	T5Ø.4X3	T5Ø.4X4	T5Ø.4X5	T5Ø.4X6
Urinary anti-infective	T37.8X1	T37.8X2	T37.8X3	T37.8X4	T37.8X5	T37.8X6
Urofollitropin	T38.811	T38.812	T38.813	T38.814	T38.815	T38.816
Urokinase	T45.611	T45.612	T45.613	T45.614	T45.615	T45.616
Urokon	T5Ø.8X1	T5Ø.8X2	T5Ø.8X3	T5Ø.8X4	T5Ø.8X5	T5Ø.8X6
Ursodeoxycholic acid	T5Ø.991	T5Ø.992	T5Ø.993	T5Ø.994	T5Ø.995	T5Ø.996
Ursodiol	T5Ø.991	T5Ø.992	T5Ø.993	T5Ø.994	T5Ø.995	T5Ø.996
Urtica	T62.2X1	T62.2X2	T62.2X3	T62.2X4	—	—
Utility gas — *see* Gas, utility						
Vaccine NEC	T5Ø.Z91	T5Ø.Z92	T5Ø.Z93	T5Ø.Z94	T5Ø.Z95	T5Ø.Z96
antineoplastic	T5Ø.Z91	T5Ø.Z92	T5Ø.Z93	T5Ø.Z94	T5Ø.Z95	T5Ø.Z96
bacterial NEC	T5Ø.A91	T5Ø.A92	T5Ø.A93	T5Ø.A94	T5Ø.A95	T5Ø.A96
with						
other bacterial component	T5Ø.A21	T5Ø.A22	T5Ø.A23	T5Ø.A24	T5Ø.A25	T5Ø.A26
pertussis component	T5Ø.A11	T5Ø.A12	T5Ø.A13	T5Ø.A14	T5Ø.A15	T5Ø.A16
viral-rickettsial component	T5Ø.A21	T5Ø.A22	T5Ø.A23	T5Ø.A24	T5Ø.A25	T5Ø.A26
mixed NEC	T5Ø.A21	T5Ø.A22	T5Ø.A23	T5Ø.A24	T5Ø.A25	T5Ø.A26
BCG	T5Ø.A91	T5Ø.A92	T5Ø.A93	T5Ø.A94	T5Ø.A95	T5Ø.A96
cholera	T5Ø.A91	T5Ø.A92	T5Ø.A93	T5Ø.A94	T5Ø.A95	T5Ø.A96
diphtheria	T5Ø.A91	T5Ø.A92	T5Ø.A93	T5Ø.A94	T5Ø.A95	T5Ø.A96
with tetanus	T5Ø.A21	T5Ø.A22	T5Ø.A23	T5Ø.A24	T5Ø.A25	T5Ø.A26
and pertussis	T5Ø.A11	T5Ø.A12	T5Ø.A13	T5Ø.A14	T5Ø.A15	T5Ø.A16
influenza	T5Ø.B91	T5Ø.B92	T5Ø.B93	T5Ø.B94	T5Ø.B95	T5Ø.B96
measles	T5Ø.B91	T5Ø.B92	T5Ø.B93	T5Ø.B94	T5Ø.B95	T5Ø.B96
with mumps and rubella	T5Ø.B91	T5Ø.B92	T5Ø.B93	T5Ø.B94	T5Ø.B95	T5Ø.B96
meningococcal	T5Ø.A91	T5Ø.A92	T5Ø.A93	T5Ø.A94	T5Ø.A95	T5Ø.A96
mumps	T5Ø.B91	T5Ø.B92	T5Ø.B93	T5Ø.B94	T5Ø.B95	T5Ø.B96
paratyphoid	T5Ø.A91	T5Ø.A92	T5Ø.A93	T5Ø.A94	T5Ø.A95	T5Ø.A96
pertussis	T5Ø.A11	T5Ø.A12	T5Ø.A13	T5Ø.A14	T5Ø.A15	T5Ø.A16
with diphtheria	T5Ø.A11	T5Ø.A12	T5Ø.A13	T5Ø.A14	T5Ø.A15	T5Ø.A16
and tetanus	T5Ø.A11	T5Ø.A12	T5Ø.A13	T5Ø.A14	T5Ø.A15	T5Ø.A16
with other component	T5Ø.A11	T5Ø.A12	T5Ø.A13	T5Ø.A14	T5Ø.A15	T5Ø.A16
plague	T5Ø.A91	T5Ø.A92	T5Ø.A93	T5Ø.A94	T5Ø.A95	T5Ø.A96
poliomyelitis	T5Ø.B91	T5Ø.B92	T5Ø.B93	T5Ø.B94	T5Ø.B95	T5Ø.B96
poliovirus	T5Ø.B91	T5Ø.B92	T5Ø.B93	T5Ø.B94	T5Ø.B95	T5Ø.B96
rabies	T5Ø.B91	T5Ø.B92	T5Ø.B93	T5Ø.B94	T5Ø.B95	T5Ø.B96
respiratory syncytial virus	T5Ø.B91	T5Ø.B92	T5Ø.B93	T5Ø.B94	T5Ø.B95	T5Ø.B96
rickettsial NEC	T5Ø.A91	T5Ø.A92	T5Ø.A93	T5Ø.A94	T5Ø.A95	T5Ø.A96
with						
bacterial component	T5Ø.A21	T5Ø.A22	T5Ø.A23	T5Ø.A24	T5Ø.A25	T5Ø.A26
Rocky Mountain spotted fever	T5Ø.A91	T5Ø.A92	T5Ø.A93	T5Ø.A94	T5Ø.A95	T5Ø.A96
rubella	T5Ø.B91	T5Ø.B92	T5Ø.B93	T5Ø.B94	T5Ø.B95	T5Ø.B96
sabin oral	T5Ø.B91	T5Ø.B92	T5Ø.B93	T5Ø.B94	T5Ø.B95	T5Ø.B96
smallpox	T5Ø.B11	T5Ø.B12	T5Ø.B13	T5Ø.B14	T5Ø.B15	T5Ø.B16
TAB	T5Ø.A91	T5Ø.A92	T5Ø.A93	T5Ø.A94	T5Ø.A95	T5Ø.A96
tetanus	T5Ø.A91	T5Ø.A92	T5Ø.A93	T5Ø.A94	T5Ø.A95	T5Ø.A96
typhoid	T5Ø.A91	T5Ø.A92	T5Ø.A93	T5Ø.A94	T5Ø.A95	T5Ø.A96
typhus	T5Ø.A91	T5Ø.A92	T5Ø.A93	T5Ø.A94	T5Ø.A95	T5Ø.A96
viral NEC	T5Ø.B91	T5Ø.B92	T5Ø.B93	T5Ø.B94	T5Ø.B95	T5Ø.B96
yellow fever	T5Ø.B91	T5Ø.B92	T5Ø.B93	T5Ø.B94	T5Ø.B95	T5Ø.B96
Vaccinia immune globulin	T5Ø.Z11	T5Ø.Z12	T5Ø.Z13	T5Ø.Z14	T5Ø.Z15	T5Ø.Z16
Vaginal contraceptives	T49.8X1	T49.8X2	T49.8X3	T49.8X4	T49.8X5	T49.8X6
Valacyclovir*	T37.5X1	T37.5X2	T37.5X3	T37.5X4	T37.5X5	T37.5X6
Valerian						
root	T42.6X1	T42.6X2	T42.6X3	T42.6X4	T42.6X5	T42.6X6
tincture	T42.6X1	T42.6X2	T42.6X3	T42.6X4	T42.6X5	T42.6X6
Valethamate bromide	T44.3X1	T44.3X2	T44.3X3	T44.3X4	T44.3X5	T44.3X6
Valisone	T49.ØX1	T49.ØX2	T49.ØX3	T49.ØX4	T49.ØX5	T49.ØX6
Valium	T42.4X1	T42.4X2	T42.4X3	T42.4X4	T42.4X5	T42.4X6
Valmid	T42.6X1	T42.6X2	T42.6X3	T42.6X4	T42.6X5	T42.6X6
Valnoctamide	T42.6X1	T42.6X2	T42.6X3	T42.6X4	T42.6X5	T42.6X6
Valproate (sodium)	T42.6X1	T42.6X2	T42.6X3	T42.6X4	T42.6X5	T42.6X6
Valproic acid	T42.6X1	T42.6X2	T42.6X3	T42.6X4	T42.6X5	T42.6X6
Valpromide	T42.6X1	T42.6X2	T42.6X3	T42.6X4	T42.6X5	T42.6X6
Vanadium	T56.891	T56.892	T56.893	T56.894	—	—
Vancomycin	T36.8X1	T36.8X2	T36.8X3	T36.8X4	T36.8X5	T36.8X6
Vandazole*	T49.ØX1	T49.ØX2	T49.ØX3	T49.ØX4	T49.ØX5	T49.ØX6
Vapor — *see also* Gas	T59.91	T59.92	T59.93	T59.94	—	—
kiln (carbon monoxide)	T58.8X1	T58.8X2	T58.8X3	T58.8X4	—	—
lead — *see* lead						
specified source NEC	T59.891	T59.892	T59.893	T59.894	—	—
Vardenafil	T46.7X1	T46.7X2	T46.7X3	T46.7X4	T46.7X5	T46.7X6
Varicose reduction drug	T46.8X1	T46.8X2	T46.8X3	T46.8X4	T46.8X5	T46.8X6
Varnish	T65.4X1	T65.4X2	T65.4X3	T65.4X4	—	—

Substance	Poisoning, Accidental (unintentional)	Poisoning, Intentional Self-harm	Poisoning, Assault	Poisoning, Undetermined	Adverse Effect	Under-dosing
Varnish — *continued*						
cleaner	T52.91	T52.92	T52.93	T52.94	—	—
Vaseline	T49.3X1	T49.3X2	T49.3X3	T49.3X4	T49.3X5	T49.3X6
Vasodilan	T46.7X1	T46.7X2	T46.7X3	T46.7X4	T46.7X5	T46.7X6
Vasodilator						
coronary NEC	T46.3X1	T46.3X2	T46.3X3	T46.3X4	T46.3X5	T46.3X6
peripheral NEC	T46.7X1	T46.7X2	T46.7X3	T46.7X4	T46.7X5	T46.7X6
Vasopressin	T38.891	T38.892	T38.893	T38.894	T38.895	T38.896
Vasopressor drugs	T38.891	T38.892	T38.893	T38.894	T38.895	T38.896
Vecuronium bromide	T48.1X1	T48.1X2	T48.1X3	T48.1X4	T48.1X5	T48.1X6
Vegetable extract, astringent	T49.2X1	T49.2X2	T49.2X3	T49.2X4	T49.2X5	T49.2X6
Venlafaxine	T43.211	T43.212	T43.213	T43.214	T43.215	T43.216
Venom, venomous (bite) (sting)	T63.91	T63.92	T63.93	T63.94	—	—
amphibian NEC	T63.831	T63.832	T63.833	T63.834	—	—
animal NEC	T63.891	T63.892	T63.893	T63.894	—	—
ant	T63.421	T63.422	T63.423	T63.424	—	—
arthropod NEC	T63.481	T63.482	T63.483	T63.484	—	—
bee	T63.441	T63.442	T63.443	T63.444	—	—
centipede	T63.411	T63.412	T63.413	T63.414	—	—
fish	T63.591	T63.592	T63.593	T63.594	—	—
frog	T63.811	T63.812	T63.813	T63.814	—	—
hornet	T63.451	T63.452	T63.453	T63.454	—	—
insect NEC	T63.481	T63.482	T63.483	T63.484	—	—
lizard	T63.121	T63.122	T63.123	T63.124	—	—
marine						
animals	T63.691	T63.692	T63.693	T63.694	—	—
bluebottle	T63.611	T63.612	T63.613	T63.614	—	—
jellyfish NEC	T63.621	T63.622	T63.623	T63.624	—	—
Portuguese Man-o-war	T63.611	T63.612	T63.613	T63.614	—	—
sea anemone	T63.631	T63.632	T63.633	T63.634	—	—
specified NEC	T63.691	T63.692	T63.693	T63.694	—	—
fish	T63.591	T63.592	T63.593	T63.594	—	—
plants	T63.711	T63.712	T63.713	T63.714	—	—
sting ray	T63.511	T63.512	T63.513	T63.514	—	—
millipede (tropical)	T63.411	T63.412	T63.413	T63.414	—	—
plant NEC	T63.791	T63.792	T63.793	T63.794	—	—
marine	T63.711	T63.712	T63.713	T63.714	—	—
reptile	T63.191	T63.192	T63.193	T63.194	—	—
gila monster	T63.111	T63.112	T63.113	T63.114	—	—
lizard NEC	T63.121	T63.122	T63.123	T63.124	—	—
scorpion	T63.2X1	T63.2X2	T63.2X3	T63.2X4	—	—
snake	T63.ØØ1	T63.ØØ2	T63.ØØ3	T63.ØØ4	—	—
African NEC	T63.Ø81	T63.Ø82	T63.Ø83	T63.Ø84	—	—
American (North) (South) NEC	T63.Ø61	T63.Ø62	T63.Ø63	T63.Ø64	—	—
Asian	T63.Ø81	T63.Ø82	T63.Ø83	T63.Ø84	—	—
Australian	T63.Ø71	T63.Ø72	T63.Ø73	T63.Ø74	—	—
cobra	T63.Ø41	T63.Ø42	T63.Ø43	T63.Ø44	—	—
coral snake	T63.Ø21	T63.Ø22	T63.Ø23	T63.Ø24	—	—
rattlesnake	T63.Ø11	T63.Ø12	T63.Ø13	T63.Ø14	—	—
specified NEC	T63.Ø91	T63.Ø92	T63.Ø93	T63.Ø94	—	—
taipan	T63.Ø31	T63.Ø32	T63.Ø33	T63.Ø34	—	—
specified NEC	T63.891	T63.892	T63.893	T63.894	—	—
spider	T63.3Ø1	T63.3Ø2	T63.3Ø3	T63.3Ø4	—	—
black widow	T63.311	T63.312	T63.313	T63.314	—	—
brown recluse	T63.331	T63.332	T63.333	T63.334	—	—
specified NEC	T63.391	T63.392	T63.393	T63.394	—	—
tarantula	T63.321	T63.322	T63.323	T63.324	—	—
sting ray	T63.511	T63.512	T63.513	T63.514	—	—
toad	T63.821	T63.822	T63.823	T63.824	—	—
wasp	T63.461	T63.462	T63.463	T63.464	—	—
Venous sclerosing drug NEC	T46.8X1	T46.8X2	T46.8X3	T46.8X4	T46.8X5	T46.8X6
Ventavis*	T46.7X1	T46.7X2	T46.7X3	T46.7X4	T46.7X5	T46.7X6
Ventolin — *see* Albuterol						
Veramon	T42.3X1	T42.3X2	T42.3X3	T42.3X4	T42.3X5	T42.3X6
Verapamil	T46.1X1	T46.1X2	T46.1X3	T46.1X4	T46.1X5	T46.1X6
Veratrine	T46.5X1	T46.5X2	T46.5X3	T46.5X4	T46.5X5	T46.5X6
Veratrum						
album	T62.2X1	T62.2X2	T62.2X3	T62.2X4	—	—
alkaloids	T46.5X1	T46.5X2	T46.5X3	T46.5X4	T46.5X5	T46.5X6
viride	T62.2X1	T62.2X2	T62.2X3	T62.2X4	—	—
Verdigris	T6Ø.3X1	T6Ø.3X2	T6Ø.3X3	T6Ø.3X4	—	—
Veronal	T42.3X1	T42.3X2	T42.3X3	T42.3X4	T42.3X5	T42.3X6
Veroxil	T37.4X1	T37.4X2	T37.4X3	T37.4X4	T37.4X5	T37.4X6
Versenate	T5Ø.6X1	T5Ø.6X2	T5Ø.6X3	T5Ø.6X4	T5Ø.6X5	T5Ø.6X6
Versidyne	T39.8X1	T39.8X2	T39.8X3	T39.8X4	T39.8X5	T39.8X6
Vetrabutine	T48.ØX1	T48.ØX2	T48.ØX3	T48.ØX4	T48.ØX5	T48.ØX6
Vexol*	T49.5X1	T49.5X2	T49.5X3	T49.5X4	T49.5X5	T49.5X6
Victrelis*	T37.5X1	T37.5X2	T37.5X3	T37.5X4	T37.5X5	T37.5X6
Vidarabine	T37.5X1	T37.5X2	T37.5X3	T37.5X4	T37.5X5	T37.5X6

Substance	Poisoning, Accidental (unintentional)	Poisoning, Intentional Self-harm	Poisoning, Assault	Poisoning, Undetermined	Adverse Effect	Under-dosing
Vienna						
green	T57.ØX1	T57.ØX2	T57.ØX3	T57.ØX4	—	—
insecticide	T6Ø.2X1	T6Ø.2X2	T6Ø.2X3	T6Ø.2X4	—	—
red	T57.ØX1	T57.ØX2	T57.ØX3	T57.ØX4	—	—
pharmaceutical dye	T5Ø.991	T5Ø.992	T5Ø.993	T5Ø.994	T5Ø.995	T5Ø.996
Vigabatrin	T42.6X1	T42.6X2	T42.6X3	T42.6X4	T42.6X5	T42.6X6
Viloxazine	T43.291	T43.292	T43.293	T43.294	T43.295	T43.296
Viminol	T39.8X1	T39.8X2	T39.8X3	T39.8X4	T39.8X5	T39.8X6
Vinbarbital, vinbarbitone	T42.3X1	T42.3X2	T42.3X3	T42.3X4	T42.3X5	T42.3X6
Vinblastine	T45.1X1	T45.1X2	T45.1X3	T45.1X4	T45.1X5	T45.1X6
Vinburnine	T46.7X1	T46.7X2	T46.7X3	T46.7X4	T46.7X5	T46.7X6
Vincamine	T45.1X1	T45.1X2	T45.1X3	T45.1X4	T45.1X5	T45.1X6
Vincristine	T45.1X1	T45.1X2	T45.1X3	T45.1X4	T45.1X5	T45.1X6
Vindesine	T45.1X1	T45.1X2	T45.1X3	T45.1X4	T45.1X5	T45.1X6
Vinesthene, vinethene	T41.ØX1	T41.ØX2	T41.ØX3	T41.ØX4	T41.ØX5	T41.ØX6
Vinorelbine tartrate	T45.1X1	T45.1X2	T45.1X3	T45.1X4	T45.1X5	T45.1X6
Vinpocetine	T46.7X1	T46.7X2	T46.7X3	T46.7X4	T46.7X5	T46.7X6
Vinyl						
acetate	T65.891	T65.892	T65.893	T65.894	—	—
bital	T42.3X1	T42.3X2	T42.3X3	T42.3X4	T42.3X5	T42.3X6
bromide	T65.891	T65.892	T65.893	T65.894	—	—
chloride	T59.891	T59.892	T59.893	T59.894	—	—
ether	T41.ØX1	T41.ØX2	T41.ØX3	T41.ØX4	T41.ØX5	T41.ØX6
Vinylbital	T42.3X1	T42.3X2	T42.3X3	T42.3X4	T42.3X5	T42.3X6
Vinylidene chloride	T65.891	T65.892	T65.893	T65.894	—	—
Vioform	T37.8X1	T37.8X2	T37.8X3	T37.8X4	T37.8X5	T37.8X6
topical	T49.ØX1	T49.ØX2	T49.ØX3	T49.ØX4	T49.ØX5	T49.ØX6
Viokase*	T47.5X1	T47.5X2	T47.5X3	T47.5X4	T47.5X5	T47.5X6
Viomycin	T36.8X1	T36.8X2	T36.8X3	T36.8X4	T36.8X5	T36.8X6
Viosterol	T45.2X1	T45.2X2	T45.2X3	T45.2X4	T45.2X5	T45.2X6
Viper (venom)	T63.Ø91	T63.Ø92	T63.Ø93	T63.Ø94		
Viprynium	T37.4X1	T37.4X2	T37.4X3	T37.4X4	T37.4X5	T37.4X6
Viquidil	T46.7X1	T46.7X2	T46.7X3	T46.7X4	T46.7X5	T46.7X6
Viral vaccine NEC	T5Ø.B91	T5Ø.B92	T5Ø.B93	T5Ø.B94	T5Ø.B95	T5Ø.B96
Virginiamycin	T36.8X1	T36.8X2	T36.8X3	T36.8X4	T36.8X5	T36.8X6
Virugon	T37.5X1	T37.5X2	T37.5X3	T37.5X4	T37.5X5	T37.5X6
Viscous agent	T5Ø.9Ø1	T5Ø.9Ø2	T5Ø.9Ø3	T5Ø.9Ø4	T5Ø.9Ø5	T5Ø.9Ø6
Visine	T49.5X1	T49.5X2	T49.5X3	T49.5X4	T49.5X5	T49.5X6
Visnadine	T46.3X1	T46.3X2	T46.3X3	T46.3X4	T46.3X5	T46.3X6
Vitamin NEC	T45.2X1	T45.2X2	T45.2X3	T45.2X4	T45.2X5	T45.2X6
A	T45.2X1	T45.2X2	T45.2X3	T45.2X4	T45.2X5	T45.2X6
B1	T45.2X1	T45.2X2	T45.2X3	T45.2X4	T45.2X5	T45.2X6
B2	T45.2X1	T45.2X2	T45.2X3	T45.2X4	T45.2X5	T45.2X6
B6	T45.2X1	T45.2X2	T45.2X3	T45.2X4	T45.2X5	T45.2X6
B12	T45.2X1	T45.2X2	T45.2X3	T45.2X4	T45.2X5	T45.2X6
B15	T45.2X1	T45.2X2	T45.2X3	T45.2X4	T45.2X5	T45.2X6
B NEC	T45.2X1	T45.2X2	T45.2X3	T45.2X4	T45.2X5	T45.2X6
nicotinic acid	T46.7X1	T46.7X2	T46.7X3	T46.7X4	T46.7X5	T46.7X6
C	T45.2X1	T45.2X2	T45.2X3	T45.2X4	T45.2X5	T45.2X6
D	T45.2X1	T45.2X2	T45.2X3	T45.2X4	T45.2X5	T45.2X6
D2	T45.2X1	T45.2X2	T45.2X3	T45.2X4	T45.2X5	T45.2X6
D3	T45.2X1	T45.2X2	T45.2X3	T45.2X4	T45.2X5	T45.2X6
E	T45.2X1	T45.2X2	T45.2X3	T45.2X4	T45.2X5	T45.2X6
E acetate	T45.2X1	T45.2X2	T45.2X3	T45.2X4	T45.2X5	T45.2X6
hematopoietic	T45.8X1	T45.8X2	T45.8X3	T45.8X4	T45.8X5	T45.8X6
K1	T45.7X1	T45.7X2	T45.7X3	T45.7X4	T45.7X5	T45.7X6
K2	T45.7X1	T45.7X2	T45.7X3	T45.7X4	T45.7X5	T45.7X6
K NEC	T45.7X1	T45.7X2	T45.7X3	T45.7X4	T45.7X5	T45.7X6
PP	T45.2X1	T45.2X2	T45.2X3	T45.2X4	T45.2X5	T45.2X6
ulceroprotectant	T47.1X1	T47.1X2	T47.1X3	T47.1X4	T47.1X5	T47.1X6
Vleminckx's solution	T49.4X1	T49.4X2	T49.4X3	T49.4X4	T49.4X5	T49.4X6
Voltaren — *see* Diclofenac sodium						
Voraxaze*	T5Ø.6X1	T5Ø.6X2	T5Ø.6X3	T5Ø.6X4	T5Ø.6X5	T5Ø.6X6
Warfarin	T45.511	T45.512	T45.513	T45.514	T45.515	T45.516
rodenticide	T6Ø.4X1-	T6Ø.4X2-	T6Ø.4X3-	T6Ø.4X4-	—	—
sodium	T45.511	T45.512	T45.513	T45.514	T45.515	T45.516
Wasp (sting)	T63.461	T63.462	T63.463	T63.464	—	—
Water						
balance drug	T5Ø.3X1	T5Ø.3X2	T5Ø.3X3	T5Ø.3X4	T5Ø.3X5	T5Ø.3X6
distilled	T5Ø.3X1	T5Ø.3X2	T5Ø.3X3	T5Ø.3X4	T5Ø.3X5	T5Ø.3X6
gas — *see* Gas, water						
incomplete combustion of — *see* Carbon, monoxide, fuel, utility						
hemlock	T62.2X1	T62.2X2	T62.2X3	T62.2X4	—	—
moccasin (venom)	T63.Ø61	T63.Ø62	T63.Ø63	T63.Ø64		
purified	T5Ø.3X1	T5Ø.3X2	T5Ø.3X3	T5Ø.3X4	T5Ø.3X5	T5Ø.3X6
Wax (paraffin) (petroleum)	T52.ØX1	T52.ØX2	T52.ØX3	T52.ØX4	—	—
automobile	T65.891	T65.892	T65.893	T65.894	—	—
floor	T52.ØX1	T52.ØX2	T52.ØX3	T52.ØX4	—	—
Weed killers NEC	T6Ø.3X1	T6Ø.3X2	T6Ø.3X3	T6Ø.3X4	—	—
Wellbutrin*	T43.291	T43.292	T43.293	T43.294	T43.295	T43.296

Substance	Poisoning, Accidental (unintentional)	Poisoning, Intentional Self-harm	Poisoning, Assault	Poisoning, Undetermined	Adverse Effect	Under-dosing
Welldorm	T42.6X1	T42.6X2	T42.6X3	T42.6X4	T42.6X5	T42.6X6
Westcort*	T49.ØX1	T49.ØX2	T49.ØX3	T49.ØX4	T49.ØX5	T49.ØX6
White						
arsenic	T57.ØX1	T57.ØX2	T57.ØX3	T57.ØX4	—	—
hellebore	T62.2X1	T62.2X2	T62.2X3	T62.2X4	—	—
lotion (keratolytic)	T49.4X1	T49.4X2	T49.4X3	T49.4X4	T49.4X5	T49.4X6
spirit	T52.ØX1	T52.ØX2	T52.ØX3	T52.ØX4	—	—
Whitewash	T65.891	T65.892	T65.893	T65.894	—	—
Whole blood (human)	T45.8X1	T45.8X2	T45.8X3	T45.8X4	T45.8X5	T45.8X6
Wild						
black cherry	T62.2X1	T62.2X2	T62.2X3	T62.2X4	—	—
poisonous plants NEC	T62.2X1	T62.2X2	T62.2X3	T62.2X4	—	—
Window cleaning fluid	T65.891	T65.892	T65.893	T65.894	—	—
Wintergreen (oil)	T49.3X1	T49.3X2	T49.3X3	T49.3X4	T49.3X5	T49.3X6
Wisterine	T62.2X1	T62.2X2	T62.2X3	T62.2X4	—	—
Witch hazel	T49.2X1	T49.2X2	T49.2X3	T49.2X4	T49.2X5	T49.2X6
Wood alcohol or spirit	T51.1X1	T51.1X2	T51.1X3	T51.1X4	—	—
Wool fat (hydrous)	T49.3X1	T49.3X2	T49.3X3	T49.3X4	T49.3X5	T49.3X6
Woorali	T48.1X1	T48.1X2	T48.1X3	T48.1X4	T48.1X5	T48.1X6
Wormseed, American	T37.4X1	T37.4X2	T37.4X3	T37.4X4	T37.4X5	T37.4X6
Xamoterol	T44.5X1	T44.5X2	T44.5X3	T44.5X4	T44.5X5	T44.5X6
Xanax*	T42.4X1	T42.4X2	T42.4X3	T42.4X4	T42.4X5	T42.4X6
Xanthine diuretics	T50.2X1	T50.2X2	T50.2X3	T50.2X4	T50.2X5	T50.2X6
Xanthinol nicotinate	T46.7X1	T46.7X2	T46.7X3	T46.7X4	T46.7X5	T46.7X6
Xanthotoxin	T49.3X1	T49.3X2	T49.3X3	T49.3X4	T49.3X5	T49.3X6
Xantinol nicotinate	T46.7X1	T46.7X2	T46.7X3	T46.7X4	T46.7X5	T46.7X6
Xantocillin	T36.ØX1	T36.ØX2	T36.ØX3	T36.ØX4	T36.ØX5	T36.ØX6
Xenon (127Xe) (133Xe)	T5Ø.8X1	T5Ø.8X2	T5Ø.8X3	T5Ø.8X4	T5Ø.8X5	T5Ø.8X6
Xenysalate	T49.4X1	T49.4X2	T49.4X3	T49.4X4	T49.4X5	T49.4X6
Xibornol	T37.8X1	T37.8X2	T37.8X3	T37.8X4	T37.8X5	T37.8X6
Xigris	T45.511	T45.512	T45.513	T45.514	T45.515	T45.516
Xipamide	T5Ø.2X1	T5Ø.2X2	T5Ø.2X3	T5Ø.2X4	T5Ø.2X5	T5Ø.2X6
Xylene (vapor)	T52.2X1	T52.2X2	T52.2X3	T52.2X4	—	—
Xylocaine (infiltration) (topical)	T41.3X1	T41.3X2	T41.3X3	T41.3X4	T41.3X5	T41.3X6
nerve block (peripheral) (plexus)	T41.3X1	T41.3X2	T41.3X3	T41.3X4	T41.3X5	T41.3X6
spinal	T41.3X1	T41.3X2	T41.3X3	T41.3X4	T41.3X5	T41.3X6
Xylol (vapor)	T52.2X1	T52.2X2	T52.2X3	T52.2X4	—	—
Xylometazoline	T48.5X1	T48.5X2	T48.5X3	T48.5X4	T48.5X5	T48.5X6
Xylose*	T5Ø.8X1	T5Ø.8X2	T5Ø.8X3	T5Ø.8X4	T5Ø.8X5	T5Ø.8X6
Yaz*	T38.4X1	T38.4X2	T38.4X3	T38.4X4	T38.4X5	T38.4X6
Yeast	T45.2X1	T45.2X2	T45.2X3	T45.2X4	T45.2X5	T45.2X6
dried	T45.2X1	T45.2X2	T45.2X3	T45.2X4	T45.2X5	T45.2X6
Yellow						
fever vaccine	T5Ø.B91	T5Ø.B92	T5Ø.B93	T5Ø.B94	T5Ø.B95	T5Ø.B96
jasmine	T62.2X1	T62.2X2	T62.2X3	T62.2X4	—	—
phenolphthalein	T47.2X1	T47.2X2	T47.2X3	T47.2X4	T47.2X5	T47.2X6
Yervoy*	T45.1X1	T45.1X2	T45.1X3	T45.1X4	T45.1X5	T45.1X6
Yew	T62.2X1	T62.2X2	T62.2X3	T62.2X4	—	—
Yohimbic acid	T4Ø.991	T4Ø.992	T4Ø.993	T4Ø.994	T4Ø.995	T4Ø.996
Zactane	T39.8X1	T39.8X2	T39.8X3	T39.8X4	T39.8X5	T39.8X6
Zalcitabine	T37.5X1	T37.5X2	T37.5X3	T37.5X4	T37.5X5	T37.5X6
Zanaflex*	T48.1X1	T48.1X2	T48.1X3	T48.1X4	T48.1X5	T48.1X6
Zaroxolyn	T5Ø.2X1	T5Ø.2X2	T5Ø.2X3	T5Ø.2X4	T5Ø.2X5	T5Ø.2X6
Zephiran (topical)	T49.ØX1	T49.ØX2	T49.ØX3	T49.ØX4	T49.ØX5	T49.ØX6
ophthalmic preparation	T49.5X1	T49.5X2	T49.5X3	T49.5X4	T49.5X5	T49.5X6
Zeranol	T38.7X1	T38.7X2	T38.7X3	T38.7X4	T38.7X5	T38.7X6
Zerone	T51.1X1	T51.1X2	T51.1X3	T51.1X4	—	—
Zidovudine	T37.5X1	T37.5X2	T37.5X3	T37.5X4	T37.5X5	T37.5X6
Zilactin*	T41.3X1	T41.3X2	T41.3X3	T41.3X4	T41.3X5	T41.3X6
Zimeldine	T43.221	T43.222	T43.223	T43.224	T43.225	T43.226
Zinc (compounds) (fumes) (vapor) NEC	T56.5X1	T56.5X2	T56.5X3	T56.5X4	—	—
anti-infectives	T49.ØX1	T49.ØX2	T49.ØX3	T49.ØX4	T49.ØX5	T49.ØX6
antivaricose	T46.8X1	T46.8X2	T46.8X3	T46.8X4	T46.8X5	T46.8X6
bacitracin	T49.ØX1	T49.ØX2	T49.ØX3	T49.ØX4	T49.ØX5	T49.ØX6
chloride (mouthwash)	T49.6X1	T49.6X2	T49.6X3	T49.6X4	T49.6X5	T49.6X6
chromate	T56.5X1	T56.5X2	T56.5X3	T56.5X4	—	—
gelatin	T49.3X1	T49.3X2	T49.3X3	T49.3X4	T49.3X5	T49.3X6
oxide	T49.3X1	T49.3X2	T49.3X3	T49.3X4	T49.3X5	T49.3X6
plaster	T49.3X1	T49.3X2	T49.3X3	T49.3X4	T49.3X5	T49.3X6
peroxide	T49.ØX1	T49.ØX2	T49.ØX3	T49.ØX4	T49.ØX5	T49.ØX6
pesticides	T56.5X1	T56.5X2	T56.5X3	T56.5X4	—	—
phosphide	T6Ø.4X1	T6Ø.4X2	T6Ø.4X3	T6Ø.4X4	—	—
pyrithionate	T49.4X1	T49.4X2	T49.4X3	T49.4X4	T49.4X5	T49.4X6
stearate	T49.3X1	T49.3X2	T49.3X3	T49.3X4	T49.3X5	T49.3X6
sulfate	T49.5X1	T49.5X2	T49.5X3	T49.5X4	T49.5X5	T49.5X6
ENT agent	T49.6X1	T49.6X2	T49.6X3	T49.6X4	T49.6X5	T49.6X6
ophthalmic solution	T49.5X1	T49.5X2	T49.5X3	T49.5X4	T49.5X5	T49.5X6
topical NEC	T49.ØX1	T49.ØX2	T49.ØX3	T49.ØX4	T49.ØX5	T49.ØX6
undecylenate	T49.ØX1	T49.ØX2	T49.ØX3	T49.ØX4	T49.ØX5	T49.ØX6
Zineb	T6Ø.ØX1	T6Ø.ØX2	T6Ø.ØX3	T6Ø.ØX4	—	—
Zinostatin	T45.1X1	T45.1X2	T45.1X3	T45.1X4	T45.1X5	T45.1X6
Zipeprol	T48.3X1	T48.3X2	T48.3X3	T48.3X4	T48.3X5	T48.3X6
Zofenopril	T46.4X1	T46.4X2	T46.4X3	T46.4X4	T46.4X5	T46.4X6
Zolpidem	T42.6X1	T42.6X2	T42.6X3	T42.6X4	T42.6X5	T42.6X6
Zomepirac	T39.391	T39.392	T39.393	T39.394	T39.395	T39.396
Zopiclone	T42.6X1	T42.6X2	T42.6X3	T42.6X4	T42.6X5	T42.6X6
Zorubicin	T45.1X1	T45.1X2	T45.1X3	T45.1X4	T45.1X5	T45.1X6
Zotepine	T43.591	T43.592	T43.593	T43.594	T43.595	T43.596
Zovant	T45.511	T45.512	T45.513	T45.514	T45.515	T45.516
Zoxazolamine	T42.8X1	T42.8X2	T42.8X3	T42.8X4	T42.8X5	T42.8X6
Zuclopenthixol	T43.4X1	T43.4X2	T43.4X3	T43.4X4	T43.4X5	T43.4X6
Zyflo*	T48.6X1	T48.6X2	T48.6X3	T48.6X4	T48.6X5	T48.6X6
Zygadenus (venenosus)	T62.2X1	T62.2X2	T62.2X3	T62.2X4	—	—
Zyprexa	T43.591	T43.592	T43.593	T43.594	T43.595	T43.596
Zyzal*	T45.ØX1	T45.ØX2	T45.ØX3	T45.ØX4	T45.ØX5	T45.ØX6

A

- **Abandonment** (causing exposure to weather conditions) (with intent to injure or kill) NEC X58 ☑
- **Abuse** (adult) (child) (mental) (physical) (sexual) X58 ☑
- **Accident** (to) X58 ☑
  - aircraft (in transit) (powered) — *see also* Accident, transport, aircraft
    - due to, caused by cataclysm — *see* Forces of nature, by type
  - animal-drawn vehicle — *see* Accident, transport, animal-drawn vehicle occupant
  - animal-rider — *see* Accident, transport, animal-rider
  - automobile — *see* Accident, transport, car occupant
  - bare foot water skier V94.4 ☑
  - boat, boating — *see also* Accident, watercraft
    - striking swimmer
      - powered V94.11 ☑
      - unpowered V94.12 ☑
  - bus — *see* Accident, transport, bus occupant
  - cable car, not on rails V98.Ø ☑
    - on rails — *see* Accident, transport, streetcar occupant
  - car — *see* Accident, transport, car occupant
  - caused by, due to
    - animal NEC W64 ☑
    - chain hoist W24.Ø ☑
    - cold (excessive) — *see* Exposure, cold
    - corrosive liquid, substance — *see* Table of Drugs and Chemicals
    - cutting or piercing instrument — *see* Contact, with, by type of instrument
    - drive belt W24.Ø ☑
    - electric
      - current — *see* Exposure, electric current
      - motor — *see also* Contact, with, by type of machine W31.3 ☑
        - current (of) W86.8 ☑
    - environmental factor NEC X58 ☑
    - explosive material — *see* Explosion
    - fire, flames — *see* Exposure, fire
    - firearm missile — *see* Discharge, firearm by type
    - heat (excessive) — *see* Heat
    - hot — *see* Contact, with, hot
    - ignition — *see* Ignition
    - lifting device W24.Ø ☑
    - lightning — *see* subcategory T75.Ø ☑
      - causing fire — *see* Exposure, fire
    - machine, machinery — *see* Contact, with, by type of machine
    - natural factor NEC X58 ☑
    - pulley (block) W24.Ø ☑
    - radiation — *see* Radiation
    - steam X13.1 ☑
      - inhalation X13.Ø ☑
      - pipe X16 ☑
    - thunderbolt — *see* subcategory T75.Ø ☑
      - causing fire — *see* Exposure, fire
    - transmission device W24.1 ☑
  - coach — *see* Accident, transport, bus occupant
  - coal car — *see* Accident, transport, industrial vehicle occupant
  - diving — *see also* Fall, into, water
    - with
      - drowning or submersion — *see* Drowning
  - forklift — *see* Accident, transport, industrial vehicle occupant
  - heavy transport vehicle NOS — *see* Accident, transport, truck occupant
  - ice yacht V98.2 ☑
  - in
    - medical, surgical procedure
      - as, or due to misadventure — *see* Misadventure
      - causing an abnormal reaction or later complication without mention of misadventure — *see also* Complication of or following, by type of procedure Y84.9
  - land yacht V98.1 ☑
  - late effect of — *see* WØØ-X58 with 7th character S
  - logging car — *see* Accident, transport, industrial vehicle occupant
  - machine, machinery — *see also* Contact, with, by type of machine
    - on board watercraft V93.69 ☑
      - explosion — *see* Explosion, in, watercraft

Accident — *continued*

  - machine, machinery — *see also* Contact, with, by type of machine — *continued*
    - on board watercraft — *continued*
      - fire — *see* Burn, on board watercraft
      - powered craft V93.63 ☑
        - ferry boat V93.61 ☑
        - fishing boat V93.62 ☑
        - jetskis V93.63 ☑
        - liner V93.61 ☑
        - merchant ship V93.6Ø ☑
        - passenger ship V93.61 ☑
        - sailboat V93.64 ☑
  - mine tram — *see* Accident, transport, industrial vehicle occupant
  - mobility scooter (motorized) — *see* Accident, transport, pedestrian, conveyance, specified type NEC
  - motor scooter — *see* Accident, transport, motorcyclist
  - motor vehicle NOS (traffic) — *see also* Accident, transport V89.2 ☑
    - nontraffic V89.Ø ☑
    - three-wheeled NOS — *see* Accident, transport, three-wheeled motor vehicle occupant
  - motorcycle NOS — *see* Accident, transport, motorcyclist
  - nonmotor vehicle NOS (nontraffic) — *see also* Accident, transport V89.1 ☑
    - traffic NOS V89.3 ☑
  - nontraffic (victim's mode of transport NOS) V88.9 ☑
    - collision (between) V88.7 ☑
      - bus and truck V88.5 ☑
      - car and:
        - bus V88.3 ☑
        - pickup V88.2 ☑
        - three-wheeled motor vehicle V88.Ø ☑
        - train V88.6 ☑
        - truck V88.4 ☑
        - two-wheeled motor vehicle V88.Ø ☑
        - van V88.2 ☑
      - specified vehicle NEC and:
        - three-wheeled motor vehicle V88.1 ☑
        - two-wheeled motor vehicle V88.1 ☑
    - known mode of transport — *see* Accident, transport, by type of vehicle
    - noncollision V88.8 ☑
  - on board watercraft V93.89 ☑
    - powered craft V93.83 ☑
      - ferry boat V93.81 ☑
      - fishing boat V93.82 ☑
      - jetskis V93.83 ☑
      - liner V93.81 ☑
      - merchant ship V93.8Ø ☑
      - passenger ship V93.81 ☑
    - unpowered craft V93.88 ☑
      - canoe V93.85 ☑
      - inflatable V93.86 ☑
        - in tow
          - recreational V94.31 ☑
          - specified NEC V94.32 ☑
      - kayak V93.85 ☑
      - sailboat V93.84 ☑
      - surf-board V93.88 ☑
      - water skis V93.87 ☑
      - windsurfer V93.88 ☑
  - parachutist V97.29 ☑
    - entangled in object V97.21 ☑
    - injured on landing V97.22 ☑
  - pedal cycle — *see* Accident, transport, pedal cyclist
  - pedestrian (on foot)
    - with
      - another pedestrian W51 ☑
        - on pedestrian conveyance NEC VØØ.Ø9 ☑
        - with fall WØ3 ☑
          - due to ice or snow WØØ.Ø ☑
      - rider of
        - hoverboard VØØ.Ø38 ☑
        - Segway VØØ.Ø38 ☑
        - standing
          - electric scooter VØØ.Ø31 ☑
          - micro-mobility pedestrian conveyance NEC VØØ.Ø38 ☑
        - roller skater (in-line) VØØ.Ø1 ☑
        - skate boarder VØØ.Ø2 ☑
      - transport vehicle — *see* Accident, transport
    - on pedestrian conveyance — *see* Accident, transport, pedestrian, conveyance

Accident — *continued*

  - pick-up truck or van — *see* Accident, transport, pickup truck occupant
  - quarry truck — *see* Accident, transport, industrial vehicle occupant
  - railway vehicle (any) (in motion) — *see* Accident, transport, railway vehicle occupant
    - due to cataclysm — *see* Forces of nature, by type
  - scooter (non-motorized) — *see* Accident, transport, pedestrian, conveyance, scooter
  - sequelae of — *see* categories WØØ-X58 with 7th character S
  - skateboard — *see* Accident, transport, pedestrian, conveyance, skateboard
  - ski(ing) — *see* Accident, transport, pedestrian, conveyance
    - lift V98.3 ☑
  - specified cause NEC X58 ☑
  - streetcar — *see* Accident, transport, streetcar occupant
  - traffic (victim's mode of transport NOS) V87.9 ☑
    - collision (between) V87.7 ☑
      - bus and truck V87.5 ☑
      - car and:
        - bus V87.3 ☑
        - pickup V87.2 ☑
        - three-wheeled motor vehicle V87.Ø ☑
        - train V87.6 ☑
        - truck V87.4 ☑
        - two-wheeled motor vehicle V87.Ø ☑
        - van V87.2 ☑
      - specified vehicle NEC V86.39 ☑
        - and
          - three-wheeled motor vehicle V87.1 ☑
          - two-wheeled motor vehicle V87.1 ☑
        - driver V86.Ø9 ☑
        - passenger V86.19 ☑
        - person on outside V86.29 ☑
        - while boarding or alighting V86.49 ☑
    - known mode of transport — *see* Accident, transport, by type of vehicle
    - noncollision V87.8 ☑
  - transport (involving injury to) V99 ☑
    - 18 wheeler — *see* Accident, transport, truck occupant
    - agricultural vehicle occupant (nontraffic) V84.9 ☑
      - driver V84.5 ☑
      - hanger-on V84.7 ☑
      - passenger V84.6 ☑
      - traffic V84.3 ☑
        - driver V84.Ø ☑
        - hanger-on V84.2 ☑
        - passenger V84.1 ☑
      - while boarding or alighting V84.4 ☑
    - aircraft NEC V97.89 ☑
      - military NEC V97.818 ☑
        - civilian injured by V97.811 ☑
        - with civilian aircraft V97.81Ø ☑
      - occupant injured (in)
        - nonpowered craft accident V96.9 ☑
          - balloon V96.ØØ ☑
            - collision V96.Ø3 ☑
            - crash V96.Ø1 ☑
            - explosion V96.Ø5 ☑
            - fire V96.Ø4 ☑
            - forced landing V96.Ø2 ☑
            - specified type NEC V96.Ø9 ☑
          - glider V96.2Ø ☑
            - collision V96.23 ☑
            - crash V96.21 ☑
            - explosion V96.25 ☑
            - fire V96.24 ☑
            - forced landing V96.22 ☑
            - specified type NEC V96.29 ☑
          - hang glider V96.1Ø ☑
            - collision V96.13 ☑
            - crash V96.11 ☑
            - explosion V96.15 ☑
            - fire V96.14 ☑
            - forced landing V96.12 ☑
            - specified type NEC V96.19 ☑
          - specified craft NEC V96.8 ☑
        - powered craft accident V95.9 ☑
          - fixed wing NEC
            - commercial V95.3Ø ☑
              - collision V95.33 ☑
              - crash V95.31 ☑

- **Accident** — *continued*
  - transport — *continued*
    - aircraft — *continued*
      - occupant injured — *continued*
        - powered craft accident — *continued*
          - fixed wing — *continued*
            - commercial — *continued*
              - explosion V95.35 ☑
              - fire V95.34 ☑
              - forced landing V95.32 ☑
              - specified type NEC V95.39 ☑
            - private V95.2Ø ☑
              - collision V95.23 ☑
              - crash V95.21 ☑
              - explosion V95.25 ☑
              - fire V95.24 ☑
              - forced landing V95.22 ☑
              - specified type NEC V95.29 ☑
          - glider V95.1Ø ☑
            - collision V95.13 ☑
            - crash V95.11 ☑
            - explosion V95.15 ☑
            - fire V95.14 ☑
            - forced landing V95.12 ☑
            - specified type NEC V95.19 ☑
          - helicopter V95.ØØ ☑
            - collision V95.Ø3 ☑
            - crash V95.Ø1 ☑
            - explosion V95.Ø5 ☑
            - fire V95.Ø4 ☑
            - forced landing V95.Ø2 ☑
            - specified type NEC V95.Ø9 ☑
          - spacecraft V95.4Ø ☑
            - collision V95.43 ☑
            - crash V95.41 ☑
            - explosion V95.45 ☑
            - fire V95.44 ☑
            - forced landing V95.42 ☑
            - specified type NEC V95.49 ☑
          - specified craft NEC V95.8 ☑
          - ultralight V95.1Ø ☑
            - collision V95.13 ☑
            - crash V95.11 ☑
            - explosion V95.15 ☑
            - fire V95.14 ☑
            - forced landing V95.12 ☑
            - specified type NEC V95.19 ☑
        - specified accident NEC V97.Ø ☑
        - while boarding or alighting V97.1 ☑
      - person (injured by)
        - falling from, in or on aircraft V97.Ø ☑
        - machinery on aircraft V97.89 ☑
        - on ground with aircraft involvement V97.39 ☑
        - rotating propeller V97.32 ☑
        - struck by object falling from aircraft V97.31 ☑
        - sucked into aircraft jet V97.33 ☑
        - while boarding or alighting aircraft V97.1 ☑
    - airport (battery-powered) passenger vehicle — *see* Accident, transport, industrial vehicle occupant
    - all-terrain vehicle occupant (nontraffic) V86.95 ☑
      - driver V86.55 ☑
      - dune buggy — *see* Accident, transport, dune buggy occupant
      - hanger-on V86.75 ☑
      - passenger V86.65 ☑
      - snowmobile — *see* Accident, transport, snowmobile occupant
      - specified type NEC V86.99 ☑
        - driver V86.59 ☑
        - passenger V86.69 ☑
        - person on outside V86.79 ☑
      - traffic V86.35 ☑
        - driver V86.Ø5 ☑
        - hanger-on V86.25 ☑
        - passenger V86.15 ☑
      - while boarding or alighting V86.45 ☑
    - ambulance occupant (traffic) V86.31 ☑
      - driver V86.Ø1 ☑
      - hanger-on V86.21 ☑
      - nontraffic V86.91 ☑
        - driver V86.51 ☑
        - hanger-on V86.71 ☑
        - passenger V86.61 ☑
      - passenger V86.11 ☑

- **Accident** — *continued*
  - transport — *continued*
    - ambulance occupant — *continued*
      - while boarding or alighting V86.41 ☑
    - animal-drawn vehicle occupant (in) V8Ø.929 ☑
      - collision (with)
        - animal V8Ø.12 ☑
          - being ridden V8Ø.711 ☑
        - animal-drawn vehicle V8Ø.721 ☑
        - bus V8Ø.42 ☑
        - car V8Ø.42 ☑
        - fixed or stationary object V8Ø.82 ☑
        - military vehicle V8Ø.92Ø ☑
        - nonmotor vehicle V8Ø.791 ☑
        - pedal cycle V8Ø.22 ☑
        - pedestrian V8Ø.12 ☑
        - pickup V8Ø.42 ☑
        - railway train or vehicle V8Ø.62 ☑
        - specified motor vehicle NEC V8Ø.52 ☑
        - streetcar V8Ø.731 ☑
        - truck V8Ø.42 ☑
        - two- or three-wheeled motor vehicle V8Ø.32 ☑
        - van V8Ø.42 ☑
      - noncollision V8Ø.Ø2 ☑
      - specified circumstance NEC V8Ø.928 ☑
    - animal-rider V8Ø.919 ☑
      - collision (with)
        - animal V8Ø.11 ☑
          - being ridden V8Ø.71Ø ☑
        - animal-drawn vehicle V8Ø.72Ø ☑
        - bus V8Ø.41 ☑
        - car V8Ø.41 ☑
        - fixed or stationary object V8Ø.81 ☑
        - military vehicle V8Ø.91Ø ☑
        - nonmotor vehicle V8Ø.79Ø ☑
        - pedal cycle V8Ø.21 ☑
        - pedestrian V8Ø.11 ☑
        - pickup V8Ø.41 ☑
        - railway train or vehicle V8Ø.61 ☑
        - specified motor vehicle NEC V8Ø.51 ☑
        - streetcar V8Ø.73Ø ☑
        - truck V8Ø.41 ☑
        - two- or three-wheeled motor vehicle V8Ø.31 ☑
        - van V8Ø.41 ☑
      - noncollision V8Ø.Ø18 ☑
        - specified as horse rider V8Ø.Ø1Ø ☑
      - specified circumstance NEC V8Ø.918 ☑
    - armored car — *see* Accident, transport, truck occupant
    - battery-powered truck (baggage) (mail) — *see* Accident, transport, industrial vehicle occupant
    - bus occupant V79.9 ☑
      - collision (with)
        - animal (traffic) V7Ø.9 ☑
          - being ridden (traffic) V76.9 ☑
            - nontraffic V76.3 ☑
              - while boarding or alighting V76.4 ☑
          - nontraffic V7Ø.3 ☑
          - while boarding or alighting V7Ø.4 ☑
        - animal-drawn vehicle (traffic) V76.9 ☑
          - nontraffic V76.3 ☑
          - while boarding or alighting V76.4 ☑
        - bus (traffic) V74.9 ☑
          - nontraffic V74.3 ☑
          - while boarding or alighting V74.4 ☑
        - car (traffic) V73.9 ☑
          - nontraffic V73.3 ☑
          - while boarding or alighting V73.4 ☑
        - motor vehicle NOS (traffic) V79.6Ø ☑
          - nontraffic V79.2Ø ☑
          - specified type NEC (traffic) V79.69 ☑
            - nontraffic V79.29 ☑
        - pedal cycle (traffic) V71.9 ☑
          - nontraffic V71.3 ☑
          - while boarding or alighting V71.4 ☑
        - pickup truck (traffic) V73.9 ☑
          - nontraffic V73.3 ☑
          - while boarding or alighting V73.4 ☑
        - railway vehicle (traffic) V75.9 ☑
          - nontraffic V75.3 ☑
          - while boarding or alighting V75.4 ☑
        - specified vehicle NEC (traffic) V76.9 ☑
          - nontraffic V76.3 ☑
          - while boarding or alighting V76.4 ☑

- **Accident** — *continued*
  - transport — *continued*
    - bus occupant — *continued*
      - collision — *continued*
        - stationary object (traffic) V77.9 ☑
          - nontraffic V77.3 ☑
          - while boarding or alighting V77.4 ☑
        - streetcar (traffic) V76.9 ☑
          - nontraffic V76.3 ☑
          - while boarding or alighting V76.4 ☑
        - three wheeled motor vehicle (traffic) V72.9 ☑
          - nontraffic V72.3 ☑
          - while boarding or alighting V72.4 ☑
        - truck (traffic) V74.9 ☑
          - nontraffic V74.3 ☑
          - while boarding or alighting V74.4 ☑
        - two wheeled motor vehicle (traffic) V72.9 ☑
          - nontraffic V72.3 ☑
          - while boarding or alighting V72.4 ☑
        - van (traffic) V73.9 ☑
          - nontraffic V73.3 ☑
          - while boarding or alighting V73.4 ☑
      - driver
        - collision (with)
          - animal (traffic) V7Ø.5 ☑
            - being ridden (traffic) V76.5 ☑
              - nontraffic V76.Ø ☑
            - nontraffic V7Ø.Ø ☑
          - animal-drawn vehicle (traffic) V76.5 ☑
            - nontraffic V76.Ø ☑
          - bus (traffic) V74.5 ☑
            - nontraffic V74.Ø ☑
          - car (traffic) V73.5 ☑
            - nontraffic V73.Ø ☑
          - motor vehicle NOS (traffic) V79.4Ø ☑
            - nontraffic V79.ØØ ☑
            - specified type NEC (traffic) V79.49 ☑
              - nontraffic V79.Ø9 ☑
          - pedal cycle (traffic) V71.5 ☑
            - nontraffic V71.Ø ☑
          - pickup truck (traffic) V73.5 ☑
            - nontraffic V73.Ø ☑
          - railway vehicle (traffic) V75.5 ☑
            - nontraffic V75.Ø ☑
          - specified vehicle NEC (traffic) V76.5 ☑
            - nontraffic V76.Ø ☑
          - stationary object (traffic) V77.5 ☑
            - nontraffic V77.Ø ☑
          - streetcar (traffic) V76.5 ☑
            - nontraffic V76.Ø ☑
          - three wheeled motor vehicle (traffic) V72.5 ☑
            - nontraffic V72.Ø ☑
          - truck (traffic) V74.5 ☑
            - nontraffic V74.Ø ☑
          - two wheeled motor vehicle (traffic) V72.5 ☑
            - nontraffic V72.Ø ☑
          - van (traffic) V73.5 ☑
            - nontraffic V73.Ø ☑
        - noncollision accident (traffic) V78.5 ☑
          - nontraffic V78.Ø ☑
      - hanger-on
        - collision (with)
          - animal (traffic) V7Ø.7 ☑
            - being ridden (traffic) V76.7 ☑
              - nontraffic V76.2 ☑
            - nontraffic V7Ø.2 ☑
          - animal-drawn vehicle (traffic) V76.7 ☑
            - nontraffic V76.2 ☑
          - bus (traffic) V74.7 ☑
            - nontraffic V74.2 ☑
          - car (traffic) V73.7 ☑
            - nontraffic V73.2 ☑
          - pedal cycle (traffic) V71.7 ☑
            - nontraffic V71.2 ☑
          - pickup truck (traffic) V73.7 ☑
            - nontraffic V73.2 ☑
          - railway vehicle (traffic) V75.7 ☑
            - nontraffic V75.2 ☑
          - specified vehicle NEC (traffic) V76.7 ☑
            - nontraffic V76.2 ☑
          - stationary object (traffic) V77.7 ☑
            - nontraffic V77.2 ☑
          - streetcar (traffic) V76.7 ☑
            - nontraffic V76.2 ☑

- **Accident** — *continued*
  - transport — *continued*
    - bus occupant — *continued*
      - hanger-on — *continued*
        - collision — *continued*
          - three wheeled motor vehicle (traffic) V72.7 ☑
            - nontraffic V72.2 ☑
          - truck (traffic) V74.7 ☑
            - nontraffic V74.2 ☑
          - two wheeled motor vehicle (traffic) V72.7 ☑
            - nontraffic V72.2 ☑
          - van (traffic) V73.7 ☑
            - nontraffic V73.2 ☑
        - noncollision accident (traffic) V78.7 ☑
          - nontraffic V78.2 ☑
      - noncollision accident (traffic) V78.9 ☑
        - nontraffic V78.3 ☑
        - while boarding or alighting V78.4 ☑
      - nontraffic V79.3 ☑
      - passenger
        - collision (with)
          - animal (traffic) V70.6 ☑
            - being ridden (traffic) V76.6 ☑
              - nontraffic V76.1 ☑
            - nontraffic V70.1 ☑
          - animal-drawn vehicle (traffic) V76.6 ☑
            - nontraffic V76.1 ☑
          - bus (traffic) V74.6 ☑
            - nontraffic V74.1 ☑
          - car (traffic) V73.6 ☑
            - nontraffic V73.1 ☑
          - motor vehicle NOS (traffic) V79.50 ☑
            - nontraffic V79.10 ☑
            - specified type NEC (traffic) V79.59 ☑
              - nontraffic V79.19 ☑
          - pedal cycle (traffic) V71.6 ☑
            - nontraffic V71.1 ☑
          - pickup truck (traffic) V73.6 ☑
            - nontraffic V73.1 ☑
          - railway vehicle (traffic) V75.6 ☑
            - nontraffic V75.1 ☑
          - specified vehicle NEC (traffic) V76.6 ☑
            - nontraffic V76.1 ☑
          - stationary object (traffic) V77.6 ☑
            - nontraffic V77.1 ☑
          - streetcar (traffic) V76.6 ☑
            - nontraffic V76.1 ☑
          - three wheeled motor vehicle (traffic) V72.6 ☑
            - nontraffic V72.1 ☑
          - truck (traffic) V74.6 ☑
            - nontraffic V74.1 ☑
          - two wheeled motor vehicle (traffic) V72.6 ☑
            - nontraffic V72.1 ☑
          - van (traffic) V73.6 ☑
            - nontraffic V73.1 ☑
        - noncollision accident (traffic) V78.6 ☑
          - nontraffic V78.1 ☑
      - specified type NEC V79.88 ☑
      - military vehicle V79.81 ☑
    - cable car, not on rails V98.0 ☑
      - on rails — *see* Accident, transport, streetcar occupant
    - car occupant V49.9 ☑
      - ambulance occupant — *see* Accident, transport, ambulance occupant
      - collision (with)
        - animal (traffic) V40.9 ☑
          - being ridden (traffic) V46.9 ☑
            - nontraffic V46.3 ☑
              - while boarding or alighting V46.4 ☑
          - nontraffic V40.3 ☑
          - while boarding or alighting V40.4 ☑
        - animal-drawn vehicle (traffic) V46.9 ☑
          - nontraffic V46.3 ☑
          - while boarding or alighting V46.4 ☑
        - bus (traffic) V44.9 ☑
          - nontraffic V44.3 ☑
          - while boarding or alighting V44.4 ☑
        - car (traffic) V43.92 ☑
          - nontraffic V43.32 ☑
          - while boarding or alighting V43.42 ☑
        - motor vehicle NOS (traffic) V49.60 ☑

- **Accident** — *continued*
  - transport — *continued*
    - car occupant — *continued*
      - collision — *continued*
        - motor vehicle — *continued*
          - nontraffic V49.20 ☑
          - specified type NEC (traffic) V49.69 ☑
            - nontraffic V49.29 ☑
        - pedal cycle (traffic) V41.9 ☑
          - nontraffic V41.3 ☑
          - while boarding or alighting V41.4 ☑
        - pickup truck (traffic) V43.93 ☑
          - nontraffic V43.33 ☑
          - while boarding or alighting V43.43 ☑
        - railway vehicle (traffic) V45.9 ☑
          - nontraffic V45.3 ☑
          - while boarding or alighting V45.4 ☑
        - specified vehicle NEC (traffic) V46.9 ☑
          - nontraffic V46.3 ☑
          - while boarding or alighting V46.4 ☑
        - sport utility vehicle (traffic) V43.91 ☑
          - nontraffic V43.31 ☑
          - while boarding or alighting V43.41 ☑
        - stationary object (traffic) V47.9 ☑
          - nontraffic V47.3 ☑
          - while boarding or alighting V47.4 ☑
        - streetcar (traffic) V46.9 ☑
          - nontraffic V46.3 ☑
          - while boarding or alighting V46.4 ☑
        - three wheeled motor vehicle (traffic) V42.9 ☑
          - nontraffic V42.3 ☑
          - while boarding or alighting V42.4 ☑
        - truck (traffic) V44.9 ☑
          - nontraffic V44.3 ☑
          - while boarding or alighting V44.4 ☑
        - two wheeled motor vehicle (traffic) V42.9 ☑
          - nontraffic V42.3 ☑
          - while boarding or alighting V42.4 ☑
        - van (traffic) V43.94 ☑
          - nontraffic V43.34 ☑
          - while boarding or alighting V43.44 ☑
      - driver
        - collision (with)
          - animal (traffic) V40.5 ☑
            - being ridden (traffic) V46.5 ☑
              - nontraffic V46.0 ☑
            - nontraffic V40.0 ☑
          - animal-drawn vehicle (traffic) V46.5 ☑
            - nontraffic V46.0 ☑
          - bus (traffic) V44.5 ☑
            - nontraffic V44.0 ☑
          - car (traffic) V43.52 ☑
            - nontraffic V43.02 ☑
          - motor vehicle NOS (traffic) V49.40 ☑
            - nontraffic V49.00 ☑
            - specified type NEC (traffic) V49.49 ☑
              - nontraffic V49.09 ☑
          - pedal cycle (traffic) V41.5 ☑
            - nontraffic V41.0 ☑
          - pickup truck (traffic) V43.53 ☑
            - nontraffic V43.03 ☑
          - railway vehicle (traffic) V45.5 ☑
            - nontraffic V45.0 ☑
          - specified vehicle NEC (traffic) V46.5 ☑
            - nontraffic V46.0 ☑
          - sport utility vehicle (traffic) V43.51 ☑
            - nontraffic V43.01 ☑
          - stationary object (traffic) V47.5 ☑
            - nontraffic V47.0 ☑
          - streetcar (traffic) V46.5 ☑
            - nontraffic V46.0 ☑
          - three wheeled motor vehicle (traffic) V42.5 ☑
            - nontraffic V42.0 ☑
          - truck (traffic) V44.5 ☑
            - nontraffic V44.0 ☑
          - two wheeled motor vehicle (traffic) V42.5 ☑
            - nontraffic V42.0 ☑
          - van (traffic) V43.54 ☑
            - nontraffic V43.04 ☑
        - noncollision accident (traffic) V48.5 ☑
          - nontraffic V48.0 ☑
      - hanger-on
        - collision (with)
          - animal (traffic) V40.7 ☑

- **Accident** — *continued*
  - transport — *continued*
    - car occupant — *continued*
      - hanger-on — *continued*
        - collision — *continued*
          - animal — *continued*
            - being ridden (traffic) V46.7 ☑
              - nontraffic V46.2 ☑
            - nontraffic V40.2 ☑
          - animal-drawn vehicle (traffic) V46.7 ☑
            - nontraffic V46.2 ☑
          - bus (traffic) V44.7 ☑
            - nontraffic V44.2 ☑
          - car (traffic) V43.72 ☑
            - nontraffic V43.22 ☑
          - pedal cycle (traffic) V41.7 ☑
            - nontraffic V41.2 ☑
          - pickup truck (traffic) V43.73 ☑
            - nontraffic V43.23 ☑
          - railway vehicle (traffic) V45.7 ☑
            - nontraffic V45.2 ☑
          - specified vehicle NEC (traffic) V46.7 ☑
            - nontraffic V46.2 ☑
          - sport utility vehicle (traffic) V43.71 ☑
            - nontraffic V43.21 ☑
          - stationary object (traffic) V47.7 ☑
            - nontraffic V47.2 ☑
          - streetcar (traffic) V46.7 ☑
            - nontraffic V46.2 ☑
          - three wheeled motor vehicle (traffic) V42.7 ☑
            - nontraffic V42.2 ☑
          - truck (traffic) V44.7 ☑
            - nontraffic V44.2 ☑
          - two wheeled motor vehicle (traffic) V42.7 ☑
            - nontraffic V42.2 ☑
          - van (traffic) V43.74 ☑
            - nontraffic V43.24 ☑
        - noncollision accident (traffic) V48.7 ☑
          - nontraffic V48.2 ☑
      - noncollision accident (traffic) V48.9 ☑
        - nontraffic V48.3 ☑
        - while boarding or alighting V48.4 ☑
      - nontraffic V49.3 ☑
      - passenger
        - collision (with)
          - animal (traffic) V40.6 ☑
            - being ridden (traffic) V46.6 ☑
              - nontraffic V46.1 ☑
            - nontraffic V40.1 ☑
          - animal-drawn vehicle (traffic) V46.6 ☑
            - nontraffic V46.1 ☑
          - bus (traffic) V44.6 ☑
            - nontraffic V44.1 ☑
          - car (traffic) V43.62 ☑
            - nontraffic V43.12 ☑
          - motor vehicle NOS (traffic) V49.50 ☑
            - nontraffic V49.10 ☑
            - specified type NEC (traffic) V49.59 ☑
              - nontraffic V49.19 ☑
          - pedal cycle (traffic) V41.6 ☑
            - nontraffic V41.1 ☑
          - pickup truck (traffic) V43.63 ☑
            - nontraffic V43.13 ☑
          - railway vehicle (traffic) V45.6 ☑
            - nontraffic V45.1 ☑
          - specified vehicle NEC (traffic) V46.6 ☑
            - nontraffic V46.1 ☑
          - sport utility vehicle (traffic) V43.61 ☑
            - nontraffic V43.11 ☑
          - stationary object (traffic) V47.6 ☑
            - nontraffic V47.1 ☑
          - streetcar (traffic) V46.6 ☑
            - nontraffic V46.1 ☑
          - three wheeled motor vehicle (traffic) V42.6 ☑
            - nontraffic V42.1 ☑
          - truck (traffic) V44.6 ☑
            - nontraffic V44.1 ☑
          - two wheeled motor vehicle (traffic) V42.6 ☑
            - nontraffic V42.1 ☑
          - van (traffic) V43.64 ☑
            - nontraffic V43.14 ☑
        - noncollision accident (traffic) V48.6 ☑

- **Accident** — *continued*
  - transport — *continued*
    - car occupant — *continued*
      - passenger — *continued*
        - noncollision accident — *continued*
          - nontraffic V48.1 ☑
      - specified type NEC V49.88 ☑
        - military vehicle V49.81 ☑
    - coal car — *see* Accident, transport, industrial vehicle occupant
    - construction vehicle occupant (nontraffic) V85.9 ☑
      - driver V85.5 ☑
      - hanger-on V85.7 ☑
      - passenger V85.6 ☑
      - traffic V85.3 ☑
        - driver V85.0 ☑
        - hanger-on V85.2 ☑
        - passenger V85.1 ☑
      - while boarding or alighting V85.4 ☑
    - dirt bike rider (nontraffic) V86.96 ☑
      - driver V86.56 ☑
      - hanger-on V86.76 ☑
      - passenger V86.66 ☑
      - traffic V86.36 ☑
        - driver V86.06 ☑
        - hanger-on V86.26 ☑
        - passenger V86.16 ☑
      - while boarding or alighting V86.46 ☑
    - due to cataclysm — *see* Forces of nature, by type
    - dune buggy occupant (nontraffic) V86.93 ☑
      - driver V86.53 ☑
      - hanger-on V86.73 ☑
      - passenger V86.63 ☑
      - traffic V86.33 ☑
        - driver V86.03 ☑
        - hanger-on V86.23 ☑
        - passenger V86.13 ☑
      - while boarding or alighting V86.43 ☑
    - e-bicycle — *see* Accident, transport, electric (assisted) bicyclist
    - e-bike — *see* Accident, transport, electric (assisted) bicyclist
    - electric (assisted) bicyclist V29.91 ☑
      - collision (with)
        - animal (traffic) V20.91 ☑
          - being ridden (traffic) V26.91 ☑
            - nontraffic V26.21 ☑
            - while boarding or alighting V26.31 ☑
          - nontraffic V20.21 ☑
          - while boarding or alighting V20.31 ☑
        - animal-drawn vehicle (traffic) V26.91 ☑
          - nontraffic V26.21 ☑
          - while boarding or alighting V26.31 ☑
        - bus (traffic) V24.91 ☑
          - nontraffic V24.21 ☑
          - while boarding or alighting V24.31 ☑
        - car (traffic) V23.91 ☑
          - nontraffic V23.21 ☑
          - while boarding or alighting V23.31 ☑
        - motor vehicle NOS (traffic) V29.601 ☑
          - nontraffic V29.201 ☑
          - specified type NEC (traffic) V29.691 ☑
            - nontraffic V29.291 ☑
        - pedal cycle (traffic) V21.91 ☑
          - nontraffic V21.21 ☑
          - while boarding or alighting V21.31 ☑
        - pedestrian V20.91 ☑
          - nontraffic V20.01 ☑
          - while boarding or alighting V20.31 ☑
        - pickup truck (traffic) V23.91 ☑
          - nontraffic V23.21 ☑
          - while boarding or alighting V23.31 ☑
        - railway vehicle (traffic) V25.91 ☑
          - nontraffic V25.21 ☑
          - while boarding or alighting V25.31 ☑
        - specified vehicle NEC (traffic) V26.91 ☑
          - nontraffic V26.21 ☑
          - while boarding or alighting V26.31 ☑
        - stationary object (traffic) V27.91 ☑
          - nontraffic V27.21 ☑
          - while boarding or alighting V27.31 ☑
        - streetcar (traffic) V26.91 ☑
          - nontraffic V26.21 ☑
          - while boarding or alighting V26.31 ☑
        - three wheeled motor vehicle (traffic) V22.91 ☑

- **Accident** — *continued*
  - transport — *continued*
    - electric bicyclist — *continued*
      - collision — *continued*
        - three wheeled motor vehicle — *continued*
          - nontraffic V22.21 ☑
          - while boarding or alighting V22.31 ☑
        - truck (traffic) V24.91 ☑
          - nontraffic V24.21 ☑
          - while boarding or alighting V24.31 ☑
        - two wheeled motor vehicle (traffic) V22.91 ☑
          - nontraffic V22.21 ☑
          - while boarding or alighting V22.31 ☑
        - van (traffic) V23.91 ☑
          - nontraffic V23.21 ☑
          - while boarding or alighting V23.31 ☑
      - driver
        - collision (with)
          - animal (traffic) V20.41 ☑
            - being ridden (traffic) V26.41 ☑
              - nontraffic V26.01 ☑
            - nontraffic V20.01 ☑
          - animal-drawn vehicle (traffic) V26.41 ☑
            - nontraffic V26.01 ☑
          - bus (traffic) V24.41 ☑
            - nontraffic V24.01 ☑
          - car (traffic) V23.41 ☑
            - nontraffic V23.01 ☑
          - motor vehicle NOS (traffic) V29.401 ☑
            - nontraffic V29.001 ☑
            - specified type NEC (traffic) V29.491 ☑
              - nontraffic V29.091 ☑
          - pedal cycle (traffic) V21.41 ☑
            - nontraffic V21.01 ☑
          - pedestrian
            - nontraffic V20.01 ☑
            - traffic V20.41 ☑
          - pickup truck (traffic) V23.41 ☑
            - nontraffic V23.01 ☑
          - railway vehicle (traffic) V25.41 ☑
            - nontraffic V25.01 ☑
          - specified vehicle NEC (traffic) V26.41 ☑
            - nontraffic V26.01 ☑
          - stationary object (traffic) V27.41 ☑
            - nontraffic V27.01 ☑
          - streetcar (traffic) V26.41 ☑
            - nontraffic V26.01 ☑
          - three wheeled motor vehicle (traffic) V22.41 ☑
            - nontraffic V22.01 ☑
          - truck (traffic) V24.41 ☑
            - nontraffic V24.01 ☑
          - two wheeled motor vehicle (traffic) V22.41 ☑
            - nontraffic V22.01 ☑
          - van (traffic) V23.41 ☑
            - nontraffic V23.01 ☑
        - noncollision accident (traffic) V28.41 ☑
          - nontraffic V28.01 ☑
      - noncollision accident (traffic) V28.91 ☑
        - nontraffic V28.21 ☑
        - while boarding or alighting V28.31 ☑
      - nontraffic V29.31 ☑
      - passenger
        - collision (with)
          - animal (traffic) V20.51 ☑
            - being ridden (traffic) V26.51 ☑
              - nontraffic V26.11 ☑
            - nontraffic V20.11 ☑
          - animal-drawn vehicle (traffic) V26.51 ☑
            - nontraffic V26.11 ☑
          - bus (traffic) V24.51 ☑
            - nontraffic V24.11 ☑
          - car (traffic) V23.51 ☑
            - nontraffic V23.11 ☑
          - motor vehicle NOS (traffic) V29.501 ☑
            - nontraffic V29.101 ☑
            - specified type NEC (traffic) V29.591 ☑
              - nontraffic V29.191 ☑
          - pedal cycle (traffic) V21.51 ☑
            - nontraffic V21.11 ☑
          - pedestrian
            - nontraffic V20.11 ☑
            - traffic V20.51 ☑
          - pickup truck (traffic) V23.51 ☑
            - nontraffic V23.11 ☑

- **Accident** — *continued*
  - transport — *continued*
    - electric bicyclist — *continued*
      - passenger — *continued*
        - collision — *continued*
          - railway vehicle (traffic) V25.51 ☑
            - nontraffic V25.11 ☑
          - specified vehicle NEC (traffic) V26.51 ☑
            - nontraffic V26.11 ☑
          - stationary object (traffic) V27.51 ☑
            - nontraffic V27.11 ☑
          - streetcar (traffic) V26.51 ☑
            - nontraffic V26.11 ☑
          - three wheeled motor vehicle (traffic) V22.51 ☑
            - nontraffic V22.11 ☑
          - truck (traffic) V24.51 ☑
            - nontraffic V24.11 ☑
          - two wheeled motor vehicle (traffic) V22.51 ☑
            - nontraffic V22.11 ☑
          - van (traffic) V23.51 ☑
            - nontraffic V23.11 ☑
        - noncollision accident (traffic) V28.51 ☑
          - nontraffic V28.11 ☑
      - specified type NEC V29.881 ☑
        - military vehicle V29.811 ☑
    - forklift — *see* Accident, transport, industrial vehicle occupant
    - go cart — *see* Accident, transport, all-terrain vehicle occupant
    - golf cart — *see* Accident, transport, all-terrain vehicle occupant
    - heavy transport vehicle occupant — *see* Accident, transport, truck occupant
    - hoverboard V00.848 ☑
    - ice yacht V98.2 ☑
    - industrial vehicle occupant (nontraffic) V83.9 ☑
      - driver V83.5 ☑
      - hanger-on V83.7 ☑
      - passenger V83.6 ☑
      - traffic V83.3 ☑
        - driver V83.0 ☑
        - hanger-on V83.2 ☑
        - passenger V83.1 ☑
      - while boarding or alighting V83.4 ☑
    - interurban electric car — *see* Accident, transport, streetcar
    - land yacht V98.1 ☑
    - logging car — *see* Accident, transport, industrial vehicle occupant
    - military vehicle occupant (traffic) V86.34 ☑
      - driver V86.04 ☑
      - hanger-on V86.24 ☑
      - nontraffic V86.94 ☑
        - driver V86.54 ☑
        - hanger-on V86.74 ☑
        - passenger V86.64 ☑
      - passenger V86.14 ☑
      - while boarding or alighting V86.44 ☑
    - mine tram — *see* Accident, transport, industrial vehicle occupant
    - motor vehicle NEC occupant (traffic) V89.2 ☑
    - motorcoach — *see* Accident, transport, bus occupant
    - motor/cross bike rider — *see also* Accident, transport, dirt bike rider V86.96 ☑
    - motorcyclist V29.99 ☑
      - collision (with)
        - animal (traffic) V20.99 ☑
          - being ridden (traffic) V26.99 ☑
            - nontraffic V26.29 ☑
            - while boarding or alighting V26.39 ☑
          - nontraffic V20.29 ☑
          - while boarding or alighting V20.39 ☑
        - animal-drawn vehicle (traffic) V26.99 ☑
          - nontraffic V26.29 ☑
          - while boarding or alighting V26.39 ☑
        - bus (traffic) V24.99 ☑
          - nontraffic V24.29 ☑
          - while boarding or alighting V24.39 ☑
        - car (traffic) V23.99 ☑
          - nontraffic V23.29 ☑
          - while boarding or alighting V23.39 ☑
        - motor vehicle NOS (traffic) V29.608 ☑
          - nontraffic V29.208 ☑

- **Accident** — *continued*
  - transport — *continued*
    - motorcyclist — *continued*
      - collision — *continued*
        - motor vehicle — *continued*
          - specified type NEC (traffic) V29.698 ☑
            - nontraffic V29.298 ☑
        - pedal cycle (traffic) V21.99 ☑
          - nontraffic V21.29 ☑
          - while boarding or alighting V21.39 ☑
        - pickup truck (traffic) V23.99 ☑
          - nontraffic V23.29 ☑
          - while boarding or alighting V23.39 ☑
        - railway vehicle (traffic) V25.99 ☑
          - nontraffic V25.29 ☑
          - while boarding or alighting V25.39 ☑
        - specified vehicle NEC (traffic) V26.99 ☑
          - nontraffic V26.29 ☑
          - while boarding or alighting V26.39 ☑
        - stationary object (traffic) V27.99 ☑
          - nontraffic V27.29 ☑
          - while boarding or alighting V27.39 ☑
        - streetcar (traffic) V26.99 ☑
          - nontraffic V26.29 ☑
          - while boarding or alighting V26.39 ☑
        - three wheeled motor vehicle (traffic) V22.99 ☑
          - nontraffic V22.29 ☑
          - while boarding or alighting V22.39 ☑
        - truck (traffic) V24.99 ☑
          - nontraffic V24.29 ☑
          - while boarding or alighting V24.39 ☑
        - two wheeled motor vehicle (traffic) V22.99 ☑
          - nontraffic V22.29 ☑
          - while boarding or alighting V22.39 ☑
        - van (traffic) V23.99 ☑
          - nontraffic V23.29 ☑
          - while boarding or alighting V23.39 ☑
      - driver
        - collision (with)
          - animal (traffic) V20.49 ☑
            - being ridden (traffic) V26.49 ☑
              - nontraffic V26.09 ☑
            - nontraffic V20.09 ☑
          - animal-drawn vehicle (traffic) V26.49 ☑
            - nontraffic V26.09 ☑
          - bus (traffic) V24.49 ☑
            - nontraffic V24.09 ☑
          - car (traffic) V23.49 ☑
            - nontraffic V23.09 ☑
          - motor vehicle NOS (traffic) V29.408 ☑
            - nontraffic V29.008 ☑
            - specified type NEC (traffic) V29.498 ☑
              - nontraffic V29.098 ☑
          - pedal cycle (traffic) V21.49 ☑
            - nontraffic V21.09 ☑
          - pedestrian
            - nontraffic V20.09 ☑
            - traffic V20.49 ☑
          - pickup truck (traffic) V23.49 ☑
            - nontraffic V23.09 ☑
          - railway vehicle (traffic) V25.49 ☑
            - nontraffic V25.09 ☑
          - specified vehicle NEC (traffic) V26.49 ☑
            - nontraffic V26.09 ☑
          - stationary object (traffic) V27.49 ☑
            - nontraffic V27.09 ☑
          - streetcar (traffic) V26.49 ☑
            - nontraffic V26.09 ☑
          - three wheeled motor vehicle (traffic) V22.49 ☑
            - nontraffic V22.09 ☑
          - truck (traffic) V24.49 ☑
            - nontraffic V24.09 ☑
          - two wheeled motor vehicle (traffic) V22.49 ☑
            - nontraffic V22.09 ☑
          - van (traffic) V23.49 ☑
            - nontraffic V23.09 ☑
        - noncollision accident (traffic) V28.49 ☑
          - nontraffic V28.09 ☑
      - noncollision accident (traffic) V28.99 ☑
        - nontraffic V28.29 ☑
        - while boarding or alighting V28.39 ☑
    - nontraffic V29.39 ☑

- **Accident** — *continued*
  - transport — *continued*
    - motorcyclist — *continued*
      - passenger
        - collision (with)
          - animal (traffic) V20.59 ☑
            - being ridden (traffic) V26.59 ☑
              - nontraffic V26.19 ☑
            - nontraffic V20.19 ☑
          - animal-drawn vehicle (traffic) V26.59 ☑
            - nontraffic V26.19 ☑
          - bus (traffic) V24.59 ☑
            - nontraffic V24.19 ☑
          - car (traffic) V23.59 ☑
            - nontraffic V23.19 ☑
          - motor vehicle NOS (traffic) V29.508 ☑
            - nontraffic V29.108 ☑
            - specified type NEC (traffic) V29.598 ☑
              - nontraffic V29.198 ☑
          - pedal cycle (traffic) V21.59 ☑
            - nontraffic V21.19 ☑
          - pedestrian
            - nontraffic V20.19 ☑
            - traffic V20.59 ☑
          - pickup truck (traffic) V23.59 ☑
            - nontraffic V23.19 ☑
          - railway vehicle (traffic) V25.59 ☑
            - nontraffic V25.19 ☑
          - specified vehicle NEC (traffic) V26.59 ☑
            - nontraffic V26.19 ☑
          - stationary object (traffic) V27.59 ☑
            - nontraffic V27.19 ☑
          - streetcar (traffic) V26.59 ☑
            - nontraffic V26.19 ☑
          - three wheeled motor vehicle (traffic) V22.59 ☑
            - nontraffic V22.19 ☑
          - truck (traffic) V24.59 ☑
            - nontraffic V24.19 ☑
          - two wheeled motor vehicle (traffic) V22.59 ☑
            - nontraffic V22.19 ☑
          - van (traffic) V23.59 ☑
            - nontraffic V23.19 ☑
        - noncollision accident (traffic) V28.59 ☑
          - nontraffic V28.19 ☑
      - specified type NEC V29.888 ☑
        - military vehicle V29.818 ☑
    - occupant (of)
      - aircraft (powered) V95.9 ☑
        - fixed wing
          - commercial — *see* Accident, transport, aircraft, occupant, powered, fixed wing, commercial
          - private — *see* Accident, transport, aircraft, occupant, powered, fixed wing, private
        - nonpowered V96.9 ☑
        - specified NEC V95.8 ☑
      - airport battery-powered vehicle — *see* Accident, transport, industrial vehicle occupant
      - all-terrain vehicle (ATV) — *see* Accident, transport, all-terrain vehicle occupant
      - animal-drawn vehicle — *see* Accident, transport, animal-drawn vehicle occupant
      - automobile — *see* Accident, transport, car occupant
      - balloon V96.00 ☑
      - battery-powered vehicle — *see* Accident, transport, industrial vehicle occupant
      - bicycle — *see* Accident, transport, pedal cyclist
        - motorized — *see* Accident, transport, motorcycle rider
      - boat NEC — *see* Accident, watercraft
      - bulldozer — *see* Accident, transport, construction vehicle occupant
      - bus — *see* Accident, transport, bus occupant
      - cable car (on rails) — *see also* Accident, transport, streetcar occupant
        - not on rails V98.0 ☑
      - car — *see also* Accident, transport, car occupant
        - cable (on rails) — *see also* Accident, transport, streetcar occupant
          - not on rails V98.0 ☑
      - coach — *see* Accident, transport, bus occupant

- **Accident** — *continued*
  - transport — *continued*
    - occupant — *continued*
      - coal-car — *see* Accident, transport, industrial vehicle occupant
      - digger — *see* Accident, transport, construction vehicle occupant
      - dump truck — *see* Accident, transport, construction vehicle occupant
      - earth-leveler — *see* Accident, transport, construction vehicle occupant
      - farm machinery (self-propelled) — *see* Accident, transport, agricultural vehicle occupant
      - forklift — *see* Accident, transport, industrial vehicle occupant
      - glider (unpowered) V96.20 ☑
        - hang V96.10 ☑
        - powered (microlight) (ultralight) — *see* Accident, transport, aircraft, occupant, powered, glider
      - glider (unpowered) NEC V96.20 ☑
      - hang-glider V96.10 ☑
      - harvester — *see* Accident, transport, agricultural vehicle occupant
      - heavy (transport) vehicle — *see* Accident, transport, truck occupant
      - helicopter — *see* Accident, transport, aircraft, occupant, helicopter
      - ice-yacht V98.2 ☑
      - kite (carrying person) V96.8 ☑
      - land-yacht V98.1 ☑
      - logging car — *see* Accident, transport, industrial vehicle occupant
      - mechanical shovel — *see* Accident, transport, construction vehicle occupant
      - microlight — *see* Accident, transport, aircraft, occupant, powered, glider
      - minibus — *see* Accident, transport, pickup truck occupant
      - minivan — *see* Accident, transport, pickup truck occupant
      - moped — *see* Accident, transport, motorcycle
      - motor scooter — *see* Accident, transport, motorcycle
      - motorcycle (with sidecar) — *see* Accident, transport, motorcycle
      - off-road motor-vehicle — *see also* Accident, transport, all-terrain vehicle occupant V86.99 ☑
      - pedal cycle — *see also* Accident, transport, pedal cyclist
      - pick-up (truck) — *see* Accident, transport, pickup truck occupant
      - railway (train) (vehicle) (subterranean) (elevated) — *see* Accident, transport, railway vehicle occupant
      - rickshaw — *see* Accident, transport, pedal cycle
        - motorized — *see* Accident, transport, three-wheeled motor vehicle
        - pedal driven — *see* Accident, transport, pedal cyclist
      - road-roller — *see* Accident, transport, construction vehicle occupant
      - ship NOS V94.9 ☑
      - ski-lift (chair) (gondola) V98.3 ☑
      - snowmobile — *see* Accident, transport, snowmobile occupant
      - spacecraft, spaceship — *see* Accident, transport, aircraft, occupant, spacecraft
      - sport utility vehicle — *see* Accident, transport, pickup truck occupant
      - streetcar (interurban) (operating on public street or highway) — *see* Accident, transport, streetcar occupant
      - SUV — *see* Accident, transport, pickup truck occupant
      - téléférique V98.0 ☑
      - three-wheeled vehicle (motorized) — *see also* Accident, transport, three-wheeled motor vehicle occupant
        - nonmotorized — *see* Accident, transport, pedal cycle
      - tractor (farm) (and trailer) — *see* Accident, transport, agricultural vehicle occupant
      - train — *see* Accident, transport, railway vehicle occupant

- **Accident** — *continued*
  - transport — *continued*
    - occupant — *continued*
      - tram — *see* Accident, transport, streetcar occupant
        - in mine or quarry — *see* Accident, transport, industrial vehicle occupant
      - tricycle — *see* Accident, transport, pedal cycle
        - motorized — *see* Accident, transport, three-wheeled motor vehicle
      - trolley — *see* Accident, transport, streetcar occupant
        - in mine or quarry — *see* Accident, transport, industrial vehicle occupant
      - tub, in mine or quarry — *see* Accident, transport, industrial vehicle occupant
      - ultralight — *see* Accident, transport, aircraft, occupant, powered, glider
      - van — *see* Accident, transport, van occupant
      - vehicle NEC V89.9 ☑
        - heavy transport — *see* Accident, transport, truck occupant
        - motor (traffic) NEC V89.2 ☑
          - nontraffic NEC V89.0 ☑
      - watercraft NOS V94.9 ☑
        - causing drowning — *see* Drowning, resulting from accident to boat
    - off-road motor-vehicle — *see also* Accident, transport, all-terrain vehicle occupant V86.99 ☑
    - parachutist V97.29 ☑
      - after accident to aircraft — *see* Accident, transport, aircraft
      - entangled in object V97.21 ☑
      - injured on landing V97.22 ☑
    - pedal cyclist V19.9 ☑
      - collision (with)
        - animal (traffic) V10.9 ☑
          - being ridden (traffic) V16.9 ☑
            - nontraffic V16.2 ☑
              - while boarding or alighting V16.3 ☑
          - nontraffic V10.2 ☑
            - while boarding or alighting V10.3 ☑
        - animal-drawn vehicle (traffic) V16.9 ☑
          - nontraffic V16.2 ☑
            - while boarding or alighting V16.3 ☑
        - bus (traffic) V14.9 ☑
          - nontraffic V14.2 ☑
            - while boarding or alighting V14.3 ☑
        - car (traffic) V13.9 ☑
          - nontraffic V13.2 ☑
            - while boarding or alighting V13.3 ☑
        - motor vehicle NOS (traffic) V19.60 ☑
          - nontraffic V19.20 ☑
          - specified type NEC (traffic) V19.69 ☑
            - nontraffic V19.29 ☑
        - pedal cycle (traffic) V11.9 ☑
          - nontraffic V11.2 ☑
            - while boarding or alighting V11.3 ☑
        - pickup truck (traffic) V13.9 ☑
          - nontraffic V13.2 ☑
            - while boarding or alighting V13.3 ☑
        - railway vehicle (traffic) V15.9 ☑
          - nontraffic V15.2 ☑
            - while boarding or alighting V15.3 ☑
        - specified vehicle NEC (traffic) V16.9 ☑
          - nontraffic V16.2 ☑
            - while boarding or alighting V16.3 ☑
        - stationary object (traffic) V17.9 ☑
          - nontraffic V17.2 ☑
            - while boarding or alighting V17.3 ☑
        - streetcar (traffic) V16.9 ☑
          - nontraffic V16.2 ☑
            - while boarding or alighting V16.3 ☑
        - three wheeled motor vehicle (traffic) V12.9 ☑
          - nontraffic V12.2 ☑
            - while boarding or alighting V12.3 ☑
        - truck (traffic) V14.9 ☑
          - nontraffic V14.2 ☑
            - while boarding or alighting V14.3 ☑
        - two wheeled motor vehicle (traffic) V12.9 ☑
          - nontraffic V12.2 ☑
            - while boarding or alighting V12.3 ☑
        - van (traffic) V13.9 ☑
          - nontraffic V13.2 ☑
            - while boarding or alighting V13.3 ☑

- **Accident** — *continued*
  - transport — *continued*
    - pedal cyclist — *continued*
      - driver
        - collision (with)
          - animal (traffic) V10.4 ☑
            - being ridden (traffic) V16.4 ☑
              - nontraffic V16.0 ☑
            - nontraffic V10.0 ☑
          - animal-drawn vehicle (traffic) V16.4 ☑
            - nontraffic V16.0 ☑
          - bus (traffic) V14.4 ☑
            - nontraffic V14.0 ☑
          - car (traffic) V13.4 ☑
            - nontraffic V13.0 ☑
          - motor vehicle NOS (traffic) V19.40 ☑
            - nontraffic V19.00 ☑
            - specified type NEC (traffic) V19.49 ☑
              - nontraffic V19.09 ☑
          - pedal cycle (traffic) V11.4 ☑
            - nontraffic V11.0 ☑
          - pickup truck (traffic) V13.4 ☑
            - nontraffic V13.0 ☑
          - railway vehicle (traffic) V15.4 ☑
            - nontraffic V15.0 ☑
          - specified vehicle NEC (traffic) V16.4 ☑
            - nontraffic V16.0 ☑
          - stationary object (traffic) V17.4 ☑
            - nontraffic V17.0 ☑
          - streetcar (traffic) V16.4 ☑
            - nontraffic V16.0 ☑
          - three wheeled motor vehicle (traffic) V12.4 ☑
            - nontraffic V12.0 ☑
          - truck (traffic) V14.4 ☑
            - nontraffic V14.0 ☑
          - two wheeled motor vehicle (traffic) V12.4 ☑
            - nontraffic V12.0 ☑
          - van (traffic) V13.4 ☑
            - nontraffic V13.0 ☑
        - noncollision accident (traffic) V18.4 ☑
          - nontraffic V18.0 ☑
      - noncollision accident (traffic) V18.9 ☑
        - nontraffic V18.2 ☑
        - while boarding or alighting V18.3 ☑
      - nontraffic V19.3 ☑
      - passenger
        - collision (with)
          - animal (traffic) V10.5 ☑
            - being ridden (traffic) V16.5 ☑
              - nontraffic V16.1 ☑
            - nontraffic V10.1 ☑
          - animal-drawn vehicle (traffic) V16.5 ☑
            - nontraffic V16.1 ☑
          - bus (traffic) V14.5 ☑
            - nontraffic V14.1 ☑
          - car (traffic) V13.5 ☑
            - nontraffic V13.1 ☑
          - motor vehicle NOS (traffic) V19.50 ☑
            - nontraffic V19.10 ☑
            - specified type NEC (traffic) V19.59 ☑
              - nontraffic V19.19 ☑
          - pedal cycle (traffic) V11.5 ☑
            - nontraffic V11.1 ☑
          - pickup truck (traffic) V13.5 ☑
            - nontraffic V13.1 ☑
          - railway vehicle (traffic) V15.5 ☑
            - nontraffic V15.1 ☑
          - specified vehicle NEC (traffic) V16.5 ☑
            - nontraffic V16.1 ☑
          - stationary object (traffic) V17.5 ☑
            - nontraffic V17.1 ☑
          - streetcar (traffic) V16.5 ☑
            - nontraffic V16.1 ☑
          - three wheeled motor vehicle (traffic) V12.5 ☑
            - nontraffic V12.1 ☑
          - truck (traffic) V14.5 ☑
            - nontraffic V14.1 ☑
          - two wheeled motor vehicle (traffic) V12.5 ☑
            - nontraffic V12.1 ☑
          - van (traffic) V13.5 ☑
            - nontraffic V13.1 ☑
        - noncollision accident (traffic) V18.5 ☑

- **Accident** — *continued*
  - transport — *continued*
    - pedal cyclist — *continued*
      - passenger — *continued*
        - noncollision accident — *continued*
          - nontraffic V18.1 ☑
      - specified type NEC V19.88 ☑
        - military vehicle V19.81 ☑
    - pedestrian
      - conveyance (occupant) V09.9 ☑
        - baby stroller V00.828 ☑
          - collision (with) V09.9 ☑
            - animal being ridden or animal drawn vehicle V06.99 ☑
              - nontraffic V06.09 ☑
              - traffic V06.19 ☑
            - bus or heavy transport V04.99 ☑
              - nontraffic V04.09 ☑
              - traffic V04.19 ☑
            - car V03.99 ☑
              - nontraffic V03.09 ☑
              - traffic V03.19 ☑
            - pedal cycle V01.99 ☑
              - nontraffic V01.09 ☑
              - traffic V01.19 ☑
            - pick-up truck or van V03.99 ☑
              - nontraffic V03.09 ☑
              - traffic V03.19 ☑
            - railway (train) (vehicle) V05.99 ☑
              - nontraffic V05.09 ☑
              - traffic V05.19 ☑
            - stationary object V00.822 ☑
            - streetcar V06.99 ☑
              - nontraffic V06.09 ☑
              - traffic V06.19 ☑
            - two- or three-wheeled motor vehicle V02.99 ☑
              - nontraffic V02.09 ☑
              - traffic V02.19 ☑
            - vehicle V09.9 ☑
              - animal-drawn V06.99 ☑
                - nontraffic V06.09 ☑
                - traffic V06.19 ☑
              - motor
                - nontraffic V09.00 ☑
                - traffic V09.20 ☑
          - fall V00.821 ☑
          - nontraffic V09.1 ☑
            - involving motor vehicle NEC V09.00 ☑
          - traffic V09.3 ☑
            - involving motor vehicle NEC V09.20 ☑
        - flat-bottomed NEC V00.388 ☑
          - collision (with) V09.9 ☑
            - animal being ridden or animal drawn vehicle V06.99 ☑
              - nontraffic V06.09 ☑
              - traffic V06.19 ☑
            - bus or heavy transport V04.99 ☑
              - nontraffic V04.09 ☑
              - traffic V04.19 ☑
            - car V03.99 ☑
              - nontraffic V03.09 ☑
              - traffic V03.19 ☑
            - pedal cycle V01.99 ☑
              - nontraffic V01.09 ☑
              - traffic V01.19 ☑
            - pick-up truck or van V03.99 ☑
              - nontraffic V03.09 ☑
              - traffic V03.19 ☑
            - railway (train) (vehicle) V05.99 ☑
              - nontraffic V05.09 ☑
              - traffic V05.19 ☑
            - stationary object V00.382 ☑
            - streetcar V06.99 ☑
              - nontraffic V06.09 ☑
              - traffic V06.19 ☑
            - two- or three-wheeled motor vehicle V02.99 ☑
              - nontraffic V02.09 ☑
              - traffic V02.19 ☑
            - vehicle V09.9 ☑
              - animal-drawn V06.99 ☑
                - nontraffic V06.09 ☑
                - traffic V06.19 ☑
              - motor
                - nontraffic V09.00 ☑

- **Accident** — *continued*
  - transport — *continued*
    - pedestrian — *continued*
      - conveyance — *continued*
        - flat-bottomed — *continued*
          - collision — *continued*
            - vehicle — *continued*
              - motor — *continued*
                - traffic V09.20 ☑
          - fall V00.381 ☑
          - nontraffic V09.1 ☑
            - involving motor vehicle NEC V09.00 ☑
          - snow
            - board — *see* Accident, transport, pedestrian, conveyance, snow board
            - ski — *see* Accident, transport, pedestrian, conveyance, skis (snow)
          - traffic V09.3 ☑
            - involving motor vehicle NEC V09.20 ☑
        - gliding type NEC V00.288 ☑
          - collision (with) V09.9 ☑
            - animal being ridden or animal drawn vehicle V06.99 ☑
              - nontraffic V06.09 ☑
              - traffic V06.19 ☑
            - bus or heavy transport V04.99 ☑
              - nontraffic V04.09 ☑
              - traffic V04.19 ☑
            - car V03.99 ☑
              - nontraffic V03.09 ☑
              - traffic V03.19 ☑
            - pedal cycle V01.99 ☑
              - nontraffic V01.09 ☑
              - traffic V01.19 ☑
            - pick-up truck or van V03.99 ☑
              - nontraffic V03.09 ☑
              - traffic V03.19 ☑
            - railway (train) (vehicle) V05.99 ☑
              - nontraffic V05.09 ☑
              - traffic V05.19 ☑
            - stationary object V00.282 ☑
            - streetcar V06.99 ☑
              - nontraffic V06.09 ☑
              - traffic V02.19 ☑
            - two- or three-wheeled motor vehicle V02.99 ☑
              - nontraffic V02.09 ☑
              - traffic V02.19 ☑
            - vehicle V09.9 ☑
              - animal-drawn V06.99 ☑
                - nontraffic V06.09 ☑
                - traffic V06.19 ☑
              - motor
                - nontraffic V09.00 ☑
                - traffic V09.20 ☑
          - fall V00.281 ☑
          - heelies — *see* Accident, transport, pedestrian, conveyance, heelies
          - ice skate — *see* Accident, transport, pedestrian, conveyance, ice skate
          - nontraffic V09.1 ☑
            - involving motor vehicle NEC V09.00 ☑
          - sled — *see* Accident, transport, pedestrian, conveyance, sled
          - traffic V09.3 ☑
            - involving motor vehicle NEC V09.20 ☑
            - wheelies — *see* Accident, transport, pedestrian, conveyance, heelies
        - heelies V00.158 ☑
          - colliding with stationary object V00.152 ☑
          - fall V00.151 ☑
        - hoverboard
          - collision with
            - animal being ridden or animal drawn vehicle V06.938 ☑
              - nontraffic V06.038 ☑
              - traffic V06.138 ☑
            - bus or heavy transport V04.938 ☑
              - nontraffic V04.038 ☑
              - traffic V04.138 ☑
            - car V03.938 ☑
              - nontraffic V03.038 ☑
              - traffic V03.138 ☑
            - pedal cycle V01.938 ☑

- **Accident** — *continued*
  - transport — *continued*
    - pedestrian — *continued*
      - conveyance — *continued*
        - hoverboard — *continued*
          - collision with — *continued*
            - pedal cycle — *continued*
              - nontraffic V01.038 ☑
              - traffic V01.138 ☑
            - pick-up or van V03.938 ☑
              - nontraffic V03.038 ☑
              - traffic V03.138 ☑
            - railway (train) (vehicle) V05.938 ☑
              - nontraffic V05.038 ☑
              - traffic V05.138 ☑
            - streetcar V06.938 ☑
              - nontraffic V06.038 ☑
              - traffic V06.138 ☑
            - three-wheeled motor vehicle V02.938 ☑
              - nontraffic V02.038 ☑
              - traffic V02.138 ☑
            - two-wheeled motor vehicle V02.938 ☑
              - nontraffic V02.038 ☑
              - traffic V02.138 ☑
            - vehicle, nonmotor, specified NEC V06.938 ☑
              - nontraffic V06.038 ☑
              - traffic V06.138 ☑
          - fall V00.848 ☑
        - ice skates V00.218 ☑
          - collision (with) V09.9 ☑
            - animal being ridden or animal drawn vehicle V06.99 ☑
              - nontraffic V06.09 ☑
              - traffic V06.19 ☑
            - bus or heavy transport V04.99 ☑
              - nontraffic V04.09 ☑
              - traffic V04.19 ☑
            - car V03.99 ☑
              - nontraffic V03.09 ☑
              - traffic V03.19 ☑
            - pedal cycle V01.99 ☑
              - nontraffic V01.09 ☑
              - traffic V01.19 ☑
            - pick-up truck or van V03.99 ☑
              - nontraffic V03.09 ☑
              - traffic V03.19 ☑
            - railway (train) (vehicle) V05.99 ☑
              - nontraffic V05.09 ☑
              - traffic V05.19 ☑
            - stationary object V00.212 ☑
            - streetcar V06.99 ☑
              - nontraffic V06.09 ☑
              - traffic V06.19 ☑
            - two- or three-wheeled motor vehicle V02.99 ☑
              - nontraffic V02.09 ☑
              - traffic V02.19 ☑
            - vehicle V09.9 ☑
              - animal-drawn V06.99 ☑
                - nontraffic V06.09 ☑
                - traffic V06.19 ☑
              - motor
                - nontraffic V09.00 ☑
                - traffic V09.20 ☑
          - fall V00.211 ☑
          - nontraffic V09.1 ☑
            - involving motor vehicle NEC V09.00 ☑
          - traffic V09.3 ☑
            - involving motor vehicle NEC V09.20 ☑
        - motorized mobility scooter V00.838 ☑
          - collision with stationary object V00.832 ☑
          - fall from V00.831 ☑
        - nontraffic V09.1 ☑
          - involving motor vehicle V09.00 ☑
            - military V09.01 ☑
            - specified type NEC V09.09 ☑
        - roller skates (non in-line) V00.128 ☑
          - collision (with) V09.9 ☑
            - animal being ridden or animal drawn vehicle V06.91 ☑
              - nontraffic V06.01 ☑
              - traffic V06.11 ☑

- **Accident** — *continued*
  - transport — *continued*
    - pedestrian — *continued*
      - conveyance — *continued*
        - roller skates — *continued*
          - collision — *continued*
            - bus or heavy transport V04.91 ☑
              - nontraffic V04.01 ☑
              - traffic V04.11 ☑
            - car V03.91 ☑
              - nontraffic V03.01 ☑
              - traffic V03.11 ☑
            - pedal cycle V01.91 ☑
              - nontraffic V01.01 ☑
              - traffic V01.11 ☑
            - pick-up truck or van V03.91 ☑
              - nontraffic V03.01 ☑
              - traffic V03.11 ☑
            - railway (train) (vehicle) V05.91 ☑
              - nontraffic V05.01 ☑
              - traffic V05.11 ☑
            - stationary object V00.122 ☑
            - streetcar V06.91 ☑
              - nontraffic V06.01 ☑
              - traffic V06.11 ☑
            - two- or three-wheeled motor vehicle V02.91 ☑
              - nontraffic V02.01 ☑
              - traffic V02.11 ☑
            - vehicle V09.9 ☑
              - animal-drawn V06.91 ☑
                - nontraffic V06.01 ☑
                - traffic V06.11 ☑
              - motor
                - nontraffic V09.00 ☑
                - traffic V09.20 ☑
          - fall V00.121 ☑
          - in-line V00.118 ☑
            - collision — *see* also Accident, transport, pedestrian, conveyance occupant, roller skates, collision
              - with stationary object V00.112 ☑
            - fall V00.111 ☑
          - nontraffic V09.1 ☑
            - involving motor vehicle NEC V09.00 ☑
          - traffic V09.3 ☑
            - involving motor vehicle NEC V09.20 ☑
        - rolling shoes V00.158 ☑
          - colliding with stationary object V00.152 ☑
          - fall V00.151 ☑
        - rolling type NEC V00.188 ☑
          - collision (with) V09.9 ☑
            - animal being ridden or animal drawn vehicle V06.99 ☑
              - nontraffic V06.09 ☑
              - traffic V06.19 ☑
            - bus or heavy transport V04.99 ☑
              - nontraffic V04.09 ☑
              - traffic V04.19 ☑
            - car V03.99 ☑
              - nontraffic V03.09 ☑
              - traffic V03.19 ☑
            - pedal cycle V01.99 ☑
              - nontraffic V01.09 ☑
              - traffic V01.19 ☑
            - pick-up truck or van V03.99 ☑
              - nontraffic V03.09 ☑
              - traffic V03.19 ☑
            - railway (train) (vehicle) V05.99 ☑
              - nontraffic V05.09 ☑
              - traffic V05.19 ☑
            - stationary object V00.182 ☑
            - streetcar V06.99 ☑
              - nontraffic V06.09 ☑
              - traffic V06.19 ☑
            - two- or three-wheeled motor vehicle V02.99 ☑
              - nontraffic V02.09 ☑
              - traffic V02.19 ☑
            - vehicle V09.9 ☑
              - animal-drawn V06.99 ☑
                - nontraffic V06.09 ☑
                - traffic V06.19 ☑
              - motor
                - nontraffic V09.00 ☑

Accident — *continued*
transport — *continued*
pedestrian — *continued*
conveyance — *continued*
rolling type — *continued*
collision — *continued*
vehicle — *continued*
motor — *continued*
traffic V09.20 ☑
fall V00.181 ☑
in-line roller skate — *see* Accident, transport, pedestrian, conveyance, roller skate, in-line
nontraffic V09.1 ☑
involving motor vehicle NEC V09.00 ☑
roller skate — *see* Accident, transport, pedestrian, conveyance, roller skate
scooter (non-motorized) — *see* Accident, transport, pedestrian, conveyance, scooter
skateboard — *see* Accident, transport, pedestrian, conveyance, skateboard
traffic V09.3 ☑
involving motor vehicle NEC V09.20 ☑
scooter (non-motorized) V00.148 ☑
collision (with) V09.9 ☑
animal being ridden or animal drawn vehicle V06.99 ☑
nontraffic V06.09 ☑
traffic V06.19 ☑
bus or heavy transport V04.99 ☑
nontraffic V04.09 ☑
traffic V04.19 ☑
car V03.99 ☑
nontraffic V03.09 ☑
traffic V03.19 ☑
pedal cycle V01.99 ☑
nontraffic V01.09 ☑
traffic V01.19 ☑
pick-up truck or van V03.99 ☑
nontraffic V03.09 ☑
traffic V03.19 ☑
railway (train) (vehicle) V05.99 ☑
nontraffic V05.09 ☑
traffic V05.19 ☑
stationary object V00.142 ☑
streetcar V06.99 ☑
nontraffic V06.09 ☑
traffic V06.19 ☑
two- or three-wheeled motor vehicle V02.99 ☑
nontraffic V02.09 ☑
traffic V02.19 ☑
vehicle V09.9 ☑
animal-drawn V06.99 ☑
nontraffic V06.09 ☑
traffic V06.19 ☑
motor
nontraffic V09.00 ☑
traffic V09.20 ☑
fall V00.141 ☑
nontraffic V09.1 ☑
involving motor vehicle NEC V09.00 ☑
traffic V09.3 ☑
involving motor vehicle NEC V09.20 ☑
Segway
collision with
animal being ridden or animal drawn vehicle V06.938 ☑
nontraffic V06.038 ☑
traffic V06.138 ☑
bus or heavy transport V04.938 ☑
nontraffic V04.038 ☑
traffic V04.138 ☑
car V03.938 ☑
nontraffic V03.038 ☑
traffic V03.138 ☑
pedal cycle V01.938 ☑
nontraffic V01.038 ☑
traffic V01.138 ☑
pick-up or van V03.938 ☑
nontraffic V03.038 ☑
traffic V03.138 ☑
railway (train) (vehicle) V05.938 ☑

Accident — *continued*
transport — *continued*
pedestrian — *continued*
conveyance — *continued*
Segway — *continued*
collision with — *continued*
railway — *continued*
nontraffic V05.038 ☑
traffic V05.138 ☑
streetcar V06.938 ☑
nontraffic V06.038 ☑
traffic V06.138 ☑
three-wheeled vehicle V02.938 ☑
nontraffic V02.038 ☑
traffic V02.138 ☑
two-wheeled vehicle V02.938 ☑
nontraffic V02.038 ☑
traffic V02.138 ☑
vehicle, nonmotor, specified NEC V06.938 ☑
nontraffic V06.038 ☑
traffic V06.138 ☑
fall V00.848 ☑
skateboard V00.138 ☑
collision (with) V09.9 ☑
animal being ridden or animal drawn vehicle V06.92 ☑
nontraffic V06.02 ☑
traffic V06.12 ☑
bus or heavy transport V04.92 ☑
nontraffic V04.02 ☑
traffic V04.12 ☑
car V03.92 ☑
nontraffic V03.02 ☑
traffic V03.12 ☑
pedal cycle V01.92 ☑
nontraffic V01.02 ☑
traffic V01.12 ☑
pick-up truck or van V03.92 ☑
nontraffic V03.02 ☑
traffic V03.12 ☑
railway (train) (vehicle) V05.92 ☑
nontraffic V05.02 ☑
traffic V05.12 ☑
stationary object V00.132 ☑
streetcar V06.92 ☑
nontraffic V06.02 ☑
traffic V06.12 ☑
two- or three-wheeled motor vehicle V02.92 ☑
nontraffic V02.02 ☑
traffic V02.12 ☑
vehicle V09.9 ☑
animal-drawn V06.92 ☑
nontraffic V06.02 ☑
traffic V06.12 ☑
motor
nontraffic V09.00 ☑
traffic V09.20 ☑
fall V00.131 ☑
nontraffic V09.1 ☑
involving motor vehicle NEC V09.00 ☑
traffic V09.3 ☑
involving motor vehicle NEC V09.20 ☑
skis (snow) V00.328 ☑
collision (with) V09.9 ☑
animal being ridden or animal drawn vehicle V06.99 ☑
nontraffic V06.09 ☑
traffic V06.19 ☑
bus or heavy transport V04.99 ☑
nontraffic V04.09 ☑
traffic V04.19 ☑
car V03.99 ☑
nontraffic V03.09 ☑
traffic V03.19 ☑
pedal cycle V01.99 ☑
nontraffic V01.09 ☑
traffic V01.19 ☑
pick-up truck or van V03.99 ☑
nontraffic V03.09 ☑
traffic V03.19 ☑
railway (train) (vehicle) V05.99 ☑
nontraffic V05.09 ☑
traffic V05.19 ☑
stationary object V00.322 ☑

Accident — *continued*
transport — *continued*
pedestrian — *continued*
conveyance — *continued*
skis — *continued*
collision — *continued*
streetcar V06.99 ☑
nontraffic V06.09 ☑
traffic V06.19 ☑
two- or three-wheeled motor vehicle V02.99 ☑
nontraffic V02.09 ☑
traffic V02.19 ☑
vehicle V09.9 ☑
animal-drawn V06.99 ☑
nontraffic V06.09 ☑
traffic V06.19 ☑
motor
nontraffic V09.00 ☑
traffic V09.20 ☑
fall V00.321 ☑
nontraffic V09.1 ☑
involving motor vehicle NEC V09.00 ☑
traffic V09.3 ☑
involving motor vehicle NEC V09.20 ☑
sled V00.228 ☑
collision (with) V09.9 ☑
animal being ridden or animal drawn vehicle V06.99 ☑
nontraffic V06.09 ☑
traffic V06.19 ☑
bus or heavy transport V04.99 ☑
nontraffic V04.09 ☑
traffic V04.19 ☑
car V03.99 ☑
nontraffic V03.09 ☑
traffic V03.19 ☑
pedal cycle V01.99 ☑
nontraffic V01.09 ☑
traffic V01.19 ☑
pick-up truck or van V03.99 ☑
nontraffic V03.09 ☑
traffic V03.19 ☑
railway (train) (vehicle) V05.99 ☑
nontraffic V05.09 ☑
traffic V05.19 ☑
stationary object V00.222 ☑
streetcar V06.99 ☑
nontraffic V06.09 ☑
traffic V06.19 ☑
two- or three-wheeled motor vehicle V02.99 ☑
nontraffic V02.09 ☑
traffic V02.19 ☑
vehicle V09.9 ☑
animal-drawn V06.99 ☑
nontraffic V06.09 ☑
traffic V06.19 ☑
motor
nontraffic V09.00 ☑
traffic V09.20 ☑
fall V00.221 ☑
nontraffic V09.1 ☑
involving motor vehicle NEC V09.00 ☑
traffic V09.3 ☑
involving motor vehicle NEC V09.20 ☑
snow board V00.318 ☑
collision (with) V09.9 ☑
animal being ridden or animal drawn vehicle V06.99 ☑
nontraffic V06.09 ☑
traffic V06.19 ☑
bus or heavy transport V04.99 ☑
nontraffic V04.09 ☑
traffic V04.19 ☑
car V03.99 ☑
nontraffic V03.09 ☑
traffic V03.19 ☑
pedal cycle V01.99 ☑
nontraffic V01.09 ☑
traffic V01.19 ☑
pick-up truck or van V03.99 ☑
nontraffic V03.09 ☑
traffic V03.19 ☑
railway (train) (vehicle) V05.99 ☑
nontraffic V05.09 ☑

- **Accident** — *continued*
  - transport — *continued*
    - pedestrian — *continued*
      - conveyance — *continued*
        - snow board — *continued*
          - collision — *continued*
            - railway — *continued*
              - traffic VØ5.19 ☑
            - stationary object VØØ.312 ☑
            - streetcar VØ6.99 ☑
              - nontraffic VØ6.Ø9 ☑
              - traffic VØ6.19 ☑
            - two- or three-wheeled motor vehicle VØ2.99 ☑
              - nontraffic VØ2.Ø9 ☑
              - traffic VØ2.19 ☑
            - vehicle VØ9.9 ☑
              - animal-drawn VØ6.99 ☑
                - nontraffic VØ6.Ø9 ☑
                - traffic VØ6.19 ☑
              - motor
                - nontraffic VØ9.ØØ ☑
                - traffic VØ9.2Ø ☑
          - fall VØØ.311 ☑
          - nontraffic VØ9.1 ☑
            - involving motor vehicle NEC VØ9.ØØ ☑
          - traffic VØ9.3 ☑
            - involving motor vehicle NEC VØ9.2Ø ☑
        - specified type NEC VØØ.898 ☑
          - collision (with) VØ9.9 ☑
            - animal being ridden or animal drawn vehicle VØ6.99 ☑
              - nontraffic VØ6.Ø9 ☑
              - traffic VØ6.19 ☑
            - bus or heavy transport VØ4.99 ☑
              - nontraffic VØ4.Ø9 ☑
              - traffic VØ4.19 ☑
            - car VØ3.99 ☑
              - nontraffic VØ3.Ø9 ☑
              - traffic VØ3.19 ☑
            - pedal cycle VØ1.99 ☑
              - nontraffic VØ1.Ø9 ☑
              - traffic VØ1.19 ☑
            - pick-up truck or van VØ3.99 ☑
              - nontraffic VØ3.Ø9 ☑
              - traffic VØ3.19 ☑
            - railway (train) (vehicle) VØ5.99 ☑
              - nontraffic VØ5.Ø9 ☑
              - traffic VØ5.19 ☑
            - stationary object VØØ.892 ☑
            - streetcar VØ6.99 ☑
              - nontraffic VØ6.Ø9 ☑
              - traffic VØ6.19 ☑
            - two- or three-wheeled motor vehicle VØ2.99 ☑
              - nontraffic VØ2.Ø9 ☑
              - traffic VØ2.19 ☑
            - vehicle VØ9.9 ☑
              - animal-drawn VØ6.99 ☑
                - nontraffic VØ6.Ø9 ☑
                - traffic VØ6.19 ☑
              - motor
                - nontraffic VØ9.ØØ ☑
                - traffic VØ9.2Ø ☑
          - fall VØØ.891 ☑
          - nontraffic VØ9.1 ☑
            - involving motor vehicle NEC VØ9.ØØ ☑
          - traffic VØ9.3 ☑
            - involving motor vehicle NEC VØ9.2Ø ☑
        - standing
          - electric scooter
            - collision with
              - animal being ridden or animal drawn vehicle VØ6.931 ☑
                - nontraffic VØ6.Ø31 ☑
                - traffic VØ6.131 ☑
              - bus or heavy transport VØ4.931 ☑
                - nontraffic VØ4.Ø31 ☑
                - traffic VØ4.131 ☑
              - car VØ3.931 ☑
                - nontraffic VØ4.Ø31 ☑
                - traffic VØ4.131 ☑
              - pedal cycle VØ1.931 ☑
                - nontraffic VØ1.Ø31 ☑
                - traffic VØ1.131 ☑
              - pick-up or van VØ3.931 ☑

- **Accident** — *continued*
  - transport — *continued*
    - pedestrian — *continued*
      - conveyance — *continued*
        - standing — *continued*
          - electric scooter — *continued*
            - collision with — *continued*
              - pick-up or van — *continued*
                - nontraffic VØ3.Ø31 ☑
                - traffic VØ3.131 ☑
              - railway (train) (vehicle) VØ5.931 ☑
                - nontraffic VØ5.Ø31 ☑
                - traffic VØ5.131 ☑
              - streetcar VØ6.931 ☑
                - nontraffic VØ6.Ø31 ☑
                - traffic VØ6.131 ☑
              - three-wheeled motor vehicle VØ2.931 ☑
                - nontraffic VØ2.Ø31 ☑
                - traffic VØ2.131 ☑
              - two-wheeled motor vehicle VØ2.931 ☑
                - nontraffic VØ2.Ø31 ☑
                - traffic VØ2.131 ☑
              - vehicle, nonmotor, specified NEC VØ6.931 ☑
                - nontraffic VØ6.Ø31 ☑
                - traffic VØ6.131 ☑
            - fall VØØ.841 ☑
          - micro-mobility pedestrian conveyance
            - collision with
              - animal being ridden or animal drawn vehicle VØ6.938 ☑
                - nontraffic VØ6.Ø38 ☑
                - traffic VØ6.138 ☑
              - bus or heavy transport VØ4.938 ☑
                - nontraffic VØ4.Ø38 ☑
                - traffic VØ4.138 ☑
              - car VØ3.938 ☑
                - nontraffic VØ3.Ø38 ☑
                - traffic VØ3.138 ☑
              - pedal cycle VØ1.938 ☑
                - nontraffic VØ1.Ø38 ☑
                - traffic VØ1.138 ☑
              - pick-up or van VØ3.938 ☑
                - nontraffic VØ3.Ø38 ☑
                - traffic VØ3.138 ☑
              - railway (train) (vehicle) VØ5.938 ☑
                - nontraffic VØ5.Ø38 ☑
                - traffic VØ5.138 ☑
              - stationary object VØØ.842 ☑
              - streetcar VØ6.938 ☑
                - nontraffic VØ6.Ø38 ☑
                - traffic VØ6.138 ☑
              - three-wheeled motor vehicle VØ2.938 ☑
                - nontraffic VØ2.Ø38 ☑
                - traffic VØ2.138 ☑
              - two-wheeled motor vehicle VØ2.938 ☑
                - nontraffic VØ2.Ø38 ☑
                - traffic VØ2.138 ☑
              - vehicle, nonmotor, specified NEC VØ6.938 ☑
                - nontraffic VØ6.Ø38 ☑
                - traffic VØ6.138 ☑
            - fall VØØ.848 ☑
        - traffic VØ9.3 ☑
          - involving motor vehicle VØ9.2Ø ☑
            - military VØ9.21 ☑
            - specified type NEC VØ9.29 ☑
        - wheelchair (powered) VØØ.818 ☑
          - collision (with) VØ9.9 ☑
            - animal being ridden or animal drawn vehicle VØ6.99 ☑
              - nontraffic VØ6.Ø9 ☑
              - traffic VØ6.19 ☑
            - bus or heavy transport VØ4.99 ☑
              - nontraffic VØ4.Ø9 ☑
              - traffic VØ4.19 ☑
            - car VØ3.99 ☑
              - nontraffic VØ3.Ø9 ☑
              - traffic VØ3.19 ☑
            - pedal cycle VØ1.99 ☑
              - nontraffic VØ1.Ø9 ☑
              - traffic VØ1.19 ☑

- **Accident** — *continued*
  - transport — *continued*
    - pedestrian — *continued*
      - conveyance — *continued*
        - wheelchair — *continued*
          - collision — *continued*
            - pick-up truck or van VØ3.99 ☑
              - nontraffic VØ3.Ø9 ☑
              - traffic VØ3.19 ☑
            - railway (train) (vehicle) VØ5.99 ☑
              - nontraffic VØ5.Ø9 ☑
              - traffic VØ5.19 ☑
            - stationary object VØØ.812 ☑
            - streetcar VØ6.99 ☑
              - nontraffic VØ6.Ø9 ☑
              - traffic VØ6.19 ☑
            - two- or three-wheeled motor vehicle VØ2.99 ☑
              - nontraffic VØ2.Ø9 ☑
              - traffic VØ2.19 ☑
            - vehicle VØ9.9 ☑
              - animal-drawn VØ6.99 ☑
                - nontraffic VØ6.Ø9 ☑
                - traffic VØ6.19 ☑
              - motor
                - nontraffic VØ9.ØØ ☑
                - traffic VØ9.2Ø ☑
          - fall VØØ.811 ☑
          - nontraffic VØ9.1 ☑
            - involving motor vehicle NEC VØ9.ØØ ☑
          - traffic VØ9.3 ☑
            - involving motor vehicle NEC VØ9.2Ø ☑
        - wheeled shoe VØØ.158 ☑
          - colliding with stationary object VØØ.152 ☑
          - fall VØØ.151 ☑
      - on foot — *see also* Accident, pedestrian
        - collision (with)
          - animal being ridden or animal drawn vehicle VØ6.9Ø ☑
            - nontraffic VØ6.ØØ ☑
            - traffic VØ6.1Ø ☑
          - bus or heavy transport VØ4.9Ø ☑
            - nontraffic VØ4.ØØ ☑
            - traffic VØ4.1Ø ☑
          - car VØ3.9Ø ☑
            - nontraffic VØ3.ØØ ☑
            - traffic VØ3.1Ø ☑
          - pedal cycle VØ1.9Ø ☑
            - nontraffic VØ1.ØØ ☑
            - traffic VØ1.1Ø ☑
          - pick-up truck or van VØ3.9Ø ☑
            - nontraffic VØ3.ØØ ☑
            - traffic VØ3.1Ø ☑
          - railway (train) (vehicle) VØ5.9Ø ☑
            - nontraffic VØ5.ØØ ☑
            - traffic VØ5.1Ø ☑
          - streetcar VØ6.9Ø ☑
            - nontraffic VØ6.ØØ ☑
            - traffic VØ6.1Ø ☑
          - two- or three-wheeled motor vehicle VØ2.9Ø ☑
            - nontraffic VØ2.ØØ ☑
            - traffic VØ2.1Ø ☑
          - vehicle VØ9.9 ☑
            - animal-drawn VØ6.9Ø ☑
              - nontraffic VØ6.ØØ ☑
              - traffic VØ6.1Ø ☑
            - motor
        - nontraffic VØ9.1 ☑
          - involving motor vehicle VØ9.ØØ ☑
            - military VØ9.Ø1 ☑
            - specified type NEC VØ9.Ø9 ☑
        - traffic VØ9.3 ☑
          - involving motor vehicle VØ9.2Ø ☑
            - military VØ9.21 ☑
            - specified type NEC VØ9.29 ☑
    - person NEC (unknown way or transportation) V99 ☑
      - collision (between)
        - bus (with)
          - heavy transport vehicle (traffic) V87.5 ☑
            - nontraffic V88.5 ☑
        - car (with)
          - bus (traffic) V87.3 ☑
            - nontraffic V88.3 ☑
          - heavy transport vehicle (traffic) V87.4 ☑

External Causes Index

Accident — Accident

- **Accident** — *continued*
  - transport — *continued*
    - person — *continued*
      - collision — *continued*
        - car — *continued*
          - heavy transport vehicle — *continued*
            - nontraffic V88.4 ☑
          - pick-up truck or van (traffic) V87.2 ☑
            - nontraffic V88.2 ☑
          - train or railway vehicle (traffic) V87.6 ☑
            - nontraffic V88.6 ☑
          - two-or three-wheeled motor vehicle (traffic) V87.0 ☑
            - nontraffic V88.0 ☑
        - motor vehicle (traffic) NEC V87.7 ☑
          - nontraffic V88.7 ☑
        - two-or three-wheeled vehicle (with) (traffic)
          - motor vehicle NEC V87.1 ☑
            - nontraffic V88.1 ☑
      - nonmotor vehicle (collision) (noncollision) (traffic) V87.9 ☑
        - nontraffic V88.9 ☑
    - pickup truck occupant V59.9 ☑
      - collision (with)
        - animal (traffic) V50.9 ☑
          - being ridden (traffic) V56.9 ☑
            - nontraffic V56.3 ☑
            - while boarding or alighting V56.4 ☑
          - nontraffic V50.3 ☑
          - while boarding or alighting V50.4 ☑
        - animal-drawn vehicle (traffic) V56.9 ☑
          - nontraffic V56.3 ☑
          - while boarding or alighting V56.4 ☑
        - bus (traffic) V54.9 ☑
          - nontraffic V54.3 ☑
          - while boarding or alighting V54.4 ☑
        - car (traffic) V53.9 ☑
          - nontraffic V53.3 ☑
          - while boarding or alighting V53.4 ☑
        - motor vehicle NOS (traffic) V59.60 ☑
          - nontraffic V59.20 ☑
          - specified type NEC (traffic) V59.69 ☑
            - nontraffic V59.29 ☑
        - pedal cycle (traffic) V51.9 ☑
          - nontraffic V51.3 ☑
          - while boarding or alighting V51.4 ☑
        - pickup truck (traffic) V53.9 ☑
          - nontraffic V53.3 ☑
          - while boarding or alighting V53.4 ☑
        - railway vehicle (traffic) V55.9 ☑
          - nontraffic V55.3 ☑
          - while boarding or alighting V55.4 ☑
        - specified vehicle NEC (traffic) V56.9 ☑
          - nontraffic V56.3 ☑
          - while boarding or alighting V56.4 ☑
        - stationary object (traffic) V57.9 ☑
          - nontraffic V57.3 ☑
          - while boarding or alighting V57.4 ☑
        - streetcar (traffic) V56.9 ☑
          - nontraffic V56.3 ☑
          - while boarding or alighting V56.4 ☑
        - three wheeled motor vehicle (traffic) V52.9 ☑
          - nontraffic V52.3 ☑
          - while boarding or alighting V52.4 ☑
        - truck (traffic) V54.9 ☑
          - nontraffic V54.3 ☑
          - while boarding or alighting V54.4 ☑
        - two wheeled motor vehicle (traffic) V52.9 ☑
          - nontraffic V52.3 ☑
          - while boarding or alighting V52.4 ☑
        - van (traffic) V53.9 ☑
          - nontraffic V53.3 ☑
          - while boarding or alighting V53.4 ☑
      - driver
        - collision (with)
          - animal (traffic) V50.5 ☑
            - being ridden (traffic) V56.5 ☑
              - nontraffic V56.0 ☑
            - nontraffic V50.0 ☑
          - animal-drawn vehicle (traffic) V56.5 ☑
            - nontraffic V56.0 ☑
          - bus (traffic) V54.5 ☑
            - nontraffic V54.0 ☑
          - car (traffic) V53.5 ☑
            - nontraffic V53.0 ☑

- **Accident** — *continued*
  - transport — *continued*
    - pickup truck occupant — *continued*
      - driver — *continued*
        - collision — *continued*
          - motor vehicle NOS (traffic) V59.40 ☑
            - nontraffic V59.00 ☑
            - specified type NEC (traffic) V59.49 ☑
              - nontraffic V59.09 ☑
          - pedal cycle (traffic) V51.5 ☑
            - nontraffic V51.0 ☑
          - pickup truck (traffic) V53.5 ☑
            - nontraffic V53.0 ☑
          - railway vehicle (traffic) V55.5 ☑
            - nontraffic V55.0 ☑
          - specified vehicle NEC (traffic) V56.5 ☑
            - nontraffic V56.0 ☑
          - stationary object (traffic) V57.5 ☑
            - nontraffic V57.0 ☑
          - streetcar (traffic) V56.5 ☑
            - nontraffic V56.0 ☑
          - three wheeled motor vehicle (traffic) V52.5 ☑
            - nontraffic V52.0 ☑
          - truck (traffic) V54.5 ☑
            - nontraffic V54.0 ☑
          - two wheeled motor vehicle (traffic) V52.5 ☑
            - nontraffic V52.0 ☑
          - van (traffic) V53.5 ☑
            - nontraffic V53.0 ☑
        - noncollision accident (traffic) V58.5 ☑
          - nontraffic V58.0 ☑
      - hanger-on
        - collision (with)
          - animal (traffic) V50.7 ☑
            - being ridden (traffic) V56.7 ☑
              - nontraffic V56.2 ☑
            - nontraffic V50.2 ☑
          - animal-drawn vehicle (traffic) V56.7 ☑
            - nontraffic V56.2 ☑
          - bus (traffic) V54.7 ☑
            - nontraffic V54.2 ☑
          - car (traffic) V53.7 ☑
            - nontraffic V53.2 ☑
          - pedal cycle (traffic) V51.7 ☑
            - nontraffic V51.2 ☑
          - pickup truck (traffic) V53.7 ☑
            - nontraffic V53.2 ☑
          - railway vehicle (traffic) V55.7 ☑
            - nontraffic V55.2 ☑
          - specified vehicle NEC (traffic) V56.7 ☑
            - nontraffic V56.2 ☑
          - stationary object (traffic) V57.7 ☑
            - nontraffic V57.2 ☑
          - streetcar (traffic) V56.7 ☑
            - nontraffic V56.2 ☑
          - three wheeled motor vehicle (traffic) V52.7 ☑
            - nontraffic V52.2 ☑
          - truck (traffic) V54.7 ☑
            - nontraffic V54.2 ☑
          - two wheeled motor vehicle (traffic) V52.7 ☑
            - nontraffic V52.2 ☑
          - van (traffic) V53.7 ☑
            - nontraffic V53.2 ☑
        - noncollision accident (traffic) V58.7 ☑
          - nontraffic V58.2 ☑
      - noncollision accident (traffic) V58.9 ☑
        - nontraffic V58.3 ☑
        - while boarding or alighting V58.4 ☑
      - nontraffic V59.3 ☑
      - passenger
        - collision (with)
          - animal (traffic) V50.6 ☑
            - being ridden (traffic) V56.6 ☑
              - nontraffic V56.1 ☑
            - nontraffic V50.1 ☑
          - animal-drawn vehicle (traffic) V56.6 ☑
            - nontraffic V56.1 ☑
          - bus (traffic) V54.6 ☑
            - nontraffic V54.1 ☑
          - car (traffic) V53.6 ☑
            - nontraffic V53.1 ☑
          - motor vehicle NOS (traffic) V59.50 ☑

- **Accident** — *continued*
  - transport — *continued*
    - pickup truck occupant — *continued*
      - passenger — *continued*
        - collision — *continued*
          - motor vehicle — *continued*
            - nontraffic V59.10 ☑
            - specified type NEC (traffic) V59.59 ☑
              - nontraffic V59.19 ☑
          - pedal cycle (traffic) V51.6 ☑
            - nontraffic V51.1 ☑
          - pickup truck (traffic) V53.6 ☑
            - nontraffic V53.1 ☑
          - railway vehicle (traffic) V55.6 ☑
            - nontraffic V55.1 ☑
          - specified vehicle NEC (traffic) V56.6 ☑
            - nontraffic V56.1 ☑
          - stationary object (traffic) V57.6 ☑
            - nontraffic V57.1 ☑
          - streetcar (traffic) V56.6 ☑
            - nontraffic V56.1 ☑
          - three wheeled motor vehicle (traffic) V52.6 ☑
            - nontraffic V52.1 ☑
          - truck (traffic) V54.6 ☑
            - nontraffic V54.1 ☑
          - two wheeled motor vehicle (traffic) V52.6 ☑
            - nontraffic V52.1 ☑
          - van (traffic) V53.6 ☑
            - nontraffic V53.1 ☑
        - noncollision accident (traffic) V58.6 ☑
          - nontraffic V58.1 ☑
      - specified type NEC V59.88 ☑
        - military vehicle V59.81 ☑
    - quarry truck — *see* Accident, transport, industrial vehicle occupant
    - race car — *see* Accident, transport, motor vehicle NEC occupant
    - railway vehicle occupant V81.9 ☑
      - collision (with) V81.3 ☑
        - motor vehicle (non-military) (traffic) V81.1 ☑
          - military V81.83 ☑
          - nontraffic V81.0 ☑
        - rolling stock V81.2 ☑
        - specified object NEC V81.3 ☑
      - during derailment V81.7 ☑
        - with antecedent collision — *see* Accident, transport, railway vehicle occupant, collision
      - explosion V81.81 ☑
      - fall (in railway vehicle) V81.5 ☑
        - during derailment V81.7 ☑
          - with antecedent collision — *see* Accident, transport, railway vehicle occupant, collision
        - from railway vehicle V81.6 ☑
          - during derailment V81.7 ☑
            - with antecedent collision — *see* Accident, transport, railway vehicle occupant, collision
        - while boarding or alighting V81.4 ☑
      - fire V81.81 ☑
      - object falling onto train V81.82 ☑
      - specified type NEC V81.89 ☑
      - while boarding or alighting V81.4 ☑
    - Segway V00.848 ☑
    - ski lift V98.3 ☑
    - snowmobile occupant (nontraffic) V86.92 ☑
      - driver V86.52 ☑
      - hanger-on V86.72 ☑
      - passenger V86.62 ☑
      - traffic V86.32 ☑
        - driver V86.02 ☑
        - hanger-on V86.22 ☑
        - passenger V86.12 ☑
      - while boarding or alighting V86.42 ☑
    - specified NEC V98.8 ☑
    - sport utility vehicle occupant — *see also* Accident, transport, pickup truck occupant
    - streetcar occupant V82.9 ☑
      - collision (with) V82.3 ☑
        - motor vehicle (traffic) V82.1 ☑
          - nontraffic V82.0 ☑
        - rolling stock V82.2 ☑
      - during derailment V82.7 ☑

- **Accident** — *continued*
  - transport — *continued*
    - streetcar occupant — *continued*
      - during derailment — *continued*
        - with antecedent collision — *see* Accident, transport, streetcar occupant, collision
      - fall (in streetcar) V82.5 ☑
        - during derailment V82.7 ☑
          - with antecedent collision — *see* Accident, transport, streetcar occupant, collision
        - from streetcar V82.6 ☑
          - during derailment V82.7 ☑
            - with antecedent collision — *see* Accident, transport, streetcar occupant, collision
          - while boarding or alighting V82.4 ☑
        - while boarding or alighting V82.4 ☑
      - specified type NEC V82.8 ☑
      - while boarding or alighting V82.4 ☑
    - three-wheeled motor vehicle occupant V39.9 ☑
      - collision (with)
        - animal (traffic) V30.9 ☑
          - being ridden (traffic) V36.9 ☑
            - nontraffic V36.3 ☑
            - while boarding or alighting V36.4 ☑
          - nontraffic V30.3 ☑
          - while boarding or alighting V30.4 ☑
        - animal-drawn vehicle (traffic) V36.9 ☑
          - nontraffic V36.3 ☑
          - while boarding or alighting V36.4 ☑
        - bus (traffic) V34.9 ☑
          - nontraffic V34.3 ☑
          - while boarding or alighting V34.4 ☑
        - car (traffic) V33.9 ☑
          - nontraffic V33.3 ☑
          - while boarding or alighting V33.4 ☑
        - motor vehicle NOS (traffic) V39.60 ☑
          - nontraffic V39.20 ☑
          - specified type NEC (traffic) V39.69 ☑
            - nontraffic V39.29 ☑
        - pedal cycle (traffic) V31.9 ☑
          - nontraffic V31.3 ☑
          - while boarding or alighting V31.4 ☑
        - pickup truck (traffic) V33.9 ☑
          - nontraffic V33.3 ☑
          - while boarding or alighting V33.4 ☑
        - railway vehicle (traffic) V35.9 ☑
          - nontraffic V35.3 ☑
          - while boarding or alighting V35.4 ☑
        - specified vehicle NEC (traffic) V36.9 ☑
          - nontraffic V36.3 ☑
          - while boarding or alighting V36.4 ☑
        - stationary object (traffic) V37.9 ☑
          - nontraffic V37.3 ☑
          - while boarding or alighting V37.4 ☑
        - streetcar (traffic) V36.9 ☑
          - nontraffic V36.3 ☑
          - while boarding or alighting V36.4 ☑
        - three wheeled motor vehicle (traffic) V32.9 ☑
          - nontraffic V32.3 ☑
          - while boarding or alighting V32.4 ☑
        - truck (traffic) V34.9 ☑
          - nontraffic V34.3 ☑
          - while boarding or alighting V34.4 ☑
        - two wheeled motor vehicle (traffic) V32.9 ☑
          - nontraffic V32.3 ☑
          - while boarding or alighting V32.4 ☑
        - van (traffic) V33.9 ☑
          - nontraffic V33.3 ☑
          - while boarding or alighting V33.4 ☑
      - driver
        - collision (with)
          - animal (traffic) V30.5 ☑
            - being ridden (traffic) V36.5 ☑
              - nontraffic V36.0 ☑
            - nontraffic V30.0 ☑
          - animal-drawn vehicle (traffic) V36.5 ☑
            - nontraffic V36.0 ☑
          - bus (traffic) V34.5 ☑
            - nontraffic V34.0 ☑
          - car (traffic) V33.5 ☑
            - nontraffic V33.0 ☑
          - motor vehicle NOS (traffic) V39.40 ☑
            - nontraffic V39.00 ☑
            - specified type NEC (traffic) V39.49 ☑

- **Accident** — *continued*
  - transport — *continued*
    - three-wheeled motor vehicle occupant — *continued*
      - driver — *continued*
        - collision — *continued*
          - motor vehicle — *continued*
            - specified type — *continued*
              - nontraffic V39.09 ☑
          - pedal cycle (traffic) V31.5 ☑
            - nontraffic V31.0 ☑
          - pickup truck (traffic) V33.5 ☑
            - nontraffic V33.0 ☑
          - railway vehicle (traffic) V35.5 ☑
            - nontraffic V35.0 ☑
          - specified vehicle NEC (traffic) V36.5 ☑
            - nontraffic V36.0 ☑
          - stationary object (traffic) V37.5 ☑
            - nontraffic V37.0 ☑
          - streetcar (traffic) V36.5 ☑
            - nontraffic V36.0 ☑
          - three wheeled motor vehicle (traffic) V32.5 ☑
            - nontraffic V32.0 ☑
          - truck (traffic) V34.5 ☑
            - nontraffic V34.0 ☑
          - two wheeled motor vehicle (traffic) V32.5 ☑
            - nontraffic V32.0 ☑
          - van (traffic) V33.5 ☑
            - nontraffic V33.0 ☑
        - noncollision accident (traffic) V38.5 ☑
          - nontraffic V38.0 ☑
      - hanger-on
        - collision (with)
          - animal (traffic) V30.7 ☑
            - being ridden (traffic) V36.7 ☑
              - nontraffic V36.2 ☑
            - nontraffic V30.2 ☑
          - animal-drawn vehicle (traffic) V36.7 ☑
            - nontraffic V36.2 ☑
          - bus (traffic) V34.7 ☑
            - nontraffic V34.2 ☑
          - car (traffic) V33.7 ☑
            - nontraffic V33.2 ☑
          - pedal cycle (traffic) V31.7 ☑
            - nontraffic V31.2 ☑
          - pickup truck (traffic) V33.7 ☑
            - nontraffic V33.2 ☑
          - railway vehicle (traffic) V35.7 ☑
            - nontraffic V35.2 ☑
          - specified vehicle NEC (traffic) V36.7 ☑
            - nontraffic V36.2 ☑
          - stationary object (traffic) V37.7 ☑
            - nontraffic V37.2 ☑
          - streetcar (traffic) V36.7 ☑
            - nontraffic V36.2 ☑
          - three wheeled motor vehicle (traffic) V32.7 ☑
            - nontraffic V32.2 ☑
          - truck (traffic) V34.7 ☑
            - nontraffic V34.2 ☑
          - two wheeled motor vehicle (traffic) V32.7 ☑
            - nontraffic V32.2 ☑
          - van (traffic) V33.7 ☑
            - nontraffic V33.2 ☑
        - noncollision accident (traffic) V38.7 ☑
          - nontraffic V38.2 ☑
      - noncollision accident (traffic) V38.9 ☑
        - nontraffic V38.3 ☑
        - while boarding or alighting V38.4 ☑
      - nontraffic V39.3 ☑
      - passenger
        - collision (with)
          - animal (traffic) V30.6 ☑
            - being ridden (traffic) V36.6 ☑
              - nontraffic V36.1 ☑
            - nontraffic V30.1 ☑
          - animal-drawn vehicle (traffic) V36.6 ☑
            - nontraffic V36.1 ☑
          - bus (traffic) V34.6 ☑
            - nontraffic V34.1 ☑
          - car (traffic) V33.6 ☑
            - nontraffic V33.1 ☑
          - motor vehicle NOS (traffic) V39.50 ☑

- **Accident** — *continued*
  - transport — *continued*
    - three-wheeled motor vehicle occupant — *continued*
      - passenger — *continued*
        - collision — *continued*
          - motor vehicle — *continued*
            - nontraffic V39.10 ☑
            - specified type NEC (traffic) V39.59 ☑
              - nontraffic V39.19 ☑
          - pedal cycle (traffic) V31.6 ☑
            - nontraffic V31.1 ☑
          - pickup truck (traffic) V33.6 ☑
            - nontraffic V33.1 ☑
          - railway vehicle (traffic) V35.6 ☑
            - nontraffic V35.1 ☑
          - specified vehicle NEC (traffic) V36.6 ☑
            - nontraffic V36.1 ☑
          - stationary object (traffic) V37.6 ☑
            - nontraffic V37.1 ☑
          - streetcar (traffic) V36.6 ☑
            - nontraffic V36.1 ☑
          - three wheeled motor vehicle (traffic) V32.6 ☑
            - nontraffic V32.1 ☑
          - truck (traffic) V34.6 ☑
            - nontraffic V34.1 ☑
          - two wheeled motor vehicle (traffic) V32.6 ☑
            - nontraffic V32.1 ☑
          - van (traffic) V33.6 ☑
            - nontraffic V33.1 ☑
        - noncollision accident (traffic) V38.6 ☑
          - nontraffic V38.1 ☑
      - specified type NEC V39.89 ☑
        - military vehicle V39.81 ☑
    - tractor (farm) (and trailer) — *see* Accident, transport, agricultural vehicle occupant
    - tram — *see* Accident, transport, streetcar
      - in mine or quarry — *see* Accident, transport, industrial vehicle occupant
    - trolley — *see* Accident, transport, streetcar
      - in mine or quarry — *see* Accident, transport, industrial vehicle occupant
    - truck (heavy) occupant V69.9 ☑
      - collision (with)
        - animal (traffic) V60.9 ☑
          - being ridden (traffic) V66.9 ☑
            - nontraffic V66.3 ☑
            - while boarding or alighting V66.4 ☑
          - nontraffic V60.3 ☑
          - while boarding or alighting V60.4 ☑
        - animal-drawn vehicle (traffic) V66.9 ☑
          - nontraffic V66.3 ☑
          - while boarding or alighting V66.4 ☑
        - bus (traffic) V64.9 ☑
          - nontraffic V64.3 ☑
          - while boarding or alighting V64.4 ☑
        - car (traffic) V63.9 ☑
          - nontraffic V63.3 ☑
          - while boarding or alighting V63.4 ☑
        - motor vehicle NOS (traffic) V69.60 ☑
          - nontraffic V69.20 ☑
          - specified type NEC (traffic) V69.69 ☑
            - nontraffic V69.29 ☑
        - pedal cycle (traffic) V61.9 ☑
          - nontraffic V61.3 ☑
          - while boarding or alighting V61.4 ☑
        - pickup truck (traffic) V63.9 ☑
          - nontraffic V63.3 ☑
          - while boarding or alighting V63.4 ☑
        - railway vehicle (traffic) V65.9 ☑
          - nontraffic V65.3 ☑
          - while boarding or alighting V65.4 ☑
        - specified vehicle NEC (traffic) V66.9 ☑
          - nontraffic V66.3 ☑
          - while boarding or alighting V66.4 ☑
        - stationary object (traffic) V67.9 ☑
          - nontraffic V67.3 ☑
          - while boarding or alighting V67.4 ☑
        - streetcar (traffic) V66.9 ☑
          - nontraffic V66.3 ☑
          - while boarding or alighting V66.4 ☑
        - three wheeled motor vehicle (traffic) V62.9 ☑
          - nontraffic V62.3 ☑
          - while boarding or alighting V62.4 ☑

- **Accident** — *continued*
  - transport — *continued*
    - truck occupant — *continued*
      - collision — *continued*
        - truck (traffic) V64.9 ☑
          - nontraffic V64.3 ☑
            - while boarding or alighting V64.4 ☑
        - two wheeled motor vehicle (traffic) V62.9 ☑
          - nontraffic V62.3 ☑
            - while boarding or alighting V62.4 ☑
        - van (traffic) V63.9 ☑
          - nontraffic V63.3 ☑
            - while boarding or alighting V63.4 ☑
      - driver
        - collision (with)
          - animal (traffic) V60.5 ☑
            - being ridden (traffic) V66.5 ☑
              - nontraffic V66.0 ☑
            - nontraffic V60.0 ☑
          - animal-drawn vehicle (traffic) V66.5 ☑
            - nontraffic V66.0 ☑
          - bus (traffic) V64.5 ☑
            - nontraffic V64.0 ☑
          - car (traffic) V63.5 ☑
            - nontraffic V63.0 ☑
          - motor vehicle NOS (traffic) V69.40 ☑
            - nontraffic V69.00 ☑
            - specified type NEC (traffic) V69.49 ☑
              - nontraffic V69.09 ☑
          - pedal cycle (traffic) V61.5 ☑
            - nontraffic V61.0 ☑
          - pickup truck (traffic) V63.5 ☑
            - nontraffic V63.0 ☑
          - railway vehicle (traffic) V65.5 ☑
            - nontraffic V65.0 ☑
          - specified vehicle NEC (traffic) V66.5 ☑
            - nontraffic V66.0 ☑
          - stationary object (traffic) V67.5 ☑
            - nontraffic V67.0 ☑
          - streetcar (traffic) V66.5 ☑
            - nontraffic V66.0 ☑
          - three wheeled motor vehicle (traffic) V62.5 ☑
            - nontraffic V62.0 ☑
          - truck (traffic) V64.5 ☑
            - nontraffic V64.0 ☑
          - two wheeled motor vehicle (traffic) V62.5 ☑
            - nontraffic V62.0 ☑
          - van (traffic) V63.5 ☑
            - nontraffic V63.0 ☑
        - noncollision accident (traffic) V68.5 ☑
          - nontraffic V68.0 ☑
      - dump — *see* Accident, transport, construction vehicle occupant
      - hanger-on
        - collision (with)
          - animal (traffic) V60.7 ☑
            - being ridden (traffic) V66.7 ☑
              - nontraffic V66.2 ☑
            - nontraffic V60.2 ☑
          - animal-drawn vehicle (traffic) V66.7 ☑
            - nontraffic V66.2 ☑
          - bus (traffic) V64.7 ☑
            - nontraffic V64.2 ☑
          - car (traffic) V63.7 ☑
            - nontraffic V63.2 ☑
          - pedal cycle (traffic) V61.7 ☑
            - nontraffic V61.2 ☑
          - pickup truck (traffic) V63.7 ☑
            - nontraffic V63.2 ☑
          - railway vehicle (traffic) V65.7 ☑
            - nontraffic V65.2 ☑
          - specified vehicle NEC (traffic) V66.7 ☑
            - nontraffic V66.2 ☑
          - stationary object (traffic) V67.7 ☑
            - nontraffic V67.2 ☑
          - streetcar (traffic) V66.7 ☑
            - nontraffic V66.2 ☑
          - three wheeled motor vehicle (traffic) V62.7 ☑
            - nontraffic V62.2 ☑
          - truck (traffic) V64.7 ☑
            - nontraffic V64.2 ☑
          - two wheeled motor vehicle (traffic) V62.7 ☑

- **Accident** — *continued*
  - transport — *continued*
    - truck occupant — *continued*
      - hanger-on — *continued*
        - collision — *continued*
          - two wheeled motor vehicle — *continued*
            - nontraffic V62.2 ☑
          - van (traffic) V63.7 ☑
            - nontraffic V63.2 ☑
        - noncollision accident (traffic) V68.7 ☑
          - nontraffic V68.2 ☑
      - noncollision accident (traffic) V68.9 ☑
        - nontraffic V68.3 ☑
          - while boarding or alighting V68.4 ☑
      - nontraffic V69.3 ☑
      - passenger
        - collision (with)
          - animal (traffic) V60.6 ☑
            - being ridden (traffic) V66.6 ☑
              - nontraffic V66.1- ☑
            - nontraffic V60.1 ☑
          - animal-drawn vehicle (traffic) V66.6 ☑
            - nontraffic V66.1 ☑
          - bus (traffic) V64.6 ☑
            - nontraffic V64.1 ☑
          - car (traffic) V63.6 ☑
            - nontraffic V63.1 ☑
          - motor vehicle NOS (traffic) V69.50 ☑
            - nontraffic V69.10 ☑
            - specified type NEC (traffic) V69.59 ☑
              - nontraffic V69.19 ☑
          - pedal cycle (traffic) V61.6 ☑
            - nontraffic V61.1 ☑
          - pickup truck (traffic) V63.6 ☑
            - nontraffic V63.1 ☑
          - railway vehicle (traffic) V65.6 ☑
            - nontraffic V65.1 ☑
          - specified vehicle NEC (traffic) V66.6 ☑
            - nontraffic V66.1 ☑
          - stationary object (traffic) V67.6 ☑
            - nontraffic V67.1 ☑
          - streetcar (traffic) V66.6 ☑
            - nontraffic V66.1 ☑
          - three wheeled motor vehicle (traffic) V62.6 ☑
            - nontraffic V62.1 ☑
          - truck (traffic) V64.6 ☑
            - nontraffic V64.1 ☑
          - two wheeled motor vehicle (traffic) V62.6 ☑
            - nontraffic V62.1 ☑
          - van (traffic) V63.6 ☑
            - nontraffic V63.1 ☑
        - noncollision accident (traffic) V68.6 ☑
          - nontraffic V68.1 ☑
    - pickup — *see* Accident, transport, pickup truck occupant
    - specified type NEC V69.88 ☑
      - military vehicle V69.81 ☑
    - van occupant V59.9 ☑
      - collision (with)
        - animal (traffic) V50.9 ☑
          - being ridden (traffic) V56.9 ☑
            - nontraffic V56.3 ☑
              - while boarding or alighting V56.4 ☑
          - nontraffic V50.3 ☑
            - while boarding or alighting V50.4 ☑
        - animal-drawn vehicle (traffic) V56.9 ☑
          - nontraffic V56.3 ☑
            - while boarding or alighting V56.4 ☑
        - bus (traffic) V54.9 ☑
          - nontraffic V54.3 ☑
            - while boarding or alighting V54.4 ☑
        - car (traffic) V53.9 ☑
          - nontraffic V53.3 ☑
            - while boarding or alighting V53.4 ☑
        - motor vehicle NOS (traffic) V59.60 ☑
          - nontraffic V59.20 ☑
          - specified type NEC (traffic) V59.69 ☑
            - nontraffic V59.29 ☑
        - pedal cycle (traffic) V51.9 ☑
          - nontraffic V51.3 ☑
            - while boarding or alighting V51.4 ☑
        - pickup truck (traffic) V53.9 ☑
          - nontraffic V53.3 ☑

- **Accident** — *continued*
  - transport — *continued*
    - van occupant — *continued*
      - collision — *continued*
        - pickup truck — *continued*
            - while boarding or alighting V53.4 ☑
        - railway vehicle (traffic) V55.9 ☑
          - nontraffic V55.3 ☑
            - while boarding or alighting V55.4 ☑
        - specified vehicle NEC (traffic) V56.9 ☑
          - nontraffic V56.3 ☑
            - while boarding or alighting V56.4 ☑
        - stationary object (traffic) V57.9 ☑
          - nontraffic V57.3 ☑
            - while boarding or alighting V57.4 ☑
        - streetcar (traffic) V56.9 ☑
          - nontraffic V56.3 ☑
            - while boarding or alighting V56.4 ☑
        - three wheeled motor vehicle (traffic) V52.9 ☑
          - nontraffic V52.3 ☑
            - while boarding or alighting V52.4 ☑
        - truck (traffic) V54.9 ☑
          - nontraffic V54.3 ☑
            - while boarding or alighting V54.4 ☑
        - two wheeled motor vehicle (traffic) V52.9 ☑
          - nontraffic V52.3 ☑
            - while boarding or alighting V52.4 ☑
        - van (traffic) V53.9 ☑
          - nontraffic V53.3 ☑
            - while boarding or alighting V53.4 ☑
      - driver
        - collision (with)
          - animal (traffic) V50.5 ☑
            - being ridden (traffic) V56.5 ☑
              - nontraffic V56.0 ☑
            - nontraffic V50.0 ☑
          - animal-drawn vehicle (traffic) V56.5 ☑
            - nontraffic V56.0 ☑
          - bus (traffic) V54.5 ☑
            - nontraffic V54.0 ☑
          - car (traffic) V53.5 ☑
            - nontraffic V53.0 ☑
          - motor vehicle NOS (traffic) V59.40 ☑
            - nontraffic V59.00 ☑
            - specified type NEC (traffic) V59.49 ☑
              - nontraffic V59.09 ☑
          - pedal cycle (traffic) V51.5 ☑
            - nontraffic V51.0 ☑
          - pickup truck (traffic) V53.5 ☑
            - nontraffic V53.0 ☑
          - railway vehicle (traffic) V55.5 ☑
            - nontraffic V55.0 ☑
          - specified vehicle NEC (traffic) V56.5 ☑
            - nontraffic V56.0 ☑
          - stationary object (traffic) V57.5 ☑
            - nontraffic V57.0 ☑
          - streetcar (traffic) V56.5 ☑
            - nontraffic V56.0 ☑
          - three wheeled motor vehicle (traffic) V52.5 ☑
            - nontraffic V52.0 ☑
          - truck (traffic) V54.5 ☑
            - nontraffic V54.0 ☑
          - two wheeled motor vehicle (traffic) V52.5 ☑
            - nontraffic V52.0 ☑
          - van (traffic) V53.5 ☑
            - nontraffic V53.0 ☑
        - noncollision accident (traffic) V58.5 ☑
          - nontraffic V58.0 ☑
      - hanger-on
        - collision (with)
          - animal (traffic) V50.7 ☑
            - being ridden (traffic) V56.7 ☑
              - nontraffic V56.2 ☑
            - nontraffic V50.2 ☑
          - animal-drawn vehicle (traffic) V56.7 ☑
            - nontraffic V56.2 ☑
          - bus (traffic) V54.7 ☑
            - nontraffic V54.2 ☑
          - car (traffic) V53.7 ☑
            - nontraffic V53.2 ☑
          - pedal cycle (traffic) V51.7 ☑
            - nontraffic V51.2 ☑
          - pickup truck (traffic) V53.7 ☑
            - nontraffic V53.2 ☑

Accident — *continued*
  transport — *continued*
    van occupant — *continued*
      hanger-on — *continued*
        collision — *continued*
          railway vehicle (traffic) V55.7 ☑
            nontraffic V55.2 ☑
          specified vehicle NEC (traffic) V56.7 ☑
            nontraffic V56.2 ☑
          stationary object (traffic) V57.7 ☑
            nontraffic V57.2 ☑
          streetcar (traffic) V56.7 ☑
            nontraffic V56.2 ☑
          three wheeled motor vehicle (traffic) V52.7 ☑
            nontraffic V52.2 ☑
          truck (traffic) V54.7 ☑
            nontraffic V54.2 ☑
          two wheeled motor vehicle (traffic) V52.7 ☑
            nontraffic V52.2 ☑
          van (traffic) V53.7 ☑
            nontraffic V53.2 ☑
        noncollision accident (traffic) V58.7 ☑
          nontraffic V58.2 ☑
      noncollision accident (traffic) V58.9 ☑
        nontraffic V58.3 ☑
        while boarding or alighting V58.4 ☑
      nontraffic V59.3 ☑
      passenger
        collision (with)
          animal (traffic) V5Ø.6 ☑
            being ridden (traffic) V56.6 ☑
              nontraffic V56.1 ☑
            nontraffic V5Ø.1 ☑
          animal-drawn vehicle (traffic) V56.6 ☑
            nontraffic V56.1 ☑
          bus (traffic) V54.6 ☑
            nontraffic V54.1 ☑
          car (traffic) V53.6 ☑
            nontraffic V53.1 ☑
          motor vehicle NOS (traffic) V59.5Ø ☑
            nontraffic V59.1Ø ☑
            specified type NEC (traffic) V59.59 ☑
              nontraffic V59.19 ☑
          pedal cycle (traffic) V51.6 ☑
            nontraffic V51.1 ☑
          pickup truck (traffic) V53.6 ☑
            nontraffic V53.1 ☑
          railway vehicle (traffic) V55.6 ☑
            nontraffic V55.1 ☑
          specified vehicle NEC (traffic) V56.6 ☑
            nontraffic V56.1 ☑
          stationary object (traffic) V57.6 ☑
            nontraffic V57.1 ☑
          streetcar (traffic) V56.6 ☑
            nontraffic V56.1 ☑
          three wheeled motor vehicle (traffic) V52.6 ☑
            nontraffic V52.1 ☑
          truck (traffic) V54.6 ☑
            nontraffic V54.1 ☑
          two wheeled motor vehicle (traffic) V52.6 ☑
            nontraffic V52.1 ☑
          van (traffic) V53.6 ☑
            nontraffic V53.1 ☑
        noncollision accident (traffic) V58.6 ☑
          nontraffic V58.1 ☑
      specified type NEC V59.88 ☑
      military vehicle V59.81 ☑
    watercraft occupant — *see* Accident, watercraft
  vehicle NEC V89.9 ☑
    animal-drawn NEC — *see* Accident, transport, animal-drawn vehicle occupant
    special
      agricultural — *see* Accident, transport, agricultural vehicle occupant
      construction — *see* Accident, transport, construction vehicle occupant
      industrial — *see* Accident, transport, industrial vehicle occupant
    three-wheeled NEC (motorized) — *see* Accident, transport, three-wheeled motor vehicle occupant
  watercraft V94.9 ☑

Accident — *continued*
  watercraft — *continued*
    causing
      drowning — *see* Drowning, due to, accident to, watercraft
      injury NEC V91.89 ☑
        crushed between craft and object V91.19 ☑
          powered craft V91.13 ☑
            ferry boat V91.11 ☑
            fishing boat V91.12 ☑
            jetskis V91.13 ☑
            liner V91.11 ☑
            merchant ship V91.1Ø ☑
            passenger ship V91.11 ☑
          unpowered craft V91.18 ☑
            canoe V91.15 ☑
            inflatable V91.16 ☑
            kayak V91.15 ☑
            sailboat V91.14 ☑
            surf-board V91.18 ☑
            windsurfer V91.18 ☑
        fall on board V91.29 ☑
          powered craft V91.23 ☑
            ferry boat V91.21 ☑
            fishing boat V91.22 ☑
            jetskis V91.23 ☑
            liner V91.21 ☑
            merchant ship V91.2Ø ☑
            passenger ship V91.21 ☑
          unpowered craft
            canoe V91.25 ☑
            inflatable V91.26 ☑
            kayak V91.25 ☑
            sailboat V91.24 ☑
        fire on board causing burn V91.Ø9 ☑
          powered craft V91.Ø3 ☑
            ferry boat V91.Ø1 ☑
            fishing boat V91.Ø2 ☑
            jetskis V91.Ø3 ☑
            liner V91.Ø1 ☑
            merchant ship V91.ØØ ☑
            passenger ship V91.Ø1 ☑
          unpowered craft V91.Ø8 ☑
            canoe V91.Ø5 ☑
            inflatable V91.Ø6 ☑
            kayak V91.Ø5 ☑
            sailboat V91.Ø4 ☑
            surf-board V91.Ø8 ☑
            water skis V91.Ø7 ☑
            windsurfer V91.Ø8 ☑
        hit by falling object V91.39 ☑
          powered craft V91.33 ☑
            ferry boat V91.31 ☑
            fishing boat V91.32 ☑
            jetskis V91.33 ☑
            liner V91.31 ☑
            merchant ship V91.3Ø ☑
            passenger ship V91.31 ☑
          unpowered craft V91.38 ☑
            canoe V91.35 ☑
            inflatable V91.36 ☑
            kayak V91.35 ☑
            sailboat V91.34 ☑
            surf-board V91.38 ☑
            water skis V91.37 ☑
            windsurfer V91.38 ☑
        specified type NEC V91.89 ☑
          powered craft V91.83 ☑
            ferry boat V91.81 ☑
            fishing boat V91.82 ☑
            jetskis V91.83 ☑
            liner V91.81 ☑
            merchant ship V91.8Ø ☑
            passenger ship V91.81 ☑
          unpowered craft V91.88 ☑
            canoe V91.85 ☑
            inflatable V91.86 ☑
            kayak V91.85 ☑
            sailboat V91.84 ☑
            surf-board V91.88 ☑
            water skis V91.87 ☑
            windsurfer V91.88 ☑
    due to, caused by cataclysm — *see* Forces of nature, by type
    military NEC V94.818 ☑
      civilian in water injured by V94.811 ☑

Accident — *continued*
  watercraft — *continued*
    military — *continued*
      with civilian watercraft V94.81Ø ☑
    nonpowered, struck by
      nonpowered vessel V94.22 ☑
      powered vessel V94.21 ☑
    specified type NEC V94.89 ☑
    striking swimmer
      powered V94.11 ☑
      unpowered V94.12 ☑
Acid throwing (assault) YØ8.89 ☑
Activity (involving) (of victim at time of event) Y93.9
  aerobic and step exercise (class) Y93.A3 (*following* Y93.7)
  alpine skiing Y93.23
  animal care NEC Y93.K9 (*following* Y93.7)
  arts and handcrafts NEC Y93.D9 (*following* Y93.7)
  athletics played as a team or group NEC Y93.69
  athletics played individually NEC Y93.59
  athletics NEC Y93.79
  baking Y93.G3 (*following* Y93.7)
  ballet Y93.41
  barbells Y93.B3 (*following* Y93.7)
  BASE (Building, Antenna, Span, Earth) jumping Y93.33
  baseball Y93.64
  basketball Y93.67
  bathing (personal) Y93.E1 (*following* Y93.7)
  beach volleyball Y93.68
  bike riding Y93.55
  blackout game Y93.85
  boogie boarding Y93.18
  bowling Y93.54
  boxing Y93.71
  brass instrument playing Y93.J4 (*following* Y93.7)
  building construction Y93.H3 (*following* Y93.7)
  bungee jumping Y93.34
  calisthenics Y93.A2 (*following* Y93.7)
  canoeing (in calm and turbulent water) Y93.16
  capture the flag Y93.6A
  cardiorespiratory exercise NEC Y93.A9 (*following* Y93.7)
  caregiving (providing) NEC Y93.F9 (*following* Y93.7)
    bathing Y93.F1 (*following* Y93.7)
    lifting Y93.F2 (*following* Y93.7)
  cellular
    communication device Y93.C2 (*following* Y93.7)
    telephone Y93.C2 (*following* Y93.7)
  challenge course Y93.A5 (*following* Y93.7)
  cheerleading Y93.45
  choking game Y93.85
  circuit training Y93.A4 (*following* Y93.7)
  cleaning
    floor Y93.E5 (*following* Y93.7)
  climbing NEC Y93.39
    mountain Y93.31
    rock Y93.31
    wall Y93.31
  clothing care and maintenance NEC Y93.E9 (*following* Y93.7)
  combatives Y93.75
  computer
    keyboarding Y93.C1 (*following* Y93.7)
    technology NEC Y93.C9 (*following* Y93.7)
  confidence course Y93.A5 (*following* Y93.7)
  construction (building) Y93.H3 (*following* Y93.7)
  cooking and baking Y93.G3 (*following* Y93.7)
  cool down exercises Y93.A2 (*following* Y93.7)
  cricket Y93.69
  crocheting Y93.D1 (*following* Y93.7)
  cross country skiing Y93.24
  dancing (all types) Y93.41
  digging
    dirt Y93.H1 (*following* Y93.7)
  dirt digging Y93.H1 (*following* Y93.7)
  dishwashing Y93.G1 (*following* Y93.7)
  diving (platform) (springboard) Y93.12
    underwater Y93.15
  dodge ball Y93.6A
  downhill skiing Y93.23
  drum playing Y93.J2 (*following* Y93.7)
  dumbbells Y93.B3 (*following* Y93.7)
  electronic
    devices NEC Y93.C9 (*following* Y93.7)
      hand held interactive Y93.C2 (*following* Y93.7)
    game playing (using) (with)
      interactive device Y93.C2 (*following* Y93.7)
      keyboard or other stationary device Y93.C1 (*following* Y93.7)

External Causes Index

Accident — Activity

Activity — *continued*
- elliptical machine Y93.A1 (*following* Y93.7)
- exercise(s)
  - machines ((primarily) for)
    - cardiorespiratory conditioning Y93.A1 (*following* Y93.7)
    - muscle strengthening Y93.B1 (*following* Y93.7)
  - muscle strengthening (non-machine) NEC Y93.B9 (*following* Y93.7)
- external motion NEC Y93.I9 (*following* Y93.7)
  - rollercoaster Y93.I1 (*following* Y93.7)
- fainting game Y93.85
- field hockey Y93.65
- figure skating (pairs) (singles) Y93.21
- flag football Y93.62
- floor mopping and cleaning Y93.E5 (*following* Y93.7)
- food preparation and clean up Y93.G1 (*following* Y93.7)
- football (American) NOS Y93.61
  - flag Y93.62
  - tackle Y93.61
  - touch Y93.62
- four square Y93.6A
- free weights Y93.B3 (*following* Y93.7)
- frisbee (ultimate) Y93.74
- furniture
  - building Y93.D3 (*following* Y93.7)
  - finishing Y93.D3 (*following* Y93.7)
  - repair Y93.D3 (*following* Y93.7)
- game playing (electronic)
  - using interactive device Y93.C2 (*following* Y93.7)
  - using keyboard or other stationary device Y93.C1 (*following* Y93.7)
- gardening Y93.H2 (*following* Y93.7)
- golf Y93.53
- grass drills Y93.A6 (*following* Y93.7)
- grilling and smoking food Y93.G2 (*following* Y93.7)
- grooming and shearing an animal Y93.K3 (*following* Y93.7)
- guerilla drills Y93.A6 (*following* Y93.7)
- gymnastics (rhythmic) Y93.43
- hand held interactive electronic device Y93.C2 (*following* Y93.7)
- handball Y93.73
- handcrafts NEC Y93.D9 (*following* Y93.7)
- hang gliding Y93.35
- hiking (on level or elevated terrain) Y93.Ø1
- hockey (ice) Y93.22
  - field Y93.65
- horseback riding Y93.52
- household (interior) maintenance NEC Y93.E9 (*following* Y93.7)
- ice NEC Y93.29
  - dancing Y93.21
  - hockey Y93.22
  - skating Y93.21
- inline roller skating Y93.51
- ironing Y93.E4 (*following* Y93.7)
- judo Y93.75
- jumping jacks Y93.A2 (*following* Y93.7)
- jumping rope Y93.56
- jumping (off) NEC Y93.39
  - BASE (Building, Antenna, Span, Earth) Y93.33
  - bungee Y93.34
  - jacks Y93.A2 (*following* Y93.7)
  - rope Y93.56
- karate Y93.75
- kayaking (in calm and turbulent water) Y93.16
- keyboarding (computer) Y93.C1 (*following* Y93.7)
- kickball Y93.6A
- knitting Y93.D1 (*following* Y93.7)
- lacrosse Y93.65
- land maintenance NEC Y93.H9 (*following* Y93.7)
- landscaping Y93.H2 (*following* Y93.7)
- laundry Y93.E2 (*following* Y93.7)
- machines (exercise)
  - primarily for cardiorespiratory conditioning Y93.A1 (*following* Y93.7)
  - primarily for muscle strengthening Y93.B1 (*following* Y93.7)
- maintenance
  - exterior building NEC Y93.H9 (*following* Y93.7)
  - household (interior) NEC Y93.E9 (*following* Y93.7)
  - land Y93.H9 (*following* Y93.7)
  - property Y93.H9 (*following* Y93.7)
- marching (on level or elevated terrain) Y93.Ø1
- martial arts Y93.75
- microwave oven Y93.G3 (*following* Y93.7)
- milking an animal Y93.K2 (*following* Y93.7)
- mopping (floor) Y93.E5 (*following* Y93.7)

Activity — *continued*
- mountain climbing Y93.31
- muscle strengthening
  - exercises (non-machine) NEC Y93.B9 (*following* Y93.7)
  - machines Y93.B1 (*following* Y93.7)
- musical keyboard (electronic) playing Y93.J1 (*following* Y93.7)
- nordic skiing Y93.24
- obstacle course Y93.A5 (*following* Y93.7)
- oven (microwave) Y93.G3 (*following* Y93.7)
- packing up and unpacking in moving to a new residence Y93.E6 (*following* Y93.7)
- parasailing Y93.19
- pass out game Y93.85
- percussion instrument playing NEC Y93.J2 (*following* Y93.7)
- personal
  - bathing and showering Y93.E1 (*following* Y93.7)
  - hygiene NEC Y93.E8 (*following* Y93.7)
  - showering Y93.E1 (*following* Y93.7)
- physical games generally associated with school recess, summer camp and children Y93.6A
- physical training NEC Y93.A9 (*following* Y93.7)
- piano playing Y93.J1 (*following* Y93.7)
- pilates Y93.B4 (*following* Y93.7)
- platform diving Y93.12
- playing musical instrument
  - brass instrument Y93.J4 (*following* Y93.7)
  - drum Y93.J2 (*following* Y93.7)
  - musical keyboard (electronic) Y93.J1 (*following* Y93.7)
  - percussion instrument NEC Y93.J2 (*following* Y93.7)
  - piano Y93.J1 (*following* Y93.7)
  - string instrument Y93.J3 (*following* Y93.7)
  - winds instrument Y93.J4 (*following* Y93.7)
- property maintenance
  - exterior NEC Y93.H9 (*following* Y93.7)
  - interior NEC Y93.E9 (*following* Y93.7)
- pruning (garden and lawn) Y93.H2 (*following* Y93.7)
- pull-ups Y93.B2 (*following* Y93.7)
- push-ups Y93.B2 (*following* Y93.7)
- racquetball Y93.73
- rafting (in calm and turbulent water) Y93.16
- raking (leaves) Y93.H1 (*following* Y93.7)
- rappelling Y93.32
- refereeing a sports activity Y93.81
- residential relocation Y93.E6 (*following* Y93.7)
- rhythmic gymnastics Y93.43
- rhythmic movement NEC Y93.49
- riding
  - horseback Y93.52
  - rollercoaster Y93.I1 (*following* Y93.7)
- rock climbing Y93.31
- roller skating (inline) Y93.51
- rollercoaster riding Y93.I1 (*following* Y93.7)
- rough housing and horseplay Y93.83
- rowing (in calm and turbulent water) Y93.16
- rugby Y93.63
- running Y93.Ø2
- SCUBA diving Y93.15
- sewing Y93.D2 (*following* Y93.7)
- shoveling Y93.H1 (*following* Y93.7)
  - dirt Y93.H1 (*following* Y93.7)
  - snow Y93.H1 (*following* Y93.7)
- showering (personal) Y93.E1 (*following* Y93.7)
- sit-ups Y93.B2 (*following* Y93.7)
- skateboarding Y93.51
- skating (ice) Y93.21
  - roller Y93.51
- skiing (alpine) (downhill) Y93.23
  - cross country Y93.24
  - nordic Y93.24
  - water Y93.17
- sledding (snow) Y93.23
- sleeping (sleep) Y93.84
- smoking and grilling food Y93.G2 (*following* Y93.7)
- snorkeling Y93.15
- snow NEC Y93.29
  - boarding Y93.23
  - shoveling Y93.H1 (*following* Y93.7)
  - sledding Y93.23
  - tubing Y93.23
- soccer Y93.66
- softball Y93.64
- specified NEC Y93.89
- spectator at an event Y93.82
- sports NEC Y93.79
  - sports played as a team or group NEC Y93.69

Activity — *continued*
- sports — *continued*
  - sports played individually NEC Y93.59
- springboard diving Y93.12
- squash Y93.73
- stationary bike Y93.A1 (*following* Y93.7)
- step (stepping) exercise (class) Y93.A3 (*following* Y93.7)
- stepper machine Y93.A1 (*following* Y93.7)
- stove Y93.G3 (*following* Y93.7)
- string instrument playing Y93.J3 (*following* Y93.7)
- surfing Y93.18
  - wind Y93.18
- swimming Y93.11
- tackle football Y93.61
- tap dancing Y93.41
- tennis Y93.73
- tobogganing Y93.23
- touch football Y93.62
- track and field events (non-running) Y93.57
  - running Y93.Ø2
- trampoline Y93.44
- treadmill Y93.A1 (*following* Y93.7)
- trimming shrubs Y93.H2 (*following* Y93.7)
- tubing (in calm and turbulent water) Y93.16
  - snow Y93.23
- ultimate frisbee Y93.74
- underwater diving Y93.15
- unpacking in moving to a new residence Y93.E6 (*following* Y93.7)
- use of stove, oven and microwave oven Y93.G3 (*following* Y93.7)
- vacuuming Y93.E3 (*following* Y93.7)
- volleyball (beach) (court) Y93.68
- wake boarding Y93.17
- walking (on level or elevated terrain) Y93.Ø1
  - an animal Y93.K1 (*following* Y93.7)
- walking an animal Y93.K1 (*following* Y93.7)
- wall climbing Y93.31
- warm up and cool down exercises Y93.A2 (*following* Y93.7)
- water NEC Y93.19
  - aerobics Y93.14
  - craft NEC Y93.19
  - exercise Y93.14
  - polo Y93.13
  - skiing Y93.17
  - sliding Y93.18
  - survival training and testing Y93.19
- weeding (garden and lawn) Y93.H2 (*following* Y93.7)
- wind instrument playing Y93.J4 (*following* Y93.7)
- windsurfing Y93.18
- wrestling Y93.72
- yoga Y93.42

Adverse effect of drugs — *see* Table of Drugs and Chemicals

Aerosinusitis — *see* Air, pressure

After-effect, late — *see* Sequelae

Air
- blast in war operations — *see* War operations, air blast
- pressure
  - change, rapid
    - during
      - ascent W94.29 ☑
        - while (in) (surfacing from)
          - aircraft W94.23 ☑
          - deep water diving W94.21 ☑
          - underground W94.22 ☑
      - descent W94.39 ☑
        - in
          - aircraft W94.31 ☑
          - water W94.32 ☑
  - high, prolonged W94.Ø ☑
  - low, prolonged W94.12 ☑
    - due to residence or long visit at high altitude W94.11 ☑

Alpine sickness W94.11 ☑

Altitude sickness W94.11 ☑

Anaphylactic shock, anaphylaxis — *see* Table of Drugs and Chemicals

Andes disease W94.11 ☑

Arachnidism, arachnoidism X58 ☑

Arson (with intent to injure or kill) X97 ☑

Asphyxia, asphyxiation
- by
  - food (bone) (seed) — *see* categories T17 and T18 ☑
  - gas — *see also* Table of Drugs and Chemicals
    - legal
      - execution — *see* Legal, intervention, gas

Asphyxia, asphyxiation — *continued*
by — *continued*
gas — *see also* Table of Drugs and Chemicals — *continued*
legal — *continued*
intervention — *see* Legal, intervention, gas
from
fire — *see also* Exposure, fire
in war operations — *see* War operations, fire
ignition — *see* Ignition
vomitus T17.81 ☑
in war operations — *see* War operations, restriction of airway
Aspiration
food (any type) (into respiratory tract) (with asphyxia, obstruction respiratory tract, suffocation) — *see* categories T17 and T18 ☑
foreign body — *see* Foreign body, aspiration
vomitus (with asphyxia, obstruction respiratory tract, suffocation) T17.81 ☑
Assassination (attempt) — *see* Assault
Assault (homicidal) (by) (in) Y09
arson X97 ☑
bite (of human being) Y04.1 ☑
bodily force Y04.8 ☑
bite Y04.1 ☑
bumping into Y04.2 ☑
sexual — *see* subcategories T74.0, T76.0 ☑
unarmed fight Y04.0 ☑
bomb X96.9 ☑
antipersonnel X96.0 ☑
fertilizer X96.3 ☑
gasoline X96.1 ☑
letter X96.2 ☑
petrol X96.1 ☑
pipe X96.3 ☑
specified NEC X96.8 ☑
brawl (hand) (fists) (foot) (unarmed) Y04.0 ☑
burning, burns (by fire) NEC X97 ☑
acid Y08.89 ☑
caustic, corrosive substance Y08.89 ☑
chemical from swallowing caustic, corrosive substance — *see* Table of Drugs and Chemicals
cigarette(s) X97 ☑
hot object X98.9 ☑
fluid NEC X98.2 ☑
household appliance X98.3 ☑
specified NEC X98.8 ☑
steam X98.0 ☑
tap water X98.1 ☑
vapors X98.0 ☑
scalding — *see* Assault, burning
steam X98.0 ☑
vitriol Y08.89 ☑
caustic, corrosive substance (gas) Y08.89 ☑
crashing of
aircraft Y08.81 ☑
motor vehicle Y03.8 ☑
pushed in front of Y02.0 ☑
run over Y03.0 ☑
specified NEC Y03.8 ☑
cutting or piercing instrument X99.9 ☑
dagger X99.2 ☑
glass X99.0 ☑
knife X99.1 ☑
specified NEC X99.8 ☑
sword X99.2 ☑
dagger X99.2 ☑
drowning (in) X92.9 ☑
bathtub X92.0 ☑
natural water X92.3 ☑
specified NEC X92.8 ☑
swimming pool X92.1 ☑
following fall X92.2 ☑
dynamite X96.8 ☑
explosive(s) (material) X96.9 ☑
fight (hand) (fists) (foot) (unarmed) Y04.0 ☑
with weapon — *see* Assault, by type of weapon
fire X97 ☑
firearm X95.9 ☑
airgun X95.01 ☑
handgun X93 ☑
hunting rifle X94.1 ☑
larger X94.9 ☑
specified NEC X94.8 ☑
machine gun X94.2 ☑

Assault — *continued*
firearm — *continued*
shotgun X94.0 ☑
specified NEC X95.8 ☑
from high place Y01 ☑
gunshot (wound) NEC — *see* Assault, firearm, by type
incendiary device X97 ☑
injury Y09
to child due to criminal abortion attempt NEC Y08.89 ☑
knife X99.1 ☑
late effect of — *see* categories X92-Y08 with 7th character S
placing before moving object NEC Y02.8 ☑
motor vehicle Y02.0 ☑
poisoning — *see* categories T36-T65 with 7th character S
puncture, any part of body — *see* Assault, cutting or piercing instrument
pushing
before moving object NEC Y02.8 ☑
motor vehicle Y02.0 ☑
subway train Y02.1 ☑
train Y02.1 ☑
from high place Y01 ☑
rape T74.2- ☑
scalding — *see* Assault, burning
sequelae of — *see* categories X92-Y08 with 7th character S
sexual (by bodily force) T74.2- ☑
shooting — *see* Assault, firearm
specified means NEC Y08.89 ☑
stab, any part of body — *see* Assault, cutting or piercing instrument
steam X98.0 ☑
striking against
other person Y04.2 ☑
sports equipment Y08.09 ☑
baseball bat Y08.02 ☑
hockey stick Y08.01 ☑
struck by
sports equipment Y08.09 ☑
baseball bat Y08.02 ☑
hockey stick Y08.01 ☑
submersion — *see* Assault, drowning
violence Y09
weapon Y09
blunt Y00 ☑
cutting or piercing — *see* Assault, cutting or piercing instrument
firearm — *see* Assault, firearm
wound Y09
cutting — *see* Assault, cutting or piercing instrument
gunshot — *see* Assault, firearm
knife X99.1 ☑
piercing — *see* Assault, cutting or piercing instrument
puncture — *see* Assault, cutting or piercing instrument
stab — *see* Assault, cutting or piercing instrument
Attack by mammals NEC W55.89 ☑
Avalanche — *see* Landslide
Aviator's disease — *see* Air, pressure

B

Barotitis, barodontalgia, barosinusitis, barotrauma (otitic) (sinus) — *see* Air, pressure
Battered (baby) (child) (person) (syndrome) X58 ☑
Bayonet wound W26.1 ☑
in
legal intervention — *see* Legal, intervention, sharp object, bayonet
war operations — *see* War operations, combat
stated as undetermined whether accidental or intentional Y28.8 ☑
suicide (attempt) X78.2 ☑
Bean in nose — *see* categories T17 and T18 ☑
Bed set on fire NEC — *see* Exposure, fire, uncontrolled, building, bed
Beheading (by guillotine)
homicide X99.9 ☑
legal execution — *see* Legal, intervention
Bending, injury in (prolonged) (static) X50.1 ☑
Bends — *see* Air, pressure, change

Bite, bitten by
alligator W58.01 ☑
arthropod (nonvenomous) NEC W57 ☑
bull W55.21 ☑
cat W55.01 ☑
cow W55.21 ☑
crocodile W58.11 ☑
dog W54.0 ☑
goat W55.31 ☑
hoof stock NEC W55.31 ☑
horse W55.11 ☑
human being (accidentally) W50.3 ☑
with intent to injure or kill Y04.1 ☑
as, or caused by, a crowd or human stampede (with fall) W52 ☑
assault Y04.1 ☑
homicide (attempt) Y04.1 ☑
in
fight Y04.1 ☑
insect (nonvenomous) W57 ☑
lizard (nonvenomous) W59.01 ☑
mammal NEC W55.81 ☑
marine W56.31 ☑
marine animal (nonvenomous) W56.81 ☑
millipede W57 ☑
moray eel W56.51 ☑
mouse W53.01 ☑
person(s) (accidentally) W50.3 ☑
with intent to injure or kill Y04.1 ☑
as, or caused by, a crowd or human stampede (with fall) W52 ☑
assault Y04.1 ☑
homicide (attempt) Y04.1 ☑
in
fight Y04.1 ☑
pig W55.41 ☑
raccoon W55.51 ☑
rat W53.11 ☑
reptile W59.81 ☑
lizard W59.01 ☑
snake W59.11 ☑
turtle W59.21 ☑
terrestrial W59.81 ☑
rodent W53.81 ☑
mouse W53.01 ☑
rat W53.11 ☑
specified NEC W53.81 ☑
squirrel W53.21 ☑
shark W56.41 ☑
sheep W55.31 ☑
snake (nonvenomous) W59.11 ☑
spider (nonvenomous) W57 ☑
squirrel W53.21 ☑
Blast (air) in war operations — *see* War operations, blast
Blizzard X37.2 ☑
Blood alcohol level Y90.9
less than 20mg/100ml Y90.0
presence in blood, level not specified Y90.9
20-39mg/100ml Y90.1
40 59mg/100ml Y90.2
60-79mg/100ml Y90.3
80-99mg/100ml Y90.4
100-119mg/100ml Y90.5
120-199mg/100ml Y90.6
200-239mg/100ml Y90.7
Blow X58 ☑
by law-enforcing agent, police (on duty) — *see* Legal, intervention, manhandling
blunt object — *see* Legal, intervention, blunt object
Blowing up — *see* Explosion
Brawl (hand) (fists) (foot) Y04.0 ☑
Breakage (accidental) (part of)
ladder (causing fall) W11 ☑
scaffolding (causing fall) W12 ☑
Broken
glass, contact with — *see* Contact, with, glass
power line (causing electric shock) W85 ☑
Bumping against, into (accidentally)
object NEC W22.8 ☑
caused by crowd or human stampede (with fall) W52 ☑
sports equipment W21.9 ☑
with fall — *see* Fall, due to, bumping against, object
person(s) W51 ☑
with fall W03 ☑
due to ice or snow W00.0 ☑

External Causes Index
Asphyxia, asphyxiation — Bumping against, into

- **Bumping against, into** — *continued*
  - person(s) — *continued*
    - assault YØ4.2 ☑
    - caused by, a crowd or human stampede (with fall) W52 ☑
    - homicide (attempt) YØ4.2 ☑
  - sports equipment W21.9 ☑
- **Burn, burned, burning** (accidental) (by) (from) (on)
  - acid NEC — *see* Table of Drugs and Chemicals
  - bed linen — *see* Exposure, fire, uncontrolled, in building, bed
  - blowtorch XØ8.8 ☑
    - with ignition of clothing NEC XØ6.2 ☑
      - nightwear XØ5 ☑
  - bonfire, campfire (controlled) — *see also* Exposure, fire, controlled, not in building)
    - uncontrolled — *see* Exposure, fire, uncontrolled, not in building
  - candle XØ8.8 ☑
    - with ignition of clothing NEC XØ6.2 ☑
      - nightwear XØ5 ☑
  - caustic liquid, substance (external) (internal) NEC — *see* Table of Drugs and Chemicals
  - chemical (external) (internal) — *see also* Table of Drugs and Chemicals
    - in war operations — *see* War operations, fire
  - cigar(s) or cigarette(s) XØ8.8 ☑
    - with ignition of clothing NEC XØ6.2 ☑
      - nightwear XØ5 ☑
  - clothes, clothing NEC (from controlled fire) XØ6.2 ☑
    - with conflagration — *see* Exposure, fire, uncontrolled, building
    - not in building or structure — *see* Exposure, fire, uncontrolled, not in building
  - cooker (hot) X15.8 ☑
    - stated as undetermined whether accidental or intentional Y27.3 ☑
    - suicide (attempt) X77.3 ☑
  - electric blanket X16 ☑
  - engine (hot) X17 ☑
  - fire, flames — *see* Exposure, fire
  - flare, Very pistol — *see* Discharge, firearm NEC
  - heat
    - from appliance (electrical) (household) X15.8 ☑
      - cooker X15.8 ☑
      - hotplate X15.2 ☑
      - kettle X15.8 ☑
      - light bulb X15.8 ☑
      - saucepan X15.3 ☑
      - skillet X15.3 ☑
      - stated as undetermined whether accidental or intentional Y27.3 ☑
      - stove X15.Ø ☑
      - suicide (attempt) X77.3 ☑
      - toaster X15.1 ☑
    - in local application or packing during medical or surgical procedure Y63.5
  - heating
    - appliance, radiator or pipe X16 ☑
  - homicide (attempt) — *see* Assault, burning
  - hot
    - air X14.1 ☑
    - cooker X15.8 ☑
    - drink X1Ø.Ø ☑
    - engine X17 ☑
    - fat X1Ø.2 ☑
    - fluid NEC X12 ☑
    - food X1Ø.1 ☑
    - gases X14.1 ☑
    - heating appliance X16 ☑
    - household appliance NEC X15.8 ☑
    - kettle X15.8 ☑
    - liquid NEC X12 ☑
    - machinery X17 ☑
    - metal (molten) (liquid) NEC X18 ☑
    - object (not producing fire or flames) NEC X19 ☑
    - oil (cooking) X1Ø.2 ☑
    - pipe(s) X16 ☑
    - radiator X16 ☑
    - saucepan (glass) (metal) X15.3 ☑
    - stove (kitchen) X15.Ø ☑
    - substance NEC X19 ☑
      - caustic or corrosive NEC — *see* Table of Drugs and Chemicals
    - toaster X15.1 ☑
    - tool X17 ☑
- **Burn, burned, burning** — *continued*
  - hot — *continued*
    - vapor X13.1 ☑
    - water (tap) — *see* Contact, with, hot, tap water
  - hotplate X15.2 ☑
    - suicide (attempt) X77.3 ☑
  - ignition — *see* Ignition
  - in war operations — *see* War operations, fire
  - inflicted by other person X97 ☑
    - by hot objects, hot vapor, and steam — *see* Assault, burning, hot object
  - internal, from swallowed caustic, corrosive liquid, substance — *see* Table of Drugs and Chemicals
  - iron (hot) X15.8 ☑
    - stated as undetermined whether accidental or intentional Y27.3 ☑
    - suicide (attempt) X77.3 ☑
  - kettle (hot) X15.8 ☑
    - stated as undetermined whether accidental or intentional Y27.3 ☑
    - suicide (attempt) X77.3 ☑
  - lamp (flame) XØ8.8 ☑
    - with ignition of clothing NEC XØ6.2 ☑
      - nightwear XØ5 ☑
  - lighter (cigar) (cigarette) XØ8.8 ☑
    - with ignition of clothing NEC XØ6.2 ☑
      - nightwear XØ5 ☑
  - lightning — *see* subcategory T75.Ø ☑
    - causing fire — *see* Exposure, fire
  - liquid (boiling) (hot) NEC X12 ☑
    - stated as undetermined whether accidental or intentional Y27.2 ☑
    - suicide (attempt) X77.2 ☑
  - local application of externally applied substance in medical or surgical care Y63.5
  - machinery (hot) X17 ☑
  - matches XØ8.8 ☑
    - with ignition of clothing NEC XØ6.2 ☑
      - nightwear XØ5 ☑
  - mattress — *see* Exposure, fire, uncontrolled, building, bed
  - medicament, externally applied Y63.5
  - metal (hot) (liquid) (molten) NEC X18 ☑
  - nightwear (nightclothes, nightdress, gown, pajamas, robe) XØ5 ☑
  - object (hot) NEC X19 ☑
  - on board watercraft
    - due to
      - accident to watercraft V91.Ø9 ☑
        - powered craft V91.Ø3 ☑
          - ferry boat V91.Ø1 ☑
          - fishing boat V91.Ø2 ☑
          - jetskis V91.Ø3 ☑
          - liner V91.Ø1 ☑
          - merchant ship V91.ØØ ☑
          - passenger ship V91.Ø1 ☑
        - unpowered craft V91.Ø8 ☑
          - canoe V91.Ø5 ☑
          - inflatable V91.Ø6 ☑
          - kayak V91.Ø5 ☑
          - sailboat V91.Ø4 ☑
          - surf-board V91.Ø8 ☑
          - water skis V91.Ø7 ☑
          - windsurfer V91.Ø8 ☑
      - fire on board V93.Ø9 ☑
        - ferry boat V93.Ø1 ☑
        - fishing boat V93.Ø2 ☑
        - jetskis V93.Ø3 ☑
        - liner V93.Ø1 ☑
        - merchant ship V93.ØØ ☑
        - passenger ship V93.Ø1 ☑
        - powered craft NEC V93.Ø3 ☑
        - sailboat V93.Ø4 ☑
      - specified heat source NEC on board V93.19 ☑
        - ferry boat V93.11 ☑
        - fishing boat V93.12 ☑
        - jetskis V93.13 ☑
        - liner V93.11 ☑
        - merchant ship V93.1Ø ☑
        - passenger ship V93.11 ☑
        - powered craft V93.13 ☑
        - sailboat V93.14 ☑
  - pipe (hot) X16 ☑
    - smoking XØ8.8 ☑
      - with ignition of clothing NEC XØ6.2 ☑
        - nightwear XØ5 ☑
- **Burn, burned, burning** — *continued*
  - powder — *see* Powder burn
  - radiator (hot) X16 ☑
  - saucepan (hot) (glass) (metal) X15.3 ☑
    - stated as undetermined whether accidental or intentional Y27.3 ☑
    - suicide (attempt) X77.3 ☑
  - self-inflicted X76 ☑
    - stated as undetermined whether accidental or intentional Y26 ☑
  - stated as undetermined whether accidental or intentional Y27.Ø ☑
  - steam X13.1 ☑
    - pipe X16 ☑
      - stated as undetermined whether accidental or intentional Y27.8 ☑
    - stated as undetermined whether accidental or intentional Y27.Ø ☑
    - suicide (attempt) X77.Ø ☑
  - stove (hot) (kitchen) X15.Ø ☑
    - stated as undetermined whether accidental or intentional Y27.3 ☑
    - suicide (attempt) X77.3 ☑
  - substance (hot) NEC X19 ☑
    - boiling X12 ☑
      - stated as undetermined whether accidental or intentional Y27.2 ☑
      - suicide (attempt) X77.2 ☑
    - molten (metal) X18 ☑
  - suicide (attempt) NEC X76 ☑
    - hot
      - household appliance X77.3 ☑
      - object X77.9 ☑
  - therapeutic misadventure
    - heat in local application or packing during medical or surgical procedure Y63.5
    - overdose of radiation Y63.2
  - toaster (hot) X15.1 ☑
    - stated as undetermined whether accidental or intentional Y27.3 ☑
    - suicide (attempt) X77.3 ☑
  - tool (hot) X17 ☑
  - torch, welding XØ8.8 ☑
    - with ignition of clothing NEC XØ6.2 ☑
      - nightwear XØ5 ☑
  - trash fire (controlled) — *see* Exposure, fire, controlled, not in building
    - uncontrolled — *see* Exposure, fire, uncontrolled, not in building
  - vapor (hot) X13.1 ☑
    - stated as undetermined whether accidental or intentional Y27.Ø ☑
    - suicide (attempt) X77.Ø ☑
  - Very pistol — *see* Discharge, firearm NEC
- **Butted by animal** W55.82 ☑
  - bull W55.22 ☑
  - cow W55.22 ☑
  - goat W55.32 ☑
  - horse W55.12 ☑
  - pig W55.42 ☑
  - sheep W55.32 ☑

C

- **Caisson disease** — *see* Air, pressure, change
- **Campfire** (exposure to) (controlled) — *see also* Exposure, fire, controlled, not in building
  - uncontrolled — *see* Exposure, fire, uncontrolled, not in building
- **Capital punishment** (any means) — *see* Legal, intervention
- **Car sickness** T75.3 ☑
- **Casualty** (not due to war) NEC X58 ☑
  - war — *see* War operations
- **Cat**
  - bite W55.Ø1 ☑
  - scratch W55.Ø3 ☑
- **Cataclysm, cataclysmic** (any injury) NEC — *see* Forces of nature
- **Catching fire** — *see* Exposure, fire
- **Caught**
  - between
    - folding object W23.Ø ☑
    - objects (moving) W23.Ø ☑

- **Caught** — *continued*
  - between — *continued*
    - objects — *continued*
      - and
        - machinery — *see* Contact, with, by type of machine
        - stationary
      - stationary W23.1 ☑
        - and moving
    - sliding door and door frame W23.Ø ☑
  - by, in
    - machinery (moving parts of) — *see* Contact, with, by type of machine
    - washing-machine wringer W23.Ø ☑
  - under packing crate (due to losing grip) W23.1 ☑
- **Cave-in caused by cataclysmic earth surface movement or eruption** — *see* Landslide
- **Change**(s) in air pressure — *see* Air, pressure, change
- **Choked, choking** (on) (any object except food or vomitus)
  - food (bone) (seed) — *see* categories T17 and T18 ☑
  - vomitus T17.81- ☑
- **Civil insurrection** — *see* War operations
- **Cloudburst** (any injury) X37.8 ☑
- **Cold, exposure to** (accidental) (excessive) (extreme) (natural) (place) NEC — *see* Exposure, cold
- **Collapse**
  - building W2Ø.1 ☑
    - burning (uncontrolled fire) XØØ.2 ☑
  - dam or man-made structure (causing earth movement) X36.Ø ☑
  - machinery — *see* Contact, with, by type of machine
  - structure W2Ø.1 ☑
    - burning (uncontrolled fire) XØØ.2 ☑
- **Collision** (accidental) NEC — *see also* Accident, transport V89.9 ☑
  - pedestrian W51 ☑
    - with fall WØ3 ☑
      - due to ice or snow WØØ.Ø ☑
      - involving pedestrian conveyance — *see* Accident, transport, pedestrian, conveyance
    - and
      - crowd or human stampede (with fall) W52 ☑
      - object W22.8 ☑
        - with fall — *see* Fall, due to, bumping against, object
  - person(s) — *see* Collision, pedestrian
  - transport vehicle NEC V89.9 ☑
    - and
      - avalanche, fallen or not moving — *see* Accident, transport
        - falling or moving — *see* Landslide
      - landslide, fallen or not moving — *see* Accident, transport
        - falling or moving — *see* Landslide
    - due to cataclysm — *see* Forces of nature, by type
    - intentional, purposeful suicide (attempt) — *see* Suicide, collision
- **Combustion, spontaneous** — *see* Ignition
- **Complication** (delayed) **of or following** (medical or surgical procedure) Y84.9
  - with misadventure — *see* Misadventure
  - amputation of limb(s) Y83.5
  - anastomosis (arteriovenous) (blood vessel) (gastrojejunal) (tendon) (natural or artificial material) Y83.2
  - aspiration (of fluid) Y84.4
    - tissue Y84.8
  - biopsy Y84.8
  - blood
    - sampling Y84.7
    - transfusion
      - procedure Y84.8
  - bypass Y83.2
  - catheterization (urinary) Y84.6
    - cardiac Y84.Ø
  - colostomy Y83.3
  - cystostomy Y83.3
  - dialysis (kidney) Y84.1
  - drug — *see* Table of Drugs and Chemicals
    - due to misadventure — *see* Misadventure
  - duodenostomy Y83.3
  - electroshock therapy Y84.3
  - external stoma, creation of Y83.3
  - formation of external stoma Y83.3
  - gastrostomy Y83.3
  - graft Y83.2
  - hypothermia (medically-induced) Y84.8

- **Complication** (delayed) **of or following** — *continued*
  - implant, implantation (of)
    - artificial
      - internal device (cardiac pacemaker) (electrodes in brain) (heart valve prosthesis) (orthopedic) Y83.1
      - material or tissue (for anastomosis or bypass) Y83.2
        - with creation of external stoma Y83.3
    - natural tissues (for anastomosis or bypass) Y83.2
      - with creation of external stoma Y83.3
  - infusion
    - procedure Y84.8
  - injection — *see* Table of Drugs and Chemicals
    - procedure Y84.8
  - insertion of gastric or duodenal sound Y84.5
  - insulin-shock therapy Y84.3
  - paracentesis (abdominal) (thoracic) (aspirative) Y84.4
  - procedures other than surgical operation — *see* Complication of or following, by type of procedure
  - radiological procedure or therapy Y84.2
  - removal of organ (partial) (total) NEC Y83.6
  - sampling
    - blood Y84.7
    - fluid NEC Y84.4
    - tissue Y84.8
  - shock therapy Y84.3
  - surgical operation NEC — *see also* Complication of or following, by type of operation Y83.9
    - reconstructive NEC Y83.4
      - with
        - anastomosis, bypass or graft Y83.2
        - formation of external stoma Y83.3
    - specified NEC Y83.8
  - transfusion — *see also* Table of Drugs and Chemicals
    - procedure Y84.8
  - transplant, transplantation (heart) (kidney) (liver) (whole organ, any) Y83.Ø
    - partial organ Y83.4
  - ureterostomy Y83.3
  - vaccination — *see also* Table of Drugs and Chemicals
    - procedure Y84.8
- **Compression**
  - divers' squeeze — *see* Air, pressure, change
  - trachea by
    - food (lodged in esophagus) — *see* categories T17 and T18 ☑
    - vomitus (lodged in esophagus) T17.81- ☑
- **Conflagration** — *see* Exposure, fire, uncontrolled
- **Constriction** (external)
  - hair W49.Ø1 ☑
  - jewelry W49.Ø4 ☑
  - ring W49.Ø4 ☑
  - rubber band W49.Ø3 ☑
  - specified item NEC W49.Ø9 ☑
  - string W49.Ø2 ☑
  - thread W49.Ø2 ☑
- **Contact** (accidental)
  - with
    - abrasive wheel (metalworking) W31.1 ☑
    - alligator W58.Ø9 ☑
      - bite W58.Ø1 ☑
      - crushing W58.Ø3 ☑
      - strike W58.Ø2 ☑
    - amphibian W62.9 ☑
      - frog W62.Ø ☑
      - toad W62.1 ☑
    - animal (nonvenomous) NEC W64 ☑
      - marine W56.89 ☑
        - bite W56.81 ☑
        - dolphin — *see* Contact, with, dolphin
        - fish NEC — *see* Contact, with, fish
        - mammal — *see* Contact, with, mammal, marine
        - orca — *see* Contact, with, orca
        - sea lion — *see* Contact, with, sea lion
        - shark — *see* Contact, with, shark
        - strike W56.82 ☑
    - animate mechanical force NEC W64 ☑
    - arrow W21.89 ☑
      - not thrown, projected or falling W45.8 ☑
    - arthropods (nonvenomous) W57 ☑
    - axe W27.Ø ☑
    - band-saw (industrial) W31.2 ☑
    - bayonet — *see* Bayonet wound
    - bee(s) X58 ☑

- **Contact** — *continued*
  - with — *continued*
    - bench-saw (industrial) W31.2 ☑
    - bird W61.99 ☑
      - bite W61.91 ☑
      - chicken — *see* Contact, with, chicken
      - duck — *see* Contact, with, duck
      - goose — *see* Contact, with, goose
      - macaw — *see* Contact, with, macaw
      - parrot — *see* Contact, with, parrot
      - psittacine — *see* Contact, with, psittacine
      - strike W61.92 ☑
      - turkey — *see* Contact, with, turkey
    - blender W29.Ø ☑
    - boiling water X12 ☑
      - stated as undetermined whether accidental or intentional Y27.2 ☑
      - suicide (attempt) X77.2 ☑
    - bore, earth-drilling or mining (land) (seabed) W31.Ø ☑
    - buffalo — *see* Contact, with, hoof stock NEC
    - bull W55.29 ☑
      - bite W55.21 ☑
      - gored W55.22 ☑
      - strike W55.22 ☑
    - bumper cars W31.81 ☑
    - camel — *see* Contact, with, hoof stock NEC
    - can
      - lid W26.8 ☑
      - opener W27.4 ☑
        - powered W29.Ø ☑
    - cat W55.Ø9 ☑
      - bite W55.Ø1 ☑
      - scratch W55.Ø3 ☑
    - caterpillar (venomous) X58 ☑
    - centipede (venomous) X58 ☑
    - chain
      - hoist W24.Ø ☑
        - agricultural operations W3Ø.89 ☑
      - saw W29.3 ☑
    - chicken W61.39 ☑
      - peck W61.33 ☑
      - strike W61.32 ☑
    - chisel W27.Ø ☑
    - circular saw W31.2 ☑
    - cobra X58 ☑
    - combine (harvester) W3Ø.Ø ☑
    - conveyer belt W24.1 ☑
    - cooker (hot) X15.8 ☑
      - stated as undetermined whether accidental or intentional Y27.3 ☑
      - suicide (attempt) X77.3 ☑
    - coral X58 ☑
    - cotton gin W31.82 ☑
    - cow W55.29 ☑
      - bite W55.21 ☑
      - strike W55.22 ☑
    - crane W24.Ø ☑
      - agricultural operations W3Ø.89 ☑
    - crocodile W58.19 ☑
      - bite W58.11 ☑
      - crushing W58.13 ☑
      - strike W58.12 ☑
    - dagger W26.1 ☑
      - stated as undetermined whether accidental or intentional Y28.2 ☑
      - suicide (attempt) X78.2 ☑
    - dairy equipment W31.82 ☑
    - dart W21.89 ☑
      - not thrown, projected or falling W45.8 ☑
    - deer — *see* Contact, with, hoof stock NEC
    - derrick W24.Ø ☑
      - agricultural operations W3Ø.89 ☑
        - hay W3Ø.2 ☑
    - dog W54.8 ☑
      - bite W54.Ø ☑
      - strike W54.1 ☑
    - dolphin W56.Ø9 ☑
      - bite W56.Ø1 ☑
      - strike W56.Ø2 ☑
    - donkey — *see* Contact, with, hoof stock NEC
    - drill (powered) W29.8 ☑
      - earth (land) (seabed) W31.Ø ☑
      - nonpowered W27.8 ☑
    - drive belt W24.Ø ☑
      - agricultural operations W3Ø.89 ☑

Contact — *continued*
with — *continued*
dry ice — *see* Exposure, cold, man-made
dryer (clothes) (powered) (spin) W29.2 ☑
duck W61.69 ☑
bite W61.61 ☑
strike W61.62 ☑
earth (-)
drilling machine (industrial) W31.Ø ☑
scraping machine in stationary use W31.83 ☑
edge of stiff paper W26.2 ☑
electric
beater W29.Ø ☑
blanket X16 ☑
fan W29.2 ☑
commercial W31.82 ☑
knife W29.1 ☑
mixer W29.Ø ☑
elevator (building) W24.Ø ☑
agricultural operations W3Ø.89 ☑
grain W3Ø.3 ☑
engine(s), hot NEC X17 ☑
excavating machine W31.Ø ☑
farm machine W3Ø.9 ☑
feces — *see* Contact, with, by type of animal
fer de lance X58 ☑
fish W56.59 ☑
bite W56.51 ☑
shark — *see* Contact, with, shark
strike W56.52 ☑
flying horses W31.81 ☑
forging (metalworking) machine W31.1 ☑
fork W27.4 ☑
forklift (truck) W24.Ø ☑
agricultural operations W3Ø.89 ☑
frog W62.Ø ☑
garden
cultivator (powered) W29.3 ☑
riding W3Ø.89 ☑
fork W27.1 ☑
gas turbine W31.3 ☑
Gila monster X58 ☑
giraffe — *see* Contact, with, hoof stock NEC
glass (sharp) (broken) W25 ☑
assault X99.Ø ☑
due to fall — *see* Fall, by type
stated as undetermined whether accidental or intentional Y28.Ø ☑
suicide (attempt) X78.Ø ☑
with subsequent fall W18.Ø2 ☑
goat W55.39 ☑
bite W55.31 ☑
strike W55.32 ☑
goose W61.59 ☑
bite W61.51 ☑
strike W61.52 ☑
hand
saw W27.Ø ☑
tool (not powered) NEC W27.8 ☑
powered W29.8 ☑
harvester W3Ø.Ø ☑
hay-derrick W3Ø.2 ☑
heating
appliance (hot) X16 ☑
pad (electric) X16 ☑
heat NEC X19 ☑
from appliance (electrical) (household) — *see* Contact, with, hot, household appliance
heating appliance X16 ☑
hedge-trimmer (powered) W29.3 ☑
hoe W27.1 ☑
hoist (chain) (shaft) NEC W24.Ø ☑
agricultural W3Ø.89 ☑
hoof stock NEC W55.39 ☑
bite W55.31 ☑
strike W55.32 ☑
hornet(s) X58 ☑
horse W55.19 ☑
bite W55.11 ☑
strike W55.12 ☑
hot
air X14.1 ☑
inhalation X14.Ø ☑
cooker X15.8 ☑
cooking
pan X15.3 ☑

Contact — *continued*
with — *continued*
hot — *continued*
cooking — *continued*
pot X15.3 ☑
drinks X1Ø.Ø ☑
engine X17 ☑
fats X1Ø.2 ☑
fluids NEC X12 ☑
assault X98.2 ☑
suicide (attempt) X77.2 ☑
undetermined whether accidental or intentional Y27.2 ☑
food X1Ø.1 ☑
gases X14.1 ☑
inhalation X14.Ø ☑
heating appliance X16 ☑
household appliance X15.8 ☑
assault X98.3 ☑
cooker X15.8 ☑
hotplate X15.2 ☑
kettle X15.8 ☑
light bulb X15.8 ☑
object NEC X19 ☑
assault X98.8 ☑
stated as undetermined whether accidental or intentional Y27.9 ☑
suicide (attempt) X77.8 ☑
saucepan X15.3 ☑
skillet X15.3 ☑
stated as undetermined whether accidental or intentional Y27.3 ☑
stove X15.Ø ☑
suicide (attempt) X77.3 ☑
toaster X15.1 ☑
kettle X15.8 ☑
light bulb X15.8 ☑
liquid NEC — *see also* Burn X12 ☑
drinks X1Ø.Ø ☑
stated as undetermined whether accidental or intentional Y27.2 ☑
suicide (attempt) X77.2 ☑
tap water X11.8 ☑
stated as undetermined whether accidental or intentional Y27.1 ☑
suicide (attempt) X77.1 ☑
machinery X17 ☑
metal (molten) (liquid) NEC X18 ☑
object (not producing fire or flames) NEC X19 ☑
oil (cooking) X1Ø.2 ☑
pipe X16 ☑
plate X15.2 ☑
radiator X16 ☑
saucepan (glass) (metal) X15.3 ☑
skillet X15.3 ☑
stove (kitchen) X15.Ø ☑
substance NEC X19 ☑
tap-water X11.8 ☑
assault X98.1 ☑
heated on stove X12 ☑
stated as undetermined whether accidental or intentional Y27.2 ☑
suicide (attempt) X77.2 ☑
in bathtub X11.Ø ☑
running X11.1 ☑
stated as undetermined whether accidental or intentional Y27.1 ☑
suicide (attempt) X77.1 ☑
toaster X15.1 ☑
tool X17 ☑
vapors X13.1 ☑
inhalation X13.Ø ☑
water (tap) X11.8 ☑
boiling X12 ☑
stated as undetermined whether accidental or intentional Y27.2 ☑
suicide (attempt) X77.2 ☑
heated on stove X12 ☑
stated as undetermined whether accidental or intentional Y27.2 ☑
suicide (attempt) X77.2 ☑
in bathtub X11.Ø ☑
running X11.1 ☑
stated as undetermined whether accidental or intentional Y27.1 ☑
suicide (attempt) X77.1 ☑

Contact — *continued*
with — *continued*
hotplate X15.2 ☑
ice-pick W27.4 ☑
insect (nonvenomous) NEC W57 ☑
kettle (hot) X15.8 ☑
knife W26.Ø ☑
assault X99.1 ☑
electric W29.1 ☑
stated as undetermined whether accidental or intentional Y28.1 ☑
suicide (attempt) X78.1 ☑
lathe (metalworking) W31.1 ☑
turnings W45.8 ☑
woodworking W31.2 ☑
lawnmower (powered) (ridden) W28 ☑
causing electrocution W86.8 ☑
suicide (attempt) X83.1 ☑
unpowered W27.1 ☑
lift, lifting (devices) W24.Ø ☑
agricultural operations W3Ø.89 ☑
shaft W24.Ø ☑
liquefied gas — *see* Exposure, cold, man-made
liquid air, hydrogen, nitrogen — *see* Exposure, cold, man-made
lizard (nonvenomous) W59.Ø9 ☑
bite W59.Ø1 ☑
strike W59.Ø2 ☑
llama — *see* Contact, with, hoof stock NEC
macaw W61.19 ☑
bite W61.11 ☑
strike W61.12 ☑
machine, machinery W31.9 ☑
abrasive wheel W31.1 ☑
agricultural including animal-powered W3Ø.9 ☑
combine harvester W3Ø.Ø ☑
grain storage elevator W3Ø.3 ☑
hay derrick W3Ø.2 ☑
power take-off device W3Ø.1 ☑
reaper W3Ø.Ø ☑
specified NEC W3Ø.89 ☑
thresher W3Ø.Ø ☑
transport vehicle, stationary W3Ø.81 ☑
band saw W31.2 ☑
bench saw W31.2 ☑
circular saw W31.2 ☑
commercial NEC W31.82 ☑
drilling, metal (industrial) W31.1 ☑
earth-drilling W31.Ø ☑
earthmoving or scraping W31.89 ☑
excavating W31.89 ☑
forging machine W31.1 ☑
gas turbine W31.3 ☑
hot X17 ☑
internal combustion engine W31.3 ☑
land drill W31.Ø ☑
lathe W31.1 ☑
lifting (devices) W24.Ø ☑
metal drill W31.1 ☑
metalworking (industrial) W31.1 ☑
milling, metal W31.1 ☑
mining W31.Ø ☑
molding W31.2 ☑
overhead plane W31.2 ☑
power press, metal W31.1 ☑
prime mover W31.3 ☑
printing W31.89 ☑
radial saw W31.2 ☑
recreational W31.81 ☑
roller-coaster W31.81 ☑
rolling mill, metal W31.1 ☑
sander W31.2 ☑
seabed drill W31.Ø ☑
shaft
hoist W31.Ø ☑
lift W31.Ø ☑
specified NEC W31.89 ☑
spinning W31.89 ☑
steam engine W31.3 ☑
transmission W24.1 ☑
undercutter W31.Ø ☑
water driven turbine W31.3 ☑
weaving W31.89 ☑
woodworking or forming (industrial) W31.2 ☑
mammal (feces) (urine) W55.89 ☑
bull — *see* Contact, with, bull

☑ **Additional Character Required — Refer to the Tabular List for Character Selection**

Contact — *continued*
- with — *continued*
  - mammal — *continued*
    - cat — *see* Contact, with, cat
    - cow — *see* Contact, with, cow
    - goat — *see* Contact, with, goat
    - hoof stock — *see* Contact, with, hoof stock
    - horse — *see* Contact, with, horse
    - marine W56.39 ☑
      - dolphin — *see* Contact, with, dolphin
      - orca — *see* Contact, with, orca
      - sea lion — *see* Contact, with, sea lion
      - specified NEC W56.39 ☑
        - bite W56.31 ☑
        - strike W56.32 ☑
    - pig — *see* Contact, with, pig
    - raccoon — *see* Contact, with, raccoon
    - rodent — *see* Contact, with, rodent
    - sheep — *see* Contact, with, sheep
    - specified NEC W55.89 ☑
      - bite W55.81 ☑
      - strike W55.82 ☑
  - marine
    - animal W56.89 ☑
      - bite W56.81 ☑
      - dolphin — *see* Contact, with, dolphin
      - fish NEC — *see* Contact, with, fish
      - mammal — *see* Contact, with, mammal, marine
      - orca — *see* Contact, with, orca
      - sea lion — *see* Contact, with, sea lion
      - shark — *see* Contact, with, shark
      - strike W56.82 ☑
  - meat
    - grinder (domestic) W29.Ø ☑
      - industrial W31.82 ☑
      - nonpowered W27.4 ☑
    - slicer (domestic) W29.Ø ☑
      - industrial W31.82 ☑
  - merry go round W31.81 ☑
  - metal, hot (liquid) (molten) NEC X18 ☑
  - millipede W57 ☑
  - nail W45.Ø ☑
    - gun W29.4 ☑
  - needle (sewing) W27.3 ☑
    - hypodermic W46.Ø ☑
      - contaminated W46.1 ☑
  - object (blunt) NEC
    - hot NEC X19 ☑
    - legal intervention — *see* Legal, intervention, blunt object
    - sharp NEC W45.8 ☑
      - inflicted by other person NEC W45.8 ☑
        - stated as
          - intentional homicide (attempt) — *see* Assault, cutting or piercing instrument
          - legal intervention — *see* Legal, intervention, sharp object
      - self-inflicted X78.9 ☑
  - orca W56.29 ☑
    - bite W56.21 ☑
    - strike W56.22 ☑
  - overhead plane W31.2 ☑
  - paper (as sharp object) W26.2 ☑
  - paper-cutter W27.5 ☑
  - parrot W61.Ø9 ☑
    - bite W61.Ø1 ☑
    - strike W61.Ø2 ☑
  - pig W55.49 ☑
    - bite W55.41 ☑
    - strike W55.42 ☑
  - pipe, hot X16 ☑
  - pitchfork W27.1 ☑
  - plane (metal) (wood) W27.Ø ☑
    - overhead W31.2 ☑
  - plant thorns, spines, sharp leaves or other mechanisms W6Ø ☑
  - powered
    - garden cultivator W29.3 ☑
    - household appliance, implement, or machine W29.8 ☑
    - saw (industrial) W31.2 ☑
      - hand W29.8 ☑
  - printing machine W31.89 ☑
  - psittacine bird W61.29 ☑

Contact — *continued*
- with — *continued*
  - psittacine bird — *continued*
    - bite W61.21 ☑
    - macaw — *see* Contact, with, macaw
    - parrot — *see* Contact, with, parrot
    - strike W61.22 ☑
  - pulley (block) (transmission) W24.Ø ☑
    - agricultural operations W3Ø.89 ☑
  - raccoon W55.59 ☑
    - bite W55.51 ☑
    - strike W55.52 ☑
  - radial-saw (industrial) W31.2 ☑
  - radiator (hot) X16 ☑
  - rake W27.1 ☑
  - rattlesnake X58 ☑
  - reaper W3Ø.Ø ☑
  - reptile W59.89 ☑
    - lizard — *see* Contact, with, lizard
    - snake — *see* Contact, with, snake
    - specified NEC W59.89 ☑
      - bite W59.81 ☑
      - crushing W59.83 ☑
      - strike W59.82 ☑
    - turtle — *see* Contact, with, turtle
  - rivet gun (powered) W29.4 ☑
  - road scraper — *see* Accident, transport, construction vehicle
  - rodent (feces) (urine) W53.89 ☑
    - bite W53.81 ☑
    - mouse W53.Ø9 ☑
      - bite W53.Ø1 ☑
    - rat W53.19 ☑
      - bite W53.11 ☑
    - specified NEC W53.89 ☑
      - bite W53.81 ☑
    - squirrel W53.29 ☑
      - bite W53.21 ☑
  - roller coaster W31.81 ☑
  - rope NEC W24.Ø ☑
    - agricultural operations W3Ø.89 ☑
  - saliva — *see* Contact, with, by type of animal
  - sander W29.8 ☑
    - industrial W31.2 ☑
  - saucepan (hot) (glass) (metal) X15.3 ☑
  - saw W27.Ø ☑
    - band (industrial) W31.2 ☑
    - bench (industrial) W31.2 ☑
    - chain W29.3 ☑
    - hand W27.Ø ☑
  - sawing machine, metal W31.1 ☑
  - scissors W27.2 ☑
  - scorpion X58 ☑
  - screwdriver W27.Ø ☑
    - powered W29.8 ☑
  - sea
    - anemone, cucumber or urchin (spine) X58 ☑
    - lion W56.19 ☑
      - bite W56.11 ☑
      - strike W56.12 ☑
  - serpent — *see* Contact, with, snake, by type
  - sewing-machine (electric) (powered) W29.2 ☑
    - not powered W27.8 ☑
  - shaft (hoist) (lift) (transmission) NEC W24.Ø ☑
    - agricultural W3Ø.89 ☑
  - shark W56.49 ☑
    - bite W56.41 ☑
    - strike W56.42 ☑
  - sharp object(s) W26.9 ☑
    - specified NEC W26.8 ☑
  - shears (hand) W27.2 ☑
    - powered (industrial) W31.1 ☑
      - domestic W29.2 ☑
  - sheep W55.39 ☑
    - bite W55.31 ☑
    - strike W55.32 ☑
  - shovel W27.8 ☑
    - steam — *see* Accident, transport, construction vehicle
  - snake (nonvenomous) W59.19 ☑
    - bite W59.11 ☑
    - crushing W59.13 ☑
    - strike W59.12 ☑
  - spade W27.1 ☑
  - spider (venomous) X58 ☑
  - spin-drier W29.2 ☑

Contact — *continued*
- with — *continued*
  - spinning machine W31.89 ☑
  - splinter W45.8 ☑
  - sports equipment W21.9 ☑
  - staple gun (powered) W29.8 ☑
  - steam X13.1 ☑
    - engine W31.3 ☑
    - inhalation X13.Ø ☑
    - pipe X16 ☑
    - shovel W31.89 ☑
  - stove (hot) (kitchen) X15.Ø ☑
  - substance, hot NEC X19 ☑
    - molten (metal) X18 ☑
  - sword W26.1 ☑
    - assault X99.2 ☑
    - stated as undetermined whether accidental or intentional Y28.2 ☑
    - suicide (attempt) X78.2 ☑
  - tarantula X58 ☑
  - thresher W3Ø.Ø ☑
  - tin can lid W26.8 ☑
  - toad W62.1 ☑
  - toaster (hot) X15.1 ☑
  - tool W27.8 ☑
    - hand (not powered) W27.8 ☑
      - auger W27.Ø ☑
      - axe W27.Ø ☑
      - can opener W27.4 ☑
      - chisel W27.Ø ☑
      - fork W27.4 ☑
      - garden W27.1 ☑
      - handsaw W27.Ø ☑
      - hoe W27.1 ☑
      - ice-pick W27.4 ☑
      - kitchen utensil W27.4 ☑
      - manual
        - lawn mower W27.1 ☑
        - sewing machine W27.8 ☑
      - meat grinder W27.4 ☑
      - needle (sewing) W27.3 ☑
        - hypodermic W46.Ø ☑
          - contaminated W46.1 ☑
      - paper cutter W27.5 ☑
      - pitchfork W27.1 ☑
      - rake W27.1 ☑
      - scissors W27.2 ☑
      - screwdriver W27.Ø ☑
      - specified NEC W27.8 ☑
      - workbench W27.Ø ☑
    - hot X17 ☑
    - powered W29.8 ☑
      - blender W29.Ø ☑
        - commercial W31.82 ☑
      - can opener W29.Ø ☑
        - commercial W31.82 ☑
      - chainsaw W29.3 ☑
      - clothes dryer W29.2 ☑
        - commercial W31.82 ☑
      - dishwasher W29.2 ☑
        - commercial W31.82 ☑
      - edger W29.3 ☑
      - electric fan W29.2 ☑
        - commercial W31.82 ☑
      - electric knife W29.1 ☑
      - food processor W29.Ø ☑
        - commercial W31.82 ☑
      - garbage disposal W29.Ø ☑
        - commercial W31.82 ☑
      - garden tool W29.3 ☑
      - hedge trimmer W29.3 ☑
      - ice maker W29.Ø ☑
        - commercial W31.82 ☑
      - kitchen appliance W29.Ø ☑
        - commercial W31.82 ☑
      - lawn mower W28 ☑
      - meat grinder W29.Ø ☑
        - commercial W31.82 ☑
      - mixer W29.Ø ☑
        - commercial W31.82 ☑
      - rototiller W29.3 ☑
      - sewing machine W29.2 ☑
        - commercial W31.82 ☑
      - washing machine W29.2 ☑
        - commercial W31.82 ☑

- **Contact** — *continued*
  - with — *continued*
    - transmission device (belt, cable, chain, gear, pinion, shaft) W24.1 ☑
      - agricultural operations W30.89 ☑
    - turbine (gas) (water-driven) W31.3 ☑
    - turkey W61.49 ☑
      - peck W61.43 ☑
      - strike W61.42 ☑
    - turtle (nonvenomous) W59.29 ☑
      - bite W59.21 ☑
      - strike W59.22 ☑
      - terrestrial W59.89 ☑
        - bite W59.81 ☑
        - crushing W59.83 ☑
        - strike W59.82 ☑
    - under-cutter W31.0 ☑
    - urine — *see* Contact, with, by type of animal
    - vehicle
      - agricultural use (transport) — *see* Accident, transport, agricultural vehicle
        - not on public highway W30.81 ☑
      - industrial use (transport) — *see* Accident, transport, industrial vehicle
        - not on public highway W31.83 ☑
      - off-road use (transport) — *see* Accident, transport, all-terrain or off-road vehicle
        - not on public highway W31.83 ☑
      - special construction use (transport) — *see* Accident, transport, construction vehicle
        - not on public highway W31.83 ☑
    - venomous
      - animal X58 ☑
      - arthropods X58 ☑
      - lizard X58 ☑
      - marine animal NEC X58 ☑
      - marine plant NEC X58 ☑
      - millipedes (tropical) X58 ☑
      - plant(s) X58 ☑
      - snake X58 ☑
      - spider X58 ☑
    - viper X58 ☑
    - washing-machine (powered) W29.2 ☑
    - wasp X58 ☑
    - weaving-machine W31.89 ☑
    - winch W24.0 ☑
      - agricultural operations W30.89 ☑
    - wire NEC W24.0 ☑
      - agricultural operations W30.89 ☑
    - wood slivers W45.8 ☑
    - yellow jacket X58 ☑
    - zebra — *see* Contact, with, hoof stock NEC
  - pressure X50.9 ☑
  - stress X50.9 ☑
- **Coup de soleil** X32 ☑
- **Crash**
  - aircraft (in transit) (powered) V95.9 ☑
    - balloon V96.01 ☑
    - fixed wing NEC (private) V95.21 ☑
      - commercial V95.31 ☑
    - glider V96.21 ☑
      - hang V96.11 ☑
      - powered V95.11 ☑
    - helicopter V95.01 ☑
    - in war operations — *see* War operations, destruction of aircraft
    - microlight V95.11 ☑
    - nonpowered V96.9 ☑
      - specified NEC V96.8 ☑
    - powered NEC V95.8 ☑
    - stated as
      - homicide (attempt) Y08.81 ☑
      - suicide (attempt) X83.0 ☑
    - ultralight V95.11 ☑
  - spacecraft V95.41 ☑
  - transport vehicle NEC — *see also* Accident, transport V89.9 ☑
    - homicide (attempt) Y03.8 ☑
    - motor NEC (traffic) V89.2 ☑
      - homicide (attempt) Y03.8 ☑
      - suicide (attempt) — *see* Suicide, collision
- **Cruelty** (mental) (physical) (sexual) X58 ☑
- **Crushed** (accidentally) X58 ☑
  - between objects (moving) (stationary and moving) W23.0 ☑
    - stationary W23.1 ☑
- **Crushed** — *continued*
  - by
    - alligator W58.03 ☑
    - avalanche NEC — *see* Landslide
    - cave-in W20.0 ☑
      - caused by cataclysmic earth surface movement — *see* Landslide
    - crocodile W58.13 ☑
    - crowd or human stampede W52 ☑
    - falling
      - aircraft V97.39 ☑
        - in war operations — *see* War operations, destruction of aircraft
      - earth, material W20.0 ☑
        - caused by cataclysmic earth surface movement — *see* Landslide
      - object NEC W20.8 ☑
    - landslide NEC — *see* Landslide
    - lizard (nonvenomous) W59.09 ☑
    - machinery — *see* Contact, with, by type of machine
    - reptile NEC W59.89 ☑
    - snake (nonvenomous) W59.13 ☑
  - in
    - machinery — *see* Contact, with, by type of machine
- **Cut, cutting** (any part of body) (accidental) — *see also* Contact, with, by object or machine
  - during medical or surgical treatment as misadventure — *see* Index to Diseases and Injuries, Complications
  - homicide (attempt) — *see* Assault, cutting or piercing instrument
  - inflicted by other person — *see* Assault, cutting or piercing instrument
  - legal
    - execution — *see* Legal, intervention
    - intervention — *see* Legal, intervention, sharp object
  - machine NEC — *see also* Contact, with, by type of machine W31.9 ☑
  - self-inflicted — *see* Suicide, cutting or piercing instrument
  - suicide (attempt) — *see* Suicide, cutting or piercing instrument
- **Cyclone** (any injury) X37.1 ☑

D

- **Decapitation** (accidental circumstances) NEC X58 ☑
  - homicide X99.9 ☑
  - legal execution — *see* Legal, intervention
- **Dehydration from lack of water** X58 ☑
- **Deprivation** X58 ☑
- **Derailment** (accidental)
  - railway (rolling stock) (train) (vehicle) (without antecedent collision) V81.7 ☑
    - with antecedent collision — *see* Accident, transport, railway vehicle occupant
  - streetcar (without antecedent collision) V82.7 ☑
    - with antecedent collision — *see* Accident, transport, streetcar occupant
- **Descent**
  - parachute (voluntary) (without accident to aircraft) V97.29 ☑
    - due to accident to aircraft — *see* Accident, transport, aircraft
- **Desertion** X58 ☑
- **Destitution** X58 ☑
- **Disability, late effect or sequela of injury** — *see* Sequelae
- **Discharge** (accidental)
  - airgun W34.010 ☑
    - assault X95.01 ☑
    - homicide (attempt) X95.01 ☑
    - stated as undetermined whether accidental or intentional Y24.0 ☑
    - suicide (attempt) X74.01 ☑
  - BB gun — *see* Discharge, airgun
  - firearm (accidental) W34.00 ☑
    - assault X95.9 ☑
    - handgun (pistol) (revolver) W32.0 ☑
      - assault X93 ☑
      - homicide (attempt) X93 ☑
      - legal intervention — *see* Legal, intervention, firearm, handgun
      - stated as undetermined whether accidental or intentional Y22 ☑
      - suicide (attempt) X72 ☑
- **Discharge** — *continued*
  - firearm — *continued*
    - homicide (attempt) X95.9 ☑
    - hunting rifle W33.02 ☑
      - assault X94.1 ☑
      - homicide (attempt) X94.1 ☑
      - legal intervention
        - injuring
          - bystander Y35.032 ☑
          - law enforcement personnel Y35.031 ☑
          - suspect Y35.033 ☑
          - unspecified person Y35.039 ☑
      - stated as undetermined whether accidental or intentional Y23.1 ☑
      - suicide (attempt) X73.1 ☑
    - larger W33.00 ☑
      - assault X94.9 ☑
      - homicide (attempt) X94.9 ☑
      - hunting rifle — *see* Discharge, firearm, hunting rifle
      - legal intervention — *see* Legal, intervention, firearm by type of firearm
      - machine gun — *see* Discharge, firearm, machine gun
      - shotgun — *see* Discharge, firearm, shotgun
      - specified NEC W33.09 ☑
        - assault X94.8 ☑
        - homicide (attempt) X94.8 ☑
        - legal intervention
          - injuring
            - bystander Y35.092 ☑
            - law enforcement personnel Y35.091 ☑
            - suspect Y35.093 ☑
            - unspecified person Y35.099 ☑
        - stated as undetermined whether accidental or intentional Y23.8 ☑
        - suicide (attempt) X73.8 ☑
      - stated as undetermined whether accidental or intentional Y23.9 ☑
      - suicide (attempt) X73.9 ☑
    - legal intervention
      - injuring
        - bystander Y35.002 ☑
        - law enforcement personnel Y35.001 ☑
        - suspect Y35.03 ☑
        - unspecified person Y35.009 ☑
      - using rubber bullet
        - injuring
          - bystander Y35.042 ☑
          - law enforcement personnel Y35.041 ☑
          - suspect Y35.043 ☑
          - unspecified person Y35.049 ☑
    - machine gun W33.03 ☑
      - assault X94.2 ☑
      - homicide (attempt) X94.2 ☑
      - legal intervention — *see* Legal, intervention, firearm, machine gun
      - stated as undetermined whether accidental or intentional Y23.3 ☑
      - suicide (attempt) X73.2 ☑
    - pellet gun — *see* Discharge, airgun
    - shotgun W33.01 ☑
      - assault X94.0 ☑
      - homicide (attempt) X94.0 ☑
      - legal intervention — *see* Legal, intervention, firearm, specified NEC
      - stated as undetermined whether accidental or intentional Y23.0 ☑
      - suicide (attempt) X73.0 ☑
    - specified NEC W34.09 ☑
      - assault X95.8 ☑
      - homicide (attempt) X95.8 ☑
      - legal intervention — *see* Legal, intervention, firearm, specified NEC
      - stated as undetermined whether accidental or intentional Y24.8 ☑
      - suicide (attempt) X74.8 ☑
    - stated as undetermined whether accidental or intentional Y24.9 ☑
    - suicide (attempt) X74.9 ☑
    - Very pistol W34.09 ☑
      - assault X95.8 ☑
      - homicide (attempt) X95.8 ☑
      - stated as undetermined whether accidental or intentional Y24.8 ☑

Discharge — *continued*
firearm — *continued*
Very pistol — *continued*
suicide (attempt) X74.8 ☑
firework(s) W39 ☑
stated as undetermined whether accidental or intentional Y25 ☑
gas-operated gun NEC W34.018 ☑
airgun — *see* Discharge, airgun
assault X95.09 ☑
homicide (attempt) X95.09 ☑
paintball gun — *see* Discharge, paintball gun
stated as undetermined whether accidental or intentional Y24.8 ☑
suicide (attempt) X74.09 ☑
gun NEC — *see also* Discharge, firearm NEC
air — *see* Discharge, airgun
BB — *see* Discharge, airgun
for single hand use — *see* Discharge, firearm, handgun
hand — *see* Discharge, firearm, handgun
machine — *see* Discharge, firearm, machine gun
other specified — *see* Discharge, firearm NEC
paintball — *see* Discharge, paintball gun
pellet — *see* Discharge, airgun
handgun — *see* Discharge, firearm, handgun
machine gun — *see* Discharge, firearm, machine gun
paintball gun W34.011 ☑
assault X95.02 ☑
homicide (attempt) X95.02 ☑
stated as undetermined whether accidental or intentional Y24.8 ☑
suicide (attempt) X74.02 ☑
pistol — *see* Discharge, firearm, handgun
flare — *see* Discharge, firearm, Very pistol
pellet — *see* Discharge, airgun
Very — *see* Discharge, firearm, Very pistol
revolver — *see* Discharge, firearm, handgun
rifle (hunting) — *see* Discharge, firearm, hunting rifle
shotgun — *see* Discharge, firearm, shotgun
spring-operated gun NEC W34.018 ☑
assault X95.09 ☑
homicide (attempt) X95.09 ☑
stated as undetermined whether accidental or intentional Y24.8 ☑
suicide (attempt) X74.09 ☑
Disease
Andes W94.11 ☑
aviator's — *see* Air, pressure
range W94.11 ☑
Diver's disease, palsy, paralysis, squeeze — *see* Air, pressure
Diving (into water) — *see* Accident, diving
Dog bite W54.0 ☑
Dragged by transport vehicle NEC — *see also* Accident, transport V09.9 ☑
Drinking poison (accidental) — *see* Table of Drugs and Chemicals
Dropped (accidentally) **while being carried or supported by other person** W04 ☑
Drowning (accidental) W74 ☑
assault X92.9 ☑
due to
accident (to)
machinery — *see* Contact, with, by type of machine
watercraft V90.89 ☑
burning V90.29 ☑
powered V90.23 ☑
fishing boat V90.22 ☑
jetskis V90.23 ☑
merchant ship V90.20 ☑
passenger ship V90.21 ☑
unpowered V90.28 ☑
canoe V90.25 ☑
inflatable V90.26 ☑
kayak V90.25 ☑
sailboat V90.24 ☑
water skis V90.27 ☑
crushed V90.39 ☑
powered V90.33 ☑
fishing boat V90.32 ☑
jetskis V90.33 ☑
merchant ship V90.30 ☑
passenger ship V90.31 ☑
unpowered V90.38 ☑

Drowning — *continued*
due to — *continued*
accident — *continued*
watercraft — *continued*
crushed — *continued*
unpowered — *continued*
canoe V90.35 ☑
inflatable V90.36 ☑
kayak V90.35 ☑
sailboat V90.34 ☑
water skis V90.37 ☑
overturning V90.09 ☑
powered V90.03 ☑
fishing boat V90.02 ☑
jetskis V90.03 ☑
merchant ship V90.00 ☑
passenger ship V90.01 ☑
unpowered V90.08 ☑
canoe V90.05 ☑
inflatable V90.06 ☑
kayak V90.05 ☑
sailboat V90.04 ☑
sinking V90.19 ☑
powered V90.13 ☑
fishing boat V90.12 ☑
jetskis V90.13 ☑
merchant ship V90.10 ☑
passenger ship V90.11 ☑
unpowered V90.18 ☑
canoe V90.15 ☑
inflatable V90.16 ☑
kayak V90.15 ☑
sailboat V90.14 ☑
specified type NEC V90.89 ☑
powered V90.83 ☑
fishing boat V90.82 ☑
jetskis V90.83 ☑
merchant ship V90.80 ☑
passenger ship V90.81 ☑
unpowered V90.88 ☑
canoe V90.85 ☑
inflatable V90.86 ☑
kayak V90.85 ☑
sailboat V90.84 ☑
water skis V90.87 ☑
avalanche — *see* Landslide
cataclysmic
earth surface movement NEC — *see* Forces of nature, earth movement
storm — *see* Forces of nature, cataclysmic storm
cloudburst X37.8 ☑
cyclone X37.1 ☑
fall overboard (from) V92.09 ☑
powered craft V92.03 ☑
ferry boat V92.01 ☑
fishing boat V92.02 ☑
jetskis V92.03 ☑
liner V92.01 ☑
merchant ship V92.00 ☑
passenger ship V92.01 ☑
resulting from
accident to watercraft — *see* Drowning, due to, accident to, watercraft
being washed overboard (from) V92.29 ☑
powered craft V92.23 ☑
ferry boat V92.21 ☑
fishing boat V92.22 ☑
jetskis V92.23 ☑
liner V92.21 ☑
merchant ship V92.20 ☑
passenger ship V92.21 ☑
unpowered craft V92.28 ☑
canoe V92.25 ☑
inflatable V92.26 ☑
kayak V92.25 ☑
sailboat V92.24 ☑
surf-board V92.28 ☑
water skis V92.27 ☑
windsurfer V92.28 ☑
motion of watercraft V92.19 ☑
powered craft V92.13 ☑
ferry boat V92.11 ☑
fishing boat V92.12 ☑
jetskis V92.13 ☑
liner V92.11 ☑
merchant ship V92.10 ☑

Drowning — *continued*
due to — *continued*
fall overboard — *continued*
resulting from — *continued*
motion of watercraft — *continued*
powered craft — *continued*
passenger ship V92.11 ☑
unpowered craft
canoe V92.15 ☑
inflatable V92.16 ☑
kayak V92.15 ☑
sailboat V92.14 ☑
unpowered craft V92.08 ☑
canoe V92.05 ☑
inflatable V92.06 ☑
kayak V92.05 ☑
sailboat V92.04 ☑
surf-board V92.08 ☑
water skis V92.07 ☑
windsurfer V92.08 ☑
hurricane X37.0 ☑
jumping into water from watercraft (involved in accident) — *see also* Drowning, due to, accident to, watercraft
without accident to or on watercraft W16.711 ☑
tidal wave NEC — *see* Forces of nature, tidal wave
torrential rain X37.8 ☑
following
fall
into
bathtub W16.211 ☑
bucket W16.221 ☑
fountain — *see* Drowning, following, fall, into, water, specified NEC
quarry — *see* Drowning, following, fall, into, water, specified NEC
reservoir — *see* Drowning, following, fall, into, water, specified NEC
swimming-pool W16.011 ☑
stated as undetermined whether accidental or intentional Y21.3 ☑
striking
bottom W16.021 ☑
wall W16.031 ☑
suicide (attempt) X71.2 ☑
water NOS W16.41 ☑
natural (lake) (open sea) (river) (stream) (pond) W16.111 ☑
striking
bottom W16.121 ☑
side W16.131 ☑
specified NEC W16.311 ☑
striking
bottom W16.321 ☑
wall W16.331 ☑
overboard NEC — *see* Drowning, due to, fall overboard
jump or dive
from boat W16.711 ☑
striking bottom W16.721 ☑
into
fountain — *see* Drowning, following, jump or dive, into, water, specified NEC
quarry — *see* Drowning, following, jump or dive, into, water, specified NEC
reservoir — *see* Drowning, following, jump or dive, into, water, specified NEC
swimming-pool W16.511 ☑
striking
bottom W16.521 ☑
wall W16.531 ☑
suicide (attempt) X71.2 ☑
water NOS W16.91 ☑
natural (lake) (open sea) (river) (stream) (pond) W16.611 ☑
specified NEC W16.811 ☑
bottom W16.821 ☑
striking
bottom W16.821 ☑
wall W16.831 ☑
striking
bottom W16.821 ☑
wall W16.831 ☑
striking bottom W16.621 ☑
homicide (attempt) X92.9 ☑
in
bathtub (accidental) W65 ☑

- **Drowning** — *continued*
  - in — *continued*
    - bathtub — *continued*
      - assault X92.Ø ☑
      - following fall W16.211 ☑
        - stated as undetermined whether accidental or intentional Y21.1 ☑
      - stated as undetermined whether accidental or intentional Y21.Ø ☑
      - suicide (attempt) X71.Ø ☑
    - lake — *see* Drowning, in, natural water
    - natural water (lake) (open sea) (river) (stream) (pond) W69 ☑
      - assault X92.3 ☑
      - following
        - dive or jump W16.611 ☑
          - striking bottom W16.621 ☑
        - fall W16.111 ☑
          - striking
            - bottom W16.121 ☑
            - side W16.131 ☑
      - stated as undetermined whether accidental or intentional Y21.4 ☑
      - suicide (attempt) X71.3 ☑
    - quarry — *see* Drowning, in, specified place NEC
    - quenching tank — *see* Drowning, in, specified place NEC
    - reservoir — *see* Drowning, in, specified place NEC
    - river — *see* Drowning, in, natural water
    - sea — *see* Drowning, in, natural water
    - specified place NEC W73 ☑
      - assault X92.8 ☑
      - following
        - dive or jump W16.811 ☑
          - striking
            - bottom W16.821 ☑
            - wall W16.831 ☑
        - fall W16.311 ☑
          - striking
            - bottom W16.321 ☑
            - wall W16.331 ☑
      - stated as undetermined whether accidental or intentional Y21.8 ☑
      - suicide (attempt) X71.8 ☑
    - stream — *see* Drowning, in, natural water
    - swimming-pool W67 ☑
      - assault X92.1 ☑
        - following fall X92.2 ☑
      - following
        - dive or jump W16.511 ☑
          - striking
            - bottom W16.521 ☑
            - wall W16.531 ☑
        - fall W16.Ø11 ☑
          - striking
            - bottom W16.Ø21 ☑
            - wall W16.Ø31 ☑
      - stated as undetermined whether accidental or intentional Y21.2 ☑
        - following fall Y21.3 ☑
      - suicide (attempt) X71.1 ☑
        - following fall X71.2 ☑
    - war operations — *see* War operations, restriction of airway
  - resulting from accident to watercraft — *see* Drowning, due to, accident, watercraft
  - self-inflicted X71.9 ☑
  - stated as undetermined whether accidental or intentional Y21.9 ☑
  - suicide (attempt) X71.9 ☑

E

- **Earth falling** (on) W20.Ø ☑
  - caused by cataclysmic earth surface movement or eruption — *see* Landslide
- **Earth** (surface) **movement NEC** — *see* Forces of nature, earth movement
- **Earthquake** (any injury) X34 ☑
- **Effect**(s) (adverse) **of**
  - air pressure (any) — *see* Air, pressure
  - cold, excessive (exposure to) — *see* Exposure, cold
  - heat (excessive) — *see* Heat
  - hot place (weather) — *see* Heat
  - insolation X3Ø ☑
  - late — *see* Sequelae
- **Effect**(s) (adverse) **of** — *continued*
  - motion — *see* Motion
  - nuclear explosion or weapon in war operations — *see* War operations, nuclear weapon
  - radiation — *see* Radiation
  - travel — *see* Travel
- **Electric shock** (accidental) (by) (in) — *see* Exposure, electric current
- **Electrocution** (accidental) — *see* Exposure, electric current
- **Endotracheal tube wrongly placed during anesthetic procedure**
- **Entanglement**
  - in
    - bed linen, causing suffocation T71 ☑
    - wheel of pedal cycle V19.88 ☑
- **Entry of foreign body or material** — *see* Foreign body
- **Environmental pollution related condition** — *see* category Z57 ☑
- **Execution, legal** (any method) — *see* Legal, intervention
- **Exhaustion**
  - cold — *see* Exposure, cold
  - due to excessive exertion — *see also* Overexertion X5Ø.9 ☑
  - heat — *see* Heat
- **Explosion** (accidental) (of) (with secondary fire) W4Ø.9 ☑
  - acetylene W4Ø.1 ☑
  - aerosol can W36.1 ☑
  - air tank (compressed) (in machinery) W36.2 ☑
  - aircraft (in transit) (powered) NEC V95.9 ☑
    - balloon V96.Ø5 ☑
    - fixed wing NEC (private) V95.25 ☑
      - commercial V95.35 ☑
    - glider V96.25 ☑
      - hang V96.15 ☑
      - powered V95.15 ☑
    - helicopter V95.Ø5 ☑
    - in war operations — *see* War operations, destruction of aircraft
    - microlight V95.15 ☑
    - nonpowered V96.9 ☑
      - specified NEC V96.8 ☑
    - powered NEC V95.8 ☑
    - stated as
      - homicide (attempt) YØ3.8 ☑
      - suicide (attempt) X83.Ø ☑
    - ultralight V95.15 ☑
  - anesthetic gas in operating room W4Ø.1 ☑
  - antipersonnel bomb W4Ø.8 ☑
    - assault X96.Ø ☑
    - homicide (attempt) X96.Ø ☑
    - suicide (attempt) X75 ☑
  - assault X96.9 ☑
  - bicycle tire W37.Ø ☑
  - blasting (cap) (materials) W4Ø.Ø ☑
  - boiler (machinery), not on transport vehicle W35 ☑
    - on watercraft — *see* Explosion, in, watercraft
  - butane W4Ø.1 ☑
  - caused by other person X96.9 ☑
  - coal gas W4Ø.1 ☑
  - detonator W4Ø.Ø ☑
  - dump (munitions) W4Ø.8 ☑
  - dynamite W4Ø.Ø ☑
    - in
      - assault X96.8 ☑
      - homicide (attempt) X96.8 ☑
      - legal intervention
        - injuring
          - bystander Y35.112 ☑
          - law enforcement personnel Y35.111 ☑
          - suspect Y35.113 ☑
          - unspecified person Y35.119 ☑
      - suicide (attempt) X75 ☑
  - explosive (material) W4Ø.9 ☑
    - gas W4Ø.1 ☑
    - in blasting operation W4Ø.Ø ☑
    - specified NEC W4Ø.8 ☑
      - in
        - assault X96.8 ☑
        - homicide (attempt) X96.8 ☑
        - legal intervention
          - injuring
            - bystander Y35.192 ☑
            - law enforcement personnel Y35.191 ☑
            - suspect Y35.193 ☑
- **Explosion** — *continued*
  - explosive — *continued*
    - specified — *continued*
      - in — *continued*
        - legal intervention — *continued*
          - injuring — *continued*
            - unspecified person Y35.199 ☑
        - suicide (attempt) X75 ☑
  - factory (munitions) W4Ø.8 ☑
  - fertilizer bomb W4Ø.8 ☑
    - assault X96.3 ☑
    - homicide (attempt) X96.3 ☑
    - suicide (attempt) X75 ☑
  - firearm (parts) NEC W34.19 ☑
    - airgun W34.11Ø ☑
    - BB gun W34.11Ø ☑
    - gas, air or spring-operated gun NEC W34.118 ☑
    - hangun W32.1 ☑
    - hunting rifle W33.12 ☑
    - larger firearm W33.1Ø ☑
      - specified NEC W33.19 ☑
    - machine gun W33.13 ☑
    - paintball gun W34.111 ☑
    - pellet gun W34.11Ø ☑
    - shotgun W33.11 ☑
    - Very pistol [flare] W34.19 ☑
  - fire-damp W4Ø.1 ☑
  - fireworks W39 ☑
  - gas (coal) (explosive) W4Ø.1 ☑
    - cylinder W36.9 ☑
      - aerosol can W36.1 ☑
      - air tank W36.2 ☑
      - pressurized W36.3 ☑
      - specified NEC W36.8 ☑
  - gasoline (fumes) (tank) not in moving motor vehicle W4Ø.1 ☑
    - bomb W4Ø.8 ☑
      - assault X96.1 ☑
      - homicide (attempt) X96.1 ☑
      - suicide (attempt) X75 ☑
    - in motor vehicle — *see* Accident, transport, by type of vehicle
  - grain store W4Ø.8 ☑
  - grenade W4Ø.8 ☑
    - in
      - assault X96.8 ☑
      - homicide (attempt) X96.8 ☑
      - legal intervention
        - injuring
          - bystander Y35.192 ☑
          - law enforcement personnel Y35.191 ☑
          - suspect Y35.193 ☑
          - unspecified person Y35.199 ☑
      - suicide (attempt) X75 ☑
  - handgun (parts) — *see* Explosion, firearm, hangun (parts)
  - homicide (attempt) X96.9 ☑
    - antipersonnel bomb — *see* Explosion, antipersonnel bomb
    - fertilizer bomb — *see* Explosion, fertilizer bomb
    - gasoline bomb — *see* Explosion, gasoline bomb
    - letter bomb — *see* Explosion, letter bomb
    - pipe bomb — *see* Explosion, pipe bomb
    - specified NEC X96.8 ☑
  - hose, pressurized W37.8 ☑
  - hot water heater, tank (in machinery) W35 ☑
    - on watercraft — *see* Explosion, in, watercraft
  - in, on
    - dump W4Ø.8 ☑
    - factory W4Ø.8 ☑
    - mine (of explosive gases) NEC W4Ø.1 ☑
    - watercraft V93.59 ☑
      - powered craft V93.53 ☑
        - ferry boat V93.51 ☑
        - fishing boat V93.52 ☑
        - jetskis V93.53 ☑
        - liner V93.51 ☑
        - merchant ship V93.5Ø ☑
        - passenger ship V93.51 ☑
        - sailboat V93.54 ☑
  - letter bomb W4Ø.8 ☑
    - assault X96.2 ☑
    - homicide (attempt) X96.2 ☑
    - suicide (attempt) X75 ☑
  - machinery — *see also* Contact, with, by type of machine

- **Explosion** — *continued*
  - machinery — *see also* Contact, with, by type of machine — *continued*
    - on board watercraft — *see* Explosion, in, watercraft
    - pressure vessel — *see* Explosion, by type of vessel
  - methane W40.1 ☑
  - mine W40.1 ☑
  - missile NEC W40.8 ☑
  - mortar bomb W40.8 ☑
    - in
      - assault X96.8 ☑
      - homicide (attempt) X96.8 ☑
      - legal intervention
        - injuring
          - bystander Y35.192 ☑
          - law enforcement personnel Y35.191 ☑
          - suspect Y35.193 ☑
          - unspecified person Y35.199 ☑
      - suicide (attempt) X75 ☑
  - munitions (dump) (factory) W40.8 ☑
  - pipe, pressurized W37.8 ☑
    - bomb W40.8 ☑
      - assault X96.4 ☑
      - homicide (attempt) X96.4 ☑
      - suicide (attempt) X75 ☑
  - pressure, pressurized
    - cooker W38 ☑
    - gas tank (in machinery) W36.3 ☑
    - hose W37.8 ☑
    - pipe W37.8 ☑
    - specified device NEC W38 ☑
    - tire W37.8 ☑
      - bicycle W37.0 ☑
    - vessel (in machinery) W38 ☑
  - propane W40.1 ☑
  - self-inflicted X75 ☑
  - shell (artillery) NEC W40.8 ☑
    - during war operations — *see* War operations, explosion
    - in
      - legal intervention
        - injuring
          - bystander Y35.122 ☑
          - law enforcement personnel Y35.121 ☑
          - suspect Y35.123 ☑
          - unspecified person Y35.129 ☑
    - war — *see* War operations, explosion
  - spacecraft V95.45 ☑
  - stated as undetermined whether accidental or intentional Y25 ☑
  - steam or water lines (in machinery) W37.8 ☑
  - stove W40.9 ☑
  - suicide (attempt) X75 ☑
  - tire, pressurized W37.8 ☑
    - bicycle W37.0 ☑
  - undetermined whether accidental or intentional Y25 ☑
  - vehicle tire NEC W37.8 ☑
    - bicycle W37.0 ☑
  - war operations — *see* War operations, explosion
- **Exposure** (to) X58 ☑
  - air pressure change — *see* Air, pressure
  - cold (accidental) (excessive) (extreme) (natural) (place) X31 ☑
    - assault Y08.89 ☑
    - due to
      - man-made conditions W93.8 ☑
        - dry ice (contact) W93.01 ☑
          - inhalation W93.02 ☑
        - liquid air (contact) (hydrogen) (nitrogen) W93.11 ☑
          - inhalation W93.12 ☑
        - refrigeration unit (deep freeze) W93.2 ☑
        - suicide (attempt) X83.2 ☑
      - weather (conditions) X31 ☑
    - homicide (attempt) Y08.89 ☑
    - self-inflicted X83.2 ☑
  - due to abandonment or neglect X58 ☑
  - electric current W86.8 ☑
    - appliance (faulty) W86.8 ☑
      - domestic W86.0 ☑
    - caused by other person Y08.89 ☑
    - conductor (faulty) W86.1 ☑
    - control apparatus (faulty) W86.1 ☑
    - electric power generating plant, distribution station W86.1 ☑

- **Exposure** — *continued*
  - electric current — *continued*
    - electroshock gun — *see* Exposure, electric current, taser
    - high-voltage cable W85 ☑
    - homicide (attempt) Y08.89 ☑
    - legal execution — *see* Legal, intervention, specified means NEC
    - lightning — *see* subcategory T75.0 ☑
    - live rail W86.8 ☑
    - misadventure in medical or surgical procedure in electroshock therapy Y63.4
    - motor (electric) (faulty) W86.8 ☑
      - domestic W86.0 ☑
    - self-inflicted X83.1 ☑
    - specified NEC W86.8 ☑
      - domestic W86.0 ☑
    - stun gun — *see* Exposure, electric current, taser
    - suicide (attempt) X83.1 ☑
    - taser W86.8 ☑
      - assault Y08.89 ☑
      - legal intervention — *see* category Y35 ☑
      - self-harm (intentional) X83.8 ☑
      - undetermined intent Y33 ☑
    - third rail W86.8 ☑
    - transformer (faulty) W86.1 ☑
    - transmission lines W85 ☑
  - environmental tobacco smoke X58 ☑
  - excessive
    - cold — *see* Exposure, cold
    - heat (natural) NEC X30 ☑
      - man-made W92 ☑
  - factor(s) NOS X58 ☑
    - environmental NEC X58 ☑
      - man-made NEC W99 ☑
      - natural NEC — *see* Forces of nature
    - specified NEC X58 ☑
  - fire, flames (accidental) X08.8 ☑
    - assault X97 ☑
    - campfire — *see* Exposure, fire, controlled, not in building
    - controlled (in)
      - with ignition (of) clothing — *see also* Ignition, clothes X06.2 ☑
        - nightwear X05 ☑
      - bonfire — *see* Exposure, fire, controlled, not in building
      - brazier (in building or structure) — *see also* Exposure, fire, controlled, building
        - not in building or structure — *see* Exposure, fire, controlled, not in building
      - building or structure X02.0 ☑
        - with
          - fall from building X02.3 ☑
          - from building X02.5 ☑
          - injury due to building collapse X02.2 ☑
          - smoke inhalation X02.1 ☑
        - hit by object from building X02.4 ☑
        - specified mode of injury NEC X02.8 ☑
      - fireplace, furnace or stove — *see* Exposure, fire, controlled, building
      - not in building or structure X03.0 ☑
        - with
          - fall X03.3 ☑
          - smoke inhalation X03.1 ☑
        - hit by object X03.4 ☑
        - specified mode of injury NEC X03.8 ☑
      - trash — *see* Exposure, fire, controlled, not in building
    - fireplace — *see* Exposure, fire, controlled, building
    - fittings or furniture (in building or structure) (uncontrolled) — *see* Exposure, fire, uncontrolled, building
    - forest (uncontrolled) — *see* Exposure, fire, uncontrolled, not in building
    - grass (uncontrolled) — *see* Exposure, fire, uncontrolled, not in building
    - hay (uncontrolled) — *see* Exposure, fire, uncontrolled, not in building
    - homicide (attempt) X97 ☑
    - ignition of highly flammable material X04 ☑
    - in, of, on, starting in
      - machinery — *see* Contact, with, by type of machine

- **Exposure** — *continued*
  - fire, flames — *continued*
    - in, of, on, starting in — *continued*
      - motor vehicle (in motion) — *see also* Accident, transport, occupant by type of vehicle V87.8 ☑
        - with collision — *see* Collision
      - railway rolling stock, train, vehicle V81.81 ☑
        - with collision — *see* Accident, transport, railway vehicle occupant
      - street car (in motion) V82.8 ☑
        - with collision — *see* Accident, transport, streetcar occupant
      - transport vehicle NEC — *see also* Accident, transport
        - with collision — *see* Collision
      - war operations — *see also* War operations, fire from nuclear explosion — *see* War operations, nuclear weapons
      - watercraft (in transit) (not in transit) V91.09 ☑
        - localized — *see* Burn, on board watercraft, due to, fire on board
        - powered craft V91.03 ☑
          - ferry boat V91.01 ☑
          - fishing boat V91.02 ☑
          - jet skis V91.03 ☑
          - liner V91.01 ☑
          - merchant ship V91.00 ☑
          - passenger ship V91.01 ☑
        - unpowered craft V91.08 ☑
          - canoe V91.05 ☑
          - inflatable V91.06 ☑
          - kayak V91.05 ☑
          - sailboat V91.04 ☑
          - surf-board V91.08 ☑
          - waterskis V91.07 ☑
          - windsurfer V91.08 ☑
    - lumber (uncontrolled) — *see* Exposure, fire, uncontrolled, not in building
    - mine (uncontrolled) — *see* Exposure, fire, uncontrolled, not in building
    - prairie (uncontrolled) — *see* Exposure, fire, uncontrolled, not in building
    - resulting from
      - explosion — *see* Explosion
      - lightning X08.8 ☑
    - self-inflicted X76 ☑
    - specified NEC X08.8 ☑
    - started by other person X97 ☑
    - stated as undetermined whether accidental or intentional Y26 ☑
    - stove — *see* Exposure, fire, controlled, building
    - suicide (attempt) X76 ☑
    - tunnel (uncontrolled) — *see* Exposure, fire, uncontrolled, not in building
    - uncontrolled
      - in building or structure X00.0 ☑
        - with
          - fall from building X00.3 ☑
          - injury due to building collapse X00.2 ☑
          - jump from building X00.5 ☑
          - smoke inhalation X00.1 ☑
        - bed X08.00 ☑
          - due to
            - cigarette X08.01 ☑
            - specified material NEC X08.09 ☑
        - furniture NEC X08.20 ☑
          - due to
            - cigarette X08.21 ☑
            - specified material NEC X08.29 ☑
        - hit by object from building X00.4 ☑
        - sofa X08.10 ☑
          - due to
            - cigarette X08.11 ☑
            - specified material NEC X08.19 ☑
        - specified mode of injury NEC X00.8 ☑
      - not in building or structure (any) X01.0 ☑
        - with
          - fall X01.3 ☑
          - smoke inhalation X01.1 ☑
        - hit by object X01.4 ☑
        - specified mode of injury NEC X01.8 ☑
    - undetermined whether accidental or intentional Y26 ☑
  - forces of nature NEC — *see* Forces of nature
  - G-forces (abnormal) W49.9 ☑

Exposure — *continued*
- gravitational forces (abnormal) W49.9 ☑
- heat (natural) NEC — *see* Heat
- high-pressure jet (hydraulic) (pneumatic) W49.9 ☑
- hydraulic jet W49.9 ☑
- inanimate mechanical force W49.9 ☑
- jet, high-pressure (hydraulic) (pneumatic) W49.9 ☑
- lightning — *see* subcategory T75.0 ☑
  - causing fire — *see* Exposure, fire
- mechanical forces NEC W49.9 ☑
  - animate NEC W64 ☑
  - inanimate NEC W49.9 ☑
- noise W42.9 ☑
  - supersonic W42.0 ☑
- noxious substance — *see* Table of Drugs and Chemicals
- pneumatic jet W49.9 ☑
- prolonged in deep-freeze unit or refrigerator W93.2 ☑
- radiation — *see* Radiation
- smoke — *see also* Exposure, fire
  - tobacco, second hand Z77.22
- specified factors NEC X58 ☑
- sunlight X32 ☑
  - man-made (sun lamp) W89.8 ☑
    - tanning bed W89.1 ☑
- supersonic waves W42.0 ☑
- transmission line(s), electric W85 ☑
- vibration W49.9 ☑
- waves
  - infrasound W49.9 ☑
  - sound W42.9 ☑
  - supersonic W42.0 ☑
- weather NEC — *see* Forces of nature

External cause status Y99.9
- child assisting in compensated work for family Y99.8
- civilian activity done for financial or other compensation Y99.0
- civilian activity done for income or pay Y99.0
- family member assisting in compensated work for other family member Y99.8
- hobby not done for income Y99.8
- leisure activity Y99.8
- military activity Y99.1
- off-duty activity of military personnel Y99.8
- recreation or sport not for income or while a student Y99.8
- specified NEC Y99.8
- student activity Y99.8
- volunteer activity Y99.2

F

Factors, supplemental
- alcohol
  - blood level
    - less than 20mg/100ml Y90.0
    - presence in blood, level not specified Y90.9
    - 20-39mg/100ml Y90.1
    - 40-59mg/100ml Y90.2
    - 60-79mg/100ml Y90.3
    - 80-99mg/100ml Y90.4
    - 100-119mg/100ml Y90.5
    - 120-199mg/100ml Y90.6
    - 200-239mg/100ml Y90.7
    - 240mg/100ml or more Y90.8
  - presence in blood, but level not specified Y90.9
- environmental-pollution-related condition- see Z57 ☑
- nosocomial condition Y95
- work-related condition Y99.0

Failure
- in suture or ligature during surgical procedure Y65.2
- mechanical, of instrument or apparatus (any) (during any medical or surgical procedure) Y65.8
- sterile precautions (during medical and surgical care) — *see* Misadventure, failure, sterile precautions, by type of procedure
- to
  - introduce tube or instrument Y65.4
    - endotracheal tube during anesthesia Y65.3
  - make curve (transport vehicle) NEC — *see* Accident, transport
  - remove tube or instrument Y65.4

Fall, falling (accidental) W19 ☑
- building W20.1 ☑
  - burning (uncontrolled fire) X00.3 ☑
- down
  - embankment W17.81 ☑
  - escalator W10.0 ☑

Fall, falling — *continued*
- down — *continued*
  - hill W17.81 ☑
  - ladder W11 ☑
  - ramp W10.2 ☑
  - stairs, steps W10.9 ☑
- due to
  - bumping against
    - object W18.00 ☑
      - sharp glass W18.02 ☑
      - specified NEC W18.09 ☑
      - sports equipment W18.01 ☑
    - person W03 ☑
      - due to ice or snow W00.0 ☑
      - on pedestrian conveyance — *see* Accident, transport, pedestrian, conveyance
  - collision with another person W03 ☑
    - due to ice or snow W00.0 ☑
    - involving pedestrian conveyance — *see* Accident, transport, pedestrian, conveyance
  - grocery cart tipping over W17.82 ☑
  - ice or snow W00.9 ☑
    - from one level to another W00.2 ☑
      - on stairs or steps W00.1 ☑
    - involving pedestrian conveyance — *see* Accident, transport, pedestrian, conveyance
    - on same level W00.0 ☑
  - slipping (on moving sidewalk) W01.0 ☑
    - with subsequent striking against object W01.10 ☑
      - furniture W01.190 ☑
      - sharp object W01.119 ☑
        - glass W01.110 ☑
        - power tool or machine W01.111 ☑
        - specified NEC W01.118 ☑
      - specified NEC W01.198 ☑
  - striking against
    - object W18.00 ☑
      - sharp glass W18.02 ☑
      - specified NEC W18.09 ☑
      - sports equipment W18.01 ☑
    - person W03 ☑
      - due to ice or snow W00.0 ☑
      - on pedestrian conveyance — *see* Accident, transport, pedestrian, conveyance
- earth (with asphyxia or suffocation (by pressure)) — *see* Earth, falling
- from, off, out of
  - aircraft NEC (with accident to aircraft NEC) V97.0 ☑
    - while boarding or alighting V97.1 ☑
  - balcony W13.0 ☑
  - bed W06 ☑
  - boat, ship, watercraft NEC (with drowning or submersion) — *see* Drowning, due to, fall overboard
    - with hitting bottom or object V94.0 ☑
  - bridge W13.1 ☑
  - building W13.9 ☑
    - burning (uncontrolled fire) X00.3 ☑
  - cavity W17.2 ☑
  - chair W07 ☑
  - cherry picker W17.89 ☑
  - cliff W15 ☑
  - dock W17.4 ☑
  - embankment W17.81 ☑
  - escalator W10.0 ☑
  - flagpole W13.8 ☑
  - furniture NEC W08 ☑
  - grocery cart W17.82 ☑
  - haystack W17.89 ☑
  - high place NEC W17.89 ☑
    - stated as undetermined whether accidental or intentional Y30 ☑
  - hole W17.2 ☑
  - incline W10.2 ☑
  - ladder W11 ☑
  - lifting device W17.89 ☑
  - machine, machinery — *see also* Contact, with, by type of machine
    - not in operation W17.89 ☑
  - manhole W17.1 ☑
  - mobile elevated work platform [MEWP] W17.89 ☑
  - motorized mobility scooter W05.2 ☑
  - one level to another NEC W17.89 ☑
    - intentional, purposeful, suicide (attempt) X80 ☑

Fall, falling — *continued*
- from, off, out of — *continued*
  - one level to another — *continued*
    - stated as undetermined whether accidental or intentional Y30 ☑
  - pit W17.2 ☑
  - playground equipment W09.8 ☑
    - jungle gym W09.2 ☑
    - slide W09.0 ☑
    - swing W09.1 ☑
  - quarry W17.89 ☑
  - railing W13.9 ☑
  - ramp W10.2 ☑
  - roof W13.2 ☑
  - scaffolding W12 ☑
  - scooter (nonmotorized) W05.1 ☑
    - motorized mobility W05.2 ☑
  - sky lift W17.89 ☑
  - stairs, steps W10.9 ☑
    - curb W10.1 ☑
    - due to ice or snow W00.1 ☑
    - escalator W10.0 ☑
    - incline W10.2 ☑
    - ramp W10.2 ☑
    - sidewalk curb W10.1 ☑
    - specified NEC W10.8 ☑
    - standing
      - electric scooter V00.841 ☑
      - micro-mobility pedestrian conveyance V00.848 ☑
  - stepladder W11 ☑
  - stool W08 ☑
  - storm drain W17.1 ☑
  - streetcar NEC V82.6 ☑
    - while boarding or alighting V82.4 ☑
    - with antecedent collision — *see* Accident, transport, streetcar occupant
  - structure NEC W13.8 ☑
    - burning (uncontrolled fire) X00.3 ☑
  - table W08 ☑
  - toilet W18.11 ☑
    - with subsequent striking against object W18.12 ☑
  - train NEC V81.6 ☑
    - during derailment (without antecedent collision) V81.7 ☑
      - with antecedent collision — *see* Accident, transport, railway vehicle occupant
    - while boarding or alighting V81.4 ☑
  - transport vehicle after collision — *see* Accident, transport, by type of vehicle, collision
  - tree W14 ☑
  - vehicle (in motion) NEC — *see also* Accident, transport V89.9 ☑
    - motor NEC — *see also* Accident, transport, occupant, by type of vehicle V87.8 ☑
    - stationary W17.89 ☑
      - while boarding or alighting — *see* Accident, transport, by type of vehicle, while boarding or alighting
  - viaduct W13.8 ☑
  - wall W13.8 ☑
  - watercraft — *see also* Drowning, due to, fall overboard
    - with hitting bottom or object V94.0 ☑
  - well W17.0 ☑
  - wheelchair, non-moving W05.0 ☑
    - powered — *see* Accident, transport, pedestrian, conveyance occupant, specified type NEC
  - window W13.4 ☑
- in, on
  - aircraft NEC V97.0 ☑
    - while boarding or alighting V97.1 ☑
    - with accident to aircraft V97.0 ☑
  - bathtub (empty) W18.2 ☑
    - filled W16.212 ☑
      - causing drowning W16.211 ☑
  - escalator W10.0 ☑
  - incline W10.2 ☑
  - ladder W11 ☑
  - machine, machinery — *see* Contact, with, by type of machine
  - object, edged, pointed or sharp (with cut) — *see* Fall, by type
  - playground equipment W09.8 ☑
    - jungle gym W09.2 ☑

- **Fall, falling** — *continued*
  - in, on — *continued*
    - playground equipment — *continued*
      - slide WØ9.Ø ☑
      - swing WØ9.1 ☑
    - ramp W1Ø.2 ☑
    - scaffolding W12 ☑
    - shower W18.2 ☑
      - causing drowning W16.211 ☑
    - staircase, stairs, steps W1Ø.9 ☑
      - curb W1Ø.1 ☑
      - due to ice or snow WØØ.1 ☑
      - escalator W1Ø.Ø ☑
      - incline W1Ø.2 ☑
      - specified NEC W1Ø.8 ☑
    - streetcar (without antecedent collision) V82.5 ☑
      - with antecedent collision — *see* Accident, transport, streetcar occupant
      - while boarding or alighting V82.4 ☑
    - train (without antecedent collision) V81.5 ☑
      - with antecedent collision — *see* Accident, transport, railway vehicle occupant
      - during derailment (without antecedent collision) V81.7 ☑
        - with antecedent collision — *see* Accident, transport, railway vehicle occupant
      - while boarding or alighting V81.4 ☑
    - transport vehicle after collision — *see* Accident, transport, by type of vehicle, collision
    - watercraft V93.39 ☑
      - due to
        - accident to craft V91.29 ☑
          - powered craft V91.23 ☑
            - ferry boat V91.21 ☑
            - fishing boat V91.22 ☑
            - jetskis V91.23 ☑
            - liner V91.21 ☑
            - merchant ship V91.2Ø ☑
            - passenger ship V91.21 ☑
          - unpowered craft
            - canoe V91.25 ☑
            - inflatable V91.26 ☑
            - kayak V91.25 ☑
            - sailboat V91.24 ☑
      - powered craft V93.33 ☑
        - ferry boat V93.31 ☑
        - fishing boat V93.32 ☑
        - jetskis V93.33 ☑
        - liner V93.31 ☑
        - merchant ship V93.3Ø ☑
        - passenger ship V93.31 ☑
      - unpowered craft V93.38 ☑
        - canoe V93.35 ☑
        - inflatable V93.36 ☑
        - kayak V93.35 ☑
        - sailboat V93.34 ☑
        - surf-board V93.38 ☑
        - windsurfer V93.38 ☑
  - into
    - cavity W17.2 ☑
    - dock W17.4 ☑
    - fire — *see* Exposure, fire, by type
    - haystack W17.89 ☑
    - hole W17.2 ☑
    - lake — *see* Fall, into, water
    - manhole W17.1 ☑
    - moving part of machinery — *see* Contact, with, by type of machine
    - ocean — *see* Fall, into, water
    - opening in surface NEC W17.89 ☑
    - pit W17.2 ☑
    - pond — *see* Fall, into, water
    - quarry W17.89 ☑
    - river — *see* Fall, into, water
    - shaft W17.89 ☑
    - storm drain W17.1 ☑
    - stream — *see* Fall, into, water
    - swimming pool — *see also* Fall, into, water, in, swimming pool
      - empty W17.3 ☑
    - tank W17.89 ☑
    - water W16.42 ☑
      - causing drowning W16.41 ☑
      - from watercraft — *see* Drowning, due to, fall overboard
      - hitting diving board W21.4 ☑

- **Fall, falling** — *continued*
  - into — *continued*
    - water — *continued*
      - in
        - bathtub W16.212 ☑
          - causing drowning W16.211 ☑
        - bucket W16.222 ☑
          - causing drowning W16.221 ☑
        - natural body of water W16.112 ☑
          - causing drowning W16.111 ☑
          - striking
            - bottom W16.122 ☑
              - causing drowning W16.121 ☑
            - side W16.132 ☑
              - causing drowning W16.131 ☑
        - specified water NEC W16.312 ☑
          - causing drowning W16.311 ☑
          - striking
            - bottom W16.322 ☑
              - causing drowning W16.321 ☑
            - wall W16.332 ☑
              - causing drowning W16.331 ☑
        - swimming pool W16.Ø12 ☑
          - causing drowning W16.Ø11 ☑
          - striking
            - bottom W16.Ø22 ☑
              - causing drowning W16.Ø31 ☑
            - wall W16.Ø32 ☑
              - causing drowning W16.Ø21 ☑
        - utility bucket W16.222 ☑
          - causing drowning W16.221 ☑
    - well W17.Ø ☑
  - involving
    - bed WØ6 ☑
    - chair WØ7 ☑
    - furniture NEC WØ8 ☑
    - glass — *see* Fall, by type
    - playground equipment WØ9.8 ☑
      - jungle gym WØ9.2 ☑
      - slide WØ9.Ø ☑
      - swing WØ9.1 ☑
    - roller blades — *see* Accident, transport, pedestrian, conveyance
    - skateboard(s) — *see* Accident, transport, pedestrian, conveyance
    - skates (ice) (in line) (roller) — *see* Accident, transport, pedestrian, conveyance
    - skis — *see* Accident, transport, pedestrian, conveyance
    - table WØ8 ☑
    - wheelchair, non-moving WØ5.Ø ☑
      - powered — *see* Accident, transport, pedestrian, conveyance, specified type NEC
  - object — *see* Struck by, object, falling
  - off
    - toilet W18.11 ☑
      - with subsequent striking against object W18.12 ☑
  - on same level W18.3Ø ☑
    - due to
      - specified NEC W18.39 ☑
      - stepping on an object W18.31 ☑
  - out of
    - bed WØ6 ☑
    - building NEC W13.8 ☑
    - chair WØ7 ☑
    - furniture NEC WØ8 ☑
    - wheelchair, non-moving WØ5.Ø ☑
      - powered — *see* Accident, transport, pedestrian, conveyance, specified type NEC
    - window W13.4 ☑
  - over
    - animal WØ1.Ø ☑
    - cliff W15 ☑
    - embankment W17.81 ☑
    - small object WØ1.Ø ☑
  - rock W2Ø.8 ☑
  - same level W18.3Ø ☑
    - from
      - being crushed, pushed, or stepped on by a crowd or human stampede W52 ☑
      - collision, pushing, shoving, by or with other person WØ3 ☑
      - slipping, stumbling, tripping WØ1.Ø ☑
    - involving ice or snow WØØ.Ø ☑

- **Fall, falling** — *continued*
  - same level — *continued*
    - involving ice or snow — *continued*
      - involving skates (ice) (roller), skateboard, skis — *see* Accident, transport, pedestrian, conveyance
  - snowslide (avalanche) — *see* Landslide
  - stone W2Ø.8 ☑
  - structure W2Ø.1 ☑
    - burning (uncontrolled fire) XØØ.3 ☑
  - through
    - bridge W13.1 ☑
    - floor W13.3 ☑
    - roof W13.2 ☑
    - wall W13.8 ☑
    - window W13.4 ☑
  - timber W2Ø.8 ☑
  - tree (caused by lightning) W2Ø.8 ☑
  - while being carried or supported by other person(s) WØ4 ☑
- **Fallen on by**
  - animal (not being ridden) NEC W55.89 ☑
- **Felo-de-se** — *see* Suicide
- **Fight** (hand) (fists) (foot) — *see* Assault, fight
- **Fire** (accidental) — *see* Exposure, fire
- **Firearm discharge** — *see* Discharge, firearm
- **Fireball effects from nuclear explosion in war operations** — *see* War operations, nuclear weapons
- **Fireworks** (explosion) W39 ☑
- **Flash burns from explosion** — *see* Explosion
- **Flood** (any injury) (caused by) X38 ☑
  - collapse of man-made structure causing earth movement X36.Ø ☑
  - tidal wave — *see* Forces of nature, tidal wave
- **Food** (any type) **in**
  - air passages (with asphyxia, obstruction, or suffocation) — *see* categories T17 and T18 ☑
  - alimentary tract causing asphyxia (due to compression of trachea) — *see* categories T17 and T18 ☑
- **Forces of nature** X39.8 ☑
  - avalanche X36.1 ☑
    - causing transport accident — *see* Accident, transport, by type of vehicle
  - blizzard X37.2 ☑
  - cataclysmic storm X37.9 ☑
    - with flood X38 ☑
    - blizzard X37.2 ☑
    - cloudburst X37.8 ☑
    - cyclone X37.1 ☑
    - dust storm X37.3 ☑
    - hurricane X37.Ø ☑
    - specified storm NEC X37.8 ☑
    - storm surge X37.Ø ☑
    - tornado X37.1 ☑
    - twister X37.1 ☑
    - typhoon X37.Ø ☑
  - cloudburst X37.8 ☑
  - cold (natural) X31 ☑
  - cyclone X37.1 ☑
  - dam collapse causing earth movement X36.Ø ☑
  - dust storm X37.3 ☑
  - earth movement X36.1 ☑
    - caused by dam or structure collapse X36.Ø ☑
    - earthquake X34 ☑
  - earthquake X34 ☑
  - flood (caused by) X38 ☑
    - dam collapse X36.Ø ☑
    - tidal wave — *see* Forces of nature, tidal wave
  - heat (natural) X3Ø ☑
  - hurricane X37.Ø ☑
  - landslide X36.1 ☑
    - causing transport accident — *see* Accident, transport, by type of vehicle
  - lightning — *see* subcategory T75.Ø ☑
    - causing fire — *see* Exposure, fire
  - mudslide X36.1 ☑
    - causing transport accident — *see* Accident, transport, by type of vehicle
  - radiation (natural) X39.Ø8 ☑
    - radon X39.Ø1 ☑
  - radon X39.Ø1 ☑
  - specified force NEC X39.8 ☑
  - storm surge X37.Ø ☑
  - structure collapse causing earth movement X36.Ø ☑
  - sunlight X32 ☑
  - tidal wave X37.41 ☑

- **Forces of nature** — *continued*
  - tidal wave — *continued*
    - due to
      - earthquake X37.41 ☑
      - landslide X37.43 ☑
      - storm X37.42 ☑
      - volcanic eruption X37.41 ☑
  - tornado X37.1 ☑
  - tsunami X37.41 ☑
  - twister X37.1 ☑
  - typhoon X37.Ø ☑
  - volcanic eruption X35 ☑
- **Foreign body**
  - aspiration — *see* Index to Diseases and Injuries, Foreign body, respiratory tract
  - embedded in skin W45 ☑
  - entering through skin W45.8 ☑
    - can lid W26.8 ☑
    - nail W45.Ø ☑
    - paper W26.2 ☑
    - specified NEC W45.8 ☑
    - splinter W45.8 ☑
- **Forest fire** (exposure to) — *see* Exposure, fire, uncontrolled, not in building
- **Found injured** X58 ☑
  - from exposure (to) — *see* Exposure
  - on
    - highway, road(way), street V89.9 ☑
    - railway right of way V81.9 ☑
- **Fracture** (circumstances unknown or unspecified) X58 ☑
  - due to specified cause NEC X58 ☑
- **Freezing** — *see* Exposure, cold
- **Frostbite** X31 ☑
  - due to man-made conditions — *see* Exposure, cold, man-made
- **Frozen** — *see* Exposure, cold

G

- **Gored by bull** W55.22 ☑
- **Gunshot wound** W34.ØØ ☑

H

- **Hailstones, injured by** X39.8 ☑
- **Hanged herself or himself** — *see* Hanging, self-inflicted
- **Hanging** (accidental) — *see also* category T71 ☑
  - legal execution — *see* Legal, intervention, specified means NEC
- **Heat** (effects of) (excessive) X3Ø ☑
  - due to
    - man-made conditions W92 ☑
      - on board watercraft V93.29 ☑
        - fishing boat V93.22 ☑
        - merchant ship V93.2Ø ☑
        - passenger ship V93.21 ☑
        - sailboat V93.24 ☑
        - specified powered craft NEC V93.23 ☑
    - weather (conditions) X3Ø ☑
  - from
    - electric heating apparatus causing burning X16 ☑
    - nuclear explosion in war operations — *see* War operations, nuclear weapons
  - inappropriate in local application or packing in medical or surgical procedure Y63.5
- **Hemorrhage**
  - delayed following medical or surgical treatment without mention of misadventure — *see* Index to Diseases and Injuries, Complication(s)
  - during medical or surgical treatment as misadventure — *see* Index to Diseases and Injuries, Complication(s)
- **High**
  - altitude (effects) — *see* Air, pressure, low
  - level of radioactivity, effects — *see* Radiation
  - pressure (effects) — *see* Air, pressure, high
  - temperature, effects — *see* Heat
- **Hit, hitting** (accidental) by — *see* Struck by
- **Hitting against** — *see* Striking against
- **Homicide** (attempt) (justifiable) — *see* Assault
- **Hot**
  - place, effects — *see also* Heat
  - weather, effects X3Ø ☑
- **House fire** (uncontrolled) — *see* Exposure, fire, uncontrolled, building
- **Humidity, causing problem** X39.8 ☑
- **Hunger** X58 ☑
- **Hurricane** (any injury) X37.Ø ☑
- **Hypobarism, hypobaropathy** — *see* Air, pressure, low

I

- **Ictus**
  - caloris — *see also* Heat
  - solaris X3Ø ☑
- **Ignition** (accidental) — *see also* Exposure, fire XØ8.8 ☑
  - anesthetic gas in operating room W4Ø.1 ☑
  - apparel XØ6.2 ☑
    - from highly flammable material XØ4 ☑
    - nightwear XØ5 ☑
  - bed linen (sheets) (spreads) (pillows) (mattress) — *see* Exposure, fire, uncontrolled, building, bed
  - benzine XØ4 ☑
  - clothes, clothing NEC (from controlled fire) XØ6.2 ☑
    - from
      - highly flammable material XØ4 ☑
  - ether XØ4 ☑
    - in operating room W4Ø.1 ☑
  - explosive material — *see* Explosion
  - gasoline XØ4 ☑
  - jewelry (plastic) (any) XØ6.Ø ☑
  - kerosene XØ4 ☑
  - material
    - explosive — *see* Explosion
    - highly flammable with secondary explosion XØ4 ☑
  - nightwear XØ5 ☑
  - paraffin XØ4 ☑
  - petrol XØ4 ☑
- **Immersion** (accidental) — *see also* Drowning
  - hand or foot due to cold (excessive) X31 ☑
- **Implantation of quills of porcupine** W55.89 ☑
- **Inanition** (from) (hunger) X58 ☑
  - thirst X58 ☑
- **Inappropriate operation performed**
  - correct operation on wrong side or body part (wrong side) (wrong site) Y65.53
  - operation intended for another patient done on wrong patient Y65.52
  - wrong operation performed on correct patient Y65.51
- **Inattention after, at birth** (homicidal intent) (infanticidal intent) X58 ☑
- **Incident, adverse**
  - device
    - anesthesiology Y7Ø.8
      - accessory Y7Ø.2
      - diagnostic Y7Ø.Ø
      - miscellaneous Y7Ø.8
      - monitoring Y7Ø.Ø
      - prosthetic Y7Ø.2
      - rehabilitative Y7Ø.1
      - surgical Y7Ø.3
      - therapeutic Y7Ø.1
    - cardiovascular Y71.8
      - accessory Y71.2
      - diagnostic Y71.Ø
      - miscellaneous Y71.8
      - monitoring Y71.Ø
      - prosthetic Y71.2
      - rehabilitative Y71.1
      - surgical Y71.3
      - therapeutic Y71.1
    - gastroenterology Y73.8
      - accessory Y73.2
      - diagnostic Y73.Ø
      - miscellaneous Y73.8
      - monitoring Y73.Ø
      - prosthetic Y73.2
      - rehabilitative Y73.1
      - surgical Y73.3
      - therapeutic Y73.1
    - general
      - hospital Y74.8
        - accessory Y74.2
        - diagnostic Y74.Ø
        - miscellaneous Y74.8
        - monitoring Y74.Ø
        - prosthetic Y74.2
        - rehabilitative Y74.1
        - surgical Y74.3
        - therapeutic Y74.1
      - surgical Y81.8
        - accessory Y81.2
        - diagnostic Y81.Ø
- **Incident, adverse** — *continued*
  - device — *continued*
    - general — *continued*
      - surgical — *continued*
        - miscellaneous Y81.8
        - monitoring Y81.Ø
        - prosthetic Y81.2
        - rehabilitative Y81.1
        - surgical Y81.3
        - therapeutic Y81.1
    - gynecological Y76.8
      - accessory Y76.2
      - diagnostic Y76.Ø
      - miscellaneous Y76.8
      - monitoring Y76.Ø
      - prosthetic Y76.2
      - rehabilitative Y76.1
      - surgical Y76.3
      - therapeutic Y76.1
    - medical Y82.9
      - specified type NEC Y82.8
    - neurological Y75.8
      - accessory Y75.2
      - diagnostic Y75.Ø
      - miscellaneous Y75.8
      - monitoring Y75.Ø
      - prosthetic Y75.2
      - rehabilitative Y75.1
      - surgical Y75.3
      - therapeutic Y75.1
    - obstetrical Y76.8
      - accessory Y76.2
      - diagnostic Y76.Ø
      - miscellaneous Y76.8
      - monitoring Y76.Ø
      - prosthetic Y76.2
      - rehabilitative Y76.1
      - surgical Y76.3
      - therapeutic Y76.1
    - ophthalmic Y77.8
      - accessory Y77.2
      - contact lens (rigid gas permeable) (soft (hydrophilic)) Y77.11
      - diagnostic Y77.Ø
      - miscellaneous Y77.8
      - monitoring Y77.Ø
      - prosthetic Y77.2
      - rehabilitative Y77.19
      - surgical Y77.3
      - therapeutic Y77.19
    - orthopedic Y79.8
      - accessory Y79.2
      - diagnostic Y79.Ø
      - miscellaneous Y79.8
      - monitoring Y79.Ø
      - prosthetic Y79.2
      - rehabilitative Y79.1
      - surgical Y79.3
      - therapeutic Y79.1
    - otorhinolaryngological Y72.8
      - accessory Y72.2
      - diagnostic Y72.Ø
      - miscellaneous Y72.8
      - monitoring Y72.Ø
      - prosthetic Y72.2
      - rehabilitative Y72.1
      - surgical Y72.3
      - therapeutic Y72.1
    - personal use Y74.8
      - accessory Y74.2
      - diagnostic Y74.Ø
      - miscellaneous Y74.8
      - monitoring Y74.Ø
      - prosthetic Y74.2
      - rehabilitative Y74.1
      - surgical Y74.3
      - therapeutic Y74.1
    - physical medicine Y8Ø.8
      - accessory Y8Ø.2
      - diagnostic Y8Ø.Ø
      - miscellaneous Y8Ø.8
      - monitoring Y8Ø.Ø
      - prosthetic Y8Ø.2
      - rehabilitative Y8Ø.1
      - surgical Y8Ø.3
      - therapeutic Y8Ø.1
    - plastic surgical Y81.8
      - accessory Y81.2
      - diagnostic Y81.Ø

- **Incident, adverse** — *continued*
  - device — *continued*
    - plastic surgical — *continued*
      - miscellaneous Y81.8
      - monitoring Y81.Ø
      - prosthetic Y81.2
      - rehabilitative Y81.1
      - surgical Y81.3
      - therapeutic Y81.1
    - radiological Y78.8
      - accessory Y78.2
      - diagnostic Y78.Ø
      - miscellaneous Y78.8
      - monitoring Y78.Ø
      - prosthetic Y78.2
      - rehabilitative Y78.1
      - surgical Y78.3
      - therapeutic Y78.1
    - urology Y73.8
      - accessory Y73.2
      - diagnostic Y73.Ø
      - miscellaneous Y73.8
      - monitoring Y73.Ø
      - prosthetic Y73.2
      - rehabilitative Y73.1
      - surgical Y73.3
      - therapeutic Y73.1
- **Incineration** (accidental) — *see* Exposure, fire
- **Infanticide** — *see* Assault
- **Infrasound waves** (causing injury) W49.9 ☑
- **Ingestion**
  - foreign body (causing injury) (with obstruction) — *see* Foreign body, alimentary canal
  - poisonous
    - plant(s) X58 ☑
    - substance NEC — *see* Table of Drugs and Chemicals
- **Inhalation**
  - excessively cold substance, man-made — *see* Exposure, cold, man-made
  - food (any type) (into respiratory tract) (with asphyxia, obstruction respiratory tract, suffocation) — *see* categories T17 and T18 ☑
  - foreign body — *see* Foreign body, aspiration
  - gastric contents (with asphyxia, obstruction respiratory passage, suffocation) T17.81- ☑
  - hot air or gases X14.Ø ☑
  - liquid air, hydrogen, nitrogen W93.12 ☑
    - suicide (attempt) X83.2 ☑
  - steam X13.Ø ☑
    - assault X98.Ø ☑
    - stated as undetermined whether accidental or intentional Y27.Ø ☑
    - suicide (attempt) X77.Ø ☑
  - toxic gas — *see* Table of Drugs and Chemicals
  - vomitus (with asphyxia, obstruction respiratory passage, suffocation) T17.81- ☑
- **Injury, injured** (accidental(ly)) NOS X58 ☑
  - by, caused by, from
    - assault — *see* Assault
    - law-enforcing agent, police, in course of legal intervention — *see* Legal intervention
    - suicide (attempt) X83.8 ☑
  - due to, in
    - civil insurrection — *see* War operations
    - fight — *see also* Assault, fight YØ4.Ø ☑
    - war operations — *see* War operations
  - homicide — *see also* Assault YØ9
  - inflicted (by)
    - in course of arrest (attempted), suppression of disturbance, maintenance of order, by law-enforcing agents — *see* Legal intervention
    - other person
      - stated as
        - accidental X58 ☑
        - intentional, homicide (attempt) — *see* Assault
        - undetermined whether accidental or intentional Y33 ☑
  - purposely (inflicted) by other person(s) — *see* Assault
  - self-inflicted X83.8 ☑
    - stated as accidental X58 ☑
  - specified cause NEC X58 ☑
  - undetermined whether accidental or intentional Y33 ☑
- **Insolation, effects** X3Ø ☑
- **Insufficient nourishment** X58 ☑
- **Interruption of respiration** (by)
  - food (lodged in esophagus) — *see* categories T17 and T18 ☑
  - vomitus (lodged in esophagus) T17.81- ☑
- **Intervention, legal** — *see* Legal intervention
- **Intoxication**
  - drug — *see* Table of Drugs and Chemicals
  - poison — *see* Table of Drugs and Chemicals

J

- **Jammed** (accidentally)
  - between objects (moving) (stationary and moving) W23.Ø ☑
    - stationary W23.1 ☑
- **Jumped, jumping**
  - before moving object NEC X81.8 ☑
    - motor vehicle X81.Ø ☑
    - subway train X81.1 ☑
    - train X81.1 ☑
    - undetermined whether accidental or intentional Y31 ☑
  - from
    - boat (into water) voluntarily, without accident (to or on boat) W16.712 ☑
      - striking bottom W16.722 ☑
        - causing drowning W16.721 ☑
      - with
        - accident to or on boat — *see* Accident, watercraft
        - drowning or submersion W16.711 ☑
          - suicide (attempt) X71.3 ☑
    - building — *see also* Jumped, from, high place W13.9 ☑
      - burning (uncontrolled fire) XØØ.5 ☑
    - high place NEC W17.89 ☑
      - suicide (attempt) X8Ø ☑
      - undetermined whether accidental or intentional Y3Ø ☑
    - structure — *see also* Jumped, from, high place W13.9 ☑
      - burning (uncontrolled fire) XØØ.5 ☑
  - into water W16.92 ☑
    - causing drowning W16.91 ☑
    - from, off watercraft — *see* Jumped, from, boat
    - in
      - natural body W16.612 ☑
        - causing drowning W16.611 ☑
        - striking bottom W16.622 ☑
          - causing drowning W16.621 ☑
      - specified place NEC W16.812 ☑
        - causing drowning W16.811 ☑
        - striking
          - bottom W16.822 ☑
            - causing drowning W16.821 ☑
          - wall W16.832 ☑
            - causing drowning W16.831 ☑
      - swimming pool W16.512 ☑
        - causing drowning W16.511 ☑
        - striking
          - bottom W16.522 ☑
            - causing drowning W16.521 ☑
          - wall W16.532 ☑
            - causing drowning W16.531 ☑
    - suicide (attempt) X71.3 ☑

K

- **Kicked by**
  - animal NEC W55.82 ☑
  - person(s) (accidentally) W5Ø.1 ☑
    - with intent to injure or kill YØ4.Ø ☑
    - as, or caused by, a crowd or human stampede (with fall) W52 ☑
    - assault YØ4.Ø ☑
    - homicide (attempt) YØ4.Ø ☑
    - in
      - fight YØ4.Ø ☑
      - legal intervention
        - injuring
          - bystander Y35.812 ☑
          - law enforcement personnel Y35.811 ☑
          - suspect Y35.813 ☑
          - unspecified person Y35.819 ☑
- **Kicking**
  - against
    - object W22.8 ☑
      - sports equipment W21.9 ☑
      - stationary W22.Ø9 ☑
        - sports equipment W21.89 ☑
    - person — *see* Striking against, person
    - sports equipment W21.9 ☑
  - carpet stretcher with knee X5Ø.3 ☑
- **Killed, killing** (accidentally) NOS — *see also* Injury X58 ☑
  - in
    - action — *see* War operations
    - brawl, fight (hand) (fists) (foot) YØ4.Ø ☑
      - by weapon — *see also* Assault
        - cutting, piercing — *see* Assault, cutting or piercing instrument
        - firearm — *see* Discharge, firearm, by type, homicide
  - self
    - stated as
      - accident NOS X58 ☑
      - suicide — *see* Suicide
      - undetermined whether accidental or intentional Y33 ☑
- **Kneeling** (prolonged (static) X5Ø.1 ☑
- **Knocked down** (accidentally) (by) NOS X58 ☑
  - animal (not being ridden) NEC — *see also* Struck by, by type of animal
  - crowd or human stampede W52 ☑
  - person W51 ☑
    - in brawl, fight YØ4.Ø ☑
  - transport vehicle NEC — *see also* Accident, transport VØ9.9 ☑

L

- **Laceration NEC** — *see* Injury
- **Lack of**
  - care (helpless person) (infant) (newborn) X58 ☑
  - food except as result of abandonment or neglect X58 ☑
    - due to abandonment or neglect X58 ☑
  - water except as result of transport accident X58 ☑
    - due to transport accident — *see* Accident, transport, by type
    - helpless person, infant, newborn X58 ☑
- **Landslide** (falling on transport vehicle) X36.1 ☑
  - caused by collapse of man-made structure X36.Ø ☑
- **Late effect** — *see* Sequelae
- **Legal**
  - execution (any method) — *see* Legal, intervention
  - intervention (by)
    - baton — *see* Legal, intervention, blunt object, baton
    - bayonet — *see* Legal, intervention, sharp object, bayonet
    - blow — *see* Legal, intervention, manhandling
    - blunt object
      - baton
        - injuring
          - bystander Y35.312 ☑
          - law enforcement personnel Y35.311 ☑
          - suspect Y35.313 ☑
          - unspecified person Y35.319 ☑
      - injuring
        - bystander Y35.3Ø2 ☑
        - law enforcement personnel Y35.3Ø1 ☑
        - suspect Y35.3Ø3 ☑
        - unspecified person Y35.3Ø9 ☑
      - specified NEC
        - injuring
          - bystander Y35.392 ☑
          - law enforcement personnel Y35.391 ☑
          - suspect Y35.393 ☑
          - unspecified person Y35.399 ☑
      - stave
        - injuring
          - bystander Y35.392 ☑
          - law enforcement personnel Y35.391 ☑
          - suspect Y35.393 ☑
          - unspecified person Y35.399 ☑
    - bomb — *see* Legal, intervention, explosive
    - conducted energy device
      - injuring
        - bystander Y35.832 ☑
        - law enforcement personnel Y35.831 ☑
        - suspect Y35.833 ☑
        - unspecified person Y35.839 ☑

External Causes Index

Incident, adverse — Legal

- **Legal** — *continued*
  - intervention — *continued*
    - cutting or piercing instrument — *see* Legal, intervention, sharp object
    - dynamite — *see* Legal, intervention, explosive, dynamite
    - electroshock device (taser)
      - injuring
        - bystander Y35.832 ☑
        - law enforcement personnel Y35.831 ☑
        - suspect Y35.833 ☑
        - unspecified person Y35.839 ☑
    - explosive(s)
      - dynamite
        - injuring
          - bystander Y35.112 ☑
          - law enforcement personnel Y35.111 ☑
          - suspect Y35.113 ☑
          - unspecified person Y35.119 ☑
      - grenade
        - injuring
          - bystander Y35.192 ☑
          - law enforcement personnel Y35.191 ☑
          - suspect Y35.193 ☑
          - unspecified person Y35.199 ☑
      - injuring
        - bystander Y35.1Ø2 ☑
        - law enforcement personnel Y35.1Ø1 ☑
        - suspect Y35.1Ø3 ☑
        - unspecified person Y35.1Ø9 ☑
      - mortar bomb
        - injuring
          - bystander Y35.192 ☑
          - law enforcement personnel Y35.191 ☑
          - suspect Y35.193 ☑
          - unspecified person Y35.199 ☑
      - shell
        - injuring
          - bystander Y35.122 ☑
          - law enforcement personnel Y35.121 ☑
          - suspect Y35.123 ☑
          - unspecified person Y35.129 ☑
      - specified NEC
        - injuring
          - bystander Y35.192 ☑
          - law enforcement personnel Y35.191 ☑
          - suspect Y35.193 ☑
          - unspecified person Y35.199 ☑
    - firearm(s) (discharge)
      - handgun
        - injuring
          - bystander Y35.Ø22 ☑
          - law enforcement personnel Y35.Ø21 ☑
          - suspect Y35.Ø23 ☑
          - unspecified person Y35.Ø29 ☑
      - injuring
        - bystander Y35.ØØ2 ☑
        - law enforcement personnel Y35.ØØ1 ☑
        - suspect Y35.ØØ3 ☑
        - unspecified person Y35.ØØ9 ☑
      - machine gun
        - injuring
          - bystander Y35.Ø12 ☑
          - law enforcement personnel Y35.Ø11 ☑
          - suspect Y35.Ø13 ☑
          - unspecified person Y35.Ø19 ☑
      - rifle pellet
        - injuring
          - bystander Y35.Ø32 ☑
          - law enforcement personnel Y35.Ø31 ☑
          - suspect Y35.Ø33 ☑
          - unspecified person Y35.Ø39 ☑
      - rubber bullet
        - injuring
          - bystander Y35.Ø42 ☑
          - law enforcement personnel Y35.Ø41 ☑
          - suspect Y35.Ø43 ☑
          - unspecified person Y35.Ø49 ☑
      - shotgun — *see* Legal, intervention, firearm, specified NEC
      - specified NEC
        - injuring
          - bystander Y35.Ø92 ☑
          - law enforcement personnel Y35.Ø91 ☑
          - suspect Y35.Ø93 ☑
          - unspecified person Y35.Ø99 ☑

- **Legal** — *continued*
  - intervention — *continued*
    - gas (asphyxiation) (poisoning)
      - injuring
        - bystander Y35.2Ø2 ☑
        - law enforcement personnel Y35.2Ø1 ☑
        - suspect Y35.2Ø3 ☑
        - unspecified person Y35.2Ø9 ☑
      - specified NEC
        - injuring
          - bystander Y35.292 ☑
          - law enforcement personnel Y35.291 ☑
          - suspect Y35.293 ☑
          - unspecified person Y35.299 ☑
      - tear gas
        - injuring
          - bystander Y35.212 ☑
          - law enforcement personnel Y35.211 ☑
          - suspect Y35.213 ☑
          - unspecified person Y35.219 ☑
    - grenade — *see* Legal, intervention, explosive, grenade
    - injuring
      - bystander Y35.92 ☑
      - law enforcement personnel Y35.91 ☑
      - suspect Y35.93 ☑
      - unspecified person Y35.99 ☑
    - late effect (of) — *see* with 7th character S Y35 ☑
    - manhandling
      - injuring
        - bystander Y35.812 ☑
        - law enforcement personnel Y35.811 ☑
        - suspect Y35.813 ☑
        - unspecified person Y35.819 ☑
    - sequelae (of) — *see* with 7th character S Y35 ☑
    - sharp objects
      - bayonet
        - injuring
          - bystander Y35.412 ☑
          - law enforcement personnel Y35.411 ☑
          - suspect Y35.413 ☑
          - unspecified person Y35.419 ☑
      - injuring
        - bystander Y35.4Ø2 ☑
        - law enforcement personnel Y35.4Ø1 ☑
        - suspect Y35.4Ø3 ☑
        - unspecified person Y35.4Ø9 ☑
      - specified NEC
        - injuring
          - bystander Y35.492 ☑
          - law enforcement personnel Y35.491 ☑
          - suspect Y35.493 ☑
          - unspecified person Y35.499 ☑
    - specified means NEC
      - injuring
        - bystander Y35.892 ☑
        - law enforcement personnel Y35.891 ☑
        - suspect Y35.893 ☑
        - unspecified person Y35.899 ☑
    - stabbing — *see* Legal, intervention, sharp object
    - stave — *see* Legal, intervention, blunt object, stave
    - stun gun
      - injuring
        - bystander Y35.832 ☑
        - law enforcement personnel Y35.831 ☑
        - suspect Y35.833 ☑
        - unspecified person Y35.839 ☑
    - taser
      - injuring
        - bystander Y35.832 ☑
        - law enforcement personnel Y35.831 ☑
        - suspect Y35.833 ☑
        - unspecified person Y35.839 ☑
    - tear gas — *see* Legal, intervention, gas, tear gas
    - truncheon — *see* Legal, intervention, blunt object, stave
- **Lifting** — *see also* Overexertion
  - heavy objects X5Ø.Ø ☑
  - weights X5Ø.Ø ☑
- **Lightning** (shock) (stroke) (struck by) — *see* subcategory T75.Ø ☑
  - causing fire — *see* Exposure, fire
- **Loss of control** (transport vehicle) NEC — *see* Accident, transport
- **Lost at sea NOS** — *see* Drowning, due to, fall overboard
- **Low**
  - pressure (effects) — *see* Air, pressure, low
  - temperature (effects) — *see* Exposure, cold
- **Lying before train, vehicle or other moving object** X81.8 ☑
  - subway train X81.1 ☑
  - train X81.1 ☑
  - undetermined whether accidental or intentional Y31 ☑
- **Lynching** — *see* Assault

M

- **Malfunction** (mechanism or component) (of)
  - firearm W34.1Ø ☑
    - airgun W34.11Ø ☑
    - BB gun W34.11Ø ☑
    - gas, air or spring-operated gun NEC W34.118 ☑
    - handgun W32.1 ☑
    - hunting rifle W33.12 ☑
    - larger firearm W33.1Ø ☑
      - specified NEC W33.19 ☑
    - machine gun W33.13 ☑
    - paintball gun W34.111 ☑
    - pellet gun W34.11Ø ☑
    - shotgun W33.11 ☑
    - specified NEC W34.19 ☑
    - Very pistol [flare] W34.19 ☑
  - handgun — *see* Malfunction, firearm, handgun
- **Maltreatment** — *see* Perpetrator
- **Mangled** (accidentally) NOS X58 ☑
- **Manhandling** (in brawl, fight) YØ4.Ø ☑
  - legal intervention — *see* Legal, intervention, manhandling
- **Manslaughter** (nonaccidental) — *see* Assault
- **Mauled by animal NEC** W55.89 ☑
- **Medical procedure, complication of** (delayed or as an abnormal reaction without mention of misadventure) — *see* Complication of or following, by specified type of procedure
  - due to or as a result of misadventure — *see* Misadventure
- **Melting** (due to fire) — *see also* Exposure, fire
  - apparel NEC XØ6.3 ☑
  - clothes, clothing NEC XØ6.3 ☑
    - nightwear XØ5 ☑
  - fittings or furniture (burning building) (uncontrolled fire) XØØ.8 ☑
  - nightwear XØ5 ☑
  - plastic jewelry XØ6.1 ☑
- **Mental cruelty** X58 ☑
- **Military operations** (injuries to military and civilians occuring during peacetime on military property and during routine military exercises and operations) (by) (from) (involving) Y37.9Ø- ☑
  - air blast Y37.2Ø- ☑
  - aircraft
    - destruction — *see* Military operations, destruction of aircraft
  - airway restriction — *see* Military operations, restriction of airways
  - asphyxiation — *see* Military operations, restriction of airways
  - biological weapons Y37.6X- ☑
  - blast Y37.2Ø- ☑
  - blast fragments Y37.2Ø- ☑
  - blast wave Y37.2Ø- ☑
  - blast wind Y37.2Ø- ☑
  - bomb Y37.2Ø- ☑
    - dirty Y37.5Ø- ☑
    - gasoline Y37.31- ☑
    - incendiary Y37.31- ☑
    - petrol Y37.31- ☑
  - bullet Y37.43- ☑
    - incendiary Y37.32- ☑
    - rubber Y37.41- ☑
  - chemical weapons Y37.7X- ☑
  - combat
    - hand to hand (unarmed) combat Y37.44- ☑
    - using blunt or piercing object Y37.45- ☑
  - conflagration — *see* Military operations, fire
  - conventional warfare NEC Y37.49- ☑
  - depth-charge Y37.Ø1- ☑
  - destruction of aircraft Y37.1Ø- ☑
    - due to
      - air to air missile Y37.11- ☑
      - collision with other aircraft Y37.12- ☑

- **Military operations** — *continued*
  - destruction of aircraft — *continued*
    - due to — *continued*
      - detonation (accidental) of onboard munitions and explosives Y37.14- ☑
      - enemy fire or explosives Y37.11- ☑
      - explosive placed on aircraft Y37.11- ☑
      - onboard fire Y37.13- ☑
      - rocket propelled grenade [RPG] Y37.11- ☑
      - small arms fire Y37.11- ☑
      - surface to air missile Y37.11- ☑
    - specified NEC Y37.19- ☑
  - detonation (accidental) of
    - onboard marine weapons Y37.Ø5- ☑
    - own munitions or munitions launch device Y37.24- ☑
  - dirty bomb Y37.5Ø- ☑
  - explosion (of) Y37.2Ø- ☑
    - aerial bomb Y37.21- ☑
    - bomb NOS — *see also* Military operations, bomb(s) Y37.2Ø- ☑
    - fragments Y37.2Ø- ☑
    - grenade Y37.29- ☑
    - guided missile Y37.22- ☑
    - improvised explosive device [IED] (person-borne) (roadside) (vehicle-borne) Y37.23- ☑
    - land mine Y37.29- ☑
    - marine mine (at sea) (in harbor) Y37.Ø2- ☑
    - marine weapon Y37.ØØ- ☑
      - specified NEC Y37.Ø9- ☑
    - own munitions or munitions launch device (accidental) Y37.24- ☑
    - sea-based artillery shell Y37.Ø3- ☑
    - specified NEC Y37.29- ☑
    - torpedo Y37.Ø4- ☑
  - fire Y37.3Ø- ☑
    - specified NEC Y37.39- ☑
  - firearms
    - discharge Y37.43- ☑
    - pellets Y37.42- ☑
  - flamethrower Y37.33- ☑
  - fragments (from) (of)
    - improvised explosive device [IED] (person-borne) (roadside) (vehicle-borne) Y37.26- ☑
    - munitions Y37.25- ☑
    - specified NEC Y37.29- ☑
    - weapons Y37.27- ☑
  - friendly fire Y37.92- ☑
  - hand to hand (unarmed) combat Y37.44- ☑
  - hot substances — *see* Military operations, fire
  - incendiary bullet Y37.32- ☑
  - nuclear weapon (effects of) Y37.5Ø- ☑
    - acute radiation exposure Y37.54- ☑
    - blast pressure Y37.51- ☑
    - direct blast Y37.51- ☑
    - direct heat Y37.53- ☑
    - fallout exposure Y37.54- ☑
    - fireball Y37.53- ☑
    - indirect blast (struck or crushed by blast debris) (being thrown by blast) Y37.52- ☑
    - ionizing radiation (immediate exposure) Y37.54- ☑
    - nuclear radiation Y37.54- ☑
    - radiation
      - ionizing (immediate exposure) Y37.54- ☑
      - nuclear Y37.54- ☑
      - thermal Y37.53- ☑
    - secondary effects Y37.54- ☑
    - specified NEC Y37.59- ☑
    - thermal radiation Y37.53- ☑
  - restriction of air (airway)
    - intentional Y37.46- ☑
    - unintentional Y37.47- ☑
  - rubber bullets Y37.41- ☑
  - shrapnel NOS Y37.29- ☑
  - suffocation — *see* Military operations, restriction of airways
  - unconventional warfare NEC Y37.7X- ☑
  - underwater blast NOS Y37.ØØ- ☑
  - warfare
    - conventional NEC Y37.49- ☑
    - unconventional NEC Y37.7X- ☑
  - weapon of mass destruction [WMD] Y37.91- ☑
  - weapons
    - biological weapons Y37.6X- ☑
    - chemical Y37.7X- ☑
    - nuclear (effects of) Y37.5Ø- ☑

- **Military operations** — *continued*
  - weapons — *continued*
    - nuclear — *continued*
      - acute radiation exposure Y37.54- ☑
      - blast pressure Y37.51- ☑
      - direct blast Y37.51- ☑
      - direct heat Y37.53- ☑
      - fallout exposure Y37.54- ☑
      - fireball Y37.53- ☑
      - radiation
        - ionizing (immediate exposure) Y37.54- ☑
        - nuclear Y37.54- ☑
        - thermal Y37.53- ☑
      - secondary effects Y37.54- ☑
      - specified NEC Y37.59- ☑
    - of mass destruction [WMD] Y37.91- ☑
- **Misadventure**(s) **to patient**(s) **during surgical or medical care** Y69
  - contaminated medical or biological substance (blood, drug, fluid) Y64.9
    - administered (by) NEC Y64.9
      - immunization Y64.1
      - infusion Y64.Ø
      - injection Y64.1
      - specified means NEC Y64.8
      - transfusion Y64.Ø
      - vaccination Y64.1
  - excessive amount of blood or other fluid during transfusion or infusion Y63.Ø
  - failure
    - in dosage Y63.9
      - electroshock therapy Y63.4
      - inappropriate temperature (too hot or too cold) in local application and packing Y63.5
      - infusion
        - excessive amount of fluid Y63.Ø
        - incorrect dilution of fluid Y63.1
      - insulin-shock therapy Y63.4
      - nonadministration of necessary drug or biological substance Y63.6
      - overdose — *see* Table of Drugs and Chemicals
        - radiation, in therapy Y63.2
      - radiation
        - overdose Y63.2
      - specified procedure NEC Y63.8
      - transfusion
        - excessive amount of blood Y63.Ø
    - mechanical, of instrument or apparatus (any) (during any procedure) Y65.8
    - sterile precautions (during procedure) Y62.9
      - aspiration of fluid or tissue (by puncture or catheterization, except heart) Y62.6
      - biopsy (except needle aspiration) Y62.8
        - needle (aspirating) Y62.6
      - blood sampling Y62.6
      - catheterization Y62.6
        - heart Y62.5
      - dialysis (kidney) Y62.2
      - endoscopic examination Y62.4
      - enema Y62.8
      - immunization Y62.3
      - infusion Y62.1
      - injection Y62.3
      - needle biopsy Y62.6
      - paracentesis (abdominal) (thoracic) Y62.6
      - perfusion Y62.2
      - puncture (lumbar) Y62.6
      - removal of catheter or packing Y62.8
      - specified procedure NEC Y62.8
      - surgical operation Y62.Ø
      - transfusion Y62.1
      - vaccination Y62.3
    - suture or ligature during surgical procedure Y65.2
    - to introduce or to remove tube or instrument — *see* Failure, to
  - hemorrhage — *see* Index to Diseases and Injuries, Complication(s)
  - inadvertent exposure of patient to radiation Y63.3
  - inappropriate
    - operation performed — *see* Inappropriate operation performed
    - temperature (too hot or too cold) in local application or packing Y63.5
  - infusion — *see also* Misadventure, by type, infusion Y69
    - excessive amount of fluid Y63.Ø
    - incorrect dilution of fluid Y63.1
    - wrong fluid Y65.1

- **Misadventure**(s) **to patient**(s) **during surgical or medical care** — *continued*
  - mismatched blood in transfusion Y65.Ø
  - nonadministration of necessary drug or biological substance Y63.6
  - overdose — *see* Table of Drugs and Chemicals
    - radiation (in therapy) Y63.2
  - perforation — *see* Index to Diseases and Injuries, Complication(s)
  - performance of inappropriate operation — *see* Inappropriate operation performed
  - puncture — *see* Index to Diseases and Injuries, Complication(s)
  - specified type NEC Y65.8
    - failure
      - suture or ligature during surgical operation Y65.2
      - to introduce or to remove tube or instrument — *see* Failure, to
    - infusion of wrong fluid Y65.1
    - performance of inappropriate operation — *see* Inappropriate operation performed
    - transfusion of mismatched blood Y65.Ø
    - wrong
      - fluid in infusion Y65.1
      - placement of endotracheal tube during anesthetic procedure Y65.3
  - transfusion — *see* Misadventure, by type, transfusion
    - excessive amount of blood Y63.Ø
    - mismatched blood Y65.Ø
  - wrong
    - drug given in error — *see* Table of Drugs and Chemicals
    - fluid in infusion Y65.1
    - placement of endotracheal tube during anesthetic procedure Y65.3
- **Mismatched blood in transfusion** Y65.Ø
- **Motion sickness** T75.3 ☑
- **Mountain sickness** W94.11 ☑
- **Mudslide** (of cataclysmic nature) — *see* Landslide
- **Murder** (attempt) — *see* Assault

N

- **Nail**
  - contact with W45.Ø ☑
    - gun W29.4 ☑
  - embedded in skin W45.Ø ☑
- **Neglect** (criminal) (homicidal intent) X58 ☑
- **Noise** (causing injury) (pollution) W42.9 ☑
  - supersonic W42.Ø ☑
- **Nonadministration** (of)
  - drug or biological substance (necessary) Y63.6
  - surgical and medical care Y66
- **Nosocomial condition** Y95

O

- **Object**
  - falling
    - from, in, on, hitting
      - machinery — *see* Contact, with, by type of machine
    - set in motion by
      - accidental explosion or rupture of pressure vessel W38 ☑
      - firearm — *see* Discharge, firearm, by type
      - machine(ry) — *see* Contact, with, by type of machine
- **Overdose** (drug) — *see* Table of Drugs and Chemicals
  - radiation Y63.2
- **Overexertion** X5Ø.9 ☑
  - from
    - prolonged static or awkward postures X5Ø.1 ☑
    - repetitive movements X5Ø.3 ☑
    - specified strenuous movements or postures NEC X5Ø.9 ☑
    - strenuous movement or load X5Ø.Ø ☑
- **Overexposure** (accidental) (to)
  - cold — *see also* Exposure, cold X31 ☑
    - due to man-made conditions — *see* Exposure, cold, man-made
  - heat — *see also* Heat X3Ø ☑
  - radiation — *see* Radiation
  - radioactivity W88.Ø ☑
  - sun (sunburn) X32 ☑
  - weather NEC — *see* Forces of nature
  - wind NEC — *see* Forces of nature

Overheated — *see* Heat
Overturning (accidental)
  machinery — *see* Contact, with, by type of machine
  transport vehicle NEC — *see also* Accident, transport V89.9 ☑
  watercraft (causing drowning, submersion) — *see also* Drowning, due to, accident to, watercraft, overturning
    causing injury except drowning or submersion — *see* Accident, watercraft, causing, injury NEC

P

Parachute descent (voluntary) (without accident to aircraft) V97.29 ☑
  due to accident to aircraft — *see* Accident, transport, aircraft
Pecked by bird W61.99 ☑
Perforation during medical or surgical treatment as misadventure — *see* Index to Diseases and Injuries, Complication(s)
Perpetrator, perpetration, of assault, maltreatment and neglect (by) YØ7.9
  boyfriend YØ7.Ø3
  brother YØ7.41Ø
    stepbrother YØ7.435
  coach YØ7.53
  cousin
    female YØ7.491
    male YØ7.49Ø
  daycare provider YØ7.519
    at-home
      adult care YØ7.512
      childcare YØ7.51Ø
    care center
      adult care YØ7.513
      childcare YØ7.511
  family member NEC YØ7.499
  father YØ7.11
    adoptive YØ7.13
    foster YØ7.42Ø
    stepfather YØ7.43Ø
  foster father YØ7.42Ø
  foster mother YØ7.421
  girl friend YØ7.Ø4
  healthcare provider YØ7.529
    mental health YØ7.521
    specified NEC YØ7.528
  husband YØ7.Ø1
  instructor YØ7.53
  mother YØ7.12
    adoptive YØ7.14
    foster YØ7.421
    stepmother YØ7.433
  multiple perpetrators YØ7.6
  nonfamily member YØ7.5Ø
    specified NEC YØ7.59
  nurse YØ7.528
  occupational therapist YØ7.528
  partner of parent
    female YØ7.434
    male YØ7.432
  physical therapist YØ7.528
  sister YØ7.411
  speech therapist YØ7.528
  stepbrother YØ7.435
  stepfather YØ7.43Ø
  stepmother YØ7.433
  stepsister YØ7.436
  teacher YØ7.53
  wife YØ7.Ø2
Piercing — *see* Contact, with, by type of object or machine
Pinched
  between objects (moving) (stationary and moving) W23.Ø ☑
    stationary W23.1 ☑
Pinned under machine(ry) — *see* Contact, with, by type of machine
Place of occurrence Y92.9
  abandoned house Y92.89
  airplane Y92.813
  airport Y92.52Ø
  ambulatory health services establishment NEC Y92.538
  ambulatory surgery center Y92.53Ø
  amusement park Y92.831
  apartment (co-op) — *see* Place of occurrence, residence, apartment

Place of occurrence — *continued*
  assembly hall Y92.29
  bank Y92.51Ø
  barn Y92.71
  baseball field Y92.32Ø
  basketball court Y92.31Ø
  beach Y92.832
  boarding house — *see* Place of occurrence, residence, boarding house
  boat Y92.814
  bowling alley Y92.39
  bridge Y92.89
  building under construction Y92.61
  bus Y92.811
    station Y92.521
  cafe Y92.511
  campsite Y92.833
  campus — *see* Place of occurrence, school
  canal Y92.89
  car Y92.81Ø
  casino Y92.59
  children's home — *see* Place of occurrence, residence, institutional, orphanage
  church Y92.22
  cinema Y92.26
  clubhouse Y92.29
  coal pit Y92.64
  college (community) Y92.214
  condominium — *see* Place of occurrence, residence, apartment
  construction area — *see* Place of occurrence, industrial and construction area
  convalescent home — *see* Place of occurrence, residence, institutional, nursing home
  court-house Y92.24Ø
  cricket ground Y92.328
  cultural building Y92.258
    art gallery Y92.25Ø
    museum Y92.251
    music hall Y92.252
    opera house Y92.253
    specified NEC Y92.258
    theater Y92.254
  dancehall Y92.252
  day nursery Y92.21Ø
  dentist office Y92.531
  derelict house Y92.89
  desert Y92.82Ø
  dockyard Y92.62
  dock NOS Y92.89
  doctor's office Y92.531
  dormitory — *see* Place of occurrence, residence, institutional, school dormitory
  dry dock Y92.62
  factory (building) (premises) Y92.63
  farm (land under cultivation) (outbuildings) Y92.79
    barn Y92.71
    chicken coop Y92.72
    field Y92.73
    hen house Y92.72
    house — *see* Place of occurrence, residence, house
    orchard Y92.74
    specified NEC Y92.79
  football field Y92.321
  forest Y92.821
  freeway Y92.411
  gallery Y92.25Ø
  garage (commercial) Y92.59
    boarding house Y92.Ø44
    military base Y92.135
    mobile home Y92.Ø25
    nursing home Y92.124
    orphanage Y92.114
    private house Y92.Ø15
    reform school Y92.155
  gas station Y92.524
  gasworks Y92.69
  golf course Y92.39
  gravel pit Y92.64
  grocery Y92.512
  gymnasium Y92.39
  handball court Y92.318
  harbor Y92.89
  harness racing course Y92.39
  healthcare provider office Y92.531
  highway Y92.41Ø
    interstate Y92.411
  hill Y92.828

Place of occurrence — *continued*
  hockey rink Y92.33Ø
  home — *see* Place of occurrence, residence
  hospice — *see* Place of occurrence, residence, institutional, nursing home
  hospital Y92.239
    cafeteria Y92.233
    corridor Y92.232
    operating room Y92.234
    patient
      bathroom Y92.231
      room Y92.23Ø
    specified NEC Y92.238
  hotel Y92.59
  house — *see also* Place of occurrence, residence
    abandoned Y92.89
    under construction Y92.61
  industrial and construction area (yard) Y92.69
    building under construction Y92.61
    dock Y92.62
    dry dock Y92.62
    factory Y92.63
    gasworks Y92.69
    mine Y92.64
    oil rig Y92.65
    pit Y92.64
    power station Y92.69
    shipyard Y92.62
    specified NEC Y92.69
    tunnel under construction Y92.69
    workshop Y92.69
  interstate Y92.411
  kindergarten Y92.211
  lacrosse field Y92.328
  lake Y92.838
    wilderness Y92.828
  library Y92.241
  mall Y92.59
  market Y92.512
  marsh Y92.828
  military
    base — *see* Place of occurrence, residence, institutional, military base
    training ground Y92.84
  mine Y92.64
  mosque Y92.22
  motel Y92.59
  motorway (interstate) Y92.411
  mountain Y92.828
  movie-house Y92.26
  museum Y92.251
  music-hall Y92.252
  not applicable Y92.9
  nuclear power station Y92.69
  nursing home — *see* Place of occurrence, residence, institutional, nursing home
  office building Y92.59
  offshore installation Y92.65
  oil rig Y92.65
  old people's home — *see* Place of occurrence, residence, institutional, specified NEC
  opera-house Y92.253
  orphanage — *see* Place of occurrence, residence, institutional, orphanage
  outpatient surgery center Y92.53Ø
  park (public) Y92.83Ø
    amusement Y92.831
  parking garage Y92.89
    lot Y92.481
  pavement Y92.48Ø
  physician office Y92.531
  polo field Y92.328
  pond Y92.828
  post office Y92.242
  power station Y92.69
  prairie Y92.828
  prison — *see* Place of occurrence, residence, institutional, prison
  public
    administration building Y92.248
      city hall Y92.243
      courthouse Y92.24Ø
      library Y92.241
      post office Y92.242
      specified NEC Y92.248
    building NEC Y92.29
    hall Y92.29
    place NOS Y92.89

Place of occurrence — *continued*
race course Y92.39
radio station Y92.59
railway line (bridge) Y92.85
ranch (outbuildings) — *see* Place of occurrence, farm
recreation area Y92.838
amusement park Y92.831
beach Y92.832
campsite Y92.833
park (public) Y92.830
seashore Y92.832
specified NEC Y92.838
reform school - — *see* Place of occurrence, residence, institutional, reform school
religious institution Y92.22
residence (non-institutional) (private) Y92.009
apartment Y92.039
bathroom Y92.031
bedroom Y92.032
kitchen Y92.030
specified NEC Y92.038
bathroom Y92.002
bedroom Y92.003
boarding house Y92.049
bathroom Y92.041
bedroom Y92.042
driveway Y92.043
garage Y92.044
garden Y92.046
kitchen Y92.040
specified NEC Y92.048
swimming pool Y92.045
yard Y92.046
dining room Y92.001
garden Y92.007
home Y92.009
house, single family Y92.019
bathroom Y92.012
bedroom Y92.013
dining room Y92.011
driveway Y92.014
garage Y92.015
garden Y92.017
kitchen Y92.010
specified NEC Y92.018
swimming pool Y92.016
yard Y92.017
institutional Y92.10
children's home — *see* Place of occurrence, residence, institutional, orphanage
hospice — *see* Place of occurrence, residence, institutional, nursing home
military base Y92.139
barracks Y92.133
garage Y92.135
garden Y92.137
kitchen Y92.130
mess hall Y92.131
specified NEC Y92.138
swimming pool Y92.136
yard Y92.137
nursing home Y92.129
bathroom Y92.121
bedroom Y92.122
driveway Y92.123
garage Y92.124
garden Y92.126
kitchen Y92.120
specified NEC Y92.128
swimming pool Y92.125
yard Y92.126
orphanage Y92.119
bathroom Y92.111
bedroom Y92.112
driveway Y92.113
garage Y92.114
garden Y92.116
kitchen Y92.110
specified NEC Y92.118
swimming pool Y92.115
yard Y92.116
prison Y92.149
bathroom Y92.142
cell Y92.143
courtyard Y92.147
dining room Y92.141
kitchen Y92.140
specified NEC Y92.148
swimming pool Y92.146

Place of occurrence — *continued*
residence — *continued*
institutional — *continued*
reform school Y92.159
bathroom Y92.152
bedroom Y92.153
dining room Y92.151
driveway Y92.154
garage Y92.155
garden Y92.157
kitchen Y92.150
specified NEC Y92.158
swimming pool Y92.156
yard Y92.157
school dormitory Y92.169
bathroom Y92.162
bedroom Y92.163
dining room Y92.161
kitchen Y92.160
specified NEC Y92.168
specified NEC Y92.199
bathroom Y92.192
bedroom Y92.193
dining room Y92.191
driveway Y92.194
garage Y92.195
garden Y92.197
kitchen Y92.190
specified NEC Y92.198
swimming pool Y92.196
yard Y92.197
kitchen Y92.000
mobile home Y92.029
bathroom Y92.022
bedroom Y92.023
dining room Y92.021
driveway Y92.024
garage Y92.025
garden Y92.027
kitchen Y92.020
specified NEC Y92.028
swimming pool Y92.026
yard Y92.027
specified place in residence NEC Y92.008
specified residence type NEC Y92.099
bathroom Y92.091
bedroom Y92.092
driveway Y92.093
garage Y92.094
garden Y92.096
kitchen Y92.090
specified NEC Y92.098
swimming pool Y92.095
yard Y92.096
restaurant Y92.511
riding school Y92.39
river Y92.828
road Y92.410
rodeo ring Y92.39
rugby field Y92.328
same day surgery center Y92.530
sand pit Y92.64
school (private) (public) (state) Y92.219
college Y92.214
daycare center Y92.210
elementary school Y92.211
high school Y92.213
kindergarten Y92.211
middle school Y92.212
specified NEC Y92.218
trace school Y92.215
university Y92.214
vocational school Y92.215
sea (shore) Y92.832
senior citizen center Y92.29
service area
airport Y92.520
bus station Y92.521
gas station Y92.524
highway rest stop Y92.523
railway station Y92.522
shipyard Y92.62
shop (commercial) Y92.513
sidewalk Y92.480
silo Y92.79
skating rink (roller) Y92.331
ice Y92.330
slaughter house Y92.86
soccer field Y92.322

Place of occurrence — *continued*
specified place NEC Y92.89
sports area Y92.39
athletic
court Y92.318
basketball Y92.310
specified NEC Y92.318
squash Y92.311
tennis Y92.312
field Y92.328
baseball Y92.320
cricket ground Y92.328
football Y92.321
hockey Y92.328
soccer Y92.322
specified NEC Y92.328
golf course Y92.39
gymnasium Y92.39
riding school Y92.39
skating rink (roller) Y92.331
ice Y92.330
stadium Y92.39
swimming pool Y92.34
squash court Y92.311
stadium Y92.39
steeplechasing course Y92.39
store Y92.512
stream Y92.828
street and highway Y92.410
bike path Y92.482
freeway Y92.411
highway ramp Y92.415
interstate highway Y92.411
local residential or business street Y92.414
motorway Y92.411
parking lot Y92.481
parkway Y92.412
sidewalk Y92.480
specified NEC Y92.488
state road Y92.413
subway car Y92.816
supermarket Y92.512
swamp Y92.828
swimming pool (public) Y92.34
private (at) Y92.095
boarding house Y92.045
military base Y92.136
mobile home Y92.026
nursing home Y92.125
orphanage Y92.115
prison Y92.146
reform school Y92.156
single family residence Y92.016
synagogue Y92.22
television station Y92.59
tennis court Y92.312
theater Y92.254
trade area Y92.59
bank Y92.510
cafe Y92.511
casino Y92.59
garage Y92.59
hotel Y92.59
market Y92.512
office building Y92.59
radio station Y92.59
restaurant Y92.511
shop Y92.513
shopping mall Y92.59
store Y92.512
supermarket Y92.512
television station Y92.59
warehouse Y92.59
trailer park, residential — *see* Place of occurrence, residence, mobile home
trailer site NOS Y92.89
train Y92.815
station Y92.522
truck Y92.812
tunnel under construction Y92.69
university Y92.214
urgent (health) care center Y92.532
vehicle (transport) Y92.818
airplane Y92.813
boat Y92.814
bus Y92.811
car Y92.810
specified NEC Y92.818
subway car Y92.816

Place of occurrence — *continued*
- vehicle — *continued*
  - train Y92.815
  - truck Y92.812
- warehouse Y92.59
- water reservoir Y92.89
- wilderness area Y92.828
  - desert Y92.82Ø
  - forest Y92.821
  - marsh Y92.828
  - mountain Y92.828
  - prairie Y92.828
  - specified NEC Y92.828
  - swamp Y92.828
- workshop Y92.69
- yard, private Y92.Ø96
  - boarding house Y92.Ø46
  - mobile home Y92.Ø27
  - single family house Y92.Ø17
- youth center Y92.29
- zoo (zoological garden) Y92.834

Plumbism — *see* Table of Drugs and Chemicals, lead

Poisoning (accidental) (by) — *see also* Table of Drugs and Chemicals
- by plant, thorns, spines, sharp leaves or other mechanisms NEC X58 ☑
- carbon monoxide
  - generated by
    - motor vehicle — *see* Accident, transport
    - watercraft (in transit) (not in transit) V93.89 ☑
      - ferry boat V93.81 ☑
      - fishing boat V93.82 ☑
      - jet skis V93.83 ☑
      - liner V93.81 ☑
      - merchant ship V93.8Ø ☑
      - passenger ship V93.81 ☑
      - powered craft NEC V93.83 ☑
- caused by injection of poisons into skin by plant thorns, spines, sharp leaves X58 ☑
  - marine or sea plants (venomous) X58 ☑
- execution — *see* Legal, intervention, gas
  - intervention
    - by gas — *see* Legal, intervention, gas
    - other specified means — *see* Legal, intervention, specified means NEC
- exhaust gas
  - generated by
    - motor vehicle — *see* Accident, transport
    - watercraft (in transit) (not in transit) V93.89 ☑
      - ferry boat V93.81 ☑
      - fishing boat V93.82 ☑
      - jet skis V93.83 ☑
      - liner V93.81 ☑
      - merchant ship V93.8Ø ☑
      - passenger ship V93.81 ☑
      - powered craft NEC V93.83 ☑
- fumes or smoke due to
  - explosion — *see also* Explosion W4Ø.9 ☑
  - fire — *see* Exposure, fire
  - ignition — *see* Ignition
- gas
  - in legal intervention — *see* Legal, intervention, gas
  - legal execution — *see* Legal, intervention, gas
- in war operations — *see* War operations
- legal

Powder burn (by) (from)
- airgun W34.11Ø ☑
- BB gun W34.11Ø ☑
- firearn NEC W34.19 ☑
- gas, air or spring-operated gun NEC W34.118 ☑
- handgun W32.1 ☑
- hunting rifle W33.12 ☑
- larger firearm W33.1Ø ☑
  - specified NEC W33.19 ☑
- machine gun W33.13 ☑
- paintball gun W34.111 ☑
- pellet gun W34.11Ø ☑
- shotgun W33.11 ☑
- Very pistol [flare] W34.19 ☑

Premature cessation (of) **surgical and medical care** Y66

Privation (food) (water) X58 ☑

Procedure (operation)
- correct, on wrong side or body part (wrong side) (wrong site) Y65.53
- intended for another patient done on wrong patient Y65.52

Procedure — *continued*
- performed on patient not scheduled for surgery Y65.52
- performed on wrong patient Y65.52
- wrong, performed on correct patient Y65.51

Prolonged
- sitting in transport vehicle — *see* Travel, by type of vehicle
- stay in
  - high altitude as cause of anoxia, barodontalgia, barotitis or hypoxia W94.11 ☑
  - weightless environment X52 ☑

Pulling, excessive — *see also* Overexertion X5Ø.9- ☑

Puncture, puncturing — *see also* Contact, with, by type of object or machine
- by
  - plant thorns, spines, sharp leaves or other mechanisms NEC W6Ø ☑
- during medical or surgical treatment as misadventure — *see* Index to Diseases and Injuries, Complication(s)

Pushed, pushing (accidental) (injury in)
- by other person(s) (accidental) W51 ☑
  - as, or caused by, a crowd or human stampede (with fall) W52 ☑
  - before moving object NEC YØ2.8 ☑
    - motor vehicle YØ2.Ø ☑
    - subway train YØ2.1 ☑
    - train YØ2.1 ☑
  - from
    - high place NEC
      - in accidental circumstances W17.89 ☑
      - stated as
        - intentional, homicide (attempt) YØ1 ☑
        - undetermined whether accidental or intentional Y3Ø ☑
    - transport vehicle NEC — *see also* Accident, transport V89.9 ☑
      - stated as
        - intentional, homicide (attempt) YØ8.89 ☑
  - with fall WØ3 ☑
    - due to ice or snow WØØ.Ø ☑
- overexertion X5Ø.9 ☑

R

Radiation (exposure to)
- arc lamps W89.Ø ☑
- atomic power plant (malfunction) NEC W88.1 ☑
- complication of or abnormal reaction to medical radiotherapy Y84.2
- electromagnetic, ionizing W88.Ø ☑
- gamma rays W88.1 ☑
- in
  - war operations (from or following nuclear explosion) — *see* War operations
- inadvertent exposure of patient (receiving test or therapy) Y63.3
- infrared (heaters and lamps) W9Ø.1 ☑
  - excessive heat from W92 ☑
- ionized, ionizing (particles, artificially accelerated)
  - radioisotopes W88.1 ☑
  - specified NEC W88.8 ☑
  - x-rays W88.Ø ☑
- isotopes, radioactive — *see* Radiation, radioactive isotopes
- laser(s) W9Ø.2 ☑
  - in war operations — *see* War operations
  - misadventure in medical care Y63.2
- light sources (man-made visible and ultraviolet) W89.9 ☑
  - natural X32 ☑
  - specified NEC W89.8 ☑
  - tanning bed W89.1 ☑
  - welding light W89.Ø ☑
- man-made visible light W89.9 ☑
  - specified NEC W89.8 ☑
  - tanning bed W89.1 ☑
  - welding light W89.Ø ☑
- microwave W9Ø.8 ☑
- misadventure in medical or surgical procedure Y63.2
- natural NEC X39.Ø8 ☑
  - radon X39.Ø1 ☑
- overdose (in medical or surgical procedure) Y63.2
- radar W9Ø.Ø ☑
- radioactive isotopes (any) W88.1 ☑
  - atomic power plant malfunction W88.1 ☑
  - misadventure in medical or surgical treatment Y63.2

Radiation — *continued*
- radiofrequency W9Ø.Ø ☑
- radium NEC W88.1 ☑
- sun X32 ☑
- ultraviolet (light) (man-made) W89.9 ☑
  - natural X32 ☑
  - specified NEC W89.8 ☑
  - tanning bed W89.1 ☑
  - welding light W89.Ø ☑
- welding arc, torch, or light W89.Ø ☑
  - excessive heat from W92 ☑
- x-rays (hard) (soft) W88.Ø ☑

Range disease W94.11 ☑

Rape (attempted) T74.2- ☑

Rat bite W53.11 ☑

Reaching (prolonged) (static) X5Ø.1 ☑

Reaction, abnormal to medical procedure — *see also* Complication of or following, by type of procedure Y84.9
- biologicals — *see* Table of Drugs and Chemicals
- drugs — *see* Table of Drugs and Chemicals
- vaccine — *see* Table of Drugs and Chemicals
- with misadventure — *see* Misadventure

Recoil
- airgun W34.11Ø ☑
- BB gun W34.11Ø ☑
- firearn NEC W34.19 ☑
- gas, air or spring-operated gun NEC W34.118 ☑
- handgun W32.1 ☑
- hunting rifle W33.12 ☑
- larger firearm W33.1Ø ☑
  - specified NEC W33.19 ☑
- machine gun W33.13 ☑
- paintball gun W34.111 ☑
- pellet W34.11Ø ☑
- shotgun W33.11 ☑
- Very pistol [flare] W34.19 ☑

Reduction in
- atmospheric pressure — *see* Air, pressure, change

Rock falling on or hitting (accidentally) (person) W2Ø.8 ☑
- in cave-in W2Ø.Ø ☑

Run over (accidentally) (by)
- animal (not being ridden) NEC W55.89 ☑
- machinery — *see* Contact, with, by specified type of machine
- transport vehicle NEC — *see also* Accident, transport VØ9.9 ☑
  - intentional homicide (attempt) YØ3.Ø ☑
  - motor NEC VØ9.2Ø ☑
    - intentional homicide (attempt) YØ3.Ø ☑

Running
- before moving object X81.8 ☑
  - motor vehicle X81.Ø ☑

Running off, away
- animal (being ridden) — *see also* Accident, transport V8Ø.918 ☑
  - not being ridden W55.89 ☑
- animal-drawn vehicle NEC — *see also* Accident, transport V8Ø.928 ☑
- highway, road(way), street
  - transport vehicle NEC — *see also* Accident, transport V89.9 ☑

Rupture pressurized devices — *see* Explosion, by type of device

S

Saturnism — *see* Table of Drugs and Chemicals, lead

Scald, scalding (accidental) (by) (from) (in) X19 ☑
- air (hot) X14.1 ☑
- gases (hot) X14.1 ☑
- homicide (attempt) — *see* Assault, burning, hot object
- inflicted by other person
  - stated as intentional, homicide (attempt) — *see* Assault, burning, hot object
- liquid (boiling) (hot) NEC X12 ☑
  - stated as undetermined whether accidental or intentional Y27.2 ☑
  - suicide (attempt) X77.2 ☑
- local application of externally applied substance in medical or surgical care Y63.5
- metal (molten) (liquid) (hot) NEC X18 ☑
- self-inflicted X77.9 ☑
- stated as undetermined whether accidental or intentional Y27.8 ☑

- **Scald, scalding** — *continued*
  - steam X13.1 ☑
    - assault X98.Ø ☑
    - stated as undetermined whether accidental or intentional Y27.Ø ☑
    - suicide (attempt) X77.Ø ☑
  - suicide (attempt) X77.9 ☑
  - vapor (hot) X13.1 ☑
    - assault X98.Ø ☑
    - stated as undetermined whether accidental or intentional Y27.Ø ☑
    - suicide (attempt) X77.Ø ☑
- **Scratched by**
  - cat W55.Ø3 ☑
  - person(s) (accidentally) W5Ø.4 ☑
    - with intent to injure or kill YØ4.Ø ☑
    - as, or caused by, a crowd or human stampede (with fall) W52 ☑
    - assault YØ4.Ø ☑
    - homicide (attempt) YØ4.Ø ☑
    - in
      - fight YØ4.Ø ☑
      - legal intervention
        - injuring
          - bystander Y35.892 ☑
          - law enforcement personnel Y35.891 ☑
          - suspect Y35.893 ☑
          - unspecified person Y35.899 ☑
- **Seasickness** T75.3 ☑
- **Self-harm NEC** — *see also* External cause by type, undetermined whether accidental or intentional
  - intentional — *see* Suicide
  - poisoning NEC — *see* Table of Drugs and Chemicals, poisoning, accidental
- **Self-inflicted** (injury) **NEC** — *see also* External cause by type, undetermined whether accidental or intentional
  - intentional — *see* Suicide
  - poisoning NEC — *see* Table of Drugs and Chemicals, poisoning, accidental
- **Sequelae** (of)
  - accident NEC — *see* WØØ-X58 with 7th character S
  - assault (homicidal) (any means) — *see* X92-YØ8 with 7th character S
  - homicide, attempt (any means) — *see* X92-YØ8 with 7th character S
  - injury undetermined whether accidentally or purposely inflicted — *see* Y21-Y33 with 7th character S
  - intentional self-harm (classifiable to X71-X83) — *see* X71-X83 with 7th character S
  - legal intervention — *see* with 7th character S Y35 ☑
  - motor vehicle accident — *see* VØØ-V99 with 7th character S
  - suicide, attempt (any means) — *see* X71-X83 with 7th character S
  - transport accident — *see* VØØ-V99 with 7th character S
  - war operations — *see* War operations
- **Shock**
  - electric — *see* Exposure, electric current
  - from electric appliance (any) (faulty) W86.8 ☑
    - domestic W86.Ø ☑
    - suicide (attempt) X83.1 ☑
- **Shooting, shot** (accidental(ly)) — *see also* Discharge, firearm, by type
  - herself or himself — *see* Discharge, firearm by type, self-inflicted
  - homicide (attempt) — *see* Discharge, firearm by type, homicide
  - in war operations — *see* War operations
  - inflicted by other person — *see* Discharge, firearm by type, homicide
    - accidental — *see* Discharge, firearm, by type of firearm
  - legal
    - execution — *see* Legal, intervention, firearm
    - intervention — *see* Legal, intervention, firearm
  - self-inflicted — *see* Discharge, firearm by type, suicide
    - accidental — *see* Discharge, firearm, by type of firearm
  - suicide (attempt) — *see* Discharge, firearm by type, suicide
- **Shoving** (accidentally) **by other person** — *see* Pushed, by other person
- **Sickness**
  - alpine W94.11 ☑
  - motion — *see* Motion
- **Sickness** — *continued*
  - mountain W94.11 ☑
- **Sinking** (accidental)
  - watercraft (causing drowning, submersion) — *see also* Drowning, due to, accident to, watercraft, sinking
    - causing injury except drowning or submersion — *see* Accident, watercraft, causing, injury NEC
- **Siriasis** X32 ☑
- **Sitting** (prolonged) (static) X5Ø.1 ☑
- **Slashed wrists** — *see* Cut, self-inflicted
- **Slipping** (accidental) (on same level) (with fall) WØ1.Ø ☑
  - on
    - ice WØØ.Ø ☑
      - with skates — *see* Accident, transport, pedestrian, conveyance
    - mud WØ1.Ø ☑
    - oil WØ1.Ø ☑
    - snow WØØ.Ø ☑
      - with skis — *see* Accident, transport, pedestrian, conveyance
    - surface (slippery) (wet) NEC WØ1.Ø ☑
  - without fall W18.4Ø ☑
    - due to
      - specified NEC W18.49 ☑
      - stepping from one level to another W18.43 ☑
      - stepping into hole or opening W18.42 ☑
      - stepping on object W18.41 ☑
- **Sliver, wood, contact with** W45.8 ☑
- **Smoldering** (due to fire) — *see* Exposure, fire
- **Sodomy** (attempted) **by force** T74.2 ☑
- **Sound waves** (causing injury) W42.9 ☑
  - supersonic W42.Ø ☑
- **Splinter, contact with** W45.8 ☑
- **Stab, stabbing** — *see* Cut
- **Standing** (prolonged) (static) X5Ø.1 ☑
- **Starvation** X58 ☑
- **Status of external cause** Y99.9
  - child assisting in compensated work for family Y99.8
  - civilian activity done for financial or other compensation Y99.Ø
  - civilian activity done for income or pay Y99.Ø
  - family member assisting in compensated work for other family member Y99.8
  - hobby not done for income Y99.8
  - leisure activity Y99.8
  - military activity Y99.1
  - off-duty activity of military personnel Y99.8
  - recreation or sport not for income or while a student Y99.8
  - specified NEC Y99.8
  - student activity Y99.8
  - volunteer activity Y99.2
- **Stepped on**
  - by
    - animal (not being ridden) NEC W55.89 ☑
    - crowd or human stampede W52 ☑
    - person W5Ø.Ø ☑
- **Stepping on**
  - object W22.8 ☑
    - sports equipment W21.9 ☑
    - stationary W22.Ø9 ☑
      - sports equipment W21.89 ☑
    - with fall W18.31 ☑
  - person W51 ☑
    - by crowd or human stampede W52 ☑
  - sports equipment W21.9 ☑
- **Sting**
  - arthropod, nonvenomous W57 ☑
  - insect, nonvenomous W57 ☑
- **Storm** (cataclysmic) — *see* Forces of nature, cataclysmic storm
- **Straining, excessive** — *see also* Overexertion X5Ø.9 ☑
- **Strangling** — *see* Strangulation
- **Strangulation** (accidental) T71 ☑
- **Strenuous movements** — *see also* Overexertion X5Ø.9 ☑
- **Striking against**
  - airbag (automobile) W22.1Ø ☑
    - driver side W22.11 ☑
    - front passenger side W22.12 ☑
    - specified NEC W22.19 ☑
  - bottom when
    - diving or jumping into water (in) W16.822 ☑
      - causing drowning W16.821 ☑
      - from boat W16.722 ☑
        - causing drowning W16.721 ☑
- **Striking against** — *continued*
  - bottom when — *continued*
    - diving or jumping into water — *continued*
      - natural body W16.622 ☑
        - causing drowning W16.821 ☑
      - swimming pool W16.522 ☑
        - causing drowning W16.521 ☑
    - falling into water (in) W16.322 ☑
      - causing drowning W16.321 ☑
      - fountain — *see* Striking against, bottom when, falling into water, specified NEC
      - natural body W16.122 ☑
        - causing drowning W16.121 ☑
      - reservoir — *see* Striking against, bottom when, falling into water, specified NEC
      - specified NEC W16.322 ☑
        - causing drowning W16.321 ☑
      - swimming pool W16.Ø22 ☑
        - causing drowning W16.Ø21 ☑
  - diving board (swimming-pool) W21.4 ☑
  - object W22.8 ☑
    - caused by crowd or human stampede (with fall) W52 ☑
    - furniture W22.Ø3 ☑
    - lamppost W22.Ø2 ☑
    - sports equipment W21.9 ☑
    - stationary W22.Ø9 ☑
      - sports equipment W21.89 ☑
    - wall W22.Ø1 ☑
    - with
      - drowning or submersion — *see* Drowning
      - fall — *see* Fall, due to, bumping against, object
  - person(s) W51 ☑
    - as, or caused by, a crowd or human stampede (with fall) W52 ☑
    - assault YØ4.2 ☑
    - homicide (attempt) YØ4.2 ☑
    - with fall WØ3 ☑
      - due to ice or snow WØØ.Ø ☑
  - sports equipment W21.9 ☑
  - wall (when) W22.Ø1 ☑
    - diving or jumping into water (in) W16.832 ☑
      - causing drowning W16.831 ☑
      - swimming pool W16.532 ☑
        - causing drowning W16.531 ☑
    - falling into water (in) W16.332 ☑
      - causing drowning W16.331 ☑
      - fountain — *see* Striking against, wall when, falling into water, specified NEC
      - natural body W16.132 ☑
        - causing drowning W16.131 ☑
      - reservoir — *see* Striking against, wall when, falling into water, specified NEC
      - specified NEC W16.332 ☑
        - causing drowning W16.331 ☑
      - swimming pool W16.Ø32 ☑
        - causing drowning W16.Ø31 ☑
    - swimming pool (when) W22.Ø42 ☑
      - causing drowning W22.Ø41 ☑
      - diving or jumping into water W16.532 ☑
        - causing drowning W16.531 ☑
      - falling into water W16.Ø32 ☑
        - causing drowning W16.Ø31 ☑
- **Struck** (accidentally) **by**
  - airbag (automobile) W22.1Ø ☑
    - driver side W22.11 ☑
    - front passenger side W22.12 ☑
    - specified NEC W22.19 ☑
  - alligator W58.Ø2 ☑
  - animal (not being ridden) NEC W55.89 ☑
  - avalanche — *see* Landslide
  - ball (hit) (thrown) W21.ØØ ☑
    - assault YØ8.Ø9 ☑
    - baseball W21.Ø3 ☑
    - basketball W21.Ø5 ☑
    - football W21.Ø1 ☑
    - golf ball W21.Ø4 ☑
    - soccer W21.Ø2 ☑
    - softball W21.Ø7 ☑
    - specified NEC W21.Ø9 ☑
    - volleyball W21.Ø6 ☑
  - bat or racquet
    - baseball bat W21.11 ☑
      - assault YØ8.Ø2 ☑
    - golf club W21.13 ☑
      - assault YØ8.Ø9 ☑

External Causes Index

Scald, scalding — Struck

- **Struck** (accidentally) **by** — *continued*
  - bat or racquet — *continued*
    - specified NEC W21.19 ☑
      - assault Y08.09 ☑
    - tennis racquet W21.12 ☑
      - assault Y08.09 ☑
  - bullet — *see also* Discharge, firearm by type
    - in war operations — *see* War operations
  - crocodile W58.12 ☑
  - dog W54.1 ☑
  - flare, Very pistol — *see* Discharge, firearm NEC
  - hailstones X39.8 ☑
  - hockey (ice)
    - field
      - puck W21.221 ☑
      - stick W21.211 ☑
    - puck W21.220 ☑
    - stick W21.210 ☑
      - assault Y08.01 ☑
  - landslide — *see* Landslide
  - law-enforcement agent (on duty) — *see* Legal, intervention, manhandling
    - with blunt object — *see* Legal, intervention, blunt object
  - lightning T75.0 ☑
    - causing fire — *see* Exposure, fire
  - machine — *see* Contact, with, by type of machine
  - mammal NEC W55.89 ☑
    - marine W56.32 ☑
  - marine animal W56.82 ☑
  - missile
    - firearm — *see* Discharge, firearm by type
    - in war operations — *see* War operations, missile
  - object W22.8 ☑
    - blunt W22.8 ☑
      - assault Y00 ☑
      - suicide (attempt) X79 ☑
      - undetermined whether accidental or intentional Y29 ☑
    - falling W20.8 ☑
      - from, in, on
        - building W20.1 ☑
          - burning (uncontrolled fire) X00.4 ☑
        - cataclysmic
          - earth surface movement NEC — *see* Landslide
          - storm — *see* Forces of nature, cataclysmic storm
        - cave-in W20.0 ☑
        - earthquake X34 ☑
        - machine (in operation) — *see* Contact, with, by type of machine
        - structure W20.1 ☑
          - burning X00.4 ☑
        - transport vehicle (in motion) — *see* Accident, transport, by type of vehicle
        - watercraft V93.49 ☑
          - due to
            - accident to craft V91.39 ☑
              - powered craft V91.33 ☑
                - ferry boat V91.31 ☑
                - fishing boat V91.32 ☑
                - jetskis V91.33 ☑
                - liner V91.31 ☑
                - merchant ship V91.30 ☑
                - passenger ship V91.31 ☑
              - unpowered craft V91.38 ☑
                - canoe V91.35 ☑
                - inflatable V91.36 ☑
                - kayak V91.35 ☑
                - sailboat V91.34 ☑
                - surf-board V91.38 ☑
                - windsurfer V91.38 ☑
          - powered craft V93.43 ☑
            - ferry boat V93.41 ☑
            - fishing boat V93.42 ☑
            - jetskis V93.43 ☑
            - liner V93.41 ☑
            - merchant ship V93.40 ☑
            - passenger ship V93.41 ☑
          - unpowered craft V93.48 ☑
            - sailboat V93.44 ☑
            - surf-board V93.48 ☑
            - windsurfer V93.48 ☑
    - moving NEC W20.8 ☑
    - projected W20.8 ☑

- **Struck** (accidentally) **by** — *continued*
  - object — *continued*
    - projected — *continued*
      - assault Y00 ☑
      - in sports W21.9 ☑
        - assault Y08.09 ☑
        - ball W21.00 ☑
          - baseball W21.03 ☑
          - basketball W21.05 ☑
          - football W21.01 ☑
          - golf ball W21.04 ☑
          - soccer W21.02 ☑
          - softball W21.07 ☑
          - specified NEC W21.09 ☑
          - volleyball W21.06 ☑
        - bat or racquet
          - baseball bat W21.11 ☑
            - assault Y08.02 ☑
          - golf club W21.13 ☑
            - assault Y08.09 ☑
          - specified NEC W21.19 ☑
            - assault Y08.09 ☑
          - tennis racquet W21.12 ☑
            - assault Y08.09 ☑
        - hockey (ice)
          - field
            - puck W21.221 ☑
            - stick W21.211 ☑
          - puck W21.220 ☑
          - stick W21.210 ☑
            - assault Y08.01 ☑
        - specified NEC W21.89 ☑
    - set in motion by explosion — *see* Explosion
    - thrown W20.8 ☑
      - assault Y00 ☑
      - in sports W21.9 ☑
        - assault Y08.09 ☑
        - ball W21.00 ☑
          - baseball W21.03 ☑
          - basketball W21.05 ☑
          - football W21.01 ☑
          - golf ball W21.04 ☑
          - soccer W21.02 ☑
          - soft ball W21.07 ☑
          - specified NEC W21.09 ☑
          - volleyball W21.06 ☑
        - bat or racquet
          - baseball bat W21.11 ☑
            - assault Y08.02 ☑
          - golf club W21.13 ☑
            - assault Y08.09 ☑
          - specified NEC W21.19 ☑
            - assault Y08.09 ☑
          - tennis racquet W21.12 ☑
            - assault Y08.09 ☑
        - hockey (ice)
          - field
            - puck W21.221 ☑
            - stick W21.211 ☑
          - puck W21.220 ☑
          - stick W21.210 ☑
            - assault Y08.01 ☑
        - specified NEC W21.89 ☑
  - other person(s) W50.0 ☑
    - with
      - blunt object W22.8 ☑
        - intentional, homicide (attempt) Y00 ☑
        - sports equipment W21.9 ☑
        - undetermined whether accidental or intentional Y29 ☑
      - fall W03 ☑
        - due to ice or snow W00.0 ☑
    - as, or caused by, a crowd or human stampede (with fall) W52 ☑
    - assault Y04.2 ☑
    - homicide (attempt) Y04.2 ☑
    - in legal intervention
      - injuring
        - bystander Y35.812 ☑
        - law enforcement personnel Y35.811 ☑
        - suspect Y35.813 ☑
        - unspecified person Y35.819 ☑
    - sports equipment W21.9 ☑
  - police (on duty) — *see* Legal, intervention, manhandling

- **Struck** (accidentally) **by** — *continued*
  - police — *see* Legal, intervention, manhandling — *continued*
    - with blunt object — *see* Legal, intervention, blunt object
  - sports equipment W21.9 ☑
    - assault Y08.09 ☑
    - ball W21.00 ☑
      - baseball W21.03 ☑
      - basketball W21.05 ☑
      - football W21.01 ☑
      - golf ball W21.04 ☑
      - soccer W21.02 ☑
      - soft ball W21.07 ☑
      - specified NEC W21.09 ☑
      - volleyball W21.06 ☑
    - bat or racquet
      - baseball bat W21.11 ☑
        - assault Y08.02 ☑
      - golf club W21.13 ☑
        - assault Y08.09 ☑
      - specified NEC W21.19 ☑
      - tennis racquet W21.12 ☑
        - assault Y08.09 ☑
    - cleats (shoe) W21.31 ☑
    - foot wear NEC W21.39 ☑
    - football helmet W21.81 ☑
    - hockey (ice)
      - field
        - puck W21.221 ☑
        - stick W21.211 ☑
      - puck W21.220 ☑
      - stick W21.210 ☑
        - assault Y08.01 ☑
    - skate blades W21.32 ☑
    - specified NEC W21.89 ☑
      - assault Y08.09 ☑
  - thunderbolt — *see* subcategory T75.0 ☑
    - causing fire — *see* Exposure, fire
  - transport vehicle NEC — *see also* Accident, transport V09.9 ☑
    - intentional, homicide (attempt) Y03.0 ☑
    - motor NEC — *see also* Accident, transport V09.20 ☑
      - homicide Y03.0 ☑
  - vehicle (transport) NEC — *see* Accident, transport, by type of vehicle
    - stationary (falling from jack, hydraulic lift, ramp) W20.8 ☑
- **Stumbling**
  - over
    - animal NEC W01.0 ☑
      - with fall W18.09 ☑
    - carpet, rug or (small) object W22.8 ☑
      - with fall W18.09 ☑
    - person W51 ☑
      - with fall W03 ☑
        - due to ice or snow W00.0 ☑
  - without fall W18.40 ☑
    - due to
      - specified NEC W18.49 ☑
      - stepping from one level to another W18.43 ☑
      - stepping into hole or opening W18.42 ☑
      - stepping on object W18.41 ☑
- **Submersion** (accidental) — *see* Drowning
- **Suffocation** (accidental) (by external means) (by pressure) (mechanical) — *see also* category T71
  - due to, by
    - avalanche — *see* Landslide
    - explosion — *see* Explosion
    - fire — *see* Exposure, fire
    - food, any type (aspiration) (ingestion) (inhalation) — *see* categories T17 and T18 ☑
    - ignition — *see* Ignition
    - landslide — *see* Landslide
    - machine(ry) — *see* Contact, with, by type of machine
    - vomitus (aspiration) (inhalation) T17.81- ☑
  - in
    - burning building X00.8 ☑
- **Suicide, suicidal** (attempted) (by) X83.8 ☑
  - blunt object X79 ☑
  - burning, burns X76 ☑
    - hot object X77.9 ☑
      - fluid NEC X77.2 ☑
      - household appliance X77.3 ☑
      - specified NEC X77.8 ☑

- **Suicide, suicidal** — *continued*
  - burning, burns — *continued*
    - hot object — *continued*
      - steam X77.0 ☑
      - tap water X77.1 ☑
      - vapors X77.0 ☑
  - caustic substance — *see* Table of Drugs and Chemicals
  - cold, extreme X83.2 ☑
  - collision of motor vehicle with
    - motor vehicle X82.0 ☑
    - specified NEC X82.8 ☑
    - train X82.1 ☑
    - tree X82.2 ☑
  - crashing of aircraft X83.0 ☑
  - cut (any part of body) X78.9 ☑
  - cutting or piercing instrument X78.9 ☑
    - dagger X78.2 ☑
    - glass X78.0 ☑
    - knife X78.1 ☑
    - specified NEC X78.8 ☑
    - sword X78.2 ☑
  - drowning (in) X71.9 ☑
    - bathtub X71.0 ☑
    - natural water X71.3 ☑
    - specified NEC X71.8 ☑
    - swimming pool X71.1 ☑
      - following fall X71.2 ☑
  - electrocution X83.1 ☑
  - explosive(s) (material) X75 ☑
  - fire, flames X76 ☑
  - firearm X74.9 ☑
    - airgun X74.01 ☑
    - handgun X72 ☑
    - hunting rifle X73.1 ☑
    - larger X73.9 ☑
      - specified NEC X73.8 ☑
    - machine gun X73.2 ☑
    - shotgun X73.0 ☑
    - specified NEC X74.8 ☑
  - hanging X83.8 ☑
  - hot object — *see* Suicide, burning, hot object
  - jumping
    - before moving object X81.8 ☑
      - motor vehicle X81.0 ☑
      - subway train X81.1 ☑
      - train X81.1 ☑
    - from high place X80 ☑
  - late effect of attempt — *see* X71-X83 with 7th character S
  - lying before moving object, train, vehicle X81.8 ☑
  - poisoning — *see* Table of Drugs and Chemicals
  - puncture (any part of body) — *see* Suicide, cutting or piercing instrument
  - scald — *see* Suicide, burning, hot object
  - sequelae of attempt — *see* X71-X83 with 7th character S
  - sharp object (any) — *see* Suicide, cutting or piercing instrument
  - shooting — *see* Suicide, firearm
  - specified means NEC X83.8 ☑
  - stab (any part of body) — *see* Suicide, cutting or piercing instrument
  - steam, hot vapors X77.0 ☑
  - strangulation X83.8 ☑
  - submersion — *see* Suicide, drowning
  - suffocation X83.8 ☑
  - wound NEC X83.8 ☑
- **Sunstroke** X32 ☑
- **Supersonic waves** (causing injury) W42.0 ☑
- **Surgical procedure, complication of** (delayed or as an abnormal reaction without mention of misadventure) — *see also* Complication of or following, by type of procedure
  - due to or as a result of misadventure — *see* Misadventure
- **Swallowed, swallowing**
  - foreign body — *see* Foreign body, alimentary canal
  - poison — *see* Table of Drugs and Chemicals
  - substance
    - caustic or corrosive — *see* Table of Drugs and Chemicals
    - poisonous — *see* Table of Drugs and Chemicals

T

- **Tackle in sport** W03 ☑
- **Terrorism** (involving) Y38.80 ☑
  - biological weapons Y38.6X- ☑
  - chemical weapons Y38.7X- ☑
  - conflagration Y38.3X- ☑
  - drowning and submersion Y38.89- ☑
  - explosion Y38.2X- ☑
    - destruction of aircraft Y38.1X- ☑
    - marine weapons Y38.0X- ☑
  - fire Y38.3X- ☑
  - firearms Y38.4X- ☑
  - hot substances Y38.3X- ☑
  - lasers Y38.89- ☑
  - nuclear weapons Y38.5X- ☑
  - piercing or stabbing instruments Y38.89- ☑
  - secondary effects Y38.9X- ☑
  - specified method NEC Y38.89- ☑
  - suicide bomber Y38.81- ☑
- **Thirst** X58 ☑
- **Threat to breathing**
  - aspiration — *see* Aspiration
  - due to cave-in, falling earth or substance NEC T71 ☑
- **Thrown** (accidentally)
  - against part (any) of or object in transport vehicle (in motion) NEC — *see also* Accident, transport
  - from
    - high place, homicide (attempt) Y01 ☑
    - machinery — *see* Contact, with, by type of machine
    - transport vehicle NEC — *see also* Accident, transport V89.9 ☑
  - off — *see* Thrown, from
- **Thunderbolt** — *see* subcategory T75.0 ☑
  - causing fire — *see* Exposure, fire
- **Tidal wave** (any injury) **NEC** — *see* Forces of nature, tidal wave
- **Took**
  - overdose (drug) — *see* Table of Drugs and Chemicals
  - poison — *see* Table of Drugs and Chemicals
- **Tornado** (any injury) X37.1 ☑
- **Torrential rain** (any injury) X37.8 ☑
- **Torture** X58 ☑
- **Trampled by animal NEC** W55.89 ☑
- **Trapped** (accidentally)
  - between objects (moving) (stationary and moving) — *see* Caught
  - by part (any) of
    - electric (assisted) bicycle V29.881 ☑
    - motorcycle V29.888 ☑
    - pedal cycle V19.88 ☑
    - transport vehicle NEC — *see also* Accident, transport V89.9 ☑
- **Travel** (effects) (sickness) T75.3 ☑
- **Tree falling on or hitting** (accidentally) (person) W20.8 ☑
- **Tripping**
  - over
    - animal W01.0 ☑
      - with fall W01.0 ☑
    - carpet, rug or (small) object W22.8 ☑
      - with fall W18.09 ☑
    - person W51 ☑
      - with fall W03 ☑
        - due to ice or snow W00.0 ☑
  - without fall W18.40 ☑
    - due to
      - specified NEC W18.49 ☑
      - stepping from one level to another W18.43 ☑
      - stepping into hole or opening W18.42 ☑
      - stepping on object W18.41 ☑
- **Twisted by person**(s) (accidentally) W50.2 ☑
  - with intent to injure or kill Y04.0 ☑
  - as, or caused by, a crowd or human stampede (with fall) W52 ☑
  - assault Y04.0 ☑
  - homicide (attempt) Y04.0 ☑
  - in
    - fight Y04.0 ☑
    - legal intervention — *see* Legal, intervention, manhandling
- **Twisting** (prolonged) (static) X50.1- ☑

U

- **Underdosing of necessary drugs, medicaments or biological substances** Y63.6
- **Undetermined intent** (contact) (exposure)
  - automobile collision Y32 ☑
  - blunt object Y29 ☑
  - drowning (submersion) (in) Y21.9 ☑
    - bathtub Y21.0 ☑
      - after fall Y21.1 ☑
    - natural water (lake) (ocean) (pond) (river) (stream) Y21.4 ☑
    - specified place NEC Y21.8 ☑
    - swimming pool Y21.2 ☑
      - after fall Y21.3 ☑
  - explosive material Y25 ☑
  - fall, jump or push from high place Y30 ☑
  - falling, lying or running before moving object Y31 ☑
  - fire Y26 ☑
  - firearm discharge Y24.9 ☑
    - airgun (BB) (pellet) Y24.0 ☑
    - handgun (pistol) (revolver) Y22 ☑
    - hunting rifle Y23.1 ☑
    - larger Y23.9 ☑
      - hunting rifle Y23.1 ☑
      - machine gun Y23.3 ☑
      - military Y23.2 ☑
      - shotgun Y23.0 ☑
      - specified type NEC Y23.8 ☑
    - machine gun Y23.3 ☑
    - military Y23.2 ☑
    - shotgun Y23.0 ☑
    - specified type NEC Y24.8 ☑
    - Very pistol Y24.8 ☑
  - hot object Y27.9 ☑
    - fluid NEC Y27.2 ☑
    - household appliance Y27.3 ☑
    - specified object NEC Y27.8 ☑
    - steam Y27.0 ☑
    - tap water Y27.1 ☑
    - vapor Y27.0 ☑
  - jump, fall or push from high place Y30 ☑
  - lying, falling or running before moving object Y31 ☑
  - motor vehicle crash Y32 ☑
  - push, fall or jump from high place Y30 ☑
  - running, falling or lying before moving object Y31 ☑
  - sharp object Y28.9 ☑
    - dagger Y28.2 ☑
    - glass Y28.0 ☑
    - knife Y28.1 ☑
    - specified object NEC Y28.8 ☑
    - sword Y28.2 ☑
  - smoke Y26 ☑
  - specified event NEC Y33 ☑
- **Use of hand as hammer** X50.3 ☑

V

- **Vibration** (causing injury) W49.9 ☑
- **Victim** (of)
  - avalanche — *see* Landslide
  - earth movements NEC — *see* Forces of nature, earth movement
  - earthquake X34 ☑
  - flood — *see* Flood
  - landslide — *see* Landslide
  - lightning — *see* subcategory T75.0 ☑
    - causing fire — *see* Exposure, fire
  - storm (cataclysmic) NEC — *see* Forces of nature, cataclysmic storm
  - volcanic eruption X35 ☑
- **Volcanic eruption** (any injury) X35 ☑
- **Vomitus, gastric contents in air passages** (with asphyxia, obstruction or suffocation) T17.81- ☑

W

- **Walked into stationary object** (any) W22.09 ☑
  - furniture W22.03 ☑
  - lamppost W22.02 ☑
  - wall W22.01 ☑
- **War operations** (injuries to military personnel and civilians during war, civil insurrection and peacekeeping missions) (by) (from) (involving) Y36.90 ☑
  - after cessation of hostilities Y36.89- ☑
    - explosion (of)
      - bomb placed during war operations Y36.82- ☑
      - mine placed during war operations Y36.81- ☑
    - specified NEC Y36.88- ☑
  - air blast Y36.20- ☑

War operations — *continued*
aircraft
destruction — *see* War operations, destruction of aircraft
airway restriction — *see* War operations, restriction of airways
asphyxiation — *see* War operations, restriction of airways
biological weapons Y36.6X- ☑
blast Y36.2Ø- ☑
blast fragments Y36.2Ø- ☑
blast wave Y36.2Ø- ☑
blast wind Y36.2Ø- ☑
bomb Y36.2Ø- ☑
dirty Y36.5Ø- ☑
gasoline Y36.31- ☑
incendiary Y36.31- ☑
petrol Y36.31- ☑
bullet Y36.43- ☑
incendiary Y36.32- ☑
rubber Y36.41- ☑
chemical weapons Y36.7X- ☑
combat
hand to hand (unarmed) combat Y36.44- ☑
using blunt or piercing object Y36.45- ☑
conflagration — *see* War operations, fire
conventional warfare NEC Y36.49- ☑
depth-charge Y36.Ø1- ☑
destruction of aircraft Y36.1Ø- ☑
due to
air to air missile Y36.11- ☑
collision with other aircraft Y36.12- ☑
detonation (accidental) of onboard munitions and explosives Y36.14- ☑
enemy fire or explosives Y36.11- ☑
explosive placed on aircraft Y36.11- ☑
onboard fire Y36.13- ☑
rocket propelled grenade [RPG] Y36.11- ☑
small arms fire Y36.11- ☑
surface to air missile Y36.11- ☑
specified NEC Y36.19- ☑
detonation (accidental) of
onboard marine weapons Y36.Ø5- ☑
own munitions or munitions launch device Y36.24- ☑
dirty bomb Y36.5Ø- ☑
explosion (of) Y36.2Ø- ☑
aerial bomb Y36.21- ☑
after cessation of hostilities
bomb placed during war operations Y36.82- ☑
mine placed during war operations Y36.81- ☑

War operations — *continued*
explosion — *continued*
bomb NOS — *see also* War operations, bomb(s) Y36.2Ø- ☑
fragments Y36.2Ø- ☑
grenade Y36.29- ☑
guided missile Y36.22- ☑
improvised explosive device [IED] (person-borne) (roadside) (vehicle-borne) Y36.23- ☑
land mine Y36.29- ☑
marine mine (at sea) (in harbor) Y36.Ø2- ☑
marine weapon Y36.ØØ- ☑
specified NEC Y36.Ø9- ☑
own munitions or munitions launch device (accidental) Y36.24- ☑
sea-based artillery shell Y36.Ø3- ☑
specified NEC Y36.29- ☑
torpedo Y36.Ø4- ☑
fire Y36.3Ø- ☑
specified NEC Y36.39- ☑
firearms
discharge Y36.43- ☑
pellets Y36.42- ☑
flamethrower Y36.33- ☑
fragments (from) (of)
improvised explosive device [IED] (person-borne) (roadside) (vehicle-borne) Y36.26- ☑
munitions Y36.25- ☑
specified NEC Y36.29- ☑
weapons Y36.27- ☑
friendly fire Y36.92 ☑
hand to hand (unarmed) combat Y36.44- ☑
hot substances — *see* War operations, fire
incendiary bullet Y36.32- ☑
nuclear weapon (effects of) Y36.5Ø- ☑
acute radiation exposure Y36.54- ☑
blast pressure Y36.51- ☑
direct blast Y36.51- ☑
direct heat Y36.53- ☑
fallout exposure Y36.54- ☑
fireball Y36.53- ☑
indirect blast (struck or crushed by blast debris) (being thrown by blast) Y36.52- ☑
ionizing radiation (immediate exposure) Y36.54- ☑
nuclear radiation Y36.54- ☑
radiation
ionizing (immediate exposure) Y36.54- ☑
nuclear Y36.54- ☑
thermal Y36.53- ☑
secondary effects Y36.54- ☑

War operations — *continued*
nuclear weapon — *continued*
specified NEC Y36.59- ☑
thermal radiation Y36.53- ☑
restriction of air (airway)
intentional Y36.46- ☑
unintentional Y36.47- ☑
rubber bullets Y36.41- ☑
shrapnel NOS Y36.29- ☑
suffocation — *see* War operations, restriction of airways
unconventional warfare NEC Y36.7X- ☑
underwater blast NOS Y36.ØØ- ☑
warfare
conventional NEC Y36.49- ☑
unconventional NEC Y36.7X- ☑
weapon of mass destruction [WMD] Y36.91 ☑
weapons
biological weapons Y36.6X- ☑
chemical Y36.7X- ☑
nuclear (effects of) Y36.5Ø- ☑
acute radiation exposure Y36.54- ☑
blast pressure Y36.51- ☑
direct blast Y36.51- ☑
direct heat Y36.53- ☑
fallout exposure Y36.54- ☑
fireball Y36.53- ☑
radiation
ionizing (immediate exposure) Y36.54- ☑
nuclear Y36.54- ☑
thermal Y36.53- ☑
secondary effects Y36.54- ☑
specified NEC Y36.59- ☑
of mass destruction [WMD] Y36.91 ☑

Washed
away by flood — *see* Flood
off road by storm (transport vehicle) — *see* Forces of nature, cataclysmic storm
Weather exposure NEC — *see* Forces of nature
Weightlessness (causing injury) (effects of) (in spacecraft, real or simulated) X52 ☑
Work related condition Y99.Ø
Wound (accidental) NEC — *see also* Injury X58 ☑
battle — *see also* War operations Y36.9Ø ☑
gunshot — *see* Discharge, firearm by type
Wreck transport vehicle NEC — *see also* Accident, transport V89.9 ☑
Wrong
device implanted into correct surgical site Y65.51
fluid in infusion Y65.1
patient, procedure performed on Y65.52
procedure (operation) on correct patient Y65.51

ICD-10-CM Tabular List of Diseases and Injuries

Chapter 1. Certain Infectious and Parasitic Diseases (AØØ–B99)

Chapter-specific Guidelines with Coding Examples

The chapter-specific guidelines from the ICD-10-CM Official Guidelines for Coding and Reporting have been provided below. Along with these guidelines are coding examples, contained in the shaded boxes, that have been developed to help illustrate the coding and/or sequencing guidance found in these guidelines.

a. Human immunodeficiency virus (HIV) infections

1) Code only confirmed cases

Code only confirmed cases of HIV infection/illness. This is an exception to the hospital inpatient guideline Section II, H.

In this context, "confirmation" does not require documentation of positive serology or culture for HIV; the provider's diagnostic statement that the patient is HIV positive or has an HIV-related illness is sufficient.

Patient being seen for hypothyroidism with possible HIV infection

EØ3.9	**Hypothyroidism, unspecified**

Explanation: Only the hypothyroidism is coded in this scenario because it has not been confirmed that an HIV infection is present.

2) Selection and sequencing of HIV codes

(a) Patient admitted for HIV-related condition

If a patient is admitted for an HIV-related condition, the principal diagnosis should be B2Ø, Human immunodeficiency virus [HIV] disease followed by additional diagnosis codes for all reported HIV-related conditions.

An exception to this guideline is if the reason for admission is hemolytic-uremic syndrome associated with HIV disease. Assign code D59.31, Infection-associated hemolytic-uremic syndrome, followed by code B2Ø, Human immunodeficiency virus [HIV] disease.

HIV with CMV

B2Ø	**Human immunodeficiency virus [HIV] disease**
B25.9	**Cytomegaloviral disease, unspecified**

Explanation: Cytomegaloviral infection is an HIV related condition, so the HIV diagnosis code is reported first, followed by the code for the CMV.

(b) Patient with HIV disease admitted for unrelated condition

If a patient with HIV disease is admitted for an unrelated condition (such as a traumatic injury), the code for the unrelated condition (e.g., the nature of injury code) should be the principal diagnosis. Other diagnoses would be B2Ø followed by additional diagnosis codes for all reported HIV-related conditions.

Sprain of the internal collateral ligament, right ankle; HIV

S93.491A	**Sprain of other ligament of right ankle, initial encounter**
B2Ø	**Human immunodeficiency virus [HIV] disease**

Explanation: The ankle sprain is not related to HIV, so it is the first-listed diagnosis code, and HIV is reported secondarily.

(c) Whether the patient is newly diagnosed

Whether the patient is newly diagnosed or has had previous admissions/encounters for HIV conditions is irrelevant to the sequencing decision.

Newly diagnosed multiple cutaneous Kaposi's sarcoma lesions in previously diagnosed HIV disease

B2Ø	**Human immunodeficiency virus [HIV] disease**
C46.Ø	**Kaposi's sarcoma of skin**

Explanation: Even though the HIV was diagnosed on a previous encounter, it is still sequenced first when coded with an HIV-related condition. Kaposi's sarcoma is an HIV-related condition.

(d) Asymptomatic human immunodeficiency virus

Z21, Asymptomatic human immunodeficiency virus [HIV] infection status, is to be applied when the patient without any documentation of symptoms is listed as being "HIV positive," "known HIV," "HIV test positive," or similar terminology. Do not use this code if the term "AIDS" or "HIV disease" is used or if the patient is treated for any HIV-related illness or is described as having any condition(s) resulting from his/her HIV positive status; use B2Ø in these cases.

(e) Patients with inconclusive HIV serology

Patients with inconclusive HIV serology, but no definitive diagnosis or manifestations of the illness, may be assigned code R75, Inconclusive laboratory evidence of human immunodeficiency virus [HIV].

(f) Previously diagnosed HIV-related illness

Patients with any known prior diagnosis of an HIV-related illness should be coded to B2Ø. Once a patient has developed an HIV-related illness, the patient should always be assigned code B2Ø on every subsequent admission/encounter. Patients previously diagnosed with any HIV illness (B2Ø) should never be assigned to R75 or Z21, Asymptomatic human immunodeficiency virus [HIV] infection status.

(g) HIV infection in pregnancy, childbirth and the puerperium

During pregnancy, childbirth or the puerperium, a patient admitted (or presenting for a health care encounter) because of an HIV-related illness should receive a principal diagnosis code of O98.7-, Human immunodeficiency [HIV] disease complicating pregnancy, childbirth and the puerperium, followed by B2Ø and the code(s) for the HIV-related illness(es). Codes from Chapter 15 always take sequencing priority.

Patients with asymptomatic HIV infection status admitted (or presenting for a health care encounter) during pregnancy, childbirth, or the puerperium should receive codes of O98.7- and Z21.

(h) Encounters for testing for HIV

If a patient is being seen to determine his/her HIV status, use code Z11.4, Encounter for screening for human immunodeficiency virus [HIV]. Use additional codes for any associated high-risk behavior, if applicable.

If a patient with signs or symptoms is being seen for HIV testing, code the signs and symptoms. An additional counseling code Z71.7, Human immunodeficiency virus [HIV] counseling, may be used if counseling is provided during the encounter for the test.

When a patient returns to be informed of his/her HIV test results and the test result is negative, use code Z71.7, Human immunodeficiency virus [HIV] counseling.

If the results are positive, see previous guidelines and assign codes as appropriate.

(i) HIV managed by antiretroviral medication

If a patient with documented HIV disease, **HIV-related illness or AIDS** is currently managed on antiretroviral medications, assign code B2Ø, Human immunodeficiency virus [HIV] disease. Code Z79.899, Other long term (current) drug therapy, may be assigned as an additional code to identify the long-term (current) use of antiretroviral medications.

b. Infectious agents as the cause of diseases classified to other chapters

Certain infections are classified in chapters other than Chapter 1 and no organism is identified as part of the infection code. In these instances, it is necessary to use an additional code from Chapter 1 to identify the organism. A code from category B95, Streptococcus, Staphylococcus, and Enterococcus as the cause of diseases classified to other chapters, B96, Other bacterial agents as the cause of diseases classified to other chapters, or B97, Viral agents as the cause of diseases classified to other chapters, is to be used as an additional code to identify the organism. An instructional note will be found at the infection code advising that an additional organism code is required.

Acute *E. coli* cystitis

N3Ø.ØØ	**Acute cystitis without hematuria**
B96.2Ø	**Unspecified Escherichia coli [E.coli] as the cause of diseases classified elsewhere**

Explanation: An instructional note under the category for the cystitis indicates to code also the specific organism.

c. Infections resistant to antibiotics

Many bacterial infections are resistant to current antibiotics. It is necessary to identify all infections documented as antibiotic resistant. Assign a code from category Z16, Resistance to antimicrobial drugs, following the infection code only if the infection code does not identify drug resistance.

Penicillin-resistant *Streptococcus pneumoniae* pneumonia

J13	**Pneumonia due to Streptococcus pneumoniae**
Z16.11	**Resistance to penicillins**

Explanation: Code Z16.11 is assigned as a secondary code to represent the penicillin resistance. This code includes resistance to amoxicillin and ampicillin.

d. Sepsis, severe sepsis, and septic shock

1) Coding of Sepsis and Severe Sepsis

(a) Sepsis

For a diagnosis of sepsis, assign the appropriate code for the underlying systemic infection. If the type of infection or causal organism is not further specified, assign code A41.9, Sepsis, unspecified organism.

A code from subcategory R65.2, Severe sepsis, should not be assigned unless severe sepsis or an associated acute organ dysfunction is documented.

Gram-negative sepsis

A41.5Ø	**Gram-negative sepsis, unspecified**

Staphylococcal sepsis

A41.2	**Sepsis due to unspecified staphylococcus**

Explanation: In both examples above the organism causing the sepsis is identified, therefore A41.9 Sepsis, unspecified organism, would not be appropriate as this code would not capture the highest degree of specificity found in the documentation. Do not use an additional code for severe sepsis unless an acute organ dysfunction was also documented as "associated with" or "due to" the sepsis or the sepsis was documented as "severe."

(i) Negative or inconclusive blood cultures and sepsis

Negative or inconclusive blood cultures do not preclude a diagnosis of sepsis in patients with clinical evidence of the condition; however, the provider should be queried.

(ii) Urosepsis

The term urosepsis is a nonspecific term. It is not to be considered synonymous with sepsis. It has no default code in the Alphabetic Index. Should a provider use this term, he/she must be queried for clarification.

(iii)Sepsis with organ dysfunction

If a patient has sepsis and associated acute organ dysfunction or multiple organ dysfunction (MOD), follow the instructions for coding severe sepsis.

(iv) Acute organ dysfunction that is not clearly associated with the sepsis

If a patient has sepsis and an acute organ dysfunction, but the medical record documentation indicates that the acute organ dysfunction is related to a medical condition other than the sepsis, do not assign a code from subcategory R65.2, Severe sepsis. An acute organ dysfunction must be associated with the sepsis in order to assign the severe sepsis code. If the documentation is not clear as to whether an acute organ dysfunction is related to the sepsis or another medical condition, query the provider.

Sepsis and acute respiratory failure due to COPD exacerbation

A41.9	**Sepsis, unspecified organism**
J44.1	**Chronic obstructive pulmonary disease with (acute) exacerbation**
J96.ØØ	**Acute respiratory failure, unspecified whether with hypoxia or hypercapnia**

Explanation: Although acute organ dysfunction is present in the form of acute respiratory failure, severe sepsis (R65.2) is not coded in this example, as the acute respiratory failure is attributed to the COPD exacerbation rather than the sepsis. Sequencing of these codes would be determined by the reason for the encounter.

(b) Severe sepsis

The coding of severe sepsis requires a minimum of 2 codes: first a code for the underlying systemic infection, followed by a code from subcategory R65.2, Severe sepsis. If the causal organism is not documented, assign code A41.9, Sepsis, unspecified organism, for the infection. Additional code(s) for the associated acute organ dysfunction are also required.

Due to the complex nature of severe sepsis, some cases may require querying the provider prior to assignment of the codes.

2) Septic shock

Septic shock generally refers to circulatory failure associated with severe sepsis, and therefore, it represents a type of acute organ dysfunction.

For cases of septic shock, the code for the systemic infection should be sequenced first, followed by code R65.21, Severe sepsis with septic shock or code T81.12, Postprocedural septic shock. Any additional codes for the other acute organ dysfunctions should also be assigned. As noted in the sequencing instructions in the Tabular List, the code for septic shock cannot be assigned as a principal diagnosis.

Sepsis with septic shock

A41.9	**Sepsis, unspecified organism**
R65.21	**Severe sepsis with septic shock**

Explanation: Documentation of septic shock automatically implies severe sepsis as it is a form of acute organ dysfunction. Septic shock is not coded as the first-listed diagnosis; it is always preceded by the code for the systemic infection.

3) Sequencing of severe sepsis

If severe sepsis is present on admission, and meets the definition of principal diagnosis, the underlying systemic infection should be assigned as principal diagnosis followed by the appropriate code from subcategory R65.2 as required by the sequencing rules in the Tabular List. A code from subcategory R65.2 can never be assigned as a principal diagnosis.

When severe sepsis develops during an encounter (it was not present on admission), the underlying systemic infection and the appropriate code from subcategory R65.2 should be assigned as secondary diagnoses.

Severe sepsis may be present on admission, but the diagnosis may not be confirmed until sometime after admission. If the documentation is not clear whether severe sepsis was present on admission, the provider should be queried.

For infection-associated hemolytic-uremic syndrome with severe sepsis, see guideline I.C.1.d.9.

4) Sepsis or severe sepsis with a localized infection

If the reason for admission is sepsis or severe sepsis and a localized infection, such as pneumonia or cellulitis, a code(s) for the underlying systemic infection should be assigned first and the code for the localized infection should be assigned as a secondary diagnosis. If the patient has severe sepsis, a code from subcategory R65.2 should also be assigned as a secondary diagnosis. If the patient is admitted with a localized infection, such as pneumonia, and sepsis/severe sepsis doesn't develop until after admission, the localized infection should be assigned first, followed by the appropriate sepsis/severe sepsis codes.

For hemolytic-uremic syndrome associated with sepsis, see guideline I. C.1.d.9.

Patient presents with acute renal failure due to severe sepsis from *Pseudomonas pneumonia*

A41.52	**Sepsis due to Pseudomonas**
J15.1	**Pneumonia due to Pseudomonas**
R65.2Ø	**Severe sepsis without septic shock**
N17.9	**Acute kidney failure, unspecified**

Explanation: If all conditions are present, the systemic infection (sepsis) is sequenced first followed by the codes for the localized infection (pneumonia), severe sepsis and any organ dysfunction.

5) Sepsis due to a postprocedural infection

(a) Documentation of causal relationship

As with all postprocedural complications, code assignment is based on the provider's documentation of the relationship between the infection and the procedure.

(b) Sepsis due to a postprocedural infection

For infections following a procedure, a code from T81.4Ø, to T81.43 Infection following a procedure, or a code from O86.ØØ to O86.Ø3, Infection of obstetric surgical wound, that identifies the site of the infection should be coded first, if known. Assign an additional code for sepsis following a procedure (T81.44) or sepsis following an obstetrical procedure (O86.Ø4). Use an additional code to identify the infectious agent. If the patient has severe sepsis, the appropriate code from subcategory R65.2 should also be assigned with the additional code(s) for any acute organ dysfunction.

For infections following infusion, transfusion, therapeutic injection, or immunization, a code from subcategory T8Ø.2, Infections following infusion, transfusion, and therapeutic injection, or code T88.Ø-, infection following immunization, should be coded first, followed by the code for the specific infection. If the patient has severe sepsis, the appropriate code from subcategory R65.2 should also be assigned, with the additional codes(s) for any acute organ dysfunction.

(c) Postprocedural infection and postprocedural septic shock

If a postprocedural infection has resulted in postprocedural septic shock, assign the codes indicated above for sepsis due to a postprocedural infection, followed by code T81.12-, Postprocedural septic shock. Do not assign code R65.21, Severe sepsis with septic shock. Additional code(s) should be assigned for any acute organ dysfunction.

6) Sepsis and severe sepsis associated with a noninfectious process (condition)

In some cases, a noninfectious process (condition) such as trauma, may lead to an infection which can result in sepsis or severe sepsis. If sepsis or severe sepsis is documented as associated with a noninfectious condition, such as a burn or serious injury, and this condition meets the definition for principal diagnosis, the code for the noninfectious condition should be sequenced first, followed by the code for the resulting infection. If severe sepsis is present, a code from subcategory R65.2 should also be assigned with any associated organ dysfunction(s) codes. It is not necessary to assign a code from subcategory R65.1, Systemic inflammatory response syndrome (SIRS) of non-infectious origin, for these cases.

If the infection meets the definition of principal diagnosis, it should be sequenced before the non-infectious condition. When both the associated non-infectious condition and the infection meet the definition of principal diagnosis, either may be assigned as principal diagnosis.

Only one code from category R65, Symptoms and signs specifically associated with systemic inflammation and infection, should be assigned. Therefore, when a non-infectious condition leads to an infection resulting in severe sepsis, assign the appropriate code from subcategory R65.2, Severe sepsis. Do not additionally assign a code from subcategory R65.1, Systemic inflammatory response syndrome (SIRS) of non-infectious origin.

See Section I.C.18. SIRS due to non-infectious process

7) Sepsis and septic shock complicating abortion, pregnancy, childbirth, and the puerperium

See Section I.C.15. Sepsis and septic shock complicating abortion, pregnancy, childbirth and the puerperium

8) Newborn sepsis

See Section I.C.16. f. Bacterial sepsis of Newborn

9) Hemolytic-uremic syndrome associated with sepsis

If the reason for admission is hemolytic-uremic syndrome that is associated with sepsis, assign code D59.31, Infection-associated hemolytic-uremic syndrome, as the principal diagnosis. Codes for the underlying systemic infection and any other conditions (such as severe sepsis) should be assigned as secondary diagnoses.

e. Methicillin resistant Staphylococcus aureus (MRSA) conditions

1) Selection and sequencing of MRSA codes

(a) Combination codes for MRSA infection

When a patient is diagnosed with an infection that is due to methicillin resistant *Staphylococcus aureus* (MRSA), and that infection has a combination code that includes the causal organism (e.g., sepsis, pneumonia) assign the appropriate combination code for the condition (e.g., code A41.Ø2, Sepsis due to Methicillin resistant Staphylococcus aureus or code J15.212, Pneumonia due to Methicillin resistant Staphylococcus aureus). Do not assign code B95.62, Methicillin resistant Staphylococcus aureus infection as the cause of diseases classified elsewhere, as an additional code, because the combination code includes the type of infection and the MRSA organism. Do not assign a code from subcategory Z16.11, Resistance to penicillins, as an additional diagnosis.

See Section C.1. for instructions on coding and sequencing of sepsis and severe sepsis.

(b) Other codes for MRSA infection

When there is documentation of a current infection (e.g., wound infection, stitch abscess, urinary tract infection) due to MRSA, and that infection does not have a combination code that includes the causal organism, assign the appropriate code to identify the condition along with code B95.62, Methicillin resistant Staphylococcus aureus infection as the cause of diseases classified elsewhere for the MRSA infection. Do not assign a code from subcategory Z16.11, Resistance to penicillins.

(c) Methicillin susceptible Staphylococcus aureus (MSSA) and MRSA colonization

The condition or state of being colonized or carrying MSSA or MRSA is called colonization or carriage, while an individual person is described as being colonized or being a carrier.

Colonization means that MSSA or MSRA is present on or in the body without necessarily causing illness. A positive MRSA colonization test might be documented by the provider as "MRSA screen positive" or "MRSA nasal swab positive".

Assign code Z22.322, Carrier or suspected carrier of Methicillin resistant Staphylococcus aureus, for patients documented as having MRSA colonization. Assign code Z22.321, Carrier or suspected carrier of Methicillin susceptible Staphylococcus aureus, for patients documented as having MSSA colonization. Colonization is not necessarily indicative of a disease process or as the cause of a specific condition the patient may have unless documented as such by the provider.

(d) MRSA colonization and infection

If a patient is documented as having both MRSA colonization and infection during a hospital admission, code Z22.322, Carrier or suspected carrier of Methicillin resistant Staphylococcus aureus, and a code for the MRSA infection may both be assigned.

f. Zika virus infections

1) Code only confirmed cases

Code only a confirmed diagnosis of Zika virus (A92.5, Zika virus disease) as documented by the provider. This is an exception to the hospital inpatient guideline Section II, H. In this context, "confirmation" does not require documentation of the type of test performed; the provider's diagnostic statement that the condition is confirmed is sufficient. This code should be assigned regardless of the stated mode of transmission.

If the provider documents "suspected", "possible" or "probable" Zika, do not assign code A92.5. Assign a code(s) explaining the reason for encounter (such as fever, rash, or joint pain) or Z2Ø.821, Contact with and (suspected) exposure to Zika virus.

g. Coronavirus infections

1) COVID-19 infection (infection due to SARS-CoV-2)

(a) Code only confirmed cases

Code only a confirmed diagnosis of the 2019 novel coronavirus disease (COVID-19) as documented by the provider, or documentation of a positive COVID-19 test result. For a confirmed diagnosis, assign code UØ7.1, COVID-19. This is an exception to the hospital inpatient guideline Section II, H. In this context, "confirmation" does not require documentation of a positive test result for COVID-19; the provider's documentation that the individual has COVID-19 is sufficient.

Physician documentation states the patient has tested positive for the 2019 novel coronavirus disease.

UØ7.1 **COVID-19**

Explanation: The type of test is not required; physician documentation that states the patient has COVID-19 or a documented positive COVID-19 test result is sufficient.

If the provider documents "suspected," "possible," "probable," or "inconclusive" COVID-19, do not assign code UØ7.1. Instead, code the signs and symptoms reported. See guideline I.C.1.g.1.g.

Patient presents with cough and a slight fever and fear they were exposed to the coronavirus. The provider documents cough, temperature of 99.4, lungs clear, rule out COVID-19.

R5Ø.9 **Fever, unspecified**

RØ5.9 **Cough, unspecified**

Z2Ø.822 **Contact with and (suspected) exposure to COVID-19**

Explanation: For patients who have been exposed or fear they have been exposed to coronavirus, report codes for signs and symptoms, followed by the Z code. Report UØ7.1 COVID-19, only when the diagnosis is confirmed through provider documentation or a documented positive test result.

(b) Sequencing of codes

When COVID-19 meets the definition of principal diagnosis, code UØ7.1, COVID-19, should be sequenced first, followed by the appropriate codes for associated manifestations, except when another guideline requires that certain codes be sequenced first, such as obstetrics, sepsis, or transplant complications.

For a COVID-19 infection that progresses to sepsis, see Section I.C.1.d. Sepsis, Severe Sepsis, and Septic Shock

See Section I.C.15.s. for COVID-19 infection in pregnancy, childbirth, and the puerperium

See Section I.C.16.h. for COVID-19 infection in newborn

For a COVID-19 infection in a lung transplant patient, see Section I.C.19.g.3.a. Transplant complications other than kidney.

(c) Acute respiratory manifestations of COVID-19

When the reason for the encounter/admission is a respiratory manifestation of COVID-19, assign code UØ7.1, COVID-19, as the principal/first-listed diagnosis and assign code(s) for the respiratory manifestation(s) as additional diagnoses.

The following conditions are examples of common respiratory manifestations of COVID-19.

(i) Pneumonia

For a patient with pneumonia confirmed as due to COVID-19, assign codes UØ7.1, COVID-19, and J12.82, Pneumonia due to coronavirus disease 2019.

(ii) Acute bronchitis

For a patient with acute bronchitis confirmed as due to COVID-19, assign codes UØ7.1, and J2Ø.8, Acute bronchitis due to other specified organisms.

Bronchitis not otherwise specified (NOS) due to COVID-19 should be coded using code UØ7.1 and J4Ø, Bronchitis, not specified as acute or chronic.

(iii) Lower respiratory infection

If the COVID-19 is documented as being associated with a lower respiratory infection, not otherwise specified (NOS), or an acute respiratory infection, NOS, codes UØ7.1 and J22, Unspecified acute lower respiratory infection, should be assigned.

If the COVID-19 is documented as being associated with a respiratory infection, NOS, codes UØ7.1 and J98.8, Other specified respiratory disorders, should be assigned.

(iv) Acute respiratory distress syndrome

For acute respiratory distress syndrome (ARDS) due to COVID-19, assign codes UØ7.1, and J8Ø, Acute respiratory distress syndrome.

(v) Acute respiratory failure

For acute respiratory failure due to COVID-19, assign code UØ7.1, and code J96.Ø-, Acute respiratory failure.

(d) Non-respiratory manifestations of COVID-19

When the reason for the encounter/admission is a non-respiratory manifestation (e.g., viral enteritis) of COVID-19, assign code UØ7.1, COVID-19, as the principal/first-listed diagnosis and assign code(s) for the manifestation(s) as additional diagnoses.

(e) Exposure to COVID-19

For asymptomatic individuals with actual or suspected exposure to COVID-19, assign code Z2Ø.822, Contact with and (suspected) exposure to COVID-19.

For symptomatic individuals with actual or suspected exposure to COVID-19 and the infection has been ruled out, or test results are inconclusive or unknown, assign code Z2Ø.822, Contact with and (suspected) exposure to COVID-19. See guideline I.C.21.c.1, Contact/Exposure, for additional guidance regarding the use of category Z2Ø codes.

If COVID-19 is confirmed, see guideline I.C.1.g.1.a.

Patient was exposed to COVID-19 by a family member. They are asymptomatic and their test result is negative.

Z2Ø.822 Contact with and (suspected) exposure to COVID-19

Explanation: Report Z2Ø.822 for patients who have a negative test result but have known exposure to someone who has tested positive for COVID-19.

(f) Screening for COVID-19

During the COVID-19 pandemic, a screening code is generally not appropriate. Do not assign code Z11.52, Encounter for screening for COVID-19. For encounters for COVID-19 testing, including preoperative testing, code as exposure to COVID-19 (guideline I.C.1.g.1.e).

Coding guidance will be updated as new information concerning any changes in the pandemic status becomes available.

(g) Signs and symptoms without definitive diagnosis of COVID-19

For patients presenting with any signs/symptoms associated with COVID-19 (such as fever, etc.) but a definitive diagnosis has not been established, assign the appropriate code(s) for each of the presenting signs and symptoms such as:

- RØ5.1, Acute cough, or RØ5.9, Cough, unspecified
- RØ6.Ø2 Shortness of breath
- R5Ø.9 Fever, unspecified

If a patient with signs/symptoms associated with COVID-19 also has an actual or suspected contact with or exposure to COVID-19, assign Z2Ø.822, Contact with and (suspected) exposure to COVID19, as an additional code.

(h) Asymptomatic individuals who test positive for COVID-19

For asymptomatic individuals who test positive for COVID-19, see guideline I.C.1.g.1.a. Although the individual is asymptomatic, the individual has tested positive and is considered to have the COVID-19 infection.

(i) Personal history of COVID-19

For patients with a history of COVID-19, assign code Z86.16, Personal history of COVID-19.

(j) Follow-up visits after COVID-19 infection has resolved

For individuals who previously had COVID-19, without residual symptom(s) or condition(s), and are being seen for follow-up evaluation, and COVID-19 test results are negative, assign codes ZØ9, Encounter for follow-up examination after completed treatment for conditions other than malignant neoplasm, and Z86.16, Personal history of COVID-19.

For follow-up visits for individuals with symptom(s) or condition(s) related to a previous COVID-19 infection, see guideline I.C.1.g.1.m.

See Section I.C.21.c.8, Factors influencing health states and contact with health services, Follow-up

(k) Encounter for antibody testing

For an encounter for antibody testing that is not being performed to confirm a current COVID-19 infection, nor is a follow-up test after resolution of COVID-19, assign ZØ1.84, Encounter for antibody response examination.

Follow the applicable guidelines above if the individual is being tested to confirm a current COVID-19 infection.

For follow-up testing after a COVID-19 infection, see guideline I.C.1.g.1.j.

(l) Multisystem inflammatory syndrome

For individuals with multisystem inflammatory syndrome (MIS) and COVID-19, assign code UØ7.1, COVID-19, as the principal/first-listed diagnosis and assign code M35.81, Multisystem inflammatory syndrome, as an additional diagnosis.

If an individual with a history of COVID-19 develops MIS, assign codes M35.81, Multisystem inflammatory syndrome, and UØ9.9, Post COVID-19 condition, unspecified.

If an individual with a known or suspected exposure to COVID- 19, and no current COVID-19 infection or history of COVID-19, develops MIS, assign codes M35.81, Multisystem inflammatory syndrome, and Z2Ø.822, Contact with and (suspected) exposure to COVID-19.

Additional codes should be assigned for any associated complications of MIS.

(m) Post COVID-19 condition

For sequela of COVID-19, or associated symptoms or conditions that develop following a previous COVID-19 infection, assign a code(s) for the specific symptom(s) or condition(s) related to the previous COVID-19 infection, if known, and code UØ9.9, Post COVID-19 condition, unspecified.

Code UØ9.9 should not be assigned for manifestations of an active (current) COVID-19 infection.

If a patient has a condition(s) associated with a previous COVID-19 infection and develops a new active (current) COVID-19 infection, code UØ9.9 may be assigned in conjunction with code UØ7.1, COVID-19, to identify that the patient also has a condition(s) associated with a previous COVID-19 infection. Code(s) for the specific condition(s) associated with the previous COVID-19 infection and code(s) for manifestation(s) of the new active (current) COVID-19 infection should also be assigned.

(n) Underimmunization for COVID-19 Status

Code Z28.31Ø, Unvaccinated for COVID-19, may be assigned when the patient has not received **a** COVID-19 vaccine **of any type.** Code Z28.311, Partially vaccinated for COVID-19, may be assigned when the patient has **been partially vaccinated for COVID-19 as per the recommendations of** the Centers for Disease Control and Prevention (CDC) in place at the time of the encounter. For information, visit the CDC's website https://www.cdc.gov/coronavirus/2019-ncov/vaccines/.

See Section I.B.14. for underimmunization documentation by clinicians other than patient's provider.

Chapter 1. Certain Infectious and Parasitic Diseases (A00-B99)

INCLUDES diseases generally recognized as communicable or transmissible

Use additional code to identify resistance to antimicrobial drugs (Z16.-)

EXCLUDES 1 *certain localized infections - see body system-related chapters*

EXCLUDES 2 *carrier or suspected carrier of infectious disease (Z22.-)*
infectious and parasitic diseases complicating pregnancy, childbirth and the puerperium (O98.-)
infectious and parasitic diseases specific to the perinatal period (P35-P39)
influenza and other acute respiratory infections (J00-J22)

This chapter contains the following blocks:

A00-A09	Intestinal infectious diseases
A15-A19	Tuberculosis
A20-A28	Certain zoonotic bacterial diseases
A30-A49	Other bacterial diseases
A50-A64	Infections with a predominantly sexual mode of transmission
A65-A69	Other spirochetal diseases
A70-A74	Other diseases caused by chlamydiae
A75-A79	Rickettsioses
A80-A89	Viral and prion infections of the central nervous system
A90-A99	Arthropod-borne viral fevers and viral hemorrhagic fevers
B00-B09	Viral infections characterized by skin and mucous membrane lesions
B10	Other human herpesviruses
B15-B19	Viral hepatitis
B20	Human immunodeficiency virus [HIV] disease
B25-B34	Other viral diseases
B35-B49	Mycoses
B50-B64	Protozoal diseases
B65-B83	Helminthiases
B85-B89	Pediculosis, acariasis and other infestations
B90-B94	Sequelae of infectious and parasitic diseases
B95-B97	Bacterial and viral infectious agents
B99	Other infectious diseases

Intestinal infectious diseases (A00-A09)

✓4th A00 Cholera

DEF: Acute infection of the bowel due to *Vibrio cholerae* that presents with profuse diarrhea, cramps, and vomiting, resulting in severe dehydration, electrolyte imbalance, and death. It is spread through ingestion of food or water contaminated with feces of infected persons.

A00.0 Cholera due to Vibrio cholerae 01, biovar cholerae
Classical cholera

A00.1 Cholera due to Vibrio cholerae 01, biovar eltor
Cholera eltor

A00.9 Cholera, unspecified

✓4th A01 Typhoid and paratyphoid fevers

DEF: Typhoid fever: Acute generalized illness caused by *Salmonella typhi*. Clinical features include fever, headache, abdominal pain, cough, toxemia, leukopenia, abnormal pulse, rose spots on the skin, bacteremia, hyperplasia of intestinal lymph nodes, mesenteric lymphadenopathy, and Peyer's patches in the intestines.

DEF: Paratyphoid fever: Prolonged febrile illness, caused by *Salmonella* serotypes other than *S. typhi*, especially *S. enterica* serotypes paratyphi A, B, and C.

✓5th A01.0 Typhoid fever
Infection due to Salmonella typhi

A01.00 Typhoid fever, unspecified

A01.01 Typhoid meningitis COM

A01.02 Typhoid fever with heart involvement COM
Typhoid endocarditis
Typhoid myocarditis

A01.03 Typhoid pneumonia HCC ESR

A01.04 Typhoid arthritis HCC ESR COM

A01.05 Typhoid osteomyelitis HCC ESR COM

A01.09 Typhoid fever with other complications

A01.1 Paratyphoid fever A

A01.2 Paratyphoid fever B

A01.3 Paratyphoid fever C

A01.4 Paratyphoid fever, unspecified
Infection due to Salmonella paratyphi NOS

✓4th A02 Other salmonella infections

INCLUDES infection or foodborne intoxication due to any Salmonella species other than S. typhi and S. paratyphi

A02.0 Salmonella enteritis
Salmonellosis

TIP: Dehydration (E86.0) is a complication of salmonella enteritis and may be reported separately.

A02.1 Salmonella sepsis HCC ESR COM

✓5th A02.2 Localized salmonella infections

A02.20 Localized salmonella infection, unspecified

A02.21 Salmonella meningitis COM

A02.22 Salmonella pneumonia HCC ESR

A02.23 Salmonella arthritis HCC ESR COM

A02.24 Salmonella osteomyelitis HCC ESR COM

A02.25 Salmonella pyelonephritis
Salmonella tubulo-interstitial nephropathy

A02.29 Salmonella with other localized infection

A02.8 Other specified salmonella infections

A02.9 Salmonella infection, unspecified

✓4th A03 Shigellosis

DEF: Infection caused by the genus *Shigella*, of the family *Enterobacteriaceae* that is known to cause an acute dysenteric infection of the bowel with fever, drowsiness, anorexia, nausea, vomiting, bloody diarrhea, abdominal cramps, and distention.

A03.0 Shigellosis due to Shigella dysenteriae
Group A shigellosis [Shiga-Kruse dysentery]

A03.1 Shigellosis due to Shigella flexneri
Group B shigellosis

A03.2 Shigellosis due to Shigella boydii
Group C shigellosis

A03.3 Shigellosis due to Shigella sonnei
Group D shigellosis

A03.8 Other shigellosis

A03.9 Shigellosis, unspecified
Bacillary dysentery NOS

✓4th A04 Other bacterial intestinal infections

EXCLUDES 1 *bacterial foodborne intoxications, NEC (A05.-)*
tuberculous enteritis (A18.32)

DEF: *Escherichia coli*: Gram-negative, anaerobic bacteria of the family *Enterobacteriaceae* found in the large intestine of warm-blooded animals, generally as a nonpathologic entity aiding in digestion. They become pathogenic when an opportunity to grow somewhere outside this relationship presents itself, such as ingestion of fecal-contaminated food or water.

A04.0 Enteropathogenic Escherichia coli infection

A04.1 Enterotoxigenic Escherichia coli infection

A04.2 Enteroinvasive Escherichia coli infection

A04.3 Enterohemorrhagic Escherichia coli infection

DEF: *E. coli* infection penetrating the intestinal mucosa, producing microscopic ulceration and bleeding.

A04.4 Other intestinal Escherichia coli infections
Escherichia coli enteritis NOS

A04.5 Campylobacter enteritis

TIP: For Guillain-Barre syndrome occurring as a sequela of *Campylobacter enteritis*, assign code G61.0 as the first-listed diagnosis followed by B94.8 for the sequelae.

A04.6 Enteritis due to Yersinia enterocolitica

EXCLUDES 1 *extraintestinal yersiniosis (A28.2)*

✓5th A04.7 Enterocolitis due to Clostridium difficile
Foodborne intoxication by Clostridium difficile
Pseudomembraneous colitis
AHA: 2017,4Q,4

A04.71 Enterocolitis due to Clostridium difficile, recurrent
AHA: 2020,1Q,18

A04.72 Enterocolitis due to Clostridium difficile, not specified as recurrent

A04.8 Other specified bacterial intestinal infections

A04.9 Bacterial intestinal infection, unspecified
Bacterial enteritis NOS

✓4th A05 Other bacterial foodborne intoxications, not elsewhere classified

EXCLUDES 1 *Clostridium difficile foodborne intoxication and infection (A04.7-)*
Escherichia coli infection (A04.0-A04.4)
listeriosis (A32.-)
salmonella foodborne intoxication and infection (A02.-)
toxic effect of noxious foodstuffs (T61-T62)

A05.0 Foodborne staphylococcal intoxication

TIP: Assign code A04.8 to report a staphylococcal infection when it is caused by the ingestion of contaminated food but not caused by *S. aureus* toxins.

A05.1 Botulism food poisoning

Botulism NOS
Classical foodborne intoxication due to Clostridium botulinum

EXCLUDES 1 *infant botulism (A48.51)*
wound botulism (A48.52)

DEF: Muscle-paralyzing neurotoxic disease caused by ingesting pre-formed toxin from the bacterium *Clostridium botulinum*. It causes vomiting and diarrhea, vision problems, slurred speech, difficulty swallowing, paralysis, and death.

A05.2 Foodborne Clostridium perfringens [Clostridium welchii] intoxication

Enteritis necroticans
Pig-bel

A05.3 Foodborne Vibrio parahaemolyticus intoxication

A05.4 Foodborne Bacillus cereus intoxication

A05.5 Foodborne Vibrio vulnificus intoxication

A05.8 Other specified bacterial foodborne intoxications

A05.9 Bacterial foodborne intoxication, unspecified

✓4th A06 Amebiasis

INCLUDES infection due to Entamoeba histolytica

EXCLUDES 1 *other protozoal intestinal diseases (A07.-)*

EXCLUDES 2 *acanthamebiasis (B60.1-)*
Naegleriasis (B60.2)

DEF: Infection with a single cell protozoan known as the amoeba. Transmission occurs through ingestion of feces, contaminated food or water, use of human feces as fertilizer, or person-to-person contact.

A06.0 Acute amebic dysentery

Acute amebiasis
Intestinal amebiasis NOS

A06.1 Chronic intestinal amebiasis

A06.2 Amebic nondysenteric colitis

A06.3 Ameboma of intestine

Ameboma NOS

A06.4 Amebic liver abscess COM

Hepatic amebiasis

A06.5 Amebic lung abscess HCC ESR COM

Amebic abscess of lung (and liver)

A06.6 Amebic brain abscess COM

Amebic abscess of brain (and liver) (and lung)

A06.7 Cutaneous amebiasis

✓5th A06.8 Amebic infection of other sites

A06.81 Amebic cystitis

A06.82 Other amebic genitourinary infections

Amebic balanitis
Amebic vesiculitis
Amebic vulvovaginitis

A06.89 Other amebic infections

Amebic appendicitis
Amebic splenic abscess

A06.9 Amebiasis, unspecified

✓4th A07 Other protozoal intestinal diseases

DEF: Protozoa: Group comprised of the simplest, single celled organisms, ranging in size from micro to macroscopic. They can live alone or in colonies, and do not show any differentiation in tissues. Most are motile and can live free in nature, but some are parasitic, causing disease in the variety of hosts they inhabit.

A07.0 Balantidiasis

Balantidial dysentery

A07.1 Giardiasis [lambliasis]

DEF: Infection caused by the flagellate protozoan *Giardia lamblia* causing gastrointestinal problems such as vomiting, chronic diarrhea, and weight loss. The most common parasite in the U.S., this is usually transmitted by ingesting contaminated water while in the cyst state, after which it latches onto the wall of the small intestine.

A07.2 Cryptosporidiosis HCC Rx ESR COM

DEF: Microscopic parasite found in water and one of the most common causes of waterborne gastrointestinal infectious disease in the United States. It is usually transmitted by ingesting contaminated drinking water or recreational water and causes profuse watery diarrhea, flatulence, abdominal pain, and cramping.

A07.3 Isosporiasis

Infection due to Isospora belli and Isospora hominis
Intestinal coccidiosis
Isosporosis

A07.4 Cyclosporiasis

A07.8 Other specified protozoal intestinal diseases

Intestinal microsporidiosis
Intestinal trichomoniasis
Sarcocystosis
Sarcosporidiosis

A07.9 Protozoal intestinal disease, unspecified

Flagellate diarrhea
Protozoal colitis
Protozoal diarrhea
Protozoal dysentery

✓4th A08 Viral and other specified intestinal infections

EXCLUDES 1 *influenza with involvement of gastrointestinal tract (J09.X3, J10.2, J11.2)*

A08.0 Rotaviral enteritis

✓5th A08.1 Acute gastroenteropathy due to Norwalk agent and other small round viruses

A08.11 Acute gastroenteropathy due to Norwalk agent

Acute gastroenteropathy due to Norovirus
Acute gastroenteropathy due to Norwalk-like agent

A08.19 Acute gastroenteropathy due to other small round viruses

Acute gastroenteropathy due to small round virus [SRV] NOS

A08.2 Adenoviral enteritis

✓5th A08.3 Other viral enteritis

A08.31 Calicivirus enteritis

A08.32 Astrovirus enteritis

A08.39 Other viral enteritis

Coxsackie virus enteritis
Echovirus enteritis
Enterovirus enteritis NEC
Torovirus enteritis

A08.4 Viral intestinal infection, unspecified

Viral enteritis NOS
Viral gastroenteritis NOS
Viral gastroenteropathy NOS

AHA: 2016,3Q,12

A08.8 Other specified intestinal infections

A09 Infectious gastroenteritis and colitis, unspecified

Infectious colitis NOS
Infectious enteritis NOS
Infectious gastroenteritis NOS

EXCLUDES 1 *colitis NOS (K52.9)*
diarrhea NOS (R19.7)
enteritis NOS (K52.9)
gastroenteritis NOS (K52.9)
noninfective gastroenteritis and colitis, unspecified (K52.9)

DEF: Colitis: Inflammation of mucous membranes of the colon.
DEF: Enteritis: Inflammation of mucous membranes of the small intestine.
DEF: Gastroenteritis: Inflammation of mucous membranes of the stomach and intestines.

Tuberculosis (A15-A19)

INCLUDES infections due to Mycobacterium tuberculosis and Mycobacterium bovis

EXCLUDES 1 *congenital tuberculosis (P37.Ø)*
nonspecific reaction to test for tuberculosis without active tuberculosis (R76.1-)
pneumoconiosis associated with tuberculosis, any type in A15 (J65)
positive PPD (R76.11)
positive tuberculin skin test without active tuberculosis (R76.11)
sequelae of tuberculosis (B9Ø.-)
silicotuberculosis (J65)

DEF: Bacterial infection that typically spreads by inhalation of an airborne agent that usually attacks the lungs, but may also affect other organs.

✓4th A15 Respiratory tuberculosis

A15.Ø Tuberculosis of lung
Tuberculous bronchiectasis
Tuberculous fibrosis of lung
Tuberculous pneumonia
Tuberculous pneumothorax

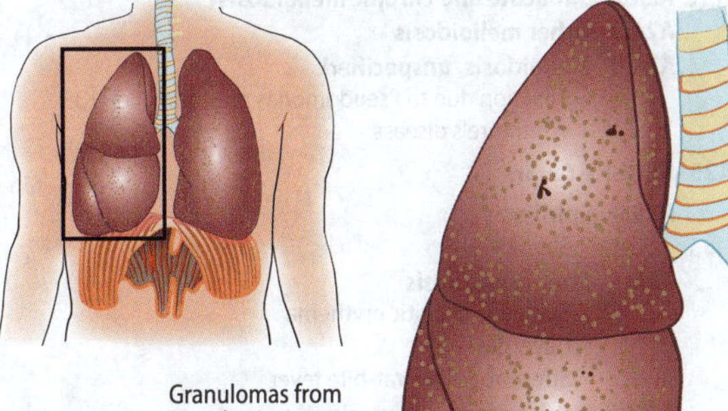

A15.4 Tuberculosis of intrathoracic lymph nodes
Tuberculosis of hilar lymph nodes
Tuberculosis of mediastinal lymph nodes
Tuberculosis of tracheobronchial lymph nodes
EXCLUDES 1 *tuberculosis specified as primary (A15.7)*

A15.5 Tuberculosis of larynx, trachea and bronchus
Tuberculosis of bronchus
Tuberculosis of glottis
Tuberculosis of larynx
Tuberculosis of trachea

A15.6 Tuberculous pleurisy
Tuberculosis of pleura Tuberculous empyema
EXCLUDES 1 *primary respiratory tuberculosis (A15.7)*

A15.7 Primary respiratory tuberculosis

A15.8 Other respiratory tuberculosis
Mediastinal tuberculosis
Nasopharyngeal tuberculosis
Tuberculosis of nose
Tuberculosis of sinus [any nasal]

A15.9 Respiratory tuberculosis unspecified

✓4th A17 Tuberculosis of nervous system

A17.Ø Tuberculous meningitis COM
Tuberculosis of meninges (cerebral)(spinal)
Tuberculous leptomeningitis
EXCLUDES 1 *tuberculous meningoencephalitis (A17.82)*

A17.1 Meningeal tuberculoma COM
Tuberculoma of meninges (cerebral) (spinal)
EXCLUDES 2 *tuberculoma of brain and spinal cord (A17.81)*

✓5th A17.8 Other tuberculosis of nervous system

A17.81 Tuberculoma of brain and spinal cord COM
Tuberculous abscess of brain and spinal cord

A17.82 Tuberculous meningoencephalitis COM
Tuberculous myelitis

A17.83 Tuberculous neuritis COM
Tuberculous mononeuropathy

A17.89 Other tuberculosis of nervous system COM
Tuberculous polyneuropathy

A17.9 Tuberculosis of nervous system, unspecified COM

✓4th A18 Tuberculosis of other organs

✓5th A18.Ø Tuberculosis of bones and joints

A18.Ø1 Tuberculosis of spine
Pott's disease or curvature of spine
Tuberculous arthritis
Tuberculous osteomyelitis of spine
Tuberculous spondylitis

A18.Ø2 Tuberculous arthritis of other joints
Tuberculosis of hip (joint)
Tuberculosis of knee (joint)

A18.Ø3 Tuberculosis of other bones
Tuberculous mastoiditis
Tuberculous osteomyelitis

A18.Ø9 Other musculoskeletal tuberculosis
Tuberculous myositis
Tuberculous synovitis
Tuberculous tenosynovitis

✓5th A18.1 Tuberculosis of genitourinary system

A18.1Ø Tuberculosis of genitourinary system, unspecified

A18.11 Tuberculosis of kidney and ureter

A18.12 Tuberculosis of bladder

A18.13 Tuberculosis of other urinary organs
Tuberculous urethritis

A18.14 Tuberculosis of prostate A ♂

A18.15 Tuberculosis of other male genital organs ♂

A18.16 Tuberculosis of cervix ♀

A18.17 Tuberculous female pelvic inflammatory disease ♀
Tuberculous endometritis
Tuberculous oophoritis and salpingitis

A18.18 Tuberculosis of other female genital organs ♀
Tuberculous ulceration of vulva

A18.2 Tuberculous peripheral lymphadenopathy
Tuberculous adenitis
EXCLUDES 2 *tuberculosis of bronchial and mediastinal lymph nodes (A15.4)*
tuberculosis of mesenteric and retroperitoneal lymph nodes (A18.39)
tuberculous tracheobronchial adenopathy (A15.4)

✓5th A18.3 Tuberculosis of intestines, peritoneum and mesenteric glands

A18.31 Tuberculous peritonitis
Tuberculous ascites
DEF: Tuberculous inflammation of the membrane lining the abdomen.

A18.32 Tuberculous enteritis
Tuberculosis of anus and rectum
Tuberculosis of intestine (large) (small)

A18.39 Retroperitoneal tuberculosis
Tuberculosis of mesenteric glands
Tuberculosis of retroperitoneal (lymph glands)

A18.4 Tuberculosis of skin and subcutaneous tissue
Erythema induratum, tuberculous
Lupus excedens
Lupus vulgaris NOS
Lupus vulgaris of eyelid
Scrofuloderma
Tuberculosis of external ear
EXCLUDES 2 *lupus erythematosus (L93.-)*
systemic lupus erythematosus (M32.-)

✓5th A18.5 Tuberculosis of eye
EXCLUDES 2 *lupus vulgaris of eyelid (A18.4)*

A18.5Ø Tuberculosis of eye, unspecified

A18.51 Tuberculous episcleritis

A18.52 Tuberculous keratitis
Tuberculous interstitial keratitis
Tuberculous keratoconjunctivitis (interstitial) (phlyctenular)

A18.53 Tuberculous chorioretinitis

A18.54 Tuberculous iridocyclitis

A18.59 Other tuberculosis of eye
Tuberculous conjunctivitis

A18.6 Tuberculosis of (inner) (middle) ear
Tuberculous otitis media
EXCLUDES 2 *tuberculosis of external ear (A18.4)*
tuberculous mastoiditis (A18.Ø3)

A18.7 Tuberculosis of adrenal glands
Tuberculous Addison's disease

✓5th **A18.8 Tuberculosis of other specified organs**

A18.81 Tuberculosis of thyroid gland

A18.82 Tuberculosis of other endocrine glands
Tuberculosis of pituitary gland
Tuberculosis of thymus gland

A18.83 Tuberculosis of digestive tract organs, not elsewhere classified
EXCLUDES 1 *tuberculosis of intestine (A18.32)*

A18.84 Tuberculosis of heart
Tuberculous cardiomyopathy
Tuberculous endocarditis
Tuberculous myocarditis
Tuberculous pericarditis

A18.85 Tuberculosis of spleen

A18.89 Tuberculosis of other sites
Tuberculosis of muscle
Tuberculous cerebral arteritis

✓4th **A19 Miliary tuberculosis**
INCLUDES disseminated tuberculosis
generalized tuberculosis
tuberculous polyserositis

A19.Ø Acute miliary tuberculosis of a single specified site

A19.1 Acute miliary tuberculosis of multiple sites

A19.2 Acute miliary tuberculosis, unspecified

A19.8 Other miliary tuberculosis

A19.9 Miliary tuberculosis, unspecified

Certain zoonotic bacterial diseases (A2Ø-A28)

✓4th **A2Ø Plague**
INCLUDES infection due to Yersinia pestis

A2Ø.Ø Bubonic plague

A2Ø.1 Cellulocutaneous plague

A2Ø.2 Pneumonic plague HCC ESR

A2Ø.3 Plague meningitis COM

A2Ø.7 Septicemic plague HCC ESR COM

A2Ø.8 Other forms of plague
Abortive plague
Asymptomatic plague
Pestis minor

A2Ø.9 Plague, unspecified

✓4th **A21 Tularemia**
INCLUDES deer-fly fever
infection due to Francisella tularensis
rabbit fever

DEF: Febrile disease transmitted to humans by the bites of deer flies, fleas, and ticks, by inhaling aerosolized *F. tularensis*, or by ingesting contaminated food or water. Patients quickly develop fever, chills, weakness, headache, backache, and malaise.

A21.Ø Ulceroglandular tularemia

A21.1 Oculoglandular tularemia
Ophthalmic tularemia

A21.2 Pulmonary tularemia HCC ESR

A21.3 Gastrointestinal tularemia
Abdominal tularemia

A21.7 Generalized tularemia

A21.8 Other forms of tularemia

A21.9 Tularemia, unspecified

✓4th **A22 Anthrax**
INCLUDES infection due to Bacillus anthracis

A22.Ø Cutaneous anthrax
Malignant carbuncle
Malignant pustule

A22.1 Pulmonary anthrax HCC ESR
Inhalation anthrax
Ragpicker's disease
Woolsorter's disease

A22.2 Gastrointestinal anthrax

A22.7 Anthrax sepsis HCC ESR COM

A22.8 Other forms of anthrax
Anthrax meningitis

A22.9 Anthrax, unspecified

✓4th **A23 Brucellosis**
INCLUDES Malta fever
Mediterranean fever
undulant fever

A23.Ø Brucellosis due to Brucella melitensis

A23.1 Brucellosis due to Brucella abortus

A23.2 Brucellosis due to Brucella suis

A23.3 Brucellosis due to Brucella canis

A23.8 Other brucellosis

A23.9 Brucellosis, unspecified

✓4th **A24 Glanders and melioidosis**

A24.Ø Glanders
Infection due to Pseudomonas mallei
Malleus

A24.1 Acute and fulminating melioidosis
Melioidosis pneumonia
Melioidosis sepsis

A24.2 Subacute and chronic melioidosis

A24.3 Other melioidosis

A24.9 Melioidosis, unspecified
Infection due to Pseudomonas pseudomallei NOS
Whitmore's disease

✓4th **A25 Rat-bite fevers**

A25.Ø Spirillosis
Sodoku

A25.1 Streptobacillosis
Epidemic arthritic erythema
Haverhill fever
Streptobacillary rat-bite fever

A25.9 Rat-bite fever, unspecified

✓4th **A26 Erysipeloid**
DEF: Acute cutaneous infection typically caused by trauma to the skin. Presenting as cellulitis, it may become systemic, affecting other organs. It is a gram-positive bacillus and mainly acquired by those who routinely handle meat.

A26.Ø Cutaneous erysipeloid
Erythema migrans

A26.7 Erysipelothrix sepsis HCC ESR COM

A26.8 Other forms of erysipeloid

A26.9 Erysipeloid, unspecified

✓4th **A27 Leptospirosis**

A27.Ø Leptospirosis icterohemorrhagica
Leptospiral or spirochetal jaundice (hemorrhagic)
Weil's disease

✓5th **A27.8 Other forms of leptospirosis**

A27.81 Aseptic meningitis in leptospirosis COM

A27.89 Other forms of leptospirosis

A27.9 Leptospirosis, unspecified

✓4th **A28 Other zoonotic bacterial diseases, not elsewhere classified**

A28.Ø Pasteurellosis

A28.1 Cat-scratch disease
Cat-scratch fever

A28.2 Extraintestinal yersiniosis
EXCLUDES 1 *enteritis due to Yersinia enterocolitica (AØ4.6)*
plague (A2Ø.-)

A28.8 Other specified zoonotic bacterial diseases, not elsewhere classified

A28.9 Zoonotic bacterial disease, unspecified

Other bacterial diseases (A3Ø-A49)

AHA: 2016,3Q,8-14

✓4th **A3Ø Leprosy [Hansen's disease]**
INCLUDES infection due to Mycobacterium leprae
EXCLUDES 1 *sequelae of leprosy (B92)*

A3Ø.Ø Indeterminate leprosy
I leprosy

A3Ø.1 Tuberculoid leprosy
TT leprosy

A30.2 Borderline tuberculoid leprosy
BT leprosy

A30.3 Borderline leprosy
BB leprosy

A30.4 Borderline lepromatous leprosy
BL leprosy

A30.5 Lepromatous leprosy
LL leprosy

A30.8 Other forms of leprosy

A30.9 Leprosy, unspecified

A31 Infection due to other mycobacteria (4th)
EXCLUDES 2 *leprosy (A30.-)*
tuberculosis (A15-A19)

A31.0 Pulmonary mycobacterial infection HCC Rx ESR COM
Infection due to Mycobacterium avium
Infection due to Mycobacterium intracellulare [Battey bacillus]
Infection due to Mycobacterium kansasii

A31.1 Cutaneous mycobacterial infection
Buruli ulcer
Infection due to Mycobacterium marinum
Infection due to Mycobacterium ulcerans

A31.2 Disseminated mycobacterium avium-intracellulare complex (DMAC) HCC Rx ESR COM
MAC sepsis

A31.8 Other mycobacterial infections

A31.9 Mycobacterial infection, unspecified
Atypical mycobacterial infection NOS
Mycobacteriosis NOS

A32 Listeriosis (4th)
INCLUDES listerial foodborne infection
EXCLUDES 1 *neonatal (disseminated) listeriosis (P37.2)*

A32.0 Cutaneous listeriosis

A32.1 Listerial meningitis and meningoencephalitis (5th)

A32.11 Listerial meningitis COM

A32.12 Listerial meningoencephalitis COM

A32.7 Listerial sepsis HCC ESR COM

A32.8 Other forms of listeriosis (5th)

A32.81 Oculoglandular listeriosis

A32.82 Listerial endocarditis COM

A32.89 Other forms of listeriosis
Listerial cerebral arteritis

A32.9 Listeriosis, unspecified

A33 Tetanus neonatorum N

A34 Obstetrical tetanus COM M ♀

A35 Other tetanus COM
Tetanus NOS
EXCLUDES 1 *obstetrical tetanus (A34)*
tetanus neonatorum (A33)

DEF: Tetanus: Acute, often fatal, infectious disease caused by the anaerobic, spore-forming bacillus *Clostridium tetani*. The bacillus enters the body through a contaminated wound, burns, surgical wounds, or cutaneous ulcers. Symptoms include lockjaw, spasms, seizures, and paralysis.

A36 Diphtheria (4th)

A36.0 Pharyngeal diphtheria
Diphtheritic membranous angina
Tonsillar diphtheria

A36.1 Nasopharyngeal diphtheria

A36.2 Laryngeal diphtheria
Diphtheritic laryngotracheitis

A36.3 Cutaneous diphtheria
EXCLUDES 2 *erythrasma (L08.1)*

A36.8 Other diphtheria (5th)

A36.81 Diphtheritic cardiomyopathy HCC Rx ESR COM
Diphtheritic myocarditis

A36.82 Diphtheritic radiculomyelitis

A36.83 Diphtheritic polyneuritis

A36.84 Diphtheritic tubulo-interstitial nephropathy

A36.85 Diphtheritic cystitis

A36.86 Diphtheritic conjunctivitis

A36.89 Other diphtheritic complications
Diphtheritic peritonitis

A36.9 Diphtheria, unspecified

A37 Whooping cough (4th)

DEF: Acute, highly contagious respiratory tract infection caused by *Bordetella pertussis* and *B. bronchiseptica.* Whooping cough is known by its characteristic paroxysmal cough.

A37.0 Whooping cough due to Bordetella pertussis (5th)

A37.00 Whooping cough due to Bordetella pertussis without pneumonia
Paroxysmal cough due to Bordetella pertussis without pneumonia

A37.01 Whooping cough due to Bordetella pertussis with pneumonia
Paroxysmal cough due to Bordetella pertussis with pneumonia

A37.1 Whooping cough due to Bordetella parapertussis (5th)

A37.10 Whooping cough due to Bordetella parapertussis without pneumonia

A37.11 Whooping cough due to Bordetella parapertussis with pneumonia

A37.8 Whooping cough due to other Bordetella species (5th)

A37.80 Whooping cough due to other Bordetella species without pneumonia

A37.81 Whooping cough due to other Bordetella species with pneumonia

A37.9 Whooping cough, unspecified species (5th)

A37.90 Whooping cough, unspecified species without pneumonia

A37.91 Whooping cough, unspecified species with pneumonia

A38 Scarlet fever (4th)
INCLUDES scarlatina
EXCLUDES 2 *streptococcal sore throat (J02.0)*

DEF: Acute contagious disease caused by Group A bacteria, the same bacterium that causes strep throat. Individuals with strep throat can develop scarlet fever particularly if the infection is not treated with antibiotics. It is characterized by a red blush to the skin of the chest and abdomen and swelling of the nose, throat, and mouth.

A38.0 Scarlet fever with otitis media

A38.1 Scarlet fever with myocarditis COM

A38.8 Scarlet fever with other complications

A38.9 Scarlet fever, uncomplicated
Scarlet fever, NOS

A39 Meningococcal infection (4th)

DEF: Condition caused by *Neisseria meningitidis*, a bacteria that may invade the spinal cord, brain, heart, joints, optic nerve, or bloodstream.

A39.0 Meningococcal meningitis COM

A39.1 Waterhouse-Friderichsen syndrome HCC Rx ESR COM
Meningococcal hemorrhagic adrenalitis
Meningococcic adrenal syndrome

A39.2 Acute meningococcemia HCC ESR COM

A39.3 Chronic meningococcemia HCC ESR COM

A39.4 Meningococcemia, unspecified HCC ESR COM

A39.5 Meningococcal heart disease (5th)

A39.50 Meningococcal carditis, unspecified COM

A39.51 Meningococcal endocarditis COM

A39.52 Meningococcal myocarditis COM

A39.53 Meningococcal pericarditis COM

A39.8 Other meningococcal infections (5th)

A39.81 Meningococcal encephalitis COM

A39.82 Meningococcal retrobulbar neuritis

A39.83 Meningococcal arthritis HCC ESR COM

A39.84 Postmeningococcal arthritis HCC ESR COM

A39.89 Other meningococcal infections
Meningococcal conjunctivitis

A39.9 Meningococcal infection, unspecified
Meningococcal disease NOS

A40 Streptococcal sepsis

Code first:
postprocedural streptococcal sepsis (T81.4-)
streptococcal sepsis during labor (O75.3)
streptococcal sepsis following abortion or ectopic or molar pregnancy (O03-O07, O08.0)
streptococcal sepsis following immunization (T88.0)
streptococcal sepsis following infusion, transfusion or therapeutic injection (T80.2-)

EXCLUDES 1 *neonatal (P36.0-P36.1)*
puerperal sepsis (O85)
sepsis due to Streptococcus, group D (A41.81)

AHA: 2020,2Q,8,28; 2019,4Q,65; 2018,4Q,89; 2018,1Q,16; 2016,1Q,32

A40.0 Sepsis due to streptococcus, group A HCC ESR COM

A40.1 Sepsis due to streptococcus, group B HCC ESR COM
AHA: 2019,1Q,14

A40.3 Sepsis due to Streptococcus pneumoniae HCC ESR COM
Pneumococcal sepsis

A40.8 Other streptococcal sepsis HCC ESR COM

A40.9 Streptococcal sepsis, unspecified HCC ESR COM

A41 Other sepsis

Code first:
postprocedural sepsis (T81.4-)
sepsis during labor (O75.3)
sepsis following abortion, ectopic or molar pregnancy (O03-O07, O08.0)
sepsis following immunization (T88.0)
sepsis following infusion, transfusion or therapeutic injection (T80.2-)

EXCLUDES 1 *bacteremia NOS (R78.81)*
neonatal (P36.-)
puerperal sepsis (O85)
streptococcal sepsis (A40.-)

EXCLUDES 2 *sepsis (due to) (in) actinomycotic (A42.7)*
sepsis (due to) (in) anthrax (A22.7)
sepsis (due to) (in) candidal (B37.7)
sepsis (due to) (in) Erysipelothrix (A26.7)
sepsis (due to) (in) extraintestinal yersiniosis (A28.2)
sepsis (due to) (in) gonococcal (A54.86)
sepsis (due to) (in) herpesviral (B00.7)
sepsis (due to) (in) listerial (A32.7)
sepsis (due to) (in) melioidosis (A24.1)
sepsis (due to) (in) meningococcal (A39.2-A39.4)
sepsis (due to) (in) plague (A20.7)
sepsis (due to) (in) tularemia (A21.7)
toxic shock syndrome (A48.3)

AHA: 2020,2Q,8,28; 2019,4Q,65; 2019,3Q,17; 2018,4Q,18; 2018,1Q,16; 2016,1Q,32; 2014,2Q,13

A41.0 Sepsis due to Staphylococcus aureus

A41.01 Sepsis due to Methicillin susceptible Staphylococcus aureus HCC ESR COM
MSSA sepsis
Staphylococcus aureus sepsis NOS
AHA: 2020,2Q,17

A41.02 Sepsis due to Methicillin resistant Staphylococcus aureus HCC ESR COM

A41.1 Sepsis due to other specified staphylococcus HCC ESR COM
Coagulase negative staphylococcus sepsis

A41.2 Sepsis due to unspecified staphylococcus HCC ESR COM

A41.3 Sepsis due to Hemophilus influenzae HCC ESR COM

A41.4 Sepsis due to anaerobes HCC ESR COM
EXCLUDES 1 *gas gangrene (A48.0)*

A41.5 Sepsis due to other Gram-negative organisms

A41.50 Gram-negative sepsis, unspecified HCC ESR COM
Gram-negative sepsis NOS
AHA: 2020,2Q,28

A41.51 Sepsis due to Escherichia coli [E. coli] HCC ESR COM
AHA: 2020,2Q,17

A41.52 Sepsis due to Pseudomonas HCC ESR COM
Pseudomonas aeroginosa

A41.53 Sepsis due to Serratia HCC ESR COM

A41.59 Other Gram-negative sepsis HCC ESR COM

A41.8 Other specified sepsis

A41.81 Sepsis due to Enterococcus HCC ESR COM
TIP: *E. faecium,* is a species of *Enterococcus* that is highly resistant to multiple antibiotics. Assign a code from category Z16 when resistance to antimicrobial drugs is documented.

A41.89 Other specified sepsis HCC ESR COM
AHA: 2020,2Q,8; 2017,1Q,51; 2016,3Q,8-14

A41.9 Sepsis, unspecified organism HCC ESR COM
Septicemia NOS
AHA: 2022,2Q,5; 2022,1Q,35; 2020,2Q,28

A42 Actinomycosis

EXCLUDES 1 *actinomycetoma (B47.1)*

A42.0 Pulmonary actinomycosis HCC ESR

A42.1 Abdominal actinomycosis

A42.2 Cervicofacial actinomycosis

A42.7 Actinomycotic sepsis HCC ESR COM

A42.8 Other forms of actinomycosis

A42.81 Actinomycotic meningitis COM

A42.82 Actinomycotic encephalitis COM

A42.89 Other forms of actinomycosis

A42.9 Actinomycosis, unspecified

A43 Nocardiosis

DEF: Rare bacterial infection occurring most often in those with weakened immune systems. Can be acquired in soil, decaying plants, or standing water. It typically begins in the lungs and has a tendency to spread to other body systems.

A43.0 Pulmonary nocardiosis HCC ESR

A43.1 Cutaneous nocardiosis

A43.8 Other forms of nocardiosis

A43.9 Nocardiosis, unspecified

A44 Bartonellosis

A44.0 Systemic bartonellosis
Oroya fever

A44.1 Cutaneous and mucocutaneous bartonellosis
Verruga peruana

A44.8 Other forms of bartonellosis

A44.9 Bartonellosis, unspecified

A46 Erysipelas

EXCLUDES 1 *postpartum or puerperal erysipelas (O86.89)*

DEF: Skin infection affecting the upper dermis and superficial dermal lymphatics. Lesion edges are well-demarcated with distinct raised borders. It is often caused by group A *Streptococci.*

A48 Other bacterial diseases, not elsewhere classified

EXCLUDES 1 *actinomycetoma (B47.1)*

A48.0 Gas gangrene HCC ESR COM
Clostridial cellulitis
Clostridial myonecrosis
AHA: 2017,4Q,102

A48.1 Legionnaires' disease HCC ESR COM
DEF: Severe and often fatal infection by *Legionella pneumophila.* Symptoms include high fever, gastrointestinal pain, headache, myalgia, dry cough, and pneumonia and it is usually transmitted through airborne water droplets via air conditioning systems or hot tubs.

A48.2 Nonpneumonic Legionnaires' disease [Pontiac fever]

A48.3 Toxic shock syndrome HCC ESR COM
Use additional code to identify the organism (B95, B96)
EXCLUDES 1 *endotoxic shock NOS (R57.8)*
sepsis NOS (A41.9)
AHA: 2022,1Q,35
DEF: Bacteria producing an endotoxin, such as *Staphylococci,* flood the body with the toxins producing a high fever, vomiting and diarrhea, decreasing blood pressure, a skin rash, and shock. ***Synonym(s):*** *TSS.*

A48.4 Brazilian purpuric fever
Systemic Hemophilus aegyptius infection

A48.5 Other specified botulism
Non-foodborne intoxication due to toxins of Clostridium botulinum [C. botulinum]
EXCLUDES 1 *food poisoning due to toxins of Clostridium botulinum (A05.1)*

A48.51 Infant botulism P

A48.52 **Wound botulism**
Non-foodborne botulism NOS
Use additional code for associated wound

A48.8 **Other specified bacterial diseases**

A49 **Bacterial infection of unspecified site**

EXCLUDES 1 *bacterial agents as the cause of diseases classified elsewhere (B95-B96)*
chlamydial infection NOS (A74.9)
meningococcal infection NOS (A39.9)
rickettsial infection NOS (A79.9)
spirochetal infection NOS (A69.9)

A49.0 **Staphylococcal infection, unspecified site**

A49.01 **Methicillin susceptible Staphylococcus aureus infection, unspecified site**
Methicillin susceptible Staphylococcus aureus (MSSA) infection
Staphylococcus aureus infection NOS

A49.02 **Methicillin resistant Staphylococcus aureus infection, unspecified site**
Methicillin resistant Staphylococcus aureus (MRSA) infection

A49.1 **Streptococcal infection, unspecified site**

A49.2 **Hemophilus influenzae infection, unspecified site**

A49.3 **Mycoplasma infection, unspecified site**

A49.8 **Other bacterial infections of unspecified site**

A49.9 **Bacterial infection, unspecified**
EXCLUDES 1 *bacteremia NOS (R78.81)*

Infections with a predominantly sexual mode of transmission (A50-A64)

EXCLUDES 1 *human immunodeficiency virus [HIV] disease (B20)*
nonspecific and nongonococcal urethritis (N34.1)
Reiter's disease (M02.3-)

AHA: 2021,2Q,6

A50 **Congenital syphilis**

A50.0 **Early congenital syphilis, symptomatic**
Any congenital syphilitic condition specified as early or manifest less than two years after birth.

A50.01 **Early congenital syphilitic oculopathy**
A50.02 **Early congenital syphilitic osteochondropathy**
A50.03 **Early congenital syphilitic pharyngitis**
Early congenital syphilitic laryngitis
A50.04 **Early congenital syphilitic pneumonia** COM
A50.05 **Early congenital syphilitic rhinitis**
A50.06 **Early cutaneous congenital syphilis**
A50.07 **Early mucocutaneous congenital syphilis**
A50.08 **Early visceral congenital syphilis**
A50.09 **Other early congenital syphilis, symptomatic**

A50.1 **Early congenital syphilis, latent**
Congenital syphilis without clinical manifestations, with positive serological reaction and negative spinal fluid test, less than two years after birth.

A50.2 **Early congenital syphilis, unspecified**
Congenital syphilis NOS less than two years after birth.

A50.3 **Late congenital syphilitic oculopathy**
EXCLUDES 1 *Hutchinson's triad (A50.53)*

A50.30 **Late congenital syphilitic oculopathy, unspecified**
A50.31 **Late congenital syphilitic interstitial keratitis**
A50.32 **Late congenital syphilitic chorioretinitis**
A50.39 **Other late congenital syphilitic oculopathy**

A50.4 **Late congenital neurosyphilis [juvenile neurosyphilis]**
Use additional code to identify any associated mental disorder
EXCLUDES 1 *Hutchinson's triad (A50.53)*

A50.40 **Late congenital neurosyphilis, unspecified** COM
Juvenile neurosyphilis NOS
A50.41 **Late congenital syphilitic meningitis** COM
A50.42 **Late congenital syphilitic encephalitis** COM
A50.43 **Late congenital syphilitic polyneuropathy** COM
A50.44 **Late congenital syphilitic optic nerve atrophy** COM
A50.45 **Juvenile general paresis** COM
Dementia paralytica juvenilis
Juvenile tabetoparetic neurosyphilis
A50.49 **Other late congenital neurosyphilis** COM
Juvenile tabes dorsalis

A50.5 **Other late congenital syphilis, symptomatic**
Any congenital syphilitic condition specified as late or manifest two years or more after birth.

A50.51 **Clutton's joints**
A50.52 **Hutchinson's teeth**
A50.53 **Hutchinson's triad**
A50.54 **Late congenital cardiovascular syphilis** COM
A50.55 **Late congenital syphilitic arthropathy** HCC ESR COM
A50.56 **Late congenital syphilitic osteochondropathy**
A50.57 **Syphilitic saddle nose**
A50.59 **Other late congenital syphilis, symptomatic**

A50.6 **Late congenital syphilis, latent**
Congenital syphilis without clinical manifestations, with positive serological reaction and negative spinal fluid test, two years or more after birth.

A50.7 **Late congenital syphilis, unspecified**
Congenital syphilis NOS two years or more after birth.

A50.9 **Congenital syphilis, unspecified**

A51 **Early syphilis**

DEF: Syphilis: Sexually transmitted disease caused by the *Treponema pallidum* spirochete. Syphilis usually exhibits cutaneous manifestations and may exist for years without symptoms.

A51.0 **Primary genital syphilis**
Syphilitic chancre NOS

A51.1 **Primary anal syphilis**

A51.2 **Primary syphilis of other sites**

A51.3 **Secondary syphilis of skin and mucous membranes**
DEF: Transitory or chronic cutaneous eruptions that present within two to 10 weeks following an initial syphilis infection that may include nontender lymphadenopathy along with alopecia and condylomata lata.

A51.31 **Condyloma latum**
A51.32 **Syphilitic alopecia**
A51.39 **Other secondary syphilis of skin**
Syphilitic leukoderma
Syphilitic mucous patch
EXCLUDES 1 *late syphilitic leukoderma (A52.79)*

A51.4 **Other secondary syphilis**

A51.41 **Secondary syphilitic meningitis** COM
A51.42 **Secondary syphilitic female pelvic disease** ♀
A51.43 **Secondary syphilitic oculopathy**
Secondary syphilitic chorioretinitis
Secondary syphilitic iridocyclitis, iritis
Secondary syphilitic uveitis
A51.44 **Secondary syphilitic nephritis**
A51.45 **Secondary syphilitic hepatitis**
A51.46 **Secondary syphilitic osteopathy**
A51.49 **Other secondary syphilitic conditions**
Secondary syphilitic lymphadenopathy
Secondary syphilitic myositis

A51.5 **Early syphilis, latent**
Syphilis (acquired) without clinical manifestations, with positive serological reaction and negative spinal fluid test, less than two years after infection.

A51.9 **Early syphilis, unspecified**

A52 **Late syphilis**

A52.0 **Cardiovascular and cerebrovascular syphilis**

A52.00 **Cardiovascular syphilis, unspecified** COM
A52.01 **Syphilitic aneurysm of aorta** COM
A52.02 **Syphilitic aortitis** COM
A52.03 **Syphilitic endocarditis** COM
Syphilitic aortic valve incompetence or stenosis
Syphilitic mitral valve stenosis
Syphilitic pulmonary valve regurgitation
A52.04 **Syphilitic cerebral arteritis**
A52.05 **Other cerebrovascular syphilis** COM
Syphilitic cerebral aneurysm (ruptured) (non-ruptured)
Syphilitic cerebral thrombosis

A52.Ø6 **Other syphilitic heart involvement** COM
Syphilitic coronary artery disease
Syphilitic myocarditis
Syphilitic pericarditis

A52.Ø9 **Other cardiovascular syphilis** COM

✓5th A52.1 **Symptomatic neurosyphilis**

A52.1Ø **Symptomatic neurosyphilis, unspecified** COM

A52.11 **Tabes dorsalis** COM
Locomotor ataxia (progressive)
Tabetic neurosyphilis

A52.12 **Other cerebrospinal syphilis** COM

A52.13 **Late syphilitic meningitis** COM

A52.14 **Late syphilitic encephalitis** COM

A52.15 **Late syphilitic neuropathy** COM
Late syphilitic acoustic neuritis
Late syphilitic optic (nerve) atrophy
Late syphilitic polyneuropathy
Late syphilitic retrobulbar neuritis

A52.16 **Charcôt's arthropathy (tabetic)** COM
DEF: Progressive neurologic arthropathy in which chronic degeneration of joints in the weight-bearing areas with peripheral hypertrophy occurs as a complication of a neuropathy disorder. Supporting structures relax from a loss of sensation resulting in chronic joint instability.

A52.17 **General paresis** COM
Dementia paralytica

A52.19 **Other symptomatic neurosyphilis** COM
Syphilitic parkinsonism

A52.2 **Asymptomatic neurosyphilis** COM

A52.3 **Neurosyphilis, unspecified** COM
Gumma (syphilitic)
Syphilis (late)
Syphiloma
AHA: 2021,2Q,6

✓5th A52.7 **Other symptomatic late syphilis**

A52.71 **Late syphilitic oculopathy**
Late syphilitic chorioretinitis
Late syphilitic episcleritis

A52.72 **Syphilis of lung and bronchus**

A52.73 **Symptomatic late syphilis of other respiratory organs**

A52.74 **Syphilis of liver and other viscera**
Late syphilitic peritonitis

A52.75 **Syphilis of kidney and ureter**
Syphilitic glomerular disease

A52.76 **Other genitourinary symptomatic late syphilis**
Late syphilitic female pelvic inflammatory disease

A52.77 **Syphilis of bone and joint**

A52.78 **Syphilis of other musculoskeletal tissue**
Late syphilitic bursitis
Syphilis [stage unspecified] of bursa
Syphilis [stage unspecified] of muscle
Syphilis [stage unspecified] of synovium
Syphilis [stage unspecified] of tendon

A52.79 **Other symptomatic late syphilis**
Late syphilitic leukoderma
Syphilis of adrenal gland
Syphilis of pituitary gland
Syphilis of thyroid gland
Syphilitic splenomegaly
EXCLUDES 1 *syphilitic leukoderma (secondary) (A51.39)*

A52.8 **Late syphilis, latent**
Syphilis (acquired) without clinical manifestations, with positive serological reaction and negative spinal fluid test, two years or more after infection

A52.9 **Late syphilis, unspecified**

✓4th **A53 Other and unspecified syphilis**

A53.Ø **Latent syphilis, unspecified as early or late**
Latent syphilis NOS
Positive serological reaction for syphilis

A53.9 **Syphilis, unspecified**
Infection due to Treponema pallidum NOS
Syphilis (acquired) NOS
EXCLUDES 1 *syphilis NOS under two years of age (A5Ø.2)*

✓4th **A54 Gonococcal infection**
DEF: Sexually transmitted bacterial infection caused by *Neisseria gonorrhoeae*. Women are often asymptomatic, while men tend to develop urinary symptoms quickly.

✓5th A54.Ø **Gonococcal infection of lower genitourinary tract without periurethral or accessory gland abscess**
EXCLUDES 1 *gonococcal infection with genitourinary gland abscess (A54.1)*
gonococcal infection with periurethral abscess (A54.1)

A54.ØØ **Gonococcal infection of lower genitourinary tract, unspecified**

A54.Ø1 **Gonococcal cystitis and urethritis, unspecified**

A54.Ø2 **Gonococcal vulvovaginitis, unspecified** ♀

A54.Ø3 **Gonococcal cervicitis, unspecified** ♀

A54.Ø9 **Other gonococcal infection of lower genitourinary tract**

A54.1 **Gonococcal infection of lower genitourinary tract with periurethral and accessory gland abscess**
Gonococcal Bartholin's gland abscess

✓5th A54.2 **Gonococcal pelviperitonitis and other gonococcal genitourinary infection**

A54.21 **Gonococcal infection of kidney and ureter**

A54.22 **Gonococcal prostatitis** ♂

A54.23 **Gonococcal infection of other male genital organs** ♂
Gonococcal epididymitis
Gonococcal orchitis

A54.24 **Gonococcal female pelvic inflammatory disease** ♀
Gonococcal pelviperitonitis
EXCLUDES 1 *gonococcal peritonitis (A54.85)*

A54.29 **Other gonococcal genitourinary infections**

✓5th A54.3 **Gonococcal infection of eye**

A54.3Ø **Gonococcal infection of eye, unspecified**

A54.31 **Gonococcal conjunctivitis**
Ophthalmia neonatorum due to gonococcus

A54.32 **Gonococcal iridocyclitis**

A54.33 **Gonococcal keratitis**

A54.39 **Other gonococcal eye infection**
Gonococcal endophthalmia

✓5th A54.4 **Gonococcal infection of musculoskeletal system**

A54.4Ø **Gonococcal infection of musculoskeletal system, unspecified** HCC ESR COM

A54.41 **Gonococcal spondylopathy** HCC ESR COM

A54.42 **Gonococcal arthritis** HCC ESR COM
EXCLUDES 2 *gonococcal infection of spine (A54.41)*

A54.43 **Gonococcal osteomyelitis** HCC ESR COM
EXCLUDES 2 *gonococcal infection of spine (A54.41)*

A54.49 **Gonococcal infection of other musculoskeletal tissue** HCC ESR COM
Gonococcal bursitis
Gonococcal myositis
Gonococcal synovitis
Gonococcal tenosynovitis

A54.5 **Gonococcal pharyngitis**

A54.6 **Gonococcal infection of anus and rectum**

✓5th A54.8 **Other gonococcal infections**

A54.81 **Gonococcal meningitis** COM

A54.82 **Gonococcal brain abscess** COM

A54.83 **Gonococcal heart infection** COM
Gonococcal endocarditis
Gonococcal myocarditis
Gonococcal pericarditis

A54.84 **Gonococcal pneumonia** HCC ESR

A54.85 **Gonococcal peritonitis** HCC ESR COM
EXCLUDES 1 *gonococcal pelviperitonitis (A54.24)*

A54.86 **Gonococcal sepsis** HCC ESR COM

A54.89 **Other gonococcal infections**
Gonococcal keratoderma
Gonococcal lymphadenitis

A54.9 **Gonococcal infection, unspecified**

A55 Chlamydial lymphogranuloma (venereum)
Climatic or tropical bubo
Durand-Nicolas-Favre disease
Esthiomene
Lymphogranuloma inguinale

A56 Other sexually transmitted chlamydial diseases
INCLUDES sexually transmitted diseases due to Chlamydia trachomatis
EXCLUDES 1 *neonatal chlamydial conjunctivitis (P39.1)*
neonatal chlamydial pneumonia (P23.1)
EXCLUDES 2 *chlamydial lymphogranuloma (A55)*
conditions classified to A74.-

DEF: *Chlamydia trachomatis*: Bacterium that causes a common venereal disease. Symptoms of chlamydia are usually mild or absent, however, serious complications may cause irreversible damage, including cystitis, pelvic inflammatory disease, and infertility in women and discharge from the penis, prostatitis, and infertility in men. Genital chlamydial infection can cause arthritis, skin lesions, and inflammation of the eye and urethra.
Synonym(s): *Reiter's syndrome.*

A56.Ø Chlamydial infection of lower genitourinary tract
A56.ØØ Chlamydial infection of lower genitourinary tract, unspecified
A56.Ø1 Chlamydial cystitis and urethritis
A56.Ø2 Chlamydial vulvovaginitis ♀
A56.Ø9 Other chlamydial infection of lower genitourinary tract
Chlamydial cervicitis

A56.1 Chlamydial infection of pelviperitoneum and other genitourinary organs
A56.11 Chlamydial female pelvic inflammatory disease ♀
A56.19 Other chlamydial genitourinary infection
Chlamydial epididymitis
Chlamydial orchitis

A56.2 Chlamydial infection of genitourinary tract, unspecified
A56.3 Chlamydial infection of anus and rectum
A56.4 Chlamydial infection of pharynx
A56.8 Sexually transmitted chlamydial infection of other sites

A57 Chancroid
Ulcus molle
DEF: Localized infection by *Haemophilus ducreyi*, causing genital ulcers and infecting the inguinal lymph nodes.

A58 Granuloma inguinale
Donovanosis

A59 Trichomoniasis
EXCLUDES 2 *intestinal trichomoniasis (AØ7.8)*
DEF: Infection with the parasitic, flagellated protozoa of the genus *Trichomonas*. This protozoon is found in the intestinal and genitourinary tracts of humans and in the mouth around tartar, cavities, and areas of periodontal disease.

A59.Ø Urogenital trichomoniasis
A59.ØØ Urogenital trichomoniasis, unspecified
Fluor (vaginalis) due to Trichomonas
Leukorrhea (vaginalis) due to Trichomonas
A59.Ø1 Trichomonal vulvovaginitis ♀
A59.Ø2 Trichomonal prostatitis ♂
A59.Ø3 Trichomonal cystitis and urethritis
A59.Ø9 Other urogenital trichomoniasis
Trichomonas cervicitis
A59.8 Trichomoniasis of other sites
A59.9 Trichomoniasis, unspecified

AØ6Ø Anogenital herpesviral [herpes simplex] infections

A6Ø.Ø Herpesviral infection of genitalia and urogenital tract
A6Ø.ØØ Herpesviral infection of urogenital system, unspecified
A6Ø.Ø1 Herpesviral infection of penis ♂
A6Ø.Ø2 Herpesviral infection of other male genital organs ♂
A6Ø.Ø3 Herpesviral cervicitis ♀
A6Ø.Ø4 Herpesviral vulvovaginitis ♀
Herpesviral [herpes simplex] ulceration
Herpesviral [herpes simplex] vaginitis
Herpesviral [herpes simplex] vulvitis
A6Ø.Ø9 Herpesviral infection of other urogenital tract
AHA: 2020,1Q,20
A6Ø.1 Herpesviral infection of perianal skin and rectum
A6Ø.9 Anogenital herpesviral infection, unspecified

A63 Other predominantly sexually transmitted diseases, not elsewhere classified
EXCLUDES 2 *molluscum contagiosum (BØ8.1)*
papilloma of cervix (D26.Ø)
A63.Ø Anogenital (venereal) warts
Anogenital warts due to (human) papillomavirus [HPV]
Condyloma acuminatum
A63.8 Other specified predominantly sexually transmitted diseases

A64 Unspecified sexually transmitted disease

Other spirochetal diseases (A65-A69)

EXCLUDES 2 *leptospirosis (A27.-)*
syphilis (A5Ø-A53)

A65 Nonvenereal syphilis
Bejel
Endemic syphilis
Njovera

A66 Yaws
INCLUDES bouba
frambesia (tropica)
pian
A66.Ø Initial lesions of yaws
Chancre of yaws
Frambesia, initial or primary
Initial frambesial ulcer
Mother yaw
A66.1 Multiple papillomata and wet crab yaws
Frambesioma
Pianoma
Plantar or palmar papilloma of yaws
A66.2 Other early skin lesions of yaws
Cutaneous yaws, less than five years after infection
Early yaws (cutaneous) (macular) (maculopapular) (micropapular) (papular)
Frambeside of early yaws
A66.3 Hyperkeratosis of yaws
Ghoul hand
Hyperkeratosis, palmar or plantar (early) (late) due to yaws
Worm-eaten soles
A66.4 Gummata and ulcers of yaws
Gummatous frambeside
Nodular late yaws (ulcerated)
A66.5 Gangosa
Rhinopharyngitis mutilans
A66.6 Bone and joint lesions of yaws HCC ESR COM
Yaws ganglion
Yaws goundou
Yaws gumma, bone
Yaws gummatous osteitis or periostitis
Yaws hydrarthrosis
Yaws osteitis
Yaws periostitis (hypertrophic)
A66.7 Other manifestations of yaws
Juxta-articular nodules of yaws
Mucosal yaws
A66.8 Latent yaws
Yaws without clinical manifestations, with positive serology
A66.9 Yaws, unspecified

A67 Pinta [carate]
A67.Ø Primary lesions of pinta
Chancre (primary) of pinta
Papule (primary) of pinta
A67.1 Intermediate lesions of pinta
Erythematous plaques of pinta
Hyperchromic lesions of pinta
Hyperkeratosis of pinta
Pintids
A67.2 Late lesions of pinta
Achromic skin lesions of pinta
Cicatricial skin lesions of pinta
Dyschromic skin lesions of pinta
A67.3 Mixed lesions of pinta
Achromic with hyperchromic skin lesions of pinta [carate]
A67.9 Pinta, unspecified

4th **A68 Relapsing fevers**

INCLUDES recurrent fever

EXCLUDES 2 *Lyme disease (A69.2-)*

A68.0 Louse-borne relapsing fever
Relapsing fever due to Borrelia recurrentis

A68.1 Tick-borne relapsing fever
Relapsing fever due to any Borrelia species other than Borrelia recurrentis

A68.9 Relapsing fever, unspecified

4th **A69 Other spirochetal infections**

A69.0 Necrotizing ulcerative stomatitis
Cancrum oris
Fusospirochetal gangrene
Noma
Stomatitis gangrenosa

A69.1 Other Vincent's infections
Fusospirochetal pharyngitis
Necrotizing ulcerative (acute) gingivitis
Necrotizing ulcerative (acute) gingivostomatitis
Spirochetal stomatitis
Trench mouth
Vincent's angina
Vincent's gingivitis

5th **A69.2 Lyme disease**
Erythema chronicum migrans due to Borrelia burgdorferi
DEF: Recurrent multisystem disorder through tick bites that begins with lesions of erythema chronicum migrans and is followed by arthritis of the large joints, myalgia, malaise, and neurological and cardiac manifestations.

A69.20 Lyme disease, unspecified
AHA: 2021,4Q,5

A69.21 Meningitis due to Lyme disease COM

A69.22 Other neurologic disorders in Lyme disease
Cranial neuritis
Meningoencephalitis
Polyneuropathy

A69.23 Arthritis due to Lyme disease HCC ESR COM

A69.29 Other conditions associated with Lyme disease
Myopericarditis due to Lyme disease
AHA: 2016,3Q,12

A69.8 Other specified spirochetal infections

A69.9 Spirochetal infection, unspecified

Other diseases caused by chlamydiae (A70-A74)

EXCLUDES 1 *sexually transmitted chlamydial diseases (A55-A56)*

A70 Chlamydia psittaci infections
Ornithosis
Parrot fever
Psittacosis

4th **A71 Trachoma**

EXCLUDES 1 *sequelae of trachoma (B94.0)*

A71.0 Initial stage of trachoma
Trachoma dubium

A71.1 Active stage of trachoma
Granular conjunctivitis (trachomatous)
Trachomatous follicular conjunctivitis
Trachomatous pannus

A71.9 Trachoma, unspecified

4th **A74 Other diseases caused by chlamydiae**

EXCLUDES 1 *neonatal chlamydial conjunctivitis (P39.1)*
neonatal chlamydial pneumonia (P23.1)
Reiter's disease (M02.3-)
sexually transmitted chlamydial diseases (A55-A56)

EXCLUDES 2 *chlamydial pneumonia (J16.0)*

A74.0 Chlamydial conjunctivitis
Paratrachoma

5th **A74.8 Other chlamydial diseases**

A74.81 Chlamydial peritonitis

A74.89 Other chlamydial diseases

A74.9 Chlamydial infection, unspecified
Chlamydiosis NOS

Rickettsioses (A75-A79)

DEF: Rickettsia: Condition caused by bacteria that live in lice/ticks transmitted to humans through bites.

4th **A75 Typhus fever**

EXCLUDES 1 *rickettsiosis due to Ehrlichia sennetsu (A79.81)*

A75.0 Epidemic louse-borne typhus fever due to Rickettsia prowazekii
Classical typhus (fever)
Epidemic (louse-borne) typhus

A75.1 Recrudescent typhus [Brill's disease]
Brill-Zinsser disease

A75.2 Typhus fever due to Rickettsia typhi
Murine (flea-borne) typhus

A75.3 Typhus fever due to Rickettsia tsutsugamushi
Scrub (mite-borne) typhus
Tsutsugamushi fever
Typhus fever due to Orientia Tsutsugamushi (scrub typhus)

A75.9 Typhus fever, unspecified
Typhus (fever) NOS

4th **A77 Spotted fever [tick-borne rickettsioses]**

A77.0 Spotted fever due to Rickettsia rickettsii
Rocky Mountain spotted fever
Sao Paulo fever

A77.1 Spotted fever due to Rickettsia conorii
African tick typhus
Boutonneuse fever
India tick typhus
Kenya tick typhus
Marseilles fever
Mediterranean tick fever

A77.2 Spotted fever due to Rickettsia siberica
North Asian tick fever
Siberian tick typhus

A77.3 Spotted fever due to Rickettsia australis
Queensland tick typhus

5th **A77.4 Ehrlichiosis**

EXCLUDES 1 *anaplasmosis [A. phagocytophilum] (A79.82)*
rickettsiosis due to Ehrlichia sennetsu (A79.81)

AHA: 2021,4Q,5

A77.40 Ehrlichiosis, unspecified

A77.41 Ehrlichiosis chafeensis [E. chafeensis]

A77.49 Other ehrlichiosis
Ehrlichiosis due to E. ewingii
Ehrlichiosis due to E. muris euclairensis

A77.8 Other spotted fevers
Rickettsia 364D/R. philipii (Pacific Coast tick fever)
Spotted fever due to Rickettsia africae (African tick bite fever)
Spotted fever due to Rickettsia parkeri

A77.9 Spotted fever, unspecified
Tick-borne typhus NOS

A78 Q fever
Infection due to Coxiella burnetii
Nine Mile fever
Quadrilateral fever

4th **A79 Other rickettsioses**

A79.0 Trench fever
Quintan fever
Wolhynian fever

A79.1 Rickettsialpox due to Rickettsia akari
Kew Garden fever
Vesicular rickettsiosis

5th **A79.8 Other specified rickettsioses**

A79.81 Rickettsiosis due to Ehrlichia sennetsu
Rickettsiosis due to Neorickettsia sennetsu

A79.82 Anaplasmosis [A. phagocytophilum]
Transfusion transmitted A. phagocytophilum
AHA: 2021,4Q,4-5

A79.89 Other specified rickettsioses

A79.9 Rickettsiosis, unspecified
Rickettsial infection NOS

Viral and prion infections of the central nervous system (A8Ø-A89)

EXCLUDES 1 *postpolio syndrome (G14)*
sequelae of poliomyelitis (B91)
sequelae of viral encephalitis (B94.1)

A8Ø Acute poliomyelitis

EXCLUDES 1 *acute flaccid myelitis (GØ4.82)*

A8Ø.Ø Acute paralytic poliomyelitis, vaccine-associated COM

A8Ø.1 Acute paralytic poliomyelitis, wild virus, imported COM

A8Ø.2 Acute paralytic poliomyelitis, wild virus, indigenous COM

A8Ø.3 Acute paralytic poliomyelitis, other and unspecified

A8Ø.3Ø Acute paralytic poliomyelitis, unspecified COM

A8Ø.39 Other acute paralytic poliomyelitis COM

A8Ø.4 Acute nonparalytic poliomyelitis COM

A8Ø.9 Acute poliomyelitis, unspecified COM

A81 Atypical virus infections of central nervous system

INCLUDES diseases of the central nervous system caused by prions

▶Use additional code, if applicable, to identify:◀
▶dementia with anxiety (FØ2.84, FØ2.A4, FØ2.B4, FØ2.C4)◀
dementia with behavioral disturbance ▶(FØ2.81-, FØ2.A1-, FØ2.B1-, FØ2.C1-)◀
▶dementia with mood disturbance (FØ2.83, FØ2.A3, FØ2.B3, FØ2.C3)◀
▶dementia with psychotic disturbance (FØ2.82, FØ2.A2, FØ2.B2, FØ2.C2)◀
dementia without behavioral disturbance ▶(FØ2.8Ø, FØ2.AØ, FØ2.BØ, FØ2.CØ)◀
▶mild neurocognitive disorder due to known physiological condition (FØ6.7-)◀

A81.Ø Creutzfeldt-Jakob disease

DEF: Communicable, rare spongiform encephalopathy occurring later in life with progressive destruction of the pyramidal and extrapyramidal systems eventually leading to death. Progressive dementia, wasting of muscles, tremor, and other symptoms are present.

A81.ØØ Creutzfeldt-Jakob disease, unspecified HCC Rx ESR
Jakob-Creutzfeldt disease, unspecified

A81.Ø1 Variant Creutzfeldt-Jakob disease HCC Rx ESR
vCJD

A81.Ø9 Other Creutzfeldt-Jakob disease HCC Rx ESR
CJD
Familial Creutzfeldt-Jakob disease
Iatrogenic Creutzfeldt-Jakob disease
Sporadic Creutzfeldt-Jakob disease
Subacute spongiform encephalopathy (with dementia)

A81.1 Subacute sclerosing panencephalitis HCC Rx ESR
Dawson's inclusion body encephalitis
Van Bogaert's sclerosing leukoencephalopathy

A81.2 Progressive multifocal leukoencephalopathy HCC Rx ESR
Multifocal leukoencephalopathy NOS

A81.8 Other atypical virus infections of central nervous system

A81.81 Kuru HCC Rx ESR

A81.82 Gerstmann-Sträussler-Scheinker syndrome HCC Rx ESR
GSS syndrome

A81.83 Fatal familial insomnia HCC Rx ESR
FFI

A81.89 Other atypical virus infections of central nervous system HCC Rx ESR

A81.9 Atypical virus infection of central nervous system, unspecified HCC Rx ESR
Prion diseases of the central nervous system NOS

A82 Rabies

A82.Ø Sylvatic rabies COM

A82.1 Urban rabies COM

A82.9 Rabies, unspecified COM

A83 Mosquito-borne viral encephalitis

INCLUDES mosquito-borne viral meningoencephalitis

EXCLUDES 2 *Venezuelan equine encephalitis (A92.2)*
West Nile fever (A92.3-)
West Nile virus (A92.3-)

A83.Ø Japanese encephalitis COM

A83.1 Western equine encephalitis COM

A83.2 Eastern equine encephalitis COM

A83.3 St Louis encephalitis COM

A83.4 Australian encephalitis COM
Kunjin virus disease

A83.5 California encephalitis COM
California meningoencephalitis
La Crosse encephalitis

A83.6 Rocio virus disease COM

A83.8 Other mosquito-borne viral encephalitis COM

A83.9 Mosquito-borne viral encephalitis, unspecified COM

A84 Tick-borne viral encephalitis

INCLUDES tick-borne viral meningoencephalitis

A84.Ø Far Eastern tick-borne encephalitis [Russian spring-summer encephalitis] COM

A84.1 Central European tick-borne encephalitis COM

A84.8 Other tick-borne viral encephalitis

AHA: 2020,4Q,4-5

A84.81 Powassan virus disease COM

A84.89 Other tick-borne viral encephalitis COM
Louping ill
Code first, if applicable, transfusion related infection (T8Ø.22-)

A84.9 Tick-borne viral encephalitis, unspecified COM

A85 Other viral encephalitis, not elsewhere classified

INCLUDES specified viral encephalomyelitis NEC
specified viral meningoencephalitis NEC

EXCLUDES 1 ~~*benign myalgic encephalomyelitis (G93.3)*~~
encephalitis due to cytomegalovirus (B25.8)
encephalitis due to herpesvirus NEC (B1Ø.Ø-)
encephalitis due to herpesvirus [herpes simplex] (BØØ.4)
encephalitis due to measles virus (BØ5.Ø)
encephalitis due to mumps virus (B26.2)
encephalitis due to poliomyelitis virus (A8Ø.-)
encephalitis due to zoster (BØ2.Ø)
lymphocytic choriomeningitis (A87.2)
▶*myalgic encephalomyelitis (G93.32)*◀

A85.Ø Enteroviral encephalitis COM
Enteroviral encephalomyelitis

A85.1 Adenoviral encephalitis COM
Adenoviral meningoencephalitis

A85.2 Arthropod-borne viral encephalitis, unspecified COM

EXCLUDES 1 *West nile virus with encephalitis (A92.31)*

A85.8 Other specified viral encephalitis COM
Encephalitis lethargica
Von Economo-Cruchet disease

A86 Unspecified viral encephalitis COM
Viral encephalomyelitis NOS
Viral meningoencephalitis NOS

A87 Viral meningitis

EXCLUDES 1 *meningitis due to herpesvirus [herpes simplex] (BØØ.3)*
meningitis due to measles virus (BØ5.1)
meningitis due to mumps virus (B26.1)
meningitis due to poliomyelitis virus (A8Ø.-)
meningitis due to zoster (BØ2.1)

DEF: Meningitis: Inflammation of the meningeal layers of the brain and spine.

A87.Ø Enteroviral meningitis COM
Coxsackievirus meningitis
Echovirus meningitis

A87.1 Adenoviral meningitis COM

A87.2 Lymphocytic choriomeningitis COM
Lymphocytic meningoencephalitis

A87.8 Other viral meningitis COM

A87.9 Viral meningitis, unspecified COM

A88 Other viral infections of central nervous system, not elsewhere classified
EXCLUDES 1 *viral encephalitis NOS (A86)*
viral meningitis NOS (A87.9)

A88.Ø Enteroviral exanthematous fever [Boston exanthem] COM
A88.1 Epidemic vertigo
A88.8 Other specified viral infections of central nervous system COM

A89 Unspecified viral infection of central nervous system COM

Arthropod-borne viral fevers and viral hemorrhagic fevers (A9Ø-A99)

A9Ø Dengue fever [classical dengue]
EXCLUDES 1 *dengue hemorrhagic fever (A91)*
AHA: 2016,3Q,13

A91 Dengue hemorrhagic fever

A92 Other mosquito-borne viral fevers
EXCLUDES 1 *Ross River disease (B33.1)*

A92.Ø Chikungunya virus disease
Chikungunya (hemorrhagic) fever
A92.1 O'nyong-nyong fever
A92.2 Venezuelan equine fever COM
Venezuelan equine encephalitis
Venezuelan equine encephalomyelitis virus disease
A92.3 West Nile virus infection
West Nile fever
AHA: 2016,3Q,12
A92.3Ø West Nile virus infection, unspecified COM
West Nile fever NOS
West Nile fever without complications
West Nile virus NOS
A92.31 West Nile virus infection with encephalitis COM
West Nile encephalitis
West Nile encephalomyelitis
A92.32 West Nile virus infection with other neurologic manifestation COM
Use additional code to specify the neurologic manifestation
A92.39 West Nile virus infection with other complications COM
Use additional code to specify the other conditions
A92.4 Rift Valley fever
A92.5 Zika virus disease
Zika virus fever
Zika virus infection
Zika NOS
EXCLUDES 1 *congenital Zika virus disease (P35.4)*
AHA: 2016,4Q,4-7
DEF: Virus transmitted via a bite from an infected Aedes species mosquito. Common symptoms of the virus include fever, rash, joint pain, and conjunctivitis; they are usually mild in nature and may last from several days to a week. Most people who have the Zika virus do not require medical attention; however, in pregnant women, the Zika virus can cause a serious birth defect called microcephaly, as well as other severe fetal brain defects.
TIP: Assign code Z71.1, when a patient requests testing for Zika virus but in the absence of symptoms or recent exposure to the virus.
TIP: Code only confirmed diagnoses of Zika virus; documentation by the physician that the disease is confirmed is sufficient.
A92.8 Other specified mosquito-borne viral fevers
A92.9 Mosquito-borne viral fever, unspecified

A93 Other arthropod-borne viral fevers, not elsewhere classified
A93.Ø Oropouche virus disease
Oropouche fever
A93.1 Sandfly fever
Pappataci fever
Phlebotomus fever
A93.2 Colorado tick fever
A93.8 Other specified arthropod-borne viral fevers
Piry virus disease
Vesicular stomatitis virus disease [Indiana fever]

A94 Unspecified arthropod-borne viral fever
Arboviral fever NOS
Arbovirus infection NOS

A95 Yellow fever
A95.Ø Sylvatic yellow fever
Jungle yellow fever
A95.1 Urban yellow fever
A95.9 Yellow fever, unspecified

A96 Arenaviral hemorrhagic fever
A96.Ø Junin hemorrhagic fever
Argentinian hemorrhagic fever
A96.1 Machupo hemorrhagic fever
Bolivian hemorrhagic fever
A96.2 Lassa fever
A96.8 Other arenaviral hemorrhagic fevers
A96.9 Arenaviral hemorrhagic fever, unspecified

A98 Other viral hemorrhagic fevers, not elsewhere classified
EXCLUDES 1 *chikungunya hemorrhagic fever (A92.Ø)*
dengue hemorrhagic fever (A91)
A98.Ø Crimean-Congo hemorrhagic fever
Central Asian hemorrhagic fever
A98.1 Omsk hemorrhagic fever
A98.2 Kyasanur Forest disease
A98.3 Marburg virus disease
A98.4 Ebola virus disease
A98.5 Hemorrhagic fever with renal syndrome
Epidemic hemorrhagic fever
Korean hemorrhagic fever
Russian hemorrhagic fever
Hantaan virus disease
Hantavirus disease with renal manifestations
Nephropathia epidemica
Songo fever
EXCLUDES 1 *hantavirus (cardio)-pulmonary syndrome (B33.4)*
A98.8 Other specified viral hemorrhagic fevers

A99 Unspecified viral hemorrhagic fever

Viral infections characterized by skin and mucous membrane lesions (BØØ-BØ9)

BØØ Herpesviral [herpes simplex] infections
EXCLUDES 1 *congenital herpesviral infections (P35.2)*
EXCLUDES 2 *anogenital herpesviral infection (A6Ø.-)*
gammaherpesviral mononucleosis (B27.Ø-)
herpangina (BØ8.5)

BØØ.Ø Eczema herpeticum
Kaposi's varicelliform eruption
BØØ.1 Herpesviral vesicular dermatitis
Herpes simplex facialis
Herpes simplex labialis
Herpes simplex otitis externa
Vesicular dermatitis of ear
Vesicular dermatitis of lip
BØØ.2 Herpesviral gingivostomatitis and pharyngotonsillitis
Herpesviral pharyngitis
BØØ.3 Herpesviral meningitis COM
BØØ.4 Herpesviral encephalitis COM
Herpesviral meningoencephalitis
Simian B disease
EXCLUDES 1 *herpesviral encephalitis due to herpesvirus 6 and 7 (B1Ø.Ø1, B1Ø.Ø9)*
non-simplex herpesviral encephalitis (B1Ø.Ø-)
BØØ.5 Herpesviral ocular disease
BØØ.5Ø Herpesviral ocular disease, unspecified
BØØ.51 Herpesviral iridocyclitis
Herpesviral iritis
Herpesviral uveitis, anterior
BØØ.52 Herpesviral keratitis
Herpesviral keratoconjunctivitis
BØØ.53 Herpesviral conjunctivitis
BØØ.59 Other herpesviral disease of eye
Herpesviral dermatitis of eyelid
BØØ.7 Disseminated herpesviral disease HCC ESR COM
Herpesviral sepsis

BØØ.8 Other forms of herpesviral infections

BØØ.81 Herpesviral hepatitis

BØØ.82 Herpes simplex myelitis HCC Rx ESR COM

BØØ.89 Other herpesviral infection
Herpesviral whitlow

BØØ.9 Herpesviral infection, unspecified
Herpes simplex infection NOS

BØ1 Varicella [chickenpox]

BØ1.Ø Varicella meningitis COM

BØ1.1 Varicella encephalitis, myelitis and encephalomyelitis
Postchickenpox encephalitis, myelitis and encephalomyelitis

BØ1.11 Varicella encephalitis and encephalomyelitis COM
Postchickenpox encephalitis and encephalomyelitis

BØ1.12 Varicella myelitis HCC Rx ESR COM
Postchickenpox myelitis

BØ1.2 Varicella pneumonia

BØ1.8 Varicella with other complications

BØ1.81 Varicella keratitis

BØ1.89 Other varicella complications

BØ1.9 Varicella without complication
Varicella NOS

BØ2 Zoster [herpes zoster]

INCLUDES shingles
zona

BØ2.Ø Zoster encephalitis COM
Zoster meningoencephalitis

BØ2.1 Zoster meningitis COM
AHA: 2019,1Q,18

BØ2.2 Zoster with other nervous system involvement

BØ2.21 Postherpetic geniculate ganglionitis Rx

BØ2.22 Postherpetic trigeminal neuralgia Rx

BØ2.23 Postherpetic polyneuropathy Rx

BØ2.24 Postherpetic myelitis HCC Rx ESR COM
Herpes zoster myelitis

BØ2.29 Other postherpetic nervous system involvement Rx
Postherpetic radiculopathy

BØ2.3 Zoster ocular disease

BØ2.30 Zoster ocular disease, unspecified

BØ2.31 Zoster conjunctivitis

BØ2.32 Zoster iridocyclitis

BØ2.33 Zoster keratitis
Herpes zoster keratoconjunctivitis

BØ2.34 Zoster scleritis

BØ2.39 Other herpes zoster eye disease
Zoster blepharitis

BØ2.7 Disseminated zoster

BØ2.8 Zoster with other complications
Herpes zoster otitis externa

BØ2.9 Zoster without complications
Zoster NOS

BØ3 Smallpox

NOTE In 198Ø the 33rd World Health Assembly declared that smallpox had been eradicated.
The classification is maintained for surveillance purposes.

BØ4 Monkeypox

BØ5 Measles

INCLUDES morbilli

EXCLUDES 1 *subacute sclerosing panencephalitis (A81.1)*

BØ5.Ø Measles complicated by encephalitis COM
Postmeasles encephalitis

BØ5.1 Measles complicated by meningitis COM
Postmeasles meningitis

BØ5.2 Measles complicated by pneumonia
Postmeasles pneumonia

BØ5.3 Measles complicated by otitis media
Postmeasles otitis media

BØ5.4 Measles with intestinal complications

BØ5.8 Measles with other complications

BØ5.81 Measles keratitis and keratoconjunctivitis

BØ5.89 Other measles complications

BØ5.9 Measles without complication
Measles NOS

BØ6 Rubella [German measles]

EXCLUDES 1 *congenital rubella (P35.Ø)*

DEF: Highly contagious virus in which the symptoms are mild and short-lived in most people. Rubella during pregnancy, however, can result in abortion, stillbirth, or congenital defects.

BØ6.Ø Rubella with neurological complications

BØ6.ØØ Rubella with neurological complication, unspecified COM

BØ6.Ø1 Rubella encephalitis
Rubella meningoencephalitis

BØ6.Ø2 Rubella meningitis COM

BØ6.Ø9 Other neurological complications of rubella

BØ6.8 Rubella with other complications

BØ6.81 Rubella pneumonia

BØ6.82 Rubella arthritis HCC ESR COM

BØ6.89 Other rubella complications

BØ6.9 Rubella without complication
Rubella NOS

BØ7 Viral warts

INCLUDES verruca simplex
verruca vulgaris
viral warts due to human papillomavirus

EXCLUDES 2 *anogenital (venereal) warts (A63.Ø)*
papilloma of bladder (D41.4)
papilloma of cervix (D26.Ø)
papilloma larynx (D14.1)

BØ7.Ø Plantar wart
Verruca plantaris

BØ7.8 Other viral warts
Common wart
Flat wart
Verruca plana

BØ7.9 Viral wart, unspecified

BØ8 Other viral infections characterized by skin and mucous membrane lesions, not elsewhere classified

EXCLUDES 1 *vesicular stomatitis virus disease (A93.8)*

BØ8.Ø Other orthopoxvirus infections

EXCLUDES 2 *monkeypox (BØ4)*

BØ8.Ø1 Cowpox and vaccinia not from vaccine

BØ8.Ø1Ø Cowpox
DEF: Disease contracted by milking infected cows. The vesicles usually appear on the fingers, hands, and adjacent areas and usually disappear without scarring. Other symptoms include local edema, lymphangitis, and regional lymphadenitis with or without fever.

BØ8.Ø11 Vaccinia not from vaccine

EXCLUDES 1 *vaccinia (from vaccination) (generalized) (T88.1)*

BØ8.Ø2 Orf virus disease
Contagious pustular dermatitis
Ecthyma contagiosum

BØ8.Ø3 Pseudocowpox [milker's node]

BØ8.Ø4 Paravaccinia, unspecified

BØ8.Ø9 Other orthopoxvirus infections
Orthopoxvirus infection NOS

BØ8.1 Molluscum contagiosum
DEF: Benign poxvirus infection causing small bumps on the skin or conjunctiva, transmitted by close contact.

BØ8.2 Exanthema subitum [sixth disease]
Roseola infantum

BØ8.2Ø Exanthema subitum [sixth disease], unspecified P
Roseola infantum, unspecified

BØ8.21 Exanthema subitum [sixth disease] due to human herpesvirus 6 P
Roseola infantum due to human herpesvirus 6

BØ8.22 Exanthema subitum [sixth disease] due to human herpesvirus 7 P
Roseola infantum due to human herpesvirus 7

BØ8.3 Erythema infectiosum [fifth disease]
DEF: Infection with human parvovirus B19, mainly occurring in children. Symptoms include a low-grade fever, malaise, or a "cold" a few days before the appearance of a mild rash illness that presents as a "slapped-cheek" rash on the face and a lacy red rash on the trunk and limbs.

BØ8.4 Enteroviral vesicular stomatitis with exanthem
Hand, foot and mouth disease

BØ8.5 Enteroviral vesicular pharyngitis
Herpangina
DEF: Acute infectious Coxsackie virus infection causing throat lesions, fever, and vomiting that generally affects children in the summer.

✓5th **BØ8.6 Parapoxvirus infections**
BØ8.6Ø Parapoxvirus infection, unspecified
BØ8.61 Bovine stomatitis
BØ8.62 Sealpox
BØ8.69 Other parapoxvirus infections

✓5th **BØ8.7 Yatapoxvirus infections**
BØ8.7Ø Yatapoxvirus infection, unspecified
BØ8.71 Tanapox virus disease
BØ8.72 Yaba pox virus disease
Yaba monkey tumor disease
BØ8.79 Other yatapoxvirus infections

BØ8.8 Other specified viral infections characterized by skin and mucous membrane lesions
Enteroviral lymphonodular pharyngitis
Foot-and-mouth disease
Poxvirus NEC

BØ9 Unspecified viral infection characterized by skin and mucous membrane lesions
Viral enanthema NOS
Viral exanthema NOS

Other human herpesviruses (B1Ø)

✓4th **B1Ø Other human herpesviruses**
EXCLUDES 2 *cytomegalovirus (B25.9)*
Epstein-Barr virus (B27.Ø-)
herpes NOS (BØØ.9)
herpes simplex (BØØ.-)
herpes zoster (BØ2.-)
human herpesvirus NOS (BØØ.-)
human herpesvirus 1 and 2 (BØØ.-)
human herpesvirus 3 (BØ1.-, BØ2.-)
human herpesvirus 4 (B27.Ø-)
human herpesvirus 5 (B25.-)
varicella (BØ1.-)
zoster (BØ2.-)

✓5th **B1Ø.Ø Other human herpesvirus encephalitis**
EXCLUDES 2 *herpes encephalitis NOS (BØØ.4)*
herpes simplex encephalitis (BØØ.4)
human herpesvirus encephalitis (BØØ.4)
simian B herpes virus encephalitis (BØØ.4)
B1Ø.Ø1 Human herpesvirus 6 encephalitis COM
B1Ø.Ø9 Other human herpesvirus encephalitis COM
Human herpesvirus 7 encephalitis

✓5th **B1Ø.8 Other human herpesvirus infection**
B1Ø.81 Human herpesvirus 6 infection
B1Ø.82 Human herpesvirus 7 infection
B1Ø.89 Other human herpesvirus infection
Human herpesvirus 8 infection
Kaposi's sarcoma-associated herpesvirus infection

Viral hepatitis (B15-B19)

EXCLUDES 1 *sequelae of viral hepatitis (B94.2)*
EXCLUDES 2 *cytomegaloviral hepatitis (B25.1)*
herpesviral [herpes simplex] hepatitis (BØØ.81)

DEF: Hepatitis A: HAV infection that is self-limiting with flulike symptoms. Transmission is fecal-oral.
DEF: Hepatitis B: HBV infection that can be chronic and systemic. Transmission is bodily fluids.
DEF: Hepatitis C: HCV infection that can be chronic and systemic. Transmission is blood transfusion and unidentified agents.
DEF: Hepatitis D (delta): HDV that occurs only in the presence of hepatitis B virus. Transmission is contaminated blood in contact with mucous membranes.
DEF: Hepatitis E: HEV is an epidemic form. Transmission is fecal-oral, most often from contaminated water.

✓4th **B15 Acute hepatitis A**
B15.Ø Hepatitis A with hepatic coma COM
B15.9 Hepatitis A without hepatic coma
Hepatitis A (acute)(viral) NOS

✓4th **B16 Acute hepatitis B**
AHA: 2016,3Q,13
B16.Ø Acute hepatitis B with delta-agent with hepatic coma COM
B16.1 Acute hepatitis B with delta-agent without hepatic coma
B16.2 Acute hepatitis B without delta-agent with hepatic coma COM
B16.9 Acute hepatitis B without delta-agent and without hepatic coma
Hepatitis B (acute) (viral) NOS

✓4th **B17 Other acute viral hepatitis**
B17.Ø Acute delta-(super) infection of hepatitis B carrier
✓5th **B17.1 Acute hepatitis C**
B17.1Ø Acute hepatitis C without hepatic coma Rx
Acute hepatitis C NOS
B17.11 Acute hepatitis C with hepatic coma Rx COM
B17.2 Acute hepatitis E
B17.8 Other specified acute viral hepatitis
Hepatitis non-A non-B (acute) (viral) NEC
B17.9 Acute viral hepatitis, unspecified
Acute hepatitis NOS
Acute infectious hepatitis NOS

✓4th **B18 Chronic viral hepatitis**
INCLUDES carrier of viral hepatitis
AHA: 2017,1Q,41
B18.Ø Chronic viral hepatitis B with delta-agent HCC Rx ESR COM
B18.1 Chronic viral hepatitis B without delta-agent HCC Rx ESR COM
Carrier of viral hepatitis B
Chronic (viral) hepatitis B
B18.2 Chronic viral hepatitis C HCC Rx ESR COM
Carrier of viral hepatitis C
AHA: 2018,1Q,4
B18.8 Other chronic viral hepatitis HCC Rx ESR COM
Carrier of other viral hepatitis
B18.9 Chronic viral hepatitis, unspecified HCC ESR COM
Carrier of unspecified viral hepatitis

✓4th **B19 Unspecified viral hepatitis**
B19.Ø Unspecified viral hepatitis with hepatic coma COM
✓5th **B19.1 Unspecified viral hepatitis B**
B19.1Ø Unspecified viral hepatitis B without hepatic coma
Unspecified viral hepatitis B NOS
B19.11 Unspecified viral hepatitis B with hepatic coma COM
✓5th **B19.2 Unspecified viral hepatitis C**
B19.2Ø Unspecified viral hepatitis C without hepatic coma Rx
Viral hepatitis C NOS
B19.21 Unspecified viral hepatitis C with hepatic coma Rx COM
B19.9 Unspecified viral hepatitis without hepatic coma
Viral hepatitis NOS

Human immunodeficiency virus [HIV] disease (B20)

B20 Human immunodeficiency virus [HIV] disease HCC Rx ESR COM

INCLUDES acquired immune deficiency syndrome [AIDS]
AIDS-related complex [ARC]
HIV infection, symptomatic

Code first Human immunodeficiency virus [HIV] disease complicating pregnancy, childbirth and the puerperium, if applicable (O98.7-)

Use additional code(s) to identify all manifestations of HIV infection

EXCLUDES 1 *asymptomatic human immunodeficiency virus [HIV] infection status (Z21)*
exposure to HIV virus (Z20.6)
inconclusive serologic evidence of HIV (R75)

AHA: 2022,1Q,36; 2021,2Q,6; 2021,1Q,52; 2020,4Q,97; 2020,2Q,12; 2019,1Q,8-11

Other viral diseases (B25-B34)

✓4th **B25 Cytomegaloviral disease**

EXCLUDES 1 *congenital cytomegalovirus infection (P35.1)*
cytomegaloviral mononucleosis (B27.1-)

B25.0 Cytomegaloviral pneumonitis HCC Rx ESR COM
B25.1 Cytomegaloviral hepatitis HCC Rx ESR COM
B25.2 Cytomegaloviral pancreatitis HCC Rx ESR COM
B25.8 Other cytomegaloviral diseases HCC Rx ESR COM
Cytomegaloviral encephalitis
B25.9 Cytomegaloviral disease, unspecified HCC Rx ESR COM

✓4th **B26 Mumps**

INCLUDES epidemic parotitis
infectious parotitis

B26.0 Mumps orchitis ♂
B26.1 Mumps meningitis COM
B26.2 Mumps encephalitis COM
B26.3 Mumps pancreatitis COM
✓5th **B26.8 Mumps with other complications**
B26.81 Mumps hepatitis
B26.82 Mumps myocarditis COM
B26.83 Mumps nephritis
B26.84 Mumps polyneuropathy
B26.85 Mumps arthritis HCC ESR COM
B26.89 Other mumps complications
B26.9 Mumps without complication
Mumps NOS
Mumps parotitis NOS

✓4th **B27 Infectious mononucleosis**

INCLUDES glandular fever
monocytic angina
Pfeiffer's disease

✓5th **B27.0 Gammaherpesviral mononucleosis**
Mononucleosis due to Epstein-Barr virus
B27.00 Gammaherpesviral mononucleosis without complication
B27.01 Gammaherpesviral mononucleosis with polyneuropathy
B27.02 Gammaherpesviral mononucleosis with meningitis COM
B27.09 Gammaherpesviral mononucleosis with other complications
Hepatomegaly in gammaherpesviral mononucleosis

✓5th **B27.1 Cytomegaloviral mononucleosis**
B27.10 Cytomegaloviral mononucleosis without complications
B27.11 Cytomegaloviral mononucleosis with polyneuropathy
B27.12 Cytomegaloviral mononucleosis with meningitis COM
B27.19 Cytomegaloviral mononucleosis with other complication
Hepatomegaly in cytomegaloviral mononucleosis

✓5th **B27.8 Other infectious mononucleosis**
B27.80 Other infectious mononucleosis without complication
B27.81 Other infectious mononucleosis with polyneuropathy
B27.82 Other infectious mononucleosis with meningitis COM
B27.89 Other infectious mononucleosis with other complication
Hepatomegaly in other infectious mononucleosis

✓5th **B27.9 Infectious mononucleosis, unspecified**
B27.90 Infectious mononucleosis, unspecified without complication
B27.91 Infectious mononucleosis, unspecified with polyneuropathy
B27.92 Infectious mononucleosis, unspecified with meningitis COM
B27.99 Infectious mononucleosis, unspecified with other complication
Hepatomegaly in unspecified infectious mononucleosis

✓4th **B30 Viral conjunctivitis**

EXCLUDES 1 *herpesviral [herpes simplex] ocular disease (B00.5)*
ocular zoster (B02.3)

Viral Conjunctivitis

B30.0 Keratoconjunctivitis due to adenovirus
Epidemic keratoconjunctivitis
Shipyard eye
B30.1 Conjunctivitis due to adenovirus
Acute adenoviral follicular conjunctivitis
Swimming-pool conjunctivitis
B30.2 Viral pharyngoconjunctivitis
B30.3 Acute epidemic hemorrhagic conjunctivitis (enteroviral)
Conjunctivitis due to coxsackievirus 24
Conjunctivitis due to enterovirus 70
Hemorrhagic conjunctivitis (acute)(epidemic)
B30.8 Other viral conjunctivitis
Newcastle conjunctivitis
B30.9 Viral conjunctivitis, unspecified

✓4th **B33 Other viral diseases, not elsewhere classified**

B33.0 Epidemic myalgia
Bornholm disease
B33.1 Ross River disease
Epidemic polyarthritis and exanthema
Ross River fever
✓5th **B33.2 Viral carditis**
Coxsackie (virus) carditis
B33.20 Viral carditis, unspecified COM
B33.21 Viral endocarditis COM
B33.22 Viral myocarditis COM
B33.23 Viral pericarditis COM
B33.24 Viral cardiomyopathy HCC Rx ESR COM
B33.3 Retrovirus infections, not elsewhere classified
Retrovirus infection NOS
B33.4 Hantavirus (cardio)-pulmonary syndrome [HPS] [HCPS]
Hantavirus disease with pulmonary manifestations
Sin nombre virus disease
Use additional code to identify any associated acute kidney failure (N17.9)

EXCLUDES 1 *hantavirus disease with renal manifestations (A98.5)*
hemorrhagic fever with renal manifestations (A98.5)

B33.8 Other specified viral diseases

EXCLUDES 1 *anogenital human papillomavirus infection (A63.0)*
viral warts due to human papillomavirus infection (B07)

B34 Viral infection of unspecified site

EXCLUDES 1 *anogenital human papillomavirus infection (A63.Ø)*
cytomegaloviral disease NOS (B25.9)
herpesvirus [herpes simplex] infection NOS (BØØ.9)
retrovirus infection NOS (B33.3)
viral agents as the cause of diseases classified elsewhere (B97.-)
viral warts due to human papillomavirus infection (BØ7)

B34.Ø Adenovirus infection, unspecified

B34.1 Enterovirus infection, unspecified
Coxsackievirus infection NOS
Echovirus infection NOS

B34.2 Coronavirus infection, unspecified
EXCLUDES 1 *COVID-19 (UØ7.1)*
pneumonia due to SARS-associated coronavirus (J12.81)
AHA: 2020,1Q,34-36

B34.3 Parvovirus infection, unspecified

B34.4 Papovavirus infection, unspecified

B34.8 Other viral infections of unspecified site

B34.9 Viral infection, unspecified
Viremia NOS
AHA: 2016,3Q,10

Mycoses (B35-B49)

EXCLUDES 2 *hypersensitivity pneumonitis due to organic dust (J67.-)*
mycosis fungoides (C84.Ø-)

B35 Dermatophytosis

INCLUDES favus
infections due to species of Epidermophyton, Micro-sporum and Trichophyton
tinea, any type except those in B36.-

DEF: Contagious superficial fungal infection of the skin that invades and grows in dead keratin.

B35.Ø Tinea barbae and tinea capitis
Beard ringworm
Kerion
Scalp ringworm
Sycosis, mycotic

B35.1 Tinea unguium
Dermatophytic onychia
Dermatophytosis of nail
Onychomycosis
Ringworm of nails

B35.2 Tinea manuum
Dermatophytosis of hand
Hand ringworm

B35.3 Tinea pedis
Athlete's foot
Dermatophytosis of foot
Foot ringworm

B35.4 Tinea corporis
Ringworm of the body

B35.5 Tinea imbricata
Tokelau

B35.6 Tinea cruris
Dhobi itch
Groin ringworm
Jock itch

B35.8 Other dermatophytoses
Disseminated dermatophytosis
Granulomatous dermatophytosis

B35.9 Dermatophytosis, unspecified
Ringworm NOS

B36 Other superficial mycoses

B36.Ø Pityriasis versicolor
Tinea flava
Tinea versicolor

B36.1 Tinea nigra
Keratomycosis nigricans palmaris
Microsporosis nigra
Pityriasis nigra

B36.2 White piedra
Tinea blanca

B36.3 Black piedra

B36.8 Other specified superficial mycoses

B36.9 Superficial mycosis, unspecified

B37 Candidiasis

INCLUDES candidosis
moniliasis

EXCLUDES 1 *neonatal candidiasis (P37.5)*

DEF: *Candida:* Genus of yeast-like fungi that are commonly found in the mouth, skin, intestinal tract, and vagina. It may cause a white, cheesy discharge.

B37.Ø Candidal stomatitis
Oral thrush

B37.1 Pulmonary candidiasis HCC Rx ESR COM
Candidal bronchitis
Candidal pneumonia

B37.2 Candidiasis of skin and nail
Candidal onychia
Candidal paronychia
EXCLUDES 2 *diaper dermatitis (L22)*

▲ **B37.3 Candidiasis of vulva and vagina**
Candidal vulvovaginitis
Monilial vulvovaginitis
Vaginal thrush

● **B37.31 Acute candidiasis of vulva and vagina**
Candidiasis of vulva and vagina NOS

● **B37.32 Chronic candidiasis of vulva and vagina**
Recurrent candidiasis of vulva and vagina

B37.4 Candidiasis of other urogenital sites

B37.41 Candidal cystitis and urethritis

B37.42 Candidal balanitis ♂

B37.49 Other urogenital candidiasis
Candidal pyelonephritis

B37.5 Candidal meningitis COM

B37.6 Candidal endocarditis COM

B37.7 Candidal sepsis HCC Rx ESR COM
Disseminated candidiasis
Systemic candidiasis
AHA: 2014,4Q,46
TIP: This code is assigned when sepsis is documented as due to any *Candida* type. If the nonspecific term "non-*Candida albicans*" is documented, code B48.8 Other specified mycoses, is assigned.

B37.8 Candidiasis of other sites

B37.81 Candidal esophagitis HCC Rx ESR COM

B37.82 Candidal enteritis
Candidal proctitis

B37.83 Candidal cheilitis

B37.84 Candidal otitis externa

B37.89 Other sites of candidiasis
Candidal osteomyelitis

B37.9 Candidiasis, unspecified
Thrush NOS

B38 Coccidioidomycosis

B38.Ø Acute pulmonary coccidioidomycosis HCC ESR COM

B38.1 Chronic pulmonary coccidioidomycosis HCC ESR COM

B38.2 Pulmonary coccidioidomycosis, unspecified HCC ESR COM

B38.3 Cutaneous coccidioidomycosis

B38.4 Coccidioidomycosis meningitis COM
DEF: *Coccidioides immitis* infection of the lining of the brain and/or spinal cord.

B38.7 Disseminated coccidioidomycosis
Generalized coccidioidomycosis

B38.8 Other forms of coccidioidomycosis

B38.81 Prostatic coccidioidomycosis ♂

B38.89 Other forms of coccidioidomycosis

B38.9 Coccidioidomycosis, unspecified

HCC CMS-HCC 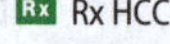 Rx Rx HCC ESR ESRD HCC COM Commercial HCC N Newborn: 0 P Pediatric: 0-17 M Maternity: 9-64 A Adult: 15-124

√4th B39 Histoplasmosis

Code first associated AIDS (B2Ø)
Use additional code for any associated manifestations, such as:
- endocarditis (I39)
- meningitis (GØ2)
- pericarditis (I32)
- retinitis (H32)

DEF: Type of lung infection caused by breathing in fungal spores often found in the droppings of bats and birds or soil contaminated by their droppings.

Histoplasmosis

Histoplasma capsulatum spores

Spores

B39.Ø **Acute pulmonary** histoplasmosis capsulati HCC ESR COM
B39.1 **Chronic pulmonary** histoplasmosis capsulati HCC ESR COM
B39.2 Pulmonary histoplasmosis capsulati, unspecified HCC ESR COM
B39.3 **Disseminated** histoplasmosis capsulati
  Generalized histoplasmosis capsulati
B39.4 Histoplasmosis capsulati, unspecified
  American histoplasmosis
B39.5 Histoplasmosis **duboisii**
  African histoplasmosis
B39.9 Histoplasmosis, unspecified

√4th B4Ø Blastomycosis

EXCLUDES 1 *Brazilian blastomycosis (B41.-)*
keloidal blastomycosis (B48.Ø)

B4Ø.Ø **Acute pulmonary** blastomycosis HCC ESR COM
B4Ø.1 **Chronic pulmonary** blastomycosis HCC ESR COM
B4Ø.2 **Pulmonary** blastomycosis, unspecified HCC ESR COM
B4Ø.3 **Cutaneous** blastomycosis
B4Ø.7 **Disseminated** blastomycosis
  Generalized blastomycosis
√5th B4Ø.8 Other forms of blastomycosis
  B4Ø.81 Blastomycotic **meningoencephalitis** COM
    Meningomyelitis due to blastomycosis
  B4Ø.89 Other forms of blastomycosis
B4Ø.9 Blastomycosis, unspecified

√4th B41 Paracoccidioidomycosis

INCLUDES Brazilian blastomycosis
Lutz' disease

B41.Ø **Pulmonary** paracoccidioidomycosis HCC ESR COM
B41.7 **Disseminated** paracoccidioidomycosis
  Generalized paracoccidioidomycosis
B41.8 Other forms of paracoccidioidomycosis
B41.9 Paracoccidioidomycosis, unspecified

√4th B42 Sporotrichosis

B42.Ø **Pulmonary** sporotrichosis
B42.1 **Lymphocutaneous** sporotrichosis
B42.7 **Disseminated** sporotrichosis
  Generalized sporotrichosis
√5th B42.8 Other forms of sporotrichosis
  B42.81 **Cerebral** sporotrichosis COM
    Meningitis due to sporotrichosis
  B42.82 Sporotrichosis **arthritis** HCC ESR COM
  B42.89 Other forms of sporotrichosis
B42.9 Sporotrichosis, unspecified

√4th B43 Chromomycosis and pheomycotic abscess

B43.Ø **Cutaneous** chromomycosis
  Dermatitis verrucosa
B43.1 Pheomycotic **brain abscess** COM
  Cerebral chromomycosis
B43.2 **Subcutaneous** pheomycotic **abscess and cyst**
B43.8 Other forms of chromomycosis
B43.9 Chromomycosis, unspecified

√4th B44 Aspergillosis

INCLUDES aspergilloma

B44.Ø **Invasive pulmonary** aspergillosis HCC Rx ESR COM
B44.1 Other pulmonary aspergillosis HCC Rx ESR COM
B44.2 **Tonsillar** aspergillosis HCC Rx ESR COM
B44.7 **Disseminated** aspergillosis HCC Rx ESR COM
  Generalized aspergillosis
√5th B44.8 Other forms of aspergillosis
  B44.81 **Allergic bronchopulmonary** aspergillosis HCC Rx ESR COM
  B44.89 Other forms of aspergillosis HCC Rx ESR COM
B44.9 Aspergillosis, unspecified HCC Rx ESR COM

√4th B45 Cryptococcosis

B45.Ø **Pulmonary** cryptococcosis HCC Rx ESR COM
B45.1 **Cerebral** cryptococcosis HCC Rx ESR COM
  Cryptococcal meningitis
  Cryptococcosis meningocerebralis
B45.2 **Cutaneous** cryptococcosis HCC Rx ESR COM
B45.3 **Osseous** cryptococcosis HCC Rx ESR COM
B45.7 **Disseminated** cryptococcosis HCC Rx ESR COM
  Generalized cryptococcosis
B45.8 Other forms of cryptococcosis HCC Rx ESR COM
B45.9 Cryptococcosis, unspecified HCC Rx ESR COM

√4th B46 Zygomycosis

B46.Ø **Pulmonary** mucormycosis HCC Rx ESR COM
B46.1 **Rhinocerebral** mucormycosis HCC Rx ESR COM
B46.2 **Gastrointestinal** mucormycosis HCC Rx ESR COM
B46.3 **Cutaneous** mucormycosis HCC Rx ESR COM
  Subcutaneous mucormycosis
B46.4 **Disseminated** mucormycosis HCC Rx ESR COM
  Generalized mucormycosis
B46.5 Mucormycosis, unspecified HCC Rx ESR COM
B46.8 Other zygomycoses HCC Rx ESR COM
  Entomophthoromycosis
B46.9 Zygomycosis, unspecified HCC Rx ESR COM
  Phycomycosis NOS

√4th B47 Mycetoma

B47.Ø Eumycetoma
  Madura foot, mycotic
  Maduromycosis
B47.1 Actinomycetoma
B47.9 Mycetoma, unspecified
  Madura foot NOS

√4th B48 Other mycoses, not elsewhere classified

B48.Ø Lobomycosis
  Keloidal blastomycosis
  Lobo's disease
B48.1 Rhinosporidiosis
B48.2 Allescheriasis
  Infection due to Pseudallescheria boydii
  EXCLUDES 1 *eumycetoma (B47.Ø)*
B48.3 Geotrichosis
  Geotrichum stomatitis

B48.4 Penicillosis HCC Rx ESR COM
Talaromycosis

B48.8 Other specified mycoses HCC Rx ESR COM
Adiaspiromycosis
Infection of tissue and organs by Alternaria
Infection of tissue and organs by Drechslera
Infection of tissue and organs by Fusarium
Infection of tissue and organs by saprophytic fungi NEC
AHA: 2014,4Q,46; 2014,2Q,13
TIP: This code is assigned when the nonspecific term "non-*Candida albicans*" sepsis is documented. If sepsis is documented as due to any *Candida* type, code B37.7 Candidal sepsis, is assigned.

B49 Unspecified mycosis
Fungemia NOS

Protozoal diseases (B50-B64)

EXCLUDES 1 *amebiasis (A06.-)*
other protozoal intestinal diseases (A07.-)

B50 Plasmodium falciparum malaria
INCLUDES mixed infections of Plasmodium falciparum with any other Plasmodium species

B50.0 Plasmodium falciparum malaria with cerebral complications
Cerebral malaria NOS

B50.8 Other severe and complicated Plasmodium falciparum malaria
Severe or complicated Plasmodium falciparum malaria NOS

B50.9 Plasmodium falciparum malaria, unspecified

B51 Plasmodium vivax malaria
INCLUDES mixed infections of Plasmodium vivax with other Plasmodium species, except Plasmodium falciparum
EXCLUDES 1 *Plasmodium vivax with Plasmodium falciparum (B50.-)*

B51.0 Plasmodium vivax malaria with rupture of spleen

B51.8 Plasmodium vivax malaria with other complications

B51.9 Plasmodium vivax malaria without complication
Plasmodium vivax malaria NOS

B52 Plasmodium malariae malaria
INCLUDES mixed infections of Plasmodium malariae with other Plasmodium species, except Plasmodium falciparum and Plasmodium vivax
EXCLUDES 1 *Plasmodium falciparum (B50.-)*
Plasmodium vivax (B51.-)

B52.0 Plasmodium malariae malaria with nephropathy

B52.8 Plasmodium malariae malaria with other complications

B52.9 Plasmodium malariae malaria without complication
Plasmodium malariae malaria NOS

B53 Other specified malaria

B53.0 Plasmodium ovale malaria
EXCLUDES 1 *Plasmodium ovale with Plasmodium falciparum (B50.-)*
Plasmodium ovale with Plasmodium malariae (B52.-)
Plasmodium ovale with Plasmodium vivax (B51.-)

B53.1 Malaria due to simian plasmodia
EXCLUDES 1 *malaria due to simian plasmodia with Plasmodium falciparum (B50.-)*
malaria due to simian plasmodia with Plasmodium malariae (B52.-)
malaria due to simian plasmodia with Plasmodium ovale (B53.0)
malaria due to simian plasmodia with Plasmodium vivax (B51.-)

B53.8 Other malaria, not elsewhere classified

B54 Unspecified malaria

B55 Leishmaniasis

B55.0 Visceral leishmaniasis
Kala-azar
Post-kala-azar dermal leishmaniasis

B55.1 Cutaneous leishmaniasis

B55.2 Mucocutaneous leishmaniasis

B55.9 Leishmaniasis, unspecified

B56 African trypanosomiasis

B56.0 Gambiense trypanosomiasis
Infection due to Trypanosoma brucei gambiense
West African sleeping sickness

B56.1 Rhodesiense trypanosomiasis
East African sleeping sickness
Infection due to Trypanosoma brucei rhodesiense

B56.9 African trypanosomiasis, unspecified
Sleeping sickness NOS

B57 Chagas' disease
INCLUDES American trypanosomiasis
infection due to Trypanosoma cruzi

B57.0 Acute Chagas' disease with heart involvement
Acute Chagas' disease with myocarditis

B57.1 Acute Chagas' disease without heart involvement
Acute Chagas' disease NOS

B57.2 Chagas' disease (chronic) with heart involvement
American trypanosomiasis NOS
Chagas' disease (chronic) NOS
Chagas' disease (chronic) with myocarditis
Trypanosomiasis NOS

B57.3 Chagas' disease (chronic) with digestive system involvement

B57.30 Chagas' disease with digestive system involvement, unspecified

B57.31 Megaesophagus in Chagas' disease

B57.32 Megacolon in Chagas' disease

B57.39 Other digestive system involvement in Chagas' disease

B57.4 Chagas' disease (chronic) with nervous system involvement

B57.40 Chagas' disease with nervous system involvement, unspecified

B57.41 Meningitis in Chagas' disease COM

B57.42 Meningoencephalitis in Chagas' disease COM

B57.49 Other nervous system involvement in Chagas' disease

B57.5 Chagas' disease (chronic) with other organ involvement

B58 Toxoplasmosis
INCLUDES infection due to Toxoplasma gondii
EXCLUDES 1 *congenital toxoplasmosis (P37.1)*

B58.0 Toxoplasma oculopathy

B58.00 Toxoplasma oculopathy, unspecified

B58.01 Toxoplasma chorioretinitis

B58.09 Other toxoplasma oculopathy
Toxoplasma uveitis

B58.1 Toxoplasma hepatitis

B58.2 Toxoplasma meningoencephalitis HCC Rx ESR COM

B58.3 Pulmonary toxoplasmosis HCC Rx ESR COM

B58.8 Toxoplasmosis with other organ involvement

B58.81 Toxoplasma myocarditis COM

B58.82 Toxoplasma myositis

B58.83 Toxoplasma tubulo-interstitial nephropathy
Toxoplasma pyelonephritis

B58.89 Toxoplasmosis with other organ involvement

B58.9 Toxoplasmosis, unspecified

B59 Pneumocystosis HCC Rx ESR COM
Pneumonia due to Pneumocystis carinii
Pneumonia due to Pneumocystis jiroveci

B60 Other protozoal diseases, not elsewhere classified
EXCLUDES 1 *cryptosporidiosis (A07.2)*
intestinal microsporidiosis (A07.8)
isosporiasis (A07.3)

B60.0 Babesiosis
AHA: 2020,4Q,5-6

B60.00 Babesiosis, unspecified
Babesiosis due to unspecified Babesia species
Piroplasmosis, unspecified

B60.01 Babesiosis due to Babesia microti
Infection due to B. microti

B60.02 Babesiosis due to Babesia duncani
Infection due to B. duncani and B. duncani-type species

B60.03 Babesiosis due to Babesia divergens
Babesiosis due to Babesia MO-1
Infection due to B. divergens and B. divergens-like strains

B60.09 Other babesiosis
Babesiosis due to Babesia KO-1
Babesiosis due to Babesia venatorum
Infection due to other Babesia species
Infection due to other protozoa of the order Piroplasmida
Other piroplasmosis

✓5th **B60.1 Acanthamebiasis**

B60.10 Acanthamebiasis, unspecified

B60.11 Meningoencephalitis due to Acanthamoeba (culbertsoni) COM

B60.12 Conjunctivitis due to Acanthamoeba

B60.13 Keratoconjunctivitis due to Acanthamoeba

B60.19 Other acanthamebic disease

B60.2 Naegleriasis
Primary amebic meningoencephalitis

B60.8 Other specified protozoal diseases
Microsporidiosis

B64 Unspecified protozoal disease

Helminthiases (B65-B83)

✓4th **B65 Schistosomiasis [bilharziasis]**
INCLUDES snail fever

B65.0 Schistosomiasis due to Schistosoma haematobium [urinary schistosomiasis]

B65.1 Schistosomiasis due to Schistosoma mansoni [intestinal schistosomiasis]

B65.2 Schistosomiasis due to Schistosoma japonicum
Asiatic schistosomiasis

B65.3 Cercarial dermatitis
Swimmer's itch

B65.8 Other schistosomiasis
Infection due to Schistosoma intercalatum
Infection due to Schistosoma mattheei
Infection due to Schistosoma mekongi

B65.9 Schistosomiasis, unspecified

✓4th **B66 Other fluke infections**

B66.0 Opisthorchiasis
Infection due to cat liver fluke
Infection due to Opisthorchis (felineus)(viverrini)

B66.1 Clonorchiasis
Chinese liver fluke disease
Infection due to Clonorchis sinensis
Oriental liver fluke disease

B66.2 Dicroceliasis
Infection due to Dicrocoelium dendriticum
Lancet fluke infection

B66.3 Fascioliasis
Infection due to Fasciola gigantica
Infection due to Fasciola hepatica
Infection due to Fasciola indica
Sheep liver fluke disease

B66.4 Paragonimiasis HCC ESR COM
Infection due to Paragonimus species
Lung fluke disease
Pulmonary distomiasis

B66.5 Fasciolopsiasis
Infection due to Fasciolopsis buski
Intestinal distomiasis

B66.8 Other specified fluke infections
Echinostomiasis
Heterophyiasis
Metagonimiasis
Nanophyetiasis
Watsoniasis

B66.9 Fluke infection, unspecified

✓4th **B67 Echinococcosis**
INCLUDES hydatidosis

B67.0 Echinococcus granulosus infection of liver

B67.1 Echinococcus granulosus infection of lung HCC ESR COM

B67.2 Echinococcus granulosus infection of bone

✓5th **B67.3 Echinococcus granulosus infection, other and multiple sites**

B67.31 Echinococcus granulosus infection, thyroid gland

B67.32 Echinococcus granulosus infection, multiple sites

B67.39 Echinococcus granulosus infection, other sites

B67.4 Echinococcus granulosus infection, unspecified
Dog tapeworm (infection)

B67.5 Echinococcus multilocularis infection of liver

✓5th **B67.6 Echinococcus multilocularis infection, other and multiple sites**

B67.61 Echinococcus multilocularis infection, multiple sites

B67.69 Echinococcus multilocularis infection, other sites

B67.7 Echinococcus multilocularis infection, unspecified

B67.8 Echinococcosis, unspecified, of liver

✓5th **B67.9 Echinococcosis, other and unspecified**

B67.90 Echinococcosis, unspecified
Echinococcosis NOS

B67.99 Other echinococcosis

✓4th **B68 Taeniasis**
EXCLUDES 1 *cysticercosis (B69.-)*

B68.0 Taenia solium taeniasis
Pork tapeworm (infection)

B68.1 Taenia saginata taeniasis
Beef tapeworm (infection)
Infection due to adult tapeworm Taenia saginata

B68.9 Taeniasis, unspecified

✓4th **B69 Cysticercosis**
INCLUDES cysticerciasis infection due to larval form of Taenia solium

DEF: Condition that is developed when larvae or eggs of the tapeworm *Taenia solium* are ingested, most commonly in fecally contaminated water or undercooked pork.

B69.0 Cysticercosis of central nervous system

B69.1 Cysticercosis of eye

✓5th **B69.8 Cysticercosis of other sites**

B69.81 Myositis in cysticercosis

B69.89 Cysticercosis of other sites

B69.9 Cysticercosis, unspecified

✓4th **B70 Diphyllobothriasis and sparganosis**

B70.0 Diphyllobothriasis
Diphyllobothrium (adult) (latum) (pacificum) infection
Fish tapeworm (infection)
EXCLUDES 2 *larval diphyllobothriasis (B70.1)*

B70.1 Sparganosis
Infection due to Sparganum (mansoni) (proliferum)
Infection due to Spirometra larva
Larval diphyllobothriasis
Spirometrosis

✓4th **B71 Other cestode infections**

B71.0 Hymenolepiasis
Dwarf tapeworm infection
Rat tapeworm (infection)

B71.1 Dipylidiasis

B71.8 Other specified cestode infections
Coenurosis

B71.9 Cestode infection, unspecified
Tapeworm (infection) NOS

B72 Dracunculiasis
INCLUDES guinea worm infection
infection due to Dracunculus medinensis

✓4th **B73 Onchocerciasis**
INCLUDES onchocerca volvulus infection
onchocercosis
river blindness

✓5th **B73.0 Onchocerciasis with eye disease**

B73.00 Onchocerciasis with eye involvement, unspecified

B73.01 Onchocerciasis with endophthalmitis

B73.02 Onchocerciasis with glaucoma

B73.09 Onchocerciasis with other eye involvement
Infestation of eyelid due to onchocerciasis

B73.1 Onchocerciasis without eye disease

B74 Filariasis

EXCLUDES 2 *onchocerciasis (B73)*
tropical (pulmonary) eosinophilia NOS (J82.89)

B74.0 Filariasis due to Wuchereria bancrofti
Bancroftian elephantiasis
Bancroftian filariasis

B74.1 Filariasis due to Brugia malayi

B74.2 Filariasis due to Brugia timori

B74.3 Loiasis
Calabar swelling
Eyeworm disease of Africa
Loa loa infection

B74.4 Mansonelliasis
Infection due to Mansonella ozzardi
Infection due to Mansonella perstans
Infection due to Mansonella streptocerca

B74.8 Other filariases
Dirofilariasis

B74.9 Filariasis, unspecified

B75 Trichinellosis

INCLUDES infection due to Trichinella species
trichiniasis

DEF: Infection by *Trichinella spiralis*, the smallest of the parasitic nematodes, that is transmitted by eating undercooked pork or bear meat. ***Synonym(s):*** *Trichinosis.*

B76 Hookworm diseases

INCLUDES uncinariasis

B76.0 Ancylostomiasis
Infection due to Ancylostoma species

B76.1 Necatoriasis
Infection due to Necator americanus

B76.8 Other hookworm diseases

B76.9 Hookworm disease, unspecified
Cutaneous larva migrans NOS

B77 Ascariasis

INCLUDES ascaridiasis
roundworm infection

B77.0 Ascariasis with intestinal complications

B77.8 Ascariasis with other complications

B77.81 Ascariasis pneumonia

B77.89 Ascariasis with other complications

B77.9 Ascariasis, unspecified

B78 Strongyloidiasis

EXCLUDES 1 *trichostrongyliasis (B81.2)*

B78.0 Intestinal strongyloidiasis

B78.1 Cutaneous strongyloidiasis

B78.7 Disseminated strongyloidiasis

B78.9 Strongyloidiasis, unspecified

B79 Trichuriasis

INCLUDES trichocephaliasis
whipworm (disease)(infection)

B80 Enterobiasis

INCLUDES oxyuriasis
pinworm infection
threadworm infection

B81 Other intestinal helminthiases, not elsewhere classified

EXCLUDES 1 *angiostrongyliasis due to:*
angiostrongylus cantonensis (B83.2)
parastrongylus cantonensis (B83.2)

B81.0 Anisakiasis
Infection due to Anisakis larva

B81.1 Intestinal capillariasis
Capillariasis NOS
Infection due to Capillaria philippinensis
EXCLUDES 2 *hepatic capillariasis (B83.8)*

B81.2 Trichostrongyliasis

B81.3 Intestinal angiostrongyliasis
Angiostrongyliasis due to:
Angiostrongylus costaricensis
Parastrongylus costaricensis

B81.4 Mixed intestinal helminthiases
Infection due to intestinal helminths classified to more than one of the categories B65.0-B81.3 and B81.8
Mixed helminthiasis NOS

B81.8 Other specified intestinal helminthiases
Infection due to Oesophagostomum species [esophagostomiasis]
Infection due to Ternidens diminutus [ternidensiasis]

B82 Unspecified intestinal parasitism

B82.0 Intestinal helminthiasis, unspecified

B82.9 Intestinal parasitism, unspecified

B83 Other helminthiases

EXCLUDES 1 *capillariasis NOS (B81.1)*
EXCLUDES 2 *intestinal capillariasis (B81.1)*

B83.0 Visceral larva migrans
Toxocariasis

B83.1 Gnathostomiasis
Wandering swelling

B83.2 Angiostrongyliasis due to Parastrongylus cantonensis
Eosinophilic meningoencephalitis due to Parastrongylus cantonensis
EXCLUDES 2 *intestinal angiostrongyliasis (B81.3)*

B83.3 Syngamiasis
Syngamosis

B83.4 Internal hirudiniasis
EXCLUDES 2 *external hirudiniasis (B88.3)*

B83.8 Other specified helminthiases
Acanthocephaliasis
Gongylonemiasis
Hepatic capillariasis
Metastrongyliasis
Thelaziasis

B83.9 Helminthiasis, unspecified
Worms NOS
EXCLUDES 1 *intestinal helminthiasis NOS (B82.0)*

Pediculosis, acariasis and other infestations (B85-B89)

B85 Pediculosis and phthiriasis

B85.0 Pediculosis due to Pediculus humanus capitis
Head-louse infestation

B85.1 Pediculosis due to Pediculus humanus corporis
Body-louse infestation

B85.2 Pediculosis, unspecified

B85.3 Phthiriasis
Infestation by crab-louse
Infestation by Phthirus pubis

B85.4 Mixed pediculosis and phthiriasis
Infestation classifiable to more than one of the categories B85.0-B85.3

B86 Scabies
Sarcoptic itch
DEF: Mite infestation that is caused by *Sarcoptes scabiei*. Scabies causes intense itching and sometimes secondary infection.

B87 Myiasis

INCLUDES infestation by larva of flies

B87.0 Cutaneous myiasis
Creeping myiasis

B87.1 Wound myiasis
Traumatic myiasis

B87.2 Ocular myiasis

B87.3 Nasopharyngeal myiasis
Laryngeal myiasis

B87.4 Aural myiasis

B87.8 Myiasis of other sites

B87.81 Genitourinary myiasis

B87.82 Intestinal myiasis

B87.89 Myiasis of other sites

B87.9 Myiasis, unspecified

B88 Other infestations

B88.Ø Other acariasis
Acarine dermatitis
Dermatitis due to Demodex species
Dermatitis due to Dermanyssus gallinae
Dermatitis due to Liponyssoides sanguineus
Trombiculosis
EXCLUDES 2 *scabies (B86)*

B88.1 Tungiasis [sandflea infestation]

B88.2 Other arthropod infestations
Scarabiasis

B88.3 External hirudiniasis
Leech infestation NOS
EXCLUDES 2 *internal hirudiniasis (B83.4)*

B88.8 Other specified infestations
Ichthyoparasitism due to Vandellia cirrhosa
Linguatulosis
Porocephaliasis

B88.9 Infestation, unspecified
Infestation (skin) NOS
Infestation by mites NOS
Skin parasites NOS

B89 Unspecified parasitic disease

Sequelae of infectious and parasitic diseases (B9Ø-B94)

NOTE Categories B9Ø-B94 are to be used to indicate conditions in categories AØØ-B89 as the cause of sequelae, which are themselves classified elsewhere. The "sequelae" include conditions specified as such; they also include residuals of diseases classifiable to the above categories if there is evidence that the disease itself is no longer present. Codes from these categories are not to be used for chronic infections. Code chronic current infections to active infectious disease as appropriate.

Code first condition resulting from (sequela) the infectious or parasitic disease

B9Ø Sequelae of tuberculosis

B9Ø.Ø Sequelae of central nervous system tuberculosis

B9Ø.1 Sequelae of genitourinary tuberculosis

B9Ø.2 Sequelae of tuberculosis of bones and joints

B9Ø.8 Sequelae of tuberculosis of other organs
EXCLUDES 2 *sequelae of respiratory tuberculosis (B9Ø.9)*

B9Ø.9 Sequelae of respiratory and unspecified tuberculosis
Sequelae of tuberculosis NOS

B91 Sequelae of poliomyelitis
EXCLUDES 1 *postpolio syndrome (G14)*

B92 Sequelae of leprosy

B94 Sequelae of other and unspecified infectious and parasitic diseases

B94.Ø Sequelae of trachoma

B94.1 Sequelae of viral encephalitis

B94.2 Sequelae of viral hepatitis

B94.8 Sequelae of other specified infectious and parasitic diseases
AHA: 2021,1Q,25-30,31-49; 2020,3Q,10-14; 2017,4Q,109

B94.9 Sequelae of unspecified infectious and parasitic disease
EXCLUDES 2 *post COVID-19 condition (UØ9.9)*

Bacterial and viral infectious agents (B95-B97)

NOTE These categories are provided for use as supplementary or additional codes to identify the infectious agent(s) in diseases classified elsewhere.

AHA: 2020,2Q,18; 2018,4Q,34; 2018,1Q,16

B95 Streptococcus, Staphylococcus, and Enterococcus as the cause of diseases classified elsewhere

B95.Ø Streptococcus, group A, as the cause of diseases classified elsewhere UPD

B95.1 Streptococcus, group B, as the cause of diseases classified elsewhere UPD
AHA: 2020,1Q,10; 2019,2Q,8-10

B95.2 Enterococcus as the cause of diseases classified elsewhere UPD

B95.3 Streptococcus pneumoniae as the cause of diseases classified elsewhere UPD

B95.4 Other streptococcus as the cause of diseases classified elsewhere UPD

B95.5 Unspecified streptococcus as the cause of diseases classified elsewhere UPD

B95.6 Staphylococcus aureus as the cause of diseases classified elsewhere

B95.61 Methicillin susceptible Staphylococcus aureus infection as the cause of diseases classified elsewhere UPD
Methicillin susceptible Staphylococcus aureus (MSSA) infection as the cause of diseases classified elsewhere
Staphylococcus aureus infection NOS as the cause of diseases classified elsewhere

B95.62 Methicillin resistant Staphylococcus aureus infection as the cause of diseases classified elsewhere UPD
Methicillin resistant staphylococcus aureus (MRSA) infection as the cause of diseases classified elsewhere
AHA: 2016,1Q,12

B95.7 Other staphylococcus as the cause of diseases classified elsewhere UPD

B95.8 Unspecified staphylococcus as the cause of diseases classified elsewhere UPD

B96 Other bacterial agents as the cause of diseases classified elsewhere

B96.Ø Mycoplasma pneumoniae [M. pneumoniae] as the cause of diseases classified elsewhere UPD
Pleuro-pneumonia-like-organism [PPLO]

B96.1 Klebsiella pneumoniae [K. pneumoniae] as the cause of diseases classified elsewhere UPD

B96.2 Escherichia coli [E. coli] as the cause of diseases classified elsewhere
AHA: 2022,1Q,31

B96.2Ø Unspecified Escherichia coli [E. coli] as the cause of diseases classified elsewhere UPD
Escherichia coli [E. coli] NOS

B96.21 Shiga toxin-producing Escherichia coli [E. coli] [STEC] O157 as the cause of diseases classified elsewhere UPD
E. coli O157:H- (nonmotile) with confirmation of Shiga toxin
E. coli O157 with confirmation of Shiga toxin when H antigen is unknown, or is not H7
O157:H7 Escherichia coli [E.coli] with or without confirmation of Shiga toxin-production
Shiga toxin-producing Escherichia coli [E.coli] O157:H7 with or without confirmation of Shiga toxin-production
STEC O157:H7 with or without confirmation of Shiga toxin-production

B96.22 Other specified Shiga toxin-producing Escherichia coli [E. coli] [STEC] as the cause of diseases classified elsewhere UPD
Non-O157 Shiga toxin-producing Escherichia coli [E.coli]
Non-O157 Shiga toxin-producing Escherichia coli [E.coli] with known O group

B96.23 Unspecified Shiga toxin-producing Escherichia coli [E. coli] [STEC] as the cause of diseases classified elsewhere UPD
Shiga toxin-producing Escherichia coli [E. coli] with unspecified O group
STEC NOS

B96.29 Other Escherichia coli [E. coli] as the cause of diseases classified elsewhere UPD
Non-Shiga toxin-producing E. coli

B96.3 Hemophilus influenzae [H. influenzae] as the cause of diseases classified elsewhere UPD

B96.4 Proteus (mirabilis) (morganii) as the cause of diseases classified elsewhere UPD

B96.5 Pseudomonas (aeruginosa) (mallei) (pseudomallei) as the cause of diseases classified elsewhere UPD
AHA: 2015,1Q,18

B96.6 Bacteroides fragilis [B. fragilis] as the cause of diseases classified elsewhere UPD

B96.7 Clostridium perfringens [C. perfringens] as the cause of diseases classified elsewhere UPD

B96.8 Other specified bacterial agents as the cause of diseases classified elsewhere

B96.81 Helicobacter pylori [H. pylori] as the cause of diseases classified elsewhere UPD

Chapter 1. Certain Infectious and Parasitic Diseases

B88–B96.81

B96.82 Vibrio vulnificus as the cause of diseases classified elsewhere UPD

B96.89 Other specified bacterial agents as the cause of diseases classified elsewhere UPD

✓4th **B97 Viral agents as the cause of diseases classified elsewhere**

AHA: 2016,3Q,8-10,14

B97.Ø Adenovirus as the cause of diseases classified elsewhere UPD

✓5th **B97.1 Enterovirus as the cause of diseases classified elsewhere**

B97.1Ø Unspecified enterovirus as the cause of diseases classified elsewhere UPD

B97.11 Coxsackievirus as the cause of diseases classified elsewhere UPD

B97.12 Echovirus as the cause of diseases classified elsewhere UPD

B97.19 Other enterovirus as the cause of diseases classified elsewhere UPD

✓5th **B97.2 Coronavirus as the cause of diseases classified elsewhere**

TIP: Do not report a code from this subcategory for COVID-19; refer to U07.1.

B97.21 SARS-associated coronavirus as the cause of diseases classified elsewhere UPD

EXCLUDES 1 *pneumonia due to SARS-associated coronavirus (J12.81)*

B97.29 Other coronavirus as the cause of diseases classified elsewhere UPD

AHA: 2020,2Q,5; 2020,1Q,34-36

✓5th **B97.3 Retrovirus as the cause of diseases classified elsewhere**

EXCLUDES 1 *human immunodeficiency virus [HIV] disease (B2Ø)*

B97.3Ø Unspecified retrovirus as the cause of diseases classified elsewhere UPD

B97.31 Lentivirus as the cause of diseases classified elsewhere UPD

B97.32 Oncovirus as the cause of diseases classified elsewhere UPD

B97.33 Human T-cell lymphotrophic virus, type I [HTLV-I] as the cause of diseases classified elsewhere UPD

B97.34 Human T-cell lymphotrophic virus, type II [HTLV-II] as the cause of diseases classified elsewhere UPD

B97.35 Human immunodeficiency virus, type 2 [HIV 2] as the cause of diseases classified elsewhere HCC Rx ESR COM UPD

B97.39 Other retrovirus as the cause of diseases classified elsewhere UPD

B97.4 Respiratory syncytial virus as the cause of diseases classified elsewhere UPD

RSV as the cause of diseases classified elsewhere

Code first related disorders, such as:
- otitis media (H65.-)
- upper respiratory infection (JØ6.9)

EXCLUDES 1 *acute bronchiolitis due to respiratory syncytial virus (RSV) (J21.Ø)*
acute bronchitis due to respiratory syncytial virus (RSV) (J2Ø.5)
respiratory syncytial virus (RSV) pneumonia (J12.1)

B97.5 Reovirus as the cause of diseases classified elsewhere UPD

B97.6 Parvovirus as the cause of diseases classified elsewhere UPD

B97.7 Papillomavirus as the cause of diseases classified elsewhere UPD

✓5th **B97.8 Other viral agents as the cause of diseases classified elsewhere**

B97.81 Human metapneumovirus as the cause of diseases classified elsewhere UPD

B97.89 Other viral agents as the cause of diseases classified elsewhere UPD

Other infectious diseases (B99)

✓4th **B99 Other and unspecified infectious diseases**

B99.8 Other infectious disease

B99.9 Unspecified infectious disease

Chapter 2. Neoplasms (CØØ–D49)

Chapter-specific Guidelines with Coding Examples

The chapter-specific guidelines from the ICD-10-CM Official Guidelines for Coding and Reporting have been provided below. Along with these guidelines are coding examples, contained in the shaded boxes, that have been developed to help illustrate the coding and/or sequencing guidance found in these guidelines.

General guidelines

Chapter 2 of the ICD-10-CM contains the codes for most benign and all malignant neoplasms. Certain benign neoplasms, such as prostatic adenomas, may be found in the specific body system chapters. To properly code a neoplasm, it is necessary to determine from the record if the neoplasm is benign, in-situ, malignant, or of uncertain histologic behavior. If malignant, any secondary (metastatic) sites should also be determined.

Primary malignant neoplasms overlapping site boundaries

A primary malignant neoplasm that overlaps two or more contiguous (next to each other) sites should be classified to the subcategory/code .8 ('overlapping lesion'), unless the combination is specifically indexed elsewhere. For multiple neoplasms of the same site that are not contiguous such as tumors in different quadrants of the same breast, codes for each site should be assigned.

A 62-year-old female with a malignant lesion of the upper lip that extends from the lipstick area to the labial frenulum

CØØ.8	**Malignant neoplasm of overlapping sites of lip**

Explanation: Because this is a single lesion that overlaps two contiguous sites, a single code for overlapping sites is assigned.

A 74-year-old male is treated for two distinct malignant lesions, one in the mucosa of the upper lip and a second in the mucosa of the lower lip.

CØØ.3	**Malignant neoplasm of upper lip, inner aspect**
CØØ.4	**Malignant neoplasm of lower lip, inner aspect**

Explanation: This patient has two distinct malignant lesions of the upper and lower lips. Because the lesions are not contiguous, two codes are reported.

Malignant neoplasm of ectopic tissue

Malignant neoplasms of ectopic tissue are to be coded to the site of origin mentioned, e.g., ectopic pancreatic malignant neoplasms involving the stomach are coded to malignant neoplasm of pancreas, unspecified (C25.9).

The neoplasm table in the Alphabetic Index should be referenced first. However, if the histological term is documented, that term should be referenced first, rather than going immediately to the Neoplasm Table, in order to determine which column in the Neoplasm Table is appropriate. For example, if the documentation indicates "adenoma," refer to the term in the Alphabetic Index to review the entries under this term and the instructional note to "see also neoplasm, by site, benign." The table provides the proper code based on the type of neoplasm and the site. It is important to select the proper column in the table that corresponds to the type of neoplasm. The Tabular List should then be referenced to verify that the correct code has been selected from the table and that a more specific site code does not exist.

See Section I.C.21. Factors influencing health status and contact with health services, Status, for information regarding Z15.Ø, codes for genetic susceptibility to cancer.

a. *Admission/Encounter for treatment of primary site*

If the malignancy **is chiefly responsible for occasioning the patient admission/encounter and treatment is directed at the primary site,** designate the **primary** malignancy as the principal/**first-listed** diagnosis.

The only exception to this guideline is if the administration of chemotherapy, immunotherapy or external beam radiation therapy **is chiefly responsible for occasioning the admission/encounter. In that case**, assign the appropriate Z51.-- code as the first-listed or principal diagnosis, and the **underlying** diagnosis or problem for which the service is being performed as a secondary diagnosis.

b. *Admission/Encounter for* treatment of secondary site

When a patient is admitted because of a primary neoplasm with metastasis and treatment is directed toward the secondary site only, the secondary neoplasm is designated as the principal diagnosis even though the primary malignancy is still present.

Patient with primary prostate cancer with metastasis to lungs presents for wedge resection of mass in right lung

C78.Ø1	**Secondary malignant neoplasm of right lung**
C61	**Malignant neoplasm of prostate**

Explanation: Since the encounter is for treatment of the lung metastasis, the secondary lung metastasis is sequenced before the primary prostate cancer.

c. Coding and sequencing of complications

Coding and sequencing of complications associated with the malignancies or with the therapy thereof are subject to the following guidelines:

1) Anemia associated with malignancy

When admission/encounter is for management of an anemia associated with the malignancy, and the treatment is only for anemia, the appropriate code for the malignancy is sequenced as the principal or first-listed diagnosis followed by the appropriate code for the anemia (such as code D63.Ø, Anemia in neoplastic disease).

Patient is seen for treatment of anemia in advanced primary liver cancer

C22.8	**Malignant neoplasm of liver, primary, unspecified as to type**
D63.Ø	**Anemia in neoplastic disease**

Explanation: Even though the admission was solely to treat the anemia, this guideline indicates that the code for the malignancy is sequenced first.

2) Anemia associated with chemotherapy, immunotherapy and radiation therapy

When the admission/encounter is for management of an anemia associated with an adverse effect of the administration of chemotherapy or immunotherapy and the only treatment is for the anemia, the anemia code is sequenced first followed by the appropriate codes for the neoplasm and the adverse effect (T45.1X5, Adverse effect of antineoplastic and immunosuppressive drugs).

When the admission/encounter is for management of an anemia associated with an adverse effect of radiotherapy, the anemia code should be sequenced first, followed by the appropriate neoplasm code and code Y84.2, Radiological procedure and radiotherapy as the cause of abnormal reaction of the patient, or of later complication, without mention of misadventure at the time of the procedure.

A 55-year-old male with a large malignant rectal tumor has been receiving external radiation therapy to shrink the tumor prior to planned surgery. He is referred today for a blood transfusion to treat anemia related to radiation therapy.

D64.89	**Other specified anemias**
C2Ø	**Malignant neoplasm of rectum**
Y84.2	**Radiological procedure and radiotherapy as the cause of abnormal reaction of the patient, or of later complication, without mention of misadventure at the time of the procedure**

Explanation: The code for the anemia is sequenced first, followed by the code for the malignancy, and lastly the code for the abnormal reaction due to radiotherapy.

3) Management of dehydration due to the malignancy

When the admission/encounter is for management of dehydration due to the malignancy and only the dehydration is being treated (intravenous rehydration), the dehydration is sequenced first, followed by the code(s) for the malignancy.

4) Treatment of a complication resulting from a surgical procedure

When the admission/encounter is for treatment of a complication resulting from a surgical procedure, designate the complication as the principal or first-listed diagnosis if treatment is directed at resolving the complication.

d. Primary malignancy previously excised

When a primary malignancy has been previously excised or eradicated from its site and there is no further treatment directed to that site and there is no evidence of any existing primary malignancy at that site, a code from category Z85, Personal history of malignant neoplasm, should be used to indicate the former site of the malignancy. Any mention of extension, invasion, or metastasis to another site is coded as a secondary malignant neoplasm to that site. The secondary site may be the principal or first-listed diagnosis with the Z85 code used as a secondary code.

See section I.C.2.t. Secondary malignant neoplasm of lymphoid tissue.

History of lung cancer, left upper lobectomy 18 months ago with no current treatment; MRI of the brain shows metastatic disease in the brain

C79.31	**Secondary malignant neoplasm of brain**
Z85.118	**Personal history of other malignant neoplasm of bronchus and lung**

Explanation: The patient has undergone a diagnostic procedure that revealed metastatic lung cancer in the brain. The code for the secondary (metastatic) site is sequenced first, followed by a personal history code to identify the former site of the primary malignancy.

e. Admissions/encounters involving chemotherapy, immunotherapy and radiation therapy

1) Episode of care involves surgical removal of neoplasm

When an episode of care involves the surgical removal of a neoplasm, primary or secondary site, followed by adjunct chemotherapy or radiation treatment during the same episode of care, the code for the neoplasm should be assigned as principal or first-listed diagnosis.

2) Patient admission/encounter solely for administration of chemotherapy, immunotherapy and radiation therapy

If a patient admission/encounter is solely for the administration of chemotherapy, immunotherapy or external beam radiation therapy assign code Z51.Ø, Encounter for antineoplastic radiation therapy, or Z51.11, Encounter for antineoplastic chemotherapy, or Z51.12, Encounter for antineoplastic immunotherapy as the first-listed or principal diagnosis. If a patient receives more than one of these therapies during the same admission more than one of these codes may be assigned, in any sequence.

The malignancy for which the therapy is being administered should be assigned as a secondary diagnosis.

If a patient admission/encounter is for the insertion or implantation of radioactive elements (e.g., brachytherapy) the appropriate code for the malignancy is sequenced as the principal or first-listed diagnosis. Code Z51.Ø should not be assigned.

Patient presents for second round of rituximab and fludarabine for his chronic B cell lymphocytic leukemia

Z51.11	**Encounter for antineoplastic chemotherapy**
Z51.12	**Encounter for antineoplastic immunotherapy**
C91.1Ø	**Chronic lymphocytic leukemia of B-cell type not having achieved remission**

Explanation: Rituximab is an antineoplastic immunotherapy while fludarabine is an antineoplastic chemotherapy. The two treatments are often used together. The encounter was solely for the purpose of administering this treatment and either can be sequenced first, before the neoplastic condition.

3) Patient admitted for radiation therapy, chemotherapy or immunotherapy and develops complications

When a patient is admitted for the purpose of external beam radiotherapy, immunotherapy or chemotherapy and develops complications such as uncontrolled nausea and vomiting or dehydration, the principal or first-listed diagnosis is Z51.Ø, Encounter for antineoplastic radiation therapy, or Z51.11, Encounter for antineoplastic chemotherapy, or Z51.12, Encounter for antineoplastic immunotherapy followed by any codes for the complications.

When a patient is admitted for the purpose of insertion or implantation of radioactive elements (e.g., brachytherapy) and develops complications such as uncontrolled nausea and vomiting or dehydration, the principal or first-listed diagnosis is the appropriate code for the malignancy followed by any codes for the complications.

f. Admission/encounter to determine extent of malignancy

When the reason for admission/encounter is to determine the extent of the malignancy, or for a procedure such as paracentesis or thoracentesis, the primary malignancy or appropriate metastatic site is designated as the principal or first-listed diagnosis, even though chemotherapy or radiotherapy is administered.

Patient with left lung cancer with malignant pleural effusion being seen for paracentesis and initiation/administration of chemotherapy

C34.92	**Malignant neoplasm of unspecified part of left bronchus or lung**
J91.Ø	**Malignant pleural effusion**
Z51.11	**Encounter for antineoplastic chemotherapy**

Explanation: The lung cancer is sequenced before the chemotherapy in this instance because the paracentesis for the malignant effusion is also being performed. An instructional note under the malignant effusion instructs that the lung cancer be sequenced first.

g. Symptoms, signs, and abnormal findings listed in Chapter 18 associated with neoplasms

Symptoms, signs, and ill-defined conditions listed in Chapter 18 characteristic of, or associated with, an existing primary or secondary site malignancy cannot be used to replace the malignancy as principal or first-listed diagnosis, regardless of the number of admissions or encounters for treatment and care of the neoplasm.

See Section I.C.21. Factors influencing health status and contact with health services, Encounter for prophylactic organ removal.

h. Admission/encounter for pain control/management

See Section I.C.6. for information on coding admission/encounter for pain control/management.

i. Malignancy in two or more noncontiguous sites

A patient may have more than one malignant tumor in the same organ. These tumors may represent different primaries or metastatic disease, depending on the site. Should the documentation be unclear, the provider should be queried as to the status of each tumor so that the correct codes can be assigned.

j. Disseminated malignant neoplasm, unspecified

Code C8Ø.Ø, Disseminated malignant neoplasm, unspecified, is for use only in those cases where the patient has advanced metastatic disease and no known primary or secondary sites are specified. It should not be used in place of assigning codes for the primary site and all known secondary sites.

k. Malignant neoplasm without specification of site

Code C8Ø.1, Malignant (primary) neoplasm, unspecified, equates to Cancer, unspecified. This code should only be used when no determination can be made as to the primary site of a malignancy. This code should rarely be used in the inpatient setting.

Evaluation of painful hip leads to diagnosis of a metastatic bone lesion from an unknown primary neoplasm source

C79.51	**Secondary malignant neoplasm of bone**
C8Ø.1	**Malignant (primary) neoplasm, unspecified**

Explanation: If only the secondary site is known, use code C8Ø.1 for the unknown primary site.

l. Sequencing of neoplasm codes

1) Encounter for treatment of primary malignancy

If the reason for the encounter is for treatment of a primary malignancy, assign the malignancy as the principal/first-listed diagnosis. The primary site is to be sequenced first, followed by any metastatic sites.

2) Encounter for treatment of secondary malignancy

When an encounter is for a primary malignancy with metastasis and treatment is directed toward the metastatic (secondary) site(s) only, the metastatic site(s) is designated as the principal/first-listed diagnosis. The primary malignancy is coded as an additional code.

Patient has primary colon cancer with metastasis to rib and is evaluated for possible excision of portion of rib bone

C79.51	**Secondary malignant neoplasm of bone**
C18.9	**Malignant neoplasm of colon, unspecified**

Explanation: The treatment for this encounter is focused on the metastasis to the rib bone rather than the primary colon cancer, thus indicating that the bone metastasis is sequenced as the first-listed code.

3) Malignant neoplasm in a pregnant patient

When a pregnant patient has a malignant neoplasm, a code from subcategory O9A.1-, Malignant neoplasm complicating pregnancy, childbirth, and the puerperium, should be sequenced first, followed by the appropriate code from Chapter 2 to indicate the type of neoplasm.

A 30-year-old pregnant female in first trimester evaluated for pituitary gland malignancy

O9A.111	**Malignant neoplasm complicating pregnancy, first trimester**
C75.1	**Malignant neoplasm of pituitary gland**

Explanation: Codes from chapter 15 describing complications of pregnancy are sequenced as first-listed codes, further specified by codes from other chapters such as neoplastic, unless the pregnancy is documented as incidental to the condition. See also guideline 1.C.15.a.1.

4) Encounter for complication associated with a neoplasm

When an encounter is for management of a complication associated with a neoplasm, such as dehydration, and the treatment is only for the complication, the complication is coded first, followed by the appropriate code(s) for the neoplasm.

The exception to this guideline is anemia. When the admission/encounter is for management of an anemia associated with the malignancy, and the treatment is only for anemia, the appropriate code for the malignancy is sequenced as the principal or first-listed diagnosis followed by code D63.Ø, Anemia in neoplastic disease.

Patient with pancreatic cancer is seen for initiation of TPN for cancer-related moderate protein-calorie malnutrition

E44.Ø	**Moderate protein-calorie malnutrition**
C25.9	**Malignant neoplasm of pancreas, unspecified**

Explanation: The encounter is to initiate treatment for malnutrition, a common complication of many types of neoplasms, and is sequenced first.

5) Complication from surgical procedure for treatment of a neoplasm

When an encounter is for treatment of a complication resulting from a surgical procedure performed for the treatment of the neoplasm, designate the complication as the principal/first-listed diagnosis. See the guideline regarding the coding of a current malignancy versus personal history to determine if the code for the neoplasm should also be assigned.

6) Pathologic fracture due to a neoplasm

When an encounter is for a pathological fracture due to a neoplasm, and the focus of treatment is the fracture, a code from subcategory M84.5, Pathological fracture in neoplastic disease, should be sequenced first, followed by the code for the neoplasm.

If the focus of treatment is the neoplasm with an associated pathological fracture, the neoplasm code should be sequenced first, followed by a code from M84.5 for the pathological fracture.

m. Current malignancy versus personal history of malignancy

When a primary malignancy has been excised but further treatment, such as an additional surgery for the malignancy, radiation therapy or chemotherapy is directed to that site, the primary malignancy code should be used until treatment is completed.

Female patient with ongoing chemotherapy after right mastectomy for breast cancer

C5Ø.911	**Malignant neoplasm of unspecified site of right female breast**
Z9Ø.11	**Acquired absence of right breast and nipple**

Explanation: Even though the breast has been removed, the breast cancer is still being treated with chemotherapy and therefore is still coded as a current condition rather than personal history.

When a primary malignancy has been previously excised or eradicated from its site, there is no further treatment (of the malignancy) directed to that site, and there is no evidence of any existing primary malignancy at that site, a code from category Z85, Personal history of malignant neoplasm, should be used to indicate the former site of the malignancy.

Codes from subcategories Z85.Ø – Z85.85 should only be assigned for the former site of a primary malignancy, not the site of a secondary malignancy. Code Z85.89 may be assigned for the former site(s) of either a primary or secondary malignancy.

See Section I.C.21. Factors influencing health status and contact with health services, History (of)

n. Leukemia, multiple myeloma, and malignant plasma cell neoplasms in remission versus personal history

The categories for leukemia, and category C9Ø, Multiple myeloma and malignant plasma cell neoplasms, have codes indicating whether or not the leukemia has achieved remission. There are also codes Z85.6, Personal history of leukemia, and Z85.79, Personal history of other malignant neoplasms of lymphoid, hematopoietic and related tissues. If the documentation is unclear as to whether the leukemia has achieved remission, the provider should be queried.

See Section I.C.21. Factors influencing health status and contact with health services, History (of)

o. Aftercare following surgery for neoplasm

See Section I.C.21. Factors influencing health status and contact with health services, Aftercare

p. Follow-up care for completed treatment of a malignancy

See Section I.C.21. Factors influencing health status and contact with health services, Follow-up

q. Prophylactic organ removal for prevention of malignancy

See Section I.C. 21, Factors influencing health status and contact with health services, Prophylactic organ removal

r. Malignant neoplasm associated with transplanted organ

A malignant neoplasm of a transplanted organ should be coded as a transplant complication. Assign first the appropriate code from category T86.-, Complications of transplanted organs and tissue, followed by code C8Ø.2, Malignant neoplasm associated with transplanted organ. Use an additional code for the specific malignancy.

s. Breast implant associated anaplastic large cell lymphoma

Breast implant associated anaplastic large cell lymphoma (BIA-ALCL) is a type of lymphoma that can develop around breast implants. Assign code C84.7A, Anaplastic large cell lymphoma, ALK-negative, breast, for BIA-ALCL. Do not assign a complication code from chapter 19.

t. Secondary malignant neoplasm of lymphoid tissue

When a malignant neoplasm of lymphoid tissue metastasizes beyond the lymph nodes, a code from categories C81-C85 with a final character "9" should be assigned identifying "extranodal and solid organ sites" rather than a code for the secondary neoplasm of the affected solid organ. For example, for metastasis of B-cell lymphoma to the lung, brain and left adrenal gland, assign code C83.39, Diffuse large B cell lymphoma, extranodal and solid organ sites.

Chapter 2. Neoplasms (C00-D49)

NOTE

Functional activity

All neoplasms are classified in this chapter, whether they are functionally active or not. An additional code from Chapter 4 may be used, to identify functional activity associated with any neoplasm.

Morphology [Histology]

Chapter 2 classifies neoplasms primarily by site (topography), with broad groupings for behavior, malignant, in situ, benign, etc. The Table of Neoplasms should be used to identify the correct topography code. In a few cases, such as for malignant melanoma and certain neuroendocrine tumors, the morphology (histologic type) is included in the category and codes.

Primary malignant neoplasms overlapping site boundaries

A primary malignant neoplasm that overlaps two or more contiguous (next to each other) sites should be classified to the subcategory/code .8 ("overlapping lesion"), unless the combination is specifically indexed elsewhere. For multiple neoplasms of the same site that are not contiguous, such as tumors in different quadrants of the same breast, codes for each site should be assigned.

Malignant neoplasm of ectopic tissue

Malignant neoplasms of ectopic tissue are to be coded to the site mentioned, e.g., ectopic pancreatic malignant neoplasms are coded to pancreas, unspecified (C25.9).

AHA: 2017,4Q,103; 2017,1Q,4,5-6,8

This chapter contains the following blocks:

- C00-C14 Malignant neoplasms of lip, oral cavity and pharynx
- C15-C26 Malignant neoplasms of digestive organs
- C30-C39 Malignant neoplasms of respiratory and intrathoracic organs
- C40-C41 Malignant neoplasms of bone and articular cartilage
- C43-C44 Melanoma and other malignant neoplasms of skin
- C45-C49 Malignant neoplasms of mesothelial and soft tissue
- C50 Malignant neoplasms of breast
- C51-C58 Malignant neoplasms of female genital organs
- C60-C63 Malignant neoplasms of male genital organs
- C64-C68 Malignant neoplasms of urinary tract
- C69-C72 Malignant neoplasms of eye, brain and other parts of central nervous system
- C73-C75 Malignant neoplasms of thyroid and other endocrine glands
- C7A Malignant neuroendocrine tumors
- C7B Secondary neuroendocrine tumors
- C76-C80 Malignant neoplasms of ill-defined, other secondary and unspecified sites
- C81-C96 Malignant neoplasms of lymphoid, hematopoietic and related tissue
- D00-D09 In situ neoplasms
- D10-D36 Benign neoplasms, except benign neuroendocrine tumors
- D3A Benign neuroendocrine tumors
- D37-D48 Neoplasms of uncertain behavior, polycythemia vera and myelodysplastic syndromes
- D49 Neoplasms of unspecified behavior

MALIGNANT NEOPLASMS (C00-C96)

Malignant neoplasms, stated or presumed to be primary (of specified sites), and certain specified histologies, except neuroendocrine, and of lymphoid, hematopoietic and related tissue (C00-C75)

AHA: 2022,1Q,16

TIP: Codes from this code block can be assigned for outpatient encounters based on the diagnosis listed in a pathology or cytology report when authenticated by a pathologist and available at the time of code assignment.

Malignant neoplasms of lip, oral cavity and pharynx (C00-C14)

4th **C00 Malignant neoplasm of lip**

Use additional code to identify:
alcohol abuse and dependence (F10.-)
history of tobacco dependence (Z87.891)
tobacco dependence (F17.-)
tobacco use (Z72.0)

EXCLUDES 1 *malignant melanoma of lip (C43.0)*
Merkel cell carcinoma of lip (C4A.0)
other and unspecified malignant neoplasm of skin of lip (C44.0-)

C00.0 Malignant neoplasm of external upper lip
Malignant neoplasm of lipstick area of upper lip
Malignant neoplasm of upper lip NOS
Malignant neoplasm of vermilion border of upper lip

C00.1 Malignant neoplasm of external lower lip
Malignant neoplasm of lower lip NOS
Malignant neoplasm of lipstick area of lower lip
Malignant neoplasm of vermilion border of lower lip

C00.2 Malignant neoplasm of external lip, unspecified
Malignant neoplasm of vermilion border of lip NOS

C00.3 Malignant neoplasm of upper lip, inner aspect
Malignant neoplasm of buccal aspect of upper lip
Malignant neoplasm of frenulum of upper lip
Malignant neoplasm of mucosa of upper lip
Malignant neoplasm of oral aspect of upper lip

C00.4 Malignant neoplasm of lower lip, inner aspect
Malignant neoplasm of buccal aspect of lower lip
Malignant neoplasm of frenulum of lower lip
Malignant neoplasm of mucosa of lower lip
Malignant neoplasm of oral aspect of lower lip

C00.5 Malignant neoplasm of lip, unspecified, inner aspect
Malignant neoplasm of buccal aspect of lip, unspecified
Malignant neoplasm of frenulum of lip, unspecified
Malignant neoplasm of mucosa of lip, unspecified
Malignant neoplasm of oral aspect of lip, unspecified

C00.6 Malignant neoplasm of commissure of lip, unspecified

C00.8 Malignant neoplasm of overlapping sites of lip

C00.9 Malignant neoplasm of lip, unspecified

C01 Malignant neoplasm of base of tongue HCC Rx ESR COM
Malignant neoplasm of dorsal surface of base of tongue
Malignant neoplasm of fixed part of tongue NOS
Malignant neoplasm of posterior third of tongue

Use additional code to identify:
alcohol abuse and dependence (F10.-)
history of tobacco dependence (Z87.891)
tobacco dependence (F17.-)
tobacco use (Z72.0)

Malignant Neoplasm of Tongue

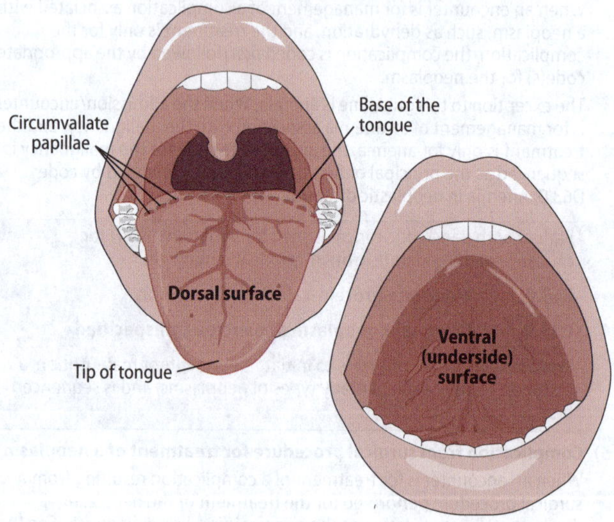

4th **C02 Malignant neoplasm of other and unspecified parts of tongue**

Use additional code to identify:
alcohol abuse and dependence (F10.-)
history of tobacco dependence (Z87.891)
tobacco dependence (F17.-)
tobacco use (Z72.0)

C02.0 Malignant neoplasm of dorsal surface of tongue HCC Rx ESR COM
Malignant neoplasm of anterior two-thirds of tongue, dorsal surface

EXCLUDES 2 *malignant neoplasm of dorsal surface of base of tongue (C01)*

C02.1 Malignant neoplasm of border of tongue HCC Rx ESR COM
Malignant neoplasm of tip of tongue

C02.2 Malignant neoplasm of ventral surface of tongue HCC Rx ESR COM
Malignant neoplasm of anterior two-thirds of tongue, ventral surface
Malignant neoplasm of frenulum linguae

C02.3 Malignant neoplasm of anterior two-thirds of tongue, part unspecified HCC Rx ESR COM
Malignant neoplasm of middle third of tongue NOS
Malignant neoplasm of mobile part of tongue NOS

C02.4 Malignant neoplasm of lingual tonsil HCC Rx ESR COM
EXCLUDES 2 *malignant neoplasm of tonsil NOS (C09.9)*

C02.8 Malignant neoplasm of overlapping sites of tongue HCC Rx ESR COM
Malignant neoplasm of two or more contiguous sites of tongue

C02.9 Malignant neoplasm of tongue, unspecified HCC Rx ESR COM

4th C03 Malignant neoplasm of gum
INCLUDES malignant neoplasm of alveolar (ridge) mucosa
malignant neoplasm of gingiva
Use additional code to identify:
alcohol abuse and dependence (F10.-)
history of tobacco dependence (Z87.891)
tobacco dependence (F17.-)
tobacco use (Z72.0)
EXCLUDES 2 *malignant odontogenic neoplasms (C41.0-C41.1)*

C03.0 Malignant neoplasm of upper gum HCC Rx ESR COM
C03.1 Malignant neoplasm of lower gum HCC Rx ESR COM
C03.9 Malignant neoplasm of gum, unspecified HCC Rx ESR COM

4th C04 Malignant neoplasm of floor of mouth
Use additional code to identify:
alcohol abuse and dependence (F10.-)
history of tobacco dependence (Z87.891)
tobacco dependence (F17.-)
tobacco use (Z72.0)

C04.0 Malignant neoplasm of anterior floor of mouth HCC Rx ESR COM
Malignant neoplasm of anterior to the premolar-canine junction

C04.1 Malignant neoplasm of lateral floor of mouth HCC Rx ESR COM
C04.8 Malignant neoplasm of overlapping sites of floor of mouth HCC Rx ESR COM
C04.9 Malignant neoplasm of floor of mouth, unspecified HCC Rx ESR COM

4th C05 Malignant neoplasm of palate
Use additional code to identify:
alcohol abuse and dependence (F10.-)
history of tobacco dependence (Z87.891)
tobacco dependence (F17.-)
tobacco use (Z72.0)
EXCLUDES 1 *Kaposi's sarcoma of palate (C46.2)*

C05.0 Malignant neoplasm of hard palate HCC Rx ESR COM
C05.1 Malignant neoplasm of soft palate HCC Rx ESR COM
EXCLUDES 2 *malignant neoplasm of nasopharyngeal surface of soft palate (C11.3)*

C05.2 Malignant neoplasm of uvula HCC Rx ESR COM
C05.8 Malignant neoplasm of overlapping sites of palate HCC Rx ESR COM
C05.9 Malignant neoplasm of palate, unspecified HCC Rx ESR COM
Malignant neoplasm of roof of mouth

4th C06 Malignant neoplasm of other and unspecified parts of mouth
Use additional code to identify:
alcohol abuse and dependence (F10.-)
history of tobacco dependence (Z87.891)
tobacco dependence (F17.-)
tobacco use (Z72.0)

C06.0 Malignant neoplasm of cheek mucosa HCC Rx ESR COM
Malignant neoplasm of buccal mucosa NOS
Malignant neoplasm of internal cheek

C06.1 Malignant neoplasm of vestibule of mouth HCC Rx ESR COM
Malignant neoplasm of buccal sulcus (upper) (lower)
Malignant neoplasm of labial sulcus (upper) (lower)

C06.2 Malignant neoplasm of retromolar area HCC Rx ESR COM

5th C06.8 Malignant neoplasm of overlapping sites of other and unspecified parts of mouth

C06.80 Malignant neoplasm of overlapping sites of unspecified parts of mouth HCC Rx ESR COM

C06.89 Malignant neoplasm of overlapping sites of other parts of mouth HCC Rx ESR COM
"book leaf" neoplasm [ventral surface of tongue and floor of mouth]

C06.9 Malignant neoplasm of mouth, unspecified HCC Rx ESR COM
Malignant neoplasm of minor salivary gland, unspecified site
Malignant neoplasm of oral cavity NOS

C07 Malignant neoplasm of parotid gland HCC Rx ESR COM
Use additional code to identify:
alcohol abuse and dependence (F10.-)
exposure to environmental tobacco smoke (Z77.22)
exposure to tobacco smoke in the perinatal period (P96.81)
history of tobacco dependence (Z87.891)
occupational exposure to environmental tobacco smoke (Z57.31)
tobacco dependence (F17.-)
tobacco use (Z72.0)

4th C08 Malignant neoplasm of other and unspecified major salivary glands
INCLUDES malignant neoplasm of salivary ducts
Use additional code to identify:
alcohol abuse and dependence (F10.-)
exposure to environmental tobacco smoke (Z77.22)
exposure to tobacco smoke in the perinatal period (P96.81)
history of tobacco dependence (Z87.891)
occupational exposure to environmental tobacco smoke (Z57.31)
tobacco dependence (F17.-)
tobacco use (Z72.0)
EXCLUDES 1 *malignant neoplasms of specified minor salivary glands which are classified according to their anatomical location*
EXCLUDES 2 *malignant neoplasms of minor salivary glands NOS (C06.9)*
malignant neoplasm of parotid gland (C07)

C08.0 Malignant neoplasm of submandibular gland HCC Rx ESR COM
Malignant neoplasm of submaxillary gland

C08.1 Malignant neoplasm of sublingual gland HCC Rx ESR COM
C08.9 Malignant neoplasm of major salivary gland, unspecified HCC Rx ESR COM
Malignant neoplasm of salivary gland (major) NOS

4th C09 Malignant neoplasm of tonsil
Use additional code to identify:
alcohol abuse and dependence (F10.-)
exposure to environmental tobacco smoke (Z77.22)
exposure to tobacco smoke in the perinatal period (P96.81)
history of tobacco dependence (Z87.891)
occupational exposure to environmental tobacco smoke (Z57.31)
tobacco dependence (F17.-)
tobacco use (Z72.0)
EXCLUDES 2 *malignant neoplasm of lingual tonsil (C02.4)*
malignant neoplasm of pharyngeal tonsil (C11.1)

C09.0 Malignant neoplasm of tonsillar fossa HCC ESR COM
C09.1 Malignant neoplasm of tonsillar pillar (anterior) (posterior) HCC ESR COM
C09.8 Malignant neoplasm of overlapping sites of tonsil HCC ESR COM
C09.9 Malignant neoplasm of tonsil, unspecified HCC ESR COM
Malignant neoplasm of tonsil NOS
Malignant neoplasm of faucial tonsils
Malignant neoplasm of palatine tonsils

4th C10 Malignant neoplasm of oropharynx
Use additional code to identify:
alcohol abuse and dependence (F10.-)
exposure to environmental tobacco smoke (Z77.22)
exposure to tobacco smoke in the perinatal period (P96.81)
history of tobacco dependence (Z87.891)
occupational exposure to environmental tobacco smoke (Z57.31)
tobacco dependence (F17.-)
tobacco use (Z72.0)
EXCLUDES 2 *malignant neoplasm of tonsil (C09.-)*
DEF: Oropharynx: Middle portion of pharynx (throat); communicates with the oral cavity, nasopharynx and laryngopharynx.

C10.0 Malignant neoplasm of vallecula HCC ESR COM
C10.1 Malignant neoplasm of anterior surface of epiglottis HCC ESR COM
Malignant neoplasm of epiglottis, free border [margin]
Malignant neoplasm of glossoepiglottic fold(s)
EXCLUDES 2 *malignant neoplasm of epiglottis (suprahyoid portion) NOS (C32.1)*

C10.2 Malignant neoplasm of lateral wall of oropharynx HCC ESR COM
C10.3 Malignant neoplasm of posterior wall of oropharynx HCC ESR COM

Chapter 2. Neoplasms
C02.4–C10.3

Additional Character Required | x7th Placeholder Alert | Manifestation | Unspecified Dx | Q QPP | UPD Unacceptable PDx

C10.4 Malignant neoplasm of branchial cleft HCC ESR COM
Malignant neoplasm of branchial cyst [site of neoplasm]

C10.8 Malignant neoplasm of overlapping sites of oropharynx HCC ESR COM
Malignant neoplasm of junctional region of oropharynx

C10.9 Malignant neoplasm of oropharynx, unspecified HCC ESR COM

C11 Malignant neoplasm of nasopharynx (4th)
Use additional code to identify:
exposure to environmental tobacco smoke (Z77.22)
exposure to tobacco smoke in the perinatal period (P96.81)
history of tobacco dependence (Z87.891)
occupational exposure to environmental tobacco smoke (Z57.31)
tobacco dependence (F17.-)
tobacco use (Z72.0)
DEF: Nasopharynx: Upper portion of pharynx (throat); communicates with the nasal cavities, oropharynx and tympanic cavities.

C11.0 Malignant neoplasm of superior wall of nasopharynx HCC ESR COM
Malignant neoplasm of roof of nasopharynx

C11.1 Malignant neoplasm of posterior wall of nasopharynx HCC ESR COM
Malignant neoplasm of adenoid
Malignant neoplasm of pharyngeal tonsil

C11.2 Malignant neoplasm of lateral wall of nasopharynx HCC ESR COM
Malignant neoplasm of fossa of Rosenmüller
Malignant neoplasm of opening of auditory tube
Malignant neoplasm of pharyngeal recess

C11.3 Malignant neoplasm of anterior wall of nasopharynx HCC ESR COM
Malignant neoplasm of floor of nasopharynx
Malignant neoplasm of nasopharyngeal (anterior) (posterior) surface of soft palate
Malignant neoplasm of posterior margin of nasal choana
Malignant neoplasm of posterior margin of nasal septum

C11.8 Malignant neoplasm of overlapping sites of nasopharynx HCC ESR COM

C11.9 Malignant neoplasm of nasopharynx, unspecified HCC ESR COM
Malignant neoplasm of nasopharyngeal wall NOS

C12 Malignant neoplasm of pyriform sinus HCC ESR COM
Malignant neoplasm of pyriform fossa
Use additional code to identify:
exposure to environmental tobacco smoke (Z77.22)
exposure to tobacco smoke in the perinatal period (P96.81)
history of tobacco dependence (Z87.891)
occupational exposure to environmental tobacco smoke (Z57.31)
tobacco dependence (F17.-)
tobacco use (Z72.0)

C13 Malignant neoplasm of hypopharynx (4th)
Use additional code to identify:
exposure to environmental tobacco smoke (Z77.22)
exposure to tobacco smoke in the perinatal period (P96.81)
history of tobacco dependence (Z87.891)
occupational exposure to environmental tobacco smoke (Z57.31)
tobacco dependence (F17.-)
tobacco use (Z72.0)
EXCLUDES 2 *malignant neoplasm of pyriform sinus (C12)*
DEF: Hypopharynx: Lower portion of pharynx (throat); communicates with the oropharynx and the esophagus. ***Synonym(s):*** *laryngopharynx.*

C13.0 Malignant neoplasm of postcricoid region HCC ESR COM

C13.1 Malignant neoplasm of aryepiglottic fold, hypopharyngeal aspect HCC ESR COM
Malignant neoplasm of aryepiglottic fold, marginal zone
Malignant neoplasm of aryepiglottic fold NOS
Malignant neoplasm of interarytenoid fold, marginal zone
Malignant neoplasm of interarytenoid fold NOS
EXCLUDES 2 *malignant neoplasm of aryepiglottic fold or interarytenoid fold, laryngeal aspect (C32.1)*

C13.2 Malignant neoplasm of posterior wall of hypopharynx HCC ESR COM

C13.8 Malignant neoplasm of overlapping sites of hypopharynx HCC ESR COM

C13.9 Malignant neoplasm of hypopharynx, unspecified HCC ESR COM
Malignant neoplasm of hypopharyngeal wall NOS

C14 Malignant neoplasm of other and ill-defined sites in the lip, oral cavity and pharynx (4th)
Use additional code to identify:
alcohol abuse and dependence (F10.-)
exposure to environmental tobacco smoke (Z77.22)
exposure to tobacco smoke in the perinatal period (P96.81)
history of tobacco dependence (Z87.891)
occupational exposure to environmental tobacco smoke (Z57.31)
tobacco dependence (F17.-)
tobacco use (Z72.0)
EXCLUDES 1 *malignant neoplasm of oral cavity NOS (C06.9)*

C14.0 Malignant neoplasm of pharynx, unspecified HCC ESR COM

C14.2 Malignant neoplasm of Waldeyer's ring HCC ESR COM
DEF: Waldeyer's ring: Ring of lymphoid tissue that is made up of the two palatine tonsils, the pharyngeal tonsil (adenoid), and the lingual tonsil. It functions as the defense against infection and assists with the development of the immune system.

C14.8 Malignant neoplasm of overlapping sites of lip, oral cavity and pharynx HCC ESR COM
Primary malignant neoplasm of two or more contiguous sites of lip, oral cavity and pharynx
EXCLUDES 1 *"book leaf" neoplasm [ventral surface of tongue and floor of mouth] (C06.89)*

Malignant neoplasms of digestive organs (C15-C26)

EXCLUDES 1 *Kaposi's sarcoma of gastrointestinal sites (C46.4)*
EXCLUDES 2 *gastrointestinal stromal tumors (C49.A-)*

C15 Malignant neoplasm of esophagus (4th)
Use additional code to identify:
alcohol abuse and dependence (F10.-)

C15.3 Malignant neoplasm of upper third of esophagus HCC ESR COM

C15.4 Malignant neoplasm of middle third of esophagus HCC ESR COM

C15.5 Malignant neoplasm of lower third of esophagus HCC ESR COM
EXCLUDES 1 *malignant neoplasm of cardio-esophageal junction (C16.0)*

C15.8 Malignant neoplasm of overlapping sites of esophagus HCC ESR COM

C15.9 Malignant neoplasm of esophagus, unspecified HCC ESR COM

C16 Malignant neoplasm of stomach (4th)
Use additional code to identify:
alcohol abuse and dependence (F10.-)
EXCLUDES 2 *malignant carcinoid tumor of the stomach (C7A.092)*

C16.0 Malignant neoplasm of cardia HCC Rx ESR COM
Malignant neoplasm of cardiac orifice
Malignant neoplasm of cardio-esophageal junction
Malignant neoplasm of esophagus and stomach
Malignant neoplasm of gastro-esophageal junction

C16.1 Malignant neoplasm of fundus of stomach HCC Rx ESR COM

C16.2 Malignant neoplasm of body of stomach HCC Rx ESR COM

C16.3 Malignant neoplasm of pyloric antrum HCC Rx ESR COM
Malignant neoplasm of gastric antrum

C16.4 Malignant neoplasm of pylorus HCC Rx ESR COM
Malignant neoplasm of prepylorus
Malignant neoplasm of pyloric canal

C16.5 Malignant neoplasm of lesser curvature of stomach, unspecified HCC Rx ESR COM
Malignant neoplasm of lesser curvature of stomach, not classifiable to C16.1-C16.4

C16.6 Malignant neoplasm of greater curvature of stomach, unspecified HCC Rx ESR COM
Malignant neoplasm of greater curvature of stomach, not classifiable to C16.0-C16.4

C16.8 Malignant neoplasm of overlapping sites of stomach HCC Rx ESR COM

C16.9 Malignant neoplasm of stomach, unspecified HCC Rx ESR COM
Gastric cancer NOS

HCC CMS-HCC Rx Rx HCC ESR ESRD HCC COM Commercial HCC N Newborn: 0 P Pediatric: 0-17 M Maternity: 9-64 A Adult: 15-124

C17 Malignant neoplasm of small intestine

EXCLUDES 1 *malignant carcinoid tumors of the small intestine (C7A.Ø1)*

AHA: 2016,1Q,19

C17.Ø Malignant neoplasm of duodenum HCC Rx ESR COM

C17.1 Malignant neoplasm of jejunum HCC Rx ESR COM

C17.2 Malignant neoplasm of ileum HCC Rx ESR COM

EXCLUDES 1 *malignant neoplasm of ileocecal valve (C18.Ø)*

C17.3 Meckel's diverticulum, malignant HCC Rx ESR COM

EXCLUDES 1 *Meckel's diverticulum, congenital (Q43.Ø)*

DEF: Congenital, abnormal remnant of embryonic digestive system development that leaves a sacculation or outpouching from the wall of the small intestine near the terminal part of the ileum made of acid-secreting tissue as in the stomach.

C17.8 Malignant neoplasm of overlapping sites of small intestine HCC Rx ESR COM

C17.9 Malignant neoplasm of small intestine, unspecified HCC Rx ESR COM

C18 Malignant neoplasm of colon

EXCLUDES 1 *malignant carcinoid tumors of the colon (C7A.Ø2-)*

Colon

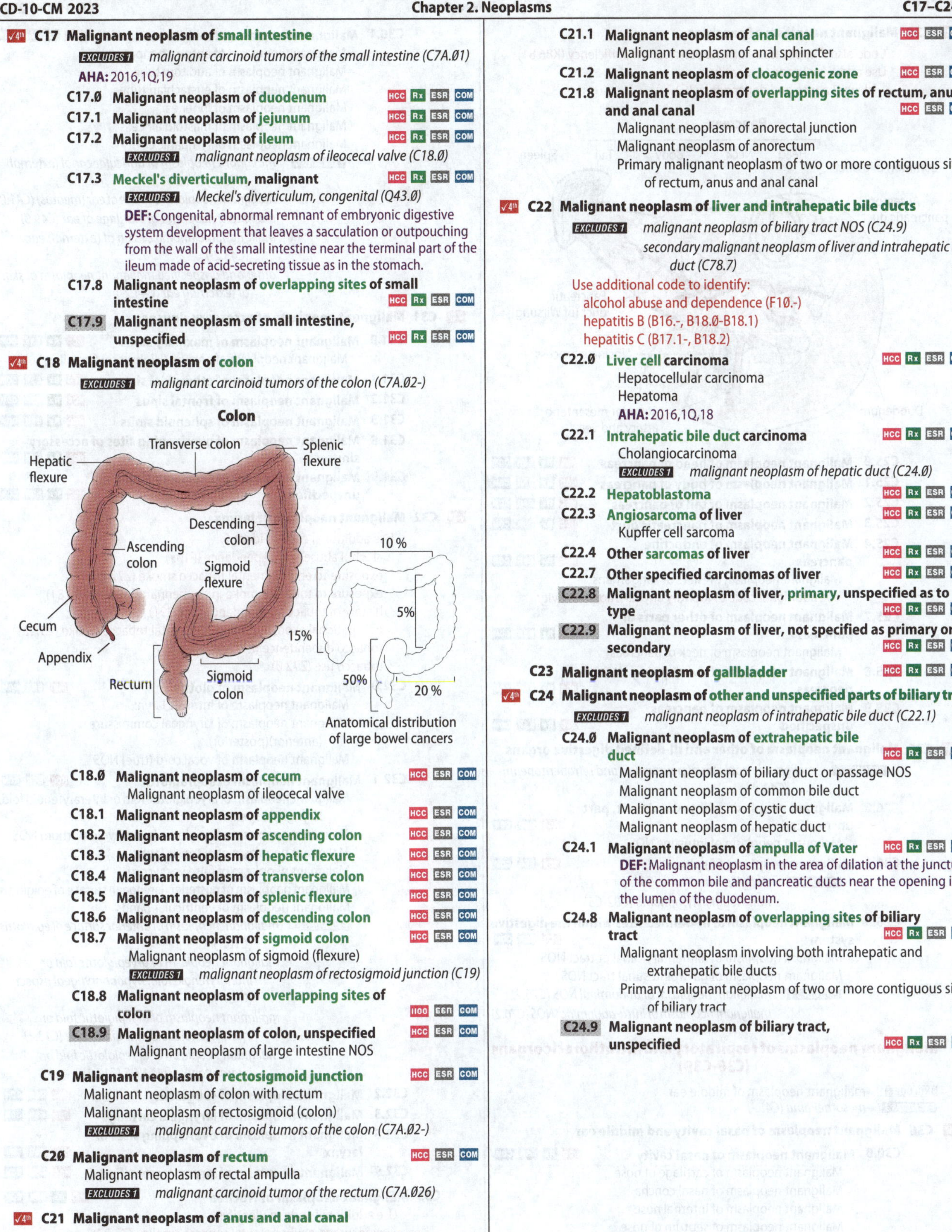

Anatomical distribution of large bowel cancers

C18.Ø Malignant neoplasm of cecum HCC ESR COM

Malignant neoplasm of ileocecal valve

C18.1 Malignant neoplasm of appendix HCC ESR COM

C18.2 Malignant neoplasm of ascending colon HCC ESR COM

C18.3 Malignant neoplasm of hepatic flexure HCC ESR COM

C18.4 Malignant neoplasm of transverse colon HCC ESR COM

C18.5 Malignant neoplasm of splenic flexure HCC ESR COM

C18.6 Malignant neoplasm of descending colon HCC ESR COM

C18.7 Malignant neoplasm of sigmoid colon HCC ESR COM

Malignant neoplasm of sigmoid (flexure)

EXCLUDES 1 *malignant neoplasm of rectosigmoid junction (C19)*

C18.8 Malignant neoplasm of overlapping sites of colon HCC ESR COM

C18.9 Malignant neoplasm of colon, unspecified HCC ESR COM

Malignant neoplasm of large intestine NOS

C19 Malignant neoplasm of rectosigmoid junction HCC ESR COM

Malignant neoplasm of colon with rectum

Malignant neoplasm of rectosigmoid (colon)

EXCLUDES 1 *malignant carcinoid tumors of the colon (C7A.Ø2-)*

C2Ø Malignant neoplasm of rectum HCC ESR COM

Malignant neoplasm of rectal ampulla

EXCLUDES 1 *malignant carcinoid tumor of the rectum (C7A.Ø26)*

C21 Malignant neoplasm of anus and anal canal

EXCLUDES 2 *malignant carcinoid tumors of the colon (C7A.Ø2-)*
malignant melanoma of anal margin (C43.51)
malignant melanoma of anal skin (C43.51)
malignant melanoma of perianal skin (C43.51)
other and unspecified malignant neoplasm of anal margin (C44.5ØØ, C44.51Ø, C44.52Ø, C44.59Ø)
other and unspecified malignant neoplasm of anal skin (C44.5ØØ, C44.51Ø, C44.52Ø, C44.59Ø)
other and unspecified malignant neoplasm of perianal skin (C44.5ØØ, C44.51Ø, C44.52Ø, C44.59Ø)

C21.Ø Malignant neoplasm of anus, unspecified HCC ESR COM

C21.1 Malignant neoplasm of anal canal HCC ESR COM

Malignant neoplasm of anal sphincter

C21.2 Malignant neoplasm of cloacogenic zone HCC ESR COM

C21.8 Malignant neoplasm of overlapping sites of rectum, anus and anal canal HCC ESR COM

Malignant neoplasm of anorectal junction

Malignant neoplasm of anorectum

Primary malignant neoplasm of two or more contiguous sites of rectum, anus and anal canal

C22 Malignant neoplasm of liver and intrahepatic bile ducts

EXCLUDES 1 *malignant neoplasm of biliary tract NOS (C24.9)*
secondary malignant neoplasm of liver and intrahepatic bile duct (C78.7)

Use additional code to identify:
alcohol abuse and dependence (F1Ø.-)
hepatitis B (B16.-, B18.Ø-B18.1)
hepatitis C (B17.1-, B18.2)

C22.Ø Liver cell carcinoma HCC Rx ESR COM

Hepatocellular carcinoma

Hepatoma

AHA: 2016,1Q,18

C22.1 Intrahepatic bile duct carcinoma HCC Rx ESR COM

Cholangiocarcinoma

EXCLUDES 1 *malignant neoplasm of hepatic duct (C24.Ø)*

C22.2 Hepatoblastoma HCC Rx ESR COM

C22.3 Angiosarcoma of liver HCC Rx ESR COM

Kupffer cell sarcoma

C22.4 Other sarcomas of liver HCC Rx ESR COM

C22.7 Other specified carcinomas of liver HCC Rx ESR COM

C22.8 Malignant neoplasm of liver, primary, unspecified as to type HCC Rx ESR COM

C22.9 Malignant neoplasm of liver, not specified as primary or secondary HCC Rx ESR COM

C23 Malignant neoplasm of gallbladder HCC Rx ESR COM

C24 Malignant neoplasm of other and unspecified parts of biliary tract

EXCLUDES 1 *malignant neoplasm of intrahepatic bile duct (C22.1)*

C24.Ø Malignant neoplasm of extrahepatic bile duct HCC Rx ESR COM

Malignant neoplasm of biliary duct or passage NOS

Malignant neoplasm of common bile duct

Malignant neoplasm of cystic duct

Malignant neoplasm of hepatic duct

C24.1 Malignant neoplasm of ampulla of Vater HCC Rx ESR COM

DEF: Malignant neoplasm in the area of dilation at the juncture of the common bile and pancreatic ducts near the opening into the lumen of the duodenum.

C24.8 Malignant neoplasm of overlapping sites of biliary tract HCC Rx ESR COM

Malignant neoplasm involving both intrahepatic and extrahepatic bile ducts

Primary malignant neoplasm of two or more contiguous sites of biliary tract

C24.9 Malignant neoplasm of biliary tract, unspecified HCC Rx ESR COM

✓4th C25 Malignant neoplasm of pancreas
Code also if applicable exocrine pancreatic insufficiency (K86.81)
Use additional code to identify:
alcohol abuse and dependence (F1Ø.-)

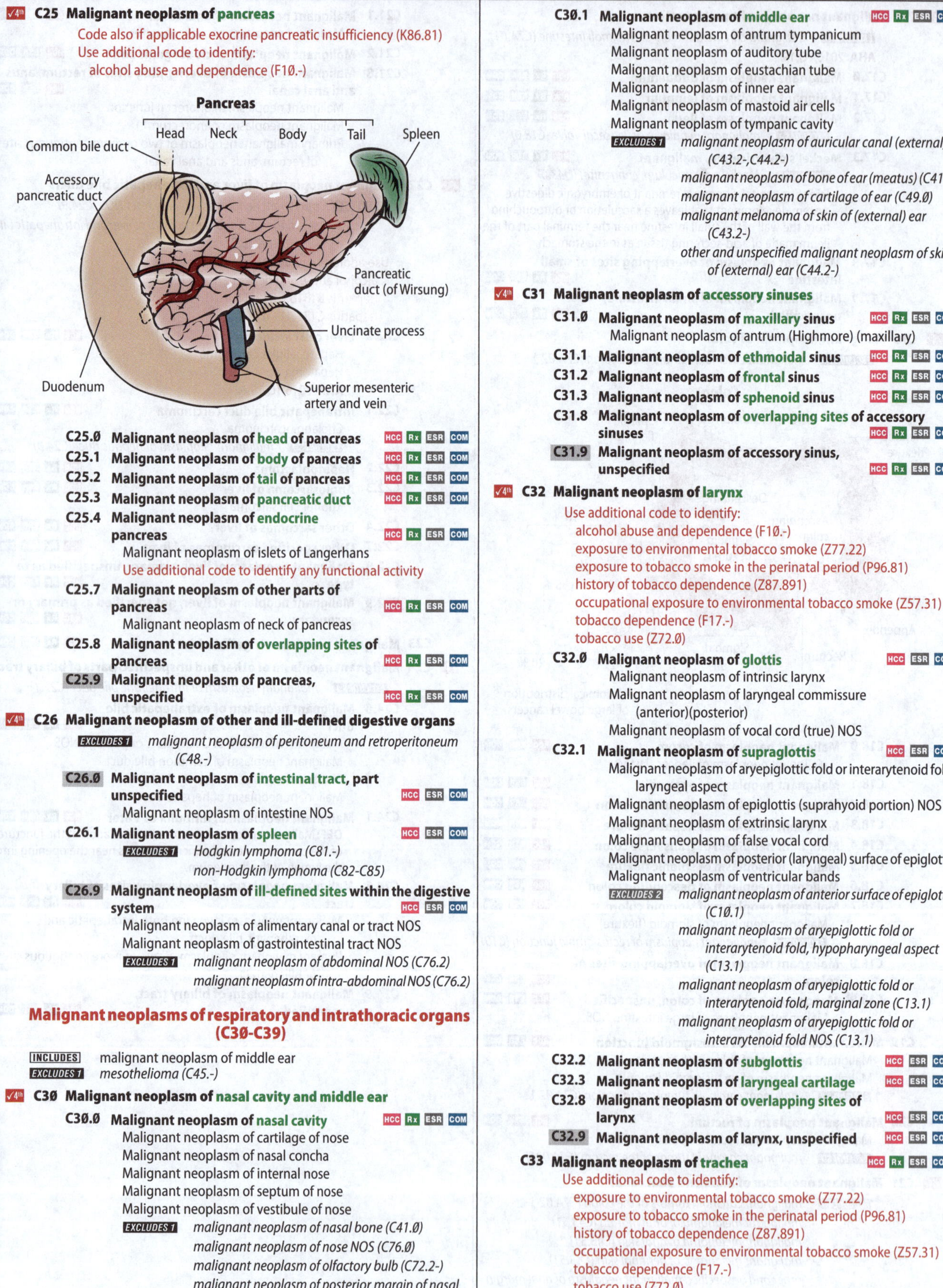

C25.Ø Malignant neoplasm of head of pancreas HCC Rx ESR COM
C25.1 Malignant neoplasm of body of pancreas HCC Rx ESR COM
C25.2 Malignant neoplasm of tail of pancreas HCC Rx ESR COM
C25.3 Malignant neoplasm of pancreatic duct HCC Rx ESR COM
C25.4 Malignant neoplasm of endocrine pancreas HCC Rx ESR COM
Malignant neoplasm of islets of Langerhans
Use additional code to identify any functional activity
C25.7 Malignant neoplasm of other parts of pancreas HCC Rx ESR COM
Malignant neoplasm of neck of pancreas
C25.8 Malignant neoplasm of overlapping sites of pancreas HCC Rx ESR COM
C25.9 Malignant neoplasm of pancreas, unspecified HCC Rx ESR COM

✓4th C26 Malignant neoplasm of other and ill-defined digestive organs
EXCLUDES 1 *malignant neoplasm of peritoneum and retroperitoneum (C48.-)*
C26.Ø Malignant neoplasm of intestinal tract, part unspecified HCC ESR COM
Malignant neoplasm of intestine NOS
C26.1 Malignant neoplasm of spleen HCC ESR COM
EXCLUDES 1 *Hodgkin lymphoma (C81.-)*
non-Hodgkin lymphoma (C82-C85)
C26.9 Malignant neoplasm of ill-defined sites within the digestive system HCC ESR COM
Malignant neoplasm of alimentary canal or tract NOS
Malignant neoplasm of gastrointestinal tract NOS
EXCLUDES 1 *malignant neoplasm of abdominal NOS (C76.2)*
malignant neoplasm of intra-abdominal NOS (C76.2)

Malignant neoplasms of respiratory and intrathoracic organs (C3Ø-C39)

INCLUDES malignant neoplasm of middle ear
EXCLUDES 1 *mesothelioma (C45.-)*

✓4th C3Ø Malignant neoplasm of nasal cavity and middle ear
C3Ø.Ø Malignant neoplasm of nasal cavity HCC Rx ESR COM
Malignant neoplasm of cartilage of nose
Malignant neoplasm of nasal concha
Malignant neoplasm of internal nose
Malignant neoplasm of septum of nose
Malignant neoplasm of vestibule of nose
EXCLUDES 1 *malignant neoplasm of nasal bone (C41.Ø)*
malignant neoplasm of nose NOS (C76.Ø)
malignant neoplasm of olfactory bulb (C72.2-)
malignant neoplasm of posterior margin of nasal septum and choana (C11.3)
malignant melanoma of skin of nose (C43.31)
malignant neoplasm of turbinates (C41.Ø)
other and unspecified malignant neoplasm of skin of nose (C44.3Ø1, C44.311, C44.321, C44.391)
C3Ø.1 Malignant neoplasm of middle ear HCC Rx ESR COM
Malignant neoplasm of antrum tympanicum
Malignant neoplasm of auditory tube
Malignant neoplasm of eustachian tube
Malignant neoplasm of inner ear
Malignant neoplasm of mastoid air cells
Malignant neoplasm of tympanic cavity
EXCLUDES 1 *malignant neoplasm of auricular canal (external) (C43.2-,C44.2-)*
malignant neoplasm of bone of ear (meatus) (C41.Ø)
malignant neoplasm of cartilage of ear (C49.Ø)
malignant melanoma of skin of (external) ear (C43.2-)
other and unspecified malignant neoplasm of skin of (external) ear (C44.2-)

✓4th C31 Malignant neoplasm of accessory sinuses
C31.Ø Malignant neoplasm of maxillary sinus HCC Rx ESR COM
Malignant neoplasm of antrum (Highmore) (maxillary)
C31.1 Malignant neoplasm of ethmoidal sinus HCC Rx ESR COM
C31.2 Malignant neoplasm of frontal sinus HCC Rx ESR COM
C31.3 Malignant neoplasm of sphenoid sinus HCC Rx ESR COM
C31.8 Malignant neoplasm of overlapping sites of accessory sinuses HCC Rx ESR COM
C31.9 Malignant neoplasm of accessory sinus, unspecified HCC Rx ESR COM

✓4th C32 Malignant neoplasm of larynx
Use additional code to identify:
alcohol abuse and dependence (F1Ø.-)
exposure to environmental tobacco smoke (Z77.22)
exposure to tobacco smoke in the perinatal period (P96.81)
history of tobacco dependence (Z87.891)
occupational exposure to environmental tobacco smoke (Z57.31)
tobacco dependence (F17.-)
tobacco use (Z72.Ø)
C32.Ø Malignant neoplasm of glottis HCC ESR COM
Malignant neoplasm of intrinsic larynx
Malignant neoplasm of laryngeal commissure (anterior)(posterior)
Malignant neoplasm of vocal cord (true) NOS
C32.1 Malignant neoplasm of supraglottis HCC ESR COM
Malignant neoplasm of aryepiglottic fold or interarytenoid fold, laryngeal aspect
Malignant neoplasm of epiglottis (suprahyoid portion) NOS
Malignant neoplasm of extrinsic larynx
Malignant neoplasm of false vocal cord
Malignant neoplasm of posterior (laryngeal) surface of epiglottis
Malignant neoplasm of ventricular bands
EXCLUDES 2 *malignant neoplasm of anterior surface of epiglottis (C1Ø.1)*
malignant neoplasm of aryepiglottic fold or interarytenoid fold, hypopharyngeal aspect (C13.1)
malignant neoplasm of aryepiglottic fold or interarytenoid fold, marginal zone (C13.1)
malignant neoplasm of aryepiglottic fold or interarytenoid fold NOS (C13.1)
C32.2 Malignant neoplasm of subglottis HCC ESR COM
C32.3 Malignant neoplasm of laryngeal cartilage HCC ESR COM
C32.8 Malignant neoplasm of overlapping sites of larynx HCC ESR COM
C32.9 Malignant neoplasm of larynx, unspecified HCC ESR COM

C33 Malignant neoplasm of trachea HCC Rx ESR COM
Use additional code to identify:
exposure to environmental tobacco smoke (Z77.22)
exposure to tobacco smoke in the perinatal period (P96.81)
history of tobacco dependence (Z87.891)
occupational exposure to environmental tobacco smoke (Z57.31)
tobacco dependence (F17.-)
tobacco use (Z72.Ø)

HCC CMS-HCC Rx Rx HCC ESR ESRD HCC COM Commercial HCC N Newborn: 0 P Pediatric: 0-17 M Maternity: 9-64 A Adult: 15-124

C34 Malignant neoplasm of bronchus and lung

Use additional code to identify:
- exposure to environmental tobacco smoke (Z77.22)
- exposure to tobacco smoke in the perinatal period (P96.81)
- history of tobacco dependence (Z87.891)
- occupational exposure to environmental tobacco smoke (Z57.31)
- tobacco dependence (F17.-)
- tobacco use (Z72.0)

EXCLUDES 1 *Kaposi's sarcoma of lung (C46.5-)*
malignant carcinoid tumor of the bronchus and lung (C7A.090)

AHA: 2019,1Q,16

TIP: When documented, assign code I31.3 for associated malignant pericardial effusion. If the sole reason for admission is to treat the effusion with no treatment of the lung malignancy rendered, code I31.3 may be sequenced first.

C34.0 Malignant neoplasm of main bronchus
Malignant neoplasm of carina
Malignant neoplasm of hilus (of lung)

C34.00 Malignant neoplasm of unspecified main bronchus HCC Rx ESR COM Q

C34.01 Malignant neoplasm of right main bronchus HCC Rx ESR COM Q

C34.02 Malignant neoplasm of left main bronchus HCC Rx ESR COM Q

C34.1 Malignant neoplasm of upper lobe, bronchus or lung

C34.10 Malignant neoplasm of upper lobe, unspecified bronchus or lung HCC Rx ESR COM Q

C34.11 Malignant neoplasm of upper lobe, right bronchus or lung HCC Rx ESR COM Q

C34.12 Malignant neoplasm of upper lobe, left bronchus or lung HCC Rx ESR COM Q

C34.2 Malignant neoplasm of middle lobe, bronchus or lung HCC Rx ESR COM Q

C34.3 Malignant neoplasm of lower lobe, bronchus or lung

C34.30 Malignant neoplasm of lower lobe, unspecified bronchus or lung HCC Rx ESR COM Q

C34.31 Malignant neoplasm of lower lobe, right bronchus or lung HCC Rx ESR COM Q

C34.32 Malignant neoplasm of lower lobe, left bronchus or lung HCC Rx ESR COM Q

C34.8 Malignant neoplasm of overlapping sites of bronchus and lung

C34.80 Malignant neoplasm of overlapping sites of unspecified bronchus and lung HCC Rx ESR COM Q

C34.81 Malignant neoplasm of overlapping sites of right bronchus and lung HCC Rx ESR COM Q

C34.82 Malignant neoplasm of overlapping sites of left bronchus and lung HCC Rx ESR COM Q

C34.9 Malignant neoplasm of unspecified part of bronchus or lung

C34.90 Malignant neoplasm of unspecified part of unspecified bronchus or lung HCC Rx ESR COM Q
Lung cancer NOS

C34.91 Malignant neoplasm of unspecified part of right bronchus or lung HCC Rx ESR COM Q

C34.92 Malignant neoplasm of unspecified part of left bronchus or lung HCC Rx ESR COM Q

C37 Malignant neoplasm of thymus HCC Rx ESR COM

EXCLUDES 1 *malignant carcinoid tumor of the thymus (C7A.091)*

C38 Malignant neoplasm of heart, mediastinum and pleura

EXCLUDES 1 *mesothelioma (C45.-)*

C38.0 Malignant neoplasm of heart HCC Rx ESR COM
Malignant neoplasm of pericardium
EXCLUDES 1 *malignant neoplasm of great vessels (C49.3)*

C38.1 Malignant neoplasm of anterior mediastinum HCC Rx ESR COM

C38.2 Malignant neoplasm of posterior mediastinum HCC Rx ESR COM

C38.3 Malignant neoplasm of mediastinum, part unspecified HCC Rx ESR COM

C38.4 Malignant neoplasm of pleura HCC Rx ESR COM

C38.8 Malignant neoplasm of overlapping sites of heart, mediastinum and pleura HCC Rx ESR COM

C39 Malignant neoplasm of other and ill-defined sites in the respiratory system and intrathoracic organs

Use additional code to identify:
- exposure to environmental tobacco smoke (Z77.22)
- exposure to tobacco smoke in the perinatal period (P96.81)
- history of tobacco dependence (Z87.891)
- occupational exposure to environmental tobacco smoke (Z57.31)
- tobacco dependence (F17.-)
- tobacco use (Z72.0)

EXCLUDES 1 *intrathoracic malignant neoplasm NOS (C76.1)*
thoracic malignant neoplasm NOS (C76.1)

C39.0 Malignant neoplasm of upper respiratory tract, part unspecified HCC Rx ESR COM

C39.9 Malignant neoplasm of lower respiratory tract, part unspecified HCC Rx ESR COM
Malignant neoplasm of respiratory tract NOS

Malignant neoplasms of bone and articular cartilage (C40-C41)

INCLUDES malignant neoplasm of cartilage (articular) (joint)
malignant neoplasm of periosteum

EXCLUDES 1 *malignant neoplasm of bone marrow NOS (C96.9)*
malignant neoplasm of synovia (C49.-)

C40 Malignant neoplasm of bone and articular cartilage of limbs

Use additional code to identify major osseous defect, if applicable (M89.7-)

C40.0 Malignant neoplasm of scapula and long bones of upper limb

C40.00 Malignant neoplasm of scapula and long bones of unspecified upper limb HCC Rx ESR COM

C40.01 Malignant neoplasm of scapula and long bones of right upper limb HCC Rx ESR COM

C40.02 Malignant neoplasm of scapula and long bones of left upper limb HCC Rx ESR COM

C40.1 Malignant neoplasm of short bones of upper limb

C40.10 Malignant neoplasm of short bones of unspecified upper limb HCC Rx ESR COM

C40.11 Malignant neoplasm of short bones of right upper limb HCC Rx ESR COM

C40.12 Malignant neoplasm of short bones of left upper limb HCC Rx ESR COM

C40.2 Malignant neoplasm of long bones of lower limb

C40.20 Malignant neoplasm of long bones of unspecified lower limb HCC Rx ESR COM

C40.21 Malignant neoplasm of long bones of right lower limb HCC Rx ESR COM

C40.22 Malignant neoplasm of long bones of left lower limb HCC Rx ESR COM

C40.3 Malignant neoplasm of short bones of lower limb

C40.30 Malignant neoplasm of short bones of unspecified lower limb HCC Rx ESR COM

C40.31 Malignant neoplasm of short bones of right lower limb HCC Rx ESR COM

C40.32 Malignant neoplasm of short bones of left lower limb HCC Rx ESR COM

C40.8 Malignant neoplasm of overlapping sites of bone and articular cartilage of limb

C40.80 Malignant neoplasm of overlapping sites of bone and articular cartilage of unspecified limb HCC Rx ESR COM

C40.81 Malignant neoplasm of overlapping sites of bone and articular cartilage of right limb HCC Rx ESR COM

C40.82 Malignant neoplasm of overlapping sites of bone and articular cartilage of left limb HCC Rx ESR COM

C40.9 Malignant neoplasm of unspecified bones and articular cartilage of limb

C40.90 Malignant neoplasm of unspecified bones and articular cartilage of unspecified limb HCC Rx ESR COM

C40.91 Malignant neoplasm of unspecified bones and articular cartilage of right limb HCC Rx ESR COM

C40.92 Malignant neoplasm of unspecified bones and articular cartilage of left limb HCC Rx ESR COM

C41 Malignant neoplasm of bone and articular cartilage of other and unspecified sites

EXCLUDES 1 *malignant neoplasm of bones of limbs (C4Ø.-)*
malignant neoplasm of cartilage of ear (C49.Ø)
malignant neoplasm of cartilage of eyelid (C49.Ø)
malignant neoplasm of cartilage of larynx (C32.3)
malignant neoplasm of cartilage of limbs (C4Ø.-)
malignant neoplasm of cartilage of nose (C3Ø.Ø)

C41.Ø Malignant neoplasm of bones of skull and face HCC Rx ESR COM
Malignant neoplasm of maxilla (superior)
Malignant neoplasm of orbital bone
EXCLUDES 2 *carcinoma, any type except intraosseous or odontogenic of:*
maxillary sinus (C31.Ø)
upper jaw (CØ3.Ø)
malignant neoplasm of jaw bone (lower) (C41.1)

C41.1 Malignant neoplasm of mandible HCC Rx ESR COM
Malignant neoplasm of inferior maxilla
Malignant neoplasm of lower jaw bone
EXCLUDES 2 *carcinoma, any type except intraosseous or odontogenic of:*
jaw NOS (CØ3.9)
lower (CØ3.1)
malignant neoplasm of upper jaw bone (C41.Ø)

C41.2 Malignant neoplasm of vertebral column HCC Rx ESR COM
EXCLUDES 1 *malignant neoplasm of sacrum and coccyx (C41.4)*

C41.3 Malignant neoplasm of ribs, sternum and clavicle HCC Rx ESR COM

C41.4 Malignant neoplasm of pelvic bones, sacrum and coccyx HCC Rx ESR COM

C41.9 Malignant neoplasm of bone and articular cartilage, unspecified HCC Rx ESR COM

Melanoma and other malignant neoplasms of skin (C43-C44)

C43 Malignant melanoma of skin

EXCLUDES 1 *melanoma in situ (DØ3.-)*
EXCLUDES 2 *malignant melanoma of skin of genital organs (C51-C52, C6Ø.-, C63.-)*
Merkel cell carcinoma (C4A.-)
sites other than skin - code to malignant neoplasm of the site

C43.Ø Malignant melanoma of lip HCC Rx ESR COM Q
EXCLUDES 1 *malignant neoplasm of vermilion border of lip (CØØ.Ø-CØØ.2)*

C43.1 Malignant melanoma of eyelid, including canthus
AHA: 2018,4Q,4

C43.1Ø Malignant melanoma of unspecified eyelid, including canthus HCC Rx ESR COM

C43.11 Malignant melanoma of right eyelid, including canthus

C43.111 Malignant melanoma of right upper eyelid, including canthus HCC Rx ESR COM

C43.112 Malignant melanoma of right lower eyelid, including canthus HCC Rx ESR COM

C43.12 Malignant melanoma of left eyelid, including canthus

C43.121 Malignant melanoma of left upper eyelid, including canthus HCC Rx ESR COM

C43.122 Malignant melanoma of left lower eyelid, including canthus HCC Rx ESR COM

C43.2 Malignant melanoma of ear and external auricular canal

C43.2Ø Malignant melanoma of unspecified ear and external auricular canal HCC Rx ESR COM Q

C43.21 Malignant melanoma of right ear and external auricular canal HCC Rx ESR COM Q

C43.22 Malignant melanoma of left ear and external auricular canal HCC Rx ESR COM Q

C43.3 Malignant melanoma of other and unspecified parts of face

C43.3Ø Malignant melanoma of unspecified part of face HCC Rx ESR COM Q

C43.31 Malignant melanoma of nose HCC Rx ESR COM Q

C43.39 Malignant melanoma of other parts of face HCC Rx ESR COM Q

C43.4 Malignant melanoma of scalp and neck HCC Rx ESR COM Q

C43.5 Malignant melanoma of trunk

EXCLUDES 2 *malignant neoplasm of anus NOS (C21.Ø)*
malignant neoplasm of scrotum (C63.2)

C43.51 Malignant melanoma of anal skin HCC Rx ESR COM Q
Malignant melanoma of anal margin
Malignant melanoma of perianal skin

C43.52 Malignant melanoma of skin of breast HCC Rx ESR COM Q

C43.59 Malignant melanoma of other part of trunk HCC Rx ESR COM Q

C43.6 Malignant melanoma of upper limb, including shoulder

C43.6Ø Malignant melanoma of unspecified upper limb, including shoulder HCC Rx ESR COM Q

C43.61 Malignant melanoma of right upper limb, including shoulder HCC Rx ESR COM Q

C43.62 Malignant melanoma of left upper limb, including shoulder HCC Rx ESR COM Q

C43.7 Malignant melanoma of lower limb, including hip

C43.7Ø Malignant melanoma of unspecified lower limb, including hip HCC Rx ESR COM Q

C43.71 Malignant melanoma of right lower limb, including hip HCC Rx ESR COM Q

C43.72 Malignant melanoma of left lower limb, including hip HCC Rx ESR COM Q

C43.8 Malignant melanoma of overlapping sites of skin HCC Rx ESR COM Q

C43.9 Malignant melanoma of skin, unspecified HCC Rx ESR COM Q
Malignant melanoma of unspecified site of skin
Melanoma (malignant) NOS

C4A Merkel cell carcinoma

DEF: Malignant cutaneous cancer predominantly found in elderly patients with sun exposure that usually presents as a flesh-colored or bluish-red lump typically seen on the neck, head, and face.

C4A.Ø Merkel cell carcinoma of lip HCC Rx ESR COM
EXCLUDES 1 *malignant neoplasm of vermilion border of lip (CØØ.Ø-CØØ.2)*

C4A.1 Merkel cell carcinoma of eyelid, including canthus
AHA: 2018,4Q,4

C4A.1Ø Merkel cell carcinoma of unspecified eyelid, including canthus HCC Rx ESR COM

C4A.11 Merkel cell carcinoma of right eyelid, including canthus

C4A.111 Merkel cell carcinoma of right upper eyelid, including canthus HCC Rx ESR COM

C4A.112 Merkel cell carcinoma of right lower eyelid, including canthus HCC Rx ESR COM

C4A.12 Merkel cell carcinoma of left eyelid, including canthus

C4A.121 Merkel cell carcinoma of left upper eyelid, including canthus HCC Rx ESR COM

C4A.122 Merkel cell carcinoma of left lower eyelid, including canthus HCC Rx ESR COM

C4A.2 Merkel cell carcinoma of ear and external auricular canal

C4A.2Ø Merkel cell carcinoma of unspecified ear and external auricular canal HCC Rx ESR COM

C4A.21 Merkel cell carcinoma of right ear and external auricular canal HCC Rx ESR COM

C4A.22 Merkel cell carcinoma of left ear and external auricular canal HCC Rx ESR COM

C4A.3 Merkel cell carcinoma of other and unspecified parts of face

C4A.3Ø Merkel cell carcinoma of unspecified part of face HCC Rx ESR COM

C4A.31 Merkel cell carcinoma of nose HCC Rx ESR COM

C4A.39 Merkel cell carcinoma of other parts of face HCC Rx ESR COM

C4A.4 Merkel cell carcinoma of scalp and neck HCC Rx ESR COM

C4A.5 Merkel cell carcinoma of trunk
EXCLUDES 2 *malignant neoplasm of anus NOS (C21.Ø)*
malignant neoplasm of scrotum (C63.2)
C4A.51 Merkel cell carcinoma of anal skin HCC Rx ESR COM
Merkel cell carcinoma of anal margin
Merkel cell carcinoma of perianal skin
C4A.52 Merkel cell carcinoma of skin of breast HCC Rx ESR COM
C4A.59 Merkel cell carcinoma of other part of trunk HCC Rx ESR COM
C4A.6 Merkel cell carcinoma of upper limb, including shoulder
C4A.6Ø Merkel cell carcinoma of unspecified upper limb, including shoulder HCC Rx ESR COM
C4A.61 Merkel cell carcinoma of right upper limb, including shoulder HCC Rx ESR COM
C4A.62 Merkel cell carcinoma of left upper limb, including shoulder HCC Rx ESR COM
C4A.7 Merkel cell carcinoma of lower limb, including hip
C4A.7Ø Merkel cell carcinoma of unspecified lower limb, including hip HCC Rx ESR COM
C4A.71 Merkel cell carcinoma of right lower limb, including hip HCC Rx ESR COM
C4A.72 Merkel cell carcinoma of left lower limb, including hip HCC Rx ESR COM
C4A.8 Merkel cell carcinoma of overlapping sites HCC Rx ESR COM
C4A.9 Merkel cell carcinoma, unspecified HCC Rx ESR COM
Merkel cell carcinoma of unspecified site
Merkel cell carcinoma NOS

C44 Other and unspecified malignant neoplasm of skin
INCLUDES malignant neoplasm of sebaceous glands
malignant neoplasm of sweat glands
EXCLUDES 1 *Kaposi's sarcoma of skin (C46.Ø)*
malignant melanoma of skin (C43.-)
malignant neoplasm of skin of genital organs (C51-C52, C6Ø.-, C63.2)
Merkel cell carcinoma (C4A.-)
DEF: Basal cell carcinoma: Abnormal growth of skin cells that arises from the deepest layer of the epidermis and may present as an open sore, red patches, pink growth, or scar. Typically caused by sun exposure, it is one of the most common forms of skin cancer.
DEF: Squamous cell carcinoma: Uncontrolled growth of abnormal skin cells that arises from the outer layers of the skin (epidermis) and may present as an open sore. It is characterized by a firm, red nodule, elevated growth with a central depression, or a flat sore with a scaly crust.

C44.Ø Other and unspecified malignant neoplasm of skin of lip
EXCLUDES 1 *malignant neoplasm of lip (CØØ.-)*
C44.ØØ Unspecified malignant neoplasm of skin of lip
C44.Ø1 Basal cell carcinoma of skin of lip
C44.Ø2 Squamous cell carcinoma of skin of lip
C44.Ø9 Other specified malignant neoplasm of skin of lip

C44.1 Other and unspecified malignant neoplasm of skin of eyelid, including canthus
EXCLUDES 1 *connective tissue of eyelid (C49.Ø)*
AHA: 2018,4Q,4
C44.1Ø Unspecified malignant neoplasm of skin of eyelid, including canthus
C44.1Ø1 Unspecified malignant neoplasm of skin of unspecified eyelid, including canthus
C44.1Ø2 Unspecified malignant neoplasm of skin of right eyelid, including canthus
C44.1Ø21 Unspecified malignant neoplasm of skin of right upper eyelid, including canthus
C44.1Ø22 Unspecified malignant neoplasm of skin of right lower eyelid, including canthus
C44.1Ø9 Unspecified malignant neoplasm of skin of left eyelid, including canthus
C44.1Ø91 Unspecified malignant neoplasm of skin of left upper eyelid, including canthus
C44.1Ø92 Unspecified malignant neoplasm of skin of left lower eyelid, including canthus
C44.11 Basal cell carcinoma of skin of eyelid, including canthus
C44.111 Basal cell carcinoma of skin of unspecified eyelid, including canthus
C44.112 Basal cell carcinoma of skin of right eyelid, including canthus
C44.1121 Basal cell carcinoma of skin of right upper eyelid, including canthus
C44.1122 Basal cell carcinoma of skin of right lower eyelid, including canthus
C44.119 Basal cell carcinoma of skin of left eyelid, including canthus
C44.1191 Basal cell carcinoma of skin of left upper eyelid, including canthus
C44.1192 Basal cell carcinoma of skin of left lower eyelid, including canthus
C44.12 Squamous cell carcinoma of skin of eyelid, including canthus
C44.121 Squamous cell carcinoma of skin of unspecified eyelid, including canthus
C44.122 Squamous cell carcinoma of skin of right eyelid, including canthus
C44.1221 Squamous cell carcinoma of skin of right upper eyelid, including canthus
C44.1222 Squamous cell carcinoma of skin of right lower eyelid, including canthus
C44.129 Squamous cell carcinoma of skin of left eyelid, including canthus
C44.1291 Squamous cell carcinoma of skin of left upper eyelid, including canthus
C44.1292 Squamous cell carcinoma of skin of left lower eyelid, including canthus
C44.13 Sebaceous cell carcinoma of skin of eyelid, including canthus
C44.131 Sebaceous cell carcinoma of skin of unspecified eyelid, including canthus
C44.132 Sebaceous cell carcinoma of skin of right eyelid, including canthus
C44.1321 Sebaceous cell carcinoma of skin of right upper eyelid, including canthus
C44.1322 Sebaceous cell carcinoma of skin of right lower eyelid, including canthus
C44.139 Sebaceous cell carcinoma of skin of left eyelid, including canthus
C44.1391 Sebaceous cell carcinoma of skin of left upper eyelid, including canthus
C44.1392 Sebaceous cell carcinoma of skin of left lower eyelid, including canthus
C44.19 Other specified malignant neoplasm of skin of eyelid, including canthus
C44.191 Other specified malignant neoplasm of skin of unspecified eyelid, including canthus
C44.192 Other specified malignant neoplasm of skin of right eyelid, including canthus
C44.1921 Other specified malignant neoplasm of skin of right upper eyelid, including canthus
C44.1922 Other specified malignant neoplasm of skin of right lower eyelid, including canthus
C44.199 Other specified malignant neoplasm of skin of left eyelid, including canthus
C44.1991 Other specified malignant neoplasm of skin of left upper eyelid, including canthus
C44.1992 Other specified malignant neoplasm of skin of left lower eyelid, including canthus

C44.2 Other and unspecified malignant neoplasm of skin of ear and external auricular canal
EXCLUDES 1 *connective tissue of ear (C49.Ø)*

C44.2Ø Unspecified malignant neoplasm of skin of ear and external auricular canal
- **C44.201 Unspecified malignant neoplasm of skin of unspecified ear and external auricular canal**
- **C44.202 Unspecified malignant neoplasm of skin of right ear and external auricular canal**
- **C44.209 Unspecified malignant neoplasm of skin of left ear and external auricular canal**

C44.21 Basal cell carcinoma of skin of ear and external auricular canal
- **C44.211 Basal cell carcinoma of skin of unspecified ear and external auricular canal**
- **C44.212 Basal cell carcinoma of skin of right ear and external auricular canal**
- **C44.219 Basal cell carcinoma of skin of left ear and external auricular canal**

C44.22 Squamous cell carcinoma of skin of ear and external auricular canal
- **C44.221 Squamous cell carcinoma of skin of unspecified ear and external auricular canal**
- **C44.222 Squamous cell carcinoma of skin of right ear and external auricular canal**
- **C44.229 Squamous cell carcinoma of skin of left ear and external auricular canal**

C44.29 Other specified malignant neoplasm of skin of ear and external auricular canal
- **C44.291 Other specified malignant neoplasm of skin of unspecified ear and external auricular canal**
- **C44.292 Other specified malignant neoplasm of skin of right ear and external auricular canal**
- **C44.299 Other specified malignant neoplasm of skin of left ear and external auricular canal**

C44.3 Other and unspecified malignant neoplasm of skin of other and unspecified parts of face

C44.3Ø Unspecified malignant neoplasm of skin of other and unspecified parts of face
- **C44.3ØØ Unspecified malignant neoplasm of skin of unspecified part of face**
- **C44.301 Unspecified malignant neoplasm of skin of nose**
- **C44.309 Unspecified malignant neoplasm of skin of other parts of face**

C44.31 Basal cell carcinoma of skin of other and unspecified parts of face
- **C44.31Ø Basal cell carcinoma of skin of unspecified parts of face**
- **C44.311 Basal cell carcinoma of skin of nose**
- **C44.319 Basal cell carcinoma of skin of other parts of face**

C44.32 Squamous cell carcinoma of skin of other and unspecified parts of face
- **C44.32Ø Squamous cell carcinoma of skin of unspecified parts of face**
- **C44.321 Squamous cell carcinoma of skin of nose**
- **C44.329 Squamous cell carcinoma of skin of other parts of face**

C44.39 Other specified malignant neoplasm of skin of other and unspecified parts of face
- **C44.39Ø Other specified malignant neoplasm of skin of unspecified parts of face**
- **C44.391 Other specified malignant neoplasm of skin of nose**
- **C44.399 Other specified malignant neoplasm of skin of other parts of face**

C44.4 Other and unspecified malignant neoplasm of skin of scalp and neck
- **C44.4Ø Unspecified malignant neoplasm of skin of scalp and neck**
- **C44.41 Basal cell carcinoma of skin of scalp and neck**
- **C44.42 Squamous cell carcinoma of skin of scalp and neck**
- **C44.49 Other specified malignant neoplasm of skin of scalp and neck**

C44.5 Other and unspecified malignant neoplasm of skin of trunk
EXCLUDES 1 *anus NOS (C21.Ø)*
scrotum (C63.2)

C44.5Ø Unspecified malignant neoplasm of skin of trunk
- **C44.5ØØ Unspecified malignant neoplasm of anal skin**
  Unspecified malignant neoplasm of anal margin
  Unspecified malignant neoplasm of perianal skin
- **C44.501 Unspecified malignant neoplasm of skin of breast**
- **C44.509 Unspecified malignant neoplasm of skin of other part of trunk**

C44.51 Basal cell carcinoma of skin of trunk
- **C44.51Ø Basal cell carcinoma of anal skin**
  Basal cell carcinoma of anal margin
  Basal cell carcinoma of perianal skin
- **C44.511 Basal cell carcinoma of skin of breast**
- **C44.519 Basal cell carcinoma of skin of other part of trunk**

C44.52 Squamous cell carcinoma of skin of trunk
- **C44.52Ø Squamous cell carcinoma of anal skin**
  Squamous cell carcinoma of anal margin
  Squamous cell carcinoma of perianal skin
- **C44.521 Squamous cell carcinoma of skin of breast**
- **C44.529 Squamous cell carcinoma of skin of other part of trunk**

C44.59 Other specified malignant neoplasm of skin of trunk
- **C44.59Ø Other specified malignant neoplasm of anal skin**
  Other specified malignant neoplasm of anal margin
  Other specified malignant neoplasm of perianal skin
- **C44.591 Other specified malignant neoplasm of skin of breast**
- **C44.599 Other specified malignant neoplasm of skin of other part of trunk**

C44.6 Other and unspecified malignant neoplasm of skin of upper limb, including shoulder

C44.6Ø Unspecified malignant neoplasm of skin of upper limb, including shoulder
- **C44.601 Unspecified malignant neoplasm of skin of unspecified upper limb, including shoulder**
- **C44.602 Unspecified malignant neoplasm of skin of right upper limb, including shoulder**
- **C44.609 Unspecified malignant neoplasm of skin of left upper limb, including shoulder**

C44.61 Basal cell carcinoma of skin of upper limb, including shoulder
- **C44.611 Basal cell carcinoma of skin of unspecified upper limb, including shoulder**
- **C44.612 Basal cell carcinoma of skin of right upper limb, including shoulder**
- **C44.619 Basal cell carcinoma of skin of left upper limb, including shoulder**

C44.62 Squamous cell carcinoma of skin of upper limb, including shoulder
- **C44.621 Squamous cell carcinoma of skin of unspecified upper limb, including shoulder**
- **C44.622 Squamous cell carcinoma of skin of right upper limb, including shoulder**
- **C44.629 Squamous cell carcinoma of skin of left upper limb, including shoulder**

C44.69 Other specified malignant neoplasm of skin of upper limb, including shoulder
- **C44.691 Other specified malignant neoplasm of skin of unspecified upper limb, including shoulder**
- **C44.692 Other specified malignant neoplasm of skin of right upper limb, including shoulder**
- **C44.699 Other specified malignant neoplasm of skin of left upper limb, including shoulder**

✓5th **C44.7 Other and unspecified malignant neoplasm of skin of lower limb, including hip**

✓6th **C44.70 Unspecified malignant neoplasm of skin of lower limb, including hip**

C44.701 Unspecified malignant neoplasm of skin of unspecified lower limb, including hip

C44.702 Unspecified malignant neoplasm of skin of right lower limb, including hip

C44.709 Unspecified malignant neoplasm of skin of left lower limb, including hip

✓6th **C44.71 Basal cell carcinoma of skin of lower limb, including hip**

C44.711 Basal cell carcinoma of skin of unspecified lower limb, including hip

C44.712 Basal cell carcinoma of skin of right lower limb, including hip

C44.719 Basal cell carcinoma of skin of left lower limb, including hip

✓6th **C44.72 Squamous cell carcinoma of skin of lower limb, including hip**

C44.721 Squamous cell carcinoma of skin of unspecified lower limb, including hip

C44.722 Squamous cell carcinoma of skin of right lower limb, including hip

C44.729 Squamous cell carcinoma of skin of left lower limb, including hip

✓6th **C44.79 Other specified malignant neoplasm of skin of lower limb, including hip**

C44.791 Other specified malignant neoplasm of skin of unspecified lower limb, including hip

C44.792 Other specified malignant neoplasm of skin of right lower limb, including hip

C44.799 Other specified malignant neoplasm of skin of left lower limb, including hip

✓5th **C44.8 Other and unspecified malignant neoplasm of overlapping sites of skin**

C44.80 Unspecified malignant neoplasm of overlapping sites of skin

C44.81 Basal cell carcinoma of overlapping sites of skin

C44.82 Squamous cell carcinoma of overlapping sites of skin

C44.89 Other specified malignant neoplasm of overlapping sites of skin

✓5th **C44.9 Other and unspecified malignant neoplasm of skin, unspecified**

C44.90 Unspecified malignant neoplasm of skin, unspecified

Malignant neoplasm of unspecified site of skin

C44.91 Basal cell carcinoma of skin, unspecified

C44.92 Squamous cell carcinoma of skin, unspecified

C44.99 Other specified malignant neoplasm of skin, unspecified

Malignant neoplasms of mesothelial and soft tissue (C45-C49)

✓4th **C45 Mesothelioma**

DEF: Rare type of cancer that forms in the thin layer of protective tissue that covers the majority of internal organs (mesothelium).

C45.0 Mesothelioma of pleura HCC Rx ESR COM

EXCLUDES 1 *other malignant neoplasm of pleura (C38.4)*

AHA: 2017,2Q,11

TIP: For pleural mesothelioma that has metastasized to the chest wall, assign this code for the primary site along with C79.89 for metastatic cancer in the chest wall.

C45.1 Mesothelioma of peritoneum HCC Rx ESR COM

Mesothelioma of cul-de-sac

Mesothelioma of mesentery

Mesothelioma of mesocolon

Mesothelioma of omentum

Mesothelioma of peritoneum (parietal) (pelvic)

EXCLUDES 1 *other malignant neoplasm of soft tissue of peritoneum (C48.-)*

C45.2 Mesothelioma of pericardium HCC Rx ESR COM

EXCLUDES 1 *other malignant neoplasm of pericardium (C38.0)*

C45.7 Mesothelioma of other sites HCC Rx ESR COM

C45.9 Mesothelioma, unspecified HCC Rx ESR COM

✓4th **C46 Kaposi's sarcoma**

Code first any human immunodeficiency virus [HIV] disease (B20)

DEF: Malignant neoplasm that causes patches of abnormal tissue to grow under the skin, in the lining of the mouth, nose, and throat, in lymph nodes, or in other visceral organs. Kaposi's sarcoma is caused by human herpesvirus8 (HHV8).

C46.0 Kaposi's sarcoma of skin HCC Rx ESR COM

C46.1 Kaposi's sarcoma of soft tissue HCC Rx ESR COM

Kaposi's sarcoma of blood vessel

Kaposi's sarcoma of connective tissue

Kaposi's sarcoma of fascia

Kaposi's sarcoma of ligament

Kaposi's sarcoma of lymphatic(s) NEC

Kaposi's sarcoma of muscle

EXCLUDES 2 *Kaposi's sarcoma of lymph glands and nodes (C46.3)*

C46.2 Kaposi's sarcoma of palate HCC Rx ESR COM

C46.3 Kaposi's sarcoma of lymph nodes HCC Rx ESR COM

C46.4 Kaposi's sarcoma of gastrointestinal sites HCC Rx ESR COM

✓5th **C46.5 Kaposi's sarcoma of lung**

AHA: 2019,1Q,16

TIP: When associated malignant pericardial effusion is documented, assign code I31.3. If the sole reason for admission is to treat the effusion with no treatment of the lung malignancy rendered, code I31.3 may be sequenced first.

C46.50 Kaposi's sarcoma of unspecified lung HCC Rx ESR COM

C46.51 Kaposi's sarcoma of right lung HCC Rx ESR COM

C46.52 Kaposi's sarcoma of left lung HCC Rx ESR COM

C46.7 Kaposi's sarcoma of other sites HCC Rx ESR COM

C46.9 Kaposi's sarcoma, unspecified HCC Rx ESR COM

Kaposi's sarcoma of unspecified site

✓4th **C47 Malignant neoplasm of peripheral nerves and autonomic nervous system**

INCLUDES malignant neoplasm of sympathetic and parasympathetic nerves and ganglia

EXCLUDES 1 *Kaposi's sarcoma of soft tissue (C46.1)*

C47.0 Malignant neoplasm of peripheral nerves of head, face and neck HCC Rx ESR COM

EXCLUDES 1 *malignant neoplasm of peripheral nerves of orbit (C69.6-)*

✓5th **C47.1 Malignant neoplasm of peripheral nerves of upper limb, including shoulder**

C47.10 Malignant neoplasm of peripheral nerves of unspecified upper limb, including shoulder HCC Rx ESR COM

C47.11 Malignant neoplasm of peripheral nerves of right upper limb, including shoulder HCC Rx ESR COM

C47.12 Malignant neoplasm of peripheral nerves of left upper limb, including shoulder HCC Rx ESR COM

✓5th **C47.2 Malignant neoplasm of peripheral nerves of lower limb, including hip**

C47.20 Malignant neoplasm of peripheral nerves of unspecified lower limb, including hip HCC Rx ESR COM

C47.21 Malignant neoplasm of peripheral nerves of right lower limb, including hip HCC Rx ESR COM

C47.22 Malignant neoplasm of peripheral nerves of left lower limb, including hip HCC Rx ESR COM

C47.3 Malignant neoplasm of peripheral nerves of thorax HCC Rx ESR COM

C47.4 Malignant neoplasm of peripheral nerves of abdomen HCC Rx ESR COM

C47.5 Malignant neoplasm of peripheral nerves of pelvis HCC Rx ESR COM

C47.6 Malignant neoplasm of peripheral nerves of trunk, unspecified HCC Rx ESR COM

Malignant neoplasm of peripheral nerves of unspecified part of trunk

C47.8 Malignant neoplasm of overlapping sites of peripheral nerves and autonomic nervous system HCC Rx ESR COM

C47.9 Malignant neoplasm of peripheral nerves and autonomic nervous system, unspecified HCC Rx ESR COM

Malignant neoplasm of unspecified site of peripheral nerves and autonomic nervous system

C48 Malignant neoplasm of retroperitoneum and peritoneum

EXCLUDES 1 *Kaposi's sarcoma of connective tissue (C46.1)*
mesothelioma (C45.-)

C48.Ø Malignant neoplasm of retroperitoneum HCC Rx ESR COM

C48.1 Malignant neoplasm of specified parts of peritoneum HCC Rx ESR COM
Malignant neoplasm of cul-de-sac
Malignant neoplasm of mesentery
Malignant neoplasm of mesocolon
Malignant neoplasm of omentum
Malignant neoplasm of parietal peritoneum
Malignant neoplasm of pelvic peritoneum

C48.2 Malignant neoplasm of peritoneum, unspecified HCC Rx ESR COM

C48.8 Malignant neoplasm of overlapping sites of retroperitoneum and peritoneum HCC Rx ESR COM

C49 Malignant neoplasm of other connective and soft tissue

INCLUDES malignant neoplasm of blood vessel
malignant neoplasm of bursa
malignant neoplasm of cartilage
malignant neoplasm of fascia
malignant neoplasm of fat
malignant neoplasm of ligament, except uterine
malignant neoplasm of lymphatic vessel
malignant neoplasm of muscle
malignant neoplasm of synovia
malignant neoplasm of tendon (sheath)

EXCLUDES 1 *malignant neoplasm of cartilage (of):*
articular (C4Ø-C41)
larynx (C32.3)
nose (C3Ø.Ø)
malignant neoplasm of connective tissue of breast (C5Ø.-)

EXCLUDES 2 *Kaposi's sarcoma of soft tissue (C46.1)*
malignant neoplasm of heart (C38.Ø)
malignant neoplasm of peripheral nerves and autonomic nervous system (C47.-)
malignant neoplasm of peritoneum (C48.2)
malignant neoplasm of retroperitoneum (C48.Ø)
malignant neoplasm of uterine ligament (C57.3)
mesothelioma (C45.-)

C49.Ø Malignant neoplasm of connective and soft tissue of head, face and neck HCC Rx ESR COM
Malignant neoplasm of connective tissue of ear
Malignant neoplasm of connective tissue of eyelid
EXCLUDES 1 *connective tissue of orbit (C69.6-)*

C49.1 Malignant neoplasm of connective and soft tissue of upper limb, including shoulder

C49.1Ø Malignant neoplasm of connective and soft tissue of unspecified upper limb, including shoulder HCC Rx ESR COM

C49.11 Malignant neoplasm of connective and soft tissue of right upper limb, including shoulder HCC Rx ESR COM

C49.12 Malignant neoplasm of connective and soft tissue of left upper limb, including shoulder HCC Rx ESR COM

C49.2 Malignant neoplasm of connective and soft tissue of lower limb, including hip

C49.2Ø Malignant neoplasm of connective and soft tissue of unspecified lower limb, including hip HCC Rx ESR COM

C49.21 Malignant neoplasm of connective and soft tissue of right lower limb, including hip HCC Rx ESR COM

C49.22 Malignant neoplasm of connective and soft tissue of left lower limb, including hip HCC Rx ESR COM

C49.3 Malignant neoplasm of connective and soft tissue of thorax HCC Rx ESR COM
Malignant neoplasm of axilla
Malignant neoplasm of diaphragm
Malignant neoplasm of great vessels
EXCLUDES 1 *malignant neoplasm of breast (C5Ø.-)*
malignant neoplasm of heart (C38.Ø)
malignant neoplasm of mediastinum (C38.1-C38.3)
malignant neoplasm of thymus (C37)
AHA: 2015,3Q,19

C49.4 Malignant neoplasm of connective and soft tissue of abdomen HCC Rx ESR COM
Malignant neoplasm of abdominal wall
Malignant neoplasm of hypochondrium

C49.5 Malignant neoplasm of connective and soft tissue of pelvis HCC Rx ESR COM
Malignant neoplasm of buttock
Malignant neoplasm of groin
Malignant neoplasm of perineum

C49.6 Malignant neoplasm of connective and soft tissue of trunk, unspecified HCC Rx ESR COM
Malignant neoplasm of back NOS

C49.8 Malignant neoplasm of overlapping sites of connective and soft tissue HCC Rx ESR COM
Primary malignant neoplasm of two or more contiguous sites of connective and soft tissue

C49.9 Malignant neoplasm of connective and soft tissue, unspecified HCC Rx ESR COM

C49.A Gastrointestinal stromal tumor
AHA: 2016,4Q,8
DEF: Uncommon malignant tumor found in the GI tract that originates from interstitial cells of the autonomic nervous system. Most occur in the stomach or small intestine but can originate anywhere in the GI tract.

C49.AØ Gastrointestinal stromal tumor, unspecified site HCC Rx ESR COM

C49.A1 Gastrointestinal stromal tumor of esophagus HCC Rx ESR COM

C49.A2 Gastrointestinal stromal tumor of stomach HCC Rx ESR COM

C49.A3 Gastrointestinal stromal tumor of small intestine HCC Rx ESR COM

C49.A4 Gastrointestinal stromal tumor of large intestine HCC Rx ESR COM

C49.A5 Gastrointestinal stromal tumor of rectum HCC Rx ESR COM

C49.A9 Gastrointestinal stromal tumor of other sites HCC Rx ESR COM

Malignant neoplasms of breast (C5Ø)

C5Ø Malignant neoplasm of breast

INCLUDES connective tissue of breast
Paget's disease of breast
Paget's disease of nipple

Use additional code to identify estrogen receptor status (Z17.Ø, Z17.1)

EXCLUDES 1 *skin of breast (C44.5Ø1, C44.511, C44.521, C44.591)*

AHA: 2017,4Q,19

Female Breast

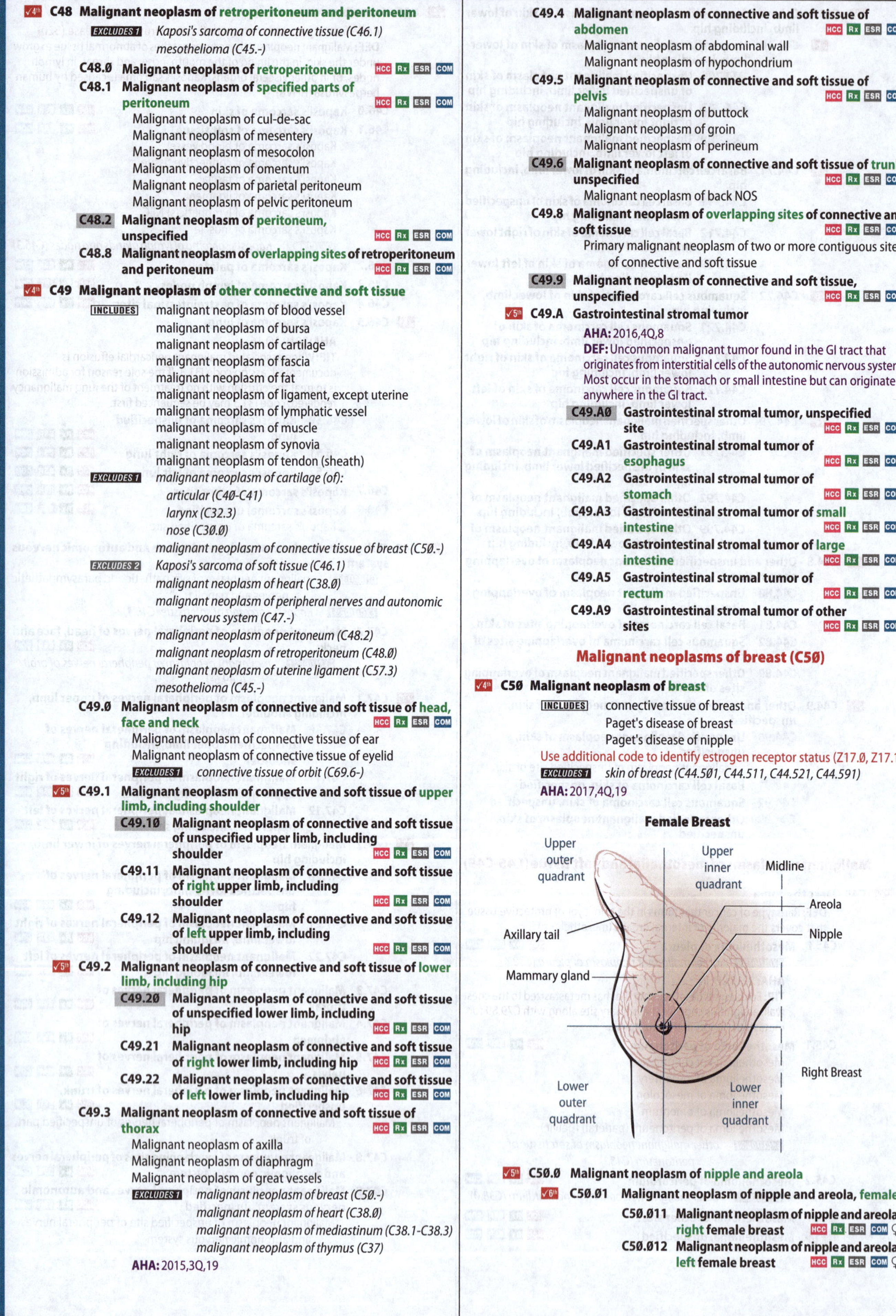

C5Ø.Ø Malignant neoplasm of nipple and areola

C5Ø.Ø1 Malignant neoplasm of nipple and areola, female

C5Ø.Ø11 Malignant neoplasm of nipple and areola, right female breast HCC Rx ESR COM ♀

C5Ø.Ø12 Malignant neoplasm of nipple and areola, left female breast HCC Rx ESR COM ♀

C50.019 Malignant neoplasm of nipple and areola, unspecified female breast HCC Rx ESR COM ♀

✓6th C50.02 Malignant neoplasm of nipple and areola, male

C50.021 Malignant neoplasm of nipple and areola, right male breast HCC Rx ESR COM ♂

C50.022 Malignant neoplasm of nipple and areola, left male breast HCC Rx ESR COM ♂

C50.029 Malignant neoplasm of nipple and areola, unspecified male breast HCC Rx ESR COM ♂

✓5th C50.1 Malignant neoplasm of central portion of breast

✓6th C50.11 Malignant neoplasm of central portion of breast, female

C50.111 Malignant neoplasm of central portion of right female breast HCC Rx ESR COM ♀

C50.112 Malignant neoplasm of central portion of left female breast HCC Rx ESR COM ♀

C50.119 Malignant neoplasm of central portion of unspecified female breast HCC Rx ESR COM ♀

✓6th C50.12 Malignant neoplasm of central portion of breast, male

C50.121 Malignant neoplasm of central portion of right male breast HCC Rx ESR COM ♂

C50.122 Malignant neoplasm of central portion of left male breast HCC Rx ESR COM ♂

C50.129 Malignant neoplasm of central portion of unspecified male breast HCC Rx ESR COM ♂

✓5th C50.2 Malignant neoplasm of upper-inner quadrant of breast

✓6th C50.21 Malignant neoplasm of upper-inner quadrant of breast, female

C50.211 Malignant neoplasm of upper-inner quadrant of right female breast HCC Rx ESR COM ♀

C50.212 Malignant neoplasm of upper-inner quadrant of left female breast HCC Rx ESR COM ♀

C50.219 Malignant neoplasm of upper-inner quadrant of unspecified female breast HCC Rx ESR COM ♀

✓6th C50.22 Malignant neoplasm of upper-inner quadrant of breast, male

C50.221 Malignant neoplasm of upper-inner quadrant of right male breast HCC Rx ESR COM ♂

C50.222 Malignant neoplasm of upper-inner quadrant of left male breast HCC Rx ESR COM ♂

C50.229 Malignant neoplasm of upper-inner quadrant of unspecified male breast HCC Rx ESR COM ♂

✓5th C50.3 Malignant neoplasm of lower-inner quadrant of breast

✓6th C50.31 Malignant neoplasm of lower-inner quadrant of breast, female

C50.311 Malignant neoplasm of lower-inner quadrant of right female breast HCC Rx ESR COM ♀

C50.312 Malignant neoplasm of lower-inner quadrant of left female breast HCC Rx ESR COM ♀

C50.319 Malignant neoplasm of lower-inner quadrant of unspecified female breast HCC Rx ESR COM ♀

✓6th C50.32 Malignant neoplasm of lower-inner quadrant of breast, male

C50.321 Malignant neoplasm of lower-inner quadrant of right male breast HCC Rx ESR COM ♂

C50.322 Malignant neoplasm of lower-inner quadrant of left male breast HCC Rx ESR COM ♂

C50.329 Malignant neoplasm of lower-inner quadrant of unspecified male breast HCC Rx ESR COM ♂

✓5th C50.4 Malignant neoplasm of upper-outer quadrant of breast

✓6th C50.41 Malignant neoplasm of upper-outer quadrant of breast, female

C50.411 Malignant neoplasm of upper-outer quadrant of right female breast HCC Rx ESR COM ♀

C50.412 Malignant neoplasm of upper-outer quadrant of left female breast HCC Rx ESR COM ♀

C50.419 Malignant neoplasm of upper-outer quadrant of unspecified female breast HCC Rx ESR COM ♀

✓6th C50.42 Malignant neoplasm of upper-outer quadrant of breast, male

C50.421 Malignant neoplasm of upper-outer quadrant of right male breast HCC Rx ESR COM ♂

C50.422 Malignant neoplasm of upper-outer quadrant of left male breast HCC Rx ESR COM ♂

C50.429 Malignant neoplasm of upper-outer quadrant of unspecified male breast HCC Rx ESR COM ♂

✓5th C50.5 Malignant neoplasm of lower-outer quadrant of breast

✓6th C50.51 Malignant neoplasm of lower-outer quadrant of breast, female

C50.511 Malignant neoplasm of lower-outer quadrant of right female breast HCC Rx ESR COM ♀

C50.512 Malignant neoplasm of lower-outer quadrant of left female breast HCC Rx ESR COM ♀

C50.519 Malignant neoplasm of lower-outer quadrant of unspecified female breast HCC Rx ESR COM ♀

✓6th C50.52 Malignant neoplasm of lower-outer quadrant of breast, male

C50.521 Malignant neoplasm of lower-outer quadrant of right male breast HCC Rx ESR COM ♂

C50.522 Malignant neoplasm of lower-outer quadrant of left male breast HCC Rx ESR COM ♂

C50.529 Malignant neoplasm of lower-outer quadrant of unspecified male breast HCC Rx ESR COM ♂

✓5th C50.6 Malignant neoplasm of axillary tail of breast

✓6th C50.61 Malignant neoplasm of axillary tail of breast, female

C50.611 Malignant neoplasm of axillary tail of right female breast HCC Rx ESR COM ♀

C50.612 Malignant neoplasm of axillary tail of left female breast HCC Rx ESR COM ♀

C50.619 Malignant neoplasm of axillary tail of unspecified female breast HCC Rx ESR COM ♀

✓6th C50.62 Malignant neoplasm of axillary tail of breast, male

C50.621 Malignant neoplasm of axillary tail of right male breast HCC Rx ESR COM ♂

C50.622 Malignant neoplasm of axillary tail of left male breast HCC Rx ESR COM ♂

C50.629 Malignant neoplasm of axillary tail of unspecified male breast HCC Rx ESR COM ♂

✓5th C50.8 Malignant neoplasm of overlapping sites of breast

✓6th C50.81 Malignant neoplasm of overlapping sites of breast, female

C50.811 Malignant neoplasm of overlapping sites of right female breast HCC Rx ESR COM ♀

C50.812 Malignant neoplasm of overlapping sites of left female breast HCC Rx ESR COM ♀

C50.819 Malignant neoplasm of overlapping sites of unspecified female breast HCC Rx ESR COM ♀

✓6th C50.82 Malignant neoplasm of overlapping sites of breast, male

C50.821 Malignant neoplasm of overlapping sites of right male breast HCC Rx ESR COM ♂

C50.822 Malignant neoplasm of overlapping sites of left male breast HCC Rx ESR COM ♂

C50.829 Malignant neoplasm of overlapping sites of unspecified male breast HCC Rx ESR COM ♂

✓5th **C50.9 Malignant neoplasm of breast of unspecified site**

✓6th **C50.91 Malignant neoplasm of breast of unspecified site, female**

C50.911 Malignant neoplasm of unspecified site of right female breast HCC Rx ESR COM ♀

C50.912 Malignant neoplasm of unspecified site of left female breast HCC Rx ESR COM ♀

C50.919 Malignant neoplasm of unspecified site of unspecified female breast HCC Rx ESR COM ♀

✓6th **C50.92 Malignant neoplasm of breast of unspecified site, male**

C50.921 Malignant neoplasm of unspecified site of right male breast HCC Rx ESR COM ♂

C50.922 Malignant neoplasm of unspecified site of left male breast HCC Rx ESR COM ♂

C50.929 Malignant neoplasm of unspecified site of unspecified male breast HCC Rx ESR COM ♂

Malignant neoplasms of female genital organs (C51-C58)

INCLUDES malignant neoplasm of skin of female genital organs

✓4th **C51 Malignant neoplasm of vulva**

EXCLUDES 1 *carcinoma in situ of vulva (D07.1)*

C51.0 Malignant neoplasm of labium majus HCC ESR COM ♀

Malignant neoplasm of Bartholin's [greater vestibular] gland

C51.1 Malignant neoplasm of labium minus HCC ESR COM ♀

C51.2 Malignant neoplasm of clitoris HCC ESR COM ♀

C51.8 Malignant neoplasm of overlapping sites of vulva HCC ESR COM ♀

C51.9 Malignant neoplasm of vulva, unspecified HCC ESR COM ♀

Malignant neoplasm of external female genitalia NOS

Malignant neoplasm of pudendum

C52 Malignant neoplasm of vagina HCC ESR COM ♀

EXCLUDES 1 *carcinoma in situ of vagina (D07.2)*

✓4th **C53 Malignant neoplasm of cervix uteri**

EXCLUDES 1 *carcinoma in situ of cervix uteri (D06.-)*

AHA: 2017,4Q,103

C53.0 Malignant neoplasm of endocervix HCC ESR COM ♀

C53.1 Malignant neoplasm of exocervix HCC ESR COM ♀

C53.8 Malignant neoplasm of overlapping sites of cervix uteri HCC ESR COM ♀

C53.9 Malignant neoplasm of cervix uteri, unspecified HCC ESR COM ♀

✓4th **C54 Malignant neoplasm of corpus uteri**

C54.0 Malignant neoplasm of isthmus uteri HCC ESR COM ♀

Malignant neoplasm of lower uterine segment

C54.1 Malignant neoplasm of endometrium HCC ESR COM ♀

C54.2 Malignant neoplasm of myometrium HCC ESR COM ♀

C54.3 Malignant neoplasm of fundus uteri HCC ESR COM ♀

C54.8 Malignant neoplasm of overlapping sites of corpus uteri HCC ESR COM ♀

C54.9 Malignant neoplasm of corpus uteri, unspecified HCC ESR COM ♀

C55 Malignant neoplasm of uterus, part unspecified HCC ESR COM ♀

✓4th **C56 Malignant neoplasm of ovary**

Use additional code to identify any functional activity

C56.1 Malignant neoplasm of right ovary HCC Rx ESR COM ♀

C56.2 Malignant neoplasm of left ovary HCC Rx ESR COM ♀

C56.3 Malignant neoplasm of bilateral ovaries HCC Rx ESR COM ♀

C56.9 Malignant neoplasm of unspecified ovary HCC Rx ESR COM ♀

✓4th **C57 Malignant neoplasm of other and unspecified female genital organs**

✓5th **C57.0 Malignant neoplasm of fallopian tube**

Malignant neoplasm of oviduct

Malignant neoplasm of uterine tube

C57.00 Malignant neoplasm of unspecified fallopian tube HCC Rx ESR COM ♀

C57.01 Malignant neoplasm of right fallopian tube HCC Rx ESR COM ♀

C57.02 Malignant neoplasm of left fallopian tube HCC Rx ESR COM ♀

✓5th **C57.1 Malignant neoplasm of broad ligament**

C57.10 Malignant neoplasm of unspecified broad ligament HCC Rx ESR COM ♀

C57.11 Malignant neoplasm of right broad ligament HCC Rx ESR COM ♀

C57.12 Malignant neoplasm of left broad ligament HCC Rx ESR COM ♀

✓5th **C57.2 Malignant neoplasm of round ligament**

C57.20 Malignant neoplasm of unspecified round ligament HCC Rx ESR COM ♀

C57.21 Malignant neoplasm of right round ligament HCC Rx ESR COM ♀

C57.22 Malignant neoplasm of left round ligament HCC Rx ESR COM ♀

C57.3 Malignant neoplasm of parametrium HCC Rx ESR COM ♀

Malignant neoplasm of uterine ligament NOS

C57.4 Malignant neoplasm of uterine adnexa, unspecified HCC Rx ESR COM ♀

C57.7 Malignant neoplasm of other specified female genital organs HCC ESR COM ♀

Malignant neoplasm of wolffian body or duct

C57.8 Malignant neoplasm of overlapping sites of female genital organs HCC ESR COM ♀

Primary malignant neoplasm of two or more contiguous sites of the female genital organs whose point of origin cannot be determined

Primary tubo-ovarian malignant neoplasm whose point of origin cannot be determined

Primary utero-ovarian malignant neoplasm whose point of origin cannot be determined

C57.9 Malignant neoplasm of female genital organ, unspecified HCC ESR COM ♀

Malignant neoplasm of female genitourinary tract NOS

C58 Malignant neoplasm of placenta HCC Rx ESR COM M ♀

INCLUDES choriocarcinoma NOS
chorionepithelioma NOS

EXCLUDES 1 *chorioadenoma (destruens) (D39.2)*
hydatidiform mole NOS (O01.9)
invasive hydatidiform mole (D39.2)
male choriocarcinoma NOS (C62.9-)
malignant hydatidiform mole (D39.2)

Malignant neoplasms of male genital organs (C60-C63)

INCLUDES malignant neoplasm of skin of male genital organs

✓4th **C60 Malignant neoplasm of penis**

C60.0 Malignant neoplasm of prepuce HCC Rx ESR COM ♂

Malignant neoplasm of foreskin

C60.1 Malignant neoplasm of glans penis HCC Rx ESR COM ♂

C60.2 Malignant neoplasm of body of penis HCC Rx ESR COM ♂

Malignant neoplasm of corpus cavernosum

C60.8 Malignant neoplasm of overlapping sites of penis HCC Rx ESR COM ♂

C60.9 Malignant neoplasm of penis, unspecified HCC Rx ESR COM ♂

Malignant neoplasm of skin of penis NOS

C61 Malignant neoplasm of prostate HCC Rx ESR COM Q ♂

▶Use additional code, if applicable, to identify:◀
hormone sensitivity status (Z19.1-Z19.2)
rising PSA following treatment for malignant neoplasm of prostate (R97.21)

EXCLUDES 1 *malignant neoplasm of seminal vesicle (C63.7)*

AHA: 2017,1Q,17

✓4th **C62 Malignant neoplasm of testis**

Use additional code to identify any functional activity

✓5th **C62.0 Malignant neoplasm of undescended testis**

Malignant neoplasm of ectopic testis

Malignant neoplasm of retained testis

C62.00 Malignant neoplasm of unspecified undescended testis HCC Rx ESR COM ♂

C62.01 Malignant neoplasm of undescended right testis HCC Rx ESR COM ♂

C62.02 **Malignant neoplasm of undescended left testis** HCC Rx ESR COM ♂

✓5th C62.1 **Malignant neoplasm of descended testis**
Malignant neoplasm of scrotal testis

C62.10 **Malignant neoplasm of unspecified descended testis** HCC Rx ESR COM ♂

C62.11 **Malignant neoplasm of descended right testis** HCC Rx ESR COM ♂

C62.12 **Malignant neoplasm of descended left testis** HCC Rx ESR COM ♂

✓5th C62.9 **Malignant neoplasm of testis, unspecified whether descended or undescended**

C62.90 **Malignant neoplasm of unspecified testis, unspecified whether descended or undescended** HCC Rx ESR COM ♂
Malignant neoplasm of testis NOS

C62.91 **Malignant neoplasm of right testis, unspecified whether descended or undescended** HCC Rx ESR COM ♂

C62.92 **Malignant neoplasm of left testis, unspecified whether descended or undescended** HCC Rx ESR COM ♂

✓4th **C63 Malignant neoplasm of other and unspecified male genital organs**

✓5th C63.0 **Malignant neoplasm of epididymis**

C63.00 **Malignant neoplasm of unspecified epididymis** HCC Rx ESR COM ♂

C63.01 **Malignant neoplasm of right epididymis** HCC Rx ESR COM ♂

C63.02 **Malignant neoplasm of left epididymis** HCC Rx ESR COM ♂

✓5th C63.1 **Malignant neoplasm of spermatic cord**

C63.10 **Malignant neoplasm of unspecified spermatic cord** HCC Rx ESR COM ♂

C63.11 **Malignant neoplasm of right spermatic cord** HCC Rx ESR COM ♂

C63.12 **Malignant neoplasm of left spermatic cord** HCC Rx ESR COM ♂

C63.2 **Malignant neoplasm of scrotum** HCC Rx ESR COM ♂
Malignant neoplasm of skin of scrotum

C63.7 **Malignant neoplasm of other specified male genital organs** HCC Rx ESR COM ♂
Malignant neoplasm of seminal vesicle
Malignant neoplasm of tunica vaginalis

C63.8 **Malignant neoplasm of overlapping sites of male genital organs** HCC Rx ESR COM ♂
Primary malignant neoplasm of two or more contiguous sites of male genital organs whose point of origin cannot be determined

C63.9 **Malignant neoplasm of male genital organ, unspecified** HCC Rx ESR COM ♂
Malignant neoplasm of male genitourinary tract NOS

Malignant neoplasms of urinary tract (C64-C68)

✓4th **C64 Malignant neoplasm of kidney, except renal pelvis**

EXCLUDES 1 *malignant carcinoid tumor of the kidney (C7A.093)*
malignant neoplasm of renal calyces (C65.-)
malignant neoplasm of renal pelvis (C65.-)

C64.1 **Malignant neoplasm of right kidney, except renal pelvis** HCC Rx ESR COM

C64.2 **Malignant neoplasm of left kidney, except renal pelvis** HCC Rx ESR COM

C64.9 **Malignant neoplasm of unspecified kidney, except renal pelvis** HCC Rx ESR COM

✓4th **C65 Malignant neoplasm of renal pelvis**

INCLUDES malignant neoplasm of pelviureteric junction
malignant neoplasm of renal calyces

C65.1 **Malignant neoplasm of right renal pelvis** HCC Rx ESR COM

C65.2 **Malignant neoplasm of left renal pelvis** HCC Rx ESR COM

C65.9 **Malignant neoplasm of unspecified renal pelvis** HCC Rx ESR COM

✓4th **C66 Malignant neoplasm of ureter**

EXCLUDES 1 *malignant neoplasm of ureteric orifice of bladder (C67.6)*

C66.1 **Malignant neoplasm of right ureter** HCC Rx ESR COM

C66.2 **Malignant neoplasm of left ureter** HCC Rx ESR COM

C66.9 **Malignant neoplasm of unspecified ureter** HCC Rx ESR COM

✓4th **C67 Malignant neoplasm of bladder**

C67.0 **Malignant neoplasm of trigone of bladder** HCC Rx ESR COM

C67.1 **Malignant neoplasm of dome of bladder** HCC Rx ESR COM

C67.2 **Malignant neoplasm of lateral wall of bladder** HCC Rx ESR COM

C67.3 **Malignant neoplasm of anterior wall of bladder** HCC Rx ESR COM

C67.4 **Malignant neoplasm of posterior wall of bladder** HCC Rx ESR COM

C67.5 **Malignant neoplasm of bladder neck** HCC Rx ESR COM
Malignant neoplasm of internal urethral orifice

C67.6 **Malignant neoplasm of ureteric orifice** HCC Rx ESR COM

C67.7 **Malignant neoplasm of urachus** HCC Rx ESR COM

C67.8 **Malignant neoplasm of overlapping sites of bladder** HCC Rx ESR COM

C67.9 **Malignant neoplasm of bladder, unspecified** HCC Rx ESR COM
AHA: 2016,1Q,19

✓4th **C68 Malignant neoplasm of other and unspecified urinary organs**

EXCLUDES 1 *malignant neoplasm of female genitourinary tract NOS (C57.9)*
malignant neoplasm of male genitourinary tract NOS (C63.9)

C68.0 **Malignant neoplasm of urethra** HCC Rx ESR COM

EXCLUDES 1 *malignant neoplasm of urethral orifice of bladder (C67.5)*

C68.1 **Malignant neoplasm of paraurethral glands** HCC Rx ESR COM

C68.8 **Malignant neoplasm of overlapping sites of urinary organs** HCC Rx ESR COM
Primary malignant neoplasm of two or more contiguous sites of urinary organs whose point of origin cannot be determined

C68.9 **Malignant neoplasm of urinary organ, unspecified** HCC Rx ESR COM
Malignant neoplasm of urinary system NOS

Malignant neoplasms of eye, brain and other parts of central nervous system (C69-C72)

✓4th **C69 Malignant neoplasm of eye and adnexa**

EXCLUDES 1 *malignant neoplasm of connective tissue of eyelid (C49.0)*
malignant neoplasm of eyelid (skin) (C43.1-, C44.1-)
malignant neoplasm of optic nerve (C72.3-)

✓5th C69.0 **Malignant neoplasm of conjunctiva**

C69.00 **Malignant neoplasm of unspecified conjunctiva** HCC Rx ESR COM

C69.01 **Malignant neoplasm of right conjunctiva** HCC Rx ESR COM

C69.02 **Malignant neoplasm of left conjunctiva** HCC Rx ESR COM

✓5th C69.1 **Malignant neoplasm of cornea**

C69.10 **Malignant neoplasm of unspecified cornea** HCC Rx ESR COM

C69.11 **Malignant neoplasm of right cornea** HCC Rx ESR COM

C69.12 **Malignant neoplasm of left cornea** HCC Rx ESR COM

✓5th C69.2 **Malignant neoplasm of retina**

EXCLUDES 1 *dark area on retina (D49.81)*
neoplasm of unspecified behavior of retina and choroid (D49.81)
retinal freckle (D49.81)

C69.20 **Malignant neoplasm of unspecified retina** HCC Rx ESR COM

C69.21 **Malignant neoplasm of right retina** HCC Rx ESR COM

C69.22 **Malignant neoplasm of left retina** HCC Rx ESR COM

✓5th C69.3 **Malignant neoplasm of choroid**

C69.30 **Malignant neoplasm of unspecified choroid** HCC Rx ESR COM

C69.31 **Malignant neoplasm of right choroid** HCC Rx ESR COM

C69.32 **Malignant neoplasm of left choroid** HCC Rx ESR COM

✓5th **C69.4 Malignant neoplasm of ciliary body**

C69.40 Malignant neoplasm of unspecified ciliary body HCC Rx ESR COM

C69.41 Malignant neoplasm of right ciliary body HCC Rx ESR COM

C69.42 Malignant neoplasm of left ciliary body HCC Rx ESR COM

✓5th **C69.5 Malignant neoplasm of lacrimal gland and duct**

Malignant neoplasm of lacrimal sac
Malignant neoplasm of nasolacrimal duct

C69.50 Malignant neoplasm of unspecified lacrimal gland and duct HCC Rx ESR COM

C69.51 Malignant neoplasm of right lacrimal gland and duct HCC Rx ESR COM

C69.52 Malignant neoplasm of left lacrimal gland and duct HCC Rx ESR COM

✓5th **C69.6 Malignant neoplasm of orbit**

Malignant neoplasm of connective tissue of orbit
Malignant neoplasm of extraocular muscle
Malignant neoplasm of peripheral nerves of orbit
Malignant neoplasm of retrobulbar tissue
Malignant neoplasm of retro-ocular tissue

EXCLUDES 1 *malignant neoplasm of orbital bone (C41.0)*

C69.60 Malignant neoplasm of unspecified orbit HCC Rx ESR COM

C69.61 Malignant neoplasm of right orbit HCC Rx ESR COM

C69.62 Malignant neoplasm of left orbit HCC Rx ESR COM

✓5th **C69.8 Malignant neoplasm of overlapping sites of eye and adnexa**

C69.80 Malignant neoplasm of overlapping sites of unspecified eye and adnexa HCC Rx ESR COM

C69.81 Malignant neoplasm of overlapping sites of right eye and adnexa HCC Rx ESR COM

C69.82 Malignant neoplasm of overlapping sites of left eye and adnexa HCC Rx ESR COM

✓5th **C69.9 Malignant neoplasm of unspecified site of eye**

Malignant neoplasm of eyeball

C69.90 Malignant neoplasm of unspecified site of unspecified eye HCC Rx ESR COM

C69.91 Malignant neoplasm of unspecified site of right eye HCC Rx ESR COM

C69.92 Malignant neoplasm of unspecified site of left eye HCC Rx ESR COM

✓4th **C70 Malignant neoplasm of meninges**

C70.0 Malignant neoplasm of cerebral meninges HCC Rx ESR COM

C70.1 Malignant neoplasm of spinal meninges HCC Rx ESR COM

C70.9 Malignant neoplasm of meninges, unspecified HCC Rx ESR COM

✓4th **C71 Malignant neoplasm of brain**

EXCLUDES 1 *malignant neoplasm of cranial nerves (C72.2-C72.5)*
retrobulbar malignant neoplasm (C69.6-)

Lobes of the Brain

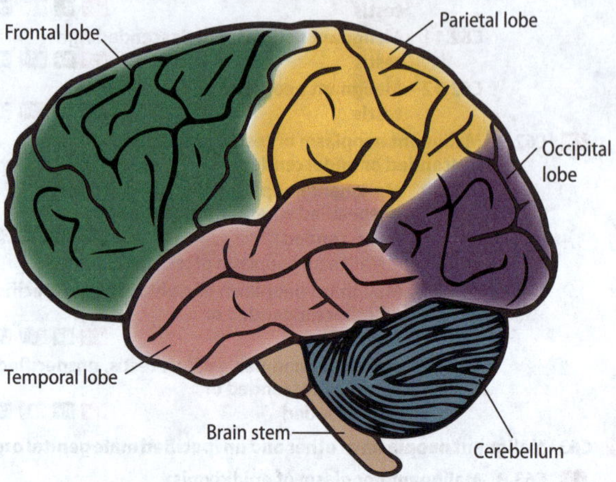

C71.0 Malignant neoplasm of cerebrum, except lobes and ventricles HCC Rx ESR COM

Malignant neoplasm of supratentorial NOS

C71.1 Malignant neoplasm of frontal lobe HCC Rx ESR COM

C71.2 Malignant neoplasm of temporal lobe HCC Rx ESR COM

C71.3 Malignant neoplasm of parietal lobe HCC Rx ESR COM

C71.4 Malignant neoplasm of occipital lobe HCC Rx ESR COM

C71.5 Malignant neoplasm of cerebral ventricle HCC Rx ESR COM

EXCLUDES 1 *malignant neoplasm of fourth cerebral ventricle (C71.7)*

C71.6 Malignant neoplasm of cerebellum HCC Rx ESR COM

C71.7 Malignant neoplasm of brain stem HCC Rx ESR COM

Malignant neoplasm of fourth cerebral ventricle
Infratentorial malignant neoplasm NOS

C71.8 Malignant neoplasm of overlapping sites of brain HCC Rx ESR COM

C71.9 Malignant neoplasm of brain, unspecified HCC Rx ESR COM

AHA: 2014,3Q,3

✓4th **C72 Malignant neoplasm of spinal cord, cranial nerves and other parts of central nervous system**

EXCLUDES 1 *malignant neoplasm of meninges (C70.-)*
malignant neoplasm of peripheral nerves and autonomic nervous system (C47.-)

C72.0 Malignant neoplasm of spinal cord HCC Rx ESR COM

C72.1 Malignant neoplasm of cauda equina HCC Rx ESR COM

✓5th **C72.2 Malignant neoplasm of olfactory nerve**

Malignant neoplasm of olfactory bulb

C72.20 Malignant neoplasm of unspecified olfactory nerve HCC Rx ESR COM

C72.21 Malignant neoplasm of right olfactory nerve HCC Rx ESR COM

C72.22 Malignant neoplasm of left olfactory nerve HCC Rx ESR COM

✓5th **C72.3 Malignant neoplasm of optic nerve**

C72.30 Malignant neoplasm of unspecified optic nerve HCC Rx ESR COM

C72.31 Malignant neoplasm of right optic nerve HCC Rx ESR COM

C72.32 Malignant neoplasm of left optic nerve HCC Rx ESR COM

✓5th **C72.4 Malignant neoplasm of acoustic nerve**

C72.40 Malignant neoplasm of unspecified acoustic nerve HCC Rx ESR COM

C72.41 Malignant neoplasm of right acoustic nerve HCC Rx ESR COM

C72.42 Malignant neoplasm of left acoustic nerve HCC Rx ESR COM

√5th **C72.5 Malignant neoplasm of other and unspecified cranial nerves**

C72.50 Malignant neoplasm of unspecified cranial nerve HCC Rx ESR COM
Malignant neoplasm of cranial nerve NOS

C72.59 Malignant neoplasm of other cranial nerves HCC Rx ESR COM

C72.9 Malignant neoplasm of central nervous system, unspecified HCC Rx ESR COM
Malignant neoplasm of unspecified site of central nervous system
Malignant neoplasm of nervous system NOS

Malignant neoplasms of thyroid and other endocrine glands (C73-C75)

C73 Malignant neoplasm of thyroid gland HCC Rx ESR COM
Use additional code to identify any functional activity

√4th **C74 Malignant neoplasm of adrenal gland**
TIP: If an adrenal gland tumor is described as functioning (producing too much of a hormone), additional codes should be assigned to report the functional activity.

√5th **C74.0 Malignant neoplasm of cortex of adrenal gland**

C74.00 Malignant neoplasm of cortex of unspecified adrenal gland HCC Rx ESR COM

C74.01 Malignant neoplasm of cortex of right adrenal gland HCC Rx ESR COM

C74.02 Malignant neoplasm of cortex of left adrenal gland HCC Rx ESR COM

√5th **C74.1 Malignant neoplasm of medulla of adrenal gland**

C74.10 Malignant neoplasm of medulla of unspecified adrenal gland HCC Rx ESR COM

C74.11 Malignant neoplasm of medulla of right adrenal gland HCC Rx ESR COM

C74.12 Malignant neoplasm of medulla of left adrenal gland HCC Rx ESR COM

√5th **C74.9 Malignant neoplasm of unspecified part of adrenal gland**

C74.90 Malignant neoplasm of unspecified part of unspecified adrenal gland HCC Rx ESR COM

C74.91 Malignant neoplasm of unspecified part of right adrenal gland HCC Rx ESR COM

C74.92 Malignant neoplasm of unspecified part of left adrenal gland HCC Rx ESR COM

√4th **C75 Malignant neoplasm of other endocrine glands and related structures**

EXCLUDES 1 *malignant carcinoid tumors (C7A.0-)*
malignant neoplasm of adrenal gland (C74.-)
malignant neoplasm of endocrine pancreas (C25.4)
malignant neoplasm of islets of Langerhans (C25.4)
malignant neoplasm of ovary (C56.-)
malignant neoplasm of testis (C62.-)
malignant neoplasm of thymus (C37)
malignant neoplasm of thyroid gland (C73)
malignant neuroendocrine tumors (C7A.-)

C75.0 Malignant neoplasm of parathyroid gland HCC Rx ESR COM

C75.1 Malignant neoplasm of pituitary gland HCC Rx ESR COM

C75.2 Malignant neoplasm of craniopharyngeal duct HCC Rx ESR COM

C75.3 Malignant neoplasm of pineal gland HCC Rx ESR COM

C75.4 Malignant neoplasm of carotid body HCC Rx ESR COM

C75.5 Malignant neoplasm of aortic body and other paraganglia HCC Rx ESR COM

C75.8 Malignant neoplasm with pluriglandular involvement, unspecified HCC Rx ESR COM

C75.9 Malignant neoplasm of endocrine gland, unspecified HCC Rx ESR COM

Malignant neuroendocrine tumors (C7A)

√4th **C7A Malignant neuroendocrine tumors**
Code also any associated multiple endocrine neoplasia [MEN] syndromes (E31.2-)
Use additional code to identify any associated endocrine syndrome, such as:
carcinoid syndrome (E34.0)

EXCLUDES 2 *malignant pancreatic islet cell tumors (C25.4)*
Merkel cell carcinoma (C4A.-)

AHA: 2019,3Q,7
DEF: Tumors comprised of cells that are capable of producing hormonal syndromes in which the normal hormonal balance required to support body system function is adversely affected.

√5th **C7A.0 Malignant carcinoid tumors**
AHA: 2019,3Q,7
DEF: Specific type of slow-growing neuroendocrine tumors. Carcinoid tumors occur most commonly in the hormone producing cells of the gastrointestinal tracts and can also occur in the pancreas, testes, ovaries, or lungs.

C7A.00 Malignant carcinoid tumor of unspecified site HCC Rx ESR COM

√6th **C7A.01 Malignant carcinoid tumors of the small intestine**

C7A.010 Malignant carcinoid tumor of the duodenum HCC Rx ESR COM

C7A.011 Malignant carcinoid tumor of the jejunum HCC Rx ESR COM

C7A.012 Malignant carcinoid tumor of the ileum HCC Rx ESR COM

C7A.019 Malignant carcinoid tumor of the small intestine, unspecified portion HCC Rx ESR COM

√6th **C7A.02 Malignant carcinoid tumors of the appendix, large intestine, and rectum**

C7A.020 Malignant carcinoid tumor of the appendix HCC Rx ESR COM

C7A.021 Malignant carcinoid tumor of the cecum HCC Rx ESR COM

C7A.022 Malignant carcinoid tumor of the ascending colon HCC Rx ESR COM

C7A.023 Malignant carcinoid tumor of the transverse colon HCC Rx ESR COM

C7A.024 Malignant carcinoid tumor of the descending colon HCC Rx ESR COM

C7A.025 Malignant carcinoid tumor of the sigmoid colon HCC Rx ESR COM

C7A.026 Malignant carcinoid tumor of the rectum HCC Rx ESR COM

C7A.029 Malignant carcinoid tumor of the large intestine, unspecified portion HCC Rx ESR COM
Malignant carcinoid tumor of the colon NOS

√6th **C7A.09 Malignant carcinoid tumors of other sites**

C7A.090 Malignant carcinoid tumor of the bronchus and lung HCC Rx ESR COM
AHA: 2019,1Q,16
TIP: When associated malignant pericardial effusion is documented, assign code I31.3. If the sole reason for admission is to treat the effusion with no treatment of the lung malignancy rendered, code I31.3 may be sequenced first.

C7A.091 Malignant carcinoid tumor of the thymus HCC Rx ESR COM

C7A.092 Malignant carcinoid tumor of the stomach HCC Rx ESR COM

C7A.093 Malignant carcinoid tumor of the kidney HCC Rx ESR COM

C7A.094 Malignant carcinoid tumor of the foregut, unspecified HCC Rx ESR COM

C7A.095 Malignant carcinoid tumor of the midgut, unspecified HCC Rx ESR COM

C7A.096 Malignant carcinoid tumor of the hindgut, unspecified HCC Rx ESR COM

C7A.098 Malignant carcinoid tumors of other sites HCC Rx ESR COM

C7A.1 Malignant poorly differentiated neuroendocrine tumors HCC Rx ESR COM
Malignant poorly differentiated neuroendocrine tumor NOS
Malignant poorly differentiated neuroendocrine carcinoma, any site
High grade neuroendocrine carcinoma, any site

C7A.8 Other malignant neuroendocrine tumors HCC Rx ESR COM
AHA: 2019,3Q,7

Secondary neuroendocrine tumors (C7B)

✓4th C7B Secondary neuroendocrine tumors
Use additional code to identify any functional activity

✓5th C7B.0 Secondary carcinoid tumors
AHA: 2019,3Q,7
DEF: Specific type of slow-growing neuroendocrine tumors. Carcinoid tumors occur most commonly in the hormone producing cells of the gastrointestinal tracts and can also occur in the pancreas, testes, ovaries, or lungs.

C7B.00 Secondary carcinoid tumors, unspecified site HCC Rx ESR COM

C7B.01 Secondary carcinoid tumors of distant lymph nodes HCC Rx ESR COM

C7B.02 Secondary carcinoid tumors of liver HCC Rx ESR COM

C7B.03 Secondary carcinoid tumors of bone HCC Rx ESR COM

C7B.04 Secondary carcinoid tumors of peritoneum HCC Rx ESR COM
Mesentary metastasis of carcinoid tumor

C7B.09 Secondary carcinoid tumors of other sites HCC Rx ESR COM

C7B.1 Secondary Merkel cell carcinoma HCC Rx ESR COM
Merkel cell carcinoma nodal presentation
Merkel cell carcinoma visceral metastatic presentation

C7B.8 Other secondary neuroendocrine tumors HCC Rx ESR COM
AHA: 2019,3Q,7

Malignant neoplasms of ill-defined, other secondary and unspecified sites (C76-C80)

✓4th C76 Malignant neoplasm of other and ill-defined sites
EXCLUDES 1 *malignant neoplasm of female genitourinary tract NOS (C57.9)*
malignant neoplasm of male genitourinary tract NOS (C63.9)
malignant neoplasm of lymphoid, hematopoietic and related tissue (C81-C96)
malignant neoplasm of skin (C44.-)
malignant neoplasm of unspecified site NOS (C80.1)

C76.0 Malignant neoplasm of head, face and neck HCC Rx ESR COM
Malignant neoplasm of cheek NOS
Malignant neoplasm of nose NOS

C76.1 Malignant neoplasm of thorax HCC Rx ESR COM
Intrathoracic malignant neoplasm NOS
Malignant neoplasm of axilla NOS
Thoracic malignant neoplasm NOS

C76.2 Malignant neoplasm of abdomen HCC Rx ESR COM

C76.3 Malignant neoplasm of pelvis HCC Rx ESR COM
Malignant neoplasm of groin NOS
Malignant neoplasm of sites overlapping systems within the pelvis
Rectovaginal (septum) malignant neoplasm
Rectovesical (septum) malignant neoplasm

✓5th C76.4 Malignant neoplasm of upper limb

C76.40 Malignant neoplasm of unspecified upper limb HCC Rx ESR COM

C76.41 Malignant neoplasm of right upper limb HCC Rx ESR COM

C76.42 Malignant neoplasm of left upper limb HCC Rx ESR COM

✓5th C76.5 Malignant neoplasm of lower limb

C76.50 Malignant neoplasm of unspecified lower limb HCC Rx ESR COM

C76.51 Malignant neoplasm of right lower limb HCC Rx ESR COM

C76.52 Malignant neoplasm of left lower limb HCC Rx ESR COM

C76.8 Malignant neoplasm of other specified ill-defined sites HCC Rx ESR COM
Malignant neoplasm of overlapping ill-defined sites

✓4th C77 Secondary and unspecified malignant neoplasm of lymph nodes
EXCLUDES 1 *malignant neoplasm of lymph nodes, specified as primary (C81-C86, C88, C96.-)*
mesentary metastasis of carcinoid tumor (C7B.04)
secondary carcinoid tumors of distant lymph nodes (C7B.01)

C77.0 Secondary and unspecified malignant neoplasm of lymph nodes of head, face and neck HCC Rx ESR COM
Secondary and unspecified malignant neoplasm of supraclavicular lymph nodes

C77.1 Secondary and unspecified malignant neoplasm of intrathoracic lymph nodes HCC Rx ESR COM

C77.2 Secondary and unspecified malignant neoplasm of intra-abdominal lymph nodes HCC Rx ESR COM

C77.3 Secondary and unspecified malignant neoplasm of axilla and upper limb lymph nodes HCC Rx ESR COM
Secondary and unspecified malignant neoplasm of pectoral lymph nodes

C77.4 Secondary and unspecified malignant neoplasm of inguinal and lower limb lymph nodes HCC Rx ESR COM

C77.5 Secondary and unspecified malignant neoplasm of intrapelvic lymph nodes HCC Rx ESR COM

C77.8 Secondary and unspecified malignant neoplasm of lymph nodes of multiple regions HCC Rx ESR COM

C77.9 Secondary and unspecified malignant neoplasm of lymph node, unspecified HCC Rx ESR COM

✓4th C78 Secondary malignant neoplasm of respiratory and digestive organs
EXCLUDES 1 *secondary carcinoid tumors of liver (C7B.02)*
secondary carcinoid tumors of peritoneum (C7B.04)
EXCLUDES 2 *lymph node metastases (C77.0)*

✓5th C78.0 Secondary malignant neoplasm of lung
AHA: 2019,1Q,16

C78.00 Secondary malignant neoplasm of unspecified lung HCC Rx ESR COM

C78.01 Secondary malignant neoplasm of right lung HCC Rx ESR COM

C78.02 Secondary malignant neoplasm of left lung HCC Rx ESR COM

C78.1 Secondary malignant neoplasm of mediastinum HCC Rx ESR COM

C78.2 Secondary malignant neoplasm of pleura HCC Rx ESR COM

✓5th C78.3 Secondary malignant neoplasm of other and unspecified respiratory organs

C78.30 Secondary malignant neoplasm of unspecified respiratory organ HCC Rx ESR COM

C78.39 Secondary malignant neoplasm of other respiratory organs HCC Rx ESR COM

C78.4 Secondary malignant neoplasm of small intestine HCC Rx ESR COM

C78.5 Secondary malignant neoplasm of large intestine and rectum HCC Rx ESR COM

C78.6 Secondary malignant neoplasm of retroperitoneum and peritoneum HCC Rx ESR COM
AHA: 2017,2Q,12

C78.7 Secondary malignant neoplasm of liver and intrahepatic bile duct HCC Rx ESR COM

✓5th C78.8 Secondary malignant neoplasm of other and unspecified digestive organs

C78.80 Secondary malignant neoplasm of unspecified digestive organ HCC Rx ESR COM

C78.89 Secondary malignant neoplasm of other digestive organs HCC Rx ESR COM
Code also exocrine pancreatic insufficiency (K86.81)

✓4th C79 Secondary malignant neoplasm of other and unspecified sites
EXCLUDES 1 *secondary carcinoid tumors (C7B.-)*
secondary neuroendocrine tumors (C7B.-)

✓5th C79.0 Secondary malignant neoplasm of kidney and renal pelvis

C79.00 Secondary malignant neoplasm of unspecified kidney and renal pelvis HCC Rx ESR COM

C79.01 Secondary malignant neoplasm of right kidney and renal pelvis HCC Rx ESR COM

C79.02 Secondary malignant neoplasm of left kidney and renal pelvis HCC Rx ESR COM

C79.1 Secondary malignant neoplasm of bladder and other and unspecified urinary organs

C79.1Ø Secondary malignant neoplasm of unspecified urinary organs HCC Rx ESR COM

C79.11 Secondary malignant neoplasm of bladder HCC Rx ESR COM

EXCLUDES 2 *lymph node metastases (C77.Ø)*

C79.19 Secondary malignant neoplasm of other urinary organs HCC Rx ESR COM

C79.2 Secondary malignant neoplasm of skin HCC Rx ESR COM

EXCLUDES 1 *secondary Merkel cell carcinoma (C7B.1)*

C79.3 Secondary malignant neoplasm of brain and cerebral meninges

C79.31 Secondary malignant neoplasm of brain HCC Rx ESR COM

C79.32 Secondary malignant neoplasm of cerebral meninges HCC Rx ESR COM

AHA: 2020,1Q,13

C79.4 Secondary malignant neoplasm of other and unspecified parts of nervous system

C79.4Ø Secondary malignant neoplasm of unspecified part of nervous system HCC Rx ESR COM

C79.49 Secondary malignant neoplasm of other parts of nervous system HCC Rx ESR COM

C79.5 Secondary malignant neoplasm of bone and bone marrow

EXCLUDES 1 *secondary carcinoid tumors of bone (C7B.Ø3)*

C79.51 Secondary malignant neoplasm of bone HCC Rx ESR COM

TIP: Do not assign in addition to a code from subcategory C90.0 when multiple myeloma is described as metastatic to the bone; bone involvement is integral to multiple myeloma.

C79.52 Secondary malignant neoplasm of bone marrow HCC Rx ESR COM

C79.6 Secondary malignant neoplasm of ovary

C79.6Ø Secondary malignant neoplasm of unspecified ovary HCC Rx ESR COM ♀

C79.61 Secondary malignant neoplasm of right ovary HCC Rx ESR COM ♀

C79.62 Secondary malignant neoplasm of left ovary HCC Rx ESR COM ♀

C79.63 Secondary malignant neoplasm of bilateral ovaries HCC Rx ESR COM ♀

C79.7 Secondary malignant neoplasm of adrenal gland

C79.7Ø Secondary malignant neoplasm of unspecified adrenal gland HCC Rx ESR COM

C79.71 Secondary malignant neoplasm of right adrenal gland HCC Rx ESR COM

C79.72 Secondary malignant neoplasm of left adrenal gland HCC Rx ESR COM

C79.8 Secondary malignant neoplasm of other specified sites

C79.81 Secondary malignant neoplasm of breast HCC Rx ESR COM

C79.82 Secondary malignant neoplasm of genital organs HCC Rx ESR COM

C79.89 Secondary malignant neoplasm of other specified sites HCC Rx ESR COM

AHA: 2017,2Q,11

C79.9 Secondary malignant neoplasm of unspecified site HCC Rx ESR COM

Metastatic cancer NOS

Metastatic disease NOS

EXCLUDES 1 *carcinomatosis NOS (C8Ø.Ø)*
generalized cancer NOS (C8Ø.Ø)
malignant (primary) neoplasm of unspecified site (C8Ø.1)

C8Ø Malignant neoplasm without specification of site

EXCLUDES 1 *malignant carcinoid tumor of unspecified site (C7A.ØØ)*
malignant neoplasm of specified multiple sites - code to each site

C8Ø.Ø Disseminated malignant neoplasm, unspecified HCC Rx ESR COM

Carcinomatosis NOS

Generalized cancer, unspecified site (primary) (secondary)

Generalized malignancy, unspecified site (primary) (secondary)

C8Ø.1 Malignant (primary) neoplasm, unspecified HCC ESR COM

Cancer NOS

Cancer unspecified site (primary)

Carcinoma unspecified site (primary)

Malignancy unspecified site (primary)

EXCLUDES 1 *secondary malignant neoplasm of unspecified site (C79.9)*

C8Ø.2 Malignant neoplasm associated with transplanted organ HCC Rx ESR COM UPD

Code first complication of transplanted organ (T86.-)

Use additional code to identify the specific malignancy

Malignant neoplasms of lymphoid, hematopoietic and related tissue (C81-C96)

EXCLUDES 2 *Kaposi's sarcoma of lymph nodes (C46.3)*
secondary and unspecified neoplasm of lymph nodes (C77.-)
secondary neoplasm of bone marrow (C79.52)
secondary neoplasm of spleen (C78.89)

C81 Hodgkin lymphoma

EXCLUDES 1 *personal history of Hodgkin lymphoma (Z85.71)*

DEF: Malignant disorder of lymphoid cells characterized by the presence of progressively swollen lymph nodes and spleen that may also involve the liver. A diagnosis of Hodgkin's lymphoma can be confirmed by the presence of Reed-Sternberg cells. ***Synonym(s):*** *Hodgkin disease.*

C81.Ø Nodular lymphocyte predominant Hodgkin lymphoma

C81.ØØ Nodular lymphocyte predominant Hodgkin lymphoma, unspecified site HCC Rx ESR COM

C81.Ø1 Nodular lymphocyte predominant Hodgkin lymphoma, lymph nodes of head, face, and neck HCC Rx ESR COM

C81.Ø2 Nodular lymphocyte predominant Hodgkin lymphoma, intrathoracic lymph nodes HCC Rx ESR COM

C81.Ø3 Nodular lymphocyte predominant Hodgkin lymphoma, intra-abdominal lymph nodes HCC Rx ESR COM

C81.Ø4 Nodular lymphocyte predominant Hodgkin lymphoma, lymph nodes of axilla and upper limb HCC Rx ESR COM

C81.Ø5 Nodular lymphocyte predominant Hodgkin lymphoma, lymph nodes of inguinal region and lower limb HCC Rx ESR COM

C81.Ø6 Nodular lymphocyte predominant Hodgkin lymphoma, intrapelvic lymph nodes HCC Rx ESR COM

C81.Ø7 Nodular lymphocyte predominant Hodgkin lymphoma, spleen HCC Rx ESR COM

C81.Ø8 Nodular lymphocyte predominant Hodgkin lymphoma, lymph nodes of multiple sites HCC Rx ESR COM

C81.Ø9 Nodular lymphocyte predominant Hodgkin lymphoma, extranodal and solid organ sites HCC Rx ESR COM

C81.1 Nodular sclerosis Hodgkin lymphoma

Nodular sclerosis classical Hodgkin lymphoma

C81.1Ø Nodular sclerosis Hodgkin lymphoma, unspecified site HCC Rx ESR COM

C81.11 Nodular sclerosis Hodgkin lymphoma, lymph nodes of head, face, and neck HCC Rx ESR COM

C81.12 Nodular sclerosis Hodgkin lymphoma, intrathoracic lymph nodes HCC Rx ESR COM

C81.13 Nodular sclerosis Hodgkin lymphoma, intra-abdominal lymph nodes HCC Rx ESR COM

C81.14 Nodular sclerosis Hodgkin lymphoma, lymph nodes of axilla and upper limb HCC Rx ESR COM

C81.15 Nodular sclerosis Hodgkin lymphoma, lymph nodes of inguinal region and lower limb HCC Rx ESR COM

C81.16 Nodular sclerosis Hodgkin lymphoma, intrapelvic lymph nodes HCC Rx ESR COM

C81.17 Nodular sclerosis Hodgkin lymphoma, spleen HCC Rx ESR COM

C81.18 Nodular sclerosis Hodgkin lymphoma, lymph nodes of multiple sites HCC Rx ESR COM

C81.19 Nodular sclerosis Hodgkin lymphoma, extranodal and solid organ sites HCC Rx ESR COM

C81.2 Mixed cellularity Hodgkin lymphoma

Mixed cellularity classical Hodgkin lymphoma

C81.2Ø Mixed cellularity Hodgkin lymphoma, unspecified site HCC Rx ESR COM

C81.21 **Mixed cellularity Hodgkin lymphoma, lymph nodes of head, face, and neck** HCC Rx ESR COM
C81.22 **Mixed cellularity Hodgkin lymphoma, intrathoracic lymph nodes** HCC Rx ESR COM
C81.23 **Mixed cellularity Hodgkin lymphoma, intra-abdominal lymph nodes** HCC Rx ESR COM
C81.24 **Mixed cellularity Hodgkin lymphoma, lymph nodes of axilla and upper limb** HCC Rx ESR COM
C81.25 **Mixed cellularity Hodgkin lymphoma, lymph nodes of inguinal region and lower limb** HCC Rx ESR COM
C81.26 **Mixed cellularity Hodgkin lymphoma, intrapelvic lymph nodes** HCC Rx ESR COM
C81.27 **Mixed cellularity Hodgkin lymphoma, spleen** HCC Rx ESR COM
C81.28 **Mixed cellularity Hodgkin lymphoma, lymph nodes of multiple sites** HCC Rx ESR COM
C81.29 **Mixed cellularity Hodgkin lymphoma, extranodal and solid organ sites** HCC Rx ESR COM

✓5th **C81.3** **Lymphocyte depleted Hodgkin lymphoma**
Lymphocyte depleted classical Hodgkin lymphoma

C81.30 **Lymphocyte depleted Hodgkin lymphoma, unspecified site** HCC Rx ESR COM
C81.31 **Lymphocyte depleted Hodgkin lymphoma, lymph nodes of head, face, and neck** HCC Rx ESR COM
C81.32 **Lymphocyte depleted Hodgkin lymphoma, intrathoracic lymph nodes** HCC Rx ESR COM
C81.33 **Lymphocyte depleted Hodgkin lymphoma, intra-abdominal lymph nodes** HCC Rx ESR COM
C81.34 **Lymphocyte depleted Hodgkin lymphoma, lymph nodes of axilla and upper limb** HCC Rx ESR COM
C81.35 **Lymphocyte depleted Hodgkin lymphoma, lymph nodes of inguinal region and lower limb** HCC Rx ESR COM
C81.36 **Lymphocyte depleted Hodgkin lymphoma, intrapelvic lymph nodes** HCC Rx ESR COM
C81.37 **Lymphocyte depleted Hodgkin lymphoma, spleen** HCC Rx ESR COM
C81.38 **Lymphocyte depleted Hodgkin lymphoma, lymph nodes of multiple sites** HCC Rx ESR COM
C81.39 **Lymphocyte depleted Hodgkin lymphoma, extranodal and solid organ sites** HCC Rx ESR COM

✓5th **C81.4** **Lymphocyte-rich Hodgkin lymphoma**
Lymphocyte-rich classical Hodgkin lymphoma
EXCLUDES 1 *nodular lymphocyte predominant Hodgkin lymphoma (C81.0-)*

C81.40 **Lymphocyte-rich Hodgkin lymphoma, unspecified site** HCC Rx ESR COM
C81.41 **Lymphocyte-rich Hodgkin lymphoma, lymph nodes of head, face, and neck** HCC Rx ESR COM
C81.42 **Lymphocyte-rich Hodgkin lymphoma, intrathoracic lymph nodes** HCC Rx ESR COM
C81.43 **Lymphocyte-rich Hodgkin lymphoma, intra-abdominal lymph nodes** HCC Rx ESR COM
C81.44 **Lymphocyte-rich Hodgkin lymphoma, lymph nodes of axilla and upper limb** HCC Rx ESR COM
C81.45 **Lymphocyte-rich Hodgkin lymphoma, lymph nodes of inguinal region and lower limb** HCC Rx ESR COM
C81.46 **Lymphocyte-rich Hodgkin lymphoma, intrapelvic lymph nodes** HCC Rx ESR COM
C81.47 **Lymphocyte-rich Hodgkin lymphoma, spleen** HCC Rx ESR COM
C81.48 **Lymphocyte-rich Hodgkin lymphoma, lymph nodes of multiple sites** HCC Rx ESR COM
C81.49 **Lymphocyte-rich Hodgkin lymphoma, extranodal and solid organ sites** HCC Rx ESR COM

✓5th **C81.7** **Other Hodgkin lymphoma**
Classical Hodgkin lymphoma NOS
Other classical Hodgkin lymphoma

C81.70 **Other Hodgkin lymphoma, unspecified site** HCC Rx ESR COM
C81.71 **Other Hodgkin lymphoma, lymph nodes of head, face, and neck** HCC Rx ESR COM
C81.72 **Other Hodgkin lymphoma, intrathoracic lymph nodes** HCC Rx ESR COM
C81.73 **Other Hodgkin lymphoma, intra-abdominal lymph nodes** HCC Rx ESR COM
C81.74 **Other Hodgkin lymphoma, lymph nodes of axilla and upper limb** HCC Rx ESR COM
C81.75 **Other Hodgkin lymphoma, lymph nodes of inguinal region and lower limb** HCC Rx ESR COM
C81.76 **Other Hodgkin lymphoma, intrapelvic lymph nodes** HCC Rx ESR COM
C81.77 **Other Hodgkin lymphoma, spleen** HCC Rx ESR COM
C81.78 **Other Hodgkin lymphoma, lymph nodes of multiple sites** HCC Rx ESR COM
C81.79 **Other Hodgkin lymphoma, extranodal and solid organ sites** HCC Rx ESR COM

✓5th **C81.9** **Hodgkin lymphoma, unspecified**

C81.90 **Hodgkin lymphoma, unspecified, unspecified site** HCC Rx ESR COM
C81.91 **Hodgkin lymphoma, unspecified, lymph nodes of head, face, and neck** HCC Rx ESR COM
C81.92 **Hodgkin lymphoma, unspecified, intrathoracic lymph nodes** HCC Rx ESR COM
C81.93 **Hodgkin lymphoma, unspecified, intra-abdominal lymph nodes** HCC Rx ESR COM
C81.94 **Hodgkin lymphoma, unspecified, lymph nodes of axilla and upper limb** HCC Rx ESR COM
C81.95 **Hodgkin lymphoma, unspecified, lymph nodes of inguinal region and lower limb** HCC Rx ESR COM
C81.96 **Hodgkin lymphoma, unspecified, intrapelvic lymph nodes** HCC Rx ESR COM
C81.97 **Hodgkin lymphoma, unspecified, spleen** HCC Rx ESR COM
C81.98 **Hodgkin lymphoma, unspecified, lymph nodes of multiple sites** HCC Rx ESR COM
C81.99 **Hodgkin lymphoma, unspecified, extranodal and solid organ sites** HCC Rx ESR COM

✓4th **C82** **Follicular lymphoma**
INCLUDES follicular lymphoma with or without diffuse areas
EXCLUDES 1 *mature T/NK-cell lymphomas (C84.-)*
personal history of non-Hodgkin lymphoma (Z85.72)

DEF: Most common subgroup of non-Hodgkin lymphomas (NHL), accounting for 20 to 30 percent of all NHLs. NHL is a B-cell lymphoma that is slow growing and characterized by the circular pattern of malignant cell growth with the cells clustered into identifiable nodules or follicles.

✓5th **C82.0** **Follicular lymphoma grade I**

C82.00 **Follicular lymphoma grade I, unspecified site** HCC Rx ESR COM
C82.01 **Follicular lymphoma grade I, lymph nodes of head, face, and neck** HCC Rx ESR COM
C82.02 **Follicular lymphoma grade I, intrathoracic lymph nodes** HCC Rx ESR COM
C82.03 **Follicular lymphoma grade I, intra-abdominal lymph nodes** HCC Rx ESR COM
C82.04 **Follicular lymphoma grade I, lymph nodes of axilla and upper limb** HCC Rx ESR COM
C82.05 **Follicular lymphoma grade I, lymph nodes of inguinal region and lower limb** HCC Rx ESR COM
C82.06 **Follicular lymphoma grade I, intrapelvic lymph nodes** HCC Rx ESR COM
C82.07 **Follicular lymphoma grade I, spleen** HCC Rx ESR COM
C82.08 **Follicular lymphoma grade I, lymph nodes of multiple sites** HCC Rx ESR COM
C82.09 **Follicular lymphoma grade I, extranodal and solid organ sites** HCC Rx ESR COM

✓5th **C82.1** **Follicular lymphoma grade II**

C82.10 **Follicular lymphoma grade II, unspecified site** HCC Rx ESR COM
C82.11 **Follicular lymphoma grade II, lymph nodes of head, face, and neck** HCC Rx ESR COM
C82.12 **Follicular lymphoma grade II, intrathoracic lymph nodes** HCC Rx ESR COM
C82.13 **Follicular lymphoma grade II, intra-abdominal lymph nodes** HCC Rx ESR COM
C82.14 **Follicular lymphoma grade II, lymph nodes of axilla and upper limb** HCC Rx ESR COM
C82.15 **Follicular lymphoma grade II, lymph nodes of inguinal region and lower limb** HCC Rx ESR COM
C82.16 **Follicular lymphoma grade II, intrapelvic lymph nodes** HCC Rx ESR COM
C82.17 **Follicular lymphoma grade II, spleen** HCC Rx ESR COM

C82.18 Follicular lymphoma grade II, lymph nodes of multiple sites HCC Rx ESR COM

C82.19 Follicular lymphoma grade II, extranodal and solid organ sites HCC Rx ESR COM

✓5th **C82.2** Follicular lymphoma grade III, unspecified

C82.2Ø Follicular lymphoma grade III, unspecified, unspecified site HCC Rx ESR COM

C82.21 Follicular lymphoma grade III, unspecified, lymph nodes of head, face, and neck HCC Rx ESR COM

C82.22 Follicular lymphoma grade III, unspecified, intrathoracic lymph nodes HCC Rx ESR COM

C82.23 Follicular lymphoma grade III, unspecified, intra-abdominal lymph nodes HCC Rx ESR COM

C82.24 Follicular lymphoma grade III, unspecified, lymph nodes of axilla and upper limb HCC Rx ESR COM

C82.25 Follicular lymphoma grade III, unspecified, lymph nodes of inguinal region and lower limb HCC Rx ESR COM

C82.26 Follicular lymphoma grade III, unspecified, intrapelvic lymph nodes HCC Rx ESR COM

C82.27 Follicular lymphoma grade III, unspecified, spleen HCC Rx ESR COM

C82.28 Follicular lymphoma grade III, unspecified, lymph nodes of multiple sites HCC Rx ESR COM

C82.29 Follicular lymphoma grade III, unspecified, extranodal and solid organ sites HCC Rx ESR COM

✓5th **C82.3** Follicular lymphoma grade IIIa

C82.3Ø Follicular lymphoma grade IIIa, unspecified site HCC Rx ESR COM

C82.31 Follicular lymphoma grade IIIa, lymph nodes of head, face, and neck HCC Rx ESR COM

C82.32 Follicular lymphoma grade IIIa, intrathoracic lymph nodes HCC Rx ESR COM

C82.33 Follicular lymphoma grade IIIa, intra-abdominal lymph nodes HCC Rx ESR COM

C82.34 Follicular lymphoma grade IIIa, lymph nodes of axilla and upper limb HCC Rx ESR COM

C82.35 Follicular lymphoma grade IIIa, lymph nodes of inguinal region and lower limb HCC Rx ESR COM

C82.36 Follicular lymphoma grade IIIa, intrapelvic lymph nodes HCC Rx ESR COM

C82.37 Follicular lymphoma grade IIIa, spleen HCC Rx ESR COM

C82.38 Follicular lymphoma grade IIIa, lymph nodes of multiple sites HCC Rx ESR COM

C82.39 Follicular lymphoma grade IIIa, extranodal and solid organ sites HCC Rx ESR COM

✓5th **C82.4** Follicular lymphoma grade IIIb

C82.4Ø Follicular lymphoma grade IIIb, unspecified site HCC Rx ESR COM

C82.41 Follicular lymphoma grade IIIb, lymph nodes of head, face, and neck HCC Rx ESR COM

C82.42 Follicular lymphoma grade IIIb, intrathoracic lymph nodes HCC Rx ESR COM

C82.43 Follicular lymphoma grade IIIb, intra-abdominal lymph nodes HCC Rx ESR COM

C82.44 Follicular lymphoma grade IIIb, lymph nodes of axilla and upper limb HCC Rx ESR COM

C82.45 Follicular lymphoma grade IIIb, lymph nodes of inguinal region and lower limb HCC Rx ESR COM

C82.46 Follicular lymphoma grade IIIb, intrapelvic lymph nodes HCC Rx ESR COM

C82.47 Follicular lymphoma grade IIIb, spleen HCC Rx ESR COM

C82.48 Follicular lymphoma grade IIIb, lymph nodes of multiple sites HCC Rx ESR COM

C82.49 Follicular lymphoma grade IIIb, extranodal and solid organ sites HCC Rx ESR COM

✓5th **C82.5** Diffuse follicle center lymphoma

C82.5Ø Diffuse follicle center lymphoma, unspecified site HCC Rx ESR COM

C82.51 Diffuse follicle center lymphoma, lymph nodes of head, face, and neck HCC Rx ESR COM

C82.52 Diffuse follicle center lymphoma, intrathoracic lymph nodes HCC Rx ESR COM

C82.53 Diffuse follicle center lymphoma, intra-abdominal lymph nodes HCC Rx ESR COM

C82.54 Diffuse follicle center lymphoma, lymph nodes of axilla and upper limb HCC Rx ESR COM

C82.55 Diffuse follicle center lymphoma, lymph nodes of inguinal region and lower limb HCC Rx ESR COM

C82.56 Diffuse follicle center lymphoma, intrapelvic lymph nodes HCC Rx ESR COM

C82.57 Diffuse follicle center lymphoma, spleen HCC Rx ESR COM

C82.58 Diffuse follicle center lymphoma, lymph nodes of multiple sites HCC Rx ESR COM

C82.59 Diffuse follicle center lymphoma, extranodal and solid organ sites HCC Rx ESR COM

✓5th **C82.6** Cutaneous follicle center lymphoma

C82.6Ø Cutaneous follicle center lymphoma, unspecified site HCC Rx ESR COM

C82.61 Cutaneous follicle center lymphoma, lymph nodes of head, face, and neck HCC Rx ESR COM

C82.62 Cutaneous follicle center lymphoma, intrathoracic lymph nodes HCC Rx ESR COM

C82.63 Cutaneous follicle center lymphoma, intra-abdominal lymph nodes HCC Rx ESR COM

C82.64 Cutaneous follicle center lymphoma, lymph nodes of axilla and upper limb HCC Rx ESR COM

C82.65 Cutaneous follicle center lymphoma, lymph nodes of inguinal region and lower limb HCC Rx ESR COM

C82.66 Cutaneous follicle center lymphoma, intrapelvic lymph nodes HCC Rx ESR COM

C82.67 Cutaneous follicle center lymphoma, spleen HCC Rx ESR COM

C82.68 Cutaneous follicle center lymphoma, lymph nodes of multiple sites HCC Rx ESR COM

C82.69 Cutaneous follicle center lymphoma, extranodal and solid organ sites HCC Rx ESR COM

✓5th **C82.8** Other types of follicular lymphoma

C82.8Ø Other types of follicular lymphoma, unspecified site HCC Rx ESR COM

C82.81 Other types of follicular lymphoma, lymph nodes of head, face, and neck HCC Rx ESR COM

C82.82 Other types of follicular lymphoma, intrathoracic lymph nodes HCC Rx ESR COM

C82.83 Other types of follicular lymphoma, intra-abdominal lymph nodes HCC Rx ESR COM

C82.84 Other types of follicular lymphoma, lymph nodes of axilla and upper limb HCC Rx ESR COM

C82.85 Other types of follicular lymphoma, lymph nodes of inguinal region and lower limb HCC Rx ESR COM

C82.86 Other types of follicular lymphoma, intrapelvic lymph nodes HCC Rx ESR COM

C82.87 Other types of follicular lymphoma, spleen HCC Rx ESR COM

C82.88 Other types of follicular lymphoma, lymph nodes of multiple sites HCC Rx ESR COM

C82.89 Other types of follicular lymphoma, extranodal and solid organ sites HCC Rx ESR COM

✓5th **C82.9** Follicular lymphoma, unspecified

C82.9Ø Follicular lymphoma, unspecified, unspecified site HCC Rx ESR COM

C82.91 Follicular lymphoma, unspecified, lymph nodes of head, face, and neck HCC Rx ESR COM

C82.92 Follicular lymphoma, unspecified, intrathoracic lymph nodes HCC Rx ESR COM

C82.93 Follicular lymphoma, unspecified, intra-abdominal lymph nodes HCC Rx ESR COM

C82.94 Follicular lymphoma, unspecified, lymph nodes of axilla and upper limb HCC Rx ESR COM

C82.95 Follicular lymphoma, unspecified, lymph nodes of inguinal region and lower limb HCC Rx ESR COM

C82.96 Follicular lymphoma, unspecified, intrapelvic lymph nodes HCC Rx ESR COM

C82.97 Follicular lymphoma, unspecified, spleen HCC Rx ESR COM

C82.98 Follicular lymphoma, unspecified, lymph nodes of multiple sites HCC Rx ESR COM

C82.99 Follicular lymphoma, unspecified, extranodal and solid organ sites HCC Rx ESR COM

C83 Non-follicular lymphoma

EXCLUDES 1 *personal history of non-Hodgkin lymphoma (Z85.72)*

C83.0 Small cell B-cell lymphoma

Lymphoplasmacytic lymphoma
Nodal marginal zone lymphoma
Non-leukemic variant of B-CLL
Splenic marginal zone lymphoma

EXCLUDES 1 *chronic lymphocytic leukemia (C91.1)*
mature T/NK-cell lymphomas (C84.-)
Waldenström macroglobulinemia (C88.0)

DEF: Nonfollicular lymphoma that is rare, slow growing, and usually found in the older population.

C83.00 Small cell B-cell lymphoma, unspecified site HCC Rx ESR COM
C83.01 Small cell B-cell lymphoma, lymph nodes of head, face, and neck HCC Rx ESR COM
C83.02 Small cell B-cell lymphoma, intrathoracic lymph nodes HCC Rx ESR COM
C83.03 Small cell B-cell lymphoma, intra-abdominal lymph nodes HCC Rx ESR COM
C83.04 Small cell B-cell lymphoma, lymph nodes of axilla and upper limb HCC Rx ESR COM
C83.05 Small cell B-cell lymphoma, lymph nodes of inguinal region and lower limb HCC Rx ESR COM
C83.06 Small cell B-cell lymphoma, intrapelvic lymph nodes HCC Rx ESR COM
C83.07 Small cell B-cell lymphoma, spleen HCC Rx ESR COM
C83.08 Small cell B-cell lymphoma, lymph nodes of multiple sites HCC Rx ESR COM
C83.09 Small cell B-cell lymphoma, extranodal and solid organ sites HCC Rx ESR COM

C83.1 Mantle cell lymphoma

Centrocytic lymphoma
Malignant lymphomatous polyposis

DEF: Rare form of B-cell non-Hodgkin lymphoma named for the location of the tumor cell production, the mantle zone of the lymph nodes.

C83.10 Mantle cell lymphoma, unspecified site HCC Rx ESR COM
C83.11 Mantle cell lymphoma, lymph nodes of head, face, and neck HCC Rx ESR COM
C83.12 Mantle cell lymphoma, intrathoracic lymph nodes HCC Rx ESR COM
C83.13 Mantle cell lymphoma, intra-abdominal lymph nodes HCC Rx ESR COM
C83.14 Mantle cell lymphoma, lymph nodes of axilla and upper limb HCC Rx ESR COM
C83.15 Mantle cell lymphoma, lymph nodes of inguinal region and lower limb HCC Rx ESR COM
C83.16 Mantle cell lymphoma, intrapelvic lymph nodes HCC Rx ESR COM
C83.17 Mantle cell lymphoma, spleen HCC Rx ESR COM
C83.18 Mantle cell lymphoma, lymph nodes of multiple sites HCC Rx ESR COM
C83.19 Mantle cell lymphoma, extranodal and solid organ sites HCC Rx ESR COM

C83.3 Diffuse large B-cell lymphoma

Anaplastic diffuse large B-cell lymphoma
CD30-positive diffuse large B-cell lymphoma
Centroblastic diffuse large B-cell lymphoma
Diffuse large B-cell lymphoma, subtype not specified
Immunoblastic diffuse large B-cell lymphoma
Plasmablastic diffuse large B-cell lymphoma
T-cell rich diffuse large B-cell lymphoma

EXCLUDES 1 *mediastinal (thymic) large B-cell lymphoma (C85.2-)*
mature T/NK-cell lymphomas (C84.-)

DEF: Nonfollicular lymphoma that is one of the more common types of lymphoma. This cancer is fast growing and affects any age but is found mostly in the older population.

C83.30 Diffuse large B-cell lymphoma, unspecified site HCC Rx ESR COM
C83.31 Diffuse large B-cell lymphoma, lymph nodes of head, face, and neck HCC Rx ESR COM
C83.32 Diffuse large B-cell lymphoma, intrathoracic lymph nodes HCC Rx ESR COM
C83.33 Diffuse large B-cell lymphoma, intra-abdominal lymph nodes HCC Rx ESR COM
C83.34 Diffuse large B-cell lymphoma, lymph nodes of axilla and upper limb HCC Rx ESR COM
C83.35 Diffuse large B-cell lymphoma, lymph nodes of inguinal region and lower limb HCC Rx ESR COM
C83.36 Diffuse large B-cell lymphoma, intrapelvic lymph nodes HCC Rx ESR COM
C83.37 Diffuse large B-cell lymphoma, spleen HCC Rx ESR COM
C83.38 Diffuse large B-cell lymphoma, lymph nodes of multiple sites HCC Rx ESR COM
C83.39 Diffuse large B-cell lymphoma, extranodal and solid organ sites HCC Rx ESR COM

C83.5 Lymphoblastic (diffuse) lymphoma

B-precursor lymphoma
Lymphoblastic B-cell lymphoma
Lymphoblastic lymphoma NOS
Lymphoblastic T-cell lymphoma
T-precursor lymphoma

DEF: Type of non-Hodgkin lymphoma considered lymphoma or leukemia—the determination is made based on the amount of bone marrow involvement. The cells are small to medium immature T-cells that often originate in the thymus where many of the T-cells are made.

C83.50 Lymphoblastic (diffuse) lymphoma, unspecified site HCC Rx ESR COM
C83.51 Lymphoblastic (diffuse) lymphoma, lymph nodes of head, face, and neck HCC Rx ESR COM
C83.52 Lymphoblastic (diffuse) lymphoma, intrathoracic lymph nodes HCC Rx ESR COM
C83.53 Lymphoblastic (diffuse) lymphoma, intra-abdominal lymph nodes HCC Rx ESR COM
C83.54 Lymphoblastic (diffuse) lymphoma, lymph nodes of axilla and upper limb HCC Rx ESR COM
C83.55 Lymphoblastic (diffuse) lymphoma, lymph nodes of inguinal region and lower limb HCC Rx ESR COM
C83.56 Lymphoblastic (diffuse) lymphoma, intrapelvic lymph nodes HCC Rx ESR COM
C83.57 Lymphoblastic (diffuse) lymphoma, spleen HCC Rx ESR COM
C83.58 Lymphoblastic (diffuse) lymphoma, lymph nodes of multiple sites HCC Rx ESR COM
C83.59 Lymphoblastic (diffuse) lymphoma, extranodal and solid organ sites HCC Rx ESR COM

C83.7 Burkitt lymphoma

Atypical Burkitt lymphoma
Burkitt-like lymphoma

EXCLUDES 1 *mature B-cell leukemia Burkitt type (C91.A-)*

DEF: Malignancy of the lymphatic system, most often seen as a large bone-deteriorating lesion within the jaw or as an abdominal mass. It is a form of non-Hodgkin's lymphoma and is recognized as the fastest growing human tumor.

C83.70 Burkitt lymphoma, unspecified site HCC Rx ESR COM
C83.71 Burkitt lymphoma, lymph nodes of head, face, and neck HCC Rx ESR COM
C83.72 Burkitt lymphoma, intrathoracic lymph nodes HCC Rx ESR COM
C83.73 Burkitt lymphoma, intra-abdominal lymph nodes HCC Rx ESR COM
C83.74 Burkitt lymphoma, lymph nodes of axilla and upper limb HCC Rx ESR COM
C83.75 Burkitt lymphoma, lymph nodes of inguinal region and lower limb HCC Rx ESR COM
C83.76 Burkitt lymphoma, intrapelvic lymph nodes HCC Rx ESR COM
C83.77 Burkitt lymphoma, spleen HCC Rx ESR COM
C83.78 Burkitt lymphoma, lymph nodes of multiple sites HCC Rx ESR COM
C83.79 Burkitt lymphoma, extranodal and solid organ sites HCC Rx ESR COM

C83.8 Other non-follicular lymphoma

Intravascular large B-cell lymphoma
Lymphoid granulomatosis
Primary effusion B-cell lymphoma

EXCLUDES 1 *mediastinal (thymic) large B-cell lymphoma (C85.2-)*
T-cell rich B-cell lymphoma (C83.3-)

C83.80 Other non-follicular lymphoma, unspecified site HCC Rx ESR COM

C83.81 Other non-follicular lymphoma, lymph nodes of head, face, and neck HCC Rx ESR COM
C83.82 Other non-follicular lymphoma, intrathoracic lymph nodes HCC Rx ESR COM
C83.83 Other non-follicular lymphoma, intra-abdominal lymph nodes HCC Rx ESR COM
C83.84 Other non-follicular lymphoma, lymph nodes of axilla and upper limb HCC Rx ESR COM
C83.85 Other non-follicular lymphoma, lymph nodes of inguinal region and lower limb HCC Rx ESR COM
C83.86 Other non-follicular lymphoma, intrapelvic lymph nodes HCC Rx ESR COM
C83.87 Other non-follicular lymphoma, spleen HCC Rx ESR COM
C83.88 Other non-follicular lymphoma, lymph nodes of multiple sites HCC Rx ESR COM
C83.89 Other non-follicular lymphoma, extranodal and solid organ sites HCC Rx ESR COM

5th C83.9 Non-follicular (diffuse) lymphoma, unspecified

C83.9Ø Non-follicular (diffuse) lymphoma, unspecified, unspecified site HCC Rx ESR COM
C83.91 Non-follicular (diffuse) lymphoma, unspecified, lymph nodes of head, face, and neck HCC Rx ESR COM
C83.92 Non-follicular (diffuse) lymphoma, unspecified, intrathoracic lymph nodes HCC Rx ESR COM
C83.93 Non-follicular (diffuse) lymphoma, unspecified, intra-abdominal lymph nodes HCC Rx ESR COM
C83.94 Non-follicular (diffuse) lymphoma, unspecified, lymph nodes of axilla and upper limb HCC Rx ESR COM
C83.95 Non-follicular (diffuse) lymphoma, unspecified, lymph nodes of inguinal region and lower limb HCC Rx ESR COM
C83.96 Non-follicular (diffuse) lymphoma, unspecified, intrapelvic lymph nodes HCC Rx ESR COM
C83.97 Non-follicular (diffuse) lymphoma, unspecified, spleen HCC Rx ESR COM
C83.98 Non-follicular (diffuse) lymphoma, unspecified, lymph nodes of multiple sites HCC Rx ESR COM
C83.99 Non-follicular (diffuse) lymphoma, unspecified, extranodal and solid organ sites HCC Rx ESR COM

4th C84 Mature T/NK-cell lymphomas

EXCLUDES 1 *personal history of non-Hodgkin lymphoma (Z85.72)*

5th C84.Ø Mycosis fungoides

EXCLUDES 1 *▶peripheral T-cell lymphoma, not elsewhere classified◀ (C84.4-)*

DEF: Most common form of cutaneous T-cell lymphoma. A type of non-Hodgkin lymphoma in which white blood cells become cancerous and affect the skin and sometimes internal organs. ***Synonym(s):*** *Alibert-Bazin syndrome.*

C84.ØØ Mycosis fungoides, unspecified site HCC Rx ESR COM
C84.Ø1 Mycosis fungoides, lymph nodes of head, face, and neck HCC Rx ESR COM
C84.Ø2 Mycosis fungoides, intrathoracic lymph nodes HCC Rx ESR COM
C84.Ø3 Mycosis fungoides, intra-abdominal lymph nodes HCC Rx ESR COM
C84.Ø4 Mycosis fungoides, lymph nodes of axilla and upper limb HCC Rx ESR COM
C84.Ø5 Mycosis fungoides, lymph nodes of inguinal region and lower limb HCC Rx ESR COM
C84.Ø6 Mycosis fungoides, intrapelvic lymph nodes HCC Rx ESR COM
C84.Ø7 Mycosis fungoides, spleen HCC Rx ESR COM
C84.Ø8 Mycosis fungoides, lymph nodes of multiple sites HCC Rx ESR COM
C84.Ø9 Mycosis fungoides, extranodal and solid organ sites HCC Rx ESR COM

5th C84.1 Sézary disease

DEF: Extension of mycosis fungoides that affects the blood and all of the skin, appearing as sunburn, rather than patches. It spreads to the lymph nodes and is often linked to a weakened immune system.

C84.1Ø Sézary disease, unspecified site HCC Rx ESR COM
C84.11 Sézary disease, lymph nodes of head, face, and neck HCC Rx ESR COM
C84.12 Sézary disease, intrathoracic lymph nodes HCC Rx ESR COM
C84.13 Sézary disease, intra-abdominal lymph nodes HCC Rx ESR COM
C84.14 Sézary disease, lymph nodes of axilla and upper limb HCC Rx ESR COM
C84.15 Sézary disease, lymph nodes of inguinal region and lower limb HCC Rx ESR COM
C84.16 Sézary disease, intrapelvic lymph nodes HCC Rx ESR COM
C84.17 Sézary disease, spleen HCC Rx ESR COM
C84.18 Sézary disease, lymph nodes of multiple sites HCC Rx ESR COM
C84.19 Sézary disease, extranodal and solid organ sites HCC Rx ESR COM

▲ 5th C84.4 Peripheral T-cell lymphoma, not elsewhere classified

Lennert's lymphoma
Lymphoepithelioid lymphoma
Mature T-cell lymphoma, not elsewhere classified

▲ C84.4Ø Peripheral T-cell lymphoma, not elsewhere classified, unspecified site HCC Rx ESR COM
▲ C84.41 Peripheral T-cell lymphoma, not elsewhere classified, lymph nodes of head, face, and neck HCC Rx ESR COM
▲ C84.42 Peripheral T-cell lymphoma, not elsewhere classified, intrathoracic lymph nodes HCC Rx ESR COM
▲ C84.43 Peripheral T-cell lymphoma, not elsewhere classified, intra-abdominal lymph nodes HCC Rx ESR COM
▲ C84.44 Peripheral T-cell lymphoma, not elsewhere classified, lymph nodes of axilla and upper limb HCC Rx ESR COM
▲ C84.45 Peripheral T-cell lymphoma, not elsewhere classified, lymph nodes of inguinal region and lower limb HCC Rx ESR COM
▲ C84.46 Peripheral T-cell lymphoma, not elsewhere classified, intrapelvic lymph nodes HCC Rx ESR COM
▲ C84.47 Peripheral T-cell lymphoma, not elsewhere classified, spleen HCC Rx ESR COM
▲ C84.48 Peripheral T-cell lymphoma, not elsewhere classified, lymph nodes of multiple sites HCC Rx ESR COM
▲ C84.49 Peripheral T-cell lymphoma, not elsewhere classified, extranodal and solid organ sites HCC Rx ESR COM

5th C84.6 Anaplastic large cell lymphoma, ALK-positive

Anaplastic large cell lymphoma, CD3Ø-positive

C84.6Ø Anaplastic large cell lymphoma, ALK-positive, unspecified site HCC Rx ESR COM
C84.61 Anaplastic large cell lymphoma, ALK-positive, lymph nodes of head, face, and neck HCC Rx ESR COM
C84.62 Anaplastic large cell lymphoma, ALK-positive, intrathoracic lymph nodes HCC Rx ESR COM
C84.63 Anaplastic large cell lymphoma, ALK-positive, intra-abdominal lymph nodes HCC Rx ESR COM
C84.64 Anaplastic large cell lymphoma, ALK-positive, lymph nodes of axilla and upper limb HCC Rx ESR COM
C84.65 Anaplastic large cell lymphoma, ALK-positive, lymph nodes of inguinal region and lower limb HCC Rx ESR COM
C84.66 Anaplastic large cell lymphoma, ALK-positive, intrapelvic lymph nodes HCC Rx ESR COM
C84.67 Anaplastic large cell lymphoma, ALK-positive, spleen HCC Rx ESR COM
C84.68 Anaplastic large cell lymphoma, ALK-positive, lymph nodes of multiple sites HCC Rx ESR COM
C84.69 Anaplastic large cell lymphoma, ALK-positive, extranodal and solid organ sites HCC Rx ESR COM

5th C84.7 Anaplastic large cell lymphoma, ALK-negative

EXCLUDES 1 *primary cutaneous CD3Ø-positive T-cell proliferations (C86.6-)*

C84.7Ø Anaplastic large cell lymphoma, ALK-negative, unspecified site HCC Rx ESR COM

C84.71 **Anaplastic large cell lymphoma, ALK-negative, lymph nodes of head, face, and neck** HCC Rx ESR COM

C84.72 **Anaplastic large cell lymphoma, ALK-negative, intrathoracic lymph nodes** HCC Rx ESR COM

C84.73 **Anaplastic large cell lymphoma, ALK-negative, intra-abdominal lymph nodes** HCC Rx ESR COM

C84.74 **Anaplastic large cell lymphoma, ALK-negative, lymph nodes of axilla and upper limb** HCC Rx ESR COM

C84.75 **Anaplastic large cell lymphoma, ALK-negative, lymph nodes of inguinal region and lower limb** HCC Rx ESR COM

C84.76 **Anaplastic large cell lymphoma, ALK-negative, intrapelvic lymph nodes** HCC Rx ESR COM

C84.77 **Anaplastic large cell lymphoma, ALK-negative, spleen** HCC Rx ESR COM

C84.78 **Anaplastic large cell lymphoma, ALK-negative, lymph nodes of multiple sites** HCC Rx ESR COM

C84.79 **Anaplastic large cell lymphoma, ALK-negative, extranodal and solid organ sites** HCC Rx ESR COM

C84.7A **Anaplastic large cell lymphoma, ALK-negative, breast** HCC Rx ESR COM

Breast implant associated anaplastic large cell lymphoma (BIA-ALCL)

Use additional code to identify:
- breast implant status (Z98.82)
- personal history of breast implant removal (Z98.86)

AHA: 2021,4Q,6

✓5th **C84.A** **Cutaneous T-cell lymphoma, unspecified**

AHA: 2021,2Q,6

C84.AØ **Cutaneous T-cell lymphoma, unspecified, unspecified site** HCC Rx ESR COM

C84.A1 **Cutaneous T-cell lymphoma, unspecified lymph nodes of head, face, and neck** HCC Rx ESR COM

C84.A2 **Cutaneous T-cell lymphoma, unspecified, intrathoracic lymph nodes** HCC Rx ESR COM

C84.A3 **Cutaneous T-cell lymphoma, unspecified, intra-abdominal lymph nodes** HCC Rx ESR COM

C84.A4 **Cutaneous T-cell lymphoma, unspecified, lymph nodes of axilla and upper limb** HCC Rx ESR COM

C84.A5 **Cutaneous T-cell lymphoma, unspecified, lymph nodes of inguinal region and lower limb** HCC Rx ESR COM

C84.A6 **Cutaneous T-cell lymphoma, unspecified, intrapelvic lymph nodes** HCC Rx ESR COM

C84.A7 **Cutaneous T-cell lymphoma, unspecified, spleen** HCC Rx ESR COM

C84.A8 **Cutaneous T-cell lymphoma, unspecified, lymph nodes of multiple sites** HCC Rx ESR COM

C84.A9 **Cutaneous T-cell lymphoma, unspecified, extranodal and solid organ sites** HCC Rx ESR COM

✓5th **C84.Z** **Other mature T/NK-cell lymphomas**

NOTE If T-cell lineage or involvement is mentioned in conjunction with a specific lymphoma, code to the more specific description.

EXCLUDES 1
- *angioimmunoblastic T-cell lymphoma (C86.5)*
- *blastic NK-cell lymphoma (C86.4)*
- *enteropathy-type T-cell lymphoma (C86.2)*
- *extranodal NK-cell lymphoma, nasal type (C86.Ø)*
- *hepatosplenic T-cell lymphoma (C86.1)*
- *primary cutaneous CD3Ø-positive T-cell proliferations (C86.6)*
- *subcutaneous panniculitis-like T-cell lymphoma (C86.3)*
- *T-cell leukemia (C91.1-)*

C84.ZØ **Other mature T/NK-cell lymphomas, unspecified site** HCC Rx ESR COM

C84.Z1 **Other mature T/NK-cell lymphomas, lymph nodes of head, face, and neck** HCC Rx ESR COM

C84.Z2 **Other mature T/NK-cell lymphomas, intrathoracic lymph nodes** HCC Rx ESR COM

C84.Z3 **Other mature T/NK-cell lymphomas, intra-abdominal lymph nodes** HCC Rx ESR COM

C84.Z4 **Other mature T/NK-cell lymphomas, lymph nodes of axilla and upper limb** HCC Rx ESR COM

C84.Z5 **Other mature T/NK-cell lymphomas, lymph nodes of inguinal region and lower limb** HCC Rx ESR COM

C84.Z6 **Other mature T/NK-cell lymphomas, intrapelvic lymph nodes** HCC Rx ESR COM

C84.Z7 **Other mature T/NK-cell lymphomas, spleen** HCC Rx ESR COM

C84.Z8 **Other mature T/NK-cell lymphomas, lymph nodes of multiple sites** HCC Rx ESR COM

C84.Z9 **Other mature T/NK-cell lymphomas, extranodal and solid organ sites** HCC Rx ESR COM

✓5th **C84.9** **Mature T/NK-cell lymphomas, unspecified**

NK/T cell lymphoma NOS

EXCLUDES 1 *mature T-cell lymphoma, not elsewhere classified (C84.4-)*

C84.9Ø **Mature T/NK-cell lymphomas, unspecified, unspecified site** HCC Rx ESR COM

C84.91 **Mature T/NK-cell lymphomas, unspecified, lymph nodes of head, face, and neck** HCC Rx ESR COM

C84.92 **Mature T/NK-cell lymphomas, unspecified, intrathoracic lymph nodes** HCC Rx ESR COM

C84.93 **Mature T/NK-cell lymphomas, unspecified, intra-abdominal lymph nodes** HCC Rx ESR COM

C84.94 **Mature T/NK-cell lymphomas, unspecified, lymph nodes of axilla and upper limb** HCC Rx ESR COM

C84.95 **Mature T/NK-cell lymphomas, unspecified, lymph nodes of inguinal region and lower limb** HCC Rx ESR COM

C84.96 **Mature T/NK-cell lymphomas, unspecified, intrapelvic lymph nodes** HCC Rx ESR COM

C84.97 **Mature T/NK-cell lymphomas, unspecified, spleen** HCC Rx ESR COM

C84.98 **Mature T/NK-cell lymphomas, unspecified, lymph nodes of multiple sites** HCC Rx ESR COM

C84.99 **Mature T/NK-cell lymphomas, unspecified, extranodal and solid organ sites** HCC Rx ESR COM

✓4th **C85** **Other specified and unspecified types of non-Hodgkin lymphoma**

EXCLUDES 1
- *other specified types of T/NK-cell lymphoma (C86.-)*
- *personal history of non-Hodgkin lymphoma (Z85.72)*

✓5th **C85.1** **Unspecified B-cell lymphoma**

NOTE If B-cell lineage or involvement is mentioned in conjunction with a specific lymphoma, code to the more specific description.

C85.1Ø **Unspecified B-cell lymphoma, unspecified site** HCC Rx ESR COM

C85.11 **Unspecified B-cell lymphoma, lymph nodes of head, face, and neck** HCC Rx ESR COM

C85.12 **Unspecified B-cell lymphoma, intrathoracic lymph nodes** HCC Rx ESR COM

C85.13 **Unspecified B-cell lymphoma, intra-abdominal lymph nodes** HCC Rx ESR COM

C85.14 **Unspecified B-cell lymphoma, lymph nodes of axilla and upper limb** HCC Rx ESR COM

C85.15 **Unspecified B-cell lymphoma, lymph nodes of inguinal region and lower limb** HCC Rx ESR COM

C85.16 **Unspecified B-cell lymphoma, intrapelvic lymph nodes** HCC Rx ESR COM

C85.17 **Unspecified B-cell lymphoma, spleen** HCC Rx ESR COM

C85.18 **Unspecified B-cell lymphoma, lymph nodes of multiple sites** HCC Rx ESR COM

C85.19 **Unspecified B-cell lymphoma, extranodal and solid organ sites** HCC Rx ESR COM

✓5th **C85.2** **Mediastinal (thymic) large B-cell lymphoma**

C85.2Ø **Mediastinal (thymic) large B-cell lymphoma, unspecified site** HCC Rx ESR COM

C85.21 **Mediastinal (thymic) large B-cell lymphoma, lymph nodes of head, face, and neck** HCC Rx ESR COM

C85.22 **Mediastinal (thymic) large B-cell lymphoma, intrathoracic lymph nodes** HCC Rx ESR COM

C85.23 **Mediastinal (thymic) large B-cell lymphoma, intra-abdominal lymph nodes** HCC Rx ESR COM

C85.24 **Mediastinal (thymic) large B-cell lymphoma, lymph nodes of axilla and upper limb** HCC Rx ESR COM

C85.25 **Mediastinal (thymic) large B-cell lymphoma, lymph nodes of inguinal region and lower limb** HCC Rx ESR COM

C85.26 **Mediastinal (thymic) large B-cell lymphoma, intrapelvic lymph nodes** HCC Rx ESR COM

C85.27 **Mediastinal (thymic) large B-cell lymphoma, spleen** HCC Rx ESR COM

C85.28 **Mediastinal (thymic) large B-cell lymphoma, lymph nodes of multiple sites** HCC Rx ESR COM

C85.29 **Mediastinal (thymic) large B-cell lymphoma, extranodal and solid organ sites** HCC Rx ESR COM

✓5th **C85.8 Other specified types of non-Hodgkin lymphoma**

C85.80 **Other specified types of non-Hodgkin lymphoma, unspecified site** HCC Rx ESR COM

C85.81 **Other specified types of non-Hodgkin lymphoma, lymph nodes of head, face, and neck** HCC Rx ESR COM

C85.82 **Other specified types of non-Hodgkin lymphoma, intrathoracic lymph nodes** HCC Rx ESR COM

C85.83 **Other specified types of non-Hodgkin lymphoma, intra-abdominal lymph nodes** HCC Rx ESR COM

C85.84 **Other specified types of non-Hodgkin lymphoma, lymph nodes of axilla and upper limb** HCC Rx ESR COM

C85.85 **Other specified types of non-Hodgkin lymphoma, lymph nodes of inguinal region and lower limb** HCC Rx ESR COM

C85.86 **Other specified types of non-Hodgkin lymphoma, intrapelvic lymph nodes** HCC Rx ESR COM

C85.87 **Other specified types of non-Hodgkin lymphoma, spleen** HCC Rx ESR COM

C85.88 **Other specified types of non-Hodgkin lymphoma, lymph nodes of multiple sites** HCC Rx ESR COM

C85.89 **Other specified types of non-Hodgkin lymphoma, extranodal and solid organ sites** HCC Rx ESR COM

✓5th **C85.9 Non-Hodgkin lymphoma, unspecified**

Lymphoma NOS
Malignant lymphoma NOS
Non-Hodgkin lymphoma NOS

C85.90 **Non-Hodgkin lymphoma, unspecified, unspecified site** HCC Rx ESR COM

C85.91 **Non-Hodgkin lymphoma, unspecified, lymph nodes of head, face, and neck** HCC Rx ESR COM

C85.92 **Non-Hodgkin lymphoma, unspecified, intrathoracic lymph nodes** HCC Rx ESR COM

C85.93 **Non-Hodgkin lymphoma, unspecified, intra-abdominal lymph nodes** HCC Rx ESR COM

C85.94 **Non-Hodgkin lymphoma, unspecified, lymph nodes of axilla and upper limb** HCC Rx ESR COM

C85.95 **Non-Hodgkin lymphoma, unspecified, lymph nodes of inguinal region and lower limb** HCC Rx ESR COM

C85.96 **Non-Hodgkin lymphoma, unspecified, intrapelvic lymph nodes** HCC Rx ESR COM

C85.97 **Non-Hodgkin lymphoma, unspecified, spleen** HCC Rx ESR COM

C85.98 **Non-Hodgkin lymphoma, unspecified, lymph nodes of multiple sites** HCC Rx ESR COM

C85.99 **Non-Hodgkin lymphoma, unspecified, extranodal and solid organ sites** HCC Rx ESR COM

✓4th **C86 Other specified types of T/NK-cell lymphoma**

EXCLUDES 1 *anaplastic large cell lymphoma, ALK negative (C84.7-)*
anaplastic large cell lymphoma, ALK positive (C84.6-)
mature T/NK-cell lymphomas (C84.-)
other specified types of non-Hodgkin lymphoma (C85.8-)

C86.0 **Extranodal NK/T-cell lymphoma, nasal type** HCC Rx ESR COM

C86.1 **Hepatosplenic T-cell lymphoma** HCC Rx ESR COM
Alpha-beta and gamma delta types

C86.2 **Enteropathy-type (intestinal) T-cell lymphoma** HCC Rx ESR COM
Enteropathy associated T-cell lymphoma

C86.3 **Subcutaneous panniculitis-like T-cell lymphoma** HCC Rx ESR COM

C86.4 **Blastic NK-cell lymphoma** HCC Rx ESR COM
Blastic plasmacytoid dendritic cell neoplasm (BPDCN)

C86.5 **Angioimmunoblastic T-cell lymphoma** HCC Rx ESR COM
Angioimmunoblastic lymphadenopathy with dysproteinemia (AILD)

C86.6 **Primary cutaneous CD30-positive T-cell proliferations** HCC Rx ESR COM
Lymphomatoid papulosis
Primary cutaneous anaplastic large cell lymphoma
Primary cutaneous CD30-positive large T-cell lymphoma

✓4th **C88 Malignant immunoproliferative diseases and certain other B-cell lymphomas**

EXCLUDES 1 *B-cell lymphoma, unspecified (C85.1-)*
personal history of other malignant neoplasms of lymphoid, hematopoietic and related tissues (Z85.79)

C88.0 **Waldenström macroglobulinemia** HCC Rx ESR COM
Lymphoplasmacytic lymphoma with IgM-production
Macroglobulinemia (idiopathic) (primary)
EXCLUDES 1 *small cell B-cell lymphoma (C83.0)*

C88.2 **Heavy chain disease** HCC Rx ESR COM
Franklin disease
Gamma heavy chain disease
Mu heavy chain disease

C88.3 **Immunoproliferative small intestinal disease** HCC Rx ESR COM
Alpha heavy chain disease
Mediterranean lymphoma

C88.4 **Extranodal marginal zone B-cell lymphoma of mucosa-associated lymphoid tissue [MALT-lymphoma]** HCC Rx ESR COM
Lymphoma of skin-associated lymphoid tissue [SALT-lymphoma]
Lymphoma of bronchial-associated lymphoid tissue [BALT-lymphoma]
EXCLUDES 1 *high malignant (diffuse large B-cell) lymphoma (C83.3-)*

C88.8 **Other malignant immunoproliferative diseases** HCC Rx ESR COM

C88.9 **Malignant immunoproliferative disease, unspecified** HCC Rx ESR COM
Immunoproliferative disease NOS

✓4th **C90 Multiple myeloma and malignant plasma cell neoplasms**

EXCLUDES 1 *personal history of other malignant neoplasms of lymphoid, hematopoietic and related tissues (Z85.79)*

AHA: 2019,2Q,30

✓5th **C90.0 Multiple myeloma**

Kahler's disease
Medullary plasmacytoma
Myelomatosis
Plasma cell myeloma
EXCLUDES 1 *solitary myeloma (C90.3-)*
solitary plasmactyoma (C90.3-)

AHA: 2021,3Q,5

TIP: Smoldering multiple myeloma (SMM) is a plasma cell disorder that has not yet progressed to active multiple myeloma. Code D47.2 should be used when only SMM is documented.

TIP: Do not assign an additional code for bone metastasis (C79.51) when multiple myeloma is described as metastatic to the bone; bone involvement is integral to this disease process.

C90.00 **Multiple myeloma not having achieved remission** HCC Rx ESR COM
Multiple myeloma with failed remission
Multiple myeloma NOS

C90.01 **Multiple myeloma in remission** HCC Rx ESR COM

C90.02 **Multiple myeloma in relapse** HCC Rx ESR COM

✓5th **C90.1 Plasma cell leukemia**

Plasmacytic leukemia

AHA: 2019,2Q,30

C90.10 **Plasma cell leukemia not having achieved remission** HCC Rx ESR COM
Plasma cell leukemia with failed remission
Plasma cell leukemia NOS

C90.11 **Plasma cell leukemia in remission** HCC Rx ESR COM

C90.12 **Plasma cell leukemia in relapse** HCC Rx ESR COM

✓5th **C90.2 Extramedullary plasmacytoma**

C90.20 **Extramedullary plasmacytoma not having achieved remission** HCC Rx ESR COM
Extramedullary plasmacytoma with failed remission
Extramedullary plasmacytoma NOS

C90.21 **Extramedullary plasmacytoma in remission** HCC Rx ESR COM

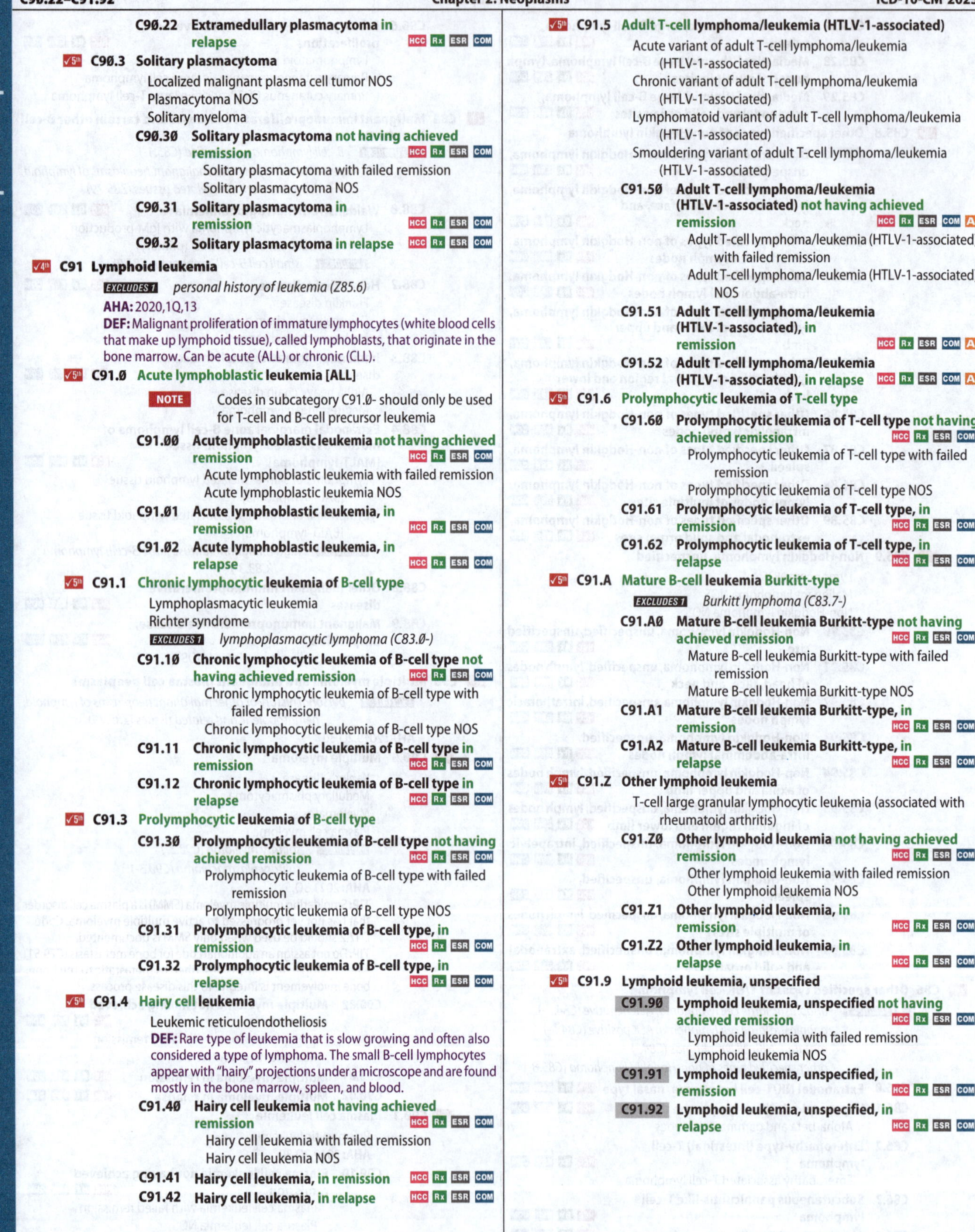

C90.22 Extramedullary plasmacytoma in relapse HCC Rx ESR COM

✓5th **C90.3 Solitary plasmacytoma**
Localized malignant plasma cell tumor NOS
Plasmacytoma NOS
Solitary myeloma

C90.30 Solitary plasmacytoma not having achieved remission HCC Rx ESR COM
Solitary plasmacytoma with failed remission
Solitary plasmacytoma NOS

C90.31 Solitary plasmacytoma in remission HCC Rx ESR COM

C90.32 Solitary plasmacytoma in relapse HCC Rx ESR COM

✓4th **C91 Lymphoid leukemia**
EXCLUDES 1 *personal history of leukemia (Z85.6)*
AHA: 2020,1Q,13
DEF: Malignant proliferation of immature lymphocytes (white blood cells that make up lymphoid tissue), called lymphoblasts, that originate in the bone marrow. Can be acute (ALL) or chronic (CLL).

✓5th **C91.0 Acute lymphoblastic leukemia [ALL]**
NOTE Codes in subcategory C91.0- should only be used for T-cell and B-cell precursor leukemia

C91.00 Acute lymphoblastic leukemia not having achieved remission HCC Rx ESR COM
Acute lymphoblastic leukemia with failed remission
Acute lymphoblastic leukemia NOS

C91.01 Acute lymphoblastic leukemia, in remission HCC Rx ESR COM

C91.02 Acute lymphoblastic leukemia, in relapse HCC Rx ESR COM

✓5th **C91.1 Chronic lymphocytic leukemia of B-cell type**
Lymphoplasmacytic leukemia
Richter syndrome
EXCLUDES 1 *lymphoplasmacytic lymphoma (C83.0-)*

C91.10 Chronic lymphocytic leukemia of B-cell type not having achieved remission HCC Rx ESR COM
Chronic lymphocytic leukemia of B-cell type with failed remission
Chronic lymphocytic leukemia of B-cell type NOS

C91.11 Chronic lymphocytic leukemia of B-cell type in remission HCC Rx ESR COM

C91.12 Chronic lymphocytic leukemia of B-cell type in relapse HCC Rx ESR COM

✓5th **C91.3 Prolymphocytic leukemia of B-cell type**

C91.30 Prolymphocytic leukemia of B-cell type not having achieved remission HCC Rx ESR COM
Prolymphocytic leukemia of B-cell type with failed remission
Prolymphocytic leukemia of B-cell type NOS

C91.31 Prolymphocytic leukemia of B-cell type, in remission HCC Rx ESR COM

C91.32 Prolymphocytic leukemia of B-cell type, in relapse HCC Rx ESR COM

✓5th **C91.4 Hairy cell leukemia**
Leukemic reticuloendotheliosis
DEF: Rare type of leukemia that is slow growing and often also considered a type of lymphoma. The small B-cell lymphocytes appear with "hairy" projections under a microscope and are found mostly in the bone marrow, spleen, and blood.

C91.40 Hairy cell leukemia not having achieved remission HCC Rx ESR COM
Hairy cell leukemia with failed remission
Hairy cell leukemia NOS

C91.41 Hairy cell leukemia, in remission HCC Rx ESR COM

C91.42 Hairy cell leukemia, in relapse HCC Rx ESR COM

✓5th **C91.5 Adult T-cell lymphoma/leukemia (HTLV-1-associated)**
Acute variant of adult T-cell lymphoma/leukemia (HTLV-1-associated)
Chronic variant of adult T-cell lymphoma/leukemia (HTLV-1-associated)
Lymphomatoid variant of adult T-cell lymphoma/leukemia (HTLV-1-associated)
Smouldering variant of adult T-cell lymphoma/leukemia (HTLV-1-associated)

C91.50 Adult T-cell lymphoma/leukemia (HTLV-1-associated) not having achieved remission HCC Rx ESR COM A
Adult T-cell lymphoma/leukemia (HTLV-1-associated) with failed remission
Adult T-cell lymphoma/leukemia (HTLV-1-associated) NOS

C91.51 Adult T-cell lymphoma/leukemia (HTLV-1-associated), in remission HCC Rx ESR COM A

C91.52 Adult T-cell lymphoma/leukemia (HTLV-1-associated), in relapse HCC Rx ESR COM A

✓5th **C91.6 Prolymphocytic leukemia of T-cell type**

C91.60 Prolymphocytic leukemia of T-cell type not having achieved remission HCC Rx ESR COM
Prolymphocytic leukemia of T-cell type with failed remission
Prolymphocytic leukemia of T-cell type NOS

C91.61 Prolymphocytic leukemia of T-cell type, in remission HCC Rx ESR COM

C91.62 Prolymphocytic leukemia of T-cell type, in relapse HCC Rx ESR COM

✓5th **C91.A Mature B-cell leukemia Burkitt-type**
EXCLUDES 1 *Burkitt lymphoma (C83.7-)*

C91.A0 Mature B-cell leukemia Burkitt-type not having achieved remission HCC Rx ESR COM
Mature B-cell leukemia Burkitt-type with failed remission
Mature B-cell leukemia Burkitt-type NOS

C91.A1 Mature B-cell leukemia Burkitt-type, in remission HCC Rx ESR COM

C91.A2 Mature B-cell leukemia Burkitt-type, in relapse HCC Rx ESR COM

✓5th **C91.Z Other lymphoid leukemia**
T-cell large granular lymphocytic leukemia (associated with rheumatoid arthritis)

C91.Z0 Other lymphoid leukemia not having achieved remission HCC Rx ESR COM
Other lymphoid leukemia with failed remission
Other lymphoid leukemia NOS

C91.Z1 Other lymphoid leukemia, in remission HCC Rx ESR COM

C91.Z2 Other lymphoid leukemia, in relapse HCC Rx ESR COM

✓5th **C91.9 Lymphoid leukemia, unspecified**

C91.90 Lymphoid leukemia, unspecified not having achieved remission HCC Rx ESR COM
Lymphoid leukemia with failed remission
Lymphoid leukemia NOS

C91.91 Lymphoid leukemia, unspecified, in remission HCC Rx ESR COM

C91.92 Lymphoid leukemia, unspecified, in relapse HCC Rx ESR COM

C92 Myeloid leukemia

INCLUDES granulocytic leukemia
myelogenous leukemia

EXCLUDES 1 *personal history of leukemia (Z85.6)*

AHA: 2020,1Q,13; 2019,1Q,16

DEF: Cancer that develops in immature myelocytes called myeloblasts. These are the cells that become white blood cells (except lymphocytes), red blood cells, or platelet-making cells. Can be acute (AML) or chronic (CML).

TIP: Pancytopenia, although common in some types of myeloid leukemias, is not always inherent. When it is documented, code D61.818 can be assigned in addition to a code from this category.

C92.0 Acute myeloblastic leukemia
Acute myeloblastic leukemia, minimal differentiation
Acute myeloblastic leukemia (with maturation)
Acute myeloblastic leukemia 1/ETO
Acute myeloblastic leukemia M0
Acute myeloblastic leukemia M1
Acute myeloblastic leukemia M2
Acute myeloblastic leukemia with t(8;21)
Acute myeloblastic leukemia (without a FAB classification) NOS
Refractory anemia with excess blasts in transformation [RAEBT]

EXCLUDES 1 *acute exacerbation of chronic myeloid leukemia (C92.10)*
refractory anemia with excess of blasts not in transformation (D46.2-)

AHA: 2018,4Q,87

C92.00 Acute myeloblastic leukemia, not having achieved remission HCC Rx ESR COM
Acute myeloblastic leukemia with failed remission
Acute myeloblastic leukemia NOS

C92.01 Acute myeloblastic leukemia, in remission HCC Rx ESR COM
AHA: 2021,3Q,4

C92.02 Acute myeloblastic leukemia, in relapse HCC Rx ESR COM

C92.1 Chronic myeloid leukemia, BCR/ABL-positive
Chronic myelogenous leukemia, Philadelphia chromosome (Ph1) positive
Chronic myelogenous leukemia, t(9;22) (q34;q11)
Chronic myelogenous leukemia with crisis of blast cells

EXCLUDES 1 *atypical chronic myeloid leukemia BCR/ABL-negative (C92.2-)*
chronic myelomonocytic leukemia (C93.1-)
chronic myeloproliferative disease (D47.1)

C92.10 Chronic myeloid leukemia, BCR/ABL-positive, not having achieved remission HCC Rx ESR COM
Chronic myeloid leukemia, BCR/ABL-positive with failed remission
Chronic myeloid leukemia, BCR/ABL-positive NOS

C92.11 Chronic myeloid leukemia, BCR/ABL-positive, in remission HCC Rx ESR COM

C92.12 Chronic myeloid leukemia, BCR/ABL-positive, in relapse HCC Rx ESR COM

C92.2 Atypical chronic myeloid leukemia, BCR/ABL-negative

C92.20 Atypical chronic myeloid leukemia, BCR/ABL-negative, not having achieved remission HCC Rx ESR COM
Atypical chronic myeloid leukemia, BCR/ABL-negative with failed remission
Atypical chronic myeloid leukemia, BCR/ABL-negative NOS

C92.21 Atypical chronic myeloid leukemia, BCR/ABL-negative, in remission HCC Rx ESR COM

C92.22 Atypical chronic myeloid leukemia, BCR/ABL-negative, in relapse HCC Rx ESR COM

C92.3 Myeloid sarcoma
A malignant tumor of immature myeloid cells
Chloroma
Granulocytic sarcoma

C92.30 Myeloid sarcoma, not having achieved remission HCC Rx ESR COM
Myeloid sarcoma with failed remission
Myeloid sarcoma NOS

C92.31 Myeloid sarcoma, in remission HCC Rx ESR COM

C92.32 Myeloid sarcoma, in relapse HCC Rx ESR COM

C92.4 Acute promyelocytic leukemia
AML M3
AML Me with t(15;17) and variants

C92.40 Acute promyelocytic leukemia, not having achieved remission HCC Rx ESR COM
Acute promyelocytic leukemia with failed remission
Acute promyelocytic leukemia NOS

C92.41 Acute promyelocytic leukemia, in remission HCC Rx ESR COM

C92.42 Acute promyelocytic leukemia, in relapse HCC Rx ESR COM

C92.5 Acute myelomonocytic leukemia
AML M4
AML M4 Eo with inv(16) or t(16;16)

C92.50 Acute myelomonocytic leukemia, not having achieved remission HCC Rx ESR COM
Acute myelomonocytic leukemia with failed remission
Acute myelomonocytic leukemia NOS

C92.51 Acute myelomonocytic leukemia, in remission HCC Rx ESR COM

C92.52 Acute myelomonocytic leukemia, in relapse HCC Rx ESR COM

C92.6 Acute myeloid leukemia with 11q23-abnormality
Acute myeloid leukemia with variation of MLL-gene

C92.60 Acute myeloid leukemia with 11q23-abnormality not having achieved remission HCC Rx ESR COM
Acute myeloid leukemia with 11q23-abnormality with failed remission
Acute myeloid leukemia with 11q23-abnormality NOS

C92.61 Acute myeloid leukemia with 11q23-abnormality in remission HCC Rx ESR COM

C92.62 Acute myeloid leukemia with 11q23-abnormality in relapse HCC Rx ESR COM

C92.A Acute myeloid leukemia with multilineage dysplasia
Acute myeloid leukemia with dysplasia of remaining hematopoesis and/or myelodysplastic disease in its history

C92.A0 Acute myeloid leukemia with multilineage dysplasia, not having achieved remission HCC Rx ESR COM
Acute myeloid leukemia with multilineage dysplasia with failed remission
Acute myeloid leukemia with multilineage dysplasia NOS

C92.A1 Acute myeloid leukemia with multilineage dysplasia, in remission HCC Rx ESR COM

C92.A2 Acute myeloid leukemia with multilineage dysplasia, in relapse HCC Rx ESR COM

C92.Z Other myeloid leukemia

C92.Z0 Other myeloid leukemia not having achieved remission HCC Rx ESR COM
Myeloid leukemia NEC with failed remission
Myeloid leukemia NEC

C92.Z1 Other myeloid leukemia, in remission HCC Rx ESR COM

C92.Z2 Other myeloid leukemia, in relapse HCC Rx ESR COM

C92.9 Myeloid leukemia, unspecified

C92.90 Myeloid leukemia, unspecified, not having achieved remission HCC Rx ESR COM
Myeloid leukemia, unspecified with failed remission
Myeloid leukemia, unspecified NOS

C92.91 Myeloid leukemia, unspecified in remission HCC Rx ESR COM

C92.92 Myeloid leukemia, unspecified in relapse HCC Rx ESR COM

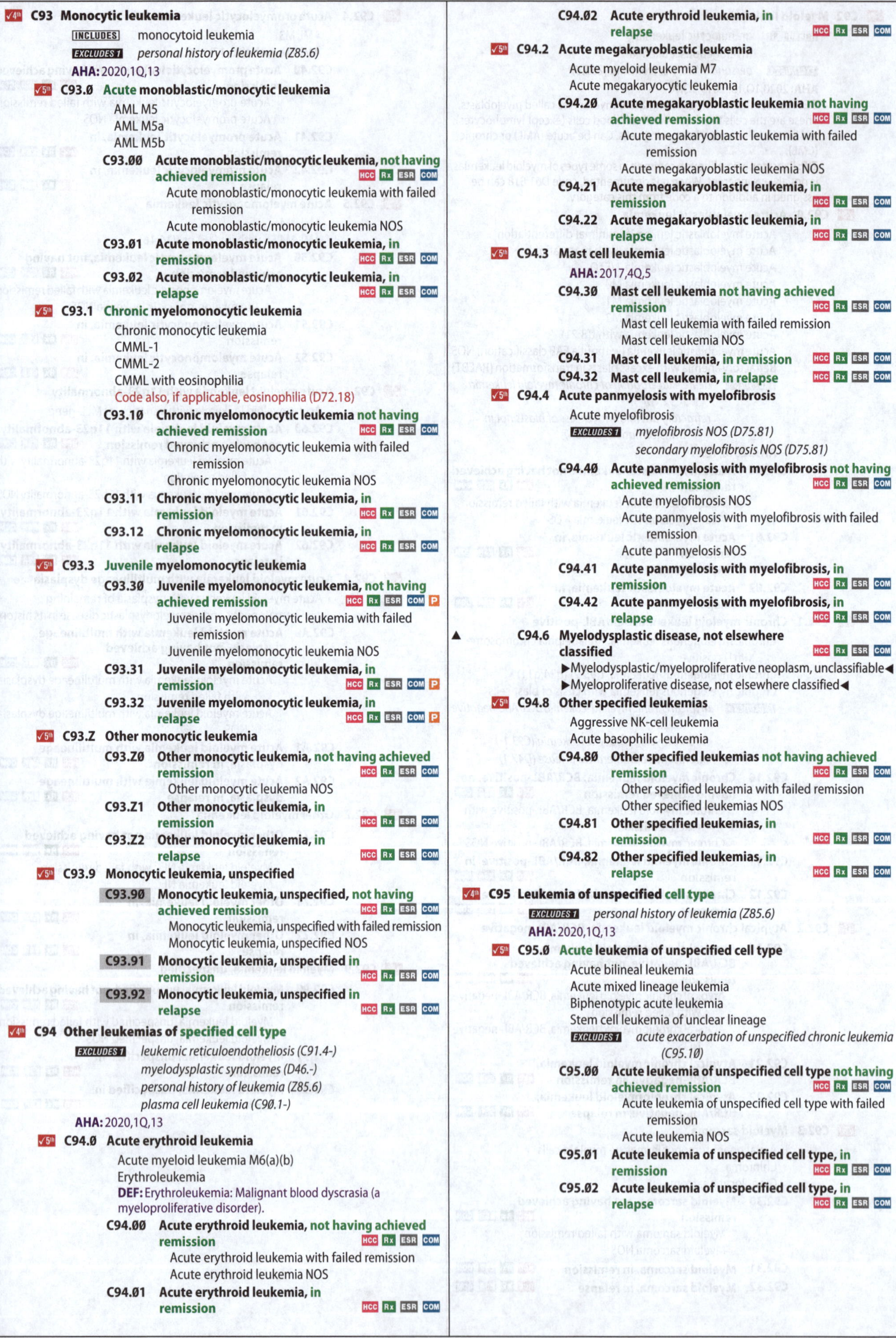

C93 Monocytic leukemia
INCLUDES monocytoid leukemia
EXCLUDES 1 *personal history of leukemia (Z85.6)*
AHA: 2020,1Q,13

C93.0 Acute monoblastic/monocytic leukemia
AML M5
AML M5a
AML M5b

C93.00 Acute monoblastic/monocytic leukemia, not having achieved remission HCC Rx ESR COM
Acute monoblastic/monocytic leukemia with failed remission
Acute monoblastic/monocytic leukemia NOS

C93.01 Acute monoblastic/monocytic leukemia, in remission HCC Rx ESR COM

C93.02 Acute monoblastic/monocytic leukemia, in relapse HCC Rx ESR COM

C93.1 Chronic myelomonocytic leukemia
Chronic monocytic leukemia
CMML-1
CMML-2
CMML with eosinophilia
Code also, if applicable, eosinophilia (D72.18)

C93.10 Chronic myelomonocytic leukemia not having achieved remission HCC Rx ESR COM
Chronic myelomonocytic leukemia with failed remission
Chronic myelomonocytic leukemia NOS

C93.11 Chronic myelomonocytic leukemia, in remission HCC Rx ESR COM

C93.12 Chronic myelomonocytic leukemia, in relapse HCC Rx ESR COM

C93.3 Juvenile myelomonocytic leukemia

C93.30 Juvenile myelomonocytic leukemia, not having achieved remission HCC Rx ESR COM P
Juvenile myelomonocytic leukemia with failed remission
Juvenile myelomonocytic leukemia NOS

C93.31 Juvenile myelomonocytic leukemia, in remission HCC Rx ESR COM P

C93.32 Juvenile myelomonocytic leukemia, in relapse HCC Rx ESR COM P

C93.Z Other monocytic leukemia

C93.Z0 Other monocytic leukemia, not having achieved remission HCC Rx ESR COM
Other monocytic leukemia NOS

C93.Z1 Other monocytic leukemia, in remission HCC Rx ESR COM

C93.Z2 Other monocytic leukemia, in relapse HCC Rx ESR COM

C93.9 Monocytic leukemia, unspecified

C93.90 Monocytic leukemia, unspecified, not having achieved remission HCC Rx ESR COM
Monocytic leukemia, unspecified with failed remission
Monocytic leukemia, unspecified NOS

C93.91 Monocytic leukemia, unspecified in remission HCC Rx ESR COM

C93.92 Monocytic leukemia, unspecified in relapse HCC Rx ESR COM

C94 Other leukemias of specified cell type
EXCLUDES 1 *leukemic reticuloendotheliosis (C91.4-)*
myelodysplastic syndromes (D46.-)
personal history of leukemia (Z85.6)
plasma cell leukemia (C90.1-)
AHA: 2020,1Q,13

C94.0 Acute erythroid leukemia
Acute myeloid leukemia M6(a)(b)
Erythroleukemia
DEF: Erythroleukemia: Malignant blood dyscrasia (a myeloproliferative disorder).

C94.00 Acute erythroid leukemia, not having achieved remission HCC Rx ESR COM
Acute erythroid leukemia with failed remission
Acute erythroid leukemia NOS

C94.01 Acute erythroid leukemia, in remission HCC Rx ESR COM

C94.02 Acute erythroid leukemia, in relapse HCC Rx ESR COM

C94.2 Acute megakaryoblastic leukemia
Acute myeloid leukemia M7
Acute megakaryocytic leukemia

C94.20 Acute megakaryoblastic leukemia not having achieved remission HCC Rx ESR COM
Acute megakaryoblastic leukemia with failed remission
Acute megakaryoblastic leukemia NOS

C94.21 Acute megakaryoblastic leukemia, in remission HCC Rx ESR COM

C94.22 Acute megakaryoblastic leukemia, in relapse HCC Rx ESR COM

C94.3 Mast cell leukemia
AHA: 2017,4Q,5

C94.30 Mast cell leukemia not having achieved remission HCC Rx ESR COM
Mast cell leukemia with failed remission
Mast cell leukemia NOS

C94.31 Mast cell leukemia, in remission HCC Rx ESR COM

C94.32 Mast cell leukemia, in relapse HCC Rx ESR COM

C94.4 Acute panmyelosis with myelofibrosis
Acute myelofibrosis
EXCLUDES 1 *myelofibrosis NOS (D75.81)*
secondary myelofibrosis NOS (D75.81)

C94.40 Acute panmyelosis with myelofibrosis not having achieved remission HCC Rx ESR COM
Acute myelofibrosis NOS
Acute panmyelosis with myelofibrosis with failed remission
Acute panmyelosis NOS

C94.41 Acute panmyelosis with myelofibrosis, in remission HCC Rx ESR COM

C94.42 Acute panmyelosis with myelofibrosis, in relapse HCC Rx ESR COM

▲ **C94.6 Myelodysplastic disease, not elsewhere classified** HCC Rx ESR COM
▶Myelodysplastic/myeloproliferative neoplasm, unclassifiable◀
▶Myeloproliferative disease, not elsewhere classified◀

C94.8 Other specified leukemias
Aggressive NK-cell leukemia
Acute basophilic leukemia

C94.80 Other specified leukemias not having achieved remission HCC Rx ESR COM
Other specified leukemia with failed remission
Other specified leukemias NOS

C94.81 Other specified leukemias, in remission HCC Rx ESR COM

C94.82 Other specified leukemias, in relapse HCC Rx ESR COM

C95 Leukemia of unspecified cell type
EXCLUDES 1 *personal history of leukemia (Z85.6)*
AHA: 2020,1Q,13

C95.0 Acute leukemia of unspecified cell type
Acute bilineal leukemia
Acute mixed lineage leukemia
Biphenotypic acute leukemia
Stem cell leukemia of unclear lineage
EXCLUDES 1 *acute exacerbation of unspecified chronic leukemia (C95.10)*

C95.00 Acute leukemia of unspecified cell type not having achieved remission HCC Rx ESR COM
Acute leukemia of unspecified cell type with failed remission
Acute leukemia NOS

C95.01 Acute leukemia of unspecified cell type, in remission HCC Rx ESR COM

C95.02 Acute leukemia of unspecified cell type, in relapse HCC Rx ESR COM

C95.1 Chronic leukemia of unspecified cell type

C95.10 Chronic leukemia of unspecified cell type not having achieved remission HCC Rx ESR COM

Chronic leukemia of unspecified cell type with failed remission

Chronic leukemia NOS

C95.11 Chronic leukemia of unspecified cell type, in remission HCC Rx ESR COM

C95.12 Chronic leukemia of unspecified cell type, in relapse HCC Rx ESR COM

C95.9 Leukemia, unspecified

C95.90 Leukemia, unspecified not having achieved remission HCC Rx ESR COM

Leukemia, unspecified with failed remission

Leukemia NOS

C95.91 Leukemia, unspecified, in remission HCC Rx ESR COM

C95.92 Leukemia, unspecified, in relapse HCC Rx ESR COM

C96 Other and unspecified malignant neoplasms of lymphoid, hematopoietic and related tissue

EXCLUDES 1 *personal history of other malignant neoplasms of lymphoid, hematopoietic and related tissues (Z85.79)*

C96.0 Multifocal and multisystemic (disseminated) Langerhans-cell histiocytosis HCC Rx ESR COM

Histiocytosis X, multisystemic

Letterer-Siwe disease

EXCLUDES 1 *adult pulmonary Langerhans cell histiocytosis (J84.82)*

multifocal and unisystemic Langerhans-cell histiocytosis (C96.5)

unifocal Langerhans-cell histiocytosis (C96.6)

C96.2 Malignant mast cell neoplasm

EXCLUDES 1 *indolent mastocytosis (D47.02)*

mast cell leukemia (C94.30)

mastocytosis (congenital) (cutaneous) (Q82.2)

AHA: 2017,4Q,5

DEF: Mast cell: Type of white blood cell found in the loose connective tissue of blood vessels and bronchioles responsible for acute hypersensitivity reactions, including anaphylactic shock. The IgE receptors on these cells bind with allergens causing cell degranulation and diffuse, widespread histamine release that results in airway constriction and vasodilation with decreased systemic blood pressure.

C96.20 Malignant mast cell neoplasm, unspecified HCC Rx ESR COM

C96.21 Aggressive systemic mastocytosis HCC Rx ESR COM

C96.22 Mast cell sarcoma HCC Rx ESR COM

C96.29 Other malignant mast cell neoplasm HCC Rx ESR COM

C96.4 Sarcoma of dendritic cells (accessory cells) HCC Rx ESR COM

Follicular dendritic cell sarcoma

Interdigitating dendritic cell sarcoma

Langerhans cell sarcoma

C96.5 Multifocal and unisystemic Langerhans-cell histiocytosis HCC Rx ESR COM

Hand-Schüller-Christian disease

Histiocytosis X, multifocal

EXCLUDES 1 *multifocal and multisystemic (disseminated) Langerhans-cell histiocytosis (C96.0)*

unifocal Langerhans-cell histiocytosis (C96.6)

C96.6 Unifocal Langerhans-cell histiocytosis HCC Rx ESR COM

Eosinophilic granuloma

Histiocytosis X, unifocal

Histiocytosis X NOS

Langerhans-cell histiocytosis NOS

EXCLUDES 1 *multifocal and multisysemic (disseminated) Langerhans-cell histiocytosis (C96.0)*

multifocal and unisystemic Langerhans-cell histiocytosis (C96.5)

C96.A Histiocytic sarcoma HCC Rx ESR COM

Malignant histiocytosis

C96.Z Other specified malignant neoplasms of lymphoid, hematopoietic and related tissue HCC Rx ESR COM

C96.9 Malignant neoplasm of lymphoid, hematopoietic and related tissue, unspecified HCC Rx ESR COM

In situ neoplasms (D00-D09)

INCLUDES Bowen's disease

erythroplasia

grade III intraepithelial neoplasia

Queyrat's erythroplasia

D00 Carcinoma in situ of oral cavity, esophagus and stomach

EXCLUDES 1 *melanoma in situ (D03.-)*

D00.0 Carcinoma in situ of lip, oral cavity and pharynx

Use additional code to identify:

exposure to environmental tobacco smoke (Z77.22)

exposure to tobacco smoke in the perinatal period (P96.81)

history of tobacco dependence (Z87.891)

occupational exposure to environmental tobacco smoke (Z57.31)

tobacco dependence (F17.-)

tobacco use (Z72.0)

EXCLUDES 1 *carcinoma in situ of aryepiglottic fold or interarytenoid fold, laryngeal aspect (D02.0)*

carcinoma in situ of epiglottis NOS (D02.0)

carcinoma in situ of epiglottis suprahyoid portion (D02.0)

carcinoma in situ of skin of lip (D03.0, D04.0)

D00.00 Carcinoma in situ of oral cavity, unspecified site

D00.01 Carcinoma in situ of labial mucosa and vermilion border

D00.02 Carcinoma in situ of buccal mucosa

D00.03 Carcinoma in situ of gingiva and edentulous alveolar ridge

D00.04 Carcinoma in situ of soft palate

D00.05 Carcinoma in situ of hard palate

D00.06 Carcinoma in situ of floor of mouth

D00.07 Carcinoma in situ of tongue

D00.08 Carcinoma in situ of pharynx

Carcinoma in situ of aryepiglottic fold NOS

Carcinoma in situ of hypopharyngeal aspect of aryepiglottic fold

Carcinoma in situ of marginal zone of aryepiglottic fold

D00.1 Carcinoma in situ of esophagus

D00.2 Carcinoma in situ of stomach

D01 Carcinoma in situ of other and unspecified digestive organs

EXCLUDES 1 *melanoma in situ (D03.-)*

D01.0 Carcinoma in situ of colon

EXCLUDES 1 *carcinoma in situ of rectosigmoid junction (D01.1)*

D01.1 Carcinoma in situ of rectosigmoid junction

D01.2 Carcinoma in situ of rectum

D01.3 Carcinoma in situ of anus and anal canal

Anal intraepithelial neoplasia III [AIN III]

Severe dysplasia of anus

EXCLUDES 1 *anal intraepithelial neoplasia I and II [AIN I and AIN II] (K62.82)*

carcinoma in situ of anal margin (D04.5)

carcinoma in situ of anal skin (D04.5)

carcinoma in situ of perianal skin (D04.5)

D01.4 Carcinoma in situ of other and unspecified parts of intestine

EXCLUDES 1 *carcinoma in situ of ampulla of Vater (D01.5)*

D01.40 Carcinoma in situ of unspecified part of intestine

D01.49 Carcinoma in situ of other parts of intestine

D01.5 Carcinoma in situ of liver, gallbladder and bile ducts

Carcinoma in situ of ampulla of Vater

D01.7 Carcinoma in situ of other specified digestive organs

Carcinoma in situ of pancreas

D01.9 Carcinoma in situ of digestive organ, unspecified

D02 Carcinoma in situ of middle ear and respiratory system
Use additional code to identify:
exposure to environmental tobacco smoke (Z77.22)
exposure to tobacco smoke in the perinatal period (P96.81)
history of tobacco dependence (Z87.891)
occupational exposure to environmental tobacco smoke (Z57.31)
tobacco dependence (F17.-)
tobacco use (Z72.0)
EXCLUDES 1 *melanoma in situ (D03.-)*

D02.0 Carcinoma in situ of larynx
Carcinoma in situ of aryepiglottic fold or interarytenoid fold, laryngeal aspect
Carcinoma in situ of epiglottis (suprahyoid portion)
EXCLUDES 1 *carcinoma in situ of aryepiglottic fold or interarytenoid fold NOS (D00.08)*
carcinoma in situ of hypopharyngeal aspect (D00.08)
carcinoma in situ of marginal zone (D00.08)

D02.1 Carcinoma in situ of trachea

D02.2 Carcinoma in situ of bronchus and lung
D02.20 Carcinoma in situ of unspecified bronchus and lung
D02.21 Carcinoma in situ of right bronchus and lung
D02.22 Carcinoma in situ of left bronchus and lung

D02.3 Carcinoma in situ of other parts of respiratory system
Carcinoma in situ of accessory sinuses
Carcinoma in situ of middle ear
Carcinoma in situ of nasal cavities
EXCLUDES 1 *carcinoma in situ of ear (external) (skin) (D04.2-)*
carcinoma in situ of nose NOS (D09.8)
carcinoma in situ of skin of nose (D04.3)

D02.4 Carcinoma in situ of respiratory system, unspecified

D03 Melanoma in situ

D03.0 Melanoma in situ of lip HCC Rx ESR COM

D03.1 Melanoma in situ of eyelid, including canthus
AHA: 2018,4Q,4
D03.10 Melanoma in situ of unspecified eyelid, including canthus HCC Rx ESR COM
D03.11 Melanoma in situ of right eyelid, including canthus
D03.111 Melanoma in situ of right upper eyelid, including canthus HCC Rx ESR COM
D03.112 Melanoma in situ of right lower eyelid, including canthus HCC Rx ESR COM
D03.12 Melanoma in situ of left eyelid, including canthus
D03.121 Melanoma in situ of left upper eyelid, including canthus HCC Rx ESR COM
D03.122 Melanoma in situ of left lower eyelid, including canthus HCC Rx ESR COM

D03.2 Melanoma in situ of ear and external auricular canal
D03.20 Melanoma in situ of unspecified ear and external auricular canal HCC Rx ESR COM
D03.21 Melanoma in situ of right ear and external auricular canal HCC Rx ESR COM
D03.22 Melanoma in situ of left ear and external auricular canal HCC Rx ESR COM

D03.3 Melanoma in situ of other and unspecified parts of face
D03.30 Melanoma in situ of unspecified part of face HCC Rx ESR COM
D03.39 Melanoma in situ of other parts of face HCC Rx ESR COM

D03.4 Melanoma in situ of scalp and neck HCC Rx ESR COM

D03.5 Melanoma in situ of trunk
D03.51 Melanoma in situ of anal skin HCC Rx ESR COM
Melanoma in situ of anal margin
Melanoma in situ of perianal skin
D03.52 Melanoma in situ of breast (skin) (soft tissue) HCC Rx ESR COM
D03.59 Melanoma in situ of other part of trunk HCC Rx ESR COM

D03.6 Melanoma in situ of upper limb, including shoulder
D03.60 Melanoma in situ of unspecified upper limb, including shoulder HCC Rx ESR COM
D03.61 Melanoma in situ of right upper limb, including shoulder HCC Rx ESR COM
D03.62 Melanoma in situ of left upper limb, including shoulder HCC Rx ESR COM

D03.7 Melanoma in situ of lower limb, including hip
D03.70 Melanoma in situ of unspecified lower limb, including hip HCC Rx ESR COM
D03.71 Melanoma in situ of right lower limb, including hip HCC Rx ESR COM
D03.72 Melanoma in situ of left lower limb, including hip HCC Rx ESR COM

D03.8 Melanoma in situ of other sites HCC Rx ESR COM
Melanoma in situ of scrotum
EXCLUDES 1 *carcinoma in situ of scrotum (D07.61)*

D03.9 Melanoma in situ, unspecified HCC Rx ESR COM

D04 Carcinoma in situ of skin
EXCLUDES 1 *erythroplasia of Queyrat (penis) NOS (D07.4)*
melanoma in situ (D03.-)

D04.0 Carcinoma in situ of skin of lip
EXCLUDES 2 *carcinoma in situ of vermilion border of lip (D00.01)*

D04.1 Carcinoma in situ of skin of eyelid, including canthus
AHA: 2018,4Q,4
D04.10 Carcinoma in situ of skin of unspecified eyelid, including canthus
D04.11 Carcinoma in situ of skin of right eyelid, including canthus
D04.111 Carcinoma in situ of skin of right upper eyelid, including canthus
D04.112 Carcinoma in situ of skin of right lower eyelid, including canthus
D04.12 Carcinoma in situ of skin of left eyelid, including canthus
D04.121 Carcinoma in situ of skin of left upper eyelid, including canthus
D04.122 Carcinoma in situ of skin of left lower eyelid, including canthus

D04.2 Carcinoma in situ of skin of ear and external auricular canal
D04.20 Carcinoma in situ of skin of unspecified ear and external auricular canal
D04.21 Carcinoma in situ of skin of right ear and external auricular canal
D04.22 Carcinoma in situ of skin of left ear and external auricular canal

D04.3 Carcinoma in situ of skin of other and unspecified parts of face
D04.30 Carcinoma in situ of skin of unspecified part of face
D04.39 Carcinoma in situ of skin of other parts of face

D04.4 Carcinoma in situ of skin of scalp and neck

D04.5 Carcinoma in situ of skin of trunk
Carcinoma in situ of anal margin
Carcinoma in situ of anal skin
Carcinoma in situ of perianal skin
Carcinoma in situ of skin of breast
EXCLUDES 1 *carcinoma in situ of anus NOS (D01.3)*
carcinoma in situ of scrotum (D07.61)
carcinoma in situ of skin of genital organs (D07.-)

D04.6 Carcinoma in situ of skin of upper limb, including shoulder
D04.60 Carcinoma in situ of skin of unspecified upper limb, including shoulder
D04.61 Carcinoma in situ of skin of right upper limb, including shoulder
D04.62 Carcinoma in situ of skin of left upper limb, including shoulder

D04.7 Carcinoma in situ of skin of lower limb, including hip
D04.70 Carcinoma in situ of skin of unspecified lower limb, including hip
D04.71 Carcinoma in situ of skin of right lower limb, including hip
D04.72 Carcinoma in situ of skin of left lower limb, including hip

D04.8 Carcinoma in situ of skin of other sites

D04.9 Carcinoma in situ of skin, unspecified

D05 Carcinoma in situ of breast
EXCLUDES 1 *carcinoma in situ of skin of breast (D04.5)*
melanoma in situ of breast (skin) (D03.5)
Paget's disease of breast or nipple (C50.-)

D05.0 Lobular carcinoma in situ of breast
D05.00 Lobular carcinoma in situ of unspecified breast
D05.01 Lobular carcinoma in situ of right breast
D05.02 Lobular carcinoma in situ of left breast

HCC CMS-HCC | Rx Rx HCC | ESR ESRD HCC | COM Commercial HCC | N Newborn: 0 | P Pediatric: 0-17 | M Maternity: 9-64 | A Adult: 15-124

D05.1 Intraductal carcinoma in situ of breast
- **D05.10 Intraductal carcinoma in situ of unspecified breast**
- **D05.11 Intraductal carcinoma in situ of right breast**
- **D05.12 Intraductal carcinoma in situ of left breast**

D05.8 Other specified type of carcinoma in situ of breast
- **D05.80 Other specified type of carcinoma in situ of unspecified breast**
- **D05.81 Other specified type of carcinoma in situ of right breast**
- **D05.82 Other specified type of carcinoma in situ of left breast**

D05.9 Unspecified type of carcinoma in situ of breast
- **D05.90 Unspecified type of carcinoma in situ of unspecified breast**
- **D05.91 Unspecified type of carcinoma in situ of right breast**
- **D05.92 Unspecified type of carcinoma in situ of left breast**

D06 Carcinoma in situ of cervix uteri

INCLUDES cervical adenocarcinoma in situ
cervical intraepithelial glandular neoplasia
cervical intraepithelial neoplasia III [CIN III]
severe dysplasia of cervix uteri

EXCLUDES 1 *cervical intraepithelial neoplasia II [CIN II] (N87.1)*
cytologic evidence of malignancy of cervix without histologic confirmation (R87.614)
high grade squamous intraepithelial lesion (HGSIL) of cervix (R87.613)
melanoma in situ of cervix (D03.5)
moderate cervical dysplasia (N87.1)

- **D06.0 Carcinoma in situ of endocervix** ♀
- **D06.1 Carcinoma in situ of exocervix** ♀
- **D06.7 Carcinoma in situ of other parts of cervix** ♀
- **D06.9 Carcinoma in situ of cervix, unspecified** ♀

D07 Carcinoma in situ of other and unspecified genital organs

EXCLUDES 1 *melanoma in situ of trunk (D03.5)*

- **D07.0 Carcinoma in situ of endometrium** ♀
- **D07.1 Carcinoma in situ of vulva** ♀
  Severe dysplasia of vulva
  Vulvar intraepithelial neoplasia III [VIN III]
  EXCLUDES 1 *moderate dysplasia of vulva (N90.1)*
  vulvar intraepithelial neoplasia II [VIN II] (N90.1)
- **D07.2 Carcinoma in situ of vagina** ♀
  Severe dysplasia of vagina
  Vaginal intraepithelial neoplasia III [VAIN III]
  EXCLUDES 1 *moderate dysplasia of vagina (N89.1)*
  vaginal intraepithelial neoplasia II [VIN II] (N89.1)
- **D07.3 Carcinoma in situ of other and unspecified female genital organs**
  - **D07.30 Carcinoma in situ of unspecified female genital organs** ♀
  - **D07.39 Carcinoma in situ of other female genital organs** ♀
- **D07.4 Carcinoma in situ of penis** ♂
  Erythroplasia of Queyrat NOS
- **D07.5 Carcinoma in situ of prostate** ♂
  Prostatic intraepithelial neoplasia III (PIN III)
  Severe dysplasia of prostate
  EXCLUDES 1 *dysplasia (mild) (moderate) of prostate (N42.3-)*
  prostatic intraepithelial neoplasia II [PIN II] (N42.3-)
- **D07.6 Carcinoma in situ of other and unspecified male genital organs**
  - **D07.60 Carcinoma in situ of unspecified male genital organs** ♂
  - **D07.61 Carcinoma in situ of scrotum** ♂
  - **D07.69 Carcinoma in situ of other male genital organs** ♂

D09 Carcinoma in situ of other and unspecified sites

EXCLUDES 1 *melanoma in situ (D03.-)*

- **D09.0 Carcinoma in situ of bladder**
- **D09.1 Carcinoma in situ of other and unspecified urinary organs**
  - **D09.10 Carcinoma in situ of unspecified urinary organ**
  - **D09.19 Carcinoma in situ of other urinary organs**
- **D09.2 Carcinoma in situ of eye**
  EXCLUDES 1 *carcinoma in situ of skin of eyelid (D04.1-)*
  - **D09.20 Carcinoma in situ of unspecified eye**
  - **D09.21 Carcinoma in situ of right eye**
  - **D09.22 Carcinoma in situ of left eye**
- **D09.3 Carcinoma in situ of thyroid and other endocrine glands**
  EXCLUDES 1 *carcinoma in situ of endocrine pancreas (D01.7)*
  carcinoma in situ of ovary (D07.39)
  carcinoma in situ of testis (D07.69)
- **D09.8 Carcinoma in situ of other specified sites**
- **D09.9 Carcinoma in situ, unspecified**

Benign neoplasms, except benign neuroendocrine tumors (D10-D36)

D10 Benign neoplasm of mouth and pharynx

- **D10.0 Benign neoplasm of lip**
  Benign neoplasm of lip (frenulum) (inner aspect) (mucosa) (vermilion border)
  EXCLUDES 1 *benign neoplasm of skin of lip (D22.0, D23.0)*
- **D10.1 Benign neoplasm of tongue**
  Benign neoplasm of lingual tonsil
- **D10.2 Benign neoplasm of floor of mouth**
- **D10.3 Benign neoplasm of other and unspecified parts of mouth**
  - **D10.30 Benign neoplasm of unspecified part of mouth**
  - **D10.39 Benign neoplasm of other parts of mouth**
    Benign neoplasm of minor salivary gland NOS
    EXCLUDES 1 *benign odontogenic neoplasms (D16.4-D16.5)*
    benign neoplasm of mucosa of lip (D10.0)
    benign neoplasm of nasopharyngeal surface of soft palate (D10.6)
- **D10.4 Benign neoplasm of tonsil**
  Benign neoplasm of tonsil (faucial) (palatine)
  EXCLUDES 1 *benign neoplasm of lingual tonsil (D10.1)*
  benign neoplasm of pharyngeal tonsil (D10.6)
  benign neoplasm of tonsillar fossa (D10.5)
  benign neoplasm of tonsillar pillars (D10.5)
- **D10.5 Benign neoplasm of other parts of oropharynx**
  Benign neoplasm of epiglottis, anterior aspect
  Benign neoplasm of tonsillar fossa
  Benign neoplasm of tonsillar pillars
  Benign neoplasm of vallecula
  EXCLUDES 1 *benign neoplasm of epiglottis NOS (D14.1)*
  benign neoplasm of epiglottis, suprahyoid portion (D14.1)
  DEF: Oropharynx: Middle portion of pharynx (throat); communicates with the oral cavity, nasopharynx and laryngopharynx.
- **D10.6 Benign neoplasm of nasopharynx**
  Benign neoplasm of pharyngeal tonsil
  Benign neoplasm of posterior margin of septum and choanae
  DEF: Nasopharynx: Upper portion of pharynx (throat); communicates with the nasal cavities, oropharynx and tympanic cavities.
- **D10.7 Benign neoplasm of hypopharynx**
  DEF: Hypopharynx: Lower portion of pharynx (throat); communicates with the oropharynx and the esophagus.
  Synonym(s): *laryngopharynx.*
- **D10.9 Benign neoplasm of pharynx, unspecified**

D11 Benign neoplasm of major salivary glands

EXCLUDES 1 *benign neoplasms of specified minor salivary glands which are classified according to their anatomical location*
benign neoplasms of minor salivary glands NOS (D10.39)

- **D11.0 Benign neoplasm of parotid gland**
- **D11.7 Benign neoplasm of other major salivary glands**
  Benign neoplasm of sublingual salivary gland
  Benign neoplasm of submandibular salivary gland
- **D11.9 Benign neoplasm of major salivary gland, unspecified**

D12 Benign neoplasm of colon, rectum, anus and anal canal

EXCLUDES 1 *benign carcinoid tumors of the large intestine, and rectum (D3A.02-)*
polyp of colon NOS (K63.5)

AHA: 2018,2Q,14; 2017,1Q,15; 2015,2Q,14

TIP: Code K63.5 Polyp of colon, is assigned when documentation states hyperplastic colon polyps, regardless of the site in the colon. Slow-growing, hyperplastic polyps are not precancerous and are classified differently from benign or adenomatous polyps.

- **D12.0 Benign neoplasm of cecum**
  Benign neoplasm of ileocecal valve

D12.1 Benign neoplasm of appendix
EXCLUDES 1 *benign carcinoid tumor of the appendix (D3A.020)*

D12.2 Benign neoplasm of ascending colon

D12.3 Benign neoplasm of transverse colon
Benign neoplasm of hepatic flexure
Benign neoplasm of splenic flexure
AHA: 2017,1Q,16

D12.4 Benign neoplasm of descending colon

D12.5 Benign neoplasm of sigmoid colon

D12.6 Benign neoplasm of colon, unspecified
Adenomatosis of colon
Benign neoplasm of large intestine NOS
Polyposis (hereditary) of colon
EXCLUDES 1 *inflammatory polyp of colon (K51.4-)*

D12.7 Benign neoplasm of rectosigmoid junction

D12.8 Benign neoplasm of rectum
EXCLUDES 1 *benign carcinoid tumor of the rectum (D3A.026)*
AHA: 2018,1Q,6

D12.9 Benign neoplasm of anus and anal canal
Benign neoplasm of anus NOS
EXCLUDES 1 *benign neoplasm of anal margin (D22.5, D23.5)*
benign neoplasm of anal skin (D22.5, D23.5)
benign neoplasm of perianal skin (D22.5, D23.5)

4th D13 Benign neoplasm of other and ill-defined parts of digestive system
EXCLUDES 1 *benign stromal tumors of digestive system (D21.4)*

D13.0 Benign neoplasm of esophagus

D13.1 Benign neoplasm of stomach
EXCLUDES 1 *benign carcinoid tumor of the stomach (D3A.092)*

D13.2 Benign neoplasm of duodenum
EXCLUDES 1 *benign carcinoid tumor of the duodenum (D3A.010)*

5th D13.3 Benign neoplasm of other and unspecified parts of small intestine
EXCLUDES 1 *benign carcinoid tumors of the small intestine (D3A.01-)*
benign neoplasm of ileocecal valve (D12.0)

D13.30 Benign neoplasm of unspecified part of small intestine

D13.39 Benign neoplasm of other parts of small intestine

D13.4 Benign neoplasm of liver
Benign neoplasm of intrahepatic bile ducts

D13.5 Benign neoplasm of extrahepatic bile ducts

D13.6 Benign neoplasm of pancreas
EXCLUDES 1 *benign neoplasm of endocrine pancreas (D13.7)*

D13.7 Benign neoplasm of endocrine pancreas
Benign neoplasm of islets of Langerhans
Islet cell tumor
Use additional code to identify any functional activity

D13.9 Benign neoplasm of ill-defined sites within the digestive system
Benign neoplasm of digestive system NOS
Benign neoplasm of intestine NOS
Benign neoplasm of spleen

4th D14 Benign neoplasm of middle ear and respiratory system

D14.0 Benign neoplasm of middle ear, nasal cavity and accessory sinuses
Benign neoplasm of cartilage of nose
EXCLUDES 1 *benign neoplasm of auricular canal (external) (D22.2-, D23.2-)*
benign neoplasm of bone of ear (D16.4)
benign neoplasm of bone of nose (D16.4)
benign neoplasm of cartilage of ear (D21.0)
benign neoplasm of ear (external)(skin) (D22.2-, D23.2-)
benign neoplasm of nose NOS (D36.7)
benign neoplasm of skin of nose (D22.39, D23.39)
benign neoplasm of olfactory bulb (D33.3)
benign neoplasm of posterior margin of septum and choanae (D10.6)
polyp of accessory sinus (J33.8)
polyp of ear (middle) (H74.4)
polyp of nasal (cavity) (J33.-)

D14.1 Benign neoplasm of larynx
Adenomatous polyp of larynx
Benign neoplasm of epiglottis (suprahyoid portion)
EXCLUDES 1 *benign neoplasm of epiglottis, anterior aspect (D10.5)*
polyp (nonadenomatous) of vocal cord or larynx (J38.1)

D14.2 Benign neoplasm of trachea

5th D14.3 Benign neoplasm of bronchus and lung
EXCLUDES 1 *benign carcinoid tumor of the bronchus and lung (D3A.090)*

D14.30 Benign neoplasm of unspecified bronchus and lung

D14.31 Benign neoplasm of right bronchus and lung

D14.32 Benign neoplasm of left bronchus and lung

D14.4 Benign neoplasm of respiratory system, unspecified

4th D15 Benign neoplasm of other and unspecified intrathoracic organs
EXCLUDES 1 *benign neoplasm of mesothelial tissue (D19.-)*

D15.0 Benign neoplasm of thymus
EXCLUDES 1 *benign carcinoid tumor of the thymus (D3A.091)*

D15.1 Benign neoplasm of heart COM
EXCLUDES 1 *benign neoplasm of great vessels (D21.3)*

D15.2 Benign neoplasm of mediastinum

D15.7 Benign neoplasm of other specified intrathoracic organs

D15.9 Benign neoplasm of intrathoracic organ, unspecified

4th D16 Benign neoplasm of bone and articular cartilage
EXCLUDES 1 *benign neoplasm of connective tissue of ear (D21.0)*
benign neoplasm of connective tissue of eyelid (D21.0)
benign neoplasm of connective tissue of larynx (D14.1)
benign neoplasm of connective tissue of nose (D14.0)
benign neoplasm of synovia (D21.-)

5th D16.0 Benign neoplasm of scapula and long bones of upper limb

D16.00 Benign neoplasm of scapula and long bones of unspecified upper limb

D16.01 Benign neoplasm of scapula and long bones of right upper limb

D16.02 Benign neoplasm of scapula and long bones of left upper limb

5th D16.1 Benign neoplasm of short bones of upper limb

D16.10 Benign neoplasm of short bones of unspecified upper limb

D16.11 Benign neoplasm of short bones of right upper limb

D16.12 Benign neoplasm of short bones of left upper limb

5th D16.2 Benign neoplasm of long bones of lower limb

D16.20 Benign neoplasm of long bones of unspecified lower limb

D16.21 Benign neoplasm of long bones of right lower limb

D16.22 Benign neoplasm of long bones of left lower limb

5th D16.3 Benign neoplasm of short bones of lower limb

D16.30 Benign neoplasm of short bones of unspecified lower limb

D16.31 Benign neoplasm of short bones of right lower limb

D16.32 Benign neoplasm of short bones of left lower limb

D16.4 Benign neoplasm of bones of skull and face
Benign neoplasm of maxilla (superior)
Benign neoplasm of orbital bone
Keratocyst of maxilla
Keratocystic odontogenic tumor of maxilla
EXCLUDES 2 *benign neoplasm of lower jaw bone (D16.5)*

D16.5 Benign neoplasm of lower jaw bone
Keratocyst of mandible
Keratocystic odontogenic tumor of mandible

D16.6 Benign neoplasm of vertebral column
EXCLUDES 1 *benign neoplasm of sacrum and coccyx (D16.8)*

D16.7 Benign neoplasm of ribs, sternum and clavicle

D16.8 Benign neoplasm of pelvic bones, sacrum and coccyx

D16.9 Benign neoplasm of bone and articular cartilage, unspecified

4th D17 Benign lipomatous neoplasm

D17.0 Benign lipomatous neoplasm of skin and subcutaneous tissue of head, face and neck

D17.1 Benign lipomatous neoplasm of skin and subcutaneous tissue of trunk

5th D17.2 Benign lipomatous neoplasm of skin and subcutaneous tissue of limb

D17.20 Benign lipomatous neoplasm of skin and subcutaneous tissue of unspecified limb

D17.21 **Benign lipomatous neoplasm of skin and subcutaneous tissue of right arm**
D17.22 **Benign lipomatous neoplasm of skin and subcutaneous tissue of left arm**
D17.23 **Benign lipomatous neoplasm of skin and subcutaneous tissue of right leg**
D17.24 **Benign lipomatous neoplasm of skin and subcutaneous tissue of left leg**

✓5th **D17.3 Benign lipomatous neoplasm of skin and subcutaneous tissue of other and unspecified sites**
D17.3Ø **Benign lipomatous neoplasm of skin and subcutaneous tissue of unspecified sites**
D17.39 **Benign lipomatous neoplasm of skin and subcutaneous tissue of other sites**

D17.4 Benign lipomatous neoplasm of intrathoracic organs
D17.5 Benign lipomatous neoplasm of intra-abdominal organs
EXCLUDES 1 *benign lipomatous neoplasm of peritoneum and retroperitoneum (D17.79)*
D17.6 Benign lipomatous neoplasm of spermatic cord ♂
✓5th **D17.7 Benign lipomatous neoplasm of other sites**
D17.71 **Benign lipomatous neoplasm of kidney**
D17.72 **Benign lipomatous neoplasm of other genitourinary organ**
D17.79 **Benign lipomatous neoplasm of other sites**
Benign lipomatous neoplasm of peritoneum
Benign lipomatous neoplasm of retroperitoneum
D17.9 Benign lipomatous neoplasm, unspecified
Lipoma NOS

✓4th **D18 Hemangioma and lymphangioma, any site**
EXCLUDES 1 *benign neoplasm of glomus jugulare (D35.6)*
blue or pigmented nevus (D22.-)
nevus NOS (D22.-)
vascular nevus (Q82.5)

✓5th **D18.Ø Hemangioma**
Angioma NOS
Cavernous nevus
DEF: Common benign tumor usually occurring in infancy that is composed of newly formed blood vessels due to malformation of the angioblastic tissue.
D18.ØØ **Hemangioma unspecified site**
D18.Ø1 **Hemangioma of skin and subcutaneous tissue**
D18.Ø2 **Hemangioma of intracranial structures** HCC Rx ESR COM
D18.Ø3 **Hemangioma of intra-abdominal structures**
D18.Ø9 **Hemangioma of other sites**
D18.1 Lymphangioma, any site
AHA: 2018,3Q,31; 2018,2Q,13

✓4th **D19 Benign neoplasm of mesothelial tissue**
D19.Ø Benign neoplasm of mesothelial tissue of pleura
D19.1 Benign neoplasm of mesothelial tissue of peritoneum
D19.7 Benign neoplasm of mesothelial tissue of other sites
D19.9 Benign neoplasm of mesothelial tissue, unspecified
Benign mesothelioma NOS

✓4th **D2Ø Benign neoplasm of soft tissue of retroperitoneum and peritoneum**
EXCLUDES 1 *benign lipomatous neoplasm of peritoneum and retroperitoneum (D17.79)*
benign neoplasm of mesothelial tissue (D19.-)
D2Ø.Ø Benign neoplasm of soft tissue of retroperitoneum
D2Ø.1 Benign neoplasm of soft tissue of peritoneum

✓4th **D21 Other benign neoplasms of connective and other soft tissue**
INCLUDES benign neoplasm of blood vessel
benign neoplasm of bursa
benign neoplasm of cartilage
benign neoplasm of fascia
benign neoplasm of fat
benign neoplasm of ligament, except uterine
benign neoplasm of lymphatic channel
benign neoplasm of muscle
benign neoplasm of synovia
benign neoplasm of tendon (sheath)
benign stromal tumors
EXCLUDES 1 *benign neoplasm of articular cartilage (D16.-)*
benign neoplasm of cartilage of larynx (D14.1)
benign neoplasm of cartilage of nose (D14.Ø)
benign neoplasm of connective tissue of breast (D24.-)
benign neoplasm of peripheral nerves and autonomic nervous system (D36.1-)
benign neoplasm of peritoneum (D2Ø.1)
benign neoplasm of retroperitoneum (D2Ø.Ø)
benign neoplasm of uterine ligament, any (D28.2)
benign neoplasm of vascular tissue (D18.-)
hemangioma (D18.Ø-)
lipomatous neoplasm (D17.-)
lymphangioma (D18.1)
uterine leiomyoma (D25.-)

D21.Ø Benign neoplasm of connective and other soft tissue of head, face and neck
Benign neoplasm of connective tissue of ear
Benign neoplasm of connective tissue of eyelid
EXCLUDES 1 *benign neoplasm of connective tissue of orbit (D31.6-)*
✓5th **D21.1 Benign neoplasm of connective and other soft tissue of upper limb, including shoulder**
D21.1Ø **Benign neoplasm of connective and other soft tissue of unspecified upper limb, including shoulder**
D21.11 **Benign neoplasm of connective and other soft tissue of right upper limb, including shoulder**
D21.12 **Benign neoplasm of connective and other soft tissue of left upper limb, including shoulder**
✓5th **D21.2 Benign neoplasm of connective and other soft tissue of lower limb, including hip**
D21.2Ø **Benign neoplasm of connective and other soft tissue of unspecified lower limb, including hip**
D21.21 **Benign neoplasm of connective and other soft tissue of right lower limb, including hip**
D21.22 **Benign neoplasm of connective and other soft tissue of left lower limb, including hip**
D21.3 Benign neoplasm of connective and other soft tissue of thorax
Benign neoplasm of axilla
Benign neoplasm of diaphragm
Benign neoplasm of great vessels
EXCLUDES 1 *benign neoplasm of heart (D15.1)*
benign neoplasm of mediastinum (D15.2)
benign neoplasm of thymus (D15.Ø)
D21.4 Benign neoplasm of connective and other soft tissue of abdomen
Benign stromal tumors of abdomen
D21.5 Benign neoplasm of connective and other soft tissue of pelvis
EXCLUDES 1 *benign neoplasm of any uterine ligament (D28.2)*
uterine leiomyoma (D25.-)
D21.6 Benign neoplasm of connective and other soft tissue of trunk, unspecified
Benign neoplasm of connective and other soft tissue of back NOS
D21.9 Benign neoplasm of connective and other soft tissue, unspecified

✓4th **D22 Melanocytic nevi**
INCLUDES atypical nevus
blue hairy pigmented nevus
nevus NOS
D22.Ø Melanocytic nevi of lip
✓5th **D22.1 Melanocytic nevi of eyelid, including canthus**
AHA: 2018,4Q,4
D22.1Ø **Melanocytic nevi of unspecified eyelid, including canthus**

D22.11 Melanocytic nevi of right eyelid, including canthus
D22.111 Melanocytic nevi of right upper eyelid, including canthus
D22.112 Melanocytic nevi of right lower eyelid, including canthus
D22.12 Melanocytic nevi of left eyelid, including canthus
D22.121 Melanocytic nevi of left upper eyelid, including canthus
D22.122 Melanocytic nevi of left lower eyelid, including canthus
D22.2 Melanocytic nevi of ear and external auricular canal
D22.20 Melanocytic nevi of unspecified ear and external auricular canal
D22.21 Melanocytic nevi of right ear and external auricular canal
D22.22 Melanocytic nevi of left ear and external auricular canal
D22.3 Melanocytic nevi of other and unspecified parts of face
D22.30 Melanocytic nevi of unspecified part of face
D22.39 Melanocytic nevi of other parts of face
D22.4 Melanocytic nevi of scalp and neck
D22.5 Melanocytic nevi of trunk
Melanocytic nevi of anal margin
Melanocytic nevi of anal skin
Melanocytic nevi of perianal skin
Melanocytic nevi of skin of breast
D22.6 Melanocytic nevi of upper limb, including shoulder
D22.60 Melanocytic nevi of unspecified upper limb, including shoulder
D22.61 Melanocytic nevi of right upper limb, including shoulder
D22.62 Melanocytic nevi of left upper limb, including shoulder
D22.7 Melanocytic nevi of lower limb, including hip
D22.70 Melanocytic nevi of unspecified lower limb, including hip
D22.71 Melanocytic nevi of right lower limb, including hip
D22.72 Melanocytic nevi of left lower limb, including hip
D22.9 Melanocytic nevi, unspecified

D23 Other benign neoplasms of skin
INCLUDES benign neoplasm of hair follicles
benign neoplasm of sebaceous glands
benign neoplasm of sweat glands
EXCLUDES 1 *benign lipomatous neoplasms of skin (D17.0-D17.3)*
EXCLUDES 2 *melanocytic nevi (D22.-)*

D23.0 Other benign neoplasm of skin of lip
EXCLUDES 1 *benign neoplasm of vermilion border of lip (D10.0)*
D23.1 Other benign neoplasm of skin of eyelid, including canthus
AHA: 2018,4Q,4
D23.10 Other benign neoplasm of skin of unspecified eyelid, including canthus
D23.11 Other benign neoplasm of skin of right eyelid, including canthus
D23.111 Other benign neoplasm of skin of right upper eyelid, including canthus
D23.112 Other benign neoplasm of skin of right lower eyelid, including canthus
D23.12 Other benign neoplasm of skin of left eyelid, including canthus
D23.121 Other benign neoplasm of skin of left upper eyelid, including canthus
D23.122 Other benign neoplasm of skin of left lower eyelid, including canthus
D23.2 Other benign neoplasm of skin of ear and external auricular canal
D23.20 Other benign neoplasm of skin of unspecified ear and external auricular canal
D23.21 Other benign neoplasm of skin of right ear and external auricular canal
D23.22 Other benign neoplasm of skin of left ear and external auricular canal
D23.3 Other benign neoplasm of skin of other and unspecified parts of face
D23.30 Other benign neoplasm of skin of unspecified part of face
D23.39 Other benign neoplasm of skin of other parts of face
D23.4 Other benign neoplasm of skin of scalp and neck
D23.5 Other benign neoplasm of skin of trunk
Other benign neoplasm of anal margin
Other benign neoplasm of anal skin
Other benign neoplasm of perianal skin
Other benign neoplasm of skin of breast
EXCLUDES 1 *benign neoplasm of anus NOS (D12.9)*
D23.6 Other benign neoplasm of skin of upper limb, including shoulder
D23.60 Other benign neoplasm of skin of unspecified upper limb, including shoulder
D23.61 Other benign neoplasm of skin of right upper limb, including shoulder
D23.62 Other benign neoplasm of skin of left upper limb, including shoulder
D23.7 Other benign neoplasm of skin of lower limb, including hip
D23.70 Other benign neoplasm of skin of unspecified lower limb, including hip
D23.71 Other benign neoplasm of skin of right lower limb, including hip
D23.72 Other benign neoplasm of skin of left lower limb, including hip
D23.9 Other benign neoplasm of skin, unspecified

D24 Benign neoplasm of breast
INCLUDES benign neoplasm of connective tissue of breast
benign neoplasm of soft parts of breast
fibroadenoma of breast
EXCLUDES 2 *adenofibrosis of breast (N60.2)*
benign cyst of breast (N60.-)
benign mammary dysplasia (N60.-)
benign neoplasm of skin of breast (D22.5, D23.5)
fibrocystic disease of breast (N60.-)
D24.1 Benign neoplasm of right breast
D24.2 Benign neoplasm of left breast
D24.9 Benign neoplasm of unspecified breast

D25 Leiomyoma of uterus
INCLUDES uterine fibroid
uterine fibromyoma
uterine myoma

Uterine Leiomyomas (Fibroids)

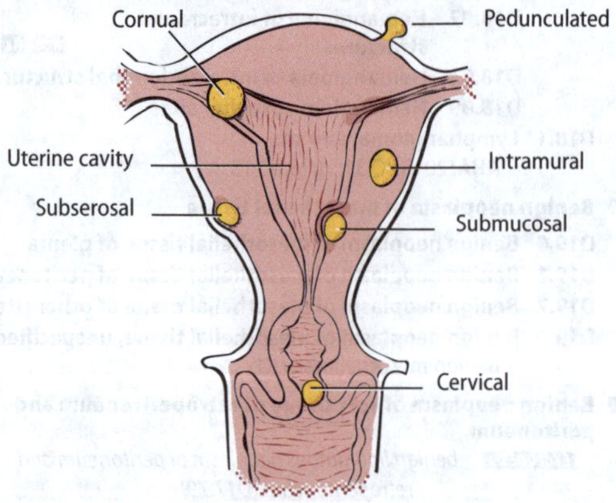

D25.0 Submucous leiomyoma of uterus ♀
D25.1 Intramural leiomyoma of uterus ♀
Interstitial leiomyoma of uterus
D25.2 Subserosal leiomyoma of uterus ♀
Subperitoneal leiomyoma of uterus
D25.9 Leiomyoma of uterus, unspecified ♀

D26 Other benign neoplasms of uterus
D26.0 Other benign neoplasm of cervix uteri ♀
D26.1 Other benign neoplasm of corpus uteri ♀
D26.7 Other benign neoplasm of other parts of uterus ♀
D26.9 Other benign neoplasm of uterus, unspecified ♀

D27 Benign neoplasm of ovary
Use additional code to identify any functional activity
EXCLUDES 2 *corpus albicans cyst (N83.2-)*
corpus luteum cyst (N83.1-)
endometrial cyst ▶(N80.1-)◀
follicular (atretic) cyst (N83.0-)
graafian follicle cyst (N83.0-)
ovarian cyst NEC (N83.2-)
ovarian retention cyst (N83.2-)
D27.0 Benign neoplasm of right ovary ♀
D27.1 Benign neoplasm of left ovary ♀
D27.9 Benign neoplasm of unspecified ovary ♀

D28 Benign neoplasm of other and unspecified female genital organs
INCLUDES adenomatous polyp
benign neoplasm of skin of female genital organs
benign teratoma
EXCLUDES 1 *epoophoron cyst (Q50.5)*
fimbrial cyst (Q50.4)
Gartner's duct cyst (Q52.4)
parovarian cyst (Q50.5)
D28.0 Benign neoplasm of vulva ♀
D28.1 Benign neoplasm of vagina ♀
D28.2 Benign neoplasm of uterine tubes and ligaments ♀
Benign neoplasm of fallopian tube
Benign neoplasm of uterine ligament (broad) (round)
D28.7 Benign neoplasm of other specified female genital organs ♀
D28.9 Benign neoplasm of female genital organ, unspecified ♀

D29 Benign neoplasm of male genital organs
INCLUDES benign neoplasm of skin of male genital organs
D29.0 Benign neoplasm of penis ♂
D29.1 Benign neoplasm of prostate ♂
EXCLUDES 1 *enlarged prostate (N40.-)*
D29.2 Benign neoplasm of testis
Use additional code to identify any functional activity
D29.20 Benign neoplasm of unspecified testis ♂
D29.21 Benign neoplasm of right testis ♂
D29.22 Benign neoplasm of left testis ♂
D29.3 Benign neoplasm of epididymis
D29.30 Benign neoplasm of unspecified epididymis ♂
D29.31 Benign neoplasm of right epididymis ♂
D29.32 Benign neoplasm of left epididymis ♂
D29.4 Benign neoplasm of scrotum ♂
Benign neoplasm of skin of scrotum
D29.8 Benign neoplasm of other specified male genital organs ♂
Benign neoplasm of seminal vesicle
Benign neoplasm of spermatic cord
Benign neoplasm of tunica vaginalis
D29.9 Benign neoplasm of male genital organ, unspecified ♂

D30 Benign neoplasm of urinary organs
D30.0 Benign neoplasm of kidney
EXCLUDES 1 *benign carcinoid tumor of the kidney (D3A.093)*
benign neoplasm of renal calyces (D30.1-)
benign neoplasm of renal pelvis (D30.1-)
D30.00 Benign neoplasm of unspecified kidney
D30.01 Benign neoplasm of right kidney
D30.02 Benign neoplasm of left kidney
D30.1 Benign neoplasm of renal pelvis
D30.10 Benign neoplasm of unspecified renal pelvis
D30.11 Benign neoplasm of right renal pelvis
D30.12 Benign neoplasm of left renal pelvis
D30.2 Benign neoplasm of ureter
EXCLUDES 1 *benign neoplasm of ureteric orifice of bladder (D30.3)*
D30.20 Benign neoplasm of unspecified ureter
D30.21 Benign neoplasm of right ureter
D30.22 Benign neoplasm of left ureter
D30.3 Benign neoplasm of bladder
Benign neoplasm of ureteric orifice of bladder
Benign neoplasm of urethral orifice of bladder
D30.4 Benign neoplasm of urethra
EXCLUDES 1 *benign neoplasm of urethral orifice of bladder (D30.3)*
D30.8 Benign neoplasm of other specified urinary organs
Benign neoplasm of paraurethral glands
D30.9 Benign neoplasm of urinary organ, unspecified
Benign neoplasm of urinary system NOS

D31 Benign neoplasm of eye and adnexa
EXCLUDES 1 *benign neoplasm of connective tissue of eyelid (D21.0)*
benign neoplasm of optic nerve (D33.3)
benign neoplasm of skin of eyelid (D22.1-, D23.1-)
D31.0 Benign neoplasm of conjunctiva
D31.00 Benign neoplasm of unspecified conjunctiva
D31.01 Benign neoplasm of right conjunctiva
D31.02 Benign neoplasm of left conjunctiva
D31.1 Benign neoplasm of cornea
D31.10 Benign neoplasm of unspecified cornea
D31.11 Benign neoplasm of right cornea
D31.12 Benign neoplasm of left cornea
D31.2 Benign neoplasm of retina
EXCLUDES 1 *dark area on retina (D49.81)*
hemangioma of retina (D49.81)
neoplasm of unspecified behavior of retina and choroid (D49.81)
retinal freckle (D49.81)
D31.20 Benign neoplasm of unspecified retina
D31.21 Benign neoplasm of right retina
D31.22 Benign neoplasm of left retina
D31.3 Benign neoplasm of choroid
D31.30 Benign neoplasm of unspecified choroid
D31.31 Benign neoplasm of right choroid
D31.32 Benign neoplasm of left choroid
D31.4 Benign neoplasm of ciliary body
D31.40 Benign neoplasm of unspecified ciliary body
D31.41 Benign neoplasm of right ciliary body
D31.42 Benign neoplasm of left ciliary body
D31.5 Benign neoplasm of lacrimal gland and duct
Benign neoplasm of lacrimal sac
Benign neoplasm of nasolacrimal duct
D31.50 Benign neoplasm of unspecified lacrimal gland and duct
D31.51 Benign neoplasm of right lacrimal gland and duct
D31.52 Benign neoplasm of left lacrimal gland and duct
D31.6 Benign neoplasm of unspecified site of orbit
Benign neoplasm of connective tissue of orbit
Benign neoplasm of extraocular muscle
Benign neoplasm of peripheral nerves of orbit
Benign neoplasm of retrobulbar tissue
Benign neoplasm of retro-ocular tissue
EXCLUDES 1 *benign neoplasm of orbital bone (D16.4)*
D31.60 Benign neoplasm of unspecified site of unspecified orbit
D31.61 Benign neoplasm of unspecified site of right orbit
D31.62 Benign neoplasm of unspecified site of left orbit
D31.9 Benign neoplasm of unspecified part of eye
Benign neoplasm of eyeball
D31.90 Benign neoplasm of unspecified part of unspecified eye
D31.91 Benign neoplasm of unspecified part of right eye
D31.92 Benign neoplasm of unspecified part of left eye

D32 Benign neoplasm of meninges
D32.0 Benign neoplasm of cerebral meninges HCC Rx ESR COM
D32.1 Benign neoplasm of spinal meninges HCC Rx ESR COM
D32.9 Benign neoplasm of meninges, unspecified HCC Rx ESR COM
Meningioma NOS

D33 Benign neoplasm of brain and other parts of central nervous system

EXCLUDES 1 *angioma (D18.Ø-)*
benign neoplasm of meninges (D32.-)
benign neoplasm of peripheral nerves and autonomic nervous system (D36.1-)
hemangioma (D18.Ø-)
neurofibromatosis (Q85.Ø-)
retro-ocular benign neoplasm (D31.6-)

D33.Ø Benign neoplasm of brain, supratentorial HCC Rx ESR COM
Benign neoplasm of cerebral ventricle
Benign neoplasm of cerebrum
Benign neoplasm of frontal lobe
Benign neoplasm of occipital lobe
Benign neoplasm of parietal lobe
Benign neoplasm of temporal lobe
EXCLUDES 1 *benign neoplasm of fourth ventricle (D33.1)*

D33.1 Benign neoplasm of brain, infratentorial HCC Rx ESR COM
Benign neoplasm of brain stem
Benign neoplasm of cerebellum
Benign neoplasm of fourth ventricle

D33.2 Benign neoplasm of brain, unspecified HCC Rx ESR COM

D33.3 Benign neoplasm of cranial nerves HCC Rx ESR COM
Benign neoplasm of olfactory bulb

D33.4 Benign neoplasm of spinal cord HCC Rx ESR COM

D33.7 Benign neoplasm of other specified parts of central nervous system HCC Rx ESR COM

D33.9 Benign neoplasm of central nervous system, unspecified HCC Rx ESR COM
Benign neoplasm of nervous system (central) NOS

D34 Benign neoplasm of thyroid gland
Use additional code to identify any functional activity

D35 Benign neoplasm of other and unspecified endocrine glands
Use additional code to identify any functional activity
EXCLUDES 1 *benign neoplasm of endocrine pancreas (D13.7)*
benign neoplasm of ovary (D27.-)
benign neoplasm of testis (D29.2.-)
benign neoplasm of thymus (D15.Ø)

D35.Ø Benign neoplasm of adrenal gland
D35.ØØ Benign neoplasm of unspecified adrenal gland
D35.Ø1 Benign neoplasm of right adrenal gland
D35.Ø2 Benign neoplasm of left adrenal gland

D35.1 Benign neoplasm of parathyroid gland

D35.2 Benign neoplasm of pituitary gland HCC Rx ESR COM
AHA: 2014,3Q,22

D35.3 Benign neoplasm of craniopharyngeal duct HCC Rx ESR COM

D35.4 Benign neoplasm of pineal gland HCC Rx ESR COM

D35.5 Benign neoplasm of carotid body

D35.6 Benign neoplasm of aortic body and other paraganglia
Benign tumor of glomus jugulare

D35.7 Benign neoplasm of other specified endocrine glands

D35.9 Benign neoplasm of endocrine gland, unspecified
Benign neoplasm of unspecified endocrine gland

D36 Benign neoplasm of other and unspecified sites

D36.Ø Benign neoplasm of lymph nodes
EXCLUDES 1 *lymphangioma (D18.1)*

D36.1 Benign neoplasm of peripheral nerves and autonomic nervous system
EXCLUDES 1 *benign neoplasm of peripheral nerves of orbit (D31.6-)*
neurofibromatosis (Q85.Ø-)

D36.1Ø Benign neoplasm of peripheral nerves and autonomic nervous system, unspecified
D36.11 Benign neoplasm of peripheral nerves and autonomic nervous system of face, head, and neck
D36.12 Benign neoplasm of peripheral nerves and autonomic nervous system, upper limb, including shoulder
D36.13 Benign neoplasm of peripheral nerves and autonomic nervous system of lower limb, including hip
D36.14 Benign neoplasm of peripheral nerves and autonomic nervous system of thorax
D36.15 Benign neoplasm of peripheral nerves and autonomic nervous system of abdomen
D36.16 Benign neoplasm of peripheral nerves and autonomic nervous system of pelvis
D36.17 Benign neoplasm of peripheral nerves and autonomic nervous system of trunk, unspecified

D36.7 Benign neoplasm of other specified sites
Benign neoplasm of back NOS
Benign neoplasm of nose NOS

D36.9 Benign neoplasm, unspecified site

Benign neuroendocrine tumors (D3A)

D3A Benign neuroendocrine tumors
Code also any associated multiple endocrine neoplasia [MEN] syndromes (E31.2-)
Use additional code to identify any associated endocrine syndrome, such as:
carcinoid syndrome (E34.Ø)
EXCLUDES 2 *benign pancreatic islet cell tumors (D13.7)*

D3A.Ø Benign carcinoid tumors
DEF: Specific type of slow-growing neuroendocrine tumors. Carcinoid tumors occur most commonly in the hormone producing cells of the gastrointestinal tracts and can also occur in the pancreas, testes, ovaries, or lungs.

D3A.ØØ Benign carcinoid tumor of unspecified site Rx
Carcinoid tumor NOS

D3A.Ø1 Benign carcinoid tumors of the small intestine
D3A.Ø1Ø Benign carcinoid tumor of the duodenum Rx
D3A.Ø11 Benign carcinoid tumor of the jejunum Rx
D3A.Ø12 Benign carcinoid tumor of the ileum Rx
D3A.Ø19 Benign carcinoid tumor of the small intestine, unspecified portion Rx

D3A.Ø2 Benign carcinoid tumors of the appendix, large intestine, and rectum
D3A.Ø2Ø Benign carcinoid tumor of the appendix Rx
D3A.Ø21 Benign carcinoid tumor of the cecum Rx
D3A.Ø22 Benign carcinoid tumor of the ascending colon Rx
D3A.Ø23 Benign carcinoid tumor of the transverse colon Rx
D3A.Ø24 Benign carcinoid tumor of the descending colon Rx
D3A.Ø25 Benign carcinoid tumor of the sigmoid colon Rx
D3A.Ø26 Benign carcinoid tumor of the rectum Rx
D3A.Ø29 Benign carcinoid tumor of the large intestine, unspecified portion Rx
Benign carcinoid tumor of the colon NOS

D3A.Ø9 Benign carcinoid tumors of other sites
D3A.Ø9Ø Benign carcinoid tumor of the bronchus and lung Rx
D3A.Ø91 Benign carcinoid tumor of the thymus Rx
D3A.Ø92 Benign carcinoid tumor of the stomach Rx
D3A.Ø93 Benign carcinoid tumor of the kidney Rx
D3A.Ø94 Benign carcinoid tumor of the foregut, unspecified Rx
D3A.Ø95 Benign carcinoid tumor of the midgut, unspecified Rx
D3A.Ø96 Benign carcinoid tumor of the hindgut, unspecified Rx
D3A.Ø98 Benign carcinoid tumors of other sites Rx

D3A.8 Other benign neuroendocrine tumors Rx
Neuroendocrine tumor NOS

Neoplasms of uncertain behavior, polycythemia vera and myelodysplastic syndromes (D37-D48)

NOTE Categories D37-D44, and D48 classify by site neoplasms of uncertain behavior, i.e., histologic confirmation whether the neoplasm is malignant or benign cannot be made.

EXCLUDES 1 *neoplasms of unspecified behavior (D49.-)*

D37 Neoplasm of uncertain behavior of oral cavity and digestive organs

EXCLUDES 1 *stromal tumors of uncertain behavior of digestive system (D48.1)*

D37.Ø Neoplasm of uncertain behavior of lip, oral cavity and pharynx

EXCLUDES 1 *neoplasm of uncertain behavior of aryepiglottic fold or interarytenoid fold, laryngeal aspect (D38.Ø)*
neoplasm of uncertain behavior of epiglottis NOS (D38.Ø)
neoplasm of uncertain behavior of skin of lip (D48.5)
neoplasm of uncertain behavior of suprahyoid portion of epiglottis (D38.Ø)

D37.Ø1 Neoplasm of uncertain behavior of lip
Neoplasm of uncertain behavior of vermilion border of lip

D37.Ø2 Neoplasm of uncertain behavior of tongue

D37.Ø3 Neoplasm of uncertain behavior of the major salivary glands

D37.Ø3Ø Neoplasm of uncertain behavior of the parotid salivary glands

D37.Ø31 Neoplasm of uncertain behavior of the sublingual salivary glands

D37.Ø32 Neoplasm of uncertain behavior of the submandibular salivary glands

D37.Ø39 Neoplasm of uncertain behavior of the major salivary glands, unspecified

D37.Ø4 Neoplasm of uncertain behavior of the minor salivary glands
Neoplasm of uncertain behavior of submucosal salivary glands of lip
Neoplasm of uncertain behavior of submucosal salivary glands of cheek
Neoplasm of uncertain behavior of submucosal salivary glands of hard palate
Neoplasm of uncertain behavior of submucosal salivary glands of soft palate

D37.Ø5 Neoplasm of uncertain behavior of pharynx
Neoplasm of uncertain behavior of aryepiglottic fold of pharynx NOS
Neoplasm of uncertain behavior of hypopharyngeal aspect of aryepiglottic fold of pharynx
Neoplasm of uncertain behavior of marginal zone of aryepiglottic fold of pharynx

D37.Ø9 Neoplasm of uncertain behavior of other specified sites of the oral cavity

D37.1 Neoplasm of uncertain behavior of stomach

D37.2 Neoplasm of uncertain behavior of small intestine

D37.3 Neoplasm of uncertain behavior of appendix

D37.4 Neoplasm of uncertain behavior of colon

D37.5 Neoplasm of uncertain behavior of rectum
Neoplasm of uncertain behavior of rectosigmoid junction

D37.6 Neoplasm of uncertain behavior of liver, gallbladder and bile ducts
Neoplasm of uncertain behavior of ampulla of Vater

D37.8 Neoplasm of uncertain behavior of other specified digestive organs
Neoplasm of uncertain behavior of anal canal
Neoplasm of uncertain behavior of anal sphincter
Neoplasm of uncertain behavior of anus NOS
Neoplasm of uncertain behavior of esophagus
Neoplasm of uncertain behavior of intestine NOS
Neoplasm of uncertain behavior of pancreas

EXCLUDES 1 *neoplasm of uncertain behavior of anal margin (D48.5)*
neoplasm of uncertain behavior of anal skin (D48.5)
neoplasm of uncertain behavior of perianal skin (D48.5)

D37.9 Neoplasm of uncertain behavior of digestive organ, unspecified

D38 Neoplasm of uncertain behavior of middle ear and respiratory and intrathoracic organs

EXCLUDES 1 *neoplasm of uncertain behavior of heart (D48.7)*

D38.Ø Neoplasm of uncertain behavior of larynx
Neoplasm of uncertain behavior of aryepiglottic fold or interarytenoid fold, laryngeal aspect
Neoplasm of uncertain behavior of epiglottis (suprahyoid portion)

EXCLUDES 1 *neoplasm of uncertain behavior of aryepiglottic fold or interarytenoid fold NOS (D37.Ø5)*
neoplasm of uncertain behavior of hypopharyngeal aspect of aryepiglottic fold (D37.Ø5)
neoplasm of uncertain behavior of marginal zone of aryepiglottic fold (D37.Ø5)

D38.1 Neoplasm of uncertain behavior of trachea, bronchus and lung

D38.2 Neoplasm of uncertain behavior of pleura

D38.3 Neoplasm of uncertain behavior of mediastinum

D38.4 Neoplasm of uncertain behavior of thymus

D38.5 Neoplasm of uncertain behavior of other respiratory organs
Neoplasm of uncertain behavior of accessory sinuses
Neoplasm of uncertain behavior of cartilage of nose
Neoplasm of uncertain behavior of middle ear
Neoplasm of uncertain behavior of nasal cavities

EXCLUDES 1 *neoplasm of uncertain behavior of ear (external) (skin) (D48.5)*
neoplasm of uncertain behavior of nose NOS (D48.7)
neoplasm of uncertain behavior of skin of nose (D48.5)

D38.6 Neoplasm of uncertain behavior of respiratory organ, unspecified

D39 Neoplasm of uncertain behavior of female genital organs

D39.Ø Neoplasm of uncertain behavior of uterus ♀

D39.1 Neoplasm of uncertain behavior of ovary
Use additional code to identify any functional activity

D39.1Ø Neoplasm of uncertain behavior of unspecified ovary ♀

D39.11 Neoplasm of uncertain behavior of right ovary ♀

D39.12 Neoplasm of uncertain behavior of left ovary ♀

D39.2 Neoplasm of uncertain behavior of placenta M ♀
Chorioadenoma destruens
Invasive hydatidiform mole
Malignant hydatidiform mole

EXCLUDES 1 *hydatidiform mole NOS (OØ1.9)*

D39.8 Neoplasm of uncertain behavior of other specified female genital organs ♀
Neoplasm of uncertain behavior of skin of female genital organs

D39.9 Neoplasm of uncertain behavior of female genital organ, unspecified ♀

D4Ø Neoplasm of uncertain behavior of male genital organs

D4Ø.Ø Neoplasm of uncertain behavior of prostate ♂

D4Ø.1 Neoplasm of uncertain behavior of testis

D4Ø.1Ø Neoplasm of uncertain behavior of unspecified testis ♂

D4Ø.11 Neoplasm of uncertain behavior of right testis ♂

D4Ø.12 Neoplasm of uncertain behavior of left testis ♂

D4Ø.8 Neoplasm of uncertain behavior of other specified male genital organs ♂
Neoplasm of uncertain behavior of skin of male genital organs

D4Ø.9 Neoplasm of uncertain behavior of male genital organ, unspecified ♂

D41 Neoplasm of uncertain behavior of urinary organs

D41.Ø Neoplasm of uncertain behavior of kidney

EXCLUDES 1 *neoplasm of uncertain behavior of renal pelvis (D41.1-)*

D41.ØØ Neoplasm of uncertain behavior of unspecified kidney

D41.Ø1 Neoplasm of uncertain behavior of right kidney

D41.Ø2 Neoplasm of uncertain behavior of left kidney

D41.1 Neoplasm of uncertain behavior of renal pelvis

D41.1Ø Neoplasm of uncertain behavior of unspecified renal pelvis

D41.11 Neoplasm of uncertain behavior of right renal pelvis

D41.12 Neoplasm of uncertain behavior of left renal pelvis

√5th **D41.2 Neoplasm of uncertain behavior of ureter**

D41.2Ø Neoplasm of uncertain behavior of unspecified ureter

D41.21 Neoplasm of uncertain behavior of right ureter

D41.22 Neoplasm of uncertain behavior of left ureter

D41.3 Neoplasm of uncertain behavior of urethra

D41.4 Neoplasm of uncertain behavior of bladder

D41.8 Neoplasm of uncertain behavior of other specified urinary organs

D41.9 Neoplasm of uncertain behavior of unspecified urinary organ

√4th **D42 Neoplasm of uncertain behavior of meninges**

D42.Ø Neoplasm of uncertain behavior of cerebral meninges HCC Rx ESR COM

D42.1 Neoplasm of uncertain behavior of spinal meninges HCC Rx ESR COM

D42.9 Neoplasm of uncertain behavior of meninges, unspecified HCC Rx ESR COM

√4th **D43 Neoplasm of uncertain behavior of brain and central nervous system**

EXCLUDES 1 *neoplasm of uncertain behavior of peripheral nerves and autonomic nervous system (D48.2)*

D43.Ø Neoplasm of uncertain behavior of brain, supratentorial HCC Rx ESR COM

Neoplasm of uncertain behavior of cerebral ventricle
Neoplasm of uncertain behavior of cerebrum
Neoplasm of uncertain behavior of frontal lobe
Neoplasm of uncertain behavior of occipital lobe
Neoplasm of uncertain behavior of parietal lobe
Neoplasm of uncertain behavior of temporal lobe

EXCLUDES 1 *neoplasm of uncertain behavior of fourth ventricle (D43.1)*

D43.1 Neoplasm of uncertain behavior of brain, infratentorial HCC Rx ESR COM

Neoplasm of uncertain behavior of brain stem
Neoplasm of uncertain behavior of cerebellum
Neoplasm of uncertain behavior of fourth ventricle

D43.2 Neoplasm of uncertain behavior of brain, unspecified HCC Rx ESR COM

D43.3 Neoplasm of uncertain behavior of cranial nerves HCC Rx ESR COM

D43.4 Neoplasm of uncertain behavior of spinal cord HCC Rx ESR COM

D43.8 Neoplasm of uncertain behavior of other specified parts of central nervous system HCC Rx ESR COM

D43.9 Neoplasm of uncertain behavior of central nervous system, unspecified HCC Rx ESR COM

Neoplasm of uncertain behavior of nervous system (central) NOS

√4th **D44 Neoplasm of uncertain behavior of endocrine glands**

EXCLUDES 1 *multiple endocrine adenomatosis (E31.2-)*
multiple endocrine neoplasia (E31.2-)
neoplasm of uncertain behavior of endocrine pancreas (D37.8)
neoplasm of uncertain behavior of ovary (D39.1-)
neoplasm of uncertain behavior of testis (D4Ø.1-)
neoplasm of uncertain behavior of thymus (D38.4)

D44.Ø Neoplasm of uncertain behavior of thyroid gland

√5th **D44.1 Neoplasm of uncertain behavior of adrenal gland**

Use additional code to identify any functional activity

D44.1Ø Neoplasm of uncertain behavior of unspecified adrenal gland

D44.11 Neoplasm of uncertain behavior of right adrenal gland

D44.12 Neoplasm of uncertain behavior of left adrenal gland

D44.2 Neoplasm of uncertain behavior of parathyroid gland

D44.3 Neoplasm of uncertain behavior of pituitary gland HCC Rx ESR COM

Use additional code to identify any functional activity

D44.4 Neoplasm of uncertain behavior of craniopharyngeal duct HCC Rx ESR COM

D44.5 Neoplasm of uncertain behavior of pineal gland HCC Rx ESR COM

D44.6 Neoplasm of uncertain behavior of carotid body HCC Rx ESR COM

D44.7 Neoplasm of uncertain behavior of aortic body and other paraganglia HCC Rx ESR COM

AHA: 2021,2Q,7; 2016,4Q,26

D44.9 Neoplasm of uncertain behavior of unspecified endocrine gland

D45 Polycythemia vera HCC Rx ESR COM

EXCLUDES 1 *familial polycythemia (D75.Ø)*
secondary polycythemia (D75.1)

DEF: Abnormal proliferation of all bone marrow elements, increased red cell mass, and total blood volume. The etiology is unknown, but it is frequently associated with splenomegaly, leukocytosis, and thrombocythemia.

√4th **D46 Myelodysplastic syndromes**

Use additional code for adverse effect, if applicable, to identify drug (T36-T5Ø with fifth or sixth character 5)

EXCLUDES 2 *drug-induced aplastic anemia (D61.1)*

D46.Ø Refractory anemia without ring sideroblasts, so stated HCC Rx ESR COM

Refractory anemia without sideroblasts, without excess of blasts

D46.1 Refractory anemia with ring sideroblasts HCC Rx ESR COM

RARS

√5th **D46.2 Refractory anemia with excess of blasts [RAEB]**

D46.2Ø Refractory anemia with excess of blasts, unspecified HCC Rx ESR COM

RAEB NOS

D46.21 Refractory anemia with excess of blasts 1 HCC Rx ESR COM

RAEB 1

D46.22 Refractory anemia with excess of blasts 2 HCC Rx ESR COM

RAEB 2

D46.A Refractory cytopenia with multilineage dysplasia HCC Rx ESR COM

D46.B Refractory cytopenia with multilineage dysplasia and ring sideroblasts HCC Rx ESR COM

RCMD RS

D46.C Myelodysplastic syndrome with isolated del(5q) chromosomal abnormality HCC Rx ESR COM

Myelodysplastic syndrome with 5q deletion
5q minus syndrome NOS

D46.4 Refractory anemia, unspecified HCC Rx ESR COM

D46.Z Other myelodysplastic syndromes HCC Rx ESR COM

EXCLUDES 1 *chronic myelomonocytic leukemia (C93.1-)*

D46.9 Myelodysplastic syndrome, unspecified HCC Rx ESR COM

Myelodysplasia NOS

√4th **D47 Other neoplasms of uncertain behavior of lymphoid, hematopoietic and related tissue**

√5th **D47.Ø Mast cell neoplasms of uncertain behavior**

EXCLUDES 1 *congenital cutaneous mastocytosis (Q82.2)*
histiocytic neoplasms of uncertain behavior (D47.Z9)
malignant mast cell neoplasm (C96.2-)

AHA: 2017,4Q,5

D47.Ø1 Cutaneous mastocytosis Rx

Diffuse cutaneous mastocytosis
Maculopapular cutaneous mastocytosis
Solitary mastocytoma
Telangiectasia macularis eruptiva perstans
Urticaria pigmentosa

EXCLUDES 1 *congenital (diffuse) (maculopapular) cutaneous mastocytosis (Q82.2)*
congenital urticaria pigmentosa (Q82.2)
extracutaneous mastocytoma (D47.Ø9)

D47.Ø2 Systemic mastocytosis Rx
Indolent systemic mastocytosis
Isolated bone marrow mastocytosis
Smoldering systemic mastocytosis
Systemic mastocytosis, with an associated hematological non-mast cell lineage disease (SM-AHNMD)
Code also, if applicable, any associated hematological non-mast cell lineage disease, such as:
acute myeloid leukemia (C92.6-, C92.A-)
chronic myelomonocytic leukemia (C93.1-)
essential thrombocytosis (D47.3)
hypereosinophilic syndrome (D72.1)
myelodysplastic syndrome (D46.9)
myeloproliferative syndrome (D47.1)
non-Hodgkin lymphoma (C82-C85)
plasma cell myeloma (C9Ø.Ø-)
polycythemia vera (D45)
EXCLUDES 1 *aggressive systemic mastocytosis (C96.21)*
mast cell leukemia (C94.3-)

D47.Ø9 Other mast cell neoplasms of uncertain behavior Rx
Extracutaneous mastocytoma
Mast cell tumor NOS
Mastocytoma NOS
Mastocytosis NOS

D47.1 Chronic myeloproliferative disease HCC Rx ESR COM
Chronic neutrophilic leukemia
Myeloproliferative disease, unspecified
EXCLUDES 1 *atypical chronic myeloid leukemia BCR/ABL-negative (C92.2-)*
chronic myeloid leukemia BCR/ABL-positive (C92.1-)
myelofibrosis NOS (D75.81)
myelophthisic anemia (D61.82)
myelophthisis (D61.82)
secondary myelofibrosis NOS (D75.81)

D47.2 Monoclonal gammopathy
Monoclonal gammopathy of undetermined significance [MGUS]
AHA: 2021,3Q,5
TIP: Smoldering multiple myeloma (SMM) is coded here.

D47.3 Essential (hemorrhagic) thrombocythemia HCC Rx ESR COM
Essential thrombocytosis
Idiopathic hemorrhagic thrombocythemia
Primary thrombocytosis
EXCLUDES 2 *reactive thrombocytosis (D75.838)*
secondary thrombocytosis (D75.838)
thrombocythemia NOS (D75.839)
thrombocytosis NOS (D75.839)
DEF: Chronic myeloproliferative neoplasm involving production of excess blood platelets that may result in abnormal clotting or hemorrhaging.

D47.4 Osteomyelofibrosis HCC Rx ESR COM
Chronic idiopathic myelofibrosis
Myelofibrosis (idiopathic) (with myeloid metaplasia)
Myelosclerosis (megakaryocytic) with myeloid metaplasia
Secondary myelofibrosis in myeloproliferative disease
EXCLUDES 1 *acute myelofibrosis (C94.4-)*

✓5th **D47.Z Other specified neoplasms of uncertain behavior of lymphoid, hematopoietic and related tissue**
AHA: 2016,4Q,8

D47.Z1 Post-transplant lymphoproliferative disorder (PTLD) HCC ESR COM UPD
Code first complications of transplanted organs and tissue (T86.-)
DEF: Excessive proliferation of B-cell lymphocytes following Epstein-Barr virus infection in organ transplant patients. It may progress to non-Hodgkin lymphoma.

D47.Z2 Castleman disease HCC Rx ESR COM
Code also, if applicable, human herpesvirus 8 infection (B1Ø.89)
EXCLUDES 2 *Kaposi's sarcoma (C46.-)*
DEF: Rare disease of the lymph nodes and lymphoid tissues that closely mimics lymphoma.

D47.Z9 Other specified neoplasms of uncertain behavior of lymphoid, hematopoietic and related tissue HCC Rx ESR COM
Histiocytic tumors of uncertain behavior

D47.9 Neoplasm of uncertain behavior of lymphoid, hematopoietic and related tissue, unspecified HCC Rx ESR COM
Lymphoproliferative disease NOS

✓4th **D48 Neoplasm of uncertain behavior of other and unspecified sites**
EXCLUDES 1 *neurofibromatosis (nonmalignant) (Q85.Ø-)*

D48.Ø Neoplasm of uncertain behavior of bone and articular cartilage
EXCLUDES 1 *neoplasm of uncertain behavior of cartilage of ear (D48.1)*
neoplasm of uncertain behavior of cartilage of larynx (D38.Ø)
neoplasm of uncertain behavior of cartilage of nose (D38.5)
neoplasm of uncertain behavior of connective tissue of eyelid (D48.1)
neoplasm of uncertain behavior of synovia (D48.1)

D48.1 Neoplasm of uncertain behavior of connective and other soft tissue
Neoplasm of uncertain behavior of connective tissue of ear
Neoplasm of uncertain behavior of connective tissue of eyelid
Stromal tumors of uncertain behavior of digestive system
EXCLUDES 1 *neoplasm of uncertain behavior of articular cartilage (D48.Ø)*
neoplasm of uncertain behavior of cartilage of larynx (D38.Ø)
neoplasm of uncertain behavior of cartilage of nose (D38.5)
neoplasm of uncertain behavior of connective tissue of breast (D48.6-)

D48.2 Neoplasm of uncertain behavior of peripheral nerves and autonomic nervous system
EXCLUDES 1 *neoplasm of uncertain behavior of peripheral nerves of orbit (D48.7)*

D48.3 Neoplasm of uncertain behavior of retroperitoneum

D48.4 Neoplasm of uncertain behavior of peritoneum

D48.5 Neoplasm of uncertain behavior of skin
Neoplasm of uncertain behavior of anal margin
Neoplasm of uncertain behavior of anal skin
Neoplasm of uncertain behavior of perianal skin
Neoplasm of uncertain behavior of skin of breast
EXCLUDES 1 *neoplasm of uncertain behavior of anus NOS (D37.8)*
neoplasm of uncertain behavior of skin of genital organs (D39.8, D4Ø.8)
neoplasm of uncertain behavior of vermilion border of lip (D37.Ø)

✓5th **D48.6 Neoplasm of uncertain behavior of breast**
Neoplasm of uncertain behavior of connective tissue of breast
Cystosarcoma phyllodes
EXCLUDES 1 *neoplasm of uncertain behavior of skin of breast (D48.5)*

D48.6Ø Neoplasm of uncertain behavior of unspecified breast

D48.61 Neoplasm of uncertain behavior of right breast

D48.62 Neoplasm of uncertain behavior of left breast

D48.7 Neoplasm of uncertain behavior of other specified sites
Neoplasm of uncertain behavior of eye
Neoplasm of uncertain behavior of heart
Neoplasm of uncertain behavior of peripheral nerves of orbit
EXCLUDES 1 *neoplasm of uncertain behavior of connective tissue (D48.1)*
neoplasm of uncertain behavior of skin of eyelid (D48.5)

D48.9 Neoplasm of uncertain behavior, unspecified

Neoplasms of unspecified behavior (D49)

✓4th **D49 Neoplasms of unspecified behavior**

NOTE Category D49 classifies by site neoplasms of unspecified morphology and behavior. The term "mass", unless otherwise stated, is not to be regarded as a neoplastic growth.

INCLUDES "growth" NOS
neoplasm NOS
new growth NOS
tumor NOS

EXCLUDES 1 *neoplasms of uncertain behavior (D37-D44, D48)*

D49.Ø Neoplasm of unspecified behavior of digestive system

EXCLUDES 1 *neoplasm of unspecified behavior of margin of anus (D49.2)*
neoplasm of unspecified behavior of perianal skin (D49.2)
neoplasm of unspecified behavior of skin of anus (D49.2)

D49.1 Neoplasm of unspecified behavior of respiratory system

D49.2 Neoplasm of unspecified behavior of bone, soft tissue, and skin

EXCLUDES 1 *neoplasm of unspecified behavior of anal canal (D49.Ø)*
neoplasm of unspecified behavior of anus NOS (D49.Ø)
neoplasm of unspecified behavior of bone marrow (D49.89)
neoplasm of unspecified behavior of cartilage of larynx (D49.1)
neoplasm of unspecified behavior of cartilage of nose (D49.1)
neoplasm of unspecified behavior of connective tissue of breast (D49.3)
neoplasm of unspecified behavior of skin of genital organs (D49.59)
neoplasm of unspecified behavior of vermilion border of lip (D49.Ø)

D49.3 Neoplasm of unspecified behavior of breast

EXCLUDES 1 *neoplasm of unspecified behavior of skin of breast (D49.2)*

D49.4 Neoplasm of unspecified behavior of bladder

✓5th **D49.5 Neoplasm of unspecified behavior of other genitourinary organs**

AHA: 2016,4Q,9

✓6th **D49.51 Neoplasm of unspecified behavior of kidney**

D49.511 Neoplasm of unspecified behavior of right kidney

D49.512 Neoplasm of unspecified behavior of left kidney

D49.519 Neoplasm of unspecified behavior of unspecified kidney

D49.59 Neoplasm of unspecified behavior of other genitourinary organ

D49.6 Neoplasm of unspecified behavior of brain HCC Rx ESR COM

EXCLUDES 1 *neoplasm of unspecified behavior of cerebral meninges (D49.7)*
neoplasm of unspecified behavior of cranial nerves (D49.7)

D49.7 Neoplasm of unspecified behavior of endocrine glands and other parts of nervous system

EXCLUDES 1 *neoplasm of unspecified behavior of peripheral, sympathetic, and parasympathetic nerves and ganglia (D49.2)*

✓5th **D49.8 Neoplasm of unspecified behavior of other specified sites**

EXCLUDES 1 *neoplasm of unspecified behavior of eyelid (skin) (D49.2)*
neoplasm of unspecified behavior of eyelid cartilage (D49.2)
neoplasm of unspecified behavior of great vessels (D49.2)
neoplasm of unspecified behavior of optic nerve (D49.7)

D49.81 Neoplasm of unspecified behavior of retina and choroid

Dark area on retina
Retinal freckle

D49.89 Neoplasm of unspecified behavior of other specified sites

D49.9 Neoplasm of unspecified behavior of unspecified site

Chapter 3. Disease of the Blood and Blood-Forming Organs and Certain Disorders Involving the Immune Mechanism (D50–D89)

Chapter-specific Guidelines with Coding Examples
Reserved for future guideline expansion.

Chapter 3. Diseases of the Blood and Blood-forming Organs and Certain Disorders Involving the Immune Mechanism (D50-D89)

EXCLUDES 2 *autoimmune disease (systemic) NOS (M35.9)*
certain conditions originating in the perinatal period (PØØ-P96)
complications of pregnancy, childbirth and the puerperium (OØØ-O9A)
congenital malformations, deformations and chromosomal abnormalities (QØØ-Q99)
endocrine, nutritional and metabolic diseases (EØØ-E88)
human immunodeficiency virus [HIV] disease (B2Ø)
injury, poisoning and certain other consequences of external causes (SØØ-T88)
neoplasms (CØØ-D49)
symptoms, signs and abnormal clinical and laboratory findings, not elsewhere classified (RØØ-R94)

This chapter contains the following blocks:

D5Ø-D53	Nutritional anemias
D55-D59	Hemolytic anemias
D6Ø-D64	Aplastic and other anemias and other bone marrow failure syndromes
D65-D69	Coagulation defects, purpura and other hemorrhagic conditions
D7Ø-D77	Other disorders of blood and blood-forming organs
D78	Intraoperative and postprocedural complications of the spleen
D8Ø-D89	Certain disorders involving the immune mechanism

Nutritional anemias (D5Ø-D53)

DEF: Nutritional anemia: The result of inadequate intake or absorption of a vitamin or mineral that impacts the production of red blood cells or causes them to develop abnormally affecting the size and shape.
TIP: Documentation must identify a link between anemia and the nutritional deficiency; low levels of a particular nutrient may occur concurrently with anemia but not cause the anemia.

✓4th **D5Ø Iron deficiency anemia**
INCLUDES asiderotic anemia
hypochromic anemia

D5Ø.Ø Iron deficiency anemia secondary to blood loss (chronic)
Posthemorrhagic anemia (chronic)
EXCLUDES 1 *acute posthemorrhagic anemia (D62)*
congenital anemia from fetal blood loss (P61.3)
AHA: 2019,3Q,17

D5Ø.1 Sideropenic dysphagia
Kelly-Paterson syndrome
Plummer-Vinson syndrome

D5Ø.8 Other iron deficiency anemias
Iron deficiency anemia due to inadequate dietary iron intake

D5Ø.9 Iron deficiency anemia, unspecified

✓4th **D51 Vitamin B12 deficiency anemia**
EXCLUDES 1 *vitamin B12 deficiency (E53.8)*

D51.Ø Vitamin B12 deficiency anemia due to intrinsic factor deficiency
Addison anemia
Biermer anemia
Pernicious (congenital) anemia
Congenital intrinsic factor deficiency
DEF: Chronic progressive anemia due to vitamin B12 malabsorption, caused by lack of secretion of intrinsic factor, which is produced by the gastric mucosa of the stomach.

D51.1 Vitamin B12 deficiency anemia due to selective vitamin B12 malabsorption with proteinuria
Imerslund (Gräsbeck) syndrome
Megaloblastic hereditary anemia

D51.2 Transcobalamin II deficiency

D51.3 Other dietary vitamin B12 deficiency anemia
Vegan anemia

D51.8 Other vitamin B12 deficiency anemias

D51.9 Vitamin B12 deficiency anemia, unspecified

✓4th **D52 Folate deficiency anemia**
EXCLUDES 1 *folate deficiency without anemia (E53.8)*
DEF: Deficiency in a B complex vitamin needed for the production of healthy red blood cells. Lack of folate, or folic acid, and other absorption conditions can cause anemia resulting in large, misshapen red blood cells called megaloblasts.

D52.Ø Dietary folate deficiency anemia
Nutritional megaloblastic anemia
DEF: Result of a poor diet with inadequate intake of folate, which is needed to produce healthy red blood cells.

D52.1 Drug-induced folate deficiency anemia
Use additional code for adverse effect, if applicable, to identify drug (T36-T5Ø with fifth or sixth character 5)

D52.8 Other folate deficiency anemias

D52.9 Folate deficiency anemia, unspecified
Folic acid deficiency anemia NOS

✓4th **D53 Other nutritional anemias**
INCLUDES megaloblastic anemia unresponsive to vitamin B12 or folate therapy

D53.Ø Protein deficiency anemia
Amino-acid deficiency anemia
Orotaciduric anemia
EXCLUDES 1 *Lesch-Nyhan syndrome (E79.1)*

D53.1 Other megaloblastic anemias, not elsewhere classified
Megaloblastic anemia NOS
EXCLUDES 1 *Di Guglielmo's disease (C94.Ø)*

D53.2 Scorbutic anemia
EXCLUDES 1 *scurvy (E54)*

D53.8 Other specified nutritional anemias
Anemia associated with deficiency of copper
Anemia associated with deficiency of molybdenum
Anemia associated with deficiency of zinc
EXCLUDES 1 *nutritional deficiencies without anemia, such as:*
copper deficiency NOS (E61.Ø)
molybdenum deficiency NOS (E61.5)
zinc deficiency NOS (E6Ø)

D53.9 Nutritional anemia, unspecified
Simple chronic anemia
EXCLUDES 1 *anemia NOS (D64.9)*
AHA: 2018,4Q,88

Hemolytic anemias (D55-D59)

✓4th **D55 Anemia due to enzyme disorders**
EXCLUDES 1 *drug-induced enzyme deficiency anemia (D59.2)*

D55.Ø Anemia due to glucose-6-phosphate dehydrogenase [G6PD] deficiency HCC ESR
Favism
G6PD deficiency anemia
EXCLUDES 1 *glucose-6-phosphate dehydrogenase (G6PD) deficiency without anemia (D75.A)*

D55.1 Anemia due to other disorders of glutathione metabolism HCC ESR
Anemia (due to) enzyme deficiencies, except G6PD, related to the hexose monophosphate [HMP] shunt pathway
Anemia (due to) hemolytic nonspherocytic (hereditary), type I

✓5th **D55.2 Anemia due to disorders of glycolytic enzymes**
EXCLUDES 1 *disorders of glycolysis not associated with anemia (E74.81-)*
AHA: 2021,4Q,6-7

D55.21 Anemia due to pyruvate kinase deficiency HCC ESR
PK deficiency anemia
Pyruvate kinase deficiency anemia

D55.29 Anemia due to other disorders of glycolytic enzymes HCC ESR
Hexokinase deficiency anemia
Triose-phosphate isomerase deficiency anemia

D55.3 Anemia due to disorders of nucleotide metabolism HCC ESR

D55.8 Other anemias due to enzyme disorders HCC ESR

D55.9 Anemia due to enzyme disorder, unspecified HCC ESR

D56 Thalassemia

EXCLUDES 1 *sickle-cell thalassemia (D57.4-)*

DEF: Group of inherited disorders of hemoglobin metabolism causing mild to severe anemia. It is usually found in people of Mediterranean, African, Chinese, or Asian descent.

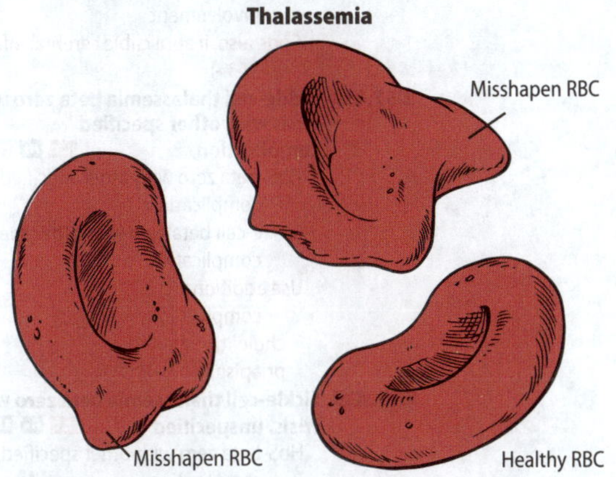

D56.Ø Alpha thalassemia HCC ESR

Alpha thalassemia major
Hemoglobin H Constant Spring
Hemoglobin H disease
Hydrops fetalis due to alpha thalassemia
Severe alpha thalassemia
Triple gene defect alpha thalassemia

Use additional code, if applicable, for hydrops fetalis due to alpha thalassemia (P56.99)

EXCLUDES 1 *alpha thalassemia trait or minor (D56.3)*
asymptomatic alpha thalassemia (D56.3)
hydrops fetalis due to isoimmunization (P56.Ø)
hydrops fetalis not due to immune hemolysis (P83.2)

DEF: HBA1 and HBA2 genetic variant of chromosome 16 prevalent among those of African and Southeast Asian descent. Alpha thalassemia is associated with a wide spectrum of anemic presentation and includes hemoglobin H disease subtypes.

D56.1 Beta thalassemia HCC ESR COM

Beta thalassemia major
Cooley's anemia
Homozygous beta thalassemia
Severe beta thalassemia
Thalassemia intermedia
Thalassemia major

EXCLUDES 1 *beta thalassemia minor (D56.3)*
beta thalassemia trait (D56.3)
delta-beta thalassemia (D56.2)
hemoglobin E-beta thalassemia (D56.5)
sickle-cell beta thalassemia (D57.4-)

D56.2 Delta-beta thalassemia HCC ESR COM

Homozygous delta-beta thalassemia

EXCLUDES 1 *delta-beta thalassemia minor (D56.3)*
delta-beta thalassemia trait (D56.3)

D56.3 Thalassemia minor

Alpha thalassemia minor
Alpha thalassemia silent carrier
Alpha thalassemia trait
Beta thalassemia minor
Beta thalassemia trait
Delta-beta thalassemia minor
Delta-beta thalassemia trait
Thalassemia trait NOS

EXCLUDES 1 *alpha thalassemia (D56.Ø)*
beta thalassemia (D56.1)
delta-beta thalassemia (D56.2)
hemoglobin E-beta thalassemia (D56.5)
sickle-cell trait (D57.3)

DEF: Solitary abnormal gene that identifies a carrier of the disease, yet with an absence of symptoms or a clinically mild anemic presentation.

D56.4 Hereditary persistence of fetal hemoglobin [HPFH] HCC ESR

D56.5 Hemoglobin E-beta thalassemia HCC ESR COM

EXCLUDES 1 *beta thalassemia (D56.1)*
beta thalassemia minor (D56.3)
beta thalassemia trait (D56.3)
delta-beta thalassemia (D56.2)
delta-beta thalassemia trait (D56.3)
hemoglobin E disease (D58.2)
other hemoglobinopathies (D58.2)
sickle-cell beta thalassemia (D57.4-)

D56.8 Other thalassemias HCC ESR

Dominant thalassemia
Hemoglobin C thalassemia
Mixed thalassemia
Thalassemia with other hemoglobinopathy

EXCLUDES 1 *hemoglobin C disease (D58.2)*
hemoglobin E disease (D58.2)
other hemoglobinopathies (D58.2)
sickle-cell anemia (D57.-)
sickle-cell thalassemia (D57.4)

D56.9 Thalassemia, unspecified

Mediterranean anemia (with other hemoglobinopathy)

D57 Sickle-cell disorders

Use additional code for any associated fever (R5Ø.81)

EXCLUDES 1 *other hemoglobinopathies (D58.-)*

AHA: 2022,2Q,28

DEF: Severe, chronic inherited diseases caused by a genetic variation in hemoglobin protein of the red blood cell. The gene mutation causes the red blood cell to become hard, sticky, and crescent or sickle shaped, making it harder for red blood cells to travel through the bloodstream, disrupting blood flow and decreasing oxygen transport to tissues.

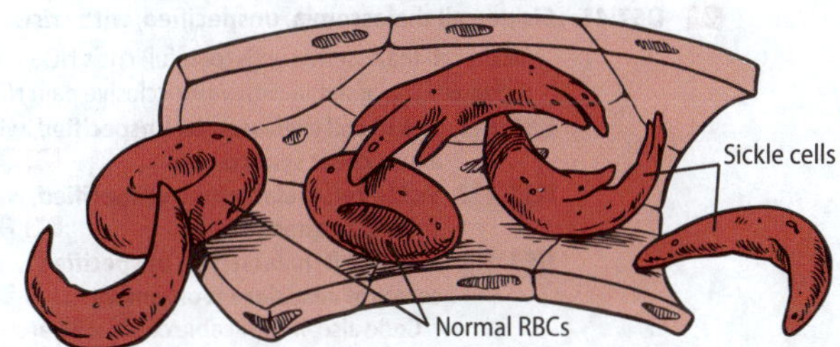

D57.Ø Hb-SS disease with crisis

Sickle-cell disease with crisis
Hb-SS disease with vasoocclusive pain

AHA: 2020,4Q,6-7

D57.ØØ Hb-SS disease with crisis, unspecified HCC Rx ESR COM

Hb-SS disease with (painful) crisis NOS
Hb-SS disease with vasoocclusive pain NOS

D57.Ø1 Hb-SS disease with acute chest syndrome HCC Rx ESR COM

D57.Ø2 Hb-SS disease with splenic sequestration HCC Rx ESR COM

D57.Ø3 Hb-SS disease with cerebral vascular involvement HCC Rx ESR COM

Code also, if applicable, cerebral infarction (I63.-)

D57.Ø9 Hb-SS disease with crisis with other specified complication HCC Rx ESR COM

Use additional code to identify complications, such as:
cholelithiasis (K8Ø.-)
priapism (N48.32)

D57.1 Sickle-cell disease without crisis HCC Rx ESR COM

Hb-SS disease without crisis
Sickle-cell anemia NOS
Sickle-cell disease NOS
Sickle-cell disorder NOS

D57.2 Sickle-cell/Hb-C disease

Hb-SC disease
Hb-S/Hb-C disease

AHA: 2020,4Q,6-7

D57.2Ø Sickle-cell/Hb-C disease without crisis HCC ESR

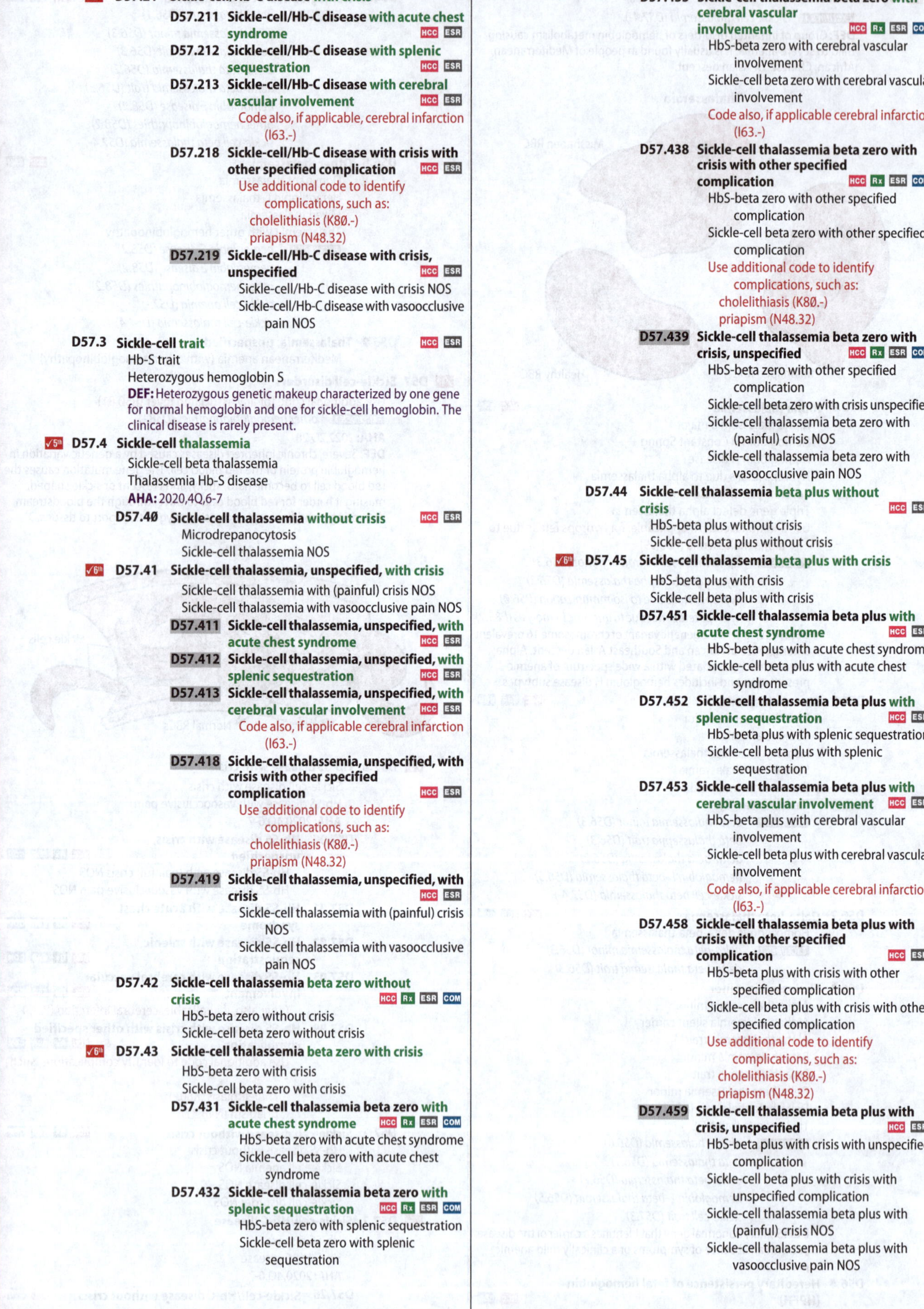

✓6th **D57.21 Sickle-cell/Hb-C disease with crisis**

D57.211 Sickle-cell/Hb-C disease with acute chest syndrome HCC ESR

D57.212 Sickle-cell/Hb-C disease with splenic sequestration HCC ESR

D57.213 Sickle-cell/Hb-C disease with cerebral vascular involvement HCC ESR

Code also, if applicable, cerebral infarction (I63.-)

D57.218 Sickle-cell/Hb-C disease with crisis with other specified complication HCC ESR

Use additional code to identify complications, such as:
cholelithiasis (K8Ø.-)
priapism (N48.32)

D57.219 Sickle-cell/Hb-C disease with crisis, unspecified HCC ESR

Sickle-cell/Hb-C disease with crisis NOS
Sickle-cell/Hb-C disease with vasoocclusive pain NOS

D57.3 Sickle-cell trait HCC ESR

Hb-S trait
Heterozygous hemoglobin S
DEF: Heterozygous genetic makeup characterized by one gene for normal hemoglobin and one for sickle-cell hemoglobin. The clinical disease is rarely present.

✓5th **D57.4 Sickle-cell thalassemia**

Sickle-cell beta thalassemia
Thalassemia Hb-S disease
AHA: 2020,4Q,6-7

D57.4Ø Sickle-cell thalassemia without crisis HCC ESR

Microdrepanocytosis
Sickle-cell thalassemia NOS

✓6th **D57.41 Sickle-cell thalassemia, unspecified, with crisis**

Sickle-cell thalassemia with (painful) crisis NOS
Sickle-cell thalassemia with vasoocclusive pain NOS

D57.411 Sickle-cell thalassemia, unspecified, with acute chest syndrome HCC ESR

D57.412 Sickle-cell thalassemia, unspecified, with splenic sequestration HCC ESR

D57.413 Sickle-cell thalassemia, unspecified, with cerebral vascular involvement HCC ESR

Code also, if applicable cerebral infarction (I63.-)

D57.418 Sickle-cell thalassemia, unspecified, with crisis with other specified complication HCC ESR

Use additional code to identify complications, such as:
cholelithiasis (K8Ø.-)
priapism (N48.32)

D57.419 Sickle-cell thalassemia, unspecified, with crisis HCC ESR

Sickle-cell thalassemia with (painful) crisis NOS
Sickle-cell thalassemia with vasoocclusive pain NOS

D57.42 Sickle-cell thalassemia beta zero without crisis HCC Rx ESR COM

HbS-beta zero without crisis
Sickle-cell beta zero without crisis

✓6th **D57.43 Sickle-cell thalassemia beta zero with crisis**

HbS-beta zero with crisis
Sickle-cell beta zero with crisis

D57.431 Sickle-cell thalassemia beta zero with acute chest syndrome HCC Rx ESR COM

HbS-beta zero with acute chest syndrome
Sickle-cell beta zero with acute chest syndrome

D57.432 Sickle-cell thalassemia beta zero with splenic sequestration HCC Rx ESR COM

HbS-beta zero with splenic sequestration
Sickle-cell beta zero with splenic sequestration

D57.433 Sickle-cell thalassemia beta zero with cerebral vascular involvement HCC Rx ESR COM

HbS-beta zero with cerebral vascular involvement
Sickle-cell beta zero with cerebral vascular involvement
Code also, if applicable cerebral infarction (I63.-)

D57.438 Sickle-cell thalassemia beta zero with crisis with other specified complication HCC Rx ESR COM

HbS-beta zero with other specified complication
Sickle-cell beta zero with other specified complication
Use additional code to identify complications, such as:
cholelithiasis (K8Ø.-)
priapism (N48.32)

D57.439 Sickle-cell thalassemia beta zero with crisis, unspecified HCC Rx ESR COM

HbS-beta zero with other specified complication
Sickle-cell beta zero with crisis unspecified
Sickle-cell thalassemia beta zero with (painful) crisis NOS
Sickle-cell thalassemia beta zero with vasoocclusive pain NOS

D57.44 Sickle-cell thalassemia beta plus without crisis HCC ESR

HbS-beta plus without crisis
Sickle-cell beta plus without crisis

✓6th **D57.45 Sickle-cell thalassemia beta plus with crisis**

HbS-beta plus with crisis
Sickle-cell beta plus with crisis

D57.451 Sickle-cell thalassemia beta plus with acute chest syndrome HCC ESR

HbS-beta plus with acute chest syndrome
Sickle-cell beta plus with acute chest syndrome

D57.452 Sickle-cell thalassemia beta plus with splenic sequestration HCC ESR

HbS-beta plus with splenic sequestration
Sickle-cell beta plus with splenic sequestration

D57.453 Sickle-cell thalassemia beta plus with cerebral vascular involvement HCC ESR

HbS-beta plus with cerebral vascular involvement
Sickle-cell beta plus with cerebral vascular involvement
Code also, if applicable cerebral infarction (I63.-)

D57.458 Sickle-cell thalassemia beta plus with crisis with other specified complication HCC ESR

HbS-beta plus with crisis with other specified complication
Sickle-cell beta plus with crisis with other specified complication
Use additional code to identify complications, such as:
cholelithiasis (K8Ø.-)
priapism (N48.32)

D57.459 Sickle-cell thalassemia beta plus with crisis, unspecified HCC ESR

HbS-beta plus with crisis with unspecified complication
Sickle-cell beta plus with crisis with unspecified complication
Sickle-cell thalassemia beta plus with (painful) crisis NOS
Sickle-cell thalassemia beta plus with vasoocclusive pain NOS

D57.8 Other sickle-cell disorders
Hb-SD disease
Hb-SE disease
AHA: 2020,4Q,6-7

D57.80 Other sickle-cell disorders without crisis HCC ESR

D57.81 Other sickle-cell disorders with crisis

D57.811 Other sickle-cell disorders with acute chest syndrome HCC ESR

D57.812 Other sickle-cell disorders with splenic sequestration HCC ESR

D57.813 Other sickle-cell disorders with cerebral vascular involvement HCC ESR
Code also, if applicable: cerebral infarction (I63.-)

D57.818 Other sickle-cell disorders with crisis with other specified complication HCC ESR
Use additional code to identify complications, such as:
cholelithiasis (K80.-)
priapism (N48.32)

D57.819 Other sickle-cell disorders with crisis, unspecified HCC ESR
Other sickle-cell disorders with crisis NOS
Other sickle-cell disorders with vasoocclusive pain NOS

D58 Other hereditary hemolytic anemias

EXCLUDES 1 *hemolytic anemia of the newborn (P55.-)*

D58.0 Hereditary spherocytosis HCC ESR
Acholuric (familial) jaundice
Congenital (spherocytic) hemolytic icterus
Minkowski-Chauffard syndrome
DEF: Inherited condition caused by mutations to genes responsible for the production of proteins that form the membranes of red blood cells. The shape and flexibility of the red blood cell membrane is altered, diminishing the cell's ability to traverse the spleen, therefore becoming trapped and destroyed before the red blood cell has reached maturity.

D58.1 Hereditary elliptocytosis HCC ESR
Elliptocytosis (congenital)
Ovalocytosis (congenital) (hereditary)

D58.2 Other hemoglobinopathies HCC ESR
Abnormal hemoglobin NOS
Congenital Heinz body anemia
Hb-C disease
Hb-D disease
Hb-E disease
Hemoglobinopathy NOS
Unstable hemoglobin hemolytic disease

EXCLUDES 1 *familial polycythemia (D75.0)*
Hb-M disease (D74.0)
hemoglobin E-beta thalassemia (D56.5)
hereditary persistence of fetal hemoglobin [HPFH] (D56.4)
high-altitude polycythemia (D75.1)
methemoglobinemia (D74.-)
other hemoglobinopathies with thalassemia (D56.8)

D58.8 Other specified hereditary hemolytic anemias HCC ESR
Stomatocytosis

D58.9 Hereditary hemolytic anemia, unspecified HCC ESR

D59 Acquired hemolytic anemia

DEF: Non-hereditary anemia characterized by premature destruction of red blood cells caused by infectious organisms, poisons, and physical agents.

D59.0 Drug-induced autoimmune hemolytic anemia HCC Rx ESR COM
Use additional code for adverse effect, if applicable, to identify drug (T36-T50 with fifth or sixth character 5)

D59.1 Other autoimmune hemolytic anemias

EXCLUDES 2 *Evans syndrome (D69.41)*
hemolytic disease of newborn (P55.-)
paroxysmal cold hemoglobinuria (D59.6)

AHA: 2020,4Q,7-8

D59.10 Autoimmune hemolytic anemia, unspecified HCC Rx ESR COM

D59.11 Warm autoimmune hemolytic anemia HCC Rx ESR COM
Warm type (primary) (secondary) (symptomatic) autoimmune hemolytic anemia
Warm type autoimmune hemolytic disease

D59.12 Cold autoimmune hemolytic anemia HCC Rx ESR COM
Chronic cold hemagglutinin disease
Cold agglutinin disease
Cold agglutinin hemoglobinuria
Cold type (primary) (secondary) (symptomatic) autoimmune hemolytic anemia
Cold type autoimmune hemolytic disease

D59.13 Mixed type autoimmune hemolytic anemia HCC Rx ESR COM
Mixed type autoimmune hemolytic disease
Mixed type, cold and warm, (primary) (secondary) (symptomatic) autoimmune hemolytic anemia

D59.19 Other autoimmune hemolytic anemia HCC Rx ESR COM

D59.2 Drug-induced nonautoimmune hemolytic anemia HCC Rx ESR COM
Drug-induced enzyme deficiency anemia
Use additional code for adverse effect, if applicable, to identify drug (T36-T50 with fifth or sixth character 5)

▲ **D59.3 Hemolytic-uremic syndrome**
~~Use additional code to identify associated:~~
~~E. coli infection (B96.2-)~~
~~Pneumococcal pneumonia (J13)~~
~~Shigella dysenteriae (A03.9)~~
▶Code also, if applicable, any associated:◀
▶acute kidney failure (N17.-)◀
▶chronic kidney disease (N18.-)◀
DEF: Condition typically precipitated by infection causing low platelets and destruction of red blood cells resulting in hemolytic anemia. This cell damage and blockage of renal capillaries lead to kidney failure. Mainly affects children.

● **D59.30 Hemolytic-uremic syndrome, unspecified**
Hemolytic-uremic syndrome NOS

● **D59.31 Infection-associated hemolytic-uremic syndrome**
Shiga toxin-producing E. coli [STEC] related hemolytic uremic syndrome
Typical hemolytic uremic syndrome
Use additional code to identify associated infection, such as:
E. coli infection (B96.2-)
human immunodeficiency virus [HIV] disease (B20)
pneumococcal meningitis (G00.1)
pneumococcal pneumonia (J13)
sepsis due to Streptococcus pneumoniae (A40.3)
Shigella dysenteriae (A03.9)
streptococcus pneumoniae as the cause of diseases classified elsewhere (B95.3)

● **D59.32 Hereditary hemolytic-uremic syndrome**
Atypical hemolytic uremic syndrome with an identified genetic cause
Code also, if applicable:
defects in the complement system (D84.1)
methylmalonic acidemia (E71.120)

● **D59.39 Other hemolytic-uremic syndrome**
Atypical (nongenetic) hemolytic uremic syndrome
Secondary hemolytic-uremic syndrome
Code first, if applicable, any associated:
COVID-19 (U07.1)
complications of kidney transplant (T86.1-)
complications of heart transplant (T86.2-)
complications of liver transplant (T86.4-)
Code also, if applicable, any associated condition, such as:
hypertensive emergency (I16.1)
malignant neoplasm (C00-C96)
systemic lupus erythematosus (M32.-)
Use additional code, if applicable, for adverse effect to identify drug (T36-T50 with fifth or sixth character 5)

D59.4 Other nonautoimmune hemolytic anemias HCC Rx ESR COM
Mechanical hemolytic anemia
Microangiopathic hemolytic anemia
Toxic hemolytic anemia

D59.5 Paroxysmal nocturnal hemoglobinuria [Marchiafava-Micheli] HCC Rx ESR COM
EXCLUDES 1 *hemoglobinuria NOS (R82.3)*

D59.6 Hemoglobinuria due to hemolysis from other external causes HCC Rx ESR COM
Hemoglobinuria from exertion
March hemoglobinuria
Paroxysmal cold hemoglobinuria
Use additional code (Chapter 2Ø) to identify external cause
EXCLUDES 1 *hemoglobinuria NOS (R82.3)*

D59.8 Other acquired hemolytic anemias HCC Rx ESR COM

D59.9 Acquired hemolytic anemia, unspecified HCC Rx ESR COM
Idiopathic hemolytic anemia, chronic

Aplastic and other anemias and other bone marrow failure syndromes (D6Ø-D64)

✓4th D6Ø Acquired pure red cell aplasia [erythroblastopenia]
INCLUDES red cell aplasia (acquired) (adult) (with thymoma)
EXCLUDES 1 *congenital red cell aplasia (D61.Ø1)*
DEF: Bone marrow failure characterized by underproduction of red blood cells while white blood cell and platelet production remains normal.

D6Ø.Ø Chronic acquired pure red cell aplasia HCC Rx ESR COM

D6Ø.1 Transient acquired pure red cell aplasia HCC Rx ESR COM

D6Ø.8 Other acquired pure red cell aplasias HCC Rx ESR COM

D6Ø.9 Acquired pure red cell aplasia, unspecified HCC Rx ESR COM

✓4th D61 Other aplastic anemias and other bone marrow failure syndromes
EXCLUDES 2 *neutropenia (D7Ø.-)*
AHA: 2020,3Q,22; 2014,4Q,22
DEF: Aplastic anemia: Bone marrow failure characterized by underproduction of red bloods cells, white blood cells and platelets.

✓5th D61.Ø Constitutional aplastic anemia

D61.Ø1 Constitutional (pure) red blood cell aplasia HCC Rx ESR COM
Blackfan-Diamond syndrome
Congenital (pure) red cell aplasia
Familial hypoplastic anemia
Primary (pure) red cell aplasia
Red cell (pure) aplasia of infants
EXCLUDES 1 *acquired red cell aplasia (D6Ø.9)*

D61.Ø9 Other constitutional aplastic anemia HCC Rx ESR COM
Fanconi's anemia
Pancytopenia with malformations

D61.1 Drug-induced aplastic anemia HCC Rx ESR COM
Use additional code for adverse effect, if applicable, to identify drug (T36-T5Ø with fifth or sixth character 5)

D61.2 Aplastic anemia due to other external agents HCC Rx ESR COM
Code first, if applicable, toxic effects of substances chiefly nonmedicinal as to source (T51-T65)

D61.3 Idiopathic aplastic anemia HCC Rx ESR COM

✓5th D61.8 Other specified aplastic anemias and other bone marrow failure syndromes

✓6th D61.81 Pancytopenia
EXCLUDES 1 *pancytopenia (due to) (with) aplastic anemia (D61.9)*
pancytopenia (due to) (with) bone marrow infiltration (D61.82)
pancytopenia (due to) (with) congenital (pure) red cell aplasia (D61.Ø1)
pancytopenia (due to) (with) hairy cell leukemia (C91.4-)
pancytopenia (due to) (with) human immunodeficiency virus disease (B2Ø)
pancytopenia (due to) (with) leukoerythroblastic anemia (D61.82)
pancytopenia (due to) (with) myeloproliferative disease (D47.1)
EXCLUDES 2 *pancytopenia (due to) (with) myelodysplastic syndromes (D46.-)*
DEF: Shortage of all three blood cells: white, red, and platelets.

D61.81Ø Antineoplastic chemotherapy induced pancytopenia HCC ESR
EXCLUDES 2 *aplastic anemia due to antineoplastic chemotherapy (D61.1)*
AHA: 2020,3Q,22

D61.811 Other drug-induced pancytopenia HCC ESR
EXCLUDES 2 *aplastic anemia due to drugs (D61.1)*

D61.818 Other pancytopenia HCC ESR
AHA: 2020,3Q,24; 2019,1Q,16
TIP: Assign this code in addition to myeloid leukemia codes (C92.-) when pancytopenia is documented. Although common in some types of myeloid leukemia, pancytopenia is not always inherent.

D61.82 Myelophthisis HCC Rx ESR COM
Leukoerythroblastic anemia
Myelophthisic anemia
Panmyelophthisis
Code also the underlying disorder, such as:
malignant neoplasm of breast (C5Ø.-)
tuberculosis (A15.-)
EXCLUDES 1 *idiopathic myelofibrosis (D47.1)*
myelofibrosis NOS (D75.81)
myelofibrosis with myeloid metaplasia (D47.4)
primary myelofibrosis (D47.1)
secondary myelofibrosis (D75.81)
DEF: Condition that occurs when normal hematopoietic tissue in the bone marrow is replaced with abnormal tissue, such as fibrous tissue or tumors. Most commonly seen during the advanced stages of cancer.

D61.89 Other specified aplastic anemias and other bone marrow failure syndromes HCC Rx ESR COM

D61.9 Aplastic anemia, unspecified HCC Rx ESR COM
Hypoplastic anemia NOS
Medullary hypoplasia

D62 Acute posthemorrhagic anemia
EXCLUDES 1 *anemia due to chronic blood loss (D5Ø.Ø)*
blood loss anemia NOS (D5Ø.Ø)
congenital anemia from fetal blood loss (P61.3)
AHA: 2019,3Q,11,17

✓4th D63 Anemia in chronic diseases classified elsewhere

***D63.Ø* Anemia in neoplastic disease**
Code first neoplasm (CØØ-D49)
EXCLUDES 1 *aplastic anemia due to antineoplastic chemotherapy (D61.1)*
EXCLUDES 2 *anemia due to antineoplastic chemotherapy (D64.81)*

***D63.1* Anemia in chronic kidney disease**
Erythropoietin resistant anemia (EPO resistant anemia)
Code first underlying chronic kidney disease (CKD) (N18.-)

HCC CMS-HCC | Rx Rx HCC | ESR ESRD HCC | COM Commercial HCC | N Newborn: 0 | P Pediatric: 0-17 | M Maternity: 9-64 | A Adult: 15-124

D63.8 Anemia in other chronic diseases classified elsewhere
Code first underlying disease, such as:
diphyllobothriasis (B70.0)
hookworm disease (B76.0-B76.9)
hypothyroidism (E00.0-E03.9)
malaria (B50.0-B54)
symptomatic late syphilis (A52.79)
tuberculosis (A18.89)

D64 Other anemias
EXCLUDES 1 *refractory anemia (D46.-)*
refractory anemia with excess blasts in transformation [RAEB T] (C92.0-)
DEF: Sideroblastic anemia: Hereditary or secondary disorder in which the red blood cells cannot effectively use iron, a nutrient needed to make hemoglobin. Although the iron can enter the red blood cell it is not assimilated into the hemoglobin molecule and builds up ringed sideroblasts around the cell nucleus.

D64.0 Hereditary sideroblastic anemia HCC Rx ESR COM
Sex-linked hypochromic sideroblastic anemia

D64.1 Secondary sideroblastic anemia due to disease HCC Rx ESR COM
Code first underlying disease

D64.2 Secondary sideroblastic anemia due to drugs and toxins HCC Rx ESR COM
Code first poisoning due to drug or toxin, if applicable (T36-T65 with fifth or sixth character 1-4 or 6)
Use additional code for adverse effect, if applicable, to identify drug (T36-T50 with fifth or sixth character 5)

D64.3 Other sideroblastic anemias HCC Rx ESR COM
Sideroblastic anemia NOS
Pyridoxine-responsive sideroblastic anemia NEC

D64.4 Congenital dyserythropoietic anemia
Dyshematopoietic anemia (congenital)
EXCLUDES 1 *Blackfan-Diamond syndrome (D61.01)*
Di Guglielmo's disease (C94.0)

D64.8 Other specified anemias

D64.81 Anemia due to antineoplastic chemotherapy
Antineoplastic chemotherapy induced anemia
EXCLUDES 2 *anemia in neoplastic disease (D63.0)*
aplastic anemia due to antineoplastic chemotherapy (D61.1)
AHA: 2021,3Q,4; 2014,4Q,22

D64.89 Other specified anemias
Infantile pseudoleukemia

D64.9 Anemia, unspecified
AHA: 2020,3Q,24; 2018,4Q,88; 2017,1Q,7

Coagulation defects, purpura and other hemorrhagic conditions (D65-D69)

D65 Disseminated intravascular coagulation [defibrination syndrome] HCC ESR COM
Afibrinogenemia, acquired
Consumption coagulopathy
Diffuse or disseminated intravascular coagulation [DIC]
Fibrinolytic hemorrhage, acquired
Fibrinolytic purpura
Purpura fulminans
EXCLUDES 1 *disseminated intravascular coagulation (complicating):*
abortion or ectopic or molar pregnancy (O00-O07, O08.1)
in newborn (P60)
pregnancy, childbirth and the puerperium (O45.0, O46.0, O67.0, O72.3)
AHA: 2021,1Q,39

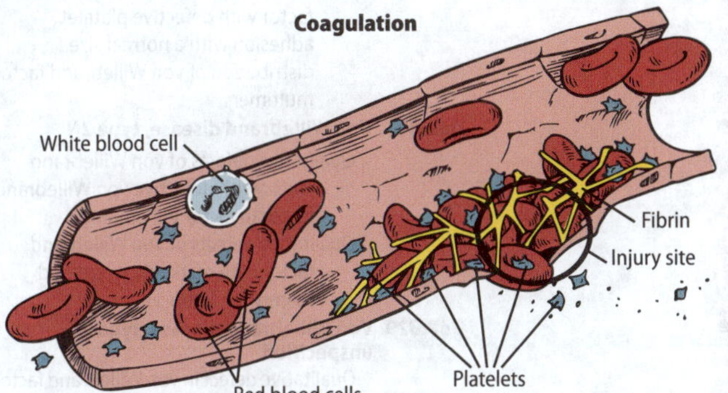

D66 Hereditary factor VIII deficiency HCC ESR COM
Classical hemophilia
Deficiency factor VIII (with functional defect)
Hemophilia NOS
Hemophilia A
EXCLUDES 1 *factor VIII deficiency with vascular defect ▶(D68.0-)◀*
DEF: Hereditary, sex-linked lack of antihemophilic globulin (AHG) (factor VIII) that causes abnormal coagulation characterized by increased bleeding; large bruises of skin; bleeding in the mouth, nose, and gastrointestinal tract; and hemorrhages into joints, resulting in swelling and impaired function.

D67 Hereditary factor IX deficiency HCC ESR COM
Christmas disease
Factor IX deficiency (with functional defect)
Hemophilia B
Plasma thromboplastin component [PTC] deficiency

D68 Other coagulation defects
EXCLUDES 1 *▶abnormal coagulation profile NOS◀ (R79.1)*
~~*coagulation defects complicating abortion or ectopic or molar pregnancy (O00-O07, O08.1)*~~
~~*coagulation defects complicating pregnancy, childbirth and the puerperium (O45.0, O46.0, O67.0, O72.3)*~~
EXCLUDES 2 *▶coagulation defects complicating abortion or ectopic or molar pregnancy (O00-O07, O08.1)◀*
▶coagulation defects complicating pregnancy, childbirth and the puerperium (O45.0, O46.0, O67.0, O72.3)◀
AHA: 2016,1Q,14

▲ **D68.0 Von Willebrand disease**
~~Angiohemophilia~~
~~Factor VIII deficiency with vascular defect~~
~~Vascular hemophilia~~
EXCLUDES 1 *capillary fragility (hereditary) (D69.8)*
factor VIII deficiency NOS (D66)
factor VIII deficiency with functional defect (D66)
DEF: Congenital, abnormal blood coagulation caused by deficient blood factor VII. Symptoms include excess or prolonged bleeding.

● **D68.00 Von Willebrand disease, unspecified**

● **D68.01 Von Willebrand disease, type 1**
Partial quantitative deficiency of von Willebrand factor
Type 1C von Willebrand disease

● 6th **D68.02 Von Willebrand disease, type 2**
Qualitative defects of von Willebrand factor

● **D68.020 Von Willebrand disease, type 2A**
Qualitative defects of von Willebrand factor with decreased platelet adhesion and selective deficiency of high-molecular-weight multimers

● **D68.021 Von Willebrand disease, type 2B**
Qualitative defects of von Willebrand factor with high-molecular-weight von Willebrand factor loss
Qualitative defects of von Willebrand factor with hyper-adhesive forms
Qualitative defects of von Willebrand factor with increased affinity for platelet glycoprotein Ib

● **D68.022 Von Willebrand disease, type 2M**
Qualitative defects of von Willebrand factor with defective platelet adhesion with a normal size distribution of von Willebrand factor multimers

● **D68.023 Von Willebrand disease, type 2N**
Qualitative defects of von Willebrand factor with defective von Willebrand factor to factor VIII binding
Qualitative defects of von Willebrand factor with markedly decreased affinity for factor VIII

● **D68.029 Von Willebrand disease, type 2, unspecified**
Qualitative defect in von Willebrand factor function, with no further subtyping

● **D68.03 Von Willebrand disease, type 3**
(Near) complete absence of von Willebrand factor
Total quantitative deficiency of von Willebrand factor

● **D68.04 Acquired von Willebrand disease**
Acquired von Willebrand syndrome

● **D68.09 Other von Willebrand disease**
Platelet-type von Willebrand disease
Pseudo-von Willebrand disease
Code also, if applicable, qualitative platelet defects (D69.1)

D68.1 Hereditary factor XI deficiency HCC ESR COM
Hemophilia C
Plasma thromboplastin antecedent [PTA] deficiency
Rosenthal's disease

D68.2 Hereditary deficiency of other clotting factors HCC ESR COM
AC globulin deficiency
Congenital afibrinogenemia
Deficiency of factor I [fibrinogen]
Deficiency of factor II [prothrombin]
Deficiency of factor V [labile]
Deficiency of factor VII [stable]
Deficiency of factor X [Stuart-Prower]
Deficiency of factor XII [Hageman]
Deficiency of factor XIII [fibrin stabilizing]
Dysfibrinogenemia (congenital)
Hypoproconvertinemia
Owren's disease
Proaccelerin deficiency

5th **D68.3 Hemorrhagic disorder due to circulating anticoagulants**

6th **D68.31 Hemorrhagic disorder due to intrinsic circulating anticoagulants, antibodies, or inhibitors**

D68.311 Acquired hemophilia HCC ESR COM
Autoimmune hemophilia
Autoimmune inhibitors to clotting factors
Secondary hemophilia

D68.312 Antiphospholipid antibody with hemorrhagic disorder HCC ESR COM
Lupus anticoagulant (LAC) with hemorrhagic disorder
Systemic lupus erythematosus [SLE] inhibitor with hemorrhagic disorder
EXCLUDES 1 *antiphospholipid antibody, finding without diagnosis (R76.0)*
antiphospholipid antibody syndrome (D68.61)
antiphospholipid antibody with hypercoagulable state (D68.61)
lupus anticoagulant (LAC) finding without diagnosis (R76.0)
lupus anticoagulant (LAC) with hypercoagulable state (D68.62)
systemic lupus erythematosus [SLE] inhibitor finding without diagnosis (R76.0)
systemic lupus erythematosus [SLE] inhibitor with hypercoagulable state (D68.62)

D68.318 Other hemorrhagic disorder due to intrinsic circulating anticoagulants, antibodies, or inhibitors HCC ESR COM
Antithromboplastinemia
Antithromboplastinogenemia
Hemorrhagic disorder due to intrinsic increase in antithrombin
Hemorrhagic disorder due to intrinsic increase in anti-VIIIa
Hemorrhagic disorder due to intrinsic increase in anti-IXa
Hemorrhagic disorder due to intrinsic increase in anti-XIa

D68.32 Hemorrhagic disorder due to extrinsic circulating anticoagulants HCC ESR COM
Drug-induced hemorrhagic disorder
Hemorrhagic disorder due to increase in anti-IIa
Hemorrhagic disorder due to increase in anti-Xa
Hyperheparinemia
Use additional code for adverse effect, if applicable, to identify drug (T45.515, T45.525)
AHA: 2021,1Q,4; 2016,1Q,14-15
TIP: Do not assign to identify routine therapeutic anticoagulation effects; assign only for documented adverse effects.

D68.4 Acquired coagulation factor deficiency HCC ESR COM
Deficiency of coagulation factor due to liver disease
Deficiency of coagulation factor due to vitamin K deficiency
EXCLUDES 1 *vitamin K deficiency of newborn (P53)*

5th **D68.5 Primary thrombophilia**
Primary hypercoagulable states
EXCLUDES 1 *antiphospholipid syndrome (D68.61)*
lupus anticoagulant (D68.62)
secondary activated protein C resistance (D68.69)
secondary antiphospholipid antibody syndrome (D68.69)
secondary lupus anticoagulant with hypercoagulable state (D68.69)
secondary systemic lupus erythematosus [SLE] inhibitor with hypercoagulable state (D68.69)
systemic lupus erythematosus [SLE] inhibitor finding without diagnosis (R76.0)
systemic lupus erythematosus [SLE] inhibitor with hemorrhagic disorder (D68.312)
thrombotic thrombocytopenic purpura (M31.19)
DEF: Thrombophilia: Increased tendency of the blood to clot, which can lead to thrombus or embolus formation.

D68.51 Activated protein C resistance HCC ESR COM
Factor V Leiden mutation

D68.52 Prothrombin gene mutation HCC ESR COM

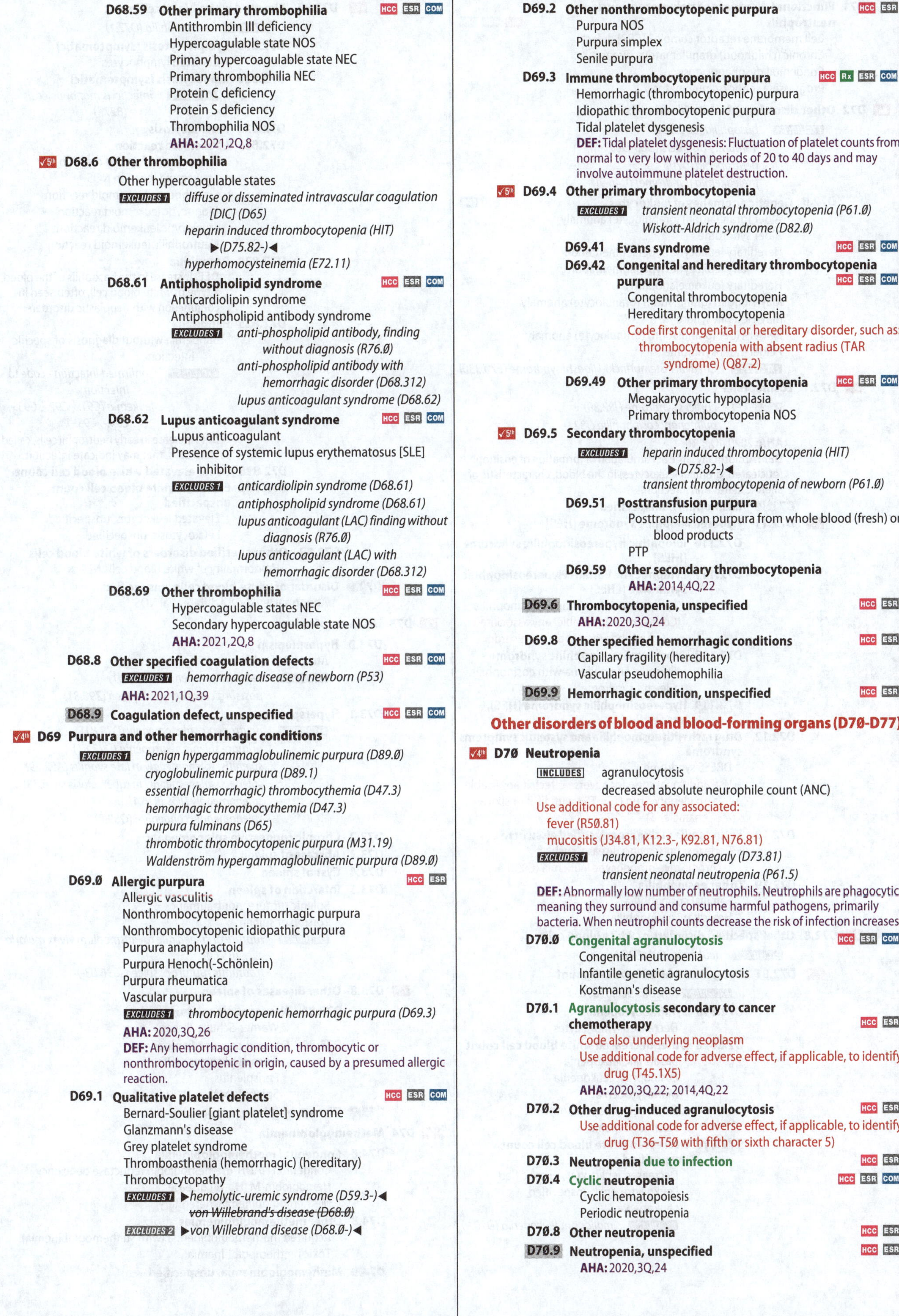

D68.59 Other primary thrombophilia HCC ESR COM
Antithrombin III deficiency
Hypercoagulable state NOS
Primary hypercoagulable state NEC
Primary thrombophilia NEC
Protein C deficiency
Protein S deficiency
Thrombophilia NOS
AHA: 2021,2Q,8

D68.6 Other thrombophilia
Other hypercoagulable states
EXCLUDES 1 *diffuse or disseminated intravascular coagulation [DIC] (D65)*
heparin induced thrombocytopenia (HIT) ▶(D75.82-)◀
hyperhomocysteinemia (E72.11)

D68.61 Antiphospholipid syndrome HCC ESR COM
Anticardiolipin syndrome
Antiphospholipid antibody syndrome
EXCLUDES 1 *anti-phospholipid antibody, finding without diagnosis (R76.0)*
anti-phospholipid antibody with hemorrhagic disorder (D68.312)
lupus anticoagulant syndrome (D68.62)

D68.62 Lupus anticoagulant syndrome HCC ESR COM
Lupus anticoagulant
Presence of systemic lupus erythematosus [SLE] inhibitor
EXCLUDES 1 *anticardiolipin syndrome (D68.61)*
antiphospholipid syndrome (D68.61)
lupus anticoagulant (LAC) finding without diagnosis (R76.0)
lupus anticoagulant (LAC) with hemorrhagic disorder (D68.312)

D68.69 Other thrombophilia HCC ESR COM
Hypercoagulable states NEC
Secondary hypercoagulable state NOS
AHA: 2021,2Q,8

D68.8 Other specified coagulation defects HCC ESR COM
EXCLUDES 1 *hemorrhagic disease of newborn (P53)*
AHA: 2021,1Q,39

D68.9 Coagulation defect, unspecified HCC ESR COM

D69 Purpura and other hemorrhagic conditions
EXCLUDES 1 *benign hypergammaglobulinemic purpura (D89.0)*
cryoglobulinemic purpura (D89.1)
essential (hemorrhagic) thrombocythemia (D47.3)
hemorrhagic thrombocythemia (D47.3)
purpura fulminans (D65)
thrombotic thrombocytopenic purpura (M31.19)
Waldenström hypergammaglobulinemic purpura (D89.0)

D69.0 Allergic purpura HCC ESR
Allergic vasculitis
Nonthrombocytopenic hemorrhagic purpura
Nonthrombocytopenic idiopathic purpura
Purpura anaphylactoid
Purpura Henoch(-Schönlein)
Purpura rheumatica
Vascular purpura
EXCLUDES 1 *thrombocytopenic hemorrhagic purpura (D69.3)*
AHA: 2020,3Q,26
DEF: Any hemorrhagic condition, thrombocytic or nonthrombocytopenic in origin, caused by a presumed allergic reaction.

D69.1 Qualitative platelet defects HCC ESR COM
Bernard-Soulier [giant platelet] syndrome
Glanzmann's disease
Grey platelet syndrome
Thromboasthenia (hemorrhagic) (hereditary)
Thrombocytopathy
EXCLUDES 1 ▶*hemolytic-uremic syndrome (D59.3-)*◀
~~*von Willebrand's disease (D68.0)*~~
EXCLUDES 2 ▶*von Willebrand disease (D68.0-)*◀

D69.2 Other nonthrombocytopenic purpura HCC ESR
Purpura NOS
Purpura simplex
Senile purpura

D69.3 Immune thrombocytopenic purpura HCC Rx ESR COM
Hemorrhagic (thrombocytopenic) purpura
Idiopathic thrombocytopenic purpura
Tidal platelet dysgenesis
DEF: Tidal platelet dysgenesis: Fluctuation of platelet counts from normal to very low within periods of 20 to 40 days and may involve autoimmune platelet destruction.

D69.4 Other primary thrombocytopenia
EXCLUDES 1 *transient neonatal thrombocytopenia (P61.0)*
Wiskott-Aldrich syndrome (D82.0)

D69.41 Evans syndrome HCC ESR COM

D69.42 Congenital and hereditary thrombocytopenia purpura HCC ESR COM
Congenital thrombocytopenia
Hereditary thrombocytopenia
Code first congenital or hereditary disorder, such as:
thrombocytopenia with absent radius (TAR syndrome) (Q87.2)

D69.49 Other primary thrombocytopenia HCC ESR COM
Megakaryocytic hypoplasia
Primary thrombocytopenia NOS

D69.5 Secondary thrombocytopenia
EXCLUDES 1 *heparin induced thrombocytopenia (HIT) ▶(D75.82-)◀*
transient thrombocytopenia of newborn (P61.0)

D69.51 Posttransfusion purpura
Posttransfusion purpura from whole blood (fresh) or blood products
PTP

D69.59 Other secondary thrombocytopenia
AHA: 2014,4Q,22

D69.6 Thrombocytopenia, unspecified HCC ESR
AHA: 2020,3Q,24

D69.8 Other specified hemorrhagic conditions HCC ESR
Capillary fragility (hereditary)
Vascular pseudohemophilia

D69.9 Hemorrhagic condition, unspecified HCC ESR

Other disorders of blood and blood-forming organs (D70-D77)

D70 Neutropenia
INCLUDES agranulocytosis
decreased absolute neurophile count (ANC)
Use additional code for any associated:
fever (R50.81)
mucositis (J34.81, K12.3-, K92.81, N76.81)
EXCLUDES 1 *neutropenic splenomegaly (D73.81)*
transient neonatal neutropenia (P61.5)
DEF: Abnormally low number of neutrophils. Neutrophils are phagocytic, meaning they surround and consume harmful pathogens, primarily bacteria. When neutrophil counts decrease the risk of infection increases.

D70.0 Congenital agranulocytosis HCC ESR COM
Congenital neutropenia
Infantile genetic agranulocytosis
Kostmann's disease

D70.1 Agranulocytosis secondary to cancer chemotherapy HCC ESR
Code also underlying neoplasm
Use additional code for adverse effect, if applicable, to identify drug (T45.1X5)
AHA: 2020,3Q,22; 2014,4Q,22

D70.2 Other drug-induced agranulocytosis HCC ESR
Use additional code for adverse effect, if applicable, to identify drug (T36-T50 with fifth or sixth character 5)

D70.3 Neutropenia due to infection HCC ESR

D70.4 Cyclic neutropenia HCC ESR COM
Cyclic hematopoiesis
Periodic neutropenia

D70.8 Other neutropenia HCC ESR

D70.9 Neutropenia, unspecified HCC ESR
AHA: 2020,3Q,24

Chapter 3. Diseases of the Blood and Blood-forming Organs

D68.59–D70.9

D71 Functional disorders of polymorphonuclear neutrophils HCC ESR COM
Cell membrane receptor complex [CR3] defect
Chronic (childhood) granulomatous disease
Congenital dysphagocytosis
Progressive septic granulomatosis

D72 Other disorders of white blood cells
EXCLUDES 1 *basophilia (D72.824)*
immunity disorders (D8Ø-D89)
neutropenia (D7Ø)
preleukemia (syndrome) (D46.9)

D72.Ø Genetic anomalies of leukocytes HCC ESR COM
Alder (granulation) (granulocyte) anomaly
Alder syndrome
Hereditary leukocytic hypersegmentation
Hereditary leukocytic hyposegmentation
Hereditary leukomelanopathy
May-Hegglin (granulation) (granulocyte) anomaly
May-Hegglin syndrome
Pelger-Huët (granulation) (granulocyte) anomaly
Pelger-Huët syndrome
EXCLUDES 1 *Chédiak (-Steinbrinck)-Higashi syndrome (E7Ø.33Ø)*

D72.1 Eosinophilia
EXCLUDES 2 *Löffler's syndrome (J82.89)*
pulmonary eosinophilia (J82.-)
AHA: 2020,4Q,8-10
DEF: Abnormally large accumulation or formation of eosinophils (nucleated, granular leukocytes) in the blood, characteristic of allergic states and infection.

D72.1Ø Eosinophilia, unspecified

D72.11 Hypereosinophilic syndrome [HES]

D72.11Ø Idiopathic hypereosinophilic syndrome [IHES]

D72.111 Lymphocytic Variant Hypereosinophilic Syndrome [LHES]
Lymphocyte variant hypereosinophilia
Code also, if applicable, any associated lymphocytic neoplastic disorder

D72.118 Other hypereosinophilic syndrome
Episodic angioedema with eosinophilia
Gleich's syndrome

D72.119 Hypereosinophilic syndrome [HES], unspecified

D72.12 Drug rash with eosinophilia and systemic symptoms syndrome
DRESS syndrome
Use additional code for adverse effect, if applicable, to identify drug (T36-T5Ø with fifth or sixth character 5)

D72.18 Eosinophilia in diseases classified elsewhere
Code first underlying disease, such as:
chronic myelomonocytic leukemia (C93.1-)

D72.19 Other eosinophilia
Familial eosinophilia
Hereditary eosinophilia

D72.8 Other specified disorders of white blood cells
EXCLUDES 1 *leukemia (C91-C95)*

D72.81 Decreased white blood cell count
EXCLUDES 1 *neutropenia (D7Ø.-)*

D72.81Ø Lymphocytopenia
Decreased lymphocytes

D72.818 Other decreased white blood cell count
Basophilic leukopenia
Eosinophilic leukopenia
Monocytopenia
Other decreased leukocytes
Plasmacytopenia

D72.819 Decreased white blood cell count, unspecified
Decreased leukocytes, unspecified
Leukocytopenia, unspecified
Leukopenia
EXCLUDES 1 *malignant leukopenia (D7Ø.9)*

D72.82 Elevated white blood cell count
EXCLUDES 1 *eosinophilia (D72.1)*

D72.82Ø Lymphocytosis (symptomatic)
Elevated lymphocytes

D72.821 Monocytosis (symptomatic)
EXCLUDES 1 *infectious mononucleosis (B27.-)*

D72.822 Plasmacytosis

D72.823 Leukemoid reaction
Basophilic leukemoid reaction
Leukemoid reaction NOS
Lymphocytic leukemoid reaction
Monocytic leukemoid reaction
Myelocytic leukemoid reaction
Neutrophilic leukemoid reaction

D72.824 Basophilia
DEF: Increase in the basophils of the blood, a type of white blood cell, often seen in conjunction with neoplastic disorders.

D72.825 Bandemia
Bandemia without diagnosis of specific infection
EXCLUDES 1 *confirmed infection - code to infection*
leukemia (C91.-, C92.-, C93.-, C94.-, C95.-)
DEF: Increase in early neutrophil cells, called band cells, that may indicate infection.

D72.828 Other elevated white blood cell count

D72.829 Elevated white blood cell count, unspecified
Elevated leukocytes, unspecified
Leukocytosis, unspecified

D72.89 Other specified disorders of white blood cells
Abnormality of white blood cells NEC

D72.9 Disorder of white blood cells, unspecified
Abnormal leukocyte differential NOS

D73 Diseases of spleen

D73.Ø Hyposplenism
Atrophy of spleen
EXCLUDES 1 *asplenia (congenital) (Q89.Ø1)*
postsurgical absence of spleen (Z9Ø.81)

D73.1 Hypersplenism
EXCLUDES 1 *neutropenic splenomegaly (D73.81)*
primary splenic neutropenia (D73.81)
splenitis, splenomegaly in late syphilis (A52.79)
splenitis, splenomegaly in tuberculosis (A18.85)
splenomegaly NOS (R16.1)
splenomegaly congenital (Q89.Ø)

D73.2 Chronic congestive splenomegaly

D73.3 Abscess of spleen

D73.4 Cyst of spleen

D73.5 Infarction of spleen
Splenic rupture, nontraumatic
Torsion of spleen
EXCLUDES 1 *rupture of spleen due to Plasmodium vivax malaria (B51.Ø)*
traumatic rupture of spleen (S36.Ø3-)

D73.8 Other diseases of spleen

D73.81 Neutropenic splenomegaly
Werner-Schultz disease

D73.89 Other diseases of spleen
Fibrosis of spleen NOS
Perisplenitis
Splenitis NOS

D73.9 Disease of spleen, unspecified

D74 Methemoglobinemia

D74.Ø Congenital methemoglobinemia
Congenital NADH-methemoglobin reductase deficiency
Hemoglobin-M [Hb-M] disease
Methemoglobinemia, hereditary

D74.8 Other methemoglobinemias
Acquired methemoglobinemia (with sulfhemoglobinemia)
Toxic methemoglobinemia

D74.9 Methemoglobinemia, unspecified

D75 Other and unspecified diseases of blood and blood-forming organs

EXCLUDES 2 *acute lymphadenitis (LØ4.-)*
chronic lymphadenitis (I88.1)
enlarged lymph nodes (R59.-)
hypergammaglobulinemia NOS (D89.2)
lymphadenitis NOS (I88.9)
mesenteric lymphadenitis (acute) (chronic) (I88.Ø)

D75.Ø Familial erythrocytosis
Benign polycythemia
Familial polycythemia
EXCLUDES 1 *hereditary ovalocytosis (D58.1)*

D75.1 Secondary polycythemia
Acquired polycythemia
Emotional polycythemia
Erythrocytosis NOS
Hypoxemic polycythemia
Nephrogenous polycythemia
Polycythemia due to erythropoietin
Polycythemia due to fall in plasma volume
Polycythemia due to high altitude
Polycythemia due to stress
Polycythemia NOS
Relative polycythemia
EXCLUDES 1 *polycythemia neonatorum (P61.1)*
polycythemia vera (D45)
DEF: Elevated number of red blood cells in circulating blood as a result of reduced oxygen supply to the tissues.

D75.8 Other specified diseases of blood and blood-forming organs

D75.81 Myelofibrosis HCC Rx ESR COM
Myelofibrosis NOS
Secondary myelofibrosis NOS
Code first the underlying disorder, such as:
malignant neoplasm of breast (C5Ø.-)
Use additional code, if applicable, for associated therapy-related myelodysplastic syndrome (D46.-)
Use additional code for adverse effect, if applicable, to identify drug (T45.1X5)
EXCLUDES 1 *acute myelofibrosis (C94.4-)*
idiopathic myelofibrosis (D47.1)
leukoerythroblastic anemia (D61.82)
myelofibrosis with myeloid metaplasia (D47.4)
myelophthisic anemia (D61.82)
myelophthisis (D61.82)
primary myelofibrosis (D47.1)

▲ **D75.82 Heparin induced thrombocytopenia (HIT)**
▶Use additional code, if applicable, for adverse effect of heparin (T45.515-)◀
DEF: Immune-mediated reaction to heparin therapy causing an abrupt fall in platelet count and serious complications such as pulmonary embolism, stroke, AMI, or DVT.

● **D75.821 Non-immune heparin-induced thrombocytopenia**
Non-immune HIT
Type 1 heparin-induced thrombocytopenia

● **D75.822 Immune-mediated heparin-induced thrombocytopenia**
Immune-mediated HIT
Type 2 heparin-induced thrombocytopenia

● **D75.828 Other heparin-induced thrombocytopenia syndrome**
Autoimmune heparin-induced thrombocytopenia syndrome
Delayed-onset heparin-induced thrombocytopenia
Persisting heparin-induced thrombocytopenia

● **D75.829 Heparin-induced thrombocytopenia, unspecified**

D75.83 Thrombocytosis
EXCLUDES 2 *essential thrombocythemia (D47.3)*
AHA: 2021,4Q,7-8

D75.838 Other thrombocytosis
Reactive thrombocytosis
Secondary thrombocytosis
Code also underlying condition, if known and applicable

D75.839 Thrombocytosis, unspecified
Thrombocythemia NOS
Thrombocytosis NOS

● **D75.84 Other platelet-activating anti-PF4 disorders**
Spontaneous heparin-induced thrombocytopenia syndrome (without heparin exposure)
Thrombosis with thrombocytopenia syndrome
Vaccine-induced thrombotic thrombocytopenia
Use additional code, if applicable, for adverse effect of other viral vaccine (T5Ø.B95-)

D75.89 Other specified diseases of blood and blood-forming organs

D75.9 Disease of blood and blood-forming organs, unspecified

D75.A Glucose-6-phosphate dehydrogenase (G6PD) deficiency without anemia
EXCLUDES 1 *glucose-6-phosphate dehydrogenase (G6PD) deficiency with anemia (D55.Ø)*
AHA: 2019,4Q,4-5

D76 Other specified diseases with participation of lymphoreticular and reticulohistiocytic tissue
EXCLUDES 1 *(Abt-) Letterer-Siwe disease (C96.Ø)*
eosinophilic granuloma (C96.6)
Hand-Schüller-Christian disease (C96.5)
histiocytic medullary reticulosis (C96.9)
histiocytic sarcoma (C96.A)
histiocytosis X, multifocal (C96.5)
histiocytosis X, unifocal (C96.6)
Langerhans-cell histiocytosis, multifocal (C96.5)
Langerhans-cell histiocytosis NOS (C96.6)
Langerhans-cell histiocytosis, unifocal (C96.6)
leukemic reticuloendotheliosis (C91.4-)
lipomelanotic reticulosis (I89.8)
malignant histiocytosis (C96.A)
malignant reticulosis (C86.Ø)
nonlipid reticuloendotheliosis (C96.Ø)

D76.1 Hemophagocytic lymphohistiocytosis HCC ESR COM
Familial hemophagocytic reticulosis
Histiocytoses of mononuclear phagocytes

D76.2 Hemophagocytic syndrome, infection-associated HCC ESR COM
Use additional code to identify infectious agent or disease

D76.3 Other histiocytosis syndromes HCC ESR COM
Reticulohistiocytoma (giant-cell)
Sinus histiocytosis with massive lymphadenopathy
Xanthogranuloma

D77 Other disorders of blood and blood-forming organs in diseases classified elsewhere
Code first underlying disease, such as:
amyloidosis (E85.-)
congenital early syphilis (A5Ø.Ø)
echinococcosis (B67.Ø-B67.9)
malaria (B5Ø.Ø-B54)
schistosomiasis [bilharziasis] (B65.Ø-B65.9)
vitamin C deficiency (E54)
EXCLUDES 1 *rupture of spleen due to Plasmodium vivax malaria (B51.Ø)*
splenitis, splenomegaly in late syphilis (A52.79)
splenitis, splenomegaly in tuberculosis (A18.85)

Intraoperative and postprocedural complications of the spleen (D78)

D78 Intraoperative and postprocedural complications of the spleen
AHA: 2016,4Q,9-10

D78.0 Intraoperative hemorrhage and hematoma of the spleen complicating a procedure
EXCLUDES 1 *intraoperative hemorrhage and hematoma of the spleen due to accidental puncture or laceration during a procedure (D78.1-)*

D78.01 Intraoperative hemorrhage and hematoma of the spleen complicating a procedure on the spleen

D78.02 Intraoperative hemorrhage and hematoma of the spleen complicating other procedure

D78.1 Accidental puncture and laceration of the spleen during a procedure

D78.11 Accidental puncture and laceration of the spleen during a procedure on the spleen

D78.12 Accidental puncture and laceration of the spleen during other procedure
AHA: 2022,1Q,22

D78.2 Postprocedural hemorrhage of the spleen following a procedure

D78.21 Postprocedural hemorrhage of the spleen following a procedure on the spleen

D78.22 Postprocedural hemorrhage of the spleen following other procedure

D78.3 Postprocedural hematoma and seroma of the spleen following a procedure

D78.31 Postprocedural hematoma of the spleen following a procedure on the spleen

D78.32 Postprocedural hematoma of the spleen following other procedure

D78.33 Postprocedural seroma of the spleen following a procedure on the spleen

D78.34 Postprocedural seroma of the spleen following other procedure

D78.8 Other intraoperative and postprocedural complications of the spleen
Use additional code, if applicable, to further specify disorder

D78.81 Other intraoperative complications of the spleen

D78.89 Other postprocedural complications of the spleen

Certain disorders involving the immune mechanism (D80-D89)

INCLUDES defects in the complement system
immunodeficiency disorders, except human immunodeficiency virus [HIV] disease
sarcoidosis

EXCLUDES 1 *autoimmune disease (systemic) NOS (M35.9)*
functional disorders of polymorphonuclear neutrophils (D71)
human immunodeficiency virus [HIV] disease (B20)

D80 Immunodeficiency with predominantly antibody defects

D80.0 Hereditary hypogammaglobulinemia HCC Rx ESR COM
Autosomal recessive agammaglobulinemia (Swiss type)
X-linked agammaglobulinemia [Bruton] (with growth hormone deficiency)

D80.1 Nonfamilial hypogammaglobulinemia HCC Rx ESR COM
Agammaglobulinemia with immunoglobulin-bearing B-lymphocytes
Common variable agammaglobulinemia [CVAgamma]
Hypogammaglobulinemia NOS

D80.2 Selective deficiency of immunoglobulin A [IgA] HCC Rx ESR COM

D80.3 Selective deficiency of immunoglobulin G [IgG] subclasses HCC Rx ESR COM

D80.4 Selective deficiency of immunoglobulin M [IgM] HCC Rx ESR COM

D80.5 Immunodeficiency with increased immunoglobulin M [IgM] HCC Rx ESR COM

D80.6 Antibody deficiency with near-normal immunoglobulins or with hyperimmunoglobulinemia HCC Rx ESR COM

D80.7 Transient hypogammaglobulinemia of infancy HCC Rx ESR COM

D80.8 Other immunodeficiencies with predominantly antibody defects HCC Rx ESR COM
Kappa light chain deficiency

D80.9 Immunodeficiency with predominantly antibody defects, unspecified HCC Rx ESR COM

D81 Combined immunodeficiencies
EXCLUDES 1 *autosomal recessive agammaglobulinemia (Swiss type) (D80.0)*

D81.0 Severe combined immunodeficiency [SCID] with reticular dysgenesis HCC Rx ESR COM

D81.1 Severe combined immunodeficiency [SCID] with low T- and B-cell numbers HCC Rx ESR COM

D81.2 Severe combined immunodeficiency [SCID] with low or normal B-cell numbers HCC Rx ESR COM

D81.3 Adenosine deaminase [ADA] deficiency
AHA: 2019,4Q,5-6

D81.30 Adenosine deaminase deficiency, unspecified HCC Rx ESR COM
ADA deficiency NOS

D81.31 Severe combined immunodeficiency due to adenosine deaminase deficiency HCC Rx ESR COM
ADA deficiency with SCID
Adenosine deaminase [ADA] deficiency with severe combined immunodeficiency

D81.32 Adenosine deaminase 2 deficiency HCC Rx ESR COM
ADA2 deficiency
Adenosine deaminase deficiency type 2
Code also, if applicable, any associated manifestations, such as:
polyarteritis nodosa (M30.0)
stroke (I63.-)

D81.39 Other adenosine deaminase deficiency HCC Rx ESR COM
Adenosine deaminase [ADA] deficiency type 1, NOS
Adenosine deaminase [ADA] deficiency type 1, without SCID
Adenosine deaminase [ADA] deficiency type 1, without severe combined immunodeficiency
Partial ADA deficiency (type 1)
Partial adenosine deaminase deficiency (type 1)

D81.4 Nezelof's syndrome HCC Rx ESR COM

D81.5 Purine nucleoside phosphorylase [PNP] deficiency HCC Rx ESR COM

D81.6 Major histocompatibility complex class I deficiency HCC Rx ESR COM
Bare lymphocyte syndrome

D81.7 Major histocompatibility complex class II deficiency HCC Rx ESR COM

D81.8 Other combined immunodeficiencies

D81.81 Biotin-dependent carboxylase deficiency
Multiple carboxylase deficiency
EXCLUDES 1 *biotin-dependent carboxylase deficiency due to dietary deficiency of biotin (E53.8)*

D81.810 Biotinidase deficiency

D81.818 Other biotin-dependent carboxylase deficiency
Holocarboxylase synthetase deficiency
Other multiple carboxylase deficiency

D81.819 Biotin-dependent carboxylase deficiency, unspecified
Multiple carboxylase deficiency, unspecified

● **D81.82 Activated Phosphoinositide 3-kinase Delta Syndrome [APDS]**
p110d-activating mutation causing senescent T cells, lymphadenopathy, and immunodeficiency [PASLI] disease
Code also, if applicable, any associated manifestations, such as:
bronchiectasis (J47.-)
herpes virus infections (B00.-)
other acute respiratory tract infections (J00-J06; J20-J22)
other infections (A00-B99)
pneumonia (J12-J18)

D81.89 Other combined immunodeficiencies HCC Rx ESR COM

D81.9 Combined immunodeficiency, unspecified HCC Rx ESR COM
Severe combined immunodeficiency disorder [SCID] NOS

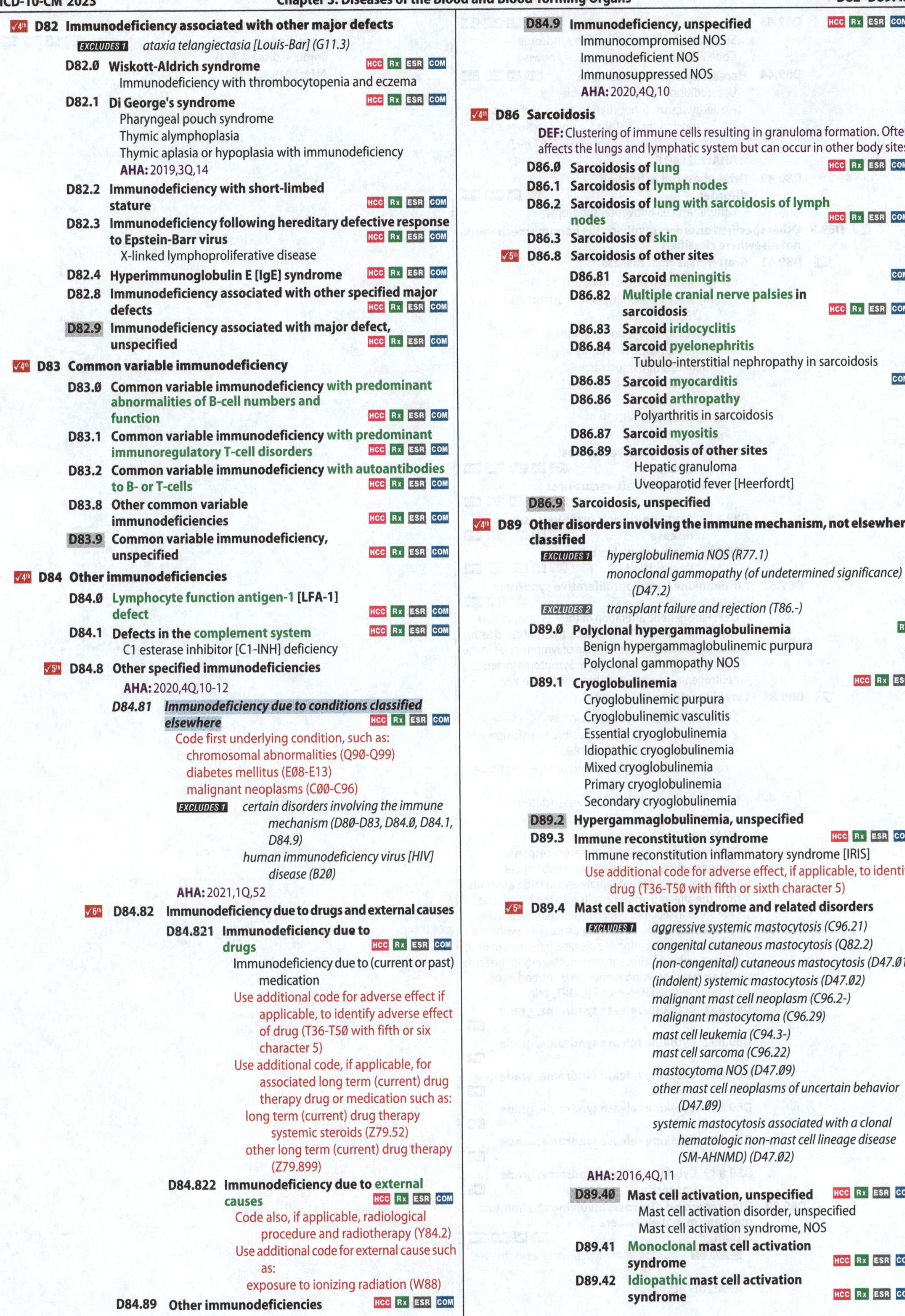

D82 Immunodeficiency associated with other major defects

EXCLUDES 1 *ataxia telangiectasia [Louis-Bar] (G11.3)*

D82.0 Wiskott-Aldrich syndrome HCC Rx ESR COM
Immunodeficiency with thrombocytopenia and eczema

D82.1 Di George's syndrome HCC Rx ESR COM
Pharyngeal pouch syndrome
Thymic alymphoplasia
Thymic aplasia or hypoplasia with immunodeficiency
AHA: 2019,3Q,14

D82.2 Immunodeficiency with short-limbed stature HCC Rx ESR COM

D82.3 Immunodeficiency following hereditary defective response to Epstein-Barr virus HCC Rx ESR COM
X-linked lymphoproliferative disease

D82.4 Hyperimmunoglobulin E [IgE] syndrome HCC Rx ESR COM

D82.8 Immunodeficiency associated with other specified major defects HCC Rx ESR COM

D82.9 Immunodeficiency associated with major defect, unspecified HCC Rx ESR COM

D83 Common variable immunodeficiency

D83.0 Common variable immunodeficiency with predominant abnormalities of B-cell numbers and function HCC Rx ESR COM

D83.1 Common variable immunodeficiency with predominant immunoregulatory T-cell disorders HCC Rx ESR COM

D83.2 Common variable immunodeficiency with autoantibodies to B- or T-cells HCC Rx ESR COM

D83.8 Other common variable immunodeficiencies HCC Rx ESR COM

D83.9 Common variable immunodeficiency, unspecified HCC Rx ESR COM

D84 Other immunodeficiencies

D84.0 Lymphocyte function antigen-1 [LFA-1] defect HCC Rx ESR COM

D84.1 Defects in the complement system HCC Rx ESR COM
C1 esterase inhibitor [C1-INH] deficiency

D84.8 Other specified immunodeficiencies
AHA: 2020,4Q,10-12

D84.81 Immunodeficiency due to conditions classified elsewhere HCC Rx ESR COM
Code first underlying condition, such as:
chromosomal abnormalities (Q90-Q99)
diabetes mellitus (E08-E13)
malignant neoplasms (C00-C96)
EXCLUDES 1 *certain disorders involving the immune mechanism (D80-D83, D84.0, D84.1, D84.9)*
human immunodeficiency virus [HIV] disease (B20)
AHA: 2021,1Q,52

D84.82 Immunodeficiency due to drugs and external causes

D84.821 Immunodeficiency due to drugs HCC Rx ESR COM
Immunodeficiency due to (current or past) medication
Use additional code for adverse effect if applicable, to identify adverse effect of drug (T36-T50 with fifth or six character 5)
Use additional code, if applicable, for associated long term (current) drug therapy drug or medication such as:
long term (current) drug therapy systemic steroids (Z79.52)
other long term (current) drug therapy (Z79.899)

D84.822 Immunodeficiency due to external causes HCC Rx ESR COM
Code also, if applicable, radiological procedure and radiotherapy (Y84.2)
Use additional code for external cause such as:
exposure to ionizing radiation (W88)

D84.89 Other immunodeficiencies HCC Rx ESR COM

D84.9 Immunodeficiency, unspecified HCC Rx ESR COM
Immunocompromised NOS
Immunodeficient NOS
Immunosuppressed NOS
AHA: 2020,4Q,10

D86 Sarcoidosis

DEF: Clustering of immune cells resulting in granuloma formation. Often affects the lungs and lymphatic system but can occur in other body sites.

D86.0 Sarcoidosis of lung HCC Rx ESR COM

D86.1 Sarcoidosis of lymph nodes

D86.2 Sarcoidosis of lung with sarcoidosis of lymph nodes HCC Rx ESR COM

D86.3 Sarcoidosis of skin

D86.8 Sarcoidosis of other sites

D86.81 Sarcoid meningitis COM

D86.82 Multiple cranial nerve palsies in sarcoidosis HCC Rx ESR COM

D86.83 Sarcoid iridocyclitis

D86.84 Sarcoid pyelonephritis
Tubulo-interstitial nephropathy in sarcoidosis

D86.85 Sarcoid myocarditis COM

D86.86 Sarcoid arthropathy
Polyarthritis in sarcoidosis

D86.87 Sarcoid myositis

D86.89 Sarcoidosis of other sites
Hepatic granuloma
Uveoparotid fever [Heerfordt]

D86.9 Sarcoidosis, unspecified

D89 Other disorders involving the immune mechanism, not elsewhere classified

EXCLUDES 1 *hyperglobulinemia NOS (R77.1)*
monoclonal gammopathy (of undetermined significance) (D47.2)

EXCLUDES 2 *transplant failure and rejection (T86.-)*

D89.0 Polyclonal hypergammaglobulinemia Rx
Benign hypergammaglobulinemic purpura
Polyclonal gammopathy NOS

D89.1 Cryoglobulinemia HCC Rx ESR
Cryoglobulinemic purpura
Cryoglobulinemic vasculitis
Essential cryoglobulinemia
Idiopathic cryoglobulinemia
Mixed cryoglobulinemia
Primary cryoglobulinemia
Secondary cryoglobulinemia

D89.2 Hypergammaglobulinemia, unspecified

D89.3 Immune reconstitution syndrome HCC Rx ESR COM
Immune reconstitution inflammatory syndrome [IRIS]
Use additional code for adverse effect, if applicable, to identify drug (T36-T50 with fifth or sixth character 5)

D89.4 Mast cell activation syndrome and related disorders

EXCLUDES 1 *aggressive systemic mastocytosis (C96.21)*
congenital cutaneous mastocytosis (Q82.2)
(non-congenital) cutaneous mastocytosis (D47.01)
(indolent) systemic mastocytosis (D47.02)
malignant mast cell neoplasm (C96.2-)
malignant mastocytoma (C96.29)
mast cell leukemia (C94.3-)
mast cell sarcoma (C96.22)
mastocytoma NOS (D47.09)
other mast cell neoplasms of uncertain behavior (D47.09)
systemic mastocytosis associated with a clonal hematologic non-mast cell lineage disease (SM-AHNMD) (D47.02)

AHA: 2016,4Q,11

D89.40 Mast cell activation, unspecified HCC Rx ESR COM
Mast cell activation disorder, unspecified
Mast cell activation syndrome, NOS

D89.41 Monoclonal mast cell activation syndrome HCC Rx ESR COM

D89.42 Idiopathic mast cell activation syndrome HCC Rx ESR COM

Chapter 3. Diseases of the Blood and Blood-forming Organs

D82–D89.42

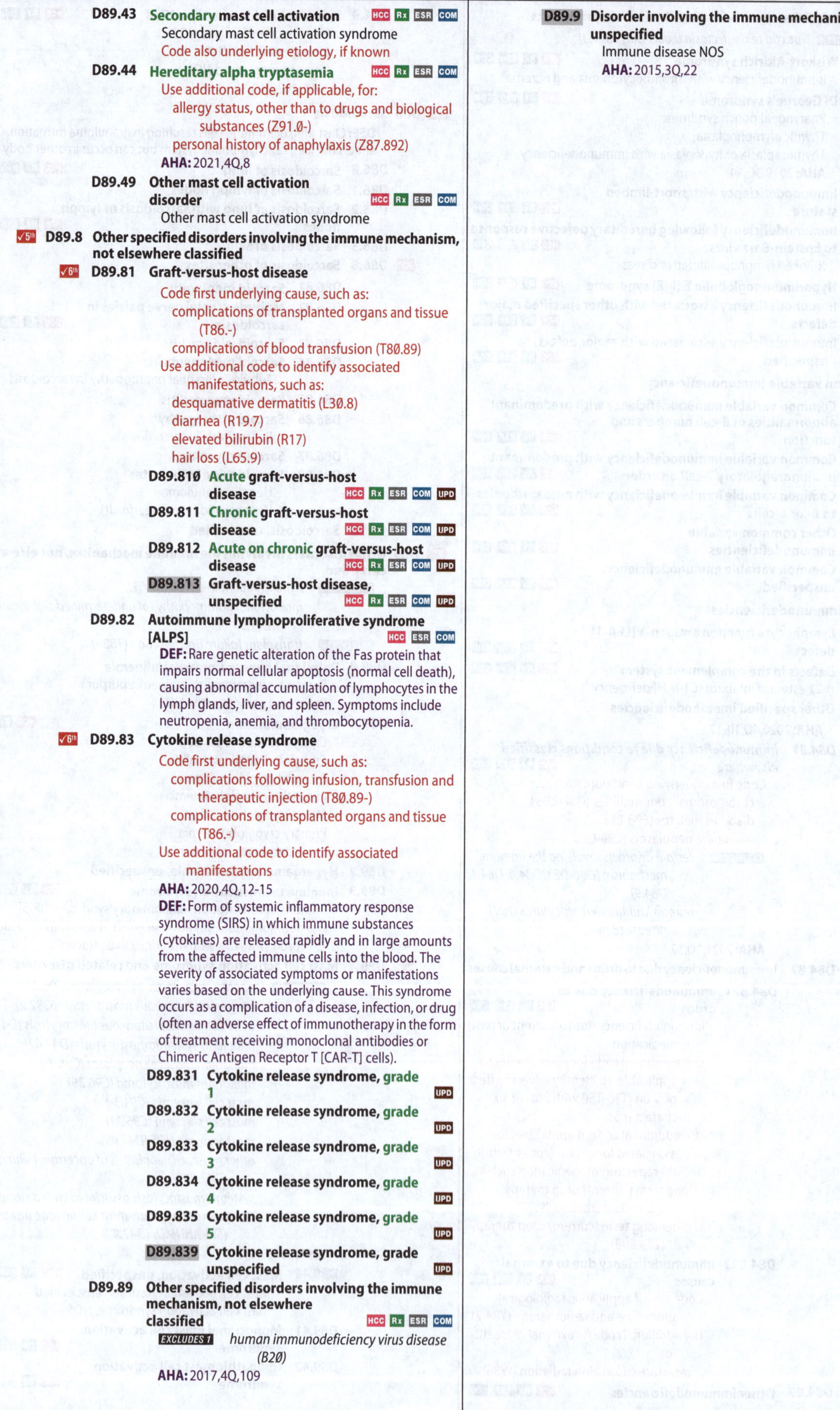

D89.43 Secondary mast cell activation HCC Rx ESR COM
Secondary mast cell activation syndrome
Code also underlying etiology, if known

D89.44 Hereditary alpha tryptasemia HCC Rx ESR COM
Use additional code, if applicable, for:
allergy status, other than to drugs and biological substances (Z91.Ø-)
personal history of anaphylaxis (Z87.892)
AHA: 2021,4Q,8

D89.49 Other mast cell activation disorder HCC Rx ESR COM
Other mast cell activation syndrome

√5th **D89.8 Other specified disorders involving the immune mechanism, not elsewhere classified**

√6th **D89.81 Graft-versus-host disease**
Code first underlying cause, such as:
complications of transplanted organs and tissue (T86.-)
complications of blood transfusion (T8Ø.89)
Use additional code to identify associated manifestations, such as:
desquamative dermatitis (L3Ø.8)
diarrhea (R19.7)
elevated bilirubin (R17)
hair loss (L65.9)

D89.81Ø Acute graft-versus-host disease HCC Rx ESR COM UPD

D89.811 Chronic graft-versus-host disease HCC Rx ESR COM UPD

D89.812 Acute on chronic graft-versus-host disease HCC Rx ESR COM UPD

D89.813 Graft-versus-host disease, unspecified HCC Rx ESR COM UPD

D89.82 Autoimmune lymphoproliferative syndrome [ALPS] HCC ESR COM
DEF: Rare genetic alteration of the Fas protein that impairs normal cellular apoptosis (normal cell death), causing abnormal accumulation of lymphocytes in the lymph glands, liver, and spleen. Symptoms include neutropenia, anemia, and thrombocytopenia.

√6th **D89.83 Cytokine release syndrome**
Code first underlying cause, such as:
complications following infusion, transfusion and therapeutic injection (T8Ø.89-)
complications of transplanted organs and tissue (T86.-)
Use additional code to identify associated manifestations
AHA: 2020,4Q,12-15
DEF: Form of systemic inflammatory response syndrome (SIRS) in which immune substances (cytokines) are released rapidly and in large amounts from the affected immune cells into the blood. The severity of associated symptoms or manifestations varies based on the underlying cause. This syndrome occurs as a complication of a disease, infection, or drug (often an adverse effect of immunotherapy in the form of treatment receiving monoclonal antibodies or Chimeric Antigen Receptor T [CAR-T] cells).

D89.831 Cytokine release syndrome, grade 1 UPD

D89.832 Cytokine release syndrome, grade 2 UPD

D89.833 Cytokine release syndrome, grade 3 UPD

D89.834 Cytokine release syndrome, grade 4 UPD

D89.835 Cytokine release syndrome, grade 5 UPD

D89.839 Cytokine release syndrome, grade unspecified UPD

D89.89 Other specified disorders involving the immune mechanism, not elsewhere classified HCC Rx ESR COM
EXCLUDES 1 *human immunodeficiency virus disease (B2Ø)*
AHA: 2017,4Q,109

D89.9 Disorder involving the immune mechanism, unspecified HCC Rx ESR COM
Immune disease NOS
AHA: 2015,3Q,22

Chapter 4. Endocrine, Nutritional, and Metabolic Diseases (EØØ–E89)

Chapter-specific Guidelines with Coding Examples

The chapter-specific guidelines from the ICD-10-CM Official Guidelines for Coding and Reporting have been provided below. Along with these guidelines are coding examples, contained in the shaded boxes, that have been developed to help illustrate the coding and/or sequencing guidance found in these guidelines.

a. Diabetes mellitus

The diabetes mellitus codes are combination codes that include the type of diabetes mellitus, the body system affected, and the complications affecting that body system. As many codes within a particular category as are necessary to describe all of the complications of the disease may be used. They should be sequenced based on the reason for a particular encounter. Assign as many codes from categories EØ8–E13 as needed to identify all of the associated conditions that the patient has.

Patient is seen for uncontrolled diabetes, type 2, with hyperglycemia diabetic nephropathy, and diabetic gastroparesis

E11.65	**Type 2 diabetes mellitus with hyperglycemia**
E11.21	**Type 2 diabetes mellitus with diabetic nephropathy**
E11.43	**Type 2 diabetes mellitus with diabetic autonomic (poly)neuropathy**
K31.84	**Gastroparesis**

Explanation: Use as many codes to describe the diabetic complications as needed. Many are combination codes that describe more than one condition. Code first the reason for the encounter. The term "uncontrolled" can refer to either hyperglycemia or hypoglycemia. In this case, "uncontrolled" is described as "with hyperglycemia."

1) Type of diabetes

The age of a patient is not the sole determining factor, though most type 1 diabetics develop the condition before reaching puberty. For this reason, type 1 diabetes mellitus is also referred to as juvenile diabetes.

A 45-year-old patient is diagnosed with type 1 diabetes

E1Ø.9	**Type 1 diabetes mellitus without complications**

Explanation: Although most type 1 diabetics are diagnosed in childhood or adolescence, it can also begin in adults.

2) Type of diabetes mellitus not documented

If the type of diabetes mellitus is not documented in the medical record the default is E11.-, Type 2 diabetes mellitus.

Office visit lists diabetic retinopathy with macular edema and hypertension on patient problem list

E11.311	**Type 2 diabetes mellitus with unspecified diabetic retinopathy with macular edema**
I1Ø	**Essential (primary) hypertension**

Explanation: Since the type of diabetes was not documented, default to category E11.

3) Diabetes mellitus and the use of insulin, oral hypoglycemics, and injectable non-insulin drugs

If the documentation in a medical record does not indicate the type of diabetes but does indicate that the patient uses insulin, code E11-, Type 2 diabetes mellitus, should be assigned. Additional code(s) should be assigned from category Z79 to identify the long-term (current) use of insulin, oral hypoglycemic drugs, or injectable non-insulin antidiabetic, as follows:

If the patient is treated with both oral **hypoglycemic drugs** and insulin, both code Z79.4, Long term (current) use of insulin, and code Z79.84, Long term (current) use of oral hypoglycemic drugs, should be assigned.

If the patient is treated with both insulin and an injectable non-insulin antidiabetic drug, assign codes Z79.4, Long term (current) use of insulin, and **Z79.85, Long-term (current) use of injectable non-insulin antidiabetic drugs.**

If the patient is treated with both oral hypoglycemic drugs and an injectable non-insulin antidiabetic drug, assign codes Z79.84, Long term (current) use of oral hypoglycemic drugs, and **Z79.85, Long-term (current) use of injectable non-insulin antidiabetic drugs.**

Code Z79.4 should not be assigned if insulin is given temporarily to bring a type 2 patient's blood sugar under control during an encounter.

Office visit lists chronic diabetes with daily insulin use on patient problem list

E11.9	**Type 2 diabetes mellitus without complications**
Z79.4	**Long term (current) use of insulin**

Explanation: Do not assume that a patient on insulin must have type 1 diabetes. The default for diabetes without further specification defaults to type 2. Add the code for long term use of insulin.

4) Diabetes mellitus in pregnancy and gestational diabetes

See Section I.C.15. Diabetes mellitus in pregnancy.

See Section I.C.15. Gestational (pregnancy induced) diabetes

5) Complications due to insulin pump malfunction

(a) Underdose of insulin due to insulin pump failure

An underdose of insulin due to an insulin pump failure should be assigned to a code from subcategory T85.6, Mechanical complication of other specified internal and external prosthetic devices, implants and grafts, that specifies the type of pump malfunction, as the principal or first-listed code, followed by code T38.3X6-, Underdosing of insulin and oral hypoglycemic [antidiabetic] drugs. Additional codes for the type of diabetes mellitus and any associated complications due to the underdosing should also be assigned.

A 24-year-old type 1 diabetic male treated in for hyperglycemia; insulin pump found to be malfunctioning and underdosing

T85.614A	**Breakdown (mechanical) of insulin pump, initial encounter**
T38.3X6A	**Underdosing of insulin and oral hypoglycemic [antidiabetic] drugs, initial encounter**
E1Ø.65	**Type 1 diabetes mellitus with hyperglycemia**

Explanation: The complication code for the mechanical breakdown of the pump is sequenced first, followed by the underdosing code and type of diabetes with complication. Code all other diabetic complication codes necessary to describe the patient's condition.

(b) Overdose of insulin due to insulin pump failure

The principal or first-listed code for an encounter due to an insulin pump malfunction resulting in an overdose of insulin, should also be T85.6-, Mechanical complication of other specified internal and external prosthetic devices, implants and grafts, followed by code T38.3X1-, Poisoning by insulin and oral hypoglycemic [antidiabetic] drugs, accidental (unintentional).

A 24-year-old type 1 diabetic male found down with diabetic coma, brought into ED and treated for hypoglycemia; insulin pump found to be malfunctioning and overdosing

T85.614A	**Breakdown (mechanical) of insulin pump, initial encounter**
T38.3X1A	**Poisoning by insulin and oral hypoglycemic [antidiabetic] drugs, accidental (unintentional), initial encounter**
E1Ø.641	**Type 1 diabetes mellitus with hypoglycemia with coma**

Explanation: The complication code for the mechanical breakdown of the pump is sequenced first, followed by the poisoning code and type of diabetes with complication. All the characters in the combination code must be used to form a valid code and to fully describe the type of diabetes, the hypoglycemia, and the coma.

6) Secondary diabetes mellitus

Codes under categories EØ8, Diabetes mellitus due to underlying condition, EØ9, Drug or chemical induced diabetes mellitus, and E13, Other specified diabetes mellitus, identify complications/manifestations associated with secondary diabetes mellitus. Secondary diabetes is always caused by another condition or event (e.g., cystic fibrosis, malignant neoplasm of pancreas, pancreatectomy, adverse effect of drug, or poisoning).

(a) Secondary diabetes mellitus and the use of insulin or oral hypoglycemic drugs

For patients with secondary diabetes mellitus who routinely use insulin, oral hypoglycemic drugs, or injectable non-insulin drugs, additional code(s) from category Z79 should be assigned to identify the long-term (current) use of insulin, oral hypoglycemic drugs, or non-injectable non-insulin drugs as follows:

If the patient is treated with both oral **hypoglycemic drugs** and insulin, both code Z79.4, Long term (current) use of insulin, and code Z79.84, Long term (current) use of oral hypoglycemic drugs, should be assigned.

If the patient is treated with both insulin and an injectable non-insulin antidiabetic drug, assign codes Z79.4, Long-term (current) use of insulin, and **Z79.85, Long-term (current) use of injectable non-insulin antidiabetic drugs.**

If the patient is treated with both oral hypoglycemic drugs and an injectable non-insulin antidiabetic drug, assign codes Z79.84, Long-term (current) use of oral hypoglycemic drugs, and **Z79.85, Long-term (current) use of injectable non-insulin antidiabetic drugs.**

Code Z79.4 should not be assigned if insulin is given temporarily to bring a secondary diabetic patient's blood sugar under control during an encounter.

Type 2 diabetic with no complications, normally only on oral metformin, is given insulin for three days to maintain glucose control while in the hospital recovering from surgery

E11.9	**Type 2 diabetes mellitus without complications**
Z79.84	**Long term (current) use of oral hypoglycemic drugs**

Explanation: Although the patient was given insulin for a short time during his hospital stay, the intent was only to maintain the patient's glucose levels while off his regular oral hypoglycemic medication, not for long term use. No code is needed for long term use of insulin, but a Z code for long term use of an oral hypoglycemic should be added to identify the chronic use of this drug.

Type 2 diabetic with diabetic polyneuropathy on insulin

E11.42	**Type 2 diabetes mellitus with diabetic polyneuropathy**
Z79.4	**Long term (current) use of insulin**

Explanation: Add a Z code for the long term use of insulin and the long term use of metformin because both are taken chronically.

(b) Assigning and sequencing secondary diabetes codes and its causes

The sequencing of the secondary diabetes codes in relationship to codes for the cause of the diabetes is based on the Tabular List instructions for categories E08, E09 and E13.

(i) Secondary diabetes mellitus due to pancreatectomy

For postpancreatectomy diabetes mellitus (lack of insulin due to the surgical removal of all or part of the pancreas), assign code E89.1, Postprocedural hypoinsulinemia. Assign a code from category E13 and a code from subcategory Z90.41-, Acquired absence of pancreas, as additional codes.

Patient with newly diagnosed diabetes after surgical removal of part of pancreas

E89.1	**Postprocedural hypoinsulinemia**
E13.9	**Other specified diabetes mellitus without complications**
Z90.411	**Acquired partial absence of pancreas**

Explanation: Sequence the postprocedural complication of the hypoinsulinemia due to the partial removal of the pancreas as the first-listed code, followed by codes for other specified diabetes (NEC) without complications and partial acquired absence of the pancreas.

(ii) Secondary diabetes due to drugs

Secondary diabetes may be caused by an adverse effect of correctly administered medications, poisoning or sequela of poisoning.

See section I.C.19.e. for coding of adverse effects and poisoning, and section I.C.20 for external cause code reporting.

Initial encounter for corticosteroid-induced diabetes mellitus

E09.9	**Drug or chemical induced diabetes mellitus without complications**
T38.0X5A	**Adverse effect of glucocorticoids and synthetic analogues, initial encounter**

Explanation: If the diabetes is caused by an adverse effect of a drug, the diabetic condition is coded first. If it occurs from a poisoning or overdose, the poisoning code causing the diabetes is sequenced first.

Chapter 4. Endocrine, Nutritional and Metabolic Diseases (EØØ-E89)

NOTE All neoplasms, whether functionally active or not, are classified in Chapter 2. Appropriate codes in this chapter (i.e. EØ5.8, EØ7.Ø, E16-E31, E34.-) may be used as additional codes to indicate either functional activity by neoplasms and ectopic endocrine tissue or hyperfunction and hypofunction of endocrine glands associated with neoplasms and other conditions classified elsewhere.

EXCLUDES 1 *transitory endocrine and metabolic disorders specific to newborn (P7Ø-P74)*

AHA: 2018,2Q,6

This chapter contains the following blocks:

EØØ-EØ7 Disorders of thyroid gland
EØ8-E13 Diabetes mellitus
E15-E16 Other disorders of glucose regulation and pancreatic internal secretion
E2Ø-E35 Disorders of other endocrine glands
E36 Intraoperative complications of endocrine system
E4Ø-E46 Malnutrition
E5Ø-E64 Other nutritional deficiencies
E65-E68 Overweight, obesity and other hyperalimentation
E7Ø-E88 Metabolic disorders
E89 Postprocedural endocrine and metabolic complications and disorders, not elsewhere classified

Disorders of thyroid gland (EØØ-EØ7)

✓4th **EØØ Congenital iodine-deficiency syndrome**

Use additional code (F7Ø-F79) to identify associated intellectual disabilities

EXCLUDES 1 *subclinical iodine-deficiency hypothyroidism (EØ2)*

EØØ.Ø Congenital iodine-deficiency syndrome, neurological type Rx
Endemic cretinism, neurological type

EØØ.1 Congenital iodine-deficiency syndrome, myxedematous type Rx
Endemic hypothyroid cretinism
Endemic cretinism, myxedematous type

EØØ.2 Congenital iodine-deficiency syndrome, mixed type Rx
Endemic cretinism, mixed type

EØØ.9 Congenital iodine-deficiency syndrome, unspecified Rx
Congenital iodine-deficiency hypothyroidism NOS
Endemic cretinism NOS

✓4th **EØ1 Iodine-deficiency related thyroid disorders and allied conditions**

EXCLUDES 1 *congenital iodine-deficiency syndrome (EØØ.-)*
subclinical iodine-deficiency hypothyroidism (EØ2)

EØ1.Ø Iodine-deficiency related diffuse (endemic) goiter Rx

EØ1.1 Iodine-deficiency related multinodular (endemic) goiter Rx
Iodine-deficiency related nodular goiter

EØ1.2 Iodine-deficiency related (endemic) goiter, unspecified Rx
Endemic goiter NOS

EØ1.8 Other iodine-deficiency related thyroid disorders and allied conditions Rx
Acquired iodine-deficiency hypothyroidism NOS

EØ2 Subclinical iodine-deficiency hypothyroidism Rx
AHA: 2021,1Q,8

✓4th **EØ3 Other hypothyroidism**

EXCLUDES 1 *iodine-deficiency related hypothyroidism (EØØ-EØ2)*
postprocedural hypothyroidism (E89.Ø)

DEF: Hypothyroidism: Underproduction of thyroid hormone.

EØ3.Ø Congenital hypothyroidism with diffuse goiter Rx
Congenital parenchymatous goiter (nontoxic)
Congenital goiter (nontoxic) NOS
EXCLUDES 1 *transitory congenital goiter with normal function (P72.Ø)*

EØ3.1 Congenital hypothyroidism without goiter Rx
Aplasia of thyroid (with myxedema)
Congenital atrophy of thyroid
Congenital hypothyroidism NOS

EØ3.2 Hypothyroidism due to medicaments and other exogenous substances Rx
Code first poisoning due to drug or toxin, if applicable (T36-T65 with fifth or sixth character 1-4 or 6)
Use additional code for adverse effect, if applicable, to identify drug (T36-T5Ø with fifth or sixth character 5)

EØ3.3 Postinfectious hypothyroidism Rx

EØ3.4 Atrophy of thyroid (acquired) Rx
EXCLUDES 1 *congenital atrophy of thyroid (EØ3.1)*

EØ3.5 Myxedema coma HCC Rx ESR COM

EØ3.8 Other specified hypothyroidism Rx
AHA: 2021,1Q,8

EØ3.9 Hypothyroidism, unspecified Rx
Myxedema NOS

✓4th **EØ4 Other nontoxic goiter**

EXCLUDES 1 *congenital goiter (NOS) (diffuse) (parenchymatous) (EØ3.Ø)*
iodine-deficiency related goiter (EØØ-EØ2)

EØ4.Ø Nontoxic diffuse goiter Rx
Diffuse (colloid) nontoxic goiter
Simple nontoxic goiter

EØ4.1 Nontoxic single thyroid nodule Rx
Colloid nodule (cystic) (thyroid)
Nontoxic uninodular goiter
Thyroid (cystic) nodule NOS
DEF: Enlarged thyroid, commonly due to decreased thyroid production, with a single nodule. No clinical hypothyroidism.

EØ4.2 Nontoxic multinodular goiter Rx
Cystic goiter NOS
Multinodular (cystic) goiter NOS
DEF: Enlarged thyroid, commonly due to decreased thyroid production with multiple nodules. No clinical hypothyroidism.

EØ4.8 Other specified nontoxic goiter Rx

EØ4.9 Nontoxic goiter, unspecified Rx
Goiter NOS
Nodular goiter (nontoxic) NOS

✓4th **EØ5 Thyrotoxicosis [hyperthyroidism]**

EXCLUDES 1 *chronic thyroiditis with transient thyrotoxicosis (EØ6.2)*
neonatal thyrotoxicosis (P72.1)

DEF: Excessive quantities of hormones from the thyroid gland caused by overproduction or loss of storage ability.

✓5th **EØ5.Ø Thyrotoxicosis with diffuse goiter**
Exophthalmic or toxic goiter NOS
Graves' disease
Toxic diffuse goiter
DEF: Diffuse thyroid enlargement accompanied by hyperthyroidism, bulging eyes, and dermopathy.

EØ5.ØØ Thyrotoxicosis with diffuse goiter without thyrotoxic crisis or storm Rx

EØ5.Ø1 Thyrotoxicosis with diffuse goiter with thyrotoxic crisis or storm Rx

Goiter

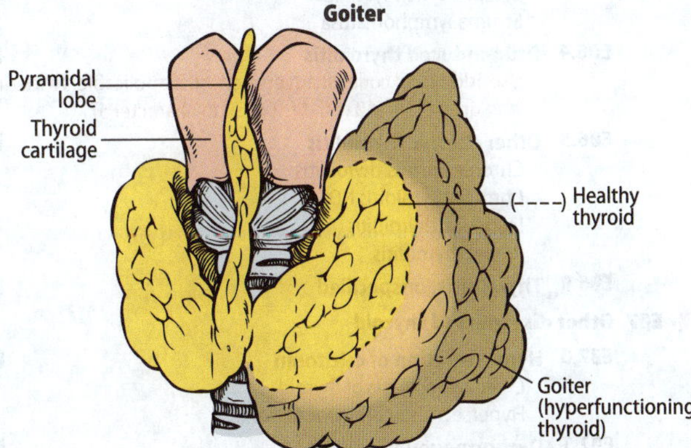

✓5th **EØ5.1 Thyrotoxicosis with toxic single thyroid nodule**
Thyrotoxicosis with toxic uninodular goiter
DEF: Symptomatic hyperthyroidism with a single nodule on the enlarged thyroid gland. Onset of symptoms can be abrupt and include extreme nervousness, insomnia, weight loss, tremors, and psychosis or coma.

EØ5.1Ø Thyrotoxicosis with toxic single thyroid nodule without thyrotoxic crisis or storm Rx

EØ5.11 Thyrotoxicosis with toxic single thyroid nodule with thyrotoxic crisis or storm Rx

✓5th **EØ5.2 Thyrotoxicosis with toxic multinodular goiter**
Toxic nodular goiter NOS

EØ5.2Ø Thyrotoxicosis with toxic multinodular goiter without thyrotoxic crisis or storm Rx

EØ5.21 Thyrotoxicosis with toxic multinodular goiter with thyrotoxic crisis or storm Rx

5th **EØ5.3 Thyrotoxicosis from ectopic thyroid tissue**
- **EØ5.3Ø Thyrotoxicosis from ectopic thyroid tissue without thyrotoxic crisis or storm** Rx
- **EØ5.31 Thyrotoxicosis from ectopic thyroid tissue with thyrotoxic crisis or storm** Rx

5th **EØ5.4 Thyrotoxicosis factitia**
- **EØ5.4Ø Thyrotoxicosis factitia without thyrotoxic crisis or storm** Rx
- **EØ5.41 Thyrotoxicosis factitia with thyrotoxic crisis or storm** Rx

5th **EØ5.8 Other thyrotoxicosis**
Overproduction of thyroid-stimulating hormone
- **EØ5.8Ø Other thyrotoxicosis without thyrotoxic crisis or storm** Rx
- **EØ5.81 Other thyrotoxicosis with thyrotoxic crisis or storm** Rx

5th **EØ5.9 Thyrotoxicosis, unspecified**
Hyperthyroidism NOS
- **EØ5.9Ø Thyrotoxicosis, unspecified without thyrotoxic crisis or storm** Rx
- **EØ5.91 Thyrotoxicosis, unspecified with thyrotoxic crisis or storm** Rx

4th **EØ6 Thyroiditis**
EXCLUDES 1 *postpartum thyroiditis (O9Ø.5)*
DEF: Inflammation of the thyroid gland.

EØ6.Ø Acute thyroiditis Rx
Abscess of thyroid
Pyogenic thyroiditis
Suppurative thyroiditis
Use additional code (B95-B97) to identify infectious agent

EØ6.1 Subacute thyroiditis Rx
de Quervain thyroiditis
Giant-cell thyroiditis
Granulomatous thyroiditis
Nonsuppurative thyroiditis
Viral thyroiditis
EXCLUDES 1 *autoimmune thyroiditis (EØ6.3)*

EØ6.2 Chronic thyroiditis with transient thyrotoxicosis Rx
EXCLUDES 1 *autoimmune thyroiditis (EØ6.3)*

EØ6.3 Autoimmune thyroiditis Rx
Hashimoto's thyroiditis
Hashitoxicosis (transient)
Lymphadenoid goiter
Lymphocytic thyroiditis
Struma lymphomatosa

EØ6.4 Drug-induced thyroiditis Rx
Use additional code for adverse effect, if applicable, to identify drug (T36-T5Ø with fifth or sixth character 5)

EØ6.5 Other chronic thyroiditis Rx
Chronic fibrous thyroiditis
Chronic thyroiditis NOS
Ligneous thyroiditis
Riedel thyroiditis

EØ6.9 Thyroiditis, unspecified Rx

4th **EØ7 Other disorders of thyroid**

EØ7.Ø Hypersecretion of calcitonin Rx
C-cell hyperplasia of thyroid
Hypersecretion of thyrocalcitonin

EØ7.1 Dyshormogenetic goiter Rx
Familial dyshormogenetic goiter
Pendred's syndrome
EXCLUDES 1 *transitory congenital goiter with normal function (P72.Ø)*

5th **EØ7.8 Other specified disorders of thyroid**
- **EØ7.81 Sick-euthyroid syndrome**
  Euthyroid sick-syndrome
  DEF: Thyroid dysfunction caused by abnormal levels of thyroid hormones T3 and/or T4. This syndrome is often associated with starvation or critical illness.
- **EØ7.89 Other specified disorders of thyroid** Rx
  Abnormality of thyroid-binding globulin
  Hemorrhage of thyroid
  Infarction of thyroid

EØ7.9 Disorder of thyroid, unspecified Rx

Diabetes mellitus (EØ8-E13)

AHA: 2020,1Q,12; 2018,2Q,6; 2017,4Q,100-101; 2016,2Q,36; 2016,1Q,11-13; 2013,4Q,114; 2013,3Q,20
TIP: There is no default code for diabetes mellitus documented only as uncontrolled. The provider must indicate whether the diabetic patient is hypoglycemic or hyperglycemic to determine the appropriate code.

4th **EØ8 Diabetes mellitus due to underlying condition**
Code first the underlying condition, such as:
- congenital rubella (P35.Ø)
- Cushing's syndrome (E24.-)
- cystic fibrosis (E84.-)
- malignant neoplasm (CØØ-C96)
- malnutrition (E4Ø-E46)
- pancreatitis and other diseases of the pancreas (K85-K86.-)

Use additional code to identify control using:
- insulin (Z79.4)
- oral antidiabetic drugs (Z79.84)
- oral hypoglycemic drugs (Z79.84)

EXCLUDES 1 *drug or chemical induced diabetes mellitus (EØ9.-)*
gestational diabetes (O24.4-)
neonatal diabetes mellitus (P7Ø.2)
postpancreatectomy diabetes mellitus (E13.-)
postprocedural diabetes mellitus (E13.-)
secondary diabetes mellitus NEC (E13.-)
type 1 diabetes mellitus (E1Ø.-)
type 2 diabetes mellitus (E11.-)

5th **EØ8.Ø Diabetes mellitus due to underlying condition with hyperosmolarity**
DEF: Diabetic hyperosmolarity: Extremely high levels of glucose in the blood without ketones.
- ***EØ8.ØØ Diabetes mellitus due to underlying condition with hyperosmolarity without nonketotic hyperglycemic-hyperosmolar coma (NKHHC)*** HCC Rx ESR COM
- ***EØ8.Ø1 Diabetes mellitus due to underlying condition with hyperosmolarity with coma*** HCC Rx ESR COM

5th **EØ8.1 Diabetes mellitus due to underlying condition with ketoacidosis**
DEF: Diabetic ketoacidosis: Potentially life-threatening complication due to a shortage of insulin in which the body switches to burning fatty acids and producing acidic ketone bodies.
- ***EØ8.1Ø Diabetes mellitus due to underlying condition with ketoacidosis without coma*** HCC Rx ESR COM
- ***EØ8.11 Diabetes mellitus due to underlying condition with ketoacidosis with coma*** HCC Rx ESR COM

5th **EØ8.2 Diabetes mellitus due to underlying condition with kidney complications**
AHA: 2019,3Q,3; 2018,4Q,88
- ***EØ8.21 Diabetes mellitus due to underlying condition with diabetic nephropathy*** HCC Rx ESR COM
  Diabetes mellitus due to underlying condition with intercapillary glomerulosclerosis
  Diabetes mellitus due to underlying condition with intracapillary glomerulonephrosis
  Diabetes mellitus due to underlying condition with Kimmelstiel-Wilson disease
- ***EØ8.22 Diabetes mellitus due to underlying condition with diabetic chronic kidney disease*** HCC Rx ESR COM
  Use additional code to identify stage of chronic kidney disease (N18.1-N18.6)
- ***EØ8.29 Diabetes mellitus due to underlying condition with other diabetic kidney complication*** HCC Rx ESR COM
  Renal tubular degeneration in diabetes mellitus due to underlying condition

E08.3 Diabetes mellitus due to underlying condition with ophthalmic complications
AHA: 2016,4Q,11-13

One of the following 7th characters is to be assigned to codes in subcategories E08.32, E08.33, E08.34, E08.35, and E08.37 to designate laterality of the disease:
1 right eye
2 left eye
3 bilateral
9 unspecified eye

E08.31 Diabetes mellitus due to underlying condition with unspecified diabetic retinopathy
DEF: Diabetic retinopathy: Diabetic complication from damage to the retinal vessels resulting in vision problems that can progress to blindness.

E08.311 Diabetes mellitus due to underlying condition with unspecified diabetic retinopathy with macular edema HCC Rx ESR COM

E08.319 Diabetes mellitus due to underlying condition with unspecified diabetic retinopathy without macular edema HCC Rx ESR COM

E08.32 Diabetes mellitus due to underlying condition with mild nonproliferative diabetic retinopathy
Diabetes mellitus due to underlying condition with nonproliferative diabetic retinopathy NOS

E08.321 Diabetes mellitus due to underlying condition with mild nonproliferative diabetic retinopathy with macular edema HCC Rx ESR COM

E08.329 Diabetes mellitus due to underlying condition with mild nonproliferative diabetic retinopathy without macular edema HCC Rx ESR COM

E08.33 Diabetes mellitus due to underlying condition with moderate nonproliferative diabetic retinopathy

E08.331 Diabetes mellitus due to underlying condition with moderate nonproliferative diabetic retinopathy with macular edema HCC Rx ESR COM

E08.339 Diabetes mellitus due to underlying condition with moderate nonproliferative diabetic retinopathy without macular edema HCC Rx ESR COM

E08.34 Diabetes mellitus due to underlying condition with severe nonproliferative diabetic retinopathy

E08.341 Diabetes mellitus due to underlying condition with severe nonproliferative diabetic retinopathy with macular edema HCC Rx ESR COM

E08.349 Diabetes mellitus due to underlying condition with severe nonproliferative diabetic retinopathy without macular edema HCC Rx ESR COM

E08.35 Diabetes mellitus due to underlying condition with proliferative diabetic retinopathy

E08.351 Diabetes mellitus due to underlying condition with proliferative diabetic retinopathy with macular edema HCC Rx ESR COM

E08.352 Diabetes mellitus due to underlying condition with proliferative diabetic retinopathy with traction retinal detachment involving the macula HCC Rx ESR COM

E08.353 Diabetes mellitus due to underlying condition with proliferative diabetic retinopathy with traction retinal detachment not involving the macula HCC Rx ESR COM

E08.354 Diabetes mellitus due to underlying condition with proliferative diabetic retinopathy with combined traction retinal detachment and rhegmatogenous retinal detachment HCC Rx ESR COM

E08.355 Diabetes mellitus due to underlying condition with stable proliferative diabetic retinopathy HCC Rx ESR COM

E08.359 Diabetes mellitus due to underlying condition with proliferative diabetic retinopathy without macular edema HCC Rx ESR COM

E08.36 Diabetes mellitus due to underlying condition with diabetic cataract HCC Rx ESR COM
AHA: 2019,2Q,30-31; 2016,4Q,142

E08.37 Diabetes mellitus due to underlying condition with diabetic macular edema, resolved following treatment HCC Rx ESR COM

E08.39 Diabetes mellitus due to underlying condition with other diabetic ophthalmic complication HCC Rx ESR COM
Use additional code to identify manifestation, such as:
diabetic glaucoma (H40-H42)

E08.4 Diabetes mellitus due to underlying condition with neurological complications

E08.40 Diabetes mellitus due to underlying condition with diabetic neuropathy, unspecified HCC Rx ESR COM

E08.41 Diabetes mellitus due to underlying condition with diabetic mononeuropathy HCC Rx ESR COM

E08.42 Diabetes mellitus due to underlying condition with diabetic polyneuropathy HCC Rx ESR COM
Diabetes mellitus due to underlying condition with diabetic neuralgia

E08.43 Diabetes mellitus due to underlying condition with diabetic autonomic (poly)neuropathy HCC Rx ESR COM
Diabetes mellitus due to underlying condition with diabetic gastroparesis
AHA: 2013,4Q,114

E08.44 Diabetes mellitus due to underlying condition with diabetic amyotrophy HCC Rx ESR COM

E08.49 Diabetes mellitus due to underlying condition with other diabetic neurological complication HCC Rx ESR COM

E08.5 Diabetes mellitus due to underlying condition with circulatory complications

E08.51 Diabetes mellitus due to underlying condition with diabetic peripheral angiopathy without gangrene HCC Rx ESR COM
AHA: 2018,3Q,3-4; 2018,2Q,7

E08.52 Diabetes mellitus due to underlying condition with diabetic peripheral angiopathy with gangrene HCC Rx ESR COM
Diabetes mellitus due to underlying condition with diabetic gangrene
AHA: 2020,2Q,18; 2018,3Q,3; 2018,2Q,7; 2017,4Q,102

E08.59 Diabetes mellitus due to underlying condition with other circulatory complications HCC Rx ESR COM

E08.6 Diabetes mellitus due to underlying condition with other specified complications

E08.61 Diabetes mellitus due to underlying condition with diabetic arthropathy

E08.610 Diabetes mellitus due to underlying condition with diabetic neuropathic arthropathy HCC Rx ESR COM
Diabetes mellitus due to underlying condition with Charcôt's joints
DEF: Charcot's joint: Progressive neurologic arthropathy in which chronic degeneration of joints in the weight-bearing areas with peripheral hypertrophy occurs as a complication of a neuropathy disorder. Supporting structures relax from a loss of sensation resulting in chronic joint instability.

E08.618 Diabetes mellitus due to underlying condition with other diabetic arthropathy HCC Rx ESR COM
AHA: 2018,2Q,6

E08.62 Diabetes mellitus due to underlying condition with skin complications

E08.620 Diabetes mellitus due to underlying condition with diabetic dermatitis HCC Rx ESR COM
Diabetes mellitus due to underlying condition with diabetic necrobiosis lipoidica

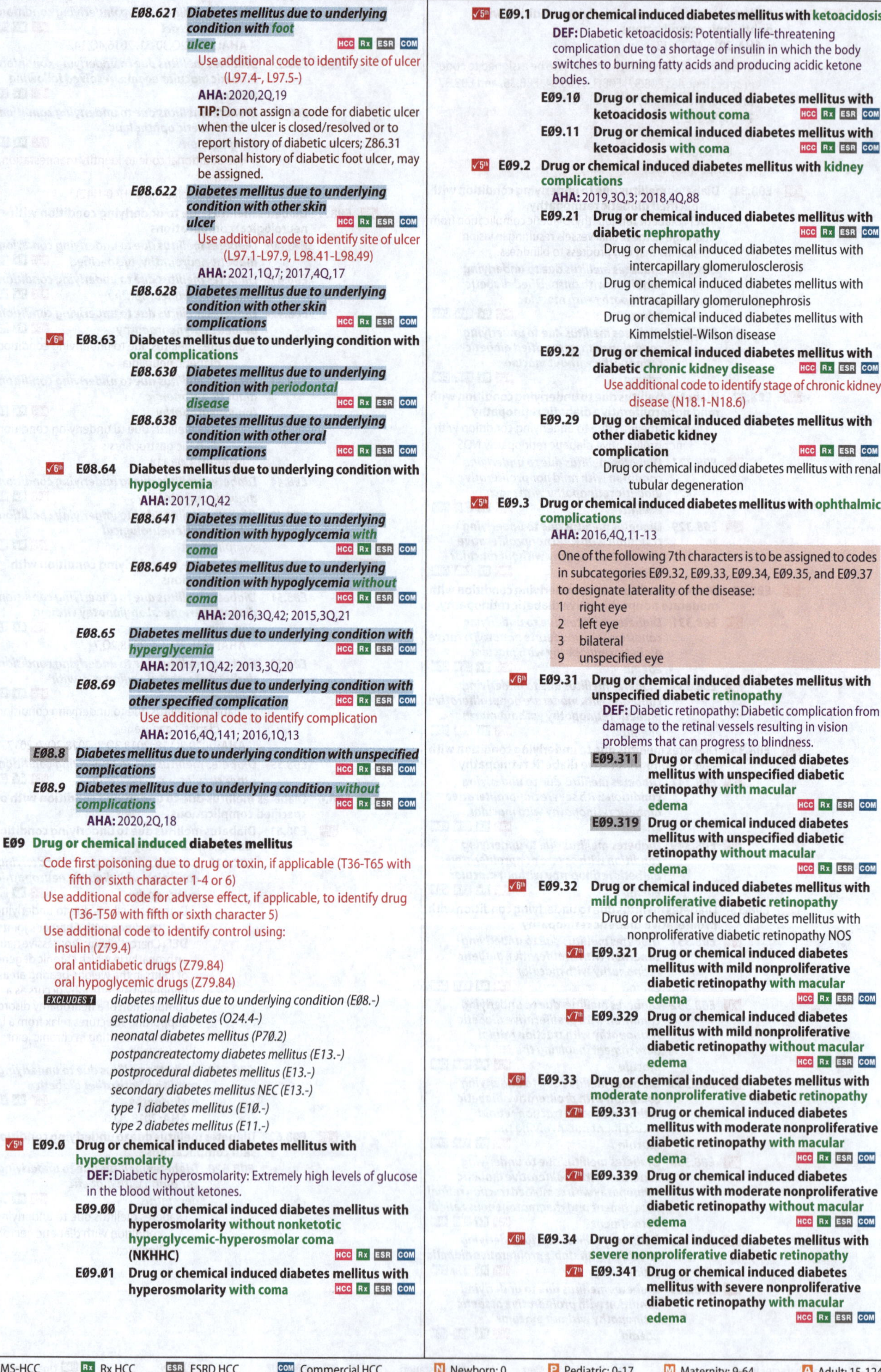

E08.621 Diabetes mellitus due to underlying condition with foot ulcer HCC Rx ESR COM
Use additional code to identify site of ulcer (L97.4-, L97.5-)
AHA: 2020,2Q,19
TIP: Do not assign a code for diabetic ulcer when the ulcer is closed/resolved or to report history of diabetic ulcers; Z86.31 Personal history of diabetic foot ulcer, may be assigned.

E08.622 Diabetes mellitus due to underlying condition with other skin ulcer HCC Rx ESR COM
Use additional code to identify site of ulcer (L97.1-L97.9, L98.41-L98.49)
AHA: 2021,1Q,7; 2017,4Q,17

E08.628 Diabetes mellitus due to underlying condition with other skin complications HCC Rx ESR COM

✓6th E08.63 Diabetes mellitus due to underlying condition with oral complications

E08.630 Diabetes mellitus due to underlying condition with periodontal disease HCC Rx ESR COM

E08.638 Diabetes mellitus due to underlying condition with other oral complications HCC Rx ESR COM

✓6th E08.64 Diabetes mellitus due to underlying condition with hypoglycemia
AHA: 2017,1Q,42

E08.641 Diabetes mellitus due to underlying condition with hypoglycemia with coma HCC Rx ESR COM

E08.649 Diabetes mellitus due to underlying condition with hypoglycemia without coma HCC Rx ESR COM
AHA: 2016,3Q,42; 2015,3Q,21

E08.65 Diabetes mellitus due to underlying condition with hyperglycemia HCC Rx ESR COM
AHA: 2017,1Q,42; 2013,3Q,20

E08.69 Diabetes mellitus due to underlying condition with other specified complication HCC Rx ESR COM
Use additional code to identify complication
AHA: 2016,4Q,141; 2016,1Q,13

E08.8 Diabetes mellitus due to underlying condition with unspecified complications HCC Rx ESR COM

E08.9 Diabetes mellitus due to underlying condition without complications HCC Rx ESR COM
AHA: 2020,2Q,18

✓4th E09 Drug or chemical induced diabetes mellitus
Code first poisoning due to drug or toxin, if applicable (T36-T65 with fifth or sixth character 1-4 or 6)
Use additional code for adverse effect, if applicable, to identify drug (T36-T50 with fifth or sixth character 5)
Use additional code to identify control using:
insulin (Z79.4)
oral antidiabetic drugs (Z79.84)
oral hypoglycemic drugs (Z79.84)
EXCLUDES 1 *diabetes mellitus due to underlying condition (E08.-)*
gestational diabetes (O24.4-)
neonatal diabetes mellitus (P70.2)
postpancreatectomy diabetes mellitus (E13.-)
postprocedural diabetes mellitus (E13.-)
secondary diabetes mellitus NEC (E13.-)
type 1 diabetes mellitus (E10.-)
type 2 diabetes mellitus (E11.-)

✓5th E09.0 Drug or chemical induced diabetes mellitus with hyperosmolarity
DEF: Diabetic hyperosmolarity: Extremely high levels of glucose in the blood without ketones.

E09.00 Drug or chemical induced diabetes mellitus with hyperosmolarity without nonketotic hyperglycemic-hyperosmolar coma (NKHHC) HCC Rx ESR COM

E09.01 Drug or chemical induced diabetes mellitus with hyperosmolarity with coma HCC Rx ESR COM

✓5th E09.1 Drug or chemical induced diabetes mellitus with ketoacidosis
DEF: Diabetic ketoacidosis: Potentially life-threatening complication due to a shortage of insulin in which the body switches to burning fatty acids and producing acidic ketone bodies.

E09.10 Drug or chemical induced diabetes mellitus with ketoacidosis without coma HCC Rx ESR COM

E09.11 Drug or chemical induced diabetes mellitus with ketoacidosis with coma HCC Rx ESR COM

✓5th E09.2 Drug or chemical induced diabetes mellitus with kidney complications
AHA: 2019,3Q,3; 2018,4Q,88

E09.21 Drug or chemical induced diabetes mellitus with diabetic nephropathy HCC Rx ESR COM
Drug or chemical induced diabetes mellitus with intercapillary glomerulosclerosis
Drug or chemical induced diabetes mellitus with intracapillary glomerulonephrosis
Drug or chemical induced diabetes mellitus with Kimmelstiel-Wilson disease

E09.22 Drug or chemical induced diabetes mellitus with diabetic chronic kidney disease HCC Rx ESR COM
Use additional code to identify stage of chronic kidney disease (N18.1-N18.6)

E09.29 Drug or chemical induced diabetes mellitus with other diabetic kidney complication HCC Rx ESR COM
Drug or chemical induced diabetes mellitus with renal tubular degeneration

✓5th E09.3 Drug or chemical induced diabetes mellitus with ophthalmic complications
AHA: 2016,4Q,11-13

One of the following 7th characters is to be assigned to codes in subcategories E09.32, E09.33, E09.34, E09.35, and E09.37 to designate laterality of the disease:
1 right eye
2 left eye
3 bilateral
9 unspecified eye

✓6th E09.31 Drug or chemical induced diabetes mellitus with unspecified diabetic retinopathy
DEF: Diabetic retinopathy: Diabetic complication from damage to the retinal vessels resulting in vision problems that can progress to blindness.

E09.311 Drug or chemical induced diabetes mellitus with unspecified diabetic retinopathy with macular edema HCC Rx ESR COM

E09.319 Drug or chemical induced diabetes mellitus with unspecified diabetic retinopathy without macular edema HCC Rx ESR COM

✓6th E09.32 Drug or chemical induced diabetes mellitus with mild nonproliferative diabetic retinopathy
Drug or chemical induced diabetes mellitus with nonproliferative diabetic retinopathy NOS

✓7th E09.321 Drug or chemical induced diabetes mellitus with mild nonproliferative diabetic retinopathy with macular edema HCC Rx ESR COM

✓7th E09.329 Drug or chemical induced diabetes mellitus with mild nonproliferative diabetic retinopathy without macular edema HCC Rx ESR COM

✓6th E09.33 Drug or chemical induced diabetes mellitus with moderate nonproliferative diabetic retinopathy

✓7th E09.331 Drug or chemical induced diabetes mellitus with moderate nonproliferative diabetic retinopathy with macular edema HCC Rx ESR COM

✓7th E09.339 Drug or chemical induced diabetes mellitus with moderate nonproliferative diabetic retinopathy without macular edema HCC Rx ESR COM

✓6th E09.34 Drug or chemical induced diabetes mellitus with severe nonproliferative diabetic retinopathy

✓7th E09.341 Drug or chemical induced diabetes mellitus with severe nonproliferative diabetic retinopathy with macular edema HCC Rx ESR COM

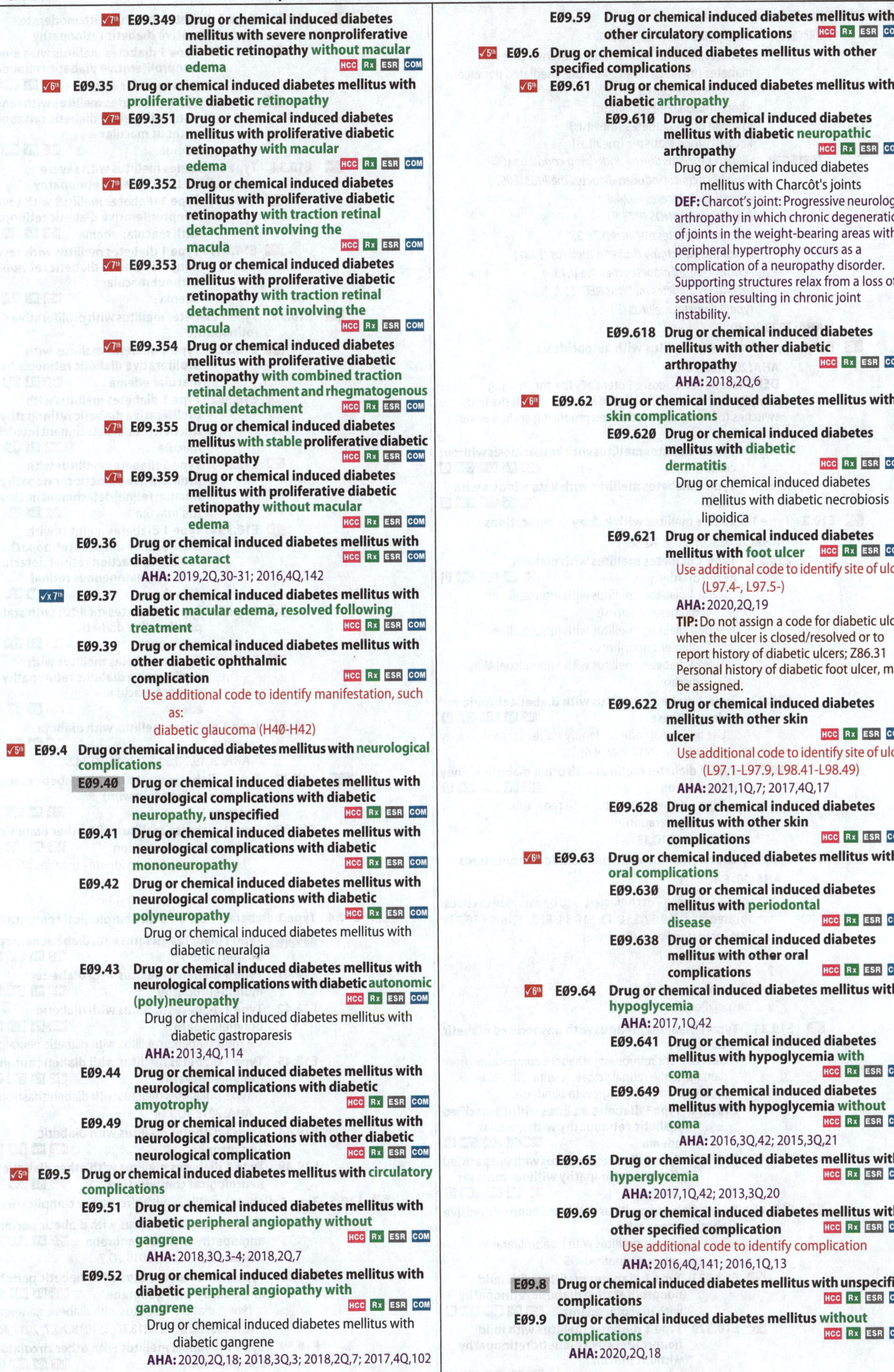

E09.349 Drug or chemical induced diabetes mellitus with severe nonproliferative diabetic retinopathy without macular edema HCC Rx ESR COM

E09.35 Drug or chemical induced diabetes mellitus with proliferative diabetic retinopathy

E09.351 Drug or chemical induced diabetes mellitus with proliferative diabetic retinopathy with macular edema HCC Rx ESR COM

E09.352 Drug or chemical induced diabetes mellitus with proliferative diabetic retinopathy with traction retinal detachment involving the macula HCC Rx ESR COM

E09.353 Drug or chemical induced diabetes mellitus with proliferative diabetic retinopathy with traction retinal detachment not involving the macula HCC Rx ESR COM

E09.354 Drug or chemical induced diabetes mellitus with proliferative diabetic retinopathy with combined traction retinal detachment and rhegmatogenous retinal detachment HCC Rx ESR COM

E09.355 Drug or chemical induced diabetes mellitus with stable proliferative diabetic retinopathy HCC Rx ESR COM

E09.359 Drug or chemical induced diabetes mellitus with proliferative diabetic retinopathy without macular edema HCC Rx ESR COM

E09.36 Drug or chemical induced diabetes mellitus with diabetic cataract HCC Rx ESR COM

AHA: 2019,2Q,30-31; 2016,4Q,142

E09.37 Drug or chemical induced diabetes mellitus with diabetic macular edema, resolved following treatment HCC Rx ESR COM

E09.39 Drug or chemical induced diabetes mellitus with other diabetic ophthalmic complication HCC Rx ESR COM

Use additional code to identify manifestation, such as:

diabetic glaucoma (H40-H42)

E09.4 Drug or chemical induced diabetes mellitus with neurological complications

E09.40 Drug or chemical induced diabetes mellitus with neurological complications with diabetic neuropathy, unspecified HCC Rx ESR COM

E09.41 Drug or chemical induced diabetes mellitus with neurological complications with diabetic mononeuropathy HCC Rx ESR COM

E09.42 Drug or chemical induced diabetes mellitus with neurological complications with diabetic polyneuropathy HCC Rx ESR COM

Drug or chemical induced diabetes mellitus with diabetic neuralgia

E09.43 Drug or chemical induced diabetes mellitus with neurological complications with diabetic autonomic (poly)neuropathy HCC Rx ESR COM

Drug or chemical induced diabetes mellitus with diabetic gastroparesis

AHA: 2013,4Q,114

E09.44 Drug or chemical induced diabetes mellitus with neurological complications with diabetic amyotrophy HCC Rx ESR COM

E09.49 Drug or chemical induced diabetes mellitus with neurological complications with other diabetic neurological complication HCC Rx ESR COM

E09.5 Drug or chemical induced diabetes mellitus with circulatory complications

E09.51 Drug or chemical induced diabetes mellitus with diabetic peripheral angiopathy without gangrene HCC Rx ESR COM

AHA: 2018,3Q,3-4; 2018,2Q,7

E09.52 Drug or chemical induced diabetes mellitus with diabetic peripheral angiopathy with gangrene HCC Rx ESR COM

Drug or chemical induced diabetes mellitus with diabetic gangrene

AHA: 2020,2Q,18; 2018,3Q,3; 2018,2Q,7; 2017,4Q,102

E09.59 Drug or chemical induced diabetes mellitus with other circulatory complications HCC Rx ESR COM

E09.6 Drug or chemical induced diabetes mellitus with other specified complications

E09.61 Drug or chemical induced diabetes mellitus with diabetic arthropathy

E09.610 Drug or chemical induced diabetes mellitus with diabetic neuropathic arthropathy HCC Rx ESR COM

Drug or chemical induced diabetes mellitus with Charcôt's joints

DEF: Charcot's joint: Progressive neurologic arthropathy in which chronic degeneration of joints in the weight-bearing areas with peripheral hypertrophy occurs as a complication of a neuropathy disorder. Supporting structures relax from a loss of sensation resulting in chronic joint instability.

E09.618 Drug or chemical induced diabetes mellitus with other diabetic arthropathy HCC Rx ESR COM

AHA: 2018,2Q,6

E09.62 Drug or chemical induced diabetes mellitus with skin complications

E09.620 Drug or chemical induced diabetes mellitus with diabetic dermatitis HCC Rx ESR COM

Drug or chemical induced diabetes mellitus with diabetic necrobiosis lipoidica

E09.621 Drug or chemical induced diabetes mellitus with foot ulcer HCC Rx ESR COM

Use additional code to identify site of ulcer (L97.4-, L97.5-)

AHA: 2020,2Q,19

TIP: Do not assign a code for diabetic ulcer when the ulcer is closed/resolved or to report history of diabetic ulcers; Z86.31 Personal history of diabetic foot ulcer, may be assigned.

E09.622 Drug or chemical induced diabetes mellitus with other skin ulcer HCC Rx ESR COM

Use additional code to identify site of ulcer (L97.1-L97.9, L98.41-L98.49)

AHA: 2021,1Q,7; 2017,4Q,17

E09.628 Drug or chemical induced diabetes mellitus with other skin complications HCC Rx ESR COM

E09.63 Drug or chemical induced diabetes mellitus with oral complications

E09.630 Drug or chemical induced diabetes mellitus with periodontal disease HCC Rx ESR COM

E09.638 Drug or chemical induced diabetes mellitus with other oral complications HCC Rx ESR COM

E09.64 Drug or chemical induced diabetes mellitus with hypoglycemia

AHA: 2017,1Q,42

E09.641 Drug or chemical induced diabetes mellitus with hypoglycemia with coma HCC Rx ESR COM

E09.649 Drug or chemical induced diabetes mellitus with hypoglycemia without coma HCC Rx ESR COM

AHA: 2016,3Q,42; 2015,3Q,21

E09.65 Drug or chemical induced diabetes mellitus with hyperglycemia HCC Rx ESR COM

AHA: 2017,1Q,42; 2013,3Q,20

E09.69 Drug or chemical induced diabetes mellitus with other specified complication HCC Rx ESR COM

Use additional code to identify complication

AHA: 2016,4Q,141; 2016,1Q,13

E09.8 Drug or chemical induced diabetes mellitus with unspecified complications HCC Rx ESR COM

E09.9 Drug or chemical induced diabetes mellitus without complications HCC Rx ESR COM

AHA: 2020,2Q,18

Chapter 4. Endocrine, Nutritional and Metabolic Diseases

E09.349–E09.9

E10 Type 1 diabetes mellitus

INCLUDES brittle diabetes (mellitus)
diabetes (mellitus) due to autoimmune process
diabetes (mellitus) due to immune mediated pancreatic islet beta-cell destruction
idiopathic diabetes (mellitus)
juvenile onset diabetes (mellitus)
ketosis-prone diabetes (mellitus)

EXCLUDES 1 *diabetes mellitus due to underlying condition (E08.-)*
drug or chemical induced diabetes mellitus (E09.-)
gestational diabetes (O24.4-)
hyperglycemia NOS (R73.9)
neonatal diabetes mellitus (P70.2)
postpancreatectomy diabetes mellitus (E13.-)
postprocedural diabetes mellitus (E13.-)
secondary diabetes mellitus NEC (E13.-)
type 2 diabetes mellitus (E11.-)

AHA: 2020,3Q,30

E10.1 Type 1 diabetes mellitus with ketoacidosis

AHA: 2013,3Q,20

DEF: Diabetic ketoacidosis: Potentially life-threatening complication due to a shortage of insulin in which the body switches to burning fatty acids and producing acidic ketone bodies.

E10.10 Type 1 diabetes mellitus with ketoacidosis without coma HCC Rx ESR COM Q

E10.11 Type 1 diabetes mellitus with ketoacidosis with coma HCC Rx ESR COM Q

E10.2 Type 1 diabetes mellitus with kidney complications

AHA: 2019,3Q,3; 2018,4Q,88

E10.21 Type 1 diabetes mellitus with diabetic nephropathy HCC Rx ESR COM Q

Type 1 diabetes mellitus with intercapillary glomerulosclerosis
Type 1 diabetes mellitus with intracapillary glomerulonephrosis
Type 1 diabetes mellitus with Kimmelstiel-Wilson disease

E10.22 Type 1 diabetes mellitus with diabetic chronic kidney disease HCC Rx ESR COM Q

Use additional code to identify stage of chronic kidney disease (N18.1-N18.6)

E10.29 Type 1 diabetes mellitus with other diabetic kidney complication HCC Rx ESR COM Q

Type 1 diabetes mellitus with renal tubular degeneration

AHA: 2016,1Q,13

E10.3 Type 1 diabetes mellitus with ophthalmic complications

AHA: 2016,4Q,11-13

One of the following 7th characters is to be assigned to codes in subcategories E10.32, E10.33, E10.34, E10.35, and E10.37 to designate laterality of the disease:
1 right eye
2 left eye
3 bilateral
9 unspecified eye

E10.31 Type 1 diabetes mellitus with unspecified diabetic retinopathy

DEF: Diabetic retinopathy: Diabetic complication from damage to the retinal vessels resulting in vision problems that can progress to blindness.

E10.311 Type 1 diabetes mellitus with unspecified diabetic retinopathy with macular edema HCC Rx ESR COM Q

E10.319 Type 1 diabetes mellitus with unspecified diabetic retinopathy without macular edema HCC Rx ESR COM Q

E10.32 Type 1 diabetes mellitus with mild nonproliferative diabetic retinopathy

Type 1 diabetes mellitus with nonproliferative diabetic retinopathy NOS

E10.321 Type 1 diabetes mellitus with mild nonproliferative diabetic retinopathy with macular edema HCC Rx ESR COM Q

E10.329 Type 1 diabetes mellitus with mild nonproliferative diabetic retinopathy without macular edema HCC Rx ESR COM Q

E10.33 Type 1 diabetes mellitus with moderate nonproliferative diabetic retinopathy

E10.331 Type 1 diabetes mellitus with moderate nonproliferative diabetic retinopathy with macular edema HCC Rx ESR COM Q

E10.339 Type 1 diabetes mellitus with moderate nonproliferative diabetic retinopathy without macular edema HCC Rx ESR COM Q

E10.34 Type 1 diabetes mellitus with severe nonproliferative diabetic retinopathy

E10.341 Type 1 diabetes mellitus with severe nonproliferative diabetic retinopathy with macular edema HCC Rx ESR COM Q

E10.349 Type 1 diabetes mellitus with severe nonproliferative diabetic retinopathy without macular edema HCC Rx ESR COM Q

E10.35 Type 1 diabetes mellitus with proliferative diabetic retinopathy

E10.351 Type 1 diabetes mellitus with proliferative diabetic retinopathy with macular edema HCC Rx ESR COM Q

E10.352 Type 1 diabetes mellitus with proliferative diabetic retinopathy with traction retinal detachment involving the macula HCC Rx ESR COM Q

E10.353 Type 1 diabetes mellitus with proliferative diabetic retinopathy with traction retinal detachment not involving the macula HCC Rx ESR COM Q

E10.354 Type 1 diabetes mellitus with proliferative diabetic retinopathy with combined traction retinal detachment and rhegmatogenous retinal detachment HCC Rx ESR COM Q

E10.355 Type 1 diabetes mellitus with stable proliferative diabetic retinopathy HCC Rx ESR COM Q

E10.359 Type 1 diabetes mellitus with proliferative diabetic retinopathy without macular edema HCC Rx ESR COM Q

E10.36 Type 1 diabetes mellitus with diabetic cataract HCC Rx ESR COM Q

AHA: 2019,2Q,30-31; 2016,4Q,142

E10.37 Type 1 diabetes mellitus with diabetic macular edema, resolved following treatment HCC Rx ESR COM Q

E10.39 Type 1 diabetes mellitus with other diabetic ophthalmic complication HCC Rx ESR COM Q

Use additional code to identify manifestation, such as:
diabetic glaucoma (H40-H42)

E10.4 Type 1 diabetes mellitus with neurological complications

E10.40 Type 1 diabetes mellitus with diabetic neuropathy, unspecified HCC Rx ESR COM Q

E10.41 Type 1 diabetes mellitus with diabetic mononeuropathy HCC Rx ESR COM Q

E10.42 Type 1 diabetes mellitus with diabetic polyneuropathy HCC Rx ESR COM Q

Type 1 diabetes mellitus with diabetic neuralgia

E10.43 Type 1 diabetes mellitus with diabetic autonomic (poly)neuropathy HCC Rx ESR COM Q

Type 1 diabetes mellitus with diabetic gastroparesis

AHA: 2013,4Q,114

E10.44 Type 1 diabetes mellitus with diabetic amyotrophy HCC Rx ESR COM Q

E10.49 Type 1 diabetes mellitus with other diabetic neurological complication HCC Rx ESR COM Q

E10.5 Type 1 diabetes mellitus with circulatory complications

E10.51 Type 1 diabetes mellitus with diabetic peripheral angiopathy without gangrene HCC Rx ESR COM Q

AHA: 2018,3Q,3-4; 2018,2Q,7

E10.52 Type 1 diabetes mellitus with diabetic peripheral angiopathy with gangrene HCC Rx ESR COM Q

Type 1 diabetes mellitus with diabetic gangrene

AHA: 2020,2Q,18; 2018,3Q,3; 2018,2Q,7; 2017,4Q,102

E10.59 Type 1 diabetes mellitus with other circulatory complications HCC Rx ESR COM Q

HCC CMS-HCC Rx Rx HCC ESR ESRD HCC COM Commercial HCC N Newborn: 0 P Pediatric: 0-17 M Maternity: 9-64 A Adult: 15-124

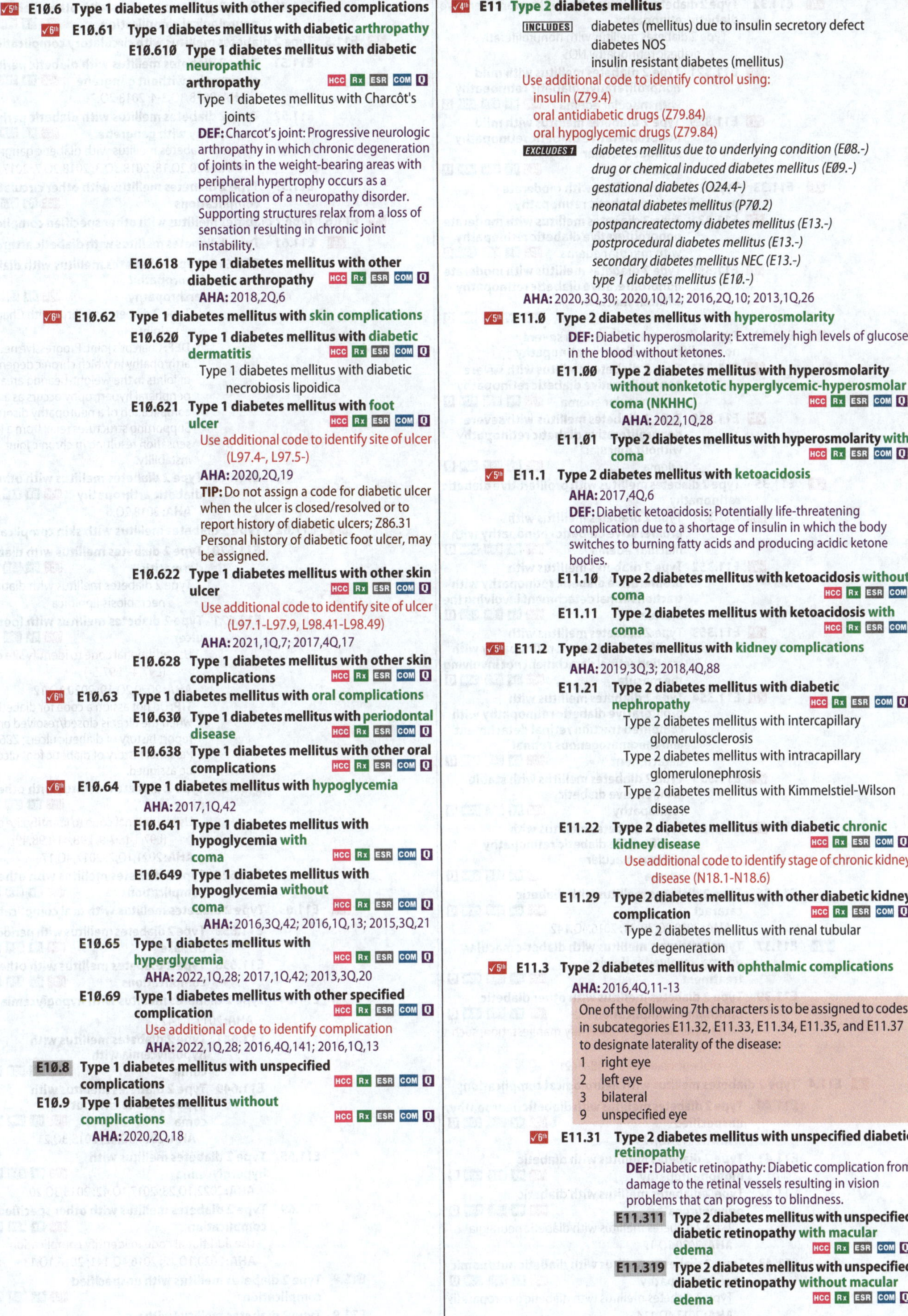

E10.6 Type 1 diabetes mellitus with other specified complications

E10.61 Type 1 diabetes mellitus with diabetic arthropathy

E10.610 Type 1 diabetes mellitus with diabetic neuropathic arthropathy HCC Rx ESR COM Q
Type 1 diabetes mellitus with Charcôt's joints
DEF: Charcot's joint: Progressive neurologic arthropathy in which chronic degeneration of joints in the weight-bearing areas with peripheral hypertrophy occurs as a complication of a neuropathy disorder. Supporting structures relax from a loss of sensation resulting in chronic joint instability.

E10.618 Type 1 diabetes mellitus with other diabetic arthropathy HCC Rx ESR COM Q
AHA: 2018,2Q,6

E10.62 Type 1 diabetes mellitus with skin complications

E10.620 Type 1 diabetes mellitus with diabetic dermatitis HCC Rx ESR COM Q
Type 1 diabetes mellitus with diabetic necrobiosis lipoidica

E10.621 Type 1 diabetes mellitus with foot ulcer HCC Rx ESR COM Q
Use additional code to identify site of ulcer (L97.4-, L97.5-)
AHA: 2020,2Q,19
TIP: Do not assign a code for diabetic ulcer when the ulcer is closed/resolved or to report history of diabetic ulcers; Z86.31 Personal history of diabetic foot ulcer, may be assigned.

E10.622 Type 1 diabetes mellitus with other skin ulcer HCC Rx ESR COM Q
Use additional code to identify site of ulcer (L97.1-L97.9, L98.41-L98.49)
AHA: 2021,1Q,7; 2017,4Q,17

E10.628 Type 1 diabetes mellitus with other skin complications HCC Rx ESR COM Q

E10.63 Type 1 diabetes mellitus with oral complications

E10.630 Type 1 diabetes mellitus with periodontal disease HCC Rx ESR COM Q

E10.638 Type 1 diabetes mellitus with other oral complications HCC Rx ESR COM Q

E10.64 Type 1 diabetes mellitus with hypoglycemia
AHA: 2017,1Q,42

E10.641 Type 1 diabetes mellitus with hypoglycemia with coma HCC Rx ESR COM Q

E10.649 Type 1 diabetes mellitus with hypoglycemia without coma HCC Rx ESR COM Q
AHA: 2016,3Q,42; 2016,1Q,13; 2015,3Q,21

E10.65 Type 1 diabetes mellitus with hyperglycemia HCC Rx ESR COM Q
AHA: 2022,1Q,28; 2017,1Q,42; 2013,3Q,20

E10.69 Type 1 diabetes mellitus with other specified complication HCC Rx ESR COM Q
Use additional code to identify complication
AHA: 2022,1Q,28; 2016,4Q,141; 2016,1Q,13

E10.8 Type 1 diabetes mellitus with unspecified complications HCC Rx ESR COM Q

E10.9 Type 1 diabetes mellitus without complications HCC Rx ESR COM Q
AHA: 2020,2Q,18

E11 Type 2 diabetes mellitus

INCLUDES diabetes (mellitus) due to insulin secretory defect
diabetes NOS
insulin resistant diabetes (mellitus)

Use additional code to identify control using:
insulin (Z79.4)
oral antidiabetic drugs (Z79.84)
oral hypoglycemic drugs (Z79.84)

EXCLUDES 1 *diabetes mellitus due to underlying condition (E08.-)*
drug or chemical induced diabetes mellitus (E09.-)
gestational diabetes (O24.4-)
neonatal diabetes mellitus (P70.2)
postpancreatectomy diabetes mellitus (E13.-)
postprocedural diabetes mellitus (E13.-)
secondary diabetes mellitus NEC (E13.-)
type 1 diabetes mellitus (E10.-)

AHA: 2020,3Q,30; 2020,1Q,12; 2016,2Q,10; 2013,1Q,26

E11.0 Type 2 diabetes mellitus with hyperosmolarity
DEF: Diabetic hyperosmolarity: Extremely high levels of glucose in the blood without ketones.

E11.00 Type 2 diabetes mellitus with hyperosmolarity without nonketotic hyperglycemic-hyperosmolar coma (NKHHC) HCC Rx ESR COM Q
AHA: 2022,1Q,28

E11.01 Type 2 diabetes mellitus with hyperosmolarity with coma HCC Rx ESR COM Q

E11.1 Type 2 diabetes mellitus with ketoacidosis
AHA: 2017,4Q,6
DEF: Diabetic ketoacidosis: Potentially life-threatening complication due to a shortage of insulin in which the body switches to burning fatty acids and producing acidic ketone bodies.

E11.10 Type 2 diabetes mellitus with ketoacidosis without coma HCC Rx ESR COM

E11.11 Type 2 diabetes mellitus with ketoacidosis with coma HCC Rx ESR COM

E11.2 Type 2 diabetes mellitus with kidney complications
AHA: 2019,3Q,3; 2018,4Q,88

E11.21 Type 2 diabetes mellitus with diabetic nephropathy HCC Rx ESR COM Q
Type 2 diabetes mellitus with intercapillary glomerulosclerosis
Type 2 diabetes mellitus with intracapillary glomerulonephrosis
Type 2 diabetes mellitus with Kimmelstiel-Wilson disease

E11.22 Type 2 diabetes mellitus with diabetic chronic kidney disease HCC Rx ESR COM Q
Use additional code to identify stage of chronic kidney disease (N18.1-N18.6)

E11.29 Type 2 diabetes mellitus with other diabetic kidney complication HCC Rx ESR COM Q
Type 2 diabetes mellitus with renal tubular degeneration

E11.3 Type 2 diabetes mellitus with ophthalmic complications
AHA: 2016,4Q,11-13

One of the following 7th characters is to be assigned to codes in subcategories E11.32, E11.33, E11.34, E11.35, and E11.37 to designate laterality of the disease:
1 right eye
2 left eye
3 bilateral
9 unspecified eye

E11.31 Type 2 diabetes mellitus with unspecified diabetic retinopathy
DEF: Diabetic retinopathy: Diabetic complication from damage to the retinal vessels resulting in vision problems that can progress to blindness.

E11.311 Type 2 diabetes mellitus with unspecified diabetic retinopathy with macular edema HCC Rx ESR COM Q

E11.319 Type 2 diabetes mellitus with unspecified diabetic retinopathy without macular edema HCC Rx ESR COM Q

✓6th **E11.32 Type 2 diabetes mellitus with mild nonproliferative diabetic retinopathy**
Type 2 diabetes mellitus with nonproliferative diabetic retinopathy NOS

✓7th **E11.321 Type 2 diabetes mellitus with mild nonproliferative diabetic retinopathy with macular edema** HCC Rx ESR COM Q

✓7th **E11.329 Type 2 diabetes mellitus with mild nonproliferative diabetic retinopathy without macular edema** HCC Rx ESR COM Q

✓6th **E11.33 Type 2 diabetes mellitus with moderate nonproliferative diabetic retinopathy**

✓7th **E11.331 Type 2 diabetes mellitus with moderate nonproliferative diabetic retinopathy with macular edema** HCC Rx ESR COM Q

✓7th **E11.339 Type 2 diabetes mellitus with moderate nonproliferative diabetic retinopathy without macular edema** HCC Rx ESR COM Q

✓6th **E11.34 Type 2 diabetes mellitus with severe nonproliferative diabetic retinopathy**

✓7th **E11.341 Type 2 diabetes mellitus with severe nonproliferative diabetic retinopathy with macular edema** HCC Rx ESR COM Q

✓7th **E11.349 Type 2 diabetes mellitus with severe nonproliferative diabetic retinopathy without macular edema** HCC Rx ESR COM Q

✓6th **E11.35 Type 2 diabetes mellitus with proliferative diabetic retinopathy**

✓7th **E11.351 Type 2 diabetes mellitus with proliferative diabetic retinopathy with macular edema** HCC Rx ESR COM Q

✓7th **E11.352 Type 2 diabetes mellitus with proliferative diabetic retinopathy with traction retinal detachment involving the macula** HCC Rx ESR COM Q

✓7th **E11.353 Type 2 diabetes mellitus with proliferative diabetic retinopathy with traction retinal detachment not involving the macula** HCC Rx ESR COM Q

✓7th **E11.354 Type 2 diabetes mellitus with proliferative diabetic retinopathy with combined traction retinal detachment and rhegmatogenous retinal detachment** HCC Rx ESR COM Q

✓7th **E11.355 Type 2 diabetes mellitus with stable proliferative diabetic retinopathy** HCC Rx ESR COM Q

✓7th **E11.359 Type 2 diabetes mellitus with proliferative diabetic retinopathy without macular edema** HCC Rx ESR COM Q

E11.36 Type 2 diabetes mellitus with diabetic cataract HCC Rx ESR COM Q
AHA: 2019,2Q,30-31; 2016,4Q,142

✓x7th **E11.37 Type 2 diabetes mellitus with diabetic macular edema, resolved following treatment** HCC Rx ESR COM Q

E11.39 Type 2 diabetes mellitus with other diabetic ophthalmic complication HCC Rx ESR COM Q
Use additional code to identify manifestation, such as:
diabetic glaucoma (H4Ø-H42)

✓5th **E11.4 Type 2 diabetes mellitus with neurological complications**

E11.4Ø Type 2 diabetes mellitus with diabetic neuropathy, unspecified HCC Rx ESR COM Q
AHA: 2013,4Q,129

E11.41 Type 2 diabetes mellitus with diabetic mononeuropathy HCC Rx ESR COM Q

E11.42 Type 2 diabetes mellitus with diabetic polyneuropathy HCC Rx ESR COM Q
Type 2 diabetes mellitus with diabetic neuralgia
AHA: 2020,1Q,12

E11.43 Type 2 diabetes mellitus with diabetic autonomic (poly)neuropathy HCC Rx ESR COM Q
Type 2 diabetes mellitus with diabetic gastroparesis
AHA: 2013,4Q,114

E11.44 Type 2 diabetes mellitus with diabetic amyotrophy HCC Rx ESR COM Q

E11.49 Type 2 diabetes mellitus with other diabetic neurological complication HCC Rx ESR COM Q

✓5th **E11.5 Type 2 diabetes mellitus with circulatory complications**

E11.51 Type 2 diabetes mellitus with diabetic peripheral angiopathy without gangrene HCC Rx ESR COM Q
AHA: 2018,3Q,3-4; 2018,2Q,7

E11.52 Type 2 diabetes mellitus with diabetic peripheral angiopathy with gangrene HCC Rx ESR COM Q
Type 2 diabetes mellitus with diabetic gangrene
AHA: 2020,2Q,18; 2018,3Q,3; 2018,2Q,7; 2017,4Q,102

E11.59 Type 2 diabetes mellitus with other circulatory complications HCC Rx ESR COM Q

✓5th **E11.6 Type 2 diabetes mellitus with other specified complications**

✓6th **E11.61 Type 2 diabetes mellitus with diabetic arthropathy**

E11.61Ø Type 2 diabetes mellitus with diabetic neuropathic arthropathy HCC Rx ESR COM Q
Type 2 diabetes mellitus with Charcôt's joints
DEF: Charcot's joint: Progressive neurologic arthropathy in which chronic degeneration of joints in the weight-bearing areas with peripheral hypertrophy occurs as a complication of a neuropathy disorder. Supporting structures relax from a loss of sensation resulting in chronic joint instability.

E11.618 Type 2 diabetes mellitus with other diabetic arthropathy HCC Rx ESR COM Q
AHA: 2018,2Q,6

✓6th **E11.62 Type 2 diabetes mellitus with skin complications**

E11.62Ø Type 2 diabetes mellitus with diabetic dermatitis HCC Rx ESR COM Q
Type 2 diabetes mellitus with diabetic necrobiosis lipoidica

E11.621 Type 2 diabetes mellitus with foot ulcer HCC Rx ESR COM Q
Use additional code to identify site of ulcer (L97.4-, L97.5-)
AHA: 2020,2Q,19; 2020,1Q,12
TIP: Do not assign a code for diabetic ulcer when the ulcer is closed/resolved or to report history of diabetic ulcers; Z86.31 Personal history of diabetic foot ulcer, may be assigned.

E11.622 Type 2 diabetes mellitus with other skin ulcer HCC Rx ESR COM Q
Use additional code to identify site of ulcer (L97.1-L97.9, L98.41-L98.49)
AHA: 2021,1Q,7; 2017,4Q,17

E11.628 Type 2 diabetes mellitus with other skin complications HCC Rx ESR COM Q

✓6th **E11.63 Type 2 diabetes mellitus with oral complications**

E11.63Ø Type 2 diabetes mellitus with periodontal disease HCC Rx ESR COM Q

E11.638 Type 2 diabetes mellitus with other oral complications HCC Rx ESR COM Q

✓6th **E11.64 Type 2 diabetes mellitus with hypoglycemia**
AHA: 2017,1Q,42

E11.641 Type 2 diabetes mellitus with hypoglycemia with coma HCC Rx ESR COM Q

E11.649 Type 2 diabetes mellitus with hypoglycemia without coma HCC Rx ESR COM Q
AHA: 2016,3Q,42; 2015,3Q,21

E11.65 Type 2 diabetes mellitus with hyperglycemia HCC Rx ESR COM Q
AHA: 2022,1Q,28; 2017,1Q,42; 2013,3Q,20

E11.69 Type 2 diabetes mellitus with other specified complication HCC Rx ESR COM Q
Use additional code to identify complication
AHA: 2020,1Q,12; 2016,4Q,141; 2016,1Q,13

E11.8 Type 2 diabetes mellitus with unspecified complications HCC Rx ESR COM Q

E11.9 Type 2 diabetes mellitus without complications HCC Rx ESR COM Q
AHA: 2020,2Q,18

E13 Other specified diabetes mellitus

INCLUDES diabetes mellitus due to genetic defects of beta-cell function
diabetes mellitus due to genetic defects in insulin action
postpancreatectomy diabetes mellitus
postprocedural diabetes mellitus
secondary diabetes mellitus NEC

Use additional code to identify control using:
insulin (Z79.4)
oral antidiabetic drugs (Z79.84)
oral hypoglycemic drugs (Z79.84)

EXCLUDES 1 *diabetes (mellitus) due to autoimmune process (E1Ø.-)*
diabetes (mellitus) due to immune mediated pancreatic islet beta-cell destruction (E1Ø.-)
diabetes mellitus due to underlying condition (EØ8.-)
drug or chemical induced diabetes mellitus (EØ9.-)
gestational diabetes (O24.4-)
neonatal diabetes mellitus (P7Ø.2)
type 1 diabetes mellitus (E1Ø.-)

AHA: 2018,3Q,4; 2016,1Q,11-13

TIP: Use this category when the diabetes is documented as diabetes type 1.5. Synonymous terms used in the documentation may also include combined diabetes type 1 and type 2, latent autoimmune diabetes of adults (LADA), slow-progressing type 1 diabetes, or double diabetes.

TIP: When postprocedural or postpancreatectomy hypoinsulinemia (E89.1) is documented with postprocedural or postpancreatectomy diabetes mellitus (E13.-), code E89.1 should be sequenced first.

E13.Ø Other specified diabetes mellitus with hyperosmolarity

DEF: Diabetic hyperosmolarity: Extremely high levels of glucose in the blood without ketones.

E13.ØØ Other specified diabetes mellitus with hyperosmolarity without nonketotic hyperglycemic-hyperosmolar coma (NKHHC) HCC Rx ESR COM Q

EXCLUDES 2 *type 2 diabetes mellitus (E11.-)*

E13.Ø1 Other specified diabetes mellitus with hyperosmolarity with coma HCC Rx ESR COM Q

E13.1 Other specified diabetes mellitus with ketoacidosis

AHA: 2016,2Q,10; 2013,1Q,26

DEF: Diabetic ketoacidosis: Potentially life-threatening complication due to a shortage of insulin in which the body switches to burning fatty acids and producing acidic ketone bodies.

E13.1Ø Other specified diabetes mellitus with ketoacidosis without coma HCC Rx ESR COM Q

E13.11 Other specified diabetes mellitus with ketoacidosis with coma HCC Rx ESR COM Q

E13.2 Other specified diabetes mellitus with kidney complications

AHA: 2019,3Q,3; 2018,4Q,88

E13.21 Other specified diabetes mellitus with diabetic nephropathy HCC Rx ESR COM Q

Other specified diabetes mellitus with intercapillary glomerulosclerosis
Other specified diabetes mellitus with intracapillary glomerulonephrosis
Other specified diabetes mellitus with Kimmelstiel-Wilson disease

E13.22 Other specified diabetes mellitus with diabetic chronic kidney disease HCC Rx ESR COM Q

Use additional code to identify stage of chronic kidney disease (N18.1-N18.6)

E13.29 Other specified diabetes mellitus with other diabetic kidney complication HCC Rx ESR COM Q

Other specified diabetes mellitus with renal tubular degeneration

E13.3 Other specified diabetes mellitus with ophthalmic complications

AHA: 2016,4Q,11-13

One of the following 7th characters is to be assigned to codes in subcategories E13.32, E13.33, E13.34, E13.35, and E13.37 to designate laterality of the disease:
1 right eye
2 left eye
3 bilateral
9 unspecified eye

E13.31 Other specified diabetes mellitus with unspecified diabetic retinopathy

DEF: Diabetic retinopathy: Diabetic complication from damage to the retinal vessels resulting in vision problems that can progress to blindness.

E13.311 Other specified diabetes mellitus with unspecified diabetic retinopathy with macular edema HCC Rx ESR COM Q

E13.319 Other specified diabetes mellitus with unspecified diabetic retinopathy without macular edema HCC Rx ESR COM Q

E13.32 Other specified diabetes mellitus with mild nonproliferative diabetic retinopathy

Other specified diabetes mellitus with nonproliferative diabetic retinopathy NOS

E13.321 Other specified diabetes mellitus with mild nonproliferative diabetic retinopathy with macular edema HCC Rx ESR COM Q

E13.329 Other specified diabetes mellitus with mild nonproliferative diabetic retinopathy without macular edema HCC Rx ESR COM Q

E13.33 Other specified diabetes mellitus with moderate nonproliferative diabetic retinopathy

E13.331 Other specified diabetes mellitus with moderate nonproliferative diabetic retinopathy with macular edema HCC Rx ESR COM Q

E13.339 Other specified diabetes mellitus with moderate nonproliferative diabetic retinopathy without macular edema HCC Rx ESR COM Q

E13.34 Other specified diabetes mellitus with severe nonproliferative diabetic retinopathy

E13.341 Other specified diabetes mellitus with severe nonproliferative diabetic retinopathy with macular edema HCC Rx ESR COM Q

E13.349 Other specified diabetes mellitus with severe nonproliferative diabetic retinopathy without macular edema HCC Rx ESR COM Q

E13.35 Other specified diabetes mellitus with proliferative diabetic retinopathy

E13.351 Other specified diabetes mellitus with proliferative diabetic retinopathy with macular edema HCC Rx ESR COM Q

E13.352 Other specified diabetes mellitus with proliferative diabetic retinopathy with traction retinal detachment involving the macula HCC Rx ESR COM Q

E13.353 Other specified diabetes mellitus with proliferative diabetic retinopathy with traction retinal detachment not involving the macula HCC Rx ESR COM Q

E13.354 Other specified diabetes mellitus with proliferative diabetic retinopathy with combined traction retinal detachment and rhegmatogenous retinal detachment HCC Rx ESR COM Q

E13.355 Other specified diabetes mellitus with stable proliferative diabetic retinopathy HCC Rx ESR COM Q

E13.359 Other specified diabetes mellitus with proliferative diabetic retinopathy without macular edema HCC Rx ESR COM Q

E13.36 Other specified diabetes mellitus with diabetic cataract HCC Rx ESR COM Q

AHA: 2019,2Q,30-31; 2016,4Q,142

√7th **E13.37 Other specified diabetes mellitus with diabetic macular edema, resolved following treatment** HCC Rx ESR COM Q

E13.39 Other specified diabetes mellitus with other diabetic ophthalmic complication HCC Rx ESR COM Q
Use additional code to identify manifestation, such as:
diabetic glaucoma (H4Ø-H42)

√5th **E13.4 Other specified diabetes mellitus with neurological complications**

E13.4Ø Other specified diabetes mellitus with diabetic neuropathy, unspecified HCC Rx ESR COM Q

E13.41 Other specified diabetes mellitus with diabetic mononeuropathy HCC Rx ESR COM Q

E13.42 Other specified diabetes mellitus with diabetic polyneuropathy HCC Rx ESR COM Q
Other specified diabetes mellitus with diabetic neuralgia

E13.43 Other specified diabetes mellitus with diabetic autonomic (poly)neuropathy HCC Rx ESR COM Q
Other specified diabetes mellitus with diabetic gastroparesis
AHA: 2013,4Q,114

E13.44 Other specified diabetes mellitus with diabetic amyotrophy HCC Rx ESR COM Q

E13.49 Other specified diabetes mellitus with other diabetic neurological complication HCC Rx ESR COM Q

√5th **E13.5 Other specified diabetes mellitus with circulatory complications**

E13.51 Other specified diabetes mellitus with diabetic peripheral angiopathy without gangrene HCC Rx ESR COM Q
AHA: 2018,3Q,3-4; 2018,2Q,7

E13.52 Other specified diabetes mellitus with diabetic peripheral angiopathy with gangrene HCC Rx ESR COM Q
Other specified diabetes mellitus with diabetic gangrene
AHA: 2020,2Q,18; 2018,3Q,3; 2018,2Q,7; 2017,4Q,102

E13.59 Other specified diabetes mellitus with other circulatory complications HCC Rx ESR COM Q

√5th **E13.6 Other specified diabetes mellitus with other specified complications**

√6th **E13.61 Other specified diabetes mellitus with diabetic arthropathy**

E13.61Ø Other specified diabetes mellitus with diabetic neuropathic arthropathy HCC Rx ESR COM Q
Other specified diabetes mellitus with Charcôt's joints
DEF: Charcot's joint: Progressive neurologic arthropathy in which chronic degeneration of joints in the weight-bearing areas with peripheral hypertrophy occurs as a complication of a neuropathy disorder. Supporting structures relax from a loss of sensation resulting in chronic joint instability.

E13.618 Other specified diabetes mellitus with other diabetic arthropathy HCC Rx ESR COM Q
AHA: 2018,2Q,6

√6th **E13.62 Other specified diabetes mellitus with skin complications**

E13.62Ø Other specified diabetes mellitus with diabetic dermatitis HCC Rx ESR COM Q
Other specified diabetes mellitus with diabetic necrobiosis lipoidica

E13.621 Other specified diabetes mellitus with foot ulcer HCC Rx ESR COM Q
Use additional code to identify site of ulcer (L97.4-, L97.5-)
AHA: 2020,2Q,19
TIP: Do not assign a code for diabetic ulcer when the ulcer is closed/resolved or to report history of diabetic ulcers; Z86.31 Personal history of diabetic foot ulcer, may be assigned.

E13.622 Other specified diabetes mellitus with other skin ulcer HCC Rx ESR COM Q
Use additional code to identify site of ulcer (L97.1-L97.9, L98.41-L98.49)
AHA: 2021,1Q,7; 2017,4Q,17

E13.628 Other specified diabetes mellitus with other skin complications HCC Rx ESR COM Q

√6th **E13.63 Other specified diabetes mellitus with oral complications**

E13.63Ø Other specified diabetes mellitus with periodontal disease HCC Rx ESR COM Q

E13.638 Other specified diabetes mellitus with other oral complications HCC Rx ESR COM Q

√6th **E13.64 Other specified diabetes mellitus with hypoglycemia**
AHA: 2017,1Q,42

E13.641 Other specified diabetes mellitus with hypoglycemia with coma HCC Rx ESR COM Q

E13.649 Other specified diabetes mellitus with hypoglycemia without coma HCC Rx ESR COM Q
AHA: 2016,3Q,42; 2015,3Q,21

E13.65 Other specified diabetes mellitus with hyperglycemia HCC Rx ESR COM Q
AHA: 2017,1Q,42; 2013,3Q,20

E13.69 Other specified diabetes mellitus with other specified complication HCC Rx ESR COM Q
Use additional code to identify complication
AHA: 2016,4Q,141; 2016,1Q,13

E13.8 Other specified diabetes mellitus with unspecified complications HCC Rx ESR COM Q

E13.9 Other specified diabetes mellitus without complications HCC Rx ESR COM Q
AHA: 2020,2Q,18

Other disorders of glucose regulation and pancreatic internal secretion (E15-E16)

E15 Nondiabetic hypoglycemic coma HCC ESR COM
INCLUDES drug-induced insulin coma in nondiabetic
hyperinsulinism with hypoglycemic coma
hypoglycemic coma NOS

√4th **E16 Other disorders of pancreatic internal secretion**

E16.Ø Drug-induced hypoglycemia without coma
EXCLUDES 1 *diabetes with hypoglycemia without coma (EØ9.649)*
Use additional code for adverse effect, if applicable, to identify drug (T36-T5Ø with fifth or sixth character 5)

E16.1 Other hypoglycemia
Functional hyperinsulinism
Functional nonhyperinsulinemic hypoglycemia
Hyperinsulinism NOS
Hyperplasia of pancreatic islet beta cells NOS
EXCLUDES 1 *diabetes with hypoglycemia (EØ8.649, E1Ø.649, E11.649, E13.649)*
hypoglycemia in infant of diabetic mother (P7Ø.1)
neonatal hypoglycemia (P7Ø.4)

E16.2 Hypoglycemia, unspecified
EXCLUDES 1 *diabetes with hypoglycemia (EØ8.649, E1Ø.649, E11.649, E13.649)*
AHA: 2016,3Q,42
TIP: Assign for nondiabetic hypoglycemic encephalopathy not further clarified in the documentation.

E16.3 Increased secretion of glucagon Rx
Hyperplasia of pancreatic endocrine cells with glucagon excess

E16.4 Increased secretion of gastrin Rx
Hypergastrinemia
Hyperplasia of pancreatic endocrine cells with gastrin excess
Zollinger-Ellison syndrome

E16.8 Other specified disorders of pancreatic internal secretion Rx
Increased secretion from endocrine pancreas of growth hormone-releasing hormone
Increased secretion from endocrine pancreas of pancreatic polypeptide
Increased secretion from endocrine pancreas of somatostatin
Increased secretion from endocrine pancreas of vasoactive-intestinal polypeptide

E16.9 Disorder of pancreatic internal secretion, unspecified Rx
Islet-cell hyperplasia NOS
Pancreatic endocrine cell hyperplasia NOS

Disorders of other endocrine glands (E2Ø-E35)

EXCLUDES 1 *galactorrhea (N64.3)*
gynecomastia (N62)

E2Ø Hypoparathyroidism
EXCLUDES 1 *Di George's syndrome (D82.1)*
postprocedural hypoparathyroidism (E89.2)
tetany NOS (R29.Ø)
transitory neonatal hypoparathyroidism (P71.4)

E2Ø.Ø Idiopathic hypoparathyroidism HCC Rx ESR COM
DEF: Abnormally low secretion of parathyroid hormones, with unknown cause, which triggers decreased calcium and increased phosphorus in the blood that can result in cataracts, muscle cramps, tetany, tingling, or burning in the lips, fingers, and toes.

E2Ø.1 Pseudohypoparathyroidism

E2Ø.8 Other hypoparathyroidism HCC Rx ESR COM

E2Ø.9 Hypoparathyroidism, unspecified HCC Rx ESR COM
Parathyroid tetany

E21 Hyperparathyroidism and other disorders of parathyroid gland
EXCLUDES 1 *adult osteomalacia (M83.-)*
ectopic hyperparathyroidism (E34.2)
hungry bone syndrome (E83.81)
infantile and juvenile osteomalacia (E55.Ø)
EXCLUDES 2 *familial hypocalciuric hypercalcemia (E83.52)*

E21.Ø Primary hyperparathyroidism HCC Rx ESR COM
Hyperplasia of parathyroid
Osteitis fibrosa cystica generalisata [von Recklinghausen's disease of bone]
DEF: Parathyroid dysfunction commonly caused by hyperplasia of two or more glands. Symptoms include hypercalcemia and increased parathyroid hormone levels.

E21.1 Secondary hyperparathyroidism, not elsewhere classified HCC Rx ESR COM
EXCLUDES 1 *secondary hyperparathyroidism of renal origin (N25.81)*

E21.2 Other hyperparathyroidism HCC Rx ESR COM
Tertiary hyperparathyroidism
EXCLUDES 1 *familial hypocalciuric hypercalcemia (E83.52)*

E21.3 Hyperparathyroidism, unspecified HCC Rx ESR COM

E21.4 Other specified disorders of parathyroid gland HCC Rx ESR COM

E21.5 Disorder of parathyroid gland, unspecified HCC Rx ESR COM

E22 Hyperfunction of pituitary gland
EXCLUDES 1 *Cushing's syndrome (E24.-)*
Nelson's syndrome (E24.1)
overproduction of ACTH not associated with Cushing's disease (E27.Ø)
overproduction of pituitary ACTH (E24.Ø)
overproduction of thyroid-stimulating hormone (EØ5.8-)

E22.Ø Acromegaly and pituitary gigantism HCC Rx ESR COM
Overproduction of growth hormone
EXCLUDES 1 *constitutional gigantism (E34.4)*
constitutional tall stature (E34.4)
increased secretion from endocrine pancreas of growth hormone-releasing hormone (E16.8)
DEF: Acromegaly: Chronic condition caused by overproduction of the pituitary growth hormone resulting in enlarged skeletal parts and facial features.

E22.1 Hyperprolactinemia HCC Rx ESR COM
Use additional code for adverse effect, if applicable, to identify drug (T36-T5Ø with fifth or sixth character 5)

E22.2 Syndrome of inappropriate secretion of antidiuretic hormone HCC Rx ESR COM

E22.8 Other hyperfunction of pituitary gland HCC Rx ESR COM
Central precocious puberty

E22.9 Hyperfunction of pituitary gland, unspecified HCC Rx ESR COM

E23 Hypofunction and other disorders of the pituitary gland
INCLUDES the listed conditions whether the disorder is in the pituitary or the hypothalamus
EXCLUDES 1 *postprocedural hypopituitarism (E89.3)*
▶*short stature due to endocrine disorder (E34.3-)*◀

E23.Ø Hypopituitarism HCC Rx ESR COM
Fertile eunuch syndrome
Hypogonadotropic hypogonadism
Idiopathic growth hormone deficiency
Isolated deficiency of gonadotropin
Isolated deficiency of growth hormone
Isolated deficiency of pituitary hormone
Kallmann's syndrome
Lorain-Levi short stature
Necrosis of pituitary gland (postpartum)
Panhypopituitarism
Pituitary cachexia
Pituitary insufficiency NOS
Pituitary short stature
Sheehan's syndrome
Simmonds' disease

E23.1 Drug-induced hypopituitarism HCC Rx ESR COM
Use additional code for adverse effect, if applicable, to identify drug (T36-T5Ø with fifth or sixth character 5)

E23.2 Diabetes insipidus HCC Rx ESR COM
EXCLUDES 1 *nephrogenic diabetes insipidus (N25.1)*

E23.3 Hypothalamic dysfunction, not elsewhere classified HCC Rx ESR COM
EXCLUDES 1 *Prader-Willi syndrome (Q87.11)*
Russell-Silver syndrome (Q87.19)

E23.6 Other disorders of pituitary gland HCC Rx ESR COM
Abscess of pituitary
Adiposogenital dystrophy

E23.7 Disorder of pituitary gland, unspecified HCC Rx ESR COM

E24 Cushing's syndrome
EXCLUDES 1 *congenital adrenal hyperplasia (E25.Ø)*
DEF: Abdominal striae, acne, hypertension, decreased carbohydrate tolerance, moon face, obesity, protein catabolism, and psychiatric disturbances resulting from increased adrenocortical secretion of cortisol caused by ACTH-dependent adrenocortical hyperplasia or tumor, or by steroid effects.

E24.Ø Pituitary-dependent Cushing's disease HCC Rx ESR COM
Overproduction of pituitary ACTH
Pituitary-dependent hypercorticalism

E24.1 Nelson's syndrome HCC Rx ESR COM

E24.2 Drug-induced Cushing's syndrome HCC Rx ESR COM
Use additional code for adverse effect, if applicable, to identify drug (T36-T5Ø with fifth or sixth character 5)

E24.3 Ectopic ACTH syndrome HCC Rx ESR COM

E24.4 Alcohol-induced pseudo-Cushing's syndrome HCC Rx ESR COM

E24.8 Other Cushing's syndrome HCC Rx ESR COM

E24.9 Cushing's syndrome, unspecified HCC Rx ESR COM

E25 Adrenogenital disorders

INCLUDES adrenogenital syndromes, virilizing or feminizing, whether acquired or due to adrenal hyperplasia consequent on inborn enzyme defects in hormone synthesis
female adrenal pseudohermaphroditism
female heterosexual precocious pseudopuberty
male isosexual precocious pseudopuberty
male macrogenitosomia praecox
male sexual precocity with adrenal hyperplasia
male virilization (female)

EXCLUDES 1 *indeterminate sex and pseudohermaphroditism (Q56)*
chromosomal abnormalities (Q9Ø-Q99)

E25.Ø Congenital adrenogenital disorders associated with enzyme deficiency HCC Rx ESR COM
Congenital adrenal hyperplasia
21-Hydroxylase deficiency
Salt-losing congenital adrenal hyperplasia

E25.8 Other adrenogenital disorders HCC Rx ESR COM
Idiopathic adrenogenital disorder
Use additional code for adverse effect, if applicable, to identify drug (T36-T5Ø with fifth or sixth character 5)

E25.9 Adrenogenital disorder, unspecified HCC Rx ESR COM
Adrenogenital syndrome NOS

E26 Hyperaldosteronism

E26.Ø Primary hyperaldosteronism

E26.Ø1 Conn's syndrome HCC Rx ESR COM
Code also adrenal adenoma (D35.Ø-)

E26.Ø2 Glucocorticoid-remediable aldosteronism HCC Rx ESR COM
Familial aldosteronism type I
DEF: Rare autosomal dominant familial form of primary aldosteronism in which the secretion of aldosterone is under the influence of adrenocorticotrophic hormone (ACTH) rather than the renin-angiotensin mechanism. Moderate hypersecretion of aldosterone and suppressed plasma renin activity that are rapidly reversed by administration of glucosteroids. Symptoms include hypertension and mild hypokalemia.

E26.Ø9 Other primary hyperaldosteronism HCC Rx ESR COM
Primary aldosteronism due to adrenal hyperplasia (bilateral)

E26.1 Secondary hyperaldosteronism HCC Rx ESR COM

E26.8 Other hyperaldosteronism

E26.81 Bartter's syndrome HCC Rx ESR COM

E26.89 Other hyperaldosteronism HCC Rx ESR COM

E26.9 Hyperaldosteronism, unspecified HCC Rx ESR COM
Aldosteronism NOS
Hyperaldosteronism NOS

E27 Other disorders of adrenal gland

E27.Ø Other adrenocortical overactivity HCC Rx ESR COM
Overproduction of ACTH, not associated with Cushing's disease
Premature adrenarche

EXCLUDES 1 *Cushing's syndrome (E24.-)*

E27.1 Primary adrenocortical insufficiency HCC Rx ESR COM
Addison's disease
Autoimmune adrenalitis

EXCLUDES 1 *Addison only phenotype adrenoleukodystrophy (E71.528)*
amyloidosis (E85.-)
tuberculous Addison's disease (A18.7)
Waterhouse-Friderichsen syndrome (A39.1)

E27.2 Addisonian crisis HCC Rx ESR COM
Adrenal crisis
Adrenocortical crisis
DEF: Life-threatening condition that occurs when there is not enough cortisol excreted from the adrenal glands. This condition may be due to injury to the adrenal glands or to the pituitary gland, which controls adrenal hormone secretion, or when a patient stops hydrocortisone treatment too quickly or too early.

E27.3 Drug-induced adrenocortical insufficiency HCC Rx ESR COM
Use additional code for adverse effect, if applicable, to identify drug (T36-T5Ø with fifth or sixth character 5)

E27.4 Other and unspecified adrenocortical insufficiency

EXCLUDES 1 *adrenoleukodystrophy [Addison-Schilder] (E71.528)*
Waterhouse-Friderichsen syndrome (A39.1)

E27.4Ø Unspecified adrenocortical insufficiency HCC Rx ESR COM
Adrenocortical insufficiency NOS
Hypoaldosteronism

E27.49 Other adrenocortical insufficiency HCC Rx ESR COM
Adrenal hemorrhage
Adrenal infarction

E27.5 Adrenomedullary hyperfunction HCC Rx ESR COM
Adrenomedullary hyperplasia
Catecholamine hypersecretion

E27.8 Other specified disorders of adrenal gland HCC Rx ESR COM
Abnormality of cortisol-binding globulin

E27.9 Disorder of adrenal gland, unspecified HCC Rx ESR COM

E28 Ovarian dysfunction

EXCLUDES 1 *isolated gonadotropin deficiency (E23.Ø)*
postprocedural ovarian failure (E89.4-)

E28.Ø Estrogen excess ♀
Use additional code for adverse effect, if applicable, to identify drug (T36-T5Ø with fifth or sixth character 5)

E28.1 Androgen excess ♀
Hypersecretion of ovarian androgens
Use additional code for adverse effect, if applicable, to identify drug (T36-T5Ø with fifth or sixth character 5)

E28.2 Polycystic ovarian syndrome ♀
Sclerocystic ovary syndrome
Stein-Leventhal syndrome
AHA: 2022,2Q,16
DEF: Common hormonal disorder among women of reproductive age that involves enlarged ovaries with numerous small cysts located along the outer ovarian edge.

E28.3 Primary ovarian failure

EXCLUDES 1 *pure gonadal dysgenesis (Q99.1)*
Turner's syndrome (Q96.-)

E28.31 Premature menopause

E28.31Ø Symptomatic premature menopause A ♀
Symptoms such as flushing, sleeplessness, headache, lack of concentration, associated with premature menopause

E28.319 Asymptomatic premature menopause A ♀
Premature menopause NOS

E28.39 Other primary ovarian failure ♀
Decreased estrogen
Resistant ovary syndrome

E28.8 Other ovarian dysfunction ♀
Ovarian hyperfunction NOS

EXCLUDES 1 *postprocedural ovarian failure (E89.4-)*

E28.9 Ovarian dysfunction, unspecified ♀

E29 Testicular dysfunction

EXCLUDES 1 *androgen insensitivity syndrome (E34.5-)*
azoospermia or oligospermia NOS (N46.Ø-N46.1)
isolated gonadotropin deficiency (E23.Ø)
Klinefelter's syndrome (Q98.Ø-Q98.1, Q98.4)

E29.Ø Testicular hyperfunction ♂
Hypersecretion of testicular hormones

E29.1 Testicular hypofunction ♂
Defective biosynthesis of testicular androgen NOS
5-delta-Reductase deficiency (with male pseudohermaphroditism)
Testicular hypogonadism NOS
Use additional code for adverse effect, if applicable, to identify drug (T36-T5Ø with fifth or sixth character 5)

EXCLUDES 1 *postprocedural testicular hypofunction (E89.5)*

E29.8 Other testicular dysfunction ♂

E29.9 Testicular dysfunction, unspecified ♂

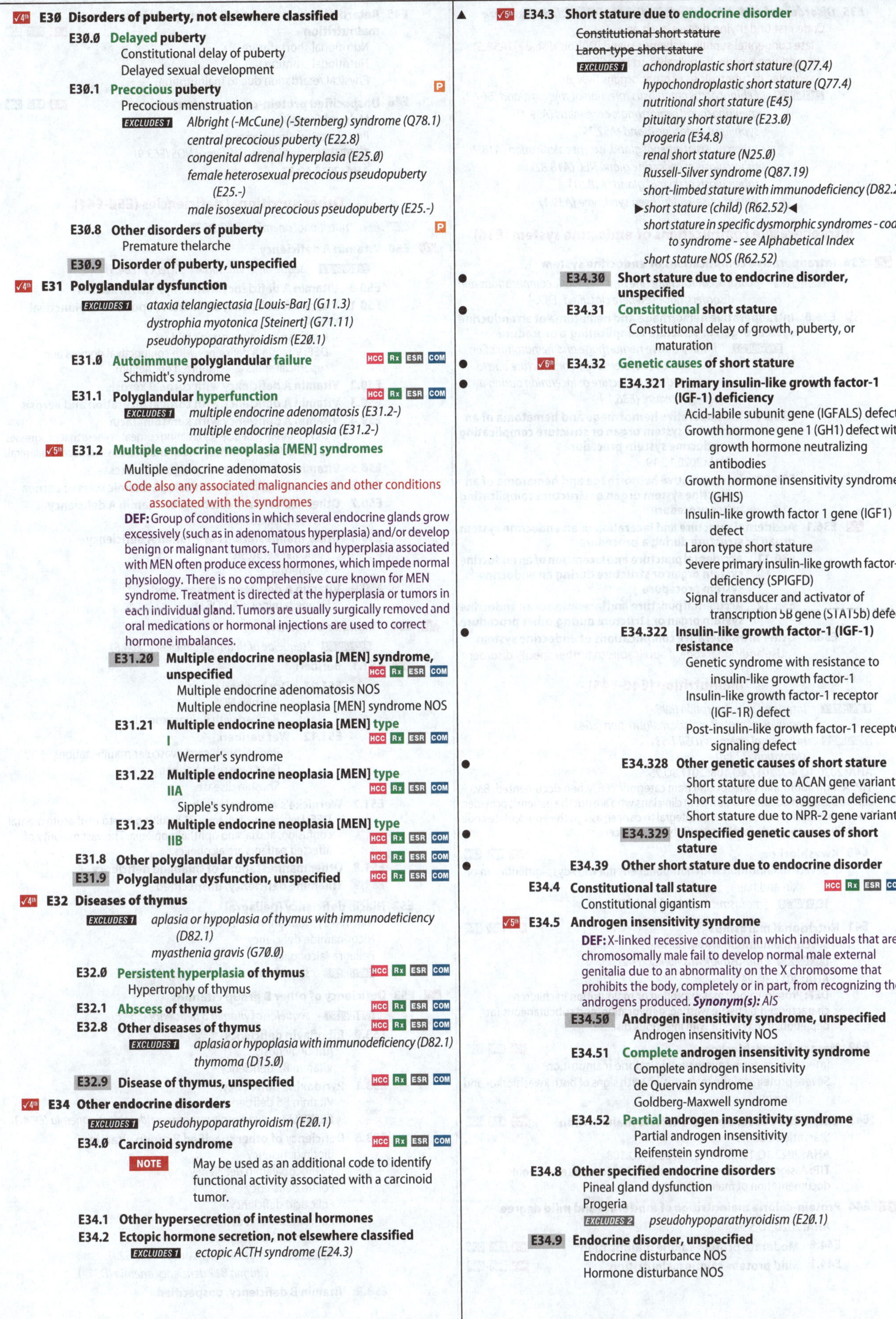

E30 Disorders of puberty, not elsewhere classified (4th)

E30.0 Delayed puberty
Constitutional delay of puberty
Delayed sexual development

E30.1 Precocious puberty (P)
Precocious menstruation
EXCLUDES 1 *Albright (-McCune) (-Sternberg) syndrome (Q78.1)*
central precocious puberty (E22.8)
congenital adrenal hyperplasia (E25.0)
female heterosexual precocious pseudopuberty (E25.-)
male isosexual precocious pseudopuberty (E25.-)

E30.8 Other disorders of puberty (P)
Premature thelarche

E30.9 Disorder of puberty, unspecified

E31 Polyglandular dysfunction (4th)
EXCLUDES 1 *ataxia telangiectasia [Louis-Bar] (G11.3)*
dystrophia myotonica [Steinert] (G71.11)
pseudohypoparathyroidism (E20.1)

E31.0 Autoimmune polyglandular failure HCC Rx ESR COM
Schmidt's syndrome

E31.1 Polyglandular hyperfunction HCC Rx ESR COM
EXCLUDES 1 *multiple endocrine adenomatosis (E31.2-)*
multiple endocrine neoplasia (E31.2-)

E31.2 Multiple endocrine neoplasia [MEN] syndromes (5th)
Multiple endocrine adenomatosis
Code also any associated malignancies and other conditions associated with the syndromes
DEF: Group of conditions in which several endocrine glands grow excessively (such as in adenomatous hyperplasia) and/or develop benign or malignant tumors. Tumors and hyperplasia associated with MEN often produce excess hormones, which impede normal physiology. There is no comprehensive cure known for MEN syndrome. Treatment is directed at the hyperplasia or tumors in each individual gland. Tumors are usually surgically removed and oral medications or hormonal injections are used to correct hormone imbalances.

E31.20 Multiple endocrine neoplasia [MEN] syndrome, unspecified HCC Rx ESR COM
Multiple endocrine adenomatosis NOS
Multiple endocrine neoplasia [MEN] syndrome NOS

E31.21 Multiple endocrine neoplasia [MEN] type I HCC Rx ESR COM
Wermer's syndrome

E31.22 Multiple endocrine neoplasia [MEN] type IIA HCC Rx ESR COM
Sipple's syndrome

E31.23 Multiple endocrine neoplasia [MEN] type IIB HCC Rx ESR COM

E31.8 Other polyglandular dysfunction HCC Rx ESR COM

E31.9 Polyglandular dysfunction, unspecified HCC Rx ESR COM

E32 Diseases of thymus (4th)
EXCLUDES 1 *aplasia or hypoplasia of thymus with immunodeficiency (D82.1)*
myasthenia gravis (G70.0)

E32.0 Persistent hyperplasia of thymus HCC Rx ESR COM
Hypertrophy of thymus

E32.1 Abscess of thymus HCC Rx ESR COM

E32.8 Other diseases of thymus HCC Rx ESR COM
EXCLUDES 1 *aplasia or hypoplasia with immunodeficiency (D82.1)*
thymoma (D15.0)

E32.9 Disease of thymus, unspecified HCC Rx ESR COM

E34 Other endocrine disorders (4th)
EXCLUDES 1 *pseudohypoparathyroidism (E20.1)*

E34.0 Carcinoid syndrome HCC Rx ESR COM
NOTE May be used as an additional code to identify functional activity associated with a carcinoid tumor.

E34.1 Other hypersecretion of intestinal hormones

E34.2 Ectopic hormone secretion, not elsewhere classified
EXCLUDES 1 *ectopic ACTH syndrome (E24.3)*

▲ **E34.3 Short stature due to endocrine disorder** (5th)
Constitutional short stature
~~Laron-type short stature~~
EXCLUDES 1 *achondroplastic short stature (Q77.4)*
hypochondroplastic short stature (Q77.4)
nutritional short stature (E45)
pituitary short stature (E23.0)
progeria (E34.8)
renal short stature (N25.0)
Russell-Silver syndrome (Q87.19)
short-limbed stature with immunodeficiency (D82.2)
▶short stature (child) (R62.52)◀
short stature in specific dysmorphic syndromes - code to syndrome - see Alphabetical Index
short stature NOS (R62.52)

● **E34.30 Short stature due to endocrine disorder, unspecified**

● **E34.31 Constitutional short stature**
Constitutional delay of growth, puberty, or maturation

● **E34.32 Genetic causes of short stature** (6th)

● **E34.321 Primary insulin-like growth factor-1 (IGF-1) deficiency**
Acid-labile subunit gene (IGFALS) defect
Growth hormone gene 1 (GH1) defect with growth hormone neutralizing antibodies
Growth hormone insensitivity syndrome (GHIS)
Insulin-like growth factor 1 gene (IGF1) defect
Laron type short stature
Severe primary insulin-like growth factor-1 deficiency (SPIGFD)
Signal transducer and activator of transcription 5B gene (STAT5b) defect

● **E34.322 Insulin-like growth factor-1 (IGF-1) resistance**
Genetic syndrome with resistance to insulin-like growth factor-1
Insulin-like growth factor-1 receptor (IGF-1R) defect
Post-insulin-like growth factor-1 receptor signaling defect

● **E34.328 Other genetic causes of short stature**
Short stature due to ACAN gene variant
Short stature due to aggrecan deficiency
Short stature due to NPR-2 gene variant

● **E34.329 Unspecified genetic causes of short stature**

● **E34.39 Other short stature due to endocrine disorder**

E34.4 Constitutional tall stature HCC Rx ESR COM
Constitutional gigantism

E34.5 Androgen insensitivity syndrome (5th)
DEF: X-linked recessive condition in which individuals that are chromosomally male fail to develop normal male external genitalia due to an abnormality on the X chromosome that prohibits the body, completely or in part, from recognizing the androgens produced. ***Synonym(s):*** *AIS*

E34.50 Androgen insensitivity syndrome, unspecified
Androgen insensitivity NOS

E34.51 Complete androgen insensitivity syndrome
Complete androgen insensitivity
de Quervain syndrome
Goldberg-Maxwell syndrome

E34.52 Partial androgen insensitivity syndrome
Partial androgen insensitivity
Reifenstein syndrome

E34.8 Other specified endocrine disorders
Pineal gland dysfunction
Progeria
EXCLUDES 2 *pseudohypoparathyroidism (E20.1)*

E34.9 Endocrine disorder, unspecified
Endocrine disturbance NOS
Hormone disturbance NOS

E35 *Disorders of endocrine glands in diseases classified elsewhere*

Code first underlying disease, such as:
late congenital syphilis of thymus gland [Dubois disease] (A5Ø.5)
Use additional code, if applicable, to identify:
sequelae of tuberculosis of other organs (B9Ø.8)

EXCLUDES 1 *Echinococcus granulosus infection of thyroid gland (B67.3)*
meningococcal hemorrhagic adrenalitis (A39.1)
syphilis of endocrine gland (A52.79)
tuberculosis of adrenal gland, except calcification (A18.7)
tuberculosis of endocrine gland NEC (A18.82)
tuberculosis of thyroid gland (A18.81)
Waterhouse-Friderichsen syndrome (A39.1)

Intraoperative complications of endocrine system (E36)

✓4th **E36 Intraoperative complications of endocrine system**

EXCLUDES 2 *postprocedural endocrine and metabolic complications and disorders, not elsewhere classified (E89.-)*

✓5th **E36.Ø Intraoperative hemorrhage and hematoma of an endocrine system organ or structure complicating a procedure**

EXCLUDES 1 *intraoperative hemorrhage and hematoma of an endocrine system organ or structure due to accidental puncture or laceration during a procedure (E36.1-)*

E36.Ø1 Intraoperative hemorrhage and hematoma of an endocrine system organ or structure complicating an endocrine system procedure
AHA: 2020,1Q,19

E36.Ø2 Intraoperative hemorrhage and hematoma of an endocrine system organ or structure complicating other procedure

✓5th **E36.1 Accidental puncture and laceration of an endocrine system organ or structure during a procedure**

E36.11 Accidental puncture and laceration of an endocrine system organ or structure during an endocrine system procedure

E36.12 Accidental puncture and laceration of an endocrine system organ or structure during other procedure

E36.8 Other intraoperative complications of endocrine system
Use additional code, if applicable, to further specify disorder

Malnutrition (E4Ø-E46)

EXCLUDES 1 *intestinal malabsorption (K9Ø.-)*
sequelae of protein-calorie malnutrition (E64.Ø)

EXCLUDES 2 *nutritional anemias (D5Ø-D53)*
starvation (T73.Ø)

AHA: 2020,1Q,4-7; 2017,4Q,108; 2017,3Q,25

TIP: Assign additional code for BMI from category Z68, when documented. BMI can be based on documentation from clinicians who are not the patient's provider.

TIP: Malnutrition is not considered integral to cancer; assign the appropriate code in addition to the code for the specific type of cancer.

E4Ø Kwashiorkor HCC ESR COM
Severe malnutrition with nutritional edema with dyspigmentation of skin and hair
EXCLUDES 1 *marasmic kwashiorkor (E42)*

E41 Nutritional marasmus HCC ESR COM
Severe malnutrition with marasmus
EXCLUDES 1 *marasmic kwashiorkor (E42)*
AHA: 2017,3Q,24
DEF: Protein-calorie malabsorption or malnutrition in children characterized by tissue wasting, dehydration, and subcutaneous fat depletion. It may occur with infectious disease.

E42 Marasmic kwashiorkor HCC ESR COM
Intermediate form severe protein-calorie malnutrition
Severe protein-calorie malnutrition with signs of both kwashiorkor and marasmus

E43 Unspecified severe protein-calorie malnutrition HCC ESR COM
Starvation edema
AHA: 2022,1Q,13; 2020,1Q,5,6; 2017,4Q,108
TIP: Assign code R64 when emaciation is documented without documentation of malnutrition.

✓4th **E44 Protein-calorie malnutrition of moderate and mild degree**
AHA: 2020,1Q,5

E44.Ø Moderate protein-calorie malnutrition HCC ESR COM

E44.1 Mild protein-calorie malnutrition HCC ESR COM

E45 Retarded development following protein-calorie malnutrition HCC ESR COM
Nutritional short stature
Nutritional stunting
Physical retardation due to malnutrition

E46 Unspecified protein-calorie malnutrition HCC ESR COM
Malnutrition NOS
Protein-calorie imbalance NOS
EXCLUDES 1 *nutritional deficiency NOS (E63.9)*
AHA: 2018,4Q,82

Other nutritional deficiencies (E5Ø-E64)

EXCLUDES 2 *nutritional anemias (D5Ø-D53)*

✓4th **E5Ø Vitamin A deficiency**

EXCLUDES 1 *sequelae of vitamin A deficiency (E64.1)*

E5Ø.Ø Vitamin A deficiency with conjunctival xerosis

E5Ø.1 Vitamin A deficiency with Bitot's spot and conjunctival xerosis
Bitot's spot in the young child
DEF: Vitamin A deficiency with conjunctival dryness and superficial spots of keratinized epithelium.

E5Ø.2 Vitamin A deficiency with corneal xerosis

E5Ø.3 Vitamin A deficiency with corneal ulceration and xerosis

E5Ø.4 Vitamin A deficiency with keratomalacia
DEF: Vitamin A deficiency creating corneal dryness that progresses to corneal insensitivity, softness, and necrosis. It is usually bilateral.

E5Ø.5 Vitamin A deficiency with night blindness

E5Ø.6 Vitamin A deficiency with xerophthalmic scars of cornea

E5Ø.7 Other ocular manifestations of vitamin A deficiency
Xerophthalmia NOS

E5Ø.8 Other manifestations of vitamin A deficiency
Follicular keratosis
Xeroderma

E5Ø.9 Vitamin A deficiency, unspecified
Hypovitaminosis A NOS

✓4th **E51 Thiamine deficiency**

EXCLUDES 1 *sequelae of thiamine deficiency (E64.8)*

✓5th **E51.1 Beriberi**

E51.11 Dry beriberi
Beriberi NOS
Beriberi with polyneuropathy

E51.12 Wet beriberi
Beriberi with cardiovascular manifestations
Cardiovascular beriberi
Shoshin disease

E51.2 Wernicke's encephalopathy
DEF: Deficiency of vitamin B1 resulting in a triad of acute mental confusion, ataxia, and ophthalmoplegia. The vast majority of affected patients are alcoholics.

E51.8 Other manifestations of thiamine deficiency

E51.9 Thiamine deficiency, unspecified

E52 Niacin deficiency [pellagra]
Niacin (-tryptophan) deficiency
Nicotinamide deficiency
Pellagra (alcoholic)
EXCLUDES 1 *sequelae of niacin deficiency (E64.8)*

✓4th **E53 Deficiency of other B group vitamins**

EXCLUDES 1 *sequelae of vitamin B deficiency (E64.8)*

E53.Ø Riboflavin deficiency
Ariboflavinosis
Vitamin B2 deficiency

E53.1 Pyridoxine deficiency
Vitamin B6 deficiency
EXCLUDES 1 *pyridoxine-responsive sideroblastic anemia (D64.3)*

E53.8 Deficiency of other specified B group vitamins
Biotin deficiency
Cyanocobalamin deficiency
Folate deficiency
Folic acid deficiency
Pantothenic acid deficiency
Vitamin B12 deficiency
EXCLUDES 1 *folate deficiency anemia (D52.-)*
vitamin B12 deficiency anemia (D51.-)

E53.9 Vitamin B deficiency, unspecified

E54 Ascorbic acid deficiency
Deficiency of vitamin C
Scurvy
EXCLUDES 1 *scorbutic anemia (D53.2)*
sequelae of vitamin C deficiency (E64.2)
DEF: Vitamin C deficiency causing swollen gums, myalgia, weight loss, and weakness.

E55 Vitamin D deficiency
EXCLUDES 1 *adult osteomalacia (M83.-)*
osteoporosis (M8Ø.-)
sequelae of rickets (E64.3)

E55.Ø Rickets, active Rx
Infantile osteomalacia
Juvenile osteomalacia
EXCLUDES 1 *celiac rickets (K9Ø.Ø)*
Crohn's rickets (K5Ø.-)
hereditary vitamin D-dependent rickets (E83.32)
inactive rickets (E64.3)
renal rickets (N25.Ø)
sequelae of rickets (E64.3)
vitamin D-resistant rickets (E83.31)
DEF: Rickets: Softening or weakening of the bones due to a lack of vitamin D, calcium, and phosphate.

E55.9 Vitamin D deficiency, unspecified
Avitaminosis D

E56 Other vitamin deficiencies
EXCLUDES 1 *sequelae of other vitamin deficiencies (E64.8)*

E56.Ø Deficiency of vitamin E
E56.1 Deficiency of vitamin K
EXCLUDES 1 *deficiency of coagulation factor due to vitamin K deficiency (D68.4)*
vitamin K deficiency of newborn (P53)
E56.8 Deficiency of other vitamins
E56.9 Vitamin deficiency, unspecified

E58 Dietary calcium deficiency
EXCLUDES 1 *disorders of calcium metabolism (E83.5-)*
sequelae of calcium deficiency (E64.8)

E59 Dietary selenium deficiency
Keshan disease
EXCLUDES 1 *sequelae of selenium deficiency (E64.8)*

E6Ø Dietary zinc deficiency

E61 Deficiency of other nutrient elements
Use additional code for adverse effect, if applicable, to identify drug (T36-T5Ø with fifth or sixth character 5)
EXCLUDES 1 *disorders of mineral metabolism (E83.-)*
iodine deficiency related thyroid disorders (EØØ-EØ2)
sequelae of malnutrition and other nutritional deficiencies (E64.-)

E61.Ø Copper deficiency
E61.1 Iron deficiency
EXCLUDES 1 *iron deficiency anemia (D5Ø.-)*
E61.2 Magnesium deficiency
E61.3 Manganese deficiency
E61.4 Chromium deficiency
E61.5 Molybdenum deficiency
E61.6 Vanadium deficiency
E61.7 Deficiency of multiple nutrient elements
E61.8 Deficiency of other specified nutrient elements
E61.9 Deficiency of nutrient element, unspecified

E63 Other nutritional deficiencies
EXCLUDES 2 *dehydration (E86.Ø)*
failure to thrive, adult (R62.7)
failure to thrive, child (R62.51)
feeding problems in newborn (P92.-)
sequelae of malnutrition and other nutritional deficiencies (E64.-)

E63.Ø Essential fatty acid [EFA] deficiency
E63.1 Imbalance of constituents of food intake
E63.8 Other specified nutritional deficiencies
E63.9 Nutritional deficiency, unspecified

E64 Sequelae of malnutrition and other nutritional deficiencies
NOTE This category is to be used to indicate conditions in categories E43, E44, E46, E5Ø-E63 as the cause of sequelae, which are themselves classified elsewhere. The 'sequelae' include conditions specified as such; they also include the late effects of diseases classifiable to the above categories if the disease itself is no longer present
Code first condition resulting from (sequela) of malnutrition and other nutritional deficiencies

E64.Ø Sequelae of protein-calorie malnutrition HCC ESR
EXCLUDES 2 *retarded development following protein-calorie malnutrition (E45)*
E64.1 Sequelae of vitamin A deficiency
E64.2 Sequelae of vitamin C deficiency
E64.3 Sequelae of rickets
E64.8 Sequelae of other nutritional deficiencies
E64.9 Sequelae of unspecified nutritional deficiency

Overweight, obesity and other hyperalimentation (E65-E68)

E65 Localized adiposity
Fat pad

E66 Overweight and obesity
Code first obesity complicating pregnancy, childbirth and the puerperium, if applicable (O99.21-)
Use additional code to identify body mass index (BMI), if known (Z68.-)
EXCLUDES 1 *adiposogenital dystrophy (E23.6)*
lipomatosis NOS (E88.2)
lipomatosis dolorosa [Dercum] (E88.2)
Prader-Willi syndrome (Q87.11)
AHA: 2018,4Q,77,79-80
TIP: Do not assign a BMI code (Z68.-) when a pregnant patient is documented as being overweight or obese. Only a code from subcategory O99.21- and a code from this category should be assigned.

E66.Ø Obesity due to excess calories
E66.Ø1 Morbid (severe) obesity due to excess calories HCC ESR
EXCLUDES 1 *morbid (severe) obesity with alveolar hypoventilation (E66.2)*
AHA: 2022,2Q,9
E66.Ø9 Other obesity due to excess calories
E66.1 Drug-induced obesity
Use additional code for adverse effect, if applicable, to identify drug (T36-T5Ø with fifth or sixth character 5)
E66.2 Morbid (severe) obesity with alveolar hypoventilation HCC ESR
Obesity hypoventilation syndrome (OHS)
Pickwickian syndrome
E66.3 Overweight
AHA: 2018,4Q,78
E66.8 Other obesity
E66.9 Obesity, unspecified
Obesity NOS
AHA: 2021,2Q,10

E67 Other hyperalimentation
EXCLUDES 1 *hyperalimentation NOS (R63.2)*
sequelae of hyperalimentation (E68)
E67.Ø Hypervitaminosis A
E67.1 Hypercarotenemia
DEF: Elevated blood carotene level as a result of excessive carotenoid ingestion or an inability to convert carotenoids to vitamin A. Characteristics often include yellow discoloration of the skin, which may follow overeating of carotenoid-rich foods such as carrots, sweet potatoes, or squash.
E67.2 Megavitamin-B6 syndrome
E67.3 Hypervitaminosis D
E67.8 Other specified hyperalimentation

E68 Sequelae of hyperalimentation
Code first condition resulting from (sequela) of hyperalimentation

Metabolic disorders (E70-E88)

EXCLUDES 1 *androgen insensitivity syndrome (E34.5-)*
congenital adrenal hyperplasia (E25.0)
hemolytic anemias attributable to enzyme disorders (D55.-)
Marfan's syndrome (Q87.4)
5-alpha-reductase deficiency (E29.1)
EXCLUDES 2 *Ehlers-Danlos syndromes (Q79.6-)*
AHA: 2018,2Q,6

✓4th E70 Disorders of aromatic amino-acid metabolism
- **E70.0 Classical phenylketonuria** HCC Rx ESR COM
- **E70.1 Other hyperphenylalaninemias** HCC Rx ESR COM
- **✓5th E70.2 Disorders of tyrosine metabolism**
  - **EXCLUDES 1** *transitory tyrosinemia of newborn (P74.5)*
  - **E70.20 Disorder of tyrosine metabolism, unspecified** HCC Rx ESR COM
  - **E70.21 Tyrosinemia** HCC Rx ESR COM
    Hypertyrosinemia
  - **E70.29 Other disorders of tyrosine metabolism** HCC Rx ESR COM
    Alkaptonuria
    Ochronosis
- **✓5th E70.3 Albinism**
  - DEF: Absence of pigment in skin, hair, and eyes. This genetic condition is often accompanied by astigmatism, photophobia, and nystagmus.
  - **E70.30 Albinism, unspecified** HCC Rx ESR COM
  - **✓6th E70.31 Ocular albinism**
    - **E70.310 X-linked ocular albinism** HCC Rx ESR COM
    - **E70.311 Autosomal recessive ocular albinism** HCC Rx ESR COM
    - **E70.318 Other ocular albinism** HCC Rx ESR COM
    - **E70.319 Ocular albinism, unspecified** HCC Rx ESR COM
  - **✓6th E70.32 Oculocutaneous albinism**
    - **EXCLUDES 1** *Chediak-Higashi syndrome (E70.330)*
      Hermansky-Pudlak syndrome (E70.331)
    - **E70.320 Tyrosinase negative oculocutaneous albinism** HCC Rx ESR COM
      Albinism I
      Oculocutaneous albinism ty-neg
    - **E70.321 Tyrosinase positive oculocutaneous albinism** HCC Rx ESR COM
      Albinism II
      Oculocutaneous albinism ty-pos
    - **E70.328 Other oculocutaneous albinism** HCC Rx ESR COM
      Cross syndrome
    - **E70.329 Oculocutaneous albinism, unspecified** HCC Rx ESR COM
  - **✓6th E70.33 Albinism with hematologic abnormality**
    - **E70.330 Chediak-Higashi syndrome** HCC Rx ESR COM
    - **E70.331 Hermansky-Pudlak syndrome** HCC Rx ESR COM
    - **E70.338 Other albinism with hematologic abnormality** HCC Rx ESR COM
    - **E70.339 Albinism with hematologic abnormality, unspecified** HCC Rx ESR COM
  - **E70.39 Other specified albinism** HCC Rx ESR COM
    Piebaldism
- **✓5th E70.4 Disorders of histidine metabolism**
  - **E70.40 Disorders of histidine metabolism, unspecified** HCC Rx ESR COM
  - **E70.41 Histidinemia** HCC Rx ESR COM
  - **E70.49 Other disorders of histidine metabolism** HCC Rx ESR COM
- **E70.5 Disorders of tryptophan metabolism** HCC Rx ESR COM
- **✓5th E70.8 Other disorders of aromatic amino-acid metabolism**
  - AHA: 2020,4Q,15-16
  - **E70.81 Aromatic L-amino acid decarboxylase deficiency** HCC Rx ESR COM
    AADC deficiency
  - **E70.89 Other disorders of aromatic amino-acid metabolism** HCC Rx ESR COM
- **E70.9 Disorder of aromatic amino-acid metabolism, unspecified** HCC Rx ESR COM

✓4th E71 Disorders of branched-chain amino-acid metabolism and fatty-acid metabolism
- **E71.0 Maple-syrup-urine disease** HCC Rx ESR COM
- **✓5th E71.1 Other disorders of branched-chain amino-acid metabolism**
  - **✓6th E71.11 Branched-chain organic acidurias**
    - **E71.110 Isovaleric acidemia** HCC Rx ESR COM
    - **E71.111 3-methylglutaconic aciduria** HCC Rx ESR COM
    - **E71.118 Other branched-chain organic acidurias** HCC Rx ESR COM
  - **✓6th E71.12 Disorders of propionate metabolism**
    - **E71.120 Methylmalonic acidemia** HCC Rx ESR COM
    - **E71.121 Propionic acidemia** HCC Rx ESR COM
    - **E71.128 Other disorders of propionate metabolism** HCC Rx ESR COM
  - **E71.19 Other disorders of branched-chain amino-acid metabolism** HCC Rx ESR COM
    Hyperleucine-isoleucinemia
    Hypervalinemia
- **E71.2 Disorder of branched-chain amino-acid metabolism, unspecified** HCC Rx ESR COM
- **✓5th E71.3 Disorders of fatty-acid metabolism**
  - **EXCLUDES 1** *peroxisomal disorders (E71.5)*
    Refsum's disease (G60.1)
    Schilder's disease (G37.0)
  - **EXCLUDES 2** *carnitine deficiency due to inborn error of metabolism (E71.42)*
  - **E71.30 Disorder of fatty-acid metabolism, unspecified** Rx COM
  - **✓6th E71.31 Disorders of fatty-acid oxidation**
    - **E71.310 Long chain/very long chain acyl CoA dehydrogenase deficiency** HCC Rx ESR COM
      LCAD
      VLCAD
    - **E71.311 Medium chain acyl CoA dehydrogenase deficiency** HCC Rx ESR COM
      MCAD
    - **E71.312 Short chain acyl CoA dehydrogenase deficiency** HCC Rx ESR COM
      SCAD
    - **E71.313 Glutaric aciduria type II** HCC Rx ESR COM
      Glutaric aciduria type II A
      Glutaric aciduria type II B
      Glutaric aciduria type II C
      EXCLUDES 1 *glutaric aciduria (type 1) NOS (E72.3)*
    - **E71.314 Muscle carnitine palmitoyltransferase deficiency** HCC Rx ESR COM
    - **E71.318 Other disorders of fatty-acid oxidation** HCC Rx ESR COM
  - **E71.32 Disorders of ketone metabolism** HCC Rx ESR COM
  - **E71.39 Other disorders of fatty-acid metabolism** HCC Rx ESR COM
- **✓5th E71.4 Disorders of carnitine metabolism**
  - **EXCLUDES 1** *muscle carnitine palmitoyltransferase deficiency (E71.314)*
  - **E71.40 Disorder of carnitine metabolism, unspecified** HCC Rx ESR COM
  - **E71.41 Primary carnitine deficiency** HCC Rx ESR COM
  - **E71.42 Carnitine deficiency due to inborn errors of metabolism** HCC Rx ESR COM
    Code also associated inborn error or metabolism
  - **E71.43 Iatrogenic carnitine deficiency** HCC Rx ESR COM
    Carnitine deficiency due to hemodialysis
    Carnitine deficiency due to Valproic acid therapy
  - **✓6th E71.44 Other secondary carnitine deficiency**
    - **E71.440 Ruvalcaba-Myhre-Smith syndrome** HCC Rx ESR COM
    - **E71.448 Other secondary carnitine deficiency** HCC Rx ESR COM

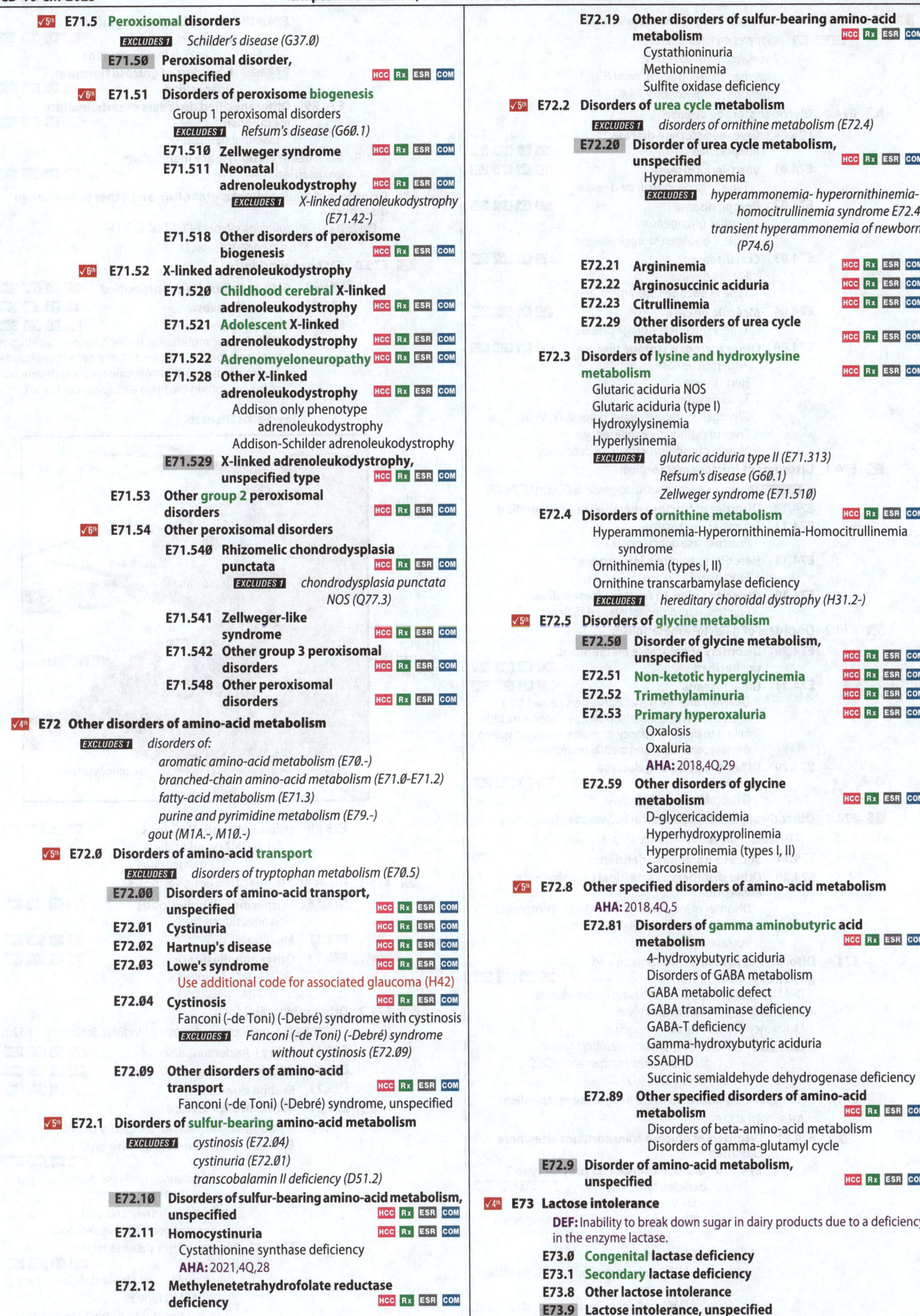

✓5th **E71.5 Peroxisomal disorders**
EXCLUDES 1 *Schilder's disease (G37.Ø)*

E71.5Ø Peroxisomal disorder, unspecified HCC Rx ESR COM

✓6th **E71.51 Disorders of peroxisome biogenesis**
Group 1 peroxisomal disorders
EXCLUDES 1 *Refsum's disease (G6Ø.1)*

E71.51Ø Zellweger syndrome HCC Rx ESR COM
E71.511 Neonatal adrenoleukodystrophy HCC Rx ESR COM
EXCLUDES 1 *X-linked adrenoleukodystrophy (E71.42-)*
E71.518 Other disorders of peroxisome biogenesis HCC Rx ESR COM

✓6th **E71.52 X-linked adrenoleukodystrophy**
E71.52Ø Childhood cerebral X-linked adrenoleukodystrophy HCC Rx ESR COM
E71.521 Adolescent X-linked adrenoleukodystrophy HCC Rx ESR COM
E71.522 Adrenomyeloneuropathy HCC Rx ESR COM
E71.528 Other X-linked adrenoleukodystrophy HCC Rx ESR COM
Addison only phenotype adrenoleukodystrophy
Addison-Schilder adrenoleukodystrophy
E71.529 X-linked adrenoleukodystrophy, unspecified type HCC Rx ESR COM

E71.53 Other group 2 peroxisomal disorders HCC Rx ESR COM

✓6th **E71.54 Other peroxisomal disorders**
E71.54Ø Rhizomelic chondrodysplasia punctata HCC Rx ESR COM
EXCLUDES 1 *chondrodysplasia punctata NOS (Q77.3)*
E71.541 Zellweger-like syndrome HCC Rx ESR COM
E71.542 Other group 3 peroxisomal disorders HCC Rx ESR COM
E71.548 Other peroxisomal disorders HCC Rx ESR COM

✓4th **E72 Other disorders of amino-acid metabolism**
EXCLUDES 1 *disorders of:*
aromatic amino-acid metabolism (E7Ø.-)
branched-chain amino-acid metabolism (E71.Ø-E71.2)
fatty-acid metabolism (E71.3)
purine and pyrimidine metabolism (E79.-)
gout (M1A.-, M1Ø.-)

✓5th **E72.Ø Disorders of amino-acid transport**
EXCLUDES 1 *disorders of tryptophan metabolism (E7Ø.5)*

E72.ØØ Disorders of amino-acid transport, unspecified HCC Rx ESR COM
E72.Ø1 Cystinuria HCC Rx ESR COM
E72.Ø2 Hartnup's disease HCC Rx ESR COM
E72.Ø3 Lowe's syndrome HCC Rx ESR COM
Use additional code for associated glaucoma (H42)
E72.Ø4 Cystinosis HCC Rx ESR COM
Fanconi (-de Toni) (-Debré) syndrome with cystinosis
EXCLUDES 1 *Fanconi (-de Toni) (-Debré) syndrome without cystinosis (E72.Ø9)*
E72.Ø9 Other disorders of amino-acid transport HCC Rx ESR COM
Fanconi (-de Toni) (-Debré) syndrome, unspecified

✓5th **E72.1 Disorders of sulfur-bearing amino-acid metabolism**
EXCLUDES 1 *cystinosis (E72.Ø4)*
cystinuria (E72.Ø1)
transcobalamin II deficiency (D51.2)

E72.1Ø Disorders of sulfur-bearing amino-acid metabolism, unspecified HCC Rx ESR COM
E72.11 Homocystinuria HCC Rx ESR COM
Cystathionine synthase deficiency
AHA: 2021,4Q,28
E72.12 Methylenetetrahydrofolate reductase deficiency HCC Rx ESR COM
E72.19 Other disorders of sulfur-bearing amino-acid metabolism HCC Rx ESR COM
Cystathioninuria
Methioninemia
Sulfite oxidase deficiency

✓5th **E72.2 Disorders of urea cycle metabolism**
EXCLUDES 1 *disorders of ornithine metabolism (E72.4)*

E72.2Ø Disorder of urea cycle metabolism, unspecified HCC Rx ESR COM
Hyperammonemia
EXCLUDES 1 *hyperammonemia- hyperornithinemia-homocitrullinemia syndrome E72.4*
transient hyperammonemia of newborn (P74.6)
E72.21 Argininemia HCC Rx ESR COM
E72.22 Arginosuccinic aciduria HCC Rx ESR COM
E72.23 Citrullinemia HCC Rx ESR COM
E72.29 Other disorders of urea cycle metabolism HCC Rx ESR COM

E72.3 Disorders of lysine and hydroxylysine metabolism HCC Rx ESR COM
Glutaric aciduria NOS
Glutaric aciduria (type I)
Hydroxylysinemia
Hyperlysinemia
EXCLUDES 1 *glutaric aciduria type II (E71.313)*
Refsum's disease (G6Ø.1)
Zellweger syndrome (E71.51Ø)

E72.4 Disorders of ornithine metabolism HCC Rx ESR COM
Hyperammonemia-Hyperornithinemia-Homocitrullinemia syndrome
Ornithinemia (types I, II)
Ornithine transcarbamylase deficiency
EXCLUDES 1 *hereditary choroidal dystrophy (H31.2-)*

✓5th **E72.5 Disorders of glycine metabolism**
E72.5Ø Disorder of glycine metabolism, unspecified HCC Rx ESR COM
E72.51 Non-ketotic hyperglycinemia HCC Rx ESR COM
E72.52 Trimethylaminuria HCC Rx ESR COM
E72.53 Primary hyperoxaluria HCC Rx ESR COM
Oxalosis
Oxaluria
AHA: 2018,4Q,29
E72.59 Other disorders of glycine metabolism HCC Rx ESR COM
D-glycericacidemia
Hyperhydroxyprolinemia
Hyperprolinemia (types I, II)
Sarcosinemia

✓5th **E72.8 Other specified disorders of amino-acid metabolism**
AHA: 2018,4Q,5
E72.81 Disorders of gamma aminobutyric acid metabolism HCC Rx ESR COM
4-hydroxybutyric aciduria
Disorders of GABA metabolism
GABA metabolic defect
GABA transaminase deficiency
GABA-T deficiency
Gamma-hydroxybutyric aciduria
SSADHD
Succinic semialdehyde dehydrogenase deficiency
E72.89 Other specified disorders of amino-acid metabolism HCC Rx ESR COM
Disorders of beta-amino-acid metabolism
Disorders of gamma-glutamyl cycle

E72.9 Disorder of amino-acid metabolism, unspecified HCC Rx ESR COM

✓4th **E73 Lactose intolerance**
DEF: Inability to break down sugar in dairy products due to a deficiency in the enzyme lactase.
E73.Ø Congenital lactase deficiency
E73.1 Secondary lactase deficiency
E73.8 Other lactose intolerance
E73.9 Lactose intolerance, unspecified

4th E74 Other disorders of carbohydrate metabolism
EXCLUDES 1 *diabetes mellitus (EØ8-E13)*
hypoglycemia NOS (E16.2)
increased secretion of glucagon (E16.3)
mucopolysaccharidosis (E76.Ø-E76.3)

5th E74.Ø Glycogen storage disease
E74.ØØ Glycogen storage disease, unspecified HCC Rx ESR COM
E74.Ø1 von Gierke disease HCC Rx ESR COM
Type I glycogen storage disease
E74.Ø2 Pompe disease HCC Rx ESR COM
Cardiac glycogenosis
Type II glycogen storage disease
E74.Ø3 Cori disease HCC Rx ESR COM
Forbes disease
Type III glycogen storage disease
E74.Ø4 McArdle disease HCC Rx ESR COM
Type V glycogen storage disease
E74.Ø9 Other glycogen storage disease HCC Rx ESR COM
Andersen disease
Hers disease
Tauri disease
Glycogen storage disease, types Ø, IV, VI-XI
Liver phosphorylase deficiency
Muscle phosphofructokinase deficiency

5th E74.1 Disorders of fructose metabolism
EXCLUDES 1 *muscle phosphofructokinase deficiency (E74.Ø9)*
E74.1Ø Disorder of fructose metabolism, unspecified
E74.11 Essential fructosuria
Fructokinase deficiency
E74.12 Hereditary fructose intolerance
Fructosemia
E74.19 Other disorders of fructose metabolism
Fructose-1, 6-diphosphatase deficiency

5th E74.2 Disorders of galactose metabolism
E74.2Ø Disorders of galactose metabolism, unspecified HCC Rx ESR COM
E74.21 Galactosemia HCC Rx ESR COM
DEF: Any of three genetic disorders caused by a defective galactose metabolism. Symptoms include failure to thrive in infancy, jaundice, liver and spleen damage, cataracts, and mental retardation.
E74.29 Other disorders of galactose metabolism HCC Rx ESR COM
Galactokinase deficiency

5th E74.3 Other disorders of intestinal carbohydrate absorption
EXCLUDES 2 *lactose intolerance (E73.-)*
E74.31 Sucrase-isomaltase deficiency Rx
E74.39 Other disorders of intestinal carbohydrate absorption
Disorder of intestinal carbohydrate absorption NOS
Glucose-galactose malabsorption
Sucrase deficiency

E74.4 Disorders of pyruvate metabolism and gluconeogenesis HCC Rx ESR COM
Deficiency of phosphoenolpyruvate carboxykinase
Deficiency of pyruvate carboxylase
Deficiency of pyruvate dehydrogenase
EXCLUDES 1 *disorders of pyruvate metabolism and gluconeogenesis with anemia (D55.-)*
Leigh's syndrome (G31.82)

5th E74.8 Other specified disorders of carbohydrate metabolism
AHA: 2020,4Q,16
6th E74.81 Disorders of glucose transport, not elsewhere classified
E74.81Ø Glucose transporter protein type 1 deficiency HCC Rx ESR COM
De Vivo syndrome
Glucose transport defect, blood-brain barrier
Glut1 deficiency
GLUT1 deficiency syndrome 1, infantile onset
GLUT1 deficiency syndrome 2, childhood onset
E74.818 Other disorders of glucose transport HCC Rx ESR COM
(Familial) renal glycosuria
E74.819 Disorders of glucose transport, unspecified HCC Rx ESR COM
E74.89 Other specified disorders of carbohydrate metabolism HCC Rx ESR COM
Essential pentosuria

E74.9 Disorder of carbohydrate metabolism, unspecified HCC Rx ESR COM

4th E75 Disorders of sphingolipid metabolism and other lipid storage disorders
EXCLUDES 1 *mucolipidosis, types I-III (E77.Ø-E77.1)*
Refsum's disease (G6Ø.1)

5th E75.Ø GM2 gangliosidosis
E75.ØØ GM2 gangliosidosis, unspecified HCC Rx ESR COM
E75.Ø1 Sandhoff disease HCC Rx ESR COM
E75.Ø2 Tay-Sachs disease HCC Rx ESR COM
DEF: Genetic mutation of the HEXA gene that inhibits the breakdown of a toxic substance called ganglioside. The accumulation of ganglioside results in destruction of the neurons in the brain and spinal cord.

Tay-Sachs Disease

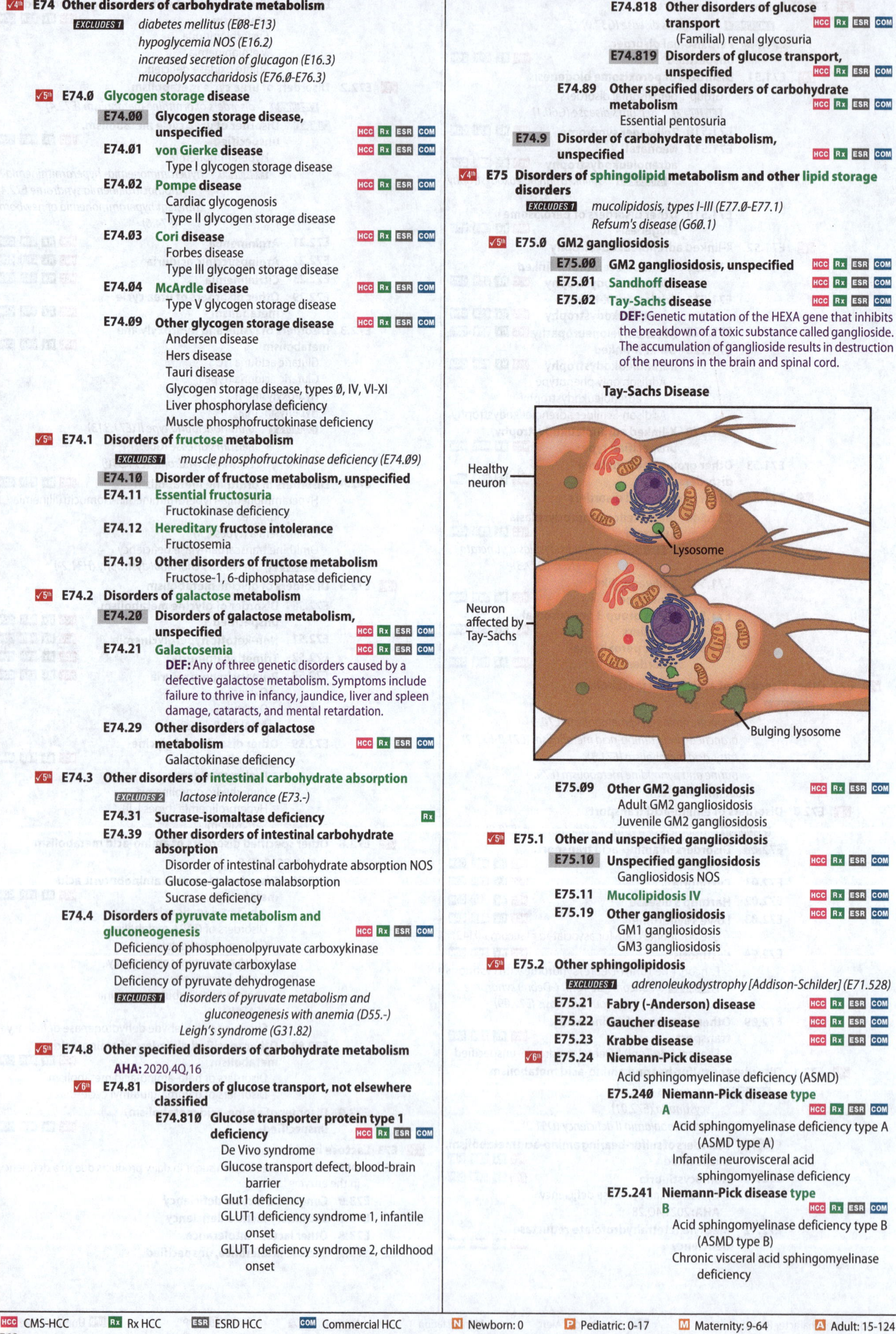

E75.Ø9 Other GM2 gangliosidosis HCC Rx ESR COM
Adult GM2 gangliosidosis
Juvenile GM2 gangliosidosis

5th E75.1 Other and unspecified gangliosidosis
E75.1Ø Unspecified gangliosidosis HCC Rx ESR COM
Gangliosidosis NOS
E75.11 Mucolipidosis IV HCC Rx ESR COM
E75.19 Other gangliosidosis HCC Rx ESR COM
GM1 gangliosidosis
GM3 gangliosidosis

5th E75.2 Other sphingolipidosis
EXCLUDES 1 *adrenoleukodystrophy [Addison-Schilder] (E71.528)*
E75.21 Fabry (-Anderson) disease HCC Rx ESR COM
E75.22 Gaucher disease HCC Rx ESR COM
E75.23 Krabbe disease HCC Rx ESR COM
6th E75.24 Niemann-Pick disease
Acid sphingomyelinase deficiency (ASMD)
E75.24Ø Niemann-Pick disease type A HCC Rx ESR COM
Acid sphingomyelinase deficiency type A (ASMD type A)
Infantile neurovisceral acid sphingomyelinase deficiency
E75.241 Niemann-Pick disease type B HCC Rx ESR COM
Acid sphingomyelinase deficiency type B (ASMD type B)
Chronic visceral acid sphingomyelinase deficiency

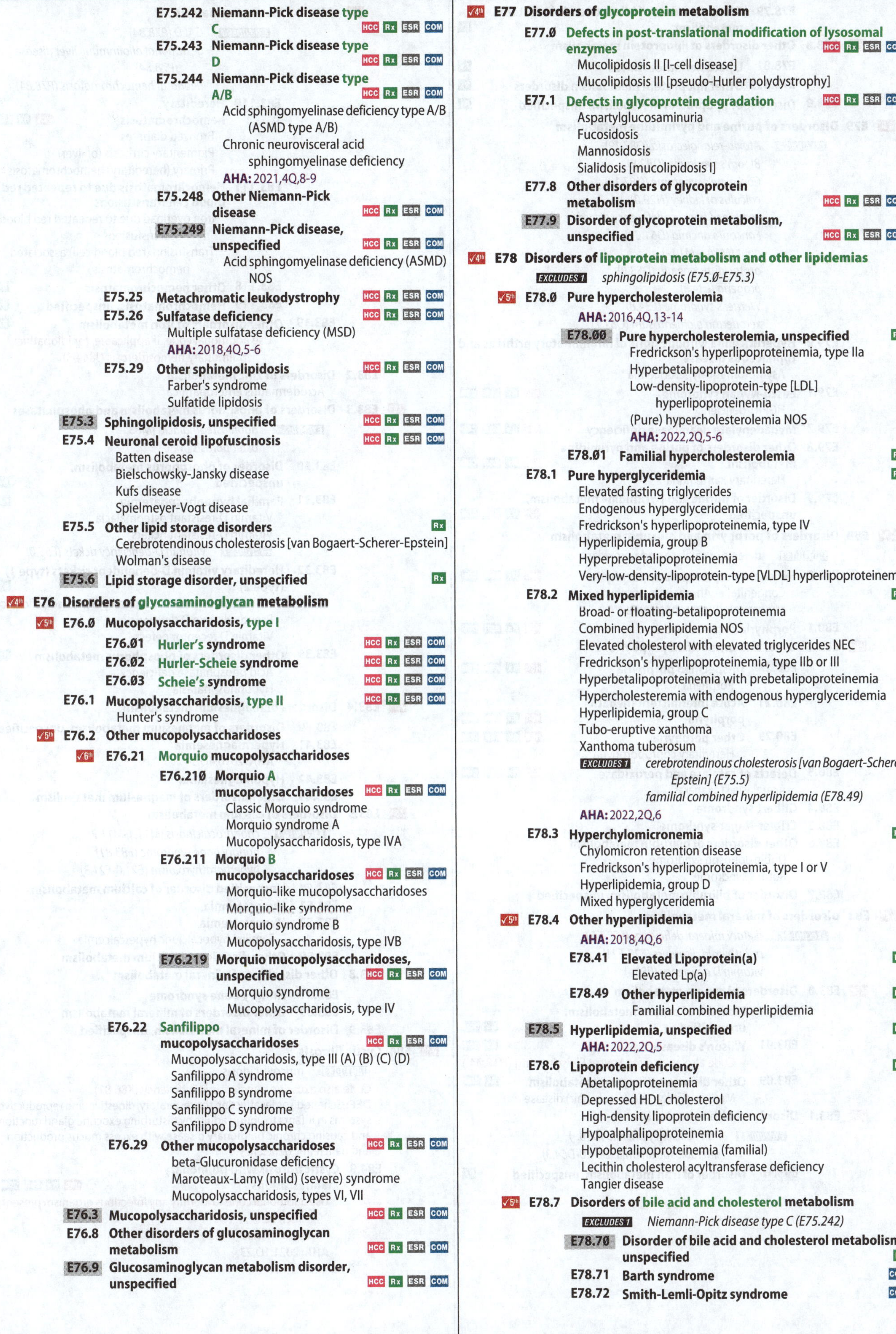

E75.242 **Niemann-Pick disease type C** HCC Rx ESR COM

E75.243 **Niemann-Pick disease type D** HCC Rx ESR COM

E75.244 **Niemann-Pick disease type A/B** HCC Rx ESR COM
Acid sphingomyelinase deficiency type A/B (ASMD type A/B)
Chronic neurovisceral acid sphingomyelinase deficiency
AHA: 2021,4Q,8-9

E75.248 **Other Niemann-Pick disease** HCC Rx ESR COM

E75.249 **Niemann-Pick disease, unspecified** HCC Rx ESR COM
Acid sphingomyelinase deficiency (ASMD) NOS

E75.25 **Metachromatic leukodystrophy** HCC Rx ESR COM

E75.26 **Sulfatase deficiency** HCC Rx ESR COM
Multiple sulfatase deficiency (MSD)
AHA: 2018,4Q,5-6

E75.29 **Other sphingolipidosis** HCC Rx ESR COM
Farber's syndrome
Sulfatide lipidosis

E75.3 **Sphingolipidosis, unspecified** HCC Rx ESR COM

E75.4 **Neuronal ceroid lipofuscinosis** HCC Rx ESR COM
Batten disease
Bielschowsky-Jansky disease
Kufs disease
Spielmeyer-Vogt disease

E75.5 **Other lipid storage disorders** Rx
Cerebrotendinous cholesterosis [van Bogaert-Scherer-Epstein]
Wolman's disease

E75.6 **Lipid storage disorder, unspecified** Rx

√4th **E76 Disorders of glycosaminoglycan metabolism**

√5th E76.0 **Mucopolysaccharidosis, type I**

E76.01 **Hurler's syndrome** HCC Rx ESR COM

E76.02 **Hurler-Scheie syndrome** HCC Rx ESR COM

E76.03 **Scheie's syndrome** HCC Rx ESR COM

E76.1 **Mucopolysaccharidosis, type II** HCC Rx ESR COM
Hunter's syndrome

√5th E76.2 **Other mucopolysaccharidoses**

√6th E76.21 **Morquio mucopolysaccharidoses**

E76.210 **Morquio A mucopolysaccharidoses** HCC Rx ESR COM
Classic Morquio syndrome
Morquio syndrome A
Mucopolysaccharidosis, type IVA

E76.211 **Morquio B mucopolysaccharidoses** HCC Rx ESR COM
Morquio-like mucopolysaccharidoses
Morquio-like syndrome
Morquio syndrome B
Mucopolysaccharidosis, type IVB

E76.219 **Morquio mucopolysaccharidoses, unspecified** HCC Rx ESR COM
Morquio syndrome
Mucopolysaccharidosis, type IV

E76.22 **Sanfilippo mucopolysaccharidoses** HCC Rx ESR COM
Mucopolysaccharidosis, type III (A) (B) (C) (D)
Sanfilippo A syndrome
Sanfilippo B syndrome
Sanfilippo C syndrome
Sanfilippo D syndrome

E76.29 **Other mucopolysaccharidoses** HCC Rx ESR COM
beta-Glucuronidase deficiency
Maroteaux-Lamy (mild) (severe) syndrome
Mucopolysaccharidosis, types VI, VII

E76.3 **Mucopolysaccharidosis, unspecified** HCC Rx ESR COM

E76.8 **Other disorders of glucosaminoglycan metabolism** HCC Rx ESR COM

E76.9 **Glucosaminoglycan metabolism disorder, unspecified** HCC Rx ESR COM

√4th **E77 Disorders of glycoprotein metabolism**

E77.0 **Defects in post-translational modification of lysosomal enzymes** HCC Rx ESR COM
Mucolipidosis II [I-cell disease]
Mucolipidosis III [pseudo-Hurler polydystrophy]

E77.1 **Defects in glycoprotein degradation** HCC Rx ESR COM
Aspartylglucosaminuria
Fucosidosis
Mannosidosis
Sialidosis [mucolipidosis I]

E77.8 **Other disorders of glycoprotein metabolism** HCC Rx ESR COM

E77.9 **Disorder of glycoprotein metabolism, unspecified** HCC Rx ESR COM

√4th **E78 Disorders of lipoprotein metabolism and other lipidemias**
EXCLUDES 1 *sphingolipidosis (E75.0-E75.3)*

√5th E78.0 **Pure hypercholesterolemia**
AHA: 2016,4Q,13-14

E78.00 **Pure hypercholesterolemia, unspecified** Rx
Fredrickson's hyperlipoproteinemia, type IIa
Hyperbetalipoproteinemia
Low-density-lipoprotein-type [LDL] hyperlipoproteinemia
(Pure) hypercholesterolemia NOS
AHA: 2022,2Q,5-6

E78.01 **Familial hypercholesterolemia** Rx

E78.1 **Pure hyperglyceridemia** Rx
Elevated fasting triglycerides
Endogenous hyperglyceridemia
Fredrickson's hyperlipoproteinemia, type IV
Hyperlipidemia, group B
Hyperprebetalipoproteinemia
Very-low-density-lipoprotein-type [VLDL] hyperlipoproteinemia

E78.2 **Mixed hyperlipidemia** Rx
Broad- or floating-betalipoproteinemia
Combined hyperlipidemia NOS
Elevated cholesterol with elevated triglycerides NEC
Fredrickson's hyperlipoproteinemia, type IIb or III
Hyperbetalipoproteinemia with prebetalipoproteinemia
Hypercholesteremia with endogenous hyperglyceridemia
Hyperlipidemia, group C
Tubo-eruptive xanthoma
Xanthoma tuberosum
EXCLUDES 1 *cerebrotendinous cholesterosis [van Bogaert-Scherer-Epstein] (E75.5)*
familial combined hyperlipidemia (E78.49)
AHA: 2022,2Q,6

E78.3 **Hyperchylomicronemia** Rx
Chylomicron retention disease
Fredrickson's hyperlipoproteinemia, type I or V
Hyperlipidemia, group D
Mixed hyperglyceridemia

√5th E78.4 **Other hyperlipidemia**
AHA: 2018,4Q,6

E78.41 **Elevated Lipoprotein(a)** Rx
Elevated Lp(a)

E78.49 **Other hyperlipidemia** Rx
Familial combined hyperlipidemia

E78.5 **Hyperlipidemia, unspecified** Rx
AHA: 2022,2Q,5

E78.6 **Lipoprotein deficiency** Rx
Abetalipoproteinemia
Depressed HDL cholesterol
High-density lipoprotein deficiency
Hypoalphalipoproteinemia
Hypobetalipoproteinemia (familial)
Lecithin cholesterol acyltransferase deficiency
Tangier disease

√5th E78.7 **Disorders of bile acid and cholesterol metabolism**
EXCLUDES 1 *Niemann-Pick disease type C (E75.242)*

E78.70 **Disorder of bile acid and cholesterol metabolism, unspecified** Rx

E78.71 **Barth syndrome** COM

E78.72 **Smith-Lemli-Opitz syndrome** COM

Chapter 4. Endocrine, Nutritional and Metabolic Diseases

E75.242–E78.72

E78.79 Other disorders of bile acid and cholesterol metabolism Rx

✓5th **E78.8 Other disorders of lipoprotein metabolism**

E78.81 Lipoid dermatoarthritis Rx

E78.89 Other lipoprotein metabolism disorders Rx

E78.9 Disorder of lipoprotein metabolism, unspecified Rx

✓4th **E79 Disorders of purine and pyrimidine metabolism**

EXCLUDES 1 *Ataxia-telangiectasia (Q87.19)*
Bloom's syndrome (Q82.8)
Cockayne's syndrome (Q87.19)
calculus of kidney (N2Ø.Ø)
combined immunodeficiency disorders (D81.-)
Fanconi's anemia (D61.Ø9)
gout (M1A.-, M1Ø.-)
orotaciduric anemia (D53.Ø)
progeria (E34.8)
Werner's syndrome (E34.8)
xeroderma pigmentosum (Q82.1)

E79.Ø Hyperuricemia without signs of inflammatory arthritis and tophaceous disease
Asymptomatic hyperuricemia

E79.1 Lesch-Nyhan syndrome HCC Rx ESR COM
HGPRT deficiency

E79.2 Myoadenylate deaminase deficiency HCC Rx ESR COM

E79.8 Other disorders of purine and pyrimidine metabolism HCC Rx ESR COM
Hereditary xanthinuria

E79.9 Disorder of purine and pyrimidine metabolism, unspecified HCC Rx ESR COM

✓4th **E8Ø Disorders of porphyrin and bilirubin metabolism**

INCLUDES defects of catalase and peroxidase

E8Ø.Ø Hereditary erythropoietic porphyria HCC Rx ESR COM
Congenital erythropoietic porphyria
Erythropoietic protoporphyria

E8Ø.1 Porphyria cutanea tarda HCC Rx ESR COM

✓5th **E8Ø.2 Other and unspecified porphyria**

E8Ø.2Ø Unspecified porphyria HCC Rx ESR COM
Porphyria NOS

E8Ø.21 Acute intermittent (hepatic) porphyria HCC Rx ESR COM

E8Ø.29 Other porphyria HCC Rx ESR COM
Hereditary coproporphyria

E8Ø.3 Defects of catalase and peroxidase HCC Rx ESR COM
Acatalasia [Takahara]

E8Ø.4 Gilbert syndrome

E8Ø.5 Crigler-Najjar syndrome

E8Ø.6 Other disorders of bilirubin metabolism
Dubin-Johnson syndrome
Rotor's syndrome

E8Ø.7 Disorder of bilirubin metabolism, unspecified

✓4th **E83 Disorders of mineral metabolism**

EXCLUDES 1 *dietary mineral deficiency (E58-E61)*
parathyroid disorders (E2Ø-E21)
vitamin D deficiency (E55.-)

✓5th **E83.Ø Disorders of copper metabolism**

E83.ØØ Disorder of copper metabolism, unspecified Rx COM

E83.Ø1 Wilson's disease Rx COM
Code also associated Kayser Fleischer ring (H18.Ø4-)

E83.Ø9 Other disorders of copper metabolism Rx COM
Menkes' (kinky hair) (steely hair) disease

✓5th **E83.1 Disorders of iron metabolism**

EXCLUDES 1 *iron deficiency anemia (D5Ø.-)*
sideroblastic anemia (D64.Ø-D64.3)

E83.1Ø Disorder of iron metabolism, unspecified Rx

✓6th **E83.11 Hemochromatosis**

EXCLUDES 1 *GALD (P78.84)*
gestational alloimmune liver disease (P78.84)
neonatal hemochromatosis (P78.84)

E83.11Ø Hereditary hemochromatosis HCC Rx ESR
Bronzed diabetes
Pigmentary cirrhosis (of liver)
Primary (hereditary) hemochromatosis

E83.111 Hemochromatosis due to repeated red blood cell transfusions
Iron overload due to repeated red blood cell transfusions
Transfusion (red blood cell) associated hemochromatosis

E83.118 Other hemochromatosis Rx

E83.119 Hemochromatosis, unspecified Rx

E83.19 Other disorders of iron metabolism Rx
Use additional code, if applicable, for idiopathic pulmonary hemosiderosis (J84.Ø3)

E83.2 Disorders of zinc metabolism
Acrodermatitis enteropathica

✓5th **E83.3 Disorders of phosphorus metabolism and phosphatases**

EXCLUDES 1 *adult osteomalacia (M83.-)*
osteoporosis (M8Ø.-)

E83.3Ø Disorder of phosphorus metabolism, unspecified Rx

E83.31 Familial hypophosphatemia Rx
Vitamin D-resistant osteomalacia
Vitamin D-resistant rickets
EXCLUDES 1 *vitamin D-deficiency rickets (E55.Ø)*

E83.32 Hereditary vitamin D-dependent rickets (type 1) (type 2) Rx
25-hydroxyvitamin D 1-alpha-hydroxylase deficiency
Pseudovitamin D deficiency
Vitamin D receptor defect

E83.39 Other disorders of phosphorus metabolism Rx
Acid phosphatase deficiency
Hypophosphatasia

✓5th **E83.4 Disorders of magnesium metabolism**

E83.4Ø Disorders of magnesium metabolism, unspecified

E83.41 Hypermagnesemia
AHA: 2016,4Q,54

E83.42 Hypomagnesemia

E83.49 Other disorders of magnesium metabolism

✓5th **E83.5 Disorders of calcium metabolism**

EXCLUDES 1 *chondrocalcinosis (M11.1-M11.2)*
hungry bone syndrome (E83.81)
hyperparathyroidism (E21.Ø-E21.3)

E83.5Ø Unspecified disorder of calcium metabolism

E83.51 Hypocalcemia

E83.52 Hypercalcemia
Familial hypocalciuric hypercalcemia

E83.59 Other disorders of calcium metabolism

✓5th **E83.8 Other disorders of mineral metabolism**

E83.81 Hungry bone syndrome

E83.89 Other disorders of mineral metabolism

E83.9 Disorder of mineral metabolism, unspecified

✓4th **E84 Cystic fibrosis**

INCLUDES mucoviscidosis

Code also exocrine pancreatic insufficiency (K86.81)

DEF: Genetic disorder affecting the respiratory, digestive, and reproductive systems in infants to young adults by disturbing exocrine gland function and causing chronic pulmonary disease with excess mucus production and pancreatic deficiency.

E84.Ø Cystic fibrosis with pulmonary manifestations HCC Rx ESR COM
Use additional code to identify any infectious organism present, such as:
Pseudomonas (B96.5)
AHA: 2021,1Q,23

✓5th **E84.1 Cystic fibrosis with intestinal manifestations**

E84.11 Meconium ileus in cystic fibrosis HCC Rx ESR COM N

EXCLUDES 1 *meconium ileus not due to cystic fibrosis (P76.Ø)*

E84.19 Cystic fibrosis with other intestinal manifestations HCC Rx ESR COM

Distal intestinal obstruction syndrome

E84.8 Cystic fibrosis with other manifestations HCC Rx ESR COM

E84.9 Cystic fibrosis, unspecified HCC Rx ESR COM

✓4th **E85 Amyloidosis**

EXCLUDES 2 *Alzheimer's disease (G3Ø.Ø-)*

DEF: Conditions of diverse etiologies characterized by the accumulation of insoluble fibrillar proteins (amyloid) in various organs and tissues of the body, compromising vital functions.

E85.Ø Non-neuropathic heredofamilial amyloidosis HCC ESR COM

Hereditary amyloid nephropathy

Code also associated disorders, such as:

autoinflammatory syndromes (MØ4.-)

EXCLUDES 2 *transthyretin-related (ATTR) familial amyloid cardiomyopathy (E85.4)*

E85.1 Neuropathic heredofamilial amyloidosis HCC ESR COM

Amyloid polyneuropathy (Portuguese)

Transthyretin-related (ATTR) familial amyloid polyneuropathy

AHA: 2012,4Q,99

E85.2 Heredofamilial amyloidosis, unspecified HCC ESR COM

E85.3 Secondary systemic amyloidosis HCC ESR COM

Hemodialysis-associated amyloidosis

E85.4 Organ-limited amyloidosis HCC ESR COM

Localized amyloidosis

Transthyretin-related (ATTR) familial amyloid cardiomyopathy

✓5th **E85.8 Other amyloidosis**

AHA: 2017,4Q,7

E85.81 Light chain (AL) amyloidosis HCC ESR COM

E85.82 Wild-type transthyretin-related (ATTR) amyloidosis HCC ESR COM

Senile systemic amyloidosis (SSA)

E85.89 Other amyloidosis HCC ESR COM

E85.9 Amyloidosis, unspecified HCC ESR COM

✓4th **E86 Volume depletion**

Use additional code(s) for any associated disorders of electrolyte and acid-base balance (E87.-)

EXCLUDES 1 *dehydration of newborn (P74.1)*
postprocedural hypovolemic shock (T81.19)
traumatic hypovolemic shock (T79.4)

EXCLUDES 2 *hypovolemic shock NOS (R57.1)*

AHA: 2019,2Q,7; 2018,2Q,6

E86.Ø Dehydration

AHA: 2019,2Q,7; 2019,1Q,12; 2014,1Q,7

TIP: Can be assigned in addition to hypernatremia (E87.0) or hyponatremia (E87.1), when documented.

E86.1 Hypovolemia

Depletion of volume of plasma

E86.9 Volume depletion, unspecified

DEF: Depletion of total body water (dehydration) and/or contraction of total intravascular plasma (hypovolemia).

✓4th **E87 Other disorders of fluid, electrolyte and acid-base balance**

EXCLUDES 1 *diabetes insipidus (E23.2)*
electrolyte imbalance associated with hyperemesis gravidarum (O21.1)
electrolyte imbalance following ectopic or molar pregnancy (OØ8.5)
familial periodic paralysis (G72.3)

AHA: 2018,2Q,6

E87.Ø Hyperosmolality and hypernatremia

Sodium [Na] excess

Sodium [Na] overload

AHA: 2022,1Q,28; 2014,1Q,7

TIP: Assign an additional code for dehydration (E86.0), when documented.

E87.1 Hypo-osmolality and hyponatremia

Sodium [Na] deficiency

EXCLUDES 1 *syndrome of inappropriate secretion of antidiuretic hormone (E22.2)*

AHA: 2014,1Q,7

TIP: Assign an additional code for dehydration (E86.0), when documented.

▲ ✓5th **E87.2 Acidosis**

~~Acidosis NOS~~

~~Lactic acidosis~~

~~Metabolic acidosis~~

~~Respiratory acidosis~~

EXCLUDES 1 *diabetic acidosis - see categories EØ8-E1Ø, E11, E13 with ketoacidosis*

AHA: 2020,3Q,30

DEF: Reduction of alkaline in the blood and tissues caused by an increase in acid and decrease in bicarbonate.

● **E87.2Ø Acidosis, unspecified**

Lactic acidosis NOS

Metabolic acidosis NOS

Code also, if applicable, respiratory failure with hypercapnia (J96. with 5th character 2)

● **E87.21 Acute metabolic acidosis**

Acute lactic acidosis

● **E87.22 Chronic metabolic acidosis**

Chronic lactic acidosis

Code first underlying etiology, if applicable

● **E87.29 Other acidosis**

Respiratory acidosis NOS

EXCLUDES 2 *acute respiratory acidosis (J96.Ø2)*
chronic respiratory acidosis (J96.12)

E87.3 Alkalosis

Alkalosis NOS

Metabolic alkalosis

Respiratory alkalosis

E87.4 Mixed disorder of acid-base balance

E87.5 Hyperkalemia

Potassium [K] excess

Potassium [K] overload

E87.6 Hypokalemia

Potassium [K] deficiency

✓5th **E87.7 Fluid overload**

EXCLUDES 1 *edema NOS (R6Ø.9)*
fluid retention (R6Ø.9)

E87.7Ø Fluid overload, unspecified

E87.71 Transfusion associated circulatory overload

Fluid overload due to transfusion (blood) (blood components)

TACO

E87.79 Other fluid overload

E87.8 Other disorders of electrolyte and fluid balance, not elsewhere classified

Electrolyte imbalance NOS

Hyperchloremia

Hypochloremia

✓4th **E88 Other and unspecified metabolic disorders**

Use additional codes for associated conditions

EXCLUDES 1 *histiocytosis X (chronic) (C96.6)*

✓5th **E88.Ø Disorders of plasma-protein metabolism, not elsewhere classified**

EXCLUDES 1 *monoclonal gammopathy (of undetermined significance) (D47.2)*
polyclonal hypergammaglobulinemia (D89.Ø)
Waldenström macroglobulinemia (C88.Ø)

EXCLUDES 2 *disorder of lipoprotein metabolism (E78.-)*

E88.Ø1 Alpha-1-antitrypsin deficiency HCC Rx ESR COM

AAT deficiency

E88.02 Plasminogen deficiency
Dysplasminogenemia
Hypoplasminogenemia
Type 1 plasminogen deficiency
Type 2 plasminogen deficiency
Code also, if applicable, ligneous conjunctivitis (H10.51)
Use additional code for associated findings, such as:
hydrocephalus (G91.4)
otitis media (H67.-)
respiratory disorder related to plasminogen deficiency (J99)
AHA: 2018,4Q,6-7

E88.09 Other disorders of plasma-protein metabolism, not elsewhere classified
Bisalbuminemia

E88.1 Lipodystrophy, not elsewhere classified
Lipodystrophy NOS
EXCLUDES 1 *Whipple's disease (K90.81)*

E88.2 Lipomatosis, not elsewhere classified Rx
Lipomatosis NOS
Lipomatosis (Check) dolorosa [Dercum]

E88.3 Tumor lysis syndrome COM
Tumor lysis syndrome (spontaneous)
Tumor lysis syndrome following antineoplastic drug chemotherapy
Use additional code for adverse effect, if applicable, to identify drug (T45.1X5)
AHA: 2020,1Q,37; 2019,2Q,24
DEF: Potentially fatal metabolic complication of tumor necrosis caused by spontaneous or treatment-related accumulation of byproducts from dying cancer cells. Symptoms include hyperkalemia, hyperphosphatemia, hypocalcemia, hyperuricemia, and hyperuricosuria.

✓5th **E88.4 Mitochondrial metabolism disorders**
EXCLUDES 1 *disorders of pyruvate metabolism (E74.4)*
Kearns-Sayre syndrome (H49.81)
Leber's disease (H47.22)
Leigh's encephalopathy (G31.82)
mitochondrial myopathy, NEC (G71.3)
Reye's syndrome (G93.7)

E88.40 Mitochondrial metabolism disorder, unspecified HCC Rx ESR COM

E88.41 MELAS syndrome HCC Rx ESR COM
Mitochondrial myopathy, encephalopathy, lactic acidosis and stroke-like episodes

E88.42 MERRF syndrome HCC Rx ESR COM
Myoclonic epilepsy associated with ragged-red fibers
Code also progressive myoclonic epilepsy (G40.3-)

E88.49 Other mitochondrial metabolism disorders HCC Rx ESR COM

✓5th **E88.8 Other specified metabolic disorders**

E88.81 Metabolic syndrome
Dysmetabolic syndrome X
Use additional codes for associated manifestations, such as:
obesity (E66.-)
DEF: Group of health risks that increase the likelihood of developing heart disease, stroke, and diabetes. These risks include certain parameters for blood pressure, cholesterol, and glucose levels.

E88.89 Other specified metabolic disorders HCC Rx ESR COM
Launois-Bensaude adenolipomatosis
EXCLUDES 1 *adult pulmonary Langerhans cell histiocytosis (J84.82)*

E88.9 Metabolic disorder, unspecified

Postprocedural endocrine and metabolic complications and disorders, not elsewhere classified (E89)

✓4th **E89 Postprocedural endocrine and metabolic complications and disorders, not elsewhere classified**
EXCLUDES 2 *intraoperative complications of endocrine system organ or structure (E36.0-, E36.1-, E36.8)*

E89.0 Postprocedural hypothyroidism Rx
Postirradiation hypothyroidism
Postsurgical hypothyroidism

E89.1 Postprocedural hypoinsulinemia
Postpancreatectomy hyperglycemia
Postsurgical hypoinsulinemia
Use additional code, if applicable, to identify:
acquired absence of pancreas (Z90.41-)
diabetes mellitus (postpancreatectomy) (postprocedural) (E13.-)
insulin use (Z79.4)
EXCLUDES 1 *transient postprocedural hyperglycemia (R73.9)*
transient postprocedural hypoglycemia (E16.2)

E89.2 Postprocedural hypoparathyroidism HCC Rx ESR COM
Parathyroprival tetany

E89.3 Postprocedural hypopituitarism HCC Rx ESR COM
Postirradiation hypopituitarism

✓5th **E89.4 Postprocedural ovarian failure**

E89.40 Asymptomatic postprocedural ovarian failure ♀
Postprocedural ovarian failure NOS

E89.41 Symptomatic postprocedural ovarian failure ♀
Symptoms such as flushing, sleeplessness, headache, lack of concentration, associated with postprocedural menopause

E89.5 Postprocedural testicular hypofunction ♂

E89.6 Postprocedural adrenocortical (-medullary) hypofunction HCC Rx ESR COM

✓5th **E89.8 Other postprocedural endocrine and metabolic complications and disorders**
AHA: 2016,4Q,9-10

✓6th **E89.81 Postprocedural hemorrhage of an endocrine system organ or structure following a procedure**

E89.810 Postprocedural hemorrhage of an endocrine system organ or structure following an endocrine system procedure

E89.811 Postprocedural hemorrhage of an endocrine system organ or structure following other procedure

✓6th **E89.82 Postprocedural hematoma and seroma of an endocrine system organ or structure**

E89.820 Postprocedural hematoma of an endocrine system organ or structure following an endocrine system procedure

E89.821 Postprocedural hematoma of an endocrine system organ or structure following other procedure

E89.822 Postprocedural seroma of an endocrine system organ or structure following an endocrine system procedure

E89.823 Postprocedural seroma of an endocrine system organ or structure following other procedure

E89.89 Other postprocedural endocrine and metabolic complications and disorders
Use additional code, if applicable, to further specify disorder

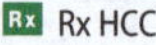

Chapter 5. Mental, Behavioral and Neurodevelopmental Disorders (FØ1–F99)

Chapter-specific Guidelines with Coding Examples

The chapter-specific guidelines from the ICD-10-CM Official Guidelines for Coding and Reporting have been provided below. Along with these guidelines are coding examples, contained in the shaded boxes, that have been developed to help illustrate the coding and/or sequencing guidance found in these guidelines.

a. Pain disorders related to psychological factors

Assign code F45.41, for pain that is exclusively related to psychological disorders. As indicated by the Excludes 1 note under category G89, a code from category G89 should not be assigned with code F45.41.

> Chest pain determined to be persistent somatoform pain disorder
>
> **F45.41 Pain disorder exclusively related to psychological factors**
>
> *Explanation*: This pain was diagnosed as being exclusively psychological; therefore, no code from category G89 is added.

Code F45.42, Pain disorders with related psychological factors, should be used with a code from category G89, Pain, not elsewhere classified, if there is documentation of a psychological component for a patient with acute or chronic pain.

See Section I.C.6. Pain

b. Mental and behavioral disorders due to psychoactive substance use

1) In remission

Selection of codes **describing** "in remission" for categories F1Ø-F19, Mental and behavioral disorders due to psychoactive substance use (categories F1Ø-F19 with -.11, -.21, **-.91**) requires the provider's clinical judgment **and** are assigned only on the basis of provider documentation (as defined in the Official Guidelines for Coding and Reporting), unless otherwise instructed by the classification.

Mild substance use disorders in early or sustained remission are classified to the appropriate codes for substance abuse in remission, and moderate or severe substance use disorders in early or sustained remission are classified to the appropriate codes for substance dependence in remission.

> Physician documentation indicates the patient is seen to monitor progress on quitting cigarette smoking. The problem list indicates mild tobacco use disorder that is currently in remission.
>
> **F17.211 Nicotine dependence, cigarettes, in remission**
>
> *Explanation*: According to the index, Disorder, tobacco use, cigarettes (mild) (moderate) (severe), in remission (early) (sustained) is categorized to dependence (F17.211). Since the physician clearly documents mild cigarette use "disorder" and that the disorder is in remission, a code for nicotine dependence "in remission" is appropriate.

2) Psychoactive substance use, abuse and dependence

When the provider documentation refers to use, abuse and dependence of the same substance (e.g. alcohol, opioid, cannabis, etc.), only one code should be assigned to identify the pattern of use based on the following hierarchy:

- If both use and abuse are documented, assign only the code for abuse
- If both abuse and dependence are documented, assign only the code for dependence
- If use, abuse and dependence are all documented, assign only the code for dependence
- If both use and dependence are documented, assign only the code for dependence.

> History and physical notes cannabis dependence and ongoing cannabis abuse
>
> **F12.2Ø Cannabis dependence, uncomplicated**
>
> *Explanation*: In the hierarchy, the dependence code is used if both abuse and dependence are documented.

> Current problem list indicates daily opioid use with opioid abuse.
>
> **F11.1Ø Opioid abuse, uncomplicated**
>
> *Explanation*: In the hierarchy, the abuse code is used if both abuse and use are documented.

3) Psychoactive substance use, unspecified

As with all other unspecified diagnoses, the codes for unspecified psychoactive substance use (F1Ø.9-, F11.9-, F12.9-, F13.9-, F14.9-, F15.9-, F16.9-, F18.9-, F19.9-) should only be assigned based on provider documentation and when they meet the definition of a reportable diagnosis (see Section III, Reporting Additional Diagnoses). These codes are to be used only when the psychoactive substance use is associated with a substance related disorder (chapter 5 disorders such as sexual dysfunction, sleep disorder, or a mental or behavioral disorder) or medical condition, and such a relationship is documented by the provider.

4) Medical conditions due to psychoactive substance use, abuse and dependence

Medical conditions due to substance use, abuse, and dependence are not classified as substance-induced disorders. Assign the diagnosis code for the medical condition as directed by the Alphabetical Index along with the appropriate psychoactive substance use, abuse or dependence code. For example, for alcoholic pancreatitis due to alcohol dependence, assign the appropriate code from subcategory K85.2, Alcohol induced acute pancreatitis, and the appropriate code from subcategory F1Ø.2, such as code F1Ø.2Ø, Alcohol dependence, uncomplicated. It would not be appropriate to assign code F1Ø.288, Alcohol dependence with other alcohol-induced disorder.

5) Blood alcohol level

A code from category Y9Ø, Evidence of alcohol involvement determined by blood alcohol level, may be assigned when this information is documented and the patient's provider has documented a condition classifiable to category F1Ø, Alcohol related disorders. The blood alcohol level does not need to be documented by the patient's provider in order for it to be coded.

See Section I.B.14. for blood alcohol level documentation by clinicians other than patient's provider.

c. Factitious disorder

Factitious disorder imposed on self or Munchausen's syndrome is a disorder in which a person falsely reports or causes his or her own physical or psychological signs or symptoms. For patients with documented factitious disorder on self or Munchausen's syndrome, assign the appropriate code from subcategory F68.1-, Factitious disorder imposed on self.

Munchausen's syndrome by proxy (MSBP) is a disorder in which a caregiver (perpetrator) falsely reports or causes an illness or injury in another person (victim) under his or her care, such as a child, an elderly adult, or a person who has a disability. The condition is also referred to as "factitious disorder imposed on another" or "factitious disorder by proxy." The perpetrator, not the victim, receives this diagnosis. Assign code F68.A, Factitious disorder imposed on another, to the perpetrator's record. For the victim of a patient suffering from MSBP, assign the appropriate code from categories T74, Adult and child abuse, neglect and other maltreatment, confirmed, or T76, Adult and child abuse, neglect and other maltreatment, suspected.

See Section I.C.19.f. Adult and child abuse, neglect and other maltreatment

d. Dementia

The ICD-10-CM classifies dementia (categories FØ1, FØ2, and FØ3) on the basis of the etiology and severity (unspecified, mild, moderate or severe). Selection of the appropriate severity level requires the provider's clinical judgment and codes should be assigned only on the basis of provider documentation (as defined in the *Official Guidelines for Coding and Reporting*), unless otherwise instructed by the classification. If the documentation does not provide information about the severity of the dementia, assign the appropriate code for unspecified severity.

If a patient is admitted to an inpatient acute care hospital or other inpatient facility setting with dementia at one severity level and it progresses to a higher severity level, assign one code for the highest severity level reported during the stay.

Chapter 5. Mental, Behavioral and Neurodevelopmental Disorders (FØ1-F99)

INCLUDES disorders of psychological development

EXCLUDES 2 *symptoms, signs and abnormal clinical laboratory findings, not elsewhere classified (RØØ-R99)*

This chapter contains the following blocks:

FØ1-FØ9 Mental disorders due to known physiological conditions
F1Ø-F19 Mental and behavioral disorders due to psychoactive substance use
F2Ø-F29 Schizophrenia, schizotypal, delusional, and other non-mood psychotic disorders
F3Ø-F39 Mood [affective] disorders
F4Ø-F48 Anxiety, dissociative, stress-related, somatoform and other nonpsychotic mental disorders
F5Ø-F59 Behavioral syndromes associated with physiological disturbances and physical factors
F6Ø-F69 Disorders of adult personality and behavior
F7Ø-F79 Intellectual disabilities
F8Ø-F89 Pervasive and specific developmental disorders
F9Ø-F98 Behavioral and emotional disorders with onset usually occurring in childhood and adolescence
F99 Unspecified mental disorder

Mental disorders due to known physiological conditions (FØ1-FØ9)

NOTE This block comprises a range of mental disorders grouped together on the basis of their having in common a demonstrable etiology in cerebral disease, brain injury, or other insult leading to cerebral dysfunction. The dysfunction may be primary, as in diseases, injuries, and insults that affect the brain directly and selectively; or secondary, as in systemic diseases and disorders that attack the brain only as one of the multiple organs or systems of the body that are involved.

✓4th FØ1 Vascular dementia

Vascular dementia as a result of infarction of the brain due to vascular disease, including hypertensive cerebrovascular disease.

INCLUDES arteriosclerotic dementia
▶major neurocognitive disorder due to vascular disease◀
▶multi-infarct dementia◀

Code first the underlying physiological condition or sequelae of cerebrovascular disease.

▲ **✓5th FØ1.5 Vascular dementia, unspecified severity**

▲ **FØ1.5Ø Vascular dementia, unspecified severity, without behavioral disturbance, psychotic disturbance, mood disturbance, and anxiety** HCC Rx ESR A
▶Major neurocognitive disorder due to vascular disease NOS◀
▶Vascular dementia NOS◀
AHA: 2021,2Q,4

▲ **✓6th FØ1.51 Vascular dementia, unspecified severity, with behavioral disturbance**
~~Major neurocognitive disorder due to vascular disease, with behavioral disturbance~~
~~Major neurocognitive disorder with aggressive behavior~~
~~Major neurocognitive disorder with combative behavior~~
~~Major neurocognitive disorder with violent behavior~~
~~Vascular dementia with aggressive behavior~~
~~Vascular dementia with combative behavior~~
~~Vascular dementia with violent behavior~~
~~Use additional code, if applicable, to identify wandering in vascular dementia (Z91.83)~~

● **FØ1.511 Vascular dementia, unspecified severity, with agitation**
Major neurocognitive disorder due to vascular disease, unspecified severity, with aberrant motor behavior such as restlessness, rocking, pacing, or exit-seeking
Major neurocognitive disorder due to vascular disease, unspecified severity, with verbal or physical behaviors such as profanity, shouting, threatening, anger, aggression, combativeness, or violence
Vascular dementia, unspecified severity, with aberrant motor behavior such as restlessness, rocking, pacing, or exit-seeking
Vascular dementia, unspecified severity, with verbal or physical behaviors such as profanity, shouting, threatening, anger, aggression, combativeness, or violence

● **FØ1.518 Vascular dementia, unspecified severity, with other behavioral disturbance**
Major neurocognitive disorder due to vascular disease, unspecified severity, with behavioral disturbances such as sleep disturbance, social disinhibition, or sexual disinhibition
Vascular dementia, unspecified severity, with behavioral disturbances such as sleep disturbance, social disinhibition, or sexual disinhibition
Use additional code, if applicable, to identify wandering in vascular dementia (Z91.83)

● **FØ1.52 Vascular dementia, unspecified severity, with psychotic disturbance**
Major neurocognitive disorder due to vascular disease, unspecified severity, with psychotic disturbance such as hallucinations, paranoia, suspiciousness, or delusional state
Vascular dementia, unspecified severity, with psychotic disturbance such as hallucinations, paranoia, suspiciousness, or delusional state

● **FØ1.53 Vascular dementia, unspecified severity, with mood disturbance**
Major neurocognitive disorder due to vascular disease, unspecified severity, with mood disturbance such as depression, apathy, or anhedonia
Vascular dementia, unspecified severity, with mood disturbance such as depression, apathy, or anhedonia

● **FØ1.54 Vascular dementia, unspecified severity, with anxiety**
Major neurocognitive disorder due to vascular disease, unspecified severity, with anxiety

● ✓5th **F01.A Vascular dementia, mild**

EXCLUDES 1 *mild neurocognitive disorder due to known physiological condition with or without behavioral disturbance (F06.7-)*

● **F01.A0 Vascular dementia, mild, without behavioral disturbance, psychotic disturbance, mood disturbance, and anxiety**

Major neurocognitive disorder due to vascular disease, mild, NOS

Vascular dementia, mild, NOS

● ✓6th **F01.A1 Vascular dementia, mild, with behavioral disturbance**

● **F01.A11 Vascular dementia, mild, with agitation**

Major neurocognitive disorder due to vascular disease, mild, with aberrant motor behavior such as restlessness, rocking, pacing, or exit-seeking

Major neurocognitive disorder due to vascular disease, mild, with verbal or physical behaviors such as profanity, shouting, threatening, anger, aggression, combativeness, or violence

Vascular dementia, mild, with aberrant motor behavior such as restlessness, rocking, pacing, or exit-seeking

Vascular dementia, mild, with verbal or physical behaviors such as profanity, shouting, threatening, anger, aggression, combativeness, or violence

● **F01.A18 Vascular dementia, mild, with other behavioral disturbance**

Major neurocognitive disorder due to vascular disease, mild, with behavioral disturbances such as sleep disturbance, social disinhibition, or sexual disinhibition

Vascular dementia, mild, with behavioral disturbances such as sleep disturbance, social disinhibition, or sexual disinhibition

Use additional code, if applicable, to identify wandering in vascular dementia (Z91.83)

● **F01.A2 Vascular dementia, mild, with psychotic disturbance**

Major neurocognitive disorder due to vascular disease, mild, with psychotic disturbance such as hallucinations, paranoia, suspiciousness, or delusional state

Vascular dementia, mild, with psychotic disturbance such as hallucinations, paranoia, suspiciousness, or delusional state

● **F01.A3 Vascular dementia, mild, with mood disturbance**

Major neurocognitive disorder due to vascular disease, mild, with mood disturbance such as depression, apathy, or anhedonia

Vascular dementia, mild, with mood disturbance such as depression, apathy, or anhedonia

● **F01.A4 Vascular dementia, mild, with anxiety**

Major neurocognitive disorder due to vascular disease, mild, with anxiety

● ✓5th **F01.B Vascular dementia, moderate**

● **F01.B0 Vascular dementia, moderate, without behavioral disturbance, psychotic disturbance, mood disturbance, and anxiety**

Major neurocognitive disorder due to vascular disease, moderate, NOS

Vascular dementia, moderate, NOS

● ✓6th **F01.B1 Vascular dementia, moderate, with behavioral disturbance**

● **F01.B11 Vascular dementia, moderate, with agitation**

Major neurocognitive disorder due to vascular disease, moderate, with aberrant motor behavior such as restlessness, rocking, pacing, or exit-seeking

Major neurocognitive disorder due to vascular disease, moderate, with verbal or physical behaviors such as profanity, shouting, threatening, anger, aggression, combativeness, or violence

Vascular dementia, moderate, with aberrant motor behavior such as restlessness, rocking, pacing, or exit-seeking

Vascular dementia, moderate, with verbal or physical behaviors such as profanity, shouting, threatening, anger, aggression, combativeness, or violence

● **F01.B18 Vascular dementia, moderate, with other behavioral disturbance**

Major neurocognitive disorder due to vascular disease, moderate, with behavioral disturbances such as sleep disturbance, social disinhibition, or sexual disinhibition

Vascular dementia, moderate, with behavioral disturbances such as sleep disturbance, social disinhibition, or sexual disinhibition

Use additional code, if applicable, to identify wandering in vascular dementia (Z91.83)

● **F01.B2 Vascular dementia, moderate, with psychotic disturbance**

Major neurocognitive disorder due to vascular disease, moderate, with psychotic disturbance such as hallucinations, paranoia, suspiciousness, or delusional state

Vascular dementia, moderate, with psychotic disturbance such as hallucinations, paranoia, suspiciousness, or delusional state

● **F01.B3 Vascular dementia, moderate, with mood disturbance**

Major neurocognitive disorder due to vascular disease, moderate, with mood disturbance such as depression, apathy, or anhedonia

Vascular dementia, moderate, with mood disturbance such as depression, apathy, or anhedonia

● **F01.B4 Vascular dementia, moderate, with anxiety**

Major neurocognitive disorder due to vascular disease, moderate, with anxiety

● ✓5th **F01.C Vascular dementia, severe**

● **F01.C0 Vascular dementia, severe, without behavioral disturbance, psychotic disturbance, mood disturbance, and anxiety**

Major neurocognitive disorder due to vascular disease, severe, NOS

Vascular dementia, severe, NOS

● ✓6th **FØ1.C1 Vascular dementia, severe, with behavioral disturbance**

● **FØ1.C11 Vascular dementia, severe, with agitation**

Major neurocognitive disorder due to vascular disease, severe, with aberrant motor behavior such as restlessness, rocking, pacing, or exit-seeking

Major neurocognitive disorder due to vascular disease, severe, with verbal or physical behaviors such as profanity, shouting, threatening, anger, aggression, combativeness, or violence

Vascular dementia, severe, with aberrant motor behavior such as restlessness, rocking, pacing, or exit-seeking

Vascular dementia, severe, with verbal or physical behaviors such as profanity, shouting, threatening, anger, aggression, combativeness, or violence

● **FØ1.C18 Vascular dementia, severe, with other behavioral disturbance**

Major neurocognitive disorder due to vascular disease, severe, with behavioral disturbances such as sleep disturbance, social disinhibition, or sexual disinhibition

Vascular dementia, severe, with behavioral disturbances such as sleep disturbance, social disinhibition, or sexual disinhibition

Use additional code, if applicable, to identify wandering in vascular dementia (Z91.83)

● **FØ1.C2 Vascular dementia, severe, with psychotic disturbance**

Major neurocognitive disorder due to vascular disease, severe, with psychotic disturbance such as hallucinations, paranoia, suspiciousness, or delusional state

Vascular dementia, severe, with psychotic disturbance such as hallucinations, paranoia, suspiciousness, or delusional state

● **FØ1.C3 Vascular dementia, severe, with mood disturbance**

Major neurocognitive disorder due to vascular disease, severe, with mood disturbance such as depression, apathy, or anhedonia

Vascular dementia, severe, with mood disturbance such as depression, apathy, or anhedonia

● **FØ1.C4 Vascular dementia, severe, with anxiety**

Major neurocognitive disorder due to vascular disease, severe, with anxiety

✓4th **FØ2 Dementia in other diseases classified elsewhere**

INCLUDES major neurocognitive disorder in other diseases classified elsewhere

Code first the underlying physiological condition, such as:
- Alzheimer's (G3Ø.-)
- cerebral lipidosis (E75.4)
- Creutzfeldt-Jakob disease (A81.Ø-)
- dementia with Lewy bodies (G31.83)
- dementia with Parkinsonism (G31.83)
- epilepsy and recurrent seizures (G4Ø.-)
- frontotemporal dementia (G31.Ø9)
- hepatolenticular degeneration (E83.Ø)
- human immunodeficiency virus [HIV] disease (B2Ø)
- Huntington's disease (G1Ø)
- hypercalcemia (E83.52)
- hypothyroidism, acquired (EØØ-EØ3.-)
- intoxications (T36-T65)
- Jakob-Creutzfeldt disease (A81.Ø-)
- multiple sclerosis (G35)
- neurosyphilis (A52.17)
- niacin deficiency [pellagra] (E52)
- Parkinson's disease (G2Ø)
- Pick's disease (G31.Ø1)
- polyarteritis nodosa (M3Ø.Ø)
- prion disease (A81.9)
- systemic lupus erythematosus (M32.-)
- traumatic brain injury (SØ6.-)
- trypanosomiasis (B56.-, B57.-)
- vitamin B deficiency (E53.8)

EXCLUDES 1 ▶*mild neurocognitive disorder due to known physiological condition with or without behavioral disturbance (FØ6.7-)*◀

EXCLUDES 2 *dementia in alcohol and psychoactive substance disorders (F1Ø-F19, with .17, .27, .97)*

vascular dementia ▶*(FØ1.5-, FØ1.A-, FØ1.B-, FØ1.C-)*◀

▲ ✓5th **FØ2.8 Dementia in other diseases classified elsewhere, unspecified severity**

AHA: 2022,1Q,25; 2017,2Q,7; 2016,4Q,141; 2016,2Q,6

TIP: A code from this subcategory should always be assigned with a code from category G30 when Alzheimer's disease is documented, even in the absence of documented dementia.

▲ ***FØ2.8Ø Dementia in other diseases classified elsewhere, unspecified severity, without behavioral disturbance, psychotic disturbance, mood disturbance, and anxiety*** HCC Rx ESR

Dementia in other diseases classified elsewhere NOS

▶Major neurocognitive disorder in other diseases classified elsewhere NOS◀

▲ ✓6th **FØ2.81 Dementia in other diseases classified elsewhere, unspecified severity, with behavioral disturbance**

~~Dementia in other diseases classified elsewhere with aggressive behavior~~

~~Dementia in other diseases classified elsewhere with combative behavior~~

~~Dementia in other diseases classified elsewhere with violent behavior~~

~~Major neurocognitive disorder in other diseases classified elsewhere with aggressive behavior~~

~~Major neurocognitive disorder in other diseases classified elsewhere with combative behavior~~

~~Major neurocognitive disorder in other diseases classified elsewhere with violent behavior~~

~~Use additional code, if applicable, to identify wandering in dementia in conditions classified elsewhere (Z91.83)~~

● **FØ2.811 Dementia in other diseases classified elsewhere, unspecified severity, with agitation**

Dementia in other diseases classified elsewhere, unspecified severity, with aberrant motor behavior such as restlessness, rocking, pacing, or exit-seeking

Dementia in other diseases classified elsewhere, unspecified severity, with verbal or physical behaviors such as profanity, shouting, threatening, anger, aggression, combativeness, or violence

Major neurocognitive disorder in other diseases classified elsewhere, unspecified severity, with aberrant motor behavior such as restlessness, rocking, pacing, or exit-seeking

Major neurocognitive disorder in other diseases classified elsewhere, unspecified severity, with verbal or physical behaviors such as profanity, shouting, threatening, anger, aggression, combativeness, or violence

● **FØ2.818 Dementia in other diseases classified elsewhere, unspecified severity, with other behavioral disturbance**

Dementia in other diseases classified elsewhere with sleep disturbance, social disinhibition, or sexual disinhibition

Major neurocognitive disorder in other diseases classified elsewhere with sleep disturbance, social disinhibition, or sexual disinhibition

Use additional code, if applicable, to identify wandering in dementia in conditions classified elsewhere (Z91.83)

● **FØ2.82 Dementia in other diseases classified elsewhere, unspecified severity, with psychotic disturbance**

Dementia in other diseases classified elsewhere, unspecified severity, with psychotic disturbance such as hallucinations, paranoia, suspiciousness, or delusional state

Major neurocognitive disorder in other diseases classified elsewhere, unspecified, with psychotic disturbance such as hallucinations, paranoia, suspiciousness, or delusional state

● **FØ2.83 Dementia in other diseases classified elsewhere, unspecified severity, with mood disturbance**

Dementia in other diseases classified elsewhere, unspecified severity, with mood disturbance such as depression, apathy, or anhedonia

Major neurocognitive disorder in other diseases classified elsewhere unspecified severity,with mood disturbance such as with depression, apathy, or anhedonia

● **FØ2.84 Dementia in other diseases classified elsewhere, unspecified severity, with anxiety**

Major neurocognitive disorder in other diseases classified elsewhere unspecified severity, with anxiety

● ✓5th **FØ2.A Dementia in other diseases classified elsewhere, mild**

EXCLUDES 1 *mild neurocognitive disorder due to known physiological condition with or without behavioral disturbance (FØ6.7-)*

● **FØ2.AØ Dementia in other diseases classified elsewhere, mild, without behavioral disturbance, psychotic disturbance, mood disturbance, and anxiety**

Dementia in other diseases classified elsewhere, mild, NOS

Major neurocognitive disorder in other diseases classified elsewhere, mild, NOS

● ✓6th **FØ2.A1 Dementia in other diseases classified elsewhere, mild, with behavioral disturbance**

● **FØ2.A11 Dementia in other diseases classified elsewhere, mild, with agitation**

Dementia in other diseases classified elsewhere, mild, with aberrant motor behavior such as restlessness, rocking, pacing, or exit-seeking

Dementia in other diseases classified elsewhere, mild, with verbal or physical behaviors such as profanity, shouting, threatening, anger, aggression, combativeness, or violence

Major neurocognitive disorder in other diseases classified elsewhere, mild, with aberrant motor behavior such as restlessness, rocking, pacing, or exit-seeking

Major neurocognitive disorder in other diseases classified elsewhere, mild, with verbal or physical behaviors such as profanity, shouting, threatening, anger, aggression, combativeness, or violence

● **FØ2.A18 Dementia in other diseases classified elsewhere, mild, with other behavioral disturbance**

Dementia in other diseases classified elsewhere, mild, with behavioral disturbances such as sleep disturbance, social disinhibition, or sexual disinhibition

Major neurocognitive disorder in other diseases classified elsewhere, mild, with behavioral disturbances such as sleep disturbance, social disinhibition, or sexual disinhibition

Use additional code, if applicable, to identify wandering in dementia in conditions classified elsewhere (Z91.83)

● **FØ2.A2 Dementia in other diseases classified elsewhere, mild, with psychotic disturbance**

Dementia in other diseases classified elsewhere, mild, with psychotic disturbance such as hallucinations, paranoia, suspiciousness, or delusional state

Major neurocognitive disorder in other diseases classified elsewhere, mild, with psychotic disturbance such as hallucinations, paranoia, suspiciousness, or delusional state

● **FØ2.A3 Dementia in other diseases classified elsewhere, mild, with mood disturbance**

Dementia in other diseases classified elsewhere, mild, with mood disturbance such as depression, apathy, or anhedonia

Major neurocognitive disorder in other diseases classified elsewhere, mild, with mood disturbance such as depression, apathy, or anhedonia

● **F02.A4 Dementia in other diseases classified elsewhere, mild, with anxiety**
Major neurocognitive disorder in other diseases classified elsewhere, mild, with anxiety

● 5th **F02.B Dementia in other diseases classified elsewhere, moderate**

● **F02.B0 Dementia in other diseases classified elsewhere, moderate, without behavioral disturbance, psychotic disturbance, mood disturbance, and anxiety**
Dementia in other diseases classified elsewhere, moderate, NOS
Major neurocognitive disorder in other diseases classified elsewhere, moderate, NOS

● 6th **F02.B1 Dementia in other diseases classified elsewhere, moderate, with behavioral disturbance**

● **F02.B11 Dementia in other diseases classified elsewhere, moderate, with agitation**
Dementia in other diseases classified elsewhere, moderate, with aberrant motor behavior such as restlessness, rocking, pacing, or exit-seeking
Dementia in other diseases classified elsewhere, moderate, with verbal or physical behaviors such as profanity, shouting, threatening, anger, aggression, combativeness, or violence
Major neurocognitive disorder in other diseases classified elsewhere, moderate, with aberrant motor behavior such as restlessness, rocking, pacing, or exit-seeking
Major neurocognitive disorder in other diseases classified elsewhere, moderate, with verbal or physical behaviors such as profanity, shouting, threatening, anger, aggression, combativeness, or violence

● **F02.B18 Dementia in other diseases classified elsewhere, moderate, with other behavioral disturbance**
Dementia in other diseases classified elsewhere, moderate, with behavioral disturbances such as sleep disturbance, social disinhibition, or sexual disinhibition
Major neurocognitive disorder in other diseases classified elsewhere, moderate, with behavioral disturbance such as sleep disturbance, social disinhibition, or sexual disinhibition
Use additional code, if applicable, to identify wandering in dementia in conditions classified elsewhere (Z91.83)

● **F02.B2 Dementia in other diseases classified elsewhere, moderate, with psychotic disturbance**
Dementia in other diseases classified elsewhere, moderate, with psychotic disturbance such as hallucinations, paranoia, suspiciousness, or delusional state
Major neurocognitive disorder in other diseases classified elsewhere, moderate, with psychotic disturbance such as hallucinations, paranoia, suspiciousness, or delusional state

● **F02.B3 Dementia in other diseases classified elsewhere, moderate, with mood disturbance**
Dementia in other diseases classified elsewhere, moderate, with mood disturbance such as depression, apathy, or anhedonia
Major neurocognitive disorder in other diseases classified elsewhere, moderate, with mood disturbance such as depression, apathy, or anhedonia

● **F02.B4 Dementia in other diseases classified elsewhere, moderate, with anxiety**
Major neurocognitive disorder in other diseases classified elsewhere, moderate, with anxiety

● 5th **F02.C Dementia in other diseases classified elsewhere, severe**

● **F02.C0 Dementia in other diseases classified elsewhere, severe, without behavioral disturbance, psychotic disturbance, mood disturbance, and anxiety**
Dementia in other diseases classified elsewhere, severe, NOS
Major neurocognitive disorder in other diseases classified elsewhere, severe, NOS

● 6th **F02.C1 Dementia in other diseases classified elsewhere, severe, with behavioral disturbance**

● **F02.C11 Dementia in other diseases classified elsewhere, severe, with agitation**
Dementia in other diseases classified elsewhere, severe, with aberrant motor behavior such as restlessness, rocking, pacing, or exit-seeking
Dementia in other diseases classified elsewhere, severe, with verbal or physical behaviors such as profanity, shouting, threatening, anger, aggression, combativeness, or violence
Major neurocognitive disorder in other diseases classified elsewhere, severe, with aberrant motor behavior such as restlessness, rocking, pacing, or exit-seeking
Major neurocognitive disorder in other diseases classified elsewhere, severe, with verbal or physical behaviors such as profanity, shouting, threatening, anger, aggression, combativeness, or violence

● **F02.C18 Dementia in other diseases classified elsewhere, severe, with other behavioral disturbance**
Dementia in other diseases classified elsewhere, severe, with behavioral disturbances such as sleep disturbance, social disinhibition, or sexual disinhibition
Major neurocognitive disorder in other diseases classified elsewhere, severe, with behavioral disturbances such as sleep disturbance, social disinhibition, or sexual disinhibition
Use additional code, if applicable, to identify wandering in dementia in conditions classified elsewhere (Z91.83)

● **F02.C2 Dementia in other diseases classified elsewhere, severe, with psychotic disturbance**
Dementia in other diseases classified elsewhere, severe, with psychotic disturbance such as hallucinations, paranoia, suspiciousness, or delusional state
Major neurocognitive disorder in other diseases classified elsewhere, severe, with psychotic disturbance such as hallucinations, paranoia, suspiciousness, or delusional state

● **F02.C3 Dementia in other diseases classified elsewhere, severe, with mood disturbance**
Dementia in other diseases classified elsewhere, severe, with mood disturbance such as depression, apathy, or anhedonia
Major neurocognitive disorder in other diseases classified elsewhere, severe, with mood disturbance such as depression, apathy, or anhedonia

● **F02.C4 Dementia in other diseases classified elsewhere, severe, with anxiety**
Major neurocognitive disorder in other diseases classified elsewhere, severe, with anxiety

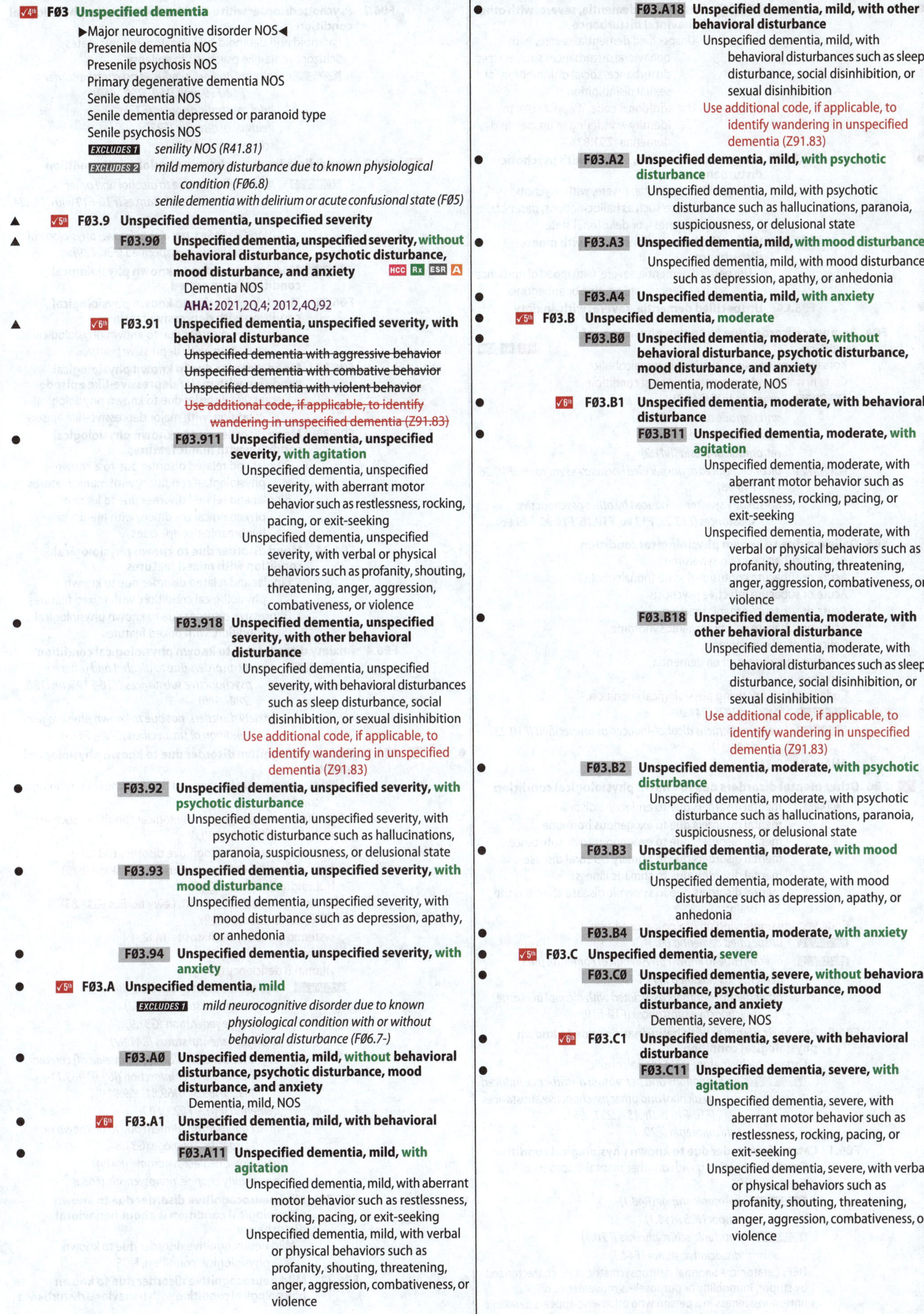

F03 Unspecified dementia
▶Major neurocognitive disorder NOS◀
Presenile dementia NOS
Presenile psychosis NOS
Primary degenerative dementia NOS
Senile dementia NOS
Senile dementia depressed or paranoid type
Senile psychosis NOS
EXCLUDES 1 *senility NOS (R41.81)*
EXCLUDES 2 *mild memory disturbance due to known physiological condition (F06.8)*
senile dementia with delirium or acute confusional state (F05)

▲ **F03.9 Unspecified dementia, unspecified severity**

▲ **F03.90 Unspecified dementia, unspecified severity, without behavioral disturbance, psychotic disturbance, mood disturbance, and anxiety** HCC Rx ESR A
Dementia NOS
AHA: 2021,2Q,4; 2012,4Q,92

▲ **F03.91 Unspecified dementia, unspecified severity, with behavioral disturbance**
~~Unspecified dementia with aggressive behavior~~
~~Unspecified dementia with combative behavior~~
~~Unspecified dementia with violent behavior~~
~~Use additional code, if applicable, to identify wandering in unspecified dementia (Z91.83)~~

● **F03.911 Unspecified dementia, unspecified severity, with agitation**
Unspecified dementia, unspecified severity, with aberrant motor behavior such as restlessness, rocking, pacing, or exit-seeking
Unspecified dementia, unspecified severity, with verbal or physical behaviors such as profanity, shouting, threatening, anger, aggression, combativeness, or violence

● **F03.918 Unspecified dementia, unspecified severity, with other behavioral disturbance**
Unspecified dementia, unspecified severity, with behavioral disturbances such as sleep disturbance, social disinhibition, or sexual disinhibition
Use additional code, if applicable, to identify wandering in unspecified dementia (Z91.83)

● **F03.92 Unspecified dementia, unspecified severity, with psychotic disturbance**
Unspecified dementia, unspecified severity, with psychotic disturbance such as hallucinations, paranoia, suspiciousness, or delusional state

● **F03.93 Unspecified dementia, unspecified severity, with mood disturbance**
Unspecified dementia, unspecified severity, with mood disturbance such as depression, apathy, or anhedonia

● **F03.94 Unspecified dementia, unspecified severity, with anxiety**

● **F03.A Unspecified dementia, mild**
EXCLUDES 1 *mild neurocognitive disorder due to known physiological condition with or without behavioral disturbance (F06.7-)*

● **F03.A0 Unspecified dementia, mild, without behavioral disturbance, psychotic disturbance, mood disturbance, and anxiety**
Dementia, mild, NOS

● **F03.A1 Unspecified dementia, mild, with behavioral disturbance**

● **F03.A11 Unspecified dementia, mild, with agitation**
Unspecified dementia, mild, with aberrant motor behavior such as restlessness, rocking, pacing, or exit-seeking
Unspecified dementia, mild, with verbal or physical behaviors such as profanity, shouting, threatening, anger, aggression, combativeness, or violence

● **F03.A18 Unspecified dementia, mild, with other behavioral disturbance**
Unspecified dementia, mild, with behavioral disturbances such as sleep disturbance, social disinhibition, or sexual disinhibition
Use additional code, if applicable, to identify wandering in unspecified dementia (Z91.83)

● **F03.A2 Unspecified dementia, mild, with psychotic disturbance**
Unspecified dementia, mild, with psychotic disturbance such as hallucinations, paranoia, suspiciousness, or delusional state

● **F03.A3 Unspecified dementia, mild, with mood disturbance**
Unspecified dementia, mild, with mood disturbance such as depression, apathy, or anhedonia

● **F03.A4 Unspecified dementia, mild, with anxiety**

● **F03.B Unspecified dementia, moderate**

● **F03.B0 Unspecified dementia, moderate, without behavioral disturbance, psychotic disturbance, mood disturbance, and anxiety**
Dementia, moderate, NOS

● **F03.B1 Unspecified dementia, moderate, with behavioral disturbance**

● **F03.B11 Unspecified dementia, moderate, with agitation**
Unspecified dementia, moderate, with aberrant motor behavior such as restlessness, rocking, pacing, or exit-seeking
Unspecified dementia, moderate, with verbal or physical behaviors such as profanity, shouting, threatening, anger, aggression, combativeness, or violence

● **F03.B18 Unspecified dementia, moderate, with other behavioral disturbance**
Unspecified dementia, moderate, with behavioral disturbances such as sleep disturbance, social disinhibition, or sexual disinhibition
Use additional code, if applicable, to identify wandering in unspecified dementia (Z91.83)

● **F03.B2 Unspecified dementia, moderate, with psychotic disturbance**
Unspecified dementia, moderate, with psychotic disturbance such as hallucinations, paranoia, suspiciousness, or delusional state

● **F03.B3 Unspecified dementia, moderate, with mood disturbance**
Unspecified dementia, moderate, with mood disturbance such as depression, apathy, or anhedonia

● **F03.B4 Unspecified dementia, moderate, with anxiety**

● **F03.C Unspecified dementia, severe**

● **F03.C0 Unspecified dementia, severe, without behavioral disturbance, psychotic disturbance, mood disturbance, and anxiety**
Dementia, severe, NOS

● **F03.C1 Unspecified dementia, severe, with behavioral disturbance**

● **F03.C11 Unspecified dementia, severe, with agitation**
Unspecified dementia, severe, with aberrant motor behavior such as restlessness, rocking, pacing, or exit-seeking
Unspecified dementia, severe, with verbal or physical behaviors such as profanity, shouting, threatening, anger, aggression, combativeness, or violence

● **F03.C18 Unspecified dementia, severe, with other behavioral disturbance**
Unspecified dementia, severe, with behavioral disturbances such as sleep disturbance, social disinhibition, or sexual disinhibition
Use additional code, if applicable, to identify wandering in unspecified dementia (Z91.83)

● **F03.C2 Unspecified dementia, severe, with psychotic disturbance**
Unspecified dementia, severe, with psychotic disturbance such as hallucinations, paranoia, suspiciousness, or delusional state

● **F03.C3 Unspecified dementia, severe, with mood disturbance**
Unspecified dementia, severe, with mood disturbance such as depression, apathy, or anhedonia

● **F03.C4 Unspecified dementia, severe, with anxiety**

F04 Amnestic disorder due to known physiological condition HCC Rx ESR
Korsakov's psychosis or syndrome, nonalcoholic
Code first the underlying physiological condition
EXCLUDES 1 *amnesia NOS (R41.3)*
anterograde amnesia (R41.1)
dissociative amnesia (F44.0)
retrograde amnesia (R41.2)
EXCLUDES 2 *alcohol-induced or unspecified Korsakov's syndrome (F10.26, F10.96)*
Korsakov's syndrome induced by other psychoactive substances (F13.26, F13.96, F19.16, F19.26, F19.96)

F05 Delirium due to known physiological condition
Acute or subacute brain syndrome
Acute or subacute confusional state (nonalcoholic)
Acute or subacute infective psychosis
Acute or subacute organic reaction
Acute or subacute psycho-organic syndrome
Delirium of mixed etiology
Delirium superimposed on dementia
Sundowning
Code first the underlying physiological condition
EXCLUDES 1 *delirium NOS (R41.0)*
EXCLUDES 2 *delirium tremens alcohol-induced or unspecified (F10.231, F10.921)*
AHA: 2019,2Q,34

4th **F06 Other mental disorders due to known physiological condition**
INCLUDES mental disorders due to endocrine disorder
mental disorders due to exogenous hormone
mental disorders due to exogenous toxic substance
mental disorders due to primary cerebral disease
mental disorders due to somatic illness
mental disorders due to systemic disease affecting the brain
Code first the underlying physiological condition
EXCLUDES 1 *unspecified dementia (F03)*
EXCLUDES 2 *delirium due to known physiological condition (F05)*
dementia as classified in F01-F02
other mental disorders associated with alcohol and other psychoactive substances (F10-F19)

F06.0 Psychotic disorder with hallucinations due to known physiological condition
Organic hallucinatory state (nonalcoholic)
EXCLUDES 2 *hallucinations and perceptual disturbance induced by alcohol and other psychoactive substances (F10-F19 with .151, .251, .951)*
schizophrenia (F20.-)

F06.1 Catatonic disorder due to known physiological condition
Catatonia associated with another mental disorder
Catatonia NOS
EXCLUDES 1 *catatonic stupor (R40.1)*
stupor NOS (R40.1)
EXCLUDES 2 *catatonic schizophrenia (F20.2)*
dissociative stupor (F44.2)

DEF: Catatonic: Abnormal neuropsychiatric state characterized by stupor, immobility or purposeless movements, or unresponsiveness in a person who otherwise appears awake.

F06.2 Psychotic disorder with delusions due to known physiological condition
Paranoid and paranoid-hallucinatory organic states
Schizophrenia-like psychosis in epilepsy
EXCLUDES 2 *alcohol and drug-induced psychotic disorder (F10-F19 with .150, .250, .950)*
brief psychotic disorder (F23)
delusional disorder (F22)
schizophrenia (F20.-)

5th **F06.3 Mood disorder due to known physiological condition**
EXCLUDES 2 *mood disorders due to alcohol and other psychoactive substances (F10-F19 with .14, .24, .94)*
mood disorders, not due to known physiological condition or unspecified (F30-F39)

F06.30 Mood disorder due to known physiological condition, unspecified

F06.31 Mood disorder due to known physiological condition with depressive features
Depressive disorder due to known physiological condition, with depressive features

F06.32 Mood disorder due to known physiological condition with major depressive-like episode
Depressive disorder due to known physiological condition, with major depressive-like episode

F06.33 Mood disorder due to known physiological condition with manic features
Bipolar and related disorder due to a known physiological condition, with manic features
Bipolar and related disorder due to known physiological condition, with manic- or hypomanic-like episodes

F06.34 Mood disorder due to known physiological condition with mixed features
Bipolar and related disorder due to known physiological condition, with mixed features
Depressive disorder due to known physiological condition, with mixed features

F06.4 Anxiety disorder due to known physiological condition
EXCLUDES 2 *anxiety disorders due to alcohol and other psychoactive substances (F10-F19 with .180, .280, .980)*
anxiety disorders, not due to known physiological condition or unspecified (F40.-, F41.-)

● 5th **F06.7 Mild neurocognitive disorder due to known physiological condition**
Mild neurocognitive impairment due to a known physiological condition
Code first the underlying physiological condition, such as:
Alzheimer's disease (G30.-)
frontotemporal neurocognitive disorder (G31.09)
human immunodeficiency virus [HIV] disease (B20)
Huntington's disease (G10)
neurocognitive disorder with Lewy bodies (G31.83)
Parkinson's disease (G20)
systemic lupus erythematosus (M32.-)
traumatic brain injury (S06.-)
vitamin B deficiency (E53-)
EXCLUDES 1 *age related cognitive decline (R41.81)*
altered mental status (R41.82)
cerebral degeneration (G31.9)
change in mental status (R41.82)
cognitive deficits following (sequelae of) cerebral hemorrhage or infarction (I69.01-I69.11-, I69.21-I69.31-, I69.81- I69.91-)
dementia (F01.-, F02.-, F03)
mild cognitive impairment due to unknown or unspecified etiology (G31.84)
neurologic neglect syndrome (R41.4)
personality change, nonpsychotic (F68.8)

● **F06.70 Mild neurocognitive disorder due to known physiological condition without behavioral disturbance**
Mild neurocognitive disorder due to known physiological condition, NOS

● **F06.71 Mild neurocognitive disorder due to known physiological condition with behavioral disturbance**

F06.8 Other specified mental disorders due to known physiological condition
Epileptic psychosis NOS
Obsessive-compulsive and related disorder due to a known physiological condition
Organic dissociative disorder
Organic emotionally labile [asthenic] disorder

F07 Personality and behavioral disorders due to known physiological condition
Code first the underlying physiological condition

F07.0 Personality change due to known physiological condition
Frontal lobe syndrome
Limbic epilepsy personality syndrome
Lobotomy syndrome
Organic personality disorder
Organic pseudopsychopathic personality
Organic pseudoretarded personality
Postleucotomy syndrome
~~Code first underlying physiological condition~~
EXCLUDES 1 *mild cognitive impairment (G31.84)*
postconcussional syndrome (F07.81)
postencephalitic syndrome (F07.89)
signs and symptoms involving emotional state (R45.-)
EXCLUDES 2 *specific personality disorder (F60.-)*

F07.8 Other personality and behavioral disorders due to known physiological condition

F07.81 Postconcussional syndrome
Postcontusional syndrome (encephalopathy)
Post-traumatic brain syndrome, nonpsychotic
Use additional code to identify associated post-traumatic headache, if applicable (G44.3-)
EXCLUDES 1 *current concussion (brain) (S06.0-)*
postencephalitic syndrome (F07.89)
DEF: Concussion symptoms that persist for weeks or months after a head injury. These symptoms may include headache, giddiness, fatigue, insomnia, mood fluctuation, and a subjective feeling of impaired intellectual function with extreme reaction to normal stressors.

F07.89 Other personality and behavioral disorders due to known physiological condition
Postencephalitic syndrome
Right hemispheric organic affective disorder

F07.9 Unspecified personality and behavioral disorder due to known physiological condition
Organic psychosyndrome

F09 Unspecified mental disorder due to known physiological condition
Mental disorder NOS due to known physiological condition
Organic brain syndrome NOS
Organic mental disorder NOS
Organic psychosis NOS
Symptomatic psychosis NOS
Code first the underlying physiological condition
EXCLUDES 1 ▶*mild neurocognitive disorder due to known physiological condition (F06.7-)*◀
psychosis NOS (F29)

Mental and behavioral disorders due to psychoactive substance use (F10-F19)

AHA: 2022,1Q,34; 2020,1Q,9; 2018,4Q,69-70; 2017,4Q,8; 2017,2Q,27
TIP: Psychoactive substance withdrawal can occur in individuals who do not have a diagnosis of dependence but who use the substance regularly (i.e., use or abuse) and then reduce or cease the use.

F10 Alcohol related disorders
Use additional code for blood alcohol level, if applicable (Y90.-)
AHA: 2019,3Q,8

F10.1 Alcohol abuse
EXCLUDES 1 *alcohol dependence (F10.2-)*
alcohol use, unspecified (F10.9-)
AHA: 2018,1Q,16; 2015,2Q,15

F10.10 Alcohol abuse, uncomplicated
Alcohol use disorder, mild

F10.11 Alcohol abuse, in remission
Alcohol use disorder, mild, in early remission
Alcohol use disorder, mild, in sustained remission
AHA: 2022,1Q,25

F10.12 Alcohol abuse with intoxication

F10.120 Alcohol abuse with intoxication, uncomplicated HCC ESR

F10.121 Alcohol abuse with intoxication delirium HCC ESR

F10.129 Alcohol abuse with intoxication, unspecified HCC ESR

F10.13 Alcohol abuse, with withdrawal
AHA: 2020,4Q,16-17

F10.130 Alcohol abuse with withdrawal, uncomplicated HCC ESR COM

F10.131 Alcohol abuse with withdrawal delirium HCC ESR COM

F10.132 Alcohol abuse with withdrawal with perceptual disturbance HCC ESR COM

F10.139 Alcohol abuse with withdrawal, unspecified HCC ESR COM

F10.14 Alcohol abuse with alcohol-induced mood disorder HCC ESR COM
Alcohol use disorder, mild, with alcohol-induced bipolar or related disorder
Alcohol use disorder, mild, with alcohol-induced depressive disorder

F10.15 Alcohol abuse with alcohol-induced psychotic disorder

F10.150 Alcohol abuse with alcohol-induced psychotic disorder with delusions HCC ESR COM

F10.151 Alcohol abuse with alcohol-induced psychotic disorder with hallucinations HCC ESR COM
DEF: Psychosis lasting less than six months with slight or no clouding of consciousness in which auditory hallucinations predominate.

F10.159 Alcohol abuse with alcohol-induced psychotic disorder, unspecified HCC ESR COM

F10.18 Alcohol abuse with other alcohol-induced disorders
AHA: 2022,1Q,33

F10.180 Alcohol abuse with alcohol-induced anxiety disorder HCC ESR COM
AHA: 2022,1Q,25,33

F10.181 Alcohol abuse with alcohol-induced sexual dysfunction HCC ESR COM

F10.182 Alcohol abuse with alcohol-induced sleep disorder HCC ESR COM

F10.188 Alcohol abuse with other alcohol-induced disorder HCC ESR COM
AHA: 2022,1Q,25

F10.19 Alcohol abuse with unspecified alcohol-induced disorder HCC ESR

F10.2 Alcohol dependence
EXCLUDES 1 *alcohol abuse (F10.1-)*
alcohol use, unspecified (F10.9-)
EXCLUDES 2 *toxic effect of alcohol (T51.0-)*

F10.20 Alcohol dependence, uncomplicated HCC ESR COM
Alcohol use disorder, moderate
Alcohol use disorder, severe
AHA: 2020,1Q,9

F10.21 Alcohol dependence, in remission HCC ESR COM
Alcohol use disorder, moderate, in early remission
Alcohol use disorder, moderate, in sustained remission
Alcohol use disorder, severe, in early remission
Alcohol use disorder, severe, in sustained remission

F10.22 Alcohol dependence with intoxication
Acute drunkenness (in alcoholism)
EXCLUDES 2 *alcohol dependence with withdrawal (F10.23-)*

F10.220 Alcohol dependence with intoxication, uncomplicated HCC ESR COM

F10.221 Alcohol dependence with intoxication delirium HCC ESR COM

F10.229 Alcohol dependence with intoxication, unspecified HCC ESR COM

Chapter 5. Mental, Behavioral and Neurodevelopmental Disorders

F06.8–F10.229

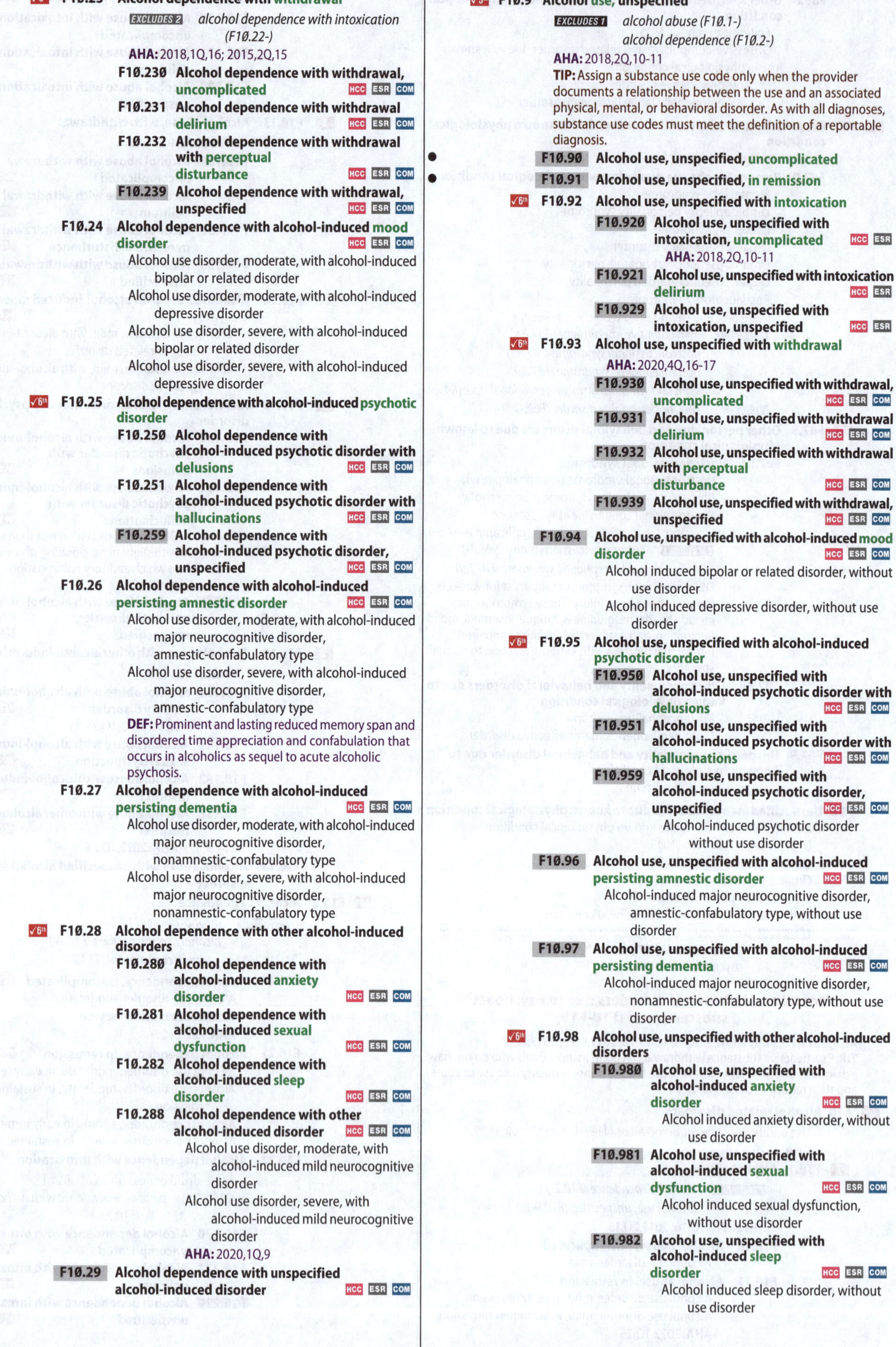

F10.23 Alcohol dependence with withdrawal

EXCLUDES 2 *alcohol dependence with intoxication (F10.22-)*

AHA: 2018,1Q,16; 2015,2Q,15

F10.230 Alcohol dependence with withdrawal, uncomplicated HCC ESR COM

F10.231 Alcohol dependence with withdrawal delirium HCC ESR COM

F10.232 Alcohol dependence with withdrawal with perceptual disturbance HCC ESR COM

F10.239 Alcohol dependence with withdrawal, unspecified HCC ESR COM

F10.24 Alcohol dependence with alcohol-induced mood disorder HCC ESR COM

Alcohol use disorder, moderate, with alcohol-induced bipolar or related disorder

Alcohol use disorder, moderate, with alcohol-induced depressive disorder

Alcohol use disorder, severe, with alcohol-induced bipolar or related disorder

Alcohol use disorder, severe, with alcohol-induced depressive disorder

F10.25 Alcohol dependence with alcohol-induced psychotic disorder

F10.250 Alcohol dependence with alcohol-induced psychotic disorder with delusions HCC ESR COM

F10.251 Alcohol dependence with alcohol-induced psychotic disorder with hallucinations HCC ESR COM

F10.259 Alcohol dependence with alcohol-induced psychotic disorder, unspecified HCC ESR COM

F10.26 Alcohol dependence with alcohol-induced persisting amnestic disorder HCC ESR COM

Alcohol use disorder, moderate, with alcohol-induced major neurocognitive disorder, amnestic-confabulatory type

Alcohol use disorder, severe, with alcohol-induced major neurocognitive disorder, amnestic-confabulatory type

DEF: Prominent and lasting reduced memory span and disordered time appreciation and confabulation that occurs in alcoholics as sequel to acute alcoholic psychosis.

F10.27 Alcohol dependence with alcohol-induced persisting dementia HCC ESR COM

Alcohol use disorder, moderate, with alcohol-induced major neurocognitive disorder, nonamnestic-confabulatory type

Alcohol use disorder, severe, with alcohol-induced major neurocognitive disorder, nonamnestic-confabulatory type

F10.28 Alcohol dependence with other alcohol-induced disorders

F10.280 Alcohol dependence with alcohol-induced anxiety disorder HCC ESR COM

F10.281 Alcohol dependence with alcohol-induced sexual dysfunction HCC ESR COM

F10.282 Alcohol dependence with alcohol-induced sleep disorder HCC ESR COM

F10.288 Alcohol dependence with other alcohol-induced disorder HCC ESR COM

Alcohol use disorder, moderate, with alcohol-induced mild neurocognitive disorder

Alcohol use disorder, severe, with alcohol-induced mild neurocognitive disorder

AHA: 2020,1Q,9

F10.29 Alcohol dependence with unspecified alcohol-induced disorder HCC ESR COM

F10.9 Alcohol use, unspecified

EXCLUDES 1 *alcohol abuse (F10.1-)*
alcohol dependence (F10.2-)

AHA: 2018,2Q,10-11

TIP: Assign a substance use code only when the provider documents a relationship between the use and an associated physical, mental, or behavioral disorder. As with all diagnoses, substance use codes must meet the definition of a reportable diagnosis.

● **F10.90 Alcohol use, unspecified, uncomplicated**

● **F10.91 Alcohol use, unspecified, in remission**

F10.92 Alcohol use, unspecified with intoxication

F10.920 Alcohol use, unspecified with intoxication, uncomplicated HCC ESR

AHA: 2018,2Q,10-11

F10.921 Alcohol use, unspecified with intoxication delirium HCC ESR

F10.929 Alcohol use, unspecified with intoxication, unspecified HCC ESR

F10.93 Alcohol use, unspecified with withdrawal

AHA: 2020,4Q,16-17

F10.930 Alcohol use, unspecified with withdrawal, uncomplicated HCC ESR COM

F10.931 Alcohol use, unspecified with withdrawal delirium HCC ESR COM

F10.932 Alcohol use, unspecified with withdrawal with perceptual disturbance HCC ESR COM

F10.939 Alcohol use, unspecified with withdrawal, unspecified HCC ESR COM

F10.94 Alcohol use, unspecified with alcohol-induced mood disorder HCC ESR COM

Alcohol induced bipolar or related disorder, without use disorder

Alcohol induced depressive disorder, without use disorder

F10.95 Alcohol use, unspecified with alcohol-induced psychotic disorder

F10.950 Alcohol use, unspecified with alcohol-induced psychotic disorder with delusions HCC ESR COM

F10.951 Alcohol use, unspecified with alcohol-induced psychotic disorder with hallucinations HCC ESR COM

F10.959 Alcohol use, unspecified with alcohol-induced psychotic disorder, unspecified HCC ESR COM

Alcohol-induced psychotic disorder without use disorder

F10.96 Alcohol use, unspecified with alcohol-induced persisting amnestic disorder HCC ESR COM

Alcohol-induced major neurocognitive disorder, amnestic-confabulatory type, without use disorder

F10.97 Alcohol use, unspecified with alcohol-induced persisting dementia HCC ESR COM

Alcohol-induced major neurocognitive disorder, nonamnestic-confabulatory type, without use disorder

F10.98 Alcohol use, unspecified with other alcohol-induced disorders

F10.980 Alcohol use, unspecified with alcohol-induced anxiety disorder HCC ESR COM

Alcohol induced anxiety disorder, without use disorder

F10.981 Alcohol use, unspecified with alcohol-induced sexual dysfunction HCC ESR COM

Alcohol induced sexual dysfunction, without use disorder

F10.982 Alcohol use, unspecified with alcohol-induced sleep disorder HCC ESR COM

Alcohol induced sleep disorder, without use disorder

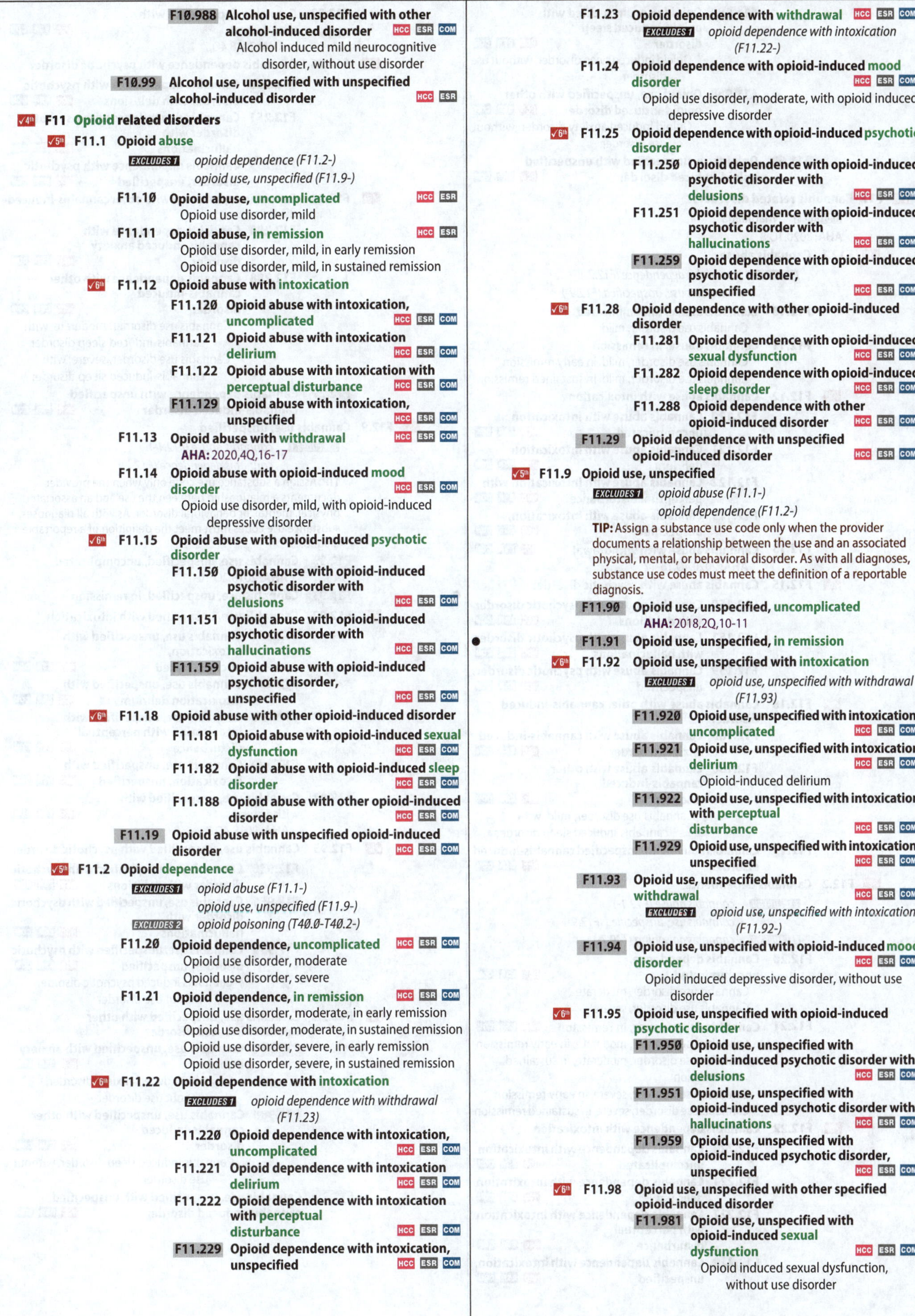

F10.988 Alcohol use, unspecified with other alcohol-induced disorder HCC ESR COM
Alcohol induced mild neurocognitive disorder, without use disorder

F10.99 Alcohol use, unspecified with unspecified alcohol-induced disorder HCC ESR

F11 Opioid related disorders

F11.1 Opioid abuse
EXCLUDES 1 *opioid dependence (F11.2-)*
opioid use, unspecified (F11.9-)

F11.10 Opioid abuse, uncomplicated HCC ESR
Opioid use disorder, mild

F11.11 Opioid abuse, in remission HCC ESR
Opioid use disorder, mild, in early remission
Opioid use disorder, mild, in sustained remission

F11.12 Opioid abuse with intoxication

F11.120 Opioid abuse with intoxication, uncomplicated HCC ESR COM

F11.121 Opioid abuse with intoxication delirium HCC ESR COM

F11.122 Opioid abuse with intoxication with perceptual disturbance HCC ESR COM

F11.129 Opioid abuse with intoxication, unspecified HCC ESR COM

F11.13 Opioid abuse with withdrawal HCC ESR COM
AHA: 2020,4Q,16-17

F11.14 Opioid abuse with opioid-induced mood disorder HCC ESR COM
Opioid use disorder, mild, with opioid-induced depressive disorder

F11.15 Opioid abuse with opioid-induced psychotic disorder

F11.150 Opioid abuse with opioid-induced psychotic disorder with delusions HCC ESR COM

F11.151 Opioid abuse with opioid-induced psychotic disorder with hallucinations HCC ESR COM

F11.159 Opioid abuse with opioid-induced psychotic disorder, unspecified HCC ESR COM

F11.18 Opioid abuse with other opioid-induced disorder

F11.181 Opioid abuse with opioid-induced sexual dysfunction HCC ESR COM

F11.182 Opioid abuse with opioid-induced sleep disorder HCC ESR COM

F11.188 Opioid abuse with other opioid-induced disorder HCC ESR COM

F11.19 Opioid abuse with unspecified opioid-induced disorder HCC ESR COM

F11.2 Opioid dependence
EXCLUDES 1 *opioid abuse (F11.1-)*
opioid use, unspecified (F11.9-)
EXCLUDES 2 *opioid poisoning (T40.0-T40.2-)*

F11.20 Opioid dependence, uncomplicated HCC ESR COM
Opioid use disorder, moderate
Opioid use disorder, severe

F11.21 Opioid dependence, in remission HCC ESR COM
Opioid use disorder, moderate, in early remission
Opioid use disorder, moderate, in sustained remission
Opioid use disorder, severe, in early remission
Opioid use disorder, severe, in sustained remission

F11.22 Opioid dependence with intoxication
EXCLUDES 1 *opioid dependence with withdrawal (F11.23)*

F11.220 Opioid dependence with intoxication, uncomplicated HCC ESR COM

F11.221 Opioid dependence with intoxication delirium HCC ESR COM

F11.222 Opioid dependence with intoxication with perceptual disturbance HCC ESR COM

F11.229 Opioid dependence with intoxication, unspecified HCC ESR COM

F11.23 Opioid dependence with withdrawal HCC ESR COM
EXCLUDES 1 *opioid dependence with intoxication (F11.22-)*

F11.24 Opioid dependence with opioid-induced mood disorder HCC ESR COM
Opioid use disorder, moderate, with opioid induced depressive disorder

F11.25 Opioid dependence with opioid-induced psychotic disorder

F11.250 Opioid dependence with opioid-induced psychotic disorder with delusions HCC ESR COM

F11.251 Opioid dependence with opioid-induced psychotic disorder with hallucinations HCC ESR COM

F11.259 Opioid dependence with opioid-induced psychotic disorder, unspecified HCC ESR COM

F11.28 Opioid dependence with other opioid-induced disorder

F11.281 Opioid dependence with opioid-induced sexual dysfunction HCC ESR COM

F11.282 Opioid dependence with opioid-induced sleep disorder HCC ESR COM

F11.288 Opioid dependence with other opioid-induced disorder HCC ESR COM

F11.29 Opioid dependence with unspecified opioid-induced disorder HCC ESR COM

F11.9 Opioid use, unspecified
EXCLUDES 1 *opioid abuse (F11.1-)*
opioid dependence (F11.2-)

TIP: Assign a substance use code only when the provider documents a relationship between the use and an associated physical, mental, or behavioral disorder. As with all diagnoses, substance use codes must meet the definition of a reportable diagnosis.

F11.90 Opioid use, unspecified, uncomplicated
AHA: 2018,2Q,10-11

● **F11.91 Opioid use, unspecified, in remission**

F11.92 Opioid use, unspecified with intoxication
EXCLUDES 1 *opioid use, unspecified with withdrawal (F11.93)*

F11.920 Opioid use, unspecified with intoxication, uncomplicated HCC ESR COM

F11.921 Opioid use, unspecified with intoxication delirium HCC ESR COM
Opioid-induced delirium

F11.922 Opioid use, unspecified with intoxication with perceptual disturbance HCC ESR COM

F11.929 Opioid use, unspecified with intoxication, unspecified HCC ESR COM

F11.93 Opioid use, unspecified with withdrawal HCC ESR COM
EXCLUDES 1 *opioid use, unspecified with intoxication (F11.92-)*

F11.94 Opioid use, unspecified with opioid-induced mood disorder HCC ESR COM
Opioid induced depressive disorder, without use disorder

F11.95 Opioid use, unspecified with opioid-induced psychotic disorder

F11.950 Opioid use, unspecified with opioid-induced psychotic disorder with delusions HCC ESR COM

F11.951 Opioid use, unspecified with opioid-induced psychotic disorder with hallucinations HCC ESR COM

F11.959 Opioid use, unspecified with opioid-induced psychotic disorder, unspecified HCC ESR COM

F11.98 Opioid use, unspecified with other specified opioid-induced disorder

F11.981 Opioid use, unspecified with opioid-induced sexual dysfunction HCC ESR COM
Opioid induced sexual dysfunction, without use disorder

Additional Character Required | Placeholder Alert | Manifestation | Unspecified Dx | QPP | Unacceptable PDx

F11.982 Opioid use, unspecified with opioid-induced sleep disorder HCC ESR COM
Opioid induced sleep disorder, without use disorder

F11.988 Opioid use, unspecified with other opioid-induced disorder HCC ESR COM
Opioid induced anxiety disorder, without use disorder

F11.99 Opioid use, unspecified with unspecified opioid-induced disorder HCC ESR COM

✓4th **F12 Cannabis related disorders**
INCLUDES marijuana
AHA: 2020,1Q,8

✓5th **F12.1 Cannabis abuse**
EXCLUDES 1 *cannabis dependence (F12.2-)*
cannabis use, unspecified (F12.9-)

F12.10 Cannabis abuse, uncomplicated
Cannabis use disorder, mild

F12.11 Cannabis abuse, in remission
Cannabis use disorder, mild, in early remission
Cannabis use disorder, mild, in sustained remission

✓6th **F12.12 Cannabis abuse with intoxication**

F12.120 Cannabis abuse with intoxication, uncomplicated HCC ESR COM

F12.121 Cannabis abuse with intoxication delirium HCC ESR COM

F12.122 Cannabis abuse with intoxication with perceptual disturbance HCC ESR COM

F12.129 Cannabis abuse with intoxication, unspecified HCC ESR COM

F12.13 Cannabis abuse with withdrawal HCC ESR COM
AHA: 2020,4Q,16-17

✓6th **F12.15 Cannabis abuse with psychotic disorder**

F12.150 Cannabis abuse with psychotic disorder with delusions HCC ESR COM

F12.151 Cannabis abuse with psychotic disorder with hallucinations HCC ESR COM

F12.159 Cannabis abuse with psychotic disorder, unspecified HCC ESR COM

✓6th **F12.18 Cannabis abuse with other cannabis-induced disorder**

F12.180 Cannabis abuse with cannabis-induced anxiety disorder HCC ESR COM

F12.188 Cannabis abuse with other cannabis-induced disorder HCC ESR COM
Cannabis use disorder, mild, with cannabis-induced sleep disorder

F12.19 Cannabis abuse with unspecified cannabis-induced disorder HCC ESR COM

✓5th **F12.2 Cannabis dependence**
EXCLUDES 1 *cannabis abuse (F12.1-)*
cannabis use, unspecified (F12.9-)
EXCLUDES 2 *cannabis poisoning (T40.7-)*

F12.20 Cannabis dependence, uncomplicated HCC ESR COM
Cannabis use disorder, moderate
Cannabis use disorder, severe

F12.21 Cannabis dependence, in remission HCC ESR COM
Cannabis use disorder, moderate, in early remission
Cannabis use disorder, moderate, in sustained remission
Cannabis use disorder, severe, in early remission
Cannabis use disorder, severe, in sustained remission

✓6th **F12.22 Cannabis dependence with intoxication**

F12.220 Cannabis dependence with intoxication, uncomplicated HCC ESR COM

F12.221 Cannabis dependence with intoxication delirium HCC ESR COM

F12.222 Cannabis dependence with intoxication with perceptual disturbance HCC ESR COM

F12.229 Cannabis dependence with intoxication, unspecified HCC ESR COM

F12.23 Cannabis dependence with withdrawal HCC ESR COM
AHA: 2018,4Q,7

✓6th **F12.25 Cannabis dependence with psychotic disorder**

F12.250 Cannabis dependence with psychotic disorder with delusions HCC ESR COM

F12.251 Cannabis dependence with psychotic disorder with hallucinations HCC ESR COM

F12.259 Cannabis dependence with psychotic disorder, unspecified HCC ESR COM

✓6th **F12.28 Cannabis dependence with other cannabis-induced disorder**

F12.280 Cannabis dependence with cannabis-induced anxiety disorder HCC ESR COM

F12.288 Cannabis dependence with other cannabis-induced disorder HCC ESR COM
Cannabis use disorder, moderate, with cannabis-induced sleep disorder
Cannabis use disorder, severe, with cannabis-induced sleep disorder

F12.29 Cannabis dependence with unspecified cannabis-induced disorder HCC ESR COM

✓5th **F12.9 Cannabis use, unspecified**
EXCLUDES 1 *cannabis abuse (F12.1-)*
cannabis dependence (F12.2-)

TIP: Assign a substance use code only when the provider documents a relationship between the use and an associated physical, mental, or behavioral disorder. As with all diagnoses, substance use codes must meet the definition of a reportable diagnosis.

F12.90 Cannabis use, unspecified, uncomplicated
AHA: 2018,2Q,10-11

● **F12.91 Cannabis use, unspecified, in remission**

✓6th **F12.92 Cannabis use, unspecified with intoxication**

F12.920 Cannabis use, unspecified with intoxication, uncomplicated HCC ESR COM

F12.921 Cannabis use, unspecified with intoxication delirium HCC ESR COM

F12.922 Cannabis use, unspecified with intoxication with perceptual disturbance HCC ESR COM

F12.929 Cannabis use, unspecified with intoxication, unspecified HCC ESR COM

F12.93 Cannabis use, unspecified with withdrawal HCC ESR COM
AHA: 2018,4Q,7

✓6th **F12.95 Cannabis use, unspecified with psychotic disorder**

F12.950 Cannabis use, unspecified with psychotic disorder with delusions HCC ESR COM

F12.951 Cannabis use, unspecified with psychotic disorder with hallucinations HCC ESR COM

F12.959 Cannabis use, unspecified with psychotic disorder, unspecified HCC ESR COM
Cannabis induced psychotic disorder, without use disorder

✓6th **F12.98 Cannabis use, unspecified with other cannabis-induced disorder**

F12.980 Cannabis use, unspecified with anxiety disorder HCC ESR COM
Cannabis induced anxiety disorder, without use disorder

F12.988 Cannabis use, unspecified with other cannabis-induced disorder HCC ESR COM
Cannabis induced sleep disorder, without use disorder

F12.99 Cannabis use, unspecified with unspecified cannabis-induced disorder HCC ESR COM

F13 Sedative, hypnotic, or anxiolytic related disorders

F13.1 Sedative, hypnotic or anxiolytic-related abuse

EXCLUDES 1 *sedative, hypnotic or anxiolytic-related dependence (F13.2-)*
sedative, hypnotic, or anxiolytic use, unspecified (F13.9-)

F13.10 Sedative, hypnotic or anxiolytic abuse, uncomplicated HCC ESR
Sedative, hypnotic, or anxiolytic use disorder, mild

F13.11 Sedative, hypnotic or anxiolytic abuse, in remission HCC ESR
Sedative, hypnotic or anxiolytic use disorder, mild, in early remission
Sedative, hypnotic or anxiolytic use disorder, mild, in sustained remission

F13.12 Sedative, hypnotic or anxiolytic abuse with intoxication

F13.120 Sedative, hypnotic or anxiolytic abuse with intoxication, uncomplicated HCC ESR COM

F13.121 Sedative, hypnotic or anxiolytic abuse with intoxication delirium HCC ESR COM

F13.129 Sedative, hypnotic or anxiolytic abuse with intoxication, unspecified HCC ESR COM

F13.13 Sedative, hypnotic or anxiolytic abuse with withdrawal
AHA: 2020,4Q,16-17

F13.130 Sedative, hypnotic or anxiolytic abuse with withdrawal, uncomplicated HCC ESR COM

F13.131 Sedative, hypnotic or anxiolytic abuse with withdrawal delirium HCC ESR COM

F13.132 Sedative, hypnotic or anxiolytic abuse with withdrawal with perceptual disturbance HCC ESR COM

F13.139 Sedative, hypnotic or anxiolytic abuse with withdrawal, unspecified HCC ESR COM

F13.14 Sedative, hypnotic or anxiolytic abuse with sedative, hypnotic or anxiolytic-induced mood disorder HCC ESR COM
Sedative, hypnotic, or anxiolytic use disorder, mild, with sedative, hypnotic, or anxiolytic-induced bipolar or related disorder
Sedative, hypnotic, or anxiolytic use disorder, mild, with sedative, hypnotic, or anxiolytic-induced depressive disorder

F13.15 Sedative, hypnotic or anxiolytic abuse with sedative, hypnotic or anxiolytic-induced psychotic disorder

F13.150 Sedative, hypnotic or anxiolytic abuse with sedative, hypnotic or anxiolytic-induced psychotic disorder with delusions HCC ESR COM

F13.151 Sedative, hypnotic or anxiolytic abuse with sedative, hypnotic or anxiolytic-induced psychotic disorder with hallucinations HCC ESR COM

F13.159 Sedative, hypnotic or anxiolytic abuse with sedative, hypnotic or anxiolytic-induced psychotic disorder, unspecified HCC ESR COM

F13.18 Sedative, hypnotic or anxiolytic abuse with other sedative, hypnotic or anxiolytic-induced disorders

F13.180 Sedative, hypnotic or anxiolytic abuse with sedative, hypnotic or anxiolytic-induced anxiety disorder HCC ESR COM

F13.181 Sedative, hypnotic or anxiolytic abuse with sedative, hypnotic or anxiolytic-induced sexual dysfunction HCC ESR COM

F13.182 Sedative, hypnotic or anxiolytic abuse with sedative, hypnotic or anxiolytic-induced sleep disorder HCC ESR COM

F13.188 Sedative, hypnotic or anxiolytic abuse with other sedative, hypnotic or anxiolytic-induced disorder HCC ESR COM

F13.19 Sedative, hypnotic or anxiolytic abuse with unspecified sedative, hypnotic or anxiolytic-induced disorder HCC ESR COM

F13.2 Sedative, hypnotic or anxiolytic-related dependence

EXCLUDES 1 *sedative, hypnotic or anxiolytic-related abuse (F13.1-)*
sedative, hypnotic, or anxiolytic use, unspecified (F13.9-)

EXCLUDES 2 *sedative, hypnotic, or anxiolytic poisoning (T42.-)*

F13.20 Sedative, hypnotic or anxiolytic dependence, uncomplicated HCC ESR COM

F13.21 Sedative, hypnotic or anxiolytic dependence, in remission HCC ESR COM
Sedative, hypnotic or anxiolytic use disorder, moderate, in early remission
Sedative, hypnotic or anxiolytic use disorder, moderate, in sustained remission
Sedative, hypnotic or anxiolytic use disorder, severe, in early remission
Sedative, hypnotic or anxiolytic use disorder, severe, in sustained remission

F13.22 Sedative, hypnotic or anxiolytic dependence with intoxication

EXCLUDES 1 *sedative, hypnotic or anxiolytic dependence with withdrawal (F13.23-)*

F13.220 Sedative, hypnotic or anxiolytic dependence with intoxication, uncomplicated HCC ESR COM

F13.221 Sedative, hypnotic or anxiolytic dependence with intoxication delirium HCC ESR COM

F13.229 Sedative, hypnotic or anxiolytic dependence with intoxication, unspecified HCC ESR COM

F13.23 Sedative, hypnotic or anxiolytic dependence with withdrawal
Sedative, hypnotic, or anxiolytic use disorder, moderate
Sedative, hypnotic, or anxiolytic use disorder, severe

EXCLUDES 1 *sedative, hypnotic or anxiolytic dependence with intoxication (F13.22-)*

F13.230 Sedative, hypnotic or anxiolytic dependence with withdrawal, uncomplicated HCC ESR COM

F13.231 Sedative, hypnotic or anxiolytic dependence with withdrawal delirium HCC ESR COM

F13.232 Sedative, hypnotic or anxiolytic dependence with withdrawal with perceptual disturbance HCC ESR COM
Sedative, hypnotic, or anxiolytic withdrawal with perceptual disturbances

F13.239 Sedative, hypnotic or anxiolytic dependence with withdrawal, unspecified HCC ESR COM
Sedative, hypnotic, or anxiolytic withdrawal without perceptual disturbances

F13.24 Sedative, hypnotic or anxiolytic dependence with sedative, hypnotic or anxiolytic-induced mood disorder HCC ESR COM
Sedative, hypnotic, or anxiolytic use disorder, moderate, with sedative, hypnotic, or anxiolytic-induced bipolar or related disorder
Sedative, hypnotic, or anxiolytic use disorder, moderate, with sedative, hypnotic, or anxiolytic-induced depressive disorder
Sedative, hypnotic, or anxiolytic use disorder, severe, with sedative, hypnotic, or anxiolytic-induced bipolar or related disorder
Sedative, hypnotic, or anxiolytic use disorder, severe, with sedative, hypnotic, or anxiolytic-induced depressive disorder

√6th **F13.25 Sedative, hypnotic or anxiolytic dependence with sedative, hypnotic or anxiolytic-induced psychotic disorder**

F13.250 Sedative, hypnotic or anxiolytic dependence with sedative, hypnotic or anxiolytic-induced psychotic disorder with delusions HCC ESR COM

F13.251 Sedative, hypnotic or anxiolytic dependence with sedative, hypnotic or anxiolytic-induced psychotic disorder with hallucinations HCC ESR COM

F13.259 Sedative, hypnotic or anxiolytic dependence with sedative, hypnotic or anxiolytic-induced psychotic disorder, unspecified HCC ESR COM

F13.26 Sedative, hypnotic or anxiolytic dependence with sedative, hypnotic or anxiolytic-induced persisting amnestic disorder HCC ESR COM

F13.27 Sedative, hypnotic or anxiolytic dependence with sedative, hypnotic or anxiolytic-induced persisting dementia HCC ESR COM

Sedative, hypnotic, or anxiolytic use disorder, moderate, with sedative, hypnotic, or anxiolytic induced major neurocognitive disorder

Sedative, hypnotic, or anxiolytic use disorder, severe, with sedative, hypnotic, or anxiolytic-induced major neurocognitive disorder

√6th **F13.28 Sedative, hypnotic or anxiolytic dependence with other sedative, hypnotic or anxiolytic-induced disorders**

F13.280 Sedative, hypnotic or anxiolytic dependence with sedative, hypnotic or anxiolytic-induced anxiety disorder HCC ESR COM

F13.281 Sedative, hypnotic or anxiolytic dependence with sedative, hypnotic or anxiolytic-induced sexual dysfunction HCC ESR COM

F13.282 Sedative, hypnotic or anxiolytic dependence with sedative, hypnotic or anxiolytic-induced sleep disorder HCC ESR COM

F13.288 Sedative, hypnotic or anxiolytic dependence with other sedative, hypnotic or anxiolytic-induced disorder HCC ESR COM

Sedative, hypnotic, or anxiolytic use disorder, moderate, with sedative, hypnotic, or anxiolytic-induced mild neurocognitive disorder

Sedative, hypnotic, or anxiolytic use disorder, severe, with sedative, hypnotic, or anxiolytic-induced mild neurocognitive disorder

F13.29 Sedative, hypnotic or anxiolytic dependence with unspecified sedative, hypnotic or anxiolytic-induced disorder HCC ESR COM

√5th **F13.9 Sedative, hypnotic or anxiolytic-related use, unspecified**

EXCLUDES 1 *sedative, hypnotic or anxiolytic-related abuse (F13.1-)*
sedative, hypnotic or anxiolytic-related dependence (F13.2-)

TIP: Assign a substance use code only when the provider documents a relationship between the use and an associated physical, mental, or behavioral disorder. As with all diagnoses, substance use codes must meet the definition of a reportable diagnosis.

F13.90 Sedative, hypnotic, or anxiolytic use, unspecified, uncomplicated

AHA: 2018,2Q,10-11

● **F13.91 Sedative, hypnotic or anxiolytic use, unspecified, in remission**

√6th **F13.92 Sedative, hypnotic or anxiolytic use, unspecified with intoxication**

EXCLUDES 1 *sedative, hypnotic or anxiolytic use, unspecified with withdrawal (F13.93-)*

F13.920 Sedative, hypnotic or anxiolytic use, unspecified with intoxication, uncomplicated HCC ESR COM

F13.921 Sedative, hypnotic or anxiolytic use, unspecified with intoxication delirium HCC ESR COM

Sedative, hypnotic, or anxiolytic-induced delirium

F13.929 Sedative, hypnotic or anxiolytic use, unspecified with intoxication, unspecified HCC ESR COM

√6th **F13.93 Sedative, hypnotic or anxiolytic use, unspecified with withdrawal**

EXCLUDES 1 *sedative, hypnotic or anxiolytic use, unspecified with intoxication (F13.92-)*

F13.930 Sedative, hypnotic or anxiolytic use, unspecified with withdrawal, uncomplicated HCC ESR COM

F13.931 Sedative, hypnotic or anxiolytic use, unspecified with withdrawal delirium HCC ESR COM

F13.932 Sedative, hypnotic or anxiolytic use, unspecified with withdrawal with perceptual disturbances HCC ESR COM

F13.939 Sedative, hypnotic or anxiolytic use, unspecified with withdrawal, unspecified HCC ESR COM

F13.94 Sedative, hypnotic or anxiolytic use, unspecified with sedative, hypnotic or anxiolytic-induced mood disorder HCC ESR COM

Sedative, hypnotic, or anxiolytic-induced bipolar or related disorder, without use disorder

Sedative, hypnotic, or anxiolytic-induced depressive disorder, without use disorder

√6th **F13.95 Sedative, hypnotic or anxiolytic use, unspecified with sedative, hypnotic or anxiolytic-induced psychotic disorder**

F13.950 Sedative, hypnotic or anxiolytic use, unspecified with sedative, hypnotic or anxiolytic-induced psychotic disorder with delusions HCC ESR COM

F13.951 Sedative, hypnotic or anxiolytic use, unspecified with sedative, hypnotic or anxiolytic-induced psychotic disorder with hallucinations HCC ESR COM

F13.959 Sedative, hypnotic or anxiolytic use, unspecified with sedative, hypnotic or anxiolytic-induced psychotic disorder, unspecified HCC ESR COM

Sedative, hypnotic, or anxiolytic-induced psychotic disorder, without use disorder

F13.96 Sedative, hypnotic or anxiolytic use, unspecified with sedative, hypnotic or anxiolytic-induced persisting amnestic disorder HCC ESR COM

F13.97 Sedative, hypnotic or anxiolytic use, unspecified with sedative, hypnotic or anxiolytic-induced persisting dementia HCC ESR COM

Sedative, hypnotic, or anxiolytic-induced major neurocognitive disorder, without use disorder

√6th **F13.98 Sedative, hypnotic or anxiolytic use, unspecified with other sedative, hypnotic or anxiolytic-induced disorders**

F13.980 Sedative, hypnotic or anxiolytic use, unspecified with sedative, hypnotic or anxiolytic-induced anxiety disorder HCC ESR COM

Sedative, hypnotic, or anxiolytic-induced anxiety disorder, without use disorder

F13.981 Sedative, hypnotic or anxiolytic use, unspecified with sedative, hypnotic or anxiolytic-induced sexual dysfunction HCC ESR COM

Sedative, hypnotic, or anxiolytic-induced sexual dysfunction disorder, without use disorder

F13.982 Sedative, hypnotic or anxiolytic use, unspecified with sedative, hypnotic or anxiolytic-induced sleep disorder HCC ESR COM

Sedative, hypnotic, or anxiolytic-induced sleep disorder, without use disorder

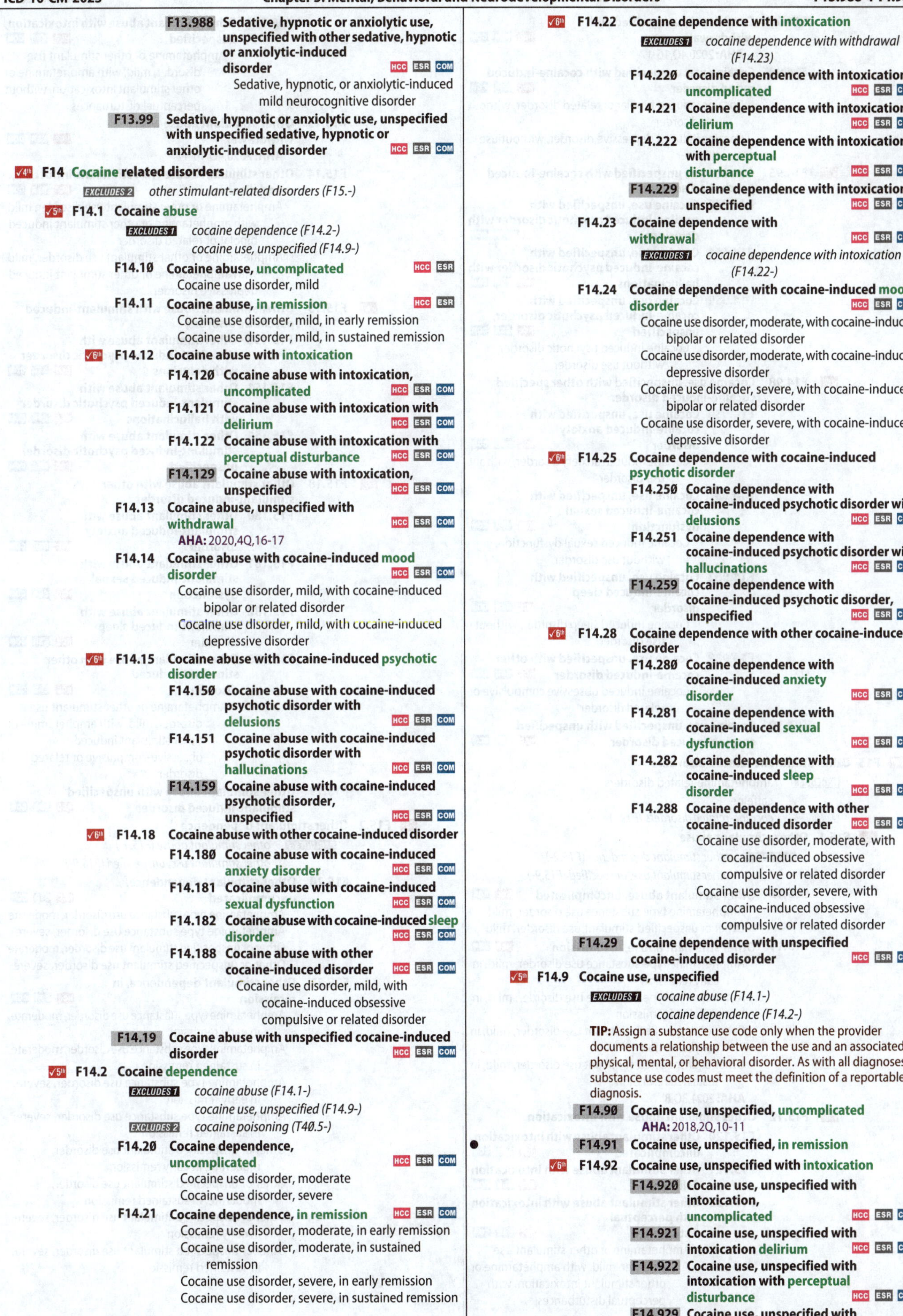

F13.988 **Sedative, hypnotic or anxiolytic use, unspecified with other sedative, hypnotic or anxiolytic-induced disorder** HCC ESR COM
Sedative, hypnotic, or anxiolytic-induced mild neurocognitive disorder

F13.99 **Sedative, hypnotic or anxiolytic use, unspecified with unspecified sedative, hypnotic or anxiolytic-induced disorder** HCC ESR COM

✓4th F14 Cocaine related disorders
EXCLUDES 2 *other stimulant-related disorders (F15.-)*

✓5th F14.1 Cocaine abuse
EXCLUDES 1 *cocaine dependence (F14.2-)*
cocaine use, unspecified (F14.9-)

F14.10 **Cocaine abuse, uncomplicated** HCC ESR
Cocaine use disorder, mild

F14.11 **Cocaine abuse, in remission** HCC ESR
Cocaine use disorder, mild, in early remission
Cocaine use disorder, mild, in sustained remission

✓6th F14.12 Cocaine abuse with intoxication

F14.120 **Cocaine abuse with intoxication, uncomplicated** HCC ESR COM

F14.121 **Cocaine abuse with intoxication with delirium** HCC ESR COM

F14.122 **Cocaine abuse with intoxication with perceptual disturbance** HCC ESR COM

F14.129 **Cocaine abuse with intoxication, unspecified** HCC ESR COM

F14.13 **Cocaine abuse, unspecified with withdrawal** HCC ESR COM
AHA: 2020,4Q,16-17

F14.14 **Cocaine abuse with cocaine-induced mood disorder** HCC ESR COM
Cocaine use disorder, mild, with cocaine-induced bipolar or related disorder
Cocaine use disorder, mild, with cocaine-induced depressive disorder

✓6th F14.15 Cocaine abuse with cocaine-induced psychotic disorder

F14.150 **Cocaine abuse with cocaine-induced psychotic disorder with delusions** HCC ESR COM

F14.151 **Cocaine abuse with cocaine-induced psychotic disorder with hallucinations** HCC ESR COM

F14.159 **Cocaine abuse with cocaine-induced psychotic disorder, unspecified** HCC ESR COM

✓6th F14.18 Cocaine abuse with other cocaine-induced disorder

F14.180 **Cocaine abuse with cocaine-induced anxiety disorder** HCC ESR COM

F14.181 **Cocaine abuse with cocaine-induced sexual dysfunction** HCC ESR COM

F14.182 **Cocaine abuse with cocaine-induced sleep disorder** HCC ESR COM

F14.188 **Cocaine abuse with other cocaine-induced disorder** HCC ESR COM
Cocaine use disorder, mild, with cocaine-induced obsessive compulsive or related disorder

F14.19 **Cocaine abuse with unspecified cocaine-induced disorder** HCC ESR COM

✓5th F14.2 Cocaine dependence
EXCLUDES 1 *cocaine abuse (F14.1-)*
cocaine use, unspecified (F14.9-)
EXCLUDES 2 *cocaine poisoning (T40.5-)*

F14.20 **Cocaine dependence, uncomplicated** HCC ESR COM
Cocaine use disorder, moderate
Cocaine use disorder, severe

F14.21 **Cocaine dependence, in remission** HCC ESR COM
Cocaine use disorder, moderate, in early remission
Cocaine use disorder, moderate, in sustained remission
Cocaine use disorder, severe, in early remission
Cocaine use disorder, severe, in sustained remission

✓6th F14.22 Cocaine dependence with intoxication
EXCLUDES 1 *cocaine dependence with withdrawal (F14.23)*

F14.220 **Cocaine dependence with intoxication, uncomplicated** HCC ESR COM

F14.221 **Cocaine dependence with intoxication delirium** HCC ESR COM

F14.222 **Cocaine dependence with intoxication with perceptual disturbance** HCC ESR COM

F14.229 **Cocaine dependence with intoxication, unspecified** HCC ESR COM

F14.23 **Cocaine dependence with withdrawal** HCC ESR COM
EXCLUDES 1 *cocaine dependence with intoxication (F14.22-)*

F14.24 **Cocaine dependence with cocaine-induced mood disorder** HCC ESR COM
Cocaine use disorder, moderate, with cocaine-induced bipolar or related disorder
Cocaine use disorder, moderate, with cocaine-induced depressive disorder
Cocaine use disorder, severe, with cocaine-induced bipolar or related disorder
Cocaine use disorder, severe, with cocaine-induced depressive disorder

✓6th F14.25 Cocaine dependence with cocaine-induced psychotic disorder

F14.250 **Cocaine dependence with cocaine-induced psychotic disorder with delusions** HCC ESR COM

F14.251 **Cocaine dependence with cocaine-induced psychotic disorder with hallucinations** HCC ESR COM

F14.259 **Cocaine dependence with cocaine-induced psychotic disorder, unspecified** HCC ESR COM

✓6th F14.28 Cocaine dependence with other cocaine-induced disorder

F14.280 **Cocaine dependence with cocaine-induced anxiety disorder** HCC ESR COM

F14.281 **Cocaine dependence with cocaine-induced sexual dysfunction** HCC ESR COM

F14.282 **Cocaine dependence with cocaine-induced sleep disorder** HCC ESR COM

F14.288 **Cocaine dependence with other cocaine-induced disorder** HCC ESR COM
Cocaine use disorder, moderate, with cocaine-induced obsessive compulsive or related disorder
Cocaine use disorder, severe, with cocaine-induced obsessive compulsive or related disorder

F14.29 **Cocaine dependence with unspecified cocaine-induced disorder** HCC ESR COM

✓5th F14.9 Cocaine use, unspecified
EXCLUDES 1 *cocaine abuse (F14.1-)*
cocaine dependence (F14.2-)

TIP: Assign a substance use code only when the provider documents a relationship between the use and an associated physical, mental, or behavioral disorder. As with all diagnoses, substance use codes must meet the definition of a reportable diagnosis.

F14.90 **Cocaine use, unspecified, uncomplicated**
AHA: 2018,2Q,10-11

● **F14.91** **Cocaine use, unspecified, in remission**

✓6th F14.92 Cocaine use, unspecified with intoxication

F14.920 **Cocaine use, unspecified with intoxication, uncomplicated** HCC ESR COM

F14.921 **Cocaine use, unspecified with intoxication delirium** HCC ESR COM

F14.922 **Cocaine use, unspecified with intoxication with perceptual disturbance** HCC ESR COM

F14.929 **Cocaine use, unspecified with intoxication, unspecified** HCC ESR COM

Chapter 5. Mental, Behavioral and Neurodevelopmental Disorders

F13.988–F14.929

F14.93 Cocaine use, unspecified with withdrawal HCC ESR COM
AHA: 2020,4Q,16-17

F14.94 Cocaine use, unspecified with cocaine-induced mood disorder HCC ESR COM
Cocaine induced bipolar or related disorder, without use disorder
Cocaine induced depressive disorder, without use disorder

√6th **F14.95 Cocaine use, unspecified with cocaine-induced psychotic disorder**

F14.950 Cocaine use, unspecified with cocaine-induced psychotic disorder with delusions HCC ESR COM

F14.951 Cocaine use, unspecified with cocaine-induced psychotic disorder with hallucinations HCC ESR COM

F14.959 Cocaine use, unspecified with cocaine-induced psychotic disorder, unspecified HCC ESR COM
Cocaine induced psychotic disorder, without use disorder

√6th **F14.98 Cocaine use, unspecified with other specified cocaine-induced disorder**

F14.980 Cocaine use, unspecified with cocaine-induced anxiety disorder HCC ESR COM
Cocaine induced anxiety disorder, without use disorder

F14.981 Cocaine use, unspecified with cocaine-induced sexual dysfunction HCC ESR COM
Cocaine induced sexual dysfunction, without use disorder

F14.982 Cocaine use, unspecified with cocaine-induced sleep disorder HCC ESR COM
Cocaine induced sleep disorder, without use disorder

F14.988 Cocaine use, unspecified with other cocaine-induced disorder HCC ESR COM
Cocaine induced obsessive compulsive or related disorder

F14.99 Cocaine use, unspecified with unspecified cocaine-induced disorder HCC ESR COM

√4th **F15 Other stimulant related disorders**

INCLUDES amphetamine-related disorders
caffeine

EXCLUDES 2 *cocaine-related disorders (F14.-)*

√5th **F15.1 Other stimulant abuse**

EXCLUDES 1 *other stimulant dependence (F15.2-)*
other stimulant use, unspecified (F15.9-)

F15.10 Other stimulant abuse, uncomplicated HCC ESR
Amphetamine type substance use disorder, mild
Other or unspecified stimulant use disorder, mild

F15.11 Other stimulant abuse, in remission HCC ESR
Amphetamine type substance use disorder, mild, in early remission
Amphetamine type substance use disorder, mild, in sustained remission
Other or unspecified stimulant use disorder, mild, in early remission
Other or unspecified stimulant use disorder, mild, in sustained remission
AHA: 2021,3Q,8

√6th **F15.12 Other stimulant abuse with intoxication**

F15.120 Other stimulant abuse with intoxication, uncomplicated HCC ESR COM

F15.121 Other stimulant abuse with intoxication delirium HCC ESR COM

F15.122 Other stimulant abuse with intoxication with perceptual disturbance HCC ESR COM
Amphetamine or other stimulant use disorder, mild, with amphetamine or other stimulant intoxication, with perceptual disturbances

F15.129 Other stimulant abuse with intoxication, unspecified HCC ESR COM
Amphetamine or other stimulant use disorder, mild, with amphetamine or other stimulant intoxication, without perceptual disturbances

F15.13 Other stimulant abuse with withdrawal HCC ESR COM
AHA: 2020,4Q,16-17

F15.14 Other stimulant abuse with stimulant-induced mood disorder HCC ESR COM
Amphetamine or other stimulant use disorder, mild, with amphetamine or other stimulant induced bipolar or related disorder
Amphetamine or other stimulant use disorder, mild, with amphetamine or other stimulant induced depressive disorder

√6th **F15.15 Other stimulant abuse with stimulant-induced psychotic disorder**

F15.150 Other stimulant abuse with stimulant-induced psychotic disorder with delusions HCC ESR COM

F15.151 Other stimulant abuse with stimulant-induced psychotic disorder with hallucinations HCC ESR COM

F15.159 Other stimulant abuse with stimulant-induced psychotic disorder, unspecified HCC ESR COM

√6th **F15.18 Other stimulant abuse with other stimulant-induced disorder**

F15.180 Other stimulant abuse with stimulant-induced anxiety disorder HCC ESR COM

F15.181 Other stimulant abuse with stimulant-induced sexual dysfunction HCC ESR COM

F15.182 Other stimulant abuse with stimulant-induced sleep disorder HCC ESR COM

F15.188 Other stimulant abuse with other stimulant-induced disorder HCC ESR COM
Amphetamine or other stimulant use disorder, mild, with amphetamine or other stimulant induced obsessive-compulsive or related disorder

F15.19 Other stimulant abuse with unspecified stimulant-induced disorder HCC ESR COM

√5th **F15.2 Other stimulant dependence**

EXCLUDES 1 *other stimulant abuse (F15.1-)*
other stimulant use, unspecified (F15.9-)

F15.20 Other stimulant dependence, uncomplicated HCC ESR COM
Amphetamine type substance use disorder, moderate
Amphetamine type substance use disorder, severe
Other or unspecified stimulant use disorder, moderate
Other or unspecified stimulant use disorder, severe

F15.21 Other stimulant dependence, in remission HCC ESR COM
Amphetamine type substance use disorder, moderate, in early remission
Amphetamine type substance use disorder, moderate, in sustained remission
Amphetamine type substance use disorder, severe, in early remission
Amphetamine type substance use disorder, severe, in sustained remission
Other or unspecified stimulant use disorder, moderate, in early remission
Other or unspecified stimulant use disorder, moderate, in sustained remission
Other or unspecified stimulant use disorder, severe, in early remission
Other or unspecified stimulant use disorder, severe, in sustained remission

F15.22 Other stimulant dependence with intoxication

EXCLUDES 1 *other stimulant dependence with withdrawal (F15.23)*

F15.220 Other stimulant dependence with intoxication, uncomplicated HCC ESR COM

F15.221 Other stimulant dependence with intoxication delirium HCC ESR COM

F15.222 Other stimulant dependence with intoxication with perceptual disturbance HCC ESR COM

Amphetamine or other stimulant use disorder, moderate, with amphetamine or other stimulant intoxication, with perceptual disturbances

Amphetamine or other stimulant use disorder, severe, with amphetamine or other stimulant intoxication, with perceptual disturbances

F15.229 Other stimulant dependence with intoxication, unspecified HCC ESR COM

Amphetamine or other stimulant use disorder, moderate, with amphetamine or other stimulant intoxication, without perceptual disturbances

Amphetamine or other stimulant use disorder, severe, with amphetamine or other stimulant intoxication, without perceptual disturbances

F15.23 Other stimulant dependence with withdrawal HCC ESR COM

Amphetamine or other stimulant withdrawal

EXCLUDES 1 *other stimulant dependence with intoxication (F15.22-)*

F15.24 Other stimulant dependence with stimulant-induced mood disorder HCC ESR COM

Amphetamine or other stimulant use disorder, moderate, with amphetamine or other stimulant-induced bipolar or related disorder

Amphetamine or other stimulant use disorder, moderate, with amphetamine or other stimulant induced depressive disorder

Amphetamine or other stimulant use disorder, severe, with amphetamine or other stimulant-induced bipolar or related disorder

Amphetamine or other stimulant use disorder, severe, with amphetamine or other stimulant-induced depressive disorder

F15.25 Other stimulant dependence with stimulant-induced psychotic disorder

F15.250 Other stimulant dependence with stimulant-induced psychotic disorder with delusions HCC ESR COM

F15.251 Other stimulant dependence with stimulant-induced psychotic disorder with hallucinations HCC ESR COM

F15.259 Other stimulant dependence with stimulant-induced psychotic disorder, unspecified HCC ESR COM

F15.28 Other stimulant dependence with other stimulant-induced disorder

F15.280 Other stimulant dependence with stimulant-induced anxiety disorder HCC ESR COM

F15.281 Other stimulant dependence with stimulant-induced sexual dysfunction HCC ESR COM

F15.282 Other stimulant dependence with stimulant-induced sleep disorder HCC ESR COM

F15.288 Other stimulant dependence with other stimulant-induced disorder HCC ESR COM

Amphetamine or other stimulant use disorder, moderate, with amphetamine orother stimulant induced obsessive compulsive or related disorder

Amphetamine or other stimulant use disorder, severe, with amphetamine or otherstimulant induced obsessive compulsive or related disorder

F15.29 Other stimulant dependence with unspecified stimulant-induced disorder HCC ESR COM

F15.9 Other stimulant use, unspecified

EXCLUDES 1 *other stimulant abuse (F15.1-)*
other stimulant dependence (F15.2-)

TIP: Assign a substance use code only when the provider documents a relationship between the use and an associated physical, mental, or behavioral disorder. As with all diagnoses, substance use codes must meet the definition of a reportable diagnosis.

F15.90 Other stimulant use, unspecified, uncomplicated

AHA: 2018,2Q,10-11

● **F15.91 Other stimulant use, unspecified, in remission**

F15.92 Other stimulant use, unspecified with intoxication

EXCLUDES 1 *other stimulant use, unspecified with withdrawal (F15.93)*

F15.920 Other stimulant use, unspecified with intoxication, uncomplicated HCC ESR COM

F15.921 Other stimulant use, unspecified with intoxication delirium HCC ESR COM

Amphetamine or other stimulant-induced delirium

F15.922 Other stimulant use, unspecified with intoxication with perceptual disturbance HCC ESR COM

F15.929 Other stimulant use, unspecified with intoxication, unspecified HCC ESR COM

Caffeine intoxication

F15.93 Other stimulant use, unspecified with withdrawal HCC ESR COM

Caffeine withdrawal

EXCLUDES 1 *other stimulant use, unspecified with intoxication (F15.92-)*

F15.94 Other stimulant use, unspecified with stimulant-induced mood disorder HCC ESR COM

Amphetamine or other stimulant-induced bipolar or related disorder, without use disorder

Amphetamine or other stimulant-induced depressive disorder, without use disorder

F15.95 Other stimulant use, unspecified with stimulant-induced psychotic disorder

F15.950 Other stimulant use, unspecified with stimulant-induced psychotic disorder with delusions HCC ESR COM

F15.951 Other stimulant use, unspecified with stimulant-induced psychotic disorder with hallucinations HCC ESR COM

F15.959 Other stimulant use, unspecified with stimulant-induced psychotic disorder, unspecified HCC ESR COM

Amphetamine or other stimulant-induced psychotic disorder, without use disorder

F15.98 Other stimulant use, unspecified with other stimulant-induced disorder

F15.980 Other stimulant use, unspecified with stimulant-induced anxiety disorder HCC ESR COM

Amphetamine or other stimulant-induced anxiety disorder, without use disorder

Caffeine induced anxiety disorder, without use disorder

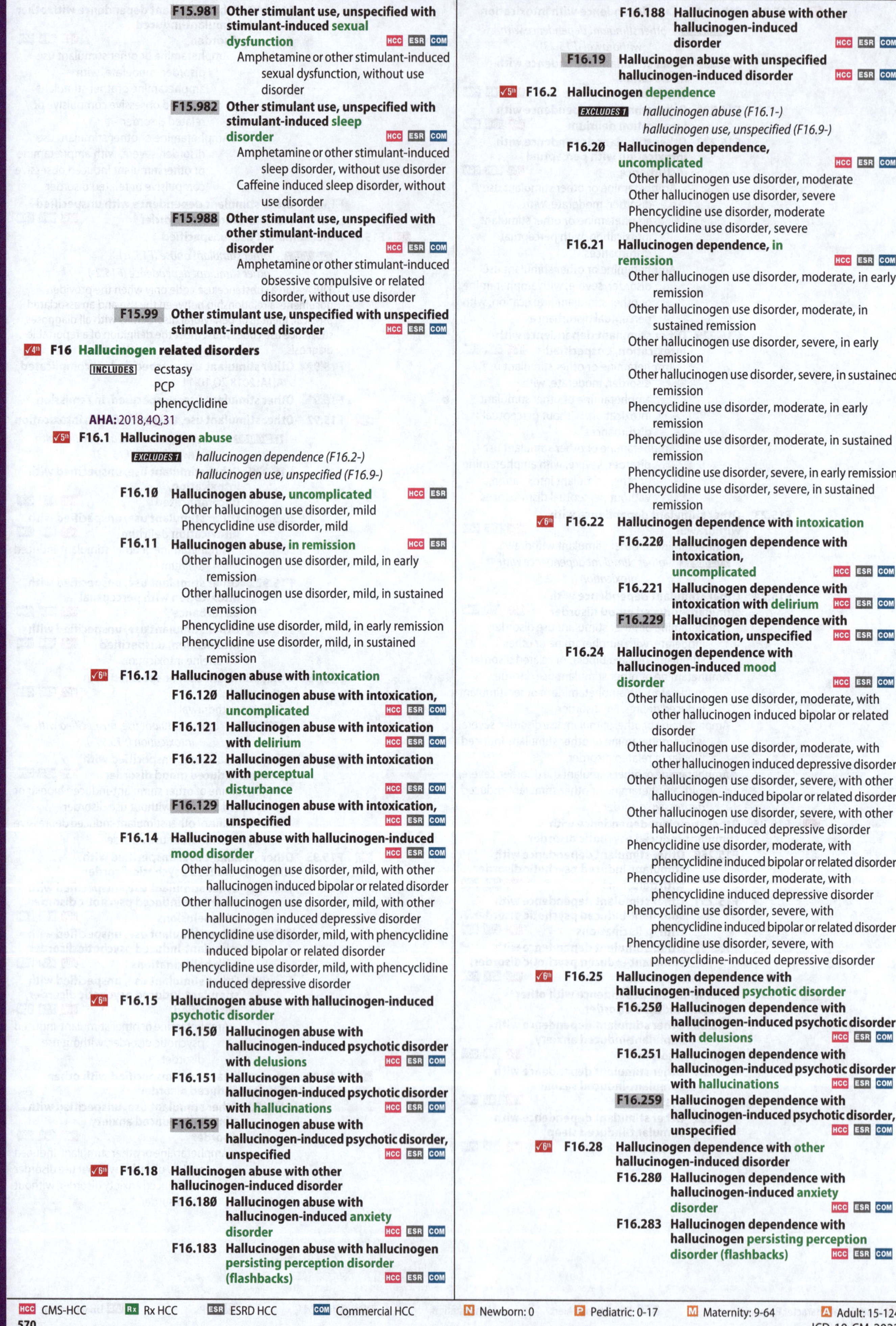

F15.981 Other stimulant use, unspecified with stimulant-induced sexual dysfunction HCC ESR COM
- Amphetamine or other stimulant-induced sexual dysfunction, without use disorder

F15.982 Other stimulant use, unspecified with stimulant-induced sleep disorder HCC ESR COM
- Amphetamine or other stimulant-induced sleep disorder, without use disorder
- Caffeine induced sleep disorder, without use disorder

F15.988 Other stimulant use, unspecified with other stimulant-induced disorder HCC ESR COM
- Amphetamine or other stimulant-induced obsessive compulsive or related disorder, without use disorder

F15.99 Other stimulant use, unspecified with unspecified stimulant-induced disorder HCC ESR COM

F16 Hallucinogen related disorders (4th)

INCLUDES ecstasy
PCP
phencyclidine

AHA: 2018,4Q,31

F16.1 Hallucinogen abuse (5th)

EXCLUDES 1 *hallucinogen dependence (F16.2-)*
hallucinogen use, unspecified (F16.9-)

F16.1Ø Hallucinogen abuse, uncomplicated HCC ESR
- Other hallucinogen use disorder, mild
- Phencyclidine use disorder, mild

F16.11 Hallucinogen abuse, in remission HCC ESR
- Other hallucinogen use disorder, mild, in early remission
- Other hallucinogen use disorder, mild, in sustained remission
- Phencyclidine use disorder, mild, in early remission
- Phencyclidine use disorder, mild, in sustained remission

F16.12 Hallucinogen abuse with intoxication (6th)

F16.12Ø Hallucinogen abuse with intoxication, uncomplicated HCC ESR COM

F16.121 Hallucinogen abuse with intoxication with delirium HCC ESR COM

F16.122 Hallucinogen abuse with intoxication with perceptual disturbance HCC ESR COM

F16.129 Hallucinogen abuse with intoxication, unspecified HCC ESR COM

F16.14 Hallucinogen abuse with hallucinogen-induced mood disorder HCC ESR COM
- Other hallucinogen use disorder, mild, with other hallucinogen induced bipolar or related disorder
- Other hallucinogen use disorder, mild, with other hallucinogen induced depressive disorder
- Phencyclidine use disorder, mild, with phencyclidine induced bipolar or related disorder
- Phencyclidine use disorder, mild, with phencyclidine induced depressive disorder

F16.15 Hallucinogen abuse with hallucinogen-induced psychotic disorder (6th)

F16.15Ø Hallucinogen abuse with hallucinogen-induced psychotic disorder with delusions HCC ESR COM

F16.151 Hallucinogen abuse with hallucinogen-induced psychotic disorder with hallucinations HCC ESR COM

F16.159 Hallucinogen abuse with hallucinogen-induced psychotic disorder, unspecified HCC ESR COM

F16.18 Hallucinogen abuse with other hallucinogen-induced disorder (6th)

F16.18Ø Hallucinogen abuse with hallucinogen-induced anxiety disorder HCC ESR COM

F16.183 Hallucinogen abuse with hallucinogen persisting perception disorder (flashbacks) HCC ESR COM

F16.188 Hallucinogen abuse with other hallucinogen-induced disorder HCC ESR COM

F16.19 Hallucinogen abuse with unspecified hallucinogen-induced disorder HCC ESR COM

F16.2 Hallucinogen dependence (5th)

EXCLUDES 1 *hallucinogen abuse (F16.1-)*
hallucinogen use, unspecified (F16.9-)

F16.2Ø Hallucinogen dependence, uncomplicated HCC ESR COM
- Other hallucinogen use disorder, moderate
- Other hallucinogen use disorder, severe
- Phencyclidine use disorder, moderate
- Phencyclidine use disorder, severe

F16.21 Hallucinogen dependence, in remission HCC ESR COM
- Other hallucinogen use disorder, moderate, in early remission
- Other hallucinogen use disorder, moderate, in sustained remission
- Other hallucinogen use disorder, severe, in early remission
- Other hallucinogen use disorder, severe, in sustained remission
- Phencyclidine use disorder, moderate, in early remission
- Phencyclidine use disorder, moderate, in sustained remission
- Phencyclidine use disorder, severe, in early remission
- Phencyclidine use disorder, severe, in sustained remission

F16.22 Hallucinogen dependence with intoxication (6th)

F16.22Ø Hallucinogen dependence with intoxication, uncomplicated HCC ESR COM

F16.221 Hallucinogen dependence with intoxication with delirium HCC ESR COM

F16.229 Hallucinogen dependence with intoxication, unspecified HCC ESR COM

F16.24 Hallucinogen dependence with hallucinogen-induced mood disorder HCC ESR COM
- Other hallucinogen use disorder, moderate, with other hallucinogen induced bipolar or related disorder
- Other hallucinogen use disorder, moderate, with other hallucinogen induced depressive disorder
- Other hallucinogen use disorder, severe, with other hallucinogen-induced bipolar or related disorder
- Other hallucinogen use disorder, severe, with other hallucinogen-induced depressive disorder
- Phencyclidine use disorder, moderate, with phencyclidine induced bipolar or related disorder
- Phencyclidine use disorder, moderate, with phencyclidine induced depressive disorder
- Phencyclidine use disorder, severe, with phencyclidine induced bipolar or related disorder
- Phencyclidine use disorder, severe, with phencyclidine-induced depressive disorder

F16.25 Hallucinogen dependence with hallucinogen-induced psychotic disorder (6th)

F16.25Ø Hallucinogen dependence with hallucinogen-induced psychotic disorder with delusions HCC ESR COM

F16.251 Hallucinogen dependence with hallucinogen-induced psychotic disorder with hallucinations HCC ESR COM

F16.259 Hallucinogen dependence with hallucinogen-induced psychotic disorder, unspecified HCC ESR COM

F16.28 Hallucinogen dependence with other hallucinogen-induced disorder (6th)

F16.28Ø Hallucinogen dependence with hallucinogen-induced anxiety disorder HCC ESR COM

F16.283 Hallucinogen dependence with hallucinogen persisting perception disorder (flashbacks) HCC ESR COM

F16.288 Hallucinogen dependence with other hallucinogen-induced disorder HCC ESR COM

F16.29 Hallucinogen dependence with unspecified hallucinogen-induced disorder HCC ESR COM

F16.9 Hallucinogen use, unspecified

EXCLUDES 1 *hallucinogen abuse (F16.1-)*
hallucinogen dependence (F16.2-)

TIP: Assign a substance use code only when the provider documents a relationship between the use and an associated physical, mental, or behavioral disorder. As with all diagnoses, substance use codes must meet the definition of a reportable diagnosis.

F16.90 Hallucinogen use, unspecified, uncomplicated
AHA: 2018,2Q,10-11

● **F16.91 Hallucinogen use, unspecified, in remission**

F16.92 Hallucinogen use, unspecified with intoxication

F16.920 Hallucinogen use, unspecified with intoxication, uncomplicated HCC ESR COM

F16.921 Hallucinogen use, unspecified with intoxication with delirium HCC ESR COM
Other hallucinogen intoxication delirium

F16.929 Hallucinogen use, unspecified with intoxication, unspecified HCC ESR COM

F16.94 Hallucinogen use, unspecified with hallucinogen-induced mood disorder HCC ESR COM
Other hallucinogen induced bipolar or related disorder, without use disorder
Other hallucinogen induced depressive disorder, without use disorder
Phencyclidine induced bipolar or related disorder, without use disorder
Phencyclidine induced depressive disorder, without use disorder

F16.95 Hallucinogen use, unspecified with hallucinogen-induced psychotic disorder

F16.950 Hallucinogen use, unspecified with hallucinogen-induced psychotic disorder with delusions HCC ESR COM

F16.951 Hallucinogen use, unspecified with hallucinogen-induced psychotic disorder with hallucinations HCC ESR COM

F16.959 Hallucinogen use, unspecified with hallucinogen-induced psychotic disorder, unspecified HCC ESR COM
Other hallucinogen induced psychotic disorder, without use disorder
Phencyclidine induced psychotic disorder, without use disorder

F16.98 Hallucinogen use, unspecified with other specified hallucinogen-induced disorder

F16.980 Hallucinogen use, unspecified with hallucinogen-induced anxiety disorder HCC ESR COM
Other hallucinogen-induced anxiety disorder, without use disorder
Phencyclidine induced anxiety disorder, without use disorder

F16.983 Hallucinogen use, unspecified with hallucinogen persisting perception disorder (flashbacks) HCC ESR COM

F16.988 Hallucinogen use, unspecified with other hallucinogen-induced disorder HCC ESR COM

F16.99 Hallucinogen use, unspecified with unspecified hallucinogen-induced disorder HCC ESR COM

F17 Nicotine dependence

EXCLUDES 1 *history of tobacco dependence (Z87.891)*
tobacco use NOS (Z72.0)

EXCLUDES 2 *tobacco use (smoking) during pregnancy, childbirth and the puerperium (O99.33-)*
toxic effect of nicotine (T65.2-)

AHA: 2013,4Q,108-109

F17.2 Nicotine dependence

F17.20 Nicotine dependence, unspecified

F17.200 Nicotine dependence, unspecified, uncomplicated
Tobacco use disorder, mild
Tobacco use disorder, moderate
Tobacco use disorder, severe
AHA: 2016,1Q,36
TIP: Assign when provider documentation indicates "smoker" without further specification.

F17.201 Nicotine dependence, unspecified, in remission
Tobacco use disorder, mild, in early remission
Tobacco use disorder, mild, in sustained remission
Tobacco use disorder, moderate, in early remission
Tobacco use disorder, moderate, in sustained remission
Tobacco use disorder, severe, in early remission
Tobacco use disorder, severe, in sustained remission

F17.203 Nicotine dependence unspecified, with withdrawal
Tobacco withdrawal

F17.208 Nicotine dependence, unspecified, with other nicotine-induced disorders

F17.209 Nicotine dependence, unspecified, with unspecified nicotine-induced disorders

F17.21 Nicotine dependence, cigarettes

F17.210 Nicotine dependence, cigarettes, uncomplicated
AHA: 2017,2Q,28-29

F17.211 Nicotine dependence, cigarettes, in remission
Tobacco use disorder, cigarettes, mild, in early remission
Tobacco use disorder, cigarettes, mild, in sustained remission
Tobacco use disorder, cigarettes, moderate, in early remission
Tobacco use disorder, cigarettes, moderate, in sustained remission
Tobacco use disorder, cigarettes, severe, in early remission
Tobacco use disorder, cigarettes, severe, in sustained remission

F17.213 Nicotine dependence, cigarettes, with withdrawal

F17.218 Nicotine dependence, cigarettes, with other nicotine-induced disorders

F17.219 Nicotine dependence, cigarettes, with unspecified nicotine-induced disorders

F17.22 Nicotine dependence, chewing tobacco

F17.220 Nicotine dependence, chewing tobacco, uncomplicated

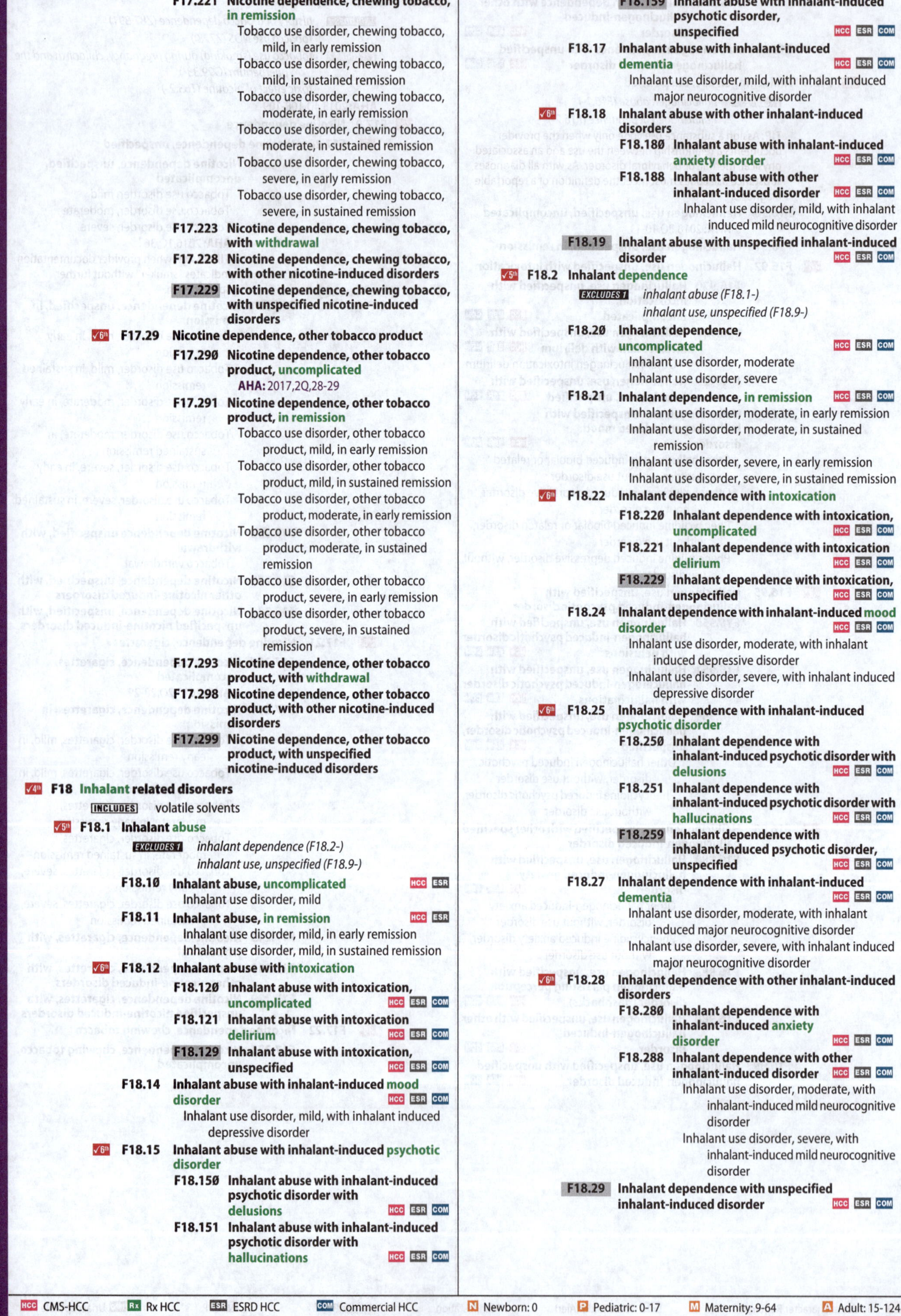

F17.221 Nicotine dependence, chewing tobacco, in remission
Tobacco use disorder, chewing tobacco, mild, in early remission
Tobacco use disorder, chewing tobacco, mild, in sustained remission
Tobacco use disorder, chewing tobacco, moderate, in early remission
Tobacco use disorder, chewing tobacco, moderate, in sustained remission
Tobacco use disorder, chewing tobacco, severe, in early remission
Tobacco use disorder, chewing tobacco, severe, in sustained remission

F17.223 Nicotine dependence, chewing tobacco, with withdrawal

F17.228 Nicotine dependence, chewing tobacco, with other nicotine-induced disorders

F17.229 Nicotine dependence, chewing tobacco, with unspecified nicotine-induced disorders

✓6th **F17.29 Nicotine dependence, other tobacco product**

F17.290 Nicotine dependence, other tobacco product, uncomplicated
AHA: 2017,2Q,28-29

F17.291 Nicotine dependence, other tobacco product, in remission
Tobacco use disorder, other tobacco product, mild, in early remission
Tobacco use disorder, other tobacco product, mild, in sustained remission
Tobacco use disorder, other tobacco product, moderate, in early remission
Tobacco use disorder, other tobacco product, moderate, in sustained remission
Tobacco use disorder, other tobacco product, severe, in early remission
Tobacco use disorder, other tobacco product, severe, in sustained remission

F17.293 Nicotine dependence, other tobacco product, with withdrawal

F17.298 Nicotine dependence, other tobacco product, with other nicotine-induced disorders

F17.299 Nicotine dependence, other tobacco product, with unspecified nicotine-induced disorders

✓4th **F18 Inhalant related disorders**

INCLUDES volatile solvents

✓5th **F18.1 Inhalant abuse**

EXCLUDES 1 *inhalant dependence (F18.2-)*
inhalant use, unspecified (F18.9-)

F18.10 Inhalant abuse, uncomplicated HCC ESR
Inhalant use disorder, mild

F18.11 Inhalant abuse, in remission HCC ESR
Inhalant use disorder, mild, in early remission
Inhalant use disorder, mild, in sustained remission

✓6th **F18.12 Inhalant abuse with intoxication**

F18.120 Inhalant abuse with intoxication, uncomplicated HCC ESR COM

F18.121 Inhalant abuse with intoxication delirium HCC ESR COM

F18.129 Inhalant abuse with intoxication, unspecified HCC ESR COM

F18.14 Inhalant abuse with inhalant-induced mood disorder HCC ESR COM
Inhalant use disorder, mild, with inhalant induced depressive disorder

✓6th **F18.15 Inhalant abuse with inhalant-induced psychotic disorder**

F18.150 Inhalant abuse with inhalant-induced psychotic disorder with delusions HCC ESR COM

F18.151 Inhalant abuse with inhalant-induced psychotic disorder with hallucinations HCC ESR COM

F18.159 Inhalant abuse with inhalant-induced psychotic disorder, unspecified HCC ESR COM

F18.17 Inhalant abuse with inhalant-induced dementia HCC ESR COM
Inhalant use disorder, mild, with inhalant induced major neurocognitive disorder

✓6th **F18.18 Inhalant abuse with other inhalant-induced disorders**

F18.180 Inhalant abuse with inhalant-induced anxiety disorder HCC ESR COM

F18.188 Inhalant abuse with other inhalant-induced disorder HCC ESR COM
Inhalant use disorder, mild, with inhalant induced mild neurocognitive disorder

F18.19 Inhalant abuse with unspecified inhalant-induced disorder HCC ESR COM

✓5th **F18.2 Inhalant dependence**

EXCLUDES 1 *inhalant abuse (F18.1-)*
inhalant use, unspecified (F18.9-)

F18.20 Inhalant dependence, uncomplicated HCC ESR COM
Inhalant use disorder, moderate
Inhalant use disorder, severe

F18.21 Inhalant dependence, in remission HCC ESR COM
Inhalant use disorder, moderate, in early remission
Inhalant use disorder, moderate, in sustained remission
Inhalant use disorder, severe, in early remission
Inhalant use disorder, severe, in sustained remission

✓6th **F18.22 Inhalant dependence with intoxication**

F18.220 Inhalant dependence with intoxication, uncomplicated HCC ESR COM

F18.221 Inhalant dependence with intoxication delirium HCC ESR COM

F18.229 Inhalant dependence with intoxication, unspecified HCC ESR COM

F18.24 Inhalant dependence with inhalant-induced mood disorder HCC ESR COM
Inhalant use disorder, moderate, with inhalant induced depressive disorder
Inhalant use disorder, severe, with inhalant induced depressive disorder

✓6th **F18.25 Inhalant dependence with inhalant-induced psychotic disorder**

F18.250 Inhalant dependence with inhalant-induced psychotic disorder with delusions HCC ESR COM

F18.251 Inhalant dependence with inhalant-induced psychotic disorder with hallucinations HCC ESR COM

F18.259 Inhalant dependence with inhalant-induced psychotic disorder, unspecified HCC ESR COM

F18.27 Inhalant dependence with inhalant-induced dementia HCC ESR COM
Inhalant use disorder, moderate, with inhalant induced major neurocognitive disorder
Inhalant use disorder, severe, with inhalant induced major neurocognitive disorder

✓6th **F18.28 Inhalant dependence with other inhalant-induced disorders**

F18.280 Inhalant dependence with inhalant-induced anxiety disorder HCC ESR COM

F18.288 Inhalant dependence with other inhalant-induced disorder HCC ESR COM
Inhalant use disorder, moderate, with inhalant-induced mild neurocognitive disorder
Inhalant use disorder, severe, with inhalant-induced mild neurocognitive disorder

F18.29 Inhalant dependence with unspecified inhalant-induced disorder HCC ESR COM

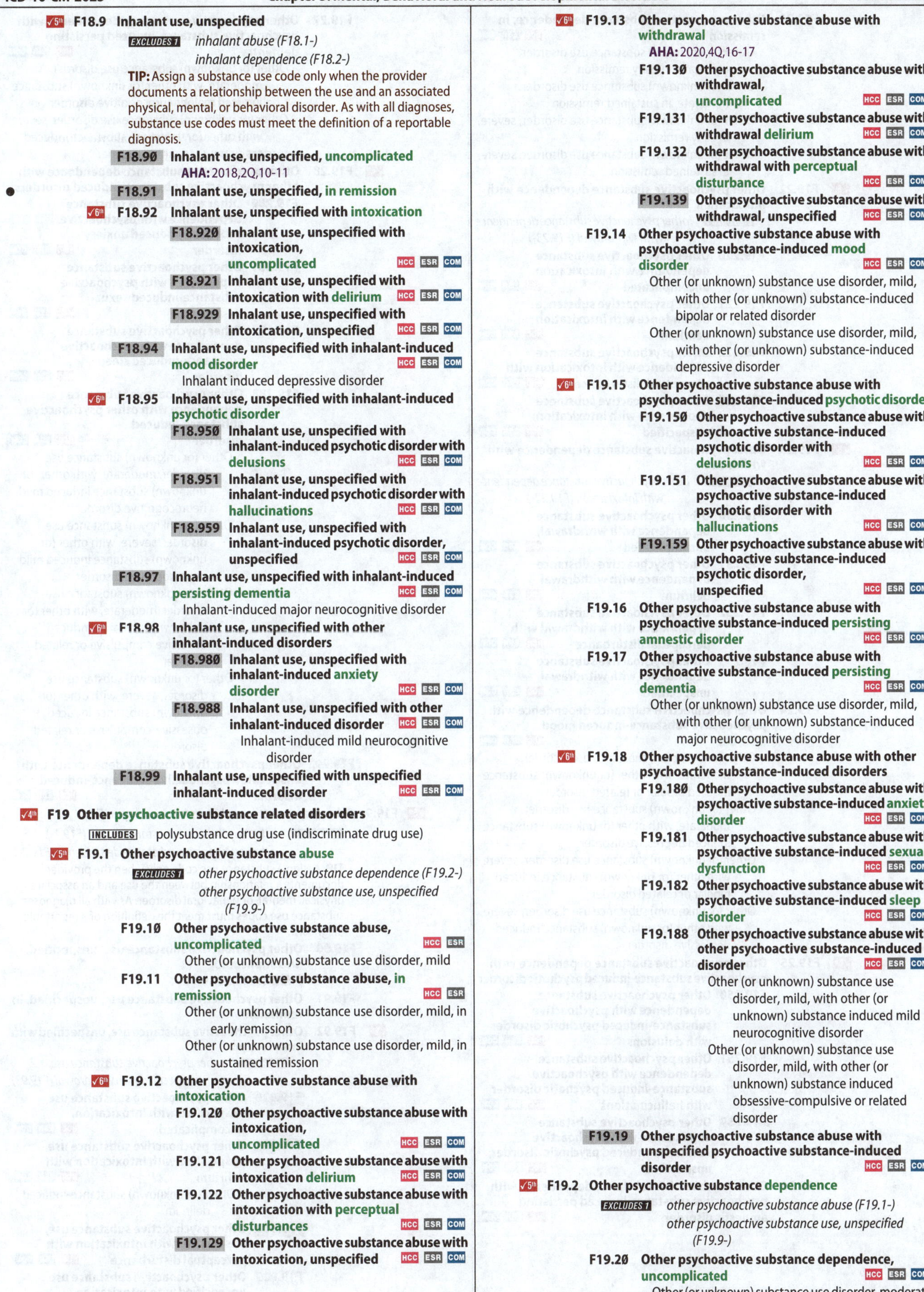

√5th **F18.9 Inhalant use, unspecified**

EXCLUDES 1 *inhalant abuse (F18.1-)*
inhalant dependence (F18.2-)

TIP: Assign a substance use code only when the provider documents a relationship between the use and an associated physical, mental, or behavioral disorder. As with all diagnoses, substance use codes must meet the definition of a reportable diagnosis.

F18.90 Inhalant use, unspecified, uncomplicated
AHA: 2018,2Q,10-11

● **F18.91 Inhalant use, unspecified, in remission**

√6th **F18.92 Inhalant use, unspecified with intoxication**

F18.920 Inhalant use, unspecified with intoxication, uncomplicated HCC ESR COM

F18.921 Inhalant use, unspecified with intoxication with delirium HCC ESR COM

F18.929 Inhalant use, unspecified with intoxication, unspecified HCC ESR COM

F18.94 Inhalant use, unspecified with inhalant-induced mood disorder HCC ESR COM
Inhalant induced depressive disorder

√6th **F18.95 Inhalant use, unspecified with inhalant-induced psychotic disorder**

F18.950 Inhalant use, unspecified with inhalant-induced psychotic disorder with delusions HCC ESR COM

F18.951 Inhalant use, unspecified with inhalant-induced psychotic disorder with hallucinations HCC ESR COM

F18.959 Inhalant use, unspecified with inhalant-induced psychotic disorder, unspecified HCC ESR COM

F18.97 Inhalant use, unspecified with inhalant-induced persisting dementia HCC ESR COM
Inhalant-induced major neurocognitive disorder

√6th **F18.98 Inhalant use, unspecified with other inhalant-induced disorders**

F18.980 Inhalant use, unspecified with inhalant-induced anxiety disorder HCC ESR COM

F18.988 Inhalant use, unspecified with other inhalant-induced disorder HCC ESR COM
Inhalant-induced mild neurocognitive disorder

F18.99 Inhalant use, unspecified with unspecified inhalant-induced disorder HCC ESR COM

√4th **F19 Other psychoactive substance related disorders**

INCLUDES polysubstance drug use (indiscriminate drug use)

√5th **F19.1 Other psychoactive substance abuse**

EXCLUDES 1 *other psychoactive substance dependence (F19.2-)*
other psychoactive substance use, unspecified (F19.9-)

F19.10 Other psychoactive substance abuse, uncomplicated HCC ESR
Other (or unknown) substance use disorder, mild

F19.11 Other psychoactive substance abuse, in remission HCC ESR
Other (or unknown) substance use disorder, mild, in early remission
Other (or unknown) substance use disorder, mild, in sustained remission

√6th **F19.12 Other psychoactive substance abuse with intoxication**

F19.120 Other psychoactive substance abuse with intoxication, uncomplicated HCC ESR COM

F19.121 Other psychoactive substance abuse with intoxication delirium HCC ESR COM

F19.122 Other psychoactive substance abuse with intoxication with perceptual disturbances HCC ESR COM

F19.129 Other psychoactive substance abuse with intoxication, unspecified HCC ESR COM

√6th **F19.13 Other psychoactive substance abuse with withdrawal**
AHA: 2020,4Q,16-17

F19.130 Other psychoactive substance abuse with withdrawal, uncomplicated HCC ESR COM

F19.131 Other psychoactive substance abuse with withdrawal delirium HCC ESR COM

F19.132 Other psychoactive substance abuse with withdrawal with perceptual disturbance HCC ESR COM

F19.139 Other psychoactive substance abuse with withdrawal, unspecified HCC ESR COM

F19.14 Other psychoactive substance abuse with psychoactive substance-induced mood disorder HCC ESR COM
Other (or unknown) substance use disorder, mild, with other (or unknown) substance-induced bipolar or related disorder
Other (or unknown) substance use disorder, mild, with other (or unknown) substance-induced depressive disorder

√6th **F19.15 Other psychoactive substance abuse with psychoactive substance-induced psychotic disorder**

F19.150 Other psychoactive substance abuse with psychoactive substance-induced psychotic disorder with delusions HCC ESR COM

F19.151 Other psychoactive substance abuse with psychoactive substance-induced psychotic disorder with hallucinations HCC ESR COM

F19.159 Other psychoactive substance abuse with psychoactive substance-induced psychotic disorder, unspecified HCC ESR COM

F19.16 Other psychoactive substance abuse with psychoactive substance-induced persisting amnestic disorder HCC ESR COM

F19.17 Other psychoactive substance abuse with psychoactive substance-induced persisting dementia HCC ESR COM
Other (or unknown) substance use disorder, mild, with other (or unknown) substance-induced major neurocognitive disorder

√6th **F19.18 Other psychoactive substance abuse with other psychoactive substance-induced disorders**

F19.180 Other psychoactive substance abuse with psychoactive substance-induced anxiety disorder HCC ESR COM

F19.181 Other psychoactive substance abuse with psychoactive substance-induced sexual dysfunction HCC ESR COM

F19.182 Other psychoactive substance abuse with psychoactive substance-induced sleep disorder HCC ESR COM

F19.188 Other psychoactive substance abuse with other psychoactive substance-induced disorder HCC ESR COM
Other (or unknown) substance use disorder, mild, with other (or unknown) substance induced mild neurocognitive disorder
Other (or unknown) substance use disorder, mild, with other (or unknown) substance induced obsessive-compulsive or related disorder

F19.19 Other psychoactive substance abuse with unspecified psychoactive substance-induced disorder HCC ESR COM

√5th **F19.2 Other psychoactive substance dependence**

EXCLUDES 1 *other psychoactive substance abuse (F19.1-)*
other psychoactive substance use, unspecified (F19.9-)

F19.20 Other psychoactive substance dependence, uncomplicated HCC ESR COM
Other (or unknown) substance use disorder, moderate
Other (or unknown) substance use disorder, severe

Chapter 5. Mental, Behavioral and Neurodevelopmental Disorders

F18.9–F19.20

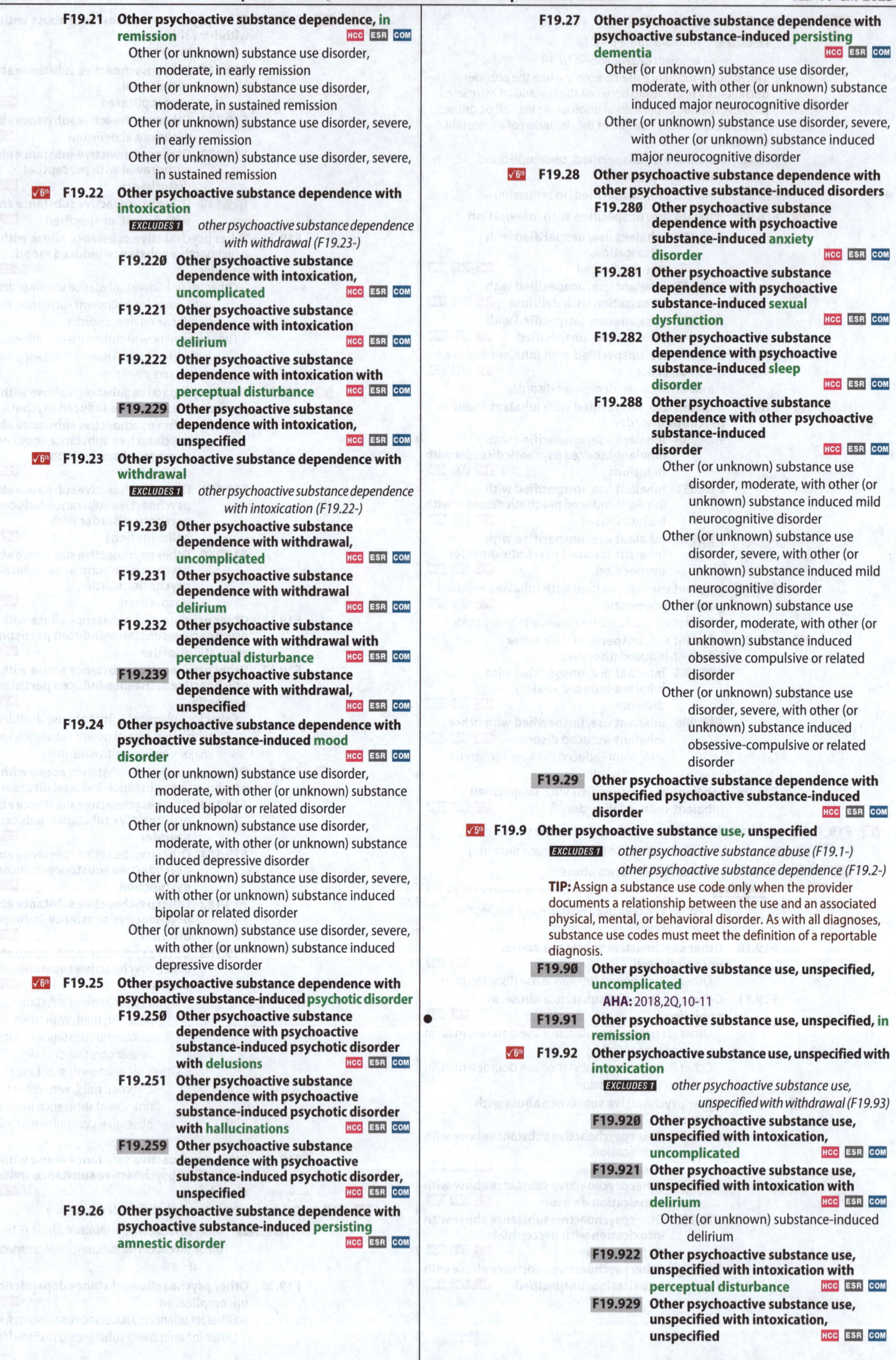

F19.21 Other psychoactive substance dependence, in remission HCC ESR COM
Other (or unknown) substance use disorder, moderate, in early remission
Other (or unknown) substance use disorder, moderate, in sustained remission
Other (or unknown) substance use disorder, severe, in early remission
Other (or unknown) substance use disorder, severe, in sustained remission

✓6th **F19.22 Other psychoactive substance dependence with intoxication**
EXCLUDES 1 *other psychoactive substance dependence with withdrawal (F19.23-)*

F19.220 Other psychoactive substance dependence with intoxication, uncomplicated HCC ESR COM

F19.221 Other psychoactive substance dependence with intoxication delirium HCC ESR COM

F19.222 Other psychoactive substance dependence with intoxication with perceptual disturbance HCC ESR COM

F19.229 Other psychoactive substance dependence with intoxication, unspecified HCC ESR COM

✓6th **F19.23 Other psychoactive substance dependence with withdrawal**
EXCLUDES 1 *other psychoactive substance dependence with intoxication (F19.22-)*

F19.230 Other psychoactive substance dependence with withdrawal, uncomplicated HCC ESR COM

F19.231 Other psychoactive substance dependence with withdrawal delirium HCC ESR COM

F19.232 Other psychoactive substance dependence with withdrawal with perceptual disturbance HCC ESR COM

F19.239 Other psychoactive substance dependence with withdrawal, unspecified HCC ESR COM

F19.24 Other psychoactive substance dependence with psychoactive substance-induced mood disorder HCC ESR COM
Other (or unknown) substance use disorder, moderate, with other (or unknown) substance induced bipolar or related disorder
Other (or unknown) substance use disorder, moderate, with other (or unknown) substance induced depressive disorder
Other (or unknown) substance use disorder, severe, with other (or unknown) substance induced bipolar or related disorder
Other (or unknown) substance use disorder, severe, with other (or unknown) substance induced depressive disorder

✓6th **F19.25 Other psychoactive substance dependence with psychoactive substance-induced psychotic disorder**

F19.250 Other psychoactive substance dependence with psychoactive substance-induced psychotic disorder with delusions HCC ESR COM

F19.251 Other psychoactive substance dependence with psychoactive substance-induced psychotic disorder with hallucinations HCC ESR COM

F19.259 Other psychoactive substance dependence with psychoactive substance-induced psychotic disorder, unspecified HCC ESR COM

F19.26 Other psychoactive substance dependence with psychoactive substance-induced persisting amnestic disorder HCC ESR COM

F19.27 Other psychoactive substance dependence with psychoactive substance-induced persisting dementia HCC ESR COM
Other (or unknown) substance use disorder, moderate, with other (or unknown) substance induced major neurocognitive disorder
Other (or unknown) substance use disorder, severe, with other (or unknown) substance induced major neurocognitive disorder

✓6th **F19.28 Other psychoactive substance dependence with other psychoactive substance-induced disorders**

F19.280 Other psychoactive substance dependence with psychoactive substance-induced anxiety disorder HCC ESR COM

F19.281 Other psychoactive substance dependence with psychoactive substance-induced sexual dysfunction HCC ESR COM

F19.282 Other psychoactive substance dependence with psychoactive substance-induced sleep disorder HCC ESR COM

F19.288 Other psychoactive substance dependence with other psychoactive substance-induced disorder HCC ESR COM
Other (or unknown) substance use disorder, moderate, with other (or unknown) substance induced mild neurocognitive disorder
Other (or unknown) substance use disorder, severe, with other (or unknown) substance induced mild neurocognitive disorder
Other (or unknown) substance use disorder, moderate, with other (or unknown) substance induced obsessive compulsive or related disorder
Other (or unknown) substance use disorder, severe, with other (or unknown) substance induced obsessive-compulsive or related disorder

F19.29 Other psychoactive substance dependence with unspecified psychoactive substance-induced disorder HCC ESR COM

✓5th **F19.9 Other psychoactive substance use, unspecified**
EXCLUDES 1 *other psychoactive substance abuse (F19.1-)*
other psychoactive substance dependence (F19.2-)

TIP: Assign a substance use code only when the provider documents a relationship between the use and an associated physical, mental, or behavioral disorder. As with all diagnoses, substance use codes must meet the definition of a reportable diagnosis.

F19.90 Other psychoactive substance use, unspecified, uncomplicated
AHA: 2018,2Q,10-11

● **F19.91 Other psychoactive substance use, unspecified, in remission**

✓6th **F19.92 Other psychoactive substance use, unspecified with intoxication**
EXCLUDES 1 *other psychoactive substance use, unspecified with withdrawal (F19.93)*

F19.920 Other psychoactive substance use, unspecified with intoxication, uncomplicated HCC ESR COM

F19.921 Other psychoactive substance use, unspecified with intoxication with delirium HCC ESR COM
Other (or unknown) substance-induced delirium

F19.922 Other psychoactive substance use, unspecified with intoxication with perceptual disturbance HCC ESR COM

F19.929 Other psychoactive substance use, unspecified with intoxication, unspecified HCC ESR COM

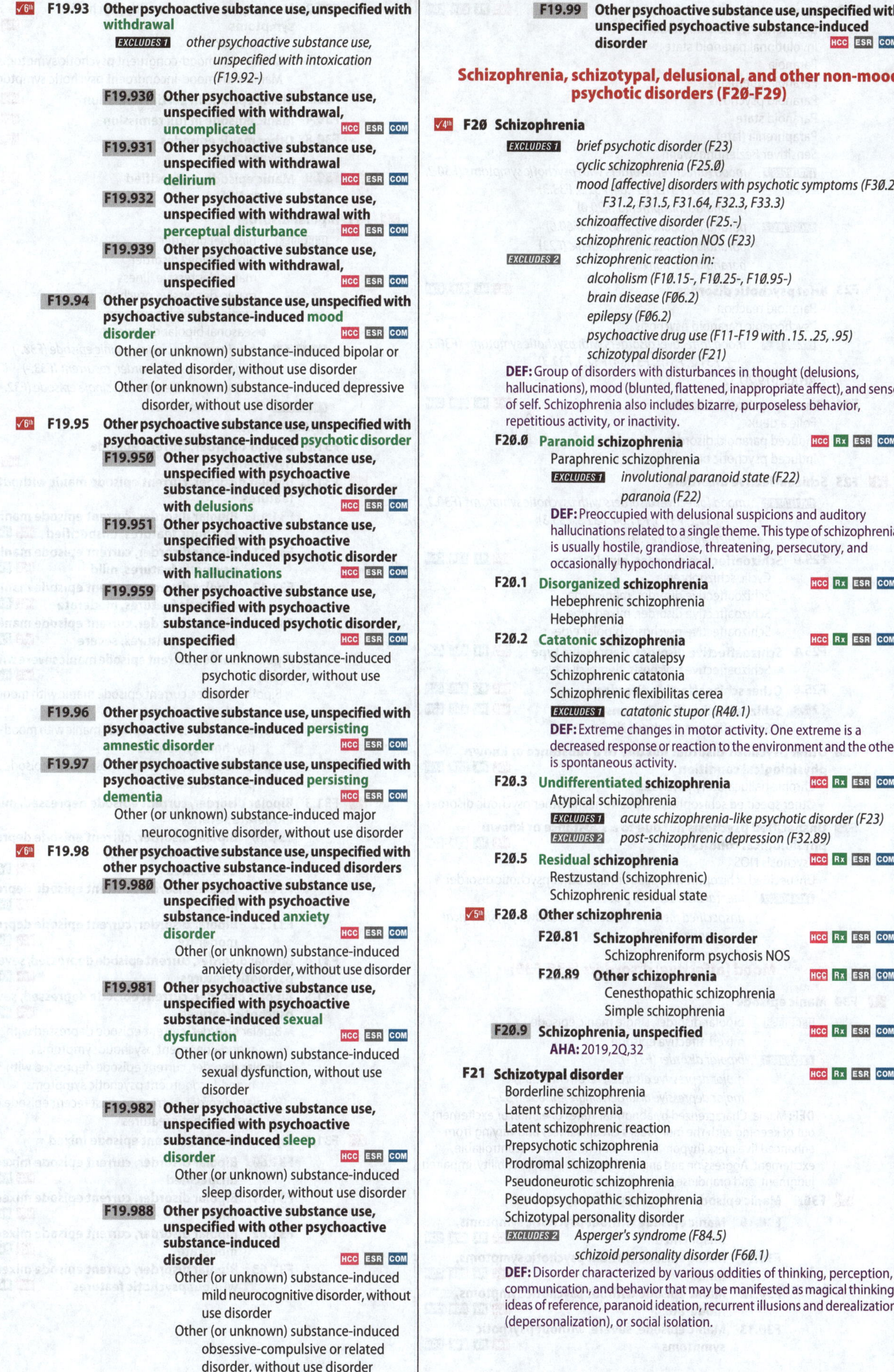

✓6th **F19.93 Other psychoactive substance use, unspecified with withdrawal**

EXCLUDES 1 *other psychoactive substance use, unspecified with intoxication (F19.92-)*

F19.930 Other psychoactive substance use, unspecified with withdrawal, uncomplicated HCC ESR COM

F19.931 Other psychoactive substance use, unspecified with withdrawal delirium HCC ESR COM

F19.932 Other psychoactive substance use, unspecified with withdrawal with perceptual disturbance HCC ESR COM

F19.939 Other psychoactive substance use, unspecified with withdrawal, unspecified HCC ESR COM

F19.94 Other psychoactive substance use, unspecified with psychoactive substance-induced mood disorder HCC ESR COM

Other (or unknown) substance-induced bipolar or related disorder, without use disorder

Other (or unknown) substance-induced depressive disorder, without use disorder

✓6th **F19.95 Other psychoactive substance use, unspecified with psychoactive substance-induced psychotic disorder**

F19.950 Other psychoactive substance use, unspecified with psychoactive substance-induced psychotic disorder with delusions HCC ESR COM

F19.951 Other psychoactive substance use, unspecified with psychoactive substance-induced psychotic disorder with hallucinations HCC ESR COM

F19.959 Other psychoactive substance use, unspecified with psychoactive substance-induced psychotic disorder, unspecified HCC ESR COM

Other or unknown substance-induced psychotic disorder, without use disorder

F19.96 Other psychoactive substance use, unspecified with psychoactive substance-induced persisting amnestic disorder HCC ESR COM

F19.97 Other psychoactive substance use, unspecified with psychoactive substance-induced persisting dementia HCC ESR COM

Other (or unknown) substance-induced major neurocognitive disorder, without use disorder

✓6th **F19.98 Other psychoactive substance use, unspecified with other psychoactive substance-induced disorders**

F19.980 Other psychoactive substance use, unspecified with psychoactive substance-induced anxiety disorder HCC ESR COM

Other (or unknown) substance-induced anxiety disorder, without use disorder

F19.981 Other psychoactive substance use, unspecified with psychoactive substance-induced sexual dysfunction HCC ESR COM

Other (or unknown) substance-induced sexual dysfunction, without use disorder

F19.982 Other psychoactive substance use, unspecified with psychoactive substance-induced sleep disorder HCC ESR COM

Other (or unknown) substance-induced sleep disorder, without use disorder

F19.988 Other psychoactive substance use, unspecified with other psychoactive substance-induced disorder HCC ESR COM

Other (or unknown) substance-induced mild neurocognitive disorder, without use disorder

Other (or unknown) substance-induced obsessive-compulsive or related disorder, without use disorder

F19.99 Other psychoactive substance use, unspecified with unspecified psychoactive substance-induced disorder HCC ESR COM

Schizophrenia, schizotypal, delusional, and other non-mood psychotic disorders (F20-F29)

✓4th **F20 Schizophrenia**

EXCLUDES 1 *brief psychotic disorder (F23)*
cyclic schizophrenia (F25.0)
mood [affective] disorders with psychotic symptoms (F30.2, F31.2, F31.5, F31.64, F32.3, F33.3)
schizoaffective disorder (F25.-)
schizophrenic reaction NOS (F23)

EXCLUDES 2 *schizophrenic reaction in:*
alcoholism (F10.15-, F10.25-, F10.95-)
brain disease (F06.2)
epilepsy (F06.2)
psychoactive drug use (F11-F19 with .15, .25, .95)
schizotypal disorder (F21)

DEF: Group of disorders with disturbances in thought (delusions, hallucinations), mood (blunted, flattened, inappropriate affect), and sense of self. Schizophrenia also includes bizarre, purposeless behavior, repetitious activity, or inactivity.

F20.0 Paranoid schizophrenia HCC Rx ESR COM

Paraphrenic schizophrenia

EXCLUDES 1 *involutional paranoid state (F22)*
paranoia (F22)

DEF: Preoccupied with delusional suspicions and auditory hallucinations related to a single theme. This type of schizophrenia is usually hostile, grandiose, threatening, persecutory, and occasionally hypochondriacal.

F20.1 Disorganized schizophrenia HCC Rx ESR COM

Hebephrenic schizophrenia
Hebephrenia

F20.2 Catatonic schizophrenia HCC Rx ESR COM

Schizophrenic catalepsy
Schizophrenic catatonia
Schizophrenic flexibilitas cerea

EXCLUDES 1 *catatonic stupor (R40.1)*

DEF: Extreme changes in motor activity. One extreme is a decreased response or reaction to the environment and the other is spontaneous activity.

F20.3 Undifferentiated schizophrenia HCC Rx ESR COM

Atypical schizophrenia

EXCLUDES 1 *acute schizophrenia-like psychotic disorder (F23)*

EXCLUDES 2 *post-schizophrenic depression (F32.89)*

F20.5 Residual schizophrenia HCC Rx ESR COM

Restzustand (schizophrenic)
Schizophrenic residual state

✓5th **F20.8 Other schizophrenia**

F20.81 Schizophreniform disorder HCC Rx ESR COM

Schizophreniform psychosis NOS

F20.89 Other schizophrenia HCC Rx ESR COM

Cenesthopathic schizophrenia
Simple schizophrenia

F20.9 Schizophrenia, unspecified HCC Rx ESR COM

AHA: 2019,2Q,32

F21 Schizotypal disorder HCC Rx ESR COM

Borderline schizophrenia
Latent schizophrenia
Latent schizophrenic reaction
Prepsychotic schizophrenia
Prodromal schizophrenia
Pseudoneurotic schizophrenia
Pseudopsychopathic schizophrenia
Schizotypal personality disorder

EXCLUDES 2 *Asperger's syndrome (F84.5)*
schizoid personality disorder (F60.1)

DEF: Disorder characterized by various oddities of thinking, perception, communication, and behavior that may be manifested as magical thinking, ideas of reference, paranoid ideation, recurrent illusions and derealization (depersonalization), or social isolation.

F22 Delusional disorders HCC Rx ESR COM
Delusional dysmorphophobia
Involutional paranoid state
Paranoia
Paranoia querulans
Paranoid psychosis
Paranoid state
Paraphrenia (late)
Sensitiver Beziehungswahn
EXCLUDES 1 *mood [affective] disorders with psychotic symptoms (F3Ø.2, F31.2, F31.5, F31.64, F32.3, F33.3)*
paranoid schizophrenia (F2Ø.Ø)
EXCLUDES 2 *paranoid personality disorder (F6Ø.Ø)*
paranoid psychosis, psychogenic (F23)
paranoid reaction (F23)

F23 Brief psychotic disorder HCC Rx ESR COM
Paranoid reaction
Psychogenic paranoid psychosis
EXCLUDES 2 *mood [affective] disorders with psychotic symptoms (F3Ø.2, F31.2, F31.5, F31.64, F32.3, F33.3)*
AHA: 2019,2Q,32

F24 Shared psychotic disorder HCC Rx ESR COM
Folie à deux
Induced paranoid disorder
Induced psychotic disorder

✓4th **F25 Schizoaffective disorders**
EXCLUDES 1 *mood [affective] disorders with psychotic symptoms (F3Ø.2, F31.2, F31.5, F31.64, F32.3, F33.3)*
schizophrenia (F2Ø.-)

F25.Ø Schizoaffective disorder, bipolar type HCC Rx ESR COM
Cyclic schizophrenia
Schizoaffective disorder, manic type
Schizoaffective disorder, mixed type
Schizoaffective psychosis, bipolar type

F25.1 Schizoaffective disorder, depressive type HCC Rx ESR COM
Schizoaffective psychosis, depressive type

F25.8 Other schizoaffective disorders HCC Rx ESR COM

F25.9 Schizoaffective disorder, unspecified HCC Rx ESR COM
Schizoaffective psychosis NOS

F28 Other psychotic disorder not due to a substance or known physiological condition HCC Rx ESR COM
Chronic hallucinatory psychosis
Other specified schizophrenia spectrum and other psychotic disorder

F29 Unspecified psychosis not due to a substance or known physiological condition HCC Rx ESR COM
Psychosis NOS
Unspecified schizophrenia spectrum and other psychotic disorder
EXCLUDES 1 *mental disorder NOS (F99)*
unspecified mental disorder due to known physiological condition (FØ9)

Mood [affective] disorders (F3Ø-F39)

✓4th **F3Ø Manic episode**
INCLUDES bipolar disorder, single manic episode
mixed affective episode
EXCLUDES 1 *bipolar disorder (F31.-)*
major depressive disorder, recurrent (F33.-)
major depressive disorder, single episode (F32.-)

DEF: Mania: Characterized by abnormal states of elation or excitement out of keeping with the individual's circumstances and varying from enhanced liveliness (hypomania) to violent, almost uncontrollable, excitement. Aggression and anger, flight of ideas, distractibility, impaired judgment, and grandiose ideas are common.

✓5th **F3Ø.1 Manic episode without psychotic symptoms**

F3Ø.1Ø Manic episode without psychotic symptoms, unspecified HCC Rx ESR COM

F3Ø.11 Manic episode without psychotic symptoms, mild HCC Rx ESR COM

F3Ø.12 Manic episode without psychotic symptoms, moderate HCC Rx ESR COM

F3Ø.13 Manic episode, severe, without psychotic symptoms HCC Rx ESR COM

F3Ø.2 Manic episode, severe with psychotic symptoms HCC Rx ESR COM
Manic stupor
Mania with mood-congruent psychotic symptoms
Mania with mood-incongruent psychotic symptoms

F3Ø.3 Manic episode in partial remission HCC Rx ESR COM

F3Ø.4 Manic episode in full remission HCC Rx ESR COM

F3Ø.8 Other manic episodes HCC Rx ESR COM
Hypomania

F3Ø.9 Manic episode, unspecified HCC Rx ESR COM
Mania NOS

✓4th **F31 Bipolar disorder**
INCLUDES bipolar I disorder
bipolar type I disorder
manic-depressive illness
manic-depressive psychosis
manic-depressive reaction
▶seasonal bipolar disorder◀
EXCLUDES 1 *bipolar disorder, single manic episode (F3Ø.-)*
major depressive disorder, recurrent (F33.-)
major depressive disorder, single episode (F32.-)
EXCLUDES 2 *cyclothymia (F34.Ø)*
AHA: 2020,1Q,23

F31.Ø Bipolar disorder, current episode hypomanic HCC Rx ESR COM

✓5th **F31.1 Bipolar disorder, current episode manic without psychotic features**

F31.1Ø Bipolar disorder, current episode manic without psychotic features, unspecified HCC Rx ESR COM Q

F31.11 Bipolar disorder, current episode manic without psychotic features, mild HCC Rx ESR COM Q

F31.12 Bipolar disorder, current episode manic without psychotic features, moderate HCC Rx ESR COM Q

F31.13 Bipolar disorder, current episode manic without psychotic features, severe HCC Rx ESR COM Q

F31.2 Bipolar disorder, current episode manic severe with psychotic features HCC Rx ESR COM Q
Bipolar disorder, current episode manic with mood-congruent psychotic symptoms
Bipolar disorder, current episode manic with mood-incongruent psychotic symptoms
Bipolar I disorder, current or most recent episode manic with psychotic features

✓5th **F31.3 Bipolar disorder, current episode depressed, mild or moderate severity**

F31.3Ø Bipolar disorder, current episode depressed, mild or moderate severity, unspecified HCC Rx ESR COM Q

F31.31 Bipolar disorder, current episode depressed, mild HCC Rx ESR COM Q

F31.32 Bipolar disorder, current episode depressed, moderate HCC Rx ESR COM Q

F31.4 Bipolar disorder, current episode depressed, severe, without psychotic features HCC Rx ESR COM Q

F31.5 Bipolar disorder, current episode depressed, severe, with psychotic features HCC Rx ESR COM Q
Bipolar disorder, current episode depressed with mood-congruent psychotic symptoms
Bipolar disorder, current episode depressed with mood-incongruent psychotic symptoms
Bipolar I disorder, current or most recent episode depressed, with psychotic features

✓5th **F31.6 Bipolar disorder, current episode mixed**

F31.6Ø Bipolar disorder, current episode mixed, unspecified HCC Rx ESR COM Q

F31.61 Bipolar disorder, current episode mixed, mild HCC Rx ESR COM Q

F31.62 Bipolar disorder, current episode mixed, moderate HCC Rx ESR COM Q

F31.63 Bipolar disorder, current episode mixed, severe, without psychotic features HCC Rx ESR COM Q

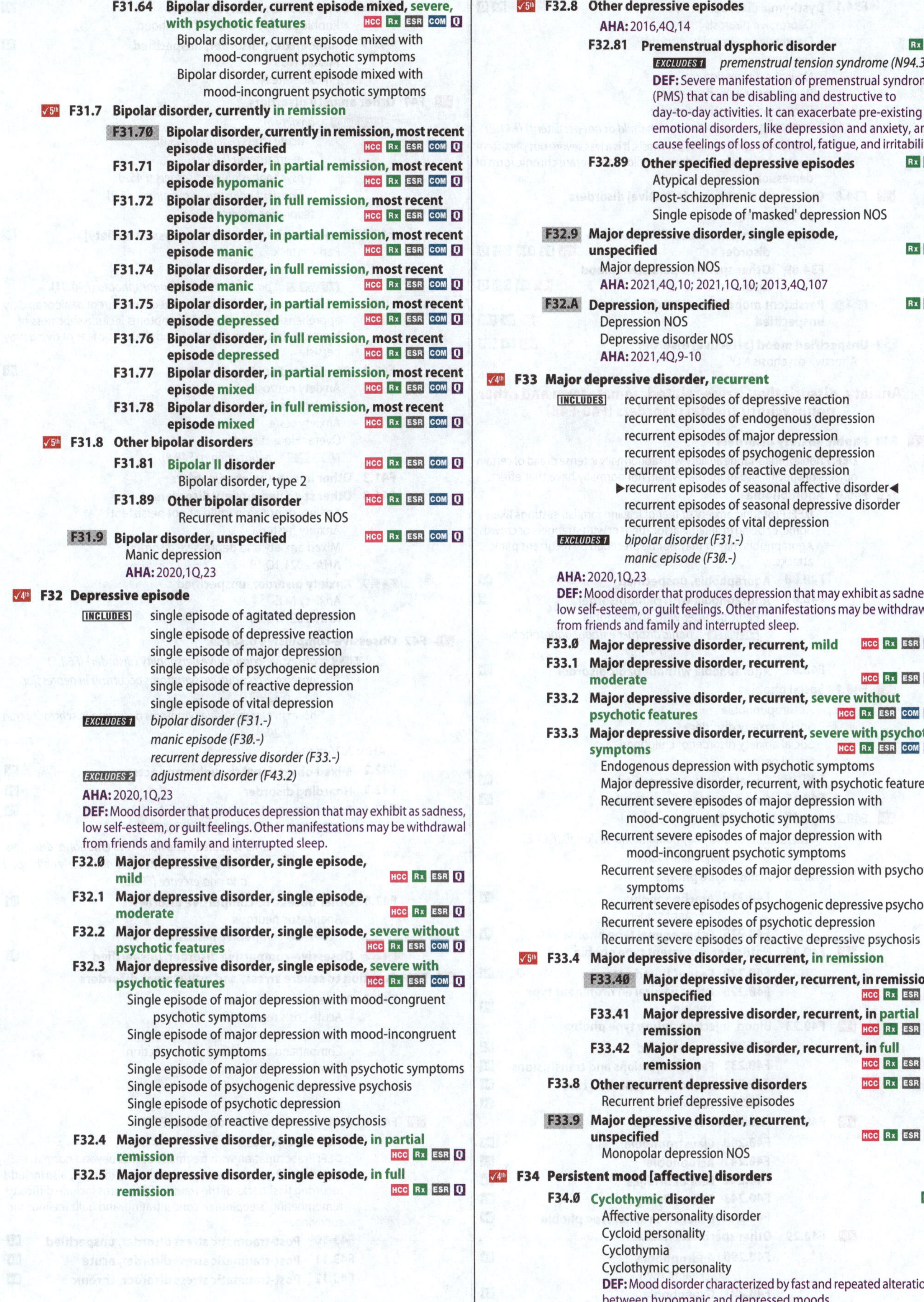

F31.64 Bipolar disorder, current episode mixed, severe, with psychotic features HCC Rx ESR COM Q
Bipolar disorder, current episode mixed with mood-congruent psychotic symptoms
Bipolar disorder, current episode mixed with mood-incongruent psychotic symptoms

F31.7 Bipolar disorder, currently in remission (5th)

F31.7Ø Bipolar disorder, currently in remission, most recent episode unspecified HCC Rx ESR COM Q

F31.71 Bipolar disorder, in partial remission, most recent episode hypomanic HCC Rx ESR COM Q

F31.72 Bipolar disorder, in full remission, most recent episode hypomanic HCC Rx ESR COM Q

F31.73 Bipolar disorder, in partial remission, most recent episode manic HCC Rx ESR COM Q

F31.74 Bipolar disorder, in full remission, most recent episode manic HCC Rx ESR COM Q

F31.75 Bipolar disorder, in partial remission, most recent episode depressed HCC Rx ESR COM Q

F31.76 Bipolar disorder, in full remission, most recent episode depressed HCC Rx ESR COM Q

F31.77 Bipolar disorder, in partial remission, most recent episode mixed HCC Rx ESR COM Q

F31.78 Bipolar disorder, in full remission, most recent episode mixed HCC Rx ESR COM Q

F31.8 Other bipolar disorders (5th)

F31.81 Bipolar II disorder HCC Rx ESR COM Q
Bipolar disorder, type 2

F31.89 Other bipolar disorder HCC Rx ESR COM Q
Recurrent manic episodes NOS

F31.9 Bipolar disorder, unspecified HCC Rx ESR COM Q
Manic depression
AHA: 2020,1Q,23

F32 Depressive episode (4th)

INCLUDES single episode of agitated depression
single episode of depressive reaction
single episode of major depression
single episode of psychogenic depression
single episode of reactive depression
single episode of vital depression

EXCLUDES 1 *bipolar disorder (F31.-)*
manic episode (F3Ø.-)
recurrent depressive disorder (F33.-)

EXCLUDES 2 *adjustment disorder (F43.2)*

AHA: 2020,1Q,23

DEF: Mood disorder that produces depression that may exhibit as sadness, low self-esteem, or guilt feelings. Other manifestations may be withdrawal from friends and family and interrupted sleep.

F32.Ø Major depressive disorder, single episode, mild HCC Rx ESR Q

F32.1 Major depressive disorder, single episode, moderate HCC Rx ESR Q

F32.2 Major depressive disorder, single episode, severe without psychotic features HCC Rx ESR COM Q

F32.3 Major depressive disorder, single episode, severe with psychotic features HCC Rx ESR COM Q
Single episode of major depression with mood-congruent psychotic symptoms
Single episode of major depression with mood-incongruent psychotic symptoms
Single episode of major depression with psychotic symptoms
Single episode of psychogenic depressive psychosis
Single episode of psychotic depression
Single episode of reactive depressive psychosis

F32.4 Major depressive disorder, single episode, in partial remission HCC Rx ESR Q

F32.5 Major depressive disorder, single episode, in full remission HCC Rx ESR Q

F32.8 Other depressive episodes (5th)
AHA: 2016,4Q,14

F32.81 Premenstrual dysphoric disorder Rx ♀
EXCLUDES 1 *premenstrual tension syndrome (N94.3)*
DEF: Severe manifestation of premenstrual syndrome (PMS) that can be disabling and destructive to day-to-day activities. It can exacerbate pre-existing emotional disorders, like depression and anxiety, and cause feelings of loss of control, fatigue, and irritability.

F32.89 Other specified depressive episodes Rx Q
Atypical depression
Post-schizophrenic depression
Single episode of 'masked' depression NOS

F32.9 Major depressive disorder, single episode, unspecified Rx Q
Major depression NOS
AHA: 2021,4Q,10; 2021,1Q,10; 2013,4Q,107

F32.A Depression, unspecified Rx Q
Depression NOS
Depressive disorder NOS
AHA: 2021,4Q,9-10

F33 Major depressive disorder, recurrent (4th)

INCLUDES recurrent episodes of depressive reaction
recurrent episodes of endogenous depression
recurrent episodes of major depression
recurrent episodes of psychogenic depression
recurrent episodes of reactive depression
▶recurrent episodes of seasonal affective disorder◀
recurrent episodes of seasonal depressive disorder
recurrent episodes of vital depression

EXCLUDES 1 *bipolar disorder (F31.-)*
manic episode (F3Ø.-)

AHA: 2020,1Q,23

DEF: Mood disorder that produces depression that may exhibit as sadness, low self-esteem, or guilt feelings. Other manifestations may be withdrawal from friends and family and interrupted sleep.

F33.Ø Major depressive disorder, recurrent, mild HCC Rx ESR Q

F33.1 Major depressive disorder, recurrent, moderate HCC Rx ESR Q

F33.2 Major depressive disorder, recurrent, severe without psychotic features HCC Rx ESR COM Q

F33.3 Major depressive disorder, recurrent, severe with psychotic symptoms HCC Rx ESR COM Q
Endogenous depression with psychotic symptoms
Major depressive disorder, recurrent, with psychotic features
Recurrent severe episodes of major depression with mood-congruent psychotic symptoms
Recurrent severe episodes of major depression with mood-incongruent psychotic symptoms
Recurrent severe episodes of major depression with psychotic symptoms
Recurrent severe episodes of psychogenic depressive psychosis
Recurrent severe episodes of psychotic depression
Recurrent severe episodes of reactive depressive psychosis

F33.4 Major depressive disorder, recurrent, in remission (5th)

F33.4Ø Major depressive disorder, recurrent, in remission, unspecified HCC Rx ESR Q

F33.41 Major depressive disorder, recurrent, in partial remission HCC Rx ESR Q

F33.42 Major depressive disorder, recurrent, in full remission HCC Rx ESR Q

F33.8 Other recurrent depressive disorders HCC Rx ESR Q
Recurrent brief depressive episodes

F33.9 Major depressive disorder, recurrent, unspecified HCC Rx ESR Q
Monopolar depression NOS

F34 Persistent mood [affective] disorders (4th)

F34.Ø Cyclothymic disorder Rx
Affective personality disorder
Cycloid personality
Cyclothymia
Cyclothymic personality
DEF: Mood disorder characterized by fast and repeated alterations between hypomanic and depressed moods.

F34.1 Dysthymic disorder Rx Q
Depressive neurosis
Depressive personality disorder
Dysthymia
Neurotic depression
Persistent anxiety depression
Persistent depressive disorder
EXCLUDES 2 *anxiety depression (mild or not persistent) (F41.8)*
DEF: Depression without psychosis. It is a less severe but persistent depression and is considered a mild to moderate chronic form of depression.

✓5th **F34.8 Other persistent mood [affective] disorders**
AHA: 2016,4Q,14

F34.81 Disruptive mood dysregulation disorder HCC Rx ESR COM Q

F34.89 Other specified persistent mood disorders HCC Rx ESR Q

F34.9 Persistent mood [affective] disorder, unspecified HCC Rx ESR

F39 Unspecified mood [affective] disorder HCC Rx ESR
Affective psychosis NOS

Anxiety, dissociative, stress-related, somatoform and other nonpsychotic mental disorders (F40-F48)

✓4th **F40 Phobic anxiety disorders**
DEF: Phobia: Broad-range anxiety with abnormally intense dread of certain objects or specific situations that would not normally have that effect.

✓5th **F40.0 Agoraphobia**
DEF: Profound anxiety or fear of leaving familiar settings like home, or being in unfamiliar locations or with strangers or crowds. Agoraphobia may or may not be preceded by recurrent panic attacks.

F40.00 Agoraphobia, unspecified Rx

F40.01 Agoraphobia with panic disorder Rx
Panic disorder with agoraphobia
EXCLUDES 1 *panic disorder without agoraphobia (F41.0)*

F40.02 Agoraphobia without panic disorder Rx

✓5th **F40.1 Social phobias**
Anthropophobia
Social anxiety disorder
Social anxiety disorder of childhood
Social neurosis

F40.10 Social phobia, unspecified Rx

F40.11 Social phobia, generalized Rx

✓5th **F40.2 Specific (isolated) phobias**
EXCLUDES 2 *dysmorphophobia (nondelusional) (F45.22)*
nosophobia (F45.22)

✓6th **F40.21 Animal type phobia**

F40.210 Arachnophobia Rx
Fear of spiders

F40.218 Other animal type phobia Rx

✓6th **F40.22 Natural environment type phobia**

F40.220 Fear of thunderstorms Rx

F40.228 Other natural environment type phobia Rx

✓6th **F40.23 Blood, injection, injury type phobia**

F40.230 Fear of blood Rx

F40.231 Fear of injections and transfusions Rx

F40.232 Fear of other medical care Rx

F40.233 Fear of injury Rx

✓6th **F40.24 Situational type phobia**

F40.240 Claustrophobia Rx

F40.241 Acrophobia Rx

F40.242 Fear of bridges Rx

F40.243 Fear of flying Rx

F40.248 Other situational type phobia Rx

✓6th **F40.29 Other specified phobia**

F40.290 Androphobia Rx
Fear of men

F40.291 Gynephobia Rx
Fear of women

F40.298 Other specified phobia Rx

F40.8 Other phobic anxiety disorders Rx
Phobic anxiety disorder of childhood

F40.9 Phobic anxiety disorder, unspecified Rx
Phobia NOS
Phobic state NOS

✓4th **F41 Other anxiety disorders**
EXCLUDES 2 *anxiety in:*
acute stress reaction (F43.0)
neurasthenia (F48.8)
psychophysiologic disorders (F45.-)
transient adjustment reaction (F43.2)
separation anxiety (F93.0)

F41.0 Panic disorder [episodic paroxysmal anxiety] Rx
Panic attack
Panic state
EXCLUDES 1 *panic disorder with agoraphobia (F40.01)*
DEF: Neurotic disorder characterized by recurrent panic or anxiety, apprehension, fear, or terror. Symptoms include shortness of breath, palpitations, dizziness, and shakiness; fear of dying may persist.

F41.1 Generalized anxiety disorder Rx
Anxiety neurosis
Anxiety reaction
Anxiety state
Overanxious disorder
EXCLUDES 2 *neurasthenia (F48.8)*

F41.3 Other mixed anxiety disorders

F41.8 Other specified anxiety disorders
Anxiety depression (mild or not persistent)
Anxiety hysteria
Mixed anxiety and depressive disorder
AHA: 2021,1Q,10

F41.9 Anxiety disorder, unspecified
Anxiety NOS
AHA: 2021,1Q,10

✓4th **F42 Obsessive-compulsive disorder**
EXCLUDES 2 *obsessive-compulsive personality (disorder) (F60.5)*
obsessive-compulsive symptoms occurring in depression (F32-F33)
obsessive-compulsive symptoms occurring in schizophrenia (F20.-)
AHA: 2016,4Q,14-15

F42.2 Mixed obsessional thoughts and acts Rx

F42.3 Hoarding disorder Rx

F42.4 Excoriation (skin-picking) disorder Rx
EXCLUDES 1 *factitial dermatitis (L98.1)*
other specified behavioral and emotional disorders with onset usually occurring in early childhood and adolescence (F98.8)

F42.8 Other obsessive-compulsive disorder Rx
Anancastic neurosis
Obsessive-compulsive neurosis

F42.9 Obsessive-compulsive disorder, unspecified Rx

✓4th **F43 Reaction to severe stress, and adjustment disorders**

F43.0 Acute stress reaction
Acute crisis reaction
Acute reaction to stress
Combat and operational stress reaction
Combat fatigue
Crisis state
Psychic shock

✓5th **F43.1 Post-traumatic stress disorder (PTSD)**
Traumatic neurosis
DEF: Preoccupation with traumatic events beyond normal experience (i.e., rape, personal assault, etc.) that may also include recurring flashbacks of the trauma. Symptoms include difficulty remembering, sleeping, or concentrating, and guilt feelings for surviving.

F43.10 Post-traumatic stress disorder, unspecified Rx

F43.11 Post-traumatic stress disorder, acute Rx

F43.12 Post-traumatic stress disorder, chronic Rx

F43.2 Adjustment disorders (5th)
Culture shock
Grief reaction
Hospitalism in children
EXCLUDES 2 *separation anxiety disorder of childhood (F93.0)*

F43.20 Adjustment disorder, unspecified Rx
F43.21 Adjustment disorder with depressed mood Rx Q
AHA: 2014,1Q,25
F43.22 Adjustment disorder with anxiety Rx
F43.23 Adjustment disorder with mixed anxiety and depressed mood Rx Q
F43.24 Adjustment disorder with disturbance of conduct Rx
F43.25 Adjustment disorder with mixed disturbance of emotions and conduct Rx
F43.29 Adjustment disorder with other symptoms Rx

▲ **F43.8 Other reactions to severe stress** (5th)
Other specified trauma and stressor-related disorder
● **F43.81 Prolonged grief disorder**
Complicated grief
Complicated grief disorder
Persistent complex bereavement disorder
● **F43.89 Other reactions to severe stress**

F43.9 Reaction to severe stress, unspecified
Trauma and stressor-related disorder, NOS
▶Unspecified trauma and stressor-related disorder◀

F44 Dissociative and conversion disorders (4th)
INCLUDES conversion hysteria
conversion reaction
hysteria
hysterical psychosis
EXCLUDES 2 *malingering [conscious simulation] (Z76.5)*

F44.0 Dissociative amnesia HCC Rx ESR COM
EXCLUDES 1 *amnesia NOS (R41.3)*
anterograde amnesia (R41.1)
dissociative amnesia with dissociative fugue (F44.1)
retrograde amnesia (R41.2)
EXCLUDES 2 *alcohol-or other psychoactive substance-induced amnestic disorder (F10, F13, F19 with .26, .96)*
amnestic disorder due to known physiological condition (F04)
postictal amnesia in epilepsy (G40.-)

F44.1 Dissociative fugue HCC Rx ESR COM
Dissociative amnesia with dissociative fugue
EXCLUDES 2 *postictal fugue in epilepsy (G40.-)*
DEF: Dissociative hysteria identified by memory loss and flight from familiar surroundings to a completely separate environment. Episodes may last hours or days. Conscious activity is not associated with perception of surroundings and there is no later memory of the episode.

F44.2 Dissociative stupor Rx
EXCLUDES 1 *catatonic stupor (R40.1)*
stupor NOS (R40.1)
EXCLUDES 2 *catatonic disorder due to known physiological condition (F06.1)*
depressive stupor (F32, F33)
manic stupor (F30, F31)

F44.4 Conversion disorder with motor symptom or deficit Rx
Conversion disorder with abnormal movement
Conversion disorder with speech symptoms
Conversion disorder with swallowing symptoms
Conversion disorder with weakness/paralysis
Dissociative motor disorders
Psychogenic aphonia
Psychogenic dysphonia

F44.5 Conversion disorder with seizures or convulsions Rx
Conversion disorder with attacks or seizures
Dissociative convulsions
AHA: 2021,1Q,3; 2019,1Q,19

F44.6 Conversion disorder with sensory symptom or deficit Rx
Conversion disorder with anesthesia or sensory loss
Conversion disorder with special sensory symptoms
Dissociative anesthesia and sensory loss
Psychogenic deafness

F44.7 Conversion disorder with mixed symptom presentation Rx

F44.8 Other dissociative and conversion disorders (5th)
F44.81 Dissociative identity disorder HCC Rx ESR COM
Multiple personality disorder
F44.89 Other dissociative and conversion disorders Rx
Ganser's syndrome
Psychogenic confusion
Psychogenic twilight state
Trance and possession disorders

F44.9 Dissociative and conversion disorder, unspecified Rx
Dissociative disorder NOS

F45 Somatoform disorders (4th)
EXCLUDES 2 *dissociative and conversion disorders (F44.-)*
factitious disorders (F68.1-, F68.A)
hair-plucking (F63.3)
lalling (F80.0)
lisping (F80.0)
malingering [conscious simulation] (Z76.5)
nail-biting (F98.8)
psychological or behavioral factors associated with disorders or diseases classified elsewhere (F54)
sexual dysfunction, not due to a substance or known physiological condition (F52.-)
thumb-sucking (F98.8)
tic disorders (in childhood and adolescence) (F95.-)
Tourette's syndrome (F95.2)
trichotillomania (F63.3)
DEF: Types of disorders causing inconsistent physical symptoms that cannot be explained.

F45.0 Somatization disorder Rx
Briquet's disorder
Multiple psychosomatic disorder

F45.1 Undifferentiated somatoform disorder Rx
Somatic symptom disorder
Undifferentiated psychosomatic disorder

F45.2 Hypochondriacal disorders (5th)
EXCLUDES 2 *delusional dysmorphophobia (F22)*
fixed delusions about bodily functions or shape (F22)
F45.20 Hypochondriacal disorder, unspecified Rx
F45.21 Hypochondriasis Rx
Hypochondriacal neurosis
Illness anxiety disorder
F45.22 Body dysmorphic disorder Rx
Dysmorphophobia (nondelusional)
Nosophobia
F45.29 Other hypochondriacal disorders Rx

F45.4 Pain disorders related to psychological factors (5th)
EXCLUDES 1 *pain NOS (R52)*
F45.41 Pain disorder exclusively related to psychological factors
Somatoform pain disorder (persistent)
F45.42 Pain disorder with related psychological factors
Code also associated acute or chronic pain (G89.-)

F45.8 Other somatoform disorders Rx
Psychogenic dysmenorrhea
Psychogenic dysphagia, including 'globus hystericus'
Psychogenic pruritus
Psychogenic torticollis
Somatoform autonomic dysfunction
Teeth grinding
EXCLUDES 1 *sleep related teeth grinding (G47.63)*

F45.9 Somatoform disorder, unspecified Rx
Psychosomatic disorder NOS

F48 Other nonpsychotic mental disorders (4th)
F48.1 Depersonalization-derealization syndrome HCC Rx ESR COM
F48.2 Pseudobulbar affect
Involuntary emotional expression disorder
Code first underlying cause, if known, such as:
amyotrophic lateral sclerosis (G12.21)
multiple sclerosis (G35)
sequelae of cerebrovascular disease (I69.-)
sequelae of traumatic intracranial injury (S06.-)

F48.8 Other specified nonpsychotic mental disorders
Dhat syndrome
Neurasthenia
Occupational neurosis, including writer's cramp
Psychasthenia
Psychasthenic neurosis
Psychogenic syncope

F48.9 Nonpsychotic mental disorder, unspecified
Neurosis NOS

Behavioral syndromes associated with physiological disturbances and physical factors (F5Ø-F59)

✓4th **F5Ø Eating disorders**
EXCLUDES 1 *anorexia NOS (R63.Ø)*
feeding problems of newborn (P92.-)
polyphagia (R63.2)
EXCLUDES 2 *feeding difficulties (R63.3)*
feeding disorder in infancy or childhood (F98.2-)
AHA: 2022,1Q,13; 2018,4Q,82
TIP: Assign additional code for BMI from category Z68, when documented. BMI can be based on documentation from clinicians who are not the patient's provider.

✓5th **F5Ø.Ø Anorexia nervosa**
EXCLUDES 1 *loss of appetite (R63.Ø)*
psychogenic loss of appetite (F5Ø.89)
DEF: Psychological eating disorder characterized by an intense fear of gaining weight and an unrealistic perception of body image that perpetuates the feeling of being fat or having too much fat. Avoidance of food and restrictive or unhealthy eating are common.

F5Ø.ØØ Anorexia nervosa, unspecified Rx COM
F5Ø.Ø1 Anorexia nervosa, restricting type Rx COM
F5Ø.Ø2 Anorexia nervosa, binge eating/purging type Rx COM
EXCLUDES 1 *bulimia nervosa (F5Ø.2)*

F5Ø.2 Bulimia nervosa Rx COM
Bulimia NOS
Hyperorexia nervosa
EXCLUDES 1 *anorexia nervosa, binge eating/purging type (F5Ø.Ø2)*
DEF: Episodic pattern of overeating (binge eating) followed by purging or extreme exercise accompanied by an awareness of the abnormal eating pattern with a fear of not being able to stop eating.

✓5th **F5Ø.8 Other eating disorders**
EXCLUDES 2 *pica of infancy and childhood (F98.3)*
AHA: 2017,4Q,9; 2016,4Q,15-16

F5Ø.81 Binge eating disorder Rx
F5Ø.82 Avoidant/restrictive food intake disorder Rx
F5Ø.89 Other specified eating disorder Rx
Pica in adults
Psychogenic loss of appetite

F5Ø.9 Eating disorder, unspecified Rx
Atypical anorexia nervosa
Atypical bulimia nervosa
Feeding or eating disorder, unspecified
Other specified feeding disorder

✓4th **F51 Sleep disorders not due to a substance or known physiological condition**
EXCLUDES 2 *organic sleep disorders (G47.-)*

✓5th **F51.Ø Insomnia not due to a substance or known physiological condition**
EXCLUDES 2 *alcohol related insomnia (F1Ø.182, F1Ø.282, F1Ø.982)*
drug-related insomnia (F11.182, F11.282, F11.982, F13.182, F13.282, F13.982, F14.182, F14.282, F14.982, F15.182, F15.282, F15.982, F19.182, F19.282, F19.982)
insomnia NOS (G47.Ø-)
insomnia due to known physiological condition (G47.Ø-)
organic insomnia (G47.Ø-)
sleep deprivation (Z72.82Ø)

F51.Ø1 Primary insomnia
Idiopathic insomnia
F51.Ø2 Adjustment insomnia
F51.Ø3 Paradoxical insomnia
F51.Ø4 Psychophysiologic insomnia
F51.Ø5 Insomnia due to other mental disorder
Code also associated mental disorder
F51.Ø9 Other insomnia not due to a substance or known physiological condition

✓5th **F51.1 Hypersomnia not due to a substance or known physiological condition**
EXCLUDES 2 *alcohol related hypersomnia (F1Ø.182, F1Ø.282, F1Ø.982)*
drug-related hypersomnia (F11.182, F11.282, F11.982, F13.182, F13.282, F13.982, F14.182, F14.282, F14.982, F15.182, F15.282, F15.982, F19.182, F19.282, F19.982)
hypersomnia NOS (G47.1Ø)
hypersomnia due to known physiological condition (G47.1Ø)
idiopathic hypersomnia (G47.11, G47.12)
narcolepsy (G47.4-)

F51.11 Primary hypersomnia
F51.12 Insufficient sleep syndrome
EXCLUDES 1 *sleep deprivation (Z72.82Ø)*
F51.13 Hypersomnia due to other mental disorder
Code also associated mental disorder
F51.19 Other hypersomnia not due to a substance or known physiological condition

F51.3 Sleepwalking [somnambulism]
Non-rapid eye movement sleep arousal disorders, sleepwalking type
F51.4 Sleep terrors [night terrors]
Non-rapid eye movement sleep arousal disorders, sleep terror type
F51.5 Nightmare disorder
Dream anxiety disorder
F51.8 Other sleep disorders not due to a substance or known physiological condition
F51.9 Sleep disorder not due to a substance or known physiological condition, unspecified
Emotional sleep disorder NOS

✓4th **F52 Sexual dysfunction not due to a substance or known physiological condition**
EXCLUDES 2 *Dhat syndrome (F48.8)*

F52.Ø Hypoactive sexual desire disorder
Lack or loss of sexual desire
Male hypoactive sexual desire disorder
Sexual anhedonia
EXCLUDES 1 *decreased libido (R68.82)*
F52.1 Sexual aversion disorder
Sexual aversion and lack of sexual enjoyment

✓5th **F52.2 Sexual arousal disorders**
Failure of genital response
F52.21 Male erectile disorder ♂
Erectile disorder
Psychogenic impotence
EXCLUDES 1 *impotence of organic origin (N52.-)*
impotence NOS (N52.-)
F52.22 Female sexual arousal disorder ♀
Female sexual interest/arousal disorder

✓5th **F52.3 Orgasmic disorder**
Inhibited orgasm
Psychogenic anorgasmy
F52.31 Female orgasmic disorder ♀
F52.32 Male orgasmic disorder ♂
Delayed ejaculation

F52.4 Premature ejaculation ♂
F52.5 Vaginismus not due to a substance or known physiological condition ♀
Psychogenic vaginismus
EXCLUDES 2 *vaginismus (due to a known physiological condition) (N94.2)*
DEF: Psychogenic response resulting in painful contractions of the vaginal canal muscles. This condition can be severe enough to prevent sexual intercourse.

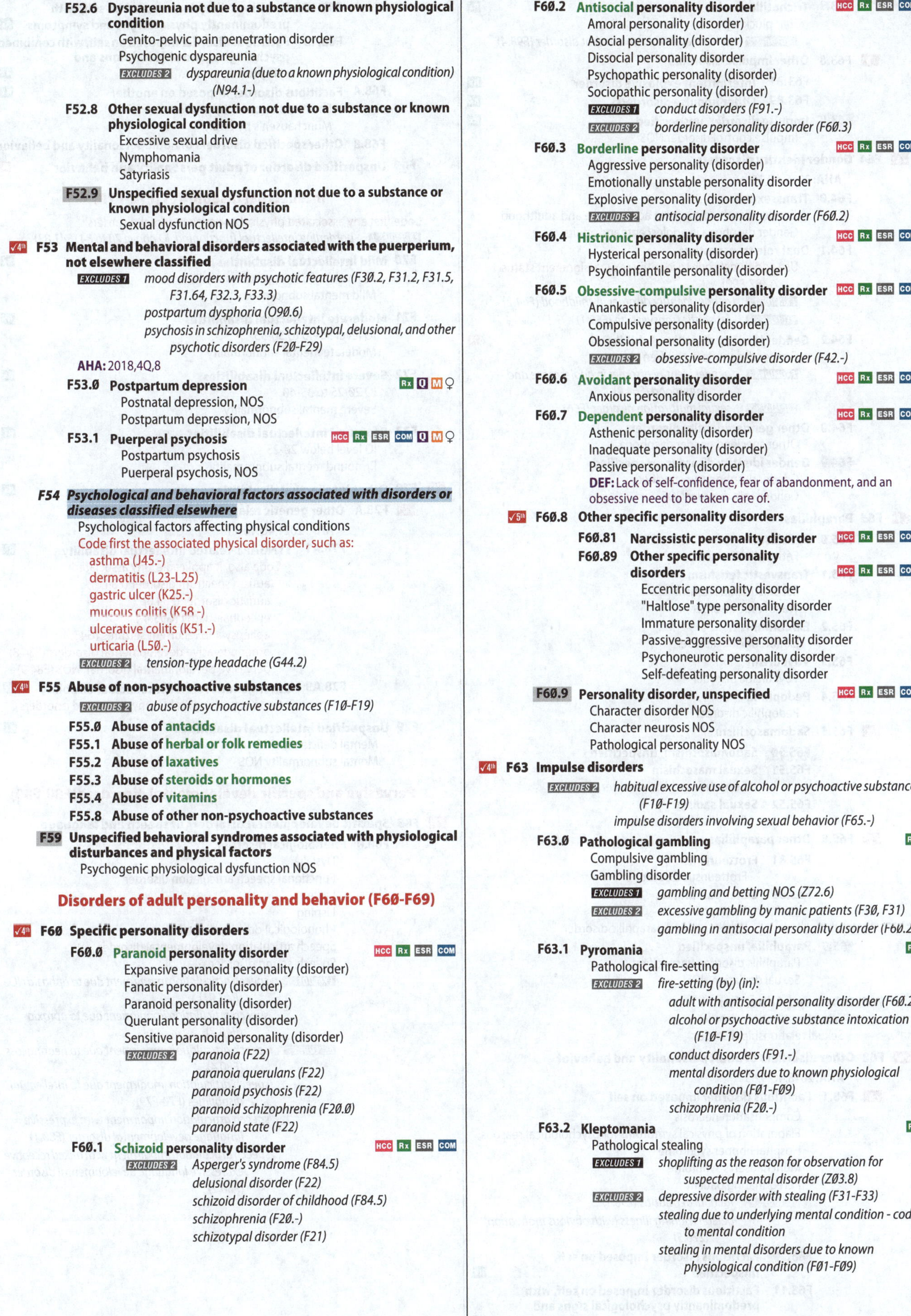

F52.6 Dyspareunia not due to a substance or known physiological condition
Genito-pelvic pain penetration disorder
Psychogenic dyspareunia
EXCLUDES 2 *dyspareunia (due to a known physiological condition) (N94.1-)*

F52.8 Other sexual dysfunction not due to a substance or known physiological condition
Excessive sexual drive
Nymphomania
Satyriasis

F52.9 Unspecified sexual dysfunction not due to a substance or known physiological condition
Sexual dysfunction NOS

F53 Mental and behavioral disorders associated with the puerperium, not elsewhere classified
EXCLUDES 1 *mood disorders with psychotic features (F30.2, F31.2, F31.5, F31.64, F32.3, F33.3)*
postpartum dysphoria (O90.6)
psychosis in schizophrenia, schizotypal, delusional, and other psychotic disorders (F20-F29)
AHA: 2018,4Q,8

F53.0 Postpartum depression Rx Q M ♀
Postnatal depression, NOS
Postpartum depression, NOS

F53.1 Puerperal psychosis HCC Rx ESR COM Q M ♀
Postpartum psychosis
Puerperal psychosis, NOS

F54 Psychological and behavioral factors associated with disorders or diseases classified elsewhere
Psychological factors affecting physical conditions
Code first the associated physical disorder, such as:
asthma (J45.-)
dermatitis (L23-L25)
gastric ulcer (K25.-)
mucous colitis (K58.-)
ulcerative colitis (K51.-)
urticaria (L50.-)
EXCLUDES 2 *tension-type headache (G44.2)*

F55 Abuse of non-psychoactive substances
EXCLUDES 2 *abuse of psychoactive substances (F10-F19)*

F55.0 Abuse of antacids
F55.1 Abuse of herbal or folk remedies
F55.2 Abuse of laxatives
F55.3 Abuse of steroids or hormones
F55.4 Abuse of vitamins
F55.8 Abuse of other non-psychoactive substances

F59 Unspecified behavioral syndromes associated with physiological disturbances and physical factors
Psychogenic physiological dysfunction NOS

Disorders of adult personality and behavior (F60-F69)

F60 Specific personality disorders

F60.0 Paranoid personality disorder HCC Rx ESR COM
Expansive paranoid personality (disorder)
Fanatic personality (disorder)
Paranoid personality (disorder)
Querulant personality (disorder)
Sensitive paranoid personality (disorder)
EXCLUDES 2 *paranoia (F22)*
paranoia querulans (F22)
paranoid psychosis (F22)
paranoid schizophrenia (F20.0)
paranoid state (F22)

F60.1 Schizoid personality disorder HCC Rx ESR COM
EXCLUDES 2 *Asperger's syndrome (F84.5)*
delusional disorder (F22)
schizoid disorder of childhood (F84.5)
schizophrenia (F20.-)
schizotypal disorder (F21)

F60.2 Antisocial personality disorder HCC Rx ESR COM
Amoral personality (disorder)
Asocial personality (disorder)
Dissocial personality disorder
Psychopathic personality (disorder)
Sociopathic personality (disorder)
EXCLUDES 1 *conduct disorders (F91.-)*
EXCLUDES 2 *borderline personality disorder (F60.3)*

F60.3 Borderline personality disorder HCC Rx ESR COM
Aggressive personality (disorder)
Emotionally unstable personality disorder
Explosive personality (disorder)
EXCLUDES 2 *antisocial personality disorder (F60.2)*

F60.4 Histrionic personality disorder HCC Rx ESR COM
Hysterical personality (disorder)
Psychoinfantile personality (disorder)

F60.5 Obsessive-compulsive personality disorder HCC Rx ESR COM
Anankastic personality (disorder)
Compulsive personality (disorder)
Obsessional personality (disorder)
EXCLUDES 2 *obsessive-compulsive disorder (F42.-)*

F60.6 Avoidant personality disorder HCC Rx ESR COM
Anxious personality disorder

F60.7 Dependent personality disorder HCC Rx ESR COM
Asthenic personality (disorder)
Inadequate personality (disorder)
Passive personality (disorder)
DEF: Lack of self-confidence, fear of abandonment, and an obsessive need to be taken care of.

F60.8 Other specific personality disorders

F60.81 Narcissistic personality disorder HCC Rx ESR COM

F60.89 Other specific personality disorders HCC Rx ESR COM
Eccentric personality disorder
"Haltlose" type personality disorder
Immature personality disorder
Passive-aggressive personality disorder
Psychoneurotic personality disorder
Self-defeating personality disorder

F60.9 Personality disorder, unspecified HCC Rx ESR COM
Character disorder NOS
Character neurosis NOS
Pathological personality NOS

F63 Impulse disorders
EXCLUDES 2 *habitual excessive use of alcohol or psychoactive substances (F10-F19)*
impulse disorders involving sexual behavior (F65.-)

F63.0 Pathological gambling Rx
Compulsive gambling
Gambling disorder
EXCLUDES 1 *gambling and betting NOS (Z72.6)*
EXCLUDES 2 *excessive gambling by manic patients (F30, F31)*
gambling in antisocial personality disorder (F60.2)

F63.1 Pyromania Rx
Pathological fire-setting
EXCLUDES 2 *fire-setting (by) (in):*
adult with antisocial personality disorder (F60.2)
alcohol or psychoactive substance intoxication (F10-F19)
conduct disorders (F91.-)
mental disorders due to known physiological condition (F01-F09)
schizophrenia (F20.-)

F63.2 Kleptomania Rx
Pathological stealing
EXCLUDES 1 *shoplifting as the reason for observation for suspected mental disorder (Z03.8)*
EXCLUDES 2 *depressive disorder with stealing (F31-F33)*
stealing due to underlying mental condition - code to mental condition
stealing in mental disorders due to known physiological condition (F01-F09)

F63.3 Trichotillomania Rx
Hair plucking
EXCLUDES 2 *other stereotyped movement disorder (F98.4)*

✓5th **F63.8 Other impulse disorders**
F63.81 Intermittent explosive disorder Rx
F63.89 Other impulse disorders Rx

F63.9 Impulse disorder, unspecified Rx
Impulse control disorder NOS

✓4th **F64 Gender identity disorders**
AHA: 2016,4Q,16

F64.0 Transsexualism
Gender identity disorder in adolescence and adulthood
Gender dysphoria in adolescents and adults

F64.1 Dual role transvestism
Use additional code to identify sex reassignment status (Z87.890)
EXCLUDES 1 *gender identity disorder in childhood (F64.2)*
EXCLUDES 2 *fetishistic transvestism (F65.1)*

F64.2 Gender identity disorder of childhood P
Gender dysphoria in children
EXCLUDES 1 *gender identity disorder in adolescence and adulthood (F64.0)*
EXCLUDES 2 *sexual maturation disorder (F66)*

F64.8 Other gender identity disorders
Other specified gender dysphoria

F64.9 Gender identity disorder, unspecified
Gender dysphoria, unspecified
Gender-role disorder NOS

✓4th **F65 Paraphilias**

F65.0 Fetishism
Fetishistic disorder

F65.1 Transvestic fetishism
Fetishistic transvestism
Transvestic disorder

F65.2 Exhibitionism
Exhibitionistic disorder

F65.3 Voyeurism
Voyeuristic disorder

F65.4 Pedophilia
Pedophilic disorder

✓5th **F65.5 Sadomasochism**
F65.50 Sadomasochism, unspecified
F65.51 Sexual masochism
Sexual masochism disorder
F65.52 Sexual sadism
Sexual sadism disorder

✓5th **F65.8 Other paraphilias**
F65.81 Frotteurism
Frotteuristic disorder
F65.89 Other paraphilias
Necrophilia
Other specified paraphilic disorder

F65.9 Paraphilia, unspecified
Paraphilic disorder, unspecified
Sexual deviation NOS

F66 Other sexual disorders
Sexual maturation disorder
Sexual relationship disorder

✓4th **F68 Other disorders of adult personality and behavior**
AHA: 2018,4Q,9,65

✓5th **F68.1 Factitious disorder imposed on self**
Compensation neurosis
Elaboration of physical symptoms for psychological reasons
Hospital hopper syndrome
Münchausen's syndrome
Peregrinating patient
EXCLUDES 2 *factitial dermatitis (L98.1)*
person feigning illness (with obvious motivation) (Z76.5)

F68.10 Factitious disorder imposed on self, unspecified Rx
F68.11 Factitious disorder imposed on self, with predominantly psychological signs and symptoms Rx
F68.12 Factitious disorder imposed on self, with predominantly physical signs and symptoms Rx
F68.13 Factitious disorder imposed on self, with combined psychological and physical signs and symptoms Rx

F68.A Factitious disorder imposed on another Rx
Factitious disorder by proxy
Münchausen's by proxy

F68.8 Other specified disorders of adult personality and behavior

F69 Unspecified disorder of adult personality and behavior A

Intellectual disabilities (F70-F79)

Code first any associated physical or developmental disorders
EXCLUDES 1 *borderline intellectual functioning, IQ above 70 to 84 (R41.83)*

F70 Mild intellectual disabilities Rx
IQ level 50-55 to approximately 70
Mild mental subnormality

F71 Moderate intellectual disabilities Rx
IQ level 35-40 to 50-55
Moderate mental subnormality

F72 Severe intellectual disabilities Rx
IQ 20-25 to 35-40
Severe mental subnormality

F73 Profound intellectual disabilities Rx
IQ level below 20-25
Profound mental subnormality

✓4th **F78 Other intellectual disabilities** Rx

✓5th **F78.A Other genetic related intellectual disabilities**
AHA: 2021,4Q,10-11

F78.A1 SYNGAP1-related intellectual disability Rx
Code also, if applicable, any associated:
autism spectrum disorder (F84.0)
autistic disorder (F84.0)
encephalopathy (G93.4-)
epilepsy and recurrent seizures (G40.-)
other pervasive developmental disorders (F84.8)
pervasive developmental disorder, NOS (F84.9)

F78.A9 Other genetic related intellectual disability Rx
Code also, if applicable, any associated disorders

F79 Unspecified intellectual disabilities Rx
Mental deficiency NOS
Mental subnormality NOS

Pervasive and specific developmental disorders (F80-F89)

✓4th **F80 Specific developmental disorders of speech and language**

F80.0 Phonological disorder
Dyslalia
Functional speech articulation disorder
Lalling
Lisping
Phonological developmental disorder
Speech articulation developmental disorder
Speech-sound disorder
EXCLUDES 1 *speech articulation impairment due to aphasia NOS (R47.01)*
speech articulation impairment due to apraxia (R48.2)
EXCLUDES 2 *speech articulation impairment due to hearing loss (F80.4)*
speech articulation impairment due to intellectual disabilities (F70-F79)
speech articulation impairment with expressive language developmental disorder (F80.1)
speech articulation impairment with mixed receptive expressive language developmental disorder (F80.2)

F8Ø.1 Expressive language disorder
Developmental dysphasia or aphasia, expressive type
EXCLUDES 1 *mixed receptive-expressive language disorder (F8Ø.2)*
dysphasia and aphasia NOS (R47.-)
EXCLUDES 2 *acquired aphasia with epilepsy [Landau-Kleffner] (G4Ø.8Ø-)*
selective mutism (F94.Ø)
intellectual disabilities (F7Ø-F79)
pervasive developmental disorders (F84.-)

F8Ø.2 Mixed receptive-expressive language disorder
Developmental dysphasia or aphasia, receptive type
Developmental Wernicke's aphasia
EXCLUDES 1 *central auditory processing disorder (H93.25)*
dysphasia or aphasia NOS (R47.-)
expressive language disorder (F8Ø.1)
expressive type dysphasia or aphasia (F8Ø.1)
word deafness (H93.25)
EXCLUDES 2 *acquired aphasia with epilepsy [Landau-Kleffner] (G4Ø.8Ø-)*
pervasive developmental disorders (F84.-)
selective mutism (F94.Ø)
intellectual disabilities (F7Ø-F79)

F8Ø.4 Speech and language development delay due to hearing loss
Code also type of hearing loss (H9Ø.-, H91.-)

✓5th **F8Ø.8 Other developmental disorders of speech and language**
AHA: 2017,1Q,27

F8Ø.81 Childhood onset fluency disorder
Cluttering NOS
Stuttering NOS
EXCLUDES 1 *adult onset fluency disorder (F98.5)*
fluency disorder in conditions classified elsewhere (R47.82)
fluency disorder (stuttering) following cerebrovascular disease (I69. with final characters -23)

F8Ø.82 Social pragmatic communication disorder
EXCLUDES 1 *Asperger's syndrome (F84.5)*
autistic disorder (F84.Ø)
AHA: 2016,4Q,16

F8Ø.89 Other developmental disorders of speech and language

F8Ø.9 Developmental disorder of speech and language, unspecified
Communication disorder NOS
Language disorder NOS

✓4th **F81 Specific developmental disorders of scholastic skills**

F81.Ø Specific reading disorder
"Backward reading"
Developmental dyslexia
Specific learning disorder, with impairment in reading
Specific reading retardation
EXCLUDES 1 *alexia NOS (R48.Ø)*
dyslexia NOS (R48.Ø)
DEF: Serious impairment of reading skills unexplained in relation to general intelligence and teaching processes.

F81.2 Mathematics disorder
Developmental acalculia
Developmental arithmetical disorder
Developmental Gerstmann's syndrome
Specific learning disorder, with impairment in mathematics
EXCLUDES 1 *acalculia NOS (R48.8)*
EXCLUDES 2 *arithmetical difficulties associated with a reading disorder (F81.Ø)*
arithmetical difficulties associated with a spelling disorder (F81.81)
arithmetical difficulties due to inadequate teaching (Z55.8)

✓5th **F81.8 Other developmental disorders of scholastic skills**

F81.81 Disorder of written expression
Specific learning disorder, with impairment in written expression
Specific spelling disorder

F81.89 Other developmental disorders of scholastic skills

F81.9 Developmental disorder of scholastic skills, unspecified
Knowledge acquisition disability NOS
Learning disability NOS
Learning disorder NOS

F82 Specific developmental disorder of motor function
Clumsy child syndrome
Developmental coordination disorder
Developmental dyspraxia
EXCLUDES 1 *abnormalities of gait and mobility (R26.-)*
lack of coordination (R27.-)
EXCLUDES 2 *lack of coordination secondary to intellectual disabilities (F7Ø-F79)*

✓4th **F84 Pervasive developmental disorders**
Code also any associated medical condition and intellectual disabilities

F84.Ø Autistic disorder Rx COM
Autism spectrum disorder
Infantile autism
Infantile psychosis
Kanner's syndrome
EXCLUDES 1 *Asperger's syndrome (F84.5)*
AHA: 2017,1Q,27
TIP: When the encounter is focused on treatment of conditions related to autism spectrum disorder, first assign codes to identify the problem or manifestation receiving therapeutic services.

F84.2 Rett's syndrome Rx COM
EXCLUDES 1 *Asperger's syndrome (F84.5)*
autistic disorder (F84.Ø)
other childhood disintegrative disorder (F84.3)

F84.3 Other childhood disintegrative disorder Rx COM P
Dementia infantilis
Disintegrative psychosis
Heller's syndrome
Symbiotic psychosis
Use additional code to identify any associated neurological condition
EXCLUDES 1 *Asperger's syndrome (F84.5)*
autistic disorder (F84.Ø)
Rett's syndrome (F84.2)

F84.5 Asperger's syndrome Rx COM
Asperger's disorder
Autistic psychopathy
Schizoid disorder of childhood
DEF: High-functioning form of autism. Children with this syndrome usually develop speech on schedule, are generally very intelligent, and communicate well, but have considerable social shortcomings. ***Synonym(s):*** *AS.*

F84.8 Other pervasive developmental disorders Rx COM
Overactive disorder associated with intellectual disabilities and stereotyped movements

F84.9 Pervasive developmental disorder, unspecified Rx COM
Atypical autism

F88 Other disorders of psychological development
Developmental agnosia
Global developmental delay
Other specified neurodevelopmental disorder

F89 Unspecified disorder of psychological development
Developmental disorder NOS
Neurodevelopmental disorder NOS

Behavioral and emotional disorders with onset usually occurring in childhood and adolescence (F9Ø-F98)

NOTE Codes within categories F9Ø-F98 may be used regardless of the age of a patient. These disorders generally have onset within the childhood or adolescent years, but may continue throughout life or not be diagnosed until adulthood

✓4th **F9Ø Attention-deficit hyperactivity disorders**

INCLUDES attention deficit disorder with hyperactivity
attention deficit syndrome with hyperactivity

EXCLUDES 2 *anxiety disorders (F4Ø.-, F41.-)*
mood [affective] disorders (F3Ø-F39)
pervasive developmental disorders (F84.-)
schizophrenia (F2Ø.-)

F9Ø.Ø Attention-deficit hyperactivity disorder, predominantly inattentive type Rx
Attention-deficit/hyperactivity disorder, predominantly inattentive presentation

F9Ø.1 Attention-deficit hyperactivity disorder, predominantly hyperactive type Rx
Attention-deficit/hyperactivity disorder, predominantly hyperactive impulsive presentation

F9Ø.2 Attention-deficit hyperactivity disorder, combined type Rx
Attention-deficit/hyperactivity disorder, combined presentation

F9Ø.8 Attention-deficit hyperactivity disorder, other type Rx

F9Ø.9 Attention-deficit hyperactivity disorder, unspecified type Rx
Attention-deficit hyperactivity disorder of childhood or adolescence NOS
Attention-deficit hyperactivity disorder NOS

✓4th **F91 Conduct disorders**

EXCLUDES 1 *antisocial behavior (Z72.81-)*
antisocial personality disorder (F6Ø.2)

EXCLUDES 2 *conduct problems associated with attention-deficit hyperactivity disorder (F9Ø.-)*
mood [affective] disorders (F3Ø-F39)
pervasive developmental disorders (F84.-)
schizophrenia (F2Ø.-)

F91.Ø Conduct disorder confined to family context Rx

F91.1 Conduct disorder, childhood-onset type Rx
Unsocialized conduct disorder
Conduct disorder, solitary aggressive type
Unsocialized aggressive disorder

F91.2 Conduct disorder, adolescent-onset type Rx
Socialized conduct disorder
Conduct disorder, group type

F91.3 Oppositional defiant disorder Rx

F91.8 Other conduct disorders Rx
Other specified conduct disorder
Other specified disruptive disorder

F91.9 Conduct disorder, unspecified Rx
Behavioral disorder NOS
Conduct disorder NOS
Disruptive behavior disorder NOS
Disruptive disorder NOS

✓4th **F93 Emotional disorders with onset specific to childhood**

F93.Ø Separation anxiety disorder of childhood Rx

EXCLUDES 2 *mood [affective] disorders (F3Ø-F39)*
nonpsychotic mental disorders (F4Ø-F48)
phobic anxiety disorder of childhood (F4Ø.8)
social phobia (F4Ø.1)

F93.8 Other childhood emotional disorders
Identity disorder

EXCLUDES 2 *gender identity disorder of childhood (F64.2)*

F93.9 Childhood emotional disorder, unspecified

✓4th **F94 Disorders of social functioning with onset specific to childhood and adolescence**

F94.Ø Selective mutism
Elective mutism

EXCLUDES 2 *pervasive developmental disorders (F84.-)*
schizophrenia (F2Ø.-)
specific developmental disorders of speech and language (F8Ø.-)
transient mutism as part of separation anxiety in young children (F93.Ø)

F94.1 Reactive attachment disorder of childhood
Use additional code to identify any associated failure to thrive or growth retardation

EXCLUDES 1 *disinhibited attachment disorder of childhood (F94.2)*
normal variation in pattern of selective attachment

EXCLUDES 2 *Asperger's syndrome (F84.5)*
maltreatment syndromes (T74.-)
sexual or physical abuse in childhood, resulting in psychosocial problems (Z62.81-)

F94.2 Disinhibited attachment disorder of childhood
Affectionless psychopathy
Institutional syndrome

EXCLUDES 1 *reactive attachment disorder of childhood (F94.1)*

EXCLUDES 2 *Asperger's syndrome (F84.5)*
attention-deficit hyperactivity disorders (F9Ø.-)
hospitalism in children (F43.2-)

F94.8 Other childhood disorders of social functioning

F94.9 Childhood disorder of social functioning, unspecified

✓4th **F95 Tic disorder**

F95.Ø Transient tic disorder Rx
Provisional tic disorder

F95.1 Chronic motor or vocal tic disorder Rx

F95.2 Tourette's disorder Rx
Combined vocal and multiple motor tic disorder [de la Tourette]
Tourette's syndrome

F95.8 Other tic disorders Rx

F95.9 Tic disorder, unspecified Rx
Tic NOS

✓4th **F98 Other behavioral and emotional disorders with onset usually occurring in childhood and adolescence**

EXCLUDES 2 *breath-holding spells (RØ6.89)*
gender identity disorder of childhood (F64.2)
Kleine-Levin syndrome (G47.13)
obsessive-compulsive disorder (F42.-)
sleep disorders not due to a substance or known physiological condition (F51.-)

F98.Ø Enuresis not due to a substance or known physiological condition
Enuresis (primary) (secondary) of nonorganic origin
Functional enuresis
Psychogenic enuresis
Urinary incontinence of nonorganic origin

EXCLUDES 1 *enuresis NOS (R32)*

F98.1 Encopresis not due to a substance or known physiological condition
Functional encopresis
Incontinence of feces of nonorganic origin
Psychogenic encopresis
Use additional code to identify the cause of any coexisting constipation

EXCLUDES 1 *encopresis NOS (R15.-)*

✓5th **F98.2 Other feeding disorders of infancy and childhood**

EXCLUDES 2 *anorexia nervosa and other eating disorders (F5Ø.-)*
feeding difficulties (R63.3)
feeding problems of newborn (P92.-)
pica of infancy or childhood (F98.3)

F98.21 Rumination disorder of infancy Rx

F98.29 Other feeding disorders of infancy and early childhood Rx

F98.3 Pica of infancy and childhood Rx

F98.4 Stereotyped movement disorders Rx

Stereotype/habit disorder

EXCLUDES 1 *abnormal involuntary movements (R25.-)*

EXCLUDES 2 *compulsions in obsessive-compulsive disorder (F42.-)*
hair plucking (F63.3)
movement disorders of organic origin (G2Ø-G25)
nail-biting (F98.8)
nose-picking (F98.8)
stereotypies that are part of a broader psychiatric condition (FØ1-F95)
thumb-sucking (F98.8)
tic disorders (F95.-)
trichotillomania (F63.3)

F98.5 Adult onset fluency disorder

EXCLUDES 1 *childhood onset fluency disorder (F8Ø.81)*
dysphasia (R47.Ø2)
fluency disorder in conditions classified elsewhere (R47.82)
fluency disorder (stuttering) following cerebrovascular disease (I69. with final characters -23)
tic disorders (F95.-)

F98.8 Other specified behavioral and emotional disorders with onset usually occurring in childhood and adolescence

Excessive masturbation
Nail-biting
Nose-picking
Thumb-sucking

F98.9 Unspecified behavioral and emotional disorders with onset usually occurring in childhood and adolescence

Unspecified mental disorder (F99)

F99 Mental disorder, not otherwise specified

Mental illness NOS

EXCLUDES 1 *unspecified mental disorder due to known physiological condition (FØ9)*

Chapter 6. Diseases of the Nervous System (GØØ-G99)

Chapter-specific Guidelines with Coding Examples

The chapter-specific guidelines from the ICD-10-CM Official Guidelines for Coding and Reporting have been provided below. Along with these guidelines are coding examples, contained in the shaded boxes, that have been developed to help illustrate the coding and/or sequencing guidance found in these guidelines.

a. Dominant/nondominant side

Codes from category G81, Hemiplegia and hemiparesis, and subcategories G83.1, Monoplegia of lower limb, G83.2, Monoplegia of upper limb, and G83.3, Monoplegia, unspecified, identify whether the dominant or nondominant side is affected. Should the affected side be documented, but not specified as dominant or nondominant, and the classification system does not indicate a default, code selection is as follows:

- For ambidextrous patients, the default should be dominant.
- If the left side is affected, the default is non-dominant.
- If the right side is affected, the default is dominant.

> Hemiplegia affecting left side of ambidextrous patient
>
> **G81.92 Hemiplegia, unspecified affecting left dominant side**
>
> *Explanation*: Documentation states that the left side is affected and dominant is used for ambidextrous persons.

> Right spastic hemiplegia, unknown whether patient is right- or left-handed
>
> **G81.11 Spastic hemiplegia affecting right dominant side**
>
> *Explanation*: Since it is unknown whether the patient is right- or left-handed, if the right side is affected, the default is dominant.

b. Pain—Category G89

1) General coding information

Codes in category G89, Pain, not elsewhere classified, may be used in conjunction with codes from other categories and chapters to provide more detail about acute or chronic pain and neoplasm-related pain, unless otherwise indicated below.

If the pain is not specified as acute or chronic, post-thoracotomy, postprocedural, or neoplasm-related, do not assign codes from category G89.

A code from category G89 should not be assigned if the underlying (definitive) diagnosis is known, unless the reason for the encounter is pain control/ management and not management of the underlying condition.

When an admission or encounter is for a procedure aimed at treating the underlying condition (e.g., spinal fusion, kyphoplasty), a code for the underlying condition (e.g., vertebral fracture, spinal stenosis) should be assigned as the principal diagnosis. No code from category G89 should be assigned.

> Elderly patient with back pain is admitted for outpatient kyphoplasty for age-related osteopathic compression fracture at vertebra T3
>
> **M8Ø.Ø8XA Age-related osteoporosis with current pathological fracture, vertebra(e), initial encounter for fracture**
>
> *Explanation*: No code is assigned for the pain as it is inherent in the underlying condition being treated.

(a) Category G89 codes as principal or first-listed diagnosis

Category G89 codes are acceptable as principal diagnosis or the first-listed code:

- When pain control or pain management is the reason for the admission/encounter (e.g., a patient with displaced intervertebral disc, nerve impingement and severe back pain presents for injection of steroid into the spinal canal). The underlying cause of the pain should be reported as an additional diagnosis, if known.

> Patient presents for steroid injection in the right elbow due to chronic pain associated with primary degenerative joint disease.
>
> **G89.29 Other chronic pain**
>
> **M19.Ø21 Primary osteoarthritis, right elbow**
>
> *Explanation*: Since the encounter is for control of pain, not treating the underlying condition, the pain code is sequenced first followed by the underlying condition. The M25 pain code is not necessary as the underlying condition code represents the specific site.

- When a patient is admitted for the insertion of a neurostimulator for pain control, assign the appropriate pain code as the principal or first-listed diagnosis. When an admission or encounter is for a procedure aimed at treating the underlying condition and a neurostimulator is inserted for pain control during the same admission/encounter, a code for the underlying condition should be assigned as the principal diagnosis and the appropriate pain code should be assigned as a secondary diagnosis.

(b) Use of category G89 codes in conjunction with site specific pain codes

(i) Assigning category G89 and site-specific pain codes

Codes from category G89 may be used in conjunction with codes that identify the site of pain (including codes from chapter 18) if the category G89 code provides additional information. For example, if the code describes the site of the pain, but does not fully describe whether the pain is acute or chronic, then both codes should be assigned.

> Patient is seen to evaluate chronic right knee pain
>
> **M25.561 Pain in right knee**
>
> **G89.29 Other chronic pain**
>
> *Explanation*: No underlying condition has been determined yet so the pain would be the reason for the visit. The M25 pain code in this instance does not fully describe the condition as it does not represent that the pain is chronic. The G89 chronic pain code is assigned to provide specificity.

(ii) Sequencing of category G89 codes with site-specific pain codes

The sequencing of category G89 codes with site-specific pain codes (including chapter 18 codes), is dependent on the circumstances of the encounter/admission as follows:

- If the encounter is for pain control or pain management, assign the code from category G89 followed by the code identifying the specific site of pain (e.g., encounter for pain management for acute neck pain from trauma is assigned code G89.11, Acute pain due to trauma, followed by code M54.2, Cervicalgia, to identify the site of pain).

> Management of acute, traumatic left shoulder pain
>
> **G89.11 Acute pain due to trauma**
>
> **M25.512 Pain in left shoulder**
>
> *Explanation*: The reason for the encounter is to manage or control the pain, not to treat or evaluate an underlying condition. The G89 pain code is assigned as the first-listed diagnosis but in this instance does not fully describe the condition as it does not include the site and laterality. The M25 pain code is added to provide this information.

- If the encounter is for any other reason except pain control or pain management, and a related definitive diagnosis has not been established (confirmed) by the provider, assign the code for the specific site of pain first, followed by the appropriate code from category G89.

Tests are performed to investigate the source of the patient's chronic epigastric abdominal pain

R1Ø.13 Epigastric pain

G89.29 Other chronic pain

Explanation: In this instance the patient's epigastric pain is not being treated; rather the source of the pain is being investigated. A code from chapter 18 for epigastric pain is sequenced before the additional specificity of the G89 code for the chronic pain.

2) Pain due to devices, implants and grafts

See Section I.C.19. Pain due to medical devices

3) Postoperative Pain

The provider's documentation should be used to guide the coding of postoperative pain, as well as *Section III. Reporting Additional Diagnoses* and *Section IV. Diagnostic Coding and Reporting in the Outpatient Setting*.

The default for post-thoracotomy and other postoperative pain not specified as acute or chronic is the code for the acute form.

Routine or expected postoperative pain immediately after surgery should not be coded.

Pain pump dose is increased for the patient's unexpected, extreme pain post-thoracotomy

G89.12 Acute post-thoracotomy pain

Explanation: When acute or chronic is not documented, default to acute. The use of "unexpected, extreme" and the increase of medication dosage indicate that the pain was more than routine or expected.

(a) Postoperative pain not associated with specific postoperative complication

Postoperative pain not associated with a specific postoperative complication is assigned to the appropriate postoperative pain code in category G89.

(b) Postoperative pain associated with specific postoperative complication

Postoperative pain associated with a specific postoperative complication (such as painful wire sutures) is assigned to the appropriate code(s) found in Chapter 19, Injury, poisoning, and certain other consequences of external causes. If appropriate, use additional code(s) from category G89 to identify acute or chronic pain (G89.18 or G89.28).

4) Chronic pain

Chronic pain is classified to subcategory G89.2. There is no time frame defining when pain becomes chronic pain. The provider's documentation should be used to guide use of these codes.

5) Neoplasm related pain

Code G89.3 is assigned to pain documented as being related, associated or due to cancer, primary or secondary malignancy, or tumor. This code is assigned regardless of whether the pain is acute or chronic.

This code may be assigned as the principal or first-listed code when the stated reason for the admission/encounter is documented as pain control/pain management. The underlying neoplasm should be reported as an additional diagnosis.

Patient referred today for pain management due to acute pain related to malignancy of the right breast.

G89.3 Neoplasm related pain (acute)(chronic)

C5Ø.911 Malignant neoplasm of unspecified site of right female breast

Explanation: Since the encounter was for pain medication management, the pain, rather than the neoplasm, was the reason for the encounter and is sequenced first. This "neoplasm-related pain" code includes both acute and chronic pain.

When the reason for the admission/encounter is management of the neoplasm and the pain associated with the neoplasm is also documented, code G89.3 may be assigned as an additional diagnosis. It is not necessary to assign an additional code for the site of the pain.

See Section I.C.2. for instructions on the sequencing of neoplasms for all other stated reasons or the admission/encounter (except for pain control/pain management).

Patient with lung cancer presents with acute hip pain and is evaluated and found to have iliac bone metastasis

C79.51 Secondary malignant neoplasm of bone

C34.9Ø Malignant neoplasm of unspecified part of unspecified bronchus or lung

G89.3 Neoplasm related pain (acute)(chronic)

Explanation: The reason for the encounter was the evaluation and diagnosis of the bone metastasis, whose code would be assigned as first-listed, followed by codes for the primary neoplasm and the pain due to the iliac bone metastasis.

6) Chronic pain syndrome

Central pain syndrome (G89.Ø) and chronic pain syndrome (G89.4) are different than the term "chronic pain," and therefore codes should only be used when the provider has specifically documented this condition.

See Section I.C.5. Pain disorders related to psychological factors

Chapter 6. Diseases of the Nervous System (G00-G99)

EXCLUDES 2 *certain conditions originating in the perinatal period (P04-P96)*
certain infectious and parasitic diseases (A00-B99)
complications of pregnancy, childbirth and the puerperium (O00-O9A)
congenital malformations, deformations, and chromosomal abnormalities (Q00-Q99)
endocrine, nutritional and metabolic diseases (E00-E88)
injury, poisoning and certain other consequences of external causes (S00-T88)
neoplasms (C00-D49)
symptoms, signs and abnormal clinical and laboratory findings, not elsewhere classified (R00-R94)

This chapter contains the following blocks:

G00-G09 Inflammatory diseases of the central nervous system
G10-G14 Systemic atrophies primarily affecting the central nervous system
G20-G26 Extrapyramidal and movement disorders
G30-G32 Other degenerative diseases of the nervous system
G35-G37 Demyelinating diseases of the central nervous system
G40-G47 Episodic and paroxysmal disorders
G50-G59 Nerve, nerve root and plexus disorders
G60-G65 Polyneuropathies and other disorders of the peripheral nervous system
G70-G73 Diseases of myoneural junction and muscle
G80-G83 Cerebral palsy and other paralytic syndromes
G89-G99 Other disorders of the nervous system

Inflammatory diseases of the central nervous system (G00-G09)

G00 Bacterial meningitis, not elsewhere classified

INCLUDES bacterial arachnoiditis
bacterial leptomeningitis
bacterial meningitis
bacterial pachymeningitis

EXCLUDES 1 *bacterial meningoencephalitis (G04.2)*
bacterial meningomyelitis (G04.2)

DEF: Inflammation of meningeal layers of the brain and spinal cord due to a bacterial infection.

G00.0 Hemophilus meningitis COM
Meningitis due to Hemophilus influenzae

G00.1 Pneumococcal meningitis COM
Meningitis due to Streptococcal pneumoniae

G00.2 Streptococcal meningitis COM
Use additional code to further identify organism (B95.0-B95.5)

G00.3 Staphylococcal meningitis COM
Use additional code to further identify organism (B95.61-B95.8)

G00.8 Other bacterial meningitis COM
Meningitis due to Escherichia coli
Meningitis due to Friedländer's bacillus
Meningitis due to Klebsiella
Use additional code to further identify organism (B96.-)

G00.9 Bacterial meningitis, unspecified COM
Meningitis due to gram-negative bacteria, unspecified
Purulent meningitis NOS
Pyogenic meningitis NOS
Suppurative meningitis NOS

G01 Meningitis in bacterial diseases classified elsewhere COM
Code first underlying disease

EXCLUDES 1 *meningitis (in):*
gonococcal (A54.81)
leptospirosis (A27.81)
listeriosis (A32.11)
Lyme disease (A69.21)
meningococcal (A39.0)
neurosyphilis (A52.13)
tuberculosis (A17.0)
meningoencephalitis and meningomyelitis in bacterial diseases classified elsewhere (G05)

G02 Meningitis in other infectious and parasitic diseases classified elsewhere COM
Code first underlying disease, such as:
African trypanosomiasis (B56.-)
poliovirus infection (A80.-)

EXCLUDES 1 *candidal meningitis (B37.5)*
coccidioidomycosis meningitis (B38.4)
cryptococcal meningitis (B45.1)
herpesviral [herpes simplex] meningitis (B00.3)
infectious mononucleosis complicated by meningitis (B27.- with fifth character 2)
measles complicated by meningitis (B05.1)
meningoencephalitis and meningomyelitis in other infectious and parasitic diseases classified elsewhere (G05)
mumps meningitis (B26.1)
rubella meningitis (B06.02)
varicella [chickenpox] meningitis (B01.0)
zoster meningitis (B02.1)

G03 Meningitis due to other and unspecified causes

INCLUDES arachnoiditis NOS
leptomeningitis NOS
meningitis NOS
pachymeningitis NOS

EXCLUDES 1 *meningoencephalitis (G04.-)*
meningomyelitis (G04.-)

G03.0 Nonpyogenic meningitis COM
Aseptic meningitis
Nonbacterial meningitis
DEF: Type of meningitis where no bacterial, viral, or other infectious source exists that explains the meningitis symptomology.

G03.1 Chronic meningitis COM

G03.2 Benign recurrent meningitis [Mollaret] COM
DEF: Aseptic or noninfectious inflammation of the meninges with the presence of Mollaret cells in the spinal fluid. The patient experiences recurrent bouts of inflammation, lasting anywhere from two to five days.

G03.8 Meningitis due to other specified causes COM

G03.9 Meningitis, unspecified COM
Arachnoiditis (spinal) NOS

G04 Encephalitis, myelitis and encephalomyelitis

INCLUDES acute ascending myelitis
meningoencephalitis
meningomyelitis

EXCLUDES 1 *encephalopathy NOS (G93.40)*

EXCLUDES 2 *acute transverse myelitis (G37.3-)*
alcoholic encephalopathy (G31.2)
~~*benign myalgic encephalomyelitis (G93.3)*~~
multiple sclerosis (G35)
▶*myalgic encephalomyelitis (G93.32)*◀
subacute necrotizing myelitis (G37.4)
toxic encephalitis (G92.8)
toxic encephalopathy (G92.8)

DEF: Encephalitis: Inflammation of the brain, often caused by viral or bacterial infection.
DEF: Encephalomyelitis: Inflammatory disease, often viral in nature, that affects the brain and spinal cord.
DEF: Myelitis: Inflammation of the spinal cord.

G04.0 Acute disseminated encephalitis and encephalomyelitis (ADEM)

EXCLUDES 1 *acute necrotizing hemorrhagic encephalopathy (G04.3-)*
other noninfectious acute disseminated encephalomyelitis (noninfectious ADEM) (G04.81)

G04.00 Acute disseminated encephalitis and encephalomyelitis, unspecified COM

G04.01 Postinfectious acute disseminated encephalitis and encephalomyelitis (postinfectious ADEM) COM

EXCLUDES 1 *post chickenpox encephalitis (B01.1)*
post measles encephalitis (B05.0)
post measles myelitis (B05.1)

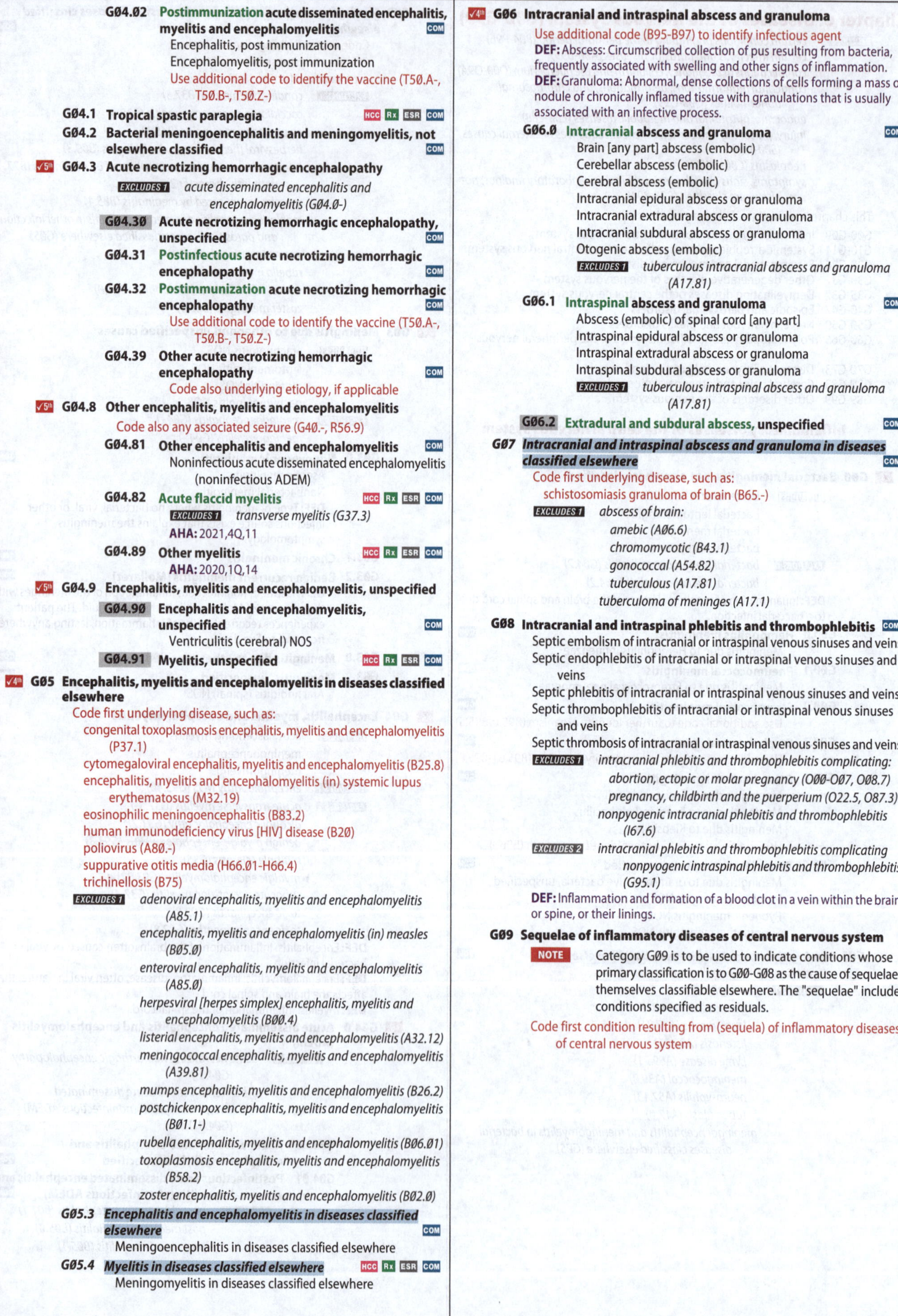

G04.02 Postimmunization acute disseminated encephalitis, myelitis and encephalomyelitis COM
Encephalitis, post immunization
Encephalomyelitis, post immunization
Use additional code to identify the vaccine (T50.A-, T50.B-, T50.Z-)

G04.1 **Tropical spastic paraplegia** HCC Rx ESR COM

G04.2 **Bacterial meningoencephalitis and meningomyelitis, not elsewhere classified** COM

✓5th G04.3 **Acute necrotizing hemorrhagic encephalopathy**
EXCLUDES 1 *acute disseminated encephalitis and encephalomyelitis (G04.0-)*

G04.30 **Acute necrotizing hemorrhagic encephalopathy, unspecified** COM

G04.31 **Postinfectious acute necrotizing hemorrhagic encephalopathy** COM

G04.32 **Postimmunization acute necrotizing hemorrhagic encephalopathy** COM
Use additional code to identify the vaccine (T50.A-, T50.B-, T50.Z-)

G04.39 **Other acute necrotizing hemorrhagic encephalopathy** COM
Code also underlying etiology, if applicable

✓5th G04.8 **Other encephalitis, myelitis and encephalomyelitis**
Code also any associated seizure (G40.-, R56.9)

G04.81 **Other encephalitis and encephalomyelitis** COM
Noninfectious acute disseminated encephalomyelitis (noninfectious ADEM)

G04.82 **Acute flaccid myelitis** HCC Rx ESR COM
EXCLUDES 1 *transverse myelitis (G37.3)*
AHA: 2021,4Q,11

G04.89 **Other myelitis** HCC Rx ESR COM
AHA: 2020,1Q,14

✓5th G04.9 **Encephalitis, myelitis and encephalomyelitis, unspecified**

G04.90 **Encephalitis and encephalomyelitis, unspecified** COM
Ventriculitis (cerebral) NOS

G04.91 **Myelitis, unspecified** HCC Rx ESR COM

✓4th G05 **Encephalitis, myelitis and encephalomyelitis in diseases classified elsewhere**
Code first underlying disease, such as:
congenital toxoplasmosis encephalitis, myelitis and encephalomyelitis (P37.1)
cytomegaloviral encephalitis, myelitis and encephalomyelitis (B25.8)
encephalitis, myelitis and encephalomyelitis (in) systemic lupus erythematosus (M32.19)
eosinophilic meningoencephalitis (B83.2)
human immunodeficiency virus [HIV] disease (B20)
poliovirus (A80.-)
suppurative otitis media (H66.01-H66.4)
trichinellosis (B75)
EXCLUDES 1 *adenoviral encephalitis, myelitis and encephalomyelitis (A85.1)*
encephalitis, myelitis and encephalomyelitis (in) measles (B05.0)
enteroviral encephalitis, myelitis and encephalomyelitis (A85.0)
herpesviral [herpes simplex] encephalitis, myelitis and encephalomyelitis (B00.4)
listerial encephalitis, myelitis and encephalomyelitis (A32.12)
meningococcal encephalitis, myelitis and encephalomyelitis (A39.81)
mumps encephalitis, myelitis and encephalomyelitis (B26.2)
postchickenpox encephalitis, myelitis and encephalomyelitis (B01.1-)
rubella encephalitis, myelitis and encephalomyelitis (B06.01)
toxoplasmosis encephalitis, myelitis and encephalomyelitis (B58.2)
zoster encephalitis, myelitis and encephalomyelitis (B02.0)

G05.3 ***Encephalitis and encephalomyelitis in diseases classified elsewhere*** COM
Meningoencephalitis in diseases classified elsewhere

G05.4 ***Myelitis in diseases classified elsewhere*** HCC Rx ESR COM
Meningomyelitis in diseases classified elsewhere

✓4th G06 **Intracranial and intraspinal abscess and granuloma**
Use additional code (B95-B97) to identify infectious agent
DEF: Abscess: Circumscribed collection of pus resulting from bacteria, frequently associated with swelling and other signs of inflammation.
DEF: Granuloma: Abnormal, dense collections of cells forming a mass or nodule of chronically inflamed tissue with granulations that is usually associated with an infective process.

G06.0 **Intracranial abscess and granuloma** COM
Brain [any part] abscess (embolic)
Cerebellar abscess (embolic)
Cerebral abscess (embolic)
Intracranial epidural abscess or granuloma
Intracranial extradural abscess or granuloma
Intracranial subdural abscess or granuloma
Otogenic abscess (embolic)
EXCLUDES 1 *tuberculous intracranial abscess and granuloma (A17.81)*

G06.1 **Intraspinal abscess and granuloma** COM
Abscess (embolic) of spinal cord [any part]
Intraspinal epidural abscess or granuloma
Intraspinal extradural abscess or granuloma
Intraspinal subdural abscess or granuloma
EXCLUDES 1 *tuberculous intraspinal abscess and granuloma (A17.81)*

G06.2 **Extradural and subdural abscess, unspecified** COM

G07 ***Intracranial and intraspinal abscess and granuloma in diseases classified elsewhere*** COM
Code first underlying disease, such as:
schistosomiasis granuloma of brain (B65.-)
EXCLUDES 1 *abscess of brain:*
amebic (A06.6)
chromomycotic (B43.1)
gonococcal (A54.82)
tuberculous (A17.81)
tuberculoma of meninges (A17.1)

G08 **Intracranial and intraspinal phlebitis and thrombophlebitis** COM
Septic embolism of intracranial or intraspinal venous sinuses and veins
Septic endophlebitis of intracranial or intraspinal venous sinuses and veins
Septic phlebitis of intracranial or intraspinal venous sinuses and veins
Septic thrombophlebitis of intracranial or intraspinal venous sinuses and veins
Septic thrombosis of intracranial or intraspinal venous sinuses and veins
EXCLUDES 1 *intracranial phlebitis and thrombophlebitis complicating:*
abortion, ectopic or molar pregnancy (O00-O07, O08.7)
pregnancy, childbirth and the puerperium (O22.5, O87.3)
nonpyogenic intracranial phlebitis and thrombophlebitis (I67.6)
EXCLUDES 2 *intracranial phlebitis and thrombophlebitis complicating nonpyogenic intraspinal phlebitis and thrombophlebitis (G95.1)*
DEF: Inflammation and formation of a blood clot in a vein within the brain or spine, or their linings.

G09 **Sequelae of inflammatory diseases of central nervous system**
NOTE Category G09 is to be used to indicate conditions whose primary classification is to G00-G08 as the cause of sequelae, themselves classifiable elsewhere. The "sequelae" include conditions specified as residuals.
Code first condition resulting from (sequela) of inflammatory diseases of central nervous system

Systemic atrophies primarily affecting the central nervous system (G10-G14)

G10 Huntington's disease HCC Rx ESR COM
Huntington's chorea
Huntington's dementia
▶Use additional code, if applicable, to identify:◀
▶dementia with anxiety (F02.84, F02.A4, F02.B4, F02.C4)◀
▶dementia with behavioral disturbance (F02.81-, F02.A1-, F02.B1-, F02.C1-)◀
▶dementia with mood disturbance (F02.83, F02.A3, F02.B3, F02.C3)◀
▶dementia with psychotic disturbance (F02.82, F02.A2, F02.B2, F02.C2)◀
▶dementia without behavioral disturbance (F02.80, F02.A0, F02.B0, F02.C0)◀
▶mild neurocognitive disorder due to known physiological condition (F06.7-)◀
~~Code also dementia in other diseases classified elsewhere without behavioral disturbance (F02.80)~~
DEF: Genetic disease caused by degeneration of nerve cells in the brain, characterized by chronic progressive mental deterioration. Dementia and death occur within 15 to 20 years of onset.

G11 Hereditary ataxia (4th)
EXCLUDES 2 *cerebral palsy (G80.-)*
hereditary and idiopathic neuropathy (G60.-)
metabolic disorders (E70-E88)
DEF: Ataxia: Defect in muscular control or coordination due to a central nervous system disorder, particularly when voluntary muscular movements are attempted.

G11.0 Congenital nonprogressive ataxia HCC ESR COM
G11.1 Early-onset cerebellar ataxia (5th)
AHA: 2020,4Q,17-18
G11.10 Early-onset cerebellar ataxia, unspecified HCC ESR COM
G11.11 Friedreich ataxia HCC ESR COM
Autosomal recessive Friedreich ataxia
Friedreich ataxia with retained reflexes
G11.19 Other early-onset cerebellar ataxia HCC ESR COM
Early-onset cerebellar ataxia with essential tremor
Early-onset cerebellar ataxia with myoclonus [Hunt's ataxia]
Early-onset cerebellar ataxia with retained tendon reflexes
X-linked recessive spinocerebellar ataxia
G11.2 Late-onset cerebellar ataxia HCC ESR COM A
G11.3 Cerebellar ataxia with defective DNA repair HCC ESR COM
Ataxia telangiectasia [Louis-Bar]
EXCLUDES 2 *Cockayne's syndrome (Q87.19)*
other disorders of purine and pyrimidine metabolism (E79.-)
xeroderma pigmentosum (Q82.1)
G11.4 Hereditary spastic paraplegia HCC ESR COM
G11.8 Other hereditary ataxias HCC ESR COM
G11.9 Hereditary ataxia, unspecified HCC ESR COM
Hereditary cerebellar ataxia NOS
Hereditary cerebellar degeneration
Hereditary cerebellar disease
Hereditary cerebellar syndrome

G12 Spinal muscular atrophy and related syndromes (4th)
G12.0 Infantile spinal muscular atrophy, type I [Werdnig-Hoffman] HCC Rx ESR COM
G12.1 Other inherited spinal muscular atrophy HCC Rx ESR COM
Adult form spinal muscular atrophy
Childhood form, type II spinal muscular atrophy
Distal spinal muscular atrophy
Juvenile form, type III spinal muscular atrophy [Kugelberg-Welander]
Progressive bulbar palsy of childhood [Fazio-Londe]
Scapuloperoneal form spinal muscular atrophy
G12.2 Motor neuron disease (5th)
AHA: 2017,4Q,9-10
G12.20 Motor neuron disease, unspecified HCC Rx ESR COM
G12.21 Amyotrophic lateral sclerosis HCC Rx ESR COM A
G12.22 Progressive bulbar palsy HCC Rx ESR COM
G12.23 Primary lateral sclerosis HCC Rx ESR COM
G12.24 Familial motor neuron disease HCC Rx ESR COM
G12.25 Progressive spinal muscle atrophy HCC Rx ESR COM
G12.29 Other motor neuron disease HCC Rx ESR COM
G12.8 Other spinal muscular atrophies and related syndromes HCC Rx ESR COM
G12.9 Spinal muscular atrophy, unspecified HCC Rx ESR COM

G13 Systemic atrophies primarily affecting central nervous system in diseases classified elsewhere (4th)
G13.0 Paraneoplastic neuromyopathy and neuropathy HCC Rx ESR COM
Carcinomatous neuromyopathy
Sensorial paraneoplastic neuropathy [Denny Brown]
Code first underlying neoplasm (C00-D49)
G13.1 Other systemic atrophy primarily affecting central nervous system in neoplastic disease HCC Rx ESR COM
Paraneoplastic limbic encephalopathy
Code first underlying neoplasm (C00-D49)
G13.2 Systemic atrophy primarily affecting the central nervous system in myxedema HCC Rx ESR
Code first underlying disease, such as:
hypothyroidism (E03.-)
myxedematous congenital iodine deficiency (E00.1)
G13.8 Systemic atrophy primarily affecting central nervous system in other diseases classified elsewhere HCC Rx ESR
Code first underlying disease

G14 Postpolio syndrome
INCLUDES postpolio myelitic syndrome
EXCLUDES 1 *sequelae of poliomyelitis (B91)*

Extrapyramidal and movement disorders (G20-G26)

G20 Parkinson's disease HCC Rx ESR COM
Hemiparkinsonism
Idiopathic Parkinsonism or Parkinson's disease
Paralysis agitans
Parkinsonism or Parkinson's disease NOS
Primary Parkinsonism or Parkinson's disease
▶Use additional code, if applicable, to identify:◀
▶dementia with anxiety (F02.84, F02.A4, F02.B4, F02.C4)◀
dementia with behavioral disturbance ▶(F02.81-, F02.A1-, F02.B1-, F02.C1-)◀
▶dementia with mood disturbance (F02.83, F02.A3, F02.B3, F02.C3)◀
▶dementia with psychotic disturbance (F02.82, F02.A2, F02.B2, F02.C2)◀
dementia without behavioral disturbance ▶(F02.80, F02.A0, F02.B0, F02.C0)◀
▶mild neurocognitive disorder due to known physiological condition (F06.7-)◀
EXCLUDES 1 ~~*dementia with Parkinsonism (G31.83)*~~
AHA: 2017,2Q,7; 2016,2Q,6
TIP: Repeated falls (R29.6) are not integral to Parkinson's disease and can be separately coded.

G21 Secondary parkinsonism (4th)
EXCLUDES 1 *dementia with Parkinsonism (G31.83)*
Huntington's disease (G10)
Shy-Drager syndrome (G90.3)
syphilitic Parkinsonism (A52.19)
G21.0 Malignant neuroleptic syndrome
Use additional code for adverse effect, if applicable, to identify drug (T43.3X5, T43.4X5, T43.505, T43.595)
EXCLUDES 1 *neuroleptic induced parkinsonism (G21.11)*
G21.1 Other drug-induced secondary parkinsonism (5th)
G21.11 Neuroleptic induced parkinsonism HCC Rx ESR COM
Use additional code for adverse effect, if applicable, to identify drug (T43.3X5, T43.4X5, T43.505, T43.595)
EXCLUDES 1 *malignant neuroleptic syndrome (G21.0)*
G21.19 Other drug induced secondary parkinsonism HCC Rx ESR COM
Other medication-induced parkinsonism
Use additional code for adverse effect, if applicable, to identify drug (T36-T50 with fifth or sixth character 5)

G21.2 Secondary parkinsonism due to other external agents HCC Rx ESR COM
Code first (T51-T65) to identify external agent

G21.3 Postencephalitic parkinsonism HCC Rx ESR COM

G21.4 Vascular parkinsonism HCC Rx ESR COM

G21.8 Other secondary parkinsonism HCC Rx ESR COM

G21.9 Secondary parkinsonism, unspecified HCC Rx ESR COM

4th G23 Other degenerative diseases of basal ganglia

EXCLUDES 2 *multi-system degeneration of the autonomic nervous system (G90.3)*

G23.0 Hallervorden-Spatz disease HCC Rx ESR COM
Pigmentary pallidal degeneration

G23.1 Progressive supranuclear ophthalmoplegia [Steele-Richardson-Olszewski] HCC Rx ESR COM
Progressive supranuclear palsy

G23.2 Striatonigral degeneration HCC Rx ESR COM

G23.8 Other specified degenerative diseases of basal ganglia HCC Rx ESR COM
Calcification of basal ganglia

G23.9 Degenerative disease of basal ganglia, unspecified HCC Rx ESR COM

4th G24 Dystonia

INCLUDES dyskinesia

EXCLUDES 2 *athetoid cerebral palsy (G80.3)*

DEF: Disorder of abnormal muscle tone, excessive or inadequate. Involuntary movements and prolonged muscle contractions result in tremors, abnormalities in posture, and twisting body motions that affect an isolated area or the whole body.

5th G24.0 Drug induced dystonia
Use additional code for adverse effect, if applicable, to identify drug (T36-T50 with fifth or sixth character 5)

G24.01 Drug induced subacute dyskinesia
Drug induced blepharospasm
Drug induced orofacial dyskinesia
Neuroleptic induced tardive dyskinesia
Tardive dyskinesia

G24.02 Drug induced acute dystonia
Acute dystonic reaction to drugs
Neuroleptic induced acute dystonia

G24.09 Other drug induced dystonia

G24.1 Genetic torsion dystonia
Dystonia deformans progressiva
Dystonia musculorum deformans
Familial torsion dystonia
Idiopathic familial dystonia
Idiopathic (torsion) dystonia NOS
(Schwalbe-) Ziehen-Oppenheim disease

G24.2 Idiopathic nonfamilial dystonia

G24.3 Spasmodic torticollis

EXCLUDES 1 *congenital torticollis (Q68.0)*
hysterical torticollis (F44.4)
ocular torticollis (R29.891)
psychogenic torticollis (F45.8)
torticollis NOS (M43.6)
traumatic recurrent torticollis (S13.4)

DEF: Twisted, unnatural position of the neck due to contracted cervical muscles that pull the head to one side or cause involuntary shaking of the head.

G24.4 Idiopathic orofacial dystonia
Orofacial dyskinesia

EXCLUDES 1 *drug induced orofacial dyskinesia (G24.01)*

G24.5 Blepharospasm

EXCLUDES 1 *drug induced blepharospasm (G24.01)*

DEF: Involuntary contraction of the orbicularis oculi muscle, resulting in the eyelids being completely closed.

G24.8 Other dystonia
Acquired torsion dystonia NOS

G24.9 Dystonia, unspecified
Dyskinesia NOS

4th G25 Other extrapyramidal and movement disorders

EXCLUDES 2 *sleep related movement disorders (G47.6-)*

G25.0 Essential tremor
Familial tremor

EXCLUDES 1 *tremor NOS (R25.1)*

G25.1 Drug-induced tremor
Use additional code for adverse effect, if applicable, to identify drug (T36-T50 with fifth or sixth character 5)

G25.2 Other specified forms of tremor
Intention tremor

G25.3 Myoclonus
Drug-induced myoclonus
Palatal myoclonus
Use additional code for adverse effect, if applicable, to identify drug (T36-T50 with fifth or sixth character 5)

EXCLUDES 1 *facial myokymia (G51.4)*
myoclonic epilepsy (G40.-)

DEF: Spasmodic, brief, involuntary muscle contractions that can be due to an undetermined etiology, drug-induced, or caused by a disease process.

G25.4 Drug-induced chorea
Use additional code for adverse effect, if applicable, to identify drug (T36-T50 with fifth or sixth character 5)

G25.5 Other chorea
Chorea NOS

EXCLUDES 1 *chorea NOS with heart involvement (I02.0)*
Huntington's chorea (G10)
rheumatic chorea (I02.-)
Sydenham's chorea (I02.-)

5th G25.6 Drug induced tics and other tics of organic origin

G25.61 Drug induced tics
Use additional code for adverse effect, if applicable, to identify drug (T36-T50 with fifth or sixth character 5)

G25.69 Other tics of organic origin

EXCLUDES 1 *habit spasm (F95.9)*
tic NOS (F95.9)
Tourette's syndrome (F95.2)

5th G25.7 Other and unspecified drug induced movement disorders
Use additional code for adverse effect, if applicable, to identify drug (T36-T50 with fifth or sixth character 5)

G25.70 Drug induced movement disorder, unspecified

G25.71 Drug induced akathisia
Drug induced acathisia
Neuroleptic induced acute akathisia
Tardive akathisia

G25.79 Other drug induced movement disorders

5th G25.8 Other specified extrapyramidal and movement disorders

G25.81 Restless legs syndrome
DEF: Neurological disorder of unknown etiology creating an irresistible urge to move the legs, which may temporarily relieve the symptoms. This syndrome is accompanied by motor restlessness and sensations of pain, burning, prickling, or tingling.

G25.82 Stiff-man syndrome

G25.83 Benign shuddering attacks

G25.89 Other specified extrapyramidal and movement disorders

G25.9 Extrapyramidal and movement disorder, unspecified

G26 *Extrapyramidal and movement disorders in diseases classified elsewhere*
Code first underlying disease

Other degenerative diseases of the nervous system (G30-G32)

G30 Alzheimer's disease

INCLUDES Alzheimer's dementia senile and presenile forms

▶Use additional code, if applicable, to identify:◀
delirium, if applicable (F05)
▶dementia with anxiety (F02.84, F02.A4, F02.B4, F02.C4)◀
dementia with behavioral disturbance ▶(F02.81-, F02.A1-, F02.B1-, F02.C1-)◀
▶dementia with mood disturbance (F02.83, F02.A3, F02.B3, F02.C3)◀
▶dementia with psychotic disturbance (F02.82, F02.A2, F02.B2, F02.C2)◀
dementia without behavioral disturbance ▶(F02.80, F02.A0, F02.B0, F02.C0)◀
▶mild neurocognitive disorder due to known physiological condition (F06.7-)◀

EXCLUDES 1 *senile degeneration of brain NEC (G31.1)*
senile dementia NOS (F03)
senility NOS (R41.81)

AHA: 2017,1Q,43
TIP: A code from subcategory F02.8 should always be assigned with a code from this category, even in the absence of documented dementia.
TIP: Functional quadriplegia (R53.2) is not integral to Alzheimer's disease and can be coded in addition to codes from category G30.

G30.0 Alzheimer's disease with early onset HCC Rx ESR
G30.1 Alzheimer's disease with late onset HCC Rx ESR A
G30.8 Other Alzheimer's disease HCC Rx ESR
G30.9 Alzheimer's disease, unspecified HCC Rx ESR
AHA: 2016,2Q,6; 2012,4Q,95

G31 Other degenerative diseases of nervous system, not elsewhere classified

For codes G31.0 - G31.83, G31.85 - G31.9, use additional code, if applicable, to identify:
▶dementia with anxiety (F02.84, F02.A4, F02.B4, F02.C4)◀
dementia with behavioral disturbance ▶(F02.81-, F02.A1-, F02.B1-, F02.C1-)◀
▶dementia with mood disturbance (F02.83, F02.A3, F02.B3, F02.C3)◀
▶dementia with psychotic disturbance (F02.82, F02.A2, F02.B2, F02.C2)◀
dementia without behavioral disturbance ▶(F02.80, F02.A0, F02.B0, F02.C0)◀
▶mild neurocognitive disorder due to known physiological condition (F06.7-)◀

EXCLUDES 2 *Reye's syndrome (G93.7)*

G31.0 Frontotemporal dementia

G31.01 Pick's disease HCC Rx ESR
Primary progressive aphasia
Progressive isolated aphasia
DEF: Progressive frontotemporal dementia with asymmetrical atrophy of the frontal and temporal regions of the cerebral cortex and abnormal rounded brain cells called Pick cells with the presence of abnormal staining of protein (called tau). Symptoms include prominent apathy, behavioral changes such as disinhibition and restlessness, echolalia, impairment of language, memory, and intellect, increased carelessness, poor personal hygiene, and decreased attention span.

▲ **G31.09 Other frontotemporal neurocognitive disorder** HCC Rx ESR
Frontal dementia
▶Use additional code, if applicable, to identify mild neurocognitive disorders due to known physiological condition (F06.7-)◀

G31.1 Senile degeneration of brain, not elsewhere classified HCC Rx ESR
EXCLUDES 1 *Alzheimer's disease (G30.-)*
senility NOS (R41.81)

G31.2 Degeneration of nervous system due to alcohol HCC Rx ESR
Alcoholic cerebellar ataxia
Alcoholic cerebellar degeneration
Alcoholic cerebral degeneration
Alcoholic encephalopathy
Dysfunction of the autonomic nervous system due to alcohol
Code also associated alcoholism (F10.-)

G31.8 Other specified degenerative diseases of nervous system

G31.81 Alpers disease HCC Rx ESR COM
Grey-matter degeneration

G31.82 Leigh's disease HCC Rx ESR COM
Subacute necrotizing encephalopathy

▲ **G31.83 Neurocognitive disorder with Lewy bodies** HCC Rx ESR
~~Dementia with Parkinsonism~~
Lewy body dementia
Lewy body disease
▶Use additional code, if applicable, to identify mild neurocognitive disorders due to known physiological condition (F06.7-)◀
AHA: 2017,2Q,7; 2016,4Q,141
DEF: Cerebral dementia with neurophysiologic changes, increased hippocampal volume, hypoperfusion in the occipital lobes, beta amyloid deposits with neurofibrillary tangles, and atrophy of the cortex and brainstem. Hallmark neuropsychological characteristics include fluctuating cognition with pronounced variation in attention and alertness, recurrent hallucinations, and Parkinsonism.

▲ **G31.84 Mild cognitive impairment of uncertain or unknown etiology**
▶Mild cognitive disorder NOS◀
~~Mild neurocognitive disorder~~
▶Mild neurocognitive disorder of uncertain or unknown etiology◀
▶Use additional code to identify presence of:◀
▶alcohol abuse and dependence (F10.-)◀
▶exposure to environmental tobacco smoke (Z77.22)◀
▶history of tobacco dependence (Z87.891)◀
▶hypertension (I10-I16)◀
▶occupational exposure to environmental tobacco smoke (Z57.31)◀
▶tobacco dependence (F17.-)◀
▶tobacco use (Z72.0)◀

EXCLUDES 1 *age related cognitive decline (R41.81)*
altered mental status (R41.82)
cerebral degeneration (G31.9)
▶cerebrovascular diseases (I60-I69)◀
change in mental status (R41.82)
cognitive deficits following (sequelae of) cerebral hemorrhage or infarction (I69.01-, I69.11-, I69.21-, I69.31-, I69.81-, I69.91-)
cognitive impairment due to intracranial or head injury (S06.-)
dementia (F01.-, F02.-, F03)
~~mild memory disturbance (F06.8)~~
▶mild neurocognitive disorder due to a known physiological condition (F06.7-)◀
neurologic neglect syndrome (R41.4)
personality change, nonpsychotic (F68.8)

AHA: 2021,3Q,3

G31.85 Corticobasal degeneration HCC Rx ESR
G31.89 Other specified degenerative diseases of nervous system HCC Rx ESR

G31.9 Degenerative disease of nervous system, unspecified HCC Rx ESR
AHA: 2021,3Q,3

G32 Other degenerative disorders of nervous system in diseases classified elsewhere

G32.0 Subacute combined degeneration of spinal cord in diseases classified elsewhere HCC Rx ESR COM
Dana-Putnam syndrome
Sclerosis of spinal cord (combined) (dorsolateral) (posterolateral)
Code first underlying disease, such as:
anemia (D51.9)
dietary (D51.3)
pernicious (D51.0)
vitamin B12 deficiency (E53.8)

EXCLUDES 1 *syphilitic combined degeneration of spinal cord (A52.11)*

√5th **G32.8 Other specified degenerative disorders of nervous system in diseases classified elsewhere**

Code first underlying disease, such as:
amyloidosis cerebral degeneration (E85.-)
cerebral degeneration (due to) hypothyroidism (E00.0-E03.9)
cerebral degeneration (due to) neoplasm (C00-D49)
cerebral degeneration (due to) vitamin B deficiency, except thiamine (E52-E53.-)

EXCLUDES 1 *superior hemorrhagic polioencephalitis [Wernicke's encephalopathy] (E51.2)*

G32.81 Cerebellar ataxia in diseases classified elsewhere HCC ESR COM

Code first underlying disease, such as:
celiac disease (with gluten ataxia) (K90.0)
cerebellar ataxia (in) neoplastic disease (paraneoplastic cerebellar degeneration) (C00-D49)
non-celiac gluten ataxia (M35.9)

EXCLUDES 1 *systemic atrophy primarily affecting the central nervous system in alcoholic cerebellar ataxia (G31.2)*
systemic atrophy primarily affecting the central nervous system in myxedema (G13.2)

G32.89 Other specified degenerative disorders of nervous system in diseases classified elsewhere

Degenerative encephalopathy in diseases classified elsewhere

Demyelinating diseases of the central nervous system (G35-G37)

G35 Multiple sclerosis HCC Rx ESR COM

Disseminated multiple sclerosis
Generalized multiple sclerosis
Multiple sclerosis NOS
Multiple sclerosis of brain stem
Multiple sclerosis of cord
AHA: 2021,1Q,7

√4th **G36 Other acute disseminated demyelination**

EXCLUDES 1 *postinfectious encephalitis and encephalomyelitis NOS (G04.01)*

DEF: Demyelination: Abnormal loss of myelin, the protective white matter that insulates nerve endings and facilitates neuroreception and neurotransmission. When this substance is damaged, the nerve is short-circuited, resulting in impaired or loss of function.

G36.0 Neuromyelitis optica [Devic] HCC Rx ESR COM

Demyelination in optic neuritis

EXCLUDES 1 *optic neuritis NOS (H46)*

G36.1 Acute and subacute hemorrhagic leukoencephalitis [Hurst] HCC ESR

G36.8 Other specified acute disseminated demyelination HCC ESR

G36.9 Acute disseminated demyelination, unspecified HCC ESR

√4th **G37 Other demyelinating diseases of central nervous system**

G37.0 Diffuse sclerosis of central nervous system HCC Rx ESR COM

Periaxial encephalitis
Schilder's disease

EXCLUDES 1 *X linked adrenoleukodystrophy (E71.52-)*

G37.1 Central demyelination of corpus callosum HCC ESR

G37.2 Central pontine myelinolysis HCC ESR

AHA: 2022,2Q,10

G37.3 Acute transverse myelitis in demyelinating disease of central nervous system HCC Rx ESR COM

Acute transverse myelitis NOS
Acute transverse myelopathy

EXCLUDES 1 *acute flaccid myelitis (G04.82)*
multiple sclerosis (G35)
neuromyelitis optica [Devic] (G36.0)

G37.4 Subacute necrotizing myelitis of central nervous system HCC Rx ESR COM

G37.5 Concentric sclerosis [Balo] of central nervous system HCC Rx ESR COM

G37.8 Other specified demyelinating diseases of central nervous system HCC ESR

G37.9 Demyelinating disease of central nervous system, unspecified HCC ESR

Episodic and paroxysmal disorders (G40-G47)

√4th **G40 Epilepsy and recurrent seizures**

NOTE The following terms are to be considered equivalent to intractable: pharmacoresistant (pharmacologically resistant), treatment resistant, refractory (medically) and poorly controlled

EXCLUDES 1 *conversion disorder with seizures (F44.5)*
convulsions NOS (R56.9)
post traumatic seizures (R56.1)
seizure (convulsive) NOS (R56.9)
seizure of newborn (P90)

EXCLUDES 2 *hippocampal sclerosis (G93.81)*
mesial temporal sclerosis (G93.81)
temporal sclerosis (G93.81)
Todd's paralysis (G83.84)

√5th **G40.0 Localization-related (focal) (partial) idiopathic epilepsy and epileptic syndromes with seizures of localized onset**

Benign childhood epilepsy with centrotemporal EEG spikes
Childhood epilepsy with occipital EEG paroxysms

EXCLUDES 1 *adult onset localization-related epilepsy (G40.1-, G40.2-)*

√6th **G40.00 Localization-related (focal) (partial) idiopathic epilepsy and epileptic syndromes with seizures of localized onset, not intractable**

Localization-related (focal) (partial) idiopathic epilepsy and epileptic syndromes with seizures of localized onset without intractability

G40.001 Localization-related (focal) (partial) idiopathic epilepsy and epileptic syndromes with seizures of localized onset, not intractable, with status epilepticus HCC Rx ESR COM

G40.009 Localization-related (focal) (partial) idiopathic epilepsy and epileptic syndromes with seizures of localized onset, not intractable, without status epilepticus HCC Rx ESR COM

Localization-related (focal) (partial) idiopathic epilepsy and epileptic syndromes with seizures of localized onset NOS

√6th **G40.01 Localization-related (focal) (partial) idiopathic epilepsy and epileptic syndromes with seizures of localized onset, intractable**

G40.011 Localization-related (focal) (partial) idiopathic epilepsy and epileptic syndromes with seizures of localized onset, intractable, with status epilepticus HCC Rx ESR COM

G40.019 Localization-related (focal) (partial) idiopathic epilepsy and epileptic syndromes with seizures of localized onset, intractable, without status epilepticus HCC Rx ESR COM

√5th **G40.1 Localization-related (focal) (partial) symptomatic epilepsy and epileptic syndromes with simple partial seizures**

Attacks without alteration of consciousness
Epilepsia partialis continua [Kozhevnikof]
Simple partial seizures developing into secondarily generalized seizures

√6th **G40.10 Localization-related (focal) (partial) symptomatic epilepsy and epileptic syndromes with simple partial seizures, not intractable**

Localization-related (focal) (partial) symptomatic epilepsy and epileptic syndromes with simple partial seizures without intractability

G40.101 Localization-related (focal) (partial) symptomatic epilepsy and epileptic syndromes with simple partial seizures, not intractable, with status epilepticus HCC Rx ESR COM

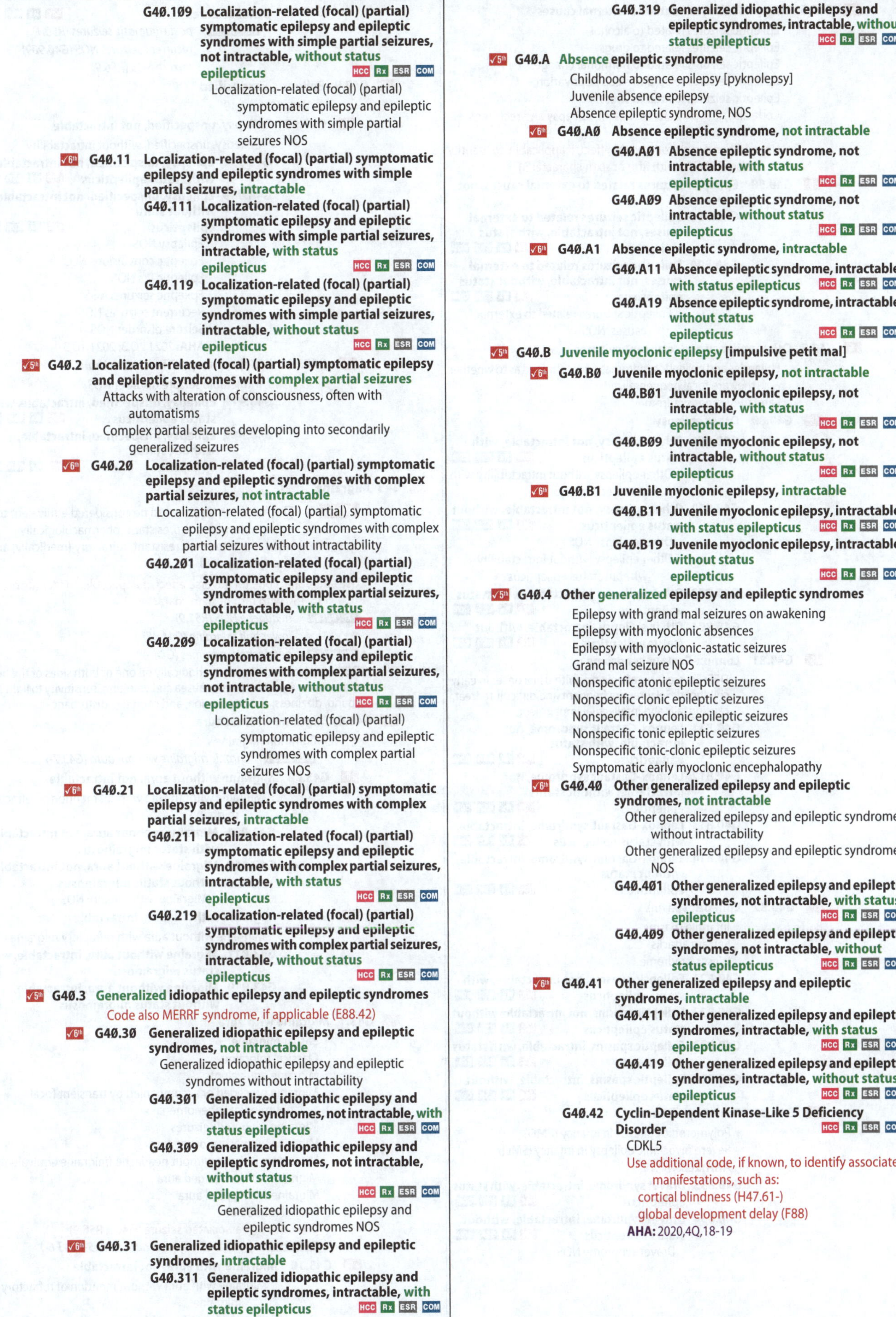

G40.109 Localization-related (focal) (partial) symptomatic epilepsy and epileptic syndromes with simple partial seizures, not intractable, without status epilepticus HCC Rx ESR COM
Localization-related (focal) (partial) symptomatic epilepsy and epileptic syndromes with simple partial seizures NOS

G40.11 Localization-related (focal) (partial) symptomatic epilepsy and epileptic syndromes with simple partial seizures, intractable

G40.111 Localization-related (focal) (partial) symptomatic epilepsy and epileptic syndromes with simple partial seizures, intractable, with status epilepticus HCC Rx ESR COM

G40.119 Localization-related (focal) (partial) symptomatic epilepsy and epileptic syndromes with simple partial seizures, intractable, without status epilepticus HCC Rx ESR COM

G40.2 Localization-related (focal) (partial) symptomatic epilepsy and epileptic syndromes with complex partial seizures
Attacks with alteration of consciousness, often with automatisms
Complex partial seizures developing into secondarily generalized seizures

G40.20 Localization-related (focal) (partial) symptomatic epilepsy and epileptic syndromes with complex partial seizures, not intractable
Localization-related (focal) (partial) symptomatic epilepsy and epileptic syndromes with complex partial seizures without intractability

G40.201 Localization-related (focal) (partial) symptomatic epilepsy and epileptic syndromes with complex partial seizures, not intractable, with status epilepticus HCC Rx ESR COM

G40.209 Localization-related (focal) (partial) symptomatic epilepsy and epileptic syndromes with complex partial seizures, not intractable, without status epilepticus HCC Rx ESR COM
Localization-related (focal) (partial) symptomatic epilepsy and epileptic syndromes with complex partial seizures NOS

G40.21 Localization-related (focal) (partial) symptomatic epilepsy and epileptic syndromes with complex partial seizures, intractable

G40.211 Localization-related (focal) (partial) symptomatic epilepsy and epileptic syndromes with complex partial seizures, intractable, with status epilepticus HCC Rx ESR COM

G40.219 Localization-related (focal) (partial) symptomatic epilepsy and epileptic syndromes with complex partial seizures, intractable, without status epilepticus HCC Rx ESR COM

G40.3 Generalized idiopathic epilepsy and epileptic syndromes
Code also MERRF syndrome, if applicable (E88.42)

G40.30 Generalized idiopathic epilepsy and epileptic syndromes, not intractable
Generalized idiopathic epilepsy and epileptic syndromes without intractability

G40.301 Generalized idiopathic epilepsy and epileptic syndromes, not intractable, with status epilepticus HCC Rx ESR COM

G40.309 Generalized idiopathic epilepsy and epileptic syndromes, not intractable, without status epilepticus HCC Rx ESR COM
Generalized idiopathic epilepsy and epileptic syndromes NOS

G40.31 Generalized idiopathic epilepsy and epileptic syndromes, intractable

G40.311 Generalized idiopathic epilepsy and epileptic syndromes, intractable, with status epilepticus HCC Rx ESR COM

G40.319 Generalized idiopathic epilepsy and epileptic syndromes, intractable, without status epilepticus HCC Rx ESR COM

G40.A Absence epileptic syndrome
Childhood absence epilepsy [pyknolepsy]
Juvenile absence epilepsy
Absence epileptic syndrome, NOS

G40.A0 Absence epileptic syndrome, not intractable

G40.A01 Absence epileptic syndrome, not intractable, with status epilepticus HCC Rx ESR COM

G40.A09 Absence epileptic syndrome, not intractable, without status epilepticus HCC Rx ESR COM

G40.A1 Absence epileptic syndrome, intractable

G40.A11 Absence epileptic syndrome, intractable, with status epilepticus HCC Rx ESR COM

G40.A19 Absence epileptic syndrome, intractable, without status epilepticus HCC Rx ESR COM

G40.B Juvenile myoclonic epilepsy [impulsive petit mal]

G40.B0 Juvenile myoclonic epilepsy, not intractable

G40.B01 Juvenile myoclonic epilepsy, not intractable, with status epilepticus HCC Rx ESR COM

G40.B09 Juvenile myoclonic epilepsy, not intractable, without status epilepticus HCC Rx ESR COM

G40.B1 Juvenile myoclonic epilepsy, intractable

G40.B11 Juvenile myoclonic epilepsy, intractable, with status epilepticus HCC Rx ESR COM

G40.B19 Juvenile myoclonic epilepsy, intractable, without status epilepticus HCC Rx ESR COM

G40.4 Other generalized epilepsy and epileptic syndromes
Epilepsy with grand mal seizures on awakening
Epilepsy with myoclonic absences
Epilepsy with myoclonic-astatic seizures
Grand mal seizure NOS
Nonspecific atonic epileptic seizures
Nonspecific clonic epileptic seizures
Nonspecific myoclonic epileptic seizures
Nonspecific tonic epileptic seizures
Nonspecific tonic-clonic epileptic seizures
Symptomatic early myoclonic encephalopathy

G40.40 Other generalized epilepsy and epileptic syndromes, not intractable
Other generalized epilepsy and epileptic syndromes without intractability
Other generalized epilepsy and epileptic syndromes NOS

G40.401 Other generalized epilepsy and epileptic syndromes, not intractable, with status epilepticus HCC Rx ESR COM

G40.409 Other generalized epilepsy and epileptic syndromes, not intractable, without status epilepticus HCC Rx ESR COM

G40.41 Other generalized epilepsy and epileptic syndromes, intractable

G40.411 Other generalized epilepsy and epileptic syndromes, intractable, with status epilepticus HCC Rx ESR COM

G40.419 Other generalized epilepsy and epileptic syndromes, intractable, without status epilepticus HCC Rx ESR COM

G40.42 Cyclin-Dependent Kinase-Like 5 Deficiency Disorder HCC Rx ESR COM
CDKL5
Use additional code, if known, to identify associated manifestations, such as:
cortical blindness (H47.61-)
global development delay (F88)
AHA: 2020,4Q,18-19

Chapter 6. Diseases of the Nervous System

G40.109–G40.42

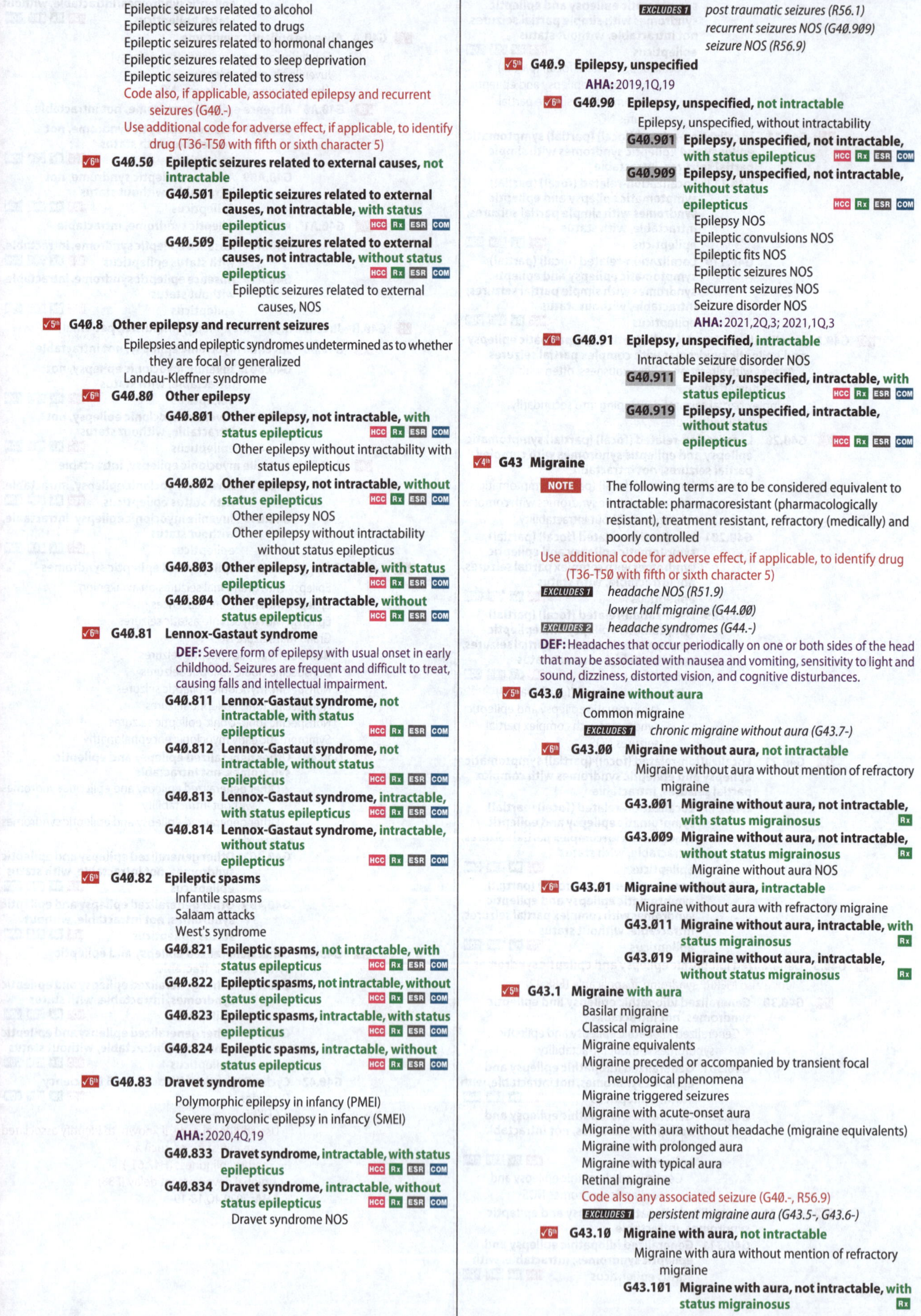

√5th **G40.5 Epileptic seizures related to external causes**
Epileptic seizures related to alcohol
Epileptic seizures related to drugs
Epileptic seizures related to hormonal changes
Epileptic seizures related to sleep deprivation
Epileptic seizures related to stress
Code also, if applicable, associated epilepsy and recurrent seizures (G40.-)
Use additional code for adverse effect, if applicable, to identify drug (T36-T50 with fifth or sixth character 5)

√6th **G40.50 Epileptic seizures related to external causes, not intractable**

G40.501 Epileptic seizures related to external causes, not intractable, with status epilepticus HCC Rx ESR COM

G40.509 Epileptic seizures related to external causes, not intractable, without status epilepticus HCC Rx ESR COM
Epileptic seizures related to external causes, NOS

√5th **G40.8 Other epilepsy and recurrent seizures**
Epilepsies and epileptic syndromes undetermined as to whether they are focal or generalized
Landau-Kleffner syndrome

√6th **G40.80 Other epilepsy**

G40.801 Other epilepsy, not intractable, with status epilepticus HCC Rx ESR COM
Other epilepsy without intractability with status epilepticus

G40.802 Other epilepsy, not intractable, without status epilepticus HCC Rx ESR COM
Other epilepsy NOS
Other epilepsy without intractability without status epilepticus

G40.803 Other epilepsy, intractable, with status epilepticus HCC Rx ESR COM

G40.804 Other epilepsy, intractable, without status epilepticus HCC Rx ESR COM

√6th **G40.81 Lennox-Gastaut syndrome**
DEF: Severe form of epilepsy with usual onset in early childhood. Seizures are frequent and difficult to treat, causing falls and intellectual impairment.

G40.811 Lennox-Gastaut syndrome, not intractable, with status epilepticus HCC Rx ESR COM

G40.812 Lennox-Gastaut syndrome, not intractable, without status epilepticus HCC Rx ESR COM

G40.813 Lennox-Gastaut syndrome, intractable, with status epilepticus HCC Rx ESR COM

G40.814 Lennox-Gastaut syndrome, intractable, without status epilepticus HCC Rx ESR COM

√6th **G40.82 Epileptic spasms**
Infantile spasms
Salaam attacks
West's syndrome

G40.821 Epileptic spasms, not intractable, with status epilepticus HCC Rx ESR COM

G40.822 Epileptic spasms, not intractable, without status epilepticus HCC Rx ESR COM

G40.823 Epileptic spasms, intractable, with status epilepticus HCC Rx ESR COM

G40.824 Epileptic spasms, intractable, without status epilepticus HCC Rx ESR COM

√6th **G40.83 Dravet syndrome**
Polymorphic epilepsy in infancy (PMEI)
Severe myoclonic epilepsy in infancy (SMEI)
AHA: 2020,4Q,19

G40.833 Dravet syndrome, intractable, with status epilepticus HCC Rx ESR COM

G40.834 Dravet syndrome, intractable, without status epilepticus HCC Rx ESR COM
Dravet syndrome NOS

G40.89 Other seizures HCC Rx ESR COM
EXCLUDES 1 *post traumatic seizures (R56.1)*
recurrent seizures NOS (G40.909)
seizure NOS (R56.9)

√5th **G40.9 Epilepsy, unspecified**
AHA: 2019,1Q,19

√6th **G40.90 Epilepsy, unspecified, not intractable**
Epilepsy, unspecified, without intractability

G40.901 Epilepsy, unspecified, not intractable, with status epilepticus HCC Rx ESR COM

G40.909 Epilepsy, unspecified, not intractable, without status epilepticus HCC Rx ESR COM
Epilepsy NOS
Epileptic convulsions NOS
Epileptic fits NOS
Epileptic seizures NOS
Recurrent seizures NOS
Seizure disorder NOS
AHA: 2021,2Q,3; 2021,1Q,3

√6th **G40.91 Epilepsy, unspecified, intractable**
Intractable seizure disorder NOS

G40.911 Epilepsy, unspecified, intractable, with status epilepticus HCC Rx ESR COM

G40.919 Epilepsy, unspecified, intractable, without status epilepticus HCC Rx ESR COM

√4th **G43 Migraine**
NOTE The following terms are to be considered equivalent to intractable: pharmacoresistant (pharmacologically resistant), treatment resistant, refractory (medically) and poorly controlled
Use additional code for adverse effect, if applicable, to identify drug (T36-T50 with fifth or sixth character 5)
EXCLUDES 1 *headache NOS (R51.9)*
lower half migraine (G44.00)
EXCLUDES 2 *headache syndromes (G44.-)*
DEF: Headaches that occur periodically on one or both sides of the head that may be associated with nausea and vomiting, sensitivity to light and sound, dizziness, distorted vision, and cognitive disturbances.

√5th **G43.0 Migraine without aura**
Common migraine
EXCLUDES 1 *chronic migraine without aura (G43.7-)*

√6th **G43.00 Migraine without aura, not intractable**
Migraine without aura without mention of refractory migraine

G43.001 Migraine without aura, not intractable, with status migrainosus Rx

G43.009 Migraine without aura, not intractable, without status migrainosus Rx
Migraine without aura NOS

√6th **G43.01 Migraine without aura, intractable**
Migraine without aura with refractory migraine

G43.011 Migraine without aura, intractable, with status migrainosus Rx

G43.019 Migraine without aura, intractable, without status migrainosus Rx

√5th **G43.1 Migraine with aura**
Basilar migraine
Classical migraine
Migraine equivalents
Migraine preceded or accompanied by transient focal neurological phenomena
Migraine triggered seizures
Migraine with acute-onset aura
Migraine with aura without headache (migraine equivalents)
Migraine with prolonged aura
Migraine with typical aura
Retinal migraine
Code also any associated seizure (G40.-, R56.9)
EXCLUDES 1 *persistent migraine aura (G43.5-, G43.6-)*

√6th **G43.10 Migraine with aura, not intractable**
Migraine with aura without mention of refractory migraine

G43.101 Migraine with aura, not intractable, with status migrainosus Rx

G43.109 Migraine with aura, not intractable, without status migrainosus Rx
Migraine with aura NOS

✓6th **G43.11 Migraine with aura, intractable**
Migraine with aura with refractory migraine

G43.111 Migraine with aura, intractable, with status migrainosus Rx

G43.119 Migraine with aura, intractable, without status migrainosus Rx

✓5th **G43.4 Hemiplegic migraine**
Familial migraine
Sporadic migraine

✓6th **G43.40 Hemiplegic migraine, not intractable**
Hemiplegic migraine without refractory migraine

G43.401 Hemiplegic migraine, not intractable, with status migrainosus Rx

G43.409 Hemiplegic migraine, not intractable, without status migrainosus Rx
Hemiplegic migraine NOS

✓6th **G43.41 Hemiplegic migraine, intractable**
Hemiplegic migraine with refractory migraine

G43.411 Hemiplegic migraine, intractable, with status migrainosus Rx

G43.419 Hemiplegic migraine, intractable, without status migrainosus Rx

✓5th **G43.5 Persistent migraine aura without cerebral infarction**

✓6th **G43.50 Persistent migraine aura without cerebral infarction, not intractable**
Persistent migraine aura without cerebral infarction, without refractory migraine

G43.501 Persistent migraine aura without cerebral infarction, not intractable, with status migrainosus Rx

G43.509 Persistent migraine aura without cerebral infarction, not intractable, without status migrainosus Rx
Persistent migraine aura NOS

✓6th **G43.51 Persistent migraine aura without cerebral infarction, intractable**
Persistent migraine aura without cerebral infarction, with refractory migraine

G43.511 Persistent migraine aura without cerebral infarction, intractable, with status migrainosus Rx

G43.519 Persistent migraine aura without cerebral infarction, intractable, without status migrainosus Rx

✓5th **G43.6 Persistent migraine aura with cerebral infarction**
Code also the type of cerebral infarction (I63.-)

✓6th **G43.60 Persistent migraine aura with cerebral infarction, not intractable**
Persistent migraine aura with cerebral infarction, without refractory migraine

G43.601 Persistent migraine aura with cerebral infarction, not intractable, with status migrainosus Rx

G43.609 Persistent migraine aura with cerebral infarction, not intractable, without status migrainosus Rx

✓6th **G43.61 Persistent migraine aura with cerebral infarction, intractable**
Persistent migraine aura with cerebral infarction, with refractory migraine

G43.611 Persistent migraine aura with cerebral infarction, intractable, with status migrainosus Rx

G43.619 Persistent migraine aura with cerebral infarction, intractable, without status migrainosus Rx

✓5th **G43.7 Chronic migraine without aura**
Transformed migraine
EXCLUDES 1 *migraine without aura (G43.0-)*

✓6th **G43.70 Chronic migraine without aura, not intractable**
Chronic migraine without aura, without refractory migraine

G43.701 Chronic migraine without aura, not intractable, with status migrainosus Rx

G43.709 Chronic migraine without aura, not intractable, without status migrainosus Rx
Chronic migraine without aura NOS

✓6th **G43.71 Chronic migraine without aura, intractable**
Chronic migraine without aura, with refractory migraine

G43.711 Chronic migraine without aura, intractable, with status migrainosus Rx

G43.719 Chronic migraine without aura, intractable, without status migrainosus Rx

✓5th **G43.A Cyclical vomiting**
EXCLUDES 1 *cyclical vomiting syndrome unrelated to migraine (R11.15)*
AHA: 2019,4Q,15

G43.A0 Cyclical vomiting, in migraine, not intractable Rx
Cyclical vomiting, without refractory migraine

G43.A1 Cyclical vomiting, in migraine, intractable Rx
Cyclical vomiting, with refractory migraine

✓5th **G43.B Ophthalmoplegic migraine**

G43.B0 Ophthalmoplegic migraine, not intractable Rx
Ophthalmoplegic migraine, without refractory migraine

G43.B1 Ophthalmoplegic migraine, intractable Rx
Ophthalmoplegic migraine, with refractory migraine

✓5th **G43.C Periodic headache syndromes in child or adult**

G43.C0 Periodic headache syndromes in child or adult, not intractable Rx
Periodic headache syndromes in child or adult, without refractory migraine

G43.C1 Periodic headache syndromes in child or adult, intractable Rx
Periodic headache syndromes in child or adult, with refractory migraine

✓5th **G43.D Abdominal migraine**

G43.D0 Abdominal migraine, not intractable Rx
Abdominal migraine, without refractory migraine

G43.D1 Abdominal migraine, intractable Rx
Abdominal migraine, with refractory migraine

✓5th **G43.8 Other migraine**

✓6th **G43.80 Other migraine, not intractable**
Other migraine, without refractory migraine

G43.801 Other migraine, not intractable, with status migrainosus Rx

G43.809 Other migraine, not intractable, without status migrainosus Rx

✓6th **G43.81 Other migraine, intractable**
Other migraine, with refractory migraine

G43.811 Other migraine, intractable, with status migrainosus Rx

G43.819 Other migraine, intractable, without status migrainosus Rx

✓6th **G43.82 Menstrual migraine, not intractable**
Menstrual headache, not intractable
Menstrual migraine, without refractory migraine
Menstrually related migraine, not intractable
Pre-menstrual headache, not intractable
Pre-menstrual migraine, not intractable
Pure menstrual migraine, not intractable
Code also associated premenstrual tension syndrome (N94.3)

G43.821 Menstrual migraine, not intractable, with status migrainosus Rx ♀

G43.829 Menstrual migraine, not intractable, without status migrainosus Rx ♀
Menstrual migraine NOS

6th G43.83 Menstrual migraine, intractable
Menstrual headache, intractable
Menstrual migraine, with refractory migraine
Menstrually related migraine, intractable
Pre-menstrual headache, intractable
Pre-menstrual migraine, intractable
Pure menstrual migraine, intractable
Code also associated premenstrual tension syndrome (N94.3)

G43.831 Menstrual migraine, intractable, with status migrainosus Rx ♀

G43.839 Menstrual migraine, intractable, without status migrainosus Rx ♀

5th G43.9 Migraine, unspecified

6th G43.90 Migraine, unspecified, not intractable
Migraine, unspecified, without refractory migraine

G43.901 Migraine, unspecified, not intractable, with status migrainosus Rx
Status migrainosus NOS

G43.909 Migraine, unspecified, not intractable, without status migrainosus Rx
Migraine NOS

6th G43.91 Migraine, unspecified, intractable
Migraine, unspecified, with refractory migraine

G43.911 Migraine, unspecified, intractable, with status migrainosus Rx

G43.919 Migraine, unspecified, intractable, without status migrainosus Rx

4th G44 Other headache syndromes
EXCLUDES 1 *headache NOS (R51.9)*
EXCLUDES 2 *atypical facial pain (G50.1)*
headache due to lumbar puncture (G97.1)
migraines (G43.-)
trigeminal neuralgia (G50.0)

5th G44.0 Cluster headaches and other trigeminal autonomic cephalgias (TAC)
DEF: Cluster headache: Characteristic grouping or clustering of headaches that can last for a number of weeks or months and then completely disappear for months or years. They are typically not associated with gastrointestinal upset or light sensitivity as experienced in migraines.

6th G44.00 Cluster headache syndrome, unspecified
Ciliary neuralgia
Cluster headache NOS
Histamine cephalgia
Lower half migraine
Migrainous neuralgia

G44.001 Cluster headache syndrome, unspecified, intractable

G44.009 Cluster headache syndrome, unspecified, not intractable
Cluster headache syndrome NOS

6th G44.01 Episodic cluster headache

G44.011 Episodic cluster headache, intractable

G44.019 Episodic cluster headache, not intractable
Episodic cluster headache NOS

6th G44.02 Chronic cluster headache

G44.021 Chronic cluster headache, intractable

G44.029 Chronic cluster headache, not intractable
Chronic cluster headache NOS

6th G44.03 Episodic paroxysmal hemicrania
Paroxysmal hemicrania NOS

G44.031 Episodic paroxysmal hemicrania, intractable

G44.039 Episodic paroxysmal hemicrania, not intractable
Episodic paroxysmal hemicrania NOS

6th G44.04 Chronic paroxysmal hemicrania

G44.041 Chronic paroxysmal hemicrania, intractable

G44.049 Chronic paroxysmal hemicrania, not intractable
Chronic paroxysmal hemicrania NOS

6th G44.05 Short lasting unilateral neuralgiform headache with conjunctival injection and tearing (SUNCT)

G44.051 Short lasting unilateral neuralgiform headache with conjunctival injection and tearing (SUNCT), intractable

G44.059 Short lasting unilateral neuralgiform headache with conjunctival injection and tearing (SUNCT), not intractable
Short lasting unilateral neuralgiform headache with conjunctival injection and tearing (SUNCT) NOS

6th G44.09 Other trigeminal autonomic cephalgias (TAC)

G44.091 Other trigeminal autonomic cephalgias (TAC), intractable

G44.099 Other trigeminal autonomic cephalgias (TAC), not intractable

G44.1 Vascular headache, not elsewhere classified
EXCLUDES 2 *cluster headache (G44.0)*
complicated headache syndromes (G44.5-)
drug-induced headache (G44.4-)
migraine (G43.-)
other specified headache syndromes (G44.8-)
post-traumatic headache (G44.3-)
tension-type headache (G44.2-)

5th G44.2 Tension-type headache

6th G44.20 Tension-type headache, unspecified

G44.201 Tension-type headache, unspecified, intractable

G44.209 Tension-type headache, unspecified, not intractable
Tension headache NOS

6th G44.21 Episodic tension-type headache

G44.211 Episodic tension-type headache, intractable

G44.219 Episodic tension-type headache, not intractable
Episodic tension-type headache NOS

6th G44.22 Chronic tension-type headache

G44.221 Chronic tension-type headache, intractable

G44.229 Chronic tension-type headache, not intractable
Chronic tension-type headache NOS

5th G44.3 Post-traumatic headache

6th G44.30 Post-traumatic headache, unspecified

G44.301 Post-traumatic headache, unspecified, intractable

G44.309 Post-traumatic headache, unspecified, not intractable
Post-traumatic headache NOS

6th G44.31 Acute post-traumatic headache

G44.311 Acute post-traumatic headache, intractable

G44.319 Acute post-traumatic headache, not intractable
Acute post-traumatic headache NOS

6th G44.32 Chronic post-traumatic headache

G44.321 Chronic post-traumatic headache, intractable

G44.329 Chronic post-traumatic headache, not intractable
Chronic post-traumatic headache NOS

5th G44.4 Drug-induced headache, not elsewhere classified
Medication overuse headache
Use additional code for adverse effect, if applicable, to identify drug (T36-T50 with fifth or sixth character 5)

G44.40 Drug-induced headache, not elsewhere classified, not intractable

G44.41 Drug-induced headache, not elsewhere classified, intractable

5th G44.5 Complicated headache syndromes

G44.51 Hemicrania continua
DEF: Persistent primary headache of unknown causation occurring on one side of the face and head. May last for more than three months, with daily and continuous pain of moderate intensity with severe exacerbations.

G44.52 New daily persistent headache (NDPH)

G44.53 Primary thunderclap headache
G44.59 Other complicated headache syndrome

G44.8 Other specified headache syndromes
EXCLUDES 2 *headache with orthostatic or positional component, not elsewhere classifed (R51.Ø)*

G44.81 Hypnic headache
G44.82 Headache associated with sexual activity
Orgasmic headache
Preorgasmic headache
G44.83 Primary cough headache
G44.84 Primary exertional headache
G44.85 Primary stabbing headache
G44.86 Cervicogenic headache
Code also associated cervical spinal condition, if known
AHA: 2021,4Q,11-12
G44.89 Other headache syndrome

G45 Transient cerebral ischemic attacks and related syndromes

EXCLUDES 1 *neonatal cerebral ischemia (P91.Ø)*
transient retinal artery occlusion (H34.Ø-)

AHA: 2018,2Q,9

DEF: Transient cerebral ischemic attack: Intermittent or brief cerebral dysfunction from lack of oxygenation with no persistent neurological deficits associated with occlusive vascular disease. TIA may denote an impending cerebrovascular accident.

G45.Ø Vertebro-basilar artery syndrome
G45.1 Carotid artery syndrome (hemispheric)
G45.2 Multiple and bilateral precerebral artery syndromes
G45.3 Amaurosis fugax
G45.4 Transient global amnesia
EXCLUDES 1 *amnesia NOS (R41.3)*
G45.8 Other transient cerebral ischemic attacks and related syndromes
G45.9 Transient cerebral ischemic attack, unspecified
Spasm of cerebral artery
TIA
Transient cerebral ischemia NOS

G46 Vascular syndromes of brain in cerebrovascular diseases

Code first underlying cerebrovascular disease (I6Ø-I69)

G46.Ø Middle cerebral artery syndrome
G46.1 Anterior cerebral artery syndrome
G46.2 Posterior cerebral artery syndrome
G46.3 Brain stem stroke syndrome
Benedikt syndrome
Claude syndrome
Foville syndrome
Millard-Gubler syndrome
Wallenberg syndrome
Weber syndrome
G46.4 Cerebellar stroke syndrome
G46.5 Pure motor lacunar syndrome
G46.6 Pure sensory lacunar syndrome
G46.7 Other lacunar syndromes
G46.8 Other vascular syndromes of brain in cerebrovascular diseases

G47 Sleep disorders

EXCLUDES 2 *nightmares (F51.5)*
nonorganic sleep disorders (F51.-)
sleep terrors (F51.4)
sleepwalking (F51.3)

G47.Ø Insomnia
EXCLUDES 2 *alcohol related insomnia (F1Ø.182, F1Ø.282, F1Ø.982)*
drug-related insomnia (F11.182, F11.282, F11.982, F13.182, F13.282, F13.982, F14.182, F14.282, F14.982, F15.182, F15.282, F15.982, F19.182, F19.282, F19.982)
idiopathic insomnia (F51.Ø1)
insomnia due to a mental disorder (F51.Ø5)
insomnia not due to a substance or known physiological condition (F51.Ø-)
nonorganic insomnia (F51.Ø-)
primary insomnia (F51.Ø1)
sleep apnea (G47.3-)

G47.ØØ Insomnia, unspecified
Insomnia NOS
G47.Ø1 Insomnia due to medical condition
Code also associated medical condition
G47.Ø9 Other insomnia

G47.1 Hypersomnia
EXCLUDES 2 *alcohol-related hypersomnia (F1Ø.182, F1Ø.282, F1Ø.982)*
drug-related hypersomnia (F11.182, F11.282, F11.982, F13.182, F13.282, F13.982, F14.182, F14.282, F14.982, F15.182, F15.282, F15.982, F19.182, F19.282, F19.982)
hypersomnia due to a mental disorder (F51.13)
hypersomnia not due to a substance or known physiological condition (F51.1-)
primary hypersomnia (F51.11)
sleep apnea (G47.3-)

G47.1Ø Hypersomnia, unspecified
Hypersomnia NOS
G47.11 Idiopathic hypersomnia with long sleep time
Idiopathic hypersomnia NOS
G47.12 Idiopathic hypersomnia without long sleep time
G47.13 Recurrent hypersomnia
Kleine-Levin syndrome
Menstrual related hypersomnia
G47.14 Hypersomnia due to medical condition
Code also associated medical condition
G47.19 Other hypersomnia

G47.2 Circadian rhythm sleep disorders
Disorders of the sleep wake schedule
Inversion of nyctohemeral rhythm
Inversion of sleep rhythm

DEF: Circadian rhythm: Daily cycle (24-hour period) of physical, mental, and behavioral changes. It is largely influenced by environmental cues, such as changes in light or temperature.
Synonym(s): sleep/wake cycle.

G47.2Ø Circadian rhythm sleep disorder, unspecified type
Sleep wake schedule disorder NOS
G47.21 Circadian rhythm sleep disorder, delayed sleep phase type
Delayed sleep phase syndrome
G47.22 Circadian rhythm sleep disorder, advanced sleep phase type
G47.23 Circadian rhythm sleep disorder, irregular sleep wake type
Irregular sleep-wake pattern
G47.24 Circadian rhythm sleep disorder, free running type
Circadian rhythm sleep disorder, non-24-hour sleep-wake type
G47.25 Circadian rhythm sleep disorder, jet lag type
G47.26 Circadian rhythm sleep disorder, shift work type
G47.27 Circadian rhythm sleep disorder in conditions classified elsewhere
Code first underlying condition
G47.29 Other circadian rhythm sleep disorder

5th G47.3 Sleep apnea

Code also any associated underlying condition

EXCLUDES 1 *apnea NOS (RØ6.81)*
Cheyne-Stokes breathing (RØ6.3)
pickwickian syndrome (E66.2)
sleep apnea of newborn ▶(P28.3-)◀

G47.3Ø Sleep apnea, unspecified
Sleep apnea NOS

G47.31 Primary central sleep apnea
Idiopathic central sleep apnea

G47.32 High altitude periodic breathing

G47.33 Obstructive sleep apnea (adult) (pediatric)
Obstructive sleep apnea hypopnea
EXCLUDES 1 *obstructive sleep apnea of newborn ▶(P28.3-)◀*

G47.34 Idiopathic sleep related nonobstructive alveolar hypoventilation
Sleep related hypoxia

G47.35 Congenital central alveolar hypoventilation syndrome

G47.36 Sleep related hypoventilation in conditions classified elsewhere
Sleep related hypoxemia in conditions classified elsewhere
Code first underlying condition

G47.37 Central sleep apnea in conditions classified elsewhere
Code first underlying condition

G47.39 Other sleep apnea

5th G47.4 Narcolepsy and cataplexy

6th G47.41 Narcolepsy

G47.411 Narcolepsy with cataplexy Rx COM

G47.419 Narcolepsy without cataplexy Rx COM
Narcolepsy NOS

6th G47.42 Narcolepsy in conditions classified elsewhere
Code first underlying condition

G47.421 Narcolepsy in conditions classified elsewhere with cataplexy Rx COM

G47.429 Narcolepsy in conditions classified elsewhere without cataplexy Rx COM

5th G47.5 Parasomnia

EXCLUDES 1 *alcohol induced parasomnia (F1Ø.182, F1Ø.282, F1Ø.982)*
drug induced parasomnia (F11.182, F11.282, F11.982, F13.182, F13.282, F13.982, F14.182, F14.282, F14.982, F15.182, F15.282, F15.982, F19.182, F19.282, F19.982)
parasomnia not due to a substance or known physiological condition (F51.8)

G47.5Ø Parasomnia, unspecified
Parasomnia NOS

G47.51 Confusional arousals

G47.52 REM sleep behavior disorder

G47.53 Recurrent isolated sleep paralysis

G47.54 Parasomnia in conditions classified elsewhere
Code first underlying condition

G47.59 Other parasomnia

5th G47.6 Sleep related movement disorders

EXCLUDES 2 *restless legs syndrome (G25.81)*

G47.61 Periodic limb movement disorder

G47.62 Sleep related leg cramps

G47.63 Sleep related bruxism
EXCLUDES 1 *psychogenic bruxism (F45.8)*

G47.69 Other sleep related movement disorders

G47.8 Other sleep disorders
Other specified sleep-wake disorder

G47.9 Sleep disorder, unspecified
Sleep disorder NOS
Unspecified sleep-wake disorder

Nerve, nerve root and plexus disorders (G5Ø-G59)

EXCLUDES 1 *current traumatic nerve, nerve root and plexus disorders - see Injury, nerve by body region*
neuralgia NOS (M79.2)
neuritis NOS (M79.2)
peripheral neuritis in pregnancy (O26.82-)
radiculitis NOS (M54.1-)

4th G5Ø Disorders of trigeminal nerve

INCLUDES disorders of 5th cranial nerve

G5Ø.Ø Trigeminal neuralgia Rx
Syndrome of paroxysmal facial pain
Tic douloureux

G5Ø.1 Atypical facial pain Rx

G5Ø.8 Other disorders of trigeminal nerve Rx

G5Ø.9 Disorder of trigeminal nerve, unspecified Rx

4th G51 Facial nerve disorders

INCLUDES disorders of 7th cranial nerve

G51.Ø Bell's palsy
Facial palsy

G51.1 Geniculate ganglionitis
EXCLUDES 1 *postherpetic geniculate ganglionitis (BØ2.21)*

G51.2 Melkersson's syndrome
Melkersson-Rosenthal syndrome

5th G51.3 Clonic hemifacial spasm
AHA: 2018,4Q,10

G51.31 Clonic hemifacial spasm, right

G51.32 Clonic hemifacial spasm, left

G51.33 Clonic hemifacial spasm, bilateral

G51.39 Clonic hemifacial spasm, unspecified

G51.4 Facial myokymia

G51.8 Other disorders of facial nerve

G51.9 Disorder of facial nerve, unspecified

4th G52 Disorders of other cranial nerves

EXCLUDES 2 *disorders of acoustic [8th] nerve (H93.3)*
disorders of optic [2nd] nerve (H46, H47.Ø)
paralytic strabismus due to nerve palsy (H49.Ø-H49.2)

G52.Ø Disorders of olfactory nerve
Disorders of 1st cranial nerve

G52.1 Disorders of glossopharyngeal nerve
Disorder of 9th cranial nerve
Glossopharyngeal neuralgia

G52.2 Disorders of vagus nerve
Disorders of pneumogastric [1Øth] nerve

G52.3 Disorders of hypoglossal nerve
Disorders of 12th cranial nerve

G52.7 Disorders of multiple cranial nerves
Polyneuritis cranialis

G52.8 Disorders of other specified cranial nerves

G52.9 Cranial nerve disorder, unspecified

G53 Cranial nerve disorders in diseases classified elsewhere

Code first underlying disease, such as:
neoplasm (CØØ-D49)

EXCLUDES 1 *multiple cranial nerve palsy in sarcoidosis (D86.82)*
multiple cranial nerve palsy in syphilis (A52.15)
postherpetic geniculate ganglionitis (BØ2.21)
postherpetic trigeminal neuralgia (BØ2.22)

G54 Nerve root and plexus disorders

EXCLUDES 1 *current traumatic nerve root and plexus disorders - see nerve injury by body region*
intervertebral disc disorders (M5Ø-M51)
neuralgia or neuritis NOS (M79.2)
neuritis or radiculitis brachial NOS (M54.13)
neuritis or radiculitis lumbar NOS (M54.16)
neuritis or radiculitis lumbosacral NOS (M54.17)
neuritis or radiculitis thoracic NOS (M54.14)
radiculitis NOS (M54.1Ø)
radiculopathy NOS (M54.1Ø)
spondylosis (M47.-)

G54.Ø Brachial plexus disorders
Thoracic outlet syndrome
DEF: Acquired disorder affecting the spinal nerves that send signals to the shoulder, arm, and hand, causing corresponding motor and sensory dysfunction. This disorder is characterized by regional paresthesia, pain, muscle weakness, and in severe cases paralysis.

G54.1 Lumbosacral plexus disorders
G54.2 Cervical root disorders, not elsewhere classified
G54.3 Thoracic root disorders, not elsewhere classified
G54.4 Lumbosacral root disorders, not elsewhere classified
G54.5 Neuralgic amyotrophy
Parsonage-Aldren-Turner syndrome
Shoulder-girdle neuritis
EXCLUDES 1 *neuralgic amyotrophy in diabetes mellitus (EØ8-E13 with .44)*

G54.6 Phantom limb syndrome with pain HCC ESR COM
G54.7 Phantom limb syndrome without pain HCC ESR COM
Phantom limb syndrome NOS
G54.8 Other nerve root and plexus disorders
G54.9 Nerve root and plexus disorder, unspecified

G55 Nerve root and plexus compressions in diseases classified elsewhere
Code first underlying disease, such as:
neoplasm (CØØ-D49)
EXCLUDES 1 *nerve root compression (due to) (in) ankylosing spondylitis (M45.-)*
nerve root compression (due to) (in) dorsopathies (M53.-, M54.-)
nerve root compression (due to) (in) intervertebral disc disorders (M5Ø.1.-, M51.1.-)
nerve root compression (due to) (in) spondylopathies (M46.-, M48.-)
nerve root compression (due to) (in) spondylosis (M47.Ø-, M47.2-)

G56 Mononeuropathies of upper limb
EXCLUDES 1 *current traumatic nerve disorder - see nerve injury by body region*
AHA: 2016,4Q,17-18

G56.Ø Carpal tunnel syndrome
DEF: Swelling and inflammation in the tendons or bursa surrounding the median nerve caused by repetitive activity. The resulting compression on the nerve causes pain, numbness, and tingling especially to the palm, index, middle finger, and thumb.
G56.ØØ Carpal tunnel syndrome, unspecified upper limb
G56.Ø1 Carpal tunnel syndrome, right upper limb
G56.Ø2 Carpal tunnel syndrome, left upper limb
G56.Ø3 Carpal tunnel syndrome, bilateral upper limbs

G56.1 Other lesions of median nerve
G56.1Ø Other lesions of median nerve, unspecified upper limb
G56.11 Other lesions of median nerve, right upper limb
G56.12 Other lesions of median nerve, left upper limb
G56.13 Other lesions of median nerve, bilateral upper limbs

G56.2 Lesion of ulnar nerve
Tardy ulnar nerve palsy
G56.2Ø Lesion of ulnar nerve, unspecified upper limb
G56.21 Lesion of ulnar nerve, right upper limb
G56.22 Lesion of ulnar nerve, left upper limb
G56.23 Lesion of ulnar nerve, bilateral upper limbs

G56.3 Lesion of radial nerve
G56.3Ø Lesion of radial nerve, unspecified upper limb
G56.31 Lesion of radial nerve, right upper limb
G56.32 Lesion of radial nerve, left upper limb
G56.33 Lesion of radial nerve, bilateral upper limbs

G56.4 Causalgia of upper limb
Complex regional pain syndrome II of upper limb
EXCLUDES 1 *complex regional pain syndrome I of lower limb (G9Ø.52-)*
complex regional pain syndrome I of upper limb (G9Ø.51-)
complex regional pain syndrome II of lower limb (G57.7-)
reflex sympathetic dystrophy of lower limb (G9Ø.52-)
reflex sympathetic dystrophy of upper limb (G9Ø.51-)
G56.4Ø Causalgia of unspecified upper limb
G56.41 Causalgia of right upper limb
G56.42 Causalgia of left upper limb
G56.43 Causalgia of bilateral upper limbs

G56.8 Other specified mononeuropathies of upper limb
Interdigital neuroma of upper limb
G56.8Ø Other specified mononeuropathies of unspecified upper limb
G56.81 Other specified mononeuropathies of right upper limb
G56.82 Other specified mononeuropathies of left upper limb
G56.83 Other specified mononeuropathies of bilateral upper limbs

G56.9 Unspecified mononeuropathy of upper limb
G56.9Ø Unspecified mononeuropathy of unspecified upper limb
G56.91 Unspecified mononeuropathy of right upper limb
G56.92 Unspecified mononeuropathy of left upper limb
G56.93 Unspecified mononeuropathy of bilateral upper limbs

G57 Mononeuropathies of lower limb
EXCLUDES 1 *current traumatic nerve disorder - see nerve injury by body region*
AHA: 2016,4Q,17-18

G57.Ø Lesion of sciatic nerve
EXCLUDES 1 *sciatica NOS (M54.3-)*
EXCLUDES 2 *sciatica attributed to intervertebral disc disorder (M51.1.-)*
G57.ØØ Lesion of sciatic nerve, unspecified lower limb
G57.Ø1 Lesion of sciatic nerve, right lower limb
G57.Ø2 Lesion of sciatic nerve, left lower limb
G57.Ø3 Lesion of sciatic nerve, bilateral lower limbs

G57.1 Meralgia paresthetica
Lateral cutaneous nerve of thigh syndrome
G57.1Ø Meralgia paresthetica, unspecified lower limb
G57.11 Meralgia paresthetica, right lower limb
G57.12 Meralgia paresthetica, left lower limb
G57.13 Meralgia paresthetica, bilateral lower limbs

G57.2 Lesion of femoral nerve
G57.2Ø Lesion of femoral nerve, unspecified lower limb
G57.21 Lesion of femoral nerve, right lower limb
G57.22 Lesion of femoral nerve, left lower limb
G57.23 Lesion of femoral nerve, bilateral lower limbs

G57.3 Lesion of lateral popliteal nerve
Peroneal nerve palsy
AHA: 2020,3Q,12
G57.3Ø Lesion of lateral popliteal nerve, unspecified lower limb
G57.31 Lesion of lateral popliteal nerve, right lower limb
G57.32 Lesion of lateral popliteal nerve, left lower limb
G57.33 Lesion of lateral popliteal nerve, bilateral lower limbs

G57.4 Lesion of medial popliteal nerve
G57.4Ø Lesion of medial popliteal nerve, unspecified lower limb
G57.41 Lesion of medial popliteal nerve, right lower limb
G57.42 Lesion of medial popliteal nerve, left lower limb
G57.43 Lesion of medial popliteal nerve, bilateral lower limbs

G57.5 Tarsal tunnel syndrome
G57.5Ø Tarsal tunnel syndrome, unspecified lower limb
G57.51 Tarsal tunnel syndrome, right lower limb
G57.52 Tarsal tunnel syndrome, left lower limb
G57.53 Tarsal tunnel syndrome, bilateral lower limbs

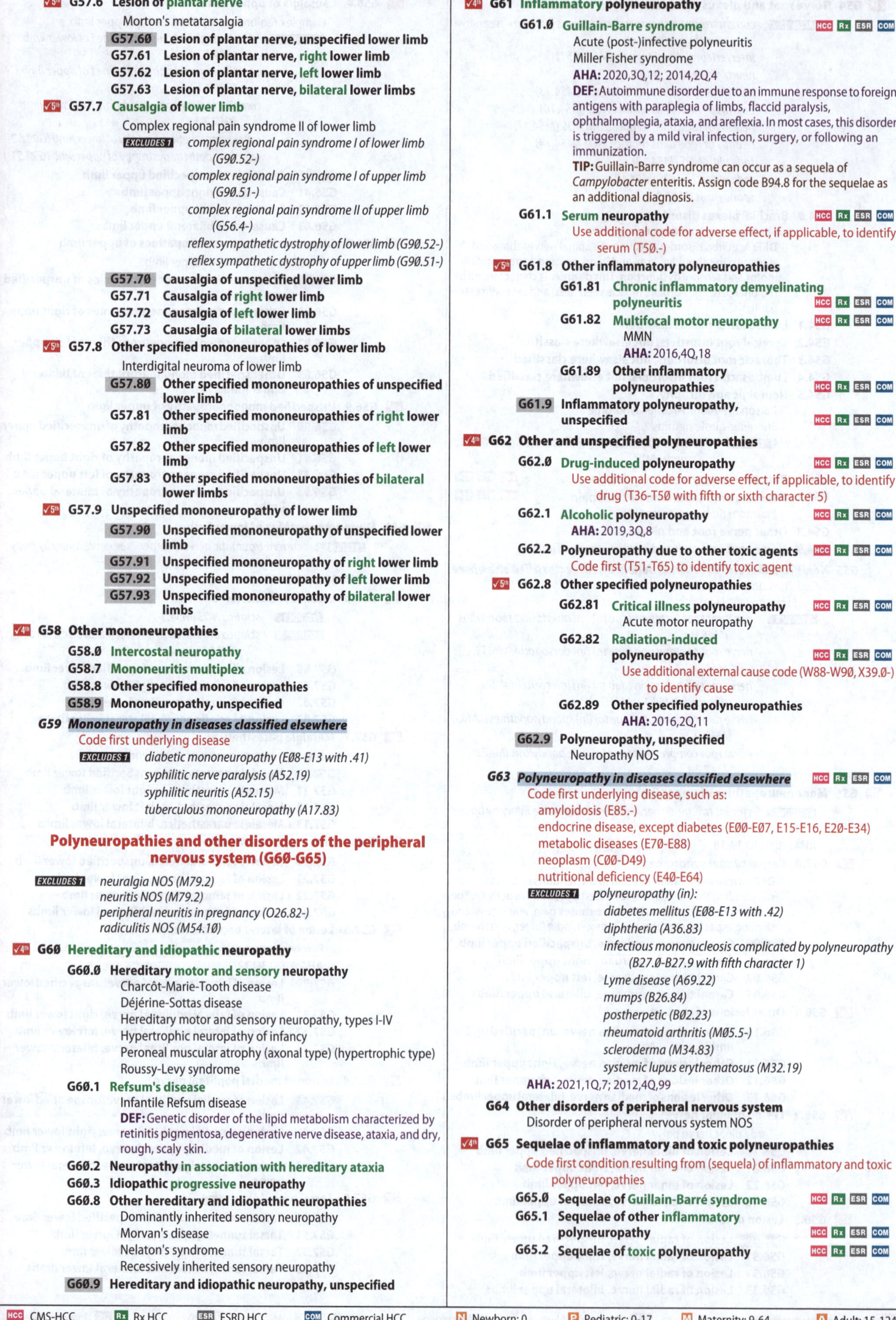

✓5th **G57.6 Lesion of plantar nerve**
Morton's metatarsalgia
G57.6Ø Lesion of plantar nerve, unspecified lower limb
G57.61 Lesion of plantar nerve, right lower limb
G57.62 Lesion of plantar nerve, left lower limb
G57.63 Lesion of plantar nerve, bilateral lower limbs

✓5th **G57.7 Causalgia of lower limb**
Complex regional pain syndrome II of lower limb
EXCLUDES 1 *complex regional pain syndrome I of lower limb (G9Ø.52-)*
complex regional pain syndrome I of upper limb (G9Ø.51-)
complex regional pain syndrome II of upper limb (G56.4-)
reflex sympathetic dystrophy of lower limb (G9Ø.52-)
reflex sympathetic dystrophy of upper limb (G9Ø.51-)
G57.7Ø Causalgia of unspecified lower limb
G57.71 Causalgia of right lower limb
G57.72 Causalgia of left lower limb
G57.73 Causalgia of bilateral lower limbs

✓5th **G57.8 Other specified mononeuropathies of lower limb**
Interdigital neuroma of lower limb
G57.8Ø Other specified mononeuropathies of unspecified lower limb
G57.81 Other specified mononeuropathies of right lower limb
G57.82 Other specified mononeuropathies of left lower limb
G57.83 Other specified mononeuropathies of bilateral lower limbs

✓5th **G57.9 Unspecified mononeuropathy of lower limb**
G57.9Ø Unspecified mononeuropathy of unspecified lower limb
G57.91 Unspecified mononeuropathy of right lower limb
G57.92 Unspecified mononeuropathy of left lower limb
G57.93 Unspecified mononeuropathy of bilateral lower limbs

✓4th **G58 Other mononeuropathies**
G58.Ø Intercostal neuropathy
G58.7 Mononeuritis multiplex
G58.8 Other specified mononeuropathies
G58.9 Mononeuropathy, unspecified

G59 Mononeuropathy in diseases classified elsewhere
Code first underlying disease
EXCLUDES 1 *diabetic mononeuropathy (EØ8-E13 with .41)*
syphilitic nerve paralysis (A52.19)
syphilitic neuritis (A52.15)
tuberculous mononeuropathy (A17.83)

Polyneuropathies and other disorders of the peripheral nervous system (G6Ø-G65)

EXCLUDES 1 *neuralgia NOS (M79.2)*
neuritis NOS (M79.2)
peripheral neuritis in pregnancy (O26.82-)
radiculitis NOS (M54.1Ø)

✓4th **G6Ø Hereditary and idiopathic neuropathy**
G6Ø.Ø Hereditary motor and sensory neuropathy
Charcôt-Marie-Tooth disease
Déjérine-Sottas disease
Hereditary motor and sensory neuropathy, types I-IV
Hypertrophic neuropathy of infancy
Peroneal muscular atrophy (axonal type) (hypertrophic type)
Roussy-Levy syndrome
G6Ø.1 Refsum's disease
Infantile Refsum disease
DEF: Genetic disorder of the lipid metabolism characterized by retinitis pigmentosa, degenerative nerve disease, ataxia, and dry, rough, scaly skin.
G6Ø.2 Neuropathy in association with hereditary ataxia
G6Ø.3 Idiopathic progressive neuropathy
G6Ø.8 Other hereditary and idiopathic neuropathies
Dominantly inherited sensory neuropathy
Morvan's disease
Nelaton's syndrome
Recessively inherited sensory neuropathy
G6Ø.9 Hereditary and idiopathic neuropathy, unspecified

✓4th **G61 Inflammatory polyneuropathy**
G61.Ø Guillain-Barre syndrome HCC Rx ESR COM
Acute (post-)infective polyneuritis
Miller Fisher syndrome
AHA: 2020,3Q,12; 2014,2Q,4
DEF: Autoimmune disorder due to an immune response to foreign antigens with paraplegia of limbs, flaccid paralysis, ophthalmoplegia, ataxia, and areflexia. In most cases, this disorder is triggered by a mild viral infection, surgery, or following an immunization.
TIP: Guillain-Barre syndrome can occur as a sequela of *Campylobacter* enteritis. Assign code B94.8 for the sequelae as an additional diagnosis.
G61.1 Serum neuropathy HCC Rx ESR COM
Use additional code for adverse effect, if applicable, to identify serum (T5Ø.-)
✓5th **G61.8 Other inflammatory polyneuropathies**
G61.81 Chronic inflammatory demyelinating polyneuritis HCC Rx ESR COM
G61.82 Multifocal motor neuropathy HCC Rx ESR COM
MMN
AHA: 2016,4Q,18
G61.89 Other inflammatory polyneuropathies HCC Rx ESR COM
G61.9 Inflammatory polyneuropathy, unspecified HCC Rx ESR COM

✓4th **G62 Other and unspecified polyneuropathies**
G62.Ø Drug-induced polyneuropathy HCC Rx ESR COM
Use additional code for adverse effect, if applicable, to identify drug (T36-T5Ø with fifth or sixth character 5)
G62.1 Alcoholic polyneuropathy HCC Rx ESR COM
AHA: 2019,3Q,8
G62.2 Polyneuropathy due to other toxic agents HCC Rx ESR COM
Code first (T51-T65) to identify toxic agent
✓5th **G62.8 Other specified polyneuropathies**
G62.81 Critical illness polyneuropathy HCC Rx ESR COM
Acute motor neuropathy
G62.82 Radiation-induced polyneuropathy HCC Rx ESR COM
Use additional external cause code (W88-W9Ø, X39.Ø-) to identify cause
G62.89 Other specified polyneuropathies
AHA: 2016,2Q,11
G62.9 Polyneuropathy, unspecified
Neuropathy NOS

G63 Polyneuropathy in diseases classified elsewhere HCC Rx ESR COM
Code first underlying disease, such as:
amyloidosis (E85.-)
endocrine disease, except diabetes (EØØ-EØ7, E15-E16, E2Ø-E34)
metabolic diseases (E7Ø-E88)
neoplasm (CØØ-D49)
nutritional deficiency (E4Ø-E64)
EXCLUDES 1 *polyneuropathy (in):*
diabetes mellitus (EØ8-E13 with .42)
diphtheria (A36.83)
infectious mononucleosis complicated by polyneuropathy (B27.Ø-B27.9 with fifth character 1)
Lyme disease (A69.22)
mumps (B26.84)
postherpetic (BØ2.23)
rheumatoid arthritis (MØ5.5-)
scleroderma (M34.83)
systemic lupus erythematosus (M32.19)
AHA: 2021,1Q,7; 2012,4Q,99

G64 Other disorders of peripheral nervous system
Disorder of peripheral nervous system NOS

✓4th **G65 Sequelae of inflammatory and toxic polyneuropathies**
Code first condition resulting from (sequela) of inflammatory and toxic polyneuropathies
G65.Ø Sequelae of Guillain-Barré syndrome HCC Rx ESR COM
G65.1 Sequelae of other inflammatory polyneuropathy HCC Rx ESR COM
G65.2 Sequelae of toxic polyneuropathy HCC Rx ESR COM

Diseases of myoneural junction and muscle (G70-G73)

G70 Myasthenia gravis and other myoneural disorders
EXCLUDES 1 *botulism (A05.1, A48.51-A48.52)*
transient neonatal myasthenia gravis (P94.0)

G70.0 Myasthenia gravis
DEF: Autoimmune neuromuscular disorder caused by antibodies to the acetylcholine receptors at the neuromuscular junction, interfering with proper binding of the neurotransmitter from the neuron to the target muscle, causing muscle weakness, fatigue, and exhaustion, without pain or atrophy.

G70.00 Myasthenia gravis without (acute) exacerbation HCC Rx ESR COM
Myasthenia gravis NOS

G70.01 Myasthenia gravis with (acute) exacerbation HCC Rx ESR COM
Myasthenia gravis in crisis

G70.1 Toxic myoneural disorders HCC Rx ESR COM
Code first (T51-T65) to identify toxic agent

G70.2 Congenital and developmental myasthenia HCC Rx ESR COM

G70.8 Other specified myoneural disorders

G70.80 Lambert-Eaton syndrome, unspecified HCC Rx ESR COM
Lambert-Eaton syndrome NOS

G70.81 Lambert-Eaton syndrome in disease classified elsewhere HCC Rx ESR COM
Code first underlying disease
EXCLUDES 1 *Lambert-Eaton syndrome in neoplastic disease (G73.1)*

G70.89 Other specified myoneural disorders HCC Rx ESR COM

G70.9 Myoneural disorder, unspecified HCC Rx ESR COM

G71 Primary disorders of muscles
EXCLUDES 2 *arthrogryposis multiplex congenita (Q74.3)*
metabolic disorders (E70-E88)
myositis (M60.-)

G71.0 Muscular dystrophy
AHA: 2018,4Q,11-12

G71.00 Muscular dystrophy, unspecified HCC ESR COM

G71.01 Duchenne or Becker muscular dystrophy HCC ESR COM
Autosomal recessive, childhood type, muscular dystrophy resembling Duchenne or Becker muscular dystrophy
Benign [Becker] muscular dystrophy
Severe [Duchenne] muscular dystrophy

G71.02 Facioscapulohumeral muscular dystrophy HCC ESR COM
Scapulohumeral muscular dystrophy

● **G71.03 Limb girdle muscular dystrophies**

● **G71.031 Autosomal dominant limb girdle muscular dystrophy**
LGMD D4 calpain-3-related
LGMD D5 collagen 6-related
Limb girdle muscular dystrophy type 1

● **G71.032 Autosomal recessive limb girdle muscular dystrophy due to calpain-3 dysfunction**
Limb girdle muscular dystrophy type 2A
LGMD R1 calpain-3-related
Primary calpainopathy

● **G71.033 Limb girdle muscular dystrophy due to dysferlin dysfunction**
Dysferlinopathy
LGMD R2 dysferlin-related
Limb girdle muscular dystrophy type 2B
Miyoshi Myopathy type 1

● **G71.034 Limb girdle muscular dystrophy due to sarcoglycan dysfunction**

● **G71.0340 Limb girdle muscular dystrophy due to sarcoglycan dysfunction, unspecified**
Sarcoglycanopathy, NOS

● **G71.0341 Limb girdle muscular dystrophy due to alpha sarcoglycan dysfunction**
Alpha sarcoglycanopathy
Limb-girdle muscular dystrophy due to alpha-sarcoglycan deficiency
Limb girdle muscular dystrophy type 2D

● **G71.0342 Limb girdle muscular dystrophy due to beta sarcoglycan dysfunction**
Beta sarcoglycanopathy
Limb girdle muscular dystrophy due to beta-sarcoglycan deficiency
Limb girdle muscular dystrophy type 2E

● **G71.0349 Limb girdle muscular dystrophy due to other sarcoglycan dysfunction**
Delta sarcoglycanopathy
Delta-sarcoglycan-related LGMD R6
Gamma sarcoglycanopathy
Gamma-sarcoglycan-related LGMD R5
Limb girdle muscular dystrophy type 2C
Limb girdle muscular dystrophy type 2F

● **G71.035 Limb girdle muscular dystrophy due to anoctamin-5 dysfunction**
Anoctamin-5-related LGMD R12
Anoctaminopathy
Autosomal recessive limb girdle muscular dystrophy type 2L
Miyoshi myopathy type 3

● **G71.038 Other limb girdle muscular dystrophy**
LGMD R9 FKRP-related
LGMD R22 collagen 6-related
Limb girdle muscular dystrophy due to fukutin related protein dysfunction
Limb girdle muscular dystrophy type 2I
Other autosomal recessive limb girdle muscular dystrophy

● **G71.039 Limb girdle muscular dystrophy, unspecified**

G71.09 Other specified muscular dystrophies HCC ESR COM
Benign scapuloperoneal muscular dystrophy with early contractures [Emery-Dreifuss]
Congenital muscular dystrophy NOS
Congenital muscular dystrophy with specific morphological abnormalities of the muscle fiber
Distal muscular dystrophy
~~Limb-girdle muscular dystrophy~~
Ocular muscular dystrophy
Oculopharyngeal muscular dystrophy
Scapuloperoneal muscular dystrophy

G71.1 Myotonic disorders

G71.11 Myotonic muscular dystrophy HCC ESR COM
Dystrophia myotonica [Steinert]
Myotonia atrophica
Myotonic dystrophy
Proximal myotonic myopathy (PROMM)
Steinert disease

G71.12 Myotonia congenita
Acetazolamide responsive myotonia congenita
Dominant myotonia congenita [Thomsen disease]
Myotonia levior
Recessive myotonia congenita [Becker disease]

G71.13 Myotonic chondrodystrophy
Chondrodystrophic myotonia
Congenital myotonic chondrodystrophy
Schwartz-Jampel disease

G71.14 Drug induced myotonia
Use additional code for adverse effect, if applicable, to identify drug (T36-T50 with fifth or sixth character 5)

G71.19 Other specified myotonic disorders
Myotonia fluctuans
Myotonia permanens
Neuromyotonia [Isaacs]
Paramyotonia congenita (of von Eulenburg)
Pseudomyotonia
Symptomatic myotonia

5th G71.2 Congenital myopathies
EXCLUDES 2 *arthrogryposis multiplex congenita (Q74.3)*
AHA: 2020,4Q,19-21

G71.20 Congenital myopathy, unspecified HCC ESR COM

G71.21 Nemaline myopathy HCC ESR COM

6th G71.22 Centronuclear myopathy

G71.220 X-linked myotubular myopathy HCC ESR COM
Myotubular (centronuclear) myopathy

G71.228 Other centronuclear myopathy HCC ESR COM
Autosomal centronuclear myopathy
Autosomal dominant centronuclear myopathy
Autosomal recessive centronuclear myopathy
Centronuclear myopathy, NOS

G71.29 Other congenital myopathy HCC ESR COM
Central core disease
Minicore disease
Multicore disease
Multiminicore disease

G71.3 Mitochondrial myopathy, not elsewhere classified
EXCLUDES 1 *Kearns-Sayre syndrome (H49.81)*
Leber's disease (H47.21)
Leigh's encephalopathy (G31.82)
mitochondrial metabolism disorders (E88.4.-)
Reye's syndrome (G93.7)

G71.8 Other primary disorders of muscles

G71.9 Primary disorder of muscle, unspecified
Hereditary myopathy NOS

4th G72 Other and unspecified myopathies
EXCLUDES 1 *arthrogryposis multiplex congenita (Q74.3)*
dermatopolymyositis (M33.-)
ischemic infarction of muscle (M62.2-)
myositis (M60.-)
polymyositis (M33.2.-)

G72.0 Drug-induced myopathy
Use additional code for adverse effect, if applicable, to identify drug (T36-T50 with fifth or sixth character 5)

G72.1 Alcoholic myopathy
Use additional code to identify alcoholism (F10.-)

G72.2 Myopathy due to other toxic agents
Code first (T51-T65) to identify toxic agent

G72.3 Periodic paralysis
Familial periodic paralysis
Hyperkalemic periodic paralysis (familial)
Hypokalemic periodic paralysis (familial)
Myotonic periodic paralysis (familial)
Normokalemic paralysis (familial)
Potassium sensitive periodic paralysis
EXCLUDES 1 *paramyotonia congenita (of von Eulenburg) (G71.19)*

5th G72.4 Inflammatory and immune myopathies, not elsewhere classified

G72.41 Inclusion body myositis [IBM]

G72.49 Other inflammatory and immune myopathies, not elsewhere classified
Inflammatory myopathy NOS

5th G72.8 Other specified myopathies

G72.81 Critical illness myopathy
Acute necrotizing myopathy
Acute quadriplegic myopathy
Intensive care (ICU) myopathy
Myopathy of critical illness
AHA: 2020,3Q,12

G72.89 Other specified myopathies

G72.9 Myopathy, unspecified

4th G73 Disorders of myoneural junction and muscle in diseases classified elsewhere

G73.1 Lambert-Eaton syndrome in neoplastic disease HCC Rx ESR COM UPD
Code first underlying neoplasm (C00-D49)
EXCLUDES 1 *Lambert-Eaton syndrome not associated with neoplasm (G70.80-G70.81)*

G73.3 Myasthenic syndromes in other diseases classified elsewhere HCC Rx ESR COM
Code first underlying disease, such as:
neoplasm (C00-D49)
thyrotoxicosis (E05.-)

G73.7 Myopathy in diseases classified elsewhere
Code first underlying disease, such as:
hyperparathyroidism (E21.0, E21.3)
hypoparathyroidism (E20.-)
glycogen storage disease (E74.0)
lipid storage disorders (E75.-)
EXCLUDES 1 *myopathy in:*
rheumatoid arthritis (M05.32)
sarcoidosis (D86.87)
scleroderma (M34.82)
Sjögren syndrome (M35.03)
systemic lupus erythematosus (M32.19)

Cerebral palsy and other paralytic syndromes (G80-G83)

4th G80 Cerebral palsy
EXCLUDES 1 *hereditary spastic paraplegia (G11.4)*

G80.0 Spastic quadriplegic cerebral palsy HCC ESR COM
Congenital spastic paralysis (cerebral)

G80.1 Spastic diplegic cerebral palsy HCC ESR COM
Spastic cerebral palsy NOS

G80.2 Spastic hemiplegic cerebral palsy HCC ESR COM

G80.3 Athetoid cerebral palsy HCC ESR COM
Double athetosis (syndrome)
Dyskinetic cerebral palsy
Dystonic cerebral palsy
Vogt disease

G80.4 Ataxic cerebral palsy HCC ESR COM

G80.8 Other cerebral palsy HCC ESR COM
Mixed cerebral palsy syndromes

G80.9 Cerebral palsy, unspecified HCC ESR COM
Cerebral palsy NOS

4th G81 Hemiplegia and hemiparesis
NOTE This category is to be used only when hemiplegia (complete)(incomplete) is reported without further specification, or is stated to be old or longstanding but of unspecified cause. The category is also for use in multiple coding to identify these types of hemiplegia resulting from any cause.
EXCLUDES 1 *congenital cerebral palsy (G80.-)*
hemiplegia and hemiparesis due to sequela of cerebrovascular disease (I69.05-, I69.15-, I69.25-, I69.35-, I69.85-, I69.95-)
AHA: 2015,1Q,25
TIP: If the documentation specifies the affected side but not whether it is the dominant or nondominant side, the default is as follows: for ambidextrous patients, the default is dominant; when the left side is affected, the default is nondominant; and when the right side is affected, the default is dominant.

5th G81.0 Flaccid hemiplegia

G81.00 Flaccid hemiplegia affecting unspecified side HCC ESR COM

G81.01 Flaccid hemiplegia affecting right dominant side HCC ESR COM

G81.02 Flaccid hemiplegia affecting left dominant side HCC ESR COM

G81.Ø3 Flaccid hemiplegia affecting right nondominant side HCC ESR COM

G81.Ø4 Flaccid hemiplegia affecting left nondominant side HCC ESR COM

✓5th G81.1 Spastic hemiplegia

G81.1Ø Spastic hemiplegia affecting unspecified side HCC Rx ESR COM

G81.11 Spastic hemiplegia affecting right dominant side HCC Rx ESR COM

G81.12 Spastic hemiplegia affecting left dominant side HCC Rx ESR COM

G81.13 Spastic hemiplegia affecting right nondominant side HCC Rx ESR COM

G81.14 Spastic hemiplegia affecting left nondominant side HCC Rx ESR COM

✓5th G81.9 Hemiplegia, unspecified

AHA: 2014,1Q,23

G81.9Ø Hemiplegia, unspecified affecting unspecified side HCC ESR COM

G81.91 Hemiplegia, unspecified affecting right dominant side HCC ESR COM

G81.92 Hemiplegia, unspecified affecting left dominant side HCC ESR COM

G81.93 Hemiplegia, unspecified affecting right nondominant side HCC ESR COM

G81.94 Hemiplegia, unspecified affecting left nondominant side HCC ESR COM

✓4th **G82 Paraplegia (paraparesis) and quadriplegia (quadriparesis)**

NOTE This category is to be used only when the listed conditions are reported without further specification, or are stated to be old or longstanding but of unspecified cause. The category is also for use in multiple coding to identify these conditions resulting from any cause

EXCLUDES 1 *congenital cerebral palsy (G8Ø.-)*
functional quadriplegia (R53.2)
hysterical paralysis (F44.4)

✓5th G82.2 Paraplegia

Paralysis of both lower limbs NOS
Paraparesis (lower) NOS
Paraplegia (lower) NOS

AHA: 2017,3Q,3

G82.2Ø Paraplegia, unspecified HCC ESR COM

G82.21 Paraplegia, complete HCC ESR COM

G82.22 Paraplegia, incomplete HCC ESR COM

✓5th G82.5 Quadriplegia

G82.5Ø Quadriplegia, unspecified HCC ESR COM

G82.51 Quadriplegia, C1-C4 complete HCC ESR COM

G82.52 Quadriplegia, C1-C4 incomplete HCC ESR COM

G82.53 Quadriplegia, C5-C7 complete HCC ESR COM

G82.54 Quadriplegia, C5-C7 incomplete HCC ESR COM

✓4th **G83 Other paralytic syndromes**

NOTE This category is to be used only when the listed conditions are reported without further specification, or are stated to be old or longstanding but of unspecified cause. The category is also for use in multiple coding to identify these conditions resulting from any cause.

INCLUDES paralysis (complete) (incomplete), except as in G8Ø-G82

G83.Ø Diplegia of upper limbs HCC ESR COM

Diplegia (upper)
Paralysis of both upper limbs

✓5th G83.1 Monoplegia of lower limb

Paralysis of lower limb

EXCLUDES 1 *monoplegia of lower limbs due to sequela of cerebrovascular disease (I69.Ø4-, I69.14-, I69.24-, I69.34-, I69.84-, I69.94-)*

TIP: If the documentation specifies the affected side but not whether it is the dominant or nondominant side, the default is as follows: for ambidextrous patients, the default is dominant; when the left side is affected, the default is nondominant; and when the right side is affected, the default is dominant.

G83.1Ø Monoplegia of lower limb affecting unspecified side HCC ESR COM

G83.11 Monoplegia of lower limb affecting right dominant side HCC ESR COM

G83.12 Monoplegia of lower limb affecting left dominant side HCC ESR COM

G83.13 Monoplegia of lower limb affecting right nondominant side HCC ESR COM

G83.14 Monoplegia of lower limb affecting left nondominant side HCC ESR COM

✓5th G83.2 Monoplegia of upper limb

Paralysis of upper limb

EXCLUDES 1 *monoplegia of upper limbs due to sequela of cerebrovascular disease (I69.Ø3-, I69.13-, I69.23-, I69.33-, I69.83-, I69.93-)*

TIP: If the documentation specifies the affected side but not whether it is the dominant or nondominant side, the default is as follows: for ambidextrous patients, the default is dominant; when the left side is affected, the default is nondominant; and when the right side is affected, the default is dominant.

G83.2Ø Monoplegia of upper limb affecting unspecified side HCC ESR COM

G83.21 Monoplegia of upper limb affecting right dominant side HCC ESR COM

G83.22 Monoplegia of upper limb affecting left dominant side HCC ESR COM

G83.23 Monoplegia of upper limb affecting right nondominant side HCC ESR COM

G83.24 Monoplegia of upper limb affecting left nondominant side HCC ESR COM

✓5th G83.3 Monoplegia, unspecified

TIP: If the documentation specifies the affected side but not whether it is the dominant or nondominant side, the default is as follows: for ambidextrous patients, the default is dominant; when the left side is affected, the default is nondominant; and when the right side is affected, the default is dominant.

G83.3Ø Monoplegia, unspecified affecting unspecified side HCC ESR COM

G83.31 Monoplegia, unspecified affecting right dominant side HCC ESR COM

G83.32 Monoplegia, unspecified affecting left dominant side HCC ESR COM

G83.33 Monoplegia, unspecified affecting right nondominant side HCC ESR COM

G83.34 Monoplegia, unspecified affecting left nondominant side HCC ESR COM

G83.4 Cauda equina syndrome HCC Rx ESR COM

Neurogenic bladder due to cauda equina syndrome

EXCLUDES 1 *cord bladder NOS (G95.89)*
neurogenic bladder NOS (N31.9)

AHA: 2020,3Q,24

DEF: Compression of the spinal nerve roots presenting with pain and tingling radiating down the buttocks, back of the thigh and calf, and into the foot in a sciatic manner with aching in the bladder, perineum, and sacrum. Loss of bowel and bladder control may also occur.

G83.5 Locked-in state HCC ESR COM

AHA: 2022,2Q,10

✓5th G83.8 Other specified paralytic syndromes

EXCLUDES 1 *paralytic syndromes due to current spinal cord injury — code to spinal cord injury (S14, S24, S34)*

G83.81 Brown-Séquard syndrome HCC ESR COM

G83.82 Anterior cord syndrome HCC ESR COM

G83.83 Posterior cord syndrome HCC ESR COM

G83.84 Todd's paralysis (postepileptic) HCC ESR COM

G83.89 Other specified paralytic syndromes HCC ESR COM

G83.9 Paralytic syndrome, unspecified HCC ESR COM

Other disorders of the nervous system (G89-G99)

✓4th G89 Pain, not elsewhere classified

Code also related psychological factors associated with pain (F45.42)

EXCLUDES 1 *generalized pain NOS (R52)*
pain disorders exclusively related to psychological factors (F45.41)
pain NOS (R52)

EXCLUDES 2 *atypical face pain (G50.1)*
headache syndromes (G44.-)
localized pain, unspecified type - code to pain by site, such as:
abdomen pain (R10.-)
back pain (M54.9)
breast pain (N64.4)
chest pain (R07.1-R07.9)
ear pain (H92.0-)
eye pain (H57.1)
headache (R51.9)
joint pain (M25.5-)
limb pain (M79.6-)
lumbar region pain (M54.5-)
painful urination (R30.9)
pelvic and perineal pain (R10.2)
renal colic (N23)
shoulder pain (M25.51-)
spine pain (M54.-)
throat pain (R07.0)
tongue pain (K14.6)
tooth pain (K08.8)
migraines (G43.-)
myalgia (M79.1-)
pain from prosthetic devices, implants, and grafts (T82.84, T83.84, T84.84, T85.84-)
phantom limb syndrome with pain (G54.6)
vulvar vestibulitis (N94.810)
vulvodynia (N94.81-)

G89.0 Central pain syndrome
Déjérine-Roussy syndrome
Myelopathic pain syndrome
Thalamic pain syndrome (hyperesthetic)

✓5th G89.1 Acute pain, not elsewhere classified

G89.11 Acute pain due to trauma

G89.12 Acute post-thoracotomy pain
Post-thoracotomy pain NOS

G89.18 Other acute postprocedural pain
Postoperative pain NOS
Postprocedural pain NOS

✓5th G89.2 Chronic pain, not elsewhere classified

EXCLUDES 1 *causalgia, lower limb (G57.7-)*
causalgia, upper limb (G56.4-)
central pain syndrome (G89.0)
chronic pain syndrome (G89.4)
complex regional pain syndrome II, lower limb (G57.7-)
complex regional pain syndrome II, upper limb (G56.4-)
neoplasm related chronic pain (G89.3)
reflex sympathetic dystrophy (G90.5-)

G89.21 Chronic pain due to trauma

G89.22 Chronic post-thoracotomy pain

G89.28 Other chronic postprocedural pain
Other chronic postoperative pain

G89.29 Other chronic pain

G89.3 Neoplasm related pain (acute) (chronic)
Cancer associated pain
Pain due to malignancy (primary) (secondary)
Tumor associated pain

G89.4 Chronic pain syndrome
Chronic pain associated with significant psychosocial dysfunction

✓4th G90 Disorders of autonomic nervous system

EXCLUDES 1 *dysfunction of the autonomic nervous system due to alcohol (G31.2)*

✓5th G90.0 Idiopathic peripheral autonomic neuropathy

G90.01 Carotid sinus syncope
Carotid sinus syndrome
DEF: Vagal activation caused by pressure on the carotid sinus baroreceptors. Sympathetic nerve impulses may cause sinus arrest or AV block.

G90.09 Other idiopathic peripheral autonomic neuropathy
Idiopathic peripheral autonomic neuropathy NOS

G90.1 Familial dysautonomia [Riley-Day] HCC Rx ESR COM

G90.2 Horner's syndrome
Bernard(-Horner) syndrome
Cervical sympathetic dystrophy or paralysis

G90.3 Multi-system degeneration of the autonomic nervous system HCC Rx ESR COM
Neurogenic orthostatic hypotension [Shy-Drager]

EXCLUDES 1 *orthostatic hypotension NOS (I95.1)*

G90.4 Autonomic dysreflexia
Use additional code to identify the cause, such as:
fecal impaction (K56.41)
pressure ulcer (pressure area) (L89.-)
urinary tract infection (N39.0)

✓5th G90.5 Complex regional pain syndrome I (CRPS I)
Reflex sympathetic dystrophy

EXCLUDES 1 *causalgia of lower limb (G57.7-)*
causalgia of upper limb (G56.4-)
complex regional pain syndrome II of lower limb (G57.7-)
complex regional pain syndrome II of upper limb (G56.4-)

G90.50 Complex regional pain syndrome I, unspecified

✓6th G90.51 Complex regional pain syndrome I of upper limb

G90.511 Complex regional pain syndrome I of right upper limb

G90.512 Complex regional pain syndrome I of left upper limb

G90.513 Complex regional pain syndrome I of upper limb, bilateral

G90.519 Complex regional pain syndrome I of unspecified upper limb

✓6th G90.52 Complex regional pain syndrome I of lower limb

G90.521 Complex regional pain syndrome I of right lower limb

G90.522 Complex regional pain syndrome I of left lower limb

G90.523 Complex regional pain syndrome I of lower limb, bilateral

G90.529 Complex regional pain syndrome I of unspecified lower limb

G90.59 Complex regional pain syndrome I of other specified site

G90.8 Other disorders of autonomic nervous system

G90.9 Disorder of the autonomic nervous system, unspecified

● **G90.A Postural orthostatic tachycardia syndrome [POTS]**
Chronic orthostatic intolerance
Postural tachycardia syndrome

G91 Hydrocephalus

INCLUDES acquired hydrocephalus

EXCLUDES 1 *Arnold-Chiari syndrome with hydrocephalus (Q07.-)*
congenital hydrocephalus (Q03.-)
spina bifida with hydrocephalus (Q05.-)

DEF: Abnormal buildup of cerebrospinal fluid in the brain causing dilation of the ventricles.

Hydrocephalus (Acquired)

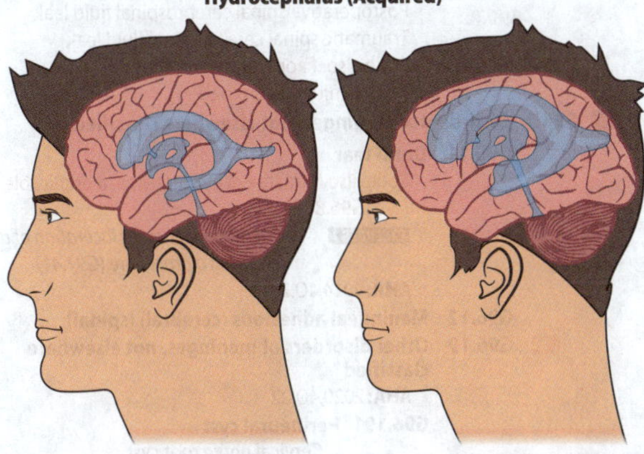

G91.0 Communicating hydrocephalus HCC ESR COM
Secondary normal pressure hydrocephalus

G91.1 Obstructive hydrocephalus HCC ESR COM
DEF: Obstruction of the cerebrospinal fluid passage from the brain into the spinal canal characterized by headaches, drowsiness, poor coordination, urinary incontinence, nausea, vomiting, and papilledema.

G91.2 (Idiopathic) normal pressure hydrocephalus HCC ESR COM
Normal pressure hydrocephalus NOS

G91.3 Post-traumatic hydrocephalus, unspecified HCC ESR COM

G91.4 Hydrocephalus in diseases classified elsewhere HCC ESR COM
Code first underlying condition, such as:
congenital syphilis (A50.4-)
neoplasm (C00-D49)
plasminogen deficiency (E88.02)

EXCLUDES 1 *hydrocephalus due to congenital toxoplasmosis (P37.1)*

AHA: 2014,3Q,3

G91.8 Other hydrocephalus HCC ESR COM

G91.9 Hydrocephalus, unspecified HCC ESR COM

G92 Toxic encephalopathy

AHA: 2022,1Q,52; 2021,4Q,12-14; 2021,1Q,13; 2017,1Q,39-40

DEF: Brain tissue degeneration due to a toxic substance.

G92.0 Immune effector cell-associated neurotoxicity syndrome
Code first underlying cause such as:
complications of immune effector cellular therapy (T80.82)
Code also associated signs and symptoms, such as seizures and cerebral edema
Code also, if applicable:
cerebral edema (G93.6)
unspecified convulsions (R56.9)

G92.00 Immune effector cell-associated neurotoxicity syndrome, grade unspecified UPD
ICANS, grade unspecified

G92.01 Immune effector cell-associated neurotoxicity syndrome, grade 1 UPD
ICANS, grade 1

G92.02 Immune effector cell-associated neurotoxicity syndrome, grade 2 UPD
ICANS, grade 2

G92.03 Immune effector cell-associated neurotoxicity syndrome, grade 3 UPD
ICANS, grade 3

G92.04 Immune effector cell-associated neurotoxicity syndrome, grade 4 UPD
ICANS, grade 4

G92.05 Immune effector cell-associated neurotoxicity syndrome, grade 5 UPD
ICANS, grade 5

G92.8 Other toxic encephalopathy
Toxic encephalitis
Toxic metabolic encephalopathy
Code first poisoning due to drug or toxin, if applicable, (T36-T65 with fifth or sixth character 1-4 or 6)
Use additional code for adverse effect, if applicable, to identify drug (T36-T50 with fifth or sixth character 5)

AHA: 2022,1Q,52

G92.9 Unspecified toxic encephalopathy
Code first poisoning due to drug or toxin, if applicable, (T36-T65 with fifth or sixth character 1-4 or 6)
Use additional code for adverse effect, if applicable, to identify drug (T36-T50 with fifth or sixth character 5)

G93 Other disorders of brain

G93.0 Cerebral cysts
Arachnoid cyst
Porencephalic cyst, acquired

EXCLUDES 1 *acquired periventricular cysts of newborn (P91.1)*
congenital cerebral cysts (Q04.6)

G93.1 Anoxic brain damage, not elsewhere classified HCC ESR COM

EXCLUDES 1 *cerebral anoxia due to anesthesia during labor and delivery (O74.3)*
cerebral anoxia due to anesthesia during the puerperium (O89.2)
neonatal anoxia (P84)

DEF: Brain injury not resulting from birth trauma that is due to lack of oxygen. Brain cells, when deprived of oxygen, begin to expire after four minutes.

G93.2 Benign intracranial hypertension
Pseudotumor

EXCLUDES 1 *hypertensive encephalopathy (I67.4)*
obstructive hydrocephalus (G91.1)

▲ **G93.3 Postviral and related fatigue syndromes**
~~Benign myalgic encephalomyelitis~~
▶Use additional code, if applicable, for post COVID-19 condition, unspecified (U09.9)◀

EXCLUDES 1 *chronic fatigue syndrome NOS (R53.82)*
▶neurasthenia (F48.8)◀

● **G93.31 Postviral fatigue syndrome**

● **G93.32 Myalgic encephalomyelitis/chronic fatigue syndrome**
Chronic fatigue syndrome
ME/CFS
Myalgic encephalomyelitis

● **G93.39 Other post infection and related fatigue syndromes**

G93.4 Other and unspecified encephalopathy

EXCLUDES 1 *alcoholic encephalopathy (G31.2)*
encephalopathy in diseases classified elsewhere (G94)
hypertensive encephalopathy (I67.4)

EXCLUDES 2 *toxic (metabolic) encephalopathy (G92.8)*

G93.40 Encephalopathy, unspecified
AHA: 2017,2Q,8

G93.41 Metabolic encephalopathy
Septic encephalopathy
AHA: 2017,2Q,8; 2016,3Q,42; 2015,3Q,21
TIP: Assign separately when documented with diabetic hypoglycemia (E08.649, E09.649, E10.649, E11.649, E13.649).

G93.49 Other encephalopathy
Encephalopathy NEC
AHA: 2021,2Q,3; 2018,4Q,16; 2018,2Q,22,24; 2017,2Q,9

G93.5 Compression of brain HCC ESR COM
Arnold-Chiari type 1 compression of brain
Compression of brain (stem)
Herniation of brain (stem)

EXCLUDES 1 *traumatic compression of brain (S06.A-)*

AHA: 2020,2Q,31

G93.6 Cerebral edema HCC ESR COM

EXCLUDES 1 *cerebral edema due to birth injury (P11.0)*
traumatic cerebral edema (S06.1-)

G93.7 Reye's syndrome HCC Rx ESR COM P

Code first poisoning due to salicylates, if applicable (T39.Ø-, with sixth character 1-4)

Use additional code for adverse effect due to salicylates, if applicable (T39.Ø-, with sixth character 5)

DEF: Rare childhood illness often developed after a viral upper respiratory infection. Symptoms include vomiting, elevated serum transaminase, brain swelling, disturbances of consciousness, seizures, and changes in liver and other viscera; it can be fatal.

✓5th **G93.8 Other specified disorders of brain**

G93.81 Temporal sclerosis
Hippocampal sclerosis
Mesial temporal sclerosis

G93.82 Brain death

G93.89 Other specified disorders of brain
Postradiation encephalopathy
AHA: 2020,2Q,24; 2019,3Q,8

G93.9 Disorder of brain, unspecified

G94 Other disorders of brain in diseases classified elsewhere

Code first underlying disease

EXCLUDES 1 *encephalopathy in congenital syphilis (A5Ø.49)*
encephalopathy in influenza (JØ9.X9, J1Ø.81, J11.81)
encephalopathy in syphilis (A52.19)
hydrocephalus in diseases classified elsewhere (G91.4)

AHA: 2018,2Q,22; 2017,2Q,8-9

✓4th **G95 Other and unspecified diseases of spinal cord**

EXCLUDES 2 *myelitis (GØ4.-)*

G95.Ø Syringomyelia and syringobulbia HCC Rx ESR COM

✓5th **G95.1 Vascular myelopathies**

EXCLUDES 2 *intraspinal phlebitis and thrombophlebitis, except non-pyogenic (GØ8)*

G95.11 Acute infarction of spinal cord (embolic) (nonembolic) HCC Rx ESR COM
Anoxia of spinal cord
Arterial thrombosis of spinal cord

G95.19 Other vascular myelopathies HCC Rx ESR COM
Edema of spinal cord
Hematomyelia
Nonpyogenic intraspinal phlebitis and thrombophlebitis
Subacute necrotic myelopathy

✓5th **G95.2 Other and unspecified cord compression**

G95.2Ø Unspecified cord compression HCC Rx ESR COM

G95.29 Other cord compression HCC Rx ESR COM

✓5th **G95.8 Other specified diseases of spinal cord**

EXCLUDES 1 *neurogenic bladder NOS (N31.9)*
neurogenic bladder due to cauda equina syndrome (G83.4)
neuromuscular dysfunction of bladder without spinal cord lesion (N31.-)

G95.81 Conus medullaris syndrome HCC Rx ESR COM

G95.89 Other specified diseases of spinal cord HCC Rx ESR COM
Cord bladder NOS
Drug-induced myelopathy
Radiation-induced myelopathy
EXCLUDES 1 *myelopathy NOS (G95.9)*

G95.9 Disease of spinal cord, unspecified HCC Rx ESR COM
Myelopathy NOS

✓4th **G96 Other disorders of central nervous system**

✓5th **G96.Ø Cerebrospinal fluid leak**

Code also if applicable:
intracranial hypotension (G96.81-)

EXCLUDES 1 *cerebrospinal fluid leak from spinal puncture (G97.Ø)*

AHA: 2020,4Q,21-22; 2018,2Q,13

G96.ØØ Cerebrospinal fluid leak, unspecified
Code also if applicable:
head injury ►(SØØ-SØ9)◄

G96.Ø1 Cranial cerebrospinal fluid leak, spontaneous
Otorrhea due to spontaneous cerebrospinal fluid CSF leak
Rhinorrhea due to spontaneous cerebrospinal fluid CSF leak
Spontaneous cerebrospinal fluid leak from skull base

G96.Ø2 Spinal cerebrospinal fluid leak, spontaneous
Spontaneous cerebrospinal fluid leak from spine

G96.Ø8 Other cranial cerebrospinal fluid leak
Postoperative cranial cerebrospinal fluid leak
Traumatic cranial cerebrospinal fluid leak
Code also if applicable:
head injury (SØØ.- to SØ9.-)

G96.Ø9 Other spinal cerebrospinal fluid leak
Other spinal CSF leak
Postoperative spinal cerebrospinal fluid leak
Traumatic spinal cerebrospinal fluid leak
Code also if applicable:
head injury (SØØ.- to SØ9.-)

✓5th **G96.1 Disorders of meninges, not elsewhere classified**

G96.11 Dural tear
Code also intracranial hypotension, if applicable (G96.81-)
EXCLUDES 1 *accidental puncture or laceration of dura during a procedure (G97.41)*
AHA: 2014,4Q,24

G96.12 Meningeal adhesions (cerebral) (spinal)

✓6th **G96.19 Other disorders of meninges, not elsewhere classified**
AHA: 2020,4Q,22

G96.191 Perineural cyst
Cervical nerve root cyst
Lumbar nerve root cyst
Sacral nerve root cyst
Tarlov cyst
Thoracic nerve root cyst

G96.198 Other disorders of meninges, not elsewhere classified

✓5th **G96.8 Other specified disorders of central nervous system**
AHA: 2020,4Q,21,23-24

✓6th **G96.81 Intracranial hypotension**
Code also any associated diagnoses, such as:
brachial amyotrophy (G54.5)
cerebrospinal fluid leak from spine (G96.Ø2)
cranial nerve disorders in diseases classified elsewhere (G53)
nerve root and compressions in diseases classified elsewhere (G55)
nonpyogenic thrombosis of intracranial venous system (I67.6)
nontraumatic intracerebral hemorrhage (I61.-)
nontraumatic subdural hemorrhage (I62.Ø-)
other and unspecified cord compression (G95.2-)
other secondary parkinsonism (G21.8)
reversible cerebrovascular vasoconstriction syndrome (I67.841)
spinal cord herniation (G95.89)
stroke (I63.-)
syringomyelia (G95.Ø)

DEF: Central nervous system disorder resulting from a loss of cerebrospinal fluid (CSF) volume. More often associated with CSF leak at the level of the spine rather than the skull base, causes can be spontaneous, iatrogenic or traumatic spinal dura defects or holes, or overdrainage of CSF shunt devices. The most common symptom is headache.

G96.81Ø Intracranial hypotension, unspecified

G96.811 Intracranial hypotension, spontaneous

G96.819 Other intracranial hypotension

G96.89 Other specified disorders of central nervous system

G96.9 Disorder of central nervous system, unspecified

G97 Intraoperative and postprocedural complications and disorders of nervous system, not elsewhere classified

EXCLUDES 2 *intraoperative and postprocedural cerebrovascular infarction (I97.81-, I97.82-)*

AHA: 2016,4Q,9-10

G97.Ø Cerebrospinal fluid leak from spinal puncture

Code also any associated diagnoses or complications, such as:
intracranial hypotension following a procedure (G97.83-G97.84)

Spinal Puncture

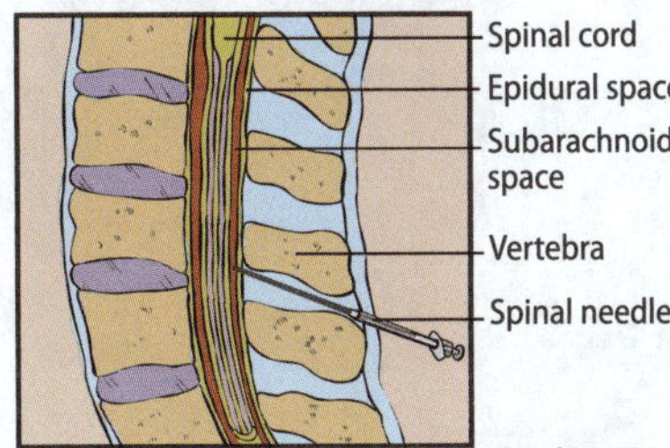

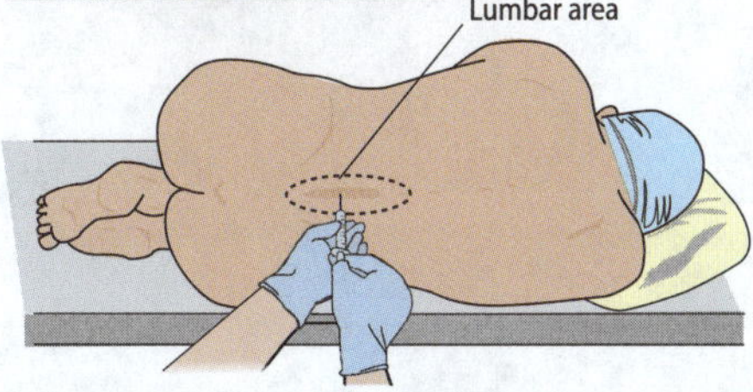

G97.1 Other reaction to spinal and lumbar puncture

Headache due to lumbar puncture
Other reaction to spinal dural puncture
Code also, if applicable, any associated headache with orthostatic component (R51.Ø)

G97.2 Intracranial hypotension following ventricular shunting

Code also any associated diagnoses or complications

G97.3 Intraoperative hemorrhage and hematoma of a nervous system organ or structure complicating a procedure

EXCLUDES 1 *intraoperative hemorrhage and hematoma of a nervous system organ or structure due to accidental puncture and laceration during a procedure (G97.4-)*

G97.31 Intraoperative hemorrhage and hematoma of a nervous system organ or structure complicating a nervous system procedure

G97.32 Intraoperative hemorrhage and hematoma of a nervous system organ or structure complicating other procedure

G97.4 Accidental puncture and laceration of a nervous system organ or structure during a procedure

G97.41 Accidental puncture or laceration of dura during a procedure

Incidental (inadvertent) durotomy
Code also any associated diagnoses or complications
AHA: 2014,4Q,24

G97.48 Accidental puncture and laceration of other nervous system organ or structure during a nervous system procedure

G97.49 Accidental puncture and laceration of other nervous system organ or structure during other procedure

G97.5 Postprocedural hemorrhage of a nervous system organ or structure following a procedure

G97.51 Postprocedural hemorrhage of a nervous system organ or structure following a nervous system procedure

G97.52 Postprocedural hemorrhage of a nervous system organ or structure following other procedure

G97.6 Postprocedural hematoma and seroma of a nervous system organ or structure following a procedure

G97.61 Postprocedural hematoma of a nervous system organ or structure following a nervous system procedure

AHA: 2020,3Q,24

G97.62 Postprocedural hematoma of a nervous system organ or structure following other procedure

G97.63 Postprocedural seroma of a nervous system organ or structure following a nervous system procedure

G97.64 Postprocedural seroma of a nervous system organ or structure following other procedure

G97.8 Other intraoperative and postprocedural complications and disorders of nervous system

Use additional code to further specify disorder
AHA: 2020,4Q,23

G97.81 Other intraoperative complications of nervous system

G97.82 Other postprocedural complications and disorders of nervous system

AHA: 2022,1Q,34

G97.83 Intracranial hypotension following lumbar cerebrospinal fluid shunting

Code also any associated diagnoses or complications

G97.84 Intracranial hypotension following other procedure

Code also, if applicable:
accidental puncture or laceration of dura during a procedure (G97.41)
cerebrospinal fluid leak from spinal puncture (G97.Ø)

G98 Other disorders of nervous system not elsewhere classified

INCLUDES nervous system disorder NOS

G98.Ø Neurogenic arthritis, not elsewhere classified

Nonsyphilitic neurogenic arthropathy NEC
Nonsyphilitic neurogenic spondylopathy NEC
EXCLUDES 1 *spondylopathy (in):*
syringomyelia and syringobulbia (G95.Ø)
tabes dorsalis (A52.11)

G98.8 Other disorders of nervous system

Nervous system disorder NOS

G99 Other disorders of nervous system in diseases classified elsewhere

G99.Ø Autonomic neuropathy in diseases classified elsewhere

Code first underlying disease, such as:
amyloidosis (E85.-)
gout (M1A.-, M1Ø.-)
hyperthyroidism (EØ5.-)
EXCLUDES 1 *diabetic autonomic neuropathy (EØ8-E13 with .43)*

G99.2 Myelopathy in diseases classified elsewhere HCC Rx ESR COM

Code first underlying disease, such as:
neoplasm (CØØ-D49)
EXCLUDES 1 *myelopathy in:*
intervertebral disease (M5Ø.Ø-, M51.Ø-)
spondylosis (M47.Ø-, M47.1-)
AHA: 2018,3Q,18-19
TIP: Use this code in addition to a spondylolisthesis code (M43.1-) or a spinal stenosis code (M48.0-) when either of these disorders is documented as the cause of the myelopathy.

G99.8 Other specified disorders of nervous system in diseases classified elsewhere

Code first underlying disorder, such as:
amyloidosis (E85.-)
avitaminosis (E56.9)
EXCLUDES 1 *nervous system involvement in:*
cysticercosis (B69.Ø)
rubella (BØ6.Ø-)
syphilis (A52.1-)

Chapter 7. Diseases of the Eye and Adnexa (H00–H59)

Chapter-specific Guidelines with Coding Examples

The chapter-specific guidelines from the ICD-10-CM Official Guidelines for Coding and Reporting have been provided below. Along with these guidelines are coding examples, contained in the shaded boxes, that have been developed to help illustrate the coding and/or sequencing guidance found in these guidelines.

a. Glaucoma

1) Assigning glaucoma codes

Assign as many codes from category H40, Glaucoma, as needed to identify the type of glaucoma, the affected eye, and the glaucoma stage.

2) Bilateral glaucoma with same type and stage

When a patient has bilateral glaucoma and both eyes are documented as being the same type and stage, and there is a code for bilateral glaucoma, report only the code for the type of glaucoma, bilateral, with the seventh character for the stage.

> Bilateral mild stage primary open-angle glaucoma
>
> **H40.1131 Primary open-angle glaucoma, bilateral, mild stage**
>
> *Explanation*: In this scenario, the patient has the same type and stage of glaucoma in both eyes. As this type of glaucoma has a code for bilateral, assign only the code for the bilateral glaucoma with the seventh character for the stage.

When a patient has bilateral glaucoma and both eyes are documented as being the same type and stage, and the classification does not provide a code for bilateral glaucoma (i.e. subcategories H40.10 and H40.20) report only one code for the type of glaucoma with the appropriate seventh character for the stage.

> Bilateral open-angle glaucoma, severe stage; not specified as to type
>
> **H40.10X3 Unspecified open-angle glaucoma, severe stage**
>
> *Explanation*: In this scenario, the patient has glaucoma of the same type and stage of both eyes, but there is no code specifically for bilateral glaucoma. Only one code is assigned with the appropriate seventh character for the stage.

3) Bilateral glaucoma stage with different types or stages

When a patient has bilateral glaucoma and each eye is documented as having a different type or stage, and the classification distinguishes laterality, assign the appropriate code for each eye rather than the code for bilateral glaucoma.

> Bilateral chronic angle-closure glaucoma; right eye is documented as mild stage and left eye as moderate stage
>
> **H40.2211 Chronic angle-closure glaucoma, right eye, mild stage**
>
> **H40.2222 Chronic angle-closure glaucoma, left eye, moderate stage**
>
> *Explanation*: In this scenario the patient has the same type of glaucoma in both eyes, but each eye is at a different stage. Because the subcategory for this condition identifies laterality, one code is assigned for the right eye and one code is assigned for the left eye, each with the appropriate seventh character for the stage appended.

When a patient has bilateral glaucoma and each eye is documented as having a different type, and the classification does not distinguish laterality (i.e. subcategories H40.10 and H40.20), assign one code for each type of glaucoma with the appropriate seventh character for the stage.

> Documentation relates mild, unspecified primary angle-closure glaucoma of the left eye with mild unspecified open-angle glaucoma of the right eye
>
> **H40.20X1 Unspecified primary angle-closure glaucoma, mild stage**
>
> **H40.10X1 Unspecified open-angle glaucoma, mild stage**
>
> *Explanation*: In this scenario the patient has a different type of glaucoma in each eye and the classification does not distinguish laterality. A code for each type of glaucoma is assigned, each with the appropriate seventh character for the stage.

When a patient has bilateral glaucoma and each eye is documented as having the same type, but different stage, and the classification does not distinguish laterality (i.e. subcategories H40.10 and H40.20), assign a code for the type of glaucoma for each eye with the seventh character for the specific glaucoma stage documented for each eye.

> Bilateral open-angle glaucoma, not specified as to type; the right eye is documented to be in mild stage and the left eye as being in moderate stage
>
> **H40.10X1 Unspecified open-angle glaucoma, mild stage**
>
> **H40.10X2 Unspecified open-angle glaucoma, moderate stage**
>
> *Explanation*: In this scenario the patient has the same type of glaucoma in each eye but each eye is at a different stage, and the classification does not distinguish laterality at this subcategory level. Two codes are assigned; both codes represent the same type of glaucoma but each has a different seventh character identifying the appropriate stage for each eye.

4) Patient admitted with glaucoma and stage evolves during the admission

If a patient is admitted with glaucoma and the stage progresses during the admission, assign the code for highest stage documented.

5) Indeterminate stage glaucoma

Assignment of the seventh character "4" for "indeterminate stage" should be based on the clinical documentation. The seventh character "4" is used for glaucomas whose stage cannot be clinically determined. This seventh character should not be confused with the seventh character "0", unspecified, which should be assigned when there is no documentation regarding the stage of the glaucoma.

b. Blindness

If "blindness" or "low vision" of both eyes is documented but the visual impairment category is not documented, assign code H54.3, Unqualified visual loss, both eyes. If "blindness" or "low vision" in one eye is documented but the visual impairment category is not documented, assign a code from H54.6-, Unqualified visual loss, one eye. If "blindness" or "visual loss" is documented without any information about whether one or both eyes are affected, assign code H54.7, Unspecified visual loss.

> Patient assessment indicates moderately impaired/low vision in the left eye with no visual impairments in the right eye
>
> **H54.62 Unqualified visual loss, left eye, normal vision right eye**
>
> Report unqualified visual loss when the visual impairment category is not specified. In this case, only the left eye is impacted by visual loss with normal vision of the right eye documented.

Chapter 7. Diseases of the Eye and Adnexa (H00-H59)

NOTE Use an external cause code following the code for the eye condition, if applicable, to identify the cause of the eye condition

EXCLUDES 2 *certain conditions originating in the perinatal period (P04-P96)*
certain infectious and parasitic diseases (A00-B99)
complications of pregnancy, childbirth and the puerperium (O00-O9A)
congenital malformations, deformations, and chromosomal abnormalities (Q00-Q99)
diabetes mellitus related eye conditions (E09.3-, E10.3-, E11.3-, E13.3-)
endocrine, nutritional and metabolic diseases (E00-E88)
injury (trauma) of eye and orbit (S05.-)
injury, poisoning and certain other consequences of external causes (S00-T88)
neoplasms (C00-D49)
symptoms, signs and abnormal clinical and laboratory findings, not elsewhere classified (R00-R94)
syphilis related eye disorders (A50.01, A50.3-, A51.43, A52.71)

This chapter contains the following blocks:

- H00-H05 Disorders of eyelid, lacrimal system and orbit
- H10-H11 Disorders of conjunctiva
- H15-H22 Disorders of sclera, cornea, iris and ciliary body
- H25-H28 Disorders of lens
- H30-H36 Disorders of choroid and retina
- H40-H42 Glaucoma
- H43-H44 Disorders of vitreous body and globe
- H46-H47 Disorders of optic nerve and visual pathways
- H49-H52 Disorders of ocular muscles, binocular movement, accommodation and refraction
- H53-H54 Visual disturbances and blindness
- H55-H57 Other disorders of eye and adnexa
- H59 Intraoperative and postprocedural complications and disorders of eye and adnexa, not elsewhere classified

Disorders of eyelid, lacrimal system and orbit (H00-H05)

EXCLUDES 2 *open wound of eyelid (S01.1-)*
superficial injury of eyelid (S00.1-, S00.2-)

4th H00 Hordeolum and chalazion

5th H00.0 Hordeolum (externum) (internum) of eyelid

DEF: Acute localized infection of the gland of Zeis (external hordeolum) or Molt or of the meibomian glands (internal hordeolum) of the orbit.

6th H00.01 Hordeolum externum

Hordeolum NOS
Stye

- **H00.011 Hordeolum externum right upper eyelid**
- **H00.012 Hordeolum externum right lower eyelid**
- **H00.013 Hordeolum externum right eye, unspecified eyelid**
- **H00.014 Hordeolum externum left upper eyelid**
- **H00.015 Hordeolum externum left lower eyelid**
- **H00.016 Hordeolum externum left eye, unspecified eyelid**
- **H00.019 Hordeolum externum unspecified eye, unspecified eyelid**

6th H00.02 Hordeolum internum

Infection of meibomian gland

- **H00.021 Hordeolum internum right upper eyelid**
- **H00.022 Hordeolum internum right lower eyelid**
- **H00.023 Hordeolum internum right eye, unspecified eyelid**
- **H00.024 Hordeolum internum left upper eyelid**
- **H00.025 Hordeolum internum left lower eyelid**
- **H00.026 Hordeolum internum left eye, unspecified eyelid**
- **H00.029 Hordeolum internum unspecified eye, unspecified eyelid**

6th H00.03 Abscess of eyelid

Furuncle of eyelid

- **H00.031 Abscess of right upper eyelid**
- **H00.032 Abscess of right lower eyelid**
- **H00.033 Abscess of eyelid right eye, unspecified eyelid**
- **H00.034 Abscess of left upper eyelid**
- **H00.035 Abscess of left lower eyelid**
- **H00.036 Abscess of eyelid left eye, unspecified eyelid**
- **H00.039 Abscess of eyelid unspecified eye, unspecified eyelid**

5th H00.1 Chalazion

Meibomian (gland) cyst

EXCLUDES 2 *infected meibomian gland (H00.02-)*

DEF: Noninfectious, obstructive mass in the oil gland of the eyelid that results in a small chronic lump or inflammation.

- **H00.11 Chalazion right upper eyelid**
- **H00.12 Chalazion right lower eyelid**
- **H00.13 Chalazion right eye, unspecified eyelid**
- **H00.14 Chalazion left upper eyelid**
- **H00.15 Chalazion left lower eyelid**
- **H00.16 Chalazion left eye, unspecified eyelid**
- **H00.19 Chalazion unspecified eye, unspecified eyelid**

4th H01 Other inflammation of eyelid

5th H01.0 Blepharitis

EXCLUDES 1 *blepharoconjunctivitis (H10.5-)*

6th H01.00 Unspecified blepharitis

AHA: 2018,4Q,13

- **H01.001 Unspecified blepharitis right upper eyelid**
- **H01.002 Unspecified blepharitis right lower eyelid**
- **H01.003 Unspecified blepharitis right eye, unspecified eyelid**
- **H01.004 Unspecified blepharitis left upper eyelid**
- **H01.005 Unspecified blepharitis left lower eyelid**
- **H01.006 Unspecified blepharitis left eye, unspecified eyelid**
- **H01.009 Unspecified blepharitis unspecified eye, unspecified eyelid**
- **H01.00A Unspecified blepharitis right eye, upper and lower eyelids**
- **H01.00B Unspecified blepharitis left eye, upper and lower eyelids**

6th H01.01 Ulcerative blepharitis

AHA: 2018,4Q,13

- **H01.011 Ulcerative blepharitis right upper eyelid**
- **H01.012 Ulcerative blepharitis right lower eyelid**
- **H01.013 Ulcerative blepharitis right eye, unspecified eyelid**
- **H01.014 Ulcerative blepharitis left upper eyelid**
- **H01.015 Ulcerative blepharitis left lower eyelid**
- **H01.016 Ulcerative blepharitis left eye, unspecified eyelid**
- **H01.019 Ulcerative blepharitis unspecified eye, unspecified eyelid**
- **H01.01A Ulcerative blepharitis right eye, upper and lower eyelids**
- **H01.01B Ulcerative blepharitis left eye, upper and lower eyelids**

6th H01.02 Squamous blepharitis

AHA: 2018,4Q,13

- **H01.021 Squamous blepharitis right upper eyelid**
- **H01.022 Squamous blepharitis right lower eyelid**
- **H01.023 Squamous blepharitis right eye, unspecified eyelid**
- **H01.024 Squamous blepharitis left upper eyelid**
- **H01.025 Squamous blepharitis left lower eyelid**
- **H01.026 Squamous blepharitis left eye, unspecified eyelid**
- **H01.029 Squamous blepharitis unspecified eye, unspecified eyelid**
- **H01.02A Squamous blepharitis right eye, upper and lower eyelids**
- **H01.02B Squamous blepharitis left eye, upper and lower eyelids**

5th H01.1 Noninfectious dermatoses of eyelid

6th H01.11 Allergic dermatitis of eyelid

Contact dermatitis of eyelid

- **H01.111 Allergic dermatitis of right upper eyelid**
- **H01.112 Allergic dermatitis of right lower eyelid**
- **H01.113 Allergic dermatitis of right eye, unspecified eyelid**
- **H01.114 Allergic dermatitis of left upper eyelid**
- **H01.115 Allergic dermatitis of left lower eyelid**
- **H01.116 Allergic dermatitis of left eye, unspecified eyelid**
- **H01.119 Allergic dermatitis of unspecified eye, unspecified eyelid**

HØ1.12 Discoid lupus erythematosus of eyelid

HØ1.121 Discoid lupus erythematosus of right upper eyelid Rx

HØ1.122 Discoid lupus erythematosus of right lower eyelid Rx

HØ1.123 Discoid lupus erythematosus of right eye, unspecified eyelid Rx

HØ1.124 Discoid lupus erythematosus of left upper eyelid Rx

HØ1.125 Discoid lupus erythematosus of left lower eyelid Rx

HØ1.126 Discoid lupus erythematosus of left eye, unspecified eyelid Rx

HØ1.129 Discoid lupus erythematosus of unspecified eye, unspecified eyelid Rx

HØ1.13 Eczematous dermatitis of eyelid

HØ1.131 Eczematous dermatitis of right upper eyelid

HØ1.132 Eczematous dermatitis of right lower eyelid

HØ1.133 Eczematous dermatitis of right eye, unspecified eyelid

HØ1.134 Eczematous dermatitis of left upper eyelid

HØ1.135 Eczematous dermatitis of left lower eyelid

HØ1.136 Eczematous dermatitis of left eye, unspecified eyelid

HØ1.139 Eczematous dermatitis of unspecified eye, unspecified eyelid

HØ1.14 Xeroderma of eyelid

HØ1.141 Xeroderma of right upper eyelid

HØ1.142 Xeroderma of right lower eyelid

HØ1.143 Xeroderma of right eye, unspecified eyelid

HØ1.144 Xeroderma of left upper eyelid

HØ1.145 Xeroderma of left lower eyelid

HØ1.146 Xeroderma of left eye, unspecified eyelid

HØ1.149 Xeroderma of unspecified eye, unspecified eyelid

HØ1.8 Other specified inflammations of eyelid

HØ1.9 Unspecified inflammation of eyelid

Inflammation of eyelid NOS

HØ2 Other disorders of eyelid

EXCLUDES 1 *congenital malformations of eyelid (Q1Ø.Ø-Q1Ø.3)*

Entropion and Ectropion

HØ2.Ø Entropion and trichiasis of eyelid

DEF: Entropion: Inversion of the eyelid, turning the edge in toward the eyeball and causing irritation from contact of the lashes with the surface of the eye.

DEF: Trichiasis: Condition wherein the eyelid is in a normal position but lashes are ingrown or misdirected in their growth so that they irritate the tissues of the eye.

HØ2.ØØ Unspecified entropion of eyelid

HØ2.ØØ1 Unspecified entropion of right upper eyelid

HØ2.ØØ2 Unspecified entropion of right lower eyelid

HØ2.ØØ3 Unspecified entropion of right eye, unspecified eyelid

HØ2.ØØ4 Unspecified entropion of left upper eyelid

HØ2.ØØ5 Unspecified entropion of left lower eyelid

HØ2.ØØ6 Unspecified entropion of left eye, unspecified eyelid

HØ2.ØØ9 Unspecified entropion of unspecified eye, unspecified eyelid

HØ2.Ø1 Cicatricial entropion of eyelid

HØ2.Ø11 Cicatricial entropion of right upper eyelid

HØ2.Ø12 Cicatricial entropion of right lower eyelid

HØ2.Ø13 Cicatricial entropion of right eye, unspecified eyelid

HØ2.Ø14 Cicatricial entropion of left upper eyelid

HØ2.Ø15 Cicatricial entropion of left lower eyelid

HØ2.Ø16 Cicatricial entropion of left eye, unspecified eyelid

HØ2.Ø19 Cicatricial entropion of unspecified eye, unspecified eyelid

HØ2.Ø2 Mechanical entropion of eyelid

HØ2.Ø21 Mechanical entropion of right upper eyelid

HØ2.Ø22 Mechanical entropion of right lower eyelid

HØ2.Ø23 Mechanical entropion of right eye, unspecified eyelid

HØ2.Ø24 Mechanical entropion of left upper eyelid

HØ2.Ø25 Mechanical entropion of left lower eyelid

HØ2.Ø26 Mechanical entropion of left eye, unspecified eyelid

HØ2.Ø29 Mechanical entropion of unspecified eye, unspecified eyelid

HØ2.Ø3 Senile entropion of eyelid

HØ2.Ø31 Senile entropion of right upper eyelid A

HØ2.Ø32 Senile entropion of right lower eyelid A

HØ2.Ø33 Senile entropion of right eye, unspecified eyelid A

HØ2.Ø34 Senile entropion of left upper eyelid A

HØ2.Ø35 Senile entropion of left lower eyelid A

HØ2.Ø36 Senile entropion of left eye, unspecified eyelid A

HØ2.Ø39 Senile entropion of unspecified eye, unspecified eyelid A

HØ2.Ø4 Spastic entropion of eyelid

HØ2.Ø41 Spastic entropion of right upper eyelid

HØ2.Ø42 Spastic entropion of right lower eyelid

HØ2.Ø43 Spastic entropion of right eye, unspecified eyelid

HØ2.Ø44 Spastic entropion of left upper eyelid

HØ2.Ø45 Spastic entropion of left lower eyelid

HØ2.Ø46 Spastic entropion of left eye, unspecified eyelid

HØ2.Ø49 Spastic entropion of unspecified eye, unspecified eyelid

HØ2.Ø5 Trichiasis without entropion

HØ2.Ø51 Trichiasis without entropion right upper eyelid

HØ2.Ø52 Trichiasis without entropion right lower eyelid

HØ2.Ø53 Trichiasis without entropion right eye, unspecified eyelid

HØ2.Ø54 Trichiasis without entropion left upper eyelid

HØ2.Ø55 Trichiasis without entropion left lower eyelid

HØ2.Ø56 Trichiasis without entropion left eye, unspecified eyelid

HØ2.Ø59 Trichiasis without entropion unspecified eye, unspecified eyelid

HØ2.1 Ectropion of eyelid

DEF: Drooping of the lower eyelid away from the eye or outward turning or eversion of the edge of the eyelid, exposing the palpebral conjunctiva and causing irritation.

HØ2.1Ø Unspecified ectropion of eyelid

HØ2.1Ø1 Unspecified ectropion of right upper eyelid

HØ2.1Ø2 Unspecified ectropion of right lower eyelid

HØ2.1Ø3 Unspecified ectropion of right eye, unspecified eyelid

HØ2.1Ø4 Unspecified ectropion of left upper eyelid

HØ2.1Ø5 Unspecified ectropion of left lower eyelid

HØ2.1Ø6 Unspecified ectropion of left eye, unspecified eyelid

HØ2.1Ø9 Unspecified ectropion of unspecified eye, unspecified eyelid

6th HØ2.11 Cicatricial ectropion of eyelid

HØ2.111 Cicatricial ectropion of right upper eyelid
HØ2.112 Cicatricial ectropion of right lower eyelid
HØ2.113 Cicatricial ectropion of right eye, unspecified eyelid
HØ2.114 Cicatricial ectropion of left upper eyelid
HØ2.115 Cicatricial ectropion of left lower eyelid
HØ2.116 Cicatricial ectropion of left eye, unspecified eyelid
HØ2.119 Cicatricial ectropion of unspecified eye, unspecified eyelid

6th HØ2.12 Mechanical ectropion of eyelid

HØ2.121 Mechanical ectropion of right upper eyelid
HØ2.122 Mechanical ectropion of right lower eyelid
HØ2.123 Mechanical ectropion of right eye, unspecified eyelid
HØ2.124 Mechanical ectropion of left upper eyelid
HØ2.125 Mechanical ectropion of left lower eyelid
HØ2.126 Mechanical ectropion of left eye, unspecified eyelid
HØ2.129 Mechanical ectropion of unspecified eye, unspecified eyelid

6th HØ2.13 Senile ectropion of eyelid

HØ2.131 Senile ectropion of right upper eyelid A
HØ2.132 Senile ectropion of right lower eyelid A
HØ2.133 Senile ectropion of right eye, unspecified eyelid A
HØ2.134 Senile ectropion of left upper eyelid A
HØ2.135 Senile ectropion of left lower eyelid A
HØ2.136 Senile ectropion of left eye, unspecified eyelid A
HØ2.139 Senile ectropion of unspecified eye, unspecified eyelid A

6th HØ2.14 Spastic ectropion of eyelid

HØ2.141 Spastic ectropion of right upper eyelid
HØ2.142 Spastic ectropion of right lower eyelid
HØ2.143 Spastic ectropion of right eye, unspecified eyelid
HØ2.144 Spastic ectropion of left upper eyelid
HØ2.145 Spastic ectropion of left lower eyelid
HØ2.146 Spastic ectropion of left eye, unspecified eyelid
HØ2.149 Spastic ectropion of unspecified eye, unspecified eyelid

6th HØ2.15 Paralytic ectropion of eyelid

AHA: 2018,4Q,13

HØ2.151 Paralytic ectropion of right upper eyelid
HØ2.152 Paralytic ectropion of right lower eyelid
HØ2.153 Paralytic ectropion of right eye, unspecified eyelid
HØ2.154 Paralytic ectropion of left upper eyelid
HØ2.155 Paralytic ectropion of left lower eyelid
HØ2.156 Paralytic ectropion of left eye, unspecified eyelid
HØ2.159 Paralytic ectropion of unspecified eye, unspecified eyelid

5th HØ2.2 Lagophthalmos

AHA: 2018,4Q,14

DEF: Condition of the eye that prevents it from closing completely.

6th HØ2.2Ø Unspecified lagophthalmos

HØ2.2Ø1 Unspecified lagophthalmos right upper eyelid
HØ2.2Ø2 Unspecified lagophthalmos right lower eyelid
HØ2.2Ø3 Unspecified lagophthalmos right eye, unspecified eyelid
HØ2.2Ø4 Unspecified lagophthalmos left upper eyelid
HØ2.2Ø5 Unspecified lagophthalmos left lower eyelid
HØ2.2Ø6 Unspecified lagophthalmos left eye, unspecified eyelid
HØ2.2Ø9 Unspecified lagophthalmos unspecified eye, unspecified eyelid
HØ2.2ØA Unspecified lagophthalmos right eye, upper and lower eyelids
HØ2.2ØB Unspecified lagophthalmos left eye, upper and lower eyelids
HØ2.2ØC Unspecified lagophthalmos, bilateral, upper and lower eyelids

6th HØ2.21 Cicatricial lagophthalmos

HØ2.211 Cicatricial lagophthalmos right upper eyelid
HØ2.212 Cicatricial lagophthalmos right lower eyelid
HØ2.213 Cicatricial lagophthalmos right eye, unspecified eyelid
HØ2.214 Cicatricial lagophthalmos left upper eyelid
HØ2.215 Cicatricial lagophthalmos left lower eyelid
HØ2.216 Cicatricial lagophthalmos left eye, unspecified eyelid
HØ2.219 Cicatricial lagophthalmos unspecified eye, unspecified eyelid
HØ2.21A Cicatricial lagophthalmos right eye, upper and lower eyelids
HØ2.21B Cicatricial lagophthalmos left eye, upper and lower eyelids
HØ2.21C Cicatricial lagophthalmos, bilateral, upper and lower eyelids

6th HØ2.22 Mechanical lagophthalmos

HØ2.221 Mechanical lagophthalmos right upper eyelid
HØ2.222 Mechanical lagophthalmos right lower eyelid
HØ2.223 Mechanical lagophthalmos right eye, unspecified eyelid
HØ2.224 Mechanical lagophthalmos left upper eyelid
HØ2.225 Mechanical lagophthalmos left lower eyelid
HØ2.226 Mechanical lagophthalmos left eye, unspecified eyelid
HØ2.229 Mechanical lagophthalmos unspecified eye, unspecified eyelid
HØ2.22A Mechanical lagophthalmos right eye, upper and lower eyelids
HØ2.22B Mechanical lagophthalmos left eye, upper and lower eyelids
HØ2.22C Mechanical lagophthalmos, bilateral, upper and lower eyelids

6th HØ2.23 Paralytic lagophthalmos

HØ2.231 Paralytic lagophthalmos right upper eyelid
HØ2.232 Paralytic lagophthalmos right lower eyelid
HØ2.233 Paralytic lagophthalmos right eye, unspecified eyelid
HØ2.234 Paralytic lagophthalmos left upper eyelid
HØ2.235 Paralytic lagophthalmos left lower eyelid
HØ2.236 Paralytic lagophthalmos left eye, unspecified eyelid
HØ2.239 Paralytic lagophthalmos unspecified eye, unspecified eyelid
HØ2.23A Paralytic lagophthalmos right eye, upper and lower eyelids
HØ2.23B Paralytic lagophthalmos left eye, upper and lower eyelids
HØ2.23C Paralytic lagophthalmos, bilateral, upper and lower eyelids

5th HØ2.3 Blepharochalasis

Pseudoptosis

DEF: Loss of elasticity and relaxation of skin of the eyelid, thickened or indurated skin on the eyelid associated with recurrent episodes of edema, and intracellular atrophy.

HØ2.3Ø Blepharochalasis unspecified eye, unspecified eyelid
HØ2.31 Blepharochalasis right upper eyelid
HØ2.32 Blepharochalasis right lower eyelid
HØ2.33 Blepharochalasis right eye, unspecified eyelid
HØ2.34 Blepharochalasis left upper eyelid
HØ2.35 Blepharochalasis left lower eyelid
HØ2.36 Blepharochalasis left eye, unspecified eyelid

H02.4 Ptosis of eyelid

H02.40 Unspecified ptosis of eyelid

H02.401 Unspecified ptosis of right eyelid

H02.402 Unspecified ptosis of left eyelid

H02.403 Unspecified ptosis of bilateral eyelids

H02.409 Unspecified ptosis of unspecified eyelid

H02.41 Mechanical ptosis of eyelid

H02.411 Mechanical ptosis of right eyelid

H02.412 Mechanical ptosis of left eyelid

H02.413 Mechanical ptosis of bilateral eyelids

H02.419 Mechanical ptosis of unspecified eyelid

H02.42 Myogenic ptosis of eyelid

H02.421 Myogenic ptosis of right eyelid

H02.422 Myogenic ptosis of left eyelid

H02.423 Myogenic ptosis of bilateral eyelids

H02.429 Myogenic ptosis of unspecified eyelid

H02.43 Paralytic ptosis of eyelid

Neurogenic ptosis of eyelid

H02.431 Paralytic ptosis of right eyelid

H02.432 Paralytic ptosis of left eyelid

H02.433 Paralytic ptosis of bilateral eyelids

H02.439 Paralytic ptosis unspecified eyelid

H02.5 Other disorders affecting eyelid function

EXCLUDES 2 *blepharospasm (G24.5)*
organic tic (G25.69)
psychogenic tic (F95.-)

H02.51 Abnormal innervation syndrome

H02.511 Abnormal innervation syndrome right upper eyelid

H02.512 Abnormal innervation syndrome right lower eyelid

H02.513 Abnormal innervation syndrome right eye, unspecified eyelid

H02.514 Abnormal innervation syndrome left upper eyelid

H02.515 Abnormal innervation syndrome left lower eyelid

H02.516 Abnormal innervation syndrome left eye, unspecified eyelid

H02.519 Abnormal innervation syndrome unspecified eye, unspecified eyelid

H02.52 Blepharophimosis

Ankyloblepharon

H02.521 Blepharophimosis right upper eyelid

H02.522 Blepharophimosis right lower eyelid

H02.523 Blepharophimosis right eye, unspecified eyelid

H02.524 Blepharophimosis left upper eyelid

H02.525 Blepharophimosis left lower eyelid

H02.526 Blepharophimosis left eye, unspecified eyelid

H02.529 Blepharophimosis unspecified eye, unspecified lid

H02.53 Eyelid retraction

Eyelid lag

H02.531 Eyelid retraction right upper eyelid

H02.532 Eyelid retraction right lower eyelid

H02.533 Eyelid retraction right eye, unspecified eyelid

H02.534 Eyelid retraction left upper eyelid

H02.535 Eyelid retraction left lower eyelid

H02.536 Eyelid retraction left eye, unspecified eyelid

H02.539 Eyelid retraction unspecified eye, unspecified lid

H02.59 Other disorders affecting eyelid function

Deficient blink reflex
Sensory disorders

H02.6 Xanthelasma of eyelid

DEF: Condition in which there are small yellow tumors that occur on the eyelid, usually appearing near the nose.

H02.60 Xanthelasma of unspecified eye, unspecified eyelid

H02.61 Xanthelasma of right upper eyelid

H02.62 Xanthelasma of right lower eyelid

H02.63 Xanthelasma of right eye, unspecified eyelid

H02.64 Xanthelasma of left upper eyelid

H02.65 Xanthelasma of left lower eyelid

H02.66 Xanthelasma of left eye, unspecified eyelid

H02.7 Other and unspecified degenerative disorders of eyelid and periocular area

H02.70 Unspecified degenerative disorders of eyelid and periocular area

H02.71 Chloasma of eyelid and periocular area

Dyspigmentation of eyelid
Hyperpigmentation of eyelid

H02.711 Chloasma of right upper eyelid and periocular area

H02.712 Chloasma of right lower eyelid and periocular area

H02.713 Chloasma of right eye, unspecified eyelid and periocular area

H02.714 Chloasma of left upper eyelid and periocular area

H02.715 Chloasma of left lower eyelid and periocular area

H02.716 Chloasma of left eye, unspecified eyelid and periocular area

H02.719 Chloasma of unspecified eye, unspecified eyelid and periocular area

H02.72 Madarosis of eyelid and periocular area

Hypotrichosis of eyelid

H02.721 Madarosis of right upper eyelid and periocular area

H02.722 Madarosis of right lower eyelid and periocular area

H02.723 Madarosis of right eye, unspecified eyelid and periocular area

H02.724 Madarosis of left upper eyelid and periocular area

H02.725 Madarosis of left lower eyelid and periocular area

H02.726 Madarosis of left eye, unspecified eyelid and periocular area

H02.729 Madarosis of unspecified eye, unspecified eyelid and periocular area

H02.73 Vitiligo of eyelid and periocular area

Hypopigmentation of eyelid

H02.731 Vitiligo of right upper eyelid and periocular area

H02.732 Vitiligo of right lower eyelid and periocular area

H02.733 Vitiligo of right eye, unspecified eyelid and periocular area

H02.734 Vitiligo of left upper eyelid and periocular area

H02.735 Vitiligo of left lower eyelid and periocular area

H02.736 Vitiligo of left eye, unspecified eyelid and periocular area

H02.739 Vitiligo of unspecified eye, unspecified eyelid and periocular area

H02.79 Other degenerative disorders of eyelid and periocular area

H02.8 Other specified disorders of eyelid

H02.81 Retained foreign body in eyelid

Use additional code to identify the type of retained foreign body (Z18.-)

EXCLUDES 1 *laceration of eyelid with foreign body (S01.12-)*
retained intraocular foreign body (H44.6-, H44.7-)
superficial foreign body of eyelid and periocular area (S00.25-)

H02.811 Retained foreign body in right upper eyelid

H02.812 Retained foreign body in right lower eyelid

H02.813 Retained foreign body in right eye, unspecified eyelid

H02.814 Retained foreign body in left upper eyelid

H02.815 Retained foreign body in left lower eyelid

H02.816 Retained foreign body in left eye, unspecified eyelid

H02.819 Retained foreign body in unspecified eye, unspecified eyelid

H02.82 Cysts of eyelid

Sebaceous cyst of eyelid

H02.821 Cysts of right upper eyelid

H02.822 Cysts of right lower eyelid

H02.823 Cysts of right eye, unspecified eyelid
H02.824 Cysts of left upper eyelid
H02.825 Cysts of left lower eyelid
H02.826 Cysts of left eye, unspecified eyelid
H02.829 Cysts of unspecified eye, unspecified eyelid

H02.83 Dermatochalasis of eyelid
DEF: Acquired form of connective tissue disorder associated with decreased elastic tissue and abnormal elastin formation, resulting in loss of elasticity of the skin of the eyelid. It is generally associated with aging.
H02.831 Dermatochalasis of right upper eyelid
H02.832 Dermatochalasis of right lower eyelid
H02.833 Dermatochalasis of right eye, unspecified eyelid
H02.834 Dermatochalasis of left upper eyelid
H02.835 Dermatochalasis of left lower eyelid
H02.836 Dermatochalasis of left eye, unspecified eyelid
H02.839 Dermatochalasis of unspecified eye, unspecified eyelid

H02.84 Edema of eyelid
Hyperemia of eyelid
H02.841 Edema of right upper eyelid
H02.842 Edema of right lower eyelid
H02.843 Edema of right eye, unspecified eyelid
H02.844 Edema of left upper eyelid
H02.845 Edema of left lower eyelid
H02.846 Edema of left eye, unspecified eyelid
H02.849 Edema of unspecified eye, unspecified eyelid

H02.85 Elephantiasis of eyelid
H02.851 Elephantiasis of right upper eyelid
H02.852 Elephantiasis of right lower eyelid
H02.853 Elephantiasis of right eye, unspecified eyelid
H02.854 Elephantiasis of left upper eyelid
H02.855 Elephantiasis of left lower eyelid
H02.856 Elephantiasis of left eye, unspecified eyelid
H02.859 Elephantiasis of unspecified eye, unspecified eyelid

H02.86 Hypertrichosis of eyelid
H02.861 Hypertrichosis of right upper eyelid
H02.862 Hypertrichosis of right lower eyelid
H02.863 Hypertrichosis of right eye, unspecified eyelid
H02.864 Hypertrichosis of left upper eyelid
H02.865 Hypertrichosis of left lower eyelid
H02.866 Hypertrichosis of left eye, unspecified eyelid
H02.869 Hypertrichosis of unspecified eye, unspecified eyelid

H02.87 Vascular anomalies of eyelid
H02.871 Vascular anomalies of right upper eyelid
H02.872 Vascular anomalies of right lower eyelid
H02.873 Vascular anomalies of right eye, unspecified eyelid
H02.874 Vascular anomalies of left upper eyelid
H02.875 Vascular anomalies of left lower eyelid
H02.876 Vascular anomalies of left eye, unspecified eyelid
H02.879 Vascular anomalies of unspecified eye, unspecified eyelid

H02.88 Meibomian gland dysfunction of eyelid
AHA: 2018,4Q,14-15
H02.881 Meibomian gland dysfunction right upper eyelid
H02.882 Meibomian gland dysfunction right lower eyelid
H02.883 Meibomian gland dysfunction of right eye, unspecified eyelid
H02.884 Meibomian gland dysfunction left upper eyelid
H02.885 Meibomian gland dysfunction left lower eyelid
H02.886 Meibomian gland dysfunction of left eye, unspecified eyelid
H02.889 Meibomian gland dysfunction of unspecified eye, unspecified eyelid
H02.88A Meibomian gland dysfunction right eye, upper and lower eyelids
H02.88B Meibomian gland dysfunction left eye, upper and lower eyelids

H02.89 Other specified disorders of eyelid
Hemorrhage of eyelid

H02.9 Unspecified disorder of eyelid
Disorder of eyelid NOS

H04 Disorders of lacrimal system

EXCLUDES 1 *congenital malformations of lacrimal system (Q10.4-Q10.6)*

H04.0 Dacryoadenitis
DEF: Inflammation of the lacrimal gland.

H04.00 Unspecified dacryoadenitis
H04.001 Unspecified dacryoadenitis, right lacrimal gland
H04.002 Unspecified dacryoadenitis, left lacrimal gland
H04.003 Unspecified dacryoadenitis, bilateral lacrimal glands
H04.009 Unspecified dacryoadenitis, unspecified lacrimal gland

H04.01 Acute dacryoadenitis
H04.011 Acute dacryoadenitis, right lacrimal gland
H04.012 Acute dacryoadenitis, left lacrimal gland
H04.013 Acute dacryoadenitis, bilateral lacrimal glands
H04.019 Acute dacryoadenitis, unspecified lacrimal gland

H04.02 Chronic dacryoadenitis
H04.021 Chronic dacryoadenitis, right lacrimal gland
H04.022 Chronic dacryoadenitis, left lacrimal gland
H04.023 Chronic dacryoadenitis, bilateral lacrimal gland
H04.029 Chronic dacryoadenitis, unspecified lacrimal gland

H04.03 Chronic enlargement of lacrimal gland
H04.031 Chronic enlargement of right lacrimal gland
H04.032 Chronic enlargement of left lacrimal gland
H04.033 Chronic enlargement of bilateral lacrimal glands
H04.039 Chronic enlargement of unspecified lacrimal gland

H04.1 Other disorders of lacrimal gland

H04.11 Dacryops
H04.111 Dacryops of right lacrimal gland
H04.112 Dacryops of left lacrimal gland
H04.113 Dacryops of bilateral lacrimal glands
H04.119 Dacryops of unspecified lacrimal gland

H04.12 Dry eye syndrome
Tear film insufficiency, NOS
H04.121 Dry eye syndrome of right lacrimal gland
H04.122 Dry eye syndrome of left lacrimal gland
H04.123 Dry eye syndrome of bilateral lacrimal glands
H04.129 Dry eye syndrome of unspecified lacrimal gland

H04.13 Lacrimal cyst
Lacrimal cystic degeneration
H04.131 Lacrimal cyst, right lacrimal gland
H04.132 Lacrimal cyst, left lacrimal gland
H04.133 Lacrimal cyst, bilateral lacrimal glands
H04.139 Lacrimal cyst, unspecified lacrimal gland

H04.14 Primary lacrimal gland atrophy
H04.141 Primary lacrimal gland atrophy, right lacrimal gland
H04.142 Primary lacrimal gland atrophy, left lacrimal gland
H04.143 Primary lacrimal gland atrophy, bilateral lacrimal glands
H04.149 Primary lacrimal gland atrophy, unspecified lacrimal gland

H04.15 Secondary lacrimal gland atrophy
H04.151 Secondary lacrimal gland atrophy, right lacrimal gland

H04.152 Secondary lacrimal gland atrophy, left lacrimal gland
H04.153 Secondary lacrimal gland atrophy, bilateral lacrimal glands
H04.159 Secondary lacrimal gland atrophy, unspecified lacrimal gland

H04.16 Lacrimal gland dislocation
H04.161 Lacrimal gland dislocation, right lacrimal gland
H04.162 Lacrimal gland dislocation, left lacrimal gland
H04.163 Lacrimal gland dislocation, bilateral lacrimal glands
H04.169 Lacrimal gland dislocation, unspecified lacrimal gland

H04.19 Other specified disorders of lacrimal gland

H04.2 Epiphora

DEF: Excessive tearing or overflow of tears down the cheeks often due to a stricture in the lacrimal passages but can be caused by other conditions.

H04.20 Unspecified epiphora
H04.201 Unspecified epiphora, right side
H04.202 Unspecified epiphora, left side
H04.203 Unspecified epiphora, bilateral
H04.209 Unspecified epiphora, unspecified side

H04.21 Epiphora due to excess lacrimation
H04.211 Epiphora due to excess lacrimation, right lacrimal gland
H04.212 Epiphora due to excess lacrimation, left lacrimal gland
H04.213 Epiphora due to excess lacrimation, bilateral lacrimal glands
H04.219 Epiphora due to excess lacrimation, unspecified lacrimal gland

H04.22 Epiphora due to insufficient drainage
H04.221 Epiphora due to insufficient drainage, right side
H04.222 Epiphora due to insufficient drainage, left side
H04.223 Epiphora due to insufficient drainage, bilateral
H04.229 Epiphora due to insufficient drainage, unspecified side

H04.3 Acute and unspecified inflammation of lacrimal passages

EXCLUDES 1 *neonatal dacryocystitis (P39.1)*

H04.30 Unspecified dacryocystitis
H04.301 Unspecified dacryocystitis of right lacrimal passage
H04.302 Unspecified dacryocystitis of left lacrimal passage
H04.303 Unspecified dacryocystitis of bilateral lacrimal passages
H04.309 Unspecified dacryocystitis of unspecified lacrimal passage

H04.31 Phlegmonous dacryocystitis
H04.311 Phlegmonous dacryocystitis of right lacrimal passage
H04.312 Phlegmonous dacryocystitis of left lacrimal passage
H04.313 Phlegmonous dacryocystitis of bilateral lacrimal passages
H04.319 Phlegmonous dacryocystitis of unspecified lacrimal passage

H04.32 Acute dacryocystitis

Acute dacryopericystitis

H04.321 Acute dacryocystitis of right lacrimal passage
H04.322 Acute dacryocystitis of left lacrimal passage
H04.323 Acute dacryocystitis of bilateral lacrimal passages
H04.329 Acute dacryocystitis of unspecified lacrimal passage

H04.33 Acute lacrimal canaliculitis
H04.331 Acute lacrimal canaliculitis of right lacrimal passage
H04.332 Acute lacrimal canaliculitis of left lacrimal passage
H04.333 Acute lacrimal canaliculitis of bilateral lacrimal passages
H04.339 Acute lacrimal canaliculitis of unspecified lacrimal passage

H04.4 Chronic inflammation of lacrimal passages

H04.41 Chronic dacryocystitis
H04.411 Chronic dacryocystitis of right lacrimal passage
H04.412 Chronic dacryocystitis of left lacrimal passage
H04.413 Chronic dacryocystitis of bilateral lacrimal passages
H04.419 Chronic dacryocystitis of unspecified lacrimal passage

H04.42 Chronic lacrimal canaliculitis
H04.421 Chronic lacrimal canaliculitis of right lacrimal passage
H04.422 Chronic lacrimal canaliculitis of left lacrimal passage
H04.423 Chronic lacrimal canaliculitis of bilateral lacrimal passages
H04.429 Chronic lacrimal canaliculitis of unspecified lacrimal passage

H04.43 Chronic lacrimal mucocele
H04.431 Chronic lacrimal mucocele of right lacrimal passage
H04.432 Chronic lacrimal mucocele of left lacrimal passage
H04.433 Chronic lacrimal mucocele of bilateral lacrimal passages
H04.439 Chronic lacrimal mucocele of unspecified lacrimal passage

H04.5 Stenosis and insufficiency of lacrimal passages

H04.51 Dacryolith
H04.511 Dacryolith of right lacrimal passage
H04.512 Dacryolith of left lacrimal passage
H04.513 Dacryolith of bilateral lacrimal passages
H04.519 Dacryolith of unspecified lacrimal passage

H04.52 Eversion of lacrimal punctum
H04.521 Eversion of right lacrimal punctum
H04.522 Eversion of left lacrimal punctum
H04.523 Eversion of bilateral lacrimal punctum
H04.529 Eversion of unspecified lacrimal punctum

H04.53 Neonatal obstruction of nasolacrimal duct

EXCLUDES 1 *congenital stenosis and stricture of lacrimal duct (Q10.5)*

H04.531 Neonatal obstruction of right nasolacrimal duct N
H04.532 Neonatal obstruction of left nasolacrimal duct N
H04.533 Neonatal obstruction of bilateral nasolacrimal duct N
H04.539 Neonatal obstruction of unspecified nasolacrimal duct N

H04.54 Stenosis of lacrimal canaliculi
H04.541 Stenosis of right lacrimal canaliculi
H04.542 Stenosis of left lacrimal canaliculi
H04.543 Stenosis of bilateral lacrimal canaliculi
H04.549 Stenosis of unspecified lacrimal canaliculi

H04.55 Acquired stenosis of nasolacrimal duct
H04.551 Acquired stenosis of right nasolacrimal duct
H04.552 Acquired stenosis of left nasolacrimal duct
H04.553 Acquired stenosis of bilateral nasolacrimal duct
H04.559 Acquired stenosis of unspecified nasolacrimal duct

H04.56 Stenosis of lacrimal punctum
H04.561 Stenosis of right lacrimal punctum
H04.562 Stenosis of left lacrimal punctum
H04.563 Stenosis of bilateral lacrimal punctum
H04.569 Stenosis of unspecified lacrimal punctum

H04.57 Stenosis of lacrimal sac
H04.571 Stenosis of right lacrimal sac
H04.572 Stenosis of left lacrimal sac
H04.573 Stenosis of bilateral lacrimal sac
H04.579 Stenosis of unspecified lacrimal sac

5th **HØ4.6 Other changes of lacrimal passages**
6th **HØ4.61 Lacrimal fistula**
HØ4.611 Lacrimal fistula right lacrimal passage
HØ4.612 Lacrimal fistula left lacrimal passage
HØ4.613 Lacrimal fistula bilateral lacrimal passages
HØ4.619 Lacrimal fistula unspecified lacrimal passage
HØ4.69 Other changes of lacrimal passages
5th **HØ4.8 Other disorders of lacrimal system**
6th **HØ4.81 Granuloma of lacrimal passages**
HØ4.811 Granuloma of right lacrimal passage
HØ4.812 Granuloma of left lacrimal passage
HØ4.813 Granuloma of bilateral lacrimal passages
HØ4.819 Granuloma of unspecified lacrimal passage
HØ4.89 Other disorders of lacrimal system
HØ4.9 Disorder of lacrimal system, unspecified

4th **HØ5 Disorders of orbit**
EXCLUDES 1 *congenital malformation of orbit (Q1Ø.7)*

5th **HØ5.Ø Acute inflammation of orbit**
HØ5.ØØ Unspecified acute inflammation of orbit
6th **HØ5.Ø1 Cellulitis of orbit**
Abscess of orbit
HØ5.Ø11 Cellulitis of right orbit
HØ5.Ø12 Cellulitis of left orbit
HØ5.Ø13 Cellulitis of bilateral orbits
HØ5.Ø19 Cellulitis of unspecified orbit
6th **HØ5.Ø2 Osteomyelitis of orbit**
HØ5.Ø21 Osteomyelitis of right orbit
HØ5.Ø22 Osteomyelitis of left orbit
HØ5.Ø23 Osteomyelitis of bilateral orbits
HØ5.Ø29 Osteomyelitis of unspecified orbit
6th **HØ5.Ø3 Periostitis of orbit**
HØ5.Ø31 Periostitis of right orbit
HØ5.Ø32 Periostitis of left orbit
HØ5.Ø33 Periostitis of bilateral orbits
HØ5.Ø39 Periostitis of unspecified orbit
6th **HØ5.Ø4 Tenonitis of orbit**
HØ5.Ø41 Tenonitis of right orbit
HØ5.Ø42 Tenonitis of left orbit
HØ5.Ø43 Tenonitis of bilateral orbits
HØ5.Ø49 Tenonitis of unspecified orbit
5th **HØ5.1 Chronic inflammatory disorders of orbit**
HØ5.1Ø Unspecified chronic inflammatory disorders of orbit
6th **HØ5.11 Granuloma of orbit**
Pseudotumor (inflammatory) of orbit
HØ5.111 Granuloma of right orbit
HØ5.112 Granuloma of left orbit
HØ5.113 Granuloma of bilateral orbits
HØ5.119 Granuloma of unspecified orbit
6th **HØ5.12 Orbital myositis**
HØ5.121 Orbital myositis, right orbit
HØ5.122 Orbital myositis, left orbit
HØ5.123 Orbital myositis, bilateral
HØ5.129 Orbital myositis, unspecified orbit
5th **HØ5.2 Exophthalmic conditions**
HØ5.2Ø Unspecified exophthalmos
6th **HØ5.21 Displacement (lateral) of globe**
HØ5.211 Displacement (lateral) of globe, right eye
HØ5.212 Displacement (lateral) of globe, left eye
HØ5.213 Displacement (lateral) of globe, bilateral
HØ5.219 Displacement (lateral) of globe, unspecified eye
6th **HØ5.22 Edema of orbit**
Orbital congestion
HØ5.221 Edema of right orbit
HØ5.222 Edema of left orbit
HØ5.223 Edema of bilateral orbit
HØ5.229 Edema of unspecified orbit
6th **HØ5.23 Hemorrhage of orbit**
HØ5.231 Hemorrhage of right orbit
HØ5.232 Hemorrhage of left orbit
HØ5.233 Hemorrhage of bilateral orbit
HØ5.239 Hemorrhage of unspecified orbit
6th **HØ5.24 Constant exophthalmos**
HØ5.241 Constant exophthalmos, right eye
HØ5.242 Constant exophthalmos, left eye
HØ5.243 Constant exophthalmos, bilateral
HØ5.249 Constant exophthalmos, unspecified eye
6th **HØ5.25 Intermittent exophthalmos**
HØ5.251 Intermittent exophthalmos, right eye
HØ5.252 Intermittent exophthalmos, left eye
HØ5.253 Intermittent exophthalmos, bilateral
HØ5.259 Intermittent exophthalmos, unspecified eye
6th **HØ5.26 Pulsating exophthalmos**
HØ5.261 Pulsating exophthalmos, right eye
HØ5.262 Pulsating exophthalmos, left eye
HØ5.263 Pulsating exophthalmos, bilateral
HØ5.269 Pulsating exophthalmos, unspecified eye
5th **HØ5.3 Deformity of orbit**
EXCLUDES 1 *congenital deformity of orbit (Q1Ø.7)*
hypertelorism (Q75.2)
HØ5.3Ø Unspecified deformity of orbit
6th **HØ5.31 Atrophy of orbit**
HØ5.311 Atrophy of right orbit
HØ5.312 Atrophy of left orbit
HØ5.313 Atrophy of bilateral orbit
HØ5.319 Atrophy of unspecified orbit
6th **HØ5.32 Deformity of orbit due to bone disease**
Code also associated bone disease
HØ5.321 Deformity of right orbit due to bone disease
HØ5.322 Deformity of left orbit due to bone disease
HØ5.323 Deformity of bilateral orbits due to bone disease
HØ5.329 Deformity of unspecified orbit due to bone disease
6th **HØ5.33 Deformity of orbit due to trauma or surgery**
HØ5.331 Deformity of right orbit due to trauma or surgery
HØ5.332 Deformity of left orbit due to trauma or surgery
HØ5.333 Deformity of bilateral orbits due to trauma or surgery
HØ5.339 Deformity of unspecified orbit due to trauma or surgery
6th **HØ5.34 Enlargement of orbit**
HØ5.341 Enlargement of right orbit
HØ5.342 Enlargement of left orbit
HØ5.343 Enlargement of bilateral orbits
HØ5.349 Enlargement of unspecified orbit
6th **HØ5.35 Exostosis of orbit**
HØ5.351 Exostosis of right orbit
HØ5.352 Exostosis of left orbit
HØ5.353 Exostosis of bilateral orbits
HØ5.359 Exostosis of unspecified orbit
5th **HØ5.4 Enophthalmos**
6th **HØ5.4Ø Unspecified enophthalmos**
HØ5.4Ø1 Unspecified enophthalmos, right eye
HØ5.4Ø2 Unspecified enophthalmos, left eye
HØ5.4Ø3 Unspecified enophthalmos, bilateral
HØ5.4Ø9 Unspecified enophthalmos, unspecified eye
6th **HØ5.41 Enophthalmos due to atrophy of orbital tissue**
HØ5.411 Enophthalmos due to atrophy of orbital tissue, right eye
HØ5.412 Enophthalmos due to atrophy of orbital tissue, left eye
HØ5.413 Enophthalmos due to atrophy of orbital tissue, bilateral
HØ5.419 Enophthalmos due to atrophy of orbital tissue, unspecified eye
6th **HØ5.42 Enophthalmos due to trauma or surgery**
HØ5.421 Enophthalmos due to trauma or surgery, right eye
HØ5.422 Enophthalmos due to trauma or surgery, left eye
HØ5.423 Enophthalmos due to trauma or surgery, bilateral

H05.429 Enophthalmos due to trauma or surgery, unspecified eye

H05.5 Retained (old) foreign body following penetrating wound of orbit

Retrobulbar foreign body

Use additional code to identify the type of retained foreign body (Z18.-)

EXCLUDES 1 *current penetrating wound of orbit (S05.4-)*

EXCLUDES 2 *retained foreign body of eyelid (H02.81-)*

retained intraocular foreign body (H44.6-, H44.7-)

H05.50 Retained (old) foreign body following penetrating wound of unspecified orbit

H05.51 Retained (old) foreign body following penetrating wound of right orbit

H05.52 Retained (old) foreign body following penetrating wound of left orbit

H05.53 Retained (old) foreign body following penetrating wound of bilateral orbits

H05.8 Other disorders of orbit

H05.81 Cyst of orbit

Encephalocele of orbit

H05.811 Cyst of right orbit

H05.812 Cyst of left orbit

H05.813 Cyst of bilateral orbits

H05.819 Cyst of unspecified orbit

H05.82 Myopathy of extraocular muscles

H05.821 Myopathy of extraocular muscles, right orbit

H05.822 Myopathy of extraocular muscles, left orbit

H05.823 Myopathy of extraocular muscles, bilateral

H05.829 Myopathy of extraocular muscles, unspecified orbit

H05.89 Other disorders of orbit

H05.9 Unspecified disorder of orbit

Disorders of conjunctiva (H10-H11)

H10 Conjunctivitis

EXCLUDES 1 *keratoconjunctivitis (H16.2-)*

H10.0 Mucopurulent conjunctivitis

H10.01 Acute follicular conjunctivitis

H10.011 Acute follicular conjunctivitis, right eye

H10.012 Acute follicular conjunctivitis, left eye

H10.013 Acute follicular conjunctivitis, bilateral

H10.019 Acute follicular conjunctivitis, unspecified eye

H10.02 Other mucopurulent conjunctivitis

H10.021 Other mucopurulent conjunctivitis, right eye

H10.022 Other mucopurulent conjunctivitis, left eye

H10.023 Other mucopurulent conjunctivitis, bilateral

H10.029 Other mucopurulent conjunctivitis, unspecified eye

H10.1 Acute atopic conjunctivitis

Acute papillary conjunctivitis

H10.10 Acute atopic conjunctivitis, unspecified eye

H10.11 Acute atopic conjunctivitis, right eye

H10.12 Acute atopic conjunctivitis, left eye

H10.13 Acute atopic conjunctivitis, bilateral

H10.2 Other acute conjunctivitis

H10.21 Acute toxic conjunctivitis

Acute chemical conjunctivitis

Code first (T51-T65) to identify chemical and intent

EXCLUDES 1 *burn and corrosion of eye and adnexa (T26.-)*

H10.211 Acute toxic conjunctivitis, right eye

H10.212 Acute toxic conjunctivitis, left eye

H10.213 Acute toxic conjunctivitis, bilateral

H10.219 Acute toxic conjunctivitis, unspecified eye

H10.22 Pseudomembranous conjunctivitis

H10.221 Pseudomembranous conjunctivitis, right eye

H10.222 Pseudomembranous conjunctivitis, left eye

H10.223 Pseudomembranous conjunctivitis, bilateral

H10.229 Pseudomembranous conjunctivitis, unspecified eye

H10.23 Serous conjunctivitis, except viral

EXCLUDES 1 *viral conjunctivitis (B30.-)*

H10.231 Serous conjunctivitis, except viral, right eye

H10.232 Serous conjunctivitis, except viral, left eye

H10.233 Serous conjunctivitis, except viral, bilateral

H10.239 Serous conjunctivitis, except viral, unspecified eye

H10.3 Unspecified acute conjunctivitis

EXCLUDES 1 *ophthalmia neonatorum NOS (P39.1)*

H10.30 Unspecified acute conjunctivitis, unspecified eye

H10.31 Unspecified acute conjunctivitis, right eye

H10.32 Unspecified acute conjunctivitis, left eye

H10.33 Unspecified acute conjunctivitis, bilateral

H10.4 Chronic conjunctivitis

H10.40 Unspecified chronic conjunctivitis

H10.401 Unspecified chronic conjunctivitis, right eye

H10.402 Unspecified chronic conjunctivitis, left eye

H10.403 Unspecified chronic conjunctivitis, bilateral

H10.409 Unspecified chronic conjunctivitis, unspecified eye

H10.41 Chronic giant papillary conjunctivitis

H10.411 Chronic giant papillary conjunctivitis, right eye

H10.412 Chronic giant papillary conjunctivitis, left eye

H10.413 Chronic giant papillary conjunctivitis, bilateral

H10.419 Chronic giant papillary conjunctivitis, unspecified eye

H10.42 Simple chronic conjunctivitis

H10.421 Simple chronic conjunctivitis, right eye

H10.422 Simple chronic conjunctivitis, left eye

H10.423 Simple chronic conjunctivitis, bilateral

H10.429 Simple chronic conjunctivitis, unspecified eye

H10.43 Chronic follicular conjunctivitis

H10.431 Chronic follicular conjunctivitis, right eye

H10.432 Chronic follicular conjunctivitis, left eye

H10.433 Chronic follicular conjunctivitis, bilateral

H10.439 Chronic follicular conjunctivitis, unspecified eye

H10.44 Vernal conjunctivitis

EXCLUDES 1 *vernal keratoconjunctivitis with limbar and corneal involvement (H16.26-)*

H10.45 Other chronic allergic conjunctivitis

H10.5 Blepharoconjunctivitis

H10.50 Unspecified blepharoconjunctivitis

H10.501 Unspecified blepharoconjunctivitis, right eye

H10.502 Unspecified blepharoconjunctivitis, left eye

H10.503 Unspecified blepharoconjunctivitis, bilateral

H10.509 Unspecified blepharoconjunctivitis, unspecified eye

H10.51 Ligneous conjunctivitis

Code also underlying condition if known, such as: plasminogen deficiency (E88.02)

H10.511 Ligneous conjunctivitis, right eye

H10.512 Ligneous conjunctivitis, left eye

H10.513 Ligneous conjunctivitis, bilateral

H10.519 Ligneous conjunctivitis, unspecified eye

H10.52 Angular blepharoconjunctivitis

H10.521 Angular blepharoconjunctivitis, right eye

H10.522 Angular blepharoconjunctivitis, left eye

H10.523 Angular blepharoconjunctivitis, bilateral

H1Ø.529 Angular blepharoconjunctivitis, unspecified eye

√6th **H1Ø.53 Contact blepharoconjunctivitis**

H1Ø.531 Contact blepharoconjunctivitis, right eye
H1Ø.532 Contact blepharoconjunctivitis, left eye
H1Ø.533 Contact blepharoconjunctivitis, bilateral
H1Ø.539 Contact blepharoconjunctivitis, unspecified eye

√5th **H1Ø.8 Other conjunctivitis**

√6th **H1Ø.81 Pingueculitis**

EXCLUDES 1 *pinguecula (H11.15-)*

H1Ø.811 Pingueculitis, right eye
H1Ø.812 Pingueculitis, left eye
H1Ø.813 Pingueculitis, bilateral
H1Ø.819 Pingueculitis, unspecified eye

√6th **H1Ø.82 Rosacea conjunctivitis**

Code first underlying rosacea dermatitis (L71.-)

AHA: 2018,4Q,15

H1Ø.821 Rosacea conjunctivitis, right eye
H1Ø.822 Rosacea conjunctivitis, left eye
H1Ø.823 Rosacea conjunctivitis, bilateral
H1Ø.829 Rosacea conjunctivitis, unspecified eye

H1Ø.89 Other conjunctivitis

H1Ø.9 Unspecified conjunctivitis

√4th **H11 Other disorders of conjunctiva**

EXCLUDES 1 *keratoconjunctivitis (H16.2-)*

√5th **H11.Ø Pterygium of eye**

EXCLUDES 1 *pseudopterygium (H11.81-)*

DEF: Benign, wedge-shaped, conjunctival thickening that advances from the inner corner of the eye toward the cornea.

Pterygium

√6th **H11.ØØ Unspecified pterygium of eye**

H11.ØØ1 Unspecified pterygium of right eye
H11.ØØ2 Unspecified pterygium of left eye
H11.ØØ3 Unspecified pterygium of eye, bilateral
H11.ØØ9 Unspecified pterygium of unspecified eye

√6th **H11.Ø1 Amyloid pterygium**

H11.Ø11 Amyloid pterygium of right eye
H11.Ø12 Amyloid pterygium of left eye
H11.Ø13 Amyloid pterygium of eye, bilateral
H11.Ø19 Amyloid pterygium of unspecified eye

√6th **H11.Ø2 Central pterygium of eye**

H11.Ø21 Central pterygium of right eye
H11.Ø22 Central pterygium of left eye
H11.Ø23 Central pterygium of eye, bilateral
H11.Ø29 Central pterygium of unspecified eye

√6th **H11.Ø3 Double pterygium of eye**

H11.Ø31 Double pterygium of right eye
H11.Ø32 Double pterygium of left eye
H11.Ø33 Double pterygium of eye, bilateral
H11.Ø39 Double pterygium of unspecified eye

√6th **H11.Ø4 Peripheral pterygium of eye, stationary**

H11.Ø41 Peripheral pterygium, stationary, right eye
H11.Ø42 Peripheral pterygium, stationary, left eye
H11.Ø43 Peripheral pterygium, stationary, bilateral
H11.Ø49 Peripheral pterygium, stationary, unspecified eye

√6th **H11.Ø5 Peripheral pterygium of eye, progressive**

H11.Ø51 Peripheral pterygium, progressive, right eye
H11.Ø52 Peripheral pterygium, progressive, left eye
H11.Ø53 Peripheral pterygium, progressive, bilateral
H11.Ø59 Peripheral pterygium, progressive, unspecified eye

√6th **H11.Ø6 Recurrent pterygium of eye**

H11.Ø61 Recurrent pterygium of right eye
H11.Ø62 Recurrent pterygium of left eye
H11.Ø63 Recurrent pterygium of eye, bilateral
H11.Ø69 Recurrent pterygium of unspecified eye

√5th **H11.1 Conjunctival degenerations and deposits**

EXCLUDES 2 *pseudopterygium (H11.81)*

H11.1Ø Unspecified conjunctival degenerations

√6th **H11.11 Conjunctival deposits**

H11.111 Conjunctival deposits, right eye
H11.112 Conjunctival deposits, left eye
H11.113 Conjunctival deposits, bilateral
H11.119 Conjunctival deposits, unspecified eye

√6th **H11.12 Conjunctival concretions**

H11.121 Conjunctival concretions, right eye
H11.122 Conjunctival concretions, left eye
H11.123 Conjunctival concretions, bilateral
H11.129 Conjunctival concretions, unspecified eye

√6th **H11.13 Conjunctival pigmentations**

Conjunctival argyrosis [argyria]

H11.131 Conjunctival pigmentations, right eye
H11.132 Conjunctival pigmentations, left eye
H11.133 Conjunctival pigmentations, bilateral
H11.139 Conjunctival pigmentations, unspecified eye

√6th **H11.14 Conjunctival xerosis, unspecified**

EXCLUDES 1 *xerosis of conjunctiva due to vitamin A deficiency (E5Ø.Ø, E5Ø.1)*

DEF: Abnormal dryness of the conjunctiva due to lack of sufficient tears or conjunctival secretions.

H11.141 Conjunctival xerosis, unspecified, right eye
H11.142 Conjunctival xerosis, unspecified, left eye
H11.143 Conjunctival xerosis, unspecified, bilateral
H11.149 Conjunctival xerosis, unspecified, unspecified eye

√6th **H11.15 Pinguecula**

EXCLUDES 1 *pingueculitis (H1Ø.81-)*

DEF: Proliferation on the conjunctiva near the sclerocorneal junction, usually of the side of the nose and usually in older patients.

Pinguecula

H11.151 Pinguecula, right eye
H11.152 Pinguecula, left eye
H11.153 Pinguecula, bilateral
H11.159 Pinguecula, unspecified eye

√5th **H11.2 Conjunctival scars**

√6th **H11.21 Conjunctival adhesions and strands (localized)**

H11.211 Conjunctival adhesions and strands (localized), right eye
H11.212 Conjunctival adhesions and strands (localized), left eye
H11.213 Conjunctival adhesions and strands (localized), bilateral
H11.219 Conjunctival adhesions and strands (localized), unspecified eye

√6th **H11.22 Conjunctival granuloma**

H11.221 Conjunctival granuloma, right eye
H11.222 Conjunctival granuloma, left eye

H11.223 Conjunctival granuloma, bilateral
H11.229 Conjunctival granuloma, unspecified

H11.23 Symblepharon
H11.231 Symblepharon, right eye
H11.232 Symblepharon, left eye
H11.233 Symblepharon, bilateral
H11.239 Symblepharon, unspecified eye

H11.24 Scarring of conjunctiva
H11.241 Scarring of conjunctiva, right eye
H11.242 Scarring of conjunctiva, left eye
H11.243 Scarring of conjunctiva, bilateral
H11.249 Scarring of conjunctiva, unspecified eye

H11.3 Conjunctival hemorrhage
Subconjunctival hemorrhage
H11.30 Conjunctival hemorrhage, unspecified eye
H11.31 Conjunctival hemorrhage, right eye
H11.32 Conjunctival hemorrhage, left eye
H11.33 Conjunctival hemorrhage, bilateral

H11.4 Other conjunctival vascular disorders and cysts

H11.41 Vascular abnormalities of conjunctiva
Conjunctival aneurysm
H11.411 Vascular abnormalities of conjunctiva, right eye
H11.412 Vascular abnormalities of conjunctiva, left eye
H11.413 Vascular abnormalities of conjunctiva, bilateral
H11.419 Vascular abnormalities of conjunctiva, unspecified eye

H11.42 Conjunctival edema
H11.421 Conjunctival edema, right eye
H11.422 Conjunctival edema, left eye
H11.423 Conjunctival edema, bilateral
H11.429 Conjunctival edema, unspecified eye

H11.43 Conjunctival hyperemia
H11.431 Conjunctival hyperemia, right eye
H11.432 Conjunctival hyperemia, left eye
H11.433 Conjunctival hyperemia, bilateral
H11.439 Conjunctival hyperemia, unspecified eye

H11.44 Conjunctival cysts
H11.441 Conjunctival cysts, right eye
H11.442 Conjunctival cysts, left eye
H11.443 Conjunctival cysts, bilateral
H11.449 Conjunctival cysts, unspecified eye

H11.8 Other specified disorders of conjunctiva

H11.81 Pseudopterygium of conjunctiva
H11.811 Pseudopterygium of conjunctiva, right eye
H11.812 Pseudopterygium of conjunctiva, left eye
H11.813 Pseudopterygium of conjunctiva, bilateral
H11.819 Pseudopterygium of conjunctiva, unspecified eye

H11.82 Conjunctivochalasis
H11.821 Conjunctivochalasis, right eye
H11.822 Conjunctivochalasis, left eye
H11.823 Conjunctivochalasis, bilateral
H11.829 Conjunctivochalasis, unspecified eye
H11.89 Other specified disorders of conjunctiva

H11.9 Unspecified disorder of conjunctiva

Disorders of sclera, cornea, iris and ciliary body (H15-H22)

H15 Disorders of sclera

H15.0 Scleritis

H15.00 Unspecified scleritis
H15.001 Unspecified scleritis, right eye
H15.002 Unspecified scleritis, left eye
H15.003 Unspecified scleritis, bilateral
H15.009 Unspecified scleritis, unspecified eye

H15.01 Anterior scleritis
H15.011 Anterior scleritis, right eye
H15.012 Anterior scleritis, left eye
H15.013 Anterior scleritis, bilateral
H15.019 Anterior scleritis, unspecified eye

H15.02 Brawny scleritis
H15.021 Brawny scleritis, right eye
H15.022 Brawny scleritis, left eye
H15.023 Brawny scleritis, bilateral
H15.029 Brawny scleritis, unspecified eye

H15.03 Posterior scleritis
Sclerotenonitis
H15.031 Posterior scleritis, right eye
H15.032 Posterior scleritis, left eye
H15.033 Posterior scleritis, bilateral
H15.039 Posterior scleritis, unspecified eye

H15.04 Scleritis with corneal involvement
H15.041 Scleritis with corneal involvement, right eye
H15.042 Scleritis with corneal involvement, left eye
H15.043 Scleritis with corneal involvement, bilateral
H15.049 Scleritis with corneal involvement, unspecified eye

H15.05 Scleromalacia perforans
H15.051 Scleromalacia perforans, right eye
H15.052 Scleromalacia perforans, left eye
H15.053 Scleromalacia perforans, bilateral
H15.059 Scleromalacia perforans, unspecified eye

H15.09 Other scleritis
Scleral abscess
H15.091 Other scleritis, right eye
H15.092 Other scleritis, left eye
H15.093 Other scleritis, bilateral
H15.099 Other scleritis, unspecified eye

H15.1 Episcleritis

H15.10 Unspecified episcleritis
H15.101 Unspecified episcleritis, right eye
H15.102 Unspecified episcleritis, left eye
H15.103 Unspecified episcleritis, bilateral
H15.109 Unspecified episcleritis, unspecified eye

H15.11 Episcleritis periodica fugax
H15.111 Episcleritis periodica fugax, right eye
H15.112 Episcleritis periodica fugax, left eye
H15.113 Episcleritis periodica fugax, bilateral
H15.119 Episcleritis periodica fugax, unspecified eye

H15.12 Nodular episcleritis
H15.121 Nodular episcleritis, right eye
H15.122 Nodular episcleritis, left eye
H15.123 Nodular episcleritis, bilateral
H15.129 Nodular episcleritis, unspecified eye

H15.8 Other disorders of sclera
EXCLUDES 2 *blue sclera (Q13.5)*
degenerative myopia (H44.2-)

H15.81 Equatorial staphyloma
H15.811 Equatorial staphyloma, right eye
H15.812 Equatorial staphyloma, left eye
H15.813 Equatorial staphyloma, bilateral
H15.819 Equatorial staphyloma, unspecified eye

H15.82 Localized anterior staphyloma
H15.821 Localized anterior staphyloma, right eye
H15.822 Localized anterior staphyloma, left eye
H15.823 Localized anterior staphyloma, bilateral
H15.829 Localized anterior staphyloma, unspecified eye

H15.83 Staphyloma posticum
H15.831 Staphyloma posticum, right eye
H15.832 Staphyloma posticum, left eye
H15.833 Staphyloma posticum, bilateral
H15.839 Staphyloma posticum, unspecified eye

H15.84 Scleral ectasia
H15.841 Scleral ectasia, right eye
H15.842 Scleral ectasia, left eye
H15.843 Scleral ectasia, bilateral
H15.849 Scleral ectasia, unspecified eye

H15.85 Ring staphyloma
H15.851 Ring staphyloma, right eye
H15.852 Ring staphyloma, left eye
H15.853 Ring staphyloma, bilateral

H15.859 Ring staphyloma, unspecified eye
H15.89 Other disorders of sclera
H15.9 Unspecified disorder of sclera

4th H16 Keratitis

DEF: Condition in which the cornea becomes inflamed and irritated.

5th H16.0 Corneal ulcer
6th H16.00 Unspecified corneal ulcer
H16.001 Unspecified corneal ulcer, right eye
H16.002 Unspecified corneal ulcer, left eye
H16.003 Unspecified corneal ulcer, bilateral
H16.009 Unspecified corneal ulcer, unspecified eye
6th H16.01 Central corneal ulcer
H16.011 Central corneal ulcer, right eye
H16.012 Central corneal ulcer, left eye
H16.013 Central corneal ulcer, bilateral
H16.019 Central corneal ulcer, unspecified eye
6th H16.02 Ring corneal ulcer
H16.021 Ring corneal ulcer, right eye
H16.022 Ring corneal ulcer, left eye
H16.023 Ring corneal ulcer, bilateral
H16.029 Ring corneal ulcer, unspecified eye
6th H16.03 Corneal ulcer with hypopyon
H16.031 Corneal ulcer with hypopyon, right eye
H16.032 Corneal ulcer with hypopyon, left eye
H16.033 Corneal ulcer with hypopyon, bilateral
H16.039 Corneal ulcer with hypopyon, unspecified eye
6th H16.04 Marginal corneal ulcer
H16.041 Marginal corneal ulcer, right eye
H16.042 Marginal corneal ulcer, left eye
H16.043 Marginal corneal ulcer, bilateral
H16.049 Marginal corneal ulcer, unspecified eye
6th H16.05 Mooren's corneal ulcer
H16.051 Mooren's corneal ulcer, right eye
H16.052 Mooren's corneal ulcer, left eye
H16.053 Mooren's corneal ulcer, bilateral
H16.059 Mooren's corneal ulcer, unspecified eye
6th H16.06 Mycotic corneal ulcer
H16.061 Mycotic corneal ulcer, right eye
H16.062 Mycotic corneal ulcer, left eye
H16.063 Mycotic corneal ulcer, bilateral
H16.069 Mycotic corneal ulcer, unspecified eye
6th H16.07 Perforated corneal ulcer
H16.071 Perforated corneal ulcer, right eye
H16.072 Perforated corneal ulcer, left eye
H16.073 Perforated corneal ulcer, bilateral
H16.079 Perforated corneal ulcer, unspecified eye

5th H16.1 Other and unspecified superficial keratitis without conjunctivitis
6th H16.10 Unspecified superficial keratitis
H16.101 Unspecified superficial keratitis, right eye
H16.102 Unspecified superficial keratitis, left eye
H16.103 Unspecified superficial keratitis, bilateral
H16.109 Unspecified superficial keratitis, unspecified eye
6th H16.11 Macular keratitis
Areolar keratitis
Nummular keratitis
Stellate keratitis
Striate keratitis
H16.111 Macular keratitis, right eye
H16.112 Macular keratitis, left eye
H16.113 Macular keratitis, bilateral
H16.119 Macular keratitis, unspecified eye
6th H16.12 Filamentary keratitis
H16.121 Filamentary keratitis, right eye
H16.122 Filamentary keratitis, left eye
H16.123 Filamentary keratitis, bilateral
H16.129 Filamentary keratitis, unspecified eye
6th H16.13 Photokeratitis
Snow blindness
Welders keratitis
H16.131 Photokeratitis, right eye
H16.132 Photokeratitis, left eye
H16.133 Photokeratitis, bilateral
H16.139 Photokeratitis, unspecified eye
6th H16.14 Punctate keratitis
H16.141 Punctate keratitis, right eye
H16.142 Punctate keratitis, left eye
H16.143 Punctate keratitis, bilateral
H16.149 Punctate keratitis, unspecified eye

5th H16.2 Keratoconjunctivitis
6th H16.20 Unspecified keratoconjunctivitis
Superficial keratitis with conjunctivitis NOS
H16.201 Unspecified keratoconjunctivitis, right eye
H16.202 Unspecified keratoconjunctivitis, left eye
H16.203 Unspecified keratoconjunctivitis, bilateral
H16.209 Unspecified keratoconjunctivitis, unspecified eye
6th H16.21 Exposure keratoconjunctivitis
H16.211 Exposure keratoconjunctivitis, right eye
H16.212 Exposure keratoconjunctivitis, left eye
H16.213 Exposure keratoconjunctivitis, bilateral
H16.219 Exposure keratoconjunctivitis, unspecified eye
6th H16.22 Keratoconjunctivitis sicca, not specified as Sjögren's
EXCLUDES 1 *Sjögren's syndrome (M35.01)*
H16.221 Keratoconjunctivitis sicca, not specified as Sjögren's, right eye
H16.222 Keratoconjunctivitis sicca, not specified as Sjögren's, left eye
H16.223 Keratoconjunctivitis sicca, not specified as Sjögren's, bilateral
H16.229 Keratoconjunctivitis sicca, not specified as Sjögren's, unspecified eye
6th H16.23 Neurotrophic keratoconjunctivitis
H16.231 Neurotrophic keratoconjunctivitis, right eye
H16.232 Neurotrophic keratoconjunctivitis, left eye
H16.233 Neurotrophic keratoconjunctivitis, bilateral
H16.239 Neurotrophic keratoconjunctivitis, unspecified eye
6th H16.24 Ophthalmia nodosa
H16.241 Ophthalmia nodosa, right eye
H16.242 Ophthalmia nodosa, left eye
H16.243 Ophthalmia nodosa, bilateral
H16.249 Ophthalmia nodosa, unspecified eye
6th H16.25 Phlyctenular keratoconjunctivitis
H16.251 Phlyctenular keratoconjunctivitis, right eye
H16.252 Phlyctenular keratoconjunctivitis, left eye
H16.253 Phlyctenular keratoconjunctivitis, bilateral
H16.259 Phlyctenular keratoconjunctivitis, unspecified eye
6th H16.26 Vernal keratoconjunctivitis, with limbar and corneal involvement
EXCLUDES 1 *vernal conjunctivitis without limbar and corneal involvement (H10.44)*
H16.261 Vernal keratoconjunctivitis, with limbar and corneal involvement, right eye
H16.262 Vernal keratoconjunctivitis, with limbar and corneal involvement, left eye
H16.263 Vernal keratoconjunctivitis, with limbar and corneal involvement, bilateral
H16.269 Vernal keratoconjunctivitis, with limbar and corneal involvement, unspecified eye
6th H16.29 Other keratoconjunctivitis
H16.291 Other keratoconjunctivitis, right eye
H16.292 Other keratoconjunctivitis, left eye
H16.293 Other keratoconjunctivitis, bilateral
H16.299 Other keratoconjunctivitis, unspecified eye

5th H16.3 Interstitial and deep keratitis
6th H16.30 Unspecified interstitial keratitis
H16.301 Unspecified interstitial keratitis, right eye
H16.302 Unspecified interstitial keratitis, left eye
H16.303 Unspecified interstitial keratitis, bilateral

H16.309 Unspecified interstitial keratitis, unspecified eye
H16.31 Corneal abscess
H16.311 Corneal abscess, right eye
H16.312 Corneal abscess, left eye
H16.313 Corneal abscess, bilateral
H16.319 Corneal abscess, unspecified eye
H16.32 Diffuse interstitial keratitis
Cogan's syndrome
H16.321 Diffuse interstitial keratitis, right eye
H16.322 Diffuse interstitial keratitis, left eye
H16.323 Diffuse interstitial keratitis, bilateral
H16.329 Diffuse interstitial keratitis, unspecified eye
H16.33 Sclerosing keratitis
H16.331 Sclerosing keratitis, right eye
H16.332 Sclerosing keratitis, left eye
H16.333 Sclerosing keratitis, bilateral
H16.339 Sclerosing keratitis, unspecified eye
H16.39 Other interstitial and deep keratitis
H16.391 Other interstitial and deep keratitis, right eye
H16.392 Other interstitial and deep keratitis, left eye
H16.393 Other interstitial and deep keratitis, bilateral
H16.399 Other interstitial and deep keratitis, unspecified eye
H16.4 Corneal neovascularization
H16.40 Unspecified corneal neovascularization
H16.401 Unspecified corneal neovascularization, right eye
H16.402 Unspecified corneal neovascularization, left eye
H16.403 Unspecified corneal neovascularization, bilateral
H16.409 Unspecified corneal neovascularization, unspecified eye
H16.41 Ghost vessels (corneal)
H16.411 Ghost vessels (corneal), right eye
H16.412 Ghost vessels (corneal), left eye
H16.413 Ghost vessels (corneal), bilateral
H16.419 Ghost vessels (corneal), unspecified eye
H16.42 Pannus (corneal)
H16.421 Pannus (corneal), right eye
H16.422 Pannus (corneal), left eye
H16.423 Pannus (corneal), bilateral
H16.429 Pannus (corneal), unspecified eye
H16.43 Localized vascularization of cornea
H16.431 Localized vascularization of cornea, right eye
H16.432 Localized vascularization of cornea, left eye
H16.433 Localized vascularization of cornea, bilateral
H16.439 Localized vascularization of cornea, unspecified eye
H16.44 Deep vascularization of cornea
H16.441 Deep vascularization of cornea, right eye
H16.442 Deep vascularization of cornea, left eye
H16.443 Deep vascularization of cornea, bilateral
H16.449 Deep vascularization of cornea, unspecified eye
H16.8 Other keratitis
H16.9 Unspecified keratitis
H17 Corneal scars and opacities
H17.0 Adherent leukoma
H17.00 Adherent leukoma, unspecified eye
H17.01 Adherent leukoma, right eye
H17.02 Adherent leukoma, left eye
H17.03 Adherent leukoma, bilateral
H17.1 Central corneal opacity
H17.10 Central corneal opacity, unspecified eye
H17.11 Central corneal opacity, right eye
H17.12 Central corneal opacity, left eye
H17.13 Central corneal opacity, bilateral
H17.8 Other corneal scars and opacities
H17.81 Minor opacity of cornea
Corneal nebula
H17.811 Minor opacity of cornea, right eye
H17.812 Minor opacity of cornea, left eye
H17.813 Minor opacity of cornea, bilateral
H17.819 Minor opacity of cornea, unspecified eye
H17.82 Peripheral opacity of cornea
H17.821 Peripheral opacity of cornea, right eye
H17.822 Peripheral opacity of cornea, left eye
H17.823 Peripheral opacity of cornea, bilateral
H17.829 Peripheral opacity of cornea, unspecified eye
H17.89 Other corneal scars and opacities
H17.9 Unspecified corneal scar and opacity
H18 Other disorders of cornea
H18.0 Corneal pigmentations and deposits
H18.00 Unspecified corneal deposit
H18.001 Unspecified corneal deposit, right eye
H18.002 Unspecified corneal deposit, left eye
H18.003 Unspecified corneal deposit, bilateral
H18.009 Unspecified corneal deposit, unspecified eye
H18.01 Anterior corneal pigmentations
Staehli's line
H18.011 Anterior corneal pigmentations, right eye
H18.012 Anterior corneal pigmentations, left eye
H18.013 Anterior corneal pigmentations, bilateral
H18.019 Anterior corneal pigmentations, unspecified eye
H18.02 Argentous corneal deposits
H18.021 Argentous corneal deposits, right eye
H18.022 Argentous corneal deposits, left eye
H18.023 Argentous corneal deposits, bilateral
H18.029 Argentous corneal deposits, unspecified eye
H18.03 Corneal deposits in metabolic disorders
Code also associated metabolic disorder
H18.031 Corneal deposits in metabolic disorders, right eye
H18.032 Corneal deposits in metabolic disorders, left eye
H18.033 Corneal deposits in metabolic disorders, bilateral
H18.039 Corneal deposits in metabolic disorders, unspecified eye
H18.04 Kayser-Fleischer ring
Code also associated Wilson's disease (E83.01)
H18.041 Kayser-Fleischer ring, right eye
H18.042 Kayser-Fleischer ring, left eye
H18.043 Kayser-Fleischer ring, bilateral
H18.049 Kayser-Fleischer ring, unspecified eye
H18.05 Posterior corneal pigmentations
Krukenberg's spindle
H18.051 Posterior corneal pigmentations, right eye
H18.052 Posterior corneal pigmentations, left eye
H18.053 Posterior corneal pigmentations, bilateral
H18.059 Posterior corneal pigmentations, unspecified eye
H18.06 Stromal corneal pigmentations
Hematocornea
H18.061 Stromal corneal pigmentations, right eye
H18.062 Stromal corneal pigmentations, left eye
H18.063 Stromal corneal pigmentations, bilateral
H18.069 Stromal corneal pigmentations, unspecified eye
H18.1 Bullous keratopathy
DEF: Corneal swelling due to a damaged corneal endothelium. Bullous keratopathy is characterized by recurring, rupturing epithelial blisters causing glaucoma, iridocyclitis, and Fuchs' dystrophy.
H18.10 Bullous keratopathy, unspecified eye
H18.11 Bullous keratopathy, right eye
H18.12 Bullous keratopathy, left eye
H18.13 Bullous keratopathy, bilateral

√5th H18.2 Other and unspecified corneal edema
H18.20 Unspecified corneal edema
√6th H18.21 Corneal edema secondary to contact lens
EXCLUDES 2 *other corneal disorders due to contact lens (H18.82-)*
H18.211 Corneal edema secondary to contact lens, right eye
H18.212 Corneal edema secondary to contact lens, left eye
H18.213 Corneal edema secondary to contact lens, bilateral
H18.219 Corneal edema secondary to contact lens, unspecified eye
√6th H18.22 Idiopathic corneal edema
H18.221 Idiopathic corneal edema, right eye
H18.222 Idiopathic corneal edema, left eye
H18.223 Idiopathic corneal edema, bilateral
H18.229 Idiopathic corneal edema, unspecified eye
√6th H18.23 Secondary corneal edema
H18.231 Secondary corneal edema, right eye
H18.232 Secondary corneal edema, left eye
H18.233 Secondary corneal edema, bilateral
H18.239 Secondary corneal edema, unspecified eye
√5th H18.3 Changes of corneal membranes
H18.30 Unspecified corneal membrane change
√6th H18.31 Folds and rupture in Bowman's membrane
H18.311 Folds and rupture in Bowman's membrane, right eye
H18.312 Folds and rupture in Bowman's membrane, left eye
H18.313 Folds and rupture in Bowman's membrane, bilateral
H18.319 Folds and rupture in Bowman's membrane, unspecified eye
√6th H18.32 Folds in Descemet's membrane
H18.321 Folds in Descemet's membrane, right eye
H18.322 Folds in Descemet's membrane, left eye
H18.323 Folds in Descemet's membrane, bilateral
H18.329 Folds in Descemet's membrane, unspecified eye
√6th H18.33 Rupture in Descemet's membrane
H18.331 Rupture in Descemet's membrane, right eye
H18.332 Rupture in Descemet's membrane, left eye
H18.333 Rupture in Descemet's membrane, bilateral
H18.339 Rupture in Descemet's membrane, unspecified eye
√5th H18.4 Corneal degeneration
EXCLUDES 1 *Mooren's ulcer (H16.Ø-)*
recurrent erosion of cornea (H18.83-)
H18.4Ø Unspecified corneal degeneration
√6th H18.41 Arcus senilis
Senile corneal changes
H18.411 Arcus senilis, right eye
H18.412 Arcus senilis, left eye
H18.413 Arcus senilis, bilateral
H18.419 Arcus senilis, unspecified eye
√6th H18.42 Band keratopathy
H18.421 Band keratopathy, right eye
H18.422 Band keratopathy, left eye
H18.423 Band keratopathy, bilateral
H18.429 Band keratopathy, unspecified eye
H18.43 Other calcerous corneal degeneration
√6th H18.44 Keratomalacia
EXCLUDES 1 *keratomalacia due to vitamin A deficiency (E5Ø.4)*
H18.441 Keratomalacia, right eye
H18.442 Keratomalacia, left eye
H18.443 Keratomalacia, bilateral
H18.449 Keratomalacia, unspecified eye
√6th H18.45 Nodular corneal degeneration
H18.451 Nodular corneal degeneration, right eye
H18.452 Nodular corneal degeneration, left eye
H18.453 Nodular corneal degeneration, bilateral
H18.459 Nodular corneal degeneration, unspecified eye
√6th H18.46 Peripheral corneal degeneration
H18.461 Peripheral corneal degeneration, right eye
H18.462 Peripheral corneal degeneration, left eye
H18.463 Peripheral corneal degeneration, bilateral
H18.469 Peripheral corneal degeneration, unspecified eye
H18.49 Other corneal degeneration
√5th H18.5 Hereditary corneal dystrophies
AHA: 2020,4Q,24
√6th H18.5Ø Unspecified hereditary corneal dystrophies
H18.5Ø1 Unspecified hereditary corneal dystrophies, right eye
H18.5Ø2 Unspecified hereditary corneal dystrophies, left eye
H18.5Ø3 Unspecified hereditary corneal dystrophies, bilateral
H18.5Ø9 Unspecified hereditary corneal dystrophies, unspecified eye
√6th H18.51 Endothelial corneal dystrophy
Fuchs' dystrophy
H18.511 Endothelial corneal dystrophy, right eye
H18.512 Endothelial corneal dystrophy, left eye
H18.513 Endothelial corneal dystrophy, bilateral
H18.519 Endothelial corneal dystrophy, unspecified eye
√6th H18.52 Epithelial (juvenile) corneal dystrophy
H18.521 Epithelial (juvenile) corneal dystrophy, right eye
H18.522 Epithelial (juvenile) corneal dystrophy, left eye
H18.523 Epithelial (juvenile) corneal dystrophy, bilateral
H18.529 Epithelial (juvenile) corneal dystrophy, unspecified eye
√6th H18.53 Granular corneal dystrophy
H18.531 Granular corneal dystrophy, right eye
H18.532 Granular corneal dystrophy, left eye
H18.533 Granular corneal dystrophy, bilateral
H18.539 Granular corneal dystrophy, unspecified eye
√6th H18.54 Lattice corneal dystrophy
H18.541 Lattice corneal dystrophy, right eye
H18.542 Lattice corneal dystrophy, left eye
H18.543 Lattice corneal dystrophy, bilateral
H18.549 Lattice corneal dystrophy, unspecified eye
√6th H18.55 Macular corneal dystrophy
H18.551 Macular corneal dystrophy, right eye
H18.552 Macular corneal dystrophy, left eye
H18.553 Macular corneal dystrophy, bilateral
H18.559 Macular corneal dystrophy, unspecified eye
√6th H18.59 Other hereditary corneal dystrophies
H18.591 Other hereditary corneal dystrophies, right eye
H18.592 Other hereditary corneal dystrophies, left eye
H18.593 Other hereditary corneal dystrophies, bilateral
H18.599 Other hereditary corneal dystrophies, unspecified eye
√5th H18.6 Keratoconus
√6th H18.6Ø Keratoconus, unspecified
H18.6Ø1 Keratoconus, unspecified, right eye
H18.6Ø2 Keratoconus, unspecified, left eye
H18.6Ø3 Keratoconus, unspecified, bilateral
H18.6Ø9 Keratoconus, unspecified, unspecified eye
√6th H18.61 Keratoconus, stable
H18.611 Keratoconus, stable, right eye
H18.612 Keratoconus, stable, left eye
H18.613 Keratoconus, stable, bilateral
H18.619 Keratoconus, stable, unspecified eye

H18.62 Keratoconus, unstable
Acute hydrops
H18.621 Keratoconus, unstable, right eye
H18.622 Keratoconus, unstable, left eye
H18.623 Keratoconus, unstable, bilateral
H18.629 Keratoconus, unstable, unspecified eye

H18.7 Other and unspecified corneal deformities
EXCLUDES 1 *congenital malformations of cornea (Q13.3-Q13.4)*
H18.70 Unspecified corneal deformity
H18.71 Corneal ectasia
H18.711 Corneal ectasia, right eye
H18.712 Corneal ectasia, left eye
H18.713 Corneal ectasia, bilateral
H18.719 Corneal ectasia, unspecified eye
H18.72 Corneal staphyloma
H18.721 Corneal staphyloma, right eye
H18.722 Corneal staphyloma, left eye
H18.723 Corneal staphyloma, bilateral
H18.729 Corneal staphyloma, unspecified eye
H18.73 Descemetocele
H18.731 Descemetocele, right eye
H18.732 Descemetocele, left eye
H18.733 Descemetocele, bilateral
H18.739 Descemetocele, unspecified eye
H18.79 Other corneal deformities
H18.791 Other corneal deformities, right eye
H18.792 Other corneal deformities, left eye
H18.793 Other corneal deformities, bilateral
H18.799 Other corneal deformities, unspecified eye

H18.8 Other specified disorders of cornea
H18.81 Anesthesia and hypoesthesia of cornea
H18.811 Anesthesia and hypoesthesia of cornea, right eye
H18.812 Anesthesia and hypoesthesia of cornea, left eye
H18.813 Anesthesia and hypoesthesia of cornea, bilateral
H18.819 Anesthesia and hypoesthesia of cornea, unspecified eye
H18.82 Corneal disorder due to contact lens
EXCLUDES 2 *corneal edema due to contact lens (H18.21-)*
H18.821 Corneal disorder due to contact lens, right eye
H18.822 Corneal disorder due to contact lens, left eye
H18.823 Corneal disorder due to contact lens, bilateral
H18.829 Corneal disorder due to contact lens, unspecified eye
H18.83 Recurrent erosion of cornea
H18.831 Recurrent erosion of cornea, right eye
H18.832 Recurrent erosion of cornea, left eye
H18.833 Recurrent erosion of cornea, bilateral
H18.839 Recurrent erosion of cornea, unspecified eye
H18.89 Other specified disorders of cornea
H18.891 Other specified disorders of cornea, right eye
H18.892 Other specified disorders of cornea, left eye
H18.893 Other specified disorders of cornea, bilateral
H18.899 Other specified disorders of cornea, unspecified eye

H18.9 Unspecified disorder of cornea

H20 Iridocyclitis

H20.0 Acute and subacute iridocyclitis
Acute anterior uveitis
Acute cyclitis
Acute iritis
Subacute anterior uveitis
Subacute cyclitis
Subacute iritis
EXCLUDES 1 *iridocyclitis, iritis, uveitis (due to) (in) diabetes mellitus (E08-E13 with .39)*
iridocyclitis, iritis, uveitis (due to) (in) diphtheria (A36.89)
iridocyclitis, iritis, uveitis (due to) (in) gonococcal (A54.32)
iridocyclitis, iritis, uveitis (due to) (in) herpes (simplex) (B00.51)
iridocyclitis, iritis, uveitis (due to) (in) herpes zoster (B02.32)
iridocyclitis, iritis, uveitis (due to) (in) late congenital syphilis (A50.39)
iridocyclitis, iritis, uveitis (due to) (in) late syphilis (A52.71)
iridocyclitis, iritis, uveitis (due to) (in) sarcoidosis (D86.83)
iridocyclitis, iritis, uveitis (due to) (in) syphilis (A51.43)
iridocyclitis, iritis, uveitis (due to) (in) toxoplasmosis (B58.09)
iridocyclitis, iritis, uveitis (due to) (in) tuberculosis (A18.54)
H20.00 Unspecified acute and subacute iridocyclitis
H20.01 Primary iridocyclitis
H20.011 Primary iridocyclitis, right eye
H20.012 Primary iridocyclitis, left eye
H20.013 Primary iridocyclitis, bilateral
H20.019 Primary iridocyclitis, unspecified eye
H20.02 Recurrent acute iridocyclitis
H20.021 Recurrent acute iridocyclitis, right eye
H20.022 Recurrent acute iridocyclitis, left eye
H20.023 Recurrent acute iridocyclitis, bilateral
H20.029 Recurrent acute iridocyclitis, unspecified eye
H20.03 Secondary infectious iridocyclitis
H20.031 Secondary infectious iridocyclitis, right eye
H20.032 Secondary infectious iridocyclitis, left eye
H20.033 Secondary infectious iridocyclitis, bilateral
H20.039 Secondary infectious iridocyclitis, unspecified eye
H20.04 Secondary noninfectious iridocyclitis
H20.041 Secondary noninfectious iridocyclitis, right eye
H20.042 Secondary noninfectious iridocyclitis, left eye
H20.043 Secondary noninfectious iridocyclitis, bilateral
H20.049 Secondary noninfectious iridocyclitis, unspecified eye
H20.05 Hypopyon
H20.051 Hypopyon, right eye
H20.052 Hypopyon, left eye
H20.053 Hypopyon, bilateral
H20.059 Hypopyon, unspecified eye

H20.1 Chronic iridocyclitis
Use additional code for any associated cataract (H26.21-)
EXCLUDES 2 *posterior cyclitis (H30.2-)*
H20.10 Chronic iridocyclitis, unspecified eye
H20.11 Chronic iridocyclitis, right eye
H20.12 Chronic iridocyclitis, left eye
H20.13 Chronic iridocyclitis, bilateral

H20.2 Lens-induced iridocyclitis
H20.20 Lens-induced iridocyclitis, unspecified eye
H20.21 Lens-induced iridocyclitis, right eye
H20.22 Lens-induced iridocyclitis, left eye
H20.23 Lens-induced iridocyclitis, bilateral

√5th H2Ø.8 Other iridocyclitis

EXCLUDES 2 *glaucomatocyclitis crises (H4Ø.4-)*
posterior cyclitis (H3Ø.2-)
sympathetic uveitis (H44.13-)

√6th H2Ø.81 Fuchs' heterochromic cyclitis

H2Ø.811 Fuchs' heterochromic cyclitis, right eye
H2Ø.812 Fuchs' heterochromic cyclitis, left eye
H2Ø.813 Fuchs' heterochromic cyclitis, bilateral
H2Ø.819 Fuchs' heterochromic cyclitis, unspecified eye

√6th H2Ø.82 Vogt-Koyanagi syndrome

H2Ø.821 Vogt-Koyanagi syndrome, right eye
H2Ø.822 Vogt-Koyanagi syndrome, left eye
H2Ø.823 Vogt-Koyanagi syndrome, bilateral
H2Ø.829 Vogt-Koyanagi syndrome, unspecified eye

H2Ø.9 Unspecified iridocyclitis

Uveitis NOS

√4th H21 Other disorders of iris and ciliary body

EXCLUDES 2 *sympathetic uveitis (H44.1-)*

√5th H21.Ø Hyphema

EXCLUDES 1 *traumatic hyphema (SØ5.1-)*

Hyphema

Iris
Cornea
Hyphema

H21.ØØ Hyphema, unspecified eye
H21.Ø1 Hyphema, right eye
H21.Ø2 Hyphema, left eye
H21.Ø3 Hyphema, bilateral

√5th H21.1 Other vascular disorders of iris and ciliary body

Neovascularization of iris or ciliary body
Rubeosis iridis
Rubeosis of iris

√6th H21.1X Other vascular disorders of iris and ciliary body

H21.1X1 Other vascular disorders of iris and ciliary body, right eye
H21.1X2 Other vascular disorders of iris and ciliary body, left eye
H21.1X3 Other vascular disorders of iris and ciliary body, bilateral
H21.1X9 Other vascular disorders of iris and ciliary body, unspecified eye

√5th H21.2 Degeneration of iris and ciliary body

√6th H21.21 Degeneration of chamber angle

H21.211 Degeneration of chamber angle, right eye
H21.212 Degeneration of chamber angle, left eye
H21.213 Degeneration of chamber angle, bilateral
H21.219 Degeneration of chamber angle, unspecified eye

√6th H21.22 Degeneration of ciliary body

H21.221 Degeneration of ciliary body, right eye
H21.222 Degeneration of ciliary body, left eye
H21.223 Degeneration of ciliary body, bilateral
H21.229 Degeneration of ciliary body, unspecified eye

√6th H21.23 Degeneration of iris (pigmentary)

Translucency of iris

H21.231 Degeneration of iris (pigmentary), right eye
H21.232 Degeneration of iris (pigmentary), left eye
H21.233 Degeneration of iris (pigmentary), bilateral
H21.239 Degeneration of iris (pigmentary), unspecified eye

√6th H21.24 Degeneration of pupillary margin

H21.241 Degeneration of pupillary margin, right eye
H21.242 Degeneration of pupillary margin, left eye
H21.243 Degeneration of pupillary margin, bilateral
H21.249 Degeneration of pupillary margin, unspecified eye

√6th H21.25 Iridoschisis

H21.251 Iridoschisis, right eye
H21.252 Iridoschisis, left eye
H21.253 Iridoschisis, bilateral
H21.259 Iridoschisis, unspecified eye

√6th H21.26 Iris atrophy (essential) (progressive)

H21.261 Iris atrophy (essential) (progressive), right eye
H21.262 Iris atrophy (essential) (progressive), left eye
H21.263 Iris atrophy (essential) (progressive), bilateral
H21.269 Iris atrophy (essential) (progressive), unspecified eye

√6th H21.27 Miotic pupillary cyst

H21.271 Miotic pupillary cyst, right eye
H21.272 Miotic pupillary cyst, left eye
H21.273 Miotic pupillary cyst, bilateral
H21.279 Miotic pupillary cyst, unspecified eye

H21.29 Other iris atrophy

√5th H21.3 Cyst of iris, ciliary body and anterior chamber

EXCLUDES 2 *miotic pupillary cyst (H21.27-)*

√6th H21.3Ø Idiopathic cysts of iris, ciliary body or anterior chamber

Cyst of iris, ciliary body or anterior chamber NOS

H21.3Ø1 Idiopathic cysts of iris, ciliary body or anterior chamber, right eye
H21.3Ø2 Idiopathic cysts of iris, ciliary body or anterior chamber, left eye
H21.3Ø3 Idiopathic cysts of iris, ciliary body or anterior chamber, bilateral
H21.3Ø9 Idiopathic cysts of iris, ciliary body or anterior chamber, unspecified eye

√6th H21.31 Exudative cysts of iris or anterior chamber

H21.311 Exudative cysts of iris or anterior chamber, right eye
H21.312 Exudative cysts of iris or anterior chamber, left eye
H21.313 Exudative cysts of iris or anterior chamber, bilateral
H21.319 Exudative cysts of iris or anterior chamber, unspecified eye

√6th H21.32 Implantation cysts of iris, ciliary body or anterior chamber

H21.321 Implantation cysts of iris, ciliary body or anterior chamber, right eye
H21.322 Implantation cysts of iris, ciliary body or anterior chamber, left eye
H21.323 Implantation cysts of iris, ciliary body or anterior chamber, bilateral
H21.329 Implantation cysts of iris, ciliary body or anterior chamber, unspecified eye

√6th H21.33 Parasitic cyst of iris, ciliary body or anterior chamber

H21.331 Parasitic cyst of iris, ciliary body or anterior chamber, right eye
H21.332 Parasitic cyst of iris, ciliary body or anterior chamber, left eye
H21.333 Parasitic cyst of iris, ciliary body or anterior chamber, bilateral
H21.339 Parasitic cyst of iris, ciliary body or anterior chamber, unspecified eye

√6th H21.34 Primary cyst of pars plana

H21.341 Primary cyst of pars plana, right eye
H21.342 Primary cyst of pars plana, left eye
H21.343 Primary cyst of pars plana, bilateral
H21.349 Primary cyst of pars plana, unspecified eye

H21.35 Exudative cyst of pars plana
DEF: Protein, fatty-filled bullous elevation of the nonpigmented outermost ciliary epithelium of pars plana, due to fluid leak from blood vessels.
H21.351 Exudative cyst of pars plana, right eye
H21.352 Exudative cyst of pars plana, left eye
H21.353 Exudative cyst of pars plana, bilateral
H21.359 Exudative cyst of pars plana, unspecified eye

H21.4 Pupillary membranes
Iris bombé
Pupillary occlusion
Pupillary seclusion
EXCLUDES 1 *congenital pupillary membranes (Q13.8)*
H21.40 Pupillary membranes, unspecified eye
H21.41 Pupillary membranes, right eye
H21.42 Pupillary membranes, left eye
H21.43 Pupillary membranes, bilateral

H21.5 Other and unspecified adhesions and disruptions of iris and ciliary body
EXCLUDES 1 *corectopia (Q13.2)*
H21.50 Unspecified adhesions of iris
Synechia (iris) NOS
H21.501 Unspecified adhesions of iris, right eye
H21.502 Unspecified adhesions of iris, left eye
H21.503 Unspecified adhesions of iris, bilateral
H21.509 Unspecified adhesions of iris and ciliary body, unspecified eye
H21.51 Anterior synechiae (iris)
H21.511 Anterior synechiae (iris), right eye
H21.512 Anterior synechiae (iris), left eye
H21.513 Anterior synechiae (iris), bilateral
H21.519 Anterior synechiae (iris), unspecified eye
H21.52 Goniosynechiae
H21.521 Goniosynechiae, right eye
H21.522 Goniosynechiae, left eye
H21.523 Goniosynechiae, bilateral
H21.529 Goniosynechiae, unspecified eye
H21.53 Iridodialysis
H21.531 Iridodialysis, right eye
H21.532 Iridodialysis, left eye
H21.533 Iridodialysis, bilateral
H21.539 Iridodialysis, unspecified eye
H21.54 Posterior synechiae (iris)
H21.541 Posterior synechiae (iris), right eye
H21.542 Posterior synechiae (iris), left eye
H21.543 Posterior synechiae (iris), bilateral
H21.549 Posterior synechiae (iris), unspecified eye
H21.55 Recession of chamber angle
H21.551 Recession of chamber angle, right eye
H21.552 Recession of chamber angle, left eye
H21.553 Recession of chamber angle, bilateral
H21.559 Recession of chamber angle, unspecified eye
H21.56 Pupillary abnormalities
Deformed pupil
Ectopic pupil
Rupture of sphincter, pupil
EXCLUDES 1 *congenital deformity of pupil (Q13.2-)*
H21.561 Pupillary abnormality, right eye
H21.562 Pupillary abnormality, left eye
H21.563 Pupillary abnormality, bilateral
H21.569 Pupillary abnormality, unspecified eye

H21.8 Other specified disorders of iris and ciliary body
H21.81 Floppy iris syndrome
Intraoperative floppy iris syndrome (IFIS)
Use additional code for adverse effect, if applicable, to identify drug (T36-T50 with fifth or sixth character 5)
H21.82 Plateau iris syndrome (post-iridectomy) (postprocedural)
H21.89 Other specified disorders of iris and ciliary body

H21.9 Unspecified disorder of iris and ciliary body

H22 Disorders of iris and ciliary body in diseases classified elsewhere
Code first underlying disease, such as:
gout (M1A.-, M10.-)
leprosy (A30.-)
parasitic disease (B89)

Disorders of lens (H25-H28)

H25 Age-related cataract
Senile cataract
EXCLUDES 2 *capsular glaucoma with pseudoexfoliation of lens (H40.1-)*

Cataracts

H25.0 Age-related incipient cataract
H25.01 Cortical age-related cataract
H25.011 Cortical age-related cataract, right eye A
H25.012 Cortical age-related cataract, left eye A
H25.013 Cortical age-related cataract, bilateral A
H25.019 Cortical age-related cataract, unspecified eye A
H25.03 Anterior subcapsular polar age-related cataract
H25.031 Anterior subcapsular polar age-related cataract, right eye A
H25.032 Anterior subcapsular polar age-related cataract, left eye A
H25.033 Anterior subcapsular polar age-related cataract, bilateral A
H25.039 Anterior subcapsular polar age-related cataract, unspecified eye A
H25.04 Posterior subcapsular polar age-related cataract
H25.041 Posterior subcapsular polar age-related cataract, right eye A
H25.042 Posterior subcapsular polar age-related cataract, left eye A
H25.043 Posterior subcapsular polar age-related cataract, bilateral A
H25.049 Posterior subcapsular polar age-related cataract, unspecified eye A
H25.09 Other age-related incipient cataract
Coronary age-related cataract
Punctate age-related cataract
Water clefts
H25.091 Other age-related incipient cataract, right eye A
H25.092 Other age-related incipient cataract, left eye A
H25.093 Other age-related incipient cataract, bilateral A
H25.099 Other age-related incipient cataract, unspecified eye A

H25.1 Age-related nuclear cataract
Cataracta brunescens
Nuclear sclerosis cataract
AHA: 2019,2Q,31; 2016,1Q,32
H25.10 Age-related nuclear cataract, unspecified eye A
H25.11 Age-related nuclear cataract, right eye A
H25.12 Age-related nuclear cataract, left eye A
H25.13 Age-related nuclear cataract, bilateral A

H25.2 Age-related cataract, morgagnian type
Age-related hypermature cataract
H25.20 Age-related cataract, morgagnian type, unspecified eye A
H25.21 Age-related cataract, morgagnian type, right eye A
H25.22 Age-related cataract, morgagnian type, left eye A
H25.23 Age-related cataract, morgagnian type, bilateral A

H25.8 Other age-related cataract
H25.81 Combined forms of age-related cataract
AHA: 2019,2Q,30
H25.811 Combined forms of age-related cataract, right eye A
H25.812 Combined forms of age-related cataract, left eye A
H25.813 Combined forms of age-related cataract, bilateral A
H25.819 Combined forms of age-related cataract, unspecified eye A
H25.89 Other age-related cataract A
H25.9 Unspecified age-related cataract A

H26 Other cataract
EXCLUDES 1 *congenital cataract (Q12.Ø)*

H26.Ø Infantile and juvenile cataract
H26.ØØ Unspecified infantile and juvenile cataract
H26.ØØ1 Unspecified infantile and juvenile cataract, right eye P
H26.ØØ2 Unspecified infantile and juvenile cataract, left eye P
H26.ØØ3 Unspecified infantile and juvenile cataract, bilateral P
H26.ØØ9 Unspecified infantile and juvenile cataract, unspecified eye P
H26.Ø1 Infantile and juvenile cortical, lamellar, or zonular cataract
H26.Ø11 Infantile and juvenile cortical, lamellar, or zonular cataract, right eye P
H26.Ø12 Infantile and juvenile cortical, lamellar, or zonular cataract, left eye P
H26.Ø13 Infantile and juvenile cortical, lamellar, or zonular cataract, bilateral P
H26.Ø19 Infantile and juvenile cortical, lamellar, or zonular cataract, unspecified eye P
H26.Ø3 Infantile and juvenile nuclear cataract
H26.Ø31 Infantile and juvenile nuclear cataract, right eye P
H26.Ø32 Infantile and juvenile nuclear cataract, left eye P
H26.Ø33 Infantile and juvenile nuclear cataract, bilateral P
H26.Ø39 Infantile and juvenile nuclear cataract, unspecified eye P
H26.Ø4 Anterior subcapsular polar infantile and juvenile cataract
H26.Ø41 Anterior subcapsular polar infantile and juvenile cataract, right eye P
H26.Ø42 Anterior subcapsular polar infantile and juvenile cataract, left eye P
H26.Ø43 Anterior subcapsular polar infantile and juvenile cataract, bilateral P
H26.Ø49 Anterior subcapsular polar infantile and juvenile cataract, unspecified eye P
H26.Ø5 Posterior subcapsular polar infantile and juvenile cataract
H26.Ø51 Posterior subcapsular polar infantile and juvenile cataract, right eye P
H26.Ø52 Posterior subcapsular polar infantile and juvenile cataract, left eye P
H26.Ø53 Posterior subcapsular polar infantile and juvenile cataract, bilateral P
H26.Ø59 Posterior subcapsular polar infantile and juvenile cataract, unspecified eye P
H26.Ø6 Combined forms of infantile and juvenile cataract
H26.Ø61 Combined forms of infantile and juvenile cataract, right eye P
H26.Ø62 Combined forms of infantile and juvenile cataract, left eye P
H26.Ø63 Combined forms of infantile and juvenile cataract, bilateral P
H26.Ø69 Combined forms of infantile and juvenile cataract, unspecified eye P
H26.Ø9 Other infantile and juvenile cataract P

H26.1 Traumatic cataract
Use additional code (Chapter 2Ø) to identify external cause
H26.1Ø Unspecified traumatic cataract
H26.1Ø1 Unspecified traumatic cataract, right eye
H26.1Ø2 Unspecified traumatic cataract, left eye
H26.1Ø3 Unspecified traumatic cataract, bilateral
H26.1Ø9 Unspecified traumatic cataract, unspecified eye
H26.11 Localized traumatic opacities
H26.111 Localized traumatic opacities, right eye
H26.112 Localized traumatic opacities, left eye
H26.113 Localized traumatic opacities, bilateral
H26.119 Localized traumatic opacities, unspecified eye
H26.12 Partially resolved traumatic cataract
H26.121 Partially resolved traumatic cataract, right eye
H26.122 Partially resolved traumatic cataract, left eye
H26.123 Partially resolved traumatic cataract, bilateral
H26.129 Partially resolved traumatic cataract, unspecified eye
H26.13 Total traumatic cataract
H26.131 Total traumatic cataract, right eye
H26.132 Total traumatic cataract, left eye
H26.133 Total traumatic cataract, bilateral
H26.139 Total traumatic cataract, unspecified eye

H26.2 Complicated cataract
H26.2Ø Unspecified complicated cataract
Cataracta complicata NOS
H26.21 Cataract with neovascularization
Code also associated condition, such as:
chronic iridocyclitis (H2Ø.1-)
H26.211 Cataract with neovascularization, right eye
H26.212 Cataract with neovascularization, left eye
H26.213 Cataract with neovascularization, bilateral
H26.219 Cataract with neovascularization, unspecified eye
H26.22 Cataract secondary to ocular disorders (degenerative) (inflammatory)
Code also associated ocular disorder
H26.221 Cataract secondary to ocular disorders (degenerative) (inflammatory), right eye
H26.222 Cataract secondary to ocular disorders (degenerative) (inflammatory), left eye
H26.223 Cataract secondary to ocular disorders (degenerative) (inflammatory), bilateral
H26.229 Cataract secondary to ocular disorders (degenerative) (inflammatory), unspecified eye
H26.23 Glaucomatous flecks (subcapsular)
Code first underlying glaucoma (H4Ø-H42)
H26.231 Glaucomatous flecks (subcapsular), right eye
H26.232 Glaucomatous flecks (subcapsular), left eye
H26.233 Glaucomatous flecks (subcapsular), bilateral
H26.239 Glaucomatous flecks (subcapsular), unspecified eye

H26.3 Drug-induced cataract
Toxic cataract
Use additional code for adverse effect, if applicable, to identify drug (T36-T5Ø with fifth or sixth character 5)
H26.3Ø Drug-induced cataract, unspecified eye
H26.31 Drug-induced cataract, right eye
H26.32 Drug-induced cataract, left eye
H26.33 Drug-induced cataract, bilateral

H26.4 Secondary cataract

H26.40 Unspecified secondary cataract

H26.41 Soemmering's ring

H26.411 Soemmering's ring, right eye

H26.412 Soemmering's ring, left eye

H26.413 Soemmering's ring, bilateral

H26.419 Soemmering's ring, unspecified eye

H26.49 Other secondary cataract

AHA: 2018,2Q,14

H26.491 Other secondary cataract, right eye

H26.492 Other secondary cataract, left eye

H26.493 Other secondary cataract, bilateral

H26.499 Other secondary cataract, unspecified eye

H26.8 Other specified cataract

H26.9 Unspecified cataract

H27 Other disorders of lens

EXCLUDES 1 *congenital lens malformations (Q12.-)*
mechanical complications of intraocular lens implant (T85.2)
pseudophakia (Z96.1)

H27.Ø Aphakia

Acquired absence of lens
Acquired aphakia
Aphakia due to trauma

EXCLUDES 1 *cataract extraction status (Z98.4-)*
congenital absence of lens (Q12.3)
congenital aphakia (Q12.3)

H27.ØØ Aphakia, unspecified eye

H27.Ø1 Aphakia, right eye

H27.Ø2 Aphakia, left eye

H27.Ø3 Aphakia, bilateral

H27.1 Dislocation of lens

H27.1Ø Unspecified dislocation of lens

H27.11 Subluxation of lens

H27.111 Subluxation of lens, right eye

H27.112 Subluxation of lens, left eye

H27.113 Subluxation of lens, bilateral

H27.119 Subluxation of lens, unspecified eye

H27.12 Anterior dislocation of lens

H27.121 Anterior dislocation of lens, right eye

H27.122 Anterior dislocation of lens, left eye

H27.123 Anterior dislocation of lens, bilateral

H27.129 Anterior dislocation of lens, unspecified eye

H27.13 Posterior dislocation of lens

H27.131 Posterior dislocation of lens, right eye

H27.132 Posterior dislocation of lens, left eye

H27.133 Posterior dislocation of lens, bilateral

H27.139 Posterior dislocation of lens, unspecified eye

H27.8 Other specified disorders of lens

H27.9 Unspecified disorder of lens

H28 Cataract in diseases classified elsewhere

Code first underlying disease, such as:
hypoparathyroidism (E2Ø.-)
myotonia (G71.1-)
myxedema (EØ3.-)
protein-calorie malnutrition (E4Ø-E46)

EXCLUDES 1 *cataract in diabetes mellitus (EØ8.36, EØ9.36, E1Ø.36, E11.36, E13.36)*

Disorders of choroid and retina (H3Ø-H36)

H3Ø Chorioretinal inflammation

H3Ø.Ø Focal chorioretinal inflammation

Focal chorioretinitis
Focal choroiditis
Focal retinitis
Focal retinochoroiditis

H3Ø.ØØ Unspecified focal chorioretinal inflammation

Focal chorioretinitis NOS
Focal choroiditis NOS
Focal retinitis NOS
Focal retinochoroiditis NOS

H3Ø.ØØ1 Unspecified focal chorioretinal inflammation, right eye

H3Ø.ØØ2 Unspecified focal chorioretinal inflammation, left eye

H3Ø.ØØ3 Unspecified focal chorioretinal inflammation, bilateral

H3Ø.ØØ9 Unspecified focal chorioretinal inflammation, unspecified eye

H3Ø.Ø1 Focal chorioretinal inflammation, juxtapapillary

H3Ø.Ø11 Focal chorioretinal inflammation, juxtapapillary, right eye

H3Ø.Ø12 Focal chorioretinal inflammation, juxtapapillary, left eye

H3Ø.Ø13 Focal chorioretinal inflammation, juxtapapillary, bilateral

H3Ø.Ø19 Focal chorioretinal inflammation, juxtapapillary, unspecified eye

H3Ø.Ø2 Focal chorioretinal inflammation of posterior pole

H3Ø.Ø21 Focal chorioretinal inflammation of posterior pole, right eye

H3Ø.Ø22 Focal chorioretinal inflammation of posterior pole, left eye

H3Ø.Ø23 Focal chorioretinal inflammation of posterior pole, bilateral

H3Ø.Ø29 Focal chorioretinal inflammation of posterior pole, unspecified eye

H3Ø.Ø3 Focal chorioretinal inflammation, peripheral

H3Ø.Ø31 Focal chorioretinal inflammation, peripheral, right eye

H3Ø.Ø32 Focal chorioretinal inflammation, peripheral, left eye

H3Ø.Ø33 Focal chorioretinal inflammation, peripheral, bilateral

H3Ø.Ø39 Focal chorioretinal inflammation, peripheral, unspecified eye

H3Ø.Ø4 Focal chorioretinal inflammation, macular or paramacular

H3Ø.Ø41 Focal chorioretinal inflammation, macular or paramacular, right eye

H3Ø.Ø42 Focal chorioretinal inflammation, macular or paramacular, left eye

H3Ø.Ø43 Focal chorioretinal inflammation, macular or paramacular, bilateral

H3Ø.Ø49 Focal chorioretinal inflammation, macular or paramacular, unspecified eye

H3Ø.1 Disseminated chorioretinal inflammation

Disseminated chorioretinitis
Disseminated choroiditis
Disseminated retinitis
Disseminated retinochoroiditis

EXCLUDES 2 *exudative retinopathy (H35.Ø2-)*

H3Ø.1Ø Unspecified disseminated chorioretinal inflammation

Disseminated chorioretinitis NOS
Disseminated choroiditis NOS
Disseminated retinitis NOS
Disseminated retinochoroiditis NOS

H3Ø.1Ø1 Unspecified disseminated chorioretinal inflammation, right eye

H3Ø.1Ø2 Unspecified disseminated chorioretinal inflammation, left eye

H3Ø.1Ø3 Unspecified disseminated chorioretinal inflammation, bilateral

H3Ø.1Ø9 Unspecified disseminated chorioretinal inflammation, unspecified eye

H3Ø.11 Disseminated chorioretinal inflammation of posterior pole

H3Ø.111 Disseminated chorioretinal inflammation of posterior pole, right eye

H3Ø.112 Disseminated chorioretinal inflammation of posterior pole, left eye

H3Ø.113 Disseminated chorioretinal inflammation of posterior pole, bilateral

H3Ø.119 Disseminated chorioretinal inflammation of posterior pole, unspecified eye

H3Ø.12 Disseminated chorioretinal inflammation, peripheral

H3Ø.121 Disseminated chorioretinal inflammation, peripheral right eye

H3Ø.122 Disseminated chorioretinal inflammation, peripheral, left eye

H3Ø.123 Disseminated chorioretinal inflammation, peripheral, bilateral

H30.129 Disseminated chorioretinal inflammation, peripheral, unspecified eye

6th H30.13 Disseminated chorioretinal inflammation, generalized
- H30.131 Disseminated chorioretinal inflammation, generalized, right eye
- H30.132 Disseminated chorioretinal inflammation, generalized, left eye
- H30.133 Disseminated chorioretinal inflammation, generalized, bilateral
- H30.139 Disseminated chorioretinal inflammation, generalized, unspecified eye

6th H30.14 Acute posterior multifocal placoid pigment epitheliopathy
- H30.141 Acute posterior multifocal placoid pigment epitheliopathy, right eye
- H30.142 Acute posterior multifocal placoid pigment epitheliopathy, left eye
- H30.143 Acute posterior multifocal placoid pigment epitheliopathy, bilateral
- H30.149 Acute posterior multifocal placoid pigment epitheliopathy, unspecified eye

5th H30.2 Posterior cyclitis

Pars planitis
- H30.20 Posterior cyclitis, unspecified eye
- H30.21 Posterior cyclitis, right eye
- H30.22 Posterior cyclitis, left eye
- H30.23 Posterior cyclitis, bilateral

5th H30.8 Other chorioretinal inflammations

6th H30.81 Harada's disease
- H30.811 Harada's disease, right eye
- H30.812 Harada's disease, left eye
- H30.813 Harada's disease, bilateral
- H30.819 Harada's disease, unspecified eye

6th H30.89 Other chorioretinal inflammations
- H30.891 Other chorioretinal inflammations, right eye
- H30.892 Other chorioretinal inflammations, left eye
- H30.893 Other chorioretinal inflammations, bilateral
- H30.899 Other chorioretinal inflammations, unspecified eye

5th H30.9 Unspecified chorioretinal inflammation

Chorioretinitis NOS
Choroiditis NOS
Neuroretinitis NOS
Retinitis NOS
Retinochoroiditis NOS
- H30.90 Unspecified chorioretinal inflammation, unspecified eye
- H30.91 Unspecified chorioretinal inflammation, right eye
- H30.92 Unspecified chorioretinal inflammation, left eye
- H30.93 Unspecified chorioretinal inflammation, bilateral

4th H31 Other disorders of choroid

5th H31.0 Chorioretinal scars

EXCLUDES 2 *postsurgical chorioretinal scars (H59.81-)*

6th H31.00 Unspecified chorioretinal scars
- H31.001 Unspecified chorioretinal scars, right eye
- H31.002 Unspecified chorioretinal scars, left eye
- H31.003 Unspecified chorioretinal scars, bilateral
- H31.009 Unspecified chorioretinal scars, unspecified eye

6th H31.01 Macula scars of posterior pole (postinflammatory) (post-traumatic)

EXCLUDES 1 *postprocedural chorioentinal scar (H59.81-)*
- H31.011 Macula scars of posterior pole (postinflammatory) (post-traumatic), right eye
- H31.012 Macula scars of posterior pole (postinflammatory) (post-traumatic), left eye
- H31.013 Macula scars of posterior pole (postinflammatory) (post-traumatic), bilateral
- H31.019 Macula scars of posterior pole (postinflammatory) (post-traumatic), unspecified eye

6th H31.02 Solar retinopathy
- H31.021 Solar retinopathy, right eye
- H31.022 Solar retinopathy, left eye
- H31.023 Solar retinopathy, bilateral
- H31.029 Solar retinopathy, unspecified eye

6th H31.09 Other chorioretinal scars
- H31.091 Other chorioretinal scars, right eye
- H31.092 Other chorioretinal scars, left eye
- H31.093 Other chorioretinal scars, bilateral
- H31.099 Other chorioretinal scars, unspecified eye

5th H31.1 Choroidal degeneration

EXCLUDES 2 *angioid streaks of macula (H35.33)*

6th H31.10 Unspecified choroidal degeneration

Choroidal sclerosis NOS
- H31.101 Choroidal degeneration, unspecified, right eye
- H31.102 Choroidal degeneration, unspecified, left eye
- H31.103 Choroidal degeneration, unspecified, bilateral
- H31.109 Choroidal degeneration, unspecified, unspecified eye

6th H31.11 Age-related choroidal atrophy
- H31.111 Age-related choroidal atrophy, right eye A
- H31.112 Age-related choroidal atrophy, left eye A
- H31.113 Age-related choroidal atrophy, bilateral A
- H31.119 Age-related choroidal atrophy, unspecified eye A

6th H31.12 Diffuse secondary atrophy of choroid
- H31.121 Diffuse secondary atrophy of choroid, right eye
- H31.122 Diffuse secondary atrophy of choroid, left eye
- H31.123 Diffuse secondary atrophy of choroid, bilateral
- H31.129 Diffuse secondary atrophy of choroid, unspecified eye

5th H31.2 Hereditary choroidal dystrophy

EXCLUDES 2 *hyperornithinemia (E72.4)*
ornithinemia (E72.4)
- H31.20 Hereditary choroidal dystrophy, unspecified
- H31.21 Choroideremia
- H31.22 Choroidal dystrophy (central areolar) (generalized) (peripapillary)
- H31.23 Gyrate atrophy, choroid
- H31.29 Other hereditary choroidal dystrophy

5th H31.3 Choroidal hemorrhage and rupture

6th H31.30 Unspecified choroidal hemorrhage
- H31.301 Unspecified choroidal hemorrhage, right eye
- H31.302 Unspecified choroidal hemorrhage, left eye
- H31.303 Unspecified choroidal hemorrhage, bilateral
- H31.309 Unspecified choroidal hemorrhage, unspecified eye

6th H31.31 Expulsive choroidal hemorrhage
- H31.311 Expulsive choroidal hemorrhage, right eye
- H31.312 Expulsive choroidal hemorrhage, left eye
- H31.313 Expulsive choroidal hemorrhage, bilateral
- H31.319 Expulsive choroidal hemorrhage, unspecified eye

6th H31.32 Choroidal rupture
- H31.321 Choroidal rupture, right eye
- H31.322 Choroidal rupture, left eye
- H31.323 Choroidal rupture, bilateral
- H31.329 Choroidal rupture, unspecified eye

5th H31.4 Choroidal detachment

6th H31.40 Unspecified choroidal detachment
- H31.401 Unspecified choroidal detachment, right eye
- H31.402 Unspecified choroidal detachment, left eye

H31.403 Unspecified choroidal detachment, bilateral
H31.409 Unspecified choroidal detachment, unspecified eye

H31.41 Hemorrhagic choroidal detachment
H31.411 Hemorrhagic choroidal detachment, right eye
H31.412 Hemorrhagic choroidal detachment, left eye
H31.413 Hemorrhagic choroidal detachment, bilateral
H31.419 Hemorrhagic choroidal detachment, unspecified eye

H31.42 Serous choroidal detachment
H31.421 Serous choroidal detachment, right eye
H31.422 Serous choroidal detachment, left eye
H31.423 Serous choroidal detachment, bilateral
H31.429 Serous choroidal detachment, unspecified eye

H31.8 Other specified disorders of choroid
H31.9 Unspecified disorder of choroid

H32 Chorioretinal disorders in diseases classified elsewhere

Code first underlying disease, such as:
congenital toxoplasmosis (P37.1)
histoplasmosis (B39.-)
leprosy (A30.-)

EXCLUDES 1 *chorioretinitis (in):*
toxoplasmosis (acquired) (B58.01)
tuberculosis (A18.53)

H33 Retinal detachments and breaks

EXCLUDES 1 *detachment of retinal pigment epithelium (H35.72-, H35.73-)*

Retinal Detachment

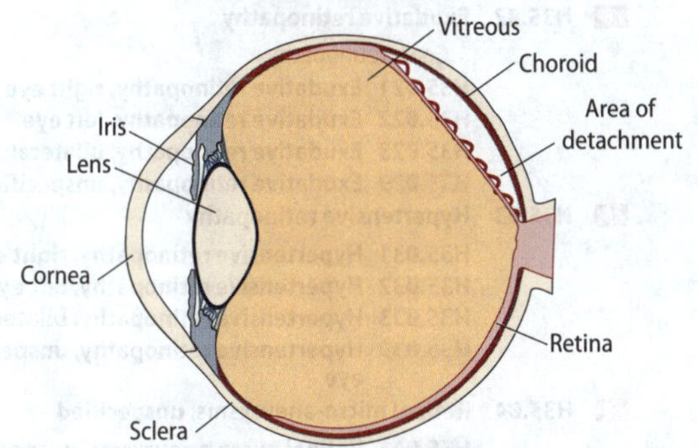

H33.0 Retinal detachment with retinal break
Rhegmatogenous retinal detachment
EXCLUDES 1 *serous retinal detachment (without retinal break) (H33.2-)*

H33.00 Unspecified retinal detachment with retinal break
H33.001 Unspecified retinal detachment with retinal break, right eye
H33.002 Unspecified retinal detachment with retinal break, left eye
H33.003 Unspecified retinal detachment with retinal break, bilateral
H33.009 Unspecified retinal detachment with retinal break, unspecified eye

H33.01 Retinal detachment with single break
H33.011 Retinal detachment with single break, right eye
H33.012 Retinal detachment with single break, left eye
H33.013 Retinal detachment with single break, bilateral
H33.019 Retinal detachment with single break, unspecified eye

H33.02 Retinal detachment with multiple breaks
H33.021 Retinal detachment with multiple breaks, right eye
H33.022 Retinal detachment with multiple breaks, left eye
H33.023 Retinal detachment with multiple breaks, bilateral
H33.029 Retinal detachment with multiple breaks, unspecified eye

H33.03 Retinal detachment with giant retinal tear
H33.031 Retinal detachment with giant retinal tear, right eye
H33.032 Retinal detachment with giant retinal tear, left eye
H33.033 Retinal detachment with giant retinal tear, bilateral
H33.039 Retinal detachment with giant retinal tear, unspecified eye

H33.04 Retinal detachment with retinal dialysis
H33.041 Retinal detachment with retinal dialysis, right eye
H33.042 Retinal detachment with retinal dialysis, left eye
H33.043 Retinal detachment with retinal dialysis, bilateral
H33.049 Retinal detachment with retinal dialysis, unspecified eye

H33.05 Total retinal detachment
H33.051 Total retinal detachment, right eye
H33.052 Total retinal detachment, left eye
H33.053 Total retinal detachment, bilateral
H33.059 Total retinal detachment, unspecified eye

H33.1 Retinoschisis and retinal cysts
EXCLUDES 1 *congenital retinoschisis (Q14.1)*
microcystoid degeneration of retina (H35.42-)

H33.10 Unspecified retinoschisis
H33.101 Unspecified retinoschisis, right eye
H33.102 Unspecified retinoschisis, left eye
H33.103 Unspecified retinoschisis, bilateral
H33.109 Unspecified retinoschisis, unspecified eye

H33.11 Cyst of ora serrata
H33.111 Cyst of ora serrata, right eye
H33.112 Cyst of ora serrata, left eye
H33.113 Cyst of ora serrata, bilateral
H33.119 Cyst of ora serrata, unspecified eye

H33.12 Parasitic cyst of retina
H33.121 Parasitic cyst of retina, right eye
H33.122 Parasitic cyst of retina, left eye
H33.123 Parasitic cyst of retina, bilateral
H33.129 Parasitic cyst of retina, unspecified eye

H33.19 Other retinoschisis and retinal cysts
Pseudocyst of retina
H33.191 Other retinoschisis and retinal cysts, right eye
H33.192 Other retinoschisis and retinal cysts, left eye
H33.193 Other retinoschisis and retinal cysts, bilateral
H33.199 Other retinoschisis and retinal cysts, unspecified eye

H33.2 Serous retinal detachment
Retinal detachment NOS
Retinal detachment without retinal break
EXCLUDES 1 *central serous chorioretinopathy (H35.71-)*

H33.20 Serous retinal detachment, unspecified eye
H33.21 Serous retinal detachment, right eye
H33.22 Serous retinal detachment, left eye
H33.23 Serous retinal detachment, bilateral

H33.3 Retinal breaks without detachment
EXCLUDES 1 *chorioretinal scars after surgery for detachment (H59.81-)*
peripheral retinal degeneration without break (H35.4-)

H33.30 Unspecified retinal break
H33.301 Unspecified retinal break, right eye
H33.302 Unspecified retinal break, left eye
H33.303 Unspecified retinal break, bilateral
H33.309 Unspecified retinal break, unspecified eye

H33.31 Horseshoe tear of retina without detachment
Operculum of retina without detachment
H33.311 Horseshoe tear of retina without detachment, right eye
H33.312 Horseshoe tear of retina without detachment, left eye

H33.313 Horseshoe tear of retina without detachment, bilateral

H33.319 Horseshoe tear of retina without detachment, unspecified eye

✓6th H33.32 Round hole of retina without detachment

H33.321 Round hole, right eye

H33.322 Round hole, left eye

H33.323 Round hole, bilateral

H33.329 Round hole, unspecified eye

✓6th H33.33 Multiple defects of retina without detachment

H33.331 Multiple defects of retina without detachment, right eye

H33.332 Multiple defects of retina without detachment, left eye

H33.333 Multiple defects of retina without detachment, bilateral

H33.339 Multiple defects of retina without detachment, unspecified eye

✓5th H33.4 Traction detachment of retina

Proliferative vitreo-retinopathy with retinal detachment

H33.4Ø Traction detachment of retina, unspecified eye

H33.41 Traction detachment of retina, right eye

H33.42 Traction detachment of retina, left eye

H33.43 Traction detachment of retina, bilateral

H33.8 Other retinal detachments

✓4th H34 Retinal vascular occlusions

EXCLUDES 1 *amaurosis fugax (G45.3)*

✓5th H34.Ø Transient retinal artery occlusion

H34.ØØ Transient retinal artery occlusion, unspecified eye

H34.Ø1 Transient retinal artery occlusion, right eye

H34.Ø2 Transient retinal artery occlusion, left eye

H34.Ø3 Transient retinal artery occlusion, bilateral

✓5th H34.1 Central retinal artery occlusion

H34.1Ø Central retinal artery occlusion, unspecified eye

H34.11 Central retinal artery occlusion, right eye

H34.12 Central retinal artery occlusion, left eye

H34.13 Central retinal artery occlusion, bilateral

✓5th H34.2 Other retinal artery occlusions

✓6th H34.21 Partial retinal artery occlusion

Hollenhorst's plaque

Retinal microembolism

H34.211 Partial retinal artery occlusion, right eye

H34.212 Partial retinal artery occlusion, left eye

H34.213 Partial retinal artery occlusion, bilateral

H34.219 Partial retinal artery occlusion, unspecified eye

✓6th H34.23 Retinal artery branch occlusion

H34.231 Retinal artery branch occlusion, right eye

H34.232 Retinal artery branch occlusion, left eye

H34.233 Retinal artery branch occlusion, bilateral

H34.239 Retinal artery branch occlusion, unspecified eye

✓5th H34.8 Other retinal vascular occlusions

AHA: 2016,4Q,19

✓6th H34.81 Central retinal vein occlusion

One of the following 7th characters is to be assigned to codes in subcategory H34.81 to designate the severity of the occlusion:
Ø with macular edema
1 with retinal neovascularization
2 stable
old central retinal vein occlusion

✓7th H34.811 Central retinal vein occlusion, right eye

✓7th H34.812 Central retinal vein occlusion, left eye

✓7th H34.813 Central retinal vein occlusion, bilateral

✓7th H34.819 Central retinal vein occlusion, unspecified eye

✓6th H34.82 Venous engorgement

Incipient retinal vein occlusion

Partial retinal vein occlusion

H34.821 Venous engorgement, right eye

H34.822 Venous engorgement, left eye

H34.823 Venous engorgement, bilateral

H34.829 Venous engorgement, unspecified eye

✓6th H34.83 Tributary (branch) retinal vein occlusion

One of the following 7th characters is to be assigned to codes in subcategory H34.83 to designate the severity of the occlusion:
Ø with macular edema
1 with retinal neovascularization
2 stable
old tributary (branch) retinal vein occlusion

✓7th H34.831 Tributary (branch) retinal vein occlusion, right eye

✓7th H34.832 Tributary (branch) retinal vein occlusion, left eye

✓7th H34.833 Tributary (branch) retinal vein occlusion, bilateral

✓7th H34.839 Tributary (branch) retinal vein occlusion, unspecified eye

H34.9 Unspecified retinal vascular occlusion

✓4th H35 Other retinal disorders

EXCLUDES 2 *diabetic retinal disorders (EØ8.311-EØ8.359, EØ9.311-EØ9.359, E1Ø.311-E1Ø.359, E11.311-E11.359, E13.311-E13.359)*

✓5th H35.Ø Background retinopathy and retinal vascular changes

Code also any associated hypertension (I1Ø)

H35.ØØ Unspecified background retinopathy

✓6th H35.Ø1 Changes in retinal vascular appearance

Retinal vascular sheathing

H35.Ø11 Changes in retinal vascular appearance, right eye

H35.Ø12 Changes in retinal vascular appearance, left eye

H35.Ø13 Changes in retinal vascular appearance, bilateral

H35.Ø19 Changes in retinal vascular appearance, unspecified eye

✓6th H35.Ø2 Exudative retinopathy

Coats retinopathy

H35.Ø21 Exudative retinopathy, right eye

H35.Ø22 Exudative retinopathy, left eye

H35.Ø23 Exudative retinopathy, bilateral

H35.Ø29 Exudative retinopathy, unspecified eye

✓6th H35.Ø3 Hypertensive retinopathy

H35.Ø31 Hypertensive retinopathy, right eye

H35.Ø32 Hypertensive retinopathy, left eye

H35.Ø33 Hypertensive retinopathy, bilateral

H35.Ø39 Hypertensive retinopathy, unspecified eye

✓6th H35.Ø4 Retinal micro-aneurysms, unspecified

H35.Ø41 Retinal micro-aneurysms, unspecified, right eye

H35.Ø42 Retinal micro-aneurysms, unspecified, left eye

H35.Ø43 Retinal micro-aneurysms, unspecified, bilateral

H35.Ø49 Retinal micro-aneurysms, unspecified, unspecified eye

✓6th H35.Ø5 Retinal neovascularization, unspecified

H35.Ø51 Retinal neovascularization, unspecified, right eye

H35.Ø52 Retinal neovascularization, unspecified, left eye

H35.Ø53 Retinal neovascularization, unspecified, bilateral

H35.Ø59 Retinal neovascularization, unspecified, unspecified eye

✓6th H35.Ø6 Retinal vasculitis

Eales disease

Retinal perivasculitis

DEF: Sight-threatening intraocular inflammation of the retinal blood vessels that causes minimal, partial, or even complete blindness.

H35.Ø61 Retinal vasculitis, right eye

H35.Ø62 Retinal vasculitis, left eye

H35.Ø63 Retinal vasculitis, bilateral

H35.Ø69 Retinal vasculitis, unspecified eye

✓6th H35.Ø7 Retinal telangiectasis

H35.Ø71 Retinal telangiectasis, right eye

H35.Ø72 Retinal telangiectasis, left eye

H35.Ø73 Retinal telangiectasis, bilateral

H35.Ø79 Retinal telangiectasis, unspecified eye

H35.Ø9 **Other intraretinal microvascular abnormalities**
Retinal varices

H35.1 **Retinopathy of prematurity**

H35.1Ø **Retinopathy of prematurity, unspecified**
Retinopathy of prematurity NOS

H35.1Ø1 **Retinopathy of prematurity, unspecified, right eye**
H35.1Ø2 **Retinopathy of prematurity, unspecified, left eye**
H35.1Ø3 **Retinopathy of prematurity, unspecified, bilateral**
H35.1Ø9 **Retinopathy of prematurity, unspecified, unspecified eye**

H35.11 **Retinopathy of prematurity, stage Ø**
H35.111 **Retinopathy of prematurity, stage Ø, right eye**
H35.112 **Retinopathy of prematurity, stage Ø, left eye**
H35.113 **Retinopathy of prematurity, stage Ø, bilateral**
H35.119 **Retinopathy of prematurity, stage Ø, unspecified eye**

H35.12 **Retinopathy of prematurity, stage 1**
H35.121 **Retinopathy of prematurity, stage 1, right eye**
H35.122 **Retinopathy of prematurity, stage 1, left eye**
H35.123 **Retinopathy of prematurity, stage 1, bilateral**
H35.129 **Retinopathy of prematurity, stage 1, unspecified eye**

H35.13 **Retinopathy of prematurity, stage 2**
H35.131 **Retinopathy of prematurity, stage 2, right eye**
H35.132 **Retinopathy of prematurity, stage 2, left eye**
H35.133 **Retinopathy of prematurity, stage 2, bilateral**
H35.139 **Retinopathy of prematurity, stage 2, unspecified eye**

H35.14 **Retinopathy of prematurity, stage 3**
H35.141 **Retinopathy of prematurity, stage 3, right eye**
H35.142 **Retinopathy of prematurity, stage 3, left eye**
H35.143 **Retinopathy of prematurity, stage 3, bilateral**
H35.149 **Retinopathy of prematurity, stage 3, unspecified eye**

H35.15 **Retinopathy of prematurity, stage 4**
H35.151 **Retinopathy of prematurity, stage 4, right eye**
H35.152 **Retinopathy of prematurity, stage 4, left eye**
H35.153 **Retinopathy of prematurity, stage 4, bilateral**
H35.159 **Retinopathy of prematurity, stage 4, unspecified eye**

H35.16 **Retinopathy of prematurity, stage 5**
H35.161 **Retinopathy of prematurity, stage 5, right eye**
H35.162 **Retinopathy of prematurity, stage 5, left eye**
H35.163 **Retinopathy of prematurity, stage 5, bilateral**
H35.169 **Retinopathy of prematurity, stage 5, unspecified eye**

H35.17 **Retrolental fibroplasia**
H35.171 **Retrolental fibroplasia, right eye**
H35.172 **Retrolental fibroplasia, left eye**
H35.173 **Retrolental fibroplasia, bilateral**
H35.179 **Retrolental fibroplasia, unspecified eye**

H35.2 **Other non-diabetic proliferative retinopathy**
Proliferative vitreo-retinopathy
EXCLUDES 1 *proliferative vitreo-retinopathy with retinal detachment (H33.4-)*

H35.2Ø **Other non-diabetic proliferative retinopathy, unspecified eye**
H35.21 **Other non-diabetic proliferative retinopathy, right eye**
H35.22 **Other non-diabetic proliferative retinopathy, left eye**
H35.23 **Other non-diabetic proliferative retinopathy, bilateral**

H35.3 **Degeneration of macula and posterior pole**

H35.3Ø **Unspecified macular degeneration** A
Age-related macular degeneration

H35.31 **Nonexudative age-related macular degeneration**
Atrophic age-related macular degeneration
Dry age-related macular degeneration
AHA: 2016,4Q,20-21

One of the following 7th characters is to be assigned to each code in subcategory H35.31 to designate the stage of the disease:
Ø stage unspecified
1 early dry stage
2 intermediate dry stage
3 advanced atrophic without subfoveal involvement
advanced dry stage
4 advanced atrophic with subfoveal involvement

H35.311 **Nonexudative age-related macular degeneration, right eye** A
H35.312 **Nonexudative age-related macular degeneration, left eye** A
H35.313 **Nonexudative age-related macular degeneration, bilateral** A
H35.319 **Nonexudative age-related macular degeneration, unspecified eye** A

H35.32 **Exudative age-related macular degeneration**
Wet age-related macular degeneration
AHA: 2016,4Q,20-21

One of the following 7th characters is to be assigned to each code in subcategory H35.32 to designate the stage of the disease:
Ø stage unspecified
1 with active choroidal neovascularization
2 with inactive choroidal neovascularization
with involuted or regressed neovascularization
3 with inactive scar

H35.321 **Exudative age-related macular degeneration, right eye** HCC ESR COM A
H35.322 **Exudative age-related macular degeneration, left eye** HCC ESR COM A
H35.323 **Exudative age-related macular degeneration, bilateral** HCC ESR COM A
H35.329 **Exudative age-related macular degeneration, unspecified eye** HCC ESR COM A

H35.33 **Angioid streaks of macula**
DEF: Degeneration of the choroid, characterized by broad, irregular, dark brown streaks radiating from the optic disc; occurs with pseudoxanthoma elasticum or Paget's disease.

H35.34 **Macular cyst, hole, or pseudohole**
H35.341 **Macular cyst, hole, or pseudohole, right eye**
H35.342 **Macular cyst, hole, or pseudohole, left eye**
H35.343 **Macular cyst, hole, or pseudohole, bilateral**
H35.349 **Macular cyst, hole, or pseudohole, unspecified eye**

H35.35 **Cystoid macular degeneration**
EXCLUDES 1 *cystoid macular edema following cataract surgery (H59.Ø3-)*
H35.351 **Cystoid macular degeneration, right eye**
H35.352 **Cystoid macular degeneration, left eye**
H35.353 **Cystoid macular degeneration, bilateral**
H35.359 **Cystoid macular degeneration, unspecified eye**

H35.36 **Drusen (degenerative) of macula**
AHA: 2017,1Q,51; 2016,4Q,21
H35.361 **Drusen (degenerative) of macula, right eye**
H35.362 **Drusen (degenerative) of macula, left eye**
H35.363 **Drusen (degenerative) of macula, bilateral**

H35.369 Drusen (degenerative) of macula, unspecified eye

H35.37 Puckering of macula

H35.371 Puckering of macula, right eye
H35.372 Puckering of macula, left eye
H35.373 Puckering of macula, bilateral
H35.379 Puckering of macula, unspecified eye

H35.38 Toxic maculopathy

Code first poisoning due to drug or toxin, if applicable (T36-T65 with fifth or sixth character 1-4 or 6)

Use additional code for adverse effect, if applicable, to identify drug (T36-T5Ø with fifth or sixth character 5)

H35.381 Toxic maculopathy, right eye
H35.382 Toxic maculopathy, left eye
H35.383 Toxic maculopathy, bilateral
H35.389 Toxic maculopathy, unspecified eye

H35.4 Peripheral retinal degeneration

EXCLUDES 1 *hereditary retinal degeneration (dystrophy) (H35.5-)*
peripheral retinal degeneration with retinal break (H33.3-)

H35.4Ø Unspecified peripheral retinal degeneration

H35.41 Lattice degeneration of retina

Palisade degeneration of retina

DEF: Degeneration of the retina, often bilateral, that is usually benign. It is characterized by lines intersecting at irregular intervals in the peripheral retina. Retinal thinning and retinal holes may occur.

H35.411 Lattice degeneration of retina, right eye
H35.412 Lattice degeneration of retina, left eye
H35.413 Lattice degeneration of retina, bilateral
H35.419 Lattice degeneration of retina, unspecified eye

H35.42 Microcystoid degeneration of retina

H35.421 Microcystoid degeneration of retina, right eye
H35.422 Microcystoid degeneration of retina, left eye
H35.423 Microcystoid degeneration of retina, bilateral
H35.429 Microcystoid degeneration of retina, unspecified eye

H35.43 Paving stone degeneration of retina

H35.431 Paving stone degeneration of retina, right eye
H35.432 Paving stone degeneration of retina, left eye
H35.433 Paving stone degeneration of retina, bilateral
H35.439 Paving stone degeneration of retina, unspecified eye

H35.44 Age-related reticular degeneration of retina

H35.441 Age-related reticular degeneration of retina, right eye A
H35.442 Age-related reticular degeneration of retina, left eye A
H35.443 Age-related reticular degeneration of retina, bilateral A
H35.449 Age-related reticular degeneration of retina, unspecified eye A

H35.45 Secondary pigmentary degeneration

H35.451 Secondary pigmentary degeneration, right eye
H35.452 Secondary pigmentary degeneration, left eye
H35.453 Secondary pigmentary degeneration, bilateral
H35.459 Secondary pigmentary degeneration, unspecified eye

H35.46 Secondary vitreoretinal degeneration

H35.461 Secondary vitreoretinal degeneration, right eye
H35.462 Secondary vitreoretinal degeneration, left eye
H35.463 Secondary vitreoretinal degeneration, bilateral
H35.469 Secondary vitreoretinal degeneration, unspecified eye

H35.5 Hereditary retinal dystrophy

EXCLUDES 1 *dystrophies primarily involving Bruch's membrane (H31.1-)*

H35.5Ø Unspecified hereditary retinal dystrophy
H35.51 Vitreoretinal dystrophy
H35.52 Pigmentary retinal dystrophy

Albipunctate retinal dystrophy
Retinitis pigmentosa
Tapetoretinal dystrophy

H35.53 Other dystrophies primarily involving the sensory retina

Stargardt's disease

H35.54 Dystrophies primarily involving the retinal pigment epithelium

Vitelliform retinal dystrophy

H35.6 Retinal hemorrhage

H35.6Ø Retinal hemorrhage, unspecified eye
H35.61 Retinal hemorrhage, right eye
H35.62 Retinal hemorrhage, left eye
H35.63 Retinal hemorrhage, bilateral

H35.7 Separation of retinal layers

EXCLUDES 1 *retinal detachment (serous) (H33.2-)*
rhegmatogenous retinal detachment (H33.Ø-)

H35.7Ø Unspecified separation of retinal layers

H35.71 Central serous chorioretinopathy

H35.711 Central serous chorioretinopathy, right eye
H35.712 Central serous chorioretinopathy, left eye
H35.713 Central serous chorioretinopathy, bilateral
H35.719 Central serous chorioretinopathy, unspecified eye

H35.72 Serous detachment of retinal pigment epithelium

H35.721 Serous detachment of retinal pigment epithelium, right eye
H35.722 Serous detachment of retinal pigment epithelium, left eye
H35.723 Serous detachment of retinal pigment epithelium, bilateral
H35.729 Serous detachment of retinal pigment epithelium, unspecified eye

H35.73 Hemorrhagic detachment of retinal pigment epithelium

H35.731 Hemorrhagic detachment of retinal pigment epithelium, right eye
H35.732 Hemorrhagic detachment of retinal pigment epithelium, left eye
H35.733 Hemorrhagic detachment of retinal pigment epithelium, bilateral
H35.739 Hemorrhagic detachment of retinal pigment epithelium, unspecified eye

H35.8 Other specified retinal disorders

EXCLUDES 2 *retinal hemorrhage (H35.6-)*

H35.81 Retinal edema

Retinal cotton wool spots

H35.82 Retinal ischemia
H35.89 Other specified retinal disorders

H35.9 Unspecified retinal disorder

H36 Retinal disorders in diseases classified elsewhere

Code first underlying disease, such as:
lipid storage disorders (E75.-)
sickle-cell disorders (D57.-)

EXCLUDES 1 *arteriosclerotic retinopathy (H35.Ø-)*
diabetic retinopathy (EØ8.3-, EØ9.3-, E1Ø.3-, E11.3-, E13.3-)

Glaucoma (H40-H42)

H40 Glaucoma

EXCLUDES 1 *absolute glaucoma (H44.51-)*
congenital glaucoma (Q15.0)
traumatic glaucoma due to birth injury (P15.3)

Open Angle/Angle Closure Glaucoma

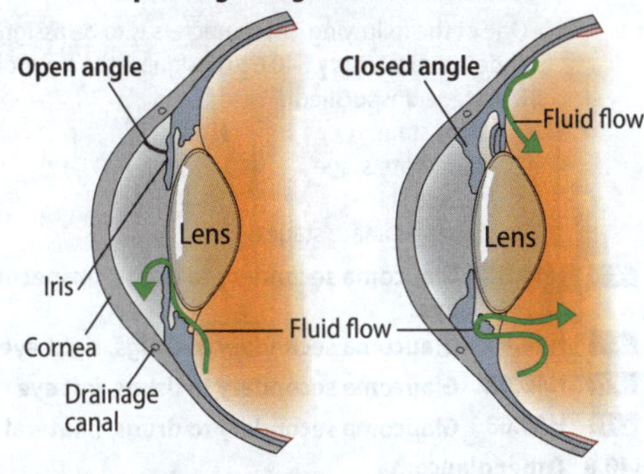

H40.0 Glaucoma suspect

H40.00 Preglaucoma, unspecified
- **H40.001 Preglaucoma, unspecified, right eye**
- **H40.002 Preglaucoma, unspecified, left eye**
- **H40.003 Preglaucoma, unspecified, bilateral**
- **H40.009 Preglaucoma, unspecified, unspecified eye**

H40.01 Open angle with borderline findings, low risk
Open angle, low risk
- **H40.011 Open angle with borderline findings, low risk, right eye**
- **H40.012 Open angle with borderline findings, low risk, left eye**
- **H40.013 Open angle with borderline findings, low risk, bilateral**
- **H40.019 Open angle with borderline findings, low risk, unspecified eye**

H40.02 Open angle with borderline findings, high risk
Open angle, high risk
- **H40.021 Open angle with borderline findings, high risk, right eye**
- **H40.022 Open angle with borderline findings, high risk, left eye**
- **H40.023 Open angle with borderline findings, high risk, bilateral**
- **H40.029 Open angle with borderline findings, high risk, unspecified eye**

H40.03 Anatomical narrow angle
Primary angle closure suspect
- **H40.031 Anatomical narrow angle, right eye**
- **H40.032 Anatomical narrow angle, left eye**
- **H40.033 Anatomical narrow angle, bilateral**
- **H40.039 Anatomical narrow angle, unspecified eye**

H40.04 Steroid responder
- **H40.041 Steroid responder, right eye**
- **H40.042 Steroid responder, left eye**
- **H40.043 Steroid responder, bilateral**
- **H40.049 Steroid responder, unspecified eye**

H40.05 Ocular hypertension
- **H40.051 Ocular hypertension, right eye**
- **H40.052 Ocular hypertension, left eye**
- **H40.053 Ocular hypertension, bilateral**
- **H40.059 Ocular hypertension, unspecified eye**

H40.06 Primary angle closure without glaucoma damage
- **H40.061 Primary angle closure without glaucoma damage, right eye**
- **H40.062 Primary angle closure without glaucoma damage, left eye**
- **H40.063 Primary angle closure without glaucoma damage, bilateral**
- **H40.069 Primary angle closure without glaucoma damage, unspecified eye**

H40.1 Open-angle glaucoma

One of the following 7th characters is to be assigned to each code in subcategories H40.10, H40.11, H40.12, H40.13, and H40.14 to designate the stage of glaucoma.
- 0 stage unspecified
- 1 mild stage
- 2 moderate stage
- 3 severe stage
- 4 indeterminate stage

H40.10 Unspecified open-angle glaucoma Rx
TIP: Only one code from this subcategory should be assigned when both left and right eyes are the same stage.

H40.11 Primary open-angle glaucoma
Chronic simple glaucoma
AHA: 2016,4Q,22
- **H40.111 Primary open-angle glaucoma, right eye** Rx Q
- **H40.112 Primary open-angle glaucoma, left eye** Rx Q
- **H40.113 Primary open-angle glaucoma, bilateral** Rx Q
- **H40.119 Primary open-angle glaucoma, unspecified eye** Rx

H40.12 Low-tension glaucoma
- **H40.121 Low-tension glaucoma, right eye** Rx Q
- **H40.122 Low-tension glaucoma, left eye** Rx Q
- **H40.123 Low-tension glaucoma, bilateral** Rx Q
- **H40.129 Low-tension glaucoma, unspecified eye** Rx

H40.13 Pigmentary glaucoma
- **H40.131 Pigmentary glaucoma, right eye** Rx
- **H40.132 Pigmentary glaucoma, left eye** Rx
- **H40.133 Pigmentary glaucoma, bilateral** Rx
- **H40.139 Pigmentary glaucoma, unspecified eye** Rx

H40.14 Capsular glaucoma with pseudoexfoliation of lens
- **H40.141 Capsular glaucoma with pseudoexfoliation of lens, right eye** Rx
- **H40.142 Capsular glaucoma with pseudoexfoliation of lens, left eye** Rx
- **H40.143 Capsular glaucoma with pseudoexfoliation of lens, bilateral** Rx
- **H40.149 Capsular glaucoma with pseudoexfoliation of lens, unspecified eye** Rx

H40.15 Residual stage of open-angle glaucoma
- **H40.151 Residual stage of open-angle glaucoma, right eye** Rx Q
- **H40.152 Residual stage of open-angle glaucoma, left eye** Rx Q
- **H40.153 Residual stage of open-angle glaucoma, bilateral** Rx Q
- **H40.159 Residual stage of open-angle glaucoma, unspecified eye** Rx

H40.2 Primary angle-closure glaucoma

EXCLUDES 1 *aqueous misdirection (H40.83-)*
malignant glaucoma (H40.83-)

One of the following 7th characters is to be assigned to code H40.20 and H40.22 to designate the stage of glaucoma.
- 0 stage unspecified
- 1 mild stage
- 2 moderate stage
- 3 severe stage
- 4 indeterminate stage

H40.20 Unspecified primary angle-closure glaucoma Rx
TIP: Only one code from this subcategory should be assigned when both left and right eyes are the same stage.

H40.21 Acute angle-closure glaucoma
Acute angle-closure glaucoma attack
Acute angle-closure glaucoma crisis
- **H40.211 Acute angle-closure glaucoma, right eye**
- **H40.212 Acute angle-closure glaucoma, left eye**

H40.213 Acute angle-closure glaucoma, bilateral
H40.219 Acute angle-closure glaucoma, unspecified eye

H40.22 Chronic angle-closure glaucoma
Chronic primary angle closure glaucoma
H40.221 Chronic angle-closure glaucoma, right eye Rx
H40.222 Chronic angle-closure glaucoma, left eye Rx
H40.223 Chronic angle-closure glaucoma, bilateral Rx
H40.229 Chronic angle-closure glaucoma, unspecified eye Rx

H40.23 Intermittent angle-closure glaucoma
H40.231 Intermittent angle-closure glaucoma, right eye Rx
H40.232 Intermittent angle-closure glaucoma, left eye Rx
H40.233 Intermittent angle-closure glaucoma, bilateral Rx
H40.239 Intermittent angle-closure glaucoma, unspecified eye Rx

H40.24 Residual stage of angle-closure glaucoma
H40.241 Residual stage of angle-closure glaucoma, right eye Rx
H40.242 Residual stage of angle-closure glaucoma, left eye Rx
H40.243 Residual stage of angle-closure glaucoma, bilateral Rx
H40.249 Residual stage of angle-closure glaucoma, unspecified eye Rx

H40.3 Glaucoma secondary to eye trauma
Code also underlying condition

One of the following 7th characters is to be assigned to each code in subcategory H40.3 to designate the stage of glaucoma.
- 0 stage unspecified
- 1 mild stage
- 2 moderate stage
- 3 severe stage
- 4 indeterminate stage

H40.30 Glaucoma secondary to eye trauma, unspecified eye Rx
H40.31 Glaucoma secondary to eye trauma, right eye Rx
H40.32 Glaucoma secondary to eye trauma, left eye Rx
H40.33 Glaucoma secondary to eye trauma, bilateral Rx

H40.4 Glaucoma secondary to eye inflammation
Code also underlying condition

One of the following 7th characters is to be assigned to each code in subcategory H40.4 to designate the stage of glaucoma.
- 0 stage unspecified
- 1 mild stage
- 2 moderate stage
- 3 severe stage
- 4 indeterminate stage

H40.40 Glaucoma secondary to eye inflammation, unspecified eye Rx
H40.41 Glaucoma secondary to eye inflammation, right eye Rx
H40.42 Glaucoma secondary to eye inflammation, left eye Rx
H40.43 Glaucoma secondary to eye inflammation, bilateral Rx

H40.5 Glaucoma secondary to other eye disorders
Code also underlying eye disorder

One of the following 7th characters is to be assigned to each code in subcategory H40.5 to designate the stage of glaucoma.
- 0 stage unspecified
- 1 mild stage
- 2 moderate stage
- 3 severe stage
- 4 indeterminate stage

H40.50 Glaucoma secondary to other eye disorders, unspecified eye Rx
H40.51 Glaucoma secondary to other eye disorders, right eye Rx
H40.52 Glaucoma secondary to other eye disorders, left eye Rx
H40.53 Glaucoma secondary to other eye disorders, bilateral Rx

H40.6 Glaucoma secondary to drugs
Use additional code for adverse effect, if applicable, to identify drug (T36-T50 with fifth or sixth character 5)

One of the following 7th characters is to be assigned to each code in subcategory H40.6 to designate the stage of glaucoma
- 0 stage unspecified
- 1 mild stage
- 2 moderate stage
- 3 severe stage
- 4 indeterminate stage

H40.60 Glaucoma secondary to drugs, unspecified eye Rx
H40.61 Glaucoma secondary to drugs, right eye Rx
H40.62 Glaucoma secondary to drugs, left eye Rx
H40.63 Glaucoma secondary to drugs, bilateral Rx

H40.8 Other glaucoma

H40.81 Glaucoma with increased episcleral venous pressure
H40.811 Glaucoma with increased episcleral venous pressure, right eye Rx
H40.812 Glaucoma with increased episcleral venous pressure, left eye Rx
H40.813 Glaucoma with increased episcleral venous pressure, bilateral Rx
H40.819 Glaucoma with increased episcleral venous pressure, unspecified eye Rx

H40.82 Hypersecretion glaucoma
H40.821 Hypersecretion glaucoma, right eye Rx
H40.822 Hypersecretion glaucoma, left eye Rx
H40.823 Hypersecretion glaucoma, bilateral Rx
H40.829 Hypersecretion glaucoma, unspecified eye Rx

H40.83 Aqueous misdirection
Malignant glaucoma
H40.831 Aqueous misdirection, right eye Rx
H40.832 Aqueous misdirection, left eye Rx
H40.833 Aqueous misdirection, bilateral Rx
H40.839 Aqueous misdirection, unspecified eye Rx

H40.89 Other specified glaucoma Rx

H40.9 Unspecified glaucoma Rx

H42 Glaucoma in diseases classified elsewhere Rx
Code first underlying condition, such as:
- amyloidosis (E85.-)
- aniridia (Q13.1)
- glaucoma (in) diabetes mellitus (E08.39, E09.39, E10.39, E11.39, E13.39)
- Lowe's syndrome (E72.03)
- Reiger's anomaly (Q13.81)
- specified metabolic disorder (E70-E88)

EXCLUDES 1 *glaucoma (in) onchocerciasis (B73.02)*
glaucoma (in) syphilis (A52.71)
glaucoma (in) tuberculous (A18.59)

Disorders of vitreous body and globe (H43-H44)

H43 Disorders of vitreous body

H43.0 Vitreous prolapse
EXCLUDES 1 *traumatic vitreous prolapse (S05.2-)*
vitreous syndrome following cataract surgery (H59.0-)
H43.00 Vitreous prolapse, unspecified eye
H43.01 Vitreous prolapse, right eye
H43.02 Vitreous prolapse, left eye
H43.03 Vitreous prolapse, bilateral

H43.1 Vitreous hemorrhage
H43.10 Vitreous hemorrhage, unspecified eye HCC ESR
H43.11 Vitreous hemorrhage, right eye HCC ESR
H43.12 Vitreous hemorrhage, left eye HCC ESR

H43.13 Vitreous hemorrhage, bilateral HCC ESR

H43.2 Crystalline deposits in vitreous body

H43.20 Crystalline deposits in vitreous body, unspecified eye

H43.21 Crystalline deposits in vitreous body, right eye

H43.22 Crystalline deposits in vitreous body, left eye

H43.23 Crystalline deposits in vitreous body, bilateral

H43.3 Other vitreous opacities

H43.31 Vitreous membranes and strands

H43.311 Vitreous membranes and strands, right eye

H43.312 Vitreous membranes and strands, left eye

H43.313 Vitreous membranes and strands, bilateral

H43.319 Vitreous membranes and strands, unspecified eye

H43.39 Other vitreous opacities

Vitreous floaters

H43.391 Other vitreous opacities, right eye

H43.392 Other vitreous opacities, left eye

H43.393 Other vitreous opacities, bilateral

H43.399 Other vitreous opacities, unspecified eye

H43.8 Other disorders of vitreous body

EXCLUDES 1 *proliferative vitreo-retinopathy with retinal detachment (H33.4-)*

EXCLUDES 2 *vitreous abscess (H44.Ø2-)*

H43.81 Vitreous degeneration

Vitreous detachment

H43.811 Vitreous degeneration, right eye

H43.812 Vitreous degeneration, left eye

H43.813 Vitreous degeneration, bilateral

H43.819 Vitreous degeneration, unspecified eye

H43.82 Vitreomacular adhesion

Vitreomacular traction

H43.821 Vitreomacular adhesion, right eye A

H43.822 Vitreomacular adhesion, left eye A

H43.823 Vitreomacular adhesion, bilateral A

H43.829 Vitreomacular adhesion, unspecified eye A

H43.89 Other disorders of vitreous body

H43.9 Unspecified disorder of vitreous body

H44 Disorders of globe

INCLUDES disorders affecting multiple structures of eye

H44.Ø Purulent endophthalmitis

Use additional code to identify organism

EXCLUDES 1 *bleb associated endophthalmitis (H59.4-)*

H44.ØØ Unspecified purulent endophthalmitis

H44.ØØ1 Unspecified purulent endophthalmitis, right eye

H44.ØØ2 Unspecified purulent endophthalmitis, left eye

H44.ØØ3 Unspecified purulent endophthalmitis, bilateral

H44.ØØ9 Unspecified purulent endophthalmitis, unspecified eye

H44.Ø1 Panophthalmitis (acute)

H44.Ø11 Panophthalmitis (acute), right eye

H44.Ø12 Panophthalmitis (acute), left eye

H44.Ø13 Panophthalmitis (acute), bilateral

H44.Ø19 Panophthalmitis (acute), unspecified eye

H44.Ø2 Vitreous abscess (chronic)

H44.Ø21 Vitreous abscess (chronic), right eye

H44.Ø22 Vitreous abscess (chronic), left eye

H44.Ø23 Vitreous abscess (chronic), bilateral

H44.Ø29 Vitreous abscess (chronic), unspecified eye

H44.1 Other endophthalmitis

EXCLUDES 1 *bleb associated endophthalmitis (H59.4-)*

EXCLUDES 2 *ophthalmia nodosa (H16.2-)*

H44.11 Panuveitis

DEF: Inflammation of all layers of the uvea of the eye, including the choroid, iris, and ciliary body. It also typically involves the lens, retina, optic nerve, and vitreous and causes reduced vision or blindness.

H44.111 Panuveitis, right eye

H44.112 Panuveitis, left eye

H44.113 Panuveitis, bilateral

H44.119 Panuveitis, unspecified eye

H44.12 Parasitic endophthalmitis, unspecified

H44.121 Parasitic endophthalmitis, unspecified, right eye

H44.122 Parasitic endophthalmitis, unspecified, left eye

H44.123 Parasitic endophthalmitis, unspecified, bilateral

H44.129 Parasitic endophthalmitis, unspecified, unspecified eye

H44.13 Sympathetic uveitis

H44.131 Sympathetic uveitis, right eye

H44.132 Sympathetic uveitis, left eye

H44.133 Sympathetic uveitis, bilateral

H44.139 Sympathetic uveitis, unspecified eye

H44.19 Other endophthalmitis

H44.2 Degenerative myopia

Malignant myopia

AHA: 2017,4Q,10-11

H44.2Ø Degenerative myopia, unspecified eye

H44.21 Degenerative myopia, right eye

H44.22 Degenerative myopia, left eye

H44.23 Degenerative myopia, bilateral

H44.2A Degenerative myopia with choroidal neovascularization

Use additional code for any associated choroid disorders (H31.-)

H44.2A1 Degenerative myopia with choroidal neovascularization, right eye

H44.2A2 Degenerative myopia with choroidal neovascularization, left eye

H44.2A3 Degenerative myopia with choroidal neovascularization, bilateral eye

H44.2A9 Degenerative myopia with choroidal neovascularization, unspecified eye

H44.2B Degenerative myopia with macular hole

H44.2B1 Degenerative myopia with macular hole, right eye

H44.2B2 Degenerative myopia with macular hole, left eye

H44.2B3 Degenerative myopia with macular hole, bilateral eye

H44.2B9 Degenerative myopia with macular hole, unspecified eye

H44.2C Degenerative myopia with retinal detachment

Use additional code to identify the retinal detachment (H33.-)

H44.2C1 Degenerative myopia with retinal detachment, right eye

H44.2C2 Degenerative myopia with retinal detachment, left eye

H44.2C3 Degenerative myopia with retinal detachment, bilateral eye

H44.2C9 Degenerative myopia with retinal detachment, unspecified eye

H44.2D Degenerative myopia with foveoschisis

H44.2D1 Degenerative myopia with foveoschisis, right eye

H44.2D2 Degenerative myopia with foveoschisis, left eye

H44.2D3 Degenerative myopia with foveoschisis, bilateral eye

H44.2D9 Degenerative myopia with foveoschisis, unspecified eye

H44.2E Degenerative myopia with other maculopathy

H44.2E1 Degenerative myopia with other maculopathy, right eye

H44.2E2 Degenerative myopia with other maculopathy, left eye

H44.2E3 Degenerative myopia with other maculopathy, bilateral eye

H44.2E9 Degenerative myopia with other maculopathy, unspecified eye

H44.3 Other and unspecified degenerative disorders of globe

H44.3Ø Unspecified degenerative disorder of globe

H44.31 Chalcosis

H44.311 Chalcosis, right eye

H44.312 Chalcosis, left eye

H44.313 Chalcosis, bilateral
H44.319 Chalcosis, unspecified eye

H44.32 Siderosis of eye
DEF: Iron pigment deposits within tissue of the eyeball caused by high iron content of the blood. Symptoms include cataracts, rust-colored anterior subcapsular deposits, iris heterochromia, pupillary mydriasis, and depressed electroretinogram amplitudes.
H44.321 Siderosis of eye, right eye
H44.322 Siderosis of eye, left eye
H44.323 Siderosis of eye, bilateral
H44.329 Siderosis of eye, unspecified eye

H44.39 Other degenerative disorders of globe
H44.391 Other degenerative disorders of globe, right eye
H44.392 Other degenerative disorders of globe, left eye
H44.393 Other degenerative disorders of globe, bilateral
H44.399 Other degenerative disorders of globe, unspecified eye

H44.4 Hypotony of eye
H44.40 Unspecified hypotony of eye

H44.41 Flat anterior chamber hypotony of eye
H44.411 Flat anterior chamber hypotony of right eye
H44.412 Flat anterior chamber hypotony of left eye
H44.413 Flat anterior chamber hypotony of eye, bilateral
H44.419 Flat anterior chamber hypotony of unspecified eye

H44.42 Hypotony of eye due to ocular fistula
H44.421 Hypotony of right eye due to ocular fistula
H44.422 Hypotony of left eye due to ocular fistula
H44.423 Hypotony of eye due to ocular fistula, bilateral
H44.429 Hypotony of unspecified eye due to ocular fistula

H44.43 Hypotony of eye due to other ocular disorders
H44.431 Hypotony of eye due to other ocular disorders, right eye
H44.432 Hypotony of eye due to other ocular disorders, left eye
H44.433 Hypotony of eye due to other ocular disorders, bilateral
H44.439 Hypotony of eye due to other ocular disorders, unspecified eye

H44.44 Primary hypotony of eye
H44.441 Primary hypotony of right eye
H44.442 Primary hypotony of left eye
H44.443 Primary hypotony of eye, bilateral
H44.449 Primary hypotony of unspecified eye

H44.5 Degenerated conditions of globe
H44.50 Unspecified degenerated conditions of globe

H44.51 Absolute glaucoma
H44.511 Absolute glaucoma, right eye
H44.512 Absolute glaucoma, left eye
H44.513 Absolute glaucoma, bilateral
H44.519 Absolute glaucoma, unspecified eye

H44.52 Atrophy of globe
Phthisis bulbi
H44.521 Atrophy of globe, right eye
H44.522 Atrophy of globe, left eye
H44.523 Atrophy of globe, bilateral
H44.529 Atrophy of globe, unspecified eye

H44.53 Leucocoria
H44.531 Leucocoria, right eye
H44.532 Leucocoria, left eye
H44.533 Leucocoria, bilateral
H44.539 Leucocoria, unspecified eye

H44.6 Retained (old) intraocular foreign body, magnetic
Use additional code to identify magnetic foreign body (Z18.11)
EXCLUDES 1 *current intraocular foreign body (S05.-)*
EXCLUDES 2 *retained foreign body in eyelid (H02.81-)*
retained (old) foreign body following penetrating wound of orbit (H05.5-)
retained (old) intraocular foreign body, nonmagnetic (H44.7-)

H44.60 Unspecified retained (old) intraocular foreign body, magnetic
H44.601 Unspecified retained (old) intraocular foreign body, magnetic, right eye
H44.602 Unspecified retained (old) intraocular foreign body, magnetic, left eye
H44.603 Unspecified retained (old) intraocular foreign body, magnetic, bilateral
H44.609 Unspecified retained (old) intraocular foreign body, magnetic, unspecified eye

H44.61 Retained (old) magnetic foreign body in anterior chamber
H44.611 Retained (old) magnetic foreign body in anterior chamber, right eye
H44.612 Retained (old) magnetic foreign body in anterior chamber, left eye
H44.613 Retained (old) magnetic foreign body in anterior chamber, bilateral
H44.619 Retained (old) magnetic foreign body in anterior chamber, unspecified eye

H44.62 Retained (old) magnetic foreign body in iris or ciliary body
H44.621 Retained (old) magnetic foreign body in iris or ciliary body, right eye
H44.622 Retained (old) magnetic foreign body in iris or ciliary body, left eye
H44.623 Retained (old) magnetic foreign body in iris or ciliary body, bilateral
H44.629 Retained (old) magnetic foreign body in iris or ciliary body, unspecified eye

H44.63 Retained (old) magnetic foreign body in lens
H44.631 Retained (old) magnetic foreign body in lens, right eye
H44.632 Retained (old) magnetic foreign body in lens, left eye
H44.633 Retained (old) magnetic foreign body in lens, bilateral
H44.639 Retained (old) magnetic foreign body in lens, unspecified eye

H44.64 Retained (old) magnetic foreign body in posterior wall of globe
H44.641 Retained (old) magnetic foreign body in posterior wall of globe, right eye
H44.642 Retained (old) magnetic foreign body in posterior wall of globe, left eye
H44.643 Retained (old) magnetic foreign body in posterior wall of globe, bilateral
H44.649 Retained (old) magnetic foreign body in posterior wall of globe, unspecified eye

H44.65 Retained (old) magnetic foreign body in vitreous body
H44.651 Retained (old) magnetic foreign body in vitreous body, right eye
H44.652 Retained (old) magnetic foreign body in vitreous body, left eye
H44.653 Retained (old) magnetic foreign body in vitreous body, bilateral
H44.659 Retained (old) magnetic foreign body in vitreous body, unspecified eye

H44.69 Retained (old) intraocular foreign body, magnetic, in other or multiple sites
H44.691 Retained (old) intraocular foreign body, magnetic, in other or multiple sites, right eye
H44.692 Retained (old) intraocular foreign body, magnetic, in other or multiple sites, left eye
H44.693 Retained (old) intraocular foreign body, magnetic, in other or multiple sites, bilateral
H44.699 Retained (old) intraocular foreign body, magnetic, in other or multiple sites, unspecified eye

H44.7 Retained (old) intraocular foreign body, nonmagnetic
Use additional code to identify nonmagnetic foreign body (Z18.01-Z18.10, Z18.12, Z18.2-Z18.9)
EXCLUDES 1 *current intraocular foreign body (S05.-)*
EXCLUDES 2 *retained foreign body in eyelid (H02.81-)*
retained (old) foreign body following penetrating wound of orbit (H05.5-)
retained (old) intraocular foreign body, magnetic (H44.6-)

H44.70 Unspecified retained (old) intraocular foreign body, nonmagnetic
H44.701 Unspecified retained (old) intraocular foreign body, nonmagnetic, right eye
H44.702 Unspecified retained (old) intraocular foreign body, nonmagnetic, left eye
H44.703 Unspecified retained (old) intraocular foreign body, nonmagnetic, bilateral
H44.709 Unspecified retained (old) intraocular foreign body, nonmagnetic, unspecified eye
Retained (old) intraocular foreign body NOS

H44.71 Retained (nonmagnetic) (old) foreign body in anterior chamber
H44.711 Retained (nonmagnetic) (old) foreign body in anterior chamber, right eye
H44.712 Retained (nonmagnetic) (old) foreign body in anterior chamber, left eye
H44.713 Retained (nonmagnetic) (old) foreign body in anterior chamber, bilateral
H44.719 Retained (nonmagnetic) (old) foreign body in anterior chamber, unspecified eye

H44.72 Retained (nonmagnetic) (old) foreign body in iris or ciliary body
H44.721 Retained (nonmagnetic) (old) foreign body in iris or ciliary body, right eye
H44.722 Retained (nonmagnetic) (old) foreign body in iris or ciliary body, left eye
H44.723 Retained (nonmagnetic) (old) foreign body in iris or ciliary body, bilateral
H44.729 Retained (nonmagnetic) (old) foreign body in iris or ciliary body, unspecified eye

H44.73 Retained (nonmagnetic) (old) foreign body in lens
H44.731 Retained (nonmagnetic) (old) foreign body in lens, right eye
H44.732 Retained (nonmagnetic) (old) foreign body in lens, left eye
H44.733 Retained (nonmagnetic) (old) foreign body in lens, bilateral
H44.739 Retained (nonmagnetic) (old) foreign body in lens, unspecified eye

H44.74 Retained (nonmagnetic) (old) foreign body in posterior wall of globe
H44.741 Retained (nonmagnetic) (old) foreign body in posterior wall of globe, right eye
H44.742 Retained (nonmagnetic) (old) foreign body in posterior wall of globe, left eye
H44.743 Retained (nonmagnetic) (old) foreign body in posterior wall of globe, bilateral
H44.749 Retained (nonmagnetic) (old) foreign body in posterior wall of globe, unspecified eye

H44.75 Retained (nonmagnetic) (old) foreign body in vitreous body
H44.751 Retained (nonmagnetic) (old) foreign body in vitreous body, right eye
H44.752 Retained (nonmagnetic) (old) foreign body in vitreous body, left eye
H44.753 Retained (nonmagnetic) (old) foreign body in vitreous body, bilateral
H44.759 Retained (nonmagnetic) (old) foreign body in vitreous body, unspecified eye

H44.79 Retained (old) intraocular foreign body, nonmagnetic, in other or multiple sites
H44.791 Retained (old) intraocular foreign body, nonmagnetic, in other or multiple sites, right eye
H44.792 Retained (old) intraocular foreign body, nonmagnetic, in other or multiple sites, left eye
H44.793 Retained (old) intraocular foreign body, nonmagnetic, in other or multiple sites, bilateral
H44.799 Retained (old) intraocular foreign body, nonmagnetic, in other or multiple sites, unspecified eye

H44.8 Other disorders of globe
H44.81 Hemophthalmos
DEF: Pool of blood within the eyeball, not from a current injury.
H44.811 Hemophthalmos, right eye
H44.812 Hemophthalmos, left eye
H44.813 Hemophthalmos, bilateral
H44.819 Hemophthalmos, unspecified eye
H44.82 Luxation of globe
H44.821 Luxation of globe, right eye
H44.822 Luxation of globe, left eye
H44.823 Luxation of globe, bilateral
H44.829 Luxation of globe, unspecified eye
H44.89 Other disorders of globe
AHA: 2022,1Q,33
H44.9 Unspecified disorder of globe

Disorders of optic nerve and visual pathways (H46-H47)

H46 Optic neuritis
EXCLUDES 2 *ischemic optic neuropathy (H47.01-)*
neuromyelitis optica [Devic] (G36.0)
H46.0 Optic papillitis
H46.00 Optic papillitis, unspecified eye
H46.01 Optic papillitis, right eye
H46.02 Optic papillitis, left eye
H46.03 Optic papillitis, bilateral
H46.1 Retrobulbar neuritis
Retrobulbar neuritis NOS
EXCLUDES 1 *syphilitic retrobulbar neuritis (A52.15)*
H46.10 Retrobulbar neuritis, unspecified eye
H46.11 Retrobulbar neuritis, right eye
H46.12 Retrobulbar neuritis, left eye
H46.13 Retrobulbar neuritis, bilateral
H46.2 Nutritional optic neuropathy
H46.3 Toxic optic neuropathy
Code first (T51-T65) to identify cause
H46.8 Other optic neuritis
H46.9 Unspecified optic neuritis

H47 Other disorders of optic [2nd] nerve and visual pathways
H47.0 Disorders of optic nerve, not elsewhere classified
H47.01 Ischemic optic neuropathy
H47.011 Ischemic optic neuropathy, right eye
H47.012 Ischemic optic neuropathy, left eye
H47.013 Ischemic optic neuropathy, bilateral
H47.019 Ischemic optic neuropathy, unspecified eye
H47.02 Hemorrhage in optic nerve sheath
H47.021 Hemorrhage in optic nerve sheath, right eye
H47.022 Hemorrhage in optic nerve sheath, left eye
H47.023 Hemorrhage in optic nerve sheath, bilateral
H47.029 Hemorrhage in optic nerve sheath, unspecified eye
H47.03 Optic nerve hypoplasia
H47.031 Optic nerve hypoplasia, right eye
H47.032 Optic nerve hypoplasia, left eye
H47.033 Optic nerve hypoplasia, bilateral
H47.039 Optic nerve hypoplasia, unspecified eye
H47.09 Other disorders of optic nerve, not elsewhere classified
Compression of optic nerve
H47.091 Other disorders of optic nerve, not elsewhere classified, right eye
H47.092 Other disorders of optic nerve, not elsewhere classified, left eye
H47.093 Other disorders of optic nerve, not elsewhere classified, bilateral

H47.099 Other disorders of optic nerve, not elsewhere classified, unspecified eye

✓5th **H47.1 Papilledema**

DEF: Swelling of the optic papilla, the raised area connected to the optic disk made up of nerves that enter the eyeball. It may be caused by increased intracranial pressure, decreased ocular pressure, or a retinal disorder.

H47.10 Unspecified papilledema

H47.11 Papilledema associated with increased intracranial pressure

H47.12 Papilledema associated with decreased ocular pressure

H47.13 Papilledema associated with retinal disorder

✓6th **H47.14** Foster-Kennedy syndrome

H47.141 Foster-Kennedy syndrome, right eye

H47.142 Foster-Kennedy syndrome, left eye

H47.143 Foster-Kennedy syndrome, bilateral

H47.149 Foster-Kennedy syndrome, unspecified eye

✓5th **H47.2 Optic atrophy**

H47.20 Unspecified optic atrophy

✓6th **H47.21** Primary optic atrophy

H47.211 Primary optic atrophy, right eye

H47.212 Primary optic atrophy, left eye

H47.213 Primary optic atrophy, bilateral

H47.219 Primary optic atrophy, unspecified eye

H47.22 Hereditary optic atrophy

Leber's optic atrophy

✓6th **H47.23** Glaucomatous optic atrophy

H47.231 Glaucomatous optic atrophy, right eye

H47.232 Glaucomatous optic atrophy, left eye

H47.233 Glaucomatous optic atrophy, bilateral

H47.239 Glaucomatous optic atrophy, unspecified eye

✓6th **H47.29** Other optic atrophy

Temporal pallor of optic disc

H47.291 Other optic atrophy, right eye

H47.292 Other optic atrophy, left eye

H47.293 Other optic atrophy, bilateral

H47.299 Other optic atrophy, unspecified eye

✓5th **H47.3 Other disorders of optic disc**

✓6th **H47.31** Coloboma of optic disc

H47.311 Coloboma of optic disc, right eye

H47.312 Coloboma of optic disc, left eye

H47.313 Coloboma of optic disc, bilateral

H47.319 Coloboma of optic disc, unspecified eye

✓6th **H47.32** Drusen of optic disc

H47.321 Drusen of optic disc, right eye

H47.322 Drusen of optic disc, left eye

H47.323 Drusen of optic disc, bilateral

H47.329 Drusen of optic disc, unspecified eye

✓6th **H47.33** Pseudopapilledema of optic disc

H47.331 Pseudopapilledema of optic disc, right eye

H47.332 Pseudopapilledema of optic disc, left eye

H47.333 Pseudopapilledema of optic disc, bilateral

H47.339 Pseudopapilledema of optic disc, unspecified eye

✓6th **H47.39** Other disorders of optic disc

H47.391 Other disorders of optic disc, right eye

H47.392 Other disorders of optic disc, left eye

H47.393 Other disorders of optic disc, bilateral

H47.399 Other disorders of optic disc, unspecified eye

✓5th **H47.4 Disorders of optic chiasm**

Code also underlying condition

H47.41 Disorders of optic chiasm in (due to) inflammatory disorders

H47.42 Disorders of optic chiasm in (due to) neoplasm

H47.43 Disorders of optic chiasm in (due to) vascular disorders

H47.49 Disorders of optic chiasm in (due to) other disorders

✓5th **H47.5 Disorders of other visual pathways**

Disorders of optic tracts, geniculate nuclei and optic radiations

Code also underlying condition

✓6th **H47.51** Disorders of visual pathways in (due to) inflammatory disorders

H47.511 Disorders of visual pathways in (due to) inflammatory disorders, right side

H47.512 Disorders of visual pathways in (due to) inflammatory disorders, left side

H47.519 Disorders of visual pathways in (due to) inflammatory disorders, unspecified side

✓6th **H47.52** Disorders of visual pathways in (due to) neoplasm

H47.521 Disorders of visual pathways in (due to) neoplasm, right side

H47.522 Disorders of visual pathways in (due to) neoplasm, left side

H47.529 Disorders of visual pathways in (due to) neoplasm, unspecified side

✓6th **H47.53** Disorders of visual pathways in (due to) vascular disorders

H47.531 Disorders of visual pathways in (due to) vascular disorders, right side

H47.532 Disorders of visual pathways in (due to) vascular disorders, left side

H47.539 Disorders of visual pathways in (due to) vascular disorders, unspecified side

✓5th **H47.6 Disorders of visual cortex**

Code also underlying condition

EXCLUDES 1 *injury to visual cortex S04.04-*

✓6th **H47.61** Cortical blindness

H47.611 Cortical blindness, right side of brain

H47.612 Cortical blindness, left side of brain

H47.619 Cortical blindness, unspecified side of brain

✓6th **H47.62** Disorders of visual cortex in (due to) inflammatory disorders

H47.621 Disorders of visual cortex in (due to) inflammatory disorders, right side of brain

H47.622 Disorders of visual cortex in (due to) inflammatory disorders, left side of brain

H47.629 Disorders of visual cortex in (due to) inflammatory disorders, unspecified side of brain

✓6th **H47.63** Disorders of visual cortex in (due to) neoplasm

H47.631 Disorders of visual cortex in (due to) neoplasm, right side of brain

H47.632 Disorders of visual cortex in (due to) neoplasm, left side of brain

H47.639 Disorders of visual cortex in (due to) neoplasm, unspecified side of brain

✓6th **H47.64** Disorders of visual cortex in (due to) vascular disorders

H47.641 Disorders of visual cortex in (due to) vascular disorders, right side of brain

H47.642 Disorders of visual cortex in (due to) vascular disorders, left side of brain

H47.649 Disorders of visual cortex in (due to) vascular disorders, unspecified side of brain

H47.9 Unspecified disorder of visual pathways

Disorders of ocular muscles, binocular movement, accommodation and refraction (H49-H52)

EXCLUDES 2 *nystagmus and other irregular eye movements (H55)*

✓4th **H49 Paralytic strabismus**

EXCLUDES 2 *internal ophthalmoplegia (H52.51-)*
internuclear ophthalmoplegia (H51.2-)
progressive supranuclear ophthalmoplegia (G23.1)

DEF: Strabismus: Misalignment of the eyes with the inability to move and focus in the same direction due to conditions affecting the muscles controlling them.

✓5th **H49.0 Third [oculomotor] nerve palsy**

H49.00 Third [oculomotor] nerve palsy, unspecified eye

H49.01 Third [oculomotor] nerve palsy, right eye

H49.02 Third [oculomotor] nerve palsy, left eye

H49.03 Third [oculomotor] nerve palsy, bilateral

✓5th **H49.1 Fourth [trochlear] nerve palsy**

H49.10 Fourth [trochlear] nerve palsy, unspecified eye

H49.11 Fourth [trochlear] nerve palsy, right eye
H49.12 Fourth [trochlear] nerve palsy, left eye
H49.13 Fourth [trochlear] nerve palsy, bilateral

5th H49.2 Sixth [abducent] nerve palsy
H49.20 Sixth [abducent] nerve palsy, unspecified eye
H49.21 Sixth [abducent] nerve palsy, right eye
H49.22 Sixth [abducent] nerve palsy, left eye
H49.23 Sixth [abducent] nerve palsy, bilateral

5th H49.3 Total (external) ophthalmoplegia
H49.30 Total (external) ophthalmoplegia, unspecified eye
H49.31 Total (external) ophthalmoplegia, right eye
H49.32 Total (external) ophthalmoplegia, left eye
H49.33 Total (external) ophthalmoplegia, bilateral

5th H49.4 Progressive external ophthalmoplegia
EXCLUDES 1 *Kearns-Sayre syndrome (H49.81-)*
H49.40 Progressive external ophthalmoplegia, unspecified eye
H49.41 Progressive external ophthalmoplegia, right eye
H49.42 Progressive external ophthalmoplegia, left eye
H49.43 Progressive external ophthalmoplegia, bilateral

5th H49.8 Other paralytic strabismus
6th H49.81 Kearns-Sayre syndrome
Progressive external ophthalmoplegia with pigmentary retinopathy
Use additional code for other manifestation, such as: heart block (I45.9)
H49.811 Kearns-Sayre syndrome, right eye HCC Rx ESR COM
H49.812 Kearns-Sayre syndrome, left eye HCC Rx ESR COM
H49.813 Kearns-Sayre syndrome, bilateral HCC Rx ESR COM
H49.819 Kearns-Sayre syndrome, unspecified eye HCC Rx ESR COM
6th H49.88 Other paralytic strabismus
External ophthalmoplegia NOS
H49.881 Other paralytic strabismus, right eye
H49.882 Other paralytic strabismus, left eye
H49.883 Other paralytic strabismus, bilateral
H49.889 Other paralytic strabismus, unspecified eye
H49.9 Unspecified paralytic strabismus

4th H50 Other strabismus
DEF: Strabismus: Misalignment of the eyes with the inability to move and focus in the same direction due to conditions affecting the muscles controlling them.

5th H50.0 Esotropia
Convergent concomitant strabismus
EXCLUDES 1 *intermittent esotropia (H50.31-, H50.32)*
H50.00 Unspecified esotropia
6th H50.01 Monocular esotropia
H50.011 Monocular esotropia, right eye
H50.012 Monocular esotropia, left eye
6th H50.02 Monocular esotropia with A pattern
H50.021 Monocular esotropia with A pattern, right eye
H50.022 Monocular esotropia with A pattern, left eye
6th H50.03 Monocular esotropia with V pattern
H50.031 Monocular esotropia with V pattern, right eye
H50.032 Monocular esotropia with V pattern, left eye
6th H50.04 Monocular esotropia with other noncomitancies
H50.041 Monocular esotropia with other noncomitancies, right eye
H50.042 Monocular esotropia with other noncomitancies, left eye
H50.05 Alternating esotropia
H50.06 Alternating esotropia with A pattern
H50.07 Alternating esotropia with V pattern
H50.08 Alternating esotropia with other noncomitancies

Eye Muscle Diseases

R. L.
Monocular (one eye only) esotropia (inward)

Monocular exotropia (outward)

Monocular hypertropia (upward)

5th H50.1 Exotropia
Divergent concomitant strabismus
EXCLUDES 1 *intermittent exotropia (H50.33-, H50.34)*
H50.10 Unspecified exotropia
6th H50.11 Monocular exotropia
H50.111 Monocular exotropia, right eye
H50.112 Monocular exotropia, left eye
6th H50.12 Monocular exotropia with A pattern
H50.121 Monocular exotropia with A pattern, right eye
H50.122 Monocular exotropia with A pattern, left eye
6th H50.13 Monocular exotropia with V pattern
H50.131 Monocular exotropia with V pattern, right eye
H50.132 Monocular exotropia with V pattern, left eye
6th H50.14 Monocular exotropia with other noncomitancies
H50.141 Monocular exotropia with other noncomitancies, right eye
H50.142 Monocular exotropia with other noncomitancies, left eye
H50.15 Alternating exotropia
H50.16 Alternating exotropia with A pattern
H50.17 Alternating exotropia with V pattern
H50.18 Alternating exotropia with other noncomitancies

5th H50.2 Vertical strabismus
Hypertropia
H50.21 Vertical strabismus, right eye
H50.22 Vertical strabismus, left eye

5th H50.3 Intermittent heterotropia
H50.30 Unspecified intermittent heterotropia
6th H50.31 Intermittent monocular esotropia
H50.311 Intermittent monocular esotropia, right eye
H50.312 Intermittent monocular esotropia, left eye
H50.32 Intermittent alternating esotropia
6th H50.33 Intermittent monocular exotropia
H50.331 Intermittent monocular exotropia, right eye
H50.332 Intermittent monocular exotropia, left eye
H50.34 Intermittent alternating exotropia

5th H50.4 Other and unspecified heterotropia
H50.40 Unspecified heterotropia
6th H50.41 Cyclotropia
H50.411 Cyclotropia, right eye
H50.412 Cyclotropia, left eye
H50.42 Monofixation syndrome
H50.43 Accommodative component in esotropia

5th H50.5 Heterophoria
H50.50 Unspecified heterophoria

H5Ø.51 Esophoria
H5Ø.52 Exophoria
H5Ø.53 Vertical heterophoria
H5Ø.54 Cyclophoria
H5Ø.55 Alternating heterophoria

5th H5Ø.6 Mechanical strabismus
H5Ø.6Ø Mechanical strabismus, unspecified
6th H5Ø.61 Brown's sheath syndrome
H5Ø.611 Brown's sheath syndrome, right eye
H5Ø.612 Brown's sheath syndrome, left eye
H5Ø.69 Other mechanical strabismus
Strabismus due to adhesions
Traumatic limitation of duction of eye muscle

5th H5Ø.8 Other specified strabismus
6th H5Ø.81 Duane's syndrome
H5Ø.811 Duane's syndrome, right eye
H5Ø.812 Duane's syndrome, left eye
H5Ø.89 Other specified strabismus

H5Ø.9 Unspecified strabismus

4th **H51 Other disorders of binocular movement**
H51.Ø Palsy (spasm) of conjugate gaze
5th H51.1 Convergence insufficiency and excess
H51.11 Convergence insufficiency
H51.12 Convergence excess
5th H51.2 Internuclear ophthalmoplegia
H51.2Ø Internuclear ophthalmoplegia, unspecified eye
H51.21 Internuclear ophthalmoplegia, right eye
H51.22 Internuclear ophthalmoplegia, left eye
H51.23 Internuclear ophthalmoplegia, bilateral
H51.8 Other specified disorders of binocular movement
H51.9 Unspecified disorder of binocular movement

4th **H52 Disorders of refraction and accommodation**
5th H52.Ø Hypermetropia
H52.ØØ Hypermetropia, unspecified eye
H52.Ø1 Hypermetropia, right eye
H52.Ø2 Hypermetropia, left eye
H52.Ø3 Hypermetropia, bilateral
5th H52.1 Myopia
EXCLUDES 1 *degenerative myopia (H44.2-)*
H52.1Ø Myopia, unspecified eye
H52.11 Myopia, right eye
H52.12 Myopia, left eye
H52.13 Myopia, bilateral
5th H52.2 Astigmatism
6th H52.2Ø Unspecified astigmatism
H52.2Ø1 Unspecified astigmatism, right eye
H52.2Ø2 Unspecified astigmatism, left eye
H52.2Ø3 Unspecified astigmatism, bilateral
H52.2Ø9 Unspecified astigmatism, unspecified eye
6th H52.21 Irregular astigmatism
H52.211 Irregular astigmatism, right eye
H52.212 Irregular astigmatism, left eye
H52.213 Irregular astigmatism, bilateral
H52.219 Irregular astigmatism, unspecified eye
6th H52.22 Regular astigmatism
H52.221 Regular astigmatism, right eye
H52.222 Regular astigmatism, left eye
H52.223 Regular astigmatism, bilateral
H52.229 Regular astigmatism, unspecified eye
5th H52.3 Anisometropia and aniseikonia
H52.31 Anisometropia
H52.32 Aniseikonia
H52.4 Presbyopia
5th H52.5 Disorders of accommodation
6th H52.51 Internal ophthalmoplegia (complete) (total)
H52.511 Internal ophthalmoplegia (complete) (total), right eye
H52.512 Internal ophthalmoplegia (complete) (total), left eye
H52.513 Internal ophthalmoplegia (complete) (total), bilateral
H52.519 Internal ophthalmoplegia (complete) (total), unspecified eye
6th H52.52 Paresis of accommodation
H52.521 Paresis of accommodation, right eye
H52.522 Paresis of accommodation, left eye
H52.523 Paresis of accommodation, bilateral
H52.529 Paresis of accommodation, unspecified eye
6th H52.53 Spasm of accommodation
H52.531 Spasm of accommodation, right eye
H52.532 Spasm of accommodation, left eye
H52.533 Spasm of accommodation, bilateral
H52.539 Spasm of accommodation, unspecified eye
H52.6 Other disorders of refraction
H52.7 Unspecified disorder of refraction

Visual disturbances and blindness (H53-H54)

4th **H53 Visual disturbances**
5th H53.Ø Amblyopia ex anopsia
EXCLUDES 1 *amblyopia due to vitamin A deficiency (E5Ø.5)*
6th H53.ØØ Unspecified amblyopia
H53.ØØ1 Unspecified amblyopia, right eye
H53.ØØ2 Unspecified amblyopia, left eye
H53.ØØ3 Unspecified amblyopia, bilateral
H53.ØØ9 Unspecified amblyopia, unspecified eye
6th H53.Ø1 Deprivation amblyopia
H53.Ø11 Deprivation amblyopia, right eye
H53.Ø12 Deprivation amblyopia, left eye
H53.Ø13 Deprivation amblyopia, bilateral
H53.Ø19 Deprivation amblyopia, unspecified eye
6th H53.Ø2 Refractive amblyopia
H53.Ø21 Refractive amblyopia, right eye
H53.Ø22 Refractive amblyopia, left eye
H53.Ø23 Refractive amblyopia, bilateral
H53.Ø29 Refractive amblyopia, unspecified eye
6th H53.Ø3 Strabismic amblyopia
EXCLUDES 1 *strabismus (H5Ø.-)*
H53.Ø31 Strabismic amblyopia, right eye
H53.Ø32 Strabismic amblyopia, left eye
H53.Ø33 Strabismic amblyopia, bilateral
H53.Ø39 Strabismic amblyopia, unspecified eye
6th H53.Ø4 Amblyopia suspect
AHA: 2016,4Q,22-23
H53.Ø41 Amblyopia suspect, right eye
H53.Ø42 Amblyopia suspect, left eye
H53.Ø43 Amblyopia suspect, bilateral
H53.Ø49 Amblyopia suspect, unspecified eye
5th H53.1 Subjective visual disturbances
EXCLUDES 1 *subjective visual disturbances due to vitamin A deficiency (E5Ø.5)*
visual hallucinations (R44.1)
H53.1Ø Unspecified subjective visual disturbances
H53.11 Day blindness
Hemeralopia
6th H53.12 Transient visual loss
Scintillating scotoma
EXCLUDES 1 *amaurosis fugax (G45.3-)*
transient retinal artery occlusion (H34.Ø-)
AHA: 2022,1Q,30
H53.121 Transient visual loss, right eye
H53.122 Transient visual loss, left eye
H53.123 Transient visual loss, bilateral
H53.129 Transient visual loss, unspecified eye
6th H53.13 Sudden visual loss
H53.131 Sudden visual loss, right eye
H53.132 Sudden visual loss, left eye
H53.133 Sudden visual loss, bilateral
H53.139 Sudden visual loss, unspecified eye
6th H53.14 Visual discomfort
Asthenopia
Photophobia
H53.141 Visual discomfort, right eye
H53.142 Visual discomfort, left eye
H53.143 Visual discomfort, bilateral
H53.149 Visual discomfort, unspecified

H53.15 Visual distortions of shape and size
Metamorphopsia

H53.16 Psychophysical visual disturbances

H53.19 Other subjective visual disturbances
Visual halos
AHA: 2022,1Q,30

H53.2 Diplopia
Double vision

H53.3 Other and unspecified disorders of binocular vision

H53.30 Unspecified disorder of binocular vision

H53.31 Abnormal retinal correspondence

H53.32 Fusion with defective stereopsis

H53.33 Simultaneous visual perception without fusion

H53.34 Suppression of binocular vision

H53.4 Visual field defects

H53.40 Unspecified visual field defects

H53.41 Scotoma involving central area
Central scotoma
AHA: 2022,1Q,30

H53.411 Scotoma involving central area, right eye

H53.412 Scotoma involving central area, left eye

H53.413 Scotoma involving central area, bilateral

H53.419 Scotoma involving central area, unspecified eye

H53.42 Scotoma of blind spot area
Enlarged blind spot

H53.421 Scotoma of blind spot area, right eye

H53.422 Scotoma of blind spot area, left eye

H53.423 Scotoma of blind spot area, bilateral

H53.429 Scotoma of blind spot area, unspecified eye

H53.43 Sector or arcuate defects
Arcuate scotoma
Bjerrum scotoma

H53.431 Sector or arcuate defects, right eye

H53.432 Sector or arcuate defects, left eye

H53.433 Sector or arcuate defects, bilateral

H53.439 Sector or arcuate defects, unspecified eye

H53.45 Other localized visual field defect
Peripheral visual field defect
Ring scotoma NOS
Scotoma NOS

H53.451 Other localized visual field defect, right eye

H53.452 Other localized visual field defect, left eye

H53.453 Other localized visual field defect, bilateral

H53.459 Other localized visual field defect, unspecified eye

H53.46 Homonymous bilateral field defects
Homonymous hemianopia
Homonymous hemianopsia
Quadrant anopia
Quadrant anopsia

H53.461 Homonymous bilateral field defects, right side

H53.462 Homonymous bilateral field defects, left side

H53.469 Homonymous bilateral field defects, unspecified side
Homonymous bilateral field defects NOS

H53.47 Heteronymous bilateral field defects
Heteronymous hemianop(s)ia

H53.48 Generalized contraction of visual field

H53.481 Generalized contraction of visual field, right eye

H53.482 Generalized contraction of visual field, left eye

H53.483 Generalized contraction of visual field, bilateral

H53.489 Generalized contraction of visual field, unspecified eye

H53.5 Color vision deficiencies
Color blindness
EXCLUDES 2 *day blindness (H53.11)*

H53.50 Unspecified color vision deficiencies
Color blindness NOS

H53.51 Achromatopsia
DEF: Nonprogressive genetic visual disorder characterized by complete color blindness, decreased vision, and light sensitivity.

H53.52 Acquired color vision deficiency

H53.53 Deuteranomaly
Deuteranopia
DEF: Male-only genetic disorder causing difficulty in distinguishing green and red; no shortened spectrum.

H53.54 Protanomaly
Protanopia

H53.55 Tritanomaly
Tritanopia

H53.59 Other color vision deficiencies

H53.6 Night blindness
EXCLUDES 1 *night blindness due to vitamin A deficiency (E50.5)*

H53.60 Unspecified night blindness

H53.61 Abnormal dark adaptation curve

H53.62 Acquired night blindness

H53.63 Congenital night blindness

H53.69 Other night blindness

H53.7 Vision sensitivity deficiencies

H53.71 Glare sensitivity

H53.72 Impaired contrast sensitivity

H53.8 Other visual disturbances

H53.9 Unspecified visual disturbance

H54 Blindness and low vision
NOTE For definition of visual impairment categories see table below
Code first any associated underlying cause of the blindness
EXCLUDES 1 *amaurosis fugax (G45.3)*
AHA: 2017,4Q,11-12

H54.0 Blindness, both eyes
Visual impairment categories 3, 4, 5 in both eyes.

H54.0X Blindness, both eyes, different category levels

H54.0X3 Blindness right eye, category 3

H54.0X33 Blindness right eye category 3, blindness left eye category 3

H54.0X34 Blindness right eye category 3, blindness left eye category 4

H54.0X35 Blindness right eye category 3, blindness left eye category 5

H54.0X4 Blindness right eye, category 4

H54.0X43 Blindness right eye category 4, blindness left eye category 3

H54.0X44 Blindness right eye category 4, blindness left eye category 4

H54.0X45 Blindness right eye category 4, blindness left eye category 5

H54.0X5 Blindness right eye, category 5

H54.0X53 Blindness right eye category 5, blindness left eye category 3

H54.0X54 Blindness right eye category 5, blindness left eye category 4

H54.0X55 Blindness right eye category 5, blindness left eye category 5

H54.1 Blindness, one eye, low vision other eye
Visual impairment categories 3, 4, 5 in one eye, with categories 1 or 2 in the other eye.

H54.10 Blindness, one eye, low vision other eye, unspecified eyes

H54.11 Blindness, right eye, low vision left eye

H54.113 Blindness right eye category 3, low vision left eye

H54.1131 Blindness right eye category 3, low vision left eye category 1

H54.1132 Blindness right eye category 3, low vision left eye category 2

H54.114 Blindness right eye category 4, low vision left eye

H54.1141 Blindness right eye category 4, low vision left eye category 1

H54.1142 **Blindness right eye category 4, low vision left eye category 2**

✓7th **H54.115** **Blindness right eye category 5, low vision left eye**

H54.1151 **Blindness right eye category 5, low vision left eye category 1**

H54.1152 **Blindness right eye category 5, low vision left eye category 2**

✓6th **H54.12** **Blindness, left eye, low vision right eye**

✓7th **H54.121** **Low vision right eye category 1, blindness left eye**

H54.1213 **Low vision right eye category 1, blindness left eye category 3**

H54.1214 **Low vision right eye category 1, blindness left eye category 4**

H54.1215 **Low vision right eye category 1, blindness left eye category 5**

✓7th **H54.122** **Low vision right eye category 2, blindness left eye**

H54.1223 **Low vision right eye category 2, blindness left eye category 3**

H54.1224 **Low vision right eye category 2, blindness left eye category 4**

H54.1225 **Low vision right eye category 2, blindness left eye category 5**

✓5th **H54.2** **Low vision, both eyes**

Visual impairment categories 1 or 2 in both eyes.

✓6th **H54.2X** **Low vision, both eyes, different category levels**

✓7th **H54.2X1** **Low vision, right eye, category 1**

H54.2X11 **Low vision right eye category 1, low vision left eye category 1**

H54.2X12 **Low vision right eye category 1, low vision left eye category 2**

✓7th **H54.2X2** **Low vision, right eye, category 2**

H54.2X21 **Low vision right eye category 2, low vision left eye category 1**

H54.2X22 **Low vision right eye category 2, low vision left eye category 2**

H54.3 **Unqualified visual loss, both eyes**

Visual impairment category 9 in both eyes.

TIP: Assign only when both eyes are documented as affected by blindness or low vision but the visual impairment category is not documented.

✓5th **H54.4** **Blindness, one eye**

Visual impairment categories 3, 4, 5 in one eye [normal vision in other eye]

H54.4Ø **Blindness, one eye, unspecified eye**

✓6th **H54.41** **Blindness, right eye, normal vision left eye**

✓7th **H54.413** **Blindness, right eye, category 3**

H54.413A **Blindness right eye category 3, normal vision left eye**

✓7th **H54.414** **Blindness, right eye, category 4**

H54.414A **Blindness right eye category 4, normal vision left eye**

✓7th **H54.415** **Blindness, right eye, category 5**

H54.415A **Blindness right eye category 5, normal vision left eye**

✓6th **H54.42** **Blindness, left eye, normal vision right eye**

✓7th **H54.42A** **Blindness, left eye, category 3-5**

H54.42A3 **Blindness left eye category 3, normal vision right eye**

H54.42A4 **Blindness left eye category 4, normal vision right eye**

H54.42A5 **Blindness left eye category 5, normal vision right eye**

✓5th **H54.5** **Low vision, one eye**

Visual impairment categories 1 or 2 in one eye [normal vision in other eye].

H54.5Ø **Low vision, one eye, unspecified eye**

✓6th **H54.51** **Low vision, right eye, normal vision left eye**

✓7th **H54.511** **Low vision, right eye, category 1-2**

H54.511A **Low vision right eye category 1, normal vision left eye**

H54.512A **Low vision right eye category 2, normal vision left eye**

✓7th **H54.52** **Low vision, left eye, normal vision right eye**

✓7th **H54.52A** **Low vision, left eye, category 1-2**

H54.52A1 **Low vision left eye category 1, normal vision right eye**

H54.52A2 **Low vision left eye category 2, normal vision right eye**

✓5th **H54.6** **Unqualified visual loss, one eye**

Visual impairment category 9 in one eye [normal vision in other eye].

TIP: Assign a code from this category only when one eye is documented as affected by blindness or low vision but the visual impairment category is not documented.

H54.6Ø **Unqualified visual loss, one eye, unspecified**

H54.61 **Unqualified visual loss, right eye, normal vision left eye**

H54.62 **Unqualified visual loss, left eye, normal vision right eye**

H54.7 **Unspecified visual loss**

Visual impairment category 9 NOS

TIP: Assign only when documentation specifies blindness, visual loss, or low vision but not whether one or both eyes are affected or the visual impairment category.

H54.8 **Legal blindness, as defined in USA**

Blindness NOS according to USA definition

EXCLUDES 1 *legal blindness with specification of impairment level (H54.Ø-H54.7)*

NOTE The table below gives a classification of severity of visual impairment recommended by a WHO Study Group on the Prevention of Blindness, Geneva, 6-1Ø November 1972.

The term "low vision" in category H54 comprises categories 1 and 2 of the table, the term "blindness" categories 3, 4 and 5, and the term "unqualified visual loss" category 9.

If the extent of the visual field is taken into account, patients with a field no greater than 1Ø but greater than 5 around central fixation should be placed in category 3 and patients with a field no greater than 5 around central fixation should be placed in category 4, even if the central acuity is not impaired.

Category of visual impairment	Visual acuity with best possible correction	
	Maximum less than:	**Minimum equal to or better than:**
1	6/18 3/1Ø (Ø.3) 2Ø/7Ø	6/6Ø 1/1Ø (Ø.1) 2Ø/2ØØ
2	6/6Ø 1/1Ø (Ø.1) 2Ø/2ØØ	3/6Ø 1/2Ø (Ø.Ø5) 2Ø/4ØØ
3	3/6Ø 1/2ØØ (Ø.Ø5) 2Ø/4ØØ	1/6Ø (finger counting at one meter) 1/5Ø (Ø.Ø2) 5/3ØØ (2Ø/12ØØ)
4	1/6Ø (finger counting at one meter) 1/5Ø (Ø.Ø2) 5/3ØØ	Light perception
5	No light perception	
9	Undetermined or unspecified	

Other disorders of eye and adnexa (H55-H57)

H55 Nystagmus and other irregular eye movements

H55.0 Nystagmus

DEF: Rapid, rhythmic, involuntary movements of the eyeball in vertical, horizontal, rotational, or mixed directions.

H55.00 Unspecified nystagmus
H55.01 Congenital nystagmus
H55.02 Latent nystagmus
H55.03 Visual deprivation nystagmus
H55.04 Dissociated nystagmus
H55.09 Other forms of nystagmus

H55.8 Other irregular eye movements

AHA: 2020,4Q,25

H55.81 Deficient saccadic eye movements
H55.82 Deficient smooth pursuit eye movements
H55.89 Other irregular eye movements

H57 Other disorders of eye and adnexa

H57.0 Anomalies of pupillary function

H57.00 Unspecified anomaly of pupillary function
H57.01 Argyll Robertson pupil, atypical

EXCLUDES 1 *syphilitic Argyll Robertson pupil (A52.19)*

H57.02 Anisocoria
H57.03 Miosis
H57.04 Mydriasis
H57.05 Tonic pupil

H57.051 Tonic pupil, right eye
H57.052 Tonic pupil, left eye
H57.053 Tonic pupil, bilateral
H57.059 Tonic pupil, unspecified eye

H57.09 Other anomalies of pupillary function

H57.1 Ocular pain

H57.10 Ocular pain, unspecified eye
H57.11 Ocular pain, right eye
H57.12 Ocular pain, left eye
H57.13 Ocular pain, bilateral

H57.8 Other specified disorders of eye and adnexa

AHA: 2018,4Q,15-16

H57.81 Brow ptosis

H57.811 Brow ptosis, right
H57.812 Brow ptosis, left
H57.813 Brow ptosis, bilateral
H57.819 Brow ptosis, unspecified

H57.89 Other specified disorders of eye and adnexa

H57.9 Unspecified disorder of eye and adnexa

Intraoperative and postprocedural complications and disorders of eye and adnexa, not elsewhere classified (H59)

H59 Intraoperative and postprocedural complications and disorders of eye and adnexa, not elsewhere classified

EXCLUDES 1 *mechanical complication of intraocular lens (T85.2)*
mechanical complication of other ocular prosthetic devices, implants and grafts (T85.3)
pseudophakia (Z96.1)
secondary cataracts (H26.4-)

H59.0 Disorders of the eye following cataract surgery

H59.01 Keratopathy (bullous aphakic) following cataract surgery

Vitreal corneal syndrome
Vitreous (touch) syndrome

H59.011 Keratopathy (bullous aphakic) following cataract surgery, right eye
H59.012 Keratopathy (bullous aphakic) following cataract surgery, left eye
H59.013 Keratopathy (bullous aphakic) following cataract surgery, bilateral
H59.019 Keratopathy (bullous aphakic) following cataract surgery, unspecified eye

H59.02 Cataract (lens) fragments in eye following cataract surgery

H59.021 Cataract (lens) fragments in eye following cataract surgery, right eye
H59.022 Cataract (lens) fragments in eye following cataract surgery, left eye
H59.023 Cataract (lens) fragments in eye following cataract surgery, bilateral
H59.029 Cataract (lens) fragments in eye following cataract surgery, unspecified eye

H59.03 Cystoid macular edema following cataract surgery

H59.031 Cystoid macular edema following cataract surgery, right eye
H59.032 Cystoid macular edema following cataract surgery, left eye
H59.033 Cystoid macular edema following cataract surgery, bilateral
H59.039 Cystoid macular edema following cataract surgery, unspecified eye

H59.09 Other disorders of the eye following cataract surgery

H59.091 Other disorders of the right eye following cataract surgery
H59.092 Other disorders of the left eye following cataract surgery
H59.093 Other disorders of the eye following cataract surgery, bilateral
H59.099 Other disorders of unspecified eye following cataract surgery

H59.1 Intraoperative hemorrhage and hematoma of eye and adnexa complicating a procedure

EXCLUDES 1 *intraoperative hemorrhage and hematoma of eye and adnexa due to accidental puncture or laceration during a procedure (H59.2-)*

H59.11 Intraoperative hemorrhage and hematoma of eye and adnexa complicating an ophthalmic procedure

H59.111 Intraoperative hemorrhage and hematoma of right eye and adnexa complicating an ophthalmic procedure
H59.112 Intraoperative hemorrhage and hematoma of left eye and adnexa complicating an ophthalmic procedure
H59.113 Intraoperative hemorrhage and hematoma of eye and adnexa complicating an ophthalmic procedure, bilateral
H59.119 Intraoperative hemorrhage and hematoma of unspecified eye and adnexa complicating an ophthalmic procedure

H59.12 Intraoperative hemorrhage and hematoma of eye and adnexa complicating other procedure

H59.121 Intraoperative hemorrhage and hematoma of right eye and adnexa complicating other procedure
H59.122 Intraoperative hemorrhage and hematoma of left eye and adnexa complicating other procedure
H59.123 Intraoperative hemorrhage and hematoma of eye and adnexa complicating other procedure, bilateral
H59.129 Intraoperative hemorrhage and hematoma of unspecified eye and adnexa complicating other procedure

H59.2 Accidental puncture and laceration of eye and adnexa during a procedure

H59.21 Accidental puncture and laceration of eye and adnexa during an ophthalmic procedure

H59.211 Accidental puncture and laceration of right eye and adnexa during an ophthalmic procedure
H59.212 Accidental puncture and laceration of left eye and adnexa during an ophthalmic procedure
H59.213 Accidental puncture and laceration of eye and adnexa during an ophthalmic procedure, bilateral
H59.219 Accidental puncture and laceration of unspecified eye and adnexa during an ophthalmic procedure

H59.22 Accidental puncture and laceration of eye and adnexa during other procedure

H59.221 Accidental puncture and laceration of right eye and adnexa during other procedure
H59.222 Accidental puncture and laceration of left eye and adnexa during other procedure
H59.223 Accidental puncture and laceration of eye and adnexa during other procedure, bilateral

H59.229 Accidental puncture and laceration of unspecified eye and adnexa during other procedure

H59.3 Postprocedural hemorrhage, hematoma, and seroma of eye and adnexa following a procedure
AHA: 2016,4Q,9-10

H59.31 Postprocedural hemorrhage of eye and adnexa following an ophthalmic procedure
H59.311 Postprocedural hemorrhage of right eye and adnexa following an ophthalmic procedure
H59.312 Postprocedural hemorrhage of left eye and adnexa following an ophthalmic procedure
H59.313 Postprocedural hemorrhage of eye and adnexa following an ophthalmic procedure, bilateral
H59.319 Postprocedural hemorrhage of unspecified eye and adnexa following an ophthalmic procedure

H59.32 Postprocedural hemorrhage of eye and adnexa following other procedure
H59.321 Postprocedural hemorrhage of right eye and adnexa following other procedure
H59.322 Postprocedural hemorrhage of left eye and adnexa following other procedure
H59.323 Postprocedural hemorrhage of eye and adnexa following other procedure, bilateral
H59.329 Postprocedural hemorrhage of unspecified eye and adnexa following other procedure

H59.33 Postprocedural hematoma of eye and adnexa following an ophthalmic procedure
H59.331 Postprocedural hematoma of right eye and adnexa following an ophthalmic procedure
H59.332 Postprocedural hematoma of left eye and adnexa following an ophthalmic procedure
H59.333 Postprocedural hematoma of eye and adnexa following an ophthalmic procedure, bilateral
H59.339 Postprocedural hematoma of unspecified eye and adnexa following an ophthalmic procedure

H59.34 Postprocedural hematoma of eye and adnexa following other procedure
H59.341 Postprocedural hematoma of right eye and adnexa following other procedure
H59.342 Postprocedural hematoma of left eye and adnexa following other procedure
H59.343 Postprocedural hematoma of eye and adnexa following other procedure, bilateral
H59.349 Postprocedural hematoma of unspecified eye and adnexa following other procedure

H59.35 Postprocedural seroma of eye and adnexa following an ophthalmic procedure
H59.351 Postprocedural seroma of right eye and adnexa following an ophthalmic procedure
H59.352 Postprocedural seroma of left eye and adnexa following an ophthalmic procedure
H59.353 Postprocedural seroma of eye and adnexa following an ophthalmic procedure, bilateral
H59.359 Postprocedural seroma of unspecified eye and adnexa following an ophthalmic procedure

H59.36 Postprocedural seroma of eye and adnexa following other procedure
H59.361 Postprocedural seroma of right eye and adnexa following other procedure
H59.362 Postprocedural seroma of left eye and adnexa following other procedure
H59.363 Postprocedural seroma of eye and adnexa following other procedure, bilateral
H59.369 Postprocedural seroma of unspecified eye and adnexa following other procedure

H59.4 Inflammation (infection) of postprocedural bleb
Postprocedural blebitis
EXCLUDES 1 *filtering (vitreous) bleb after glaucoma surgery status (Z98.83)*

H59.40 Inflammation (infection) of postprocedural bleb, unspecified
H59.41 Inflammation (infection) of postprocedural bleb, stage 1
H59.42 Inflammation (infection) of postprocedural bleb, stage 2
H59.43 Inflammation (infection) of postprocedural bleb, stage 3
Bleb endophthalmitis

H59.8 Other intraoperative and postprocedural complications and disorders of eye and adnexa, not elsewhere classified

H59.81 Chorioretinal scars after surgery for detachment
H59.811 Chorioretinal scars after surgery for detachment, right eye
H59.812 Chorioretinal scars after surgery for detachment, left eye
H59.813 Chorioretinal scars after surgery for detachment, bilateral
H59.819 Chorioretinal scars after surgery for detachment, unspecified eye

H59.88 Other intraoperative complications of eye and adnexa, not elsewhere classified

H59.89 Other postprocedural complications and disorders of eye and adnexa, not elsewhere classified
AHA: 2020,3Q,29

Chapter 8. Diseases of the Ear and Mastoid Process (H6Ø–H95)

Chapter-specific Guidelines with Coding Examples
Reserved for future guideline expansion.

Chapter 8. Diseases of the Ear and Mastoid Process (H60-H95)

NOTE Use an external cause code following the code for the ear condition, if applicable, to identify the cause of the ear condition

EXCLUDES 2 *certain conditions originating in the perinatal period (P04-P96)*
certain infectious and parasitic diseases (A00-B99)
complications of pregnancy, childbirth and the puerperium (O00-O9A)
congenital malformations, deformations and chromosomal abnormalities (Q00-Q99)
endocrine, nutritional and metabolic diseases (E00-E88)
injury, poisoning and certain other consequences of external causes (S00-T88)
neoplasms (C00-D49)
symptoms, signs and abnormal clinical and laboratory findings, not elsewhere classified (R00-R94)

This chapter contains the following blocks:

H60-H62 Diseases of external ear
H65-H75 Diseases of middle ear and mastoid
H80-H83 Diseases of inner ear
H90-H94 Other disorders of ear
H95 Intraoperative and postprocedural complications and disorders of ear and mastoid process, not elsewhere classified

Diseases of external ear (H60-H62)

✓4th **H60 Otitis externa**

TIP: When the specific infectious agent is identified, a code from Chapter 1 is assigned instead of a code from this category.

✓5th **H60.0 Abscess of external ear**

Boil of external ear
Carbuncle of auricle or external auditory canal
Furuncle of external ear

H60.00 Abscess of external ear, unspecified ear
H60.01 Abscess of right external ear
H60.02 Abscess of left external ear
H60.03 Abscess of external ear, bilateral

✓5th **H60.1 Cellulitis of external ear**

Cellulitis of auricle
Cellulitis of external auditory canal

H60.10 Cellulitis of external ear, unspecified ear
H60.11 Cellulitis of right external ear
H60.12 Cellulitis of left external ear
H60.13 Cellulitis of external ear, bilateral

✓5th **H60.2 Malignant otitis externa**

H60.20 Malignant otitis externa, unspecified ear
H60.21 Malignant otitis externa, right ear
H60.22 Malignant otitis externa, left ear
H60.23 Malignant otitis externa, bilateral

✓5th **H60.3 Other infective otitis externa**

✓6th **H60.31 Diffuse otitis externa**

H60.311 Diffuse otitis externa, right ear
H60.312 Diffuse otitis externa, left ear
H60.313 Diffuse otitis externa, bilateral
H60.319 Diffuse otitis externa, unspecified ear

✓6th **H60.32 Hemorrhagic otitis externa**

H60.321 Hemorrhagic otitis externa, right ear
H60.322 Hemorrhagic otitis externa, left ear
H60.323 Hemorrhagic otitis externa, bilateral
H60.329 Hemorrhagic otitis externa, unspecified ear

✓6th **H60.33 Swimmer's ear**

DEF: Commonly occurs when water gets trapped in the ear after swimming.

H60.331 Swimmer's ear, right ear
H60.332 Swimmer's ear, left ear
H60.333 Swimmer's ear, bilateral
H60.339 Swimmer's ear, unspecified ear

✓6th **H60.39 Other infective otitis externa**

H60.391 Other infective otitis externa, right ear
H60.392 Other infective otitis externa, left ear
H60.393 Other infective otitis externa, bilateral
H60.399 Other infective otitis externa, unspecified ear

✓5th **H60.4 Cholesteatoma of external ear**

Keratosis obturans of external ear (canal)

EXCLUDES 2 *cholesteatoma of middle ear (H71.-)*
recurrent cholesteatoma of postmastoidectomy cavity (H95.0-)

DEF: Cholesteatoma: Noncancerous cyst-like mass of cell debris, including cholesterol and epithelial cells resulting from trauma, repeated or improperly healed infections, and congenital enclosure of epidermal cells.

H60.40 Cholesteatoma of external ear, unspecified ear
H60.41 Cholesteatoma of right external ear
H60.42 Cholesteatoma of left external ear
H60.43 Cholesteatoma of external ear, bilateral

✓5th **H60.5 Acute noninfective otitis externa**

✓6th **H60.50 Unspecified acute noninfective otitis externa**

Acute otitis externa NOS

H60.501 Unspecified acute noninfective otitis externa, right ear
H60.502 Unspecified acute noninfective otitis externa, left ear
H60.503 Unspecified acute noninfective otitis externa, bilateral
H60.509 Unspecified acute noninfective otitis externa, unspecified ear

✓6th **H60.51 Acute actinic otitis externa**

H60.511 Acute actinic otitis externa, right ear
H60.512 Acute actinic otitis externa, left ear
H60.513 Acute actinic otitis externa, bilateral
H60.519 Acute actinic otitis externa, unspecified ear

✓6th **H60.52 Acute chemical otitis externa**

H60.521 Acute chemical otitis externa, right ear
H60.522 Acute chemical otitis externa, left ear
H60.523 Acute chemical otitis externa, bilateral
H60.529 Acute chemical otitis externa, unspecified ear

✓6th **H60.53 Acute contact otitis externa**

H60.531 Acute contact otitis externa, right ear
H60.532 Acute contact otitis externa, left ear
H60.533 Acute contact otitis externa, bilateral
H60.539 Acute contact otitis externa, unspecified ear

✓6th **H60.54 Acute eczematoid otitis externa**

H60.541 Acute eczematoid otitis externa, right ear
H60.542 Acute eczematoid otitis externa, left ear
H60.543 Acute eczematoid otitis externa, bilateral
H60.549 Acute eczematoid otitis externa, unspecified ear

✓6th **H60.55 Acute reactive otitis externa**

H60.551 Acute reactive otitis externa, right ear
H60.552 Acute reactive otitis externa, left ear
H60.553 Acute reactive otitis externa, bilateral
H60.559 Acute reactive otitis externa, unspecified ear

✓6th **H60.59 Other noninfective acute otitis externa**

H60.591 Other noninfective acute otitis externa, right ear
H60.592 Other noninfective acute otitis externa, left ear
H60.593 Other noninfective acute otitis externa, bilateral
H60.599 Other noninfective acute otitis externa, unspecified ear

✓5th **H60.6 Unspecified chronic otitis externa**

H60.60 Unspecified chronic otitis externa, unspecified ear
H60.61 Unspecified chronic otitis externa, right ear
H60.62 Unspecified chronic otitis externa, left ear
H60.63 Unspecified chronic otitis externa, bilateral

✓5th **H60.8 Other otitis externa**

✓6th **H60.8X Other otitis externa**

H60.8X1 Other otitis externa, right ear
H60.8X2 Other otitis externa, left ear
H60.8X3 Other otitis externa, bilateral
H60.8X9 Other otitis externa, unspecified ear

✓5th **H60.9 Unspecified otitis externa**

H60.90 Unspecified otitis externa, unspecified ear
H60.91 Unspecified otitis externa, right ear

H60.92 Unspecified otitis externa, left ear
H60.93 Unspecified otitis externa, bilateral

H61 Other disorders of external ear

H61.0 Chondritis and perichondritis of external ear
Chondrodermatitis nodularis chronica helicis
Perichondritis of auricle
Perichondritis of pinna

H61.00 Unspecified perichondritis of external ear
H61.001 Unspecified perichondritis of right external ear
H61.002 Unspecified perichondritis of left external ear
H61.003 Unspecified perichondritis of external ear, bilateral
H61.009 Unspecified perichondritis of external ear, unspecified ear

H61.01 Acute perichondritis of external ear
H61.011 Acute perichondritis of right external ear
H61.012 Acute perichondritis of left external ear
H61.013 Acute perichondritis of external ear, bilateral
H61.019 Acute perichondritis of external ear, unspecified ear

H61.02 Chronic perichondritis of external ear
H61.021 Chronic perichondritis of right external ear
H61.022 Chronic perichondritis of left external ear
H61.023 Chronic perichondritis of external ear, bilateral
H61.029 Chronic perichondritis of external ear, unspecified ear

H61.03 Chondritis of external ear
Chondritis of auricle
Chondritis of pinna
AHA: 2015,1Q,18
DEF: Infection that has progressed into the cartilage and presents as indurated and edematous skin over the pinna. Vascular compromise occurs with tissue necrosis and deformity.
H61.031 Chondritis of right external ear
H61.032 Chondritis of left external ear
H61.033 Chondritis of external ear, bilateral
H61.039 Chondritis of external ear, unspecified ear

H61.1 Noninfective disorders of pinna
EXCLUDES 2 *cauliflower ear (M95.1-)*
gouty tophi of ear (M1A.-)

H61.10 Unspecified noninfective disorders of pinna
Disorder of pinna NOS
H61.101 Unspecified noninfective disorders of pinna, right ear
H61.102 Unspecified noninfective disorders of pinna, left ear
H61.103 Unspecified noninfective disorders of pinna, bilateral
H61.109 Unspecified noninfective disorders of pinna, unspecified ear

H61.11 Acquired deformity of pinna
Acquired deformity of auricle
EXCLUDES 2 *cauliflower ear (M95.1-)*
H61.111 Acquired deformity of pinna, right ear
H61.112 Acquired deformity of pinna, left ear
H61.113 Acquired deformity of pinna, bilateral
H61.119 Acquired deformity of pinna, unspecified ear

H61.12 Hematoma of pinna
Hematoma of auricle
H61.121 Hematoma of pinna, right ear
H61.122 Hematoma of pinna, left ear
H61.123 Hematoma of pinna, bilateral
H61.129 Hematoma of pinna, unspecified ear

H61.19 Other noninfective disorders of pinna
H61.191 Noninfective disorders of pinna, right ear
H61.192 Noninfective disorders of pinna, left ear
H61.193 Noninfective disorders of pinna, bilateral
H61.199 Noninfective disorders of pinna, unspecified ear

H61.2 Impacted cerumen
Wax in ear
H61.20 Impacted cerumen, unspecified ear
H61.21 Impacted cerumen, right ear
H61.22 Impacted cerumen, left ear
H61.23 Impacted cerumen, bilateral

H61.3 Acquired stenosis of external ear canal
Collapse of external ear canal
EXCLUDES 1 *postprocedural stenosis of external ear canal (H95.81-)*

H61.30 Acquired stenosis of external ear canal, unspecified
H61.301 Acquired stenosis of right external ear canal, unspecified
H61.302 Acquired stenosis of left external ear canal, unspecified
H61.303 Acquired stenosis of external ear canal, unspecified, bilateral
H61.309 Acquired stenosis of external ear canal, unspecified, unspecified ear

H61.31 Acquired stenosis of external ear canal secondary to trauma
H61.311 Acquired stenosis of right external ear canal secondary to trauma
H61.312 Acquired stenosis of left external ear canal secondary to trauma
H61.313 Acquired stenosis of external ear canal secondary to trauma, bilateral
H61.319 Acquired stenosis of external ear canal secondary to trauma, unspecified ear

H61.32 Acquired stenosis of external ear canal secondary to inflammation and infection
DEF: Narrowing of the external ear canal due to chronic inflammation or infection.
H61.321 Acquired stenosis of right external ear canal secondary to inflammation and infection
H61.322 Acquired stenosis of left external ear canal secondary to inflammation and infection
H61.323 Acquired stenosis of external ear canal secondary to inflammation and infection, bilateral
H61.329 Acquired stenosis of external ear canal secondary to inflammation and infection, unspecified ear

H61.39 Other acquired stenosis of external ear canal
H61.391 Other acquired stenosis of right external ear canal
H61.392 Other acquired stenosis of left external ear canal
H61.393 Other acquired stenosis of external ear canal, bilateral
H61.399 Other acquired stenosis of external ear canal, unspecified ear

H61.8 Other specified disorders of external ear

H61.81 Exostosis of external canal
H61.811 Exostosis of right external canal
H61.812 Exostosis of left external canal
H61.813 Exostosis of external canal, bilateral
H61.819 Exostosis of external canal, unspecified ear

H61.89 Other specified disorders of external ear
H61.891 Other specified disorders of right external ear
H61.892 Other specified disorders of left external ear
H61.893 Other specified disorders of external ear, bilateral
H61.899 Other specified disorders of external ear, unspecified ear

H61.9 Disorder of external ear, unspecified
H61.90 Disorder of external ear, unspecified, unspecified ear
H61.91 Disorder of right external ear, unspecified
H61.92 Disorder of left external ear, unspecified
H61.93 Disorder of external ear, unspecified, bilateral

H62 Disorders of external ear in diseases classified elsewhere

H62.4 Otitis externa in other diseases classified elsewhere

Code first underlying disease, such as:
erysipelas (A46)
impetigo (LØ1.Ø)

EXCLUDES 1 *otitis externa (in):*
candidiasis (B37.84)
herpes viral [herpes simplex] (BØØ.1)
herpes zoster (BØ2.8)

H62.4Ø Otitis externa in other diseases classified elsewhere, unspecified ear
H62.41 Otitis externa in other diseases classified elsewhere, right ear
H62.42 Otitis externa in other diseases classified elsewhere, left ear
H62.43 Otitis externa in other diseases classified elsewhere, bilateral

H62.8 Other disorders of external ear in diseases classified elsewhere

Code first underlying disease, such as:
gout (M1A.-, M1Ø.-)

H62.8X Other disorders of external ear in diseases classified elsewhere
H62.8X1 Other disorders of right external ear in diseases classified elsewhere
H62.8X2 Other disorders of left external ear in diseases classified elsewhere
H62.8X3 Other disorders of external ear in diseases classified elsewhere, bilateral
H62.8X9 Other disorders of external ear in diseases classified elsewhere, unspecified ear

Diseases of middle ear and mastoid (H65-H75)

H65 Nonsuppurative otitis media

INCLUDES nonsuppurative otitis media with myringitis

Use additional code for any associated perforated tympanic membrane (H72.-)

Use additional code, if applicable, to identify:
exposure to environmental tobacco smoke (Z77.22)
exposure to tobacco smoke in the perinatal period (P96.81)
history of tobacco dependence (Z87.891)
infectious agent (B95-B97)
occupational exposure to environmental tobacco smoke (Z57.31)
tobacco dependence (F17.-)
tobacco use (Z72.Ø)

H65.Ø Acute serous otitis media

Acute and subacute secretory otitis

H65.ØØ Acute serous otitis media, unspecified ear
H65.Ø1 Acute serous otitis media, right ear
H65.Ø2 Acute serous otitis media, left ear
H65.Ø3 Acute serous otitis media, bilateral
H65.Ø4 Acute serous otitis media, recurrent, right ear
H65.Ø5 Acute serous otitis media, recurrent, left ear
H65.Ø6 Acute serous otitis media, recurrent, bilateral
H65.Ø7 Acute serous otitis media, recurrent, unspecified ear

H65.1 Other acute nonsuppurative otitis media

EXCLUDES 1 *otitic barotrauma (T7Ø.Ø)*
otitis media (acute) NOS (H66.9)

H65.11 Acute and subacute allergic otitis media (mucoid) (sanguinous) (serous)
H65.111 Acute and subacute allergic otitis media (mucoid) (sanguinous) (serous), right ear
H65.112 Acute and subacute allergic otitis media (mucoid) (sanguinous) (serous), left ear
H65.113 Acute and subacute allergic otitis media (mucoid) (sanguinous) (serous), bilateral
H65.114 Acute and subacute allergic otitis media (mucoid) (sanguinous) (serous), recurrent, right ear
H65.115 Acute and subacute allergic otitis media (mucoid) (sanguinous) (serous), recurrent, left ear
H65.116 Acute and subacute allergic otitis media (mucoid) (sanguinous) (serous), recurrent, bilateral
H65.117 Acute and subacute allergic otitis media (mucoid) (sanguinous) (serous), recurrent, unspecified ear
H65.119 Acute and subacute allergic otitis media (mucoid) (sanguinous) (serous), unspecified ear

H65.19 Other acute nonsuppurative otitis media

Acute and subacute mucoid otitis media
Acute and subacute nonsuppurative otitis media NOS
Acute and subacute sanguinous otitis media
Acute and subacute seromucinous otitis media

H65.191 Other acute nonsuppurative otitis media, right ear
H65.192 Other acute nonsuppurative otitis media, left ear
H65.193 Other acute nonsuppurative otitis media, bilateral
H65.194 Other acute nonsuppurative otitis media, recurrent, right ear
H65.195 Other acute nonsuppurative otitis media, recurrent, left ear
H65.196 Other acute nonsuppurative otitis media, recurrent, bilateral
H65.197 Other acute nonsuppurative otitis media recurrent, unspecified ear
H65.199 Other acute nonsuppurative otitis media, unspecified ear

H65.2 Chronic serous otitis media

Chronic tubotympanal catarrh

H65.2Ø Chronic serous otitis media, unspecified ear
H65.21 Chronic serous otitis media, right ear
H65.22 Chronic serous otitis media, left ear
H65.23 Chronic serous otitis media, bilateral

H65.3 Chronic mucoid otitis media

Chronic mucinous otitis media
Chronic secretory otitis media
Chronic transudative otitis media
Glue ear

EXCLUDES 1 *adhesive middle ear disease (H74.1)*

H65.3Ø Chronic mucoid otitis media, unspecified ear
H65.31 Chronic mucoid otitis media, right ear
H65.32 Chronic mucoid otitis media, left ear
H65.33 Chronic mucoid otitis media, bilateral

H65.4 Other chronic nonsuppurative otitis media

H65.41 Chronic allergic otitis media
H65.411 Chronic allergic otitis media, right ear
H65.412 Chronic allergic otitis media, left ear
H65.413 Chronic allergic otitis media, bilateral
H65.419 Chronic allergic otitis media, unspecified ear

H65.49 Other chronic nonsuppurative otitis media

Chronic exudative otitis media
Chronic nonsuppurative otitis media NOS
Chronic otitis media with effusion (nonpurulent)
Chronic seromucinous otitis media

H65.491 Other chronic nonsuppurative otitis media, right ear
H65.492 Other chronic nonsuppurative otitis media, left ear
H65.493 Other chronic nonsuppurative otitis media, bilateral
H65.499 Other chronic nonsuppurative otitis media, unspecified ear

H65.9 Unspecified nonsuppurative otitis media

Allergic otitis media NOS
Catarrhal otitis media NOS
Exudative otitis media NOS
Mucoid otitis media NOS
Otitis media with effusion (nonpurulent) NOS
Secretory otitis media NOS
Seromucinous otitis media NOS
Serous otitis media NOS
Transudative otitis media NOS

H65.9Ø Unspecified nonsuppurative otitis media, unspecified ear
H65.91 Unspecified nonsuppurative otitis media, right ear
H65.92 Unspecified nonsuppurative otitis media, left ear
H65.93 Unspecified nonsuppurative otitis media, bilateral

H66 Suppurative and unspecified otitis media

INCLUDES suppurative and unspecified otitis media with myringitis

Use additional code to identify:
- exposure to environmental tobacco smoke (Z77.22)
- exposure to tobacco smoke in the perinatal period (P96.81)
- history of tobacco dependence (Z87.891)
- occupational exposure to environmental tobacco smoke (Z57.31)
- tobacco dependence (F17.-)
- tobacco use (Z72.Ø)

AHA: 2016,1Q,34

H66.Ø Acute suppurative otitis media

H66.ØØ Acute suppurative otitis media without spontaneous rupture of ear drum

H66.ØØ1 Acute suppurative otitis media without spontaneous rupture of ear drum, right ear
H66.ØØ2 Acute suppurative otitis media without spontaneous rupture of ear drum, left ear
H66.ØØ3 Acute suppurative otitis media without spontaneous rupture of ear drum, bilateral
H66.ØØ4 Acute suppurative otitis media without spontaneous rupture of ear drum, recurrent, right ear
H66.ØØ5 Acute suppurative otitis media without spontaneous rupture of ear drum, recurrent, left ear
H66.ØØ6 Acute suppurative otitis media without spontaneous rupture of ear drum, recurrent, bilateral
H66.ØØ7 Acute suppurative otitis media without spontaneous rupture of ear drum, recurrent, unspecified ear
H66.ØØ9 Acute suppurative otitis media without spontaneous rupture of ear drum, unspecified ear

H66.Ø1 Acute suppurative otitis media with spontaneous rupture of ear drum

DEF: Sudden, severe inflammation of the middle ear, causing pressure that perforates the ear drum tissue.

H66.Ø11 Acute suppurative otitis media with spontaneous rupture of ear drum, right ear
H66.Ø12 Acute suppurative otitis media with spontaneous rupture of ear drum, left ear
H66.Ø13 Acute suppurative otitis media with spontaneous rupture of ear drum, bilateral
H66.Ø14 Acute suppurative otitis media with spontaneous rupture of ear drum, recurrent, right ear
H66.Ø15 Acute suppurative otitis media with spontaneous rupture of ear drum, recurrent, left ear
H66.Ø16 Acute suppurative otitis media with spontaneous rupture of ear drum, recurrent, bilateral
H66.Ø17 Acute suppurative otitis media with spontaneous rupture of ear drum, recurrent, unspecified ear
H66.Ø19 Acute suppurative otitis media with spontaneous rupture of ear drum, unspecified ear

H66.1 Chronic tubotympanic suppurative otitis media

Benign chronic suppurative otitis media
Chronic tubotympanic disease

Use additional code for any associated perforated tympanic membrane (H72.-)

H66.1Ø Chronic tubotympanic suppurative otitis media, unspecified
H66.11 Chronic tubotympanic suppurative otitis media, right ear
H66.12 Chronic tubotympanic suppurative otitis media, left ear
H66.13 Chronic tubotympanic suppurative otitis media, bilateral

H66.2 Chronic atticoantral suppurative otitis media

Chronic atticoantral disease

Use additional code for any associated perforated tympanic membrane (H72.-)

H66.2Ø Chronic atticoantral suppurative otitis media, unspecified ear
H66.21 Chronic atticoantral suppurative otitis media, right ear
H66.22 Chronic atticoantral suppurative otitis media, left ear
H66.23 Chronic atticoantral suppurative otitis media, bilateral

H66.3 Other chronic suppurative otitis media

Chronic suppurative otitis media NOS

Use additional code for any associated perforated tympanic membrane (H72.-)

EXCLUDES 1 *tuberculous otitis media (A18.6)*

H66.3X Other chronic suppurative otitis media

H66.3X1 Other chronic suppurative otitis media, right ear
H66.3X2 Other chronic suppurative otitis media, left ear
H66.3X3 Other chronic suppurative otitis media, bilateral
H66.3X9 Other chronic suppurative otitis media, unspecified ear

H66.4 Suppurative otitis media, unspecified

Purulent otitis media NOS

Use additional code for any associated perforated tympanic membrane (H72.-)

H66.4Ø Suppurative otitis media, unspecified, unspecified ear
H66.41 Suppurative otitis media, unspecified, right ear
H66.42 Suppurative otitis media, unspecified, left ear
H66.43 Suppurative otitis media, unspecified, bilateral

H66.9 Otitis media, unspecified

Otitis media NOS
Acute otitis media NOS
Chronic otitis media NOS

Use additional code for any associated perforated tympanic membrane (H72.-)

H66.9Ø Otitis media, unspecified, unspecified ear
H66.91 Otitis media, unspecified, right ear
H66.92 Otitis media, unspecified, left ear
H66.93 Otitis media, unspecified, bilateral

H67 Otitis media in diseases classified elsewhere

Code first underlying disease, such as:
- plasminogen deficiency (E88.Ø2)
- viral disease NEC (BØØ-B34)

Use additional code for any associated perforated tympanic membrane (H72.-)

EXCLUDES 1 *otitis media in:*
- *influenza (JØ9.X9, J1Ø.83, J11.83)*
- *measles (BØ5.3)*
- *scarlet fever (A38.Ø)*
- *tuberculosis (A18.6)*

H67.1 *Otitis media in diseases classified elsewhere, right ear*
H67.2 *Otitis media in diseases classified elsewhere, left ear*
H67.3 *Otitis media in diseases classified elsewhere, bilateral*
H67.9 *Otitis media in diseases classified elsewhere, unspecified ear*

H68 Eustachian salpingitis and obstruction

DEF: Eustachian tube: Internal channel between the tympanic cavity and the nasopharynx that equalizes internal pressure to the outside pressure and drains mucous production from the middle ear.

H68.Ø Eustachian salpingitis

H68.ØØ Unspecified Eustachian salpingitis

H68.ØØ1 Unspecified Eustachian salpingitis, right ear
H68.ØØ2 Unspecified Eustachian salpingitis, left ear
H68.ØØ3 Unspecified Eustachian salpingitis, bilateral
H68.ØØ9 Unspecified Eustachian salpingitis, unspecified ear

H68.Ø1 Acute Eustachian salpingitis

H68.Ø11 Acute Eustachian salpingitis, right ear
H68.Ø12 Acute Eustachian salpingitis, left ear
H68.Ø13 Acute Eustachian salpingitis, bilateral
H68.Ø19 Acute Eustachian salpingitis, unspecified ear

H68.Ø2 Chronic Eustachian salpingitis

H68.Ø21 Chronic Eustachian salpingitis, right ear
H68.Ø22 Chronic Eustachian salpingitis, left ear

Chapter 8. Diseases of the Ear and Mastoid Process

H66–H68.Ø22

H68.023 Chronic Eustachian salpingitis, bilateral
H68.029 Chronic Eustachian salpingitis, unspecified ear

H68.1 Obstruction of Eustachian tube
Stenosis of Eustachian tube
Stricture of Eustachian tube

H68.10 Unspecified obstruction of Eustachian tube
H68.101 Unspecified obstruction of Eustachian tube, right ear
H68.102 Unspecified obstruction of Eustachian tube, left ear
H68.103 Unspecified obstruction of Eustachian tube, bilateral
H68.109 Unspecified obstruction of Eustachian tube, unspecified ear

H68.11 Osseous obstruction of Eustachian tube
H68.111 Osseous obstruction of Eustachian tube, right ear
H68.112 Osseous obstruction of Eustachian tube, left ear
H68.113 Osseous obstruction of Eustachian tube, bilateral
H68.119 Osseous obstruction of Eustachian tube, unspecified ear

H68.12 Intrinsic cartilagenous obstruction of Eustachian tube
H68.121 Intrinsic cartilagenous obstruction of Eustachian tube, right ear
H68.122 Intrinsic cartilagenous obstruction of Eustachian tube, left ear
H68.123 Intrinsic cartilagenous obstruction of Eustachian tube, bilateral
H68.129 Intrinsic cartilagenous obstruction of Eustachian tube, unspecified ear

H68.13 Extrinsic cartilagenous obstruction of Eustachian tube
Compression of Eustachian tube
H68.131 Extrinsic cartilagenous obstruction of Eustachian tube, right ear
H68.132 Extrinsic cartilagenous obstruction of Eustachian tube, left ear
H68.133 Extrinsic cartilagenous obstruction of Eustachian tube, bilateral
H68.139 Extrinsic cartilagenous obstruction of Eustachian tube, unspecified ear

H69 Other and unspecified disorders of Eustachian tube
DEF: Eustachian tube: Internal channel between the tympanic cavity and the nasopharynx that equalizes internal pressure to the outside pressure and drains mucous production from the middle ear.

H69.0 Patulous Eustachian tube
H69.00 Patulous Eustachian tube, unspecified ear
H69.01 Patulous Eustachian tube, right ear
H69.02 Patulous Eustachian tube, left ear
H69.03 Patulous Eustachian tube, bilateral

H69.8 Other specified disorders of Eustachian tube
H69.80 Other specified disorders of Eustachian tube, unspecified ear
H69.81 Other specified disorders of Eustachian tube, right ear
H69.82 Other specified disorders of Eustachian tube, left ear
H69.83 Other specified disorders of Eustachian tube, bilateral

H69.9 Unspecified Eustachian tube disorder
H69.90 Unspecified Eustachian tube disorder, unspecified ear
H69.91 Unspecified Eustachian tube disorder, right ear
H69.92 Unspecified Eustachian tube disorder, left ear
H69.93 Unspecified Eustachian tube disorder, bilateral

H70 Mastoiditis and related conditions

H70.0 Acute mastoiditis
Abscess of mastoid
Empyema of mastoid

H70.00 Acute mastoiditis without complications
H70.001 Acute mastoiditis without complications, right ear
H70.002 Acute mastoiditis without complications, left ear
H70.003 Acute mastoiditis without complications, bilateral
H70.009 Acute mastoiditis without complications, unspecified ear

H70.01 Subperiosteal abscess of mastoid
H70.011 Subperiosteal abscess of mastoid, right ear
H70.012 Subperiosteal abscess of mastoid, left ear
H70.013 Subperiosteal abscess of mastoid, bilateral
H70.019 Subperiosteal abscess of mastoid, unspecified ear

H70.09 Acute mastoiditis with other complications
H70.091 Acute mastoiditis with other complications, right ear
H70.092 Acute mastoiditis with other complications, left ear
H70.093 Acute mastoiditis with other complications, bilateral
H70.099 Acute mastoiditis with other complications, unspecified ear

H70.1 Chronic mastoiditis
Caries of mastoid
Fistula of mastoid
EXCLUDES 1 *tuberculous mastoiditis (A18.03)*
H70.10 Chronic mastoiditis, unspecified ear
H70.11 Chronic mastoiditis, right ear
H70.12 Chronic mastoiditis, left ear
H70.13 Chronic mastoiditis, bilateral

H70.2 Petrositis
Inflammation of petrous bone

H70.20 Unspecified petrositis
H70.201 Unspecified petrositis, right ear
H70.202 Unspecified petrositis, left ear
H70.203 Unspecified petrositis, bilateral
H70.209 Unspecified petrositis, unspecified ear

H70.21 Acute petrositis
DEF: Sudden, severe inflammation of the petrous temporal bone behind the ear, associated with a middle ear infection.
H70.211 Acute petrositis, right ear
H70.212 Acute petrositis, left ear
H70.213 Acute petrositis, bilateral
H70.219 Acute petrositis, unspecified ear

H70.22 Chronic petrositis
H70.221 Chronic petrositis, right ear
H70.222 Chronic petrositis, left ear
H70.223 Chronic petrositis, bilateral
H70.229 Chronic petrositis, unspecified ear

H70.8 Other mastoiditis and related conditions
EXCLUDES 1 *preauricular sinus and cyst (Q18.1)*
sinus, fistula, and cyst of branchial cleft (Q18.0)

H70.81 Postauricular fistula
H70.811 Postauricular fistula, right ear
H70.812 Postauricular fistula, left ear
H70.813 Postauricular fistula, bilateral
H70.819 Postauricular fistula, unspecified ear

H70.89 Other mastoiditis and related conditions
H70.891 Other mastoiditis and related conditions, right ear
H70.892 Other mastoiditis and related conditions, left ear
H70.893 Other mastoiditis and related conditions, bilateral
H70.899 Other mastoiditis and related conditions, unspecified ear

H70.9 Unspecified mastoiditis
H70.90 Unspecified mastoiditis, unspecified ear
H70.91 Unspecified mastoiditis, right ear
H70.92 Unspecified mastoiditis, left ear
H70.93 Unspecified mastoiditis, bilateral

4th H71 Cholesteatoma of middle ear

EXCLUDES 2 *cholesteatoma of external ear (H60.4-)*
recurrent cholesteatoma of postmastoidectomy cavity (H95.0-)

AHA: 2021,3Q,8

DEF: Cholesteatoma: Noncancerous cyst-like mass of cell debris, including cholesterol and epithelial cells resulting from trauma, repeated or improperly healed infections, and congenital enclosure of epidermal cells.

Cholesteatoma of Middle Ear

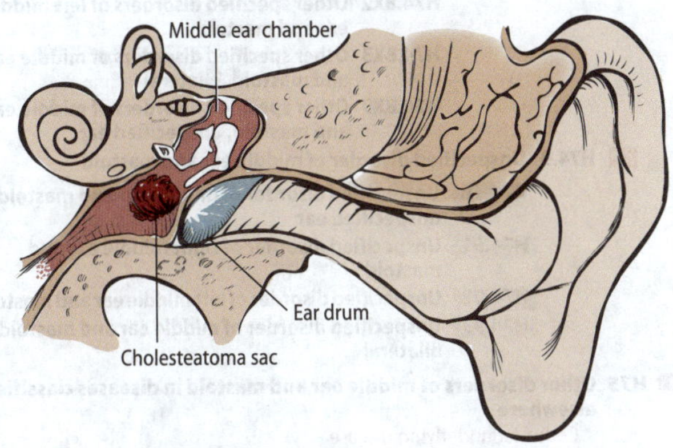

5th H71.0 Cholesteatoma of attic
- **H71.00 Cholesteatoma of attic, unspecified ear**
- **H71.01 Cholesteatoma of attic, right ear**
- **H71.02 Cholesteatoma of attic, left ear**
- **H71.03 Cholesteatoma of attic, bilateral**

5th H71.1 Cholesteatoma of tympanum
- **H71.10 Cholesteatoma of tympanum, unspecified ear**
- **H71.11 Cholesteatoma of tympanum, right ear**
- **H71.12 Cholesteatoma of tympanum, left ear**
- **H71.13 Cholesteatoma of tympanum, bilateral**

5th H71.2 Cholesteatoma of mastoid
- **H71.20 Cholesteatoma of mastoid, unspecified ear**
- **H71.21 Cholesteatoma of mastoid, right ear**
- **H71.22 Cholesteatoma of mastoid, left ear**
- **H71.23 Cholesteatoma of mastoid, bilateral**

5th H71.3 Diffuse cholesteatosis

AHA: 2021,3Q,8
- **H71.30 Diffuse cholesteatosis, unspecified ear**
- **H71.31 Diffuse cholesteatosis, right ear**
- **H71.32 Diffuse cholesteatosis, left ear**
- **H71.33 Diffuse cholesteatosis, bilateral**

5th H71.9 Unspecified cholesteatoma
- **H71.90 Unspecified cholesteatoma, unspecified ear**
- **H71.91 Unspecified cholesteatoma, right ear**
- **H71.92 Unspecified cholesteatoma, left ear**
- **H71.93 Unspecified cholesteatoma, bilateral**

4th H72 Perforation of tympanic membrane

INCLUDES persistent post-traumatic perforation of ear drum
postinflammatory perforation of ear drum

Code first any associated otitis media (H65.-, H66.1-, H66.2-, H66.3-, H66.4-, H66.9-, H67.-)

EXCLUDES 1 *acute suppurative otitis media with rupture of the tympanic membrane (H66.01-)*
traumatic rupture of ear drum (S09.2-)

5th H72.0 Central perforation of tympanic membrane
- **H72.00 Central perforation of tympanic membrane, unspecified ear**
- **H72.01 Central perforation of tympanic membrane, right ear**
- **H72.02 Central perforation of tympanic membrane, left ear**
- **H72.03 Central perforation of tympanic membrane, bilateral**

5th H72.1 Attic perforation of tympanic membrane

Perforation of pars flaccida
- **H72.10 Attic perforation of tympanic membrane, unspecified ear**
- **H72.11 Attic perforation of tympanic membrane, right ear**
- **H72.12 Attic perforation of tympanic membrane, left ear**
- **H72.13 Attic perforation of tympanic membrane, bilateral**

5th H72.2 Other marginal perforations of tympanic membrane

6th H72.2X Other marginal perforations of tympanic membrane
- **H72.2X1 Other marginal perforations of tympanic membrane, right ear**
- **H72.2X2 Other marginal perforations of tympanic membrane, left ear**
- **H72.2X3 Other marginal perforations of tympanic membrane, bilateral**
- **H72.2X9 Other marginal perforations of tympanic membrane, unspecified ear**

5th H72.8 Other perforations of tympanic membrane

6th H72.81 Multiple perforations of tympanic membrane
- **H72.811 Multiple perforations of tympanic membrane, right ear**
- **H72.812 Multiple perforations of tympanic membrane, left ear**
- **H72.813 Multiple perforations of tympanic membrane, bilateral**
- **H72.819 Multiple perforations of tympanic membrane, unspecified ear**

6th H72.82 Total perforations of tympanic membrane
- **H72.821 Total perforations of tympanic membrane, right ear**
- **H72.822 Total perforations of tympanic membrane, left ear**
- **H72.823 Total perforations of tympanic membrane, bilateral**
- **H72.829 Total perforations of tympanic membrane, unspecified ear**

5th H72.9 Unspecified perforation of tympanic membrane
- **H72.90 Unspecified perforation of tympanic membrane, unspecified ear**
- **H72.91 Unspecified perforation of tympanic membrane, right ear**
- **H72.92 Unspecified perforation of tympanic membrane, left ear**
- **H72.93 Unspecified perforation of tympanic membrane, bilateral**

4th H73 Other disorders of tympanic membrane

5th H73.0 Acute myringitis

EXCLUDES 1 *acute myringitis with otitis media (H65, H66)*

6th H73.00 Unspecified acute myringitis

Acute tympanitis NOS
- **H73.001 Acute myringitis, right ear**
- **H73.002 Acute myringitis, left ear**
- **H73.003 Acute myringitis, bilateral**
- **H73.009 Acute myringitis, unspecified ear**

6th H73.01 Bullous myringitis

DEF: Bacterial or viral otitis media that is characterized by the appearance of serous or hemorrhagic blebs on the ear drum and sudden onset of severe pain in ear.
- **H73.011 Bullous myringitis, right ear**
- **H73.012 Bullous myringitis, left ear**
- **H73.013 Bullous myringitis, bilateral**
- **H73.019 Bullous myringitis, unspecified ear**

6th H73.09 Other acute myringitis
- **H73.091 Other acute myringitis, right ear**
- **H73.092 Other acute myringitis, left ear**
- **H73.093 Other acute myringitis, bilateral**
- **H73.099 Other acute myringitis, unspecified ear**

5th H73.1 Chronic myringitis

Chronic tympanitis

EXCLUDES 1 *chronic myringitis with otitis media (H65, H66)*
- **H73.10 Chronic myringitis, unspecified ear**
- **H73.11 Chronic myringitis, right ear**
- **H73.12 Chronic myringitis, left ear**
- **H73.13 Chronic myringitis, bilateral**

5th H73.2 Unspecified myringitis
- **H73.20 Unspecified myringitis, unspecified ear**
- **H73.21 Unspecified myringitis, right ear**
- **H73.22 Unspecified myringitis, left ear**
- **H73.23 Unspecified myringitis, bilateral**

5th H73.8 Other specified disorders of tympanic membrane

6th H73.81 Atrophic flaccid tympanic membrane
- **H73.811 Atrophic flaccid tympanic membrane, right ear**

H73.812 Atrophic flaccid tympanic membrane, left ear

H73.813 Atrophic flaccid tympanic membrane, bilateral

H73.819 Atrophic flaccid tympanic membrane, unspecified ear

6th H73.82 Atrophic nonflaccid tympanic membrane

H73.821 Atrophic nonflaccid tympanic membrane, right ear

H73.822 Atrophic nonflaccid tympanic membrane, left ear

H73.823 Atrophic nonflaccid tympanic membrane, bilateral

H73.829 Atrophic nonflaccid tympanic membrane, unspecified ear

6th H73.89 Other specified disorders of tympanic membrane

H73.891 Other specified disorders of tympanic membrane, right ear

H73.892 Other specified disorders of tympanic membrane, left ear

H73.893 Other specified disorders of tympanic membrane, bilateral

H73.899 Other specified disorders of tympanic membrane, unspecified ear

5th H73.9 Unspecified disorder of tympanic membrane

H73.90 Unspecified disorder of tympanic membrane, unspecified ear

H73.91 Unspecified disorder of tympanic membrane, right ear

H73.92 Unspecified disorder of tympanic membrane, left ear

H73.93 Unspecified disorder of tympanic membrane, bilateral

4th **H74 Other disorders of middle ear mastoid**

EXCLUDES 2 *mastoiditis (H70.-)*

5th H74.0 Tympanosclerosis

DEF: Calcification of tissue in the ear drum, middle ear bones, and middle ear canal.

H74.01 Tympanosclerosis, right ear

H74.02 Tympanosclerosis, left ear

H74.03 Tympanosclerosis, bilateral

H74.09 Tympanosclerosis, unspecified ear

5th H74.1 Adhesive middle ear disease

Adhesive otitis

EXCLUDES 1 *glue ear (H65.3-)*

H74.11 Adhesive right middle ear disease

H74.12 Adhesive left middle ear disease

H74.13 Adhesive middle ear disease, bilateral

H74.19 Adhesive middle ear disease, unspecified ear

5th H74.2 Discontinuity and dislocation of ear ossicles

H74.20 Discontinuity and dislocation of ear ossicles, unspecified ear

H74.21 Discontinuity and dislocation of right ear ossicles

H74.22 Discontinuity and dislocation of left ear ossicles

H74.23 Discontinuity and dislocation of ear ossicles, bilateral

5th H74.3 Other acquired abnormalities of ear ossicles

6th H74.31 Ankylosis of ear ossicles

H74.311 Ankylosis of ear ossicles, right ear

H74.312 Ankylosis of ear ossicles, left ear

H74.313 Ankylosis of ear ossicles, bilateral

H74.319 Ankylosis of ear ossicles, unspecified ear

6th H74.32 Partial loss of ear ossicles

H74.321 Partial loss of ear ossicles, right ear

H74.322 Partial loss of ear ossicles, left ear

H74.323 Partial loss of ear ossicles, bilateral

H74.329 Partial loss of ear ossicles, unspecified ear

6th H74.39 Other acquired abnormalities of ear ossicles

H74.391 Other acquired abnormalities of right ear ossicles

H74.392 Other acquired abnormalities of left ear ossicles

H74.393 Other acquired abnormalities of ear ossicles, bilateral

H74.399 Other acquired abnormalities of ear ossicles, unspecified ear

5th H74.4 Polyp of middle ear

H74.40 Polyp of middle ear, unspecified ear

H74.41 Polyp of right middle ear

H74.42 Polyp of left middle ear

H74.43 Polyp of middle ear, bilateral

5th H74.8 Other specified disorders of middle ear and mastoid

6th H74.8X Other specified disorders of middle ear and mastoid

H74.8X1 Other specified disorders of right middle ear and mastoid

H74.8X2 Other specified disorders of left middle ear and mastoid

H74.8X3 Other specified disorders of middle ear and mastoid, bilateral

H74.8X9 Other specified disorders of middle ear and mastoid, unspecified ear

5th H74.9 Unspecified disorder of middle ear and mastoid

H74.90 Unspecified disorder of middle ear and mastoid, unspecified ear

H74.91 Unspecified disorder of right middle ear and mastoid

H74.92 Unspecified disorder of left middle ear and mastoid

H74.93 Unspecified disorder of middle ear and mastoid, bilateral

4th **H75 Other disorders of middle ear and mastoid in diseases classified elsewhere**

Code first underlying disease

5th H75.0 Mastoiditis in infectious and parasitic diseases classified elsewhere

EXCLUDES 1 *mastoiditis (in):*
syphilis (A52.77)
tuberculosis (A18.03)

H75.00 Mastoiditis in infectious and parasitic diseases classified elsewhere, unspecified ear

H75.01 Mastoiditis in infectious and parasitic diseases classified elsewhere, right ear

H75.02 Mastoiditis in infectious and parasitic diseases classified elsewhere, left ear

H75.03 Mastoiditis in infectious and parasitic diseases classified elsewhere, bilateral

5th H75.8 Other specified disorders of middle ear and mastoid in diseases classified elsewhere

H75.80 Other specified disorders of middle ear and mastoid in diseases classified elsewhere, unspecified ear

H75.81 Other specified disorders of right middle ear and mastoid in diseases classified elsewhere

H75.82 Other specified disorders of left middle ear and mastoid in diseases classified elsewhere

H75.83 Other specified disorders of middle ear and mastoid in diseases classified elsewhere, bilateral

Diseases of inner ear (H80-H83)

4th **H80 Otosclerosis**

INCLUDES otospongiosis

5th H80.0 Otosclerosis involving oval window, nonobliterative

H80.00 Otosclerosis involving oval window, nonobliterative, unspecified ear

H80.01 Otosclerosis involving oval window, nonobliterative, right ear

H80.02 Otosclerosis involving oval window, nonobliterative, left ear

H80.03 Otosclerosis involving oval window, nonobliterative, bilateral

5th H80.1 Otosclerosis involving oval window, obliterative

H80.10 Otosclerosis involving oval window, obliterative, unspecified ear

H80.11 Otosclerosis involving oval window, obliterative, right ear

H80.12 Otosclerosis involving oval window, obliterative, left ear

H80.13 Otosclerosis involving oval window, obliterative, bilateral

5th H80.2 Cochlear otosclerosis

Otosclerosis involving otic capsule
Otosclerosis involving round window

H80.20 Cochlear otosclerosis, unspecified ear

H80.21 Cochlear otosclerosis, right ear

H80.22 Cochlear otosclerosis, left ear

H80.23 Cochlear otosclerosis, bilateral

H80.8 Other otosclerosis
- **H80.80 Other otosclerosis, unspecified ear**
- **H80.81 Other otosclerosis, right ear**
- **H80.82 Other otosclerosis, left ear**
- **H80.83 Other otosclerosis, bilateral**

H80.9 Unspecified otosclerosis
- **H80.90 Unspecified otosclerosis, unspecified ear**
- **H80.91 Unspecified otosclerosis, right ear**
- **H80.92 Unspecified otosclerosis, left ear**
- **H80.93 Unspecified otosclerosis, bilateral**

H81 Disorders of vestibular function

EXCLUDES 1 *epidemic vertigo (A88.1)*
vertigo NOS (R42)

H81.0 Ménière's disease

Labyrinthine hydrops
Ménière's syndrome or vertigo

DEF: Distended membranous labyrinth of the middle ear from fluctuating pressure of fluid (hydrops) that causes vertigo, tinnitus, pressure, and hearing loss that may last on and off for several hours. Episodes may occur in clusters or may subside for weeks, months, or even years.

- **H81.01 Ménière's disease, right ear**
- **H81.02 Ménière's disease, left ear**
- **H81.03 Ménière's disease, bilateral**
- **H81.09 Ménière's disease, unspecified ear**

H81.1 Benign paroxysmal vertigo
- **H81.10 Benign paroxysmal vertigo, unspecified ear** Q
- **H81.11 Benign paroxysmal vertigo, right ear** Q
- **H81.12 Benign paroxysmal vertigo, left ear** Q
- **H81.13 Benign paroxysmal vertigo, bilateral** Q

H81.2 Vestibular neuronitis

DEF: Transient benign vertigo caused by inflammation of the vestibular nerve. It is characterized by response to caloric stimulation on one side and nystagmus with rhythmic movement of the eyes. Normal auditory function is present.

- **H81.20 Vestibular neuronitis, unspecified ear**
- **H81.21 Vestibular neuronitis, right ear**
- **H81.22 Vestibular neuronitis, left ear**
- **H81.23 Vestibular neuronitis, bilateral**

H81.3 Other peripheral vertigo

H81.31 Aural vertigo
- **H81.311 Aural vertigo, right ear**
- **H81.312 Aural vertigo, left ear**
- **H81.313 Aural vertigo, bilateral**
- **H81.319 Aural vertigo, unspecified ear**

H81.39 Other peripheral vertigo

Lermoyez' syndrome
Otogenic vertigo
Peripheral vertigo NOS

- **H81.391 Other peripheral vertigo, right ear**
- **H81.392 Other peripheral vertigo, left ear**
- **H81.393 Other peripheral vertigo, bilateral**
- **H81.399 Other peripheral vertigo, unspecified ear**

H81.4 Vertigo of central origin

Central positional nystagmus

H81.8 Other disorders of vestibular function

H81.8X Other disorders of vestibular function
- **H81.8X1 Other disorders of vestibular function, right ear**
- **H81.8X2 Other disorders of vestibular function, left ear**
- **H81.8X3 Other disorders of vestibular function, bilateral**
- **H81.8X9 Other disorders of vestibular function, unspecified ear**

AHA: 2022,2Q,12

H81.9 Unspecified disorder of vestibular function

Vertiginous syndrome NOS

- **H81.90 Unspecified disorder of vestibular function, unspecified ear**
- **H81.91 Unspecified disorder of vestibular function, right ear**
- **H81.92 Unspecified disorder of vestibular function, left ear**
- **H81.93 Unspecified disorder of vestibular function, bilateral**

H82 Vertiginous syndromes in diseases classified elsewhere

Code first underlying disease

EXCLUDES 1 *epidemic vertigo (A88.1)*

- *H82.1* **Vertiginous syndromes in diseases classified elsewhere, right ear**
- *H82.2* **Vertiginous syndromes in diseases classified elsewhere, left ear**
- *H82.3* **Vertiginous syndromes in diseases classified elsewhere, bilateral**
- *H82.9* **Vertiginous syndromes in diseases classified elsewhere, unspecified ear**

H83 Other diseases of inner ear

H83.0 Labyrinthitis

DEF: Inflammation of the inner ear, or labyrinth, characterized by pus, vertigo, dizziness, nausea, and hearing loss.

- **H83.01 Labyrinthitis, right ear**
- **H83.02 Labyrinthitis, left ear**
- **H83.03 Labyrinthitis, bilateral**
- **H83.09 Labyrinthitis, unspecified ear**

H83.1 Labyrinthine fistula
- **H83.11 Labyrinthine fistula, right ear**
- **H83.12 Labyrinthine fistula, left ear**
- **H83.13 Labyrinthine fistula, bilateral**
- **H83.19 Labyrinthine fistula, unspecified ear**

H83.2 Labyrinthine dysfunction

Labyrinthine hypersensitivity
Labyrinthine hypofunction
Labyrinthine loss of function

DEF: Decreased function of the labyrinth sensors.

H83.2X Labyrinthine dysfunction
- **H83.2X1 Labyrinthine dysfunction, right ear**
- **H83.2X2 Labyrinthine dysfunction, left ear**
- **H83.2X3 Labyrinthine dysfunction, bilateral**
- **H83.2X9 Labyrinthine dysfunction, unspecified ear**

H83.3 Noise effects on inner ear

Acoustic trauma of inner ear
Noise-induced hearing loss of inner ear

H83.3X Noise effects on inner ear
- **H83.3X1 Noise effects on right inner ear**
- **H83.3X2 Noise effects on left inner ear**
- **H83.3X3 Noise effects on inner ear, bilateral**
- **H83.3X9 Noise effects on inner ear, unspecified ear**

H83.8 Other specified diseases of inner ear

H83.8X Other specified diseases of inner ear
- **H83.8X1 Other specified diseases of right inner ear**
- **H83.8X2 Other specified diseases of left inner ear**
- **H83.8X3 Other specified diseases of inner ear, bilateral**
- **H83.8X9 Other specified diseases of inner ear, unspecified ear**

H83.9 Unspecified disease of inner ear
- **H83.90 Unspecified disease of inner ear, unspecified ear**
- **H83.91 Unspecified disease of right inner ear**
- **H83.92 Unspecified disease of left inner ear**
- **H83.93 Unspecified disease of inner ear, bilateral**

Other disorders of ear (H90-H94)

H90 Conductive and sensorineural hearing loss

EXCLUDES 1 *deaf nonspeaking NEC (H91.3)*
deafness NOS (H91.9-)
hearing loss NOS (H91.9-)
noise-induced hearing loss (H83.3-)
ototoxic hearing loss (H91.0-)
sudden (idiopathic) hearing loss (H91.2-)

AHA: 2015,2Q,7

DEF: Conductive hearing loss: Hearing loss due to the inability of soundwaves to move from the outer (external) ear to the inner ear.
DEF: Sensorineural hearing loss: Hearing loss that occurs from damage to the hair cells of the inner ear or problems with the nerve pathways from the inner ear to the brain.

H90.0 Conductive hearing loss, bilateral

H90.1 **Conductive hearing loss, unilateral with unrestricted hearing on the contralateral side**

H90.11 **Conductive hearing loss, unilateral, right ear, with unrestricted hearing on the contralateral side**

H90.12 **Conductive hearing loss, unilateral, left ear, with unrestricted hearing on the contralateral side**

H90.2 **Conductive hearing loss, unspecified**

Conductive deafness NOS

H90.3 **Sensorineural hearing loss, bilateral**

H90.4 **Sensorineural hearing loss, unilateral with unrestricted hearing on the contralateral side**

H90.41 **Sensorineural hearing loss, unilateral, right ear, with unrestricted hearing on the contralateral side**

H90.42 **Sensorineural hearing loss, unilateral, left ear, with unrestricted hearing on the contralateral side**

H90.5 **Unspecified sensorineural hearing loss**

Central hearing loss NOS
Congenital deafness NOS
Neural hearing loss NOS
Perceptive hearing loss NOS
Sensorineural deafness NOS
Sensory hearing loss NOS

EXCLUDES 1 *abnormal auditory perception (H93.2-)*
psychogenic deafness (F44.6)

H90.6 **Mixed conductive and sensorineural hearing loss, bilateral**

AHA: 2015,2Q,7

H90.7 **Mixed conductive and sensorineural hearing loss, unilateral with unrestricted hearing on the contralateral side**

H90.71 **Mixed conductive and sensorineural hearing loss, unilateral, right ear, with unrestricted hearing on the contralateral side**

H90.72 **Mixed conductive and sensorineural hearing loss, unilateral, left ear, with unrestricted hearing on the contralateral side**

H90.8 **Mixed conductive and sensorineural hearing loss, unspecified**

H90.A **Conductive and sensorineural hearing loss with restricted hearing on the contralateral side**

AHA: 2016,4Q,23-25

H90.A1 **Conductive hearing loss, unilateral, with restricted hearing on the contralateral side**

H90.A11 **Conductive hearing loss, unilateral, right ear with restricted hearing on the contralateral side**

H90.A12 **Conductive hearing loss, unilateral, left ear with restricted hearing on the contralateral side**

H90.A2 **Sensorineural hearing loss, unilateral, with restricted hearing on the contralateral side**

H90.A21 **Sensorineural hearing loss, unilateral, right ear, with restricted hearing on the contralateral side**

H90.A22 **Sensorineural hearing loss, unilateral, left ear, with restricted hearing on the contralateral side**

H90.A3 **Mixed conductive and sensorineural hearing loss, unilateral with restricted hearing on the contralateral side**

H90.A31 **Mixed conductive and sensorineural hearing loss, unilateral, right ear with restricted hearing on the contralateral side**

H90.A32 **Mixed conductive and sensorineural hearing, unilateral, left ear with restricted hearing on the contralateral side**

H91 **Other and unspecified hearing loss**

EXCLUDES 1 *abnormal auditory perception (H93.2-)*
hearing loss as classified in H90.-
impacted cerumen (H61.2-)
noise-induced hearing loss (H83.3-)
psychogenic deafness (F44.6)
transient ischemic deafness (H93.01-)

H91.0 **Ototoxic hearing loss**

Code first poisoning due to drug or toxin, if applicable (T36-T65 with fifth or sixth character 1-4 or 6)

Use additional code for adverse effect, if applicable, to identify drug (T36-T50 with fifth or sixth character 5)

H91.01 **Ototoxic hearing loss, right ear**

H91.02 **Ototoxic hearing loss, left ear**

H91.03 **Ototoxic hearing loss, bilateral**

H91.09 **Ototoxic hearing loss, unspecified ear**

H91.1 **Presbycusis**

Presbyacusia

H91.10 **Presbycusis, unspecified ear**

H91.11 **Presbycusis, right ear**

H91.12 **Presbycusis, left ear**

H91.13 **Presbycusis, bilateral**

H91.2 **Sudden idiopathic hearing loss**

Sudden hearing loss NOS

H91.20 **Sudden idiopathic hearing loss, unspecified ear**

H91.21 **Sudden idiopathic hearing loss, right ear**

H91.22 **Sudden idiopathic hearing loss, left ear**

H91.23 **Sudden idiopathic hearing loss, bilateral**

H91.3 **Deaf nonspeaking, not elsewhere classified**

H91.8 **Other specified hearing loss**

H91.8X **Other specified hearing loss**

H91.8X1 **Other specified hearing loss, right ear**

H91.8X2 **Other specified hearing loss, left ear**

H91.8X3 **Other specified hearing loss, bilateral**

H91.8X9 **Other specified hearing loss, unspecified ear**

H91.9 **Unspecified hearing loss**

Deafness NOS
High frequency deafness
Low frequency deafness

H91.90 **Unspecified hearing loss, unspecified ear**

H91.91 **Unspecified hearing loss, right ear**

H91.92 **Unspecified hearing loss, left ear**

H91.93 **Unspecified hearing loss, bilateral**

H92 **Otalgia and effusion of ear**

H92.0 **Otalgia**

H92.01 **Otalgia, right ear**

H92.02 **Otalgia, left ear**

H92.03 **Otalgia, bilateral**

H92.09 **Otalgia, unspecified ear**

H92.1 **Otorrhea**

EXCLUDES 1 *leakage of cerebrospinal fluid through ear (G96.0)*

H92.10 **Otorrhea, unspecified ear**

H92.11 **Otorrhea, right ear**

H92.12 **Otorrhea, left ear**

H92.13 **Otorrhea, bilateral**

H92.2 **Otorrhagia**

EXCLUDES 1 *traumatic otorrhagia - code to injury*

H92.20 **Otorrhagia, unspecified ear**

H92.21 **Otorrhagia, right ear**

H92.22 **Otorrhagia, left ear**

H92.23 **Otorrhagia, bilateral**

H93 **Other disorders of ear, not elsewhere classified**

H93.0 **Degenerative and vascular disorders of ear**

EXCLUDES 1 *presbycusis (H91.1)*

H93.01 **Transient ischemic deafness**

H93.011 **Transient ischemic deafness, right ear**

H93.012 **Transient ischemic deafness, left ear**

H93.013 **Transient ischemic deafness, bilateral**

H93.019 **Transient ischemic deafness, unspecified ear**

H93.09 **Unspecified degenerative and vascular disorders of ear**

H93.091 **Unspecified degenerative and vascular disorders of right ear**

H93.092 **Unspecified degenerative and vascular disorders of left ear**

H93.093 **Unspecified degenerative and vascular disorders of ear, bilateral**

H93.099 **Unspecified degenerative and vascular disorders of unspecified ear**

H93.1 **Tinnitus**

H93.11 **Tinnitus, right ear**

H93.12 **Tinnitus, left ear**

H93.13 **Tinnitus, bilateral**

H93.19 **Tinnitus, unspecified ear**

H93.A **Pulsatile tinnitus**

AHA: 2016,4Q,25-26

H93.A1 **Pulsatile tinnitus, right ear**

H93.A2 **Pulsatile tinnitus, left ear**

H93.A3 **Pulsatile tinnitus, bilateral**

H93.A9 Pulsatile tinnitus, unspecified ear

H93.2 Other abnormal auditory perceptions

EXCLUDES 2 *auditory hallucinations (R44.Ø)*

H93.21 Auditory recruitment

H93.211 Auditory recruitment, right ear

H93.212 Auditory recruitment, left ear

H93.213 Auditory recruitment, bilateral

H93.219 Auditory recruitment, unspecified ear

H93.22 Diplacusis

H93.221 Diplacusis, right ear

H93.222 Diplacusis, left ear

H93.223 Diplacusis, bilateral

H93.229 Diplacusis, unspecified ear

H93.23 Hyperacusis

DEF: Exceptionally acute sense of hearing caused by such conditions as Bell's palsy. This term may also refer to painful sensitivity to sounds.

H93.231 Hyperacusis, right ear

H93.232 Hyperacusis, left ear

H93.233 Hyperacusis, bilateral

H93.239 Hyperacusis, unspecified ear

H93.24 Temporary auditory threshold shift

H93.241 Temporary auditory threshold shift, right ear

H93.242 Temporary auditory threshold shift, left ear

H93.243 Temporary auditory threshold shift, bilateral

H93.249 Temporary auditory threshold shift, unspecified ear

H93.25 Central auditory processing disorder

Congenital auditory imperception

Word deafness

EXCLUDES 1 *mixed receptive-expressive language disorder (F8Ø.2)*

H93.29 Other abnormal auditory perceptions

H93.291 Other abnormal auditory perceptions, right ear

H93.292 Other abnormal auditory perceptions, left ear

H93.293 Other abnormal auditory perceptions, bilateral

H93.299 Other abnormal auditory perceptions, unspecified ear

H93.3 Disorders of acoustic nerve

Disorder of 8th cranial nerve

EXCLUDES 1 *acoustic neuroma (D33.3)*

syphilitic acoustic neuritis (A52.15)

H93.3X Disorders of acoustic nerve

H93.3X1 Disorders of right acoustic nerve

H93.3X2 Disorders of left acoustic nerve

H93.3X3 Disorders of bilateral acoustic nerves

H93.3X9 Disorders of unspecified acoustic nerve

H93.8 Other specified disorders of ear

H93.8X Other specified disorders of ear

H93.8X1 Other specified disorders of right ear

H93.8X2 Other specified disorders of left ear

H93.8X3 Other specified disorders of ear, bilateral

H93.8X9 Other specified disorders of ear, unspecified ear

H93.9 Unspecified disorder of ear

H93.9Ø Unspecified disorder of ear, unspecified ear

H93.91 Unspecified disorder of right ear

H93.92 Unspecified disorder of left ear

H93.93 Unspecified disorder of ear, bilateral

H94 Other disorders of ear in diseases classified elsewhere

H94.Ø Acoustic neuritis in infectious and parasitic diseases classified elsewhere

Code first underlying disease, such as:
parasitic disease (B65-B89)

EXCLUDES 1 *acoustic neuritis (in):*

herpes zoster (BØ2.29)

syphilis (A52.15)

H94.ØØ Acoustic neuritis in infectious and parasitic diseases classified elsewhere, unspecified ear

H94.Ø1 Acoustic neuritis in infectious and parasitic diseases classified elsewhere, right ear

H94.Ø2 Acoustic neuritis in infectious and parasitic diseases classified elsewhere, left ear

H94.Ø3 Acoustic neuritis in infectious and parasitic diseases classified elsewhere, bilateral

H94.8 Other specified disorders of ear in diseases classified elsewhere

Code first underlying disease, such as:
congenital syphilis (A5Ø.Ø)

EXCLUDES 1 *aural myiasis (B87.4)*

syphilitic labyrinthitis (A52.79)

H94.8Ø Other specified disorders of ear in diseases classified elsewhere, unspecified ear

H94.81 Other specified disorders of right ear in diseases classified elsewhere

H94.82 Other specified disorders of left ear in diseases classified elsewhere

H94.83 Other specified disorders of ear in diseases classified elsewhere, bilateral

Intraoperative and postprocedural complications and disorders of ear and mastoid process, not elsewhere classified (H95)

H95 Intraoperative and postprocedural complications and disorders of ear and mastoid process, not elsewhere classified

AHA: 2016,4Q,9-10

H95.Ø Recurrent cholesteatoma of postmastoidectomy cavity

H95.ØØ Recurrent cholesteatoma of postmastoidectomy cavity, unspecified ear

H95.Ø1 Recurrent cholesteatoma of postmastoidectomy cavity, right ear

H95.Ø2 Recurrent cholesteatoma of postmastoidectomy cavity, left ear

H95.Ø3 Recurrent cholesteatoma of postmastoidectomy cavity, bilateral ears

H95.1 Other disorders of ear and mastoid process following mastoidectomy

H95.11 Chronic inflammation of postmastoidectomy cavity

H95.111 Chronic inflammation of postmastoidectomy cavity, right ear

H95.112 Chronic inflammation of postmastoidectomy cavity, left ear

H95.113 Chronic inflammation of postmastoidectomy cavity, bilateral ears

H95.119 Chronic inflammation of postmastoidectomy cavity, unspecified ear

H95.12 Granulation of postmastoidectomy cavity

H95.121 Granulation of postmastoidectomy cavity, right ear

H95.122 Granulation of postmastoidectomy cavity, left ear

H95.123 Granulation of postmastoidectomy cavity, bilateral ears

H95.129 Granulation of postmastoidectomy cavity, unspecified ear

H95.13 Mucosal cyst of postmastoidectomy cavity

H95.131 Mucosal cyst of postmastoidectomy cavity, right ear

H95.132 Mucosal cyst of postmastoidectomy cavity, left ear

H95.133 Mucosal cyst of postmastoidectomy cavity, bilateral ears

H95.139 Mucosal cyst of postmastoidectomy cavity, unspecified ear

H95.19 Other disorders following mastoidectomy

H95.191 Other disorders following mastoidectomy, right ear

H95.192 Other disorders following mastoidectomy, left ear

H95.193 Other disorders following mastoidectomy, bilateral ears

H95.199 Other disorders following mastoidectomy, unspecified ear

H95.2 Intraoperative hemorrhage and hematoma of ear and mastoid process complicating a procedure

EXCLUDES 1 *intraoperative hemorrhage and hematoma of ear and mastoid process due to accidental puncture or laceration during a procedure (H95.3-)*

H95.21 Intraoperative hemorrhage and hematoma of ear and mastoid process complicating a procedure on the ear and mastoid process

H95.22 Intraoperative hemorrhage and hematoma of ear and mastoid process complicating other procedure

H95.3 Accidental puncture and laceration of ear and mastoid process during a procedure

H95.31 Accidental puncture and laceration of the ear and mastoid process during a procedure on the ear and mastoid process

H95.32 Accidental puncture and laceration of the ear and mastoid process during other procedure

H95.4 Postprocedural hemorrhage of ear and mastoid process following a procedure

H95.41 Postprocedural hemorrhage of ear and mastoid process following a procedure on the ear and mastoid process

H95.42 Postprocedural hemorrhage of ear and mastoid process following other procedure

H95.5 Postprocedural hematoma and seroma of ear and mastoid process following a procedure

H95.51 Postprocedural hematoma of ear and mastoid process following a procedure on the ear and mastoid process

H95.52 Postprocedural hematoma of ear and mastoid process following other procedure

H95.53 Postprocedural seroma of ear and mastoid process following a procedure on the ear and mastoid process

H95.54 Postprocedural seroma of ear and mastoid process following other procedure

H95.8 Other intraoperative and postprocedural complications and disorders of the ear and mastoid process, not elsewhere classified

EXCLUDES 2 *postprocedural complications and disorders following mastoidectomy (H95.Ø-, H95.1-)*

H95.81 Postprocedural stenosis of external ear canal

H95.811 Postprocedural stenosis of right external ear canal

H95.812 Postprocedural stenosis of left external ear canal

H95.813 Postprocedural stenosis of external ear canal, bilateral

H95.819 Postprocedural stenosis of unspecified external ear canal

H95.88 Other intraoperative complications and disorders of the ear and mastoid process, not elsewhere classified

Use additional code, if applicable, to further specify disorder

H95.89 Other postprocedural complications and disorders of the ear and mastoid process, not elsewhere classified

Use additional code, if applicable, to further specify disorder

Chapter 9. Diseases of the Circulatory System (I00–I99)

Chapter-specific Guidelines with Coding Examples

The chapter-specific guidelines from the ICD-10-CM Official Guidelines for Coding and Reporting have been provided below. Along with these guidelines are coding examples, contained in the shaded boxes, that have been developed to help illustrate the coding and/or sequencing guidance found in these guidelines.

a. Hypertension

The classification presumes a causal relationship between hypertension and heart involvement and between hypertension and kidney involvement, as the two conditions are linked by the term "with" in the Alphabetic Index. These conditions should be coded as related even in the absence of provider documentation explicitly linking them, unless the documentation clearly states the conditions are unrelated.

For hypertension and conditions not specifically linked by relational terms such as "with," "associated with" or "due to" in the classification, provider documentation must link the conditions in order to code them as related.

1) Hypertension with heart disease

Hypertension with heart conditions classified to I50.- or I51.4-I51.7, I51.89, I51.9, are assigned to a code from category I11, Hypertensive heart disease. Use additional code(s) from category I50, Heart failure, to identify the type(s) of heart failure in those patients with heart failure.

The same heart conditions (I50.-, I51.4-I51.7, I51.89, I51.9) with hypertension are coded separately if the provider has documented they are unrelated to the hypertension. Sequence according to the circumstances of the admission/encounter.

2) Hypertensive chronic kidney disease

Assign codes from category I12, Hypertensive chronic kidney disease, when both hypertension and a condition classifiable to category N18, Chronic kidney disease (CKD), are present. CKD should not be coded as hypertensive if the provider indicates the CKD is not related to the hypertension.

The appropriate code from category N18 should be used as a secondary code with a code from category I12 to identify the stage of chronic kidney disease.

See Section I.C.14. Chronic kidney disease.

If a patient has hypertensive chronic kidney disease and acute renal failure, the acute renal failure should also be coded. Sequence according to the circumstances of the admission/encounter.

Patient is admitted with stage IV chronic kidney disease (CKD) due to polycystic kidney disease. Patient also is on lisinopril for hypertension.

N18.4	**Chronic kidney disease, stage 4 (severe)**
Q61.3	**Polycystic kidney, unspecified**
I10	**Essential (primary) hypertension**

Explanation: A combination code describing a relationship between hypertension and CKD is not used because the physician documentation identifies the polycystic kidney disease as the cause for the CKD.

3) Hypertensive heart and chronic kidney disease

Assign codes from combination category I13, Hypertensive heart and chronic kidney disease, when there is hypertension with both heart and kidney involvement. If heart failure is present, assign an additional code from category I50 to identify the type of heart failure.

The appropriate code from category N18, Chronic kidney disease, should be used as a secondary code with a code from category I13 to identify the stage of chronic kidney disease.

See Section I.C.14. Chronic kidney disease.

The codes in category I13, Hypertensive heart and chronic kidney disease, are combination codes that include hypertension, heart disease and chronic kidney disease. The Includes note at I13 specifies that the conditions included at I11 and I12 are included together in I13. If a patient has hypertension, heart disease and chronic kidney disease, then a code from I13 should be used, not individual codes for hypertension, heart disease and chronic kidney disease, or codes from I11 or I12.

For patients with both acute renal failure and chronic kidney disease, the acute renal failure should also be coded. Sequence according to the circumstances of the admission/encounter.

Hypertensive heart and kidney disease with congestive heart failure and stage 2 chronic kidney disease

I13.0	**Hypertensive heart and chronic kidney disease with heart failure and stage 1 through stage 4 chronic kidney disease, or unspecified chronic kidney disease**
I50.9	**Heart failure, unspecified**
N18.2	**Chronic kidney disease, stage 2 (mild)**

Explanation: Combination codes in category I13 are used to report conditions classifiable to *both* categories I11 and I12. Do not report conditions classifiable to I11 and I12 separately. Use additional codes to report type of heart failure and stage of CKD.

4) Hypertensive cerebrovascular disease

For hypertensive cerebrovascular disease, first assign the appropriate code from categories I60-I69, followed by the appropriate hypertension code.

Rupture of cerebral aneurysm caused by malignant hypertension

I60.7	**Nontraumatic subarachnoid hemorrhage from unspecified intracranial artery**
I10	**Essential (primary) hypertension**

Explanation: Hypertensive cerebrovascular disease requires two codes: the appropriate I60–I69 code followed by the appropriate hypertension code.

5) Hypertensive retinopathy

Subcategory H35.0, Background retinopathy and retinal vascular changes, should be used along with a code from categories I10-I15, in the Hypertensive diseases section, to include the systemic hypertension. The sequencing is based on the reason for the encounter.

6) Hypertension, secondary

Secondary hypertension is due to an underlying condition. Two codes are required: one to identify the underlying etiology and one from category I15 to identify the hypertension. Sequencing of codes is determined by the reason for admission/encounter.

Renovascular hypertension due to renal artery atherosclerosis

I15.0	**Renovascular hypertension**
I70.1	**Atherosclerosis of renal artery**

Explanation: Secondary hypertension requires two codes: a code to identify the etiology and the appropriate I15 code.

7) Hypertension, transient

Assign code R03.0, Elevated blood pressure reading without diagnosis of hypertension, unless patient has an established diagnosis of hypertension. Assign code O13.-, Gestational [pregnancy-induced] hypertension without significant proteinuria, or O14.-, Pre-eclampsia, for transient hypertension of pregnancy.

8) Hypertension, controlled

This diagnostic statement usually refers to an existing state of hypertension under control by therapy. Assign the appropriate code from categories I10-I15, Hypertensive diseases.

9) Hypertension, uncontrolled

Uncontrolled hypertension may refer to untreated hypertension or hypertension not responding to current therapeutic regimen. In either case, assign the appropriate code from categories I10-I15, Hypertensive diseases.

10) Hypertensive crisis

Assign a code from category I16, Hypertensive crisis, for documented hypertensive urgency, hypertensive emergency or unspecified hypertensive crisis. Code also any identified hypertensive disease (I10-I15). The sequencing is based on the reason for the encounter.

11) Pulmonary hypertension

Pulmonary hypertension is classified to category I27, Other pulmonary heart diseases. For secondary pulmonary hypertension (I27.1, I27.2-), code also any associated conditions or adverse effects of drugs or toxins. The sequencing is based on the reason for the encounter, except for adverse effects of drugs (See Section I.C.19.e.).

b. Atherosclerotic coronary artery disease and angina

ICD-10-CM has combination codes for atherosclerotic heart disease with angina pectoris. The subcategories for these codes are I25.11, Atherosclerotic heart disease of native coronary artery with angina pectoris and I25.7, Atherosclerosis of coronary artery bypass graft(s) and coronary artery of transplanted heart with angina pectoris.

When using one of these combination codes it is not necessary to use an additional code for angina pectoris. A causal relationship can be assumed in a patient with both atherosclerosis and angina pectoris, unless the documentation indicates the angina is due to something other than the atherosclerosis.

If a patient with coronary artery disease is admitted due to an acute myocardial infarction (AMI), the AMI should be sequenced before the coronary artery disease.

See Section I.C.9. Acute myocardial infarction (AMI)

> Patient is being seen for spastic angina pectoris. She also has a documented history of progressive coronary artery disease of the native vessels.
>
> **I25.111 Atherosclerotic heart disease of native coronary artery with angina pectoris with documented spasm**
>
> *Explanation*: Report the combination code for atherosclerotic heart disease (coronary artery disease) with angina pectoris. A causal relationship is assumed in a patient with both atherosclerosis and angina pectoris, unless the documentation indicates the angina is due to something other than the atherosclerosis. When using one of these combination codes, it is not necessary to use an additional code for angina pectoris.

c. Intraoperative and postprocedural cerebrovascular accident

Medical record documentation should clearly specify the cause- and- effect relationship between the medical intervention and the cerebrovascular accident in order to assign a code for intraoperative or postprocedural cerebrovascular accident.

Proper code assignment depends on whether it was an infarction or hemorrhage and whether it occurred intraoperatively or postoperatively. If it was a cerebral hemorrhage, code assignment depends on the type of procedure performed.

> Embolic cerebral infarction of the right middle cerebral artery that occurred during hip replacement surgery. The surgeon documented as due to the surgery.
>
> **I97.811 Intraoperative cerebrovascular infarction during other surgery**
>
> **I63.411 Cerebral infarction due to embolism of right middle cerebral artery**
>
> *Explanation*: Code assignment for intraoperative or postprocedural cerebrovascular accident is based on the provider's documentation of a cause-and-effect relationship between the condition and the procedure. Proper code assignment also depends on whether the cerebrovascular accident was an infarction or hemorrhage, occurred intraoperatively or postoperatively, and the type of procedure performed.

d. Sequelae of cerebrovascular disease

1) Category I69, Sequelae of cerebrovascular disease

Category I69 is used to indicate conditions classifiable to categories I60-I67 as the causes of sequela (neurologic deficits), themselves classified elsewhere. These "late effects" include neurologic deficits that persist after initial onset of conditions classifiable to categories I60-I67. The neurologic deficits caused by cerebrovascular disease may be present from the onset or may arise at any time after the onset of the condition classifiable to categories I60-I67.

Codes from category I69, Sequelae of cerebrovascular disease, that specify hemiplegia, hemiparesis and monoplegia identify whether the dominant or nondominant side is affected. Should the affected side be documented, but not specified as dominant or nondominant, and the classification system does not indicate a default, code selection is as follows:

- For ambidextrous patients, the default should be dominant.
- If the left side is affected, the default is non-dominant.
- If the right side is affected, the default is dominant.

2) Codes from category I69 with codes from I60–I67

Codes from category I69 may be assigned on a health care record with codes from I60-I67, if the patient has a current cerebrovascular disease and deficits from an old cerebrovascular disease.

3) Codes from category I69 and personal history of transient ischemic attack (TIA) and cerebral infarction (Z86.73)

Codes from category I69 should not be assigned if the patient does not have neurologic deficits.

See Section I.C.21. 4. History (of) for use of personal history codes

e. Acute myocardial infarction (AMI)

1) Type 1 ST elevation myocardial infarction (STEMI) and non-ST elevation myocardial infarction (NSTEMI)

The ICD-10-CM codes for type 1 acute myocardial infarction (AMI) identify the site, such as anterolateral wall or true posterior wall. Subcategories I21.Ø-I21.2 and code I21.3 are used for type 1 ST elevation myocardial infarction (STEMI). Code I21.4, Non-ST elevation (NSTEMI) myocardial infarction, is used for type 1 non-ST elevation myocardial infarction (NSTEMI) and nontransmural MIs.

If a type 1 NSTEMI evolves to STEMI, assign the STEMI code. If a type 1 STEMI converts to NSTEMI due to thrombolytic therapy, it is still coded as STEMI.

For encounters occurring while the myocardial infarction is equal to, or less than, four weeks old, including transfers to another acute setting or a postacute setting, and the myocardial infarction meets the definition for "other diagnoses" (see Section III, Reporting Additional Diagnoses), codes from category I21 may continue to be reported. For encounters after the 4-week time frame and the patient is still receiving care related to the myocardial infarction, the appropriate aftercare code should be assigned, rather than a code from category I21. For old or healed myocardial infarctions not requiring further care, code I25.2, Old myocardial infarction, may be assigned.

2) Acute myocardial infarction, unspecified

Code I21.9, Acute myocardial infarction, unspecified, is the default for unspecified acute myocardial infarction or unspecified type. If only type 1 STEMI or transmural MI without the site is documented, assign code I21.3, ST elevation (STEMI) myocardial infarction of unspecified site.

3) AMI documented as nontransmural or subendocardial but site provided

If an AMI is documented as nontransmural or subendocardial, but the site is provided, it is still coded as a subendocardial AMI.

See Section I.C.21.3.for information on coding status post administration of tPA in a different facility within the last 24 hours.

> Acute inferior subendocardial myocardial infarction (NSTEMI)
>
> **I21.4 Non-ST elevation (NSTEMI) myocardial infarction**
>
> *Explanation*: An AMI documented as subendocardial or nontransmural is coded as such (I21.4, I22.2), even if the site of infarction is specified.

4) Subsequent acute myocardial infarction

A code from category I22, Subsequent ST elevation (STEMI) and non-ST elevation (NSTEMI) myocardial infarction, is to be used when a patient who has suffered a type 1 or unspecified AMI has a new AMI within the 4-week time frame of the initial AMI. A code from category I22 must be used in conjunction with a code from category I21. The sequencing of the I22 and I21 codes depends on the circumstances of the encounter.

Do not assign code I22 for subsequent myocardial infarctions other than type 1 or unspecified. For subsequent type 2 AMI assign only code I21.A1. For subsequent type 4 or type 5 AMI, assign only code I21.A9.

If a subsequent myocardial infarction of one type occurs within 4 weeks of a myocardial infarction of a different type, assign the appropriate codes from category I21 to identify each type. Do not assign a code from I22. Codes from category I22 should only be assigned if both the initial and subsequent myocardial infarctions are type 1 or unspecified.

> Patient suffered an acute NSTEMI 14 days ago and is now seen for an inferior STEMI.
>
> **I22.1 Subsequent ST elevation (STEMI) myocardial infarction of inferior wall**
>
> **I21.4 Non-ST elevation (NSTEMI) myocardial infarction**
>
> *Explanation*: Both MIs were type 1, and the current MI occurred within the four-week time frame; therefore a code for the current/subsequent STEMI (I22.1) is reported as well as a code for the previous NSTEMI (I21.4).

5) Other Types of Myocardial Infarction

The ICD-10-CM provides codes for different types of myocardial infarction. Type 1 myocardial infarctions are assigned to codes I21.Ø-I21.4.

Type 2 myocardial infarction (myocardial infarction due to demand ischemia or secondary to ischemic imbalance) is assigned to code I21.A1, Myocardial infarction type 2 with the underlying cause coded first. Do not assign code I24.8, Other forms of acute ischemic heart disease, for the demand ischemia. If a type 2 AMI is described as NSTEMI or STEMI, only assign code I21.A1. Codes I21.Ø1-I21.4 should only be assigned for type 1 AMIs.

Acute myocardial infarctions type 3, 4a, 4b, 4c and 5 are assigned to code I21.A9, Other myocardial infarction type.

The "Code also" and "Code first" notes should be followed related to complications, and for coding of postprocedural myocardial infarctions during or following cardiac surgery.

Chapter 9. Diseases of the Circulatory System (I00-I99)

EXCLUDES 2 *certain conditions originating in the perinatal period (P04-P96)*
certain infectious and parasitic diseases (A00-B99)
complications of pregnancy, childbirth and the puerperium (O00-O9A)
congenital malformations, deformations, and chromosomal abnormalities (Q00-Q99)
endocrine, nutritional and metabolic diseases (E00-E88)
injury, poisoning and certain other consequences of external causes (S00-T88)
neoplasms (C00-D49)
symptoms, signs and abnormal clinical and laboratory findings, not elsewhere classified (R00-R94)
systemic connective tissue disorders (M30-M36)
transient cerebral ischemic attacks and related syndromes (G45.-)

This chapter contains the following blocks:

- I00-I02 Acute rheumatic fever
- I05-I09 Chronic rheumatic heart diseases
- I10-I16 Hypertensive diseases
- I20-I25 Ischemic heart diseases
- I26-I28 Pulmonary heart disease and diseases of pulmonary circulation
- I30-I5A Other forms of heart disease
- I60-I69 Cerebrovascular diseases
- I70-I79 Diseases of arteries, arterioles and capillaries
- I80-I89 Diseases of veins, lymphatic vessels and lymph nodes, not elsewhere classified
- I95-I99 Other and unspecified disorders of the circulatory system

Acute rheumatic fever (I00-I02)

DEF: Rheumatic fever: Inflammatory disease that can follow a throat infection by group A *streptococci*. Complications can involve the joints (arthritis), subcutaneous tissue (nodules), skin (erythema marginatum), heart (carditis), or brain (chorea).

I00 Rheumatic fever without heart involvement
INCLUDES arthritis, rheumatic, acute or subacute
EXCLUDES 1 *rheumatic fever with heart involvement (I01.0-I01.9)*

✓4th **I01 Rheumatic fever with heart involvement**
EXCLUDES 1 *chronic diseases of rheumatic origin (I05-I09) unless rheumatic fever is also present or there is evidence of reactivation or activity of the rheumatic process*

I01.0 Acute rheumatic pericarditis
Any condition in I00 with pericarditis
Rheumatic pericarditis (acute)
EXCLUDES 1 *acute pericarditis not specified as rheumatic (I30.-)*

I01.1 Acute rheumatic endocarditis
Any condition in I00 with endocarditis or valvulitis
Acute rheumatic valvulitis

I01.2 Acute rheumatic myocarditis
Any condition in I00 with myocarditis

I01.8 Other acute rheumatic heart disease
Any condition in I00 with other or multiple types of heart involvement
Acute rheumatic pancarditis

I01.9 Acute rheumatic heart disease, unspecified
Any condition in I00 with unspecified type of heart involvement
Rheumatic carditis, acute
Rheumatic heart disease, active or acute

✓4th **I02 Rheumatic chorea**
INCLUDES Sydenham's chorea
EXCLUDES 1 *chorea NOS (G25.5)*
Huntington's chorea (G10)

I02.0 Rheumatic chorea with heart involvement
Chorea NOS with heart involvement
Rheumatic chorea with heart involvement of any type classifiable under I01.-

I02.9 Rheumatic chorea without heart involvement
Rheumatic chorea NOS

Chronic rheumatic heart diseases (I05-I09)

✓4th **I05 Rheumatic mitral valve diseases**
INCLUDES conditions classifiable to both I05.0 and I05.2-I05.9, whether specified as rheumatic or not
EXCLUDES 1 *mitral valve disease specified as nonrheumatic (I34.-)*
mitral valve disease with aortic and/or tricuspid valve involvement (I08.-)

I05.0 Rheumatic mitral stenosis
Mitral (valve) obstruction (rheumatic)

I05.1 Rheumatic mitral insufficiency
Rheumatic mitral incompetence
Rheumatic mitral regurgitation
EXCLUDES 1 *mitral insufficiency not specified as rheumatic (I34.0)*

I05.2 Rheumatic mitral stenosis with insufficiency
Rheumatic mitral stenosis with incompetence or regurgitation

I05.8 Other rheumatic mitral valve diseases
Rheumatic mitral (valve) failure

I05.9 Rheumatic mitral valve disease, unspecified
Rheumatic mitral (valve) disorder (chronic) NOS

✓4th **I06 Rheumatic aortic valve diseases**
EXCLUDES 1 *aortic valve disease not specified as rheumatic (I35.-)*
aortic valve disease with mitral and/or tricuspid valve involvement (I08.-)

I06.0 Rheumatic aortic stenosis
Rheumatic aortic (valve) obstruction

I06.1 Rheumatic aortic insufficiency
Rheumatic aortic incompetence
Rheumatic aortic regurgitation

I06.2 Rheumatic aortic stenosis with insufficiency
Rheumatic aortic stenosis with incompetence or regurgitation

I06.8 Other rheumatic aortic valve diseases

I06.9 Rheumatic aortic valve disease, unspecified
Rheumatic aortic (valve) disease NOS

✓4th **I07 Rheumatic tricuspid valve diseases**
INCLUDES rheumatic tricuspid valve diseases specified as rheumatic or unspecified
EXCLUDES 1 *tricuspid valve disease specified as nonrheumatic (I36.-)*
tricuspid valve disease with aortic and/or mitral valve involvement (I08.-)

I07.0 Rheumatic tricuspid stenosis
Tricuspid (valve) stenosis (rheumatic)

I07.1 Rheumatic tricuspid insufficiency
Tricuspid (valve) insufficiency (rheumatic)

I07.2 Rheumatic tricuspid stenosis and insufficiency

I07.8 Other rheumatic tricuspid valve diseases

I07.9 Rheumatic tricuspid valve disease, unspecified
Rheumatic tricuspid valve disorder NOS

✓4th **I08 Multiple valve diseases**
INCLUDES multiple valve diseases specified as rheumatic or unspecified
EXCLUDES 1 *endocarditis, valve unspecified (I38)*
multiple valve disease specified a nonrheumatic (I34.-, I35.-, I36.-, I37.-, I38.-, Q22.-, Q23.-, Q24.8-)
rheumatic valve disease NOS (I09.1)

I08.0 Rheumatic disorders of both mitral and aortic valves
Involvement of both mitral and aortic valves specified as rheumatic or unspecified
AHA: 2019,2Q,5

I08.1 Rheumatic disorders of both mitral and tricuspid valves

I08.2 Rheumatic disorders of both aortic and tricuspid valves

I08.3 Combined rheumatic disorders of mitral, aortic and tricuspid valves

I08.8 Other rheumatic multiple valve diseases

I08.9 Rheumatic multiple valve disease, unspecified

✓4th **I09 Other rheumatic heart diseases**

I09.0 Rheumatic myocarditis
EXCLUDES 1 *myocarditis not specified as rheumatic (I51.4)*

I09.1 Rheumatic diseases of endocardium, valve unspecified
Rheumatic endocarditis (chronic)
Rheumatic valvulitis (chronic)
EXCLUDES 1 *endocarditis, valve unspecified (I38)*

I09.2 Chronic rheumatic pericarditis
Adherent pericardium, rheumatic
Chronic rheumatic mediastinopericarditis
Chronic rheumatic myopericarditis
EXCLUDES 1 *chronic pericarditis not specified as rheumatic (I31.-)*

✓5th **I09.8 Other specified rheumatic heart diseases**

I09.81 Rheumatic heart failure HCC Rx ESR COM
Use additional code to identify type of heart failure (I50.-)

I09.89 Other specified rheumatic heart diseases
Rheumatic disease of pulmonary valve

I09.9 Rheumatic heart disease, unspecified
Rheumatic carditis
EXCLUDES 1 *rheumatoid carditis (M05.31)*

Hypertensive diseases (I10-I16)

Use additional code to identify:
exposure to environmental tobacco smoke (Z77.22)
history of tobacco dependence (Z87.891)
occupational exposure to environmental tobacco smoke (Z57.31)
tobacco dependence (F17.-)
tobacco use (Z72.0)

EXCLUDES 1 *neonatal hypertension (P29.2)*
primary pulmonary hypertension (I27.0)

EXCLUDES 2 *hypertensive disease complicating pregnancy, childbirth and the puerperium (O10-O11, O13-O16)*

I10 Essential (primary) hypertension Rx Q
INCLUDES high blood pressure
hypertension (arterial) (benign) (essential) (malignant) (primary) (systemic)
EXCLUDES 1 *hypertensive disease complicating pregnancy, childbirth and the puerperium (O10-O11, O13-O16)*
EXCLUDES 2 *essential (primary) hypertension involving vessels of brain (I60-I69)*
essential (primary) hypertension involving vessels of eye (H35.0-)
AHA: 2022,1Q,36; 2020,1Q,12; 2018,2Q,9; 2016,4Q,27

I11 Hypertensive heart disease
INCLUDES any condition in I50.- or I51.4-I51.7, I51.89, I51.9 due to hypertension
AHA: 2018,2Q,9
TIP: Do not assign a code from this category when provider documentation indicates the heart disease is attributable to another cause.

I11.0 Hypertensive heart disease with heart failure HCC Rx ESR COM
Hypertensive heart failure
Use additional code to identify type of heart failure (I50.-)
AHA: 2017,1Q,47

I11.9 Hypertensive heart disease without heart failure Rx
Hypertensive heart disease NOS

I12 Hypertensive chronic kidney disease
INCLUDES any condition in N18 and N26 — due to hypertension
arteriosclerosis of kidney
arteriosclerotic nephritis (chronic) (interstitial)
hypertensive nephropathy
nephrosclerosis
EXCLUDES 1 *hypertension due to kidney disease (I15.0, I15.1)*
renovascular hypertension (I15.0)
secondary hypertension (I15.-)
EXCLUDES 2 *acute kidney failure (N17.-)*
AHA: 2019,3Q,3; 2018,4Q,88; 2016,3Q,22
TIP: Do not assign a code from this category when provider documentation indicates the chronic kidney disease (CKD) is attributable to another cause.

I12.0 Hypertensive chronic kidney disease with stage 5 chronic kidney disease or end stage renal disease HCC Rx ESR COM
Use additional code to identify the stage of chronic kidney disease (N18.5, N18.6)

I12.9 Hypertensive chronic kidney disease with stage 1 through stage 4 chronic kidney disease, or unspecified chronic kidney disease Rx
Hypertensive chronic kidney disease NOS
Hypertensive renal disease NOS
Use additional code to identify the stage of chronic kidney disease (N18.1-N18.4, N18.9)

I13 Hypertensive heart and chronic kidney disease
INCLUDES any condition in I11.- with any condition in I12.-
cardiorenal disease
cardiovascular renal disease
TIP: Do not assign a code from this category when provider documentation indicates the heart and/or chronic kidney disease is attributable to another cause.

I13.0 Hypertensive heart and chronic kidney disease with heart failure and stage 1 through stage 4 chronic kidney disease, or unspecified chronic kidney disease HCC Rx ESR COM
Use additional code to identify type of heart failure (I50.-)
Use additional code to identify stage of chronic kidney disease (N18.1-N18.4, N18.9)

I13.1 Hypertensive heart and chronic kidney disease without heart failure

I13.10 Hypertensive heart and chronic kidney disease without heart failure, with stage 1 through stage 4 chronic kidney disease, or unspecified chronic kidney disease Rx
Hypertensive heart disease and hypertensive chronic kidney disease NOS
Use additional code to identify the stage of chronic kidney disease (N18.1-N18.4, N18.9)

I13.11 Hypertensive heart and chronic kidney disease without heart failure, with stage 5 chronic kidney disease, or end stage renal disease HCC Rx ESR COM
Use additional code to identify the stage of chronic kidney disease (N18.5, N18.6)

I13.2 Hypertensive heart and chronic kidney disease with heart failure and with stage 5 chronic kidney disease, or end stage renal disease HCC Rx ESR COM
Use additional code to identify type of heart failure (I50.-)
Use additional code to identify the stage of chronic kidney disease (N18.5, N18.6)

I15 Secondary hypertension
Code also underlying condition
EXCLUDES 1 *postprocedural hypertension (I97.3)*
EXCLUDES 2 *secondary hypertension involving vessels of brain (I60-I69)*
secondary hypertension involving vessels of eye (H35.0-)

I15.0 Renovascular hypertension Rx
I15.1 Hypertension secondary to other renal disorders Rx
AHA: 2016,3Q,22
I15.2 Hypertension secondary to endocrine disorders Rx
I15.8 Other secondary hypertension Rx
I15.9 Secondary hypertension, unspecified Rx

I16 Hypertensive crisis
Code also any identified hypertensive disease (I10-I15)
AHA: 2016,4Q,26-28
I16.0 Hypertensive urgency Rx
I16.1 Hypertensive emergency Rx
I16.9 Hypertensive crisis, unspecified Rx

Ischemic heart diseases (I20-I25)

Code also the presence of hypertension (I10-I16)

I20 Angina pectoris
Use additional code to identify:
exposure to environmental tobacco smoke (Z77.22)
history of tobacco dependence (Z87.891)
occupational exposure to environmental tobacco smoke (Z57.31)
tobacco dependence (F17.-)
tobacco use (Z72.0)
EXCLUDES 1 *angina pectoris with atherosclerotic heart disease of native coronary arteries (I25.1-)*
atherosclerosis of coronary artery bypass graft(s) and coronary artery of transplanted heart with angina pectoris (I25.7-)
postinfarction angina (I23.7)
DEF: Chest pain due to reduced blood flow resulting in a lack of oxygen to the heart muscles.

I20.0 Unstable angina HCC Rx ESR COM
Accelerated angina
Crescendo angina
De novo effort angina
Intermediate coronary syndrome
Preinfarction syndrome
Worsening effort angina

I20.1 Angina pectoris with documented spasm HCC Rx ESR
Angiospastic angina
Prinzmetal angina
Spasm-induced angina
Variant angina

● **I20.2 Refractory angina pectoris**

I20.8 Other forms of angina pectoris HCC Rx ESR
Angina equivalent
Angina of effort
Coronary slow flow syndrome
Stable angina
Stenocardia
Use additional code(s) for symptoms associated with angina equivalent

I20.9 Angina pectoris, unspecified HCC Rx ESR
Angina NOS
Anginal syndrome
Cardiac angina
Ischemic chest pain

✓4th I21 Acute myocardial infarction
INCLUDES cardiac infarction
coronary (artery) embolism
coronary (artery) occlusion
coronary (artery) rupture
coronary (artery) thrombosis
infarction of heart, myocardium, or ventricle
myocardial infarction specified as acute or with a stated duration of 4 weeks (28 days) or less from onset

Use additional code, if applicable, to identify:
exposure to environmental tobacco smoke (Z77.22)
history of tobacco dependence (Z87.891)
occupational exposure to environmental tobacco smoke (Z57.31)
status post administration of tPA (rtPA) in a different facility within the last 24 hours prior to admission to current facility (Z92.82)
tobacco dependence (F17.-)
tobacco use (Z72.0)

EXCLUDES 2 *old myocardial infarction (I25.2)*
postmyocardial infarction syndrome (I24.1)
subsequent type 1 myocardial infarction (I22.-)

AHA: 2019,2Q,5; 2018,4Q,68; 2018,3Q,5; 2017,4Q,12-14; 2017,1Q,44-45; 2016,4Q,140; 2015,2Q,16; 2013,1Q,25; 2012,4Q,96,102-103
TIP: When chronic total occlusion and myocardial infarction are documented as being in different vessels, assign code I25.82 Chronic total occlusion of coronary artery, in addition to the myocardial infarction code.

✓5th I21.0 ST elevation (STEMI) myocardial infarction of anterior wall
Type 1 ST elevation myocardial infarction of anterior wall
DEF: ST elevation myocardial infarction: Complete obstruction of one or more coronary arteries causing decreased blood flow (ischemia) and necrosis of myocardial muscle cells.

I21.01 ST elevation (STEMI) myocardial infarction involving left main coronary artery HCC Rx ESR COM

I21.02 ST elevation (STEMI) myocardial infarction involving left anterior descending coronary artery HCC Rx ESR COM
ST elevation (STEMI) myocardial infarction involving diagonal coronary artery
AHA: 2013,1Q,25

I21.09 ST elevation (STEMI) myocardial infarction involving other coronary artery of anterior wall HCC Rx ESR COM
Acute transmural myocardial infarction of anterior wall
Anteroapical transmural (Q wave) infarction (acute)
Anterolateral transmural (Q wave) infarction (acute)
Anteroseptal transmural (Q wave) infarction (acute)
Transmural (Q wave) infarction (acute) (of) anterior (wall) NOS
AHA: 2012,4Q,102-103

✓5th I21.1 ST elevation (STEMI) myocardial infarction of inferior wall
Type 1 ST elevation myocardial infarction of inferior wall
DEF: ST elevation myocardial infarction: Complete obstruction of one or more coronary arteries causing decreased blood flow (ischemia) and necrosis of myocardial muscle cells.

I21.11 ST elevation (STEMI) myocardial infarction involving right coronary artery HCC Rx ESR COM
Inferoposterior transmural (Q wave) infarction (acute)

I21.19 ST elevation (STEMI) myocardial infarction involving other coronary artery of inferior wall HCC Rx ESR COM
Acute transmural myocardial infarction of inferior wall
Inferolateral transmural (Q wave) infarction (acute)
Transmural (Q wave) infarction (acute) (of) diaphragmatic wall
Transmural (Q wave) infarction (acute) (of) inferior (wall) NOS
EXCLUDES 2 *ST elevation (STEMI) myocardial infarction involving left circumflex coronary artery (I21.21)*
AHA: 2012,4Q,96

✓5th I21.2 ST elevation (STEMI) myocardial infarction of other sites
Type 1 ST elevation myocardial infarction of other sites
DEF: ST elevation myocardial infarction: Complete obstruction of one or more coronary arteries causing decreased blood flow (ischemia) and necrosis of myocardial muscle cells.

I21.21 ST elevation (STEMI) myocardial infarction involving left circumflex coronary artery HCC Rx ESR COM
ST elevation (STEMI) myocardial infarction involving oblique marginal coronary artery

I21.29 ST elevation (STEMI) myocardial infarction involving other sites HCC Rx ESR COM
Acute transmural myocardial infarction of other sites
Apical-lateral transmural (Q wave) infarction (acute)
Basal-lateral transmural (Q wave) infarction (acute)
High lateral transmural (Q wave) infarction (acute)
Lateral (wall) NOS transmural (Q wave) infarction (acute)
Posterior (true) transmural (Q wave) infarction (acute)
Posterobasal transmural (Q wave) infarction (acute)
Posterolateral transmural (Q wave) infarction (acute)
Posteroseptal transmural (Q wave) infarction (acute)
Septal transmural (Q wave) infarction (acute) NOS

I21.3 ST elevation (STEMI) myocardial infarction of unspecified site HCC Rx ESR COM
Acute transmural myocardial infarction of unspecified site
Transmural (Q wave) myocardial infarction NOS
Type 1 ST elevation myocardial infarction of unspecified site
DEF: ST elevation myocardial infarction: Complete obstruction of one or more coronary arteries causing decreased blood flow (ischemia) and necrosis of myocardial muscle cells.

I21.4 Non-ST elevation (NSTEMI) myocardial infarction HCC Rx ESR COM
Acute subendocardial myocardial infarction
Non-Q wave myocardial infarction NOS
Nontransmural myocardial infarction NOS
Type 1 non-ST elevation myocardial infarction
AHA: 2021,3Q,6; 2019,2Q,33; 2017,1Q,44-45
DEF: Partial obstruction of one or more coronary arteries that causes decreased blood flow (ischemia) and may cause partial thickness necrosis of myocardial muscle cells.

I21.9 Acute myocardial infarction, unspecified HCC Rx ESR COM
Myocardial infarction (acute) NOS

✓5th I21.A Other type of myocardial infarction
AHA: 2019,2Q,5

I21.A1 Myocardial infarction type 2 HCC Rx ESR COM
Myocardial infarction due to demand ischemia
Myocardial infarction secondary to ischemic imbalance
Code first the underlying cause, such as:
anemia (D50.0-D64.9)
chronic obstructive pulmonary disease (J44.-)
paroxysmal tachycardia (I47.0-I47.9)
shock (R57.0-R57.9)
AHA: 2019,4Q,53; 2017,4Q,13-14
DEF: Often referred to as due to demand ischemia, myocardial infarction (MI) type 2 refers to an MI due to ischemia and necrosis resulting from an oxygen imbalance to the heart. This mismatch between oxygen decreased supply and increased demand is caused by conditions other than coronary artery disease such as vasospasm, embolism, anemia, hypertension, hypotension, or arrhythmias.

I21.A9 Other myocardial infarction type HCC Rx ESR COM

Myocardial infarction associated with revascularization procedure
Myocardial infarction type 3
Myocardial infarction type 4a
Myocardial infarction type 4b
Myocardial infarction type 4c
Myocardial infarction type 5

Code first, if applicable, postprocedural myocardial infarction following cardiac surgery (I97.19Ø), or postprocedural myocardial infarction during cardiac surgery (I97.79Ø)

Code also complication, if known and applicable, such as:
(acute) stent occlusion (T82.897-)
(acute) stent stenosis (T82.855-)
(acute) stent thrombosis (T82.867-)
cardiac arrest due to underlying cardiac condition (I46.2)
complication of percutaneous coronary intervention (PCI) (I97.89)
occlusion of coronary artery bypass graft (T82.218-)

AHA: 2021,3Q,6; 2019,2Q,33

✓4th **I22 Subsequent ST elevation (STEMI) and non-ST elevation (NSTEMI) myocardial infarction**

INCLUDES acute myocardial infarction occurring within four weeks (28 days) of a previous acute myocardial infarction, regardless of site
cardiac infarction
coronary (artery) embolism
coronary (artery) occlusion
coronary (artery) rupture
coronary (artery) thrombosis
infarction of heart, myocardium, or ventricle
recurrent myocardial infarction
reinfarction of myocardium
rupture of heart, myocardium, or ventricle
subsequent type 1 myocardial infarction

Use additional code, if applicable, to identify:
exposure to environmental tobacco smoke (Z77.22)
history of tobacco dependence (Z87.891)
occupational exposure to environmental tobacco smoke (Z57.31)
status post administration of tPA (rtPA) in a different facility within the last 24 hours prior to admission to current facility (Z92.82)
tobacco dependence (F17.-)
tobacco use (Z72.Ø)

EXCLUDES1 *subsequent myocardial infarction, type 2 (I21.A1)*
subsequent myocardial infarction of other type (type 3) (type 4) (type 5) (I21.A9)

AHA: 2018,4Q,68; 2018,3Q,5; 2017,4Q,12-13; 2017,2Q,11; 2013,1Q,25; 2012,4Q,97,102-103

DEF: Non-ST elevation myocardial infarction: Partial obstruction of one or more coronary arteries that causes decreased blood flow (ischemia) and may cause partial thickness necrosis of myocardial muscle cells.

DEF: ST elevation myocardial infarction: Complete obstruction of one or more coronary arteries causing decreased blood flow (ischemia) and necrosis of myocardial muscle cells.

TIP: When chronic total occlusion and myocardial infarction are documented as being in different vessels, assign code I25.82 Chronic total occlusion of coronary artery, in addition to the myocardial infarction code.

I22.Ø Subsequent ST elevation (STEMI) myocardial infarction of anterior wall HCC Rx ESR COM

Subsequent acute transmural myocardial infarction of anterior wall
Subsequent transmural (Q wave) infarction (acute)(of) anterior (wall) NOS
Subsequent anteroapical transmural (Q wave) infarction (acute)
Subsequent anterolateral transmural (Q wave) infarction (acute)
Subsequent anteroseptal transmural (Q wave) infarction (acute)

I22.1 Subsequent ST elevation (STEMI) myocardial infarction of inferior wall HCC Rx ESR COM

Subsequent acute transmural myocardial infarction of inferior wall
Subsequent transmural (Q wave) infarction (acute)(of) diaphragmatic wall
Subsequent transmural (Q wave) infarction (acute)(of) inferior (wall) NOS
Subsequent inferolateral transmural (Q wave) infarction (acute)
Subsequent inferoposterior transmural (Q wave) infarction (acute)

AHA: 2012,4Q,102

I22.2 Subsequent non-ST elevation (NSTEMI) myocardial infarction HCC Rx ESR COM

Subsequent acute subendocardial myocardial infarction
Subsequent non-Q wave myocardial infarction NOS
Subsequent nontransmural myocardial infarction NOS

I22.8 Subsequent ST elevation (STEMI) myocardial infarction of other sites HCC Rx ESR COM

Subsequent acute transmural myocardial infarction of other sites
Subsequent apical-lateral transmural (Q wave) myocardial infarction (acute)
Subsequent basal-lateral transmural (Q wave) myocardial infarction (acute)
Subsequent high lateral transmural (Q wave) myocardial infarction (acute)
Subsequent transmural (Q wave) myocardial infarction (acute)(of) lateral (wall) NOS
Subsequent posterior (true) transmural (Q wave) myocardial infarction (acute)
Subsequent posterobasal transmural (Q wave) myocardial infarction (acute)
Subsequent posterolateral transmural (Q wave) myocardial infarction (acute)
Subsequent posteroseptal transmural (Q wave) myocardial infarction (acute)
Subsequent septal NOS transmural (Q wave) myocardial infarction (acute)

I22.9 Subsequent ST elevation (STEMI) myocardial infarction of unspecified site HCC Rx ESR COM

Subsequent acute myocardial infarction of unspecified site
Subsequent myocardial infarction (acute) NOS

✓4th **I23 Certain current complications following ST elevation (STEMI) and non-ST elevation (NSTEMI) myocardial infarction (within the 28 day period)**

AHA: 2017,2Q,11

DEF: ST elevation myocardial infarction: Complete obstruction of one or more coronary arteries causing decreased blood flow (ischemia) and necrosis of myocardial muscle cells.

DEF: Non-ST elevation myocardial infarction: Partial obstruction of one or more coronary arteries that causes decreased blood flow (ischemia) and may cause partial thickness necrosis of myocardial muscle cells.

I23.Ø Hemopericardium as current complication following acute myocardial infarction HCC Rx ESR COM A

EXCLUDES1 *hemopericardium not specified as current complication following acute myocardial infarction (I31.2)*

I23.1 Atrial septal defect as current complication following acute myocardial infarction HCC Rx ESR COM A

EXCLUDES1 *acquired atrial septal defect not specified as current complication following acute myocardial infarction (I51.Ø)*

I23.2 Ventricular septal defect as current complication following acute myocardial infarction HCC Rx ESR COM A

EXCLUDES1 *acquired ventricular septal defect not specified as current complication following acute myocardial infarction (I51.Ø)*

I23.3 Rupture of cardiac wall without hemopericardium as current complication following acute myocardial infarction HCC Rx ESR COM A

I23.4 Rupture of chordae tendineae as current complication following acute myocardial infarction HCC Rx ESR COM

EXCLUDES1 *rupture of chordae tendineae not specified as current complication following acute myocardial infarction (I51.1)*

I23.5 Rupture of papillary muscle as current complication following acute myocardial infarction HCC Rx ESR COM

EXCLUDES 1 *rupture of papillary muscle not specified as current complication following acute myocardial infarction (I51.2)*

I23.6 Thrombosis of atrium, auricular appendage, and ventricle as current complications following acute myocardial infarction HCC Rx ESR COM A

EXCLUDES 1 *thrombosis of atrium, auricular appendage, and ventricle not specified as current complication following acute myocardial infarction (I51.3)*

I23.7 Postinfarction angina HCC Rx ESR COM A

AHA: 2015,2Q,16

TIP: When postinfarction angina occurs with atherosclerotic coronary artery disease, code both I23.7 and I25.118 for atherosclerotic disease with other forms of angina pectoris.

I23.8 Other current complications following acute myocardial infarction HCC Rx ESR COM A

I24 Other acute ischemic heart diseases (4th)

EXCLUDES 1 *angina pectoris (I2Ø.-)*
transient myocardial ischemia in newborn (P29.4)

EXCLUDES 2 *non-ischemic myocardial injury (I5A)*

I24.Ø Acute coronary thrombosis not resulting in myocardial infarction HCC Rx ESR COM

Acute coronary (artery) (vein) embolism not resulting in myocardial infarction

Acute coronary (artery) (vein) occlusion not resulting in myocardial infarction

Acute coronary (artery) (vein) thromboembolism not resulting in myocardial infarction

EXCLUDES 1 *atherosclerotic heart disease (I25.1-)*

AHA: 2013,1Q,24

I24.1 Dressler's syndrome HCC Rx ESR COM

Postmyocardial infarction syndrome

EXCLUDES 1 *postinfarction angina (I23.7)*

DEF: Fever, leukocytosis, chest pain, evidence of pericarditis, pleurisy, and pneumonia occurring days or weeks after a myocardial infarction.

I24.8 Other forms of acute ischemic heart disease HCC Rx ESR COM

EXCLUDES 1 *myocardial infarction due to demand ischemia (I21.A1)*

AHA: 2019,4Q,53; 2017,4Q,13

I24.9 Acute ischemic heart disease, unspecified HCC Rx ESR COM

EXCLUDES 1 *ischemic heart disease (chronic) NOS (I25.9)*

I25 Chronic ischemic heart disease (4th)

Use additional code to identify:
chronic total occlusion of coronary artery (I25.82)
exposure to environmental tobacco smoke (Z77.22)
history of tobacco dependence (Z87.891)
occupational exposure to environmental tobacco smoke (Z57.31)
tobacco dependence (F17.-)
tobacco use (Z72.Ø)

EXCLUDES 2 *non-ischemic myocardial injury (I5A)*

I25.1 Atherosclerotic heart disease of native coronary artery (5th)

Atherosclerotic cardiovascular disease
Coronary (artery) atheroma
Coronary (artery) atherosclerosis
Coronary (artery) disease
Coronary (artery) sclerosis

Use additional code, if applicable, to identify:
coronary atherosclerosis due to calcified coronary lesion (I25.84)
coronary atherosclerosis due to lipid rich plaque (I25.83)

EXCLUDES 2 *atheroembolism (I75.-)*
atherosclerosis of coronary artery bypass graft(s) and transplanted heart (I25.7-)

Atheromas

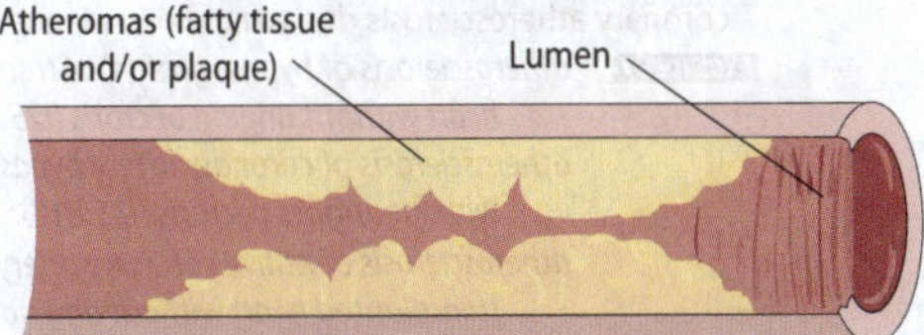

I25.1Ø Atherosclerotic heart disease of native coronary artery without angina pectoris Rx A

Atherosclerotic heart disease NOS

AHA: 2021,3Q,6-7; 2015,2Q,16; 2012,4Q,92

I25.11 Atherosclerotic heart disease of native coronary artery with angina pectoris (6th)

I25.11Ø Atherosclerotic heart disease of native coronary artery with unstable angina pectoris HCC Rx ESR COM A

EXCLUDES 1 *unstable angina without atherosclerotic heart disease (I2Ø.Ø)*

I25.111 Atherosclerotic heart disease of native coronary artery with angina pectoris with documented spasm HCC Rx ESR A

EXCLUDES 1 *angina pectoris with documented spasm without atherosclerotic heart disease (I2Ø.1)*

● **I25.112 Atherosclersic heart disease of native coronary artery with refractory angina pectoris**

I25.118 Atherosclerotic heart disease of native coronary artery with other forms of angina pectoris HCC Rx ESR A

EXCLUDES 1 *other forms of angina pectoris without atherosclerotic heart disease (I2Ø.8)*

AHA: 2015,2Q,16

TIP: When postinfarction angina occurs with atherosclerotic coronary artery disease, code both I23.7 and I25.118 for atherosclerotic disease with other forms of angina pectoris.

I25.119 Atherosclerotic heart disease of native coronary artery with unspecified angina pectoris HCC Rx ESR A

Atherosclerotic heart disease with angina NOS

Atherosclerotic heart disease with ischemic chest pain

EXCLUDES 1 *unspecified angina pectoris without atherosclerotic heart disease (I2Ø.9)*

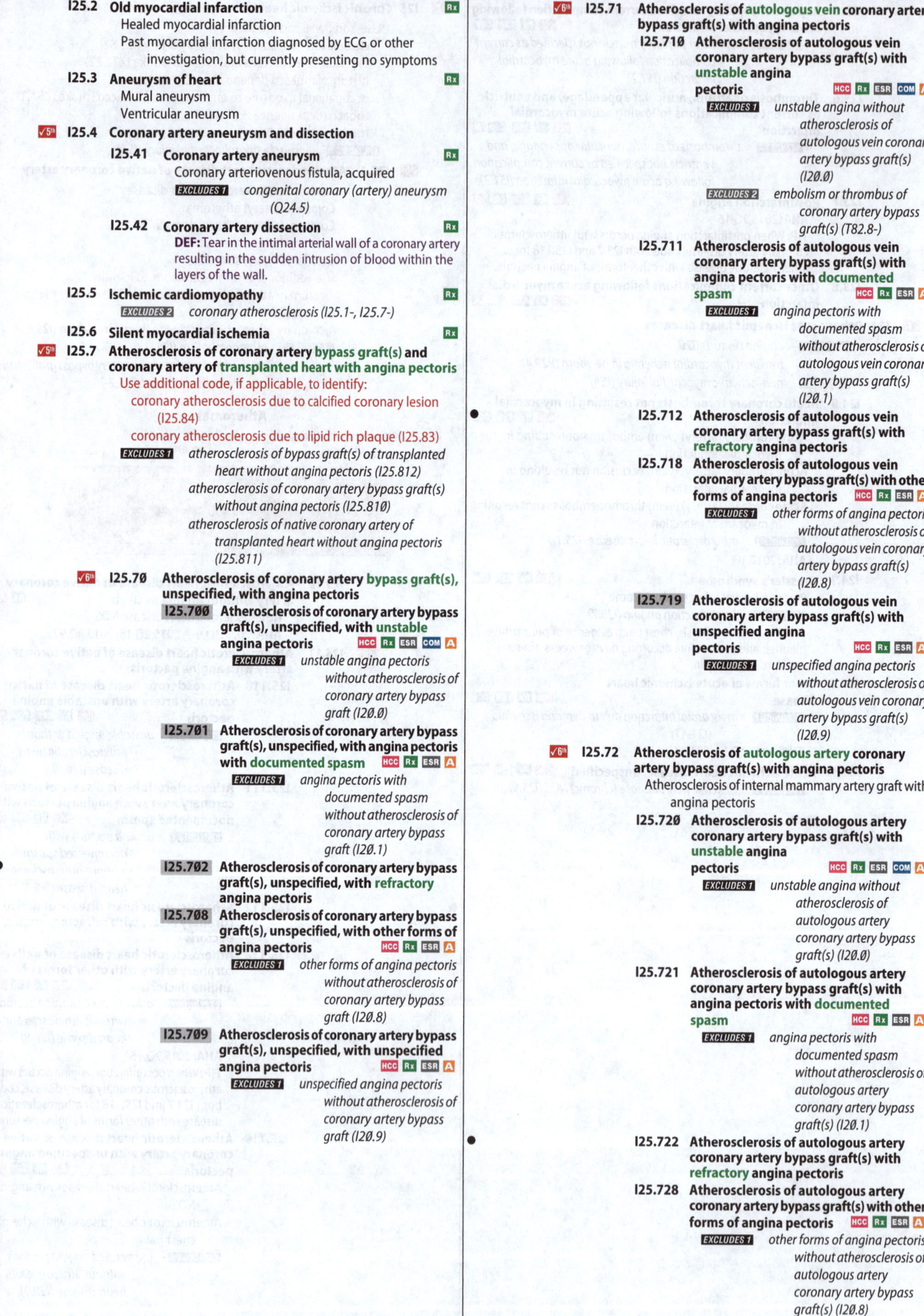

I25.2 Old myocardial infarction Rx
Healed myocardial infarction
Past myocardial infarction diagnosed by ECG or other investigation, but currently presenting no symptoms

I25.3 Aneurysm of heart Rx
Mural aneurysm
Ventricular aneurysm

√5th **I25.4 Coronary artery aneurysm and dissection**

I25.41 Coronary artery aneurysm Rx
Coronary arteriovenous fistula, acquired
EXCLUDES 1 *congenital coronary (artery) aneurysm (Q24.5)*

I25.42 Coronary artery dissection Rx
DEF: Tear in the intimal arterial wall of a coronary artery resulting in the sudden intrusion of blood within the layers of the wall.

I25.5 Ischemic cardiomyopathy Rx
EXCLUDES 2 *coronary atherosclerosis (I25.1-, I25.7-)*

I25.6 Silent myocardial ischemia Rx

√5th **I25.7 Atherosclerosis of coronary artery bypass graft(s) and coronary artery of transplanted heart with angina pectoris**
Use additional code, if applicable, to identify:
coronary atherosclerosis due to calcified coronary lesion (I25.84)
coronary atherosclerosis due to lipid rich plaque (I25.83)
EXCLUDES 1 *atherosclerosis of bypass graft(s) of transplanted heart without angina pectoris (I25.812)*
atherosclerosis of coronary artery bypass graft(s) without angina pectoris (I25.810)
atherosclerosis of native coronary artery of transplanted heart without angina pectoris (I25.811)

√6th **I25.70 Atherosclerosis of coronary artery bypass graft(s), unspecified, with angina pectoris**

I25.700 Atherosclerosis of coronary artery bypass graft(s), unspecified, with unstable angina pectoris HCC Rx ESR COM A
EXCLUDES 1 *unstable angina pectoris without atherosclerosis of coronary artery bypass graft (I20.0)*

I25.701 Atherosclerosis of coronary artery bypass graft(s), unspecified, with angina pectoris with documented spasm HCC Rx ESR A
EXCLUDES 1 *angina pectoris with documented spasm without atherosclerosis of coronary artery bypass graft (I20.1)*

● **I25.702 Atherosclerosis of coronary artery bypass graft(s), unspecified, with refractory angina pectoris**

I25.708 Atherosclerosis of coronary artery bypass graft(s), unspecified, with other forms of angina pectoris HCC Rx ESR A
EXCLUDES 1 *other forms of angina pectoris without atherosclerosis of coronary artery bypass graft (I20.8)*

I25.709 Atherosclerosis of coronary artery bypass graft(s), unspecified, with unspecified angina pectoris HCC Rx ESR A
EXCLUDES 1 *unspecified angina pectoris without atherosclerosis of coronary artery bypass graft (I20.9)*

√6th **I25.71 Atherosclerosis of autologous vein coronary artery bypass graft(s) with angina pectoris**

I25.710 Atherosclerosis of autologous vein coronary artery bypass graft(s) with unstable angina pectoris HCC Rx ESR COM A
EXCLUDES 1 *unstable angina without atherosclerosis of autologous vein coronary artery bypass graft(s) (I20.0)*
EXCLUDES 2 *embolism or thrombus of coronary artery bypass graft(s) (T82.8-)*

I25.711 Atherosclerosis of autologous vein coronary artery bypass graft(s) with angina pectoris with documented spasm HCC Rx ESR A
EXCLUDES 1 *angina pectoris with documented spasm without atherosclerosis of autologous vein coronary artery bypass graft(s) (I20.1)*

● **I25.712 Atherosclerosis of autologous vein coronary artery bypass graft(s) with refractory angina pectoris**

I25.718 Atherosclerosis of autologous vein coronary artery bypass graft(s) with other forms of angina pectoris HCC Rx ESR A
EXCLUDES 1 *other forms of angina pectoris without atherosclerosis of autologous vein coronary artery bypass graft(s) (I20.8)*

I25.719 Atherosclerosis of autologous vein coronary artery bypass graft(s) with unspecified angina pectoris HCC Rx ESR A
EXCLUDES 1 *unspecified angina pectoris without atherosclerosis of autologous vein coronary artery bypass graft(s) (I20.9)*

√6th **I25.72 Atherosclerosis of autologous artery coronary artery bypass graft(s) with angina pectoris**
Atherosclerosis of internal mammary artery graft with angina pectoris

I25.720 Atherosclerosis of autologous artery coronary artery bypass graft(s) with unstable angina pectoris HCC Rx ESR COM A
EXCLUDES 1 *unstable angina without atherosclerosis of autologous artery coronary artery bypass graft(s) (I20.0)*

I25.721 Atherosclerosis of autologous artery coronary artery bypass graft(s) with angina pectoris with documented spasm HCC Rx ESR A
EXCLUDES 1 *angina pectoris with documented spasm without atherosclerosis of autologous artery coronary artery bypass graft(s) (I20.1)*

● **I25.722 Atherosclerosis of autologous artery coronary artery bypass graft(s) with refractory angina pectoris**

I25.728 Atherosclerosis of autologous artery coronary artery bypass graft(s) with other forms of angina pectoris HCC Rx ESR A
EXCLUDES 1 *other forms of angina pectoris without atherosclerosis of autologous artery coronary artery bypass graft(s) (I20.8)*

HCC CMS-HCC | Rx Rx HCC | ESR ESRD HCC | COM Commercial HCC | N Newborn: 0 | P Pediatric: 0-17 | M Maternity: 9-64 | A Adult: 15-124

I25.729 Atherosclerosis of autologous artery coronary artery bypass graft(s) with unspecified angina pectoris HCC Rx ESR A

EXCLUDES 1 *unspecified angina pectoris without atherosclerosis of autologous artery coronary artery bypass graft(s) (I20.9)*

✓6th **I25.73 Atherosclerosis of nonautologous biological coronary artery bypass graft(s) with angina pectoris**

I25.730 Atherosclerosis of nonautologous biological coronary artery bypass graft(s) with unstable angina pectoris HCC Rx ESR COM A

EXCLUDES 1 *unstable angina without atherosclerosis of nonautologous biological coronary artery bypass graft(s) (I20.0)*

I25.731 Atherosclerosis of nonautologous biological coronary artery bypass graft(s) with angina pectoris with documented spasm HCC Rx ESR A

EXCLUDES 1 *angina pectoris with documented spasm without atherosclerosis of nonautologous biological coronary artery bypass graft(s) (I20.1)*

● **I25.732 Atherosclerosis of nonautologous biological coronary artery bypass graft(s) with refractory angina pectoris**

I25.738 Atherosclerosis of nonautologous biological coronary artery bypass graft(s) with other forms of angina pectoris HCC Rx ESR A

EXCLUDES 1 *other forms of angina pectoris without atherosclerosis of nonautologous biological coronary artery bypass graft(s) (I20.8)*

I25.739 Atherosclerosis of nonautologous biological coronary artery bypass graft(s) with unspecified angina pectoris HCC Rx ESR A

EXCLUDES 1 *unspecified angina pectoris without atherosclerosis of nonautologous biological coronary artery bypass graft(s) (I20.9)*

✓6th **I25.75 Atherosclerosis of native coronary artery of transplanted heart with angina pectoris**

EXCLUDES 1 *atherosclerosis of native coronary artery of transplanted heart without angina pectoris (I25.811)*

I25.750 Atherosclerosis of native coronary artery of transplanted heart with unstable angina HCC Rx ESR COM

I25.751 Atherosclerosis of native coronary artery of transplanted heart with angina pectoris with documented spasm HCC Rx ESR

● **I25.752 Atherosclerosis of native coronary artery of transplanted heart with refractory angina pectoris**

I25.758 Atherosclerosis of native coronary artery of transplanted heart with other forms of angina pectoris HCC Rx ESR

I25.759 Atherosclerosis of native coronary artery of transplanted heart with unspecified angina pectoris HCC Rx ESR

✓6th **I25.76 Atherosclerosis of bypass graft of coronary artery of transplanted heart with angina pectoris**

EXCLUDES 1 *atherosclerosis of bypass graft of coronary artery of transplanted heart without angina pectoris (I25.812)*

I25.760 Atherosclerosis of bypass graft of coronary artery of transplanted heart with unstable angina HCC Rx ESR COM A

I25.761 Atherosclerosis of bypass graft of coronary artery of transplanted heart with angina pectoris with documented spasm HCC Rx ESR A

● **I25.762 Atherosclerosis of bypass graft of coronary artery of transplanted heart with refractory angina pectoris**

I25.768 Atherosclerosis of bypass graft of coronary artery of transplanted heart with other forms of angina pectoris HCC Rx ESR A

I25.769 Atherosclerosis of bypass graft of coronary artery of transplanted heart with unspecified angina pectoris HCC Rx ESR A

✓6th **I25.79 Atherosclerosis of other coronary artery bypass graft(s) with angina pectoris**

I25.790 Atherosclerosis of other coronary artery bypass graft(s) with unstable angina pectoris HCC Rx ESR COM A

EXCLUDES 1 *unstable angina without atherosclerosis of other coronary artery bypass graft(s) (I20.0)*

I25.791 Atherosclerosis of other coronary artery bypass graft(s) with angina pectoris with documented spasm HCC Rx ESR A

EXCLUDES 1 *angina pectoris with documented spasm without atherosclerosis of other coronary artery bypass graft(s) (I20.1)*

● **I25.792 Atherosclerosis of other coronary artery bypass graft(s) with refractory angina pectoris**

I25.798 Atherosclerosis of other coronary artery bypass graft(s) with other forms of angina pectoris HCC Rx ESR A

EXCLUDES 1 *other forms of angina pectoris without atherosclerosis of other coronary artery bypass graft(s) (I20.8)*

I25.799 Atherosclerosis of other coronary artery bypass graft(s) with unspecified angina pectoris HCC Rx ESR A

EXCLUDES 1 *unspecified angina pectoris without atherosclerosis of other coronary artery bypass graft(s) (I20.9)*

✓5th **I25.8 Other forms of chronic ischemic heart disease**

✓6th **I25.81 Atherosclerosis of other coronary vessels without angina pectoris**

Use additional code, if applicable, to identify:

coronary atherosclerosis due to calcified coronary lesion (I25.84)

coronary atherosclerosis due to lipid rich plaque (I25.83)

EXCLUDES 2 *atherosclerotic heart disease of native coronary artery without angina pectoris (I25.10)*

I25.810 Atherosclerosis of coronary artery bypass graft(s) without angina pectoris Rx A

Atherosclerosis of coronary artery bypass graft NOS

EXCLUDES 1 *atherosclerosis of coronary bypass graft(s) with angina pectoris (I25.70-I25.73-, I25.79-)*

I25.811 Atherosclerosis of native coronary artery of transplanted heart without angina pectoris Rx

Atherosclerosis of native coronary artery of transplanted heart NOS

EXCLUDES 1 *atherosclerosis of native coronary artery of transplanted heart with angina pectoris (I25.75-)*

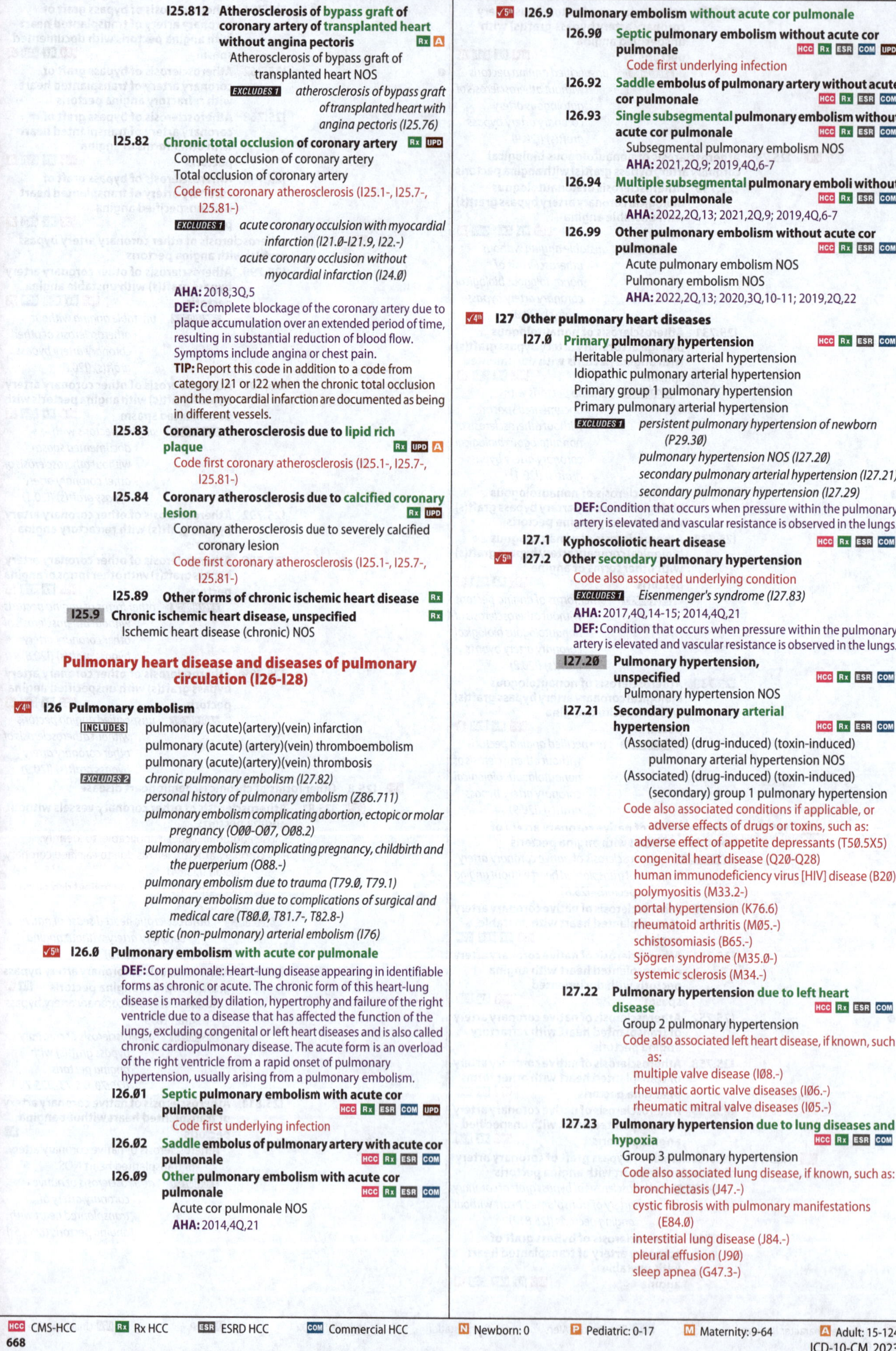

I25.812 Atherosclerosis of bypass graft of coronary artery of transplanted heart without angina pectoris Rx A
Atherosclerosis of bypass graft of transplanted heart NOS
EXCLUDES 1 *atherosclerosis of bypass graft of transplanted heart with angina pectoris (I25.76)*

I25.82 Chronic total occlusion of coronary artery Rx UPD
Complete occlusion of coronary artery
Total occlusion of coronary artery
Code first coronary atherosclerosis (I25.1-, I25.7-, I25.81-)
EXCLUDES 1 *acute coronary occulsion with myocardial infarction (I21.Ø-I21.9, I22.-)*
acute coronary occlusion without myocardial infarction (I24.Ø)
AHA: 2018,3Q,5
DEF: Complete blockage of the coronary artery due to plaque accumulation over an extended period of time, resulting in substantial reduction of blood flow. Symptoms include angina or chest pain.
TIP: Report this code in addition to a code from category I21 or I22 when the chronic total occlusion and the myocardial infarction are documented as being in different vessels.

I25.83 Coronary atherosclerosis due to lipid rich plaque Rx UPD A
Code first coronary atherosclerosis (I25.1-, I25.7-, I25.81-)

I25.84 Coronary atherosclerosis due to calcified coronary lesion Rx UPD
Coronary atherosclerosis due to severely calcified coronary lesion
Code first coronary atherosclerosis (I25.1-, I25.7-, I25.81-)

I25.89 Other forms of chronic ischemic heart disease Rx

I25.9 Chronic ischemic heart disease, unspecified Rx
Ischemic heart disease (chronic) NOS

Pulmonary heart disease and diseases of pulmonary circulation (I26-I28)

4th I26 Pulmonary embolism
INCLUDES pulmonary (acute)(artery)(vein) infarction
pulmonary (acute) (artery)(vein) thromboembolism
pulmonary (acute)(artery)(vein) thrombosis
EXCLUDES 2 *chronic pulmonary embolism (I27.82)*
personal history of pulmonary embolism (Z86.711)
pulmonary embolism complicating abortion, ectopic or molar pregnancy (OØØ-OØ7, OØ8.2)
pulmonary embolism complicating pregnancy, childbirth and the puerperium (O88.-)
pulmonary embolism due to trauma (T79.Ø, T79.1)
pulmonary embolism due to complications of surgical and medical care (T8Ø.Ø, T81.7-, T82.8-)
septic (non-pulmonary) arterial embolism (I76)

5th I26.Ø Pulmonary embolism with acute cor pulmonale
DEF: Cor pulmonale: Heart-lung disease appearing in identifiable forms as chronic or acute. The chronic form of this heart-lung disease is marked by dilation, hypertrophy and failure of the right ventricle due to a disease that has affected the function of the lungs, excluding congenital or left heart diseases and is also called chronic cardiopulmonary disease. The acute form is an overload of the right ventricle from a rapid onset of pulmonary hypertension, usually arising from a pulmonary embolism.

I26.Ø1 Septic pulmonary embolism with acute cor pulmonale HCC Rx ESR COM UPD
Code first underlying infection

I26.Ø2 Saddle embolus of pulmonary artery with acute cor pulmonale HCC Rx ESR COM

I26.Ø9 Other pulmonary embolism with acute cor pulmonale HCC Rx ESR COM
Acute cor pulmonale NOS
AHA: 2014,4Q,21

5th I26.9 Pulmonary embolism without acute cor pulmonale

I26.9Ø Septic pulmonary embolism without acute cor pulmonale HCC Rx ESR COM UPD
Code first underlying infection

I26.92 Saddle embolus of pulmonary artery without acute cor pulmonale HCC Rx ESR COM

I26.93 Single subsegmental pulmonary embolism without acute cor pulmonale HCC Rx ESR COM
Subsegmental pulmonary embolism NOS
AHA: 2021,2Q,9; 2019,4Q,6-7

I26.94 Multiple subsegmental pulmonary emboli without acute cor pulmonale HCC Rx ESR COM
AHA: 2022,2Q,13; 2021,2Q,9; 2019,4Q,6-7

I26.99 Other pulmonary embolism without acute cor pulmonale HCC Rx ESR COM
Acute pulmonary embolism NOS
Pulmonary embolism NOS
AHA: 2022,2Q,13; 2020,3Q,10-11; 2019,2Q,22

4th I27 Other pulmonary heart diseases

I27.Ø Primary pulmonary hypertension HCC Rx ESR COM
Heritable pulmonary arterial hypertension
Idiopathic pulmonary arterial hypertension
Primary group 1 pulmonary hypertension
Primary pulmonary arterial hypertension
EXCLUDES 1 *persistent pulmonary hypertension of newborn (P29.3Ø)*
pulmonary hypertension NOS (I27.2Ø)
secondary pulmonary arterial hypertension (I27.21)
secondary pulmonary hypertension (I27.29)
DEF: Condition that occurs when pressure within the pulmonary artery is elevated and vascular resistance is observed in the lungs.

I27.1 Kyphoscoliotic heart disease HCC Rx ESR COM

5th I27.2 Other secondary pulmonary hypertension
Code also associated underlying condition
EXCLUDES 1 *Eisenmenger's syndrome (I27.83)*
AHA: 2017,4Q,14-15; 2014,4Q,21
DEF: Condition that occurs when pressure within the pulmonary artery is elevated and vascular resistance is observed in the lungs.

I27.2Ø Pulmonary hypertension, unspecified HCC Rx ESR COM
Pulmonary hypertension NOS

I27.21 Secondary pulmonary arterial hypertension HCC Rx ESR COM
(Associated) (drug-induced) (toxin-induced) pulmonary arterial hypertension NOS
(Associated) (drug-induced) (toxin-induced) (secondary) group 1 pulmonary hypertension
Code also associated conditions if applicable, or adverse effects of drugs or toxins, such as:
adverse effect of appetite depressants (T5Ø.5X5)
congenital heart disease (Q2Ø-Q28)
human immunodeficiency virus [HIV] disease (B2Ø)
polymyositis (M33.2-)
portal hypertension (K76.6)
rheumatoid arthritis (MØ5.-)
schistosomiasis (B65.-)
Sjögren syndrome (M35.Ø-)
systemic sclerosis (M34.-)

I27.22 Pulmonary hypertension due to left heart disease HCC Rx ESR COM
Group 2 pulmonary hypertension
Code also associated left heart disease, if known, such as:
multiple valve disease (IØ8.-)
rheumatic aortic valve diseases (IØ6.-)
rheumatic mitral valve diseases (IØ5.-)

I27.23 Pulmonary hypertension due to lung diseases and hypoxia HCC Rx ESR COM
Group 3 pulmonary hypertension
Code also associated lung disease, if known, such as:
bronchiectasis (J47.-)
cystic fibrosis with pulmonary manifestations (E84.Ø)
interstitial lung disease (J84.-)
pleural effusion (J9Ø)
sleep apnea (G47.3-)

I27.24 Chronic thromboembolic pulmonary hypertension HCC Rx ESR COM
Group 4 pulmonary hypertension
Code also associated pulmonary embolism, if applicable (I26.-, I27.82)

I27.29 Other secondary pulmonary hypertension HCC Rx ESR COM
Group 5 pulmonary hypertension
Pulmonary hypertension with unclear multifactorial mechanisms
Pulmonary hypertension due to hematologic disorders
Pulmonary hypertension due to metabolic disorders
Pulmonary hypertension due to other systemic disorders
Code also other associated disorders, if known, such as:
chronic myeloid leukemia (C92.1Ø-C92.22)
essential thrombocythemia (D47.3)
Gaucher disease (E75.22)
hypertensive chronic kidney disease with end stage renal disease (I12.Ø, I13.11, I13.2)
hyperthyroidism (EØ5.-)
hypothyroidism (EØØ-EØ3)
polycythemia vera (D45)
sarcoidosis (D86.-)
AHA: 2016,2Q,8

√5th **I27.8 Other specified pulmonary heart diseases**

I27.81 Cor pulmonale (chronic) HCC Rx ESR COM
Cor pulmonale NOS
EXCLUDES 1 *acute cor pulmonale (I26.Ø-)*
AHA: 2014,4Q,21
DEF: Heart-lung disease appearing in identifiable forms as chronic or acute. The chronic form of this heart-lung disease is marked by dilation, hypertrophy and failure of the right ventricle due to a disease that has affected the function of the lungs, excluding congenital or left heart diseases and is also called chronic cardiopulmonary disease. The acute form is an overload of the right ventricle from a rapid onset of pulmonary hypertension, usually arising from a pulmonary embolism.

I27.82 Chronic pulmonary embolism HCC Rx ESR COM
Use additional code, if applicable, for associated long-term (current) use of anticoagulants (Z79.Ø1)
EXCLUDES 1 *personal history of pulmonary embolism (Z86.711)*
AHA: 2021,2Q,9
DEF: Long-standing condition commonly associated with pulmonary hypertension in which small blood clots travel to the lungs repeatedly over many weeks, months, or years, requiring continuation of established anticoagulant or thrombolytic therapy.

I27.83 Eisenmenger's syndrome HCC Rx ESR COM
Eisenmenger's complex
(Irreversible) Eisenmenger's disease
Pulmonary hypertension with right to left shunt related to congenital heart disease
Code also underlying heart defect, if known, such as:
atrial septal defect ►(Q21.1-)◄
Eisenmenger's defect (Q21.8)
patent ductus arteriosus (Q25.Ø)
ventricular septal defect (Q21.Ø)
DEF: Pulmonary hypertension with congenital communication between two circulations resulting in a right to left shunt. This causes reduced oxygen saturation in the arterial blood, leading to cyanosis and organ damage. Once it develops, this life-threating condition is irreversible.

I27.89 Other specified pulmonary heart diseases HCC Rx ESR COM

I27.9 Pulmonary heart disease, unspecified HCC Rx ESR COM
Chronic cardiopulmonary disease

√4th **I28 Other diseases of pulmonary vessels**

I28.Ø Arteriovenous fistula of pulmonary vessels HCC Rx ESR COM
EXCLUDES 1 *congenital arteriovenous fistula (Q25.72)*

I28.1 Aneurysm of pulmonary artery HCC Rx ESR COM
EXCLUDES 1 *congenital aneurysm (Q25.79)*
congenital arteriovenous aneurysm (Q25.72)

I28.8 Other diseases of pulmonary vessels HCC Rx ESR COM
Pulmonary arteritis
Pulmonary endarteritis
Rupture of pulmonary vessels
Stenosis of pulmonary vessels
Stricture of pulmonary vessels

I28.9 Disease of pulmonary vessels, unspecified HCC Rx ESR COM

Other forms of heart disease (I3Ø-I5A)

√4th **I3Ø Acute pericarditis**
INCLUDES acute mediastinopericarditis
acute myopericarditis
acute pericardial effusion
acute pleuropericarditis
acute pneumopericarditis
EXCLUDES 1 *Dressler's syndrome (I24.1)*
rheumatic pericarditis (acute) (IØ1.Ø)
viral pericarditis due to Coxsakie virus (B33.23)
DEF: Pericarditis: Inflammation affecting the pericardium, the fibroserous membrane that surrounds the heart.

I3Ø.Ø Acute nonspecific idiopathic pericarditis COM

I3Ø.1 Infective pericarditis COM
Pneumococcal pericarditis
Pneumopyopericardium
Purulent pericarditis
Pyopericarditis
Pyopericardium
Pyopneumopericardium
Staphylococcal pericarditis
Streptococcal pericarditis
Suppurative pericarditis
Viral pericarditis
Use additional code (B95-B97) to identify infectious agent

I3Ø.8 Other forms of acute pericarditis COM

I3Ø.9 Acute pericarditis, unspecified COM

√4th **I31 Other diseases of pericardium**
EXCLUDES 1 *diseases of pericardium specified as rheumatic (IØ9.2)*
postcardiotomy syndrome (I97.Ø)
traumatic injury to pericardium (S26.-)

I31.Ø Chronic adhesive pericarditis COM
Accretio cordis
Adherent pericardium
Adhesive mediastinopericarditis

I31.1 Chronic constrictive pericarditis COM
Concretio cordis
Pericardial calcification

I31.2 Hemopericardium, not elsewhere classified COM
EXCLUDES 1 *hemopericardium as current complication following acute myocardial infarction (I23.Ø)*
►malignant pericardial effusion (I31.31)◄
DEF: Presence of blood in the pericardial sac (pericardium). It can lead to potentially fatal cardiac tamponade if enough blood enters the pericardial cavity.

▲ √5th **I31.3 Pericardial effusion (noninflammatory)**
~~Chylopericardium~~
EXCLUDES 1 *acute pericardial effusion (I3Ø.9)*
AHA: 2019,1Q,16

● **I31.31 Malignant pericardial effusion in diseases classified elsewhere**
Code first underlying neoplasm (CØØ-D49)

● **I31.39 Other pericardial effusion (noninflammatory)**
Chylopericardium

I31.4 Cardiac tamponade COM UPD
Code first underlying cause
DEF: Life-threatening condition in which fluid or blood accumulates in the space between the muscle of the heart (myocardium) and the outer sac that covers the heart (pericardium), resulting in compression of the heart.

Cardiac Tamponade

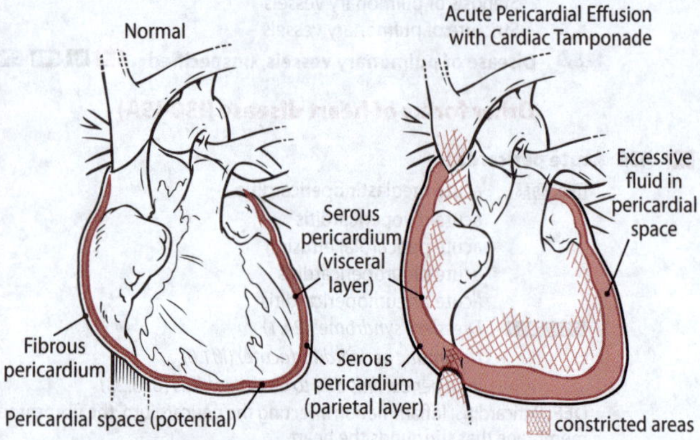

Normal
Acute Pericardial Effusion with Cardiac Tamponade
Excessive fluid in pericardial space
Serous pericardium (visceral layer)
Fibrous pericardium
Serous pericardium (parietal layer)
Pericardial space (potential)
constricted areas

I31.8 Other specified diseases of pericardium COM
Epicardial plaques
Focal pericardial adhesions

I31.9 Disease of pericardium, unspecified COM
Pericarditis (chronic) NOS

I32 Pericarditis in diseases classified elsewhere COM
Code first underlying disease
EXCLUDES 1 *pericarditis (in):*
coxsackie (virus) (B33.23)
gonococcal (A54.83)
meningococcal (A39.53)
rheumatoid (arthritis) (MØ5.31)
syphilitic (A52.Ø6)
systemic lupus erythematosus (M32.12)
tuberculosis (A18.84)
DEF: Pericarditis: Inflammation affecting the pericardium, the fibroserous membrane that surrounds the heart.

✓4th **I33 Acute and subacute endocarditis**
EXCLUDES 1 *acute rheumatic endocarditis (IØ1.1)*
endocarditis NOS (I38)
DEF: Endocarditis: Inflammatory disease of the interior lining of the heart chamber and heart valves.

I33.Ø Acute and subacute infective endocarditis COM
Bacterial endocarditis (acute) (subacute)
Infective endocarditis (acute) (subacute) NOS
Endocarditis lenta (acute) (subacute)
Malignant endocarditis (acute) (subacute)
Purulent endocarditis (acute) (subacute)
Septic endocarditis (acute) (subacute)
Ulcerative endocarditis (acute) (subacute)
Vegetative endocarditis (acute) (subacute)
Use additional code (B95-B97) to identify infectious agent

I33.9 Acute and subacute endocarditis, unspecified COM
Acute endocarditis NOS
Acute myoendocarditis NOS
Acute periendocarditis NOS
Subacute endocarditis NOS
Subacute myoendocarditis NOS
Subacute periendocarditis NOS

✓4th **I34 Nonrheumatic mitral valve disorders**
EXCLUDES 1 *mitral valve disease (IØ5.9)*
mitral valve failure (IØ5.8)
mitral valve stenosis (IØ5.Ø)
mitral valve disorder of unspecified cause with diseases of aortic and/or tricuspid valve(s) (IØ8.-)
mitral valve disorder of unspecified cause with mitral stenosis or obstruction (IØ5.Ø)
mitral valve disorder specified as congenital (Q23.2, Q23.9)
mitral valve disorder specified as rheumatic (IØ5.-)

I34.Ø Nonrheumatic mitral (valve) insufficiency
Nonrheumatic mitral (valve) incompetence NOS
Nonrheumatic mitral (valve) regurgitation NOS
▶Code also, if applicable:◀
▶nonrheumatic mitral (valve) annulus calcification (I34.81)◀

I34.1 Nonrheumatic mitral (valve) prolapse
Floppy nonrheumatic mitral valve syndrome
EXCLUDES 1 *Marfan's syndrome (Q87.4-)*

I34.2 Nonrheumatic mitral (valve) stenosis
▶Code also, if applicable:◀
▶nonrheumatic mitral (valve) annulus calcification (I34.81)◀

▲ ✓5th **I34.8 Other nonrheumatic mitral valve disorders**

● **I34.81 Nonrheumatic mitral (valve) annulus calcification**
Nonrheumatic mitral (valve) annular calcification
Mitral (valve) annulus calcification NOS
Code also, if applicable:
nonrheumatic mitral (valve) insufficiency (I34.Ø)
nonrheumatic mitral (valve) stenosis (I34.2)

● **I34.89 Other nonrheumatic mitral valve disorders**

I34.9 Nonrheumatic mitral valve disorder, unspecified

✓4th **I35 Nonrheumatic aortic valve disorders**
EXCLUDES 1 *aortic valve disorder of unspecified cause but with diseases of mitral and/or tricuspid valve(s) (IØ8.-)*
aortic valve disorder specified as congenital (Q23.Ø, Q23.1)
aortic valve disorder specified as rheumatic (IØ6.-)
hypertrophic subaortic stenosis (I42.1)

I35.Ø Nonrheumatic aortic (valve) stenosis

I35.1 Nonrheumatic aortic (valve) insufficiency
Nonrheumatic aortic (valve) incompetence NOS
Nonrheumatic aortic (valve) regurgitation NOS

I35.2 Nonrheumatic aortic (valve) stenosis with insufficiency

I35.8 Other nonrheumatic aortic valve disorders

I35.9 Nonrheumatic aortic valve disorder, unspecified

✓4th **I36 Nonrheumatic tricuspid valve disorders**
EXCLUDES 1 *tricuspid valve disorders of unspecified cause (IØ7.-)*
tricuspid valve disorders specified as congenital (Q22.4, Q22.8, Q22.9)
tricuspid valve disorders specified as rheumatic (IØ7.-)
tricuspid valve disorders with aortic and/or mitral valve involvement (IØ8.-)

I36.Ø Nonrheumatic tricuspid (valve) stenosis

I36.1 Nonrheumatic tricuspid (valve) insufficiency
Nonrheumatic tricuspid (valve) incompetence
Nonrheumatic tricuspid (valve) regurgitation

I36.2 Nonrheumatic tricuspid (valve) stenosis with insufficiency

I36.8 Other nonrheumatic tricuspid valve disorders

I36.9 Nonrheumatic tricuspid valve disorder, unspecified

✓4th **I37 Nonrheumatic pulmonary valve disorders**
EXCLUDES 1 *pulmonary valve disorder specified as congenital (Q22.1, Q22.2, Q22.3)*
pulmonary valve disorder specified as rheumatic (IØ9.89)

I37.Ø Nonrheumatic pulmonary valve stenosis

I37.1 Nonrheumatic pulmonary valve insufficiency
Nonrheumatic pulmonary valve incompetence
Nonrheumatic pulmonary valve regurgitation

I37.2 Nonrheumatic pulmonary valve stenosis with insufficiency

I37.8 Other nonrheumatic pulmonary valve disorders

I37.9 Nonrheumatic pulmonary valve disorder, unspecified

I38 Endocarditis, valve unspecified

INCLUDES endocarditis (chronic) NOS
valvular incompetence NOS
valvular insufficiency NOS
valvular regurgitation NOS
valvular stenosis NOS
valvulitis (chronic) NOS

EXCLUDES 1 *congenital insufficiency of cardiac valve NOS (Q24.8)*
congenital stenosis of cardiac valve NOS (Q24.8)
endocardial fibroelastosis (I42.4)
endocarditis specified as rheumatic (I09.1)

DEF: Endocarditis: Inflammatory disease of the interior lining of the heart chamber and heart valves.

I39 Endocarditis and heart valve disorders in diseases classified elsewhere

Code first underlying disease, such as:
Q fever (A78)

EXCLUDES 1 *endocardial involvement in:*
candidiasis (B37.6)
gonococcal infection (A54.83)
Libman-Sacks disease (M32.11)
listerosis (A32.82)
meningococcal infection (A39.51)
rheumatoid arthritis (M05.31)
syphilis (A52.03)
tuberculosis (A18.84)
typhoid fever (A01.02)

DEF: Endocarditis: Inflammatory disease of the interior lining of the heart chamber and heart valves.

✓4th **I40 Acute myocarditis**

INCLUDES subacute myocarditis

EXCLUDES 1 *acute rheumatic myocarditis (I01.2)*

DEF: Myocarditis: Inflammation of the middle layer of the heart, which is composed of muscle tissue.

I40.0 Infective myocarditis COM
Septic myocarditis
Use additional code (B95-B97) to identify infectious agent

I40.1 Isolated myocarditis COM
Fiedler's myocarditis
Giant cell myocarditis
Idiopathic myocarditis

I40.8 Other acute myocarditis COM

I40.9 Acute myocarditis, unspecified COM

I41 Myocarditis in diseases classified elsewhere COM

Code first underlying disease, such as:
typhus (A75.0-A75.9)

EXCLUDES 1 *myocarditis (in):*
Chagas' disease (chronic) (B57.2)
acute (B57.0)
coxsackie (virus) infection (B33.22)
diphtheritic (A36.81)
gonococcal (A54.83)
influenzal (J09.X9, J10.82, J11.82)
meningococcal (A39.52)
mumps (B26.82)
rheumatoid arthritis (M05.31)
sarcoid (D86.85)
syphilis (A52.06)
toxoplasmosis (B58.81)
tuberculous (A18.84)

DEF: Myocarditis: Inflammation of the middle layer of the heart, which is composed of muscle tissue.

✓4th **I42 Cardiomyopathy**

INCLUDES myocardiopathy

Code first pre-existing cardiomyopathy complicating pregnancy and puerperium (O99.4)

EXCLUDES 2 *ischemic cardiomyopathy (I25.5)*
peripartum cardiomyopathy (O90.3)
ventricular hypertrophy (I51.7)

I42.0 Dilated cardiomyopathy HCC Rx ESR COM
Congestive cardiomyopathy

I42.1 Obstructive hypertrophic cardiomyopathy HCC Rx ESR COM
Hypertrophic subaortic stenosis (idiopathic)
DEF: Cardiomyopathy marked by left ventricle hypertrophy and an enlarged septum that result in obstructed blood flow, arrhythmias, mitral regurgitation, and sudden cardiac death.
TIP: When this condition is described as inherited, assign code Q24.8.

I42.2 Other hypertrophic cardiomyopathy HCC Rx ESR COM
Nonobstructive hypertrophic cardiomyopathy

I42.3 Endomyocardial (eosinophilic) disease HCC Rx ESR COM
Endomyocardial (tropical) fibrosis
Löffler's endocarditis

I42.4 Endocardial fibroelastosis HCC Rx ESR COM
Congenital cardiomyopathy
Elastomyofibrosis

I42.5 Other restrictive cardiomyopathy HCC Rx ESR COM
Constrictive cardiomyopathy NOS

I42.6 Alcoholic cardiomyopathy HCC Rx ESR COM
Code also presence of alcoholism (F10.-)

I42.7 Cardiomyopathy due to drug and external agent HCC Rx ESR COM
Code first poisoning due to drug or toxin, if applicable (T36-T65 with fifth or sixth character 1-4 or 6)
Use additional code for adverse effect, if applicable, to identify drug (T36-T50 with fifth or sixth character 5)
AHA: 2021,3Q,8

I42.8 Other cardiomyopathies HCC Rx ESR COM

I42.9 Cardiomyopathy, unspecified HCC Rx ESR COM
Cardiomyopathy (primary) (secondary) NOS

I43 Cardiomyopathy in diseases classified elsewhere HCC Rx ESR COM

Code first underlying disease, such as:
amyloidosis (E85.-)
glycogen storage disease (E74.0)
gout (M10.0-)
thyrotoxicosis (E05.0-E05.9-)

EXCLUDES 1 *cardiomyopathy (in):*
coxsackie (virus) (B33.24)
diphtheria (A36.81)
sarcoidosis (D86.85)
tuberculosis (A18.84)

✓4th **I44 Atrioventricular and left bundle-branch block**

I44.0 Atrioventricular block, first degree

I44.1 Atrioventricular block, second degree
Atrioventricular block, type I and II
Möbitz block, type I and II
Second degree block, type I and II
Wenckebach's block

I44.2 Atrioventricular block, complete HCC ESR COM
Complete heart block NOS
Third degree block
AHA: 2019,2Q,4

✓5th **I44.3 Other and unspecified atrioventricular block**
Atrioventricular block NOS

I44.30 Unspecified atrioventricular block

I44.39 Other atrioventricular block

I44.4 Left anterior fascicular block

I44.5 Left posterior fascicular block

✓5th **I44.6 Other and unspecified fascicular block**

I44.60 Unspecified fascicular block
Left bundle-branch hemiblock NOS

I44.69 Other fascicular block

I44.7 **Left bundle-branch block, unspecified**

Conduction Disorders

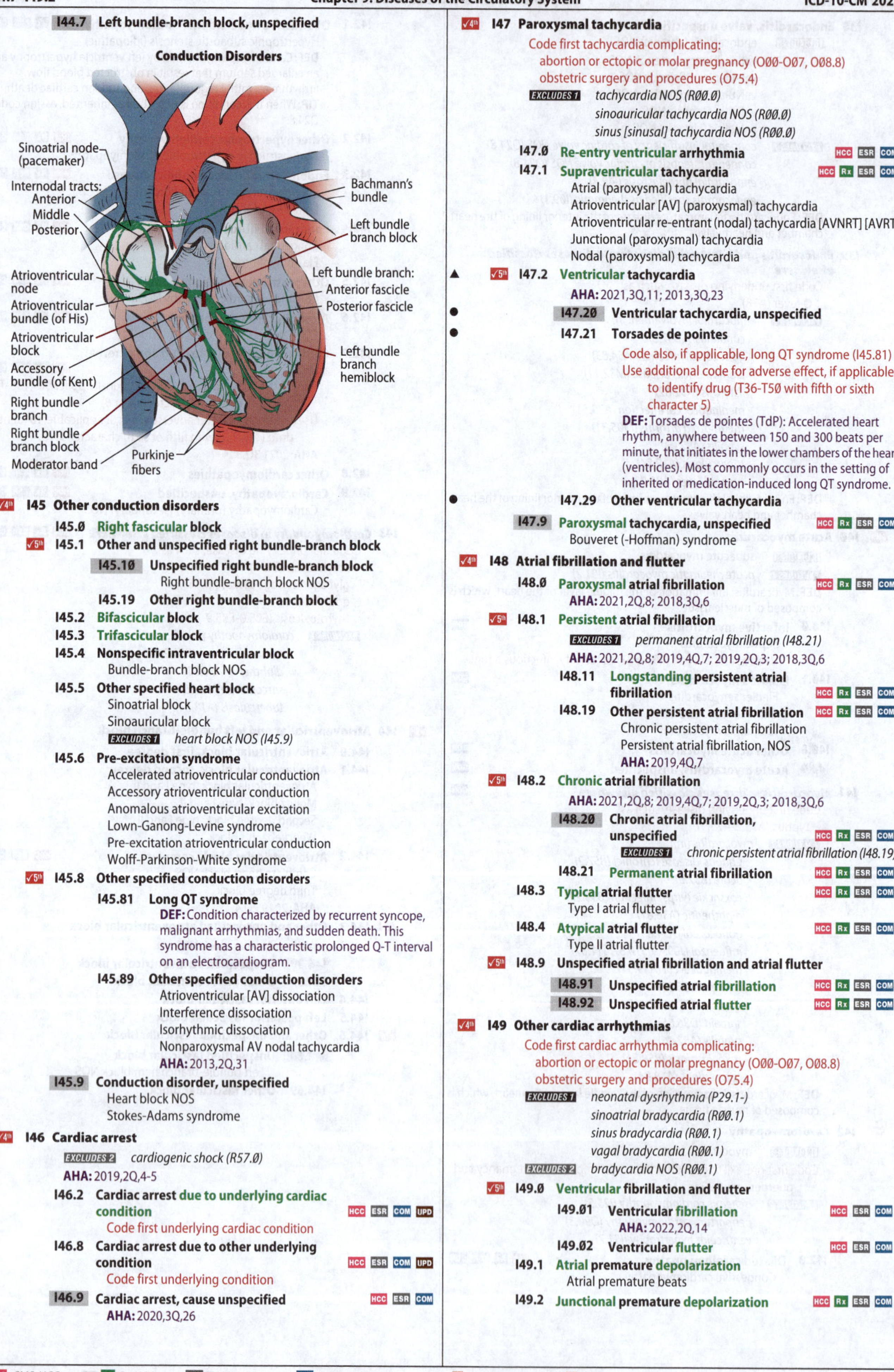

✓4th **I45 Other conduction disorders**

I45.Ø **Right fascicular block**

✓5th **I45.1** **Other and unspecified right bundle-branch block**

I45.1Ø **Unspecified right bundle-branch block**
Right bundle-branch block NOS

I45.19 **Other right bundle-branch block**

I45.2 **Bifascicular block**

I45.3 **Trifascicular block**

I45.4 **Nonspecific intraventricular block**
Bundle-branch block NOS

I45.5 **Other specified heart block**
Sinoatrial block
Sinoauricular block
EXCLUDES 1 *heart block NOS (I45.9)*

I45.6 **Pre-excitation syndrome**
Accelerated atrioventricular conduction
Accessory atrioventricular conduction
Anomalous atrioventricular excitation
Lown-Ganong-Levine syndrome
Pre-excitation atrioventricular conduction
Wolff-Parkinson-White syndrome

✓5th **I45.8** **Other specified conduction disorders**

I45.81 **Long QT syndrome**
DEF: Condition characterized by recurrent syncope, malignant arrhythmias, and sudden death. This syndrome has a characteristic prolonged Q-T interval on an electrocardiogram.

I45.89 **Other specified conduction disorders**
Atrioventricular [AV] dissociation
Interference dissociation
Isorhythmic dissociation
Nonparoxysmal AV nodal tachycardia
AHA: 2013,2Q,31

I45.9 **Conduction disorder, unspecified**
Heart block NOS
Stokes-Adams syndrome

✓4th **I46 Cardiac arrest**
EXCLUDES 2 *cardiogenic shock (R57.Ø)*
AHA: 2019,2Q,4-5

I46.2 **Cardiac arrest due to underlying cardiac condition** HCC ESR COM UPD
Code first underlying cardiac condition

I46.8 **Cardiac arrest due to other underlying condition** HCC ESR COM UPD
Code first underlying condition

I46.9 **Cardiac arrest, cause unspecified** HCC ESR COM
AHA: 2020,3Q,26

✓4th **I47 Paroxysmal tachycardia**
Code first tachycardia complicating:
abortion or ectopic or molar pregnancy (OØØ-OØ7, OØ8.8)
obstetric surgery and procedures (O75.4)
EXCLUDES 1 *tachycardia NOS (RØØ.Ø)*
sinoauricular tachycardia NOS (RØØ.Ø)
sinus [sinusal] tachycardia NOS (RØØ.Ø)

I47.Ø **Re-entry ventricular arrhythmia** HCC ESR COM

I47.1 **Supraventricular tachycardia** HCC Rx ESR COM
Atrial (paroxysmal) tachycardia
Atrioventricular [AV] (paroxysmal) tachycardia
Atrioventricular re-entrant (nodal) tachycardia [AVNRT] [AVRT]
Junctional (paroxysmal) tachycardia
Nodal (paroxysmal) tachycardia

▲ ✓5th **I47.2** **Ventricular tachycardia**
AHA: 2021,3Q,11; 2013,3Q,23

● **I47.2Ø** **Ventricular tachycardia, unspecified**

● **I47.21** **Torsades de pointes**
Code also, if applicable, long QT syndrome (I45.81)
Use additional code for adverse effect, if applicable, to identify drug (T36-T5Ø with fifth or sixth character 5)
DEF: Torsades de pointes (TdP): Accelerated heart rhythm, anywhere between 150 and 300 beats per minute, that initiates in the lower chambers of the heart (ventricles). Most commonly occurs in the setting of inherited or medication-induced long QT syndrome.

● **I47.29** **Other ventricular tachycardia**

I47.9 **Paroxysmal tachycardia, unspecified** HCC Rx ESR COM
Bouveret (-Hoffman) syndrome

✓4th **I48 Atrial fibrillation and flutter**

I48.Ø **Paroxysmal atrial fibrillation** HCC Rx ESR COM
AHA: 2021,2Q,8; 2018,3Q,6

✓5th **I48.1** **Persistent atrial fibrillation**
EXCLUDES 1 *permanent atrial fibrillation (I48.21)*
AHA: 2021,2Q,8; 2019,4Q,7; 2019,2Q,3; 2018,3Q,6

I48.11 **Longstanding persistent atrial fibrillation** HCC Rx ESR COM

I48.19 **Other persistent atrial fibrillation** HCC Rx ESR COM
Chronic persistent atrial fibrillation
Persistent atrial fibrillation, NOS
AHA: 2019,4Q,7

✓5th **I48.2** **Chronic atrial fibrillation**
AHA: 2021,2Q,8; 2019,4Q,7; 2019,2Q,3; 2018,3Q,6

I48.2Ø **Chronic atrial fibrillation, unspecified** HCC Rx ESR COM
EXCLUDES 1 *chronic persistent atrial fibrillation (I48.19)*

I48.21 **Permanent atrial fibrillation** HCC Rx ESR COM

I48.3 **Typical atrial flutter** HCC Rx ESR COM
Type I atrial flutter

I48.4 **Atypical atrial flutter** HCC Rx ESR COM
Type II atrial flutter

✓5th **I48.9** **Unspecified atrial fibrillation and atrial flutter**

I48.91 **Unspecified atrial fibrillation** HCC Rx ESR COM

I48.92 **Unspecified atrial flutter** HCC Rx ESR COM

✓4th **I49 Other cardiac arrhythmias**
Code first cardiac arrhythmia complicating:
abortion or ectopic or molar pregnancy (OØØ-OØ7, OØ8.8)
obstetric surgery and procedures (O75.4)
EXCLUDES 1 *neonatal dysrhythmia (P29.1-)*
sinoatrial bradycardia (RØØ.1)
sinus bradycardia (RØØ.1)
vagal bradycardia (RØØ.1)
EXCLUDES 2 *bradycardia NOS (RØØ.1)*

✓5th **I49.Ø** **Ventricular fibrillation and flutter**

I49.Ø1 **Ventricular fibrillation** HCC ESR COM
AHA: 2022,2Q,14

I49.Ø2 **Ventricular flutter** HCC ESR COM

I49.1 **Atrial premature depolarization**
Atrial premature beats

I49.2 **Junctional premature depolarization** HCC Rx ESR COM

I49.3 Ventricular premature depolarization
AHA: 2020,2Q,23

✓5th I49.4 Other and unspecified premature depolarization

I49.4Ø Unspecified premature depolarization
Premature beats NOS

I49.49 Other premature depolarization
Ectopic beats
Extrasystoles
Extrasystolic arrhythmias
Premature contractions

I49.5 Sick sinus syndrome HCC ESR COM
Tachycardia-bradycardia syndrome
AHA: 2019,1Q,33
TIP: The presence of a pacemaker controls but does not cure sick sinus syndrome and therefore is considered a reportable chronic condition. When a pacemaker is evaluated by a provider, this code and code Z95.0 Presence of cardiac pacemaker, should be reported, even in the absence of any notable changes or management.

I49.8 Other specified cardiac arrhythmias
Brugada syndrome
Coronary sinus rhythm disorder
Ectopic rhythm disorder
Nodal rhythm disorder

I49.9 Cardiac arrhythmia, unspecified
Arrhythmia (cardiac) NOS

✓4th I5Ø Heart failure
Code first:
heart failure complicating abortion or ectopic or molar pregnancy (OØØ-OØ7, OØ8.8)
heart failure due to hypertension (I11.Ø)
heart failure due to hypertension with chronic kidney disease (I13.-)
heart failure following surgery (I97.13-)
obstetric surgery and procedures (O75.4)
rheumatic heart failure (IØ9.81)
EXCLUDES 2 *cardiac arrest (I46.-)*
neonatal cardiac failure (P29.Ø)
AHA: 2018,4Q,67; 2018,2Q,9; 2017,1Q,47; 2014,1Q,25; 2013,2Q,33

I5Ø.1 Left ventricular failure, unspecified HCC Rx ESR COM
Cardiac asthma
Edema of lung with heart disease NOS
Edema of lung with heart failure
Left heart failure
Pulmonary edema with heart disease NOS
Pulmonary edema with heart failure
EXCLUDES 1 *edema of lung without heart disease or heart failure (J81.-)*
pulmonary edema without heart disease or failure (J81.-)

✓5th I5Ø.2 Systolic (congestive) heart failure
Heart failure with reduced ejection fraction [HFrEF]
Systolic left ventricular heart failure
Code also end stage heart failure, if applicable (I5Ø.84)
EXCLUDES 1 *combined systolic (congestive) and diastolic (congestive) heart failure (I5Ø.4-)*
AHA: 2020,3Q,32; 2017,1Q,46; 2016,1Q,10

I5Ø.2Ø Unspecified systolic (congestive) heart failure HCC Rx ESR COM

I5Ø.21 Acute systolic (congestive) heart failure HCC Rx ESR COM

I5Ø.22 Chronic systolic (congestive) heart failure HCC Rx ESR COM

I5Ø.23 Acute on chronic systolic (congestive) heart failure HCC Rx ESR COM

✓5th I5Ø.3 Diastolic (congestive) heart failure
Diastolic left ventricular heart failure
Heart failure with normal ejection fraction
Heart failure with preserved ejection fraction [HFpEF]
Code also end stage heart failure, if applicable (I5Ø.84)
EXCLUDES 1 *combined systolic (congestive) and diastolic (congestive) heart failure (I5Ø.4-)*
AHA: 2020,3Q,32; 2017,1Q,46; 2016,1Q,10

I5Ø.3Ø Unspecified diastolic (congestive) heart failure HCC Rx ESR COM

I5Ø.31 Acute diastolic (congestive) heart failure HCC Rx ESR COM

I5Ø.32 Chronic diastolic (congestive) heart failure HCC Rx ESR COM

I5Ø.33 Acute on chronic diastolic (congestive) heart failure HCC Rx ESR COM

✓5th I5Ø.4 Combined systolic (congestive) and diastolic (congestive) heart failure
Combined systolic and diastolic left ventricular heart failure
Heart failure with reduced ejection fraction and diastolic dysfunction
Code also end stage heart failure, if applicable (I5Ø.84)
AHA: 2017,1Q,46; 2016,1Q,10

I5Ø.4Ø Unspecified combined systolic (congestive) and diastolic (congestive) heart failure HCC Rx ESR COM

I5Ø.41 Acute combined systolic (congestive) and diastolic (congestive) heart failure HCC Rx ESR COM

I5Ø.42 Chronic combined systolic (congestive) and diastolic (congestive) heart failure HCC Rx ESR COM

I5Ø.43 Acute on chronic combined systolic (congestive) and diastolic (congestive) heart failure HCC Rx ESR COM

✓5th I5Ø.8 Other heart failure
AHA: 2017,4Q,15-16

✓6th I5Ø.81 Right heart failure
Right ventricular failure

I5Ø.81Ø Right heart failure, unspecified HCC Rx ESR COM
Right heart failure without mention of left heart failure
Right ventricular failure NOS

I5Ø.811 Acute right heart failure HCC Rx ESR COM
Acute isolated right heart failure
Acute (isolated) right ventricular failure

I5Ø.812 Chronic right heart failure HCC Rx ESR COM
Chronic isolated right heart failure
Chronic (isolated) right ventricular failure

I5Ø.813 Acute on chronic right heart failure HCC Rx ESR COM
Acute on chronic isolated right heart failure
Acute on chronic (isolated) right ventricular failure
Acute decompensation of chronic (isolated) right ventricular failure
Acute exacerbation of chronic (isolated) right ventricular failure

I5Ø.814 Right heart failure due to left heart failure HCC Rx ESR COM
Right ventricular failure secondary to left ventricular failure
Code also the type of left ventricular failure, if known (I5Ø.2-I5Ø.43)
EXCLUDES 1 *right heart failure with but not due to left heart failure (I5Ø.82)*

I5Ø.82 Biventricular heart failure HCC Rx ESR COM
Code also the type of left ventricular failure as systolic, diastolic, or combined, if known (I5Ø.2-I5Ø.43)

I5Ø.83 High output heart failure HCC Rx ESR COM
DEF: Occurs when the high demand for blood exceeds the capacity of a normally functioning heart to meet the demand.

I5Ø.84 End stage heart failure HCC Rx ESR COM
Stage D heart failure
Code also the type of heart failure as systolic, diastolic, or combined, if known (I5Ø.2-I5Ø.43)

I5Ø.89 Other heart failure HCC Rx ESR COM

I5Ø.9 Heart failure, unspecified HCC Rx ESR COM
Cardiac, heart or myocardial failure NOS
Congestive heart disease
Congestive heart failure NOS
EXCLUDES 2 *fluid overload unrelated to congestive heart failure (E87.7Ø)*
AHA: 2017,4Q,15-16; 2017,1Q,45-46; 2014,4Q,21; 2012,4Q,92

✓4th **I51 Complications and ill-defined descriptions of heart disease**

EXCLUDES 1 *any condition in I51.4-I51.9 due to hypertension (I11.-)*
any condition in I51.4-I51.9 due to hypertension and chronic kidney disease (I13.-)
heart disease specified as rheumatic (I00-I09)

I51.0 Cardiac septal defect, acquired A

Acquired septal atrial defect (old)
Acquired septal auricular defect (old)
Acquired septal ventricular defect (old)

EXCLUDES 1 *cardiac septal defect as current complication following acute myocardial infarction (I23.1, I23.2)*

DEF: Abnormal communication between opposite heart chambers due to a defect of the septum. It is not present at birth.

I51.1 Rupture of chordae tendineae, not elsewhere classified HCC Rx ESR COM

EXCLUDES 1 *rupture of chordae tendineae as current complication following acute myocardial infarction (I23.4)*

I51.2 Rupture of papillary muscle, not elsewhere classified HCC Rx ESR COM

EXCLUDES 1 *rupture of papillary muscle as current complication following acute myocardial infarction (I23.5)*

I51.3 Intracardiac thrombosis, not elsewhere classified

Apical thrombosis (old)
Atrial thrombosis (old)
Auricular thrombosis (old)
Mural thrombosis (old)
Ventricular thrombosis (old)

EXCLUDES 1 *intracardiac thrombosis as current complication following acute myocardial infarction (I23.6)*

AHA: 2013,1Q,24

I51.4 Myocarditis, unspecified HCC Rx ESR COM

Chronic (interstitial) myocarditis
Myocardial fibrosis
Myocarditis NOS

EXCLUDES 1 *acute or subacute myocarditis (I40.-)*

AHA: 2018,4Q,67; 2018,2Q,9

I51.5 Myocardial degeneration HCC Rx ESR COM

Fatty degeneration of heart or myocardium
Myocardial disease
Senile degeneration of heart or myocardium

AHA: 2018,4Q,67; 2018,2Q,9

I51.7 Cardiomegaly

Cardiac dilatation
Cardiac hypertrophy
Ventricular dilatation

AHA: 2018,4Q,67; 2018,2Q,9

✓5th **I51.8 Other ill-defined heart diseases**

AHA: 2018,2Q,9

I51.81 Takotsubo syndrome

Reversible left ventricular dysfunction following sudden emotional stress
Stress induced cardiomyopathy
Takotsubo cardiomyopathy
Transient left ventricular apical ballooning syndrome

DEF: Complex of symptoms mimicking myocardial infarct in absence of heart disease, with the majority of cases occurring in postmenopausal women. Heart muscles are temporarily weakened, and a sudden, massive surge of adrenalin stuns the heart, greatly reducing the ability to pump blood.

I51.89 Other ill-defined heart diseases

Carditis (acute)(chronic)
Pancarditis (acute)(chronic)

AHA: 2019,2Q,5; 2018,4Q,67

I51.9 Heart disease, unspecified

AHA: 2018,4Q,67; 2018,2Q,9

I52 Other heart disorders in diseases classified elsewhere

Code first underlying disease, such as:
congenital syphilis (A50.5)
mucopolysaccharidosis (E76.3)
schistosomiasis (B65.0-B65.9)

EXCLUDES 1 *heart disease (in):*
gonococcal infection (A54.83)
meningococcal infection (A39.50)
rheumatoid arthritis (M05.31)
syphilis (A52.06)

I5A Non-ischemic myocardial injury (non-traumatic)

Acute (non-ischemic) myocardial injury
Chronic (non-ischemic) myocardial injury
Unspecified (non-ischemic) myocardial injury

Code first the underlying cause, if known and applicable, such as:
acute kidney failure (N17.-)
acute myocarditis (I40.-)
cardiomyopathy (I42.-)
chronic kidney disease (CKD) (N18.-)
heart failure (I50.-)
hypertensive urgency (I16.0)
nonrheumatic aortic valve disorders (I35.-)
paroxysmal tachycardia (I47.-)
pulmonary embolism (I26.-)
pulmonary hypertension (I27.0, I27.2-)
sepsis (A41.-)
takotsubo syndrome (I51.81)

EXCLUDES 1 *acute myocardial infarction (I21.-)*
injury of heart (S26.-)

EXCLUDES 2 *other acute ischemic heart diseases (I24.-)*

AHA: 2021,4Q,14-15

Cerebrovascular diseases (I60-I69)

Use additional code to identify presence of:
alcohol abuse and dependence (F10.-)
exposure to environmental tobacco smoke (Z77.22)
history of tobacco dependence (Z87.891)
hypertension (I10-I16)
occupational exposure to environmental tobacco smoke (Z57.31)
tobacco dependence (F17.-)
tobacco use (Z72.0)

EXCLUDES 1 *traumatic intracranial hemorrhage (S06.-)*

AHA: 2014,3Q,5; 2012,4Q,91-92

✓4th **I60 Nontraumatic subarachnoid hemorrhage**

EXCLUDES 1 *syphilitic ruptured cerebral aneurysm (A52.05)*

EXCLUDES 2 *sequelae of subarachnoid hemorrhage (I69.0-)*

✓5th **I60.0 Nontraumatic subarachnoid hemorrhage from carotid siphon and bifurcation**

I60.00 Nontraumatic subarachnoid hemorrhage from unspecified carotid siphon and bifurcation HCC ESR COM

I60.01 Nontraumatic subarachnoid hemorrhage from right carotid siphon and bifurcation HCC ESR COM

I60.02 Nontraumatic subarachnoid hemorrhage from left carotid siphon and bifurcation HCC ESR COM

✓5th **I60.1 Nontraumatic subarachnoid hemorrhage from middle cerebral artery**

I60.10 Nontraumatic subarachnoid hemorrhage from unspecified middle cerebral artery HCC ESR COM

I60.11 Nontraumatic subarachnoid hemorrhage from right middle cerebral artery HCC ESR COM

I60.12 Nontraumatic subarachnoid hemorrhage from left middle cerebral artery HCC ESR COM

I60.2 Nontraumatic subarachnoid hemorrhage from anterior communicating artery HCC ESR COM

✓5th **I60.3 Nontraumatic subarachnoid hemorrhage from posterior communicating artery**

I60.30 Nontraumatic subarachnoid hemorrhage from unspecified posterior communicating artery HCC ESR COM

I60.31 Nontraumatic subarachnoid hemorrhage from right posterior communicating artery HCC ESR COM

I60.32 Nontraumatic subarachnoid hemorrhage from left posterior communicating artery HCC ESR COM

I60.4 Nontraumatic subarachnoid hemorrhage from basilar artery HCC ESR COM

5th **I6Ø.5 Nontraumatic subarachnoid hemorrhage from vertebral artery**

I6Ø.5Ø Nontraumatic subarachnoid hemorrhage from unspecified vertebral artery HCC ESR COM

I6Ø.51 Nontraumatic subarachnoid hemorrhage from right vertebral artery HCC ESR COM

I6Ø.52 Nontraumatic subarachnoid hemorrhage from left vertebral artery HCC ESR COM

I6Ø.6 Nontraumatic subarachnoid hemorrhage from other intracranial arteries HCC ESR COM

I6Ø.7 Nontraumatic subarachnoid hemorrhage from unspecified intracranial artery HCC ESR COM

Ruptured (congenital) berry aneurysm

Ruptured (congenital) cerebral aneurysm

Subarachnoid hemorrhage (nontraumatic) from cerebral artery NOS

Subarachnoid hemorrhage (nontraumatic) from communicating artery NOS

EXCLUDES 1 *berry aneurysm, nonruptured (I67.1)*

I6Ø.8 Other nontraumatic subarachnoid hemorrhage HCC ESR COM

Meningeal hemorrhage

Rupture of cerebral arteriovenous malformation

I6Ø.9 Nontraumatic subarachnoid hemorrhage, unspecified HCC ESR COM

4th **I61 Nontraumatic intracerebral hemorrhage**

EXCLUDES 2 *sequelae of intracerebral hemorrhage (I69.1-)*

AHA: 2017,2Q,9-10

I61.Ø Nontraumatic intracerebral hemorrhage in hemisphere, subcortical HCC ESR COM

Deep intracerebral hemorrhage (nontraumatic)

AHA: 2016,4Q,27

I61.1 Nontraumatic intracerebral hemorrhage in hemisphere, cortical HCC ESR COM

Cerebral lobe hemorrhage (nontraumatic)

Superficial intracerebral hemorrhage (nontraumatic)

I61.2 Nontraumatic intracerebral hemorrhage in hemisphere, unspecified HCC ESR COM

I61.3 Nontraumatic intracerebral hemorrhage in brain stem HCC ESR COM

I61.4 Nontraumatic intracerebral hemorrhage in cerebellum HCC ESR COM

I61.5 Nontraumatic intracerebral hemorrhage, intraventricular HCC ESR COM

I61.6 Nontraumatic intracerebral hemorrhage, multiple localized HCC ESR COM

I61.8 Other nontraumatic intracerebral hemorrhage HCC ESR COM

I61.9 Nontraumatic intracerebral hemorrhage, unspecified HCC ESR COM

4th **I62 Other and unspecified nontraumatic intracranial hemorrhage**

EXCLUDES 2 *sequelae of intracranial hemorrhage (I69.2)*

5th **I62.Ø Nontraumatic subdural hemorrhage**

I62.ØØ Nontraumatic subdural hemorrhage, unspecified HCC ESR COM

I62.Ø1 Nontraumatic acute subdural hemorrhage HCC ESR COM

I62.Ø2 Nontraumatic subacute subdural hemorrhage HCC ESR COM

I62.Ø3 Nontraumatic chronic subdural hemorrhage HCC ESR COM

I62.1 Nontraumatic extradural hemorrhage HCC ESR COM

Nontraumatic epidural hemorrhage

I62.9 Nontraumatic intracranial hemorrhage, unspecified HCC ESR COM

4th **I63 Cerebral infarction**

INCLUDES occlusion and stenosis of cerebral and precerebral arteries, resulting in cerebral infarction

Use additional code, if applicable, to identify status post administration of tPA (rtPA) in a different facility within the last 24 hours prior to admission to current facility (Z92.82)

Use additional code, if known, to indicate National Institutes of Health Stroke Scale (NIHSS) score (R29.7-)

EXCLUDES 1 *neonatal cerebral infarction (P91.82-)*

EXCLUDES 2 *sequelae of cerebral infarction (I69.3-)*

AHA: 2017,2Q,9-10; 2016,4Q,28,61-62; 2015,1Q,25; 2014,1Q,23

TIP: Weakness on one side of the body documented as secondary to stroke is synonymous with hemiparesis/hemiplegia (G81.-). Weakness of one limb documented as secondary to stroke is synonymous with monoplegia (G83.1-, G83.2-, G83.3-).

5th **I63.Ø Cerebral infarction due to thrombosis of precerebral arteries**

I63.ØØ Cerebral infarction due to thrombosis of unspecified precerebral artery HCC ESR COM

6th **I63.Ø1 Cerebral infarction due to thrombosis of vertebral artery**

I63.Ø11 Cerebral infarction due to thrombosis of right vertebral artery HCC ESR COM

I63.Ø12 Cerebral infarction due to thrombosis of left vertebral artery HCC ESR COM

I63.Ø13 Cerebral infarction due to thrombosis of bilateral vertebral arteries HCC ESR COM

I63.Ø19 Cerebral infarction due to thrombosis of unspecified vertebral artery HCC ESR COM

I63.Ø2 Cerebral infarction due to thrombosis of basilar artery HCC ESR COM

6th **I63.Ø3 Cerebral infarction due to thrombosis of carotid artery**

I63.Ø31 Cerebral infarction due to thrombosis of right carotid artery HCC ESR COM

I63.Ø32 Cerebral infarction due to thrombosis of left carotid artery HCC ESR COM

I63.Ø33 Cerebral infarction due to thrombosis of bilateral carotid arteries HCC ESR COM

I63.Ø39 Cerebral infarction due to thrombosis of unspecified carotid artery HCC ESR COM

I63.Ø9 Cerebral infarction due to thrombosis of other precerebral artery HCC ESR COM

5th **I63.1 Cerebral infarction due to embolism of precerebral arteries**

I63.1Ø Cerebral infarction due to embolism of unspecified precerebral artery HCC ESR COM

6th **I63.11 Cerebral infarction due to embolism of vertebral artery**

I63.111 Cerebral infarction due to embolism of right vertebral artery HCC ESR COM

I63.112 Cerebral infarction due to embolism of left vertebral artery HCC ESR COM

I63.113 Cerebral infarction due to embolism of bilateral vertebral arteries HCC ESR COM

I63.119 Cerebral infarction due to embolism of unspecified vertebral artery HCC ESR COM

I63.12 Cerebral infarction due to embolism of basilar artery HCC ESR COM

6th **I63.13 Cerebral infarction due to embolism of carotid artery**

I63.131 Cerebral infarction due to embolism of right carotid artery HCC ESR COM

I63.132 Cerebral infarction due to embolism of left carotid artery HCC ESR COM

I63.133 Cerebral infarction due to embolism of bilateral carotid arteries HCC ESR COM

I63.139 Cerebral infarction due to embolism of unspecified carotid artery HCC ESR COM

I63.19 Cerebral infarction due to embolism of other precerebral artery HCC ESR COM

5th **I63.2 Cerebral infarction due to unspecified occlusion or stenosis of precerebral arteries**

AHA: 2020,3Q,27-28

I63.2Ø Cerebral infarction due to unspecified occlusion or stenosis of unspecified precerebral arteries HCC ESR COM

Chapter 9. Diseases of the Circulatory System

√6th **I63.21 Cerebral infarction due to unspecified occlusion or stenosis of vertebral arteries**

I63.211 Cerebral infarction due to unspecified occlusion or stenosis of right vertebral artery HCC ESR COM

I63.212 Cerebral infarction due to unspecified occlusion or stenosis of left vertebral artery HCC ESR COM

I63.213 Cerebral infarction due to unspecified occlusion or stenosis of bilateral vertebral arteries HCC ESR COM

I63.219 Cerebral infarction due to unspecified occlusion or stenosis of unspecified vertebral artery HCC ESR COM

I63.22 Cerebral infarction due to unspecified occlusion or stenosis of basilar artery HCC ESR COM

√6th **I63.23 Cerebral infarction due to unspecified occlusion or stenosis of carotid arteries**

I63.231 Cerebral infarction due to unspecified occlusion or stenosis of right carotid arteries HCC ESR COM

I63.232 Cerebral infarction due to unspecified occlusion or stenosis of left carotid arteries HCC ESR COM

I63.233 Cerebral infarction due to unspecified occlusion or stenosis of bilateral carotid arteries HCC ESR COM

I63.239 Cerebral infarction due to unspecified occlusion or stenosis of unspecified carotid artery HCC ESR COM

I63.29 Cerebral infarction due to unspecified occlusion or stenosis of other precerebral arteries HCC ESR COM

√5th **I63.3 Cerebral infarction due to thrombosis of cerebral arteries**

I63.30 Cerebral infarction due to thrombosis of unspecified cerebral artery HCC ESR COM

√6th **I63.31 Cerebral infarction due to thrombosis of middle cerebral artery**

I63.311 Cerebral infarction due to thrombosis of right middle cerebral artery HCC ESR COM

I63.312 Cerebral infarction due to thrombosis of left middle cerebral artery HCC ESR COM

I63.313 Cerebral infarction due to thrombosis of bilateral middle cerebral arteries HCC ESR COM

I63.319 Cerebral infarction due to thrombosis of unspecified middle cerebral artery HCC ESR COM

√6th **I63.32 Cerebral infarction due to thrombosis of anterior cerebral artery**

I63.321 Cerebral infarction due to thrombosis of right anterior cerebral artery HCC ESR COM

I63.322 Cerebral infarction due to thrombosis of left anterior cerebral artery HCC ESR COM

I63.323 Cerebral infarction due to thrombosis of bilateral anterior cerebral arteries HCC ESR COM

I63.329 Cerebral infarction due to thrombosis of unspecified anterior cerebral artery HCC ESR COM

√6th **I63.33 Cerebral infarction due to thrombosis of posterior cerebral artery**

I63.331 Cerebral infarction due to thrombosis of right posterior cerebral artery HCC ESR COM

I63.332 Cerebral infarction due to thrombosis of left posterior cerebral artery HCC ESR COM

I63.333 Cerebral infarction due to thrombosis of bilateral posterior cerebral arteries HCC ESR COM

I63.339 Cerebral infarction due to thrombosis of unspecified posterior cerebral artery HCC ESR COM

√6th **I63.34 Cerebral infarction due to thrombosis of cerebellar artery**

I63.341 Cerebral infarction due to thrombosis of right cerebellar artery HCC ESR COM

I63.342 Cerebral infarction due to thrombosis of left cerebellar artery HCC ESR COM

I63.343 Cerebral infarction due to thrombosis of bilateral cerebellar arteries HCC ESR COM

I63.349 Cerebral infarction due to thrombosis of unspecified cerebellar artery HCC ESR COM

I63.39 Cerebral infarction due to thrombosis of other cerebral artery HCC ESR COM

√5th **I63.4 Cerebral infarction due to embolism of cerebral arteries**

I63.40 Cerebral infarction due to embolism of unspecified cerebral artery HCC ESR COM

√6th **I63.41 Cerebral infarction due to embolism of middle cerebral artery**

I63.411 Cerebral infarction due to embolism of right middle cerebral artery HCC ESR COM

I63.412 Cerebral infarction due to embolism of left middle cerebral artery HCC ESR COM

I63.413 Cerebral infarction due to embolism of bilateral middle cerebral arteries HCC ESR COM

I63.419 Cerebral infarction due to embolism of unspecified middle cerebral artery HCC ESR COM

√6th **I63.42 Cerebral infarction due to embolism of anterior cerebral artery**

I63.421 Cerebral infarction due to embolism of right anterior cerebral artery HCC ESR COM

I63.422 Cerebral infarction due to embolism of left anterior cerebral artery HCC ESR COM

I63.423 Cerebral infarction due to embolism of bilateral anterior cerebral arteries HCC ESR COM

I63.429 Cerebral infarction due to embolism of unspecified anterior cerebral artery HCC ESR COM

√6th **I63.43 Cerebral infarction due to embolism of posterior cerebral artery**

I63.431 Cerebral infarction due to embolism of right posterior cerebral artery HCC ESR COM

I63.432 Cerebral infarction due to embolism of left posterior cerebral artery HCC ESR COM

I63.433 Cerebral infarction due to embolism of bilateral posterior cerebral arteries HCC ESR COM

I63.439 Cerebral infarction due to embolism of unspecified posterior cerebral artery HCC ESR COM

√6th **I63.44 Cerebral infarction due to embolism of cerebellar artery**

I63.441 Cerebral infarction due to embolism of right cerebellar artery HCC ESR COM

I63.442 Cerebral infarction due to embolism of left cerebellar artery HCC ESR COM

I63.443 Cerebral infarction due to embolism of bilateral cerebellar arteries HCC ESR COM

I63.449 Cerebral infarction due to embolism of unspecified cerebellar artery HCC ESR COM

I63.49 Cerebral infarction due to embolism of other cerebral artery HCC ESR COM

√5th **I63.5 Cerebral infarction due to unspecified occlusion or stenosis of cerebral arteries**

I63.50 Cerebral infarction due to unspecified occlusion or stenosis of unspecified cerebral artery HCC ESR COM

√6th **I63.51 Cerebral infarction due to unspecified occlusion or stenosis of middle cerebral artery**

I63.511 Cerebral infarction due to unspecified occlusion or stenosis of right middle cerebral artery HCC ESR COM

I63.512 Cerebral infarction due to unspecified occlusion or stenosis of left middle cerebral artery HCC ESR COM

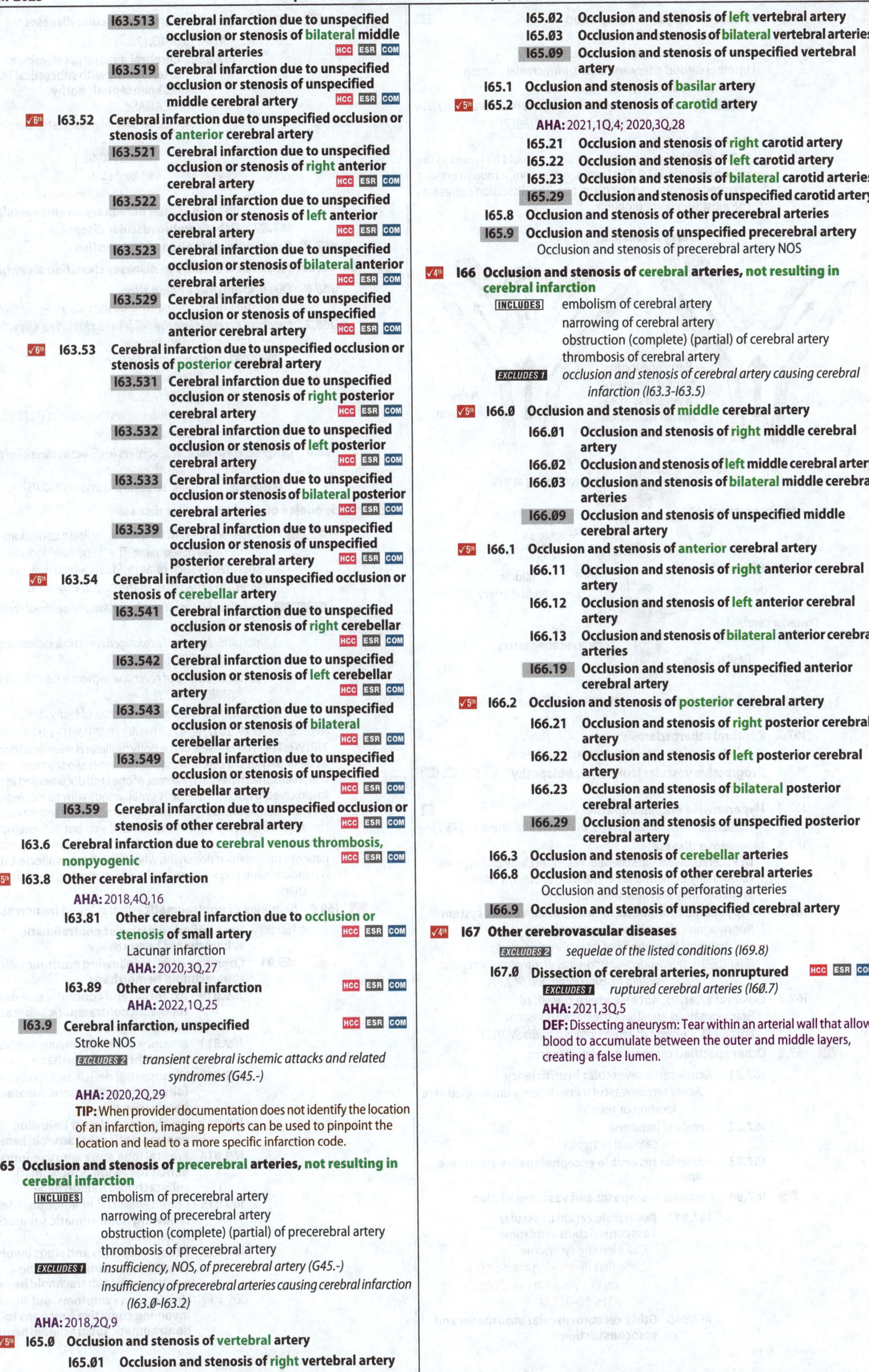

I63.513 Cerebral infarction due to unspecified occlusion or stenosis of bilateral middle cerebral arteries HCC ESR COM

I63.519 Cerebral infarction due to unspecified occlusion or stenosis of unspecified middle cerebral artery HCC ESR COM

✓6th **I63.52 Cerebral infarction due to unspecified occlusion or stenosis of anterior cerebral artery**

I63.521 Cerebral infarction due to unspecified occlusion or stenosis of right anterior cerebral artery HCC ESR COM

I63.522 Cerebral infarction due to unspecified occlusion or stenosis of left anterior cerebral artery HCC ESR COM

I63.523 Cerebral infarction due to unspecified occlusion or stenosis of bilateral anterior cerebral arteries HCC ESR COM

I63.529 Cerebral infarction due to unspecified occlusion or stenosis of unspecified anterior cerebral artery HCC ESR COM

✓6th **I63.53 Cerebral infarction due to unspecified occlusion or stenosis of posterior cerebral artery**

I63.531 Cerebral infarction due to unspecified occlusion or stenosis of right posterior cerebral artery HCC ESR COM

I63.532 Cerebral infarction due to unspecified occlusion or stenosis of left posterior cerebral artery HCC ESR COM

I63.533 Cerebral infarction due to unspecified occlusion or stenosis of bilateral posterior cerebral arteries HCC ESR COM

I63.539 Cerebral infarction due to unspecified occlusion or stenosis of unspecified posterior cerebral artery HCC ESR COM

✓6th **I63.54 Cerebral infarction due to unspecified occlusion or stenosis of cerebellar artery**

I63.541 Cerebral infarction due to unspecified occlusion or stenosis of right cerebellar artery HCC ESR COM

I63.542 Cerebral infarction due to unspecified occlusion or stenosis of left cerebellar artery HCC ESR COM

I63.543 Cerebral infarction due to unspecified occlusion or stenosis of bilateral cerebellar arteries HCC ESR COM

I63.549 Cerebral infarction due to unspecified occlusion or stenosis of unspecified cerebellar artery HCC ESR COM

I63.59 Cerebral infarction due to unspecified occlusion or stenosis of other cerebral artery HCC ESR COM

I63.6 Cerebral infarction due to cerebral venous thrombosis, nonpyogenic HCC ESR COM

✓5th **I63.8 Other cerebral infarction**

AHA: 2018,4Q,16

I63.81 Other cerebral infarction due to occlusion or stenosis of small artery HCC ESR COM

Lacunar infarction

AHA: 2020,3Q,27

I63.89 Other cerebral infarction HCC ESR COM

AHA: 2022,1Q,25

I63.9 Cerebral infarction, unspecified HCC ESR COM

Stroke NOS

EXCLUDES 2 *transient cerebral ischemic attacks and related syndromes (G45.-)*

AHA: 2020,2Q,29

TIP: When provider documentation does not identify the location of an infarction, imaging reports can be used to pinpoint the location and lead to a more specific infarction code.

✓4th **I65 Occlusion and stenosis of precerebral arteries, not resulting in cerebral infarction**

INCLUDES embolism of precerebral artery
narrowing of precerebral artery
obstruction (complete) (partial) of precerebral artery
thrombosis of precerebral artery

EXCLUDES 1 *insufficiency, NOS, of precerebral artery (G45.-)*
insufficiency of precerebral arteries causing cerebral infarction (I63.Ø-I63.2)

AHA: 2018,2Q,9

✓5th **I65.Ø Occlusion and stenosis of vertebral artery**

I65.Ø1 Occlusion and stenosis of right vertebral artery

I65.Ø2 Occlusion and stenosis of left vertebral artery

I65.Ø3 Occlusion and stenosis of bilateral vertebral arteries

I65.Ø9 Occlusion and stenosis of unspecified vertebral artery

I65.1 Occlusion and stenosis of basilar artery

✓5th **I65.2 Occlusion and stenosis of carotid artery**

AHA: 2021,1Q,4; 2020,3Q,28

I65.21 Occlusion and stenosis of right carotid artery

I65.22 Occlusion and stenosis of left carotid artery

I65.23 Occlusion and stenosis of bilateral carotid arteries

I65.29 Occlusion and stenosis of unspecified carotid artery

I65.8 Occlusion and stenosis of other precerebral arteries

I65.9 Occlusion and stenosis of unspecified precerebral artery

Occlusion and stenosis of precerebral artery NOS

✓4th **I66 Occlusion and stenosis of cerebral arteries, not resulting in cerebral infarction**

INCLUDES embolism of cerebral artery
narrowing of cerebral artery
obstruction (complete) (partial) of cerebral artery
thrombosis of cerebral artery

EXCLUDES 1 *occlusion and stenosis of cerebral artery causing cerebral infarction (I63.3-I63.5)*

✓5th **I66.Ø Occlusion and stenosis of middle cerebral artery**

I66.Ø1 Occlusion and stenosis of right middle cerebral artery

I66.Ø2 Occlusion and stenosis of left middle cerebral artery

I66.Ø3 Occlusion and stenosis of bilateral middle cerebral arteries

I66.Ø9 Occlusion and stenosis of unspecified middle cerebral artery

✓5th **I66.1 Occlusion and stenosis of anterior cerebral artery**

I66.11 Occlusion and stenosis of right anterior cerebral artery

I66.12 Occlusion and stenosis of left anterior cerebral artery

I66.13 Occlusion and stenosis of bilateral anterior cerebral arteries

I66.19 Occlusion and stenosis of unspecified anterior cerebral artery

✓5th **I66.2 Occlusion and stenosis of posterior cerebral artery**

I66.21 Occlusion and stenosis of right posterior cerebral artery

I66.22 Occlusion and stenosis of left posterior cerebral artery

I66.23 Occlusion and stenosis of bilateral posterior cerebral arteries

I66.29 Occlusion and stenosis of unspecified posterior cerebral artery

I66.3 Occlusion and stenosis of cerebellar arteries

I66.8 Occlusion and stenosis of other cerebral arteries

Occlusion and stenosis of perforating arteries

I66.9 Occlusion and stenosis of unspecified cerebral artery

✓4th **I67 Other cerebrovascular diseases**

EXCLUDES 2 *sequelae of the listed conditions (I69.8)*

I67.Ø Dissection of cerebral arteries, nonruptured HCC ESR COM

EXCLUDES 1 *ruptured cerebral arteries (I6Ø.7)*

AHA: 2021,3Q,5

DEF: Dissecting aneurysm: Tear within an arterial wall that allows blood to accumulate between the outer and middle layers, creating a false lumen.

I67.1 Cerebral aneurysm, nonruptured COM
Cerebral aneurysm NOS
Cerebral arteriovenous fistula, acquired
Internal carotid artery aneurysm, intracranial portion
Internal carotid artery aneurysm, NOS
EXCLUDES 1 *congenital cerebral aneurysm, nonruptured (Q28.-)*
ruptured cerebral aneurysm (I60.7)

AHA: 2021,3Q,5
TIP: A diagnosis of dissecting aneurysm should be coded to the dissection code, I67.0. The bulging/aneurysm, although present, occurred secondary to the dissection. The dissection represents the most significant problem.

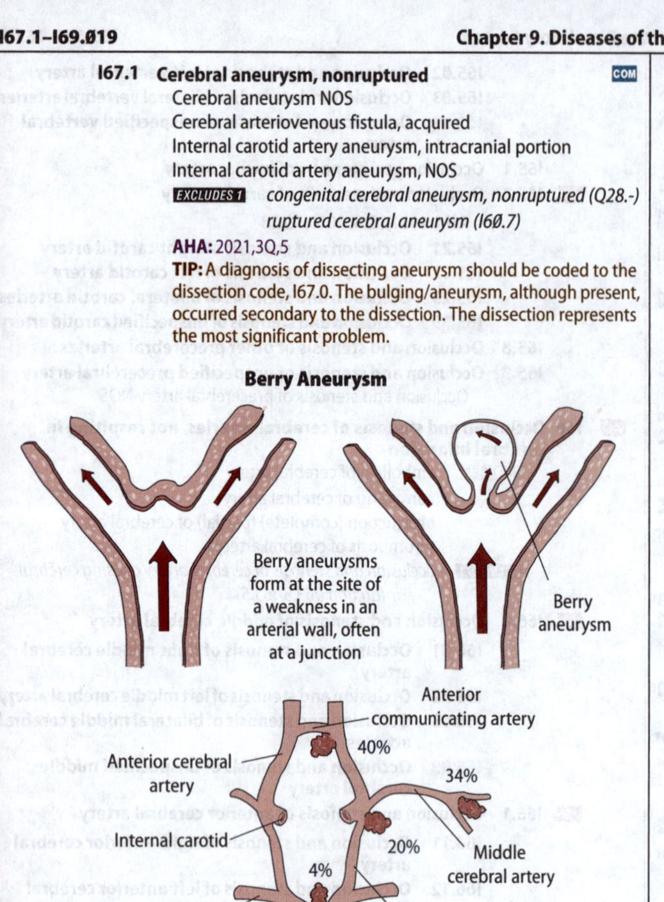

Common sites of berry aneurysms in the circle of Willis arteries

I67.2 Cerebral atherosclerosis A
Atheroma of cerebral and precerebral arteries

I67.3 Progressive vascular leukoencephalopathy HCC Rx ESR
Binswanger's disease

I67.4 Hypertensive encephalopathy Rx
EXCLUDES 2 *insufficiency, NOS, of precerebral arteries (G45.2)*

I67.5 Moyamoya disease
DEF: Cerebrovascular ischemia. Vessels occlude and rupture, causing tiny hemorrhages at the base of brain. It affects predominantly Japanese people.

I67.6 Nonpyogenic thrombosis of intracranial venous system
Nonpyogenic thrombosis of cerebral vein
Nonpyogenic thrombosis of intracranial venous sinus
EXCLUDES 1 *nonpyogenic thrombosis of intracranial venous system causing infarction (I63.6)*

I67.7 Cerebral arteritis, not elsewhere classified
Granulomatous angiitis of the nervous system
EXCLUDES 1 *allergic granulomatous angiitis (M30.1)*

√5th **I67.8 Other specified cerebrovascular diseases**

I67.81 Acute cerebrovascular insufficiency
Acute cerebrovascular insufficiency unspecified as to location or reversibility

I67.82 Cerebral ischemia
Chronic cerebral ischemia

I67.83 Posterior reversible encephalopathy syndrome
PRES

√6th **I67.84 Cerebral vasospasm and vasoconstriction**

I67.841 Reversible cerebrovascular vasoconstriction syndrome
Call-Fleming syndrome
Code first underlying condition, if applicable, such as eclampsia (O15.00-O15.9)

I67.848 Other cerebrovascular vasospasm and vasoconstriction

√6th **I67.85 Hereditary cerebrovascular diseases**
AHA: 2018,4Q,17

I67.850 Cerebral autosomal dominant arteriopathy with subcortical infarcts and leukoencephalopathy
CADASIL
Code also any associated diagnoses, such as:
epilepsy (G40.-)
stroke (I63.-)
vascular dementia (F01.-)

I67.858 Other hereditary cerebrovascular disease

I67.89 Other cerebrovascular disease

I67.9 Cerebrovascular disease, unspecified

√4th **I68 Cerebrovascular disorders in diseases classified elsewhere**

I68.0 Cerebral amyloid angiopathy
Code first underlying amyloidosis (E85.-)

I68.2 Cerebral arteritis in other diseases classified elsewhere
Code first underlying disease
EXCLUDES 1 *cerebral arteritis (in):*
listerosis (A32.89)
syphilis (A52.04)
systemic lupus erythematosus (M32.19)
tuberculosis (A18.89)

I68.8 Other cerebrovascular disorders in diseases classified elsewhere
Code first underlying disease
EXCLUDES 1 *syphilitic cerebral aneurysm (A52.05)*

√4th **I69 Sequelae of cerebrovascular disease**

NOTE Category I69 is to be used to indicate conditions in I60-I67 as the cause of sequelae. The "sequelae" include conditions specified as such or as residuals which may occur at any time after the onset of the causal condition

EXCLUDES 1 *personal history of cerebral infarction without residual deficit (Z86.73)*
personal history of prolonged reversible ischemic neurologic deficit (PRIND) (Z86.73)
personal history of reversible ischemic neurologcial deficit (RIND) (Z86.73)
sequelae of traumatic intracranial injury (S06.-)

AHA: 2020,2Q,29; 2017,1Q,47; 2016,4Q,28; 2015,1Q,25; 2012,4Q,106
TIP: Weakness on one side of the body (unilateral weakness) documented as secondary to old cerebrovascular disease is synonymous with hemiparesis/hemiplegia. Weakness of one limb documented as secondary to old cerebrovascular disease is synonymous with monoplegia.
TIP: For codes describing hemiplegia, hemiparesis, and monoplegia; if the documentation identifies the affected side but not whether it is the dominant or nondominant side, the default is as follows: for ambidextrous patients, the default is dominant; when the left side is affected, the default is nondominant; and when the right side is affected, the default is dominant.

√5th **I69.0 Sequelae of nontraumatic subarachnoid hemorrhage**

I69.00 Unspecified sequelae of nontraumatic subarachnoid hemorrhage

√6th **I69.01 Cognitive deficits following nontraumatic subarachnoid hemorrhage**

I69.010 Attention and concentration deficit following nontraumatic subarachnoid hemorrhage

I69.011 Memory deficit following nontraumatic subarachnoid hemorrhage

I69.012 Visuospatial deficit and spatial neglect following nontraumatic subarachnoid hemorrhage

I69.013 Psychomotor deficit following nontraumatic subarachnoid hemorrhage

I69.014 Frontal lobe and executive function deficit following nontraumatic subarachnoid hemorrhage

I69.015 Cognitive social or emotional deficit following nontraumatic subarachnoid hemorrhage

I69.018 Other symptoms and signs involving cognitive functions following nontraumatic subarachnoid hemorrhage

I69.019 Unspecified symptoms and signs involving cognitive functions following nontraumatic subarachnoid hemorrhage

I69.02 Speech and language deficits following nontraumatic subarachnoid hemorrhage

I69.020 Aphasia following nontraumatic subarachnoid hemorrhage

I69.021 Dysphasia following nontraumatic subarachnoid hemorrhage

I69.022 Dysarthria following nontraumatic subarachnoid hemorrhage

I69.023 Fluency disorder following nontraumatic subarachnoid hemorrhage

Stuttering following nontraumatic subarachnoid hemorrhage

I69.028 Other speech and language deficits following nontraumatic subarachnoid hemorrhage

I69.03 Monoplegia of upper limb following nontraumatic subarachnoid hemorrhage

AHA: 2017,1Q,47

I69.031 Monoplegia of upper limb following nontraumatic subarachnoid hemorrhage affecting right dominant side HCC ESR COM

I69.032 Monoplegia of upper limb following nontraumatic subarachnoid hemorrhage affecting left dominant side HCC ESR COM

I69.033 Monoplegia of upper limb following nontraumatic subarachnoid hemorrhage affecting right non-dominant side HCC ESR COM

I69.034 Monoplegia of upper limb following nontraumatic subarachnoid hemorrhage affecting left non-dominant side HCC ESR COM

I69.039 Monoplegia of upper limb following nontraumatic subarachnoid hemorrhage affecting unspecified side HCC ESR COM

I69.04 Monoplegia of lower limb following nontraumatic subarachnoid hemorrhage

AHA: 2017,1Q,47

I69.041 Monoplegia of lower limb following nontraumatic subarachnoid hemorrhage affecting right dominant side HCC ESR COM

I69.042 Monoplegia of lower limb following nontraumatic subarachnoid hemorrhage affecting left dominant side HCC ESR COM

I69.043 Monoplegia of lower limb following nontraumatic subarachnoid hemorrhage affecting right non-dominant side HCC ESR COM

I69.044 Monoplegia of lower limb following nontraumatic subarachnoid hemorrhage affecting left non-dominant side HCC ESR COM

I69.049 Monoplegia of lower limb following nontraumatic subarachnoid hemorrhage affecting unspecified side HCC ESR COM

I69.05 Hemiplegia and hemiparesis following nontraumatic subarachnoid hemorrhage

AHA: 2015,1Q,25

I69.051 Hemiplegia and hemiparesis following nontraumatic subarachnoid hemorrhage affecting right dominant side HCC ESR COM

I69.052 Hemiplegia and hemiparesis following nontraumatic subarachnoid hemorrhage affecting left dominant side HCC ESR COM

I69.053 Hemiplegia and hemiparesis following nontraumatic subarachnoid hemorrhage affecting right non-dominant side HCC ESR COM

I69.054 Hemiplegia and hemiparesis following nontraumatic subarachnoid hemorrhage affecting left non-dominant side HCC ESR COM

I69.059 Hemiplegia and hemiparesis following nontraumatic subarachnoid hemorrhage affecting unspecified side HCC ESR COM

I69.06 Other paralytic syndrome following nontraumatic subarachnoid hemorrhage

Use additional code to identify type of paralytic syndrome, such as:
locked-in state (G83.5)
quadriplegia (G82.5-)

EXCLUDES 1 *hemiplegia/hemiparesis following nontraumatic subarachnoid hemorrhage (I69.05-)*
monoplegia of lower limb following nontraumatic subarachnoid hemorrhage (I69.04-)
monoplegia of upper limb following nontraumatic subarachnoid hemorrhage (I69.03-)

I69.061 Other paralytic syndrome following nontraumatic subarachnoid hemorrhage affecting right dominant side HCC ESR COM

I69.062 Other paralytic syndrome following nontraumatic subarachnoid hemorrhage affecting left dominant side HCC ESR COM

I69.063 Other paralytic syndrome following nontraumatic subarachnoid hemorrhage affecting right non-dominant side HCC ESR COM

I69.064 Other paralytic syndrome following nontraumatic subarachnoid hemorrhage affecting left non-dominant side HCC ESR COM

I69.065 Other paralytic syndrome following nontraumatic subarachnoid hemorrhage, bilateral HCC ESR COM

I69.069 Other paralytic syndrome following nontraumatic subarachnoid hemorrhage affecting unspecified side HCC ESR COM

I69.09 Other sequelae of nontraumatic subarachnoid hemorrhage

I69.090 Apraxia following nontraumatic subarachnoid hemorrhage

I69.091 Dysphagia following nontraumatic subarachnoid hemorrhage

Use additional code to identify the type of dysphagia, if known ►(R13.11-R13.19)◄

I69.092 Facial weakness following nontraumatic subarachnoid hemorrhage

Facial droop following nontraumatic subarachnoid hemorrhage

I69.093 Ataxia following nontraumatic subarachnoid hemorrhage

I69.098 Other sequelae following nontraumatic subarachnoid hemorrhage

Alterations of sensation following nontraumatic subarachnoid hemorrhage
Disturbance of vision following nontraumatic subarachnoid hemorrhage
Use additional code to identify the sequelae

I69.1 Sequelae of nontraumatic intracerebral hemorrhage

I69.10 Unspecified sequelae of nontraumatic intracerebral hemorrhage

I69.11 Cognitive deficits following nontraumatic intracerebral hemorrhage

I69.110 Attention and concentration deficit following nontraumatic intracerebral hemorrhage

I69.111 Memory deficit following nontraumatic intracerebral hemorrhage

I69.112 Visuospatial deficit and spatial neglect following nontraumatic intracerebral hemorrhage

I69.113 Psychomotor deficit following nontraumatic intracerebral hemorrhage

I69.114 Frontal lobe and executive function deficit following nontraumatic intracerebral hemorrhage

I69.115 Cognitive social or emotional deficit following nontraumatic intracerebral hemorrhage

I69.118 Other symptoms and signs involving cognitive functions following nontraumatic intracerebral hemorrhage

I69.119 Unspecified symptoms and signs involving cognitive functions following nontraumatic intracerebral hemorrhage

6th **I69.12 Speech and language deficits following nontraumatic intracerebral hemorrhage**

I69.120 Aphasia following nontraumatic intracerebral hemorrhage

I69.121 Dysphasia following nontraumatic intracerebral hemorrhage

I69.122 Dysarthria following nontraumatic intracerebral hemorrhage

I69.123 Fluency disorder following nontraumatic intracerebral hemorrhage

Stuttering following nontraumatic intracerebral hemorrhage

I69.128 Other speech and language deficits following nontraumatic intracerebral hemorrhage

6th **I69.13 Monoplegia of upper limb following nontraumatic intracerebral hemorrhage**

AHA: 2017,1Q,47

I69.131 Monoplegia of upper limb following nontraumatic intracerebral hemorrhage affecting right dominant side HCC ESR COM

I69.132 Monoplegia of upper limb following nontraumatic intracerebral hemorrhage affecting left dominant side HCC ESR COM

I69.133 Monoplegia of upper limb following nontraumatic intracerebral hemorrhage affecting right non-dominant side HCC ESR COM

I69.134 Monoplegia of upper limb following nontraumatic intracerebral hemorrhage affecting left non-dominant side HCC ESR COM

I69.139 Monoplegia of upper limb following nontraumatic intracerebral hemorrhage affecting unspecified side HCC ESR COM

6th **I69.14 Monoplegia of lower limb following nontraumatic intracerebral hemorrhage**

AHA: 2017,1Q,47

I69.141 Monoplegia of lower limb following nontraumatic intracerebral hemorrhage affecting right dominant side HCC ESR COM

I69.142 Monoplegia of lower limb following nontraumatic intracerebral hemorrhage affecting left dominant side HCC ESR COM

I69.143 Monoplegia of lower limb following nontraumatic intracerebral hemorrhage affecting right non-dominant side HCC ESR COM

I69.144 Monoplegia of lower limb following nontraumatic intracerebral hemorrhage affecting left non-dominant side HCC ESR COM

I69.149 Monoplegia of lower limb following nontraumatic intracerebral hemorrhage affecting unspecified side HCC ESR COM

6th **I69.15 Hemiplegia and hemiparesis following nontraumatic intracerebral hemorrhage**

AHA: 2015,1Q,25

I69.151 Hemiplegia and hemiparesis following nontraumatic intracerebral hemorrhage affecting right dominant side HCC ESR COM

I69.152 Hemiplegia and hemiparesis following nontraumatic intracerebral hemorrhage affecting left dominant side HCC ESR COM

I69.153 Hemiplegia and hemiparesis following nontraumatic intracerebral hemorrhage affecting right non-dominant side HCC ESR COM

I69.154 Hemiplegia and hemiparesis following nontraumatic intracerebral hemorrhage affecting left non-dominant side HCC ESR COM

I69.159 Hemiplegia and hemiparesis following nontraumatic intracerebral hemorrhage affecting unspecified side HCC ESR COM

6th **I69.16 Other paralytic syndrome following nontraumatic intracerebral hemorrhage**

Use additional code to identify type of paralytic syndrome, such as:
locked-in state (G83.5)
quadriplegia (G82.5-)

EXCLUDES 1 *hemiplegia/hemiparesis following nontraumatic intracerebral hemorrhage (I69.15-)*
monoplegia of lower limb following nontraumatic intracerebral hemorrhage (I69.14-)
monoplegia of upper limb following nontraumatic intracerebral hemorrhage (I69.13-)

I69.161 Other paralytic syndrome following nontraumatic intracerebral hemorrhage affecting right dominant side HCC ESR COM

I69.162 Other paralytic syndrome following nontraumatic intracerebral hemorrhage affecting left dominant side HCC ESR COM

I69.163 Other paralytic syndrome following nontraumatic intracerebral hemorrhage affecting right non-dominant side HCC ESR COM

I69.164 Other paralytic syndrome following nontraumatic intracerebral hemorrhage affecting left non-dominant side HCC ESR COM

I69.165 Other paralytic syndrome following nontraumatic intracerebral hemorrhage, bilateral HCC ESR COM

I69.169 Other paralytic syndrome following nontraumatic intracerebral hemorrhage affecting unspecified side HCC ESR COM

6th **I69.19 Other sequelae of nontraumatic intracerebral hemorrhage**

I69.190 Apraxia following nontraumatic intracerebral hemorrhage

I69.191 Dysphagia following nontraumatic intracerebral hemorrhage

Use additional code to identify the type of dysphagia, if known ►(R13.11-R13.19)◄

I69.192 Facial weakness following nontraumatic intracerebral hemorrhage

Facial droop following nontraumatic intracerebral hemorrhage

I69.193 Ataxia following nontraumatic intracerebral hemorrhage

I69.198 Other sequelae of nontraumatic intracerebral hemorrhage

Alteration of sensations following nontraumatic intracerebral hemorrhage
Disturbance of vision following nontraumatic intracerebral hemorrhage

Use additional code to identify the sequelae

5th **I69.2 Sequelae of other nontraumatic intracranial hemorrhage**

I69.20 Unspecified sequelae of other nontraumatic intracranial hemorrhage

6th **I69.21 Cognitive deficits following other nontraumatic intracranial hemorrhage**

I69.210 Attention and concentration deficit following other nontraumatic intracranial hemorrhage

I69.211 Memory deficit following other nontraumatic intracranial hemorrhage

I69.212 Visuospatial deficit and spatial neglect following other nontraumatic intracranial hemorrhage

I69.213 Psychomotor deficit following other nontraumatic intracranial hemorrhage
I69.214 Frontal lobe and executive function deficit following other nontraumatic intracranial hemorrhage
I69.215 Cognitive social or emotional deficit following other nontraumatic intracranial hemorrhage
I69.218 Other symptoms and signs involving cognitive functions following other nontraumatic intracranial hemorrhage
I69.219 Unspecified symptoms and signs involving cognitive functions following other nontraumatic intracranial hemorrhage

I69.22 Speech and language deficits following other nontraumatic intracranial hemorrhage
I69.220 Aphasia following other nontraumatic intracranial hemorrhage
I69.221 Dysphasia following other nontraumatic intracranial hemorrhage
I69.222 Dysarthria following other nontraumatic intracranial hemorrhage
I69.223 Fluency disorder following other nontraumatic intracranial hemorrhage
Stuttering following other nontraumatic intracranial hemorrhage
I69.228 Other speech and language deficits following other nontraumatic intracranial hemorrhage

I69.23 Monoplegia of upper limb following other nontraumatic intracranial hemorrhage
AHA: 2017,1Q,47
I69.231 Monoplegia of upper limb following other nontraumatic intracranial hemorrhage affecting right dominant side HCC ESR COM
I69.232 Monoplegia of upper limb following other nontraumatic intracranial hemorrhage affecting left dominant side HCC ESR COM
I69.233 Monoplegia of upper limb following other nontraumatic intracranial hemorrhage affecting right non-dominant side HCC ESR COM
I69.234 Monoplegia of upper limb following other nontraumatic intracranial hemorrhage affecting left non-dominant side HCC ESR COM
I69.239 Monoplegia of upper limb following other nontraumatic intracranial hemorrhage affecting unspecified side HCC ESR COM

I69.24 Monoplegia of lower limb following other nontraumatic intracranial hemorrhage
AHA: 2017,1Q,47
I69.241 Monoplegia of lower limb following other nontraumatic intracranial hemorrhage affecting right dominant side HCC ESR COM
I69.242 Monoplegia of lower limb following other nontraumatic intracranial hemorrhage affecting left dominant side HCC ESR COM
I69.243 Monoplegia of lower limb following other nontraumatic intracranial hemorrhage affecting right non-dominant side HCC ESR COM
I69.244 Monoplegia of lower limb following other nontraumatic intracranial hemorrhage affecting left non-dominant side HCC ESR COM
I69.249 Monoplegia of lower limb following other nontraumatic intracranial hemorrhage affecting unspecified side HCC ESR COM

I69.25 Hemiplegia and hemiparesis following other nontraumatic intracranial hemorrhage
AHA: 2015,1Q,25
I69.251 Hemiplegia and hemiparesis following other nontraumatic intracranial hemorrhage affecting right dominant side HCC ESR COM
I69.252 Hemiplegia and hemiparesis following other nontraumatic intracranial hemorrhage affecting left dominant side HCC ESR COM
I69.253 Hemiplegia and hemiparesis following other nontraumatic intracranial hemorrhage affecting right non-dominant side HCC ESR COM
I69.254 Hemiplegia and hemiparesis following other nontraumatic intracranial hemorrhage affecting left non-dominant side HCC ESR COM
I69.259 Hemiplegia and hemiparesis following other nontraumatic intracranial hemorrhage affecting unspecified side HCC ESR COM

I69.26 Other paralytic syndrome following other nontraumatic intracranial hemorrhage
Use additional code to identify type of paralytic syndrome, such as:
locked-in state (G83.5)
quadriplegia (G82.5-)
EXCLUDES 1 *hemiplegia/hemiparesis following other nontraumatic intracranial hemorrhage (I69.25-)*
monoplegia of lower limb following other nontraumatic intracranial hemorrhage (I69.24-)
monoplegia of upper limb following other nontraumatic intracranial hemorrhage (I69.23-)
I69.261 Other paralytic syndrome following other nontraumatic intracranial hemorrhage affecting right dominant side HCC ESR COM
I69.262 Other paralytic syndrome following other nontraumatic intracranial hemorrhage affecting left dominant side HCC ESR COM
I69.263 Other paralytic syndrome following other nontraumatic intracranial hemorrhage affecting right non-dominant side HCC ESR COM
I69.264 Other paralytic syndrome following other nontraumatic intracranial hemorrhage affecting left non-dominant side HCC ESR COM
I69.265 Other paralytic syndrome following other nontraumatic intracranial hemorrhage, bilateral HCC ESR COM
I69.269 Other paralytic syndrome following other nontraumatic intracranial hemorrhage affecting unspecified side HCC ESR COM

I69.29 Other sequelae of other nontraumatic intracranial hemorrhage
I69.290 Apraxia following other nontraumatic intracranial hemorrhage
I69.291 Dysphagia following other nontraumatic intracranial hemorrhage
Use additional code to identify the type of dysphagia, if known ►(R13.11-R13.19)◄
I69.292 Facial weakness following other nontraumatic intracranial hemorrhage
Facial droop following other nontraumatic intracranial hemorrhage
I69.293 Ataxia following other nontraumatic intracranial hemorrhage
I69.298 Other sequelae of other nontraumatic intracranial hemorrhage
Alteration of sensation following other nontraumatic intracranial hemorrhage
Disturbance of vision following other nontraumatic intracranial hemorrhage
Use additional code to identify the sequelae

I69.3 Sequelae of cerebral infarction
Sequelae of stroke NOS
AHA: 2013,4Q,127-128; 2012,4Q,92,94

I69.30 Unspecified sequelae of cerebral infarction

I69.31 Cognitive deficits following cerebral infarction

I69.310 Attention and concentration deficit following cerebral infarction

I69.311 Memory deficit following cerebral infarction

I69.312 Visuospatial deficit and spatial neglect following cerebral infarction

I69.313 Psychomotor deficit following cerebral infarction

I69.314 Frontal lobe and executive function deficit following cerebral infarction

I69.315 Cognitive social or emotional deficit following cerebral infarction

I69.318 Other symptoms and signs involving cognitive functions following cerebral infarction

I69.319 Unspecified symptoms and signs involving cognitive functions following cerebral infarction

I69.32 Speech and language deficits following cerebral infarction

I69.320 Aphasia following cerebral infarction

I69.321 Dysphasia following cerebral infarction
AHA: 2012,4Q,91

I69.322 Dysarthria following cerebral infarction
EXCLUDES 2 *transient ischemic attack (TIA) (G45.9)*

I69.323 Fluency disorder following cerebral infarction
Stuttering following cerebral infarction

I69.328 Other speech and language deficits following cerebral infarction

I69.33 Monoplegia of upper limb following cerebral infarction
AHA: 2017,1Q,47

I69.331 Monoplegia of upper limb following cerebral infarction affecting right dominant side HCC ESR COM

I69.332 Monoplegia of upper limb following cerebral infarction affecting left dominant side HCC ESR COM

I69.333 Monoplegia of upper limb following cerebral infarction affecting right non-dominant side HCC ESR COM

I69.334 Monoplegia of upper limb following cerebral infarction affecting left non-dominant side HCC ESR COM

I69.339 Monoplegia of upper limb following cerebral infarction affecting unspecified side HCC ESR COM

I69.34 Monoplegia of lower limb following cerebral infarction
AHA: 2017,1Q,47

I69.341 Monoplegia of lower limb following cerebral infarction affecting right dominant side HCC ESR COM

I69.342 Monoplegia of lower limb following cerebral infarction affecting left dominant side HCC ESR COM

I69.343 Monoplegia of lower limb following cerebral infarction affecting right non-dominant side HCC ESR COM

I69.344 Monoplegia of lower limb following cerebral infarction affecting left non-dominant side HCC ESR COM

I69.349 Monoplegia of lower limb following cerebral infarction affecting unspecified side HCC ESR COM

I69.35 Hemiplegia and hemiparesis following cerebral infarction
AHA: 2015,1Q,25

I69.351 Hemiplegia and hemiparesis following cerebral infarction affecting right dominant side HCC ESR COM
EXCLUDES 2 *transient ischemic attack (TIA) (G45.9)*

I69.352 Hemiplegia and hemiparesis following cerebral infarction affecting left dominant side HCC ESR COM

I69.353 Hemiplegia and hemiparesis following cerebral infarction affecting right non-dominant side HCC ESR COM

I69.354 Hemiplegia and hemiparesis following cerebral infarction affecting left non-dominant side HCC ESR COM
AHA: 2012,4Q,91

I69.359 Hemiplegia and hemiparesis following cerebral infarction affecting unspecified side HCC ESR COM

I69.36 Other paralytic syndrome following cerebral infarction
Use additional code to identify type of paralytic syndrome, such as:
locked-in state (G83.5)
quadriplegia (G82.5-)
EXCLUDES 1 *hemiplegia/hemiparesis following cerebral infarction (I69.35-)*
monoplegia of lower limb following cerebral infarction (I69.34-)
monoplegia of upper limb following cerebral infarction (I69.33-)

I69.361 Other paralytic syndrome following cerebral infarction affecting right dominant side HCC ESR COM

I69.362 Other paralytic syndrome following cerebral infarction affecting left dominant side HCC ESR COM

I69.363 Other paralytic syndrome following cerebral infarction affecting right non-dominant side HCC ESR COM

I69.364 Other paralytic syndrome following cerebral infarction affecting left non-dominant side HCC ESR COM

I69.365 Other paralytic syndrome following cerebral infarction, bilateral HCC ESR COM

I69.369 Other paralytic syndrome following cerebral infarction affecting unspecified side HCC ESR COM

I69.39 Other sequelae of cerebral infarction

I69.390 Apraxia following cerebral infarction

I69.391 Dysphagia following cerebral infarction
Use additional code to identify the type of dysphagia, if known ▶(R13.11-R13.19)◀

I69.392 Facial weakness following cerebral infarction
Facial droop following cerebral infarction

I69.393 Ataxia following cerebral infarction

I69.398 Other sequelae of cerebral infarction
Alteration of sensation following cerebral infarction
Disturbance of vision following cerebral infarction
Use additional code to identify the sequelae
AHA: 2020,2Q,29

I69.8 Sequelae of other cerebrovascular diseases
EXCLUDES 1 *sequelae of traumatic intracranial injury (S06.-)*

I69.80 Unspecified sequelae of other cerebrovascular disease

I69.81 Cognitive deficits following other cerebrovascular disease

I69.810 Attention and concentration deficit following other cerebrovascular disease

I69.811 Memory deficit following other cerebrovascular disease

I69.812 Visuospatial deficit and spatial neglect following other cerebrovascular disease

I69.813 Psychomotor deficit following other cerebrovascular disease

I69.814 Frontal lobe and executive function deficit following other cerebrovascular disease

I69.815 Cognitive social or emotional deficit following other cerebrovascular disease

I69.818 Other symptoms and signs involving cognitive functions following other cerebrovascular disease

I69.819 Unspecified symptoms and signs involving cognitive functions following other cerebrovascular disease

✓6th **I69.82 Speech and language deficits following other cerebrovascular disease**

I69.820 Aphasia following other cerebrovascular disease

I69.821 Dysphasia following other cerebrovascular disease

I69.822 Dysarthria following other cerebrovascular disease

I69.823 Fluency disorder following other cerebrovascular disease

Stuttering following other cerebrovascular disease

I69.828 Other speech and language deficits following other cerebrovascular disease

AHA: 2019,3Q,8

✓6th **I69.83 Monoplegia of upper limb following other cerebrovascular disease**

AHA: 2017,1Q,47

I69.831 Monoplegia of upper limb following other cerebrovascular disease affecting right dominant side HCC ESR COM

I69.832 Monoplegia of upper limb following other cerebrovascular disease affecting left dominant side HCC ESR COM

I69.833 Monoplegia of upper limb following other cerebrovascular disease affecting right non-dominant side HCC ESR COM

I69.834 Monoplegia of upper limb following other cerebrovascular disease affecting left non-dominant side HCC ESR COM

I69.839 Monoplegia of upper limb following other cerebrovascular disease affecting unspecified side HCC ESR COM

✓6th **I69.84 Monoplegia of lower limb following other cerebrovascular disease**

AHA: 2017,1Q,47

I69.841 Monoplegia of lower limb following other cerebrovascular disease affecting right dominant side HCC ESR COM

I69.842 Monoplegia of lower limb following other cerebrovascular disease affecting left dominant side HCC ESR COM

I69.843 Monoplegia of lower limb following other cerebrovascular disease affecting right non-dominant side HCC ESR COM

I69.844 Monoplegia of lower limb following other cerebrovascular disease affecting left non-dominant side HCC ESR COM

I69.849 Monoplegia of lower limb following other cerebrovascular disease affecting unspecified side HCC ESR COM

✓6th **I69.85 Hemiplegia and hemiparesis following other cerebrovascular disease**

AHA: 2015,1Q,25

I69.851 Hemiplegia and hemiparesis following other cerebrovascular disease affecting right dominant side HCC ESR COM

I69.852 Hemiplegia and hemiparesis following other cerebrovascular disease affecting left dominant side HCC ESR COM

I69.853 Hemiplegia and hemiparesis following other cerebrovascular disease affecting right non-dominant side HCC ESR COM

I69.854 Hemiplegia and hemiparesis following other cerebrovascular disease affecting left non-dominant side HCC ESR COM

I69.859 Hemiplegia and hemiparesis following other cerebrovascular disease affecting unspecified side HCC ESR COM

✓6th **I69.86 Other paralytic syndrome following other cerebrovascular disease**

Use additional code to identify type of paralytic syndrome, such as:
locked-in state (G83.5)
quadriplegia (G82.5-)

EXCLUDES 1 *hemiplegia/hemiparesis following other cerebrovascular disease (I69.85-)*
monoplegia of lower limb following other cerebrovascular disease (I69.84-)
monoplegia of upper limb following other cerebrovascular disease (I69.83-)

I69.861 Other paralytic syndrome following other cerebrovascular disease affecting right dominant side HCC ESR COM

I69.862 Other paralytic syndrome following other cerebrovascular disease affecting left dominant side HCC ESR COM

I69.863 Other paralytic syndrome following other cerebrovascular disease affecting right non-dominant side HCC ESR COM

I69.864 Other paralytic syndrome following other cerebrovascular disease affecting left non-dominant side HCC ESR COM

I69.865 Other paralytic syndrome following other cerebrovascular disease, bilateral HCC ESR COM

I69.869 Other paralytic syndrome following other cerebrovascular disease affecting unspecified side HCC ESR COM

✓6th **I69.89 Other sequelae of other cerebrovascular disease**

I69.890 Apraxia following other cerebrovascular disease

I69.891 Dysphagia following other cerebrovascular disease

Use additional code to identify the type of dysphagia, if known
▶(R13.11-R13.19)◀

I69.892 Facial weakness following other cerebrovascular disease

Facial droop following other cerebrovascular disease

I69.893 Ataxia following other cerebrovascular disease

I69.898 Other sequelae of other cerebrovascular disease

Alteration of sensation following other cerebrovascular disease
Disturbance of vision following other cerebrovascular disease

Use additional code to identify the sequelae

✓5th **I69.9 Sequelae of unspecified cerebrovascular diseases**

EXCLUDES 1 *sequelae of stroke (I69.3)*
sequelae of traumatic intracranial injury (S06.-)

I69.90 Unspecified sequelae of unspecified cerebrovascular disease

✓6th **I69.91 Cognitive deficits following unspecified cerebrovascular disease**

I69.910 Attention and concentration deficit following unspecified cerebrovascular disease

I69.911 Memory deficit following unspecified cerebrovascular disease

I69.912 Visuospatial deficit and spatial neglect following unspecified cerebrovascular disease

I69.913 Psychomotor deficit following unspecified cerebrovascular disease

I69.914 Frontal lobe and executive function deficit following unspecified cerebrovascular disease

I69.915 Cognitive social or emotional deficit following unspecified cerebrovascular disease

I69.918 Other symptoms and signs involving cognitive functions following unspecified cerebrovascular disease

I69.919 Unspecified symptoms and signs involving cognitive functions following unspecified cerebrovascular disease

✓6th I69.92 **Speech and language deficits following unspecified cerebrovascular disease**

I69.920 **Aphasia following unspecified cerebrovascular disease**

I69.921 **Dysphasia following unspecified cerebrovascular disease**

I69.922 **Dysarthria following unspecified cerebrovascular disease**

I69.923 **Fluency disorder following unspecified cerebrovascular disease**

Stuttering following unspecified cerebrovascular disease

I69.928 **Other speech and language deficits following unspecified cerebrovascular disease**

✓6th I69.93 **Monoplegia of upper limb following unspecified cerebrovascular disease**

AHA: 2017,1Q,47

I69.931 **Monoplegia of upper limb following unspecified cerebrovascular disease affecting right dominant side** HCC ESR COM

I69.932 **Monoplegia of upper limb following unspecified cerebrovascular disease affecting left dominant side** HCC ESR COM

I69.933 **Monoplegia of upper limb following unspecified cerebrovascular disease affecting right non-dominant side** HCC ESR COM

I69.934 **Monoplegia of upper limb following unspecified cerebrovascular disease affecting left non-dominant side** HCC ESR COM

I69.939 **Monoplegia of upper limb following unspecified cerebrovascular disease affecting unspecified side** HCC ESR COM

✓6th I69.94 **Monoplegia of lower limb following unspecified cerebrovascular disease**

AHA: 2017,1Q,47

I69.941 **Monoplegia of lower limb following unspecified cerebrovascular disease affecting right dominant side** HCC ESR COM

I69.942 **Monoplegia of lower limb following unspecified cerebrovascular disease affecting left dominant side** HCC ESR COM

I69.943 **Monoplegia of lower limb following unspecified cerebrovascular disease affecting right non-dominant side** HCC ESR COM

I69.944 **Monoplegia of lower limb following unspecified cerebrovascular disease affecting left non-dominant side** HCC ESR COM

I69.949 **Monoplegia of lower limb following unspecified cerebrovascular disease affecting unspecified side** HCC ESR COM

✓6th I69.95 **Hemiplegia and hemiparesis following unspecified cerebrovascular disease**

AHA: 2015,1Q,25

I69.951 **Hemiplegia and hemiparesis following unspecified cerebrovascular disease affecting right dominant side** HCC ESR COM

I69.952 **Hemiplegia and hemiparesis following unspecified cerebrovascular disease affecting left dominant side** HCC ESR COM

I69.953 **Hemiplegia and hemiparesis following unspecified cerebrovascular disease affecting right non-dominant side** HCC ESR COM

I69.954 **Hemiplegia and hemiparesis following unspecified cerebrovascular disease affecting left non-dominant side** HCC ESR COM

I69.959 **Hemiplegia and hemiparesis following unspecified cerebrovascular disease affecting unspecified side** HCC ESR COM

✓6th I69.96 **Other paralytic syndrome following unspecified cerebrovascular disease**

Use additional code to identify type of paralytic syndrome, such as:
locked-in state (G83.5)
quadriplegia (G82.5-)

EXCLUDES 1 *hemiplegia/hemiparesis following unspecified cerebrovascular disease (I69.95-)*
monoplegia of lower limb following unspecified cerebrovascular disease (I69.94-)
monoplegia of upper limb following unspecified cerebrovascular disease (I69.93-)

I69.961 **Other paralytic syndrome following unspecified cerebrovascular disease affecting right dominant side** HCC ESR COM

I69.962 **Other paralytic syndrome following unspecified cerebrovascular disease affecting left dominant side** HCC ESR COM

I69.963 **Other paralytic syndrome following unspecified cerebrovascular disease affecting right non-dominant side** HCC ESR COM

I69.964 **Other paralytic syndrome following unspecified cerebrovascular disease affecting left non-dominant side** HCC ESR COM

I69.965 **Other paralytic syndrome following unspecified cerebrovascular disease, bilateral** HCC ESR COM

I69.969 **Other paralytic syndrome following unspecified cerebrovascular disease affecting unspecified side** HCC ESR COM

✓6th I69.99 **Other sequelae of unspecified cerebrovascular disease**

I69.990 **Apraxia following unspecified cerebrovascular disease**

I69.991 **Dysphagia following unspecified cerebrovascular disease**

Use additional code to identify the type of dysphagia, if known ►(R13.11-R13.19)◄

I69.992 **Facial weakness following unspecified cerebrovascular disease**

Facial droop following unspecified cerebrovascular disease

I69.993 **Ataxia following unspecified cerebrovascular disease**

I69.998 **Other sequelae following unspecified cerebrovascular disease**

Alteration in sensation following unspecified cerebrovascular disease
Disturbance of vision following unspecified cerebrovascular disease

Use additional code to identify the sequelae

Diseases of arteries, arterioles and capillaries (I70-I79)

I70 Atherosclerosis

INCLUDES arterial degeneration
arteriolosclerosis
arteriosclerosis
arteriosclerotic vascular disease
arteriovascular degeneration
atheroma
endarteritis deformans or obliterans
senile arteritis
senile endarteritis
vascular degeneration

Use additional code to identify:
exposure to environmental tobacco smoke (Z77.22)
history of tobacco dependence (Z87.891)
occupational exposure to environmental tobacco smoke (Z57.31)
tobacco dependence (F17.-)
tobacco use (Z72.0)

EXCLUDES 2 *arteriosclerotic cardiovascular disease (I25.1-)*
arteriosclerotic heart disease (I25.1-)
atheroembolism (I75.-)
cerebral atherosclerosis (I67.2)
coronary atherosclerosis (I25.1-)
mesenteric atherosclerosis (K55.1)
precerebral atherosclerosis (I67.2)
primary pulmonary atherosclerosis (I27.0)

I70.0 Atherosclerosis of aorta HCC ESR A

I70.1 Atherosclerosis of renal artery HCC ESR A
Goldblatt's kidney
EXCLUDES 2 *atherosclerosis of renal arterioles (I12.-)*

I70.2 Atherosclerosis of native arteries of the extremities
Mönckeberg's (medial) sclerosis
Use additional code, if applicable, to identify chronic total occlusion of artery of extremity (I70.92)
EXCLUDES 2 *atherosclerosis of bypass graft of extremities (I70.30-I70.79)*
AHA: 2020,4Q,98; 2018,3Q,4; 2018,2Q,7

I70.20 Unspecified atherosclerosis of native arteries of extremities

I70.201 Unspecified atherosclerosis of native arteries of extremities, right leg HCC ESR A

I70.202 Unspecified atherosclerosis of native arteries of extremities, left leg HCC ESR A

I70.203 Unspecified atherosclerosis of native arteries of extremities, bilateral legs HCC ESR A

I70.208 Unspecified atherosclerosis of native arteries of extremities, other extremity HCC ESR A

I70.209 Unspecified atherosclerosis of native arteries of extremities, unspecified extremity HCC ESR A

I70.21 Atherosclerosis of native arteries of extremities with intermittent claudication

I70.211 Atherosclerosis of native arteries of extremities with intermittent claudication, right leg HCC ESR A

I70.212 Atherosclerosis of native arteries of extremities with intermittent claudication, left leg HCC ESR A

I70.213 Atherosclerosis of native arteries of extremities with intermittent claudication, bilateral legs HCC ESR A

I70.218 Atherosclerosis of native arteries of extremities with intermittent claudication, other extremity HCC ESR A

I70.219 Atherosclerosis of native arteries of extremities with intermittent claudication, unspecified extremity HCC ESR A

I70.22 Atherosclerosis of native arteries of extremities with rest pain

INCLUDES any condition classifiable to I70.21-
chronic limb-threatening ischemia NOS of native arteries of extremities
chronic limb-threatening ischemia of native arteries of extremities with rest pain
critical limb ischemia NOS of native arteries of extremities
critical limb ischemia of native arteries of extremities with rest pain

I70.221 Atherosclerosis of native arteries of extremities with rest pain, right leg HCC ESR A

I70.222 Atherosclerosis of native arteries of extremities with rest pain, left leg HCC ESR A

I70.223 Atherosclerosis of native arteries of extremities with rest pain, bilateral legs HCC ESR A

I70.228 Atherosclerosis of native arteries of extremities with rest pain, other extremity HCC ESR A

I70.229 Atherosclerosis of native arteries of extremities with rest pain, unspecified extremity HCC ESR A

I70.23 Atherosclerosis of native arteries of right leg with ulceration

INCLUDES any condition classifiable to I70.211 and I70.221
chronic limb-threatening ischemia of native arteries of right leg with ulceration
critical limb ischemia of native arteries of right leg with ulceration

Use additional code to identify severity of ulcer (L97.-)

I70.231 Atherosclerosis of native arteries of right leg with ulceration of thigh HCC Rx ESR COM A

I70.232 Atherosclerosis of native arteries of right leg with ulceration of calf HCC Rx ESR COM A

I70.233 Atherosclerosis of native arteries of right leg with ulceration of ankle HCC Rx ESR COM A

I70.234 Atherosclerosis of native arteries of right leg with ulceration of heel and midfoot HCC Rx ESR COM A
Atherosclerosis of native arteries of right leg with ulceration of plantar surface of midfoot

I70.235 Atherosclerosis of native arteries of right leg with ulceration of other part of foot HCC Rx ESR COM A
Atherosclerosis of native arteries of right leg extremities with ulceration of toe

I70.238 Atherosclerosis of native arteries of right leg with ulceration of other part of lower leg HCC Rx ESR COM A

I70.239 Atherosclerosis of native arteries of right leg with ulceration of unspecified site HCC Rx ESR COM A

I70.24 Atherosclerosis of native arteries of left leg with ulceration

INCLUDES any condition classifiable to I70.212 and I70.222
chronic limb-threatening ischemia of native arteries of left leg with ulceration
critical limb ischemia of native arteries of left leg with ulceration

Use additional code to identify severity of ulcer (L97.-)

I70.241 Atherosclerosis of native arteries of left leg with ulceration of thigh HCC Rx ESR COM A

I70.242 Atherosclerosis of native arteries of left leg with ulceration of calf HCC Rx ESR COM A

I70.243 Atherosclerosis of native arteries of left leg with ulceration of ankle HCC Rx ESR COM A

I70.244 Atherosclerosis of native arteries of left leg with ulceration of heel and midfoot HCC Rx ESR COM A

Atherosclerosis of native arteries of left leg with ulceration of plantar surface of midfoot

I70.245 Atherosclerosis of native arteries of left leg with ulceration of other part of foot HCC Rx ESR COM A

Atherosclerosis of native arteries of left leg extremities with ulceration of toe

I70.248 Atherosclerosis of native arteries of left leg with ulceration of other part of lower leg HCC Rx ESR COM A

I70.249 Atherosclerosis of native arteries of left leg with ulceration of unspecified site HCC Rx ESR COM A

I70.25 Atherosclerosis of native arteries of other extremities with ulceration HCC Rx ESR COM A

INCLUDES any condition classifiable to I70.218 and I70.228

Use additional code to identify the severity of the ulcer (L98.49-)

✓6th **I70.26 Atherosclerosis of native arteries of extremities with gangrene**

INCLUDES any condition classifiable to I70.21-, I70.22-, I70.23-, I70.24-, and I70.25-

chronic limb-threatening ischemia of native arteries of extremities with gangrene

critical limb ischemia of native arteries of extremities with gangrene

Use additional code to identify the severity of any ulcer (L97.-, L98.49-), if applicable

I70.261 Atherosclerosis of native arteries of extremities with gangrene, right leg HCC ESR COM A

I70.262 Atherosclerosis of native arteries of extremities with gangrene, left leg HCC ESR COM A

I70.263 Atherosclerosis of native arteries of extremities with gangrene, bilateral legs HCC ESR COM A

I70.268 Atherosclerosis of native arteries of extremities with gangrene, other extremity HCC ESR COM A

I70.269 Atherosclerosis of native arteries of extremities with gangrene, unspecified extremity HCC ESR COM A

✓6th **I70.29 Other atherosclerosis of native arteries of extremities**

I70.291 Other atherosclerosis of native arteries of extremities, right leg HCC ESR A

I70.292 Other atherosclerosis of native arteries of extremities, left leg HCC ESR A

I70.293 Other atherosclerosis of native arteries of extremities, bilateral legs HCC ESR A

I70.298 Other atherosclerosis of native arteries of extremities, other extremity HCC ESR A

I70.299 Other atherosclerosis of native arteries of extremities, unspecified extremity HCC ESR A

✓5th **I70.3 Atherosclerosis of unspecified type of bypass graft(s) of the extremities**

Use additional code, if applicable, to identify chronic total occlusion of artery of extremity (I70.92)

EXCLUDES 1 *embolism or thrombus of bypass graft(s) of extremities (T82.8-)*

AHA: 2020,4Q,98

✓6th **I70.30 Unspecified atherosclerosis of unspecified type of bypass graft(s) of the extremities**

I70.301 Unspecified atherosclerosis of unspecified type of bypass graft(s) of the extremities, right leg HCC ESR A

I70.302 Unspecified atherosclerosis of unspecified type of bypass graft(s) of the extremities, left leg HCC ESR A

I70.303 Unspecified atherosclerosis of unspecified type of bypass graft(s) of the extremities, bilateral legs HCC ESR A

I70.308 Unspecified atherosclerosis of unspecified type of bypass graft(s) of the extremities, other extremity HCC ESR A

I70.309 Unspecified atherosclerosis of unspecified type of bypass graft(s) of the extremities, unspecified extremity HCC ESR A

✓6th **I70.31 Atherosclerosis of unspecified type of bypass graft(s) of the extremities with intermittent claudication**

I70.311 Atherosclerosis of unspecified type of bypass graft(s) of the extremities with intermittent claudication, right leg HCC ESR A

I70.312 Atherosclerosis of unspecified type of bypass graft(s) of the extremities with intermittent claudication, left leg HCC ESR A

I70.313 Atherosclerosis of unspecified type of bypass graft(s) of the extremities with intermittent claudication, bilateral legs HCC ESR A

I70.318 Atherosclerosis of unspecified type of bypass graft(s) of the extremities with intermittent claudication, other extremity HCC ESR A

I70.319 Atherosclerosis of unspecified type of bypass graft(s) of the extremities with intermittent claudication, unspecified extremity HCC ESR A

✓6th **I70.32 Atherosclerosis of unspecified type of bypass graft(s) of the extremities with rest pain**

INCLUDES any condition classifiable to I70.31-

chronic limb-threatening ischemia NOS of unspecified type of bypass graft(s) of the extremities

▶chronic limb-threatening ischemia of unspecified type of bypass graft(s) of the extremities with rest pain◀

critical limb ischemia NOS of unspecified type of bypass graft(s) of the extremities

critical limb ischemia of unspecified type of bypass graft(s) of the extremities with rest pain

I70.321 Atherosclerosis of unspecified type of bypass graft(s) of the extremities with rest pain, right leg HCC ESR A

I70.322 Atherosclerosis of unspecified type of bypass graft(s) of the extremities with rest pain, left leg HCC ESR A

I70.323 Atherosclerosis of unspecified type of bypass graft(s) of the extremities with rest pain, bilateral legs HCC ESR A

I70.328 Atherosclerosis of unspecified type of bypass graft(s) of the extremities with rest pain, other extremity HCC ESR A

I70.329 Atherosclerosis of unspecified type of bypass graft(s) of the extremities with rest pain, unspecified extremity HCC ESR A

✓6th **I70.33 Atherosclerosis of unspecified type of bypass graft(s) of the right leg with ulceration**

INCLUDES any condition classifiable to I70.311 and I70.321

chronic limb-threatening ischemia of unspecified type of bypass graft(s) of the right leg with ulceration

critical limb ischemia of unspecified type of bypass graft(s) of the right leg with ulceration

Use additional code to identify severity of ulcer (L97.-)

I70.331 Atherosclerosis of unspecified type of bypass graft(s) of the right leg with ulceration of thigh HCC Rx ESR COM A

I70.332 **Atherosclerosis of unspecified type of bypass graft(s) of the right leg with ulceration of calf** HCC Rx ESR COM A

I70.333 **Atherosclerosis of unspecified type of bypass graft(s) of the right leg with ulceration of ankle** HCC Rx ESR COM A

I70.334 **Atherosclerosis of unspecified type of bypass graft(s) of the right leg with ulceration of heel and midfoot** HCC Rx ESR COM A
Atherosclerosis of unspecified type of bypass graft(s) of right leg with ulceration of plantar surface of midfoot

I70.335 **Atherosclerosis of unspecified type of bypass graft(s) of the right leg with ulceration of other part of foot** HCC Rx ESR COM A
Atherosclerosis of unspecified type of bypass graft(s) of the right leg with ulceration of toe

I70.338 **Atherosclerosis of unspecified type of bypass graft(s) of the right leg with ulceration of other part of lower leg** HCC Rx ESR COM A

I70.339 **Atherosclerosis of unspecified type of bypass graft(s) of the right leg with ulceration of unspecified site** HCC Rx ESR COM A

✓6th I70.34 **Atherosclerosis of unspecified type of bypass graft(s) of the left leg with ulceration**
INCLUDES any condition classifiable to I70.312 and I70.322
chronic limb-threatening ischemia of unspecified type of bypass graft(s) of the left leg with ulceration
critical limb ischemia of unspecified type of bypass graft(s) of the left leg with ulceration
Use additional code to identify severity of ulcer (L97.-)

I70.341 **Atherosclerosis of unspecified type of bypass graft(s) of the left leg with ulceration of thigh** HCC Rx ESR COM A

I70.342 **Atherosclerosis of unspecified type of bypass graft(s) of the left leg with ulceration of calf** HCC Rx ESR COM A

I70.343 **Atherosclerosis of unspecified type of bypass graft(s) of the left leg with ulceration of ankle** HCC Rx ESR COM A

I70.344 **Atherosclerosis of unspecified type of bypass graft(s) of the left leg with ulceration of heel and midfoot** HCC Rx ESR COM A
Atherosclerosis of unspecified type of bypass graft(s) of left leg with ulceration of plantar surface of midfoot

I70.345 **Atherosclerosis of unspecified type of bypass graft(s) of the left leg with ulceration of other part of foot** HCC Rx ESR COM A
Atherosclerosis of unspecified type of bypass graft(s) of the left leg with ulceration of toe

I70.348 **Atherosclerosis of unspecified type of bypass graft(s) of the left leg with ulceration of other part of lower leg** HCC Rx ESR COM A

I70.349 **Atherosclerosis of unspecified type of bypass graft(s) of the left leg with ulceration of unspecified site** HCC Rx ESR COM A

I70.35 **Atherosclerosis of unspecified type of bypass graft(s) of other extremity with ulceration** HCC Rx ESR COM A
INCLUDES any condition classifiable to I70.318 and I70.328
Use additional code to identify severity of ulcer (L98.49-)

✓6th I70.36 **Atherosclerosis of unspecified type of bypass graft(s) of the extremities with gangrene**
INCLUDES any condition classifiable to I70.31-, I70.32-, I70.33-, I70.34-, I70.35
chronic limb-threatening ischemia of unspecified type of bypass graft(s) of the extremities with gangrene
critical limb ischemia of unspecified type of bypass graft(s) of the extremities with gangrene
Use additional code to identify the severity of any ulcer (L97.-, L98.49-), if applicable

I70.361 **Atherosclerosis of unspecified type of bypass graft(s) of the extremities with gangrene, right leg** HCC ESR COM A

I70.362 **Atherosclerosis of unspecified type of bypass graft(s) of the extremities with gangrene, left leg** HCC ESR COM A

I70.363 **Atherosclerosis of unspecified type of bypass graft(s) of the extremities with gangrene, bilateral legs** HCC ESR COM A

I70.368 **Atherosclerosis of unspecified type of bypass graft(s) of the extremities with gangrene, other extremity** HCC ESR COM A

I70.369 **Atherosclerosis of unspecified type of bypass graft(s) of the extremities with gangrene, unspecified extremity** HCC ESR COM A

✓6th I70.39 **Other atherosclerosis of unspecified type of bypass graft(s) of the extremities**

I70.391 **Other atherosclerosis of unspecified type of bypass graft(s) of the extremities, right leg** HCC ESR A

I70.392 **Other atherosclerosis of unspecified type of bypass graft(s) of the extremities, left leg** HCC ESR A

I70.393 **Other atherosclerosis of unspecified type of bypass graft(s) of the extremities, bilateral legs** HCC ESR A

I70.398 **Other atherosclerosis of unspecified type of bypass graft(s) of the extremities, other extremity** HCC ESR A

I70.399 **Other atherosclerosis of unspecified type of bypass graft(s) of the extremities, unspecified extremity** HCC ESR A

✓5th I70.4 **Atherosclerosis of autologous vein bypass graft(s) of the extremities**
Use additional code, if applicable, to identify chronic total occlusion of artery of extremity (I70.92)
AHA: 2020,4Q,98

✓6th I70.40 **Unspecified atherosclerosis of autologous vein bypass graft(s) of the extremities**

I70.401 **Unspecified atherosclerosis of autologous vein bypass graft(s) of the extremities, right leg** HCC ESR A

I70.402 **Unspecified atherosclerosis of autologous vein bypass graft(s) of the extremities, left leg** HCC ESR A

I70.403 **Unspecified atherosclerosis of autologous vein bypass graft(s) of the extremities, bilateral legs** HCC ESR A

I70.408 **Unspecified atherosclerosis of autologous vein bypass graft(s) of the extremities, other extremity** HCC ESR A

I70.409 **Unspecified atherosclerosis of autologous vein bypass graft(s) of the extremities, unspecified extremity** HCC ESR A

✓6th I70.41 **Atherosclerosis of autologous vein bypass graft(s) of the extremities with intermittent claudication**

I70.411 **Atherosclerosis of autologous vein bypass graft(s) of the extremities with intermittent claudication, right leg** HCC ESR A

I70.412 **Atherosclerosis of autologous vein bypass graft(s) of the extremities with intermittent claudication, left leg** HCC ESR A

I70.413 **Atherosclerosis of autologous vein bypass graft(s) of the extremities with intermittent claudication, bilateral legs** HCC ESR A

I7Ø.418 **Atherosclerosis of autologous vein bypass graft(s) of the extremities with intermittent claudication, other extremity** HCC ESR A

I7Ø.419 **Atherosclerosis of autologous vein bypass graft(s) of the extremities with intermittent claudication, unspecified extremity** HCC ESR A

6th I7Ø.42 **Atherosclerosis of autologous vein bypass graft(s) of the extremities with rest pain**

INCLUDES any condition classifiable to I7Ø.41-
chronic limb-threatening ischemia NOS of autologous vein bypass graft(s) of the extremities
chronic limb-threatening ischemia of autologous vein bypass graft(s) of the extremities with rest pain
critical limb ischemia NOS of autologous vein bypass graft(s) of the extremities
critical limb ischemia of autologous vein bypass graft(s) of the extremities with rest pain

I7Ø.421 **Atherosclerosis of autologous vein bypass graft(s) of the extremities with rest pain, right leg** HCC ESR A

I7Ø.422 **Atherosclerosis of autologous vein bypass graft(s) of the extremities with rest pain, left leg** HCC ESR A

I7Ø.423 **Atherosclerosis of autologous vein bypass graft(s) of the extremities with rest pain, bilateral legs** HCC ESR A

I7Ø.428 **Atherosclerosis of autologous vein bypass graft(s) of the extremities with rest pain, other extremity** HCC ESR A

I7Ø.429 **Atherosclerosis of autologous vein bypass graft(s) of the extremities with rest pain, unspecified extremity** HCC ESR A

6th I7Ø.43 **Atherosclerosis of autologous vein bypass graft(s) of the right leg with ulceration**

INCLUDES any condition classifiable to I7Ø.411 and I7Ø.421
chronic limb-threatening ischemia of autologous vein bypass graft(s) of the right leg with ulceration
critical limb ischemia of autologous vein bypass graft(s) of the right leg with ulceration

Use additional code to identify severity of ulcer (L97.-)

I7Ø.431 **Atherosclerosis of autologous vein bypass graft(s) of the right leg with ulceration of thigh** HCC Rx ESR COM A

I7Ø.432 **Atherosclerosis of autologous vein bypass graft(s) of the right leg with ulceration of calf** HCC Rx ESR COM A

I7Ø.433 **Atherosclerosis of autologous vein bypass graft(s) of the right leg with ulceration of ankle** HCC Rx ESR COM A

I7Ø.434 **Atherosclerosis of autologous vein bypass graft(s) of the right leg with ulceration of heel and midfoot** HCC Rx ESR COM A
Atherosclerosis of autologous vein bypass graft(s) of right leg with ulceration of plantar surface of midfoot

I7Ø.435 **Atherosclerosis of autologous vein bypass graft(s) of the right leg with ulceration of other part of foot** HCC Rx ESR COM A
Atherosclerosis of autologous vein bypass graft(s) of right leg with ulceration of toe

I7Ø.438 **Atherosclerosis of autologous vein bypass graft(s) of the right leg with ulceration of other part of lower leg** HCC Rx ESR COM A

I7Ø.439 **Atherosclerosis of autologous vein bypass graft(s) of the right leg with ulceration of unspecified site** HCC Rx ESR COM A

6th I7Ø.44 **Atherosclerosis of autologous vein bypass graft(s) of the left leg with ulceration**

INCLUDES any condition classifiable to I7Ø.412 and I7Ø.422
chronic limb-threatening ischemia of autologous vein bypass graft(s) of the left leg with ulceration
critical limb ischemia of autologous vein bypass graft(s) of the left leg with ulceration

Use additional code to identify severity of ulcer (L97.-)

I7Ø.441 **Atherosclerosis of autologous vein bypass graft(s) of the left leg with ulceration of thigh** HCC Rx ESR COM A

I7Ø.442 **Atherosclerosis of autologous vein bypass graft(s) of the left leg with ulceration of calf** HCC Rx ESR COM A

I7Ø.443 **Atherosclerosis of autologous vein bypass graft(s) of the left leg with ulceration of ankle** HCC Rx ESR COM A

I7Ø.444 **Atherosclerosis of autologous vein bypass graft(s) of the left leg with ulceration of heel and midfoot** HCC Rx ESR COM A
Atherosclerosis of autologous vein bypass graft(s) of left leg with ulceration of plantar surface of midfoot

I7Ø.445 **Atherosclerosis of autologous vein bypass graft(s) of the left leg with ulceration of other part of foot** HCC Rx ESR COM A
Atherosclerosis of autologous vein bypass graft(s) of left leg with ulceration of toe

I7Ø.448 **Atherosclerosis of autologous vein bypass graft(s) of the left leg with ulceration of other part of lower leg** HCC Rx ESR COM A

I7Ø.449 **Atherosclerosis of autologous vein bypass graft(s) of the left leg with ulceration of unspecified site** HCC Rx ESR COM A

I7Ø.45 **Atherosclerosis of autologous vein bypass graft(s) of other extremity with ulceration** HCC Rx ESR COM A

INCLUDES any condition classifiable to I7Ø.418, I7Ø.428, and I7Ø.438

Use additional code to identify severity of ulcer (L98.49)

6th I7Ø.46 **Atherosclerosis of autologous vein bypass graft(s) of the extremities with gangrene**

INCLUDES any condition classifiable to I7Ø.41-, I7Ø.42-, and I7Ø.43-, I7Ø.44-, I7Ø.45
chronic limb-threatening ischemia of autologous vein bypass graft(s) of the extremities with gangrene
critical limb ischemia of autologous vein bypass graft(s) of the extremities with gangrene

Use additional code to identify the severity of any ulcer (L97.-, L98.49-), if applicable

I7Ø.461 **Atherosclerosis of autologous vein bypass graft(s) of the extremities with gangrene, right leg** HCC ESR COM A

I7Ø.462 **Atherosclerosis of autologous vein bypass graft(s) of the extremities with gangrene, left leg** HCC ESR COM A

I7Ø.463 **Atherosclerosis of autologous vein bypass graft(s) of the extremities with gangrene, bilateral legs** HCC ESR COM A

I7Ø.468 **Atherosclerosis of autologous vein bypass graft(s) of the extremities with gangrene, other extremity** HCC ESR COM A

I7Ø.469 **Atherosclerosis of autologous vein bypass graft(s) of the extremities with gangrene, unspecified extremity** HCC ESR COM A

6th I7Ø.49 **Other atherosclerosis of autologous vein bypass graft(s) of the extremities**

I7Ø.491 **Other atherosclerosis of autologous vein bypass graft(s) of the extremities, right leg** HCC ESR A

I7Ø.492 **Other atherosclerosis of autologous vein bypass graft(s) of the extremities, left leg** HCC ESR A

I70.493 **Other atherosclerosis of autologous vein bypass graft(s) of the extremities, bilateral legs** HCC ESR A

I70.498 **Other atherosclerosis of autologous vein bypass graft(s) of the extremities, other extremity** HCC ESR A

I70.499 **Other atherosclerosis of autologous vein bypass graft(s) of the extremities, unspecified extremity** HCC ESR A

I70.5 **Atherosclerosis of nonautologous biological bypass graft(s) of the extremities**

Use additional code, if applicable, to identify chronic total occlusion of artery of extremity (I70.92)

AHA: 2020,4Q,98

I70.50 **Unspecified atherosclerosis of nonautologous biological bypass graft(s) of the extremities**

I70.501 **Unspecified atherosclerosis of nonautologous biological bypass graft(s) of the extremities, right leg** HCC ESR A

I70.502 **Unspecified atherosclerosis of nonautologous biological bypass graft(s) of the extremities, left leg** HCC ESR A

I70.503 **Unspecified atherosclerosis of nonautologous biological bypass graft(s) of the extremities, bilateral legs** HCC ESR A

I70.508 **Unspecified atherosclerosis of nonautologous biological bypass graft(s) of the extremities, other extremity** HCC ESR A

I70.509 **Unspecified atherosclerosis of nonautologous biological bypass graft(s) of the extremities, unspecified extremity** HCC ESR A

I70.51 **Atherosclerosis of nonautologous biological bypass graft(s) of the extremities intermittent claudication**

I70.511 **Atherosclerosis of nonautologous biological bypass graft(s) of the extremities with intermittent claudication, right leg** HCC ESR A

I70.512 **Atherosclerosis of nonautologous biological bypass graft(s) of the extremities with intermittent claudication, left leg** HCC ESR A

I70.513 **Atherosclerosis of nonautologous biological bypass graft(s) of the extremities with intermittent claudication, bilateral legs** HCC ESR A

I70.518 **Atherosclerosis of nonautologous biological bypass graft(s) of the extremities with intermittent claudication, other extremity** HCC ESR A

I70.519 **Atherosclerosis of nonautologous biological bypass graft(s) of the extremities with intermittent claudication, unspecified extremity** HCC ESR A

I70.52 **Atherosclerosis of nonautologous biological bypass graft(s) of the extremities with rest pain**

INCLUDES any condition classifiable to I70.51-

chronic limb-threatening ischemia NOS of nonautologous biological bypass graft(s) of the extremities

chronic limb-threatening ischemia of nonautologous biological bypass graft(s) of the extremities with rest pain

critical limb ischemia NOS of nonautologous biological bypass graft(s) of the extremities

critical limb ischemia of nonautologous biological bypass graft(s) of the extremities with rest pain

I70.521 **Atherosclerosis of nonautologous biological bypass graft(s) of the extremities with rest pain, right leg** HCC ESR A

I70.522 **Atherosclerosis of nonautologous biological bypass graft(s) of the extremities with rest pain, left leg** HCC ESR A

I70.523 **Atherosclerosis of nonautologous biological bypass graft(s) of the extremities with rest pain, bilateral legs** HCC ESR A

I70.528 **Atherosclerosis of nonautologous biological bypass graft(s) of the extremities with rest pain, other extremity** HCC ESR A

I70.529 **Atherosclerosis of nonautologous biological bypass graft(s) of the extremities with rest pain, unspecified extremity** HCC ESR A

I70.53 **Atherosclerosis of nonautologous biological bypass graft(s) of the right leg with ulceration**

INCLUDES any condition classifiable to I70.511 and I70.521

chronic limb-threatening ischemia of nonautologous biological bypass graft(s) of the right leg with ulceration

critical limb ischemia of nonautologous biological bypass graft(s) of the right leg with ulceration

Use additional code to identify severity of ulcer (L97.-)

I70.531 **Atherosclerosis of nonautologous biological bypass graft(s) of the right leg with ulceration of thigh** HCC Rx ESR COM A

I70.532 **Atherosclerosis of nonautologous biological bypass graft(s) of the right leg with ulceration of calf** HCC Rx ESR COM A

I70.533 **Atherosclerosis of nonautologous biological bypass graft(s) of the right leg with ulceration of ankle** HCC Rx ESR COM A

I70.534 **Atherosclerosis of nonautologous biological bypass graft(s) of the right leg with ulceration of heel and midfoot** HCC Rx ESR COM A

Atherosclerosis of nonautologous biological bypass graft(s) of right leg with ulceration of plantar surface of midfoot

I70.535 **Atherosclerosis of nonautologous biological bypass graft(s) of the right leg with ulceration of other part of foot** HCC Rx ESR COM A

Atherosclerosis of nonautologous biological bypass graft(s) of the right leg with ulceration of toe

I70.538 **Atherosclerosis of nonautologous biological bypass graft(s) of the right leg with ulceration of other part of lower leg** HCC Rx ESR COM A

I70.539 **Atherosclerosis of nonautologous biological bypass graft(s) of the right leg with ulceration of unspecified site** HCC Rx ESR COM A

I70.54 **Atherosclerosis of nonautologous biological bypass graft(s) of the left leg with ulceration**

INCLUDES any condition classifiable to I70.512 and I70.522

chronic limb-threatening ischemia of nonautologous biological bypass graft(s) of the left leg with ulceration

critical limb ischemia of nonautologous biological bypass graft(s) of the left leg with ulceration

Use additional code to identify severity of ulcer (L97.-)

I70.541 **Atherosclerosis of nonautologous biological bypass graft(s) of the left leg with ulceration of thigh** HCC Rx ESR COM A

I70.542 **Atherosclerosis of nonautologous biological bypass graft(s) of the left leg with ulceration of calf** HCC Rx ESR COM A

Chapter 9. Diseases of the Circulatory System

I70.493–I70.542

I70.543 Atherosclerosis of nonautologous biological bypass graft(s) of the left leg with ulceration of ankle HCC Rx ESR COM A

I70.544 Atherosclerosis of nonautologous biological bypass graft(s) of the left leg with ulceration of heel and midfoot HCC Rx ESR COM A

Atherosclerosis of nonautologous biological bypass graft(s) of left leg with ulceration of plantar surface of midfoot

I70.545 Atherosclerosis of nonautologous biological bypass graft(s) of the left leg with ulceration of other part of foot HCC Rx ESR COM A

Atherosclerosis of nonautologous biological bypass graft(s) of the left leg with ulceration of toe

I70.548 Atherosclerosis of nonautologous biological bypass graft(s) of the left leg with ulceration of other part of lower leg HCC Rx ESR COM A

I70.549 Atherosclerosis of nonautologous biological bypass graft(s) of the left leg with ulceration of unspecified site HCC Rx ESR COM A

I70.55 Atherosclerosis of nonautologous biological bypass graft(s) of other extremity with ulceration HCC Rx ESR COM A

INCLUDES any condition classifiable to I70.518, I70.528, and I70.538

Use additional code to identify severity of ulcer (L98.49)

√6th **I70.56 Atherosclerosis of nonautologous biological bypass graft(s) of the extremities with gangrene**

INCLUDES any condition classifiable to I70.51-, I70.52-, and I70.53-, I70.54-, I70.55

chronic limb-threatening ischemia of nonautologous biological bypass graft(s) of the extremities with gangrene

critical limb ischemia of nonautologous biological bypass graft(s) of the extremities with gangrene

Use additional code to identify the severity of any ulcer (L97.-, L98.49-), if applicable

I70.561 Atherosclerosis of nonautologous biological bypass graft(s) of the extremities with gangrene, right leg HCC ESR COM A

I70.562 Atherosclerosis of nonautologous biological bypass graft(s) of the extremities with gangrene, left leg HCC ESR COM A

I70.563 Atherosclerosis of nonautologous biological bypass graft(s) of the extremities with gangrene, bilateral legs HCC ESR COM A

I70.568 Atherosclerosis of nonautologous biological bypass graft(s) of the extremities with gangrene, other extremity HCC ESR COM A

I70.569 Atherosclerosis of nonautologous biological bypass graft(s) of the extremities with gangrene, unspecified extremity HCC ESR COM A

√6th **I70.59 Other atherosclerosis of nonautologous biological bypass graft(s) of the extremities**

I70.591 Other atherosclerosis of nonautologous biological bypass graft(s) of the extremities, right leg HCC ESR A

I70.592 Other atherosclerosis of nonautologous biological bypass graft(s) of the extremities, left leg HCC ESR A

I70.593 Other atherosclerosis of nonautologous biological bypass graft(s) of the extremities, bilateral legs HCC ESR A

I70.598 Other atherosclerosis of nonautologous biological bypass graft(s) of the extremities, other extremity HCC ESR A

I70.599 Other atherosclerosis of nonautologous biological bypass graft(s) of the extremities, unspecified extremity HCC ESR A

√5th **I70.6 Atherosclerosis of nonbiological bypass graft(s) of the extremities**

Use additional code, if applicable, to identify chronic total occlusion of artery of extremity (I70.92)

AHA: 2020,4Q,98

√6th **I70.60 Unspecified atherosclerosis of nonbiological bypass graft(s) of the extremities**

I70.601 Unspecified atherosclerosis of nonbiological bypass graft(s) of the extremities, right leg HCC ESR A

I70.602 Unspecified atherosclerosis of nonbiological bypass graft(s) of the extremities, left leg HCC ESR A

I70.603 Unspecified atherosclerosis of nonbiological bypass graft(s) of the extremities, bilateral legs HCC ESR A

I70.608 Unspecified atherosclerosis of nonbiological bypass graft(s) of the extremities, other extremity HCC ESR A

I70.609 Unspecified atherosclerosis of nonbiological bypass graft(s) of the extremities, unspecified extremity HCC ESR A

√6th **I70.61 Atherosclerosis of nonbiological bypass graft(s) of the extremities with intermittent claudication**

I70.611 Atherosclerosis of nonbiological bypass graft(s) of the extremities with intermittent claudication, right leg HCC ESR A

I70.612 Atherosclerosis of nonbiological bypass graft(s) of the extremities with intermittent claudication, left leg HCC ESR A

I70.613 Atherosclerosis of nonbiological bypass graft(s) of the extremities with intermittent claudication, bilateral legs HCC ESR A

I70.618 Atherosclerosis of nonbiological bypass graft(s) of the extremities with intermittent claudication, other extremity HCC ESR A

I70.619 Atherosclerosis of nonbiological bypass graft(s) of the extremities with intermittent claudication, unspecified extremity HCC ESR A

√6th **I70.62 Atherosclerosis of nonbiological bypass graft(s) of the extremities with rest pain**

INCLUDES any condition classifiable to I70.61-

chronic limb-threatening ischemia NOS of nonbiological bypass graft(s) of the extremities

chronic limb-threatening ischemia of nonbiological bypass graft(s) of the extremities with rest pain

critical limb ischemia NOS of nonbiological bypass graft(s) of the extremities

critical limb ischemia of nonbiological bypass graft(s) of the extremities with rest pain

I70.621 Atherosclerosis of nonbiological bypass graft(s) of the extremities with rest pain, right leg HCC ESR A

I70.622 Atherosclerosis of nonbiological bypass graft(s) of the extremities with rest pain, left leg HCC ESR A

I70.623 Atherosclerosis of nonbiological bypass graft(s) of the extremities with rest pain, bilateral legs HCC ESR A

I70.628 Atherosclerosis of nonbiological bypass graft(s) of the extremities with rest pain, other extremity HCC ESR A

I70.629 Atherosclerosis of nonbiological bypass graft(s) of the extremities with rest pain, unspecified extremity HCC ESR A

HCC CMS-HCC Rx Rx HCC ESR ESRD HCC COM Commercial HCC N Newborn: 0 P Pediatric: 0-17 M Maternity: 9-64 A Adult: 15-124

√6th **I70.63 Atherosclerosis of nonbiological bypass graft(s) of the right leg with ulceration**
INCLUDES any condition classifiable to I70.611 and I70.621
chronic limb-threatening ischemia of nonbiological bypass graft(s) of the right leg with ulceration
critical limb ischemia of nonbiological bypass graft(s) of the right leg with ulceration
Use additional code to identify severity of ulcer (L97.-)

I70.631 Atherosclerosis of nonbiological bypass graft(s) of the right leg with ulceration of thigh HCC Rx ESR COM A

I70.632 Atherosclerosis of nonbiological bypass graft(s) of the right leg with ulceration of calf HCC Rx ESR COM A

I70.633 Atherosclerosis of nonbiological bypass graft(s) of the right leg with ulceration of ankle HCC Rx ESR COM A

I70.634 Atherosclerosis of nonbiological bypass graft(s) of the right leg with ulceration of heel and midfoot HCC Rx ESR COM A
Atherosclerosis of nonbiological bypass graft(s) of right leg with ulceration of plantar surface of midfoot

I70.635 Atherosclerosis of nonbiological bypass graft(s) of the right leg with ulceration of other part of foot HCC Rx ESR COM A
Atherosclerosis of nonbiological bypass graft(s) of the right leg with ulceration of toe

I70.638 Atherosclerosis of nonbiological bypass graft(s) of the right leg with ulceration of other part of lower leg HCC Rx ESR COM A

I70.639 Atherosclerosis of nonbiological bypass graft(s) of the right leg with ulceration of unspecified site HCC Rx ESR COM A

√6th **I70.64 Atherosclerosis of nonbiological bypass graft(s) of the left leg with ulceration**
INCLUDES any condition classifiable to I70.612 and I70.622
chronic limb-threatening ischemia of nonbiological bypass graft(s) of the left leg with ulceration
critical limb ischemia of nonbiological bypass graft(s) of the left leg with ulceration
Use additional code to identify severity of ulcer (L97.-)

I70.641 Atherosclerosis of nonbiological bypass graft(s) of the left leg with ulceration of thigh HCC Rx ESR COM A

I70.642 Atherosclerosis of nonbiological bypass graft(s) of the left leg with ulceration of calf HCC Rx ESR COM A

I70.643 Atherosclerosis of nonbiological bypass graft(s) of the left leg with ulceration of ankle HCC Rx ESR COM A

I70.644 Atherosclerosis of nonbiological bypass graft(s) of the left leg with ulceration of heel and midfoot HCC Rx ESR COM A
Atherosclerosis of nonbiological bypass graft(s) of left leg with ulceration of plantar surface of midfoot

I70.645 Atherosclerosis of nonbiological bypass graft(s) of the left leg with ulceration of other part of foot HCC Rx ESR COM A
Atherosclerosis of nonbiological bypass graft(s) of the left leg with ulceration of toe

I70.648 Atherosclerosis of nonbiological bypass graft(s) of the left leg with ulceration of other part of lower leg HCC Rx ESR COM A

I70.649 Atherosclerosis of nonbiological bypass graft(s) of the left leg with ulceration of unspecified site HCC Rx ESR COM A

I70.65 Atherosclerosis of nonbiological bypass graft(s) of other extremity with ulceration HCC Rx ESR COM A
INCLUDES any condition classifiable to I70.618 and I70.628
Use additional code to identify severity of ulcer (L98.49)

√6th **I70.66 Atherosclerosis of nonbiological bypass graft(s) of the extremities with gangrene**
INCLUDES any condition classifiable to I70.61-, I70.62-, I70.63-, I70.64-, I70.65
chronic limb-threatening ischemia of nonbiological bypass graft(s) of the extremities with gangrene
critical limb ischemia of nonbiological bypass graft(s) of the extremities with gangrene
Use additional code to identify the severity of any ulcer (L97.-, L98.49-), if applicable

I70.661 Atherosclerosis of nonbiological bypass graft(s) of the extremities with gangrene, right leg HCC ESR COM A

I70.662 Atherosclerosis of nonbiological bypass graft(s) of the extremities with gangrene, left leg HCC ESR COM A

I70.663 Atherosclerosis of nonbiological bypass graft(s) of the extremities with gangrene, bilateral legs HCC ESR COM A

I70.668 Atherosclerosis of nonbiological bypass graft(s) of the extremities with gangrene, other extremity HCC ESR COM A

I70.669 Atherosclerosis of nonbiological bypass graft(s) of the extremities with gangrene, unspecified extremity HCC ESR COM A

√6th **I70.69 Other atherosclerosis of nonbiological bypass graft(s) of the extremities**

I70.691 Other atherosclerosis of nonbiological bypass graft(s) of the extremities, right leg HCC ESR A

I70.692 Other atherosclerosis of nonbiological bypass graft(s) of the extremities, left leg HCC ESR A

I70.693 Other atherosclerosis of nonbiological bypass graft(s) of the extremities, bilateral legs HCC ESR A

I70.698 Other atherosclerosis of nonbiological bypass graft(s) of the extremities, other extremity HCC ESR A

I70.699 Other atherosclerosis of nonbiological bypass graft(s) of the extremities, unspecified extremity HCC ESR A

√5th **I70.7 Atherosclerosis of other type of bypass graft(s) of the extremities**
Use additional code, if applicable, to identify chronic total occlusion of artery of extremity (I70.92)
AHA: 2020,4Q,98

√6th **I70.70 Unspecified atherosclerosis of other type of bypass graft(s) of the extremities**

I70.701 Unspecified atherosclerosis of other type of bypass graft(s) of the extremities, right leg HCC ESR A

I70.702 Unspecified atherosclerosis of other type of bypass graft(s) of the extremities, left leg HCC ESR A

I70.703 Unspecified atherosclerosis of other type of bypass graft(s) of the extremities, bilateral legs HCC ESR A

I70.708 Unspecified atherosclerosis of other type of bypass graft(s) of the extremities, other extremity HCC ESR A

I70.709 Unspecified atherosclerosis of other type of bypass graft(s) of the extremities, unspecified extremity HCC ESR A

√6th **I70.71 Atherosclerosis of other type of bypass graft(s) of the extremities with intermittent claudication**

I70.711 Atherosclerosis of other type of bypass graft(s) of the extremities with intermittent claudication, right leg HCC ESR A

I70.712 Atherosclerosis of other type of bypass graft(s) of the extremities with intermittent claudication, left leg HCC ESR A

I70.713 Atherosclerosis of other type of bypass graft(s) of the extremities with intermittent claudication, bilateral legs HCC ESR A

I70.718 Atherosclerosis of other type of bypass graft(s) of the extremities with intermittent claudication, other extremity HCC ESR A

I70.719 Atherosclerosis of other type of bypass graft(s) of the extremities with intermittent claudication, unspecified extremity HCC ESR A

√6th **I70.72 Atherosclerosis of other type of bypass graft(s) of the extremities with rest pain**

INCLUDES any condition classifiable to I70.71-
chronic limb-threatening ischemia NOS of other type of bypass graft(s) of the extremities
chronic limb-threatening ischemia of other type of bypass graft(s) of the extremities with rest pain
critical limb ischemia NOS of other type of bypass graft(s) of the extremities
critical limb ischemia of other type of bypass graft(s) of the extremities with rest pain

I70.721 Atherosclerosis of other type of bypass graft(s) of the extremities with rest pain, right leg HCC ESR A

I70.722 Atherosclerosis of other type of bypass graft(s) of the extremities with rest pain, left leg HCC ESR A

I70.723 Atherosclerosis of other type of bypass graft(s) of the extremities with rest pain, bilateral legs HCC ESR A

I70.728 Atherosclerosis of other type of bypass graft(s) of the extremities with rest pain, other extremity HCC ESR A

I70.729 Atherosclerosis of other type of bypass graft(s) of the extremities with rest pain, unspecified extremity HCC ESR A

√6th **I70.73 Atherosclerosis of other type of bypass graft(s) of the right leg with ulceration**

INCLUDES any condition classifiable to I70.711 and I70.721
chronic limb-threatening ischemia of other type of bypass graft(s) of the right leg with ulceration
critical limb ischemia of other type of bypass graft(s) of the right leg with ulceration

Use additional code to identify severity of ulcer (L97.-)

I70.731 Atherosclerosis of other type of bypass graft(s) of the right leg with ulceration of thigh HCC Rx ESR COM A

I70.732 Atherosclerosis of other type of bypass graft(s) of the right leg with ulceration of calf HCC Rx ESR COM A

I70.733 Atherosclerosis of other type of bypass graft(s) of the right leg with ulceration of ankle HCC Rx ESR COM A

I70.734 Atherosclerosis of other type of bypass graft(s) of the right leg with ulceration of heel and midfoot HCC Rx ESR COM A

Atherosclerosis of other type of bypass graft(s) of right leg with ulceration of plantar surface of midfoot

I70.735 Atherosclerosis of other type of bypass graft(s) of the right leg with ulceration of other part of foot HCC Rx ESR COM A

Atherosclerosis of other type of bypass graft(s) of right leg with ulceration of toe

I70.738 Atherosclerosis of other type of bypass graft(s) of the right leg with ulceration of other part of lower leg HCC Rx ESR COM A

I70.739 Atherosclerosis of other type of bypass graft(s) of the right leg with ulceration of unspecified site HCC Rx ESR COM A

√6th **I70.74 Atherosclerosis of other type of bypass graft(s) of the left leg with ulceration**

INCLUDES any condition classifiable to I70.712 and I70.722
chronic limb-threatening ischemia of other type of bypass graft(s) of the left leg with ulceration
critical limb ischemia of other type of bypass graft(s) of the left leg with ulceration

Use additional code to identify severity of ulcer (L97.-)

I70.741 Atherosclerosis of other type of bypass graft(s) of the left leg with ulceration of thigh HCC Rx ESR COM A

I70.742 Atherosclerosis of other type of bypass graft(s) of the left leg with ulceration of calf HCC Rx ESR COM A

I70.743 Atherosclerosis of other type of bypass graft(s) of the left leg with ulceration of ankle HCC Rx ESR COM A

I70.744 Atherosclerosis of other type of bypass graft(s) of the left leg with ulceration of heel and midfoot HCC Rx ESR COM A

Atherosclerosis of other type of bypass graft(s) of left leg with ulceration of plantar surface of midfoot

I70.745 Atherosclerosis of other type of bypass graft(s) of the left leg with ulceration of other part of foot HCC Rx ESR COM A

Atherosclerosis of other type of bypass graft(s) of left leg with ulceration of toe

I70.748 Atherosclerosis of other type of bypass graft(s) of the left leg with ulceration of other part of lower leg HCC Rx ESR COM A

I70.749 Atherosclerosis of other type of bypass graft(s) of the left leg with ulceration of unspecified site HCC Rx ESR COM A

I70.75 Atherosclerosis of other type of bypass graft(s) of other extremity with ulceration HCC Rx ESR COM A

INCLUDES any condition classifiable to I70.718 and I70.728

Use additional code to identify severity of ulcer (L98.49)

√6th **I70.76 Atherosclerosis of other type of bypass graft(s) of the extremities with gangrene**

INCLUDES any condition classifiable to I70.71-, I70.72-, I70.73-, I70.74-, I70.75
chronic limb-threatening ischemia of other type of bypass graft(s) of the extremities with gangrene
critical limb ischemia of other type of bypass graft(s) of the extremities with gangrene

Use additional code to identify the severity of any ulcer (L97.-, L98.49-), if applicable

I70.761 Atherosclerosis of other type of bypass graft(s) of the extremities with gangrene, right leg HCC ESR COM A

I70.762 Atherosclerosis of other type of bypass graft(s) of the extremities with gangrene, left leg HCC ESR COM A

I70.763 Atherosclerosis of other type of bypass graft(s) of the extremities with gangrene, bilateral legs HCC ESR COM A

I70.768 Atherosclerosis of other type of bypass graft(s) of the extremities with gangrene, other extremity HCC ESR COM A

I70.769 Atherosclerosis of other type of bypass graft(s) of the extremities with gangrene, unspecified extremity HCC ESR COM A

√6th **I70.79 Other atherosclerosis of other type of bypass graft(s) of the extremities**

I70.791 Other atherosclerosis of other type of bypass graft(s) of the extremities, right leg HCC ESR A

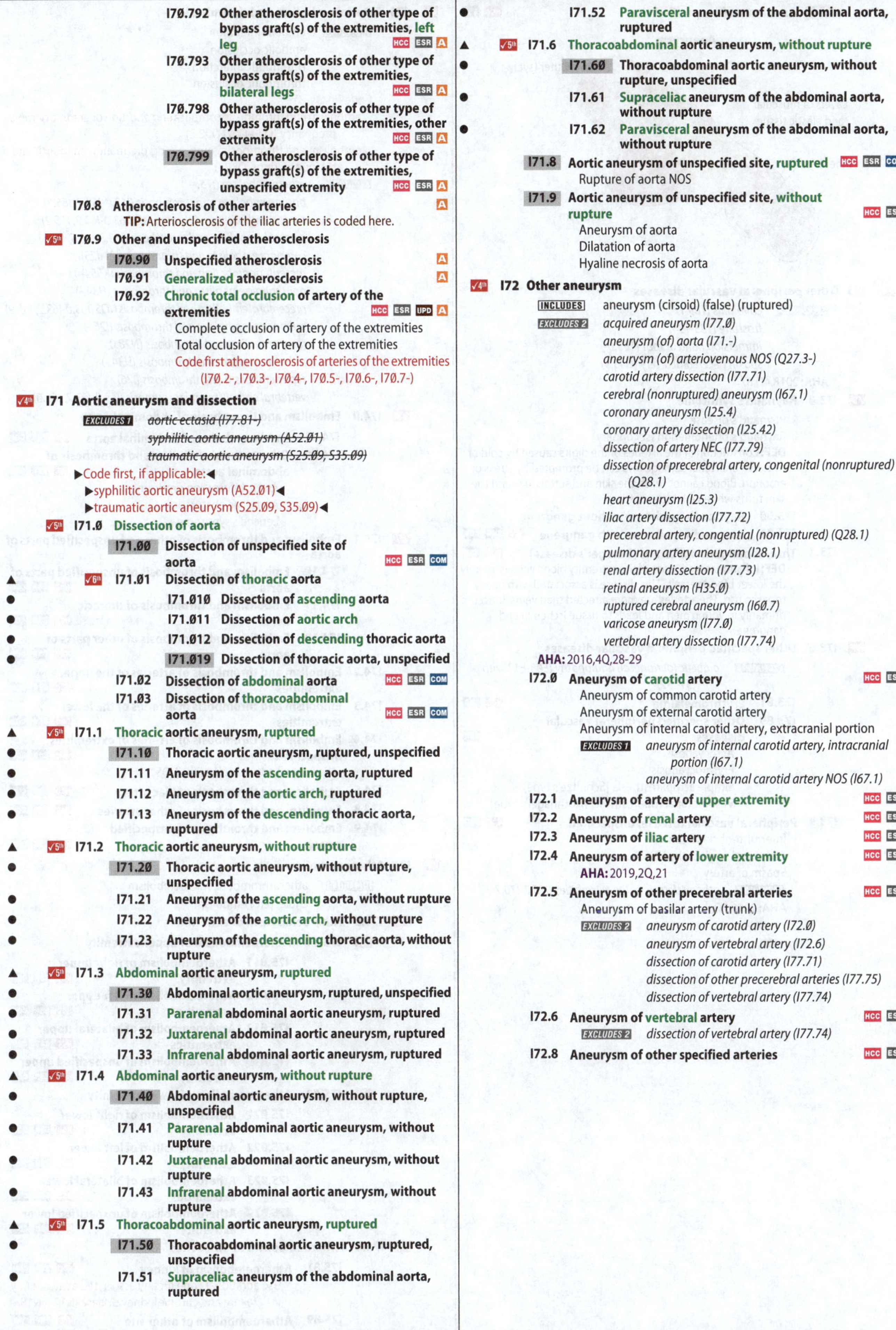

I7Ø.792 **Other atherosclerosis of other type of bypass graft(s) of the extremities, left leg** HCC ESR A

I7Ø.793 **Other atherosclerosis of other type of bypass graft(s) of the extremities, bilateral legs** HCC ESR A

I7Ø.798 **Other atherosclerosis of other type of bypass graft(s) of the extremities, other extremity** HCC ESR A

I7Ø.799 **Other atherosclerosis of other type of bypass graft(s) of the extremities, unspecified extremity** HCC ESR A

I7Ø.8 **Atherosclerosis of other arteries** A

TIP: Arteriosclerosis of the iliac arteries is coded here.

✓5th I7Ø.9 **Other and unspecified atherosclerosis**

I7Ø.9Ø **Unspecified atherosclerosis** A

I7Ø.91 **Generalized atherosclerosis** A

I7Ø.92 **Chronic total occlusion of artery of the extremities** HCC ESR UPD A

Complete occlusion of artery of the extremities

Total occlusion of artery of the extremities

Code first atherosclerosis of arteries of the extremities (I7Ø.2-, I7Ø.3-, I7Ø.4-, I7Ø.5-, I7Ø.6-, I7Ø.7-)

✓4th **I71 Aortic aneurysm and dissection**

EXCLUDES 1 ~~*aortic ectasia (I77.81-)*~~

~~*syphilitic aortic aneurysm (A52.Ø1)*~~

~~*traumatic aortic aneurysm (S25.Ø9, S35.Ø9)*~~

▶Code first, if applicable:◀

▶syphilitic aortic aneurysm (A52.Ø1)◀

▶traumatic aortic aneurysm (S25.Ø9, S35.Ø9)◀

✓5th I71.Ø **Dissection of aorta**

I71.ØØ **Dissection of unspecified site of aorta** HCC ESR COM

▲ ✓6th I71.Ø1 **Dissection of thoracic aorta**

● I71.Ø1Ø **Dissection of ascending aorta**

● I71.Ø11 **Dissection of aortic arch**

● I71.Ø12 **Dissection of descending thoracic aorta**

● I71.Ø19 **Dissection of thoracic aorta, unspecified**

I71.Ø2 **Dissection of abdominal aorta** HCC ESR COM

I71.Ø3 **Dissection of thoracoabdominal aorta** HCC ESR COM

▲ ✓5th I71.1 **Thoracic aortic aneurysm, ruptured**

● I71.1Ø **Thoracic aortic aneurysm, ruptured, unspecified**

● I71.11 **Aneurysm of the ascending aorta, ruptured**

● I71.12 **Aneurysm of the aortic arch, ruptured**

● I71.13 **Aneurysm of the descending thoracic aorta, ruptured**

▲ ✓5th I71.2 **Thoracic aortic aneurysm, without rupture**

● I71.2Ø **Thoracic aortic aneurysm, without rupture, unspecified**

● I71.21 **Aneurysm of the ascending aorta, without rupture**

● I71.22 **Aneurysm of the aortic arch, without rupture**

● I71.23 **Aneurysm of the descending thoracic aorta, without rupture**

▲ ✓5th I71.3 **Abdominal aortic aneurysm, ruptured**

● I71.3Ø **Abdominal aortic aneurysm, ruptured, unspecified**

● I71.31 **Pararenal abdominal aortic aneurysm, ruptured**

● I71.32 **Juxtarenal abdominal aortic aneurysm, ruptured**

● I71.33 **Infrarenal abdominal aortic aneurysm, ruptured**

▲ ✓5th I71.4 **Abdominal aortic aneurysm, without rupture**

● I71.4Ø **Abdominal aortic aneurysm, without rupture, unspecified**

● I71.41 **Pararenal abdominal aortic aneurysm, without rupture**

● I71.42 **Juxtarenal abdominal aortic aneurysm, without rupture**

● I71.43 **Infrarenal abdominal aortic aneurysm, without rupture**

▲ ✓5th I71.5 **Thoracoabdominal aortic aneurysm, ruptured**

● I71.5Ø **Thoracoabdominal aortic aneurysm, ruptured, unspecified**

● I71.51 **Supraceliac aneurysm of the abdominal aorta, ruptured**

● I71.52 **Paravisceral aneurysm of the abdominal aorta, ruptured**

▲ ✓5th I71.6 **Thoracoabdominal aortic aneurysm, without rupture**

● I71.6Ø **Thoracoabdominal aortic aneurysm, without rupture, unspecified**

● I71.61 **Supraceliac aneurysm of the abdominal aorta, without rupture**

● I71.62 **Paravisceral aneurysm of the abdominal aorta, without rupture**

I71.8 **Aortic aneurysm of unspecified site, ruptured** HCC ESR COM

Rupture of aorta NOS

I71.9 **Aortic aneurysm of unspecified site, without rupture** HCC ESR

Aneurysm of aorta

Dilatation of aorta

Hyaline necrosis of aorta

✓4th **I72 Other aneurysm**

INCLUDES aneurysm (cirsoid) (false) (ruptured)

EXCLUDES 2 *acquired aneurysm (I77.Ø)*

aneurysm (of) aorta (I71.-)

aneurysm (of) arteriovenous NOS (Q27.3-)

carotid artery dissection (I77.71)

cerebral (nonruptured) aneurysm (I67.1)

coronary aneurysm (I25.4)

coronary artery dissection (I25.42)

dissection of artery NEC (I77.79)

dissection of precerebral artery, congenital (nonruptured) (Q28.1)

heart aneurysm (I25.3)

iliac artery dissection (I77.72)

precerebral artery, congential (nonruptured) (Q28.1)

pulmonary artery aneurysm (I28.1)

renal artery dissection (I77.73)

retinal aneurysm (H35.Ø)

ruptured cerebral aneurysm (I6Ø.7)

varicose aneurysm (I77.Ø)

vertebral artery dissection (I77.74)

AHA: 2016,4Q,28-29

I72.Ø **Aneurysm of carotid artery** HCC ESR

Aneurysm of common carotid artery

Aneurysm of external carotid artery

Aneurysm of internal carotid artery, extracranial portion

EXCLUDES 1 *aneurysm of internal carotid artery, intracranial portion (I67.1)*

aneurysm of internal carotid artery NOS (I67.1)

I72.1 **Aneurysm of artery of upper extremity** HCC ESR

I72.2 **Aneurysm of renal artery** HCC ESR

I72.3 **Aneurysm of iliac artery** HCC ESR

I72.4 **Aneurysm of artery of lower extremity** HCC ESR

AHA: 2019,2Q,21

I72.5 **Aneurysm of other precerebral arteries** HCC ESR

Aneurysm of basilar artery (trunk)

EXCLUDES 2 *aneurysm of carotid artery (I72.Ø)*

aneurysm of vertebral artery (I72.6)

dissection of carotid artery (I77.71)

dissection of other precerebral arteries (I77.75)

dissection of vertebral artery (I77.74)

I72.6 **Aneurysm of vertebral artery** HCC ESR

EXCLUDES 2 *dissection of vertebral artery (I77.74)*

I72.8 **Aneurysm of other specified arteries** HCC ESR

I72.9 Aneurysm of unspecified site HCC ESR

Aneurysm
Outer layer 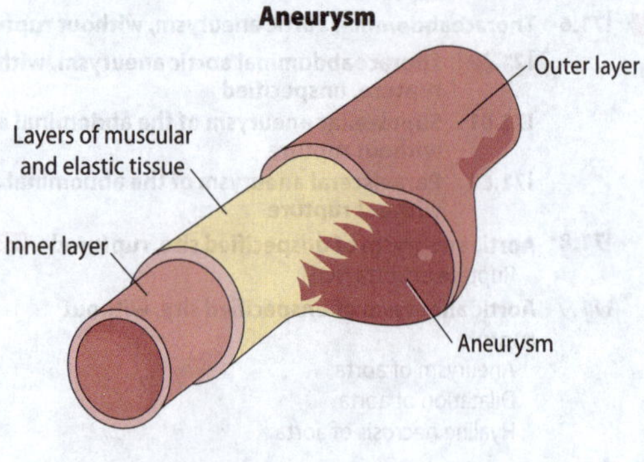
Layers of muscular and elastic tissue
Inner layer
Aneurysm

I73 Other peripheral vascular diseases

EXCLUDES 2 *chilblains (T69.1)*
frostbite (T33-T34)
immersion hand or foot (T69.0-)
spasm of cerebral artery (G45.9)

AHA: 2018,4Q,87

I73.0 Raynaud's syndrome

Raynaud's disease
Raynaud's phenomenon (secondary)

DEF: Constriction of the arteries of the digits caused by cold or by nerve or arterial damage and can be prompted by stress or emotion. Blood cannot reach the skin and soft tissues and the skin turns white with blue mottling.

I73.00 Raynaud's syndrome without gangrene

I73.01 Raynaud's syndrome with gangrene HCC ESR COM

I73.1 Thromboangiitis obliterans [Buerger's disease] HCC ESR

DEF: Inflammatory disease of the extremity blood vessels, mainly the lower blood vessels. This disease is associated with heavy tobacco use. The arteries are more affected than veins. It occurs primarily in young men and leads to tissue ischemia and gangrene.

I73.8 Other specified peripheral vascular diseases

EXCLUDES 1 *diabetic (peripheral) angiopathy (E08-E13 with .51-.52)*

I73.81 Erythromelalgia HCC ESR

I73.89 Other specified peripheral vascular diseases HCC ESR

Acrocyanosis
Erythrocyanosis
Simple acroparesthesia [Schultze's type]
Vasomotor acroparesthesia [Nothnagel's type]

I73.9 Peripheral vascular disease, unspecified HCC ESR

Intermittent claudication
Peripheral angiopathy NOS
Spasm of artery

EXCLUDES 1 *atherosclerosis of the extremities (I70.2-I70.7-)*

AHA: 2018,2Q,7

I74 Arterial embolism and thrombosis

INCLUDES embolic infarction
embolic occlusion
thrombotic infarction
thrombotic occlusion

Code first:
embolism and thrombosis complicating abortion or ectopic or molar pregnancy (O00-O07, O08.2)
embolism and thrombosis complicating pregnancy, childbirth and the puerperium (O88.-)

EXCLUDES 2 *atheroembolism (I75.-)*
basilar embolism and thrombosis (I63.0-I63.2, I65.1)
carotid embolism and thrombosis (I63.0-I63.2, I65.2)
cerebral embolism and thrombosis (I63.3-I63.5, I66.-)
coronary embolism and thrombosis (I21-I25)
mesenteric embolism and thrombosis (K55.0-)
ophthalmic embolism and thrombosis (H34.-)
precerebral embolism and thrombosis NOS (I63.0-I63.2, I65.9)
pulmonary embolism and thrombosis (I26.-)
renal embolism and thrombosis (N28.0)
retinal embolism and thrombosis (H34.-)
septic embolism and thrombosis (I76)
vertebral embolism and thrombosis (I63.0-I63.2, I65.0)

I74.0 Embolism and thrombosis of abdominal aorta

I74.01 Saddle embolus of abdominal aorta HCC ESR COM

I74.09 Other arterial embolism and thrombosis of abdominal aorta HCC ESR COM

Aortic bifurcation syndrome
Aortoiliac obstruction
Leriche's syndrome

I74.1 Embolism and thrombosis of other and unspecified parts of aorta

I74.10 Embolism and thrombosis of unspecified parts of aorta HCC ESR COM

I74.11 Embolism and thrombosis of thoracic aorta HCC ESR COM

I74.19 Embolism and thrombosis of other parts of aorta HCC ESR COM

I74.2 Embolism and thrombosis of arteries of the upper extremities HCC ESR COM

I74.3 Embolism and thrombosis of arteries of the lower extremities HCC ESR COM

I74.4 Embolism and thrombosis of arteries of extremities, unspecified HCC ESR COM

Peripheral arterial embolism NOS

I74.5 Embolism and thrombosis of iliac artery HCC ESR COM

I74.8 Embolism and thrombosis of other arteries HCC ESR COM

I74.9 Embolism and thrombosis of unspecified artery HCC ESR COM

I75 Atheroembolism

INCLUDES atherothrombotic microembolism
cholesterol embolism

I75.0 Atheroembolism of extremities

I75.01 Atheroembolism of upper extremity

I75.011 Atheroembolism of right upper extremity HCC ESR COM

I75.012 Atheroembolism of left upper extremity HCC ESR COM

I75.013 Atheroembolism of bilateral upper extremities HCC ESR COM

I75.019 Atheroembolism of unspecified upper extremity HCC ESR COM

I75.02 Atheroembolism of lower extremity

I75.021 Atheroembolism of right lower extremity HCC ESR COM

I75.022 Atheroembolism of left lower extremity HCC ESR COM

I75.023 Atheroembolism of bilateral lower extremities HCC ESR COM

I75.029 Atheroembolism of unspecified lower extremity HCC ESR COM

I75.8 Atheroembolism of other sites

I75.81 Atheroembolism of kidney HCC ESR COM

Use additional code for any associated acute kidney failure and chronic kidney disease (N17.-, N18.-)

I75.89 Atheroembolism of other site HCC ESR COM

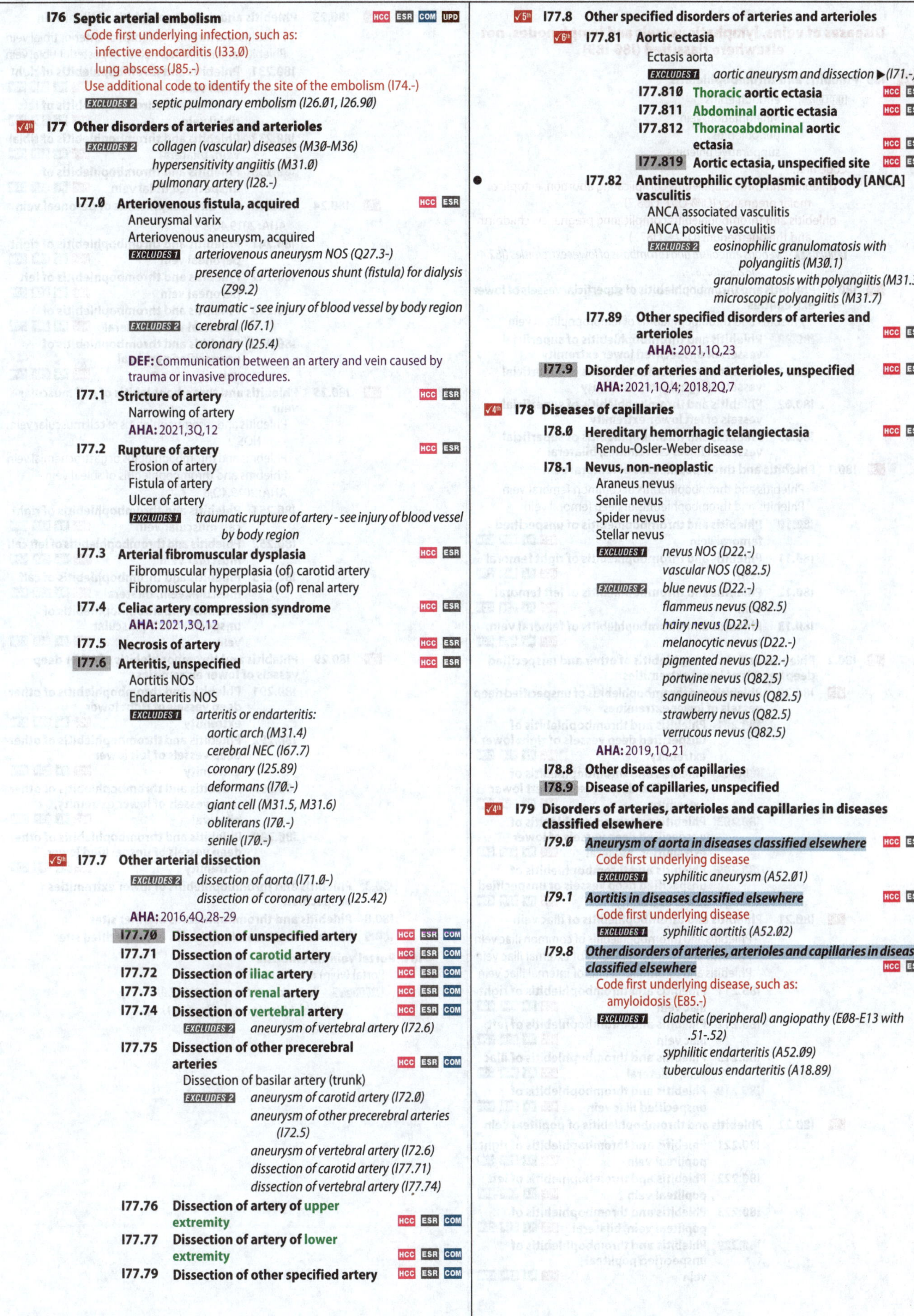

I76 Septic arterial embolism HCC ESR COM UPD

Code first underlying infection, such as:
infective endocarditis (I33.Ø)
lung abscess (J85.-)

Use additional code to identify the site of the embolism (I74.-)

EXCLUDES 2 *septic pulmonary embolism (I26.Ø1, I26.9Ø)*

I77 Other disorders of arteries and arterioles

EXCLUDES 2 *collagen (vascular) diseases (M3Ø-M36)*
hypersensitivity angiitis (M31.Ø)
pulmonary artery (I28.-)

I77.Ø Arteriovenous fistula, acquired HCC ESR
Aneurysmal varix
Arteriovenous aneurysm, acquired
EXCLUDES 1 *arteriovenous aneurysm NOS (Q27.3-)*
presence of arteriovenous shunt (fistula) for dialysis (Z99.2)
traumatic - see injury of blood vessel by body region
EXCLUDES 2 *cerebral (I67.1)*
coronary (I25.4)
DEF: Communication between an artery and vein caused by trauma or invasive procedures.

I77.1 Stricture of artery HCC ESR
Narrowing of artery
AHA: 2021,3Q,12

I77.2 Rupture of artery HCC ESR
Erosion of artery
Fistula of artery
Ulcer of artery
EXCLUDES 1 *traumatic rupture of artery - see injury of blood vessel by body region*

I77.3 Arterial fibromuscular dysplasia HCC ESR
Fibromuscular hyperplasia (of) carotid artery
Fibromuscular hyperplasia (of) renal artery

I77.4 Celiac artery compression syndrome HCC ESR
AHA: 2021,3Q,12

I77.5 Necrosis of artery HCC ESR

I77.6 Arteritis, unspecified HCC ESR
Aortitis NOS
Endarteritis NOS
EXCLUDES 1 *arteritis or endarteritis:*
aortic arch (M31.4)
cerebral NEC (I67.7)
coronary (I25.89)
deformans (I7Ø.-)
giant cell (M31.5, M31.6)
obliterans (I7Ø.-)
senile (I7Ø.-)

I77.7 Other arterial dissection
EXCLUDES 2 *dissection of aorta (I71.Ø-)*
dissection of coronary artery (I25.42)
AHA: 2016,4Q,28-29

I77.7Ø Dissection of unspecified artery HCC ESR COM
I77.71 Dissection of carotid artery HCC ESR COM
I77.72 Dissection of iliac artery HCC ESR COM
I77.73 Dissection of renal artery HCC ESR COM
I77.74 Dissection of vertebral artery HCC ESR COM
EXCLUDES 2 *aneurysm of vertebral artery (I72.6)*
I77.75 Dissection of other precerebral arteries HCC ESR COM
Dissection of basilar artery (trunk)
EXCLUDES 2 *aneurysm of carotid artery (I72.Ø)*
aneurysm of other precerebral arteries (I72.5)
aneurysm of vertebral artery (I72.6)
dissection of carotid artery (I77.71)
dissection of vertebral artery (I77.74)
I77.76 Dissection of artery of upper extremity HCC ESR COM
I77.77 Dissection of artery of lower extremity HCC ESR COM
I77.79 Dissection of other specified artery HCC ESR COM

I77.8 Other specified disorders of arteries and arterioles

I77.81 Aortic ectasia
Ectasis aorta
EXCLUDES 1 *aortic aneurysm and dissection ▶(I71.-)◀*
I77.81Ø Thoracic aortic ectasia HCC ESR
I77.811 Abdominal aortic ectasia HCC ESR
I77.812 Thoracoabdominal aortic ectasia HCC ESR
I77.819 Aortic ectasia, unspecified site HCC ESR

● **I77.82 Antineutrophilic cytoplasmic antibody [ANCA] vasculitis**
ANCA associated vasculitis
ANCA positive vasculitis
EXCLUDES 2 *eosinophilic granulomatosis with polyangiitis (M3Ø.1)*
granulomatosis with polyangiitis (M31.3-)
microscopic polyangiitis (M31.7)

I77.89 Other specified disorders of arteries and arterioles HCC ESR
AHA: 2021,1Q,23

I77.9 Disorder of arteries and arterioles, unspecified HCC ESR
AHA: 2021,1Q,4; 2018,2Q,7

I78 Diseases of capillaries

I78.Ø Hereditary hemorrhagic telangiectasia HCC ESR
Rendu-Osler-Weber disease

I78.1 Nevus, non-neoplastic
Araneus nevus
Senile nevus
Spider nevus
Stellar nevus
EXCLUDES 1 *nevus NOS (D22.-)*
vascular NOS (Q82.5)
EXCLUDES 2 *blue nevus (D22.-)*
flammeus nevus (Q82.5)
hairy nevus (D22.-)
melanocytic nevus (D22.-)
pigmented nevus (D22.-)
portwine nevus (Q82.5)
sanguineous nevus (Q82.5)
strawberry nevus (Q82.5)
verrucous nevus (Q82.5)
AHA: 2019,1Q,21

I78.8 Other diseases of capillaries

I78.9 Disease of capillaries, unspecified

I79 Disorders of arteries, arterioles and capillaries in diseases classified elsewhere

I79.Ø Aneurysm of aorta in diseases classified elsewhere HCC ESR
Code first underlying disease
EXCLUDES 1 *syphilitic aneurysm (A52.Ø1)*

I79.1 Aortitis in diseases classified elsewhere HCC ESR
Code first underlying disease
EXCLUDES 1 *syphilitic aortitis (A52.Ø2)*

I79.8 Other disorders of arteries, arterioles and capillaries in diseases classified elsewhere HCC ESR
Code first underlying disease, such as:
amyloidosis (E85.-)
EXCLUDES 1 *diabetic (peripheral) angiopathy (EØ8-E13 with .51-.52)*
syphilitic endarteritis (A52.Ø9)
tuberculous endarteritis (A18.89)

Diseases of veins, lymphatic vessels and lymph nodes, not elsewhere classified (I8Ø-I89)

I8Ø Phlebitis and thrombophlebitis

INCLUDES endophlebitis
inflammation, vein
periphlebitis
suppurative phlebitis

Code first:
phlebitis and thrombophlebitis complicating abortion, ectopic or molar pregnancy (OØØ-OØ7, OØ8.7)
phlebitis and thrombophlebitis complicating pregnancy, childbirth and the puerperium (O22.-, O87.-)

EXCLUDES 1 *venous embolism and thrombosis of lower extremities (I82.4-, I82.5-, I82.81-)*

I8Ø.Ø Phlebitis and thrombophlebitis of superficial vessels of lower extremities
Phlebitis and thrombophlebitis of femoropopliteal vein

I8Ø.ØØ Phlebitis and thrombophlebitis of superficial vessels of unspecified lower extremity
I8Ø.Ø1 Phlebitis and thrombophlebitis of superficial vessels of right lower extremity
I8Ø.Ø2 Phlebitis and thrombophlebitis of superficial vessels of left lower extremity
I8Ø.Ø3 Phlebitis and thrombophlebitis of superficial vessels of lower extremities, bilateral

I8Ø.1 Phlebitis and thrombophlebitis of femoral vein
Phlebitis and thrombophlebitis of common femoral vein
Phlebitis and thrombophlebitis of deep femoral vein

I8Ø.1Ø Phlebitis and thrombophlebitis of unspecified femoral vein HCC Rx ESR COM
I8Ø.11 Phlebitis and thrombophlebitis of right femoral vein HCC Rx ESR COM
I8Ø.12 Phlebitis and thrombophlebitis of left femoral vein HCC Rx ESR COM
I8Ø.13 Phlebitis and thrombophlebitis of femoral vein, bilateral HCC Rx ESR COM

I8Ø.2 Phlebitis and thrombophlebitis of other and unspecified deep vessels of lower extremities

I8Ø.2Ø Phlebitis and thrombophlebitis of unspecified deep vessels of lower extremities
I8Ø.2Ø1 Phlebitis and thrombophlebitis of unspecified deep vessels of right lower extremity HCC Rx ESR COM
I8Ø.2Ø2 Phlebitis and thrombophlebitis of unspecified deep vessels of left lower extremity HCC Rx ESR COM
I8Ø.2Ø3 Phlebitis and thrombophlebitis of unspecified deep vessels of lower extremities, bilateral HCC Rx ESR COM
I8Ø.2Ø9 Phlebitis and thrombophlebitis of unspecified deep vessels of unspecified lower extremity HCC Rx ESR COM

I8Ø.21 Phlebitis and thrombophlebitis of iliac vein
Phlebitis and thrombophlebitis of common iliac vein
Phlebitis and thrombophlebitis of external iliac vein
Phlebitis and thrombophlebitis of internal iliac vein
I8Ø.211 Phlebitis and thrombophlebitis of right iliac vein HCC Rx ESR COM
I8Ø.212 Phlebitis and thrombophlebitis of left iliac vein HCC Rx ESR COM
I8Ø.213 Phlebitis and thrombophlebitis of iliac vein, bilateral HCC Rx ESR COM
I8Ø.219 Phlebitis and thrombophlebitis of unspecified iliac vein HCC Rx ESR COM

I8Ø.22 Phlebitis and thrombophlebitis of popliteal vein
I8Ø.221 Phlebitis and thrombophlebitis of right popliteal vein HCC Rx ESR COM
I8Ø.222 Phlebitis and thrombophlebitis of left popliteal vein HCC Rx ESR COM
I8Ø.223 Phlebitis and thrombophlebitis of popliteal vein, bilateral HCC Rx ESR COM
I8Ø.229 Phlebitis and thrombophlebitis of unspecified popliteal vein HCC Rx ESR COM

I8Ø.23 Phlebitis and thrombophlebitis of tibial vein
Phlebitis and thrombophlebitis of anterior tibial vein
Phlebitis and thrombophlebitis of posterior tibial vein
I8Ø.231 Phlebitis and thrombophlebitis of right tibial vein HCC Rx ESR COM
I8Ø.232 Phlebitis and thrombophlebitis of left tibial vein HCC Rx ESR COM
I8Ø.233 Phlebitis and thrombophlebitis of tibial vein, bilateral HCC Rx ESR COM
I8Ø.239 Phlebitis and thrombophlebitis of unspecified tibial vein HCC Rx ESR COM

I8Ø.24 Phlebitis and thrombophlebitis of peroneal vein
AHA: 2019,4Q,8
I8Ø.241 Phlebitis and thrombophlebitis of right peroneal vein HCC Rx ESR COM
I8Ø.242 Phlebitis and thrombophlebitis of left peroneal vein HCC Rx ESR COM
I8Ø.243 Phlebitis and thrombophlebitis of peroneal vein, bilateral HCC Rx ESR COM
I8Ø.249 Phlebitis and thrombophlebitis of unspecified peroneal vein HCC Rx ESR COM

I8Ø.25 Phlebitis and thrombophlebitis of calf muscular vein
Phlebitis and thrombophlebitis of calf muscular vein, NOS
Phlebitis and thrombophlebitis of gastrocnemial vein
Phlebitis and thrombophlebitis of soleal vein
AHA: 2019,4Q,8
I8Ø.251 Phlebitis and thrombophlebitis of right calf muscular vein HCC Rx ESR COM
I8Ø.252 Phlebitis and thrombophlebitis of left calf muscular vein HCC Rx ESR COM
I8Ø.253 Phlebitis and thrombophlebitis of calf muscular vein, bilateral HCC Rx ESR COM
I8Ø.259 Phlebitis and thrombophlebitis of unspecified calf muscular vein HCC Rx ESR COM

I8Ø.29 Phlebitis and thrombophlebitis of other deep vessels of lower extremities
I8Ø.291 Phlebitis and thrombophlebitis of other deep vessels of right lower extremity HCC Rx ESR COM
I8Ø.292 Phlebitis and thrombophlebitis of other deep vessels of left lower extremity HCC Rx ESR COM
I8Ø.293 Phlebitis and thrombophlebitis of other deep vessels of lower extremity, bilateral HCC Rx ESR COM
I8Ø.299 Phlebitis and thrombophlebitis of other deep vessels of unspecified lower extremity HCC Rx ESR COM

I8Ø.3 Phlebitis and thrombophlebitis of lower extremities, unspecified
I8Ø.8 Phlebitis and thrombophlebitis of other sites
I8Ø.9 Phlebitis and thrombophlebitis of unspecified site

I81 Portal vein thrombosis
Portal (vein) obstruction
EXCLUDES 2 *hepatic vein thrombosis (I82.Ø)*
phlebitis of portal vein (K75.1)
AHA: 2019,4Q,68

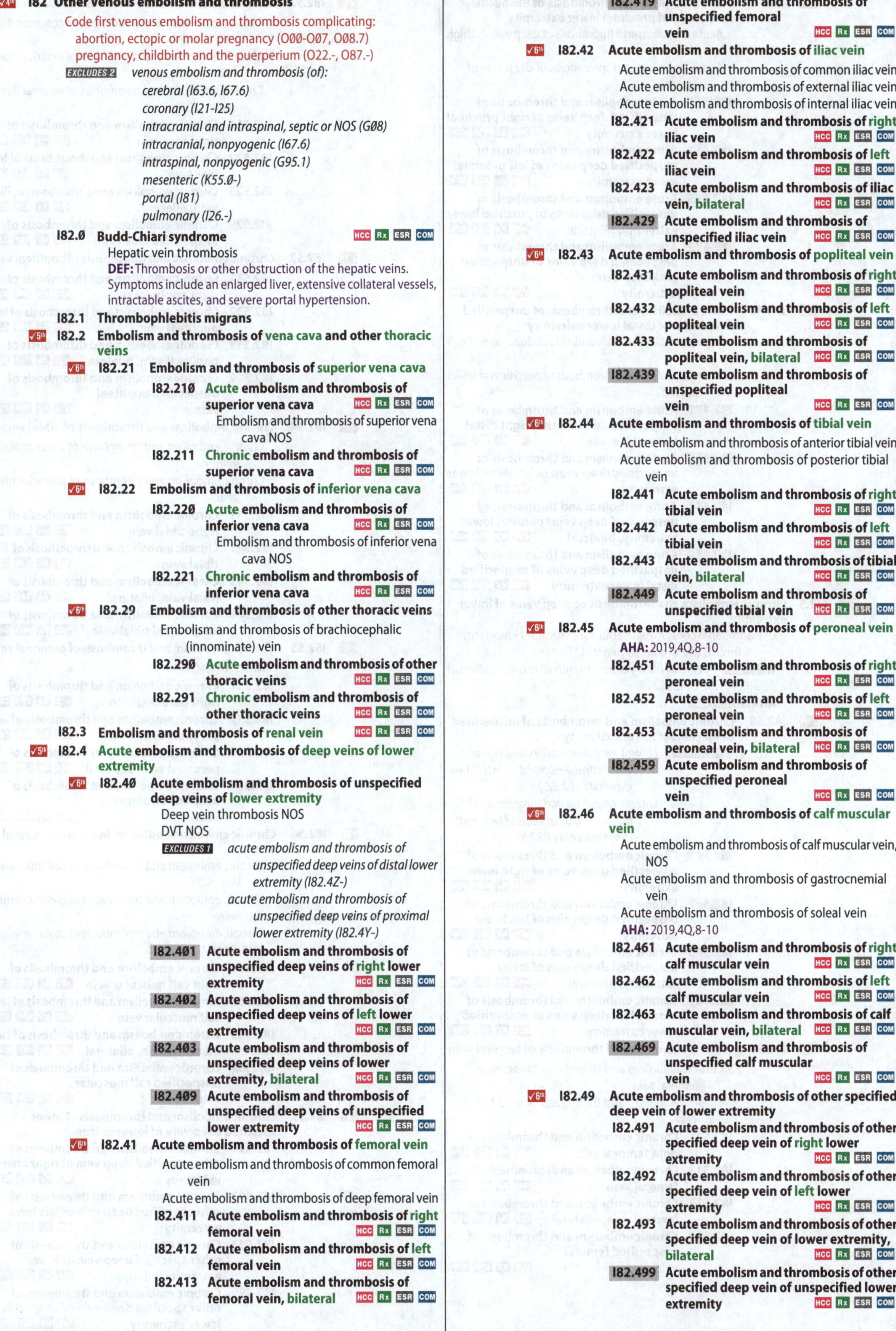

✓4th I82 Other venous embolism and thrombosis

Code first venous embolism and thrombosis complicating:
- abortion, ectopic or molar pregnancy (O00-O07, O08.7)
- pregnancy, childbirth and the puerperium (O22.-, O87.-)

EXCLUDES 2 *venous embolism and thrombosis (of):*
- *cerebral (I63.6, I67.6)*
- *coronary (I21-I25)*
- *intracranial and intraspinal, septic or NOS (G08)*
- *intracranial, nonpyogenic (I67.6)*
- *intraspinal, nonpyogenic (G95.1)*
- *mesenteric (K55.0-)*
- *portal (I81)*
- *pulmonary (I26.-)*

I82.0 Budd-Chiari syndrome HCC Rx ESR COM
Hepatic vein thrombosis
DEF: Thrombosis or other obstruction of the hepatic veins. Symptoms include an enlarged liver, extensive collateral vessels, intractable ascites, and severe portal hypertension.

I82.1 Thrombophlebitis migrans

✓5th I82.2 Embolism and thrombosis of vena cava and other thoracic veins

✓6th I82.21 Embolism and thrombosis of superior vena cava

I82.210 Acute embolism and thrombosis of superior vena cava HCC Rx ESR COM
Embolism and thrombosis of superior vena cava NOS

I82.211 Chronic embolism and thrombosis of superior vena cava HCC Rx ESR COM

✓6th I82.22 Embolism and thrombosis of inferior vena cava

I82.220 Acute embolism and thrombosis of inferior vena cava HCC Rx ESR COM
Embolism and thrombosis of inferior vena cava NOS

I82.221 Chronic embolism and thrombosis of inferior vena cava HCC Rx ESR COM

✓6th I82.29 Embolism and thrombosis of other thoracic veins
Embolism and thrombosis of brachiocephalic (innominate) vein

I82.290 Acute embolism and thrombosis of other thoracic veins HCC Rx ESR COM

I82.291 Chronic embolism and thrombosis of other thoracic veins HCC Rx ESR COM

I82.3 Embolism and thrombosis of renal vein HCC Rx ESR COM

✓5th I82.4 Acute embolism and thrombosis of deep veins of lower extremity

✓6th I82.40 Acute embolism and thrombosis of unspecified deep veins of lower extremity
Deep vein thrombosis NOS
DVT NOS

EXCLUDES 1 *acute embolism and thrombosis of unspecified deep veins of distal lower extremity (I82.4Z-)*
acute embolism and thrombosis of unspecified deep veins of proximal lower extremity (I82.4Y-)

I82.401 Acute embolism and thrombosis of unspecified deep veins of right lower extremity HCC Rx ESR COM

I82.402 Acute embolism and thrombosis of unspecified deep veins of left lower extremity HCC Rx ESR COM

I82.403 Acute embolism and thrombosis of unspecified deep veins of lower extremity, bilateral HCC Rx ESR COM

I82.409 Acute embolism and thrombosis of unspecified deep veins of unspecified lower extremity HCC Rx ESR COM

✓6th I82.41 Acute embolism and thrombosis of femoral vein
Acute embolism and thrombosis of common femoral vein
Acute embolism and thrombosis of deep femoral vein

I82.411 Acute embolism and thrombosis of right femoral vein HCC Rx ESR COM

I82.412 Acute embolism and thrombosis of left femoral vein HCC Rx ESR COM

I82.413 Acute embolism and thrombosis of femoral vein, bilateral HCC Rx ESR COM

I82.419 Acute embolism and thrombosis of unspecified femoral vein HCC Rx ESR COM

✓6th I82.42 Acute embolism and thrombosis of iliac vein
Acute embolism and thrombosis of common iliac vein
Acute embolism and thrombosis of external iliac vein
Acute embolism and thrombosis of internal iliac vein

I82.421 Acute embolism and thrombosis of right iliac vein HCC Rx ESR COM

I82.422 Acute embolism and thrombosis of left iliac vein HCC Rx ESR COM

I82.423 Acute embolism and thrombosis of iliac vein, bilateral HCC Rx ESR COM

I82.429 Acute embolism and thrombosis of unspecified iliac vein HCC Rx ESR COM

✓6th I82.43 Acute embolism and thrombosis of popliteal vein

I82.431 Acute embolism and thrombosis of right popliteal vein HCC Rx ESR COM

I82.432 Acute embolism and thrombosis of left popliteal vein HCC Rx ESR COM

I82.433 Acute embolism and thrombosis of popliteal vein, bilateral HCC Rx ESR COM

I82.439 Acute embolism and thrombosis of unspecified popliteal vein HCC Rx ESR COM

✓6th I82.44 Acute embolism and thrombosis of tibial vein
Acute embolism and thrombosis of anterior tibial vein
Acute embolism and thrombosis of posterior tibial vein

I82.441 Acute embolism and thrombosis of right tibial vein HCC Rx ESR COM

I82.442 Acute embolism and thrombosis of left tibial vein HCC Rx ESR COM

I82.443 Acute embolism and thrombosis of tibial vein, bilateral HCC Rx ESR COM

I82.449 Acute embolism and thrombosis of unspecified tibial vein HCC Rx ESR COM

✓6th I82.45 Acute embolism and thrombosis of peroneal vein
AHA: 2019,4Q,8-10

I82.451 Acute embolism and thrombosis of right peroneal vein HCC Rx ESR COM

I82.452 Acute embolism and thrombosis of left peroneal vein HCC Rx ESR COM

I82.453 Acute embolism and thrombosis of peroneal vein, bilateral HCC Rx ESR COM

I82.459 Acute embolism and thrombosis of unspecified peroneal vein HCC Rx ESR COM

✓6th I82.46 Acute embolism and thrombosis of calf muscular vein
Acute embolism and thrombosis of calf muscular vein, NOS
Acute embolism and thrombosis of gastrocnemial vein
Acute embolism and thrombosis of soleal vein
AHA: 2019,4Q,8-10

I82.461 Acute embolism and thrombosis of right calf muscular vein HCC Rx ESR COM

I82.462 Acute embolism and thrombosis of left calf muscular vein HCC Rx ESR COM

I82.463 Acute embolism and thrombosis of calf muscular vein, bilateral HCC Rx ESR COM

I82.469 Acute embolism and thrombosis of unspecified calf muscular vein HCC Rx ESR COM

✓6th I82.49 Acute embolism and thrombosis of other specified deep vein of lower extremity

I82.491 Acute embolism and thrombosis of other specified deep vein of right lower extremity HCC Rx ESR COM

I82.492 Acute embolism and thrombosis of other specified deep vein of left lower extremity HCC Rx ESR COM

I82.493 Acute embolism and thrombosis of other specified deep vein of lower extremity, bilateral HCC Rx ESR COM

I82.499 Acute embolism and thrombosis of other specified deep vein of unspecified lower extremity HCC Rx ESR COM

✓6th **I82.4Y Acute embolism and thrombosis of unspecified deep veins of proximal lower extremity**
Acute embolism and thrombosis of deep vein of thigh NOS
Acute embolism and thrombosis of deep vein of upper leg NOS

I82.4Y1 Acute embolism and thrombosis of unspecified deep veins of right proximal lower extremity HCC Rx ESR COM

I82.4Y2 Acute embolism and thrombosis of unspecified deep veins of left proximal lower extremity HCC Rx ESR COM

I82.4Y3 Acute embolism and thrombosis of unspecified deep veins of proximal lower extremity, bilateral HCC Rx ESR COM

I82.4Y9 Acute embolism and thrombosis of unspecified deep veins of unspecified proximal lower extremity HCC Rx ESR COM

✓6th **I82.4Z Acute embolism and thrombosis of unspecified deep veins of distal lower extremity**
Acute embolism and thrombosis of deep vein of calf NOS
Acute embolism and thrombosis of deep vein of lower leg NOS

I82.4Z1 Acute embolism and thrombosis of unspecified deep veins of right distal lower extremity HCC Rx ESR COM

I82.4Z2 Acute embolism and thrombosis of unspecified deep veins of left distal lower extremity HCC Rx ESR COM

I82.4Z3 Acute embolism and thrombosis of unspecified deep veins of distal lower extremity, bilateral HCC Rx ESR COM

I82.4Z9 Acute embolism and thrombosis of unspecified deep veins of unspecified distal lower extremity HCC Rx ESR COM

✓5th **I82.5 Chronic embolism and thrombosis of deep veins of lower extremity**
Use additional code, if applicable, for associated long-term (current) use of anticoagulants (Z79.01)
EXCLUDES 1 *personal history of venous embolism and thrombosis (Z86.718)*
AHA: 2020,2Q,20

✓6th **I82.50 Chronic embolism and thrombosis of unspecified deep veins of lower extremity**
EXCLUDES 1 *chronic embolism and thrombosis of unspecified deep veins of distal lower extremity (I82.5Z-)*
chronic embolism and thrombosis of unspecified deep veins of proximal lower extremity (I82.5Y-)

I82.501 Chronic embolism and thrombosis of unspecified deep veins of right lower extremity HCC Rx ESR COM

I82.502 Chronic embolism and thrombosis of unspecified deep veins of left lower extremity HCC Rx ESR COM

I82.503 Chronic embolism and thrombosis of unspecified deep veins of lower extremity, bilateral HCC Rx ESR COM

I82.509 Chronic embolism and thrombosis of unspecified deep veins of unspecified lower extremity HCC Rx ESR COM

✓6th **I82.51 Chronic embolism and thrombosis of femoral vein**
Chronic embolism and thrombosis of common femoral vein
Chronic embolism and thrombosis of deep femoral vein

I82.511 Chronic embolism and thrombosis of right femoral vein HCC Rx ESR COM

I82.512 Chronic embolism and thrombosis of left femoral vein HCC Rx ESR COM

I82.513 Chronic embolism and thrombosis of femoral vein, bilateral HCC Rx ESR COM

I82.519 Chronic embolism and thrombosis of unspecified femoral vein HCC Rx ESR COM

✓6th **I82.52 Chronic embolism and thrombosis of iliac vein**
Chronic embolism and thrombosis of common iliac vein
Chronic embolism and thrombosis of external iliac vein
Chronic embolism and thrombosis of internal iliac vein

I82.521 Chronic embolism and thrombosis of right iliac vein HCC Rx ESR COM

I82.522 Chronic embolism and thrombosis of left iliac vein HCC Rx ESR COM

I82.523 Chronic embolism and thrombosis of iliac vein, bilateral HCC Rx ESR COM

I82.529 Chronic embolism and thrombosis of unspecified iliac vein HCC Rx ESR COM

✓6th **I82.53 Chronic embolism and thrombosis of popliteal vein**

I82.531 Chronic embolism and thrombosis of right popliteal vein HCC Rx ESR COM

I82.532 Chronic embolism and thrombosis of left popliteal vein HCC Rx ESR COM

I82.533 Chronic embolism and thrombosis of popliteal vein, bilateral HCC Rx ESR COM

I82.539 Chronic embolism and thrombosis of unspecified popliteal vein HCC Rx ESR COM

✓6th **I82.54 Chronic embolism and thrombosis of tibial vein**
Chronic embolism and thrombosis of anterior tibial vein
Chronic embolism and thrombosis of posterior tibial vein

I82.541 Chronic embolism and thrombosis of right tibial vein HCC Rx ESR COM

I82.542 Chronic embolism and thrombosis of left tibial vein HCC Rx ESR COM

I82.543 Chronic embolism and thrombosis of tibial vein, bilateral HCC Rx ESR COM

I82.549 Chronic embolism and thrombosis of unspecified tibial vein HCC Rx ESR COM

✓6th **I82.55 Chronic embolism and thrombosis of peroneal vein**
AHA: 2019,4Q,8-10

I82.551 Chronic embolism and thrombosis of right peroneal vein HCC Rx ESR COM

I82.552 Chronic embolism and thrombosis of left peroneal vein HCC Rx ESR COM

I82.553 Chronic embolism and thrombosis of peroneal vein, bilateral HCC Rx ESR COM

I82.559 Chronic embolism and thrombosis of unspecified peroneal vein HCC Rx ESR COM

✓6th **I82.56 Chronic embolism and thrombosis of calf muscular vein**
Chronic embolism and thrombosis of calf muscular vein NOS
Chronic embolism and thrombosis of gastrocnemial vein
Chronic embolism and thrombosis of soleal vein
AHA: 2019,4Q,8-10

I82.561 Chronic embolism and thrombosis of right calf muscular vein HCC Rx ESR COM

I82.562 Chronic embolism and thrombosis of left calf muscular vein HCC Rx ESR COM

I82.563 Chronic embolism and thrombosis of calf muscular vein, bilateral HCC Rx ESR COM

I82.569 Chronic embolism and thrombosis of unspecified calf muscular vein HCC Rx ESR COM

✓6th **I82.59 Chronic embolism and thrombosis of other specified deep vein of lower extremity**

I82.591 Chronic embolism and thrombosis of other specified deep vein of right lower extremity HCC Rx ESR COM

I82.592 Chronic embolism and thrombosis of other specified deep vein of left lower extremity HCC Rx ESR COM

I82.593 Chronic embolism and thrombosis of other specified deep vein of lower extremity, bilateral HCC Rx ESR COM

I82.599 Chronic embolism and thrombosis of other specified deep vein of unspecified lower extremity HCC Rx ESR COM

I82.5Y Chronic embolism and thrombosis of unspecified deep veins of proximal lower extremity
Chronic embolism and thrombosis of deep veins of thigh NOS
Chronic embolism and thrombosis of deep veins of upper leg NOS

I82.5Y1 Chronic embolism and thrombosis of unspecified deep veins of right proximal lower extremity HCC Rx ESR COM

I82.5Y2 Chronic embolism and thrombosis of unspecified deep veins of left proximal lower extremity HCC Rx ESR COM

I82.5Y3 Chronic embolism and thrombosis of unspecified deep veins of proximal lower extremity, bilateral HCC Rx ESR COM

I82.5Y9 Chronic embolism and thrombosis of unspecified deep veins of unspecified proximal lower extremity HCC Rx ESR COM

I82.5Z Chronic embolism and thrombosis of unspecified deep veins of distal lower extremity
Chronic embolism and thrombosis of deep veins of calf NOS
Chronic embolism and thrombosis of deep veins of lower leg NOS

I82.5Z1 Chronic embolism and thrombosis of unspecified deep veins of right distal lower extremity HCC Rx ESR COM

I82.5Z2 Chronic embolism and thrombosis of unspecified deep veins of left distal lower extremity HCC Rx ESR COM

I82.5Z3 Chronic embolism and thrombosis of unspecified deep veins of distal lower extremity, bilateral HCC Rx ESR COM

I82.5Z9 Chronic embolism and thrombosis of unspecified deep veins of unspecified distal lower extremity HCC Rx ESR COM

I82.6 Acute embolism and thrombosis of veins of upper extremity

I82.60 Acute embolism and thrombosis of unspecified veins of upper extremity

I82.601 Acute embolism and thrombosis of unspecified veins of right upper extremity

I82.602 Acute embolism and thrombosis of unspecified veins of left upper extremity

I82.603 Acute embolism and thrombosis of unspecified veins of upper extremity, bilateral

I82.609 Acute embolism and thrombosis of unspecified veins of unspecified upper extremity

I82.61 Acute embolism and thrombosis of superficial veins of upper extremity
Acute embolism and thrombosis of antecubital vein
Acute embolism and thrombosis of basilic vein
Acute embolism and thrombosis of cephalic vein

I82.611 Acute embolism and thrombosis of superficial veins of right upper extremity

I82.612 Acute embolism and thrombosis of superficial veins of left upper extremity

I82.613 Acute embolism and thrombosis of superficial veins of upper extremity, bilateral

I82.619 Acute embolism and thrombosis of superficial veins of unspecified upper extremity

I82.62 Acute embolism and thrombosis of deep veins of upper extremity
Acute embolism and thrombosis of brachial vein
Acute embolism and thrombosis of radial vein
Acute embolism and thrombosis of ulnar vein

I82.621 Acute embolism and thrombosis of deep veins of right upper extremity HCC Rx ESR COM

I82.622 Acute embolism and thrombosis of deep veins of left upper extremity HCC Rx ESR COM

I82.623 Acute embolism and thrombosis of deep veins of upper extremity, bilateral HCC Rx ESR COM

I82.629 Acute embolism and thrombosis of deep veins of unspecified upper extremity HCC Rx ESR COM

I82.7 Chronic embolism and thrombosis of veins of upper extremity
Use additional code, if applicable, for associated long-term (current) use of anticoagulants (Z79.01)
EXCLUDES 1 *personal history of venous embolism and thrombosis (Z86.718)*

I82.70 Chronic embolism and thrombosis of unspecified veins of upper extremity

I82.701 Chronic embolism and thrombosis of unspecified veins of right upper extremity

I82.702 Chronic embolism and thrombosis of unspecified veins of left upper extremity

I82.703 Chronic embolism and thrombosis of unspecified veins of upper extremity, bilateral

I82.709 Chronic embolism and thrombosis of unspecified veins of unspecified upper extremity

I82.71 Chronic embolism and thrombosis of superficial veins of upper extremity
Chronic embolism and thrombosis of antecubital vein
Chronic embolism and thrombosis of basilic vein
Chronic embolism and thrombosis of cephalic vein

I82.711 Chronic embolism and thrombosis of superficial veins of right upper extremity

I82.712 Chronic embolism and thrombosis of superficial veins of left upper extremity

I82.713 Chronic embolism and thrombosis of superficial veins of upper extremity, bilateral

I82.719 Chronic embolism and thrombosis of superficial veins of unspecified upper extremity

I82.72 Chronic embolism and thrombosis of deep veins of upper extremity
Chronic embolism and thrombosis of brachial vein
Chronic embolism and thrombosis of radial vein
Chronic embolism and thrombosis of ulnar vein

I82.721 Chronic embolism and thrombosis of deep veins of right upper extremity HCC Rx ESR COM

I82.722 Chronic embolism and thrombosis of deep veins of left upper extremity HCC Rx ESR COM

I82.723 Chronic embolism and thrombosis of deep veins of upper extremity, bilateral HCC Rx ESR COM

I82.729 Chronic embolism and thrombosis of deep veins of unspecified upper extremity HCC Rx ESR COM

I82.A Embolism and thrombosis of axillary vein

I82.A1 Acute embolism and thrombosis of axillary vein

I82.A11 Acute embolism and thrombosis of right axillary vein HCC Rx ESR COM

I82.A12 Acute embolism and thrombosis of left axillary vein HCC Rx ESR COM

I82.A13 Acute embolism and thrombosis of axillary vein, bilateral HCC Rx ESR COM

I82.A19 Acute embolism and thrombosis of unspecified axillary vein HCC Rx ESR COM

I82.A2 Chronic embolism and thrombosis of axillary vein

I82.A21 Chronic embolism and thrombosis of right axillary vein HCC Rx ESR COM

I82.A22 Chronic embolism and thrombosis of left axillary vein HCC Rx ESR COM

I82.A23 Chronic embolism and thrombosis of axillary vein, bilateral HCC Rx ESR COM

I82.A29 Chronic embolism and thrombosis of unspecified axillary vein HCC Rx ESR COM

I82.B Embolism and thrombosis of subclavian vein

I82.B1 Acute embolism and thrombosis of subclavian vein

I82.B11 Acute embolism and thrombosis of right subclavian vein HCC Rx ESR COM

I82.B12 Acute embolism and thrombosis of left subclavian vein HCC Rx ESR COM

I82.B13 Acute embolism and thrombosis of subclavian vein, bilateral HCC Rx ESR COM

I82.B19 Acute embolism and thrombosis of unspecified subclavian vein HCC Rx ESR COM

6th **I82.B2 Chronic embolism and thrombosis of subclavian vein**

I82.B21 Chronic embolism and thrombosis of right subclavian vein HCC Rx ESR COM

I82.B22 Chronic embolism and thrombosis of left subclavian vein HCC Rx ESR COM

I82.B23 Chronic embolism and thrombosis of subclavian vein, bilateral HCC Rx ESR COM

I82.B29 Chronic embolism and thrombosis of unspecified subclavian vein HCC Rx ESR COM

5th **I82.C Embolism and thrombosis of internal jugular vein**

6th **I82.C1 Acute embolism and thrombosis of internal jugular vein**

I82.C11 Acute embolism and thrombosis of right internal jugular vein HCC Rx ESR COM

I82.C12 Acute embolism and thrombosis of left internal jugular vein HCC Rx ESR COM

I82.C13 Acute embolism and thrombosis of internal jugular vein, bilateral HCC Rx ESR COM

I82.C19 Acute embolism and thrombosis of unspecified internal jugular vein HCC Rx ESR COM

6th **I82.C2 Chronic embolism and thrombosis of internal jugular vein**

I82.C21 Chronic embolism and thrombosis of right internal jugular vein HCC Rx ESR COM

I82.C22 Chronic embolism and thrombosis of left internal jugular vein HCC Rx ESR COM

I82.C23 Chronic embolism and thrombosis of internal jugular vein, bilateral HCC Rx ESR COM

I82.C29 Chronic embolism and thrombosis of unspecified internal jugular vein HCC Rx ESR COM

5th **I82.8 Embolism and thrombosis of other specified veins**

Use additional code, if applicable, for associated long-term (current) use of anticoagulants (Z79.01)

6th **I82.81 Embolism and thrombosis of superficial veins of lower extremities**

Embolism and thrombosis of saphenous vein (greater) (lesser)

I82.811 Embolism and thrombosis of superficial veins of right lower extremity

I82.812 Embolism and thrombosis of superficial veins of left lower extremity

I82.813 Embolism and thrombosis of superficial veins of lower extremities, bilateral

I82.819 Embolism and thrombosis of superficial veins of unspecified lower extremity

6th **I82.89 Embolism and thrombosis of other specified veins**

I82.890 Acute embolism and thrombosis of other specified veins

I82.891 Chronic embolism and thrombosis of other specified veins

5th **I82.9 Embolism and thrombosis of unspecified vein**

I82.90 Acute embolism and thrombosis of unspecified vein

Embolism of vein NOS

Thrombosis (vein) NOS

I82.91 Chronic embolism and thrombosis of unspecified vein

4th **I83 Varicose veins of lower extremities**

EXCLUDES 2 *varicose veins complicating pregnancy (O22.0-)*

varicose veins complicating the puerperium (O87.4)

5th **I83.0 Varicose veins of lower extremities with ulcer**

Use additional code to identify severity of ulcer (L97.-)

6th **I83.00 Varicose veins of unspecified lower extremity with ulcer**

I83.001 Varicose veins of unspecified lower extremity with ulcer of thigh HCC ESR COM A

I83.002 Varicose veins of unspecified lower extremity with ulcer of calf HCC ESR COM A

I83.003 Varicose veins of unspecified lower extremity with ulcer of ankle HCC ESR COM A

I83.004 Varicose veins of unspecified lower extremity with ulcer of heel and midfoot HCC ESR COM A

Varicose veins of unspecified lower extremity with ulcer of plantar surface of midfoot

I83.005 Varicose veins of unspecified lower extremity with ulcer other part of foot HCC ESR COM A

Varicose veins of unspecified lower extremity with ulcer of toe

I83.008 Varicose veins of unspecified lower extremity with ulcer other part of lower leg HCC ESR COM A

I83.009 Varicose veins of unspecified lower extremity with ulcer of unspecified site HCC ESR COM A

6th **I83.01 Varicose veins of right lower extremity with ulcer**

I83.011 Varicose veins of right lower extremity with ulcer of thigh HCC ESR COM A

I83.012 Varicose veins of right lower extremity with ulcer of calf HCC ESR COM A

I83.013 Varicose veins of right lower extremity with ulcer of ankle HCC ESR COM A

I83.014 Varicose veins of right lower extremity with ulcer of heel and midfoot HCC ESR COM A

Varicose veins of right lower extremity with ulcer of plantar surface of midfoot

I83.015 Varicose veins of right lower extremity with ulcer other part of foot HCC ESR COM A

Varicose veins of right lower extremity with ulcer of toe

I83.018 Varicose veins of right lower extremity with ulcer other part of lower leg HCC ESR COM A

I83.019 Varicose veins of right lower extremity with ulcer of unspecified site HCC ESR COM A

6th **I83.02 Varicose veins of left lower extremity with ulcer**

I83.021 Varicose veins of left lower extremity with ulcer of thigh HCC ESR COM A

I83.022 Varicose veins of left lower extremity with ulcer of calf HCC ESR COM A

I83.023 Varicose veins of left lower extremity with ulcer of ankle HCC ESR COM A

I83.024 Varicose veins of left lower extremity with ulcer of heel and midfoot HCC ESR COM A

Varicose veins of left lower extremity with ulcer of plantar surface of midfoot

I83.025 Varicose veins of left lower extremity with ulcer other part of foot HCC ESR COM A

Varicose veins of left lower extremity with ulcer of toe

I83.028 Varicose veins of left lower extremity with ulcer other part of lower leg HCC ESR COM A

I83.029 Varicose veins of left lower extremity with ulcer of unspecified site HCC ESR COM A

5th **I83.1 Varicose veins of lower extremities with inflammation**

I83.10 Varicose veins of unspecified lower extremity with inflammation A

I83.11 Varicose veins of right lower extremity with inflammation A

I83.12 Varicose veins of left lower extremity with inflammation A

I83.2 Varicose veins of lower extremities with both ulcer and inflammation
Use additional code to identify severity of ulcer (L97.-)

I83.20 Varicose veins of unspecified lower extremity with both ulcer and inflammation

I83.201 Varicose veins of unspecified lower extremity with both ulcer of thigh and inflammation HCC ESR COM A

I83.202 Varicose veins of unspecified lower extremity with both ulcer of calf and inflammation HCC ESR COM A

I83.203 Varicose veins of unspecified lower extremity with both ulcer of ankle and inflammation HCC ESR COM A

I83.204 Varicose veins of unspecified lower extremity with both ulcer of heel and midfoot and inflammation HCC ESR COM A
Varicose veins of unspecified lower extremity with both ulcer of plantar surface of midfoot and inflammation

I83.205 Varicose veins of unspecified lower extremity with both ulcer of other part of foot and inflammation HCC ESR COM A
Varicose veins of unspecified lower extremity with both ulcer of toe and inflammation

I83.208 Varicose veins of unspecified lower extremity with both ulcer of other part of lower extremity and inflammation HCC ESR COM A

I83.209 Varicose veins of unspecified lower extremity with both ulcer of unspecified site and inflammation HCC ESR COM A

I83.21 Varicose veins of right lower extremity with both ulcer and inflammation

I83.211 Varicose veins of right lower extremity with both ulcer of thigh and inflammation HCC ESR COM A

I83.212 Varicose veins of right lower extremity with both ulcer of calf and inflammation HCC ESR COM A

I83.213 Varicose veins of right lower extremity with both ulcer of ankle and inflammation HCC ESR COM A

I83.214 Varicose veins of right lower extremity with both ulcer of heel and midfoot and inflammation HCC ESR COM A
Varicose veins of right lower extremity with both ulcer of plantar surface of midfoot and inflammation

I83.215 Varicose veins of right lower extremity with both ulcer other part of foot and inflammation HCC ESR COM A
Varicose veins of right lower extremity with both ulcer of toe and inflammation

I83.218 Varicose veins of right lower extremity with both ulcer of other part of lower extremity and inflammation HCC ESR COM A

I83.219 Varicose veins of right lower extremity with both ulcer of unspecified site and inflammation HCC ESR COM A

I83.22 Varicose veins of left lower extremity with both ulcer and inflammation

I83.221 Varicose veins of left lower extremity with both ulcer of thigh and inflammation HCC ESR COM A

I83.222 Varicose veins of left lower extremity with both ulcer of calf and inflammation HCC ESR COM A

I83.223 Varicose veins of left lower extremity with both ulcer of ankle and inflammation HCC ESR COM A

I83.224 Varicose veins of left lower extremity with both ulcer of heel and midfoot and inflammation HCC ESR COM A
Varicose veins of left lower extremity with both ulcer of plantar surface of midfoot and inflammation

I83.225 Varicose veins of left lower extremity with both ulcer other part of foot and inflammation HCC ESR COM A
Varicose veins of left lower extremity with both ulcer of toe and inflammation

I83.228 Varicose veins of left lower extremity with both ulcer of other part of lower extremity and inflammation HCC ESR COM A

I83.229 Varicose veins of left lower extremity with both ulcer of unspecified site and inflammation HCC ESR COM A

I83.8 Varicose veins of lower extremities with other complications

I83.81 Varicose veins of lower extremities with pain

I83.811 Varicose veins of right lower extremity with pain A

I83.812 Varicose veins of left lower extremity with pain A

I83.813 Varicose veins of bilateral lower extremities with pain A

I83.819 Varicose veins of unspecified lower extremity with pain A

I83.89 Varicose veins of lower extremities with other complications
Varicose veins of lower extremities with edema
Varicose veins of lower extremities with swelling

I83.891 Varicose veins of right lower extremity with other complications A

I83.892 Varicose veins of left lower extremity with other complications A

I83.893 Varicose veins of bilateral lower extremities with other complications A

I83.899 Varicose veins of unspecified lower extremity with other complications A

I83.9 Asymptomatic varicose veins of lower extremities
Phlebectasia of lower extremities
Varicose veins of lower extremities
Varix of lower extremities

I83.90 Asymptomatic varicose veins of unspecified lower extremity A
Varicose veins NOS

I83.91 Asymptomatic varicose veins of right lower extremity A

I83.92 Asymptomatic varicose veins of left lower extremity A

I83.93 Asymptomatic varicose veins of bilateral lower extremities A

I85 Esophageal varices
Use additional code to identify:
alcohol abuse and dependence (F10.-)

I85.0 Esophageal varices
Idiopathic esophageal varices
Primary esophageal varices

I85.00 Esophageal varices without bleeding HCC ESR COM
Esophageal varices NOS

I85.01 Esophageal varices with bleeding HCC ESR COM

I85.1 Secondary esophageal varices
Esophageal varices secondary to alcoholic liver disease
Esophageal varices secondary to cirrhosis of liver
Esophageal varices secondary to schistosomiasis
Esophageal varices secondary to toxic liver disease
Code first underlying disease

I85.10 Secondary esophageal varices without bleeding HCC ESR COM

I85.11 Secondary esophageal varices with bleeding HCC ESR COM

I86 Varicose veins of other sites
EXCLUDES 1 *varicose veins of unspecified site (I83.9-)*
EXCLUDES 2 *retinal varices (H35.0-)*

I86.0 Sublingual varices
DEF: Distended, tortuous veins beneath the tongue.

I86.1 Scrotal varices ♂
Varicocele

I86.2 Pelvic varices

I86.3 Vulval varices ♀
EXCLUDES 1 *vulval varices complicating childbirth and the puerperium (O87.8)*
vulval varices complicating pregnancy (O22.1-)

I86.4 Gastric varices

I86.8 Varicose veins of other specified sites A
Varicose ulcer of nasal septum

✓4th I87 Other disorders of veins

✓5th I87.0 Postthrombotic syndrome
Chronic venous hypertension due to deep vein thrombosis
Postphlebitic syndrome
EXCLUDES 1 *chronic venous hypertension without deep vein thrombosis (I87.3-)*

✓6th I87.00 Postthrombotic syndrome without complications
Asymptomatic postthrombotic syndrome

I87.001 Postthrombotic syndrome without complications of right lower extremity

I87.002 Postthrombotic syndrome without complications of left lower extremity

I87.003 Postthrombotic syndrome without complications of bilateral lower extremity

I87.009 Postthrombotic syndrome without complications of unspecified extremity
Postthrombotic syndrome NOS

✓6th I87.01 Postthrombotic syndrome with ulcer
Use additional code to specify site and severity of ulcer (L97.-)

I87.011 Postthrombotic syndrome with ulcer of right lower extremity HCC ESR COM

I87.012 Postthrombotic syndrome with ulcer of left lower extremity HCC ESR COM

I87.013 Postthrombotic syndrome with ulcer of bilateral lower extremity HCC ESR COM

I87.019 Postthrombotic syndrome with ulcer of unspecified lower extremity HCC ESR COM

✓6th I87.02 Postthrombotic syndrome with inflammation

I87.021 Postthrombotic syndrome with inflammation of right lower extremity

I87.022 Postthrombotic syndrome with inflammation of left lower extremity

I87.023 Postthrombotic syndrome with inflammation of bilateral lower extremity

I87.029 Postthrombotic syndrome with inflammation of unspecified lower extremity

✓6th I87.03 Postthrombotic syndrome with ulcer and inflammation
Use additional code to specify site and severity of ulcer (L97.-)

I87.031 Postthrombotic syndrome with ulcer and inflammation of right lower extremity HCC ESR COM

I87.032 Postthrombotic syndrome with ulcer and inflammation of left lower extremity HCC ESR COM

I87.033 Postthrombotic syndrome with ulcer and inflammation of bilateral lower extremity HCC ESR COM

I87.039 Postthrombotic syndrome with ulcer and inflammation of unspecified lower extremity HCC ESR COM

✓6th I87.09 Postthrombotic syndrome with other complications

I87.091 Postthrombotic syndrome with other complications of right lower extremity

I87.092 Postthrombotic syndrome with other complications of left lower extremity

I87.093 Postthrombotic syndrome with other complications of bilateral lower extremity

I87.099 Postthrombotic syndrome with other complications of unspecified lower extremity

I87.1 Compression of vein
Stricture of vein
Vena cava syndrome (inferior) (superior)
EXCLUDES 2 *compression of pulmonary vein (I28.8)*

I87.2 Venous insufficiency (chronic) (peripheral)
Stasis dermatitis
EXCLUDES 1 *stasis dermatitis with varicose veins of lower extremities (I83.1-, I83.2-)*
DEF: Insufficient drainage of venous blood in any part of the body that results in edema or dermatosis.

✓5th I87.3 Chronic venous hypertension (idiopathic)
Stasis edema
EXCLUDES 1 *chronic venous hypertension due to deep vein thrombosis (I87.0-)*
varicose veins of lower extremities (I83.-)

✓6th I87.30 Chronic venous hypertension (idiopathic) without complications
Asymptomatic chronic venous hypertension (idiopathic)

I87.301 Chronic venous hypertension (idiopathic) without complications of right lower extremity

I87.302 Chronic venous hypertension (idiopathic) without complications of left lower extremity

I87.303 Chronic venous hypertension (idiopathic) without complications of bilateral lower extremity

I87.309 Chronic venous hypertension (idiopathic) without complications of unspecified lower extremity
Chronic venous hypertension NOS

✓6th I87.31 Chronic venous hypertension (idiopathic) with ulcer
Use additional code to specify site and severity of ulcer (L97.-)

I87.311 Chronic venous hypertension (idiopathic) with ulcer of right lower extremity HCC ESR COM

I87.312 Chronic venous hypertension (idiopathic) with ulcer of left lower extremity HCC ESR COM

I87.313 Chronic venous hypertension (idiopathic) with ulcer of bilateral lower extremity HCC ESR COM

I87.319 Chronic venous hypertension (idiopathic) with ulcer of unspecified lower extremity HCC ESR COM

✓6th I87.32 Chronic venous hypertension (idiopathic) with inflammation

I87.321 Chronic venous hypertension (idiopathic) with inflammation of right lower extremity

I87.322 Chronic venous hypertension (idiopathic) with inflammation of left lower extremity

I87.323 Chronic venous hypertension (idiopathic) with inflammation of bilateral lower extremity

I87.329 Chronic venous hypertension (idiopathic) with inflammation of unspecified lower extremity

✓6th I87.33 Chronic venous hypertension (idiopathic) with ulcer and inflammation
Use additional code to specify site and severity of ulcer (L97.-)

I87.331 Chronic venous hypertension (idiopathic) with ulcer and inflammation of right lower extremity HCC ESR COM

I87.332 Chronic venous hypertension (idiopathic) with ulcer and inflammation of left lower extremity HCC ESR COM

I87.333 Chronic venous hypertension (idiopathic) with ulcer and inflammation of bilateral lower extremity HCC ESR COM

I87.339 Chronic venous hypertension (idiopathic) with ulcer and inflammation of unspecified lower extremity HCC ESR COM

✓6th I87.39 Chronic venous hypertension (idiopathic) with other complications

I87.391 Chronic venous hypertension (idiopathic) with other complications of right lower extremity

I87.392 Chronic venous hypertension (idiopathic) with other complications of left lower extremity

I87.393 **Chronic venous hypertension (idiopathic) with other complications of bilateral lower extremity**

I87.399 **Chronic venous hypertension (idiopathic) with other complications of unspecified lower extremity**

I87.8 **Other specified disorders of veins**
Phlebosclerosis
Venofibrosis

I87.9 **Disorder of vein, unspecified**

I88 Nonspecific lymphadenitis

EXCLUDES 1 *acute lymphadenitis, except mesenteric (LØ4.-)*
enlarged lymph nodes NOS (R59.-)
human immunodeficiency virus [HIV] disease resulting in generalized lymphadenopathy (B2Ø)

I88.Ø **Nonspecific mesenteric lymphadenitis**
Mesenteric lymphadenitis (acute)(chronic)

I88.1 **Chronic lymphadenitis, except mesenteric**
Adenitis
Lymphadenitis

I88.8 **Other nonspecific lymphadenitis**

I88.9 **Nonspecific lymphadenitis, unspecified**
Lymphadenitis NOS

I89 Other noninfective disorders of lymphatic vessels and lymph nodes

EXCLUDES 1 *chylocele, tunica vaginalis (nonfilarial) NOS (N5Ø.89)*
enlarged lymph nodes NOS (R59.-)
filarial chylocele (B74.-)
hereditary lymphedema (Q82.Ø)

I89.Ø **Lymphedema, not elsewhere classified**
Elephantiasis (nonfilarial) NOS
Lymphangiectasis
Obliteration, lymphatic vessel
Praecox lymphedema
Secondary lymphedema

EXCLUDES 1 *postmastectomy lymphedema (I97.2)*

I89.1 **Lymphangitis**
Chronic lymphangitis
Lymphangitis NOS
Subacute lymphangitis

EXCLUDES 1 *acute lymphangitis (LØ3.-)*

I89.8 **Other specified noninfective disorders of lymphatic vessels and lymph nodes**
Chylocele (nonfilarial)
Chylous ascites
Chylous cyst
Lipomelanotic reticulosis
Lymph node or vessel fistula
Lymph node or vessel infarction
Lymph node or vessel rupture

I89.9 **Noninfective disorder of lymphatic vessels and lymph nodes, unspecified**
Disease of lymphatic vessels NOS

Other and unspecified disorders of the circulatory system (I95-I99)

I95 Hypotension

EXCLUDES 1 *cardiovascular collapse (R57.9) (~R57.9)*
maternal hypotension syndrome (O26.5-)
nonspecific low blood pressure reading NOS (RØ3.1)

I95.Ø **Idiopathic hypotension**

I95.1 **Orthostatic hypotension**
Hypotension, postural

EXCLUDES 1 *neurogenic orthostatic hypotension [Shy-Drager] (G9Ø.3)*
orthostatic hypotension due to drugs (I95.2)

I95.2 **Hypotension due to drugs**
Orthostatic hypotension due to drugs
Use additional code for adverse effect, if applicable, to identify drug (T36-T5Ø with fifth or sixth character 5)

I95.3 **Hypotension of hemodialysis**
Intra-dialytic hypotension

I95.8 **Other hypotension**

I95.81 **Postprocedural hypotension**

I95.89 **Other hypotension**
Chronic hypotension

I95.9 **Hypotension, unspecified**

I96 Gangrene, not elsewhere classified HCC ESR COM
Gangrenous cellulitis

EXCLUDES 1 *gangrene in atherosclerosis of native arteries of the extremities (I7Ø.26)*
gangrene in hernia (K4Ø.1, K4Ø.4, K41.1, K41.4, K42.1, K43.1-, K44.1, K45.1, K46.1)
gangrene in other peripheral vascular diseases (I73.-)
gangrene of certain specified sites - see Alphabetical Index
gas gangrene (A48.Ø)
pyoderma gangrenosum (L88)

EXCLUDES 2 *gangrene in diabetes mellitus (EØ8-E13 with .52)*

AHA: 2018,4Q,87; 2018,3Q,3; 2017,3Q,6; 2013,2Q,34

I97 Intraoperative and postprocedural complications and disorders of circulatory system, not elsewhere classified

EXCLUDES 2 *postprocedural shock (T81.1-)*

AHA: 2021,1Q,13; 2019,2Q,21

I97.Ø **Postcardiotomy syndrome**

I97.1 **Other postprocedural cardiac functional disturbances**

EXCLUDES 2 *acute pulmonary insufficiency following thoracic surgery (J95.1)*
intraoperative cardiac functional disturbances (I97.7-)

I97.11 **Postprocedural cardiac insufficiency**

I97.11Ø **Postprocedural cardiac insufficiency following cardiac surgery**

I97.111 **Postprocedural cardiac insufficiency following other surgery**

I97.12 **Postprocedural cardiac arrest**

I97.12Ø **Postprocedural cardiac arrest following cardiac surgery**

I97.121 **Postprocedural cardiac arrest following other surgery**

I97.13 **Postprocedural heart failure**
Use additional code to identify the heart failure (I5Ø.-)

I97.13Ø **Postprocedural heart failure following cardiac surgery**

I97.131 **Postprocedural heart failure following other surgery**

I97.19 **Other postprocedural cardiac functional disturbances**
Use additional code, if applicable, to further specify disorder

I97.19Ø **Other postprocedural cardiac functional disturbances following cardiac surgery**
Use additional code, if applicable, for type 4 or type 5 myocardial infarction, to further specify disorder
AHA: 2019,2Q,33

I97.191 **Other postprocedural cardiac functional disturbances following other surgery**

I97.2 **Postmastectomy lymphedema syndrome** A
Elephantiasis due to mastectomy
Obliteration of lymphatic vessels

I97.3 **Postprocedural hypertension**

I97.4 **Intraoperative hemorrhage and hematoma of a circulatory system organ or structure complicating a procedure**

EXCLUDES 1 *intraoperative hemorrhage and hematoma of a circulatory system organ or structure due to accidental puncture and laceration during a procedure (I97.5-)*

EXCLUDES 2 *intraoperative cerebrovascular hemorrhage complicating a procedure (G97.3-)*

I97.41 **Intraoperative hemorrhage and hematoma of a circulatory system organ or structure complicating a circulatory system procedure**

I97.41Ø **Intraoperative hemorrhage and hematoma of a circulatory system organ or structure complicating a cardiac catheterization**

I97.411 **Intraoperative hemorrhage and hematoma of a circulatory system organ or structure complicating a cardiac bypass**

I97.418 Intraoperative hemorrhage and hematoma of a circulatory system organ or structure complicating other circulatory system procedure

I97.42 Intraoperative hemorrhage and hematoma of a circulatory system organ or structure complicating other procedure
AHA: 2020,1Q,19

✓5th I97.5 Accidental puncture and laceration of a circulatory system organ or structure during a procedure
EXCLUDES 2 *accidental puncture and laceration of brain during a procedure (G97.4-)*

I97.51 Accidental puncture and laceration of a circulatory system organ or structure during a circulatory system procedure
AHA: 2019,2Q,24

I97.52 Accidental puncture and laceration of a circulatory system organ or structure during other procedure

✓5th I97.6 Postprocedural hemorrhage, hematoma and seroma of a circulatory system organ or structure following a procedure
EXCLUDES 2 *postprocedural cerebrovascular hemorrhage complicating a procedure (G97.5-)*
AHA: 2016,4Q,9-10

✓6th I97.61 Postprocedural hemorrhage of a circulatory system organ or structure following a circulatory system procedure

I97.610 Postprocedural hemorrhage of a circulatory system organ or structure following a cardiac catheterization

I97.611 Postprocedural hemorrhage of a circulatory system organ or structure following cardiac bypass

I97.618 Postprocedural hemorrhage of a circulatory system organ or structure following other circulatory system procedure

✓6th I97.62 Postprocedural hemorrhage, hematoma and seroma of a circulatory system organ or structure following other procedure

I97.620 Postprocedural hemorrhage of a circulatory system organ or structure following other procedure

I97.621 Postprocedural hematoma of a circulatory system organ or structure following other procedure

I97.622 Postprocedural seroma of a circulatory system organ or structure following other procedure

✓6th I97.63 Postprocedural hematoma of a circulatory system organ or structure following a circulatory system procedure

I97.630 Postprocedural hematoma of a circulatory system organ or structure following a cardiac catheterization

I97.631 Postprocedural hematoma of a circulatory system organ or structure following cardiac bypass

I97.638 Postprocedural hematoma of a circulatory system organ or structure following other circulatory system procedure

✓6th I97.64 Postprocedural seroma of a circulatory system organ or structure following a circulatory system procedure

I97.640 Postprocedural seroma of a circulatory system organ or structure following a cardiac catheterization

I97.641 Postprocedural seroma of a circulatory system organ or structure following cardiac bypass

I97.648 Postprocedural seroma of a circulatory system organ or structure following other circulatory system procedure

✓5th I97.7 Intraoperative cardiac functional disturbances
EXCLUDES 2 *acute pulmonary insufficiency following thoracic surgery (J95.1)*
postprocedural cardiac functional disturbances (I97.1-)

✓6th I97.71 Intraoperative cardiac arrest

I97.710 Intraoperative cardiac arrest during cardiac surgery

I97.711 Intraoperative cardiac arrest during other surgery

✓6th I97.79 Other intraoperative cardiac functional disturbances
Use additional code, if applicable, to further specify disorder

I97.790 Other intraoperative cardiac functional disturbances during cardiac surgery

I97.791 Other intraoperative cardiac functional disturbances during other surgery

✓5th I97.8 Other intraoperative and postprocedural complications and disorders of the circulatory system, not elsewhere classified
Use additional code, if applicable, to further specify disorder

✓6th I97.81 Intraoperative cerebrovascular infarction

I97.810 Intraoperative cerebrovascular infarction during cardiac surgery HCC ESR

I97.811 Intraoperative cerebrovascular infarction during other surgery HCC ESR

✓6th I97.82 Postprocedural cerebrovascular infarction

I97.820 Postprocedural cerebrovascular infarction following cardiac surgery HCC ESR

I97.821 Postprocedural cerebrovascular infarction following other surgery HCC ESR

I97.88 Other intraoperative complications of the circulatory system, not elsewhere classified

I97.89 Other postprocedural complications and disorders of the circulatory system, not elsewhere classified
AHA: 2021,3Q,33; 2020,3Q,3-8; 2019,2Q,33

✓4th I99 Other and unspecified disorders of circulatory system

I99.8 Other disorder of circulatory system
AHA: 2020,4Q,98

I99.9 Unspecified disorder of circulatory system

Chapter 10. Diseases of the Respiratory System (JØØ–J99)

Chapter-specific Guidelines with Coding Examples

The chapter-specific guidelines from the ICD-10-CM Official Guidelines for Coding and Reporting have been provided below. Along with these guidelines are coding examples, contained in the shaded boxes, that have been developed to help illustrate the coding and/or sequencing guidance found in these guidelines.

a. Chronic obstructive pulmonary disease [COPD] and asthma

1) Acute exacerbation of chronic obstructive bronchitis and asthma

The codes in categories J44 and J45 distinguish between uncomplicated cases and those in acute exacerbation. An acute exacerbation is a worsening or a decompensation of a chronic condition. An acute exacerbation is not equivalent to an infection superimposed on a chronic condition, though an exacerbation may be triggered by an infection.

Acute streptococcal bronchitis with acute exacerbation of COPD

J2Ø.2 **Acute bronchitis due to streptococcus**

J44.Ø **Chronic obstructive pulmonary disease with (acute) lower respiratory infection**

J44.1 **Chronic obstructive pulmonary disease with (acute) exacerbation**

Explanation: ICD-10-CM uses combination codes to create organism-specific classifications for acute bronchitis. Category J44 codes include combination codes with severity components, which differentiate between COPD with acute lower respiratory infection (acute bronchitis), COPD with acute exacerbation, and COPD without mention of a complication (unspecified).

An acute exacerbation is a worsening or a decompensation of a chronic condition. An acute exacerbation is not equivalent to an infection superimposed on a chronic condition, though an exacerbation may be triggered by an infection, as in this example.

Exacerbation of moderate persistent asthma with status asthmaticus

J45.42 **Moderate persistent asthma with status asthmaticus**

Explanation: Category J45 Asthma includes severity-specific subcategories and fifth-character codes to distinguish between uncomplicated cases, those in acute exacerbation, and those with status asthmaticus.

b. Acute respiratory failure

1) Acute respiratory failure as principal diagnosis

A code from subcategory J96.Ø, Acute respiratory failure, or subcategory J96.2, Acute and chronic respiratory failure, may be assigned as a principal diagnosis when it is the condition established after study to be chiefly responsible for occasioning the admission to the hospital, and the selection is supported by the Alphabetic Index and Tabular List. However, chapter-specific coding guidelines (such as obstetrics, poisoning, HIV, newborn) that provide sequencing direction take precedence.

Acute hypoxic respiratory failure due to exacerbation of chronic obstructive bronchitis

J96.Ø1 **Acute respiratory failure with hypoxia**

J44.1 **Chronic obstructive pulmonary disease with (acute) exacerbation**

Explanation: Category J96 classifies respiratory failure with combination codes that designate the severity and the presence of hypoxia and hypercapnia. Code J96.Ø1 is sequenced as the first-listed diagnosis, as the reason for the encounter. Respiratory failure may be assigned as a principal diagnosis when it is the condition established after study to be chiefly responsible for occasioning the encounter and the selection is supported by the Alphabetic Index and Tabular List.

2) Acute respiratory failure as secondary diagnosis

Respiratory failure may be listed as a secondary diagnosis if it occurs after admission, or if it is present on admission, but does not meet the definition of principal diagnosis.

Acute respiratory failure due to accidental oxycodone overdose

T4Ø.2X1A **Poisoning by other opioids, accidental (unintentional), initial encounter**

J96.ØØ **Acute respiratory failure, unspecified whether with hypoxia or hypercapnia**

Explanation: Respiratory failure may be assigned as a principal diagnosis when it is the condition established after study to be chiefly responsible for occasioning the encounter, and the selection is supported by the Alphabetic Index and Tabular List. However, chapter-specific coding guidelines, such as poisoning, that provide sequencing direction take precedence. When coding a poisoning or reaction to the improper use of a medication (e.g., overdose, wrong substance given or taken in error, wrong route of administration), first assign the appropriate code from categories T36–T5Ø. Use additional code(s) for all manifestations of the poisoning. In this instance, the respiratory failure is a manifestation of the poisoning and is sequenced as a secondary diagnosis.

3) Sequencing of acute respiratory failure and another acute condition

When a patient is admitted with respiratory failure and another acute condition, (e.g., myocardial infarction, cerebrovascular accident, aspiration pneumonia), the principal diagnosis will not be the same in every situation. This applies whether the other acute condition is a respiratory or nonrespiratory condition. Selection of the principal diagnosis will be dependent on the circumstances of admission. If both the respiratory failure and the other acute condition are equally responsible for occasioning the admission to the hospital, and there are no chapter-specific sequencing rules, the guideline regarding two or more diagnoses that equally meet the definition for principal diagnosis (*Section II, C.*) may be applied in these situations.

If the documentation is not clear as to whether acute respiratory failure and another condition are equally responsible for occasioning the admission, query the provider for clarification.

Patient presents with acute pneumococcal pneumonia and acute respiratory failure

J96.ØØ **Acute respiratory failure, unspecified whether with hypoxia or hypercapnia**

J13 **Pneumonia due to Streptococcus pneumoniae**

Explanation: When a patient is seen for respiratory failure and another acute condition, such as a bacterial pneumonia, the principal or first-listed diagnosis is not the same in every situation. This applies whether the other acute condition is a respiratory or nonrespiratory condition. The principal diagnosis depends on the problem chiefly responsible for the encounter.

c. Influenza due to certain identified influenza viruses

Code only confirmed cases of influenza due to certain identified influenza viruses (category JØ9), and due to other identified influenza virus (category J1Ø). This is an exception to the hospital inpatient guideline Section II, H. (Uncertain Diagnosis).

In this context, "confirmation" does not require documentation of positive laboratory testing specific for avian or other novel influenza A or other identified influenza virus. However, coding should be based on the provider's diagnostic statement that the patient has avian influenza, or other novel influenza A, for category JØ9, or has another particular identified strain of influenza, such as H1N1 or H3N2, but not identified as novel or variant, for category J1Ø.

If the provider records "suspected" or "possible" or "probable" avian influenza, or novel influenza, or other identified influenza, then the appropriate influenza code from category J11, Influenza due to unidentified influenza virus, should be assigned. A code from category JØ9, Influenza due to certain identified influenza viruses, should not be assigned nor should a code from category J1Ø, Influenza due to other identified influenza virus.

Influenza due to avian influenza virus with pneumonia

J09.X1 Influenza due to identified novel influenza A virus with pneumonia

Explanation: Codes in category J09 Influenza due to certain identified influenza viruses should be assigned only for confirmed cases. "Confirmation" does not require positive laboratory testing of a specific influenza virus but does need to be based on the provider's diagnostic statement, which should not include terms such as "possible," "probable," or "suspected."

d. Ventilator associated pneumonia

1) Documentation of ventilator associated pneumonia

As with all procedural or postprocedural complications, code assignment is based on the provider's documentation of the relationship between the condition and the procedure.

Code J95.851, Ventilator associated pneumonia, should be assigned only when the provider has documented ventilator associated pneumonia (VAP). An additional code to identify the organism (e.g., Pseudomonas aeruginosa, code B96.5) should also be assigned. Do not assign an additional code from categories J12-J18 to identify the type of pneumonia.

Code J95.851 should not be assigned for cases where the patient has pneumonia and is on a mechanical ventilator and the provider has not specifically stated that the pneumonia is ventilator-associated pneumonia. If the documentation is unclear as to whether the patient has a pneumonia that is a complication attributable to the mechanical ventilator, query the provider.

2) Ventilator associated pneumonia develops after admission

A patient may be admitted with one type of pneumonia (e.g., code J13, Pneumonia due to Streptococcus pneumonia) and subsequently develop VAP. In this instance, the principal diagnosis would be the appropriate code from categories J12-J18 for the pneumonia diagnosed at the time of admission. Code J95.851, Ventilator associated pneumonia, would be assigned as an additional diagnosis when the provider has also documented the presence of ventilator associated pneumonia.

e. Vaping-related disorders

For patients presenting with condition(s) related to vaping, assign code U07.0, Vaping-related disorder, as the principal diagnosis. For lung injury due to vaping, assign only code U07.0. Assign additional codes for other manifestations, such as acute respiratory failure (subcategory J96.0-) or pneumonitis (code J68.0).

Associated respiratory signs and symptoms due to vaping, such as cough, shortness of breath, etc., are not coded separately, when a definitive diagnosis has been established. However, it would be appropriate to code separately any gastrointestinal symptoms, such as diarrhea and abdominal pain.

See Section I.C.1.g.1.c.i. for Pneumonia confirmed as due to COVID-19

Chapter 10. Diseases of the Respiratory System (J00-J99)

NOTE When a respiratory condition is described as occurring in more than one site and is not specifically indexed, it should be classified to the lower anatomic site (e.g., tracheobronchitis to bronchitis in J40).

Use additional code, where applicable, to identify:
- exposure to environmental tobacco smoke (Z77.22)
- exposure to tobacco smoke in the perinatal period (P96.81)
- history of tobacco dependence (Z87.891)
- occupational exposure to environmental tobacco smoke (Z57.31)
- tobacco dependence (F17.-)
- tobacco use (Z72.0)

EXCLUDES 2
certain conditions originating in the perinatal period (P04-P96)
certain infectious and parasitic diseases (A00-B99)
complications of pregnancy, childbirth and the puerperium (O00-O9A)
congenital malformations, deformations and chromosomal abnormalities (Q00-Q99)
endocrine, nutritional and metabolic diseases (E00-E88)
injury, poisoning and certain other consequences of external causes (S00-T88)
neoplasms (C00-D49)
smoke inhalation (T59.81-)
symptoms, signs and abnormal clinical and laboratory findings, not elsewhere classified (R00-R94)

This chapter contains the following blocks:

J00-J06	Acute upper respiratory infections
J09-J18	Influenza and pneumonia
J20-J22	Other acute lower respiratory infections
J30-J39	Other diseases of upper respiratory tract
J40-J47	Chronic lower respiratory diseases
J60-J70	Lung diseases due to external agents
J80-J84	Other respiratory diseases principally affecting the interstitium
J85-J86	Suppurative and necrotic conditions of the lower respiratory tract
J90-J94	Other diseases of the pleura
J95	Intraoperative and postprocedural complications and disorders of respiratory system, not elsewhere classified
J96-J99	Other diseases of the respiratory system

Acute upper respiratory infections (J00-J06)

EXCLUDES 1 *chronic obstructive pulmonary disease with acute lower respiratory infection (J44.0)*

J00 Acute nasopharyngitis [common cold]

Acute rhinitis
Coryza (acute)
Infective nasopharyngitis NOS
Infective rhinitis
Nasal catarrh, acute
Nasopharyngitis NOS

EXCLUDES 1
acute pharyngitis (J02.-)
acute sore throat NOS (J02.9)
influenza virus with other respiratory manifestations (J09.X2, J10.1, J11.1)
pharyngitis NOS (J02.9)
rhinitis NOS (J31.0)
sore throat NOS (J02.9)

EXCLUDES 2
allergic rhinitis (J30.1-J30.9)
chronic pharyngitis (J31.2)
chronic rhinitis (J31.0)
chronic sore throat (J31.2)
nasopharyngitis, chronic (J31.1)
vasomotor rhinitis (J30.0)

✓4th J01 Acute sinusitis

INCLUDES
acute abscess of sinus
acute empyema of sinus
acute infection of sinus
acute inflammation of sinus
acute suppuration of sinus

Use additional code (B95-B97) to identify infectious agent

EXCLUDES 1 *sinusitis NOS (J32.9)*

EXCLUDES 2 *chronic sinusitis (J32.0-J32.8)*

✓5th **J01.0 Acute maxillary sinusitis**
Acute antritis

J01.00 Acute maxillary sinusitis, unspecified
J01.01 Acute recurrent maxillary sinusitis

✓5th **J01.1 Acute frontal sinusitis**

J01.10 Acute frontal sinusitis, unspecified
J01.11 Acute recurrent frontal sinusitis

✓5th **J01.2 Acute ethmoidal sinusitis**

J01.20 Acute ethmoidal sinusitis, unspecified
J01.21 Acute recurrent ethmoidal sinusitis

✓5th **J01.3 Acute sphenoidal sinusitis**

J01.30 Acute sphenoidal sinusitis, unspecified
J01.31 Acute recurrent sphenoidal sinusitis

✓5th **J01.4 Acute pansinusitis**

J01.40 Acute pansinusitis, unspecified
J01.41 Acute recurrent pansinusitis

✓5th **J01.8 Other acute sinusitis**

J01.80 Other acute sinusitis
Acute sinusitis involving more than one sinus but not pansinusitis

J01.81 Other acute recurrent sinusitis
Acute recurrent sinusitis involving more than one sinus but not pansinusitis

✓5th **J01.9 Acute sinusitis, unspecified**

J01.90 Acute sinusitis, unspecified
J01.91 Acute recurrent sinusitis, unspecified

✓4th J02 Acute pharyngitis

INCLUDES acute sore throat

EXCLUDES 1
acute laryngopharyngitis (J06.0)
peritonsillar abscess (J36)
pharyngeal abscess (J39.1)
retropharyngeal abscess (J39.0)

EXCLUDES 2 *chronic pharyngitis (J31.2)*

J02.0 Streptococcal pharyngitis
Septic pharyngitis
Streptococcal sore throat

EXCLUDES 2 *scarlet fever (A38.-)*

J02.8 Acute pharyngitis due to other specified organisms
Use additional code (B95-B97) to identify infectious agent

EXCLUDES 1
acute pharyngitis due to coxsackie virus (B08.5)
acute pharyngitis due to gonococcus (A54.5)
acute pharyngitis due to herpes [simplex] virus (B00.2)
acute pharyngitis due to infectious mononucleosis (B27.-)
enteroviral vesicular pharyngitis (B08.5)

J02.9 Acute pharyngitis, unspecified
Gangrenous pharyngitis (acute)
Infective pharyngitis (acute) NOS
Pharyngitis (acute) NOS
Sore throat (acute) NOS
Suppurative pharyngitis (acute)
Ulcerative pharyngitis (acute)

EXCLUDES 1 *influenza virus with other respiratory manifestations (J09.X2, J10.1, J11.1)*

✓4th J03 Acute tonsillitis

EXCLUDES 1
acute sore throat (J02.-)
hypertrophy of tonsils (J35.1)
peritonsillar abscess (J36)
sore throat NOS (J02.9)
streptococcal sore throat (J02.0)

EXCLUDES 2 *chronic tonsillitis (J35.0)*

✓5th **J03.0 Streptococcal tonsillitis**

J03.00 Acute streptococcal tonsillitis, unspecified
J03.01 Acute recurrent streptococcal tonsillitis

✓5th **J03.8 Acute tonsillitis due to other specified organisms**
Use additional code (B95-B97) to identify infectious agent

EXCLUDES 1
diphtheritic tonsillitis (A36.0)
herpesviral pharyngotonsillitis (B00.2)
streptococcal tonsillitis (J03.0)
tuberculous tonsillitis (A15.8)
Vincent's tonsillitis (A69.1)

J03.80 Acute tonsillitis due to other specified organisms
J03.81 Acute recurrent tonsillitis due to other specified organisms

5th **J03.9 Acute tonsillitis, unspecified**
Follicular tonsillitis (acute)
Gangrenous tonsillitis (acute)
Infective tonsillitis (acute)
Tonsillitis (acute) NOS
Ulcerative tonsillitis (acute)
EXCLUDES 1 *influenza virus with other respiratory manifestations (J09.X2, J10.1, J11.1)*

J03.90 Acute tonsillitis, unspecified
J03.91 Acute recurrent tonsillitis, unspecified

4th **J04 Acute laryngitis and tracheitis**
Code also influenza, if present, such as:
influenza due to identified novel influenza A virus with other respiratory manifestations (J09.X2)
influenza due to other identified influenza virus with other respiratory manifestations (J10.1)
influenza due to unidentified influenza virus with other respiratory manifestations (J11.1)
Use additional code (B95-B97) to identify infectious agent
EXCLUDES 1 *acute obstructive laryngitis [croup] and epiglottitis (J05.-)*
EXCLUDES 2 *laryngismus (stridulus) (J38.5)*

J04.0 Acute laryngitis
Edematous laryngitis (acute)
Laryngitis (acute) NOS
Subglottic laryngitis (acute)
Suppurative laryngitis (acute)
Ulcerative laryngitis (acute)
EXCLUDES 1 *acute obstructive laryngitis (J05.0)*
EXCLUDES 2 *chronic laryngitis (J37.0)*

5th **J04.1 Acute tracheitis**
Acute viral tracheitis
Catarrhal tracheitis (acute)
Tracheitis (acute) NOS
EXCLUDES 2 *chronic tracheitis (J42)*

J04.10 Acute tracheitis without obstruction
J04.11 Acute tracheitis with obstruction

J04.2 Acute laryngotracheitis
Laryngotracheitis NOS
Tracheitis (acute) with laryngitis (acute)
EXCLUDES 1 *acute obstructive laryngotracheitis (J05.0)*
EXCLUDES 2 *chronic laryngotracheitis (J37.1)*

5th **J04.3 Supraglottitis, unspecified**
J04.30 Supraglottitis, unspecified, without obstruction
J04.31 Supraglottitis, unspecified, with obstruction

4th **J05 Acute obstructive laryngitis [croup] and epiglottitis**
Code also, influenza, if present, such as:
influenza due to identified novel influenza A virus with other respiratory manifestations (J09.X2)
influenza due to other identified influenza virus with other respiratory manifestations (J10.1)
influenza due to unidentified influenza virus with other respiratory manifestations (J11.1)
Use additional code (B95-B97) to identify infectious agent

J05.0 Acute obstructive laryngitis [croup]
Obstructive laryngitis (acute) NOS
Obstructive laryngotracheitis NOS
DEF: Acute laryngeal obstruction due to allergies, foreign bodies, or in the majority of cases a viral infection. Symptoms include a harsh, barking cough, hoarseness, and a persistent, high-pitched respiratory sound (stridor).

5th **J05.1 Acute epiglottitis**
EXCLUDES 2 *epiglottitis, chronic (J37.0)*
J05.10 Acute epiglottitis without obstruction
Epiglottitis NOS
J05.11 Acute epiglottitis with obstruction

4th **J06 Acute upper respiratory infections of multiple and unspecified sites**
EXCLUDES 1 *acute respiratory infection NOS (J22)*
influenza virus with other respiratory manifestations (J09.X2, J10.1, J11.1)
streptococcal pharyngitis (J02.0)

J06.0 Acute laryngopharyngitis

J06.9 Acute upper respiratory infection, unspecified
Upper respiratory disease, acute
Upper respiratory infection NOS
Use additional code (B95-B97) to identify infectious agent, if known, such as:
respiratory syncytial virus (RSV) (B97.4)
AHA: 2020,1Q,22

Influenza and pneumonia (J09-J18)

EXCLUDES 2 *allergic or eosinophilic pneumonia (J82)*
aspiration pneumonia NOS (J69.0)
meconium pneumonia (P24.01)
neonatal aspiration pneumonia (P24.-)
pneumonia due to solids and liquids (J69.-)
congenital pneumonia (P23.9)
lipid pneumonia (J69.1)
rheumatic pneumonia (I00)
ventilator associated pneumonia (J95.851)

AHA: 2017,4Q,96
TIP: Hemoptysis (R04.2) is not customarily associated with pneumonia and may be reported separately.

4th **J09 Influenza due to certain identified influenza viruses**
EXCLUDES 1 *influenza A/H1N1 (J10.-)*
influenza due to other identified influenza virus (J10.-)
influenza due to unidentified influenza virus (J11.-)
seasonal influenza due to other identified influenza virus (J10.-)
seasonal influenza due to unidentified influenza virus (J11.-)

5th **J09.X Influenza due to identified novel influenza A virus**
Avian influenza
Bird influenza
Influenza A/H5N1
Influenza of other animal origin, not bird or swine
Swine influenza virus (viruses that normally cause infections in pigs)
AHA: 2016,3Q,10

J09.X1 Influenza due to identified novel influenza A virus with pneumonia
Code also, if applicable, associated:
lung abscess (J85.1)
other specified type of pneumonia

J09.X2 Influenza due to identified novel influenza A virus with other respiratory manifestations
Influenza due to identified novel influenza A virus NOS
Influenza due to identified novel influenza A virus with laryngitis
Influenza due to identified novel influenza A virus with pharyngitis
Influenza due to identified novel influenza A virus with upper respiratory symptoms
Use additional code, if applicable, for associated:
pleural effusion (J91.8)
sinusitis (J01.-)

J09.X3 Influenza due to identified novel influenza A virus with gastrointestinal manifestations
Influenza due to identified novel influenza A virus gastroenteritis
EXCLUDES 1 *'intestinal flu' [viral gastroenteritis] (A08.-)*

J09.X9 Influenza due to identified novel influenza A virus with other manifestations
Influenza due to identified novel influenza A virus with encephalopathy
Influenza due to identified novel influenza A virus with myocarditis
Influenza due to identified novel influenza A virus with otitis media
Use additional code to identify manifestation

J10 Influenza due to other identified influenza virus

INCLUDES influenza A (non-novel)
influenza B
influenza C

EXCLUDES 1 *influenza due to avian influenza virus (J09.X-)*
influenza due to swine flu (J09.X-)
influenza due to unidentifed influenza virus (J11.-)

J10.0 Influenza due to other identified influenza virus with pneumonia
Code also associated lung abscess, if applicable (J85.1)

J10.00 Influenza due to other identified influenza virus with unspecified type of pneumonia

J10.01 Influenza due to other identified influenza virus with the same other identified influenza virus pneumonia

J10.08 Influenza due to other identified influenza virus with other specified pneumonia
Code also other specified type of pneumonia

J10.1 Influenza due to other identified influenza virus with other respiratory manifestations
Influenza due to other identified influenza virus NOS
Influenza due to other identified influenza virus with laryngitis
Influenza due to other identified influenza virus with pharyngitis
Influenza due to other identified influenza virus with upper respiratory symptoms
Use additional code for associated pleural effusion, if applicable (J91.8)
Use additional code for associated sinusitis, if applicable (J01.-)
AHA: 2016,3Q,10-11

J10.2 Influenza due to other identified influenza virus with gastrointestinal manifestations
Influenza due to other identified influenza virus gastroenteritis
EXCLUDES 1 *"intestinal flu" [viral gastroenteritis] (A08.-)*

J10.8 Influenza due to other identified influenza virus with other manifestations

J10.81 Influenza due to other identified influenza virus with encephalopathy

J10.82 Influenza due to other identified influenza virus with myocarditis

J10.83 Influenza due to other identified influenza virus with otitis media
Use additional code for any associated perforated tympanic membrane (H72.-)

J10.89 Influenza due to other identified influenza virus with other manifestations
Use additional codes to identify the manifestations

J11 Influenza due to unidentified influenza virus

J11.0 Influenza due to unidentified influenza virus with pneumonia
Code also associated lung abscess, if applicable (J85.1)
AHA: 2016,3Q,11

J11.00 Influenza due to unidentified influenza virus with unspecified type of pneumonia
Influenza with pneumonia NOS

J11.08 Influenza due to unidentified influenza virus with specified pneumonia
Code also other specified type of pneumonia

J11.1 Influenza due to unidentified influenza virus with other respiratory manifestations
Influenza NOS
Influenzal laryngitis NOS
Influenzal pharyngitis NOS
Influenza with upper respiratory symptoms NOS
Use additional code for associated pleural effusion, if applicable (J91.8)
Use additional code for associated sinusitis, if applicable (J01.-)

J11.2 Influenza due to unidentified influenza virus with gastrointestinal manifestations
Influenza gastroenteritis NOS
EXCLUDES 1 *"intestinal flu" [viral gastroenteritis] (A08.-)*

J11.8 Influenza due to unidentified influenza virus with other manifestations

J11.81 Influenza due to unidentified influenza virus with encephalopathy
Influenzal encephalopathy NOS

J11.82 Influenza due to unidentified influenza virus with myocarditis
Influenzal myocarditis NOS

J11.83 Influenza due to unidentified influenza virus with otitis media
Influenzal otitis media NOS
Use additional code for any associated perforated tympanic membrane (H72.-)

J11.89 Influenza due to unidentified influenza virus with other manifestations
Use additional codes to identify the manifestations

J12 Viral pneumonia, not elsewhere classified

INCLUDES bronchopneumonia due to viruses other than influenza viruses
Code first associated influenza, if applicable (J09.X1, J10.0-, J11.0-)
Code also associated abscess, if applicable (J85.1)

EXCLUDES 1 *aspiration pneumonia due to anesthesia during labor and delivery (O74.0)*
aspiration pneumonia due to anesthesia during pregnancy (O29)
aspiration pneumonia due to anesthesia during puerperium (O89.0)
aspiration pneumonia due to solids and liquids (J69.-)
aspiration pneumonia NOS (J69.0)
congenital pneumonia (P23.0)
congenital rubella pneumonitis (P35.0)
interstitial pneumonia NOS (J84.9)
lipid pneumonia (J69.1)
neonatal aspiration pneumonia (P24.-)

AHA: 2020,2Q,28; 2019,1Q,35; 2018,3Q,24; 2016,3Q,15; 2013,4Q,118

J12.0 Adenoviral pneumonia

J12.1 Respiratory syncytial virus pneumonia
RSV pneumonia

J12.2 Parainfluenza virus pneumonia

J12.3 Human metapneumovirus pneumonia

J12.8 Other viral pneumonia

J12.81 Pneumonia due to SARS-associated coronavirus
Severe acute respiratory syndrome NOS
DEF: Inflammation of the lungs with consolidation, caused by the severe adult respiratory syndrome (SARS)-associated coronavirus or SARS-CoV. This pneumonia should not be confused with that caused by SARS-CoV-2 (COVID-19).

J12.82 Pneumonia due to coronavirus disease 2019 UPD
Pneumonia due to 2019 novel coronavirus (SARS-CoV-2)
Pneumonia due to COVID-19
Code first COVID-19 (U07.1)
AHA: 2021,1Q,25-30,31-49

J12.89 Other viral pneumonia
AHA: 2021,1Q,33-34; 2020,2Q,8,11; 2020,1Q,34-36

J12.9 Viral pneumonia, unspecified

J13 Pneumonia due to Streptococcus pneumoniae HCC ESR
Bronchopneumonia due to S. pneumoniae
Code first associated influenza, if applicable (J09.X1, J10.0-, J11.0-)
Code also associated abscess, if applicable (J85.1)

EXCLUDES 1 *congenital pneumonia due to S. pneumoniae (P23.6)*
lobar pneumonia, unspecified organism (J18.1)
pneumonia due to other streptococci (J15.3-J15.4)

AHA: 2020,2Q,28; 2019,1Q,35; 2018,3Q,24; 2016,3Q,15; 2013,4Q,118

J14 Pneumonia due to Hemophilus influenzae HCC ESR
Bronchopneumonia due to H. influenzae
Code first associated influenza, if applicable (J09.X1, J10.0-, J11.0-)
Code also associated abscess, if applicable (J85.1)

EXCLUDES 1 *congenital pneumonia due to H. influenzae (P23.6)*

AHA: 2020,2Q,28; 2019,1Q,35; 2018,3Q,24; 2016,3Q,15; 2013,4Q,118

J15 Bacterial pneumonia, not elsewhere classified

INCLUDES Bronchopneumonia due to bacteria other than S. pneumoniae and H. influenzae
Code first associated influenza, if applicable (J09.X1, J10.0-, -J11.0-)
Code also associated abscess, if applicable (J85.1)

EXCLUDES 1 *chlamydial pneumonia (J16.0)*
congenital pneumonia (P23.-)
Legionnaires' disease (A48.1)
spirochetal pneumonia (A69.8)

AHA: 2020,2Q,28; 2019,1Q,35; 2018,3Q,24; 2016,3Q,15; 2013,4Q,118

J15.0 Pneumonia due to Klebsiella pneumoniae HCC ESR COM

J15.1 Pneumonia due to Pseudomonas HCC ESR COM

√5th **J15.2 Pneumonia due to staphylococcus**

J15.20 Pneumonia due to staphylococcus, unspecified HCC ESR COM

√6th **J15.21 Pneumonia due to Staphylococcus aureus**

J15.211 Pneumonia due to methicillin susceptible Staphylococcus aureus HCC ESR COM
MSSA pneumonia
Pneumonia due to Staphylococcus aureus NOS

J15.212 Pneumonia due to methicillin resistant Staphylococcus aureus HCC ESR COM

J15.29 Pneumonia due to other staphylococcus HCC ESR COM

J15.3 Pneumonia due to streptococcus, group B HCC ESR

J15.4 Pneumonia due to other streptococci HCC ESR
EXCLUDES 1 *pneumonia due to streptococcus, group B (J15.3)*
pneumonia due to Streptococcus pneumoniae (J13)

J15.5 Pneumonia due to Escherichia coli HCC ESR COM

J15.6 Pneumonia due to other Gram-negative bacteria HCC ESR COM
Pneumonia due to other aerobic Gram-negative bacteria
Pneumonia due to Serratia marcescens
AHA: 2020,2Q,28

J15.7 Pneumonia due to Mycoplasma pneumoniae

J15.8 Pneumonia due to other specified bacteria HCC ESR COM

J15.9 Unspecified bacterial pneumonia
Pneumonia due to gram-positive bacteria

√4th **J16 Pneumonia due to other infectious organisms, not elsewhere classified**
Code first associated influenza, if applicable (J09.X1, J10.0-, J11.0-)
Code also associated abscess, if applicable (J85.1)
EXCLUDES 1 *congenital pneumonia (P23.-)*
ornithosis (A70)
pneumocystosis (B59)
pneumonia NOS (J18.9)
AHA: 2020,2Q,28; 2019,1Q,35; 2018,3Q,24; 2016,3Q,15; 2013,4Q,118

J16.0 Chlamydial pneumonia

J16.8 Pneumonia due to other specified infectious organisms

J17 Pneumonia in diseases classified elsewhere
Code first underlying disease, such as:
Q fever (A78)
rheumatic fever (I00)
schistosomiasis (B65.0-B65.9)
EXCLUDES 1 *candidial pneumonia (B37.1)*
chlamydial pneumonia (J16.0)
gonorrheal pneumonia (A54.84)
histoplasmosis pneumonia (B39.0-B39.2)
measles pneumonia (B05.2)
nocardiosis pneumonia (A43.0)
pneumocystosis (B59)
pneumonia due to Pneumocystis carinii (B59)
pneumonia due to Pneumocystis jiroveci (B59)
pneumonia in actinomycosis (A42.0)
pneumonia in anthrax (A22.1)
pneumonia in ascariasis (B77.81)
pneumonia in aspergillosis (B44.0-B44.1)
pneumonia in coccidioidomycosis (B38.0-B38.2)
pneumonia in cytomegalovirus disease (B25.0)
pneumonia in toxoplasmosis (B58.3)
rubella pneumonia (B06.81)
salmonella pneumonia (A02.22)
spirochetal infection NEC with pneumonia (A69.8)
tularemia pneumonia (A21.2)
typhoid fever with pneumonia (A01.03)
varicella pneumonia (B01.2)
whooping cough with pneumonia (A37 with fifth character 1)
AHA: 2020,2Q,28; 2019,1Q,35; 2016,3Q,15; 2013,4Q,118

√4th **J18 Pneumonia, unspecified organism**
Code first associated influenza, if applicable (J09.X1, J10.0-, J11.0-)
EXCLUDES 1 *abscess of lung with pneumonia (J85.1)*
aspiration pneumonia due to anesthesia during labor and delivery (O74.0)
aspiration pneumonia due to anesthesia during pregnancy (O29)
aspiration pneumonia due to anesthesia during puerperium (O89.0)
aspiration pneumonia due to solids and liquids (J69.-)
aspiration pneumonia NOS (J69.0)
congenital pneumonia (P23.0)
drug-induced interstitial lung disorder (J70.2-J70.4)
interstitial pneumonia NOS (J84.9)
lipid pneumonia (J69.1)
neonatal aspiration pneumonia (P24.-)
pneumonitis due to external agents (J67-J70)
pneumonitis due to fumes and vapors (J68.0)
usual interstitial pneumonia (J84.178)
AHA: 2020,2Q,28; 2019,1Q,35; 2016,3Q,15; 2013,4Q,118

J18.0 Bronchopneumonia, unspecified organism
EXCLUDES 1 *hypostatic bronchopneumonia (J18.2)*
lipid pneumonia (J69.1)
EXCLUDES 2 *acute bronchiolitis (J21.-)*
chronic bronchiolitis (J44.9)

J18.1 Lobar pneumonia, unspecified organism HCC ESR
AHA: 2019,3Q,37; 2018,3Q,24
DEF: Lobar pneumonia is characterized by consolidated inflammation confined or localized to only one or a few lobes of the lung. The consolidation affects primarily the alveolar air spaces, unlike bronchopneumonia, which arises from the bronchi or bronchioles and affects a wide area without any localization.
TIP: Documentation of right upper lobe, left upper lobe, right lower lobe, left lower lobe, or right middle lobe pneumonia alone is not synonymous with "lobar pneumonia," nor should a diagnosis of lobar pneumonia be assumed based on an imaging report that identifies pneumonia in a specific lobe. Assign J18.1 only when the provider specifically documents "lobar pneumonia" without specifying a causal organism.

J18.2 Hypostatic pneumonia, unspecified organism COM
Hypostatic bronchopneumonia
Passive pneumonia

J18.8 Other pneumonia, unspecified organism

J18.9 Pneumonia, unspecified organism
AHA: 2020,2Q,28; 2019,3Q,15; 2019,2Q,28; 2014,3Q,4; 2013,4Q,119; 2012,4Q,94

Other acute lower respiratory infections (J20-J22)

EXCLUDES 2 *chronic obstructive pulmonary disease with acute lower respiratory infection (J44.0)*

J20 Acute bronchitis

INCLUDES acute and subacute bronchitis (with) bronchospasm
acute and subacute bronchitis (with) tracheitis
acute and subacute bronchitis (with) tracheobronchitis, acute
acute and subacute fibrinous bronchitis
acute and subacute membranous bronchitis
acute and subacute purulent bronchitis
acute and subacute septic bronchitis

EXCLUDES 1 *bronchitis NOS (J40)*
tracheobronchitis NOS (J40)

EXCLUDES 2 *acute bronchitis with bronchiectasis (J47.0)*
acute bronchitis with chronic obstructive asthma (J44.0)
acute bronchitis with chronic obstructive pulmonary disease (J44.0)
allergic bronchitis NOS (J45.909-)
bronchitis due to chemicals, fumes and vapors (J68.0)
chronic bronchitis NOS (J42)
chronic mucopurulent bronchitis (J41.1)
chronic obstructive bronchitis (J44.-)
chronic obstructive tracheobronchitis (J44.-)
chronic simple bronchitis (J41.0)
chronic tracheobronchitis (J42)

AHA: 2019,1Q,35; 2016,3Q,10,16

DEF: Acute inflammation of the main branches of the bronchial tree due to infectious or irritant agents. Symptoms include cough with a varied production of sputum, fever, substernal soreness, and lung rales. Bronchitis usually lasts three to 10 days.

J20.0 Acute bronchitis due to Mycoplasma pneumoniae

J20.1 Acute bronchitis due to Hemophilus influenzae

J20.2 Acute bronchitis due to streptococcus

J20.3 Acute bronchitis due to coxsackievirus

J20.4 Acute bronchitis due to parainfluenza virus

J20.5 Acute bronchitis due to respiratory syncytial virus
Acute bronchitis due to RSV

J20.6 Acute bronchitis due to rhinovirus

J20.7 Acute bronchitis due to echovirus

J20.8 Acute bronchitis due to other specified organisms
AHA: 2020,1Q,34-36
TIP: Assign as a secondary code for a patient with acute bronchitis confirmed as due to COVID-19; assign U07.1 as the principal or first-listed code.

J20.9 Acute bronchitis, unspecified

J21 Acute bronchiolitis

INCLUDES acute bronchiolitis with bronchospasm

EXCLUDES 2 *respiratory bronchiolitis interstitial lung disease (J84.115)*

J21.0 Acute bronchiolitis due to respiratory syncytial virus
Acute bronchiolitis due to RSV

J21.1 Acute bronchiolitis due to human metapneumovirus

J21.8 Acute bronchiolitis due to other specified organisms

J21.9 Acute bronchiolitis, unspecified
Bronchiolitis (acute)
EXCLUDES 1 *chronic bronchiolitis (J44.-)*

J22 Unspecified acute lower respiratory infection
Acute (lower) respiratory (tract) infection NOS
EXCLUDES 1 *upper respiratory infection (acute) (J06.9)*
AHA: 2020,1Q,22,34-36
TIP: Assign as a secondary code for a patient with a respiratory infection specified as acute or lower that is documented as being associated with COVID-19; assign U07.1 as the principal or first-listed code. If the respiratory infection documentation does not specify acute or lower, assign J98.8.

Other diseases of upper respiratory tract (J30-J39)

J30 Vasomotor and allergic rhinitis

INCLUDES spasmodic rhinorrhea

EXCLUDES 1 *allergic rhinitis with asthma (bronchial) (J45.909)*
rhinitis NOS (J31.0)

J30.0 Vasomotor rhinitis
DEF: Noninfectious and nonallergic type of rhinitis for which the cause is often unknown. Symptoms often mimic those of allergic rhinitis with a diagnosis of vasomotor rhinitis typically made after ruling out allergens as the cause.

J30.1 Allergic rhinitis due to pollen
Allergy NOS due to pollen
Hay fever
Pollinosis

J30.2 Other seasonal allergic rhinitis

J30.5 Allergic rhinitis due to food

J30.8 Other allergic rhinitis

J30.81 Allergic rhinitis due to animal (cat) (dog) hair and dander

J30.89 Other allergic rhinitis
Perennial allergic rhinitis

J30.9 Allergic rhinitis, unspecified

J31 Chronic rhinitis, nasopharyngitis and pharyngitis

Use additional code to identify:
exposure to environmental tobacco smoke (Z77.22)
exposure to tobacco smoke in the perinatal period (P96.81)
history of tobacco dependence (Z87.891)
occupational exposure to environmental tobacco smoke (Z57.31)
tobacco dependence (F17.-)
tobacco use (Z72.0)

J31.0 Chronic rhinitis
Atrophic rhinitis (chronic)
Granulomatous rhinitis (chronic)
Hypertrophic rhinitis (chronic)
Obstructive rhinitis (chronic)
Ozena
Purulent rhinitis (chronic)
Rhinitis (chronic) NOS
Ulcerative rhinitis (chronic)
EXCLUDES 1 *allergic rhinitis (J30.1-J30.9)*
vasomotor rhinitis (J30.0)
DEF: Persistent inflammation of the mucous membranes of the nose, characterized by a postnasal drip.

J31.1 Chronic nasopharyngitis
EXCLUDES 2 *acute nasopharyngitis (J00)*
DEF: Persistent inflammation of the mucous membranes extending from the nares to the pharynx. It is characterized by constant irritation in the nasopharynx and postnasal drip.

J31.2 Chronic pharyngitis
Atrophic pharyngitis (chronic)
Chronic sore throat
Granular pharyngitis (chronic)
Hypertrophic pharyngitis (chronic)
EXCLUDES 2 *acute pharyngitis (J02.9)*

J32 Chronic sinusitis

INCLUDES sinus abscess
sinus empyema
sinus infection
sinus suppuration

Use additional code to identify:
exposure to environmental tobacco smoke (Z77.22)
exposure to tobacco smoke in the perinatal period (P96.81)
history of tobacco dependence (Z87.891)
infectious agent (B95-B97)
occupational exposure to environmental tobacco smoke (Z57.31)
tobacco dependence (F17.-)
tobacco use (Z72.0)

EXCLUDES 2 *acute sinusitis (J01.-)*

J32.0 Chronic maxillary sinusitis
Antritis (chronic)
Maxillary sinusitis NOS

J32.1 Chronic frontal sinusitis
Frontal sinusitis NOS

J32.2 Chronic ethmoidal sinusitis
Ethmoidal sinusitis NOS
EXCLUDES 1 *Woakes' ethmoiditis (J33.1)*

J32.3 Chronic sphenoidal sinusitis
Sphenoidal sinusitis NOS

J32.4 Chronic pansinusitis
Pansinusitis NOS

J32.8 Other chronic sinusitis
Sinusitis (chronic) involving more than one sinus but not pansinusitis

J32.9 Chronic sinusitis, unspecified
Sinusitis (chronic) NOS

✓4th **J33 Nasal polyp**
Use additional code to identify:
exposure to environmental tobacco smoke (Z77.22)
exposure to tobacco smoke in the perinatal period (P96.81)
history of tobacco dependence (Z87.891)
occupational exposure to environmental tobacco smoke (Z57.31)
tobacco dependence (F17.-)
tobacco use (Z72.Ø)
EXCLUDES 1 *adenomatous polyps (D14.Ø)*

J33.Ø Polyp of nasal cavity
Choanal polyp
Nasopharyngeal polyp

J33.1 Polypoid sinus degeneration
Woakes' syndrome or ethmoiditis

J33.8 Other polyp of sinus
Accessory polyp of sinus
Ethmoidal polyp of sinus
Maxillary polyp of sinus
Sphenoidal polyp of sinus

J33.9 Nasal polyp, unspecified

✓4th **J34 Other and unspecified disorders of nose and nasal sinuses**
EXCLUDES 2 *varicose ulcer of nasal septum (I86.8)*

J34.Ø Abscess, furuncle and carbuncle of nose
Cellulitis of nose
Necrosis of nose
Ulceration of nose

J34.1 Cyst and mucocele of nose and nasal sinus

J34.2 Deviated nasal septum
Deflection or deviation of septum (nasal) (acquired)
EXCLUDES 1 *congenital deviated nasal septum (Q67.4)*
DEF: Condition in which the nasal septum, a thin wall composed of cartilage and bone that separates the two nostrils, is crooked or displaced from the midline.

J34.3 Hypertrophy of nasal turbinates
DEF: Overgrowth of bones within the nasal turbinate, which are ridges of bone and soft tissue that project from the sidewalls of the nasal passages. Hypertrophy can cause obstruction of the nasal passages.

✓5th **J34.8 Other specified disorders of nose and nasal sinuses**

J34.81 Nasal mucositis (ulcerative)
Code also type of associated therapy, such as:
antineoplastic and immunosuppressive drugs (T45.1X-)
radiological procedure and radiotherapy (Y84.2)
EXCLUDES 2 *gastrointestinal mucositis (ulcerative) (K92.81)*
mucositis (ulcerative) of vagina and vulva (N76.81)
oral mucositis (ulcerative) (K12.3-)

J34.89 Other specified disorders of nose and nasal sinuses
Perforation of nasal septum NOS
Rhinolith

J34.9 Unspecified disorder of nose and nasal sinuses

✓4th **J35 Chronic diseases of tonsils and adenoids**
Use additional code to identify:
exposure to environmental tobacco smoke (Z77.22)
exposure to tobacco smoke in the perinatal period (P96.81)
history of tobacco dependence (Z87.891)
occupational exposure to environmental tobacco smoke (Z57.31)
tobacco dependence (F17.-)
tobacco use (Z72.Ø)

✓5th **J35.Ø Chronic tonsillitis and adenoiditis**
EXCLUDES 2 *acute tonsillitis (JØ3.-)*

J35.Ø1 Chronic tonsillitis

J35.Ø2 Chronic adenoiditis

J35.Ø3 Chronic tonsillitis and adenoiditis

J35.1 Hypertrophy of tonsils
Enlargement of tonsils
EXCLUDES 1 *hypertrophy of tonsils with tonsillitis (J35.Ø-)*

J35.2 Hypertrophy of adenoids
Enlargement of adenoids
EXCLUDES 1 *hypertrophy of adenoids with adenoiditis (J35.Ø-)*

J35.3 Hypertrophy of tonsils with hypertrophy of adenoids
EXCLUDES 1 *hypertrophy of tonsils and adenoids with tonsillitis and adenoiditis (J35.Ø3)*

J35.8 Other chronic diseases of tonsils and adenoids
Adenoid vegetations
Amygdalolith
Calculus, tonsil
Cicatrix of tonsil (and adenoid)
Tonsillar tag
Ulcer of tonsil

J35.9 Chronic disease of tonsils and adenoids, unspecified
Disease (chronic) of tonsils and adenoids NOS

J36 Peritonsillar abscess
INCLUDES abscess of tonsil
peritonsillar cellulitis
quinsy
Use additional code (B95-B97) to identify infectious agent
EXCLUDES 1 *acute tonsillitis (JØ3.-)*
chronic tonsillitis (J35.Ø)
retropharyngeal abscess (J39.Ø)
tonsillitis NOS (JØ3.9-)

✓4th **J37 Chronic laryngitis and laryngotracheitis**
Use additional code to identify:
exposure to environmental tobacco smoke (Z77.22)
exposure to tobacco smoke in the perinatal period (P96.81)
history of tobacco dependence (Z87.891)
infectious agent (B95-B97)
occupational exposure to environmental tobacco smoke (Z57.31)
tobacco dependence (F17.-)
tobacco use (Z72.Ø)

J37.Ø Chronic laryngitis
Catarrhal laryngitis
Hypertrophic laryngitis
Sicca laryngitis
EXCLUDES 2 *acute laryngitis (JØ4.Ø)*
obstructive (acute) laryngitis (JØ5.Ø)

J37.1 Chronic laryngotracheitis
Laryngitis, chronic, with tracheitis (chronic)
Tracheitis, chronic, with laryngitis
EXCLUDES 1 *chronic tracheitis (J42)*
EXCLUDES 2 *acute laryngotracheitis (JØ4.2)*
acute tracheitis (JØ4.1)

✓4th **J38 Diseases of vocal cords and larynx, not elsewhere classified**
Use additional code to identify:
exposure to environmental tobacco smoke (Z77.22)
exposure to tobacco smoke in the perinatal period (P96.81)
history of tobacco dependence (Z87.891)
occupational exposure to environmental tobacco smoke (Z57.31)
tobacco dependence (F17.-)
tobacco use (Z72.Ø)
EXCLUDES 1 *congenital laryngeal stridor (P28.89)*
obstructive laryngitis (acute) (JØ5.Ø)
postprocedural subglottic stenosis (J95.5)
stridor (RØ6.1)
ulcerative laryngitis (JØ4.Ø)

✓5th **J38.Ø Paralysis of vocal cords and larynx**
Laryngoplegia
Paralysis of glottis

J38.ØØ Paralysis of vocal cords and larynx, unspecified

J38.Ø1 Paralysis of vocal cords and larynx, unilateral

J38.Ø2 Paralysis of vocal cords and larynx, bilateral

J38.1 Polyp of vocal cord and larynx
EXCLUDES 1 *adenomatous polyps (D14.1)*

J38.2 Nodules of vocal cords
Chorditis (fibrinous)(nodosa)(tuberosa)
Singer's nodes
Teacher's nodes

J38.3 Other diseases of vocal cords
Abscess of vocal cords
Cellulitis of vocal cords
Granuloma of vocal cords
Leukokeratosis of vocal cords
Leukoplakia of vocal cords

J38.4 Edema of larynx
Edema (of) glottis
Subglottic edema
Supraglottic edema
EXCLUDES 1 *acute obstructive laryngitis [croup] (JØ5.Ø)*
edematous laryngitis (JØ4.Ø)

J38.5 Laryngeal spasm
Laryngismus (stridulus)

J38.6 Stenosis of larynx

J38.7 Other diseases of larynx
Abscess of larynx
Cellulitis of larynx
Disease of larynx NOS
Necrosis of larynx
Pachyderma of larynx
Perichondritis of larynx
Ulcer of larynx

4th **J39 Other diseases of upper respiratory tract**
EXCLUDES 1 *acute respiratory infection NOS (J22)*
acute upper respiratory infection (JØ6.9)
upper respiratory inflammation due to chemicals, gases, fumes or vapors (J68.2)

J39.Ø Retropharyngeal and parapharyngeal abscess
Peripharyngeal abscess
EXCLUDES 1 *peritonsillar abscess (J36)*
DEF: Purulent infection behind the pharynx and the front of the precerebral fascia, characterized by neck stiffness, cervical lymphadenopathy, sore throat, fever, and stridor.

J39.1 Other abscess of pharynx
Cellulitis of pharynx
Nasopharyngeal abscess

J39.2 Other diseases of pharynx
Cyst of pharynx
Edema of pharynx
EXCLUDES 2 *chronic pharyngitis (J31.2)*
ulcerative pharyngitis (JØ2.9)

J39.3 Upper respiratory tract hypersensitivity reaction, site unspecified
EXCLUDES 1 *hypersensitivity reaction of upper respiratory tract, such as:*
extrinsic allergic alveolitis (J67.9)
pneumoconiosis (J6Ø-J67.9)

J39.8 Other specified diseases of upper respiratory tract

J39.9 Disease of upper respiratory tract, unspecified

Chronic lower respiratory diseases (J4Ø-J47)

EXCLUDES 1 *bronchitis due to chemicals, gases, fumes and vapors (J68.Ø)*
EXCLUDES 2 *cystic fibrosis (E84.-)*

J4Ø Bronchitis, not specified as acute or chronic
Bronchitis NOS
Bronchitis with tracheitis NOS
Catarrhal bronchitis
Tracheobronchitis NOS
Use additional code to identify:
exposure to environmental tobacco smoke (Z77.22)
exposure to tobacco smoke in the perinatal period (P96.81)
history of tobacco dependence (Z87.891)
occupational exposure to environmental tobacco smoke (Z57.31)
tobacco dependence (F17.-)
tobacco use (Z72.Ø)
EXCLUDES 1 *acute bronchitis (J2Ø.-)*
allergic bronchitis NOS (J45.9Ø9-)
asthmatic bronchitis NOS (J45.9-)
bronchitis due to chemicals, gases, fumes and vapors (J68.Ø)
AHA: 2020,1Q,34-36
TIP: Assign as a secondary code for a patient with bronchitis of unspecified acuity due to COVID-19; assign U07.1 as the principal or first-listed code.

4th **J41 Simple and mucopurulent chronic bronchitis**
Use additional code to identify:
exposure to environmental tobacco smoke (Z77.22)
exposure to tobacco smoke in the perinatal period (P96.81)
history of tobacco dependence (Z87.891)
occupational exposure to environmental tobacco smoke (Z57.31)
tobacco dependence (F17.-)
tobacco use (Z72.Ø)
EXCLUDES 1 *chronic bronchitis NOS (J42)*
chronic obstructive bronchitis (J44.-)

J41.Ø Simple chronic bronchitis HCC Rx ESR COM

J41.1 Mucopurulent chronic bronchitis HCC Rx ESR COM

J41.8 Mixed simple and mucopurulent chronic bronchitis HCC Rx ESR COM

J42 Unspecified chronic bronchitis HCC Rx ESR COM
Chronic bronchitis NOS
Chronic tracheitis
Chronic tracheobronchitis
Use additional code to identify:
exposure to environmental tobacco smoke (Z77.22)
exposure to tobacco smoke in the perinatal period (P96.81)
history of tobacco dependence (Z87.891)
occupational exposure to environmental tobacco smoke (Z57.31)
tobacco dependence (F17.-)
tobacco use (Z72.Ø)
EXCLUDES 1 *chronic asthmatic bronchitis (J44.-)*
chronic bronchitis with airways obstruction (J44.-)
chronic emphysematous bronchitis (J44.-)
chronic obstructive pulmonary disease NOS (J44.9)
simple and mucopurulent chronic bronchitis (J41.-)

✓4th J43 Emphysema

Use additional code to identify:
- exposure to environmental tobacco smoke (Z77.22)
- history of tobacco dependence (Z87.891)
- occupational exposure to environmental tobacco smoke (Z57.31)
- tobacco dependence (F17.-)
- tobacco use (Z72.Ø)

EXCLUDES 1 *compensatory emphysema (J98.3)*
emphysema due to inhalation of chemicals, gases, fumes or vapors (J68.4)
emphysema with chronic (obstructive) bronchitis (J44.-)
emphysematous (obstructive) bronchitis (J44.-)
interstitial emphysema (J98.2)
mediastinal emphysema (J98.2)
neonatal interstitial emphysema (P25.Ø)
surgical (subcutaneous) emphysema (T81.82)

EXCLUDES 2 *traumatic subcutaneous emphysema (T79.7)*

DEF: Pathological condition in which there is destructive enlargement of the air sacs in the lungs resulting in damage and lack of elasticity to the alveolar walls, commonly seen in long-term smokers.

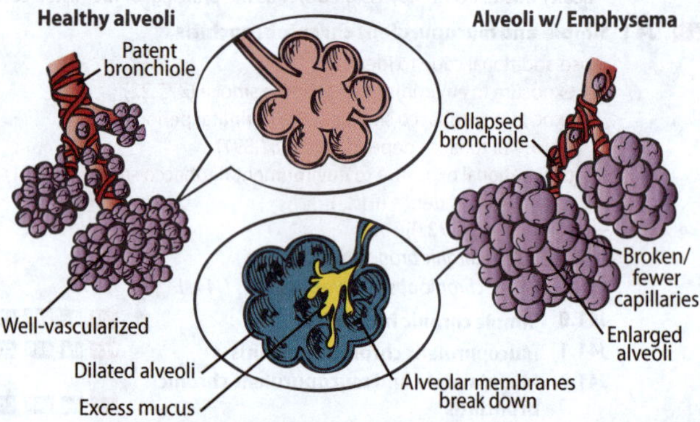

J43.Ø Unilateral pulmonary emphysema [MacLeod's syndrome] HCC Rx ESR COM
- Swyer-James syndrome
- Unilateral emphysema
- Unilateral hyperlucent lung
- Unilateral pulmonary artery functional hypoplasia
- Unilateral transparency of lung

J43.1 Panlobular emphysema HCC Rx ESR COM
- Panacinar emphysema

J43.2 Centrilobular emphysema HCC Rx ESR COM

J43.8 Other emphysema HCC Rx ESR COM

J43.9 Emphysema, unspecified HCC Rx ESR COM
- Bullous emphysema (lung)(pulmonary)
- Emphysema (lung)(pulmonary) NOS
- Emphysematous bleb
- Vesicular emphysema (lung)(pulmonary)

AHA: 2019,1Q,34-36; 2017,4Q,97-98

✓4th J44 Other chronic obstructive pulmonary disease

INCLUDES asthma with chronic obstructive pulmonary disease
chronic asthmatic (obstructive) bronchitis
chronic bronchitis with airway obstruction
chronic bronchitis with emphysema
chronic emphysematous bronchitis
chronic obstructive asthma
chronic obstructive bronchitis
chronic obstructive tracheobronchitis

Code also type of asthma, if applicable (J45.-)

Use additional code to identify:
- exposure to environmental tobacco smoke (Z77.22)
- history of tobacco dependence (Z87.891)
- occupational exposure to environmental tobacco smoke (Z57.31)
- tobacco dependence (F17.-)
- tobacco use (Z72.Ø)

EXCLUDES 1 *bronchiectasis (J47.-)*
chronic bronchitis NOS (J42)
chronic simple and mucopurulent bronchitis (J41.-)
chronic tracheitis (J42)
chronic tracheobronchitis (J42)
emphysema without chronic bronchitis (J43.-)

AHA: 2019,1Q,34-36; 2017,4Q,97-98; 2017,1Q,25-26; 2016,3Q,15-16; 2013,4Q,109

J44.Ø Chronic obstructive pulmonary disease with (acute) lower respiratory infection HCC Rx ESR COM

Code also to identify the infection

AHA: 2019,1Q,35; 2017,4Q,96; 2017,1Q,24-25

TIP: Do not assign when only aspiration pneumonia is present. Aspiration pneumonia is not classified as a respiratory infection.

J44.1 Chronic obstructive pulmonary disease with (acute) exacerbation HCC Rx ESR COM
- Decompensated COPD
- Decompensated COPD with (acute) exacerbation

EXCLUDES 2 *chronic obstructive pulmonary disease [COPD] with acute bronchitis (J44.Ø)*
lung diseases due to external agents (J6Ø-J7Ø)

AHA: 2019,1Q,34; 2017,4Q,96; 2017,1Q,26; 2016,1Q,36

TIP: Exacerbation of COPD should not be assumed based upon worsening of a concomitant respiratory disease or when COPD is described as end-stage.

TIP: Assign J43.9 when COPD exacerbation with emphysema is documented.

J44.9 Chronic obstructive pulmonary disease, unspecified HCC Rx ESR COM
- Chronic obstructive airway disease NOS
- Chronic obstructive lung disease NOS

EXCLUDES 2 *lung diseases due to external agents (J6Ø-J7Ø)*

AHA: 2019,1Q,36; 2017,4Q,96-97; 2016,1Q,36; 2014,4Q,21; 2013,4Q,109

J45 Asthma

INCLUDES allergic (predominantly) asthma
allergic bronchitis NOS
allergic rhinitis with asthma
atopic asthma
extrinsic allergic asthma
hay fever with asthma
idiosyncratic asthma
intrinsic nonallergic asthma
nonallergic asthma

Use additional code to identify:
eosinophilic asthma (J82.83)
exposure to environmental tobacco smoke (Z77.22)
exposure to tobacco smoke in the perinatal period (P96.81)
history of tobacco dependence (Z87.891)
occupational exposure to environmental tobacco smoke (Z57.31)
tobacco dependence (F17.-)
tobacco use (Z72.Ø)

EXCLUDES 1 *detergent asthma (J69.8)*
~~eosinophilic asthma (J82)~~
miner's asthma (J6Ø)
wheezing NOS (RØ6.2)
wood asthma (J67.8)

EXCLUDES 2 *asthma with chronic obstructive pulmonary disease (J44.9)*
chronic asthmatic (obstructive) bronchitis (J44.9)
chronic obstructive asthma (J44.9)

AHA: 2019,1Q,36; 2017,1Q,25-26; 2012,4Q,99

DEF: Status asthmaticus: Severe, intractable episode of asthma that is unresponsive to normal therapeutic measures.

J45.2 Mild intermittent asthma

J45.2Ø Mild intermittent asthma, uncomplicated Rx COM
Mild intermittent asthma NOS

J45.21 Mild intermittent asthma with (acute) exacerbation Rx COM

J45.22 Mild intermittent asthma with status asthmaticus Rx COM

J45.3 Mild persistent asthma

J45.3Ø Mild persistent asthma, uncomplicated Rx COM
Mild persistent asthma NOS

J45.31 Mild persistent asthma with (acute) exacerbation Rx COM
AHA: 2016,1Q,35

J45.32 Mild persistent asthma with status asthmaticus Rx COM

J45.4 Moderate persistent asthma

J45.4Ø Moderate persistent asthma, uncomplicated Rx COM
Moderate persistent asthma NOS

J45.41 Moderate persistent asthma with (acute) exacerbation Rx COM
AHA: 2017,1Q,26

J45.42 Moderate persistent asthma with status asthmaticus Rx COM

J45.5 Severe persistent asthma

J45.5Ø Severe persistent asthma, uncomplicated Rx COM
Severe persistent asthma NOS

J45.51 Severe persistent asthma with (acute) exacerbation Rx COM

J45.52 Severe persistent asthma with status asthmaticus Rx COM

J45.9 Other and unspecified asthma

J45.9Ø Unspecified asthma
Asthmatic bronchitis NOS
Childhood asthma NOS
Late onset asthma
AHA: 2017,4Q,96; 2017,1Q,25

J45.9Ø1 Unspecified asthma with (acute) exacerbation Rx COM

J45.9Ø2 Unspecified asthma with status asthmaticus Rx COM

J45.9Ø9 Unspecified asthma, uncomplicated Rx COM
Asthma NOS
EXCLUDES 2 *lung diseases due to external agents (J6Ø-J7Ø)*
AHA: 2017,1Q,25

J45.99 Other asthma

J45.99Ø Exercise induced bronchospasm Rx COM

J45.991 Cough variant asthma Rx COM

J45.998 Other asthma Rx COM

J47 Bronchiectasis

INCLUDES bronchiolectasis

Use additional code to identify:
exposure to environmental tobacco smoke (Z77.22)
exposure to tobacco smoke in the perinatal period (P96.81)
history of tobacco dependence (Z87.891)
occupational exposure to environmental tobacco smoke (Z57.31)
tobacco dependence (F17.-)
tobacco use (Z72.Ø)

EXCLUDES 1 *congenital bronchiectasis (Q33.4)*
tuberculous bronchiectasis (current disease) (A15.Ø)

DEF: Dilation of the bronchi with mucus production and persistent cough due to infection or chronic conditions that causes diminished lung capacity and frequent infections of the lung.

J47.Ø Bronchiectasis with acute lower respiratory infection HCC Rx ESR COM
Bronchiectasis with acute bronchitis
Code also to identify infection, if applicable

J47.1 Bronchiectasis with (acute) exacerbation HCC Rx ESR COM
AHA: 2021,1Q,23

J47.9 Bronchiectasis, uncomplicated HCC Rx ESR COM
Bronchiectasis NOS

Lung diseases due to external agents (J6Ø-J7Ø)

EXCLUDES 2 *asthma (J45.-)*
malignant neoplasm of bronchus and lung (C34.-)

DEF: Pneumoconiosis: Condition caused by inhaling inorganic dust particles, typically associated with occupations that require regular exposure to mineral dusts. A form of interstitial lung disease that contributes to the inflammation of the air sacs, causing the lung tissue to harden.

J6Ø Coalworker's pneumoconiosis HCC ESR COM A
Anthracosilicosis
Anthracosis
Black lung disease
Coalworker's lung
EXCLUDES 1 *coalworker pneumoconiosis with tuberculosis, any type in A15 (J65)*

J61 Pneumoconiosis due to asbestos and other mineral fibers HCC ESR COM A
Asbestosis
EXCLUDES 1 *pleural plaque with asbestosis (J92.Ø)*
pneumoconiosis with tuberculosis, any type in A15 (J65)

J62 Pneumoconiosis due to dust containing silica

INCLUDES silicotic fibrosis (massive) of lung

EXCLUDES 1 *pneumoconiosis with tuberculosis, any type in A15 (J65)*

J62.Ø Pneumoconiosis due to talc dust HCC ESR COM

J62.8 Pneumoconiosis due to other dust containing silica HCC ESR COM
Silicosis NOS

J63 Pneumoconiosis due to other inorganic dusts

EXCLUDES 1 *pneumoconiosis with tuberculosis, any type in A15 (J65)*

J63.Ø Aluminosis (of lung) HCC ESR COM

J63.1 Bauxite fibrosis (of lung) HCC ESR COM

J63.2 Berylliosis HCC ESR COM

J63.3 Graphite fibrosis (of lung) HCC ESR COM

J63.4 Siderosis HCC ESR COM
AHA: 2019,3Q,8

J63.5 Stannosis HCC ESR COM

J63.6 Pneumoconiosis due to other specified inorganic dusts HCC ESR COM

J64 Unspecified pneumoconiosis HCC ESR COM
EXCLUDES 1 *pneumonoconiosis with tuberculosis, any type in A15 (J65)*

J65 Pneumoconiosis associated with tuberculosis HCC ESR COM
Any condition in J60-J64 with tuberculosis, any type in A15
Silicotuberculosis

J66 Airway disease due to specific organic dust
EXCLUDES 2 *allergic alveolitis (J67.-)*
asbestosis (J61)
bagassosis (J67.1)
farmer's lung (J67.0)
hypersensitivity pneumonitis due to organic dust (J67.-)
reactive airways dysfunction syndrome (J68.3)

J66.0 Byssinosis HCC ESR COM
Airway disease due to cotton dust

J66.1 Flax-dressers' disease HCC ESR COM

J66.2 Cannabinosis HCC ESR COM

J66.8 Airway disease due to other specific organic dusts HCC ESR COM

J67 Hypersensitivity pneumonitis due to organic dust
INCLUDES allergic alveolitis and pneumonitis due to inhaled organic dust and particles of fungal, actinomycetic or other origin
EXCLUDES 1 *pneumonitis due to inhalation of chemicals, gases, fumes or vapors (J68.0)*

J67.0 Farmer's lung HCC ESR COM
Harvester's lung
Haymaker's lung
Moldy hay disease

J67.1 Bagassosis HCC ESR COM
Bagasse disease
Bagasse pneumonitis

J67.2 Bird fancier's lung HCC ESR COM
Budgerigar fancier's disease or lung
Pigeon fancier's disease or lung

J67.3 Suberosis HCC ESR COM
Corkhandler's disease or lung
Corkworker's disease or lung

J67.4 Maltworker's lung HCC ESR COM
Alveolitis due to Aspergillus clavatus

J67.5 Mushroom-worker's lung HCC ESR COM

J67.6 Maple-bark-stripper's lung HCC ESR COM
Alveolitis due to Cryptostroma corticale
Cryptostromosis

J67.7 Air conditioner and humidifier lung HCC ESR COM
Allergic alveolitis due to fungal, thermophilic actinomycetes and other organisms growing in ventilation [air conditioning] systems

J67.8 Hypersensitivity pneumonitis due to other organic dusts HCC ESR COM
Cheese-washer's lung
Coffee-worker's lung
Fish-meal worker's lung
Furrier's lung
Sequoiosis

J67.9 Hypersensitivity pneumonitis due to unspecified organic dust HCC ESR COM
Allergic alveolitis (extrinsic) NOS
Hypersensitivity pneumonitis NOS

J68 Respiratory conditions due to inhalation of chemicals, gases, fumes and vapors
Code first (T51-T65) to identify cause
Use additional code to identify associated respiratory conditions, such as:
acute respiratory failure (J96.0-)

J68.0 Bronchitis and pneumonitis due to chemicals, gases, fumes and vapors HCC ESR COM
Chemical bronchitis (acute)
AHA: 2019,2Q,31

J68.1 Pulmonary edema due to chemicals, gases, fumes and vapors HCC ESR COM
Chemical pulmonary edema (acute) (chronic)
EXCLUDES 1 *pulmonary edema (acute) (chronic) NOS (J81.-)*

J68.2 Upper respiratory inflammation due to chemicals, gases, fumes and vapors, not elsewhere classified HCC ESR COM

J68.3 Other acute and subacute respiratory conditions due to chemicals, gases, fumes and vapors HCC ESR COM
Reactive airways dysfunction syndrome

J68.4 Chronic respiratory conditions due to chemicals, gases, fumes and vapors HCC ESR COM
Emphysema (diffuse) (chronic) due to inhalation of chemicals, gases, fumes and vapors
Obliterative bronchiolitis (chronic) (subacute) due to inhalation of chemicals, gases, fumes and vapors
Pulmonary fibrosis (chronic) due to inhalation of chemicals, gases, fumes and vapors
EXCLUDES 1 *chronic pulmonary edema due to chemicals, gases, fumes and vapors (J68.1)*

J68.8 Other respiratory conditions due to chemicals, gases, fumes and vapors HCC ESR COM

J68.9 Unspecified respiratory condition due to chemicals, gases, fumes and vapors HCC ESR COM

J69 Pneumonitis due to solids and liquids
EXCLUDES 1 *neonatal aspiration syndromes (P24.-)*
postprocedural pneumonitis (J95.4)
AHA: 2017,1Q,24
DEF: Pneumonitis: Noninfectious inflammation of the walls of the alveoli in the lung tissue due to inhalation of food, vomit, oils, essences, or other solids or liquids.

J69.0 Pneumonitis due to inhalation of food and vomit HCC ESR COM
Aspiration pneumonia NOS
Aspiration pneumonia (due to) food (regurgitated)
Aspiration pneumonia (due to) gastric secretions
Aspiration pneumonia (due to) milk
Aspiration pneumonia (due to) vomit
Code also any associated foreign body in respiratory tract (T17.-)
EXCLUDES 1 *chemical pneumonitis due to anesthesia (J95.4)*
obstetric aspiration pneumonitis (O74.0)
AHA: 2020,2Q,11,28; 2019,3Q,17; 2019,2Q,6,31

J69.1 Pneumonitis due to inhalation of oils and essences HCC ESR COM
Exogenous lipoid pneumonia
Lipid pneumonia NOS
Code first (T51-T65) to identify substance
EXCLUDES 1 *endogenous lipoid pneumonia (J84.89)*

J69.8 Pneumonitis due to inhalation of other solids and liquids HCC ESR COM
Pneumonitis due to aspiration of blood
Pneumonitis due to aspiration of detergent
Code first (T51-T65) to identify substance

J70 Respiratory conditions due to other external agents

J70.0 Acute pulmonary manifestations due to radiation HCC ESR COM
Radiation pneumonitis
Use additional code (W88-W90, X39.0-) to identify the external cause

J70.1 Chronic and other pulmonary manifestations due to radiation HCC ESR COM
Fibrosis of lung following radiation
Use additional code (W88-W90, X39.0-) to identify the external cause

J70.2 Acute drug-induced interstitial lung disorders HCC ESR
Use additional code for adverse effect, if applicable, to identify drug (T36-T50 with fifth or sixth character 5)
EXCLUDES 1 *interstitial pneumonia NOS (J84.9)*
lymphoid interstitial pneumonia (J84.2)
AHA: 2019,2Q,28

J70.3 Chronic drug-induced interstitial lung disorders HCC ESR
Use additional code for adverse effect, if applicable, to identify drug (T36-T50 with fifth or sixth character 5)
EXCLUDES 1 *interstitial pneumonia NOS (J84.9)*
lymphoid interstitial pneumonia (J84.2)

J70.4 Drug-induced interstitial lung disorders, unspecified HCC ESR
Use additional code for adverse effect, if applicable, to identify drug (T36-T50 with fifth or sixth character 5)
EXCLUDES 1 *interstitial pneumonia NOS (J84.9)*
lymphoid interstitial pneumonia (J84.2)
AHA: 2019,2Q,28

J70.5 Respiratory conditions due to smoke inhalation HCC ESR
Code first smoke inhalation (T59.81-)
EXCLUDES 2 *smoke inhalation due to chemicals, gases, fumes and vapors (J68.9)*
AHA: 2013,4Q,121

J70.8 Respiratory conditions due to other specified external agents HCC ESR
Code first (T51-T65) to identify the external agent

J70.9 Respiratory conditions due to unspecified external agent HCC ESR
Code first (T51-T65) to identify the external agent

Other respiratory diseases principally affecting the interstitium (J80-J84)

J80 Acute respiratory distress syndrome HCC ESR COM
Acute respiratory distress syndrome in adult or child
Adult hyaline membrane disease
EXCLUDES 1 *respiratory distress syndrome in newborn (perinatal) (P22.0)*
AHA: 2021,1Q,23; 2020,4Q,96; 2020,1Q,34-36; 2017,1Q,26
DEF: Lung inflammation or injury resulting in a build-up of fluid in the air sacs, preventing the passage of oxygen from the air into the bloodstream.
TIP: Assign as a secondary code for a patient with acute respiratory distress syndrome (ARDS) due to COVID-19; assign code U07.1 as the principal or first-listed code.

✓4th **J81 Pulmonary edema**
Use additional code to identify:
exposure to environmental tobacco smoke (Z77.22)
history of tobacco dependence (Z87.891)
occupational exposure to environmental tobacco smoke (Z57.31)
tobacco dependence (F17.-)
tobacco use (Z72.0)
EXCLUDES 1 *chemical (acute) pulmonary edema (J68.1)*
hypostatic pneumonia (J18.2)
passive pneumonia (J18.2)
pulmonary edema due to external agents (J60-J70)
pulmonary edema with heart disease NOS (I50.1)
pulmonary edema with heart failure (I50.1)
DEF: Accumulation of fluid in the air sacs of the lungs, making it difficult to breathe.

J81.0 Acute pulmonary edema HCC ESR COM
Acute edema of lung
AHA: 2020,3Q,27

J81.1 Chronic pulmonary edema COM
Pulmonary congestion (chronic) (passive)
Pulmonary edema NOS

✓4th **J82 Pulmonary eosinophilia, not elsewhere classified**
EXCLUDES 2 *pulmonary eosinophilia due to aspergillosis (B44.-)*
pulmonary eosinophilia due to drugs (J70.2-J70.4)
pulmonary eosinophilia due to specified parasitic infection (B50-B83)
pulmonary eosinophilia due to systemic connective tissue disorders (M30-M36)
pulmonary infiltrate NOS (R91.8)
DEF: Infiltration of eosinophils (white blood cells of the immune system) into the parenchyma of the lungs, resulting in cough, fever, and dyspnea.

✓5th **J82.8 Pulmonary eosinophilia, not elsewhere classified**
AHA: 2020,4Q,25-27

J82.81 Chronic eosinophilic pneumonia HCC Rx ESR COM
Eosinophilic pneumonia, NOS

J82.82 Acute eosinophilic pneumonia

J82.83 Eosinophilic asthma Rx COM
Code first asthma, by type, such as:
mild intermittent asthma (J45.2-)
mild persistent asthma (J45.3-)
moderate persistent asthma (J45.4-)
severe persistent asthma (J45.5-)

J82.89 Other pulmonary eosinophilia, not elsewhere classified HCC ESR COM
Allergic pneumonia
Löffler's pneumonia
Tropical (pulmonary) eosinophilia NOS

✓4th **J84 Other interstitial pulmonary diseases**
EXCLUDES 1 *drug-induced interstitial lung disorders (J70.2-J70.4)*
interstitial emphysema (J98.2)
EXCLUDES 2 *lung diseases due to external agents (J60-J70)*
DEF: Interstitial: Within the small spaces or gaps occurring in tissue or organs.

✓5th **J84.0 Alveolar and parieto-alveolar conditions**

J84.01 Alveolar proteinosis HCC Rx ESR COM
DEF: Reduced ventilation due to proteinaceous deposits on alveoli. Symptoms include dyspnea, cough, chest pain, weakness, weight loss, and hemoptysis.

J84.02 Pulmonary alveolar microlithiasis HCC Rx ESR COM

J84.03 Idiopathic pulmonary hemosiderosis HCC Rx ESR COM
Essential brown induration of lung
Code first underlying disease, such as:
disorders of iron metabolism (E83.1-)
EXCLUDES 1 *acute idiopathic pulmonary hemorrhage in infants [AIPHI] (R04.81)*
DEF: Fibrosis of the alveolar walls marked by abnormal accumulation of iron as hemosiderin in the lungs. It primarily affects children and symptoms include anemia, fluid in the lungs, and blood in the sputum. Etiology is unknown.

J84.09 Other alveolar and parieto-alveolar conditions HCC Rx ESR COM

✓5th **J84.1 Other interstitial pulmonary diseases with fibrosis**
EXCLUDES 1 *pulmonary fibrosis (chronic) due to inhalation of chemicals, gases, fumes or vapors (J68.4)*
pulmonary fibrosis (chronic) following radiation (J70.1)

J84.10 Pulmonary fibrosis, unspecified HCC Rx ESR COM
Capillary fibrosis of lung
Cirrhosis of lung (chronic) NOS
Fibrosis of lung (atrophic) (chronic) (confluent) (massive) (perialveolar) (peribronchial) NOS
Induration of lung (chronic) NOS
Postinflammatory pulmonary fibrosis

✓6th **J84.11 Idiopathic interstitial pneumonia**
EXCLUDES 1 *lymphoid interstitial pneumonia (J84.2)*
pneumocystis pneumonia (B59)

J84.111 Idiopathic interstitial pneumonia, not otherwise specified HCC Rx ESR COM

J84.112 Idiopathic pulmonary fibrosis HCC Rx ESR COM
Cryptogenic fibrosing alveolitis
Idiopathic fibrosing alveolitis

J84.113 Idiopathic non-specific interstitial pneumonitis HCC Rx ESR COM
EXCLUDES 1 *non-specific interstitial pneumonia NOS, or due to known underlying cause (J84.89)*

J84.114 Acute interstitial pneumonitis HCC Rx ESR COM
Hamman-Rich syndrome
EXCLUDES 1 *pneumocystis pneumonia (B59)*

J84.115 Respiratory bronchiolitis interstitial lung disease HCC Rx ESR COM

J84.116 Cryptogenic organizing pneumonia HCC Rx ESR COM
EXCLUDES 1 *organizing pneumonia NOS, or due to known underlying cause (J84.89)*

J84.117 Desquamative interstitial pneumonia HCC Rx ESR COM

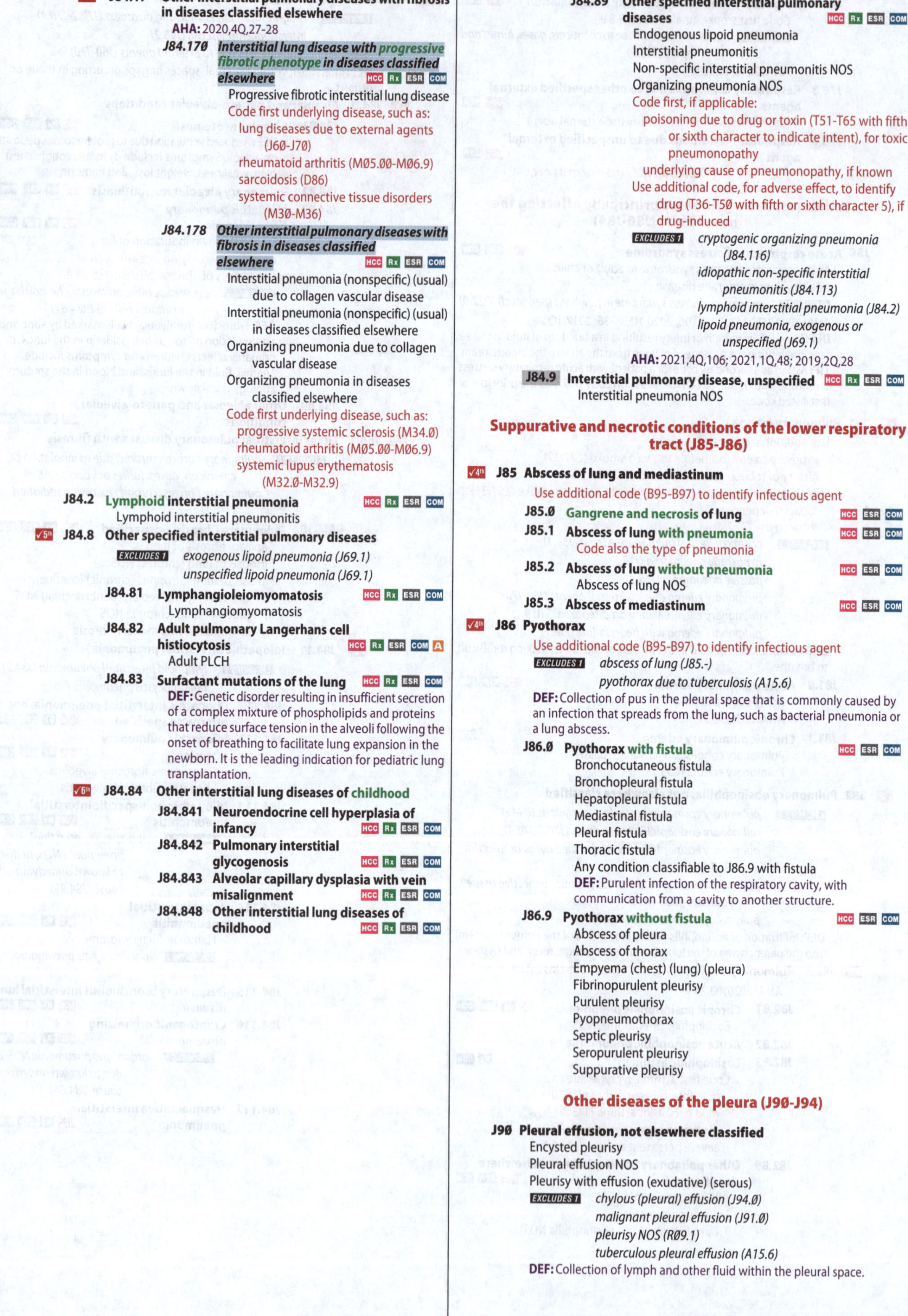

✓6th **J84.17 Other interstitial pulmonary diseases with fibrosis in diseases classified elsewhere**
AHA: 2020,4Q,27-28

J84.170 *Interstitial lung disease with progressive fibrotic phenotype in diseases classified elsewhere* HCC Rx ESR COM
Progressive fibrotic interstitial lung disease
Code first underlying disease, such as:
lung diseases due to external agents (J60-J70)
rheumatoid arthritis (M05.00-M06.9)
sarcoidosis (D86)
systemic connective tissue disorders (M30-M36)

J84.178 *Other interstitial pulmonary diseases with fibrosis in diseases classified elsewhere* HCC Rx ESR COM
Interstitial pneumonia (nonspecific) (usual) due to collagen vascular disease
Interstitial pneumonia (nonspecific) (usual) in diseases classified elsewhere
Organizing pneumonia due to collagen vascular disease
Organizing pneumonia in diseases classified elsewhere
Code first underlying disease, such as:
progressive systemic sclerosis (M34.0)
rheumatoid arthritis (M05.00-M06.9)
systemic lupus erythematosis (M32.0-M32.9)

J84.2 Lymphoid interstitial pneumonia HCC Rx ESR COM
Lymphoid interstitial pneumonitis

✓5th **J84.8 Other specified interstitial pulmonary diseases**
EXCLUDES 1 *exogenous lipoid pneumonia (J69.1)*
unspecified lipoid pneumonia (J69.1)

J84.81 Lymphangioleiomyomatosis HCC Rx ESR COM
Lymphangiomyomatosis

J84.82 Adult pulmonary Langerhans cell histiocytosis HCC Rx ESR COM A
Adult PLCH

J84.83 Surfactant mutations of the lung HCC Rx ESR COM
DEF: Genetic disorder resulting in insufficient secretion of a complex mixture of phospholipids and proteins that reduce surface tension in the alveoli following the onset of breathing to facilitate lung expansion in the newborn. It is the leading indication for pediatric lung transplantation.

✓6th **J84.84 Other interstitial lung diseases of childhood**

J84.841 Neuroendocrine cell hyperplasia of infancy HCC Rx ESR COM

J84.842 Pulmonary interstitial glycogenosis HCC Rx ESR COM

J84.843 Alveolar capillary dysplasia with vein misalignment HCC Rx ESR COM

J84.848 Other interstitial lung diseases of childhood HCC Rx ESR COM

J84.89 Other specified interstitial pulmonary diseases HCC Rx ESR COM
Endogenous lipoid pneumonia
Interstitial pneumonitis
Non-specific interstitial pneumonitis NOS
Organizing pneumonia NOS
Code first, if applicable:
poisoning due to drug or toxin (T51-T65 with fifth or sixth character to indicate intent), for toxic pneumonopathy
underlying cause of pneumonopathy, if known
Use additional code, for adverse effect, to identify drug (T36-T50 with fifth or sixth character 5), if drug-induced
EXCLUDES 1 *cryptogenic organizing pneumonia (J84.116)*
idiopathic non-specific interstitial pneumonitis (J84.113)
lymphoid interstitial pneumonia (J84.2)
lipoid pneumonia, exogenous or unspecified (J69.1)
AHA: 2021,4Q,106; 2021,1Q,48; 2019,2Q,28

J84.9 Interstitial pulmonary disease, unspecified HCC Rx ESR COM
Interstitial pneumonia NOS

Suppurative and necrotic conditions of the lower respiratory tract (J85-J86)

✓4th **J85 Abscess of lung and mediastinum**
Use additional code (B95-B97) to identify infectious agent

J85.0 Gangrene and necrosis of lung HCC ESR COM

J85.1 Abscess of lung with pneumonia HCC ESR COM
Code also the type of pneumonia

J85.2 Abscess of lung without pneumonia HCC ESR COM
Abscess of lung NOS

J85.3 Abscess of mediastinum HCC ESR COM

✓4th **J86 Pyothorax**
Use additional code (B95-B97) to identify infectious agent
EXCLUDES 1 *abscess of lung (J85.-)*
pyothorax due to tuberculosis (A15.6)
DEF: Collection of pus in the pleural space that is commonly caused by an infection that spreads from the lung, such as bacterial pneumonia or a lung abscess.

J86.0 Pyothorax with fistula HCC ESR COM
Bronchocutaneous fistula
Bronchopleural fistula
Hepatopleural fistula
Mediastinal fistula
Pleural fistula
Thoracic fistula
Any condition classifiable to J86.9 with fistula
DEF: Purulent infection of the respiratory cavity, with communication from a cavity to another structure.

J86.9 Pyothorax without fistula HCC ESR COM
Abscess of pleura
Abscess of thorax
Empyema (chest) (lung) (pleura)
Fibrinopurulent pleurisy
Purulent pleurisy
Pyopneumothorax
Septic pleurisy
Seropurulent pleurisy
Suppurative pleurisy

Other diseases of the pleura (J90-J94)

J90 Pleural effusion, not elsewhere classified
Encysted pleurisy
Pleural effusion NOS
Pleurisy with effusion (exudative) (serous)
EXCLUDES 1 *chylous (pleural) effusion (J94.0)*
malignant pleural effusion (J91.0)
pleurisy NOS (R09.1)
tuberculous pleural effusion (A15.6)
DEF: Collection of lymph and other fluid within the pleural space.

J91 Pleural effusion in conditions classified elsewhere

EXCLUDES 2 *pleural effusion in heart failure (I5Ø.-)*
pleural effusion in systemic lupus erythematosus (M32.13)

DEF: Collection of lymph and other fluid within the pleural space.

J91.Ø Malignant pleural effusion
Code first underlying neoplasm ▶(CØØ-D49)◀

J91.8 Pleural effusion in other conditions classified elsewhere
Code first underlying disease, such as:
filariasis (B74.Ø-B74.9)
influenza (JØ9.X2, J1Ø.1, J11.1)
AHA: 2015,2Q,15
TIP: Assign this code as a secondary diagnosis to congestive heart failure (I50.-) only if pleural effusion is specifically evaluated or treated.

Pleural Effusion

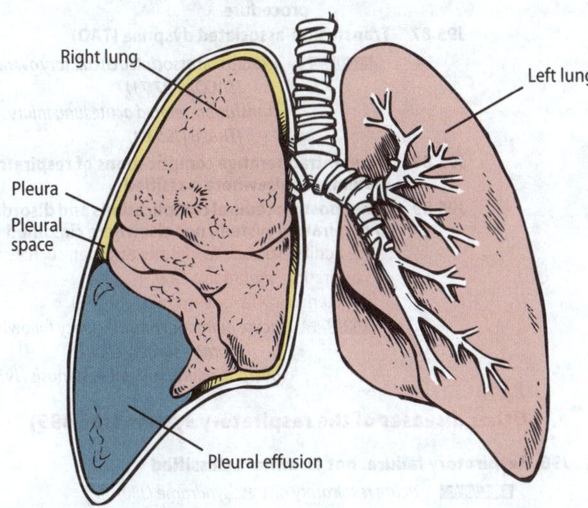

J92 Pleural plaque

INCLUDES pleural thickening

DEF: Areas of fibrous thickening that form on the parietal or visceral pleura, the membranes that line the ribs and lungs.

J92.Ø Pleural plaque with presence of asbestos
J92.9 Pleural plaque without asbestos
Pleural plaque NOS

J93 Pneumothorax and air leak

EXCLUDES 1 *congenital or perinatal pneumothorax (P25.1)*
postprocedural air leak (J95.812)
postprocedural pneumothorax (J95.811)
pyopneumothorax (J86.-)
traumatic pneumothorax (S27.Ø)
tuberculous (current disease) pneumothorax (A15.-)

DEF: Pneumothorax: Lung displacement due to abnormal leakage of air or gas that is trapped in the pleural space formed by the membrane that encloses the lungs and lines the thoracic cavity.

J93.Ø Spontaneous tension pneumothorax
DEF: Leaking air from the lung into the lining, causing collapse.

J93.1 Other spontaneous pneumothorax
J93.11 Primary spontaneous pneumothorax
J93.12 Secondary spontaneous pneumothorax UPD
Code first underlying condition, such as:
catamenial pneumothorax due to endometriosis ▶(N8Ø.B-)◀
cystic fibrosis (E84.-)
eosinophilic pneumonia (J82)
lymphangioleiomyomatosis (J84.81)
malignant neoplasm of bronchus and lung (C34.-)
Marfan's syndrome (Q87.4)
pneumonia due to Pneumocystis carinii (B59)
secondary malignant neoplasm of lung (C78.Ø-)
spontaneous rupture of the esophagus (K22.3)

J93.8 Other pneumothorax and air leak
J93.81 Chronic pneumothorax
J93.82 Other air leak
Persistent air leak
J93.83 Other pneumothorax
Acute pneumothorax
Spontaneous pneumothorax NOS
AHA: 2020,3Q,9-10

J93.9 Pneumothorax, unspecified
Pneumothorax NOS

J94 Other pleural conditions

EXCLUDES 1 *pleurisy NOS (RØ9.1)*
traumatic hemopneumothorax (S27.2)
traumatic hemothorax (S27.1)
tuberculous pleural conditions (current disease) (A15.-)

J94.Ø Chylous effusion
Chyliform effusion
DEF: Fluid within the pleural space due to the leaking of lymph contents into the space, usually as a result of thoracic duct damage or injury or mediastinal lymphoma.

J94.1 Fibrothorax
DEF: Fibrosis within the pleural lining of the lungs commonly seen as a stiff layer surrounding the lung typically attributed to traumatic hemothorax or pleural effusion.

J94.2 Hemothorax
Hemopneumothorax

J94.8 Other specified pleural conditions
Hydropneumothorax
Hydrothorax
AHA: 2021,1Q,48

J94.9 Pleural condition, unspecified

Intraoperative and postprocedural complications and disorders of respiratory system, not elsewhere classified (J95)

J95 Intraoperative and postprocedural complications and disorders of respiratory system, not elsewhere classified

EXCLUDES 2 *aspiration pneumonia (J69.-)*
emphysema (subcutaneous) resulting from a procedure (T81.82)
hypostatic pneumonia (J18.2)
pulmonary manifestations due to radiation (J7Ø.Ø-J7Ø.1)

J95.Ø Tracheostomy complications
DEF: Tracheostomy: Formation of a tracheal opening on the neck surface with tube insertion to allow for respiration in cases of obstruction or decreased patency. A tracheostomy may be planned or performed on an emergency basis for temporary or long-term use.

J95.ØØ Unspecified tracheostomy complication HCC ESR COM
J95.Ø1 Hemorrhage from tracheostomy stoma HCC ESR COM
J95.Ø2 Infection of tracheostomy stoma HCC ESR COM
Use additional code to identify type of infection, such as:
cellulitis of neck (LØ3.221)
sepsis (A4Ø, A41.-)
J95.Ø3 Malfunction of tracheostomy stoma HCC ESR COM
Mechanical complication of tracheostomy stoma
Obstruction of tracheostomy airway
Tracheal stenosis due to tracheostomy
J95.Ø4 Tracheo-esophageal fistula following tracheostomy HCC ESR COM
J95.Ø9 Other tracheostomy complication HCC ESR COM

J95.1 Acute pulmonary insufficiency following thoracic surgery HCC ESR
EXCLUDES 2 *functional disturbances following cardiac surgery (I97.Ø, I97.1-)*

J95.2 Acute pulmonary insufficiency following nonthoracic surgery HCC ESR
EXCLUDES 2 *functional disturbances following cardiac surgery (I97.Ø, I97.1-)*

J95.3 Chronic pulmonary insufficiency following surgery HCC ESR
EXCLUDES 2 *functional disturbances following cardiac surgery (I97.Ø, I97.1-)*

J95.4 **Chemical pneumonitis due to anesthesia**
Mendelson's syndrome
Postprocedural aspiration pneumonia
Use additional code for adverse effect, if applicable, to identify drug (T41.- with fifth or sixth character 5)
EXCLUDES 1 *aspiration pneumonitis due to anesthesia complicating labor and delivery (O74.0)*
aspiration pneumonitis due to anesthesia complicating pregnancy (O29)
aspiration pneumonitis due to anesthesia complicating the puerperium (O89.01)

J95.5 **Postprocedural subglottic stenosis**

✓5th J95.6 **Intraoperative hemorrhage and hematoma of a respiratory system organ or structure complicating a procedure**
EXCLUDES 1 *intraoperative hemorrhage and hematoma of a respiratory system organ or structure due to accidental puncture and laceration during procedure (J95.7-)*
J95.61 **Intraoperative hemorrhage and hematoma of a respiratory system organ or structure complicating a respiratory system procedure**
J95.62 **Intraoperative hemorrhage and hematoma of a respiratory system organ or structure complicating other procedure**

✓5th J95.7 **Accidental puncture and laceration of a respiratory system organ or structure during a procedure**
EXCLUDES 2 *postprocedural pneumothorax (J95.811)*
J95.71 **Accidental puncture and laceration of a respiratory system organ or structure during a respiratory system procedure**
J95.72 **Accidental puncture and laceration of a respiratory system organ or structure during other procedure**

✓5th J95.8 **Other intraoperative and postprocedural complications and disorders of respiratory system, not elsewhere classified**
AHA: 2016,4Q,9-10
✓6th J95.81 **Postprocedural pneumothorax and air leak**
J95.811 **Postprocedural pneumothorax**
AHA: 2021,1Q,48
J95.812 **Postprocedural air leak**
✓6th J95.82 **Postprocedural respiratory failure**
EXCLUDES 1 *respiratory failure in other conditions (J96.-)*
J95.821 **Acute postprocedural respiratory failure** HCC ESR
Postprocedural respiratory failure NOS
J95.822 **Acute and chronic postprocedural respiratory failure** HCC ESR
✓6th J95.83 **Postprocedural hemorrhage of a respiratory system organ or structure following a procedure**
J95.830 **Postprocedural hemorrhage of a respiratory system organ or structure following a respiratory system procedure**
J95.831 **Postprocedural hemorrhage of a respiratory system organ or structure following other procedure**
J95.84 **Transfusion-related acute lung injury (TRALI)**
DEF: Relatively rare, but serious, pulmonary complication of blood transfusion, with acute respiratory distress, noncardiogenic pulmonary edema, cyanosis, hypoxemia, hypotension, fever, and chills.
✓6th J95.85 **Complication of respirator [ventilator]**
J95.850 **Mechanical complication of respirator** HCC ESR COM
EXCLUDES 1 *encounter for respirator [ventilator] dependence during power failure (Z99.12)*
J95.851 **Ventilator associated pneumonia** HCC ESR
Ventilator associated pneumonitis
Use additional code to identify the organism, if known (B95.-, B96.-, B97.-)
EXCLUDES 1 *ventilator lung in newborn (P27.8)*
AHA: 2020,2Q,17; 2017,1Q,25
J95.859 **Other complication of respirator [ventilator]** HCC ESR COM
AHA: 2021,1Q,48
✓6th J95.86 **Postprocedural hematoma and seroma of a respiratory system organ or structure following a procedure**
J95.860 **Postprocedural hematoma of a respiratory system organ or structure following a respiratory system procedure**
J95.861 **Postprocedural hematoma of a respiratory system organ or structure following other procedure**
J95.862 **Postprocedural seroma of a respiratory system organ or structure following a respiratory system procedure**
J95.863 **Postprocedural seroma of a respiratory system organ or structure following other procedure**
● J95.87 **Transfusion-associated dyspnea (TAD)**
EXCLUDES 1 *transfusion associated circulatory overload (TACO) (E87.71)*
transfusion-related acute lung injury (TRALI) (J95.84)
J95.88 **Other intraoperative complications of respiratory system, not elsewhere classified**
J95.89 **Other postprocedural complications and disorders of respiratory system, not elsewhere classified**
Use additional code to identify disorder, such as:
aspiration pneumonia (J69.-)
bacterial or viral pneumonia (J12-J18)
EXCLUDES 2 *acute pulmonary insufficiency following thoracic surgery (J95.1)*
postprocedural subglottic stenosis (J95.5)

Other diseases of the respiratory system (J96-J99)

✓4th J96 **Respiratory failure, not elsewhere classified**
EXCLUDES 1 *acute respiratory distress syndrome (J80)*
cardiorespiratory failure (R09.2)
newborn respiratory distress syndrome (P22.0)
postprocedural respiratory failure (J95.82-)
respiratory arrest (R09.2)
respiratory arrest of newborn (P28.81)
respiratory failure of newborn (P28.5)
AHA: 2021,1Q,27,44-45; 2020,4Q,96
✓5th J96.0 **Acute respiratory failure**
J96.00 **Acute respiratory failure, unspecified whether with hypoxia or hypercapnia** HCC ESR COM
AHA: 2016,3Q,14; 2013,4Q,121
J96.01 **Acute respiratory failure with hypoxia** HCC ESR COM
AHA: 2020,3Q,12
J96.02 **Acute respiratory failure with hypercapnia** HCC ESR COM
▶Acute respiratory acidosis◀
✓5th J96.1 **Chronic respiratory failure**
J96.10 **Chronic respiratory failure, unspecified whether with hypoxia or hypercapnia** HCC ESR COM
AHA: 2016,1Q,38; 2015,1Q,21
J96.11 **Chronic respiratory failure with hypoxia** HCC ESR COM
AHA: 2013,4Q,129
J96.12 **Chronic respiratory failure with hypercapnia** HCC ESR COM
▶Chronic respiratory acidosis◀
✓5th J96.2 **Acute and chronic respiratory failure**
Acute on chronic respiratory failure
J96.20 **Acute and chronic respiratory failure, unspecified whether with hypoxia or hypercapnia** HCC ESR COM
J96.21 **Acute and chronic respiratory failure with hypoxia** HCC ESR COM
J96.22 **Acute and chronic respiratory failure with hypercapnia** HCC ESR COM
✓5th J96.9 **Respiratory failure, unspecified**
J96.90 **Respiratory failure, unspecified, unspecified whether with hypoxia or hypercapnia** HCC ESR COM

J96.91 Respiratory failure, unspecified with hypoxia HCC ESR COM

J96.92 Respiratory failure, unspecified with hypercapnia HCC ESR COM

✓4th **J98 Other respiratory disorders**

Use additional code to identify:
- exposure to environmental tobacco smoke (Z77.22)
- exposure to tobacco smoke in the perinatal period (P96.81)
- history of tobacco dependence (Z87.891)
- occupational exposure to environmental tobacco smoke (Z57.31)
- tobacco dependence (F17.-)
- tobacco use (Z72.Ø)

EXCLUDES 1 *newborn apnea ▶(P28.4-)◀*
newborn sleep apnea ▶(P28.3-)◀

EXCLUDES 2 *apnea NOS (RØ6.81)*
sleep apnea (G47.3-)

✓5th **J98.Ø Diseases of bronchus, not elsewhere classified**

J98.Ø1 Acute bronchospasm

EXCLUDES 1 *acute bronchiolitis with bronchospasm (J21.-)*
acute bronchitis with bronchospasm (J2Ø.-)
asthma (J45.-)
exercise induced bronchospasm (J45.99Ø)

J98.Ø9 Other diseases of bronchus, not elsewhere classified
Broncholithiasis
Calcification of bronchus
Stenosis of bronchus
Tracheobronchial collapse
Tracheobronchial dyskinesia
Ulcer of bronchus

✓5th **J98.1 Pulmonary collapse**

EXCLUDES 1 *therapeutic collapse of lung status (Z98.3)*

J98.11 Atelectasis

EXCLUDES 1 *newborn atelectasis*
tuberculous atelectasis (current disease) (A15)

DEF: Collapse of lung tissue affecting part or all of one lung, preventing normal oxygen absorption to healthy tissues.

J98.19 Other pulmonary collapse

J98.2 Interstitial emphysema HCC Rx ESR COM
Mediastinal emphysema

EXCLUDES 1 *emphysema NOS (J43.9)*
emphysema in newborn (P25.Ø)
surgical emphysema (subcutaneous) (T81.82)
traumatic subcutaneous emphysema (T79.7)

J98.3 Compensatory emphysema HCC Rx ESR COM

DEF: Distention of all or part of the lung caused by disease processes or surgical intervention that decreased volume in another part of the lung, causing an overcompensation reaction. Compensatory emphysema occurs in association with pneumonias, pleural effusions, atelectasis, empyema, and pneumothorax.

J98.4 Other disorders of lung
Calcification of lung
Cystic lung disease (acquired)
Lung disease NOS
Pulmolithiasis

EXCLUDES 1 *acute interstitial pneumonitis (J84.114)*
pulmonary insufficiency following surgery (J95.1-J95.2)

✓5th **J98.5 Diseases of mediastinum, not elsewhere classified**

EXCLUDES 2 *abscess of mediastinum (J85.3)*

AHA: 2016,4Q,29

J98.51 Mediastinitis

Code first underlying condition, if applicable, such as postoperative mediastinitis (T81.-)

J98.59 Other diseases of mediastinum, not elsewhere classified
Fibrosis of mediastinum
Hernia of mediastinum
Retraction of mediastinum

J98.6 Disorders of diaphragm
Diaphragmatitis
Paralysis of diaphragm
Relaxation of diaphragm

EXCLUDES 1 *congenital malformation of diaphragm NEC (Q79.1)*
congenital diaphragmatic hernia (Q79.Ø)

EXCLUDES 2 *diaphragmatic hernia (K44.-)*

J98.8 Other specified respiratory disorders

AHA: 2020,1Q,34-36

TIP: Assign as a secondary code for a patient with a respiratory infection that is not further specified but is documented as being associated with COVID-19; assign U07.1 as the principal or first-listed code. If the respiratory infection documentation specifies acute or lower respiratory infection (NOS), assign J22 instead.

J98.9 Respiratory disorder, unspecified
Respiratory disease (chronic) NOS

J99 Respiratory disorders in diseases classified elsewhere HCC Rx ESR COM

Code first underlying disease, such as:
- amyloidosis (E85.-)
- ankylosing spondylitis (M45)
- congenital syphilis (A5Ø.5)
- cryoglobulinemia (D89.1)
- early congenital syphilis (A5Ø.Ø)
- plasminogen deficiency (E88.Ø2)
- schistosomiasis (B65.Ø-B65.9)

EXCLUDES 1 *respiratory disorders in:*
amebiasis (AØ6.5)
blastomycosis (B4Ø.Ø-B4Ø.2)
candidiasis (B37.1)
coccidioidomycosis (B38.Ø-B38.2)
cystic fibrosis with pulmonary manifestations (E84.Ø)
dermatomyositis (M33.Ø1, M33.11)
histoplasmosis (B39.Ø-B39.2)
late syphilis (A52.72, A52.73)
polymyositis (M33.21)
Sjögren syndrome (M35.Ø2)
systemic lupus erythematosus (M32.13)
systemic sclerosis (M34.81)
Wegener's granulomatosis (M31.3Ø-M31.31)

Chapter 11. Diseases of the Digestive System (KØØ–K95)

Chapter-specific Guidelines with Coding Examples
Reserved for future guideline expansion.

Chapter 11. Diseases of the Digestive System (KØØ-K95)

EXCLUDES 2 *certain conditions originating in the perinatal period (PØ4-P96)*
certain infectious and parasitic diseases (AØØ-B99)
complications of pregnancy, childbirth and the puerperium (OØØ-O9A)
congenital malformations, deformations and chromosomal abnormalities (QØØ-Q99)
endocrine, nutritional and metabolic diseases (EØØ-E88)
injury, poisoning and certain other consequences of external causes (SØØ-T88)
neoplasms (CØØ-D49)
symptoms, signs and abnormal clinical and laboratory findings, not elsewhere classified (RØØ-R94)

This chapter contains the following blocks:

KØØ-K14 Diseases of oral cavity and salivary glands
K2Ø-K31 Diseases of esophagus, stomach and duodenum
K35-K38 Diseases of appendix
K4Ø-K46 Hernia
K5Ø-K52 Noninfective enteritis and colitis
K55-K64 Other diseases of intestines
K65-K68 Diseases of peritoneum and retroperitoneum
K7Ø-K77 Diseases of liver
K8Ø-K87 Disorders of gallbladder, biliary tract and pancreas
K9Ø-K95 Other diseases of the digestive system

Diseases of oral cavity and salivary glands (KØØ-K14)

✓4th **KØØ Disorders of tooth development and eruption**
EXCLUDES 2 *embedded and impacted teeth (KØ1.-)*

KØØ.Ø Anodontia
Hypodontia
Oligodontia
EXCLUDES 1 *acquired absence of teeth (KØ8.1-)*
DEF: Partial or complete absence of teeth due to a congenital defect involving the tooth bud.

KØØ.1 Supernumerary teeth
Distomolar
Fourth molar
Mesiodens
Paramolar
Supplementary teeth
EXCLUDES 2 *supernumerary roots (KØØ.2)*

KØØ.2 Abnormalities of size and form of teeth
Concrescence of teeth
Fusion of teeth
Gemination of teeth
Dens evaginatus
Dens in dente
Dens invaginatus
Enamel pearls
Macrodontia
Microdontia
Peg-shaped [conical] teeth
Supernumerary roots
Taurodontism
Tuberculum paramolare
EXCLUDES 1 *abnormalities of teeth due to congenital syphilis (A5Ø.5)*
tuberculum Carabelli, which is regarded as a normal variation and should not be coded

KØØ.3 Mottled teeth
Dental fluorosis
Mottling of enamel
Nonfluoride enamel opacities
EXCLUDES 2 *deposits [accretions] on teeth (KØ3.6)*

KØØ.4 Disturbances in tooth formation
Aplasia and hypoplasia of cementum
Dilaceration of tooth
Enamel hypoplasia (neonatal) (postnatal) (prenatal)
Regional odontodysplasia
Turner's tooth
EXCLUDES 1 *Hutchinson's teeth and mulberry molars in congenital syphilis (A5Ø.5)*
EXCLUDES 2 *mottled teeth (KØØ.3)*

KØØ.5 Hereditary disturbances in tooth structure, not elsewhere classified
Amelogenesis imperfecta
Dentinogenesis imperfecta
Odontogenesis imperfecta
Dentinal dysplasia
Shell teeth

KØØ.6 Disturbances in tooth eruption
Dentia praecox
Natal tooth
Neonatal tooth
Premature eruption of tooth
Premature shedding of primary [deciduous] tooth
Prenatal teeth
Retained [persistent] primary tooth
EXCLUDES 2 *embedded and impacted teeth (KØ1.-)*

KØØ.7 Teething syndrome

KØØ.8 Other disorders of tooth development
Color changes during tooth formation
Intrinsic staining of teeth NOS
EXCLUDES 2 *posteruptive color changes (KØ3.7)*

KØØ.9 Disorder of tooth development, unspecified
Disorder of odontogenesis NOS

✓4th **KØ1 Embedded and impacted teeth**
EXCLUDES 1 *abnormal position of fully erupted teeth (M26.3-)*

KØ1.Ø Embedded teeth

KØ1.1 Impacted teeth

✓4th **KØ2 Dental caries**
INCLUDES caries of dentine
dental cavities
early childhood caries
pre-eruptive caries
recurrent caries (dentino enamel junction) (enamel) (to the pulp)
tooth decay

Tooth Anatomy

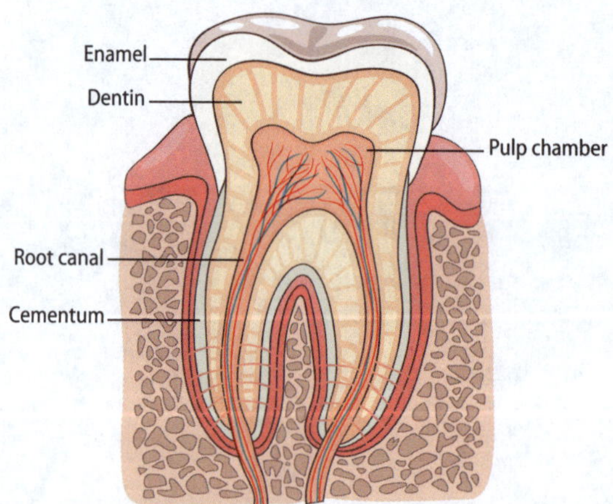

KØ2.3 Arrested dental caries
Arrested coronal and root caries

✓5th **KØ2.5 Dental caries on pit and fissure surface**
Dental caries on chewing surface of tooth

KØ2.51 Dental caries on pit and fissure surface limited to enamel
White spot lesions [initial caries] on pit and fissure surface of tooth

KØ2.52 Dental caries on pit and fissure surface penetrating into dentin
Primary dental caries, cervical origin

KØ2.53 Dental caries on pit and fissure surface penetrating into pulp

✓5th **KØ2.6 Dental caries on smooth surface**

KØ2.61 Dental caries on smooth surface limited to enamel
White spot lesions [initial caries] on smooth surface of tooth

KØ2.62 Dental caries on smooth surface penetrating into dentin

KØ2.63 Dental caries on smooth surface penetrating into pulp

KØ2.7 Dental root caries

KØ2.9 Dental caries, unspecified

KØ3 Other diseases of hard tissues of teeth

EXCLUDES 2 *bruxism (F45.8)*
dental caries (KØ2.-)
teeth-grinding NOS (F45.8)

KØ3.Ø Excessive attrition of teeth
Approximal wear of teeth
Occlusal wear of teeth
DEF: Attrition: In dentistry, wearing away or erosion of tooth surface from abrasive food or grinding teeth.

KØ3.1 Abrasion of teeth
Dentifrice abrasion of teeth
Habitual abrasion of teeth
Occupational abrasion of teeth
Ritual abrasion of teeth
Traditional abrasion of teeth
Wedge defect NOS

KØ3.2 Erosion of teeth
Erosion of teeth due to diet
Erosion of teeth due to drugs and medicaments
Erosion of teeth due to persistent vomiting
Erosion of teeth NOS
Idiopathic erosion of teeth
Occupational erosion of teeth

KØ3.3 Pathological resorption of teeth
Internal granuloma of pulp
Resorption of teeth (external)

KØ3.4 Hypercementosis
Cementation hyperplasia

KØ3.5 Ankylosis of teeth

KØ3.6 Deposits [accretions] on teeth
Betel deposits [accretions] on teeth
Black deposits [accretions] on teeth
Extrinsic staining of teeth NOS
Green deposits [accretions] on teeth
Materia alba deposits [accretions] on teeth
Orange deposits [accretions] on teeth
Staining of teeth NOS
Subgingival dental calculus
Supragingival dental calculus
Tobacco deposits [accretions] on teeth

KØ3.7 Posteruptive color changes of dental hard tissues
EXCLUDES 2 *deposits [accretions] on teeth (KØ3.6)*

KØ3.8 Other specified diseases of hard tissues of teeth

KØ3.81 Cracked tooth
EXCLUDES 1 *asymptomatic craze lines in enamel - omit code*
broken or fractured tooth due to trauma (SØ2.5)

KØ3.89 Other specified diseases of hard tissues of teeth

KØ3.9 Disease of hard tissues of teeth, unspecified

KØ4 Diseases of pulp and periapical tissues
AHA: 2016,4Q,29-30

KØ4.Ø Pulpitis
Acute pulpitis
Chronic (hyperplastic) (ulcerative) pulpitis

KØ4.Ø1 Reversible pulpitis

KØ4.Ø2 Irreversible pulpitis

KØ4.1 Necrosis of pulp
Pulpal gangrene

KØ4.2 Pulp degeneration
Denticles
Pulpal calcifications
Pulpal stones

KØ4.3 Abnormal hard tissue formation in pulp
Secondary or irregular dentine

KØ4.4 Acute apical periodontitis of pulpal origin
Acute apical periodontitis NOS
EXCLUDES 1 *acute periodontitis (KØ5.2-)*
DEF: Severe inflammation of the area surrounding the tip of a tooth's root that is often secondary to infection or trauma.

KØ4.5 Chronic apical periodontitis
Apical or periapical granuloma
Apical periodontitis NOS
EXCLUDES 1 *chronic periodontitis (KØ5.3-)*

KØ4.6 Periapical abscess with sinus
Dental abscess with sinus
Dentoalveolar abscess with sinus

KØ4.7 Periapical abscess without sinus
Dental abscess without sinus
Dentoalveolar abscess without sinus

KØ4.8 Radicular cyst
Apical (periodontal) cyst
Periapical cyst
Residual radicular cyst
EXCLUDES 2 *lateral periodontal cyst (KØ9.Ø)*
DEF: Most common odontogenic cyst in tissue around the tooth apex due to chronic inflammation of dental pulp.

KØ4.9 Other and unspecified diseases of pulp and periapical tissues

KØ4.9Ø Unspecified diseases of pulp and periapical tissues

KØ4.99 Other diseases of pulp and periapical tissues

KØ5 Gingivitis and periodontal diseases
Use additional code to identify:
alcohol abuse and dependence (F1Ø.-)
exposure to environmental tobacco smoke (Z77.22)
exposure to tobacco smoke in the perinatal period (P96.81)
history of tobacco dependence (Z87.891)
occupational exposure to environmental tobacco smoke (Z57.31)
tobacco dependence (F17.-)
tobacco use (Z72.Ø)
AHA: 2016,4Q,29-30

KØ5.Ø Acute gingivitis
EXCLUDES 1 *acute necrotizing ulcerative gingivitis (A69.1)*
herpesviral [herpes simplex] gingivostomatitis (BØØ.2)

KØ5.ØØ Acute gingivitis, plaque induced
Acute gingivitis NOS
Plaque induced gingival disease

KØ5.Ø1 Acute gingivitis, non-plaque induced

KØ5.1 Chronic gingivitis
Desquamative gingivitis (chronic)
Gingivitis (chronic) NOS
Hyperplastic gingivitis (chronic)
Pregnancy associated gingivitis
Simple marginal gingivitis (chronic)
Ulcerative gingivitis (chronic)
Code first, if applicable, diseases of the digestive system complicating pregnacy (O99.61-)

KØ5.1Ø Chronic gingivitis, plaque induced
Chronic gingivitis NOS
Gingivitis NOS

KØ5.11 Chronic gingivitis, non-plaque induced

KØ5.2 Aggressive periodontitis
Acute pericoronitis
EXCLUDES 1 *acute apical periodontitis (KØ4.4)*
periapical abscess (KØ4.7)
periapical abscess with sinus (KØ4.6)

KØ5.2Ø Aggressive periodontitis, unspecified

KØ5.21 Aggressive periodontitis, localized
Periodontal abscess

KØ5.211 Aggressive periodontitis, localized, slight

KØ5.212 Aggressive periodontitis, localized, moderate

KØ5.213 Aggressive periodontitis, localized, severe

KØ5.219 Aggressive periodontitis, localized, unspecified severity

KØ5.22 Aggressive periodontitis, generalized

KØ5.221 Aggressive periodontitis, generalized, slight

KØ5.222 Aggressive periodontitis, generalized, moderate

KØ5.223 Aggressive periodontitis, generalized, severe

KØ5.229 Aggressive periodontitis, generalized, unspecified severity

KØ5.3 Chronic periodontitis
Chronic pericoronitis
Complex periodontitis
Periodontitis NOS
Simplex periodontitis
EXCLUDES 1 *chronic apical periodontitis (KØ4.5)*

KØ5.3Ø Chronic periodontitis, unspecified

KØ5.31 Chronic periodontitis, localized
- **KØ5.311 Chronic periodontitis, localized, slight**
- **KØ5.312 Chronic periodontitis, localized, moderate**
- **KØ5.313 Chronic periodontitis, localized, severe**
- **KØ5.319 Chronic periodontitis, localized, unspecified severity**

KØ5.32 Chronic periodontitis, generalized
- **KØ5.321 Chronic periodontitis, generalized, slight**
- **KØ5.322 Chronic periodontitis, generalized, moderate**
- **KØ5.323 Chronic periodontitis, generalized, severe**
- **KØ5.329 Chronic periodontitis, generalized, unspecified**

KØ5.4 Periodontosis
Juvenile periodontosis

KØ5.5 Other periodontal diseases
Combined periodontic-endodontic lesion
Narrow gingival width (of periodontal soft tissue)
EXCLUDES 2 *leukoplakia of gingiva (K13.21)*

KØ5.6 Periodontal disease, unspecified

KØ6 Other disorders of gingiva and edentulous alveolar ridge
EXCLUDES 2 *acute gingivitis (KØ5.Ø)*
atrophy of edentulous alveolar ridge (KØ8.2)
chronic gingivitis (KØ5.1)
gingivitis NOS (KØ5.1)
AHA: 2016,4Q,29-30

KØ6.Ø Gingival recession
Gingival recession (postinfective) (postprocedural)
AHA: 2017,4Q,16

KØ6.Ø1 Gingival recession, localized
- **KØ6.Ø1Ø Localized gingival recession, unspecified**
  Localized gingival recession, NOS
- **KØ6.Ø11 Localized gingival recession, minimal**
- **KØ6.Ø12 Localized gingival recession, moderate**
- **KØ6.Ø13 Localized gingival recession, severe**

KØ6.Ø2 Gingival recession, generalized
- **KØ6.Ø2Ø Generalized gingival recession, unspecified**
  Generalized gingival recession, NOS
- **KØ6.Ø21 Generalized gingival recession, minimal**
- **KØ6.Ø22 Generalized gingival recession, moderate**
- **KØ6.Ø23 Generalized gingival recession, severe**

KØ6.1 Gingival enlargement
Gingival fibromatosis

KØ6.2 Gingival and edentulous alveolar ridge lesions associated with trauma
Irritative hyperplasia of edentulous ridge [denture hyperplasia]
Use additional code (Chapter 2Ø) to identify external cause or denture status (Z97.2)

KØ6.3 Horizontal alveolar bone loss

KØ6.8 Other specified disorders of gingiva and edentulous alveolar ridge
Fibrous epulis
Flabby alveolar ridge
Giant cell epulis
Peripheral giant cell granuloma of gingiva
Pyogenic granuloma of gingiva
Vertical ridge deficiency
EXCLUDES 2 *gingival cyst (KØ9.Ø)*

KØ6.9 Disorder of gingiva and edentulous alveolar ridge, unspecified

KØ8 Other disorders of teeth and supporting structures
EXCLUDES 2 *dentofacial anomalies [including malocclusion] (M26.-)*
disorders of jaw (M27.-)
AHA: 2016,4Q,29-30

KØ8.Ø Exfoliation of teeth due to systemic causes
Code also underlying systemic condition

KØ8.1 Complete loss of teeth
Acquired loss of teeth, complete
EXCLUDES 1 *congenital absence of teeth (KØØ.Ø)*
exfoliation of teeth due to systemic causes (KØ8.Ø)
partial loss of teeth (KØ8.4-)

KØ8.1Ø Complete loss of teeth, unspecified cause
- **KØ8.1Ø1 Complete loss of teeth, unspecified cause, class I**
- **KØ8.1Ø2 Complete loss of teeth, unspecified cause, class II**
- **KØ8.1Ø3 Complete loss of teeth, unspecified cause, class III**
- **KØ8.1Ø4 Complete loss of teeth, unspecified cause, class IV**
- **KØ8.1Ø9 Complete loss of teeth, unspecified cause, unspecified class**
  Edentulism NOS

KØ8.11 Complete loss of teeth due to trauma
- **KØ8.111 Complete loss of teeth due to trauma, class I**
- **KØ8.112 Complete loss of teeth due to trauma, class II**
- **KØ8.113 Complete loss of teeth due to trauma, class III**
- **KØ8.114 Complete loss of teeth due to trauma, class IV**
- **KØ8.119 Complete loss of teeth due to trauma, unspecified class**

KØ8.12 Complete loss of teeth due to periodontal diseases
- **KØ8.121 Complete loss of teeth due to periodontal diseases, class I**
- **KØ8.122 Complete loss of teeth due to periodontal diseases, class II**
- **KØ8.123 Complete loss of teeth due to periodontal diseases, class III**
- **KØ8.124 Complete loss of teeth due to periodontal diseases, class IV**
- **KØ8.129 Complete loss of teeth due to periodontal diseases, unspecified class**

KØ8.13 Complete loss of teeth due to caries
- **KØ8.131 Complete loss of teeth due to caries, class I**
- **KØ8.132 Complete loss of teeth due to caries, class II**
- **KØ8.133 Complete loss of teeth due to caries, class III**
- **KØ8.134 Complete loss of teeth due to caries, class IV**
- **KØ8.139 Complete loss of teeth due to caries, unspecified class**

KØ8.19 Complete loss of teeth due to other specified cause
- **KØ8.191 Complete loss of teeth due to other specified cause, class I**
- **KØ8.192 Complete loss of teeth due to other specified cause, class II**
- **KØ8.193 Complete loss of teeth due to other specified cause, class III**
- **KØ8.194 Complete loss of teeth due to other specified cause, class IV**
- **KØ8.199 Complete loss of teeth due to other specified cause, unspecified class**

KØ8.2 Atrophy of edentulous alveolar ridge
- **KØ8.2Ø Unspecified atrophy of edentulous alveolar ridge**
  Atrophy of the mandible NOS
  Atrophy of the maxilla NOS
- **KØ8.21 Minimal atrophy of the mandible**
  Minimal atrophy of the edentulous mandible
- **KØ8.22 Moderate atrophy of the mandible**
  Moderate atrophy of the edentulous mandible
- **KØ8.23 Severe atrophy of the mandible**
  Severe atrophy of the edentulous mandible
- **KØ8.24 Minimal atrophy of maxilla**
  Minimal atrophy of the edentulous maxilla
- **KØ8.25 Moderate atrophy of the maxilla**
  Moderate atrophy of the edentulous maxilla
- **KØ8.26 Severe atrophy of the maxilla**
  Severe atrophy of the edentulous maxilla

KØ8.3 Retained dental root

K08.4 Partial loss of teeth
Acquired loss of teeth, partial
EXCLUDES 1 *complete loss of teeth (K08.1-)*
congenital absence of teeth (K00.0)
EXCLUDES 2 *exfoliation of teeth due to systemic causes (K08.0)*

K08.40 Partial loss of teeth, unspecified cause
K08.401 Partial loss of teeth, unspecified cause, class I
K08.402 Partial loss of teeth, unspecified cause, class II
K08.403 Partial loss of teeth, unspecified cause, class III
K08.404 Partial loss of teeth, unspecified cause, class IV
K08.409 Partial loss of teeth, unspecified cause, unspecified class
Tooth extraction status NOS

K08.41 Partial loss of teeth due to trauma
K08.411 Partial loss of teeth due to trauma, class I
K08.412 Partial loss of teeth due to trauma, class II
K08.413 Partial loss of teeth due to trauma, class III
K08.414 Partial loss of teeth due to trauma, class IV
K08.419 Partial loss of teeth due to trauma, unspecified class

K08.42 Partial loss of teeth due to periodontal diseases
K08.421 Partial loss of teeth due to periodontal diseases, class I
K08.422 Partial loss of teeth due to periodontal diseases, class II
K08.423 Partial loss of teeth due to periodontal diseases, class III
K08.424 Partial loss of teeth due to periodontal diseases, class IV
K08.429 Partial loss of teeth due to periodontal diseases, unspecified class

K08.43 Partial loss of teeth due to caries
K08.431 Partial loss of teeth due to caries, class I
K08.432 Partial loss of teeth due to caries, class II
K08.433 Partial loss of teeth due to caries, class III
K08.434 Partial loss of teeth due to caries, class IV
K08.439 Partial loss of teeth due to caries, unspecified class

K08.49 Partial loss of teeth due to other specified cause
K08.491 Partial loss of teeth due to other specified cause, class I
K08.492 Partial loss of teeth due to other specified cause, class II
K08.493 Partial loss of teeth due to other specified cause, class III
K08.494 Partial loss of teeth due to other specified cause, class IV
K08.499 Partial loss of teeth due to other specified cause, unspecified class

K08.5 Unsatisfactory restoration of tooth
Defective bridge, crown, filling
Defective dental restoration
EXCLUDES 1 *dental restoration status (Z98.811)*
EXCLUDES 2 *endosseous dental implant failure (M27.6-)*
unsatisfactory endodontic treatment (M27.5-)

K08.50 Unsatisfactory restoration of tooth, unspecified
Defective dental restoration NOS

K08.51 Open restoration margins of tooth
Dental restoration failure of marginal integrity
Open margin on tooth restoration
Poor gingival margin to tooth restoration

K08.52 Unrepairable overhanging of dental restorative materials
Overhanging of tooth restoration

K08.53 Fractured dental restorative material
EXCLUDES 1 *cracked tooth (K03.81)*
traumatic fracture of tooth (S02.5)
K08.530 Fractured dental restorative material without loss of material
K08.531 Fractured dental restorative material with loss of material
K08.539 Fractured dental restorative material, unspecified

K08.54 Contour of existing restoration of tooth biologically incompatible with oral health
Dental restoration failure of periodontal anatomical integrity
Unacceptable contours of existing restoration of tooth
Unacceptable morphology of existing restoration of tooth

K08.55 Allergy to existing dental restorative material
Use additional code to identify the specific type of allergy

K08.56 Poor aesthetic of existing restoration of tooth
Dental restoration aesthetically inadequate or displeasing

K08.59 Other unsatisfactory restoration of tooth
Other defective dental restoration

K08.8 Other specified disorders of teeth and supporting structures
K08.81 Primary occlusal trauma
K08.82 Secondary occlusal trauma
K08.89 Other specified disorders of teeth and supporting structures
Enlargement of alveolar ridge NOS
Insufficient anatomic crown height
Insufficient clinical crown length
Irregular alveolar process
Toothache NOS

K08.9 Disorder of teeth and supporting structures, unspecified

K09 Cysts of oral region, not elsewhere classified
INCLUDES lesions showing histological features both of aneurysmal cyst and of another fibro-osseous lesion
EXCLUDES 2 *cysts of jaw (M27.0-, M27.4-)*
radicular cyst (K04.8)

K09.0 Developmental odontogenic cysts
Dentigerous cyst
Eruption cyst
Follicular cyst
Gingival cyst
Lateral periodontal cyst
Primordial cyst
EXCLUDES 2 *keratocysts (D16.4, D16.5)*
odontogenic keratocystic tumors (D16.4, D16.5)

K09.1 Developmental (nonodontogenic) cysts of oral region
Cyst (of) incisive canal
Cyst (of) palatine of papilla
Globulomaxillary cyst
Median palatal cyst
Nasoalveolar cyst
Nasolabial cyst
Nasopalatine duct cyst

K09.8 Other cysts of oral region, not elsewhere classified
Dermoid cyst
Epidermoid cyst
Lymphoepithelial cyst
Epstein's pearl

K09.9 Cyst of oral region, unspecified

K11 Diseases of salivary glands
Use additional code to identify:
alcohol abuse and dependence (F10.-)
exposure to environmental tobacco smoke (Z77.22)
exposure to tobacco smoke in the perinatal period (P96.81)
history of tobacco dependence (Z87.891)
occupational exposure to environmental tobacco smoke (Z57.31)
tobacco dependence (F17.-)
tobacco use (Z72.0)

K11.0 Atrophy of salivary gland
K11.1 Hypertrophy of salivary gland
DEF: Overgrowth of or enlarged salivary gland tissue caused by infection, salivary duct blockage, autoimmune diseases, and benign and malignant tumors.

K11.2 Sialoadenitis
Parotitis
EXCLUDES 1 *epidemic parotitis (B26.-)*
mumps (B26.-)
uveoparotid fever [Heerfordt] (D86.89)
DEF: Inflammation of the salivary gland.
K11.20 Sialoadenitis, unspecified

Additional Character Required | Placeholder Alert | Manifestation | Unspecified Dx | QPP | UPD Unacceptable PDx

K11.21 Acute sialoadenitis
EXCLUDES 1 *acute recurrent sialoadenitis (K11.22)*

K11.22 Acute recurrent sialoadenitis

K11.23 Chronic sialoadenitis

K11.3 Abscess of salivary gland

K11.4 Fistula of salivary gland
EXCLUDES 1 *congenital fistula of salivary gland (Q38.4)*

K11.5 Sialolithiasis
Calculus of salivary gland or duct
Stone of salivary gland or duct

K11.6 Mucocele of salivary gland
Mucous extravasation cyst of salivary gland
Mucous retention cyst of salivary gland
Ranula

K11.7 Disturbances of salivary secretion
Hypoptyalism
Ptyalism
Xerostomia
EXCLUDES 2 *dry mouth NOS (R68.2)*

K11.8 Other diseases of salivary glands
Benign lymphoepithelial lesion of salivary gland
Mikulicz' disease
Necrotizing sialometaplasia
Sialectasia
Stenosis of salivary duct
Stricture of salivary duct
EXCLUDES 1 *Sjögren syndrome (M35.Ø-)*

K11.9 Disease of salivary gland, unspecified
Sialoadenopathy NOS

4th K12 Stomatitis and related lesions
Use additional code to identify:
alcohol abuse and dependence (F1Ø.-)
exposure to environmental tobacco smoke (Z77.22)
exposure to tobacco smoke in the perinatal period (P96.81)
history of tobacco dependence (Z87.891)
occupational exposure to environmental tobacco smoke (Z57.31)
tobacco dependence (F17.-)
tobacco use (Z72.Ø)
EXCLUDES 1 *cancrum oris (A69.Ø)*
cheilitis (K13.Ø)
gangrenous stomatitis (A69.Ø)
herpesviral [herpes simplex] gingivostomatitis (BØØ.2)
noma (A69.Ø)

K12.Ø Recurrent oral aphthae
Aphthous stomatitis (major) (minor)
Bednar's aphthae
Periadenitis mucosa necrotica recurrens
Recurrent aphthous ulcer
Stomatitis herpetiformis
DEF: Disorder of unknown etiology with small oval or round painful ulcers of the mouth marked by a grayish exudate and a red halo effect.

K12.1 Other forms of stomatitis
Stomatitis NOS
Denture stomatitis
Ulcerative stomatitis
Vesicular stomatitis
EXCLUDES 1 *acute necrotizing ulcerative stomatitis (A69.1)*
Vincent's stomatitis (A69.1)

K12.2 Cellulitis and abscess of mouth
Cellulitis of mouth (floor)
Submandibular abscess
EXCLUDES 2 *abscess of salivary gland (K11.3)*
abscess of tongue (K14.Ø)
periapical abscess (KØ4.6-KØ4.7)
periodontal abscess (KØ5.21)
peritonsillar abscess (J36)

5th K12.3 Oral mucositis (ulcerative)
Mucositis (oral) (oropharyneal)
EXCLUDES 2 *gastrointestinal mucositis (ulcerative) (K92.81)*
mucositis (ulcerative) of vagina and vulva (N76.81)
nasal mucositis (ulcerative) (J34.81)

K12.3Ø Oral mucositis (ulcerative), unspecified

K12.31 Oral mucositis (ulcerative) due to antineoplastic therapy
Use additional code for adverse effect, if applicable, to identify antineoplastic and immunosuppressive drugs (T45.1X5)
Use additional code for other antineoplastic therapy, such as:
radiological procedure and radiotherapy (Y84.2)

K12.32 Oral mucositis (ulcerative) due to other drugs
Use additional code for adverse effect, if applicable, to identify drug (T36-T5Ø with fifth or sixth character 5)

K12.33 Oral mucositis (ulcerative) due to radiation
Use additional external cause code (W88-W9Ø, X39.Ø-) to identify cause

K12.39 Other oral mucositis (ulcerative)
Viral oral mucositis (ulcerative)

4th K13 Other diseases of lip and oral mucosa
INCLUDES epithelial disturbances of tongue
Use additional code to identify:
alcohol abuse and dependence (F1Ø.-)
exposure to environmental tobacco smoke (Z77.22)
exposure to tobacco smoke in the perinatal period (P96.81)
history of tobacco dependence (Z87.891)
occupational exposure to environmental tobacco smoke (Z57.31)
tobacco dependence (F17.-)
tobacco use (Z72.Ø)
EXCLUDES 2 *certain disorders of gingiva and edentulous alveolar ridge (KØ5-KØ6)*
cysts of oral region (KØ9.-)
diseases of tongue (K14.-)
stomatitis and related lesions (K12.-)

K13.Ø Diseases of lips
Abscess of lips
Angular cheilitis
Cellulitis of lips
Cheilitis NOS
Cheilodynia
Cheilosis
Exfoliative cheilitis
Fistula of lips
Glandular cheilitis
Hypertrophy of lips
Perlèche NEC
EXCLUDES 1 *ariboflavinosis (E53.Ø)*
cheilitis due to radiation-related disorders (L55-L59)
congenital fistula of lips (Q38.Ø)
congenital hypertrophy of lips (Q18.6)
perlèche due to candidiasis (B37.83)
perlèche due to riboflavin deficiency (E53.Ø)

K13.1 Cheek and lip biting

5th K13.2 Leukoplakia and other disturbances of oral epithelium, including tongue
EXCLUDES 1 *carcinoma in situ of oral epithelium (DØØ.Ø-)*
hairy leukoplakia (K13.3)
DEF: Leukoplakia: Thickened white patches or lesions appearing on a mucous membrane, such as oral mucosa or tongue.

K13.21 Leukoplakia of oral mucosa, including tongue
Leukokeratosis of oral mucosa
Leukoplakia of gingiva, lips, tongue
EXCLUDES 1 *hairy leukoplakia (K13.3)*
leukokeratosis nicotina palati (K13.24)

K13.22 Minimal keratinized residual ridge mucosa
Minimal keratinization of alveolar ridge mucosa

K13.23 Excessive keratinized residual ridge mucosa
Excessive keratinization of alveolar ridge mucosa

K13.24 Leukokeratosis nicotina palati
Smoker's palate

K13.29 Other disturbances of oral epithelium, including tongue
Erythroplakia of mouth or tongue
Focal epithelial hyperplasia of mouth or tongue
Leukoedema of mouth or tongue
Other oral epithelium disturbances

K13.3 Hairy leukoplakia

K13.4 Granuloma and granuloma-like lesions of oral mucosa
Eosinophilic granuloma
Granuloma pyogenicum
Verrucous xanthoma

K13.5 Oral submucous fibrosis
Submucous fibrosis of tongue

K13.6 Irritative hyperplasia of oral mucosa
EXCLUDES 2 *irritative hyperplasia of edentulous ridge [denture hyperplasia] (K06.2)*

K13.7 Other and unspecified lesions of oral mucosa

K13.70 Unspecified lesions of oral mucosa

K13.79 Other lesions of oral mucosa
Focal oral mucinosis
AHA: 2022,2Q,7

K14 Diseases of tongue
Use additional code to identify:
alcohol abuse and dependence (F10.-)
exposure to environmental tobacco smoke (Z77.22)
history of tobacco dependence (Z87.891)
occupational exposure to environmental tobacco smoke (Z57.31)
tobacco dependence (F17.-)
tobacco use (Z72.0)
EXCLUDES 2 *erythroplakia (K13.29)*
focal epithelial hyperplasia (K13.29)
leukedema of tongue (K13.29)
leukoplakia of tongue (K13.21)
hairy leukoplakia (K13.3)
macroglossia (congenital) (Q38.2)
submucous fibrosis of tongue (K13.5)

K14.0 Glossitis
Abscess of tongue
Ulceration (traumatic) of tongue
EXCLUDES 1 *atrophic glossitis (K14.4)*
DEF: Inflammation and swelling of the tongue that may be associated with infection, adverse drug reactions, smoking, or injury.

K14.1 Geographic tongue
Benign migratory glossitis
Glossitis areata exfoliativa

K14.2 Median rhomboid glossitis

K14.3 Hypertrophy of tongue papillae
Black hairy tongue
Coated tongue
Hypertrophy of foliate papillae
Lingua villosa nigra

K14.4 Atrophy of tongue papillae
Atrophic glossitis

K14.5 Plicated tongue
Fissured tongue
Furrowed tongue
Scrotal tongue
EXCLUDES 1 *fissured tongue, congenital (Q38.3)*

K14.6 Glossodynia
Glossopyrosis
Painful tongue

K14.8 Other diseases of tongue
Atrophy of tongue
Crenated tongue
Enlargement of tongue
Glossocele
Glossoptosis
Hypertrophy of tongue

K14.9 Disease of tongue, unspecified
Glossopathy NOS

Diseases of esophagus, stomach and duodenum (K20-K31)

EXCLUDES 2 *hiatus hernia (K44.-)*

K20 Esophagitis
Use additional code to identify:
alcohol abuse and dependence (F10.-)
EXCLUDES 1 *erosion of esophagus (K22.1-)*
esophagitis with gastro-esophageal reflux disease (K21.0-)
reflux esophagitis (K21.0-)
ulcerative esophagitis (K22.1-)
EXCLUDES 2 *eosinophilic gastritis or gastroenteritis (K52.81)*

K20.0 Eosinophilic esophagitis
AHA: 2020,4Q,9

K20.8 Other esophagitis
AHA: 2020,4Q,28-29

K20.80 Other esophagitis without bleeding
Abscess of esophagus
Other esophagitis NOS

K20.81 Other esophagitis with bleeding

K20.9 Esophagitis, unspecified
AHA: 2020,4Q,28-29

K20.90 Esophagitis, unspecified without bleeding
Esophagitis NOS

K20.91 Esophagitis, unspecified with bleeding

K21 Gastro-esophageal reflux disease
EXCLUDES 1 *newborn esophageal reflux (P78.83)*

K21.0 Gastro-esophageal reflux disease with esophagitis
AHA: 2020,4Q,28-29

K21.00 Gastro-esophageal reflux disease with esophagitis, without bleeding
Reflux esophagitis

K21.01 Gastro-esophageal reflux disease with esophagitis, with bleeding

K21.9 Gastro-esophageal reflux disease without esophagitis
Esophageal reflux NOS
AHA: 2016,1Q,18

K22 Other diseases of esophagus
EXCLUDES 2 *esophageal varices (I85.-)*

K22.0 Achalasia of cardia
Achalasia NOS
Cardiospasm
EXCLUDES 1 *congenital cardiospasm (Q39.5)*
DEF: Esophageal motility disorder that is caused by absence of the esophageal peristalsis and impaired relaxation of the lower esophageal sphincter. It is characterized by dysphagia, regurgitation, and heartburn.

K22.1 Ulcer of esophagus
Barrett's ulcer
Erosion of esophagus
Fungal ulcer of esophagus
Peptic ulcer of esophagus
Ulcer of esophagus due to ingestion of chemicals
Ulcer of esophagus due to ingestion of drugs and medicaments
Ulcerative esophagitis
Code first poisoning due to drug or toxin, if applicable (T36-T65 with fifth or sixth character 1-4 or 6)
Use additional code for adverse effect, if applicable, to identify drug (T36-T50 with fifth or sixth character 5)
EXCLUDES 1 *Barrett's esophagus (K22.7-)*
AHA: 2018,3Q,22; 2017,3Q,27
TIP: Assign a code for "with bleeding" when an esophageal ulcer and bleeding (hematemesis) are documented. The ICD-10-CM classification assumes the two are related without the provider linking the two conditions. Evidence of bleeding during a procedure is not required.

K22.10 Ulcer of esophagus without bleeding
Ulcer of esophagus NOS

K22.11 Ulcer of esophagus with bleeding
EXCLUDES 2 *bleeding esophageal varices (I85.01, I85.11)*
TIP: For bleeding esophageal ulcers resulting from anticoagulant therapy, assign this code, code D68.32 Hemorrhagic disorder due to extrinsic circulating anticoagulant, and adverse effect code T45.515- with the appropriate seventh character.

K22.2 Esophageal obstruction
Compression of esophagus
Constriction of esophagus
Stenosis of esophagus
Stricture of esophagus
EXCLUDES 1 *congenital stenosis or stricture of esophagus (Q39.3)*

K22.3 Perforation of esophagus
Rupture of esophagus
EXCLUDES 1 *traumatic perforation of (thoracic) esophagus (S27.8-)*

K22.4 Dyskinesia of esophagus
Corkscrew esophagus
Diffuse esophageal spasm
Spasm of esophagus
EXCLUDES 1 *cardiospasm (K22.Ø)*

K22.5 Diverticulum of esophagus, acquired
Esophageal pouch, acquired
EXCLUDES 1 *diverticulum of esophagus (congenital) (Q39.6)*

K22.6 Gastro-esophageal laceration-hemorrhage syndrome
Mallory-Weiss syndrome

✓5th **K22.7 Barrett's esophagus**
Barrett's disease
Barrett's syndrome
EXCLUDES 1 *Barrett's ulcer (K22.1)*
malignant neoplasm of esophagus (C15.-)
DEF: Metaplastic disorder in which specialized columnar epithelial cells replace the normal squamous epithelial cells. Secondary to chronic gastroesophageal reflux damage to the mucosa, this disorder increases the risk of developing adenocarcinoma.

K22.7Ø Barrett's esophagus without dysplasia Q
Barrett's esophagus NOS

✓6th **K22.71 Barrett's esophagus with dysplasia**

K22.71Ø Barrett's esophagus with low grade dysplasia Q

K22.711 Barrett's esophagus with high grade dysplasia Q

K22.719 Barrett's esophagus with dysplasia, unspecified Q

✓5th **K22.8 Other specified diseases of esophagus**
EXCLUDES 2 *esophageal varices (I85.-)*
Paterson-Kelly syndrome (D5Ø.1)
AHA: 2021,4Q,15; 2020,1Q,16

K22.81 Esophageal polyp
EXCLUDES 1 *benign neoplasm of esophagus (D13.Ø)*

K22.82 Esophagogastric junction polyp
EXCLUDES 1 *benign neoplasm of stomach (D13.1)*

K22.89 Other specified disease of esophagus
Hemorrhage of esophagus NOS

K22.9 Disease of esophagus, unspecified

K23 Disorders of esophagus in diseases classified elsewhere
Code first underlying disease, such as:
congenital syphilis (A5Ø.5)
EXCLUDES 1 *late syphilis (A52.79)*
megaesophagus due to Chagas' disease (B57.31)
tuberculosis (A18.83)

✓4th **K25 Gastric ulcer**
INCLUDES erosion (acute) of stomach
pylorus ulcer (peptic)
stomach ulcer (peptic)
Use additional code to identify:
alcohol abuse and dependence (F1Ø.-)
EXCLUDES 1 *acute gastritis (K29.Ø-)*
peptic ulcer NOS (K27.-)
AHA: 2021,1Q,9,11; 2017,3Q,27
TIP: Assign a code for "with hemorrhage" when a gastric ulcer and GI bleeding are documented. The ICD-10-CM classification assumes the two are related without the provider linking the two conditions. Evidence of bleeding during a procedure is not required.
TIP: For bleeding ulcers resulting from anticoagulant therapy, assign the appropriate "with hemorrhage" ulcer code from this category, code D68.32 Hemorrhagic disorder due to extrinsic circulating anticoagulant, and adverse effect code T45.515- with the appropriate seventh character.

K25.Ø Acute gastric ulcer with hemorrhage

K25.1 Acute gastric ulcer with perforation HCC ESR COM

K25.2 Acute gastric ulcer with both hemorrhage and perforation HCC ESR COM

K25.3 Acute gastric ulcer without hemorrhage or perforation

K25.4 Chronic or unspecified gastric ulcer with hemorrhage

K25.5 Chronic or unspecified gastric ulcer with perforation HCC ESR COM

K25.6 Chronic or unspecified gastric ulcer with both hemorrhage and perforation HCC ESR COM

K25.7 Chronic gastric ulcer without hemorrhage or perforation

K25.9 Gastric ulcer, unspecified as acute or chronic, without hemorrhage or perforation

Gastrointestinal Ulcers

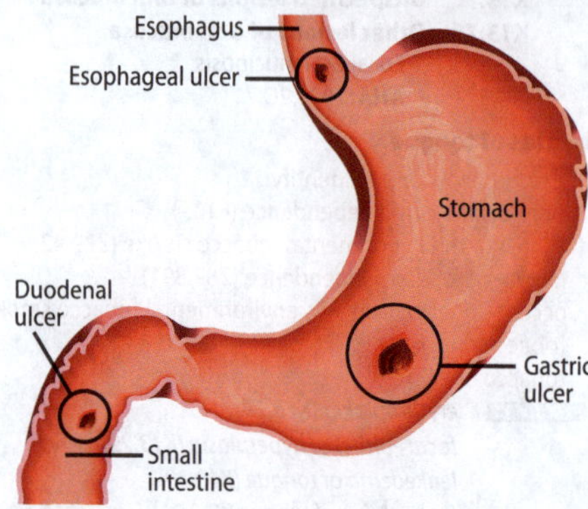

✓4th **K26 Duodenal ulcer**
INCLUDES erosion (acute) of duodenum
duodenum ulcer (peptic)
postpyloric ulcer (peptic)
Use additional code to identify:
alcohol abuse and dependence (F1Ø.-)
EXCLUDES 1 *peptic ulcer NOS (K27.-)*
AHA: 2017,3Q,27
TIP: Assign a code for "with hemorrhage" when a duodenal ulcer and GI bleeding are documented. The ICD-10-CM classification assumes the two are related without the provider linking the two conditions. Evidence of bleeding during a procedure is not required.
TIP: For bleeding ulcers resulting from anticoagulant therapy, assign the appropriate "with hemorrhage" ulcer code from this category, code D68.32 Hemorrhagic disorder due to extrinsic circulating anticoagulant, and adverse effect code T45.515- with the appropriate seventh character.

K26.Ø Acute duodenal ulcer with hemorrhage

K26.1 Acute duodenal ulcer with perforation HCC ESR COM

K26.2 Acute duodenal ulcer with both hemorrhage and perforation HCC ESR COM

K26.3 Acute duodenal ulcer without hemorrhage or perforation

K26.4 Chronic or unspecified duodenal ulcer with hemorrhage
AHA: 2016,1Q,14

K26.5 Chronic or unspecified duodenal ulcer with perforation HCC ESR COM

K26.6 Chronic or unspecified duodenal ulcer with both hemorrhage and perforation HCC ESR COM

K26.7 Chronic duodenal ulcer without hemorrhage or perforation

K26.9 Duodenal ulcer, unspecified as acute or chronic, without hemorrhage or perforation

✓4th **K27 Peptic ulcer, site unspecified**
INCLUDES gastroduodenal ulcer NOS
peptic ulcer NOS
Use additional code to identify:
alcohol abuse and dependence (F1Ø.-)
EXCLUDES 1 *peptic ulcer of newborn (P78.82)*
AHA: 2017,3Q,27
TIP: Assign a code for "with hemorrhage" when a peptic ulcer and GI bleeding are documented. The ICD-10-CM classification assumes the two are related without the provider linking the two conditions. Evidence of bleeding during a procedure is not required.
TIP: For bleeding ulcers resulting from anticoagulant therapy, assign the appropriate "with hemorrhage" ulcer code from this category, code D68.32 Hemorrhagic disorder due to extrinsic circulating anticoagulant, and adverse effect code T45.515- with the appropriate seventh character.

K27.Ø Acute peptic ulcer, site unspecified, with hemorrhage

K27.1 Acute peptic ulcer, site unspecified, with perforation HCC ESR COM

K27.2 Acute peptic ulcer, site unspecified, with both hemorrhage and perforation HCC ESR COM

K27.3 **Acute peptic ulcer, site unspecified, without hemorrhage or perforation**

K27.4 **Chronic or unspecified peptic ulcer, site unspecified, with hemorrhage**

K27.5 **Chronic or unspecified peptic ulcer, site unspecified, with perforation** HCC ESR COM

K27.6 **Chronic or unspecified peptic ulcer, site unspecified, with both hemorrhage and perforation** HCC ESR COM

K27.7 **Chronic peptic ulcer, site unspecified, without hemorrhage or perforation**

K27.9 **Peptic ulcer, site unspecified, unspecified as acute or chronic, without hemorrhage or perforation**

✓4th **K28 Gastrojejunal ulcer**

INCLUDES anastomotic ulcer (peptic) or erosion
gastrocolic ulcer (peptic) or erosion
gastrointestinal ulcer (peptic) or erosion
gastrojejunal ulcer (peptic) or erosion
jejunal ulcer (peptic) or erosion
marginal ulcer (peptic) or erosion
stomal ulcer (peptic) or erosion

Use additional code to identify:
alcohol abuse and dependence (F10.-)

EXCLUDES 1 *primary ulcer of small intestine (K63.3)*

AHA: 2017,3Q,27

TIP: Assign a code for "with hemorrhage" when a gastrojejunal ulcer and GI bleeding are documented. The ICD-10-CM classification assumes the two are related without the provider linking the two conditions. Evidence of bleeding during a procedure is not required.

TIP: For bleeding ulcers resulting from anticoagulant therapy, assign the appropriate "with hemorrhage" ulcer code from this category, code D68.32 Hemorrhagic disorder due to extrinsic circulating anticoagulant, and adverse effect code T45.515- with the appropriate seventh character.

K28.0 **Acute gastrojejunal ulcer with hemorrhage**

K28.1 **Acute gastrojejunal ulcer with perforation** HCC ESR COM

K28.2 **Acute gastrojejunal ulcer with both hemorrhage and perforation** HCC ESR COM

K28.3 **Acute gastrojejunal ulcer without hemorrhage or perforation**

K28.4 **Chronic or unspecified gastrojejunal ulcer with hemorrhage**

K28.5 **Chronic or unspecified gastrojejunal ulcer with perforation** HCC ESR COM

K28.6 **Chronic or unspecified gastrojejunal ulcer with both hemorrhage and perforation** HCC ESR COM

K28.7 **Chronic gastrojejunal ulcer without hemorrhage or perforation**

K28.9 **Gastrojejunal ulcer, unspecified as acute or chronic, without hemorrhage or perforation**

✓4th **K29 Gastritis and duodenitis**

EXCLUDES 1 *eosinophilic gastritis or gastroenteritis (K52.81)*
Zollinger-Ellison syndrome (E16.4)

AHA: 2018,3Q,22

TIP: Assign a code for "with bleeding" when gastritis or duodenitis and GI bleeding are documented. The ICD-10-CM classification assumes the two are related without the provider linking the two conditions. Evidence of bleeding during a procedure is not required.

TIP: For bleeding ulcers resulting from anticoagulant therapy, assign the appropriate "with hemorrhage" ulcer code from this category, code D68.32 Hemorrhagic disorder due to extrinsic circulating anticoagulant, and adverse effect code T45.515- with the appropriate seventh character.

✓5th **K29.0** **Acute gastritis**

Use additional code to identify:
alcohol abuse and dependence (F10.-)

EXCLUDES 1 *erosion (acute) of stomach (K25.-)*

K29.00 **Acute gastritis without bleeding**

K29.01 **Acute gastritis with bleeding**

✓5th **K29.2** **Alcoholic gastritis**

Use additional code to identify:
alcohol abuse and dependence (F10.-)

K29.20 **Alcoholic gastritis without bleeding**

K29.21 **Alcoholic gastritis with bleeding**

✓5th **K29.3** **Chronic superficial gastritis**

K29.30 **Chronic superficial gastritis without bleeding**

K29.31 **Chronic superficial gastritis with bleeding**

✓5th **K29.4** **Chronic atrophic gastritis**

Gastric atrophy

K29.40 **Chronic atrophic gastritis without bleeding**

K29.41 **Chronic atrophic gastritis with bleeding**

✓5th **K29.5** **Unspecified chronic gastritis**

Chronic antral gastritis
Chronic fundal gastritis

K29.50 **Unspecified chronic gastritis without bleeding**

K29.51 **Unspecified chronic gastritis with bleeding**

✓5th **K29.6** **Other gastritis**

Giant hypertrophic gastritis
Granulomatous gastritis
Ménétrier's disease

K29.60 **Other gastritis without bleeding**

K29.61 **Other gastritis with bleeding**

✓5th **K29.7** **Gastritis, unspecified**

K29.70 **Gastritis, unspecified, without bleeding**

K29.71 **Gastritis, unspecified, with bleeding**

✓5th **K29.8** **Duodenitis**

K29.80 **Duodenitis without bleeding**

K29.81 **Duodenitis with bleeding**

✓5th **K29.9** **Gastroduodenitis, unspecified**

K29.90 **Gastroduodenitis, unspecified, without bleeding**

K29.91 **Gastroduodenitis, unspecified, with bleeding**

K30 Functional dyspepsia

Indigestion

EXCLUDES 1 *dyspepsia NOS (R10.13)*
heartburn (R12)
nervous dyspepsia (F45.8)
neurotic dyspepsia (F45.8)
psychogenic dyspepsia (F45.8)

✓4th **K31 Other diseases of stomach and duodenum**

INCLUDES functional disorders of stomach

EXCLUDES 2 *diabetic gastroparesis (E08.43, E09.43, E10.43, E11.43, E13.43)*
diverticulum of duodenum (K57.00-K57.13)

K31.0 **Acute dilatation of stomach**

Acute distention of stomach

K31.1 **Adult hypertrophic pyloric stenosis** COM A

Pyloric stenosis NOS

EXCLUDES 1 *congenital or infantile pyloric stenosis (Q40.0)*

K31.2 **Hourglass stricture and stenosis of stomach**

EXCLUDES 1 *congenital hourglass stomach (Q40.2)*
hourglass contraction of stomach (K31.89)

K31.3 **Pylorospasm, not elsewhere classified** COM

EXCLUDES 1 *congenital or infantile pylorospasm (Q40.0)*
neurotic pylorospasm (F45.8)
psychogenic pylorospasm (F45.8)

K31.4 **Gastric diverticulum**

EXCLUDES 1 *congenital diverticulum of stomach (Q40.2)*

K31.5 **Obstruction of duodenum** COM

Constriction of duodenum
Duodenal ileus (chronic)
Stenosis of duodenum
Stricture of duodenum
Volvulus of duodenum

EXCLUDES 1 *congenital stenosis of duodenum (Q41.0)*

K31.6 **Fistula of stomach and duodenum**

Gastrocolic fistula
Gastrojejunocolic fistula

K31.7 **Polyp of stomach and duodenum**

EXCLUDES 1 *adenomatous polyp of stomach (D13.1)*

AHA: 2020,1Q,16

✓5th **K31.8** **Other specified diseases of stomach and duodenum**

✓6th **K31.81** **Angiodysplasia of stomach and duodenum**

TIP: Assign a code for "with bleeding" when angiodysplasia of the stomach or the duodenum and GI bleeding are documented. The ICD-10-CM classification assumes the two are related without the provider linking the two conditions. Evidence of bleeding during a procedure is not required.

K31.811 **Angiodysplasia of stomach and duodenum with bleeding**

K31.819 **Angiodysplasia of stomach and duodenum without bleeding**

Angiodysplasia of stomach and duodenum NOS

K31.82 Dieulafoy lesion (hemorrhagic) of stomach and duodenum

EXCLUDES 2 *Dieulafoy lesion of intestine (K63.81)*

DEF: Abnormally large submucosal artery protruding through a defect in the stomach mucosa or intestines that can cause massive and life-threatening hemorrhaging.

K31.83 Achlorhydria

DEF: Absence of hydrochloric acid in gastric secretions due to gastric mucosa atrophy. Achlorhydria is unresponsive to histamines.

K31.84 Gastroparesis

Gastroparalysis

Code first underlying disease, if known, such as:

anorexia nervosa (F50.0-)

diabetes mellitus (E08.43, E09.43, E10.43, E11.43, E13.43)

scleroderma (M34.-)

AHA: 2013,4Q,114

K31.89 Other diseases of stomach and duodenum

AHA: 2020,1Q,15; 2017,1Q,28

K31.9 Disease of stomach and duodenum, unspecified

K31.A Gastric intestinal metaplasia

AHA: 2021,4Q,15-16

K31.A0 Gastric intestinal metaplasia, unspecified

Gastric intestinal metaplasia indefinite for dysplasia

Gastric intestinal metaplasia NOS

K31.A1 Gastric intestinal metaplasia without dysplasia

K31.A11 Gastric intestinal metaplasia without dysplasia, involving the antrum

K31.A12 Gastric intestinal metaplasia without dysplasia, involving the body (corpus)

K31.A13 Gastric intestinal metaplasia without dysplasia, involving the fundus

K31.A14 Gastric intestinal metaplasia without dysplasia, involving the cardia

K31.A15 Gastric intestinal metaplasia without dysplasia, involving multiple sites

K31.A19 Gastric intestinal metaplasia without dysplasia, unspecified site

K31.A2 Gastric intestinal metaplasia with dysplasia

K31.A21 Gastric intestinal metaplasia with low grade dysplasia

K31.A22 Gastric intestinal metaplasia with high grade dysplasia

K31.A29 Gastric intestinal metaplasia with dysplasia, unspecified

Diseases of appendix (K35-K38)

K35 Acute appendicitis

AHA: 2018,4Q,17-18

K35.2 Acute appendicitis with generalized peritonitis

Appendicitis (acute) with generalized (diffuse) peritonitis following rupture or perforation of appendix

K35.20 Acute appendicitis with generalized peritonitis, without abscess

(Acute) appendicitis with generalized peritonitis NOS

K35.21 Acute appendicitis with generalized peritonitis, with abscess

K35.3 Acute appendicitis with localized peritonitis

K35.30 Acute appendicitis with localized peritonitis, without perforation or gangrene

Acute appendicitis with localized peritonitis NOS

K35.31 Acute appendicitis with localized peritonitis and gangrene, without perforation

▲ **K35.32 Acute appendicitis with perforation, localized peritonitis, and gangrene, without abscess**

(Acute) appendicitis with perforation NOS

Perforated appendix NOS

Ruptured appendix (with localized peritonitis) NOS

AHA: 2020,1Q,16

▲ **K35.33 Acute appendicitis with perforation, localized peritonitis, and gangrene, with abscess**

(Acute) appendicitis with (peritoneal) abscess NOS

Ruptured appendix with localized peritonitis and abscess

K35.8 Other and unspecified acute appendicitis

K35.80 Unspecified acute appendicitis

Acute appendicitis NOS

Acute appendicitis without (localized) (generalized) peritonitis

K35.89 Other acute appendicitis

AHA: 2020,1Q,16

K35.890 Other acute appendicitis without perforation or gangrene

K35.891 Other acute appendicitis without perforation, with gangrene

(Acute) appendicitis with gangrene NOS

K36 Other appendicitis

Chronic appendicitis

Recurrent appendicitis

K37 Unspecified appendicitis

EXCLUDES 1 *unspecified appendicitis with peritonitis (K35.2-, K35.3-)*

K38 Other diseases of appendix

K38.0 Hyperplasia of appendix

K38.1 Appendicular concretions

Fecalith of appendix

Stercolith of appendix

K38.2 Diverticulum of appendix

K38.3 Fistula of appendix

K38.8 Other specified diseases of appendix

Intussusception of appendix

K38.9 Disease of appendix, unspecified

Hernia (K40-K46)

NOTE Hernia with both gangrene and obstruction is classified to hernia with gangrene.

INCLUDES acquired hernia

congenital [except diaphragmatic or hiatus] hernia

recurrent hernia

AHA: 2021,3Q,30-31

TIP: Do not assign a code for bilateral hernia when the right and left sides have differing pathology. For example, two codes would be assigned for bilateral femoral hernia in which the left side is incarcerated (with obstruction) but the right side is not incarcerated; the code for bilateral would not apply in this case.

K40 Inguinal hernia

INCLUDES bubonocele

direct inguinal hernia

double inguinal hernia

indirect inguinal hernia

inguinal hernia NOS

oblique inguinal hernia

scrotal hernia

DEF: Within the groin region.

K40.0 Bilateral inguinal hernia, with obstruction, without gangrene

Inguinal hernia (bilateral) causing obstruction without gangrene

Incarcerated inguinal hernia (bilateral) without gangrene

Irreducible inguinal hernia (bilateral) without gangrene

Strangulated inguinal hernia (bilateral) without gangrene

K40.00 Bilateral inguinal hernia, with obstruction, without gangrene, not specified as recurrent

Bilateral inguinal hernia, with obstruction, without gangrene NOS

K40.01 Bilateral inguinal hernia, with obstruction, without gangrene, recurrent

K40.1 Bilateral inguinal hernia, with gangrene

K40.10 Bilateral inguinal hernia, with gangrene, not specified as recurrent

Bilateral inguinal hernia, with gangrene NOS

K40.11 Bilateral inguinal hernia, with gangrene, recurrent

K40.2 Bilateral inguinal hernia, without obstruction or gangrene

K40.20 Bilateral inguinal hernia, without obstruction or gangrene, not specified as recurrent

Bilateral inguinal hernia NOS

K40.21 Bilateral inguinal hernia, without obstruction or gangrene, recurrent

K40.3 Unilateral inguinal hernia, with obstruction, without gangrene
Inguinal hernia (unilateral) causing obstruction without gangrene
Incarcerated inguinal hernia (unilateral) without gangrene
Irreducible inguinal hernia (unilateral) without gangrene
Strangulated inguinal hernia (unilateral) without gangrene

K40.30 Unilateral inguinal hernia, with obstruction, without gangrene, not specified as recurrent
Inguinal hernia, with obstruction NOS
Unilateral inguinal hernia, with obstruction, without gangrene NOS

K40.31 Unilateral inguinal hernia, with obstruction, without gangrene, recurrent

K40.4 Unilateral inguinal hernia, with gangrene

K40.40 Unilateral inguinal hernia, with gangrene, not specified as recurrent
Inguinal hernia with gangrene NOS
Unilateral inguinal hernia with gangrene NOS

K40.41 Unilateral inguinal hernia, with gangrene, recurrent

K40.9 Unilateral inguinal hernia, without obstruction or gangrene

K40.90 Unilateral inguinal hernia, without obstruction or gangrene, not specified as recurrent
Inguinal hernia NOS
Unilateral inguinal hernia NOS

K40.91 Unilateral inguinal hernia, without obstruction or gangrene, recurrent

Hernia Sites

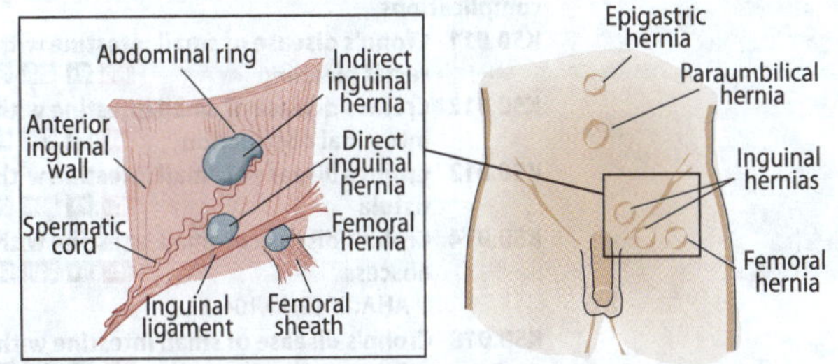

K41 Femoral hernia

K41.0 Bilateral femoral hernia, with obstruction, without gangrene
Femoral hernia (bilateral) causing obstruction, without gangrene
Incarcerated femoral hernia (bilateral), without gangrene
Irreducible femoral hernia (bilateral), without gangrene
Strangulated femoral hernia (bilateral), without gangrene

K41.00 Bilateral femoral hernia, with obstruction, without gangrene, not specified as recurrent
Bilateral femoral hernia, with obstruction, without gangrene NOS

K41.01 Bilateral femoral hernia, with obstruction, without gangrene, recurrent

K41.1 Bilateral femoral hernia, with gangrene

K41.10 Bilateral femoral hernia, with gangrene, not specified as recurrent
Bilateral femoral hernia, with gangrene NOS

K41.11 Bilateral femoral hernia, with gangrene, recurrent

K41.2 Bilateral femoral hernia, without obstruction or gangrene

K41.20 Bilateral femoral hernia, without obstruction or gangrene, not specified as recurrent
Bilateral femoral hernia NOS

K41.21 Bilateral femoral hernia, without obstruction or gangrene, recurrent

K41.3 Unilateral femoral hernia, with obstruction, without gangrene
Femoral hernia (unilateral) causing obstruction, without gangrene
Incarcerated femoral hernia (unilateral), without gangrene
Irreducible femoral hernia (unilateral), without gangrene
Strangulated femoral hernia (unilateral), without gangrene

K41.30 Unilateral femoral hernia, with obstruction, without gangrene, not specified as recurrent
Femoral hernia, with obstruction NOS
Unilateral femoral hernia, with obstruction NOS

K41.31 Unilateral femoral hernia, with obstruction, without gangrene, recurrent

K41.4 Unilateral femoral hernia, with gangrene

K41.40 Unilateral femoral hernia, with gangrene, not specified as recurrent
Femoral hernia, with gangrene NOS
Unilateral femoral hernia, with gangrene NOS

K41.41 Unilateral femoral hernia, with gangrene, recurrent

K41.9 Unilateral femoral hernia, without obstruction or gangrene

K41.90 Unilateral femoral hernia, without obstruction or gangrene, not specified as recurrent
Femoral hernia NOS
Unilateral femoral hernia NOS

K41.91 Unilateral femoral hernia, without obstruction or gangrene, recurrent

K42 Umbilical hernia
INCLUDES paraumbilical hernia
EXCLUDES 1 *omphalocele (Q79.2)*

K42.0 Umbilical hernia with obstruction, without gangrene
Umbilical hernia causing obstruction, without gangrene
Incarcerated umbilical hernia, without gangrene
Irreducible umbilical hernia, without gangrene
Strangulated umbilical hernia, without gangrene

K42.1 Umbilical hernia with gangrene
Gangrenous umbilical hernia

K42.9 Umbilical hernia without obstruction or gangrene
Umbilical hernia NOS

K43 Ventral hernia
DEF: Condition in which a loop of bowel protrudes through a weakness in the abdominal wall muscles that may occur as a birth defect, past surgical site (incisional), or form at a stomal site (parastomal).

K43.0 Incisional hernia with obstruction, without gangrene
Incisional hernia causing obstruction, without gangrene
Incarcerated incisional hernia, without gangrene
Irreducible incisional hernia, without gangrene
Strangulated incisional hernia, without gangrene

K43.1 Incisional hernia with gangrene
Gangrenous incisional hernia
AHA: 2020,2Q,22

K43.2 Incisional hernia without obstruction or gangrene
Incisional hernia NOS

K43.3 Parastomal hernia with obstruction, without gangrene
Incarcerated parastomal hernia, without gangrene
Irreducible parastomal hernia, without gangrene
Parastomal hernia causing obstruction, without gangrene
Strangulated parastomal hernia, without gangrene

K43.4 Parastomal hernia with gangrene
Gangrenous parastomal hernia

K43.5 Parastomal hernia without obstruction or gangrene
Parastomal hernia NOS

K43.6 Other and unspecified ventral hernia with obstruction, without gangrene
Epigastric hernia causing obstruction, without gangrene
Hypogastric hernia causing obstruction, without gangrene
Incarcerated epigastric hernia without gangrene
Incarcerated hypogastric hernia without gangrene
Incarcerated midline hernia without gangrene
Incarcerated spigelian hernia without gangrene
Incarcerated subxiphoid hernia without gangrene
Irreducible epigastric hernia without gangrene
Irreducible hypogastric hernia without gangrene
Irreducible midline hernia without gangrene
Irreducible spigelian hernia without gangrene
Irreducible subxiphoid hernia without gangrene
Midline hernia causing obstruction, without gangrene
Spigelian hernia causing obstruction, without gangrene
Strangulated epigastric hernia without gangrene
Strangulated hypogastric hernia without gangrene
Strangulated midline hernia without gangrene
Strangulated spigelian hernia without gangrene
Strangulated subxiphoid hernia without gangrene
Subxiphoid hernia causing obstruction, without gangrene

K43.7 Other and unspecified ventral hernia with gangrene
Any condition listed under K43.6 specified as gangrenous

K43.9 Ventral hernia without obstruction or gangrene
Epigastric hernia
Ventral hernia NOS

K44 Diaphragmatic hernia

INCLUDES hiatus hernia (esophageal) (sliding)
paraesophageal hernia

EXCLUDES 1 *congenital diaphragmatic hernia (Q79.Ø)*
congenital hiatus hernia (Q4Ø.1)

DEF: Protrusion of an abdominal organ, usually the stomach, through the esophageal opening within the diaphragm and occurring in two types: the sliding hiatal hernia and the paraesophageal hernia.

Hiatal Hernia

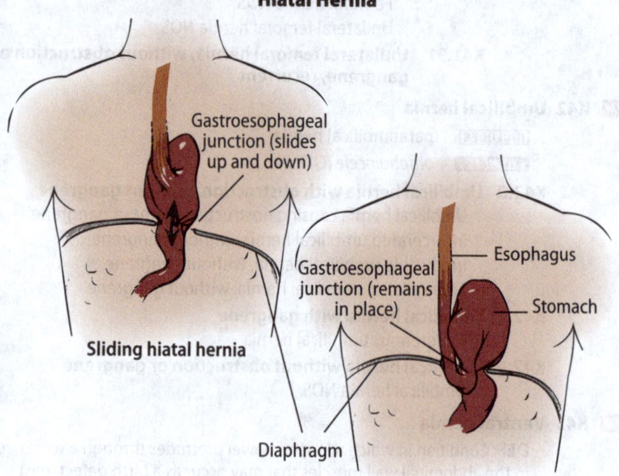

K44.Ø Diaphragmatic hernia with obstruction, without gangrene
Diaphragmatic hernia causing obstruction
Incarcerated diaphragmatic hernia
Irreducible diaphragmatic hernia
Strangulated diaphragmatic hernia
AHA: 2022,2Q,13

K44.1 Diaphragmatic hernia with gangrene
Gangrenous diaphragmatic hernia

K44.9 Diaphragmatic hernia without obstruction or gangrene
Diaphragmatic hernia NOS

K45 Other abdominal hernia

INCLUDES abdominal hernia, specified site NEC
lumbar hernia
obturator hernia
pudendal hernia
retroperitoneal hernia
sciatic hernia

K45.Ø Other specified abdominal hernia with obstruction, without gangrene
Other specified abdominal hernia causing obstruction
Other specified incarcerated abdominal hernia
Other specified irreducible abdominal hernia
Other specified strangulated abdominal hernia

K45.1 Other specified abdominal hernia with gangrene
Any condition listed under K45 specified as gangrenous

K45.8 Other specified abdominal hernia without obstruction or gangrene

K46 Unspecified abdominal hernia

INCLUDES enterocele
epiplocele
hernia NOS
interstitial hernia
intestinal hernia
intra-abdominal hernia

EXCLUDES 1 *vaginal enterocele (N81.5)*

K46.Ø Unspecified abdominal hernia with obstruction, without gangrene
Unspecified abdominal hernia causing obstruction
Unspecified incarcerated abdominal hernia
Unspecified irreducible abdominal hernia
Unspecified strangulated abdominal hernia

K46.1 Unspecified abdominal hernia with gangrene
Any condition listed under K46 specified as gangrenous

K46.9 Unspecified abdominal hernia without obstruction or gangrene
Abdominal hernia NOS

Noninfective enteritis and colitis (K5Ø-K52)

INCLUDES noninfective inflammatory bowel disease

EXCLUDES 1 *irritable bowel syndrome (K58.-)*
megacolon (K59.3-)

K5Ø Crohn's disease [regional enteritis]

INCLUDES granulomatous enteritis

Use additional code to identify manifestations, such as:
pyoderma gangrenosum (L88)

EXCLUDES 1 *ulcerative colitis (K51.-)*

AHA: 2019,3Q,5; 2012,4Q,104

DEF: Chronic inflammation of the gastrointestinal tract characterized by chronic granulomatous disease, most commonly affecting the intestines and the terminal ileum.

K5Ø.Ø Crohn's disease of small intestine
Crohn's disease [regional enteritis] of duodenum
Crohn's disease [regional enteritis] of ileum
Crohn's disease [regional enteritis] of jejunum
Regional ileitis
Terminal ileitis

EXCLUDES 1 *Crohn's disease of both small and large intestine (K5Ø.8-)*

K5Ø.ØØ Crohn's disease of small intestine without complications HCC Rx ESR COM

K5Ø.Ø1 Crohn's disease of small intestine with complications

K5Ø.Ø11 Crohn's disease of small intestine with rectal bleeding HCC Rx ESR COM

K5Ø.Ø12 Crohn's disease of small intestine with intestinal obstruction HCC Rx ESR COM

K5Ø.Ø13 Crohn's disease of small intestine with fistula HCC Rx ESR COM

K5Ø.Ø14 Crohn's disease of small intestine with abscess HCC Rx ESR COM
AHA: 2012,4Q,104

K5Ø.Ø18 Crohn's disease of small intestine with other complication HCC Rx ESR COM

K5Ø.Ø19 Crohn's disease of small intestine with unspecified complications HCC Rx ESR COM

K5Ø.1 Crohn's disease of large intestine
Crohn's disease [regional enteritis] of colon
Crohn's disease [regional enteritis] of large bowel
Crohn's disease [regional enteritis] of rectum
Granulomatous colitis
Regional colitis

EXCLUDES 1 *Crohn's disease of both small and large intestine (K5Ø.8)*

K5Ø.1Ø Crohn's disease of large intestine without complications HCC Rx ESR COM

K5Ø.11 Crohn's disease of large intestine with complications

K5Ø.111 Crohn's disease of large intestine with rectal bleeding HCC Rx ESR COM

K5Ø.112 Crohn's disease of large intestine with intestinal obstruction HCC Rx ESR COM

K5Ø.113 Crohn's disease of large intestine with fistula HCC Rx ESR COM

K5Ø.114 Crohn's disease of large intestine with abscess HCC Rx ESR COM

K5Ø.118 Crohn's disease of large intestine with other complication HCC Rx ESR COM

K5Ø.119 Crohn's disease of large intestine with unspecified complications HCC Rx ESR COM

K5Ø.8 Crohn's disease of both small and large intestine

K5Ø.8Ø Crohn's disease of both small and large intestine without complications HCC Rx ESR COM

K5Ø.81 Crohn's disease of both small and large intestine with complications

K5Ø.811 Crohn's disease of both small and large intestine with rectal bleeding HCC Rx ESR COM

K50.812 Crohn's disease of both small and large intestine with intestinal obstruction HCC Rx ESR COM

K50.813 Crohn's disease of both small and large intestine with fistula HCC Rx ESR COM

K50.814 Crohn's disease of both small and large intestine with abscess HCC Rx ESR COM

K50.818 Crohn's disease of both small and large intestine with other complication HCC Rx ESR COM

K50.819 Crohn's disease of both small and large intestine with unspecified complications HCC Rx ESR COM

✓5th K50.9 Crohn's disease, unspecified

K50.90 Crohn's disease, unspecified, without complications HCC Rx ESR COM
Crohn's disease NOS
Regional enteritis NOS

✓6th K50.91 Crohn's disease, unspecified, with complications

K50.911 Crohn's disease, unspecified, with rectal bleeding HCC Rx ESR COM

K50.912 Crohn's disease, unspecified, with intestinal obstruction HCC Rx ESR COM

K50.913 Crohn's disease, unspecified, with fistula HCC Rx ESR COM

K50.914 Crohn's disease, unspecified, with abscess HCC Rx ESR COM

K50.918 Crohn's disease, unspecified, with other complication HCC Rx ESR COM

K50.919 Crohn's disease, unspecified, with unspecified complications HCC Rx ESR COM

✓4th K51 Ulcerative colitis

Use additional code to identify manifestations, such as:
pyoderma gangrenosum (L88)

EXCLUDES 1 *Crohn's disease [regional enteritis] (K50.-)*

✓5th K51.0 Ulcerative (chronic) pancolitis
Backwash ileitis

K51.00 Ulcerative (chronic) pancolitis without complications HCC Rx ESR COM
Ulcerative (chronic) pancolitis NOS

✓6th K51.01 Ulcerative (chronic) pancolitis with complications

K51.011 Ulcerative (chronic) pancolitis with rectal bleeding HCC Rx ESR COM

K51.012 Ulcerative (chronic) pancolitis with intestinal obstruction HCC Rx ESR COM

K51.013 Ulcerative (chronic) pancolitis with fistula HCC Rx ESR COM

K51.014 Ulcerative (chronic) pancolitis with abscess HCC Rx ESR COM

K51.018 Ulcerative (chronic) pancolitis with other complication HCC Rx ESR COM

K51.019 Ulcerative (chronic) pancolitis with unspecified complications HCC Rx ESR COM

✓5th K51.2 Ulcerative (chronic) proctitis

K51.20 Ulcerative (chronic) proctitis without complications HCC Rx ESR COM
Ulcerative (chronic) proctitis NOS

✓6th K51.21 Ulcerative (chronic) proctitis with complications

K51.211 Ulcerative (chronic) proctitis with rectal bleeding HCC Rx ESR COM

K51.212 Ulcerative (chronic) proctitis with intestinal obstruction HCC Rx ESR COM

K51.213 Ulcerative (chronic) proctitis with fistula HCC Rx ESR COM

K51.214 Ulcerative (chronic) proctitis with abscess HCC Rx ESR COM

K51.218 Ulcerative (chronic) proctitis with other complication HCC Rx ESR COM

K51.219 Ulcerative (chronic) proctitis with unspecified complications HCC Rx ESR COM

✓5th K51.3 Ulcerative (chronic) rectosigmoiditis

K51.30 Ulcerative (chronic) rectosigmoiditis without complications HCC Rx ESR COM
Ulcerative (chronic) rectosigmoiditis NOS

✓6th K51.31 Ulcerative (chronic) rectosigmoiditis with complications

K51.311 Ulcerative (chronic) rectosigmoiditis with rectal bleeding HCC Rx ESR COM

K51.312 Ulcerative (chronic) rectosigmoiditis with intestinal obstruction HCC Rx ESR COM

K51.313 Ulcerative (chronic) rectosigmoiditis with fistula HCC Rx ESR COM

K51.314 Ulcerative (chronic) rectosigmoiditis with abscess HCC Rx ESR COM

K51.318 Ulcerative (chronic) rectosigmoiditis with other complication HCC Rx ESR COM

K51.319 Ulcerative (chronic) rectosigmoiditis with unspecified complications HCC Rx ESR COM

✓5th K51.4 Inflammatory polyps of colon

EXCLUDES 1 *adenomatous polyp of colon (D12.6)*
polyposis of colon (D12.6)
polyps of colon NOS (K63.5)

K51.40 Inflammatory polyps of colon without complications HCC Rx ESR COM
Inflammatory polyps of colon NOS

✓6th K51.41 Inflammatory polyps of colon with complications

K51.411 Inflammatory polyps of colon with rectal bleeding HCC Rx ESR COM

K51.412 Inflammatory polyps of colon with intestinal obstruction HCC Rx ESR COM

K51.413 Inflammatory polyps of colon with fistula HCC Rx ESR COM

K51.414 Inflammatory polyps of colon with abscess HCC Rx ESR COM

K51.418 Inflammatory polyps of colon with other complication HCC Rx ESR COM

K51.419 Inflammatory polyps of colon with unspecified complications HCC Rx ESR COM

✓5th K51.5 Left sided colitis
Left hemicolitis

K51.50 Left sided colitis without complications HCC Rx ESR COM
Left sided colitis NOS

✓6th K51.51 Left sided colitis with complications

K51.511 Left sided colitis with rectal bleeding HCC Rx ESR COM

K51.512 Left sided colitis with intestinal obstruction HCC Rx ESR COM

K51.513 Left sided colitis with fistula HCC Rx ESR COM

K51.514 Left sided colitis with abscess HCC Rx ESR COM

K51.518 Left sided colitis with other complication HCC Rx ESR COM

K51.519 Left sided colitis with unspecified complications HCC Rx ESR COM

✓5th K51.8 Other ulcerative colitis

K51.80 Other ulcerative colitis without complications HCC Rx ESR COM

✓6th K51.81 Other ulcerative colitis with complications

K51.811 Other ulcerative colitis with rectal bleeding HCC Rx ESR COM

K51.812 Other ulcerative colitis with intestinal obstruction HCC Rx ESR COM

K51.813 Other ulcerative colitis with fistula HCC Rx ESR COM

K51.814 Other ulcerative colitis with abscess HCC Rx ESR COM

K51.818 Other ulcerative colitis with other complication HCC Rx ESR COM

K51.819 Other ulcerative colitis with unspecified complications HCC Rx ESR COM

✓5th K51.9 Ulcerative colitis, unspecified

K51.90 Ulcerative colitis, unspecified, without complications HCC Rx ESR COM

✓6th K51.91 Ulcerative colitis, unspecified, with complications

K51.911 Ulcerative colitis, unspecified with rectal bleeding HCC Rx ESR COM

K51.912 Ulcerative colitis, unspecified with intestinal obstruction HCC Rx ESR COM

K51.913 Ulcerative colitis, unspecified with fistula HCC Rx ESR COM

K51.914 Ulcerative colitis, unspecified with abscess HCC Rx ESR COM

K51.918 Ulcerative colitis, unspecified with other complication HCC Rx ESR COM

K51.919 Ulcerative colitis, unspecified with unspecified complications HCC Rx ESR COM

K52 Other and unspecified noninfective gastroenteritis and colitis

AHA: 2016,4Q,30-31

K52.Ø Gastroenteritis and colitis due to radiation

K52.1 Toxic gastroenteritis and colitis

Drug-induced gastroenteritis and colitis

Code first (T51-T65) to identify toxic agent

Use additional code for adverse effect, if applicable, to identify drug (T36-T5Ø with fifth or sixth character 5)

AHA: 2019,1Q,17

K52.2 Allergic and dietetic gastroenteritis and colitis

Food hypersensitivity gastroenteritis or colitis

Use additional code to identify type of food allergy (Z91.Ø1-, Z91.Ø2-)

EXCLUDES 2 *allergic eosinophilic colitis (K52.82)*
allergic eosinophilic esophagitis (K2Ø.Ø)
allergic eosinophilic gastritis (K52.81)
allergic eosinophilic gastroenteritis (K52.81)

DEF: True immunoglobulin E (IgE)-mediated allergic reaction of the stomach, intestines, or colon to food proteins. It causes nausea, vomiting, diarrhea, and abdominal cramping.

K52.21 Food protein-induced enterocolitis syndrome

FPIES

Use additional code for hypovolemic shock, if present (R57.1)

K52.22 Food protein-induced enteropathy

K52.29 Other allergic and dietetic gastroenteritis and colitis

Allergic proctocolitis
Food hypersensitivity gastroenteritis or colitis
Food-induced eosinophilic proctocolitis
Food protein-induced proctocolitis
Immediate gastrointestinal hypersensitivity
Milk protein-induced proctocolitis

K52.3 Indeterminate colitis

Colonic inflammatory bowel disease unclassified (IBDU)

EXCLUDES 1 *unspecified colitis (K52.9)*

K52.8 Other specified noninfective gastroenteritis and colitis

K52.81 Eosinophilic gastritis or gastroenteritis

Eosinophilic enteritis

EXCLUDES 2 *eosinophilic esophagitis (K2Ø.Ø)*

DEF: Disorder involving the accumulation of eosinophil in the lining of the stomach or multiple levels of the gastrointestinal tract, but without a known cause such as connective tissue disease, drug reaction, malignancy, or parasitic infection.

K52.82 Eosinophilic colitis

EXCLUDES 2 *allergic proctocolitis (K52.29)*
food-induced eosinophilic proctocolitis (K52.29)
food protein-induced enterocolitis syndrome (FPIES) (K52.21)
food protein-induced proctocolitis (K52.29)
milk protein-induced proctocolitis (K52.29)

DEF: Disorder involving the accumulation of eosinophil in the tissues lining the colon, but without a known cause such as connective tissue disease, drug reaction, malignancy, or parasitic infection. The resultant inflammation may cause extreme abdominal pain, diarrhea, or bloody stool.

K52.83 Microscopic colitis

K52.831 Collagenous colitis Rx

K52.832 Lymphocytic colitis Rx

K52.838 Other microscopic colitis Rx

K52.839 Microscopic colitis, unspecified Rx

K52.89 Other specified noninfective gastroenteritis and colitis

AHA: 2019,1Q,20

K52.9 Noninfective gastroenteritis and colitis, unspecified

Colitis NOS
Enteritis NOS
Gastroenteritis NOS
Ileitis NOS
Jejunitis NOS
Sigmoiditis NOS

EXCLUDES 1 *diarrhea NOS (R19.7)*
functional diarrhea (K59.1)
infectious gastroenteritis and colitis NOS (AØ9)
neonatal diarrhea (noninfective) (P78.3)
psychogenic diarrhea (F45.8)

AHA: 2021,3Q,3

Other diseases of intestines (K55-K64)

K55 Vascular disorders of intestine

EXCLUDES 1 *necrotizing enterocolitis of newborn (P77.-)*

AHA: 2016,4Q,32

K55.Ø Acute vascular disorders of intestine

Infarction of appendices epiploicae
Mesenteric (artery) (vein) embolism
Mesenteric (artery) (vein) infarction
Mesenteric (artery) (vein) thrombosis

AHA: 2019,4Q,68

K55.Ø1 Acute (reversible) ischemia of small intestine

K55.Ø11 Focal (segmental) acute (reversible) ischemia of small intestine HCC ESR COM

K55.Ø12 Diffuse acute (reversible) ischemia of small intestine HCC ESR COM

K55.Ø19 Acute (reversible) ischemia of small intestine, extent unspecified HCC ESR COM

K55.Ø2 Acute infarction of small intestine

Gangrene of small intestine
Necrosis of small intestine

K55.Ø21 Focal (segmental) acute infarction of small intestine HCC ESR COM

K55.Ø22 Diffuse acute infarction of small intestine HCC ESR COM

K55.Ø29 Acute infarction of small intestine, extent unspecified HCC ESR COM

K55.Ø3 Acute (reversible) ischemia of large intestine

Acute fulminant ischemic colitis
Subacute ischemic colitis

K55.Ø31 Focal (segmental) acute (reversible) ischemia of large intestine HCC ESR COM

K55.Ø32 Diffuse acute (reversible) ischemia of large intestine HCC ESR COM

K55.Ø39 Acute (reversible) ischemia of large intestine, extent unspecified HCC ESR COM

AHA: 2019,4Q,68

K55.Ø4 Acute infarction of large intestine

Gangrene of large intestine
Necrosis of large intestine

K55.Ø41 Focal (segmental) acute infarction of large intestine HCC ESR COM

K55.Ø42 Diffuse acute infarction of large intestine HCC ESR COM

K55.Ø49 Acute infarction of large intestine, extent unspecified HCC ESR COM

K55.Ø5 Acute (reversible) ischemia of intestine, part unspecified

K55.Ø51 Focal (segmental) acute (reversible) ischemia of intestine, part unspecified HCC ESR COM

K55.Ø52 Diffuse acute (reversible) ischemia of intestine, part unspecified HCC ESR COM

K55.Ø59 Acute (reversible) ischemia of intestine, part and extent unspecified HCC ESR COM

✓6th **K55.Ø6 Acute infarction of intestine, part unspecified**

Acute intestinal infarction
Gangrene of intestine
Necrosis of intestine

K55.Ø61 Focal (segmental) acute infarction of intestine, part unspecified HCC ESR COM

K55.Ø62 Diffuse acute infarction of intestine, part unspecified HCC ESR COM

K55.Ø69 Acute infarction of intestine, part and extent unspecified HCC ESR COM

K55.1 Chronic vascular disorders of intestine HCC ESR COM

Chronic ischemic colitis
Chronic ischemic enteritis
Chronic ischemic enterocolitis
Ischemic stricture of intestine
Mesenteric atherosclerosis
Mesenteric vascular insufficiency

✓5th **K55.2 Angiodysplasia of colon**

AHA: 2018,3Q,21

TIP: Assign a code for "with hemorrhage" when angiodysplasia and GI bleeding are documented. The ICD-10-CM classification assumes the two are related without the provider linking the two conditions. Evidence of bleeding during a procedure is not required.

K55.2Ø Angiodysplasia of colon without hemorrhage

K55.21 Angiodysplasia of colon with hemorrhage

DEF: Small vascular abnormalities due to fragile blood vessels in the colon, resulting in blood loss from the gastrointestinal (GI) tract.

✓5th **K55.3 Necrotizing enterocolitis**

EXCLUDES 1 *necrotizing enterocolitis of newborn (P77.-)*

EXCLUDES 2 *necrotizing enterocolitis due to Clostridium difficile (AØ4.7-)*

K55.3Ø Necrotizing enterocolitis, unspecified HCC ESR COM

Necrotizing enterocolitis, NOS

K55.31 Stage 1 necrotizing enterocolitis HCC ESR COM

Necrotizing enterocolitis without pneumatosis, without perforation

K55.32 Stage 2 necrotizing enterocolitis HCC ESR COM

Necrotizing enterocolitis with pneumatosis, without perforation

K55.33 Stage 3 necrotizing enterocolitis HCC ESR COM

Necrotizing enterocolitis with perforation
Necrotizing enterocolitis with pneumatosis and perforation

K55.8 Other vascular disorders of intestine HCC ESR COM

K55.9 Vascular disorder of intestine, unspecified HCC ESR COM

Ischemic colitis
Ischemic enteritis
Ischemic enterocolitis

✓4th **K56 Paralytic ileus and intestinal obstruction without hernia**

EXCLUDES 1 *congenital stricture or stenosis of intestine (Q41-Q42)*
cystic fibrosis with meconium ileus (E84.11)
ischemic stricture of intestine (K55.1)
meconium ileus NOS (P76.Ø)
neonatal intestinal obstructions classifiable to P76.-
obstruction of duodenum (K31.5)
postprocedural intestinal obstruction (K91.3-)

EXCLUDES 2 *stenosis of anus or rectum (K62.4)*

K56.Ø Paralytic ileus HCC ESR COM

Paralysis of bowel
Paralysis of colon
Paralysis of intestine

EXCLUDES 1 *gallstone ileus (K56.3)*
ileus NOS (K56.7)
obstructive ileus NOS (K56.69-)

DEF: Intestinal obstruction due to paralysis of bowel motility or peristalsis.

K56.1 Intussusception HCC ESR COM

Intussusception or invagination of bowel
Intussusception or invagination of colon
Intussusception or invagination of intestine
Intussusception or invagination of rectum

EXCLUDES 2 *intussusception of appendix (K38.8)*

DEF: Intestinal obstruction due to prolapse of a bowel section into an adjacent section. It occurs primarily in children and symptoms include acute abdominal pain, vomiting, and passage of blood and mucus from the rectum.

K56.2 Volvulus HCC ESR COM

Strangulation of colon or intestine
Torsion of colon or intestine
Twist of colon or intestine

EXCLUDES 2 *volvulus of duodenum (K31.5)*

DEF: Twisting, knotting, or entanglement of the bowel on itself that may quickly compromise oxygen supply to the intestinal tissues. A volvulus usually occurs at the sigmoid and ileocecal areas of the intestines.

Volvulus

Knotted intestine (volvulus)

K56.3 Gallstone ileus HCC ESR COM

Obstruction of intestine by gallstone

✓5th **K56.4 Other impaction of intestine**

K56.41 Fecal impaction HCC ESR COM

EXCLUDES 1 *constipation (K59.Ø-)*
incomplete defecation (R15.Ø)

K56.49 Other impaction of intestine HCC ESR COM

✓5th **K56.5 Intestinal adhesions [bands] with obstruction (postinfection)**

Abdominal hernia due to adhesions with obstruction
Peritoneal adhesions [bands] with intestinal obstruction (postinfection)

AHA: 2017,4Q,16-17

K56.5Ø Intestinal adhesions [bands], unspecified as to partial versus complete obstruction HCC ESR COM

Intestinal adhesions with obstruction NOS

K56.51 Intestinal adhesions [bands], with partial obstruction HCC ESR COM

Intestinal adhesions with incomplete obstruction

K56.52 Intestinal adhesions [bands] with complete obstruction HCC ESR COM

✓5th **K56.6 Other and unspecified intestinal obstruction**

AHA: 2017,4Q,16-17; 2017,2Q,12

✓6th **K56.6Ø Unspecified intestinal obstruction**

K56.6ØØ Partial intestinal obstruction, unspecified as to cause HCC ESR COM

Incomplete intestinal obstruction, NOS

K56.6Ø1 Complete intestinal obstruction, unspecified as to cause HCC ESR COM

K56.6Ø9 Unspecified intestinal obstruction, unspecified as to partial versus complete obstruction HCC ESR COM

Intestinal obstruction NOS

6th **K56.69 Other intestinal obstruction**
Enterostenosis NOS
Obstructive ileus NOS
Occlusion of colon or intestine NOS
Stenosis of colon or intestine NOS
Stricture of colon or intestine NOS
EXCLUDES 1 *intestinal obstruction due to specified condition - code to condition*

K56.690 Other partial intestinal obstruction HCC ESR COM
Other incomplete intestinal obstruction

K56.691 Other complete intestinal obstruction HCC ESR COM

K56.699 Other intestinal obstruction unspecified as to partial versus complete obstruction HCC ESR COM
Other intestinal obstruction, NEC

K56.7 Ileus, unspecified HCC ESR COM
EXCLUDES 1 *obstructive ileus (K56.69-)*
EXCLUDES 2 *intestinal obstruction with hernia (K40-K46)*
AHA: 2017,1Q,40

4th **K57 Diverticular disease of intestine**
Code also if applicable peritonitis K65.-
EXCLUDES 1 *congenital diverticulum of intestine (Q43.8)*
Meckel's diverticulum (Q43.0)
EXCLUDES 2 *diverticulum of appendix (K38.2)*
AHA: 2022,1Q,26-27; 2021,1Q,9,11; 2018,3Q,21
TIP: Assign a code for "with bleeding" when diverticular disease of the intestine and GI bleeding are documented. The ICD-10-CM classification assumes the two are related without the provider linking the two conditions. Evidence of bleeding during a procedure is not required.

5th **K57.0 Diverticulitis of small intestine with perforation and abscess**
EXCLUDES 1 *diverticulitis of both small and large intestine with perforation and abscess (K57.4-)*

K57.00 Diverticulitis of small intestine with perforation and abscess without bleeding

K57.01 Diverticulitis of small intestine with perforation and abscess with bleeding

5th **K57.1 Diverticular disease of small intestine without perforation or abscess**
EXCLUDES 1 *diverticular disease of both small and large intestine without perforation or abscess (K57.5-)*

K57.10 Diverticulosis of small intestine without perforation or abscess without bleeding
Diverticular disease of small intestine NOS

K57.11 Diverticulosis of small intestine without perforation or abscess with bleeding

K57.12 Diverticulitis of small intestine without perforation or abscess without bleeding

K57.13 Diverticulitis of small intestine without perforation or abscess with bleeding

5th **K57.2 Diverticulitis of large intestine with perforation and abscess**
EXCLUDES 1 *diverticulitis of both small and large intestine with perforation and abscess (K57.4-)*

K57.20 Diverticulitis of large intestine with perforation and abscess without bleeding

K57.21 Diverticulitis of large intestine with perforation and abscess with bleeding

5th **K57.3 Diverticular disease of large intestine without perforation or abscess**
EXCLUDES 1 *diverticular disease of both small and large intestine without perforation or abscess (K57.5-)*

K57.30 Diverticulosis of large intestine without perforation or abscess without bleeding
Diverticular disease of colon NOS

K57.31 Diverticulosis of large intestine without perforation or abscess with bleeding

K57.32 Diverticulitis of large intestine without perforation or abscess without bleeding

K57.33 Diverticulitis of large intestine without perforation or abscess with bleeding

5th **K57.4 Diverticulitis of both small and large intestine with perforation and abscess**

K57.40 Diverticulitis of both small and large intestine with perforation and abscess without bleeding

K57.41 Diverticulitis of both small and large intestine with perforation and abscess with bleeding

5th **K57.5 Diverticular disease of both small and large intestine without perforation or abscess**

K57.50 Diverticulosis of both small and large intestine without perforation or abscess without bleeding
Diverticular disease of both small and large intestine NOS

K57.51 Diverticulosis of both small and large intestine without perforation or abscess with bleeding

K57.52 Diverticulitis of both small and large intestine without perforation or abscess without bleeding

K57.53 Diverticulitis of both small and large intestine without perforation or abscess with bleeding

5th **K57.8 Diverticulitis of intestine, part unspecified, with perforation and abscess**

K57.80 Diverticulitis of intestine, part unspecified, with perforation and abscess without bleeding

K57.81 Diverticulitis of intestine, part unspecified, with perforation and abscess with bleeding

5th **K57.9 Diverticular disease of intestine, part unspecified, without perforation or abscess**

K57.90 Diverticulosis of intestine, part unspecified, without perforation or abscess without bleeding
Diverticular disease of intestine NOS

K57.91 Diverticulosis of intestine, part unspecified, without perforation or abscess with bleeding

K57.92 Diverticulitis of intestine, part unspecified, without perforation or abscess without bleeding

K57.93 Diverticulitis of intestine, part unspecified, without perforation or abscess with bleeding

4th **K58 Irritable bowel syndrome**
INCLUDES irritable colon
spastic colon
AHA: 2016,4Q,32-33

K58.0 Irritable bowel syndrome with diarrhea
K58.1 Irritable bowel syndrome with constipation
K58.2 Mixed irritable bowel syndrome
K58.8 Other irritable bowel syndrome
K58.9 Irritable bowel syndrome without diarrhea
Irritable bowel syndrome NOS

4th **K59 Other functional intestinal disorders**
EXCLUDES 1 *change in bowel habit NOS (R19.4)*
intestinal malabsorption (K90.-)
psychogenic intestinal disorders (F45.8)
EXCLUDES 2 *functional disorders of stomach (K31.-)*

5th **K59.0 Constipation**
EXCLUDES 1 *fecal impaction (K56.41)*
incomplete defecation (R15.0)
AHA: 2016,4Q,33

K59.00 Constipation, unspecified
K59.01 Slow transit constipation
DEF: Delay in the transit of fecal material through the colon secondary to smooth muscle dysfunction or decreased peristaltic contractions along the colon.
K59.02 Outlet dysfunction constipation
K59.03 Drug induced constipation
Use additional code for adverse effect, if applicable, to identify drug (T36-T50 with fifth or sixth character 5)
K59.04 Chronic idiopathic constipation
Functional constipation
K59.09 Other constipation
Chronic constipation

K59.1 Functional diarrhea
EXCLUDES 1 *diarrhea NOS (R19.7)*
irritable bowel syndrome with diarrhea (K58.0)

K59.2 Neurogenic bowel, not elsewhere classified
DEF: Disorder of bowel due to a spinal cord lesion because of injury or as a complication of conditions such as multiple sclerosis (MS) or spina bifida. Loss of bowel control is the primary symptom, manifested as constipation or bowel incontinence.

✓5th **K59.3 Megacolon, not elsewhere classified**
Dilatation of colon
Code first, if applicable (T51-T65) to identify toxic agent
EXCLUDES 1 *congenital megacolon (aganglionic) (Q43.1)*
megacolon (due to) (in) Chagas' disease (B57.32)
megacolon (due to) (in) Clostridium difficile (AØ4.7-)
megacolon (due to) (in) Hirschsprung's disease (Q43.1)
AHA: 2016,4Q,33-34

K59.31 Toxic megacolon HCC ESR COM

K59.39 Other megacolon
Megacolon NOS

K59.4 Anal spasm
Proctalgia fugax

✓5th **K59.8 Other specified functional intestinal disorders**
AHA: 2020,4Q,29-30

K59.81 Ogilvie syndrome
Acute colonic pseudo-obstruction (ACPO)

K59.89 Other specified functional intestinal disorders
Atony of colon
Pseudo-obstruction (acute) (chronic) of intestine

K59.9 Functional intestinal disorder, unspecified

✓4th **K6Ø Fissure and fistula of anal and rectal regions**
EXCLUDES 1 *fissure and fistula of anal and rectal regions with abscess or cellulitis (K61.-)*
EXCLUDES 2 *anal sphincter tear (healed) (nontraumatic) (old) (K62.81)*

K6Ø.Ø Acute anal fissure

K6Ø.1 Chronic anal fissure

K6Ø.2 Anal fissure, unspecified

K6Ø.3 Anal fistula

K6Ø.4 Rectal fistula
Fistula of rectum to skin
EXCLUDES 1 *rectovaginal fistula (N82.3)*
vesicorectal fistual (N32.1)

K6Ø.5 Anorectal fistula

✓4th **K61 Abscess of anal and rectal regions**
INCLUDES abscess of anal and rectal regions
cellulitis of anal and rectal regions

K61.Ø Anal abscess
Perianal abscess
EXCLUDES 2 *intrasphincteric abscess (K61.4)*

K61.1 Rectal abscess
Perirectal abscess
EXCLUDES 1 *ischiorectal abscess (K61.39)*
AHA: 2012,4Q,104

K61.2 Anorectal abscess

✓5th **K61.3 Ischiorectal abscess**
AHA: 2018,4Q,19

K61.31 Horseshoe abscess

K61.39 Other ischiorectal abscess
Abscess of ischiorectal fossa
Ischiorectal abscess, NOS

K61.4 Intrasphincteric abscess
Intersphincteric abscess

K61.5 Supralevator abscess
AHA: 2018,4Q,19

✓4th **K62 Other diseases of anus and rectum**
INCLUDES anal canal
EXCLUDES 2 *colostomy and enterostomy malfunction (K94.Ø-, K94.1-)*
fecal incontinence (R15.-)
hemorrhoids (K64.-)

K62.Ø Anal polyp

K62.1 Rectal polyp
EXCLUDES 1 *adenomatous polyp (D12.8)*
AHA: 2018,1Q,6

K62.2 Anal prolapse
Prolapse of anal canal

K62.3 Rectal prolapse
Prolapse of rectal mucosa

K62.4 Stenosis of anus and rectum
Stricture of anus (sphincter)
AHA: 2019,2Q,13

K62.5 Hemorrhage of anus and rectum
EXCLUDES 1 *gastrointestinal bleeding NOS (K92.2)*
melena (K92.1)
neonatal rectal hemorrhage (P54.2)
AHA: 2019,1Q,21

K62.6 Ulcer of anus and rectum
Solitary ulcer of anus and rectum
Stercoral ulcer of anus and rectum
EXCLUDES 1 *fissure and fistula of anus and rectum (K6Ø.-)*
ulcerative colitis (K51.-)

K62.7 Radiation proctitis
Use additional code to identify the type of radiation (W88.-) or radiation therapy (Y84.2)
AHA: 2019,1Q,21

✓5th **K62.8 Other specified diseases of anus and rectum**
EXCLUDES 2 *ulcerative proctitis (K51.2)*

K62.81 Anal sphincter tear (healed) (nontraumatic) (old)
Tear of anus, nontraumatic
Use additional code for any associated fecal incontinence (R15.-)
EXCLUDES 2 *anal fissure (K6Ø.-)*
anal sphincter tear (healed) (old) complicating delivery (O34.7-)
traumatic tear of anal sphincter (S31.831)

K62.82 Dysplasia of anus
Anal intraepithelial neoplasia I and II (AIN I and II) (histologically confirmed)
Dysplasia of anus NOS
Mild and moderate dysplasia of anus (histologically confirmed)
EXCLUDES 1 *abnormal results from anal cytologic examination without histologic confirmation (R85.61-)*
anal intraepithelial neoplasia III (DØ1.3)
carcinoma in situ of anus (DØ1.3)
HGSIL of anus (R85.613)
severe dysplasia of anus (DØ1.3)

K62.89 Other specified diseases of anus and rectum
Proctitis NOS
Use additional code for any associated fecal incontinence (R15.-)

K62.9 Disease of anus and rectum, unspecified

✓4th **K63 Other diseases of intestine**

K63.Ø Abscess of intestine
EXCLUDES 1 *abscess of intestine with Crohn's disease (K5Ø.Ø14, K5Ø.114, K5Ø.814, K5Ø.914)*
abscess of intestine with diverticular disease (K57.Ø, K57.2, K57.4, K57.8)
abscess of intestine with ulcerative colitis (K51.Ø14, K51.214, K51.314, K51.414, K51.514, K51.814, K51.914)
EXCLUDES 2 *abscess of anal and rectal regions (K61.-)*
abscess of appendix (K35.3-)

K63.1 Perforation of intestine (nontraumatic) HCC ESR COM
Perforation (nontraumatic) of rectum
EXCLUDES 1 *perforation (nontraumatic) of duodenum (K26.-)*
perforation (nontraumatic) of intestine with diverticular disease (K57.Ø, K57.2, K57.4, K57.8)
EXCLUDES 2 *perforation (nontraumatic) of appendix (K35.2-, K35.3-)*
AHA: 2020,2Q,22

K63.2 Fistula of intestine
EXCLUDES 1 *fistula of duodenum (K31.6)*
fistula of intestine with Crohn's disease (K5Ø.Ø13, K5Ø.113, K5Ø.813, K5Ø.913)
fistula of intestine with ulcerative colitis (K51.Ø13, K51.213, K51.313, K51.413, K51.513, K51.813, K51.913)
EXCLUDES 2 *fistula of anal and rectal regions (K6Ø.-)*
fistula of appendix (K38.3)
intestinal-genital fistula, female (N82.2-N82.4)
vesicointestinal fistula (N32.1)
AHA: 2017,3Q,4

K63.3 Ulcer of intestine
Primary ulcer of small intestine
EXCLUDES 1 *duodenal ulcer (K26.-)*
gastrointestinal ulcer (K28.-)
gastrojejunal ulcer (K28.-)
jejunal ulcer (K28.-)
peptic ulcer, site unspecified (K27.-)
ulcer of intestine with perforation (K63.1)
ulcer of anus or rectum (K62.6)
ulcerative colitis (K51.-)

K63.4 Enteroptosis

K63.5 Polyp of colon
EXCLUDES 1 *adenomatous polyp of colon (D12.-)*
inflammatory polyp of colon (K51.4-)
polyposis of colon (D12.6)
AHA: 2019,1Q,33; 2018,2Q,14; 2017,1Q,15; 2015,2Q,14
TIP: Assign this code when documentation states hyperplastic colon polyp regardless of the site in the colon. Slow-growing, hyperplastic polyps are not precancerous and are classified differently from benign or adenomatous polyps.

✓5th **K63.8 Other specified diseases of intestine**

K63.81 Dieulafoy lesion of intestine
EXCLUDES 2 *Dieulafoy lesion of stomach and duodenum (K31.82)*
DEF: Abnormally large submucosal artery protruding through a defect in the stomach mucosa or intestines that can cause massive and life-threatening hemorrhaging.

K63.89 Other specified diseases of intestine
AHA: 2013,2Q,31

K63.9 Disease of intestine, unspecified

✓4th **K64 Hemorrhoids and perianal venous thrombosis**
INCLUDES piles
EXCLUDES 1 *hemorrhoids complicating childbirth and the puerperium (O87.2)*
hemorrhoids complicating pregnancy (O22.4)

Hemorrhoids

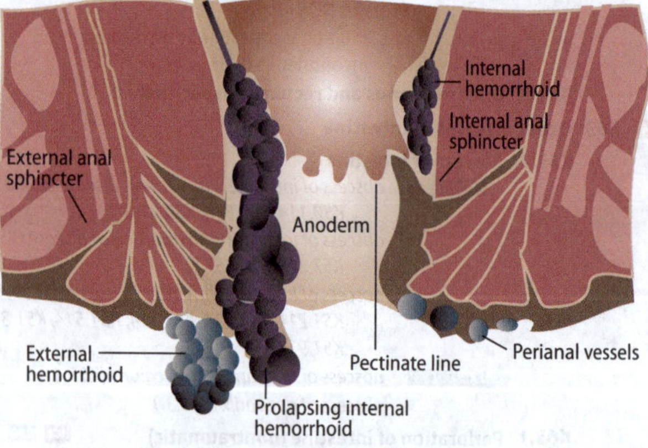

K64.0 First degree hemorrhoids
Grade/stage I hemorrhoids
Hemorrhoids (bleeding) without prolapse outside of anal canal

K64.1 Second degree hemorrhoids
Grade/stage II hemorrhoids
Hemorrhoids (bleeding) that prolapse with straining, but retract spontaneously

K64.2 Third degree hemorrhoids
Grade/stage III hemorrhoids
Hemorrhoids (bleeding) that prolapse with straining and require manual replacement back inside anal canal

K64.3 Fourth degree hemorrhoids
Grade/stage IV hemorrhoids
Hemorrhoids (bleeding) with prolapsed tissue that cannot be manually replaced

K64.4 Residual hemorrhoidal skin tags
External hemorrhoids, NOS
Skin tags of anus

K64.5 Perianal venous thrombosis
External hemorrhoids with thrombosis
Perianal hematoma
Thrombosed hemorrhoids NOS

K64.8 Other hemorrhoids
Internal hemorrhoids, without mention of degree
Prolapsed hemorrhoids, degree not specified

K64.9 Unspecified hemorrhoids
Hemorrhoids (bleeding) NOS
Hemorrhoids (bleeding) without mention of degree

Diseases of peritoneum and retroperitoneum (K65-K68)

✓4th **K65 Peritonitis**
Use additional code (B95-B97), to identify infectious agent, if known
Code also if applicable diverticular disease of intestine (K57.-)
EXCLUDES 1 *acute appendicitis with generalized peritonitis (K35.2-)*
aseptic peritonitis (T81.6)
benign paroxysmal peritonitis (E85.0)
chemical peritonitis (T81.6)
gonococcal peritonitis (A54.85)
neonatal peritonitis (P78.0-P78.1)
pelvic peritonitis, female (N73.3-N73.5)
periodic familial peritonitis (E85.0)
peritonitis due to talc or other foreign substance (T81.6)
peritonitis in chlamydia (A74.81)
peritonitis in diphtheria (A36.89)
peritonitis in syphilis (late) (A52.74)
peritonitis in tuberculosis (A18.31)
peritonitis with or following abortion or ectopic or molar pregnancy (O00-O07, O08.0)
peritonitis with or following appendicitis (K35.-)
puerperal peritonitis (O85)
retroperitoneal infections (K68.-)

K65.0 Generalized (acute) peritonitis HCC ESR COM
Pelvic peritonitis (acute), male
Subphrenic peritonitis (acute)
Suppurative peritonitis (acute)

K65.1 Peritoneal abscess HCC ESR COM
Abdominopelvic abscess
Abscess (of) omentum
Abscess (of) peritoneum
Mesenteric abscess
Retrocecal abscess
Subdiaphragmatic abscess
Subhepatic abscess
Subphrenic abscess
AHA: 2022,1Q,26; 2019,1Q,15

K65.2 Spontaneous bacterial peritonitis HCC ESR COM
EXCLUDES 1 *bacterial peritonitis NOS (K65.9)*

K65.3 Choleperitonitis HCC ESR COM
Peritonitis due to bile
DEF: Inflammation of the peritoneum due to leakage of bile into the peritoneal cavity resulting from rupture of the bile passages or gallbladder.

K65.4 Sclerosing mesenteritis HCC ESR COM
Fat necrosis of peritoneum
(Idiopathic) sclerosing mesenteric fibrosis
Mesenteric lipodystrophy
Mesenteric panniculitis
Retractile mesenteritis

K65.8 Other peritonitis HCC ESR COM
Chronic proliferative peritonitis
Peritonitis due to urine

K65.9 Peritonitis, unspecified HCC ESR COM
Bacterial peritonitis NOS
AHA: 2022,1Q,27; 2013,2Q,31

K66 Other disorders of peritoneum

EXCLUDES 2 *ascites (R18.-)*
peritoneal effusion (chronic) (R18.8)

K66.0 Peritoneal adhesions (postprocedural) (postinfection)
Adhesions (of) abdominal (wall)
Adhesions (of) diaphragm
Adhesions (of) intestine
Adhesions (of) male pelvis
Adhesions (of) omentum
Adhesions (of) stomach
Adhesive bands
Mesenteric adhesions
EXCLUDES 1 *female pelvic adhesions [bands] (N73.6)*
peritoneal adhesions with intestinal obstruction (K56.5-)

K66.1 Hemoperitoneum
EXCLUDES 1 *traumatic hemoperitoneum (S36.8-)*
AHA: 2022,1Q,22-23

K66.8 Other specified disorders of peritoneum

K66.9 Disorder of peritoneum, unspecified

K67 Disorders of peritoneum in infectious diseases classified elsewhere HCC ESR COM
Code first underlying disease, such as:
congenital syphilis (A50.0)
helminthiasis (B65.0-B83.9)
EXCLUDES 1 *peritonitis in chlamydia (A74.81)*
peritonitis in diphtheria (A36.89)
peritonitis in gonococcal (A54.85)
peritonitis in syphilis (late) (A52.74)
peritonitis in tuberculosis (A18.31)

K68 Disorders of retroperitoneum

K68.1 Retroperitoneal abscess

K68.11 Postprocedural retroperitoneal abscess
EXCLUDES 2 *infection following procedure (T81.4-)*

K68.12 Psoas muscle abscess HCC ESR COM

K68.19 Other retroperitoneal abscess HCC ESR COM
AHA: 2019,1Q,15
TIP: This code should be used for a diagnosis of internal presacral abscess. If an intra-abdominal abscess is also present, code K65.1 can also be assigned; sequencing depends on the circumstances of admission.

K68.9 Other disorders of retroperitoneum

Diseases of liver (K70-K77)

EXCLUDES 1 *jaundice NOS (R17)*
EXCLUDES 2 *hemochromatosis (E83.11-)*
Reye's syndrome (G93.7)
viral hepatitis (B15-B19)
Wilson's disease (E83.0)

K70 Alcoholic liver disease
Use additional code to identify:
alcohol abuse and dependence (F10.-)

K70.0 Alcoholic fatty liver A

K70.1 Alcoholic hepatitis

K70.10 Alcoholic hepatitis without ascites COM A

K70.11 Alcoholic hepatitis with ascites COM A

K70.2 Alcoholic fibrosis and sclerosis of liver A

K70.3 Alcoholic cirrhosis of liver
Alcoholic cirrhosis NOS

K70.30 Alcoholic cirrhosis of liver without ascites HCC ESR COM A

K70.31 Alcoholic cirrhosis of liver with ascites HCC ESR COM A
AHA: 2018,1Q,4

K70.4 Alcoholic hepatic failure
Acute alcoholic hepatic failure
Alcoholic hepatic failure NOS
Chronic alcoholic hepatic failure
Subacute alcoholic hepatic failure

K70.40 Alcoholic hepatic failure without coma HCC ESR COM A

K70.41 Alcoholic hepatic failure with coma HCC ESR COM A

K70.9 Alcoholic liver disease, unspecified HCC ESR A

K71 Toxic liver disease

INCLUDES drug-induced idiosyncratic (unpredictable) liver disease
drug-induced toxic (predictable) liver disease
Code first poisoning due to drug or toxin, if applicable (T36-T65 with fifth or sixth character 1-4 or 6)
Use additional code for adverse effect, if applicable, to identify drug (T36-T50 with fifth or sixth character 5)
EXCLUDES 2 *alcoholic liver disease (K70.-)*
Budd-Chiari syndrome (I82.0)

K71.0 Toxic liver disease with cholestasis
Cholestasis with hepatocyte injury
"Pure" cholestasis

K71.1 Toxic liver disease with hepatic necrosis
Hepatic failure (acute) (chronic) due to drugs

K71.10 Toxic liver disease with hepatic necrosis, without coma COM

K71.11 Toxic liver disease with hepatic necrosis, with coma HCC ESR COM

K71.2 Toxic liver disease with acute hepatitis

K71.3 Toxic liver disease with chronic persistent hepatitis COM

K71.4 Toxic liver disease with chronic lobular hepatitis COM

K71.5 Toxic liver disease with chronic active hepatitis
Toxic liver disease with lupoid hepatitis

K71.50 Toxic liver disease with chronic active hepatitis without ascites COM

K71.51 Toxic liver disease with chronic active hepatitis with ascites COM
AHA: 2018,1Q,4

K71.6 Toxic liver disease with hepatitis, not elsewhere classified

K71.7 Toxic liver disease with fibrosis and cirrhosis of liver COM

K71.8 Toxic liver disease with other disorders of liver
Toxic liver disease with focal nodular hyperplasia
Toxic liver disease with hepatic granulomas
Toxic liver disease with peliosis hepatis
Toxic liver disease with veno-occlusive disease of liver

K71.9 Toxic liver disease, unspecified

K72 Hepatic failure, not elsewhere classified

INCLUDES fulminant hepatitis NEC, with hepatic failure
~~hepatic encephalopathy NOS~~
liver (cell) necrosis with hepatic failure
malignant hepatitis NEC, with hepatic failure
yellow liver atrophy or dystrophy
EXCLUDES 1 *alcoholic hepatic failure (K70.4)*
hepatic failure with toxic liver disease (K71.1-)
icterus of newborn (P55-P59)
postprocedural hepatic failure (K91.82)
EXCLUDES 2 *hepatic failure complicating abortion or ectopic or molar pregnancy (O00-O07, O08.8)*
hepatic failure complicating pregnancy, childbirth and the puerperium (O26.6-)
viral hepatitis with hepatic coma (B15-B19)
AHA: 2017,1Q,41

K72.0 Acute and subacute hepatic failure
Acute non-viral hepatitis NOS
AHA: 2015,2Q,17; 2014,2Q,13

K72.00 Acute and subacute hepatic failure without coma COM
AHA: 2021,1Q,13

K72.01 Acute and subacute hepatic failure with coma HCC ESR COM

K72.1 Chronic hepatic failure
End stage liver disease

K72.10 Chronic hepatic failure without coma HCC ESR COM
AHA: 2021,1Q,13

K72.11 Chronic hepatic failure with coma HCC ESR COM

K72.9 Hepatic failure, unspecified

K72.90 Hepatic failure, unspecified without coma HCC ESR COM
AHA: 2022,1Q,52; 2018,4Q,20; 2016,2Q,35

K72.91 Hepatic failure, unspecified with coma HCC ESR COM
Hepatic coma NOS

K73 Chronic hepatitis, not elsewhere classified
EXCLUDES 1 *alcoholic hepatitis (chronic) (K70.1-)*
drug-induced hepatitis (chronic) (K71.-)
granulomatous hepatitis (chronic) NEC (K75.3)
reactive, nonspecific hepatitis (chronic) (K75.2)
viral hepatitis (chronic) (B15-B19)

K73.0 Chronic persistent hepatitis, not elsewhere classified HCC ESR COM
K73.1 Chronic lobular hepatitis, not elsewhere classified HCC ESR COM
K73.2 Chronic active hepatitis, not elsewhere classified HCC ESR COM
K73.8 Other chronic hepatitis, not elsewhere classified HCC ESR COM
K73.9 Chronic hepatitis, unspecified HCC ESR COM

K74 Fibrosis and cirrhosis of liver
Code also, if applicable, viral hepatitis (acute) (chronic) (B15-B19)
EXCLUDES 1 *alcoholic cirrhosis (of liver) (K70.3)*
alcoholic fibrosis of liver (K70.2)
cardiac sclerosis of liver (K76.1)
cirrhosis (of liver) with toxic liver disease (K71.7)
congenital cirrhosis (of liver) (P78.81)
pigmentary cirrhosis (of liver) (E83.110)

K74.0 Hepatic fibrosis
Code first underlying liver disease, such as:
nonalcoholic steatohepatitis (NASH) (K75.81)
AHA: 2020,4Q,30-31
K74.00 Hepatic fibrosis, unspecified
K74.01 Hepatic fibrosis, early fibrosis
Hepatic fibrosis, stage F1 or stage F2
K74.02 Hepatic fibrosis, advanced fibrosis
Hepatic fibrosis, stage F3
EXCLUDES 1 *cirrhosis of liver (K74.6-)*
hepatic fibrosis, stage F4 (K74.6-)

K74.1 Hepatic sclerosis
K74.2 Hepatic fibrosis with hepatic sclerosis
K74.3 Primary biliary cirrhosis HCC Rx ESR COM
Chronic nonsuppurative destructive cholangitis
Primary biliary cholangitis
EXCLUDES 2 *primary sclerosing cholangitis (K83.01)*
K74.4 Secondary biliary cirrhosis HCC ESR COM
K74.5 Biliary cirrhosis, unspecified HCC ESR COM
K74.6 Other and unspecified cirrhosis of liver
AHA: 2020,4Q,30-31
K74.60 Unspecified cirrhosis of liver HCC ESR COM
Cirrhosis (of liver) NOS
AHA: 2018,1Q,4
K74.69 Other cirrhosis of liver HCC ESR COM
Cryptogenic cirrhosis (of liver)
Macronodular cirrhosis (of liver)
Micronodular cirrhosis (of liver)
Mixed type cirrhosis (of liver)
Portal cirrhosis (of liver)
Postnecrotic cirrhosis (of liver)

K75 Other inflammatory liver diseases
EXCLUDES 2 *toxic liver disease (K71.-)*

K75.0 Abscess of liver COM
Cholangitic hepatic abscess
Hematogenic hepatic abscess
Hepatic abscess NOS
Lymphogenic hepatic abscess
Pylephlebitic hepatic abscess
EXCLUDES 1 *amebic liver abscess (A06.4)*
cholangitis without liver abscess (K83.09)
pylephlebitis without liver abscess (K75.1)
EXCLUDES 2 *acute or subacute hepatitis NOS (B17.9)*
acute or subacute non-viral hepatitis (K72.0)
chronic hepatitis NEC (K73.8)

K75.1 Phlebitis of portal vein COM
Pylephlebitis
EXCLUDES 1 *pylephlebitic liver abscess (K75.0)*
DEF: Inflammation of the portal vein or branches due to diverticulitis, perforated appendicitis, or peritonitis. Symptoms include fever, chills, jaundice, sweating, and abscess in various body parts.

K75.2 Nonspecific reactive hepatitis
EXCLUDES 1 *acute or subacute hepatitis (K72.0-)*
chronic hepatitis NEC (K73.-)
viral hepatitis (B15-B19)

K75.3 Granulomatous hepatitis, not elsewhere classified
EXCLUDES 1 *acute or subacute hepatitis (K72.0-)*
chronic hepatitis NEC (K73.-)
viral hepatitis (B15-B19)

K75.4 Autoimmune hepatitis HCC ESR COM
Lupoid hepatitis NEC

K75.8 Other specified inflammatory liver diseases
K75.81 Nonalcoholic steatohepatitis (NASH)
Use additional code, if applicable, hepatic fibrosis (K74.0-)
K75.89 Other specified inflammatory liver diseases

K75.9 Inflammatory liver disease, unspecified
Hepatitis NOS
EXCLUDES 1 *acute or subacute hepatitis (K72.0-)*
chronic hepatitis NEC (K73.-)
viral hepatitis (B15-B19)
AHA: 2015,2Q,17

K76 Other diseases of liver
EXCLUDES 2 *alcoholic liver disease (K70.-)*
amyloid degeneration of liver (E85.-)
cystic disease of liver (congenital) (Q44.6)
hepatic vein thrombosis (I82.0)
hepatomegaly NOS (R16.0)
pigmentary cirrhosis (of liver) (E83.110)
portal vein thrombosis (I81)
toxic liver disease (K71.-)

K76.0 Fatty (change of) liver, not elsewhere classified
Nonalcoholic fatty liver disease (NAFLD)
EXCLUDES 1 *nonalcoholic steatohepatitis (NASH) (K75.81)*
K76.1 Chronic passive congestion of liver
Cardiac cirrhosis
Cardiac sclerosis
K76.2 Central hemorrhagic necrosis of liver COM
EXCLUDES 1 *liver necrosis with hepatic failure (K72.-)*
K76.3 Infarction of liver COM
K76.4 Peliosis hepatis
Hepatic angiomatosis
K76.5 Hepatic veno-occlusive disease
EXCLUDES 1 *Budd-Chiari syndrome (I82.0)*
K76.6 Portal hypertension HCC ESR COM
Use additional code for any associated complications, such as:
portal hypertensive gastropathy (K31.89)
AHA: 2020,1Q,15
K76.7 Hepatorenal syndrome HCC ESR COM
EXCLUDES 1 *hepatorenal syndrome following labor and delivery (O90.4)*
postprocedural hepatorenal syndrome (K91.83)
K76.8 Other specified diseases of liver
K76.81 Hepatopulmonary syndrome HCC ESR COM
Code first underlying liver disease, such as:
alcoholic cirrhosis of liver (K70.3-)
cirrhosis of liver without mention of alcohol (K74.6-)

● **K76.82 Hepatic encephalopathy**
Hepatic encephalopathy, NOS
Hepatic encephalopathy without coma
Hepatocerebral intoxication
Portal-systemic encephalopathy
Code also underlying liver disease, such as:
acute and subacute hepatic failure without coma (K72.00)
alcoholic hepatic failure without coma (K70.40)
chronic hepatic failure without coma (K72.10)
hepatic failure with toxic liver disease without coma (K71.10)
hepatic failure without coma (K72.90)
icterus of newborn (P55-P59)
postprocedural hepatic failure (K91.82)
viral hepatitis without hepatic coma (B15.9, B16.1, B16.9, B17.10, B19.10, B19.20, B19.9)
EXCLUDES 1 *acute and subacute hepatic failure with coma (K72.01)*
alcoholic hepatic failure with coma (K70.41)
chronic hepatic failure with coma (K72.11)
hepatic failure with coma (K72.91)

K76.89 Other specified diseases of liver
Cyst (simple) of liver
Focal nodular hyperplasia of liver
Hepatoptosis

K76.9 Liver disease, unspecified

K77 Liver disorders in diseases classified elsewhere
Code first underlying disease, such as:
amyloidosis (E85.-)
congenital syphilis (A50.0, A50.5)
congenital toxoplasmosis (P37.1)
infectious mononucleosis with liver disease ▶(B27.0-B27.9 with fifth character 9)◀
schistosomiasis (B65.0-B65.9)
EXCLUDES 1 *alcoholic hepatitis (K70.1-)*
alcoholic liver disease (K70.-)
cytomegaloviral hepatitis (B25.1)
herpesviral [herpes simplex] hepatitis (B00.81)
mumps hepatitis (B26.81)
sarcoidosis with liver disease (D86.89)
secondary syphilis with liver disease (A51.45)
syphilis (late) with liver disease (A52.74)
toxoplasmosis (acquired) hepatitis (B58.1)
tuberculosis with liver disease (A18.83)

Disorders of gallbladder, biliary tract and pancreas (K80-K87)

✓4th **K80 Cholelithiasis**
EXCLUDES 1 *retained cholelithiasis following cholecystectomy (K91.86)*
AHA: 2018,4Q,20
DEF: Presence or formation of concretions (calculi or "gallstones") in the gallbladder. The stones contain cholesterol, calcium carbonate, or calcium bilirubinate in pure forms or in various combinations.

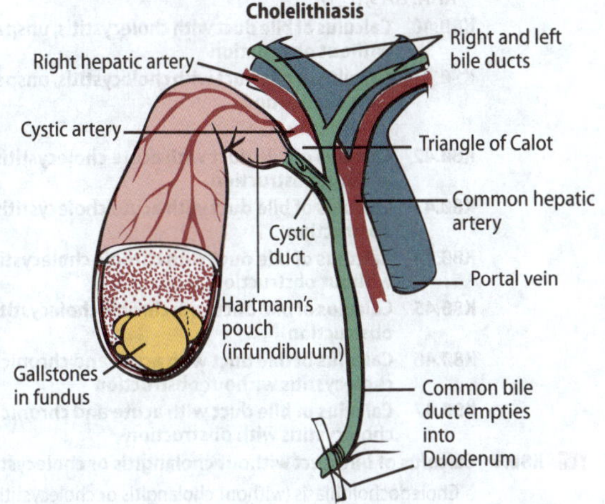

✓5th **K80.0 Calculus of gallbladder with acute cholecystitis**
Any condition listed in K80.2 with acute cholecystitis
Use additional code if applicable for associated gangrene of gallbladder (K82.A1), or perforation of gallbladder (K82.A2)

K80.00 Calculus of gallbladder with acute cholecystitis without obstruction

K80.01 Calculus of gallbladder with acute cholecystitis with obstruction

✓5th **K80.1 Calculus of gallbladder with other cholecystitis**
Use additional code if applicable for associated gangrene of gallbladder (K82.A1), or perforation of gallbladder (K82.A2)

K80.10 Calculus of gallbladder with chronic cholecystitis without obstruction
Cholelithiasis with cholecystitis NOS

K80.11 Calculus of gallbladder with chronic cholecystitis with obstruction

K80.12 Calculus of gallbladder with acute and chronic cholecystitis without obstruction

K80.13 Calculus of gallbladder with acute and chronic cholecystitis with obstruction

K80.18 Calculus of gallbladder with other cholecystitis without obstruction

K80.19 Calculus of gallbladder with other cholecystitis with obstruction

✓5th **K80.2 Calculus of gallbladder without cholecystitis**
Cholecystolithiasis without cholecystitis
Cholelithiasis (without cholecystitis)
Colic (recurrent) of gallbladder (without cholecystitis)
Gallstone (impacted) of cystic duct (without cholecystitis)
Gallstone (impacted) of gallbladder (without cholecystitis)

K80.20 Calculus of gallbladder without cholecystitis without obstruction

K80.21 Calculus of gallbladder without cholecystitis with obstruction

✓5th **K80.3 Calculus of bile duct with cholangitis**
Any condition listed in K80.5 with cholangitis
DEF: Cholangitis: Inflammation of the bile ducts.

K80.30 Calculus of bile duct with cholangitis, unspecified, without obstruction

K80.31 Calculus of bile duct with cholangitis, unspecified, with obstruction

K80.32 Calculus of bile duct with acute cholangitis without obstruction

K80.33 Calculus of bile duct with acute cholangitis with obstruction

K80.34 Calculus of bile duct with chronic cholangitis without obstruction

K80.35 Calculus of bile duct with chronic cholangitis with obstruction

K80.36 **Calculus of bile duct with acute and chronic cholangitis without obstruction**

K80.37 **Calculus of bile duct with acute and chronic cholangitis with obstruction**

K80.4 **Calculus of bile duct with cholecystitis**

Any condition listed in K80.5 with cholecystitis (with cholangitis)

▶Code also fistula of bile duct◀ (K83.3)

Use additional code if applicable for associated gangrene of gallbladder (K82.A1), or perforation of gallbladder (K82.A2)

AHA: 2019,1Q,17

K80.40 **Calculus of bile duct with cholecystitis, unspecified, without obstruction**

K80.41 **Calculus of bile duct with cholecystitis, unspecified, with obstruction**

AHA: 2019,1Q,17

K80.42 **Calculus of bile duct with acute cholecystitis without obstruction**

K80.43 **Calculus of bile duct with acute cholecystitis with obstruction**

K80.44 **Calculus of bile duct with chronic cholecystitis without obstruction**

K80.45 **Calculus of bile duct with chronic cholecystitis with obstruction**

K80.46 **Calculus of bile duct with acute and chronic cholecystitis without obstruction**

K80.47 **Calculus of bile duct with acute and chronic cholecystitis with obstruction**

K80.5 **Calculus of bile duct without cholangitis or cholecystitis**

Choledocholithiasis (without cholangitis or cholecystitis)

Gallstone (impacted) of bile duct NOS (without cholangitis or cholecystitis)

Gallstone (impacted) of common duct (without cholangitis or cholecystitis)

Gallstone (impacted) of hepatic duct (without cholangitis or cholecystitis)

Hepatic cholelithiasis (without cholangitis or cholecystitis)

Hepatic colic (recurrent) (without cholangitis or cholecystitis)

DEF: Cholangitis: Inflammation of the bile ducts.

K80.50 **Calculus of bile duct without cholangitis or cholecystitis without obstruction**

K80.51 **Calculus of bile duct without cholangitis or cholecystitis with obstruction**

K80.6 **Calculus of gallbladder and bile duct with cholecystitis**

Use additional code if applicable for associated gangrene of gallbladder (K82.A1), or perforation of gallbladder (K82.A2)

K80.60 **Calculus of gallbladder and bile duct with cholecystitis, unspecified, without obstruction**

K80.61 **Calculus of gallbladder and bile duct with cholecystitis, unspecified, with obstruction**

K80.62 **Calculus of gallbladder and bile duct with acute cholecystitis without obstruction**

K80.63 **Calculus of gallbladder and bile duct with acute cholecystitis with obstruction**

K80.64 **Calculus of gallbladder and bile duct with chronic cholecystitis without obstruction**

K80.65 **Calculus of gallbladder and bile duct with chronic cholecystitis with obstruction**

K80.66 **Calculus of gallbladder and bile duct with acute and chronic cholecystitis without obstruction**

K80.67 **Calculus of gallbladder and bile duct with acute and chronic cholecystitis with obstruction**

K80.7 **Calculus of gallbladder and bile duct without cholecystitis**

K80.70 **Calculus of gallbladder and bile duct without cholecystitis without obstruction**

K80.71 **Calculus of gallbladder and bile duct without cholecystitis with obstruction**

K80.8 **Other cholelithiasis**

K80.80 **Other cholelithiasis without obstruction**

K80.81 **Other cholelithiasis with obstruction**

K81 **Cholecystitis**

Use additional code if applicable for associated gangrene of gallbladder (K82.A1), or perforation of gallbladder (K82.A2)

EXCLUDES 1 *cholecystitis with cholelithiasis (K80.-)*

AHA: 2018,4Q,20

K81.0 **Acute cholecystitis**

Abscess of gallbladder

Angiocholecystitis

Emphysematous (acute) cholecystitis

Empyema of gallbladder

Gangrene of gallbladder

Gangrenous cholecystitis

Suppurative cholecystitis

K81.1 **Chronic cholecystitis**

K81.2 **Acute cholecystitis with chronic cholecystitis**

K81.9 **Cholecystitis, unspecified**

K82 **Other diseases of gallbladder**

EXCLUDES 1 *nonvisualization of gallbladder (R93.2)*

postcholecystectomy syndrome (K91.5)

K82.0 **Obstruction of gallbladder**

Occlusion of cystic duct or gallbladder without cholelithiasis

Stenosis of cystic duct or gallbladder without cholelithiasis

Stricture of cystic duct or gallbladder without cholelithiasis

EXCLUDES 1 *obstruction of gallbladder with cholelithiasis (K80.-)*

K82.1 **Hydrops of gallbladder**

Mucocele of gallbladder

K82.2 **Perforation of gallbladder**

Rupture of cystic duct or gallbladder

EXCLUDES 1 *perforation of gallbladder in cholecystitis (K82.A2)*

K82.3 **Fistula of gallbladder**

Cholecystocolic fistula

Cholecystoduodenal fistula

K82.4 **Cholesterolosis of gallbladder**

Strawberry gallbladder

EXCLUDES 1 *cholesterolosis of gallbladder with cholecystitis (K81.-)*

cholesterolosis of gallbladder with cholelithiasis (K80.-)

K82.8 **Other specified diseases of gallbladder**

Adhesions of cystic duct or gallbladder

Atrophy of cystic duct or gallbladder

Cyst of cystic duct or gallbladder

Dyskinesia of cystic duct or gallbladder

Hypertrophy of cystic duct or gallbladder

Nonfunctioning of cystic duct or gallbladder

Ulcer of cystic duct or gallbladder

K82.9 **Disease of gallbladder, unspecified**

K82.A **Disorders of gallbladder in diseases classified elsewhere**

Code first the type of cholecystitis (K81.-), or cholelithiasis with cholecystitis (K80.00-K80.19, K80.40-K80.47, K80.60-K80.67)

AHA: 2018,4Q,19-20

K82.A1 ***Gangrene of gallbladder in cholecystitis***

K82.A2 ***Perforation of gallbladder in cholecystitis***

K83 **Other diseases of biliary tract**

EXCLUDES 1 *postcholecystectomy syndrome (K91.5)*

EXCLUDES 2 *conditions involving the gallbladder (K81-K82)*

conditions involving the cystic duct (K81-K82)

K83.0 **Cholangitis**

EXCLUDES 1 *cholangitic liver abscess (K75.0)*

cholangitis with choledocholithiasis (K80.3-, K80.4-)

EXCLUDES 2 *chronic nonsuppurative destructive cholangitis (K74.3)*

primary biliary cholangitis (K74.3)

primary biliary cirrhosis (K74.3)

AHA: 2018,4Q,20

K83.01 **Primary sclerosing cholangitis**

K83.Ø9 Other cholangitis
Ascending cholangitis
Cholangitis NOS
Primary cholangitis
Recurrent cholangitis
Sclerosing cholangitis
Secondary cholangitis
Stenosing cholangitis
Suppurative cholangitis

K83.1 Obstruction of bile duct
Occlusion of bile duct without cholelithiasis
Stenosis of bile duct without cholelithiasis
Stricture of bile duct without cholelithiasis
EXCLUDES 1 *congenital obstruction of bile duct (Q44.3)*
obstruction of bile duct with cholelithiasis (K8Ø.-)
AHA: 2016,1Q,18

K83.2 Perforation of bile duct
Rupture of bile duct

K83.3 Fistula of bile duct
Choledochoduodenal fistula
AHA: 2019,1Q,17

K83.4 Spasm of sphincter of Oddi

K83.5 Biliary cyst

K83.8 Other specified diseases of biliary tract
Adhesions of biliary tract
Atrophy of biliary tract
Hypertrophy of biliary tract
Ulcer of biliary tract

K83.9 Disease of biliary tract, unspecified

K85 Acute pancreatitis (4th)
INCLUDES acute (recurrent) pancreatitis
subacute pancreatitis
AHA: 2016,4Q,34

K85.Ø Idiopathic acute pancreatitis (5th)

K85.ØØ Idiopathic acute pancreatitis without necrosis or infection COM

K85.Ø1 Idiopathic acute pancreatitis with uninfected necrosis COM

K85.Ø2 Idiopathic acute pancreatitis with infected necrosis COM

K85.1 Biliary acute pancreatitis (5th)
Gallstone pancreatitis

K85.1Ø Biliary acute pancreatitis without necrosis or infection COM

K85.11 Biliary acute pancreatitis with uninfected necrosis COM

K85.12 Biliary acute pancreatitis with infected necrosis COM

K85.2 Alcohol induced acute pancreatitis (5th)
EXCLUDES 2 *alcohol induced chronic pancreatitis (K86.Ø)*

K85.2Ø Alcohol induced acute pancreatitis without necrosis or infection COM
AHA: 2020,1Q,9

K85.21 Alcohol induced acute pancreatitis with uninfected necrosis COM

K85.22 Alcohol induced acute pancreatitis with infected necrosis COM

K85.3 Drug induced acute pancreatitis (5th)
Use additional code for adverse effect, if applicable, to identify drug (T36-T5Ø with fifth or sixth character 5)
Use additional code to identify drug abuse and dependence (F11.- F17.-)

K85.3Ø Drug induced acute pancreatitis without necrosis or infection COM

K85.31 Drug induced acute pancreatitis with uninfected necrosis COM

K85.32 Drug induced acute pancreatitis with infected necrosis COM

K85.8 Other acute pancreatitis (5th)

K85.8Ø Other acute pancreatitis without necrosis or infection COM

K85.81 Other acute pancreatitis with uninfected necrosis COM

K85.82 Other acute pancreatitis with infected necrosis COM

K85.9 Acute pancreatitis, unspecified (5th)
Pancreatitis NOS

K85.9Ø Acute pancreatitis without necrosis or infection, unspecified COM

K85.91 Acute pancreatitis with uninfected necrosis, unspecified COM

K85.92 Acute pancreatitis with infected necrosis, unspecified COM

K86 Other diseases of pancreas (4th)
EXCLUDES 2 *fibrocystic disease of pancreas (E84.-)*
islet cell tumor (of pancreas) (D13.7)
pancreatic steatorrhea (K9Ø.3)

K86.Ø Alcohol-induced chronic pancreatitis HCC Rx ESR COM
Use additional code to identify:
alcohol abuse and dependence (F1Ø.-)
Code also exocrine pancreatic insufficiency (K86.81)
EXCLUDES 2 *alcohol induced acute pancreatitis (K85.2-)*

K86.1 Other chronic pancreatitis HCC Rx ESR COM
Chronic pancreatitis NOS
Infectious chronic pancreatitis
Recurrent chronic pancreatitis
Relapsing chronic pancreatitis
Code also exocrine pancreatic insufficiency (K86.81)

K86.2 Cyst of pancreas Rx

K86.3 Pseudocyst of pancreas Rx

K86.8 Other specified diseases of pancreas (5th)
AHA: 2016,4Q,34-35

K86.81 Exocrine pancreatic insufficiency Rx

K86.89 Other specified diseases of pancreas Rx
Aseptic pancreatic necrosis, unrelated to acute pancreatitis
Atrophy of pancreas
Calculus of pancreas
Cirrhosis of pancreas
Fibrosis of pancreas
Pancreatic fat necrosis, unrelated to acute pancreatitis
Pancreatic infantilism
Pancreatic necrosis NOS, unrelated to acute pancreatitis

K86.9 Disease of pancreas, unspecified Rx

K87 Disorders of gallbladder, biliary tract and pancreas in diseases classified elsewhere Rx
Code first underlying disease
EXCLUDES 1 *cytomegaloviral pancreatitis (B25.2)*
mumps pancreatitis (B26.3)
syphilitic gallbladder (A52.74)
syphilitic pancreas (A52.74)
tuberculosis of gallbladder (A18.83)
tuberculosis of pancreas (A18.83)

Other diseases of the digestive system (K9Ø-K95)

K9Ø Intestinal malabsorption (4th)
EXCLUDES 1 *intestinal malabsorption following gastrointestinal surgery (K91.2)*
AHA: 2017,4Q,108

K9Ø.Ø Celiac disease Rx
Celiac disease with steatorrhea
Celiac gluten-sensitive enteropathy
Nontropical sprue
Use additional code for associated disorders including:
dermatitis herpetiformis (L13.Ø)
gluten ataxia (G32.81)
Code also exocrine pancreatic insufficiency (K86.81)
DEF: Malabsorption syndrome due to gluten consumption. Symptoms include fetid, bulky, frothy, oily stools; a distended abdomen; gas; asthenia; electrolyte depletion; and vitamin B, D, and K deficiency.

K9Ø.1 Tropical sprue Rx
Sprue NOS
Tropical steatorrhea

K9Ø.2 Blind loop syndrome, not elsewhere classified Rx
Blind loop syndrome NOS
EXCLUDES 1 *congenital blind loop syndrome (Q43.8)*
postsurgical blind loop syndrome (K91.2)

K9Ø.3 Pancreatic steatorrhea Rx

Chapter 11. Diseases of the Digestive System
K83.Ø9–K9Ø.3

K90.4 Other malabsorption due to intolerance
EXCLUDES 2 *celiac gluten-sensitive enteropathy (K90.0)*
lactose intolerance (E73.-)
AHA: 2016,4Q,35-36

K90.41 Non-celiac gluten sensitivity
Gluten sensitivity NOS
Non-celiac gluten sensitive enteropathy

K90.49 Malabsorption due to intolerance, not elsewhere classified Rx
Malabsorption due to intolerance to carbohydrate
Malabsorption due to intolerance to fat
Malabsorption due to intolerance to protein
Malabsorption due to intolerance to starch

K90.8 Other intestinal malabsorption

K90.81 Whipple's disease Rx

K90.89 Other intestinal malabsorption Rx

K90.9 Intestinal malabsorption, unspecified Rx

K91 Intraoperative and postprocedural complications and disorders of digestive system, not elsewhere classified
EXCLUDES 2 *complications of artificial opening of digestive system (K94.-)*
complications of bariatric procedures (K95.-)
gastrojejunal ulcer (K28.-)
postprocedural (radiation) retroperitoneal abscess (K68.11)
radiation colitis (K52.0)
radiation gastroenteritis (K52.0)
radiation proctitis (K62.7)
AHA: 2016,4Q,9-10

K91.0 Vomiting following gastrointestinal surgery

K91.1 Postgastric surgery syndromes
Dumping syndrome
Postgastrectomy syndrome
Postvagotomy syndrome

K91.2 Postsurgical malabsorption, not elsewhere classified Rx
Postsurgical blind loop syndrome
EXCLUDES 1 *malabsorption osteomalacia in adults (M83.2)*
malabsorption osteoporosis, postsurgical (M80.8-, M81.8)

K91.3 Postprocedural intestinal obstruction
AHA: 2017,4Q,16-17; 2017,1Q,40

K91.30 Postprocedural intestinal obstruction, unspecified as to partial versus complete
Postprocedural intestinal obstruction NOS

K91.31 Postprocedural partial intestinal obstruction
Postprocedural incomplete intestinal obstruction

K91.32 Postprocedural complete intestinal obstruction

K91.5 Postcholecystectomy syndrome

K91.6 Intraoperative hemorrhage and hematoma of a digestive system organ or structure complicating a procedure
EXCLUDES 1 *intraoperative hemorrhage and hematoma of a digestive system organ or structure due to accidental puncture and laceration during a procedure (K91.7-)*

K91.61 Intraoperative hemorrhage and hematoma of a digestive system organ or structure complicating a digestive system procedure
AHA: 2020,1Q,19

K91.62 Intraoperative hemorrhage and hematoma of a digestive system organ or structure complicating other procedure

K91.7 Accidental puncture and laceration of a digestive system organ or structure during a procedure
AHA: 2022,1Q,51

K91.71 Accidental puncture and laceration of a digestive system organ or structure during a digestive system procedure
AHA: 2021,2Q,11

K91.72 Accidental puncture and laceration of a digestive system organ or structure during other procedure
AHA: 2019,2Q,23

K91.8 Other intraoperative and postprocedural complications and disorders of digestive system

K91.81 Other intraoperative complications of digestive system

K91.82 Postprocedural hepatic failure

K91.83 Postprocedural hepatorenal syndrome

K91.84 Postprocedural hemorrhage of a digestive system organ or structure following a procedure

K91.840 Postprocedural hemorrhage of a digestive system organ or structure following a digestive system procedure
AHA: 2016,1Q,15

K91.841 Postprocedural hemorrhage of a digestive system organ or structure following other procedure

K91.85 Complications of intestinal pouch

K91.850 Pouchitis HCC ESR COM
Inflammation of internal ileoanal pouch
DEF: Inflammatory complication of an existing surgically created ileoanal pouch, resulting in multiple GI complaints, including diarrhea, abdominal pain, rectal bleeding, fecal urgency, or incontinence.

K91.858 Other complications of intestinal pouch HCC ESR COM
AHA: 2019,2Q,13

K91.86 Retained cholelithiasis following cholecystectomy

K91.87 Postprocedural hematoma and seroma of a digestive system organ or structure following a procedure

K91.870 Postprocedural hematoma of a digestive system organ or structure following a digestive system procedure
AHA: 2022,1Q,24

K91.871 Postprocedural hematoma of a digestive system organ or structure following other procedure

K91.872 Postprocedural seroma of a digestive system organ or structure following a digestive system procedure

K91.873 Postprocedural seroma of a digestive system organ or structure following other procedure

K91.89 Other postprocedural complications and disorders of digestive system
Use additional code, if applicable, to further specify disorder
EXCLUDES 2 *postprocedural retroperitoneal abscess (K68.11)*
AHA: 2020,2Q,22; 2017,1Q,40

K92 Other diseases of digestive system
EXCLUDES 1 *neonatal gastrointestinal hemorrhage (P54.0-P54.3)*

K92.0 Hematemesis

K92.1 Melena
EXCLUDES 1 *occult blood in feces (R19.5)*

K92.2 Gastrointestinal hemorrhage, unspecified
Gastric hemorrhage NOS
Intestinal hemorrhage NOS
EXCLUDES 1 *acute hemorrhagic gastritis (K29.01)*
hemorrhage of anus and rectum (K62.5)
angiodysplasia of stomach with hemorrhage (K31.811)
diverticular disease with hemorrhage (K57.-)
gastritis and duodenitis with hemorrhage (K29.-)
peptic ulcer with hemorrhage (K25-K28)
AHA: 2021,1Q,11

K92.8 Other specified diseases of the digestive system

K92.81 Gastrointestinal mucositis (ulcerative)
Code also type of associated therapy, such as:
antineoplastic and immunosuppressive drugs (T45.1X-)
radiological procedure and radiotherapy (Y84.2)
EXCLUDES 2 *mucositis (ulcerative) of vagina and vulva (N76.81)*
nasal mucositis (ulcerative) (J34.81)
oral mucositis (ulcerative) (K12.3-)

K92.89 Other specified diseases of the digestive system

K92.9 Disease of digestive system, unspecified

K94 Complications of artificial openings of the digestive system

K94.0 Colostomy complications

K94.00 Colostomy complication, unspecified HCC ESR COM

K94.01 Colostomy hemorrhage HCC ESR COM

K94.Ø2 Colostomy infection HCC ESR COM
Use additional code to specify type of infection, such as:
cellulitis of abdominal wall (LØ3.311)
sepsis (A4Ø.-, A41.-)

K94.Ø3 Colostomy malfunction HCC ESR COM
Mechanical complication of colostomy

K94.Ø9 Other complications of colostomy HCC ESR COM

✓5th **K94.1 Enterostomy complications**

K94.1Ø Enterostomy complication, unspecified HCC ESR COM

K94.11 Enterostomy hemorrhage HCC ESR COM

K94.12 Enterostomy infection HCC ESR COM
Use additional code to specify type of infection, such as:
cellulitis of abdominal wall (LØ3.311)
sepsis (A4Ø.-, A41.-)

K94.13 Enterostomy malfunction HCC ESR COM
Mechanical complication of enterostomy

K94.19 Other complications of enterostomy HCC ESR COM

✓5th **K94.2 Gastrostomy complications**

K94.2Ø Gastrostomy complication, unspecified HCC ESR COM

K94.21 Gastrostomy hemorrhage HCC ESR COM

K94.22 Gastrostomy infection HCC ESR COM
Use additional code to specify type of infection, such as:
cellulitis of abdominal wall (LØ3.311)
sepsis (A4Ø.-, A41.-)

K94.23 Gastrostomy malfunction HCC ESR COM
Mechanical complication of gastrostomy
AHA: 2019,1Q,26

K94.29 Other complications of gastrostomy HCC ESR COM

✓5th **K94.3 Esophagostomy complications**

K94.3Ø Esophagostomy complications, unspecified HCC ESR COM

K94.31 Esophagostomy hemorrhage HCC ESR COM

K94.32 Esophagostomy infection HCC ESR COM
Use additional code to identify the infection

K94.33 Esophagostomy malfunction HCC ESR COM
Mechanical complication of esophagostomy

K94.39 Other complications of esophagostomy HCC ESR COM

✓4th **K95 Complications of bariatric procedures**

✓5th **K95.Ø Complications of gastric band procedure**

K95.Ø1 Infection due to gastric band procedure
Use additional code to specify type of infection or organism, such as:
bacterial and viral infectious agents (B95.-, B96.-)
cellulitis of abdominal wall (LØ3.311)
sepsis (A4Ø.-, A41.-)

K95.Ø9 Other complications of gastric band procedure
Use additional code, if applicable, to further specify complication

✓5th **K95.8 Complications of other bariatric procedure**

EXCLUDES 1 *complications of gastric band surgery (K95.Ø-)*

K95.81 Infection due to other bariatric procedure
Use additional code to specify type of infection or organism, such as:
bacterial and viral infectious agents (B95.-, B96.-)
cellulitis of abdominal wall (LØ3.311)
sepsis (A4Ø.-, A41.-)

K95.89 Other complications of other bariatric procedure
Use additional code, if applicable, to further specify complication

Chapter 12. Diseases of the Skin and Subcutaneous Tissue (LØØ–L99)

Chapter-specific Guidelines with Coding Examples

The chapter-specific guidelines from the ICD-10-CM Official Guidelines for Coding and Reporting have been provided below. Along with these guidelines are coding examples, contained in the shaded boxes, that have been developed to help illustrate the coding and/or sequencing guidance found in these guidelines.

a. Pressure ulcer stage codes

1) Pressure ulcer stages

Codes in category L89, Pressure ulcer, identify the site and stage of the pressure ulcer.

The ICD-1Ø-CM classifies pressure ulcer stages based on severity, which is designated by stages 1-4, deep tissue pressure injury, unspecified stage, and unstageable.

Assign as many codes from category L89 as needed to identify all the pressure ulcers the patient has, if applicable.

See Section I.B.14. for pressure ulcer stage documentation by clinicians other than patient's provider.

> Stage 3 pressure ulcer left ankle, 6 x 7 cm that invades the fascia; stage 2 pressure ulcer of left hip
>
> **L89.523 Pressure ulcer of left ankle, stage 3**
>
> **L89.222 Pressure ulcer of left hip, stage 2**
>
> *Explanation:* Patient has a left ankle pressure ulcer documented as stage 3 and a left hip pressure ulcer documented as stage 2. Combination codes from category L89 Pressure ulcer, identify the site of the pressure ulcer as well as the stage. Assign as many codes from category L89 as needed to identify all the pressure ulcers the patient has.

2) Unstageable pressure ulcers

Assignment of the code for unstageable pressure ulcer (L89.--Ø) should be based on the clinical documentation. These codes are used for pressure ulcers whose stage cannot be clinically determined (e.g., the ulcer is covered by eschar or has been treated with a skin or muscle graft). This code should not be confused with the codes for unspecified stage (L89.--9). When there is no documentation regarding the stage of the pressure ulcer, assign the appropriate code for unspecified stage (L89.--9).

> Pressure ulcer of the right lower back documented as unstageable due to the presence of thick eschar covering the ulcer
>
> **L89.13Ø Pressure ulcer of right lower back, unstageable**
>
> *Explanation:* Codes for unstageable pressure ulcers are assigned when the stage cannot be clinically determined (e.g., the ulcer is covered by eschar or has been treated with a skin or muscle graft).

If during an encounter, the stage of an unstageable pressure ulcer is revealed after debridement, assign only the code for the stage revealed following debridement.

3) Documented pressure ulcer stage

Assignment of the pressure ulcer stage code should be guided by clinical documentation of the stage or documentation of the terms found in the Alphabetic Index. For clinical terms describing the stage that are not found in the Alphabetic Index, and there is no documentation of the stage, the provider should be queried.

> Left heel pressure ulcer with partial thickness skin loss involving the dermis
>
> **L89.622 Pressure ulcer of left heel, stage 2**
>
> *Explanation:* Code assignment for the pressure ulcer stage should be guided by either the clinical documentation of the stage or the documentation of terms found in the Alphabetic Index. The clinical documentation describing the left heel pressure ulcer "partial thickness skin loss involving the dermis" matches the ICD-10-CM index parenthetical description for stage 2 "(abrasion, blister, partial thickness skin loss involving epidermis and/or dermis)."

4) Patients admitted with pressure ulcers documented as healed

No code is assigned if the documentation states that the pressure ulcer is completely healed at the time of admission.

> Patient receiving follow-up examination of a completely healed pressure ulcer of the foot
>
> **Z09 Encounter for follow-up examination after completed treatment for conditions other than malignant neoplasm**
>
> **Z87.2 Personal history of diseases of the skin and subcutaneous tissue**
>
> *Explanation:* Assign only codes for the reason for the encounter and the personal history of the pressure ulcer. Personal history code Z87.2 includes conditions classifiable to LØØ–L99 such as pressure ulcer. No code is assigned for a pressure ulcer documented as completely healed.

5) Pressure ulcers documented as healing

Pressure ulcers described as healing should be assigned the appropriate pressure ulcer stage code based on the documentation in the medical record. If the documentation does not provide information about the stage of the healing pressure ulcer, assign the appropriate code for unspecified stage.

If the documentation is unclear as to whether the patient has a current (new) pressure ulcer or if the patient is being treated for a healing pressure ulcer, query the provider.

For ulcers that were present on admission but healed at the time of discharge, assign the code for the site and stage of the pressure ulcer at the time of admission.

6) Patient admitted with pressure ulcer evolving into another stage during the admission

If a patient is admitted to an inpatient hospital with a pressure ulcer at one stage and it progresses to a higher stage, two separate codes should be assigned: one code for the site and stage of the ulcer on admission and a second code for the same ulcer site and the highest stage reported during the stay.

7) Pressure-induced deep tissue damage

For pressure-induced deep tissue damage or deep tissue pressure injury, assign only the appropriate code for pressure-induced deep tissue damage (L89.--6).

b. Non-pressure chronic ulcers

1) Patients admitted with non-pressure ulcers documented as healed

No code is assigned if the documentation states that the non-pressure ulcer is completely healed at the time of admission.

2) Non-pressure ulcers documented as healing

Non-pressure ulcers described as healing should be assigned the appropriate non-pressure ulcer code based on the documentation in the medical record. If the documentation does not provide information about the severity of the healing non-pressure ulcer, assign the appropriate code for unspecified severity.

If the documentation is unclear as to whether the patient has a current (new) non-pressure ulcer or if the patient is being treated for a healing non-pressure ulcer, query the provider.

For ulcers that were present on admission but healed at the time of discharge, assign the code for the site and severity of the non-pressure ulcer at the time of admission.

3) Patient admitted with non-pressure ulcer that progresses to another severity level during the admission

If a patient is admitted to an inpatient hospital with a non-pressure ulcer at one severity level and it progresses to a higher severity level, two separate codes should be assigned: one code for the site and severity level of the ulcer on admission and a second code for the same ulcer site and the highest severity level reported during the stay.

See Section I.B.14. for pressure ulcer stage documentation by clinicians other than patient's provider.

Chapter 12. Diseases of the Skin and Subcutaneous Tissue (L00-L99)

EXCLUDES 2 *certain conditions originating in the perinatal period (P04-P96)*
certain infectious and parasitic diseases (A00-B99)
complications of pregnancy, childbirth and the puerperium (O00-O9A)
congenital malformations, deformations, and chromosomal abnormalities (Q00-Q99)
endocrine, nutritional and metabolic diseases (E00-E88)
lipomelanotic reticulosis (I89.8)
neoplasms (C00-D49)
symptoms, signs and abnormal clinical and laboratory findings, not elsewhere classified (R00-R94)
systemic connective tissue disorders (M30-M36)
viral warts (B07.-)

AHA: 2022,2Q,7

This chapter contains the following blocks:

L00-L08 Infections of the skin and subcutaneous tissue
L10-L14 Bullous disorders
L20-L30 Dermatitis and eczema
L40-L45 Papulosquamous disorders
L49-L54 Urticaria and erythema
L55-L59 Radiation-related disorders of the skin and subcutaneous tissue
L60-L75 Disorders of skin appendages
L76 Intraoperative and postprocedural complications of skin and subcutaneous tissue
L80-L99 Other disorders of the skin and subcutaneous tissue

Infections of the skin and subcutaneous tissue (L00-L08)

Use additional code (B95-B97) to identify infectious agent

EXCLUDES 2 *hordeolum (H00.0)*
infective dermatitis (L30.3)
local infections of skin classified in Chapter 1
lupus panniculitis (L93.2)
panniculitis NOS (M79.3)
panniculitis of neck and back (M54.0-)
perlèche NOS (K13.0)
perlèche due to candidiasis (B37.0)
perlèche due to riboflavin deficiency (E53.0)
pyogenic granuloma (L98.0)
relapsing panniculitis [Weber-Christian] (M35.6)
viral warts (B07.-)
zoster (B02.-)

L00 Staphylococcal scalded skin syndrome COM
Ritter's disease
Use additional code to identify percentage of skin exfoliation (L49.-)
EXCLUDES 1 *bullous impetigo (L01.03)*
pemphigus neonatorum (L01.03)
toxic epidermal necrolysis [Lyell] (L51.2)

DEF: Infectious skin disease of children younger than 5 years marked by eruptions ranging from a few localized blisters to widespread, easily ruptured, fine vesicles and bullae affecting almost the entire body. It results in exfoliation of large planes of skin and leaves raw areas.

4th **L01 Impetigo**
EXCLUDES 1 *impetigo herpetiformis (L40.1)*

DEF: Acute, superficial, highly contagious skin infection commonly occurring in children. Skin lesions usually appear on the face and consist of vesicles and bullae that burst and form yellow crusts.

5th **L01.0 Impetigo**
Impetigo contagiosa
Impetigo vulgaris

L01.00 Impetigo, unspecified
Impetigo NOS

L01.01 Non-bullous impetigo

L01.02 Bockhart's impetigo
Impetigo follicularis
Perifolliculitis NOS
Superficial pustular perifolliculitis

DEF: Superficial inflammation of the hair follicles commonly caused by *Staphylococcus aureus* that manifests as rounded, sphere-shaped, pustular eruptions in the areas of the scalp, beard, underarms, extremities, and buttocks.

L01.03 Bullous impetigo
Impetigo neonatorum
Pemphigus neonatorum

L01.09 Other impetigo
Ulcerative impetigo

L01.1 Impetiginization of other dermatoses

4th **L02 Cutaneous abscess, furuncle and carbuncle**
Use additional code to identify organism (B95-B96)
EXCLUDES 2 *abscess of anus and rectal regions (K61.-)*
abscess of female genital organs (external) (N76.4)
abscess of male genital organs (external) (N48.2, N49.-)

DEF: Carbuncle: Infection of the skin that arises from a collection of interconnected infected boils or furuncles, usually from hair follicles infected by *Staphylococcus*. This condition can produce pus and form drainage cavities.

DEF: Furuncle: Inflamed, painful abscess, cyst, or nodule on the skin caused by bacteria, often *Staphylococcus*, entering along the hair follicle.

5th **L02.0 Cutaneous abscess, furuncle and carbuncle of face**
EXCLUDES 2 *abscess of ear, external (H60.0)*
abscess of eyelid (H00.0)
abscess of head [any part, except face] (L02.8)
abscess of lacrimal gland (H04.0)
abscess of lacrimal passages (H04.3)
abscess of mouth (K12.2)
abscess of nose (J34.0)
abscess of orbit (H05.0)
submandibular abscess (K12.2)

L02.01 Cutaneous abscess of face

L02.02 Furuncle of face
Boil of face
Folliculitis of face

L02.03 Carbuncle of face

5th **L02.1 Cutaneous abscess, furuncle and carbuncle of neck**

L02.11 Cutaneous abscess of neck

L02.12 Furuncle of neck
Boil of neck
Folliculitis of neck

L02.13 Carbuncle of neck

5th **L02.2 Cutaneous abscess, furuncle and carbuncle of trunk**
EXCLUDES 1 *non-newborn omphalitis (L08.82)*
omphalitis of newborn (P38.-)
EXCLUDES 2 *abscess of breast (N61.1)*
abscess of buttocks (L02.3)
abscess of female external genital organs (N76.4)
abscess of hip (L02.4)
abscess of male external genital organs (N48.2, N49.-)

6th **L02.21 Cutaneous abscess of trunk**

L02.211 Cutaneous abscess of abdominal wall
L02.212 Cutaneous abscess of back [any part, except buttock]
L02.213 Cutaneous abscess of chest wall
L02.214 Cutaneous abscess of groin
L02.215 Cutaneous abscess of perineum
L02.216 Cutaneous abscess of umbilicus
L02.219 Cutaneous abscess of trunk, unspecified

6th **L02.22 Furuncle of trunk**
Boil of trunk
Folliculitis of trunk

L02.221 Furuncle of abdominal wall
L02.222 Furuncle of back [any part, except buttock]
L02.223 Furuncle of chest wall
L02.224 Furuncle of groin
L02.225 Furuncle of perineum
L02.226 Furuncle of umbilicus
L02.229 Furuncle of trunk, unspecified

6th **L02.23 Carbuncle of trunk**

L02.231 Carbuncle of abdominal wall
L02.232 Carbuncle of back [any part, except buttock]
L02.233 Carbuncle of chest wall
L02.234 Carbuncle of groin
L02.235 Carbuncle of perineum
L02.236 Carbuncle of umbilicus
L02.239 Carbuncle of trunk, unspecified

5th **L02.3 Cutaneous abscess, furuncle and carbuncle of buttock**
EXCLUDES 1 *pilonidal cyst with abscess (L05.01)*

L02.31 Cutaneous abscess of buttock
Cutaneous abscess of gluteal region

LØ2.32 Furuncle of buttock
Boil of buttock
Folliculitis of buttock
Furuncle of gluteal region
LØ2.33 Carbuncle of buttock
Carbuncle of gluteal region

√5th **LØ2.4 Cutaneous abscess, furuncle and carbuncle of limb**
EXCLUDES 2 *cutaneous abscess, furuncle and carbuncle of groin (LØ2.214, LØ2.224, LØ2.234)*
cutaneous abscess, furuncle and carbuncle of hand (LØ2.5-)
cutaneous abscess, furuncle and carbuncle of foot (LØ2.6-)

√6th **LØ2.41 Cutaneous abscess of limb**
LØ2.411 Cutaneous abscess of right axilla
LØ2.412 Cutaneous abscess of left axilla
LØ2.413 Cutaneous abscess of right upper limb
LØ2.414 Cutaneous abscess of left upper limb
LØ2.415 Cutaneous abscess of right lower limb
LØ2.416 Cutaneous abscess of left lower limb
LØ2.419 Cutaneous abscess of limb, unspecified

√6th **LØ2.42 Furuncle of limb**
Boil of limb
Folliculitis of limb
LØ2.421 Furuncle of right axilla
LØ2.422 Furuncle of left axilla
LØ2.423 Furuncle of right upper limb
LØ2.424 Furuncle of left upper limb
LØ2.425 Furuncle of right lower limb
LØ2.426 Furuncle of left lower limb
LØ2.429 Furuncle of limb, unspecified

√6th **LØ2.43 Carbuncle of limb**
LØ2.431 Carbuncle of right axilla
LØ2.432 Carbuncle of left axilla
LØ2.433 Carbuncle of right upper limb
LØ2.434 Carbuncle of left upper limb
LØ2.435 Carbuncle of right lower limb
LØ2.436 Carbuncle of left lower limb
LØ2.439 Carbuncle of limb, unspecified

√5th **LØ2.5 Cutaneous abscess, furuncle and carbuncle of hand**

√6th **LØ2.51 Cutaneous abscess of hand**
LØ2.511 Cutaneous abscess of right hand
LØ2.512 Cutaneous abscess of left hand
LØ2.519 Cutaneous abscess of unspecified hand

√6th **LØ2.52 Furuncle hand**
Boil of hand
Folliculitis of hand
LØ2.521 Furuncle right hand
LØ2.522 Furuncle left hand
LØ2.529 Furuncle unspecified hand

√6th **LØ2.53 Carbuncle of hand**
LØ2.531 Carbuncle of right hand
LØ2.532 Carbuncle of left hand
LØ2.539 Carbuncle of unspecified hand

√5th **LØ2.6 Cutaneous abscess, furuncle and carbuncle of foot**

√6th **LØ2.61 Cutaneous abscess of foot**
LØ2.611 Cutaneous abscess of right foot
LØ2.612 Cutaneous abscess of left foot
LØ2.619 Cutaneous abscess of unspecified foot

√6th **LØ2.62 Furuncle of foot**
Boil of foot
Folliculitis of foot
LØ2.621 Furuncle of right foot
LØ2.622 Furuncle of left foot
LØ2.629 Furuncle of unspecified foot

√6th **LØ2.63 Carbuncle of foot**
LØ2.631 Carbuncle of right foot
LØ2.632 Carbuncle of left foot
LØ2.639 Carbuncle of unspecified foot

√5th **LØ2.8 Cutaneous abscess, furuncle and carbuncle of other sites**

√6th **LØ2.81 Cutaneous abscess of other sites**
LØ2.811 Cutaneous abscess of head [any part, except face]
LØ2.818 Cutaneous abscess of other sites

√6th **LØ2.82 Furuncle of other sites**
Boil of other sites
Folliculitis of other sites
LØ2.821 Furuncle of head [any part, except face]
LØ2.828 Furuncle of other sites

√6th **LØ2.83 Carbuncle of other sites**
LØ2.831 Carbuncle of head [any part, except face]
LØ2.838 Carbuncle of other sites

√5th **LØ2.9 Cutaneous abscess, furuncle and carbuncle, unspecified**
LØ2.91 Cutaneous abscess, unspecified
LØ2.92 Furuncle, unspecified
Boil NOS
Furunculosis NOS
LØ2.93 Carbuncle, unspecified

√4th **LØ3 Cellulitis and acute lymphangitis**
EXCLUDES 2 *cellulitis of anal and rectal region (K61.-)*
cellulitis of external auditory canal (H6Ø.1)
cellulitis of eyelid (HØØ.Ø)
cellulitis of female external genital organs (N76.4)
cellulitis of lacrimal apparatus (HØ4.3)
cellulitis of male external genital organs (N48.2, N49.-)
cellulitis of mouth (K12.2)
cellulitis of nose (J34.Ø)
eosinophilic cellulitis [Wells] (L98.3)
febrile neutrophilic dermatosis [Sweet] (L98.2)
lymphangitis (chronic) (subacute) (I89.1)

AHA: 2017,4Q,100

DEF: Cellulitis: Infection of the skin and subcutaneous tissues, most often caused by *Staphylococcus* or *Streptococcus* bacteria secondary to a cutaneous lesion. Progression of the inflammation may lead to abscess and tissue death, or even systemic infection-like bacteremia.

DEF: Lymphangitis: Inflammation of the lymph channels most often caused by *Streptococcus*.

√5th **LØ3.Ø Cellulitis and acute lymphangitis of finger and toe**
Infection of nail
Onychia
Paronychia
Perionychia

√6th **LØ3.Ø1 Cellulitis of finger**
Felon
Whitlow
EXCLUDES 1 *herpetic whitlow (BØØ.89)*

DEF: Felon: Superficial bacterial skin infection at the tip of the finger.

LØ3.Ø11 Cellulitis of right finger
LØ3.Ø12 Cellulitis of left finger
LØ3.Ø19 Cellulitis of unspecified finger

√6th **LØ3.Ø2 Acute lymphangitis of finger**
Hangnail with lymphangitis of finger
LØ3.Ø21 Acute lymphangitis of right finger
LØ3.Ø22 Acute lymphangitis of left finger
LØ3.Ø29 Acute lymphangitis of unspecified finger

√6th **LØ3.Ø3 Cellulitis of toe**
LØ3.Ø31 Cellulitis of right toe
LØ3.Ø32 Cellulitis of left toe
LØ3.Ø39 Cellulitis of unspecified toe

√6th **LØ3.Ø4 Acute lymphangitis of toe**
Hangnail with lymphangitis of toe
LØ3.Ø41 Acute lymphangitis of right toe
LØ3.Ø42 Acute lymphangitis of left toe
LØ3.Ø49 Acute lymphangitis of unspecified toe

√5th **LØ3.1 Cellulitis and acute lymphangitis of other parts of limb**

√6th **LØ3.11 Cellulitis of other parts of limb**
EXCLUDES 2 *cellulitis of fingers (LØ3.Ø1-)*
cellulitis of toes (LØ3.Ø3-)
groin (LØ3.314)
LØ3.111 Cellulitis of right axilla
LØ3.112 Cellulitis of left axilla
LØ3.113 Cellulitis of right upper limb
LØ3.114 Cellulitis of left upper limb
LØ3.115 Cellulitis of right lower limb
LØ3.116 Cellulitis of left lower limb
LØ3.119 Cellulitis of unspecified part of limb

Chapter 12. Diseases of the Skin and Subcutaneous Tissue

√6th LØ3.12 Acute lymphangitis of other parts of limb
EXCLUDES 2 *acute lymphangitis of fingers (LØ3.2-)*
acute lymphangitis of groin (LØ3.324)
acute lymphangitis of toes (LØ3.Ø4-)
LØ3.121 Acute lymphangitis of right axilla
LØ3.122 Acute lymphangitis of left axilla
LØ3.123 Acute lymphangitis of right upper limb
LØ3.124 Acute lymphangitis of left upper limb
LØ3.125 Acute lymphangitis of right lower limb
LØ3.126 Acute lymphangitis of left lower limb
LØ3.129 Acute lymphangitis of unspecified part of limb

√5th LØ3.2 Cellulitis and acute lymphangitis of face and neck
√6th LØ3.21 Cellulitis and acute lymphangitis of face
LØ3.211 Cellulitis of face
EXCLUDES 2 *abscess of orbit (HØ5.Ø1-)*
cellulitis of ear (H6Ø.1-)
cellulitis of eyelid (HØØ.Ø-)
cellulitis of head (LØ3.81)
cellulitis of lacrimal apparatus (HØ4.3)
cellulitis of lip (K13.Ø)
cellulitis of mouth (K12.2)
cellulitis of nose (internal) (J34.Ø)
cellulitis of orbit (HØ5.Ø1-)
cellulitis of scalp (LØ3.81)
AHA: 2013,4Q,123
LØ3.212 Acute lymphangitis of face
LØ3.213 Periorbital cellulitis
Preseptal cellulitis
AHA: 2016,4Q,36
√6th LØ3.22 Cellulitis and acute lymphangitis of neck
LØ3.221 Cellulitis of neck
LØ3.222 Acute lymphangitis of neck

√5th LØ3.3 Cellulitis and acute lymphangitis of trunk
√6th LØ3.31 Cellulitis of trunk
EXCLUDES 2 *cellulitis of anal and rectal regions (K61.-)*
cellulitis of breast NOS (N61.Ø)
cellulitis of female external genital organs (N76.4)
cellulitis of male external genital organs (N48.2, N49.-)
omphalitis of newborn (P38.-)
puerperal cellulitis of breast (O91.2)
LØ3.311 Cellulitis of abdominal wall
EXCLUDES 2 *cellulitis of umbilicus (LØ3.316)*
cellulitis of groin (LØ3.314)
LØ3.312 Cellulitis of back [any part except buttock]
LØ3.313 Cellulitis of chest wall
LØ3.314 Cellulitis of groin
LØ3.315 Cellulitis of perineum
LØ3.316 Cellulitis of umbilicus
LØ3.317 Cellulitis of buttock
LØ3.319 Cellulitis of trunk, unspecified
√6th LØ3.32 Acute lymphangitis of trunk
LØ3.321 Acute lymphangitis of abdominal wall
LØ3.322 Acute lymphangitis of back [any part except buttock]
LØ3.323 Acute lymphangitis of chest wall
LØ3.324 Acute lymphangitis of groin
LØ3.325 Acute lymphangitis of perineum
LØ3.326 Acute lymphangitis of umbilicus
LØ3.327 Acute lymphangitis of buttock
LØ3.329 Acute lymphangitis of trunk, unspecified

√5th LØ3.8 Cellulitis and acute lymphangitis of other sites
√6th LØ3.81 Cellulitis of other sites
LØ3.811 Cellulitis of head [any part, except face]
Cellulitis of scalp
EXCLUDES 2 *cellulitis of face (LØ3.211)*
LØ3.818 Cellulitis of other sites
√6th LØ3.89 Acute lymphangitis of other sites
LØ3.891 Acute lymphangitis of head [any part, except face]
LØ3.898 Acute lymphangitis of other sites

√5th LØ3.9 Cellulitis and acute lymphangitis, unspecified
LØ3.9Ø Cellulitis, unspecified
LØ3.91 Acute lymphangitis, unspecified
EXCLUDES 1 *lymphangitis NOS (I89.1)*

√4th LØ4 Acute lymphadenitis
INCLUDES abscess (acute) of lymph nodes, except mesenteric
acute lymphadenitis, except mesenteric
EXCLUDES 1 *chronic or subacute lymphadenitis, except mesenteric (I88.1)*
enlarged lymph nodes (R59.-)
human immunodeficiency virus [HIV] disease resulting in generalized lymphadenopathy (B2Ø)
lymphadenitis NOS (I88.9)
nonspecific mesenteric lymphadenitis (I88.Ø)
DEF: Inflammation or enlargement of the lymph nodes.
LØ4.Ø Acute lymphadenitis of face, head and neck
LØ4.1 Acute lymphadenitis of trunk
LØ4.2 Acute lymphadenitis of upper limb
Acute lymphadenitis of axilla
Acute lymphadenitis of shoulder
LØ4.3 Acute lymphadenitis of lower limb
Acute lymphadenitis of hip
EXCLUDES 2 *acute lymphadenitis of groin (LØ4.1)*
LØ4.8 Acute lymphadenitis of other sites
LØ4.9 Acute lymphadenitis, unspecified

√4th LØ5 Pilonidal cyst and sinus
DEF: Pilonidal cyst: Sac or sinus cavity of trapped epithelial tissues in the sacrococcygeal region, usually associated with ingrown hair.
DEF: Pilonidal sinus: Fistula, tract, or channel that extends from an infected area of ingrown hair to another site within the skin or out to the skin surface.

Pilonidal Cyst

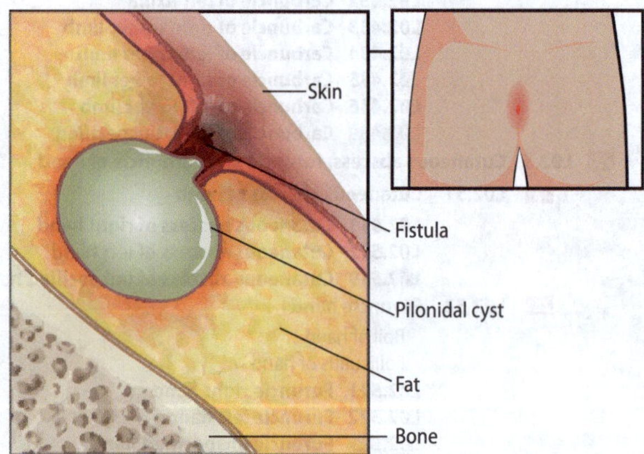

√5th LØ5.Ø Pilonidal cyst and sinus with abscess
LØ5.Ø1 Pilonidal cyst with abscess
Pilonidal abscess
Pilonidal dimple with abscess
Postanal dimple with abscess
EXCLUDES 2 *congenital sacral dimple (Q82.6)*
parasacral dimple (Q82.6)
LØ5.Ø2 Pilonidal sinus with abscess
Coccygeal fistula with abscess
Coccygeal sinus with abscess
Pilonidal fistula with abscess

√5th LØ5.9 Pilonidal cyst and sinus without abscess
LØ5.91 Pilonidal cyst without abscess
Pilonidal dimple
Postanal dimple
Pilonidal cyst NOS
EXCLUDES 2 *congenital sacral dimple (Q82.6)*
parasacral dimple (Q82.6)
LØ5.92 Pilonidal sinus without abscess
Coccygeal fistula
Coccygeal sinus without abscess
Pilonidal fistula

L08 Other local infections of skin and subcutaneous tissue

L08.0 Pyoderma
Dermatitis gangrenosa
Purulent dermatitis
Septic dermatitis
Suppurative dermatitis
EXCLUDES 1 *pyoderma gangrenosum (L88)*
pyoderma vegetans (L08.81)
DEF: Any superficial skin disease commonly characterized by the discharging of pus not attributed to another condition.

L08.1 Erythrasma
DEF: Chronic, superficial skin infection of brown scaly patches, commonly found in skin folds most prevalent in the overweight or diabetic population.

L08.8 Other specified local infections of the skin and subcutaneous tissue

L08.81 Pyoderma vegetans
EXCLUDES 1 *pyoderma gangrenosum (L88)*
pyoderma NOS (L08.0)

L08.82 Omphalitis not of newborn
EXCLUDES 1 *omphalitis of newborn (P38.-)*

L08.89 Other specified local infections of the skin and subcutaneous tissue

L08.9 Local infection of the skin and subcutaneous tissue, unspecified

Bullous disorders (L10-L14)

EXCLUDES 1 *benign familial pemphigus [Hailey-Hailey] (Q82.8)*
staphylococcal scalded skin syndrome (L00)
toxic epidermal necrolysis [Lyell] (L51.2)

L10 Pemphigus
EXCLUDES 1 *pemphigus neonatorum (L01.03)*

L10.0 Pemphigus vulgaris Rx COM
L10.1 Pemphigus vegetans Rx COM
L10.2 Pemphigus foliaceous Rx COM
L10.3 Brazilian pemphigus [fogo selvagem] Rx COM
L10.4 Pemphigus erythematosus Rx COM
Senear-Usher syndrome
L10.5 Drug-induced pemphigus Rx COM
Use additional code for adverse effect, if applicable, to identify drug (T36-T50 with fifth or sixth character 5)

L10.8 Other pemphigus
L10.81 Paraneoplastic pemphigus Rx COM
L10.89 Other pemphigus Rx COM
L10.9 Pemphigus, unspecified Rx COM

L11 Other acantholytic disorders

L11.0 Acquired keratosis follicularis
EXCLUDES 1 *keratosis follicularis (congenital) [Darier-White] (Q82.8)*
AHA: 2021,3Q,10
L11.1 Transient acantholytic dermatosis [Grover]
L11.8 Other specified acantholytic disorders
L11.9 Acantholytic disorder, unspecified

L12 Pemphigoid
EXCLUDES 1 *herpes gestationis (O26.4-)*
impetigo herpetiformis (L40.1)

L12.0 Bullous pemphigoid Rx COM
L12.1 Cicatricial pemphigoid Rx COM
Benign mucous membrane pemphigoid
DEF: Chronic autoimmune disease characterized by subepidermal blistering lesions of the mucosa, including the conjunctiva. It is seen predominantly in the elderly and produces adhesions and scarring.
L12.2 Chronic bullous disease of childhood Rx P
Juvenile dermatitis herpetiformis

L12.3 Acquired epidermolysis bullosa
EXCLUDES 1 *epidermolysis bullosa (congenital) (Q81.-)*
L12.30 Acquired epidermolysis bullosa, unspecified HCC ESR COM
L12.31 Epidermolysis bullosa due to drug HCC ESR COM
Use additional code for adverse effect, if applicable, to identify drug (T36-T50 with fifth or sixth character 5)
L12.35 Other acquired epidermolysis bullosa HCC ESR COM

L12.8 Other pemphigoid Rx COM
L12.9 Pemphigoid, unspecified Rx COM

L13 Other bullous disorders

L13.0 Dermatitis herpetiformis Rx
Duhring's disease
Hydroa herpetiformis
EXCLUDES 1 *juvenile dermatitis herpetiformis (L12.2)*
senile dermatitis herpetiformis (L12.0)
DEF: Skin disease to which people are genetically predisposed resulting from an immunological response to gluten. Dermatitis herpetiformis is an extremely pruritic eruption of various lesions that frequently heal, leaving hyperpigmentation or hypopigmentation and occasionally scarring. It is usually associated with asymptomatic gluten-sensitive enteropathy.
L13.1 Subcorneal pustular dermatitis Rx
Sneddon-Wilkinson disease
L13.8 Other specified bullous disorders Rx
L13.9 Bullous disorder, unspecified Rx

L14 Bullous disorders in diseases classified elsewhere Rx
Code first underlying disease

Dermatitis and eczema (L20-L30)

NOTE In this block the terms dermatitis and eczema are used synonymously and interchangeably.

EXCLUDES 2 *chronic (childhood) granulomatous disease (D71)*
dermatitis gangrenosa (L08.0)
dermatitis herpetiformis (L13.0)
dry skin dermatitis (L85.3)
factitial dermatitis (L98.1)
perioral dermatitis (L71.0)
radiation-related disorders of the skin and subcutaneous tissue (L55-L59)
stasis dermatitis (I87.2)

L20 Atopic dermatitis

L20.0 Besnier's prurigo
L20.8 Other atopic dermatitis
EXCLUDES 2 *circumscribed neurodermatitis (L28.0)*
L20.81 Atopic neurodermatitis
Diffuse neurodermatitis
L20.82 Flexural eczema
L20.83 Infantile (acute) (chronic) eczema P
L20.84 Intrinsic (allergic) eczema
L20.89 Other atopic dermatitis
L20.9 Atopic dermatitis, unspecified

L21 Seborrheic dermatitis
EXCLUDES 2 *infective dermatitis (L30.3)*
seborrheic keratosis (L82.-)

L21.0 Seborrhea capitis
Cradle cap
AHA: 2018,1Q,6
TIP: Assign for dandruff in an adult patient.
L21.1 Seborrheic infantile dermatitis P
L21.8 Other seborrheic dermatitis
L21.9 Seborrheic dermatitis, unspecified
Seborrhea NOS

L22 Diaper dermatitis
Diaper erythema
Diaper rash
Psoriasiform diaper rash
AHA: 2021,4Q,18

L23 Allergic contact dermatitis
EXCLUDES 1 *allergy NOS (T78.4Ø)*
contact dermatitis NOS (L25.9)
dermatitis NOS (L3Ø.9)
EXCLUDES 2 *dermatitis due to substances taken internally (L27.-)*
dermatitis of eyelid (HØ1.1-)
diaper dermatitis (L22)
eczema of external ear (H6Ø.5-)
irritant contact dermatitis (L24.-)
perioral dermatitis (L71.Ø)
radiation-related disorders of the skin and subcutaneous tissue (L55-L59)

L23.Ø Allergic contact dermatitis due to metals
Allergic contact dermatitis due to chromium
Allergic contact dermatitis due to nickel
L23.1 Allergic contact dermatitis due to adhesives
L23.2 Allergic contact dermatitis due to cosmetics
L23.3 Allergic contact dermatitis due to drugs in contact with skin
Use additional code for adverse effect, if applicable, to identify drug (T36-T5Ø with fifth or sixth character 5)
EXCLUDES 2 *dermatitis due to ingested drugs and medicaments (L27.Ø-L27.1)*
L23.4 Allergic contact dermatitis due to dyes
L23.5 Allergic contact dermatitis due to other chemical products
Allergic contact dermatitis due to cement
Allergic contact dermatitis due to insecticide
Allergic contact dermatitis due to plastic
Allergic contact dermatitis due to rubber
L23.6 Allergic contact dermatitis due to food in contact with the skin
EXCLUDES 2 *dermatitis due to ingested food (L27.2)*
L23.7 Allergic contact dermatitis due to plants, except food
EXCLUDES 2 *allergy NOS due to pollen (J3Ø.1)*
L23.8 Allergic contact dermatitis due to other agents
L23.81 Allergic contact dermatitis due to animal (cat) (dog) dander
Allergic contact dermatitis due to animal (cat) (dog) hair
L23.89 Allergic contact dermatitis due to other agents
L23.9 Allergic contact dermatitis, unspecified cause
Allergic contact eczema NOS

L24 Irritant contact dermatitis
EXCLUDES 1 *allergy NOS (T78.4Ø)*
contact dermatitis NOS (L25.9)
dermatitis NOS (L3Ø.9)
EXCLUDES 2 *allergic contact dermatitis (L23.-)*
dermatitis due to substances taken internally (L27.-)
dermatitis of eyelid (HØ1.1-)
diaper dermatitis (L22)
eczema of external ear (H6Ø.5-)
perioral dermatitis (L71.Ø)
radiation-related disorders of the skin and subcutaneous tissue (L55-L59)

L24.Ø Irritant contact dermatitis due to detergents
L24.1 Irritant contact dermatitis due to oils and greases
L24.2 Irritant contact dermatitis due to solvents
Irritant contact dermatitis due to chlorocompound
Irritant contact dermatitis due to cyclohexane
Irritant contact dermatitis due to ester
Irritant contact dermatitis due to glycol
Irritant contact dermatitis due to hydrocarbon
Irritant contact dermatitis due to ketone
L24.3 Irritant contact dermatitis due to cosmetics
L24.4 Irritant contact dermatitis due to drugs in contact with skin
Use additional code for adverse effect, if applicable, to identify drug (T36-T5Ø with fifth or sixth character 5)
L24.5 Irritant contact dermatitis due to other chemical products
Irritant contact dermatitis due to cement
Irritant contact dermatitis due to insecticide
Irritant contact dermatitis due to plastic
Irritant contact dermatitis due to rubber
L24.6 Irritant contact dermatitis due to food in contact with skin
EXCLUDES 2 *dermatitis due to ingested food (L27.2)*
L24.7 Irritant contact dermatitis due to plants, except food
EXCLUDES 2 *allergy NOS to pollen (J3Ø.1)*
L24.8 Irritant contact dermatitis due to other agents
L24.81 Irritant contact dermatitis due to metals
Irritant contact dermatitis due to chromium
Irritant contact dermatitis due to nickel
L24.89 Irritant contact dermatitis due to other agents
Irritant contact dermatitis due to dyes
L24.9 Irritant contact dermatitis, unspecified cause
Irritant contact eczema NOS
L24.A Irritant contact dermatitis due to friction or contact with body fluids
EXCLUDES 1 *irritant contact dermatitis related to stoma or fistula (L24.B-)*
EXCLUDES 2 *erythema intertrigo (L3Ø.4)*
AHA: 2021,4Q,16-18
L24.AØ Irritant contact dermatitis due to friction or contact with body fluids, unspecified
L24.A1 Irritant contact dermatitis due to saliva
L24.A2 Irritant contact dermatitis due to fecal, urinary or dual incontinence
EXCLUDES 1 *diaper dermatitis (L22)*
L24.A9 Irritant contact dermatitis due friction or contact with other specified body fluids
Irritant contact dermatitis related to endotracheal tube
Wound fluids, exudate
L24.B Irritant contact dermatitis related to stoma or fistula
Use additional code to identify any artificial opening status (Z93.-), if applicable, for contact dermatitis related to stoma secretions
AHA: 2021,4Q,16-18
L24.BØ Irritant contact dermatitis related to unspecified stoma or fistula
Irritant contact dermatitis related to fistula NOS
Irritant contact dermatitis related to stoma NOS
L24.B1 Irritant contact dermatitis related to digestive stoma or fistula
Irritant contact dermatitis related to gastrostomy
Irritant contact dermatitis related to jejunostomy
Irritant contact dermatitis related to saliva or spit fistula
L24.B2 Irritant contact dermatitis related to respiratory stoma or fistula
Irritant contact dermatitis related to tracheostomy
L24.B3 Irritant contact dermatitis related to fecal or urinary stoma or fistula
Irritant contact dermatitis related to colostomy
Irritant contact dermatitis related to enterocutaneous fistula
Irritant contact dermatitis related to ileostomy

L25 Unspecified contact dermatitis
EXCLUDES 1 *allergic contact dermatitis (L23.-)*
allergy NOS (T78.4Ø)
dermatitis NOS (L3Ø.9)
irritant contact dermatitis (L24.-)
EXCLUDES 2 *dermatitis due to ingested substances (L27.-)*
dermatitis of eyelid (HØ1.1-)
eczema of external ear (H6Ø.5-)
perioral dermatitis (L71.Ø)
radiation-related disorders of the skin and subcutaneous tissue (L55-L59)

L25.Ø Unspecified contact dermatitis due to cosmetics
L25.1 Unspecified contact dermatitis due to drugs in contact with skin
Use additional code for adverse effect, if applicable, to identify drug (T36-T5Ø with fifth or sixth character 5)
EXCLUDES 2 *dermatitis due to ingested drugs and medicaments (L27.Ø-L27.1)*
L25.2 Unspecified contact dermatitis due to dyes
L25.3 Unspecified contact dermatitis due to other chemical products
Unspecified contact dermatitis due to cement
Unspecified contact dermatitis due to insecticide

L25.4 Unspecified contact dermatitis due to food in contact with skin
EXCLUDES 2 *dermatitis due to ingested food (L27.2)*

L25.5 Unspecified contact dermatitis due to plants, except food
EXCLUDES 1 *nettle rash (L50.9)*
EXCLUDES 2 *allergy NOS due to pollen (J30.1)*

L25.8 Unspecified contact dermatitis due to other agents

L25.9 Unspecified contact dermatitis, unspecified cause
Contact dermatitis (occupational) NOS
Contact eczema (occupational) NOS

L26 Exfoliative dermatitis
Hebra's pityriasis
EXCLUDES 1 *Ritter's disease (L00)*

L27 Dermatitis due to substances taken internally
EXCLUDES 1 *allergy NOS (T78.40)*
EXCLUDES 2 *adverse food reaction, except dermatitis (T78.0-T78.1)*
contact dermatitis (L23-L25)
drug photoallergic response (L56.1)
drug phototoxic response (L56.0)
urticaria (L50.-)

L27.0 Generalized skin eruption due to drugs and medicaments taken internally
Use additional code for adverse effect, if applicable, to identify drug (T36-T50 with fifth or sixth character 5)

L27.1 Localized skin eruption due to drugs and medicaments taken internally
Use additional code for adverse effect, if applicable, to identify drug (T36-T50 with fifth or sixth character 5)

L27.2 Dermatitis due to ingested food
EXCLUDES 2 *dermatitis due to food in contact with skin (L23.6, L24.6, L25.4)*

L27.8 Dermatitis due to other substances taken internally

L27.9 Dermatitis due to unspecified substance taken internally

L28 Lichen simplex chronicus and prurigo

L28.0 Lichen simplex chronicus
Circumscribed neurodermatitis
Lichen NOS

L28.1 Prurigo nodularis

L28.2 Other prurigo
Prurigo NOS
Prurigo Hebra
Prurigo mitis
Urticaria papulosa

L29 Pruritus
EXCLUDES 1 *neurotic excoriation (L98.1)*
psychogenic pruritus (F45.8)

L29.0 Pruritus ani

L29.1 Pruritus scroti ♂

L29.2 Pruritus vulvae ♀

L29.3 Anogenital pruritus, unspecified

L29.8 Other pruritus

L29.9 Pruritus, unspecified
Itch NOS

L30 Other and unspecified dermatitis
EXCLUDES 2 *contact dermatitis (L23-L25)*
dry skin dermatitis (L85.3)
small plaque parapsoriasis (L41.3)
stasis dermatitis (I87.2)

L30.0 Nummular dermatitis

L30.1 Dyshidrosis [pompholyx]

L30.2 Cutaneous autosensitization
Candidid [levurid]
Dermatophytid
Eczematid

L30.3 Infective dermatitis
Infectious eczematoid dermatitis

L30.4 Erythema intertrigo

L30.5 Pityriasis alba
AHA: 2018,1Q,6

L30.8 Other specified dermatitis

L30.9 Dermatitis, unspecified
Eczema NOS

Papulosquamous disorders (L40-L45)

L40 Psoriasis
DEF: Chronic autoimmune condition that speeds up skin cell growth, causing excessive immature skin cells to form raised, rounded erythematous lesions covered by dry, silvery scaling patches. Most commonly found on the scalp, elbows, knees, hands, feet, and genitals, it can also affect the joints with stiffness and swelling.

L40.0 Psoriasis vulgaris Rx
Nummular psoriasis
Plaque psoriasis

L40.1 Generalized pustular psoriasis Rx
Impetigo herpetiformis
Von Zumbusch's disease

L40.2 Acrodermatitis continua Rx

L40.3 Pustulosis palmaris et plantaris Rx

L40.4 Guttate psoriasis Rx

L40.5 Arthropathic psoriasis

L40.50 Arthropathic psoriasis, unspecified HCC Rx ESR COM

L40.51 Distal interphalangeal psoriatic arthropathy HCC Rx ESR COM

L40.52 Psoriatic arthritis mutilans HCC Rx ESR COM

L40.53 Psoriatic spondylitis HCC Rx ESR COM

L40.54 Psoriatic juvenile arthropathy HCC Rx ESR COM

L40.59 Other psoriatic arthropathy HCC Rx ESR COM

L40.8 Other psoriasis Rx
Flexural psoriasis

L40.9 Psoriasis, unspecified Rx

L41 Parapsoriasis
EXCLUDES 1 *poikiloderma vasculare atrophicans (L94.5)*

L41.0 Pityriasis lichenoides et varioliformis acuta Rx
Mucha-Habermann disease

L41.1 Pityriasis lichenoides chronica Rx

L41.3 Small plaque parapsoriasis Rx

L41.4 Large plaque parapsoriasis Rx

L41.5 Retiform parapsoriasis Rx

L41.8 Other parapsoriasis Rx

L41.9 Parapsoriasis, unspecified Rx

L42 Pityriasis rosea

L43 Lichen planus
EXCLUDES 1 *lichen planopilaris (L66.1)*

L43.0 Hypertrophic lichen planus

L43.1 Bullous lichen planus

L43.2 Lichenoid drug reaction
Use additional code for adverse effect, if applicable, to identify drug (T36-T50 with fifth or sixth character 5)

L43.3 Subacute (active) lichen planus
Lichen planus tropicus

L43.8 Other lichen planus

L43.9 Lichen planus, unspecified

L44 Other papulosquamous disorders

L44.0 Pityriasis rubra pilaris

L44.1 Lichen nitidus
DEF: Chronic, inflammatory, asymptomatic skin disorder, characterized by numerous glistening, flat-topped, discrete, skin-colored micropapules, most often on the penis, lower abdomen, inner thighs, wrists, forearms, breasts, and buttocks.

L44.2 Lichen striatus

L44.3 Lichen ruber moniliformis

L44.4 Infantile papular acrodermatitis [Gianotti-Crosti] P

L44.8 Other specified papulosquamous disorders

L44.9 Papulosquamous disorder, unspecified

L45 Papulosquamous disorders in diseases classified elsewhere
Code first underlying disease

Urticaria and erythema (L49-L54)

EXCLUDES 1 *Lyme disease (A69.2-)*
rosacea (L71.-)

✓4th **L49 Exfoliation due to erythematous conditions according to extent of body surface involved**

Code first erythematous condition causing exfoliation, such as:
Ritter's disease (LØØ)
(Staphylococcal) scalded skin syndrome (LØØ)
Stevens-Johnson syndrome (L51.1)
Stevens-Johnson syndrome-toxic epidermal necrolysis overlap syndrome (L51.3)
toxic epidermal necrolysis (L51.2)

DEF: Exfoliation: Falling or sloughing off skin in layers.

L49.Ø Exfoliation due to erythematous condition involving less than 1Ø percent of body surface UPD
Exfoliation due to erythematous condition NOS

L49.1 Exfoliation due to erythematous condition involving 1Ø-19 percent of body surface COM UPD

L49.2 Exfoliation due to erythematous condition involving 2Ø-29 percent of body surface COM UPD

L49.3 Exfoliation due to erythematous condition involving 3Ø-39 percent of body surface COM UPD

L49.4 Exfoliation due to erythematous condition involving 4Ø-49 percent of body surface COM UPD

L49.5 Exfoliation due to erythematous condition involving 5Ø-59 percent of body surface COM UPD

L49.6 Exfoliation due to erythematous condition involving 6Ø-69 percent of body surface COM UPD

L49.7 Exfoliation due to erythematous condition involving 7Ø-79 percent of body surface COM UPD

L49.8 Exfoliation due to erythematous condition involving 8Ø-89 percent of body surface COM UPD

L49.9 Exfoliation due to erythematous condition involving 9Ø or more percent of body surface COM UPD

✓4th **L5Ø Urticaria**

EXCLUDES 1 *allergic contact dermatitis (L23.-)*
angioneurotic edema (T78.3)
giant urticaria (T78.3)
hereditary angio-edema (D84.1)
Quincke's edema (T78.3)
serum urticaria (T8Ø.6-)
solar urticaria (L56.3)
urticaria neonatorum (P83.8)
urticaria papulosa (L28.2)
urticaria pigmentosa (D47.Ø1)

DEF: Eruption of itching edema of the skin. ***Synonym(s):*** *hives.*

L5Ø.Ø Allergic urticaria

L5Ø.1 Idiopathic urticaria

L5Ø.2 Urticaria due to cold and heat
EXCLUDES 2 *familial cold urticaria (MØ4.2)*

L5Ø.3 Dermatographic urticaria

L5Ø.4 Vibratory urticaria

L5Ø.5 Cholinergic urticaria

L5Ø.6 Contact urticaria

L5Ø.8 Other urticaria
Chronic urticaria
Recurrent periodic urticaria

L5Ø.9 Urticaria, unspecified

✓4th **L51 Erythema multiforme**

Use additional code for adverse effect, if applicable, to identify drug (T36-T5Ø with fifth or sixth character 5)
Use additional code to identify associated manifestations, such as:
arthropathy associated with dermatological disorders (M14.8-)
conjunctival edema (H11.42)
conjunctivitis (H1Ø.22-)
corneal scars and opacities (H17.-)
corneal ulcer (H16.Ø-)
edema of eyelid (HØ2.84-)
inflammation of eyelid (HØ1.8)
keratoconjunctivitis sicca (H16.22-)
mechanical lagophthalmos (HØ2.22-)
stomatitis (K12.-)
symblepharon (H11.23-)
Use additional code to identify percentage of skin exfoliation (L49.-)

EXCLUDES 1 *staphylococcal scalded skin syndrome (LØØ)*
Ritter's disease (LØØ)

DEF: Acute complex of symptoms with a varied pattern of skin eruptions, such as macular, bullous, papular, nodose, or vesicular lesions on the neck, face, and legs. Erythema (redness of skin and mucous membranes) multiforme (multiple forms) is a hypersensitivity (allergic) reaction that can occur at any age but primarily affects children or young adults.

L51.Ø Nonbullous erythema multiforme

L51.1 Stevens-Johnson syndrome HCC ESR COM

L51.2 Toxic epidermal necrolysis [Lyell] HCC ESR COM

L51.3 Stevens-Johnson syndrome-toxic epidermal necrolysis overlap syndrome HCC ESR COM
SJS-TEN overlap syndrome

L51.8 Other erythema multiforme

L51.9 Erythema multiforme, unspecified
Erythema iris
Erythema multiforme major NOS
Erythema multiforme minor NOS
Herpes iris

L52 Erythema nodosum

EXCLUDES 1 *tuberculous erythema nodosum (A18.4)*

DEF: Form of panniculitis (inflammation of the fat layer beneath the skin) most often occurring in women. Commonly seen as a hypersensitivity reaction to infections, drugs, sarcoidosis, and specific enteropathies. The acute stage is associated with fever, malaise, and arthralgia. The lesions are pink to blue in color as tender nodules and are found on the front of the legs below the knees.

✓4th **L53 Other erythematous conditions**

EXCLUDES 1 *erythema ab igne (L59.Ø)*
erythema due to external agents in contact with skin (L23-L25)
erythema intertrigo (L3Ø.4)

L53.Ø Toxic erythema
Code first poisoning due to drug or toxin, if applicable (T36-T65 with fifth or sixth character 1-4 or 6)
Use additional code for adverse effect, if applicable, to identify drug (T36-T5Ø with fifth or sixth character 5)
EXCLUDES 1 *neonatal erythema toxicum (P83.1)*

L53.1 Erythema annulare centrifugum

L53.2 Erythema marginatum

L53.3 Other chronic figurate erythema

L53.8 Other specified erythematous conditions

L53.9 Erythematous condition, unspecified
Erythema NOS
Erythroderma NOS

L54 Erythema in diseases classified elsewhere
Code first underlying disease

Radiation-related disorders of the skin and subcutaneous tissue (L55-L59)

✓4th **L55 Sunburn**

L55.Ø Sunburn of first degree

L55.1 Sunburn of second degree

L55.2 Sunburn of third degree COM

L55.9 Sunburn, unspecified

L56 Other acute skin changes due to ultraviolet radiation
Use additional code to identify the source of the ultraviolet radiation (W89, X32)

L56.0 Drug phototoxic response
Use additional code for adverse effect, if applicable, to identify drug (T36-T50 with fifth or sixth character 5)

L56.1 Drug photoallergic response
Use additional code for adverse effect, if applicable, to identify drug (T36-T50 with fifth or sixth character 5)

L56.2 Photocontact dermatitis [berloque dermatitis]

L56.3 Solar urticaria

L56.4 Polymorphous light eruption

L56.5 Disseminated superficial actinic porokeratosis (DSAP)
DEF: Autosomal dominant skin condition occurring in sun-exposed areas of the skin (particularly the arms and legs), characterized by superficial annular, keratotic, brownish-red spots or thickenings with depressed centers and sharp, ridged borders. It may evolve into squamous cell carcinoma.

L56.8 Other specified acute skin changes due to ultraviolet radiation

L56.9 Acute skin change due to ultraviolet radiation, unspecified

L57 Skin changes due to chronic exposure to nonionizing radiation
Use additional code to identify the source of the ultraviolet radiation (W89), or other nonionizing radiation (W90)

L57.0 Actinic keratosis
Keratosis NOS
Senile keratosis
Solar keratosis

L57.1 Actinic reticuloid

L57.2 Cutis rhomboidalis nuchae

L57.3 Poikiloderma of Civatte

L57.4 Cutis laxa senilis
Elastosis senilis

L57.5 Actinic granuloma

L57.8 Other skin changes due to chronic exposure to nonionizing radiation
Farmer's skin
Sailor's skin
Solar dermatitis

L57.9 Skin changes due to chronic exposure to nonionizing radiation, unspecified

L58 Radiodermatitis
Use additional code to identify the source of the radiation (W88, W90)

L58.0 Acute radiodermatitis

L58.1 Chronic radiodermatitis

L58.9 Radiodermatitis, unspecified

L59 Other disorders of skin and subcutaneous tissue related to radiation

L59.0 Erythema ab igne [dermatitis ab igne]

L59.8 Other specified disorders of the skin and subcutaneous tissue related to radiation
AHA: 2017,1Q,33

L59.9 Disorder of the skin and subcutaneous tissue related to radiation, unspecified

Disorders of skin appendages (L60-L75)

EXCLUDES 1 *congenital malformations of integument (Q84.-)*

L60 Nail disorders
EXCLUDES 2 *clubbing of nails (R68.3)*
onychia and paronychia (L03.0-)

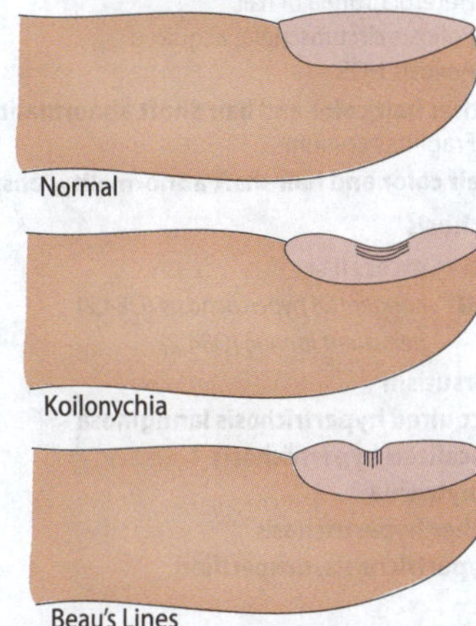

L60.0 Ingrowing nail

L60.1 Onycholysis

L60.2 Onychogryphosis

L60.3 Nail dystrophy

L60.4 Beau's lines

L60.5 Yellow nail syndrome

L60.8 Other nail disorders

L60.9 Nail disorder, unspecified

L62 Nail disorders in diseases classified elsewhere
Code first underlying disease, such as:
pachydermoperiostosis (M89.4-)

L63 Alopecia areata

L63.0 Alopecia (capitis) totalis

L63.1 Alopecia universalis

L63.2 Ophiasis

L63.8 Other alopecia areata

L63.9 Alopecia areata, unspecified

L64 Androgenic alopecia
INCLUDES male-pattern baldness

L64.0 Drug-induced androgenic alopecia
Use additional code for adverse effect, if applicable, to identify drug (T36-T50 with fifth or sixth character 5)

L64.8 Other androgenic alopecia

L64.9 Androgenic alopecia, unspecified

L65 Other nonscarring hair loss
Use additional code for adverse effect, if applicable, to identify drug (T36-T50 with fifth or sixth character 5)
EXCLUDES 1 *trichotillomania (F63.3)*

L65.0 Telogen effluvium
DEF: Form of nonscarring alopecia characterized by shedding of hair from premature telogen development in follicles due to stress, including shock, childbirth, surgery, drugs, or weight loss.

L65.1 Anagen effluvium

L65.2 Alopecia mucinosa

L65.8 Other specified nonscarring hair loss

L65.9 Nonscarring hair loss, unspecified
Alopecia NOS

L66 Cicatricial alopecia [scarring hair loss]

L66.0 Pseudopelade

L66.1 Lichen planopilaris
Follicular lichen planus

L66.2 Folliculitis decalvans

L66.3 Perifolliculitis capitis abscedens

L66.4 Folliculitis ulerythematosa reticulata

L66.8 Other cicatricial alopecia
AHA: 2015,1Q,19

L66.9 Cicatricial alopecia, unspecified

✓4th L67 Hair color and hair shaft abnormalities

EXCLUDES 1 *monilethrix (Q84.1)*
pili annulati (Q84.1)
telogen effluvium (L65.Ø)

L67.Ø Trichorrhexis nodosa

L67.1 Variations in hair color
Canities
Greyness, hair (premature)
Heterochromia of hair
Poliosis circumscripta, acquired
Poliosis NOS

L67.8 Other hair color and hair shaft abnormalities
Fragilitas crinium

L67.9 Hair color and hair shaft abnormality, unspecified

✓4th L68 Hypertrichosis

INCLUDES excess hair
EXCLUDES 1 *congenital hypertrichosis (Q84.2)*
persistent lanugo (Q84.2)

L68.Ø Hirsutism
L68.1 Acquired hypertrichosis lanuginosa
L68.2 Localized hypertrichosis
L68.3 Polytrichia
L68.8 Other hypertrichosis
L68.9 Hypertrichosis, unspecified

✓4th L7Ø Acne

EXCLUDES 2 *acne keloid (L73.Ø)*

L7Ø.Ø Acne vulgaris
L7Ø.1 Acne conglobata
L7Ø.2 Acne varioliformis
Acne necrotica miliaris
DEF: Rare form of acne characterized by development of persistent brown papulopustules followed by scar formation. This type of acne usually presents on the brow and temporoparietal part of the scalp.

L7Ø.3 Acne tropica
L7Ø.4 Infantile acne P
L7Ø.5 Acné excoriée
Acné excoriée des jeunes filles
Picker's acne
L7Ø.8 Other acne
L7Ø.9 Acne, unspecified

✓4th L71 Rosacea

Use additional code for adverse effect, if applicable, to identify drug (T36-T5Ø with fifth or sixth character 5)

L71.Ø Perioral dermatitis
L71.1 Rhinophyma
L71.8 Other rosacea
AHA: 2018,4Q,15
L71.9 Rosacea, unspecified

✓4th L72 Follicular cysts of skin and subcutaneous tissue

L72.Ø Epidermal cyst
✓5th L72.1 Pilar and trichodermal cyst
L72.11 Pilar cyst
L72.12 Trichodermal cyst
Trichilemmal (proliferating) cyst
L72.2 Steatocystoma multiplex
L72.3 Sebaceous cyst
EXCLUDES 2 *pilar cyst (L72.11)*
trichilemmal (proliferating) cyst (L72.12)
L72.8 Other follicular cysts of the skin and subcutaneous tissue
L72.9 Follicular cyst of the skin and subcutaneous tissue, unspecified

✓4th L73 Other follicular disorders

L73.Ø Acne keloid
L73.1 Pseudofolliculitis barbae
L73.2 Hidradenitis suppurativa
L73.8 Other specified follicular disorders
Sycosis barbae
L73.9 Follicular disorder, unspecified

✓4th L74 Eccrine sweat disorders

EXCLUDES 2 *generalized hyperhidrosis (R61)*

DEF: Eccrine sweat glands: Glands found in the dermal and hypodermal layer of the skin throughout the body, particularly on the forehead, scalp, axillae, palms, and soles. These glands produce watery and neutral or slightly acidic sweat.

L74.Ø Miliaria rubra
L74.1 Miliaria crystallina
L74.2 Miliaria profunda
Miliaria tropicalis
L74.3 Miliaria, unspecified
L74.4 Anhidrosis
Hypohidrosis
DEF: Inability to sweat normally. When the body can't cool itself through perspiration it can lead to heatstroke, a life-threatening condition.
✓5th L74.5 Focal hyperhidrosis
✓6th L74.51 Primary focal hyperhidrosis
L74.51Ø Primary focal hyperhidrosis, axilla
L74.511 Primary focal hyperhidrosis, face
L74.512 Primary focal hyperhidrosis, palms
L74.513 Primary focal hyperhidrosis, soles
L74.519 Primary focal hyperhidrosis, unspecified
L74.52 Secondary focal hyperhidrosis
Frey's syndrome
L74.8 Other eccrine sweat disorders
L74.9 Eccrine sweat disorder, unspecified
Sweat gland disorder NOS

✓4th L75 Apocrine sweat disorders

EXCLUDES 1 *dyshidrosis (L3Ø.1)*
hidradenitis suppurativa (L73.2)

DEF: Apocrine sweat glands: Found in the axilla, areola, and circumanal region, these glands begin to function in puberty and produce viscid milky secretions in response to external stimuli.

L75.Ø Bromhidrosis
L75.1 Chromhidrosis
L75.2 Apocrine miliaria
Fox-Fordyce disease
DEF: Chronic, usually pruritic disease evidenced by small follicular papular eruptions, especially in the axillary and pubic areas. Apocrine miliaria develops from the closure and rupture of the affected apocrine glands' intraepidermal portion of the ducts.
L75.8 Other apocrine sweat disorders
L75.9 Apocrine sweat disorder, unspecified

Intraoperative and postprocedural complications of skin and subcutaneous tissue (L76)

✓4th L76 Intraoperative and postprocedural complications of skin and subcutaneous tissue

AHA: 2016,4Q,9-10

✓5th L76.Ø Intraoperative hemorrhage and hematoma of skin and subcutaneous tissue complicating a procedure
EXCLUDES 1 *intraoperative hemorrhage and hematoma of skin and subcutaneous tissue due to accidental puncture and laceration during a procedure (L76.1-)*
L76.Ø1 Intraoperative hemorrhage and hematoma of skin and subcutaneous tissue complicating a dermatologic procedure
L76.Ø2 Intraoperative hemorrhage and hematoma of skin and subcutaneous tissue complicating other procedure

✓5th L76.1 Accidental puncture and laceration of skin and subcutaneous tissue during a procedure
L76.11 Accidental puncture and laceration of skin and subcutaneous tissue during a dermatologic procedure
L76.12 Accidental puncture and laceration of skin and subcutaneous tissue during other procedure

✓5th L76.2 Postprocedural hemorrhage of skin and subcutaneous tissue following a procedure
L76.21 Postprocedural hemorrhage of skin and subcutaneous tissue following a dermatologic procedure
L76.22 Postprocedural hemorrhage of skin and subcutaneous tissue following other procedure

✓5th **L76.3 Postprocedural hematoma and seroma of skin and subcutaneous tissue following a procedure**

L76.31 Postprocedural hematoma of skin and subcutaneous tissue following a dermatologic procedure

L76.32 Postprocedural hematoma of skin and subcutaneous tissue following other procedure

L76.33 Postprocedural seroma of skin and subcutaneous tissue following a dermatologic procedure

L76.34 Postprocedural seroma of skin and subcutaneous tissue following other procedure

✓5th **L76.8 Other intraoperative and postprocedural complications of skin and subcutaneous tissue**

Use additional code, if applicable, to further specify disorder

L76.81 Other intraoperative complications of skin and subcutaneous tissue

L76.82 Other postprocedural complications of skin and subcutaneous tissue

AHA: 2017,3Q,6

Other disorders of the skin and subcutaneous tissue (L80-L99)

L80 Vitiligo

EXCLUDES 2 *vitiligo of eyelids (H02.73-)*
vitiligo of vulva (N90.89)

DEF: Persistent, progressive development of nonpigmented white patches on otherwise normal skin.

✓4th **L81 Other disorders of pigmentation**

EXCLUDES 1 *birthmark NOS (Q82.5)*
Peutz-Jeghers syndrome ►(Q85.89)◄

EXCLUDES 2 *nevus - see Alphabetical Index*

L81.0 Postinflammatory hyperpigmentation

L81.1 Chloasma

L81.2 Freckles

L81.3 Café au lait spots

L81.4 Other melanin hyperpigmentation
Lentigo

L81.5 Leukoderma, not elsewhere classified

L81.6 Other disorders of diminished melanin formation

L81.7 Pigmented purpuric dermatosis
Angioma serpiginosum

L81.8 Other specified disorders of pigmentation
Iron pigmentation
Tattoo pigmentation

L81.9 Disorder of pigmentation, unspecified

✓4th **L82 Seborrheic keratosis**

INCLUDES basal cell papilloma
dermatosis papulosa nigra
Leser-Trélat disease

EXCLUDES 2 *seborrheic dermatitis (L21.-)*

DEF: Common, benign, noninvasive, lightly pigmented, warty growth composed of basaloid cells that usually appear at middle age as soft, easily crumbling plaques on the face, trunk, and extremities.

L82.0 Inflamed seborrheic keratosis
AHA: 2021,3Q,10

L82.1 Other seborrheic keratosis
Seborrheic keratosis NOS

L83 Acanthosis nigricans
Confluent and reticulated papillomatosis

DEF: Diffuse, velvety hyperplasia of the spinous skin layer of the axilla and other body folds marked by gray, brown, or black pigmentation. In adult form, it is often associated with malignant acanthosis nigricans in a benign, nevoid form relatively generalized.

L84 Corns and callosities
Callus
Clavus

✓4th **L85 Other epidermal thickening**

EXCLUDES 2 *hypertrophic disorders of the skin (L91.-)*

L85.0 Acquired ichthyosis

EXCLUDES 1 *congenital ichthyosis (Q80.-)*

L85.1 Acquired keratosis [keratoderma] palmaris et plantaris

EXCLUDES 1 *inherited keratosis palmaris et plantaris (Q82.8)*

L85.2 Keratosis punctata (palmaris et plantaris)

L85.3 Xerosis cutis
Dry skin dermatitis

L85.8 Other specified epidermal thickening
Cutaneous horn

L85.9 Epidermal thickening, unspecified

L86 Keratoderma in diseases classified elsewhere

Code first underlying disease, such as:
Reiter's disease (M02.3-)

EXCLUDES 1 *gonococcal keratoderma (A54.89)*
gonococcal keratosis (A54.89)
keratoderma due to vitamin A deficiency (E50.8)
keratosis due to vitamin A deficiency (E50.8)
xeroderma due to vitamin A deficiency (E50.8)

✓4th **L87 Transepidermal elimination disorders**

EXCLUDES 1 *granuloma annulare (perforating) (L92.0)*

L87.0 Keratosis follicularis et parafollicularis in cutem penetrans
Hyperkeratosis follicularis penetrans
Kyrle disease

L87.1 Reactive perforating collagenosis

L87.2 Elastosis perforans serpiginosa

L87.8 Other transepidermal elimination disorders

L87.9 Transepidermal elimination disorder, unspecified

L88 Pyoderma gangrenosum Rx COM
Phagedenic pyoderma

EXCLUDES 1 *dermatitis gangrenosa (L08.0)*

DEF: Persistent debilitating skin disease characterized by irregular, boggy, blue-red ulcerations, with central healing and undermined edges.

✓4th **L89 Pressure ulcer**

INCLUDES bed sore
decubitus ulcer
plaster ulcer
pressure area
pressure sore

Code first any associated gangrene (I96)

EXCLUDES 2 *decubitus (trophic) ulcer of cervix (uteri) (N86)*
diabetic ulcers (E08.621, E08.622, E09.621, E09.622, E10.621, E10.622, E11.621, E11.622, E13.621, E13.622)
non-pressure chronic ulcer of skin (L97.-)
skin infections (L00-L08)
varicose ulcer (I83.0, I83.2)

AHA: 2022,2Q,8; 2021,1Q,24; 2019,4Q,10-11,54; 2018,4Q,69; 2018,3Q,3; 2018,2Q,21; 2017,4Q,109; 2017,1Q,49; 2016,4Q,143

TIP: The stage of a diagnosed pressure ulcer can be based on documentation from clinicians who are not the patient's provider.

Four Stages of Pressure Ulcer

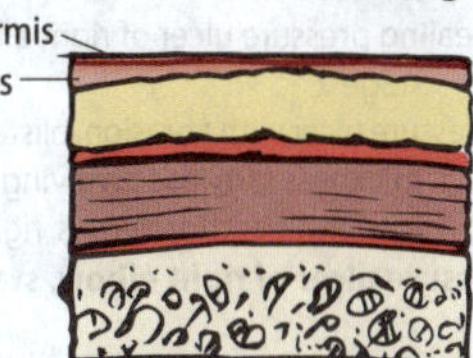

Stage 1
Persistent focal edema

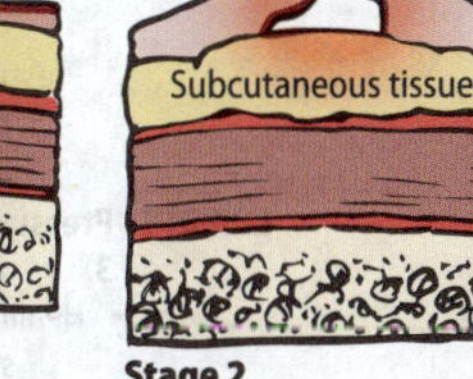

Stage 2
Abrasion, blister, partial thickness skin loss involving epidermis and/or dermis

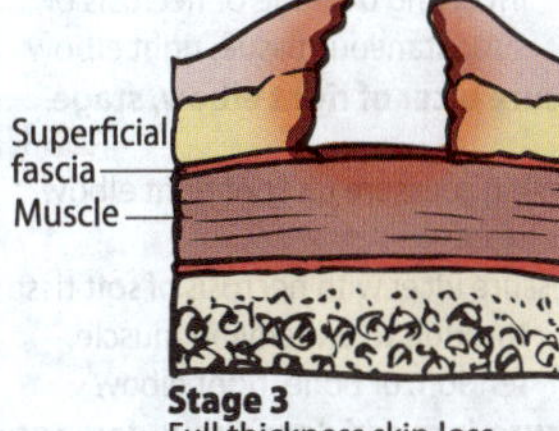

Stage 3
Full thickness skin loss involving damage or necrosis of subcutaneous tissue

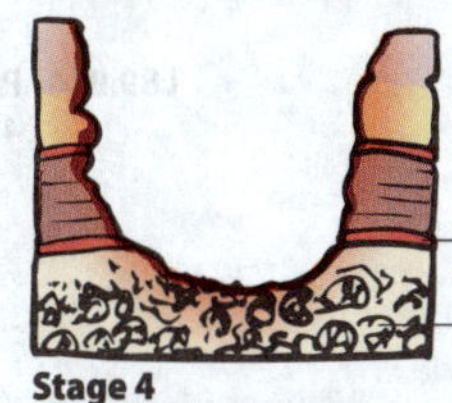

Stage 4
Necrosis of soft tissues through to underlying muscle, tendon, or bone

✓5th **L89.0 Pressure ulcer of elbow**

✓6th **L89.00 Pressure ulcer of unspecified elbow**

L89.000 Pressure ulcer of unspecified elbow, unstageable

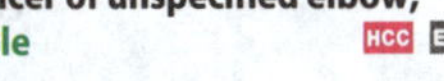

L89.001 Pressure ulcer of unspecified elbow, stage 1
Healing pressure ulcer of unspecified elbow, stage 1
Pressure pre-ulcer skin changes limited to persistent focal edema, unspecified elbow

L89.002 Pressure ulcer of unspecified elbow, stage 2 HCC ESR
Healing pressure ulcer of unspecified elbow, stage 2
Pressure ulcer with abrasion, blister, partial thickness skin loss involving epidermis and/or dermis, unspecified elbow

L89.003 Pressure ulcer of unspecified elbow, stage 3 HCC ESR
Healing pressure ulcer of unspecified elbow, stage 3
Pressure ulcer with full thickness skin loss involving damage or necrosis of subcutaneous tissue, unspecified elbow

L89.004 Pressure ulcer of unspecified elbow, stage 4 HCC ESR
Healing pressure ulcer of unspecified elbow, stage 4
Pressure ulcer with necrosis of soft tissues through to underlying muscle, tendon, or bone, unspecified elbow

L89.006 Pressure-induced deep tissue damage of unspecified elbow

L89.009 Pressure ulcer of unspecified elbow, unspecified stage
Healing pressure ulcer of elbow NOS
Healing pressure ulcer of unspecified elbow, unspecified stage

√6th **L89.01 Pressure ulcer of right elbow**

L89.010 Pressure ulcer of right elbow, unstageable HCC ESR

L89.011 Pressure ulcer of right elbow, stage 1
Healing pressure ulcer of right elbow, stage 1
Pressure pre-ulcer skin changes limited to persistent focal edema, right elbow

L89.012 Pressure ulcer of right elbow, stage 2 HCC ESR
Healing pressure ulcer of right elbow, stage 2
Pressure ulcer with abrasion, blister, partial thickness skin loss involving epidermis and/or dermis, right elbow

L89.013 Pressure ulcer of right elbow, stage 3 HCC ESR
Healing pressure ulcer of right elbow, stage 3
Pressure ulcer with full thickness skin loss involving damage or necrosis of subcutaneous tissue, right elbow

L89.014 Pressure ulcer of right elbow, stage 4 HCC ESR
Healing pressure ulcer of right elbow, stage 4
Pressure ulcer with necrosis of soft tissues through to underlying muscle, tendon, or bone, right elbow

L89.016 Pressure-induced deep tissue damage of right elbow

L89.019 Pressure ulcer of right elbow, unspecified stage
Healing pressure ulcer of right elbow NOS

√6th **L89.02 Pressure ulcer of left elbow**

L89.020 Pressure ulcer of left elbow, unstageable HCC ESR

L89.021 Pressure ulcer of left elbow, stage 1
Healing pressure ulcer of left elbow, stage 1
Pressure pre-ulcer skin changes limited to persistent focal edema, left elbow

L89.022 Pressure ulcer of left elbow, stage 2 HCC ESR
Healing pressure ulcer of left elbow, stage 2
Pressure ulcer with abrasion, blister, partial thickness skin loss involving epidermis and/or dermis, left elbow

L89.023 Pressure ulcer of left elbow, stage 3 HCC ESR
Healing pressure ulcer of left elbow, stage 3
Pressure ulcer with full thickness skin loss involving damage or necrosis of subcutaneous tissue, left elbow

L89.024 Pressure ulcer of left elbow, stage 4 HCC ESR
Healing pressure ulcer of left elbow, stage 4
Pressure ulcer with necrosis of soft tissues through to underlying muscle, tendon, or bone, left elbow

L89.026 Pressure-induced deep tissue damage of left elbow

L89.029 Pressure ulcer of left elbow, unspecified stage
Healing pressure ulcer of left elbow NOS

√5th **L89.1 Pressure ulcer of back**

√6th **L89.10 Pressure ulcer of unspecified part of back**

L89.100 Pressure ulcer of unspecified part of back, unstageable HCC ESR

L89.101 Pressure ulcer of unspecified part of back, stage 1
Healing pressure ulcer of unspecified part of back, stage 1
Pressure pre-ulcer skin changes limited to persistent focal edema, unspecified part of back

L89.102 Pressure ulcer of unspecified part of back, stage 2 HCC ESR
Healing pressure ulcer of unspecified part of back, stage 2
Pressure ulcer with abrasion, blister, partial thickness skin loss involving epidermis and/or dermis, unspecified part of back

L89.103 Pressure ulcer of unspecified part of back, stage 3 HCC ESR
Healing pressure ulcer of unspecified part of back, stage 3
Pressure ulcer with full thickness skin loss involving damage or necrosis of subcutaneous tissue, unspecified part of back

L89.104 Pressure ulcer of unspecified part of back, stage 4 HCC ESR
Healing pressure ulcer of unspecified part of back, stage 4
Pressure ulcer with necrosis of soft tissues through to underlying muscle, tendon, or bone, unspecified part of back

L89.106 Pressure-induced deep tissue damage of unspecified part of back

L89.109 Pressure ulcer of unspecified part of back, unspecified stage
Healing pressure ulcer of unspecified part of back NOS
Healing pressure ulcer of unspecified part of back, unspecified stage

√6th **L89.11 Pressure ulcer of right upper back**
Pressure ulcer of right shoulder blade

L89.110 Pressure ulcer of right upper back, unstageable HCC ESR

L89.111 Pressure ulcer of right upper back, stage 1
Healing pressure ulcer of right upper back, stage 1
Pressure pre-ulcer skin changes limited to persistent focal edema, right upper back

L89.112 Pressure ulcer of right upper back, stage 2 HCC ESR
Healing pressure ulcer of right upper back, stage 2
Pressure ulcer with abrasion, blister, partial thickness skin loss involving epidermis and/or dermis, right upper back

L89.113 Pressure ulcer of right upper back, stage 3 HCC ESR
Healing pressure ulcer of right upper back, stage 3
Pressure ulcer with full thickness skin loss involving damage or necrosis of subcutaneous tissue, right upper back

L89.114 Pressure ulcer of right upper back, stage 4 HCC ESR
Healing pressure ulcer of right upper back, stage 4
Pressure ulcer with necrosis of soft tissues through to underlying muscle, tendon, or bone, right upper back

L89.116 Pressure-induced deep tissue damage of right upper back

L89.119 Pressure ulcer of right upper back, unspecified stage
Healing pressure ulcer of right upper back NOS
Healing pressure ulcer of right upper back, unspecified stage

✓6th **L89.12 Pressure ulcer of left upper back**
Pressure ulcer of left shoulder blade

L89.120 Pressure ulcer of left upper back, unstageable HCC ESR

L89.121 Pressure ulcer of left upper back, stage 1
Healing pressure ulcer of left upper back, stage 1
Pressure pre-ulcer skin changes limited to persistent focal edema, left upper back

L89.122 Pressure ulcer of left upper back, stage 2 HCC ESR
Healing pressure ulcer of left upper back, stage 2
Pressure ulcer with abrasion, blister, partial thickness skin loss involving epidermis and/or dermis, left upper back

L89.123 Pressure ulcer of left upper back, stage 3 HCC ESR
Healing pressure ulcer of left upper back, stage 3
Pressure ulcer with full thickness skin loss involving damage or necrosis of subcutaneous tissue, left upper back

L89.124 Pressure ulcer of left upper back, stage 4 HCC ESR
Healing pressure ulcer of left upper back, stage 4
Pressure ulcer with necrosis of soft tissues through to underlying muscle, tendon, or bone, left upper back

L89.126 Pressure-induced deep tissue damage of left upper back

L89.129 Pressure ulcer of left upper back, unspecified stage
Healing pressure ulcer of left upper back NOS
Healing pressure ulcer of left upper back, unspecified stage

✓6th **L89.13 Pressure ulcer of right lower back**

L89.130 Pressure ulcer of right lower back, unstageable HCC ESR

L89.131 Pressure ulcer of right lower back, stage 1
Healing pressure ulcer of right lower back, stage 1
Pressure pre-ulcer skin changes limited to persistent focal edema, right lower back

L89.132 Pressure ulcer of right lower back, stage 2 HCC ESR
Healing pressure ulcer of right lower back, stage 2
Pressure ulcer with abrasion, blister, partial thickness skin loss involving epidermis and/or dermis, right lower back

L89.133 Pressure ulcer of right lower back, stage 3 HCC ESR
Healing pressure ulcer of right lower back, stage 3
Pressure ulcer with full thickness skin loss involving damage or necrosis of subcutaneous tissue, right lower back

L89.134 Pressure ulcer of right lower back, stage 4 HCC ESR
Healing pressure ulcer of right lower back, stage 4
Pressure ulcer with necrosis of soft tissues through to underlying muscle, tendon, or bone, right lower back

L89.136 Pressure-induced deep tissue damage of right lower back

L89.139 Pressure ulcer of right lower back, unspecified stage
Healing pressure ulcer of right lower back NOS
Healing pressure ulcer of right lower back, unspecified stage

✓6th **L89.14 Pressure ulcer of left lower back**

L89.140 Pressure ulcer of left lower back, unstageable HCC ESR

L89.141 Pressure ulcer of left lower back, stage 1
Healing pressure ulcer of left lower back, stage 1
Pressure pre-ulcer skin changes limited to persistent focal edema, left lower back

L89.142 Pressure ulcer of left lower back, stage 2 HCC ESR
Healing pressure ulcer of left lower back, stage 2
Pressure ulcer with abrasion, blister, partial thickness skin loss involving epidermis and/or dermis, left lower back

L89.143 Pressure ulcer of left lower back, stage 3 HCC ESR
Healing pressure ulcer of left lower back, stage 3
Pressure ulcer with full thickness skin loss involving damage or necrosis of subcutaneous tissue, left lower back

L89.144 Pressure ulcer of left lower back, stage 4 HCC ESR
Healing pressure ulcer of left lower back, stage 4
Pressure ulcer with necrosis of soft tissues through to underlying muscle, tendon, or bone, left lower back

L89.146 Pressure-induced deep tissue damage of left lower back

L89.149 Pressure ulcer of left lower back, unspecified stage
Healing pressure ulcer of left lower back NOS
Healing pressure ulcer of left lower back, unspecified stage

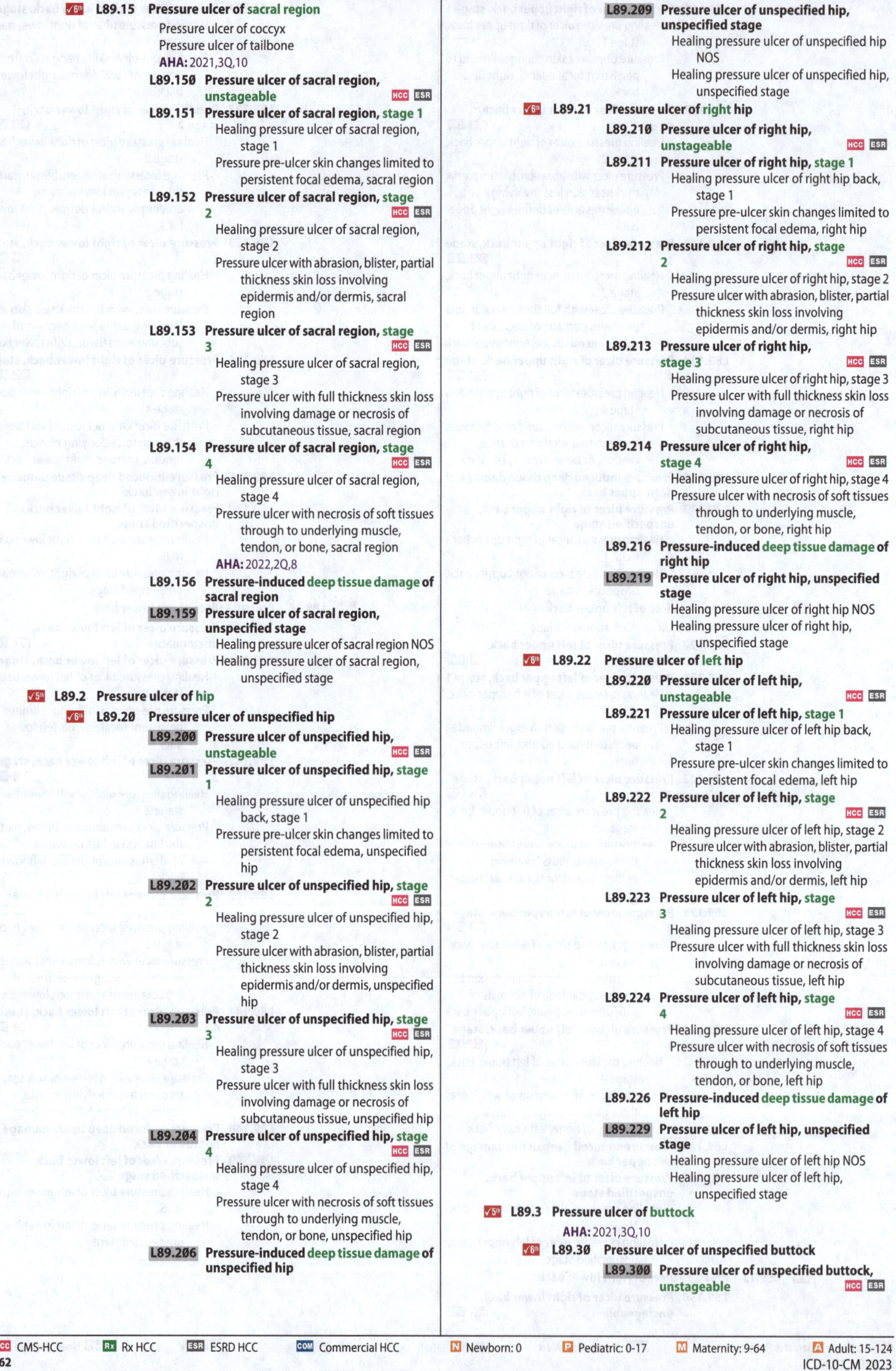

✓6th **L89.15 Pressure ulcer of sacral region**
Pressure ulcer of coccyx
Pressure ulcer of tailbone
AHA: 2021,3Q,10

L89.150 Pressure ulcer of sacral region, unstageable HCC ESR

L89.151 Pressure ulcer of sacral region, stage 1
Healing pressure ulcer of sacral region, stage 1
Pressure pre-ulcer skin changes limited to persistent focal edema, sacral region

L89.152 Pressure ulcer of sacral region, stage 2 HCC ESR
Healing pressure ulcer of sacral region, stage 2
Pressure ulcer with abrasion, blister, partial thickness skin loss involving epidermis and/or dermis, sacral region

L89.153 Pressure ulcer of sacral region, stage 3 HCC ESR
Healing pressure ulcer of sacral region, stage 3
Pressure ulcer with full thickness skin loss involving damage or necrosis of subcutaneous tissue, sacral region

L89.154 Pressure ulcer of sacral region, stage 4 HCC ESR
Healing pressure ulcer of sacral region, stage 4
Pressure ulcer with necrosis of soft tissues through to underlying muscle, tendon, or bone, sacral region
AHA: 2022,2Q,8

L89.156 Pressure-induced deep tissue damage of sacral region

L89.159 Pressure ulcer of sacral region, unspecified stage
Healing pressure ulcer of sacral region NOS
Healing pressure ulcer of sacral region, unspecified stage

✓5th **L89.2 Pressure ulcer of hip**

✓6th **L89.20 Pressure ulcer of unspecified hip**

L89.200 Pressure ulcer of unspecified hip, unstageable HCC ESR

L89.201 Pressure ulcer of unspecified hip, stage 1
Healing pressure ulcer of unspecified hip back, stage 1
Pressure pre-ulcer skin changes limited to persistent focal edema, unspecified hip

L89.202 Pressure ulcer of unspecified hip, stage 2 HCC ESR
Healing pressure ulcer of unspecified hip, stage 2
Pressure ulcer with abrasion, blister, partial thickness skin loss involving epidermis and/or dermis, unspecified hip

L89.203 Pressure ulcer of unspecified hip, stage 3 HCC ESR
Healing pressure ulcer of unspecified hip, stage 3
Pressure ulcer with full thickness skin loss involving damage or necrosis of subcutaneous tissue, unspecified hip

L89.204 Pressure ulcer of unspecified hip, stage 4 HCC ESR
Healing pressure ulcer of unspecified hip, stage 4
Pressure ulcer with necrosis of soft tissues through to underlying muscle, tendon, or bone, unspecified hip

L89.206 Pressure-induced deep tissue damage of unspecified hip

L89.209 Pressure ulcer of unspecified hip, unspecified stage
Healing pressure ulcer of unspecified hip NOS
Healing pressure ulcer of unspecified hip, unspecified stage

✓6th **L89.21 Pressure ulcer of right hip**

L89.210 Pressure ulcer of right hip, unstageable HCC ESR

L89.211 Pressure ulcer of right hip, stage 1
Healing pressure ulcer of right hip back, stage 1
Pressure pre-ulcer skin changes limited to persistent focal edema, right hip

L89.212 Pressure ulcer of right hip, stage 2 HCC ESR
Healing pressure ulcer of right hip, stage 2
Pressure ulcer with abrasion, blister, partial thickness skin loss involving epidermis and/or dermis, right hip

L89.213 Pressure ulcer of right hip, stage 3 HCC ESR
Healing pressure ulcer of right hip, stage 3
Pressure ulcer with full thickness skin loss involving damage or necrosis of subcutaneous tissue, right hip

L89.214 Pressure ulcer of right hip, stage 4 HCC ESR
Healing pressure ulcer of right hip, stage 4
Pressure ulcer with necrosis of soft tissues through to underlying muscle, tendon, or bone, right hip

L89.216 Pressure-induced deep tissue damage of right hip

L89.219 Pressure ulcer of right hip, unspecified stage
Healing pressure ulcer of right hip NOS
Healing pressure ulcer of right hip, unspecified stage

✓6th **L89.22 Pressure ulcer of left hip**

L89.220 Pressure ulcer of left hip, unstageable HCC ESR

L89.221 Pressure ulcer of left hip, stage 1
Healing pressure ulcer of left hip back, stage 1
Pressure pre-ulcer skin changes limited to persistent focal edema, left hip

L89.222 Pressure ulcer of left hip, stage 2 HCC ESR
Healing pressure ulcer of left hip, stage 2
Pressure ulcer with abrasion, blister, partial thickness skin loss involving epidermis and/or dermis, left hip

L89.223 Pressure ulcer of left hip, stage 3 HCC ESR
Healing pressure ulcer of left hip, stage 3
Pressure ulcer with full thickness skin loss involving damage or necrosis of subcutaneous tissue, left hip

L89.224 Pressure ulcer of left hip, stage 4 HCC ESR
Healing pressure ulcer of left hip, stage 4
Pressure ulcer with necrosis of soft tissues through to underlying muscle, tendon, or bone, left hip

L89.226 Pressure-induced deep tissue damage of left hip

L89.229 Pressure ulcer of left hip, unspecified stage
Healing pressure ulcer of left hip NOS
Healing pressure ulcer of left hip, unspecified stage

✓5th **L89.3 Pressure ulcer of buttock**
AHA: 2021,3Q,10

✓6th **L89.30 Pressure ulcer of unspecified buttock**

L89.300 Pressure ulcer of unspecified buttock, unstageable HCC ESR

L89.301 Pressure ulcer of unspecified buttock, stage 1
Healing pressure ulcer of unspecified buttock, stage 1
Pressure pre-ulcer skin changes limited to persistent focal edema, unspecified buttock

L89.302 Pressure ulcer of unspecified buttock, stage 2 HCC ESR
Healing pressure ulcer of unspecified buttock, stage 2
Pressure ulcer with abrasion, blister, partial thickness skin loss involving epidermis and/or dermis, unspecified buttock

L89.303 Pressure ulcer of unspecified buttock, stage 3 HCC ESR
Healing pressure ulcer of unspecified buttock, stage 3
Pressure ulcer with full thickness skin loss involving damage or necrosis of subcutaneous tissue, unspecified buttock

L89.304 Pressure ulcer of unspecified buttock, stage 4 HCC ESR
Healing pressure ulcer of unspecified buttock, stage 4
Pressure ulcer with necrosis of soft tissues through to underlying muscle, tendon, or bone, unspecified buttock

L89.306 Pressure-induced deep tissue damage of unspecified buttock

L89.309 Pressure ulcer of unspecified buttock, unspecified stage
Healing pressure ulcer of unspecified buttock NOS
Healing pressure ulcer of unspecified buttock, unspecified stage

✓6th **L89.31 Pressure ulcer of right buttock**

L89.310 Pressure ulcer of right buttock, unstageable HCC ESR

L89.311 Pressure ulcer of right buttock, stage 1
Healing pressure ulcer of right buttock, stage 1
Pressure pre-ulcer skin changes limited to persistent focal edema, right buttock

L89.312 Pressure ulcer of right buttock, stage 2 HCC ESR
Healing pressure ulcer of right buttock, stage 2
Pressure ulcer with abrasion, blister, partial thickness skin loss involving epidermis and/or dermis, right buttock

L89.313 Pressure ulcer of right buttock, stage 3 HCC ESR
Healing pressure ulcer of right buttock, stage 3
Pressure ulcer with full thickness skin loss involving damage or necrosis of subcutaneous tissue, right buttock

L89.314 Pressure ulcer of right buttock, stage 4 HCC ESR
Healing pressure ulcer of right buttock, stage 4
Pressure ulcer with necrosis of soft tissues through to underlying muscle, tendon, or bone, right buttock

L89.316 Pressure-induced deep tissue damage of right buttock

L89.319 Pressure ulcer of right buttock, unspecified stage
Healing pressure ulcer of right buttock NOS
Healing pressure ulcer of right buttock, unspecified stage

✓6th **L89.32 Pressure ulcer of left buttock**

L89.320 Pressure ulcer of left buttock, unstageable HCC ESR

L89.321 Pressure ulcer of left buttock, stage 1
Healing pressure ulcer of left buttock, stage 1
Pressure pre-ulcer skin changes limited to persistent focal edema, left buttock

L89.322 Pressure ulcer of left buttock, stage 2 HCC ESR
Healing pressure ulcer of left buttock, stage 2
Pressure ulcer with abrasion, blister, partial thickness skin loss involving epidermis and/or dermis, left buttock

L89.323 Pressure ulcer of left buttock, stage 3 HCC ESR
Healing pressure ulcer of left buttock, stage 3
Pressure ulcer with full thickness skin loss involving damage or necrosis of subcutaneous tissue, left buttock

L89.324 Pressure ulcer of left buttock, stage 4 HCC ESR
Healing pressure ulcer of left buttock, stage 4
Pressure ulcer with necrosis of soft tissues through to underlying muscle, tendon, or bone, left buttock

L89.326 Pressure-induced deep tissue damage of left buttock

L89.329 Pressure ulcer of left buttock, unspecified stage
Healing pressure ulcer of left buttock NOS
Healing pressure ulcer of left buttock, unspecified stage

✓5th **L89.4 Pressure ulcer of contiguous site of back, buttock and hip**

L89.40 Pressure ulcer of contiguous site of back, buttock and hip, unspecified stage
Healing pressure ulcer of contiguous site of back, buttock and hip NOS
Healing pressure ulcer of contiguous site of back, buttock and hip, unspecified stage

L89.41 Pressure ulcer of contiguous site of back, buttock and hip, stage 1
Healing pressure ulcer of contiguous site of back, buttock and hip, stage 1
Pressure pre-ulcer skin changes limited to persistent focal edema, contiguous site of back, buttock and hip

L89.42 Pressure ulcer of contiguous site of back, buttock and hip, stage 2 HCC ESR
Healing pressure ulcer of contiguous site of back, buttock and hip, stage 2
Pressure ulcer with abrasion, blister, partial thickness skin loss involving epidermis and/or dermis, contiguous site of back, buttock and hip

L89.43 Pressure ulcer of contiguous site of back, buttock and hip, stage 3 HCC ESR
Healing pressure ulcer of contiguous site of back, buttock and hip, stage 3
Pressure ulcer with full thickness skin loss involving damage or necrosis of subcutaneous tissue, contiguous site of back, buttock and hip

L89.44 Pressure ulcer of contiguous site of back, buttock and hip, stage 4 HCC ESR
Healing pressure ulcer of contiguous site of back, buttock and hip, stage 4
Pressure ulcer with necrosis of soft tissues through to underlying muscle, tendon, or bone, contiguous site of back, buttock and hip

L89.45 Pressure ulcer of contiguous site of back, buttock and hip, unstageable HCC ESR

L89.46 Pressure-induced deep tissue damage of contiguous site of back, buttock and hip

✓5th **L89.5 Pressure ulcer of ankle**

✓6th **L89.50 Pressure ulcer of unspecified ankle**

L89.500 Pressure ulcer of unspecified ankle, unstageable HCC ESR

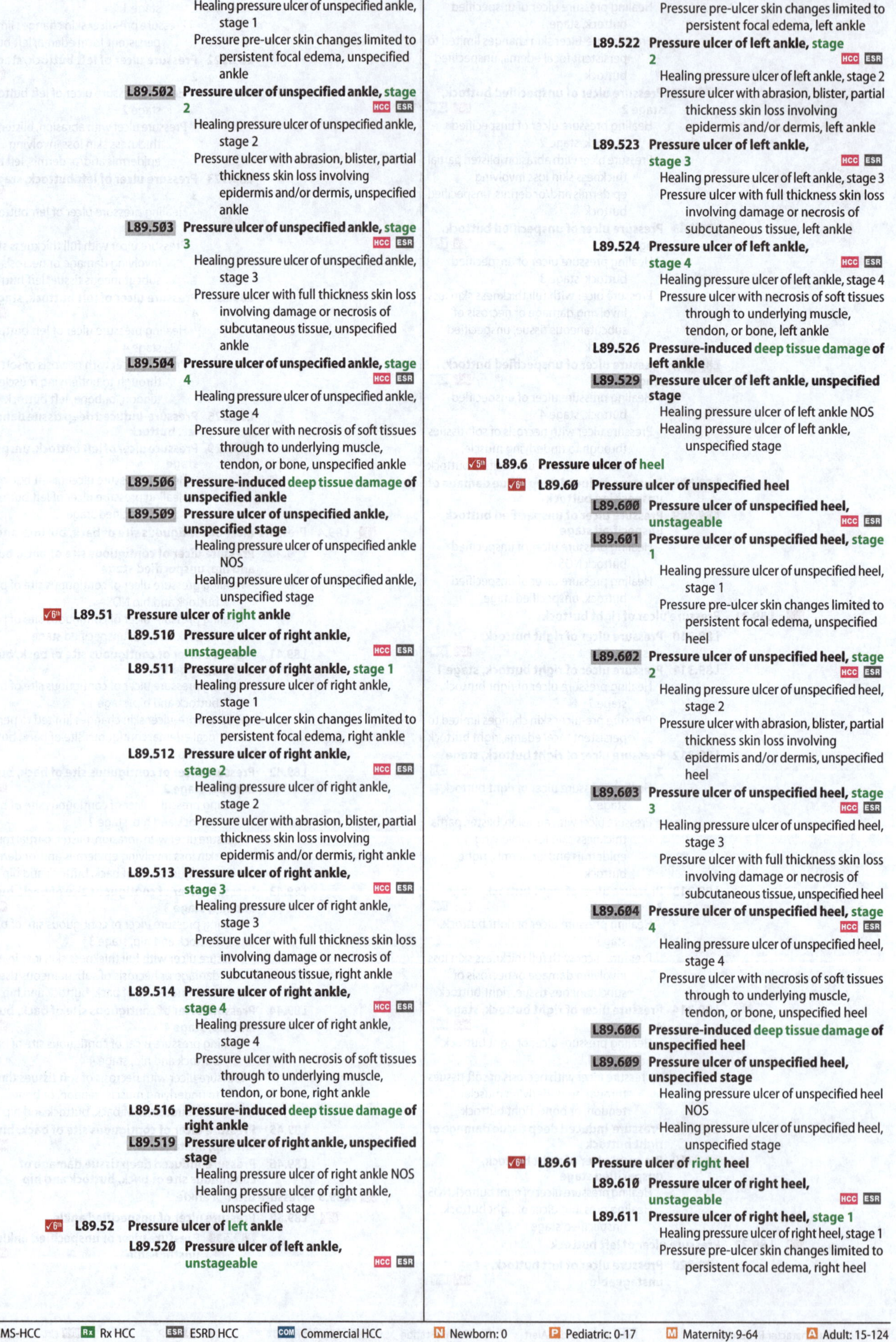

L89.5Ø1 Pressure ulcer of unspecified ankle, stage 1
- Healing pressure ulcer of unspecified ankle, stage 1
- Pressure pre-ulcer skin changes limited to persistent focal edema, unspecified ankle

L89.5Ø2 Pressure ulcer of unspecified ankle, stage 2 HCC ESR
- Healing pressure ulcer of unspecified ankle, stage 2
- Pressure ulcer with abrasion, blister, partial thickness skin loss involving epidermis and/or dermis, unspecified ankle

L89.5Ø3 Pressure ulcer of unspecified ankle, stage 3 HCC ESR
- Healing pressure ulcer of unspecified ankle, stage 3
- Pressure ulcer with full thickness skin loss involving damage or necrosis of subcutaneous tissue, unspecified ankle

L89.5Ø4 Pressure ulcer of unspecified ankle, stage 4 HCC ESR
- Healing pressure ulcer of unspecified ankle, stage 4
- Pressure ulcer with necrosis of soft tissues through to underlying muscle, tendon, or bone, unspecified ankle

L89.5Ø6 Pressure-induced deep tissue damage of unspecified ankle

L89.5Ø9 Pressure ulcer of unspecified ankle, unspecified stage
- Healing pressure ulcer of unspecified ankle NOS
- Healing pressure ulcer of unspecified ankle, unspecified stage

✓6th **L89.51 Pressure ulcer of right ankle**

L89.51Ø Pressure ulcer of right ankle, unstageable HCC ESR

L89.511 Pressure ulcer of right ankle, stage 1
- Healing pressure ulcer of right ankle, stage 1
- Pressure pre-ulcer skin changes limited to persistent focal edema, right ankle

L89.512 Pressure ulcer of right ankle, stage 2 HCC ESR
- Healing pressure ulcer of right ankle, stage 2
- Pressure ulcer with abrasion, blister, partial thickness skin loss involving epidermis and/or dermis, right ankle

L89.513 Pressure ulcer of right ankle, stage 3 HCC ESR
- Healing pressure ulcer of right ankle, stage 3
- Pressure ulcer with full thickness skin loss involving damage or necrosis of subcutaneous tissue, right ankle

L89.514 Pressure ulcer of right ankle, stage 4 HCC ESR
- Healing pressure ulcer of right ankle, stage 4
- Pressure ulcer with necrosis of soft tissues through to underlying muscle, tendon, or bone, right ankle

L89.516 Pressure-induced deep tissue damage of right ankle

L89.519 Pressure ulcer of right ankle, unspecified stage
- Healing pressure ulcer of right ankle NOS
- Healing pressure ulcer of right ankle, unspecified stage

✓6th **L89.52 Pressure ulcer of left ankle**

L89.52Ø Pressure ulcer of left ankle, unstageable HCC ESR

L89.521 Pressure ulcer of left ankle, stage 1
- Healing pressure ulcer of left ankle, stage 1
- Pressure pre-ulcer skin changes limited to persistent focal edema, left ankle

L89.522 Pressure ulcer of left ankle, stage 2 HCC ESR
- Healing pressure ulcer of left ankle, stage 2
- Pressure ulcer with abrasion, blister, partial thickness skin loss involving epidermis and/or dermis, left ankle

L89.523 Pressure ulcer of left ankle, stage 3 HCC ESR
- Healing pressure ulcer of left ankle, stage 3
- Pressure ulcer with full thickness skin loss involving damage or necrosis of subcutaneous tissue, left ankle

L89.524 Pressure ulcer of left ankle, stage 4 HCC ESR
- Healing pressure ulcer of left ankle, stage 4
- Pressure ulcer with necrosis of soft tissues through to underlying muscle, tendon, or bone, left ankle

L89.526 Pressure-induced deep tissue damage of left ankle

L89.529 Pressure ulcer of left ankle, unspecified stage
- Healing pressure ulcer of left ankle NOS
- Healing pressure ulcer of left ankle, unspecified stage

✓5th **L89.6 Pressure ulcer of heel**

✓6th **L89.6Ø Pressure ulcer of unspecified heel**

L89.6ØØ Pressure ulcer of unspecified heel, unstageable HCC ESR

L89.6Ø1 Pressure ulcer of unspecified heel, stage 1
- Healing pressure ulcer of unspecified heel, stage 1
- Pressure pre-ulcer skin changes limited to persistent focal edema, unspecified heel

L89.6Ø2 Pressure ulcer of unspecified heel, stage 2 HCC ESR
- Healing pressure ulcer of unspecified heel, stage 2
- Pressure ulcer with abrasion, blister, partial thickness skin loss involving epidermis and/or dermis, unspecified heel

L89.6Ø3 Pressure ulcer of unspecified heel, stage 3 HCC ESR
- Healing pressure ulcer of unspecified heel, stage 3
- Pressure ulcer with full thickness skin loss involving damage or necrosis of subcutaneous tissue, unspecified heel

L89.6Ø4 Pressure ulcer of unspecified heel, stage 4 HCC ESR
- Healing pressure ulcer of unspecified heel, stage 4
- Pressure ulcer with necrosis of soft tissues through to underlying muscle, tendon, or bone, unspecified heel

L89.6Ø6 Pressure-induced deep tissue damage of unspecified heel

L89.6Ø9 Pressure ulcer of unspecified heel, unspecified stage
- Healing pressure ulcer of unspecified heel NOS
- Healing pressure ulcer of unspecified heel, unspecified stage

✓6th **L89.61 Pressure ulcer of right heel**

L89.61Ø Pressure ulcer of right heel, unstageable HCC ESR

L89.611 Pressure ulcer of right heel, stage 1
- Healing pressure ulcer of right heel, stage 1
- Pressure pre-ulcer skin changes limited to persistent focal edema, right heel

L89.612 **Pressure ulcer of right heel, stage 2** HCC ESR
Healing pressure ulcer of right heel, stage 2
Pressure ulcer with abrasion, blister, partial thickness skin loss involving epidermis and/or dermis, right heel

L89.613 **Pressure ulcer of right heel, stage 3** HCC ESR
Healing pressure ulcer of right heel, stage 3
Pressure ulcer with full thickness skin loss involving damage or necrosis of subcutaneous tissue, right heel

L89.614 **Pressure ulcer of right heel, stage 4** HCC ESR
Healing pressure ulcer of right heel, stage 4
Pressure ulcer with necrosis of soft tissues through to underlying muscle, tendon, or bone, right heel

L89.616 **Pressure-induced deep tissue damage of right heel**

L89.619 **Pressure ulcer of right heel, unspecified stage**
Healing pressure ulcer of right heel NOS
Healing pressure ulcer of right heel, unspecified stage

✓6th L89.62 **Pressure ulcer of left heel**

L89.620 **Pressure ulcer of left heel, unstageable** HCC ESR

L89.621 **Pressure ulcer of left heel, stage 1**
Healing pressure ulcer of left heel, stage 1
Pressure pre-ulcer skin changes limited to persistent focal edema, left heel

L89.622 **Pressure ulcer of left heel, stage 2** HCC ESR
Healing pressure ulcer of left heel, stage 2
Pressure ulcer with abrasion, blister, partial thickness skin loss involving epidermis and/or dermis, left heel

L89.623 **Pressure ulcer of left heel, stage 3** HCC ESR
Healing pressure ulcer of left heel, stage 3
Pressure ulcer with full thickness skin loss involving damage or necrosis of subcutaneous tissue, left heel

L89.624 **Pressure ulcer of left heel, stage 4** HCC ESR
Healing pressure ulcer of left heel, stage 4
Pressure ulcer with necrosis of soft tissues through to underlying muscle, tendon, or bone, left heel

L89.626 **Pressure-induced deep tissue damage of left heel**

L89.629 **Pressure ulcer of left heel, unspecified stage**
Healing pressure ulcer of left heel NOS
Healing pressure ulcer of left heel, unspecified stage

✓5th L89.8 **Pressure ulcer of other site**

✓6th L89.81 **Pressure ulcer of head**
Pressure ulcer of face

L89.810 **Pressure ulcer of head, unstageable** HCC ESR

L89.811 **Pressure ulcer of head, stage 1**
Healing pressure ulcer of head, stage 1
Pressure pre-ulcer skin changes limited to persistent focal edema, head

L89.812 **Pressure ulcer of head, stage 2** HCC ESR
Healing pressure ulcer of head, stage 2
Pressure ulcer with abrasion, blister, partial thickness skin loss involving epidermis and/or dermis, head

L89.813 **Pressure ulcer of head, stage 3** HCC ESR
Healing pressure ulcer of head, stage 3
Pressure ulcer with full thickness skin loss involving damage or necrosis of subcutaneous tissue, head

L89.814 **Pressure ulcer of head, stage 4** HCC ESR
Healing pressure ulcer of head, stage 4
Pressure ulcer with necrosis of soft tissues through to underlying muscle, tendon, or bone, head

L89.816 **Pressure-induced deep tissue damage of head**

L89.819 **Pressure ulcer of head, unspecified stage**
Healing pressure ulcer of head NOS
Healing pressure ulcer of head, unspecified stage

✓6th L89.89 **Pressure ulcer of other site**

L89.890 **Pressure ulcer of other site, unstageable** HCC ESR

L89.891 **Pressure ulcer of other site, stage 1**
Healing pressure ulcer of other site, stage 1
Pressure pre-ulcer skin changes limited to persistent focal edema, other site

L89.892 **Pressure ulcer of other site, stage 2** HCC ESR
Healing pressure ulcer of other site, stage 2
Pressure ulcer with abrasion, blister, partial thickness skin loss involving epidermis and/or dermis, other site

L89.893 **Pressure ulcer of other site, stage 3** HCC ESR
Healing pressure ulcer of other site, stage 3
Pressure ulcer with full thickness skin loss involving damage or necrosis of subcutaneous tissue, other site

L89.894 **Pressure ulcer of other site, stage 4** HCC ESR
Healing pressure ulcer of other site, stage 4
Pressure ulcer with necrosis of soft tissues through to underlying muscle, tendon, or bone, other site

L89.896 **Pressure-induced deep tissue damage of other site**

L89.899 **Pressure ulcer of other site, unspecified stage**
Healing pressure ulcer of other site NOS
Healing pressure ulcer of other site, unspecified stage

✓5th L89.9 **Pressure ulcer of unspecified site**

L89.90 **Pressure ulcer of unspecified site, unspecified stage**
Healing pressure ulcer of unspecified site NOS
Healing pressure ulcer of unspecified site, unspecified stage

L89.91 **Pressure ulcer of unspecified site, stage 1**
Healing pressure ulcer of unspecified site, stage 1
Pressure pre-ulcer skin changes limited to persistent focal edema, unspecified site

L89.92 **Pressure ulcer of unspecified site, stage 2** HCC ESR
Healing pressure ulcer of unspecified site, stage 2
Pressure ulcer with abrasion, blister, partial thickness skin loss involving epidermis and/or dermis, unspecified site

L89.93 **Pressure ulcer of unspecified site, stage 3** HCC ESR
Healing pressure ulcer of unspecified site, stage 3
Pressure ulcer with full thickness skin loss involving damage or necrosis of subcutaneous tissue, unspecified site

L89.94 **Pressure ulcer of unspecified site, stage 4** HCC ESR
Healing pressure ulcer of unspecified site, stage 4
Pressure ulcer with necrosis of soft tissues through to underlying muscle, tendon, or bone, unspecified site

L89.95 **Pressure ulcer of unspecified site, unstageable** HCC ESR

L89.96 **Pressure-induced deep tissue damage of unspecified site**

√4th L90 Atrophic disorders of skin

L90.0 Lichen sclerosus et atrophicus
EXCLUDES 2 *lichen sclerosus of external female genital organs (N90.4)*
lichen sclerosus of external male genital organs (N48.0)

L90.1 Anetoderma of Schweninger-Buzzi
L90.2 Anetoderma of Jadassohn-Pellizzari
L90.3 Atrophoderma of Pasini and Pierini
L90.4 Acrodermatitis chronica atrophicans
L90.5 Scar conditions and fibrosis of skin
Adherent scar (skin)
Cicatrix
Disfigurement of skin due to scar
Fibrosis of skin NOS
Scar NOS
EXCLUDES 2 *hypertrophic scar (L91.0)*
keloid scar (L91.0)
AHA: 2016,2Q,5; 2015,1Q,19

L90.6 Striae atrophicae
L90.8 Other atrophic disorders of skin
L90.9 Atrophic disorder of skin, unspecified

√4th L91 Hypertrophic disorders of skin

L91.0 Hypertrophic scar
Keloid
Keloid scar
EXCLUDES 2 *acne keloid (L73.0)*
scar NOS (L90.5)
DEF: Overgrowth of scar tissue due to excess amounts of collagen during connective tissue repair, occurring mainly on the upper trunk and face.

L91.8 Other hypertrophic disorders of the skin
L91.9 Hypertrophic disorder of the skin, unspecified

√4th L92 Granulomatous disorders of skin and subcutaneous tissue
EXCLUDES 2 *actinic granuloma (L57.5)*

L92.0 Granuloma annulare
Perforating granuloma annulare

L92.1 Necrobiosis lipoidica, not elsewhere classified
EXCLUDES 1 *necrobiosis lipoidica associated with diabetes mellitus (E08-E13 with .620)*

L92.2 Granuloma faciale [eosinophilic granuloma of skin]
L92.3 Foreign body granuloma of the skin and subcutaneous tissue
Use additional code to identify the type of retained foreign body (Z18.-)

L92.8 Other granulomatous disorders of the skin and subcutaneous tissue
L92.9 Granulomatous disorder of the skin and subcutaneous tissue, unspecified
EXCLUDES 2 *umbilical granuloma (P83.81)*
AHA: 2017,4Q,21-22

√4th L93 Lupus erythematosus
Use additional code for adverse effect, if applicable, to identify drug (T36-T50 with fifth or sixth character 5)
EXCLUDES 1 *lupus exedens (A18.4)*
lupus vulgaris (A18.4)
scleroderma (M34.-)
systemic lupus erythematosus (M32.-)
DEF: Inflammatory, autoimmune skin condition in which the body's autoimmune system attacks healthy tissue of the integumentary system.

L93.0 Discoid lupus erythematosus Rx
Lupus erythematosus NOS
L93.1 Subacute cutaneous lupus erythematosus Rx
L93.2 Other local lupus erythematosus Rx
Lupus erythematosus profundus
Lupus panniculitis

√4th L94 Other localized connective tissue disorders
EXCLUDES 1 *systemic connective tissue disorders (M30-M36)*

L94.0 Localized scleroderma [morphea]
Circumscribed scleroderma
L94.1 Linear scleroderma
En coup de sabre lesion
L94.2 Calcinosis cutis
L94.3 Sclerodactyly
L94.4 Gottron's papules
L94.5 Poikiloderma vasculare atrophicans Rx
L94.6 Ainhum
L94.8 Other specified localized connective tissue disorders
L94.9 Localized connective tissue disorder, unspecified

√4th L95 Vasculitis limited to skin, not elsewhere classified
EXCLUDES 1 *angioma serpiginosum (L81.7)*
Henoch(-Schönlein) purpura (D69.0)
hypersensitivity angiitis (M31.0)
lupus panniculitis (L93.2)
panniculitis NOS (M79.3)
panniculitis of neck and back (M54.0-)
polyarteritis nodosa (M30.0)
relapsing panniculitis (M35.6)
rheumatoid vasculitis (M05.2)
serum sickness (T80.6-)
urticaria (L50.-)
Wegener's granulomatosis (M31.3-)

L95.0 Livedoid vasculitis
Atrophie blanche (en plaque)
L95.1 Erythema elevatum diutinum
L95.8 Other vasculitis limited to the skin
L95.9 Vasculitis limited to the skin, unspecified

√4th L97 Non-pressure chronic ulcer of lower limb, not elsewhere classified
INCLUDES chronic ulcer of skin of lower limb NOS
non-healing ulcer of skin
non-infected sinus of skin
trophic ulcer NOS
tropical ulcer NOS
ulcer of skin of lower limb NOS
Code first any associated underlying condition, such as:
any associated gangrene (I96)
atherosclerosis of the lower extremities (I70.23-, I70.24-, I70.33-, I70.34-, I70.43-, I70.44-, I70.53-, I70.54-, I70.63-, I70.64-, I70.73-, I70.74-)
chronic venous hypertension (I87.31-, I87.33-)
diabetic ulcers (E08.621, E08.622, E09.621, E09.622, E10.621, E10.622, E11.621, E11.622, E13.621, E13.622)
postphlebitic syndrome (I87.01-, I87.03-)
postthrombotic syndrome (I87.01-, I87.03-)
varicose ulcer (I83.0-, I83.2-)
EXCLUDES 2 *pressure ulcer (pressure area) (L89.-)*
skin infections (L00-L08)
specific infections classified to A00-B99
AHA: 2021,1Q,7; 2020,2Q,19; 2018,4Q,69; 2017,4Q,17
TIP: Assign a code from this category/subcategory for nonpressure ulcers documented as acute.
TIP: The depth and/or severity of a diagnosed nonpressure ulcer can be determined based on medical record documentation from clinicians who are not the patient's provider.

√5th L97.1 Non-pressure chronic ulcer of thigh

√6th L97.10 Non-pressure chronic ulcer of unspecified thigh

L97.101 Non-pressure chronic ulcer of unspecified thigh limited to breakdown of skin HCC Rx ESR COM
L97.102 Non-pressure chronic ulcer of unspecified thigh with fat layer exposed HCC Rx ESR COM
L97.103 Non-pressure chronic ulcer of unspecified thigh with necrosis of muscle HCC Rx ESR COM
L97.104 Non-pressure chronic ulcer of unspecified thigh with necrosis of bone HCC Rx ESR COM
L97.105 Non-pressure chronic ulcer of unspecified thigh with muscle involvement without evidence of necrosis HCC Rx ESR COM
L97.106 Non-pressure chronic ulcer of unspecified thigh with bone involvement without evidence of necrosis HCC Rx ESR COM
L97.108 Non-pressure chronic ulcer of unspecified thigh with other specified severity HCC Rx ESR COM
L97.109 Non-pressure chronic ulcer of unspecified thigh with unspecified severity HCC Rx ESR COM

✓6th L97.11 Non-pressure chronic ulcer of right thigh
L97.111 Non-pressure chronic ulcer of right thigh limited to breakdown of skin HCC Rx ESR COM
L97.112 Non-pressure chronic ulcer of right thigh with fat layer exposed HCC Rx ESR COM
L97.113 Non-pressure chronic ulcer of right thigh with necrosis of muscle HCC Rx ESR COM
L97.114 Non-pressure chronic ulcer of right thigh with necrosis of bone HCC Rx ESR COM
L97.115 Non-pressure chronic ulcer of right thigh with muscle involvement without evidence of necrosis HCC Rx ESR COM
L97.116 Non-pressure chronic ulcer of right thigh with bone involvement without evidence of necrosis HCC Rx ESR COM
L97.118 Non-pressure chronic ulcer of right thigh with other specified severity HCC Rx ESR COM
L97.119 Non-pressure chronic ulcer of right thigh with unspecified severity HCC Rx ESR COM

✓6th L97.12 Non-pressure chronic ulcer of left thigh
L97.121 Non-pressure chronic ulcer of left thigh limited to breakdown of skin HCC Rx ESR COM
L97.122 Non-pressure chronic ulcer of left thigh with fat layer exposed HCC Rx ESR COM
L97.123 Non-pressure chronic ulcer of left thigh with necrosis of muscle HCC Rx ESR COM
L97.124 Non-pressure chronic ulcer of left thigh with necrosis of bone HCC Rx ESR COM
L97.125 Non-pressure chronic ulcer of left thigh with muscle involvement without evidence of necrosis HCC Rx ESR COM
L97.126 Non-pressure chronic ulcer of left thigh with bone involvement without evidence of necrosis HCC Rx ESR COM
L97.128 Non-pressure chronic ulcer of left thigh with other specified severity HCC Rx ESR COM
L97.129 Non-pressure chronic ulcer of left thigh with unspecified severity HCC Rx ESR COM

✓5th L97.2 Non-pressure chronic ulcer of calf

✓6th L97.20 Non-pressure chronic ulcer of unspecified calf
L97.201 Non-pressure chronic ulcer of unspecified calf limited to breakdown of skin HCC Rx ESR COM
L97.202 Non-pressure chronic ulcer of unspecified calf with fat layer exposed HCC Rx ESR COM
L97.203 Non-pressure chronic ulcer of unspecified calf with necrosis of muscle HCC Rx ESR COM
L97.204 Non-pressure chronic ulcer of unspecified calf with necrosis of bone HCC Rx ESR COM
L97.205 Non-pressure chronic ulcer of unspecified calf with muscle involvement without evidence of necrosis HCC Rx ESR COM
L97.206 Non-pressure chronic ulcer of unspecified calf with bone involvement without evidence of necrosis HCC Rx ESR COM
L97.208 Non-pressure chronic ulcer of unspecified calf with other specified severity HCC Rx ESR COM
L97.209 Non-pressure chronic ulcer of unspecified calf with unspecified severity HCC Rx ESR COM

✓6th L97.21 Non-pressure chronic ulcer of right calf
L97.211 Non-pressure chronic ulcer of right calf limited to breakdown of skin HCC Rx ESR COM
L97.212 Non-pressure chronic ulcer of right calf with fat layer exposed HCC Rx ESR COM
L97.213 Non-pressure chronic ulcer of right calf with necrosis of muscle HCC Rx ESR COM
L97.214 Non-pressure chronic ulcer of right calf with necrosis of bone HCC Rx ESR COM
L97.215 Non-pressure chronic ulcer of right calf with muscle involvement without evidence of necrosis HCC Rx ESR COM
L97.216 Non-pressure chronic ulcer of right calf with bone involvement without evidence of necrosis HCC Rx ESR COM
L97.218 Non-pressure chronic ulcer of right calf with other specified severity HCC Rx ESR COM
L97.219 Non-pressure chronic ulcer of right calf with unspecified severity HCC Rx ESR COM

✓6th L97.22 Non-pressure chronic ulcer of left calf
L97.221 Non-pressure chronic ulcer of left calf limited to breakdown of skin HCC Rx ESR COM
L97.222 Non-pressure chronic ulcer of left calf with fat layer exposed HCC Rx ESR COM
L97.223 Non-pressure chronic ulcer of left calf with necrosis of muscle HCC Rx ESR COM
L97.224 Non-pressure chronic ulcer of left calf with necrosis of bone HCC Rx ESR COM
L97.225 Non-pressure chronic ulcer of left calf with muscle involvement without evidence of necrosis HCC Rx ESR COM
L97.226 Non-pressure chronic ulcer of left calf with bone involvement without evidence of necrosis HCC Rx ESR COM
L97.228 Non-pressure chronic ulcer of left calf with other specified severity HCC Rx ESR COM
L97.229 Non-pressure chronic ulcer of left calf with unspecified severity HCC Rx ESR COM

✓5th L97.3 Non-pressure chronic ulcer of ankle

✓6th L97.30 Non-pressure chronic ulcer of unspecified ankle
L97.301 Non-pressure chronic ulcer of unspecified ankle limited to breakdown of skin HCC Rx ESR COM
L97.302 Non-pressure chronic ulcer of unspecified ankle with fat layer exposed HCC Rx ESR COM
L97.303 Non-pressure chronic ulcer of unspecified ankle with necrosis of muscle HCC Rx ESR COM
L97.304 Non-pressure chronic ulcer of unspecified ankle with necrosis of bone HCC Rx ESR COM
L97.305 Non-pressure chronic ulcer of unspecified ankle with muscle involvement without evidence of necrosis HCC Rx ESR COM
L97.306 Non-pressure chronic ulcer of unspecified ankle with bone involvement without evidence of necrosis HCC Rx ESR COM
L97.308 Non-pressure chronic ulcer of unspecified ankle with other specified severity HCC Rx ESR COM
L97.309 Non-pressure chronic ulcer of unspecified ankle with unspecified severity HCC Rx ESR COM

✓6th L97.31 Non-pressure chronic ulcer of right ankle
L97.311 Non-pressure chronic ulcer of right ankle limited to breakdown of skin HCC Rx ESR COM
L97.312 Non-pressure chronic ulcer of right ankle with fat layer exposed HCC Rx ESR COM
L97.313 Non-pressure chronic ulcer of right ankle with necrosis of muscle HCC Rx ESR COM
L97.314 Non-pressure chronic ulcer of right ankle with necrosis of bone HCC Rx ESR COM
L97.315 Non-pressure chronic ulcer of right ankle with muscle involvement without evidence of necrosis HCC Rx ESR COM
L97.316 Non-pressure chronic ulcer of right ankle with bone involvement without evidence of necrosis HCC Rx ESR COM
L97.318 Non-pressure chronic ulcer of right ankle with other specified severity HCC Rx ESR COM

L97.319 Non-pressure chronic ulcer of right ankle with unspecified severity HCC Rx ESR COM

✓6th L97.32 Non-pressure chronic ulcer of left ankle

L97.321 Non-pressure chronic ulcer of left ankle limited to breakdown of skin HCC Rx ESR COM

L97.322 Non-pressure chronic ulcer of left ankle with fat layer exposed HCC Rx ESR COM

L97.323 Non-pressure chronic ulcer of left ankle with necrosis of muscle HCC Rx ESR COM

L97.324 Non-pressure chronic ulcer of left ankle with necrosis of bone HCC Rx ESR COM

L97.325 Non-pressure chronic ulcer of left ankle with muscle involvement without evidence of necrosis HCC Rx ESR COM

L97.326 Non-pressure chronic ulcer of left ankle with bone involvement without evidence of necrosis HCC Rx ESR COM

L97.328 Non-pressure chronic ulcer of left ankle with other specified severity HCC Rx ESR COM

L97.329 Non-pressure chronic ulcer of left ankle with unspecified severity HCC Rx ESR COM

✓5th L97.4 Non-pressure chronic ulcer of heel and midfoot

Non-pressure chronic ulcer of plantar surface of midfoot

✓6th L97.40 Non-pressure chronic ulcer of unspecified heel and midfoot

L97.401 Non-pressure chronic ulcer of unspecified heel and midfoot limited to breakdown of skin HCC Rx ESR COM

L97.402 Non-pressure chronic ulcer of unspecified heel and midfoot with fat layer exposed HCC Rx ESR COM

L97.403 Non-pressure chronic ulcer of unspecified heel and midfoot with necrosis of muscle HCC Rx ESR COM

L97.404 Non-pressure chronic ulcer of unspecified heel and midfoot with necrosis of bone HCC Rx ESR COM

L97.405 Non-pressure chronic ulcer of unspecified heel and midfoot with muscle involvement without evidence of necrosis HCC Rx ESR COM

L97.406 Non-pressure chronic ulcer of unspecified heel and midfoot with bone involvement without evidence of necrosis HCC Rx ESR COM

L97.408 Non-pressure chronic ulcer of unspecified heel and midfoot with other specified severity HCC Rx ESR COM

L97.409 Non-pressure chronic ulcer of unspecified heel and midfoot with unspecified severity HCC Rx ESR COM

✓6th L97.41 Non-pressure chronic ulcer of right heel and midfoot

L97.411 Non-pressure chronic ulcer of right heel and midfoot limited to breakdown of skin HCC Rx ESR COM

L97.412 Non-pressure chronic ulcer of right heel and midfoot with fat layer exposed HCC Rx ESR COM

AHA: 2020,2Q,19

L97.413 Non-pressure chronic ulcer of right heel and midfoot with necrosis of muscle HCC Rx ESR COM

L97.414 Non-pressure chronic ulcer of right heel and midfoot with necrosis of bone HCC Rx ESR COM

L97.415 Non-pressure chronic ulcer of right heel and midfoot with muscle involvement without evidence of necrosis HCC Rx ESR COM

L97.416 Non-pressure chronic ulcer of right heel and midfoot with bone involvement without evidence of necrosis HCC Rx ESR COM

L97.418 Non-pressure chronic ulcer of right heel and midfoot with other specified severity HCC Rx ESR COM

L97.419 Non-pressure chronic ulcer of right heel and midfoot with unspecified severity HCC Rx ESR COM

✓6th L97.42 Non-pressure chronic ulcer of left heel and midfoot

L97.421 Non-pressure chronic ulcer of left heel and midfoot limited to breakdown of skin HCC Rx ESR COM

AHA: 2016,1Q,12

L97.422 Non-pressure chronic ulcer of left heel and midfoot with fat layer exposed HCC Rx ESR COM

AHA: 2020,2Q,19

L97.423 Non-pressure chronic ulcer of left heel and midfoot with necrosis of muscle HCC Rx ESR COM

L97.424 Non-pressure chronic ulcer of left heel and midfoot with necrosis of bone HCC Rx ESR COM

L97.425 Non-pressure chronic ulcer of left heel and midfoot with muscle involvement without evidence of necrosis HCC Rx ESR COM

L97.426 Non-pressure chronic ulcer of left heel and midfoot with bone involvement without evidence of necrosis HCC Rx ESR COM

L97.428 Non-pressure chronic ulcer of left heel and midfoot with other specified severity HCC Rx ESR COM

L97.429 Non-pressure chronic ulcer of left heel and midfoot with unspecified severity HCC Rx ESR COM

✓5th L97.5 Non-pressure chronic ulcer of other part of foot

Non-pressure chronic ulcer of toe

✓6th L97.50 Non-pressure chronic ulcer of other part of unspecified foot

L97.501 Non-pressure chronic ulcer of other part of unspecified foot limited to breakdown of skin HCC Rx ESR COM

L97.502 Non-pressure chronic ulcer of other part of unspecified foot with fat layer exposed HCC Rx ESR COM

L97.503 Non-pressure chronic ulcer of other part of unspecified foot with necrosis of muscle HCC Rx ESR COM

L97.504 Non-pressure chronic ulcer of other part of unspecified foot with necrosis of bone HCC Rx ESR COM

L97.505 Non-pressure chronic ulcer of other part of unspecified foot with muscle involvement without evidence of necrosis HCC Rx ESR COM

L97.506 Non-pressure chronic ulcer of other part of unspecified foot with bone involvement without evidence of necrosis HCC Rx ESR COM

L97.508 Non-pressure chronic ulcer of other part of unspecified foot with other specified severity HCC Rx ESR COM

L97.509 Non-pressure chronic ulcer of other part of unspecified foot with unspecified severity HCC Rx ESR COM

✓6th L97.51 Non-pressure chronic ulcer of other part of right foot

AHA: 2020,1Q,12

L97.511 Non-pressure chronic ulcer of other part of right foot limited to breakdown of skin HCC Rx ESR COM

L97.512 Non-pressure chronic ulcer of other part of right foot with fat layer exposed HCC Rx ESR COM

AHA: 2020,2Q,19

L97.513 Non-pressure chronic ulcer of other part of right foot with necrosis of muscle HCC Rx ESR COM

L97.514 Non-pressure chronic ulcer of other part of right foot with necrosis of bone HCC Rx ESR COM

L97.515 Non-pressure chronic ulcer of other part of right foot with muscle involvement without evidence of necrosis HCC Rx ESR COM

L97.516 Non-pressure chronic ulcer of other part of right foot with bone involvement without evidence of necrosis HCC Rx ESR COM

L97.518 Non-pressure chronic ulcer of other part of right foot with other specified severity HCC Rx ESR COM

L97.519 Non-pressure chronic ulcer of other part of right foot with unspecified severity HCC Rx ESR COM

✓6th L97.52 Non-pressure chronic ulcer of other part of left foot

AHA: 2020,1Q,12

L97.521 Non-pressure chronic ulcer of other part of left foot limited to breakdown of skin HCC Rx ESR COM

L97.522 Non-pressure chronic ulcer of other part of left foot with fat layer exposed HCC Rx ESR COM

AHA: 2020,2Q,19

L97.523 Non-pressure chronic ulcer of other part of left foot with necrosis of muscle HCC Rx ESR COM

L97.524 Non-pressure chronic ulcer of other part of left foot with necrosis of bone HCC Rx ESR COM

L97.525 Non-pressure chronic ulcer of other part of left foot with muscle involvement without evidence of necrosis HCC Rx ESR COM

L97.526 Non-pressure chronic ulcer of other part of left foot with bone involvement without evidence of necrosis HCC Rx ESR COM

L97.528 Non-pressure chronic ulcer of other part of left foot with other specified severity HCC Rx ESR COM

L97.529 Non-pressure chronic ulcer of other part of left foot with unspecified severity HCC Rx ESR COM

✓5th L97.8 Non-pressure chronic ulcer of other part of lower leg

✓6th L97.80 Non-pressure chronic ulcer of other part of unspecified lower leg

L97.801 Non-pressure chronic ulcer of other part of unspecified lower leg limited to breakdown of skin HCC Rx ESR COM

L97.802 Non-pressure chronic ulcer of other part of unspecified lower leg with fat layer exposed HCC Rx ESR COM

L97.803 Non-pressure chronic ulcer of other part of unspecified lower leg with necrosis of muscle HCC Rx ESR COM

L97.804 Non-pressure chronic ulcer of other part of unspecified lower leg with necrosis of bone HCC Rx ESR COM

L97.805 Non-pressure chronic ulcer of other part of unspecified lower leg with muscle involvement without evidence of necrosis HCC Rx ESR COM

L97.806 Non-pressure chronic ulcer of other part of unspecified lower leg with bone involvement without evidence of necrosis HCC Rx ESR COM

L97.808 Non-pressure chronic ulcer of other part of unspecified lower leg with other specified severity HCC Rx ESR COM

L97.809 Non-pressure chronic ulcer of other part of unspecified lower leg with unspecified severity HCC Rx ESR COM

✓6th L97.81 Non-pressure chronic ulcer of other part of right lower leg

L97.811 Non-pressure chronic ulcer of other part of right lower leg limited to breakdown of skin HCC Rx ESR COM

L97.812 Non-pressure chronic ulcer of other part of right lower leg with fat layer exposed HCC Rx ESR COM

L97.813 Non-pressure chronic ulcer of other part of right lower leg with necrosis of muscle HCC Rx ESR COM

L97.814 Non-pressure chronic ulcer of other part of right lower leg with necrosis of bone HCC Rx ESR COM

L97.815 Non-pressure chronic ulcer of other part of right lower leg with muscle involvement without evidence of necrosis HCC Rx ESR COM

L97.816 Non-pressure chronic ulcer of other part of right lower leg with bone involvement without evidence of necrosis HCC Rx ESR COM

L97.818 Non-pressure chronic ulcer of other part of right lower leg with other specified severity HCC Rx ESR COM

L97.819 Non-pressure chronic ulcer of other part of right lower leg with unspecified severity HCC Rx ESR COM

✓6th L97.82 Non-pressure chronic ulcer of other part of left lower leg

L97.821 Non-pressure chronic ulcer of other part of left lower leg limited to breakdown of skin HCC Rx ESR COM

L97.822 Non-pressure chronic ulcer of other part of left lower leg with fat layer exposed HCC Rx ESR COM

L97.823 Non-pressure chronic ulcer of other part of left lower leg with necrosis of muscle HCC Rx ESR COM

L97.824 Non-pressure chronic ulcer of other part of left lower leg with necrosis of bone HCC Rx ESR COM

L97.825 Non-pressure chronic ulcer of other part of left lower leg with muscle involvement without evidence of necrosis HCC Rx ESR COM

L97.826 Non-pressure chronic ulcer of other part of left lower leg with bone involvement without evidence of necrosis HCC Rx ESR COM

L97.828 Non-pressure chronic ulcer of other part of left lower leg with other specified severity HCC Rx ESR COM

L97.829 Non-pressure chronic ulcer of other part of left lower leg with unspecified severity HCC Rx ESR COM

✓5th L97.9 Non-pressure chronic ulcer of unspecified part of lower leg

✓6th L97.90 Non-pressure chronic ulcer of unspecified part of unspecified lower leg

L97.901 Non-pressure chronic ulcer of unspecified part of unspecified lower leg limited to breakdown of skin HCC Rx ESR COM

L97.902 Non-pressure chronic ulcer of unspecified part of unspecified lower leg with fat layer exposed HCC Rx ESR COM

L97.903 Non-pressure chronic ulcer of unspecified part of unspecified lower leg with necrosis of muscle HCC Rx ESR COM

L97.904 Non-pressure chronic ulcer of unspecified part of unspecified lower leg with necrosis of bone HCC Rx ESR COM

L97.905 Non-pressure chronic ulcer of unspecified part of unspecified lower leg with muscle involvement without evidence of necrosis HCC Rx ESR COM

L97.906 Non-pressure chronic ulcer of unspecified part of unspecified lower leg with bone involvement without evidence of necrosis HCC Rx ESR COM

L97.908 Non-pressure chronic ulcer of unspecified part of unspecified lower leg with other specified severity HCC Rx ESR COM

L97.909 Non-pressure chronic ulcer of unspecified part of unspecified lower leg with unspecified severity HCC Rx ESR COM

✓6th L97.91 Non-pressure chronic ulcer of unspecified part of right lower leg

L97.911 Non-pressure chronic ulcer of unspecified part of right lower leg limited to breakdown of skin HCC Rx ESR COM

L97.912 Non-pressure chronic ulcer of unspecified part of right lower leg with fat layer exposed HCC Rx ESR COM

L97.913 Non-pressure chronic ulcer of unspecified part of right lower leg with necrosis of muscle HCC Rx ESR COM

L97.914 Non-pressure chronic ulcer of unspecified part of right lower leg with necrosis of bone HCC Rx ESR COM

L97.915 Non-pressure chronic ulcer of unspecified part of right lower leg with muscle involvement without evidence of necrosis HCC Rx ESR COM

L97.916 Non-pressure chronic ulcer of unspecified part of right lower leg with bone involvement without evidence of necrosis HCC Rx ESR COM

L97.918 Non-pressure chronic ulcer of unspecified part of right lower leg with other specified severity HCC Rx ESR COM

L97.919 Non-pressure chronic ulcer of unspecified part of right lower leg with unspecified severity HCC Rx ESR COM

√6th L97.92 Non-pressure chronic ulcer of unspecified part of left lower leg

L97.921 Non-pressure chronic ulcer of unspecified part of left lower leg limited to breakdown of skin HCC Rx ESR COM

L97.922 Non-pressure chronic ulcer of unspecified part of left lower leg with fat layer exposed HCC Rx ESR COM

L97.923 Non-pressure chronic ulcer of unspecified part of left lower leg with necrosis of muscle HCC Rx ESR COM

L97.924 Non-pressure chronic ulcer of unspecified part of left lower leg with necrosis of bone HCC Rx ESR COM

L97.925 Non-pressure chronic ulcer of unspecified part of left lower leg with muscle involvement without evidence of necrosis HCC Rx ESR COM

L97.926 Non-pressure chronic ulcer of unspecified part of left lower leg with bone involvement without evidence of necrosis HCC Rx ESR COM

L97.928 Non-pressure chronic ulcer of unspecified part of left lower leg with other specified severity HCC Rx ESR COM

L97.929 Non-pressure chronic ulcer of unspecified part of left lower leg with unspecified severity HCC Rx ESR COM

√4th **L98 Other disorders of skin and subcutaneous tissue, not elsewhere classified**

L98.0 Pyogenic granuloma

EXCLUDES 2 *pyogenic granuloma of gingiva (K06.8)*
pyogenic granuloma of maxillary alveolar ridge (K04.5)
pyogenic granuloma of oral mucosa (K13.4)

DEF: Solitary polypoid capillary hemangioma often associated with local irritation, trauma, and superimposed inflammation. Located on the skin and gingival or oral mucosa, they bleed easily and may ulcerate and form crusted sores.

L98.1 Factitial dermatitis

Neurotic excoriation

EXCLUDES 1 *excoriation (skin-picking) disorder (F42.4)*

AHA: 2016,4Q,15

DEF: Self-inflicted skin lesions to satisfy an unconscious psychological or emotional need. Methods used to injure the skin include deep excoriations with a sharp instrument, scarification with a knife, or the application of caustic chemicals and burning, sometimes with a cigarette.

L98.2 Febrile neutrophilic dermatosis [Sweet]

L98.3 Eosinophilic cellulitis [Wells]

√5th **L98.4 Non-pressure chronic ulcer of skin, not elsewhere classified**

Chronic ulcer of skin NOS
Tropical ulcer NOS
Ulcer of skin NOS

EXCLUDES 2 *gangrene (I96)*
pressure ulcer (pressure area) (L89.-)
skin infections (L00-L08)
specific infections classified to A00-B99
ulcer of lower limb NEC (L97.-)
varicose ulcer (I83.0-I83.93)

AHA: 2017,4Q,17

TIP: The depth and/or severity of a diagnosed nonpressure ulcer can be determined based on medical record documentation from clinicians who are not the patient's provider.

TIP: Assign a code from this category/subcategory for nonpressure ulcers documented as acute.

√6th L98.41 Non-pressure chronic ulcer of buttock

L98.411 Non-pressure chronic ulcer of buttock limited to breakdown of skin HCC Rx ESR COM

L98.412 Non-pressure chronic ulcer of buttock with fat layer exposed HCC Rx ESR COM

L98.413 Non-pressure chronic ulcer of buttock with necrosis of muscle HCC Rx ESR COM

L98.414 Non-pressure chronic ulcer of buttock with necrosis of bone HCC Rx ESR COM

L98.415 Non-pressure chronic ulcer of buttock with muscle involvement without evidence of necrosis HCC Rx ESR COM

L98.416 Non-pressure chronic ulcer of buttock with bone involvement without evidence of necrosis HCC Rx ESR COM

L98.418 Non-pressure chronic ulcer of buttock with other specified severity HCC Rx ESR COM

L98.419 Non-pressure chronic ulcer of buttock with unspecified severity HCC Rx ESR COM

√6th L98.42 Non-pressure chronic ulcer of back

L98.421 Non-pressure chronic ulcer of back limited to breakdown of skin HCC Rx ESR COM

L98.422 Non-pressure chronic ulcer of back with fat layer exposed HCC Rx ESR COM

L98.423 Non-pressure chronic ulcer of back with necrosis of muscle HCC Rx ESR COM

L98.424 Non-pressure chronic ulcer of back with necrosis of bone HCC Rx ESR COM

L98.425 Non-pressure chronic ulcer of back with muscle involvement without evidence of necrosis HCC Rx ESR COM

L98.426 Non-pressure chronic ulcer of back with bone involvement without evidence of necrosis HCC Rx ESR COM

L98.428 Non-pressure chronic ulcer of back with other specified severity HCC Rx ESR COM

L98.429 Non-pressure chronic ulcer of back with unspecified severity HCC Rx ESR COM

√6th L98.49 Non-pressure chronic ulcer of skin of other sites

Non-pressure chronic ulcer of skin NOS

L98.491 Non-pressure chronic ulcer of skin of other sites limited to breakdown of skin HCC Rx ESR COM

L98.492 Non-pressure chronic ulcer of skin of other sites with fat layer exposed HCC Rx ESR COM

L98.493 Non-pressure chronic ulcer of skin of other sites with necrosis of muscle HCC Rx ESR COM

L98.494 Non-pressure chronic ulcer of skin of other sites with necrosis of bone HCC Rx ESR COM

L98.495 Non-pressure chronic ulcer of skin of other sites with muscle involvement without evidence of necrosis HCC Rx ESR COM

L98.496 Non-pressure chronic ulcer of skin of other sites with bone involvement without evidence of necrosis HCC Rx ESR COM

L98.498 Non-pressure chronic ulcer of skin of other sites with other specified severity HCC Rx ESR COM

L98.499 Non-pressure chronic ulcer of skin of other sites with unspecified severity HCC Rx ESR COM

L98.5 Mucinosis of the skin
Focal mucinosis
Lichen myxedematosus
Reticular erythematous mucinosis
EXCLUDES 1 *focal oral mucinosis (K13.79)*
myxedema (EØ3.9)

L98.6 Other infiltrative disorders of the skin and subcutaneous tissue
EXCLUDES 1 *hyalinosis cutis et mucosae (E78.89)*

L98.7 Excessive and redundant skin and subcutaneous tissue
Loose or sagging skin, following bariatric surgery weight loss
Loose or sagging skin following dietary weight loss
Loose or sagging skin, NOS
EXCLUDES 2 *acquired excess or redundant skin of eyelid (HØ2.3-)*
congenital excess or redundant skin of eyelid (Q1Ø.3)
skin changes due to chronic exposure to nonionizing radiation (L57.-)
AHA: 2016,4Q,36

L98.8 Other specified disorders of the skin and subcutaneous tissue
AHA: 2013,2Q,32

L98.9 Disorder of the skin and subcutaneous tissue, unspecified

L99 Other disorders of skin and subcutaneous tissue in diseases classified elsewhere
Code first underlying disease, such as:
amyloidosis (E85.-)
EXCLUDES 1 *skin disorders in diabetes (EØ8-E13 with .62-)*
skin disorders in gonorrhea (A54.89)
skin disorders in syphilis (A51.31, A52.79)
AHA: 2021,1Q,39

Chapter 13. Diseases of the Musculoskeletal System and Connective Tissue (MØØ–M99)

Chapter-specific Guidelines with Coding Examples

The chapter-specific guidelines from the ICD-10-CM Official Guidelines for Coding and Reporting have been provided below. Along with these guidelines are coding examples, contained in the shaded boxes, that have been developed to help illustrate the coding and/or sequencing guidance found in these guidelines.

a. Site and laterality

Most of the codes within Chapter 13 have site and laterality designations. The site represents the bone, joint or the muscle involved. For some conditions where more than one bone, joint or muscle is usually involved, such as osteoarthritis, there is a "multiple sites" code available. For categories where no multiple site code is provided and more than one bone, joint or muscle is involved, multiple codes should be used to indicate the different sites involved.

> Rheumatoid arthritis of multiple sites without rheumatoid factor
>
> **MØ6.Ø9 Rheumatoid arthritis without rheumatoid factor, multiple sites**
>
> *Explanation:* For some conditions where more than one bone, joint or muscle is usually involved, such as osteoarthritis, there is a "multiple sites" code available.

> Adolescent scoliosis in the upper thoracic region and the lumbar vertebrae
>
> **M41.124 Adolescent idiopathic scoliosis, thoracic region**
>
> **M41.126 Adolescent idiopathic scoliosis, lumbar region**
>
> *Explanation:* For categories without a multiple site code and more than one bone, joint, or muscle is involved, multiple codes should be used to indicate the different sites involved.

1) Bone versus joint

For certain conditions, the bone may be affected at the upper or lower end, (e.g., avascular necrosis of bone, M87, Osteoporosis, M8Ø, M81). Though the portion of the bone affected may be at the joint, the site designation will be the bone, not the joint.

> Idiopathic avascular necrosis of the femoral head of the left hip joint
>
> **M87.Ø52 Idiopathic aseptic necrosis of left femur**
>
> *Explanation:* For certain conditions such as avascular necrosis, the bone may be affected at the joint, but the site designation is the bone, not the joint.

b. Acute traumatic versus chronic or recurrent musculoskeletal conditions

Many musculoskeletal conditions are a result of previous injury or trauma to a site, or are recurrent conditions. Bone, joint or muscle conditions that are the result of a healed injury are usually found in chapter 13. Recurrent bone, joint or muscle conditions are also usually found in chapter 13. Any current, acute injury should be coded to the appropriate injury code from chapter 19. Chronic or recurrent conditions should generally be coded with a code from chapter 13. If it is difficult to determine from the documentation in the record which code is best to describe a condition, query the provider.

> Acute traumatic bucket handle tear of right medial meniscus
>
> **S83.211A Bucket-handle tear of medial meniscus, current injury, right knee, initial encounter**
>
> *Explanation:* Any current, acute injury is not coded in chapter 13. It should instead be coded to the appropriate injury code from chapter 19.

> Old bucket handle tear of right medial meniscus
>
> **M23.2Ø3 Derangement of unspecified medial meniscus due to old tear or injury, right knee**
>
> *Explanation:* Chronic or recurrent conditions should generally be coded with a code from chapter 13.

c. Coding of Pathologic Fractures

7th character A is for use as long as the patient is receiving active treatment for the fracture. Examples of active treatment are: surgical treatment, emergency department encounter, evaluation and continuing treatment by the same or a different physician. While the patient may be seen by a new or different provider over the course of treatment for a pathological fracture, assignment of the 7th character is based on whether the patient is undergoing active treatment and not whether the provider is seeing the patient for the first time.

> Pathologic fracture of left foot, unknown cause, currently under active treatment by a follow-up provider
>
> **M84.475A Pathological fracture, left foot, initial encounter for fracture**
>
> *Explanation:* Seventh character A is for use as long as the patient is receiving active treatment for a pathologic fracture. Examples of active treatment are surgical treatment, emergency department encounter, evaluation, and continuing treatment by the same or a different physician.
>
> The seventh character is based on whether the patient is undergoing active treatment and not whether the provider is seeing the patient for the first time.

7th character D is to be used for encounters after the patient has completed active treatment for the fracture and is receiving routine care for the fracture during the healing or recovery phase. The other 7th characters, listed under each subcategory in the Tabular List, are to be used for subsequent encounters for treatment of problems associated with the healing, such as malunions, nonunions, and sequelae.

Care for complications of surgical treatment for fracture repairs during the healing or recovery phase should be coded with the appropriate complication codes.

See Section I.C.19. Coding of traumatic fractures.

d. Osteoporosis

Osteoporosis is a systemic condition, meaning that all bones of the musculoskeletal system are affected. Therefore, site is not a component of the codes under category M81, Osteoporosis without current pathological fracture. The site codes under category M8Ø, Osteoporosis with current pathological fracture, identify the site of the fracture, not the osteoporosis.

1) Osteoporosis without pathological fracture

Category M81, Osteoporosis without current pathological fracture, is for use for patients with osteoporosis who do not currently have a pathologic fracture due to the osteoporosis, even if they have had a fracture in the past. For patients with a history of osteoporosis fractures, status code Z87.31Ø, Personal history of (healed) osteoporosis fracture, should follow the code from M81.

> Age-related osteoporosis with healed osteoporotic fracture of the lumbar vertebra
>
> **M81.Ø Age-related osteoporosis without current pathological fracture**
>
> **Z87.31Ø Personal history of (healed) osteoporosis fracture**
>
> *Explanation:* Category M81 is used for patients with osteoporosis who do not currently have a pathologic fracture due to the osteoporosis. To report a previous (healed) fracture, status code Z87.31Ø Personal history of (healed) osteoporosis fracture, should follow the code from M81.

2) Osteoporosis with current pathological fracture

Category M8Ø, Osteoporosis with current pathological fracture, is for patients who have a current pathologic fracture at the time of an encounter. The codes under M8Ø identify the site of the fracture. A code from category M8Ø, not a traumatic fracture code, should be used for any patient with known osteoporosis who suffers a fracture, even if the patient had a minor fall or trauma, if that fall or trauma would not usually break a normal, healthy bone.

> Disuse osteoporosis with current fracture of right shoulder sustained lifting a grocery bag, initial encounter
>
> **M8Ø.811A Other osteoporosis with current pathological fracture, right shoulder, initial encounter for fracture**
>
> *Explanation:* A code from category M8Ø, not a traumatic fracture code, should be used for any patient with known osteoporosis who suffers a fracture, even if the patient had a minor fall or trauma, if that fall or trauma would not usually break a normal, healthy bone.

e. Multisystem inflammatory syndrome

See Section I.C.1.g.1.l. for Multisystem Inflammatory Syndrome

Muscle/Tendon Table

ICD-10-CM categorizes certain muscles and tendons in the upper and lower extremities by their action (e.g., extension, flexion), their anatomical location (e.g., posterior, anterior), and/or whether they are intrinsic or extrinsic to a certain anatomical area. The Muscle/Tendon Table is provided at the beginning of chapters 13 and 19 as a resource to help users when code selection depends on one or more of these characteristics. A **TIP** has been placed at those categories and/or subcategories that relate to this table. Please note that this table is not all-inclusive, and proper code assignment should be based on the provider's documentation.

Body Region	Muscle	Extensor Tendon	Flexor Tendon	Other Tendon
Shoulder				
	Deltoid	Posterior deltoid	Anterior deltoid	
	Rotator cuff			
	Infraspinatus			Infraspinatus
	Subscapularis			Subscapularis
	Supraspinatus			Supraspinatus
	Teres minor			Teres minor
	Teres major	Teres major		
Upper arm				
	Anterior muscles			
	Biceps brachii — long head		Biceps brachii — long head	
	Biceps brachii — short head		Biceps brachii — short head	
	Brachialis		Brachialis	
	Coracobrachialis		Coracobrachialis	
	Posterior muscles			
	Triceps brachii	Triceps brachii		
Forearm				
	Anterior muscles			
	Flexors			
	Deep			
	Flexor digitorum profundus		Flexor digitorum profundus	
	Flexor pollicis longus		Flexor pollicis longus	
	Intermediate			
	Flexor digitorum superficialis		Flexor digitorum superficialis	
	Superficial			
	Flexor carpi radialis		Flexor carpi radialis	
	Flexor carpi ulnaris		Flexor carpi ulnaris	
	Palmaris longus		Palmaris longus	
	Pronators			
	Pronator quadratus			Pronator quadratus
	Pronator teres			Pronator teres
	Posterior muscles			
	Extensors			
	Deep			
	Abductor pollicis longus			Abductor pollicis longus
	Extensor indicis	Extensor indicis		
	Extensor pollicis brevis	Extensor pollicis brevis		
	Extensor pollicis longus	Extensor pollicis longus		
	Superficial			
	Brachioradialis			Brachioradialis
	Extensor carpi radialis brevis	Extensor carpi radialis brevis		
	Extensor carpi radialis longus	Extensor carpi radialis longus		
	Extensor carpi ulnaris	Extensor carpi ulnaris		
	Extensor digiti minimi	Extensor digiti minimi		
	Extensor digitorum	Extensor digitorum		
	Anconeus	Anconeus		
	Supinator			Supinator

Body Region	Muscle	Extensor Tendon	Flexor Tendon	Other Tendon
Hand				
Extrinsic — attach to a site in the forearm as well as a site in the hand with action related to hand movement at the wrist				
	Extensor carpi radialis brevis	Extensor carpi radialis brevis		
	Extensor carpi radialis longus	Extensor carpi radialis longus		
	Extensor carpi ulnaris	Extensor carpi ulnaris		
	Flexor carpi radialis		Flexor carpi radialis	
	Flexor carpi ulnaris		Flexor carpi ulnaris	
	Flexor digitorum superficialis		Flexor digitorum superficialis	
	Palmaris longus		Palmaris longus	
Extrinsic — attach to a site in the forearm as well as a site in the hand with action in the hand related to finger movement				
	Adductor pollicis longus			Adductor pollicis longus
	Extensor digiti minimi	Extensor digiti minimi		
	Extensor digitorum	Extensor digitorum		
	Extensor indicis	Extensor indicis		
	Flexor digitorum profundus		Flexor digitorum profundus	
	Flexor digitorum superficialis		Flexor digitorum superficialis	
Extrinsic — attach to a site in the forearm as well as a site in the hand with action in the hand related to thumb movement				
	Extensor pollicis brevis	Extensor pollicis brevis		
	Extensor pollicis longus	Extensor pollicis longus		
	Flexor pollicis longus		Flexor pollicis longus	
Intrinsic — found within the hand only				
	Adductor pollicis			Adductor pollicis
	Dorsal interossei	Dorsal interossei	Dorsal interossei	
	Lumbricals	Lumbricals	Lumbricals	
	Palmaris brevis			Palmaris brevis
	Palmar interossei	Palmar interossei	Palmar interossei	
	Hypothenar muscles			
	Abductor digiti minimi			Abductor digiti minimi
	Flexor digiti minimi brevis		Flexor digiti minimi brevis	
	Opponens digiti minimi		Opponens digiti minimi	
	Thenar muscles			
	Abductor pollicis brevis			Abductor pollicis brevis
	Flexor pollicis brevis		Flexor pollicis brevis	
	Opponens pollicis		Opponens pollicis	
Thigh				
	Anterior muscles			
	Iliopsoas		Iliopsoas	
	Pectineus		Pectineus	
	Quadriceps	Quadriceps		
	Rectus femoris	Rectus femoris — Extends knee	Rectus femoris — Flexes hip	
	Vastus intermedius	Vastus intermedius		
	Vastus lateralis	Vastus lateralis		
	Vastus medialis	Vastus medialis		
	Sartorius		Sartorius	
	Medial muscles			
	Adductor brevis			Adductor brevis
	Adductor longus			Adductor longus
	Adductor magnus			Adductor magnus
	Gracilis			Gracilis
	Obturator externus			Obturator externus
	Posterior muscles			
	Hamstring	Hamstring — Extends hip	Hamstring — Flexes knee	
	Biceps femoris	Biceps femoris	Biceps femoris	
	Semimembranosus	Semimembranosus	Semimembranosus	
	Semitendinosus	Semitendinosus	Semitendinosus	

Body Region	Muscle	Extensor Tendon	Flexor Tendon	Other Tendon
Lower leg				
	Anterior muscles			
	Extensor digitorum longus	Extensor digitorum longus		
	Extensor hallucis longus	Extensor hallucis longus		
	Fibularis (peroneus) tertius	Fibularis (peroneus) tertius		
	Tibialis anterior	Tibialis anterior		Tibialis anterior
	Lateral muscles			
	Fibularis (peroneus) brevis		Fibularis (peroneus) brevis	
	Fibularis (peroneus) longus		Fibularis (peroneus) longus	
	Posterior muscles			
	Deep			
	Flexor digitorum longus		Flexor digitorum longus	
	Flexor hallucis longus		Flexor hallucis longus	
	Popliteus		Popliteus	
	Tibialis posterior		Tibialis posterior	
	Superficial			
	Gastrocnemius		Gastrocnemius	
	Plantaris		Plantaris	
	Soleus		Soleus	
				Calcaneal (Achilles)
Ankle/Foot				
Extrinsic — attach to a site in the lower leg as well as a site in the foot with action related to foot movement at the ankle				
	Plantaris		Plantaris	
	Soleus		Soleus	
	Tibialis anterior	Tibialis anterior		
	Tibialis posterior		Tibialis posterior	
Extrinsic — attach to a site in the lower leg as well as a site in the foot with action in the foot related to toe movement				
	Extensor digitorum longus	Extensor digitorum longus		
	Extensor hallucis longus	Extensor hallucis longus		
	Flexor digitorum longus		Flexor digitorum longus	
	Flexor hallucis longus		Flexor hallucis longus	
Intrinsic — found within the ankle/foot only				
	Dorsal muscles			
	Extensor digitorum brevis	Extensor digitorum brevis		
	Extensor hallucis brevis	Extensor hallucis brevis		
	Plantar muscles			
	Abductor digiti minimi		Abductor digiti minimi	
	Abductor hallucis		Abductor hallucis	
	Dorsal interossei	Dorsal interossei	Dorsal interossei	
	Flexor digiti minimi brevis		Flexor digiti minimi brevis	
	Flexor digitorum brevis		Flexor digitorum brevis	
	Flexor hallucis brevis		Flexor hallucis brevis	
	Lumbricals	Lumbricals	Lumbricals	
	Quadratus plantae		Quadratus plantae	
	Plantar interossei	Plantar interossei	Plantar interossei	

Chapter 13. Diseases of the Musculoskeletal System and Connective Tissue (M00-M99)

NOTE Use an external cause code following the code for the musculoskeletal condition, if applicable, to identify the cause of the musculoskeletal condition

EXCLUDES 2 *arthropathic psoriasis (L40.5-)*
certain conditions originating in the perinatal period (P04-P96)
certain infectious and parasitic diseases (A00-B99)
compartment syndrome (traumatic) (T79.A-)
complications of pregnancy, childbirth and the puerperium (O00-O9A)
congenital malformations, deformations, and chromosomal abnormalities (Q00-Q99)
endocrine, nutritional and metabolic diseases (E00-E88)
injury, poisoning and certain other consequences of external causes (S00-T88)
neoplasms (C00-D49)
symptoms, signs and abnormal clinical and laboratory findings, not elsewhere classified (R00-R94)

This chapter contains the following blocks:

- M00-M02 Infectious arthropathies
- M04 Autoinflammatory syndromes
- M05-M14 Inflammatory polyarthropathies
- M15-M19 Osteoarthritis
- M20-M25 Other joint disorders
- M26-M27 Dentofacial anomalies [including malocclusion] and other disorders of jaw
- M30-M36 Systemic connective tissue disorders
- M40-M43 Deforming dorsopathies
- M45-M49 Spondylopathies
- M50-M54 Other dorsopathies
- M60-M63 Disorders of muscles
- M65-M67 Disorders of synovium and tendon
- M70-M79 Other soft tissue disorders
- M80-M85 Disorders of bone density and structure
- M86-M90 Other osteopathies
- M91-M94 Chondropathies
- M95 Other disorders of the musculoskeletal system and connective tissue
- M96 Intraoperative and postprocedural complications and disorders of musculoskeletal system, not elsewhere classified
- M97 Periprosthetic fracture around internal prosthetic joint
- M99 Biomechanical lesions, not elsewhere classified

ARTHROPATHIES (M00-M25)

INCLUDES disorders affecting predominantly peripheral (limb) joints

Infectious arthropathies (M00-M02)

NOTE This block comprises arthropathies due to microbiological agents. Distinction is made between the following types of etiological relationship:

a) direct infection of joint, where organisms invade synovial tissue and microbial antigen is present in the joint;

b) indirect infection, which may be of two types: a reactive arthropathy, where microbial infection of the body is established but neither organisms nor antigens can be identified in the joint, and a postinfective arthropathy, where microbial antigen is present but recovery of an organism is inconstant and evidence of local multiplication is lacking.

AHA: 2019,3Q,16

✓4th **M00 Pyogenic arthritis**

EXCLUDES 2 *infection and inflammatory reaction due to internal joint prosthesis (T84.5-)*

AHA: 2022,1Q,31

DEF: Pyogenic: Relating to or involving pus production, often referred to as suppurative or purulent.

✓5th **M00.0 Staphylococcal arthritis and polyarthritis**

Use additional code (B95.61-B95.8) to identify bacterial agent

M00.00 Staphylococcal arthritis, unspecified joint HCC ESR COM

✓6th **M00.01 Staphylococcal arthritis, shoulder**

M00.011 Staphylococcal arthritis, right shoulder HCC ESR COM

M00.012 Staphylococcal arthritis, left shoulder HCC ESR COM

M00.019 Staphylococcal arthritis, unspecified shoulder HCC ESR COM

✓6th **M00.02 Staphylococcal arthritis, elbow**

M00.021 Staphylococcal arthritis, right elbow HCC ESR COM

M00.022 Staphylococcal arthritis, left elbow HCC ESR COM

M00.029 Staphylococcal arthritis, unspecified elbow HCC ESR COM

✓6th **M00.03 Staphylococcal arthritis, wrist**

Staphylococcal arthritis of carpal bones

M00.031 Staphylococcal arthritis, right wrist HCC ESR COM

M00.032 Staphylococcal arthritis, left wrist HCC ESR COM

M00.039 Staphylococcal arthritis, unspecified wrist HCC ESR COM

✓6th **M00.04 Staphylococcal arthritis, hand**

Staphylococcal arthritis of metacarpus and phalanges

M00.041 Staphylococcal arthritis, right hand HCC ESR COM

M00.042 Staphylococcal arthritis, left hand HCC ESR COM

M00.049 Staphylococcal arthritis, unspecified hand HCC ESR COM

✓6th **M00.05 Staphylococcal arthritis, hip**

M00.051 Staphylococcal arthritis, right hip HCC ESR COM

M00.052 Staphylococcal arthritis, left hip HCC ESR COM

M00.059 Staphylococcal arthritis, unspecified hip HCC ESR COM

✓6th **M00.06 Staphylococcal arthritis, knee**

M00.061 Staphylococcal arthritis, right knee HCC ESR COM

M00.062 Staphylococcal arthritis, left knee HCC ESR COM

M00.069 Staphylococcal arthritis, unspecified knee HCC ESR COM

✓6th **M00.07 Staphylococcal arthritis, ankle and foot**

Staphylococcal arthritis, tarsus, metatarsus and phalanges

M00.071 Staphylococcal arthritis, right ankle and foot HCC ESR COM

M00.072 Staphylococcal arthritis, left ankle and foot HCC ESR COM

M00.079 Staphylococcal arthritis, unspecified ankle and foot HCC ESR COM

M00.08 Staphylococcal arthritis, vertebrae HCC ESR COM

M00.09 Staphylococcal polyarthritis HCC ESR COM

✓5th **M00.1 Pneumococcal arthritis and polyarthritis**

M00.10 Pneumococcal arthritis, unspecified joint HCC ESR COM

✓6th **M00.11 Pneumococcal arthritis, shoulder**

M00.111 Pneumococcal arthritis, right shoulder HCC ESR COM

M00.112 Pneumococcal arthritis, left shoulder HCC ESR COM

M00.119 Pneumococcal arthritis, unspecified shoulder HCC ESR COM

✓6th **M00.12 Pneumococcal arthritis, elbow**

M00.121 Pneumococcal arthritis, right elbow HCC ESR COM

M00.122 Pneumococcal arthritis, left elbow HCC ESR COM

M00.129 Pneumococcal arthritis, unspecified elbow HCC ESR COM

✓6th **M00.13 Pneumococcal arthritis, wrist**

Pneumococcal arthritis of carpal bones

M00.131 Pneumococcal arthritis, right wrist HCC ESR COM

M00.132 Pneumococcal arthritis, left wrist HCC ESR COM

M00.139 Pneumococcal arthritis, unspecified wrist HCC ESR COM

✓6th **M00.14 Pneumococcal arthritis, hand**

Pneumococcal arthritis of metacarpus and phalanges

M00.141 Pneumococcal arthritis, right hand HCC ESR COM

M00.142 Pneumococcal arthritis, left hand HCC ESR COM

M00.149 Pneumococcal arthritis, unspecified hand HCC ESR COM

✓6th MØØ.15 Pneumococcal arthritis, hip
MØØ.151 Pneumococcal arthritis, right hip HCC ESR COM
MØØ.152 Pneumococcal arthritis, left hip HCC ESR COM
MØØ.159 Pneumococcal arthritis, unspecified hip HCC ESR COM

✓6th MØØ.16 Pneumococcal arthritis, knee
MØØ.161 Pneumococcal arthritis, right knee HCC ESR COM
MØØ.162 Pneumococcal arthritis, left knee HCC ESR COM
MØØ.169 Pneumococcal arthritis, unspecified knee HCC ESR COM

✓6th MØØ.17 Pneumococcal arthritis, ankle and foot
Pneumococcal arthritis, tarsus, metatarsus and phalanges
MØØ.171 Pneumococcal arthritis, right ankle and foot HCC ESR COM
MØØ.172 Pneumococcal arthritis, left ankle and foot HCC ESR COM
MØØ.179 Pneumococcal arthritis, unspecified ankle and foot HCC ESR COM

MØØ.18 Pneumococcal arthritis, vertebrae HCC ESR COM
MØØ.19 Pneumococcal polyarthritis HCC ESR COM

✓5th MØØ.2 Other streptococcal arthritis and polyarthritis
Use additional code (B95.Ø-B95.2, B95.4-B95.5) to identify bacterial agent

MØØ.20 Other streptococcal arthritis, unspecified joint HCC ESR COM

✓6th MØØ.21 Other streptococcal arthritis, shoulder
MØØ.211 Other streptococcal arthritis, right shoulder HCC ESR COM
MØØ.212 Other streptococcal arthritis, left shoulder HCC ESR COM
MØØ.219 Other streptococcal arthritis, unspecified shoulder HCC ESR COM

✓6th MØØ.22 Other streptococcal arthritis, elbow
MØØ.221 Other streptococcal arthritis, right elbow HCC ESR COM
MØØ.222 Other streptococcal arthritis, left elbow HCC ESR COM
MØØ.229 Other streptococcal arthritis, unspecified elbow HCC ESR COM

✓6th MØØ.23 Other streptococcal arthritis, wrist
Other streptococcal arthritis of carpal bones
MØØ.231 Other streptococcal arthritis, right wrist HCC ESR COM
MØØ.232 Other streptococcal arthritis, left wrist HCC ESR COM
MØØ.239 Other streptococcal arthritis, unspecified wrist HCC ESR COM

✓6th MØØ.24 Other streptococcal arthritis, hand
Other streptococcal arthritis metacarpus and phalanges
MØØ.241 Other streptococcal arthritis, right hand HCC ESR COM
MØØ.242 Other streptococcal arthritis, left hand HCC ESR COM
MØØ.249 Other streptococcal arthritis, unspecified hand HCC ESR COM

✓6th MØØ.25 Other streptococcal arthritis, hip
MØØ.251 Other streptococcal arthritis, right hip HCC ESR COM
MØØ.252 Other streptococcal arthritis, left hip HCC ESR COM
MØØ.259 Other streptococcal arthritis, unspecified hip HCC ESR COM

✓6th MØØ.26 Other streptococcal arthritis, knee
MØØ.261 Other streptococcal arthritis, right knee HCC ESR COM
MØØ.262 Other streptococcal arthritis, left knee HCC ESR COM
MØØ.269 Other streptococcal arthritis, unspecified knee HCC ESR COM

✓6th MØØ.27 Other streptococcal arthritis, ankle and foot
Other streptococcal arthritis, tarsus, metatarsus and phalanges
MØØ.271 Other streptococcal arthritis, right ankle and foot HCC ESR COM
MØØ.272 Other streptococcal arthritis, left ankle and foot HCC ESR COM
MØØ.279 Other streptococcal arthritis, unspecified ankle and foot HCC ESR COM

MØØ.28 Other streptococcal arthritis, vertebrae HCC ESR COM
MØØ.29 Other streptococcal polyarthritis HCC ESR COM

✓5th MØØ.8 Arthritis and polyarthritis due to other bacteria
Use additional code (B96) to identify bacteria

MØØ.80 Arthritis due to other bacteria, unspecified joint HCC ESR COM

✓6th MØØ.81 Arthritis due to other bacteria, shoulder
MØØ.811 Arthritis due to other bacteria, right shoulder HCC ESR COM
MØØ.812 Arthritis due to other bacteria, left shoulder HCC ESR COM
MØØ.819 Arthritis due to other bacteria, unspecified shoulder HCC ESR COM

✓6th MØØ.82 Arthritis due to other bacteria, elbow
MØØ.821 Arthritis due to other bacteria, right elbow HCC ESR COM
MØØ.822 Arthritis due to other bacteria, left elbow HCC ESR COM
MØØ.829 Arthritis due to other bacteria, unspecified elbow HCC ESR COM

✓6th MØØ.83 Arthritis due to other bacteria, wrist
Arthritis due to other bacteria, carpal bones
MØØ.831 Arthritis due to other bacteria, right wrist HCC ESR COM
MØØ.832 Arthritis due to other bacteria, left wrist HCC ESR COM
MØØ.839 Arthritis due to other bacteria, unspecified wrist HCC ESR COM

✓6th MØØ.84 Arthritis due to other bacteria, hand
Arthritis due to other bacteria, metacarpus and phalanges
MØØ.841 Arthritis due to other bacteria, right hand HCC ESR COM
MØØ.842 Arthritis due to other bacteria, left hand HCC ESR COM
MØØ.849 Arthritis due to other bacteria, unspecified hand HCC ESR COM

✓6th MØØ.85 Arthritis due to other bacteria, hip
MØØ.851 Arthritis due to other bacteria, right hip HCC ESR COM
MØØ.852 Arthritis due to other bacteria, left hip HCC ESR COM
MØØ.859 Arthritis due to other bacteria, unspecified hip HCC ESR COM

✓6th MØØ.86 Arthritis due to other bacteria, knee
AHA: 2019,3Q,16
MØØ.861 Arthritis due to other bacteria, right knee HCC ESR COM
MØØ.862 Arthritis due to other bacteria, left knee HCC ESR COM
MØØ.869 Arthritis due to other bacteria, unspecified knee HCC ESR COM

✓6th MØØ.87 Arthritis due to other bacteria, ankle and foot
Arthritis due to other bacteria, tarsus, metatarsus, and phalanges
MØØ.871 Arthritis due to other bacteria, right ankle and foot HCC ESR COM
MØØ.872 Arthritis due to other bacteria, left ankle and foot HCC ESR COM
MØØ.879 Arthritis due to other bacteria, unspecified ankle and foot HCC ESR COM

MØØ.88 Arthritis due to other bacteria, vertebrae HCC ESR COM
MØØ.89 Polyarthritis due to other bacteria HCC ESR COM

M00.9 Pyogenic arthritis, unspecified HCC ESR COM
Infective arthritis NOS

M01 Direct infections of joint in infectious and parasitic diseases classified elsewhere
Code first underlying disease, such as:
leprosy [Hansen's disease] (A30.-)
mycoses (B35-B49)
O'nyong-nyong fever (A92.1)
paratyphoid fever (A01.1-A01.4)

EXCLUDES 1 *arthropathy in Lyme disease (A69.23)*
gonococcal arthritis (A54.42)
meningococcal arthritis (A39.83)
mumps arthritis (B26.85)
postinfective arthropathy (M02.-)
postmeningococcal arthritis (A39.84)
reactive arthritis (M02.3)
rubella arthritis (B06.82)
sarcoidosis arthritis (D86.86)
typhoid fever arthritis (A01.04)
tuberculosis arthritis (A18.01-A18.02)

M01.X Direct infection of joint in infectious and parasitic diseases classified elsewhere

M01.X0 Direct infection of unspecified joint in infectious and parasitic diseases classified elsewhere HCC ESR COM

M01.X1 Direct infection of shoulder joint in infectious and parasitic diseases classified elsewhere
M01.X11 Direct infection of right shoulder in infectious and parasitic diseases classified elsewhere HCC ESR COM
M01.X12 Direct infection of left shoulder in infectious and parasitic diseases classified elsewhere HCC ESR COM
M01.X19 Direct infection of unspecified shoulder in infectious and parasitic diseases classified elsewhere HCC ESR COM

M01.X2 Direct infection of elbow in infectious and parasitic diseases classified elsewhere
M01.X21 Direct infection of right elbow in infectious and parasitic diseases classified elsewhere HCC ESR COM
M01.X22 Direct infection of left elbow in infectious and parasitic diseases classified elsewhere HCC ESR COM
M01.X29 Direct infection of unspecified elbow in infectious and parasitic diseases classified elsewhere HCC ESR COM

M01.X3 Direct infection of wrist in infectious and parasitic diseases classified elsewhere
Direct infection of carpal bones in infectious and parasitic diseases classified elsewhere
M01.X31 Direct infection of right wrist in infectious and parasitic diseases classified elsewhere HCC ESR COM
M01.X32 Direct infection of left wrist in infectious and parasitic diseases classified elsewhere HCC ESR COM
M01.X39 Direct infection of unspecified wrist in infectious and parasitic diseases classified elsewhere HCC ESR COM

M01.X4 Direct infection of hand in infectious and parasitic diseases classified elsewhere
Direct infection of metacarpus and phalanges in infectious and parasitic diseases classified elsewhere
M01.X41 Direct infection of right hand in infectious and parasitic diseases classified elsewhere HCC ESR COM
M01.X42 Direct infection of left hand in infectious and parasitic diseases classified elsewhere HCC ESR COM
M01.X49 Direct infection of unspecified hand in infectious and parasitic diseases classified elsewhere HCC ESR COM

M01.X5 Direct infection of hip in infectious and parasitic diseases classified elsewhere
M01.X51 Direct infection of right hip in infectious and parasitic diseases classified elsewhere HCC ESR COM
M01.X52 Direct infection of left hip in infectious and parasitic diseases classified elsewhere HCC ESR COM
M01.X59 Direct infection of unspecified hip in infectious and parasitic diseases classified elsewhere HCC ESR COM

M01.X6 Direct infection of knee in infectious and parasitic diseases classified elsewhere
M01.X61 Direct infection of right knee in infectious and parasitic diseases classified elsewhere HCC ESR COM
M01.X62 Direct infection of left knee in infectious and parasitic diseases classified elsewhere HCC ESR COM
M01.X69 Direct infection of unspecified knee in infectious and parasitic diseases classified elsewhere HCC ESR COM

M01.X7 Direct infection of ankle and foot in infectious and parasitic diseases classified elsewhere
Direct infection of tarsus, metatarsus and phalanges in infectious and parasitic diseases classified elsewhere
M01.X71 Direct infection of right ankle and foot in infectious and parasitic diseases classified elsewhere HCC ESR COM
M01.X72 Direct infection of left ankle and foot in infectious and parasitic diseases classified elsewhere HCC ESR COM
M01.X79 Direct infection of unspecified ankle and foot in infectious and parasitic diseases classified elsewhere HCC ESR COM

M01.X8 Direct infection of vertebrae in infectious and parasitic diseases classified elsewhere HCC ESR COM
M01.X9 Direct infection of multiple joints in infectious and parasitic diseases classified elsewhere HCC ESR COM

M02 Postinfective and reactive arthropathies
Code first underlying disease, such as:
congenital syphilis [Clutton's joints] (A50.5)
enteritis due to Yersinia enterocolitica (A04.6)
infective endocarditis (I33.0)
viral hepatitis (B15-B19)

EXCLUDES 1 *Behçet's disease (M35.2)*
direct infections of joint in infectious and parasitic diseases classified elsewhere (M01.-)
mumps arthritis (B26.85)
postmeningococcal arthritis (A39.84)
rheumatic fever (I00)
rubella arthritis (B06.82)
syphilis arthritis (late) (A52.77)
tabetic arthropathy [Charcôt's] (A52.16)

M02.0 Arthropathy following intestinal bypass
M02.00 Arthropathy following intestinal bypass, unspecified site
M02.01 Arthropathy following intestinal bypass, shoulder
M02.011 Arthropathy following intestinal bypass, right shoulder
M02.012 Arthropathy following intestinal bypass, left shoulder
M02.019 Arthropathy following intestinal bypass, unspecified shoulder
M02.02 Arthropathy following intestinal bypass, elbow
M02.021 Arthropathy following intestinal bypass, right elbow
M02.022 Arthropathy following intestinal bypass, left elbow
M02.029 Arthropathy following intestinal bypass, unspecified elbow
M02.03 Arthropathy following intestinal bypass, wrist
Arthropathy following intestinal bypass, carpal bones
M02.031 Arthropathy following intestinal bypass, right wrist
M02.032 Arthropathy following intestinal bypass, left wrist
M02.039 Arthropathy following intestinal bypass, unspecified wrist

√6th MØ2.Ø4 Arthropathy following intestinal bypass, hand
Arthropathy following intestinal bypass, metacarpals and phalanges
MØ2.Ø41 Arthropathy following intestinal bypass, right hand
MØ2.Ø42 Arthropathy following intestinal bypass, left hand
MØ2.Ø49 Arthropathy following intestinal bypass, unspecified hand
√6th MØ2.Ø5 Arthropathy following intestinal bypass, hip
MØ2.Ø51 Arthropathy following intestinal bypass, right hip
MØ2.Ø52 Arthropathy following intestinal bypass, left hip
MØ2.Ø59 Arthropathy following intestinal bypass, unspecified hip
√6th MØ2.Ø6 Arthropathy following intestinal bypass, knee
MØ2.Ø61 Arthropathy following intestinal bypass, right knee
MØ2.Ø62 Arthropathy following intestinal bypass, left knee
MØ2.Ø69 Arthropathy following intestinal bypass, unspecified knee
√6th MØ2.Ø7 Arthropathy following intestinal bypass, ankle and foot
Arthropathy following intestinal bypass, tarsus, metatarsus and phalanges
MØ2.Ø71 Arthropathy following intestinal bypass, right ankle and foot
MØ2.Ø72 Arthropathy following intestinal bypass, left ankle and foot
MØ2.Ø79 Arthropathy following intestinal bypass, unspecified ankle and foot
MØ2.Ø8 Arthropathy following intestinal bypass, vertebrae
MØ2.Ø9 Arthropathy following intestinal bypass, multiple sites

√5th MØ2.1 Postdysenteric arthropathy
MØ2.1Ø Postdysenteric arthropathy, unspecified site HCC ESR COM
√6th MØ2.11 Postdysenteric arthropathy, shoulder
MØ2.111 Postdysenteric arthropathy, right shoulder HCC ESR COM
MØ2.112 Postdysenteric arthropathy, left shoulder HCC ESR COM
MØ2.119 Postdysenteric arthropathy, unspecified shoulder HCC ESR COM
√6th MØ2.12 Postdysenteric arthropathy, elbow
MØ2.121 Postdysenteric arthropathy, right elbow HCC ESR COM
MØ2.122 Postdysenteric arthropathy, left elbow HCC ESR COM
MØ2.129 Postdysenteric arthropathy, unspecified elbow HCC ESR COM
√6th MØ2.13 Postdysenteric arthropathy, wrist
Postdysenteric arthropathy, carpal bones
MØ2.131 Postdysenteric arthropathy, right wrist HCC ESR COM
MØ2.132 Postdysenteric arthropathy, left wrist HCC ESR COM
MØ2.139 Postdysenteric arthropathy, unspecified wrist HCC ESR COM
√6th MØ2.14 Postdysenteric arthropathy, hand
Postdysenteric arthropathy, metacarpus and phalanges
MØ2.141 Postdysenteric arthropathy, right hand HCC ESR COM
MØ2.142 Postdysenteric arthropathy, left hand HCC ESR COM
MØ2.149 Postdysenteric arthropathy, unspecified hand HCC ESR COM
√6th MØ2.15 Postdysenteric arthropathy, hip
MØ2.151 Postdysenteric arthropathy, right hip HCC ESR COM
MØ2.152 Postdysenteric arthropathy, left hip HCC ESR COM
MØ2.159 Postdysenteric arthropathy, unspecified hip HCC ESR COM
√6th MØ2.16 Postdysenteric arthropathy, knee
MØ2.161 Postdysenteric arthropathy, right knee HCC ESR COM
MØ2.162 Postdysenteric arthropathy, left knee HCC ESR COM
MØ2.169 Postdysenteric arthropathy, unspecified knee HCC ESR COM
√6th MØ2.17 Postdysenteric arthropathy, ankle and foot
Postdysenteric arthropathy, tarsus, metatarsus and phalanges
MØ2.171 Postdysenteric arthropathy, right ankle and foot HCC ESR COM
MØ2.172 Postdysenteric arthropathy, left ankle and foot HCC ESR COM
MØ2.179 Postdysenteric arthropathy, unspecified ankle and foot HCC ESR COM
MØ2.18 Postdysenteric arthropathy, vertebrae HCC ESR COM
MØ2.19 Postdysenteric arthropathy, multiple sites HCC ESR COM

√5th MØ2.2 Postimmunization arthropathy
MØ2.2Ø Postimmunization arthropathy, unspecified site
√6th MØ2.21 Postimmunization arthropathy, shoulder
MØ2.211 Postimmunization arthropathy, right shoulder
MØ2.212 Postimmunization arthropathy, left shoulder
MØ2.219 Postimmunization arthropathy, unspecified shoulder
√6th MØ2.22 Postimmunization arthropathy, elbow
MØ2.221 Postimmunization arthropathy, right elbow
MØ2.222 Postimmunization arthropathy, left elbow
MØ2.229 Postimmunization arthropathy, unspecified elbow
√6th MØ2.23 Postimmunization arthropathy, wrist
Postimmunization arthropathy, carpal bones
MØ2.231 Postimmunization arthropathy, right wrist
MØ2.232 Postimmunization arthropathy, left wrist
MØ2.239 Postimmunization arthropathy, unspecified wrist
√6th MØ2.24 Postimmunization arthropathy, hand
Postimmunization arthropathy, metacarpus and phalanges
MØ2.241 Postimmunization arthropathy, right hand
MØ2.242 Postimmunization arthropathy, left hand
MØ2.249 Postimmunization arthropathy, unspecified hand
√6th MØ2.25 Postimmunization arthropathy, hip
MØ2.251 Postimmunization arthropathy, right hip
MØ2.252 Postimmunization arthropathy, left hip
MØ2.259 Postimmunization arthropathy, unspecified hip
√6th MØ2.26 Postimmunization arthropathy, knee
MØ2.261 Postimmunization arthropathy, right knee
MØ2.262 Postimmunization arthropathy, left knee
MØ2.269 Postimmunization arthropathy, unspecified knee
√6th MØ2.27 Postimmunization arthropathy, ankle and foot
Postimmunization arthropathy, tarsus, metatarsus and phalanges
MØ2.271 Postimmunization arthropathy, right ankle and foot
MØ2.272 Postimmunization arthropathy, left ankle and foot
MØ2.279 Postimmunization arthropathy, unspecified ankle and foot
MØ2.28 Postimmunization arthropathy, vertebrae
MØ2.29 Postimmunization arthropathy, multiple sites

√5th MØ2.3 Reiter's disease
Reactive arthritis
DEF: Arthritis, iridocyclitis, and urethritis, sometimes with diarrhea. While symptoms may recur, arthritis is constant.
MØ2.3Ø Reiter's disease, unspecified site HCC Rx ESR COM

✓6th **M02.31 Reiter's disease, shoulder**
- **M02.311 Reiter's disease, right shoulder** HCC Rx ESR COM
- **M02.312 Reiter's disease, left shoulder** HCC Rx ESR COM
- **M02.319 Reiter's disease, unspecified shoulder** HCC Rx ESR COM

✓6th **M02.32 Reiter's disease, elbow**
- **M02.321 Reiter's disease, right elbow** HCC Rx ESR COM
- **M02.322 Reiter's disease, left elbow** HCC Rx ESR COM
- **M02.329 Reiter's disease, unspecified elbow** HCC Rx ESR COM

✓6th **M02.33 Reiter's disease, wrist**
Reiter's disease, carpal bones
- **M02.331 Reiter's disease, right wrist** HCC Rx ESR COM
- **M02.332 Reiter's disease, left wrist** HCC Rx ESR COM
- **M02.339 Reiter's disease, unspecified wrist** HCC Rx ESR COM

✓6th **M02.34 Reiter's disease, hand**
Reiter's disease, metacarpus and phalanges
- **M02.341 Reiter's disease, right hand** HCC Rx ESR COM
- **M02.342 Reiter's disease, left hand** HCC Rx ESR COM
- **M02.349 Reiter's disease, unspecified hand** HCC Rx ESR COM

✓6th **M02.35 Reiter's disease, hip**
- **M02.351 Reiter's disease, right hip** HCC Rx ESR COM
- **M02.352 Reiter's disease, left hip** HCC Rx ESR COM
- **M02.359 Reiter's disease, unspecified hip** HCC Rx ESR COM

✓6th **M02.36 Reiter's disease, knee**
- **M02.361 Reiter's disease, right knee** HCC Rx ESR COM
- **M02.362 Reiter's disease, left knee** HCC Rx ESR COM
- **M02.369 Reiter's disease, unspecified knee** HCC Rx ESR COM

✓6th **M02.37 Reiter's disease, ankle and foot**
Reiter's disease, tarsus, metatarsus and phalanges
- **M02.371 Reiter's disease, right ankle and foot** HCC Rx ESR COM
- **M02.372 Reiter's disease, left ankle and foot** HCC Rx ESR COM
- **M02.379 Reiter's disease, unspecified ankle and foot** HCC Rx ESR COM

M02.38 Reiter's disease, vertebrae HCC Rx ESR COM
M02.39 Reiter's disease, multiple sites HCC Rx ESR COM

✓5th **M02.8 Other reactive arthropathies**
- ***M02.80 Other reactive arthropathies, unspecified site*** HCC ESR COM

✓6th **M02.81 Other reactive arthropathies, shoulder**
- ***M02.811 Other reactive arthropathies, right shoulder*** HCC ESR COM
- ***M02.812 Other reactive arthropathies, left shoulder*** HCC ESR COM
- ***M02.819 Other reactive arthropathies, unspecified shoulder*** HCC ESR COM

✓6th **M02.82 Other reactive arthropathies, elbow**
- ***M02.821 Other reactive arthropathies, right elbow*** HCC ESR COM
- ***M02.822 Other reactive arthropathies, left elbow*** HCC ESR COM
- ***M02.829 Other reactive arthropathies, unspecified elbow*** HCC ESR COM

✓6th **M02.83 Other reactive arthropathies, wrist**
Other reactive arthropathies, carpal bones
- ***M02.831 Other reactive arthropathies, right wrist*** HCC ESR COM
- ***M02.832 Other reactive arthropathies, left wrist*** HCC ESR COM
- ***M02.839 Other reactive arthropathies, unspecified wrist*** HCC ESR COM

✓6th **M02.84 Other reactive arthropathies, hand**
Other reactive arthropathies, metacarpus and phalanges
- ***M02.841 Other reactive arthropathies, right hand*** HCC ESR COM
- ***M02.842 Other reactive arthropathies, left hand*** HCC ESR COM
- ***M02.849 Other reactive arthropathies, unspecified hand*** HCC ESR COM

✓6th **M02.85 Other reactive arthropathies, hip**
- ***M02.851 Other reactive arthropathies, right hip*** HCC ESR COM
- ***M02.852 Other reactive arthropathies, left hip*** HCC ESR COM
- ***M02.859 Other reactive arthropathies, unspecified hip*** HCC ESR COM

✓6th **M02.86 Other reactive arthropathies, knee**
- ***M02.861 Other reactive arthropathies, right knee*** HCC ESR COM
- ***M02.862 Other reactive arthropathies, left knee*** HCC ESR COM
- ***M02.869 Other reactive arthropathies, unspecified knee*** HCC ESR COM

✓6th **M02.87 Other reactive arthropathies, ankle and foot**
Other reactive arthropathies, tarsus, metatarsus and phalanges
- ***M02.871 Other reactive arthropathies, right ankle and foot*** HCC ESR COM
- ***M02.872 Other reactive arthropathies, left ankle and foot*** HCC ESR COM
- ***M02.879 Other reactive arthropathies, unspecified ankle and foot*** HCC ESR COM

M02.88 Other reactive arthropathies, vertebrae HCC ESR COM
M02.89 Other reactive arthropathies, multiple sites HCC ESR COM

M02.9 Reactive arthropathy, unspecified HCC ESR COM

Autoinflammatory syndromes (M04)

✓4th **M04 Autoinflammatory syndromes**
EXCLUDES 2 *Crohn's disease (K50.-)*
AHA: 2016,4Q,37

M04.1 Periodic fever syndromes HCC Rx ESR COM
Familial Mediterranean fever
Hyperimmunoglobin D syndrome
Mevalonate kinase deficiency
Tumor necrosis factor receptor associated periodic syndrome [TRAPS]

M04.2 Cryopyrin-associated periodic syndromes HCC Rx ESR COM
Chronic infantile neurological, cutaneous and articular syndrome [CINCA]
Familial cold autoinflammatory syndrome
Familial cold urticaria
Muckle-Wells syndrome
Neonatal onset multisystemic inflammatory disorder [NOMID]

M04.8 Other autoinflammatory syndromes HCC Rx ESR COM
Blau syndrome
Deficiency of interleukin 1 receptor antagonist [DIRA]
Majeed syndrome
Periodic fever, aphthous stomatitis, pharyngitis, and adenopathy syndrome [PFAPA]
Pyogenic arthritis, pyoderma gangrenosum, and acne syndrome [PAPA]

M04.9 Autoinflammatory syndrome, unspecified HCC Rx ESR COM

Inflammatory polyarthropathies (M05-M14)

M05 Rheumatoid arthritis with rheumatoid factor

EXCLUDES 1 *rheumatic fever (I00)*
juvenile rheumatoid arthritis (M08.-)
rheumatoid arthritis of spine (M45.-)

AHA: 2020,4Q,31-32

DEF: Rheumatoid arthritis: Autoimmune systemic disease that causes chronic inflammation of the joints and other areas of the body, manifested by inflammatory changes in articular structures and synovial membranes, atrophy, and loss in bone density.

M05.0 Felty's syndrome
Rheumatoid arthritis with splenoadenomegaly and leukopenia

- **M05.00 Felty's syndrome, unspecified site** HCC Rx ESR COM
- **M05.01 Felty's syndrome, shoulder**
  - **M05.011 Felty's syndrome, right shoulder** HCC Rx ESR COM
  - **M05.012 Felty's syndrome, left shoulder** HCC Rx ESR COM
  - **M05.019 Felty's syndrome, unspecified shoulder** HCC Rx ESR COM
- **M05.02 Felty's syndrome, elbow**
  - **M05.021 Felty's syndrome, right elbow** HCC Rx ESR COM
  - **M05.022 Felty's syndrome, left elbow** HCC Rx ESR COM
  - **M05.029 Felty's syndrome, unspecified elbow** HCC Rx ESR COM
- **M05.03 Felty's syndrome, wrist**
  Felty's syndrome, carpal bones
  - **M05.031 Felty's syndrome, right wrist** HCC Rx ESR COM
  - **M05.032 Felty's syndrome, left wrist** HCC Rx ESR COM
  - **M05.039 Felty's syndrome, unspecified wrist** HCC Rx ESR COM
- **M05.04 Felty's syndrome, hand**
  Felty's syndrome, metacarpus and phalanges
  - **M05.041 Felty's syndrome, right hand** HCC Rx ESR COM
  - **M05.042 Felty's syndrome, left hand** HCC Rx ESR COM
  - **M05.049 Felty's syndrome, unspecified hand** HCC Rx ESR COM
- **M05.05 Felty's syndrome, hip**
  - **M05.051 Felty's syndrome, right hip** HCC Rx ESR COM
  - **M05.052 Felty's syndrome, left hip** HCC Rx ESR COM
  - **M05.059 Felty's syndrome, unspecified hip** HCC Rx ESR COM
- **M05.06 Felty's syndrome, knee**
  - **M05.061 Felty's syndrome, right knee** HCC Rx ESR COM
  - **M05.062 Felty's syndrome, left knee** HCC Rx ESR COM
  - **M05.069 Felty's syndrome, unspecified knee** HCC Rx ESR COM
- **M05.07 Felty's syndrome, ankle and foot**
  Felty's syndrome, tarsus, metatarsus and phalanges
  - **M05.071 Felty's syndrome, right ankle and foot** HCC Rx ESR COM
  - **M05.072 Felty's syndrome, left ankle and foot** HCC Rx ESR COM
  - **M05.079 Felty's syndrome, unspecified ankle and foot** HCC Rx ESR COM
- **M05.09 Felty's syndrome, multiple sites** HCC Rx ESR COM

M05.1 Rheumatoid lung disease with rheumatoid arthritis

- **M05.10 Rheumatoid lung disease with rheumatoid arthritis of unspecified site** HCC Rx ESR COM
- **M05.11 Rheumatoid lung disease with rheumatoid arthritis of shoulder**
  - **M05.111 Rheumatoid lung disease with rheumatoid arthritis of right shoulder** HCC Rx ESR COM
  - **M05.112 Rheumatoid lung disease with rheumatoid arthritis of left shoulder** HCC Rx ESR COM
  - **M05.119 Rheumatoid lung disease with rheumatoid arthritis of unspecified shoulder** HCC Rx ESR COM
- **M05.12 Rheumatoid lung disease with rheumatoid arthritis of elbow**
  - **M05.121 Rheumatoid lung disease with rheumatoid arthritis of right elbow** HCC Rx ESR COM
  - **M05.122 Rheumatoid lung disease with rheumatoid arthritis of left elbow** HCC Rx ESR COM
  - **M05.129 Rheumatoid lung disease with rheumatoid arthritis of unspecified elbow** HCC Rx ESR COM
- **M05.13 Rheumatoid lung disease with rheumatoid arthritis of wrist**
  Rheumatoid lung disease with rheumatoid arthritis, carpal bones
  - **M05.131 Rheumatoid lung disease with rheumatoid arthritis of right wrist** HCC Rx ESR COM
  - **M05.132 Rheumatoid lung disease with rheumatoid arthritis of left wrist** HCC Rx ESR COM
  - **M05.139 Rheumatoid lung disease with rheumatoid arthritis of unspecified wrist** HCC Rx ESR COM
- **M05.14 Rheumatoid lung disease with rheumatoid arthritis of hand**
  Rheumatoid lung disease with rheumatoid arthritis, metacarpus and phalanges
  - **M05.141 Rheumatoid lung disease with rheumatoid arthritis of right hand** HCC Rx ESR COM
  - **M05.142 Rheumatoid lung disease with rheumatoid arthritis of left hand** HCC Rx ESR COM
  - **M05.149 Rheumatoid lung disease with rheumatoid arthritis of unspecified hand** HCC Rx ESR COM
- **M05.15 Rheumatoid lung disease with rheumatoid arthritis of hip**
  - **M05.151 Rheumatoid lung disease with rheumatoid arthritis of right hip** HCC Rx ESR COM
  - **M05.152 Rheumatoid lung disease with rheumatoid arthritis of left hip** HCC Rx ESR COM
  - **M05.159 Rheumatoid lung disease with rheumatoid arthritis of unspecified hip** HCC Rx ESR COM
- **M05.16 Rheumatoid lung disease with rheumatoid arthritis of knee**
  - **M05.161 Rheumatoid lung disease with rheumatoid arthritis of right knee** HCC Rx ESR COM
  - **M05.162 Rheumatoid lung disease with rheumatoid arthritis of left knee** HCC Rx ESR COM
  - **M05.169 Rheumatoid lung disease with rheumatoid arthritis of unspecified knee** HCC Rx ESR COM
- **M05.17 Rheumatoid lung disease with rheumatoid arthritis of ankle and foot**
  Rheumatoid lung disease with rheumatoid arthritis, tarsus, metatarsus and phalanges
  - **M05.171 Rheumatoid lung disease with rheumatoid arthritis of right ankle and foot** HCC Rx ESR COM
  - **M05.172 Rheumatoid lung disease with rheumatoid arthritis of left ankle and foot** HCC Rx ESR COM
  - **M05.179 Rheumatoid lung disease with rheumatoid arthritis of unspecified ankle and foot** HCC Rx ESR COM
- **M05.19 Rheumatoid lung disease with rheumatoid arthritis of multiple sites** HCC Rx ESR COM

M05.2 Rheumatoid vasculitis with rheumatoid arthritis
- **M05.20 Rheumatoid vasculitis with rheumatoid arthritis of unspecified site** HCC Rx ESR COM
- **M05.21 Rheumatoid vasculitis with rheumatoid arthritis of shoulder**
  - **M05.211 Rheumatoid vasculitis with rheumatoid arthritis of right shoulder** HCC Rx ESR COM
  - **M05.212 Rheumatoid vasculitis with rheumatoid arthritis of left shoulder** HCC Rx ESR COM
  - **M05.219 Rheumatoid vasculitis with rheumatoid arthritis of unspecified shoulder** HCC Rx ESR COM
- **M05.22 Rheumatoid vasculitis with rheumatoid arthritis of elbow**
  - **M05.221 Rheumatoid vasculitis with rheumatoid arthritis of right elbow** HCC Rx ESR COM
  - **M05.222 Rheumatoid vasculitis with rheumatoid arthritis of left elbow** HCC Rx ESR COM
  - **M05.229 Rheumatoid vasculitis with rheumatoid arthritis of unspecified elbow** HCC Rx ESR COM
- **M05.23 Rheumatoid vasculitis with rheumatoid arthritis of wrist**
  Rheumatoid vasculitis with rheumatoid arthritis, carpal bones
  - **M05.231 Rheumatoid vasculitis with rheumatoid arthritis of right wrist** HCC Rx ESR COM
  - **M05.232 Rheumatoid vasculitis with rheumatoid arthritis of left wrist** HCC Rx ESR COM
  - **M05.239 Rheumatoid vasculitis with rheumatoid arthritis of unspecified wrist** HCC Rx ESR COM
- **M05.24 Rheumatoid vasculitis with rheumatoid arthritis of hand**
  Rheumatoid vasculitis with rheumatoid arthritis, metacarpus and phalanges
  - **M05.241 Rheumatoid vasculitis with rheumatoid arthritis of right hand** HCC Rx ESR COM
  - **M05.242 Rheumatoid vasculitis with rheumatoid arthritis of left hand** HCC Rx ESR COM
  - **M05.249 Rheumatoid vasculitis with rheumatoid arthritis of unspecified hand** HCC Rx ESR COM
- **M05.25 Rheumatoid vasculitis with rheumatoid arthritis of hip**
  - **M05.251 Rheumatoid vasculitis with rheumatoid arthritis of right hip** HCC Rx ESR COM
  - **M05.252 Rheumatoid vasculitis with rheumatoid arthritis of left hip** HCC Rx ESR COM
  - **M05.259 Rheumatoid vasculitis with rheumatoid arthritis of unspecified hip** HCC Rx ESR COM
- **M05.26 Rheumatoid vasculitis with rheumatoid arthritis of knee**
  - **M05.261 Rheumatoid vasculitis with rheumatoid arthritis of right knee** HCC Rx ESR COM
  - **M05.262 Rheumatoid vasculitis with rheumatoid arthritis of left knee** HCC Rx ESR COM
  - **M05.269 Rheumatoid vasculitis with rheumatoid arthritis of unspecified knee** HCC Rx ESR COM
- **M05.27 Rheumatoid vasculitis with rheumatoid arthritis of ankle and foot**
  Rheumatoid vasculitis with rheumatoid arthritis, tarsus, metatarsus and phalanges
  - **M05.271 Rheumatoid vasculitis with rheumatoid arthritis of right ankle and foot** HCC Rx ESR COM
  - **M05.272 Rheumatoid vasculitis with rheumatoid arthritis of left ankle and foot** HCC Rx ESR COM
  - **M05.279 Rheumatoid vasculitis with rheumatoid arthritis of unspecified ankle and foot** HCC Rx ESR COM
- **M05.29 Rheumatoid vasculitis with rheumatoid arthritis of multiple sites** HCC Rx ESR COM

M05.3 Rheumatoid heart disease with rheumatoid arthritis
Rheumatoid carditis
Rheumatoid endocarditis
Rheumatoid myocarditis
Rheumatoid pericarditis
- **M05.30 Rheumatoid heart disease with rheumatoid arthritis of unspecified site** HCC Rx ESR COM
- **M05.31 Rheumatoid heart disease with rheumatoid arthritis of shoulder**
  - **M05.311 Rheumatoid heart disease with rheumatoid arthritis of right shoulder** HCC Rx ESR COM
  - **M05.312 Rheumatoid heart disease with rheumatoid arthritis of left shoulder** HCC Rx ESR COM
  - **M05.319 Rheumatoid heart disease with rheumatoid arthritis of unspecified shoulder** HCC Rx ESR COM
- **M05.32 Rheumatoid heart disease with rheumatoid arthritis of elbow**
  - **M05.321 Rheumatoid heart disease with rheumatoid arthritis of right elbow** HCC Rx ESR COM
  - **M05.322 Rheumatoid heart disease with rheumatoid arthritis of left elbow** HCC Rx ESR COM
  - **M05.329 Rheumatoid heart disease with rheumatoid arthritis of unspecified elbow** HCC Rx ESR COM
- **M05.33 Rheumatoid heart disease with rheumatoid arthritis of wrist**
  Rheumatoid heart disease with rheumatoid arthritis, carpal bones
  - **M05.331 Rheumatoid heart disease with rheumatoid arthritis of right wrist** HCC Rx ESR COM
  - **M05.332 Rheumatoid heart disease with rheumatoid arthritis of left wrist** HCC Rx ESR COM
  - **M05.339 Rheumatoid heart disease with rheumatoid arthritis of unspecified wrist** HCC Rx ESR COM
- **M05.34 Rheumatoid heart disease with rheumatoid arthritis of hand**
  Rheumatoid heart disease with rheumatoid arthritis, metacarpus and phalanges
  - **M05.341 Rheumatoid heart disease with rheumatoid arthritis of right hand** HCC Rx ESR COM
  - **M05.342 Rheumatoid heart disease with rheumatoid arthritis of left hand** HCC Rx ESR COM
  - **M05.349 Rheumatoid heart disease with rheumatoid arthritis of unspecified hand** HCC Rx ESR COM
- **M05.35 Rheumatoid heart disease with rheumatoid arthritis of hip**
  - **M05.351 Rheumatoid heart disease with rheumatoid arthritis of right hip** HCC Rx ESR COM
  - **M05.352 Rheumatoid heart disease with rheumatoid arthritis of left hip** HCC Rx ESR COM
  - **M05.359 Rheumatoid heart disease with rheumatoid arthritis of unspecified hip** HCC Rx ESR COM
- **M05.36 Rheumatoid heart disease with rheumatoid arthritis of knee**
  - **M05.361 Rheumatoid heart disease with rheumatoid arthritis of right knee** HCC Rx ESR COM
  - **M05.362 Rheumatoid heart disease with rheumatoid arthritis of left knee** HCC Rx ESR COM
  - **M05.369 Rheumatoid heart disease with rheumatoid arthritis of unspecified knee** HCC Rx ESR COM

√6th **MØ5.37 Rheumatoid heart disease with rheumatoid arthritis of ankle and foot**
Rheumatoid heart disease with rheumatoid arthritis, tarsus, metatarsus and phalanges

MØ5.371 Rheumatoid heart disease with rheumatoid arthritis of right ankle and foot HCC Rx ESR COM

MØ5.372 Rheumatoid heart disease with rheumatoid arthritis of left ankle and foot HCC Rx ESR COM

MØ5.379 Rheumatoid heart disease with rheumatoid arthritis of unspecified ankle and foot HCC Rx ESR COM

MØ5.39 Rheumatoid heart disease with rheumatoid arthritis of multiple sites HCC Rx ESR COM

√5th **MØ5.4 Rheumatoid myopathy with rheumatoid arthritis**

MØ5.4Ø Rheumatoid myopathy with rheumatoid arthritis of unspecified site HCC Rx ESR COM

√6th **MØ5.41 Rheumatoid myopathy with rheumatoid arthritis of shoulder**

MØ5.411 Rheumatoid myopathy with rheumatoid arthritis of right shoulder HCC Rx ESR COM

MØ5.412 Rheumatoid myopathy with rheumatoid arthritis of left shoulder HCC Rx ESR COM

MØ5.419 Rheumatoid myopathy with rheumatoid arthritis of unspecified shoulder HCC Rx ESR COM

√6th **MØ5.42 Rheumatoid myopathy with rheumatoid arthritis of elbow**

MØ5.421 Rheumatoid myopathy with rheumatoid arthritis of right elbow HCC Rx ESR COM

MØ5.422 Rheumatoid myopathy with rheumatoid arthritis of left elbow HCC Rx ESR COM

MØ5.429 Rheumatoid myopathy with rheumatoid arthritis of unspecified elbow HCC Rx ESR COM

√6th **MØ5.43 Rheumatoid myopathy with rheumatoid arthritis of wrist**
Rheumatoid myopathy with rheumatoid arthritis, carpal bones

MØ5.431 Rheumatoid myopathy with rheumatoid arthritis of right wrist HCC Rx ESR COM

MØ5.432 Rheumatoid myopathy with rheumatoid arthritis of left wrist HCC Rx ESR COM

MØ5.439 Rheumatoid myopathy with rheumatoid arthritis of unspecified wrist HCC Rx ESR COM

√6th **MØ5.44 Rheumatoid myopathy with rheumatoid arthritis of hand**
Rheumatoid myopathy with rheumatoid arthritis, metacarpus and phalanges

MØ5.441 Rheumatoid myopathy with rheumatoid arthritis of right hand HCC Rx ESR COM

MØ5.442 Rheumatoid myopathy with rheumatoid arthritis of left hand HCC Rx ESR COM

MØ5.449 Rheumatoid myopathy with rheumatoid arthritis of unspecified hand HCC Rx ESR COM

√6th **MØ5.45 Rheumatoid myopathy with rheumatoid arthritis of hip**

MØ5.451 Rheumatoid myopathy with rheumatoid arthritis of right hip HCC Rx ESR COM

MØ5.452 Rheumatoid myopathy with rheumatoid arthritis of left hip HCC Rx ESR COM

MØ5.459 Rheumatoid myopathy with rheumatoid arthritis of unspecified hip HCC Rx ESR COM

√6th **MØ5.46 Rheumatoid myopathy with rheumatoid arthritis of knee**

MØ5.461 Rheumatoid myopathy with rheumatoid arthritis of right knee HCC Rx ESR COM

MØ5.462 Rheumatoid myopathy with rheumatoid arthritis of left knee HCC Rx ESR COM

MØ5.469 Rheumatoid myopathy with rheumatoid arthritis of unspecified knee HCC Rx ESR COM

√6th **MØ5.47 Rheumatoid myopathy with rheumatoid arthritis of ankle and foot**
Rheumatoid myopathy with rheumatoid arthritis, tarsus, metatarsus and phalanges

MØ5.471 Rheumatoid myopathy with rheumatoid arthritis of right ankle and foot HCC Rx ESR COM

MØ5.472 Rheumatoid myopathy with rheumatoid arthritis of left ankle and foot HCC Rx ESR COM

MØ5.479 Rheumatoid myopathy with rheumatoid arthritis of unspecified ankle and foot HCC Rx ESR COM

MØ5.49 Rheumatoid myopathy with rheumatoid arthritis of multiple sites HCC Rx ESR COM

√5th **MØ5.5 Rheumatoid polyneuropathy with rheumatoid arthritis**

MØ5.5Ø Rheumatoid polyneuropathy with rheumatoid arthritis of unspecified site HCC Rx ESR COM

√6th **MØ5.51 Rheumatoid polyneuropathy with rheumatoid arthritis of shoulder**

MØ5.511 Rheumatoid polyneuropathy with rheumatoid arthritis of right shoulder HCC Rx ESR COM

MØ5.512 Rheumatoid polyneuropathy with rheumatoid arthritis of left shoulder HCC Rx ESR COM

MØ5.519 Rheumatoid polyneuropathy with rheumatoid arthritis of unspecified shoulder HCC Rx ESR COM

√6th **MØ5.52 Rheumatoid polyneuropathy with rheumatoid arthritis of elbow**

MØ5.521 Rheumatoid polyneuropathy with rheumatoid arthritis of right elbow HCC Rx ESR COM

MØ5.522 Rheumatoid polyneuropathy with rheumatoid arthritis of left elbow HCC Rx ESR COM

MØ5.529 Rheumatoid polyneuropathy with rheumatoid arthritis of unspecified elbow HCC Rx ESR COM

√6th **MØ5.53 Rheumatoid polyneuropathy with rheumatoid arthritis of wrist**
Rheumatoid polyneuropathy with rheumatoid arthritis, carpal bones

MØ5.531 Rheumatoid polyneuropathy with rheumatoid arthritis of right wrist HCC Rx ESR COM

MØ5.532 Rheumatoid polyneuropathy with rheumatoid arthritis of left wrist HCC Rx ESR COM

MØ5.539 Rheumatoid polyneuropathy with rheumatoid arthritis of unspecified wrist HCC Rx ESR COM

√6th **MØ5.54 Rheumatoid polyneuropathy with rheumatoid arthritis of hand**
Rheumatoid polyneuropathy with rheumatoid arthritis, metacarpus and phalanges

MØ5.541 Rheumatoid polyneuropathy with rheumatoid arthritis of right hand HCC Rx ESR COM

MØ5.542 Rheumatoid polyneuropathy with rheumatoid arthritis of left hand HCC Rx ESR COM

MØ5.549 Rheumatoid polyneuropathy with rheumatoid arthritis of unspecified hand HCC Rx ESR COM

√6th **MØ5.55 Rheumatoid polyneuropathy with rheumatoid arthritis of hip**

MØ5.551 Rheumatoid polyneuropathy with rheumatoid arthritis of right hip HCC Rx ESR COM

MØ5.552 Rheumatoid polyneuropathy with rheumatoid arthritis of left hip HCC Rx ESR COM

MØ5.559 Rheumatoid polyneuropathy with rheumatoid arthritis of unspecified hip HCC Rx ESR COM

√6th **MØ5.56 Rheumatoid polyneuropathy with rheumatoid arthritis of knee**

MØ5.561 Rheumatoid polyneuropathy with rheumatoid arthritis of right knee HCC Rx ESR COM

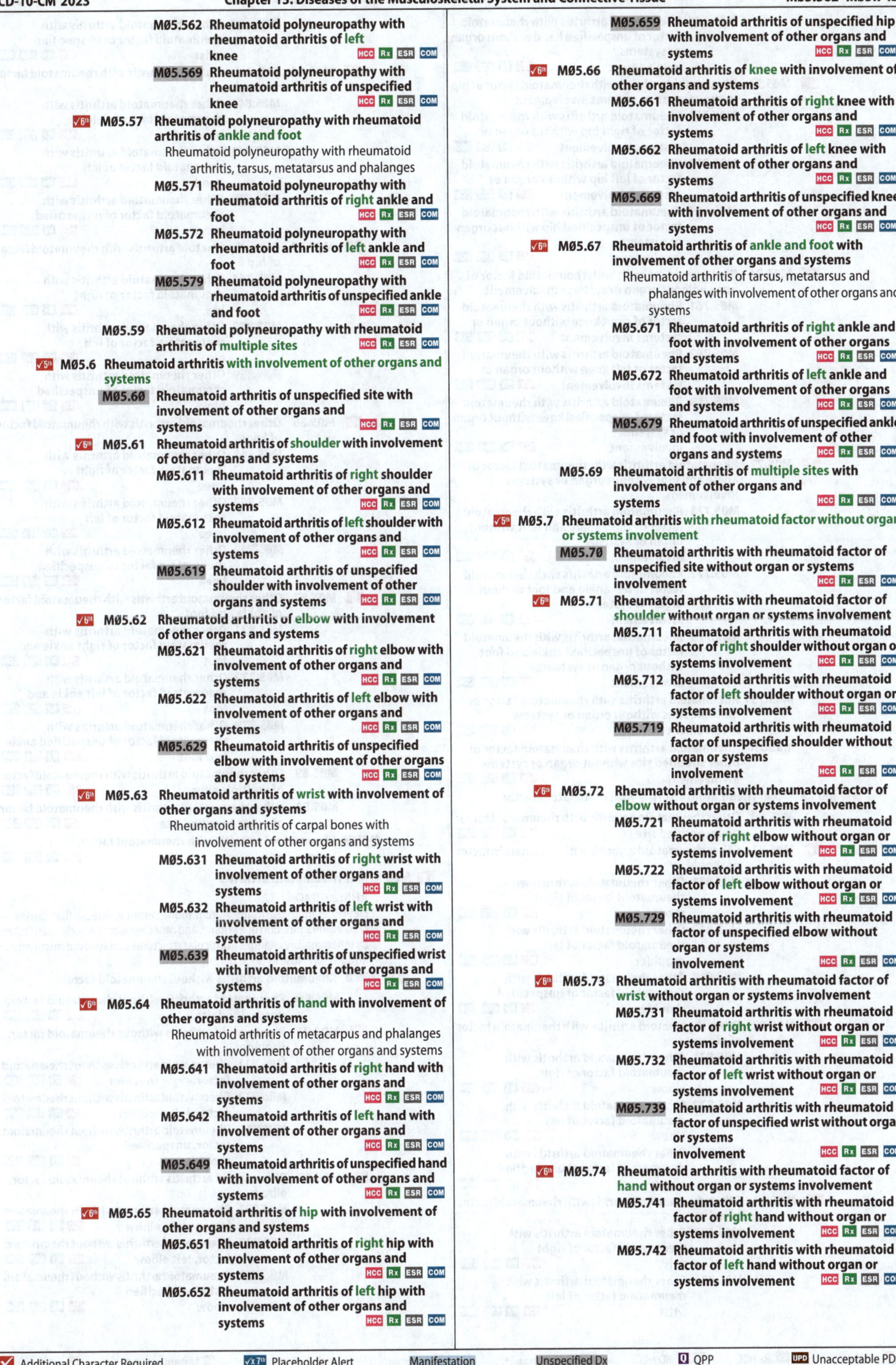

MØ5.562 Rheumatoid polyneuropathy with rheumatoid arthritis of left knee HCC Rx ESR COM

MØ5.569 Rheumatoid polyneuropathy with rheumatoid arthritis of unspecified knee HCC Rx ESR COM

✓6th MØ5.57 Rheumatoid polyneuropathy with rheumatoid arthritis of ankle and foot

Rheumatoid polyneuropathy with rheumatoid arthritis, tarsus, metatarsus and phalanges

MØ5.571 Rheumatoid polyneuropathy with rheumatoid arthritis of right ankle and foot HCC Rx ESR COM

MØ5.572 Rheumatoid polyneuropathy with rheumatoid arthritis of left ankle and foot HCC Rx ESR COM

MØ5.579 Rheumatoid polyneuropathy with rheumatoid arthritis of unspecified ankle and foot HCC Rx ESR COM

MØ5.59 Rheumatoid polyneuropathy with rheumatoid arthritis of multiple sites HCC Rx ESR COM

✓5th MØ5.6 Rheumatoid arthritis with involvement of other organs and systems

MØ5.60 Rheumatoid arthritis of unspecified site with involvement of other organs and systems HCC Rx ESR COM

✓6th MØ5.61 Rheumatoid arthritis of shoulder with involvement of other organs and systems

MØ5.611 Rheumatoid arthritis of right shoulder with involvement of other organs and systems HCC Rx ESR COM

MØ5.612 Rheumatoid arthritis of left shoulder with involvement of other organs and systems HCC Rx ESR COM

MØ5.619 Rheumatoid arthritis of unspecified shoulder with involvement of other organs and systems HCC Rx ESR COM

✓6th MØ5.62 Rheumatoid arthritis of elbow with involvement of other organs and systems

MØ5.621 Rheumatoid arthritis of right elbow with involvement of other organs and systems HCC Rx ESR COM

MØ5.622 Rheumatoid arthritis of left elbow with involvement of other organs and systems HCC Rx ESR COM

MØ5.629 Rheumatoid arthritis of unspecified elbow with involvement of other organs and systems HCC Rx ESR COM

✓6th MØ5.63 Rheumatoid arthritis of wrist with involvement of other organs and systems

Rheumatoid arthritis of carpal bones with involvement of other organs and systems

MØ5.631 Rheumatoid arthritis of right wrist with involvement of other organs and systems HCC Rx ESR COM

MØ5.632 Rheumatoid arthritis of left wrist with involvement of other organs and systems HCC Rx ESR COM

MØ5.639 Rheumatoid arthritis of unspecified wrist with involvement of other organs and systems HCC Rx ESR COM

✓6th MØ5.64 Rheumatoid arthritis of hand with involvement of other organs and systems

Rheumatoid arthritis of metacarpus and phalanges with involvement of other organs and systems

MØ5.641 Rheumatoid arthritis of right hand with involvement of other organs and systems HCC Rx ESR COM

MØ5.642 Rheumatoid arthritis of left hand with involvement of other organs and systems HCC Rx ESR COM

MØ5.649 Rheumatoid arthritis of unspecified hand with involvement of other organs and systems HCC Rx ESR COM

✓6th MØ5.65 Rheumatoid arthritis of hip with involvement of other organs and systems

MØ5.651 Rheumatoid arthritis of right hip with involvement of other organs and systems HCC Rx ESR COM

MØ5.652 Rheumatoid arthritis of left hip with involvement of other organs and systems HCC Rx ESR COM

MØ5.659 Rheumatoid arthritis of unspecified hip with involvement of other organs and systems HCC Rx ESR COM

✓6th MØ5.66 Rheumatoid arthritis of knee with involvement of other organs and systems

MØ5.661 Rheumatoid arthritis of right knee with involvement of other organs and systems HCC Rx ESR COM

MØ5.662 Rheumatoid arthritis of left knee with involvement of other organs and systems HCC Rx ESR COM

MØ5.669 Rheumatoid arthritis of unspecified knee with involvement of other organs and systems HCC Rx ESR COM

✓6th MØ5.67 Rheumatoid arthritis of ankle and foot with involvement of other organs and systems

Rheumatoid arthritis of tarsus, metatarsus and phalanges with involvement of other organs and systems

MØ5.671 Rheumatoid arthritis of right ankle and foot with involvement of other organs and systems HCC Rx ESR COM

MØ5.672 Rheumatoid arthritis of left ankle and foot with involvement of other organs and systems HCC Rx ESR COM

MØ5.679 Rheumatoid arthritis of unspecified ankle and foot with involvement of other organs and systems HCC Rx ESR COM

MØ5.69 Rheumatoid arthritis of multiple sites with involvement of other organs and systems HCC Rx ESR COM

✓5th MØ5.7 Rheumatoid arthritis with rheumatoid factor without organ or systems involvement

MØ5.70 Rheumatoid arthritis with rheumatoid factor of unspecified site without organ or systems involvement HCC Rx ESR COM

✓6th MØ5.71 Rheumatoid arthritis with rheumatoid factor of shoulder without organ or systems involvement

MØ5.711 Rheumatoid arthritis with rheumatoid factor of right shoulder without organ or systems involvement HCC Rx ESR COM

MØ5.712 Rheumatoid arthritis with rheumatoid factor of left shoulder without organ or systems involvement HCC Rx ESR COM

MØ5.719 Rheumatoid arthritis with rheumatoid factor of unspecified shoulder without organ or systems involvement HCC Rx ESR COM

✓6th MØ5.72 Rheumatoid arthritis with rheumatoid factor of elbow without organ or systems involvement

MØ5.721 Rheumatoid arthritis with rheumatoid factor of right elbow without organ or systems involvement HCC Rx ESR COM

MØ5.722 Rheumatoid arthritis with rheumatoid factor of left elbow without organ or systems involvement HCC Rx ESR COM

MØ5.729 Rheumatoid arthritis with rheumatoid factor of unspecified elbow without organ or systems involvement HCC Rx ESR COM

✓6th MØ5.73 Rheumatoid arthritis with rheumatoid factor of wrist without organ or systems involvement

MØ5.731 Rheumatoid arthritis with rheumatoid factor of right wrist without organ or systems involvement HCC Rx ESR COM

MØ5.732 Rheumatoid arthritis with rheumatoid factor of left wrist without organ or systems involvement HCC Rx ESR COM

MØ5.739 Rheumatoid arthritis with rheumatoid factor of unspecified wrist without organ or systems involvement HCC Rx ESR COM

✓6th MØ5.74 Rheumatoid arthritis with rheumatoid factor of hand without organ or systems involvement

MØ5.741 Rheumatoid arthritis with rheumatoid factor of right hand without organ or systems involvement HCC Rx ESR COM

MØ5.742 Rheumatoid arthritis with rheumatoid factor of left hand without organ or systems involvement HCC Rx ESR COM

MØ5.749 Rheumatoid arthritis with rheumatoid factor of unspecified hand without organ or systems involvement HCC Rx ESR COM

✓6th MØ5.75 Rheumatoid arthritis with rheumatoid factor of hip without organ or systems involvement

MØ5.751 Rheumatoid arthritis with rheumatoid factor of right hip without organ or systems involvement HCC Rx ESR COM

MØ5.752 Rheumatoid arthritis with rheumatoid factor of left hip without organ or systems involvement HCC Rx ESR COM

MØ5.759 Rheumatoid arthritis with rheumatoid factor of unspecified hip without organ or systems involvement HCC Rx ESR COM

✓6th MØ5.76 Rheumatoid arthritis with rheumatoid factor of knee without organ or systems involvement

MØ5.761 Rheumatoid arthritis with rheumatoid factor of right knee without organ or systems involvement HCC Rx ESR COM

MØ5.762 Rheumatoid arthritis with rheumatoid factor of left knee without organ or systems involvement HCC Rx ESR COM

MØ5.769 Rheumatoid arthritis with rheumatoid factor of unspecified knee without organ or systems involvement HCC Rx ESR COM

✓6th MØ5.77 Rheumatoid arthritis with rheumatoid factor of ankle and foot without organ or systems involvement

MØ5.771 Rheumatoid arthritis with rheumatoid factor of right ankle and foot without organ or systems involvement HCC Rx ESR COM

MØ5.772 Rheumatoid arthritis with rheumatoid factor of left ankle and foot without organ or systems involvement HCC Rx ESR COM

MØ5.779 Rheumatoid arthritis with rheumatoid factor of unspecified ankle and foot without organ or systems involvement HCC Rx ESR COM

MØ5.79 Rheumatoid arthritis with rheumatoid factor of multiple sites without organ or systems involvement HCC Rx ESR COM

MØ5.7A Rheumatoid arthritis with rheumatoid factor of other specified site without organ or systems involvement HCC Rx ESR COM

✓5th MØ5.8 Other rheumatoid arthritis with rheumatoid factor

MØ5.8Ø Other rheumatoid arthritis with rheumatoid factor of unspecified site HCC Rx ESR COM

✓6th MØ5.81 Other rheumatoid arthritis with rheumatoid factor of shoulder

MØ5.811 Other rheumatoid arthritis with rheumatoid factor of right shoulder HCC Rx ESR COM

MØ5.812 Other rheumatoid arthritis with rheumatoid factor of left shoulder HCC Rx ESR COM

MØ5.819 Other rheumatoid arthritis with rheumatoid factor of unspecified shoulder HCC Rx ESR COM

✓6th MØ5.82 Other rheumatoid arthritis with rheumatoid factor of elbow

MØ5.821 Other rheumatoid arthritis with rheumatoid factor of right elbow HCC Rx ESR COM

MØ5.822 Other rheumatoid arthritis with rheumatoid factor of left elbow HCC Rx ESR COM

MØ5.829 Other rheumatoid arthritis with rheumatoid factor of unspecified elbow HCC Rx ESR COM

✓6th MØ5.83 Other rheumatoid arthritis with rheumatoid factor of wrist

MØ5.831 Other rheumatoid arthritis with rheumatoid factor of right wrist HCC Rx ESR COM

MØ5.832 Other rheumatoid arthritis with rheumatoid factor of left wrist HCC Rx ESR COM

MØ5.839 Other rheumatoid arthritis with rheumatoid factor of unspecified wrist HCC Rx ESR COM

✓6th MØ5.84 Other rheumatoid arthritis with rheumatoid factor of hand

MØ5.841 Other rheumatoid arthritis with rheumatoid factor of right hand HCC Rx ESR COM

MØ5.842 Other rheumatoid arthritis with rheumatoid factor of left hand HCC Rx ESR COM

MØ5.849 Other rheumatoid arthritis with rheumatoid factor of unspecified hand HCC Rx ESR COM

✓6th MØ5.85 Other rheumatoid arthritis with rheumatoid factor of hip

MØ5.851 Other rheumatoid arthritis with rheumatoid factor of right hip HCC Rx ESR COM

MØ5.852 Other rheumatoid arthritis with rheumatoid factor of left hip HCC Rx ESR COM

MØ5.859 Other rheumatoid arthritis with rheumatoid factor of unspecified hip HCC Rx ESR COM

✓6th MØ5.86 Other rheumatoid arthritis with rheumatoid factor of knee

MØ5.861 Other rheumatoid arthritis with rheumatoid factor of right knee HCC Rx ESR COM

MØ5.862 Other rheumatoid arthritis with rheumatoid factor of left knee HCC Rx ESR COM

MØ5.869 Other rheumatoid arthritis with rheumatoid factor of unspecified knee HCC Rx ESR COM

✓6th MØ5.87 Other rheumatoid arthritis with rheumatoid factor of ankle and foot

MØ5.871 Other rheumatoid arthritis with rheumatoid factor of right ankle and foot HCC Rx ESR COM

MØ5.872 Other rheumatoid arthritis with rheumatoid factor of left ankle and foot HCC Rx ESR COM

MØ5.879 Other rheumatoid arthritis with rheumatoid factor of unspecified ankle and foot HCC Rx ESR COM

MØ5.89 Other rheumatoid arthritis with rheumatoid factor of multiple sites HCC Rx ESR COM

MØ5.8A Other rheumatoid arthritis with rheumatoid factor of other specified site HCC Rx ESR COM

MØ5.9 Rheumatoid arthritis with rheumatoid factor, unspecified HCC Rx ESR COM

✓4th **MØ6 Other rheumatoid arthritis**

AHA: 2020,4Q,31-32

DEF: Rheumatoid arthritis: Autoimmune systemic disease that causes chronic inflammation of the joints and other areas of the body, manifested by inflammatory changes in articular structures and synovial membranes, atrophy, and loss in bone density.

✓5th MØ6.Ø Rheumatoid arthritis without rheumatoid factor

MØ6.ØØ Rheumatoid arthritis without rheumatoid factor, unspecified site HCC Rx ESR COM

✓6th MØ6.Ø1 Rheumatoid arthritis without rheumatoid factor, shoulder

MØ6.Ø11 Rheumatoid arthritis without rheumatoid factor, right shoulder HCC Rx ESR COM

MØ6.Ø12 Rheumatoid arthritis without rheumatoid factor, left shoulder HCC Rx ESR COM

MØ6.Ø19 Rheumatoid arthritis without rheumatoid factor, unspecified shoulder HCC Rx ESR COM

✓6th MØ6.Ø2 Rheumatoid arthritis without rheumatoid factor, elbow

MØ6.Ø21 Rheumatoid arthritis without rheumatoid factor, right elbow HCC Rx ESR COM

MØ6.Ø22 Rheumatoid arthritis without rheumatoid factor, left elbow HCC Rx ESR COM

MØ6.Ø29 Rheumatoid arthritis without rheumatoid factor, unspecified elbow HCC Rx ESR COM

✓6th **M06.03 Rheumatoid arthritis without rheumatoid factor, wrist**
M06.031 Rheumatoid arthritis without rheumatoid factor, right wrist HCC Rx ESR COM
M06.032 Rheumatoid arthritis without rheumatoid factor, left wrist HCC Rx ESR COM
M06.039 Rheumatoid arthritis without rheumatoid factor, unspecified wrist HCC Rx ESR COM

✓6th **M06.04 Rheumatoid arthritis without rheumatoid factor, hand**
M06.041 Rheumatoid arthritis without rheumatoid factor, right hand HCC Rx ESR COM
M06.042 Rheumatoid arthritis without rheumatoid factor, left hand HCC Rx ESR COM
M06.049 Rheumatoid arthritis without rheumatoid factor, unspecified hand HCC Rx ESR COM

✓6th **M06.05 Rheumatoid arthritis without rheumatoid factor, hip**
M06.051 Rheumatoid arthritis without rheumatoid factor, right hip HCC Rx ESR COM
M06.052 Rheumatoid arthritis without rheumatoid factor, left hip HCC Rx ESR COM
M06.059 Rheumatoid arthritis without rheumatoid factor, unspecified hip HCC Rx ESR COM

✓6th **M06.06 Rheumatoid arthritis without rheumatoid factor, knee**
M06.061 Rheumatoid arthritis without rheumatoid factor, right knee HCC Rx ESR COM
M06.062 Rheumatoid arthritis without rheumatoid factor, left knee HCC Rx ESR COM
M06.069 Rheumatoid arthritis without rheumatoid factor, unspecified knee HCC Rx ESR COM

✓6th **M06.07 Rheumatoid arthritis without rheumatoid factor, ankle and foot**
M06.071 Rheumatoid arthritis without rheumatoid factor, right ankle and foot HCC Rx ESR COM
M06.072 Rheumatoid arthritis without rheumatoid factor, left ankle and foot HCC Rx ESR COM
M06.079 Rheumatoid arthritis without rheumatoid factor, unspecified ankle and foot HCC Rx ESR COM

M06.08 Rheumatoid arthritis without rheumatoid factor, vertebrae HCC Rx ESR COM

M06.09 Rheumatoid arthritis without rheumatoid factor, multiple sites HCC Rx ESR COM

M06.0A Rheumatoid arthritis without rheumatoid factor, other specified site HCC Rx ESR COM

M06.1 Adult-onset Still's disease HCC Rx ESR COM A

EXCLUDES 1 *Still's disease NOS (M08.2-)*

DEF: Type of systemic arthritis characterized by a transient rash and spiking fevers. This condition may resolve or develop into a chronic condition and may affect internal organs, as well as joints.

Synonym(s): *AOSD*

✓5th **M06.2 Rheumatoid bursitis**

M06.20 Rheumatoid bursitis, unspecified site HCC Rx ESR COM

✓6th **M06.21 Rheumatoid bursitis, shoulder**
M06.211 Rheumatoid bursitis, right shoulder HCC Rx ESR COM
M06.212 Rheumatoid bursitis, left shoulder HCC Rx ESR COM
M06.219 Rheumatoid bursitis, unspecified shoulder HCC Rx ESR COM

✓6th **M06.22 Rheumatoid bursitis, elbow**
M06.221 Rheumatoid bursitis, right elbow HCC Rx ESR COM
M06.222 Rheumatoid bursitis, left elbow HCC Rx ESR COM
M06.229 Rheumatoid bursitis, unspecified elbow HCC Rx ESR COM

✓6th **M06.23 Rheumatoid bursitis, wrist**
M06.231 Rheumatoid bursitis, right wrist HCC Rx ESR COM
M06.232 Rheumatoid bursitis, left wrist HCC Rx ESR COM
M06.239 Rheumatoid bursitis, unspecified wrist HCC Rx ESR COM

✓6th **M06.24 Rheumatoid bursitis, hand**
M06.241 Rheumatoid bursitis, right hand HCC Rx ESR COM
M06.242 Rheumatoid bursitis, left hand HCC Rx ESR COM
M06.249 Rheumatoid bursitis, unspecified hand HCC Rx ESR COM

✓6th **M06.25 Rheumatoid bursitis, hip**
M06.251 Rheumatoid bursitis, right hip HCC Rx ESR COM
M06.252 Rheumatoid bursitis, left hip HCC Rx ESR COM
M06.259 Rheumatoid bursitis, unspecified hip HCC Rx ESR COM

✓6th **M06.26 Rheumatoid bursitis, knee**
M06.261 Rheumatoid bursitis, right knee HCC Rx ESR COM
M06.262 Rheumatoid bursitis, left knee HCC Rx ESR COM
M06.269 Rheumatoid bursitis, unspecified knee HCC Rx ESR COM

✓6th **M06.27 Rheumatoid bursitis, ankle and foot**
M06.271 Rheumatoid bursitis, right ankle and foot HCC Rx ESR COM
M06.272 Rheumatoid bursitis, left ankle and foot HCC Rx ESR COM
M06.279 Rheumatoid bursitis, unspecified ankle and foot HCC Rx ESR COM

M06.28 Rheumatoid bursitis, vertebrae HCC Rx ESR COM

M06.29 Rheumatoid bursitis, multiple sites HCC Rx ESR COM

✓5th **M06.3 Rheumatoid nodule**

M06.30 Rheumatoid nodule, unspecified site HCC Rx ESR COM

✓6th **M06.31 Rheumatoid nodule, shoulder**
M06.311 Rheumatoid nodule, right shoulder HCC Rx ESR COM
M06.312 Rheumatoid nodule, left shoulder HCC Rx ESR COM
M06.319 Rheumatoid nodule, unspecified shoulder HCC Rx ESR COM

✓6th **M06.32 Rheumatoid nodule, elbow**
M06.321 Rheumatoid nodule, right elbow HCC Rx ESR COM
M06.322 Rheumatoid nodule, left elbow HCC Rx ESR COM
M06.329 Rheumatoid nodule, unspecified elbow HCC Rx ESR COM

✓6th **M06.33 Rheumatoid nodule, wrist**
M06.331 Rheumatoid nodule, right wrist HCC Rx ESR COM
M06.332 Rheumatoid nodule, left wrist HCC Rx ESR COM
M06.339 Rheumatoid nodule, unspecified wrist HCC Rx ESR COM

✓6th **M06.34 Rheumatoid nodule, hand**
M06.341 Rheumatoid nodule, right hand HCC Rx ESR COM
M06.342 Rheumatoid nodule, left hand HCC Rx ESR COM
M06.349 Rheumatoid nodule, unspecified hand HCC Rx ESR COM

✓6th **M06.35 Rheumatoid nodule, hip**
M06.351 Rheumatoid nodule, right hip HCC Rx ESR COM
M06.352 Rheumatoid nodule, left hip HCC Rx ESR COM
M06.359 Rheumatoid nodule, unspecified hip HCC Rx ESR COM

✓6th **M06.36 Rheumatoid nodule, knee**
M06.361 Rheumatoid nodule, right knee HCC Rx ESR COM
M06.362 Rheumatoid nodule, left knee HCC Rx ESR COM

M06.369 Rheumatoid nodule, unspecified knee HCC Rx ESR COM

M06.37 Rheumatoid nodule, ankle and foot

M06.371 Rheumatoid nodule, right ankle and foot HCC Rx ESR COM

M06.372 Rheumatoid nodule, left ankle and foot HCC Rx ESR COM

M06.379 Rheumatoid nodule, unspecified ankle and foot HCC Rx ESR COM

M06.38 Rheumatoid nodule, vertebrae HCC Rx ESR COM

M06.39 Rheumatoid nodule, multiple sites HCC Rx ESR COM

M06.4 Inflammatory polyarthropathy HCC Rx ESR COM

EXCLUDES 1 *polyarthritis NOS (M13.0)*

M06.8 Other specified rheumatoid arthritis

M06.80 Other specified rheumatoid arthritis, unspecified site HCC Rx ESR COM

M06.81 Other specified rheumatoid arthritis, shoulder

M06.811 Other specified rheumatoid arthritis, right shoulder HCC Rx ESR COM

M06.812 Other specified rheumatoid arthritis, left shoulder HCC Rx ESR COM

M06.819 Other specified rheumatoid arthritis, unspecified shoulder HCC Rx ESR COM

M06.82 Other specified rheumatoid arthritis, elbow

M06.821 Other specified rheumatoid arthritis, right elbow HCC Rx ESR COM

M06.822 Other specified rheumatoid arthritis, left elbow HCC Rx ESR COM

M06.829 Other specified rheumatoid arthritis, unspecified elbow HCC Rx ESR COM

M06.83 Other specified rheumatoid arthritis, wrist

M06.831 Other specified rheumatoid arthritis, right wrist HCC Rx ESR COM

M06.832 Other specified rheumatoid arthritis, left wrist HCC Rx ESR COM

M06.839 Other specified rheumatoid arthritis, unspecified wrist HCC Rx ESR COM

M06.84 Other specified rheumatoid arthritis, hand

M06.841 Other specified rheumatoid arthritis, right hand HCC Rx ESR COM

M06.842 Other specified rheumatoid arthritis, left hand HCC Rx ESR COM

M06.849 Other specified rheumatoid arthritis, unspecified hand HCC Rx ESR COM

M06.85 Other specified rheumatoid arthritis, hip

M06.851 Other specified rheumatoid arthritis, right hip HCC Rx ESR COM

M06.852 Other specified rheumatoid arthritis, left hip HCC Rx ESR COM

M06.859 Other specified rheumatoid arthritis, unspecified hip HCC Rx ESR COM

M06.86 Other specified rheumatoid arthritis, knee

M06.861 Other specified rheumatoid arthritis, right knee HCC Rx ESR COM

M06.862 Other specified rheumatoid arthritis, left knee HCC Rx ESR COM

M06.869 Other specified rheumatoid arthritis, unspecified knee HCC Rx ESR COM

M06.87 Other specified rheumatoid arthritis, ankle and foot

M06.871 Other specified rheumatoid arthritis, right ankle and foot HCC Rx ESR COM

M06.872 Other specified rheumatoid arthritis, left ankle and foot HCC Rx ESR COM

M06.879 Other specified rheumatoid arthritis, unspecified ankle and foot HCC Rx ESR COM

M06.88 Other specified rheumatoid arthritis, vertebrae HCC Rx ESR COM

M06.89 Other specified rheumatoid arthritis, multiple sites HCC Rx ESR COM

M06.8A Other specified rheumatoid arthritis, other specified site HCC Rx ESR COM

M06.9 Rheumatoid arthritis, unspecified HCC Rx ESR COM

M07 Enteropathic arthropathies

Code also associated enteropathy, such as:
regional enteritis [Crohn's disease] (K50.-)
ulcerative colitis (K51.-)

EXCLUDES 1 *psoriatic arthropathies (L40.5-)*

M07.6 Enteropathic arthropathies

M07.60 Enteropathic arthropathies, unspecified site

M07.61 Enteropathic arthropathies, shoulder

M07.611 Enteropathic arthropathies, right shoulder

M07.612 Enteropathic arthropathies, left shoulder

M07.619 Enteropathic arthropathies, unspecified shoulder

M07.62 Enteropathic arthropathies, elbow

M07.621 Enteropathic arthropathies, right elbow

M07.622 Enteropathic arthropathies, left elbow

M07.629 Enteropathic arthropathies, unspecified elbow

M07.63 Enteropathic arthropathies, wrist

M07.631 Enteropathic arthropathies, right wrist

M07.632 Enteropathic arthropathies, left wrist

M07.639 Enteropathic arthropathies, unspecified wrist

M07.64 Enteropathic arthropathies, hand

M07.641 Enteropathic arthropathies, right hand

M07.642 Enteropathic arthropathies, left hand

M07.649 Enteropathic arthropathies, unspecified hand

M07.65 Enteropathic arthropathies, hip

M07.651 Enteropathic arthropathies, right hip

M07.652 Enteropathic arthropathies, left hip

M07.659 Enteropathic arthropathies, unspecified hip

M07.66 Enteropathic arthropathies, knee

M07.661 Enteropathic arthropathies, right knee

M07.662 Enteropathic arthropathies, left knee

M07.669 Enteropathic arthropathies, unspecified knee

M07.67 Enteropathic arthropathies, ankle and foot

M07.671 Enteropathic arthropathies, right ankle and foot

M07.672 Enteropathic arthropathies, left ankle and foot

M07.679 Enteropathic arthropathies, unspecified ankle and foot

M07.68 Enteropathic arthropathies, vertebrae

M07.69 Enteropathic arthropathies, multiple sites

M08 Juvenile arthritis

Code also any associated underlying condition, such as:
regional enteritis [Crohn's disease] (K50.-)
ulcerative colitis (K51.-)

EXCLUDES 1 *arthropathy in Whipple's disease (M14.8)*
Felty's syndrome (M05.0)
juvenile dermatomyositis (M33.0-)
psoriatic juvenile arthropathy (L40.54)

AHA: 2020,4Q,31-32

M08.0 Unspecified juvenile rheumatoid arthritis

Juvenile rheumatoid arthritis with or without rheumatoid factor

M08.00 Unspecified juvenile rheumatoid arthritis of unspecified site HCC Rx ESR COM

M08.01 Unspecified juvenile rheumatoid arthritis, shoulder

M08.011 Unspecified juvenile rheumatoid arthritis, right shoulder HCC Rx ESR COM

M08.012 Unspecified juvenile rheumatoid arthritis, left shoulder HCC Rx ESR COM

M08.019 Unspecified juvenile rheumatoid arthritis, unspecified shoulder HCC Rx ESR COM

M08.02 Unspecified juvenile rheumatoid arthritis of elbow

M08.021 Unspecified juvenile rheumatoid arthritis, right elbow HCC Rx ESR COM

M08.022 Unspecified juvenile rheumatoid arthritis, left elbow HCC Rx ESR COM

M08.029 Unspecified juvenile rheumatoid arthritis, unspecified elbow HCC Rx ESR COM

√6th **M08.03 Unspecified juvenile rheumatoid arthritis, wrist**
- **M08.031 Unspecified juvenile rheumatoid arthritis, right wrist** HCC Rx ESR COM
- **M08.032 Unspecified juvenile rheumatoid arthritis, left wrist** HCC Rx ESR COM
- **M08.039 Unspecified juvenile rheumatoid arthritis, unspecified wrist** HCC Rx ESR COM

√6th **M08.04 Unspecified juvenile rheumatoid arthritis, hand**
- **M08.041 Unspecified juvenile rheumatoid arthritis, right hand** HCC Rx ESR COM
- **M08.042 Unspecified juvenile rheumatoid arthritis, left hand** HCC Rx ESR COM
- **M08.049 Unspecified juvenile rheumatoid arthritis, unspecified hand** HCC Rx ESR COM

√6th **M08.05 Unspecified juvenile rheumatoid arthritis, hip**
- **M08.051 Unspecified juvenile rheumatoid arthritis, right hip** HCC Rx ESR COM
- **M08.052 Unspecified juvenile rheumatoid arthritis, left hip** HCC Rx ESR COM
- **M08.059 Unspecified juvenile rheumatoid arthritis, unspecified hip** HCC Rx ESR COM

√6th **M08.06 Unspecified juvenile rheumatoid arthritis, knee**
- **M08.061 Unspecified juvenile rheumatoid arthritis, right knee** HCC Rx ESR COM
- **M08.062 Unspecified juvenile rheumatoid arthritis, left knee** HCC Rx ESR COM
- **M08.069 Unspecified juvenile rheumatoid arthritis, unspecified knee** HCC Rx ESR COM

√6th **M08.07 Unspecified juvenile rheumatoid arthritis, ankle and foot**
- **M08.071 Unspecified juvenile rheumatoid arthritis, right ankle and foot** HCC Rx ESR COM
- **M08.072 Unspecified juvenile rheumatoid arthritis, left ankle and foot** HCC Rx ESR COM
- **M08.079 Unspecified juvenile rheumatoid arthritis, unspecified ankle and foot** HCC Rx ESR COM

M08.08 Unspecified juvenile rheumatoid arthritis, vertebrae HCC Rx ESR COM

M08.09 Unspecified juvenile rheumatoid arthritis, multiple sites HCC Rx ESR COM

M08.0A Unspecified juvenile rheumatoid arthritis, other specified site HCC Rx ESR COM

M08.1 Juvenile ankylosing spondylitis HCC Rx ESR COM

EXCLUDES 1 *ankylosing spondylitis in adults (M45.0-)*

√5th **M08.2 Juvenile rheumatoid arthritis with systemic onset**

Still's disease NOS

EXCLUDES 1 *adult-onset Still's disease (M06.1-)*

DEF: Systemic juvenile rheumatoid arthritis characterized by a transient rash and spiking fevers that may affect internal organs, as well as joints.

M08.20 Juvenile rheumatoid arthritis with systemic onset, unspecified site HCC Rx ESR COM

√6th **M08.21 Juvenile rheumatoid arthritis with systemic onset, shoulder**
- **M08.211 Juvenile rheumatoid arthritis with systemic onset, right shoulder** HCC Rx ESR COM
- **M08.212 Juvenile rheumatoid arthritis with systemic onset, left shoulder** HCC Rx ESR COM
- **M08.219 Juvenile rheumatoid arthritis with systemic onset, unspecified shoulder** HCC Rx ESR COM

√6th **M08.22 Juvenile rheumatoid arthritis with systemic onset, elbow**
- **M08.221 Juvenile rheumatoid arthritis with systemic onset, right elbow** HCC Rx ESR COM
- **M08.222 Juvenile rheumatoid arthritis with systemic onset, left elbow** HCC Rx ESR COM
- **M08.229 Juvenile rheumatoid arthritis with systemic onset, unspecified elbow** HCC Rx ESR COM

√6th **M08.23 Juvenile rheumatoid arthritis with systemic onset, wrist**
- **M08.231 Juvenile rheumatoid arthritis with systemic onset, right wrist** HCC Rx ESR COM
- **M08.232 Juvenile rheumatoid arthritis with systemic onset, left wrist** HCC Rx ESR COM
- **M08.239 Juvenile rheumatoid arthritis with systemic onset, unspecified wrist** HCC Rx ESR COM

√6th **M08.24 Juvenile rheumatoid arthritis with systemic onset, hand**
- **M08.241 Juvenile rheumatoid arthritis with systemic onset, right hand** HCC Rx ESR COM
- **M08.242 Juvenile rheumatoid arthritis with systemic onset, left hand** HCC Rx ESR COM
- **M08.249 Juvenile rheumatoid arthritis with systemic onset, unspecified hand** HCC Rx ESR COM

√6th **M08.25 Juvenile rheumatoid arthritis with systemic onset, hip**
- **M08.251 Juvenile rheumatoid arthritis with systemic onset, right hip** HCC Rx ESR COM
- **M08.252 Juvenile rheumatoid arthritis with systemic onset, left hip** HCC Rx ESR COM
- **M08.259 Juvenile rheumatoid arthritis with systemic onset, unspecified hip** HCC Rx ESR COM

√6th **M08.26 Juvenile rheumatoid arthritis with systemic onset, knee**
- **M08.261 Juvenile rheumatoid arthritis with systemic onset, right knee** HCC Rx ESR COM
- **M08.262 Juvenile rheumatoid arthritis with systemic onset, left knee** HCC Rx ESR COM
- **M08.269 Juvenile rheumatoid arthritis with systemic onset, unspecified knee** HCC Rx ESR COM

√6th **M08.27 Juvenile rheumatoid arthritis with systemic onset, ankle and foot**
- **M08.271 Juvenile rheumatoid arthritis with systemic onset, right ankle and foot** HCC Rx ESR COM
- **M08.272 Juvenile rheumatoid arthritis with systemic onset, left ankle and foot** HCC Rx ESR COM
- **M08.279 Juvenile rheumatoid arthritis with systemic onset, unspecified ankle and foot** HCC Rx ESR COM

M08.28 Juvenile rheumatoid arthritis with systemic onset, vertebrae HCC Rx ESR COM

M08.29 Juvenile rheumatoid arthritis with systemic onset, multiple sites HCC Rx ESR COM

M08.2A Juvenile rheumatoid arthritis with systemic onset, other specified site HCC Rx ESR COM

M08.3 Juvenile rheumatoid polyarthritis (seronegative) HCC Rx ESR COM

√5th **M08.4 Pauciarticular juvenile rheumatoid arthritis**

M08.40 Pauciarticular juvenile rheumatoid arthritis, unspecified site HCC Rx ESR COM

√6th **M08.41 Pauciarticular juvenile rheumatoid arthritis, shoulder**
- **M08.411 Pauciarticular juvenile rheumatoid arthritis, right shoulder** HCC Rx ESR COM
- **M08.412 Pauciarticular juvenile rheumatoid arthritis, left shoulder** HCC Rx ESR COM
- **M08.419 Pauciarticular juvenile rheumatoid arthritis, unspecified shoulder** HCC Rx ESR COM

√6th **M08.42 Pauciarticular juvenile rheumatoid arthritis, elbow**
- **M08.421 Pauciarticular juvenile rheumatoid arthritis, right elbow** HCC Rx ESR COM
- **M08.422 Pauciarticular juvenile rheumatoid arthritis, left elbow** HCC Rx ESR COM
- **M08.429 Pauciarticular juvenile rheumatoid arthritis, unspecified elbow** HCC Rx ESR COM

√6th **M08.43 Pauciarticular juvenile rheumatoid arthritis, wrist**
- **M08.431 Pauciarticular juvenile rheumatoid arthritis, right wrist** HCC Rx ESR COM

MØ8.432 Pauciarticular juvenile rheumatoid arthritis, left wrist HCC Rx ESR COM

MØ8.439 Pauciarticular juvenile rheumatoid arthritis, unspecified wrist HCC Rx ESR COM

6th MØ8.44 Pauciarticular juvenile rheumatoid arthritis, hand

MØ8.441 Pauciarticular juvenile rheumatoid arthritis, right hand HCC Rx ESR COM

MØ8.442 Pauciarticular juvenile rheumatoid arthritis, left hand HCC Rx ESR COM

MØ8.449 Pauciarticular juvenile rheumatoid arthritis, unspecified hand HCC Rx ESR COM

6th MØ8.45 Pauciarticular juvenile rheumatoid arthritis, hip

MØ8.451 Pauciarticular juvenile rheumatoid arthritis, right hip HCC Rx ESR COM

MØ8.452 Pauciarticular juvenile rheumatoid arthritis, left hip HCC Rx ESR COM

MØ8.459 Pauciarticular juvenile rheumatoid arthritis, unspecified hip HCC Rx ESR COM

6th MØ8.46 Pauciarticular juvenile rheumatoid arthritis, knee

MØ8.461 Pauciarticular juvenile rheumatoid arthritis, right knee HCC Rx ESR COM

MØ8.462 Pauciarticular juvenile rheumatoid arthritis, left knee HCC Rx ESR COM

MØ8.469 Pauciarticular juvenile rheumatoid arthritis, unspecified knee HCC Rx ESR COM

6th MØ8.47 Pauciarticular juvenile rheumatoid arthritis, ankle and foot

MØ8.471 Pauciarticular juvenile rheumatoid arthritis, right ankle and foot HCC Rx ESR COM

MØ8.472 Pauciarticular juvenile rheumatoid arthritis, left ankle and foot HCC Rx ESR COM

MØ8.479 Pauciarticular juvenile rheumatoid arthritis, unspecified ankle and foot HCC Rx ESR COM

MØ8.48 Pauciarticular juvenile rheumatoid arthritis, vertebrae HCC Rx ESR COM

MØ8.4A Pauciarticular juvenile rheumatoid arthritis, other specified site HCC Rx ESR COM

5th MØ8.8 Other juvenile arthritis

MØ8.80 Other juvenile arthritis, unspecified site HCC Rx ESR COM

6th MØ8.81 Other juvenile arthritis, shoulder

MØ8.811 Other juvenile arthritis, right shoulder HCC Rx ESR COM

MØ8.812 Other juvenile arthritis, left shoulder HCC Rx ESR COM

MØ8.819 Other juvenile arthritis, unspecified shoulder HCC Rx ESR COM

6th MØ8.82 Other juvenile arthritis, elbow

MØ8.821 Other juvenile arthritis, right elbow HCC Rx ESR COM

MØ8.822 Other juvenile arthritis, left elbow HCC Rx ESR COM

MØ8.829 Other juvenile arthritis, unspecified elbow HCC Rx ESR COM

6th MØ8.83 Other juvenile arthritis, wrist

MØ8.831 Other juvenile arthritis, right wrist HCC Rx ESR COM

MØ8.832 Other juvenile arthritis, left wrist HCC Rx ESR COM

MØ8.839 Other juvenile arthritis, unspecified wrist HCC Rx ESR COM

6th MØ8.84 Other juvenile arthritis, hand

MØ8.841 Other juvenile arthritis, right hand HCC Rx ESR COM

MØ8.842 Other juvenile arthritis, left hand HCC Rx ESR COM

MØ8.849 Other juvenile arthritis, unspecified hand HCC Rx ESR COM

6th MØ8.85 Other juvenile arthritis, hip

MØ8.851 Other juvenile arthritis, right hip HCC Rx ESR COM

MØ8.852 Other juvenile arthritis, left hip HCC Rx ESR COM

MØ8.859 Other juvenile arthritis, unspecified hip HCC Rx ESR COM

6th MØ8.86 Other juvenile arthritis, knee

MØ8.861 Other juvenile arthritis, right knee HCC Rx ESR COM

MØ8.862 Other juvenile arthritis, left knee HCC Rx ESR COM

MØ8.869 Other juvenile arthritis, unspecified knee HCC Rx ESR COM

6th MØ8.87 Other juvenile arthritis, ankle and foot

MØ8.871 Other juvenile arthritis, right ankle and foot HCC Rx ESR COM

MØ8.872 Other juvenile arthritis, left ankle and foot HCC Rx ESR COM

MØ8.879 Other juvenile arthritis, unspecified ankle and foot HCC Rx ESR COM

MØ8.88 Other juvenile arthritis, other specified site HCC Rx ESR COM

Other juvenile arthritis, vertebrae

MØ8.89 Other juvenile arthritis, multiple sites HCC Rx ESR COM

5th MØ8.9 Juvenile arthritis, unspecified

EXCLUDES 1 *juvenile rheumatoid arthritis, unspecified (MØ8.Ø-)*

MØ8.90 Juvenile arthritis, unspecified, unspecified site HCC Rx ESR COM

6th MØ8.91 Juvenile arthritis, unspecified, shoulder

MØ8.911 Juvenile arthritis, unspecified, right shoulder HCC Rx ESR COM

MØ8.912 Juvenile arthritis, unspecified, left shoulder HCC Rx ESR COM

MØ8.919 Juvenile arthritis, unspecified, unspecified shoulder HCC Rx ESR COM

6th MØ8.92 Juvenile arthritis, unspecified, elbow

MØ8.921 Juvenile arthritis, unspecified, right elbow HCC Rx ESR COM

MØ8.922 Juvenile arthritis, unspecified, left elbow HCC Rx ESR COM

MØ8.929 Juvenile arthritis, unspecified, unspecified elbow HCC Rx ESR COM

6th MØ8.93 Juvenile arthritis, unspecified, wrist

MØ8.931 Juvenile arthritis, unspecified, right wrist HCC Rx ESR COM

MØ8.932 Juvenile arthritis, unspecified, left wrist HCC Rx ESR COM

MØ8.939 Juvenile arthritis, unspecified, unspecified wrist HCC Rx ESR COM

6th MØ8.94 Juvenile arthritis, unspecified, hand

MØ8.941 Juvenile arthritis, unspecified, right hand HCC Rx ESR COM

MØ8.942 Juvenile arthritis, unspecified, left hand HCC Rx ESR COM

MØ8.949 Juvenile arthritis, unspecified, unspecified hand HCC Rx ESR COM

6th MØ8.95 Juvenile arthritis, unspecified, hip

MØ8.951 Juvenile arthritis, unspecified, right hip HCC Rx ESR COM

MØ8.952 Juvenile arthritis, unspecified, left hip HCC Rx ESR COM

MØ8.959 Juvenile arthritis, unspecified, unspecified hip HCC Rx ESR COM

6th MØ8.96 Juvenile arthritis, unspecified, knee

MØ8.961 Juvenile arthritis, unspecified, right knee HCC Rx ESR COM

MØ8.962 Juvenile arthritis, unspecified, left knee HCC Rx ESR COM

MØ8.969 Juvenile arthritis, unspecified, unspecified knee HCC Rx ESR COM

6th MØ8.97 Juvenile arthritis, unspecified, ankle and foot

MØ8.971 Juvenile arthritis, unspecified, right ankle and foot HCC Rx ESR COM

MØ8.972 Juvenile arthritis, unspecified, left ankle and foot HCC Rx ESR COM

MØ8.979 Juvenile arthritis, unspecified, unspecified ankle and foot HCC Rx ESR COM

HCC CMS-HCC Rx Rx HCC ESR ESRD HCC COM Commercial HCC N Newborn: 0 P Pediatric: 0-17 M Maternity: 9-64 A Adult: 15-124

M08.98 Juvenile arthritis, unspecified, vertebrae HCC Rx ESR COM

M08.99 Juvenile arthritis, unspecified, multiple sites HCC Rx ESR COM

M08.9A Juvenile arthritis, unspecified, other specified site HCC Rx ESR COM

✓4th **M1A Chronic gout**

Use additional code to identify:
- autonomic neuropathy in diseases classified elsewhere (G99.0)
- calculus of urinary tract in diseases classified elsewhere (N22)
- cardiomyopathy in diseases classified elsewhere (I43)
- disorders of external ear in diseases classified elsewhere (H61.1-, H62.8-)
- disorders of iris and ciliary body in diseases classified elsewhere (H22)
- glomerular disorders in diseases classified elsewhere (N08)

EXCLUDES 1 *gout NOS (M10.-)*

EXCLUDES 2 *acute gout (M10.-)*

The appropriate 7th character is to be added to each code from category M1A.
- 0 without tophus (tophi)
- 1 with tophus (tophi)

✓5th **M1A.0 Idiopathic chronic gout**
Chronic gouty bursitis
Primary chronic gout

✓x7th **M1A.00** Idiopathic chronic gout, unspecified site

✓6th **M1A.01** Idiopathic chronic gout, shoulder

✓7th **M1A.011** Idiopathic chronic gout, right shoulder

✓7th **M1A.012** Idiopathic chronic gout, left shoulder

✓7th **M1A.019** Idiopathic chronic gout, unspecified shoulder

✓6th **M1A.02** Idiopathic chronic gout, elbow

✓7th **M1A.021** Idiopathic chronic gout, right elbow

✓7th **M1A.022** Idiopathic chronic gout, left elbow

✓7th **M1A.029** Idiopathic chronic gout, unspecified elbow

✓6th **M1A.03** Idiopathic chronic gout, wrist

✓7th **M1A.031** Idiopathic chronic gout, right wrist

✓7th **M1A.032** Idiopathic chronic gout, left wrist

✓7th **M1A.039** Idiopathic chronic gout, unspecified wrist

✓6th **M1A.04** Idiopathic chronic gout, hand

✓7th **M1A.041** Idiopathic chronic gout, right hand

✓7th **M1A.042** Idiopathic chronic gout, left hand

✓7th **M1A.049** Idiopathic chronic gout, unspecified hand

✓6th **M1A.05** Idiopathic chronic gout, hip

✓7th **M1A.051** Idiopathic chronic gout, right hip

✓7th **M1A.052** Idiopathic chronic gout, left hip

✓7th **M1A.059** Idiopathic chronic gout, unspecified hip

✓6th **M1A.06** Idiopathic chronic gout, knee

✓7th **M1A.061** Idiopathic chronic gout, right knee

✓7th **M1A.062** Idiopathic chronic gout, left knee

✓7th **M1A.069** Idiopathic chronic gout, unspecified knee

✓6th **M1A.07** Idiopathic chronic gout, ankle and foot

✓7th **M1A.071** Idiopathic chronic gout, right ankle and foot

✓7th **M1A.072** Idiopathic chronic gout, left ankle and foot

✓7th **M1A.079** Idiopathic chronic gout, unspecified ankle and foot

✓x7th **M1A.08** Idiopathic chronic gout, vertebrae

✓x7th **M1A.09** Idiopathic chronic gout, multiple sites

✓5th **M1A.1 Lead-induced chronic gout**

Code first toxic effects of lead and its compounds (T56.0-)

✓x7th **M1A.10** Lead-induced chronic gout, unspecified site

✓6th **M1A.11** Lead-induced chronic gout, shoulder

✓7th **M1A.111** Lead-induced chronic gout, right shoulder

✓7th **M1A.112** Lead-induced chronic gout, left shoulder

✓7th **M1A.119** Lead-induced chronic gout, unspecified shoulder

✓6th **M1A.12** Lead-induced chronic gout, elbow

✓7th **M1A.121** Lead-induced chronic gout, right elbow

✓7th **M1A.122** Lead-induced chronic gout, left elbow

✓7th **M1A.129** Lead-induced chronic gout, unspecified elbow

✓6th **M1A.13** Lead-induced chronic gout, wrist

✓7th **M1A.131** Lead-induced chronic gout, right wrist

✓7th **M1A.132** Lead-induced chronic gout, left wrist

✓7th **M1A.139** Lead-induced chronic gout, unspecified wrist

✓6th **M1A.14** Lead-induced chronic gout, hand

✓7th **M1A.141** Lead-induced chronic gout, right hand

✓7th **M1A.142** Lead-induced chronic gout, left hand

✓7th **M1A.149** Lead-induced chronic gout, unspecified hand

✓6th **M1A.15** Lead-induced chronic gout, hip

✓7th **M1A.151** Lead-induced chronic gout, right hip

✓7th **M1A.152** Lead-induced chronic gout, left hip

✓7th **M1A.159** Lead-induced chronic gout, unspecified hip

✓6th **M1A.16** Lead-induced chronic gout, knee

✓7th **M1A.161** Lead-induced chronic gout, right knee

✓7th **M1A.162** Lead-induced chronic gout, left knee

✓7th **M1A.169** Lead-induced chronic gout, unspecified knee

✓6th **M1A.17** Lead-induced chronic gout, ankle and foot

✓7th **M1A.171** Lead-induced chronic gout, right ankle and foot

✓7th **M1A.172** Lead-induced chronic gout, left ankle and foot

✓7th **M1A.179** Lead-induced chronic gout, unspecified ankle and foot

✓x7th **M1A.18** Lead-induced chronic gout, vertebrae

✓x7th **M1A.19** Lead-induced chronic gout, multiple sites

✓5th **M1A.2 Drug-induced chronic gout**

Use additional code for adverse effect, if applicable, to identify drug (T36-T50 with fifth or sixth character 5)

✓x7th **M1A.20** Drug-induced chronic gout, unspecified site

✓6th **M1A.21** Drug-induced chronic gout, shoulder

✓7th **M1A.211** Drug-induced chronic gout, right shoulder

✓7th **M1A.212** Drug-induced chronic gout, left shoulder

✓7th **M1A.219** Drug-induced chronic gout, unspecified shoulder

✓6th **M1A.22** Drug-induced chronic gout, elbow

✓7th **M1A.221** Drug-induced chronic gout, right elbow

✓7th **M1A.222** Drug-induced chronic gout, left elbow

✓7th **M1A.229** Drug-induced chronic gout, unspecified elbow

✓6th **M1A.23** Drug-induced chronic gout, wrist

✓7th **M1A.231** Drug-induced chronic gout, right wrist

✓7th **M1A.232** Drug-induced chronic gout, left wrist

✓7th **M1A.239** Drug-induced chronic gout, unspecified wrist

✓6th **M1A.24** Drug-induced chronic gout, hand

✓7th **M1A.241** Drug-induced chronic gout, right hand

✓7th **M1A.242** Drug-induced chronic gout, left hand

✓7th **M1A.249** Drug-induced chronic gout, unspecified hand

✓6th **M1A.25** Drug-induced chronic gout, hip

✓7th **M1A.251** Drug-induced chronic gout, right hip

✓7th **M1A.252** Drug-induced chronic gout, left hip

✓7th **M1A.259** Drug-induced chronic gout, unspecified hip

✓6th **M1A.26** Drug-induced chronic gout, knee

✓7th **M1A.261** Drug-induced chronic gout, right knee

✓7th **M1A.262** Drug-induced chronic gout, left knee

✓7th **M1A.269** Drug-induced chronic gout, unspecified knee

✓6th **M1A.27** Drug-induced chronic gout, ankle and foot

✓7th **M1A.271** Drug-induced chronic gout, right ankle and foot

✓7th **M1A.272** Drug-induced chronic gout, left ankle and foot

M1A.279 Drug-induced chronic gout, unspecified ankle and foot
M1A.28 Drug-induced chronic gout, vertebrae
M1A.29 Drug-induced chronic gout, multiple sites
M1A.3 Chronic gout due to renal impairment
Code first associated renal disease
M1A.3Ø Chronic gout due to renal impairment, unspecified site
M1A.31 Chronic gout due to renal impairment, shoulder
M1A.311 Chronic gout due to renal impairment, right shoulder
M1A.312 Chronic gout due to renal impairment, left shoulder
M1A.319 Chronic gout due to renal impairment, unspecified shoulder
M1A.32 Chronic gout due to renal impairment, elbow
M1A.321 Chronic gout due to renal impairment, right elbow
M1A.322 Chronic gout due to renal impairment, left elbow
M1A.329 Chronic gout due to renal impairment, unspecified elbow
M1A.33 Chronic gout due to renal impairment, wrist
M1A.331 Chronic gout due to renal impairment, right wrist
M1A.332 Chronic gout due to renal impairment, left wrist
M1A.339 Chronic gout due to renal impairment, unspecified wrist
M1A.34 Chronic gout due to renal impairment, hand
M1A.341 Chronic gout due to renal impairment, right hand
M1A.342 Chronic gout due to renal impairment, left hand
M1A.349 Chronic gout due to renal impairment, unspecified hand
M1A.35 Chronic gout due to renal impairment, hip
M1A.351 Chronic gout due to renal impairment, right hip
M1A.352 Chronic gout due to renal impairment, left hip
M1A.359 Chronic gout due to renal impairment, unspecified hip
M1A.36 Chronic gout due to renal impairment, knee
M1A.361 Chronic gout due to renal impairment, right knee
M1A.362 Chronic gout due to renal impairment, left knee
M1A.369 Chronic gout due to renal impairment, unspecified knee
M1A.37 Chronic gout due to renal impairment, ankle and foot
M1A.371 Chronic gout due to renal impairment, right ankle and foot
M1A.372 Chronic gout due to renal impairment, left ankle and foot
M1A.379 Chronic gout due to renal impairment, unspecified ankle and foot
M1A.38 Chronic gout due to renal impairment, vertebrae
M1A.39 Chronic gout due to renal impairment, multiple sites
M1A.4 Other secondary chronic gout
Code first associated condition
M1A.4Ø Other secondary chronic gout, unspecified site
M1A.41 Other secondary chronic gout, shoulder
M1A.411 Other secondary chronic gout, right shoulder
M1A.412 Other secondary chronic gout, left shoulder
M1A.419 Other secondary chronic gout, unspecified shoulder
M1A.42 Other secondary chronic gout, elbow
M1A.421 Other secondary chronic gout, right elbow
M1A.422 Other secondary chronic gout, left elbow
M1A.429 Other secondary chronic gout, unspecified elbow
M1A.43 Other secondary chronic gout, wrist
M1A.431 Other secondary chronic gout, right wrist
M1A.432 Other secondary chronic gout, left wrist
M1A.439 Other secondary chronic gout, unspecified wrist
M1A.44 Other secondary chronic gout, hand
M1A.441 Other secondary chronic gout, right hand
M1A.442 Other secondary chronic gout, left hand
M1A.449 Other secondary chronic gout, unspecified hand
M1A.45 Other secondary chronic gout, hip
M1A.451 Other secondary chronic gout, right hip
M1A.452 Other secondary chronic gout, left hip
M1A.459 Other secondary chronic gout, unspecified hip
M1A.46 Other secondary chronic gout, knee
M1A.461 Other secondary chronic gout, right knee
M1A.462 Other secondary chronic gout, left knee
M1A.469 Other secondary chronic gout, unspecified knee
M1A.47 Other secondary chronic gout, ankle and foot
M1A.471 Other secondary chronic gout, right ankle and foot
M1A.472 Other secondary chronic gout, left ankle and foot
M1A.479 Other secondary chronic gout, unspecified ankle and foot
M1A.48 Other secondary chronic gout, vertebrae
M1A.49 Other secondary chronic gout, multiple sites
M1A.9 Chronic gout, unspecified

M1Ø Gout
Acute gout
Gout attack
Gout flare
Podagra
Use additional code to identify:
autonomic neuropathy in diseases classified elsewhere (G99.Ø)
calculus of urinary tract in diseases classified elsewhere (N22)
cardiomyopathy in diseases classified elsewhere (I43)
disorders of external ear in diseases classified elsewhere (H61.1-, H62.8-)
disorders of iris and ciliary body in diseases classified elsewhere (H22)
glomerular disorders in diseases classified elsewhere (NØ8)
EXCLUDES 2 *chronic gout (M1A.-)*
DEF: Purine and pyrimidine metabolic disorders, manifested by hyperuricemia and recurrent acute inflammatory arthritis. Monosodium urate or monohydrate crystals may be deposited in and around the joints, leading to joint destruction and severe crippling.
M1Ø.Ø Idiopathic gout
Gouty bursitis
Primary gout
M1Ø.ØØ Idiopathic gout, unspecified site
M1Ø.Ø1 Idiopathic gout, shoulder
M1Ø.Ø11 Idiopathic gout, right shoulder
M1Ø.Ø12 Idiopathic gout, left shoulder
M1Ø.Ø19 Idiopathic gout, unspecified shoulder
M1Ø.Ø2 Idiopathic gout, elbow
M1Ø.Ø21 Idiopathic gout, right elbow
M1Ø.Ø22 Idiopathic gout, left elbow
M1Ø.Ø29 Idiopathic gout, unspecified elbow
M1Ø.Ø3 Idiopathic gout, wrist
M1Ø.Ø31 Idiopathic gout, right wrist
M1Ø.Ø32 Idiopathic gout, left wrist
M1Ø.Ø39 Idiopathic gout, unspecified wrist
M1Ø.Ø4 Idiopathic gout, hand
M1Ø.Ø41 Idiopathic gout, right hand
M1Ø.Ø42 Idiopathic gout, left hand
M1Ø.Ø49 Idiopathic gout, unspecified hand
M1Ø.Ø5 Idiopathic gout, hip
M1Ø.Ø51 Idiopathic gout, right hip
M1Ø.Ø52 Idiopathic gout, left hip
M1Ø.Ø59 Idiopathic gout, unspecified hip
M1Ø.Ø6 Idiopathic gout, knee
M1Ø.Ø61 Idiopathic gout, right knee

M10.062 Idiopathic gout, left knee
M10.069 Idiopathic gout, unspecified knee
M10.07 Idiopathic gout, ankle and foot
M10.071 Idiopathic gout, right ankle and foot
M10.072 Idiopathic gout, left ankle and foot
M10.079 Idiopathic gout, unspecified ankle and foot
M10.08 Idiopathic gout, vertebrae
M10.09 Idiopathic gout, multiple sites
M10.1 Lead-induced gout
Code first toxic effects of lead and its compounds (T56.0-)
M10.10 Lead-induced gout, unspecified site
M10.11 Lead-induced gout, shoulder
M10.111 Lead-induced gout, right shoulder
M10.112 Lead-induced gout, left shoulder
M10.119 Lead-induced gout, unspecified shoulder
M10.12 Lead-induced gout, elbow
M10.121 Lead-induced gout, right elbow
M10.122 Lead-induced gout, left elbow
M10.129 Lead-induced gout, unspecified elbow
M10.13 Lead-induced gout, wrist
M10.131 Lead-induced gout, right wrist
M10.132 Lead-induced gout, left wrist
M10.139 Lead-induced gout, unspecified wrist
M10.14 Lead-induced gout, hand
M10.141 Lead-induced gout, right hand
M10.142 Lead-induced gout, left hand
M10.149 Lead-induced gout, unspecified hand
M10.15 Lead-induced gout, hip
M10.151 Lead-induced gout, right hip
M10.152 Lead-induced gout, left hip
M10.159 Lead-induced gout, unspecified hip
M10.16 Lead-induced gout, knee
M10.161 Lead-induced gout, right knee
M10.162 Lead-induced gout, left knee
M10.169 Lead-induced gout, unspecified knee
M10.17 Lead-induced gout, ankle and foot
M10.171 Lead-induced gout, right ankle and foot
M10.172 Lead-induced gout, left ankle and foot
M10.179 Lead-induced gout, unspecified ankle and foot
M10.18 Lead-induced gout, vertebrae
M10.19 Lead-induced gout, multiple sites
M10.2 Drug-induced gout
Use additional code for adverse effect, if applicable, to identify drug (T36-T50 with fifth or sixth character 5)
M10.20 Drug-induced gout, unspecified site
M10.21 Drug-induced gout, shoulder
M10.211 Drug-induced gout, right shoulder
M10.212 Drug-induced gout, left shoulder
M10.219 Drug-induced gout, unspecified shoulder
M10.22 Drug-induced gout, elbow
M10.221 Drug-induced gout, right elbow
M10.222 Drug-induced gout, left elbow
M10.229 Drug-induced gout, unspecified elbow
M10.23 Drug-induced gout, wrist
M10.231 Drug-induced gout, right wrist
M10.232 Drug-induced gout, left wrist
M10.239 Drug-induced gout, unspecified wrist
M10.24 Drug-induced gout, hand
M10.241 Drug-induced gout, right hand
M10.242 Drug-induced gout, left hand
M10.249 Drug-induced gout, unspecified hand
M10.25 Drug-induced gout, hip
M10.251 Drug-induced gout, right hip
M10.252 Drug-induced gout, left hip
M10.259 Drug-induced gout, unspecified hip
M10.26 Drug-induced gout, knee
M10.261 Drug-induced gout, right knee
M10.262 Drug-induced gout, left knee
M10.269 Drug-induced gout, unspecified knee
M10.27 Drug-induced gout, ankle and foot
M10.271 Drug-induced gout, right ankle and foot
M10.272 Drug-induced gout, left ankle and foot
M10.279 Drug-induced gout, unspecified ankle and foot
M10.28 Drug-induced gout, vertebrae
M10.29 Drug-induced gout, multiple sites
M10.3 Gout due to renal impairment
Code first associated renal disease
M10.30 Gout due to renal impairment, unspecified site
M10.31 Gout due to renal impairment, shoulder
M10.311 Gout due to renal impairment, right shoulder
M10.312 Gout due to renal impairment, left shoulder
M10.319 Gout due to renal impairment, unspecified shoulder
M10.32 Gout due to renal impairment, elbow
M10.321 Gout due to renal impairment, right elbow
M10.322 Gout due to renal impairment, left elbow
M10.329 Gout due to renal impairment, unspecified elbow
M10.33 Gout due to renal impairment, wrist
M10.331 Gout due to renal impairment, right wrist
M10.332 Gout due to renal impairment, left wrist
M10.339 Gout due to renal impairment, unspecified wrist
M10.34 Gout due to renal impairment, hand
M10.341 Gout due to renal impairment, right hand
M10.342 Gout due to renal impairment, left hand
M10.349 Gout due to renal impairment, unspecified hand
M10.35 Gout due to renal impairment, hip
M10.351 Gout due to renal impairment, right hip
M10.352 Gout due to renal impairment, left hip
M10.359 Gout due to renal impairment, unspecified hip
M10.36 Gout due to renal impairment, knee
M10.361 Gout due to renal impairment, right knee
M10.362 Gout due to renal impairment, left knee
M10.369 Gout due to renal impairment, unspecified knee
M10.37 Gout due to renal impairment, ankle and foot
M10.371 Gout due to renal impairment, right ankle and foot
M10.372 Gout due to renal impairment, left ankle and foot
M10.379 Gout due to renal impairment, unspecified ankle and foot
M10.38 Gout due to renal impairment, vertebrae
M10.39 Gout due to renal impairment, multiple sites
M10.4 Other secondary gout
Code first associated condition
M10.40 Other secondary gout, unspecified site
M10.41 Other secondary gout, shoulder
M10.411 Other secondary gout, right shoulder
M10.412 Other secondary gout, left shoulder
M10.419 Other secondary gout, unspecified shoulder
M10.42 Other secondary gout, elbow
M10.421 Other secondary gout, right elbow
M10.422 Other secondary gout, left elbow
M10.429 Other secondary gout, unspecified elbow
M10.43 Other secondary gout, wrist
M10.431 Other secondary gout, right wrist
M10.432 Other secondary gout, left wrist
M10.439 Other secondary gout, unspecified wrist
M10.44 Other secondary gout, hand
M10.441 Other secondary gout, right hand
M10.442 Other secondary gout, left hand
M10.449 Other secondary gout, unspecified hand
M10.45 Other secondary gout, hip
M10.451 Other secondary gout, right hip
M10.452 Other secondary gout, left hip
M10.459 Other secondary gout, unspecified hip
M10.46 Other secondary gout, knee
M10.461 Other secondary gout, right knee
M10.462 Other secondary gout, left knee
M10.469 Other secondary gout, unspecified knee

M10.47 Other secondary gout, ankle and foot
M10.471 Other secondary gout, right ankle and foot
M10.472 Other secondary gout, left ankle and foot
M10.479 Other secondary gout, unspecified ankle and foot
M10.48 Other secondary gout, vertebrae
M10.49 Other secondary gout, multiple sites
M10.9 Gout, unspecified
Gout NOS

M11 Other crystal arthropathies

M11.0 Hydroxyapatite deposition disease
DEF: Disease caused by deposits of calcium phosphate crystals in the soft tissues close to the joint (especially tendons) or in the joints. These calcifications can be mono or polyarticular and can cause destruction of the joint involved.
M11.00 Hydroxyapatite deposition disease, unspecified site
M11.01 Hydroxyapatite deposition disease, shoulder
M11.011 Hydroxyapatite deposition disease, right shoulder
M11.012 Hydroxyapatite deposition disease, left shoulder
M11.019 Hydroxyapatite deposition disease, unspecified shoulder
M11.02 Hydroxyapatite deposition disease, elbow
M11.021 Hydroxyapatite deposition disease, right elbow
M11.022 Hydroxyapatite deposition disease, left elbow
M11.029 Hydroxyapatite deposition disease, unspecified elbow
M11.03 Hydroxyapatite deposition disease, wrist
M11.031 Hydroxyapatite deposition disease, right wrist
M11.032 Hydroxyapatite deposition disease, left wrist
M11.039 Hydroxyapatite deposition disease, unspecified wrist
M11.04 Hydroxyapatite deposition disease, hand
M11.041 Hydroxyapatite deposition disease, right hand
M11.042 Hydroxyapatite deposition disease, left hand
M11.049 Hydroxyapatite deposition disease, unspecified hand
M11.05 Hydroxyapatite deposition disease, hip
M11.051 Hydroxyapatite deposition disease, right hip
M11.052 Hydroxyapatite deposition disease, left hip
M11.059 Hydroxyapatite deposition disease, unspecified hip
M11.06 Hydroxyapatite deposition disease, knee
M11.061 Hydroxyapatite deposition disease, right knee
M11.062 Hydroxyapatite deposition disease, left knee
M11.069 Hydroxyapatite deposition disease, unspecified knee
M11.07 Hydroxyapatite deposition disease, ankle and foot
M11.071 Hydroxyapatite deposition disease, right ankle and foot
M11.072 Hydroxyapatite deposition disease, left ankle and foot
M11.079 Hydroxyapatite deposition disease, unspecified ankle and foot
M11.08 Hydroxyapatite deposition disease, vertebrae
M11.09 Hydroxyapatite deposition disease, multiple sites

M11.1 Familial chondrocalcinosis
M11.10 Familial chondrocalcinosis, unspecified site
M11.11 Familial chondrocalcinosis, shoulder
M11.111 Familial chondrocalcinosis, right shoulder
M11.112 Familial chondrocalcinosis, left shoulder
M11.119 Familial chondrocalcinosis, unspecified shoulder
M11.12 Familial chondrocalcinosis, elbow
M11.121 Familial chondrocalcinosis, right elbow
M11.122 Familial chondrocalcinosis, left elbow
M11.129 Familial chondrocalcinosis, unspecified elbow
M11.13 Familial chondrocalcinosis, wrist
M11.131 Familial chondrocalcinosis, right wrist
M11.132 Familial chondrocalcinosis, left wrist
M11.139 Familial chondrocalcinosis, unspecified wrist
M11.14 Familial chondrocalcinosis, hand
M11.141 Familial chondrocalcinosis, right hand
M11.142 Familial chondrocalcinosis, left hand
M11.149 Familial chondrocalcinosis, unspecified hand
M11.15 Familial chondrocalcinosis, hip
M11.151 Familial chondrocalcinosis, right hip
M11.152 Familial chondrocalcinosis, left hip
M11.159 Familial chondrocalcinosis, unspecified hip
M11.16 Familial chondrocalcinosis, knee
M11.161 Familial chondrocalcinosis, right knee
M11.162 Familial chondrocalcinosis, left knee
M11.169 Familial chondrocalcinosis, unspecified knee
M11.17 Familial chondrocalcinosis, ankle and foot
M11.171 Familial chondrocalcinosis, right ankle and foot
M11.172 Familial chondrocalcinosis, left ankle and foot
M11.179 Familial chondrocalcinosis, unspecified ankle and foot
M11.18 Familial chondrocalcinosis, vertebrae
M11.19 Familial chondrocalcinosis, multiple sites

M11.2 Other chondrocalcinosis
Chondrocalcinosis NOS
AHA: 2018,3Q,20
TIP: Pseudogout is captured with codes in this subcategory.
M11.20 Other chondrocalcinosis, unspecified site
M11.21 Other chondrocalcinosis, shoulder
M11.211 Other chondrocalcinosis, right shoulder
M11.212 Other chondrocalcinosis, left shoulder
M11.219 Other chondrocalcinosis, unspecified shoulder
M11.22 Other chondrocalcinosis, elbow
M11.221 Other chondrocalcinosis, right elbow
M11.222 Other chondrocalcinosis, left elbow
M11.229 Other chondrocalcinosis, unspecified elbow
M11.23 Other chondrocalcinosis, wrist
M11.231 Other chondrocalcinosis, right wrist
M11.232 Other chondrocalcinosis, left wrist
M11.239 Other chondrocalcinosis, unspecified wrist
M11.24 Other chondrocalcinosis, hand
M11.241 Other chondrocalcinosis, right hand
M11.242 Other chondrocalcinosis, left hand
M11.249 Other chondrocalcinosis, unspecified hand
M11.25 Other chondrocalcinosis, hip
M11.251 Other chondrocalcinosis, right hip
M11.252 Other chondrocalcinosis, left hip
M11.259 Other chondrocalcinosis, unspecified hip
M11.26 Other chondrocalcinosis, knee
M11.261 Other chondrocalcinosis, right knee
M11.262 Other chondrocalcinosis, left knee
M11.269 Other chondrocalcinosis, unspecified knee
M11.27 Other chondrocalcinosis, ankle and foot
M11.271 Other chondrocalcinosis, right ankle and foot
M11.272 Other chondrocalcinosis, left ankle and foot
M11.279 Other chondrocalcinosis, unspecified ankle and foot
M11.28 Other chondrocalcinosis, vertebrae
M11.29 Other chondrocalcinosis, multiple sites

M11.8 Other specified crystal arthropathies
M11.80 Other specified crystal arthropathies, unspecified site

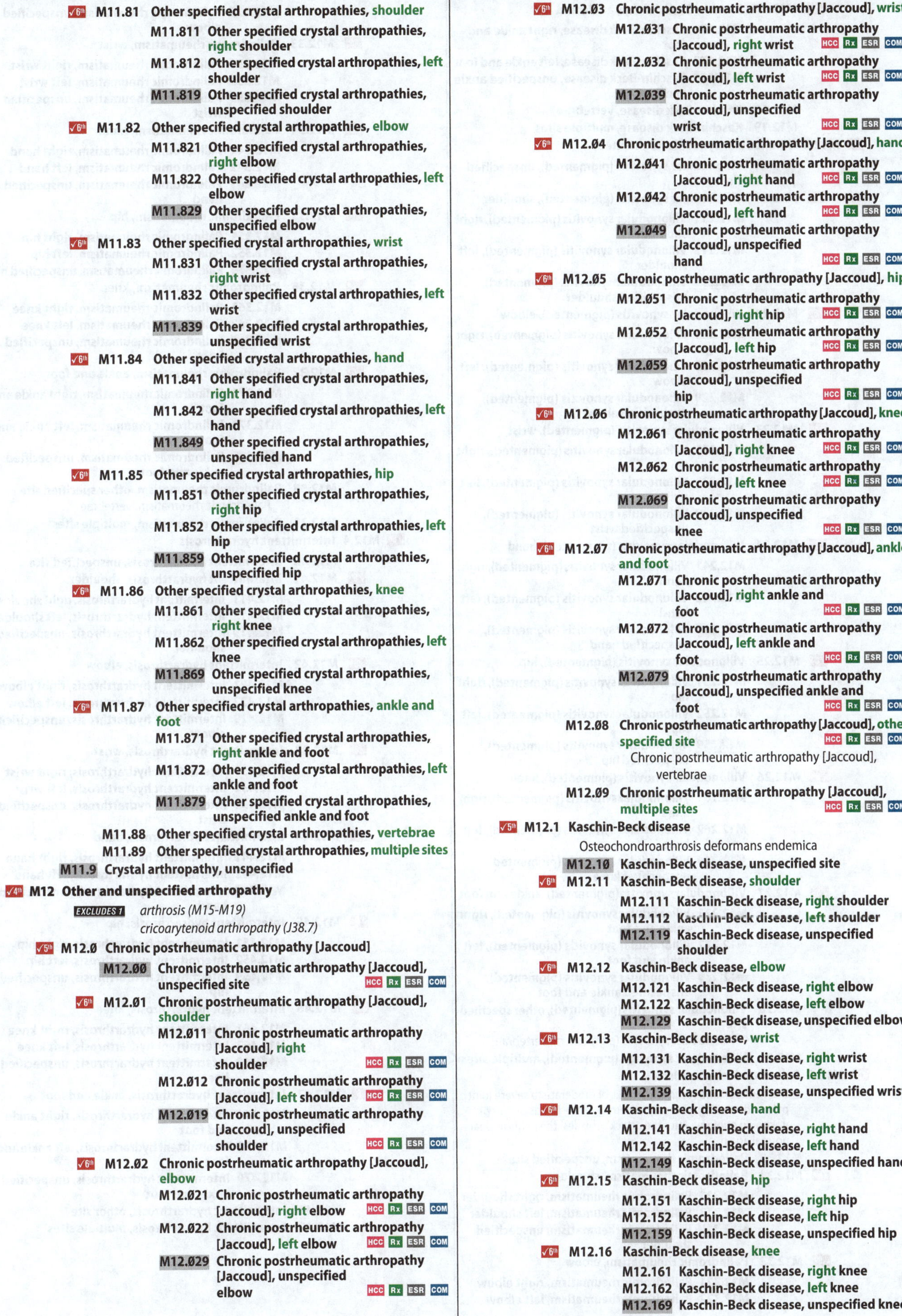

✓6th **M11.81 Other specified crystal arthropathies, shoulder**
- **M11.811 Other specified crystal arthropathies, right shoulder**
- **M11.812 Other specified crystal arthropathies, left shoulder**
- **M11.819 Other specified crystal arthropathies, unspecified shoulder**

✓6th **M11.82 Other specified crystal arthropathies, elbow**
- **M11.821 Other specified crystal arthropathies, right elbow**
- **M11.822 Other specified crystal arthropathies, left elbow**
- **M11.829 Other specified crystal arthropathies, unspecified elbow**

✓6th **M11.83 Other specified crystal arthropathies, wrist**
- **M11.831 Other specified crystal arthropathies, right wrist**
- **M11.832 Other specified crystal arthropathies, left wrist**
- **M11.839 Other specified crystal arthropathies, unspecified wrist**

✓6th **M11.84 Other specified crystal arthropathies, hand**
- **M11.841 Other specified crystal arthropathies, right hand**
- **M11.842 Other specified crystal arthropathies, left hand**
- **M11.849 Other specified crystal arthropathies, unspecified hand**

✓6th **M11.85 Other specified crystal arthropathies, hip**
- **M11.851 Other specified crystal arthropathies, right hip**
- **M11.852 Other specified crystal arthropathies, left hip**
- **M11.859 Other specified crystal arthropathies, unspecified hip**

✓6th **M11.86 Other specified crystal arthropathies, knee**
- **M11.861 Other specified crystal arthropathies, right knee**
- **M11.862 Other specified crystal arthropathies, left knee**
- **M11.869 Other specified crystal arthropathies, unspecified knee**

✓6th **M11.87 Other specified crystal arthropathies, ankle and foot**
- **M11.871 Other specified crystal arthropathies, right ankle and foot**
- **M11.872 Other specified crystal arthropathies, left ankle and foot**
- **M11.879 Other specified crystal arthropathies, unspecified ankle and foot**

M11.88 Other specified crystal arthropathies, vertebrae

M11.89 Other specified crystal arthropathies, multiple sites

M11.9 Crystal arthropathy, unspecified

✓4th **M12 Other and unspecified arthropathy**

EXCLUDES 1 *arthrosis (M15-M19)*
cricoarytenoid arthropathy (J38.7)

✓5th **M12.Ø Chronic postrheumatic arthropathy [Jaccoud]**

M12.ØØ Chronic postrheumatic arthropathy [Jaccoud], unspecified site HCC Rx ESR COM

✓6th **M12.Ø1 Chronic postrheumatic arthropathy [Jaccoud], shoulder**
- **M12.Ø11 Chronic postrheumatic arthropathy [Jaccoud], right shoulder** HCC Rx ESR COM
- **M12.Ø12 Chronic postrheumatic arthropathy [Jaccoud], left shoulder** HCC Rx ESR COM
- **M12.Ø19 Chronic postrheumatic arthropathy [Jaccoud], unspecified shoulder** HCC Rx ESR COM

✓6th **M12.Ø2 Chronic postrheumatic arthropathy [Jaccoud], elbow**
- **M12.Ø21 Chronic postrheumatic arthropathy [Jaccoud], right elbow** HCC Rx ESR COM
- **M12.Ø22 Chronic postrheumatic arthropathy [Jaccoud], left elbow** HCC Rx ESR COM
- **M12.Ø29 Chronic postrheumatic arthropathy [Jaccoud], unspecified elbow** HCC Rx ESR COM

✓6th **M12.Ø3 Chronic postrheumatic arthropathy [Jaccoud], wrist**
- **M12.Ø31 Chronic postrheumatic arthropathy [Jaccoud], right wrist** HCC Rx ESR COM
- **M12.Ø32 Chronic postrheumatic arthropathy [Jaccoud], left wrist** HCC Rx ESR COM
- **M12.Ø39 Chronic postrheumatic arthropathy [Jaccoud], unspecified wrist** HCC Rx ESR COM

✓6th **M12.Ø4 Chronic postrheumatic arthropathy [Jaccoud], hand**
- **M12.Ø41 Chronic postrheumatic arthropathy [Jaccoud], right hand** HCC Rx ESR COM
- **M12.Ø42 Chronic postrheumatic arthropathy [Jaccoud], left hand** HCC Rx ESR COM
- **M12.Ø49 Chronic postrheumatic arthropathy [Jaccoud], unspecified hand** HCC Rx ESR COM

✓6th **M12.Ø5 Chronic postrheumatic arthropathy [Jaccoud], hip**
- **M12.Ø51 Chronic postrheumatic arthropathy [Jaccoud], right hip** HCC Rx ESR COM
- **M12.Ø52 Chronic postrheumatic arthropathy [Jaccoud], left hip** HCC Rx ESR COM
- **M12.Ø59 Chronic postrheumatic arthropathy [Jaccoud], unspecified hip** HCC Rx ESR COM

✓6th **M12.Ø6 Chronic postrheumatic arthropathy [Jaccoud], knee**
- **M12.Ø61 Chronic postrheumatic arthropathy [Jaccoud], right knee** HCC Rx ESR COM
- **M12.Ø62 Chronic postrheumatic arthropathy [Jaccoud], left knee** HCC Rx ESR COM
- **M12.Ø69 Chronic postrheumatic arthropathy [Jaccoud], unspecified knee** HCC Rx ESR COM

✓6th **M12.Ø7 Chronic postrheumatic arthropathy [Jaccoud], ankle and foot**
- **M12.Ø71 Chronic postrheumatic arthropathy [Jaccoud], right ankle and foot** HCC Rx ESR COM
- **M12.Ø72 Chronic postrheumatic arthropathy [Jaccoud], left ankle and foot** HCC Rx ESR COM
- **M12.Ø79 Chronic postrheumatic arthropathy [Jaccoud], unspecified ankle and foot** HCC Rx ESR COM

M12.Ø8 Chronic postrheumatic arthropathy [Jaccoud], other specified site HCC Rx ESR COM
Chronic postrheumatic arthropathy [Jaccoud], vertebrae

M12.Ø9 Chronic postrheumatic arthropathy [Jaccoud], multiple sites HCC Rx ESR COM

✓5th **M12.1 Kaschin-Beck disease**
Osteochondroarthrosis deformans endemica

M12.1Ø Kaschin-Beck disease, unspecified site

✓6th **M12.11 Kaschin-Beck disease, shoulder**
- **M12.111 Kaschin-Beck disease, right shoulder**
- **M12.112 Kaschin-Beck disease, left shoulder**
- **M12.119 Kaschin-Beck disease, unspecified shoulder**

✓6th **M12.12 Kaschin-Beck disease, elbow**
- **M12.121 Kaschin-Beck disease, right elbow**
- **M12.122 Kaschin-Beck disease, left elbow**
- **M12.129 Kaschin-Beck disease, unspecified elbow**

✓6th **M12.13 Kaschin-Beck disease, wrist**
- **M12.131 Kaschin-Beck disease, right wrist**
- **M12.132 Kaschin-Beck disease, left wrist**
- **M12.139 Kaschin-Beck disease, unspecified wrist**

✓6th **M12.14 Kaschin-Beck disease, hand**
- **M12.141 Kaschin-Beck disease, right hand**
- **M12.142 Kaschin-Beck disease, left hand**
- **M12.149 Kaschin-Beck disease, unspecified hand**

✓6th **M12.15 Kaschin-Beck disease, hip**
- **M12.151 Kaschin-Beck disease, right hip**
- **M12.152 Kaschin-Beck disease, left hip**
- **M12.159 Kaschin-Beck disease, unspecified hip**

✓6th **M12.16 Kaschin-Beck disease, knee**
- **M12.161 Kaschin-Beck disease, right knee**
- **M12.162 Kaschin-Beck disease, left knee**
- **M12.169 Kaschin-Beck disease, unspecified knee**

6th M12.17 Kaschin-Beck disease, ankle and foot
M12.171 Kaschin-Beck disease, right ankle and foot
M12.172 Kaschin-Beck disease, left ankle and foot
M12.179 Kaschin-Beck disease, unspecified ankle and foot
M12.18 Kaschin-Beck disease, vertebrae
M12.19 Kaschin-Beck disease, multiple sites
5th M12.2 Villonodular synovitis (pigmented)
M12.20 Villonodular synovitis (pigmented), unspecified site
6th M12.21 Villonodular synovitis (pigmented), shoulder
M12.211 Villonodular synovitis (pigmented), right shoulder
M12.212 Villonodular synovitis (pigmented), left shoulder
M12.219 Villonodular synovitis (pigmented), unspecified shoulder
6th M12.22 Villonodular synovitis (pigmented), elbow
M12.221 Villonodular synovitis (pigmented), right elbow
M12.222 Villonodular synovitis (pigmented), left elbow
M12.229 Villonodular synovitis (pigmented), unspecified elbow
6th M12.23 Villonodular synovitis (pigmented), wrist
M12.231 Villonodular synovitis (pigmented), right wrist
M12.232 Villonodular synovitis (pigmented), left wrist
M12.239 Villonodular synovitis (pigmented), unspecified wrist
6th M12.24 Villonodular synovitis (pigmented), hand
M12.241 Villonodular synovitis (pigmented), right hand
M12.242 Villonodular synovitis (pigmented), left hand
M12.249 Villonodular synovitis (pigmented), unspecified hand
6th M12.25 Villonodular synovitis (pigmented), hip
M12.251 Villonodular synovitis (pigmented), right hip
M12.252 Villonodular synovitis (pigmented), left hip
M12.259 Villonodular synovitis (pigmented), unspecified hip
6th M12.26 Villonodular synovitis (pigmented), knee
M12.261 Villonodular synovitis (pigmented), right knee
M12.262 Villonodular synovitis (pigmented), left knee
M12.269 Villonodular synovitis (pigmented), unspecified knee
6th M12.27 Villonodular synovitis (pigmented), ankle and foot
M12.271 Villonodular synovitis (pigmented), right ankle and foot
M12.272 Villonodular synovitis (pigmented), left ankle and foot
M12.279 Villonodular synovitis (pigmented), unspecified ankle and foot
M12.28 Villonodular synovitis (pigmented), other specified site
Villonodular synovitis (pigmented), vertebrae
M12.29 Villonodular synovitis (pigmented), multiple sites
5th M12.3 Palindromic rheumatism
DEF: Sudden and recurring attacks of moderate to severe joint pain and swelling generally occurring in the hands or feet of unknown etiology. After the attack subsides, the joints appear normal again.
M12.30 Palindromic rheumatism, unspecified site
6th M12.31 Palindromic rheumatism, shoulder
M12.311 Palindromic rheumatism, right shoulder
M12.312 Palindromic rheumatism, left shoulder
M12.319 Palindromic rheumatism, unspecified shoulder
6th M12.32 Palindromic rheumatism, elbow
M12.321 Palindromic rheumatism, right elbow
M12.322 Palindromic rheumatism, left elbow
M12.329 Palindromic rheumatism, unspecified elbow
6th M12.33 Palindromic rheumatism, wrist
M12.331 Palindromic rheumatism, right wrist
M12.332 Palindromic rheumatism, left wrist
M12.339 Palindromic rheumatism, unspecified wrist
6th M12.34 Palindromic rheumatism, hand
M12.341 Palindromic rheumatism, right hand
M12.342 Palindromic rheumatism, left hand
M12.349 Palindromic rheumatism, unspecified hand
6th M12.35 Palindromic rheumatism, hip
M12.351 Palindromic rheumatism, right hip
M12.352 Palindromic rheumatism, left hip
M12.359 Palindromic rheumatism, unspecified hip
6th M12.36 Palindromic rheumatism, knee
M12.361 Palindromic rheumatism, right knee
M12.362 Palindromic rheumatism, left knee
M12.369 Palindromic rheumatism, unspecified knee
6th M12.37 Palindromic rheumatism, ankle and foot
M12.371 Palindromic rheumatism, right ankle and foot
M12.372 Palindromic rheumatism, left ankle and foot
M12.379 Palindromic rheumatism, unspecified ankle and foot
M12.38 Palindromic rheumatism, other specified site
Palindromic rheumatism, vertebrae
M12.39 Palindromic rheumatism, multiple sites
5th M12.4 Intermittent hydrarthrosis
M12.40 Intermittent hydrarthrosis, unspecified site
6th M12.41 Intermittent hydrarthrosis, shoulder
M12.411 Intermittent hydrarthrosis, right shoulder
M12.412 Intermittent hydrarthrosis, left shoulder
M12.419 Intermittent hydrarthrosis, unspecified shoulder
6th M12.42 Intermittent hydrarthrosis, elbow
M12.421 Intermittent hydrarthrosis, right elbow
M12.422 Intermittent hydrarthrosis, left elbow
M12.429 Intermittent hydrarthrosis, unspecified elbow
6th M12.43 Intermittent hydrarthrosis, wrist
M12.431 Intermittent hydrarthrosis, right wrist
M12.432 Intermittent hydrarthrosis, left wrist
M12.439 Intermittent hydrarthrosis, unspecified wrist
6th M12.44 Intermittent hydrarthrosis, hand
M12.441 Intermittent hydrarthrosis, right hand
M12.442 Intermittent hydrarthrosis, left hand
M12.449 Intermittent hydrarthrosis, unspecified hand
6th M12.45 Intermittent hydrarthrosis, hip
M12.451 Intermittent hydrarthrosis, right hip
M12.452 Intermittent hydrarthrosis, left hip
M12.459 Intermittent hydrarthrosis, unspecified hip
6th M12.46 Intermittent hydrarthrosis, knee
M12.461 Intermittent hydrarthrosis, right knee
M12.462 Intermittent hydrarthrosis, left knee
M12.469 Intermittent hydrarthrosis, unspecified knee
6th M12.47 Intermittent hydrarthrosis, ankle and foot
M12.471 Intermittent hydrarthrosis, right ankle and foot
M12.472 Intermittent hydrarthrosis, left ankle and foot
M12.479 Intermittent hydrarthrosis, unspecified ankle and foot
M12.48 Intermittent hydrarthrosis, other site
M12.49 Intermittent hydrarthrosis, multiple sites

M12.5 Traumatic arthropathy

EXCLUDES 1 *current injury-see Alphabetic Index*
post-traumatic osteoarthritis of first carpometacarpal joint (M18.2-M18.3)
post-traumatic osteoarthritis of hip (M16.4-M16.5)
post-traumatic osteoarthritis of knee (M17.2-M17.3)
post-traumatic osteoarthritis NOS (M19.1-)
post-traumatic osteoarthritis of other single joints (M19.1-)

AHA: 2015,1Q,17

M12.50 Traumatic arthropathy, unspecified site
M12.51 Traumatic arthropathy, shoulder
M12.511 Traumatic arthropathy, right shoulder
M12.512 Traumatic arthropathy, left shoulder
M12.519 Traumatic arthropathy, unspecified shoulder
M12.52 Traumatic arthropathy, elbow
M12.521 Traumatic arthropathy, right elbow
M12.522 Traumatic arthropathy, left elbow
M12.529 Traumatic arthropathy, unspecified elbow
M12.53 Traumatic arthropathy, wrist
M12.531 Traumatic arthropathy, right wrist
M12.532 Traumatic arthropathy, left wrist
M12.539 Traumatic arthropathy, unspecified wrist
M12.54 Traumatic arthropathy, hand
M12.541 Traumatic arthropathy, right hand
M12.542 Traumatic arthropathy, left hand
M12.549 Traumatic arthropathy, unspecified hand
M12.55 Traumatic arthropathy, hip
M12.551 Traumatic arthropathy, right hip
M12.552 Traumatic arthropathy, left hip
M12.559 Traumatic arthropathy, unspecified hip
M12.56 Traumatic arthropathy, knee
M12.561 Traumatic arthropathy, right knee
M12.562 Traumatic arthropathy, left knee
M12.569 Traumatic arthropathy, unspecified knee
M12.57 Traumatic arthropathy, ankle and foot
M12.571 Traumatic arthropathy, right ankle and foot
M12.572 Traumatic arthropathy, left ankle and foot
M12.579 Traumatic arthropathy, unspecified ankle and foot
M12.58 Traumatic arthropathy, other specified site
Traumatic arthropathy, vertebrae
M12.59 Traumatic arthropathy, multiple sites

M12.8 Other specific arthropathies, not elsewhere classified
Transient arthropathy

M12.80 Other specific arthropathies, not elsewhere classified, unspecified site
M12.81 Other specific arthropathies, not elsewhere classified, shoulder
M12.811 Other specific arthropathies, not elsewhere classified, right shoulder
M12.812 Other specific arthropathies, not elsewhere classified, left shoulder
M12.819 Other specific arthropathies, not elsewhere classified, unspecified shoulder
M12.82 Other specific arthropathies, not elsewhere classified, elbow
M12.821 Other specific arthropathies, not elsewhere classified, right elbow
M12.822 Other specific arthropathies, not elsewhere classified, left elbow
M12.829 Other specific arthropathies, not elsewhere classified, unspecified elbow
M12.83 Other specific arthropathies, not elsewhere classified, wrist
M12.831 Other specific arthropathies, not elsewhere classified, right wrist
M12.832 Other specific arthropathies, not elsewhere classified, left wrist
M12.839 Other specific arthropathies, not elsewhere classified, unspecified wrist
M12.84 Other specific arthropathies, not elsewhere classified, hand
M12.841 Other specific arthropathies, not elsewhere classified, right hand
M12.842 Other specific arthropathies, not elsewhere classified, left hand
M12.849 Other specific arthropathies, not elsewhere classified, unspecified hand
M12.85 Other specific arthropathies, not elsewhere classified, hip
M12.851 Other specific arthropathies, not elsewhere classified, right hip
M12.852 Other specific arthropathies, not elsewhere classified, left hip
M12.859 Other specific arthropathies, not elsewhere classified, unspecified hip
M12.86 Other specific arthropathies, not elsewhere classified, knee
M12.861 Other specific arthropathies, not elsewhere classified, right knee
M12.862 Other specific arthropathies, not elsewhere classified, left knee
M12.869 Other specific arthropathies, not elsewhere classified, unspecified knee
M12.87 Other specific arthropathies, not elsewhere classified, ankle and foot
M12.871 Other specific arthropathies, not elsewhere classified, right ankle and foot
M12.872 Other specific arthropathies, not elsewhere classified, left ankle and foot
M12.879 Other specific arthropathies, not elsewhere classified, unspecified ankle and foot
M12.88 Other specific arthropathies, not elsewhere classified, other specified site
Other specific arthropathies, not elsewhere classified, vertebrae
M12.89 Other specific arthropathies, not elsewhere classified, multiple sites

M12.9 Arthropathy, unspecified

M13 Other arthritis

EXCLUDES 1 *arthrosis (M15-M19)*
osteoarthritis (M15-M19)

M13.0 Polyarthritis, unspecified

M13.1 Monoarthritis, not elsewhere classified

M13.10 Monoarthritis, not elsewhere classified, unspecified site
M13.11 Monoarthritis, not elsewhere classified, shoulder
M13.111 Monoarthritis, not elsewhere classified, right shoulder
M13.112 Monoarthritis, not elsewhere classified, left shoulder
M13.119 Monoarthritis, not elsewhere classified, unspecified shoulder
M13.12 Monoarthritis, not elsewhere classified, elbow
M13.121 Monoarthritis, not elsewhere classified, right elbow
M13.122 Monoarthritis, not elsewhere classified, left elbow
M13.129 Monoarthritis, not elsewhere classified, unspecified elbow
M13.13 Monoarthritis, not elsewhere classified, wrist
M13.131 Monoarthritis, not elsewhere classified, right wrist
M13.132 Monoarthritis, not elsewhere classified, left wrist
M13.139 Monoarthritis, not elsewhere classified, unspecified wrist
M13.14 Monoarthritis, not elsewhere classified, hand
M13.141 Monoarthritis, not elsewhere classified, right hand
M13.142 Monoarthritis, not elsewhere classified, left hand
M13.149 Monoarthritis, not elsewhere classified, unspecified hand
M13.15 Monoarthritis, not elsewhere classified, hip
M13.151 Monoarthritis, not elsewhere classified, right hip
M13.152 Monoarthritis, not elsewhere classified, left hip

M13.159 Monoarthritis, not elsewhere classified, unspecified hip

√6th M13.16 Monoarthritis, not elsewhere classified, knee

M13.161 Monoarthritis, not elsewhere classified, right knee

M13.162 Monoarthritis, not elsewhere classified, left knee

M13.169 Monoarthritis, not elsewhere classified, unspecified knee

√6th M13.17 Monoarthritis, not elsewhere classified, ankle and foot

M13.171 Monoarthritis, not elsewhere classified, right ankle and foot

M13.172 Monoarthritis, not elsewhere classified, left ankle and foot

M13.179 Monoarthritis, not elsewhere classified, unspecified ankle and foot

√5th **M13.8 Other specified arthritis**

Allergic arthritis

EXCLUDES 1 *osteoarthritis (M15-M19)*

M13.80 Other specified arthritis, unspecified site

√6th M13.81 Other specified arthritis, shoulder

M13.811 Other specified arthritis, right shoulder

M13.812 Other specified arthritis, left shoulder

M13.819 Other specified arthritis, unspecified shoulder

√6th M13.82 Other specified arthritis, elbow

M13.821 Other specified arthritis, right elbow

M13.822 Other specified arthritis, left elbow

M13.829 Other specified arthritis, unspecified elbow

√6th M13.83 Other specified arthritis, wrist

M13.831 Other specified arthritis, right wrist

M13.832 Other specified arthritis, left wrist

M13.839 Other specified arthritis, unspecified wrist

√6th M13.84 Other specified arthritis, hand

M13.841 Other specified arthritis, right hand

M13.842 Other specified arthritis, left hand

M13.849 Other specified arthritis, unspecified hand

√6th M13.85 Other specified arthritis, hip

M13.851 Other specified arthritis, right hip

M13.852 Other specified arthritis, left hip

M13.859 Other specified arthritis, unspecified hip

√6th M13.86 Other specified arthritis, knee

M13.861 Other specified arthritis, right knee

M13.862 Other specified arthritis, left knee

M13.869 Other specified arthritis, unspecified knee

√6th M13.87 Other specified arthritis, ankle and foot

M13.871 Other specified arthritis, right ankle and foot

M13.872 Other specified arthritis, left ankle and foot

M13.879 Other specified arthritis, unspecified ankle and foot

M13.88 Other specified arthritis, other site

M13.89 Other specified arthritis, multiple sites

√4th **M14 Arthropathies in other diseases classified elsewhere**

EXCLUDES 1 *arthropathy in:*

diabetes mellitus (EØ8-E13 with .61-)

hematological disorders (M36.2-M36.3)

hypersensitivity reactions (M36.4)

neoplastic disease (M36.1)

neurosyphillis (A52.16)

sarcoidosis (D86.86)

enteropathic arthropathies (MØ7.-)

juvenile psoriatic arthropathy (L4Ø.54)

lipoid dermatoarthritis (E78.81)

√5th **M14.6 Charcôt's joint**

Neuropathic arthropathy

EXCLUDES 1 *Charcôt's joint in diabetes mellitus (EØ8-E13 with .61Ø)*

Charcôt's joint in tabes dorsalis (A52.16)

DEF: Progressive neurologic arthropathy in which chronic degeneration of joints in the weight-bearing areas with peripheral hypertrophy occurs as a complication of a neuropathy disorder. Supporting structures relax from a loss of sensation resulting in chronic joint instability.

M14.60 Charcôt's joint, unspecified site

√6th M14.61 Charcôt's joint, shoulder

M14.611 Charcôt's joint, right shoulder

M14.612 Charcôt's joint, left shoulder

M14.619 Charcôt's joint, unspecified shoulder

√6th M14.62 Charcôt's joint, elbow

M14.621 Charcôt's joint, right elbow

M14.622 Charcôt's joint, left elbow

M14.629 Charcôt's joint, unspecified elbow

√6th M14.63 Charcôt's joint, wrist

M14.631 Charcôt's joint, right wrist

M14.632 Charcôt's joint, left wrist

M14.639 Charcôt's joint, unspecified wrist

√6th M14.64 Charcôt's joint, hand

M14.641 Charcôt's joint, right hand

M14.642 Charcôt's joint, left hand

M14.649 Charcôt's joint, unspecified hand

√6th M14.65 Charcôt's joint, hip

M14.651 Charcôt's joint, right hip

M14.652 Charcôt's joint, left hip

M14.659 Charcôt's joint, unspecified hip

√6th M14.66 Charcôt's joint, knee

M14.661 Charcôt's joint, right knee

M14.662 Charcôt's joint, left knee

M14.669 Charcôt's joint, unspecified knee

√6th M14.67 Charcôt's joint, ankle and foot

M14.671 Charcôt's joint, right ankle and foot

M14.672 Charcôt's joint, left ankle and foot

M14.679 Charcôt's joint, unspecified ankle and foot

M14.68 Charcôt's joint, vertebrae

M14.69 Charcôt's joint, multiple sites

√5th **M14.8 Arthropathies in other specified diseases classified elsewhere**

Code first underlying disease, such as:

amyloidosis (E85.-)

erythema multiforme (L51.-)

erythema nodosum (L52)

hemochromatosis (E83.11-)

hyperparathyroidism (E21.-)

hypothyroidism (EØØ-EØ3)

sickle-cell disorders (D57.-)

thyrotoxicosis [hyperthyroidism] (EØ5.-)

Whipple's disease (K9Ø.81)

M14.8Ø Arthropathies in other specified diseases classified elsewhere, unspecified site

√6th M14.81 Arthropathies in other specified diseases classified elsewhere, shoulder

M14.811 Arthropathies in other specified diseases classified elsewhere, right shoulder

M14.812 Arthropathies in other specified diseases classified elsewhere, left shoulder

M14.819 Arthropathies in other specified diseases classified elsewhere, unspecified shoulder

M14.82 Arthropathies in other specified diseases classified elsewhere, elbow
- *M14.821 Arthropathies in other specified diseases classified elsewhere, right elbow*
- *M14.822 Arthropathies in other specified diseases classified elsewhere, left elbow*
- *M14.829 Arthropathies in other specified diseases classified elsewhere, unspecified elbow*

M14.83 Arthropathies in other specified diseases classified elsewhere, wrist
- *M14.831 Arthropathies in other specified diseases classified elsewhere, right wrist*
- *M14.832 Arthropathies in other specified diseases classified elsewhere, left wrist*
- *M14.839 Arthropathies in other specified diseases classified elsewhere, unspecified wrist*

M14.84 Arthropathies in other specified diseases classified elsewhere, hand
- *M14.841 Arthropathies in other specified diseases classified elsewhere, right hand*
- *M14.842 Arthropathies in other specified diseases classified elsewhere, left hand*
- *M14.849 Arthropathies in other specified diseases classified elsewhere, unspecified hand*

M14.85 Arthropathies in other specified diseases classified elsewhere, hip
- *M14.851 Arthropathies in other specified diseases classified elsewhere, right hip*
- *M14.852 Arthropathies in other specified diseases classified elsewhere, left hip*
- *M14.859 Arthropathies in other specified diseases classified elsewhere, unspecified hip*

M14.86 Arthropathies in other specified diseases classified elsewhere, knee
- *M14.861 Arthropathies in other specified diseases classified elsewhere, right knee*
- *M14.862 Arthropathies in other specified diseases classified elsewhere, left knee*
- *M14.869 Arthropathies in other specified diseases classified elsewhere, unspecified knee*

M14.87 Arthropathies in other specified diseases classified elsewhere, ankle and foot
- *M14.871 Arthropathies in other specified diseases classified elsewhere, right ankle and foot*
- *M14.872 Arthropathies in other specified diseases classified elsewhere, left ankle and foot*
- *M14.879 Arthropathies in other specified diseases classified elsewhere, unspecified ankle and foot*

M14.88 Arthropathies in other specified diseases classified elsewhere, vertebrae

M14.89 Arthropathies in other specified diseases classified elsewhere, multiple sites

Osteoarthritis (M15-M19)

EXCLUDES 2 *osteoarthritis of spine (M47.-)*

AHA: 2020,2Q,14; 2016,4Q,147

TIP: Assign a primary osteoarthritis code when the site of the osteoarthritis is documented but the type of osteoarthritis — primary, secondary, generalized, or post-traumatic — is not documented. Primary is considered the default.

M15 Polyosteoarthritis

INCLUDES arthritis of multiple sites

EXCLUDES 1 *bilateral involvement of single joint (M16-M19)*

- **M15.Ø Primary generalized (osteo)arthritis**
- **M15.1 Heberden's nodes (with arthropathy)**
  Interphalangeal distal osteoarthritis
- **M15.2 Bouchard's nodes (with arthropathy)**
  Juxtaphalangeal distal osteoarthritis
- **M15.3 Secondary multiple arthritis**
  Post-traumatic polyosteoarthritis
- **M15.4 Erosive (osteo)arthritis**
- **M15.8 Other polyosteoarthritis**
- **M15.9 Polyosteoarthritis, unspecified**
  Generalized osteoarthritis NOS

M16 Osteoarthritis of hip

AHA: 2016,4Q,146

- **M16.Ø Bilateral primary osteoarthritis of hip**
  AHA: 2018,2Q,15
- **M16.1 Unilateral primary osteoarthritis of hip**
  Primary osteoarthritis of hip NOS
  AHA: 2018,2Q,15
  - **M16.1Ø Unilateral primary osteoarthritis, unspecified hip**
  - **M16.11 Unilateral primary osteoarthritis, right hip**
  - **M16.12 Unilateral primary osteoarthritis, left hip**
- **M16.2 Bilateral osteoarthritis resulting from hip dysplasia**
- **M16.3 Unilateral osteoarthritis resulting from hip dysplasia**
  Dysplastic osteoarthritis of hip NOS
  - **M16.3Ø Unilateral osteoarthritis resulting from hip dysplasia, unspecified hip**
  - **M16.31 Unilateral osteoarthritis resulting from hip dysplasia, right hip**
  - **M16.32 Unilateral osteoarthritis resulting from hip dysplasia, left hip**
- **M16.4 Bilateral post-traumatic osteoarthritis of hip**
- **M16.5 Unilateral post-traumatic osteoarthritis of hip**
  Post-traumatic osteoarthritis of hip NOS
  - **M16.5Ø Unilateral post-traumatic osteoarthritis, unspecified hip**
  - **M16.51 Unilateral post-traumatic osteoarthritis, right hip**
  - **M16.52 Unilateral post-traumatic osteoarthritis, left hip**
- **M16.6 Other bilateral secondary osteoarthritis of hip**
- **M16.7 Other unilateral secondary osteoarthritis of hip**
  Secondary osteoarthritis of hip NOS
- **M16.9 Osteoarthritis of hip, unspecified**

M17 Osteoarthritis of knee

AHA: 2016,4Q,146-147

- **M17.Ø Bilateral primary osteoarthritis of knee**
  AHA: 2018,2Q,15
- **M17.1 Unilateral primary osteoarthritis of knee**
  Primary osteoarthritis of knee NOS
  AHA: 2018,2Q,15
  - **M17.1Ø Unilateral primary osteoarthritis, unspecified knee**
  - **M17.11 Unilateral primary osteoarthritis, right knee**
  - **M17.12 Unilateral primary osteoarthritis, left knee**
- **M17.2 Bilateral post-traumatic osteoarthritis of knee**
- **M17.3 Unilateral post-traumatic osteoarthritis of knee**
  Post-traumatic osteoarthritis of knee NOS
  - **M17.3Ø Unilateral post-traumatic osteoarthritis, unspecified knee**
  - **M17.31 Unilateral post-traumatic osteoarthritis, right knee**
  - **M17.32 Unilateral post-traumatic osteoarthritis, left knee**
- **M17.4 Other bilateral secondary osteoarthritis of knee**
- **M17.5 Other unilateral secondary osteoarthritis of knee**
  Secondary osteoarthritis of knee NOS
- **M17.9 Osteoarthritis of knee, unspecified**

M18 Osteoarthritis of first carpometacarpal joint

- **M18.Ø Bilateral primary osteoarthritis of first carpometacarpal joints**
- **M18.1 Unilateral primary osteoarthritis of first carpometacarpal joint**
  Primary osteoarthritis of first carpometacarpal joint NOS
  - **M18.1Ø Unilateral primary osteoarthritis of first carpometacarpal joint, unspecified hand**
  - **M18.11 Unilateral primary osteoarthritis of first carpometacarpal joint, right hand**
  - **M18.12 Unilateral primary osteoarthritis of first carpometacarpal joint, left hand**
- **M18.2 Bilateral post-traumatic osteoarthritis of first carpometacarpal joints**
- **M18.3 Unilateral post-traumatic osteoarthritis of first carpometacarpal joint**
  Post-traumatic osteoarthritis of first carpometacarpal joint NOS
  - **M18.3Ø Unilateral post-traumatic osteoarthritis of first carpometacarpal joint, unspecified hand**
  - **M18.31 Unilateral post-traumatic osteoarthritis of first carpometacarpal joint, right hand**
  - **M18.32 Unilateral post-traumatic osteoarthritis of first carpometacarpal joint, left hand**
- **M18.4 Other bilateral secondary osteoarthritis of first carpometacarpal joints**
- **M18.5 Other unilateral secondary osteoarthritis of first carpometacarpal joint**
  Secondary osteoarthritis of first carpometacarpal joint NOS
  - **M18.5Ø Other unilateral secondary osteoarthritis of first carpometacarpal joint, unspecified hand**

M18.51 Other unilateral secondary osteoarthritis of first carpometacarpal joint, right hand
M18.52 Other unilateral secondary osteoarthritis of first carpometacarpal joint, left hand
M18.9 Osteoarthritis of first carpometacarpal joint, unspecified

✓4th M19 Other and unspecified osteoarthritis

EXCLUDES 1 *polyarthritis (M15.-)*

EXCLUDES 2 *arthrosis of spine (M47.-)*
hallux rigidus (M20.2)
osteoarthritis of spine (M47.-)

AHA: 2020,4Q,31-32

✓5th M19.0 Primary osteoarthritis of other joints

AHA: 2018,2Q,15; 2016,4Q,145

✓6th M19.01 Primary osteoarthritis, shoulder
M19.011 Primary osteoarthritis, right shoulder
M19.012 Primary osteoarthritis, left shoulder
M19.019 Primary osteoarthritis, unspecified shoulder

✓6th M19.02 Primary osteoarthritis, elbow
M19.021 Primary osteoarthritis, right elbow
M19.022 Primary osteoarthritis, left elbow
M19.029 Primary osteoarthritis, unspecified elbow

✓6th M19.03 Primary osteoarthritis, wrist
M19.031 Primary osteoarthritis, right wrist
M19.032 Primary osteoarthritis, left wrist
M19.039 Primary osteoarthritis, unspecified wrist

✓6th M19.04 Primary osteoarthritis, hand

EXCLUDES 2 *primary osteoarthritis of first carpometacarpal joint (M18.0-, M18.1-)*

M19.041 Primary osteoarthritis, right hand
M19.042 Primary osteoarthritis, left hand
M19.049 Primary osteoarthritis, unspecified hand

✓6th M19.07 Primary osteoarthritis ankle and foot
M19.071 Primary osteoarthritis, right ankle and foot
M19.072 Primary osteoarthritis, left ankle and foot
M19.079 Primary osteoarthritis, unspecified ankle and foot

M19.09 Primary osteoarthritis, other specified site

✓5th M19.1 Post-traumatic osteoarthritis of other joints

✓6th M19.11 Post-traumatic osteoarthritis, shoulder
M19.111 Post-traumatic osteoarthritis, right shoulder
M19.112 Post-traumatic osteoarthritis, left shoulder
M19.119 Post-traumatic osteoarthritis, unspecified shoulder

✓6th M19.12 Post-traumatic osteoarthritis, elbow
M19.121 Post-traumatic osteoarthritis, right elbow
M19.122 Post-traumatic osteoarthritis, left elbow
M19.129 Post-traumatic osteoarthritis, unspecified elbow

✓6th M19.13 Post-traumatic osteoarthritis, wrist
M19.131 Post-traumatic osteoarthritis, right wrist
M19.132 Post-traumatic osteoarthritis, left wrist
M19.139 Post-traumatic osteoarthritis, unspecified wrist

✓6th M19.14 Post-traumatic osteoarthritis, hand

EXCLUDES 2 *post-traumatic osteoarthritis of first carpometacarpal joint (M18.2-, M18.3-)*

M19.141 Post-traumatic osteoarthritis, right hand
M19.142 Post-traumatic osteoarthritis, left hand
M19.149 Post-traumatic osteoarthritis, unspecified hand

✓6th M19.17 Post-traumatic osteoarthritis, ankle and foot
M19.171 Post-traumatic osteoarthritis, right ankle and foot
M19.172 Post-traumatic osteoarthritis, left ankle and foot
M19.179 Post-traumatic osteoarthritis, unspecified ankle and foot

M19.19 Post-traumatic osteoarthritis, other specified site

✓5th M19.2 Secondary osteoarthritis of other joints

✓6th M19.21 Secondary osteoarthritis, shoulder
M19.211 Secondary osteoarthritis, right shoulder
M19.212 Secondary osteoarthritis, left shoulder
M19.219 Secondary osteoarthritis, unspecified shoulder

✓6th M19.22 Secondary osteoarthritis, elbow
M19.221 Secondary osteoarthritis, right elbow
M19.222 Secondary osteoarthritis, left elbow
M19.229 Secondary osteoarthritis, unspecified elbow

✓6th M19.23 Secondary osteoarthritis, wrist
M19.231 Secondary osteoarthritis, right wrist
M19.232 Secondary osteoarthritis, left wrist
M19.239 Secondary osteoarthritis, unspecified wrist

✓6th M19.24 Secondary osteoarthritis, hand
M19.241 Secondary osteoarthritis, right hand
M19.242 Secondary osteoarthritis, left hand
M19.249 Secondary osteoarthritis, unspecified hand

✓6th M19.27 Secondary osteoarthritis, ankle and foot
M19.271 Secondary osteoarthritis, right ankle and foot
M19.272 Secondary osteoarthritis, left ankle and foot
M19.279 Secondary osteoarthritis, unspecified ankle and foot

M19.29 Secondary osteoarthritis, other specified site

✓5th M19.9 Osteoarthritis, unspecified site

TIP: Assign M19.90 when neither the site nor the type of osteoarthritis — primary, secondary, or post-traumatic — is documented.

M19.90 Unspecified osteoarthritis, unspecified site
Arthrosis NOS
Arthritis NOS
Osteoarthritis NOS
AHA: 2016,4Q,145-147

M19.91 Primary osteoarthritis, unspecified site
Primary osteoarthritis NOS

M19.92 Post-traumatic osteoarthritis, unspecified site
Post-traumatic osteoarthritis NOS

M19.93 Secondary osteoarthritis, unspecified site
Secondary osteoarthritis NOS

Other joint disorders (M20-M25)

EXCLUDES 2 *joints of the spine (M40-M54)*

✓4th M20 Acquired deformities of fingers and toes

EXCLUDES 1 *acquired absence of fingers and toes (Z89.-)*
congenital absence of fingers and toes (Q71.3-, Q72.3-)
congenital deformities and malformations of fingers and toes (Q66.-, Q68-Q70, Q74.-)

✓5th M20.0 Deformity of finger(s)

EXCLUDES 1 *clubbing of fingers (R68.3)*
palmar fascial fibromatosis [Dupuytren] (M72.0)
trigger finger (M65.3)

✓6th M20.00 Unspecified deformity of finger(s)
M20.001 Unspecified deformity of right finger(s)
M20.002 Unspecified deformity of left finger(s)
M20.009 Unspecified deformity of unspecified finger(s)

✓6th M20.01 Mallet finger
M20.011 Mallet finger of right finger(s)
M20.012 Mallet finger of left finger(s)
M20.019 Mallet finger of unspecified finger(s)

✓6th M20.02 Boutonnière deformity

DEF: Deformity of the finger caused by flexion of the proximal interphalangeal joint and hyperextension of the distal joint. The deformity results from rheumatoid arthritis, osteoarthritis, or injury.

M20.021 Boutonnière deformity of right finger(s)
M20.022 Boutonnière deformity of left finger(s)
M20.029 Boutonnière deformity of unspecified finger(s)

M2Ø.Ø3 Swan-neck deformity

DEF: Flexed distal and hyperextended proximal interphalangeal joint most commonly caused by rheumatoid arthritis.

M2Ø.Ø31 Swan-neck deformity of right finger(s)
M2Ø.Ø32 Swan-neck deformity of left finger(s)
M2Ø.Ø39 Swan-neck deformity of unspecified finger(s)

M2Ø.Ø9 Other deformity of finger(s)

M2Ø.Ø91 Other deformity of right finger(s)
M2Ø.Ø92 Other deformity of left finger(s)
M2Ø.Ø99 Other deformity of finger(s), unspecified finger(s)

M2Ø.1 Hallux valgus (acquired)

EXCLUDES 2 *bunion (M21.6-)*

AHA: 2016,4Q,38

DEF: Deformity in which the great toe deviates toward the other toes and may even be positioned over or under the second toe.

Hallux Valgus

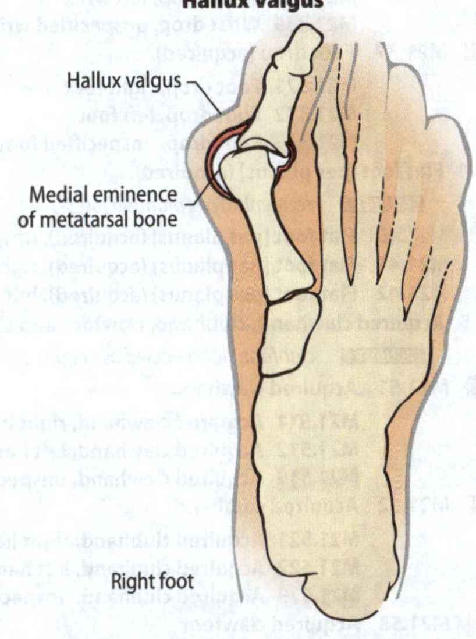

M2Ø.1Ø Hallux valgus (acquired), unspecified foot
M2Ø.11 Hallux valgus (acquired), right foot
M2Ø.12 Hallux valgus (acquired), left foot

M2Ø.2 Hallux rigidus

M2Ø.2Ø Hallux rigidus, unspecified foot
M2Ø.21 Hallux rigidus, right foot
M2Ø.22 Hallux rigidus, left foot

M2Ø.3 Hallux varus (acquired)

DEF: Deformity in which the great toe deviates away from the other toes.

M2Ø.3Ø Hallux varus (acquired), unspecified foot
M2Ø.31 Hallux varus (acquired), right foot
M2Ø.32 Hallux varus (acquired), left foot

M2Ø.4 Other hammer toe(s) (acquired)

M2Ø.4Ø Other hammer toe(s) (acquired), unspecified foot
M2Ø.41 Other hammer toe(s) (acquired), right foot
M2Ø.42 Other hammer toe(s) (acquired), left foot

M2Ø.5 Other deformities of toe(s) (acquired)

M2Ø.5X Other deformities of toe(s) (acquired)

M2Ø.5X1 Other deformities of toe(s) (acquired), right foot
M2Ø.5X2 Other deformities of toe(s) (acquired), left foot
M2Ø.5X9 Other deformities of toe(s) (acquired), unspecified foot

M2Ø.6 Acquired deformities of toe(s), unspecified

M2Ø.6Ø Acquired deformities of toe(s), unspecified, unspecified foot
M2Ø.61 Acquired deformities of toe(s), unspecified, right foot
M2Ø.62 Acquired deformities of toe(s), unspecified, left foot

M21 Other acquired deformities of limbs

EXCLUDES 1 *acquired absence of limb (Z89.-)*
congenital absence of limbs (Q71-Q73)
congenital deformities and malformations of limbs (Q65-Q66, Q68-Q74)

EXCLUDES 2 *acquired deformities of fingers or toes (M2Ø.-)*
coxa plana (M91.2)

M21.Ø Valgus deformity, not elsewhere classified

EXCLUDES 1 *metatarsus valgus (Q66.6)*
talipes calcaneovalgus (Q66.4-)

M21.ØØ Valgus deformity, not elsewhere classified, unspecified site

M21.Ø2 Valgus deformity, not elsewhere classified, elbow

Cubitus valgus

M21.Ø21 Valgus deformity, not elsewhere classified, right elbow
M21.Ø22 Valgus deformity, not elsewhere classified, left elbow
M21.Ø29 Valgus deformity, not elsewhere classified, unspecified elbow

M21.Ø5 Valgus deformity, not elsewhere classified, hip

M21.Ø51 Valgus deformity, not elsewhere classified, right hip
M21.Ø52 Valgus deformity, not elsewhere classified, left hip
M21.Ø59 Valgus deformity, not elsewhere classified, unspecified hip

M21.Ø6 Valgus deformity, not elsewhere classified, knee

Genu valgum
Knock knee

DEF: Genu valga/valgum: Condition in which the thighs slant inward, causing the knees to be angled abnormally close together, leaving the space between the ankles wider than normal.

Genu Valga (knock-knee)

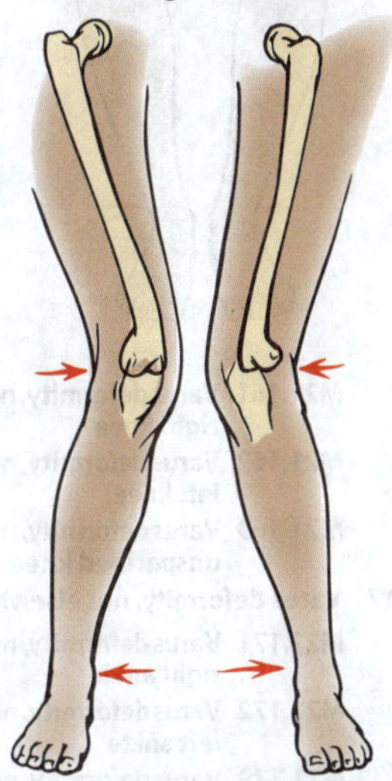

M21.Ø61 Valgus deformity, not elsewhere classified, right knee
M21.Ø62 Valgus deformity, not elsewhere classified, left knee
M21.Ø69 Valgus deformity, not elsewhere classified, unspecified knee

M21.Ø7 Valgus deformity, not elsewhere classified, ankle

M21.Ø71 Valgus deformity, not elsewhere classified, right ankle
M21.Ø72 Valgus deformity, not elsewhere classified, left ankle
M21.Ø79 Valgus deformity, not elsewhere classified, unspecified ankle

M21.1 Varus deformity, not elsewhere classified

EXCLUDES 1 *metatarsus varus (Q66.22-)*
tibia vara (M92.51-)

M21.1Ø Varus deformity, not elsewhere classified, unspecified site

✓6th **M21.12 Varus deformity, not elsewhere classified, elbow**
Cubitus varus, elbow
M21.121 Varus deformity, not elsewhere classified, right elbow
M21.122 Varus deformity, not elsewhere classified, left elbow
M21.129 Varus deformity, not elsewhere classified, unspecified elbow

✓6th **M21.15 Varus deformity, not elsewhere classified, hip**
M21.151 Varus deformity, not elsewhere classified, right hip
M21.152 Varus deformity, not elsewhere classified, left hip
M21.159 Varus deformity, not elsewhere classified, unspecified

✓6th **M21.16 Varus deformity, not elsewhere classified, knee**
Bow leg
Genu varum
DEF: Genu varus/varum: Condition in which the thighs and/or legs are bowed in an outward curve with an abnormally increased space between the knees.

Genu Varus (bowleg)

M21.161 Varus deformity, not elsewhere classified, right knee
M21.162 Varus deformity, not elsewhere classified, left knee
M21.169 Varus deformity, not elsewhere classified, unspecified knee

✓6th **M21.17 Varus deformity, not elsewhere classified, ankle**
M21.171 Varus deformity, not elsewhere classified, right ankle
M21.172 Varus deformity, not elsewhere classified, left ankle
M21.179 Varus deformity, not elsewhere classified, unspecified ankle

✓5th **M21.2 Flexion deformity**
M21.2Ø Flexion deformity, unspecified site

✓6th **M21.21 Flexion deformity, shoulder**
M21.211 Flexion deformity, right shoulder
M21.212 Flexion deformity, left shoulder
M21.219 Flexion deformity, unspecified shoulder

✓6th **M21.22 Flexion deformity, elbow**
M21.221 Flexion deformity, right elbow
M21.222 Flexion deformity, left elbow
M21.229 Flexion deformity, unspecified elbow

✓6th **M21.23 Flexion deformity, wrist**
M21.231 Flexion deformity, right wrist
M21.232 Flexion deformity, left wrist
M21.239 Flexion deformity, unspecified wrist

✓6th **M21.24 Flexion deformity, finger joints**
M21.241 Flexion deformity, right finger joints
M21.242 Flexion deformity, left finger joints
M21.249 Flexion deformity, unspecified finger joints

✓6th **M21.25 Flexion deformity, hip**
M21.251 Flexion deformity, right hip
M21.252 Flexion deformity, left hip
M21.259 Flexion deformity, unspecified hip

✓6th **M21.26 Flexion deformity, knee**
M21.261 Flexion deformity, right knee
M21.262 Flexion deformity, left knee
M21.269 Flexion deformity, unspecified knee

✓6th **M21.27 Flexion deformity, ankle and toes**
M21.271 Flexion deformity, right ankle and toes
M21.272 Flexion deformity, left ankle and toes
M21.279 Flexion deformity, unspecified ankle and toes

✓5th **M21.3 Wrist or foot drop (acquired)**

✓6th **M21.33 Wrist drop (acquired)**
M21.331 Wrist drop, right wrist
M21.332 Wrist drop, left wrist
M21.339 Wrist drop, unspecified wrist

✓6th **M21.37 Foot drop (acquired)**
M21.371 Foot drop, right foot
M21.372 Foot drop, left foot
M21.379 Foot drop, unspecified foot

✓5th **M21.4 Flat foot [pes planus] (acquired)**
EXCLUDES 1 *congenital pes planus (Q66.5-)*
M21.4Ø Flat foot [pes planus] (acquired), unspecified foot
M21.41 Flat foot [pes planus] (acquired), right foot
M21.42 Flat foot [pes planus] (acquired), left foot

✓5th **M21.5 Acquired clawhand, clubhand, clawfoot and clubfoot**
EXCLUDES 1 *clubfoot, not specified as acquired (Q66.89)*

✓6th **M21.51 Acquired clawhand**
M21.511 Acquired clawhand, right hand
M21.512 Acquired clawhand, left hand
M21.519 Acquired clawhand, unspecified hand

✓6th **M21.52 Acquired clubhand**
M21.521 Acquired clubhand, right hand
M21.522 Acquired clubhand, left hand
M21.529 Acquired clubhand, unspecified hand

✓6th **M21.53 Acquired clawfoot**
DEF: High foot arch with hyperextended toes at the metatarsophalangeal joint and flexed toes at the distal joints.
M21.531 Acquired clawfoot, right foot
M21.532 Acquired clawfoot, left foot
M21.539 Acquired clawfoot, unspecified foot

✓6th **M21.54 Acquired clubfoot**
DEF: Acquired anomaly of the foot with the heel elevated and rotated outward and the toes pointing inward.
M21.541 Acquired clubfoot, right foot
M21.542 Acquired clubfoot, left foot
M21.549 Acquired clubfoot, unspecified foot

✓5th **M21.6 Other acquired deformities of foot**
EXCLUDES 2 *deformities of toe (acquired) (M2Ø.1-M2Ø.6-)*
AHA: 2016,4Q,38

✓6th **M21.61 Bunion**
M21.611 Bunion of right foot
M21.612 Bunion of left foot
M21.619 Bunion of unspecified foot

✓6th **M21.62 Bunionette**
M21.621 Bunionette of right foot
M21.622 Bunionette of left foot
M21.629 Bunionette of unspecified foot

✓6th **M21.6X Other acquired deformities of foot**
M21.6X1 Other acquired deformities of right foot
M21.6X2 Other acquired deformities of left foot
M21.6X9 Other acquired deformities of unspecified foot

✓5th **M21.7 Unequal limb length (acquired)**
NOTE The site used should correspond to the shorter limb
M21.7Ø Unequal limb length (acquired), unspecified site

✓6th **M21.72 Unequal limb length (acquired), humerus**
M21.721 Unequal limb length (acquired), right humerus

M21.722 Unequal limb length (acquired), left humerus
M21.729 Unequal limb length (acquired), unspecified humerus

M21.73 Unequal limb length (acquired), ulna and radius
M21.731 Unequal limb length (acquired), right ulna
M21.732 Unequal limb length (acquired), left ulna
M21.733 Unequal limb length (acquired), right radius
M21.734 Unequal limb length (acquired), left radius
M21.739 Unequal limb length (acquired), unspecified ulna and radius

M21.75 Unequal limb length (acquired), femur
M21.751 Unequal limb length (acquired), right femur
M21.752 Unequal limb length (acquired), left femur
M21.759 Unequal limb length (acquired), unspecified femur

M21.76 Unequal limb length (acquired), tibia and fibula
M21.761 Unequal limb length (acquired), right tibia
M21.762 Unequal limb length (acquired), left tibia
M21.763 Unequal limb length (acquired), right fibula
M21.764 Unequal limb length (acquired), left fibula
M21.769 Unequal limb length (acquired), unspecified tibia and fibula

M21.8 Other specified acquired deformities of limbs
EXCLUDES 2 *coxa plana (M91.2)*
M21.80 Other specified acquired deformities of unspecified limb

M21.82 Other specified acquired deformities of upper arm
M21.821 Other specified acquired deformities of right upper arm
M21.822 Other specified acquired deformities of left upper arm
M21.829 Other specified acquired deformities of unspecified upper arm

M21.83 Other specified acquired deformities of forearm
M21.831 Other specified acquired deformities of right forearm
M21.832 Other specified acquired deformities of left forearm
M21.839 Other specified acquired deformities of unspecified forearm

M21.85 Other specified acquired deformities of thigh
M21.851 Other specified acquired deformities of right thigh
M21.852 Other specified acquired deformities of left thigh
M21.859 Other specified acquired deformities of unspecified thigh

M21.86 Other specified acquired deformities of lower leg
M21.861 Other specified acquired deformities of right lower leg
M21.862 Other specified acquired deformities of left lower leg
M21.869 Other specified acquired deformities of unspecified lower leg

M21.9 Unspecified acquired deformity of limb and hand
M21.90 Unspecified acquired deformity of unspecified limb

M21.92 Unspecified acquired deformity of upper arm
M21.921 Unspecified acquired deformity of right upper arm
M21.922 Unspecified acquired deformity of left upper arm
M21.929 Unspecified acquired deformity of unspecified upper arm

M21.93 Unspecified acquired deformity of forearm
M21.931 Unspecified acquired deformity of right forearm
M21.932 Unspecified acquired deformity of left forearm
M21.939 Unspecified acquired deformity of unspecified forearm

M21.94 Unspecified acquired deformity of hand
M21.941 Unspecified acquired deformity of hand, right hand
M21.942 Unspecified acquired deformity of hand, left hand
M21.949 Unspecified acquired deformity of hand, unspecified hand

M21.95 Unspecified acquired deformity of thigh
M21.951 Unspecified acquired deformity of right thigh
M21.952 Unspecified acquired deformity of left thigh
M21.959 Unspecified acquired deformity of unspecified thigh

M21.96 Unspecified acquired deformity of lower leg
M21.961 Unspecified acquired deformity of right lower leg
M21.962 Unspecified acquired deformity of left lower leg
M21.969 Unspecified acquired deformity of unspecified lower leg

M22 Disorder of patella
EXCLUDES 2 *traumatic dislocation of patella (S83.0-)*

M22.0 Recurrent dislocation of patella
M22.00 Recurrent dislocation of patella, unspecified knee
M22.01 Recurrent dislocation of patella, right knee
M22.02 Recurrent dislocation of patella, left knee

M22.1 Recurrent subluxation of patella
Incomplete dislocation of patella
M22.10 Recurrent subluxation of patella, unspecified knee
M22.11 Recurrent subluxation of patella, right knee
M22.12 Recurrent subluxation of patella, left knee

M22.2 Patellofemoral disorders
M22.2X Patellofemoral disorders
M22.2X1 Patellofemoral disorders, right knee
M22.2X2 Patellofemoral disorders, left knee
M22.2X9 Patellofemoral disorders, unspecified knee

M22.3 Other derangements of patella
M22.3X Other derangements of patella
M22.3X1 Other derangements of patella, right knee
M22.3X2 Other derangements of patella, left knee
M22.3X9 Other derangements of patella, unspecified knee

M22.4 Chondromalacia patellae
M22.40 Chondromalacia patellae, unspecified knee
M22.41 Chondromalacia patellae, right knee
M22.42 Chondromalacia patellae, left knee

M22.8 Other disorders of patella
M22.8X Other disorders of patella
M22.8X1 Other disorders of patella, right knee
M22.8X2 Other disorders of patella, left knee
M22.8X9 Other disorders of patella, unspecified knee

M22.9 Unspecified disorder of patella
M22.90 Unspecified disorder of patella, unspecified knee
M22.91 Unspecified disorder of patella, right knee
M22.92 Unspecified disorder of patella, left knee

M23 Internal derangement of knee
EXCLUDES 1 *ankylosis (M24.66)*
deformity of knee (M21.-)
osteochondritis dissecans (M93.2)
EXCLUDES 2 *current injury - see injury of knee and lower leg (S80-S89)*
recurrent dislocation or subluxation of joints (M24.4)
recurrent dislocation or subluxation of patella (M22.0-M22.1)

M23.0 Cystic meniscus
M23.00 Cystic meniscus, unspecified meniscus
Cystic meniscus, unspecified lateral meniscus
Cystic meniscus, unspecified medial meniscus
M23.000 Cystic meniscus, unspecified lateral meniscus, right knee
M23.001 Cystic meniscus, unspecified lateral meniscus, left knee

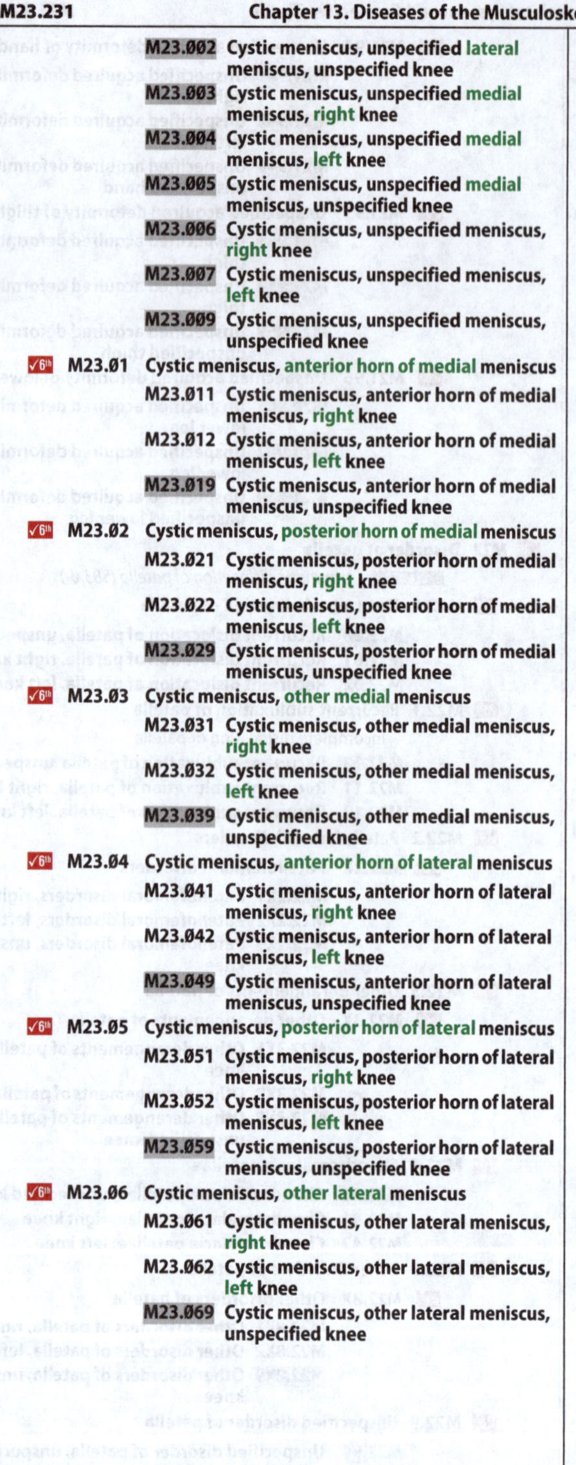

M23.002 Cystic meniscus, unspecified lateral meniscus, unspecified knee

M23.003 Cystic meniscus, unspecified medial meniscus, right knee

M23.004 Cystic meniscus, unspecified medial meniscus, left knee

M23.005 Cystic meniscus, unspecified medial meniscus, unspecified knee

M23.006 Cystic meniscus, unspecified meniscus, right knee

M23.007 Cystic meniscus, unspecified meniscus, left knee

M23.009 Cystic meniscus, unspecified meniscus, unspecified knee

✓6th **M23.01** Cystic meniscus, anterior horn of medial meniscus

- **M23.011** Cystic meniscus, anterior horn of medial meniscus, right knee
- **M23.012** Cystic meniscus, anterior horn of medial meniscus, left knee
- **M23.019** Cystic meniscus, anterior horn of medial meniscus, unspecified knee

✓6th **M23.02** Cystic meniscus, posterior horn of medial meniscus

- **M23.021** Cystic meniscus, posterior horn of medial meniscus, right knee
- **M23.022** Cystic meniscus, posterior horn of medial meniscus, left knee
- **M23.029** Cystic meniscus, posterior horn of medial meniscus, unspecified knee

✓6th **M23.03** Cystic meniscus, other medial meniscus

- **M23.031** Cystic meniscus, other medial meniscus, right knee
- **M23.032** Cystic meniscus, other medial meniscus, left knee
- **M23.039** Cystic meniscus, other medial meniscus, unspecified knee

✓6th **M23.04** Cystic meniscus, anterior horn of lateral meniscus

- **M23.041** Cystic meniscus, anterior horn of lateral meniscus, right knee
- **M23.042** Cystic meniscus, anterior horn of lateral meniscus, left knee
- **M23.049** Cystic meniscus, anterior horn of lateral meniscus, unspecified knee

✓6th **M23.05** Cystic meniscus, posterior horn of lateral meniscus

- **M23.051** Cystic meniscus, posterior horn of lateral meniscus, right knee
- **M23.052** Cystic meniscus, posterior horn of lateral meniscus, left knee
- **M23.059** Cystic meniscus, posterior horn of lateral meniscus, unspecified knee

✓6th **M23.06** Cystic meniscus, other lateral meniscus

- **M23.061** Cystic meniscus, other lateral meniscus, right knee
- **M23.062** Cystic meniscus, other lateral meniscus, left knee
- **M23.069** Cystic meniscus, other lateral meniscus, unspecified knee

✓5th **M23.2 Derangement of meniscus due to old tear or injury**

Old bucket-handle tear

AHA: 2019,2Q,26

Derangement of Meniscus

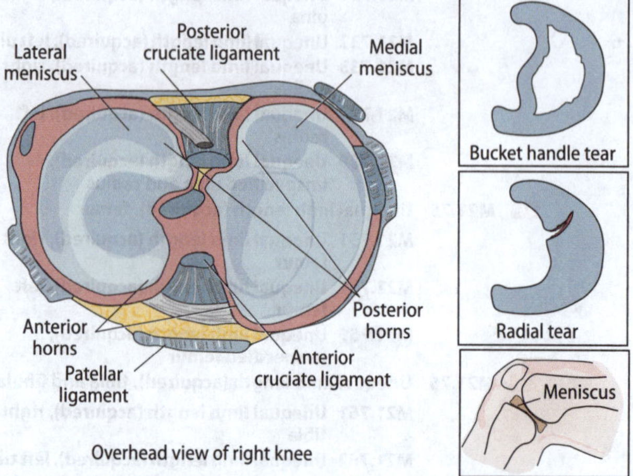

Overhead view of right knee

✓6th **M23.20** Derangement of unspecified meniscus due to old tear or injury

Derangement of unspecified lateral meniscus due to old tear or injury

Derangement of unspecified medial meniscus due to old tear or injury

- **M23.200** Derangement of unspecified lateral meniscus due to old tear or injury, right knee
- **M23.201** Derangement of unspecified lateral meniscus due to old tear or injury, left knee
- **M23.202** Derangement of unspecified lateral meniscus due to old tear or injury, unspecified knee
- **M23.203** Derangement of unspecified medial meniscus due to old tear or injury, right knee
- **M23.204** Derangement of unspecified medial meniscus due to old tear or injury, left knee
- **M23.205** Derangement of unspecified medial meniscus due to old tear or injury, unspecified knee
- **M23.206** Derangement of unspecified meniscus due to old tear or injury, right knee
- **M23.207** Derangement of unspecified meniscus due to old tear or injury, left knee
- **M23.209** Derangement of unspecified meniscus due to old tear or injury, unspecified knee

✓6th **M23.21** Derangement of anterior horn of medial meniscus due to old tear or injury

- **M23.211** Derangement of anterior horn of medial meniscus due to old tear or injury, right knee
- **M23.212** Derangement of anterior horn of medial meniscus due to old tear or injury, left knee
- **M23.219** Derangement of anterior horn of medial meniscus due to old tear or injury, unspecified knee

✓6th **M23.22** Derangement of posterior horn of medial meniscus due to old tear or injury

- **M23.221** Derangement of posterior horn of medial meniscus due to old tear or injury, right knee
- **M23.222** Derangement of posterior horn of medial meniscus due to old tear or injury, left knee
- **M23.229** Derangement of posterior horn of medial meniscus due to old tear or injury, unspecified knee

✓6th **M23.23** Derangement of other medial meniscus due to old tear or injury

- **M23.231** Derangement of other medial meniscus due to old tear or injury, right knee

M23.232 Derangement of other medial meniscus due to old tear or injury, left knee
M23.239 Derangement of other medial meniscus due to old tear or injury, unspecified knee
M23.24 Derangement of anterior horn of lateral meniscus due to old tear or injury
M23.241 Derangement of anterior horn of lateral meniscus due to old tear or injury, right knee
M23.242 Derangement of anterior horn of lateral meniscus due to old tear or injury, left knee
M23.249 Derangement of anterior horn of lateral meniscus due to old tear or injury, unspecified knee
M23.25 Derangement of posterior horn of lateral meniscus due to old tear or injury
M23.251 Derangement of posterior horn of lateral meniscus due to old tear or injury, right knee
M23.252 Derangement of posterior horn of lateral meniscus due to old tear or injury, left knee
M23.259 Derangement of posterior horn of lateral meniscus due to old tear or injury, unspecified knee
M23.26 Derangement of other lateral meniscus due to old tear or injury
M23.261 Derangement of other lateral meniscus due to old tear or injury, right knee
M23.262 Derangement of other lateral meniscus due to old tear or injury, left knee
M23.269 Derangement of other lateral meniscus due to old tear or injury, unspecified knee
M23.3 Other meniscus derangements
Degenerate meniscus
Detached meniscus
Retained meniscus
M23.30 Other meniscus derangements, unspecified meniscus
Other meniscus derangements, unspecified lateral meniscus
Other meniscus derangements, unspecified medial meniscus
M23.300 Other meniscus derangements, unspecified lateral meniscus, right knee
M23.301 Other meniscus derangements, unspecified lateral meniscus, left knee
M23.302 Other meniscus derangements, unspecified lateral meniscus, unspecified knee
M23.303 Other meniscus derangements, unspecified medial meniscus, right knee
M23.304 Other meniscus derangements, unspecified medial meniscus, left knee
M23.305 Other meniscus derangements, unspecified medial meniscus, unspecified knee
M23.306 Other meniscus derangements, unspecified meniscus, right knee
M23.307 Other meniscus derangements, unspecified meniscus, left knee
M23.309 Other meniscus derangements, unspecified meniscus, unspecified knee
M23.31 Other meniscus derangements, anterior horn of medial meniscus
M23.311 Other meniscus derangements, anterior horn of medial meniscus, right knee
M23.312 Other meniscus derangements, anterior horn of medial meniscus, left knee
M23.319 Other meniscus derangements, anterior horn of medial meniscus, unspecified knee
M23.32 Other meniscus derangements, posterior horn of medial meniscus
M23.321 Other meniscus derangements, posterior horn of medial meniscus, right knee
M23.322 Other meniscus derangements, posterior horn of medial meniscus, left knee
M23.329 Other meniscus derangements, posterior horn of medial meniscus, unspecified knee
M23.33 Other meniscus derangements, other medial meniscus
M23.331 Other meniscus derangements, other medial meniscus, right knee
M23.332 Other meniscus derangements, other medial meniscus, left knee
M23.339 Other meniscus derangements, other medial meniscus, unspecified knee
M23.34 Other meniscus derangements, anterior horn of lateral meniscus
M23.341 Other meniscus derangements, anterior horn of lateral meniscus, right knee
M23.342 Other meniscus derangements, anterior horn of lateral meniscus, left knee
M23.349 Other meniscus derangements, anterior horn of lateral meniscus, unspecified knee
M23.35 Other meniscus derangements, posterior horn of lateral meniscus
M23.351 Other meniscus derangements, posterior horn of lateral meniscus, right knee
M23.352 Other meniscus derangements, posterior horn of lateral meniscus, left knee
M23.359 Other meniscus derangements, posterior horn of lateral meniscus, unspecified knee
M23.36 Other meniscus derangements, other lateral meniscus
M23.361 Other meniscus derangements, other lateral meniscus, right knee
M23.362 Other meniscus derangements, other lateral meniscus, left knee
M23.369 Other meniscus derangements, other lateral meniscus, unspecified knee
M23.4 Loose body in knee
M23.40 Loose body in knee, unspecified knee
M23.41 Loose body in knee, right knee
M23.42 Loose body in knee, left knee
M23.5 Chronic instability of knee
M23.50 Chronic instability of knee, unspecified knee
M23.51 Chronic instability of knee, right knee
M23.52 Chronic instability of knee, left knee
M23.6 Other spontaneous disruption of ligament(s) of knee
M23.60 Other spontaneous disruption of unspecified ligament of knee
M23.601 Other spontaneous disruption of unspecified ligament of right knee
M23.602 Other spontaneous disruption of unspecified ligament of left knee
M23.609 Other spontaneous disruption of unspecified ligament of unspecified knee
M23.61 Other spontaneous disruption of anterior cruciate ligament of knee
M23.611 Other spontaneous disruption of anterior cruciate ligament of right knee
M23.612 Other spontaneous disruption of anterior cruciate ligament of left knee
M23.619 Other spontaneous disruption of anterior cruciate ligament of unspecified knee
M23.62 Other spontaneous disruption of posterior cruciate ligament of knee
M23.621 Other spontaneous disruption of posterior cruciate ligament of right knee
M23.622 Other spontaneous disruption of posterior cruciate ligament of left knee
M23.629 Other spontaneous disruption of posterior cruciate ligament of unspecified knee
M23.63 Other spontaneous disruption of medial collateral ligament of knee
M23.631 Other spontaneous disruption of medial collateral ligament of right knee
M23.632 Other spontaneous disruption of medial collateral ligament of left knee
M23.639 Other spontaneous disruption of medial collateral ligament of unspecified knee
M23.64 Other spontaneous disruption of lateral collateral ligament of knee
M23.641 Other spontaneous disruption of lateral collateral ligament of right knee
M23.642 Other spontaneous disruption of lateral collateral ligament of left knee

M23.649 Other spontaneous disruption of lateral collateral ligament of unspecified knee

M23.67 Other spontaneous disruption of capsular ligament of knee

M23.671 Other spontaneous disruption of capsular ligament of right knee

M23.672 Other spontaneous disruption of capsular ligament of left knee

M23.679 Other spontaneous disruption of capsular ligament of unspecified knee

M23.8 Other internal derangements of knee

Laxity of ligament of knee
Snapping knee

M23.8X Other internal derangements of knee

M23.8X1 Other internal derangements of right knee

M23.8X2 Other internal derangements of left knee

M23.8X9 Other internal derangements of unspecified knee

M23.9 Unspecified internal derangement of knee

M23.90 Unspecified internal derangement of unspecified knee

M23.91 Unspecified internal derangement of right knee

M23.92 Unspecified internal derangement of left knee

M24 Other specific joint derangements

EXCLUDES 1 *current injury - see injury of joint by body region*

EXCLUDES 2 *ganglion (M67.4)*
snapping knee (M23.8-)
temporomandibular joint disorders (M26.6-)

AHA: 2020,4Q,31-32

M24.0 Loose body in joint

EXCLUDES 2 *loose body in knee (M23.4)*

M24.00 Loose body in unspecified joint

M24.01 Loose body in shoulder

M24.011 Loose body in right shoulder

M24.012 Loose body in left shoulder

M24.019 Loose body in unspecified shoulder

M24.02 Loose body in elbow

M24.021 Loose body in right elbow

M24.022 Loose body in left elbow

M24.029 Loose body in unspecified elbow

M24.03 Loose body in wrist

M24.031 Loose body in right wrist

M24.032 Loose body in left wrist

M24.039 Loose body in unspecified wrist

M24.04 Loose body in finger joints

M24.041 Loose body in right finger joint(s)

M24.042 Loose body in left finger joint(s)

M24.049 Loose body in unspecified finger joint(s)

M24.05 Loose body in hip

M24.051 Loose body in right hip

M24.052 Loose body in left hip

M24.059 Loose body in unspecified hip

M24.07 Loose body in ankle and toe joints

M24.071 Loose body in right ankle

M24.072 Loose body in left ankle

M24.073 Loose body in unspecified ankle

M24.074 Loose body in right toe joint(s)

M24.075 Loose body in left toe joint(s)

M24.076 Loose body in unspecified toe joints

M24.08 Loose body, other site

M24.1 Other articular cartilage disorders

EXCLUDES 2 *chondrocalcinosis (M11.1, M11.2-)*
internal derangement of knee (M23.-)
metastatic calcification (E83.5)
ochronosis (E70.2)

M24.10 Other articular cartilage disorders, unspecified site

M24.11 Other articular cartilage disorders, shoulder

M24.111 Other articular cartilage disorders, right shoulder

M24.112 Other articular cartilage disorders, left shoulder

M24.119 Other articular cartilage disorders, unspecified shoulder

M24.12 Other articular cartilage disorders, elbow

M24.121 Other articular cartilage disorders, right elbow

M24.122 Other articular cartilage disorders, left elbow

M24.129 Other articular cartilage disorders, unspecified elbow

M24.13 Other articular cartilage disorders, wrist

M24.131 Other articular cartilage disorders, right wrist

M24.132 Other articular cartilage disorders, left wrist

M24.139 Other articular cartilage disorders, unspecified wrist

M24.14 Other articular cartilage disorders, hand

M24.141 Other articular cartilage disorders, right hand

M24.142 Other articular cartilage disorders, left hand

M24.149 Other articular cartilage disorders, unspecified hand

M24.15 Other articular cartilage disorders, hip

M24.151 Other articular cartilage disorders, right hip

M24.152 Other articular cartilage disorders, left hip

M24.159 Other articular cartilage disorders, unspecified hip

M24.17 Other articular cartilage disorders, ankle and foot

M24.171 Other articular cartilage disorders, right ankle

M24.172 Other articular cartilage disorders, left ankle

M24.173 Other articular cartilage disorders, unspecified ankle

M24.174 Other articular cartilage disorders, right foot

M24.175 Other articular cartilage disorders, left foot

M24.176 Other articular cartilage disorders, unspecified foot

M24.19 Other articular cartilage disorders, other specified site

M24.2 Disorder of ligament

Instability secondary to old ligament injury
Ligamentous laxity NOS

EXCLUDES 1 *familial ligamentous laxity (M35.7)*

EXCLUDES 2 *internal derangement of knee (M23.5-M23.8X9)*

M24.20 Disorder of ligament, unspecified site

M24.21 Disorder of ligament, shoulder

M24.211 Disorder of ligament, right shoulder

M24.212 Disorder of ligament, left shoulder

M24.219 Disorder of ligament, unspecified shoulder

M24.22 Disorder of ligament, elbow

M24.221 Disorder of ligament, right elbow

M24.222 Disorder of ligament, left elbow

M24.229 Disorder of ligament, unspecified elbow

M24.23 Disorder of ligament, wrist

M24.231 Disorder of ligament, right wrist

M24.232 Disorder of ligament, left wrist

M24.239 Disorder of ligament, unspecified wrist

M24.24 Disorder of ligament, hand

M24.241 Disorder of ligament, right hand

M24.242 Disorder of ligament, left hand

M24.249 Disorder of ligament, unspecified hand

M24.25 Disorder of ligament, hip

M24.251 Disorder of ligament, right hip

M24.252 Disorder of ligament, left hip

M24.259 Disorder of ligament, unspecified hip

M24.27 Disorder of ligament, ankle and foot

M24.271 Disorder of ligament, right ankle

M24.272 Disorder of ligament, left ankle

M24.273 Disorder of ligament, unspecified ankle

M24.274 Disorder of ligament, right foot

M24.275 Disorder of ligament, left foot

M24.276 Disorder of ligament, unspecified foot

M24.28 Disorder of ligament, vertebrae

M24.29 Disorder of ligament, other specified site

✓5th M24.3 Pathological dislocation of joint, not elsewhere classified

EXCLUDES 1 *congenital dislocation or displacement of joint - see congenital malformations and deformations of the musculoskeletal system (Q65-Q79)*
current injury - see injury of joints and ligaments by body region
recurrent dislocation of joint (M24.4-)

M24.30 Pathological dislocation of unspecified joint, not elsewhere classified

✓6th M24.31 Pathological dislocation of shoulder, not elsewhere classified
- M24.311 Pathological dislocation of right shoulder, not elsewhere classified
- M24.312 Pathological dislocation of left shoulder, not elsewhere classified
- M24.319 Pathological dislocation of unspecified shoulder, not elsewhere classified

✓6th M24.32 Pathological dislocation of elbow, not elsewhere classified
- M24.321 Pathological dislocation of right elbow, not elsewhere classified
- M24.322 Pathological dislocation of left elbow, not elsewhere classified
- M24.329 Pathological dislocation of unspecified elbow, not elsewhere classified

✓6th M24.33 Pathological dislocation of wrist, not elsewhere classified
- M24.331 Pathological dislocation of right wrist, not elsewhere classified
- M24.332 Pathological dislocation of left wrist, not elsewhere classified
- M24.339 Pathological dislocation of unspecified wrist, not elsewhere classified

✓6th M24.34 Pathological dislocation of hand, not elsewhere classified
- M24.341 Pathological dislocation of right hand, not elsewhere classified
- M24.342 Pathological dislocation of left hand, not elsewhere classified
- M24.349 Pathological dislocation of unspecified hand, not elsewhere classified

✓6th M24.35 Pathological dislocation of hip, not elsewhere classified
AHA: 2022,1Q,32
- M24.351 Pathological dislocation of right hip, not elsewhere classified
- M24.352 Pathological dislocation of left hip, not elsewhere classified
- M24.359 Pathological dislocation of unspecified hip, not elsewhere classified

✓6th M24.36 Pathological dislocation of knee, not elsewhere classified
- M24.361 Pathological dislocation of right knee, not elsewhere classified
- M24.362 Pathological dislocation of left knee, not elsewhere classified
- M24.369 Pathological dislocation of unspecified knee, not elsewhere classified

✓6th M24.37 Pathological dislocation of ankle and foot, not elsewhere classified
- M24.371 Pathological dislocation of right ankle, not elsewhere classified
- M24.372 Pathological dislocation of left ankle, not elsewhere classified
- M24.373 Pathological dislocation of unspecified ankle, not elsewhere classified
- M24.374 Pathological dislocation of right foot, not elsewhere classified
- M24.375 Pathological dislocation of left foot, not elsewhere classified
- M24.376 Pathological dislocation of unspecified foot, not elsewhere classified

M24.39 Pathological dislocation of other specified joint, not elsewhere classified

✓5th M24.4 Recurrent dislocation of joint

Recurrent subluxation of joint

EXCLUDES 2 *recurrent dislocation of patella (M22.0-M22.1)*
recurrent vertebral dislocation (M43.3-, M43.4, M43.5-)

M24.40 Recurrent dislocation, unspecified joint

✓6th M24.41 Recurrent dislocation, shoulder
- M24.411 Recurrent dislocation, right shoulder
- M24.412 Recurrent dislocation, left shoulder
- M24.419 Recurrent dislocation, unspecified shoulder

✓6th M24.42 Recurrent dislocation, elbow
- M24.421 Recurrent dislocation, right elbow
- M24.422 Recurrent dislocation, left elbow
- M24.429 Recurrent dislocation, unspecified elbow

✓6th M24.43 Recurrent dislocation, wrist
- M24.431 Recurrent dislocation, right wrist
- M24.432 Recurrent dislocation, left wrist
- M24.439 Recurrent dislocation, unspecified wrist

✓6th M24.44 Recurrent dislocation, hand and finger(s)
- M24.441 Recurrent dislocation, right hand
- M24.442 Recurrent dislocation, left hand
- M24.443 Recurrent dislocation, unspecified hand
- M24.444 Recurrent dislocation, right finger
- M24.445 Recurrent dislocation, left finger
- M24.446 Recurrent dislocation, unspecified finger

✓6th M24.45 Recurrent dislocation, hip
- M24.451 Recurrent dislocation, right hip
- M24.452 Recurrent dislocation, left hip
- M24.459 Recurrent dislocation, unspecified hip

✓6th M24.46 Recurrent dislocation, knee
- M24.461 Recurrent dislocation, right knee
- M24.462 Recurrent dislocation, left knee
- M24.469 Recurrent dislocation, unspecified knee

✓6th M24.47 Recurrent dislocation, ankle, foot and toes
- M24.471 Recurrent dislocation, right ankle
- M24.472 Recurrent dislocation, left ankle
- M24.473 Recurrent dislocation, unspecified ankle
- M24.474 Recurrent dislocation, right foot
- M24.475 Recurrent dislocation, left foot
- M24.476 Recurrent dislocation, unspecified foot
- M24.477 Recurrent dislocation, right toe(s)
- M24.478 Recurrent dislocation, left toe(s)
- M24.479 Recurrent dislocation, unspecified toe(s)

M24.49 Recurrent dislocation, other specified joint

✓5th M24.5 Contracture of joint

EXCLUDES 1 *contracture of muscle without contracture of joint (M62.4-)*
contracture of tendon (sheath) without contracture of joint (M62.4-)
Dupuytren's contracture (M72.0)

EXCLUDES 2 *acquired deformities of limbs (M20-M21)*

AHA: 2016,2Q,6

M24.50 Contracture, unspecified joint

✓6th M24.51 Contracture, shoulder
- M24.511 Contracture, right shoulder
- M24.512 Contracture, left shoulder
- M24.519 Contracture, unspecified shoulder

✓6th M24.52 Contracture, elbow
- M24.521 Contracture, right elbow
- M24.522 Contracture, left elbow
- M24.529 Contracture, unspecified elbow

✓6th M24.53 Contracture, wrist
- M24.531 Contracture, right wrist
- M24.532 Contracture, left wrist
- M24.539 Contracture, unspecified wrist

✓6th M24.54 Contracture, hand
- M24.541 Contracture, right hand
- M24.542 Contracture, left hand
- M24.549 Contracture, unspecified hand

✓6th M24.55 Contracture, hip
- M24.551 Contracture, right hip
- M24.552 Contracture, left hip
- M24.559 Contracture, unspecified hip

✓6th M24.56 Contracture, knee
- M24.561 Contracture, right knee
- M24.562 Contracture, left knee
- M24.569 Contracture, unspecified knee

✓6th M24.57 Contracture, ankle and foot
- M24.571 Contracture, right ankle
- M24.572 Contracture, left ankle

M24.573 Contracture, unspecified ankle
M24.574 Contracture, right foot
M24.575 Contracture, left foot
M24.576 Contracture, unspecified foot
M24.59 Contracture, other specified joint

M24.6 Ankylosis of joint
EXCLUDES 1 *stiffness of joint without ankylosis (M25.6-)*
EXCLUDES 2 *spine (M43.2-)*
DEF: Ankylosis: Abnormal union or fusion of bones in a joint, which is normally moveable.

M24.60 Ankylosis, unspecified joint
M24.61 Ankylosis, shoulder
M24.611 Ankylosis, right shoulder
M24.612 Ankylosis, left shoulder
M24.619 Ankylosis, unspecified shoulder
M24.62 Ankylosis, elbow
M24.621 Ankylosis, right elbow
M24.622 Ankylosis, left elbow
M24.629 Ankylosis, unspecified elbow
M24.63 Ankylosis, wrist
M24.631 Ankylosis, right wrist
M24.632 Ankylosis, left wrist
M24.639 Ankylosis, unspecified wrist
M24.64 Ankylosis, hand
M24.641 Ankylosis, right hand
M24.642 Ankylosis, left hand
M24.649 Ankylosis, unspecified hand
M24.65 Ankylosis, hip
M24.651 Ankylosis, right hip
M24.652 Ankylosis, left hip
M24.659 Ankylosis, unspecified hip
M24.66 Ankylosis, knee
M24.661 Ankylosis, right knee
M24.662 Ankylosis, left knee
M24.669 Ankylosis, unspecified knee
M24.67 Ankylosis, ankle and foot
M24.671 Ankylosis, right ankle
M24.672 Ankylosis, left ankle
M24.673 Ankylosis, unspecified ankle
M24.674 Ankylosis, right foot
M24.675 Ankylosis, left foot
M24.676 Ankylosis, unspecified foot
M24.69 Ankylosis, other specified joint

M24.7 Protrusio acetabuli
DEF: Intrapelvic protrusion of the acetabulum characterized by the sinking of the floor of the acetabulum, causing the femoral head to protrude. It limits hip movement and is of unknown etiology. ***Synonym(s):*** *Otto's pelvis.*

M24.8 Other specific joint derangements, not elsewhere classified
EXCLUDES 2 *iliotibial band syndrome (M76.3)*

M24.80 Other specific joint derangements of unspecified joint, not elsewhere classified
M24.81 Other specific joint derangements of shoulder, not elsewhere classified
M24.811 Other specific joint derangements of right shoulder, not elsewhere classified
M24.812 Other specific joint derangements of left shoulder, not elsewhere classified
M24.819 Other specific joint derangements of unspecified shoulder, not elsewhere classified
M24.82 Other specific joint derangements of elbow, not elsewhere classified
M24.821 Other specific joint derangements of right elbow, not elsewhere classified
M24.822 Other specific joint derangements of left elbow, not elsewhere classified
M24.829 Other specific joint derangements of unspecified elbow, not elsewhere classified
M24.83 Other specific joint derangements of wrist, not elsewhere classified
M24.831 Other specific joint derangements of right wrist, not elsewhere classified
M24.832 Other specific joint derangements of left wrist, not elsewhere classified
M24.839 Other specific joint derangements of unspecified wrist, not elsewhere classified
M24.84 Other specific joint derangements of hand, not elsewhere classified
M24.841 Other specific joint derangements of right hand, not elsewhere classified
M24.842 Other specific joint derangements of left hand, not elsewhere classified
M24.849 Other specific joint derangements of unspecified hand, not elsewhere classified
M24.85 Other specific joint derangements of hip, not elsewhere classified
Irritable hip
M24.851 Other specific joint derangements of right hip, not elsewhere classified
M24.852 Other specific joint derangements of left hip, not elsewhere classified
M24.859 Other specific joint derangements of unspecified hip, not elsewhere classified
M24.87 Other specific joint derangements of ankle and foot, not elsewhere classified
M24.871 Other specific joint derangements of right ankle, not elsewhere classified
M24.872 Other specific joint derangements of left ankle, not elsewhere classified
M24.873 Other specific joint derangements of unspecified ankle, not elsewhere classified
M24.874 Other specific joint derangements of right foot, not elsewhere classified
M24.875 Other specific joint derangements left foot, not elsewhere classified
M24.876 Other specific joint derangements of unspecified foot, not elsewhere classified
M24.89 Other specific joint derangement of other specified joint, not elsewhere classified

M24.9 Joint derangement, unspecified

M25 Other joint disorder, not elsewhere classified
EXCLUDES 2 *abnormality of gait and mobility (R26.-)*
acquired deformities of limb (M2Ø-M21)
calcification of bursa (M71.4-)
calcification of shoulder (joint) (M75.3)
calcification of tendon (M65.2-)
difficulty in walking (R26.2)
temporomandibular joint disorder (M26.6-)
AHA: 2020,4Q,31-32

M25.Ø Hemarthrosis
EXCLUDES 1 *current injury - see injury of joint by body region*
hemophilic arthropathy (M36.2)

M25.ØØ Hemarthrosis, unspecified joint
M25.Ø1 Hemarthrosis, shoulder
M25.Ø11 Hemarthrosis, right shoulder
M25.Ø12 Hemarthrosis, left shoulder
M25.Ø19 Hemarthrosis, unspecified shoulder
M25.Ø2 Hemarthrosis, elbow
M25.Ø21 Hemarthrosis, right elbow
M25.Ø22 Hemarthrosis, left elbow
M25.Ø29 Hemarthrosis, unspecified elbow
M25.Ø3 Hemarthrosis, wrist
M25.Ø31 Hemarthrosis, right wrist
M25.Ø32 Hemarthrosis, left wrist
M25.Ø39 Hemarthrosis, unspecified wrist
M25.Ø4 Hemarthrosis, hand
M25.Ø41 Hemarthrosis, right hand
M25.Ø42 Hemarthrosis, left hand
M25.Ø49 Hemarthrosis, unspecified hand
M25.Ø5 Hemarthrosis, hip
M25.Ø51 Hemarthrosis, right hip
M25.Ø52 Hemarthrosis, left hip
M25.Ø59 Hemarthrosis, unspecified hip
M25.Ø6 Hemarthrosis, knee
M25.Ø61 Hemarthrosis, right knee
M25.Ø62 Hemarthrosis, left knee
M25.Ø69 Hemarthrosis, unspecified knee
M25.Ø7 Hemarthrosis, ankle and foot
M25.Ø71 Hemarthrosis, right ankle
M25.Ø72 Hemarthrosis, left ankle
M25.Ø73 Hemarthrosis, unspecified ankle
M25.Ø74 Hemarthrosis, right foot

M25.Ø75 Hemarthrosis, left foot
M25.Ø76 Hemarthrosis, unspecified foot
M25.Ø8 Hemarthrosis, other specified site
Hemarthrosis, vertebrae

✓5th M25.1 Fistula of joint
M25.1Ø Fistula, unspecified joint
✓6th M25.11 Fistula, shoulder
M25.111 Fistula, right shoulder
M25.112 Fistula, left shoulder
M25.119 Fistula, unspecified shoulder
✓6th M25.12 Fistula, elbow
M25.121 Fistula, right elbow
M25.122 Fistula, left elbow
M25.129 Fistula, unspecified elbow
✓6th M25.13 Fistula, wrist
M25.131 Fistula, right wrist
M25.132 Fistula, left wrist
M25.139 Fistula, unspecified wrist
✓6th M25.14 Fistula, hand
M25.141 Fistula, right hand
M25.142 Fistula, left hand
M25.149 Fistula, unspecified hand
✓6th M25.15 Fistula, hip
M25.151 Fistula, right hip
M25.152 Fistula, left hip
M25.159 Fistula, unspecified hip
✓6th M25.16 Fistula, knee
M25.161 Fistula, right knee
M25.162 Fistula, left knee
M25.169 Fistula, unspecified knee
✓6th M25.17 Fistula, ankle and foot
M25.171 Fistula, right ankle
M25.172 Fistula, left ankle
M25.173 Fistula, unspecified ankle
M25.174 Fistula, right foot
M25.175 Fistula, left foot
M25.176 Fistula, unspecified foot
M25.18 Fistula, other specified site
Fistula, vertebrae

✓5th M25.2 Flail joint
DEF: Hinged joint that exhibits an abnormal or excessive degree of range and mobility.
M25.2Ø Flail joint, unspecified joint
✓6th M25.21 Flail joint, shoulder
M25.211 Flail joint, right shoulder
M25.212 Flail joint, left shoulder
M25.219 Flail joint, unspecified shoulder
✓6th M25.22 Flail joint, elbow
M25.221 Flail joint, right elbow
M25.222 Flail joint, left elbow
M25.229 Flail joint, unspecified elbow
✓6th M25.23 Flail joint, wrist
M25.231 Flail joint, right wrist
M25.232 Flail joint, left wrist
M25.239 Flail joint, unspecified wrist
✓6th M25.24 Flail joint, hand
M25.241 Flail joint, right hand
M25.242 Flail joint, left hand
M25.249 Flail joint, unspecified hand
✓6th M25.25 Flail joint, hip
M25.251 Flail joint, right hip
M25.252 Flail joint, left hip
M25.259 Flail joint, unspecified hip
✓6th M25.26 Flail joint, knee
M25.261 Flail joint, right knee
M25.262 Flail joint, left knee
M25.269 Flail joint, unspecified knee
✓6th M25.27 Flail joint, ankle and foot
M25.271 Flail joint, right ankle and foot
M25.272 Flail joint, left ankle and foot
M25.279 Flail joint, unspecified ankle and foot
M25.28 Flail joint, other site

✓5th M25.3 Other instability of joint
EXCLUDES 1 *instability of joint secondary to old ligament injury (M24.2-)*
instability of joint secondary to removal of joint prosthesis (M96.8-)
EXCLUDES 2 *spinal instabilities (M53.2-)*
M25.3Ø Other instability, unspecified joint
✓6th M25.31 Other instability, shoulder
M25.311 Other instability, right shoulder
M25.312 Other instability, left shoulder
M25.319 Other instability, unspecified shoulder
✓6th M25.32 Other instability, elbow
M25.321 Other instability, right elbow
M25.322 Other instability, left elbow
M25.329 Other instability, unspecified elbow
✓6th M25.33 Other instability, wrist
M25.331 Other instability, right wrist
M25.332 Other instability, left wrist
M25.339 Other instability, unspecified wrist
✓6th M25.34 Other instability, hand
M25.341 Other instability, right hand
M25.342 Other instability, left hand
M25.349 Other instability, unspecified hand
✓6th M25.35 Other instability, hip
M25.351 Other instability, right hip
M25.352 Other instability, left hip
M25.359 Other instability, unspecified hip
✓6th M25.36 Other instability, knee
M25.361 Other instability, right knee
M25.362 Other instability, left knee
M25.369 Other instability, unspecified knee
✓6th M25.37 Other instability, ankle and foot
M25.371 Other instability, right ankle
M25.372 Other instability, left ankle
M25.373 Other instability, unspecified ankle
M25.374 Other instability, right foot
M25.375 Other instability, left foot
M25.376 Other instability, unspecified foot
M25.39 Other instability, other specified joint

✓5th M25.4 Effusion of joint
EXCLUDES 1 *hydrarthrosis in yaws (A66.6)*
intermittent hydrarthrosis (M12.4-)
other infective (teno)synovitis (M65.1-)
M25.4Ø Effusion, unspecified joint
✓6th M25.41 Effusion, shoulder
M25.411 Effusion, right shoulder
M25.412 Effusion, left shoulder
M25.419 Effusion, unspecified shoulder
✓6th M25.42 Effusion, elbow
M25.421 Effusion, right elbow
M25.422 Effusion, left elbow
M25.429 Effusion, unspecified elbow
✓6th M25.43 Effusion, wrist
M25.431 Effusion, right wrist
M25.432 Effusion, left wrist
M25.439 Effusion, unspecified wrist
✓6th M25.44 Effusion, hand
M25.441 Effusion, right hand
M25.442 Effusion, left hand
M25.449 Effusion, unspecified hand
✓6th M25.45 Effusion, hip
M25.451 Effusion, right hip
M25.452 Effusion, left hip
M25.459 Effusion, unspecified hip
✓6th M25.46 Effusion, knee
M25.461 Effusion, right knee
M25.462 Effusion, left knee
M25.469 Effusion, unspecified knee
✓6th M25.47 Effusion, ankle and foot
M25.471 Effusion, right ankle
M25.472 Effusion, left ankle
M25.473 Effusion, unspecified ankle
M25.474 Effusion, right foot
M25.475 Effusion, left foot
M25.476 Effusion, unspecified foot

M25.48 Effusion, other site

✓5th **M25.5 Pain in joint**

EXCLUDES 2 *pain in hand (M79.64-)*
pain in fingers (M79.64-)
pain in foot (M79.67-)
pain in limb (M79.6-)
pain in toes (M79.67-)

M25.50 Pain in unspecified joint

✓6th **M25.51 Pain in shoulder**
M25.511 Pain in right shoulder
M25.512 Pain in left shoulder
M25.519 Pain in unspecified shoulder

✓6th **M25.52 Pain in elbow**
M25.521 Pain in right elbow
M25.522 Pain in left elbow
M25.529 Pain in unspecified elbow

✓6th **M25.53 Pain in wrist**
M25.531 Pain in right wrist
M25.532 Pain in left wrist
M25.539 Pain in unspecified wrist

✓6th **M25.54 Pain in joints of hand**
AHA: 2016,4Q,38
M25.541 Pain in joints of right hand
M25.542 Pain in joints of left hand
M25.549 Pain in joints of unspecified hand
Pain in joints of hand NOS

✓6th **M25.55 Pain in hip**
M25.551 Pain in right hip
M25.552 Pain in left hip
M25.559 Pain in unspecified hip

✓6th **M25.56 Pain in knee**
M25.561 Pain in right knee
M25.562 Pain in left knee
M25.569 Pain in unspecified knee

✓6th **M25.57 Pain in ankle and joints of foot**
M25.571 Pain in right ankle and joints of right foot
M25.572 Pain in left ankle and joints of left foot
M25.579 Pain in unspecified ankle and joints of unspecified foot

M25.59 Pain in other specified joint

✓5th **M25.6 Stiffness of joint, not elsewhere classified**

EXCLUDES 1 *ankylosis of joint (M24.6-)*
contracture of joint (M24.5-)

M25.60 Stiffness of unspecified joint, not elsewhere classified

✓6th **M25.61 Stiffness of shoulder, not elsewhere classified**
M25.611 Stiffness of right shoulder, not elsewhere classified
M25.612 Stiffness of left shoulder, not elsewhere classified
M25.619 Stiffness of unspecified shoulder, not elsewhere classified

✓6th **M25.62 Stiffness of elbow, not elsewhere classified**
M25.621 Stiffness of right elbow, not elsewhere classified
M25.622 Stiffness of left elbow, not elsewhere classified
M25.629 Stiffness of unspecified elbow, not elsewhere classified

✓6th **M25.63 Stiffness of wrist, not elsewhere classified**
M25.631 Stiffness of right wrist, not elsewhere classified
M25.632 Stiffness of left wrist, not elsewhere classified
M25.639 Stiffness of unspecified wrist, not elsewhere classified

✓6th **M25.64 Stiffness of hand, not elsewhere classified**
M25.641 Stiffness of right hand, not elsewhere classified
M25.642 Stiffness of left hand, not elsewhere classified
M25.649 Stiffness of unspecified hand, not elsewhere classified

✓6th **M25.65 Stiffness of hip, not elsewhere classified**
M25.651 Stiffness of right hip, not elsewhere classified
M25.652 Stiffness of left hip, not elsewhere classified
M25.659 Stiffness of unspecified hip, not elsewhere classified

✓6th **M25.66 Stiffness of knee, not elsewhere classified**
M25.661 Stiffness of right knee, not elsewhere classified
M25.662 Stiffness of left knee, not elsewhere classified
M25.669 Stiffness of unspecified knee, not elsewhere classified

✓6th **M25.67 Stiffness of ankle and foot, not elsewhere classified**
M25.671 Stiffness of right ankle, not elsewhere classified
M25.672 Stiffness of left ankle, not elsewhere classified
M25.673 Stiffness of unspecified ankle, not elsewhere classified
M25.674 Stiffness of right foot, not elsewhere classified
M25.675 Stiffness of left foot, not elsewhere classified
M25.676 Stiffness of unspecified foot, not elsewhere classified

M25.69 Stiffness of other specified joint, not elsewhere classified

✓5th **M25.7 Osteophyte**

M25.70 Osteophyte, unspecified joint

✓6th **M25.71 Osteophyte, shoulder**
M25.711 Osteophyte, right shoulder
M25.712 Osteophyte, left shoulder
M25.719 Osteophyte, unspecified shoulder

✓6th **M25.72 Osteophyte, elbow**
M25.721 Osteophyte, right elbow
M25.722 Osteophyte, left elbow
M25.729 Osteophyte, unspecified elbow

✓6th **M25.73 Osteophyte, wrist**
M25.731 Osteophyte, right wrist
M25.732 Osteophyte, left wrist
M25.739 Osteophyte, unspecified wrist

✓6th **M25.74 Osteophyte, hand**
M25.741 Osteophyte, right hand
M25.742 Osteophyte, left hand
M25.749 Osteophyte, unspecified hand

✓6th **M25.75 Osteophyte, hip**
M25.751 Osteophyte, right hip
M25.752 Osteophyte, left hip
M25.759 Osteophyte, unspecified hip

✓6th **M25.76 Osteophyte, knee**
M25.761 Osteophyte, right knee
M25.762 Osteophyte, left knee
M25.769 Osteophyte, unspecified knee

✓6th **M25.77 Osteophyte, ankle and foot**
M25.771 Osteophyte, right ankle
M25.772 Osteophyte, left ankle
M25.773 Osteophyte, unspecified ankle
M25.774 Osteophyte, right foot
M25.775 Osteophyte, left foot
M25.776 Osteophyte, unspecified foot

M25.78 Osteophyte, vertebrae

✓5th **M25.8 Other specified joint disorders**

M25.80 Other specified joint disorders, unspecified joint

✓6th **M25.81 Other specified joint disorders, shoulder**
M25.811 Other specified joint disorders, right shoulder
M25.812 Other specified joint disorders, left shoulder
M25.819 Other specified joint disorders, unspecified shoulder

✓6th **M25.82 Other specified joint disorders, elbow**
M25.821 Other specified joint disorders, right elbow
M25.822 Other specified joint disorders, left elbow
M25.829 Other specified joint disorders, unspecified elbow

✓6th **M25.83 Other specified joint disorders, wrist**
M25.831 Other specified joint disorders, right wrist

M25.832 Other specified joint disorders, left wrist
M25.839 Other specified joint disorders, unspecified wrist
✓6th M25.84 Other specified joint disorders, hand
M25.841 Other specified joint disorders, right hand
M25.842 Other specified joint disorders, left hand
M25.849 Other specified joint disorders, unspecified hand
✓6th M25.85 Other specified joint disorders, hip
AHA: 2014,4Q,25
M25.851 Other specified joint disorders, right hip
M25.852 Other specified joint disorders, left hip
M25.859 Other specified joint disorders, unspecified hip
✓6th M25.86 Other specified joint disorders, knee
M25.861 Other specified joint disorders, right knee
M25.862 Other specified joint disorders, left knee
M25.869 Other specified joint disorders, unspecified knee
✓6th M25.87 Other specified joint disorders, ankle and foot
M25.871 Other specified joint disorders, right ankle and foot
M25.872 Other specified joint disorders, left ankle and foot
M25.879 Other specified joint disorders, unspecified ankle and foot
M25.9 Joint disorder, unspecified

Dentofacial anomalies [including malocclusion] and other disorders of jaw (M26-M27)

EXCLUDES 1 *hemifacial atrophy or hypertrophy (Q67.4)*
unilateral condylar hyperplasia or hypoplasia (M27.8)

✓4th M26 Dentofacial anomalies [including malocclusion]
✓5th M26.0 Major anomalies of jaw size
EXCLUDES 1 *acromegaly (E22.0)*
Robin's syndrome (Q87.0)
M26.00 Unspecified anomaly of jaw size
M26.01 Maxillary hyperplasia
M26.02 Maxillary hypoplasia
AHA: 2014,3Q,23
M26.03 Mandibular hyperplasia
M26.04 Mandibular hypoplasia
M26.05 Macrogenia
M26.06 Microgenia
M26.07 Excessive tuberosity of jaw
Entire maxillary tuberosity
M26.09 Other specified anomalies of jaw size
✓5th M26.1 Anomalies of jaw-cranial base relationship
M26.10 Unspecified anomaly of jaw-cranial base relationship
M26.11 Maxillary asymmetry
M26.12 Other jaw asymmetry
M26.19 Other specified anomalies of jaw-cranial base relationship
AHA: 2020,1Q,21
✓5th M26.2 Anomalies of dental arch relationship
M26.20 Unspecified anomaly of dental arch relationship
✓6th M26.21 Malocclusion, Angle's class
M26.211 Malocclusion, Angle's class I
Neutro-occlusion
M26.212 Malocclusion, Angle's class II
Disto-occlusion Division I
Disto-occlusion Division II
M26.213 Malocclusion, Angle's class III
Mesio-occlusion
M26.219 Malocclusion, Angle's class, unspecified
✓6th M26.22 Open occlusal relationship
M26.220 Open anterior occlusal relationship
Anterior open bite
M26.221 Open posterior occlusal relationship
Posterior open bite
M26.23 Excessive horizontal overlap
Excessive horizontal overjet
M26.24 Reverse articulation
Crossbite (anterior) (posterior)
M26.25 Anomalies of interarch distance
M26.29 Other anomalies of dental arch relationship
Midline deviation of dental arch
Overbite (excessive) deep
Overbite (excessive) horizontal
Overbite (excessive) vertical
Posterior lingual occlusion of mandibular teeth
✓5th M26.3 Anomalies of tooth position of fully erupted tooth or teeth
EXCLUDES 2 *embedded and impacted teeth (K01.-)*
M26.30 Unspecified anomaly of tooth position of fully erupted tooth or teeth
Abnormal spacing of fully erupted tooth or teeth NOS
Displacement of fully erupted tooth or teeth NOS
Transposition of fully erupted tooth or teeth NOS
M26.31 Crowding of fully erupted teeth
M26.32 Excessive spacing of fully erupted teeth
Diastema of fully erupted tooth or teeth NOS
M26.33 Horizontal displacement of fully erupted tooth or teeth
Tipped tooth or teeth
Tipping of fully erupted tooth
M26.34 Vertical displacement of fully erupted tooth or teeth
Extruded tooth
Infraeruption of tooth or teeth
Supraeruption of tooth or teeth
M26.35 Rotation of fully erupted tooth or teeth
M26.36 Insufficient interocclusal distance of fully erupted teeth (ridge)
Lack of adequate intermaxillary vertical dimension of fully erupted teeth
M26.37 Excessive interocclusal distance of fully erupted teeth
Excessive intermaxillary vertical dimension of fully erupted teeth
Loss of occlusal vertical dimension of fully erupted teeth
M26.39 Other anomalies of tooth position of fully erupted tooth or teeth
M26.4 Malocclusion, unspecified
✓5th M26.5 Dentofacial functional abnormalities
EXCLUDES 1 *bruxism (F45.8)*
teeth-grinding NOS (F45.8)
M26.50 Dentofacial functional abnormalities, unspecified
M26.51 Abnormal jaw closure
M26.52 Limited mandibular range of motion
M26.53 Deviation in opening and closing of the mandible
M26.54 Insufficient anterior guidance
Insufficient anterior occlusal guidance
M26.55 Centric occlusion maximum intercuspation discrepancy
EXCLUDES 1 *centric occlusion NOS (M26.59)*
M26.56 Non-working side interference
Balancing side interference
M26.57 Lack of posterior occlusal support
M26.59 Other dentofacial functional abnormalities
Centric occlusion (of teeth) NOS
Malocclusion due to abnormal swallowing
Malocclusion due to mouth breathing
Malocclusion due to tongue, lip or finger habits

M26.6 Temporomandibular joint disorders (5th)

EXCLUDES 2 *current temporomandibular joint dislocation (S03.0)*
current temporomandibular joint sprain (S03.4)

AHA: 2016,4Q,38-39

Temporomandibular Joint

Cutaway detail
Upper joint space
Articular disc (meniscus)
Lower joint space
Condyle
Mandible

Cutaway view of temporomandibular joint (TMJ)

M26.60 Temporomandibular joint disorder, unspecified (6th)

M26.601 Right temporomandibular joint disorder, unspecified

M26.602 Left temporomandibular joint disorder, unspecified

M26.603 Bilateral temporomandibular joint disorder, unspecified

M26.609 Unspecified temporomandibular joint disorder, unspecified side
Temporomandibular joint disorder NOS

M26.61 Adhesions and ankylosis of temporomandibular joint (6th)

M26.611 Adhesions and ankylosis of right temporomandibular joint

M26.612 Adhesions and ankylosis of left temporomandibular joint

M26.613 Adhesions and ankylosis of bilateral temporomandibular joint

M26.619 Adhesions and ankylosis of temporomandibular joint, unspecified side

M26.62 Arthralgia of temporomandibular joint (6th)

M26.621 Arthralgia of right temporomandibular joint

M26.622 Arthralgia of left temporomandibular joint

M26.623 Arthralgia of bilateral temporomandibular joint

M26.629 Arthralgia of temporomandibular joint, unspecified side

M26.63 Articular disc disorder of temporomandibular joint (6th)

M26.631 Articular disc disorder of right temporomandibular joint

M26.632 Articular disc disorder of left temporomandibular joint

M26.633 Articular disc disorder of bilateral temporomandibular joint

M26.639 Articular disc disorder of temporomandibular joint, unspecified side

M26.64 Arthritis of temporomandibular joint (6th)

AHA: 2020,4Q,32

M26.641 Arthritis of right temporomandibular joint

M26.642 Arthritis of left temporomandibular joint

M26.643 Arthritis of bilateral temporomandibular joint

M26.649 Arthritis of unspecified temporomandibular joint

M26.65 Arthropathy of temporomandibular joint (6th)

AHA: 2020,4Q,32

M26.651 Arthropathy of right temporomandibular joint

M26.652 Arthropathy of left temporomandibular joint

M26.653 Arthropathy of bilateral temporomandibular joint

M26.659 Arthropathy of unspecified temporomandibular joint

M26.69 Other specified disorders of temporomandibular joint

M26.7 Dental alveolar anomalies (5th)

M26.70 Unspecified alveolar anomaly

M26.71 Alveolar maxillary hyperplasia

M26.72 Alveolar mandibular hyperplasia

M26.73 Alveolar maxillary hypoplasia

M26.74 Alveolar mandibular hypoplasia

M26.79 Other specified alveolar anomalies

M26.8 Other dentofacial anomalies (5th)

M26.81 Anterior soft tissue impingement
Anterior soft tissue impingement on teeth

M26.82 Posterior soft tissue impingement
Posterior soft tissue impingement on teeth

M26.89 Other dentofacial anomalies

M26.9 Dentofacial anomaly, unspecified

M27 Other diseases of jaws (4th)

M27.0 Developmental disorders of jaws
Latent bone cyst of jaw
Stafne's cyst
Torus mandibularis
Torus palatinus

M27.1 Giant cell granuloma, central
Giant cell granuloma NOS

EXCLUDES 1 *peripheral giant cell granuloma (K06.8)*

M27.2 Inflammatory conditions of jaws
Osteitis of jaw(s)
Osteomyelitis (neonatal) jaw(s)
Osteoradionecrosis jaw(s)
Periostitis jaw(s)
Sequestrum of jaw bone
Use additional code (W88-W90, X39.0) to identify radiation, if radiation-induced

EXCLUDES 2 *osteonecrosis of jaw due to drug (M87.180)*

M27.3 Alveolitis of jaws
Alveolar osteitis
Dry socket

M27.4 Other and unspecified cysts of jaw (5th)

EXCLUDES 1 *cysts of oral region (K09.-)*
latent bone cyst of jaw (M27.0)
Stafne's cyst (M27.0)

M27.40 Unspecified cyst of jaw
Cyst of jaw NOS

M27.49 Other cysts of jaw
Aneurysmal cyst of jaw
Hemorrhagic cyst of jaw
Traumatic cyst of jaw

M27.5 Periradicular pathology associated with previous endodontic treatment (5th)

M27.51 Perforation of root canal space due to endodontic treatment

M27.52 Endodontic overfill

M27.53 Endodontic underfill

M27.59 Other periradicular pathology associated with previous endodontic treatment

M27.6 Endosseous dental implant failure (5th)

M27.61 Osseointegration failure of dental implant
Hemorrhagic complication of dental implant placement
Iatrogenic osseointegration failure of dental implant
Osseointegration failure of dental implant due to complications of systemic disease
Osseointegration failure of dental implant due to poor bone quality
Pre-integration failure of dental implant NOS
Pre-osseointegration failure of dental implant

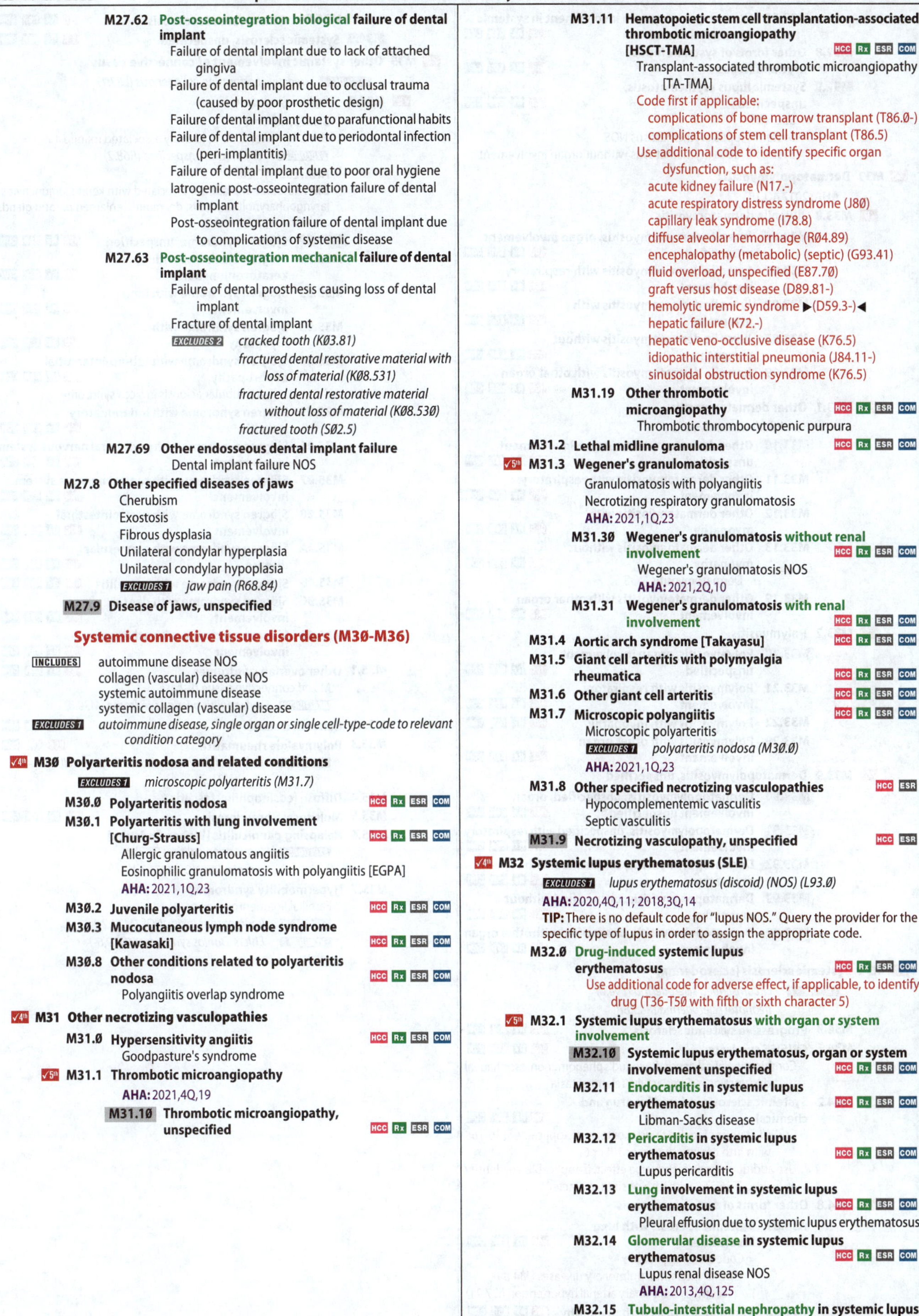

M27.62 Post-osseointegration biological failure of dental implant
Failure of dental implant due to lack of attached gingiva
Failure of dental implant due to occlusal trauma (caused by poor prosthetic design)
Failure of dental implant due to parafunctional habits
Failure of dental implant due to periodontal infection (peri-implantitis)
Failure of dental implant due to poor oral hygiene
Iatrogenic post-osseointegration failure of dental implant
Post-osseointegration failure of dental implant due to complications of systemic disease

M27.63 Post-osseointegration mechanical failure of dental implant
Failure of dental prosthesis causing loss of dental implant
Fracture of dental implant
EXCLUDES 2 *cracked tooth (KØ3.81)*
fractured dental restorative material with loss of material (KØ8.531)
fractured dental restorative material without loss of material (KØ8.53Ø)
fractured tooth (SØ2.5)

M27.69 Other endosseous dental implant failure
Dental implant failure NOS

M27.8 Other specified diseases of jaws
Cherubism
Exostosis
Fibrous dysplasia
Unilateral condylar hyperplasia
Unilateral condylar hypoplasia
EXCLUDES 1 *jaw pain (R68.84)*

M27.9 Disease of jaws, unspecified

Systemic connective tissue disorders (M3Ø-M36)

INCLUDES autoimmune disease NOS
collagen (vascular) disease NOS
systemic autoimmune disease
systemic collagen (vascular) disease

EXCLUDES 1 *autoimmune disease, single organ or single cell-type-code to relevant condition category*

M3Ø Polyarteritis nodosa and related conditions
EXCLUDES 1 *microscopic polyarteritis (M31.7)*

M3Ø.Ø Polyarteritis nodosa HCC Rx ESR COM

M3Ø.1 Polyarteritis with lung involvement [Churg-Strauss] HCC Rx ESR COM
Allergic granulomatous angiitis
Eosinophilic granulomatosis with polyangiitis [EGPA]
AHA: 2021,1Q,23

M3Ø.2 Juvenile polyarteritis HCC Rx ESR COM

M3Ø.3 Mucocutaneous lymph node syndrome [Kawasaki] HCC Rx ESR COM

M3Ø.8 Other conditions related to polyarteritis nodosa HCC Rx ESR COM
Polyangiitis overlap syndrome

M31 Other necrotizing vasculopathies

M31.Ø Hypersensitivity angiitis HCC Rx ESR COM
Goodpasture's syndrome

M31.1 Thrombotic microangiopathy
AHA: 2021,4Q,19

M31.1Ø Thrombotic microangiopathy, unspecified HCC Rx ESR COM

M31.11 Hematopoietic stem cell transplantation-associated thrombotic microangiopathy [HSCT-TMA] HCC Rx ESR COM
Transplant-associated thrombotic microangiopathy [TA-TMA]
Code first if applicable:
complications of bone marrow transplant (T86.Ø-)
complications of stem cell transplant (T86.5)
Use additional code to identify specific organ dysfunction, such as:
acute kidney failure (N17.-)
acute respiratory distress syndrome (J8Ø)
capillary leak syndrome (I78.8)
diffuse alveolar hemorrhage (RØ4.89)
encephalopathy (metabolic) (septic) (G93.41)
fluid overload, unspecified (E87.7Ø)
graft versus host disease (D89.81-)
hemolytic uremic syndrome ▶(D59.3-)◀
hepatic failure (K72.-)
hepatic veno-occlusive disease (K76.5)
idiopathic interstitial pneumonia (J84.11-)
sinusoidal obstruction syndrome (K76.5)

M31.19 Other thrombotic microangiopathy HCC Rx ESR COM
Thrombotic thrombocytopenic purpura

M31.2 Lethal midline granuloma HCC Rx ESR COM

M31.3 Wegener's granulomatosis
Granulomatosis with polyangiitis
Necrotizing respiratory granulomatosis
AHA: 2021,1Q,23

M31.3Ø Wegener's granulomatosis without renal involvement HCC Rx ESR COM
Wegener's granulomatosis NOS
AHA: 2021,2Q,10

M31.31 Wegener's granulomatosis with renal involvement HCC Rx ESR COM

M31.4 Aortic arch syndrome [Takayasu] HCC Rx ESR COM

M31.5 Giant cell arteritis with polymyalgia rheumatica HCC Rx ESR COM

M31.6 Other giant cell arteritis HCC Rx ESR COM

M31.7 Microscopic polyangiitis HCC Rx ESR COM
Microscopic polyarteritis
EXCLUDES 1 *polyarteritis nodosa (M3Ø.Ø)*
AHA: 2021,1Q,23

M31.8 Other specified necrotizing vasculopathies HCC ESR
Hypocomplementemic vasculitis
Septic vasculitis

M31.9 Necrotizing vasculopathy, unspecified HCC ESR

M32 Systemic lupus erythematosus (SLE)
EXCLUDES 1 *lupus erythematosus (discoid) (NOS) (L93.Ø)*
AHA: 2020,4Q,11; 2018,3Q,14
TIP: There is no default code for "lupus NOS." Query the provider for the specific type of lupus in order to assign the appropriate code.

M32.Ø Drug-induced systemic lupus erythematosus HCC Rx ESR COM
Use additional code for adverse effect, if applicable, to identify drug (T36-T5Ø with fifth or sixth character 5)

M32.1 Systemic lupus erythematosus with organ or system involvement

M32.1Ø Systemic lupus erythematosus, organ or system involvement unspecified HCC Rx ESR COM

M32.11 Endocarditis in systemic lupus erythematosus HCC Rx ESR COM
Libman-Sacks disease

M32.12 Pericarditis in systemic lupus erythematosus HCC Rx ESR COM
Lupus pericarditis

M32.13 Lung involvement in systemic lupus erythematosus HCC Rx ESR COM
Pleural effusion due to systemic lupus erythematosus

M32.14 Glomerular disease in systemic lupus erythematosus HCC Rx ESR COM
Lupus renal disease NOS
AHA: 2013,4Q,125

M32.15 Tubulo-interstitial nephropathy in systemic lupus erythematosus HCC Rx ESR COM

M32.19 Other organ or system involvement in systemic lupus erythematosus HCC Rx ESR COM

M32.8 Other forms of systemic lupus erythematosus HCC Rx ESR COM

M32.9 Systemic lupus erythematosus, unspecified HCC Rx ESR COM
SLE NOS
Systemic lupus erythematosus NOS
Systemic lupus erythematosus without organ involvement

✓4th M33 Dermatopolymyositis
AHA: 2017,4Q,18

✓5th M33.0 Juvenile dermatomyositis

M33.00 Juvenile dermatomyositis, organ involvement unspecified HCC Rx ESR COM

M33.01 Juvenile dermatomyositis with respiratory involvement HCC Rx ESR COM

M33.02 Juvenile dermatomyositis with myopathy HCC Rx ESR COM

M33.03 Juvenile dermatomyositis without myopathy HCC Rx ESR COM

M33.09 Juvenile dermatomyositis with other organ involvement HCC Rx ESR COM

✓5th M33.1 Other dermatomyositis
Adult dermatomyositis

M33.10 Other dermatomyositis, organ involvement unspecified HCC Rx ESR COM

M33.11 Other dermatomyositis with respiratory involvement HCC Rx ESR COM

M33.12 Other dermatomyositis with myopathy HCC Rx ESR COM

M33.13 Other dermatomyositis without myopathy HCC Rx ESR COM
Dermatomyositis NOS

M33.19 Other dermatomyositis with other organ involvement HCC Rx ESR COM

✓5th M33.2 Polymyositis

M33.20 Polymyositis, organ involvement unspecified HCC Rx ESR COM

M33.21 Polymyositis with respiratory involvement HCC Rx ESR COM

M33.22 Polymyositis with myopathy HCC Rx ESR COM

M33.29 Polymyositis with other organ involvement HCC Rx ESR COM

✓5th M33.9 Dermatopolymyositis, unspecified

M33.90 Dermatopolymyositis, unspecified, organ involvement unspecified HCC Rx ESR COM

M33.91 Dermatopolymyositis, unspecified with respiratory involvement HCC Rx ESR COM

M33.92 Dermatopolymyositis, unspecified with myopathy HCC Rx ESR COM

M33.93 Dermatopolymyositis, unspecified without myopathy HCC Rx ESR COM

M33.99 Dermatopolymyositis, unspecified with other organ involvement HCC Rx ESR COM

✓4th M34 Systemic sclerosis [scleroderma]
EXCLUDES 1 *circumscribed scleroderma (L94.0)*
neonatal scleroderma (P83.88)

M34.0 Progressive systemic sclerosis HCC Rx ESR COM

M34.1 CR(E)ST syndrome HCC Rx ESR COM
Combination of calcinosis, Raynaud's phenomenon, esophageal dysfunction, sclerodactyly, telangiectasia

M34.2 Systemic sclerosis induced by drug and chemical HCC Rx ESR COM
Code first poisoning due to drug or toxin, if applicable (T36-T65 with fifth or sixth character 1-4 or 6)
Use additional code for adverse effect, if applicable, to identify drug (T36-T50 with fifth or sixth character 5)

✓5th M34.8 Other forms of systemic sclerosis

M34.81 Systemic sclerosis with lung involvement HCC Rx ESR COM
Code also if applicable:
other interstitial pulmonary diseases (J84.89)
secondary pulmonary arterial hypertension (I27.21)

M34.82 Systemic sclerosis with myopathy HCC Rx ESR COM

M34.83 Systemic sclerosis with polyneuropathy HCC Rx ESR COM

M34.89 Other systemic sclerosis HCC Rx ESR COM

M34.9 Systemic sclerosis, unspecified HCC Rx ESR COM

✓4th M35 Other systemic involvement of connective tissue
EXCLUDES 1 *reactive perforating collagenosis (L87.1)*

✓5th M35.0 Sjögren syndrome
Sicca syndrome
Use additional code to identify associated manifestations
EXCLUDES 1 *dry mouth, unspecified (R68.2)*
AHA: 2021,4Q,20
DEF: Autoimmune disease associated with keratoconjunctivitis, laryngopharyngitis, rhinitis, dry mouth, enlarged parotid gland, and chronic polyarthritis.

M35.00 Sjögren syndrome, unspecified HCC Rx ESR COM

M35.01 Sjögren syndrome with keratoconjunctivitis HCC Rx ESR COM

M35.02 Sjögren syndrome with lung involvement HCC Rx ESR COM

M35.03 Sjögren syndrome with myopathy HCC Rx ESR COM

M35.04 Sjögren syndrome with tubulo-interstitial nephropathy HCC Rx ESR COM
Renal tubular acidosis in sicca syndrome

M35.05 Sjögren syndrome with inflammatory arthritis HCC Rx ESR COM

M35.06 Sjögren syndrome with peripheral nervous system involvement HCC Rx ESR COM

M35.07 Sjögren syndrome with central nervous system involvement HCC Rx ESR COM

M35.08 Sjögren syndrome with gastrointestinal involvement HCC Rx ESR COM

M35.0A Sjögren syndrome with glomerular disease HCC Rx ESR COM

M35.0B Sjögren syndrome with vasculitis HCC Rx ESR COM

M35.0C Sjögren syndrome with dental involvement HCC Rx ESR COM

M35.09 Sjögren syndrome with other organ involvement HCC Rx ESR COM

M35.1 Other overlap syndromes HCC Rx ESR COM
Mixed connective tissue disease
EXCLUDES 1 *polyangiitis overlap syndrome (M30.8)*

M35.2 Behçet's disease HCC Rx ESR COM

M35.3 Polymyalgia rheumatica HCC ESR COM
EXCLUDES 1 *polymyalgia rheumatica with giant cell arteritis (M31.5)*

M35.4 Diffuse (eosinophilic) fasciitis

M35.5 Multifocal fibrosclerosis HCC Rx ESR COM

M35.6 Relapsing panniculitis [Weber-Christian]
EXCLUDES 1 *lupus panniculitis (L93.2)*
panniculitis NOS (M79.3-)

M35.7 Hypermobility syndrome
Familial ligamentous laxity
EXCLUDES 1 *ligamentous laxity, NOS (M24.2-)*
EXCLUDES 2 *Ehlers-Danlos syndromes (Q79.6-)*

M35.8 Other specified systemic involvement of connective tissue
AHA: 2021,1Q,36; 2020,3Q,13-14

M35.81 Multisystem inflammatory syndrome HCC ESR COM
MIS-A
MIS-C
Multisystem inflammatory syndrome in adults
Multisystem inflammatory syndrome in children
Pediatric inflammatory multisystem syndrome
PIMS
Code first, if applicable, COVID-19 (UØ7.1)
Code also any associated complications such as:
- acute hepatic failure (K72.Ø-)
- acute kidney failure (N17.-)
- acute myocarditis (I4Ø.-)
- acute respiratory distress syndrome (J8Ø)
- cardiac arrhythmia (I47-I49.-)
- pneumonia due to COVID-19 (J12.82)
- severe sepsis (R65.2-)
- viral cardiomyopathy (B33.24)
- viral pericarditis (B33.23)

Use additional code, if applicable, for:
- exposure to COVID-19 or SARS-CoV-2 infection (Z2Ø.822)
- personal history of COVID-19 (Z86.16)
- post COVID-19 condition (UØ9.9)

AHA: 2021,4Q,102; 2021,1Q,29,36,41
DEF: Hyperinflammatory condition that seems to be largely associated with past or present coronavirus disease 2019 (COVID-19) infection. Predominantly occurring in children, with less frequent occurrences in adults, symptoms often include fever, laboratory evidence of inflammation, and evidence of clinically severe illness requiring hospitalization with multisystem (two or more) organ involvement. ***Synonym(s): MIS, MIS-C.***

M35.89 Other specified systemic involvement of connective tissue HCC Rx ESR COM

M35.9 Systemic involvement of connective tissue, unspecified HCC Rx ESR COM
Autoimmune disease (systemic) NOS
Collagen (vascular) disease NOS

M36 Systemic disorders of connective tissue in diseases classified elsewhere
EXCLUDES 2 *arthropathies in diseases classified elsewhere (M14.-)*

M36.Ø Dermato(poly)myositis in neoplastic disease HCC Rx ESR COM
Code first underlying neoplasm (CØØ-D49)

M36.1 Arthropathy in neoplastic disease
Code first underlying neoplasm, such as:
- leukemia (C91-C95)
- malignant histiocytosis (C96.A)
- multiple myeloma (C9Ø.Ø)

M36.2 Hemophilic arthropathy
Hemarthrosis in hemophilic arthropathy
Code first underlying disease, such as:
- factor VIII deficiency (D66)
  - with vascular defect ▶(D68.Ø-)◀
- factor IX deficiency (D67)
- hemophilia (classical) (D66)
- hemophilia B (D67)
- hemophilia C (D68.1)

M36.3 Arthropathy in other blood disorders

M36.4 Arthropathy in hypersensitivity reactions classified elsewhere
Code first underlying disease, such as:
- Henoch (-Schönlein) purpura (D69.Ø)
- serum sickness (T8Ø.6-)

M36.8 Systemic disorders of connective tissue in other diseases classified elsewhere HCC Rx ESR COM
Code first underlying disease, such as:
- alkaptonuria (E7Ø.2)
- hypogammaglobulinemia (D8Ø.-)
- ochronosis (E7Ø.2)

DORSOPATHIES (M4Ø-M54)

Deforming dorsopathies (M4Ø-M43)

M4Ø Kyphosis and lordosis
Code first underlying disease
EXCLUDES 1 *congenital kyphosis and lordosis (Q76.4)*
kyphoscoliosis (M41.-)
postprocedural kyphosis and lordosis (M96.-)

Kyphosis and Lordosis

M4Ø.Ø Postural kyphosis
EXCLUDES 1 *osteochondrosis of spine (M42.-)*

M4Ø.ØØ Postural kyphosis, site unspecified
M4Ø.Ø3 Postural kyphosis, cervicothoracic region
M4Ø.Ø4 Postural kyphosis, thoracic region
M4Ø.Ø5 Postural kyphosis, thoracolumbar region

M4Ø.1 Other secondary kyphosis
M4Ø.1Ø Other secondary kyphosis, site unspecified UPD
M4Ø.12 Other secondary kyphosis, cervical region UPD
M4Ø.13 Other secondary kyphosis, cervicothoracic region UPD
M4Ø.14 Other secondary kyphosis, thoracic region UPD
M4Ø.15 Other secondary kyphosis, thoracolumbar region UPD

M4Ø.2 Other and unspecified kyphosis
M4Ø.2Ø Unspecified kyphosis
M4Ø.2Ø2 Unspecified kyphosis, cervical region
M4Ø.2Ø3 Unspecified kyphosis, cervicothoracic region
M4Ø.2Ø4 Unspecified kyphosis, thoracic region
M4Ø.2Ø5 Unspecified kyphosis, thoracolumbar region
M4Ø.2Ø9 Unspecified kyphosis, site unspecified
M4Ø.29 Other kyphosis
M4Ø.292 Other kyphosis, cervical region
M4Ø.293 Other kyphosis, cervicothoracic region
M4Ø.294 Other kyphosis, thoracic region
M4Ø.295 Other kyphosis, thoracolumbar region
M4Ø.299 Other kyphosis, site unspecified

M4Ø.3 Flatback syndrome
M4Ø.3Ø Flatback syndrome, site unspecified
M4Ø.35 Flatback syndrome, thoracolumbar region
M4Ø.36 Flatback syndrome, lumbar region
M4Ø.37 Flatback syndrome, lumbosacral region

M4Ø.4 Postural lordosis
Acquired lordosis
M4Ø.4Ø Postural lordosis, site unspecified
M4Ø.45 Postural lordosis, thoracolumbar region
M4Ø.46 Postural lordosis, lumbar region
M4Ø.47 Postural lordosis, lumbosacral region

M4Ø.5 Lordosis, unspecified
M4Ø.5Ø Lordosis, unspecified, site unspecified
M4Ø.55 Lordosis, unspecified, thoracolumbar region
M4Ø.56 Lordosis, unspecified, lumbar region
M4Ø.57 Lordosis, unspecified, lumbosacral region

✓4th M41 Scoliosis

INCLUDES kyphoscoliosis

EXCLUDES 1 *congenital scoliosis due to bony malformation (Q76.3)*
congenital scoliosis NOS (Q67.5)
kyphoscoliotic heart disease (I27.1)
postural congenital scoliosis (Q67.5)

EXCLUDES 2 *postprocedural scoliosis (M96.-)*

AHA: 2022,1Q,30

Scoliosis

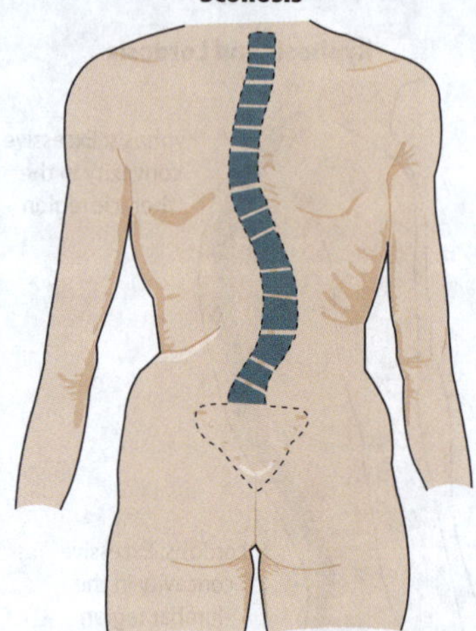

Lateral curvature of spine

✓5th M41.Ø Infantile idiopathic scoliosis

AHA: 2014,4Q,26

- **M41.ØØ** Infantile idiopathic scoliosis, site unspecified
- **M41.Ø2** Infantile idiopathic scoliosis, cervical region
- **M41.Ø3** Infantile idiopathic scoliosis, cervicothoracic region
- **M41.Ø4** Infantile idiopathic scoliosis, thoracic region
- **M41.Ø5** Infantile idiopathic scoliosis, thoracolumbar region
- **M41.Ø6** Infantile idiopathic scoliosis, lumbar region
- **M41.Ø7** Infantile idiopathic scoliosis, lumbosacral region
- **M41.Ø8** Infantile idiopathic scoliosis, sacral and sacrococcygeal region

✓5th M41.1 Juvenile and adolescent idiopathic scoliosis

✓6th M41.11 Juvenile idiopathic scoliosis

AHA: 2014,4Q,28

- **M41.112** Juvenile idiopathic scoliosis, cervical region
- **M41.113** Juvenile idiopathic scoliosis, cervicothoracic region
- **M41.114** Juvenile idiopathic scoliosis, thoracic region
- **M41.115** Juvenile idiopathic scoliosis, thoracolumbar region
- **M41.116** Juvenile idiopathic scoliosis, lumbar region
- **M41.117** Juvenile idiopathic scoliosis, lumbosacral region
- **M41.119** Juvenile idiopathic scoliosis, site unspecified

✓6th M41.12 Adolescent scoliosis

- **M41.122** Adolescent idiopathic scoliosis, cervical region
- **M41.123** Adolescent idiopathic scoliosis, cervicothoracic region
- **M41.124** Adolescent idiopathic scoliosis, thoracic region
- **M41.125** Adolescent idiopathic scoliosis, thoracolumbar region
- **M41.126** Adolescent idiopathic scoliosis, lumbar region
- **M41.127** Adolescent idiopathic scoliosis, lumbosacral region
- **M41.129** Adolescent idiopathic scoliosis, site unspecified

✓5th M41.2 Other idiopathic scoliosis

- **M41.2Ø** Other idiopathic scoliosis, site unspecified
- **M41.22** Other idiopathic scoliosis, cervical region
- **M41.23** Other idiopathic scoliosis, cervicothoracic region
- **M41.24** Other idiopathic scoliosis, thoracic region
- **M41.25** Other idiopathic scoliosis, thoracolumbar region
- **M41.26** Other idiopathic scoliosis, lumbar region
- **M41.27** Other idiopathic scoliosis, lumbosacral region

✓5th M41.3 Thoracogenic scoliosis

- **M41.3Ø** Thoracogenic scoliosis, site unspecified
- **M41.34** Thoracogenic scoliosis, thoracic region
- **M41.35** Thoracogenic scoliosis, thoracolumbar region

✓5th M41.4 Neuromuscular scoliosis

Scoliosis secondary to cerebral palsy, Friedreich's ataxia, poliomyelitis and other neuromuscular disorders

Code also underlying condition

AHA: 2014,4Q,27

- **M41.4Ø** Neuromuscular scoliosis, site unspecified
- **M41.41** Neuromuscular scoliosis, occipito-atlanto-axial region
- **M41.42** Neuromuscular scoliosis, cervical region
- **M41.43** Neuromuscular scoliosis, cervicothoracic region
- **M41.44** Neuromuscular scoliosis, thoracic region
- **M41.45** Neuromuscular scoliosis, thoracolumbar region
- **M41.46** Neuromuscular scoliosis, lumbar region
- **M41.47** Neuromuscular scoliosis, lumbosacral region

✓5th M41.5 Other secondary scoliosis

Code first underlying disease

AHA: 2019,1Q,19

- **M41.5Ø** Other secondary scoliosis, site unspecified UPD
- **M41.52** Other secondary scoliosis, cervical region UPD
- **M41.53** Other secondary scoliosis, cervicothoracic region UPD
- **M41.54** Other secondary scoliosis, thoracic region UPD
- **M41.55** Other secondary scoliosis, thoracolumbar region UPD
- **M41.56** Other secondary scoliosis, lumbar region UPD
- **M41.57** Other secondary scoliosis, lumbosacral region UPD

✓5th M41.8 Other forms of scoliosis

AHA: 2022,1Q,30

- **M41.8Ø** Other forms of scoliosis, site unspecified
- **M41.82** Other forms of scoliosis, cervical region
- **M41.83** Other forms of scoliosis, cervicothoracic region
- **M41.84** Other forms of scoliosis, thoracic region
- **M41.85** Other forms of scoliosis, thoracolumbar region
- **M41.86** Other forms of scoliosis, lumbar region
- **M41.87** Other forms of scoliosis, lumbosacral region

M41.9 Scoliosis, unspecified

AHA: 2022,1Q,30

✓4th M42 Spinal osteochondrosis

✓5th M42.Ø Juvenile osteochondrosis of spine

Calvé's disease
Scheuermann's disease

EXCLUDES 1 *postural kyphosis (M4Ø.Ø)*

- **M42.ØØ** Juvenile osteochondrosis of spine, site unspecified COM
- **M42.Ø1** Juvenile osteochondrosis of spine, occipito-atlanto-axial region COM
- **M42.Ø2** Juvenile osteochondrosis of spine, cervical region COM
- **M42.Ø3** Juvenile osteochondrosis of spine, cervicothoracic region COM
- **M42.Ø4** Juvenile osteochondrosis of spine, thoracic region COM
- **M42.Ø5** Juvenile osteochondrosis of spine, thoracolumbar region COM
- **M42.Ø6** Juvenile osteochondrosis of spine, lumbar region COM
- **M42.Ø7** Juvenile osteochondrosis of spine, lumbosacral region COM
- **M42.Ø8** Juvenile osteochondrosis of spine, sacral and sacrococcygeal region COM
- **M42.Ø9** Juvenile osteochondrosis of spine, multiple sites in spine COM

✓5th M42.1 Adult osteochondrosis of spine

- **M42.1Ø** Adult osteochondrosis of spine, site unspecified A
- **M42.11** Adult osteochondrosis of spine, occipito-atlanto-axial region A

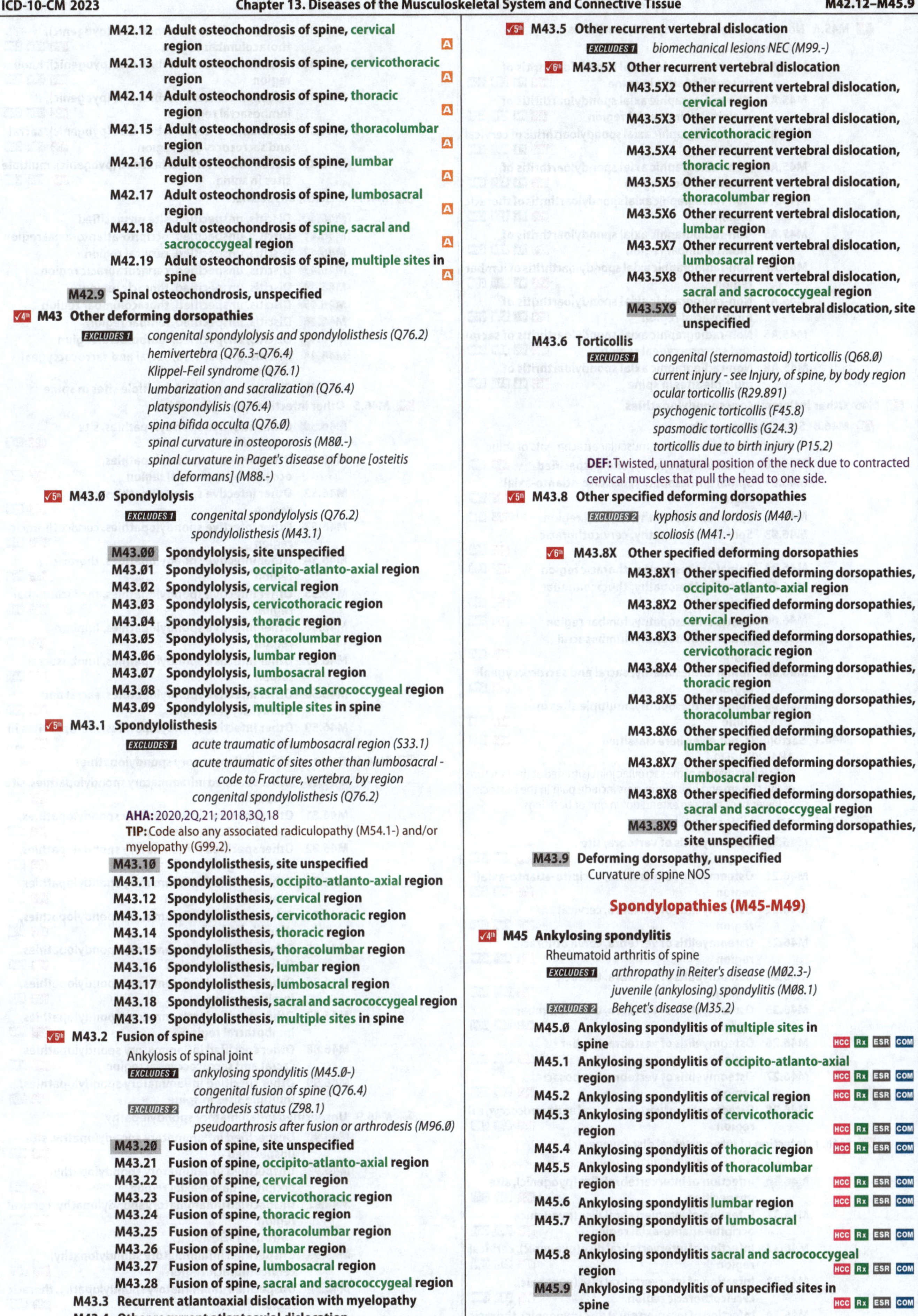

M42.12 Adult osteochondrosis of spine, cervical region A

M42.13 Adult osteochondrosis of spine, cervicothoracic region A

M42.14 Adult osteochondrosis of spine, thoracic region A

M42.15 Adult osteochondrosis of spine, thoracolumbar region A

M42.16 Adult osteochondrosis of spine, lumbar region A

M42.17 Adult osteochondrosis of spine, lumbosacral region A

M42.18 Adult osteochondrosis of spine, sacral and sacrococcygeal region A

M42.19 Adult osteochondrosis of spine, multiple sites in spine A

M42.9 Spinal osteochondrosis, unspecified

M43 Other deforming dorsopathies

EXCLUDES 1 *congenital spondylolysis and spondylolisthesis (Q76.2)*
hemivertebra (Q76.3-Q76.4)
Klippel-Feil syndrome (Q76.1)
lumbarization and sacralization (Q76.4)
platyspondylisis (Q76.4)
spina bifida occulta (Q76.Ø)
spinal curvature in osteoporosis (M8Ø.-)
spinal curvature in Paget's disease of bone [osteitis deformans] (M88.-)

M43.Ø Spondylolysis

EXCLUDES 1 *congenital spondylolysis (Q76.2)*
spondylolisthesis (M43.1)

M43.ØØ Spondylolysis, site unspecified
M43.Ø1 Spondylolysis, occipito-atlanto-axial region
M43.Ø2 Spondylolysis, cervical region
M43.Ø3 Spondylolysis, cervicothoracic region
M43.Ø4 Spondylolysis, thoracic region
M43.Ø5 Spondylolysis, thoracolumbar region
M43.Ø6 Spondylolysis, lumbar region
M43.Ø7 Spondylolysis, lumbosacral region
M43.Ø8 Spondylolysis, sacral and sacrococcygeal region
M43.Ø9 Spondylolysis, multiple sites in spine

M43.1 Spondylolisthesis

EXCLUDES 1 *acute traumatic of lumbosacral region (S33.1)*
acute traumatic of sites other than lumbosacral - code to Fracture, vertebra, by region
congenital spondylolisthesis (Q76.2)

AHA: 2020,2Q,21; 2018,3Q,18

TIP: Code also any associated radiculopathy (M54.1-) and/or myelopathy (G99.2).

M43.1Ø Spondylolisthesis, site unspecified
M43.11 Spondylolisthesis, occipito-atlanto-axial region
M43.12 Spondylolisthesis, cervical region
M43.13 Spondylolisthesis, cervicothoracic region
M43.14 Spondylolisthesis, thoracic region
M43.15 Spondylolisthesis, thoracolumbar region
M43.16 Spondylolisthesis, lumbar region
M43.17 Spondylolisthesis, lumbosacral region
M43.18 Spondylolisthesis, sacral and sacrococcygeal region
M43.19 Spondylolisthesis, multiple sites in spine

M43.2 Fusion of spine

Ankylosis of spinal joint

EXCLUDES 1 *ankylosing spondylitis (M45.Ø-)*
congenital fusion of spine (Q76.4)

EXCLUDES 2 *arthrodesis status (Z98.1)*
pseudoarthrosis after fusion or arthrodesis (M96.Ø)

M43.2Ø Fusion of spine, site unspecified
M43.21 Fusion of spine, occipito-atlanto-axial region
M43.22 Fusion of spine, cervical region
M43.23 Fusion of spine, cervicothoracic region
M43.24 Fusion of spine, thoracic region
M43.25 Fusion of spine, thoracolumbar region
M43.26 Fusion of spine, lumbar region
M43.27 Fusion of spine, lumbosacral region
M43.28 Fusion of spine, sacral and sacrococcygeal region

M43.3 Recurrent atlantoaxial dislocation with myelopathy

M43.4 Other recurrent atlantoaxial dislocation

M43.5 Other recurrent vertebral dislocation

EXCLUDES 1 *biomechanical lesions NEC (M99.-)*

M43.5X Other recurrent vertebral dislocation

M43.5X2 Other recurrent vertebral dislocation, cervical region
M43.5X3 Other recurrent vertebral dislocation, cervicothoracic region
M43.5X4 Other recurrent vertebral dislocation, thoracic region
M43.5X5 Other recurrent vertebral dislocation, thoracolumbar region
M43.5X6 Other recurrent vertebral dislocation, lumbar region
M43.5X7 Other recurrent vertebral dislocation, lumbosacral region
M43.5X8 Other recurrent vertebral dislocation, sacral and sacrococcygeal region
M43.5X9 Other recurrent vertebral dislocation, site unspecified

M43.6 Torticollis

EXCLUDES 1 *congenital (sternomastoid) torticollis (Q68.Ø)*
current injury - see Injury, of spine, by body region
ocular torticollis (R29.891)
psychogenic torticollis (F45.8)
spasmodic torticollis (G24.3)
torticollis due to birth injury (P15.2)

DEF: Twisted, unnatural position of the neck due to contracted cervical muscles that pull the head to one side.

M43.8 Other specified deforming dorsopathies

EXCLUDES 2 *kyphosis and lordosis (M4Ø.-)*
scoliosis (M41.-)

M43.8X Other specified deforming dorsopathies

M43.8X1 Other specified deforming dorsopathies, occipito-atlanto-axial region
M43.8X2 Other specified deforming dorsopathies, cervical region
M43.8X3 Other specified deforming dorsopathies, cervicothoracic region
M43.8X4 Other specified deforming dorsopathies, thoracic region
M43.8X5 Other specified deforming dorsopathies, thoracolumbar region
M43.8X6 Other specified deforming dorsopathies, lumbar region
M43.8X7 Other specified deforming dorsopathies, lumbosacral region
M43.8X8 Other specified deforming dorsopathies, sacral and sacrococcygeal region
M43.8X9 Other specified deforming dorsopathies, site unspecified

M43.9 Deforming dorsopathy, unspecified

Curvature of spine NOS

Spondylopathies (M45-M49)

M45 Ankylosing spondylitis

Rheumatoid arthritis of spine

EXCLUDES 1 *arthropathy in Reiter's disease (MØ2.3-)*
juvenile (ankylosing) spondylitis (MØ8.1)

EXCLUDES 2 *Behçet's disease (M35.2)*

M45.Ø Ankylosing spondylitis of multiple sites in spine HCC Rx ESR COM
M45.1 Ankylosing spondylitis of occipito-atlanto-axial region HCC Rx ESR COM
M45.2 Ankylosing spondylitis of cervical region HCC Rx ESR COM
M45.3 Ankylosing spondylitis of cervicothoracic region HCC Rx ESR COM
M45.4 Ankylosing spondylitis of thoracic region HCC Rx ESR COM
M45.5 Ankylosing spondylitis of thoracolumbar region HCC Rx ESR COM
M45.6 Ankylosing spondylitis lumbar region HCC Rx ESR COM
M45.7 Ankylosing spondylitis of lumbosacral region HCC Rx ESR COM
M45.8 Ankylosing spondylitis sacral and sacrococcygeal region HCC Rx ESR COM
M45.9 Ankylosing spondylitis of unspecified sites in spine HCC Rx ESR COM

M45.A Non-radiographic axial spondyloarthritis
AHA: 2021,4Q,21-22
- **M45.A0** Non-radiographic axial spondyloarthritis of unspecified sites in spine HCC Rx ESR COM
- **M45.A1** Non-radiographic axial spondyloarthritis of occipito-atlanto-axial region HCC Rx ESR COM
- **M45.A2** Non-radiographic axial spondyloarthritis of cervical region HCC Rx ESR COM
- **M45.A3** Non-radiographic axial spondyloarthritis of cervicothoracic region HCC Rx ESR COM
- **M45.A4** Non-radiographic axial spondyloarthritis of thoracic region HCC Rx ESR COM
- **M45.A5** Non-radiographic axial spondyloarthritis of thoracolumbar region HCC Rx ESR COM
- **M45.A6** Non-radiographic axial spondyloarthritis of lumbar region HCC Rx ESR COM
- **M45.A7** Non-radiographic axial spondyloarthritis of lumbosacral region HCC Rx ESR COM
- **M45.A8** Non-radiographic axial spondyloarthritis of sacral and sacrococcygeal region HCC Rx ESR COM
- **M45.AB** Non-radiographic axial spondyloarthritis of multiple sites in spine HCC Rx ESR COM

M46 Other inflammatory spondylopathies

M46.0 Spinal enthesopathy
Disorder of ligamentous or muscular attachments of spine
- **M46.00** Spinal enthesopathy, site unspecified HCC ESR
- **M46.01** Spinal enthesopathy, occipito-atlanto-axial region HCC ESR
- **M46.02** Spinal enthesopathy, cervical region HCC ESR
- **M46.03** Spinal enthesopathy, cervicothoracic region HCC ESR
- **M46.04** Spinal enthesopathy, thoracic region HCC ESR
- **M46.05** Spinal enthesopathy, thoracolumbar region HCC ESR
- **M46.06** Spinal enthesopathy, lumbar region HCC ESR
- **M46.07** Spinal enthesopathy, lumbosacral region HCC ESR
- **M46.08** Spinal enthesopathy, sacral and sacrococcygeal region HCC ESR
- **M46.09** Spinal enthesopathy, multiple sites in spine HCC ESR

M46.1 Sacroiliitis, not elsewhere classified HCC ESR
AHA: 2020,2Q,14
DEF: Inflammation of the sacroiliac joint (situated at the juncture of the sacrum and hip). Symptoms include pain in the buttocks or lower back that can extend down one or both legs.

M46.2 Osteomyelitis of vertebra
- **M46.20** Osteomyelitis of vertebra, site unspecified HCC ESR COM
- **M46.21** Osteomyelitis of vertebra, occipito-atlanto-axial region HCC ESR COM
- **M46.22** Osteomyelitis of vertebra, cervical region HCC ESR COM
- **M46.23** Osteomyelitis of vertebra, cervicothoracic region HCC ESR COM
- **M46.24** Osteomyelitis of vertebra, thoracic region HCC ESR COM
- **M46.25** Osteomyelitis of vertebra, thoracolumbar region HCC ESR COM
- **M46.26** Osteomyelitis of vertebra, lumbar region HCC ESR COM
- **M46.27** Osteomyelitis of vertebra, lumbosacral region HCC ESR COM
- **M46.28** Osteomyelitis of vertebra, sacral and sacrococcygeal region HCC ESR COM

M46.3 Infection of intervertebral disc (pyogenic)
Use additional code (B95-B97) to identify infectious agent
- **M46.30** Infection of intervertebral disc (pyogenic), site unspecified HCC ESR COM
- **M46.31** Infection of intervertebral disc (pyogenic), occipito-atlanto-axial region HCC ESR COM
- **M46.32** Infection of intervertebral disc (pyogenic), cervical region HCC ESR COM
- **M46.33** Infection of intervertebral disc (pyogenic), cervicothoracic region HCC ESR COM
- **M46.34** Infection of intervertebral disc (pyogenic), thoracic region HCC ESR COM
- **M46.35** Infection of intervertebral disc (pyogenic), thoracolumbar region HCC ESR COM
- **M46.36** Infection of intervertebral disc (pyogenic), lumbar region HCC ESR COM
- **M46.37** Infection of intervertebral disc (pyogenic), lumbosacral region HCC ESR COM
- **M46.38** Infection of intervertebral disc (pyogenic), sacral and sacrococcygeal region HCC ESR COM
- **M46.39** Infection of intervertebral disc (pyogenic), multiple sites in spine HCC ESR COM

M46.4 Discitis, unspecified
- **M46.40** Discitis, unspecified, site unspecified
- **M46.41** Discitis, unspecified, occipito-atlanto-axial region
- **M46.42** Discitis, unspecified, cervical region
- **M46.43** Discitis, unspecified, cervicothoracic region
- **M46.44** Discitis, unspecified, thoracic region
- **M46.45** Discitis, unspecified, thoracolumbar region
- **M46.46** Discitis, unspecified, lumbar region
- **M46.47** Discitis, unspecified, lumbosacral region
- **M46.48** Discitis, unspecified, sacral and sacrococcygeal region
- **M46.49** Discitis, unspecified, multiple sites in spine

M46.5 Other infective spondylopathies
- **M46.50** Other infective spondylopathies, site unspecified HCC ESR
- **M46.51** Other infective spondylopathies, occipito-atlanto-axial region HCC ESR
- **M46.52** Other infective spondylopathies, cervical region HCC ESR
- **M46.53** Other infective spondylopathies, cervicothoracic region HCC ESR
- **M46.54** Other infective spondylopathies, thoracic region HCC ESR
- **M46.55** Other infective spondylopathies, thoracolumbar region HCC ESR
- **M46.56** Other infective spondylopathies, lumbar region HCC ESR
- **M46.57** Other infective spondylopathies, lumbosacral region HCC ESR
- **M46.58** Other infective spondylopathies, sacral and sacrococcygeal region HCC ESR
- **M46.59** Other infective spondylopathies, multiple sites in spine HCC ESR

M46.8 Other specified inflammatory spondylopathies
- **M46.80** Other specified inflammatory spondylopathies, site unspecified HCC ESR
- **M46.81** Other specified inflammatory spondylopathies, occipito-atlanto-axial region HCC ESR
- **M46.82** Other specified inflammatory spondylopathies, cervical region HCC ESR
- **M46.83** Other specified inflammatory spondylopathies, cervicothoracic region HCC ESR
- **M46.84** Other specified inflammatory spondylopathies, thoracic region HCC ESR
- **M46.85** Other specified inflammatory spondylopathies, thoracolumbar region HCC ESR
- **M46.86** Other specified inflammatory spondylopathies, lumbar region HCC ESR
- **M46.87** Other specified inflammatory spondylopathies, lumbosacral region HCC ESR
- **M46.88** Other specified inflammatory spondylopathies, sacral and sacrococcygeal region HCC ESR
- **M46.89** Other specified inflammatory spondylopathies, multiple sites in spine HCC ESR

M46.9 Unspecified inflammatory spondylopathy
- **M46.90** Unspecified inflammatory spondylopathy, site unspecified HCC ESR
- **M46.91** Unspecified inflammatory spondylopathy, occipito-atlanto-axial region HCC ESR
- **M46.92** Unspecified inflammatory spondylopathy, cervical region HCC ESR
  AHA: 2019,3Q,10
- **M46.93** Unspecified inflammatory spondylopathy, cervicothoracic region HCC ESR
- **M46.94** Unspecified inflammatory spondylopathy, thoracic region HCC ESR
- **M46.95** Unspecified inflammatory spondylopathy, thoracolumbar region HCC ESR

M46.96 **Unspecified inflammatory spondylopathy, lumbar region** HCC ESR

M46.97 **Unspecified inflammatory spondylopathy, lumbosacral region** HCC ESR

M46.98 **Unspecified inflammatory spondylopathy, sacral and sacrococcygeal region** HCC ESR

M46.99 **Unspecified inflammatory spondylopathy, multiple sites in spine** HCC ESR

4th **M47 Spondylosis**

INCLUDES arthrosis or osteoarthritis of spine
degeneration of facet joints

AHA: 2020,1Q,17; 2019,3Q,10-11; 2016,4Q,147

5th **M47.0** **Anterior spinal and vertebral artery compression syndromes**

6th **M47.01** **Anterior spinal artery compression syndromes**

M47.011 **Anterior spinal artery compression syndromes, occipito-atlanto-axial region**

M47.012 **Anterior spinal artery compression syndromes, cervical region**

M47.013 **Anterior spinal artery compression syndromes, cervicothoracic region**

M47.014 **Anterior spinal artery compression syndromes, thoracic region**

M47.015 **Anterior spinal artery compression syndromes, thoracolumbar region**

M47.016 **Anterior spinal artery compression syndromes, lumbar region**

M47.019 **Anterior spinal artery compression syndromes, site unspecified**

6th **M47.02** **Vertebral artery compression syndromes**

M47.021 **Vertebral artery compression syndromes, occipito-atlanto-axial region**

M47.022 **Vertebral artery compression syndromes, cervical region**

M47.029 **Vertebral artery compression syndromes, site unspecified**

5th **M47.1** **Other spondylosis with myelopathy**

Spondylogenic compression of spinal cord

EXCLUDES 1 *vertebral subluxation (M43.3-M43.5X9)*

AHA: 2020,1Q,17

M47.10 **Other spondylosis with myelopathy, site unspecified**

M47.11 **Other spondylosis with myelopathy, occipito-atlanto-axial region**

M47.12 **Other spondylosis with myelopathy, cervical region**

M47.13 **Other spondylosis with myelopathy, cervicothoracic region**

M47.14 **Other spondylosis with myelopathy, thoracic region**

M47.15 **Other spondylosis with myelopathy, thoracolumbar region**

M47.16 **Other spondylosis with myelopathy, lumbar region**

5th **M47.2** **Other spondylosis with radiculopathy**

AHA: 2020,1Q,17

M47.20 **Other spondylosis with radiculopathy, site unspecified**

M47.21 **Other spondylosis with radiculopathy, occipito-atlanto-axial region**

M47.22 **Other spondylosis with radiculopathy, cervical region**

M47.23 **Other spondylosis with radiculopathy, cervicothoracic region**

M47.24 **Other spondylosis with radiculopathy, thoracic region**

M47.25 **Other spondylosis with radiculopathy, thoracolumbar region**

M47.26 **Other spondylosis with radiculopathy, lumbar region**

M47.27 **Other spondylosis with radiculopathy, lumbosacral region**

M47.28 **Other spondylosis with radiculopathy, sacral and sacrococcygeal region**

5th **M47.8** **Other spondylosis**

6th **M47.81** **Spondylosis without myelopathy or radiculopathy**

AHA: 2019,3Q,10-11; 2018,2Q,14

M47.811 **Spondylosis without myelopathy or radiculopathy, occipito-atlanto-axial region**

M47.812 **Spondylosis without myelopathy or radiculopathy, cervical region**

M47.813 **Spondylosis without myelopathy or radiculopathy, cervicothoracic region**

M47.814 **Spondylosis without myelopathy or radiculopathy, thoracic region**

M47.815 **Spondylosis without myelopathy or radiculopathy, thoracolumbar region**

M47.816 **Spondylosis without myelopathy or radiculopathy, lumbar region**

M47.817 **Spondylosis without myelopathy or radiculopathy, lumbosacral region**

M47.818 **Spondylosis without myelopathy or radiculopathy, sacral and sacrococcygeal region**

M47.819 **Spondylosis without myelopathy or radiculopathy, site unspecified**

6th **M47.89** **Other spondylosis**

M47.891 **Other spondylosis, occipito-atlanto-axial region**

M47.892 **Other spondylosis, cervical region**

M47.893 **Other spondylosis, cervicothoracic region**

M47.894 **Other spondylosis, thoracic region**

M47.895 **Other spondylosis, thoracolumbar region**

M47.896 **Other spondylosis, lumbar region**

M47.897 **Other spondylosis, lumbosacral region**

M47.898 **Other spondylosis, sacral and sacrococcygeal region**

M47.899 **Other spondylosis, site unspecified**

M47.9 **Spondylosis, unspecified**

4th **M48 Other spondylopathies**

5th **M48.0** **Spinal stenosis**

Caudal stenosis

AHA: 2020,1Q,17; 2018,3Q,18-19

TIP: Code also any associated radiculopathy (M54.1-) and/or myelopathy (G99.2).

M48.00 **Spinal stenosis, site unspecified**

M48.01 **Spinal stenosis, occipito-atlanto-axial region**

M48.02 **Spinal stenosis, cervical region**

M48.03 **Spinal stenosis, cervicothoracic region**

M48.04 **Spinal stenosis, thoracic region**

M48.05 **Spinal stenosis, thoracolumbar region**

6th **M48.06** **Spinal stenosis, lumbar region**

AHA: 2018,3Q,19; 2017,4Q,18-19

M48.061 **Spinal stenosis, lumbar region without neurogenic claudication**

Spinal stenosis, lumbar region NOS

M48.062 **Spinal stenosis, lumbar region with neurogenic claudication**

M48.07 **Spinal stenosis, lumbosacral region**

M48.08 **Spinal stenosis, sacral and sacrococcygeal region**

5th **M48.1** **Ankylosing hyperostosis [Forestier]**

Diffuse idiopathic skeletal hyperostosis [DISH]

M48.10 **Ankylosing hyperostosis [Forestier], site unspecified**

M48.11 **Ankylosing hyperostosis [Forestier], occipito-atlanto-axial region**

M48.12 **Ankylosing hyperostosis [Forestier], cervical region**

M48.13 **Ankylosing hyperostosis [Forestier], cervicothoracic region**

M48.14 **Ankylosing hyperostosis [Forestier], thoracic region**

M48.15 **Ankylosing hyperostosis [Forestier], thoracolumbar region**

M48.16 **Ankylosing hyperostosis [Forestier], lumbar region**

M48.17 **Ankylosing hyperostosis [Forestier], lumbosacral region**

M48.18 **Ankylosing hyperostosis [Forestier], sacral and sacrococcygeal region**

M48.19 **Ankylosing hyperostosis [Forestier], multiple sites in spine**

5th **M48.2** **Kissing spine**

M48.20 **Kissing spine, site unspecified**

M48.21 **Kissing spine, occipito-atlanto-axial region**

M48.22 **Kissing spine, cervical region**

M48.23 **Kissing spine, cervicothoracic region**

M48.24 **Kissing spine, thoracic region**

M48.25 **Kissing spine, thoracolumbar region**

M48.26 **Kissing spine, lumbar region**

M48.27 **Kissing spine, lumbosacral region**

5th M48.3 Traumatic spondylopathy

M48.30 Traumatic spondylopathy, site unspecified
M48.31 Traumatic spondylopathy, occipito-atlanto-axial region
M48.32 Traumatic spondylopathy, cervical region
M48.33 Traumatic spondylopathy, cervicothoracic region
M48.34 Traumatic spondylopathy, thoracic region
M48.35 Traumatic spondylopathy, thoracolumbar region
M48.36 Traumatic spondylopathy, lumbar region
M48.37 Traumatic spondylopathy, lumbosacral region
M48.38 Traumatic spondylopathy, sacral and sacrococcygeal region

5th M48.4 Fatigue fracture of vertebra

Stress fracture of vertebra

EXCLUDES 1 *pathological fracture NOS (M84.4-)*
pathological fracture of vertebra due to neoplasm (M84.58)
pathological fracture of vertebra due to osteoporosis (M80.-)
pathological fracture of vertebra due to other diagnosis (M84.68)
traumatic fracture of vertebrae (S12.0-S12.3-, S22.0-, S32.0-)

The appropriate 7th character is to be added to each code from subcategory M48.4.
- A initial encounter for fracture
- D subsequent encounter for fracture with routine healing
- G subsequent encounter for fracture with delayed healing
- S sequela of fracture

x7th **M48.40 Fatigue fracture of vertebra, site unspecified** Q
x7th **M48.41 Fatigue fracture of vertebra, occipito-atlanto-axial region** Q
x7th **M48.42 Fatigue fracture of vertebra, cervical region** Q
x7th **M48.43 Fatigue fracture of vertebra, cervicothoracic region** Q
x7th **M48.44 Fatigue fracture of vertebra, thoracic region** Q
x7th **M48.45 Fatigue fracture of vertebra, thoracolumbar region** Q
x7th **M48.46 Fatigue fracture of vertebra, lumbar region** Q
x7th **M48.47 Fatigue fracture of vertebra, lumbosacral region** Q
x7th **M48.48 Fatigue fracture of vertebra, sacral and sacrococcygeal region** Q

5th M48.5 Collapsed vertebra, not elsewhere classified

Collapsed vertebra NOS
Compression fracture of vertebra NOS
Wedging of vertebra NOS

EXCLUDES 1 *current injury - see Injury of spine, by body region*
fatigue fracture of vertebra (M48.4)
pathological fracture NOS (M84.4-)
pathological fracture of vertebra due to neoplasm (M84.58)
pathological fracture of vertebra due to osteoporosis (M80.-)
pathological fracture of vertebra due to other diagnosis (M84.68)
stress fracture of vertebra (M48.4-)
traumatic fracture of vertebra (S12.-, S22.-, S32.-)

The appropriate 7th character is to be added to each code from subcategory M48.5.
- A initial encounter for fracture
- D subsequent encounter for fracture with routine healing
- G subsequent encounter for fracture with delayed healing
- S sequela of fracture

1 x7th **M48.50 Collapsed vertebra, not elsewhere classified, site unspecified** HCC Rx ESR COM
1 x7th **M48.51 Collapsed vertebra, not elsewhere classified, occipito-atlanto-axial region** HCC Rx ESR COM
1 x7th **M48.52 Collapsed vertebra, not elsewhere classified, cervical region** HCC Rx ESR COM
1 x7th **M48.53 Collapsed vertebra, not elsewhere classified, cervicothoracic region** HCC Rx ESR COM
1 x7th **M48.54 Collapsed vertebra, not elsewhere classified, thoracic region** HCC Rx ESR COM
1 x7th **M48.55 Collapsed vertebra, not elsewhere classified, thoracolumbar region** HCC Rx ESR COM
1 x7th **M48.56 Collapsed vertebra, not elsewhere classified, lumbar region** HCC Rx ESR COM
1 x7th **M48.57 Collapsed vertebra, not elsewhere classified, lumbosacral region** HCC Rx ESR COM
1 x7th **M48.58 Collapsed vertebra, not elsewhere classified, sacral and sacrococcygeal region** HCC Rx ESR COM

5th M48.8 Other specified spondylopathies

Ossification of posterior longitudinal ligament

6th M48.8X Other specified spondylopathies

M48.8X1 Other specified spondylopathies, occipito-atlanto-axial region HCC Rx ESR COM
M48.8X2 Other specified spondylopathies, cervical region HCC Rx ESR COM
M48.8X3 Other specified spondylopathies, cervicothoracic region HCC Rx ESR COM
M48.8X4 Other specified spondylopathies, thoracic region HCC Rx ESR COM
M48.8X5 Other specified spondylopathies, thoracolumbar region HCC Rx ESR COM
M48.8X6 Other specified spondylopathies, lumbar region HCC Rx ESR COM
M48.8X7 Other specified spondylopathies, lumbosacral region HCC Rx ESR COM
M48.8X8 Other specified spondylopathies, sacral and sacrococcygeal region HCC Rx ESR COM
M48.8X9 Other specified spondylopathies, site unspecified HCC Rx ESR COM

M48.9 Spondylopathy, unspecified

4th M49 Spondylopathies in diseases classified elsewhere

INCLUDES curvature of spine in diseases classified elsewhere
deformity of spine in diseases classified elsewhere
kyphosis in diseases classified elsewhere
scoliosis in diseases classified elsewhere
spondylopathy in diseases classified elsewhere

Code first underlying disease, such as:
brucellosis (A23.-)
Charcôt-Marie-Tooth disease (G60.0)
enterobacterial infections (A01-A04)
osteitis fibrosa cystica (E21.0)

EXCLUDES 1 *curvature of spine in tuberculosis [Pott's] (A18.01)*
enteropathic arthropathies (M07.-)
gonococcal spondylitis (A54.41)
neuropathic spondylopathy in syringomyelia (G95.0)
neuropathic spondylopathy in tabes dorsalis (A52.11)
neuropathic [tabes dorsalis] spondylitis (A52.11)
nonsyphilitic neuropathic spondylopathy NEC (G98.0)
spondylitis in syphilis (acquired) (A52.77)
tuberculous spondylitis (A18.01)
typhoid fever spondylitis (A01.05)

5th M49.8 Spondylopathy in diseases classified elsewhere

M49.80 Spondylopathy in diseases classified elsewhere, site unspecified HCC ESR
M49.81 Spondylopathy in diseases classified elsewhere, occipito-atlanto-axial region HCC ESR
M49.82 Spondylopathy in diseases classified elsewhere, cervical region HCC ESR
M49.83 Spondylopathy in diseases classified elsewhere, cervicothoracic region HCC ESR
M49.84 Spondylopathy in diseases classified elsewhere, thoracic region HCC ESR
M49.85 Spondylopathy in diseases classified elsewhere, thoracolumbar region HCC ESR
M49.86 Spondylopathy in diseases classified elsewhere, lumbar region HCC ESR
M49.87 Spondylopathy in diseases classified elsewhere, lumbosacral region HCC ESR
M49.88 Spondylopathy in diseases classified elsewhere, sacral and sacrococcygeal region HCC ESR
M49.89 Spondylopathy in diseases classified elsewhere, multiple sites in spine HCC ESR

Other dorsopathies (M50-M54)

EXCLUDES 1 *current injury - see injury of spine by body region*
discitis NOS (M46.4-)

M50 Cervical disc disorders

NOTE Code to the most superior level of disorder

INCLUDES cervicothoracic disc disorders
cervicothoracic disc disorders with cervicalgia

AHA: 2016,4Q,39-40; 2016,1Q,17

M50.0 Cervical disc disorder with myelopathy

AHA: 2018,3Q,19

M50.00 Cervical disc disorder with myelopathy, unspecified cervical region

M50.01 Cervical disc disorder with myelopathy, high cervical region
C2-C3 disc disorder with myelopathy
C3-C4 disc disorder with myelopathy

M50.02 Cervical disc disorder with myelopathy, mid-cervical region

M50.020 Cervical disc disorder with myelopathy, mid-cervical region, unspecified level

M50.021 Cervical disc disorder at C4-C5 level with myelopathy
C4-C5 disc disorder with myelopathy

M50.022 Cervical disc disorder at C5-C6 level with myelopathy
C5-C6 disc disorder with myelopathy

M50.023 Cervical disc disorder at C6-C7 level with myelopathy
C6-C7 disc disorder with myelopathy

M50.03 Cervical disc disorder with myelopathy, cervicothoracic region
C7-T1 disc disorder with myelopathy

M50.1 Cervical disc disorder with radiculopathy

EXCLUDES 2 *brachial radiculitis NOS (M54.13)*

AHA: 2018,3Q,19

M50.10 Cervical disc disorder with radiculopathy, unspecified cervical region

M50.11 Cervical disc disorder with radiculopathy, high cervical region
C2-C3 disc disorder with radiculopathy
C3 radiculopathy due to disc disorder
C3-C4 disc disorder with radiculopathy
C4 radiculopathy due to disc disorder

M50.12 Cervical disc disorder with radiculopathy, mid-cervical region

M50.120 Mid-cervical disc disorder, unspecified level

M50.121 Cervical disc disorder at C4-C5 level with radiculopathy
C4-C5 disc disorder with radiculopathy
C5 radiculopathy due to disc disorder

M50.122 Cervical disc disorder at C5-C6 level with radiculopathy
C5-C6 disc disorder with radiculopathy
C6 radiculopathy due to disc disorder

M50.123 Cervical disc disorder at C6-C7 level with radiculopathy
C6-C7 disc disorder with radiculopathy
C7 radiculopathy due to disc disorder

M50.13 Cervical disc disorder with radiculopathy, cervicothoracic region
C7-T1 disc disorder with radiculopathy
C8 radiculopathy due to disc disorder

M50.2 Other cervical disc displacement

M50.20 Other cervical disc displacement, unspecified cervical region

M50.21 Other cervical disc displacement, high cervical region
Other C2-C3 cervical disc displacement
Other C3-C4 cervical disc displacement

M50.22 Other cervical disc displacement, mid-cervical region

M50.220 Other cervical disc displacement, mid-cervical region, unspecified level

M50.221 Other cervical disc displacement at C4-C5 level
Other C4-C5 cervical disc displacement

M50.222 Other cervical disc displacement at C5-C6 level
Other C5-C6 cervical disc displacement

M50.223 Other cervical disc displacement at C6-C7 level
Other C6-C7 cervical disc displacement

M50.23 Other cervical disc displacement, cervicothoracic region
Other C7-T1 cervical disc displacement

M50.3 Other cervical disc degeneration

M50.30 Other cervical disc degeneration, unspecified cervical region

M50.31 Other cervical disc degeneration, high cervical region
Other C2-C3 cervical disc degeneration
Other C3-C4 cervical disc degeneration

M50.32 Other cervical disc degeneration, mid-cervical region

M50.320 Other cervical disc degeneration, mid-cervical region, unspecified level

M50.321 Other cervical disc degeneration at C4-C5 level
Other C4-C5 cervical disc degeneration

M50.322 Other cervical disc degeneration at C5-C6 level
Other C5-C6 cervical disc degeneration

M50.323 Other cervical disc degeneration at C6-C7 level
Other C6-C7 cervical disc degeneration

M50.33 Other cervical disc degeneration, cervicothoracic region
Other C7-T1 cervical disc degeneration

M50.8 Other cervical disc disorders

M50.80 Other cervical disc disorders, unspecified cervical region

M50.81 Other cervical disc disorders, high cervical region
Other C2-C3 cervical disc disorders
Other C3-C4 cervical disc disorders

M50.82 Other cervical disc disorders, mid-cervical region

M50.820 Other cervical disc disorders, mid-cervical region, unspecified level

M50.821 Other cervical disc disorders at C4-C5 level
Other C4-C5 cervical disc disorders

M50.822 Other cervical disc disorders at C5-C6 level
Other C5-C6 cervical disc disorders

M50.823 Other cervical disc disorders at C6-C7 level
Other C6-C7 cervical disc disorders

M50.83 Other cervical disc disorders, cervicothoracic region
Other C7-T1 cervical disc disorders

M50.9 Cervical disc disorder, unspecified

M50.90 Cervical disc disorder, unspecified, unspecified cervical region

M50.91 Cervical disc disorder, unspecified, high cervical region
C2-C3 cervical disc disorder, unspecified
C3-C4 cervical disc disorder, unspecified

M50.92 Cervical disc disorder, unspecified, mid-cervical region

M50.920 Unspecified cervical disc disorder, mid-cervical region, unspecified level

M50.921 Unspecified cervical disc disorder at C4-C5 level
Unspecified C4-C5 cervical disc disorder

M50.922 Unspecified cervical disc disorder at C5-C6 level
Unspecified C5-C6 cervical disc disorder

M50.923 Unspecified cervical disc disorder at C6-C7 level
Unspecified C6-C7 cervical disc disorder

M50.93 Cervical disc disorder, unspecified, cervicothoracic region
C7-T1 cervical disc disorder, unspecified

M51 Thoracic, thoracolumbar, and lumbosacral intervertebral disc disorders
EXCLUDES 2 *cervical and cervicothoracic disc disorders (M50.-)*
sacral and sacrococcygeal disorders (M53.3)

M51.0 Thoracic, thoracolumbar and lumbosacral intervertebral disc disorders with myelopathy
M51.04 Intervertebral disc disorders with myelopathy, thoracic region
M51.05 Intervertebral disc disorders with myelopathy, thoracolumbar region
M51.06 Intervertebral disc disorders with myelopathy, lumbar region

M51.1 Thoracic, thoracolumbar and lumbosacral intervertebral disc disorders with radiculopathy
Sciatica due to intervertebral disc disorder
EXCLUDES 1 *lumbar radiculitis NOS (M54.16)*
sciatica NOS (M54.3)
AHA: 2018,3Q,18
M51.14 Intervertebral disc disorders with radiculopathy, thoracic region
M51.15 Intervertebral disc disorders with radiculopathy, thoracolumbar region
M51.16 Intervertebral disc disorders with radiculopathy, lumbar region
M51.17 Intervertebral disc disorders with radiculopathy, lumbosacral region

M51.2 Other thoracic, thoracolumbar and lumbosacral intervertebral disc displacement
Lumbago due to displacement of intervertebral disc
AHA: 2022,1Q,26

Displacement Intervertebral Disc

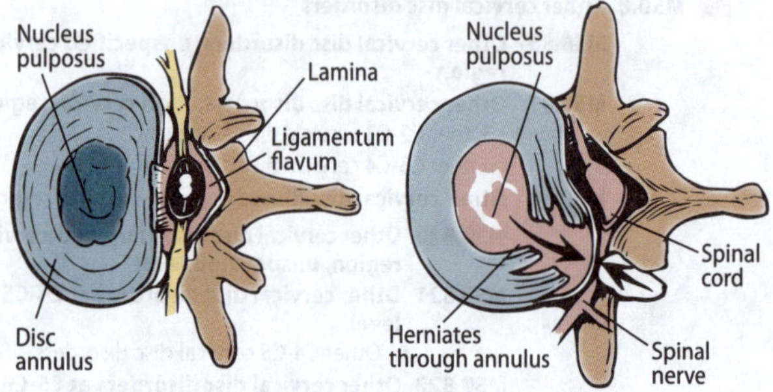

M51.24 Other intervertebral disc displacement, thoracic region
M51.25 Other intervertebral disc displacement, thoracolumbar region
M51.26 Other intervertebral disc displacement, lumbar region
M51.27 Other intervertebral disc displacement, lumbosacral region

M51.3 Other thoracic, thoracolumbar and lumbosacral intervertebral disc degeneration
AHA: 2022,1Q,26; 2018,2Q,15; 2013,3Q,22
M51.34 Other intervertebral disc degeneration, thoracic region
M51.35 Other intervertebral disc degeneration, thoracolumbar region
M51.36 Other intervertebral disc degeneration, lumbar region
M51.37 Other intervertebral disc degeneration, lumbosacral region

M51.4 Schmorl's nodes
DEF: Irregular bone defect in the margin of the vertebral body that causes herniation into the end plate of the vertebral body.
M51.44 Schmorl's nodes, thoracic region
M51.45 Schmorl's nodes, thoracolumbar region
M51.46 Schmorl's nodes, lumbar region
M51.47 Schmorl's nodes, lumbosacral region

M51.8 Other thoracic, thoracolumbar and lumbosacral intervertebral disc disorders
M51.84 Other intervertebral disc disorders, thoracic region
M51.85 Other intervertebral disc disorders, thoracolumbar region
M51.86 Other intervertebral disc disorders, lumbar region
M51.87 Other intervertebral disc disorders, lumbosacral region

M51.9 Unspecified thoracic, thoracolumbar and lumbosacral intervertebral disc disorder

● **M51.A Other lumbar and lumbosacral annulus fibrosus disc defects**
● **M51.A0 Intervertebral annulus fibrosus defect, lumbar region, unspecified size**
Code first, if applicable, lumbar disc herniation (M51.06, M51.16, M51.26)
● **M51.A1 Intervertebral annulus fibrosus defect, small, lumbar region**
Code first, if applicable, lumbar disc herniation (M51.06, M51.16, M51.26)
● **M51.A2 Intervertebral annulus fibrosus defect, large, lumbar region**
Code first, if applicable, lumbar disc herniation (M51.06, M51.16, M51.26)
● **M51.A3 Intervertebral annulus fibrosus defect, lumbosacral region, unspecified size**
Code first, if applicable, lumbosacral disc herniation (M51.17, M51.27)
● **M51.A4 Intervertebral annulus fibrosus defect, small, lumbosacral region**
Code first, if applicable, lumbosacral disc herniation (M51.17, M51.27)
● **M51.A5 Intervertebral annulus fibrosus defect, large, lumbosacral region**
Code first, if applicable, lumbosacral disc herniation (M51.17, M51.27)

M53 Other and unspecified dorsopathies, not elsewhere classified
M53.0 Cervicocranial syndrome
Posterior cervical sympathetic syndrome
M53.1 Cervicobrachial syndrome
EXCLUDES 2 *cervical disc disorder (M50.-)*
thoracic outlet syndrome (G54.0)
M53.2 Spinal instabilities
M53.2X Spinal instabilities
M53.2X1 Spinal instabilities, occipito-atlanto-axial region
M53.2X2 Spinal instabilities, cervical region
M53.2X3 Spinal instabilities, cervicothoracic region
M53.2X4 Spinal instabilities, thoracic region
M53.2X5 Spinal instabilities, thoracolumbar region
M53.2X6 Spinal instabilities, lumbar region
M53.2X7 Spinal instabilities, lumbosacral region
M53.2X8 Spinal instabilities, sacral and sacrococcygeal region
M53.2X9 Spinal instabilities, site unspecified
M53.3 Sacrococcygeal disorders, not elsewhere classified
Coccygodynia
M53.8 Other specified dorsopathies
M53.80 Other specified dorsopathies, site unspecified
M53.81 Other specified dorsopathies, occipito-atlanto-axial region
M53.82 Other specified dorsopathies, cervical region
M53.83 Other specified dorsopathies, cervicothoracic region
M53.84 Other specified dorsopathies, thoracic region
M53.85 Other specified dorsopathies, thoracolumbar region
M53.86 Other specified dorsopathies, lumbar region
M53.87 Other specified dorsopathies, lumbosacral region
M53.88 Other specified dorsopathies, sacral and sacrococcygeal region
M53.9 Dorsopathy, unspecified

M54 Dorsalgia
EXCLUDES 1 *psychogenic dorsalgia (F45.41)*
M54.0 Panniculitis affecting regions of neck and back
EXCLUDES 1 *lupus panniculitis (L93.2)*
panniculitis NOS (M79.3)
relapsing [Weber-Christian] panniculitis (M35.6)
M54.00 Panniculitis affecting regions of neck and back, site unspecified
M54.01 Panniculitis affecting regions of neck and back, occipito-atlanto-axial region
M54.02 Panniculitis affecting regions of neck and back, cervical region

M54.Ø3 Panniculitis affecting regions of neck and back, cervicothoracic region
M54.Ø4 Panniculitis affecting regions of neck and back, thoracic region
M54.Ø5 Panniculitis affecting regions of neck and back, thoracolumbar region
M54.Ø6 Panniculitis affecting regions of neck and back, lumbar region
M54.Ø7 Panniculitis affecting regions of neck and back, lumbosacral region
M54.Ø8 Panniculitis affecting regions of neck and back, sacral and sacrococcygeal region
M54.Ø9 Panniculitis affecting regions, neck and back, multiple sites in spine

✓5th **M54.1 Radiculopathy**
Brachial neuritis or radiculitis NOS
Lumbar neuritis or radiculitis NOS
Lumbosacral neuritis or radiculitis NOS
Thoracic neuritis or radiculitis NOS
Radiculitis NOS
EXCLUDES 1 *neuralgia and neuritis NOS (M79.2)*
radiculopathy with cervical disc disorder (M5Ø.1)
radiculopathy with lumbar and other intervertebral disc disorder (M51.1-)
radiculopathy with spondylosis (M47.2-)
AHA: 2018,3Q,18
TIP: A code from this subcategory can be used in addition to a spondylolisthesis code (M43.1-) or a spinal stenosis code (M48.Ø-) when either condition is documented as the cause of the radiculopathy.
M54.1Ø Radiculopathy, site unspecified
M54.11 Radiculopathy, occipito-atlanto-axial region
M54.12 Radiculopathy, cervical region
M54.13 Radiculopathy, cervicothoracic region
M54.14 Radiculopathy, thoracic region
M54.15 Radiculopathy, thoracolumbar region
M54.16 Radiculopathy, lumbar region
M54.17 Radiculopathy, lumbosacral region
M54.18 Radiculopathy, sacral and sacrococcygeal region

M54.2 Cervicalgia
EXCLUDES 1 *cervicalgia due to intervertebral cervical disc disorder (M5Ø.-)*

✓5th **M54.3 Sciatica**
EXCLUDES 1 *lesion of sciatic nerve (G57.Ø)*
sciatica due to intervertebral disc disorder (M51.1-)
sciatica with lumbago (M54.4-)
M54.3Ø Sciatica, unspecified side
M54.31 Sciatica, right side
M54.32 Sciatica, left side

✓5th **M54.4 Lumbago with sciatica**
EXCLUDES 1 *lumbago with sciatica due to intervertebral disc disorder (M51.1-)*
AHA: 2016,2Q,7
M54.4Ø Lumbago with sciatica, unspecified side
M54.41 Lumbago with sciatica, right side
M54.42 Lumbago with sciatica, left side

✓5th **M54.5 Low back pain**
EXCLUDES 1 *low back strain (S39.Ø12)*
lumbago due to intervertebral disc displacement (M51.2-)
lumbago with sciatica (M54.4-)
AHA: 2021,4Q,22
M54.5Ø Low back pain, unspecified
Loin pain
Lumbago NOS
M54.51 Vertebrogenic low back pain
Low back vertebral endplate pain
M54.59 Other low back pain

M54.6 Pain in thoracic spine
EXCLUDES 1 *pain in thoracic spine due to intervertebral disc disorder (M51.-)*

✓5th **M54.8 Other dorsalgia**
EXCLUDES 1 *dorsalgia in thoracic region (M54.6)*
low back pain (M54.5-)
M54.81 Occipital neuralgia
M54.89 Other dorsalgia

M54.9 Dorsalgia, unspecified
Backache NOS
Back pain NOS

SOFT TISSUE DISORDERS (M6Ø-M79)

Disorders of muscles (M6Ø-M63)

EXCLUDES 1 *dermatopolymyositis (M33.-)*
~~muscular dystrophies and myopathies (G71-G72)~~
myopathy in amyloidosis (E85.-)
myopathy in polyarteritis nodosa (M3Ø.Ø)
myopathy in rheumatoid arthritis (MØ5.32)
myopathy in scleroderma (M34.-)
myopathy in Sjögren's syndrome (M35.Ø3)
myopathy in systemic lupus erythematosus (M32.-)
EXCLUDES 2 ►*muscular dystrophies and myopathies (G71-G72)*◄

✓4th **M6Ø Myositis**
EXCLUDES 2 *inclusion body myositis [IBM] (G72.41)*

✓5th **M6Ø.Ø Infective myositis**
Tropical pyomyositis
Use additional code (B95-B97) to identify infectious agent

✓6th **M6Ø.ØØ Infective myositis, unspecified site**
M6Ø.ØØØ Infective myositis, unspecified right arm
Infective myositis, right upper limb NOS
M6Ø.ØØ1 Infective myositis, unspecified left arm
Infective myositis, left upper limb NOS
M6Ø.ØØ2 Infective myositis, unspecified arm
Infective myositis, upper limb NOS
M6Ø.ØØ3 Infective myositis, unspecified right leg
Infective myositis, right lower limb NOS
M6Ø.ØØ4 Infective myositis, unspecified left leg
Infective myositis, left lower limb NOS
M6Ø.ØØ5 Infective myositis, unspecified leg
Infective myositis, lower limb NOS
M6Ø.ØØ9 Infective myositis, unspecified site

✓6th **M6Ø.Ø1 Infective myositis, shoulder**
M6Ø.Ø11 Infective myositis, right shoulder
M6Ø.Ø12 Infective myositis, left shoulder
M6Ø.Ø19 Infective myositis, unspecified shoulder

✓6th **M6Ø.Ø2 Infective myositis, upper arm**
M6Ø.Ø21 Infective myositis, right upper arm
M6Ø.Ø22 Infective myositis, left upper arm
M6Ø.Ø29 Infective myositis, unspecified upper arm

✓6th **M6Ø.Ø3 Infective myositis, forearm**
M6Ø.Ø31 Infective myositis, right forearm
M6Ø.Ø32 Infective myositis, left forearm
M6Ø.Ø39 Infective myositis, unspecified forearm

✓6th **M6Ø.Ø4 Infective myositis, hand and fingers**
M6Ø.Ø41 Infective myositis, right hand
M6Ø.Ø42 Infective myositis, left hand
M6Ø.Ø43 Infective myositis, unspecified hand
M6Ø.Ø44 Infective myositis, right finger(s)
M6Ø.Ø45 Infective myositis, left finger(s)
M6Ø.Ø46 Infective myositis, unspecified finger(s)

✓6th **M6Ø.Ø5 Infective myositis, thigh**
M6Ø.Ø51 Infective myositis, right thigh
M6Ø.Ø52 Infective myositis, left thigh
M6Ø.Ø59 Infective myositis, unspecified thigh

✓6th **M6Ø.Ø6 Infective myositis, lower leg**
M6Ø.Ø61 Infective myositis, right lower leg
M6Ø.Ø62 Infective myositis, left lower leg
M6Ø.Ø69 Infective myositis, unspecified lower leg

✓6th **M6Ø.Ø7 Infective myositis, ankle, foot and toes**
M6Ø.Ø7Ø Infective myositis, right ankle
M6Ø.Ø71 Infective myositis, left ankle
M6Ø.Ø72 Infective myositis, unspecified ankle
M6Ø.Ø73 Infective myositis, right foot
M6Ø.Ø74 Infective myositis, left foot
M6Ø.Ø75 Infective myositis, unspecified foot
M6Ø.Ø76 Infective myositis, right toe(s)
M6Ø.Ø77 Infective myositis, left toe(s)
M6Ø.Ø78 Infective myositis, unspecified toe(s)

M6Ø.Ø8 Infective myositis, other site
M6Ø.Ø9 Infective myositis, multiple sites

✓5th **M6Ø.1 Interstitial myositis**
M6Ø.1Ø Interstitial myositis of unspecified site

Chapter 13. Diseases of the Musculoskeletal System and Connective Tissue

✓6th M60.11 Interstitial myositis, shoulder
M60.111 Interstitial myositis, right shoulder
M60.112 Interstitial myositis, left shoulder
M60.119 Interstitial myositis, unspecified shoulder

✓6th M60.12 Interstitial myositis, upper arm
M60.121 Interstitial myositis, right upper arm
M60.122 Interstitial myositis, left upper arm
M60.129 Interstitial myositis, unspecified upper arm

✓6th M60.13 Interstitial myositis, forearm
M60.131 Interstitial myositis, right forearm
M60.132 Interstitial myositis, left forearm
M60.139 Interstitial myositis, unspecified forearm

✓6th M60.14 Interstitial myositis, hand
M60.141 Interstitial myositis, right hand
M60.142 Interstitial myositis, left hand
M60.149 Interstitial myositis, unspecified hand

✓6th M60.15 Interstitial myositis, thigh
M60.151 Interstitial myositis, right thigh
M60.152 Interstitial myositis, left thigh
M60.159 Interstitial myositis, unspecified thigh

✓6th M60.16 Interstitial myositis, lower leg
M60.161 Interstitial myositis, right lower leg
M60.162 Interstitial myositis, left lower leg
M60.169 Interstitial myositis, unspecified lower leg

✓6th M60.17 Interstitial myositis, ankle and foot
M60.171 Interstitial myositis, right ankle and foot
M60.172 Interstitial myositis, left ankle and foot
M60.179 Interstitial myositis, unspecified ankle and foot

M60.18 Interstitial myositis, other site
M60.19 Interstitial myositis, multiple sites

✓5th M60.2 Foreign body granuloma of soft tissue, not elsewhere classified
Use additional code to identify the type of retained foreign body (Z18.-)
EXCLUDES 1 *foreign body granuloma of skin and subcutaneous tissue (L92.3)*

M60.20 Foreign body granuloma of soft tissue, not elsewhere classified, unspecified site

✓6th M60.21 Foreign body granuloma of soft tissue, not elsewhere classified, shoulder
M60.211 Foreign body granuloma of soft tissue, not elsewhere classified, right shoulder
M60.212 Foreign body granuloma of soft tissue, not elsewhere classified, left shoulder
M60.219 Foreign body granuloma of soft tissue, not elsewhere classified, unspecified shoulder

✓6th M60.22 Foreign body granuloma of soft tissue, not elsewhere classified, upper arm
M60.221 Foreign body granuloma of soft tissue, not elsewhere classified, right upper arm
M60.222 Foreign body granuloma of soft tissue, not elsewhere classified, left upper arm
M60.229 Foreign body granuloma of soft tissue, not elsewhere classified, unspecified upper arm

✓6th M60.23 Foreign body granuloma of soft tissue, not elsewhere classified, forearm
M60.231 Foreign body granuloma of soft tissue, not elsewhere classified, right forearm
M60.232 Foreign body granuloma of soft tissue, not elsewhere classified, left forearm
M60.239 Foreign body granuloma of soft tissue, not elsewhere classified, unspecified forearm

✓6th M60.24 Foreign body granuloma of soft tissue, not elsewhere classified, hand
M60.241 Foreign body granuloma of soft tissue, not elsewhere classified, right hand
M60.242 Foreign body granuloma of soft tissue, not elsewhere classified, left hand
M60.249 Foreign body granuloma of soft tissue, not elsewhere classified, unspecified hand

✓6th M60.25 Foreign body granuloma of soft tissue, not elsewhere classified, thigh
M60.251 Foreign body granuloma of soft tissue, not elsewhere classified, right thigh
M60.252 Foreign body granuloma of soft tissue, not elsewhere classified, left thigh
M60.259 Foreign body granuloma of soft tissue, not elsewhere classified, unspecified thigh

✓6th M60.26 Foreign body granuloma of soft tissue, not elsewhere classified, lower leg
M60.261 Foreign body granuloma of soft tissue, not elsewhere classified, right lower leg
M60.262 Foreign body granuloma of soft tissue, not elsewhere classified, left lower leg
M60.269 Foreign body granuloma of soft tissue, not elsewhere classified, unspecified lower leg

✓6th M60.27 Foreign body granuloma of soft tissue, not elsewhere classified, ankle and foot
M60.271 Foreign body granuloma of soft tissue, not elsewhere classified, right ankle and foot
M60.272 Foreign body granuloma of soft tissue, not elsewhere classified, left ankle and foot
M60.279 Foreign body granuloma of soft tissue, not elsewhere classified, unspecified ankle and foot

M60.28 Foreign body granuloma of soft tissue, not elsewhere classified, other site

✓5th M60.8 Other myositis
M60.80 Other myositis, unspecified site

✓6th M60.81 Other myositis shoulder
M60.811 Other myositis, right shoulder
M60.812 Other myositis, left shoulder
M60.819 Other myositis, unspecified shoulder

✓6th M60.82 Other myositis, upper arm
M60.821 Other myositis, right upper arm
M60.822 Other myositis, left upper arm
M60.829 Other myositis, unspecified upper arm

✓6th M60.83 Other myositis, forearm
M60.831 Other myositis, right forearm
M60.832 Other myositis, left forearm
M60.839 Other myositis, unspecified forearm

✓6th M60.84 Other myositis, hand
M60.841 Other myositis, right hand
M60.842 Other myositis, left hand
M60.849 Other myositis, unspecified hand

✓6th M60.85 Other myositis, thigh
M60.851 Other myositis, right thigh
M60.852 Other myositis, left thigh
M60.859 Other myositis, unspecified thigh

✓6th M60.86 Other myositis, lower leg
M60.861 Other myositis, right lower leg
M60.862 Other myositis, left lower leg
M60.869 Other myositis, unspecified lower leg

✓6th M60.87 Other myositis, ankle and foot
M60.871 Other myositis, right ankle and foot
M60.872 Other myositis, left ankle and foot
M60.879 Other myositis, unspecified ankle and foot

M60.88 Other myositis, other site
M60.89 Other myositis, multiple sites

M60.9 Myositis, unspecified

✓4th M61 Calcification and ossification of muscle

✓5th M61.0 Myositis ossificans traumatica
M61.00 Myositis ossificans traumatica, unspecified site

✓6th M61.01 Myositis ossificans traumatica, shoulder
M61.011 Myositis ossificans traumatica, right shoulder
M61.012 Myositis ossificans traumatica, left shoulder
M61.019 Myositis ossificans traumatica, unspecified shoulder

✓6th M61.02 Myositis ossificans traumatica, upper arm
M61.021 Myositis ossificans traumatica, right upper arm

M61.Ø22 Myositis ossificans traumatica, left upper arm
M61.Ø29 Myositis ossificans traumatica, unspecified upper arm
✓6th M61.Ø3 Myositis ossificans traumatica, forearm
M61.Ø31 Myositis ossificans traumatica, right forearm
M61.Ø32 Myositis ossificans traumatica, left forearm
M61.Ø39 Myositis ossificans traumatica, unspecified forearm
✓6th M61.Ø4 Myositis ossificans traumatica, hand
M61.Ø41 Myositis ossificans traumatica, right hand
M61.Ø42 Myositis ossificans traumatica, left hand
M61.Ø49 Myositis ossificans traumatica, unspecified hand
✓6th M61.Ø5 Myositis ossificans traumatica, thigh
M61.Ø51 Myositis ossificans traumatica, right thigh
M61.Ø52 Myositis ossificans traumatica, left thigh
M61.Ø59 Myositis ossificans traumatica, unspecified thigh
✓6th M61.Ø6 Myositis ossificans traumatica, lower leg
M61.Ø61 Myositis ossificans traumatica, right lower leg
M61.Ø62 Myositis ossificans traumatica, left lower leg
M61.Ø69 Myositis ossificans traumatica, unspecified lower leg
✓6th M61.Ø7 Myositis ossificans traumatica, ankle and foot
M61.Ø71 Myositis ossificans traumatica, right ankle and foot
M61.Ø72 Myositis ossificans traumatica, left ankle and foot
M61.Ø79 Myositis ossificans traumatica, unspecified ankle and foot
M61.Ø8 Myositis ossificans traumatica, other site
M61.Ø9 Myositis ossificans traumatica, multiple sites

✓5th M61.1 Myositis ossificans progressiva
Fibrodysplasia ossificans progressiva
M61.1Ø Myositis ossificans progressiva, unspecified site
✓6th M61.11 Myositis ossificans progressiva, shoulder
M61.111 Myositis ossificans progressiva, right shoulder
M61.112 Myositis ossificans progressiva, left shoulder
M61.119 Myositis ossificans progressiva, unspecified shoulder
✓6th M61.12 Myositis ossificans progressiva, upper arm
M61.121 Myositis ossificans progressiva, right upper arm
M61.122 Myositis ossificans progressiva, left upper arm
M61.129 Myositis ossificans progressiva, unspecified arm
✓6th M61.13 Myositis ossificans progressiva, forearm
M61.131 Myositis ossificans progressiva, right forearm
M61.132 Myositis ossificans progressiva, left forearm
M61.139 Myositis ossificans progressiva, unspecified forearm
✓6th M61.14 Myositis ossificans progressiva, hand and finger(s)
M61.141 Myositis ossificans progressiva, right hand
M61.142 Myositis ossificans progressiva, left hand
M61.143 Myositis ossificans progressiva, unspecified hand
M61.144 Myositis ossificans progressiva, right finger(s)
M61.145 Myositis ossificans progressiva, left finger(s)
M61.146 Myositis ossificans progressiva, unspecified finger(s)
✓6th M61.15 Myositis ossificans progressiva, thigh
M61.151 Myositis ossificans progressiva, right thigh
M61.152 Myositis ossificans progressiva, left thigh
M61.159 Myositis ossificans progressiva, unspecified thigh
✓6th M61.16 Myositis ossificans progressiva, lower leg
M61.161 Myositis ossificans progressiva, right lower leg
M61.162 Myositis ossificans progressiva, left lower leg
M61.169 Myositis ossificans progressiva, unspecified lower leg
✓6th M61.17 Myositis ossificans progressiva, ankle, foot and toe(s)
M61.171 Myositis ossificans progressiva, right ankle
M61.172 Myositis ossificans progressiva, left ankle
M61.173 Myositis ossificans progressiva, unspecified ankle
M61.174 Myositis ossificans progressiva, right foot
M61.175 Myositis ossificans progressiva, left foot
M61.176 Myositis ossificans progressiva, unspecified foot
M61.177 Myositis ossificans progressiva, right toe(s)
M61.178 Myositis ossificans progressiva, left toe(s)
M61.179 Myositis ossificans progressiva, unspecified toe(s)
M61.18 Myositis ossificans progressiva, other site
M61.19 Myositis ossificans progressiva, multiple sites

✓5th M61.2 Paralytic calcification and ossification of muscle
Myositis ossificans associated with quadriplegia or paraplegia
M61.2Ø Paralytic calcification and ossification of muscle, unspecified site
✓6th M61.21 Paralytic calcification and ossification of muscle, shoulder
M61.211 Paralytic calcification and ossification of muscle, right shoulder
M61.212 Paralytic calcification and ossification of muscle, left shoulder
M61.219 Paralytic calcification and ossification of muscle, unspecified shoulder
✓6th M61.22 Paralytic calcification and ossification of muscle, upper arm
M61.221 Paralytic calcification and ossification of muscle, right upper arm
M61.222 Paralytic calcification and ossification of muscle, left upper arm
M61.229 Paralytic calcification and ossification of muscle, unspecified upper arm
✓6th M61.23 Paralytic calcification and ossification of muscle, forearm
M61.231 Paralytic calcification and ossification of muscle, right forearm
M61.232 Paralytic calcification and ossification of muscle, left forearm
M61.239 Paralytic calcification and ossification of muscle, unspecified forearm
✓6th M61.24 Paralytic calcification and ossification of muscle, hand
M61.241 Paralytic calcification and ossification of muscle, right hand
M61.242 Paralytic calcification and ossification of muscle, left hand
M61.249 Paralytic calcification and ossification of muscle, unspecified hand
✓6th M61.25 Paralytic calcification and ossification of muscle, thigh
M61.251 Paralytic calcification and ossification of muscle, right thigh
M61.252 Paralytic calcification and ossification of muscle, left thigh
M61.259 Paralytic calcification and ossification of muscle, unspecified thigh
✓6th M61.26 Paralytic calcification and ossification of muscle, lower leg
M61.261 Paralytic calcification and ossification of muscle, right lower leg
M61.262 Paralytic calcification and ossification of muscle, left lower leg
M61.269 Paralytic calcification and ossification of muscle, unspecified lower leg
✓6th M61.27 Paralytic calcification and ossification of muscle, ankle and foot
M61.271 Paralytic calcification and ossification of muscle, right ankle and foot

M61.272 Paralytic calcification and ossification of muscle, left ankle and foot

M61.279 Paralytic calcification and ossification of muscle, unspecified ankle and foot

M61.28 Paralytic calcification and ossification of muscle, other site

M61.29 Paralytic calcification and ossification of muscle, multiple sites

5th M61.3 Calcification and ossification of muscles associated with burns

Myositis ossificans associated with burns

M61.30 Calcification and ossification of muscles associated with burns, unspecified site

6th M61.31 Calcification and ossification of muscles associated with burns, shoulder

M61.311 Calcification and ossification of muscles associated with burns, right shoulder

M61.312 Calcification and ossification of muscles associated with burns, left shoulder

M61.319 Calcification and ossification of muscles associated with burns, unspecified shoulder

6th M61.32 Calcification and ossification of muscles associated with burns, upper arm

M61.321 Calcification and ossification of muscles associated with burns, right upper arm

M61.322 Calcification and ossification of muscles associated with burns, left upper arm

M61.329 Calcification and ossification of muscles associated with burns, unspecified upper arm

6th M61.33 Calcification and ossification of muscles associated with burns, forearm

M61.331 Calcification and ossification of muscles associated with burns, right forearm

M61.332 Calcification and ossification of muscles associated with burns, left forearm

M61.339 Calcification and ossification of muscles associated with burns, unspecified forearm

6th M61.34 Calcification and ossification of muscles associated with burns, hand

M61.341 Calcification and ossification of muscles associated with burns, right hand

M61.342 Calcification and ossification of muscles associated with burns, left hand

M61.349 Calcification and ossification of muscles associated with burns, unspecified hand

6th M61.35 Calcification and ossification of muscles associated with burns, thigh

M61.351 Calcification and ossification of muscles associated with burns, right thigh

M61.352 Calcification and ossification of muscles associated with burns, left thigh

M61.359 Calcification and ossification of muscles associated with burns, unspecified thigh

6th M61.36 Calcification and ossification of muscles associated with burns, lower leg

M61.361 Calcification and ossification of muscles associated with burns, right lower leg

M61.362 Calcification and ossification of muscles associated with burns, left lower leg

M61.369 Calcification and ossification of muscles associated with burns, unspecified lower leg

6th M61.37 Calcification and ossification of muscles associated with burns, ankle and foot

M61.371 Calcification and ossification of muscles associated with burns, right ankle and foot

M61.372 Calcification and ossification of muscles associated with burns, left ankle and foot

M61.379 Calcification and ossification of muscles associated with burns, unspecified ankle and foot

M61.38 Calcification and ossification of muscles associated with burns, other site

M61.39 Calcification and ossification of muscles associated with burns, multiple sites

5th M61.4 Other calcification of muscle

EXCLUDES 1 *calcific tendinitis NOS (M65.2-)*
calcific tendinitis of shoulder (M75.3)

M61.40 Other calcification of muscle, unspecified site

6th M61.41 Other calcification of muscle, shoulder

M61.411 Other calcification of muscle, right shoulder

M61.412 Other calcification of muscle, left shoulder

M61.419 Other calcification of muscle, unspecified shoulder

6th M61.42 Other calcification of muscle, upper arm

M61.421 Other calcification of muscle, right upper arm

M61.422 Other calcification of muscle, left upper arm

M61.429 Other calcification of muscle, unspecified upper arm

6th M61.43 Other calcification of muscle, forearm

M61.431 Other calcification of muscle, right forearm

M61.432 Other calcification of muscle, left forearm

M61.439 Other calcification of muscle, unspecified forearm

6th M61.44 Other calcification of muscle, hand

M61.441 Other calcification of muscle, right hand

M61.442 Other calcification of muscle, left hand

M61.449 Other calcification of muscle, unspecified hand

6th M61.45 Other calcification of muscle, thigh

M61.451 Other calcification of muscle, right thigh

M61.452 Other calcification of muscle, left thigh

M61.459 Other calcification of muscle, unspecified thigh

6th M61.46 Other calcification of muscle, lower leg

M61.461 Other calcification of muscle, right lower leg

M61.462 Other calcification of muscle, left lower leg

M61.469 Other calcification of muscle, unspecified lower leg

6th M61.47 Other calcification of muscle, ankle and foot

M61.471 Other calcification of muscle, right ankle and foot

M61.472 Other calcification of muscle, left ankle and foot

M61.479 Other calcification of muscle, unspecified ankle and foot

M61.48 Other calcification of muscle, other site

M61.49 Other calcification of muscle, multiple sites

5th M61.5 Other ossification of muscle

M61.50 Other ossification of muscle, unspecified site

6th M61.51 Other ossification of muscle, shoulder

M61.511 Other ossification of muscle, right shoulder

M61.512 Other ossification of muscle, left shoulder

M61.519 Other ossification of muscle, unspecified shoulder

6th M61.52 Other ossification of muscle, upper arm

M61.521 Other ossification of muscle, right upper arm

M61.522 Other ossification of muscle, left upper arm

M61.529 Other ossification of muscle, unspecified upper arm

6th M61.53 Other ossification of muscle, forearm

M61.531 Other ossification of muscle, right forearm

M61.532 Other ossification of muscle, left forearm

M61.539 Other ossification of muscle, unspecified forearm

6th M61.54 Other ossification of muscle, hand

M61.541 Other ossification of muscle, right hand

M61.542 Other ossification of muscle, left hand

M61.549 Other ossification of muscle, unspecified hand

6th M61.55 Other ossification of muscle, thigh

M61.551 Other ossification of muscle, right thigh

M61.552 Other ossification of muscle, left thigh

M61.559 Other ossification of muscle, unspecified thigh

✓6th **M61.56 Other ossification of muscle, lower leg**
M61.561 Other ossification of muscle, right lower leg
M61.562 Other ossification of muscle, left lower leg
M61.569 Other ossification of muscle, unspecified lower leg

✓6th **M61.57 Other ossification of muscle, ankle and foot**
M61.571 Other ossification of muscle, right ankle and foot
M61.572 Other ossification of muscle, left ankle and foot
M61.579 Other ossification of muscle, unspecified ankle and foot

M61.58 Other ossification of muscle, other site
M61.59 Other ossification of muscle, multiple sites

M61.9 Calcification and ossification of muscle, unspecified

✓4th **M62 Other disorders of muscle**

EXCLUDES 1 *alcoholic myopathy (G72.1)*
cramp and spasm (R25.2)
drug-induced myopathy (G72.Ø)
myalgia (M79.1-)
stiff-man syndrome (G25.82)

EXCLUDES 2 *nontraumatic hematoma of muscle (M79.81)*

✓5th **M62.Ø Separation of muscle (nontraumatic)**
Diastasis of muscle

EXCLUDES 1 *diastasis recti complicating pregnancy, labor and delivery (O71.8)*
traumatic separation of muscle - see strain of muscle by body region

M62.ØØ Separation of muscle (nontraumatic), unspecified site

✓6th **M62.Ø1 Separation of muscle (nontraumatic), shoulder**
M62.Ø11 Separation of muscle (nontraumatic), right shoulder
M62.Ø12 Separation of muscle (nontraumatic), left shoulder
M62.Ø19 Separation of muscle (nontraumatic), unspecified shoulder

✓6th **M62.Ø2 Separation of muscle (nontraumatic), upper arm**
M62.Ø21 Separation of muscle (nontraumatic), right upper arm
M62.Ø22 Separation of muscle (nontraumatic), left upper arm
M62.Ø29 Separation of muscle (nontraumatic), unspecified upper arm

✓6th **M62.Ø3 Separation of muscle (nontraumatic), forearm**
M62.Ø31 Separation of muscle (nontraumatic), right forearm
M62.Ø32 Separation of muscle (nontraumatic), left forearm
M62.Ø39 Separation of muscle (nontraumatic), unspecified forearm

✓6th **M62.Ø4 Separation of muscle (nontraumatic), hand**
M62.Ø41 Separation of muscle (nontraumatic), right hand
M62.Ø42 Separation of muscle (nontraumatic), left hand
M62.Ø49 Separation of muscle (nontraumatic), unspecified hand

✓6th **M62.Ø5 Separation of muscle (nontraumatic), thigh**
M62.Ø51 Separation of muscle (nontraumatic), right thigh
M62.Ø52 Separation of muscle (nontraumatic), left thigh
M62.Ø59 Separation of muscle (nontraumatic), unspecified thigh

✓6th **M62.Ø6 Separation of muscle (nontraumatic), lower leg**
M62.Ø61 Separation of muscle (nontraumatic), right lower leg
M62.Ø62 Separation of muscle (nontraumatic), left lower leg
M62.Ø69 Separation of muscle (nontraumatic), unspecified lower leg

✓6th **M62.Ø7 Separation of muscle (nontraumatic), ankle and foot**
M62.Ø71 Separation of muscle (nontraumatic), right ankle and foot
M62.Ø72 Separation of muscle (nontraumatic), left ankle and foot
M62.Ø79 Separation of muscle (nontraumatic), unspecified ankle and foot

M62.Ø8 Separation of muscle (nontraumatic), other site

✓5th **M62.1 Other rupture of muscle (nontraumatic)**

EXCLUDES 1 *traumatic rupture of muscle - see strain of muscle by body region*

EXCLUDES 2 *rupture of tendon (M66.-)*

M62.1Ø Other rupture of muscle (nontraumatic), unspecified site

✓6th **M62.11 Other rupture of muscle (nontraumatic), shoulder**
M62.111 Other rupture of muscle (nontraumatic), right shoulder
M62.112 Other rupture of muscle (nontraumatic), left shoulder
M62.119 Other rupture of muscle (nontraumatic), unspecified shoulder

✓6th **M62.12 Other rupture of muscle (nontraumatic), upper arm**
M62.121 Other rupture of muscle (nontraumatic), right upper arm
M62.122 Other rupture of muscle (nontraumatic), left upper arm
M62.129 Other rupture of muscle (nontraumatic), unspecified upper arm

✓6th **M62.13 Other rupture of muscle (nontraumatic), forearm**
M62.131 Other rupture of muscle (nontraumatic), right forearm
M62.132 Other rupture of muscle (nontraumatic), left forearm
M62.139 Other rupture of muscle (nontraumatic), unspecified forearm

✓6th **M62.14 Other rupture of muscle (nontraumatic), hand**
M62.141 Other rupture of muscle (nontraumatic), right hand
M62.142 Other rupture of muscle (nontraumatic), left hand
M62.149 Other rupture of muscle (nontraumatic), unspecified hand

✓6th **M62.15 Other rupture of muscle (nontraumatic), thigh**
M62.151 Other rupture of muscle (nontraumatic), right thigh
M62.152 Other rupture of muscle (nontraumatic), left thigh
M62.159 Other rupture of muscle (nontraumatic), unspecified thigh

✓6th **M62.16 Other rupture of muscle (nontraumatic), lower leg**
M62.161 Other rupture of muscle (nontraumatic), right lower leg
M62.162 Other rupture of muscle (nontraumatic), left lower leg
M62.169 Other rupture of muscle (nontraumatic), unspecified lower leg

✓6th **M62.17 Other rupture of muscle (nontraumatic), ankle and foot**
M62.171 Other rupture of muscle (nontraumatic), right ankle and foot
M62.172 Other rupture of muscle (nontraumatic), left ankle and foot
M62.179 Other rupture of muscle (nontraumatic), unspecified ankle and foot

M62.18 Other rupture of muscle (nontraumatic), other site

✓5th **M62.2 Nontraumatic ischemic infarction of muscle**

EXCLUDES 1 *compartment syndrome (traumatic) (T79.A-)*
nontraumatic compartment syndrome (M79.A-)
rhabdomyolysis (M62.82)
traumatic ischemia of muscle (T79.6)
Volkmann's ischemic contracture (T79.6)

M62.2Ø Nontraumatic ischemic infarction of muscle, unspecified site

✓6th **M62.21 Nontraumatic ischemic infarction of muscle, shoulder**
M62.211 Nontraumatic ischemic infarction of muscle, right shoulder
M62.212 Nontraumatic ischemic infarction of muscle, left shoulder
M62.219 Nontraumatic ischemic infarction of muscle, unspecified shoulder

√6th **M62.22 Nontraumatic ischemic infarction of muscle, upper arm**
- **M62.221 Nontraumatic ischemic infarction of muscle, right upper arm**
- **M62.222 Nontraumatic ischemic infarction of muscle, left upper arm**
- **M62.229 Nontraumatic ischemic infarction of muscle, unspecified upper arm**

√6th **M62.23 Nontraumatic ischemic infarction of muscle, forearm**
- **M62.231 Nontraumatic ischemic infarction of muscle, right forearm**
- **M62.232 Nontraumatic ischemic infarction of muscle, left forearm**
- **M62.239 Nontraumatic ischemic infarction of muscle, unspecified forearm**

√6th **M62.24 Nontraumatic ischemic infarction of muscle, hand**
- **M62.241 Nontraumatic ischemic infarction of muscle, right hand**
- **M62.242 Nontraumatic ischemic infarction of muscle, left hand**
- **M62.249 Nontraumatic ischemic infarction of muscle, unspecified hand**

√6th **M62.25 Nontraumatic ischemic infarction of muscle, thigh**
- **M62.251 Nontraumatic ischemic infarction of muscle, right thigh**
- **M62.252 Nontraumatic ischemic infarction of muscle, left thigh**
- **M62.259 Nontraumatic ischemic infarction of muscle, unspecified thigh**

√6th **M62.26 Nontraumatic ischemic infarction of muscle, lower leg**
- **M62.261 Nontraumatic ischemic infarction of muscle, right lower leg**
- **M62.262 Nontraumatic ischemic infarction of muscle, left lower leg**
- **M62.269 Nontraumatic ischemic infarction of muscle, unspecified lower leg**

√6th **M62.27 Nontraumatic ischemic infarction of muscle, ankle and foot**
- **M62.271 Nontraumatic ischemic infarction of muscle, right ankle and foot**
- **M62.272 Nontraumatic ischemic infarction of muscle, left ankle and foot**
- **M62.279 Nontraumatic ischemic infarction of muscle, unspecified ankle and foot**

M62.28 Nontraumatic ischemic infarction of muscle, other site

M62.3 Immobility syndrome (paraplegic)

√5th **M62.4 Contracture of muscle**

Contracture of tendon (sheath)

EXCLUDES 1 *contracture of joint (M24.5-)*

M62.40 Contracture of muscle, unspecified site

√6th **M62.41 Contracture of muscle, shoulder**
- **M62.411 Contracture of muscle, right shoulder**
- **M62.412 Contracture of muscle, left shoulder**
- **M62.419 Contracture of muscle, unspecified shoulder**

√6th **M62.42 Contracture of muscle, upper arm**
- **M62.421 Contracture of muscle, right upper arm**
- **M62.422 Contracture of muscle, left upper arm**
- **M62.429 Contracture of muscle, unspecified upper arm**

√6th **M62.43 Contracture of muscle, forearm**
- **M62.431 Contracture of muscle, right forearm**
- **M62.432 Contracture of muscle, left forearm**
- **M62.439 Contracture of muscle, unspecified forearm**

√6th **M62.44 Contracture of muscle, hand**
- **M62.441 Contracture of muscle, right hand**
- **M62.442 Contracture of muscle, left hand**
- **M62.449 Contracture of muscle, unspecified hand**

√6th **M62.45 Contracture of muscle, thigh**
- **M62.451 Contracture of muscle, right thigh**
- **M62.452 Contracture of muscle, left thigh**
- **M62.459 Contracture of muscle, unspecified thigh**

√6th **M62.46 Contracture of muscle, lower leg**
- **M62.461 Contracture of muscle, right lower leg**
- **M62.462 Contracture of muscle, left lower leg**
- **M62.469 Contracture of muscle, unspecified lower leg**

√6th **M62.47 Contracture of muscle, ankle and foot**
- **M62.471 Contracture of muscle, right ankle and foot**
- **M62.472 Contracture of muscle, left ankle and foot**
- **M62.479 Contracture of muscle, unspecified ankle and foot**

M62.48 Contracture of muscle, other site

M62.49 Contracture of muscle, multiple sites

√5th **M62.5 Muscle wasting and atrophy, not elsewhere classified**

Disuse atrophy NEC

EXCLUDES 1 *neuralgic amyotrophy (G54.5)*
progressive muscular atrophy (G12.21)
sarcopenia (M62.84)

EXCLUDES 2 *pelvic muscle wasting (N81.84)*

M62.50 Muscle wasting and atrophy, not elsewhere classified, unspecified site

√6th **M62.51 Muscle wasting and atrophy, not elsewhere classified, shoulder**
- **M62.511 Muscle wasting and atrophy, not elsewhere classified, right shoulder**
- **M62.512 Muscle wasting and atrophy, not elsewhere classified, left shoulder**
- **M62.519 Muscle wasting and atrophy, not elsewhere classified, unspecified shoulder**

√6th **M62.52 Muscle wasting and atrophy, not elsewhere classified, upper arm**
- **M62.521 Muscle wasting and atrophy, not elsewhere classified, right upper arm**
- **M62.522 Muscle wasting and atrophy, not elsewhere classified, left upper arm**
- **M62.529 Muscle wasting and atrophy, not elsewhere classified, unspecified upper arm**

√6th **M62.53 Muscle wasting and atrophy, not elsewhere classified, forearm**
- **M62.531 Muscle wasting and atrophy, not elsewhere classified, right forearm**
- **M62.532 Muscle wasting and atrophy, not elsewhere classified, left forearm**
- **M62.539 Muscle wasting and atrophy, not elsewhere classified, unspecified forearm**

√6th **M62.54 Muscle wasting and atrophy, not elsewhere classified, hand**
- **M62.541 Muscle wasting and atrophy, not elsewhere classified, right hand**
- **M62.542 Muscle wasting and atrophy, not elsewhere classified, left hand**
- **M62.549 Muscle wasting and atrophy, not elsewhere classified, unspecified hand**

√6th **M62.55 Muscle wasting and atrophy, not elsewhere classified, thigh**
- **M62.551 Muscle wasting and atrophy, not elsewhere classified, right thigh**
- **M62.552 Muscle wasting and atrophy, not elsewhere classified, left thigh**
- **M62.559 Muscle wasting and atrophy, not elsewhere classified, unspecified thigh**

√6th **M62.56 Muscle wasting and atrophy, not elsewhere classified, lower leg**
- **M62.561 Muscle wasting and atrophy, not elsewhere classified, right lower leg**
- **M62.562 Muscle wasting and atrophy, not elsewhere classified, left lower leg**
- **M62.569 Muscle wasting and atrophy, not elsewhere classified, unspecified lower leg**

√6th **M62.57 Muscle wasting and atrophy, not elsewhere classified, ankle and foot**
- **M62.571 Muscle wasting and atrophy, not elsewhere classified, right ankle and foot**
- **M62.572 Muscle wasting and atrophy, not elsewhere classified, left ankle and foot**
- **M62.579 Muscle wasting and atrophy, not elsewhere classified, unspecified ankle and foot**

M62.58 Muscle wasting and atrophy, not elsewhere classified, other site

M62.59 Muscle wasting and atrophy, not elsewhere classified, multiple sites

● ✓6th M62.5A Muscle wasting and atrophy, not elsewhere classified, back

● M62.5A0 Muscle wasting and atrophy, not elsewhere classified, back, cervical

● M62.5A1 Muscle wasting and atrophy, not elsewhere classified, back, thoracic

● M62.5A2 Muscle wasting and atrophy, not elsewhere classified, back, lumbosacral

● M62.5A9 Muscle wasting and atrophy, not elsewhere classified, back, unspecified level

✓5th M62.8 Other specified disorders of muscle

EXCLUDES 2 *nontraumatic hematoma of muscle (M79.81)*

M62.81 Muscle weakness (generalized)

EXCLUDES 1 *muscle weakness in sarcopenia (M62.84)*

M62.82 Rhabdomyolysis

EXCLUDES 1 *traumatic rhabdomyolysis (T79.6)*

AHA: 2019,2Q,12

DEF: Rapid disintegration or destruction of skeletal muscle caused by direct or indirect injury, resulting in the excretion of muscle protein myoglobin into the urine.

✓6th M62.83 Muscle spasm

M62.830 Muscle spasm of back

M62.831 Muscle spasm of calf

Charley-horse

M62.838 Other muscle spasm

M62.84 Sarcopenia

Age-related sarcopenia

Code first underlying disease, if applicable, such as:

disorders of myoneural junction and muscle disease in diseases classified elsewhere (G73.-)

other and unspecified myopathies (G72.-)

primary disorders of muscles (G71.-)

AHA: 2016,4Q,41

M62.89 Other specified disorders of muscle

Muscle (sheath) hernia

M62.9 Disorder of muscle, unspecified

✓4th M63 Disorders of muscle in diseases classified elsewhere

Code first underlying disease, such as:

leprosy (A30.-)

neoplasm (C49.-, C79.89, D21.-, D48.1)

schistosomiasis (B65.-)

trichinellosis (B75)

EXCLUDES 1 *myopathy in cysticercosis (B69.81)*

myopathy in endocrine diseases (G73.7)

myopathy in metabolic diseases (G73.7)

myopathy in sarcoidosis (D86.87)

myopathy in secondary syphilis (A51.49)

myopathy in syphilis (late) (A52.78)

myopathy in toxoplasmosis (B58.82)

myopathy in tuberculosis (A18.09)

✓5th M63.8 Disorders of muscle in diseases classified elsewhere

M63.80 Disorders of muscle in diseases classified elsewhere, unspecified site

✓6th M63.81 Disorders of muscle in diseases classified elsewhere, shoulder

M63.811 Disorders of muscle in diseases classified elsewhere, right shoulder

M63.812 Disorders of muscle in diseases classified elsewhere, left shoulder

M63.819 Disorders of muscle in diseases classified elsewhere, unspecified shoulder

✓6th M63.82 Disorders of muscle in diseases classified elsewhere, upper arm

M63.821 Disorders of muscle in diseases classified elsewhere, right upper arm

M63.822 Disorders of muscle in diseases classified elsewhere, left upper arm

M63.829 Disorders of muscle in diseases classified elsewhere, unspecified upper arm

✓6th M63.83 Disorders of muscle in diseases classified elsewhere, forearm

M63.831 Disorders of muscle in diseases classified elsewhere, right forearm

M63.832 Disorders of muscle in diseases classified elsewhere, left forearm

M63.839 Disorders of muscle in diseases classified elsewhere, unspecified forearm

✓6th M63.84 Disorders of muscle in diseases classified elsewhere, hand

M63.841 Disorders of muscle in diseases classified elsewhere, right hand

M63.842 Disorders of muscle in diseases classified elsewhere, left hand

M63.849 Disorders of muscle in diseases classified elsewhere, unspecified hand

✓6th M63.85 Disorders of muscle in diseases classified elsewhere, thigh

M63.851 Disorders of muscle in diseases classified elsewhere, right thigh

M63.852 Disorders of muscle in diseases classified elsewhere, left thigh

M63.859 Disorders of muscle in diseases classified elsewhere, unspecified thigh

✓6th M63.86 Disorders of muscle in diseases classified elsewhere, lower leg

M63.861 Disorders of muscle in diseases classified elsewhere, right lower leg

M63.862 Disorders of muscle in diseases classified elsewhere, left lower leg

M63.869 Disorders of muscle in diseases classified elsewhere, unspecified lower leg

✓6th M63.87 Disorders of muscle in diseases classified elsewhere, ankle and foot

M63.871 Disorders of muscle in diseases classified elsewhere, right ankle and foot

M63.872 Disorders of muscle in diseases classified elsewhere, left ankle and foot

M63.879 Disorders of muscle in diseases classified elsewhere, unspecified ankle and foot

M63.88 Disorders of muscle in diseases classified elsewhere, other site

M63.89 Disorders of muscle in diseases classified elsewhere, multiple sites

Disorders of synovium and tendon (M65-M67)

✓4th M65 Synovitis and tenosynovitis

EXCLUDES 1 *chronic crepitant synovitis of hand and wrist (M70.0-)*

current injury - see injury of ligament or tendon by body region

soft tissue disorders related to use, overuse and pressure (M70.-)

✓5th M65.0 Abscess of tendon sheath

Use additional code (B95-B96) to identify bacterial agent.

M65.00 Abscess of tendon sheath, unspecified site

✓6th M65.01 Abscess of tendon sheath, shoulder

M65.011 Abscess of tendon sheath, right shoulder

M65.012 Abscess of tendon sheath, left shoulder

M65.019 Abscess of tendon sheath, unspecified shoulder

✓6th M65.02 Abscess of tendon sheath, upper arm

M65.021 Abscess of tendon sheath, right upper arm

M65.022 Abscess of tendon sheath, left upper arm

M65.029 Abscess of tendon sheath, unspecified upper arm

✓6th M65.03 Abscess of tendon sheath, forearm

M65.031 Abscess of tendon sheath, right forearm

M65.032 Abscess of tendon sheath, left forearm

M65.039 Abscess of tendon sheath, unspecified forearm

✓6th M65.04 Abscess of tendon sheath, hand

M65.041 Abscess of tendon sheath, right hand

M65.042 Abscess of tendon sheath, left hand

M65.049 Abscess of tendon sheath, unspecified hand

✓6th M65.05 Abscess of tendon sheath, thigh

M65.051 Abscess of tendon sheath, right thigh

M65.052 Abscess of tendon sheath, left thigh

M65.059 Abscess of tendon sheath, unspecified thigh

✓6th M65.06 Abscess of tendon sheath, lower leg

M65.061 Abscess of tendon sheath, right lower leg

M65.062 Abscess of tendon sheath, left lower leg

M65.069 Abscess of tendon sheath, unspecified lower leg

M65.07 **Abscess of tendon sheath, ankle and foot**
- **M65.071** **Abscess of tendon sheath, right ankle and foot**
- **M65.072** **Abscess of tendon sheath, left ankle and foot**
- **M65.079** **Abscess of tendon sheath, unspecified ankle and foot**

M65.08 **Abscess of tendon sheath, other site**

M65.1 **Other infective (teno)synovitis**
- **M65.10** **Other infective (teno)synovitis, unspecified site**

M65.11 **Other infective (teno)synovitis, shoulder**
- **M65.111** **Other infective (teno)synovitis, right shoulder**
- **M65.112** **Other infective (teno)synovitis, left shoulder**
- **M65.119** **Other infective (teno)synovitis, unspecified shoulder**

M65.12 **Other infective (teno)synovitis, elbow**
- **M65.121** **Other infective (teno)synovitis, right elbow**
- **M65.122** **Other infective (teno)synovitis, left elbow**
- **M65.129** **Other infective (teno)synovitis, unspecified elbow**

M65.13 **Other infective (teno)synovitis, wrist**
- **M65.131** **Other infective (teno)synovitis, right wrist**
- **M65.132** **Other infective (teno)synovitis, left wrist**
- **M65.139** **Other infective (teno)synovitis, unspecified wrist**

M65.14 **Other infective (teno)synovitis, hand**
- **M65.141** **Other infective (teno)synovitis, right hand**
- **M65.142** **Other infective (teno)synovitis, left hand**
- **M65.149** **Other infective (teno)synovitis, unspecified hand**

M65.15 **Other infective (teno)synovitis, hip**
- **M65.151** **Other infective (teno)synovitis, right hip**
- **M65.152** **Other infective (teno)synovitis, left hip**
- **M65.159** **Other infective (teno)synovitis, unspecified hip**

M65.16 **Other infective (teno)synovitis, knee**
- **M65.161** **Other infective (teno)synovitis, right knee**
- **M65.162** **Other infective (teno)synovitis, left knee**
- **M65.169** **Other infective (teno)synovitis, unspecified knee**

M65.17 **Other infective (teno)synovitis, ankle and foot**
- **M65.171** **Other infective (teno)synovitis, right ankle and foot**
- **M65.172** **Other infective (teno)synovitis, left ankle and foot**
- **M65.179** **Other infective (teno)synovitis, unspecified ankle and foot**

M65.18 **Other infective (teno)synovitis, other site**

M65.19 **Other infective (teno)synovitis, multiple sites**

M65.2 **Calcific tendinitis**

EXCLUDES 1 *tendinitis as classified in M75-M77*
calcified tendinitis of shoulder (M75.3)

- **M65.20** **Calcific tendinitis, unspecified site**

M65.22 **Calcific tendinitis, upper arm**
- **M65.221** **Calcific tendinitis, right upper arm**
- **M65.222** **Calcific tendinitis, left upper arm**
- **M65.229** **Calcific tendinitis, unspecified upper arm**

M65.23 **Calcific tendinitis, forearm**
- **M65.231** **Calcific tendinitis, right forearm**
- **M65.232** **Calcific tendinitis, left forearm**
- **M65.239** **Calcific tendinitis, unspecified forearm**

M65.24 **Calcific tendinitis, hand**
- **M65.241** **Calcific tendinitis, right hand**
- **M65.242** **Calcific tendinitis, left hand**
- **M65.249** **Calcific tendinitis, unspecified hand**

M65.25 **Calcific tendinitis, thigh**
- **M65.251** **Calcific tendinitis, right thigh**
- **M65.252** **Calcific tendinitis, left thigh**
- **M65.259** **Calcific tendinitis, unspecified thigh**

M65.26 **Calcific tendinitis, lower leg**
- **M65.261** **Calcific tendinitis, right lower leg**
- **M65.262** **Calcific tendinitis, left lower leg**
- **M65.269** **Calcific tendinitis, unspecified lower leg**

M65.27 **Calcific tendinitis, ankle and foot**
- **M65.271** **Calcific tendinitis, right ankle and foot**
- **M65.272** **Calcific tendinitis, left ankle and foot**
- **M65.279** **Calcific tendinitis, unspecified ankle and foot**

M65.28 **Calcific tendinitis, other site**

M65.29 **Calcific tendinitis, multiple sites**

M65.3 **Trigger finger**

Nodular tendinous disease

- **M65.30** **Trigger finger, unspecified finger**

M65.31 **Trigger thumb**
- **M65.311** **Trigger thumb, right thumb**
- **M65.312** **Trigger thumb, left thumb**
- **M65.319** **Trigger thumb, unspecified thumb**

M65.32 **Trigger finger, index finger**
- **M65.321** **Trigger finger, right index finger**
- **M65.322** **Trigger finger, left index finger**
- **M65.329** **Trigger finger, unspecified index finger**

M65.33 **Trigger finger, middle finger**
- **M65.331** **Trigger finger, right middle finger**
- **M65.332** **Trigger finger, left middle finger**
- **M65.339** **Trigger finger, unspecified middle finger**

M65.34 **Trigger finger, ring finger**
- **M65.341** **Trigger finger, right ring finger**
- **M65.342** **Trigger finger, left ring finger**
- **M65.349** **Trigger finger, unspecified ring finger**

M65.35 **Trigger finger, little finger**
- **M65.351** **Trigger finger, right little finger**
- **M65.352** **Trigger finger, left little finger**
- **M65.359** **Trigger finger, unspecified little finger**

M65.4 **Radial styloid tenosynovitis [de Quervain]**

M65.8 **Other synovitis and tenosynovitis**
- **M65.80** **Other synovitis and tenosynovitis, unspecified site**

M65.81 **Other synovitis and tenosynovitis, shoulder**
- **M65.811** **Other synovitis and tenosynovitis, right shoulder**
- **M65.812** **Other synovitis and tenosynovitis, left shoulder**
- **M65.819** **Other synovitis and tenosynovitis, unspecified shoulder**

M65.82 **Other synovitis and tenosynovitis, upper arm**
- **M65.821** **Other synovitis and tenosynovitis, right upper arm**
- **M65.822** **Other synovitis and tenosynovitis, left upper arm**
- **M65.829** **Other synovitis and tenosynovitis, unspecified upper arm**

M65.83 **Other synovitis and tenosynovitis, forearm**
- **M65.831** **Other synovitis and tenosynovitis, right forearm**
- **M65.832** **Other synovitis and tenosynovitis, left forearm**
- **M65.839** **Other synovitis and tenosynovitis, unspecified forearm**

M65.84 **Other synovitis and tenosynovitis, hand**
- **M65.841** **Other synovitis and tenosynovitis, right hand**
- **M65.842** **Other synovitis and tenosynovitis, left hand**
- **M65.849** **Other synovitis and tenosynovitis, unspecified hand**

M65.85 **Other synovitis and tenosynovitis, thigh**
- **M65.851** **Other synovitis and tenosynovitis, right thigh**
- **M65.852** **Other synovitis and tenosynovitis, left thigh**
- **M65.859** **Other synovitis and tenosynovitis, unspecified thigh**

M65.86 **Other synovitis and tenosynovitis, lower leg**
- **M65.861** **Other synovitis and tenosynovitis, right lower leg**
- **M65.862** **Other synovitis and tenosynovitis, left lower leg**
- **M65.869** **Other synovitis and tenosynovitis, unspecified lower leg**

M65.87 **Other synovitis and tenosynovitis, ankle and foot**
- **M65.871** **Other synovitis and tenosynovitis, right ankle and foot**

M65.872 Other synovitis and tenosynovitis, left ankle and foot
M65.879 Other synovitis and tenosynovitis, unspecified ankle and foot
M65.88 Other synovitis and tenosynovitis, other site
M65.89 Other synovitis and tenosynovitis, multiple sites
M65.9 Synovitis and tenosynovitis, unspecified

M66 Spontaneous rupture of synovium and tendon

INCLUDES rupture that occurs when a normal force is applied to tissues that are inferred to have less than normal strength

EXCLUDES 2 *rotator cuff syndrome (M75.1-)*
rupture where an abnormal force is applied to normal tissue - see injury of tendon by body region

M66.0 Rupture of popliteal cyst
M66.1 Rupture of synovium
Rupture of synovial cyst
EXCLUDES 2 *rupture of popliteal cyst (M66.0)*
M66.10 Rupture of synovium, unspecified joint
M66.11 Rupture of synovium, shoulder
M66.111 Rupture of synovium, right shoulder
M66.112 Rupture of synovium, left shoulder
M66.119 Rupture of synovium, unspecified shoulder
M66.12 Rupture of synovium, elbow
M66.121 Rupture of synovium, right elbow
M66.122 Rupture of synovium, left elbow
M66.129 Rupture of synovium, unspecified elbow
M66.13 Rupture of synovium, wrist
M66.131 Rupture of synovium, right wrist
M66.132 Rupture of synovium, left wrist
M66.139 Rupture of synovium, unspecified wrist
M66.14 Rupture of synovium, hand and fingers
M66.141 Rupture of synovium, right hand
M66.142 Rupture of synovium, left hand
M66.143 Rupture of synovium, unspecified hand
M66.144 Rupture of synovium, right finger(s)
M66.145 Rupture of synovium, left finger(s)
M66.146 Rupture of synovium, unspecified finger(s)
M66.15 Rupture of synovium, hip
M66.151 Rupture of synovium, right hip
M66.152 Rupture of synovium, left hip
M66.159 Rupture of synovium, unspecified hip
M66.17 Rupture of synovium, ankle, foot and toes
M66.171 Rupture of synovium, right ankle
M66.172 Rupture of synovium, left ankle
M66.173 Rupture of synovium, unspecified ankle
M66.174 Rupture of synovium, right foot
M66.175 Rupture of synovium, left foot
M66.176 Rupture of synovium, unspecified foot
M66.177 Rupture of synovium, right toe(s)
M66.178 Rupture of synovium, left toe(s)
M66.179 Rupture of synovium, unspecified toe(s)
M66.18 Rupture of synovium, other site
M66.2 Spontaneous rupture of extensor tendons
TIP: Refer to the Muscle/Tendon table at the beginning of this chapter.
M66.20 Spontaneous rupture of extensor tendons, unspecified site
M66.21 Spontaneous rupture of extensor tendons, shoulder
M66.211 Spontaneous rupture of extensor tendons, right shoulder
M66.212 Spontaneous rupture of extensor tendons, left shoulder
M66.219 Spontaneous rupture of extensor tendons, unspecified shoulder
M66.22 Spontaneous rupture of extensor tendons, upper arm
M66.221 Spontaneous rupture of extensor tendons, right upper arm
M66.222 Spontaneous rupture of extensor tendons, left upper arm
M66.229 Spontaneous rupture of extensor tendons, unspecified upper arm
M66.23 Spontaneous rupture of extensor tendons, forearm
M66.231 Spontaneous rupture of extensor tendons, right forearm
M66.232 Spontaneous rupture of extensor tendons, left forearm
M66.239 Spontaneous rupture of extensor tendons, unspecified forearm
M66.24 Spontaneous rupture of extensor tendons, hand
M66.241 Spontaneous rupture of extensor tendons, right hand
M66.242 Spontaneous rupture of extensor tendons, left hand
M66.249 Spontaneous rupture of extensor tendons, unspecified hand
M66.25 Spontaneous rupture of extensor tendons, thigh
M66.251 Spontaneous rupture of extensor tendons, right thigh
M66.252 Spontaneous rupture of extensor tendons, left thigh
M66.259 Spontaneous rupture of extensor tendons, unspecified thigh
M66.26 Spontaneous rupture of extensor tendons, lower leg
M66.261 Spontaneous rupture of extensor tendons, right lower leg
M66.262 Spontaneous rupture of extensor tendons, left lower leg
M66.269 Spontaneous rupture of extensor tendons, unspecified lower leg
M66.27 Spontaneous rupture of extensor tendons, ankle and foot
M66.271 Spontaneous rupture of extensor tendons, right ankle and foot
M66.272 Spontaneous rupture of extensor tendons, left ankle and foot
M66.279 Spontaneous rupture of extensor tendons, unspecified ankle and foot
M66.28 Spontaneous rupture of extensor tendons, other site
M66.29 Spontaneous rupture of extensor tendons, multiple sites
M66.3 Spontaneous rupture of flexor tendons
TIP: Refer to the Muscle/Tendon table at the beginning of this chapter.
M66.30 Spontaneous rupture of flexor tendons, unspecified site
M66.31 Spontaneous rupture of flexor tendons, shoulder
M66.311 Spontaneous rupture of flexor tendons, right shoulder
M66.312 Spontaneous rupture of flexor tendons, left shoulder
M66.319 Spontaneous rupture of flexor tendons, unspecified shoulder
M66.32 Spontaneous rupture of flexor tendons, upper arm
M66.321 Spontaneous rupture of flexor tendons, right upper arm
M66.322 Spontaneous rupture of flexor tendons, left upper arm
M66.329 Spontaneous rupture of flexor tendons, unspecified upper arm
M66.33 Spontaneous rupture of flexor tendons, forearm
M66.331 Spontaneous rupture of flexor tendons, right forearm
M66.332 Spontaneous rupture of flexor tendons, left forearm
M66.339 Spontaneous rupture of flexor tendons, unspecified forearm
M66.34 Spontaneous rupture of flexor tendons, hand
M66.341 Spontaneous rupture of flexor tendons, right hand
M66.342 Spontaneous rupture of flexor tendons, left hand
M66.349 Spontaneous rupture of flexor tendons, unspecified hand
M66.35 Spontaneous rupture of flexor tendons, thigh
M66.351 Spontaneous rupture of flexor tendons, right thigh
M66.352 Spontaneous rupture of flexor tendons, left thigh
M66.359 Spontaneous rupture of flexor tendons, unspecified thigh

M66.36 Spontaneous rupture of flexor tendons, lower leg
- **M66.361 Spontaneous rupture of flexor tendons, right lower leg**
- **M66.362 Spontaneous rupture of flexor tendons, left lower leg**
- **M66.369 Spontaneous rupture of flexor tendons, unspecified lower leg**

M66.37 Spontaneous rupture of flexor tendons, ankle and foot
- **M66.371 Spontaneous rupture of flexor tendons, right ankle and foot**
- **M66.372 Spontaneous rupture of flexor tendons, left ankle and foot**
- **M66.379 Spontaneous rupture of flexor tendons, unspecified ankle and foot**

M66.38 Spontaneous rupture of flexor tendons, other site

M66.39 Spontaneous rupture of flexor tendons, multiple sites

M66.8 Spontaneous rupture of other tendons

TIP: Refer to the Muscle/Tendon table at the beginning of this chapter.

M66.80 Spontaneous rupture of other tendons, unspecified site

M66.81 Spontaneous rupture of other tendons, shoulder
- **M66.811 Spontaneous rupture of other tendons, right shoulder**
- **M66.812 Spontaneous rupture of other tendons, left shoulder**
- **M66.819 Spontaneous rupture of other tendons, unspecified shoulder**

M66.82 Spontaneous rupture of other tendons, upper arm
- **M66.821 Spontaneous rupture of other tendons, right upper arm**
- **M66.822 Spontaneous rupture of other tendons, left upper arm**
- **M66.829 Spontaneous rupture of other tendons, unspecified upper arm**

M66.83 Spontaneous rupture of other tendons, forearm
- **M66.831 Spontaneous rupture of other tendons, right forearm**
- **M66.832 Spontaneous rupture of other tendons, left forearm**
- **M66.839 Spontaneous rupture of other tendons, unspecified forearm**

M66.84 Spontaneous rupture of other tendons, hand
- **M66.841 Spontaneous rupture of other tendons, right hand**
- **M66.842 Spontaneous rupture of other tendons, left hand**
- **M66.849 Spontaneous rupture of other tendons, unspecified hand**

M66.85 Spontaneous rupture of other tendons, thigh
- **M66.851 Spontaneous rupture of other tendons, right thigh**
- **M66.852 Spontaneous rupture of other tendons, left thigh**
- **M66.859 Spontaneous rupture of other tendons, unspecified thigh**

M66.86 Spontaneous rupture of other tendons, lower leg
- **M66.861 Spontaneous rupture of other tendons, right lower leg**
- **M66.862 Spontaneous rupture of other tendons, left lower leg**
- **M66.869 Spontaneous rupture of other tendons, unspecified lower leg**

M66.87 Spontaneous rupture of other tendons, ankle and foot
- **M66.871 Spontaneous rupture of other tendons, right ankle and foot**
- **M66.872 Spontaneous rupture of other tendons, left ankle and foot**
- **M66.879 Spontaneous rupture of other tendons, unspecified ankle and foot**

M66.88 Spontaneous rupture of other tendons, other sites

M66.89 Spontaneous rupture of other tendons, multiple sites

M66.9 Spontaneous rupture of unspecified tendon

Rupture at musculotendinous junction, nontraumatic

M67 Other disorders of synovium and tendon

EXCLUDES 1 *palmar fascial fibromatosis [Dupuytren] (M72.Ø)*
tendinitis NOS (M77.9-)
xanthomatosis localized to tendons (E78.2)

M67.Ø Short Achilles tendon (acquired)
- **M67.ØØ Short Achilles tendon (acquired), unspecified ankle**
- **M67.Ø1 Short Achilles tendon (acquired), right ankle**
- **M67.Ø2 Short Achilles tendon (acquired), left ankle**

M67.2 Synovial hypertrophy, not elsewhere classified

EXCLUDES 1 *villonodular synovitis (pigmented) (M12.2-)*

M67.2Ø Synovial hypertrophy, not elsewhere classified, unspecified site

M67.21 Synovial hypertrophy, not elsewhere classified, shoulder
- **M67.211 Synovial hypertrophy, not elsewhere classified, right shoulder**
- **M67.212 Synovial hypertrophy, not elsewhere classified, left shoulder**
- **M67.219 Synovial hypertrophy, not elsewhere classified, unspecified shoulder**

M67.22 Synovial hypertrophy, not elsewhere classified, upper arm
- **M67.221 Synovial hypertrophy, not elsewhere classified, right upper arm**
- **M67.222 Synovial hypertrophy, not elsewhere classified, left upper arm**
- **M67.229 Synovial hypertrophy, not elsewhere classified, unspecified upper arm**

M67.23 Synovial hypertrophy, not elsewhere classified, forearm
- **M67.231 Synovial hypertrophy, not elsewhere classified, right forearm**
- **M67.232 Synovial hypertrophy, not elsewhere classified, left forearm**
- **M67.239 Synovial hypertrophy, not elsewhere classified, unspecified forearm**

M67.24 Synovial hypertrophy, not elsewhere classified, hand
- **M67.241 Synovial hypertrophy, not elsewhere classified, right hand**
- **M67.242 Synovial hypertrophy, not elsewhere classified, left hand**
- **M67.249 Synovial hypertrophy, not elsewhere classified, unspecified hand**

M67.25 Synovial hypertrophy, not elsewhere classified, thigh
- **M67.251 Synovial hypertrophy, not elsewhere classified, right thigh**
- **M67.252 Synovial hypertrophy, not elsewhere classified, left thigh**
- **M67.259 Synovial hypertrophy, not elsewhere classified, unspecified thigh**

M67.26 Synovial hypertrophy, not elsewhere classified, lower leg
- **M67.261 Synovial hypertrophy, not elsewhere classified, right lower leg**
- **M67.262 Synovial hypertrophy, not elsewhere classified, left lower leg**
- **M67.269 Synovial hypertrophy, not elsewhere classified, unspecified lower leg**

M67.27 Synovial hypertrophy, not elsewhere classified, ankle and foot
- **M67.271 Synovial hypertrophy, not elsewhere classified, right ankle and foot**
- **M67.272 Synovial hypertrophy, not elsewhere classified, left ankle and foot**
- **M67.279 Synovial hypertrophy, not elsewhere classified, unspecified ankle and foot**

M67.28 Synovial hypertrophy, not elsewhere classified, other site

M67.29 Synovial hypertrophy, not elsewhere classified, multiple sites

M67.3 Transient synovitis

Toxic synovitis

EXCLUDES 1 *palindromic rheumatism (M12.3-)*

M67.3Ø Transient synovitis, unspecified site

M67.31 Transient synovitis, shoulder
- **M67.311 Transient synovitis, right shoulder**
- **M67.312 Transient synovitis, left shoulder**
- **M67.319 Transient synovitis, unspecified shoulder**

M67.32 Transient synovitis, elbow
M67.321 Transient synovitis, right elbow
M67.322 Transient synovitis, left elbow
M67.329 Transient synovitis, unspecified elbow
M67.33 Transient synovitis, wrist
M67.331 Transient synovitis, right wrist
M67.332 Transient synovitis, left wrist
M67.339 Transient synovitis, unspecified wrist
M67.34 Transient synovitis, hand
M67.341 Transient synovitis, right hand
M67.342 Transient synovitis, left hand
M67.349 Transient synovitis, unspecified hand
M67.35 Transient synovitis, hip
M67.351 Transient synovitis, right hip
M67.352 Transient synovitis, left hip
M67.359 Transient synovitis, unspecified hip
M67.36 Transient synovitis, knee
M67.361 Transient synovitis, right knee
M67.362 Transient synovitis, left knee
M67.369 Transient synovitis, unspecified knee
M67.37 Transient synovitis, ankle and foot
M67.371 Transient synovitis, right ankle and foot
M67.372 Transient synovitis, left ankle and foot
M67.379 Transient synovitis, unspecified ankle and foot
M67.38 Transient synovitis, other site
M67.39 Transient synovitis, multiple sites
M67.4 Ganglion
Ganglion of joint or tendon (sheath)
EXCLUDES 1 *ganglion in yaws (A66.6)*
EXCLUDES 2 *cyst of bursa (M71.2-M71.3)*
cyst of synovium (M71.2-M71.3)
DEF: Fluid-filled, benign cyst appearing on a tendon sheath or aponeurosis, frequently connecting to an underlying joint.
M67.40 Ganglion, unspecified site
M67.41 Ganglion, shoulder
M67.411 Ganglion, right shoulder
M67.412 Ganglion, left shoulder
M67.419 Ganglion, unspecified shoulder
M67.42 Ganglion, elbow
M67.421 Ganglion, right elbow
M67.422 Ganglion, left elbow
M67.429 Ganglion, unspecified elbow
M67.43 Ganglion, wrist

Ganglion of Wrist

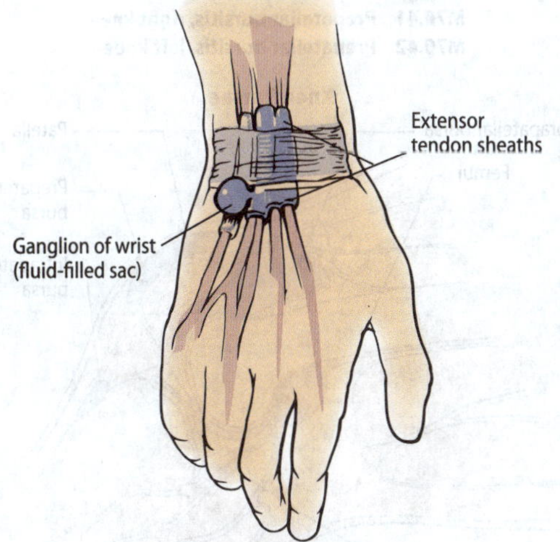

M67.431 Ganglion, right wrist
M67.432 Ganglion, left wrist
M67.439 Ganglion, unspecified wrist
M67.44 Ganglion, hand
M67.441 Ganglion, right hand
M67.442 Ganglion, left hand
M67.449 Ganglion, unspecified hand
M67.45 Ganglion, hip
M67.451 Ganglion, right hip
M67.452 Ganglion, left hip
M67.459 Ganglion, unspecified hip
M67.46 Ganglion, knee
M67.461 Ganglion, right knee
M67.462 Ganglion, left knee
M67.469 Ganglion, unspecified knee
M67.47 Ganglion, ankle and foot
M67.471 Ganglion, right ankle and foot
M67.472 Ganglion, left ankle and foot
M67.479 Ganglion, unspecified ankle and foot
M67.48 Ganglion, other site
M67.49 Ganglion, multiple sites
M67.5 Plica syndrome
Plica knee
M67.50 Plica syndrome, unspecified knee
M67.51 Plica syndrome, right knee
M67.52 Plica syndrome, left knee
M67.8 Other specified disorders of synovium and tendon
M67.80 Other specified disorders of synovium and tendon, unspecified site
M67.81 Other specified disorders of synovium and tendon, shoulder
M67.811 Other specified disorders of synovium, right shoulder
M67.812 Other specified disorders of synovium, left shoulder
M67.813 Other specified disorders of tendon, right shoulder
M67.814 Other specified disorders of tendon, left shoulder
M67.819 Other specified disorders of synovium and tendon, unspecified shoulder
M67.82 Other specified disorders of synovium and tendon, elbow
M67.821 Other specified disorders of synovium, right elbow
M67.822 Other specified disorders of synovium, left elbow
M67.823 Other specified disorders of tendon, right elbow
M67.824 Other specified disorders of tendon, left elbow
M67.829 Other specified disorders of synovium and tendon, unspecified elbow
M67.83 Other specified disorders of synovium and tendon, wrist
M67.831 Other specified disorders of synovium, right wrist
M67.832 Other specified disorders of synovium, left wrist
M67.833 Other specified disorders of tendon, right wrist
M67.834 Other specified disorders of tendon, left wrist
M67.839 Other specified disorders of synovium and tendon, unspecified wrist
M67.84 Other specified disorders of synovium and tendon, hand
M67.841 Other specified disorders of synovium, right hand
M67.842 Other specified disorders of synovium, left hand
M67.843 Other specified disorders of tendon, right hand
M67.844 Other specified disorders of tendon, left hand
M67.849 Other specified disorders of synovium and tendon, unspecified hand
M67.85 Other specified disorders of synovium and tendon, hip
M67.851 Other specified disorders of synovium, right hip
M67.852 Other specified disorders of synovium, left hip
M67.853 Other specified disorders of tendon, right hip
M67.854 Other specified disorders of tendon, left hip
M67.859 Other specified disorders of synovium and tendon, unspecified hip

✓6th **M67.86** **Other specified disorders of synovium and tendon, knee**
- **M67.861** **Other specified disorders of synovium, right knee**
- **M67.862** **Other specified disorders of synovium, left knee**
- **M67.863** **Other specified disorders of tendon, right knee**
- **M67.864** **Other specified disorders of tendon, left knee**
- **M67.869** **Other specified disorders of synovium and tendon, unspecified knee**

✓6th **M67.87** **Other specified disorders of synovium and tendon, ankle and foot**
- **M67.871** **Other specified disorders of synovium, right ankle and foot**
- **M67.872** **Other specified disorders of synovium, left ankle and foot**
- **M67.873** **Other specified disorders of tendon, right ankle and foot**
- **M67.874** **Other specified disorders of tendon, left ankle and foot**
- **M67.879** **Other specified disorders of synovium and tendon, unspecified ankle and foot**

M67.88 **Other specified disorders of synovium and tendon, other site**

M67.89 **Other specified disorders of synovium and tendon, multiple sites**

✓5th **M67.9** **Unspecified disorder of synovium and tendon**

M67.9Ø **Unspecified disorder of synovium and tendon, unspecified site**

✓6th **M67.91** **Unspecified disorder of synovium and tendon, shoulder**
- **M67.911** **Unspecified disorder of synovium and tendon, right shoulder**
- **M67.912** **Unspecified disorder of synovium and tendon, left shoulder**
- **M67.919** **Unspecified disorder of synovium and tendon, unspecified shoulder**

✓6th **M67.92** **Unspecified disorder of synovium and tendon, upper arm**
- **M67.921** **Unspecified disorder of synovium and tendon, right upper arm**
- **M67.922** **Unspecified disorder of synovium and tendon, left upper arm**
- **M67.929** **Unspecified disorder of synovium and tendon, unspecified upper arm**

✓6th **M67.93** **Unspecified disorder of synovium and tendon, forearm**
- **M67.931** **Unspecified disorder of synovium and tendon, right forearm**
- **M67.932** **Unspecified disorder of synovium and tendon, left forearm**
- **M67.939** **Unspecified disorder of synovium and tendon, unspecified forearm**

✓6th **M67.94** **Unspecified disorder of synovium and tendon, hand**
- **M67.941** **Unspecified disorder of synovium and tendon, right hand**
- **M67.942** **Unspecified disorder of synovium and tendon, left hand**
- **M67.949** **Unspecified disorder of synovium and tendon, unspecified hand**

✓6th **M67.95** **Unspecified disorder of synovium and tendon, thigh**
- **M67.951** **Unspecified disorder of synovium and tendon, right thigh**
- **M67.952** **Unspecified disorder of synovium and tendon, left thigh**
- **M67.959** **Unspecified disorder of synovium and tendon, unspecified thigh**

✓6th **M67.96** **Unspecified disorder of synovium and tendon, lower leg**
- **M67.961** **Unspecified disorder of synovium and tendon, right lower leg**
- **M67.962** **Unspecified disorder of synovium and tendon, left lower leg**
- **M67.969** **Unspecified disorder of synovium and tendon, unspecified lower leg**

✓6th **M67.97** **Unspecified disorder of synovium and tendon, ankle and foot**
- **M67.971** **Unspecified disorder of synovium and tendon, right ankle and foot**
- **M67.972** **Unspecified disorder of synovium and tendon, left ankle and foot**
- **M67.979** **Unspecified disorder of synovium and tendon, unspecified ankle and foot**

M67.98 **Unspecified disorder of synovium and tendon, other site**

M67.99 **Unspecified disorder of synovium and tendon, multiple sites**

Other soft tissue disorders (M7Ø-M79)

✓4th **M7Ø** **Soft tissue disorders related to use, overuse and pressure**

INCLUDES soft tissue disorders of occupational origin

Use additional external cause code to identify activity causing disorder (Y93.-)

EXCLUDES 1 *bursitis NOS (M71.9-)*

EXCLUDES 2 *bursitis of shoulder (M75.5)*
enthesopathies (M76-M77)
pressure ulcer (pressure area) (L89.-)

✓5th **M7Ø.Ø** **Crepitant synovitis (acute) (chronic) of hand and wrist**

✓6th **M7Ø.Ø3** **Crepitant synovitis (acute) (chronic), wrist**
- **M7Ø.Ø31** **Crepitant synovitis (acute) (chronic), right wrist**
- **M7Ø.Ø32** **Crepitant synovitis (acute) (chronic), left wrist**
- **M7Ø.Ø39** **Crepitant synovitis (acute) (chronic), unspecified wrist**

✓6th **M7Ø.Ø4** **Crepitant synovitis (acute) (chronic), hand**
- **M7Ø.Ø41** **Crepitant synovitis (acute) (chronic), right hand**
- **M7Ø.Ø42** **Crepitant synovitis (acute) (chronic), left hand**
- **M7Ø.Ø49** **Crepitant synovitis (acute) (chronic), unspecified hand**

✓5th **M7Ø.1** **Bursitis of hand**
- **M7Ø.1Ø** **Bursitis, unspecified hand**
- **M7Ø.11** **Bursitis, right hand**
- **M7Ø.12** **Bursitis, left hand**

✓5th **M7Ø.2** **Olecranon bursitis**
- **M7Ø.2Ø** **Olecranon bursitis, unspecified elbow**
- **M7Ø.21** **Olecranon bursitis, right elbow**
- **M7Ø.22** **Olecranon bursitis, left elbow**

✓5th **M7Ø.3** **Other bursitis of elbow**
- **M7Ø.3Ø** **Other bursitis of elbow, unspecified elbow**
- **M7Ø.31** **Other bursitis of elbow, right elbow**
- **M7Ø.32** **Other bursitis of elbow, left elbow**

✓5th **M7Ø.4** **Prepatellar bursitis**
- **M7Ø.4Ø** **Prepatellar bursitis, unspecified knee**
- **M7Ø.41** **Prepatellar bursitis, right knee**
- **M7Ø.42** **Prepatellar bursitis, left knee**

Knee Bursae

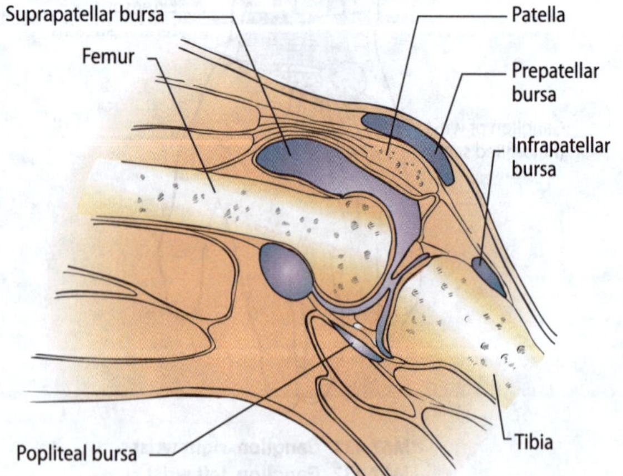

✓5th **M7Ø.5** **Other bursitis of knee**
- **M7Ø.5Ø** **Other bursitis of knee, unspecified knee**
- **M7Ø.51** **Other bursitis of knee, right knee**
- **M7Ø.52** **Other bursitis of knee, left knee**

M70.6 Trochanteric bursitis
Trochanteric tendinitis
M70.60 Trochanteric bursitis, unspecified hip
M70.61 Trochanteric bursitis, right hip
M70.62 Trochanteric bursitis, left hip
M70.7 Other bursitis of hip
Ischial bursitis
M70.70 Other bursitis of hip, unspecified hip
M70.71 Other bursitis of hip, right hip
M70.72 Other bursitis of hip, left hip
M70.8 Other soft tissue disorders related to use, overuse and pressure
M70.80 Other soft tissue disorders related to use, overuse and pressure of unspecified site
M70.81 Other soft tissue disorders related to use, overuse and pressure of shoulder
M70.811 Other soft tissue disorders related to use, overuse and pressure, right shoulder
M70.812 Other soft tissue disorders related to use, overuse and pressure, left shoulder
M70.819 Other soft tissue disorders related to use, overuse and pressure, unspecified shoulder
M70.82 Other soft tissue disorders related to use, overuse and pressure of upper arm
M70.821 Other soft tissue disorders related to use, overuse and pressure, right upper arm
M70.822 Other soft tissue disorders related to use, overuse and pressure, left upper arm
M70.829 Other soft tissue disorders related to use, overuse and pressure, unspecified upper arms
M70.83 Other soft tissue disorders related to use, overuse and pressure of forearm
M70.831 Other soft tissue disorders related to use, overuse and pressure, right forearm
M70.832 Other soft tissue disorders related to use, overuse and pressure, left forearm
M70.839 Other soft tissue disorders related to use, overuse and pressure, unspecified forearm
M70.84 Other soft tissue disorders related to use, overuse and pressure of hand
M70.841 Other soft tissue disorders related to use, overuse and pressure, right hand
M70.842 Other soft tissue disorders related to use, overuse and pressure, left hand
M70.849 Other soft tissue disorders related to use, overuse and pressure, unspecified hand
M70.85 Other soft tissue disorders related to use, overuse and pressure of thigh
M70.851 Other soft tissue disorders related to use, overuse and pressure, right thigh
M70.852 Other soft tissue disorders related to use, overuse and pressure, left thigh
M70.859 Other soft tissue disorders related to use, overuse and pressure, unspecified thigh
M70.86 Other soft tissue disorders related to use, overuse and pressure lower leg
M70.861 Other soft tissue disorders related to use, overuse and pressure, right lower leg
M70.862 Other soft tissue disorders related to use, overuse and pressure, left lower leg
M70.869 Other soft tissue disorders related to use, overuse and pressure, unspecified leg
M70.87 Other soft tissue disorders related to use, overuse and pressure of ankle and foot
M70.871 Other soft tissue disorders related to use, overuse and pressure, right ankle and foot
M70.872 Other soft tissue disorders related to use, overuse and pressure, left ankle and foot
M70.879 Other soft tissue disorders related to use, overuse and pressure, unspecified ankle and foot
M70.88 Other soft tissue disorders related to use, overuse and pressure other site
M70.89 Other soft tissue disorders related to use, overuse and pressure multiple sites
M70.9 Unspecified soft tissue disorder related to use, overuse and pressure
M70.90 Unspecified soft tissue disorder related to use, overuse and pressure of unspecified site
M70.91 Unspecified soft tissue disorder related to use, overuse and pressure of shoulder
M70.911 Unspecified soft tissue disorder related to use, overuse and pressure, right shoulder
M70.912 Unspecified soft tissue disorder related to use, overuse and pressure, left shoulder
M70.919 Unspecified soft tissue disorder related to use, overuse and pressure, unspecified shoulder
M70.92 Unspecified soft tissue disorder related to use, overuse and pressure of upper arm
M70.921 Unspecified soft tissue disorder related to use, overuse and pressure, right upper arm
M70.922 Unspecified soft tissue disorder related to use, overuse and pressure, left upper arm
M70.929 Unspecified soft tissue disorder related to use, overuse and pressure, unspecified upper arm
M70.93 Unspecified soft tissue disorder related to use, overuse and pressure of forearm
M70.931 Unspecified soft tissue disorder related to use, overuse and pressure, right forearm
M70.932 Unspecified soft tissue disorder related to use, overuse and pressure, left forearm
M70.939 Unspecified soft tissue disorder related to use, overuse and pressure, unspecified forearm
M70.94 Unspecified soft tissue disorder related to use, overuse and pressure of hand
M70.941 Unspecified soft tissue disorder related to use, overuse and pressure, right hand
M70.942 Unspecified soft tissue disorder related to use, overuse and pressure, left hand
M70.949 Unspecified soft tissue disorder related to use, overuse and pressure, unspecified hand
M70.95 Unspecified soft tissue disorder related to use, overuse and pressure of thigh
M70.951 Unspecified soft tissue disorder related to use, overuse and pressure, right thigh
M70.952 Unspecified soft tissue disorder related to use, overuse and pressure, left thigh
M70.959 Unspecified soft tissue disorder related to use, overuse and pressure, unspecified thigh
M70.96 Unspecified soft tissue disorder related to use, overuse and pressure lower leg
M70.961 Unspecified soft tissue disorder related to use, overuse and pressure, right lower leg
M70.962 Unspecified soft tissue disorder related to use, overuse and pressure, left lower leg
M70.969 Unspecified soft tissue disorder related to use, overuse and pressure, unspecified lower leg
M70.97 Unspecified soft tissue disorder related to use, overuse and pressure of ankle and foot
M70.971 Unspecified soft tissue disorder related to use, overuse and pressure, right ankle and foot
M70.972 Unspecified soft tissue disorder related to use, overuse and pressure, left ankle and foot
M70.979 Unspecified soft tissue disorder related to use, overuse and pressure, unspecified ankle and foot
M70.98 Unspecified soft tissue disorder related to use, overuse and pressure other
M70.99 Unspecified soft tissue disorder related to use, overuse and pressure multiple sites

M71 Other bursopathies
EXCLUDES 1 *bunion (M20.1)*
bursitis related to use, overuse or pressure (M70.-)
enthesopathies (M76-M77)

M71.0 Abscess of bursa
Use additional code (B95.-, B96.-) to identify causative organism
M71.00 Abscess of bursa, unspecified site
M71.01 Abscess of bursa, shoulder
M71.011 Abscess of bursa, right shoulder
M71.012 Abscess of bursa, left shoulder
M71.019 Abscess of bursa, unspecified shoulder
M71.02 Abscess of bursa, elbow
M71.021 Abscess of bursa, right elbow
M71.022 Abscess of bursa, left elbow
M71.029 Abscess of bursa, unspecified elbow
M71.03 Abscess of bursa, wrist
M71.031 Abscess of bursa, right wrist
M71.032 Abscess of bursa, left wrist
M71.039 Abscess of bursa, unspecified wrist
M71.04 Abscess of bursa, hand
M71.041 Abscess of bursa, right hand
M71.042 Abscess of bursa, left hand
M71.049 Abscess of bursa, unspecified hand
M71.05 Abscess of bursa, hip
M71.051 Abscess of bursa, right hip
M71.052 Abscess of bursa, left hip
M71.059 Abscess of bursa, unspecified hip
M71.06 Abscess of bursa, knee
M71.061 Abscess of bursa, right knee
M71.062 Abscess of bursa, left knee
M71.069 Abscess of bursa, unspecified knee
M71.07 Abscess of bursa, ankle and foot
M71.071 Abscess of bursa, right ankle and foot
M71.072 Abscess of bursa, left ankle and foot
M71.079 Abscess of bursa, unspecified ankle and foot
M71.08 Abscess of bursa, other site
M71.09 Abscess of bursa, multiple sites

M71.1 Other infective bursitis
Use additional code (B95.-, B96.-) to identify causative organism
M71.10 Other infective bursitis, unspecified site
M71.11 Other infective bursitis, shoulder
M71.111 Other infective bursitis, right shoulder
M71.112 Other infective bursitis, left shoulder
M71.119 Other infective bursitis, unspecified shoulder
M71.12 Other infective bursitis, elbow
M71.121 Other infective bursitis, right elbow
M71.122 Other infective bursitis, left elbow
M71.129 Other infective bursitis, unspecified elbow
M71.13 Other infective bursitis, wrist
M71.131 Other infective bursitis, right wrist
M71.132 Other infective bursitis, left wrist
M71.139 Other infective bursitis, unspecified wrist
M71.14 Other infective bursitis, hand
M71.141 Other infective bursitis, right hand
M71.142 Other infective bursitis, left hand
M71.149 Other infective bursitis, unspecified hand
M71.15 Other infective bursitis, hip
M71.151 Other infective bursitis, right hip
M71.152 Other infective bursitis, left hip
M71.159 Other infective bursitis, unspecified hip
M71.16 Other infective bursitis, knee
M71.161 Other infective bursitis, right knee
M71.162 Other infective bursitis, left knee
M71.169 Other infective bursitis, unspecified knee
M71.17 Other infective bursitis, ankle and foot
M71.171 Other infective bursitis, right ankle and foot
M71.172 Other infective bursitis, left ankle and foot
M71.179 Other infective bursitis, unspecified ankle and foot
M71.18 Other infective bursitis, other site
M71.19 Other infective bursitis, multiple sites

M71.2 Synovial cyst of popliteal space [Baker]
EXCLUDES 1 *synovial cyst of popliteal space with rupture (M66.0)*
DEF: Sac filled with clear synovial fluid in adults, usually secondary to disease inside the joint, located on the back of the knee in the popliteal fossa area. In children, the cyst usually represents a ganglion of one of the tendons in the knee.

Baker's Cyst

M71.20 Synovial cyst of popliteal space [Baker], unspecified knee
M71.21 Synovial cyst of popliteal space [Baker], right knee
M71.22 Synovial cyst of popliteal space [Baker], left knee

M71.3 Other bursal cyst
Synovial cyst NOS
EXCLUDES 1 *synovial cyst with rupture (M66.1-)*
M71.30 Other bursal cyst, unspecified site
M71.31 Other bursal cyst, shoulder
M71.311 Other bursal cyst, right shoulder
M71.312 Other bursal cyst, left shoulder
M71.319 Other bursal cyst, unspecified shoulder
M71.32 Other bursal cyst, elbow
M71.321 Other bursal cyst, right elbow
M71.322 Other bursal cyst, left elbow
M71.329 Other bursal cyst, unspecified elbow
M71.33 Other bursal cyst, wrist
M71.331 Other bursal cyst, right wrist
M71.332 Other bursal cyst, left wrist
M71.339 Other bursal cyst, unspecified wrist
M71.34 Other bursal cyst, hand
M71.341 Other bursal cyst, right hand
M71.342 Other bursal cyst, left hand
M71.349 Other bursal cyst, unspecified hand
M71.35 Other bursal cyst, hip
M71.351 Other bursal cyst, right hip
M71.352 Other bursal cyst, left hip
M71.359 Other bursal cyst, unspecified hip
M71.37 Other bursal cyst, ankle and foot
M71.371 Other bursal cyst, right ankle and foot
M71.372 Other bursal cyst, left ankle and foot
M71.379 Other bursal cyst, unspecified ankle and foot
M71.38 Other bursal cyst, other site
M71.39 Other bursal cyst, multiple sites

M71.4 Calcium deposit in bursa
EXCLUDES 2 *calcium deposit in bursa of shoulder (M75.3)*
M71.40 Calcium deposit in bursa, unspecified site
M71.42 Calcium deposit in bursa, elbow
M71.421 Calcium deposit in bursa, right elbow
M71.422 Calcium deposit in bursa, left elbow
M71.429 Calcium deposit in bursa, unspecified elbow
M71.43 Calcium deposit in bursa, wrist
M71.431 Calcium deposit in bursa, right wrist
M71.432 Calcium deposit in bursa, left wrist

M71.439 Calcium deposit in bursa, unspecified wrist

✓6th M71.44 Calcium deposit in bursa, **hand**
M71.441 Calcium deposit in bursa, **right** hand
M71.442 Calcium deposit in bursa, **left** hand
M71.449 Calcium deposit in bursa, unspecified hand

✓6th M71.45 Calcium deposit in bursa, **hip**
M71.451 Calcium deposit in bursa, **right** hip
M71.452 Calcium deposit in bursa, **left** hip
M71.459 Calcium deposit in bursa, unspecified hip

✓6th M71.46 Calcium deposit in bursa, **knee**
M71.461 Calcium deposit in bursa, **right** knee
M71.462 Calcium deposit in bursa, **left** knee
M71.469 Calcium deposit in bursa, unspecified knee

✓6th M71.47 Calcium deposit in bursa, **ankle and foot**
M71.471 Calcium deposit in bursa, **right** ankle and foot
M71.472 Calcium deposit in bursa, **left** ankle and foot
M71.479 Calcium deposit in bursa, unspecified ankle and foot

M71.48 Calcium deposit in bursa, other site
M71.49 Calcium deposit in bursa, **multiple sites**

✓5th M71.5 Other bursitis, not elsewhere classified
EXCLUDES 1 *bursitis NOS (M71.9-)*
EXCLUDES 2 *bursitis of shoulder (M75.5)*
bursitis of tibial collateral [Pellegrini-Stieda] (M76.4-)

M71.50 Other bursitis, not elsewhere classified, unspecified site

✓6th M71.52 Other bursitis, not elsewhere classified, **elbow**
M71.521 Other bursitis, not elsewhere classified, **right** elbow
M71.522 Other bursitis, not elsewhere classified, **left** elbow
M71.529 Other bursitis, not elsewhere classified, unspecified elbow

✓6th M71.53 Other bursitis, not elsewhere classified, **wrist**
M71.531 Other bursitis, not elsewhere classified, **right** wrist
M71.532 Other bursitis, not elsewhere classified, **left** wrist
M71.539 Other bursitis, not elsewhere classified, unspecified wrist

✓6th M71.54 Other bursitis, not elsewhere classified, **hand**
M71.541 Other bursitis, not elsewhere classified, **right** hand
M71.542 Other bursitis, not elsewhere classified, **left** hand
M71.549 Other bursitis, not elsewhere classified, unspecified hand

✓6th M71.55 Other bursitis, not elsewhere classified, **hip**
M71.551 Other bursitis, not elsewhere classified, **right** hip
M71.552 Other bursitis, not elsewhere classified, **left** hip
M71.559 Other bursitis, not elsewhere classified, unspecified hip

✓6th M71.56 Other bursitis, not elsewhere classified, **knee**
M71.561 Other bursitis, not elsewhere classified, **right** knee
M71.562 Other bursitis, not elsewhere classified, **left** knee
M71.569 Other bursitis, not elsewhere classified, unspecified knee

✓6th M71.57 Other bursitis, not elsewhere classified, **ankle and foot**
M71.571 Other bursitis, not elsewhere classified, **right** ankle and foot
M71.572 Other bursitis, not elsewhere classified, **left** ankle and foot
M71.579 Other bursitis, not elsewhere classified, unspecified ankle and foot

M71.58 Other bursitis, not elsewhere classified, other site

✓5th M71.8 Other specified bursopathies
M71.80 Other specified bursopathies, unspecified site

✓6th M71.81 Other specified bursopathies, **shoulder**
M71.811 Other specified bursopathies, **right** shoulder
M71.812 Other specified bursopathies, **left** shoulder
M71.819 Other specified bursopathies, unspecified shoulder

✓6th M71.82 Other specified bursopathies, **elbow**
M71.821 Other specified bursopathies, **right** elbow
M71.822 Other specified bursopathies, **left** elbow
M71.829 Other specified bursopathies, unspecified elbow

✓6th M71.83 Other specified bursopathies, **wrist**
M71.831 Other specified bursopathies, **right** wrist
M71.832 Other specified bursopathies, **left** wrist
M71.839 Other specified bursopathies, unspecified wrist

✓6th M71.84 Other specified bursopathies, **hand**
M71.841 Other specified bursopathies, **right** hand
M71.842 Other specified bursopathies, **left** hand
M71.849 Other specified bursopathies, unspecified hand

✓6th M71.85 Other specified bursopathies, **hip**
M71.851 Other specified bursopathies, **right** hip
M71.852 Other specified bursopathies, **left** hip
M71.859 Other specified bursopathies, unspecified hip

✓6th M71.86 Other specified bursopathies, **knee**
M71.861 Other specified bursopathies, **right** knee
M71.862 Other specified bursopathies, **left** knee
M71.869 Other specified bursopathies, unspecified knee

✓6th M71.87 Other specified bursopathies, **ankle and foot**
M71.871 Other specified bursopathies, **right** ankle and foot
M71.872 Other specified bursopathies, **left** ankle and foot
M71.879 Other specified bursopathies, unspecified ankle and foot

M71.88 Other specified bursopathies, other site
M71.89 Other specified bursopathies, **multiple sites**

M71.9 Bursopathy, unspecified
Bursitis NOS

✓4th **M72 Fibroblastic disorders**
EXCLUDES 2 *retroperitoneal fibromatosis (D48.3)*

M72.0 Palmar fascial fibromatosis [Dupuytren] A
DEF: Dupuytren's contracture: Flexion deformity of a finger, due to shortened, thickened fibrosing of palmar fascia. The cause is unknown, but it is associated with long-standing epilepsy.

M72.1 Knuckle pads

M72.2 Plantar fascial fibromatosis
Plantar fasciitis
DEF: Rapid-growing and multiplanar nodular swellings and pain in the foot that is not associated with contractures.

M72.4 Pseudosarcomatous fibromatosis
Nodular fasciitis

M72.6 Necrotizing fasciitis HCC ESR COM
Use additional code (B95.-, B96.-) to identify causative organism

M72.8 Other fibroblastic disorders
Abscess of fascia
Fasciitis NEC
Other infective fasciitis
Use additional code to (B95.-, B96.-) identify causative organism
EXCLUDES 1 *diffuse (eosinophilic) fasciitis (M35.4)*
necrotizing fasciitis (M72.6)
nodular fasciitis (M72.4)
perirenal fasciitis NOS (N13.5)
perirenal fasciitis with infection (N13.6)
plantar fasciitis (M72.2)

M72.9 Fibroblastic disorder, unspecified
Fasciitis NOS
Fibromatosis NOS

M75 Shoulder lesions
EXCLUDES 2 *shoulder-hand syndrome (M89.Ø-)*

M75.Ø Adhesive capsulitis of shoulder
Frozen shoulder
Periarthritis of shoulder
AHA: 2015,2Q,23
- **M75.ØØ Adhesive capsulitis of unspecified shoulder**
- **M75.Ø1 Adhesive capsulitis of right shoulder**
- **M75.Ø2 Adhesive capsulitis of left shoulder**

M75.1 Rotator cuff tear or rupture, not specified as traumatic
Rotator cuff syndrome
Supraspinatus syndrome
Supraspinatus tear or rupture, not specified as traumatic
EXCLUDES 1 *tear of rotator cuff, traumatic (S46.Ø1-)*

M75.1Ø Unspecified rotator cuff tear or rupture, not specified as traumatic
- **M75.1ØØ Unspecified rotator cuff tear or rupture of unspecified shoulder, not specified as traumatic**
- **M75.1Ø1 Unspecified rotator cuff tear or rupture of right shoulder, not specified as traumatic**
- **M75.1Ø2 Unspecified rotator cuff tear or rupture of left shoulder, not specified as traumatic**

M75.11 Incomplete rotator cuff tear or rupture not specified as traumatic
- **M75.11Ø Incomplete rotator cuff tear or rupture of unspecified shoulder, not specified as traumatic**
- **M75.111 Incomplete rotator cuff tear or rupture of right shoulder, not specified as traumatic**
- **M75.112 Incomplete rotator cuff tear or rupture of left shoulder, not specified as traumatic**

M75.12 Complete rotator cuff tear or rupture not specified as traumatic
- **M75.12Ø Complete rotator cuff tear or rupture of unspecified shoulder, not specified as traumatic**
- **M75.121 Complete rotator cuff tear or rupture of right shoulder, not specified as traumatic**
- **M75.122 Complete rotator cuff tear or rupture of left shoulder, not specified as traumatic**

M75.2 Bicipital tendinitis
- **M75.2Ø Bicipital tendinitis, unspecified shoulder**
- **M75.21 Bicipital tendinitis, right shoulder**
- **M75.22 Bicipital tendinitis, left shoulder**

M75.3 Calcific tendinitis of shoulder
Calcified bursa of shoulder
- **M75.3Ø Calcific tendinitis of unspecified shoulder**
- **M75.31 Calcific tendinitis of right shoulder**
- **M75.32 Calcific tendinitis of left shoulder**

M75.4 Impingement syndrome of shoulder
- **M75.4Ø Impingement syndrome of unspecified shoulder**
- **M75.41 Impingement syndrome of right shoulder**
- **M75.42 Impingement syndrome of left shoulder**

M75.5 Bursitis of shoulder
- **M75.5Ø Bursitis of unspecified shoulder**
- **M75.51 Bursitis of right shoulder**
- **M75.52 Bursitis of left shoulder**

M75.8 Other shoulder lesions
- **M75.8Ø Other shoulder lesions, unspecified shoulder**
- **M75.81 Other shoulder lesions, right shoulder**
- **M75.82 Other shoulder lesions, left shoulder**

M75.9 Shoulder lesion, unspecified
- **M75.9Ø Shoulder lesion, unspecified, unspecified shoulder**
- **M75.91 Shoulder lesion, unspecified, right shoulder**
- **M75.92 Shoulder lesion, unspecified, left shoulder**

M76 Enthesopathies, lower limb, excluding foot
EXCLUDES 2 *bursitis due to use, overuse and pressure (M7Ø.-)*
enthesopathies of ankle and foot (M77.5-)

M76.Ø Gluteal tendinitis
- **M76.ØØ Gluteal tendinitis, unspecified hip**
- **M76.Ø1 Gluteal tendinitis, right hip**
- **M76.Ø2 Gluteal tendinitis, left hip**

M76.1 Psoas tendinitis
- **M76.1Ø Psoas tendinitis, unspecified hip**
- **M76.11 Psoas tendinitis, right hip**
- **M76.12 Psoas tendinitis, left hip**

M76.2 Iliac crest spur
- **M76.2Ø Iliac crest spur, unspecified hip**
- **M76.21 Iliac crest spur, right hip**
- **M76.22 Iliac crest spur, left hip**

M76.3 Iliotibial band syndrome
- **M76.3Ø Iliotibial band syndrome, unspecified leg**
- **M76.31 Iliotibial band syndrome, right leg**
- **M76.32 Iliotibial band syndrome, left leg**

M76.4 Tibial collateral bursitis [Pellegrini-Stieda]
- **M76.4Ø Tibial collateral bursitis [Pellegrini-Stieda], unspecified leg**
- **M76.41 Tibial collateral bursitis [Pellegrini-Stieda], right leg**
- **M76.42 Tibial collateral bursitis [Pellegrini-Stieda], left leg**

M76.5 Patellar tendinitis
- **M76.5Ø Patellar tendinitis, unspecified knee**
- **M76.51 Patellar tendinitis, right knee**
- **M76.52 Patellar tendinitis, left knee**

M76.6 Achilles tendinitis
Achilles bursitis
- **M76.6Ø Achilles tendinitis, unspecified leg**
- **M76.61 Achilles tendinitis, right leg**
- **M76.62 Achilles tendinitis, left leg**

M76.7 Peroneal tendinitis
- **M76.7Ø Peroneal tendinitis, unspecified leg**
- **M76.71 Peroneal tendinitis, right leg**
- **M76.72 Peroneal tendinitis, left leg**

M76.8 Other specified enthesopathies of lower limb, excluding foot

M76.81 Anterior tibial syndrome
- **M76.811 Anterior tibial syndrome, right leg**
- **M76.812 Anterior tibial syndrome, left leg**
- **M76.819 Anterior tibial syndrome, unspecified leg**

M76.82 Posterior tibial tendinitis
- **M76.821 Posterior tibial tendinitis, right leg**
- **M76.822 Posterior tibial tendinitis, left leg**
- **M76.829 Posterior tibial tendinitis, unspecified leg**

M76.89 Other specified enthesopathies of lower limb, excluding foot
- **M76.891 Other specified enthesopathies of right lower limb, excluding foot**
- **M76.892 Other specified enthesopathies of left lower limb, excluding foot**
- **M76.899 Other specified enthesopathies of unspecified lower limb, excluding foot**

M76.9 Unspecified enthesopathy, lower limb, excluding foot

M77 Other enthesopathies
EXCLUDES 1 *bursitis NOS (M71.9-)*
EXCLUDES 2 *bursitis due to use, overuse and pressure (M7Ø.-)*
osteophyte (M25.7)
spinal enthesopathy (M46.Ø-)

M77.Ø Medial epicondylitis
- **M77.ØØ Medial epicondylitis, unspecified elbow**
- **M77.Ø1 Medial epicondylitis, right elbow**
- **M77.Ø2 Medial epicondylitis, left elbow**

M77.1 Lateral epicondylitis
Tennis elbow
- **M77.1Ø Lateral epicondylitis, unspecified elbow**
- **M77.11 Lateral epicondylitis, right elbow**
- **M77.12 Lateral epicondylitis, left elbow**

M77.2 Periarthritis of wrist
- **M77.2Ø Periarthritis, unspecified wrist**
- **M77.21 Periarthritis, right wrist**
- **M77.22 Periarthritis, left wrist**

M77.3 Calcaneal spur
DEF: Overgrowth of calcaneus bone on the underside of the heel that causes pain on walking. Calcaneal spur is due to a chronic avulsion injury of the plantar fascia from the calcaneus.
- **M77.3Ø Calcaneal spur, unspecified foot**
- **M77.31 Calcaneal spur, right foot**
- **M77.32 Calcaneal spur, left foot**

✓5th **M77.4 Metatarsalgia**

EXCLUDES 1 *Morton's metatarsalgia (G57.6)*

M77.40 Metatarsalgia, unspecified foot

M77.41 Metatarsalgia, right foot

M77.42 Metatarsalgia, left foot

✓5th **M77.5 Other enthesopathy of foot and ankle**

M77.50 Other enthesopathy of unspecified foot and ankle

M77.51 Other enthesopathy of right foot and ankle

M77.52 Other enthesopathy of left foot and ankle

M77.8 Other enthesopathies, not elsewhere classified

M77.9 Enthesopathy, unspecified

Bone spur NOS
Capsulitis NOS
Periarthritis NOS
Tendinitis NOS

✓4th **M79 Other and unspecified soft tissue disorders, not elsewhere classified**

EXCLUDES 1 *psychogenic rheumatism (F45.8)*
soft tissue pain, psychogenic (F45.41)

M79.0 Rheumatism, unspecified

EXCLUDES 1 *fibromyalgia (M79.7)*
palindromic rheumatism (M12.3-)

✓5th **M79.1 Myalgia**

Myofascial pain syndrome

EXCLUDES 1 *fibromyalgia (M79.7)*
myositis (M60.-)

AHA: 2018,4Q,21

M79.10 Myalgia, unspecified site

M79.11 Myalgia of mastication muscle

M79.12 Myalgia of auxiliary muscles, head and neck

M79.18 Myalgia, other site

M79.2 Neuralgia and neuritis, unspecified

EXCLUDES 1 *brachial radiculitis NOS (M54.1)*
lumbosacral radiculitis NOS (M54.1)
mononeuropathies (G56-G58)
radiculitis NOS (M54.1)
sciatica (M54.3-M54.4)

TIP: Assign for documented neuropathic pain.

M79.3 Panniculitis, unspecified

EXCLUDES 1 *lupus panniculitis (L93.2)*
neck and back panniculitis (M54.0-)
relapsing [Weber-Christian] panniculitis (M35.6)

M79.4 Hypertrophy of (infrapatellar) fat pad

M79.5 Residual foreign body in soft tissue

EXCLUDES 1 *foreign body granuloma of skin and subcutaneous tissue (L92.3)*
foreign body granuloma of soft tissue (M60.2-)

✓5th **M79.6 Pain in limb, hand, foot, fingers and toes**

EXCLUDES 2 *pain in joint (M25.5-)*

✓6th **M79.60 Pain in limb, unspecified**

M79.601 Pain in right arm
Pain in right upper limb NOS

M79.602 Pain in left arm
Pain in left upper limb NOS

M79.603 Pain in arm, unspecified
Pain in upper limb NOS

M79.604 Pain in right leg
Pain in right lower limb NOS

M79.605 Pain in left leg
Pain in left lower limb NOS

M79.606 Pain in leg, unspecified
Pain in lower limb NOS

M79.609 Pain in unspecified limb
Pain in limb NOS

✓6th **M79.62 Pain in upper arm**

Pain in axillary region

M79.621 Pain in right upper arm

M79.622 Pain in left upper arm

M79.629 Pain in unspecified upper arm

✓6th **M79.63 Pain in forearm**

M79.631 Pain in right forearm

M79.632 Pain in left forearm

M79.639 Pain in unspecified forearm

✓6th **M79.64 Pain in hand and fingers**

M79.641 Pain in right hand

M79.642 Pain in left hand

M79.643 Pain in unspecified hand

M79.644 Pain in right finger(s)

M79.645 Pain in left finger(s)

M79.646 Pain in unspecified finger(s)

✓6th **M79.65 Pain in thigh**

M79.651 Pain in right thigh

M79.652 Pain in left thigh

M79.659 Pain in unspecified thigh

✓6th **M79.66 Pain in lower leg**

M79.661 Pain in right lower leg

M79.662 Pain in left lower leg

M79.669 Pain in unspecified lower leg

✓6th **M79.67 Pain in foot and toes**

M79.671 Pain in right foot

M79.672 Pain in left foot

M79.673 Pain in unspecified foot

M79.674 Pain in right toe(s)

M79.675 Pain in left toe(s)

M79.676 Pain in unspecified toe(s)

M79.7 Fibromyalgia

Fibromyositis
Fibrositis
Myofibrositis

✓5th **M79.A Nontraumatic compartment syndrome**

Code first, if applicable, associated postprocedural complication

EXCLUDES 1 *compartment syndrome NOS (T79.A-)*
fibromyalgia (M79.7)
nontraumatic ischemic infarction of muscle (M62.2-)
traumatic compartment syndrome (T79.A-)

✓6th **M79.A1 Nontraumatic compartment syndrome of upper extremity**

Nontraumatic compartment syndrome of shoulder, arm, forearm, wrist, hand, and fingers

M79.A11 Nontraumatic compartment syndrome of right upper extremity

M79.A12 Nontraumatic compartment syndrome of left upper extremity

M79.A19 Nontraumatic compartment syndrome of unspecified upper extremity

✓6th **M79.A2 Nontraumatic compartment syndrome of lower extremity**

Nontraumatic compartment syndrome of hip, buttock, thigh, leg, foot, and toes

M79.A21 Nontraumatic compartment syndrome of right lower extremity

M79.A22 Nontraumatic compartment syndrome of left lower extremity

M79.A29 Nontraumatic compartment syndrome of unspecified lower extremity

M79.A3 Nontraumatic compartment syndrome of abdomen

M79.A9 Nontraumatic compartment syndrome of other sites

✓5th **M79.8 Other specified soft tissue disorders**

M79.81 Nontraumatic hematoma of soft tissue
Nontraumatic hematoma of muscle
Nontraumatic seroma of muscle and soft tissue

M79.89 Other specified soft tissue disorders
Polyalgia

M79.9 Soft tissue disorder, unspecified

OSTEOPATHIES AND CHONDROPATHIES (M80-M94)

Disorders of bone density and structure (M80-M85)

M80 Osteoporosis with current pathological fracture

INCLUDES osteoporosis with current fragility fracture

Use additional code to identify major osseous defect, if applicable (M89.7-)

EXCLUDES 1 *collapsed vertebra NOS (M48.5)*
pathological fracture NOS (M84.4)
wedging of vertebra NOS (M48.5)

EXCLUDES 2 *personal history of (healed) osteoporosis fracture (Z87.310)*

AHA: 2018,2Q,12

TIP: The site codes in this category identify the site of the fracture, not the site of the osteoporosis.

The appropriate 7th character is to be added to each code from category M80:
- A initial encounter for fracture
- D subsequent encounter for fracture with routine healing
- G subsequent encounter for fracture with delayed healing
- K subsequent encounter for fracture with nonunion
- P subsequent encounter for fracture with malunion
- S sequela

M80.0 Age-related osteoporosis with current pathological fracture
Involutional osteoporosis with current pathological fracture
Osteoporosis NOS with current pathological fracture
Postmenopausal osteoporosis with current pathological fracture
Senile osteoporosis with current pathological fracture

M80.00 Age-related osteoporosis with current pathological fracture, unspecified site Rx Q A

M80.01 Age-related osteoporosis with current pathological fracture, shoulder

M80.011 Age-related osteoporosis with current pathological fracture, right shoulder Rx Q A

M80.012 Age-related osteoporosis with current pathological fracture, left shoulder Rx Q A

M80.019 Age-related osteoporosis with current pathological fracture, unspecified shoulder Rx Q A

M80.02 Age-related osteoporosis with current pathological fracture, humerus

M80.021 Age-related osteoporosis with current pathological fracture, right humerus Rx Q A

M80.022 Age-related osteoporosis with current pathological fracture, left humerus Rx Q A

M80.029 Age-related osteoporosis with current pathological fracture, unspecified humerus Rx Q A

M80.03 Age-related osteoporosis with current pathological fracture, forearm
Age-related osteoporosis with current pathological fracture of wrist

M80.031 Age-related osteoporosis with current pathological fracture, right forearm Rx Q A

M80.032 Age-related osteoporosis with current pathological fracture, left forearm Rx Q A

M80.039 Age-related osteoporosis with current pathological fracture, unspecified forearm Rx Q A

M80.04 Age-related osteoporosis with current pathological fracture, hand

M80.041 Age-related osteoporosis with current pathological fracture, right hand Rx Q A

M80.042 Age-related osteoporosis with current pathological fracture, left hand Rx Q A

M80.049 Age-related osteoporosis with current pathological fracture, unspecified hand Rx Q A

M80.05 Age-related osteoporosis with current pathological fracture, femur
Age-related osteoporosis with current pathological fracture of hip

1 **M80.051 Age-related osteoporosis with current pathological fracture, right femur** HCC Rx ESR COM Q A

1 **M80.052 Age-related osteoporosis with current pathological fracture, left femur** HCC Rx ESR COM Q A

1 **M80.059 Age-related osteoporosis with current pathological fracture, unspecified femur** HCC Rx ESR COM Q A

M80.06 Age-related osteoporosis with current pathological fracture, lower leg

M80.061 Age-related osteoporosis with current pathological fracture, right lower leg Rx Q A

M80.062 Age-related osteoporosis with current pathological fracture, left lower leg Rx Q A

M80.069 Age-related osteoporosis with current pathological fracture, unspecified lower leg Rx Q A

M80.07 Age-related osteoporosis with current pathological fracture, ankle and foot

M80.071 Age-related osteoporosis with current pathological fracture, right ankle and foot Rx Q A

M80.072 Age-related osteoporosis with current pathological fracture, left ankle and foot Rx Q A

M80.079 Age-related osteoporosis with current pathological fracture, unspecified ankle and foot Rx Q A

1 **M80.08 Age-related osteoporosis with current pathological fracture, vertebra(e)** HCC Rx ESR COM Q A

M80.0A Age-related osteoporosis with current pathological fracture, other site Rx Q A
AHA: 2020,4Q,32-33

M80.8 Other osteoporosis with current pathological fracture
Drug-induced osteoporosis with current pathological fracture
Idiopathic osteoporosis with current pathological fracture
Osteoporosis of disuse with current pathological fracture
Postoophorectomy osteoporosis with current pathological fracture
Postsurgical malabsorption osteoporosis with current pathological fracture
Post-traumatic osteoporosis with current pathological fracture
Use additional code for adverse effect, if applicable, to identify drug (T36-T50 with fifth or sixth character 5)

M80.80 Other osteoporosis with current pathological fracture, unspecified site Rx Q

M80.81 Other osteoporosis with pathological fracture, shoulder

M80.811 Other osteoporosis with current pathological fracture, right shoulder Rx Q

M80.812 Other osteoporosis with current pathological fracture, left shoulder Rx Q

M80.819 Other osteoporosis with current pathological fracture, unspecified shoulder Rx Q

M80.82 Other osteoporosis with current pathological fracture, humerus

M80.821 Other osteoporosis with current pathological fracture, right humerus Rx Q

M80.822 Other osteoporosis with current pathological fracture, left humerus Rx Q

M80.829 Other osteoporosis with current pathological fracture, unspecified humerus Rx Q

M80.83 Other osteoporosis with current pathological fracture, forearm
Other osteoporosis with current pathological fracture of wrist
M80.831 Other osteoporosis with current pathological fracture, right forearm Rx Q
M80.832 Other osteoporosis with current pathological fracture, left forearm Rx Q
M80.839 Other osteoporosis with current pathological fracture, unspecified forearm Rx Q
M80.84 Other osteoporosis with current pathological fracture, hand
M80.841 Other osteoporosis with current pathological fracture, right hand Rx Q
M80.842 Other osteoporosis with current pathological fracture, left hand Rx Q
M80.849 Other osteoporosis with current pathological fracture, unspecified hand Rx Q
M80.85 Other osteoporosis with current pathological fracture, femur
Other osteoporosis with current pathological fracture of hip
1 M80.851 Other osteoporosis with current pathological fracture, right femur HCC Rx ESR COM Q
1 M80.852 Other osteoporosis with current pathological fracture, left femur HCC Rx ESR COM Q
1 M80.859 Other osteoporosis with current pathological fracture, unspecified femur HCC Rx ESR COM Q
M80.86 Other osteoporosis with current pathological fracture, lower leg
M80.861 Other osteoporosis with current pathological fracture, right lower leg Rx Q
M80.862 Other osteoporosis with current pathological fracture, left lower leg Rx Q
M80.869 Other osteoporosis with current pathological fracture, unspecified lower leg Rx Q
M80.87 Other osteoporosis with current pathological fracture, ankle and foot
M80.871 Other osteoporosis with current pathological fracture, right ankle and foot Rx Q
M80.872 Other osteoporosis with current pathological fracture, left ankle and foot Rx Q
M80.879 Other osteoporosis with current pathological fracture, unspecified ankle and foot Rx Q
1 M80.88 Other osteoporosis with current pathological fracture, vertebra(e) HCC Rx ESR COM Q
M80.8A Other osteoporosis with current pathological fracture, other site Rx Q
AHA: 2020,4Q,32

M81 Osteoporosis without current pathological fracture
Use additional code to identify:
major osseous defect, if applicable (M89.7-)
personal history of (healed) osteoporosis fracture, if applicable (Z87.310)
EXCLUDES 1 *osteoporosis with current pathological fracture (M80.-)*
Sudeck's atrophy (M89.0)
M81.0 Age-related osteoporosis without current pathological fracture Rx Q A
Involutional osteoporosis without current pathological fracture
Osteoporosis NOS
Postmenopausal osteoporosis without current pathological fracture
Senile osteoporosis without current pathological fracture
M81.6 Localized osteoporosis [Lequesne] Rx Q
EXCLUDES 1 *Sudeck's atrophy (M89.0)*
M81.8 Other osteoporosis without current pathological fracture Rx Q
Drug-induced osteoporosis without current pathological fracture
Idiopathic osteoporosis without current pathological fracture
Osteoporosis of disuse without current pathological fracture
Postoophorectomy osteoporosis without current pathological fracture
Postsurgical malabsorption osteoporosis without current pathological fracture
Post-traumatic osteoporosis without current pathological fracture
Use additional code for adverse effect, if applicable, to identify drug (T36-T50 with fifth or sixth character 5)

M83 Adult osteomalacia
EXCLUDES 1 *infantile and juvenile osteomalacia (E55.0)*
renal osteodystrophy (N25.0)
rickets (active) (E55.0)
rickets (active) sequelae (E64.3)
vitamin D-resistant osteomalacia (E83.3)
vitamin D-resistant rickets (active) (E83.3)
M83.0 Puerperal osteomalacia Rx M ♀
M83.1 Senile osteomalacia Rx A
M83.2 Adult osteomalacia due to malabsorption Rx A
Postsurgical malabsorption osteomalacia in adults
M83.3 Adult osteomalacia due to malnutrition Rx A
M83.4 Aluminum bone disease Rx
M83.5 Other drug-induced osteomalacia in adults Rx A
Use additional code for adverse effect, if applicable, to identify drug (T36-T50 with fifth or sixth character 5)
M83.8 Other adult osteomalacia Rx A
M83.9 Adult osteomalacia, unspecified Rx A

M84 Disorder of continuity of bone
EXCLUDES 2 *traumatic fracture of bone-see fracture, by site*
M84.3 Stress fracture
Fatigue fracture
March fracture
Stress fracture NOS
Stress reaction
Use additional external cause code(s) to identify the cause of the stress fracture
EXCLUDES 1 *pathological fracture due to osteoporosis (M80.-)*
pathological fracture NOS (M84.4.-)
traumatic fracture (S12.-, S22.-, S32.-, S42.-, S52.-, S62.-, S72.-, S82.-, S92.-)
EXCLUDES 2 *personal history of (healed) stress (fatigue) fracture (Z87.312)*
stress fracture of vertebra (M48.4-)

The appropriate 7th character is to be added to each code from subcategory M84.3.
A initial encounter for fracture
D subsequent encounter for fracture with routine healing
G subsequent encounter for fracture with delayed healing
K subsequent encounter for fracture with nonunion
P subsequent encounter for fracture with malunion
S sequela

M84.30 Stress fracture, unspecified site
M84.31 Stress fracture, shoulder
M84.311 Stress fracture, right shoulder Q
M84.312 Stress fracture, left shoulder Q
M84.319 Stress fracture, unspecified shoulder Q
M84.32 Stress fracture, humerus
M84.321 Stress fracture, right humerus Q
M84.322 Stress fracture, left humerus Q
M84.329 Stress fracture, unspecified humerus Q
M84.33 Stress fracture, ulna and radius
M84.331 Stress fracture, right ulna Q
M84.332 Stress fracture, left ulna Q
M84.333 Stress fracture, right radius Q
M84.334 Stress fracture, left radius Q

M84.339 Stress fracture, unspecified ulna and radius
M84.34 Stress fracture, hand and fingers
M84.341 Stress fracture, right hand
M84.342 Stress fracture, left hand
M84.343 Stress fracture, unspecified hand
M84.344 Stress fracture, right finger(s)
M84.345 Stress fracture, left finger(s)
M84.346 Stress fracture, unspecified finger(s)
M84.35 Stress fracture, pelvis and femur
Stress fracture, hip
M84.350 Stress fracture, pelvis
M84.351 Stress fracture, right femur
M84.352 Stress fracture, left femur
M84.353 Stress fracture, unspecified femur
M84.359 Stress fracture, hip, unspecified
M84.36 Stress fracture, tibia and fibula
M84.361 Stress fracture, right tibia
M84.362 Stress fracture, left tibia
M84.363 Stress fracture, right fibula
M84.364 Stress fracture, left fibula
M84.369 Stress fracture, unspecified tibia and fibula
M84.37 Stress fracture, ankle, foot and toes
M84.371 Stress fracture, right ankle
M84.372 Stress fracture, left ankle
M84.373 Stress fracture, unspecified ankle
M84.374 Stress fracture, right foot
M84.375 Stress fracture, left foot
M84.376 Stress fracture, unspecified foot
M84.377 Stress fracture, right toe(s)
M84.378 Stress fracture, left toe(s)
M84.379 Stress fracture, unspecified toe(s)
M84.38 Stress fracture, other site
EXCLUDES 2 *stress fracture of vertebra (M48.4-)*

M84.4 Pathological fracture, not elsewhere classified
Chronic fracture
Pathological fracture NOS
EXCLUDES 1 *collapsed vertebra NEC (M48.5)*
pathological fracture in neoplastic disease (M84.5-)
pathological fracture in osteoporosis (M80.-)
pathological fracture in other disease (M84.6-)
stress fracture (M84.3-)
traumatic fracture (S12.-, S22.-, S32.-, S42.-, S52.-, S62.-, S72.-, S82.-, S92.-)
EXCLUDES 2 *personal history of (healed) pathological fracture (Z87.311)*

The appropriate 7th character is to be added to each code from subcategory M84.4.
A initial encounter for fracture
D subsequent encounter for fracture with routine healing
G subsequent encounter for fracture with delayed healing
K subsequent encounter for fracture with nonunion
P subsequent encounter for fracture with malunion
S sequela

M84.40 Pathological fracture, unspecified site
M84.41 Pathological fracture, shoulder
M84.411 Pathological fracture, right shoulder
M84.412 Pathological fracture, left shoulder
M84.419 Pathological fracture, unspecified shoulder
M84.42 Pathological fracture, humerus
M84.421 Pathological fracture, right humerus
M84.422 Pathological fracture, left humerus
M84.429 Pathological fracture, unspecified humerus
M84.43 Pathological fracture, ulna and radius
M84.431 Pathological fracture, right ulna
M84.432 Pathological fracture, left ulna
M84.433 Pathological fracture, right radius
M84.434 Pathological fracture, left radius
M84.439 Pathological fracture, unspecified ulna and radius
M84.44 Pathological fracture, hand and fingers
M84.441 Pathological fracture, right hand
M84.442 Pathological fracture, left hand
M84.443 Pathological fracture, unspecified hand
M84.444 Pathological fracture, right finger(s)
M84.445 Pathological fracture, left finger(s)
M84.446 Pathological fracture, unspecified finger(s)
M84.45 Pathological fracture, femur and pelvis
AHA: 2016,4Q,43
1 M84.451 Pathological fracture, right femur
1 M84.452 Pathological fracture, left femur
1 M84.453 Pathological fracture, unspecified femur
M84.454 Pathological fracture, pelvis
1 M84.459 Pathological fracture, hip, unspecified
M84.46 Pathological fracture, tibia and fibula
M84.461 Pathological fracture, right tibia
M84.462 Pathological fracture, left tibia
M84.463 Pathological fracture, right fibula
M84.464 Pathological fracture, left fibula
M84.469 Pathological fracture, unspecified tibia and fibula
M84.47 Pathological fracture, ankle, foot and toes
M84.471 Pathological fracture, right ankle
M84.472 Pathological fracture, left ankle
M84.473 Pathological fracture, unspecified ankle
M84.474 Pathological fracture, right foot
M84.475 Pathological fracture, left foot
M84.476 Pathological fracture, unspecified foot
M84.477 Pathological fracture, right toe(s)
M84.478 Pathological fracture, left toe(s)
M84.479 Pathological fracture, unspecified toe(s)
M84.48 Pathological fracture, other site

M84.5 Pathological fracture in neoplastic disease
Code also underlying neoplasm

The appropriate 7th character is to be added to each code from subcategory M84.5.
A initial encounter for fracture
D subsequent encounter for fracture with routine healing
G subsequent encounter for fracture with delayed healing
K subsequent encounter for fracture with nonunion
P subsequent encounter for fracture with malunion
S sequela

M84.50 Pathological fracture in neoplastic disease, unspecified site
M84.51 Pathological fracture in neoplastic disease, shoulder
M84.511 Pathological fracture in neoplastic disease, right shoulder
M84.512 Pathological fracture in neoplastic disease, left shoulder
M84.519 Pathological fracture in neoplastic disease, unspecified shoulder
M84.52 Pathological fracture in neoplastic disease, humerus
M84.521 Pathological fracture in neoplastic disease, right humerus
M84.522 Pathological fracture in neoplastic disease, left humerus

M84.529 Pathological fracture in neoplastic disease, unspecified humerus Rx

M84.53 Pathological fracture in neoplastic disease, ulna and radius

M84.531 Pathological fracture in neoplastic disease, right ulna Rx

M84.532 Pathological fracture in neoplastic disease, left ulna Rx

M84.533 Pathological fracture in neoplastic disease, right radius Rx

M84.534 Pathological fracture in neoplastic disease, left radius Rx

M84.539 Pathological fracture in neoplastic disease, unspecified ulna and radius Rx

M84.54 Pathological fracture in neoplastic disease, hand

M84.541 Pathological fracture in neoplastic disease, right hand Rx

M84.542 Pathological fracture in neoplastic disease, left hand Rx

M84.549 Pathological fracture in neoplastic disease, unspecified hand Rx

M84.55 Pathological fracture in neoplastic disease, pelvis and femur

M84.550 Pathological fracture in neoplastic disease, pelvis Rx

1 M84.551 Pathological fracture in neoplastic disease, right femur HCC Rx ESR COM

1 M84.552 Pathological fracture in neoplastic disease, left femur HCC Rx ESR COM

1 M84.553 Pathological fracture in neoplastic disease, unspecified femur HCC Rx ESR COM

1 M84.559 Pathological fracture in neoplastic disease, hip, unspecified HCC Rx ESR COM

M84.56 Pathological fracture in neoplastic disease, tibia and fibula

M84.561 Pathological fracture in neoplastic disease, right tibia Rx

M84.562 Pathological fracture in neoplastic disease, left tibia Rx

M84.563 Pathological fracture in neoplastic disease, right fibula Rx

M84.564 Pathological fracture in neoplastic disease, left fibula Rx

M84.569 Pathological fracture in neoplastic disease, unspecified tibia and fibula Rx

M84.57 Pathological fracture in neoplastic disease, ankle and foot

M84.571 Pathological fracture in neoplastic disease, right ankle Rx

M84.572 Pathological fracture in neoplastic disease, left ankle Rx

M84.573 Pathological fracture in neoplastic disease, unspecified ankle Rx

M84.574 Pathological fracture in neoplastic disease, right foot Rx

M84.575 Pathological fracture in neoplastic disease, left foot Rx

M84.576 Pathological fracture in neoplastic disease, unspecified foot Rx

M84.58 Pathological fracture in neoplastic disease, other specified site Rx

Pathological fracture in neoplastic disease, vertebrae

M84.6 Pathological fracture in other disease

Code also underlying condition

EXCLUDES 1 *pathological fracture in osteoporosis (M8Ø.-)*

The appropriate 7th character is to be added to each code from subcategory M84.6.
A initial encounter for fracture
D subsequent encounter for fracture with routine healing
G subsequent encounter for fracture with delayed healing
K subsequent encounter for fracture with nonunion
P subsequent encounter for fracture with malunion
S sequela

M84.6Ø Pathological fracture in other disease, unspecified site Rx

M84.61 Pathological fracture in other disease, shoulder

M84.611 Pathological fracture in other disease, right shoulder Rx

M84.612 Pathological fracture in other disease, left shoulder Rx

M84.619 Pathological fracture in other disease, unspecified shoulder Rx

M84.62 Pathological fracture in other disease, humerus

M84.621 Pathological fracture in other disease, right humerus Rx

M84.622 Pathological fracture in other disease, left humerus Rx

M84.629 Pathological fracture in other disease, unspecified humerus Rx

M84.63 Pathological fracture in other disease, ulna and radius

M84.631 Pathological fracture in other disease, right ulna Rx

M84.632 Pathological fracture in other disease, left ulna Rx

M84.633 Pathological fracture in other disease, right radius Rx

M84.634 Pathological fracture in other disease, left radius Rx

M84.639 Pathological fracture in other disease, unspecified ulna and radius Rx

M84.64 Pathological fracture in other disease, hand

M84.641 Pathological fracture in other disease, right hand Rx

M84.642 Pathological fracture in other disease, left hand Rx

M84.649 Pathological fracture in other disease, unspecified hand Rx

M84.65 Pathological fracture in other disease, pelvis and femur

M84.650 Pathological fracture in other disease, pelvis Rx

1 M84.651 Pathological fracture in other disease, right femur HCC Rx ESR COM

1 M84.652 Pathological fracture in other disease, left femur HCC Rx ESR COM

1 M84.653 Pathological fracture in other disease, unspecified femur HCC Rx ESR COM

1 M84.659 Pathological fracture in other disease, hip, unspecified HCC Rx ESR COM

M84.66 Pathological fracture in other disease, tibia and fibula

M84.661 Pathological fracture in other disease, right tibia Rx

M84.662 Pathological fracture in other disease, left tibia Rx

M84.663 Pathological fracture in other disease, right fibula Rx

M84.664 Pathological fracture in other disease, left fibula Rx

M84.669 Pathological fracture in other disease, unspecified tibia and fibula Rx

M84.67 Pathological fracture in other disease, ankle and foot

M84.671 Pathological fracture in other disease, right ankle Rx

M84.672 Pathological fracture in other disease, left ankle Rx

M84.673 Pathological fracture in other disease, unspecified ankle Rx

M84.674 Pathological fracture in other disease, right foot Rx

M84.675 Pathological fracture in other disease, left foot Rx

M84.676 Pathological fracture in other disease, unspecified foot Rx

M84.68 Pathological fracture in other disease, other site Rx

M84.7 Nontraumatic fracture, not elsewhere classified

M84.75 Atypical femoral fracture

AHA: 2016,4Q,41-42

The appropriate 7th character is to be added to each code from M84.75.
- A initial encounter for fracture
- D subsequent encounter for fracture with routine healing
- G subsequent encounter for fracture with delayed healing
- K subsequent encounter for fracture with nonunion
- P subsequent encounter for fracture with malunion
- S sequela

M84.750 Atypical femoral fracture, unspecified Q

M84.751 Incomplete atypical femoral fracture, right leg Q

M84.752 Incomplete atypical femoral fracture, left leg Q

M84.753 Incomplete atypical femoral fracture, unspecified leg Q

1 **M84.754 Complete transverse atypical femoral fracture, right leg** HCC ESR COM Q

1 **M84.755 Complete transverse atypical femoral fracture, left leg** HCC ESR COM Q

1 **M84.756 Complete transverse atypical femoral fracture, unspecified leg** HCC ESR COM Q

1 **M84.757 Complete oblique atypical femoral fracture, right leg** HCC ESR COM Q

1 **M84.758 Complete oblique atypical femoral fracture, left leg** HCC ESR COM

1 **M84.759 Complete oblique atypical femoral fracture, unspecified leg** HCC ESR COM Q

M84.8 Other disorders of continuity of bone

M84.80 Other disorders of continuity of bone, unspecified site

M84.81 Other disorders of continuity of bone, shoulder

M84.811 Other disorders of continuity of bone, right shoulder

M84.812 Other disorders of continuity of bone, left shoulder

M84.819 Other disorders of continuity of bone, unspecified shoulder

M84.82 Other disorders of continuity of bone, humerus

M84.821 Other disorders of continuity of bone, right humerus

M84.822 Other disorders of continuity of bone, left humerus

M84.829 Other disorders of continuity of bone, unspecified humerus

M84.83 Other disorders of continuity of bone, ulna and radius

M84.831 Other disorders of continuity of bone, right ulna

M84.832 Other disorders of continuity of bone, left ulna

M84.833 Other disorders of continuity of bone, right radius

M84.834 Other disorders of continuity of bone, left radius

M84.839 Other disorders of continuity of bone, unspecified ulna and radius

M84.84 Other disorders of continuity of bone, hand

M84.841 Other disorders of continuity of bone, right hand

M84.842 Other disorders of continuity of bone, left hand

M84.849 Other disorders of continuity of bone, unspecified hand

M84.85 Other disorders of continuity of bone, pelvic region and thigh

M84.851 Other disorders of continuity of bone, right pelvic region and thigh

M84.852 Other disorders of continuity of bone, left pelvic region and thigh

M84.859 Other disorders of continuity of bone, unspecified pelvic region and thigh

M84.86 Other disorders of continuity of bone, tibia and fibula

M84.861 Other disorders of continuity of bone, right tibia

M84.862 Other disorders of continuity of bone, left tibia

M84.863 Other disorders of continuity of bone, right fibula

M84.864 Other disorders of continuity of bone, left fibula

M84.869 Other disorders of continuity of bone, unspecified tibia and fibula

M84.87 Other disorders of continuity of bone, ankle and foot

M84.871 Other disorders of continuity of bone, right ankle and foot

M84.872 Other disorders of continuity of bone, left ankle and foot

M84.879 Other disorders of continuity of bone, unspecified ankle and foot

M84.88 Other disorders of continuity of bone, other site

M84.9 Disorder of continuity of bone, unspecified

M85 Other disorders of bone density and structure

EXCLUDES 1 *osteogenesis imperfecta (Q78.0)*
osteopetrosis (Q78.2)
osteopoikilosis (Q78.8)
polyostotic fibrous dysplasia (Q78.1)

M85.0 Fibrous dysplasia (monostotic)

EXCLUDES 2 *fibrous dysplasia of jaw (M27.8)*

M85.00 Fibrous dysplasia (monostotic), unspecified site

M85.01 Fibrous dysplasia (monostotic), shoulder

M85.011 Fibrous dysplasia (monostotic), right shoulder

M85.012 Fibrous dysplasia (monostotic), left shoulder

M85.019 Fibrous dysplasia (monostotic), unspecified shoulder

M85.02 Fibrous dysplasia (monostotic), upper arm

M85.021 Fibrous dysplasia (monostotic), right upper arm

M85.022 Fibrous dysplasia (monostotic), left upper arm

M85.029 Fibrous dysplasia (monostotic), unspecified upper arm

M85.03 Fibrous dysplasia (monostotic), forearm

M85.031 Fibrous dysplasia (monostotic), right forearm

M85.032 Fibrous dysplasia (monostotic), left forearm

M85.039 Fibrous dysplasia (monostotic), unspecified forearm

M85.04 Fibrous dysplasia (monostotic), hand

M85.041 Fibrous dysplasia (monostotic), right hand

M85.042 Fibrous dysplasia (monostotic), left hand

M85.049 Fibrous dysplasia (monostotic), unspecified hand

M85.05 Fibrous dysplasia (monostotic), thigh

M85.051 Fibrous dysplasia (monostotic), right thigh

M85.052 Fibrous dysplasia (monostotic), left thigh

M85.059 Fibrous dysplasia (monostotic), unspecified thigh

M85.06 Fibrous dysplasia (monostotic), lower leg

M85.061 Fibrous dysplasia (monostotic), right lower leg

M85.062 Fibrous dysplasia (monostotic), left lower leg

M85.069 Fibrous dysplasia (monostotic), unspecified lower leg

M85.07 Fibrous dysplasia (monostotic), ankle and foot

M85.071 Fibrous dysplasia (monostotic), right ankle and foot

M85.072 Fibrous dysplasia (monostotic), left ankle and foot

M85.079 Fibrous dysplasia (monostotic), unspecified ankle and foot

M85.Ø8 Fibrous dysplasia (monostotic), other site
M85.Ø9 Fibrous dysplasia (monostotic), multiple sites

√5th M85.1 Skeletal fluorosis
M85.1Ø Skeletal fluorosis, unspecified site
√6th M85.11 Skeletal fluorosis, shoulder
M85.111 Skeletal fluorosis, right shoulder
M85.112 Skeletal fluorosis, left shoulder
M85.119 Skeletal fluorosis, unspecified shoulder
√6th M85.12 Skeletal fluorosis, upper arm
M85.121 Skeletal fluorosis, right upper arm
M85.122 Skeletal fluorosis, left upper arm
M85.129 Skeletal fluorosis, unspecified upper arm
√6th M85.13 Skeletal fluorosis, forearm
M85.131 Skeletal fluorosis, right forearm
M85.132 Skeletal fluorosis, left forearm
M85.139 Skeletal fluorosis, unspecified forearm
√6th M85.14 Skeletal fluorosis, hand
M85.141 Skeletal fluorosis, right hand
M85.142 Skeletal fluorosis, left hand
M85.149 Skeletal fluorosis, unspecified hand
√6th M85.15 Skeletal fluorosis, thigh
M85.151 Skeletal fluorosis, right thigh
M85.152 Skeletal fluorosis, left thigh
M85.159 Skeletal fluorosis, unspecified thigh
√6th M85.16 Skeletal fluorosis, lower leg
M85.161 Skeletal fluorosis, right lower leg
M85.162 Skeletal fluorosis, left lower leg
M85.169 Skeletal fluorosis, unspecified lower leg
√6th M85.17 Skeletal fluorosis, ankle and foot
M85.171 Skeletal fluorosis, right ankle and foot
M85.172 Skeletal fluorosis, left ankle and foot
M85.179 Skeletal fluorosis, unspecified ankle and foot
M85.18 Skeletal fluorosis, other site
M85.19 Skeletal fluorosis, multiple sites

M85.2 Hyperostosis of skull
DEF: Abnormal bone growth on the inner aspect of the cranial bones.

√5th M85.3 Osteitis condensans
M85.3Ø Osteitis condensans, unspecified site
√6th M85.31 Osteitis condensans, shoulder
M85.311 Osteitis condensans, right shoulder
M85.312 Osteitis condensans, left shoulder
M85.319 Osteitis condensans, unspecified shoulder
√6th M85.32 Osteitis condensans, upper arm
M85.321 Osteitis condensans, right upper arm
M85.322 Osteitis condensans, left upper arm
M85.329 Osteitis condensans, unspecified upper arm
√6th M85.33 Osteitis condensans, forearm
M85.331 Osteitis condensans, right forearm
M85.332 Osteitis condensans, left forearm
M85.339 Osteitis condensans, unspecified forearm
√6th M85.34 Osteitis condensans, hand
M85.341 Osteitis condensans, right hand
M85.342 Osteitis condensans, left hand
M85.349 Osteitis condensans, unspecified hand
√6th M85.35 Osteitis condensans, thigh
M85.351 Osteitis condensans, right thigh
M85.352 Osteitis condensans, left thigh
M85.359 Osteitis condensans, unspecified thigh
√6th M85.36 Osteitis condensans, lower leg
M85.361 Osteitis condensans, right lower leg
M85.362 Osteitis condensans, left lower leg
M85.369 Osteitis condensans, unspecified lower leg
√6th M85.37 Osteitis condensans, ankle and foot
M85.371 Osteitis condensans, right ankle and foot
M85.372 Osteitis condensans, left ankle and foot
M85.379 Osteitis condensans, unspecified ankle and foot
M85.38 Osteitis condensans, other site
M85.39 Osteitis condensans, multiple sites

√5th M85.4 Solitary bone cyst
EXCLUDES 2 *solitary cyst of jaw (M27.4)*
M85.4Ø Solitary bone cyst, unspecified site
√6th M85.41 Solitary bone cyst, shoulder
M85.411 Solitary bone cyst, right shoulder
M85.412 Solitary bone cyst, left shoulder
M85.419 Solitary bone cyst, unspecified shoulder
√6th M85.42 Solitary bone cyst, humerus
M85.421 Solitary bone cyst, right humerus
M85.422 Solitary bone cyst, left humerus
M85.429 Solitary bone cyst, unspecified humerus
√6th M85.43 Solitary bone cyst, ulna and radius
M85.431 Solitary bone cyst, right ulna and radius
M85.432 Solitary bone cyst, left ulna and radius
M85.439 Solitary bone cyst, unspecified ulna and radius
√6th M85.44 Solitary bone cyst, hand
M85.441 Solitary bone cyst, right hand
M85.442 Solitary bone cyst, left hand
M85.449 Solitary bone cyst, unspecified hand
√6th M85.45 Solitary bone cyst, pelvis
M85.451 Solitary bone cyst, right pelvis
M85.452 Solitary bone cyst, left pelvis
M85.459 Solitary bone cyst, unspecified pelvis
√6th M85.46 Solitary bone cyst, tibia and fibula
M85.461 Solitary bone cyst, right tibia and fibula
M85.462 Solitary bone cyst, left tibia and fibula
M85.469 Solitary bone cyst, unspecified tibia and fibula
√6th M85.47 Solitary bone cyst, ankle and foot
M85.471 Solitary bone cyst, right ankle and foot
M85.472 Solitary bone cyst, left ankle and foot
M85.479 Solitary bone cyst, unspecified ankle and foot
M85.48 Solitary bone cyst, other site

√5th M85.5 Aneurysmal bone cyst
EXCLUDES 2 *aneurysmal cyst of jaw (M27.4)*
DEF: Solitary bone lesion that bulges into the periosteum and is marked by a calcified rim.
M85.5Ø Aneurysmal bone cyst, unspecified site
√6th M85.51 Aneurysmal bone cyst, shoulder
M85.511 Aneurysmal bone cyst, right shoulder
M85.512 Aneurysmal bone cyst, left shoulder
M85.519 Aneurysmal bone cyst, unspecified shoulder
√6th M85.52 Aneurysmal bone cyst, upper arm
M85.521 Aneurysmal bone cyst, right upper arm
M85.522 Aneurysmal bone cyst, left upper arm
M85.529 Aneurysmal bone cyst, unspecified upper arm
√6th M85.53 Aneurysmal bone cyst, forearm
M85.531 Aneurysmal bone cyst, right forearm
M85.532 Aneurysmal bone cyst, left forearm
M85.539 Aneurysmal bone cyst, unspecified forearm
√6th M85.54 Aneurysmal bone cyst, hand
M85.541 Aneurysmal bone cyst, right hand
M85.542 Aneurysmal bone cyst, left hand
M85.549 Aneurysmal bone cyst, unspecified hand
√6th M85.55 Aneurysmal bone cyst, thigh
M85.551 Aneurysmal bone cyst, right thigh
M85.552 Aneurysmal bone cyst, left thigh
M85.559 Aneurysmal bone cyst, unspecified thigh
√6th M85.56 Aneurysmal bone cyst, lower leg
M85.561 Aneurysmal bone cyst, right lower leg
M85.562 Aneurysmal bone cyst, left lower leg
M85.569 Aneurysmal bone cyst, unspecified lower leg
√6th M85.57 Aneurysmal bone cyst, ankle and foot
M85.571 Aneurysmal bone cyst, right ankle and foot
M85.572 Aneurysmal bone cyst, left ankle and foot
M85.579 Aneurysmal bone cyst, unspecified ankle and foot
M85.58 Aneurysmal bone cyst, other site
M85.59 Aneurysmal bone cyst, multiple sites

M85.6 Other cyst of bone
EXCLUDES 1 *cyst of jaw NEC (M27.4)*
osteitis fibrosa cystica generalisata [von Recklinghausen's disease of bone] (E21.Ø)
M85.6Ø Other cyst of bone, unspecified site
M85.61 Other cyst of bone, shoulder
M85.611 Other cyst of bone, right shoulder
M85.612 Other cyst of bone, left shoulder
M85.619 Other cyst of bone, unspecified shoulder
M85.62 Other cyst of bone, upper arm
M85.621 Other cyst of bone, right upper arm
M85.622 Other cyst of bone, left upper arm
M85.629 Other cyst of bone, unspecified upper arm
M85.63 Other cyst of bone, forearm
M85.631 Other cyst of bone, right forearm
M85.632 Other cyst of bone, left forearm
M85.639 Other cyst of bone, unspecified forearm
M85.64 Other cyst of bone, hand
M85.641 Other cyst of bone, right hand
M85.642 Other cyst of bone, left hand
M85.649 Other cyst of bone, unspecified hand
M85.65 Other cyst of bone, thigh
M85.651 Other cyst of bone, right thigh
M85.652 Other cyst of bone, left thigh
M85.659 Other cyst of bone, unspecified thigh
M85.66 Other cyst of bone, lower leg
M85.661 Other cyst of bone, right lower leg
M85.662 Other cyst of bone, left lower leg
M85.669 Other cyst of bone, unspecified lower leg
M85.67 Other cyst of bone, ankle and foot
M85.671 Other cyst of bone, right ankle and foot
M85.672 Other cyst of bone, left ankle and foot
M85.679 Other cyst of bone, unspecified ankle and foot
M85.68 Other cyst of bone, other site
M85.69 Other cyst of bone, multiple sites

M85.8 Other specified disorders of bone density and structure
Hyperostosis of bones, except skull
Osteosclerosis, acquired
EXCLUDES 1 *diffuse idiopathic skeletal hyperostosis [DISH] (M48.1)*
osteosclerosis congenita (Q77.4)
osteosclerosis fragilitas (generalista) (Q78.2)
osteosclerosis myelofibrosis (D75.81)
M85.8Ø Other specified disorders of bone density and structure, unspecified site
M85.81 Other specified disorders of bone density and structure, shoulder
M85.811 Other specified disorders of bone density and structure, right shoulder
M85.812 Other specified disorders of bone density and structure, left shoulder
M85.819 Other specified disorders of bone density and structure, unspecified shoulder
M85.82 Other specified disorders of bone density and structure, upper arm
M85.821 Other specified disorders of bone density and structure, right upper arm
M85.822 Other specified disorders of bone density and structure, left upper arm
M85.829 Other specified disorders of bone density and structure, unspecified upper arm
M85.83 Other specified disorders of bone density and structure, forearm
M85.831 Other specified disorders of bone density and structure, right forearm
M85.832 Other specified disorders of bone density and structure, left forearm
M85.839 Other specified disorders of bone density and structure, unspecified forearm
M85.84 Other specified disorders of bone density and structure, hand
M85.841 Other specified disorders of bone density and structure, right hand
M85.842 Other specified disorders of bone density and structure, left hand
M85.849 Other specified disorders of bone density and structure, unspecified hand
M85.85 Other specified disorders of bone density and structure, thigh
M85.851 Other specified disorders of bone density and structure, right thigh
M85.852 Other specified disorders of bone density and structure, left thigh
M85.859 Other specified disorders of bone density and structure, unspecified thigh
M85.86 Other specified disorders of bone density and structure, lower leg
M85.861 Other specified disorders of bone density and structure, right lower leg
M85.862 Other specified disorders of bone density and structure, left lower leg
M85.869 Other specified disorders of bone density and structure, unspecified lower leg
M85.87 Other specified disorders of bone density and structure, ankle and foot
M85.871 Other specified disorders of bone density and structure, right ankle and foot
M85.872 Other specified disorders of bone density and structure, left ankle and foot
M85.879 Other specified disorders of bone density and structure, unspecified ankle and foot
M85.88 Other specified disorders of bone density and structure, other site
M85.89 Other specified disorders of bone density and structure, multiple sites
M85.9 Disorder of bone density and structure, unspecified
AHA: 2021,3Q,11

Other osteopathies (M86-M9Ø)

EXCLUDES 1 *postprocedural osteopathies (M96.-)*

M86 Osteomyelitis
Use additional code (B95-B97) to identify infectious agent
Use additional code to identify major osseous defect, if applicable (M89.7-)
EXCLUDES 1 *osteomyelitis due to:*
echinococcus (B67.2)
gonococcus (A54.43)
salmonella (AØ2.24)
EXCLUDES 2 *ostemyelitis of:*
orbit (HØ5.Ø-)
petrous bone (H7Ø.2-)
vertebra (M46.2-)

M86.Ø Acute hematogenous osteomyelitis
M86.ØØ Acute hematogenous osteomyelitis, unspecified site HCC ESR COM
M86.Ø1 Acute hematogenous osteomyelitis, shoulder
M86.Ø11 Acute hematogenous osteomyelitis, right shoulder HCC ESR COM
M86.Ø12 Acute hematogenous osteomyelitis, left shoulder HCC ESR COM
M86.Ø19 Acute hematogenous osteomyelitis, unspecified shoulder HCC ESR COM
M86.Ø2 Acute hematogenous osteomyelitis, humerus
M86.Ø21 Acute hematogenous osteomyelitis, right humerus HCC ESR COM
M86.Ø22 Acute hematogenous osteomyelitis, left humerus HCC ESR COM
M86.Ø29 Acute hematogenous osteomyelitis, unspecified humerus HCC ESR COM
M86.Ø3 Acute hematogenous osteomyelitis, radius and ulna
M86.Ø31 Acute hematogenous osteomyelitis, right radius and ulna HCC ESR COM
M86.Ø32 Acute hematogenous osteomyelitis, left radius and ulna HCC ESR COM
M86.Ø39 Acute hematogenous osteomyelitis, unspecified radius and ulna HCC ESR COM
M86.Ø4 Acute hematogenous osteomyelitis, hand
M86.Ø41 Acute hematogenous osteomyelitis, right hand HCC ESR COM
M86.Ø42 Acute hematogenous osteomyelitis, left hand HCC ESR COM
M86.Ø49 Acute hematogenous osteomyelitis, unspecified hand HCC ESR COM

M86.Ø5 Acute hematogenous osteomyelitis, femur
M86.Ø51 Acute hematogenous osteomyelitis, right femur HCC ESR COM
M86.Ø52 Acute hematogenous osteomyelitis, left femur HCC ESR COM
M86.Ø59 Acute hematogenous osteomyelitis, unspecified femur HCC ESR COM
M86.Ø6 Acute hematogenous osteomyelitis, tibia and fibula
M86.Ø61 Acute hematogenous osteomyelitis, right tibia and fibula HCC ESR COM
M86.Ø62 Acute hematogenous osteomyelitis, left tibia and fibula HCC ESR COM
M86.Ø69 Acute hematogenous osteomyelitis, unspecified tibia and fibula HCC ESR COM
M86.Ø7 Acute hematogenous osteomyelitis, ankle and foot
M86.Ø71 Acute hematogenous osteomyelitis, right ankle and foot HCC ESR COM
M86.Ø72 Acute hematogenous osteomyelitis, left ankle and foot HCC ESR COM
M86.Ø79 Acute hematogenous osteomyelitis, unspecified ankle and foot HCC ESR COM
M86.Ø8 Acute hematogenous osteomyelitis, other sites HCC ESR COM
M86.Ø9 Acute hematogenous osteomyelitis, multiple sites HCC ESR COM
M86.1 Other acute osteomyelitis
M86.1Ø Other acute osteomyelitis, unspecified site HCC ESR COM
M86.11 Other acute osteomyelitis, shoulder
M86.111 Other acute osteomyelitis, right shoulder HCC ESR COM
M86.112 Other acute osteomyelitis, left shoulder HCC ESR COM
M86.119 Other acute osteomyelitis, unspecified shoulder HCC ESR COM
M86.12 Other acute osteomyelitis, humerus
M86.121 Other acute osteomyelitis, right humerus HCC ESR COM
M86.122 Other acute osteomyelitis, left humerus HCC ESR COM
M86.129 Other acute osteomyelitis, unspecified humerus HCC ESR COM
M86.13 Other acute osteomyelitis, radius and ulna
M86.131 Other acute osteomyelitis, right radius and ulna HCC ESR COM
M86.132 Other acute osteomyelitis, left radius and ulna HCC ESR COM
M86.139 Other acute osteomyelitis, unspecified radius and ulna HCC ESR COM
M86.14 Other acute osteomyelitis, hand
M86.141 Other acute osteomyelitis, right hand HCC ESR COM
M86.142 Other acute osteomyelitis, left hand HCC ESR COM
M86.149 Other acute osteomyelitis, unspecified hand HCC ESR COM
M86.15 Other acute osteomyelitis, femur
M86.151 Other acute osteomyelitis, right femur HCC ESR COM
M86.152 Other acute osteomyelitis, left femur HCC ESR COM
M86.159 Other acute osteomyelitis, unspecified femur HCC ESR COM
M86.16 Other acute osteomyelitis, tibia and fibula
M86.161 Other acute osteomyelitis, right tibia and fibula HCC ESR COM
M86.162 Other acute osteomyelitis, left tibia and fibula HCC ESR COM
M86.169 Other acute osteomyelitis, unspecified tibia and fibula HCC ESR COM
M86.17 Other acute osteomyelitis, ankle and foot
AHA: 2020,1Q,12
M86.171 Other acute osteomyelitis, right ankle and foot HCC ESR COM
M86.172 Other acute osteomyelitis, left ankle and foot HCC ESR COM
M86.179 Other acute osteomyelitis, unspecified ankle and foot HCC ESR COM
M86.18 Other acute osteomyelitis, other site HCC ESR COM
M86.19 Other acute osteomyelitis, multiple sites HCC ESR COM
M86.2 Subacute osteomyelitis
M86.2Ø Subacute osteomyelitis, unspecified site HCC ESR COM
M86.21 Subacute osteomyelitis, shoulder
M86.211 Subacute osteomyelitis, right shoulder HCC ESR COM
M86.212 Subacute osteomyelitis, left shoulder HCC ESR COM
M86.219 Subacute osteomyelitis, unspecified shoulder HCC ESR COM
M86.22 Subacute osteomyelitis, humerus
M86.221 Subacute osteomyelitis, right humerus HCC ESR COM
M86.222 Subacute osteomyelitis, left humerus HCC ESR COM
M86.229 Subacute osteomyelitis, unspecified humerus HCC ESR COM
M86.23 Subacute osteomyelitis, radius and ulna
M86.231 Subacute osteomyelitis, right radius and ulna HCC ESR COM
M86.232 Subacute osteomyelitis, left radius and ulna HCC ESR COM
M86.239 Subacute osteomyelitis, unspecified radius and ulna HCC ESR COM
M86.24 Subacute osteomyelitis, hand
M86.241 Subacute osteomyelitis, right hand HCC ESR COM
M86.242 Subacute osteomyelitis, left hand HCC ESR COM
M86.249 Subacute osteomyelitis, unspecified hand HCC ESR COM
M86.25 Subacute osteomyelitis, femur
M86.251 Subacute osteomyelitis, right femur HCC ESR COM
M86.252 Subacute osteomyelitis, left femur HCC ESR COM
M86.259 Subacute osteomyelitis, unspecified femur HCC ESR COM
M86.26 Subacute osteomyelitis, tibia and fibula
M86.261 Subacute osteomyelitis, right tibia and fibula HCC ESR COM
M86.262 Subacute osteomyelitis, left tibia and fibula HCC ESR COM
M86.269 Subacute osteomyelitis, unspecified tibia and fibula HCC ESR COM
M86.27 Subacute osteomyelitis, ankle and foot
M86.271 Subacute osteomyelitis, right ankle and foot HCC ESR COM
M86.272 Subacute osteomyelitis, left ankle and foot HCC ESR COM
M86.279 Subacute osteomyelitis, unspecified ankle and foot HCC ESR COM
M86.28 Subacute osteomyelitis, other site HCC ESR COM
M86.29 Subacute osteomyelitis, multiple sites HCC ESR COM
M86.3 Chronic multifocal osteomyelitis
M86.3Ø Chronic multifocal osteomyelitis, unspecified site HCC ESR COM
M86.31 Chronic multifocal osteomyelitis, shoulder
M86.311 Chronic multifocal osteomyelitis, right shoulder HCC ESR COM
M86.312 Chronic multifocal osteomyelitis, left shoulder HCC ESR COM
M86.319 Chronic multifocal osteomyelitis, unspecified shoulder HCC ESR COM
M86.32 Chronic multifocal osteomyelitis, humerus
M86.321 Chronic multifocal osteomyelitis, right humerus HCC ESR COM
M86.322 Chronic multifocal osteomyelitis, left humerus HCC ESR COM

M86.329 Chronic multifocal osteomyelitis, unspecified humerus HCC ESR COM

✓6th M86.33 Chronic multifocal osteomyelitis, radius and ulna
M86.331 Chronic multifocal osteomyelitis, right radius and ulna HCC ESR COM
M86.332 Chronic multifocal osteomyelitis, left radius and ulna HCC ESR COM
M86.339 Chronic multifocal osteomyelitis, unspecified radius and ulna HCC ESR COM

✓6th M86.34 Chronic multifocal osteomyelitis, hand
M86.341 Chronic multifocal osteomyelitis, right hand HCC ESR COM
M86.342 Chronic multifocal osteomyelitis, left hand HCC ESR COM
M86.349 Chronic multifocal osteomyelitis, unspecified hand HCC ESR COM

✓6th M86.35 Chronic multifocal osteomyelitis, femur
M86.351 Chronic multifocal osteomyelitis, right femur HCC ESR COM
M86.352 Chronic multifocal osteomyelitis, left femur HCC ESR COM
M86.359 Chronic multifocal osteomyelitis, unspecified femur HCC ESR COM

✓6th M86.36 Chronic multifocal osteomyelitis, tibia and fibula
M86.361 Chronic multifocal osteomyelitis, right tibia and fibula HCC ESR COM
M86.362 Chronic multifocal osteomyelitis, left tibia and fibula HCC ESR COM
M86.369 Chronic multifocal osteomyelitis, unspecified tibia and fibula HCC ESR COM

✓6th M86.37 Chronic multifocal osteomyelitis, ankle and foot
M86.371 Chronic multifocal osteomyelitis, right ankle and foot HCC ESR COM
M86.372 Chronic multifocal osteomyelitis, left ankle and foot HCC ESR COM
M86.379 Chronic multifocal osteomyelitis, unspecified ankle and foot HCC ESR COM

M86.38 Chronic multifocal osteomyelitis, other site HCC ESR COM

M86.39 Chronic multifocal osteomyelitis, multiple sites HCC ESR COM

✓5th M86.4 Chronic osteomyelitis with draining sinus

M86.40 Chronic osteomyelitis with draining sinus, unspecified site HCC ESR COM

✓6th M86.41 Chronic osteomyelitis with draining sinus, shoulder
M86.411 Chronic osteomyelitis with draining sinus, right shoulder HCC ESR COM
M86.412 Chronic osteomyelitis with draining sinus, left shoulder HCC ESR COM
M86.419 Chronic osteomyelitis with draining sinus, unspecified shoulder HCC ESR COM

✓6th M86.42 Chronic osteomyelitis with draining sinus, humerus
M86.421 Chronic osteomyelitis with draining sinus, right humerus HCC ESR COM
M86.422 Chronic osteomyelitis with draining sinus, left humerus HCC ESR COM
M86.429 Chronic osteomyelitis with draining sinus, unspecified humerus HCC ESR COM

✓6th M86.43 Chronic osteomyelitis with draining sinus, radius and ulna
M86.431 Chronic osteomyelitis with draining sinus, right radius and ulna HCC ESR COM
M86.432 Chronic osteomyelitis with draining sinus, left radius and ulna HCC ESR COM
M86.439 Chronic osteomyelitis with draining sinus, unspecified radius and ulna HCC ESR COM

✓6th M86.44 Chronic osteomyelitis with draining sinus, hand
M86.441 Chronic osteomyelitis with draining sinus, right hand HCC ESR COM
M86.442 Chronic osteomyelitis with draining sinus, left hand HCC ESR COM
M86.449 Chronic osteomyelitis with draining sinus, unspecified hand HCC ESR COM

✓6th M86.45 Chronic osteomyelitis with draining sinus, femur
M86.451 Chronic osteomyelitis with draining sinus, right femur HCC ESR COM
M86.452 Chronic osteomyelitis with draining sinus, left femur HCC ESR COM
M86.459 Chronic osteomyelitis with draining sinus, unspecified femur HCC ESR COM

✓6th M86.46 Chronic osteomyelitis with draining sinus, tibia and fibula
M86.461 Chronic osteomyelitis with draining sinus, right tibia and fibula HCC ESR COM
M86.462 Chronic osteomyelitis with draining sinus, left tibia and fibula HCC ESR COM
M86.469 Chronic osteomyelitis with draining sinus, unspecified tibia and fibula HCC ESR COM

✓6th M86.47 Chronic osteomyelitis with draining sinus, ankle and foot
M86.471 Chronic osteomyelitis with draining sinus, right ankle and foot HCC ESR COM
M86.472 Chronic osteomyelitis with draining sinus, left ankle and foot HCC ESR COM
M86.479 Chronic osteomyelitis with draining sinus, unspecified ankle and foot HCC ESR COM

M86.48 Chronic osteomyelitis with draining sinus, other site HCC ESR COM

M86.49 Chronic osteomyelitis with draining sinus, multiple sites HCC ESR COM

✓5th M86.5 Other chronic hematogenous osteomyelitis

M86.50 Other chronic hematogenous osteomyelitis, unspecified site HCC ESR COM

✓6th M86.51 Other chronic hematogenous osteomyelitis, shoulder
M86.511 Other chronic hematogenous osteomyelitis, right shoulder HCC ESR COM
M86.512 Other chronic hematogenous osteomyelitis, left shoulder HCC ESR COM
M86.519 Other chronic hematogenous osteomyelitis, unspecified shoulder HCC ESR COM

✓6th M86.52 Other chronic hematogenous osteomyelitis, humerus
M86.521 Other chronic hematogenous osteomyelitis, right humerus HCC ESR COM
M86.522 Other chronic hematogenous osteomyelitis, left humerus HCC ESR COM
M86.529 Other chronic hematogenous osteomyelitis, unspecified humerus HCC ESR COM

✓6th M86.53 Other chronic hematogenous osteomyelitis, radius and ulna
M86.531 Other chronic hematogenous osteomyelitis, right radius and ulna HCC ESR COM
M86.532 Other chronic hematogenous osteomyelitis, left radius and ulna HCC ESR COM
M86.539 Other chronic hematogenous osteomyelitis, unspecified radius and ulna HCC ESR COM

✓6th M86.54 Other chronic hematogenous osteomyelitis, hand
M86.541 Other chronic hematogenous osteomyelitis, right hand HCC ESR COM
M86.542 Other chronic hematogenous osteomyelitis, left hand HCC ESR COM
M86.549 Other chronic hematogenous osteomyelitis, unspecified hand HCC ESR COM

✓6th M86.55 Other chronic hematogenous osteomyelitis, femur
M86.551 Other chronic hematogenous osteomyelitis, right femur HCC ESR COM
M86.552 Other chronic hematogenous osteomyelitis, left femur HCC ESR COM
M86.559 Other chronic hematogenous osteomyelitis, unspecified femur HCC ESR COM

HCC CMS-HCC Rx Rx HCC ESR ESRD HCC COM Commercial HCC N Newborn: 0 P Pediatric: 0-17 M Maternity: 9-64 A Adult: 15-124

M86.56 Other chronic hematogenous osteomyelitis, tibia and fibula
- **M86.561 Other chronic hematogenous osteomyelitis, right tibia and fibula** HCC ESR COM
- **M86.562 Other chronic hematogenous osteomyelitis, left tibia and fibula** HCC ESR COM
- **M86.569 Other chronic hematogenous osteomyelitis, unspecified tibia and fibula** HCC ESR COM

M86.57 Other chronic hematogenous osteomyelitis, ankle and foot
- **M86.571 Other chronic hematogenous osteomyelitis, right ankle and foot** HCC ESR COM
- **M86.572 Other chronic hematogenous osteomyelitis, left ankle and foot** HCC ESR COM
- **M86.579 Other chronic hematogenous osteomyelitis, unspecified ankle and foot** HCC ESR COM

M86.58 Other chronic hematogenous osteomyelitis, other site HCC ESR COM

M86.59 Other chronic hematogenous osteomyelitis, multiple sites HCC ESR COM

M86.6 Other chronic osteomyelitis

M86.60 Other chronic osteomyelitis, unspecified site HCC ESR COM

M86.61 Other chronic osteomyelitis, shoulder
- **M86.611 Other chronic osteomyelitis, right shoulder** HCC ESR COM
- **M86.612 Other chronic osteomyelitis, left shoulder** HCC ESR COM
- **M86.619 Other chronic osteomyelitis, unspecified shoulder** HCC ESR COM

M86.62 Other chronic osteomyelitis, humerus
- **M86.621 Other chronic osteomyelitis, right humerus** HCC ESR COM
- **M86.622 Other chronic osteomyelitis, left humerus** HCC ESR COM
- **M86.629 Other chronic osteomyelitis, unspecified humerus** HCC ESR COM

M86.63 Other chronic osteomyelitis, radius and ulna
- **M86.631 Other chronic osteomyelitis, right radius and ulna** HCC ESR COM
- **M86.632 Other chronic osteomyelitis, left radius and ulna** HCC ESR COM
- **M86.639 Other chronic osteomyelitis, unspecified radius and ulna** HCC ESR COM

M86.64 Other chronic osteomyelitis, hand
- **M86.641 Other chronic osteomyelitis, right hand** HCC ESR COM
- **M86.642 Other chronic osteomyelitis, left hand** HCC ESR COM
- **M86.649 Other chronic osteomyelitis, unspecified hand** HCC ESR COM

M86.65 Other chronic osteomyelitis, thigh
- **M86.651 Other chronic osteomyelitis, right thigh** HCC ESR COM
- **M86.652 Other chronic osteomyelitis, left thigh** HCC ESR COM
- **M86.659 Other chronic osteomyelitis, unspecified thigh** HCC ESR COM

M86.66 Other chronic osteomyelitis, tibia and fibula
- **M86.661 Other chronic osteomyelitis, right tibia and fibula** HCC ESR COM
- **M86.662 Other chronic osteomyelitis, left tibia and fibula** HCC ESR COM
- **M86.669 Other chronic osteomyelitis, unspecified tibia and fibula** HCC ESR COM

M86.67 Other chronic osteomyelitis, ankle and foot
- **M86.671 Other chronic osteomyelitis, right ankle and foot** HCC ESR COM
  AHA: 2016,1Q,13
- **M86.672 Other chronic osteomyelitis, left ankle and foot** HCC ESR COM
- **M86.679 Other chronic osteomyelitis, unspecified ankle and foot** HCC ESR COM

M86.68 Other chronic osteomyelitis, other site HCC ESR COM

M86.69 Other chronic osteomyelitis, multiple sites HCC ESR COM

M86.8 Other osteomyelitis
Brodie's abscess
AHA: 2022,1Q,31

M86.8X Other osteomyelitis
- **M86.8X0 Other osteomyelitis, multiple sites** HCC ESR COM
- **M86.8X1 Other osteomyelitis, shoulder** HCC ESR COM
- **M86.8X2 Other osteomyelitis, upper arm** HCC ESR COM
- **M86.8X3 Other osteomyelitis, forearm** HCC ESR COM
- **M86.8X4 Other osteomyelitis, hand** HCC ESR COM
- **M86.8X5 Other osteomyelitis, thigh** HCC ESR COM
- **M86.8X6 Other osteomyelitis, lower leg** HCC ESR COM
- **M86.8X7 Other osteomyelitis, ankle and foot** HCC ESR COM
- **M86.8X8 Other osteomyelitis, other site** HCC ESR COM
- **M86.8X9 Other osteomyelitis, unspecified sites** HCC ESR COM

M86.9 Osteomyelitis, unspecified HCC ESR COM
Infection of bone NOS
Periostitis without osteomyelitis

M87 Osteonecrosis

INCLUDES avascular necrosis of bone

Use additional code to identify major osseous defect, if applicable (M89.7-)

EXCLUDES 1 *juvenile osteonecrosis (M91-M92)*
osteochondropathies (M90-M93)

M87.0 Idiopathic aseptic necrosis of bone

M87.00 Idiopathic aseptic necrosis of unspecified bone HCC Rx ESR COM

M87.01 Idiopathic aseptic necrosis of shoulder
Idiopathic aseptic necrosis of clavicle and scapula
- **M87.011 Idiopathic aseptic necrosis of right shoulder** HCC Rx ESR COM
- **M87.012 Idiopathic aseptic necrosis of left shoulder** HCC Rx ESR COM
- **M87.019 Idiopathic aseptic necrosis of unspecified shoulder** HCC Rx ESR COM

M87.02 Idiopathic aseptic necrosis of humerus
- **M87.021 Idiopathic aseptic necrosis of right humerus** HCC Rx ESR COM
- **M87.022 Idiopathic aseptic necrosis of left humerus** HCC Rx ESR COM
- **M87.029 Idiopathic aseptic necrosis of unspecified humerus** HCC Rx ESR COM

M87.03 Idiopathic aseptic necrosis of radius, ulna and carpus
- **M87.031 Idiopathic aseptic necrosis of right radius** HCC Rx ESR COM
- **M87.032 Idiopathic aseptic necrosis of left radius** HCC Rx ESR COM
- **M87.033 Idiopathic aseptic necrosis of unspecified radius** HCC Rx ESR COM
- **M87.034 Idiopathic aseptic necrosis of right ulna** HCC Rx ESR COM
- **M87.035 Idiopathic aseptic necrosis of left ulna** HCC Rx ESR COM
- **M87.036 Idiopathic aseptic necrosis of unspecified ulna** HCC Rx ESR COM
- **M87.037 Idiopathic aseptic necrosis of right carpus** HCC Rx ESR COM
- **M87.038 Idiopathic aseptic necrosis of left carpus** HCC Rx ESR COM
- **M87.039 Idiopathic aseptic necrosis of unspecified carpus** HCC Rx ESR COM

6th **M87.04 Idiopathic aseptic necrosis of hand and fingers**
Idiopathic aseptic necrosis of metacarpals and phalanges of hands
M87.041 Idiopathic aseptic necrosis of right hand HCC Rx ESR COM
M87.042 Idiopathic aseptic necrosis of left hand HCC Rx ESR COM
M87.043 Idiopathic aseptic necrosis of unspecified hand HCC Rx ESR COM
M87.044 Idiopathic aseptic necrosis of right finger(s) HCC Rx ESR COM
M87.045 Idiopathic aseptic necrosis of left finger(s) HCC Rx ESR COM
M87.046 Idiopathic aseptic necrosis of unspecified finger(s) HCC Rx ESR COM
6th **M87.05 Idiopathic aseptic necrosis of pelvis and femur**
M87.050 Idiopathic aseptic necrosis of pelvis HCC Rx ESR COM
M87.051 Idiopathic aseptic necrosis of right femur HCC Rx ESR COM
M87.052 Idiopathic aseptic necrosis of left femur HCC Rx ESR COM
M87.059 Idiopathic aseptic necrosis of unspecified femur HCC Rx ESR COM
6th **M87.06 Idiopathic aseptic necrosis of tibia and fibula**
M87.061 Idiopathic aseptic necrosis of right tibia HCC Rx ESR COM
M87.062 Idiopathic aseptic necrosis of left tibia HCC Rx ESR COM
M87.063 Idiopathic aseptic necrosis of unspecified tibia HCC Rx ESR COM
M87.064 Idiopathic aseptic necrosis of right fibula HCC Rx ESR COM
M87.065 Idiopathic aseptic necrosis of left fibula HCC Rx ESR COM
M87.066 Idiopathic aseptic necrosis of unspecified fibula HCC Rx ESR COM
6th **M87.07 Idiopathic aseptic necrosis of ankle, foot and toes**
Idiopathic aseptic necrosis of metatarsus, tarsus, and phalanges of toes
M87.071 Idiopathic aseptic necrosis of right ankle HCC Rx ESR COM
M87.072 Idiopathic aseptic necrosis of left ankle HCC Rx ESR COM
M87.073 Idiopathic aseptic necrosis of unspecified ankle HCC Rx ESR COM
M87.074 Idiopathic aseptic necrosis of right foot HCC Rx ESR COM
M87.075 Idiopathic aseptic necrosis of left foot HCC Rx ESR COM
M87.076 Idiopathic aseptic necrosis of unspecified foot HCC Rx ESR COM
M87.077 Idiopathic aseptic necrosis of right toe(s) HCC Rx ESR COM
M87.078 Idiopathic aseptic necrosis of left toe(s) HCC Rx ESR COM
M87.079 Idiopathic aseptic necrosis of unspecified toe(s) HCC Rx ESR COM
M87.08 Idiopathic aseptic necrosis of bone, other site HCC Rx ESR COM
M87.09 Idiopathic aseptic necrosis of bone, multiple sites HCC Rx ESR COM
5th **M87.1 Osteonecrosis due to drugs**
Use additional code for adverse effect, if applicable, to identify drug (T36-T50 with fifth or sixth character 5)
M87.10 Osteonecrosis due to drugs, unspecified bone HCC Rx ESR COM
6th **M87.11 Osteonecrosis due to drugs, shoulder**
M87.111 Osteonecrosis due to drugs, right shoulder HCC Rx ESR COM
M87.112 Osteonecrosis due to drugs, left shoulder HCC Rx ESR COM
M87.119 Osteonecrosis due to drugs, unspecified shoulder HCC Rx ESR COM
6th **M87.12 Osteonecrosis due to drugs, humerus**
M87.121 Osteonecrosis due to drugs, right humerus HCC Rx ESR COM
M87.122 Osteonecrosis due to drugs, left humerus HCC Rx ESR COM
M87.129 Osteonecrosis due to drugs, unspecified humerus HCC Rx ESR COM
6th **M87.13 Osteonecrosis due to drugs of radius, ulna and carpus**
M87.131 Osteonecrosis due to drugs of right radius HCC Rx ESR COM
M87.132 Osteonecrosis due to drugs of left radius HCC Rx ESR COM
M87.133 Osteonecrosis due to drugs of unspecified radius HCC Rx ESR COM
M87.134 Osteonecrosis due to drugs of right ulna HCC Rx ESR COM
M87.135 Osteonecrosis due to drugs of left ulna HCC Rx ESR COM
M87.136 Osteonecrosis due to drugs of unspecified ulna HCC Rx ESR COM
M87.137 Osteonecrosis due to drugs of right carpus HCC Rx ESR COM
M87.138 Osteonecrosis due to drugs of left carpus HCC Rx ESR COM
M87.139 Osteonecrosis due to drugs of unspecified carpus HCC Rx ESR COM
6th **M87.14 Osteonecrosis due to drugs, hand and fingers**
M87.141 Osteonecrosis due to drugs, right hand HCC Rx ESR COM
M87.142 Osteonecrosis due to drugs, left hand HCC Rx ESR COM
M87.143 Osteonecrosis due to drugs, unspecified hand HCC Rx ESR COM
M87.144 Osteonecrosis due to drugs, right finger(s) HCC Rx ESR COM
M87.145 Osteonecrosis due to drugs, left finger(s) HCC Rx ESR COM
M87.146 Osteonecrosis due to drugs, unspecified finger(s) HCC Rx ESR COM
6th **M87.15 Osteonecrosis due to drugs, pelvis and femur**
M87.150 Osteonecrosis due to drugs, pelvis HCC Rx ESR COM
M87.151 Osteonecrosis due to drugs, right femur HCC Rx ESR COM
M87.152 Osteonecrosis due to drugs, left femur HCC Rx ESR COM
M87.159 Osteonecrosis due to drugs, unspecified femur HCC Rx ESR COM
6th **M87.16 Osteonecrosis due to drugs, tibia and fibula**
M87.161 Osteonecrosis due to drugs, right tibia HCC Rx ESR COM
M87.162 Osteonecrosis due to drugs, left tibia HCC Rx ESR COM
M87.163 Osteonecrosis due to drugs, unspecified tibia HCC Rx ESR COM
M87.164 Osteonecrosis due to drugs, right fibula HCC Rx ESR COM
M87.165 Osteonecrosis due to drugs, left fibula HCC Rx ESR COM
M87.166 Osteonecrosis due to drugs, unspecified fibula HCC Rx ESR COM
6th **M87.17 Osteonecrosis due to drugs, ankle, foot and toes**
M87.171 Osteonecrosis due to drugs, right ankle HCC Rx ESR COM
M87.172 Osteonecrosis due to drugs, left ankle HCC Rx ESR COM
M87.173 Osteonecrosis due to drugs, unspecified ankle HCC Rx ESR COM
M87.174 Osteonecrosis due to drugs, right foot HCC Rx ESR COM
M87.175 Osteonecrosis due to drugs, left foot HCC Rx ESR COM
M87.176 Osteonecrosis due to drugs, unspecified foot HCC Rx ESR COM
M87.177 Osteonecrosis due to drugs, right toe(s) HCC Rx ESR COM
M87.178 Osteonecrosis due to drugs, left toe(s) HCC Rx ESR COM
M87.179 Osteonecrosis due to drugs, unspecified toe(s) HCC Rx ESR COM

M87.18 Osteonecrosis due to drugs, other site
M87.180 Osteonecrosis due to drugs, jaw HCC Rx ESR COM
M87.188 Osteonecrosis due to drugs, other site HCC Rx ESR COM
M87.19 Osteonecrosis due to drugs, multiple sites HCC Rx ESR COM
M87.2 Osteonecrosis due to previous trauma
M87.20 Osteonecrosis due to previous trauma, unspecified bone HCC Rx ESR COM
M87.21 Osteonecrosis due to previous trauma, shoulder
M87.211 Osteonecrosis due to previous trauma, right shoulder HCC Rx ESR COM
M87.212 Osteonecrosis due to previous trauma, left shoulder HCC Rx ESR COM
M87.219 Osteonecrosis due to previous trauma, unspecified shoulder HCC Rx ESR COM
M87.22 Osteonecrosis due to previous trauma, humerus
M87.221 Osteonecrosis due to previous trauma, right humerus HCC Rx ESR COM
M87.222 Osteonecrosis due to previous trauma, left humerus HCC Rx ESR COM
M87.229 Osteonecrosis due to previous trauma, unspecified humerus HCC Rx ESR COM
M87.23 Osteonecrosis due to previous trauma of radius, ulna and carpus
M87.231 Osteonecrosis due to previous trauma of right radius HCC Rx ESR COM
M87.232 Osteonecrosis due to previous trauma of left radius HCC Rx ESR COM
M87.233 Osteonecrosis due to previous trauma of unspecified radius HCC Rx ESR COM
M87.234 Osteonecrosis due to previous trauma of right ulna HCC Rx ESR COM
M87.235 Osteonecrosis due to previous trauma of left ulna HCC Rx ESR COM
M87.236 Osteonecrosis due to previous trauma of unspecified ulna HCC Rx ESR COM
M87.237 Osteonecrosis due to previous trauma of right carpus HCC Rx ESR COM
M87.238 Osteonecrosis due to previous trauma of left carpus HCC Rx ESR COM
M87.239 Osteonecrosis due to previous trauma of unspecified carpus HCC Rx ESR COM
M87.24 Osteonecrosis due to previous trauma, hand and fingers
M87.241 Osteonecrosis due to previous trauma, right hand HCC Rx ESR COM
M87.242 Osteonecrosis due to previous trauma, left hand HCC Rx ESR COM
M87.243 Osteonecrosis due to previous trauma, unspecified hand HCC Rx ESR COM
M87.244 Osteonecrosis due to previous trauma, right finger(s) HCC Rx ESR COM
M87.245 Osteonecrosis due to previous trauma, left finger(s) HCC Rx ESR COM
M87.246 Osteonecrosis due to previous trauma, unspecified finger(s) HCC Rx ESR COM
M87.25 Osteonecrosis due to previous trauma, pelvis and femur
M87.250 Osteonecrosis due to previous trauma, pelvis HCC Rx ESR COM
M87.251 Osteonecrosis due to previous trauma, right femur HCC Rx ESR COM
M87.252 Osteonecrosis due to previous trauma, left femur HCC Rx ESR COM
M87.256 Osteonecrosis due to previous trauma, unspecified femur HCC Rx ESR COM
M87.26 Osteonecrosis due to previous trauma, tibia and fibula
M87.261 Osteonecrosis due to previous trauma, right tibia HCC Rx ESR COM
M87.262 Osteonecrosis due to previous trauma, left tibia HCC Rx ESR COM
M87.263 Osteonecrosis due to previous trauma, unspecified tibia HCC Rx ESR COM
M87.264 Osteonecrosis due to previous trauma, right fibula HCC Rx ESR COM
M87.265 Osteonecrosis due to previous trauma, left fibula HCC Rx ESR COM
M87.266 Osteonecrosis due to previous trauma, unspecified fibula HCC Rx ESR COM
M87.27 Osteonecrosis due to previous trauma, ankle, foot and toes
M87.271 Osteonecrosis due to previous trauma, right ankle HCC Rx ESR COM
M87.272 Osteonecrosis due to previous trauma, left ankle HCC Rx ESR COM
M87.273 Osteonecrosis due to previous trauma, unspecified ankle HCC Rx ESR COM
M87.274 Osteonecrosis due to previous trauma, right foot HCC Rx ESR COM
M87.275 Osteonecrosis due to previous trauma, left foot HCC Rx ESR COM
M87.276 Osteonecrosis due to previous trauma, unspecified foot HCC Rx ESR COM
M87.277 Osteonecrosis due to previous trauma, right toe(s) HCC Rx ESR COM
M87.278 Osteonecrosis due to previous trauma, left toe(s) HCC Rx ESR COM
M87.279 Osteonecrosis due to previous trauma, unspecified toe(s) HCC Rx ESR COM
M87.28 Osteonecrosis due to previous trauma, other site HCC Rx ESR COM
M87.29 Osteonecrosis due to previous trauma, multiple sites HCC Rx ESR COM
M87.3 Other secondary osteonecrosis
M87.30 Other secondary osteonecrosis, unspecified bone HCC Rx ESR COM
M87.31 Other secondary osteonecrosis, shoulder
M87.311 Other secondary osteonecrosis, right shoulder HCC Rx ESR COM
M87.312 Other secondary osteonecrosis, left shoulder HCC Rx ESR COM
M87.319 Other secondary osteonecrosis, unspecified shoulder HCC Rx ESR COM
M87.32 Other secondary osteonecrosis, humerus
M87.321 Other secondary osteonecrosis, right humerus HCC Rx ESR COM
M87.322 Other secondary osteonecrosis, left humerus HCC Rx ESR COM
M87.329 Other secondary osteonecrosis, unspecified humerus HCC Rx ESR COM
M87.33 Other secondary osteonecrosis of radius, ulna and carpus
M87.331 Other secondary osteonecrosis of right radius HCC Rx ESR COM
M87.332 Other secondary osteonecrosis of left radius HCC Rx ESR COM
M87.333 Other secondary osteonecrosis of unspecified radius HCC Rx ESR COM
M87.334 Other secondary osteonecrosis of right ulna HCC Rx ESR COM
M87.335 Other secondary osteonecrosis of left ulna HCC Rx ESR COM
M87.336 Other secondary osteonecrosis of unspecified ulna HCC Rx ESR COM
M87.337 Other secondary osteonecrosis of right carpus HCC Rx ESR COM
M87.338 Other secondary osteonecrosis of left carpus HCC Rx ESR COM
M87.339 Other secondary osteonecrosis of unspecified carpus HCC Rx ESR COM
M87.34 Other secondary osteonecrosis, hand and fingers
M87.341 Other secondary osteonecrosis, right hand HCC Rx ESR COM
M87.342 Other secondary osteonecrosis, left hand HCC Rx ESR COM
M87.343 Other secondary osteonecrosis, unspecified hand HCC Rx ESR COM
M87.344 Other secondary osteonecrosis, right finger(s) HCC Rx ESR COM
M87.345 Other secondary osteonecrosis, left finger(s) HCC Rx ESR COM
M87.346 Other secondary osteonecrosis, unspecified finger(s) HCC Rx ESR COM

√6th **M87.35 Other secondary osteonecrosis, pelvis and femur**
- **M87.350 Other secondary osteonecrosis, pelvis** HCC Rx ESR COM
- **M87.351 Other secondary osteonecrosis, right femur** HCC Rx ESR COM
- **M87.352 Other secondary osteonecrosis, left femur** HCC Rx ESR COM
- **M87.353 Other secondary osteonecrosis, unspecified femur** HCC Rx ESR COM

√6th **M87.36 Other secondary osteonecrosis, tibia and fibula**
- **M87.361 Other secondary osteonecrosis, right tibia** HCC Rx ESR COM
- **M87.362 Other secondary osteonecrosis, left tibia** HCC Rx ESR COM
- **M87.363 Other secondary osteonecrosis, unspecified tibia** HCC Rx ESR COM
- **M87.364 Other secondary osteonecrosis, right fibula** HCC Rx ESR COM
- **M87.365 Other secondary osteonecrosis, left fibula** HCC Rx ESR COM
- **M87.366 Other secondary osteonecrosis, unspecified fibula** HCC Rx ESR COM

√6th **M87.37 Other secondary osteonecrosis, ankle and foot**
- **M87.371 Other secondary osteonecrosis, right ankle** HCC Rx ESR COM
- **M87.372 Other secondary osteonecrosis, left ankle** HCC Rx ESR COM
- **M87.373 Other secondary osteonecrosis, unspecified ankle** HCC Rx ESR COM
- **M87.374 Other secondary osteonecrosis, right foot** HCC Rx ESR COM
- **M87.375 Other secondary osteonecrosis, left foot** HCC Rx ESR COM
- **M87.376 Other secondary osteonecrosis, unspecified foot** HCC Rx ESR COM
- **M87.377 Other secondary osteonecrosis, right toe(s)** HCC Rx ESR COM
- **M87.378 Other secondary osteonecrosis, left toe(s)** HCC Rx ESR COM
- **M87.379 Other secondary osteonecrosis, unspecified toe(s)** HCC Rx ESR COM

M87.38 Other secondary osteonecrosis, other site HCC Rx ESR COM

M87.39 Other secondary osteonecrosis, multiple sites HCC Rx ESR COM

√5th **M87.8 Other osteonecrosis**

M87.80 Other osteonecrosis, unspecified bone HCC Rx ESR COM

√6th **M87.81 Other osteonecrosis, shoulder**
- **M87.811 Other osteonecrosis, right shoulder** HCC Rx ESR COM
- **M87.812 Other osteonecrosis, left shoulder** HCC Rx ESR COM
- **M87.819 Other osteonecrosis, unspecified shoulder** HCC Rx ESR COM

√6th **M87.82 Other osteonecrosis, humerus**
- **M87.821 Other osteonecrosis, right humerus** HCC Rx ESR COM
- **M87.822 Other osteonecrosis, left humerus** HCC Rx ESR COM
- **M87.829 Other osteonecrosis, unspecified humerus** HCC Rx ESR COM

√6th **M87.83 Other osteonecrosis of radius, ulna and carpus**
- **M87.831 Other osteonecrosis of right radius** HCC Rx ESR COM
- **M87.832 Other osteonecrosis of left radius** HCC Rx ESR COM
- **M87.833 Other osteonecrosis of unspecified radius** HCC Rx ESR COM
- **M87.834 Other osteonecrosis of right ulna** HCC Rx ESR COM
- **M87.835 Other osteonecrosis of left ulna** HCC Rx ESR COM
- **M87.836 Other osteonecrosis of unspecified ulna** HCC Rx ESR COM
- **M87.837 Other osteonecrosis of right carpus** HCC Rx ESR COM
- **M87.838 Other osteonecrosis of left carpus** HCC Rx ESR COM
- **M87.839 Other osteonecrosis of unspecified carpus** HCC Rx ESR COM

√6th **M87.84 Other osteonecrosis, hand and fingers**
- **M87.841 Other osteonecrosis, right hand** HCC Rx ESR COM
- **M87.842 Other osteonecrosis, left hand** HCC Rx ESR COM
- **M87.843 Other osteonecrosis, unspecified hand** HCC Rx ESR COM
- **M87.844 Other osteonecrosis, right finger(s)** HCC Rx ESR COM
- **M87.845 Other osteonecrosis, left finger(s)** HCC Rx ESR COM
- **M87.849 Other osteonecrosis, unspecified finger(s)** HCC Rx ESR COM

√6th **M87.85 Other osteonecrosis, pelvis and femur**
- **M87.850 Other osteonecrosis, pelvis** HCC Rx ESR COM
- **M87.851 Other osteonecrosis, right femur** HCC Rx ESR COM
- **M87.852 Other osteonecrosis, left femur** HCC Rx ESR COM
- **M87.859 Other osteonecrosis, unspecified femur** HCC Rx ESR COM

√6th **M87.86 Other osteonecrosis, tibia and fibula**
- **M87.861 Other osteonecrosis, right tibia** HCC Rx ESR COM
- **M87.862 Other osteonecrosis, left tibia** HCC Rx ESR COM
- **M87.863 Other osteonecrosis, unspecified tibia** HCC Rx ESR COM
- **M87.864 Other osteonecrosis, right fibula** HCC Rx ESR COM
- **M87.865 Other osteonecrosis, left fibula** HCC Rx ESR COM
- **M87.869 Other osteonecrosis, unspecified fibula** HCC Rx ESR COM

√6th **M87.87 Other osteonecrosis, ankle, foot and toes**
- **M87.871 Other osteonecrosis, right ankle** HCC Rx ESR COM
- **M87.872 Other osteonecrosis, left ankle** HCC Rx ESR COM
- **M87.873 Other osteonecrosis, unspecified ankle** HCC Rx ESR COM
- **M87.874 Other osteonecrosis, right foot** HCC Rx ESR COM
- **M87.875 Other osteonecrosis, left foot** HCC Rx ESR COM
- **M87.876 Other osteonecrosis, unspecified foot** HCC Rx ESR COM
- **M87.877 Other osteonecrosis, right toe(s)** HCC Rx ESR COM
- **M87.878 Other osteonecrosis, left toe(s)** HCC Rx ESR COM
- **M87.879 Other osteonecrosis, unspecified toe(s)** HCC Rx ESR COM

M87.88 Other osteonecrosis, other site HCC Rx ESR COM

M87.89 Other osteonecrosis, multiple sites HCC Rx ESR COM

M87.9 Osteonecrosis, unspecified HCC Rx ESR COM
Necrosis of bone NOS

√4th **M88 Osteitis deformans [Paget's disease of bone]**

EXCLUDES 1 *osteitis deformans in neoplastic disease (M90.6)*

DEF: Bone disease characterized by numerous cycles of bone resorption by the body. Resorption is followed by accelerated repair attempts, causing bone deformities and bowing, with associated fractures and pain.

M88.0 Osteitis deformans of skull

M88.1 Osteitis deformans of vertebrae

√5th **M88.8 Osteitis deformans of other bones**

√6th **M88.81 Osteitis deformans of shoulder**
- **M88.811 Osteitis deformans of right shoulder**
- **M88.812 Osteitis deformans of left shoulder**
- **M88.819 Osteitis deformans of unspecified shoulder**

M88.82 Osteitis deformans of upper arm
- **M88.821 Osteitis deformans of right upper arm**
- **M88.822 Osteitis deformans of left upper arm**
- **M88.829 Osteitis deformans of unspecified upper arm**

M88.83 Osteitis deformans of forearm
- **M88.831 Osteitis deformans of right forearm**
- **M88.832 Osteitis deformans of left forearm**
- **M88.839 Osteitis deformans of unspecified forearm**

M88.84 Osteitis deformans of hand
- **M88.841 Osteitis deformans of right hand**
- **M88.842 Osteitis deformans of left hand**
- **M88.849 Osteitis deformans of unspecified hand**

M88.85 Osteitis deformans of thigh
- **M88.851 Osteitis deformans of right thigh**
- **M88.852 Osteitis deformans of left thigh**
- **M88.859 Osteitis deformans of unspecified thigh**

M88.86 Osteitis deformans of lower leg
- **M88.861 Osteitis deformans of right lower leg**
- **M88.862 Osteitis deformans of left lower leg**
- **M88.869 Osteitis deformans of unspecified lower leg**

M88.87 Osteitis deformans of ankle and foot
- **M88.871 Osteitis deformans of right ankle and foot**
- **M88.872 Osteitis deformans of left ankle and foot**
- **M88.879 Osteitis deformans of unspecified ankle and foot**

M88.88 Osteitis deformans of other bones

EXCLUDES 2 *osteitis deformans of skull (M88.Ø)*
osteitis deformans of vertebrae (M88.1)

M88.89 Osteitis deformans of multiple sites

M88.9 Osteitis deformans of unspecified bone

M89 Other disorders of bone

M89.Ø Algoneurodystrophy

Shoulder-hand syndrome
Sudeck's atrophy

EXCLUDES 1 *causalgia, lower limb (G57.7-)*
causalgia, upper limb (G56.4-)
complex regional pain syndrome II, lower limb (G57.7-)
complex regional pain syndrome II, upper limb (G56.4-)
reflex sympathetic dystrophy (G9Ø.5-)

M89.ØØ Algoneurodystrophy, unspecified site

M89.Ø1 Algoneurodystrophy, shoulder
- **M89.Ø11 Algoneurodystrophy, right shoulder**
- **M89.Ø12 Algoneurodystrophy, left shoulder**
- **M89.Ø19 Algoneurodystrophy, unspecified shoulder**

M89.Ø2 Algoneurodystrophy, upper arm
- **M89.Ø21 Algoneurodystrophy, right upper arm**
- **M89.Ø22 Algoneurodystrophy, left upper arm**
- **M89.Ø29 Algoneurodystrophy, unspecified upper arm**

M89.Ø3 Algoneurodystrophy, forearm
- **M89.Ø31 Algoneurodystrophy, right forearm**
- **M89.Ø32 Algoneurodystrophy, left forearm**
- **M89.Ø39 Algoneurodystrophy, unspecified forearm**

M89.Ø4 Algoneurodystrophy, hand
- **M89.Ø41 Algoneurodystrophy, right hand**
- **M89.Ø42 Algoneurodystrophy, left hand**
- **M89.Ø49 Algoneurodystrophy, unspecified hand**

M89.Ø5 Algoneurodystrophy, thigh
- **M89.Ø51 Algoneurodystrophy, right thigh**
- **M89.Ø52 Algoneurodystrophy, left thigh**
- **M89.Ø59 Algoneurodystrophy, unspecified thigh**

M89.Ø6 Algoneurodystrophy, lower leg
- **M89.Ø61 Algoneurodystrophy, right lower leg**
- **M89.Ø62 Algoneurodystrophy, left lower leg**
- **M89.Ø69 Algoneurodystrophy, unspecified lower leg**

M89.Ø7 Algoneurodystrophy, ankle and foot
- **M89.Ø71 Algoneurodystrophy, right ankle and foot**
- **M89.Ø72 Algoneurodystrophy, left ankle and foot**
- **M89.Ø79 Algoneurodystrophy, unspecified ankle and foot**

M89.Ø8 Algoneurodystrophy, other site

M89.Ø9 Algoneurodystrophy, multiple sites

M89.1 Physeal arrest

Arrest of growth plate
Epiphyseal arrest
Growth plate arrest

M89.12 Physeal arrest, humerus
- **M89.121 Complete physeal arrest, right proximal humerus**
- **M89.122 Complete physeal arrest, left proximal humerus**
- **M89.123 Partial physeal arrest, right proximal humerus**
- **M89.124 Partial physeal arrest, left proximal humerus**
- **M89.125 Complete physeal arrest, right distal humerus**
- **M89.126 Complete physeal arrest, left distal humerus**
- **M89.127 Partial physeal arrest, right distal humerus**
- **M89.128 Partial physeal arrest, left distal humerus**
- **M89.129 Physeal arrest, humerus, unspecified**

M89.13 Physeal arrest, forearm
- **M89.131 Complete physeal arrest, right distal radius**
- **M89.132 Complete physeal arrest, left distal radius**
- **M89.133 Partial physeal arrest, right distal radius**
- **M89.134 Partial physeal arrest, left distal radius**
- **M89.138 Other physeal arrest of forearm**
- **M89.139 Physeal arrest, forearm, unspecified**

M89.15 Physeal arrest, femur
- **M89.151 Complete physeal arrest, right proximal femur**
- **M89.152 Complete physeal arrest, left proximal femur**
- **M89.153 Partial physeal arrest, right proximal femur**
- **M89.154 Partial physeal arrest, left proximal femur**
- **M89.155 Complete physeal arrest, right distal femur**
- **M89.156 Complete physeal arrest, left distal femur**
- **M89.157 Partial physeal arrest, right distal femur**
- **M89.158 Partial physeal arrest, left distal femur**
- **M89.159 Physeal arrest, femur, unspecified**

M89.16 Physeal arrest, lower leg
- **M89.16Ø Complete physeal arrest, right proximal tibia**
- **M89.161 Complete physeal arrest, left proximal tibia**
- **M89.162 Partial physeal arrest, right proximal tibia**
- **M89.163 Partial physeal arrest, left proximal tibia**
- **M89.164 Complete physeal arrest, right distal tibia**
- **M89.165 Complete physeal arrest, left distal tibia**
- **M89.166 Partial physeal arrest, right distal tibia**
- **M89.167 Partial physeal arrest, left distal tibia**
- **M89.168 Other physeal arrest of lower leg**
- **M89.169 Physeal arrest, lower leg, unspecified**

M89.18 Physeal arrest, other site

M89.2 Other disorders of bone development and growth

M89.2Ø Other disorders of bone development and growth, unspecified site

M89.21 Other disorders of bone development and growth, shoulder
- **M89.211 Other disorders of bone development and growth, right shoulder**
- **M89.212 Other disorders of bone development and growth, left shoulder**
- **M89.219 Other disorders of bone development and growth, unspecified shoulder**

M89.22 Other disorders of bone development and growth, humerus
- **M89.221 Other disorders of bone development and growth, right humerus**
- **M89.222 Other disorders of bone development and growth, left humerus**
- **M89.229 Other disorders of bone development and growth, unspecified humerus**

Chapter 13. Diseases of the Musculoskeletal System and Connective Tissue

M88.82–M89.229

M89.23 Other disorders of bone development and growth, ulna and radius
- **M89.231** Other disorders of bone development and growth, right ulna
- **M89.232** Other disorders of bone development and growth, left ulna
- **M89.233** Other disorders of bone development and growth, right radius
- **M89.234** Other disorders of bone development and growth, left radius
- **M89.239** Other disorders of bone development and growth, unspecified ulna and radius

M89.24 Other disorders of bone development and growth, hand
- **M89.241** Other disorders of bone development and growth, right hand
- **M89.242** Other disorders of bone development and growth, left hand
- **M89.249** Other disorders of bone development and growth, unspecified hand

M89.25 Other disorders of bone development and growth, femur
- **M89.251** Other disorders of bone development and growth, right femur
- **M89.252** Other disorders of bone development and growth, left femur
- **M89.259** Other disorders of bone development and growth, unspecified femur

M89.26 Other disorders of bone development and growth, tibia and fibula
- **M89.261** Other disorders of bone development and growth, right tibia
- **M89.262** Other disorders of bone development and growth, left tibia
- **M89.263** Other disorders of bone development and growth, right fibula
- **M89.264** Other disorders of bone development and growth, left fibula
- **M89.269** Other disorders of bone development and growth, unspecified lower leg

M89.27 Other disorders of bone development and growth, ankle and foot
- **M89.271** Other disorders of bone development and growth, right ankle and foot
- **M89.272** Other disorders of bone development and growth, left ankle and foot
- **M89.279** Other disorders of bone development and growth, unspecified ankle and foot

M89.28 Other disorders of bone development and growth, other site

M89.29 Other disorders of bone development and growth, multiple sites

M89.3 Hypertrophy of bone

M89.3Ø Hypertrophy of bone, unspecified site

M89.31 Hypertrophy of bone, shoulder
- **M89.311** Hypertrophy of bone, right shoulder
- **M89.312** Hypertrophy of bone, left shoulder
- **M89.319** Hypertrophy of bone, unspecified shoulder

M89.32 Hypertrophy of bone, humerus
- **M89.321** Hypertrophy of bone, right humerus
- **M89.322** Hypertrophy of bone, left humerus
- **M89.329** Hypertrophy of bone, unspecified humerus

M89.33 Hypertrophy of bone, ulna and radius
- **M89.331** Hypertrophy of bone, right ulna
- **M89.332** Hypertrophy of bone, left ulna
- **M89.333** Hypertrophy of bone, right radius
- **M89.334** Hypertrophy of bone, left radius
- **M89.339** Hypertrophy of bone, unspecified ulna and radius

M89.34 Hypertrophy of bone, hand
- **M89.341** Hypertrophy of bone, right hand
- **M89.342** Hypertrophy of bone, left hand
- **M89.349** Hypertrophy of bone, unspecified hand

M89.35 Hypertrophy of bone, femur
- **M89.351** Hypertrophy of bone, right femur
- **M89.352** Hypertrophy of bone, left femur
- **M89.359** Hypertrophy of bone, unspecified femur

M89.36 Hypertrophy of bone, tibia and fibula
- **M89.361** Hypertrophy of bone, right tibia
- **M89.362** Hypertrophy of bone, left tibia
- **M89.363** Hypertrophy of bone, right fibula
- **M89.364** Hypertrophy of bone, left fibula
- **M89.369** Hypertrophy of bone, unspecified tibia and fibula

M89.37 Hypertrophy of bone, ankle and foot
- **M89.371** Hypertrophy of bone, right ankle and foot
- **M89.372** Hypertrophy of bone, left ankle and foot
- **M89.379** Hypertrophy of bone, unspecified ankle and foot

M89.38 Hypertrophy of bone, other site

M89.39 Hypertrophy of bone, multiple sites

M89.4 Other hypertrophic osteoarthropathy

Marie-Bamberger disease
Pachydermoperiostosis

M89.4Ø Other hypertrophic osteoarthropathy, unspecified site

M89.41 Other hypertrophic osteoarthropathy, shoulder
- **M89.411** Other hypertrophic osteoarthropathy, right shoulder
- **M89.412** Other hypertrophic osteoarthropathy, left shoulder
- **M89.419** Other hypertrophic osteoarthropathy, unspecified shoulder

M89.42 Other hypertrophic osteoarthropathy, upper arm
- **M89.421** Other hypertrophic osteoarthropathy, right upper arm
- **M89.422** Other hypertrophic osteoarthropathy, left upper arm
- **M89.429** Other hypertrophic osteoarthropathy, unspecified upper arm

M89.43 Other hypertrophic osteoarthropathy, forearm
- **M89.431** Other hypertrophic osteoarthropathy, right forearm
- **M89.432** Other hypertrophic osteoarthropathy, left forearm
- **M89.439** Other hypertrophic osteoarthropathy, unspecified forearm

M89.44 Other hypertrophic osteoarthropathy, hand
- **M89.441** Other hypertrophic osteoarthropathy, right hand
- **M89.442** Other hypertrophic osteoarthropathy, left hand
- **M89.449** Other hypertrophic osteoarthropathy, unspecified hand

M89.45 Other hypertrophic osteoarthropathy, thigh
- **M89.451** Other hypertrophic osteoarthropathy, right thigh
- **M89.452** Other hypertrophic osteoarthropathy, left thigh
- **M89.459** Other hypertrophic osteoarthropathy, unspecified thigh

M89.46 Other hypertrophic osteoarthropathy, lower leg
- **M89.461** Other hypertrophic osteoarthropathy, right lower leg
- **M89.462** Other hypertrophic osteoarthropathy, left lower leg
- **M89.469** Other hypertrophic osteoarthropathy, unspecified lower leg

M89.47 Other hypertrophic osteoarthropathy, ankle and foot
- **M89.471** Other hypertrophic osteoarthropathy, right ankle and foot
- **M89.472** Other hypertrophic osteoarthropathy, left ankle and foot
- **M89.479** Other hypertrophic osteoarthropathy, unspecified ankle and foot

M89.48 Other hypertrophic osteoarthropathy, other site

M89.49 Other hypertrophic osteoarthropathy, multiple sites

M89.5 Osteolysis

Use additional code to identify major osseous defect, if applicable (M89.7-)

EXCLUDES 2 *periprosthetic osteolysis of internal prosthetic joint (T84.Ø5-)*

M89.5Ø Osteolysis, unspecified site

M89.51 Osteolysis, shoulder
M89.511 Osteolysis, right shoulder
M89.512 Osteolysis, left shoulder
M89.519 Osteolysis, unspecified shoulder
M89.52 Osteolysis, upper arm
M89.521 Osteolysis, right upper arm
M89.522 Osteolysis, left upper arm
M89.529 Osteolysis, unspecified upper arm
M89.53 Osteolysis, forearm
M89.531 Osteolysis, right forearm
M89.532 Osteolysis, left forearm
M89.539 Osteolysis, unspecified forearm
M89.54 Osteolysis, hand
M89.541 Osteolysis, right hand
M89.542 Osteolysis, left hand
M89.549 Osteolysis, unspecified hand
M89.55 Osteolysis, thigh
M89.551 Osteolysis, right thigh
M89.552 Osteolysis, left thigh
M89.559 Osteolysis, unspecified thigh
M89.56 Osteolysis, lower leg
M89.561 Osteolysis, right lower leg
M89.562 Osteolysis, left lower leg
M89.569 Osteolysis, unspecified lower leg
M89.57 Osteolysis, ankle and foot
M89.571 Osteolysis, right ankle and foot
M89.572 Osteolysis, left ankle and foot
M89.579 Osteolysis, unspecified ankle and foot
M89.58 Osteolysis, other site
M89.59 Osteolysis, multiple sites
M89.6 Osteopathy after poliomyelitis
Use additional code (B91) to identify previous poliomyelitis
EXCLUDES 1 postpolio syndrome (G14)
M89.60 Osteopathy after poliomyelitis, unspecified site HCC ESR COM
M89.61 Osteopathy after poliomyelitis, shoulder
M89.611 Osteopathy after poliomyelitis, right shoulder HCC ESR COM
M89.612 Osteopathy after poliomyelitis, left shoulder HCC ESR COM
M89.619 Osteopathy after poliomyelitis, unspecified shoulder HCC ESR COM
M89.62 Osteopathy after poliomyelitis, upper arm
M89.621 Osteopathy after poliomyelitis, right upper arm HCC ESR COM
M89.622 Osteopathy after poliomyelitis, left upper arm HCC ESR COM
M89.629 Osteopathy after poliomyelitis, unspecified upper arm HCC ESR COM
M89.63 Osteopathy after poliomyelitis, forearm
M89.631 Osteopathy after poliomyelitis, right forearm HCC ESR COM
M89.632 Osteopathy after poliomyelitis, left forearm HCC ESR COM
M89.639 Osteopathy after poliomyelitis, unspecified forearm HCC ESR COM
M89.64 Osteopathy after poliomyelitis, hand
M89.641 Osteopathy after poliomyelitis, right hand HCC ESR COM
M89.642 Osteopathy after poliomyelitis, left hand HCC ESR COM
M89.649 Osteopathy after poliomyelitis, unspecified hand HCC ESR COM
M89.65 Osteopathy after poliomyelitis, thigh
M89.651 Osteopathy after poliomyelitis, right thigh HCC ESR COM
M89.652 Osteopathy after poliomyelitis, left thigh HCC ESR COM
M89.659 Osteopathy after poliomyelitis, unspecified thigh HCC ESR COM
M89.66 Osteopathy after poliomyelitis, lower leg
M89.661 Osteopathy after poliomyelitis, right lower leg HCC ESR COM
M89.662 Osteopathy after poliomyelitis, left lower leg HCC ESR COM
M89.669 Osteopathy after poliomyelitis, unspecified lower leg HCC ESR COM
M89.67 Osteopathy after poliomyelitis, ankle and foot
M89.671 Osteopathy after poliomyelitis, right ankle and foot HCC ESR COM
M89.672 Osteopathy after poliomyelitis, left ankle and foot HCC ESR COM
M89.679 Osteopathy after poliomyelitis, unspecified ankle and foot HCC ESR COM
M89.68 Osteopathy after poliomyelitis, other site HCC ESR COM
M89.69 Osteopathy after poliomyelitis, multiple sites HCC ESR COM
M89.7 Major osseous defect
Code first underlying disease, if known, such as:
aseptic necrosis of bone (M87.-)
malignant neoplasm of bone (C4Ø.-)
osteolysis (M89.5)
osteomyelitis (M86.-)
osteonecrosis (M87.-)
osteoporosis (M8Ø.-, M81.-)
periprosthetic osteolysis (T84.Ø5-)
M89.7Ø Major osseous defect, unspecified site
M89.71 Major osseous defect, shoulder region
Major osseous defect clavicle or scapula
M89.711 Major osseous defect, right shoulder region
M89.712 Major osseous defect, left shoulder region
M89.719 Major osseous defect, unspecified shoulder region
M89.72 Major osseous defect, humerus
M89.721 Major osseous defect, right humerus
M89.722 Major osseous defect, left humerus
M89.729 Major osseous defect, unspecified humerus
M89.73 Major osseous defect, forearm
Major osseous defect of radius and ulna
M89.731 Major osseous defect, right forearm
M89.732 Major osseous defect, left forearm
M89.739 Major osseous defect, unspecified forearm
M89.74 Major osseous defect, hand
Major osseous defect of carpus, fingers, metacarpus
M89.741 Major osseous defect, right hand
M89.742 Major osseous defect, left hand
M89.749 Major osseous defect, unspecified hand
M89.75 Major osseous defect, pelvic region and thigh
Major osseous defect of femur and pelvis
M89.751 Major osseous defect, right pelvic region and thigh
M89.752 Major osseous defect, left pelvic region and thigh
M89.759 Major osseous defect, unspecified pelvic region and thigh
M89.76 Major osseous defect, lower leg
Major osseous defect of fibula and tibia
M89.761 Major osseous defect, right lower leg
M89.762 Major osseous defect, left lower leg
M89.769 Major osseous defect, unspecified lower leg
M89.77 Major osseous defect, ankle and foot
Major osseous defect of metatarsus, tarsus, toes
M89.771 Major osseous defect, right ankle and foot
M89.772 Major osseous defect, left ankle and foot
M89.779 Major osseous defect, unspecified ankle and foot
M89.78 Major osseous defect, other site
M89.79 Major osseous defect, multiple sites
M89.8 Other specified disorders of bone
Infantile cortical hyperostoses
Post-traumatic subperiosteal ossification
AHA: 2022,2Q,10
M89.8X Other specified disorders of bone
M89.8XØ Other specified disorders of bone, multiple sites

M89.8X1 Other specified disorders of bone, shoulder

M89.8X2 Other specified disorders of bone, upper arm

M89.8X3 Other specified disorders of bone, forearm
AHA: 2019,3Q,9

M89.8X4 Other specified disorders of bone, hand

M89.8X5 Other specified disorders of bone, thigh

M89.8X6 Other specified disorders of bone, lower leg

M89.8X7 Other specified disorders of bone, ankle and foot

M89.8X8 Other specified disorders of bone, other site

M89.8X9 Other specified disorders of bone, unspecified site

M89.9 Disorder of bone, unspecified

4th M90 Osteopathies in diseases classified elsewhere

EXCLUDES 1 *osteochondritis, osteomyelitis, and osteopathy (in):*
cryptococcosis (B45.3)
diabetes mellitus (E08-E13 with .69-)
gonococcal (A54.43)
neurogenic syphilis (A52.11)
renal osteodystrophy (N25.0)
salmonellosis (A02.24)
secondary syphilis (A51.46)
syphilis (late) (A52.77)

5th M90.5 Osteonecrosis in diseases classified elsewhere

Code first underlying disease, such as:
caisson disease (T70.3)
hemoglobinopathy (D50-D64)

M90.50 Osteonecrosis in diseases classified elsewhere, unspecified site HCC Rx ESR COM

6th M90.51 Osteonecrosis in diseases classified elsewhere, shoulder

M90.511 Osteonecrosis in diseases classified elsewhere, right shoulder HCC Rx ESR COM

M90.512 Osteonecrosis in diseases classified elsewhere, left shoulder HCC Rx ESR COM

M90.519 Osteonecrosis in diseases classified elsewhere, unspecified shoulder HCC Rx ESR COM

6th M90.52 Osteonecrosis in diseases classified elsewhere, upper arm

M90.521 Osteonecrosis in diseases classified elsewhere, right upper arm HCC Rx ESR COM

M90.522 Osteonecrosis in diseases classified elsewhere, left upper arm HCC Rx ESR COM

M90.529 Osteonecrosis in diseases classified elsewhere, unspecified upper arm HCC Rx ESR COM

6th M90.53 Osteonecrosis in diseases classified elsewhere, forearm

M90.531 Osteonecrosis in diseases classified elsewhere, right forearm HCC Rx ESR COM

M90.532 Osteonecrosis in diseases classified elsewhere, left forearm HCC Rx ESR COM

M90.539 Osteonecrosis in diseases classified elsewhere, unspecified forearm HCC Rx ESR COM

6th M90.54 Osteonecrosis in diseases classified elsewhere, hand

M90.541 Osteonecrosis in diseases classified elsewhere, right hand HCC Rx ESR COM

M90.542 Osteonecrosis in diseases classified elsewhere, left hand HCC Rx ESR COM

M90.549 Osteonecrosis in diseases classified elsewhere, unspecified hand HCC Rx ESR COM

6th M90.55 Osteonecrosis in diseases classified elsewhere, thigh

M90.551 Osteonecrosis in diseases classified elsewhere, right thigh HCC Rx ESR COM

M90.552 Osteonecrosis in diseases classified elsewhere, left thigh HCC Rx ESR COM

M90.559 Osteonecrosis in diseases classified elsewhere, unspecified thigh HCC Rx ESR COM

6th M90.56 Osteonecrosis in diseases classified elsewhere, lower leg

M90.561 Osteonecrosis in diseases classified elsewhere, right lower leg HCC Rx ESR COM

M90.562 Osteonecrosis in diseases classified elsewhere, left lower leg HCC Rx ESR COM

M90.569 Osteonecrosis in diseases classified elsewhere, unspecified lower leg HCC Rx ESR COM

6th M90.57 Osteonecrosis in diseases classified elsewhere, ankle and foot

M90.571 Osteonecrosis in diseases classified elsewhere, right ankle and foot HCC Rx ESR COM

M90.572 Osteonecrosis in diseases classified elsewhere, left ankle and foot HCC Rx ESR COM

M90.579 Osteonecrosis in diseases classified elsewhere, unspecified ankle and foot HCC Rx ESR COM

M90.58 Osteonecrosis in diseases classified elsewhere, other site HCC Rx ESR COM

M90.59 Osteonecrosis in diseases classified elsewhere, multiple sites HCC Rx ESR COM

5th M90.6 Osteitis deformans in neoplastic diseases

Osteitis deformans in malignant neoplasm of bone
Code first the neoplasm (C40.-, C41.-)

EXCLUDES 1 *osteitis deformans [Paget's disease of bone] (M88.-)*

M90.60 Osteitis deformans in neoplastic diseases, unspecified site

6th M90.61 Osteitis deformans in neoplastic diseases, shoulder

M90.611 Osteitis deformans in neoplastic diseases, right shoulder

M90.612 Osteitis deformans in neoplastic diseases, left shoulder

M90.619 Osteitis deformans in neoplastic diseases, unspecified shoulder

6th M90.62 Osteitis deformans in neoplastic diseases, upper arm

M90.621 Osteitis deformans in neoplastic diseases, right upper arm

M90.622 Osteitis deformans in neoplastic diseases, left upper arm

M90.629 Osteitis deformans in neoplastic diseases, unspecified upper arm

6th M90.63 Osteitis deformans in neoplastic diseases, forearm

M90.631 Osteitis deformans in neoplastic diseases, right forearm

M90.632 Osteitis deformans in neoplastic diseases, left forearm

M90.639 Osteitis deformans in neoplastic diseases, unspecified forearm

6th M90.64 Osteitis deformans in neoplastic diseases, hand

M90.641 Osteitis deformans in neoplastic diseases, right hand

M90.642 Osteitis deformans in neoplastic diseases, left hand

M90.649 Osteitis deformans in neoplastic diseases, unspecified hand

6th M90.65 Osteitis deformans in neoplastic diseases, thigh

M90.651 Osteitis deformans in neoplastic diseases, right thigh

M90.652 Osteitis deformans in neoplastic diseases, left thigh

M90.659 Osteitis deformans in neoplastic diseases, unspecified thigh

6th M90.66 Osteitis deformans in neoplastic diseases, lower leg

M90.661 Osteitis deformans in neoplastic diseases, right lower leg

M90.662 Osteitis deformans in neoplastic diseases, left lower leg

M90.669 Osteitis deformans in neoplastic diseases, unspecified lower leg

M90.67 Osteitis deformans in neoplastic diseases, ankle and foot
- M90.671 Osteitis deformans in neoplastic diseases, right ankle and foot
- M90.672 Osteitis deformans in neoplastic diseases, left ankle and foot
- M90.679 Osteitis deformans in neoplastic diseases, unspecified ankle and foot

M90.68 Osteitis deformans in neoplastic diseases, other site

M90.69 Osteitis deformans in neoplastic diseases, multiple sites

M90.8 Osteopathy in diseases classified elsewhere

Code first underlying disease, such as:
- rickets (E55.0)
- vitamin-D-resistant rickets (E83.3)

M90.80 Osteopathy in diseases classified elsewhere, unspecified site

M90.81 Osteopathy in diseases classified elsewhere, shoulder
- M90.811 Osteopathy in diseases classified elsewhere, right shoulder
- M90.812 Osteopathy in diseases classified elsewhere, left shoulder
- M90.819 Osteopathy in diseases classified elsewhere, unspecified shoulder

M90.82 Osteopathy in diseases classified elsewhere, upper arm
- M90.821 Osteopathy in diseases classified elsewhere, right upper arm
- M90.822 Osteopathy in diseases classified elsewhere, left upper arm
- M90.829 Osteopathy in diseases classified elsewhere, unspecified upper arm

M90.83 Osteopathy in diseases classified elsewhere, forearm
- M90.831 Osteopathy in diseases classified elsewhere, right forearm
- M90.832 Osteopathy in diseases classified elsewhere, left forearm
- M90.839 Osteopathy in diseases classified elsewhere, unspecified forearm

M90.84 Osteopathy in diseases classified elsewhere, hand
- M90.841 Osteopathy in diseases classified elsewhere, right hand
- M90.842 Osteopathy in diseases classified elsewhere, left hand
- M90.849 Osteopathy in diseases classified elsewhere, unspecified hand

M90.85 Osteopathy in diseases classified elsewhere, thigh
- M90.851 Osteopathy in diseases classified elsewhere, right thigh
- M90.852 Osteopathy in diseases classified elsewhere, left thigh
- M90.859 Osteopathy in diseases classified elsewhere, unspecified thigh

M90.86 Osteopathy in diseases classified elsewhere, lower leg
- M90.861 Osteopathy in diseases classified elsewhere, right lower leg
- M90.862 Osteopathy in diseases classified elsewhere, left lower leg
- M90.869 Osteopathy in diseases classified elsewhere, unspecified lower leg

M90.87 Osteopathy in diseases classified elsewhere, ankle and foot
- M90.871 Osteopathy in diseases classified elsewhere, right ankle and foot
- M90.872 Osteopathy in diseases classified elsewhere, left ankle and foot
- M90.879 Osteopathy in diseases classified elsewhere, unspecified ankle and foot

M90.88 Osteopathy in diseases classified elsewhere, other site

M90.89 Osteopathy in diseases classified elsewhere, multiple sites

Chondropathies (M91-M94)

EXCLUDES 1 postprocedural chondropathies (M96.-)

M91 Juvenile osteochondrosis of hip and pelvis

EXCLUDES 1 slipped upper femoral epiphysis (nontraumatic) ►(M93.0-)◄

M91.0 Juvenile osteochondrosis of pelvis COM
- Osteochondrosis (juvenile) of acetabulum
- Osteochondrosis (juvenile) of iliac crest [Buchanan]
- Osteochondrosis (juvenile) of ischiopubic synchondrosis [van Neck]
- Osteochondrosis (juvenile) of symphysis pubis [Pierson]

M91.1 Juvenile osteochondrosis of head of femur [Legg-Calvé-Perthes]
- M91.10 Juvenile osteochondrosis of head of femur [Legg-Calvé-Perthes], unspecified leg COM
- M91.11 Juvenile osteochondrosis of head of femur [Legg-Calvé-Perthes], right leg COM
- M91.12 Juvenile osteochondrosis of head of femur [Legg-Calvé-Perthes], left leg COM

M91.2 Coxa plana

Hip deformity due to previous juvenile osteochondrosis
- M91.20 Coxa plana, unspecified hip COM
- M91.21 Coxa plana, right hip COM
- M91.22 Coxa plana, left hip COM

M91.3 Pseudocoxalgia
- M91.30 Pseudocoxalgia, unspecified hip COM
- M91.31 Pseudocoxalgia, right hip COM
- M91.32 Pseudocoxalgia, left hip COM

M91.4 Coxa magna
- M91.40 Coxa magna, unspecified hip COM
- M91.41 Coxa magna, right hip COM
- M91.42 Coxa magna, left hip COM

M91.8 Other juvenile osteochondrosis of hip and pelvis

Juvenile osteochondrosis after reduction of congenital dislocation of hip
- M91.80 Other juvenile osteochondrosis of hip and pelvis, unspecified leg COM
- M91.81 Other juvenile osteochondrosis of hip and pelvis, right leg COM
- M91.82 Other juvenile osteochondrosis of hip and pelvis, left leg COM

M91.9 Juvenile osteochondrosis of hip and pelvis, unspecified
- M91.90 Juvenile osteochondrosis of hip and pelvis, unspecified, unspecified leg COM
- M91.91 Juvenile osteochondrosis of hip and pelvis, unspecified, right leg COM
- M91.92 Juvenile osteochondrosis of hip and pelvis, unspecified, left leg COM

M92 Other juvenile osteochondrosis

M92.0 Juvenile osteochondrosis of humerus
- Osteochondrosis (juvenile) of capitulum of humerus [Panner]
- Osteochondrosis (juvenile) of head of humerus [Haas]
- M92.00 Juvenile osteochondrosis of humerus, unspecified arm
- M92.01 Juvenile osteochondrosis of humerus, right arm
- M92.02 Juvenile osteochondrosis of humerus, left arm

M92.1 Juvenile osteochondrosis of radius and ulna
- Osteochondrosis (juvenile) of lower ulna [Burns]
- Osteochondrosis (juvenile) of radial head [Brailsford]
- M92.10 Juvenile osteochondrosis of radius and ulna, unspecified arm
- M92.11 Juvenile osteochondrosis of radius and ulna, right arm
- M92.12 Juvenile osteochondrosis of radius and ulna, left arm

M92.2 Juvenile osteochondrosis, hand

M92.20 Unspecified juvenile osteochondrosis, hand
- M92.201 Unspecified juvenile osteochondrosis, right hand
- M92.202 Unspecified juvenile osteochondrosis, left hand
- M92.209 Unspecified juvenile osteochondrosis, unspecified hand

M92.21 Osteochondrosis (juvenile) of carpal lunate [Kienböck]

M92.211 Osteochondrosis (juvenile) of carpal lunate [Kienböck], right hand

M92.212 Osteochondrosis (juvenile) of carpal lunate [Kienböck], left hand

M92.219 Osteochondrosis (juvenile) of carpal lunate [Kienböck], unspecified hand

M92.22 Osteochondrosis (juvenile) of metacarpal heads [Mauclaire]

M92.221 Osteochondrosis (juvenile) of metacarpal heads [Mauclaire], right hand

M92.222 Osteochondrosis (juvenile) of metacarpal heads [Mauclaire], left hand

M92.229 Osteochondrosis (juvenile) of metacarpal heads [Mauclaire], unspecified hand

M92.29 Other juvenile osteochondrosis, hand

M92.291 Other juvenile osteochondrosis, right hand

M92.292 Other juvenile osteochondrosis, left hand

M92.299 Other juvenile osteochondrosis, unspecified hand

M92.3 Other juvenile osteochondrosis, upper limb

M92.30 Other juvenile osteochondrosis, unspecified upper limb

M92.31 Other juvenile osteochondrosis, right upper limb

M92.32 Other juvenile osteochondrosis, left upper limb

M92.4 Juvenile osteochondrosis of patella

Osteochondrosis (juvenile) of primary patellar center [Köhler]
Osteochondrosis (juvenile) of secondary patellar centre [Sinding Larsen]

M92.40 Juvenile osteochondrosis of patella, unspecified knee

M92.41 Juvenile osteochondrosis of patella, right knee

M92.42 Juvenile osteochondrosis of patella, left knee

M92.5 Juvenile osteochondrosis of tibia and fibula

AHA: 2020,4Q,33-34

M92.50 Unspecified juvenile osteochondrosis of tibia and fibula

M92.501 Unspecified juvenile osteochondrosis, right leg

M92.502 Unspecified juvenile osteochondrosis, left leg

● **M92.503 Unspecified juvenile osteochondrosis, bilateral leg**

▲ **M92.509 Unspecified juvenile osteochondrosis, unspecified leg**

▲ **M92.51 Juvenile osteochondrosis of proximal tibia**

Blount disease
Tibia vara

▲ **M92.511 Juvenile osteochondrosis of proximal tibia, right leg**

▲ **M92.512 Juvenile osteochondrosis of proximal tibia, left leg**

● **M92.513 Juvenile osteochondrosis of proximal tibia, bilateral**

▲ **M92.519 Juvenile osteochondrosis of proximal tibia, unspecified leg**

▲ **M92.52 Juvenile osteochondrosis of tibia tubercle**

Osgood-Schlatter disease

▲ **M92.521 Juvenile osteochondrosis of tibia tubercle, right leg**

▲ **M92.522 Juvenile osteochondrosis of tibia tubercle, left leg**

● **M92.523 Juvenile osteochondrosis of tibia tubercle, bilateral**

▲ **M92.529 Juvenile osteochondrosis of tibia tubercle, unspecified leg**

▲ **M92.59 Other juvenile osteochondrosis of tibia and fibula**

▲ **M92.591 Other juvenile osteochondrosis of tibia and fibula, right leg**

▲ **M92.592 Other juvenile osteochondrosis of tibia and fibula, left leg**

● **M92.593 Other juvenile osteochondrosis of tibia and fibula, bilateral**

▲ **M92.599 Other juvenile osteochondrosis of tibia and fibula, unspecified leg**

M92.6 Juvenile osteochondrosis of tarsus

Osteochondrosis (juvenile) of calcaneum [Sever]
Osteochondrosis (juvenile) of os tibiale externum [Haglund]
Osteochondrosis (juvenile) of talus [Diaz]
Osteochondrosis (juvenile) of tarsal navicular [Köhler]

M92.60 Juvenile osteochondrosis of tarsus, unspecified ankle

M92.61 Juvenile osteochondrosis of tarsus, right ankle

M92.62 Juvenile osteochondrosis of tarsus, left ankle

M92.7 Juvenile osteochondrosis of metatarsus

Osteochondrosis (juvenile) of fifth metatarsus [Iselin]
Osteochondrosis (juvenile) of second metatarsus [Freiberg]

M92.70 Juvenile osteochondrosis of metatarsus, unspecified foot

M92.71 Juvenile osteochondrosis of metatarsus, right foot

M92.72 Juvenile osteochondrosis of metatarsus, left foot

M92.8 Other specified juvenile osteochondrosis

Calcaneal apophysitis

DEF: Calcaneal apophysitis: Inflammation of the calcaneus at the point of Achilles tendon insertion usually occurring in boys ages 8 to 14. Pain, tenderness, and localized swelling are present.

M92.9 Juvenile osteochondrosis, unspecified

Juvenile apophysitis NOS
Juvenile epiphysitis NOS
Juvenile osteochondritis NOS
Juvenile osteochondrosis NOS

M93 Other osteochondropathies

EXCLUDES 2 *osteochondrosis of spine (M42.-)*

M93.0 Slipped upper femoral epiphysis (nontraumatic)

▶Slipped capital femoral epiphysis (SCFE)◀
▶Slipped upper femoral epiphysis (SUFE)◀

Use additional code for associated chondrolysis (M94.3)

M93.00 Unspecified slipped upper femoral epiphysis (nontraumatic)

M93.001 Unspecified slipped upper femoral epiphysis (nontraumatic), right hip COM

M93.002 Unspecified slipped upper femoral epiphysis (nontraumatic), left hip COM

M93.003 Unspecified slipped upper femoral epiphysis (nontraumatic), unspecified hip COM

M93.004 Unspecified slipped upper femoral epiphysis (nontraumatic), bilateral hips

M93.01 Acute slipped upper femoral epiphysis, stable (nontraumatic)

M93.011 Acute slipped upper femoral epiphysis, stable (nontraumatic), right hip COM

M93.012 Acute slipped upper femoral epiphysis, stable (nontraumatic), left hip COM

M93.013 Acute slipped upper femoral epiphysis, stable (nontraumatic), unspecified hip COM

M93.014 Acute slipped upper femoral epiphysis, stable (nontraumatic), bilateral hips

M93.02 Chronic slipped upper femoral epiphysis, stable (nontraumatic)

M93.021 Chronic slipped upper femoral epiphysis, stable (nontraumatic), right hip COM

M93.022 Chronic slipped upper femoral epiphysis, stable (nontraumatic), left hip COM

M93.023 Chronic slipped upper femoral epiphysis, stable (nontraumatic), unspecified hip COM

M93.024 Chronic slipped upper femoral epiphysis, stable (nontraumatic), bilateral hips

M93.03 Acute on chronic slipped upper femoral epiphysis, stable (nontraumatic)

M93.031 Acute on chronic slipped upper femoral epiphysis, stable (nontraumatic), right hip COM

M93.032 Acute on chronic slipped upper femoral epiphysis, stable (nontraumatic), left hip COM

M93.033 Acute on chronic slipped upper femoral epiphysis, stable (nontraumatic), unspecified hip COM

M93.034 Acute on chronic slipped upper femoral epiphysis, stable (nontraumatic), bilateral hips

● ✓6th M93.04 Acute slipped upper femoral epiphysis, unstable (nontraumatic)
● M93.041 Acute slipped upper femoral epiphysis, unstable (nontraumatic), right hip
● M93.042 Acute slipped upper femoral epiphysis, unstable (nontraumatic), left hip
● M93.043 Acute slipped upper femoral epiphysis, unstable (nontraumatic), unspecified hip
● M93.044 Acute slipped upper femoral epiphysis, unstable (nontraumatic), bilateral hips
● ✓6th M93.05 Acute on chronic slipped upper femoral epiphysis, unstable (nontraumatic)
● M93.051 Acute on chronic slipped upper femoral epiphysis, unstable (nontraumatic), right hip
● M93.052 Acute on chronic slipped upper femoral epiphysis, unstable (nontraumatic), left hip
● M93.053 Acute on chronic slipped upper femoral epiphysis, unstable (nontraumatic), unspecified hip
● M93.054 Acute on chronic slipped upper femoral epiphysis, unstable (nontraumatic), bilateral hips
● ✓6th M93.06 Acute slipped upper femoral epiphysis, unspecified stability (nontraumatic)
● M93.061 Acute slipped upper femoral epiphysis, unspecified stability (nontraumatic), right hip
● M93.062 Acute slipped upper femoral epiphysis, unspecified stability (nontraumatic), left hip
● M93.063 Acute slipped upper femoral epiphysis, unspecified stability (nontraumatic), unspecified hip
● M93.064 Acute slipped upper femoral epiphysis, unspecified stability (nontraumatic), bilateral hips
● ✓6th M93.07 Acute on chronic slipped upper femoral epiphysis, unspecified stability (nontraumatic)
● M93.071 Acute on chronic slipped upper femoral epiphysis, unspecified stability (nontraumatic), right hip
● M93.072 Acute on chronic slipped upper femoral epiphysis, unspecified stability (nontraumatic), left hip
● M93.073 Acute on chronic slipped upper femoral epiphysis, unspecified stability (nontraumatic), unspecified hip
● M93.074 Acute on chronic slipped upper femoral epiphysis, unspecified stability (nontraumatic), bilateral hips

M93.1 Kienböck's disease of adults A
Adult osteochondrosis of carpal lunates

✓5th M93.2 Osteochondritis dissecans
DEF: Avascular necrosis caused by lack of blood flow to the bone and cartilage of a joint causing the bone to die. This can result in splinters or pieces of cartilage breaking off in the joint.
M93.20 Osteochondritis dissecans of unspecified site
✓6th M93.21 Osteochondritis dissecans of shoulder
M93.211 Osteochondritis dissecans, right shoulder
M93.212 Osteochondritis dissecans, left shoulder
M93.219 Osteochondritis dissecans, unspecified shoulder
✓6th M93.22 Osteochondritis dissecans of elbow
M93.221 Osteochondritis dissecans, right elbow
M93.222 Osteochondritis dissecans, left elbow
M93.229 Osteochondritis dissecans, unspecified elbow
✓6th M93.23 Osteochondritis dissecans of wrist
M93.231 Osteochondritis dissecans, right wrist
M93.232 Osteochondritis dissecans, left wrist
M93.239 Osteochondritis dissecans, unspecified wrist
✓6th M93.24 Osteochondritis dissecans of joints of hand
M93.241 Osteochondritis dissecans, joints of right hand
M93.242 Osteochondritis dissecans, joints of left hand
M93.249 Osteochondritis dissecans, joints of unspecified hand
✓6th M93.25 Osteochondritis dissecans of hip
M93.251 Osteochondritis dissecans, right hip
M93.252 Osteochondritis dissecans, left hip
M93.259 Osteochondritis dissecans, unspecified hip
✓6th M93.26 Osteochondritis dissecans knee
M93.261 Osteochondritis dissecans, right knee
M93.262 Osteochondritis dissecans, left knee
M93.269 Osteochondritis dissecans, unspecified knee
✓6th M93.27 Osteochondritis dissecans of ankle and joints of foot
M93.271 Osteochondritis dissecans, right ankle and joints of right foot
M93.272 Osteochondritis dissecans, left ankle and joints of left foot
M93.279 Osteochondritis dissecans, unspecified ankle and joints of foot
M93.28 Osteochondritis dissecans other site
M93.29 Osteochondritis dissecans multiple sites

✓5th M93.8 Other specified osteochondropathies
M93.80 Other specified osteochondropathies of unspecified site
✓6th M93.81 Other specified osteochondropathies of shoulder
M93.811 Other specified osteochondropathies, right shoulder
M93.812 Other specified osteochondropathies, left shoulder
M93.819 Other specified osteochondropathies, unspecified shoulder
✓6th M93.82 Other specified osteochondropathies of upper arm
M93.821 Other specified osteochondropathies, right upper arm
M93.822 Other specified osteochondropathies, left upper arm
M93.829 Other specified osteochondropathies, unspecified upper arm
✓6th M93.83 Other specified osteochondropathies of forearm
M93.831 Other specified osteochondropathies, right forearm
M93.832 Other specified osteochondropathies, left forearm
M93.839 Other specified osteochondropathies, unspecified forearm
✓6th M93.84 Other specified osteochondropathies of hand
M93.841 Other specified osteochondropathies, right hand
M93.842 Other specified osteochondropathies, left hand
M93.849 Other specified osteochondropathies, unspecified hand
✓6th M93.85 Other specified osteochondropathies of thigh
M93.851 Other specified osteochondropathies, right thigh
M93.852 Other specified osteochondropathies, left thigh
M93.859 Other specified osteochondropathies, unspecified thigh
✓6th M93.86 Other specified osteochondropathies lower leg
M93.861 Other specified osteochondropathies, right lower leg
M93.862 Other specified osteochondropathies, left lower leg
M93.869 Other specified osteochondropathies, unspecified lower leg
✓6th M93.87 Other specified osteochondropathies of ankle and foot
M93.871 Other specified osteochondropathies, right ankle and foot
M93.872 Other specified osteochondropathies, left ankle and foot
M93.879 Other specified osteochondropathies, unspecified ankle and foot
M93.88 Other specified osteochondropathies other site
M93.89 Other specified osteochondropathies multiple sites

5th **M93.9 Osteochondropathy, unspecified**
Apophysitis NOS
Epiphysitis NOS
Osteochondritis NOS
Osteochondrosis NOS

M93.90 Osteochondropathy, unspecified of unspecified site

6th **M93.91 Osteochondropathy, unspecified of shoulder**
M93.911 Osteochondropathy, unspecified, right shoulder
M93.912 Osteochondropathy, unspecified, left shoulder
M93.919 Osteochondropathy, unspecified, unspecified shoulder

6th **M93.92 Osteochondropathy, unspecified of upper arm**
M93.921 Osteochondropathy, unspecified, right upper arm
M93.922 Osteochondropathy, unspecified, left upper arm
M93.929 Osteochondropathy, unspecified, unspecified upper arm

6th **M93.93 Osteochondropathy, unspecified of forearm**
M93.931 Osteochondropathy, unspecified, right forearm
M93.932 Osteochondropathy, unspecified, left forearm
M93.939 Osteochondropathy, unspecified, unspecified forearm

6th **M93.94 Osteochondropathy, unspecified of hand**
M93.941 Osteochondropathy, unspecified, right hand
M93.942 Osteochondropathy, unspecified, left hand
M93.949 Osteochondropathy, unspecified, unspecified hand

6th **M93.95 Osteochondropathy, unspecified of thigh**
M93.951 Osteochondropathy, unspecified, right thigh
M93.952 Osteochondropathy, unspecified, left thigh
M93.959 Osteochondropathy, unspecified, unspecified thigh

6th **M93.96 Osteochondropathy, unspecified lower leg**
M93.961 Osteochondropathy, unspecified, right lower leg
M93.962 Osteochondropathy, unspecified, left lower leg
M93.969 Osteochondropathy, unspecified, unspecified lower leg

6th **M93.97 Osteochondropathy, unspecified of ankle and foot**
M93.971 Osteochondropathy, unspecified, right ankle and foot
M93.972 Osteochondropathy, unspecified, left ankle and foot
M93.979 Osteochondropathy, unspecified, unspecified ankle and foot

M93.98 Osteochondropathy, unspecified other site
M93.99 Osteochondropathy, unspecified multiple sites

4th **M94 Other disorders of cartilage**

M94.Ø Chondrocostal junction syndrome [Tietze]
Costochondritis

M94.1 Relapsing polychondritis

5th **M94.2 Chondromalacia**
EXCLUDES 1 *chondromalacia patellae (M22.4)*

M94.20 Chondromalacia, unspecified site

6th **M94.21 Chondromalacia, shoulder**
M94.211 Chondromalacia, right shoulder
M94.212 Chondromalacia, left shoulder
M94.219 Chondromalacia, unspecified shoulder

6th **M94.22 Chondromalacia, elbow**
M94.221 Chondromalacia, right elbow
M94.222 Chondromalacia, left elbow
M94.229 Chondromalacia, unspecified elbow

6th **M94.23 Chondromalacia, wrist**
M94.231 Chondromalacia, right wrist
M94.232 Chondromalacia, left wrist
M94.239 Chondromalacia, unspecified wrist

6th **M94.24 Chondromalacia, joints of hand**
M94.241 Chondromalacia, joints of right hand
M94.242 Chondromalacia, joints of left hand
M94.249 Chondromalacia, joints of unspecified hand

6th **M94.25 Chondromalacia, hip**
M94.251 Chondromalacia, right hip
M94.252 Chondromalacia, left hip
M94.259 Chondromalacia, unspecified hip

6th **M94.26 Chondromalacia, knee**
M94.261 Chondromalacia, right knee
M94.262 Chondromalacia, left knee
M94.269 Chondromalacia, unspecified knee

6th **M94.27 Chondromalacia, ankle and joints of foot**
M94.271 Chondromalacia, right ankle and joints of right foot
M94.272 Chondromalacia, left ankle and joints of left foot
M94.279 Chondromalacia, unspecified ankle and joints of foot

M94.28 Chondromalacia, other site
M94.29 Chondromalacia, multiple sites

5th **M94.3 Chondrolysis**
Code first any associated slipped upper femoral epiphysis (nontraumatic) (M93.Ø-)

6th **M94.35 Chondrolysis, hip**
M94.351 Chondrolysis, right hip
M94.352 Chondrolysis, left hip
M94.359 Chondrolysis, unspecified hip

5th **M94.8 Other specified disorders of cartilage**

6th **M94.8X Other specified disorders of cartilage**
M94.8XØ Other specified disorders of cartilage, multiple sites
M94.8X1 Other specified disorders of cartilage, shoulder
M94.8X2 Other specified disorders of cartilage, upper arm
M94.8X3 Other specified disorders of cartilage, forearm
M94.8X4 Other specified disorders of cartilage, hand
M94.8X5 Other specified disorders of cartilage, thigh
M94.8X6 Other specified disorders of cartilage, lower leg
M94.8X7 Other specified disorders of cartilage, ankle and foot
M94.8X8 Other specified disorders of cartilage, other site
M94.8X9 Other specified disorders of cartilage, unspecified sites

M94.9 Disorder of cartilage, unspecified

Other disorders of the musculoskeletal system and connective tissue (M95)

4th **M95 Other acquired deformities of musculoskeletal system and connective tissue**
EXCLUDES 2 *acquired absence of limbs and organs (Z89-Z9Ø)*
acquired deformities of limbs (M2Ø-M21)
congenital malformations and deformations of the musculoskeletal system (Q65-Q79)
deforming dorsopathies (M4Ø-M43)
dentofacial anomalies [including malocclusion] (M26.-)
postprocedural musculoskeletal disorders (M96.-)

M95.Ø Acquired deformity of nose
EXCLUDES 2 *deviated nasal septum (J34.2)*

5th **M95.1 Cauliflower ear**
EXCLUDES 2 *other acquired deformities of ear (H61.1)*
DEF: Acquired deformity of the external ear due to injury or subsequent perichondritis.

M95.1Ø Cauliflower ear, unspecified ear
M95.11 Cauliflower ear, right ear
M95.12 Cauliflower ear, left ear

M95.2 Other acquired deformity of head
AHA: 2022,1Q,34

M95.3 Acquired deformity of neck

M95.4 Acquired deformity of chest and rib
AHA: 2022,2Q,14; 2014,4Q,26-27

M95.5 Acquired deformity of pelvis
EXCLUDES 1 *maternal care for known or suspected disproportion (O33.-)*

M95.8 Other specified acquired deformities of musculoskeletal system

M95.9 Acquired deformity of musculoskeletal system, unspecified

Intraoperative and postprocedural complications and disorders of musculoskeletal system, not elsewhere classified (M96)

M96 Intraoperative and postprocedural complications and disorders of musculoskeletal system, not elsewhere classified
EXCLUDES 2 *arthropathy following intestinal bypass (M02.0-)*
complications of internal orthopedic prosthetic devices, implants and grafts (T84.-)
disorders associated with osteoporosis (M80)
periprosthetic fracture around internal prosthetic joint (M97.-)
presence of functional implants and other devices (Z96-Z97)

M96.0 Pseudarthrosis after fusion or arthrodesis

M96.1 Postlaminectomy syndrome, not elsewhere classified

M96.2 Postradiation kyphosis

M96.3 Postlaminectomy kyphosis

M96.4 Postsurgical lordosis

M96.5 Postradiation scoliosis

M96.6 Fracture of bone following insertion of orthopedic implant, joint prosthesis, or bone plate
Intraoperative fracture of bone during insertion of orthopedic implant, joint prosthesis, or bone plate
EXCLUDES 2 *complication of internal orthopedic devices, implants or grafts (T84.-)*

M96.62 Fracture of humerus following insertion of orthopedic implant, joint prosthesis, or bone plate

M96.621 Fracture of humerus following insertion of orthopedic implant, joint prosthesis, or bone plate, right arm HCC ESR

M96.622 Fracture of humerus following insertion of orthopedic implant, joint prosthesis, or bone plate, left arm HCC ESR

M96.629 Fracture of humerus following insertion of orthopedic implant, joint prosthesis, or bone plate, unspecified arm HCC ESR

M96.63 Fracture of radius or ulna following insertion of orthopedic implant, joint prosthesis, or bone plate

M96.631 Fracture of radius or ulna following insertion of orthopedic implant, joint prosthesis, or bone plate, right arm HCC ESR

M96.632 Fracture of radius or ulna following insertion of orthopedic implant, joint prosthesis, or bone plate, left arm HCC ESR

M96.639 Fracture of radius or ulna following insertion of orthopedic implant, joint prosthesis, or bone plate, unspecified arm HCC ESR

M96.65 Fracture of pelvis following insertion of orthopedic implant, joint prosthesis, or bone plate HCC ESR

M96.66 Fracture of femur following insertion of orthopedic implant, joint prosthesis, or bone plate

M96.661 Fracture of femur following insertion of orthopedic implant, joint prosthesis, or bone plate, right leg HCC ESR

M96.662 Fracture of femur following insertion of orthopedic implant, joint prosthesis, or bone plate, left leg HCC ESR

M96.669 Fracture of femur following insertion of orthopedic implant, joint prosthesis, or bone plate, unspecified leg HCC ESR

M96.67 Fracture of tibia or fibula following insertion of orthopedic implant, joint prosthesis, or bone plate

M96.671 Fracture of tibia or fibula following insertion of orthopedic implant, joint prosthesis, or bone plate, right leg HCC ESR

M96.672 Fracture of tibia or fibula following insertion of orthopedic implant, joint prosthesis, or bone plate, left leg HCC ESR

M96.679 Fracture of tibia or fibula following insertion of orthopedic implant, joint prosthesis, or bone plate, unspecified leg HCC ESR

M96.69 Fracture of other bone following insertion of orthopedic implant, joint prosthesis, or bone plate HCC ESR

M96.8 Other intraoperative and postprocedural complications and disorders of musculoskeletal system, not elsewhere classified
AHA: 2016,4Q,9-10

M96.81 Intraoperative hemorrhage and hematoma of a musculoskeletal structure complicating a procedure
EXCLUDES 1 *intraoperative hemorrhage and hematoma of a musculoskeletal structure due to accidental puncture and laceration during a procedure (M96.82-)*

M96.810 Intraoperative hemorrhage and hematoma of a musculoskeletal structure complicating a musculoskeletal system procedure

M96.811 Intraoperative hemorrhage and hematoma of a musculoskeletal structure complicating other procedure

M96.82 Accidental puncture and laceration of a musculoskeletal structure during a procedure

M96.820 Accidental puncture and laceration of a musculoskeletal structure during a musculoskeletal system procedure

M96.821 Accidental puncture and laceration of a musculoskeletal structure during other procedure

M96.83 Postprocedural hemorrhage of a musculoskeletal structure following a procedure

M96.830 Postprocedural hemorrhage of a musculoskeletal structure following a musculoskeletal system procedure

M96.831 Postprocedural hemorrhage of a musculoskeletal structure following other procedure

M96.84 Postprocedural hematoma and seroma of a musculoskeletal structure following a procedure

M96.840 Postprocedural hematoma of a musculoskeletal structure following a musculoskeletal system procedure

M96.841 Postprocedural hematoma of a musculoskeletal structure following other procedure
AHA: 2016,4Q,10

M96.842 Postprocedural seroma of a musculoskeletal structure following a musculoskeletal system procedure

M96.843 Postprocedural seroma of a musculoskeletal structure following other procedure
AHA: 2018,3Q,6

M96.89 Other intraoperative and postprocedural complications and disorders of the musculoskeletal system
Instability of joint secondary to removal of joint prosthesis
Use additional code, if applicable, to further specify disorder
AHA: 2022,2Q,14; 2021,1Q,5

● **M96.A Fracture of ribs, sternum and thorax associated with compression of the chest and cardiopulmonary resuscitation**

● **M96.A1 Fracture of sternum associated with chest compression and cardiopulmonary resuscitation**
Fracture of xiphoid process associated with chest compression and cardiopulmonary resuscitation

● **M96.A2 Fracture of one rib associated with chest compression and cardiopulmonary resuscitation**

● **M96.A3 Multiple fractures of ribs associated with chest compression and cardiopulmonary resuscitation**

● **M96.A4 Flail chest associated with chest compression and cardiopulmonary resuscitation**

● **M96.A9 Other fracture associated with chest compression and cardiopulmonary resuscitation**

Periprosthetic fractures around internal prosthetic joint (M97)

M97 Periprosthetic fracture around internal prosthetic joint

EXCLUDES 2 *breakage (fracture) of prosthetic joint (T84.01-)*
fracture of bone following insertion of orthopedic implant, joint prosthesis or bone plate (M96.6-)

AHA: 2016,4Q,42-43

The appropriate 7th character is to be added to each code from category M97.
A initial encounter
D subsequent encounter
S sequela

M97.0 Periprosthetic fracture around internal prosthetic hip joint
AHA: 2018,1Q,21; 2016,4Q,42
1 **M97.01 Periprosthetic fracture around internal prosthetic right hip joint** HCC ESR Q
1 **M97.02 Periprosthetic fracture around internal prosthetic left hip joint** HCC ESR Q

M97.1 Periprosthetic fracture around internal prosthetic knee joint
M97.11 Periprosthetic fracture around internal prosthetic right knee joint Q
M97.12 Periprosthetic fracture around internal prosthetic left knee joint Q

M97.2 Periprosthetic fracture around internal prosthetic ankle joint
M97.21 Periprosthetic fracture around internal prosthetic right ankle joint Q
M97.22 Periprosthetic fracture around internal prosthetic left ankle joint Q

M97.3 Periprosthetic fracture around internal prosthetic shoulder joint
M97.31 Periprosthetic fracture around internal prosthetic right shoulder joint Q
M97.32 Periprosthetic fracture around internal prosthetic left shoulder joint Q

M97.4 Periprosthetic fracture around internal prosthetic elbow joint
M97.41 Periprosthetic fracture around internal prosthetic right elbow joint Q
M97.42 Periprosthetic fracture around internal prosthetic left elbow joint Q

M97.8 Periprosthetic fracture around other internal prosthetic joint
Periprosthetic fracture around internal prosthetic finger joint
Periprosthetic fracture around internal prosthetic spinal joint
Periprosthetic fracture around internal prosthetic toe joint
Periprosthetic fracture around internal prosthetic wrist joint
Use additional code to identify the joint (Z96.6-)

M97.9 Periprosthetic fracture around unspecified internal prosthetic joint

Biomechanical lesions, not elsewhere classified (M99)

M99 Biomechanical lesions, not elsewhere classified

NOTE This category should not be used if the condition can be classified elsewhere.

DEF: Biomechanical lesion: Term used by osteopathic and chiropractic physicians to describe musculoskeletal conditions treated that are not more appropriately classified elsewhere.

M99.0 Segmental and somatic dysfunction
M99.00 Segmental and somatic dysfunction of head region
M99.01 Segmental and somatic dysfunction of cervical region
M99.02 Segmental and somatic dysfunction of thoracic region
M99.03 Segmental and somatic dysfunction of lumbar region
M99.04 Segmental and somatic dysfunction of sacral region
M99.05 Segmental and somatic dysfunction of pelvic region
M99.06 Segmental and somatic dysfunction of lower extremity
M99.07 Segmental and somatic dysfunction of upper extremity
M99.08 Segmental and somatic dysfunction of rib cage
M99.09 Segmental and somatic dysfunction of abdomen and other regions

M99.1 Subluxation complex (vertebral)
M99.10 Subluxation complex (vertebral) of head region
M99.11 Subluxation complex (vertebral) of cervical region
M99.12 Subluxation complex (vertebral) of thoracic region
M99.13 Subluxation complex (vertebral) of lumbar region
M99.14 Subluxation complex (vertebral) of sacral region
M99.15 Subluxation complex (vertebral) of pelvic region
M99.16 Subluxation complex (vertebral) of lower extremity
M99.17 Subluxation complex (vertebral) of upper extremity
M99.18 Subluxation complex (vertebral) of rib cage
M99.19 Subluxation complex (vertebral) of abdomen and other regions

M99.2 Subluxation stenosis of neural canal
M99.20 Subluxation stenosis of neural canal of head region
M99.21 Subluxation stenosis of neural canal of cervical region
M99.22 Subluxation stenosis of neural canal of thoracic region
M99.23 Subluxation stenosis of neural canal of lumbar region
M99.24 Subluxation stenosis of neural canal of sacral region
M99.25 Subluxation stenosis of neural canal of pelvic region
M99.26 Subluxation stenosis of neural canal of lower extremity
M99.27 Subluxation stenosis of neural canal of upper extremity
M99.28 Subluxation stenosis of neural canal of rib cage
M99.29 Subluxation stenosis of neural canal of abdomen and other regions

M99.3 Osseous stenosis of neural canal
M99.30 Osseous stenosis of neural canal of head region
M99.31 Osseous stenosis of neural canal of cervical region
M99.32 Osseous stenosis of neural canal of thoracic region
M99.33 Osseous stenosis of neural canal of lumbar region
M99.34 Osseous stenosis of neural canal of sacral region
M99.35 Osseous stenosis of neural canal of pelvic region
M99.36 Osseous stenosis of neural canal of lower extremity
M99.37 Osseous stenosis of neural canal of upper extremity
M99.38 Osseous stenosis of neural canal of rib cage
M99.39 Osseous stenosis of neural canal of abdomen and other regions

M99.4 Connective tissue stenosis of neural canal
M99.40 Connective tissue stenosis of neural canal of head region
M99.41 Connective tissue stenosis of neural canal of cervical region
M99.42 Connective tissue stenosis of neural canal of thoracic region
M99.43 Connective tissue stenosis of neural canal of lumbar region
M99.44 Connective tissue stenosis of neural canal of sacral region
M99.45 Connective tissue stenosis of neural canal of pelvic region
M99.46 Connective tissue stenosis of neural canal of lower extremity
M99.47 Connective tissue stenosis of neural canal of upper extremity
M99.48 Connective tissue stenosis of neural canal of rib cage
M99.49 Connective tissue stenosis of neural canal of abdomen and other regions

M99.5 Intervertebral disc stenosis of neural canal
M99.50 Intervertebral disc stenosis of neural canal of head region
M99.51 Intervertebral disc stenosis of neural canal of cervical region
M99.52 Intervertebral disc stenosis of neural canal of thoracic region
M99.53 Intervertebral disc stenosis of neural canal of lumbar region
M99.54 Intervertebral disc stenosis of neural canal of sacral region
M99.55 Intervertebral disc stenosis of neural canal of pelvic region
M99.56 Intervertebral disc stenosis of neural canal of lower extremity
M99.57 Intervertebral disc stenosis of neural canal of upper extremity
M99.58 Intervertebral disc stenosis of neural canal of rib cage

M99.59 Intervertebral disc stenosis of neural canal of abdomen and other regions

✓5th M99.6 Osseous and subluxation stenosis of intervertebral foramina

M99.60 Osseous and subluxation stenosis of intervertebral foramina of head region

M99.61 Osseous and subluxation stenosis of intervertebral foramina of cervical region

M99.62 Osseous and subluxation stenosis of intervertebral foramina of thoracic region

M99.63 Osseous and subluxation stenosis of intervertebral foramina of lumbar region

M99.64 Osseous and subluxation stenosis of intervertebral foramina of sacral region

M99.65 Osseous and subluxation stenosis of intervertebral foramina of pelvic region

M99.66 Osseous and subluxation stenosis of intervertebral foramina of lower extremity

M99.67 Osseous and subluxation stenosis of intervertebral foramina of upper extremity

M99.68 Osseous and subluxation stenosis of intervertebral foramina of rib cage

M99.69 Osseous and subluxation stenosis of intervertebral foramina of abdomen and other regions

✓5th M99.7 Connective tissue and disc stenosis of intervertebral foramina

M99.70 Connective tissue and disc stenosis of intervertebral foramina of head region

M99.71 Connective tissue and disc stenosis of intervertebral foramina of cervical region

M99.72 Connective tissue and disc stenosis of intervertebral foramina of thoracic region

M99.73 Connective tissue and disc stenosis of intervertebral foramina of lumbar region

M99.74 Connective tissue and disc stenosis of intervertebral foramina of sacral region

M99.75 Connective tissue and disc stenosis of intervertebral foramina of pelvic region

M99.76 Connective tissue and disc stenosis of intervertebral foramina of lower extremity

M99.77 Connective tissue and disc stenosis of intervertebral foramina of upper extremity

M99.78 Connective tissue and disc stenosis of intervertebral foramina of rib cage

M99.79 Connective tissue and disc stenosis of intervertebral foramina of abdomen and other regions

✓5th M99.8 Other biomechanical lesions

M99.80 Other biomechanical lesions of head region

M99.81 Other biomechanical lesions of cervical region

M99.82 Other biomechanical lesions of thoracic region

M99.83 Other biomechanical lesions of lumbar region

M99.84 Other biomechanical lesions of sacral region

M99.85 Other biomechanical lesions of pelvic region

M99.86 Other biomechanical lesions of lower extremity

M99.87 Other biomechanical lesions of upper extremity

M99.88 Other biomechanical lesions of rib cage

M99.89 Other biomechanical lesions of abdomen and other regions

M99.9 Biomechanical lesion, unspecified

Chapter 14. Diseases of Genitourinary System (NØØ–N99)

Chapter-specific Guidelines with Coding Examples

The chapter-specific guidelines from the ICD-10-CM Official Guidelines for Coding and Reporting have been provided below. Along with these guidelines are coding examples, contained in the shaded boxes, that have been developed to help illustrate the coding and/or sequencing guidance found in these guidelines.

a. Chronic kidney disease

1) Stages of chronic kidney disease (CKD)

The ICD-10-CM classifies CKD based on severity. The severity of CKD is designated by stages 1-5. Stage 2, code N18.2, equates to mild CKD; stage 3, codes N18.3Ø-N18.32, equate to moderate CKD; and stage 4, code N18.4, equates to severe CKD. Code N18.6, End stage renal disease (ESRD), is assigned when the provider has documented end-stage renal disease (ESRD).

If both a stage of CKD and ESRD are documented, assign code N18.6 only.

Stage 5 chronic kidney disease with ESRD requiring chronic dialysis

N18.6 **End stage renal disease**

Z99.2 **Dependence on renal dialysis**

Explanation: The diagnostic statement indicates the patient has chronic kidney disease, documented both as stage 5 and as ESRD requiring chronic dialysis. Code N18.6 End stage renal disease (ESRD), is assigned when the provider has documented end-stage-renal disease (ESRD). If both a stage of CKD and ESRD are documented, assign code N18.6 only.

2) Chronic kidney disease and kidney transplant status

Patients who have undergone kidney transplant may still have some form of chronic kidney disease (CKD) because the kidney transplant may not fully restore kidney function. Therefore, the presence of CKD alone does not constitute a transplant complication. Assign the appropriate N18 code for the patient's stage of CKD and code Z94.Ø, Kidney transplant status. If a transplant complication such as failure or rejection or other transplant complication is documented, see section I.C.19.g for information on coding complications of a kidney transplant. If the documentation is unclear as to whether the patient has a complication of the transplant, query the provider.

Patient with residual chronic kidney disease stage 1 after kidney transplant

N18.1 **Chronic kidney disease, stage 1**

Z94.Ø **Kidney transplant status**

Explanation: Patients who have undergone kidney transplant may still have some form of chronic kidney disease (CKD) because the kidney transplant may not fully restore kidney function. The presence of CKD alone does not constitute a transplant complication. Assign the appropriate N18 code for the patient's stage of CKD and code Z94.Ø Kidney transplant status.

3) Chronic kidney disease with other conditions

Patients with CKD may also suffer from other serious conditions, most commonly diabetes mellitus and hypertension. The sequencing of the CKD code in relationship to codes for other contributing conditions is based on the conventions in the Tabular List.

See I.C.9. Hypertensive chronic kidney disease.

See I.C.19. Chronic kidney disease and kidney transplant complications.

Type 1 diabetic chronic kidney disease, stage 2

E1Ø.22 **Type 1 diabetes mellitus with diabetic chronic kidney disease**

N18.2 **Chronic kidney disease, stage 2 (mild)**

Explanation: Patients with CKD may also suffer from other serious conditions such as diabetes mellitus. The sequencing of the CKD code in relationship to codes for other contributing conditions is based on the conventions in the Tabular List. Diabetic CKD code E1Ø.22 includes an instructional note to "Use additional code to identify stage of chronic kidney disease (N18.1–N18.6)," thus providing sequencing direction.

Chapter 14. Diseases of the Genitourinary System (NØØ-N99)

EXCLUDES 2 *certain conditions originating in the perinatal period (PØ4-P96)*
certain infectious and parasitic diseases (AØØ-B99)
complications of pregnancy, childbirth and the puerperium (OØØ-O9A)
congenital malformations, deformations and chromosomal abnormalities (QØØ-Q99)
endocrine, nutritional and metabolic diseases (EØØ-E88)
injury, poisoning and certain other consequences of external causes (SØØ-T88)
neoplasms (CØØ-D49)
symptoms, signs and abnormal clinical and laboratory findings, not elsewhere classified (RØØ-R94)

This chapter contains the following blocks:

NØØ-NØ8 Glomerular diseases
N1Ø-N16 Renal tubulo-interstitial diseases
N17-N19 Acute kidney failure and chronic kidney disease
N2Ø-N23 Urolithiasis
N25-N29 Other disorders of kidney and ureter
N3Ø-N39 Other diseases of the urinary system
N4Ø-N53 Diseases of male genital organs
N6Ø-N65 Disorders of breast
N7Ø-N77 Inflammatory diseases of female pelvic organs
N8Ø-N98 Noninflammatory disorders of female genital tract
N99 Intraoperative and postprocedural complications and disorders of genitourinary system, not elsewhere classified

Glomerular diseases (NØØ-NØ8)

Code also any associated kidney failure (N17-N19).

EXCLUDES 1 *hypertensive chronic kidney disease (I12.-)*

AHA: 2020,4Q,34-35

DEF: Glomeruli: Clusters of microscopic blood vessels located within the kidneys containing small pores through which waste products are filtered from the blood and urine is formed.

DEF: Glomerulonephritis: Disease of the kidney with diffuse inflammation of the capillary loops of the glomeruli.

✓4th NØØ Acute nephritic syndrome

INCLUDES acute glomerular disease
acute glomerulonephritis
acute nephritis

EXCLUDES 1 *acute tubulo-interstitial nephritis (N1Ø)*
nephritic syndrome NOS (NØ5.-)

AHA: 2021,1Q,23

NØØ.Ø Acute nephritic syndrome with minor glomerular abnormality
Acute nephritic syndrome with minimal change lesion

NØØ.1 Acute nephritic syndrome with focal and segmental glomerular lesions
Acute nephritic syndrome with focal and segmental hyalinosis
Acute nephritic syndrome with focal and segmental sclerosis
Acute nephritic syndrome with focal glomerulonephritis

NØØ.2 Acute nephritic syndrome with diffuse membranous glomerulonephritis

NØØ.3 Acute nephritic syndrome with diffuse mesangial proliferative glomerulonephritis

NØØ.4 Acute nephritic syndrome with diffuse endocapillary proliferative glomerulonephritis

NØØ.5 Acute nephritic syndrome with diffuse mesangiocapillary glomerulonephritis
Acute nephritic syndrome with membranoproliferative glomerulonephritis, types 1 and 3, or NOS

EXCLUDES 1 *acute nephritic syndrome with C3 glomerulonephritis (NØØ.A)*
acute nephritic syndrome with C3 glomerulopathy (NØØ.A)

NØØ.6 Acute nephritic syndrome with dense deposit disease
Acute nephritic syndrome with C3 glomerulopathy with dense deposit disease
Acute nephritic syndrome with membranoproliferative glomerulonephritis, type 2

NØØ.7 Acute nephritic syndrome with diffuse crescentic glomerulonephritis
Acute nephritic syndrome with extracapillary glomerulonephritis

NØØ.8 Acute nephritic syndrome with other morphologic changes
Acute nephritic syndrome with proliferative glomerulonephritis NOS

NØØ.9 Acute nephritic syndrome with unspecified morphologic changes

NØØ.A Acute nephritic syndrome with C3 glomerulonephritis
Acute nephritic syndrome with C3 glomerulopathy, NOS

EXCLUDES 1 *acute nephritic syndrome (with C3 glomerulopathy) with dense deposit disease (NØØ.6)*

✓4th NØ1 Rapidly progressive nephritic syndrome

INCLUDES rapidly progressive glomerular disease
rapidly progressive glomerulonephritis
rapidly progressive nephritis

EXCLUDES 1 *nephritic syndrome NOS (NØ5.-)*

AHA: 2021,1Q,23

NØ1.Ø Rapidly progressive nephritic syndrome with minor glomerular abnormality
Rapidly progressive nephritic syndrome with minimal change lesion

NØ1.1 Rapidly progressive nephritic syndrome with focal and segmental glomerular lesions
Rapidly progressive nephritic syndrome with focal and segmental hyalinosis
Rapidly progressive nephritic syndrome with focal and segmental sclerosis
Rapidly progressive nephritic syndrome with focal glomerulonephritis

NØ1.2 Rapidly progressive nephritic syndrome with diffuse membranous glomerulonephritis

NØ1.3 Rapidly progressive nephritic syndrome with diffuse mesangial proliferative glomerulonephritis

NØ1.4 Rapidly progressive nephritic syndrome with diffuse endocapillary proliferative glomerulonephritis

NØ1.5 Rapidly progressive nephritic syndrome with diffuse mesangiocapillary glomerulonephritis
Rapidly progressive nephritic syndrome with membranoproliferative glomerulonephritis, types 1 and 3, or NOS

EXCLUDES 1 *rapidly progressive nephritic syndrome with C3 glomerulonephritis (NØ1.A)*
rapidly progressive nephritic syndrome with C3 glomerulopathy (NØ1.A)

NØ1.6 Rapidly progressive nephritic syndrome with dense deposit disease
Rapidly progressive nephritic syndrome with C3 glomerulopathy with dense deposit disease
Rapidly progressive nephritic syndrome with membranoproliferative glomerulonephritis, type 2

NØ1.7 Rapidly progressive nephritic syndrome with diffuse crescentic glomerulonephritis
Rapidly progressive nephritic syndrome with extracapillary glomerulonephritis

NØ1.8 Rapidly progressive nephritic syndrome with other morphologic changes
Rapidly progressive nephritic syndrome with proliferative glomerulonephritis NOS

NØ1.9 Rapidly progressive nephritic syndrome with unspecified morphologic changes

NØ1.A Rapidly progressive nephritic syndrome with C3 glomerulonephritis
Rapidly progressive nephritic syndrome with C3 glomerulopathy, NOS

EXCLUDES 1 *rapidly progressive nephritic syndrome (with C3 glomerulopathy) with dense deposit disease (NØ1.6)*

✓4th NØ2 Recurrent and persistent hematuria

EXCLUDES 1 *acute cystitis with hematuria (N3Ø.Ø1)*
hematuria NOS (R31.9)
hematuria not associated with specified morphologic lesions (R31.-)

NØ2.Ø Recurrent and persistent hematuria with minor glomerular abnormality
Recurrent and persistent hematuria with minimal change lesion

NØ2.1 Recurrent and persistent hematuria with focal and segmental glomerular lesions
Recurrent and persistent hematuria with focal and segmental hyalinosis
Recurrent and persistent hematuria with focal and segmental sclerosis
Recurrent and persistent hematuria with focal glomerulonephritis

NØ2.2 Recurrent and persistent hematuria with diffuse membranous glomerulonephritis

NØ2.3 Recurrent and persistent hematuria with diffuse mesangial proliferative glomerulonephritis

NØ2.4 Recurrent and persistent hematuria with diffuse endocapillary proliferative glomerulonephritis

NØ2.5 Recurrent and persistent hematuria with diffuse mesangiocapillary glomerulonephritis

Recurrent and persistent hematuria with membranoproliferative glomerulonephritis, types 1 and 3, or NOS

EXCLUDES 1 *recurrent and persistent hematuria with C3 glomerulonephritis (NØ2.A)*

recurrent and persistent hematuria with C3 glomerulopathy (NØ2.A)

NØ2.6 Recurrent and persistent hematuria with dense deposit disease

Recurrent and persistent hematuria with C3 glomerulopathy with dense deposit disease

Recurrent and persistent hematuria with membranoproliferative glomerulonephritis, type 2

NØ2.7 Recurrent and persistent hematuria with diffuse crescentic glomerulonephritis

Recurrent and persistent hematuria with extracapillary glomerulonephritis

NØ2.8 Recurrent and persistent hematuria with other morphologic changes

Recurrent and persistent hematuria with proliferative glomerulonephritis NOS

NØ2.9 Recurrent and persistent hematuria with unspecified morphologic changes

AHA: 2017,2Q,5

NØ2.A Recurrent and persistent hematuria with C3 glomerulonephritis

Recurrent and persistent hematuria with C3 glomerulopathy

EXCLUDES 1 *recurrent and persistent hematuria (with C3 glomerulopathy) with dense deposit disease (NØ2.6)*

4th NØ3 Chronic nephritic syndrome

INCLUDES chronic glomerular disease

chronic glomerulonephritis

chronic nephritis

EXCLUDES 1 *chronic tubulo-interstitial nephritis (N11.-)*

diffuse sclerosing glomerulonephritis (NØ5.8-)

nephritic syndrome NOS (NØ5.-)

AHA: 2021,1Q,23

DEF: Slow, progressive type of nephritis characterized by inflammation of the capillary loops in the glomeruli of the kidney, which leads to renal failure.

NØ3.Ø Chronic nephritic syndrome with minor glomerular abnormality

Chronic nephritic syndrome with minimal change lesion

NØ3.1 Chronic nephritic syndrome with focal and segmental glomerular lesions

Chronic nephritic syndrome with focal and segmental hyalinosis

Chronic nephritic syndrome with focal and segmental sclerosis

Chronic nephritic syndrome with focal glomerulonephritis

NØ3.2 Chronic nephritic syndrome with diffuse membranous glomerulonephritis

NØ3.3 Chronic nephritic syndrome with diffuse mesangial proliferative glomerulonephritis

NØ3.4 Chronic nephritic syndrome with diffuse endocapillary proliferative glomerulonephritis

NØ3.5 Chronic nephritic syndrome with diffuse mesangiocapillary glomerulonephritis

Chronic nephritic syndrome with membranoproliferative glomerulonephritis, types 1 and 3, or NOS

EXCLUDES 1 *chronic nephritic syndrome with C3 glomerulonephritis (NØ3.A)*

chronic nephritic syndrome with C3 glomerulopathy (NØ3.A)

NØ3.6 Chronic nephritic syndrome with dense deposit disease

Chronic nephritic syndrome with C3 glomerulopathy with dense deposit disease

Chronic nephritic syndrome with membranoproliferative glomerulonephritis, type 2

NØ3.7 Chronic nephritic syndrome with diffuse crescentic glomerulonephritis

Chronic nephritic syndrome with extracapillary glomerulonephritis

NØ3.8 Chronic nephritic syndrome with other morphologic changes

Chronic nephritic syndrome with proliferative glomerulonephritis NOS

NØ3.9 Chronic nephritic syndrome with unspecified morphologic changes

NØ3.A Chronic nephritic syndrome with C3 glomerulonephritis

Chronic nephritic syndrome with C3 glomerulopathy

EXCLUDES 1 *chronic nephritic syndrome (with C3 glomerulopathy) with dense deposit disease (NØ3.6)*

4th NØ4 Nephrotic syndrome

INCLUDES congenital nephrotic syndrome

lipoid nephrosis

NØ4.Ø Nephrotic syndrome with minor glomerular abnormality

Nephrotic syndrome with minimal change lesion

NØ4.1 Nephrotic syndrome with focal and segmental glomerular lesions

Nephrotic syndrome with focal and segmental hyalinosis

Nephrotic syndrome with focal and segmental sclerosis

Nephrotic syndrome with focal glomerulonephritis

NØ4.2 Nephrotic syndrome with diffuse membranous glomerulonephritis

NØ4.3 Nephrotic syndrome with diffuse mesangial proliferative glomerulonephritis

NØ4.4 Nephrotic syndrome with diffuse endocapillary proliferative glomerulonephritis

NØ4.5 Nephrotic syndrome with diffuse mesangiocapillary glomerulonephritis

Nephrotic syndrome with membranoproliferative glomerulonephritis, types 1 and 3, or NOS

EXCLUDES 1 *nephrotic syndrome with C3 glomerulonephritis (NØ4.A)*

nephrotic syndrome with C3 glomerulopathy (NØ4.A)

NØ4.6 Nephrotic syndrome with dense deposit disease

Nephrotic syndrome with C3 glomerulopathy with dense deposit disease

Nephrotic syndrome with membranoproliferative glomerulonephritis, type 2

NØ4.7 Nephrotic syndrome with diffuse crescentic glomerulonephritis

Nephrotic syndrome with extracapillary glomerulonephritis

NØ4.8 Nephrotic syndrome with other morphologic changes

Nephrotic syndrome with proliferative glomerulonephritis NOS

NØ4.9 Nephrotic syndrome with unspecified morphologic changes

NØ4.A Nephrotic syndrome with C3 glomerulonephritis

Nephrotic syndrome with C3 glomerulopathy

EXCLUDES 1 *nephrotic syndrome (with C3 glomerulopathy) with dense deposit disease (NØ4.6)*

4th NØ5 Unspecified nephritic syndrome

INCLUDES glomerular disease NOS

glomerulonephritis NOS

nephritis NOS

nephropathy NOS and renal disease NOS with morphological lesion specified in .Ø-.8

EXCLUDES 1 *nephropathy NOS with no stated morphological lesion (N28.9)*

renal disease NOS with no stated morphological lesion (N28.9)

tubulo-interstitial nephritis NOS (N12)

NØ5.Ø Unspecified nephritic syndrome with minor glomerular abnormality

Unspecified nephritic syndrome with minimal change lesion

NØ5.1 Unspecified nephritic syndrome with focal and segmental glomerular lesions

Unspecified nephritic syndrome with focal and segmental hyalinosis

Unspecified nephritic syndrome with focal and segmental sclerosis

Unspecified nephritic syndrome with focal glomerulonephritis

NØ5.2 Unspecified nephritic syndrome with diffuse membranous glomerulonephritis

NØ5.3 Unspecified nephritic syndrome with diffuse mesangial proliferative glomerulonephritis

NØ5.4 Unspecified nephritic syndrome with diffuse endocapillary proliferative glomerulonephritis

NØ5.5 Unspecified nephritic syndrome with diffuse mesangiocapillary glomerulonephritis
Unspecified nephritic syndrome with membranoproliferative glomerulonephritis, types 1 and 3, or NOS
EXCLUDES 1 *unspecified nephritic syndrome with C3 glomerulonephritis (NØ5.A)*
unspecified nephritic syndrome with C3 glomerulopathy (NØ5.A)

NØ5.6 Unspecified nephritic syndrome with dense deposit disease
Unspecified nephritic syndrome with C3 glomerulopathy with dense deposit disease
Unspecified nephritic syndrome with membranoproliferative glomerulonephritis, type 2

NØ5.7 Unspecified nephritic syndrome with diffuse crescentic glomerulonephritis
Unspecified nephritic syndrome with extracapillary glomerulonephritis

NØ5.8 Unspecified nephritic syndrome with other morphologic changes
Unspecified nephritic syndrome with proliferative glomerulonephritis NOS

NØ5.9 Unspecified nephritic syndrome with unspecified morphologic changes

NØ5.A Unspecified nephritic syndrome with C3 glomerulonephritis
Unspecified nephritic syndrome with C3 glomerulopathy
EXCLUDES 1 *unspecified nephritic syndrome (with C3 glomerulopathy) with dense deposit disease (NØ5.6)*

✓4th NØ6 Isolated proteinuria with specified morphological lesion
EXCLUDES 1 *proteinuria not associated with specific morphologic lesions (R8Ø.Ø)*

NØ6.Ø Isolated proteinuria with minor glomerular abnormality
Isolated proteinuria with minimal change lesion

NØ6.1 Isolated proteinuria with focal and segmental glomerular lesions
Isolated proteinuria with focal and segmental hyalinosis
Isolated proteinuria with focal and segmental sclerosis
Isolated proteinuria with focal glomerulonephritis

NØ6.2 Isolated proteinuria with diffuse membranous glomerulonephritis

NØ6.3 Isolated proteinuria with diffuse mesangial proliferative glomerulonephritis

NØ6.4 Isolated proteinuria with diffuse endocapillary proliferative glomerulonephritis

NØ6.5 Isolated proteinuria with diffuse mesangiocapillary glomerulonephritis
Isolated proteinuria with membranoproliferative glomerulonephritis, types 1 and 3, or NOS
EXCLUDES 1 *isolated proteinuria with C3 glomerulonephritis (NØ6.A)*
isolated proteinuria with C3 glomerulopathy (NØ6.A)

NØ6.6 Isolated proteinuria with dense deposit disease
Isolated proteinuria with C3 glomerulopathy with dense deposit disease
Isolated proteinuria with membranoproliferative glomerulonephritis, type 2

NØ6.7 Isolated proteinuria with diffuse crescentic glomerulonephritis
Isolated proteinuria with extracapillary glomerulonephritis

NØ6.8 Isolated proteinuria with other morphologic lesion
Isolated proteinuria with proliferative glomerulonephritis NOS

NØ6.9 Isolated proteinuria with unspecified morphologic lesion

NØ6.A Isolated proteinuria with C3 glomerulonephritis
Isolated proteinuria with C3 glomerulopathy
EXCLUDES 1 *isolated proteinuria (with C3 glomerulopathy) with dense deposit disease (NØ6.6)*

✓4th NØ7 Hereditary nephropathy, not elsewhere classified
EXCLUDES 2 *Alport's syndrome (Q87.81-)*
hereditary amyloid nephropathy (E85.-)
nail patella syndrome (Q87.2)
non-neuropathic heredofamilial amyloidosis (E85.-)

NØ7.Ø Hereditary nephropathy, not elsewhere classified with minor glomerular abnormality
Hereditary nephropathy, not elsewhere classified with minimal change lesion

NØ7.1 Hereditary nephropathy, not elsewhere classified with focal and segmental glomerular lesions
Hereditary nephropathy, not elsewhere classified with focal and segmental hyalinosis
Hereditary nephropathy, not elsewhere classified with focal and segmental sclerosis
Hereditary nephropathy, not elsewhere classified with focal glomerulonephritis

NØ7.2 Hereditary nephropathy, not elsewhere classified with diffuse membranous glomerulonephritis

NØ7.3 Hereditary nephropathy, not elsewhere classified with diffuse mesangial proliferative glomerulonephritis

NØ7.4 Hereditary nephropathy, not elsewhere classified with diffuse endocapillary proliferative glomerulonephritis

NØ7.5 Hereditary nephropathy, not elsewhere classified with diffuse mesangiocapillary glomerulonephritis
Hereditary nephropathy, not elsewhere classified with membranoproliferative glomerulonephritis, types 1 and 3, or NOS
EXCLUDES 1 *hereditary nephropathy, not elsewhere classified with C3 glomerulonephritis (NØ7.A)*
hereditary nephropathy, not elsewhere classified with C3 glomerulopathy (NØ7.A)

NØ7.6 Hereditary nephropathy, not elsewhere classified with dense deposit disease
Hereditary nephropathy, not elsewhere classified with C3 glomerulopathy with dense deposit disease
Hereditary nephropathy, not elsewhere classified with membranoproliferative glomerulonephritis, type 2

NØ7.7 Hereditary nephropathy, not elsewhere classified with diffuse crescentic glomerulonephritis
Hereditary nephropathy, not elsewhere classified with extracapillary glomerulonephritis

NØ7.8 Hereditary nephropathy, not elsewhere classified with other morphologic lesions
Hereditary nephropathy, not elsewhere classified with proliferative glomerulonephritis NOS

NØ7.9 Hereditary nephropathy, not elsewhere classified with unspecified morphologic lesions

NØ7.A Hereditary nephropathy, not elsewhere classified with C3 glomerulonephritis
Hereditary nephropathy, not elsewhere classified with C3 glomerulopathy
EXCLUDES 1 *hereditary nephropathy, not elsewhere classified (with C3 glomerulopathy) with dense deposit disease (NØ7.6)*

NØ8 Glomerular disorders in diseases classified elsewhere
Glomerulonephritis
Nephritis
Nephropathy
Code first underlying disease, such as:
amyloidosis (E85.-)
congenital syphilis (A5Ø.5)
cryoglobulinemia (D89.1)
disseminated intravascular coagulation (D65)
gout (M1A.-, M1Ø.-)
microscopic polyangiitis (M31.7)
multiple myeloma (C9Ø.Ø-)
sepsis (A4Ø.Ø-A41.9)
sickle-cell disease (D57.Ø-D57.8)
EXCLUDES 1 *glomerulonephritis, nephritis and nephropathy (in):*
antiglomerular basement membrane disease (M31.Ø)
diabetes (EØ8-E13 with .21)
gonococcal (A54.21)
Goodpasture's syndrome (M31.Ø)
hemolytic-uremic syndrome ▶(D59.3-)◀
lupus (M32.14)
mumps (B26.83)
syphilis (A52.75)
systemic lupus erythematosus (M32.14)
Wegener's granulomatosis (M31.31)
pyelonephritis in diseases classified elsewhere (N16)
renal tubulo-interstitial disorders classified elsewhere (N16)

Renal tubulo-interstitial diseases (N10-N16)

INCLUDES pyelonephritis

EXCLUDES 1 *pyeloureteritis cystica (N28.85)*

N10 Acute pyelonephritis

Acute infectious interstitial nephritis
Acute pyelitis
Acute tubulo-interstitial nephritis
Hemoglobin nephrosis
Myoglobin nephrosis
Use additional code (B95-B97), to identify infectious agent
AHA: 2020,3Q,25; 2019,3Q,13

✓4th **N11 Chronic tubulo-interstitial nephritis**

INCLUDES chronic infectious interstitial nephritis
chronic pyelitis
chronic pyelonephritis
Use additional code (B95-B97), to identify infectious agent

N11.0 Nonobstructive reflux-associated chronic pyelonephritis

Pyelonephritis (chronic) associated with (vesicoureteral) reflux
EXCLUDES 1 *vesicoureteral reflux NOS (N13.70)*

N11.1 Chronic obstructive pyelonephritis

Pyelonephritis (chronic) associated with anomaly of pelviureteric junction
Pyelonephritis (chronic) associated with anomaly of pyeloureteric junction
Pyelonephritis (chronic) associated with crossing of vessel
Pyelonephritis (chronic) associated with kinking of ureter
Pyelonephritis (chronic) associated with obstruction of ureter
Pyelonephritis (chronic) associated with stricture of pelviureteric junction
Pyelonephritis (chronic) associated with stricture of ureter
EXCLUDES 1 *calculous pyelonephritis (N20.9)*
obstructive uropathy (N13.-)

N11.8 Other chronic tubulo-interstitial nephritis

Nonobstructive chronic pyelonephritis NOS

N11.9 Chronic tubulo-interstitial nephritis, unspecified

Chronic interstitial nephritis NOS
Chronic pyelitis NOS
Chronic pyelonephritis NOS

N12 Tubulo-interstitial nephritis, not specified as acute or chronic

Interstitial nephritis NOS
Pyelitis NOS
Pyelonephritis NOS
EXCLUDES 1 *calculous pyelonephritis (N20.9)*

✓4th **N13 Obstructive and reflux uropathy**

EXCLUDES 2 *calculus of kidney and ureter without hydronephrosis (N20.-)*
congenital obstructive defects of renal pelvis and ureter (Q62.0-Q62.3)
hydronephrosis with ureteropelvic junction obstruction (Q62.11)
obstructive pyelonephritis (N11.1)

DEF: Hydronephrosis: Distension of the kidney caused by an accumulation of urine that cannot flow out due to an obstruction that may be caused by conditions such as kidney stones or vesicoureteral reflux.

N13.0 Hydronephrosis with ureteropelvic junction obstruction

Hydronephrosis due to acquired occlusion of ureteropelvic junction
EXCLUDES 2 *hydronephrosis with ureteropelvic junction obstruction due to calculus (N13.2)*
AHA: 2016,4Q,43

Hydronephrosis/UPJ Obstruction

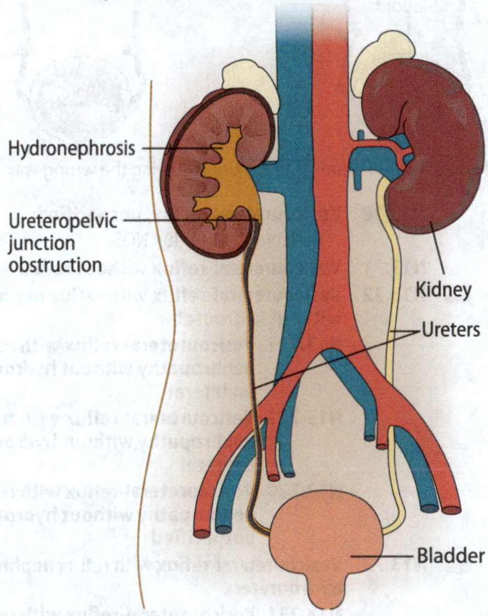

N13.1 Hydronephrosis with ureteral stricture, not elsewhere classified

EXCLUDES 1 *hydronephrosis with ureteral stricture with infection (N13.6)*

N13.2 Hydronephrosis with renal and ureteral calculous obstruction

EXCLUDES 1 *hydronephrosis with renal and ureteral calculous obstruction with infection (N13.6)*

✓5th **N13.3 Other and unspecified hydronephrosis**

EXCLUDES 1 *hydronephrosis with infection (N13.6)*

N13.30 Unspecified hydronephrosis

N13.39 Other hydronephrosis

N13.4 Hydroureter

EXCLUDES 1 *congenital hydroureter (Q62.3-)*
hydroureter with infection (N13.6)
vesicoureteral-reflux with hydroureter (N13.73-)

DEF: Abnormal enlargement or distension of the ureter with water or urine caused by an obstruction.

N13.5 Crossing vessel and stricture of ureter without hydronephrosis

Kinking and stricture of ureter without hydronephrosis
EXCLUDES 1 *crossing vessel and stricture of ureter without hydronephrosis with infection (N13.6)*

N13.6 Pyonephrosis

Conditions in N13.0-N13.5 with infection
Obstructive uropathy with infection
Use additional code (B95-B97), to identify infectious agent
AHA: 2018,2Q,21

N13.7 Vesicoureteral-reflux

EXCLUDES 1 *reflux-associated pyelonephritis (N11.Ø)*

DEF: Urine passage from the bladder flows backward up into the ureter and kidneys that can lead to bacterial infection and an increase in hydrostatic pressure, causing kidney damage.

Vesicoureteral Reflux

N13.7Ø Vesicoureteral-reflux, unspecified
Vesicoureteral-reflux NOS

N13.71 Vesicoureteral-reflux without reflux nephropathy

N13.72 Vesicoureteral-reflux with reflux nephropathy without hydroureter

N13.721 Vesicoureteral-reflux with reflux nephropathy without hydroureter, unilateral

N13.722 Vesicoureteral-reflux with reflux nephropathy without hydroureter, bilateral

N13.729 Vesicoureteral-reflux with reflux nephropathy without hydroureter, unspecified

N13.73 Vesicoureteral-reflux with reflux nephropathy with hydroureter

N13.731 Vesicoureteral-reflux with reflux nephropathy with hydroureter, unilateral

N13.732 Vesicoureteral-reflux with reflux nephropathy with hydroureter, bilateral

N13.739 Vesicoureteral-reflux with reflux nephropathy with hydroureter, unspecified

N13.8 Other obstructive and reflux uropathy
Urinary tract obstruction due to specified cause
Code first, if applicable, any causal condition, such as:
enlarged prostate (N4Ø.1)

N13.9 Obstructive and reflux uropathy, unspecified
Urinary tract obstruction NOS

N14 Drug- and heavy-metal-induced tubulo-interstitial and tubular conditions
Code first poisoning due to drug or toxin, if applicable (T36-T65 with fifth or sixth character 1-4 or 6)
Use additional code for adverse effect, if applicable, to identify drug (T36-T5Ø with fifth or sixth character 5)

N14.Ø Analgesic nephropathy

▲ **N14.1 Nephropathy induced by other drugs, medicaments and biological substances**
AHA: 2021,3Q,9-10

● **N14.11 Contrast-induced nephropathy**
Contrast medium, radiography nephropathy
EXCLUDES 2 *acute kidney failure (N17.-)*

● **N14.19 Nephropathy induced by other drugs, medicaments and biological substances**

N14.2 Nephropathy induced by unspecified drug, medicament or biological substance

N14.3 Nephropathy induced by heavy metals

N14.4 Toxic nephropathy, not elsewhere classified

N15 Other renal tubulo-interstitial diseases

N15.Ø Balkan nephropathy
Balkan endemic nephropathy

N15.1 Renal and perinephric abscess

N15.8 Other specified renal tubulo-interstitial diseases

N15.9 Renal tubulo-interstitial disease, unspecified
Infection of kidney NOS
EXCLUDES 1 *urinary tract infection NOS (N39.Ø)*

N16 Renal tubulo-interstitial disorders in diseases classified elsewhere
Pyelonephritis
Tubulo-interstitial nephritis
Code first underlying disease, such as:
brucellosis (A23.Ø-A23.9)
cryoglobulinemia (D89.1)
glycogen storage disease (E74.Ø)
leukemia (C91-C95)
lymphoma (C81.Ø-C85.9, C96.Ø-C96.9)
multiple myeloma (C9Ø.Ø-)
sepsis (A4Ø.Ø-A41.9)
Wilson's disease (E83.Ø)

EXCLUDES 1 *diphtheritic pyelonephritis and tubulo-interstitial nephritis (A36.84)*
pyelonephritis and tubulo-interstitial nephritis in candidiasis (B37.49)
pyelonephritis and tubulo-interstitial nephritis in cystinosis (E72.Ø4)
pyelonephritis and tubulo-interstitial nephritis in salmonella infection (AØ2.25)
pyelonephritis and tubulo-interstitial nephritis in sarcoidosis (D86.84)
pyelonephritis and tubulo-interstitial nephritis in Sjögren syndrome (M35.Ø4)
pyelonephritis and tubulo-interstitial nephritis in systemic lupus erythematosus (M32.15)
pyelonephritis and tubulo-interstitial nephritis in toxoplasmosis (B58.83)
renal tubular degeneration in diabetes (EØ8-E13 with .29)
syphilitic pyelonephritis and tubulo-interstitial nephritis (A52.75)

Acute kidney failure and chronic kidney disease (N17-N19)

EXCLUDES 2 *congenital renal failure (P96.Ø)*
drug- and heavy-metal-induced tubulo-interstitial and tubular conditions (N14.-)
extrarenal uremia (R39.2)
hemolytic-uremic syndrome ►(D59.3-)◄
hepatorenal syndrome (K76.7)
postpartum hepatorenal syndrome (O9Ø.4)
posttraumatic renal failure (T79.5)
prerenal uremia (R39.2)
renal failure complicating abortion or ectopic or molar pregnancy (OØØ-OØ7, OØ8.4)
renal failure following labor and delivery (O9Ø.4)
renal failure postprocedural (N99.Ø)

N17 Acute kidney failure
Code also associated underlying condition
EXCLUDES 1 *posttraumatic renal failure (T79.5)*
AHA: 2020,3Q,22; 2019,2Q,7; 2019,1Q,12; 2013,4Q,124

N17.Ø Acute kidney failure with tubular necrosis HCC ESR
Acute tubular necrosis
Renal tubular necrosis
Tubular necrosis NOS
AHA: 2021,3Q,10

N17.1 Acute kidney failure with acute cortical necrosis HCC ESR
Acute cortical necrosis
Cortical necrosis NOS
Renal cortical necrosis

N17.2 Acute kidney failure with medullary necrosis HCC ESR
Medullary [papillary] necrosis NOS
Acute medullary [papillary] necrosis
Renal medullary [papillary] necrosis

N17.8 Other acute kidney failure HCC ESR

N17.9 Acute kidney failure, unspecified HCC ESR
Acute kidney injury (nontraumatic)
EXCLUDES 2 *traumatic kidney injury (S37.Ø-)*

N18 Chronic kidney disease (CKD)
Code first any associated:
diabetic chronic kidney disease (E08.22, E09.22, E10.22, E11.22, E13.22)
hypertensive chronic kidney disease (I12.-, I13.-)
Use additional code to identify kidney transplant status, if applicable, (Z94.0)
AHA: 2019,3Q,3; 2018,4Q,88; 2013,1Q,24
TIP: CKD/ESRD occurring in an individual with a history of kidney transplant should not be assumed to be a transplant complication unless specifically indicated as such by provider documentation.

N18.1 Chronic kidney disease, stage 1
N18.2 Chronic kidney disease, stage 2 (mild)
N18.3 Chronic kidney disease, stage 3 (moderate)
AHA: 2020,4Q,35
N18.30 Chronic kidney disease, stage 3 unspecified HCC ESR
N18.31 Chronic kidney disease, stage 3a HCC ESR
N18.32 Chronic kidney disease, stage 3b HCC ESR
N18.4 Chronic kidney disease, stage 4 (severe) HCC Rx ESR COM
N18.5 Chronic kidney disease, stage 5 HCC Rx ESR COM
EXCLUDES 1 *chronic kidney disease, stage 5 requiring chronic dialysis (N18.6)*
DEF: End-stage renal disease (ESRD) with a GFR value of 15 ml/min or less not yet requiring chronic dialysis.
TIP: When both ESRD and CKD 5 are documented, code only for ESRD.
N18.6 End stage renal disease HCC Rx ESR COM
Chronic kidney disease requiring chronic dialysis
Use additional code to identify dialysis status (Z99.2)
AHA: 2016,3Q,22; 2016,1Q,12; 2013,4Q,124-125
TIP: When both ESRD and CKD 5 are documented, code only for ESRD.
N18.9 Chronic kidney disease, unspecified
Chronic renal disease
Chronic renal failure NOS
Chronic renal insufficiency
Chronic uremia NOS
Diffuse sclerosing glomerulonephritis NOS

N19 Unspecified kidney failure
Uremia NOS
EXCLUDES 1 *acute kidney failure (N17.-)*
chronic kidney disease (N18.-)
chronic uremia (N18.9)
extrarenal uremia (R39.2)
prerenal uremia (R39.2)
renal insufficiency (acute) (N28.9)
uremia of newborn (P96.0)

Urolithiasis (N20-N23)

AHA: 2017,1Q,5; 2015,2Q,8
TIP: Codes from this code block can be assigned based on the diagnosis listed in a radiology report when authenticated by a radiologist and available at the time of code assignment.

N20 Calculus of kidney and ureter
Calculous pyelonephritis
EXCLUDES 1 *nephrocalcinosis (E83.5)*
that with hydronephrosis (N13.2)
AHA: 2019,3Q,13
N20.0 Calculus of kidney
Nephrolithiasis NOS
Renal calculus
Renal stone
Staghorn calculus
Stone in kidney
AHA: 2019,3Q,13
N20.1 Calculus of ureter
Calculus of the ureteropelvic junction
Ureteric stone
AHA: 2016,3Q,22
N20.2 Calculus of kidney with calculus of ureter
N20.9 Urinary calculus, unspecified

N21 Calculus of lower urinary tract
INCLUDES calculus of lower urinary tract with cystitis and urethritis
N21.0 Calculus in bladder
Calculus in diverticulum of bladder
Urinary bladder stone
EXCLUDES 2 *staghorn calculus (N20.0)*
N21.1 Calculus in urethra
EXCLUDES 2 *calculus of prostate (N42.0)*
N21.8 Other lower urinary tract calculus
N21.9 Calculus of lower urinary tract, unspecified
EXCLUDES 1 *calculus of urinary tract NOS (N20.9)*

N22 Calculus of urinary tract in diseases classified elsewhere
Code first underlying disease, such as:
gout (M1A.-, M10.-)
schistosomiasis (B65.0-B65.9)

N23 Unspecified renal colic

Other disorders of kidney and ureter (N25-N29)

EXCLUDES 2 *disorders of kidney and ureter with urolithiasis (N20-N23)*

N25 Disorders resulting from impaired renal tubular function
N25.0 Renal osteodystrophy Rx
Azotemic osteodystrophy
Phosphate-losing tubular disorders
Renal rickets
Renal short stature
EXCLUDES 2 *metabolic disorders classifiable to E70-E88*
DEF: Various bone diseases occurring when kidney function is impaired or fails. Abnormal levels of phosphorous and calcium can lead to osteomalacia, osteoporosis, or osteosclerosis.
N25.1 Nephrogenic diabetes insipidus HCC Rx ESR COM
EXCLUDES 1 *diabetes insipidus NOS (E23.2)*
DEF: Type of diabetes due to the inability of renal tubules to reabsorb water back into the body. It is not responsive to vasopressin (antidiuretic hormone) and it is characterized by excessive thirst and excessive urine production. It may develop into chronic renal insufficiency.
N25.8 Other disorders resulting from impaired renal tubular function
N25.81 Secondary hyperparathyroidism of renal origin HCC Rx ESR COM
EXCLUDES 1 *secondary hyperparathyroidism, non-renal (E21.1)*
EXCLUDES 2 *metabolic disorders classifiable to E70-E88*
DEF: Parathyroid dysfunction caused by chronic renal failure. Phosphate clearance and vitamin D production is impaired resulting in lowered calcium blood levels and an excessive production of parathyroid hormone.
N25.89 Other disorders resulting from impaired renal tubular function
Hypokalemic nephropathy
Lightwood-Albright syndrome
Renal tubular acidosis NOS
N25.9 Disorder resulting from impaired renal tubular function, unspecified

N26 Unspecified contracted kidney
EXCLUDES 1 *contracted kidney due to hypertension (I12.-)*
diffuse sclerosing glomerulonephritis (N05.8.-)
hypertensive nephrosclerosis (arteriolar) (arteriosclerotic) (I12.-)
small kidney of unknown cause (N27.-)
N26.1 Atrophy of kidney (terminal)
N26.2 Page kidney Rx
N26.9 Renal sclerosis, unspecified

N27 Small kidney of unknown cause
INCLUDES oligonephronia
N27.0 Small kidney, unilateral
N27.1 Small kidney, bilateral
N27.9 Small kidney, unspecified

✓4th N28 Other disorders of kidney and ureter, not elsewhere classified

N28.Ø Ischemia and infarction of kidney HCC ESR COM

Renal artery embolism
Renal artery obstruction
Renal artery occlusion
Renal artery thrombosis
Renal infarct

EXCLUDES 1 *atherosclerosis of renal artery (extrarenal part) (I7Ø.1)*
congenital stenosis of renal artery (Q27.1)
Goldblatt's kidney (I7Ø.1)

N28.1 Cyst of kidney, acquired

Cyst (multiple) (solitary) of kidney (acquired)

EXCLUDES 1 *cystic kidney disease (congenital) (Q61.-)*

✓5th N28.8 Other specified disorders of kidney and ureter

EXCLUDES 1 *hydroureter (N13.4)*
ureteric stricture with hydronephrosis (N13.1)
ureteric stricture without hydronephrosis (N13.5)

N28.81 Hypertrophy of kidney
N28.82 Megaloureter
N28.83 Nephroptosis
N28.84 Pyelitis cystica
N28.85 Pyeloureteritis cystica
N28.86 Ureteritis cystica
N28.89 Other specified disorders of kidney and ureter

N28.9 Disorder of kidney and ureter, unspecified

Nephropathy NOS
Renal disease (acute) NOS
Renal insufficiency (acute)

EXCLUDES 1 *chronic renal insufficiency (N18.9)*
unspecified nephritic syndrome (NØ5.-)

AHA: 2016,1Q,13

N29 Other disorders of kidney and ureter in diseases classified elsewhere

Code first underlying disease, such as:
amyloidosis (E85.-)
nephrocalcinosis (E83.5)
schistosomiasis (B65.Ø-B65.9)

EXCLUDES 1 *disorders of kidney and ureter in:*
cystinosis (E72.Ø)
gonorrhea (A54.21)
syphilis (A52.75)
tuberculosis (A18.11)

Other diseases of the urinary system (N3Ø-N39)

EXCLUDES 2 *urinary infection (complicating):*
abortion or ectopic or molar pregnancy (OØØ-OØ7, OØ8.8)
pregnancy, childbirth and the puerperium (O23.-, O75.3, O86.2-)

✓4th N3Ø Cystitis

Use additional code to identify infectious agent (B95-B97)

EXCLUDES 1 *prostatocystitis (N41.3)*

AHA: 2017,1Q,6

DEF: Inflammation of the urinary bladder. Symptoms include dysuria, frequency of urination, urgency, and hematuria.

✓5th N3Ø.Ø Acute cystitis

EXCLUDES 1 *irradiation cystitis (N3Ø.4-)*
trigonitis (N3Ø.3-)

N3Ø.ØØ Acute cystitis without hematuria
N3Ø.Ø1 Acute cystitis with hematuria

✓5th N3Ø.1 Interstitial cystitis (chronic)

N3Ø.1Ø Interstitial cystitis (chronic) without hematuria
N3Ø.11 Interstitial cystitis (chronic) with hematuria

✓5th N3Ø.2 Other chronic cystitis

N3Ø.2Ø Other chronic cystitis without hematuria
N3Ø.21 Other chronic cystitis with hematuria

✓5th N3Ø.3 Trigonitis

Urethrotrigonitis

N3Ø.3Ø Trigonitis without hematuria
N3Ø.31 Trigonitis with hematuria

✓5th N3Ø.4 Irradiation cystitis

N3Ø.4Ø Irradiation cystitis without hematuria
N3Ø.41 Irradiation cystitis with hematuria

✓5th N3Ø.8 Other cystitis

Abscess of bladder

N3Ø.8Ø Other cystitis without hematuria
N3Ø.81 Other cystitis with hematuria

✓5th N3Ø.9 Cystitis, unspecified

N3Ø.9Ø Cystitis, unspecified without hematuria
N3Ø.91 Cystitis, unspecified with hematuria

✓4th N31 Neuromuscular dysfunction of bladder, not elsewhere classified

Use additional code to identify any associated urinary incontinence (N39.3-N39.4-)

EXCLUDES 1 *cord bladder NOS (G95.89)*
neurogenic bladder due to cauda equina syndrome (G83.4)
neuromuscular dysfunction due to spinal cord lesion (G95.89)

N31.Ø Uninhibited neuropathic bladder, not elsewhere classified
N31.1 Reflex neuropathic bladder, not elsewhere classified
N31.2 Flaccid neuropathic bladder, not elsewhere classified

Atonic (motor) (sensory) neuropathic bladder
Autonomous neuropathic bladder
Nonreflex neuropathic bladder

N31.8 Other neuromuscular dysfunction of bladder
N31.9 Neuromuscular dysfunction of bladder, unspecified

Neurogenic bladder dysfunction NOS

✓4th N32 Other disorders of bladder

EXCLUDES 2 *calculus of bladder (N21.Ø)*
cystocele (N81.1-)
hernia or prolapse of bladder, female (N81.1-)

N32.Ø Bladder-neck obstruction

Bladder-neck stenosis (acquired)

EXCLUDES 1 *congenital bladder-neck obstruction (Q64.3-)*

DEF: Bladder outlet and vesicourethral obstruction that occurs as a consequence of benign prostatic hypertrophy or prostatic cancer. It may also occur in either sex due to strictures, radiation, cystoscopy, catheterization, injury, infection, blood clots, bladder cancer, impaction, or other disease that compresses the bladder neck.

N32.1 Vesicointestinal fistula

Vesicorectal fistula

N32.2 Vesical fistula, not elsewhere classified

EXCLUDES 1 *fistula between bladder and female genital tract (N82.Ø-N82.1)*

N32.3 Diverticulum of bladder

EXCLUDES 1 *congenital diverticulum of bladder (Q64.6)*
diverticulitis of bladder (N3Ø.8-)

✓5th N32.8 Other specified disorders of bladder

N32.81 Overactive bladder

Detrusor muscle hyperactivity

EXCLUDES 1 *frequent urination due to specified bladder condition — code to condition*

DEF: Sudden involuntary contractions of the muscular wall of the bladder that results in a sudden, strong urge to urinate.

N32.89 Other specified disorders of bladder

Bladder hemorrhage
Bladder hypertrophy
Calcified bladder
Contracted bladder

N32.9 Bladder disorder, unspecified

N33 Bladder disorders in diseases classified elsewhere

Code first underlying disease, such as:
schistosomiasis (B65.Ø-B65.9)

EXCLUDES 1 *bladder disorder in syphilis (A52.76)*
bladder disorder in tuberculosis (A18.12)
candidal cystitis (B37.41)
chlamydial cystitis (A56.Ø1)
cystitis in gonorrhea (A54.Ø1)
cystitis in neurogenic bladder (N31.-)
diphtheritic cystitis (A36.85)
neurogenic bladder (N31.-)
syphilitic cystitis (A52.76)
trichomonal cystitis (A59.Ø3)

N34 Urethritis and urethral syndrome

Use additional code (B95-B97), to identify infectious agent

EXCLUDES 2 *Reiter's disease (M02.3-)*
urethritis in diseases with a predominantly sexual mode of transmission (A50-A64)
urethrotrigonitis (N30.3-)

AHA: 2017,1Q,6

N34.0 Urethral abscess
Abscess (of) Cowper's gland
Abscess (of) Littré's gland
Abscess (of) urethral (gland)
Periurethral abscess
EXCLUDES 1 *urethral caruncle (N36.2)*

N34.1 Nonspecific urethritis
Nongonococcal urethritis
Nonvenereal urethritis

N34.2 Other urethritis
Meatitis, urethral
Postmenopausal urethritis
Ulcer of urethra (meatus)
Urethritis NOS

N34.3 Urethral syndrome, unspecified

N35 Urethral stricture

EXCLUDES 1 *congenital urethral stricture (Q64.3-)*
postprocedural urethral stricture (N99.1-)

AHA: 2018,4Q,21-22

N35.0 Post-traumatic urethral stricture
Urethral stricture due to injury
EXCLUDES 1 *postprocedural urethral stricture (N99.1-)*

N35.01 Post-traumatic urethral stricture, male
N35.010 Post-traumatic urethral stricture, male, meatal ♂
N35.011 Post-traumatic bulbous urethral stricture ♂
N35.012 Post-traumatic membranous urethral stricture ♂
N35.013 Post-traumatic anterior urethral stricture ♂
N35.014 Post-traumatic urethral stricture, male, unspecified ♂
N35.016 Post-traumatic urethral stricture, male, overlapping sites ♂

N35.02 Post-traumatic urethral stricture, female
N35.021 Urethral stricture due to childbirth ♀
N35.028 Other post-traumatic urethral stricture, female ♀

N35.1 Postinfective urethral stricture, not elsewhere classified
EXCLUDES 1 *gonococcal urethral stricture (A54.01)*
syphilitic urethral stricture (A52.76)
urethral stricture associated with schistosomiasis (B65.-, N29)

N35.11 Postinfective urethral stricture, not elsewhere classified, male
N35.111 Postinfective urethral stricture, not elsewhere classified, male, meatal ♂
N35.112 Postinfective bulbous urethral stricture, not elsewhere classified, male ♂
N35.113 Postinfective membranous urethral stricture, not elsewhere classified, male ♂
N35.114 Postinfective anterior urethral stricture, not elsewhere classified, male ♂
N35.116 Postinfective urethral stricture, not elsewhere classified, male, overlapping sites ♂
N35.119 Postinfective urethral stricture, not elsewhere classified, male, unspecified ♂

N35.12 Postinfective urethral stricture, not elsewhere classified, female ♀

N35.8 Other urethral stricture
EXCLUDES 1 *postprocedural urethral stricture (N99.1-)*

N35.81 Other urethral stricture, male
N35.811 Other urethral stricture, male, meatal ♂
N35.812 Other urethral bulbous stricture, male ♂
N35.813 Other membranous urethral stricture, male ♂
N35.814 Other anterior urethral stricture, male ♂
N35.816 Other urethral stricture, male, overlapping sites ♂
N35.819 Other urethral stricture, male, unspecified site ♂

N35.82 Other urethral stricture, female ♀

N35.9 Urethral stricture, unspecified

N35.91 Urethral stricture, unspecified, male
N35.911 Unspecified urethral stricture, male, meatal ♂
N35.912 Unspecified bulbous urethral stricture, male ♂
N35.913 Unspecified membranous urethral stricture, male ♂
N35.914 Unspecified anterior urethral stricture, male ♂
N35.916 Unspecified urethral stricture, male, overlapping sites ♂
N35.919 Unspecified urethral stricture, male, unspecified site ♂
Pinhole meatus NOS
Urethral stricture NOS

N35.92 Unspecified urethral stricture, female ♀

N36 Other disorders of urethra

N36.0 Urethral fistula
Urethroperineal fistula
Urethrorectal fistula
Urinary fistula NOS
EXCLUDES 1 *urethroscrotal fistula (N50.89)*
urethrovaginal fistula (N82.1)
urethrovesicovaginal fistula (N82.1)

N36.1 Urethral diverticulum

N36.2 Urethral caruncle

N36.4 Urethral functional and muscular disorders
Use additional code to identify associated urinary stress incontinence (N39.3)

N36.41 Hypermobility of urethra
N36.42 Intrinsic sphincter deficiency (ISD)
N36.43 Combined hypermobility of urethra and intrinsic sphincter deficiency
N36.44 Muscular disorders of urethra
Bladder sphincter dyssynergy

N36.5 Urethral false passage

N36.8 Other specified disorders of urethra
EXCLUDES 1 *congenital urethrocele (Q64.7)*
female urethrocele (N81.0)

AHA: 2022,2Q,7

N36.9 Urethral disorder, unspecified

N37 Urethral disorders in diseases classified elsewhere

Code first underlying disease

EXCLUDES 1 *urethritis (in):*
candidal infection (B37.41)
chlamydial (A56.01)
gonorrhea (A54.01)
syphilis (A52.76)
trichomonal infection (A59.03)
tuberculosis (A18.13)

N39 Other disorders of urinary system

EXCLUDES 2 *hematuria NOS (R31.-)*
recurrent or persistent hematuria (NØ2.-)
recurrent or persistent hematuria with specified morphological lesion (NØ2.-)
proteinuria NOS (R8Ø.-)

N39.Ø Urinary tract infection, site not specified
Use additional code (B95-B97), to identify infectious agent
EXCLUDES 1 *candidiasis of urinary tract (B37.4-)*
neonatal urinary tract infection (P39.3)
pyuria (R82.81)
urinary tract infection of specified site, such as:
cystitis (N3Ø.-)
urethritis (N34.-)
AHA: 2019,3Q,17; 2018,2Q,21,22; 2018,1Q,16; 2017,1Q,6; 2012,4Q,94

N39.3 Stress incontinence (female) (male)
Code also any associated overactive bladder (N32.81)
EXCLUDES 1 *mixed incontinence (N39.46)*

N39.4 Other specified urinary incontinence
Code also any associated overactive bladder (N32.81)
EXCLUDES 1 *enuresis NOS (R32)*
functional urinary incontinence (R39.81)
urinary incontinence associated with cognitive impairment (R39.81)
urinary incontinence NOS (R32)
urinary incontinence of nonorganic origin (F98.Ø)

N39.41 Urge incontinence
EXCLUDES 1 *mixed incontinence (N39.46)*

N39.42 Incontinence without sensory awareness
Insensible (urinary) incontinence

N39.43 Post-void dribbling

N39.44 Nocturnal enuresis
EXCLUDES 2 *nocturnal polyuria (R35.81)*

N39.45 Continuous leakage

N39.46 Mixed incontinence
Urge and stress incontinence

N39.49 Other specified urinary incontinence
AHA: 2016,4Q,44

N39.49Ø Overflow incontinence

N39.491 Coital incontinence

N39.492 Postural (urinary) incontinence

N39.498 Other specified urinary incontinence
Reflex incontinence
Total incontinence

N39.8 Other specified disorders of urinary system

N39.9 Disorder of urinary system, unspecified

Diseases of male genital organs (N4Ø-N53)

N4Ø Benign prostatic hyperplasia

INCLUDES adenofibromatous hypertrophy of prostate
benign hypertrophy of the prostate
benign prostatic hypertrophy
BPH
enlarged prostate
nodular prostate
polyp of prostate

EXCLUDES 1 *benign neoplasms of prostate (adenoma, benign) (fibroadenoma) (fibroma) (myoma) (D29.1)*

EXCLUDES 2 *malignant neoplasm of prostate (C61)*

DEF: Enlargement of the prostate gland due to an abnormal proliferation of fibrostromal tissue in the paraurethral glands. This condition causes impingement of the urethra resulting in obstructed urinary flow.

N4Ø.Ø Benign prostatic hyperplasia without lower urinary tract symptoms A ♂
Enlarged prostate NOS
Enlarged prostate without LUTS

N4Ø.1 Benign prostatic hyperplasia with lower urinary tract symptoms A ♂
Enlarged prostate with LUTS
Use additional code for associated symptoms, when specified:
incomplete bladder emptying (R39.14)
nocturia (R35.1)
straining on urination (R39.16)
urinary frequency (R35.Ø)
urinary hesitancy (R39.11)
urinary incontinence (N39.4-)
urinary obstruction (N13.8)
urinary retention (R33.8)
urinary urgency (R39.15)
weak urinary stream (R39.12)
AHA: 2018,4Q,55

N4Ø.2 Nodular prostate without lower urinary tract symptoms A ♂
Nodular prostate without LUTS

N4Ø.3 Nodular prostate with lower urinary tract symptoms A ♂
Use additional code for associated symptoms, when specified:
incomplete bladder emptying (R39.14)
nocturia (R35.1)
straining on urination (R39.16)
urinary frequency (R35.Ø)
urinary hesitancy (R39.11)
urinary incontinence (N39.4-)
urinary obstruction (N13.8)
urinary retention (R33.8)
urinary urgency (R39.15)
weak urinary stream (R39.12)

N41 Inflammatory diseases of prostate
Use additional code (B95-B97), to identify infectious agent

N41.Ø Acute prostatitis A ♂

N41.1 Chronic prostatitis A ♂

N41.2 Abscess of prostate A ♂

N41.3 Prostatocystitis A ♂

N41.4 Granulomatous prostatitis A ♂

N41.8 Other inflammatory diseases of prostate A ♂

N41.9 Inflammatory disease of prostate, unspecified A ♂
Prostatitis NOS

N42 Other and unspecified disorders of prostate

N42.Ø Calculus of prostate A ♂
Prostatic stone
DEF: Formation of a small, solid stone often composed of calcium carbonate or calcium phosphate in the prostate gland.

N42.1 Congestion and hemorrhage of prostate A ♂
EXCLUDES 1 *enlarged prostate (N4Ø.-)*
hematuria (R31.-)
hyperplasia of prostate (N4Ø.-)
inflammatory diseases of prostate (N41.-)

N42.3 Dysplasia of prostate
AHA: 2016,4Q,44

N42.3Ø Unspecified dysplasia of prostate ♂

N42.31 Prostatic intraepithelial neoplasia ♂
PIN
Prostatic intraepithelial neoplasia I (PIN I)
Prostatic intraepithelial neoplasia II (PIN II)
EXCLUDES 1 *prostatic intraepithelial neoplasia III (PIN III) (DØ7.5)*
DEF: Abnormality of shape and size of the intraepithelial tissues of the prostate. It is a premalignant condition characterized by stalks and absence of a basilar cell layer.

N42.32 Atypical small acinar proliferation of prostate ♂

N42.39 Other dysplasia of prostate ♂

N42.8 Other specified disorders of prostate

N42.81 Prostatodynia syndrome A ♂
Painful prostate syndrome

N42.82 Prostatosis syndrome A ♂

N42.83 Cyst of prostate A ♂

N42.89 Other specified disorders of prostate A ♂

N42.9 Disorder of prostate, unspecified A ♂

N43 Hydrocele and spermatocele
INCLUDES hydrocele of spermatic cord, testis or tunica vaginalis
EXCLUDES 1 *congenital hydrocele (P83.5)*
DEF: Hydrocele: Serous fluid that collects in the tunica vaginalis of the scrotum along the spermatic cord in males.

N43.Ø Encysted hydrocele ♂
N43.1 Infected hydrocele ♂
Use additional code (B95-B97), to identify infectious agent
N43.2 Other hydrocele ♂

Hydrocele

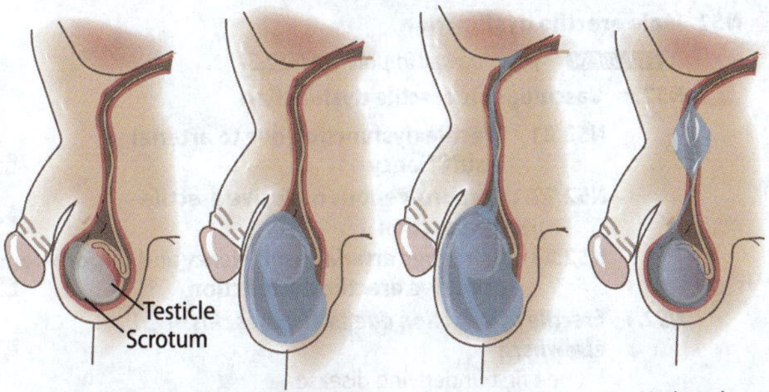

N43.3 Hydrocele, unspecified ♂
N43.4 Spermatocele of epididymis
Spermatic cyst
DEF: Spermatocele: Noncancerous accumulation of fluid and dead sperm cells normally located at the head of the epididymis that exhibits itself as a hard, smooth scrotal mass and do not normally require treatment unless they become enlarged or cause pain.
N43.4Ø Spermatocele of epididymis, unspecified ♂
N43.41 Spermatocele of epididymis, single ♂
N43.42 Spermatocele of epididymis, multiple ♂

N44 Noninflammatory disorders of testis
N44.Ø Torsion of testis
N44.ØØ Torsion of testis, unspecified ♂
N44.Ø1 Extravaginal torsion of spermatic cord ♂
DEF: Torsion of the spermatic cord just below the tunica vaginalis attachments.
N44.Ø2 Intravaginal torsion of spermatic cord ♂
Torsion of spermatic cord NOS
N44.Ø3 Torsion of appendix testis ♂
N44.Ø4 Torsion of appendix epididymis ♂
N44.1 Cyst of tunica albuginea testis ♂
N44.2 Benign cyst of testis ♂
N44.8 Other noninflammatory disorders of the testis ♂

N45 Orchitis and epididymitis
Use additional code (B95-B97), to identify infectious agent
N45.1 Epididymitis ♂
N45.2 Orchitis ♂
N45.3 Epididymo-orchitis ♂
N45.4 Abscess of epididymis or testis ♂

N46 Male infertility
EXCLUDES 1 *vasectomy status (Z98.52)*
N46.Ø Azoospermia
Absolute male infertility
Male infertility due to germinal (cell) aplasia
Male infertility due to spermatogenic arrest (complete)
DEF: Failure of the development of sperm or the absence of sperm in semen.
N46.Ø1 Organic azoospermia A ♂
Azoospermia NOS
N46.Ø2 Azoospermia due to extratesticular causes
Code also associated cause
N46.Ø21 Azoospermia due to drug therapy A ♂
N46.Ø22 Azoospermia due to infection A ♂
N46.Ø23 Azoospermia due to obstruction of efferent ducts A ♂
N46.Ø24 Azoospermia due to radiation A ♂
N46.Ø25 Azoospermia due to systemic disease A ♂
N46.Ø29 Azoospermia due to other extratesticular causes A ♂
N46.1 Oligospermia
Male infertility due to germinal cell desquamation
Male infertility due to hypospermatogenesis
Male infertility due to incomplete spermatogenic arrest
DEF: Insufficient production of sperm in semen.
N46.11 Organic oligospermia A ♂
Oligospermia NOS
N46.12 Oligospermia due to extratesticular causes
Code also associated cause
N46.121 Oligospermia due to drug therapy A ♂
N46.122 Oligospermia due to infection A ♂
N46.123 Oligospermia due to obstruction of efferent ducts A ♂
N46.124 Oligospermia due to radiation A ♂
N46.125 Oligospermia due to systemic disease A ♂
N46.129 Oligospermia due to other extratesticular causes A ♂
N46.8 Other male infertility A ♂
N46.9 Male infertility, unspecified A ♂

N47 Disorders of prepuce
N47.Ø Adherent prepuce, newborn N ♂
N47.1 Phimosis ♂
DEF: Condition in which the foreskin is contracted and cannot be drawn back behind the glans penis.
N47.2 Paraphimosis ♂
N47.3 Deficient foreskin ♂
N47.4 Benign cyst of prepuce ♂
N47.5 Adhesions of prepuce and glans penis ♂
N47.6 Balanoposthitis ♂
Use additional code (B95-B97), to identify infectious agent
EXCLUDES 1 *balanitis (N48.1)*
N47.7 Other inflammatory diseases of prepuce ♂
Use additional code (B95-B97), to identify infectious agent
N47.8 Other disorders of prepuce ♂

N48 Other disorders of penis
N48.Ø Leukoplakia of penis ♂
Balanitis xerotica obliterans
Kraurosis of penis
Lichen sclerosus of external male genital organs
EXCLUDES 1 *carcinoma in situ of penis (DØ7.4)*
N48.1 Balanitis ♂
Use additional code (B95-B97), to identify infectious agent
EXCLUDES 1 *amebic balanitis (AØ6.8)*
balanitis xerotica obliterans (N48.Ø)
candidal balanitis (B37.42)
gonococcal balanitis (A54.23)
herpesviral [herpes simplex] balanitis (A6Ø.Ø1)
DEF: Inflammation of the glans penis, most often affecting uncircumcised males.
N48.2 Other inflammatory disorders of penis
Use additional code (B95-B97), to identify infectious agent
EXCLUDES 1 *balanitis (N48.1)*
balanitis xerotica obliterans (N48.Ø)
balanoposthitis (N47.6)
N48.21 Abscess of corpus cavernosum and penis ♂
N48.22 Cellulitis of corpus cavernosum and penis ♂
N48.29 Other inflammatory disorders of penis ♂
N48.3 Priapism
Painful erection
Code first underlying cause
N48.3Ø Priapism, unspecified ♂
N48.31 Priapism due to trauma ♂
N48.32 Priapism due to disease classified elsewhere ♂
N48.33 Priapism, drug-induced ♂
N48.39 Other priapism ♂
N48.5 Ulcer of penis ♂

N48.6 Induration penis plastica ♂
Peyronie's disease
Plastic induration of penis

5th **N48.8 Other specified disorders of penis**

N48.81 Thrombosis of superficial vein of penis ♂

N48.82 Acquired torsion of penis ♂
Acquired torsion of penis NOS
EXCLUDES 1 *congenital torsion of penis (Q55.63)*

N48.83 Acquired buried penis ♂
EXCLUDES 1 *congenital hidden penis (Q55.64)*

N48.89 Other specified disorders of penis ♂

N48.9 Disorder of penis, unspecified ♂

4th **N49 Inflammatory disorders of male genital organs, not elsewhere classified**
Use additional code (B95-B97), to identify infectious agent
EXCLUDES 1 *inflammation of penis (N48.1, N48.2-)*
orchitis and epididymitis (N45.-)

N49.0 Inflammatory disorders of seminal vesicle ♂
Vesiculitis NOS

N49.1 Inflammatory disorders of spermatic cord, tunica vaginalis and vas deferens ♂
Vasitis

N49.2 Inflammatory disorders of scrotum ♂

N49.3 Fournier gangrene ♂
AHA: 2020,2Q,18

N49.8 Inflammatory disorders of other specified male genital organs ♂
Inflammation of multiple sites in male genital organs

N49.9 Inflammatory disorder of unspecified male genital organ ♂
Abscess of unspecified male genital organ
Boil of unspecified male genital organ
Carbuncle of unspecified male genital organ
Cellulitis of unspecified male genital organ

4th **N50 Other and unspecified disorders of male genital organs**
EXCLUDES 2 *torsion of testis (N44.0-)*

N50.0 Atrophy of testis ♂

N50.1 Vascular disorders of male genital organs ♂
Hematocele, NOS, of male genital organs
Hemorrhage of male genital organs
Thrombosis of male genital organs

N50.3 Cyst of epididymis ♂

5th **N50.8 Other specified disorders of male genital organs**
AHA: 2016,4Q,45

6th **N50.81 Testicular pain**

N50.811 Right testicular pain ♂

N50.812 Left testicular pain ♂

N50.819 Testicular pain, unspecified ♂

N50.82 Scrotal pain ♂

N50.89 Other specified disorders of the male genital organs ♂
Atrophy of scrotum, seminal vesicle, spermatic cord, tunica vaginalis and vas deferens
Chylocele, tunica vaginalis (nonfilarial) NOS
Edema of scrotum, seminal vesicle, spermatic cord, tunica vaginalis and vas deferens
Hypertrophy of scrotum, seminal vesicle, spermatic cord, tunica vaginalis and vas deferens
Stricture of spermatic cord, tunica vaginalis, and vas deferens
Ulcer of scrotum, seminal vesicle, spermatic cord, testis, tunica vaginalis and vas deferens
Urethroscrotal fistula

N50.9 Disorder of male genital organs, unspecified ♂

N51 Disorders of male genital organs in diseases classified elsewhere ♂
Code first underlying disease, such as:
filariasis (B74.0-B74.9)
EXCLUDES 1 *amebic balanitis (A06.8)*
candidal balanitis (B37.42)
gonococcal balanitis (A54.23)
gonococcal prostatitis (A54.22)
herpesviral [herpes simplex] balanitis (A60.01)
trichomonal prostatitis (A59.02)
tuberculous prostatitis (A18.14)

4th **N52 Male erectile dysfunction**
EXCLUDES 1 *psychogenic impotence (F52.21)*

5th **N52.0 Vasculogenic erectile dysfunction**

N52.01 Erectile dysfunction due to arterial insufficiency A ♂

N52.02 Corporo-venous occlusive erectile dysfunction A ♂

N52.03 Combined arterial insufficiency and corporo-venous occlusive erectile dysfunction A ♂

N52.1 Erectile dysfunction due to diseases classified elsewhere A ♂
Code first underlying disease

N52.2 Drug-induced erectile dysfunction A ♂

5th **N52.3 Postprocedural erectile dysfunction**
AHA: 2016,4Q,45

N52.31 Erectile dysfunction following radical prostatectomy A ♂

N52.32 Erectile dysfunction following radical cystectomy A ♂

N52.33 Erectile dysfunction following urethral surgery A ♂

N52.34 Erectile dysfunction following simple prostatectomy A ♂

N52.35 Erectile dysfunction following radiation therapy A ♂

N52.36 Erectile dysfunction following interstitial seed therapy A ♂

N52.37 Erectile dysfunction following prostate ablative therapy A ♂
Erectile dysfunction following cryotherapy
Erectile dysfunction following other prostate ablative therapies
Erectile dysfunction following ultrasound ablative therapies

N52.39 Other and unspecified postprocedural erectile dysfunction A ♂

N52.8 Other male erectile dysfunction A ♂

N52.9 Male erectile dysfunction, unspecified A ♂
Impotence NOS

4th **N53 Other male sexual dysfunction**
EXCLUDES 1 *psychogenic sexual dysfunction (F52.-)*

5th **N53.1 Ejaculatory dysfunction**
EXCLUDES 1 *premature ejaculation (F52.4)*

N53.11 Retarded ejaculation ♂

N53.12 Painful ejaculation ♂

N53.13 Anejaculatory orgasm ♂

N53.14 Retrograde ejaculation ♂
DEF: Form of male sexual dysfunction in which the semen enters the bladder instead of going out through the urethra during ejaculation.

N53.19 Other ejaculatory dysfunction ♂
Ejaculatory dysfunction NOS

N53.8 Other male sexual dysfunction ♂

N53.9 Unspecified male sexual dysfunction ♂

Disorders of breast (N60-N65)

EXCLUDES 1 *disorders of breast associated with childbirth (O91-O92)*

4th **N60 Benign mammary dysplasia**
INCLUDES fibrocystic mastopathy

5th **N60.0 Solitary cyst of breast**
Cyst of breast

N60.01 Solitary cyst of right breast

N60.02 Solitary cyst of left breast

N60.09 Solitary cyst of unspecified breast

N6Ø.1 Diffuse cystic mastopathy
Cystic breast
Fibrocystic disease of breast
EXCLUDES 1 *diffuse cystic mastopathy with epithelial proliferation (N6Ø.3-)*
N6Ø.11 Diffuse cystic mastopathy of right breast
N6Ø.12 Diffuse cystic mastopathy of left breast
N6Ø.19 Diffuse cystic mastopathy of unspecified breast

N6Ø.2 Fibroadenosis of breast
Adenofibrosis of breast
EXCLUDES 2 *fibroadenoma of breast (D24.-)*
N6Ø.21 Fibroadenosis of right breast
N6Ø.22 Fibroadenosis of left breast
N6Ø.29 Fibroadenosis of unspecified breast

N6Ø.3 Fibrosclerosis of breast
Cystic mastopathy with epithelial proliferation
N6Ø.31 Fibrosclerosis of right breast
N6Ø.32 Fibrosclerosis of left breast
N6Ø.39 Fibrosclerosis of unspecified breast

N6Ø.4 Mammary duct ectasia
N6Ø.41 Mammary duct ectasia of right breast
N6Ø.42 Mammary duct ectasia of left breast
N6Ø.49 Mammary duct ectasia of unspecified breast

N6Ø.8 Other benign mammary dysplasias
N6Ø.81 Other benign mammary dysplasias of right breast
N6Ø.82 Other benign mammary dysplasias of left breast
N6Ø.89 Other benign mammary dysplasias of unspecified breast

N6Ø.9 Unspecified benign mammary dysplasia
N6Ø.91 Unspecified benign mammary dysplasia of right breast
N6Ø.92 Unspecified benign mammary dysplasia of left breast
N6Ø.99 Unspecified benign mammary dysplasia of unspecified breast

N61 Inflammatory disorders of breast
EXCLUDES 1 *inflammatory carcinoma of breast (C5Ø.9)*
inflammatory disorder of breast associated with childbirth (O91.-)
neonatal infective mastitis (P39.Ø)
thrombophlebitis of breast [Mondor's disease] (I8Ø.8)

N61.Ø Mastitis without abscess
Infective mastitis (acute) (nonpuerperal) (subacute)
Mastitis (acute) (nonpuerperal) (subacute) NOS
Cellulitis (acute) (nonpuerperal) (subacute) of breast NOS
Cellulitis (acute) (nonpuerperal) (subacute) of nipple NOS

N61.1 Abscess of the breast and nipple
Abscess (acute) (chronic) (nonpuerperal) of areola
Abscess (acute) (chronic) (nonpuerperal) of breast
Carbuncle of breast
Mastitis with abscess

N61.2 Granulomatous mastitis
AHA: 2020,4Q,35
N61.2Ø Granulomatous mastitis, unspecified breast
N61.21 Granulomatous mastitis, right breast
N61.22 Granulomatous mastitis, left breast
N61.23 Granulomatous mastitis, bilateral breast

N62 Hypertrophy of breast
Gynecomastia
Hypertrophy of breast NOS
Massive pubertal hypertrophy of breast
EXCLUDES 1 *breast engorgement of newborn (P83.4)*
disproportion of reconstructed breast (N65.1)

N63 Unspecified lump in breast
Nodule(s) NOS in breast
AHA: 2019,4Q,12; 2017,4Q,19
N63.Ø Unspecified lump in unspecified breast

N63.1 Unspecified lump in the right breast
N63.1Ø Unspecified lump in the right breast, unspecified quadrant
N63.11 Unspecified lump in the right breast, upper outer quadrant
N63.12 Unspecified lump in the right breast, upper inner quadrant
N63.13 Unspecified lump in the right breast, lower outer quadrant
N63.14 Unspecified lump in the right breast, lower inner quadrant
N63.15 Unspecified lump in the right breast, overlapping quadrants

N63.2 Unspecified lump in the left breast
N63.2Ø Unspecified lump in the left breast, unspecified quadrant
N63.21 Unspecified lump in the left breast, upper outer quadrant
N63.22 Unspecified lump in the left breast, upper inner quadrant
N63.23 Unspecified lump in the left breast, lower outer quadrant
N63.24 Unspecified lump in the left breast, lower inner quadrant
N63.25 Unspecified lump in the left breast, overlapping quadrants

N63.3 Unspecified lump in axillary tail
N63.31 Unspecified lump in axillary tail of the right breast
N63.32 Unspecified lump in axillary tail of the left breast

N63.4 Unspecified lump in breast, subareolar
N63.41 Unspecified lump in right breast, subareolar
N63.42 Unspecified lump in left breast, subareolar

N64 Other disorders of breast
EXCLUDES 2 *mechanical complication of breast prosthesis and implant (T85.4-)*
N64.Ø Fissure and fistula of nipple
N64.1 Fat necrosis of breast
Fat necrosis (segmental) of breast
Code first breast necrosis due to breast graft (T85.898)
N64.2 Atrophy of breast
N64.3 Galactorrhea not associated with childbirth
N64.4 Mastodynia

N64.5 Other signs and symptoms in breast
EXCLUDES 2 *abnormal findings on diagnostic imaging of breast (R92.-)*
N64.51 Induration of breast
N64.52 Nipple discharge
EXCLUDES 1 *abnormal findings in nipple discharge (R89.-)*
N64.53 Retraction of nipple
N64.59 Other signs and symptoms in breast

N64.8 Other specified disorders of breast
N64.81 Ptosis of breast
EXCLUDES 1 *ptosis of native breast in relation to reconstructed breast (N65.1)*
N64.82 Hypoplasia of breast
Micromastia
EXCLUDES 1 *congenital absence of breast (Q83.Ø)*
hypoplasia of native breast in relation to reconstructed breast (N65.1)
N64.89 Other specified disorders of breast
Galactocele
Subinvolution of breast (postlactational)
AHA: 2019,1Q,32; 2018,1Q,3
N64.9 Disorder of breast, unspecified

N65 Deformity and disproportion of reconstructed breast
N65.Ø Deformity of reconstructed breast
Contour irregularity in reconstructed breast
Excess tissue in reconstructed breast
Misshapen reconstructed breast
N65.1 Disproportion of reconstructed breast
Breast asymmetry between native breast and reconstructed breast
Disproportion between native breast and reconstructed breast

Inflammatory diseases of female pelvic organs (N70-N77)

EXCLUDES 1 *inflammatory diseases of female pelvic organs complicating:*
abortion or ectopic or molar pregnancy (O00-O07, O08.0)
pregnancy, childbirth and the puerperium (O23.-, O75.3, O85, O86.-)

N70 Salpingitis and oophoritis
INCLUDES abscess (of) fallopian tube
abscess (of) ovary
pyosalpinx
salpingo-oophoritis
tubo-ovarian abscess
tubo-ovarian inflammatory disease
Use additional code (B95-B97), to identify infectious agent
EXCLUDES 1 *gonococcal infection (A54.24)*
tuberculous infection (A18.17)

N70.0 Acute salpingitis and oophoritis
N70.01 Acute salpingitis ♀
N70.02 Acute oophoritis ♀
N70.03 Acute salpingitis and oophoritis ♀

N70.1 Chronic salpingitis and oophoritis
Hydrosalpinx
N70.11 Chronic salpingitis ♀
N70.12 Chronic oophoritis ♀
N70.13 Chronic salpingitis and oophoritis ♀

N70.9 Salpingitis and oophoritis, unspecified
N70.91 Salpingitis, unspecified ♀
N70.92 Oophoritis, unspecified ♀
N70.93 Salpingitis and oophoritis, unspecified ♀

N71 Inflammatory disease of uterus, except cervix
INCLUDES endo (myo) metritis
metritis
myometritis
pyometra
uterine abscess
Use additional code (B95-B97), to identify infectious agent
EXCLUDES 1 *hyperplastic endometritis (N85.0-)*
infection of uterus following delivery (O85, O86.-)

N71.0 Acute inflammatory disease of uterus ♀
N71.1 Chronic inflammatory disease of uterus ♀
N71.9 Inflammatory disease of uterus, unspecified ♀

N72 Inflammatory disease of cervix uteri ♀
INCLUDES cervicitis (with or without erosion or ectropion)
endocervicitis (with or without erosion or ectropion)
exocervicitis (with or without erosion or ectropion)
Use additional code (B95-B97), to identify infectious agent
EXCLUDES 1 *erosion and ectropion of cervix without cervicitis (N86)*

N73 Other female pelvic inflammatory diseases
Use additional code (B95-B97), to identify infectious agent

N73.0 Acute parametritis and pelvic cellulitis ♀
Abscess of broad ligament
Abscess of parametrium
Pelvic cellulitis, female
DEF: Parametritis: Inflammation of the parametrium.

N73.1 Chronic parametritis and pelvic cellulitis ♀
Any condition in N73.0 specified as chronic
EXCLUDES 1 *tuberculous parametritis and pelvic cellulitis (A18.17)*

N73.2 Unspecified parametritis and pelvic cellulitis ♀
Any condition in N73.0 unspecified whether acute or chronic

N73.3 Female acute pelvic peritonitis ♀
N73.4 Female chronic pelvic peritonitis ♀
EXCLUDES 1 *tuberculous pelvic (female) peritonitis (A18.17)*

N73.5 Female pelvic peritonitis, unspecified ♀
N73.6 Female pelvic peritoneal adhesions (postinfective) ♀
EXCLUDES 2 *postprocedural pelvic peritoneal adhesions (N99.4)*
AHA: 2014,1Q,6

N73.8 Other specified female pelvic inflammatory diseases ♀
N73.9 Female pelvic inflammatory disease, unspecified ♀
Female pelvic infection or inflammation NOS

N74 Female pelvic inflammatory disorders in diseases classified elsewhere ♀
Code first underlying disease
EXCLUDES 1 *chlamydial cervicitis (A56.02)*
chlamydial pelvic inflammatory disease (A56.11)
gonococcal cervicitis (A54.03)
gonococcal pelvic inflammatory disease (A54.24)
herpesviral [herpes simplex] cervicitis (A60.03)
herpesviral [herpes simplex] pelvic inflammatory disease (A60.09)
syphilitic cervicitis (A52.76)
syphilitic pelvic inflammatory disease (A52.76)
trichomonal cervicitis (A59.09)
tuberculous cervicitis (A18.16)
tuberculous pelvic inflammatory disease (A18.17)

N75 Diseases of Bartholin's gland
DEF: Bartholin's gland: Mucous-producing gland found in the vestibular bulbs on either side of the vaginal orifice and connected to the mucosal membrane at the opening by a duct.

N75.0 Cyst of Bartholin's gland ♀
N75.1 Abscess of Bartholin's gland ♀
N75.8 Other diseases of Bartholin's gland ♀
Bartholinitis
N75.9 Disease of Bartholin's gland, unspecified ♀

N76 Other inflammation of vagina and vulva
Use additional code (B95-B97), to identify infectious agent
EXCLUDES 2 *senile (atrophic) vaginitis (N95.2)*
vulvar vestibulitis (N94.810)

N76.0 Acute vaginitis ♀
Acute vulvovaginitis
Vaginitis NOS
Vulvovaginitis NOS

N76.1 Subacute and chronic vaginitis ♀
Chronic vulvovaginitis
Subacute vulvovaginitis

N76.2 Acute vulvitis ♀
Vulvitis NOS

N76.3 Subacute and chronic vulvitis ♀
N76.4 Abscess of vulva ♀
Furuncle of vulva
N76.5 Ulceration of vagina ♀
N76.6 Ulceration of vulva ♀

N76.8 Other specified inflammation of vagina and vulva
N76.81 Mucositis (ulcerative) of vagina and vulva ♀
Code also type of associated therapy, such as:
antineoplastic and immunosuppressive drugs (T45.1X-)
radiological procedure and radiotherapy (Y84.2)
EXCLUDES 2 *gastrointestinal mucositis (ulcerative) (K92.81)*
nasal mucositis (ulcerative) (J34.81)
oral mucositis (ulcerative) (K12.3-)

● **N76.82 Fournier disease of vagina and vulva**
Fournier gangrene of vagina and vulva
Code also, if applicable, diabetes mellitus (E08-E13 with 9)
EXCLUDES 1 *gangrene in diabetes mellitus (E08-E13 with .52)*

N76.89 Other specified inflammation of vagina and vulva ♀

N77 Vulvovaginal ulceration and inflammation in diseases classified elsewhere
N77.0 Ulceration of vulva in diseases classified elsewhere ♀
Code first underlying disease, such as:
Behçet's disease (M35.2)
EXCLUDES 1 *ulceration of vulva in gonococcal infection (A54.02)*
ulceration of vulva in herpesviral [herpes simplex] infection (A60.04)
ulceration of vulva in syphilis (A51.0)
ulceration of vulva in tuberculosis (A18.18)

N77.1 ***Vaginitis, vulvitis and vulvovaginitis in diseases classified elsewhere*** ♀

Code first underlying disease, such as:
pinworm (B80)

EXCLUDES 1 *candidal vulvovaginitis* ►*(B37.3-)*◄
chlamydial vulvovaginitis (A56.02)
gonococcal vulvovaginitis (A54.02)
herpesviral [herpes simplex] vulvovaginitis (A60.04)
trichomonal vulvovaginitis (A59.01)
tuberculous vulvovaginitis (A18.18)
vulvovaginitis in early syphilis (A51.0)
vulvovaginitis in late syphilis (A52.76)

Noninflammatory disorders of female genital tract (N80-N98)

N80 Endometriosis

DEF: Aberrant uterine mucosal tissue appearing in areas of the pelvic cavity outside of its normal location, lining the uterus, and inflaming surrounding tissues often resulting in infertility or spontaneous abortion.

▲ **N80.0 Endometriosis of uterus**
Adenomyosis
►Endometriosis of the cervix◄
EXCLUDES 1 *stromal endometriosis (D39.0)*

- **N80.00 Endometriosis of the uterus, unspecified**
- **N80.01 Superficial endometriosis of the uterus**
- **N80.02 Deep endometriosis of the uterus**
  Deep retrocervical endometriosis
- **N80.03 Adenomyosis of the uterus**
  Adenomyosis NOS

▲ **N80.1 Endometriosis of ovary**

- **N80.10 Endometriosis of ovary, unspecified depth**
  - **N80.101 Endometriosis of right ovary, unspecified depth**
  - **N80.102 Endometriosis of left ovary, unspecified depth**
  - **N80.103 Endometriosis of bilateral ovaries, unspecified depth**
  - **N80.109 Endometriosis of ovary, unspecified side, unspecified depth**
    Endometriosis of ovary NOS
- **N80.11 Superficial endometriosis of the ovary**
  - **N80.111 Superficial endometriosis of right ovary**
  - **N80.112 Superficial endometriosis of left ovary**
  - **N80.113 Superficial endometriosis of bilateral ovaries**
  - **N80.119 Superficial endometriosis of ovary, unspecified ovary**
- **N80.12 Deep endometriosis of ovary**
  Deep ovarian endometriosis
  Endometrioma
  - **N80.121 Deep endometriosis of right ovary**
  - **N80.122 Deep endometriosis of left ovary**
  - **N80.123 Deep endometriosis of bilateral ovaries**
  - **N80.129 Deep endometriosis of ovary, unspecified ovary**

▲ **N80.2 Endometriosis of fallopian tube**

- **N80.20 Endometriosis of fallopian tube, unspecified depth**
  - **N80.201 Endometriosis of right fallopian tube, unspecified depth**
  - **N80.202 Endometriosis of left fallopian tube, unspecified depth**
  - **N80.203 Endometriosis of bilateral fallopian tubes, unspecified depth**
  - **N80.209 Endometriosis of unspecified fallopian tube, unspecified depth**
    Endometriosis fallopian tube NOS
- **N80.21 Superficial endometriosis of fallopian tube**
  - **N80.211 Superficial endometriosis of right fallopian tube**
  - **N80.212 Superficial endometriosis of left fallopian tube**
  - **N80.213 Superficial endometriosis of bilateral fallopian tubes**
  - **N80.219 Superficial endometriosis of unspecified fallopian tube**
- **N80.22 Deep endometriosis of the fallopian tube**
  Deep endometriosis involving muscular wall of fallopian tube
  - **N80.221 Deep endometriosis of right fallopian tube**
  - **N80.222 Deep endometriosis of left fallopian tube**
  - **N80.223 Deep endometriosis of bilateral fallopian tubes**
  - **N80.229 Deep endometriosis of unspecified fallopian tube**

▲ **N80.3 Endometriosis of pelvic peritoneum**

- **N80.30 Endometriosis of pelvic peritoneum, unspecified**
  Endometriosis of the retroperitoneum NOS
- **N80.31 Endometriosis of the anterior cul-de-sac**
  - **N80.311 Superficial endometriosis of the anterior cul-de-sac**
  - **N80.312 Deep endometriosis of the anterior cul-de-sac**
  - **N80.319 Endometriosis of the anterior cul-de-sac, unspecified depth**
    Endometriosis of the anterior cul-de-sac NOS
- **N80.32 Endometriosis of the posterior cul-de-sac**
  - **N80.321 Superficial endometriosis of the posterior cul-de-sac**
  - **N80.322 Deep endometriosis of the posterior cul-de-sac**
  - **N80.329 Endometriosis of the posterior cul-de-sac, unspecified depth**
    Endometriosis of the posterior cul-de-sac NOS
- **N80.33 Superficial endometriosis of the pelvic sidewall**
  - **N80.331 Superficial endometriosis of the right pelvic sidewall**
  - **N80.332 Superficial endometriosis of the left pelvic sidewall**
  - **N80.333 Superficial endometriosis of bilateral pelvic sidewall**
  - **N80.339 Superficial endometriosis of pelvic sidewall, unspecified side**
- **N80.34 Deep endometriosis of the pelvic sidewall**
  - **N80.341 Deep endometriosis of the right pelvic sidewall**
  - **N80.342 Deep endometriosis of the left pelvic sidewall**
  - **N80.343 Deep endometriosis of the bilateral pelvic sidewall**
  - **N80.349 Deep endometriosis of the pelvic sidewall, unspecified side**
- **N80.35 Endometriosis of the pelvic sidewall, unspecified depth**
  - **N80.351 Endometriosis of the right pelvic sidewall, unspecified depth**
  - **N80.352 Endometriosis of the left pelvic sidewall, unspecified depth**
  - **N80.353 Endometriosis of bilateral pelvic sidewall, unspecified depth**
  - **N80.359 Endometriosis of pelvic sidewall, unspecified side, unspecified depth**
    Endometriosis of the pelvic sidewall NOS
- **N80.36 Superficial endometriosis of the pelvic brim**
  - **N80.361 Superficial endometriosis of the right pelvic brim**
  - **N80.362 Superficial endometriosis of the left pelvic brim**
  - **N80.363 Superficial endometriosis of bilateral pelvic brim**
  - **N80.369 Superficial endometriosis of the pelvic brim, unspecified side**
- **N80.37 Deep endometriosis of the pelvic brim**
  - **N80.371 Deep endometriosis of the right pelvic brim**
  - **N80.372 Deep endometriosis of the left pelvic brim**
  - **N80.373 Deep endometriosis of bilateral pelvic brim**
  - **N80.379 Deep endometriosis of the pelvic brim, unspecified side**
- **N80.38 Endometriosis of the pelvic brim, unspecified depth**
  - **N80.381 Endometriosis of the right pelvic brim, unspecified depth**

- N80.382 Endometriosis of the left pelvic brim, unspecified depth
- N80.383 Endometriosis of bilateral pelvic brim, unspecified depth
- N80.389 Endometriosis of the pelvic brim, unspecified side, unspecified depth
  - Endometriosis of the pelvic brim NOS
- 6th N80.3A Superficial endometriosis of the uterosacral ligament(s)
  - N80.3A1 Superficial endometriosis of the right uterosacral ligament
  - N80.3A2 Superficial endometriosis of the left uterosacral ligament
  - N80.3A3 Superficial endometriosis of the bilateral uterosacral ligament(s)
  - N80.3A9 Superficial endometriosis of the uterosacral ligament(s), unspecified side
- 6th N80.3B Deep endometriosis of the uterosacral ligament(s)
  - N80.3B1 Deep endometriosis of the right uterosacral ligament
  - N80.3B2 Deep endometriosis of the left uterosacral ligament
  - N80.3B3 Deep endometriosis of bilateral uterosacral ligament(s)
  - N80.3B9 Deep endometriosis of the uterosacral ligament(s), unspecified side
- 6th N80.3C Endometriosis of the uterosacral ligament(s), unspecified depth
  - N80.3C1 Endometriosis of the right uterosacral ligament, unspecified depth
  - N80.3C2 Endometriosis of the left uterosacral ligament, unspecified depth
  - N80.3C3 Endometriosis of bilateral uterosacral ligament(s), unspecified depth
  - N80.3C9 Endometriosis of the uterosacral ligament(s), unspecified side, unspecified depth
    - Endometriosis of the uterosacral ligament(s) NOS
- 6th N80.39 Endometriosis of other pelvic peritoneum
  - N80.391 Superficial endometriosis of the pelvic peritoneum, other specified sites
  - N80.392 Deep endometriosis of the pelvic peritoneum, other specified sites
  - N80.399 Endometriosis of the pelvic peritoneum, other specified sites, unspecified depth

▲ 5th N80.4 Endometriosis of rectovaginal septum and vagina
- N80.40 Endometriosis of rectovaginal septum, unspecified involvement of vagina
  - Endometriosis of the rectovaginal septum, NOS
- N80.41 Endometriosis of rectovaginal septum without involvement of vagina
- N80.42 Endometriosis of rectovaginal septum with involvement of vagina

▲ 5th N80.5 Endometriosis of intestine
- N80.50 Endometriosis of intestine, unspecified
- 6th N80.51 Endometriosis of the rectum
  - N80.511 Superficial endometriosis of the rectum
  - N80.512 Deep endometriosis of the rectum
    - Deep endometriosis of the rectum, multifocal
  - N80.519 Endometriosis of the rectum, unspecified depth
    - Endometriosis of the rectum NOS
- 6th N80.52 Endometriosis of the sigmoid colon
  - N80.521 Superficial endometriosis of the sigmoid colon
  - N80.522 Deep endometriosis of the sigmoid colon
  - N80.529 Endometriosis of the sigmoid colon, unspecified depth
    - Endometriosis of the sigmoid colon NOS
- 6th N80.53 Endometriosis of the cecum
  - N80.531 Superficial endometriosis of the cecum
  - N80.532 Deep endometriosis of the cecum
  - N80.539 Endometriosis of the cecum, unspecified depth
    - Endometriosis of the cecum NOS
- 6th N80.54 Endometriosis of the appendix
  - N80.541 Superficial endometriosis of the appendix
  - N80.542 Deep endometriosis of the appendix
  - N80.549 Endometriosis of the appendix, unspecified depth
    - Endometriosis of the appendix NOS
- 6th N80.55 Endometriosis of other parts of the colon
  - Endometriosis of descending colon
  - Endometriosis of transverse colon
  - N80.551 Superficial endometriosis of other parts of the colon
  - N80.552 Deep endometriosis of other parts of the colon
  - N80.559 Endometriosis of other parts of the colon, unspecified depth
    - Endometriosis of colon NOS
- 6th N80.56 Endometriosis of the small intestine
  - N80.561 Superficial endometriosis of the small intestine
  - N80.562 Deep endometriosis of the small intestine
    - Deep endometriosis of the small intestine, multifocal
  - N80.569 Endometriosis of the small intestine, unspecified depth
    - Endometriosis of the small intestine NOS

N80.6 Endometriosis in cutaneous scar ♀

5th N80.A Endometriosis of bladder and ureters
- N80.A0 Endometriosis of bladder, unspecified depth
  - Endometriosis of bladder NOS
- N80.A1 Superficial endometriosis of bladder
- N80.A2 Deep endometriosis of bladder
- 6th N80.A4 Superficial endometriosis of ureter
  - Extrinsic endometriosis of ureter
  - Code also, if applicable, obstructive and reflux uropathy (N13.-)
  - N80.A41 Superficial endometriosis of right ureter
  - N80.A42 Superficial endometriosis of left ureter
  - N80.A43 Superficial endometriosis of bilateral ureters
  - N80.A49 Superficial endometriosis of unspecified ureter
- 6th N80.A5 Deep endometriosis of ureter
  - Intrinsic endometriosis of ureter
  - Code also, if applicable, obstructive and reflux uropathy (N13.-)
  - N80.A51 Deep endometriosis of right ureter
  - N80.A52 Deep endometriosis of left ureter
  - N80.A53 Deep endometriosis of bilateral ureters
  - N80.A59 Deep endometriosis of unspecified ureter
- 6th N80.A6 Endometriosis of ureter, unspecified depth
  - Code also, if applicable, obstructive and reflux uropathy (N13.-)
  - N80.A61 Endometriosis of right ureter, unspecified depth
  - N80.A62 Endometriosis of left ureter, unspecified depth
  - N80.A63 Endometriosis of bilateral ureters, unspecified depth
  - N80.A69 Endometriosis of unspecified ureter, unspecified depth

5th N80.B Endometriosis of cardiothoracic space
- Endometriosis of thorax
- Code also, if applicable:
  - catamenial hemothorax (J94.2)
  - catamenial pneumothorax (J93.12)
- N80.B1 Endometriosis of pleura
- N80.B2 Endometriosis of lung
- 6th N80.B3 Endometriosis of diaphragm
  - N80.B31 Superficial endometriosis of diaphragm
  - N80.B32 Deep endometriosis of diaphragm
  - N80.B39 Endometriosis of diaphragm, unspecified depth
    - Endometriosis of the diaphragm NOS
- N80.B4 Endometriosis of the pericardial space
- N80.B5 Endometriosis of the mediastinal space
- N80.B6 Endometriosis of cardiothoracic space

● ✓5th **N8Ø.C Endometriosis of the abdomen**

● **N8Ø.CØ Endometriosis of the abdomen, unspecified**
Endometriosis of the abdomen NOS

● ✓6th **N8Ø.C1 Endometriosis of the anterior abdominal wall**

● **N8Ø.C1Ø Endometriosis of the anterior abdominal wall, subcutaneous tissue**

● **N8Ø.C11 Endometriosis of the anterior abdominal wall, fascia and muscular layers**

● **N8Ø.C19 Endometriosis of the anterior abdominal wall, unspecified depth**
Endometriosis of the anterior abdominal wall NOS

● **N8Ø.C2 Endometriosis of the umbilicus**

● **N8Ø.C3 Endometriosis of the inguinal canal**

● **N8Ø.C4 Endometriosis of extra-pelvic abdominal peritoneum**

● **N8Ø.C9 Endometriosis of other site of abdomen**

● ✓5th **N8Ø.D Endometriosis of the pelvic nerves**
Endometriosis of the nerves of the retroperitoneum

● **N8Ø.DØ Endometriosis of the pelvic nerves, unspecified**
Endometriosis of nerve of the retroperitoneum, NOS

● **N8Ø.D1 Endometriosis of the sacral splanchnic nerves**
Endometriosis of the pelvic splanchnic nerves

● **N8Ø.D2 Endometriosis of the sacral nerve roots**

● **N8Ø.D3 Endometriosis of the obturator nerve**

● **N8Ø.D4 Endometriosis of the sciatic nerve**

● **N8Ø.D5 Endometriosis of the pudendal nerve**

● **N8Ø.D6 Endometriosis of the femoral nerve**

● **N8Ø.D9 Endometriosis of other pelvic nerve**
Endometriosis of the other nerves of the retroperitoneum

N8Ø.8 Other endometriosis ♀
▶Endometriosis of other site◀

N8Ø.9 Endometriosis, unspecified ♀

✓4th **N81 Female genital prolapse**

EXCLUDES 1 *genital prolapse complicating pregnancy, labor or delivery (O34.5-)*
prolapse and hernia of ovary and fallopian tube (N83.4-)
prolapse of vaginal vault after hysterectomy (N99.3)

Types of Pelvic Organ Prolapse

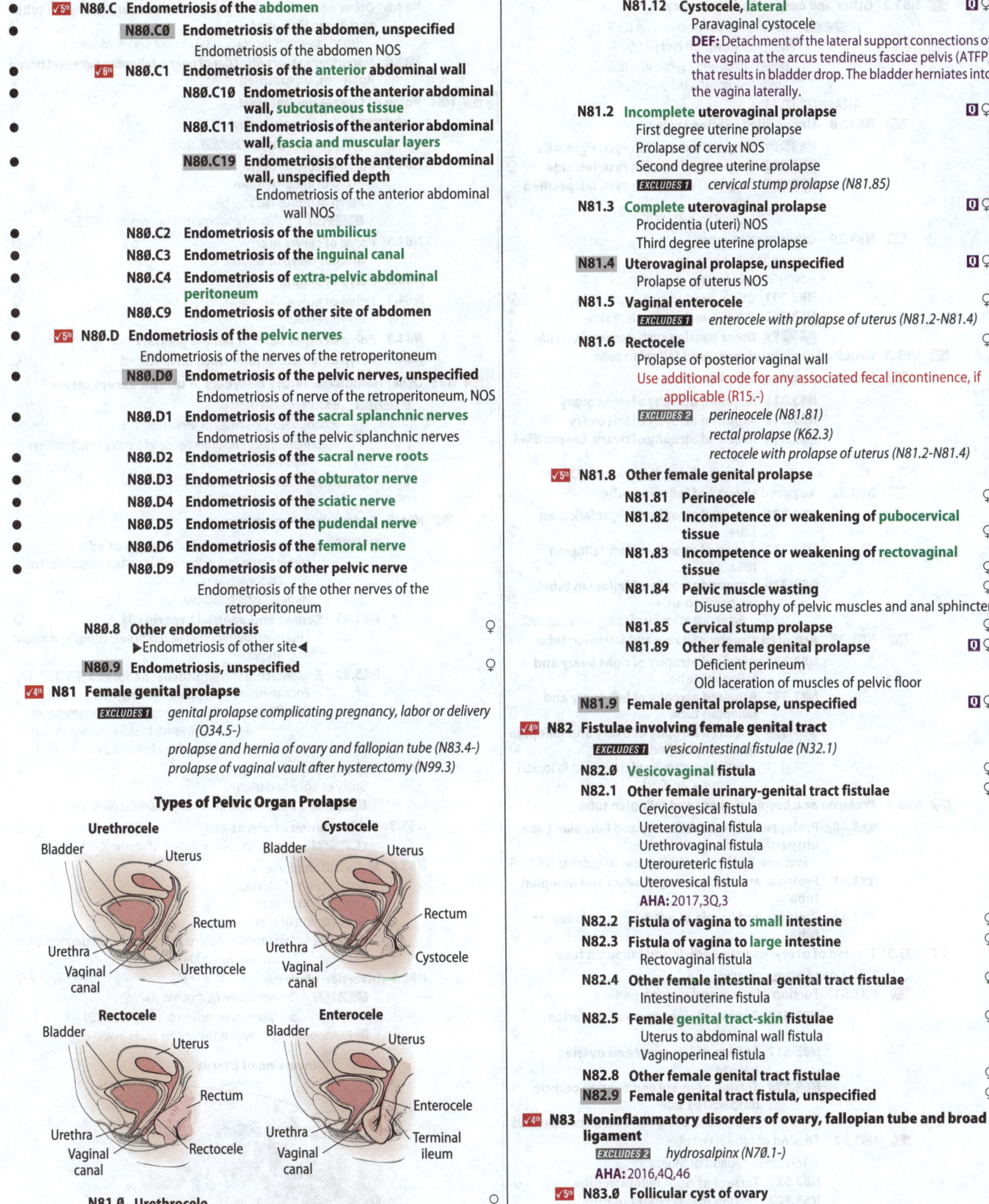

N81.Ø Urethrocele ♀
EXCLUDES 1 *urethrocele with cystocele (N81.1-)*
urethrocele with prolapse of uterus (N81.2-N81.4)

✓5th **N81.1 Cystocele**
Cystocele with urethrocele
Cystourethrocele
EXCLUDES 1 *cystocele with prolapse of uterus (N81.2-N81.4)*

N81.1Ø Cystocele, unspecified Q ♀
Prolapse of (anterior) vaginal wall NOS

N81.11 Cystocele, midline Q ♀

N81.12 Cystocele, lateral Q ♀
Paravaginal cystocele
DEF: Detachment of the lateral support connections of the vagina at the arcus tendineus fasciae pelvis (ATFP) that results in bladder drop. The bladder herniates into the vagina laterally.

N81.2 Incomplete uterovaginal prolapse Q ♀
First degree uterine prolapse
Prolapse of cervix NOS
Second degree uterine prolapse
EXCLUDES 1 *cervical stump prolapse (N81.85)*

N81.3 Complete uterovaginal prolapse Q ♀
Procidentia (uteri) NOS
Third degree uterine prolapse

N81.4 Uterovaginal prolapse, unspecified Q ♀
Prolapse of uterus NOS

N81.5 Vaginal enterocele ♀
EXCLUDES 1 *enterocele with prolapse of uterus (N81.2-N81.4)*

N81.6 Rectocele ♀
Prolapse of posterior vaginal wall
Use additional code for any associated fecal incontinence, if applicable (R15.-)
EXCLUDES 2 *perineocele (N81.81)*
rectal prolapse (K62.3)
rectocele with prolapse of uterus (N81.2-N81.4)

✓5th **N81.8 Other female genital prolapse**

N81.81 Perineocele ♀

N81.82 Incompetence or weakening of pubocervical tissue ♀

N81.83 Incompetence or weakening of rectovaginal tissue ♀

N81.84 Pelvic muscle wasting ♀
Disuse atrophy of pelvic muscles and anal sphincter

N81.85 Cervical stump prolapse ♀

N81.89 Other female genital prolapse Q ♀
Deficient perineum
Old laceration of muscles of pelvic floor

N81.9 Female genital prolapse, unspecified Q ♀

✓4th **N82 Fistulae involving female genital tract**
EXCLUDES 1 *vesicointestinal fistulae (N32.1)*

N82.Ø Vesicovaginal fistula ♀

N82.1 Other female urinary-genital tract fistulae ♀
Cervicovesical fistula
Ureterovaginal fistula
Urethrovaginal fistula
Uteroureteric fistula
Uterovesical fistula
AHA: 2017,3Q,3

N82.2 Fistula of vagina to small intestine ♀

N82.3 Fistula of vagina to large intestine ♀
Rectovaginal fistula

N82.4 Other female intestinal-genital tract fistulae ♀
Intestinouterine fistula

N82.5 Female genital tract-skin fistulae ♀
Uterus to abdominal wall fistula
Vaginoperineal fistula

N82.8 Other female genital tract fistulae ♀

N82.9 Female genital tract fistula, unspecified ♀

✓4th **N83 Noninflammatory disorders of ovary, fallopian tube and broad ligament**
EXCLUDES 2 *hydrosalpinx (N7Ø.1-)*
AHA: 2016,4Q,46

✓5th **N83.Ø Follicular cyst of ovary**
Cyst of graafian follicle
Hemorrhagic follicular cyst (of ovary)

N83.ØØ Follicular cyst of ovary, unspecified side ♀

N83.Ø1 Follicular cyst of right ovary ♀

N83.Ø2 Follicular cyst of left ovary ♀

✓5th **N83.1 Corpus luteum cyst**
Hemorrhagic corpus luteum cyst
AHA: 2022,1Q,23

N83.1Ø Corpus luteum cyst of ovary, unspecified side ♀

N83.11 Corpus luteum cyst of right ovary ♀

N83.12 Corpus luteum cyst of left ovary ♀

Chapter 14. Diseases of the Genitourinary System

√5th **N83.2 Other and unspecified ovarian cysts**
EXCLUDES 1 *developmental ovarian cyst (Q5Ø.1)*
neoplastic ovarian cyst (D27.-)
polycystic ovarian syndrome (E28.2)
Stein-Leventhal syndrome (E28.2)
AHA: 2022,1Q,23

√6th **N83.2Ø Unspecified ovarian cysts**
N83.2Ø1 Unspecified ovarian cyst, right side ♀
N83.2Ø2 Unspecified ovarian cyst, left side ♀
N83.2Ø9 Unspecified ovarian cyst, unspecified side ♀
Ovarian cyst, NOS

√6th **N83.29 Other ovarian cysts**
Retention cyst of ovary
Simple cyst of ovary
N83.291 Other ovarian cyst, right side ♀
N83.292 Other ovarian cyst, left side ♀
N83.299 Other ovarian cyst, unspecified side ♀

√5th **N83.3 Acquired atrophy of ovary and fallopian tube**

√6th **N83.31 Acquired atrophy of ovary**
N83.311 Acquired atrophy of right ovary ♀
N83.312 Acquired atrophy of left ovary ♀
N83.319 Acquired atrophy of ovary, unspecified side ♀
Acquired atrophy of ovary, NOS

√6th **N83.32 Acquired atrophy of fallopian tube**
N83.321 Acquired atrophy of right fallopian tube ♀
N83.322 Acquired atrophy of left fallopian tube ♀
N83.329 Acquired atrophy of fallopian tube, unspecified side ♀
Acquired atrophy of fallopian tube, NOS

√6th **N83.33 Acquired atrophy of ovary and fallopian tube**
N83.331 Acquired atrophy of right ovary and fallopian tube ♀
N83.332 Acquired atrophy of left ovary and fallopian tube ♀
N83.339 Acquired atrophy of ovary and fallopian tube, unspecified side ♀
Acquired atrophy of ovary and fallopian tube, NOS

√5th **N83.4 Prolapse and hernia of ovary and fallopian tube**
N83.4Ø Prolapse and hernia of ovary and fallopian tube, unspecified side ♀
Prolapse and hernia of ovary and fallopian tube, NOS
N83.41 Prolapse and hernia of right ovary and fallopian tube ♀
N83.42 Prolapse and hernia of left ovary and fallopian tube ♀

√5th **N83.5 Torsion of ovary, ovarian pedicle and fallopian tube**
Torsion of accessory tube

√6th **N83.51 Torsion of ovary and ovarian pedicle**
N83.511 Torsion of right ovary and ovarian pedicle ♀
N83.512 Torsion of left ovary and ovarian pedicle ♀
N83.519 Torsion of ovary and ovarian pedicle, unspecified side ♀
Torsion of ovary and ovarian pedicle, NOS

√6th **N83.52 Torsion of fallopian tube**
Torsion of hydatid of Morgagni
N83.521 Torsion of right fallopian tube ♀
N83.522 Torsion of left fallopian tube ♀
N83.529 Torsion of fallopian tube, unspecified side ♀
Torsion of fallopian tube, NOS

N83.53 Torsion of ovary, ovarian pedicle and fallopian tube ♀

N83.6 Hematosalpinx ♀
EXCLUDES 1 *hematosalpinx (with) (in):*
hematocolpos (N89.7)
hematometra (N85.7)
tubal pregnancy (OØØ.1-)

N83.7 Hematoma of broad ligament ♀

N83.8 Other noninflammatory disorders of ovary, fallopian tube and broad ligament ♀
Broad ligament laceration syndrome [Allen-Masters]

N83.9 Noninflammatory disorder of ovary, fallopian tube and broad ligament, unspecified ♀

√4th **N84 Polyp of female genital tract**
EXCLUDES 1 *adenomatous polyp (D28.-)*
placental polyp (O9Ø.89)

N84.Ø Polyp of corpus uteri ♀
Polyp of endometrium
Polyp of uterus NOS
EXCLUDES 1 *polypoid endometrial hyperplasia (N85.Ø-)*

N84.1 Polyp of cervix uteri ♀
Mucous polyp of cervix

N84.2 Polyp of vagina ♀

N84.3 Polyp of vulva ♀
Polyp of labia

N84.8 Polyp of other parts of female genital tract ♀

N84.9 Polyp of female genital tract, unspecified ♀

√4th **N85 Other noninflammatory disorders of uterus, except cervix**
EXCLUDES 1 *endometriosis (N8Ø.-)*
inflammatory diseases of uterus (N71.-)
noninflammatory disorders of cervix, except malposition (N86-N88)
polyp of corpus uteri (N84.Ø)
uterine prolapse (N81.-)

√5th **N85.Ø Endometrial hyperplasia**
N85.ØØ Endometrial hyperplasia, unspecified ♀
Hyperplasia (adenomatous) (cystic) (glandular) of endometrium
Hyperplastic endometritis
N85.Ø1 Benign endometrial hyperplasia ♀
Endometrial hyperplasia (complex) (simple) without atypia
N85.Ø2 Endometrial intraepithelial neoplasia [EIN] ♀
Endometrial hyperplasia with atypia
EXCLUDES 1 *malignant neoplasm of endometrium (with endometrial intraepithelial neoplasia [EIN]) (C54.1)*

N85.2 Hypertrophy of uterus ♀
Bulky or enlarged uterus
EXCLUDES 1 *puerperal hypertrophy of uterus (O9Ø.89)*

N85.3 Subinvolution of uterus ♀
EXCLUDES 1 *puerperal subinvolution of uterus (O9Ø.89)*

N85.4 Malposition of uterus ♀
Anteversion of uterus
Retroflexion of uterus
Retroversion of uterus
EXCLUDES 1 *malposition of uterus complicating pregnancy, labor or delivery (O34.5-, O65.5)*

N85.5 Inversion of uterus ♀
EXCLUDES 1 *current obstetric trauma (O71.2)*
postpartum inversion of uterus (O71.2)
DEF: Abnormality in which the uterus turns inside out.

Inversion of Uterus

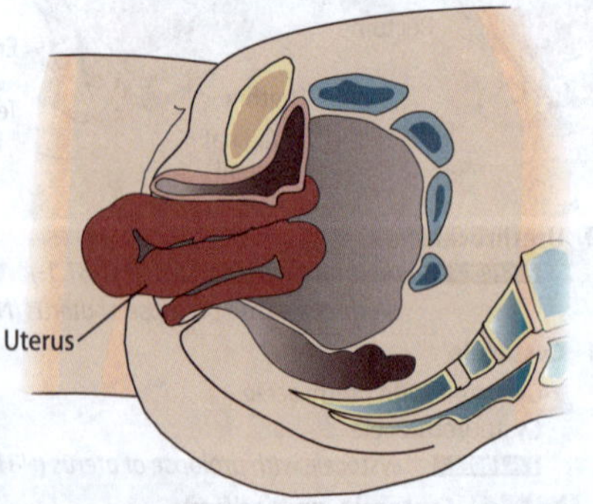

Uterus

N85.6 Intrauterine synechiae ♀

N83.2–N85.6

N85.7 Hematometra ♀
Hematosalpinx with hematometra
EXCLUDES 1 *hematometra with hematocolpos (N89.7)*
DEF: Accumulation of blood within the uterus.

N85.8 Other specified noninflammatory disorders of uterus ♀
Atrophy of uterus, acquired
Fibrosis of uterus NOS

N85.9 Noninflammatory disorder of uterus, unspecified ♀
Disorder of uterus NOS

● **N85.A Isthmocele**
Isthmocele (non-pregnant state)
Code also any associated conditions such as:
abnormal uterine and vaginal bleeding, unspecified (N93.9)
female infertility of uterine origin (N97.2)
pelvic and perineal pain (R1Ø.2)
EXCLUDES 1 *maternal care for cesarean scar defect (isthmocele) (O34.22)*

N86 Erosion and ectropion of cervix uteri ♀
Decubitus (trophic) ulcer of cervix
Eversion of cervix
EXCLUDES 1 *erosion and ectropion of cervix with cervicitis (N72)*

✓4th **N87 Dysplasia of cervix uteri**
EXCLUDES 1 *abnormal results from cervical cytologic examination without histologic confirmation (R87.61-)*
carcinoma in situ of cervix uteri (DØ6.-)
cervical intraepithelial neoplasia III [CIN III] (DØ6.-)
HGSIL of cervix (R87.613)
severe dysplasia of cervix uteri (DØ6.-)

N87.Ø Mild cervical dysplasia ♀
Cervical intraepithelial neoplasia I [CIN I]

N87.1 Moderate cervical dysplasia ♀
Cervical intraepithelial neoplasia II [CIN II]

N87.9 Dysplasia of cervix uteri, unspecified ♀
Anaplasia of cervix
Cervical atypism
Cervical dysplasia NOS

✓4th **N88 Other noninflammatory disorders of cervix uteri**
EXCLUDES 2 *inflammatory disease of cervix (N72)*
polyp of cervix (N84.1)

N88.Ø Leukoplakia of cervix uteri ♀

N88.1 Old laceration of cervix uteri ♀
Adhesions of cervix
EXCLUDES 1 *current obstetric trauma (O71.3)*

N88.2 Stricture and stenosis of cervix uteri ♀
EXCLUDES 1 *stricture and stenosis of cervix uteri complicating labor (O65.5)*

N88.3 Incompetence of cervix uteri ♀
Investigation and management of (suspected) cervical incompetence in a nonpregnant woman
EXCLUDES 1 *cervical incompetence complicating pregnancy (O34.3-)*
DEF: Inadequate functioning of the cervix marked by abnormal widening during pregnancy and causing premature birth or miscarriage.

N88.4 Hypertrophic elongation of cervix uteri ♀

N88.8 Other specified noninflammatory disorders of cervix uteri ♀
EXCLUDES 1 *current obstetric trauma (O71.3)*

N88.9 Noninflammatory disorder of cervix uteri, unspecified ♀

✓4th **N89 Other noninflammatory disorders of vagina**
EXCLUDES 1 *abnormal results from vaginal cytologic examination without histologic confirmation (R87.62-)*
carcinoma in situ of vagina (DØ7.2)
HGSIL of vagina (R87.623)
inflammation of vagina (N76.-)
senile (atrophic) vaginitis (N95.2)
severe dysplasia of vagina (DØ7.2)
trichomonal leukorrhea (A59.ØØ)
vaginal intraepithelial neoplasia [VAIN], grade III (DØ7.2)

N89.Ø Mild vaginal dysplasia ♀
Vaginal intraepithelial neoplasia [VAIN], grade I

N89.1 Moderate vaginal dysplasia ♀
Vaginal intraepithelial neoplasia [VAIN], grade II

N89.3 Dysplasia of vagina, unspecified ♀

N89.4 Leukoplakia of vagina ♀

N89.5 Stricture and atresia of vagina ♀
Vaginal adhesions
Vaginal stenosis
EXCLUDES 1 *congenital atresia or stricture (Q52.4)*
postprocedural adhesions of vagina (N99.2)

N89.6 Tight hymenal ring ♀
Rigid hymen
Tight introitus
EXCLUDES 1 *imperforate hymen (Q52.3)*

N89.7 Hematocolpos ♀
Hematocolpos with hematometra or hematosalpinx
AHA: 2016,4Q,58

N89.8 Other specified noninflammatory disorders of vagina ♀
Leukorrhea NOS
Old vaginal laceration
Pessary ulcer of vagina
EXCLUDES 1 *current obstetric trauma (O7Ø.-, O71.4, O71.7-O71.8)*
old laceration involving muscles of pelvic floor (N81.8)

N89.9 Noninflammatory disorder of vagina, unspecified ♀

✓4th **N9Ø Other noninflammatory disorders of vulva and perineum**
EXCLUDES 1 *anogenital (venereal) warts (A63.Ø)*
carcinoma in situ of vulva (DØ7.1)
condyloma acuminatum (A63.Ø)
current obstetric trauma (O7Ø.-, O71.7-O71.8)
inflammation of vulva (N76.-)
severe dysplasia of vulva (DØ7.1)
vulvar intraepithelial neoplasm III [VIN III] (DØ7.1)

N9Ø.Ø Mild vulvar dysplasia ♀
Vulvar intraepithelial neoplasia [VIN], grade I

N9Ø.1 Moderate vulvar dysplasia ♀
Vulvar intraepithelial neoplasia [VIN], grade II

N9Ø.3 Dysplasia of vulva, unspecified ♀

N9Ø.4 Leukoplakia of vulva ♀
Dystrophy of vulva
Kraurosis of vulva
Lichen sclerosus of external female genital organs

N9Ø.5 Atrophy of vulva ♀
Stenosis of vulva

✓5th **N9Ø.6 Hypertrophy of vulva**
AHA: 2016,4Q,46

N9Ø.6Ø Unspecified hypertrophy of vulva ♀
Unspecified hypertrophy of labia

N9Ø.61 Childhood asymmetric labium majus enlargement ♀
CALME

N9Ø.69 Other specified hypertrophy of vulva ♀
Other specified hypertrophy of labia

N9Ø.7 Vulvar cyst ♀

✓5th **N9Ø.8 Other specified noninflammatory disorders of vulva and perineum**

✓6th **N9Ø.81 Female genital mutilation status**
Female genital cutting status

N9Ø.81Ø Female genital mutilation status, unspecified ♀
Female genital cutting status, unspecified
Female genital mutilation status NOS

N9Ø.811 Female genital mutilation Type I status ♀
Clitorectomy status
Female genital cutting Type I status

N9Ø.812 Female genital mutilation Type II status ♀
Clitorectomy with excision of labia minora status
Female genital cutting Type II status

N9Ø.813 Female genital mutilation Type III status ♀
Female genital cutting Type III status
Infibulation status

N90.818 Other female genital mutilation status ♀
Female genital cutting Type IV status
Female genital mutilation Type IV status
Other female genital cutting status

N90.89 Other specified noninflammatory disorders of vulva and perineum ♀
Adhesions of vulva
Hypertrophy of clitoris

N90.9 Noninflammatory disorder of vulva and perineum, unspecified ♀

✓4th N91 Absent, scanty and rare menstruation
EXCLUDES 1 *ovarian dysfunction (E28.-)*

N91.0 Primary amenorrhea ♀
N91.1 Secondary amenorrhea ♀
N91.2 Amenorrhea, unspecified ♀
N91.3 Primary oligomenorrhea ♀
N91.4 Secondary oligomenorrhea ♀
N91.5 Oligomenorrhea, unspecified ♀
Hypomenorrhea NOS

✓4th N92 Excessive, frequent and irregular menstruation
EXCLUDES 1 *postmenopausal bleeding (N95.0)*
precocious puberty (menstruation) (E30.1)

N92.0 Excessive and frequent menstruation with regular cycle ♀
Heavy periods NOS
Menorrhagia NOS
Polymenorrhea

N92.1 Excessive and frequent menstruation with irregular cycle ♀
Irregular intermenstrual bleeding
Irregular, shortened intervals between menstrual bleeding
Menometrorrhagia
Metrorrhagia

N92.2 Excessive menstruation at puberty P ♀
Excessive bleeding associated with onset of menstrual periods
Pubertal menorrhagia
Puberty bleeding

N92.3 Ovulation bleeding ♀
Regular intermenstrual bleeding

N92.4 Excessive bleeding in the premenopausal period ♀
Climacteric menorrhagia or metrorrhagia
Menopausal menorrhagia or metrorrhagia
Perimenopausal bleeding
Perimenopausal menorrhagia or metrorrhagia
Preclimacteric menorrhagia or metrorrhagia
Premenopausal menorrhagia or metrorrhagia

N92.5 Other specified irregular menstruation ♀

N92.6 Irregular menstruation, unspecified ♀
Irregular bleeding NOS
Irregular periods NOS
EXCLUDES 1 *irregular menstruation with:*
lengthened intervals or scanty bleeding (N91.3-N91.5)
shortened intervals or excessive bleeding (N92.1)

✓4th N93 Other abnormal uterine and vaginal bleeding
EXCLUDES 1 *neonatal vaginal hemorrhage (P54.6)*
precocious puberty (menstruation) (E30.1)
pseudomenses (P54.6)

N93.0 Postcoital and contact bleeding ♀

N93.1 Pre-pubertal vaginal bleeding ♀
AHA: 2016,4Q,47

N93.8 Other specified abnormal uterine and vaginal bleeding ♀
Dysfunctional or functional uterine or vaginal bleeding NOS

N93.9 Abnormal uterine and vaginal bleeding, unspecified ♀

✓4th N94 Pain and other conditions associated with female genital organs and menstrual cycle

N94.0 Mittelschmerz ♀
DEF: One-sided, lower abdominal pain occurring between menstrual periods that is associated with ovulation.

✓5th N94.1 Dyspareunia
EXCLUDES 1 *psychogenic dyspareunia (F52.6)*
AHA: 2016,4Q,47

N94.10 Unspecified dyspareunia ♀
N94.11 Superficial (introital) dyspareunia ♀
N94.12 Deep dyspareunia ♀
N94.19 Other specified dyspareunia ♀

N94.2 Vaginismus ♀
EXCLUDES 1 *psychogenic vaginismus (F52.5)*
DEF: Spontaneous contractions of the muscles surrounding the vagina, causing it to constrict or close.

N94.3 Premenstrual tension syndrome ♀
Code also associated menstrual migraine (G43.82-, G43.83-)
EXCLUDES 1 *premenstrual dysphoric disorder (F32.81)*

N94.4 Primary dysmenorrhea ♀
N94.5 Secondary dysmenorrhea ♀
N94.6 Dysmenorrhea, unspecified ♀
EXCLUDES 1 *psychogenic dysmenorrhea (F45.8)*

✓5th N94.8 Other specified conditions associated with female genital organs and menstrual cycle

✓6th N94.81 Vulvodynia

N94.810 Vulvar vestibulitis ♀
N94.818 Other vulvodynia ♀
N94.819 Vulvodynia, unspecified ♀
Vulvodynia NOS

N94.89 Other specified conditions associated with female genital organs and menstrual cycle ♀
DEF: Hydrocele: Serous fluid that collects in the canal of Nuck in females.

N94.9 Unspecified condition associated with female genital organs and menstrual cycle ♀

✓4th N95 Menopausal and other perimenopausal disorders
Menopausal and other perimenopausal disorders due to naturally occurring (age-related) menopause and perimenopause
EXCLUDES 1 *excessive bleeding in the premenopausal period (N92.4)*
menopausal and perimenopausal disorders due to artificial or premature menopause (E89.4-, E28.31-)
premature menopause (E28.31-)
EXCLUDES 2 *postmenopausal osteoporosis (M81.0-)*
postmenopausal osteoporosis with current pathological fracture (M80.0-)
postmenopausal urethritis (N34.2)

N95.0 Postmenopausal bleeding ♀

N95.1 Menopausal and female climacteric states ♀
Symptoms such as flushing, sleeplessness, headache, lack of concentration, associated with natural (age-related) menopause
Use additional code for associated symptoms
EXCLUDES 1 *asymptomatic menopausal state (Z78.0)*
symptoms associated with artificial menopause (E89.41)
symptoms associated with premature menopause (E28.310)

N95.2 Postmenopausal atrophic vaginitis ♀
Senile (atrophic) vaginitis

N95.8 Other specified menopausal and perimenopausal disorders ♀

N95.9 Unspecified menopausal and perimenopausal disorder ♀

N96 Recurrent pregnancy loss ♀
Investigation or care in a nonpregnant woman with history of recurrent pregnancy loss
EXCLUDES 1 *recurrent pregnancy loss with current pregnancy (O26.2-)*

✓4th N97 Female infertility
INCLUDES inability to achieve a pregnancy
sterility, female NOS
EXCLUDES 2 *female infertility associated with:*
hypopituitarism (E23.0)
Stein-Leventhal syndrome (E28.2)
incompetence of cervix uteri (N88.3)
DEF: Infertility: Inability to conceive for at least one year with regular intercourse.
DEF: Primary infertility: Infertility occurring in patients who have never conceived.
DEF: Secondary infertility: Infertility occurring in patients who have previously conceived.

N97.0 Female infertility associated with anovulation ♀
AHA: 2022,2Q,16

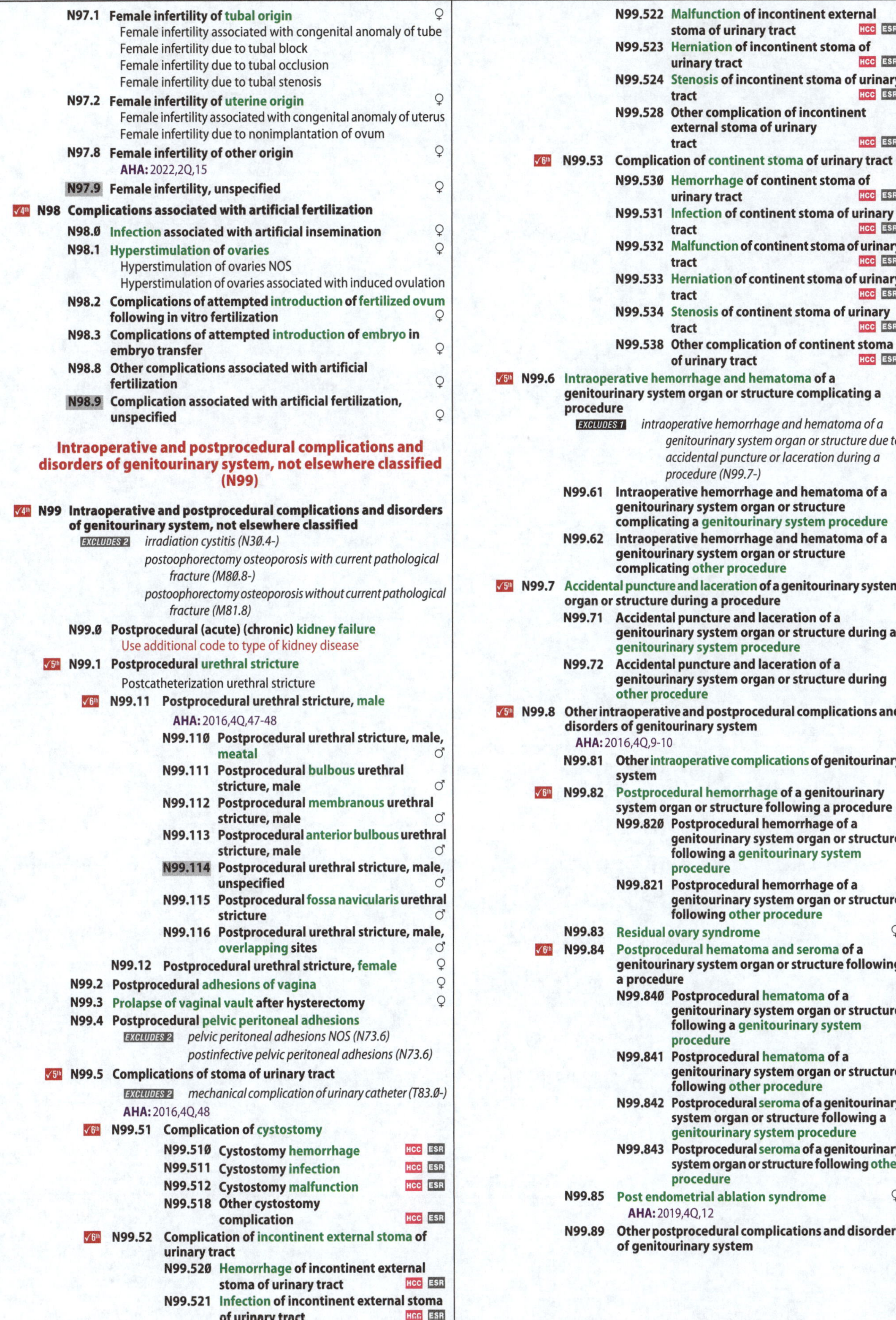

N97.1 **Female infertility of tubal origin** ♀
Female infertility associated with congenital anomaly of tube
Female infertility due to tubal block
Female infertility due to tubal occlusion
Female infertility due to tubal stenosis

N97.2 **Female infertility of uterine origin** ♀
Female infertility associated with congenital anomaly of uterus
Female infertility due to nonimplantation of ovum

N97.8 **Female infertility of other origin** ♀
AHA: 2022,2Q,15

N97.9 **Female infertility, unspecified** ♀

✓4th **N98 Complications associated with artificial fertilization**

N98.0 **Infection associated with artificial insemination** ♀

N98.1 **Hyperstimulation of ovaries** ♀
Hyperstimulation of ovaries NOS
Hyperstimulation of ovaries associated with induced ovulation

N98.2 **Complications of attempted introduction of fertilized ovum following in vitro fertilization** ♀

N98.3 **Complications of attempted introduction of embryo in embryo transfer** ♀

N98.8 **Other complications associated with artificial fertilization** ♀

N98.9 **Complication associated with artificial fertilization, unspecified** ♀

Intraoperative and postprocedural complications and disorders of genitourinary system, not elsewhere classified (N99)

✓4th **N99 Intraoperative and postprocedural complications and disorders of genitourinary system, not elsewhere classified**
EXCLUDES 2 *irradiation cystitis (N30.4-)*
postoophorectomy osteoporosis with current pathological fracture (M80.8-)
postoophorectomy osteoporosis without current pathological fracture (M81.8)

N99.0 **Postprocedural (acute) (chronic) kidney failure**
Use additional code to type of kidney disease

✓5th N99.1 **Postprocedural urethral stricture**
Postcatheterization urethral stricture

✓6th N99.11 **Postprocedural urethral stricture, male**
AHA: 2016,4Q,47-48

N99.110 **Postprocedural urethral stricture, male, meatal** ♂
N99.111 **Postprocedural bulbous urethral stricture, male** ♂
N99.112 **Postprocedural membranous urethral stricture, male** ♂
N99.113 **Postprocedural anterior bulbous urethral stricture, male** ♂
N99.114 **Postprocedural urethral stricture, male, unspecified** ♂
N99.115 **Postprocedural fossa navicularis urethral stricture** ♂
N99.116 **Postprocedural urethral stricture, male, overlapping sites** ♂

N99.12 **Postprocedural urethral stricture, female** ♀

N99.2 **Postprocedural adhesions of vagina** ♀

N99.3 **Prolapse of vaginal vault after hysterectomy** ♀

N99.4 **Postprocedural pelvic peritoneal adhesions**
EXCLUDES 2 *pelvic peritoneal adhesions NOS (N73.6)*
postinfective pelvic peritoneal adhesions (N73.6)

✓5th N99.5 **Complications of stoma of urinary tract**
EXCLUDES 2 *mechanical complication of urinary catheter (T83.0-)*
AHA: 2016,4Q,48

✓6th N99.51 **Complication of cystostomy**

N99.510 **Cystostomy hemorrhage** HCC ESR
N99.511 **Cystostomy infection** HCC ESR
N99.512 **Cystostomy malfunction** HCC ESR
N99.518 **Other cystostomy complication** HCC ESR

✓6th N99.52 **Complication of incontinent external stoma of urinary tract**

N99.520 **Hemorrhage of incontinent external stoma of urinary tract** HCC ESR
N99.521 **Infection of incontinent external stoma of urinary tract** HCC ESR
N99.522 **Malfunction of incontinent external stoma of urinary tract** HCC ESR
N99.523 **Herniation of incontinent stoma of urinary tract** HCC ESR
N99.524 **Stenosis of incontinent stoma of urinary tract** HCC ESR
N99.528 **Other complication of incontinent external stoma of urinary tract** HCC ESR

✓6th N99.53 **Complication of continent stoma of urinary tract**

N99.530 **Hemorrhage of continent stoma of urinary tract** HCC ESR
N99.531 **Infection of continent stoma of urinary tract** HCC ESR
N99.532 **Malfunction of continent stoma of urinary tract** HCC ESR
N99.533 **Herniation of continent stoma of urinary tract** HCC ESR
N99.534 **Stenosis of continent stoma of urinary tract** HCC ESR
N99.538 **Other complication of continent stoma of urinary tract** HCC ESR

✓5th N99.6 **Intraoperative hemorrhage and hematoma of a genitourinary system organ or structure complicating a procedure**
EXCLUDES 1 *intraoperative hemorrhage and hematoma of a genitourinary system organ or structure due to accidental puncture or laceration during a procedure (N99.7-)*

N99.61 **Intraoperative hemorrhage and hematoma of a genitourinary system organ or structure complicating a genitourinary system procedure**

N99.62 **Intraoperative hemorrhage and hematoma of a genitourinary system organ or structure complicating other procedure**

✓5th N99.7 **Accidental puncture and laceration of a genitourinary system organ or structure during a procedure**

N99.71 **Accidental puncture and laceration of a genitourinary system organ or structure during a genitourinary system procedure**

N99.72 **Accidental puncture and laceration of a genitourinary system organ or structure during other procedure**

✓5th N99.8 **Other intraoperative and postprocedural complications and disorders of genitourinary system**
AHA: 2016,4Q,9-10

N99.81 **Other intraoperative complications of genitourinary system**

✓6th N99.82 **Postprocedural hemorrhage of a genitourinary system organ or structure following a procedure**

N99.820 **Postprocedural hemorrhage of a genitourinary system organ or structure following a genitourinary system procedure**
N99.821 **Postprocedural hemorrhage of a genitourinary system organ or structure following other procedure**

N99.83 **Residual ovary syndrome** ♀

✓6th N99.84 **Postprocedural hematoma and seroma of a genitourinary system organ or structure following a procedure**

N99.840 **Postprocedural hematoma of a genitourinary system organ or structure following a genitourinary system procedure**
N99.841 **Postprocedural hematoma of a genitourinary system organ or structure following other procedure**
N99.842 **Postprocedural seroma of a genitourinary system organ or structure following a genitourinary system procedure**
N99.843 **Postprocedural seroma of a genitourinary system organ or structure following other procedure**

N99.85 **Post endometrial ablation syndrome** ♀
AHA: 2019,4Q,12

N99.89 **Other postprocedural complications and disorders of genitourinary system**

Chapter 15. Pregnancy, Childbirth, and the Puerperium (O00–O9A)

Chapter-specific Guidelines with Coding Examples

The chapter-specific guidelines from the ICD-10-CM Official Guidelines for Coding and Reporting have been provided below. Along with these guidelines are coding examples, contained in the shaded boxes, that have been developed to help illustrate the coding and/or sequencing guidance found in these guidelines.

a. General rules for obstetric cases

1) Codes from Chapter 15 and sequencing priority

Obstetric cases require codes from chapter 15, codes in the range O00-O9A, Pregnancy, Childbirth, and the Puerperium. Chapter 15 codes have sequencing priority over codes from other chapters. Additional codes from other chapters may be used in conjunction with chapter 15 codes to further specify conditions. Should the provider document that the pregnancy is incidental to the encounter, then code Z33.1, Pregnant state, incidental, should be used in place of any chapter 15 codes. It is the provider's responsibility to state that the condition being treated is not affecting the pregnancy.

Bladder abscess in pregnant patient at 25 weeks' gestation

O23.12	**Infections of bladder in pregnancy, second trimester**
N30.80	**Other cystitis without hematuria**
Z3A.25	**25 weeks gestation of pregnancy**

Explanation: The documentation does not indicate that the pregnancy is incidental or in any way unaffected by the bladder abscess; therefore, an obstetrics code should be sequenced first. An additional code was provided to identify the specific bladder condition as this information is not called out specifically in the obstetrics code.

2) Chapter 15 codes used only on the maternal record

Chapter 15 codes are to be used only on the maternal record, never on the record of the newborn.

3) Final character for trimester

The majority of codes in Chapter 15 have a final character indicating the trimester of pregnancy. The timeframes for the trimesters are indicated at the beginning of the chapter. If trimester is not a component of a code, it is because the condition always occurs in a specific trimester, or the concept of trimester of pregnancy is not applicable. Certain codes have characters for only certain trimesters because the condition does not occur in all trimesters, but it may occur in more than just one. Assignment of the final character for trimester should be based on the provider's documentation of the trimester (or number of weeks) for the current admission/encounter. This applies to the assignment of trimester for pre-existing conditions as well as those that develop during or are due to the pregnancy. The provider's documentation of the number of weeks may be used to assign the appropriate code identifying the trimester.

Pregnant patient at 21 weeks' gestation admitted with excessive vomiting

O21.2	**Late vomiting of pregnancy**
Z3A.21	**21 weeks gestation of pregnancy**

Explanation: Category O21 classifies vomiting in pregnancy. Although code selection is based on whether the vomiting is before or after 20 completed weeks, these codes are not further classified by trimester. If vomiting only in the second trimester was documented, the provider should be queried for the specific week of gestation, as this will affect code selection.

Whenever delivery occurs during the current admission, and there is an "in childbirth" option for the obstetric complication being coded, the "in childbirth" code should be assigned. When the classification does not provide an obstetric code with an "in childbirth" option, it is appropriate to assign a code describing the current trimester.

4) Selection of trimester for inpatient admissions that encompass more than one trimester

In instances when a patient is admitted to a hospital for complications of pregnancy during one trimester and remains in the hospital into a subsequent trimester, the trimester character for the antepartum complication code should be assigned on the basis of the trimester when the complication developed, not the trimester of the discharge. If the condition developed prior to the current admission/encounter or represents a pre-existing condition, the trimester character for the trimester at the time of the admission/encounter should be assigned.

5) Unspecified trimester

Each category that includes codes for trimester has a code for "unspecified trimester." The "unspecified trimester" code should rarely be used, such as when the documentation in the record is insufficient to determine the trimester and it is not possible to obtain clarification.

6) 7th character for fetus identification

Where applicable, a 7th character is to be assigned for certain categories (O31, O32, O33.3 - O33.6, O35, O36, O40, O41, O60.1, O60.2, O64, and O69) to identify the fetus for which the complication code applies.

Assign 7th character "0":

- For single gestations.
- When the documentation in the record is insufficient to determine the fetus affected and it is not possible to obtain clarification.
- When it is not possible to clinically determine which fetus is affected.

Maternal patient with twin gestations is seen after ultrasound identifies fetus B to be in breech presentation

O32.1XX2	**Maternal care for breech presentation, fetus 2**

Explanation: The documentation indicates that although there are two fetuses, only one fetus is determined to be in breech presentation. Whether fetus 2 or fetus B is used, the coder can assign the seventh character of 2 to identify the second fetus as the one in breech.

7) Completed weeks of gestation

In ICD-10-CM, "completed" weeks of gestation refers to full weeks. For example, if the provider documents gestation at 39 weeks and 6 days, the code for 39 weeks of gestation should be assigned, as the patient has not yet reached 40 completed weeks.

b. Selection of OB principal or first-listed diagnosis

1) Routine outpatient prenatal visits

For routine outpatient prenatal visits when no complications are present, a code from category Z34, Encounter for supervision of normal pregnancy, should be used as the first-listed diagnosis. These codes should not be used in conjunction with chapter 15 codes.

2) Supervision of high-risk pregnancy

Codes from category O09, Supervision of high-risk pregnancy, are intended for use only during the prenatal period. For complications during the labor or delivery episode as a result of a high-risk pregnancy, assign the applicable complication codes from Chapter 15. If there are no complications during the labor or delivery episode, assign code O80, Encounter for full-term uncomplicated delivery.

For routine prenatal outpatient visits for patients with high-risk pregnancies, a code from category O09, Supervision of high-risk pregnancy, should be used as the first-listed diagnosis. Secondary chapter 15 codes may be used in conjunction with these codes if appropriate.

36-year-old seen in labor with second child at 39 weeks' gestation, delivered a healthy baby, delivery complicated by tear of fourchette that was repaired

O70.0	**First degree perineal laceration during delivery**
Z3A.39	**39 weeks gestation of pregnancy**
Z37.0	**Single live birth**

Explanation: Although this patient is over 35 and having her second child (elderly multigravida), do not append a code from subcategory O09.52-. A code describing the tear of the fourchette, which complicated the delivery, should be used in addition to the applicable Z codes.

3) Episodes when no delivery occurs

In episodes when no delivery occurs, the principal diagnosis should correspond to the principal complication of the pregnancy which necessitated the encounter. Should more than one complication exist, all of which are treated or monitored, any of the complication codes may be sequenced first.

4) When a delivery occurs

When an obstetric patient is admitted and delivers during that admission, the condition that prompted the admission should be sequenced as the principal diagnosis. If multiple conditions prompted the admission, sequence the one most related to the delivery as the principal diagnosis. A code for any complication of the delivery should be assigned as an additional diagnosis. In cases of cesarean delivery, if the patient was admitted with a condition that resulted in the performance of a cesarean procedure, that condition should be selected as the principal diagnosis. If the reason for the admission was unrelated to the condition resulting in the cesarean delivery, the condition related to the reason for the admission should be selected as the principal diagnosis.

Maternal patient with diet-controlled gestational diabetes was seen at 38 weeks' gestation in obstructed labor due to footling presentation; cesarean performed for the malpresentation

O64.8XXØ	**Obstructed labor due to other malposition and malpresentation, not applicable or unspecified**
O24.42Ø	**Gestational diabetes mellitus in childbirth, diet controlled**
Z3A.38	**38 weeks gestation of pregnancy**
Z37.Ø	**Single live birth**

Explanation: The obstructed labor necessitated the cesarean procedure.

5) Outcome of delivery

A code from category Z37, Outcome of delivery, should be included on every maternal record when a delivery has occurred. These codes are not to be used on subsequent records or on the newborn record.

c. Pre-existing conditions versus conditions due to the pregnancy

Certain categories in Chapter 15 distinguish between conditions of the mother that existed prior to pregnancy (pre-existing) and those that are a direct result of pregnancy. When assigning codes from Chapter 15, it is important to assess if a condition was pre-existing prior to pregnancy or developed during or due to the pregnancy in order to assign the correct code.

Categories that do not distinguish between pre-existing and pregnancy-related conditions may be used for either. It is acceptable to use codes specifically for the puerperium with codes complicating pregnancy and childbirth if a condition arises postpartum during the delivery encounter.

Type 2 diabetic patient presents at 19 weeks gestation for glucose check. Patient has been taking oral metformin for several years and currently is experiencing no diabetic complications.

O24.112	**Pre-existing type 2 diabetes mellitus, in pregnancy, second trimester**
E11.9	**Type 2 diabetes mellitus without complications**
Z79.84	**Long term (current) use of oral hypoglycemic drugs**

Explanation: The documentation states that the patient has been on a diabetic medication (oral metformin) for several years, indicating the patient was diabetic prior to becoming pregnant. Reporting pre-existing Type 2 diabetes in a pregnant patient requires two codes to capture the condition, a code from category O24 and a code from category E11. A note at E11 indicates that the code for long-term use of oral hypoglycemic drugs should also be reported.

d. Pre-existing hypertension in pregnancy

Category O1Ø, Pre-existing hypertension complicating pregnancy, childbirth and the puerperium, includes codes for hypertensive heart and hypertensive chronic kidney disease. When assigning one of the O1Ø codes that includes hypertensive heart disease or hypertensive chronic kidney disease, it is necessary to add a secondary code from the appropriate hypertension category to specify the type of heart failure or chronic kidney disease.

See Section I.C.9. Hypertension.

e. Fetal conditions affecting the management of the mother

1) Codes from categories O35 and O36

Codes from categories O35, Maternal care for known or suspected fetal abnormality and damage, and O36, Maternal care for other fetal problems, are assigned only when the fetal condition is actually responsible for modifying the management of the mother, i.e., by requiring diagnostic studies, additional observation, special care, or termination of pregnancy. The fact that the fetal condition exists does not justify assigning a code from this series to the mother's record.

A patient with twin gestation is seen for spotting 15 weeks into her pregnancy; the doctors also suspect fetal hydrocephalus. Patient is instructed to return in one week for additional diagnostic testing, sooner if the problem worsens.

O35.ØØXØ	**Maternal care for (suspected) central nervous system malformation or damage in fetus, unspecified, not applicable or unspecified**
O26.852	**Spotting complicating pregnancy, second trimester**
Z3A.15	**15 weeks gestation of pregnancy**

Explanation: Whether the fetal hydrocephalus was suspected or confirmed, an additional code is warranted for this condition since documentation indicates the patient is to return sooner than her routine visit for further testing.

2) In utero surgery

In cases when surgery is performed on the fetus, a diagnosis code from category O35, Maternal care for known or suspected fetal abnormality and damage, should be assigned identifying the fetal condition. Assign the appropriate procedure code for the procedure performed.

No code from Chapter 16, the perinatal codes, should be used on the mother's record to identify fetal conditions. Surgery performed in utero on a fetus is still to be coded as an obstetric encounter.

f. HIV infection in pregnancy, childbirth and the puerperium

During pregnancy, childbirth or the puerperium, a patient admitted because of an HIV-related illness should receive a principal diagnosis from subcategory O98.7-, Human immunodeficiency [HIV] disease complicating pregnancy, childbirth and the puerperium, followed by the code(s) for the HIV-related illness(es).

Patients with asymptomatic HIV infection status admitted during pregnancy, childbirth, or the puerperium should receive codes of O98.7- and Z21, Asymptomatic human immunodeficiency virus [HIV] infection status.

A previously asymptomatic HIV patient who is 13 weeks pregnant is evaluated for HIV-related candidal bronchitis

O98.711	**Human immunodeficiency virus [HIV] disease complicating pregnancy, first trimester**
B2Ø	**Human immunodeficiency virus [HIV] disease**
B37.1	**Pulmonary candidiasis**
Z3A.13	**13 weeks gestation of pregnancy**

Explanation: Because candidal bronchitis is an AIDS-related condition, this patient is now considered to have HIV disease. An obstetrics code indicating that HIV is complicating the pregnancy is coded first, followed by B2Ø for HIV disease as well as a code for the candidal bronchitis.

g. Diabetes mellitus in pregnancy

Diabetes mellitus is a significant complicating factor in pregnancy. Pregnant patients who are diabetic should be assigned a code from category O24, Diabetes mellitus in pregnancy, childbirth, and the puerperium, first, followed by the appropriate diabetes code(s) (EØ8-E13) from Chapter 4.

h. Long term use of insulin and oral hypoglycemics

See section I.C.4.a.3 for information on the long term-use of insulin and oral hypoglycemics.

i. Gestational (pregnancy induced) diabetes

Gestational (pregnancy induced) diabetes can occur during the second and third trimester of pregnancy in patients who were not diabetic prior to pregnancy. Gestational diabetes can cause complications in the pregnancy similar to those of pre-existing diabetes mellitus. It also puts the patient at greater risk of developing diabetes after the pregnancy.

Codes for gestational diabetes are in subcategory O24.4, Gestational diabetes mellitus. No other code from category O24, Diabetes mellitus in pregnancy, childbirth, and the puerperium, should be used with a code from O24.4.

The codes under subcategory O24.4 include diet controlled, insulin controlled, and controlled by oral hypoglycemic drugs. If a patient with gestational diabetes is treated with both diet and insulin, only the code for insulin-controlled is required. If a patient with gestational diabetes is treated with both diet and oral hypoglycemic medications, only the code for "controlled by oral hypoglycemic drugs" is required. Codes Z79.4, Long-term (current) use of insulin, Z79.84, Long-term (current) use of oral hypoglycemic drugs, **and Z79.85, Long-term (current) use of injectable non-insulin antidiabetic drugs,** should not be assigned with codes from subcategory O24.4.

An abnormal glucose tolerance in pregnancy is assigned a code from subcategory O99.81, Abnormal glucose complicating pregnancy, childbirth, and the puerperium.

j. Sepsis and septic shock complicating abortion, pregnancy, childbirth and the puerperium

When assigning a chapter 15 code for sepsis complicating abortion, pregnancy, childbirth, and the puerperium, a code for the specific type of infection should be assigned as an additional diagnosis. If severe sepsis is present, a code from subcategory R65.2, Severe sepsis, and code(s) for associated organ dysfunction(s) should also be assigned as additional diagnoses.

Patient is seen several days after a miscarriage with sepsis; cultures return MSSA

O03.87	**Sepsis following complete or unspecified spontaneous abortion**
B95.61	**Methicillin susceptible Staphylococcus aureus infection as the cause of diseases classified elsewhere**

Explanation: The type of infection that caused this patient to become septic was methicillin susceptible *Staphylococcus aureus* (MSSA), which as a secondary code helps capture all aspects related to this patient's septic condition.

k. Puerperal sepsis

Code O85, Puerperal sepsis, should be assigned with a secondary code to identify the causal organism (e.g., for a bacterial infection, assign a code from category B95-B96, Bacterial infections in conditions classified elsewhere). A code from category A40, Streptococcal sepsis, or A41, Other sepsis, should not be used for puerperal sepsis. If applicable, use additional codes to identify severe sepsis (R65.2-) and any associated acute organ dysfunction.

Code O85 should not be assigned for sepsis following an obstetrical procedure (See Section I.C.1.d.5.b., Sepsis due to a postprocedural infection).

l. Alcohol, tobacco and drug use during pregnancy, childbirth and the puerperium

1) Alcohol use during pregnancy, childbirth and the puerperium

Codes under subcategory O99.31, Alcohol use complicating pregnancy, childbirth, and the puerperium, should be assigned for any pregnancy case when a patient uses alcohol during the pregnancy or postpartum. A secondary code from category F10, Alcohol related disorders, should also be assigned to identify manifestations of the alcohol use.

2) Tobacco use during pregnancy, childbirth and the puerperium

Codes under subcategory O99.33, Smoking (tobacco) complicating pregnancy, childbirth, and the puerperium, should be assigned for any pregnancy case when a patient uses any type of tobacco product during the pregnancy or postpartum.

A secondary code from category F17, Nicotine dependence, should also be assigned to identify the type of nicotine dependence.

3) Drug use during pregnancy, childbirth and the puerperium

Codes under subcategory O99.32, Drug use complicating pregnancy, childbirth, and the puerperium, should be assigned for any pregnancy case when a patient uses drugs during the pregnancy or postpartum. This can involve illegal drugs, or inappropriate use or abuse of prescription drugs. Secondary code(s) from categories F11-F16 and F18-F19 should also be assigned to identify manifestations of the drug use.

m. Poisoning, toxic effects, adverse effects and underdosing in a pregnant patient

A code from subcategory O9A.2, Injury, poisoning and certain other consequences of external causes complicating pregnancy, childbirth, and the puerperium, should be sequenced first, followed by the appropriate injury, poisoning, toxic effect, adverse effect or underdosing code, and then the additional code(s) that specifies the condition caused by the poisoning, toxic effect, adverse effect or underdosing.

See Section I.C.19. Adverse effects, poisoning, underdosing and toxic effects.

Patient treated for accidental carbon monoxide poisoning from a gas heating implement; the patient is 18 weeks' pregnant

O9A.212	**Injury, poisoning and certain other consequences of external causes complicating pregnancy, second trimester**
T58.11XA	**Toxic effect of carbon monoxide from utility gas, accidental (unintentional), initial encounter**
Z3A.18	**18 weeks gestation of pregnancy**

Explanation: Although the carbon monoxide poisoning is the reason for the encounter, a code from the obstetrics chapter must be sequenced first. Chapter 15 codes have sequencing priority over codes from other chapters.

n. Normal delivery, code O80

1) Encounter for full term uncomplicated delivery

Code O80 should be assigned when a patient is admitted for a full-term normal delivery and delivers a single, healthy infant without any complications antepartum, during the delivery, or postpartum during the delivery episode. Code O80 is always a principal diagnosis. It is not to be used if any other code from chapter 15 is needed to describe a current complication of the antenatal, delivery, or postnatal period. Additional codes from other chapters may be used with code O80 if they are not related to or are in any way complicating the pregnancy.

2) Uncomplicated delivery with resolved antepartum complication

Code O80 may be used if the patient had a complication at some point during the pregnancy, but the complication is not present at the time of the admission for delivery.

Patient presents in labor at 39 weeks' gestation and delivers a healthy newborn; patient had abnormal glucose levels in her first trimester, which have since resolved

O80	**Encounter for full-term uncomplicated delivery**
Z37.0	**Single live birth**

Explanation: The abnormal glucose levels during the first trimester cannot be coded if they are not affecting the patient's current trimester. Without additional complications associated with the pregnancy, fetus, or mother, code O80 is appropriate.

3) Outcome of delivery for O80

Z37.0, Single live birth, is the only outcome of delivery code appropriate for use with O80.

o. The peripartum and postpartum periods

1) Peripartum and postpartum periods

The postpartum period begins immediately after delivery and continues for six weeks following delivery. The peripartum period is defined as the last month of pregnancy to five months postpartum.

2) Peripartum and postpartum complication

A postpartum complication is any complication occurring within the six-week period.

3) Pregnancy-related complications after 6-week period

Chapter 15 codes may also be used to describe pregnancy-related complications after the peripartum or postpartum period if the provider documents that a condition is pregnancy related.

Patient referred for varicose veins. She had a baby boy three months ago; the varicose veins started to appear one month ago. The doctor attributes the patient's pregnancy as the cause of the varicose veins, which continue to be painful and bother the patient. She is seeking surgical relief.

O87.4	**Varicose veins of the lower extremity in the puerperium**

Explanation: Although the varicose veins occurred several months after the delivery of the newborn, the doctor attributed the varicose veins to pregnancy and therefore a code from chapter 15 is appropriate.

4) Admission for routine postpartum care following delivery outside hospital

When the mother delivers outside the hospital prior to admission and is admitted for routine postpartum care and no complications are noted, code Z39.0, Encounter for care and examination of mother immediately after delivery, should be assigned as the principal diagnosis.

5) Pregnancy associated cardiomyopathy

Pregnancy associated cardiomyopathy, code O90.3, is unique in that it may be diagnosed in the third trimester of pregnancy but may continue to progress months after delivery. For this reason, it is referred to as peripartum cardiomyopathy. Code O90.3 is only for use when the cardiomyopathy develops as a result of pregnancy in a patient who did not have pre-existing heart disease.

p. Code O94, Sequelae of complication of pregnancy, childbirth, and the puerperium

1) Code O94

Code O94, Sequelae of complication of pregnancy, childbirth, and the puerperium, is for use in those cases when an initial complication of a pregnancy develops a sequela or sequelae requiring care or treatment at a future date.

2) After the initial postpartum period

This code may be used at any time after the initial postpartum period.

3) Sequencing of code O94

This code, like all sequela codes, is to be sequenced following the code describing the sequelae of the complication.

q. Termination of pregnancy and spontaneous abortions

1) Abortion with Liveborn Fetus

When an attempted termination of pregnancy results in a liveborn fetus, assign code Z33.2, Encounter for elective termination of pregnancy and a code from category Z37, Outcome of Delivery.

2) Retained Products of Conception following an abortion

Subsequent encounters for retained products of conception following a spontaneous abortion or elective termination of pregnancy, without complications are assigned O03.4, Incomplete spontaneous abortion without complication, or code O07.4, Failed attempted termination of pregnancy without complication. This advice is appropriate even when the patient was discharged previously with a discharge diagnosis of complete abortion. If the patient has a specific complication associated with the spontaneous abortion or elective termination of pregnancy in addition to retained products of conception, assign the appropriate complication code (e.g., O03.-, O04.-, O07.-) instead of code O03.4 or O07.4.

Patient was seen two days ago for complete spontaneous abortion but returns today for urinary tract infection (UTI) with ultrasound showing retained products of conception

O03.38 Urinary tract infection following incomplete spontaneous abortion

Explanation: Although the diagnosis from the patient's previous stay indicated that the patient had a complete abortion, it is now determined that there were actually retained products of conception (POC). An abortion with retained POC is considered incomplete and in this case resulted in the patient developing a UTI.

3) Complications leading to abortion

Codes from Chapter 15 may be used as additional codes to identify any documented complications of the pregnancy in conjunction with codes in categories in O04, O07 and O08.

4) Hemorrhage following elective abortion

For hemorrhage post elective abortion, assign code O04.6, Delayed or excessive hemorrhage following (induced) termination of pregnancy. Do not assign code O72.1, Other immediate postpartum hemorrhage, as this code should not be assigned for post abortion conditions. Do not assign code Z33.2, Encounter for elective termination of pregnancy, when the patient experiences a complication post elective abortion.

r. Abuse in a pregnant patient

For suspected or confirmed cases of abuse of a pregnant patient, a code(s) from subcategories O9A.3, Physical abuse complicating pregnancy, childbirth, and the puerperium, O9A.4, Sexual abuse complicating pregnancy, childbirth, and the puerperium, and O9A.5, Psychological abuse complicating pregnancy, childbirth, and the puerperium, should be sequenced first, followed by the appropriate codes (if applicable) to identify any associated current injury due to physical abuse, sexual abuse, and the perpetrator of abuse.

See Section I.C.19. Adult and child abuse, neglect and other maltreatment.

s. COVID-19 infection in pregnancy, childbirth, and the puerperium

During pregnancy, childbirth or the puerperium, when COVID-19 is the reason for admission/encounter, code O98.5-, Other viral diseases complicating pregnancy, childbirth and the puerperium, should be sequenced as the principal/first-listed diagnosis, and code U07.1, COVID-19, and the appropriate codes for associated manifestation(s) should be assigned as additional diagnoses. Codes from Chapter 15 always take sequencing priority.

If the reason for admission/encounter is unrelated to COVID-19 but the patient tests positive for COVID-19 during the admission/encounter, the appropriate code for the reason for admission/encounter should be sequenced as the principal/first-listed diagnosis, and codes O98.5-and U07.1, as well as the appropriate codes for associated COVID-19 manifestations, should be assigned as additional diagnoses.

Chapter 15. Pregnancy, Childbirth and the Puerperium (O00-O9A)

NOTE CODES FROM THIS CHAPTER ARE FOR USE ONLY ON MATERNAL RECORDS, NEVER ON NEWBORN RECORDS

Codes from this chapter are for use for conditions related to or aggravated by the pregnancy, childbirth, or by the puerperium (maternal causes or obstetric causes)

NOTE Trimesters are counted from the first day of the last menstrual period. They are defined as follows:

1st trimester- less than 14 weeks 0 days

2nd trimester- 14 weeks 0 days to less than 28 weeks 0 days

3rd trimester- 28 weeks 0 days until delivery

Use additional code from category Z3A, Weeks of gestation, to identify the specific week of the pregnancy, if known.

EXCLUDES 1 *supervision of normal pregnancy (Z34.-)*

EXCLUDES 2 *mental and behavioral disorders associated with the puerperium (F53.-)*
obstetrical tetanus (A34)
postpartum necrosis of pituitary gland (E23.0)
puerperal osteomalacia (M83.0)

AHA: 2016,1Q,3-5; 2014,3Q,17

This chapter contains the following blocks:

- O00-O08 Pregnancy with abortive outcome
- O09 Supervision of high risk pregnancy
- O10-O16 Edema, proteinuria and hypertensive disorders in pregnancy, childbirth and the puerperium
- O20-O29 Other maternal disorders predominantly related to pregnancy
- O30-O48 Maternal care related to the fetus and amniotic cavity and possible delivery problems
- O60-O77 Complications of labor and delivery
- O80-O82 Encounter for delivery
- O85-O92 Complications predominantly related to the puerperium
- O94-O9A Other obstetric conditions, not elsewhere classified

Pregnancy with abortive outcome (O00-O08)

EXCLUDES 1 *continuing pregnancy in multiple gestation after abortion of one fetus or more (O31.1-, O31.3-)*

TIP: Do not assign a code from category Z3A with codes in this code block.

✓4th O00 Ectopic pregnancy

INCLUDES ruptured ectopic pregnancy

Use additional code from category O08 to identify any associated complication

AHA: 2016,4Q,48-50; 2014,3Q,17

DEF: Implantation of a fertilized egg outside the uterus, usually in the fallopian tube or abdomen that requires emergency treatment.

✓5th **O00.0 Abdominal pregnancy**

EXCLUDES 1 *maternal care for viable fetus in abdominal pregnancy (O36.7-)*

O00.00 Abdominal pregnancy without intrauterine pregnancy COM M ♀
Abdominal pregnancy NOS

O00.01 Abdominal pregnancy with intrauterine pregnancy COM M ♀

✓5th **O00.1 Tubal pregnancy**
Fallopian pregnancy
Rupture of (fallopian) tube due to pregnancy
Tubal abortion
AHA: 2017,4Q,20

✓6th **O00.10 Tubal pregnancy without intrauterine pregnancy**
Tubal pregnancy NOS

O00.101 Right tubal pregnancy without intrauterine pregnancy COM M ♀

O00.102 Left tubal pregnancy without intrauterine pregnancy COM M ♀

O00.109 Unspecified tubal pregnancy without intrauterine pregnancy COM M ♀

✓6th **O00.11 Tubal pregnancy with intrauterine pregnancy**

O00.111 Right tubal pregnancy with intrauterine pregnancy COM M ♀

O00.112 Left tubal pregnancy with intrauterine pregnancy COM M ♀

O00.119 Unspecified tubal pregnancy with intrauterine pregnancy COM M ♀

✓5th **O00.2 Ovarian pregnancy**
AHA: 2017,4Q,20

✓6th **O00.20 Ovarian pregnancy without intrauterine pregnancy**
Ovarian pregnancy NOS

O00.201 Right ovarian pregnancy without intrauterine pregnancy COM M ♀

O00.202 Left ovarian pregnancy without intrauterine pregnancy COM M ♀

O00.209 Unspecified ovarian pregnancy without intrauterine pregnancy COM M ♀

✓6th **O00.21 Ovarian pregnancy with intrauterine pregnancy**

O00.211 Right ovarian pregnancy with intrauterine pregnancy COM M ♀

O00.212 Left ovarian pregnancy with intrauterine pregnancy COM M ♀

O00.219 Unspecified ovarian pregnancy with intrauterine pregnancy COM M ♀

✓5th **O00.8 Other ectopic pregnancy**
Cervical pregnancy
Cornual pregnancy
Intraligamentous pregnancy
Mural pregnancy

O00.80 Other ectopic pregnancy without intrauterine pregnancy COM M ♀
Other ectopic pregnancy NOS

O00.81 Other ectopic pregnancy with intrauterine pregnancy COM M ♀

✓5th **O00.9 Ectopic pregnancy, unspecified**

O00.90 Unspecified ectopic pregnancy without intrauterine pregnancy COM M ♀
Ectopic pregnancy NOS

O00.91 Unspecified ectopic pregnancy with intrauterine pregnancy COM M ♀

✓4th O01 Hydatidiform mole

Use additional code from category O08 to identify any associated complication

EXCLUDES 1 *chorioadenoma (destruens) (D39.2)*
malignant hydatidiform mole (D39.2)

AHA: 2014,3Q,17

DEF: Abnormal product of pregnancy, marked by a mass of cysts resembling a bunch of grapes due to chorionic villi proliferation and dissolution. It must be surgically removed.

O01.0 Classical hydatidiform mole COM M ♀
Complete hydatidiform mole

O01.1 Incomplete and partial hydatidiform mole COM M ♀

O01.9 Hydatidiform mole, unspecified COM M ♀
Trophoblastic disease NOS
Vesicular mole NOS

✓4th O02 Other abnormal products of conception

Use additional code from category O08 to identify any associated complication

EXCLUDES 1 *papyraceous fetus (O31.0-)*

AHA: 2014,3Q,17

O02.0 Blighted ovum and nonhydatidiform mole COM M ♀
Carneous mole
Fleshy mole
Intrauterine mole NOS
Molar pregnancy NEC
Pathological ovum

O02.1 Missed abortion COM M ♀
Early fetal death, before completion of 20 weeks of gestation, with retention of dead fetus

EXCLUDES 1 *failed induced abortion (O07.-)*
fetal death (intrauterine) (late) (O36.4)
missed abortion with blighted ovum (O02.0)
missed abortion with hydatidiform mole (O01.-)
missed abortion with nonhydatidiform (O02.0)
missed abortion with other abnormal products of conception (O02.8-)
missed delivery (O36.4)
stillbirth (P95)

AHA: 2022,2Q,3; 2019,3Q,11

✓5th O02.8 Other specified abnormal products of conception

EXCLUDES 1 *abnormal products of conception with blighted ovum (O02.0)*
abnormal products of conception with hydatidiform mole (O01.-)
abnormal products of conception with nonhydatidiform mole (O02.0)

O02.81 Inappropriate change in quantitative human chorionic gonadotropin (hCG) in early pregnancy COM M ♀

Biochemical pregnancy
Chemical pregnancy
Inappropriate level of quantitative human chorionic gonadotropin (hCG) for gestational age in early pregnancy

O02.89 Other abnormal products of conception COM M ♀

O02.9 Abnormal product of conception, unspecified COM M ♀

✓4th O03 Spontaneous abortion

NOTE Incomplete abortion includes retained products of conception following spontaneous abortion

INCLUDES miscarriage

O03.0 Genital tract and pelvic infection following incomplete spontaneous abortion COM M ♀

Endometritis following incomplete spontaneous abortion
Oophoritis following incomplete spontaneous abortion
Parametritis following incomplete spontaneous abortion
Pelvic peritonitis following incomplete spontaneous abortion
Salpingitis following incomplete spontaneous abortion
Salpingo-oophoritis following incomplete spontaneous abortion

EXCLUDES 1 *sepsis following incomplete spontaneous abortion (O03.37)*
urinary tract infection following incomplete spontaneous abortion (O03.38)

O03.1 Delayed or excessive hemorrhage following incomplete spontaneous abortion COM M ♀

Afibrinogenemia following incomplete spontaneous abortion
Defibrination syndrome following incomplete spontaneous abortion
Hemolysis following incomplete spontaneous abortion
Intravascular coagulation following incomplete spontaneous abortion

AHA: 2022,1Q,19

O03.2 Embolism following incomplete spontaneous abortion COM M ♀

Air embolism following incomplete spontaneous abortion
Amniotic fluid embolism following incomplete spontaneous abortion
Blood-clot embolism following incomplete spontaneous abortion
Embolism NOS following incomplete spontaneous abortion
Fat embolism following incomplete spontaneous abortion
Pulmonary embolism following incomplete spontaneous abortion
Pyemic embolism following incomplete spontaneous abortion
Septic or septicopyemic embolism following incomplete spontaneous abortion
Soap embolism following incomplete spontaneous abortion

✓5th O03.3 Other and unspecified complications following incomplete spontaneous abortion

O03.30 Unspecified complication following incomplete spontaneous abortion COM M ♀

O03.31 Shock following incomplete spontaneous abortion COM M ♀

Circulatory collapse following incomplete spontaneous abortion
Shock (postprocedural) following incomplete spontaneous abortion

EXCLUDES 1 *shock due to infection following incomplete spontaneous abortion (O03.37)*

O03.32 Renal failure following incomplete spontaneous abortion COM M ♀

Kidney failure (acute) following incomplete spontaneous abortion
Oliguria following incomplete spontaneous abortion
Renal shutdown following incomplete spontaneous abortion
Renal tubular necrosis following incomplete spontaneous abortion
Uremia following incomplete spontaneous abortion

O03.33 Metabolic disorder following incomplete spontaneous abortion COM M ♀

O03.34 Damage to pelvic organs following incomplete spontaneous abortion COM M ♀

Laceration, perforation, tear or chemical damage of bladder following incomplete spontaneous abortion
Laceration, perforation, tear or chemical damage of bowel following incomplete spontaneous abortion
Laceration, perforation, tear or chemical damage of broad ligament following incomplete spontaneous abortion
Laceration, perforation, tear or chemical damage of cervix following incomplete spontaneous abortion
Laceration, perforation, tear or chemical damage of periurethral tissue following incomplete spontaneous abortion
Laceration, perforation, tear or chemical damage of uterus following incomplete spontaneous abortion
Laceration, perforation, tear or chemical damage of vagina following incomplete spontaneous abortion

O03.35 Other venous complications following incomplete spontaneous abortion COM M ♀

O03.36 Cardiac arrest following incomplete spontaneous abortion COM M ♀

O03.37 Sepsis following incomplete spontaneous abortion COM M ♀

Use additional code to identify infectious agent (B95-B97)
Use additional code to identify severe sepsis, if applicable (R65.2-)

EXCLUDES 1 *septic or septicopyemic embolism following incomplete spontaneous abortion (O03.2)*

O03.38 Urinary tract infection following incomplete spontaneous abortion COM M ♀

Cystitis following incomplete spontaneous abortion

O03.39 Incomplete spontaneous abortion with other complications COM M ♀

O03.4 Incomplete spontaneous abortion without complication COM M ♀

O03.5 Genital tract and pelvic infection following complete or unspecified spontaneous abortion COM M ♀

Endometritis following complete or unspecified spontaneous abortion
Oophoritis following complete or unspecified spontaneous abortion
Parametritis following complete or unspecified spontaneous abortion
Pelvic peritonitis following complete or unspecified spontaneous abortion
Salpingitis following complete or unspecified spontaneous abortion
Salpingo-oophoritis following complete or unspecified spontaneous abortion

EXCLUDES 1 *sepsis following complete or unspecified spontaneous abortion (O03.87)*
urinary tract infection following complete or unspecified spontaneous abortion (O03.88)

O03.6 Delayed or excessive hemorrhage following complete or unspecified spontaneous abortion COM M ♀
Afibrinogenemia following complete or unspecified spontaneous abortion
Defibrination syndrome following complete or unspecified spontaneous abortion
Hemolysis following complete or unspecified spontaneous abortion
Intravascular coagulation following complete or unspecified spontaneous abortion
AHA: 2022,1Q,19

O03.7 Embolism following complete or unspecified spontaneous abortion COM M ♀
Air embolism following complete or unspecified spontaneous abortion
Amniotic fluid embolism following complete or unspecified spontaneous abortion
Blood-clot embolism following complete or unspecified spontaneous abortion
Embolism NOS following complete or unspecified spontaneous abortion
Fat embolism following complete or unspecified spontaneous abortion
Pulmonary embolism following complete or unspecified spontaneous abortion
Pyemic embolism following complete or unspecified spontaneous abortion
Septic or septicopyemic embolism following complete or unspecified spontaneous abortion
Soap embolism following complete or unspecified spontaneous abortion

√5th **O03.8 Other and unspecified complications following complete or unspecified spontaneous abortion**

O03.80 Unspecified complication following complete or unspecified spontaneous abortion COM M ♀

O03.81 Shock following complete or unspecified spontaneous abortion COM M ♀
Circulatory collapse following complete or unspecified spontaneous abortion
Shock (postprocedural) following complete or unspecified spontaneous abortion
EXCLUDES 1 *shock due to infection following complete or unspecified spontaneous abortion (O03.87)*

O03.82 Renal failure following complete or unspecified spontaneous abortion COM M ♀
Kidney failure (acute) following complete or unspecified spontaneous abortion
Oliguria following complete or unspecified spontaneous abortion
Renal shutdown following complete or unspecified spontaneous abortion
Renal tubular necrosis following complete or unspecified spontaneous abortion
Uremia following complete or unspecified spontaneous abortion

O03.83 Metabolic disorder following complete or unspecified spontaneous abortion COM M ♀

O03.84 Damage to pelvic organs following complete or unspecified spontaneous abortion COM M ♀
Laceration, perforation, tear or chemical damage of bladder following complete or unspecified spontaneous abortion
Laceration, perforation, tear or chemical damage of bowel following complete or unspecified spontaneous abortion
Laceration, perforation, tear or chemical damage of broad ligament following complete or unspecified spontaneous abortion
Laceration, perforation, tear or chemical damage of cervix following complete or unspecified spontaneous abortion
Laceration, perforation, tear or chemical damage of periurethral tissue following complete or unspecified spontaneous abortion
Laceration, perforation, tear or chemical damage of uterus following complete or unspecified spontaneous abortion
Laceration, perforation, tear or chemical damage of vagina following complete or unspecified spontaneous abortion

O03.85 Other venous complications following complete or unspecified spontaneous abortion COM M ♀

O03.86 Cardiac arrest following complete or unspecified spontaneous abortion COM M ♀

O03.87 Sepsis following complete or unspecified spontaneous abortion COM M ♀
Use additional code to identify infectious agent (B95-B97)
Use additional code to identify severe sepsis, if applicable (R65.2-)
EXCLUDES 1 *septic or septicopyemic embolism following complete or unspecified spontaneous abortion (O03.7)*

O03.88 Urinary tract infection following complete or unspecified spontaneous abortion COM M ♀
Cystitis following complete or unspecified spontaneous abortion

O03.89 Complete or unspecified spontaneous abortion with other complications COM M ♀

O03.9 Complete or unspecified spontaneous abortion without complication COM M ♀
Miscarriage NOS
Spontaneous abortion NOS

√4th **O04 Complications following (induced) termination of pregnancy**
INCLUDES complications following (induced) termination of pregnancy
EXCLUDES 1 *encounter for elective termination of pregnancy, uncomplicated (Z33.2)*
failed attempted termination of pregnancy (O07.-)

O04.5 Genital tract and pelvic infection following (induced) termination of pregnancy M ♀
Endometritis following (induced) termination of pregnancy
Oophoritis following (induced) termination of pregnancy
Parametritis following (induced) termination of pregnancy
Pelvic peritonitis following (induced) termination of pregnancy
Salpingitis following (induced) termination of pregnancy
Salpingo-oophoritis following (induced) termination of pregnancy
EXCLUDES 1 *sepsis following (induced) termination of pregnancy (O04.87)*
urinary tract infection following (induced) termination of pregnancy (O04.88)

O04.6 Delayed or excessive hemorrhage following (induced) termination of pregnancy M ♀
Afibrinogenemia following (induced) termination of pregnancy
Defibrination syndrome following (induced) termination of pregnancy
Hemolysis following (induced) termination of pregnancy
Intravascular coagulation following (induced) termination of pregnancy
AHA: 2019,3Q,11

O04.7 Embolism following (induced) termination of pregnancy M ♀
Air embolism following (induced) termination of pregnancy
Amniotic fluid embolism following (induced) termination of pregnancy
Blood-clot embolism following (induced) termination of pregnancy
Embolism NOS following (induced) termination of pregnancy
Fat embolism following (induced) termination of pregnancy
Pulmonary embolism following (induced) termination of pregnancy
Pyemic embolism following (induced) termination of pregnancy
Septic or septicopyemic embolism following (induced) termination of pregnancy
Soap embolism following (induced) termination of pregnancy

5th O04.8 (Induced) termination of pregnancy with other and unspecified complications

O04.80 (Induced) termination of pregnancy with unspecified complications M ♀

O04.81 Shock following (induced) termination of pregnancy M ♀
Circulatory collapse following (induced) termination of pregnancy
Shock (postprocedural) following (induced) termination of pregnancy
EXCLUDES 1 *shock due to infection following (induced) termination of pregnancy (O04.87)*

O04.82 Renal failure following (induced) termination of pregnancy M ♀
Kidney failure (acute) following (induced) termination of pregnancy
Oliguria following (induced) termination of pregnancy
Renal shutdown following (induced) termination of pregnancy
Renal tubular necrosis following (induced) termination of pregnancy
Uremia following (induced) termination of pregnancy

O04.83 Metabolic disorder following (induced) termination of pregnancy M ♀

O04.84 Damage to pelvic organs following (induced) termination of pregnancy M ♀
Laceration, perforation, tear or chemical damage of bladder following (induced) termination of pregnancy
Laceration, perforation, tear or chemical damage of bowel following (induced) termination of pregnancy
Laceration, perforation, tear or chemical damage of broad ligament following (induced) termination of pregnancy
Laceration, perforation, tear or chemical damage of cervix following (induced) termination of pregnancy
Laceration, perforation, tear or chemical damage of periurethral tissue following (induced) termination of pregnancy
Laceration, perforation, tear or chemical damage of uterus following (induced) termination of pregnancy
Laceration, perforation, tear or chemical damage of vagina following (induced) termination of pregnancy

O04.85 Other venous complications following (induced) termination of pregnancy M ♀

O04.86 Cardiac arrest following (induced) termination of pregnancy M ♀

O04.87 Sepsis following (induced) termination of pregnancy M ♀
Use additional code to identify infectious agent (B95-B97)
Use additional code to identify severe sepsis, if applicable (R65.2-)
EXCLUDES 1 *septic or septicopyemic embolism following (induced) termination of pregnancy (O04.7)*

O04.88 Urinary tract infection following (induced) termination of pregnancy M ♀
Cystitis following (induced) termination of pregnancy

O04.89 (Induced) termination of pregnancy with other complications M ♀

4th O07 Failed attempted termination of pregnancy

INCLUDES failure of attempted induction of termination of pregnancy
incomplete elective abortion
EXCLUDES 1 *incomplete spontaneous abortion (O03.0-)*

O07.0 Genital tract and pelvic infection following failed attempted termination of pregnancy M ♀
Endometritis following failed attempted termination of pregnancy
Oophoritis following failed attempted termination of pregnancy
Parametritis following failed attempted termination of pregnancy
Pelvic peritonitis following failed attempted termination of pregnancy
Salpingitis following failed attempted termination of pregnancy
Salpingo-oophoritis following failed attempted termination of pregnancy
EXCLUDES 1 *sepsis following failed attempted termination of pregnancy (O07.37)*
urinary tract infection following failed attempted termination of pregnancy (O07.38)

O07.1 Delayed or excessive hemorrhage following failed attempted termination of pregnancy M ♀
Afibrinogenemia following failed attempted termination of pregnancy
Defibrination syndrome following failed attempted termination of pregnancy
Hemolysis following failed attempted termination of pregnancy
Intravascular coagulation following failed attempted termination of pregnancy

O07.2 Embolism following failed attempted termination of pregnancy M ♀
Air embolism following failed attempted termination of pregnancy
Amniotic fluid embolism following failed attempted termination of pregnancy
Blood-clot embolism following failed attempted termination of pregnancy
Embolism NOS following failed attempted termination of pregnancy
Fat embolism following failed attempted termination of pregnancy
Pulmonary embolism following failed attempted termination of pregnancy
Pyemic embolism following failed attempted termination of pregnancy
Septic or septicopyemic embolism following failed attempted termination of pregnancy
Soap embolism following failed attempted termination of pregnancy

5th O07.3 Failed attempted termination of pregnancy with other and unspecified complications

O07.30 Failed attempted termination of pregnancy with unspecified complications M ♀

O07.31 Shock following failed attempted termination of pregnancy M ♀
Circulatory collapse following failed attempted termination of pregnancy
Shock (postprocedural) following failed attempted termination of pregnancy
EXCLUDES 1 *shock due to infection following failed attempted termination of pregnancy (O07.37)*

O07.32 Renal failure following failed attempted termination of pregnancy M ♀
Kidney failure (acute) following failed attempted termination of pregnancy
Oliguria following failed attempted termination of pregnancy
Renal shutdown following failed attempted termination of pregnancy
Renal tubular necrosis following failed attempted termination of pregnancy
Uremia following failed attempted termination of pregnancy

O07.33 Metabolic disorder following failed attempted termination of pregnancy M ♀

O07.34 Damage to pelvic organs following failed attempted termination of pregnancy M ♀
Laceration, perforation, tear or chemical damage of bladder following failed attempted termination of pregnancy
Laceration, perforation, tear or chemical damage of bowel following failed attempted termination of pregnancy
Laceration, perforation, tear or chemical damage of broad ligament following failed attempted termination of pregnancy
Laceration, perforation, tear or chemical damage of cervix following failed attempted termination of pregnancy
Laceration, perforation, tear or chemical damage of periurethral tissue following failed attempted termination of pregnancy
Laceration, perforation, tear or chemical damage of uterus following failed attempted termination of pregnancy
Laceration, perforation, tear or chemical damage of vagina following failed attempted termination of pregnancy

O07.35 Other venous complications following failed attempted termination of pregnancy M ♀

O07.36 Cardiac arrest following failed attempted termination of pregnancy M ♀

O07.37 Sepsis following failed attempted termination of pregnancy M ♀
Use additional code (B95-B97), to identify infectious agent
Use additional code (R65.2-) to identify severe sepsis, if applicable
EXCLUDES 1 *septic or septicopyemic embolism following failed attempted termination of pregnancy (O07.2)*

O07.38 Urinary tract infection following failed attempted termination of pregnancy M ♀
Cystitis following failed attempted termination of pregnancy

O07.39 Failed attempted termination of pregnancy with other complications M ♀

O07.4 Failed attempted termination of pregnancy without complication M ♀

✓4th **O08 Complications following ectopic and molar pregnancy**
This category is for use with categories O00-O02 to identify any associated complications

O08.0 Genital tract and pelvic infection following ectopic and molar pregnancy COM M ♀
Endometritis following ectopic and molar pregnancy
Oophoritis following ectopic and molar pregnancy
Parametritis following ectopic and molar pregnancy
Pelvic peritonitis following ectopic and molar pregnancy
Salpingitis following ectopic and molar pregnancy
Salpingo-oophoritis following ectopic and molar pregnancy
EXCLUDES 1 *sepsis following ectopic and molar pregnancy (O08.82)*
urinary tract infection (O08.83)

O08.1 Delayed or excessive hemorrhage following ectopic and molar pregnancy COM M ♀
Afibrinogenemia following ectopic and molar pregnancy
Defibrination syndrome following ectopic and molar pregnancy
Hemolysis following ectopic and molar pregnancy
Intravascular coagulation following ectopic and molar pregnancy
EXCLUDES 1 *delayed or excessive hemorrhage due to incomplete abortion (O03.1)*

O08.2 Embolism following ectopic and molar pregnancy COM M ♀
Air embolism following ectopic and molar pregnancy
Amniotic fluid embolism following ectopic and molar pregnancy
Blood-clot embolism following ectopic and molar pregnancy
Embolism NOS following ectopic and molar pregnancy
Fat embolism following ectopic and molar pregnancy
Pulmonary embolism following ectopic and molar pregnancy
Pyemic embolism following ectopic and molar pregnancy
Septic or septicopyemic embolism following ectopic and molar pregnancy
Soap embolism following ectopic and molar pregnancy

O08.3 Shock following ectopic and molar pregnancy COM M ♀
Circulatory collapse following ectopic and molar pregnancy
Shock (postprocedural) following ectopic and molar pregnancy
EXCLUDES 1 *shock due to infection following ectopic and molar pregnancy (O08.82)*

O08.4 Renal failure following ectopic and molar pregnancy COM M ♀
Kidney failure (acute) following ectopic and molar pregnancy
Oliguria following ectopic and molar pregnancy
Renal shutdown following ectopic and molar pregnancy
Renal tubular necrosis following ectopic and molar pregnancy
Uremia following ectopic and molar pregnancy

O08.5 Metabolic disorders following an ectopic and molar pregnancy COM M ♀

O08.6 Damage to pelvic organs and tissues following an ectopic and molar pregnancy COM M ♀
Laceration, perforation, tear or chemical damage of bladder following an ectopic and molar pregnancy
Laceration, perforation, tear or chemical damage of bowel following an ectopic and molar pregnancy
Laceration, perforation, tear or chemical damage of broad ligament following an ectopic and molar pregnancy
Laceration, perforation, tear or chemical damage of cervix following an ectopic and molar pregnancy
Laceration, perforation, tear or chemical damage of periurethral tissue following an ectopic and molar pregnancy
Laceration, perforation, tear or chemical damage of uterus following an ectopic and molar pregnancy
Laceration, perforation, tear or chemical damage of vagina following an ectopic and molar pregnancy

O08.7 Other venous complications following an ectopic and molar pregnancy COM M ♀

✓5th **O08.8 Other complications following an ectopic and molar pregnancy**

O08.81 Cardiac arrest following an ectopic and molar pregnancy COM M ♀

O08.82 Sepsis following ectopic and molar pregnancy COM M ♀
Use additional code (B95-B97), to identify infectious agent
Use additional code (R65.2-) to identify severe sepsis, if applicable
EXCLUDES 1 *septic or septicopyemic embolism following ectopic and molar pregnancy (O08.2)*

O08.83 Urinary tract infection following an ectopic and molar pregnancy COM M ♀
Cystitis following an ectopic and molar pregnancy

O08.89 Other complications following an ectopic and molar pregnancy COM M ♀

O08.9 Unspecified complication following an ectopic and molar pregnancy COM M ♀

Supervision of high risk pregnancy (O09)

✓4th **O09 Supervision of high risk pregnancy**
AHA: 2019,3Q,5; 2016,4Q,48-50,150

✓5th **O09.0 Supervision of pregnancy with history of infertility**

O09.00 Supervision of pregnancy with history of infertility, unspecified trimester COM M ♀

O09.01 Supervision of pregnancy with history of infertility, first trimester COM M ♀

O09.02 Supervision of pregnancy with history of infertility, second trimester COM M ♀

O09.03 Supervision of pregnancy with history of infertility, third trimester COM M ♀

Chapter 15. Pregnancy, Childbirth and the Puerperium
O07.34–O09.03

✓5th **O09.1 Supervision of pregnancy with history of ectopic pregnancy**

O09.10 Supervision of pregnancy with history of ectopic pregnancy, unspecified trimester COM M ♀

O09.11 Supervision of pregnancy with history of ectopic pregnancy, first trimester COM M ♀

O09.12 Supervision of pregnancy with history of ectopic pregnancy, second trimester COM M ♀

O09.13 Supervision of pregnancy with history of ectopic pregnancy, third trimester COM M ♀

✓5th **O09.A Supervision of pregnancy with history of molar pregnancy**

DEF: Molar pregnancy: Trophoblastic neoplasm that mimics pregnancy by proliferating from a pathologic ovum and resulting only in a mass of cysts resembling grapes, 80 percent of which are benign, but require surgical removal.

O09.A0 Supervision of pregnancy with history of molar pregnancy, unspecified trimester COM M ♀

O09.A1 Supervision of pregnancy with history of molar pregnancy, first trimester COM M ♀

O09.A2 Supervision of pregnancy with history of molar pregnancy, second trimester COM M ♀

O09.A3 Supervision of pregnancy with history of molar pregnancy, third trimester COM M ♀

✓5th **O09.2 Supervision of pregnancy with other poor reproductive or obstetric history**

EXCLUDES 2 *pregnancy care for patient with history of recurrent pregnancy loss (O26.2-)*

✓6th **O09.21 Supervision of pregnancy with history of pre-term labor**

O09.211 Supervision of pregnancy with history of pre-term labor, first trimester COM M ♀

O09.212 Supervision of pregnancy with history of pre-term labor, second trimester COM M ♀

O09.213 Supervision of pregnancy with history of pre-term labor, third trimester COM M ♀

O09.219 Supervision of pregnancy with history of pre-term labor, unspecified trimester COM M ♀

✓6th **O09.29 Supervision of pregnancy with other poor reproductive or obstetric history**

Supervision of pregnancy with history of neonatal death

Supervision of pregnancy with history of stillbirth

O09.291 Supervision of pregnancy with other poor reproductive or obstetric history, first trimester COM M ♀

O09.292 Supervision of pregnancy with other poor reproductive or obstetric history, second trimester COM M ♀

O09.293 Supervision of pregnancy with other poor reproductive or obstetric history, third trimester COM M ♀

O09.299 Supervision of pregnancy with other poor reproductive or obstetric history, unspecified trimester COM M ♀

✓5th **O09.3 Supervision of pregnancy with insufficient antenatal care**

Supervision of concealed pregnancy

Supervision of hidden pregnancy

O09.30 Supervision of pregnancy with insufficient antenatal care, unspecified trimester COM M ♀

O09.31 Supervision of pregnancy with insufficient antenatal care, first trimester COM M ♀

O09.32 Supervision of pregnancy with insufficient antenatal care, second trimester COM M ♀

O09.33 Supervision of pregnancy with insufficient antenatal care, third trimester COM M ♀

✓5th **O09.4 Supervision of pregnancy with grand multiparity**

O09.40 Supervision of pregnancy with grand multiparity, unspecified trimester COM M ♀

O09.41 Supervision of pregnancy with grand multiparity, first trimester COM M ♀

O09.42 Supervision of pregnancy with grand multiparity, second trimester COM M ♀

O09.43 Supervision of pregnancy with grand multiparity, third trimester COM M ♀

✓5th **O09.5 Supervision of elderly primigravida and multigravida**

Pregnancy for a female 35 years and older at expected date of delivery

✓6th **O09.51 Supervision of elderly primigravida**

O09.511 Supervision of elderly primigravida, first trimester COM M ♀

O09.512 Supervision of elderly primigravida, second trimester COM M ♀

O09.513 Supervision of elderly primigravida, third trimester COM M ♀

O09.519 Supervision of elderly primigravida, unspecified trimester COM M ♀

✓6th **O09.52 Supervision of elderly multigravida**

O09.521 Supervision of elderly multigravida, first trimester COM M ♀

O09.522 Supervision of elderly multigravida, second trimester COM M ♀

O09.523 Supervision of elderly multigravida, third trimester COM M ♀

O09.529 Supervision of elderly multigravida, unspecified trimester COM M ♀

✓5th **O09.6 Supervision of young primigravida and multigravida**

Supervision of pregnancy for a female less than 16 years old at expected date of delivery

✓6th **O09.61 Supervision of young primigravida**

O09.611 Supervision of young primigravida, first trimester COM M ♀

O09.612 Supervision of young primigravida, second trimester COM M ♀

O09.613 Supervision of young primigravida, third trimester COM M ♀

O09.619 Supervision of young primigravida, unspecified trimester COM M ♀

✓6th **O09.62 Supervision of young multigravida**

O09.621 Supervision of young multigravida, first trimester COM M ♀

O09.622 Supervision of young multigravida, second trimester COM M ♀

O09.623 Supervision of young multigravida, third trimester COM M ♀

O09.629 Supervision of young multigravida, unspecified trimester COM M ♀

✓5th **O09.7 Supervision of high risk pregnancy due to social problems**

O09.70 Supervision of high risk pregnancy due to social problems, unspecified trimester COM M ♀

O09.71 Supervision of high risk pregnancy due to social problems, first trimester COM M ♀

O09.72 Supervision of high risk pregnancy due to social problems, second trimester COM M ♀

O09.73 Supervision of high risk pregnancy due to social problems, third trimester COM M ♀

✓5th **O09.8 Supervision of other high risk pregnancies**

✓6th **O09.81 Supervision of pregnancy resulting from assisted reproductive technology**

Supervision of pregnancy resulting from in-vitro fertilization

EXCLUDES 2 *gestational carrier status (Z33.3)*

O09.811 Supervision of pregnancy resulting from assisted reproductive technology, first trimester COM M ♀

O09.812 Supervision of pregnancy resulting from assisted reproductive technology, second trimester COM M ♀

O09.813 Supervision of pregnancy resulting from assisted reproductive technology, third trimester COM M ♀

O09.819 Supervision of pregnancy resulting from assisted reproductive technology, unspecified trimester COM M ♀

✓6th **O09.82 Supervision of pregnancy with history of in utero procedure during previous pregnancy**

O09.821 Supervision of pregnancy with history of in utero procedure during previous pregnancy, first trimester COM M ♀

O09.822 Supervision of pregnancy with history of in utero procedure during previous pregnancy, second trimester COM M ♀

O09.823 Supervision of pregnancy with history of in utero procedure during previous pregnancy, third trimester COM M ♀

O09.829 Supervision of pregnancy with history of in utero procedure during previous pregnancy, unspecified trimester COM M ♀

EXCLUDES 1 *supervision of pregnancy affected by in utero procedure during current pregnancy (O35.7)*

O09.89 Supervision of other high risk pregnancies

O09.891 Supervision of other high risk pregnancies, first trimester COM M ♀

O09.892 Supervision of other high risk pregnancies, second trimester COM M ♀

O09.893 Supervision of other high risk pregnancies, third trimester COM M ♀

O09.899 Supervision of other high risk pregnancies, unspecified trimester COM M ♀

O09.9 Supervision of high risk pregnancy, unspecified

O09.90 Supervision of high risk pregnancy, unspecified, unspecified trimester COM M ♀

O09.91 Supervision of high risk pregnancy, unspecified, first trimester COM M ♀

O09.92 Supervision of high risk pregnancy, unspecified, second trimester COM M ♀

O09.93 Supervision of high risk pregnancy, unspecified, third trimester COM M ♀

Edema, proteinuria and hypertensive disorders in pregnancy, childbirth and the puerperium (O10-O16)

AHA: 2016,4Q,50

O10 Pre-existing hypertension complicating pregnancy, childbirth and the puerperium

INCLUDES pre-existing hypertension with pre-existing proteinuria complicating pregnancy, childbirth and the puerperium

EXCLUDES 2 *pre-existing hypertension with superimposed pre-eclampsia complicating pregnancy, childbirth and the puerperium (O11.-)*

O10.0 Pre-existing essential hypertension complicating pregnancy, childbirth and the puerperium

Any condition in I10 specified as a reason for obstetric care during pregnancy, childbirth or the puerperium

O10.01 Pre-existing essential hypertension complicating pregnancy

O10.011 Pre-existing essential hypertension complicating pregnancy, first trimester COM M ♀

O10.012 Pre-existing essential hypertension complicating pregnancy, second trimester COM M ♀

O10.013 Pre-existing essential hypertension complicating pregnancy, third trimester COM M ♀

O10.019 Pre-existing essential hypertension complicating pregnancy, unspecified trimester COM M ♀

O10.02 Pre-existing essential hypertension complicating childbirth COM M ♀

O10.03 Pre-existing essential hypertension complicating the puerperium COM M ♀

O10.1 Pre-existing hypertensive heart disease complicating pregnancy, childbirth and the puerperium

Any condition in I11 specified as a reason for obstetric care during pregnancy, childbirth or the puerperium

Use additional code from I11 to identify the type of hypertensive heart disease

O10.11 Pre-existing hypertensive heart disease complicating pregnancy

O10.111 Pre-existing hypertensive heart disease complicating pregnancy, first trimester COM M ♀

O10.112 Pre-existing hypertensive heart disease complicating pregnancy, second trimester COM M ♀

O10.113 Pre-existing hypertensive heart disease complicating pregnancy, third trimester COM M ♀

O10.119 Pre-existing hypertensive heart disease complicating pregnancy, unspecified trimester COM M ♀

O10.12 Pre-existing hypertensive heart disease complicating childbirth COM M ♀

O10.13 Pre-existing hypertensive heart disease complicating the puerperium COM M ♀

O10.2 Pre-existing hypertensive chronic kidney disease complicating pregnancy, childbirth and the puerperium

Any condition in I12 specified as a reason for obstetric care during pregnancy, childbirth or the puerperium

Use additional code from I12 to identify the type of hypertensive chronic kidney disease

O10.21 Pre-existing hypertensive chronic kidney disease complicating pregnancy

O10.211 Pre-existing hypertensive chronic kidney disease complicating pregnancy, first trimester COM M ♀

O10.212 Pre-existing hypertensive chronic kidney disease complicating pregnancy, second trimester COM M ♀

O10.213 Pre-existing hypertensive chronic kidney disease complicating pregnancy, third trimester COM M ♀

O10.219 Pre-existing hypertensive chronic kidney disease complicating pregnancy, unspecified trimester COM M ♀

O10.22 Pre-existing hypertensive chronic kidney disease complicating childbirth COM M ♀

O10.23 Pre-existing hypertensive chronic kidney disease complicating the puerperium COM M ♀

O10.3 Pre-existing hypertensive heart and chronic kidney disease complicating pregnancy, childbirth and the puerperium

Any condition in I13 specified as a reason for obstetric care during pregnancy, childbirth or the puerperium

Use additional code from I13 to identify the type of hypertensive heart and chronic kidney disease

O10.31 Pre-existing hypertensive heart and chronic kidney disease complicating pregnancy

O10.311 Pre-existing hypertensive heart and chronic kidney disease complicating pregnancy, first trimester COM M ♀

O10.312 Pre-existing hypertensive heart and chronic kidney disease complicating pregnancy, second trimester COM M ♀

O10.313 Pre-existing hypertensive heart and chronic kidney disease complicating pregnancy, third trimester COM M ♀

O10.319 Pre-existing hypertensive heart and chronic kidney disease complicating pregnancy, unspecified trimester COM M ♀

O10.32 Pre-existing hypertensive heart and chronic kidney disease complicating childbirth COM M ♀

O10.33 Pre-existing hypertensive heart and chronic kidney disease complicating the puerperium COM M ♀

O10.4 Pre-existing secondary hypertension complicating pregnancy, childbirth and the puerperium

Any condition in I15 specified as a reason for obstetric care during pregnancy, childbirth or the puerperium

Use additional code from I15 to identify the type of secondary hypertension

O10.41 Pre-existing secondary hypertension complicating pregnancy

O10.411 Pre-existing secondary hypertension complicating pregnancy, first trimester COM M ♀

O10.412 Pre-existing secondary hypertension complicating pregnancy, second trimester COM M ♀

O10.413 Pre-existing secondary hypertension complicating pregnancy, third trimester COM M ♀

O10.419 Pre-existing secondary hypertension complicating pregnancy, unspecified trimester COM M ♀

O10.42 Pre-existing secondary hypertension complicating childbirth COM M ♀

O10.43 Pre-existing secondary hypertension complicating the puerperium COM M ♀

O10.9 Unspecified pre-existing hypertension complicating pregnancy, childbirth and the puerperium

O10.91 Unspecified pre-existing hypertension complicating pregnancy

O10.911 Unspecified pre-existing hypertension complicating pregnancy, first trimester COM M ♀

O10.912 Unspecified pre-existing hypertension complicating pregnancy, second trimester COM M ♀

O10.913 Unspecified pre-existing hypertension complicating pregnancy, third trimester COM M ♀

O10.919 Unspecified pre-existing hypertension complicating pregnancy, unspecified trimester COM M ♀

O10.92 Unspecified pre-existing hypertension complicating childbirth COM M ♀

O10.93 Unspecified pre-existing hypertension complicating the puerperium COM M ♀

O11 Pre-existing hypertension with pre-eclampsia

INCLUDES conditions in O10 complicated by pre-eclampsia
pre-eclampsia superimposed pre-existing in hypertension

Use additional code from O10 to identify the type of hypertension

DEF: Complication of pregnancy manifesting in the development of borderline hypertension, protein in the urine, and unresponsive swelling between the 20th week of pregnancy and the end of the first week following birth in mild to moderate cases. Severe preeclampsia presents with hypertension, associated with marked swelling, proteinuria, abdominal pain, and/or visual changes.

O11.1 Pre-existing hypertension with pre-eclampsia, first trimester COM M ♀

O11.2 Pre-existing hypertension with pre-eclampsia, second trimester COM M ♀

O11.3 Pre-existing hypertension with pre-eclampsia, third trimester COM M ♀

O11.4 Pre-existing hypertension with pre-eclampsia, complicating childbirth COM M ♀

O11.5 Pre-existing hypertension with pre-eclampsia, complicating the puerperium COM M ♀

O11.9 Pre-existing hypertension with pre-eclampsia, unspecified trimester COM M ♀

O12 Gestational [pregnancy-induced] edema and proteinuria without hypertension

O12.0 Gestational edema

O12.00 Gestational edema, unspecified trimester COM M ♀

O12.01 Gestational edema, first trimester COM M ♀

O12.02 Gestational edema, second trimester COM M ♀

O12.03 Gestational edema, third trimester COM M ♀

O12.04 Gestational edema, complicating childbirth COM M ♀

O12.05 Gestational edema, complicating the puerperium COM M ♀

O12.1 Gestational proteinuria

O12.10 Gestational proteinuria, unspecified trimester COM M ♀

O12.11 Gestational proteinuria, first trimester COM M ♀

O12.12 Gestational proteinuria, second trimester COM M ♀

O12.13 Gestational proteinuria, third trimester COM M ♀

O12.14 Gestational proteinuria, complicating childbirth COM M ♀

O12.15 Gestational proteinuria, complicating the puerperium COM M ♀

O12.2 Gestational edema with proteinuria

O12.20 Gestational edema with proteinuria, unspecified trimester COM M ♀

O12.21 Gestational edema with proteinuria, first trimester COM M ♀

O12.22 Gestational edema with proteinuria, second trimester COM M ♀

O12.23 Gestational edema with proteinuria, third trimester COM M ♀

O12.24 Gestational edema with proteinuria, complicating childbirth COM M ♀

O12.25 Gestational edema with proteinuria, complicating the puerperium COM M ♀

O13 Gestational [pregnancy-induced] hypertension without significant proteinuria

INCLUDES gestational hypertension NOS
transient hypertension of pregnancy

AHA: 2016,1Q,5

O13.1 Gestational [pregnancy-induced] hypertension without significant proteinuria, first trimester COM M ♀

O13.2 Gestational [pregnancy-induced] hypertension without significant proteinuria, second trimester COM M ♀

O13.3 Gestational [pregnancy-induced] hypertension without significant proteinuria, third trimester COM M ♀

O13.4 Gestational [pregnancy-induced] hypertension without significant proteinuria, complicating childbirth COM M ♀

O13.5 Gestational [pregnancy-induced] hypertension without significant proteinuria, complicating the puerperium COM M ♀

O13.9 Gestational [pregnancy-induced] hypertension without significant proteinuria, unspecified trimester COM M ♀

O14 Pre-eclampsia

EXCLUDES 1 *pre-existing hypertension with pre-eclampsia (O11)*

DEF: Complication of pregnancy manifesting in the development of borderline hypertension, protein in the urine, and unresponsive swelling between the 20th week of pregnancy and the end of the first week following birth in mild to moderate cases. Severe preeclampsia presents with hypertension, associated with marked swelling, proteinuria, abdominal pain, and/or visual changes.

O14.0 Mild to moderate pre-eclampsia

AHA: 2019,3Q,12; 2019,2Q,8

O14.00 Mild to moderate pre-eclampsia, unspecified trimester COM M ♀

O14.02 Mild to moderate pre-eclampsia, second trimester COM M ♀

O14.03 Mild to moderate pre-eclampsia, third trimester COM M ♀

O14.04 Mild to moderate pre-eclampsia, complicating childbirth COM M ♀

AHA: 2019,2Q,8

O14.05 Mild to moderate pre-eclampsia, complicating the puerperium COM M ♀

O14.1 Severe pre-eclampsia

EXCLUDES 1 *HELLP syndrome (O14.2-)*

AHA: 2019,3Q,12

O14.10 Severe pre-eclampsia, unspecified trimester COM M ♀

O14.12 Severe pre-eclampsia, second trimester COM M ♀

O14.13 Severe pre-eclampsia, third trimester COM M ♀

O14.14 Severe pre-eclampsia complicating childbirth COM M ♀

O14.15 Severe pre-eclampsia, complicating the puerperium COM M ♀

O14.2 HELLP syndrome

Severe pre-eclampsia with hemolysis, elevated liver enzymes and low platelet count (HELLP)

AHA: 2019,3Q,12

O14.20 HELLP syndrome (HELLP), unspecified trimester COM M ♀

O14.22 HELLP syndrome (HELLP), second trimester COM M ♀

O14.23 HELLP syndrome (HELLP), third trimester COM M ♀

O14.24 HELLP syndrome, complicating childbirth COM M ♀

O14.25 HELLP syndrome, complicating the puerperium COM M ♀

O14.9 Unspecified pre-eclampsia

O14.90 Unspecified pre-eclampsia, unspecified trimester COM M ♀

O14.92 Unspecified pre-eclampsia, second trimester COM M ♀

O14.93 Unspecified pre-eclampsia, third trimester COM M ♀

O14.94 Unspecified pre-eclampsia, complicating childbirth COM M ♀

O14.95 Unspecified pre-eclampsia, complicating the puerperium COM M ♀

O15 Eclampsia

INCLUDES convulsions following conditions in O10-O14 and O16

DEF: Tetany and toxemia producing seizure activity or coma in a pregnant patient who most often has presented with prior preeclampsia (i.e., hypertension, albuminuria, and edema).

O15.0 Eclampsia complicating pregnancy

O15.00 Eclampsia complicating pregnancy, unspecified trimester COM M ♀

O15.02 Eclampsia complicating pregnancy, second trimester COM M ♀

O15.03 Eclampsia complicating pregnancy, third trimester COM M ♀

O15.1 Eclampsia complicating labor COM M ♀

O15.2 Eclampsia complicating the puerperium COM M ♀

O15.9 Eclampsia, unspecified as to time period COM M ♀

Eclampsia NOS

O16 Unspecified maternal hypertension

O16.1 Unspecified maternal hypertension, first trimester COM M ♀

O16.2 Unspecified maternal hypertension, second trimester COM M ♀

O16.3 Unspecified maternal hypertension, third trimester COM M ♀

O16.4 Unspecified maternal hypertension, complicating childbirth COM M ♀

O16.5 Unspecified maternal hypertension, complicating the puerperium COM M ♀

O16.9 Unspecified maternal hypertension, unspecified trimester COM M ♀

Other maternal disorders predominantly related to pregnancy (O20-O29)

EXCLUDES 2 *maternal care related to the fetus and amniotic cavity and possible delivery problems (O30-O48)*

maternal diseases classifiable elsewhere but complicating pregnancy, labor and delivery, and the puerperium (O98-O99)

O20 Hemorrhage in early pregnancy

INCLUDES hemorrhage before completion of 20 weeks gestation

EXCLUDES 1 *pregnancy with abortive outcome (O00-O08)*

O20.0 Threatened abortion COM M ♀

Hemorrhage specified as due to threatened abortion

DEF: Bloody discharge during pregnancy. The cervix may be dilated and pregnancy threatened, but the pregnancy is not terminated.

O20.8 Other hemorrhage in early pregnancy COM M ♀

O20.9 Hemorrhage in early pregnancy, unspecified COM M ♀

O21 Excessive vomiting in pregnancy

O21.0 Mild hyperemesis gravidarum COM M ♀

Hyperemesis gravidarum, mild or unspecified, starting before the end of the 20th week of gestation

O21.1 Hyperemesis gravidarum with metabolic disturbance COM M ♀

Hyperemesis gravidarum, starting before the end of the 20th week of gestation, with metabolic disturbance such as carbohydrate depletion

Hyperemesis gravidarum, starting before the end of the 20th week of gestation, with metabolic disturbance such as dehydration

Hyperemesis gravidarum, starting before the end of the 20th week of gestation, with metabolic disturbance such as electrolyte imbalance

O21.2 Late vomiting of pregnancy COM M ♀

Excessive vomiting starting after 20 completed weeks of gestation

O21.8 Other vomiting complicating pregnancy COM M ♀

Vomiting due to diseases classified elsewhere, complicating pregnancy

Use additional code, to identify cause

O21.9 Vomiting of pregnancy, unspecified COM M ♀

O22 Venous complications and hemorrhoids in pregnancy

EXCLUDES 1 *venous complications of:*

abortion NOS (O03.9)

ectopic or molar pregnancy (O08.7)

failed attempted abortion (O07.35)

induced abortion (O04.85)

spontaneous abortion (O03.89)

EXCLUDES 2 *obstetric pulmonary embolism (O88.-)*

venous complications and hemorrhoids of childbirth and the puerperium (O87.-)

O22.0 Varicose veins of lower extremity in pregnancy

Varicose veins NOS in pregnancy

DEF: Distended, tortuous veins of the lower extremities associated with pregnancy.

O22.00 Varicose veins of lower extremity in pregnancy, unspecified trimester COM M ♀

O22.01 Varicose veins of lower extremity in pregnancy, first trimester COM M ♀

O22.02 Varicose veins of lower extremity in pregnancy, second trimester COM M ♀

O22.03 Varicose veins of lower extremity in pregnancy, third trimester COM M ♀

O22.1 Genital varices in pregnancy

Perineal varices in pregnancy

Vaginal varices in pregnancy

Vulval varices in pregnancy

O22.10 Genital varices in pregnancy, unspecified trimester COM M ♀

O22.11 Genital varices in pregnancy, first trimester COM M ♀

O22.12 Genital varices in pregnancy, second trimester COM M ♀

O22.13 Genital varices in pregnancy, third trimester COM M ♀

O22.2 Superficial thrombophlebitis in pregnancy

Phlebitis in pregnancy NOS

Thrombophlebitis of legs in pregnancy

Thrombosis in pregnancy NOS

Use additional code to identify the superficial thrombophlebitis (I80.0-)

O22.20 Superficial thrombophlebitis in pregnancy, unspecified trimester COM M ♀

O22.21 Superficial thrombophlebitis in pregnancy, first trimester COM M ♀

O22.22 Superficial thrombophlebitis in pregnancy, second trimester COM M ♀

O22.23 Superficial thrombophlebitis in pregnancy, third trimester COM M ♀

O22.3 Deep phlebothrombosis in pregnancy

Deep vein thrombosis, antepartum

Use additional code to identify the deep vein thrombosis (I82.4-, I82.5-, I82.62-, I82.72-)

Use additional code, if applicable, for associated long-term (current) use of anticoagulants (Z79.01)

O22.30 Deep phlebothrombosis in pregnancy, unspecified trimester COM M ♀

O22.31 Deep phlebothrombosis in pregnancy, first trimester COM M ♀

O22.32 Deep phlebothrombosis in pregnancy, second trimester COM M ♀

O22.33 Deep phlebothrombosis in pregnancy, third trimester COM M ♀

O22.4 Hemorrhoids in pregnancy

O22.40 Hemorrhoids in pregnancy, unspecified trimester COM M ♀

O22.41 Hemorrhoids in pregnancy, first trimester COM M ♀

O22.42 Hemorrhoids in pregnancy, second trimester COM M ♀

O22.43 Hemorrhoids in pregnancy, third trimester COM M ♀

O22.5 Cerebral venous thrombosis in pregnancy

Cerebrovenous sinus thrombosis in pregnancy

O22.50 Cerebral venous thrombosis in pregnancy, unspecified trimester COM M ♀

O22.51 Cerebral venous thrombosis in pregnancy, first trimester COM M ♀

O22.52 **Cerebral venous thrombosis in pregnancy, second trimester** COM M ♀

O22.53 **Cerebral venous thrombosis in pregnancy, third trimester** COM M ♀

5th O22.8 **Other venous complications in pregnancy**

6th O22.8X **Other venous complications in pregnancy**

O22.8X1 **Other venous complications in pregnancy, first trimester** COM M ♀

O22.8X2 **Other venous complications in pregnancy, second trimester** COM M ♀

O22.8X3 **Other venous complications in pregnancy, third trimester** COM M ♀

O22.8X9 **Other venous complications in pregnancy, unspecified trimester** COM M ♀

5th O22.9 **Venous complication in pregnancy, unspecified**

Gestational phlebitis NOS

Gestational phlebopathy NOS

Gestational thrombosis NOS

O22.90 **Venous complication in pregnancy, unspecified, unspecified trimester** COM M ♀

O22.91 **Venous complication in pregnancy, unspecified, first trimester** COM M ♀

O22.92 **Venous complication in pregnancy, unspecified, second trimester** COM M ♀

O22.93 **Venous complication in pregnancy, unspecified, third trimester** COM M ♀

4th O23 **Infections of genitourinary tract in pregnancy**

Use additional code to identify organism (B95.-, B96.-)

EXCLUDES 2 *gonococcal infections complicating pregnancy, childbirth and the puerperium (O98.2)*

infections with a predominantly sexual mode of transmission NOS complicating pregnancy, childbirth and the puerperium (O98.3)

syphilis complicating pregnancy, childbirth and the puerperium (O98.1)

tuberculosis of genitourinary system complicating pregnancy, childbirth and the puerperium (O98.0)

venereal disease NOS complicating pregnancy, childbirth and the puerperium (O98.3)

AHA: 2018,2Q,20

5th O23.0 **Infections of kidney in pregnancy**

Pyelonephritis in pregnancy

O23.00 **Infections of kidney in pregnancy, unspecified trimester** COM M ♀

O23.01 **Infections of kidney in pregnancy, first trimester** COM M ♀

O23.02 **Infections of kidney in pregnancy, second trimester** COM M ♀

O23.03 **Infections of kidney in pregnancy, third trimester** COM M ♀

5th O23.1 **Infections of bladder in pregnancy**

O23.10 **Infections of bladder in pregnancy, unspecified trimester** COM M ♀

O23.11 **Infections of bladder in pregnancy, first trimester** COM M ♀

O23.12 **Infections of bladder in pregnancy, second trimester** COM M ♀

O23.13 **Infections of bladder in pregnancy, third trimester** COM M ♀

5th O23.2 **Infections of urethra in pregnancy**

O23.20 **Infections of urethra in pregnancy, unspecified trimester** COM M ♀

O23.21 **Infections of urethra in pregnancy, first trimester** COM M ♀

O23.22 **Infections of urethra in pregnancy, second trimester** COM M ♀

O23.23 **Infections of urethra in pregnancy, third trimester** COM M ♀

5th O23.3 **Infections of other parts of urinary tract in pregnancy**

O23.30 **Infections of other parts of urinary tract in pregnancy, unspecified trimester** COM M ♀

O23.31 **Infections of other parts of urinary tract in pregnancy, first trimester** COM M ♀

O23.32 **Infections of other parts of urinary tract in pregnancy, second trimester** COM M ♀

O23.33 **Infections of other parts of urinary tract in pregnancy, third trimester** COM M ♀

5th O23.4 **Unspecified infection of urinary tract in pregnancy**

O23.40 **Unspecified infection of urinary tract in pregnancy, unspecified trimester** COM M ♀

O23.41 **Unspecified infection of urinary tract in pregnancy, first trimester** COM M ♀

O23.42 **Unspecified infection of urinary tract in pregnancy, second trimester** COM M ♀

O23.43 **Unspecified infection of urinary tract in pregnancy, third trimester** COM M ♀

5th O23.5 **Infections of the genital tract in pregnancy**

6th O23.51 **Infection of cervix in pregnancy**

O23.511 **Infections of cervix in pregnancy, first trimester** COM M ♀

O23.512 **Infections of cervix in pregnancy, second trimester** COM M ♀

O23.513 **Infections of cervix in pregnancy, third trimester** COM M ♀

O23.519 **Infections of cervix in pregnancy, unspecified trimester** COM M ♀

6th O23.52 **Salpingo-oophoritis in pregnancy**

Oophoritis in pregnancy

Salpingitis in pregnancy

O23.521 **Salpingo-oophoritis in pregnancy, first trimester** COM M ♀

O23.522 **Salpingo-oophoritis in pregnancy, second trimester** COM M ♀

O23.523 **Salpingo-oophoritis in pregnancy, third trimester** COM M ♀

O23.529 **Salpingo-oophoritis in pregnancy, unspecified trimester** COM M ♀

6th O23.59 **Infection of other part of genital tract in pregnancy**

AHA: 2022,1Q,20

O23.591 **Infection of other part of genital tract in pregnancy, first trimester** COM M ♀

O23.592 **Infection of other part of genital tract in pregnancy, second trimester** COM M ♀

O23.593 **Infection of other part of genital tract in pregnancy, third trimester** COM M ♀

O23.599 **Infection of other part of genital tract in pregnancy, unspecified trimester** COM M ♀

5th O23.9 **Unspecified genitourinary tract infection in pregnancy**

Genitourinary tract infection in pregnancy NOS

O23.90 **Unspecified genitourinary tract infection in pregnancy, unspecified trimester** COM M ♀

O23.91 **Unspecified genitourinary tract infection in pregnancy, first trimester** COM M ♀

O23.92 **Unspecified genitourinary tract infection in pregnancy, second trimester** COM M ♀

O23.93 **Unspecified genitourinary tract infection in pregnancy, third trimester** COM M ♀

4th O24 **Diabetes mellitus in pregnancy, childbirth and the puerperium**

5th O24.0 **Pre-existing type 1 diabetes mellitus, in pregnancy, childbirth and the puerperium**

Juvenile onset diabetes mellitus, in pregnancy, childbirth and the puerperium

Ketosis-prone diabetes mellitus in pregnancy, childbirth and the puerperium

Use additional code from category E10 to further identify any manifestations

6th O24.01 **Pre-existing type 1 diabetes mellitus, in pregnancy**

O24.011 **Pre-existing type 1 diabetes mellitus, in pregnancy, first trimester** COM Q M ♀

O24.012 **Pre-existing type 1 diabetes mellitus, in pregnancy, second trimester** COM Q M ♀

O24.013 **Pre-existing type 1 diabetes mellitus, in pregnancy, third trimester** COM Q M ♀

O24.019 **Pre-existing type 1 diabetes mellitus, in pregnancy, unspecified trimester** COM Q M ♀

O24.02 **Pre-existing type 1 diabetes mellitus, in childbirth** COM Q M ♀

O24.03 **Pre-existing type 1 diabetes mellitus, in the puerperium** COM Q M ♀

O24.1 **Pre-existing type 2 diabetes mellitus, in pregnancy, childbirth and the puerperium**
Insulin-resistant diabetes mellitus in pregnancy, childbirth and the puerperium
Use additional code (for):
from category E11 to further identify any manifestations
long-term (current) use of insulin (Z79.4)

O24.11 **Pre-existing type 2 diabetes mellitus, in pregnancy**
O24.111 **Pre-existing type 2 diabetes mellitus, in pregnancy, first trimester** COM Q M ♀
O24.112 **Pre-existing type 2 diabetes mellitus, in pregnancy, second trimester** COM Q M ♀
O24.113 **Pre-existing type 2 diabetes mellitus, in pregnancy, third trimester** COM Q M ♀
O24.119 **Pre-existing type 2 diabetes mellitus, in pregnancy, unspecified trimester** COM Q M ♀
O24.12 **Pre-existing type 2 diabetes mellitus, in childbirth** COM Q M ♀
O24.13 **Pre-existing type 2 diabetes mellitus, in the puerperium** COM Q M ♀

O24.3 **Unspecified pre-existing diabetes mellitus in pregnancy, childbirth and the puerperium**
Use additional code (for):
from category E11 to further identify any manifestation
long-term (current) use of insulin (Z79.4)

O24.31 **Unspecified pre-existing diabetes mellitus in pregnancy**
O24.311 **Unspecified pre-existing diabetes mellitus in pregnancy, first trimester** COM Q M ♀
O24.312 **Unspecified pre-existing diabetes mellitus in pregnancy, second trimester** COM Q M ♀
O24.313 **Unspecified pre-existing diabetes mellitus in pregnancy, third trimester** COM Q M ♀
O24.319 **Unspecified pre-existing diabetes mellitus in pregnancy, unspecified trimester** COM Q M ♀
O24.32 **Unspecified pre-existing diabetes mellitus in childbirth** COM Q M ♀
O24.33 **Unspecified pre-existing diabetes mellitus in the puerperium** COM Q M ♀

O24.4 **Gestational diabetes mellitus**
Diabetes mellitus arising in pregnancy
Gestational diabetes mellitus NOS
AHA: 2020,3Q,30; 2016,4Q,50; 2015,4Q,34

O24.41 **Gestational diabetes mellitus in pregnancy**
O24.410 **Gestational diabetes mellitus in pregnancy, diet controlled** COM M ♀
O24.414 **Gestational diabetes mellitus in pregnancy, insulin controlled** COM M ♀
O24.415 **Gestational diabetes mellitus in pregnancy, controlled by oral hypoglycemic drugs** COM M ♀
Gestational diabetes mellitus in pregnancy, controlled by oral antidiabetic drugs
O24.419 **Gestational diabetes mellitus in pregnancy, unspecified control** COM M ♀

O24.42 **Gestational diabetes mellitus in childbirth**
AHA: 2016,1Q,5
O24.420 **Gestational diabetes mellitus in childbirth, diet controlled** COM M ♀
O24.424 **Gestational diabetes mellitus in childbirth, insulin controlled** COM M ♀
O24.425 **Gestational diabetes mellitus in childbirth, controlled by oral hypoglycemic drugs** COM M ♀
Gestational diabetes mellitus in childbirth, controlled by oral antidiabetic drugs
O24.429 **Gestational diabetes mellitus in childbirth, unspecified control** COM M ♀

O24.43 **Gestational diabetes mellitus in the puerperium**
O24.430 **Gestational diabetes mellitus in the puerperium, diet controlled** COM M ♀
O24.434 **Gestational diabetes mellitus in the puerperium, insulin controlled** COM M ♀
O24.435 **Gestational diabetes mellitus in puerperium, controlled by oral hypoglycemic drugs** COM M ♀
Gestational diabetes mellitus in puerperium, controlled by oral antidiabetic drugs
O24.439 **Gestational diabetes mellitus in the puerperium, unspecified control** COM M ♀

O24.8 **Other pre-existing diabetes mellitus in pregnancy, childbirth, and the puerperium**
Use additional code (for):
from categories E08, E09 and E13 to further identify any manifestation
long-term (current) use of insulin (Z79.4)

O24.81 **Other pre-existing diabetes mellitus in pregnancy**
O24.811 **Other pre-existing diabetes mellitus in pregnancy, first trimester** COM Q M ♀
O24.812 **Other pre-existing diabetes mellitus in pregnancy, second trimester** COM Q M ♀
O24.813 **Other pre-existing diabetes mellitus in pregnancy, third trimester** COM Q M ♀
O24.819 **Other pre-existing diabetes mellitus in pregnancy, unspecified trimester** COM Q M ♀
O24.82 **Other pre-existing diabetes mellitus in childbirth** COM Q M ♀
O24.83 **Other pre-existing diabetes mellitus in the puerperium** COM Q M ♀

O24.9 **Unspecified diabetes mellitus in pregnancy, childbirth and the puerperium**
Use additional code for long-term (current) use of insulin (Z79.4)

O24.91 **Unspecified diabetes mellitus in pregnancy**
O24.911 **Unspecified diabetes mellitus in pregnancy, first trimester** COM M ♀
O24.912 **Unspecified diabetes mellitus in pregnancy, second trimester** COM M ♀
O24.913 **Unspecified diabetes mellitus in pregnancy, third trimester** COM M ♀
O24.919 **Unspecified diabetes mellitus in pregnancy, unspecified trimester** COM M ♀
O24.92 **Unspecified diabetes mellitus in childbirth** COM M ♀
O24.93 **Unspecified diabetes mellitus in the puerperium** COM M ♀

O25 **Malnutrition in pregnancy, childbirth and the puerperium**
O25.1 **Malnutrition in pregnancy**
O25.10 **Malnutrition in pregnancy, unspecified trimester** COM M ♀
O25.11 **Malnutrition in pregnancy, first trimester** COM M ♀
O25.12 **Malnutrition in pregnancy, second trimester** COM M ♀
O25.13 **Malnutrition in pregnancy, third trimester** COM M ♀
O25.2 **Malnutrition in childbirth** COM M ♀
O25.3 **Malnutrition in the puerperium** COM M ♀

O26 **Maternal care for other conditions predominantly related to pregnancy**
O26.0 **Excessive weight gain in pregnancy**
EXCLUDES 2 *gestational edema (O12.0, O12.2)*
O26.00 **Excessive weight gain in pregnancy, unspecified trimester** COM M ♀
O26.01 **Excessive weight gain in pregnancy, first trimester** COM M ♀
O26.02 **Excessive weight gain in pregnancy, second trimester** COM M ♀
O26.03 **Excessive weight gain in pregnancy, third trimester** COM M ♀
O26.1 **Low weight gain in pregnancy**
O26.10 **Low weight gain in pregnancy, unspecified trimester** COM M ♀

Chapter 15. Pregnancy, Childbirth and the Puerperium

O26.11 Low weight gain in pregnancy, first trimester COM M ♀
O26.12 Low weight gain in pregnancy, second trimester COM M ♀
O26.13 Low weight gain in pregnancy, third trimester COM M ♀

✓5th O26.2 Pregnancy care for patient with recurrent pregnancy loss
O26.20 Pregnancy care for patient with recurrent pregnancy loss, unspecified trimester COM M ♀
O26.21 Pregnancy care for patient with recurrent pregnancy loss, first trimester COM M ♀
O26.22 Pregnancy care for patient with recurrent pregnancy loss, second trimester COM M ♀
O26.23 Pregnancy care for patient with recurrent pregnancy loss, third trimester COM M ♀

✓5th O26.3 Retained intrauterine contraceptive device in pregnancy
O26.30 Retained intrauterine contraceptive device in pregnancy, unspecified trimester COM M ♀
O26.31 Retained intrauterine contraceptive device in pregnancy, first trimester COM M ♀
O26.32 Retained intrauterine contraceptive device in pregnancy, second trimester COM M ♀
O26.33 Retained intrauterine contraceptive device in pregnancy, third trimester COM M ♀

✓5th O26.4 Herpes gestationis
DEF: Rare skin disorder of unknown origin that appears on the abdomen in the second and third trimester as intensely itchy blisters that spread to other sites.
O26.40 Herpes gestationis, unspecified trimester COM M ♀
O26.41 Herpes gestationis, first trimester COM M ♀
O26.42 Herpes gestationis, second trimester COM M ♀
O26.43 Herpes gestationis, third trimester COM M ♀

✓5th O26.5 Maternal hypotension syndrome
Supine hypotensive syndrome
O26.50 Maternal hypotension syndrome, unspecified trimester COM M ♀
O26.51 Maternal hypotension syndrome, first trimester COM M ♀
O26.52 Maternal hypotension syndrome, second trimester COM M ♀
O26.53 Maternal hypotension syndrome, third trimester COM M ♀

✓5th O26.6 Liver and biliary tract disorders in pregnancy, childbirth and the puerperium
Use additional code to identify the specific disorder
EXCLUDES 2 *hepatorenal syndrome following labor and delivery (O90.4)*

✓6th O26.61 Liver and biliary tract disorders in pregnancy
O26.611 Liver and biliary tract disorders in pregnancy, first trimester COM M ♀
O26.612 Liver and biliary tract disorders in pregnancy, second trimester COM M ♀
O26.613 Liver and biliary tract disorders in pregnancy, third trimester COM M ♀
O26.619 Liver and biliary tract disorders in pregnancy, unspecified trimester COM M ♀
O26.62 Liver and biliary tract disorders in childbirth COM M ♀
O26.63 Liver and biliary tract disorders in the puerperium COM M ♀

✓5th O26.7 Subluxation of symphysis (pubis) in pregnancy, childbirth and the puerperium
EXCLUDES 1 *traumatic separation of symphysis (pubis) during childbirth (O71.6)*

✓6th O26.71 Subluxation of symphysis (pubis) in pregnancy
O26.711 Subluxation of symphysis (pubis) in pregnancy, first trimester COM M ♀
O26.712 Subluxation of symphysis (pubis) in pregnancy, second trimester COM M ♀
O26.713 Subluxation of symphysis (pubis) in pregnancy, third trimester COM M ♀
O26.719 Subluxation of symphysis (pubis) in pregnancy, unspecified trimester COM M ♀
O26.72 Subluxation of symphysis (pubis) in childbirth COM M ♀
O26.73 Subluxation of symphysis (pubis) in the puerperium COM M ♀

✓5th O26.8 Other specified pregnancy related conditions

✓6th O26.81 Pregnancy related exhaustion and fatigue
O26.811 Pregnancy related exhaustion and fatigue, first trimester COM M ♀
O26.812 Pregnancy related exhaustion and fatigue, second trimester COM M ♀
O26.813 Pregnancy related exhaustion and fatigue, third trimester COM M ♀
O26.819 Pregnancy related exhaustion and fatigue, unspecified trimester COM M ♀

✓6th O26.82 Pregnancy related peripheral neuritis
O26.821 Pregnancy related peripheral neuritis, first trimester COM M ♀
O26.822 Pregnancy related peripheral neuritis, second trimester COM M ♀
O26.823 Pregnancy related peripheral neuritis, third trimester COM M ♀
O26.829 Pregnancy related peripheral neuritis, unspecified trimester COM M ♀

✓6th O26.83 Pregnancy related renal disease
Use additional code to identify the specific disorder
O26.831 Pregnancy related renal disease, first trimester COM M ♀
O26.832 Pregnancy related renal disease, second trimester COM M ♀
O26.833 Pregnancy related renal disease, third trimester COM M ♀
O26.839 Pregnancy related renal disease, unspecified trimester COM M ♀

✓6th O26.84 Uterine size-date discrepancy complicating pregnancy
EXCLUDES 1 *encounter for suspected problem with fetal growth ruled out (Z03.74)*
O26.841 Uterine size-date discrepancy, first trimester COM M ♀
O26.842 Uterine size-date discrepancy, second trimester COM M ♀
O26.843 Uterine size-date discrepancy, third trimester COM M ♀
O26.849 Uterine size-date discrepancy, unspecified trimester COM M ♀

✓6th O26.85 Spotting complicating pregnancy
O26.851 Spotting complicating pregnancy, first trimester COM M ♀
O26.852 Spotting complicating pregnancy, second trimester COM M ♀
O26.853 Spotting complicating pregnancy, third trimester COM M ♀
O26.859 Spotting complicating pregnancy, unspecified trimester COM M ♀
O26.86 Pruritic urticarial papules and plaques of pregnancy (PUPPP) COM M ♀
Polymorphic eruption of pregnancy

✓6th O26.87 Cervical shortening
EXCLUDES 1 *encounter for suspected cervical shortening ruled out (Z03.75)*
DEF: Cervix that has shortened to less than 25 mm before the 24th week of pregnancy. A shortened cervix is a warning sign for impending premature delivery and is treated by cervical cerclage placement or progesterone.
O26.872 Cervical shortening, second trimester COM M ♀
O26.873 Cervical shortening, third trimester COM M ♀
O26.879 Cervical shortening, unspecified trimester COM M ♀

✓6th O26.89 Other specified pregnancy related conditions
AHA: 2015,3Q,40
O26.891 Other specified pregnancy related conditions, first trimester COM M ♀
O26.892 Other specified pregnancy related conditions, second trimester COM M ♀
O26.893 Other specified pregnancy related conditions, third trimester COM M ♀

O26.899 Other specified pregnancy related conditions, unspecified trimester COM M ♀

O26.9 Pregnancy related conditions, unspecified

O26.90 Pregnancy related conditions, unspecified, unspecified trimester COM M ♀

O26.91 Pregnancy related conditions, unspecified, first trimester COM M ♀

O26.92 Pregnancy related conditions, unspecified, second trimester COM M ♀

O26.93 Pregnancy related conditions, unspecified, third trimester COM M ♀

O28 Abnormal findings on antenatal screening of mother

EXCLUDES 1 *diagnostic findings classified elsewhere - see Alphabetical Index*

O28.0 Abnormal hematological finding on antenatal screening of mother M ♀

O28.1 Abnormal biochemical finding on antenatal screening of mother M ♀

O28.2 Abnormal cytological finding on antenatal screening of mother M ♀

O28.3 Abnormal ultrasonic finding on antenatal screening of mother M ♀

O28.4 Abnormal radiological finding on antenatal screening of mother M ♀

O28.5 Abnormal chromosomal and genetic finding on antenatal screening of mother M ♀

O28.8 Other abnormal findings on antenatal screening of mother M ♀

O28.9 Unspecified abnormal findings on antenatal screening of mother M ♀

O29 Complications of anesthesia during pregnancy

INCLUDES maternal complications arising from the administration of a general, regional or local anesthetic, analgesic or other sedation during pregnancy

Use additional code, if necessary, to identify the complication

EXCLUDES 2 *complications of anesthesia during labor and delivery (O74.-)*
complications of anesthesia during the puerperium (O89.-)

O29.0 Pulmonary complications of anesthesia during pregnancy

O29.01 Aspiration pneumonitis due to anesthesia during pregnancy
Inhalation of stomach contents or secretions NOS due to anesthesia during pregnancy
Mendelson's syndrome due to anesthesia during pregnancy

O29.011 Aspiration pneumonitis due to anesthesia during pregnancy, first trimester COM M ♀

O29.012 Aspiration pneumonitis due to anesthesia during pregnancy, second trimester COM M ♀

O29.013 Aspiration pneumonitis due to anesthesia during pregnancy, third trimester COM M ♀

O29.019 Aspiration pneumonitis due to anesthesia during pregnancy, unspecified trimester COM M ♀

O29.02 Pressure collapse of lung due to anesthesia during pregnancy

O29.021 Pressure collapse of lung due to anesthesia during pregnancy, first trimester COM M ♀

O29.022 Pressure collapse of lung due to anesthesia during pregnancy, second trimester COM M ♀

O29.023 Pressure collapse of lung due to anesthesia during pregnancy, third trimester COM M ♀

O29.029 Pressure collapse of lung due to anesthesia during pregnancy, unspecified trimester COM M ♀

O29.09 Other pulmonary complications of anesthesia during pregnancy

O29.091 Other pulmonary complications of anesthesia during pregnancy, first trimester COM M ♀

O29.092 Other pulmonary complications of anesthesia during pregnancy, second trimester COM M ♀

O29.093 Other pulmonary complications of anesthesia during pregnancy, third trimester COM M ♀

O29.099 Other pulmonary complications of anesthesia during pregnancy, unspecified trimester COM M ♀

O29.1 Cardiac complications of anesthesia during pregnancy

O29.11 Cardiac arrest due to anesthesia during pregnancy

O29.111 Cardiac arrest due to anesthesia during pregnancy, first trimester COM M ♀

O29.112 Cardiac arrest due to anesthesia during pregnancy, second trimester COM M ♀

O29.113 Cardiac arrest due to anesthesia during pregnancy, third trimester COM M ♀

O29.119 Cardiac arrest due to anesthesia during pregnancy, unspecified trimester COM M ♀

O29.12 Cardiac failure due to anesthesia during pregnancy

O29.121 Cardiac failure due to anesthesia during pregnancy, first trimester COM M ♀

O29.122 Cardiac failure due to anesthesia during pregnancy, second trimester COM M ♀

O29.123 Cardiac failure due to anesthesia during pregnancy, third trimester COM M ♀

O29.129 Cardiac failure due to anesthesia during pregnancy, unspecified trimester COM M ♀

O29.19 Other cardiac complications of anesthesia during pregnancy

O29.191 Other cardiac complications of anesthesia during pregnancy, first trimester COM M ♀

O29.192 Other cardiac complications of anesthesia during pregnancy, second trimester COM M ♀

O29.193 Other cardiac complications of anesthesia during pregnancy, third trimester COM M ♀

O29.199 Other cardiac complications of anesthesia during pregnancy, unspecified trimester COM M ♀

O29.2 Central nervous system complications of anesthesia during pregnancy

O29.21 Cerebral anoxia due to anesthesia during pregnancy

O29.211 Cerebral anoxia due to anesthesia during pregnancy, first trimester COM M ♀

O29.212 Cerebral anoxia due to anesthesia during pregnancy, second trimester COM M ♀

O29.213 Cerebral anoxia due to anesthesia during pregnancy, third trimester COM M ♀

O29.219 Cerebral anoxia due to anesthesia during pregnancy, unspecified trimester COM M ♀

O29.29 Other central nervous system complications of anesthesia during pregnancy

O29.291 Other central nervous system complications of anesthesia during pregnancy, first trimester COM M ♀

O29.292 Other central nervous system complications of anesthesia during pregnancy, second trimester COM M ♀

O29.293 Other central nervous system complications of anesthesia during pregnancy, third trimester COM M ♀

O29.299 Other central nervous system complications of anesthesia during pregnancy, unspecified trimester COM M ♀

O29.3 Toxic reaction to local anesthesia during pregnancy

O29.3X Toxic reaction to local anesthesia during pregnancy

O29.3X1 Toxic reaction to local anesthesia during pregnancy, first trimester COM M ♀

O29.3X2 Toxic reaction to local anesthesia during pregnancy, second trimester COM M ♀

O29.3X3 Toxic reaction to local anesthesia during pregnancy, third trimester COM M ♀

O29.3X9 Toxic reaction to local anesthesia during pregnancy, unspecified trimester COM M ♀

O29.4 Spinal and epidural anesthesia induced headache during pregnancy

O29.40 Spinal and epidural anesthesia induced headache during pregnancy, unspecified trimester COM M ♀

O29.41 Spinal and epidural anesthesia induced headache during pregnancy, first trimester COM M ♀

O29.42 Spinal and epidural anesthesia induced headache during pregnancy, second trimester COM M ♀

O29.43 Spinal and epidural anesthesia induced headache during pregnancy, third trimester COM M ♀

O29.5 Other complications of spinal and epidural anesthesia during pregnancy

O29.5X Other complications of spinal and epidural anesthesia during pregnancy

O29.5X1 Other complications of spinal and epidural anesthesia during pregnancy, first trimester COM M ♀

O29.5X2 Other complications of spinal and epidural anesthesia during pregnancy, second trimester COM M ♀

O29.5X3 Other complications of spinal and epidural anesthesia during pregnancy, third trimester COM M ♀

O29.5X9 Other complications of spinal and epidural anesthesia during pregnancy, unspecified trimester COM M ♀

O29.6 Failed or difficult intubation for anesthesia during pregnancy

O29.60 Failed or difficult intubation for anesthesia during pregnancy, unspecified trimester COM M ♀

O29.61 Failed or difficult intubation for anesthesia during pregnancy, first trimester COM M ♀

O29.62 Failed or difficult intubation for anesthesia during pregnancy, second trimester COM M ♀

O29.63 Failed or difficult intubation for anesthesia during pregnancy, third trimester COM M ♀

O29.8 Other complications of anesthesia during pregnancy

O29.8X Other complications of anesthesia during pregnancy

O29.8X1 Other complications of anesthesia during pregnancy, first trimester COM M ♀

O29.8X2 Other complications of anesthesia during pregnancy, second trimester COM M ♀

O29.8X3 Other complications of anesthesia during pregnancy, third trimester COM M ♀

O29.8X9 Other complications of anesthesia during pregnancy, unspecified trimester COM M ♀

O29.9 Unspecified complication of anesthesia during pregnancy

O29.90 Unspecified complication of anesthesia during pregnancy, unspecified trimester COM M ♀

O29.91 Unspecified complication of anesthesia during pregnancy, first trimester COM M ♀

O29.92 Unspecified complication of anesthesia during pregnancy, second trimester COM M ♀

O29.93 Unspecified complication of anesthesia during pregnancy, third trimester COM M ♀

Maternal care related to the fetus and amniotic cavity and possible delivery problems (O30-O48)

O30 Multiple gestation

Code also any complications specific to multiple gestation

AHA: 2016,4Q,51

O30.0 Twin pregnancy

O30.00 Twin pregnancy, unspecified number of placenta and unspecified number of amniotic sacs

O30.001 Twin pregnancy, unspecified number of placenta and unspecified number of amniotic sacs, first trimester COM M ♀

O30.002 Twin pregnancy, unspecified number of placenta and unspecified number of amniotic sacs, second trimester COM M ♀

O30.003 Twin pregnancy, unspecified number of placenta and unspecified number of amniotic sacs, third trimester COM M ♀

O30.009 Twin pregnancy, unspecified number of placenta and unspecified number of amniotic sacs, unspecified trimester COM M ♀

O30.01 Twin pregnancy, monochorionic/monoamniotic

Twin pregnancy, one placenta, one amniotic sac

EXCLUDES 1 *conjoined twins (O30.02-)*

O30.011 Twin pregnancy, monochorionic/monoamniotic, first trimester COM M ♀

O30.012 Twin pregnancy, monochorionic/monoamniotic, second trimester COM M ♀

O30.013 Twin pregnancy, monochorionic/monoamniotic, third trimester COM M ♀

O30.019 Twin pregnancy, monochorionic/monoamniotic, unspecified trimester COM M ♀

O30.02 Conjoined twin pregnancy

O30.021 Conjoined twin pregnancy, first trimester COM M ♀

O30.022 Conjoined twin pregnancy, second trimester COM M ♀

O30.023 Conjoined twin pregnancy, third trimester COM M ♀

O30.029 Conjoined twin pregnancy, unspecified trimester COM M ♀

O30.03 Twin pregnancy, monochorionic/diamniotic

Twin pregnancy, one placenta, two amniotic sacs

O30.031 Twin pregnancy, monochorionic/diamniotic, first trimester COM M ♀

O30.032 Twin pregnancy, monochorionic/diamniotic, second trimester COM M ♀

O30.033 Twin pregnancy, monochorionic/diamniotic, third trimester COM M ♀

O30.039 Twin pregnancy, monochorionic/diamniotic, unspecified trimester COM M ♀

O30.04 Twin pregnancy, dichorionic/diamniotic

Twin pregnancy, two placentae, two amniotic sacs

O30.041 Twin pregnancy, dichorionic/diamniotic, first trimester COM M ♀

O30.042 Twin pregnancy, dichorionic/diamniotic, second trimester COM M ♀

O30.043 Twin pregnancy, dichorionic/diamniotic, third trimester COM M ♀

O30.049 Twin pregnancy, dichorionic/diamniotic, unspecified trimester COM M ♀

O30.09 Twin pregnancy, unable to determine number of placenta and number of amniotic sacs

O30.091 Twin pregnancy, unable to determine number of placenta and number of amniotic sacs, first trimester COM M ♀

O30.092 Twin pregnancy, unable to determine number of placenta and number of amniotic sacs, second trimester COM M ♀

O30.093 Twin pregnancy, unable to determine number of placenta and number of amniotic sacs, third trimester COM M ♀

O30.099 Twin pregnancy, unable to determine number of placenta and number of amniotic sacs, unspecified trimester COM M ♀

O30.1 Triplet pregnancy

O30.10 Triplet pregnancy, unspecified number of placenta and unspecified number of amniotic sacs

AHA: 2016,2Q,8

O30.101 Triplet pregnancy, unspecified number of placenta and unspecified number of amniotic sacs, first trimester COM M ♀

O30.102 Triplet pregnancy, unspecified number of placenta and unspecified number of amniotic sacs, second trimester COM M ♀

O30.103 Triplet pregnancy, unspecified number of placenta and unspecified number of amniotic sacs, third trimester COM M ♀

O30.109 Triplet pregnancy, unspecified number of placenta and unspecified number of amniotic sacs, unspecified trimester COM M ♀

✓6th **O30.11** Triplet pregnancy with two or more monochorionic fetuses

O30.111 Triplet pregnancy with two or more monochorionic fetuses, first trimester COM M ♀

O30.112 Triplet pregnancy with two or more monochorionic fetuses, second trimester COM M ♀

O30.113 Triplet pregnancy with two or more monochorionic fetuses, third trimester COM M ♀

O30.119 Triplet pregnancy with two or more monochorionic fetuses, unspecified trimester COM M ♀

✓6th **O30.12** Triplet pregnancy with two or more monoamniotic fetuses

O30.121 Triplet pregnancy with two or more monoamniotic fetuses, first trimester COM M ♀

O30.122 Triplet pregnancy with two or more monoamniotic fetuses, second trimester COM M ♀

O30.123 Triplet pregnancy with two or more monoamniotic fetuses, third trimester COM M ♀

O30.129 Triplet pregnancy with two or more monoamniotic fetuses, unspecified trimester COM M ♀

✓6th **O30.13** Triplet pregnancy, trichorionic/triamniotic

AHA: 2018,4Q,22

O30.131 Triplet pregnancy, trichorionic/triamniotic, first trimester COM M ♀

O30.132 Triplet pregnancy, trichorionic/triamniotic, second trimester COM M ♀

O30.133 Triplet pregnancy, trichorionic/triamniotic, third trimester COM M ♀

O30.139 Triplet pregnancy, trichorionic/triamniotic, unspecified trimester COM M ♀

✓6th **O30.19** Triplet pregnancy, unable to determine number of placenta and number of amniotic sacs

O30.191 Triplet pregnancy, unable to determine number of placenta and number of amniotic sacs, first trimester COM M ♀

O30.192 Triplet pregnancy, unable to determine number of placenta and number of amniotic sacs, second trimester COM M ♀

O30.193 Triplet pregnancy, unable to determine number of placenta and number of amniotic sacs, third trimester COM M ♀

O30.199 Triplet pregnancy, unable to determine number of placenta and number of amniotic sacs, unspecified trimester COM M ♀

✓5th **O30.2 Quadruplet pregnancy**

✓6th **O30.20** Quadruplet pregnancy, unspecified number of placenta and unspecified number of amniotic sacs

O30.201 Quadruplet pregnancy, unspecified number of placenta and unspecified number of amniotic sacs, first trimester COM M ♀

O30.202 Quadruplet pregnancy, unspecified number of placenta and unspecified number of amniotic sacs, second trimester COM M ♀

O30.203 Quadruplet pregnancy, unspecified number of placenta and unspecified number of amniotic sacs, third trimester COM M ♀

O30.209 Quadruplet pregnancy, unspecified number of placenta and unspecified number of amniotic sacs, unspecified trimester COM M ♀

✓6th **O30.21** Quadruplet pregnancy with two or more monochorionic fetuses

O30.211 Quadruplet pregnancy with two or more monochorionic fetuses, first trimester COM M ♀

O30.212 Quadruplet pregnancy with two or more monochorionic fetuses, second trimester COM M ♀

O30.213 Quadruplet pregnancy with two or more monochorionic fetuses, third trimester COM M ♀

O30.219 Quadruplet pregnancy with two or more monochorionic fetuses, unspecified trimester COM M ♀

✓6th **O30.22** Quadruplet pregnancy with two or more monoamniotic fetuses

O30.221 Quadruplet pregnancy with two or more monoamniotic fetuses, first trimester COM M ♀

O30.222 Quadruplet pregnancy with two or more monoamniotic fetuses, second trimester COM M ♀

O30.223 Quadruplet pregnancy with two or more monoamniotic fetuses, third trimester COM M ♀

O30.229 Quadruplet pregnancy with two or more monoamniotic fetuses, unspecified trimester COM M ♀

✓6th **O30.23** Quadruplet pregnancy, quadrachorionic/quadra-amniotic

AHA: 2018,4Q,22

O30.231 Quadruplet pregnancy, quadrachorionic/quadra-amniotic, first trimester COM M ♀

O30.232 Quadruplet pregnancy, quadrachorionic/quadra-amniotic, second trimester COM M ♀

O30.233 Quadruplet pregnancy, quadrachorionic/quadra-amniotic, third trimester COM M ♀

O30.239 Quadruplet pregnancy, quadrachorionic/quadra-amniotic, unspecified trimester COM M ♀

✓6th **O30.29** Quadruplet pregnancy, unable to determine number of placenta and number of amniotic sacs

O30.291 Quadruplet pregnancy, unable to determine number of placenta and number of amniotic sacs, first trimester COM M ♀

O30.292 Quadruplet pregnancy, unable to determine number of placenta and number of amniotic sacs, second trimester COM M ♀

O30.293 Quadruplet pregnancy, unable to determine number of placenta and number of amniotic sacs, third trimester COM M ♀

O30.299 Quadruplet pregnancy, unable to determine number of placenta and number of amniotic sacs, unspecified trimester COM M ♀

✓5th **O30.8 Other specified multiple gestation**

Multiple gestation pregnancy greater then quadruplets

✓6th **O30.80** Other specified multiple gestation, unspecified number of placenta and unspecified number of amniotic sacs

O30.801 Other specified multiple gestation, unspecified number of placenta and unspecified number of amniotic sacs, first trimester COM M ♀

O30.802 Other specified multiple gestation, unspecified number of placenta and unspecified number of amniotic sacs, second trimester COM M ♀

O30.803 Other specified multiple gestation, unspecified number of placenta and unspecified number of amniotic sacs, third trimester COM M ♀

O30.809 Other specified multiple gestation, unspecified number of placenta and unspecified number of amniotic sacs, unspecified trimester COM M ♀

6th **O30.81 Other specified multiple gestation with two or more monochorionic fetuses**

O30.811 Other specified multiple gestation with two or more monochorionic fetuses, first trimester COM M ♀

O30.812 Other specified multiple gestation with two or more monochorionic fetuses, second trimester COM M ♀

O30.813 Other specified multiple gestation with two or more monochorionic fetuses, third trimester COM M ♀

O30.819 Other specified multiple gestation with two or more monochorionic fetuses, unspecified trimester COM M ♀

6th **O30.82 Other specified multiple gestation with two or more monoamniotic fetuses**

O30.821 Other specified multiple gestation with two or more monoamniotic fetuses, first trimester COM M ♀

O30.822 Other specified multiple gestation with two or more monoamniotic fetuses, second trimester COM M ♀

O30.823 Other specified multiple gestation with two or more monoamniotic fetuses, third trimester COM M ♀

O30.829 Other specified multiple gestation with two or more monoamniotic fetuses, unspecified trimester COM M ♀

6th **O30.83 Other specified multiple gestation, number of chorions and amnions are both equal to the number of fetuses**

Pentachorionic, penta-amniotic pregnancy (quintuplets)

Hexachorionic, hexa-amniotic pregnancy (sextuplets)

Heptachorionic, hepta-amniotic pregnancy (septuplets)

AHA: 2018,4Q,22

O30.831 Other specified multiple gestation, number of chorions and amnions are both equal to the number of fetuses, first trimester COM M ♀

O30.832 Other specified multiple gestation, number of chorions and amnions are both equal to the number of fetuses, second trimester COM M ♀

O30.833 Other specified multiple gestation, number of chorions and amnions are both equal to the number of fetuses, third trimester COM M ♀

O30.839 Other specified multiple gestation, number of chorions and amnions are both equal to the number of fetuses, unspecified trimester COM M ♀

6th **O30.89 Other specified multiple gestation, unable to determine number of placenta and number of amniotic sacs**

O30.891 Other specified multiple gestation, unable to determine number of placenta and number of amniotic sacs, first trimester COM M ♀

O30.892 Other specified multiple gestation, unable to determine number of placenta and number of amniotic sacs, second trimester COM M ♀

O30.893 Other specified multiple gestation, unable to determine number of placenta and number of amniotic sacs, third trimester COM M ♀

O30.899 Other specified multiple gestation, unable to determine number of placenta and number of amniotic sacs, unspecified trimester COM M ♀

5th **O30.9 Multiple gestation, unspecified**

Multiple pregnancy NOS

O30.90 Multiple gestation, unspecified, unspecified trimester COM M ♀

O30.91 Multiple gestation, unspecified, first trimester COM M ♀

O30.92 Multiple gestation, unspecified, second trimester COM M ♀

O30.93 Multiple gestation, unspecified, third trimester COM M ♀

4th **O31 Complications specific to multiple gestation**

EXCLUDES 2 *delayed delivery of second twin, triplet, etc. (O63.2)*
malpresentation of one fetus or more (O32.9)
placental transfusion syndromes (O43.0-)

AHA: 2012,4Q,107

One of the following 7th characters is to be assigned to each code under category O31. 7th character 0 is for single gestations and multiple gestations where the fetus is unspecified. 7th characters 1 through 9 are for cases of multiple gestations to identify the fetus for which the code applies. The appropriate code from category O30, Multiple gestation, must also be assigned when assigning a code from category O31 that has a 7th character of 1 through 9.

- 0 not applicable or unspecified
- 1 fetus 1
- 2 fetus 2
- 3 fetus 3
- 4 fetus 4
- 5 fetus 5
- 9 other fetus

5th **O31.0 Papyraceous fetus**

Fetus compressus

DEF: Fetus that has died, but remains in utero for weeks before delivery, becoming compacted and mummified in appearance, with skin resembling parchment. Occurs most commonly in multigestational pregnancies. ***Synonym(s):*** *paper doll fetus.*

x7th **O31.00 Papyraceous fetus, unspecified trimester** COM M ♀

x7th **O31.01 Papyraceous fetus, first trimester** COM M ♀

x7th **O31.02 Papyraceous fetus, second trimester** COM M ♀

x7th **O31.03 Papyraceous fetus, third trimester** COM M ♀

5th **O31.1 Continuing pregnancy after spontaneous abortion of one fetus or more**

x7th **O31.10 Continuing pregnancy after spontaneous abortion of one fetus or more, unspecified trimester** COM M ♀

x7th **O31.11 Continuing pregnancy after spontaneous abortion of one fetus or more, first trimester** COM M ♀

x7th **O31.12 Continuing pregnancy after spontaneous abortion of one fetus or more, second trimester** COM M ♀

x7th **O31.13 Continuing pregnancy after spontaneous abortion of one fetus or more, third trimester** COM M ♀

5th **O31.2 Continuing pregnancy after intrauterine death of one fetus or more**

x7th **O31.20 Continuing pregnancy after intrauterine death of one fetus or more, unspecified trimester** COM M ♀

x7th **O31.21 Continuing pregnancy after intrauterine death of one fetus or more, first trimester** COM M ♀

x7th **O31.22 Continuing pregnancy after intrauterine death of one fetus or more, second trimester** COM M ♀

x7th **O31.23 Continuing pregnancy after intrauterine death of one fetus or more, third trimester** COM M ♀

5th **O31.3 Continuing pregnancy after elective fetal reduction of one fetus or more**

Continuing pregnancy after selective termination of one fetus or more

x7th **O31.30 Continuing pregnancy after elective fetal reduction of one fetus or more, unspecified trimester** COM M ♀

x7th **O31.31 Continuing pregnancy after elective fetal reduction of one fetus or more, first trimester** COM M ♀

x7th **O31.32 Continuing pregnancy after elective fetal reduction of one fetus or more, second trimester** COM M ♀

x7th **O31.33 Continuing pregnancy after elective fetal reduction of one fetus or more, third trimester** COM M ♀

5th **O31.8 Other complications specific to multiple gestation** COM

6th **O31.8X Other complications specific to multiple gestation**

7th **O31.8X1 Other complications specific to multiple gestation, first trimester** M ♀

7th **O31.8X2 Other complications specific to multiple gestation, second trimester** M ♀

7th **O31.8X3 Other complications specific to multiple gestation, third trimester** M ♀

✓7th **O31.8X9 Other complications specific to multiple gestation, unspecified trimester** M ♀

✓4th **O32 Maternal care for malpresentation of fetus**

INCLUDES the listed conditions as a reason for observation, hospitalization or other obstetric care of the mother, or for cesarean delivery before onset of labor

EXCLUDES 1 *malpresentation of fetus with obstructed labor (O64.-)*

AHA: 2012,4Q,107

One of the following 7th characters is to be assigned to each code under category O32. 7th character Ø is for single gestations and multiple gestations where the fetus is unspecified. 7th characters 1 through 9 are for cases of multiple gestations to identify the fetus for which the code applies. The appropriate code from category O3Ø, Multiple gestation, must also be assigned when assigning a code from category O32 that has a 7th character of 1 through 9.

Ø not applicable or unspecified
1 fetus 1
2 fetus 2
3 fetus 3
4 fetus 4
5 fetus 5
9 other fetus

Fetal Malpresentation

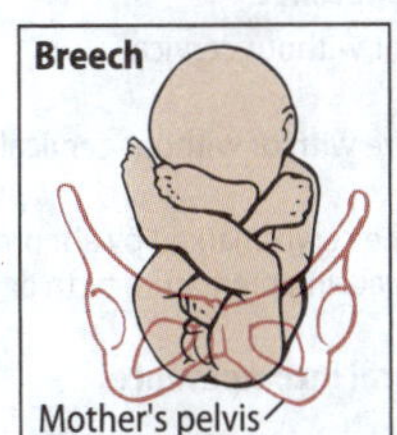

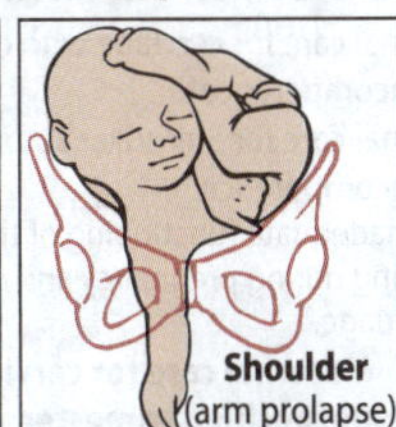

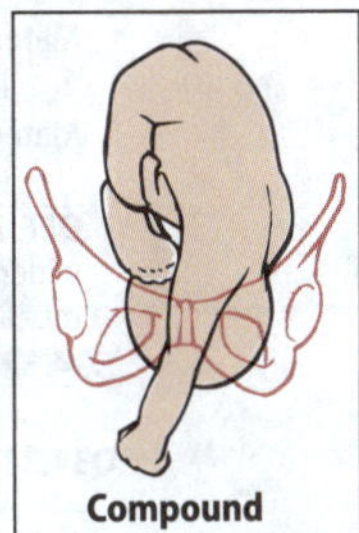

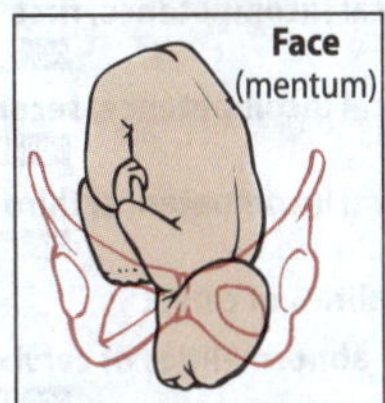

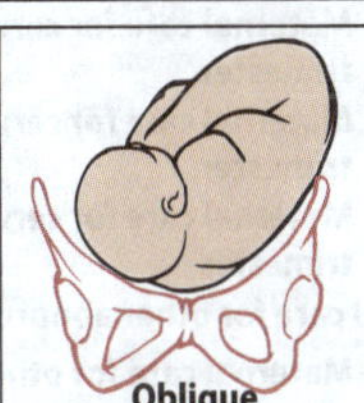

✓x7th **O32.Ø Maternal care for unstable lie** COM M ♀

✓x7th **O32.1 Maternal care for breech presentation** COM M ♀

Maternal care for buttocks presentation
Maternal care for complete breech
Maternal care for frank breech

EXCLUDES 1 *footling presentation (O32.8)*
incomplete breech (O32.8)

DEF: Fetus presentation in a longitudinal lie with the buttocks or feet closest to birth canal that may require external cephalic version or cesarean delivery.

✓x7th **O32.2 Maternal care for transverse and oblique lie** COM M ♀

Maternal care for oblique presentation
Maternal care for transverse presentation

✓x7th **O32.3 Maternal care for face, brow and chin presentation** COM M ♀

✓x7th **O32.4 Maternal care for high head at term** COM M ♀

Maternal care for failure of head to enter pelvic brim

✓x7th **O32.6 Maternal care for compound presentation** COM M ♀

✓x7th **O32.8 Maternal care for other malpresentation of fetus** COM M ♀

Maternal care for footling presentation
Maternal care for incomplete breech

✓x7th **O32.9 Maternal care for malpresentation of fetus, unspecified** COM M ♀

✓4th **O33 Maternal care for disproportion**

INCLUDES the listed conditions as a reason for observation, hospitalization or other obstetric care of the mother, or for cesarean delivery before onset of labor

EXCLUDES 1 *disproportion with obstructed labor (O65-O66)*

O33.Ø Maternal care for disproportion due to deformity of maternal pelvic bones COM M ♀

Maternal care for disproportion due to pelvic deformity causing disproportion NOS

O33.1 Maternal care for disproportion due to generally contracted pelvis COM M ♀

Maternal care for disproportion due to contracted pelvis NOS causing disproportion

O33.2 Maternal care for disproportion due to inlet contraction of pelvis COM M ♀

Maternal care for disproportion due to inlet contraction (pelvis) causing disproportion

✓x7th **O33.3 Maternal care for disproportion due to outlet contraction of pelvis** COM M ♀

Maternal care for disproportion due to mid-cavity contraction (pelvis)
Maternal care for disproportion due to outlet contraction (pelvis)

One of the following 7th characters is to be assigned to code O33.3. 7th character Ø is for single gestations and multiple gestations where the fetus is unspecified. 7th characters 1 through 9 are for cases of multiple gestations to identify the fetus for which the code applies. The appropriate code from category O3Ø, Multiple gestation, must also be assigned when assigning code O33.3 with a 7th character of 1 through 9.

Ø not applicable or unspecified
1 fetus 1
2 fetus 2
3 fetus 3
4 fetus 4
5 fetus 5
9 other fetus

✓x7th **O33.4 Maternal care for disproportion of mixed maternal and fetal origin** COM M ♀

One of the following 7th characters is to be assigned to code O33.4. 7th character Ø is for single gestations and multiple gestations where the fetus is unspecified. 7th characters 1 through 9 are for cases of multiple gestations to identify the fetus for which the code applies. The appropriate code from category O3Ø, Multiple gestation, must also be assigned when assigning code O33.4 with a 7th character of 1 through 9.

Ø not applicable or unspecified
1 fetus 1
2 fetus 2
3 fetus 3
4 fetus 4
5 fetus 5
9 other fetus

✓x7th **O33.5 Maternal care for disproportion due to unusually large fetus** COM M ♀

Maternal care for disproportion due to disproportion of fetal origin with normally formed fetus
Maternal care for disproportion due to fetal disproportion NOS

One of the following 7th characters is to be assigned to code O33.5. 7th character Ø is for single gestations and multiple gestations where the fetus is unspecified. 7th characters 1 through 9 are for cases of multiple gestations to identify the fetus for which the code applies. The appropriate code from category O3Ø, Multiple gestation, must also be assigned when assigning code O33.5 with a 7th character of 1 through 9.

Ø not applicable or unspecified
1 fetus 1
2 fetus 2
3 fetus 3
4 fetus 4
5 fetus 5
9 other fetus

√x7th **O33.6 Maternal care for disproportion due to hydrocephalic fetus** COM M ♀

One of the following 7th characters is to be assigned to code O33.6. 7th character Ø is for single gestations and multiple gestations where the fetus is unspecified. 7th characters 1 through 9 are for cases of multiple gestations to identify the fetus for which the code applies. The appropriate code from category O3Ø, Multiple gestation, must also be assigned when assigning code O33.6 with a 7th character of 1 through 9.

- Ø not applicable or unspecified
- 1 fetus 1
- 2 fetus 2
- 3 fetus 3
- 4 fetus 4
- 5 fetus 5
- 9 other fetus

√x7th **O33.7 Maternal care for disproportion due to other fetal deformities** COM M ♀

Maternal care for disproportion due to fetal ascites
Maternal care for disproportion due to fetal hydrops
Maternal care for disproportion due to fetal meningomyelocele
Maternal care for disproportion due to fetal sacral teratoma
Maternal care for disproportion due to fetal tumor

EXCLUDES 1 *obstructed labor due to other fetal deformities (O66.3)*

AHA: 2016,4Q,51

One of the following 7th characters is to be assigned to code O33.7. 7th character Ø is for single gestations and multiple gestations where the fetus is unspecified. 7th characters 1 through 9 are for cases of multiple gestations to identify the fetus for which the code applies. The appropriate code from category O3Ø, Multiple gestation, must also be assigned when assigning code O33.7 with a 7th character of 1 through 9.

- Ø not applicable or unspecified
- 1 fetus 1
- 2 fetus 2
- 3 fetus 3
- 4 fetus 4
- 5 fetus 5
- 9 other fetus

O33.8 Maternal care for disproportion of other origin COM M ♀

O33.9 Maternal care for disproportion, unspecified COM M ♀

Maternal care for disproportion due to cephalopelvic disproportion NOS
Maternal care for disproportion due to fetopelvic disproportion NOS

√4th **O34 Maternal care for abnormality of pelvic organs**

INCLUDES the listed conditions as a reason for hospitalization or other obstetric care of the mother, or for cesarean delivery before onset of labor

Code first any associated obstructed labor (O65.5)
Use additional code for specific condition

√5th **O34.Ø Maternal care for congenital malformation of uterus**

Maternal care for double uterus
Maternal care for uterus bicornis

O34.ØØ Maternal care for unspecified congenital malformation of uterus, unspecified trimester COM M ♀

O34.Ø1 Maternal care for unspecified congenital malformation of uterus, first trimester COM M ♀

O34.Ø2 Maternal care for unspecified congenital malformation of uterus, second trimester COM M ♀

O34.Ø3 Maternal care for unspecified congenital malformation of uterus, third trimester COM M ♀

√5th **O34.1 Maternal care for benign tumor of corpus uteri**

EXCLUDES 2 *maternal care for benign tumor of cervix (O34.4-)*
maternal care for malignant neoplasm of uterus (O9A.1-)

O34.1Ø Maternal care for benign tumor of corpus uteri, unspecified trimester COM M ♀

O34.11 Maternal care for benign tumor of corpus uteri, first trimester COM M ♀

O34.12 Maternal care for benign tumor of corpus uteri, second trimester COM M ♀

O34.13 Maternal care for benign tumor of corpus uteri, third trimester COM M ♀

√5th **O34.2 Maternal care due to uterine scar from previous surgery**

AHA: 2020,4Q,36; 2016,4Q,76

√6th **O34.21 Maternal care for scar from previous cesarean delivery**

AHA: 2018,3Q,23; 2016,4Q,51-52

O34.211 Maternal care for low transverse scar from previous cesarean delivery COM M ♀

O34.212 Maternal care for vertical scar from previous cesarean delivery COM M ♀

Maternal care for classical scar from previous cesarean delivery

O34.218 Maternal care for other type scar from previous cesarean delivery COM M ♀

Mid-transverse T incision

O34.219 Maternal care for unspecified type scar from previous cesarean delivery COM M ♀

O34.22 Maternal care for cesarean scar defect (isthmocele) COM M ♀

O34.29 Maternal care due to uterine scar from other previous surgery COM M ♀

Maternal care due to uterine scar from other transmural uterine incision

√5th **O34.3 Maternal care for cervical incompetence**

Maternal care for cerclage with or without cervical incompetence
Maternal care for Shirodkar suture with or without cervical incompetence

DEF: Inadequate functioning of the cervix marked by abnormal widening during pregnancy and causing premature birth or miscarriage.

O34.3Ø Maternal care for cervical incompetence, unspecified trimester COM M ♀

O34.31 Maternal care for cervical incompetence, first trimester COM M ♀

O34.32 Maternal care for cervical incompetence, second trimester COM M ♀

O34.33 Maternal care for cervical incompetence, third trimester COM M ♀

√5th **O34.4 Maternal care for other abnormalities of cervix**

O34.4Ø Maternal care for other abnormalities of cervix, unspecified trimester COM M ♀

O34.41 Maternal care for other abnormalities of cervix, first trimester COM M ♀

O34.42 Maternal care for other abnormalities of cervix, second trimester COM M ♀

O34.43 Maternal care for other abnormalities of cervix, third trimester COM M ♀

√5th **O34.5 Maternal care for other abnormalities of gravid uterus**

√6th **O34.51 Maternal care for incarceration of gravid uterus**

O34.511 Maternal care for incarceration of gravid uterus, first trimester COM M ♀

O34.512 Maternal care for incarceration of gravid uterus, second trimester COM M ♀

O34.513 Maternal care for incarceration of gravid uterus, third trimester COM M ♀

O34.519 Maternal care for incarceration of gravid uterus, unspecified trimester COM M ♀

√6th **O34.52 Maternal care for prolapse of gravid uterus**

O34.521 Maternal care for prolapse of gravid uterus, first trimester COM M ♀

O34.522 Maternal care for prolapse of gravid uterus, second trimester COM M ♀

O34.523 Maternal care for prolapse of gravid uterus, third trimester COM M ♀

O34.529 Maternal care for prolapse of gravid uterus, unspecified trimester COM M ♀

√6th **O34.53 Maternal care for retroversion of gravid uterus**

O34.531 Maternal care for retroversion of gravid uterus, first trimester COM M ♀

O34.532 Maternal care for retroversion of gravid uterus, second trimester COM M ♀

O34.533 Maternal care for retroversion of gravid uterus, third trimester COM M ♀

O34.539 Maternal care for retroversion of gravid uterus, unspecified trimester COM M ♀

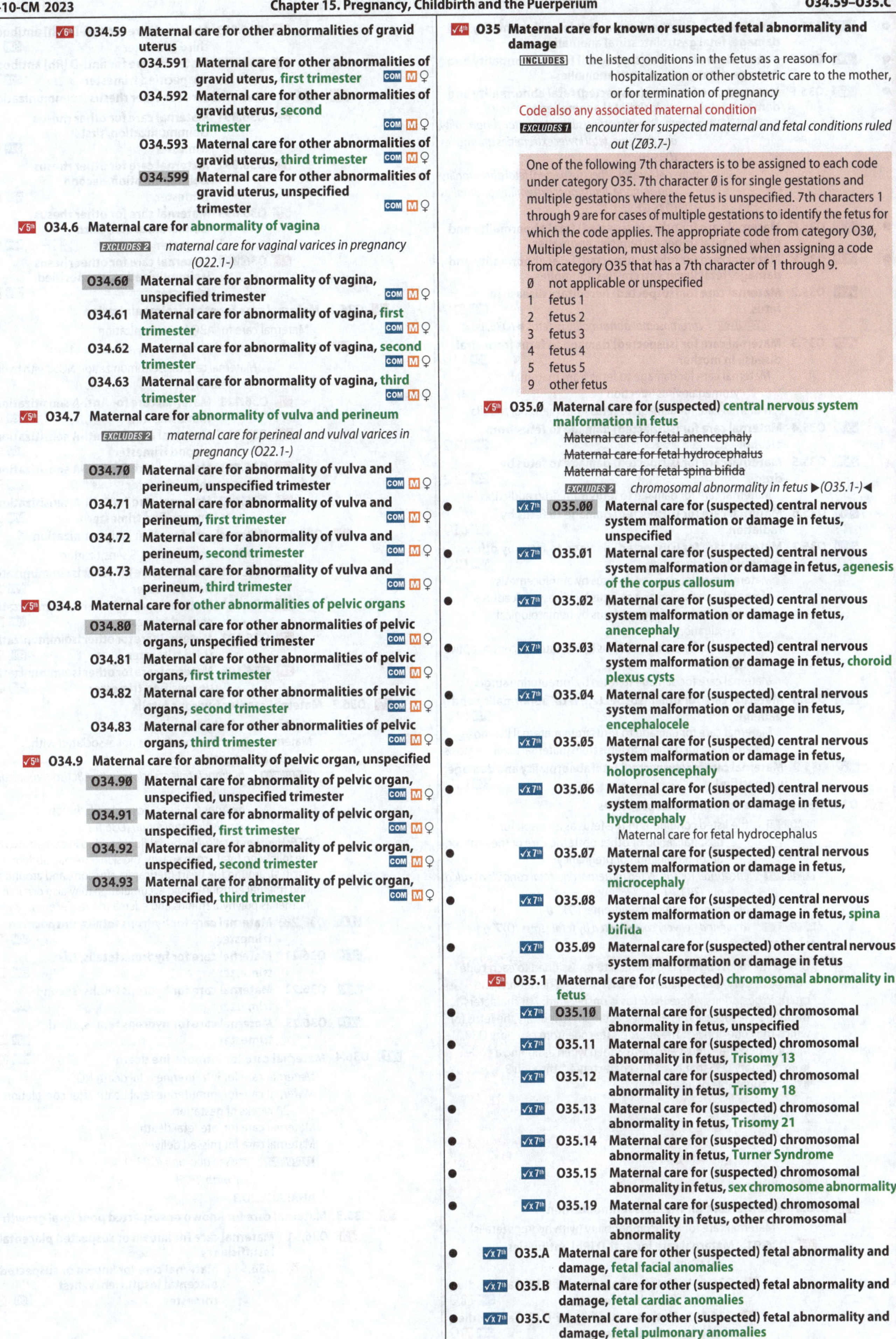

O34.59 Maternal care for other abnormalities of gravid uterus
- **O34.591 Maternal care for other abnormalities of gravid uterus, first trimester** COM M ♀
- **O34.592 Maternal care for other abnormalities of gravid uterus, second trimester** COM M ♀
- **O34.593 Maternal care for other abnormalities of gravid uterus, third trimester** COM M ♀
- **O34.599 Maternal care for other abnormalities of gravid uterus, unspecified trimester** COM M ♀

O34.6 Maternal care for abnormality of vagina

EXCLUDES 2 *maternal care for vaginal varices in pregnancy (O22.1-)*

- **O34.60 Maternal care for abnormality of vagina, unspecified trimester** COM M ♀
- **O34.61 Maternal care for abnormality of vagina, first trimester** COM M ♀
- **O34.62 Maternal care for abnormality of vagina, second trimester** COM M ♀
- **O34.63 Maternal care for abnormality of vagina, third trimester** COM M ♀

O34.7 Maternal care for abnormality of vulva and perineum

EXCLUDES 2 *maternal care for perineal and vulval varices in pregnancy (O22.1-)*

- **O34.70 Maternal care for abnormality of vulva and perineum, unspecified trimester** COM M ♀
- **O34.71 Maternal care for abnormality of vulva and perineum, first trimester** COM M ♀
- **O34.72 Maternal care for abnormality of vulva and perineum, second trimester** COM M ♀
- **O34.73 Maternal care for abnormality of vulva and perineum, third trimester** COM M ♀

O34.8 Maternal care for other abnormalities of pelvic organs
- **O34.80 Maternal care for other abnormalities of pelvic organs, unspecified trimester** COM M ♀
- **O34.81 Maternal care for other abnormalities of pelvic organs, first trimester** COM M ♀
- **O34.82 Maternal care for other abnormalities of pelvic organs, second trimester** COM M ♀
- **O34.83 Maternal care for other abnormalities of pelvic organs, third trimester** COM M ♀

O34.9 Maternal care for abnormality of pelvic organ, unspecified
- **O34.90 Maternal care for abnormality of pelvic organ, unspecified, unspecified trimester** COM M ♀
- **O34.91 Maternal care for abnormality of pelvic organ, unspecified, first trimester** COM M ♀
- **O34.92 Maternal care for abnormality of pelvic organ, unspecified, second trimester** COM M ♀
- **O34.93 Maternal care for abnormality of pelvic organ, unspecified, third trimester** COM M ♀

O35 Maternal care for known or suspected fetal abnormality and damage

INCLUDES the listed conditions in the fetus as a reason for hospitalization or other obstetric care to the mother, or for termination of pregnancy

Code also any associated maternal condition

EXCLUDES 1 *encounter for suspected maternal and fetal conditions ruled out (Z03.7-)*

One of the following 7th characters is to be assigned to each code under category O35. 7th character 0 is for single gestations and multiple gestations where the fetus is unspecified. 7th characters 1 through 9 are for cases of multiple gestations to identify the fetus for which the code applies. The appropriate code from category O30, Multiple gestation, must also be assigned when assigning a code from category O35 that has a 7th character of 1 through 9.
- 0 not applicable or unspecified
- 1 fetus 1
- 2 fetus 2
- 3 fetus 3
- 4 fetus 4
- 5 fetus 5
- 9 other fetus

O35.0 Maternal care for (suspected) central nervous system malformation in fetus

~~Maternal care for fetal anencephaly~~
~~Maternal care for fetal hydrocephalus~~
~~Maternal care for fetal spina bifida~~

EXCLUDES 2 *chromosomal abnormality in fetus* ▶(O35.1-)◀

- ● **O35.00 Maternal care for (suspected) central nervous system malformation or damage in fetus, unspecified**
- ● **O35.01 Maternal care for (suspected) central nervous system malformation or damage in fetus, agenesis of the corpus callosum**
- ● **O35.02 Maternal care for (suspected) central nervous system malformation or damage in fetus, anencephaly**
- ● **O35.03 Maternal care for (suspected) central nervous system malformation or damage in fetus, choroid plexus cysts**
- ● **O35.04 Maternal care for (suspected) central nervous system malformation or damage in fetus, encephalocele**
- ● **O35.05 Maternal care for (suspected) central nervous system malformation or damage in fetus, holoprosencephaly**
- ● **O35.06 Maternal care for (suspected) central nervous system malformation or damage in fetus, hydrocephaly**
  Maternal care for fetal hydrocephalus
- ● **O35.07 Maternal care for (suspected) central nervous system malformation or damage in fetus, microcephaly**
- ● **O35.08 Maternal care for (suspected) central nervous system malformation or damage in fetus, spina bifida**
- ● **O35.09 Maternal care for (suspected) other central nervous system malformation or damage in fetus**

O35.1 Maternal care for (suspected) chromosomal abnormality in fetus
- ● **O35.10 Maternal care for (suspected) chromosomal abnormality in fetus, unspecified**
- ● **O35.11 Maternal care for (suspected) chromosomal abnormality in fetus, Trisomy 13**
- ● **O35.12 Maternal care for (suspected) chromosomal abnormality in fetus, Trisomy 18**
- ● **O35.13 Maternal care for (suspected) chromosomal abnormality in fetus, Trisomy 21**
- ● **O35.14 Maternal care for (suspected) chromosomal abnormality in fetus, Turner Syndrome**
- ● **O35.15 Maternal care for (suspected) chromosomal abnormality in fetus, sex chromosome abnormality**
- ● **O35.19 Maternal care for (suspected) chromosomal abnormality in fetus, other chromosomal abnormality**

- ● **O35.A Maternal care for other (suspected) fetal abnormality and damage, fetal facial anomalies**
- ● **O35.B Maternal care for other (suspected) fetal abnormality and damage, fetal cardiac anomalies**
- ● **O35.C Maternal care for other (suspected) fetal abnormality and damage, fetal pulmonary anomalies**

● ✓x7th **O35.D Maternal care for other (suspected) fetal abnormality and damage, fetal gastrointestinal anomalies**

● ✓x7th **O35.E Maternal care for other (suspected) fetal abnormality and damage, fetal genitourinary anomalies**

● ✓x7th **O35.F Maternal care for other (suspected) fetal abnormality and damage, fetal musculoskeletal anomalies of trunk**

EXCLUDES 2 *maternal care for other (suspected) fetal abnormality and damage, fetal lower extremities anomalies (O35.H)*
maternal care for other (suspected) fetal abnormality and damage, fetal upper extremities anomalies (O35.G)

● ✓x7th **O35.G Maternal care for other (suspected) fetal abnormality and damage, fetal upper extremities anomalies**

● ✓x7th **O35.H Maternal care for other (suspected) fetal abnormality and damage, fetal lower extremities anomalies**

✓x7th **O35.2 Maternal care for (suspected) hereditary disease in fetus** COM M ♀

EXCLUDES 2 *chromosomal abnormality in fetus ▶(O35.1-)◀*

✓x7th **O35.3 Maternal care for (suspected) damage to fetus from viral disease in mother** COM M ♀

Maternal care for damage to fetus from maternal cytomegalovirus infection
Maternal care for damage to fetus from maternal rubella

✓x7th **O35.4 Maternal care for (suspected) damage to fetus from alcohol** COM M ♀

✓x7th **O35.5 Maternal care for (suspected) damage to fetus by drugs** COM M ♀

Maternal care for damage to fetus from drug addiction

✓x7th **O35.6 Maternal care for (suspected) damage to fetus by radiation** COM M ♀

✓x7th **O35.7 Maternal care for (suspected) damage to fetus by other medical procedures** COM M ♀

Maternal care for damage to fetus by amniocentesis
Maternal care for damage to fetus by biopsy procedures
Maternal care for damage to fetus by hematological investigation
Maternal care for damage to fetus by intrauterine contraceptive device
Maternal care for damage to fetus by intrauterine surgery

✓x7th **O35.8 Maternal care for other (suspected) fetal abnormality and damage** COM M ♀

Maternal care for damage to fetus from maternal listeriosis
Maternal care for damage to fetus from maternal toxoplasmosis

✓x7th **O35.9 Maternal care for (suspected) fetal abnormality and damage, unspecified** COM M ♀

✓4th **O36 Maternal care for other fetal problems**

INCLUDES the listed conditions in the fetus as a reason for hospitalization or other obstetric care of the mother, or for termination of pregnancy

EXCLUDES 1 *encounter for suspected maternal and fetal conditions ruled out (Z03.7-)*
placental transfusion syndromes (O43.0-)

EXCLUDES 2 *labor and delivery complicated by fetal stress (O77.-)*

AHA: 2015,3Q,40

One of the following 7th characters is to be assigned to each code under category O36. 7th character 0 is for single gestations and multiple gestations where the fetus is unspecified. 7th characters 1 through 9 are for cases of multiple gestations to identify the fetus for which the code applies. The appropriate code from category O30, Multiple gestation, must also be assigned when assigning a code from category O36 that has a 7th character of 1 through 9.
0 not applicable or unspecified
1 fetus 1
2 fetus 2
3 fetus 3
4 fetus 4
5 fetus 5
9 other fetus

✓5th **O36.0 Maternal care for rhesus isoimmunization**

Maternal care for Rh incompatibility (with hydrops fetalis)

✓6th **O36.01 Maternal care for anti-D [Rh] antibodies**

AHA: 2014,4Q,17

✓7th **O36.011 Maternal care for anti-D [Rh] antibodies, first trimester** COM M ♀

✓7th **O36.012 Maternal care for anti-D [Rh] antibodies, second trimester** COM M ♀

✓7th **O36.013 Maternal care for anti-D [Rh] antibodies, third trimester** COM M ♀

✓7th **O36.019 Maternal care for anti-D [Rh] antibodies, unspecified trimester** COM M ♀

✓6th **O36.09 Maternal care for other rhesus isoimmunization**

✓7th **O36.091 Maternal care for other rhesus isoimmunization, first trimester** COM M ♀

✓7th **O36.092 Maternal care for other rhesus isoimmunization, second trimester** COM M ♀

✓7th **O36.093 Maternal care for other rhesus isoimmunization, third trimester** COM M ♀

✓7th **O36.099 Maternal care for other rhesus isoimmunization, unspecified trimester** COM M ♀

✓5th **O36.1 Maternal care for other isoimmunization**

Maternal care for ABO isoimmunization

✓6th **O36.11 Maternal care for Anti-A sensitization**

Maternal care for isoimmunization NOS (with hydrops fetalis)

✓7th **O36.111 Maternal care for Anti-A sensitization, first trimester** COM M ♀

✓7th **O36.112 Maternal care for Anti-A sensitization, second trimester** COM M ♀

✓7th **O36.113 Maternal care for Anti-A sensitization, third trimester** COM M ♀

✓7th **O36.119 Maternal care for Anti-A sensitization, unspecified trimester** COM M ♀

✓6th **O36.19 Maternal care for other isoimmunization**

Maternal care for Anti-B sensitization

✓7th **O36.191 Maternal care for other isoimmunization, first trimester** COM M ♀

✓7th **O36.192 Maternal care for other isoimmunization, second trimester** COM M ♀

✓7th **O36.193 Maternal care for other isoimmunization, third trimester** COM M ♀

✓7th **O36.199 Maternal care for other isoimmunization, unspecified trimester** COM M ♀

✓5th **O36.2 Maternal care for hydrops fetalis**

Maternal care for hydrops fetalis NOS
Maternal care for hydrops fetalis not associated with isoimmunization

EXCLUDES 1 *hydrops fetalis associated with ABO isoimmunization (O36.1-)*
hydrops fetalis associated with rhesus isoimmunization (O36.0-)

DEF: Hydrops fetalis: Abnormal fluid buildup in at least two of the following fetal organ spaces: the skin (edema), abdomen (ascites), around the heart (pericardia effusion), and around the lung (pleural effusion). Fluid accumulation may also occur in the mother as polyhydramnios and edema of the placenta.

✓x7th **O36.20 Maternal care for hydrops fetalis, unspecified trimester** COM M ♀

✓x7th **O36.21 Maternal care for hydrops fetalis, first trimester** COM M ♀

✓x7th **O36.22 Maternal care for hydrops fetalis, second trimester** COM M ♀

✓x7th **O36.23 Maternal care for hydrops fetalis, third trimester** COM M ♀

✓x7th **O36.4 Maternal care for intrauterine death** COM M ♀

Maternal care for intrauterine fetal death NOS
Maternal care for intrauterine fetal death after completion of 20 weeks of gestation
Maternal care for late fetal death
Maternal care for missed delivery

EXCLUDES 1 *missed abortion (O02.1)*
stillbirth (P95)

AHA: 2022,2Q,3

✓5th **O36.5 Maternal care for known or suspected poor fetal growth**

✓6th **O36.51 Maternal care for known or suspected placental insufficiency**

✓7th **O36.511 Maternal care for known or suspected placental insufficiency, first trimester** COM M ♀

O36.512 **Maternal care for known or suspected placental insufficiency, second trimester**

O36.513 **Maternal care for known or suspected placental insufficiency, third trimester**

O36.519 **Maternal care for known or suspected placental insufficiency, unspecified trimester**

O36.59 **Maternal care for other known or suspected poor fetal growth**
Maternal care for known or suspected light-for-dates NOS
Maternal care for known or suspected small-for-dates NOS

O36.591 **Maternal care for other known or suspected poor fetal growth, first trimester**

O36.592 **Maternal care for other known or suspected poor fetal growth, second trimester**

O36.593 **Maternal care for other known or suspected poor fetal growth, third trimester**

O36.599 **Maternal care for other known or suspected poor fetal growth, unspecified trimester**

O36.6 **Maternal care for excessive fetal growth**
Maternal care for known or suspected large-for-dates

O36.6Ø **Maternal care for excessive fetal growth, unspecified trimester**

O36.61 **Maternal care for excessive fetal growth, first trimester**

O36.62 **Maternal care for excessive fetal growth, second trimester**

O36.63 **Maternal care for excessive fetal growth, third trimester**

O36.7 **Maternal care for viable fetus in abdominal pregnancy**

O36.7Ø **Maternal care for viable fetus in abdominal pregnancy, unspecified trimester**

O36.71 **Maternal care for viable fetus in abdominal pregnancy, first trimester**

O36.72 **Maternal care for viable fetus in abdominal pregnancy, second trimester**

O36.73 **Maternal care for viable fetus in abdominal pregnancy, third trimester**

O36.8 **Maternal care for other specified fetal problems**

O36.8Ø **Pregnancy with inconclusive fetal viability**
Encounter to determine fetal viability of pregnancy
AHA: 2019,2Q,29

O36.81 **Decreased fetal movements**

O36.812 **Decreased fetal movements, second trimester**

O36.813 **Decreased fetal movements, third trimester**

O36.819 **Decreased fetal movements, unspecified trimester**

O36.82 **Fetal anemia and thrombocytopenia**

O36.821 **Fetal anemia and thrombocytopenia, first trimester**

O36.822 **Fetal anemia and thrombocytopenia, second trimester**

O36.823 **Fetal anemia and thrombocytopenia, third trimester**

O36.829 **Fetal anemia and thrombocytopenia, unspecified trimester**

O36.83 **Maternal care for abnormalities of the fetal heart rate or rhythm**
Maternal care for depressed fetal heart rate tones
Maternal care for fetal bradycardia
Maternal care for fetal heart rate abnormal variability
Maternal care for fetal heart rate decelerations
Maternal care for fetal heart rate irregularity
Maternal care for fetal tachycardia
Maternal care for non-reassuring fetal heart rate or rhythm
AHA: 2017,4Q,20
TIP: Assign for documented fetal tachycardia, bradycardia, decelerations, or loss of variability detected during antenatal testing.

O36.831 **Maternal care for abnormalities of the fetal heart rate or rhythm, first trimester**

O36.832 **Maternal care for abnormalities of the fetal heart rate or rhythm, second trimester**

O36.833 **Maternal care for abnormalities of the fetal heart rate or rhythm, third trimester**

O36.839 **Maternal care for abnormalities of the fetal heart rate or rhythm, unspecified trimester**

O36.89 **Maternal care for other specified fetal problems**

O36.891 **Maternal care for other specified fetal problems, first trimester**

O36.892 **Maternal care for other specified fetal problems, second trimester**

O36.893 **Maternal care for other specified fetal problems, third trimester**

O36.899 **Maternal care for other specified fetal problems, unspecified trimester**

O36.9 **Maternal care for fetal problem, unspecified**

O36.9Ø **Maternal care for fetal problem, unspecified, unspecified trimester**

O36.91 **Maternal care for fetal problem, unspecified, first trimester**

O36.92 **Maternal care for fetal problem, unspecified, second trimester**

O36.93 **Maternal care for fetal problem, unspecified, third trimester**

O4Ø Polyhydramnios

INCLUDES hydramnios

EXCLUDES 1 *encounter for suspected maternal and fetal conditions ruled out (ZØ3.7-)*

AHA: 2016,1Q,4
DEF: Excess amniotic fluid surrounding the fetus, typically defined as a total fluid volume of greater than 24 cm.

One of the following 7th characters is to be assigned to each code under category O4Ø. 7th character Ø is for single gestations and multiple gestations where the fetus is unspecified. 7th characters 1 through 9 are for cases of multiple gestations to identify the fetus for which the code applies. The appropriate code from category O3Ø, Multiple gestation, must also be assigned when assigning a code from category O4Ø that has a 7th character of 1 through 9.
Ø not applicable or unspecified
1 fetus 1
2 fetus 2
3 fetus 3
4 fetus 4
5 fetus 5
9 other fetus

O4Ø.1 **Polyhydramnios, first trimester**

O4Ø.2 **Polyhydramnios, second trimester**

O4Ø.3 **Polyhydramnios, third trimester**

O4Ø.9 **Polyhydramnios, unspecified trimester**

Additional Character Required 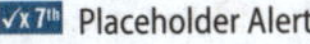 Placeholder Alert Manifestation Unspecified Dx QPP UPD Unacceptable PDx

O41 Other disorders of amniotic fluid and membranes

EXCLUDES 1 *encounter for suspected maternal and fetal conditions ruled out (Z03.7-)*

One of the following 7th characters is to be assigned to each code under category O41. 7th character 0 is for single gestations and multiple gestations where the fetus is unspecified. 7th characters 1 through 9 are for cases of multiple gestations to identify the fetus for which the code applies. The appropriate code from category O30, Multiple gestation, must also be assigned when assigning a code from category O41 that has a 7th character of 1 through 9.

- 0 not applicable or unspecified
- 1 fetus 1
- 2 fetus 2
- 3 fetus 3
- 4 fetus 4
- 5 fetus 5
- 9 other fetus

O41.0 Oligohydramnios

Oligohydramnios without rupture of membranes

DEF: Low amniotic fluid, occurring most frequently in the last trimester.

- **O41.00 Oligohydramnios, unspecified trimester** COM M ♀
- **O41.01 Oligohydramnios, first trimester** COM M ♀
- **O41.02 Oligohydramnios, second trimester** COM M ♀
- **O41.03 Oligohydramnios, third trimester** COM M ♀

O41.1 Infection of amniotic sac and membranes

O41.10 Infection of amniotic sac and membranes, unspecified

- **O41.101 Infection of amniotic sac and membranes, unspecified, first trimester** COM M ♀
- **O41.102 Infection of amniotic sac and membranes, unspecified, second trimester** COM M ♀
- **O41.103 Infection of amniotic sac and membranes, unspecified, third trimester** COM M ♀
- **O41.109 Infection of amniotic sac and membranes, unspecified, unspecified trimester** COM M ♀

O41.12 Chorioamnionitis

AHA: 2019,2Q,34

- **O41.121 Chorioamnionitis, first trimester** COM M ♀
- **O41.122 Chorioamnionitis, second trimester** COM M ♀
- **O41.123 Chorioamnionitis, third trimester** COM M ♀
- **O41.129 Chorioamnionitis, unspecified trimester** COM M ♀

O41.14 Placentitis

- **O41.141 Placentitis, first trimester** COM M ♀
- **O41.142 Placentitis, second trimester** COM M ♀
- **O41.143 Placentitis, third trimester** COM M ♀
- **O41.149 Placentitis, unspecified trimester** COM M ♀

O41.8 Other specified disorders of amniotic fluid and membranes

O41.8X Other specified disorders of amniotic fluid and membranes

- **O41.8X1 Other specified disorders of amniotic fluid and membranes, first trimester** COM M ♀
- **O41.8X2 Other specified disorders of amniotic fluid and membranes, second trimester** COM M ♀
- **O41.8X3 Other specified disorders of amniotic fluid and membranes, third trimester** COM M ♀
- **O41.8X9 Other specified disorders of amniotic fluid and membranes, unspecified trimester** COM M ♀

O41.9 Disorder of amniotic fluid and membranes, unspecified

- **O41.90 Disorder of amniotic fluid and membranes, unspecified, unspecified trimester** COM M ♀
- **O41.91 Disorder of amniotic fluid and membranes, unspecified, first trimester** COM M ♀
- **O41.92 Disorder of amniotic fluid and membranes, unspecified, second trimester** COM M ♀
- **O41.93 Disorder of amniotic fluid and membranes, unspecified, third trimester** COM M ♀

O42 Premature rupture of membranes

AHA: 2016,1Q,3

O42.0 Premature rupture of membranes, onset of labor within 24 hours of rupture

- **O42.00 Premature rupture of membranes, onset of labor within 24 hours of rupture, unspecified weeks of gestation** COM M ♀

O42.01 Preterm premature rupture of membranes, onset of labor within 24 hours of rupture

Premature rupture of membranes before 37 completed weeks of gestation

- **O42.011 Preterm premature rupture of membranes, onset of labor within 24 hours of rupture, first trimester** COM M ♀
- **O42.012 Preterm premature rupture of membranes, onset of labor within 24 hours of rupture, second trimester** COM M ♀
- **O42.013 Preterm premature rupture of membranes, onset of labor within 24 hours of rupture, third trimester** COM M ♀
- **O42.019 Preterm premature rupture of membranes, onset of labor within 24 hours of rupture, unspecified trimester** COM M ♀

O42.02 Full-term premature rupture of membranes, onset of labor within 24 hours of rupture COM M ♀

Premature rupture of membranes at or after 37 completed weeks of gestation, onset of labor within 24 hours of rupture

O42.1 Premature rupture of membranes, onset of labor more than 24 hours following rupture

AHA: 2016,1Q,5

- **O42.10 Premature rupture of membranes, onset of labor more than 24 hours following rupture, unspecified weeks of gestation** COM M ♀

O42.11 Preterm premature rupture of membranes, onset of labor more than 24 hours following rupture

Premature rupture of membranes before 37 completed weeks of gestation

- **O42.111 Preterm premature rupture of membranes, onset of labor more than 24 hours following rupture, first trimester** COM M ♀
- **O42.112 Preterm premature rupture of membranes, onset of labor more than 24 hours following rupture, second trimester** COM M ♀
- **O42.113 Preterm premature rupture of membranes, onset of labor more than 24 hours following rupture, third trimester** COM M ♀
- **O42.119 Preterm premature rupture of membranes, onset of labor more than 24 hours following rupture, unspecified trimester** COM M ♀

O42.12 Full-term premature rupture of membranes, onset of labor more than 24 hours following rupture COM M ♀

Premature rupture of membranes at or after 37 completed weeks of gestation, onset of labor more than 24 hours following rupture

O42.9 Premature rupture of membranes, unspecified as to length of time between rupture and onset of labor

- **O42.90 Premature rupture of membranes, unspecified as to length of time between rupture and onset of labor, unspecified weeks of gestation** COM M ♀

O42.91 Preterm premature rupture of membranes, unspecified as to length of time between rupture and onset of labor

Premature rupture of membranes before 37 completed weeks of gestation

- **O42.911 Preterm premature rupture of membranes, unspecified as to length of time between rupture and onset of labor, first trimester** COM M ♀

O42.912 Preterm premature rupture of membranes, unspecified as to length of time between rupture and onset of labor, second trimester COM M ♀

O42.913 Preterm premature rupture of membranes, unspecified as to length of time between rupture and onset of labor, third trimester COM M ♀

O42.919 Preterm premature rupture of membranes, unspecified as to length of time between rupture and onset of labor, unspecified trimester COM M ♀

O42.92 Full-term premature rupture of membranes, unspecified as to length of time between rupture and onset of labor COM M ♀

Premature rupture of membranes at or after 37 completed weeks of gestation, unspecified as to length of time between rupture and onset of labor

4th O43 Placental disorders

EXCLUDES 2 *maternal care for poor fetal growth due to placental insufficiency (O36.5-)*
placenta previa (O44.-)
placental polyp (O90.89)
placentitis (O41.14-)
premature separation of placenta [abruptio placentae] (O45.-)

5th O43.0 Placental transfusion syndromes

6th O43.01 Fetomaternal placental transfusion syndrome

Maternofetal placental transfusion syndrome

O43.011 Fetomaternal placental transfusion syndrome, first trimester COM M ♀

O43.012 Fetomaternal placental transfusion syndrome, second trimester COM M ♀

O43.013 Fetomaternal placental transfusion syndrome, third trimester COM M ♀

O43.019 Fetomaternal placental transfusion syndrome, unspecified trimester COM M ♀

6th O43.02 Fetus-to-fetus placental transfusion syndrome

DEF: Condition in which an imbalance in amniotic fluid occurs due to uneven blood flow between twins sharing a placenta.

Twin to Twin Transfusion Syndrome (TTTS)

Healthy twins Twins with TTTS

O43.021 Fetus-to-fetus placental transfusion syndrome, first trimester COM M ♀

O43.022 Fetus-to-fetus placental transfusion syndrome, second trimester COM M ♀

O43.023 Fetus-to-fetus placental transfusion syndrome, third trimester COM M ♀

O43.029 Fetus-to-fetus placental transfusion syndrome, unspecified trimester COM M ♀

5th O43.1 Malformation of placenta

6th O43.10 Malformation of placenta, unspecified

Abnormal placenta NOS

O43.101 Malformation of placenta, unspecified, first trimester COM M ♀

O43.102 Malformation of placenta, unspecified, second trimester COM M ♀

O43.103 Malformation of placenta, unspecified, third trimester COM M ♀

O43.109 Malformation of placenta, unspecified, unspecified trimester COM M ♀

6th O43.11 Circumvallate placenta

O43.111 Circumvallate placenta, first trimester COM M ♀

O43.112 Circumvallate placenta, second trimester COM M ♀

O43.113 Circumvallate placenta, third trimester COM M ♀

O43.119 Circumvallate placenta, unspecified trimester COM M ♀

6th O43.12 Velamentous insertion of umbilical cord

O43.121 Velamentous insertion of umbilical cord, first trimester COM M ♀

O43.122 Velamentous insertion of umbilical cord, second trimester COM M ♀

O43.123 Velamentous insertion of umbilical cord, third trimester COM M ♀

O43.129 Velamentous insertion of umbilical cord, unspecified trimester COM M ♀

6th O43.19 Other malformation of placenta

O43.191 Other malformation of placenta, first trimester COM M ♀

O43.192 Other malformation of placenta, second trimester COM M ♀

O43.193 Other malformation of placenta, third trimester COM M ♀

O43.199 Other malformation of placenta, unspecified trimester COM M ♀

5th O43.2 Morbidly adherent placenta

Code also associated third stage postpartum hemorrhage, if applicable (O72.0)

EXCLUDES 1 *retained placenta (O73.-)*

6th O43.21 Placenta accreta

DEF: Condition where the placenta adheres too deeply to the uterine wall; often associated with placenta previa.

O43.211 Placenta accreta, first trimester COM M ♀

O43.212 Placenta accreta, second trimester COM M ♀

O43.213 Placenta accreta, third trimester COM M ♀

O43.219 Placenta accreta, unspecified trimester COM M ♀

6th O43.22 Placenta increta

AHA: 2022,1Q,20

DEF: Condition where the placenta adheres too deeply to the uterine wall and penetrates the muscle; often associated with placenta previa.

O43.221 Placenta increta, first trimester COM M ♀

O43.222 Placenta increta, second trimester COM M ♀

O43.223 Placenta increta, third trimester COM M ♀

O43.229 Placenta increta, unspecified trimester COM M ♀

6th O43.23 Placenta percreta

DEF: Condition where the placenta attaches through the uterine muscle and may invade other organs, resulting in antenatal complications, premature delivery, retention of all or a portion of the placenta, or postpartum bleeding.

O43.231 Placenta percreta, first trimester COM M ♀

O43.232 Placenta percreta, second trimester COM M ♀

O43.233 Placenta percreta, third trimester COM M ♀

O43.239 Placenta percreta, unspecified trimester COM M ♀

5th O43.8 Other placental disorders

6th O43.81 Placental infarction

O43.811 Placental infarction, first trimester COM M ♀

O43.812 Placental infarction, second trimester COM M ♀

O43.813 **Placental infarction, third trimester** COM M ♀
O43.819 **Placental infarction, unspecified trimester** COM M ♀

✓6th O43.89 **Other placental disorders**
Placental dysfunction
O43.891 **Other placental disorders, first trimester** COM M ♀
O43.892 **Other placental disorders, second trimester** COM M ♀
O43.893 **Other placental disorders, third trimester** COM M ♀
O43.899 **Other placental disorders, unspecified trimester** COM M ♀

✓5th O43.9 **Unspecified placental disorder**
O43.90 **Unspecified placental disorder, unspecified trimester** COM M ♀
O43.91 **Unspecified placental disorder, first trimester** COM M ♀
O43.92 **Unspecified placental disorder, second trimester** COM M ♀
O43.93 **Unspecified placental disorder, third trimester** COM M ♀

✓4th **O44 Placenta previa**
AHA: 2016,4Q,52-53
DEF: Placenta implanted in the lower segment of the uterus, which commonly causes hemorrhage in the last trimester of pregnancy.

✓5th O44.0 **Complete placenta previa NOS or without hemorrhage**
Placenta previa NOS
O44.00 **Complete placenta previa NOS or without hemorrhage, unspecified trimester** COM M ♀
O44.01 **Complete placenta previa NOS or without hemorrhage, first trimester** COM M ♀
O44.02 **Complete placenta previa NOS or without hemorrhage, second trimester** COM M ♀
O44.03 **Complete placenta previa NOS or without hemorrhage, third trimester** COM M ♀

✓5th O44.1 **Complete placenta previa with hemorrhage**
EXCLUDES 1 *labor and delivery complicated by hemorrhage from vasa previa (O69.4)*
O44.10 **Complete placenta previa with hemorrhage, unspecified trimester** COM M ♀
O44.11 **Complete placenta previa with hemorrhage, first trimester** COM M ♀
O44.12 **Complete placenta previa with hemorrhage, second trimester** COM M ♀
O44.13 **Complete placenta previa with hemorrhage, third trimester** COM M ♀

✓5th O44.2 **Partial placenta previa without hemorrhage**
Marginal placenta previa, NOS or without hemorrhage
O44.20 **Partial placenta previa NOS or without hemorrhage, unspecified trimester** COM M ♀
O44.21 **Partial placenta previa NOS or without hemorrhage, first trimester** COM M ♀
O44.22 **Partial placenta previa NOS or without hemorrhage, second trimester** COM M ♀
O44.23 **Partial placenta previa NOS or without hemorrhage, third trimester** COM M ♀

✓5th O44.3 **Partial placenta previa with hemorrhage**
Marginal placenta previa with hemorrhage
O44.30 **Partial placenta previa with hemorrhage, unspecified trimester** COM M ♀
O44.31 **Partial placenta previa with hemorrhage, first trimester** COM M ♀
O44.32 **Partial placenta previa with hemorrhage, second trimester** COM M ♀
O44.33 **Partial placenta previa with hemorrhage, third trimester** COM M ♀

✓5th O44.4 **Low lying placenta NOS or without hemorrhage**
Low implantation of placenta NOS or without hemorrhage
O44.40 **Low lying placenta NOS or without hemorrhage, unspecified trimester** COM M ♀
O44.41 **Low lying placenta NOS or without hemorrhage, first trimester** COM M ♀
O44.42 **Low lying placenta NOS or without hemorrhage, second trimester** COM M ♀
O44.43 **Low lying placenta NOS or without hemorrhage, third trimester** COM M ♀

✓5th O44.5 **Low lying placenta with hemorrhage**
Low implantation of placenta with hemorrhage
O44.50 **Low lying placenta with hemorrhage, unspecified trimester** COM M ♀
O44.51 **Low lying placenta with hemorrhage, first trimester** COM M ♀
O44.52 **Low lying placenta with hemorrhage, second trimester** COM M ♀
O44.53 **Low lying placenta with hemorrhage, third trimester** COM M ♀

✓4th **O45 Premature separation of placenta [abruptio placentae]**

✓5th O45.0 **Premature separation of placenta with coagulation defect**

✓6th O45.00 **Premature separation of placenta with coagulation defect, unspecified**
O45.001 **Premature separation of placenta with coagulation defect, unspecified, first trimester** COM M ♀
O45.002 **Premature separation of placenta with coagulation defect, unspecified, second trimester** COM M ♀
O45.003 **Premature separation of placenta with coagulation defect, unspecified, third trimester** COM M ♀
O45.009 **Premature separation of placenta with coagulation defect, unspecified, unspecified trimester** COM M ♀

✓6th O45.01 **Premature separation of placenta with afibrinogenemia**
Premature separation of placenta with hypofibrinogenemia
O45.011 **Premature separation of placenta with afibrinogenemia, first trimester** COM M ♀
O45.012 **Premature separation of placenta with afibrinogenemia, second trimester** COM M ♀
O45.013 **Premature separation of placenta with afibrinogenemia, third trimester** COM M ♀
O45.019 **Premature separation of placenta with afibrinogenemia, unspecified trimester** COM M ♀

✓6th O45.02 **Premature separation of placenta with disseminated intravascular coagulation**
O45.021 **Premature separation of placenta with disseminated intravascular coagulation, first trimester** COM M ♀
O45.022 **Premature separation of placenta with disseminated intravascular coagulation, second trimester** COM M ♀
O45.023 **Premature separation of placenta with disseminated intravascular coagulation, third trimester** COM M ♀
O45.029 **Premature separation of placenta with disseminated intravascular coagulation, unspecified trimester** COM M ♀

✓6th O45.09 **Premature separation of placenta with other coagulation defect**
O45.091 **Premature separation of placenta with other coagulation defect, first trimester** COM M ♀
O45.092 **Premature separation of placenta with other coagulation defect, second trimester** COM M ♀
O45.093 **Premature separation of placenta with other coagulation defect, third trimester** COM M ♀
O45.099 **Premature separation of placenta with other coagulation defect, unspecified trimester** COM M ♀

✓5th O45.8 **Other premature separation of placenta**

✓6th O45.8X **Other premature separation of placenta**
O45.8X1 **Other premature separation of placenta, first trimester** COM M ♀
O45.8X2 **Other premature separation of placenta, second trimester** COM M ♀
O45.8X3 **Other premature separation of placenta, third trimester** COM M ♀

O45.8X9 Other premature separation of placenta, unspecified trimester COM M ♀

✓5th O45.9 Premature separation of placenta, unspecified
Abruptio placentae NOS

O45.90 Premature separation of placenta, unspecified, unspecified trimester COM M ♀

O45.91 Premature separation of placenta, unspecified, first trimester COM M ♀

O45.92 Premature separation of placenta, unspecified, second trimester COM M ♀

O45.93 Premature separation of placenta, unspecified, third trimester COM M ♀

✓4th **O46 Antepartum hemorrhage, not elsewhere classified**

EXCLUDES 1 *hemorrhage in early pregnancy (O20.-)*
intrapartum hemorrhage NEC (O67.-)
placenta previa (O44.-)
premature separation of placenta [abruptio placentae] (O45.-)

DEF: Uterine hemorrhage prior to delivery that is not related to placenta previa or abruptio placentae.

✓5th O46.0 Antepartum hemorrhage with coagulation defect

✓6th O46.00 Antepartum hemorrhage with coagulation defect, unspecified

O46.001 Antepartum hemorrhage with coagulation defect, unspecified, first trimester COM M ♀

O46.002 Antepartum hemorrhage with coagulation defect, unspecified, second trimester COM M ♀

O46.003 Antepartum hemorrhage with coagulation defect, unspecified, third trimester COM M ♀

O46.009 Antepartum hemorrhage with coagulation defect, unspecified, unspecified trimester COM M ♀

✓6th O46.01 Antepartum hemorrhage with afibrinogenemia
Antepartum hemorrhage with hypofibrinogenemia

O46.011 Antepartum hemorrhage with afibrinogenemia, first trimester COM M ♀

O46.012 Antepartum hemorrhage with afibrinogenemia, second trimester COM M ♀

O46.013 Antepartum hemorrhage with afibrinogenemia, third trimester COM M ♀

O46.019 Antepartum hemorrhage with afibrinogenemia, unspecified trimester COM M ♀

✓6th O46.02 Antepartum hemorrhage with disseminated intravascular coagulation

O46.021 Antepartum hemorrhage with disseminated intravascular coagulation, first trimester COM M ♀

O46.022 Antepartum hemorrhage with disseminated intravascular coagulation, second trimester COM M ♀

O46.023 Antepartum hemorrhage with disseminated intravascular coagulation, third trimester COM M ♀

O46.029 Antepartum hemorrhage with disseminated intravascular coagulation, unspecified trimester COM M ♀

✓6th O46.09 Antepartum hemorrhage with other coagulation defect

O46.091 Antepartum hemorrhage with other coagulation defect, first trimester COM M ♀

O46.092 Antepartum hemorrhage with other coagulation defect, second trimester COM M ♀

O46.093 Antepartum hemorrhage with other coagulation defect, third trimester COM M ♀

O46.099 Antepartum hemorrhage with other coagulation defect, unspecified trimester COM M ♀

✓5th O46.8 Other antepartum hemorrhage

✓6th O46.8X Other antepartum hemorrhage

O46.8X1 Other antepartum hemorrhage, first trimester COM M ♀

O46.8X2 Other antepartum hemorrhage, second trimester COM M ♀

O46.8X3 Other antepartum hemorrhage, third trimester COM M ♀

O46.8X9 Other antepartum hemorrhage, unspecified trimester COM M ♀

✓5th O46.9 Antepartum hemorrhage, unspecified

O46.90 Antepartum hemorrhage, unspecified, unspecified trimester COM M ♀

O46.91 Antepartum hemorrhage, unspecified, first trimester COM M ♀

O46.92 Antepartum hemorrhage, unspecified, second trimester COM M ♀

O46.93 Antepartum hemorrhage, unspecified, third trimester COM M ♀

✓4th **O47 False labor**

INCLUDES Braxton Hicks contractions
threatened labor

EXCLUDES 1 *preterm labor (O60.-)*

AHA: 2021,1Q,10

✓5th O47.0 False labor before 37 completed weeks of gestation

O47.00 False labor before 37 completed weeks of gestation, unspecified trimester COM M ♀

O47.02 False labor before 37 completed weeks of gestation, second trimester COM M ♀

O47.03 False labor before 37 completed weeks of gestation, third trimester COM M ♀

O47.1 False labor at or after 37 completed weeks of gestation COM M ♀

O47.9 False labor, unspecified COM M ♀

✓4th **O48 Late pregnancy**

AHA: 2022,2Q,3

O48.0 Post-term pregnancy COM M ♀
Pregnancy over 40 completed weeks to 42 completed weeks gestation

O48.1 Prolonged pregnancy COM M ♀
Pregnancy which has advanced beyond 42 completed weeks gestation
AHA: 2016,1Q,5

Complications of labor and delivery (O60-O77)

✓4th **O60 Preterm labor**

INCLUDES onset (spontaneous) of labor before 37 completed weeks of gestation

EXCLUDES 1 *false labor (O47.0-)*
threatened labor NOS (O47.0-)

✓5th O60.0 Preterm labor without delivery

O60.00 Preterm labor without delivery, unspecified trimester COM M ♀

O60.02 Preterm labor without delivery, second trimester COM M ♀

O60.03 Preterm labor without delivery, third trimester COM M ♀

✓5th O60.1 Preterm labor with preterm delivery

AHA: 2016,2Q,10

One of the following 7th characters is to be assigned to each code under subcategory O60.1. 7th character 0 is for single gestations and multiple gestations where the fetus is unspecified. 7th characters 1 through 9 are for cases of multiple gestations to identify the fetus for which the code applies. The appropriate code from category O30, Multiple gestation, must also be assigned when assigning a code from subcategory O60.1 that has a 7th character of 1 through 9.

0 not applicable or unspecified
1 fetus 1
2 fetus 2
3 fetus 3
4 fetus 4
5 fetus 5
9 other fetus

✓x7th O60.10 Preterm labor with preterm delivery, unspecified trimester COM M ♀
Preterm labor with delivery NOS

✓x7th O60.12 Preterm labor second trimester with preterm delivery second trimester COM M ♀

✓x7th **O6Ø.13 Preterm labor second trimester with preterm delivery third trimester** COM M ♀

✓x7th **O6Ø.14 Preterm labor third trimester with preterm delivery third trimester** COM M ♀

✓5th **O6Ø.2 Term delivery with preterm labor**

One of the following 7th characters is to be assigned to each code under subcategory O6Ø.2. 7th character Ø is for single gestations and multiple gestations where the fetus is unspecified. 7th characters 1 through 9 are for cases of multiple gestations to identify the fetus for which the code applies. The appropriate code from category O3Ø, Multiple gestation, must also be assigned when assigning a code from subcategory O6Ø.2 that has a 7th character of 1 through 9.

- Ø not applicable or unspecified
- 1 fetus 1
- 2 fetus 2
- 3 fetus 3
- 4 fetus 4
- 5 fetus 5
- 9 other fetus

✓x7th **O6Ø.2Ø Term delivery with preterm labor, unspecified trimester** COM M ♀

✓x7th **O6Ø.22 Term delivery with preterm labor, second trimester** COM M ♀

✓x7th **O6Ø.23 Term delivery with preterm labor, third trimester** COM M ♀

✓4th **O61 Failed induction of labor**

O61.Ø Failed medical induction of labor COM M ♀
- Failed induction (of labor) by oxytocin
- Failed induction (of labor) by prostaglandins

O61.1 Failed instrumental induction of labor COM M ♀
- Failed mechanical induction (of labor)
- Failed surgical induction (of labor)

O61.8 Other failed induction of labor COM M ♀

O61.9 Failed induction of labor, unspecified COM M ♀

✓4th **O62 Abnormalities of forces of labor**

DEF: Uterine inertia: Weak or poorly coordinated contractions of the uterus during labor.

O62.Ø Primary inadequate contractions COM M ♀
- Failure of cervical dilatation
- Primary hypotonic uterine dysfunction
- Uterine inertia during latent phase of labor

O62.1 Secondary uterine inertia COM M ♀
- Arrested active phase of labor
- Secondary hypotonic uterine dysfunction

O62.2 Other uterine inertia COM M ♀
- Atony of uterus without hemorrhage
- Atony of uterus NOS
- Desultory labor
- Hypotonic uterine dysfunction NOS
- Irregular labor
- Poor contractions
- Slow slope active phase of labor
- Uterine inertia NOS

EXCLUDES 1 *atony of uterus with hemorrhage (postpartum) (O72.1)*
postpartum atony of uterus without hemorrhage (O75.89)

DEF: Uterine atony: Failure of the uterine muscles to contract after the fetus and placenta are delivered.

O62.3 Precipitate labor COM M ♀

DEF: Rapid labor with delivery occurring in three hours or less from the onset of contractions.

O62.4 Hypertonic, incoordinate, and prolonged uterine contractions COM M ♀
- Cervical spasm
- Contraction ring dystocia
- Dyscoordinate labor
- Hour-glass contraction of uterus
- Hypertonic uterine dysfunction
- Incoordinate uterine action
- Tetanic contractions
- Uterine dystocia NOS
- Uterine spasm

EXCLUDES 1 *dystocia (fetal) (maternal) NOS (O66.9)*

O62.8 Other abnormalities of forces of labor COM M ♀

O62.9 Abnormality of forces of labor, unspecified COM M ♀

✓4th **O63 Long labor**

O63.Ø Prolonged first stage (of labor) COM M ♀

O63.1 Prolonged second stage (of labor) COM M ♀

O63.2 Delayed delivery of second twin, triplet, etc. COM M ♀

O63.9 Long labor, unspecified COM M ♀
- Prolonged labor NOS

✓4th **O64 Obstructed labor due to malposition and malpresentation of fetus**

One of the following 7th characters is to be assigned to each code under category O64. 7th character Ø is for single gestations and multiple gestations where the fetus is unspecified. 7th characters 1 through 9 are for cases of multiple gestations to identify the fetus for which the code applies. The appropriate code from category O3Ø, Multiple gestation, must also be assigned when assigning a code from category O64 that has a 7th character of 1 through 9.

- Ø not applicable or unspecified
- 1 fetus 1
- 2 fetus 2
- 3 fetus 3
- 4 fetus 4
- 5 fetus 5
- 9 other fetus

Fetal Malposition

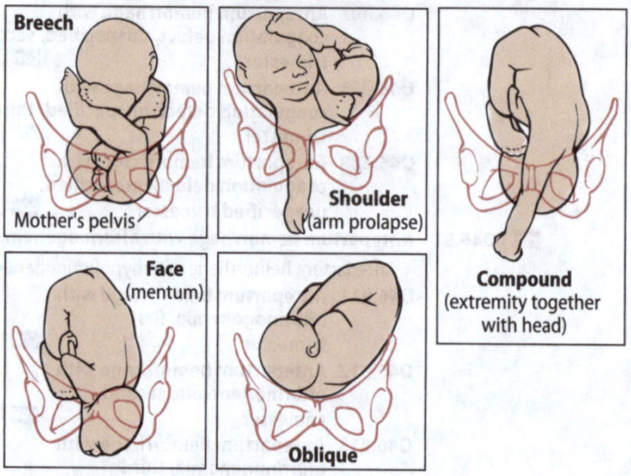

✓x7th **O64.Ø Obstructed labor due to incomplete rotation of fetal head** COM M ♀
- Deep transverse arrest
- Obstructed labor due to persistent occipitoiliac (position)
- Obstructed labor due to persistent occipitoposterior (position)
- Obstructed labor due to persistent occipitosacral (position)
- Obstructed labor due to persistent occipitotransverse (position)

✓x7th **O64.1 Obstructed labor due to breech presentation** COM M ♀
- Obstructed labor due to buttocks presentation
- Obstructed labor due to complete breech presentation
- Obstructed labor due to frank breech presentation

✓x7th **O64.2 Obstructed labor due to face presentation** COM M ♀
- Obstructed labor due to chin presentation

✓x7th **O64.3 Obstructed labor due to brow presentation** COM M ♀

✓x7th **O64.4 Obstructed labor due to shoulder presentation** COM M ♀
- Prolapsed arm

EXCLUDES 1 *impacted shoulders (O66.Ø)*
shoulder dystocia (O66.Ø)

✓x7th **O64.5 Obstructed labor due to compound presentation** COM M ♀

✓x7th **O64.8 Obstructed labor due to other malposition and malpresentation** COM M ♀
- Obstructed labor due to footling presentation
- Obstructed labor due to incomplete breech presentation

✓x7th **O64.9 Obstructed labor due to malposition and malpresentation, unspecified** COM M ♀

✓4th **O65 Obstructed labor due to maternal pelvic abnormality**

O65.Ø Obstructed labor due to deformed pelvis COM M ♀

O65.1 Obstructed labor due to generally contracted pelvis COM M ♀

O65.2 Obstructed labor due to pelvic inlet contraction COM M ♀

O65.3 Obstructed labor due to pelvic outlet and mid-cavity contraction COM M ♀

HCC CMS-HCC | Rx Rx HCC | ESR ESRD HCC | COM Commercial HCC | N Newborn: 0 | P Pediatric: 0-17 | M Maternity: 9-64 | A Adult: 15-124

O65.4 Obstructed labor due to fetopelvic disproportion, unspecified COM M ♀
EXCLUDES 1 *dystocia due to abnormality of fetus (O66.2-O66.3)*

O65.5 Obstructed labor due to abnormality of maternal pelvic organs COM M ♀
Obstructed labor due to conditions listed in O34.-
Use additional code to identify abnormality of pelvic organs O34.-

O65.8 Obstructed labor due to other maternal pelvic abnormalities COM M ♀

O65.9 Obstructed labor due to maternal pelvic abnormality, unspecified COM M ♀

O66 Other obstructed labor (4th)

O66.0 Obstructed labor due to shoulder dystocia COM M ♀
Impacted shoulders
DEF: Obstructed labor due to impacted fetal shoulders. It is an emergency condition that may require cesarean section, forceps delivery, vacuum extraction, or symphysiotomy.

O66.1 Obstructed labor due to locked twins COM M ♀

O66.2 Obstructed labor due to unusually large fetus COM M ♀

O66.3 Obstructed labor due to other abnormalities of fetus COM M ♀
Dystocia due to fetal ascites
Dystocia due to fetal hydrops
Dystocia due to fetal meningomyelocele
Dystocia due to fetal sacral teratoma
Dystocia due to fetal tumor
Dystocia due to hydrocephalic fetus
Use additional code to identify cause of obstruction

O66.4 Failed trial of labor (5th)

O66.40 Failed trial of labor, unspecified COM M ♀

O66.41 Failed attempted vaginal birth after previous cesarean delivery COM M ♀
Code first rupture of uterus, if applicable (O71.0-, O71.1)

O66.5 Attempted application of vacuum extractor and forceps COM M ♀
Attempted application of vacuum or forceps, with subsequent delivery by forceps or cesarean delivery

O66.6 Obstructed labor due to other multiple fetuses COM M ♀

O66.8 Other specified obstructed labor COM M ♀
Use additional code to identify cause of obstruction

O66.9 Obstructed labor, unspecified COM M ♀
Dystocia NOS
Fetal dystocia NOS
Maternal dystocia NOS

O67 Labor and delivery complicated by intrapartum hemorrhage, not elsewhere classified (4th)
EXCLUDES 1 *antepartum hemorrhage NEC (O46.-)*
placenta previa (O44.-)
premature separation of placenta [abruptio placentae] (O45.-)
EXCLUDES 2 *postpartum hemorrhage (O72.-)*

O67.0 Intrapartum hemorrhage with coagulation defect COM M ♀
Intrapartum hemorrhage (excessive) associated with afibrinogenemia
Intrapartum hemorrhage (excessive) associated with disseminated intravascular coagulation
Intrapartum hemorrhage (excessive) associated with hyperfibrinolysis
Intrapartum hemorrhage (excessive) associated with hypofibrinogenemia

O67.8 Other intrapartum hemorrhage COM M ♀
Excessive intrapartum hemorrhage

O67.9 Intrapartum hemorrhage, unspecified COM M ♀

O68 Labor and delivery complicated by abnormality of fetal acid-base balance COM M ♀
Fetal acidemia complicating labor and delivery
Fetal acidosis complicating labor and delivery
Fetal alkalosis complicating labor and delivery
Fetal metabolic acidemia complicating labor and delivery
EXCLUDES 1 *fetal stress NOS (O77.9)*
labor and delivery complicated by electrocardiographic evidence of fetal stress (O77.8)
labor and delivery complicated by ultrasonic evidence of fetal stress (O77.8)
EXCLUDES 2 *abnormality in fetal heart rate or rhythm (O76)*
labor and delivery complicated by meconium in amniotic fluid (O77.0)

O69 Labor and delivery complicated by umbilical cord complications (4th)
AHA: 2016,1Q,5

One of the following 7th characters is to be assigned to each code under category O69. 7th character 0 is for single gestations and multiple gestations where the fetus is unspecified. 7th characters 1 through 9 are for cases of multiple gestations to identify the fetus for which the code applies. The appropriate code from category O30, Multiple gestation, must also be assigned when assigning a code from category O69 that has a 7th character of 1 through 9.
0 not applicable or unspecified
1 fetus 1
2 fetus 2
3 fetus 3
4 fetus 4
5 fetus 5
9 other fetus

O69.0 Labor and delivery complicated by prolapse of cord (x7th) COM M ♀
DEF: Abnormal presentation of the fetus marked by a protruding umbilical cord during labor. It can cause fetal death.

O69.1 Labor and delivery complicated by cord around neck, with compression (x7th) COM M ♀
EXCLUDES 1 *labor and delivery complicated by cord around neck, without compression (O69.81)*

O69.2 Labor and delivery complicated by other cord entanglement, with compression (x7th) COM M ♀
Labor and delivery complicated by compression of cord NOS
Labor and delivery complicated by entanglement of cords of twins in monoamniotic sac
Labor and delivery complicated by knot in cord
EXCLUDES 1 *labor and delivery complicated by other cord entanglement, without compression (O69.82)*

O69.3 Labor and delivery complicated by short cord (x7th) COM M ♀

O69.4 Labor and delivery complicated by vasa previa (x7th) COM M ♀
Labor and delivery complicated by hemorrhage from vasa previa

O69.5 Labor and delivery complicated by vascular lesion of cord (x7th) COM M ♀
Labor and delivery complicated by cord bruising
Labor and delivery complicated by cord hematoma
Labor and delivery complicated by thrombosis of umbilical vessels

O69.8 Labor and delivery complicated by other cord complications (5th)

O69.81 Labor and delivery complicated by cord around neck, without compression (x7th) COM M ♀
AHA: 2016,1Q,5

O69.82 Labor and delivery complicated by other cord entanglement, without compression (x7th) COM M ♀

O69.89 Labor and delivery complicated by other cord complications (x7th) COM M ♀

O69.9 Labor and delivery complicated by cord complication, unspecified (x7th) COM M ♀

O70 Perineal laceration during delivery

INCLUDES episiotomy extended by laceration

EXCLUDES 1 *obstetric high vaginal laceration alone (O71.4)*

AHA: 2016,2Q,34; 2016,1Q,3-4,5

O70.0 First degree perineal laceration during delivery COM M ♀

Perineal laceration, rupture or tear involving fourchette during delivery

Perineal laceration, rupture or tear involving labia during delivery

Perineal laceration, rupture or tear involving skin during delivery

Perineal laceration, rupture or tear involving vagina during delivery

Perineal laceration, rupture or tear involving vulva during delivery

Slight perineal laceration, rupture or tear during delivery

O70.1 Second degree perineal laceration during delivery COM M ♀

Perineal laceration, rupture or tear during delivery as in O70.0, also involving pelvic floor

Perineal laceration, rupture or tear during delivery as in O70.0, also involving perineal muscles

Perineal laceration, rupture or tear during delivery as in O70.0, also involving vaginal muscles

EXCLUDES 1 *perineal laceration involving anal sphincter (O70.2)*

O70.2 Third degree perineal laceration during delivery

Perineal laceration, rupture or tear during delivery as in O70.1, also involving anal sphincter

Perineal laceration, rupture or tear during delivery as in O70.1, also involving rectovaginal septum

Perineal laceration, rupture or tear during delivery as in O70.1, also involving sphincter NOS

EXCLUDES 1 *anal sphincter tear during delivery without third degree perineal laceration (O70.4)*

perineal laceration involving anal or rectal mucosa (O70.3)

AHA: 2016,4Q,53-54

O70.20 Third degree perineal laceration during delivery, unspecified COM M ♀

O70.21 Third degree perineal laceration during delivery, IIIa COM M ♀

Third degree perineal laceration during delivery with less than 50% of external anal sphincter (EAS) thickness torn

O70.22 Third degree perineal laceration during delivery, IIIb COM M ♀

Third degree perineal laceration during delivery with more than 50% external anal sphincter (EAS) thickness torn

O70.23 Third degree perineal laceration during delivery, IIIc COM M ♀

Third degree perineal laceration during delivery with both external anal sphincter (EAS) and internal anal sphincter (IAS) torn

O70.3 Fourth degree perineal laceration during delivery COM M ♀

Perineal laceration, rupture or tear during delivery as in O70.2, also involving anal mucosa

Perineal laceration, rupture or tear during delivery as in O70.2, also involving rectal mucosa

O70.4 Anal sphincter tear complicating delivery, not associated with third degree laceration COM M ♀

EXCLUDES 1 *anal sphincter tear with third degree perineal laceration (O70.2)*

O70.9 Perineal laceration during delivery, unspecified COM M ♀

O71 Other obstetric trauma

INCLUDES obstetric damage from instruments

O71.0 Rupture of uterus (spontaneous) before onset of labor

EXCLUDES 1 *disruption of (current) cesarean delivery wound (O90.0)*

laceration of uterus, NEC (O71.81)

O71.00 Rupture of uterus before onset of labor, unspecified trimester COM M ♀

O71.02 Rupture of uterus before onset of labor, second trimester COM M ♀

O71.03 Rupture of uterus before onset of labor, third trimester COM M ♀

O71.1 Rupture of uterus during labor COM M ♀

Rupture of uterus not stated as occurring before onset of labor

EXCLUDES 1 *disruption of cesarean delivery wound (O90.0)*

laceration of uterus, NEC (O71.81)

O71.2 Postpartum inversion of uterus COM M ♀

O71.3 Obstetric laceration of cervix COM M ♀

Annular detachment of cervix

O71.4 Obstetric high vaginal laceration alone COM M ♀

Laceration of vaginal wall without perineal laceration

EXCLUDES 1 *obstetric high vaginal laceration with perineal laceration (O70.-)*

AHA: 2016,1Q,5

O71.5 Other obstetric injury to pelvic organs COM M ♀

Obstetric injury to bladder

Obstetric injury to urethra

EXCLUDES 2 *obstetric periurethral trauma (O71.82)*

AHA: 2014,4Q,18

O71.6 Obstetric damage to pelvic joints and ligaments COM M ♀

Obstetric avulsion of inner symphyseal cartilage

Obstetric damage to coccyx

Obstetric traumatic separation of symphysis (pubis)

O71.7 Obstetric hematoma of pelvis COM M ♀

Obstetric hematoma of perineum

Obstetric hematoma of vagina

Obstetric hematoma of vulva

O71.8 Other specified obstetric trauma

O71.81 Laceration of uterus, not elsewhere classified COM M ♀

O71.82 Other specified trauma to perineum and vulva COM M ♀

Obstetric periurethral trauma

AHA: 2016,1Q,4; 2014,4Q,18

O71.89 Other specified obstetric trauma COM M ♀

O71.9 Obstetric trauma, unspecified COM M ♀

O72 Postpartum hemorrhage

INCLUDES hemorrhage after delivery of fetus or infant

O72.0 Third-stage hemorrhage COM M ♀

Hemorrhage associated with retained, trapped or adherent placenta

Retained placenta NOS

Code also type of adherent placenta (O43.2-)

AHA: 2019,3Q,11

O72.1 Other immediate postpartum hemorrhage COM M ♀

Hemorrhage following delivery of placenta

Postpartum hemorrhage (atonic) NOS

Uterine atony with hemorrhage

EXCLUDES 1 *uterine atony NOS (O62.2)*

uterine atony without hemorrhage (O62.2)

postpartum atony of uterus without hemorrhage (O75.89)

AHA: 2016,1Q,4

DEF: Uterine atony: Failure of the uterine muscles to contract after the fetus and placenta are delivered.

O72.2 Delayed and secondary postpartum hemorrhage COM M ♀

Hemorrhage associated with retained portions of placenta or membranes after the first 24 hours following delivery of placenta

Retained products of conception NOS, following delivery

O72.3 Postpartum coagulation defects COM M ♀

Postpartum afibrinogenemia

Postpartum fibrinolysis

O73 Retained placenta and membranes, without hemorrhage

EXCLUDES 1 *placenta accreta (O43.21-)*

placenta increta (O43.22-)

placenta percreta (O43.23-)

DEF: Postpartum condition resulting from failure to expel placental membrane tissues due to failed contractions of the uterine wall.

O73.0 Retained placenta without hemorrhage COM M ♀

Adherent placenta, without hemorrhage

Trapped placenta without hemorrhage

O73.1 Retained portions of placenta and membranes, without hemorrhage COM M ♀

Retained products of conception following delivery, without hemorrhage

O74 Complications of anesthesia during labor and delivery

INCLUDES maternal complications arising from the administration of a general, regional or local anesthetic, analgesic or other sedation during labor and delivery

Use additional code, if applicable, to identify specific complication

O74.Ø Aspiration pneumonitis due to anesthesia during labor and delivery COM M ♀

Inhalation of stomach contents or secretions NOS due to anesthesia during labor and delivery

Mendelson's syndrome due to anesthesia during labor and delivery

O74.1 Other pulmonary complications of anesthesia during labor and delivery COM M ♀

O74.2 Cardiac complications of anesthesia during labor and delivery COM M ♀

O74.3 Central nervous system complications of anesthesia during labor and delivery COM M ♀

O74.4 Toxic reaction to local anesthesia during labor and delivery COM M ♀

O74.5 Spinal and epidural anesthesia-induced headache during labor and delivery COM M ♀

O74.6 Other complications of spinal and epidural anesthesia during labor and delivery COM M ♀

O74.7 Failed or difficult intubation for anesthesia during labor and delivery COM M ♀

O74.8 Other complications of anesthesia during labor and delivery COM M ♀

O74.9 Complication of anesthesia during labor and delivery, unspecified COM ♀

O75 Other complications of labor and delivery, not elsewhere classified

EXCLUDES 2 *puerperal (postpartum) infection (O86.-)*
puerperal (postpartum) sepsis (O85)

O75.Ø Maternal distress during labor and delivery COM M ♀

O75.1 Shock during or following labor and delivery COM M ♀

Obstetric shock following labor and delivery

O75.2 Pyrexia during labor, not elsewhere classified COM M ♀

O75.3 Other infection during labor COM M ♀

Sepsis during labor

Use additional code (B95-B97), to identify infectious agent

O75.4 Other complications of obstetric surgery and procedures COM M ♀

Cardiac arrest following obstetric surgery or procedures

Cardiac failure following obstetric surgery or procedures

Cerebral anoxia following obstetric surgery or procedures

Pulmonary edema following obstetric surgery or procedures

Use additional code to identify specific complication

EXCLUDES 2 *complications of anesthesia during labor and delivery (O74.-)*
disruption of obstetrical (surgical) wound (O9Ø.Ø-O9Ø.1)
hematoma of obstetrical (surgical) wound (O9Ø.2)
infection of obstetrical (surgical) wound (O86.Ø-)

O75.5 Delayed delivery after artificial rupture of membranes COM M ♀

O75.8 Other specified complications of labor and delivery

O75.81 Maternal exhaustion complicating labor and delivery COM M ♀

O75.82 Onset (spontaneous) of labor after 37 completed weeks of gestation but before 39 completed weeks gestation, with delivery by (planned) cesarean section COM M ♀

Delivery by (planned) cesarean section occurring after 37 completed weeks of gestation but before 39 completed weeks gestation due to (spontaneous) onset of labor

Code first to specify reason for planned cesarean section such as:
cephalopelvic disproportion (normally formed fetus) (O33.9)
previous cesarean delivery (O34.21)

AHA: 2022,2Q,3

O75.89 Other specified complications of labor and delivery COM M ♀

O75.9 Complication of labor and delivery, unspecified COM M ♀

O76 Abnormality in fetal heart rate and rhythm complicating labor and delivery COM M ♀

Depressed fetal heart rate tones complicating labor and delivery

Fetal bradycardia complicating labor and delivery

Fetal heart rate decelerations complicating labor and delivery

Fetal heart rate irregularity complicating labor and delivery

Fetal heart rate abnormal variability complicating labor and delivery

Fetal tachycardia complicating labor and delivery

Non-reassuring fetal heart rate or rhythm complicating labor and delivery

EXCLUDES 1 *fetal stress NOS (O77.9)*
labor and delivery complicated by electrocardiographic evidence of fetal stress (O77.8)
labor and delivery complicated by ultrasonic evidence of fetal stress (O77.8)

EXCLUDES 2 *fetal metabolic acidemia (O68)*
other fetal stress (O77.Ø-O77.1)

AHA: 2013,4Q,118

O77 Other fetal stress complicating labor and delivery

O77.Ø Labor and delivery complicated by meconium in amniotic fluid COM M ♀

AHA: 2022,2Q,16; 2013,4Q,117-118

O77.1 Fetal stress in labor or delivery due to drug administration COM M ♀

O77.8 Labor and delivery complicated by other evidence of fetal stress COM M ♀

Labor and delivery complicated by electrocardiographic evidence of fetal stress

Labor and delivery complicated by ultrasonic evidence of fetal stress

EXCLUDES 1 *abnormality of fetal acid-base balance (O68)*
abnormality in fetal heart rate or rhythm (O76)
fetal metabolic acidemia (O68)

O77.9 Labor and delivery complicated by fetal stress, unspecified COM M ♀

EXCLUDES 1 *abnormality of fetal acid-base balance (O68)*
abnormality in fetal heart rate or rhythm (O76)
fetal metabolic acidemia (O68)

Encounter for delivery (O8Ø-O82)

O8Ø Encounter for full-term uncomplicated delivery COM M ♀

NOTE Delivery requiring minimal or no assistance, with or without episiotomy, without fetal manipulation [e.g., rotation version] or instrumentation [forceps] of a spontaneous, cephalic, vaginal, full-term, single, live-born infant. This code is for use as a single diagnosis code and is not to be used with any other code from chapter 15.

Use additional code to indicate outcome of delivery (Z37.Ø)

AHA: 2016,4Q,150; 2014,2Q,9

O82 Encounter for cesarean delivery without indication COM M ♀

Use additional code to indicate outcome of delivery (Z37.Ø)

Complications predominantly related to the puerperium (O85-O92)

EXCLUDES 2 *mental and behavioral disorders associated with the puerperium (F53.-)*
obstetrical tetanus (A34)
puerperal osteomalacia (M83.Ø)

O85 Puerperal sepsis COM M ♀

Postpartum sepsis

Puerperal peritonitis

Puerperal pyemia

Use additional code (B95-B97), to identify infectious agent

Use additional code (R65.2-) to identify severe sepsis, if applicable

EXCLUDES 1 *fever of unknown origin following delivery (O86.4)*
genital tract infection following delivery (O86.1-)
obstetric pyemic and septic embolism (O88.3-)
puerperal septic thrombophlebitis (O86.81)
urinary tract infection following delivery (O86.2-)

EXCLUDES 2 *sepsis during labor (O75.3)*

AHA: 2022,2Q,5; 2020,2Q,32; 2019,2Q,39; 2018,4Q,23

O86 Other puerperal infections

Use additional code (B95-B97), to identify infectious agent

EXCLUDES 2 *infection during labor (O75.3)*
obstetrical tetanus (A34)

O86.Ø Infection of obstetric surgical wound

Infected cesarean delivery wound following delivery
Infected perineal repair following delivery

EXCLUDES 1 *complications of procedures, not elsewhere classified (T81.4-)*
postprocedural fever NOS (R5Ø.82)
postprocedural retroperitoneal abscess (K68.11)

AHA: 2020,2Q,32; 2018,4Q,22-23,62

O86.ØØ Infection of obstetric surgical wound, unspecified COM M ♀

O86.Ø1 Infection of obstetric surgical wound, superficial incisional site COM M ♀
Subcutaneous abscess following an obstetrical procedure
Stitch abscess following an obstetrical procedure

O86.Ø2 Infection of obstetric surgical wound, deep incisional site COM M ♀
Intramuscular abscess following an obstetrical procedure
Sub-fascial abscess following an obstetrical procedure
AHA: 2020,2Q,32

O86.Ø3 Infection of obstetric surgical wound, organ and space site COM M ♀
Intraabdominal abscess following an obstetrical procedure
Subphrenic abscess following an obstetrical procedure

O86.Ø4 Sepsis following an obstetrical procedure COM M ♀
Use additional code to identify the sepsis
AHA: 2020,2Q,32; 2019,2Q,39

O86.Ø9 Infection of obstetric surgical wound, other surgical site COM M ♀

O86.1 Other infection of genital tract following delivery

O86.11 Cervicitis following delivery COM M ♀

O86.12 Endometritis following delivery COM M ♀

O86.13 Vaginitis following delivery COM M ♀

O86.19 Other infection of genital tract following delivery COM M ♀

O86.2 Urinary tract infection following delivery

O86.2Ø Urinary tract infection following delivery, unspecified COM M ♀
Puerperal urinary tract infection NOS
AHA: 2022,2Q,5

O86.21 Infection of kidney following delivery COM M ♀

O86.22 Infection of bladder following delivery COM M ♀
Infection of urethra following delivery

O86.29 Other urinary tract infection following delivery COM M ♀

O86.4 Pyrexia of unknown origin following delivery COM M ♀
Puerperal infection NOS following delivery
Puerperal pyrexia NOS following delivery

EXCLUDES 2 *pyrexia during labor (O75.2)*

DEF: Fever of unknown origin experienced by the mother after childbirth.

O86.8 Other specified puerperal infections

O86.81 Puerperal septic thrombophlebitis COM M ♀

O86.89 Other specified puerperal infections COM M ♀

O87 Venous complications and hemorrhoids in the puerperium

INCLUDES venous complications in labor, delivery and the puerperium

EXCLUDES 2 *obstetric embolism (O88.-)*
puerperal septic thrombophlebitis (O86.81)
venous complications in pregnancy (O22.-)

O87.Ø Superficial thrombophlebitis in the puerperium COM M ♀
Puerperal phlebitis NOS
Puerperal thrombosis NOS

O87.1 Deep phlebothrombosis in the puerperium COM M ♀
Deep vein thrombosis, postpartum
Pelvic thrombophlebitis, postpartum
Use additional code to identify the deep vein thrombosis (I82.4-, I82.5-, I82.62-, I82.72-)
Use additional code, if applicable, for associated long-term (current) use of anticoagulants (Z79.Ø1)

O87.2 Hemorrhoids in the puerperium COM M ♀

O87.3 Cerebral venous thrombosis in the puerperium COM M ♀
Cerebrovenous sinus thrombosis in the puerperium

O87.4 Varicose veins of lower extremity in the puerperium COM M ♀

O87.8 Other venous complications in the puerperium COM M ♀
Genital varices in the puerperium

O87.9 Venous complication in the puerperium, unspecified COM M ♀
Puerperal phlebopathy NOS

O88 Obstetric embolism

EXCLUDES 1 *embolism complicating abortion NOS (OØ3.2)*
embolism complicating ectopic or molar pregnancy (OØ8.2)
embolism complicating failed attempted abortion (OØ7.2)
embolism complicating induced abortion (OØ4.7)
embolism complicating spontaneous abortion (OØ3.2, OØ3.7)

O88.Ø Obstetric air embolism

DEF: Sudden blocking of the pulmonary artery or right ventricle with air or nitrogen bubbles.

O88.Ø1 Obstetric air embolism in pregnancy

O88.Ø11 Air embolism in pregnancy, first trimester COM M ♀

O88.Ø12 Air embolism in pregnancy, second trimester COM M ♀

O88.Ø13 Air embolism in pregnancy, third trimester COM M ♀

O88.Ø19 Air embolism in pregnancy, unspecified trimester COM M ♀

O88.Ø2 Air embolism in childbirth COM M ♀

O88.Ø3 Air embolism in the puerperium COM M ♀

O88.1 Amniotic fluid embolism
Anaphylactoid syndrome in pregnancy

O88.11 Amniotic fluid embolism in pregnancy

O88.111 Amniotic fluid embolism in pregnancy, first trimester COM M ♀

O88.112 Amniotic fluid embolism in pregnancy, second trimester COM M ♀

O88.113 Amniotic fluid embolism in pregnancy, third trimester COM M ♀

O88.119 Amniotic fluid embolism in pregnancy, unspecified trimester COM M ♀

O88.12 Amniotic fluid embolism in childbirth COM M ♀

O88.13 Amniotic fluid embolism in the puerperium COM M ♀

O88.2 Obstetric thromboembolism

O88.21 Thromboembolism in pregnancy
Obstetric (pulmonary) embolism NOS

O88.211 Thromboembolism in pregnancy, first trimester COM M ♀

O88.212 Thromboembolism in pregnancy, second trimester COM M ♀

O88.213 Thromboembolism in pregnancy, third trimester COM M ♀

O88.219 Thromboembolism in pregnancy, unspecified trimester COM M ♀

O88.22 Thromboembolism in childbirth COM M ♀

O88.23 Thromboembolism in the puerperium COM M ♀
Puerperal (pulmonary) embolism NOS

O88.3 Obstetric pyemic and septic embolism

O88.31 Pyemic and septic embolism in pregnancy

O88.311 Pyemic and septic embolism in pregnancy, first trimester COM M ♀

O88.312 Pyemic and septic embolism in pregnancy, second trimester COM M ♀

O88.313 Pyemic and septic embolism in pregnancy, third trimester COM M ♀

O88.319 Pyemic and septic embolism in pregnancy, unspecified trimester COM M ♀

O88.32 Pyemic and septic embolism in childbirth COM M ♀

O88.33 Pyemic and septic embolism in the puerperium COM M ♀

O88.8 Other obstetric embolism
Obstetric fat embolism

O88.81 Other embolism in pregnancy

O88.811 Other embolism in pregnancy, first trimester COM M ♀

O88.812 Other embolism in pregnancy, second trimester COM M ♀

O88.813 Other embolism in pregnancy, third trimester COM M ♀

O88.819 Other embolism in pregnancy, unspecified trimester COM M ♀

O88.82 Other embolism in childbirth COM M ♀

O88.83 Other embolism in the puerperium COM M ♀

O89 Complications of anesthesia during the puerperium

INCLUDES maternal complications arising from the administration of a general, regional or local anesthetic, analgesic or other sedation during the puerperium

Use additional code, if applicable, to identify specific complication

O89.0 Pulmonary complications of anesthesia during the puerperium

O89.01 Aspiration pneumonitis due to anesthesia during the puerperium COM M ♀
Inhalation of stomach contents or secretions NOS due to anesthesia during the puerperium
Mendelson's syndrome due to anesthesia during the puerperium

O89.09 Other pulmonary complications of anesthesia during the puerperium COM M ♀

O89.1 Cardiac complications of anesthesia during the puerperium COM M ♀

O89.2 Central nervous system complications of anesthesia during the puerperium COM M ♀

O89.3 Toxic reaction to local anesthesia during the puerperium COM M ♀

O89.4 Spinal and epidural anesthesia-induced headache during the puerperium COM M ♀

O89.5 Other complications of spinal and epidural anesthesia during the puerperium COM M ♀

O89.6 Failed or difficult intubation for anesthesia during the puerperium COM M ♀

O89.8 Other complications of anesthesia during the puerperium COM M ♀

O89.9 Complication of anesthesia during the puerperium, unspecified COM M ♀

O90 Complications of the puerperium, not elsewhere classified

O90.0 Disruption of cesarean delivery wound COM M ♀
Dehiscence of cesarean delivery wound
EXCLUDES 1 *rupture of uterus (spontaneous) before onset of labor (O71.0-)*
rupture of uterus during labor (O71.1)

O90.1 Disruption of perineal obstetric wound COM M ♀
Disruption of wound of episiotomy
Disruption of wound of perineal laceration
Secondary perineal tear

O90.2 Hematoma of obstetric wound COM M ♀

O90.3 Peripartum cardiomyopathy COM M ♀
Conditions in I42- arising during pregnancy and the puerperium
EXCLUDES 1 *pre-existing heart disease complicating pregnancy and the puerperium (O99.4-)*
DEF: Any structural or functional abnormality of the ventricular myocardium. It is a noninflammatory disease of obscure or unknown etiology with onset during the postpartum period.

O90.4 Postpartum acute kidney failure COM M ♀
Hepatorenal syndrome following labor and delivery

O90.5 Postpartum thyroiditis COM M ♀

O90.6 Postpartum mood disturbance COM Q M ♀
Postpartum blues
Postpartum dysphoria
Postpartum sadness
EXCLUDES 1 *postpartum depression (F53.0)*
puerperal psychosis (F53.1)

O90.8 Other complications of the puerperium, not elsewhere classified

O90.81 Anemia of the puerperium COM M ♀
Postpartum anemia NOS
EXCLUDES 1 *pre-existing anemia complicating the puerperium (O99.03)*
AHA: 2019,3Q,11

O90.89 Other complications of the puerperium, not elsewhere classified COM M ♀
Placental polyp

O90.9 Complication of the puerperium, unspecified COM M ♀

O91 Infections of breast associated with pregnancy, the puerperium and lactation

Use additional code to identify infection

O91.0 Infection of nipple associated with pregnancy, the puerperium and lactation

O91.01 Infection of nipple associated with pregnancy
Gestational abscess of nipple

O91.011 Infection of nipple associated with pregnancy, first trimester COM M ♀

O91.012 Infection of nipple associated with pregnancy, second trimester COM M ♀

O91.013 Infection of nipple associated with pregnancy, third trimester COM M ♀

O91.019 Infection of nipple associated with pregnancy, unspecified trimester COM M ♀

O91.02 Infection of nipple associated with the puerperium M ♀
Puerperal abscess of nipple

O91.03 Infection of nipple associated with lactation M ♀
Abscess of nipple associated with lactation

O91.1 Abscess of breast associated with pregnancy, the puerperium and lactation

O91.11 Abscess of breast associated with pregnancy
Gestational mammary abscess
Gestational purulent mastitis
Gestational subareolar abscess

O91.111 Abscess of breast associated with pregnancy, first trimester COM M ♀

O91.112 Abscess of breast associated with pregnancy, second trimester COM M ♀

O91.113 Abscess of breast associated with pregnancy, third trimester COM M ♀

O91.119 Abscess of breast associated with pregnancy, unspecified trimester COM M ♀

O91.12 Abscess of breast associated with the puerperium M ♀
Puerperal mammary abscess
Puerperal purulent mastitis
Puerperal subareolar abscess

O91.13 Abscess of breast associated with lactation M ♀
Mammary abscess associated with lactation
Purulent mastitis associated with lactation
Subareolar abscess associated with lactation

O91.2 Nonpurulent mastitis associated with pregnancy, the puerperium and lactation

O91.21 Nonpurulent mastitis associated with pregnancy
Gestational interstitial mastitis
Gestational lymphangitis of breast
Gestational mastitis NOS
Gestational parenchymatous mastitis

O91.211 Nonpurulent mastitis associated with pregnancy, first trimester COM M ♀

O91.212 Nonpurulent mastitis associated with pregnancy, second trimester COM M ♀

O91.213 Nonpurulent mastitis associated with pregnancy, third trimester COM M ♀

O91.219 Nonpurulent mastitis associated with pregnancy, unspecified trimester COM M ♀

O91.22 **Nonpurulent mastitis associated with the puerperium** M ♀
Puerperal interstitial mastitis
Puerperal lymphangitis of breast
Puerperal mastitis NOS
Puerperal parenchymatous mastitis

O91.23 **Nonpurulent mastitis associated with lactation** M ♀
Interstitial mastitis associated with lactation
Lymphangitis of breast associated with lactation
Mastitis NOS associated with lactation
Parenchymatous mastitis associated with lactation

✓4th **O92 Other disorders of breast and disorders of lactation associated with pregnancy and the puerperium**

✓5th **O92.Ø Retracted nipple associated with pregnancy, the puerperium, and lactation**

✓6th O92.Ø1 **Retracted nipple associated with pregnancy**

O92.Ø11 **Retracted nipple associated with pregnancy, first trimester** COM M ♀

O92.Ø12 **Retracted nipple associated with pregnancy, second trimester** COM M ♀

O92.Ø13 **Retracted nipple associated with pregnancy, third trimester** COM M ♀

O92.Ø19 **Retracted nipple associated with pregnancy, unspecified trimester** COM M ♀

O92.Ø2 **Retracted nipple associated with the puerperium** M ♀

O92.Ø3 **Retracted nipple associated with lactation** M ♀

✓5th **O92.1 Cracked nipple associated with pregnancy, the puerperium, and lactation**
Fissure of nipple, gestational or puerperal

✓6th O92.11 **Cracked nipple associated with pregnancy**

O92.111 **Cracked nipple associated with pregnancy, first trimester** COM M ♀

O92.112 **Cracked nipple associated with pregnancy, second trimester** COM M ♀

O92.113 **Cracked nipple associated with pregnancy, third trimester** COM M ♀

O92.119 **Cracked nipple associated with pregnancy, unspecified trimester** COM M ♀

O92.12 **Cracked nipple associated with the puerperium** M ♀

O92.13 **Cracked nipple associated with lactation** M ♀

✓5th **O92.2 Other and unspecified disorders of breast associated with pregnancy and the puerperium**

O92.2Ø **Unspecified disorder of breast associated with pregnancy and the puerperium** M ♀

O92.29 **Other disorders of breast associated with pregnancy and the puerperium** M ♀

O92.3 Agalactia M ♀
Primary agalactia
EXCLUDES 1 *elective agalactia (O92.5)*
secondary agalactia (O92.5)
therapeutic agalactia (O92.5)
DEF: Absence of milk secretion in a female after delivery.

O92.4 Hypogalactia M ♀

O92.5 Suppressed lactation M ♀
Elective agalactia
Secondary agalactia
Therapeutic agalactia
EXCLUDES 1 *primary agalactia (O92.3)*

O92.6 Galactorrhea M ♀
DEF: Excessive or persistent milk secretion by the breast that may occur in the absence of nursing.

✓5th **O92.7 Other and unspecified disorders of lactation**

O92.7Ø **Unspecified disorders of lactation** M ♀

O92.79 **Other disorders of lactation** M ♀
Puerperal galactocele

Other obstetric conditions, not elsewhere classified (O94-O9A)

O94 Sequelae of complication of pregnancy, childbirth, and the puerperium UPD M ♀
NOTE This category is to be used to indicate conditions in OØØ-O77.-, O85-O94 and O98-O9A.- as the cause of late effects. The sequelae include conditions specified as such, or as late effects, which may occur at any time after the puerperium
Code first condition resulting from (sequela) of complication of pregnancy, childbirth, and the puerperium

✓4th **O98 Maternal infectious and parasitic diseases classifiable elsewhere but complicating pregnancy, childbirth and the puerperium**
INCLUDES the listed conditions when complicating the pregnant state, when aggravated by the pregnancy, or as a reason for obstetric care
Use additional code (Chapter 1), to identify specific infectious or parasitic disease
EXCLUDES 2 *herpes gestationis (O26.4-)*
infectious carrier state (O99.82-, O99.83-)
obstetrical tetanus (A34)
puerperal infection (O86.-)
puerperal sepsis (O85)
when the reason for maternal care is that the disease is known or suspected to have affected the fetus (O35-O36)

✓5th **O98.Ø Tuberculosis complicating pregnancy, childbirth and the puerperium**
Conditions in A15-A19

✓6th O98.Ø1 **Tuberculosis complicating pregnancy**

O98.Ø11 **Tuberculosis complicating pregnancy, first trimester** COM M ♀

O98.Ø12 **Tuberculosis complicating pregnancy, second trimester** COM M ♀

O98.Ø13 **Tuberculosis complicating pregnancy, third trimester** COM M ♀

O98.Ø19 **Tuberculosis complicating pregnancy, unspecified trimester** COM M ♀

O98.Ø2 **Tuberculosis complicating childbirth** COM M ♀

O98.Ø3 **Tuberculosis complicating the puerperium** COM M ♀

✓5th **O98.1 Syphilis complicating pregnancy, childbirth and the puerperium**
Conditions in A5Ø-A53

✓6th O98.11 **Syphilis complicating pregnancy**

O98.111 **Syphilis complicating pregnancy, first trimester** COM M ♀

O98.112 **Syphilis complicating pregnancy, second trimester** COM M ♀

O98.113 **Syphilis complicating pregnancy, third trimester** COM M ♀

O98.119 **Syphilis complicating pregnancy, unspecified trimester** COM M ♀

O98.12 **Syphilis complicating childbirth** COM M ♀

O98.13 **Syphilis complicating the puerperium** COM M ♀

✓5th **O98.2 Gonorrhea complicating pregnancy, childbirth and the puerperium**
Conditions in A54.-

✓6th O98.21 **Gonorrhea complicating pregnancy**

O98.211 **Gonorrhea complicating pregnancy, first trimester** COM M ♀

O98.212 **Gonorrhea complicating pregnancy, second trimester** COM M ♀

O98.213 **Gonorrhea complicating pregnancy, third trimester** COM M ♀

O98.219 **Gonorrhea complicating pregnancy, unspecified trimester** COM M ♀

O98.22 **Gonorrhea complicating childbirth** COM M ♀

O98.23 **Gonorrhea complicating the puerperium** COM M ♀

O98.3 Other infections with a predominantly sexual mode of transmission complicating pregnancy, childbirth and the puerperium
Conditions in A55-A64
AHA: 2020,1Q,20

O98.31 Other infections with a predominantly sexual mode of transmission complicating pregnancy
- **O98.311 Other infections with a predominantly sexual mode of transmission complicating pregnancy, first trimester** COM M ♀
- **O98.312 Other infections with a predominantly sexual mode of transmission complicating pregnancy, second trimester** COM M ♀
- **O98.313 Other infections with a predominantly sexual mode of transmission complicating pregnancy, third trimester** COM M ♀
- **O98.319 Other infections with a predominantly sexual mode of transmission complicating pregnancy, unspecified trimester** COM M ♀

O98.32 Other infections with a predominantly sexual mode of transmission complicating childbirth COM M ♀

O98.33 Other infections with a predominantly sexual mode of transmission complicating the puerperium COM M ♀

O98.4 Viral hepatitis complicating pregnancy, childbirth and the puerperium
Conditions in B15-B19

O98.41 Viral hepatitis complicating pregnancy
- **O98.411 Viral hepatitis complicating pregnancy, first trimester** COM M ♀
- **O98.412 Viral hepatitis complicating pregnancy, second trimester** COM M ♀
- **O98.413 Viral hepatitis complicating pregnancy, third trimester** COM M ♀
- **O98.419 Viral hepatitis complicating pregnancy, unspecified trimester** COM M ♀

O98.42 Viral hepatitis complicating childbirth COM M ♀

O98.43 Viral hepatitis complicating the puerperium COM M ♀

O98.5 Other viral diseases complicating pregnancy, childbirth and the puerperium
Conditions in A8Ø-BØ9, B25-B34, R87.81-, R87.82-

EXCLUDES 1 *human immunodeficiency virus [HIV] disease complicating pregnancy, childbirth and the puerperium (O98.7-)*

TIP: Assign a code from this subcategory as the principal or first-listed diagnosis for a patient admitted/presenting during pregnancy, childbirth, or the puerperium because of COVID-19; assign U07.1 and codes for associated manifestations as secondary codes.

O98.51 Other viral diseases complicating pregnancy
- **O98.511 Other viral diseases complicating pregnancy, first trimester** COM M ♀
- **O98.512 Other viral diseases complicating pregnancy, second trimester** COM M ♀
- **O98.513 Other viral diseases complicating pregnancy, third trimester** COM M ♀
- **O98.519 Other viral diseases complicating pregnancy, unspecified trimester** COM M ♀

O98.52 Other viral diseases complicating childbirth COM M ♀

O98.53 Other viral diseases complicating the puerperium COM M ♀

O98.6 Protozoal diseases complicating pregnancy, childbirth and the puerperium
Conditions in B5Ø-B64

O98.61 Protozoal diseases complicating pregnancy
- **O98.611 Protozoal diseases complicating pregnancy, first trimester** COM M ♀
- **O98.612 Protozoal diseases complicating pregnancy, second trimester** COM M ♀
- **O98.613 Protozoal diseases complicating pregnancy, third trimester** COM M ♀
- **O98.619 Protozoal diseases complicating pregnancy, unspecified trimester** COM M ♀

O98.62 Protozoal diseases complicating childbirth COM M ♀

O98.63 Protozoal diseases complicating the puerperium COM M ♀

O98.7 Human immunodeficiency virus [HIV] disease complicating pregnancy, childbirth and the puerperium
Use additional code to identify the type of HIV disease:
- acquired immune deficiency syndrome (AIDS) (B2Ø)
- asymptomatic HIV status (Z21)
- HIV positive NOS (Z21)
- symptomatic HIV disease (B2Ø)

O98.71 Human immunodeficiency virus [HIV] disease complicating pregnancy
- **O98.711 Human immunodeficiency virus [HIV] disease complicating pregnancy, first trimester** COM M ♀
- **O98.712 Human immunodeficiency virus [HIV] disease complicating pregnancy, second trimester** COM M ♀
- **O98.713 Human immunodeficiency virus [HIV] disease complicating pregnancy, third trimester** COM M ♀
- **O98.719 Human immunodeficiency virus [HIV] disease complicating pregnancy, unspecified trimester** COM M ♀

O98.72 Human immunodeficiency virus [HIV] disease complicating childbirth COM M ♀

O98.73 Human immunodeficiency virus [HIV] disease complicating the puerperium COM M ♀

O98.8 Other maternal infectious and parasitic diseases complicating pregnancy, childbirth and the puerperium
AHA: 2020,1Q,10

O98.81 Other maternal infectious and parasitic diseases complicating pregnancy
- **O98.811 Other maternal infectious and parasitic diseases complicating pregnancy, first trimester** COM M ♀
- **O98.812 Other maternal infectious and parasitic diseases complicating pregnancy, second trimester** COM M ♀
- **O98.813 Other maternal infectious and parasitic diseases complicating pregnancy, third trimester** COM M ♀
- **O98.819 Other maternal infectious and parasitic diseases complicating pregnancy, unspecified trimester** COM M ♀

O98.82 Other maternal infectious and parasitic diseases complicating childbirth COM M ♀

O98.83 Other maternal infectious and parasitic diseases complicating the puerperium COM M ♀
AHA: 2022,2Q,5

O98.9 Unspecified maternal infectious and parasitic disease complicating pregnancy, childbirth and the puerperium

O98.91 Unspecified maternal infectious and parasitic disease complicating pregnancy
- **O98.911 Unspecified maternal infectious and parasitic disease complicating pregnancy, first trimester** COM M ♀
- **O98.912 Unspecified maternal infectious and parasitic disease complicating pregnancy, second trimester** COM M ♀
- **O98.913 Unspecified maternal infectious and parasitic disease complicating pregnancy, third trimester** COM M ♀
- **O98.919 Unspecified maternal infectious and parasitic disease complicating pregnancy, unspecified trimester** COM M ♀

O98.92 Unspecified maternal infectious and parasitic disease complicating childbirth COM M ♀

O98.93 Unspecified maternal infectious and parasitic disease complicating the puerperium COM M ♀

✓4th **O99 Other maternal diseases classifiable elsewhere but complicating pregnancy, childbirth and the puerperium**

INCLUDES conditions which complicate the pregnant state, are aggravated by the pregnancy or are a main reason for obstetric care

Use additional code to identify specific condition

EXCLUDES 2 *when the reason for maternal care is that the condition is known or suspected to have affected the fetus (O35-O36)*

✓5th **O99.Ø Anemia complicating pregnancy, childbirth and the puerperium**

Conditions in D5Ø-D64

EXCLUDES 1 *anemia arising in the puerperium (O9Ø.81)*
postpartum anemia NOS (O9Ø.81)

AHA: 2019,3Q,11

✓6th **O99.Ø1 Anemia complicating pregnancy**

AHA: 2016,1Q,4

O99.Ø11 Anemia complicating pregnancy, first trimester COM M ♀

O99.Ø12 Anemia complicating pregnancy, second trimester COM M ♀

O99.Ø13 Anemia complicating pregnancy, third trimester COM M ♀

O99.Ø19 Anemia complicating pregnancy, unspecified trimester COM M ♀

O99.Ø2 Anemia complicating childbirth COM M ♀

O99.Ø3 Anemia complicating the puerperium COM M ♀

EXCLUDES 1 *postpartum anemia not pre-existing prior to delivery (O9Ø.81)*

✓5th **O99.1 Other diseases of the blood and blood-forming organs and certain disorders involving the immune mechanism complicating pregnancy, childbirth and the puerperium**

Conditions in D65-D89

EXCLUDES 1 *hemorrhage with coagulation defects (O45.-, O46.Ø-, O67.Ø, O72.3)*

✓6th **O99.11 Other diseases of the blood and blood-forming organs and certain disorders involving the immune mechanism complicating pregnancy**

O99.111 Other diseases of the blood and blood-forming organs and certain disorders involving the immune mechanism complicating pregnancy, first trimester COM M ♀

O99.112 Other diseases of the blood and blood-forming organs and certain disorders involving the immune mechanism complicating pregnancy, second trimester COM M ♀

O99.113 Other diseases of the blood and blood-forming organs and certain disorders involving the immune mechanism complicating pregnancy, third trimester COM M ♀

O99.119 Other diseases of the blood and blood-forming organs and certain disorders involving the immune mechanism complicating pregnancy, unspecified trimester COM M ♀

O99.12 Other diseases of the blood and blood-forming organs and certain disorders involving the immune mechanism complicating childbirth COM M ♀

O99.13 Other diseases of the blood and blood-forming organs and certain disorders involving the immune mechanism complicating the puerperium COM M ♀

✓5th **O99.2 Endocrine, nutritional and metabolic diseases complicating pregnancy, childbirth and the puerperium**

Conditions in EØØ-E89

EXCLUDES 2 *diabetes mellitus (O24.-)*
malnutrition (O25.-)
postpartum thyroiditis (O9Ø.5)

✓6th **O99.21 Obesity complicating pregnancy, childbirth, and the puerperium**

Use additional code to identify the type of obesity (E66.-)

AHA: 2021,2Q,10; 2018,4Q,80

TIP: Do not assign a BMI code (Z68.-) for obese or overweight patients who are pregnant.

O99.21Ø Obesity complicating pregnancy, unspecified trimester COM M ♀

O99.211 Obesity complicating pregnancy, first trimester COM M ♀

O99.212 Obesity complicating pregnancy, second trimester COM M ♀

O99.213 Obesity complicating pregnancy, third trimester COM M ♀

O99.214 Obesity complicating childbirth COM M ♀

O99.215 Obesity complicating the puerperium COM M ♀

✓6th **O99.28 Other endocrine, nutritional and metabolic diseases complicating pregnancy, childbirth and the puerperium**

AHA: 2021,1Q,8

O99.28Ø Endocrine, nutritional and metabolic diseases complicating pregnancy, unspecified trimester COM M ♀

O99.281 Endocrine, nutritional and metabolic diseases complicating pregnancy, first trimester COM M ♀

O99.282 Endocrine, nutritional and metabolic diseases complicating pregnancy, second trimester COM M ♀

O99.283 Endocrine, nutritional and metabolic diseases complicating pregnancy, third trimester COM M ♀

O99.284 Endocrine, nutritional and metabolic diseases complicating childbirth COM M ♀

O99.285 Endocrine, nutritional and metabolic diseases complicating the puerperium COM M ♀

✓5th **O99.3 Mental disorders and diseases of the nervous system complicating pregnancy, childbirth and the puerperium**

✓6th **O99.31 Alcohol use complicating pregnancy, childbirth, and the puerperium**

Use additional code(s) from F1Ø to identify manifestations of the alcohol use

O99.31Ø Alcohol use complicating pregnancy, unspecified trimester COM M ♀

O99.311 Alcohol use complicating pregnancy, first trimester COM M ♀

O99.312 Alcohol use complicating pregnancy, second trimester COM M ♀

O99.313 Alcohol use complicating pregnancy, third trimester COM M ♀

O99.314 Alcohol use complicating childbirth COM M ♀

O99.315 Alcohol use complicating the puerperium COM M ♀

✓6th **O99.32 Drug use complicating pregnancy, childbirth, and the puerperium**

Use additional code(s) from F11-F16 and F18-F19 to identify manifestations of the drug use

AHA: 2018,4Q,69-70; 2018,2Q,10

TIP: When drug use is documented during pregnancy, assign first a code from this subcategory followed by an additional code from F11-F16 and F18-F19 identifying the specific drug use even if not documented as associated with a physical, mental, or behavioral disorder. According to chapter 15 guidelines, it is the provider's responsibility to state that the condition being treated is *not* affecting the pregnancy.

O99.32Ø Drug use complicating pregnancy, unspecified trimester COM M ♀

O99.321 Drug use complicating pregnancy, first trimester COM M ♀

O99.322 Drug use complicating pregnancy, second trimester COM M ♀

O99.323 Drug use complicating pregnancy, third trimester COM M ♀

O99.324 Drug use complicating childbirth COM M ♀

O99.325 Drug use complicating the puerperium COM M ♀

O99.33 Tobacco use disorder complicating pregnancy, childbirth, and the puerperium
Smoking complicating pregnancy, childbirth, and the puerperium
Use additional code from category F17 to identify type of tobacco nicotine dependence

O99.330 Smoking (tobacco) complicating pregnancy, unspecified trimester COM M ♀
O99.331 Smoking (tobacco) complicating pregnancy, first trimester COM M ♀
O99.332 Smoking (tobacco) complicating pregnancy, second trimester COM M ♀
O99.333 Smoking (tobacco) complicating pregnancy, third trimester COM M ♀
O99.334 Smoking (tobacco) complicating childbirth COM M ♀
O99.335 Smoking (tobacco) complicating the puerperium COM M ♀

O99.34 Other mental disorders complicating pregnancy, childbirth, and the puerperium
Conditions in F01-F09, F20-F52 and F54-F99
EXCLUDES 2 *postpartum mood disturbance (O90.6)*
postnatal psychosis (F53.1)
puerperal psychosis (F53.1)

O99.340 Other mental disorders complicating pregnancy, unspecified trimester COM Q M ♀
O99.341 Other mental disorders complicating pregnancy, first trimester COM Q M ♀
O99.342 Other mental disorders complicating pregnancy, second trimester COM Q M ♀
O99.343 Other mental disorders complicating pregnancy, third trimester COM Q M ♀
O99.344 Other mental disorders complicating childbirth COM M ♀
O99.345 Other mental disorders complicating the puerperium COM Q M ♀
AHA: 2018,4Q,8

O99.35 Diseases of the nervous system complicating pregnancy, childbirth, and the puerperium
Conditions in G00-G99
EXCLUDES 2 *pregnancy related peripheral neuritis (O26.8-)*

O99.350 Diseases of the nervous system complicating pregnancy, unspecified trimester COM M ♀
O99.351 Diseases of the nervous system complicating pregnancy, first trimester COM M ♀
O99.352 Diseases of the nervous system complicating pregnancy, second trimester COM M ♀
O99.353 Diseases of the nervous system complicating pregnancy, third trimester COM M ♀
O99.354 Diseases of the nervous system complicating childbirth COM M ♀
O99.355 Diseases of the nervous system complicating the puerperium COM M ♀

O99.4 Diseases of the circulatory system complicating pregnancy, childbirth and the puerperium
Conditions in I00-I99
EXCLUDES 1 *peripartum cardiomyopathy (O90.3)*
EXCLUDES 2 *hypertensive disorders (O10-O16)*
obstetric embolism (O88.-)
venous complications and cerebrovenous sinus thrombosis in labor, childbirth and the puerperium (O87.-)
venous complications and cerebrovenous sinus thrombosis in pregnancy (O22.-)
AHA: 2016,2Q,8

O99.41 Diseases of the circulatory system complicating pregnancy
O99.411 Diseases of the circulatory system complicating pregnancy, first trimester COM M ♀
O99.412 Diseases of the circulatory system complicating pregnancy, second trimester COM M ♀
O99.413 Diseases of the circulatory system complicating pregnancy, third trimester COM M ♀
O99.419 Diseases of the circulatory system complicating pregnancy, unspecified trimester COM M ♀
O99.42 Diseases of the circulatory system complicating childbirth COM M ♀
O99.43 Diseases of the circulatory system complicating the puerperium COM M ♀

O99.5 Diseases of the respiratory system complicating pregnancy, childbirth and the puerperium
Conditions in J00-J99

O99.51 Diseases of the respiratory system complicating pregnancy
O99.511 Diseases of the respiratory system complicating pregnancy, first trimester COM M ♀
O99.512 Diseases of the respiratory system complicating pregnancy, second trimester COM M ♀
O99.513 Diseases of the respiratory system complicating pregnancy, third trimester COM M ♀
O99.519 Diseases of the respiratory system complicating pregnancy, unspecified trimester COM M ♀
O99.52 Diseases of the respiratory system complicating childbirth COM M ♀
O99.53 Diseases of the respiratory system complicating the puerperium COM M ♀

O99.6 Diseases of the digestive system complicating pregnancy, childbirth and the puerperium
Conditions in K00-K93
EXCLUDES 2 *hemorrhoids in pregnancy (O22.4-)*
liver and biliary tract disorders in pregnancy, childbirth and the puerperium (O26.6-)

O99.61 Diseases of the digestive system complicating pregnancy
AHA: 2016,1Q,4
O99.611 Diseases of the digestive system complicating pregnancy, first trimester COM M ♀
O99.612 Diseases of the digestive system complicating pregnancy, second trimester COM M ♀
O99.613 Diseases of the digestive system complicating pregnancy, third trimester COM M ♀
O99.619 Diseases of the digestive system complicating pregnancy, unspecified trimester COM M ♀
O99.62 Diseases of the digestive system complicating childbirth COM M ♀
O99.63 Diseases of the digestive system complicating the puerperium COM M ♀

O99.7 Diseases of the skin and subcutaneous tissue complicating pregnancy, childbirth and the puerperium
Conditions in L00-L99
EXCLUDES 2 *herpes gestationis (O26.4)*
pruritic urticarial papules and plaques of pregnancy (PUPPP) (O26.86)

O99.71 Diseases of the skin and subcutaneous tissue complicating pregnancy
O99.711 Diseases of the skin and subcutaneous tissue complicating pregnancy, first trimester COM M ♀
O99.712 Diseases of the skin and subcutaneous tissue complicating pregnancy, second trimester COM M ♀
O99.713 Diseases of the skin and subcutaneous tissue complicating pregnancy, third trimester COM M ♀
O99.719 Diseases of the skin and subcutaneous tissue complicating pregnancy, unspecified trimester COM M ♀
O99.72 Diseases of the skin and subcutaneous tissue complicating childbirth COM M ♀

O99.73 Diseases of the skin and subcutaneous tissue complicating the puerperium COM M ♀

✓5th **O99.8 Other specified diseases and conditions complicating pregnancy, childbirth and the puerperium**
Conditions in DØØ-D48, HØØ-H95, MØØ-N99, and QØØ-Q99
Use additional code to identify condition
EXCLUDES 2 *genitourinary infections in pregnancy (O23.-)*
infection of genitourinary tract following delivery (O86.1-O86.4)
malignant neoplasm complicating pregnancy, childbirth and the puerperium (O9A.1-)
maternal care for known or suspected abnormality of maternal pelvic organs (O34.-)
postpartum acute kidney failure (O9Ø.4)
traumatic injuries in pregnancy (O9A.2-)

✓6th **O99.81 Abnormal glucose complicating pregnancy, childbirth and the puerperium**
EXCLUDES 1 *gestational diabetes (O24.4-)*

O99.81Ø Abnormal glucose complicating pregnancy COM M ♀

O99.814 Abnormal glucose complicating childbirth COM M ♀

O99.815 Abnormal glucose complicating the puerperium COM M ♀

✓6th **O99.82 Streptococcus B carrier state complicating pregnancy, childbirth and the puerperium**
EXCLUDES 1 *carrier of streptococcus group B (GBS) in a nonpregnant woman (Z22.33Ø)*
DEF: *Streptococcus* group B colonization: Bacteria normally found in the vagina or lower intestine of many healthy adult women that may infect the fetus during childbirth, causing mental or physical handicaps or death. Women who test positive for *Streptococcus* group B during pregnancy are considered a "colonized" status and are treated with IV antibiotics at the time of delivery and may also be treated with oral antibiotics during the pregnancy.

O99.82Ø Streptococcus B carrier state complicating pregnancy COM M ♀

O99.824 Streptococcus B carrier state complicating childbirth COM M ♀
AHA: 2019,2Q,8

O99.825 Streptococcus B carrier state complicating the puerperium COM M ♀

✓6th **O99.83 Other infection carrier state complicating pregnancy, childbirth and the puerperium**
Use additional code to identify the carrier state (Z22.-)

O99.83Ø Other infection carrier state complicating pregnancy COM M ♀

O99.834 Other infection carrier state complicating childbirth COM M ♀

O99.835 Other infection carrier state complicating the puerperium COM M ♀

✓6th **O99.84 Bariatric surgery status complicating pregnancy, childbirth and the puerperium**
Gastric banding status complicating pregnancy, childbirth and the puerperium
Gastric bypass status for obesity complicating pregnancy, childbirth and the puerperium
Obesity surgery status complicating pregnancy, childbirth and the puerperium

O99.84Ø Bariatric surgery status complicating pregnancy, unspecified trimester COM M ♀

O99.841 Bariatric surgery status complicating pregnancy, first trimester COM M ♀

O99.842 Bariatric surgery status complicating pregnancy, second trimester COM M ♀

O99.843 Bariatric surgery status complicating pregnancy, third trimester COM M ♀

O99.844 Bariatric surgery status complicating childbirth COM M ♀

O99.845 Bariatric surgery status complicating the puerperium COM M ♀

✓6th **O99.89 Other specified diseases and conditions complicating pregnancy, childbirth and the puerperium**
AHA: 2020,4Q,36-37

O99.891 Other specified diseases and conditions complicating pregnancy COM M ♀

O99.892 Other specified diseases and conditions complicating childbirth COM M ♀

O99.893 Other specified diseases and conditions complicating puerperium COM M ♀

✓4th **O9A Maternal malignant neoplasms, traumatic injuries and abuse classifiable elsewhere but complicating pregnancy, childbirth and the puerperium**

✓5th **O9A.1 Malignant neoplasm complicating pregnancy, childbirth and the puerperium**
Conditions in CØØ-C96
Use additional code to identify neoplasm
EXCLUDES 2 *maternal care for benign tumor of corpus uteri (O34.1-)*
maternal care for benign tumor of cervix (O34.4-)
AHA: 2015,3Q,19

✓6th **O9A.11 Malignant neoplasm complicating pregnancy**

O9A.111 Malignant neoplasm complicating pregnancy, first trimester COM M ♀

O9A.112 Malignant neoplasm complicating pregnancy, second trimester COM M ♀

O9A.113 Malignant neoplasm complicating pregnancy, third trimester COM M ♀

O9A.119 Malignant neoplasm complicating pregnancy, unspecified trimester COM M ♀

O9A.12 Malignant neoplasm complicating childbirth COM M ♀

O9A.13 Malignant neoplasm complicating the puerperium COM M ♀

✓5th **O9A.2 Injury, poisoning and certain other consequences of external causes complicating pregnancy, childbirth and the puerperium**
Conditions in SØØ-T88, except T74 and T76
Use additional code(s) to identify the injury or poisoning
EXCLUDES 2 *physical, sexual and psychological abuse complicating pregnancy, childbirth and the puerperium (O9A.3-, O9A.4-, O9A.5-)*

✓6th **O9A.21 Injury, poisoning and certain other consequences of external causes complicating pregnancy**

O9A.211 Injury, poisoning and certain other consequences of external causes complicating pregnancy, first trimester COM M ♀

O9A.212 Injury, poisoning and certain other consequences of external causes complicating pregnancy, second trimester COM M ♀

O9A.213 Injury, poisoning and certain other consequences of external causes complicating pregnancy, third trimester COM M ♀

O9A.219 Injury, poisoning and certain other consequences of external causes complicating pregnancy, unspecified trimester COM M ♀

O9A.22 Injury, poisoning and certain other consequences of external causes complicating childbirth COM M ♀

O9A.23 Injury, poisoning and certain other consequences of external causes complicating the puerperium COM M ♀

✓5th **O9A.3 Physical abuse complicating pregnancy, childbirth and the puerperium**
Conditions in T74.11 or T76.11
Use additional code (if applicable):
to identify any associated current injury due to physical abuse
to identify the perpetrator of abuse (YØ7.-)
EXCLUDES 2 *sexual abuse complicating pregnancy, childbirth and the puerperium (O9A.4)*

✓6th **O9A.31 Physical abuse complicating pregnancy**

O9A.311 Physical abuse complicating pregnancy, first trimester COM M ♀

O9A.312 Physical abuse complicating pregnancy, second trimester COM M ♀

O9A.313 Physical abuse complicating pregnancy, third trimester COM M ♀

O9A.319 Physical abuse complicating pregnancy, unspecified trimester COM M ♀

O9A.32 Physical abuse complicating childbirth COM M ♀

O9A.33 **Physical abuse complicating the puerperium** COM M ♀

✓5th **O9A.4 Sexual abuse complicating pregnancy, childbirth and the puerperium**
Conditions in T74.21 or T76.21
Use additional code (if applicable):
to identify any associated current injury due to sexual abuse
to identify the perpetrator of abuse (YØ7.-)

✓6th **O9A.41 Sexual abuse complicating pregnancy**

O9A.411 **Sexual abuse complicating pregnancy, first trimester** COM M ♀

O9A.412 **Sexual abuse complicating pregnancy, second trimester** COM M ♀

O9A.413 **Sexual abuse complicating pregnancy, third trimester** COM M ♀

O9A.419 **Sexual abuse complicating pregnancy, unspecified trimester** COM M ♀

O9A.42 **Sexual abuse complicating childbirth** COM M ♀

O9A.43 **Sexual abuse complicating the puerperium** COM M ♀

✓5th **O9A.5 Psychological abuse complicating pregnancy, childbirth and the puerperium**
Conditions in T74.31 or T76.31
Use additional code to identify the perpetrator of abuse (YØ7.-)

✓6th **O9A.51 Psychological abuse complicating pregnancy**

O9A.511 **Psychological abuse complicating pregnancy, first trimester** COM M ♀

O9A.512 **Psychological abuse complicating pregnancy, second trimester** COM M ♀

O9A.513 **Psychological abuse complicating pregnancy, third trimester** COM M ♀

O9A.519 **Psychological abuse complicating pregnancy, unspecified trimester** COM M ♀

O9A.52 **Psychological abuse complicating childbirth** COM M ♀

O9A.53 **Psychological abuse complicating the puerperium** COM M ♀

Chapter 16. Certain Conditions Originating in the Perinatal Period (PØØ–P96)

Chapter-specific Guidelines with Coding Examples

The chapter-specific guidelines from the ICD-10-CM Official Guidelines for Coding and Reporting have been provided below. Along with these guidelines are coding examples, contained in the shaded boxes, that have been developed to help illustrate the coding and/or sequencing guidance found in these guidelines.

For coding and reporting purposes the perinatal period is defined as before birth through the 28th day following birth. The following guidelines are provided for reporting purposes

a. General perinatal rules

1) Use of Chapter 16 codes

Codes in this chapter are never for use on the maternal record. Codes from Chapter 15, the obstetric chapter, are never permitted on the newborn record. Chapter 16 codes may be used throughout the life of the patient if the condition is still present.

2) Principal diagnosis for birth record

When coding the birth episode in a newborn record, assign a code from category Z38, Liveborn infants according to place of birth and type of delivery, as the principal diagnosis. A code from category Z38 is assigned only once, to a newborn at the time of birth. If a newborn is transferred to another institution, a code from category Z38 should not be used at the receiving hospital.

A code from category Z38 is used only on the newborn record, not on the mother's record.

3) Use of codes from other chapters with codes from Chapter 16

Codes from other chapters may be used with codes from chapter 16 if the codes from the other chapters provide more specific detail. Codes for signs and symptoms may be assigned when a definitive diagnosis has not been established. If the reason for the encounter is a perinatal condition, the code from chapter 16 should be sequenced first.

4) Use of Chapter 16 codes after the perinatal period

Should a condition originate in the perinatal period, and continue throughout the life of the patient, the perinatal code should continue to be used regardless of the patient's age.

A 7-year-old patient with history of birth injury that resulted in Erb's palsy is seen for subscapularis release

P14.Ø	**Erb's paralysis due to birth injury**

Explanation: Although in this instance Erb's palsy is specifically related to a birth injury, it has not resolved and continues to be a health concern. A perinatal code is appropriate even though this patient is beyond the perinatal period.

5) Birth process or community acquired conditions

If a newborn has a condition that may be either due to the birth process or community acquired and the documentation does not indicate which it is, the default is due to the birth process and the code from Chapter 16 should be used. If the condition is community-acquired, a code from Chapter 16 should not be assigned.

For COVID-19 infection in a newborn, see guideline I.C.16.h.

6) Code all clinically significant conditions

All clinically significant conditions noted on routine newborn examination should be coded. A condition is clinically significant if it requires:

clinical evaluation; or

therapeutic treatment; or

diagnostic procedures; or

extended length of hospital stay; or

increased nursing care and/or monitoring; or

has implications for future health care needs

Note: The perinatal guidelines listed above are the same as the general coding guidelines for "additional diagnoses", except for the final point regarding implications for future health care needs. Codes should be assigned for conditions that have been specified by the provider as having implications for future health care needs.

b. Observation and evaluation of newborns for suspected conditions not found

1) Use of Z05 codes

Assign a code from category ZØ5, Observation and evaluation of newborn for suspected **diseases and** conditions ruled out, to identify those instances when a healthy newborn is evaluated for a suspected condition/**disease** that is determined after study not to be present. Do not use a code from category ZØ5 when the patient **is documented to have** signs or symptoms of a suspected problem; in such cases code the sign or symptom.

2) Z05 on other than the birth record

A code from category ZØ5 may also be assigned as a principal or first-listed code for readmissions or encounters when the code from category Z38 code no longer applies. Codes from category ZØ5 are for use only for healthy newborns and infants for which no condition after study is found to be present.

3) Z05 on a birth record

A code from category ZØ5 is to be used as a secondary code after the code from category Z38, Liveborn infants according to place of birth and type of delivery.

Newborn delivered via vaginal delivery; previous ultrasounds showed what appeared to be an abnormality of the right kidney. Kidney function tests were performed and ultrasounds taken and any genitourinary conditions ruled out.

Z38.ØØ	**Single liveborn infant, delivered vaginally**
ZØ5.6	**Observation and evaluation of newborn for suspected genitourinary condition ruled out**

Explanation: The newborn had no signs or symptoms of kidney or other genitourinary condition but was evaluated after delivery due to the abnormal prenatal ultrasound findings. A Z code describing the type and place of birth should be coded first, followed by a ZØ5 category code for the work performed to rule out a suspected genitourinary condition.

c. Coding additional perinatal diagnoses

1) Assigning codes for conditions that require treatment

Assign codes for conditions that require treatment or further investigation, prolong the length of stay, or require resource utilization.

2) Codes for conditions specified as having implications for future health care needs

Assign codes for conditions that have been specified by the provider as having implications for future health care needs.

Note: This guideline should not be used for adult patients.

An abnormal noise was heard in the left hip of a post-term newborn during a physical examination. The pediatrician would like to follow the patient after discharge as a hip click can be an early sign of hip dysplasia. The newborn was delivered via cesarean at 41 weeks.

Z38.Ø1	**Single liveborn infant, delivered by cesarean**
PØ8.21	**Post-term newborn**
R29.4	**Clicking hip**

Explanation: The abnormal hip noise or click is appended as a secondary diagnosis not only because it is an abnormal finding upon examination, but also due to its potential to be part of a bigger health issue. The hip dysplasia has not yet been diagnosed and does not warrant a code at this time.

d. Prematurity and fetal growth retardation

Providers utilize different criteria in determining prematurity. A code for prematurity should not be assigned unless it is documented. Assignment of codes in categories PØ5, Disorders of newborn related to slow fetal growth and fetal malnutrition, and PØ7, Disorders of newborn related to short gestation and low birth weight, not elsewhere classified, should be based on the recorded birth weight and estimated gestational age.

When both birth weight and gestational age are available, two codes from category PØ7 should be assigned, with the code for birth weight sequenced before the code for gestational age.

e. Low birth weight and immaturity status

Codes from category PØ7, Disorders of newborn related to short gestation and low birth weight, not elsewhere classified, are for use for a child or adult who was premature or had a low birth weight as a newborn and this is affecting the patient's current health status.

See Section I.C.21. Factors influencing health status and contact with health services, Status.

A 35-year-old patient, who weighed 659 grams at birth, is seen for heart disease documented as being a consequence of the low birth weight

I51.9	**Heart disease, unspecified**
PØ7.Ø2	**Extremely low birth weight newborn, 5ØØ–749 grams**

Explanation: A code from subcategories PØ7.Ø- and PØ7.1- is appropriate, regardless of the age of the patient, as long as the documentation provides a clear link between the patient's current illness and the low birth weight.

f. Bacterial sepsis of newborn

Category P36, Bacterial sepsis of newborn, includes congenital sepsis. If a perinate is documented as having sepsis without documentation of congenital or community acquired, the default is congenital and a code from category P36 should be assigned. If the P36 code includes the causal organism, an additional code from category B95, Streptococcus, Staphylococcus, and Enterococcus as the cause of diseases classified elsewhere, or B96, Other bacterial agents as the cause of diseases classified elsewhere, should not be assigned. If the P36 code does not include the causal organism, assign an additional code from category B96. If applicable, use additional codes to identify severe sepsis (R65.2-) and any associated acute organ dysfunction.

A full-term infant develops severe sepsis 24 hours after discharge from the hospital and is readmitted; cultures identified *E. coli* as the infective agent

P36.4	**Sepsis of newborn due to Escherichia coli**
R65.2Ø	**Severe sepsis without septic shock**

Explanation: Even though this newborn was discharged and could have acquired *E. coli* from his/her external environment, due to the lack of documentation specifying specifically how this pathogen was acquired, the default is to code the *E. coli* sepsis as congenital. A code from chapter 1, "Certain Infectious and Parasitic Diseases," is not required because the perinatal sepsis code identifies both the sepsis and the bacteria causing the sepsis.

g. Stillbirth

Code P95, Stillbirth, is only for use in institutions that maintain separate records for stillbirths. No other code should be used with P95. Code P95 should not be used on the mother's record.

h. COVID-19 infection in newborn

For a newborn that tests positive for COVID-19, assign code UØ7.1, COVID-19, and the appropriate codes for associated manifestation(s) in neonates/newborns in the absence of documentation indicating a specific type of transmission. For a newborn that tests positive for COVID-19 and the provider documents the condition was contracted in utero or during the birth process, assign codes P35.8, Other congenital viral diseases, and UØ7.1, COVID-19. When coding the birth episode in a newborn record, the appropriate code from category Z38, Liveborn infants according to place of birth and type of delivery, should be assigned as the principal diagnosis.

Chapter 16. Certain Conditions Originating in the Perinatal Period (P00-P96)

NOTE Codes from this chapter are for use on newborn records only, never on maternal records

INCLUDES conditions that have their origin in the fetal or perinatal period (before birth through the first 28 days after birth) even if morbidity occurs later

EXCLUDES 2 *congenital malformations, deformations and chromosomal abnormalities (Q00-Q99)*
endocrine, nutritional and metabolic diseases (E00-E88)
injury, poisoning and certain other consequences of external causes (S00-T88)
neoplasms (C00-D49)
tetanus neonatorum (A33)

This chapter contains the following blocks:

- P00-P04 Newborn affected by maternal factors and by complications of pregnancy, labor, and delivery
- P05-P08 Disorders of newborn related to length of gestation and fetal growth
- P09 Abnormal findings on neonatal screening
- P10-P15 Birth trauma
- P19-P29 Respiratory and cardiovascular disorders specific to the perinatal period
- P35-P39 Infections specific to the perinatal period
- P50-P61 Hemorrhagic and hematological disorders of newborn
- P70-P74 Transitory endocrine and metabolic disorders specific to newborn
- P76-P78 Digestive system disorders of newborn
- P80-P83 Conditions involving the integument and temperature regulation of newborn
- P84 Other problems with newborn
- P90-P96 Other disorders originating in the perinatal period

Newborn affected by maternal factors and by complications of pregnancy, labor, and delivery (P00-P04)

NOTE These codes are for use when the listed maternal conditions are specified as the cause of confirmed morbidity or potential morbidity which have their origin in the perinatal period (before birth through the first 28 days after birth).

AHA: 2016,4Q,54-55

P00 Newborn affected by maternal conditions that may be unrelated to present pregnancy

Code first any current condition in newborn

EXCLUDES 2 *encounter for observation of newborn for suspected diseases and conditions ruled out (Z05.-)*
newborn affected by maternal complications of pregnancy (P01.-)
newborn affected by maternal endocrine and metabolic disorders (P70-P74)
newborn affected by noxious substances transmitted via placenta or breast milk (P04.-)

P00.0 Newborn affected by maternal hypertensive disorders
Newborn affected by maternal conditions classifiable to O10-O11, O13-O16

P00.1 Newborn affected by maternal renal and urinary tract diseases
Newborn affected by maternal conditions classifiable to N00-N39

P00.2 Newborn affected by maternal infectious and parasitic diseases
Newborn affected by maternal infectious disease classifiable to A00-B99, J09 and J10

EXCLUDES 1 *maternal genital tract or other localized infections (P00.8)*

EXCLUDES 2 *infections specific to the perinatal period (P35-P39)*
newborn affected by (positive) maternal group B streptococcus (GBS) colonization (P00.82)

AHA: 2019,2Q,10; 2015,3Q,20

P00.3 Newborn affected by other maternal circulatory and respiratory diseases
Newborn affected by maternal conditions classifiable to I00-I99, J00-J99, Q20-Q34 and not included in P00.0, P00.2

P00.4 Newborn affected by maternal nutritional disorders
Newborn affected by maternal disorders classifiable to E40-E64
Maternal malnutrition NOS

P00.5 Newborn affected by maternal injury
Newborn affected by maternal conditions classifiable to O9A.2-

P00.6 Newborn affected by surgical procedure on mother
Newborn affected by amniocentesis

EXCLUDES 1 *Cesarean delivery for present delivery (P03.4)*
damage to placenta from amniocentesis, Cesarean delivery or surgical induction (P02.1)
previous surgery to uterus or pelvic organs (P03.89)

EXCLUDES 2 *newborn affected by complication of (fetal) intrauterine procedure (P96.5)*

P00.7 Newborn affected by other medical procedures on mother, not elsewhere classified
Newborn affected by radiation to mother

EXCLUDES 1 *damage to placenta from amniocentesis, cesarean delivery or surgical induction (P02.1)*
newborn affected by other complications of labor and delivery (P03.-)

P00.8 Newborn affected by other maternal conditions

P00.81 Newborn affected by periodontal disease in mother

P00.82 Newborn affected by (positive) maternal group B streptococcus (GBS) colonization
Contact with positive maternal group B streptococcus

AHA: 2021,4Q,23

P00.89 Newborn affected by other maternal conditions
Newborn affected by conditions classifiable to T80-T88
Newborn affected by maternal genital tract or other localized infections
Newborn affected by maternal systemic lupus erythematosus
Use additional code to identify infectious agent, if known

EXCLUDES 2 *newborn affected by positive maternal group B streptococcus (GBS) colonization (P00.82)*

AHA: 2019,2Q,9

P00.9 Newborn affected by unspecified maternal condition

P01 Newborn affected by maternal complications of pregnancy

Code first any current condition in newborn

EXCLUDES 2 *encounter for observation of newborn for suspected diseases and conditions ruled out (Z05.-)*

P01.0 Newborn affected by incompetent cervix

P01.1 Newborn affected by premature rupture of membranes

P01.2 Newborn affected by oligohydramnios

EXCLUDES 1 *oligohydramnios due to premature rupture of membranes (P01.1)*

DEF: Low amniotic fluid level, resulting in underdeveloped organs in the fetus.

P01.3 Newborn affected by polyhydramnios
Newborn affected by hydramnios

DEF: Excess amniotic fluid surrounding the fetus, typically defined as a total fluid volume of greater than 24 cm.

P01.4 Newborn affected by ectopic pregnancy
Newborn affected by abdominal pregnancy

P01.5 Newborn affected by multiple pregnancy
Newborn affected by triplet (pregnancy)
Newborn affected by twin (pregnancy)

P01.6 Newborn affected by maternal death

P01.7 Newborn affected by malpresentation before labor
Newborn affected by breech presentation before labor
Newborn affected by external version before labor
Newborn affected by face presentation before labor
Newborn affected by transverse lie before labor
Newborn affected by unstable lie before labor

P01.8 Newborn affected by other maternal complications of pregnancy

P01.9 Newborn affected by maternal complication of pregnancy, unspecified

P02 Newborn affected by complications of placenta, cord and membranes

Code first any current condition in newborn

EXCLUDES 2 *encounter for observation of newborn for suspected diseases and conditions ruled out (Z05.-)*

P02.0 Newborn affected by placenta previa

DEF: Placenta developed in the lower segment of the uterus that can cause hemorrhaging leading to preterm delivery.

PØ2.1 Newborn affected by other forms of placental separation and hemorrhage
Newborn affected by abruptio placenta
Newborn affected by accidental hemorrhage
Newborn affected by antepartum hemorrhage
Newborn affected by damage to placenta from amniocentesis, cesarean delivery or surgical induction
Newborn affected by maternal blood loss
Newborn affected by premature separation of placenta

√5th PØ2.2 Newborn affected by other and unspecified morphological and functional abnormalities of placenta

PØ2.2Ø Newborn affected by unspecified morphological and functional abnormalities of placenta

PØ2.29 Newborn affected by other morphological and functional abnormalities of placenta
Newborn affected by placental dysfunction
Newborn affected by placental infarction
Newborn affected by placental insufficiency

PØ2.3 Newborn affected by placental transfusion syndromes
Newborn affected by placental and cord abnormalities resulting in twin-to-twin or other transplacental transfusion

PØ2.4 Newborn affected by prolapsed cord

PØ2.5 Newborn affected by other compression of umbilical cord
Newborn affected by umbilical cord (tightly) around neck
Newborn affected by entanglement of umbilical cord
Newborn affected by knot in umbilical cord
AHA: 2022,1Q,22

√5th PØ2.6 Newborn affected by other and unspecified conditions of umbilical cord

PØ2.6Ø Newborn affected by unspecified conditions of umbilical cord

PØ2.69 Newborn affected by other conditions of umbilical cord
Newborn affected by short umbilical cord
Newborn affected by vasa previa
EXCLUDES 1 *newborn affected by single umbilical artery (Q27.Ø)*

√5th PØ2.7 Newborn affected by chorioamnionitis
AHA: 2018,4Q,23-24
DEF: Inflammation of the fetal membranes due to maternal infection characterized by fetal tachycardia, respiratory distress, apnea, weak cries, and poor sucking.

PØ2.7Ø Newborn affected by fetal inflammatory response syndrome HCC ESR COM
Newborn affected by FIRS

PØ2.78 Newborn affected by other conditions from chorioamnionitis
Newborn affected by amnionitis
Newborn affected by membranitis
Newborn affected by placentitis

PØ2.8 Newborn affected by other abnormalities of membranes

PØ2.9 Newborn affected by abnormality of membranes, unspecified

√4th PØ3 Newborn affected by other complications of labor and delivery
Code first any current condition in newborn
EXCLUDES 2 *encounter for observation of newborn for suspected diseases and conditions ruled out (ZØ5.-)*

PØ3.Ø Newborn affected by breech delivery and extraction

PØ3.1 Newborn affected by other malpresentation, malposition and disproportion during labor and delivery
Newborn affected by contracted pelvis
Newborn affected by conditions classifiable to O64-O66
Newborn affected by persistent occipitoposterior
Newborn affected by transverse lie

PØ3.2 Newborn affected by forceps delivery

Forceps Assisted Birth

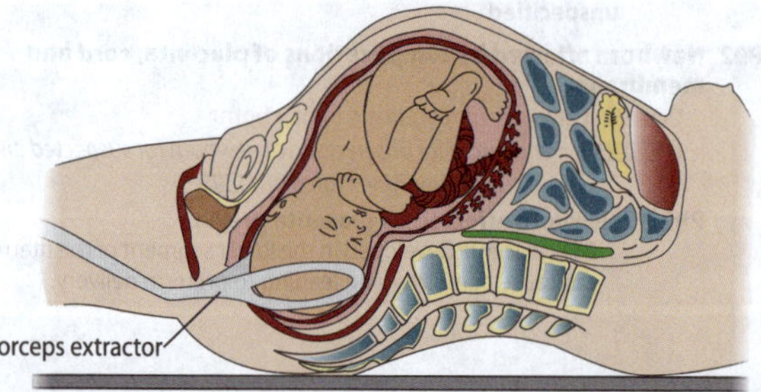

PØ3.3 Newborn affected by delivery by vacuum extractor [ventouse]

Vacuum Assisted Birth

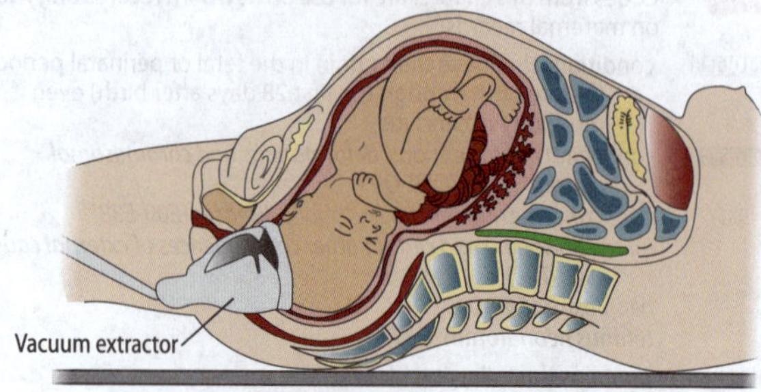

PØ3.4 Newborn affected by Cesarean delivery

PØ3.5 Newborn affected by precipitate delivery
Newborn affected by rapid second stage

PØ3.6 Newborn affected by abnormal uterine contractions
Newborn affected by conditions classifiable to O62.-, except O62.3
Newborn affected by hypertonic labor
Newborn affected by uterine inertia

√5th PØ3.8 Newborn affected by other specified complications of labor and delivery

√6th PØ3.81 Newborn affected by abnormality in fetal (intrauterine) heart rate or rhythm
EXCLUDES 1 *neonatal cardiac dysrhythmia (P29.1-)*

PØ3.81Ø Newborn affected by abnormality in fetal (intrauterine) heart rate or rhythm before the onset of labor

PØ3.811 Newborn affected by abnormality in fetal (intrauterine) heart rate or rhythm during labor

PØ3.819 Newborn affected by abnormality in fetal (intrauterine) heart rate or rhythm, unspecified as to time of onset

PØ3.82 Meconium passage during delivery
EXCLUDES 1 *meconium aspiration (P24.ØØ, P24.Ø1)*
meconium staining (P96.83)
DEF: Fetal intestinal activity that increases in response to a fetomaternal distressed state during delivery. The anal sphincter relaxes and meconium is passed into the amniotic fluid.

PØ3.89 Newborn affected by other specified complications of labor and delivery
Newborn affected by abnormality of maternal soft tissues
Newborn affected by conditions classifiable to O6Ø-O75 and by procedures used in labor and delivery not included in PØ2.- and PØ3.Ø-PØ3.6
Newborn affected by induction of labor

PØ3.9 Newborn affected by complication of labor and delivery, unspecified

√4th PØ4 Newborn affected by noxious substances transmitted via placenta or breast milk
INCLUDES nonteratogenic effects of substances transmitted via placenta
Code first any current condition in newborn, if applicable
EXCLUDES 2 *congenital malformations (QØØ-Q99)*
encounter for observation of newborn for suspected diseases and conditions ruled out (ZØ5.-)
neonatal jaundice from excessive hemolysis due to drugs or toxins transmitted from mother (P58.4)
newborn in contact with and (suspected) exposures hazardous to health not transmitted via placenta or breast milk (Z77.-)

PØ4.Ø Newborn affected by maternal anesthesia and analgesia in pregnancy, labor and delivery COM
Newborn affected by reactions and intoxications from maternal opiates and tranquilizers administered for procedures during pregnancy or labor and delivery
EXCLUDES 2 *newborn affected by other maternal medication (PØ4.1-)*

P04.1 **Newborn affected by other maternal medication**

Code first withdrawal symptoms from maternal use of drugs of addiction, if applicable (P96.1)

EXCLUDES 1 *dysmorphism due to warfarin (Q86.2)*
fetal hydantoin syndrome (Q86.1)

EXCLUDES 2 *maternal anesthesia and analgesia in pregnancy, labor and delivery (P04.0)*
maternal use of drugs of addiction (P04.4-)

AHA: 2018,4Q,24-25

P04.11 **Newborn affected by maternal antineoplastic chemotherapy** COM

P04.12 **Newborn affected by maternal cytotoxic drugs** COM

P04.13 **Newborn affected by maternal use of anticonvulsants** COM

P04.14 **Newborn affected by maternal use of opiates** COM

P04.15 **Newborn affected by maternal use of antidepressants** COM

P04.16 **Newborn affected by maternal use of amphetamines** COM

P04.17 **Newborn affected by maternal use of sedative-hypnotics** COM

P04.1A **Newborn affected by maternal use of anxiolytics** COM

P04.18 **Newborn affected by other maternal medication** COM

P04.19 **Newborn affected by maternal use of unspecified medication** COM

P04.2 **Newborn affected by maternal use of tobacco** COM

Newborn affected by exposure in utero to tobacco smoke

EXCLUDES 2 *newborn exposure to environmental tobacco smoke (P96.81)*

P04.3 **Newborn affected by maternal use of alcohol** COM

EXCLUDES 1 *fetal alcohol syndrome (Q86.0)*

P04.4 **Newborn affected by maternal use of drugs of addiction**

AHA: 2018,4Q,25

P04.40 **Newborn affected by maternal use of unspecified drugs of addiction** COM

P04.41 **Newborn affected by maternal use of cocaine** COM

P04.42 **Newborn affected by maternal use of hallucinogens** COM

EXCLUDES 2 *newborn affected by other maternal medication (P04.1-)*

P04.49 **Newborn affected by maternal use of other drugs of addiction** COM

EXCLUDES 2 *newborn affected by maternal anesthesia and analgesia (P04.0)*
withdrawal symptoms from maternal use of drugs of addiction (P96.1)

P04.5 **Newborn affected by maternal use of nutritional chemical substances** COM

P04.6 **Newborn affected by maternal exposure to environmental chemical substances** COM

P04.8 **Newborn affected by other maternal noxious substances**

AHA: 2018,4Q,25

P04.81 **Newborn affected by maternal use of cannabis** COM

P04.89 **Newborn affected by other maternal noxious substances** COM

P04.9 **Newborn affected by maternal noxious substance, unspecified** COM

Disorders of newborn related to length of gestation and fetal growth (P05-P08)

P05 **Disorders of newborn related to slow fetal growth and fetal malnutrition**

AHA: 2016,4Q,55-56

P05.0 **Newborn light for gestational age**

Newborn light-for-dates

Weight below but length above 10th percentile for gestational age

P05.00 **Newborn light for gestational age, unspecified weight** COM

P05.01 **Newborn light for gestational age, less than 500 grams** COM

P05.02 **Newborn light for gestational age, 500-749 grams** COM

P05.03 **Newborn light for gestational age, 750-999 grams** COM

P05.04 **Newborn light for gestational age, 1000-1249 grams** COM

P05.05 **Newborn light for gestational age, 1250-1499 grams** COM

P05.06 **Newborn light for gestational age, 1500-1749 grams** COM

P05.07 **Newborn light for gestational age, 1750-1999 grams** COM

P05.08 **Newborn light for gestational age, 2000-2499 grams** COM

P05.09 **Newborn light for gestational age, 2500 grams and over** COM

Newborn light for gestational age, other

P05.1 **Newborn small for gestational age**

Newborn small-and-light-for-dates

Newborn small-for-dates

Weight and length below 10th percentile for gestational age

P05.10 **Newborn small for gestational age, unspecified weight** COM

P05.11 **Newborn small for gestational age, less than 500 grams** COM

P05.12 **Newborn small for gestational age, 500-749 grams** COM

P05.13 **Newborn small for gestational age, 750-999 grams** COM

P05.14 **Newborn small for gestational age, 1000-1249 grams** COM

P05.15 **Newborn small for gestational age, 1250-1499 grams** COM

P05.16 **Newborn small for gestational age, 1500-1749 grams** COM

P05.17 **Newborn small for gestational age, 1750-1999 grams** COM

P05.18 **Newborn small for gestational age, 2000-2499 grams** COM

P05.19 **Newborn small for gestational age, other** COM

Newborn small for gestational age, 2500 grams and over

P05.2 **Newborn affected by fetal (intrauterine) malnutrition not light or small for gestational age** COM

Infant, not light or small for gestational age, showing signs of fetal malnutrition, such as dry, peeling skin and loss of subcutaneous tissue

EXCLUDES 1 *newborn affected by fetal malnutrition with light for gestational age (P05.0-)*
newborn affected by fetal malnutrition with small for gestational age (P05.1-)

P05.9 **Newborn affected by slow intrauterine growth, unspecified** COM

Newborn affected by fetal growth retardation NOS

P07 **Disorders of newborn related to short gestation and low birth weight, not elsewhere classified**

NOTE When both birth weight and gestational age of the newborn are available, both should be coded with birth weight sequenced before gestational age

INCLUDES the listed conditions, without further specification, as the cause of morbidity or additional care, in newborn

P07.0 **Extremely low birth weight newborn**

Newborn birth weight 999 g. or less

EXCLUDES 1 *low birth weight due to slow fetal growth and fetal malnutrition (P05.-)*

P07.00 **Extremely low birth weight newborn, unspecified weight** COM

P07.01 **Extremely low birth weight newborn, less than 500 grams** COM

P07.02 **Extremely low birth weight newborn, 500-749 grams** COM

P07.03 **Extremely low birth weight newborn, 750-999 grams** COM

P07.1 Other low birth weight newborn

Newborn birth weight 1000-2499 g.

EXCLUDES 1 *low birth weight due to slow fetal growth and fetal malnutrition (P05.-)*

P07.10 Other low birth weight newborn, unspecified weight COM

P07.14 Other low birth weight newborn, 1000-1249 grams COM

P07.15 Other low birth weight newborn, 1250-1499 grams COM

P07.16 Other low birth weight newborn, 1500-1749 grams COM

P07.17 Other low birth weight newborn, 1750-1999 grams COM

P07.18 Other low birth weight newborn, 2000-2499 grams COM

P07.2 Extreme immaturity of newborn

Less than 28 completed weeks (less than 196 completed days) of gestation.

P07.20 Extreme immaturity of newborn, unspecified weeks of gestation COM

Gestational age less than 28 completed weeks NOS

P07.21 Extreme immaturity of newborn, gestational age less than 23 completed weeks COM

Extreme immaturity of newborn, gestational age less than 23 weeks, 0 days

P07.22 Extreme immaturity of newborn, gestational age 23 completed weeks COM

Extreme immaturity of newborn, gestational age 23 weeks, 0 days through 23 weeks, 6 days

P07.23 Extreme immaturity of newborn, gestational age 24 completed weeks COM

Extreme immaturity of newborn, gestational age 24 weeks, 0 days through 24 weeks, 6 days

P07.24 Extreme immaturity of newborn, gestational age 25 completed weeks COM

Extreme immaturity of newborn, gestational age 25 weeks, 0 days through 25 weeks, 6 days

P07.25 Extreme immaturity of newborn, gestational age 26 completed weeks COM

Extreme immaturity of newborn, gestational age 26 weeks, 0 days through 26 weeks, 6 days

P07.26 Extreme immaturity of newborn, gestational age 27 completed weeks COM

Extreme immaturity of newborn, gestational age 27 weeks, 0 days through 27 weeks, 6 days

P07.3 Preterm [premature] newborn [other]

28 completed weeks or more but less than 37 completed weeks (196 completed days but less than 259 completed days) of gestation

Prematurity NOS

AHA: 2017,3Q,26

P07.30 Preterm newborn, unspecified weeks of gestation COM

P07.31 Preterm newborn, gestational age 28 completed weeks COM

Preterm newborn, gestational age 28 weeks, 0 days through 28 weeks, 6 days

P07.32 Preterm newborn, gestational age 29 completed weeks COM

Preterm newborn, gestational age 29 weeks, 0 days through 29 weeks, 6 days

P07.33 Preterm newborn, gestational age 30 completed weeks COM

Preterm newborn, gestational age 30 weeks, 0 days through 30 weeks, 6 days

P07.34 Preterm newborn, gestational age 31 completed weeks COM

Preterm newborn, gestational age 31 weeks, 0 days through 31 weeks, 6 days

P07.35 Preterm newborn, gestational age 32 completed weeks COM

Preterm newborn, gestational age 32 weeks, 0 days through 32 weeks, 6 days

P07.36 Preterm newborn, gestational age 33 completed weeks COM

Preterm newborn, gestational age 33 weeks, 0 days through 33 weeks, 6 days

P07.37 Preterm newborn, gestational age 34 completed weeks COM

Preterm newborn, gestational age 34 weeks, 0 days through 34 weeks, 6 days

P07.38 Preterm newborn, gestational age 35 completed weeks COM

Preterm newborn, gestational age 35 weeks, 0 days through 35 weeks, 6 days

P07.39 Preterm newborn, gestational age 36 completed weeks COM

Preterm newborn, gestational age 36 weeks, 0 days through 36 weeks, 6 days

P08 Disorders of newborn related to long gestation and high birth weight

NOTE When both birth weight and gestational age of the newborn are available, priority of assignment should be given to birth weight

INCLUDES the listed conditions, without further specification, as causes of morbidity or additional care, in newborn

P08.0 Exceptionally large newborn baby COM

Usually implies a birth weight of 4500 g. or more

EXCLUDES 1 *syndrome of infant of diabetic mother (P70.1)*
syndrome of infant of mother with gestational diabetes (P70.0)

P08.1 Other heavy for gestational age newborn COM

Other newborn heavy- or large-for-dates regardless of period of gestation

Usually implies a birth weight of 4000 g. to 4499 g.

EXCLUDES 1 *newborn with a birth weight of 4500 or more (P08.0)*
syndrome of infant of diabetic mother (P70.1)
syndrome of infant of mother with gestational diabetes (P70.0)

P08.2 Late newborn, not heavy for gestational age

AHA: 2014,1Q,14

P08.21 Post-term newborn COM

Newborn with gestation period over 40 completed weeks to 42 completed weeks

P08.22 Prolonged gestation of newborn COM

Newborn with gestation period over 42 completed weeks (294 days or more), not heavy- or large-for-dates.

Postmaturity NOS

Abnormal findings on neonatal screening (P09)

P09 Abnormal findings on neonatal screening

INCLUDES abnormal findings on state mandated newborn screens
failed newborn screening

EXCLUDES 2 *nonspecific serologic evidence of human immunodeficiency virus [HIV] (R75)*

AHA: 2021,4Q,24

P09.1 Abnormal findings on neonatal screening for inborn errors of metabolism

P09.2 Abnormal findings on neonatal screening for congenital endocrine disease

Abnormal findings on neonatal screening for congenital adrenal hyperplasia

Abnormal findings on neonatal screening for hypothyroidism screen

P09.3 Abnormal findings on neonatal screening for congenital hematologic disorders

Abnormal findings for hemoglobinothies screen

Abnormal findings on red cell membrane defects screen

Abnormal findings on sickle cell screen

P09.4 Abnormal findings on neonatal screening for cystic fibrosis

P09.5 Abnormal findings on neonatal screening for critical congenital heart disease

Neonatal congenital heart disease screening failure

P09.6 Abnormal findings on neonatal screening for neonatal hearing loss

EXCLUDES 2 *encounter for hearing examination following failed hearing screening (Z01.110)*

P09.8 Other abnormal findings on neonatal screening

P09.9 Abnormal findings on neonatal screening, unspecified

Birth trauma (P10-P15)

P10 Intracranial laceration and hemorrhage due to birth injury
EXCLUDES 1 *intracranial hemorrhage of newborn NOS (P52.9)*
intracranial hemorrhage of newborn due to anoxia or hypoxia (P52.-)
nontraumatic intracranial hemorrhage of newborn (P52.-)

P10.0 Subdural hemorrhage due to birth injury COM
Subdural hematoma (localized) due to birth injury
EXCLUDES 1 *subdural hemorrhage accompanying tentorial tear (P10.4)*

P10.1 Cerebral hemorrhage due to birth injury COM

P10.2 Intraventricular hemorrhage due to birth injury COM

P10.3 Subarachnoid hemorrhage due to birth injury COM

P10.4 Tentorial tear due to birth injury COM

P10.8 Other intracranial lacerations and hemorrhages due to birth injury COM

P10.9 Unspecified intracranial laceration and hemorrhage due to birth injury COM

P11 Other birth injuries to central nervous system

P11.0 Cerebral edema due to birth injury COM

P11.1 Other specified brain damage due to birth injury COM

P11.2 Unspecified brain damage due to birth injury COM

P11.3 Birth injury to facial nerve
Facial palsy due to birth injury

P11.4 Birth injury to other cranial nerves

P11.5 Birth injury to spine and spinal cord COM
Fracture of spine due to birth injury

P11.9 Birth injury to central nervous system, unspecified

P12 Birth injury to scalp

Birth Injuries to Scalp

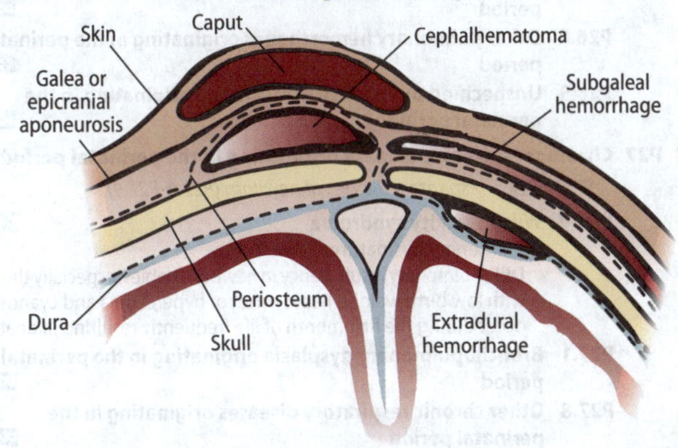

P12.0 Cephalhematoma due to birth injury
DEF: Condition that occurs in a neonate when blood vessels between the skull and periosteum rupture and blood collects in the subperiosteal space (below the periosteum). It is typically caused by prolonged labor or trauma due to instrument-assisted delivery (e.g., forceps, vacuum extraction), although in rare circumstances, it may indicate a linear skull fracture with intracranial hemorrhage.

P12.1 Chignon (from vacuum extraction) due to birth injury
DEF: Artificial swelling of the scalp that occurs when a collection of interstitial fluid and blood forms in the area of the scalp where the suction cup was applied during a vacuum-assisted delivery.

P12.2 Epicranial subaponeurotic hemorrhage due to birth injury
Subgaleal hemorrhage

P12.3 Bruising of scalp due to birth injury

P12.4 Injury of scalp of newborn due to monitoring equipment
Sampling incision of scalp of newborn
Scalp clip (electrode) injury of newborn

P12.8 Other birth injuries to scalp

P12.81 Caput succedaneum
DEF: Swelling of the scalp as a result of pressure being exerted on the head from the vaginal walls, uterus, or instrumentation used in assisting a delivery (e.g., vacuum).

P12.89 Other birth injuries to scalp

P12.9 Birth injury to scalp, unspecified

P13 Birth injury to skeleton
EXCLUDES 2 *birth injury to spine (P11.5)*

P13.0 Fracture of skull due to birth injury

P13.1 Other birth injuries to skull
EXCLUDES 1 *cephalhematoma (P12.0)*

P13.2 Birth injury to femur

P13.3 Birth injury to other long bones

P13.4 Fracture of clavicle due to birth injury

P13.8 Birth injuries to other parts of skeleton

P13.9 Birth injury to skeleton, unspecified

P14 Birth injury to peripheral nervous system

P14.0 Erb's paralysis due to birth injury
DEF: Erb's paralysis: Most common type of brachial plexus (peripheral nerve) injury in a neonate that involves nerve damage at the level of C5-C6. ***Synonym(s):*** *Erb's palsy*

P14.1 Klumpke's paralysis due to birth injury

P14.2 Phrenic nerve paralysis due to birth injury

P14.3 Other brachial plexus birth injuries

P14.8 Birth injuries to other parts of peripheral nervous system

P14.9 Birth injury to peripheral nervous system, unspecified

P15 Other birth injuries

P15.0 Birth injury to liver
Rupture of liver due to birth injury

P15.1 Birth injury to spleen
Rupture of spleen due to birth injury

P15.2 Sternomastoid injury due to birth injury

P15.3 Birth injury to eye
Subconjunctival hemorrhage due to birth injury
Traumatic glaucoma due to birth injury

P15.4 Birth injury to face
Facial congestion due to birth injury

P15.5 Birth injury to external genitalia

P15.6 Subcutaneous fat necrosis due to birth injury

P15.8 Other specified birth injuries

P15.9 Birth injury, unspecified

Respiratory and cardiovascular disorders specific to the perinatal period (P19-P29)

P19 Metabolic acidemia in newborn
INCLUDES metabolic acidemia in newborn

P19.0 Metabolic acidemia in newborn first noted before onset of labor

P19.1 Metabolic acidemia in newborn first noted during labor

P19.2 Metabolic acidemia noted at birth

P19.9 Metabolic acidemia, unspecified

P22 Respiratory distress of newborn
AHA: 2019,2Q,29

P22.0 Respiratory distress syndrome of newborn COM
Cardiorespiratory distress syndrome of newborn
Hyaline membrane disease
Idiopathic respiratory distress syndrome [IRDS or RDS] of newborn
Pulmonary hypoperfusion syndrome
Respiratory distress syndrome, type I
EXCLUDES 2 *respiratory arrest of newborn (P28.81)*
respiratory failure of newborn NOS (P28.5)
AHA: 2019,2Q,29
DEF: Severe chest contractions upon air intake and expiratory grunting. The infant appears blue due to oxygen deficiency and has a rapid respiratory rate, formerly called hyaline membrane disease.

P22.1 Transient tachypnea of newborn
Idiopathic tachypnea of newborn
Respiratory distress syndrome, type II
Wet lung syndrome
DEF: Rapid, labored breathing of a newborn. It is a short-term problem that begins after birth and lasts about three days.

P22.8 Other respiratory distress of newborn
EXCLUDES 1 *respiratory arrest of newborn (P28.81)*
respiratory failure of newborn NOS (P28.5)

P22.9 Respiratory distress of newborn, unspecified
EXCLUDES 1 *respiratory arrest of newborn (P28.81)*
respiratory failure of newborn NOS (P28.5)

✓4th P23 Congenital pneumonia

INCLUDES infective pneumonia acquired in utero or during birth

EXCLUDES 1 *neonatal pneumonia resulting from aspiration (P24.-)*

P23.Ø Congenital pneumonia due to viral agent COM

Use additional code (B97) to identify organism

EXCLUDES 1 *congenital rubella pneumonitis (P35.Ø)*

P23.1 Congenital pneumonia due to Chlamydia COM

P23.2 Congenital pneumonia due to staphylococcus COM

P23.3 Congenital pneumonia due to streptococcus, group B COM

P23.4 Congenital pneumonia due to Escherichia coli COM

P23.5 Congenital pneumonia due to Pseudomonas COM

P23.6 Congenital pneumonia due to other bacterial agents COM

Congenital pneumonia due to Hemophilus influenzae

Congenital pneumonia due to Klebsiella pneumoniae

Congenital pneumonia due to Mycoplasma

Congenital pneumonia due to Streptococcus, except group B

Use additional code (B95-B96) to identify organism

P23.8 Congenital pneumonia due to other organisms COM

P23.9 Congenital pneumonia, unspecified COM

✓4th P24 Neonatal aspiration

INCLUDES aspiration in utero and during delivery

✓5th P24.Ø Meconium aspiration

EXCLUDES 1 *meconium passage (without aspiration) during delivery (PØ3.82)*
meconium staining (P96.83)

DEF: Meconium in the trachea or seen on chest x-ray after birth.

P24.ØØ Meconium aspiration without respiratory symptoms

Meconium aspiration NOS

P24.Ø1 Meconium aspiration with respiratory symptoms COM

Meconium aspiration pneumonia

Meconium aspiration pneumonitis

Meconium aspiration syndrome NOS

Use additional code to identify any secondary pulmonary hypertension, if applicable (I27.2-)

DEF: Aspiration of fetal intestinal material during or prior to delivery. It is usually a complication of placental insufficiency, causing pneumonitis and bronchial obstruction (inflammatory reaction of lungs).

✓5th P24.1 Neonatal aspiration of (clear) amniotic fluid and mucus

Neonatal aspiration of liquor (amnii)

P24.1Ø Neonatal aspiration of (clear) amniotic fluid and mucus without respiratory symptoms

Neonatal aspiration of amniotic fluid and mucus NOS

P24.11 Neonatal aspiration of (clear) amniotic fluid and mucus with respiratory symptoms COM

Neonatal aspiration of amniotic fluid and mucus with pneumonia

Neonatal aspiration of amniotic fluid and mucus with pneumonitis

Use additional code to identify any secondary pulmonary hypertension, if applicable (I27.2-)

✓5th P24.2 Neonatal aspiration of blood

P24.2Ø Neonatal aspiration of blood without respiratory symptoms

Neonatal aspiration of blood NOS

P24.21 Neonatal aspiration of blood with respiratory symptoms COM

Neonatal aspiration of blood with pneumonia

Neonatal aspiration of blood with pneumonitis

Use additional code to identify any secondary pulmonary hypertension, if applicable (I27.2-)

✓5th P24.3 Neonatal aspiration of milk and regurgitated food

Neonatal aspiration of stomach contents

P24.3Ø Neonatal aspiration of milk and regurgitated food without respiratory symptoms

Neonatal aspiration of milk and regurgitated food NOS

P24.31 Neonatal aspiration of milk and regurgitated food with respiratory symptoms COM

Neonatal aspiration of milk and regurgitated food with pneumonia

Neonatal aspiration of milk and regurgitated food with pneumonitis

Use additional code to identify any secondary pulmonary hypertension, if applicable (I27.2-)

✓5th P24.8 Other neonatal aspiration

P24.8Ø Other neonatal aspiration without respiratory symptoms

Neonatal aspiration NEC

P24.81 Other neonatal aspiration with respiratory symptoms COM

Neonatal aspiration pneumonia NEC

Neonatal aspiration with pneumonitis NEC

Neonatal aspiration with pneumonia NOS

Neonatal aspiration with pneumonitis NOS

Use additional code to identify any secondary pulmonary hypertension, if applicable (I27.2-)

P24.9 Neonatal aspiration, unspecified

✓4th P25 Interstitial emphysema and related conditions originating in the perinatal period

P25.Ø Interstitial emphysema originating in the perinatal period

P25.1 Pneumothorax originating in the perinatal period

P25.2 Pneumomediastinum originating in the perinatal period

P25.3 Pneumopericardium originating in the perinatal period

P25.8 Other conditions related to interstitial emphysema originating in the perinatal period

✓4th P26 Pulmonary hemorrhage originating in the perinatal period

EXCLUDES 1 *acute idiopathic hemorrhage in infants over 28 days old (RØ4.81)*

P26.Ø Tracheobronchial hemorrhage originating in the perinatal period COM

P26.1 Massive pulmonary hemorrhage originating in the perinatal period COM

P26.8 Other pulmonary hemorrhages originating in the perinatal period COM

P26.9 Unspecified pulmonary hemorrhage originating in the perinatal period COM

✓4th P27 Chronic respiratory disease originating in the perinatal period

EXCLUDES 2 *respiratory distress of newborn (P22.Ø-P22.9)*

P27.Ø Wilson-Mikity syndrome COM

Pulmonary dysmaturity

DEF: Pulmonary insufficiency in newborn babies, especially those with low birth weight. Rapid onset of hypercapnia and cyanosis occur during the first month of life frequently resulting in death.

P27.1 Bronchopulmonary dysplasia originating in the perinatal period COM

P27.8 Other chronic respiratory diseases originating in the perinatal period COM

Congenital pulmonary fibrosis

Ventilator lung in newborn

P27.9 Unspecified chronic respiratory disease originating in the perinatal period COM

✓4th P28 Other respiratory conditions originating in the perinatal period

▶Code also, if applicable, congenital malformations of the respiratory system (Q3Ø-Q34)◀

EXCLUDES 1 ~~*congenital malformations of the respiratory system (Q3Ø-Q34)*~~

P28.Ø Primary atelectasis of newborn COM

Primary failure to expand terminal respiratory units

Pulmonary hypoplasia associated with short gestation

Pulmonary immaturity NOS

✓5th P28.1 Other and unspecified atelectasis of newborn

P28.1Ø Unspecified atelectasis of newborn COM

Atelectasis of newborn NOS

P28.11 Resorption atelectasis without respiratory distress syndrome COM

EXCLUDES 1 *resorption atelectasis with respiratory distress syndrome (P22.Ø)*

P28.19 Other atelectasis of newborn COM

Partial atelectasis of newborn

Secondary atelectasis of newborn

P28.2 Cyanotic attacks of newborn

EXCLUDES 1 *apnea of newborn ▶(P28.3- - P28.4-)◀*

▲ P28.3 Primary sleep apnea of newborn
Central sleep apnea of newborn
Obstructive sleep apnea of newborn
Sleep apnea of newborn NOS
EXCLUDES 2 ►*other apnea of newborn (P28.4-)*◄
DEF: Unexplained cessation of breathing when a neonate makes no respiratory effort for 20 seconds or longer or when a neonate's breathing cessation is accompanied by cyanosis, bradycardia, or hypotonia.

● **P28.30 Primary sleep apnea of newborn, unspecified**
Transient oxygen desaturation spells of newborn during sleep

● **P28.31 Primary central sleep apnea of newborn**

● **P28.32 Primary obstructive sleep apnea of newborn**

● **P28.33 Primary mixed sleep apnea of newborn**

● **P28.39 Other primary sleep apnea of newborn**

▲ **P28.4 Other apnea of newborn**
~~Apnea of prematurity~~
~~Obstructive apnea of newborn~~
~~EXCLUDES 1 *obstructive sleep apnea of newborn (P28.3)*~~
EXCLUDES 2 ►*primary sleep apnea of newborn (P28.3-)*◄

● **P28.40 Unspecified apnea of newborn**
Apnea of newborn, NOS
Transient oxygen desaturation spells of newborn

● **P28.41 Central neonatal apnea of newborn**

● **P28.42 Obstructive apnea of newborn**

● **P28.43 Mixed neonatal apnea of newborn**

● **P28.49 Other apnea of newborn**
Apnea of prematurity

P28.5 Respiratory failure of newborn COM
EXCLUDES 1 *respiratory arrest of newborn (P28.81)*
respiratory distress of newborn (P22.0-)
AHA: 2019,2Q,29

P28.8 Other specified respiratory conditions of newborn

P28.81 Respiratory arrest of newborn COM

P28.89 Other specified respiratory conditions of newborn
Congenital laryngeal stridor
Sniffles in newborn
Snuffles in newborn
EXCLUDES 1 *early congenital syphilitic rhinitis (A50.05)*

P28.9 Respiratory condition of newborn, unspecified
Respiratory depression in newborn

P29 Cardiovascular disorders originating in the perinatal period
EXCLUDES 2 *congenital malformations of the circulatory system (Q20-Q28)*

P29.0 Neonatal cardiac failure COM

P29.1 Neonatal cardiac dysrhythmia

P29.11 Neonatal tachycardia

P29.12 Neonatal bradycardia

P29.2 Neonatal hypertension

P29.3 Persistent fetal circulation
AHA: 2017,4Q,20-21

P29.30 Pulmonary hypertension of newborn COM
Persistent pulmonary hypertension of newborn
DEF: Condition that occurs when pressure within the pulmonary artery is elevated and vascular resistance is observed in the lungs.

P29.38 Other persistent fetal circulation COM
Delayed closure of ductus arteriosus

P29.4 Transient myocardial ischemia in newborn

P29.8 Other cardiovascular disorders originating in the perinatal period

P29.81 Cardiac arrest of newborn COM

P29.89 Other cardiovascular disorders originating in the perinatal period
AHA: 2014,4Q,23

P29.9 Cardiovascular disorder originating in the perinatal period, unspecified

Infections specific to the perinatal period (P35-P39)

Infections acquired in utero, during birth via the umbilicus, or during the first 28 days after birth
EXCLUDES 2 *asymptomatic human immunodeficiency virus [HIV] infection status (Z21)*
congenital gonococcal infection (A54.-)
congenital pneumonia (P23.-)
congenital syphilis (A50.-)
human immunodeficiency virus [HIV] disease (B20)
infant botulism (A48.51)
infectious diseases not specific to the perinatal period (A00-B99, J09, J10.-)
intestinal infectious disease (A00-A09)
laboratory evidence of human immunodeficiency virus [HIV] (R75)
tetanus neonatorum (A33)

P35 Congenital viral diseases
INCLUDES infections acquired in utero or during birth

P35.0 Congenital rubella syndrome
Congenital rubella pneumonitis

P35.1 Congenital cytomegalovirus infection COM

P35.2 Congenital herpesviral [herpes simplex] infection

P35.3 Congenital viral hepatitis

P35.4 Congenital Zika virus disease
Use additional code to identify manifestations of congenital Zika virus disease
AHA: 2018,4Q,25-26

P35.8 Other congenital viral diseases
Congenital varicella [chickenpox]
AHA: 2020,2Q,13

P35.9 Congenital viral disease, unspecified

P36 Bacterial sepsis of newborn
INCLUDES congenital sepsis
Use additional code(s), if applicable, to identify severe sepsis (R65.2-) and associated acute organ dysfunction(s)

P36.0 Sepsis of newborn due to streptococcus, group B HCC ESR COM

P36.1 Sepsis of newborn due to other and unspecified streptococci

P36.10 Sepsis of newborn due to unspecified streptococci HCC ESR COM

P36.19 Sepsis of newborn due to other streptococci HCC ESR COM

P36.2 Sepsis of newborn due to Staphylococcus aureus HCC ESR COM

P36.3 Sepsis of newborn due to other and unspecified staphylococci

P36.30 Sepsis of newborn due to unspecified staphylococci HCC ESR COM

P36.39 Sepsis of newborn due to other staphylococci HCC ESR COM

P36.4 Sepsis of newborn due to Escherichia coli HCC ESR COM

P36.5 Sepsis of newborn due to anaerobes HCC ESR COM

P36.8 Other bacterial sepsis of newborn HCC ESR COM
Use additional code from category B96 to identify organism

P36.9 Bacterial sepsis of newborn, unspecified HCC ESR COM

P37 Other congenital infectious and parasitic diseases
EXCLUDES 2 *congenital syphilis (A50.-)*
infectious neonatal diarrhea (A00-A09)
necrotizing enterocolitis in newborn (P77.-)
noninfectious neonatal diarrhea (P78.3)
ophthalmia neonatorum due to gonococcus (A54.31)
tetanus neonatorum (A33)

P37.0 Congenital tuberculosis

P37.1 Congenital toxoplasmosis
Hydrocephalus due to congenital toxoplasmosis

P37.2 Neonatal (disseminated) listeriosis

P37.3 Congenital falciparum malaria

P37.4 Other congenital malaria

P37.5 Neonatal candidiasis

P37.8 Other specified congenital infectious and parasitic diseases

P37.9 Congenital infectious or parasitic disease, unspecified

P38 Omphalitis of newborn

EXCLUDES 1 *omphalitis not of newborn (L08.82)*
tetanus omphalitis (A33)
umbilical hemorrhage of newborn (P51.-)

DEF: Omphalitis: Infection and inflammation of the umbilical stump, often due to bacteria that can spread beyond the umbilical stump to the fascia, muscle, or even the umbilical vessels.

P38.1 Omphalitis with mild hemorrhage
P38.9 Omphalitis without hemorrhage
Omphalitis of newborn NOS

P39 Other infections specific to the perinatal period
Use additional code to identify organism or specific infection

P39.0 Neonatal infective mastitis
EXCLUDES 1 *breast engorgement of newborn (P83.4)*
noninfective mastitis of newborn (P83.4)

P39.1 Neonatal conjunctivitis and dacryocystitis
Neonatal chlamydial conjunctivitis
Ophthalmia neonatorum NOS
EXCLUDES 1 *gonococcal conjunctivitis (A54.31)*

P39.2 Intra-amniotic infection affecting newborn, not elsewhere classified
P39.3 Neonatal urinary tract infection
P39.4 Neonatal skin infection
Neonatal pyoderma
EXCLUDES 1 *pemphigus neonatorum (L00)*
staphylococcal scalded skin syndrome (L00)

P39.8 Other specified infections specific to the perinatal period
P39.9 Infection specific to the perinatal period, unspecified

Hemorrhagic and hematological disorders of newborn (P50-P61)

EXCLUDES 1 *congenital stenosis and stricture of bile ducts (Q44.3)*
Crigler-Najjar syndrome (E80.5)
Dubin-Johnson syndrome (E80.6)
Gilbert syndrome (E80.4)
hereditary hemolytic anemias (D55-D58)

P50 Newborn affected by intrauterine (fetal) blood loss
EXCLUDES 1 *congenital anemia from intrauterine (fetal) blood loss (P61.3)*

P50.0 Newborn affected by intrauterine (fetal) blood loss from vasa previa
P50.1 Newborn affected by intrauterine (fetal) blood loss from ruptured cord
P50.2 Newborn affected by intrauterine (fetal) blood loss from placenta
P50.3 Newborn affected by hemorrhage into co-twin
P50.4 Newborn affected by hemorrhage into maternal circulation
P50.5 Newborn affected by intrauterine (fetal) blood loss from cut end of co-twin's cord
P50.8 Newborn affected by other intrauterine (fetal) blood loss
P50.9 Newborn affected by intrauterine (fetal) blood loss, unspecified
Newborn affected by fetal hemorrhage NOS

P51 Umbilical hemorrhage of newborn
EXCLUDES 1 *omphalitis with mild hemorrhage (P38.1)*
umbilical hemorrhage from cut end of co-twins cord (P50.5)

P51.0 Massive umbilical hemorrhage of newborn
P51.8 Other umbilical hemorrhages of newborn
Slipped umbilical ligature NOS
P51.9 Umbilical hemorrhage of newborn, unspecified

P52 Intracranial nontraumatic hemorrhage of newborn
INCLUDES intracranial hemorrhage due to anoxia or hypoxia
EXCLUDES 1 *intracranial hemorrhage due to birth injury (P10.-)*
intracranial hemorrhage due to other injury (S06.-)

P52.0 Intraventricular (nontraumatic) hemorrhage, grade 1, of newborn COM
Subependymal hemorrhage (without intraventricular extension)
Bleeding into germinal matrix

P52.1 Intraventricular (nontraumatic) hemorrhage, grade 2, of newborn COM
Subependymal hemorrhage with intraventricular extension
Bleeding into ventricle

P52.2 Intraventricular (nontraumatic) hemorrhage, grade 3 and grade 4, of newborn

P52.21 Intraventricular (nontraumatic) hemorrhage, grade 3, of newborn COM
Subependymal hemorrhage with intraventricular extension with enlargement of ventricle

P52.22 Intraventricular (nontraumatic) hemorrhage, grade 4, of newborn COM
Bleeding into cerebral cortex
Subependymal hemorrhage with intracerebral extension

P52.3 Unspecified intraventricular (nontraumatic) hemorrhage of newborn COM
P52.4 Intracerebral (nontraumatic) hemorrhage of newborn COM
P52.5 Subarachnoid (nontraumatic) hemorrhage of newborn COM
P52.6 Cerebellar (nontraumatic) and posterior fossa hemorrhage of newborn COM
P52.8 Other intracranial (nontraumatic) hemorrhages of newborn COM
P52.9 Intracranial (nontraumatic) hemorrhage of newborn, unspecified COM

P53 Hemorrhagic disease of newborn COM
Vitamin K deficiency of newborn

P54 Other neonatal hemorrhages
EXCLUDES 1 *newborn affected by (intrauterine) blood loss (P50.-)*
pulmonary hemorrhage originating in the perinatal period (P26.-)

P54.0 Neonatal hematemesis
EXCLUDES 1 *neonatal hematemesis due to swallowed maternal blood (P78.2)*

P54.1 Neonatal melena
EXCLUDES 1 *neonatal melena due to swallowed maternal blood (P78.2)*

P54.2 Neonatal rectal hemorrhage
P54.3 Other neonatal gastrointestinal hemorrhage
P54.4 Neonatal adrenal hemorrhage
P54.5 Neonatal cutaneous hemorrhage
Neonatal bruising
Neonatal ecchymoses
Neonatal petechiae
Neonatal superficial hematomata
EXCLUDES 2 *bruising of scalp due to birth injury (P12.3)*
cephalhematoma due to birth injury (P12.0)

P54.6 Neonatal vaginal hemorrhage ♀
Neonatal pseudomenses

P54.8 Other specified neonatal hemorrhages
P54.9 Neonatal hemorrhage, unspecified

P55 Hemolytic disease of newborn

P55.0 Rh isoimmunization of newborn COM
DEF: Incompatible Rh fetal-maternal blood grouping that prematurely destroys red blood cells. Symptoms include jaundice, asphyxia, pulmonary hypertension, edema, respiratory distress, kernicterus, and coagulopathies. It is detected by a Coombs test.
TIP: A positive Coombs test without documentation of associated Rh isoimmunization should be coded to R79.89 Other specified abnormal findings of blood chemistry.

P55.1 ABO isoimmunization of newborn COM
AHA: 2015,3Q,20

P55.8 Other hemolytic diseases of newborn COM
AHA: 2018,3Q,24

P55.9 Hemolytic disease of newborn, unspecified COM

P56 Hydrops fetalis due to hemolytic disease
EXCLUDES 1 *hydrops fetalis NOS (P83.2)*

P56.0 Hydrops fetalis due to isoimmunization COM
P56.9 Hydrops fetalis due to other and unspecified hemolytic disease

P56.90 Hydrops fetalis due to unspecified hemolytic disease COM
P56.99 Hydrops fetalis due to other hemolytic disease COM

P57 Kernicterus

P57.0 Kernicterus due to isoimmunization COM

DEF: Complication of erythroblastosis fetalis associated with severe neural symptoms, high blood bilirubin levels, and nerve cell destruction. It results in bilirubin-pigmented gray matter of the central nervous system.

P57.8 Other specified kernicterus COM

EXCLUDES 1 *Crigler-Najjar syndrome (E80.5)*

P57.9 Kernicterus, unspecified COM

P58 Neonatal jaundice due to other excessive hemolysis

EXCLUDES 1 *jaundice due to isoimmunization (P55-P57)*

P58.0 Neonatal jaundice due to bruising

P58.1 Neonatal jaundice due to bleeding

P58.2 Neonatal jaundice due to infection

P58.3 Neonatal jaundice due to polycythemia

P58.4 Neonatal jaundice due to drugs or toxins transmitted from mother or given to newborn

Code first poisoning due to drug or toxin, if applicable (T36-T65 with fifth or sixth character 1-4 or 6)

Use additional code for adverse effect, if applicable, to identify drug (T36-T50 with fifth or sixth character 5)

P58.41 Neonatal jaundice due to drugs or toxins transmitted from mother

P58.42 Neonatal jaundice due to drugs or toxins given to newborn

P58.5 Neonatal jaundice due to swallowed maternal blood

P58.8 Neonatal jaundice due to other specified excessive hemolysis

P58.9 Neonatal jaundice due to excessive hemolysis, unspecified

P59 Neonatal jaundice from other and unspecified causes

EXCLUDES 1 *jaundice due to inborn errors of metabolism (E70-E88)*
kernicterus (P57.-)

P59.0 Neonatal jaundice associated with preterm delivery

Hyperbilirubinemia of prematurity
Jaundice due to delayed conjugation associated with preterm delivery

P59.1 Inspissated bile syndrome COM

DEF: Biliary obstruction in newborn resulting from obstruction of outflow tract.

P59.2 Neonatal jaundice from other and unspecified hepatocellular damage

EXCLUDES 1 *congenital viral hepatitis (P35.3)*

P59.20 Neonatal jaundice from unspecified hepatocellular damage COM

P59.29 Neonatal jaundice from other hepatocellular damage COM

Neonatal giant cell hepatitis
Neonatal (idiopathic) hepatitis

P59.3 Neonatal jaundice from breast milk inhibitor

P59.8 Neonatal jaundice from other specified causes

P59.9 Neonatal jaundice, unspecified

Neonatal physiological jaundice (intense)(prolonged) NOS
AHA: 2015,3Q,20

P60 Disseminated intravascular coagulation of newborn COM

Defibrination syndrome of newborn

P61 Other perinatal hematological disorders

EXCLUDES 1 *transient hypogammaglobulinemia of infancy (D80.7)*

P61.0 Transient neonatal thrombocytopenia COM

Neonatal thrombocytopenia due to exchange transfusion
Neonatal thrombocytopenia due to idiopathic maternal thrombocytopenia
Neonatal thrombocytopenia due to isoimmunization

DEF: Temporary decrease in blood platelets of a newborn that is secondary to placental insufficiency.

P61.1 Polycythemia neonatorum

DEF: Abnormal increase of total red blood cells of a newborn that results in hyperviscosity, which slows the flow of blood through small blood vessels.

P61.2 Anemia of prematurity

P61.3 Congenital anemia from fetal blood loss

P61.4 Other congenital anemias, not elsewhere classified

Congenital anemia NOS

P61.5 Transient neonatal neutropenia COM

EXCLUDES 1 *congenital neutropenia (nontransient) (D70.0)*

DEF: Low blood neutrophil counts of newborn that occurs due to maternal hypertension, sepsis, twin-twin transfusion, alloimmunization, and hemolytic disease.

P61.6 Other transient neonatal disorders of coagulation COM

P61.8 Other specified perinatal hematological disorders

P61.9 Perinatal hematological disorder, unspecified

Transitory endocrine and metabolic disorders specific to newborn (P70-P74)

INCLUDES transitory endocrine and metabolic disturbances caused by the infant's response to maternal endocrine and metabolic factors, or its adjustment to extrauterine environment

AHA: 2018,2Q,6

P70 Transitory disorders of carbohydrate metabolism specific to newborn

P70.0 Syndrome of infant of mother with gestational diabetes

Newborn (with hypoglycemia) affected by maternal gestational diabetes

EXCLUDES 1 *newborn (with hypoglycemia) affected by maternal (pre-existing) diabetes mellitus (P70.1)*
syndrome of infant of a diabetic mother (P70.1)

P70.1 Syndrome of infant of a diabetic mother

Newborn (with hypoglycemia) affected by maternal (pre-existing) diabetes mellitus

EXCLUDES 1 *newborn (with hypoglycemia) affected by maternal gestational diabetes (P70.0)*
syndrome of infant of mother with gestational diabetes (P70.0)

P70.2 Neonatal diabetes mellitus

P70.3 Iatrogenic neonatal hypoglycemia

P70.4 Other neonatal hypoglycemia

Transitory neonatal hypoglycemia

P70.8 Other transitory disorders of carbohydrate metabolism of newborn

P70.9 Transitory disorder of carbohydrate metabolism of newborn, unspecified

P71 Transitory neonatal disorders of calcium and magnesium metabolism

P71.0 Cow's milk hypocalcemia in newborn

P71.1 Other neonatal hypocalcemia

EXCLUDES 1 *neonatal hypoparathyroidism (P71.4)*

P71.2 Neonatal hypomagnesemia

P71.3 Neonatal tetany without calcium or magnesium deficiency

Neonatal tetany NOS

P71.4 Transitory neonatal hypoparathyroidism

P71.8 Other transitory neonatal disorders of calcium and magnesium metabolism

AHA: 2016,4Q,54

P71.9 Transitory neonatal disorder of calcium and magnesium metabolism, unspecified

P72 Other transitory neonatal endocrine disorders

EXCLUDES 1 *congenital hypothyroidism with or without goiter (E03.0-E03.1)*
dyshormogenetic goiter (E07.1)
Pendred's syndrome (E07.1)

P72.0 Neonatal goiter, not elsewhere classified

Transitory congenital goiter with normal functioning

P72.1 Transitory neonatal hyperthyroidism

Neonatal thyrotoxicosis

P72.2 Other transitory neonatal disorders of thyroid function, not elsewhere classified

Transitory neonatal hypothyroidism

P72.8 Other specified transitory neonatal endocrine disorders

P72.9 Transitory neonatal endocrine disorder, unspecified

P74 Other transitory neonatal electrolyte and metabolic disturbances

AHA: 2018,4Q,26-27

P74.0 Late metabolic acidosis of newborn

EXCLUDES 1 *(fetal) metabolic acidosis of newborn (P19)*

P74.1 Dehydration of newborn

P74.2 Disturbances of sodium balance of newborn

P74.21 Hypernatremia of newborn

P74.22 Hyponatremia of newborn

P74.3 Disturbances of potassium balance of newborn

P74.31 Hyperkalemia of newborn

P74.32 **Hypokalemia of newborn**

√5th **P74.4 Other transitory electrolyte disturbances of newborn**

P74.41 **Alkalosis of newborn**
Hyperbicarbonatemia

√6th **P74.42 Disturbances of chlorine balance of newborn**

P74.421 **Hyperchloremia of newborn**
Hyperchloremic metabolic acidosis
EXCLUDES 2 *late metabolic acidosis of the newborn (P74.Ø)*

P74.422 **Hypochloremia of newborn**

P74.49 **Other transitory electrolyte disturbance of newborn**

P74.5 Transitory tyrosinemia of newborn

P74.6 Transitory hyperammonemia of newborn

P74.8 Other transitory metabolic disturbances of newborn
Amino-acid metabolic disorders described as transitory

P74.9 Transitory metabolic disturbance of newborn, unspecified

Digestive system disorders of newborn (P76-P78)

√4th **P76 Other intestinal obstruction of newborn**

P76.Ø Meconium plug syndrome
Meconium ileus NOS
EXCLUDES 1 *meconium ileus in cystic fibrosis (E84.11)*
DEF: Meconium obstruction of a newborn's intestines, resulting from unusually thick or hard meconium.

P76.1 Transitory ileus of newborn
EXCLUDES 1 *Hirschsprung's disease (Q43.1)*

P76.2 Intestinal obstruction due to inspissated milk

P76.8 Other specified intestinal obstruction of newborn
EXCLUDES 1 *intestinal obstruction classifiable to K56.-*

P76.9 Intestinal obstruction of newborn, unspecified

√4th **P77 Necrotizing enterocolitis of newborn**
DEF: Serious intestinal infection and inflammation in preterm infants. Severity is measured by stages and may progress to life-threatening perforation or peritonitis. Resection surgical treatment may be necessary.

P77.1 Stage 1 necrotizing enterocolitis in newborn COM
Necrotizing enterocolitis without pneumatosis, without perforation
DEF: Broad-spectrum symptoms with nonspecific signs, including feeding intolerance, abdominal distention, bradycardia, and metabolic abnormalities.

P77.2 Stage 2 necrotizing enterocolitis in newborn COM
Necrotizing enterocolitis with pneumatosis, without perforation
DEF: Radiographic confirmation of necrotizing enterocolitis showing intestinal dilatation, fixed loops of bowels, pneumatosis intestinalis, metabolic acidosis, and thrombocytopenia.

P77.3 Stage 3 necrotizing enterocolitis in newborn COM
Necrotizing enterocolitis with perforation
Necrotizing enterocolitis with pneumatosis and perforation
DEF: Advanced stage in which an infant demonstrates signs of bowel perforation, septic shock, metabolic acidosis, ascites, disseminated intravascular coagulopathy, and neutropenia.

P77.9 Necrotizing enterocolitis in newborn, unspecified COM
Necrotizing enterocolitis in newborn, NOS

√4th **P78 Other perinatal digestive system disorders**
EXCLUDES 1 *cystic fibrosis (E84.Ø-E84.9)*
neonatal gastrointestinal hemorrhages (P54.Ø-P54.3)

P78.Ø Perinatal intestinal perforation COM
Meconium peritonitis

P78.1 Other neonatal peritonitis
Neonatal peritonitis NOS

P78.2 Neonatal hematemesis and melena due to swallowed maternal blood

P78.3 Noninfective neonatal diarrhea
Neonatal diarrhea NOS

√5th **P78.8 Other specified perinatal digestive system disorders**

P78.81 **Congenital cirrhosis (of liver)**

P78.82 **Peptic ulcer of newborn**

P78.83 **Newborn esophageal reflux**
Neonatal esophageal reflux

P78.84 **Gestational alloimmune liver disease** COM
GALD
Neonatal hemochromatosis
EXCLUDES 1 *hemochromatosis (E83.11-)*
AHA: 2017,4Q,21
DEF: Severe hepatic injury with onset during fetal development with manifestations beginning during fetal life. It is due to maternal antibodies to fetal hepatic cells (hepatocytes) that cross the placenta into the fetal circulation, causing hepatic cell necrosis.

P78.89 **Other specified perinatal digestive system disorders**

P78.9 Perinatal digestive system disorder, unspecified

Conditions involving the integument and temperature regulation of newborn (P8Ø-P83)

√4th **P8Ø Hypothermia of newborn**
DEF: Decrease in newborn body temperature due to their larger ratio of surface area to body weight, thin skin with blood vessels close to the surface, and a limited amount of subcutaneous fat.

P8Ø.Ø Cold injury syndrome
Severe and usually chronic hypothermia associated with a pink flushed appearance, edema and neurological and biochemical abnormalities.
EXCLUDES 1 *mild hypothermia of newborn (P8Ø.8)*

P8Ø.8 Other hypothermia of newborn
Mild hypothermia of newborn

P8Ø.9 Hypothermia of newborn, unspecified

√4th **P81 Other disturbances of temperature regulation of newborn**

P81.Ø Environmental hyperthermia of newborn

P81.8 Other specified disturbances of temperature regulation of newborn

P81.9 Disturbance of temperature regulation of newborn, unspecified
Fever of newborn NOS

√4th **P83 Other conditions of integument specific to newborn**
EXCLUDES 1 *congenital malformations of skin and integument (Q8Ø-Q84)*
hydrops fetalis due to hemolytic disease (P56.-)
neonatal skin infection (P39.4)
staphylococcal scalded skin syndrome (LØØ)
EXCLUDES 2 *cradle cap (L21.Ø)*
diaper [napkin] dermatitis (L22)

P83.Ø Sclerema neonatorum
DEF: Diffuse, rapidly progressing white, waxy, nonpitting hardening of tissue, usually of legs and feet that is life-threatening. It is found in preterm or debilitated infants. Etiology is unknown.

P83.1 Neonatal erythema toxicum

P83.2 Hydrops fetalis not due to hemolytic disease
Hydrops fetalis NOS
DEF: Severe, life-threatening problem of a newborn characterized by severe edema of the entire body. It is unrelated to immune response.

√5th **P83.3 Other and unspecified edema specific to newborn**

P83.3Ø **Unspecified edema specific to newborn**

P83.39 **Other edema specific to newborn**

P83.4 Breast engorgement of newborn
Noninfective mastitis of newborn

P83.5 Congenital hydrocele ♂
DEF: Hydrocele: Serous fluid that collects in the tunica vaginalis of the scrotum along the spermatic cord in males.

P83.6 Umbilical polyp of newborn

√5th **P83.8 Other specified conditions of integument specific to newborn**
AHA: 2017,4Q,21-22

P83.81 **Umbilical granuloma**
EXCLUDES 2 *granulomatous disorder of the skin and subcutaneous tissue, unspecified (L92.9)*

P83.88 **Other specified conditions of integument specific to newborn**
Bronze baby syndrome
Neonatal scleroderma
Urticaria neonatorum

P83.9 Condition of the integument specific to newborn, unspecified

Other problems with newborn (P84)

P84 Other problems with newborn
Acidemia of newborn
Acidosis of newborn
Anoxia of newborn NOS
Asphyxia of newborn NOS
Hypercapnia of newborn
Hypoxemia of newborn
Hypoxia of newborn NOS
Mixed metabolic and respiratory acidosis of newborn
EXCLUDES 1 *intracranial hemorrhage due to anoxia or hypoxia (P52.-)*
hypoxic ischemic encephalopathy [HIE] (P91.6-)
late metabolic acidosis of newborn (P74.Ø)

Other disorders originating in the perinatal period (P9Ø-P96)

P9Ø Convulsions of newborn COM
EXCLUDES 1 *benign myoclonic epilepsy in infancy (G4Ø.3-)*
benign neonatal convulsions (familial) (G4Ø.3-)

✓4th **P91 Other disturbances of cerebral status of newborn**
P91.Ø Neonatal cerebral ischemia COM
EXCLUDES 1 *neonatal cerebral infarction (P91.82-)*
P91.1 Acquired periventricular cysts of newborn COM
P91.2 Neonatal cerebral leukomalacia COM
Periventricular leukomalacia
P91.3 Neonatal cerebral irritability COM
P91.4 Neonatal cerebral depression COM
P91.5 Neonatal coma COM
✓5th **P91.6 Hypoxic ischemic encephalopathy [HIE]**
EXCLUDES 1 *neonatal cerebral depression (P91.4)*
neonatal cerebral irritability (P91.3)
neonatal coma (P91.5)
AHA: 2017,4Q,22
P91.6Ø Hypoxic ischemic encephalopathy [HIE], unspecified COM
P91.61 Mild hypoxic ischemic encephalopathy [HIE] COM
P91.62 Moderate hypoxic ischemic encephalopathy [HIE] COM
P91.63 Severe hypoxic ischemic encephalopathy [HIE] COM
✓5th **P91.8 Other specified disturbances of cerebral status of newborn**
AHA: 2017,4Q,22
✓6th **P91.81 Neonatal encephalopathy**
P91.811 ***Neonatal encephalopathy in diseases classified elsewhere*** COM
Code first underlying condition, if known, such as:
congenital cirrhosis (of liver) (P78.81)
intracranial nontraumatic hemorrhage of newborn (P52.-)
kernicterus (P57.-)
P91.819 Neonatal encephalopathy, unspecified COM
✓6th **P91.82 Neonatal cerebral infarction**
Neonatal stroke
Perinatal arterial ischemic stroke
Perinatal cerebral infarction
EXCLUDES 1 *cerebral infarction (I63.-)*
EXCLUDES 2 *intracranial hemorrhage of newborn (P52.-)*
AHA: 2020,4Q,37-38
P91.821 Neonatal cerebral infarction, right side of brain HCC ESR COM
P91.822 Neonatal cerebral infarction, left side of brain HCC ESR COM
P91.823 Neonatal cerebral infarction, bilateral HCC ESR COM
P91.829 Neonatal cerebral infarction, unspecified side HCC ESR COM
P91.88 Other specified disturbances of cerebral status of newborn COM
P91.9 Disturbance of cerebral status of newborn, unspecified COM

✓4th **P92 Feeding problems of newborn**
EXCLUDES 1 *eating disorders (F5Ø.-)*
EXCLUDES 2 *feeding problems in child over 28 days old (R63.3)*
AHA: 2016,3Q,19
✓5th **P92.Ø Vomiting of newborn**
EXCLUDES 1 *vomiting of child over 28 days old (R11.-)*
P92.Ø1 Bilious vomiting of newborn
EXCLUDES 1 *bilious vomiting in child over 28 days old (R11.14)*
P92.Ø9 Other vomiting of newborn
EXCLUDES 1 *regurgitation of food in newborn (P92.1)*
P92.1 Regurgitation and rumination of newborn
P92.2 Slow feeding of newborn
P92.3 Underfeeding of newborn
P92.4 Overfeeding of newborn
P92.5 Neonatal difficulty in feeding at breast
AHA: 2017,1Q,28
P92.6 Failure to thrive in newborn
EXCLUDES 1 *failure to thrive in child over 28 days old (R62.51)*
P92.8 Other feeding problems of newborn
P92.9 Feeding problem of newborn, unspecified

✓4th **P93 Reactions and intoxications due to drugs administered to newborn**
INCLUDES reactions and intoxications due to drugs administered to fetus affecting newborn
EXCLUDES 1 *jaundice due to drugs or toxins transmitted from mother or given to newborn (P58.4-)*
reactions and intoxications from maternal opiates, tranquilizers and other medication (PØ4.Ø-PØ4.1, PØ4.4-)
withdrawal symptoms from maternal use of drugs of addiction (P96.1)
withdrawal symptoms from therapeutic use of drugs in newborn (P96.2)
P93.Ø Grey baby syndrome COM
Grey syndrome from chloramphenicol administration in newborn
P93.8 Other reactions and intoxications due to drugs administered to newborn COM
Use additional code for adverse effect, if applicable, to identify drug (T36-T5Ø with fifth or sixth character 5)

✓4th **P94 Disorders of muscle tone of newborn**
P94.Ø Transient neonatal myasthenia gravis
EXCLUDES 1 *myasthenia gravis (G7Ø.Ø)*
P94.1 Congenital hypertonia
P94.2 Congenital hypotonia
Floppy baby syndrome, unspecified
P94.8 Other disorders of muscle tone of newborn
P94.9 Disorder of muscle tone of newborn, unspecified

P95 Stillbirth
Deadborn fetus NOS
Fetal death of unspecified cause
Stillbirth NOS
EXCLUDES 1 *maternal care for intrauterine death (O36.4)*
missed abortion (OØ2.1)
outcome of delivery, stillbirth (Z37.1, Z37.3, Z37.4, Z37.7)

✓4th **P96 Other conditions originating in the perinatal period**
P96.Ø Congenital renal failure
Uremia of newborn
P96.1 Neonatal withdrawal symptoms from maternal use of drugs of addiction COM
Drug withdrawal syndrome in infant of dependent mother
Neonatal abstinence syndrome
EXCLUDES 1 *reactions and intoxications from maternal opiates and tranquilizers administered during labor and delivery (PØ4.Ø)*
AHA: 2018,4Q,24-25
P96.2 Withdrawal symptoms from therapeutic use of drugs in newborn COM
P96.3 Wide cranial sutures of newborn
Neonatal craniotabes
P96.5 Complication to newborn due to (fetal) intrauterine procedure
EXCLUDES 2 *newborn affected by amniocentesis (PØØ.6)*

√5th **P96.8 Other specified conditions originating in the perinatal period**

P96.81 Exposure to (parental) (environmental) tobacco smoke in the perinatal period

EXCLUDES 2 *newborn affected by in utero exposure to tobacco (P04.2)*
exposure to environmental tobacco smoke after the perinatal period (Z77.22)

P96.82 Delayed separation of umbilical cord

P96.83 Meconium staining

EXCLUDES 1 *meconium aspiration (P24.00, P24.01)*
meconium passage during delivery (P03.82)

DEF: Meconium passed in utero causing discoloration on the fetal skin and nails or on the umbilicus. This staining may be incidental or may be an indicator of significant fetal stress that could affect outcomes.

P96.89 Other specified conditions originating in the perinatal period

Use additional code to specify condition

P96.9 Condition originating in the perinatal period, unspecified

Congenital debility NOS

Chapter 17. Congenital Malformations, Deformations, and Chromosomal Abnormalities (Q00–Q99)

Chapter-specific Guidelines with Coding Examples

The chapter-specific guidelines from the ICD-10-CM Official Guidelines for Coding and Reporting have been provided below. Along with these guidelines are coding examples, contained in the shaded boxes, that have been developed to help illustrate the coding and/or sequencing guidance found in these guidelines.

Assign an appropriate code(s) from categories Q00-Q99, Congenital malformations, deformations, and chromosomal abnormalities when a malformation/deformation or chromosomal abnormality is documented. A malformation/deformation/or chromosomal abnormality may be the principal/first-listed diagnosis on a record or a secondary diagnosis.

When a malformation/deformation/or chromosomal abnormality does not have a unique code assignment, assign additional code(s) for any manifestations that may be present.

When the code assignment specifically identifies the malformation/deformation/or chromosomal abnormality, manifestations that are an inherent component of the anomaly should not be coded separately. Additional codes should be assigned for manifestations that are not an inherent component.

8-day-old infant with tetralogy of Fallot and pulmonary stenosis

Q21.3 Tetralogy of Fallot

Explanation: Pulmonary stenosis is inherent in the disease process of tetralogy of Fallot. When the code assignment specifically identifies the malformation/deformation/or chromosomal abnormality, manifestations that are inherent components of the anomaly should not be coded separately.

7-month-old infant with Down syndrome and common atrioventricular canal

Q90.9 Down syndrome, unspecified

Q21.23 Complete atrioventricular septal defect

Explanation: While a common atrioventricular canal is often associated with patients with Down syndrome, this manifestation is not an inherent component and may be reported separately. When the code assignment specifically identifies the anomaly, manifestations that are inherent components of the condition should not be coded separately. Additional codes should be assigned for manifestations that are not inherent components.

Codes from Chapter 17 may be used throughout the life of the patient. If a congenital malformation or deformity has been corrected, a personal history code should be used to identify the history of the malformation or deformity. Although present at birth, a malformation/deformation/or chromosomal abnormality may not be identified until later in life. Whenever the condition is diagnosed by the provider, it is appropriate to assign a code from codes Q00-Q99. For the birth admission, the appropriate code from category Z38, Liveborn infants, according to place of birth and type of delivery, should be sequenced as the principal diagnosis, followed by any congenital anomaly codes, Q00- Q99.

Three-year-old with history of corrected ventricular septal defect

Z87.74 Personal history of (corrected) congenital malformations of heart and circulatory system

Explanation: If a congenital malformation or deformity has been corrected, a personal history code should be used to identify the history of the malformation or deformity.

Forty-year-old man with headaches diagnosed with congenital arteriovenous malformation of cerebral vessels by brain scan

Q28.2 Arteriovenous malformation of cerebral vessels

Explanation: Although present at birth, malformations may not be identified until later in life. Whenever a congenital condition is diagnosed by the physician, it is appropriate to assign a code from the range Q00–Q99.

Chapter 17. Congenital Malformations, Deformations and Chromosomal Abnormalities (Q00-Q99)

NOTE Codes from this chapter are not for use on maternal records

EXCLUDES 2 *inborn errors of metabolism (E70-E88)*

This chapter contains the following blocks:

Q00-Q07 Congenital malformations of the nervous system
Q10-Q18 Congenital malformations of eye, ear, face and neck
Q20-Q28 Congenital malformations of the circulatory system
Q30-Q34 Congenital malformations of the respiratory system
Q35-Q37 Cleft lip and cleft palate
Q38-Q45 Other congenital malformations of the digestive system
Q50-Q56 Congenital malformations of genital organs
Q60-Q64 Congenital malformations of the urinary system
Q65-Q79 Congenital malformations and deformations of the musculoskeletal system
Q80-Q89 Other congenital malformations
Q90-Q99 Chromosomal abnormalities, not elsewhere classified

Congenital malformations of the nervous system (Q00-Q07)

Q00 Anencephaly and similar malformations

Q00.0 Anencephaly HCC Rx ESR COM
- Acephaly
- Acrania
- Amyelencephaly
- Hemianencephaly
- Hemicephaly

Q00.1 Craniorachischisis HCC Rx ESR COM

Q00.2 Iniencephaly HCC Rx ESR COM

Q01 Encephalocele

INCLUDES Arnold-Chiari syndrome, type III
encephalocystocele
encephalomyelocele
hydroencephalocele
hydromeningocele, cranial
meningocele, cerebral
meningoencephalocele

EXCLUDES 1 *Meckel-Gruber syndrome (Q61.9)*

DEF: Congenital protrusion of brain tissue through a defect in the skull.

Q01.0 Frontal encephalocele HCC Rx ESR COM

Q01.1 Nasofrontal encephalocele HCC Rx ESR COM

Q01.2 Occipital encephalocele HCC Rx ESR COM

Q01.8 Encephalocele of other sites HCC Rx ESR COM

Q01.9 Encephalocele, unspecified HCC Rx ESR COM

Q02 Microcephaly HCC Rx ESR COM

INCLUDES hydromicrocephaly
micrencephalon

Code first, if applicable, congenital Zika virus disease

EXCLUDES 1 *Meckel-Gruber syndrome (Q61.9)*

AHA: 2018,4Q,26

DEF: Congenital disorder in which the head circumference is more than two standard deviations below the mean for age, sex, race, and gestation and associated with a decreased life expectancy.

Q03 Congenital hydrocephalus

INCLUDES hydrocephalus in newborn

EXCLUDES 1 *Arnold-Chiari syndrome, type II (Q07.0-)*
acquired hydrocephalus (G91.-)
hydrocephalus due to congenital toxoplasmosis (P37.1)
hydrocephalus with spina bifida (Q05.0-Q05.4)

DEF: Hydrocephalus: Abnormal buildup of cerebrospinal fluid in the brain causing dilation of the ventricles.

Congenital Hydrocephalus

Q03.0 Malformations of aqueduct of Sylvius HCC Rx ESR COM
- Anomaly of aqueduct of Sylvius
- Obstruction of aqueduct of Sylvius, congenital
- Stenosis of aqueduct of Sylvius

Q03.1 Atresia of foramina of Magendie and Luschka HCC Rx ESR COM
- Dandy-Walker syndrome

Q03.8 Other congenital hydrocephalus HCC Rx ESR COM

Q03.9 Congenital hydrocephalus, unspecified HCC Rx ESR COM

Q04 Other congenital malformations of brain

EXCLUDES 1 *cyclopia (Q87.0)*
macrocephaly (Q75.3)

Q04.0 Congenital malformations of corpus callosum HCC Rx ESR COM
- Agenesis of corpus callosum

Q04.1 Arhinencephaly HCC Rx ESR COM

Q04.2 Holoprosencephaly HCC Rx ESR COM

Q04.3 Other reduction deformities of brain HCC Rx ESR COM
- Absence of part of brain
- Agenesis of part of brain
- Agyria
- Aplasia of part of brain
- Hydranencephaly
- Hypoplasia of part of brain
- Lissencephaly
- Microgyria
- Pachygyria

EXCLUDES 1 *congenital malformations of corpus callosum (Q04.0)*

Q04.4 Septo-optic dysplasia of brain HCC Rx ESR COM

Q04.5 Megalencephaly HCC Rx ESR COM

Q04.6 Congenital cerebral cysts HCC Rx ESR COM
- Porencephaly
- Schizencephaly

EXCLUDES 1 *acquired porencephalic cyst (G93.0)*

Q04.8 Other specified congenital malformations of brain HCC Rx ESR COM
- Arnold-Chiari syndrome, type IV
- Macrogyria

Q04.9 Congenital malformation of brain, unspecified HCC Rx ESR COM
- Congenital anomaly NOS of brain
- Congenital deformity NOS of brain
- Congenital disease or lesion NOS of brain
- Multiple anomalies NOS of brain, congenital

Q05 Spina bifida

INCLUDES hydromeningocele (spinal)
meningocele (spinal)
meningomyelocele
myelocele
myelomeningocele
rachischisis
spina bifida (aperta)(cystica)
syringomyelocele

Use additional code for any associated paraplegia (paraparesis) (G82.2-)

EXCLUDES 1 *Arnold-Chiari syndrome, type II (Q07.0-)*
spina bifida occulta (Q76.0)

DEF: Lack of closure in the vertebral column with protrusion of the spinal cord through the defect, often in the lumbosacral area. This condition can be recognized by the presence of alpha-fetoproteins in the amniotic fluid.

Spina Bifida

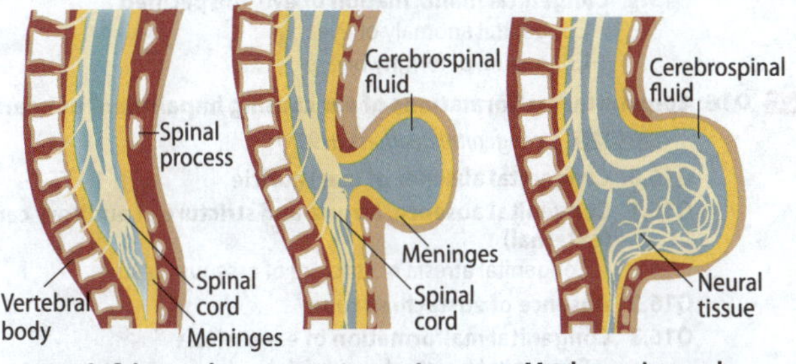

Q05.0 Cervical spina bifida with hydrocephalus HCC Rx ESR COM

Q05.1 Thoracic spina bifida with hydrocephalus HCC Rx ESR COM
Dorsal spina bifida with hydrocephalus
Thoracolumbar spina bifida with hydrocephalus

Q05.2 Lumbar spina bifida with hydrocephalus HCC Rx ESR COM
Lumbosacral spina bifida with hydrocephalus

Q05.3 Sacral spina bifida with hydrocephalus HCC Rx ESR COM

Q05.4 Unspecified spina bifida with hydrocephalus HCC Rx ESR COM

Q05.5 Cervical spina bifida without hydrocephalus HCC Rx ESR COM

Q05.6 Thoracic spina bifida without hydrocephalus HCC Rx ESR COM
Dorsal spina bifida NOS
Thoracolumbar spina bifida NOS

Q05.7 Lumbar spina bifida without hydrocephalus HCC Rx ESR COM
Lumbosacral spina bifida NOS

Q05.8 Sacral spina bifida without hydrocephalus HCC Rx ESR COM

Q05.9 Spina bifida, unspecified HCC Rx ESR COM

Q06 Other congenital malformations of spinal cord

Q06.0 Amyelia HCC Rx ESR COM

Q06.1 Hypoplasia and dysplasia of spinal cord HCC Rx ESR COM
Atelomyelia
Myelatelia
Myelodysplasia of spinal cord

Q06.2 Diastematomyelia HCC Rx ESR COM
DEF: Rare congenital anomaly often associated with spina bifida. The spinal cord is separated into longitudinal halves by a bony, cartilaginous or fibrous septum, each half surrounded by a dural sac.

Q06.3 Other congenital cauda equina malformations HCC Rx ESR COM

Q06.4 Hydromyelia HCC Rx ESR COM
Hydrorachis

Q06.8 Other specified congenital malformations of spinal cord HCC Rx ESR COM

Q06.9 Congenital malformation of spinal cord, unspecified HCC Rx ESR COM
Congenital anomaly NOS of spinal cord
Congenital deformity NOS of spinal cord
Congenital disease or lesion NOS of spinal cord

Q07 Other congenital malformations of nervous system

EXCLUDES 2 *congenital central alveolar hypoventilation syndrome (G47.35)*
familial dysautonomia [Riley-Day] (G90.1)
neurofibromatosis (nonmalignant) (Q85.0-)

Q07.0 Arnold-Chiari syndrome
Arnold-Chiari syndrome, type II
EXCLUDES 1 *Arnold-Chiari syndrome, type III (Q01.-)*
Arnold-Chiari syndrome, type IV (Q04.8)
DEF: Congenital malformation of the brain in which the cerebellum protrudes through the foramen magnum into the spinal canal.

Q07.00 Arnold-Chiari syndrome without spina bifida or hydrocephalus HCC Rx ESR COM

Q07.01 Arnold-Chiari syndrome with spina bifida HCC Rx ESR COM

Q07.02 Arnold-Chiari syndrome with hydrocephalus HCC Rx ESR COM

Q07.03 Arnold-Chiari syndrome with spina bifida and hydrocephalus HCC Rx ESR COM

Q07.8 Other specified congenital malformations of nervous system HCC Rx ESR COM
Agenesis of nerve
Displacement of brachial plexus
Jaw-winking syndrome
Marcus Gunn's syndrome

Q07.9 Congenital malformation of nervous system, unspecified HCC Rx ESR COM
Congenital anomaly NOS of nervous system
Congenital deformity NOS of nervous system
Congenital disease or lesion NOS of nervous system

Congenital malformations of eye, ear, face and neck (Q10-Q18)

EXCLUDES 2 *cleft lip and cleft palate (Q35-Q37)*
congenital malformation of cervical spine (Q05.0, Q05.5, Q67.5, Q76.0-Q76.4)
congenital malformation of larynx (Q31.-)
congenital malformation of lip NEC (Q38.0)
congenital malformation of nose (Q30.-)
congenital malformation of parathyroid gland (Q89.2)
congenital malformation of thyroid gland (Q89.2)

Q10 Congenital malformations of eyelid, lacrimal apparatus and orbit

EXCLUDES 1 *cryptophthalmos NOS (Q11.2)*
cryptophthalmos syndrome (Q87.0)

Q10.0 Congenital ptosis
DEF: Congenital drooping of the eyelid. Ptosis is mostly idiopathic, but may occur genetically.

Q10.1 Congenital ectropion

Q10.2 Congenital entropion

Q10.3 Other congenital malformations of eyelid
Ablepharon
Blepharophimosis, congenital
Coloboma of eyelid
Congenital absence or agenesis of cilia
Congenital absence or agenesis of eyelid
Congenital accessory eyelid
Congenital accessory eye muscle
Congenital malformation of eyelid NOS

Q10.4 Absence and agenesis of lacrimal apparatus
Congenital absence of punctum lacrimale

Q10.5 Congenital stenosis and stricture of lacrimal duct

Q10.6 Other congenital malformations of lacrimal apparatus
Congenital malformation of lacrimal apparatus NOS

Q10.7 Congenital malformation of orbit

Q11 Anophthalmos, microphthalmos and macrophthalmos

Q11.0 Cystic eyeball

Q11.1 Other anophthalmos
Anophthalmos NOS
Agenesis of eye
Aplasia of eye

Q11.2 Microphthalmos
Cryptophthalmos NOS
Dysplasia of eye
Hypoplasia of eye
Rudimentary eye
EXCLUDES 1 *cryptophthalmos syndrome (Q87.0)*

Q11.3 Macrophthalmos

EXCLUDES 1 *macrophthalmos in congenital glaucoma (Q15.Ø)*

4th **Q12 Congenital lens malformations**

Q12.Ø Congenital cataract

Q12.1 Congenital displaced lens

Q12.2 Coloboma of lens

Coloboma of Lens

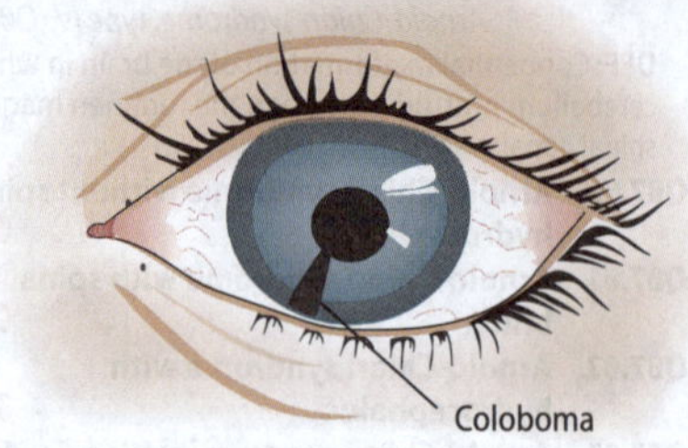

Coloboma

Q12.3 Congenital aphakia

Q12.4 Spherophakia

Q12.8 Other congenital lens malformations

Microphakia

Q12.9 Congenital lens malformation, unspecified

4th **Q13 Congenital malformations of anterior segment of eye**

Q13.Ø Coloboma of iris

Coloboma NOS

DEF: Defective or absent section of ocular tissue that may present as mild cupping or a small pit in the ocular disc due to extensive defects in the iris, ciliary body, choroids, and retina.

Q13.1 Absence of iris

Aniridia

Use additional code for associated glaucoma (H42)

DEF: Incompletely formed or absent iris. It affects both eyes and is a dominant trait.

Q13.2 Other congenital malformations of iris

Anisocoria, congenital
Atresia of pupil
Congenital malformation of iris NOS
Corectopia

Q13.3 Congenital corneal opacity

Q13.4 Other congenital corneal malformations

Congenital malformation of cornea NOS
Microcornea
Peter's anomaly

Q13.5 Blue sclera

5th **Q13.8 Other congenital malformations of anterior segment of eye**

Q13.81 Rieger's anomaly

Use additional code for associated glaucoma (H42)

Q13.89 Other congenital malformations of anterior segment of eye

Q13.9 Congenital malformation of anterior segment of eye, unspecified

4th **Q14 Congenital malformations of posterior segment of eye**

EXCLUDES 2 *optic nerve hypoplasia (H47.Ø3-)*

Q14.Ø Congenital malformation of vitreous humor

Congenital vitreous opacity

Q14.1 Congenital malformation of retina

Congenital retinal aneurysm

Q14.2 Congenital malformation of optic disc

Coloboma of optic disc

Q14.3 Congenital malformation of choroid

Q14.8 Other congenital malformations of posterior segment of eye

Coloboma of the fundus

Q14.9 Congenital malformation of posterior segment of eye, unspecified

4th **Q15 Other congenital malformations of eye**

EXCLUDES 1 *congenital nystagmus (H55.Ø1)*
ocular albinism (E7Ø.31-)
optic nerve hypoplasia (H47.Ø3-)
retinitis pigmentosa (H35.52)

Q15.Ø Congenital glaucoma

Axenfeld's anomaly
Buphthalmos
Glaucoma of childhood
Glaucoma of newborn
Hydrophthalmos
Keratoglobus, congenital, with glaucoma
Macrocornea with glaucoma
Macrophthalmos in congenital glaucoma
Megalocornea with glaucoma

Q15.8 Other specified congenital malformations of eye

Q15.9 Congenital malformation of eye, unspecified

Congenital anomaly of eye
Congenital deformity of eye

4th **Q16 Congenital malformations of ear causing impairment of hearing**

EXCLUDES 1 *congenital deafness (H9Ø.-)*

Q16.Ø Congenital absence of (ear) auricle

Q16.1 Congenital absence, atresia and stricture of auditory canal (external)

Congenital atresia or stricture of osseous meatus

Q16.2 Absence of eustachian tube

Q16.3 Congenital malformation of ear ossicles

Congenital fusion of ear ossicles

Q16.4 Other congenital malformations of middle ear

Congenital malformation of middle ear NOS

Q16.5 Congenital malformation of inner ear

Congenital anomaly of membranous labyrinth
Congenital anomaly of organ of Corti

Q16.9 Congenital malformation of ear causing impairment of hearing, unspecified

Congenital absence of ear NOS

4th **Q17 Other congenital malformations of ear**

EXCLUDES 1 *congenital malformations of ear with impairment of hearing (Q16.Ø-Q16.9)*
preauricular sinus (Q18.1)

Q17.Ø Accessory auricle

Accessory tragus
Polyotia
Preauricular appendage or tag
Supernumerary ear
Supernumerary lobule

Q17.1 Macrotia

DEF: Birth defect characterized by abnormal enlargement of the pinna of the ear.

Q17.2 Microtia

Q17.3 Other misshapen ear

Pointed ear

Q17.4 Misplaced ear

Low-set ears

EXCLUDES 1 *cervical auricle (Q18.2)*

Q17.5 Prominent ear

Bat ear

Q17.8 Other specified congenital malformations of ear

Congenital absence of lobe of ear

Q17.9 Congenital malformation of ear, unspecified

Congenital anomaly of ear NOS

4th **Q18 Other congenital malformations of face and neck**

EXCLUDES 1 *cleft lip and cleft palate (Q35-Q37)*
conditions classified to Q67.Ø-Q67.4
congenital malformations of skull and face bones (Q75.-)
cyclopia (Q87.Ø)
dentofacial anomalies [including malocclusion] (M26.-)
malformation syndromes affecting facial appearance (Q87.Ø)
persistent thyroglossal duct (Q89.2)

Q18.Ø Sinus, fistula and cyst of branchial cleft

Branchial vestige

Q18.1 Preauricular sinus and cyst

Fistula of auricle, congenital
Cervicoaural fistula

Q18.2 Other branchial cleft malformations
Branchial cleft malformation NOS
Cervical auricle
Otocephaly

Q18.3 Webbing of neck
Pterygium colli
DEF: Congenital malformation characterized by a thick, triangular skinfold that stretches from the lateral side of the neck across the shoulder. It is associated with genetic conditions such as Turner's and Noonan's syndromes.

Q18.4 Macrostomia
DEF: Rare congenital craniofacial bilateral or unilateral anomaly of the mouth due to malformed maxillary and mandibular processes. It results in an abnormally large mouth extending toward the ear.

Q18.5 Microstomia

Q18.6 Macrocheilia
Hypertrophy of lip, congenital

Q18.7 Microcheilia

Q18.8 Other specified congenital malformations of face and neck
Medial cyst of face and neck
Medial fistula of face and neck
Medial sinus of face and neck

Q18.9 Congenital malformation of face and neck, unspecified
Congenital anomaly NOS of face and neck

Congenital malformations of the circulatory system (Q2Ø-Q28)

✓4th Q2Ø Congenital malformations of cardiac chambers and connections
EXCLUDES 1 *dextrocardia with situs inversus (Q89.3)*
mirror-image atrial arrangement with situs inversus (Q89.3)

Q2Ø.Ø Common arterial trunk Rx COM
Persistent truncus arteriosus
EXCLUDES 1 *aortic septal defect (Q21.4)*

Q2Ø.1 Double outlet right ventricle Rx COM
Taussig-Bing syndrome

Q2Ø.2 Double outlet left ventricle Rx COM

Q2Ø.3 Discordant ventriculoarterial connection Rx COM
Dextrotransposition of aorta
Transposition of great vessels (complete)

Q2Ø.4 Double inlet ventricle Rx COM
Common ventricle
Cor triloculare biatriatum
Single ventricle

Q2Ø.5 Discordant atrioventricular connection Rx COM
Corrected transposition
Levotransposition
Ventricular inversion

Q2Ø.6 Isomerism of atrial appendages COM
Isomerism of atrial appendages with asplenia or polysplenia

Q2Ø.8 Other congenital malformations of cardiac chambers and connections Rx COM
Cor binoculare

Q2Ø.9 Congenital malformation of cardiac chambers and connections, unspecified COM

✓4th Q21 Congenital malformations of cardiac septa
EXCLUDES 1 *acquired cardiac septal defect (I51.Ø)*

Q21.Ø Ventricular septal defect Rx COM
Roger's disease

Ventricular Septal Defect

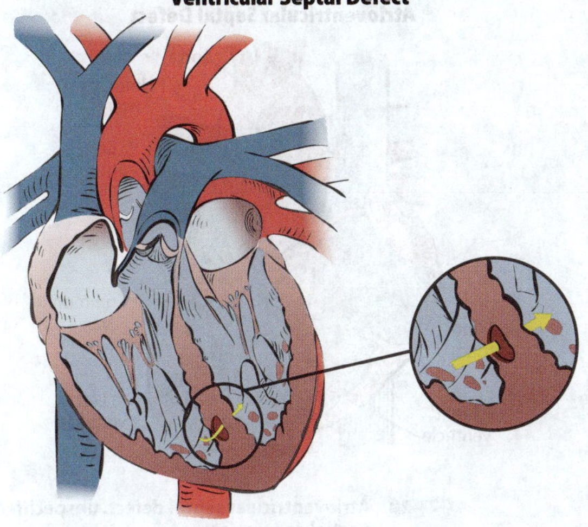

▲ **✓5th Q21.1 Atrial septal defect**
~~Coronary sinus defect~~
~~Patent or persistent foramen ovale~~
~~Patent or persistent ostium secundum defect (type II)~~
~~Patent or persistent sinus venosus defect~~
EXCLUDES 2 ▶*ostium primum atrial septal defect (type I) (Q21.2Ø)*◀

Atrial Septal Defect

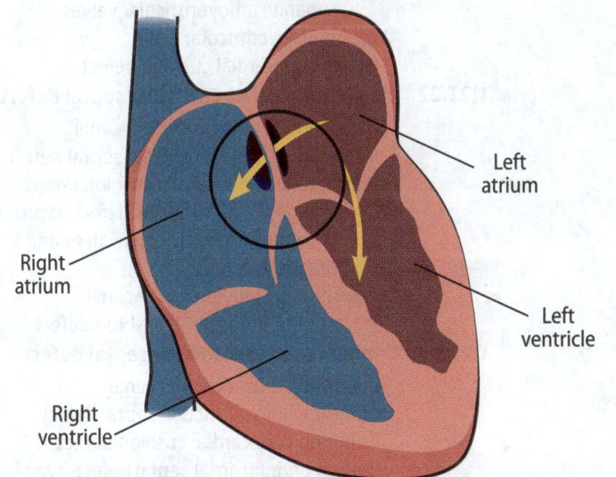

● **Q21.1Ø Atrial septal defect, unspecified**

● **Q21.11 Secundum atrial septal defect**
Fenestrated atrial septum
Patent or persistent ostium secundum defect (type II)

● **Q21.12 Patent foramen ovale**
Persistent foramen ovale

● **Q21.13 Coronary sinus atrial septal defect**
Coronary sinus defect
Unroofed coronary sinus

● **Q21.14 Superior sinus venosus atrial septal defect**
Superior vena cava type atrial septal defect

● **Q21.15 Inferior sinus venosus atrial septal defect**
Inferior vena cava type atrial septal defect

● **Q21.16 Sinus venosus atrial septal defect, unspecified**
Sinus venosus defect, NOS

● **Q21.19 Other specified atrial septal defect**
Common atrium
Other specified atrial septal abnormality

▲ ✓5th **Q21.2 Atrioventricular septal defect**
▶Atrioventricular canal defect◀
~~Common atrioventricular canal~~
Endocardial cushion defect
Ostium primum atrial septal defect (type I)

Atrioventricular Septal Defect

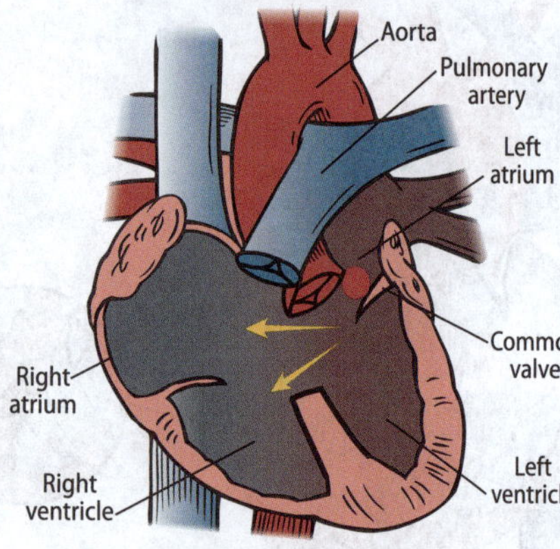

● **Q21.2Ø Atrioventricular septal defect, unspecified as to partial or complete**
Atrioventricular canal, NOS
Endocardial cushion defect NOS
Ostium primum atrial septal defect (type I) NOS

● **Q21.21 Partial atrioventricular septal defect**
Incomplete atrioventricular canal
Incomplete atrioventricular septal defect
Incomplete endocardial cushion defect
Ostium primum atrial septal defect (type I) with separate atrioventricular valves
Partial atrioventricular canal
Partial endocardial cushion defect

● **Q21.22 Transitional atrioventricular septal defect**
Intermediate atrioventricular canal
Intermediate atrioventricular septal defect
Intermediate endocardial cushion defect
Ostium primum atrial septal defect (type I) with separate atrioventricular valves and a small or restrictive inlet VSD
Transitional atrioventricular canal
Transitional endocardial cushion defect

● **Q21.23 Complete atrioventricular septal defect**
Common atrioventricular canal
Common atrioventricular septal defect
Common endocardial cushion defect
Ostium primum atrial septal defect (type I) with common atrioventricular valve and a moderate or larger inlet VSD

Q21.3 Tetralogy of Fallot Rx COM
Ventricular septal defect with pulmonary stenosis or atresia, dextroposition of aorta and hypertrophy of right ventricle.
AHA: 2014,3Q,16

Q21.4 Aortopulmonary septal defect COM
Aortic septal defect
Aortopulmonary window

Q21.8 Other congenital malformations of cardiac septa COM
Eisenmenger's defect
Pentalogy of Fallot
Code also, if applicable:
Eisenmenger's complex (I27.83)
Eisenmenger's syndrome (I27.83)

Q21.9 Congenital malformation of cardiac septum, unspecified COM
Septal (heart) defect NOS

✓4th **Q22 Congenital malformations of pulmonary and tricuspid valves**

Q22.Ø Pulmonary valve atresia Rx COM

Q22.1 Congenital pulmonary valve stenosis COM

Q22.2 Congenital pulmonary valve insufficiency COM
Congenital pulmonary valve regurgitation

Q22.3 Other congenital malformations of pulmonary valve COM
Congenital malformation of pulmonary valve NOS
Supernumerary cusps of pulmonary valve

Q22.4 Congenital tricuspid stenosis COM
Congenital tricuspid atresia

Q22.5 Ebstein's anomaly COM
DEF: Malformation of the tricuspid valve characterized by septal and posterior leaflets attaching to the wall of the right ventricle. Ebstein's anomaly causes the right ventricle to fuse with the atrium into a large right atrium and a small ventricle and leads to heart failure and abnormal cardiac rhythm.

Q22.6 Hypoplastic right heart syndrome COM

Q22.8 Other congenital malformations of tricuspid valve COM

Q22.9 Congenital malformation of tricuspid valve, unspecified COM

✓4th **Q23 Congenital malformations of aortic and mitral valves**

Q23.Ø Congenital stenosis of aortic valve COM
Congenital aortic atresia
Congenital aortic stenosis NOS
EXCLUDES 1 *congenital stenosis of aortic valve in hypoplastic left heart syndrome (Q23.4)*
congenital subaortic stenosis (Q24.4)
supravalvular aortic stenosis (congenital) (Q25.3)

Q23.1 Congenital insufficiency of aortic valve COM
Bicuspid aortic valve
Congenital aortic insufficiency

Q23.2 Congenital mitral stenosis COM
Congenital mitral atresia

Q23.3 Congenital mitral insufficiency COM

Q23.4 Hypoplastic left heart syndrome Rx COM

Q23.8 Other congenital malformations of aortic and mitral valves COM

Q23.9 Congenital malformation of aortic and mitral valves, unspecified COM

✓4th **Q24 Other congenital malformations of heart**
EXCLUDES 1 *endocardial fibroelastosis (I42.4)*

Q24.Ø Dextrocardia COM
EXCLUDES 1 *dextrocardia with situs inversus (Q89.3)*
isomerism of atrial appendages (with asplenia or polysplenia) (Q2Ø.6)
mirror-image atrial arrangement with situs inversus (Q89.3)
DEF: Congenital condition in which the heart is located on the right side of the chest rather than in its normal position on the left.

Q24.1 Levocardia COM

Q24.2 Cor triatriatum COM

Q24.3 Pulmonary infundibular stenosis COM
Subvalvular pulmonic stenosis

Q24.4 Congenital subaortic stenosis COM
DEF: Congenital heart defect characterized by stenosis of the left ventricular outflow tract due to a fibrous tissue ring or septal hypertrophy below the aortic valve.

Q24.5 Malformation of coronary vessels Rx COM
Congenital coronary (artery) aneurysm

Q24.6 Congenital heart block COM

Q24.8 Other specified congenital malformations of heart COM
Congenital diverticulum of left ventricle
Congenital malformation of myocardium
Congenital malformation of pericardium
Malposition of heart
Uhl's disease

Q24.9 Congenital malformation of heart, unspecified COM
Congenital anomaly of heart
Congenital disease of heart

✓4th **Q25 Congenital malformations of great arteries**

Q25.Ø Patent ductus arteriosus Rx COM
Patent ductus Botallo
Persistent ductus arteriosus
DEF: Condition in which the normal channel between the pulmonary artery and the aorta fails to close at birth, causing arterial blood to recirculate in the lungs and inhibiting the blood supply to the aorta. ***Synonym(s):*** *PDA.*

Q25.1 Coarctation of aorta COM
Coarctation of aorta (preductal) (postductal)
Stenosis of aorta
AHA: 2016,4Q,56-57

✓5th **Q25.2 Atresia of aorta**
AHA: 2016,4Q,56-57

Q25.21 Interruption of aortic arch COM
Atresia of aortic arch

Q25.29 Other atresia of aorta COM
Atresia of aorta

Q25.3 Supravalvular aortic stenosis COM
EXCLUDES 1 *congenital aortic stenosis NOS (Q23.Ø)*
congenital stenosis of aortic valve (Q23.Ø)

✓5th **Q25.4 Other congenital malformations of aorta**
EXCLUDES 1 *hypoplasia of aorta in hypoplastic left heart syndrome (Q23.4)*
AHA: 2016,4Q,57

Q25.4Ø Congenital malformation of aorta unspecified COM

Q25.41 Absence and aplasia of aorta COM

Q25.42 Hypoplasia of aorta COM

Q25.43 Congenital aneurysm of aorta COM
Congenital aneurysm of aortic root
Congenital aneurysm of aortic sinus

Q25.44 Congenital dilation of aorta COM

Q25.45 Double aortic arch COM
Vascular ring of aorta

Aortic Arch Anomalies

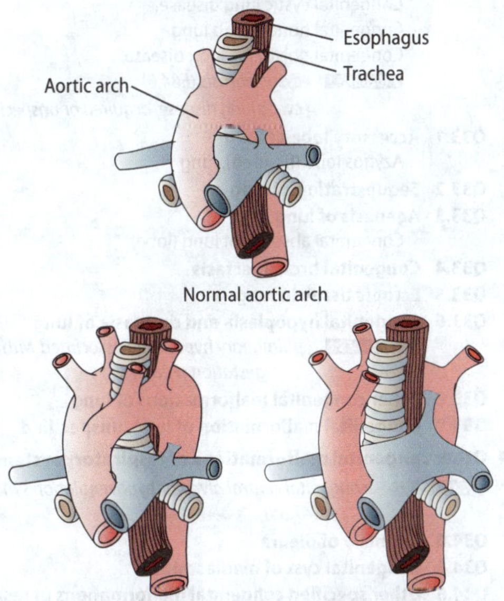

Q25.46 Tortuous aortic arch COM
Persistent convolutions of aortic arch

Q25.47 Right aortic arch COM
Persistent right aortic arch

Q25.48 Anomalous origin of subclavian artery COM

Q25.49 Other congenital malformations of aorta COM
Aortic arch
Bovine arch

Q25.5 Atresia of pulmonary artery Rx COM

Q25.6 Stenosis of pulmonary artery COM
Supravalvular pulmonary stenosis

✓5th **Q25.7 Other congenital malformations of pulmonary artery**

Q25.71 Coarctation of pulmonary artery Rx COM

Q25.72 Congenital pulmonary arteriovenous malformation COM
Congenital pulmonary arteriovenous aneurysm

Q25.79 Other congenital malformations of pulmonary artery COM
Aberrant pulmonary artery
Agenesis of pulmonary artery
Congenital aneurysm of pulmonary artery
Congenital anomaly of pulmonary artery
Hypoplasia of pulmonary artery

Q25.8 Other congenital malformations of other great arteries COM

Q25.9 Congenital malformation of great arteries, unspecified COM

✓4th **Q26 Congenital malformations of great veins**

Q26.Ø Congenital stenosis of vena cava Rx COM
Congenital stenosis of vena cava (inferior)(superior)

Q26.1 Persistent left superior vena cava Rx COM

Q26.2 Total anomalous pulmonary venous connection Rx COM
Total anomalous pulmonary venous return [TAPVR], subdiaphragmatic
Total anomalous pulmonary venous return [TAPVR], supradiaphragmatic

Q26.3 Partial anomalous pulmonary venous connection Rx COM
Partial anomalous pulmonary venous return

Q26.4 Anomalous pulmonary venous connection, unspecified Rx COM

Q26.5 Anomalous portal venous connection COM

Q26.6 Portal vein-hepatic artery fistula COM

Q26.8 Other congenital malformations of great veins Rx COM
Absence of vena cava (inferior) (superior)
Azygos continuation of inferior vena cava
Persistent left posterior cardinal vein
Scimitar syndrome

Q26.9 Congenital malformation of great vein, unspecified Rx COM
Congenital anomaly of vena cava (inferior) (superior) NOS

✓4th **Q27 Other congenital malformations of peripheral vascular system**
EXCLUDES 2 *anomalies of cerebral and precerebral vessels (Q28.Ø-Q28.3)*
anomalies of coronary vessels (Q24.5)
anomalies of pulmonary artery (Q25.5-Q25.7)
congenital retinal aneurysm (Q14.1)
hemangioma and lymphangioma (D18.-)

Q27.Ø Congenital absence and hypoplasia of umbilical artery COM
Single umbilical artery

Q27.1 Congenital renal artery stenosis COM

Q27.2 Other congenital malformations of renal artery COM
Congenital malformation of renal artery NOS
Multiple renal arteries

✓5th **Q27.3 Arteriovenous malformation (peripheral)**
Arteriovenous aneurysm
EXCLUDES 1 *acquired arteriovenous aneurysm (I77.Ø)*
EXCLUDES 2 *arteriovenous malformation of cerebral vessels (Q28.2)*
arteriovenous malformation of precerebral vessels (Q28.Ø)
DEF: Arteriovenous malformation: Connecting passage between an artery and a vein.

Q27.3Ø Arteriovenous malformation, site unspecified COM

Q27.31 Arteriovenous malformation of vessel of upper limb COM

Q27.32 Arteriovenous malformation of vessel of lower limb COM

Q27.33 Arteriovenous malformation of digestive system vessel COM
AHA: 2018,3Q,21

Q27.34 Arteriovenous malformation of renal vessel COM

Q27.39 Arteriovenous malformation, other site COM

Q27.4 Congenital phlebectasia COM

Q27.8 Other specified congenital malformations of peripheral vascular system COM
Absence of peripheral vascular system
Atresia of peripheral vascular system
Congenital aneurysm (peripheral)
Congenital stricture, artery
Congenital varix
EXCLUDES 1 *arteriovenous malformation (Q27.3-)*

Q27.9 Congenital malformation of peripheral vascular system, unspecified COM
Anomaly of artery or vein NOS

✓4th Q28 Other congenital malformations of circulatory system
EXCLUDES 1 *congenital aneurysm NOS (Q27.8)*
congenital coronary aneurysm (Q24.5)
ruptured cerebral arteriovenous malformation (I6Ø.8)
ruptured malformation of precerebral vessels (I72.Ø)
EXCLUDES 2 *congenital peripheral aneurysm (Q27.8)*
congenital pulmonary aneurysm (Q25.79)
congenital retinal aneurysm (Q14.1)

Q28.Ø Arteriovenous malformation of precerebral vessels COM
Congenital arteriovenous precerebral aneurysm (nonruptured)

Q28.1 Other malformations of precerebral vessels COM
Congenital malformation of precerebral vessels NOS
Congenital precerebral aneurysm (nonruptured)

Q28.2 Arteriovenous malformation of cerebral vessels COM
Arteriovenous malformation of brain NOS
Congenital arteriovenous cerebral aneurysm (nonruptured)

Q28.3 Other malformations of cerebral vessels COM
Congenital cerebral aneurysm (nonruptured)
Congenital malformation of cerebral vessels NOS
Developmental venous anomaly

Q28.8 Other specified congenital malformations of circulatory system COM
Congenital aneurysm, specified site NEC
Spinal vessel anomaly

Q28.9 Congenital malformation of circulatory system, unspecified COM

Congenital malformations of the respiratory system (Q3Ø-Q34)

✓4th Q3Ø Congenital malformations of nose
EXCLUDES 1 *congenital deviation of nasal septum (Q67.4)*

Q3Ø.Ø Choanal atresia
Atresia of nares (anterior) (posterior)
Congenital stenosis of nares (anterior) (posterior)

Q3Ø.1 Agenesis and underdevelopment of nose
Congenital absent of nose

Q3Ø.2 Fissured, notched and cleft nose

Q3Ø.3 Congenital perforated nasal septum

Q3Ø.8 Other congenital malformations of nose
Accessory nose
Congenital anomaly of nasal sinus wall
AHA: 2022,2Q,17

Q3Ø.9 Congenital malformation of nose, unspecified

✓4th Q31 Congenital malformations of larynx
EXCLUDES 1 *congenital laryngeal stridor NOS (P28.89)*

Q31.Ø Web of larynx
Glottic web of larynx
Subglottic web of larynx
Web of larynx NOS
DEF: Congenital malformation of the larynx marked by thin, translucent, or thick fibrotic membrane-like structure between the vocal folds. It is characterized by shortness of breath and stridor.

Q31.1 Congenital subglottic stenosis

Q31.2 Laryngeal hypoplasia

Q31.3 Laryngocele

Q31.5 Congenital laryngomalacia

Q31.8 Other congenital malformations of larynx
Absence of larynx
Agenesis of larynx
Atresia of larynx
Congenital cleft thyroid cartilage
Congenital fissure of epiglottis
Congenital stenosis of larynx NEC
Posterior cleft of cricoid cartilage

Q31.9 Congenital malformation of larynx, unspecified

✓4th Q32 Congenital malformations of trachea and bronchus
EXCLUDES 1 *congenital bronchiectasis (Q33.4)*

Q32.Ø Congenital tracheomalacia

Q32.1 Other congenital malformations of trachea
Atresia of trachea
Congenital anomaly of tracheal cartilage
Congenital dilatation of trachea
Congenital malformation of trachea
Congenital stenosis of trachea
Congenital tracheocele

Q32.2 Congenital bronchomalacia

Q32.3 Congenital stenosis of bronchus

Q32.4 Other congenital malformations of bronchus
Absence of bronchus
Agenesis of bronchus
Atresia of bronchus
Congenital diverticulum of bronchus
Congenital malformation of bronchus NOS

✓4th Q33 Congenital malformations of lung

Q33.Ø Congenital cystic lung
Congenital cystic lung disease
Congenital honeycomb lung
Congenital polycystic lung disease
EXCLUDES 1 *cystic fibrosis (E84.Ø)*
cystic lung disease, acquired or unspecified (J98.4)

Q33.1 Accessory lobe of lung
Azygos lobe (fissured), lung

Q33.2 Sequestration of lung

Q33.3 Agenesis of lung
Congenital absence of lung (lobe)

Q33.4 Congenital bronchiectasis

Q33.5 Ectopic tissue in lung

Q33.6 Congenital hypoplasia and dysplasia of lung
EXCLUDES 1 *pulmonary hypoplasia associated with short gestation (P28.Ø)*

Q33.8 Other congenital malformations of lung

Q33.9 Congenital malformation of lung, unspecified

✓4th Q34 Other congenital malformations of respiratory system
EXCLUDES 2 *congenital central alveolar hypoventilation syndrome (G47.35)*

Q34.Ø Anomaly of pleura

Q34.1 Congenital cyst of mediastinum

Q34.8 Other specified congenital malformations of respiratory system
Atresia of nasopharynx

Q34.9 Congenital malformation of respiratory system, unspecified
Congenital absence of respiratory system
Congenital anomaly of respiratory system NOS

Cleft lip and cleft palate (Q35-Q37)

Use additional code to identify associated malformation of the nose (Q3Ø.2)

EXCLUDES 2 *Robin's syndrome (Q87.Ø)*

✓4th **Q35 Cleft palate**

INCLUDES fissure of palate
palatoschisis

EXCLUDES 1 *cleft palate with cleft lip (Q37.-)*

DEF: Congenital fissure or defect of the roof of the mouth opening to the nasal cavity due to failure of embryonic cells to fuse completely.

Cleft Palate

Cleft in soft palate
Cleft in hard and soft palate
Hard palate
Soft palate
Cleft
Cleft

Q35.1 Cleft hard palate COM

Q35.3 Cleft soft palate COM

Q35.5 Cleft hard palate with cleft soft palate COM

Q35.7 Cleft uvula COM

Q35.9 Cleft palate, unspecified COM
Cleft palate NOS

✓4th **Q36 Cleft lip**

INCLUDES cheiloschisis
congenital fissure of lip
harelip
labium leporinum

EXCLUDES 1 *cleft lip with cleft palate (Q37.-)*

DEF: Congenital fissure or opening in the upper lip due to failure of embryonic cells to fuse completely.

Cleft Lip

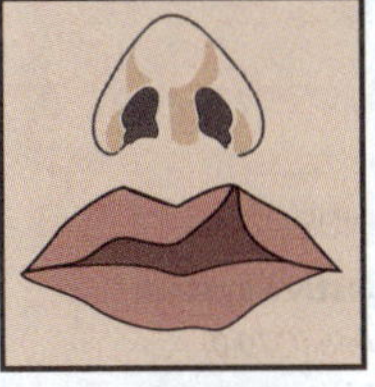
Unilateral incomplete

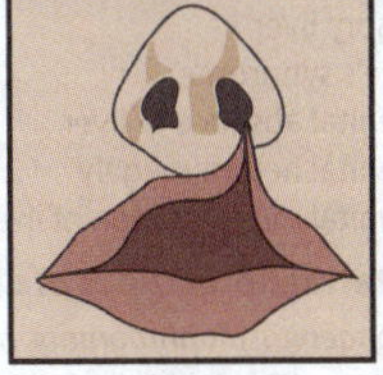
Unilateral complete

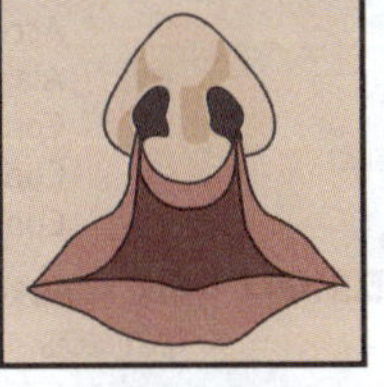
Bilateral complete

Q36.Ø Cleft lip, bilateral COM

Q36.1 Cleft lip, median COM

Q36.9 Cleft lip, unilateral COM
Cleft lip NOS

✓4th **Q37 Cleft palate with cleft lip**

INCLUDES cheilopalatoschisis

Q37.Ø Cleft hard palate with bilateral cleft lip COM

Q37.1 Cleft hard palate with unilateral cleft lip COM
Cleft hard palate with cleft lip NOS

Q37.2 Cleft soft palate with bilateral cleft lip COM

Q37.3 Cleft soft palate with unilateral cleft lip COM
Cleft soft palate with cleft lip NOS

Q37.4 Cleft hard and soft palate with bilateral cleft lip COM

Q37.5 Cleft hard and soft palate with unilateral cleft lip COM
Cleft hard and soft palate with cleft lip NOS

Q37.8 Unspecified cleft palate with bilateral cleft lip COM

Q37.9 Unspecified cleft palate with unilateral cleft lip COM
Cleft palate with cleft lip NOS

Other congenital malformations of the digestive system (Q38-Q45)

✓4th **Q38 Other congenital malformations of tongue, mouth and pharynx**

EXCLUDES 1 *dentofacial anomalies (M26.-)*
macrostomia (Q18.4)
microstomia (Q18.5)

Q38.Ø Congenital malformations of lips, not elsewhere classified
Congenital fistula of lip
Congenital malformation of lip NOS
Van der Woude's syndrome

EXCLUDES 1 *cleft lip (Q36.-)*
cleft lip with cleft palate (Q37.-)
macrocheilia (Q18.6)
microcheilia (Q18.7)

Q38.1 Ankyloglossia
Tongue tie

Q38.2 Macroglossia
Congenital hypertrophy of tongue

Q38.3 Other congenital malformations of tongue
Aglossia
Bifid tongue
Congenital adhesion of tongue
Congenital fissure of tongue
Congenital malformation of tongue NOS
Double tongue
Hypoglossia
Hypoplasia of tongue
Microglossia

Q38.4 Congenital malformations of salivary glands and ducts
Atresia of salivary glands and ducts
Congenital absence of salivary glands and ducts
Congenital accessory salivary glands and ducts
Congenital fistula of salivary gland

Q38.5 Congenital malformations of palate, not elsewhere classified
Congenital absence of uvula
Congenital malformation of palate NOS
Congenital high arched palate

EXCLUDES 1 *cleft palate (Q35.-)*
cleft palate with cleft lip (Q37.-)

Q38.6 Other congenital malformations of mouth
Congenital malformation of mouth NOS

Q38.7 Congenital pharyngeal pouch
Congenital diverticulum of pharynx

EXCLUDES 1 *pharyngeal pouch syndrome (D82.1)*

Q38.8 Other congenital malformations of pharynx
Congenital malformation of pharynx NOS
Imperforate pharynx

✓4th **Q39 Congenital malformations of esophagus**

Q39.Ø Atresia of esophagus without fistula COM
Atresia of esophagus NOS

Q39.1 Atresia of esophagus with tracheo-esophageal fistula COM
Atresia of esophagus with broncho-esophageal fistula

Q39.2 Congenital tracheo-esophageal fistula without atresia COM
Congenital tracheo-esophageal fistula NOS

Q39.3 Congenital stenosis and stricture of esophagus COM

Q39.4 Esophageal web COM

Q39.5 Congenital dilatation of esophagus
Congenital cardiospasm

Q39.6 Congenital diverticulum of esophagus
Congenital esophageal pouch

Q39.8 Other congenital malformations of esophagus
Congenital absence of esophagus
Congenital displacement of esophagus
Congenital duplication of esophagus

Q39.9 Congenital malformation of esophagus, unspecified

✓4th **Q4Ø Other congenital malformations of upper alimentary tract**

Q4Ø.Ø Congenital hypertrophic pyloric stenosis COM
Congenital or infantile constriction
Congenital or infantile hypertrophy
Congenital or infantile spasm
Congenital or infantile stenosis
Congenital or infantile stricture

Q40.1 Congenital hiatus hernia
Congenital displacement of cardia through esophageal hiatus
EXCLUDES 1 *congenital diaphragmatic hernia (Q79.0)*

Q40.2 Other specified congenital malformations of stomach
Congenital displacement of stomach
Congenital diverticulum of stomach
Congenital hourglass stomach
Congenital duplication of stomach
Megalogastria
Microgastria

Q40.3 Congenital malformation of stomach, unspecified

Q40.8 Other specified congenital malformations of upper alimentary tract

Q40.9 Congenital malformation of upper alimentary tract, unspecified
Congenital anomaly of upper alimentary tract
Congenital deformity of upper alimentary tract

Q41 Congenital absence, atresia and stenosis of small intestine
INCLUDES congenital obstruction, occlusion or stricture of small intestine or intestine NOS
EXCLUDES 1 *cystic fibrosis with intestinal manifestation (E84.11)*
meconium ileus NOS (without cystic fibrosis) (P76.0)

Q41.0 Congenital absence, atresia and stenosis of duodenum COM

Q41.1 Congenital absence, atresia and stenosis of jejunum COM
Apple peel syndrome
Imperforate jejunum

Q41.2 Congenital absence, atresia and stenosis of ileum COM

Q41.8 Congenital absence, atresia and stenosis of other specified parts of small intestine COM

Q41.9 Congenital absence, atresia and stenosis of small intestine, part unspecified COM
Congenital absence, atresia and stenosis of intestine NOS

Q42 Congenital absence, atresia and stenosis of large intestine
INCLUDES congenital obstruction, occlusion and stricture of large intestine

Q42.0 Congenital absence, atresia and stenosis of rectum with fistula COM

Q42.1 Congenital absence, atresia and stenosis of rectum without fistula COM
Imperforate rectum

Q42.2 Congenital absence, atresia and stenosis of anus with fistula COM

Q42.3 Congenital absence, atresia and stenosis of anus without fistula COM
Imperforate anus

Q42.8 Congenital absence, atresia and stenosis of other parts of large intestine COM

Q42.9 Congenital absence, atresia and stenosis of large intestine, part unspecified COM

Q43 Other congenital malformations of intestine

Q43.0 Meckel's diverticulum (displaced) (hypertrophic)
Persistent omphalomesenteric duct
Persistent vitelline duct
DEF: Congenital, abnormal remnant of embryonic digestive system development that leaves a sacculation or outpouching from the wall of the small intestine near the terminal part of the ileum made of acid-secreting tissue as in the stomach.

Q43.1 Hirschsprung's disease COM
Aganglionosis
Congenital (aganglionic) megacolon
DEF: Congenital enlargement or dilation of the colon, with the absence of nerve cells in a segment of colon distally that causes the inability to defecate.

Q43.2 Other congenital functional disorders of colon COM
Congenital dilatation of colon

Q43.3 Congenital malformations of intestinal fixation COM
Congenital omental, anomalous adhesions [bands]
Congenital peritoneal adhesions [bands]
Incomplete rotation of cecum and colon
Insufficient rotation of cecum and colon
Jackson's membrane
Malrotation of colon
Rotation failure of cecum and colon
Universal mesentery

Q43.4 Duplication of intestine

Q43.5 Ectopic anus

Q43.6 Congenital fistula of rectum and anus
EXCLUDES 1 *congenital fistula of anus with absence, atresia and stenosis (Q42.2)*
congenital fistula of rectum with absence, atresia and stenosis (Q42.0)
congenital rectovaginal fistula (Q52.2)
congenital urethrorectal fistula (Q64.73)
pilonidal fistula or sinus (L05.-)

Q43.7 Persistent cloaca
Cloaca NOS

Q43.8 Other specified congenital malformations of intestine
Congenital blind loop syndrome
Congenital diverticulitis, colon
Congenital diverticulum, intestine
Dolichocolon
Megaloappendix
Megaloduodenum
Microcolon
Transposition of appendix
Transposition of colon
Transposition of intestine
AHA: 2013,2Q,31

Q43.9 Congenital malformation of intestine, unspecified

Q44 Congenital malformations of gallbladder, bile ducts and liver

Q44.0 Agenesis, aplasia and hypoplasia of gallbladder
Congenital absence of gallbladder

Q44.1 Other congenital malformations of gallbladder
Congenital malformation of gallbladder NOS
Intrahepatic gallbladder

Q44.2 Atresia of bile ducts

Q44.3 Congenital stenosis and stricture of bile ducts

Q44.4 Choledochal cyst

Q44.5 Other congenital malformations of bile ducts
Accessory hepatic duct
Biliary duct duplication
Congenital malformation of bile duct NOS
Cystic duct duplication

Q44.6 Cystic disease of liver
Fibrocystic disease of liver

Q44.7 Other congenital malformations of liver
Accessory liver
Alagille's syndrome
Congenital absence of liver
Congenital hepatomegaly
Congenital malformation of liver NOS

Q45 Other congenital malformations of digestive system
EXCLUDES 2 *congenital diaphragmatic hernia (Q79.0)*
congenital hiatus hernia (Q40.1)

Q45.0 Agenesis, aplasia and hypoplasia of pancreas
Congenital absence of pancreas

Q45.1 Annular pancreas

Q45.2 Congenital pancreatic cyst

Q45.3 Other congenital malformations of pancreas and pancreatic duct
Accessory pancreas
Congenital malformation of pancreas or pancreatic duct NOS
EXCLUDES 1 *congenital diabetes mellitus (E10.-)*
cystic fibrosis (E84.0-E84.9)
fibrocystic disease of pancreas (E84.-)
neonatal diabetes mellitus (P70.2)

Q45.8 Other specified congenital malformations of digestive system
Absence (complete) (partial) of alimentary tract NOS
Duplication of digestive system
Malposition, congenital of digestive system

Q45.9 Congenital malformation of digestive system, unspecified
Congenital anomaly of digestive system
Congenital deformity of digestive system

Congenital malformations of genital organs (Q50-Q56)

EXCLUDES 1 *androgen insensitivity syndrome (E34.5-)*
syndromes associated with anomalies in the number and form of chromosomes (Q90-Q99)

Q50 Congenital malformations of ovaries, fallopian tubes and broad ligaments

Q50.0 Congenital absence of ovary

EXCLUDES 1 *Turner's syndrome (Q96.-)*

Q50.01 Congenital absence of ovary, unilateral ♀

Q50.02 Congenital absence of ovary, bilateral ♀

Q50.1 Developmental ovarian cyst ♀

Q50.2 Congenital torsion of ovary ♀

Q50.3 Other congenital malformations of ovary

Q50.31 Accessory ovary ♀

Q50.32 Ovarian streak ♀
46, XX with streak gonads

Q50.39 Other congenital malformation of ovary ♀
Congenital malformation of ovary NOS

Q50.4 Embryonic cyst of fallopian tube ♀
Fimbrial cyst

Q50.5 Embryonic cyst of broad ligament ♀
Epoophoron cyst
Parovarian cyst

Q50.6 Other congenital malformations of fallopian tube and broad ligament ♀
Absence of fallopian tube and broad ligament
Accessory fallopian tube and broad ligament
Atresia of fallopian tube and broad ligament
Congenital malformation of fallopian tube or broad ligament NOS

Q51 Congenital malformations of uterus and cervix

Q51.0 Agenesis and aplasia of uterus ♀
Congenital absence of uterus

Q51.1 Doubling of uterus with doubling of cervix and vagina

Q51.10 Doubling of uterus with doubling of cervix and vagina without obstruction ♀
Doubling of uterus with doubling of cervix and vagina NOS

Q51.11 Doubling of uterus with doubling of cervix and vagina with obstruction ♀

Q51.2 Other doubling of uterus
Doubling of uterus NOS
Septate uterus
AHA: 2018,4Q,27

Q51.21 Complete doubling of uterus ♀
Complete septate uterus

Q51.22 Partial doubling of uterus ♀
Partial septate uterus

Q51.28 Other and unspecified doubling of uterus ♀
Septate uterus NOS

Q51.3 Bicornate uterus ♀
Bicornate uterus, complete or partial

Q51.4 Unicornate uterus ♀
Unicornate uterus with or without a separate uterine horn
Uterus with only one functioning horn

Q51.5 Agenesis and aplasia of cervix ♀
Congenital absence of cervix

Q51.6 Embryonic cyst of cervix ♀

Q51.7 Congenital fistulae between uterus and digestive and urinary tracts ♀

Q51.8 Other congenital malformations of uterus and cervix

Q51.81 Other congenital malformations of uterus

Q51.810 Arcuate uterus ♀
Arcuatus uterus

Q51.811 Hypoplasia of uterus ♀

Q51.818 Other congenital malformations of uterus ♀
Müllerian anomaly of uterus NEC

Q51.82 Other congenital malformations of cervix

Q51.820 Cervical duplication ♀

Q51.821 Hypoplasia of cervix ♀

Q51.828 Other congenital malformations of cervix ♀

Q51.9 Congenital malformation of uterus and cervix, unspecified ♀

Q52 Other congenital malformations of female genitalia

Q52.0 Congenital absence of vagina ♀
Vaginal agenesis, total or partial

Q52.1 Doubling of vagina

EXCLUDES 1 *doubling of vagina with doubling of uterus and cervix (Q51.1-)*

Q52.10 Doubling of vagina, unspecified ♀
Septate vagina NOS

Q52.11 Transverse vaginal septum ♀

Q52.12 Longitudinal vaginal septum
AHA: 2016,4Q,58-59

Q52.120 Longitudinal vaginal septum, nonobstructing ♀

Q52.121 Longitudinal vaginal septum, obstructing, right side ♀

Q52.122 Longitudinal vaginal septum, obstructing, left side ♀

Q52.123 Longitudinal vaginal septum, microperforate, right side ♀

Q52.124 Longitudinal vaginal septum, microperforate, left side ♀

Q52.129 Other and unspecified longitudinal vaginal septum ♀

Q52.2 Congenital rectovaginal fistula ♀

EXCLUDES 1 *cloaca (Q43.7)*

Q52.3 Imperforate hymen ♀
DEF: Obstructive anomaly of vagina, characterized by complete closure of the membranous fold around the external opening of the vagina, obstructing the vaginal introitus.

Q52.4 Other congenital malformations of vagina ♀
Canal of Nuck cyst, congenital
Congenital malformation of vagina NOS
Embryonic vaginal cyst
Gartner's duct cyst
AHA: 2022,2Q,15

Q52.5 Fusion of labia ♀

Q52.6 Congenital malformation of clitoris ♀

Q52.7 Other and unspecified congenital malformations of vulva

Q52.70 Unspecified congenital malformations of vulva ♀
Congenital malformation of vulva NOS

Q52.71 Congenital absence of vulva ♀

Q52.79 Other congenital malformations of vulva ♀
Congenital cyst of vulva

Q52.8 Other specified congenital malformations of female genitalia ♀

Q52.9 Congenital malformation of female genitalia, unspecified ♀

Q53 Undescended and ectopic testicle

Q53.0 Ectopic testis

Q53.00 Ectopic testis, unspecified ♂

Q53.01 Ectopic testis, unilateral ♂

Q53.02 Ectopic testes, bilateral ♂

Q53.1 Undescended testicle, unilateral
AHA: 2017,4Q,22-23

Q53.10 Unspecified undescended testicle, unilateral ♂

Q53.11 Abdominal testis, unilateral

Q53.111 Unilateral intraabdominal testis ♂

Q53.112 Unilateral inguinal testis ♂

Q53.12 Ectopic perineal testis, unilateral ♂

Q53.13 Unilateral high scrotal testis ♂

Q53.2 Undescended testicle, bilateral
AHA: 2017,4Q,22-23

Q53.20 Undescended testicle, unspecified, bilateral ♂

Q53.21 Abdominal testis, bilateral

Q53.211 Bilateral intraabdominal testes ♂

Q53.212 Bilateral inguinal testes ♂

Q53.22 Ectopic perineal testis, bilateral ♂

Q53.23 Bilateral high scrotal testes ♂

Q53.9 Undescended testicle, unspecified ♂
Cryptorchism NOS

Q54 Hypospadias

EXCLUDES 1 *epispadias (Q64.Ø)*

DEF: Abnormal opening of the urethra on the ventral (underside) surface of the penis.

Hypospadias

Balanic (glanular, coronal) hypospadias
Subcoronal hypospadias
Penile hypospadias
Penile raphe
Scrotal hypospadias
Penoscrotal hypospadias
Scrotum
Scrotal raphe
Perineal hypospadias

Hypospadias (ventral view)

Q54.Ø Hypospadias, balanic ♂
Hypospadias, coronal
Hypospadias, glandular

Q54.1 Hypospadias, penile ♂

Q54.2 Hypospadias, penoscrotal ♂

Q54.3 Hypospadias, perineal ♂

Q54.4 Congenital chordee ♂
Chordee without hypospadias

Q54.8 Other hypospadias ♂
Hypospadias with intersex state

Q54.9 Hypospadias, unspecified ♂

Q55 Other congenital malformations of male genital organs

EXCLUDES 1 *congenital hydrocele (P83.5)*
hypospadias (Q54.-)

Q55.Ø Absence and aplasia of testis ♂
Monorchism

Q55.1 Hypoplasia of testis and scrotum ♂
Fusion of testes

Q55.2 Other and unspecified congenital malformations of testis and scrotum

Q55.2Ø Unspecified congenital malformations of testis and scrotum ♂
Congenital malformation of testis or scrotum NOS

Q55.21 Polyorchism ♂
DEF: Congenital anomaly in which there are more than two testes.

Q55.22 Retractile testis ♂

Q55.23 Scrotal transposition ♂

Q55.29 Other congenital malformations of testis and scrotum ♂

Q55.3 Atresia of vas deferens ♂
Code first any associated cystic fibrosis (E84.-)

Q55.4 Other congenital malformations of vas deferens, epididymis, seminal vesicles and prostate ♂
Absence or aplasia of prostate
Absence or aplasia of spermatic cord
Congenital malformation of vas deferens, epididymis, seminal vesicles or prostate NOS

Q55.5 Congenital absence and aplasia of penis ♂

Q55.6 Other congenital malformations of penis

Q55.61 Curvature of penis (lateral) ♂

Q55.62 Hypoplasia of penis ♂
Micropenis

Q55.63 Congenital torsion of penis ♂
EXCLUDES 1 *acquired torsion of penis (N48.82)*

Q55.64 Hidden penis ♂
Buried penis
Concealed penis
EXCLUDES 1 *acquired buried penis (N48.83)*

Q55.69 Other congenital malformation of penis ♂
Congenital malformation of penis NOS

Q55.7 Congenital vasocutaneous fistula ♂

Q55.8 Other specified congenital malformations of male genital organs ♂

Q55.9 Congenital malformation of male genital organ, unspecified ♂
Congenital anomaly of male genital organ
Congenital deformity of male genital organ

Q56 Indeterminate sex and pseudohermaphroditism

EXCLUDES 1 *46, XX true hermaphrodite (Q99.1)*
androgen insensitivity syndrome (E34.5-)
chimera 46, XX/46, XY true hermaphrodite (Q99.Ø)
female pseudohermaphroditism with adrenocortical disorder (E25.-)
pseudohermaphroditism with specified chromosomal anomaly (Q96-Q99)
pure gonadal dysgenesis (Q99.1)

DEF: Indeterminate sex: External genitalia that is nondescript, lacking the physical appearance specific to either sex.

DEF: Pseudohermaphroditism: Presence of gonads of one sex and external genitalia of another sex.

Q56.Ø Hermaphroditism, not elsewhere classified
Ovotestis

Q56.1 Male pseudohermaphroditism, not elsewhere classified ♂
46, XY with streak gonads
Male pseudohermaphroditism NOS

Q56.2 Female pseudohermaphroditism, not elsewhere classified ♀
Female pseudohermaphroditism NOS

Q56.3 Pseudohermaphroditism, unspecified

Q56.4 Indeterminate sex, unspecified
Ambiguous genitalia

Congenital malformations of the urinary system (Q6Ø-Q64)

Q6Ø Renal agenesis and other reduction defects of kidney

INCLUDES congenital absence of kidney
congenital atrophy of kidney
infantile atrophy of kidney

Q6Ø.Ø Renal agenesis, unilateral

Q6Ø.1 Renal agenesis, bilateral

Q6Ø.2 Renal agenesis, unspecified

Q6Ø.3 Renal hypoplasia, unilateral

Q6Ø.4 Renal hypoplasia, bilateral

Q6Ø.5 Renal hypoplasia, unspecified

Q6Ø.6 Potter's syndrome

Q61 Cystic kidney disease

EXCLUDES 1 *acquired cyst of kidney (N28.1)*
Potter's syndrome (Q6Ø.6)

Q61.Ø Congenital renal cyst

Q61.ØØ Congenital renal cyst, unspecified
Cyst of kidney NOS (congenital)

Q61.Ø1 Congenital single renal cyst

Q61.Ø2 Congenital multiple renal cysts

Q61.1 Polycystic kidney, infantile type
Polycystic kidney, autosomal recessive

Q61.11 Cystic dilatation of collecting ducts COM

Q61.19 Other polycystic kidney, infantile type COM

Q61.2 Polycystic kidney, adult type
Polycystic kidney, autosomal dominant

Q61.3 Polycystic kidney, unspecified
AHA: 2016,3Q,22

Q61.4 Renal dysplasia
Multicystic dysplastic kidney
Multicystic kidney (development)
Multicystic kidney disease
Multicystic renal dysplasia
EXCLUDES 1 *polycystic kidney disease (Q61.11-Q61.3)*

Q61.5 Medullary cystic kidney
Nephronophthisis
Sponge kidney NOS
DEF: Sponge kidney: Dilated collecting tubules that are usually asymptomatic. Calcinosis in tubules may cause renal insufficiency.

Q61.8 Other cystic kidney diseases
Fibrocystic kidney
Fibrocystic renal degeneration or disease

Q61.9 Cystic kidney disease, unspecified
Meckel-Gruber syndrome

Q62 Congenital obstructive defects of renal pelvis and congenital malformations of ureter

Q62.Ø Congenital hydronephrosis

Q62.1 Congenital occlusion of ureter

Atresia and stenosis of ureter

Q62.1Ø Congenital occlusion of ureter, unspecified

Q62.11 Congenital occlusion of ureteropelvic junction

Q62.12 Congenital occlusion of ureterovesical orifice

Q62.2 Congenital megaureter

Congenital dilatation of ureter

Q62.3 Other obstructive defects of renal pelvis and ureter

Q62.31 Congenital ureterocele, orthotopic

Q62.32 Cecoureterocele

Ectopic ureterocele

Q62.39 Other obstructive defects of renal pelvis and ureter

Ureteropelvic junction obstruction NOS

Q62.4 Agenesis of ureter

Congenital absence ureter

Q62.5 Duplication of ureter

Accessory ureter

Double ureter

Q62.6 Malposition of ureter

Q62.6Ø Malposition of ureter, unspecified

Q62.61 Deviation of ureter

Q62.62 Displacement of ureter

Q62.63 Anomalous implantation of ureter

Ectopia of ureter

Ectopic ureter

Q62.69 Other malposition of ureter

Q62.7 Congenital vesico-uretero-renal reflux

Q62.8 Other congenital malformations of ureter

Anomaly of ureter NOS

Q63 Other congenital malformations of kidney

EXCLUDES 1 *congenital nephrotic syndrome (NØ4.-)*

Q63.Ø Accessory kidney

Q63.1 Lobulated, fused and horseshoe kidney

Q63.2 Ectopic kidney

Congenital displaced kidney

Malrotation of kidney

Q63.3 Hyperplastic and giant kidney

Compensatory hypertrophy of kidney

Q63.8 Other specified congenital malformations of kidney

Congenital renal calculi

Q63.9 Congenital malformation of kidney, unspecified

Q64 Other congenital malformations of urinary system

Q64.Ø Epispadias

EXCLUDES 1 *hypospadias (Q54.-)*

Epispadias

Epispadias (dorsal view)

Q64.1 Exstrophy of urinary bladder

Q64.1Ø Exstrophy of urinary bladder, unspecified COM

Ectopia vesicae

Q64.11 Supravesical fissure of urinary bladder COM

Q64.12 Cloacal exstrophy of urinary bladder COM

Q64.19 Other exstrophy of urinary bladder COM

Extroversion of bladder

Q64.2 Congenital posterior urethral valves

Q64.3 Other atresia and stenosis of urethra and bladder neck

Q64.31 Congenital bladder neck obstruction

Congenital obstruction of vesicourethral orifice

Q64.32 Congenital stricture of urethra

Q64.33 Congenital stricture of urinary meatus

Q64.39 Other atresia and stenosis of urethra and bladder neck

Atresia and stenosis of urethra and bladder neck NOS

Q64.4 Malformation of urachus

Cyst of urachus

Patent urachus

Prolapse of urachus

Q64.5 Congenital absence of bladder and urethra

Q64.6 Congenital diverticulum of bladder

Q64.7 Other and unspecified congenital malformations of bladder and urethra

EXCLUDES 1 *congenital prolapse of bladder (mucosa) (Q79.4)*

Q64.7Ø Unspecified congenital malformation of bladder and urethra

Malformation of bladder or urethra NOS

Q64.71 Congenital prolapse of urethra

Q64.72 Congenital prolapse of urinary meatus

Q64.73 Congenital urethrorectal fistula

Q64.74 Double urethra

Q64.75 Double urinary meatus

Q64.79 Other congenital malformations of bladder and urethra

Q64.8 Other specified congenital malformations of urinary system

Q64.9 Congenital malformation of urinary system, unspecified

Congenital anomaly NOS of urinary system

Congenital deformity NOS of urinary system

Congenital malformations and deformations of the musculoskeletal system (Q65-Q79)

Q65 Congenital deformities of hip

EXCLUDES 1 *clicking hip (R29.4)*

Q65.Ø Congenital dislocation of hip, unilateral

Q65.ØØ Congenital dislocation of unspecified hip, unilateral COM

Q65.Ø1 Congenital dislocation of right hip, unilateral COM

Q65.Ø2 Congenital dislocation of left hip, unilateral COM

Q65.1 Congenital dislocation of hip, bilateral COM

Q65.2 Congenital dislocation of hip, unspecified COM

Q65.3 Congenital partial dislocation of hip, unilateral

Q65.3Ø Congenital partial dislocation of unspecified hip, unilateral COM

Q65.31 Congenital partial dislocation of right hip, unilateral COM

Q65.32 Congenital partial dislocation of left hip, unilateral COM

Q65.4 Congenital partial dislocation of hip, bilateral COM

Q65.5 Congenital partial dislocation of hip, unspecified COM

Q65.6 Congenital unstable hip COM

Congenital dislocatable hip

Q65.8 Other congenital deformities of hip

Q65.81 Congenital coxa valga COM

Q65.82 Congenital coxa vara COM

Q65.89 Other specified congenital deformities of hip COM

Anteversion of femoral neck

Congenital acetabular dysplasia

Q65.9 Congenital deformity of hip, unspecified COM

Q66 Congenital deformities of feet

EXCLUDES 1 *reduction defects of feet (Q72.-)*
valgus deformities (acquired) (M21.Ø-)
varus deformities (acquired) (M21.1-)

AHA: 2019,4Q,13

Q66.Ø Congenital talipes equinovarus

Q66.ØØ Congenital talipes equinovarus, unspecified foot

Q66.Ø1 Congenital talipes equinovarus, right foot

Q66.Ø2 Congenital talipes equinovarus, left foot

Q66.1 Congenital talipes calcaneovarus

Q66.1Ø Congenital talipes calcaneovarus, unspecified foot

Q66.11 Congenital talipes calcaneovarus, right foot

Q66.12 Congenital talipes calcaneovarus, left foot

5th **Q66.2 Congenital metatarsus (primus) varus**
AHA: 2016,4Q,59
6th **Q66.21 Congenital metatarsus primus varus**
Q66.211 Congenital metatarsus primus varus, right foot
Q66.212 Congenital metatarsus primus varus, left foot
Q66.219 Congenital metatarsus primus varus, unspecified foot
6th **Q66.22 Congenital metatarsus adductus**
Congenital metatarsus varus
Q66.221 Congenital metatarsus adductus, right foot
Q66.222 Congenital metatarsus adductus, left foot
Q66.229 Congenital metatarsus adductus, unspecified foot
5th **Q66.3 Other congenital varus deformities of feet**
Hallux varus, congenital
Q66.30 Other congenital varus deformities of feet, unspecified foot
Q66.31 Other congenital varus deformities of feet, right foot
Q66.32 Other congenital varus deformities of feet, left foot
5th **Q66.4 Congenital talipes calcaneovalgus**
Q66.40 Congenital talipes calcaneovalgus, unspecified foot
Q66.41 Congenital talipes calcaneovalgus, right foot
Q66.42 Congenital talipes calcaneovalgus, left foot
5th **Q66.5 Congenital pes planus**
Congenital flat foot
Congenital rigid flat foot
Congenital spastic (everted) flat foot
EXCLUDES 1 *pes planus, acquired (M21.4)*
Q66.50 Congenital pes planus, unspecified foot
Q66.51 Congenital pes planus, right foot
Q66.52 Congenital pes planus, left foot
Q66.6 Other congenital valgus deformities of feet
Congenital metatarsus valgus
5th **Q66.7 Congenital pes cavus**
Q66.70 Congenital pes cavus, unspecified foot
Q66.71 Congenital pes cavus, right foot
Q66.72 Congenital pes cavus, left foot
5th **Q66.8 Other congenital deformities of feet**
Q66.80 Congenital vertical talus deformity, unspecified foot
Q66.81 Congenital vertical talus deformity, right foot
Q66.82 Congenital vertical talus deformity, left foot
Q66.89 Other specified congenital deformities of feet
Congenital asymmetric talipes
Congenital clubfoot NOS
Congenital talipes NOS
Congenital tarsal coalition
Hammer toe, congenital
DEF: Clubfoot: Congenital anomaly of the foot with the heel elevated and rotated outward and the toes pointing inward.
5th **Q66.9 Congenital deformity of feet, unspecified**
Q66.90 Congenital deformity of feet, unspecified, unspecified foot
Q66.91 Congenital deformity of feet, unspecified, right foot
Q66.92 Congenital deformity of feet, unspecified, left foot
4th **Q67 Congenital musculoskeletal deformities of head, face, spine and chest**
EXCLUDES 1 *congenital malformation syndromes classified to Q87.-*
Potter's syndrome (Q60.6)
Q67.0 Congenital facial asymmetry
Q67.1 Congenital compression facies
Q67.2 Dolichocephaly
Q67.3 Plagiocephaly
Q67.4 Other congenital deformities of skull, face and jaw
Congenital depressions in skull
Congenital hemifacial atrophy or hypertrophy
Deviation of nasal septum, congenital
Squashed or bent nose, congenital
EXCLUDES 1 *dentofacial anomalies [including malocclusion] (M26.-)*
syphilitic saddle nose (A50.5)
DEF: Deviated septum: Condition in which the nasal septum, a thin wall composed of cartilage and bone that separates the two nostrils, is crooked or displaced from the midline.
Q67.5 Congenital deformity of spine
Congenital postural scoliosis
Congenital scoliosis NOS
EXCLUDES 1 *infantile idiopathic scoliosis (M41.0)*
scoliosis due to congenital bony malformation (Q76.3)
AHA: 2014,4Q,26
Q67.6 Pectus excavatum
Congenital funnel chest
Q67.7 Pectus carinatum
Congenital pigeon chest
Q67.8 Other congenital deformities of chest
Congenital deformity of chest wall NOS
4th **Q68 Other congenital musculoskeletal deformities**
EXCLUDES 1 *reduction defects of limb(s) (Q71-Q73)*
EXCLUDES 2 *congenital myotonic chondrodystrophy (G71.13)*
Q68.0 Congenital deformity of sternocleidomastoid muscle
Congenital contracture of sternocleidomastoid (muscle)
Congenital (sternomastoid) torticollis
Sternomastoid tumor (congenital)
Q68.1 Congenital deformity of finger(s) and hand
Congenital clubfinger
Spade-like hand (congenital)
Q68.2 Congenital deformity of knee
Congenital dislocation of knee
Congenital genu recurvatum
Q68.3 Congenital bowing of femur
EXCLUDES 1 *anteversion of femur (neck) (Q65.89)*
Q68.4 Congenital bowing of tibia and fibula
Q68.5 Congenital bowing of long bones of leg, unspecified
Q68.6 Discoid meniscus
Q68.8 Other specified congenital musculoskeletal deformities
Congenital deformity of clavicle
Congenital deformity of elbow
Congenital deformity of forearm
Congenital deformity of scapula
Congenital deformity of wrist
Congenital dislocation of elbow
Congenital dislocation of shoulder
Congenital dislocation of wrist
4th **Q69 Polydactyly**
Q69.0 Accessory finger(s)
Q69.1 Accessory thumb(s)
Q69.2 Accessory toe(s)
Accessory hallux
Q69.9 Polydactyly, unspecified
Supernumerary digit(s) NOS
4th **Q70 Syndactyly**
5th **Q70.0 Fused fingers**
Complex syndactyly of fingers with synostosis
Q70.00 Fused fingers, unspecified hand
Q70.01 Fused fingers, right hand
Q70.02 Fused fingers, left hand
Q70.03 Fused fingers, bilateral
5th **Q70.1 Webbed fingers**
Simple syndactyly of fingers without synostosis
Q70.10 Webbed fingers, unspecified hand
Q70.11 Webbed fingers, right hand
Q70.12 Webbed fingers, left hand
Q70.13 Webbed fingers, bilateral
5th **Q70.2 Fused toes**
Complex syndactyly of toes with synostosis
Q70.20 Fused toes, unspecified foot
Q70.21 Fused toes, right foot

Q70.22 Fused toes, left foot
Q70.23 Fused toes, bilateral

Q70.3 Webbed toes
Simple syndactyly of toes without synostosis
Q70.30 Webbed toes, unspecified foot
Q70.31 Webbed toes, right foot
Q70.32 Webbed toes, left foot
Q70.33 Webbed toes, bilateral

Q70.4 Polysyndactyly, unspecified
EXCLUDES 1 *specified syndactyly of hand and feet - code to specified conditions (Q70.0-Q70.3-)*

Q70.9 Syndactyly, unspecified
Symphalangy NOS

Q71 Reduction defects of upper limb

Q71.0 Congenital complete absence of upper limb
Q71.00 Congenital complete absence of unspecified upper limb
Q71.01 Congenital complete absence of right upper limb
Q71.02 Congenital complete absence of left upper limb
Q71.03 Congenital complete absence of upper limb, bilateral

Q71.1 Congenital absence of upper arm and forearm with hand present
Q71.10 Congenital absence of unspecified upper arm and forearm with hand present
Q71.11 Congenital absence of right upper arm and forearm with hand present
Q71.12 Congenital absence of left upper arm and forearm with hand present
Q71.13 Congenital absence of upper arm and forearm with hand present, bilateral

Q71.2 Congenital absence of both forearm and hand
Q71.20 Congenital absence of both forearm and hand, unspecified upper limb
Q71.21 Congenital absence of both forearm and hand, right upper limb
Q71.22 Congenital absence of both forearm and hand, left upper limb
Q71.23 Congenital absence of both forearm and hand, bilateral

Q71.3 Congenital absence of hand and finger
Q71.30 Congenital absence of unspecified hand and finger
Q71.31 Congenital absence of right hand and finger
Q71.32 Congenital absence of left hand and finger
Q71.33 Congenital absence of hand and finger, bilateral

Q71.4 Longitudinal reduction defect of radius
Clubhand (congenital)
Radial clubhand
Q71.40 Longitudinal reduction defect of unspecified radius
Q71.41 Longitudinal reduction defect of right radius
Q71.42 Longitudinal reduction defect of left radius
Q71.43 Longitudinal reduction defect of radius, bilateral

Q71.5 Longitudinal reduction defect of ulna
Q71.50 Longitudinal reduction defect of unspecified ulna
Q71.51 Longitudinal reduction defect of right ulna
Q71.52 Longitudinal reduction defect of left ulna
Q71.53 Longitudinal reduction defect of ulna, bilateral

Q71.6 Lobster-claw hand
Q71.60 Lobster-claw hand, unspecified hand
Q71.61 Lobster-claw right hand
Q71.62 Lobster-claw left hand
Q71.63 Lobster-claw hand, bilateral

Q71.8 Other reduction defects of upper limb
Q71.81 Congenital shortening of upper limb
Q71.811 Congenital shortening of right upper limb
Q71.812 Congenital shortening of left upper limb
Q71.813 Congenital shortening of upper limb, bilateral
Q71.819 Congenital shortening of unspecified upper limb
Q71.89 Other reduction defects of upper limb
Q71.891 Other reduction defects of right upper limb
Q71.892 Other reduction defects of left upper limb
Q71.893 Other reduction defects of upper limb, bilateral
Q71.899 Other reduction defects of unspecified upper limb

Q71.9 Unspecified reduction defect of upper limb
Q71.90 Unspecified reduction defect of unspecified upper limb
Q71.91 Unspecified reduction defect of right upper limb
Q71.92 Unspecified reduction defect of left upper limb
Q71.93 Unspecified reduction defect of upper limb, bilateral

Q72 Reduction defects of lower limb

Q72.0 Congenital complete absence of lower limb
Q72.00 Congenital complete absence of unspecified lower limb
Q72.01 Congenital complete absence of right lower limb
Q72.02 Congenital complete absence of left lower limb
Q72.03 Congenital complete absence of lower limb, bilateral

Q72.1 Congenital absence of thigh and lower leg with foot present
Q72.10 Congenital absence of unspecified thigh and lower leg with foot present
Q72.11 Congenital absence of right thigh and lower leg with foot present
Q72.12 Congenital absence of left thigh and lower leg with foot present
Q72.13 Congenital absence of thigh and lower leg with foot present, bilateral

Q72.2 Congenital absence of both lower leg and foot
Q72.20 Congenital absence of both lower leg and foot, unspecified lower limb
Q72.21 Congenital absence of both lower leg and foot, right lower limb
Q72.22 Congenital absence of both lower leg and foot, left lower limb
Q72.23 Congenital absence of both lower leg and foot, bilateral

Q72.3 Congenital absence of foot and toe(s)
Q72.30 Congenital absence of unspecified foot and toe(s)
Q72.31 Congenital absence of right foot and toe(s)
Q72.32 Congenital absence of left foot and toe(s)
Q72.33 Congenital absence of foot and toe(s), bilateral

Q72.4 Longitudinal reduction defect of femur
Proximal femoral focal deficiency
Q72.40 Longitudinal reduction defect of unspecified femur
Q72.41 Longitudinal reduction defect of right femur
Q72.42 Longitudinal reduction defect of left femur
Q72.43 Longitudinal reduction defect of femur, bilateral

Q72.5 Longitudinal reduction defect of tibia
Q72.50 Longitudinal reduction defect of unspecified tibia
Q72.51 Longitudinal reduction defect of right tibia
Q72.52 Longitudinal reduction defect of left tibia
Q72.53 Longitudinal reduction defect of tibia, bilateral

Q72.6 Longitudinal reduction defect of fibula
Q72.60 Longitudinal reduction defect of unspecified fibula
Q72.61 Longitudinal reduction defect of right fibula
Q72.62 Longitudinal reduction defect of left fibula
Q72.63 Longitudinal reduction defect of fibula, bilateral

Q72.7 Split foot
Q72.70 Split foot, unspecified lower limb
Q72.71 Split foot, right lower limb
Q72.72 Split foot, left lower limb
Q72.73 Split foot, bilateral

Q72.8 Other reduction defects of lower limb
Q72.81 Congenital shortening of lower limb
Q72.811 Congenital shortening of right lower limb
Q72.812 Congenital shortening of left lower limb
Q72.813 Congenital shortening of lower limb, bilateral
Q72.819 Congenital shortening of unspecified lower limb
Q72.89 Other reduction defects of lower limb
Q72.891 Other reduction defects of right lower limb
Q72.892 Other reduction defects of left lower limb
Q72.893 Other reduction defects of lower limb, bilateral

Q72.899 Other reduction defects of unspecified lower limb

Q72.9 Unspecified reduction defect of lower limb

Q72.90 Unspecified reduction defect of unspecified lower limb

Q72.91 Unspecified reduction defect of right lower limb

Q72.92 Unspecified reduction defect of left lower limb

Q72.93 Unspecified reduction defect of lower limb, bilateral

Q73 Reduction defects of unspecified limb

Q73.Ø Congenital absence of unspecified limb(s)
Amelia NOS

Q73.1 Phocomelia, unspecified limb(s)
Phocomelia NOS

Q73.8 Other reduction defects of unspecified limb(s)
Longitudinal reduction deformity of unspecified limb(s)
Ectromelia of limb NOS
Hemimelia of limb NOS
Reduction defect of limb NOS

Q74 Other congenital malformations of limb(s)
EXCLUDES 1 *polydactyly (Q69.-)*
reduction defect of limb (Q71-Q73)
syndactyly (Q7Ø.-)

Q74.Ø Other congenital malformations of upper limb(s), including shoulder girdle
Accessory carpal bones
Cleidocranial dysostosis
Congenital pseudarthrosis of clavicle
Macrodactylia (fingers)
Madelung's deformity
Radioulnar synostosis
Sprengel's deformity
Triphalangeal thumb

Q74.1 Congenital malformation of knee
Congenital absence of patella
Congenital dislocation of patella
Congenital genu valgum
Congenital genu varum
Rudimentary patella
EXCLUDES 1 *congenital dislocation of knee (Q68.2)*
congenital genu recurvatum (Q68.2)
nail patella syndrome (Q87.2)

Q74.2 Other congenital malformations of lower limb(s), including pelvic girdle
Congenital fusion of sacroiliac joint
Congenital malformation of ankle joint
Congenital malformation of sacroiliac joint
EXCLUDES 1 *anteversion of femur (neck) (Q65.89)*

Q74.3 Arthrogryposis multiplex congenita

Q74.8 Other specified congenital malformations of limb(s)

Q74.9 Unspecified congenital malformation of limb(s)
Congenital anomaly of limb(s) NOS

Q75 Other congenital malformations of skull and face bones
EXCLUDES 1 *congenital malformation of face NOS (Q18.-)*
congenital malformation syndromes classified to Q87.-
dentofacial anomalies [including malocclusion] (M26.-)
musculoskeletal deformities of head and face (Q67.Ø-Q67.4)
skull defects associated with congenital anomalies of brain such as:
anencephaly (QØØ.Ø)
encephalocele (QØ1.-)
hydrocephalus (QØ3.-)
microcephaly (QØ2)

Q75.Ø Craniosynostosis
Acrocephaly
Imperfect fusion of skull
Oxycephaly
Trigonocephaly
DEF: Congenital condition in which one or more of the cranial sutures fuse prematurely, creating a deformed or aberrant head shape.

Q75.1 Craniofacial dysostosis
Crouzon's disease

Q75.2 Hypertelorism

Q75.3 Macrocephaly

Q75.4 Mandibulofacial dysostosis
Franceschetti syndrome
Treacher Collins syndrome

Q75.5 Oculomandibular dysostosis

Q75.8 Other specified congenital malformations of skull and face bones
Absence of skull bone, congenital
Congenital deformity of forehead
Platybasia

Q75.9 Congenital malformation of skull and face bones, unspecified
Congenital anomaly of face bones NOS
Congenital anomaly of skull NOS

Q76 Congenital malformations of spine and bony thorax
EXCLUDES 1 *congenital musculoskeletal deformities of spine and chest (Q67.5-Q67.8)*

Q76.Ø Spina bifida occulta
EXCLUDES 1 *meningocele (spinal) (QØ5.-)*
spina bifida (aperta) (cystica) (QØ5.-)

Q76.1 Klippel-Feil syndrome
Cervical fusion syndrome

Q76.2 Congenital spondylolisthesis
Congenital spondylolysis
EXCLUDES 1 *spondylolisthesis (acquired) (M43.1-)*
spondylolysis (acquired) (M43.Ø-)

Q76.3 Congenital scoliosis due to congenital bony malformation
Hemivertebra fusion or failure of segmentation with scoliosis

Q76.4 Other congenital malformations of spine, not associated with scoliosis

Q76.41 Congenital kyphosis

Q76.411 Congenital kyphosis, occipito-atlanto-axial region

Q76.412 Congenital kyphosis, cervical region

Q76.413 Congenital kyphosis, cervicothoracic region

Q76.414 Congenital kyphosis, thoracic region

Q76.415 Congenital kyphosis, thoracolumbar region

Q76.419 Congenital kyphosis, unspecified region

Q76.42 Congenital lordosis

Q76.425 Congenital lordosis, thoracolumbar region

Q76.426 Congenital lordosis, lumbar region

Q76.427 Congenital lordosis, lumbosacral region

Q76.428 Congenital lordosis, sacral and sacrococcygeal region

Q76.429 Congenital lordosis, unspecified region

Q76.49 Other congenital malformations of spine, not associated with scoliosis
Congenital absence of vertebra NOS
Congenital fusion of spine NOS
Congenital malformation of lumbosacral (joint) (region) NOS
Congenital malformation of spine NOS
Hemivertebra NOS
Malformation of spine NOS
Platyspondylisis NOS
Supernumerary vertebra NOS

Q76.5 Cervical rib
Supernumerary rib in cervical region

Q76.6 Other congenital malformations of ribs
Accessory rib
Congenital absence of rib
Congenital fusion of ribs
Congenital malformation of ribs NOS
EXCLUDES 1 *short rib syndrome (Q77.2)*

Q76.7 Congenital malformation of sternum
Congenital absence of sternum
Sternum bifidum

Q76.8 Other congenital malformations of bony thorax

Q76.9 Congenital malformation of bony thorax, unspecified

Q77 Osteochondrodysplasia with defects of growth of tubular bones and spine
EXCLUDES 1 *mucopolysaccharidosis (E76.Ø-E76.3)*
EXCLUDES 2 *congenital myotonic chondrodystrophy (G71.13)*

Q77.Ø Achondrogenesis COM
Hypochondrogenesis

Q77.1 Thanatophoric short stature COM

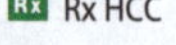 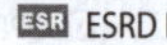  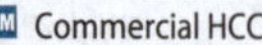 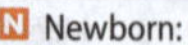 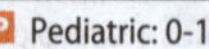 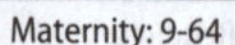
HCC CMS-HCC | Rx Rx HCC | ESR ESRD HCC | COM Commercial HCC | N Newborn: 0 | P Pediatric: 0-17 | M Maternity: 9-64 | A Adult: 15-124

Q77.2 Short rib syndrome COM
Asphyxiating thoracic dysplasia [Jeune]

Q77.3 Chondrodysplasia punctata COM
EXCLUDES 1 *Rhizomelic chondrodysplasia punctata (E71.43)*

Q77.4 Achondroplasia COM
Hypochondroplasia
Osteosclerosis congenita

Q77.5 Diastrophic dysplasia COM

Q77.6 Chondroectodermal dysplasia COM
Ellis-van Creveld syndrome

Q77.7 Spondyloepiphyseal dysplasia COM

Q77.8 Other osteochondrodysplasia with defects of growth of tubular bones and spine COM

Q77.9 Osteochondrodysplasia with defects of growth of tubular bones and spine, unspecified COM

✓4th **Q78 Other osteochondrodysplasias**
EXCLUDES 2 *congenital myotonic chondrodystrophy (G71.13)*

Q78.0 Osteogenesis imperfecta COM
Fragilitas ossium
Osteopsathyrosis

Q78.1 Polyostotic fibrous dysplasia COM
Albright(-McCune)(-Sternberg) syndrome

Q78.2 Osteopetrosis COM
Albers-Schönberg syndrome
Osteosclerosis NOS
DEF: Rare congenital condition in which the bones are excessively dense, resulting from a discrepancy in the formation and breakdown of bone.

Q78.3 Progressive diaphyseal dysplasia COM
Camurati-Engelmann syndrome

Q78.4 Enchondromatosis COM
Maffucci's syndrome
Ollier's disease

Q78.5 Metaphyseal dysplasia COM
Pyle's syndrome

Q78.6 Multiple congenital exostoses COM
Diaphyseal aclasis

Q78.8 Other specified osteochondrodysplasias COM
Osteopoikilosis

Q78.9 Osteochondrodysplasia, unspecified COM
Chondrodystrophy NOS
Osteodystrophy NOS

✓4th **Q79 Congenital malformations of musculoskeletal system, not elsewhere classified**
EXCLUDES 2 *congenital (sternomastoid) torticollis (Q68.0)*

Q79.0 Congenital diaphragmatic hernia COM
EXCLUDES 1 *congenital hiatus hernia (Q40.1)*

Q79.1 Other congenital malformations of diaphragm COM
Absence of diaphragm
Congenital malformation of diaphragm NOS
Eventration of diaphragm

Q79.2 Exomphalos COM
Omphalocele
EXCLUDES 1 *umbilical hernia (K42.-)*

Q79.3 Gastroschisis COM

Gastroschisis

Q79.4 Prune belly syndrome COM
Congenital prolapse of bladder mucosa
Eagle-Barrett syndrome

✓5th **Q79.5 Other congenital malformations of abdominal wall**
EXCLUDES 1 *umbilical hernia (K42.-)*

Q79.51 Congenital hernia of bladder COM

Q79.59 Other congenital malformations of abdominal wall COM

✓5th **Q79.6 Ehlers-Danlos syndromes**
AHA: 2019,4Q,13-14
DEF: Connective tissue disorder that causes hyperextended skin and joints and results in fragile blood vessels with bleeding, poor wound healing, and subcutaneous pseudotumors.

Q79.60 Ehlers-Danlos syndrome, unspecified Rx COM

Q79.61 Classical Ehlers-Danlos syndrome Rx COM
Classical EDS (cEDS)

Q79.62 Hypermobile Ehlers-Danlos syndrome Rx COM
Hypermobile EDS (hEDS)

Q79.63 Vascular Ehlers-Danlos syndrome Rx COM
Vascular EDS (vEDS)

Q79.69 Other Ehlers-Danlos syndromes Rx COM

Q79.8 Other congenital malformations of musculoskeletal system
Absence of muscle
Absence of tendon
Accessory muscle
Amyotrophia congenita
Congenital constricting bands
Congenital shortening of tendon
Poland syndrome

Q79.9 Congenital malformation of musculoskeletal system, unspecified
Congenital anomaly of musculoskeletal system NOS
Congenital deformity of musculoskeletal system NOS

Other congenital malformations (Q80-Q89)

✓4th **Q80 Congenital ichthyosis**
EXCLUDES 1 *Refsum's disease (G60.1)*
DEF: Excessive production of skin cells resulting in red, dry, scaly skin.

Q80.0 Ichthyosis vulgaris

Q80.1 X-linked ichthyosis

Q80.2 Lamellar ichthyosis
Collodion baby

Q80.3 Congenital bullous ichthyosiform erythroderma

Q80.4 Harlequin fetus

Q80.8 Other congenital ichthyosis

Q80.9 Congenital ichthyosis, unspecified

✓4th **Q81 Epidermolysis bullosa**

Q81.0 Epidermolysis bullosa simplex COM
EXCLUDES 1 *Cockayne's syndrome (Q87.19)*

Q81.1 Epidermolysis bullosa letalis COM
Herlitz' syndrome

Q81.2 Epidermolysis bullosa dystrophica COM

Q81.8 Other epidermolysis bullosa COM

Q81.9 Epidermolysis bullosa, unspecified COM

✓4th **Q82 Other congenital malformations of skin**
EXCLUDES 1 *acrodermatitis enteropathica (E83.2)*
congenital erythropoietic porphyria (E80.0)
pilonidal cyst or sinus (L05.-)
Sturge-Weber (-Dimitri) syndrome ▶(Q85.89)◀

Q82.0 Hereditary lymphedema

Q82.1 Xeroderma pigmentosum

Q82.2 Congenital cutaneous mastocytosis
Congenital diffuse cutaneous mastocytosis
Congenital maculopapular cutaneous mastocytosis
Congenital urticaria pigmentosa
EXCLUDES 1 *cutaneous mastocytosis NOS (D47.01)*
diffuse cutaneous mastocytosis (with onset after newborn period) (D47.01)
malignant mastocytosis (C96.2-)
systemic mastocytosis (D47.02)
urticaria pigmentosa (non-congenital) (with onset after newborn period) (D47.01)
AHA: 2017,4Q,5

Q82.3 Incontinentia pigmenti

Q82.4 Ectodermal dysplasia (anhidrotic)
EXCLUDES 1 *Ellis-van Creveld syndrome (Q77.6)*

Q82.5 Congenital non-neoplastic nevus
Birthmark NOS
Flammeus Nevus
Portwine Nevus
Sanguineous Nevus
Strawberry Nevus
Vascular Nevus NOS
Verrucous Nevus
EXCLUDES 2 *araneus nevus (I78.1)*
Café au lait spots (L81.3)
lentigo (L81.4)
melanocytic nevus (D22.-)
nevus NOS (D22.-)
pigmented nevus (D22.-)
spider nevus (I78.1)
stellar nevus (I78.1)

Q82.6 Congenital sacral dimple
Parasacral dimple
EXCLUDES 2 *pilonidal cyst with abscess (LØ5.Ø1)*
pilonidal cyst without abscess (LØ5.91)
AHA: 2016,4Q,60

Q82.8 Other specified congenital malformations of skin
Abnormal palmar creases
Accessory skin tags
Benign familial pemphigus [Hailey-Hailey]
Congenital poikiloderma
Cutis laxa (hyperelastica)
Dermatoglyphic anomalies
Inherited keratosis palmaris et plantaris
Keratosis follicularis [Darier-White]
EXCLUDES 1 *Ehlers-Danlos syndromes (Q79.6-)*
AHA: 2021,3Q,10; 2016,1Q,17

Q82.9 Congenital malformation of skin, unspecified

✓4th Q83 Congenital malformations of breast
EXCLUDES 2 *absence of pectoral muscle (Q79.8)*
hypoplasia of breast (N64.82)
micromastia (N64.82)

Q83.Ø Congenital absence of breast with absent nipple

Q83.1 Accessory breast
Supernumerary breast

Q83.2 Absent nipple

Q83.3 Accessory nipple
Supernumerary nipple

Q83.8 Other congenital malformations of breast

Q83.9 Congenital malformation of breast, unspecified

✓4th Q84 Other congenital malformations of integument

Q84.Ø Congenital alopecia
Congenital atrichosis

Q84.1 Congenital morphological disturbances of hair, not elsewhere classified
Beaded hair
Monilethrix
Pili annulati
EXCLUDES 1 *Menkes' kinky hair syndrome (E83.Ø)*

Q84.2 Other congenital malformations of hair
Congenital hypertrichosis
Congenital malformation of hair NOS
Persistent lanugo

Q84.3 Anonychia
EXCLUDES 1 *nail patella syndrome (Q87.2)*

Q84.4 Congenital leukonychia

Q84.5 Enlarged and hypertrophic nails
Congenital onychauxis
Pachyonychia

Q84.6 Other congenital malformations of nails
Congenital clubnail
Congenital koilonychia
Congenital malformation of nail NOS

Q84.8 Other specified congenital malformations of integument
Aplasia cutis congenita

Q84.9 Congenital malformation of integument, unspecified
Congenital anomaly of integument NOS
Congenital deformity of integument NOS

✓4th Q85 Phakomatoses, not elsewhere classified
EXCLUDES 1 *ataxia telangiectasia [Louis-Bar] (G11.3)*
familial dysautonomia [Riley-Day] (G9Ø.1)

✓5th Q85.Ø Neurofibromatosis (nonmalignant)

Q85.ØØ Neurofibromatosis, unspecified HCC ESR COM

Q85.Ø1 Neurofibromatosis, type 1 HCC ESR COM
Von Recklinghausen disease

Q85.Ø2 Neurofibromatosis, type 2 HCC ESR COM
Acoustic neurofibromatosis
DEF: Inherited condition with cutaneous lesions, benign tumors of peripheral nerves, and bilateral 8th nerve masses.

Q85.Ø3 Schwannomatosis HCC ESR COM
DEF: Genetic mutation (SMARCB1/INI1) causing multiple benign tumors along the nerve pathways, except on the 8th cranial (vestibular) nerve.

Q85.Ø9 Other neurofibromatosis HCC ESR COM

Q85.1 Tuberous sclerosis HCC Rx ESR COM
Bourneville's disease
Epiloia

▲ **✓5th Q85.8 Other phakomatoses, not elsewhere classified**
~~Peutz-Jeghers Syndrome~~
~~Sturge-Weber(-Dimitri) syndrome~~
~~von Hippel-Lindau syndrome~~
EXCLUDES 1 *Meckel-Gruber syndrome (Q61.9)*
AHA: 2021,3Q,12

● **Q85.81 PTEN tumor syndrome**
PHTS
PTEN hamartoma tumor syndrome
PTEN related Cowden syndrome
Code also, if applicable, genetic susceptibility to malignant neoplasm (Z15.Ø-)

● **Q85.82 Other Cowden syndrome**

● **Q85.83 Von Hippel-Lindau syndrome**
Code also manifestations

● **Q85.89 Other phakomatoses, not elsewhere classified**
Peutz-Jeghers syndrome
Sturge-Weber(-Dimitri) syndrome

Q85.9 Phakomatosis, unspecified HCC Rx ESR COM
Hamartosis NOS

✓4th Q86 Congenital malformation syndromes due to known exogenous causes, not elsewhere classified
EXCLUDES 2 *iodine-deficiency-related hypothyroidism (EØØ-EØ2)*
nonteratogenic effects of substances transmitted via placenta or breast milk (PØ4.-)

Q86.Ø Fetal alcohol syndrome (dysmorphic) COM

Q86.1 Fetal hydantoin syndrome COM
Meadow's syndrome

Q86.2 Dysmorphism due to warfarin COM

Q86.8 Other congenital malformation syndromes due to known exogenous causes COM

✓4th Q87 Other specified congenital malformation syndromes affecting multiple systems
Use additional code(s) to identify all associated manifestations

Q87.Ø Congenital malformation syndromes predominantly affecting facial appearance
Acrocephalopolysyndactyly
Acrocephalosyndactyly [Apert]
Cryptophthalmos syndrome
Cyclopia
Goldenhar syndrome
Moebius syndrome
Oro-facial-digital syndrome
Robin syndrome
Whistling face

✓5th Q87.1 Congenital malformation syndromes predominantly associated with short stature
EXCLUDES 1 *Ellis-van Creveld syndrome (Q77.6)*
Smith-Lemli-Opitz syndrome (E78.72)
AHA: 2019,4Q,14-15

Q87.11 Prader-Willi syndrome Rx COM

Q87.19 Other congenital malformation syndromes predominantly associated with short stature COM
Aarskog syndrome
Cockayne syndrome
De Lange syndrome
Dubowitz syndrome
Noonan syndrome
Robinow-Silverman-Smith syndrome
Russell-Silver syndrome
Seckel syndrome

Q87.2 Congenital malformation syndromes predominantly involving limbs COM
Holt-Oram syndrome
Klippel-Trenaunay-Weber syndrome
Nail patella syndrome
Rubinstein-Taybi syndrome
Sirenomelia syndrome
Thrombocytopenia with absent radius [TAR] syndrome
VATER syndrome

Q87.3 Congenital malformation syndromes involving early overgrowth COM
Beckwith-Wiedemann syndrome
Sotos syndrome
Weaver syndrome

√5th **Q87.4 Marfan's syndrome**
DEF: Disorder that affects the connective tissue of multiple systems, including disproportionally long or abnormal bone structure and eye and cardiovascular complications.

Q87.40 Marfan's syndrome, unspecified Rx COM

√6th **Q87.41 Marfan's syndrome with cardiovascular manifestations**

Q87.410 Marfan's syndrome with aortic dilation Rx COM

Q87.418 Marfan's syndrome with other cardiovascular manifestations Rx COM

Q87.42 Marfan's syndrome with ocular manifestations Rx COM

Q87.43 Marfan's syndrome with skeletal manifestation Rx COM

Q87.5 Other congenital malformation syndromes with other skeletal changes COM

√5th **Q87.8 Other specified congenital malformation syndromes, not elsewhere classified**
EXCLUDES 1 *Zellweger syndrome (E71.510)*

Q87.81 Alport syndrome COM
Use additional code to identify stage of chronic kidney disease (N18.1-N18.6)

Q87.82 Arterial tortuosity syndrome Rx COM
AHA: 2016,4Q,60-61

Q87.89 Other specified congenital malformation syndromes, not elsewhere classified COM
Laurence-Moon (-Bardet)-Biedl syndrome

√4th **Q89 Other congenital malformations, not elsewhere classified**

√5th **Q89.0 Congenital absence and malformations of spleen**
EXCLUDES 1 *isomerism of atrial appendages (with asplenia or polysplenia) (Q20.6)*

Q89.01 Asplenia (congenital)

Q89.09 Congenital malformations of spleen
Congenital splenomegaly

Q89.1 Congenital malformations of adrenal gland
EXCLUDES 1 *adrenogenital disorders (E25.-)*
congenital adrenal hyperplasia (E25.0)

Q89.2 Congenital malformations of other endocrine glands
Congenital malformation of parathyroid or thyroid gland
Persistent thyroglossal duct
Thyroglossal cyst
EXCLUDES 1 *congenital goiter (E03.0)*
congenital hypothyroidism (E03.1)

Q89.3 Situs inversus COM
Dextrocardia with situs inversus
Mirror-image atrial arrangement with situs inversus
Situs inversus or transversus abdominalis
Situs inversus or transversus thoracis
Transposition of abdominal viscera
Transposition of thoracic viscera
EXCLUDES 1 *dextrocardia NOS (Q24.0)*
DEF: Congenital anomaly in which the internal thoracic and abdominal organs are transposed laterally and found on the opposite side from the normal position.

Q89.4 Conjoined twins COM
Craniopagus
Dicephaly
Pygopagus
Thoracopagus

Q89.7 Multiple congenital malformations, not elsewhere classified
Multiple congenital anomalies NOS
Multiple congenital deformities NOS
EXCLUDES 1 *congenital malformation syndromes affecting multiple systems (Q87.-)*

Q89.8 Other specified congenital malformations COM
Use additional code(s) to identify all associated manifestations
AHA: 2021,3Q,12

Q89.9 Congenital malformation, unspecified
Congenital anomaly NOS
Congenital deformity NOS

Chromosomal abnormalities, not elsewhere classified (Q90-Q99)

EXCLUDES 2 *mitochondrial metabolic disorders (E88.4-)*

√4th **Q90 Down syndrome**
Use additional code(s) to identify any associated physical conditions and degree of intellectual disabilities (F70-F79)

Q90.0 Trisomy 21, nonmosaicism (meiotic nondisjunction) COM

Q90.1 Trisomy 21, mosaicism (mitotic nondisjunction) COM

Q90.2 Trisomy 21, translocation COM

Q90.9 Down syndrome, unspecified COM
Trisomy 21 NOS

√4th **Q91 Trisomy 18 and Trisomy 13**

Q91.0 Trisomy 18, nonmosaicism (meiotic nondisjunction) Rx COM

Q91.1 Trisomy 18, mosaicism (mitotic nondisjunction) Rx COM

Q91.2 Trisomy 18, translocation Rx COM

Q91.3 Trisomy 18, unspecified Rx COM

Q91.4 Trisomy 13, nonmosaicism (meiotic nondisjunction) Rx COM

Q91.5 Trisomy 13, mosaicism (mitotic nondisjunction) Rx COM

Q91.6 Trisomy 13, translocation Rx COM

Q91.7 Trisomy 13, unspecified Rx COM

√4th **Q92 Other trisomies and partial trisomies of the autosomes, not elsewhere classified**
INCLUDES unbalanced translocations and insertions
EXCLUDES 1 *trisomies of chromosomes 13, 18, 21 (Q90-Q91)*

Q92.0 Whole chromosome trisomy, nonmosaicism (meiotic nondisjunction) Rx COM

Q92.1 Whole chromosome trisomy, mosaicism (mitotic nondisjunction) Rx COM

Q92.2 Partial trisomy Rx COM
Less than whole arm duplicated
Whole arm or more duplicated
EXCLUDES 1 *partial trisomy due to unbalanced translocation (Q92.5)*

Q92.5 Duplications with other complex rearrangements Rx COM
Partial trisomy due to unbalanced translocations
Code also any associated deletions due to unbalanced translocations, inversions and insertions (Q93.7)

√5th **Q92.6 Marker chromosomes**
Trisomies due to dicentrics
Trisomies due to extra rings
Trisomies due to isochromosomes
Individual with marker heterochromatin

Q92.61 Marker chromosomes in normal individual Rx COM

Q92.62 Marker chromosomes in abnormal individual Rx COM

Q92.7 Triploidy and polyploidy Rx COM

Q92.8 Other specified trisomies and partial trisomies of autosomes Rx COM

Duplications identified by fluorescence in situ hybridization (FISH)

Duplications identified by in situ hybridization (ISH)

Duplications seen only at prometaphase

Q92.9 Trisomy and partial trisomy of autosomes, unspecified Rx COM

✓4th Q93 Monosomies and deletions from the autosomes, not elsewhere classified

Q93.Ø Whole chromosome monosomy, nonmosaicism (meiotic nondisjunction) Rx COM

Q93.1 Whole chromosome monosomy, mosaicism (mitotic nondisjunction) Rx COM

Q93.2 Chromosome replaced with ring, dicentric or isochromosome Rx COM

Q93.3 Deletion of short arm of chromosome 4 Rx COM

Wolff-Hirschorn syndrome

Q93.4 Deletion of short arm of chromosome 5 Rx COM

Cri-du-chat syndrome

✓5th Q93.5 Other deletions of part of a chromosome

AHA: 2018,4Q,28

Q93.51 Angelman syndrome Rx COM

Q93.59 Other deletions of part of a chromosome Rx COM

Q93.7 Deletions with other complex rearrangements Rx COM

Deletions due to unbalanced translocations, inversions and insertions

Code also any associated duplications due to unbalanced translocations, inversions and insertions (Q92.5)

✓5th Q93.8 Other deletions from the autosomes

Q93.81 Velo-cardio-facial syndrome Rx COM

Deletion 22q11.2

AHA: 2019,3Q,14

DEF: Microdeletion syndrome affecting multiple organs characterized by a cleft palate, heart defects, an elongated face with almond-shaped eyes, wide nose, small ears, weak immune system, weak musculature, hypothyroidism, short stature, and scoliosis. The deletion occurs at q11.2 on the long arm of the chromosome 22.

Q93.82 Williams syndrome Rx COM

AHA: 2018,4Q,28-29

Q93.88 Other microdeletions Rx COM

Miller-Dieker syndrome

Smith-Magenis syndrome

Q93.89 Other deletions from the autosomes Rx COM

Deletions identified by fluorescence in situ hybridization (FISH)

Deletions identified by in situ hybridization (ISH)

Deletions seen only at prometaphase

Q93.9 Deletion from autosomes, unspecified Rx COM

✓4th Q95 Balanced rearrangements and structural markers, not elsewhere classified

INCLUDES Robertsonian and balanced reciprocal translocations and insertions

Q95.Ø Balanced translocation and insertion in normal individual

Q95.1 Chromosome inversion in normal individual

Q95.2 Balanced autosomal rearrangement in abnormal individual Rx COM

Q95.3 Balanced sex/autosomal rearrangement in abnormal individual Rx COM

Q95.5 Individual with autosomal fragile site

Q95.8 Other balanced rearrangements and structural markers

Q95.9 Balanced rearrangement and structural marker, unspecified

✓4th Q96 Turner's syndrome

EXCLUDES 1 *Noonan syndrome (Q87.19)*

Q96.Ø Karyotype 45, X COM ♀

Q96.1 Karyotype 46, X iso (Xq) COM ♀

Karyotype 46, isochromosome Xq

Q96.2 Karyotype 46, X with abnormal sex chromosome, except iso (Xq) COM ♀

Karyotype 46, X with abnormal sex chromosome, except isochromosome Xq

Q96.3 Mosaicism, 45, X/46, XX or XY COM ♀

Q96.4 Mosaicism, 45, X/other cell line(s) with abnormal sex chromosome COM ♀

Q96.8 Other variants of Turner's syndrome COM ♀

Q96.9 Turner's syndrome, unspecified COM ♀

✓4th Q97 Other sex chromosome abnormalities, female phenotype, not elsewhere classified

EXCLUDES 1 *Turner's syndrome (Q96.-)*

Q97.Ø Karyotype 47, XXX COM ♀

Q97.1 Female with more than three X chromosomes COM ♀

Q97.2 Mosaicism, lines with various numbers of X chromosomes COM ♀

Q97.3 Female with 46, XY karyotype COM ♀

Q97.8 Other specified sex chromosome abnormalities, female phenotype COM ♀

Q97.9 Sex chromosome abnormality, female phenotype, unspecified COM ♀

✓4th Q98 Other sex chromosome abnormalities, male phenotype, not elsewhere classified

Q98.Ø Klinefelter syndrome karyotype 47, XXY COM ♂

Q98.1 Klinefelter syndrome, male with more than two X chromosomes COM ♂

Q98.3 Other male with 46, XX karyotype COM ♂

Q98.4 Klinefelter syndrome, unspecified COM ♂

Q98.5 Karyotype 47, XYY COM

Q98.6 Male with structurally abnormal sex chromosome COM ♂

Q98.7 Male with sex chromosome mosaicism COM ♂

Q98.8 Other specified sex chromosome abnormalities, male phenotype COM ♂

Q98.9 Sex chromosome abnormality, male phenotype, unspecified COM ♂

✓4th Q99 Other chromosome abnormalities, not elsewhere classified

Q99.Ø Chimera 46, XX/46, XY COM

Chimera 46, XX/46, XY true hermaphrodite

Q99.1 46, XX true hermaphrodite COM

46, XX with streak gonads

46, XY with streak gonads

Pure gonadal dysgenesis

Q99.2 Fragile X chromosome Rx COM

Fragile X syndrome

Q99.8 Other specified chromosome abnormalities COM

Q99.9 Chromosomal abnormality, unspecified COM

Chapter 18. Symptoms, Signs and Abnormal Clinical and Laboratory Findings (RØØ–R99)

Chapter-specific Guidelines with Coding Examples

The chapter-specific guidelines from the ICD-10-CM Official Guidelines for Coding and Reporting have been provided below. Along with these guidelines are coding examples, contained in the shaded boxes, that have been developed to help illustrate the coding and/or sequencing guidance found in these guidelines.

Chapter 18 includes symptoms, signs, abnormal results of clinical or other investigative procedures, and ill-defined conditions regarding which no diagnosis classifiable elsewhere is recorded. Signs and symptoms that point to a specific diagnosis have been assigned to a category in other chapters of the classification.

a. Use of symptom codes

Codes that describe symptoms and signs are acceptable for reporting purposes when a related definitive diagnosis has not been established (confirmed) by the provider.

Tenderness and localized pain in the right upper quadrant; based on presentation, probable gallstones

R1Ø.11 **Right upper quadrant pain**

R1Ø.811 **Right upper quadrant abdominal tenderness**

Explanation: Codes that describe symptoms such as abdominal pain are acceptable for reporting purposes when the provider has not established (confirmed) a definitive diagnosis.

b. Use of a symptom code with a definitive diagnosis code

Codes for signs and symptoms may be reported in addition to a related definitive diagnosis when the sign or symptom is not routinely associated with that diagnosis, such as the various signs and symptoms associated with complex syndromes. The definitive diagnosis code should be sequenced before the symptom code.

Signs or symptoms that are associated routinely with a disease process should not be assigned as additional codes, unless otherwise instructed by the classification.

Pneumonia with hemoptysis

J18.9 **Pneumonia, unspecified organism**

RØ4.2 **Hemoptysis**

Explanation: Codes for signs and symptoms may be reported in addition to a related definitive diagnosis when the sign or symptom is not routinely associated with that diagnosis.

Abdominal pain due to acute appendicitis

K35.8Ø **Unspecified acute appendicitis**

Explanation: Codes for signs or symptoms routinely associated with a disease process should not be assigned unless the classification instructs otherwise.

c. Combination codes that include symptoms

ICD-10-CM contains a number of combination codes that identify both the definitive diagnosis and common symptoms of that diagnosis. When using one of these combination codes, an additional code should not be assigned for the symptom.

IBS with diarrhea

K58.Ø **Irritable bowel syndrome with diarrhea**

Explanation: When a combination code identifies both the definitive diagnosis and the symptom, an additional code should not be assigned for the symptom.

d. Repeated falls

Code R29.6, Repeated falls, is for use for encounters when a patient has recently fallen and the reason for the fall is being investigated.

Code Z91.81, History of falling, is for use when a patient has fallen in the past and is at risk for future falls. When appropriate, both codes R29.6 and Z91.81 may be assigned together.

e. Coma

Code R4Ø.2Ø, Unspecified coma, may be assigned in conjunction with codes for any medical condition.

Do not report codes for unspecified coma, individual or total Glasgow coma scale scores for a patient with a medically induced coma or a sedated patient.

1) Coma scale

The coma scale codes (R4Ø.21- to R4Ø.24-) can be used in conjunction with traumatic brain injury codes. These codes are primarily for use by trauma registries, but they may be used in any setting where this information is collected. The coma scale codes should be sequenced after the diagnosis code(s).

These codes, one from each subcategory, are needed to complete the scale. The 7th character indicates when the scale was recorded. The 7th character should match for all three codes.

At a minimum, report the initial score documented on presentation at your facility. This may be a score from the emergency medicine technician (EMT) or in the emergency department. If desired, a facility may choose to capture multiple coma scale scores.

Assign code R4Ø.24-, Glasgow coma scale, total score, when only the total score is documented in the medical record and not the individual score(s).

If multiple coma scores are captured within the first 24 hours after hospital admission, assign only the code for the score at the time of admission. ICD-1Ø-CM does not classify coma scores that are reported after admission but less than 24 hours later.

See Section I.B.14. for coma scale documentation by clinicians other than patient's provider

36-year-old man found down after unknown injury with skull fracture and with concussion and loss of consciousness of unknown duration. Upon hospital admission, the patient was evaluated with the following Glasgow coma scores:

Eye-opening response—3: eyes open to speech

Verbal response—3: random speech with no conversational exchange

Motor response—4: pulls limb away from painful stimulus

SØ2.ØXXA **Fracture of vault of skull, initial encounter for closed fracture**

SØ6.ØX9A **Concussion with loss of consciousness of unspecified duration, initial encounter**

R4Ø.2133 **Coma scale, eyes open, to sound, at hospital admission**

R4Ø.2233 **Coma scale, best verbal response, inappropriate words, at hospital admission**

R4Ø.2343 **Coma scale, best motor response, flexion withdrawal, at hospital admission**

Explanation: When individual scores for the Glasgow coma scale are documented, one code from each category is needed to complete the scale. The seventh character indicates when the scale was recorded and should match for all three codes. Assign a code from subcategory R4Ø.24- Glasgow coma scale, total score, when only the total and not the individual score(s) is documented.

f. Functional quadriplegia

GUIDELINE HAS BEEN DELETED EFFECTIVE OCTOBER 1, 2017

g. SIRS due to non-infectious process

The systemic inflammatory response syndrome (SIRS) can develop as a result of certain non-infectious disease processes, such as trauma, malignant neoplasm, or pancreatitis. When SIRS is documented with a noninfectious condition, and no subsequent infection is documented, the code for the underlying condition, such as an injury, should be assigned, followed by code R65.1Ø, Systemic inflammatory response syndrome (SIRS) of non-infectious origin without acute organ dysfunction, or code R65.11, Systemic inflammatory response syndrome (SIRS) of non-infectious origin with acute organ dysfunction. If an associated acute organ dysfunction is documented, the appropriate code(s) for the specific type of organ dysfunction(s) should be assigned in addition to code R65.11. If acute organ dysfunction is documented, but it cannot be determined if the acute organ dysfunction is associated with SIRS or due to another condition (e.g., directly due to the trauma), the provider should be queried.

Systemic inflammatory response syndrome (SIRS) due to acute gallstone pancreatitis

K85.10 **Biliary acute pancreatitis without necrosis or infection**

R65.10 **Systemic inflammatory response syndrome [SIRS] of non-infectious origin without acute organ dysfunction**

Explanation: When SIRS is documented with a non-infectious condition without subsequent infection documented, the code for the underlying condition such as pancreatitis should be assigned followed by the appropriate code for SIRS of noninfectious origin, either with or without associated organ dysfunction.

h. Death NOS

Code R99, Ill-defined and unknown cause of mortality, is only for use in the very limited circumstance when a patient who has already died is brought into an emergency department or other healthcare facility and is pronounced dead upon arrival. It does not represent the discharge disposition of death.

i. NIHSS stroke scale

The NIH stroke scale (NIHSS) codes (R29.7- -) can be used in conjunction with acute stroke codes (I63) to identify the patient's neurological status and the severity of the stroke. The stroke scale codes should be sequenced after the acute stroke diagnosis code(s).

At a minimum, report the initial score documented. If desired, a facility may choose to capture multiple stroke scale scores.

See Section I.B.14. for NIHSS stroke scale documentation by clinicians other than patient's provider

Chapter 18. Symptoms, Signs and Abnormal Clinical and Laboratory Findings, Not Elsewhere Classified (RØØ-R99)

NOTE This chapter includes symptoms, signs, abnormal results of clinical or other investigative procedures, and ill-defined conditions regarding which no diagnosis classifiable elsewhere is recorded.

Signs and symptoms that point rather definitely to a given diagnosis have been assigned to a category in other chapters of the classification. In general, categories in this chapter include the less well-defined conditions and symptoms that, without the necessary study of the case to establish a final diagnosis, point perhaps equally to two or more diseases or to two or more systems of the body. Practically all categories in the chapter could be designated 'not otherwise specified', 'unknown etiology' or 'transient'. The Alphabetical Index should be consulted to determine which symptoms and signs are to be allocated here and which to other chapters. The residual subcategories, numbered .8, are generally provided for other relevant symptoms that cannot be allocated elsewhere in the classification.

The conditions and signs or symptoms included in categories RØØ-R94 consist of:

(a) cases for which no more specific diagnosis can be made even after all the facts bearing on the case have been investigated;

(b) signs or symptoms existing at the time of initial encounter that proved to be transient and whose causes could not be determined;

(c) provisional diagnosis in a patient who failed to return for further investigation or care;

(d) cases referred elsewhere for investigation or treatment before the diagnosis was made;

(e) cases in which a more precise diagnosis was not available for any other reason;

(f) certain symptoms, for which supplementary information is provided, that represent important problems in medical care in their own right.

EXCLUDES 2 *abnormal findings on antenatal screening of mother (O28.-)*
certain conditions originating in the perinatal period (PØ4-P96)
signs and symptoms classified in the body system chapters
signs and symptoms of breast (N63, N64.5)

AHA: 2017,1Q,6,7

This chapter contains the following blocks:

RØØ-RØ9 Symptoms and signs involving the circulatory and respiratory systems
R1Ø-R19 Symptoms and signs involving the digestive system and abdomen
R2Ø-R23 Symptoms and signs involving the skin and subcutaneous tissue
R25-R29 Symptoms and signs involving the nervous and musculoskeletal systems
R3Ø-R39 Symptoms and signs involving the genitourinary system
R4Ø-R46 Symptoms and signs involving cognition, perception, emotional state and behavior
R47-R49 Symptoms and signs involving speech and voice
R5Ø-R69 General symptoms and signs
R7Ø-R79 Abnormal findings on examination of blood, without diagnosis
R8Ø-R82 Abnormal findings on examination of urine, without diagnosis
R83-R89 Abnormal findings on examination of other body fluids, substances and tissues, without diagnosis
R9Ø-R94 Abnormal findings on diagnostic imaging and in function studies, without diagnosis
R97 Abnormal tumor markers
R99 Ill-defined and unknown cause of mortality

Symptoms and signs involving the circulatory and respiratory systems (RØØ-RØ9)

✓4th RØØ Abnormalities of heart beat

EXCLUDES 1 *abnormalities originating in the perinatal period (P29.1-)*
EXCLUDES 2 *specified arrhythmias (I47-I49)*

RØØ.Ø Tachycardia, unspecified
Rapid heart beat
Sinoauricular tachycardia NOS
Sinus [sinusal] tachycardia NOS
EXCLUDES 1 *neonatal tachycardia (P29.11)*
paroxysmal tachycardia (I47.-)
DEF: Excessively rapid heart rate of more than 100 beats per minute.

RØØ.1 Bradycardia, unspecified
Sinoatrial bradycardia
Sinus bradycardia
Slow heart beat
Vagal bradycardia
Use additional code for adverse effect, if applicable, to identify drug (T36-T5Ø with fifth or sixth character 5)
EXCLUDES 1 *neonatal bradycardia (P29.12)*
AHA: 2020,2Q,23
DEF: Slowed heartbeat, usually defined as a rate fewer than 60 beats per minute. Heart rhythm may be slow as a result of a congenital defect or an acquired problem.

RØØ.2 Palpitations
Awareness of heart beat

RØØ.8 Other abnormalities of heart beat

RØØ.9 Unspecified abnormalities of heart beat

✓4th RØ1 Cardiac murmurs and other cardiac sounds

EXCLUDES 1 *cardiac murmurs and sounds originating in the perinatal period (P29.8)*

RØ1.Ø Benign and innocent cardiac murmurs
Functional cardiac murmur

RØ1.1 Cardiac murmur, unspecified
Cardiac bruit NOS
Heart murmur NOS
Systolic murmur NOS

RØ1.2 Other cardiac sounds
Cardiac dullness, increased or decreased
Precordial friction

✓4th RØ3 Abnormal blood-pressure reading, without diagnosis

RØ3.Ø Elevated blood-pressure reading, without diagnosis of hypertension
NOTE This category is to be used to record an episode of elevated blood pressure in a patient in whom no formal diagnosis of hypertension has been made, or as an isolated incidental finding.

RØ3.1 Nonspecific low blood-pressure reading
EXCLUDES 1 *hypotension (I95.-)*
maternal hypotension syndrome (O26.5-)
neurogenic orthostatic hypotension (G9Ø.3)

✓4th RØ4 Hemorrhage from respiratory passages

RØ4.Ø Epistaxis
Hemorrhage from nose
Nosebleed

RØ4.1 Hemorrhage from throat
EXCLUDES 2 *hemoptysis (RØ4.2)*

RØ4.2 Hemoptysis
Blood-stained sputum
Cough with hemorrhage
AHA: 2013,4Q,118

✓5th RØ4.8 Hemorrhage from other sites in respiratory passages

RØ4.81 Acute idiopathic pulmonary hemorrhage in infants P
AIPHI
Acute idiopathic hemorrhage in infants over 28 days old
EXCLUDES 1 *perinatal pulmonary hemorrhage (P26.-)*
▶*von Willebrand disease (D68.Ø-)*◀

RØ4.89 Hemorrhage from other sites in respiratory passages
Pulmonary hemorrhage NOS

RØ4.9 Hemorrhage from respiratory passages, unspecified

✓4th RØ5 Cough

EXCLUDES 1 *paroxysmal cough due to Bordetella pertussis (A37.Ø-)*
smoker's cough (J41.Ø)
EXCLUDES 2 *cough with hemorrhage (RØ4.2)*
AHA: 2021,4Q,24-25; 2016,2Q,33

RØ5.1 Acute cough

RØ5.2 Subacute cough

RØ5.3 Chronic cough
Persistent cough
Refractory cough
Unexplained cough

RØ5.4 Cough syncope UPD
Code first syncope and collapse (R55)

RØ5.8 Other specified cough

RØ5.9 Cough, unspecified

RØ6 Abnormalities of breathing

EXCLUDES 1 *acute respiratory distress syndrome (J8Ø)*
respiratory arrest (RØ9.2)
respiratory arrest of newborn (P28.81)
respiratory distress syndrome of newborn (P22.-)
respiratory failure (J96.-)
respiratory failure of newborn (P28.5)

RØ6.Ø Dyspnea

EXCLUDES 1 *tachypnea NOS (RØ6.82)*
transient tachypnea of newborn (P22.1)

RØ6.ØØ Dyspnea, unspecified
AHA: 2017,1Q,26

RØ6.Ø1 Orthopnea

RØ6.Ø2 Shortness of breath

RØ6.Ø3 Acute respiratory distress
AHA: 2017,4Q,23

RØ6.Ø9 Other forms of dyspnea

RØ6.1 Stridor

EXCLUDES 1 *congenital laryngeal stridor (P28.89)*
laryngismus (stridulus) (J38.5)

DEF: Certain type of wheezing described as a loud, constant, musical sound produced when breathing with an obstructed airway, like the inspiratory sound heard when laryngeal or esophageal obstruction is present.

RØ6.2 Wheezing

EXCLUDES 1 *asthma (J45.-)*

AHA: 2016,2Q,33
DEF: High-pitched whistling sound during breathing due to stenosis of the respiratory passageway. Wheezing is associated with asthma, sleep apnea, bronchiectasis, bronchiolitis, COPD, and pleural effusion.

RØ6.3 Periodic breathing
Cheyne-Stokes breathing

RØ6.4 Hyperventilation

EXCLUDES 1 *psychogenic hyperventilation (F45.8)*

RØ6.5 Mouth breathing

EXCLUDES 2 *dry mouth NOS (R68.2)*

RØ6.6 Hiccough

EXCLUDES 1 *psychogenic hiccough (F45.8)*

RØ6.7 Sneezing

RØ6.8 Other abnormalities of breathing

RØ6.81 Apnea, not elsewhere classified
Apnea NOS

EXCLUDES 1 *apnea (of) newborn ▶(P28.4-)◀*
sleep apnea (G47.3-)
sleep apnea of newborn (primary) ▶(P28.3-)◀

RØ6.82 Tachypnea, not elsewhere classified
Tachypnea NOS

EXCLUDES 1 *transitory tachypnea of newborn (P22.1)*

RØ6.83 Snoring

RØ6.89 Other abnormalities of breathing
Breath-holding (spells)
Sighing

RØ6.9 Unspecified abnormalities of breathing

RØ7 Pain in throat and chest

EXCLUDES 1 *epidemic myalgia (B33.Ø)*

EXCLUDES 2 *jaw pain R68.84*
pain in breast (N64.4)

RØ7.Ø Pain in throat

EXCLUDES 1 *chronic sore throat (J31.2)*
sore throat (acute) NOS (JØ2.9)

EXCLUDES 2 *dysphagia (R13.1-)*
pain in neck (M54.2)

RØ7.1 Chest pain on breathing
Painful respiration

RØ7.2 Precordial pain
DEF: Pain felt in the anterior (front) chest wall over the region of the heart. This type of pain is generally felt slightly to the left of the sternum, but may also extend into the surrounding chest wall region.

RØ7.8 Other chest pain

RØ7.81 Pleurodynia
Pleurodynia NOS

EXCLUDES 1 *epidemic pleurodynia (B33.Ø)*

RØ7.82 Intercostal pain

RØ7.89 Other chest pain
Anterior chest-wall pain NOS
AHA: 2021,1Q,42

RØ7.9 Chest pain, unspecified

RØ9 Other symptoms and signs involving the circulatory and respiratory system

EXCLUDES 1 *acute respiratory distress syndrome (J8Ø)*
respiratory arrest of newborn (P28.81)
respiratory distress syndrome of newborn (P22.Ø)
respiratory failure (J96.-)
respiratory failure of newborn (P28.5)

RØ9.Ø Asphyxia and hypoxemia

EXCLUDES 1 *asphyxia due to carbon monoxide (T58.-)*
asphyxia due to foreign body in respiratory tract (T17.-)
birth (intrauterine) asphyxia (P84)
hyperventilation (RØ6.4)
traumatic asphyxia (T71.-)

EXCLUDES 2 *hypercapnia (RØ6.89)*

RØ9.Ø1 Asphyxia
DEF: Interference of oxygen intake due to obstruction or injury of airways resulting in a lack of oxygen perfusion to the tissues or excessive carbon dioxide in the blood. Can cause unconsciousness or death.

RØ9.Ø2 Hypoxemia
AHA: 2019,3Q,15
DEF: Insufficient oxygen in the arterial blood resulting in inadequate delivery of oxygen to the body tissues.

RØ9.1 Pleurisy

EXCLUDES 1 *pleurisy with effusion (J9Ø)*

RØ9.2 Respiratory arrest HCC ESR COM
Cardiorespiratory failure

EXCLUDES 1 *cardiac arrest (I46.-)*
respiratory arrest of newborn (P28.81)
respiratory distress of newborn (P22.Ø)
respiratory failure (J96.-)
respiratory failure of newborn (P28.5)
respiratory insufficiency (RØ6.89)
respiratory insufficiency of newborn (P28.5)

RØ9.3 Abnormal sputum
Abnormal amount of sputum
Abnormal color of sputum
Abnormal odor of sputum
Excessive sputum

EXCLUDES 1 *blood-stained sputum (RØ4.2)*

RØ9.8 Other specified symptoms and signs involving the circulatory and respiratory systems

RØ9.81 Nasal congestion

RØ9.82 Postnasal drip

RØ9.89 Other specified symptoms and signs involving the circulatory and respiratory systems
Abnormal chest percussion
Bruit (arterial)
Chest tympany
Choking sensation
Feeling of foreign body in throat
Friction sounds in chest
Rales
Weak pulse

EXCLUDES 2 *foreign body in throat (T17.2-)*
wheezing (RØ6.2)

AHA: 2021,1Q,42

Symptoms and signs involving the digestive system and abdomen (R1Ø-R19)

EXCLUDES 2 *congenital or infantile pylorospasm (Q4Ø.Ø)*
gastrointestinal hemorrhage (K92.Ø-K92.2)
intestinal obstruction (K56.-)
newborn gastrointestinal hemorrhage (P54.Ø-P54.3)
newborn intestinal obstruction (P76.-)
pylorospasm (K31.3)
signs and symptoms involving the urinary system (R3Ø-R39)
symptoms referable to female genital organs (N94.-)
symptoms referable to male genital organs (N48-N5Ø)

R1Ø Abdominal and pelvic pain
EXCLUDES 1 *renal colic (N23)*
EXCLUDES 2 *dorsalgia (M54.-)*
flatulence and related conditions (R14.-)

R1Ø.Ø Acute abdomen
Severe abdominal pain (generalized) (with abdominal rigidity)
EXCLUDES 1 *abdominal rigidity NOS (R19.3)*
generalized abdominal pain NOS (R1Ø.84)
localized abdominal pain (R1Ø.1-R1Ø.3-)

R1Ø.1 Pain localized to upper abdomen
R1Ø.1Ø Upper abdominal pain, unspecified
R1Ø.11 Right upper quadrant pain
R1Ø.12 Left upper quadrant pain
R1Ø.13 Epigastric pain
Dyspepsia
EXCLUDES 1 *functional dyspepsia (K3Ø)*

Abdominal Pain

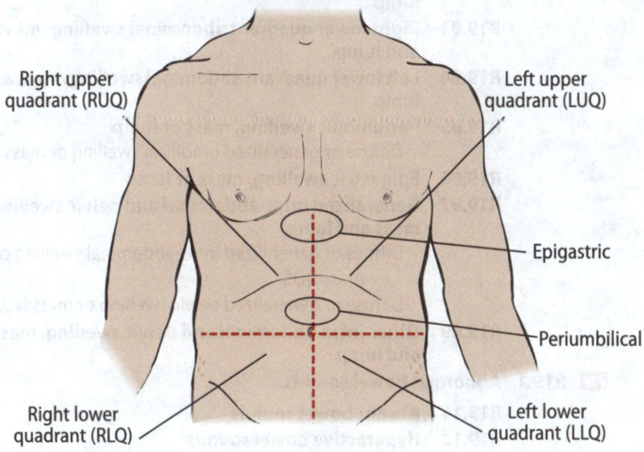

R1Ø.2 Pelvic and perineal pain
EXCLUDES 1 *vulvodynia (N94.81)*

R1Ø.3 Pain localized to other parts of lower abdomen
R1Ø.3Ø Lower abdominal pain, unspecified
R1Ø.31 Right lower quadrant pain
R1Ø.32 Left lower quadrant pain
R1Ø.33 Periumbilical pain

R1Ø.8 Other abdominal pain
R1Ø.81 Abdominal tenderness
Abdominal tenderness NOS
R1Ø.811 Right upper quadrant abdominal tenderness
R1Ø.812 Left upper quadrant abdominal tenderness
R1Ø.813 Right lower quadrant abdominal tenderness
R1Ø.814 Left lower quadrant abdominal tenderness
R1Ø.815 Periumbilic abdominal tenderness
R1Ø.816 Epigastric abdominal tenderness
R1Ø.817 Generalized abdominal tenderness
R1Ø.819 Abdominal tenderness, unspecified site
R1Ø.82 Rebound abdominal tenderness
R1Ø.821 Right upper quadrant rebound abdominal tenderness
R1Ø.822 Left upper quadrant rebound abdominal tenderness
R1Ø.823 Right lower quadrant rebound abdominal tenderness
R1Ø.824 Left lower quadrant rebound abdominal tenderness
R1Ø.825 Periumbilic rebound abdominal tenderness
R1Ø.826 Epigastric rebound abdominal tenderness
R1Ø.827 Generalized rebound abdominal tenderness
R1Ø.829 Rebound abdominal tenderness, unspecified site

R1Ø.83 Colic P
Colic NOS
Infantile colic
EXCLUDES 1 *colic in adult and child over 12 months old (R1Ø.84)*
DEF: Inconsolable crying in an otherwise well-fed and healthy infant for more than three hours a day, three days a week, for more than three weeks.

R1Ø.84 Generalized abdominal pain
EXCLUDES 1 *generalized abdominal pain associated with acute abdomen (R1Ø.Ø)*

R1Ø.9 Unspecified abdominal pain

R11 Nausea and vomiting
EXCLUDES 1 *cyclical vomiting associated with migraine (G43.A-)*
excessive vomiting in pregnancy (O21.-)
hematemesis (K92.Ø)
neonatal hematemesis (P54.Ø)
newborn vomiting (P92.Ø-)
psychogenic vomiting (F5Ø.89)
vomiting associated with bulimia nervosa (F5Ø.2)
vomiting following gastrointestinal surgery (K91.Ø)
AHA: 2017,1Q,28

R11.Ø Nausea
Nausea NOS
Nausea without vomiting

R11.1 Vomiting
R11.1Ø Vomiting, unspecified
Vomiting NOS
R11.11 Vomiting without nausea
R11.12 Projectile vomiting
R11.13 Vomiting of fecal matter
R11.14 Bilious vomiting
Bilious emesis
R11.15 Cyclical vomiting syndrome unrelated to migraine
Cyclic vomiting syndrome NOS
Persistent vomiting
EXCLUDES 1 *cyclical vomiting in migraine (G43.A-)*
EXCLUDES 2 *bulimia nervosa (F5Ø.2)*
diabetes mellitus due to underlying condition (EØ8.-)
AHA: 2019,4Q,15

R11.2 Nausea with vomiting, unspecified
Persistent nausea with vomiting NOS
AHA: 2020,1Q,8

R12 Heartburn
EXCLUDES 1 *dyspepsia NOS (R1Ø.13)*
functional dyspepsia (K3Ø)

R13 Aphagia and dysphagia
R13.Ø Aphagia
Inability to swallow
EXCLUDES 1 *psychogenic aphagia (F5Ø.9)*

R13.1 Dysphagia
Code first, if applicable, dysphagia following cerebrovascular disease (I69. with final characters -91)
EXCLUDES 1 *psychogenic dysphagia (F45.8)*

Swallowing Function

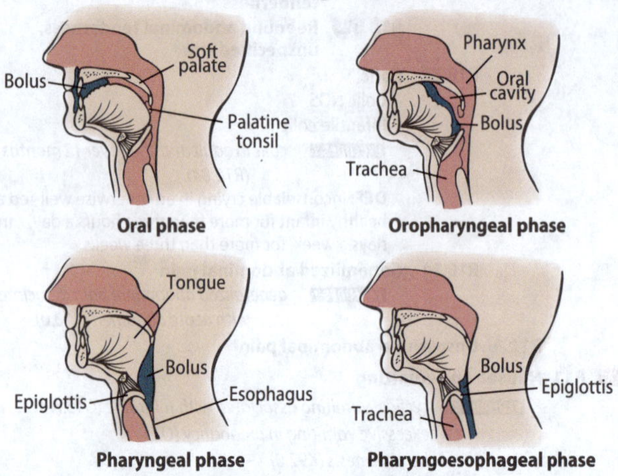

R13.10 Dysphagia, unspecified
Difficulty in swallowing NOS
R13.11 Dysphagia, oral phase
R13.12 Dysphagia, oropharyngeal phase
R13.13 Dysphagia, pharyngeal phase
R13.14 Dysphagia, pharyngoesophageal phase
R13.19 Other dysphagia
Cervical dysphagia
Neurogenic dysphagia

R14 Flatulence and related conditions
EXCLUDES 1 *psychogenic aerophagy (F45.8)*
R14.Ø Abdominal distension (gaseous)
Bloating
Tympanites (abdominal) (intestinal)
R14.1 Gas pain
R14.2 Eructation
R14.3 Flatulence

R15 Fecal incontinence
INCLUDES encopresis NOS
EXCLUDES 1 *fecal incontinence of nonorganic origin (F98.1)*
R15.Ø Incomplete defecation
EXCLUDES 1 *constipation (K59.Ø-)*
fecal impaction (K56.41)
R15.1 Fecal smearing
Fecal soiling
R15.2 Fecal urgency
R15.9 Full incontinence of feces
Fecal incontinence NOS

R16 Hepatomegaly and splenomegaly, not elsewhere classified
R16.Ø Hepatomegaly, not elsewhere classified
Hepatomegaly NOS
R16.1 Splenomegaly, not elsewhere classified
Splenomegaly NOS
R16.2 Hepatomegaly with splenomegaly, not elsewhere classified
Hepatosplenomegaly NOS

R17 Unspecified jaundice
EXCLUDES 1 *neonatal jaundice (P55, P57-P59)*

R18 Ascites
INCLUDES fluid in peritoneal cavity
EXCLUDES 1 *ascites in alcoholic cirrhosis (K7Ø.31)*
ascites in alcoholic hepatitis (K7Ø.11)
ascites in toxic liver disease with chronic active hepatitis (K71.51)
DEF: Abnormal accumulation of free fluid in the abdominal cavity, causing distention and tightness in addition to shortness of breath as the fluid accumulates. Ascites is usually an underlying disorder and can be a manifestation of any number of diseases.
R18.Ø Malignant ascites UPD
Code first malignancy, such as:
malignant neoplasm of ovary (C56.-)
secondary malignant neoplasm of retroperitoneum and peritoneum (C78.6)
R18.8 Other ascites
Ascites NOS
Peritoneal effusion (chronic)
AHA: 2018,1Q,4

R19 Other symptoms and signs involving the digestive system and abdomen
EXCLUDES 1 *acute abdomen (R1Ø.Ø)*
R19.Ø Intra-abdominal and pelvic swelling, mass and lump
EXCLUDES 1 *abdominal distension (gaseous) (R14.-)*
ascites (R18.-)
R19.ØØ Intra-abdominal and pelvic swelling, mass and lump, unspecified site
R19.Ø1 Right upper quadrant abdominal swelling, mass and lump
R19.Ø2 Left upper quadrant abdominal swelling, mass and lump
R19.Ø3 Right lower quadrant abdominal swelling, mass and lump
R19.Ø4 Left lower quadrant abdominal swelling, mass and lump
R19.Ø5 Periumbilic swelling, mass or lump
Diffuse or generalized umbilical swelling or mass
R19.Ø6 Epigastric swelling, mass or lump
R19.Ø7 Generalized intra-abdominal and pelvic swelling, mass and lump
Diffuse or generalized intra-abdominal swelling or mass NOS
Diffuse or generalized pelvic swelling or mass NOS
R19.Ø9 Other intra-abdominal and pelvic swelling, mass and lump
R19.1 Abnormal bowel sounds
R19.11 Absent bowel sounds
R19.12 Hyperactive bowel sounds
R19.15 Other abnormal bowel sounds
Abnormal bowel sounds NOS
R19.2 Visible peristalsis
Hyperperistalsis
DEF: Visible movements of muscular attempts to move food through the digestive tract due to pyloric obstruction, stomach obstruction, or intestinal obstruction.
R19.3 Abdominal rigidity
EXCLUDES 1 *abdominal rigidity with severe abdominal pain (R1Ø.Ø)*
R19.3Ø Abdominal rigidity, unspecified site
R19.31 Right upper quadrant abdominal rigidity
R19.32 Left upper quadrant abdominal rigidity
R19.33 Right lower quadrant abdominal rigidity
R19.34 Left lower quadrant abdominal rigidity
R19.35 Periumbilic abdominal rigidity
R19.36 Epigastric abdominal rigidity
R19.37 Generalized abdominal rigidity
R19.4 Change in bowel habit
EXCLUDES 1 *constipation (K59.Ø-)*
functional diarrhea (K59.1)

R19.5 Other fecal abnormalities
Abnormal stool color
Bulky stools
Mucus in stools
Occult blood in feces
Occult blood in stools
EXCLUDES 1 *melena (K92.1)*
neonatal melena (P54.1)
AHA: 2021,1Q,9; 2019,1Q,32

R19.6 Halitosis

R19.7 Diarrhea, unspecified
Diarrhea NOS
EXCLUDES 1 *functional diarrhea (K59.1)*
neonatal diarrhea (P78.3)
psychogenic diarrhea (F45.8)
AHA: 2021,3Q,3

R19.8 Other specified symptoms and signs involving the digestive system and abdomen

Symptoms and signs involving the skin and subcutaneous tissue (R2Ø-R23)

EXCLUDES 2 *symptoms relating to breast (N64.4-N64.5)*

✓4th **R2Ø Disturbances of skin sensation**
EXCLUDES 1 *dissociative anesthesia and sensory loss (F44.6)*
psychogenic disturbances (F45.8)

R2Ø.Ø Anesthesia of skin
R2Ø.1 Hypoesthesia of skin
R2Ø.2 Paresthesia of skin
Formication
Pins and needles
Tingling skin
EXCLUDES 1 *acroparesthesia (I73.8)*
R2Ø.3 Hyperesthesia
R2Ø.8 Other disturbances of skin sensation
R2Ø.9 Unspecified disturbances of skin sensation

R21 Rash and other nonspecific skin eruption
INCLUDES rash NOS
EXCLUDES 1 *specified type of rash - code to condition*
vesicular eruption (R23.8)

✓4th **R22 Localized swelling, mass and lump of skin and subcutaneous tissue**
INCLUDES subcutaneous nodules (localized)(superficial)
EXCLUDES 1 *abnormal findings on diagnostic imaging (R9Ø-R93)*
edema (R6Ø.-)
enlarged lymph nodes (R59.-)
localized adiposity (E65)
swelling of joint (M25.4-)

R22.Ø Localized swelling, mass and lump, head
R22.1 Localized swelling, mass and lump, neck
R22.2 Localized swelling, mass and lump, trunk
EXCLUDES 1 *intra-abdominal or pelvic mass and lump (R19.Ø-)*
intra abdominal or pelvic swelling (R19.Ø-)
EXCLUDES 2 *breast mass and lump (N63)*

✓5th **R22.3 Localized swelling, mass and lump, upper limb**
R22.3Ø Localized swelling, mass and lump, unspecified upper limb
R22.31 Localized swelling, mass and lump, right upper limb
R22.32 Localized swelling, mass and lump, left upper limb
R22.33 Localized swelling, mass and lump, upper limb, bilateral

✓5th **R22.4 Localized swelling, mass and lump, lower limb**
R22.4Ø Localized swelling, mass and lump, unspecified lower limb
R22.41 Localized swelling, mass and lump, right lower limb
R22.42 Localized swelling, mass and lump, left lower limb
R22.43 Localized swelling, mass and lump, lower limb, bilateral

R22.9 Localized swelling, mass and lump, unspecified

✓4th **R23 Other skin changes**
R23.Ø Cyanosis
EXCLUDES 1 *acrocyanosis (I73.8)*
cyanotic attacks of newborn (P28.2)
DEF: Bluish or purplish discoloration of the skin due to an inadequate oxygen blood level.

R23.1 Pallor
Clammy skin
R23.2 Flushing
Excessive blushing
Code first, if applicable, menopausal and female climacteric states (N95.1)
R23.3 Spontaneous ecchymoses
Petechiae
EXCLUDES 1 *ecchymoses of newborn (P54.5)*
purpura (D69.-)
R23.4 Changes in skin texture
Desquamation of skin
Induration of skin
Scaling of skin
EXCLUDES 1 *epidermal thickening NOS (L85.9)*
R23.8 Other skin changes
R23.9 Unspecified skin changes

Symptoms and signs involving the nervous and musculoskeletal systems (R25-R29)

✓4th **R25 Abnormal involuntary movements**
EXCLUDES 1 *specific movement disorders (G2Ø-G26)*
stereotyped movement disorders (F98.4)
tic disorders (F95.-)

R25.Ø Abnormal head movements
R25.1 Tremor, unspecified
EXCLUDES 1 *chorea NOS (G25.5)*
essential tremor (G25.Ø)
hysterical tremor (F44.4)
intention tremor (G25.2)
R25.2 Cramp and spasm
EXCLUDES 2 *carpopedal spasm (R29.Ø)*
charley-horse (M62.831)
infantile spasms (G4Ø.4-)
muscle spasm of back (M62.83Ø)
muscle spasm of calf (M62.831)
R25.3 Fasciculation
Twitching NOS
R25.8 Other abnormal involuntary movements
R25.9 Unspecified abnormal involuntary movements

✓4th **R26 Abnormalities of gait and mobility**
EXCLUDES 1 *ataxia NOS (R27.Ø)*
hereditary ataxia (G11.-)
locomotor (syphilitic) ataxia (A52.11)
immobility syndrome (paraplegic) (M62.3)

R26.Ø Ataxic gait
Staggering gait
AHA: 2022,2Q,12
R26.1 Paralytic gait
Spastic gait
R26.2 Difficulty in walking, not elsewhere classified
EXCLUDES 1 *falling (R29.6)*
unsteadiness on feet (R26.81)
AHA: 2016,2Q,7

✓5th **R26.8 Other abnormalities of gait and mobility**
R26.81 Unsteadiness on feet
R26.89 Other abnormalities of gait and mobility
AHA: 2020,2Q,29

R26.9 Unspecified abnormalities of gait and mobility

✓4th **R27 Other lack of coordination**
EXCLUDES 1 *ataxic gait (R26.Ø)*
hereditary ataxia (G11.-)
vertigo NOS (R42)

R27.Ø Ataxia, unspecified
EXCLUDES 1 *ataxia following cerebrovascular disease (I69. with final characters -93)*
R27.8 Other lack of coordination
R27.9 Unspecified lack of coordination

R29 Other symptoms and signs involving the nervous and musculoskeletal systems

R29.Ø Tetany

Carpopedal spasm

EXCLUDES 1 *hysterical tetany (F44.5)*
neonatal tetany (P71.3)
parathyroid tetany (E2Ø.9)
post-thyroidectomy tetany (E89.2)

DEF: Calcium or other mineral imbalance causing voluntary muscles such as hands, feet, or larynx to spasm rhythmically.

R29.1 Meningismus

R29.2 Abnormal reflex

EXCLUDES 2 *abnormal pupillary reflex (H57.Ø)*
hyperactive gag reflex (J39.2)
vasovagal reaction or syncope (R55)

R29.3 Abnormal posture

R29.4 Clicking hip

EXCLUDES 1 *congenital deformities of hip (Q65.-)*

R29.5 Transient paralysis

Code first any associated spinal cord injury (S14.Ø, S14.1-, S24.Ø, S24.1-, S34.Ø-, S34.1-)

EXCLUDES 1 *transient ischemic attack (G45.9)*

R29.6 Repeated falls

Falling
Tendency to fall

EXCLUDES 2 *at risk for falling (Z91.81)*
history of falling (Z91.81)

AHA: 2016,2Q,6

TIP: Code in addition to Parkinson's disease (G20), when documented.

R29.7 National Institutes of Health Stroke Scale (NIHSS) score

Code first the type of cerebral infarction (I63.-)

AHA: 2016,4Q,61-62

TIP: Codes from this subcategory may be assigned based on medical record documentation from clinicians who are not the patient's provider.

R29.7Ø NIHSS score Ø-9

R29.7ØØ NIHSS score Ø UPD
R29.7Ø1 NIHSS score 1 UPD
R29.7Ø2 NIHSS score 2 UPD
R29.7Ø3 NIHSS score 3 UPD
R29.7Ø4 NIHSS score 4 UPD
R29.7Ø5 NIHSS score 5 UPD
R29.7Ø6 NIHSS score 6 UPD
R29.7Ø7 NIHSS score 7 UPD
R29.7Ø8 NIHSS score 8 UPD
R29.7Ø9 NIHSS score 9 UPD

R29.71 NIHSS score 1Ø-19

R29.71Ø NIHSS score 1Ø UPD
R29.711 NIHSS score 11 UPD
R29.712 NIHSS score 12 UPD
R29.713 NIHSS score 13 UPD
R29.714 NIHSS score 14 UPD
R29.715 NIHSS score 15 UPD
R29.716 NIHSS score 16 UPD
R29.717 NIHSS score 17 UPD
R29.718 NIHSS score 18 UPD
R29.719 NIHSS score 19 UPD

R29.72 NIHSS score 2Ø-29

R29.72Ø NIHSS score 2Ø UPD
R29.721 NIHSS score 21 UPD
R29.722 NIHSS score 22 UPD
R29.723 NIHSS score 23 UPD
R29.724 NIHSS score 24 UPD
R29.725 NIHSS score 25 UPD
R29.726 NIHSS score 26 UPD
R29.727 NIHSS score 27 UPD
R29.728 NIHSS score 28 UPD
R29.729 NIHSS score 29 UPD

R29.73 NIHSS score 3Ø-39

R29.73Ø NIHSS score 3Ø UPD
R29.731 NIHSS score 31 UPD
R29.732 NIHSS score 32 UPD
R29.733 NIHSS score 33 UPD
R29.734 NIHSS score 34 UPD
R29.735 NIHSS score 35 UPD
R29.736 NIHSS score 36 UPD
R29.737 NIHSS score 37 UPD
R29.738 NIHSS score 38 UPD
R29.739 NIHSS score 39 UPD

R29.74 NIHSS score 4Ø-42

R29.74Ø NIHSS score 4Ø UPD
R29.741 NIHSS score 41 UPD
R29.742 NIHSS score 42 UPD

R29.8 Other symptoms and signs involving the nervous and musculoskeletal systems

R29.81 Other symptoms and signs involving the nervous system

R29.81Ø Facial weakness

Facial droop

EXCLUDES 1 *Bell's palsy (G51.Ø)*
facial weakness following cerebrovascular disease (I69. with final characters -92)

R29.818 Other symptoms and signs involving the nervous system

R29.89 Other symptoms and signs involving the musculoskeletal system

EXCLUDES 2 *pain in limb (M79.6-)*

R29.89Ø Loss of height

EXCLUDES 1 *osteoporosis (M8Ø-M81)*

R29.891 Ocular torticollis

EXCLUDES 1 *congenital (sternomastoid) torticollis Q68.Ø*
psychogenic torticollis (F45.8)
spasmodic torticollis (G24.3)
torticollis due to birth injury (P15.8)
torticollis NOS M43.6

DEF: Abnormal head posture as a result of a contracted state of cervical muscles to correct a visual disturbance, either double vision or a visual field defect.

R29.898 Other symptoms and signs involving the musculoskeletal system

R29.9 Unspecified symptoms and signs involving the nervous and musculoskeletal systems

R29.9Ø Unspecified symptoms and signs involving the nervous system

R29.91 Unspecified symptoms and signs involving the musculoskeletal system

Symptoms and signs involving the genitourinary system (R3Ø-R39)

R3Ø Pain associated with micturition

EXCLUDES 1 *psychogenic pain associated with micturition (F45.8)*

R3Ø.Ø Dysuria

Strangury

R3Ø.1 Vesical tenesmus

DEF: Feeling of a full bladder even when there is little or no urine in the bladder.

R3Ø.9 Painful micturition, unspecified

Painful urination NOS

R31 Hematuria

EXCLUDES 1 *hematuria included with underlying conditions, such as:*
acute cystitis with hematuria (N3Ø.Ø1)
recurrent and persistent hematuria in glomerular diseases (NØ2.-)

AHA: 2017,1Q,17

R31.Ø Gross hematuria

R31.1 Benign essential microscopic hematuria

R31.2 Other microscopic hematuria

AHA: 2016,4Q,62

R31.21 Asymptomatic microscopic hematuria

AMH

R31.29 Other microscopic hematuria

R31.9 Hematuria, unspecified

R32 Unspecified urinary incontinence
Enuresis NOS
EXCLUDES 1 *functional urinary incontinence (R39.81)*
nonorganic enuresis (F98.0)
stress incontinence and other specified urinary incontinence (N39.3-N39.4-)
urinary incontinence associated with cognitive impairment (R39.81)

R33 Retention of urine
EXCLUDES 1 *psychogenic retention of urine (F45.8)*

R33.0 Drug induced retention of urine
Use additional code for adverse effect, if applicable, to identify drug (T36-T50 with fifth or sixth character 5)

R33.8 Other retention of urine
Code first, if applicable, any causal condition, such as:
enlarged prostate (N40.1)
AHA: 2018,4Q,55

R33.9 Retention of urine, unspecified

R34 Anuria and oliguria
EXCLUDES 1 *anuria and oliguria complicating abortion or ectopic or molar pregnancy (O00-O07, O08.4)*
anuria and oliguria complicating pregnancy (O26.83-)
anuria and oliguria complicating the puerperium (O90.4)

R35 Polyuria
Code first, if applicable, any causal condition, such as:
enlarged prostate (N40.1)
EXCLUDES 1 *psychogenic polyuria (F45.8)*

R35.0 Frequency of micturition

R35.1 Nocturia

R35.8 Other polyuria
AHA: 2021,4Q,26

R35.81 Nocturnal polyuria
EXCLUDES 2 *nocturnal enuresis (N39.44)*

R35.89 Other polyuria
Polyuria NOS

R36 Urethral discharge

R36.0 Urethral discharge without blood

R36.1 Hematospermia ♂

R36.9 Urethral discharge, unspecified
Penile discharge NOS
Urethrorrhea

R37 Sexual dysfunction, unspecified

R39 Other and unspecified symptoms and signs involving the genitourinary system

R39.0 Extravasation of urine

R39.1 Other difficulties with micturition
Code first, if applicable, any causal condition, such as:
enlarged prostate (N40.1)

R39.11 Hesitancy of micturition

R39.12 Poor urinary stream
Weak urinary steam

R39.13 Splitting of urinary stream

R39.14 Feeling of incomplete bladder emptying

R39.15 Urgency of urination
EXCLUDES 1 *urge incontinence (N39.41, N39.46)*

R39.16 Straining to void

R39.19 Other difficulties with micturition
AHA: 2016,4Q,63

R39.191 Need to immediately re-void

R39.192 Position dependent micturition

R39.198 Other difficulties with micturition

R39.2 Extrarenal uremia
Prerenal uremia
EXCLUDES 1 *uremia NOS (N19)*

R39.8 Other symptoms and signs involving the genitourinary system
AHA: 2017,4Q,22-23

R39.81 Functional urinary incontinence
Urinary incontinence due to cognitive impairment, or severe physical disability or immobility
EXCLUDES 1 *stress incontinence and other specified urinary incontinence (N39.3-N39.4-)*
urinary incontinence NOS (R32)

R39.82 Chronic bladder pain
AHA: 2016,4Q,64

R39.83 Unilateral non-palpable testicle ♂

R39.84 Bilateral non-palpable testicles ♂

R39.89 Other symptoms and signs involving the genitourinary system

R39.9 Unspecified symptoms and signs involving the genitourinary system

Symptoms and signs involving cognition, perception, emotional state and behavior (R40-R46)

EXCLUDES 2 *symptoms and signs constituting part of a pattern of mental disorder (F01-F99)*

R40 Somnolence, stupor and coma
EXCLUDES 1 *neonatal coma (P91.5)*
somnolence, stupor and coma in diabetes (E08-E13)
somnolence, stupor and coma in hepatic failure (K72.-)
somnolence, stupor and coma in hypoglycemia (nondiabetic) (E15)

R40.0 Somnolence
Drowsiness
EXCLUDES 1 *coma (R40.2-)*

R40.1 Stupor
Catatonic stupor
Semicoma
EXCLUDES 1 *catatonic schizophrenia (F20.2)*
coma (R40.2-)
depressive stupor (F31-F33)
dissociative stupor (F44.2)
manic stupor (F30.2)

R40.2 Coma
Code first any associated:
fracture of skull (S02.-)
intracranial injury (S06.-)

NOTE One code from each subcategory, R40.21-R40.23, is required to complete the coma scale

AHA: 2020,3Q,46; 2019,2Q,12; 2018,4Q,70; 2017,4Q,23-25,95; 2015,2Q,17; 2014,1Q,19

TIP: Codes for individual (R40.21-, R40.22-, R40.23-) or total (R40.24-) coma scale scores may be assigned based on medical record documentation from clinicians who are not the patient's provider.

TIP: It is not appropriate to assign individual (R40.21- , R40.22-, R40.23-) or total (R40.24-) coma scale score codes for patients who are sedated or in medically induced comas.

R40.20 Unspecified coma HCC ESR COM
Coma NOS
Unconsciousness NOS
AHA: 2021,4Q,112-113; 2021,2Q,5

R40.21 Coma scale, eyes open

The following appropriate 7th character is to be added to subcategory R40.21-, R40.22-, R40.23-, and R40.24-.
0 unspecified time
1 in the field [EMT or ambulance]
2 at arrival to emergency department
3 at hospital admission
4 24 hours or more after hospital admission

R40.211 Coma scale, eyes open, never HCC ESR COM UPD
Coma scale eye opening score of 1

R40.212 Coma scale, eyes open, to pain HCC ESR COM UPD
Coma scale eye opening score of 2

R40.213 Coma scale, eyes open, to sound UPD
Coma scale eye opening score of 3

R40.214 Coma scale, eyes open, spontaneous UPD
Coma scale eye opening score of 4

R40.22 Coma scale, best verbal response

R40.221 Coma scale, best verbal response, none HCC ESR COM UPD
Coma scale verbal score of 1

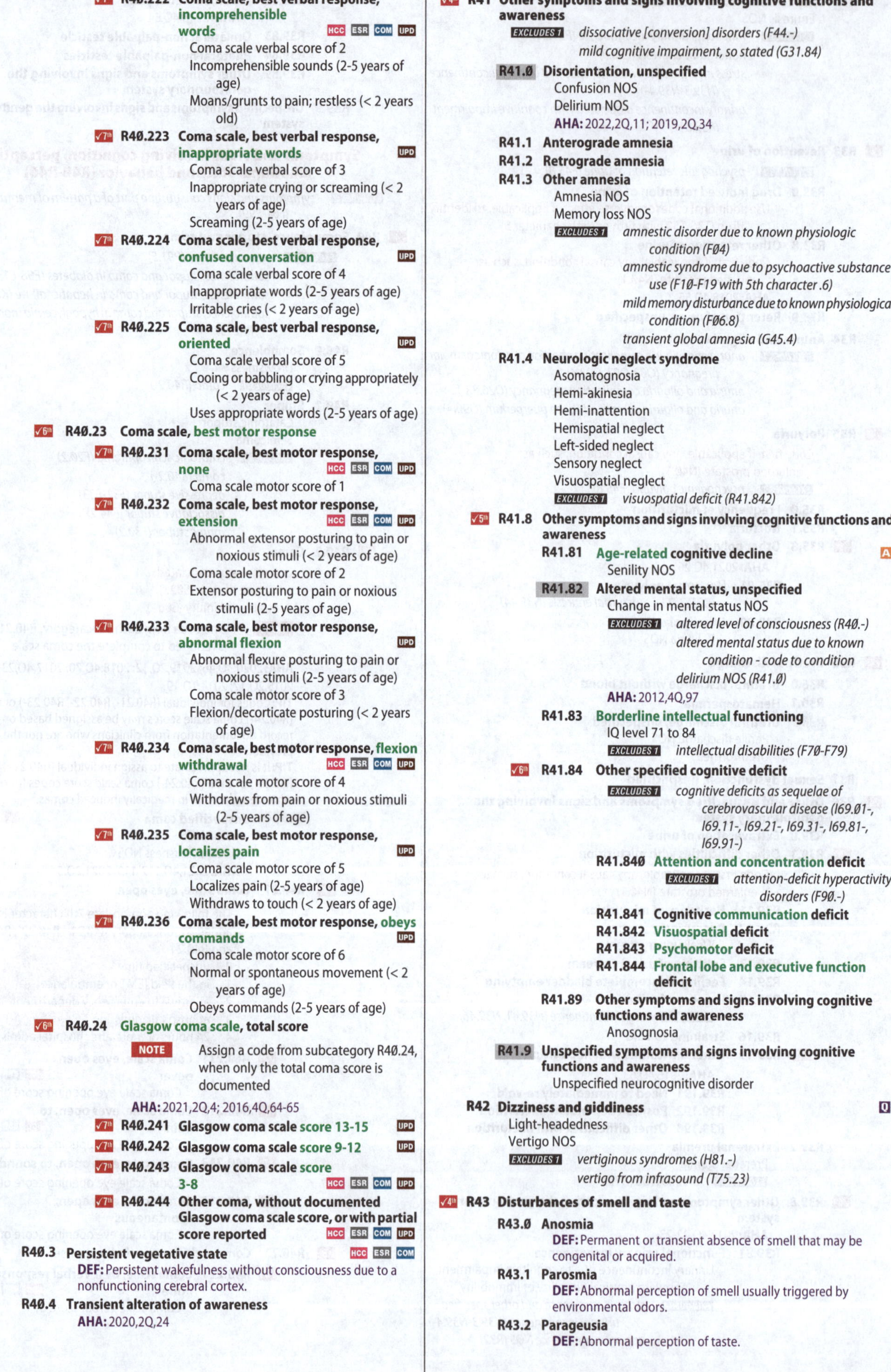

√7th **R40.222 Coma scale, best verbal response, incomprehensible words** HCC ESR COM UPD
Coma scale verbal score of 2
Incomprehensible sounds (2-5 years of age)
Moans/grunts to pain; restless (< 2 years old)

√7th **R40.223 Coma scale, best verbal response, inappropriate words** UPD
Coma scale verbal score of 3
Inappropriate crying or screaming (< 2 years of age)
Screaming (2-5 years of age)

√7th **R40.224 Coma scale, best verbal response, confused conversation** UPD
Coma scale verbal score of 4
Inappropriate words (2-5 years of age)
Irritable cries (< 2 years of age)

√7th **R40.225 Coma scale, best verbal response, oriented** UPD
Coma scale verbal score of 5
Cooing or babbling or crying appropriately (< 2 years of age)
Uses appropriate words (2-5 years of age)

√6th **R40.23 Coma scale, best motor response**

√7th **R40.231 Coma scale, best motor response, none** HCC ESR COM UPD
Coma scale motor score of 1

√7th **R40.232 Coma scale, best motor response, extension** HCC ESR COM UPD
Abnormal extensor posturing to pain or noxious stimuli (< 2 years of age)
Coma scale motor score of 2
Extensor posturing to pain or noxious stimuli (2-5 years of age)

√7th **R40.233 Coma scale, best motor response, abnormal flexion** UPD
Abnormal flexure posturing to pain or noxious stimuli (2-5 years of age)
Coma scale motor score of 3
Flexion/decorticate posturing (< 2 years of age)

√7th **R40.234 Coma scale, best motor response, flexion withdrawal** HCC ESR COM UPD
Coma scale motor score of 4
Withdraws from pain or noxious stimuli (2-5 years of age)

√7th **R40.235 Coma scale, best motor response, localizes pain** UPD
Coma scale motor score of 5
Localizes pain (2-5 years of age)
Withdraws to touch (< 2 years of age)

√7th **R40.236 Coma scale, best motor response, obeys commands** UPD
Coma scale motor score of 6
Normal or spontaneous movement (< 2 years of age)
Obeys commands (2-5 years of age)

√6th **R40.24 Glasgow coma scale, total score**
NOTE Assign a code from subcategory R40.24, when only the total coma score is documented
AHA: 2021,2Q,4; 2016,4Q,64-65

√7th **R40.241 Glasgow coma scale score 13-15** UPD
√7th **R40.242 Glasgow coma scale score 9-12** UPD
√7th **R40.243 Glasgow coma scale score 3-8** HCC ESR COM UPD
√7th **R40.244 Other coma, without documented Glasgow coma scale score, or with partial score reported** HCC ESR COM UPD

R40.3 Persistent vegetative state HCC ESR COM
DEF: Persistent wakefulness without consciousness due to a nonfunctioning cerebral cortex.

R40.4 Transient alteration of awareness
AHA: 2020,2Q,24

√4th **R41 Other symptoms and signs involving cognitive functions and awareness**
EXCLUDES 1 *dissociative [conversion] disorders (F44.-)*
mild cognitive impairment, so stated (G31.84)

R41.0 Disorientation, unspecified
Confusion NOS
Delirium NOS
AHA: 2022,2Q,11; 2019,2Q,34

R41.1 Anterograde amnesia

R41.2 Retrograde amnesia

R41.3 Other amnesia
Amnesia NOS
Memory loss NOS
EXCLUDES 1 *amnestic disorder due to known physiologic condition (F04)*
amnestic syndrome due to psychoactive substance use (F10-F19 with 5th character .6)
mild memory disturbance due to known physiological condition (F06.8)
transient global amnesia (G45.4)

R41.4 Neurologic neglect syndrome
Asomatognosia
Hemi-akinesia
Hemi-inattention
Hemispatial neglect
Left-sided neglect
Sensory neglect
Visuospatial neglect
EXCLUDES 1 *visuospatial deficit (R41.842)*

√5th **R41.8 Other symptoms and signs involving cognitive functions and awareness**

R41.81 Age-related cognitive decline A
Senility NOS

R41.82 Altered mental status, unspecified
Change in mental status NOS
EXCLUDES 1 *altered level of consciousness (R40.-)*
altered mental status due to known condition - code to condition
delirium NOS (R41.0)
AHA: 2012,4Q,97

R41.83 Borderline intellectual functioning
IQ level 71 to 84
EXCLUDES 1 *intellectual disabilities (F70-F79)*

√6th **R41.84 Other specified cognitive deficit**
EXCLUDES 1 *cognitive deficits as sequelae of cerebrovascular disease (I69.01-, I69.11-, I69.21-, I69.31-, I69.81-, I69.91-)*

R41.840 Attention and concentration deficit
EXCLUDES 1 *attention-deficit hyperactivity disorders (F90.-)*

R41.841 Cognitive communication deficit

R41.842 Visuospatial deficit

R41.843 Psychomotor deficit

R41.844 Frontal lobe and executive function deficit

R41.89 Other symptoms and signs involving cognitive functions and awareness
Anosognosia

R41.9 Unspecified symptoms and signs involving cognitive functions and awareness
Unspecified neurocognitive disorder

R42 Dizziness and giddiness O
Light-headedness
Vertigo NOS
EXCLUDES 1 *vertiginous syndromes (H81.-)*
vertigo from infrasound (T75.23)

√4th **R43 Disturbances of smell and taste**

R43.0 Anosmia
DEF: Permanent or transient absence of smell that may be congenital or acquired.

R43.1 Parosmia
DEF: Abnormal perception of smell usually triggered by environmental odors.

R43.2 Parageusia
DEF: Abnormal perception of taste.

R43.8 Other disturbances of smell and taste
Mixed disturbance of smell and taste

R43.9 Unspecified disturbances of smell and taste

R44 Other symptoms and signs involving general sensations and perceptions
EXCLUDES 1 *alcoholic hallucinations (F10.151, F10.251, F10.951)*
hallucinations in drug psychosis (F11-F19 with fifth to sixth characters 51)
hallucinations in mood disorders with psychotic symptoms (F30.2, F31.5, F32.3, F33.3)
hallucinations in schizophrenia, schizotypal and delusional disorders (F20-F29)
EXCLUDES 2 *disturbances of skin sensation (R20.-)*

R44.0 Auditory hallucinations

R44.1 Visual hallucinations

R44.2 Other hallucinations

R44.3 Hallucinations, unspecified
AHA: 2022,2Q,11

R44.8 Other symptoms and signs involving general sensations and perceptions

R44.9 Unspecified symptoms and signs involving general sensations and perceptions

R45 Symptoms and signs involving emotional state

R45.0 Nervousness
Nervous tension

R45.1 Restlessness and agitation

R45.2 Unhappiness

R45.3 Demoralization and apathy
EXCLUDES 1 *anhedonia (R45.84)*

R45.4 Irritability and anger

R45.5 Hostility

R45.6 Violent behavior

R45.7 State of emotional shock and stress, unspecified

R45.8 Other symptoms and signs involving emotional state

R45.81 Low self-esteem

R45.82 Worries

R45.83 Excessive crying of child, adolescent or adult
EXCLUDES 1 *excessive crying of infant (baby) R68.11*

R45.84 Anhedonia

R45.85 Homicidal and suicidal ideations
EXCLUDES 1 *suicide attempt (T14.91)*

R45.850 Homicidal ideations

R45.851 Suicidal ideations
AHA: 2022,1Q,29
DEF: Thoughts of committing suicide but no actual attempt of suicide has been made.

R45.86 Emotional lability

R45.87 Impulsiveness

R45.88 Nonsuicidal self-harm HCC Rx ESR COM
Nonsuicidal self-injury
Nonsuicidal self-mutilation
Self-inflicted injury without suicidal intent
Code also injury, if known
AHA: 2021,4Q,26-27

R45.89 Other symptoms and signs involving emotional state

R46 Symptoms and signs involving appearance and behavior
EXCLUDES 1 *appearance and behavior in schizophrenia, schizotypal and delusional disorders (F20-F29)*
mental and behavioral disorders (F01-F99)

R46.0 Very low level of personal hygiene

R46.1 Bizarre personal appearance

R46.2 Strange and inexplicable behavior

R46.3 Overactivity

R46.4 Slowness and poor responsiveness
EXCLUDES 1 *stupor (R40.1)*

R46.5 Suspiciousness and marked evasiveness

R46.6 Undue concern and preoccupation with stressful events

R46.7 Verbosity and circumstantial detail obscuring reason for contact

R46.8 Other symptoms and signs involving appearance and behavior

R46.81 Obsessive-compulsive behavior
EXCLUDES 1 *obsessive-compulsive disorder (F42.-)*

R46.89 Other symptoms and signs involving appearance and behavior

Symptoms and signs involving speech and voice (R47-R49)

R47 Speech disturbances, not elsewhere classified
EXCLUDES 1 *autism (F84.0)*
cluttering (F80.81)
specific developmental disorders of speech and language (F80.-)
stuttering (F80.81)

R47.0 Dysphasia and aphasia

R47.01 Aphasia
EXCLUDES 1 *aphasia following cerebrovascular disease (I69. with final characters -20)*
progressive isolated aphasia (G31.01)

R47.02 Dysphasia
EXCLUDES 1 *dysphasia following cerebrovascular disease (I69. with final characters -21)*

R47.1 Dysarthria and anarthria
EXCLUDES 1 *dysarthria following cerebrovascular disease (I69. with final characters -22)*

R47.8 Other speech disturbances
EXCLUDES 1 *dysarthria following cerebrovascular disease (I69. with final characters -28)*

R47.81 Slurred speech

R47.82 Fluency disorder in conditions classified elsewhere
Stuttering in conditions classified elsewhere
Code first underlying disease or condition, such as:
Parkinson's disease (G20)
EXCLUDES 1 *adult onset fluency disorder (F98.5)*
childhood onset fluency disorder (F80.81)
fluency disorder (stuttering) following cerebrovascular disease (I69. with final characters -23)

R47.89 Other speech disturbances

R47.9 Unspecified speech disturbances

R48 Dyslexia and other symbolic dysfunctions, not elsewhere classified
EXCLUDES 1 *specific developmental disorders of scholastic skills (F81.-)*

R48.0 Dyslexia and alexia

R48.1 Agnosia
Astereognosia (astereognosis)
Autotopagnosia
EXCLUDES 1 *visual object agnosia (R48.3)*
DEF: Inability to recognize common things such as faces, objects, smells, or voices.

R48.2 Apraxia
EXCLUDES 1 *apraxia following cerebrovascular disease (I69. with final characters -90)*

R48.3 Visual agnosia
Prosopagnosia
Simultanagnosia (asimultagnosia)

R48.8 Other symbolic dysfunctions
Acalculia
Agraphia
AHA: 2017,1Q,27

R48.9 Unspecified symbolic dysfunctions

R49 Voice and resonance disorders
EXCLUDES 1 *psychogenic voice and resonance disorders (F44.4)*

R49.0 Dysphonia
Hoarseness

R49.1 Aphonia
Loss of voice

R49.2 Hypernasality and hyponasality

R49.21 Hypernasality

R49.22 Hyponasality

R49.8 Other voice and resonance disorders

R49.9 Unspecified voice and resonance disorder
Change in voice NOS
Resonance disorder NOS

General symptoms and signs (R5Ø-R69)

R5Ø Fever of other and unknown origin

EXCLUDES 1 *chills without fever (R68.83)*
febrile convulsions (R56.Ø-)
fever of unknown origin during labor (O75.2)
fever of unknown origin in newborn (P81.9)
hypothermia due to illness (R68.Ø)
malignant hyperthermia due to anesthesia (T88.3)
puerperal pyrexia NOS (O86.4)

R5Ø.2 Drug induced fever
Use additional code for adverse effect, if applicable, to identify drug (T36-T5Ø with fifth or sixth character 5)
EXCLUDES 1 *postvaccination (postimmunization) fever (R5Ø.83)*

R5Ø.8 Other specified fever

R5Ø.81 Fever presenting with conditions classified elsewhere
Code first underlying condition when associated fever is present, such as with:
leukemia (C91-C95)
neutropenia (D7Ø.-)
sickle-cell disease (D57.-)
AHA: 2020,3Q,22; 2014,4Q,22

R5Ø.82 Postprocedural fever
EXCLUDES 1 *postprocedural infection (T81.4-)*
posttransfusion fever (R5Ø.84)
postvaccination (postimmunization) fever (R5Ø.83)

R5Ø.83 Postvaccination fever
Postimmunization fever

R5Ø.84 Febrile nonhemolytic transfusion reaction
FNHTR
Posttransfusion fever

R5Ø.9 Fever, unspecified
Fever NOS
Fever of unknown origin [FUO]
Fever with chills
Fever with rigors
Hyperpyrexia NOS
Persistent fever
Pyrexia NOS

R51 Headache

EXCLUDES 2 *atypical face pain (G5Ø.1)*
migraine and other headache syndromes (G43-G44)
trigeminal neuralgia (G5Ø.Ø)
AHA: 2020,4Q,38-39

R51.Ø Headache with orthostatic component, not elsewhere classified
Headache with positional component, not elsewhere classified

R51.9 Headache, unspecified
Facial pain NOS

R52 Pain, unspecified
Acute pain NOS
Generalized pain NOS
Pain NOS
EXCLUDES 1 *acute and chronic pain, not elsewhere classified (G89.-)*
localized pain, unspecified type - code to pain by site, such as:
abdomen pain (R1Ø.-)
back pain (M54.9)
breast pain (N64.4)
chest pain (RØ7.1-RØ7.9)
ear pain (H92.Ø-)
eye pain (H57.1)
headache (R51.9)
joint pain (M25.5-)
limb pain (M79.6-)
lumbar region pain (M54.5-)
pelvic and perineal pain (R1Ø.2)
renal colic (N23)
shoulder pain (M25.51-)
spine pain (M54.-)
throat pain (RØ7.Ø)
tongue pain (K14.6)
tooth pain (KØ8.8)
pain disorders exclusively related to psychological factors (F45.41)

R53 Malaise and fatigue

R53.Ø Neoplastic (malignant) related fatigue
Code first associated neoplasm

R53.1 Weakness
Asthenia NOS
EXCLUDES 1 *age-related weakness (R54)*
muscle weakness (generalized) (M62.81)
sarcopenia (M62.84)
senile asthenia (R54)
AHA: 2017,1Q,7; 2015,1Q,25

R53.2 Functional quadriplegia HCC ESR COM
Complete immobility due to severe physical disability or frailty
EXCLUDES 1 *frailty NOS (R54)*
hysterical paralysis (F44.4)
immobility syndrome (M62.3)
neurologic quadriplegia (G82.5-)
quadriplegia (G82.5Ø)
AHA: 2016,2Q,6
DEF: Inability to move due to a nonphysiological condition, such as dementia. The patient has no mental ability to move independently.

R53.8 Other malaise and fatigue
EXCLUDES 1 *combat exhaustion and fatigue (F43.Ø)*
congenital debility (P96.9)
exhaustion and fatigue due to excessive exertion (T73.3)
exhaustion and fatigue due to exposure (T73.2)
exhaustion and fatigue due to heat (T67.-)
exhaustion and fatigue due to pregnancy (O26.8-)
exhaustion and fatigue due to recurrent depressive episode (F33)
exhaustion and fatigue due to senile debility (R54)

R53.81 Other malaise
Chronic debility
Debility NOS
General physical deterioration
Malaise NOS
Nervous debility
EXCLUDES 1 *age-related physical debility (R54)*
AHA: 2021,1Q,43

R53.82 Chronic fatigue, unspecified
~~Chronic fatigue syndrome NOS~~
EXCLUDES 1 ►*chronic fatigue syndrome (G93.32)*◄
►*myalgic encephalomyelitis (G93.32)*◄
►*post infection and related fatigue syndromes (G93.39)*◄
postviral fatigue syndrome ►*(G93.31)*◄

R53.83 Other fatigue
Fatigue NOS
Lack of energy
Lethargy
Tiredness
EXCLUDES 2 *exhaustion and fatigue due to depressive episode (F32.-)*

R54 Age-related physical debility A
Frailty
Old age
Senescence
Senile asthenia
Senile debility
EXCLUDES 1 *age-related cognitive decline (R41.81)*
sarcopenia (M62.84)
senile psychosis (FØ3)
senility NOS (R41.81)

R55 Syncope and collapse
Blackout
Fainting
Vasovagal attack
EXCLUDES 1 *cardiogenic shock (R57.Ø)*
carotid sinus syncope (G9Ø.Ø1)
heat syncope (T67.1)
neurocirculatory asthenia (F45.8)
neurogenic orthostatic hypotension (G9Ø.3)
orthostatic hypotension (I95.1)
postprocedural shock (T81.1-)
psychogenic syncope (F48.8)
shock NOS (R57.9)
shock complicating or following abortion or ectopic or molar pregnancy (OØØ-OØ7, OØ8.3)
shock complicating or following labor and delivery (O75.1)
Stokes-Adams attack (I45.9)
unconsciousness NOS (R4Ø.2-)

✓4th **R56 Convulsions, not elsewhere classified**
EXCLUDES 1 *dissociative convulsions and seizures (F44.5)*
epileptic convulsions and seizures (G4Ø.-)
newborn convulsions and seizures (P9Ø)

✓5th **R56.Ø Febrile convulsions**

R56.ØØ Simple febrile convulsions HCC ESR COM
Febrile convulsion NOS
Febrile seizure NOS

R56.Ø1 Complex febrile convulsions HCC ESR COM
Atypical febrile seizure
Complex febrile seizure
Complicated febrile seizure
EXCLUDES 1 *status epilepticus (G4Ø.9Ø1)*

R56.1 Post traumatic seizures HCC ESR COM
EXCLUDES 1 *post traumatic epilepsy (G4Ø.-)*

R56.9 Unspecified convulsions HCC ESR COM
Convulsion disorder
Fit NOS
Recurrent convulsions
Seizure(s) (convulsive) NOS
AHA: 2021,1Q,3; 2019,1Q,19

✓4th **R57 Shock, not elsewhere classified**
EXCLUDES 1 *anaphylactic shock NOS (T78.2)*
anaphylactic reaction or shock due to adverse food reaction (T78.Ø-)
anaphylactic shock due to adverse effect of correct drug or medicament properly administered (T88.6)
anaphylactic shock due to serum (T8Ø.5-)
electric shock (T75.4)
obstetric shock (O75.1)
postprocedural shock (T81.1-)
psychic shock (F43.Ø)
shock complicating or following ectopic or molar pregnancy (OØØ-OØ7, OØ8.3)
shock due to anesthesia (T88.2)
shock due to lightning (T75.Ø1)
toxic shock syndrome (A48.3)
traumatic shock (T79.4)

R57.Ø Cardiogenic shock HCC ESR COM
EXCLUDES 2 *septic shock (R65.21)*
AHA: 2020,3Q,26
DEF: Associated with myocardial infarction, cardiac tamponade, and massive pulmonary embolism. Symptoms include mental confusion, reduced blood pressure, tachycardia, pallor, and cold, clammy skin.

R57.1 Hypovolemic shock HCC ESR COM
AHA: 2019,2Q,7

R57.8 Other shock HCC ESR COM

R57.9 Shock, unspecified HCC ESR COM
Failure of peripheral circulation NOS

R58 Hemorrhage, not elsewhere classified
Hemorrhage NOS
EXCLUDES 1 *hemorrhage included with underlying conditions, such as:*
acute duodenal ulcer with hemorrhage (K26.Ø)
acute gastritis with bleeding (K29.Ø1)
ulcerative enterocolitis with rectal bleeding (K51.Ø1)

✓4th **R59 Enlarged lymph nodes**
INCLUDES swollen glands
EXCLUDES 1 *acute lymphadenitis (LØ4.-)*
chronic lymphadenitis (I88.1)
lymphadenitis NOS (I88.9)
mesenteric (acute) (chronic) lymphadenitis (I88.Ø)

R59.Ø Localized enlarged lymph nodes

R59.1 Generalized enlarged lymph nodes
Lymphadenopathy NOS

R59.9 Enlarged lymph nodes, unspecified

✓4th **R6Ø Edema, not elsewhere classified**
EXCLUDES 1 *angioneurotic edema (T78.3)*
ascites (R18.-)
cerebral edema (G93.6)
cerebral edema due to birth injury (P11.Ø)
edema of larynx (J38.4)
edema of nasopharynx (J39.2)
edema of pharynx (J39.2)
gestational edema (O12.Ø-)
hereditary edema (Q82.Ø)
hydrops fetalis NOS (P83.2)
hydrothorax (J94.8)
newborn edema (P83.3)
pulmonary edema (J81.-)

R6Ø.Ø Localized edema

R6Ø.1 Generalized edema
EXCLUDES 2 *nutritional edema (E4Ø-E46)*

R6Ø.9 Edema, unspecified
Fluid retention NOS

R61 Generalized hyperhidrosis
Excessive sweating
Night sweats
Secondary hyperhidrosis
Code first, if applicable, menopausal and female climacteric states (N95.1)
EXCLUDES 1 *focal (primary) (secondary) hyperhidrosis (L74.5-)*
Frey's syndrome (L74.52)
localized (primary) (secondary) hyperhidrosis (L74.5-)

Chapter 18. Symptoms, Signs and Abnormal Clinical and Laboratory Findings

4th R62 Lack of expected normal physiological development in childhood and adults

EXCLUDES 1 *delayed puberty (E30.0)*
gonadal dysgenesis (Q99.1)
hypopituitarism (E23.0)

R62.0 Delayed milestone in childhood P

Delayed attainment of expected physiological developmental stage
Late talker
Late walker

5th R62.5 Other and unspecified lack of expected normal physiological development in childhood

EXCLUDES 1 *HIV disease resulting in failure to thrive (B20)*
physical retardation due to malnutrition (E45)

R62.50 Unspecified lack of expected normal physiological development in childhood

Infantilism NOS

R62.51 Failure to thrive (child) P

Failure to gain weight

EXCLUDES 1 *failure to thrive in child under 28 days old (P92.6)*

AHA: 2018,4Q,82

DEF: Organic failure to thrive (FTT): Acute or chronic illness that interferes with nutritional intake, absorption, metabolism excretion, and energy requirements.

DEF: Nonorganic failure to thrive (FTT): Symptom of neglect or abuse.

R62.52 Short stature (child)

Lack of growth
Physical retardation
Short stature NOS

EXCLUDES 1 *short stature due to endocrine disorder ▶(E34.3-)◀*

R62.59 Other lack of expected normal physiological development in childhood

R62.7 Adult failure to thrive A

4th R63 Symptoms and signs concerning food and fluid intake

EXCLUDES 1 *bulimia NOS (F50.2)*

R63.0 Anorexia

Loss of appetite

EXCLUDES 1 *anorexia nervosa (F50.0-)*
loss of appetite of nonorganic origin (F50.89)

AHA: 2018,4Q,82

TIP: Assign an additional code from category Z68 when BMI is documented. BMI can be based on documentation from clinicians who are not the patient's provider.

R63.1 Polydipsia

Excessive thirst

R63.2 Polyphagia

Excessive eating
Hyperalimentation NOS

5th R63.3 Feeding difficulties

EXCLUDES 2 *eating disorders (F50.-)*
feeding problems of newborn (P92.-)
infant feeding disorder of nonorganic origin (F98.2-)

AHA: 2021,4Q,27-28; 2017,1Q,28; 2016,3Q,19

R63.30 Feeding difficulties, unspecified

R63.31 Pediatric feeding disorder, acute P

Pediatric feeding dysfunction, acute
Code also, if applicable, associated conditions such as:
aspiration pneumonia (J69.0)
dysphagia (R13.1-)
gastro-esophageal reflux disease (K21.-)
malnutrition (E40-E46)

R63.32 Pediatric feeding disorder, chronic P

Pediatric feeding dysfunction, chronic
Code also, if applicable, associated conditions such as:
aspiration pneumonia (J69.0)
dysphagia (R13.1-)
gastro-esophageal reflux disease (K21.-)
malnutrition (E40-E46)

R63.39 Other feeding difficulties

Feeding problem (elderly) (infant) NOS
Picky eater

R63.4 Abnormal weight loss

AHA: 2018,4Q,82

TIP: Assign an additional code from category Z68 when BMI is documented. BMI can be based on documentation from clinicians who are not the patient's provider.

R63.5 Abnormal weight gain

EXCLUDES 1 *excessive weight gain in pregnancy (O26.0-)*
obesity (E66.-)

AHA: 2018,4Q,82

TIP: Assign an additional code from category Z68 when BMI is documented. BMI can be based on documentation from clinicians who are not the patient's provider.

R63.6 Underweight

Use additional code to identify body mass index (BMI), if known (Z68.-)

EXCLUDES 1 *abnormal weight loss (R63.4)*
anorexia nervosa (F50.0-)
malnutrition (E40-E46)

AHA: 2018,4Q,82

R63.8 Other symptoms and signs concerning food and fluid intake

R64 Cachexia HCC ESR COM

Wasting syndrome
Code first underlying condition, if known

EXCLUDES 1 *abnormal weight loss (R63.4)*
nutritional marasmus (E41)

AHA: 2018,4Q,82; 2017,3Q,24

TIP: Assign code E43 when emaciated or emaciation is documented in relation to malnutrition.

4th R65 Symptoms and signs specifically associated with systemic inflammation and infection

AHA: 2019,2Q,38

TIP: When documentation states SIRS with an infection, assign only a code for the infection. ICD-10-CM does not offer a code for SIRS due to infectious process. If sepsis is suspected, query the provider.

5th R65.1 Systemic inflammatory response syndrome [SIRS] of non-infectious origin

Code first underlying condition, such as:
heatstroke (T67.0-)
injury and trauma (S00-T88)

EXCLUDES 1 *sepsis - code to infection*
severe sepsis (R65.2)

R65.10 Systemic inflammatory response syndrome [SIRS] of non-infectious origin without acute organ dysfunction HCC ESR COM UPD

Systemic inflammatory response syndrome (SIRS) NOS

AHA: 2019,2Q,24

R65.11 Systemic inflammatory response syndrome [SIRS] of non-infectious origin with acute organ dysfunction HCC ESR COM UPD

Use additional code to identify specific acute organ dysfunction, such as:
acute kidney failure (N17.-)
acute respiratory failure (J96.0-)
critical illness myopathy (G72.81)
critical illness polyneuropathy (G62.81)
disseminated intravascular coagulopathy [DIC] (D65)
encephalopathy (metabolic) (septic) (G93.41)
hepatic failure (K72.0-)

R65.2 Severe sepsis

Infection with associated acute organ dysfunction
Sepsis with acute organ dysfunction
Sepsis with multiple organ dysfunction
Systemic inflammatory response syndrome due to infectious process with acute organ dysfunction

Code first underlying infection, such as:
- infection following a procedure (T81.4-)
- infections following infusion, transfusion and therapeutic injection (T80.2-)
- puerperal sepsis (O85)
- sepsis following complete or unspecified spontaneous abortion (O03.87)
- sepsis following ectopic and molar pregnancy (O08.82)
- sepsis following incomplete spontaneous abortion (O03.37)
- sepsis following (induced) termination of pregnancy (O04.87)
- sepsis NOS (A41.9)

Use additional code to identify specific acute organ dysfunction, such as:
- acute kidney failure (N17.-)
- acute respiratory failure (J96.0-)
- critical illness myopathy (G72.81)
- critical illness polyneuropathy (G62.81)
- disseminated intravascular coagulopathy [DIC] (D65)
- encephalopathy (metabolic) (septic) (G93.41)
- hepatic failure (K72.0-)

AHA: 2020,2Q,17; 2018,4Q,62-63; 2017,4Q,98-99; 2016,3Q,8

R65.20 Severe sepsis without septic shock HCC ESR COM UPD
Severe sepsis NOS
AHA: 2020,2Q,17; 2016,3Q,14; 2013,4Q,119

R65.21 Severe sepsis with septic shock HCC ESR COM UPD
AHA: 2018,4Q,63

R68 Other general symptoms and signs

R68.0 Hypothermia, not associated with low environmental temperature

EXCLUDES 1 *hypothermia NOS (accidental) (T68)*
hypothermia due to anesthesia (T88.51)
hypothermia due to low environmental temperature (T68)
newborn hypothermia (P80.-)

R68.1 Nonspecific symptoms peculiar to infancy

EXCLUDES 1 *colic, infantile (R10.83)*
neonatal cerebral irritability (P91.3)
teething syndrome (K00.7)

R68.11 Excessive crying of infant (baby) P
EXCLUDES 1 *excessive crying of child, adolescent, or adult (R45.83)*

R68.12 Fussy infant (baby) P
Irritable infant

R68.13 Apparent life threatening event in infant (ALTE) P
Apparent life threatening event in newborn
Brief resolved unexplained event (BRUE)
Code first confirmed diagnosis, if known
Use additional code(s) for associated signs and symptoms if no confirmed diagnosis established, or if signs and symptoms are not associated routinely with confirmed diagnosis, or provide additional information for cause of ALTE

R68.19 Other nonspecific symptoms peculiar to infancy P

R68.2 Dry mouth, unspecified

EXCLUDES 1 *dry mouth due to dehydration (E86.0)*
dry mouth due to Sjögren syndrome (M35.0-)
salivary gland hyposecretion (K11.7)

R68.3 Clubbing of fingers
Clubbing of nails
EXCLUDES 1 *congenital clubfinger (Q68.1)*
DEF: Enlarged soft tissue of the distal fingers that usually occurs in heart and lung diseases.

R68.8 Other general symptoms and signs

R68.81 Early satiety
DEF: Premature feeling of being full after eating only a small amount of food. The mechanism of satiety is multifactorial.

R68.82 Decreased libido A
Decreased sexual desire

R68.83 Chills (without fever)
Chills NOS
EXCLUDES 1 *chills with fever (R50.9)*

R68.84 Jaw pain
Mandibular pain
Maxilla pain
EXCLUDES 1 *temporomandibular joint arthralgia (M26.62-)*

R68.89 Other general symptoms and signs

R69 Illness, unspecified
Unknown and unspecified cases of morbidity

Abnormal findings on examination of blood, without diagnosis (R70-R79)

EXCLUDES 2 *abnormal findings on antenatal screening of mother (O28.-)*
abnormalities of lipids (E78.-)
abnormalities of platelets and thrombocytes (D69.-)
abnormalities of white blood cells classified elsewhere (D70-D72)
coagulation hemorrhagic disorders (D65-D68)
diagnostic abnormal findings classified elsewhere - see Alphabetical Index
hemorrhagic and hematological disorders of newborn (P50-P61)

R70 Elevated erythrocyte sedimentation rate and abnormality of plasma viscosity

R70.0 Elevated erythrocyte sedimentation rate

R70.1 Abnormal plasma viscosity

R71 Abnormality of red blood cells

EXCLUDES 1 *anemias (D50-D64)*
anemia of premature infant (P61.2)
benign (familial) polycythemia (D75.0)
congenital anemias (P61.2-P61.4)
newborn anemia due to isoimmunization (P55.-)
polycythemia neonatorum (P61.1)
polycythemia NOS (D75.1)
polycythemia vera (D45)
secondary polycythemia (D75.1)

R71.0 Precipitous drop in hematocrit
Drop (precipitous) in hemoglobin
Drop in hematocrit

R71.8 Other abnormality of red blood cells
Abnormal red-cell morphology NOS
Abnormal red-cell volume NOS
Anisocytosis
Poikilocytosis

R73 Elevated blood glucose level

EXCLUDES 1 *diabetes mellitus (E08-E13)*
diabetes mellitus in pregnancy, childbirth and the puerperium (O24.-)
neonatal disorders (P70.0-P70.2)
postsurgical hypoinsulinemia (E89.1)

R73.0 Abnormal glucose

EXCLUDES 1 *abnormal glucose in pregnancy (O99.81-)*
diabetes mellitus (E08-E13)
dysmetabolic syndrome X (E88.81)
gestational diabetes (O24.4-)
glycosuria (R81)
hypoglycemia (E16.2)

R73.01 Impaired fasting glucose
Elevated fasting glucose

R73.02 Impaired glucose tolerance (oral)
Elevated glucose tolerance

R73.03 Prediabetes
Latent diabetes
AHA: 2016,4Q,65

R73.09 Other abnormal glucose
Abnormal glucose NOS
Abnormal non-fasting glucose tolerance

R73.9 Hyperglycemia, unspecified

R74 Abnormal serum enzyme levels

R74.0 Nonspecific elevation of levels of transaminase and lactic acid dehydrogenase [LDH]
AHA: 2020,4Q,39

R74.01 Elevation of levels of liver transaminase levels
Elevation of levels of alanine transaminase (ALT)
Elevation of levels of aspartate transaminase (AST)

R74.02 Elevation of levels of lactic acid dehydrogenase [LDH]

R74.8 Abnormal levels of other serum enzymes
Abnormal level of acid phosphatase
Abnormal level of alkaline phosphatase
Abnormal level of amylase
Abnormal level of lipase [triacylglycerol lipase]
AHA: 2019,2Q,6

R74.9 Abnormal serum enzyme level, unspecified

R75 Inconclusive laboratory evidence of human immunodeficiency virus [HIV]
Nonconclusive HIV-test finding in infants
EXCLUDES 1 *asymptomatic human immunodeficiency virus [HIV] infection status (Z21)*
human immunodeficiency virus [HIV] disease (B20)

R76 Other abnormal immunological findings in serum

R76.0 Raised antibody titer
EXCLUDES 1 *isoimmunization in pregnancy (O36.0-O36.1)*
isoimmunization affecting newborn (P55.-)
AHA: 2021,1Q,6

R76.1 Nonspecific reaction to test for tuberculosis

R76.11 Nonspecific reaction to tuberculin skin test without active tuberculosis
Abnormal result of Mantoux test
PPD positive
Tuberculin (skin test) positive
Tuberculin (skin test) reactor
EXCLUDES 1 *nonspecific reaction to cell mediated immunity measurement of gamma interferon antigen response without active tuberculosis (R76.12)*

R76.12 Nonspecific reaction to cell mediated immunity measurement of gamma interferon antigen response without active tuberculosis
Nonspecific reaction to QuantiFERON-TB test (QFT) without active tuberculosis
EXCLUDES 1 *nonspecific reaction to tuberculin skin test without active tuberculosis (R76.11)*
positive tuberculin skin test (R76.11)

R76.8 Other specified abnormal immunological findings in serum
Raised level of immunoglobulins NOS
AHA: 2021,1Q,6

R76.9 Abnormal immunological finding in serum, unspecified

R77 Other abnormalities of plasma proteins
EXCLUDES 1 *disorders of plasma-protein metabolism (E88.0-)*

R77.0 Abnormality of albumin

R77.1 Abnormality of globulin
Hyperglobulinemia NOS

R77.2 Abnormality of alphafetoprotein

R77.8 Other specified abnormalities of plasma proteins

R77.9 Abnormality of plasma protein, unspecified
AHA: 2019,2Q,6

R78 Findings of drugs and other substances, not normally found in blood
Use additional code to identify the any retained foreign body, if applicable (Z18.-)
EXCLUDES 1 *mental or behavioral disorders due to psychoactive substance use (F10-F19)*

R78.0 Finding of alcohol in blood
Use additional external cause code (Y90.-), for detail regarding alcohol level

R78.1 Finding of opiate drug in blood

R78.2 Finding of cocaine in blood

R78.3 Finding of hallucinogen in blood

R78.4 Finding of other drugs of addictive potential in blood

R78.5 Finding of other psychotropic drug in blood

R78.6 Finding of steroid agent in blood

R78.7 Finding of abnormal level of heavy metals in blood

R78.71 Abnormal lead level in blood
EXCLUDES 1 *lead poisoning (T56.0-)*

R78.79 Finding of abnormal level of heavy metals in blood

R78.8 Finding of other specified substances, not normally found in blood

R78.81 Bacteremia
EXCLUDES 1 *sepsis — code to specified infection*
DEF: Laboratory finding of bacteria in the blood in the absence of two or more signs of sepsis. Transient in nature, it can progress to septicemia with a severe infectious process.

R78.89 Finding of other specified substances, not normally found in blood
Finding of abnormal level of lithium in blood

R78.9 Finding of unspecified substance, not normally found in blood

R79 Other abnormal findings of blood chemistry
Use additional code to identify any retained foreign body, if applicable (Z18.-)
EXCLUDES 1 *asymptomatic hyperuricemia (E79.0)*
hyperglycemia NOS (R73.9)
hypoglycemia NOS (E16.2)
neonatal hypoglycemia (P70.3-P70.4)
specific findings indicating disorder of amino-acid metabolism (E70-E72)
specific findings indicating disorder of carbohydrate metabolism (E73-E74)
specific findings indicating disorder of lipid metabolism (E75.-)

R79.0 Abnormal level of blood mineral
Abnormal blood level of cobalt
Abnormal blood level of copper
Abnormal blood level of iron
Abnormal blood level of magnesium
Abnormal blood level of mineral NEC
Abnormal blood level of zinc
EXCLUDES 1 *abnormal level of lithium (R78.89)*
disorders of mineral metabolism (E83.-)
neonatal hypomagnesemia (P71.2)
nutritional mineral deficiency (E58-E61)

R79.1 Abnormal coagulation profile
Abnormal or prolonged bleeding time
Abnormal or prolonged coagulation time
Abnormal or prolonged partial thromboplastin time [PTT]
Abnormal or prolonged prothrombin time [PT]
►Low von Willebrand factor◄
EXCLUDES 1 *coagulation defects (D68.-)*
EXCLUDES 2 *abnormality of fluid, electrolyte or acid-base balance (E86-E87)*

R79.8 Other specified abnormal findings of blood chemistry

R79.81 Abnormal blood-gas level

R79.82 Elevated C-reactive protein [CRP]

R79.83 Abnormal findings of blood amino-acid level
Homocysteinemia
EXCLUDES 1 *disorders of amino-acid metabolism (E70-E72)*
AHA: 2021,4Q,28

R79.89 Other specified abnormal findings of blood chemistry
AHA: 2019,2Q,6
TIP: Assign for positive Coombs test when not further clarified in the documentation.

R79.9 Abnormal finding of blood chemistry, unspecified

Chapter 18. Symptoms, Signs and Abnormal Clinical and Laboratory Findings

R74–R79.9

Abnormal findings on examination of urine, without diagnosis (R80-R82)

EXCLUDES 1 *abnormal findings on antenatal screening of mother (O28.-)*
diagnostic abnormal findings classified elsewhere - see Alphabetical Index
specific findings indicating disorder of amino-acid metabolism (E70-E72)
specific findings indicating disorder of carbohydrate metabolism (E73-E74)

R80 Proteinuria
EXCLUDES 1 *gestational proteinuria (O12.1-)*

R80.0 Isolated proteinuria
Idiopathic proteinuria
EXCLUDES 1 *isolated proteinuria with specific morphological lesion (N06.-)*

R80.1 Persistent proteinuria, unspecified

R80.2 Orthostatic proteinuria, unspecified
Postural proteinuria

R80.3 Bence Jones proteinuria

R80.8 Other proteinuria

R80.9 Proteinuria, unspecified
Albuminuria NOS

R81 Glycosuria
EXCLUDES 1 *renal glycosuria (E74.818)*

R82 Other and unspecified abnormal findings in urine
INCLUDES chromoabnormalities in urine
Use additional code to identify any retained foreign body, if applicable (Z18.-)
EXCLUDES 2 *hematuria (R31.-)*

R82.0 Chyluria
EXCLUDES 1 *filarial chyluria (B74.-)*

R82.1 Myoglobinuria

R82.2 Biliuria

R82.3 Hemoglobinuria
EXCLUDES 1 *hemoglobinuria due to hemolysis from external causes NEC (D59.6)*
hemoglobinuria due to paroxysmal nocturnal [Marchiafava-Micheli] (D59.5)
DEF: Free hemoglobin in blood due to rapid hemolysis of red blood cells. Causes include burns, crushed injury, sickle cell anemia, thalassemia, parasitic infections, or kidney infections.

R82.4 Acetonuria
Ketonuria
DEF: Excessive excretion of acetone in urine that commonly occurs in diabetic acidosis.

R82.5 Elevated urine levels of drugs, medicaments and biological substances
Elevated urine levels of catecholamines
Elevated urine levels of indoleacetic acid
Elevated urine levels of 17-ketosteroids
Elevated urine levels of steroids

R82.6 Abnormal urine levels of substances chiefly nonmedicinal as to source
Abnormal urine level of heavy metals

R82.7 Abnormal findings on microbiological examination of urine
EXCLUDES 1 *colonization status (Z22.-)*
AHA: 2016,4Q,65

R82.71 Bacteriuria

R82.79 Other abnormal findings on microbiological examination of urine
Positive culture findings of urine

R82.8 Abnormal findings on cytological and histological examination of urine
AHA: 2019,4Q,16

R82.81 Pyuria
Sterile pyuria

R82.89 Other abnormal findings on cytological and histological examination of urine

R82.9 Other and unspecified abnormal findings in urine

R82.90 Unspecified abnormal findings in urine

R82.91 Other chromoabnormalities of urine
Chromoconversion (dipstick)
Idiopathic dipstick converts positive for blood with no cellular forms in sediment
EXCLUDES 1 *hemoglobinuria (R82.3)*
myoglobinuria (R82.1)

R82.99 Other abnormal findings in urine
AHA: 2018,4Q,29-30

R82.991 Hypocitraturia

R82.992 Hyperoxaluria
EXCLUDES 1 *primary hyperoxaluria (E72.53)*

R82.993 Hyperuricosuria

R82.994 Hypercalciuria
Idiopathic hypercalciuria

R82.998 Other abnormal findings in urine
Cells and casts in urine
Crystalluria
Melanuria

Abnormal findings on examination of other body fluids, substances and tissues, without diagnosis (R83-R89)

EXCLUDES 1 *abnormal findings on antenatal screening of mother (O28.-)*
diagnostic abnormal findings classified elsewhere - see Alphabetical Index
EXCLUDES 2 *abnormal findings on examination of blood, without diagnosis (R70-R79)*
abnormal findings on examination of urine, without diagnosis (R80-R82)
abnormal tumor markers (R97.-)

R83 Abnormal findings in cerebrospinal fluid

R83.0 Abnormal level of enzymes in cerebrospinal fluid

R83.1 Abnormal level of hormones in cerebrospinal fluid

R83.2 Abnormal level of other drugs, medicaments and biological substances in cerebrospinal fluid

R83.3 Abnormal level of substances chiefly nonmedicinal as to source in cerebrospinal fluid

R83.4 Abnormal immunological findings in cerebrospinal fluid

R83.5 Abnormal microbiological findings in cerebrospinal fluid
Positive culture findings in cerebrospinal fluid
EXCLUDES 1 *colonization status (Z22.-)*

R83.6 Abnormal cytological findings in cerebrospinal fluid

R83.8 Other abnormal findings in cerebrospinal fluid
Abnormal chromosomal findings in cerebrospinal fluid

R83.9 Unspecified abnormal finding in cerebrospinal fluid

R84 Abnormal findings in specimens from respiratory organs and thorax
INCLUDES abnormal findings in bronchial washings
abnormal findings in nasal secretions
abnormal findings in pleural fluid
abnormal findings in sputum
abnormal findings in throat scrapings
EXCLUDES 1 *blood-stained sputum (R04.2)*

R84.0 Abnormal level of enzymes in specimens from respiratory organs and thorax

R84.1 Abnormal level of hormones in specimens from respiratory organs and thorax

R84.2 Abnormal level of other drugs, medicaments and biological substances in specimens from respiratory organs and thorax

R84.3 Abnormal level of substances chiefly nonmedicinal as to source in specimens from respiratory organs and thorax

R84.4 Abnormal immunological findings in specimens from respiratory organs and thorax

R84.5 Abnormal microbiological findings in specimens from respiratory organs and thorax
Positive culture findings in specimens from respiratory organs and thorax
EXCLUDES 1 *colonization status (Z22.-)*

R84.6 Abnormal cytological findings in specimens from respiratory organs and thorax

R84.7 Abnormal histological findings in specimens from respiratory organs and thorax

R84.8 Other abnormal findings in specimens from respiratory organs and thorax
Abnormal chromosomal findings in specimens from respiratory organs and thorax

R84.9 Unspecified abnormal finding in specimens from respiratory organs and thorax

R85 Abnormal findings in specimens from digestive organs and abdominal cavity

INCLUDES abnormal findings in peritoneal fluid
abnormal findings in saliva

EXCLUDES 1 *cloudy peritoneal dialysis effluent (R88.Ø)*
fecal abnormalities (R19.5)

R85.Ø Abnormal level of enzymes in specimens from digestive organs and abdominal cavity

R85.1 Abnormal level of hormones in specimens from digestive organs and abdominal cavity

R85.2 Abnormal level of other drugs, medicaments and biological substances in specimens from digestive organs and abdominal cavity

R85.3 Abnormal level of substances chiefly nonmedicinal as to source in specimens from digestive organs and abdominal cavity

R85.4 Abnormal immunological findings in specimens from digestive organs and abdominal cavity

R85.5 Abnormal microbiological findings in specimens from digestive organs and abdominal cavity

Positive culture findings in specimens from digestive organs and abdominal cavity

EXCLUDES 1 *colonization status (Z22.-)*

R85.6 Abnormal cytological findings in specimens from digestive organs and abdominal cavity

R85.61 Abnormal cytologic smear of anus

EXCLUDES 1 *abnormal cytological findings in specimens from other digestive organs and abdominal cavity (R85.69)*
anal intraepithelial neoplasia I [AIN I] (K62.82)
anal intraepithelial neoplasia II [AIN II] (K62.82)
anal intraepithelial neoplasia III [AIN III] (DØ1.3)
carcinoma in situ of anus (histologically confirmed) (DØ1.3)
dysplasia (mild) (moderate) of anus (histologically confirmed) (K62.82)
severe dysplasia of anus (histologically confirmed) (DØ1.3)

EXCLUDES 2 *anal high risk human papillomavirus (HPV) DNA test positive (R85.81)*
anal low risk human papillomavirus (HPV) DNA test positive (R85.82)

R85.61Ø Atypical squamous cells of undetermined significance on cytologic smear of anus [ASC-US]

R85.611 Atypical squamous cells cannot exclude high grade squamous intraepithelial lesion on cytologic smear of anus [ASC-H]

R85.612 Low grade squamous intraepithelial lesion on cytologic smear of anus [LGSIL]

R85.613 High grade squamous intraepithelial lesion on cytologic smear of anus [HGSIL]

R85.614 Cytologic evidence of malignancy on smear of anus

R85.615 Unsatisfactory cytologic smear of anus

Inadequate sample of cytologic smear of anus

R85.616 Satisfactory anal smear but lacking transformation zone

R85.618 Other abnormal cytological findings on specimens from anus

R85.619 Unspecified abnormal cytological findings in specimens from anus

Abnormal anal cytology NOS
Atypical glandular cells of anus NOS

R85.69 Abnormal cytological findings in specimens from other digestive organs and abdominal cavity

R85.7 Abnormal histological findings in specimens from digestive organs and abdominal cavity

R85.8 Other abnormal findings in specimens from digestive organs and abdominal cavity

R85.81 Anal high risk human papillomavirus [HPV] DNA test positive

EXCLUDES 1 *anogenital warts due to human papillomavirus (HPV) (A63.Ø)*
condyloma acuminatum (A63.Ø)

R85.82 Anal low risk human papillomavirus [HPV] DNA test positive

Use additional code for associated human papillomavirus (B97.7)

R85.89 Other abnormal findings in specimens from digestive organs and abdominal cavity

Abnormal chromosomal findings in specimens from digestive organs and abdominal cavity

R85.9 Unspecified abnormal finding in specimens from digestive organs and abdominal cavity

R86 Abnormal findings in specimens from male genital organs

INCLUDES abnormal findings in prostatic secretions
abnormal findings in semen, seminal fluid
abnormal spermatozoa

EXCLUDES 1 *azoospermia (N46.Ø-)*
oligospermia (N46.1-)

R86.Ø Abnormal level of enzymes in specimens from male genital organs ♂

R86.1 Abnormal level of hormones in specimens from male genital organs ♂

R86.2 Abnormal level of other drugs, medicaments and biological substances in specimens from male genital organs ♂

R86.3 Abnormal level of substances chiefly nonmedicinal as to source in specimens from male genital organs ♂

R86.4 Abnormal immunological findings in specimens from male genital organs ♂

R86.5 Abnormal microbiological findings in specimens from male genital organs ♂

Positive culture findings in specimens from male genital organs

EXCLUDES 1 *colonization status (Z22.-)*

R86.6 Abnormal cytological findings in specimens from male genital organs ♂

R86.7 Abnormal histological findings in specimens from male genital organs ♂

R86.8 Other abnormal findings in specimens from male genital organs ♂

Abnormal chromosomal findings in specimens from male genital organs

R86.9 Unspecified abnormal finding in specimens from male genital organs ♂

R87 Abnormal findings in specimens from female genital organs

INCLUDES abnormal findings in secretion and smears from cervix uteri
abnormal findings in secretion and smears from vagina
abnormal findings in secretion and smears from vulva

R87.Ø Abnormal level of enzymes in specimens from female genital organs ♀

R87.1 Abnormal level of hormones in specimens from female genital organs ♀

R87.2 Abnormal level of other drugs, medicaments and biological substances in specimens from female genital organs ♀

R87.3 Abnormal level of substances chiefly nonmedicinal as to source in specimens from female genital organs ♀

R87.4 Abnormal immunological findings in specimens from female genital organs ♀

R87.5 Abnormal microbiological findings in specimens from female genital organs ♀

Positive culture findings in specimens from female genital organs

EXCLUDES 1 *colonization status (Z22.-)*

R87.6 Abnormal cytological findings in specimens from female genital organs

R87.61 Abnormal cytological findings in specimens from cervix uteri

EXCLUDES 1 *abnormal cytological findings in specimens from other female genital organs (R87.69)*
abnormal cytological findings in specimens from vagina (R87.62-)
carcinoma in situ of cervix uteri (histologically confirmed) (DØ6.-)
cervical intraepithelial neoplasia I [CIN I] (N87.Ø)
cervical intraepithelial neoplasia II [CIN II] (N87.1)
cervical intraepithelial neoplasia III [CIN III] (DØ6.-)
dysplasia (mild) (moderate) of cervix uteri (histologically confirmed) (N87.-)
severe dysplasia of cervix uteri (histologically confirmed) (DØ6.-)

EXCLUDES 2 *cervical high risk human papillomavirus (HPV) DNA test positive (R87.81Ø)*
cervical low risk human papillomavirus (HPV) DNA test positive (R87.82Ø)

R87.61Ø Atypical squamous cells of undetermined significance on cytologic smear of cervix [ASC-US] ♀

R87.611 Atypical squamous cells cannot exclude high grade squamous intraepithelial lesion on cytologic smear of cervix [ASC-H] ♀

R87.612 Low grade squamous intraepithelial lesion on cytologic smear of cervix [LGSIL] ♀

R87.613 High grade squamous intraepithelial lesion on cytologic smear of cervix [HGSIL] ♀

R87.614 Cytologic evidence of malignancy on smear of cervix ♀

R87.615 Unsatisfactory cytologic smear of cervix ♀
Inadequate sample of cytologic smear of cervix

R87.616 Satisfactory cervical smear but lacking transformation zone ♀

R87.618 Other abnormal cytological findings on specimens from cervix uteri ♀

R87.619 Unspecified abnormal cytological findings in specimens from cervix uteri ♀
Abnormal cervical cytology NOS
Abnormal Papanicolaou smear of cervix NOS
Abnormal thin preparation smear of cervix NOS
Atypical endocervial cells of cervix NOS
Atypical endometrial cells of cervix NOS
Atypical glandular cells of cervix NOS

R87.62 Abnormal cytological findings in specimens from vagina
Use additional code to identify acquired absence of uterus and cervix, if applicable (Z9Ø.71-)

EXCLUDES 1 *abnormal cytological findings in specimens from cervix uteri (R87.61-)*
abnormal cytological findings in specimens from other female genital organs (R87.69)
carcinoma in situ of vagina (histologically confirmed) (DØ7.2)
dysplasia (mild) (moderate) of vagina (histologically confirmed) (N89.-)
severe dysplasia of vagina (histologically confirmed) (DØ7.2)
vaginal intraepithelial neoplasia I [VAIN I] (N89.Ø)
vaginal intraepithelial neoplasia II [VAIN II] (N89.1)
vaginal intraepithelial neoplasia III [VAIN III] (DØ7.2)

EXCLUDES 2 *vaginal high risk human papillomavirus (HPV) DNA test positive (R87.811)*
vaginal low risk human papillomavirus (HPV) DNA test positive (R87.821)

R87.62Ø Atypical squamous cells of undetermined significance on cytologic smear of vagina [ASC-US] ♀

R87.621 Atypical squamous cells cannot exclude high grade squamous intraepithelial lesion on cytologic smear of vagina [ASC-H] ♀

R87.622 Low grade squamous intraepithelial lesion on cytologic smear of vagina [LGSIL] ♀

R87.623 High grade squamous intraepithelial lesion on cytologic smear of vagina [HGSIL] ♀

R87.624 Cytologic evidence of malignancy on smear of vagina ♀

R87.625 Unsatisfactory cytologic smear of vagina ♀
Inadequate sample of cytologic smear of vagina

R87.628 Other abnormal cytological findings on specimens from vagina ♀

R87.629 Unspecified abnormal cytological findings in specimens from vagina ♀
Abnormal Papanicolaou smear of vagina NOS
Abnormal thin preparation smear of vagina NOS
Abnormal vaginal cytology NOS
Atypical endocervical cells of vagina NOS
Atypical endometrial cells of vagina NOS
Atypical glandular cells of vagina NOS

R87.69 Abnormal cytological findings in specimens from other female genital organs ♀
Abnormal cytological findings in specimens from female genital organs NOS

EXCLUDES 1 *dysplasia of vulva (histologically confirmed) (N9Ø.Ø-N9Ø.3)*

R87.7 Abnormal histological findings in specimens from female genital organs ♀

EXCLUDES 1 *carcinoma in situ (histologically confirmed) of female genital organs (DØ6-DØ7.3)*
cervical intraepithelial neoplasia I [CIN I] (N87.Ø)
cervical intraepithelial neoplasia II [CIN II] (N87.1)
cervical intraepithelial neoplasia III [CIN III] (DØ6.-)
dysplasia (mild) (moderate) of cervix uteri (histologically confirmed) (N87.-)
dysplasia (mild) (moderate) of vagina (histologically confirmed) (N89.-)
severe dysplasia of cervix uteri (histologically confirmed) (DØ6.-)
severe dysplasia of vagina (histologically confirmed) (DØ7.2)
vaginal intraepithelial neoplasia I [VAIN I] (N89.Ø)
vaginal intraepithelial neoplasia II [VAIN II] (N89.1)
vaginal intraepithelial neoplasia III [VAIN III] (DØ7.2)

5th **R87.8 Other abnormal findings in specimens from female genital organs**

6th **R87.81 High risk human papillomavirus [HPV] DNA test positive from female genital organs**

EXCLUDES 1 *anogenital warts due to human papillomavirus (HPV) (A63.Ø)*
condyloma acuminatum (A63.Ø)

R87.81Ø Cervical high risk human papillomavirus [HPV] DNA test positive ♀

R87.811 Vaginal high risk human papillomavirus [HPV] DNA test positive ♀

6th **R87.82 Low risk human papillomavirus [HPV] DNA test positive from female genital organs**

Use additional code for associated human papillomavirus (B97.7)

R87.82Ø Cervical low risk human papillomavirus [HPV] DNA test positive ♀

R87.821 Vaginal low risk human papillomavirus [HPV] DNA test positive ♀

R87.89 Other abnormal findings in specimens from female genital organs ♀

Abnormal chromosomal findings in specimens from female genital organs

R87.9 Unspecified abnormal finding in specimens from female genital organs ♀

4th **R88 Abnormal findings in other body fluids and substances**

R88.Ø Cloudy (hemodialysis) (peritoneal) dialysis effluent

R88.8 Abnormal findings in other body fluids and substances

4th **R89 Abnormal findings in specimens from other organs, systems and tissues**

INCLUDES abnormal findings in nipple discharge
abnormal findings in synovial fluid
abnormal findings in wound secretions

R89.Ø Abnormal level of enzymes in specimens from other organs, systems and tissues

R89.1 Abnormal level of hormones in specimens from other organs, systems and tissues

R89.2 Abnormal level of other drugs, medicaments and biological substances in specimens from other organs, systems and tissues

R89.3 Abnormal level of substances chiefly nonmedicinal as to source in specimens from other organs, systems and tissues

R89.4 Abnormal immunological findings in specimens from other organs, systems and tissues

R89.5 Abnormal microbiological findings in specimens from other organs, systems and tissues

Positive culture findings in specimens from other organs, systems and tissues

EXCLUDES 1 *colonization status (Z22.-)*

R89.6 Abnormal cytological findings in specimens from other organs, systems and tissues

R89.7 Abnormal histological findings in specimens from other organs, systems and tissues

R89.8 Other abnormal findings in specimens from other organs, systems and tissues

Abnormal chromosomal findings in specimens from other organs, systems and tissues

R89.9 Unspecified abnormal finding in specimens from other organs, systems and tissues

Abnormal findings on diagnostic imaging and in function studies, without diagnosis (R9Ø-R94)

INCLUDES nonspecific abnormal findings on diagnostic imaging by computerized axial tomography [CAT scan]
nonspecific abnormal findings on diagnostic imaging by magnetic resonance imaging [MRI][NMR]
nonspecific abnormal findings on diagnostic imaging by positron emission tomography [PET scan]
nonspecific abnormal findings on diagnostic imaging by thermography
nonspecific abnormal findings on diagnostic imaging by ultrasound [echogram]
nonspecific abnormal findings on diagnostic imaging by X-ray examination

EXCLUDES 1 *abnormal findings on antenatal screening of mother (O28.-)*
diagnostic abnormal findings classified elsewhere - see Alphabetical Index

4th **R9Ø Abnormal findings on diagnostic imaging of central nervous system**

R9Ø.Ø Intracranial space-occupying lesion found on diagnostic imaging of central nervous system

5th **R9Ø.8 Other abnormal findings on diagnostic imaging of central nervous system**

R9Ø.81 Abnormal echoencephalogram

R9Ø.82 White matter disease, unspecified

R9Ø.89 Other abnormal findings on diagnostic imaging of central nervous system

Other cerebrovascular abnormality found on diagnostic imaging of central nervous system

4th **R91 Abnormal findings on diagnostic imaging of lung**

R91.1 Solitary pulmonary nodule

Coin lesion lung
Solitary pulmonary nodule, subsegmental branch of the bronchial tree

R91.8 Other nonspecific abnormal finding of lung field

Lung mass NOS found on diagnostic imaging of lung
Pulmonary infiltrate NOS
Shadow, lung

4th **R92 Abnormal and inconclusive findings on diagnostic imaging of breast**

R92.Ø Mammographic microcalcification found on diagnostic imaging of breast

EXCLUDES 2 *mammographic calcification (calculus) found on diagnostic imaging of breast (R92.1)*

DEF: Calcium and cellular debris deposits in the breast that cannot be felt but can be detected on a mammogram. The deposits can be a sign of cancer, benign conditions, or changes in the breast tissue as a result of inflammation, injury, or an obstructed duct.

R92.1 Mammographic calcification found on diagnostic imaging of breast

Mammographic calculus found on diagnostic imaging of breast

R92.2 Inconclusive mammogram

Dense breasts NOS
Inconclusive mammogram NEC
Inconclusive mammography due to dense breasts
Inconclusive mammography NEC
AHA: 2015,1Q,24

R92.8 Other abnormal and inconclusive findings on diagnostic imaging of breast

4th **R93 Abnormal findings on diagnostic imaging of other body structures**

R93.Ø Abnormal findings on diagnostic imaging of skull and head, not elsewhere classified

EXCLUDES 1 *intracranial space-occupying lesion found on diagnostic imaging (R9Ø.Ø)*

R93.1 Abnormal findings on diagnostic imaging of heart and coronary circulation

Abnormal echocardiogram NOS
Abnormal heart shadow

R93.2 Abnormal findings on diagnostic imaging of liver and biliary tract

Nonvisualization of gallbladder

R93.3 Abnormal findings on diagnostic imaging of other parts of digestive tract

✓5th **R93.4 Abnormal findings on diagnostic imaging of urinary organs**
EXCLUDES 2 *hypertrophy of kidney (N28.81)*
AHA: 2016,4Q,66

R93.41 Abnormal radiologic findings on diagnostic imaging of renal pelvis, ureter, or bladder
Filling defect of bladder found on diagnostic imaging
Filling defect of renal pelvis found on diagnostic imaging
Filling defect of ureter found on diagnostic imaging

✓6th **R93.42 Abnormal radiologic findings on diagnostic imaging of kidney**
R93.421 Abnormal radiologic findings on diagnostic imaging of right kidney
R93.422 Abnormal radiologic findings on diagnostic imaging of left kidney
R93.429 Abnormal radiologic findings on diagnostic imaging of unspecified kidney

R93.49 Abnormal radiologic findings on diagnostic imaging of other urinary organs

R93.5 Abnormal findings on diagnostic imaging of other abdominal regions, including retroperitoneum

R93.6 Abnormal findings on diagnostic imaging of limbs
EXCLUDES 2 *abnormal finding in skin and subcutaneous tissue (R93.8-)*
AHA: 2020,1Q,14

R93.7 Abnormal findings on diagnostic imaging of other parts of musculoskeletal system
EXCLUDES 2 *abnormal findings on diagnostic imaging of skull (R93.Ø)*

✓5th **R93.8 Abnormal findings on diagnostic imaging of other specified body structures**
AHA: 2018,4Q,30

✓6th **R93.81 Abnormal radiologic findings on diagnostic imaging of testis**
R93.811 Abnormal radiologic findings on diagnostic imaging of right testicle ♂
R93.812 Abnormal radiologic findings on diagnostic imaging of left testicle ♂
R93.813 Abnormal radiologic findings on diagnostic imaging of testicles, bilateral ♂
R93.819 Abnormal radiologic findings on diagnostic imaging of unspecified testicle ♂

R93.89 Abnormal findings on diagnostic imaging of other specified body structures
Abnormal finding by radioisotope localization of placenta
Abnormal radiological finding in skin and subcutaneous tissue
Mediastinal shift

R93.9 Diagnostic imaging inconclusive due to excess body fat of patient

✓4th **R94 Abnormal results of function studies**
INCLUDES abnormal results of radionuclide [radioisotope] uptake studies
abnormal results of scintigraphy

✓5th **R94.Ø Abnormal results of function studies of central nervous system**
R94.Ø1 Abnormal electroencephalogram [EEG]
R94.Ø2 Abnormal brain scan
R94.Ø9 Abnormal results of other function studies of central nervous system

✓5th **R94.1 Abnormal results of function studies of peripheral nervous system and special senses**

✓6th **R94.11 Abnormal results of function studies of eye**
R94.11Ø Abnormal electro-oculogram [EOG]
R94.111 Abnormal electroretinogram [ERG]
Abnormal retinal function study
R94.112 Abnormal visually evoked potential [VEP]
R94.113 Abnormal oculomotor study
R94.118 Abnormal results of other function studies of eye

✓6th **R94.12 Abnormal results of function studies of ear and other special senses**
AHA: 2016,3Q,17
R94.12Ø Abnormal auditory function study
R94.121 Abnormal vestibular function study
R94.128 Abnormal results of other function studies of ear and other special senses

✓6th **R94.13 Abnormal results of function studies of peripheral nervous system**
R94.13Ø Abnormal response to nerve stimulation, unspecified
R94.131 Abnormal electromyogram [EMG]
EXCLUDES 1 *electromyogram of eye (R94.113)*
R94.138 Abnormal results of other function studies of peripheral nervous system

R94.2 Abnormal results of pulmonary function studies
Reduced ventilatory capacity
Reduced vital capacity

✓5th **R94.3 Abnormal results of cardiovascular function studies**
R94.3Ø Abnormal result of cardiovascular function study, unspecified
R94.31 Abnormal electrocardiogram [ECG] [EKG]
EXCLUDES 1 *long QT syndrome (I45.81)*
R94.39 Abnormal result of other cardiovascular function study
Abnormal electrophysiological intracardiac studies
Abnormal phonocardiogram
Abnormal vectorcardiogram

R94.4 Abnormal results of kidney function studies
Abnormal renal function test

R94.5 Abnormal results of liver function studies

R94.6 Abnormal results of thyroid function studies

R94.7 Abnormal results of other endocrine function studies
EXCLUDES 2 *abnormal glucose (R73.Ø-)*

R94.8 Abnormal results of function studies of other organs and systems
Abnormal basal metabolic rate [BMR]
Abnormal bladder function test
Abnormal splenic function test

Abnormal tumor markers (R97)

✓4th **R97 Abnormal tumor markers**
Elevated tumor associated antigens [TAA]
Elevated tumor specific antigens [TSA]

R97.Ø Elevated carcinoembryonic antigen [CEA]
R97.1 Elevated cancer antigen 125 [CA 125]
✓5th **R97.2 Elevated prostate specific antigen [PSA]**
AHA: 2016,4Q,66
R97.2Ø Elevated prostate specific antigen [PSA] A ♂
R97.21 Rising PSA following treatment for malignant neoplasm of prostate A ♂
R97.8 Other abnormal tumor markers

Ill-defined and unknown cause of mortality (R99)

R99 Ill-defined and unknown cause of mortality
Death (unexplained) NOS
Unspecified cause of mortality

Chapter 19. Injury, Poisoning, and Certain Other Consequences of External Causes (S00–T88)

Chapter-specific Guidelines with Coding Examples

The chapter-specific guidelines from the ICD-10-CM Official Guidelines for Coding and Reporting have been provided below. Along with these guidelines are coding examples, contained in the shaded boxes, that have been developed to help illustrate the coding and/or sequencing guidance found in these guidelines.

a. Application of 7th characters in Chapter 19

Most categories in chapter 19 have a 7th character requirement for each applicable code. Most categories in this chapter have three 7th character values (with the exception of fractures): A, initial encounter, D, subsequent encounter and S, sequela. Categories for traumatic fractures have additional 7th character values. While the patient may be seen by a new or different provider over the course of treatment for an injury, assignment of the 7th character is based on whether the patient is undergoing active treatment and not whether the provider is seeing the patient for the first time.

For complication codes, active treatment refers to treatment for the condition described by the code, even though it may be related to an earlier precipitating problem. For example, code T84.50XA, Infection and inflammatory reaction due to unspecified internal joint prosthesis, initial encounter, is used when active treatment is provided for the infection, even though the condition relates to the prosthetic device, implant or graft that was placed at a previous encounter.

7th character "A", initial encounter is used for each encounter where the patient is receiving active treatment for the condition.

Patient evaluated after fall from a skateboard onto the sidewalk, x-rays identify a nondisplaced fracture to the distal pole of the right scaphoid bone. The patient is placed in a cast.

S62.014A	**Nondisplaced fracture of distal pole of navicular [scaphoid] bone of right wrist, initial encounter for closed fracture**
V00.131A	**Fall from skateboard, initial encounter**
Y93.51	**Activity, roller skating (inline) and skateboarding**
Y92.480	**Sidewalk as the place of occurrence of the external cause**
Y99.8	**Other external cause status**

Explanation: This fracture would be coded with a seventh character A for initial encounter because the patient received x-rays to identify the site of the fracture and treatment was rendered; this would be considered active treatment.

7th character "D" subsequent encounter is used for encounters after the patient has completed active treatment of the condition and is receiving routine care for the condition during the healing or recovery phase.

Patient seen in follow-up after fall from a skateboard onto the sidewalk resulted in casting of the right arm. X-rays are taken to evaluate how well the nondisplaced fracture to the distal pole of the right scaphoid bone is healing. The physician feels the fracture is healing appropriately; no adjustments to the cast are made.

S62.014D	**Nondisplaced fracture of distal pole of navicular [scaphoid] bone of right wrist, subsequent encounter for fracture with routine healing**
V00.131D	**Fall from skateboard, subsequent encounter**

Explanation: This fracture would be coded with a seventh character D for subsequent encounter, whether the same physician who provided the initial cast application or a different physician is now seeing the patient. Although the patient received x-rays, the intent of the x-rays was to assess how the fracture was healing. There was no active treatment rendered and the visit is therefore considered a subsequent encounter.

The aftercare Z codes should not be used for aftercare for conditions such as injuries or poisonings, where 7th characters are provided to identify subsequent care. For example, for aftercare of an injury, assign the acute injury code with the 7th character "D" (subsequent encounter).

7th character "S", sequela, is for use for complications or conditions that arise as a direct result of a condition, such as scar formation after a burn. The scars are sequelae of the burn. When using 7th character "S", it is necessary to use both the injury code that precipitated the sequela and the code for the sequela itself. The "S" is added only to the injury code, not the sequela code. The 7th character "S" identifies the injury responsible for the sequela. The specific type of sequela (e.g. scar) is sequenced first, followed by the injury code.

See Section I.B.10. Sequelae, (Late Effects)

Patient with a history of a nondisplaced fracture to the distal pole of the right scaphoid bone due to a fall from a skateboard is seen for evaluation of arthritis to the right wrist that has developed as a consequence of the traumatic fracture.

M12.531	**Traumatic arthropathy, right wrist**
S62.014S	**Nondisplaced fracture of distal pole of navicular [scaphoid] bone of right wrist, sequela**
V00.131S	**Fall from skateboard, sequela**

Explanation: The code identifying the specific sequela condition (traumatic arthritis) should be coded first followed by the injury that instigated the development of the sequela (fracture). The scaphoid fracture injury code is given a 7th character S for sequela to represent its role as the inciting injury. The fracture has healed and is not being managed or treated on this admit and therefore is not applicable as a first listed or principal diagnosis. However, it is directly related to the development of the arthritis and should be appended as a secondary code to signify this cause and effect relationship.

b. Coding of injuries

When coding injuries, assign separate codes for each injury unless a combination code is provided, in which case the combination code is assigned. Codes from category T07, Unspecified multiple injuries should not be assigned in the inpatient setting unless information for a more specific code is not available. Traumatic injury codes (S00-T14.9) are not to be used for normal, healing surgical wounds or to identify complications of surgical wounds.

11-year-old girl fell from her horse, resulting in a laceration to her right forearm with several large pieces of wooden fragments embedded in the wound as well as abrasions to her right ear; in addition, her right shoulder was dislocated.

S43.004A	**Unspecified dislocation of right shoulder joint, initial encounter**
S51.821A	**Laceration with foreign body of right forearm, initial encounter**
S00.411A	**Abrasion of right ear, initial encounter**
V80.010A	**Animal-rider injured by fall from or being thrown from horse in noncollision accident, initial encounter**
Y93.52	**Activity, horseback riding**

Explanation: Each separate injury should be reported. The patient's injury to the forearm is reported with one combination code that captures both the laceration and the foreign body.

The code for the most serious injury, as determined by the provider and the focus of treatment, is sequenced first.

1) Superficial injuries

Superficial injuries such as abrasions or contusions are not coded when associated with more severe injuries of the same site.

2) Primary injury with damage to nerves/blood vessels

When a primary injury results in minor damage to peripheral nerves or blood vessels, the primary injury is sequenced first with additional code(s) for injuries to nerves and spinal cord (such as category S04), and/or injury to blood vessels (such as category S15). When the primary injury is to the blood vessels or nerves, that injury should be sequenced first.

3) Iatrogenic injuries

Injury codes from Chapter 19 should not be assigned for injuries that occur during, or as a result of, a medical intervention. Assign the appropriate complication code(s).

c. Coding of traumatic fractures

The principles of multiple coding of injuries should be followed in coding fractures. Fractures of specified sites are coded individually by site in accordance with both the provisions within categories S02, S12, S22, S32, S42, S49, S52, S59, S62, S72, S79, S82, S89, S92 and the level of detail furnished by medical record content.

A fracture not indicated as open or closed should be coded to closed. A fracture not indicated whether displaced or not displaced should be coded to displaced.

More specific guidelines are as follows:

1) Initial vs. subsequent encounter for fractures

Traumatic fractures are coded using the appropriate 7th character for initial encounter (A, B, C) for each encounter where the patient is receiving active treatment for the fracture. The appropriate 7th character for initial encounter should also be assigned for a patient who delayed seeking treatment for the fracture or nonunion.

Fractures are coded using the appropriate 7th character for subsequent care for encounters after the patient has completed active treatment of the fracture and is receiving routine care for the fracture during the healing or recovery phase.

Care for complications of surgical treatment for fracture repairs during the healing or recovery phase should be coded with the appropriate complication codes.

Care of complications of fractures, such as malunion and nonunion, should be reported with the appropriate 7th character for subsequent care with nonunion (K, M, N,) or subsequent care with malunion (P, Q, R).

Malunion/nonunion: The appropriate 7th character for initial encounter should also be assigned for a patient who delayed seeking treatment for the fracture or nonunion.

Female patient fell during a forest hiking excursion almost six months ago and until recently did not feel she needed to seek medical attention for her left ankle pain; x-rays show nonunion of lateral malleolus and surgery has been scheduled

S82.62XA	**Displaced fracture of lateral malleolus of left fibula, initial encounter for closed fracture**
W01.0XXA	**Fall on same level from slipping, tripping and stumbling without subsequent striking against object, initial encounter**
Y92.821	**Forest as place of occurrence of the external cause**
Y93.01	**Activity, walking, marching and hiking**
Y99.8	**Other external cause status**

Explanation: A seventh character of A is used for the lateral malleolus nonunion fracture to signify that the fracture is receiving active treatment. The delayed care for the fracture has resulted in a nonunion, but capturing the nonunion in the seventh character is trumped by the provision of active care.

The open fracture designations in the assignment of the 7th character for fractures of the forearm, femur and lower leg, including ankle are based on the Gustilo open fracture classification. When the Gustilo classification type is not specified for an open fracture, the 7th character for open fracture type I or II should be assigned (B, E, H, M, Q).

A code from category M80, not a traumatic fracture code, should be used for any patient with known osteoporosis who suffers a fracture, even if the patient had a minor fall or trauma, if that fall or trauma would not usually break a normal, healthy bone.

See Section I.C.13. Osteoporosis.

The aftercare Z codes should not be used for aftercare for traumatic fractures. For aftercare of a traumatic fracture, assign the acute fracture code with the appropriate 7th character.

2) Multiple fractures sequencing

Multiple fractures are sequenced in accordance with the severity of the fracture.

3) Physeal fractures

For physeal fractures, assign only the code identifying the type of physeal fracture. Do not assign a separate code to identify the specific bone that is fractured.

d. Coding of burns and corrosions

The ICD-10-CM makes a distinction between burns and corrosions. The burn codes are for thermal burns, except sunburns, that come from a heat source, such as a fire or hot appliance. The burn codes are also for burns resulting from electricity and radiation. Corrosions are burns due to chemicals. The guidelines are the same for burns and corrosions.

Current burns (T20-T25) are classified by depth, extent and by agent (X code). Burns are classified by depth as first degree (erythema), second degree (blistering), and third degree (full-thickness involvement). Burns of the eye and internal organs (T26-T28) are classified by site, but not by degree.

1) Sequencing of burn and related condition codes

Sequence first the code that reflects the highest degree of burn when more than one burn is present.

a. When the reason for the admission or encounter is for treatment of external multiple burns, sequence first the code that reflects the burn of the highest degree.

b. When a patient has both internal and external burns, the circumstances of admission govern the selection of the principal diagnosis or first-listed diagnosis.

c. When a patient is admitted for burn injuries and other related conditions such as smoke inhalation and/or respiratory failure, the circumstances of admission govern the selection of the principal or first-listed diagnosis.

Patient referred for minor first-degree burns to multiple sites of her right and left hands as well as severe smoke inhalation. While she was sleeping at home, a candle on her dresser lit the bedroom curtains on fire.

T59.811A	**Toxic effect of smoke, accidental (unintentional), initial encounter**
J70.5	**Respiratory conditions due to smoke inhalation**
T23.191A	**Burn of first degree of multiple sites of right wrist and hand, initial encounter**
T23.192A	**Burn of first degree of multiple sites of left wrist and hand, initial encounter**
X08.8XXA	**Exposure to other specified smoke, fire and flames, initial encounter**
Y99.8	**Other external cause status**
Y92.003	**Bedroom of unspecified non-institutional (private) residence as the place of occurrence of the external cause**
Y93.84	**Activity, sleeping**

Explanation: Based on the documentation, the inhalation injury is more severe than the first-degree burns and is sequenced first. The burns to the hands are appended as secondary diagnoses.

2) Burns of the same anatomic site

Classify burns of the same anatomic site and on the same side but of different degrees to the subcategory identifying the highest degree recorded in the diagnosis (e.g., for second and third degree burns of right thigh, assign only code T24.311-).

3) Non-healing burns

Non-healing burns are coded as acute burns.

Necrosis of burned skin should be coded as a non-healed burn.

4) Infected burn

For any documented infected burn site, use an additional code for the infection.

5) Assign separate codes for each burn site

When coding burns, assign separate codes for each burn site. Category T30, Burn and corrosion, body region unspecified is extremely vague and should rarely be used.

Codes for burns of "multiple sites" should only be assigned when the medical record documentation does not specify the individual sites.

6) Burns and corrosions classified according to extent of body surface involved

Assign codes from category T31, Burns classified according to extent of body surface involved, or T32, Corrosions classified according to extent of body surface involved, for acute burns or corrosions when the site of the burn or corrosion is not specified or when there is a need for additional data. It is advisable to use category T31 as additional coding when needed to provide data for evaluating burn mortality, such as that needed by burn units. It is also advisable to use category T31 as an additional code for reporting purposes when there is mention of a third- degree burn involving 20 percent or more of the body surface. Codes from categories T31 and T32 should not be used for sequelae of burns or corrosions.

Categories T31 and T32 are based on the classic "rule of nines" in estimating body surface involved: head and neck are assigned nine percent, each arm nine percent, each leg 18 percent, the anterior trunk 18 percent, posterior trunk 18 percent, and genitalia one percent. Providers may change these percentage assignments where necessary to accommodate infants and children who have proportionately larger heads than adults, and patients who have large buttocks, thighs, or abdomen that involve burns.

Patient seen for dressing change after he accidentally spilled acetic acid on himself two days ago. The second-degree burns to his right thigh, covering about 3 percent of his body surface, are healing appropriately.

T54.2X1D	**Toxic effect of corrosive acids and acid-like substances, accidental (unintentional), subsequent encounter**
T24.611D	**Corrosion of second degree of right thigh, subsequent encounter**
T32.Ø	**Corrosions involving less than 1Ø% of body surface**

Explanation: Code T32.Ø provides additional information as to how much of the patient's body was affected by the corrosive substance.

7) **Encounters for treatment of sequela of burns**
Encounters for the treatment of the late effects of burns or corrosions (i.e., scars or joint contractures) should be coded with a burn or corrosion code with the 7th character "S" for sequela.

8) **Sequelae with a late effect code and current burn**
When appropriate, both a code for a current burn or corrosion with 7th character "A" or "D" and a burn or corrosion code with 7th character "S" may be assigned on the same record (when both a current burn and sequelae of an old burn exist). Burns and corrosions do not heal at the same rate and a current healing wound may still exist with sequela of a healed burn or corrosion.
See Section I.B.1Ø. Sequela (Late Effects)

Female patient seen for second-degree burn to the left ear; she also has significant scarring on her left elbow from a third-degree burn from childhood

T2Ø.212A	**Burn of second degree of left ear [any part, except ear drum], initial encounter**
L9Ø.5	**Scar conditions and fibrosis of skin**
T22.322S	**Burn of third degree of left elbow, sequela**

Explanation: The patient is being seen for management of a current second-degree burn, which is reflected in the code by appending the seventh character of A, indicating active treatment or management of this burn. The elbow scarring is a sequela of a previous third-degree burn. The sequela condition precedes the original burn injury, which is appended with a seventh character of S.

9) **Use of an external cause code with burns and corrosions**
An external cause code should be used with burns and corrosions to identify the source and intent of the burn, as well as the place where it occurred.

e. **Adverse effects, poisoning, underdosing and toxic effects**
Codes in categories T36-T65 are combination codes that include the substance that was taken as well as the intent. No additional external cause code is required for poisonings, toxic effects, adverse effects and underdosing codes.

1) **Do not code directly from the Table of Drugs**
Do not code directly from the Table of Drugs and Chemicals. Always refer back to the Tabular List.

2) **Use as many codes as necessary to describe**
Use as many codes as necessary to describe completely all drugs, medicinal or biological substances.

3) **If the same code would describe the causative agent**
If the same code would describe the causative agent for more than one adverse reaction, poisoning, toxic effect or underdosing, assign the code only once.

4) **If two or more drugs, medicinal or biological substances**
If two or more drugs, medicinal or biological substances are taken, code each individually unless a combination code is listed in the Table of Drugs and Chemicals.

If multiple unspecified drugs, medicinal or biological substances were taken, assign the appropriate code from subcategory T5Ø.91, Poisoning by, adverse effect of and underdosing of multiple unspecified drugs, medicaments and biological substances.

5) **The occurrence of drug toxicity is classified in ICD-10-CM as follows:**

(a) **Adverse effect**
When coding an adverse effect of a drug that has been correctly prescribed and properly administered, assign the appropriate code for the nature of the adverse effect followed by the appropriate code for the adverse effect of the drug (T36-T5Ø). The code for the drug should have a 5th or 6th character "5" (for example T36.ØX5-) Examples of the nature of an adverse effect are tachycardia, delirium, gastrointestinal hemorrhaging, vomiting, hypokalemia, hepatitis, renal failure, or respiratory failure.

(b) **Poisoning**
When coding a poisoning or reaction to the improper use of a medication (e.g., overdose, wrong substance given or taken in error, wrong route of administration), first assign the appropriate code from categories T36-T5Ø. The poisoning codes have an associated intent as their 5th or 6th character (accidental, intentional self-harm, assault and undetermined). If the intent of the poisoning is unknown or unspecified, code the intent as accidental intent. The undetermined intent is only for use if the documentation in the record specifies that the intent cannot be determined. Use additional code(s) for all manifestations of poisonings.

If there is also a diagnosis of abuse or dependence of the substance, the abuse or dependence is assigned as an additional code.

Examples of poisoning include:

(i) Error was made in drug prescription
Errors made in drug prescription or in the administration of the drug by provider, nurse, patient, or other person.

(ii Overdose of a drug intentionally taken
If an overdose of a drug was intentionally taken or administered and resulted in drug toxicity, it would be coded as a poisoning.

(iii) Nonprescribed drug taken with correctly prescribed and properly administered drug
If a nonprescribed drug or medicinal agent was taken in combination with a correctly prescribed and properly administered drug, any drug toxicity or other reaction resulting from the interaction of the two drugs would be classified as a poisoning.

(iv) Interaction of drug(s) and alcohol
When a reaction results from the interaction of a drug(s) and alcohol, this would be classified as poisoning.
See Section I.C.4. if poisoning is the result of insulin pump malfunctions.

(c) **Underdosing**
Underdosing refers to taking less of a medication than is prescribed by a provider or a manufacturer's instruction. Discontinuing the use of a prescribed medication on the patient's own initiative (not directed by the patient's provider) is also classified as an underdosing. For underdosing, assign the code from categories T36-T5Ø (fifth or sixth character "6"). **Documentation of a change in the patient's condition is not required in order to assign an underdosing code. Documentation that the patient is taking less of a medication than is prescribed or discontinued the prescribed medication is sufficient for code assignment.**

Codes for underdosing should never be assigned as principal or first-listed codes. If a patient has a relapse or exacerbation of the medical condition for which the drug is prescribed because of the reduction in dose, then the medical condition itself should be coded.

Noncompliance (Z91.12-, Z91.13- and Z91.14-) or complication of care (Y63.6-Y63.9) codes are to be used with an underdosing code to indicate intent, if known.

Patient referred for atrial fibrillation with history of chronic atrial fibrillation for which she is prescribed amiodarone. Financial concerns have left the patient unable to pay for her prescriptions and she has been skipping her amiodarone dose every other day to offset the cost.

I48.2Ø	**Chronic atrial fibrillation, unspecified**
T46.2X6A	**Underdosing of other antidysrhythmic drugs, initial encounter**
Z91.12Ø	**Patient's intentional underdosing of medication regimen due to financial hardship**

Explanation: By skipping her amiodarone pill every other day, the patient's atrial fibrillation returned. The condition for which the drug was being taken is reported first, followed by an underdosing code to show that the patient was not adhering to her prescription regiment. The Z code helps elaborate on the patient's social and/or economic circumstances that led to the patient taking less then what she was prescribed.

(d) **Toxic effects**
When a harmful substance is ingested or comes in contact with a person, this is classified as a toxic effect. The toxic effect codes are in categories T51-T65.

Toxic effect codes have an associated intent: accidental, intentional self-harm, assault and undetermined.

f. Adult and child abuse, neglect and other maltreatment

Sequence first the appropriate code from categories T74, Adult and child abuse, neglect and other maltreatment, confirmed, or T76, Adult and child abuse, neglect and other maltreatment, suspected, for abuse, neglect and other maltreatment, followed by any accompanying mental health or injury code(s).

If the documentation in the medical record states abuse or neglect, it is coded as confirmed (T74.-). It is coded as suspected if it is documented as suspected (T76.-).

For cases of confirmed abuse or neglect an external cause code from the assault section (X92-YØ9) should be added to identify the cause of any physical injuries. A perpetrator code (YØ7) should be added when the perpetrator of the abuse is known. For suspected cases of abuse or neglect, do not report external cause or perpetrator code.

If a suspected case of abuse, neglect or mistreatment is ruled out during an encounter code ZØ4.71, Encounter for examination and observation following alleged physical adult abuse, ruled out, or code ZØ4.72, Encounter for examination and observation following alleged child physical abuse, ruled out, should be used, not a code from T76.

If a suspected case of alleged rape or sexual abuse is ruled out during an encounter code ZØ4.41, Encounter for examination and observation following alleged adult rape or code ZØ4.42, Encounter for examination and observation following alleged child rape, should be used, not a code from T76.

If a suspected case of forced sexual exploitation or forced labor exploitation is ruled out during an encounter, code ZØ4.81, Encounter for examination and observation of victim following forced sexual exploitation, or code ZØ4.82, Encounter for examination and observation of victim following forced labor exploitation, should be used, not a code from T76.

See Section I.C.15. Abuse in a pregnant patient.

g. Complications of care

1) General guidelines for complications of care

(a) Documentation of complications of care

See Section I.B.16. for information on documentation of complications of care.

2) Pain due to medical devices

Pain associated with devices, implants or grafts left in a surgical site (for example painful hip prosthesis) is assigned to the appropriate code(s) found in Chapter 19, Injury, poisoning, and certain other consequences of external causes. Specific codes for pain due to medical devices are found in the T code section of the ICD-1Ø-CM. Use additional code(s) from category G89 to identify acute or chronic pain due to presence of the device, implant or graft (G89.18 or G89.28).

Chronic left breast pain secondary to breast implant

T85.848A	**Pain due to other internal prosthetic devices, implants and grafts, initial encounter**
N64.4	**Mastodynia**
G89.28	**Other chronic postprocedural pain**

Explanation: As the pain is a complication related to the breast implant, the complication code is sequenced first. The T code does not describe the site or type of pain, so additional codes may be appended to indicate that the patient is experiencing chronic pain in the breast.

3) Transplant complications

(a) Transplant complications other than kidney

Codes under category T86, Complications of transplanted organs and tissues, are for use for both complications and rejection of transplanted organs. A transplant complication code is only assigned if the complication affects the function of the transplanted organ. Two codes are required to fully describe a transplant complication: the appropriate code from category T86 and a secondary code that identifies the complication.

Pre-existing conditions or conditions that develop after the transplant are not coded as complications unless they affect the function of the transplanted organs.

See I.C.21. for transplant organ removal status

See I.C.2. for malignant neoplasm associated with transplanted organ.

(b) Kidney transplant complications

Patients who have undergone kidney transplant may still have some form of chronic kidney disease (CKD) because the kidney transplant may not fully restore kidney function. Code T86.1- should be assigned for documented complications of a kidney transplant, such as transplant failure or rejection or other transplant complication. Code T86.1- should not be assigned for post kidney transplant patients who have chronic kidney (CKD) unless a transplant complication such as transplant failure or rejection is documented. If the documentation is unclear as to whether the patient has a complication of the transplant, query the provider.

Conditions that affect the function of the transplanted kidney, other than CKD, should be assigned a code from subcategory T86.1, Complications of transplanted organ, Kidney, and a secondary code that identifies the complication.

For patients with CKD following a kidney transplant, but who do not have a complication such as failure or rejection, *see section I.C.14. Chronic kidney disease and kidney transplant status.*

Patient seen for chronic kidney disease stage 2; history of successful kidney transplant with no complications identified

N18.2	**Chronic kidney disease, stage 2 (mild)**
Z94.Ø	**Kidney transplant status**

Explanation: This patient's stage 2 CKD is not indicated as being due to the transplanted kidney but instead is just the residual disease the patient had prior to the transplant.

4) Complication codes that include the external cause

As with certain other T codes, some of the complications of care codes have the external cause included in the code. The code includes the nature of the complication as well as the type of procedure that caused the complication. No external cause code indicating the type of procedure is necessary for these codes.

5) Complications of care codes within the body system chapters

Intraoperative and postprocedural complication codes are found within the body system chapters with codes specific to the organs and structures of that body system. These codes should be sequenced first, followed by a code(s) for the specific complication, if applicable.

Postprocedural ischemic infarction of the left middle cerebral artery due to cardiac surgery

I97.82Ø	**Postprocedural cerebrovascular infarction following cardiac surgery**
I63.512	**Cerebral infarction due to unspecified occlusion or stenosis of left middle cerebral artery**

Explanation: The infarction was caused by the cardiac procedure and is coded as a postprocedural complication. The postprocedural cerebrovascular infarction is the first-listed diagnosis, followed by the code for the infarction itself.

Complication codes from the body system chapters should be assigned for intraoperative and postprocedural complications (e.g., the appropriate complication code from chapter 9 would be assigned for a vascular intraoperative or postprocedural complication) unless the complication is specifically indexed to a T code in chapter 19.

Muscle/Tendon Table

ICD-10-CM categorizes certain muscles and tendons in the upper and lower extremities by their action (e.g., extension, flexion), their anatomical location (e.g., posterior, anterior), and/or whether they are intrinsic or extrinsic to a certain anatomical area. The Muscle/Tendon Table is provided at the beginning of chapters 13 and 19 as a resource to help users when code selection depends on one or more of these characteristics. A **TIP** has been placed at those categories and/or subcategories that relate to this table. Please note that this table is not all-inclusive, and proper code assignment should be based on the provider's documentation.

Body Region	Muscle	Extensor Tendon	Flexor Tendon	Other Tendon
Shoulder				
	Deltoid	Posterior deltoid	Anterior deltoid	
	Rotator cuff			
	Infraspinatus			Infraspinatus
	Subscapularis			Subscapularis
	Supraspinatus			Supraspinatus
	Teres minor			Teres minor
	Teres major	Teres major		
Upper arm				
	Anterior muscles			
	Biceps brachii — long head		Biceps brachii — long head	
	Biceps brachii — short head		Biceps brachii — short head	
	Brachialis		Brachialis	
	Coracobrachialis		Coracobrachialis	
	Posterior muscles			
	Triceps brachii	Triceps brachii		
Forearm				
	Anterior muscles			
	Flexors			
	Deep			
	Flexor digitorum profundus		Flexor digitorum profundus	
	Flexor pollicis longus		Flexor pollicis longus	
	Intermediate			
	Flexor digitorum superficialis		Flexor digitorum superficialis	
	Superficial			
	Flexor carpi radialis		Flexor carpi radialis	
	Flexor carpi ulnaris		Flexor carpi ulnaris	
	Palmaris longus		Palmaris longus	
	Pronators			
	Pronator quadratus			Pronator quadratus
	Pronator teres			Pronator teres
	Posterior muscles			
	Extensors			
	Deep			
	Abductor pollicis longus			Abductor pollicis longus
	Extensor indicis	Extensor indicis		
	Extensor pollicis brevis	Extensor pollicis brevis		
	Extensor pollicis longus	Extensor pollicis longus		
	Superficial			
	Brachioradialis			Brachioradialis
	Extensor carpi radialis brevis	Extensor carpi radialis brevis		
	Extensor carpi radialis longus	Extensor carpi radialis longus		
	Extensor carpi ulnaris	Extensor carpi ulnaris		
	Extensor digiti minimi	Extensor digiti minimi		
	Extensor digitorum	Extensor digitorum		
	Anconeus	Anconeus		
	Supinator			Supinator

Body Region	Muscle	Extensor Tendon	Flexor Tendon	Other Tendon
Hand				
Extrinsic — attach to a site in the forearm as well as a site in the hand with action related to hand movement at the wrist				
	Extensor carpi radialis brevis	Extensor carpi radialis brevis		
	Extensor carpi radialis longus	Extensor carpi radialis longus		
	Extensor carpi ulnaris	Extensor carpi ulnaris		
	Flexor carpi radialis		Flexor carpi radialis	
	Flexor carpi ulnaris		Flexor carpi ulnaris	
	Flexor digitorum superficialis		Flexor digitorum superficialis	
	Palmaris longus		Palmaris longus	
Extrinsic — attach to a site in the forearm as well as a site in the hand with action in the hand related to finger movement				
	Adductor pollicis longus			Adductor pollicis longus
	Extensor digiti minimi	Extensor digiti minimi		
	Extensor digitorum	Extensor digitorum		
	Extensor indicis	Extensor indicis		
	Flexor digitorum profundus		Flexor digitorum profundus	
	Flexor digitorum superficialis		Flexor digitorum superficialis	
Extrinsic — attach to a site in the forearm as well as a site in the hand with action in the hand related to thumb movement				
	Extensor pollicis brevis	Extensor pollicis brevis		
	Extensor pollicis longus	Extensor pollicis longus		
	Flexor pollicis longus		Flexor pollicis longus	
Intrinsic — found within the hand only				
	Adductor pollicis			Adductor pollicis
	Dorsal interossei	Dorsal interossei	Dorsal interossei	
	Lumbricals	Lumbricals	Lumbricals	
	Palmaris brevis			Palmaris brevis
	Palmar interossei	Palmar interossei	Palmar interossei	
	Hypothenar muscles			
	Abductor digiti minimi			Abductor digiti minimi
	Flexor digiti minimi brevis		Flexor digiti minimi brevis	
	Opponens digiti minimi		Opponens digiti minimi	
	Thenar muscles			
	Abductor pollicis brevis			Abductor pollicis brevis
	Flexor pollicis brevis		Flexor pollicis brevis	
	Opponens pollicis		Opponens pollicis	
Thigh				
	Anterior muscles			
	Iliopsoas		Iliopsoas	
	Pectineus		Pectineus	
	Quadriceps	Quadriceps		
	Rectus femoris	Rectus femoris — Extends knee	Rectus femoris — Flexes hip	
	Vastus intermedius	Vastus intermedius		
	Vastus lateralis	Vastus lateralis		
	Vastus medialis	Vastus medialis		
	Sartorius		Sartorius	
	Medial muscles			
	Adductor brevis			Adductor brevis
	Adductor longus			Adductor longus
	Adductor magnus			Adductor magnus
	Gracilis			Gracilis
	Obturator externus			Obturator externus
	Posterior muscles			
	Hamstring	Hamstring — Extends hip	Hamstring — Flexes knee	
	Biceps femoris	Biceps femoris	Biceps femoris	
	Semimembranosus	Semimembranosus	Semimembranosus	
	Semitendinosus	Semitendinosus	Semitendinosus	

Body Region	Muscle	Extensor Tendon	Flexor Tendon	Other Tendon
Lower leg				
	Anterior muscles			
	Extensor digitorum longus	Extensor digitorum longus		
	Extensor hallucis longus	Extensor hallucis longus		
	Fibularis (peroneus) tertius	Fibularis (peroneus) tertius		
	Tibialis anterior	Tibialis anterior		Tibialis anterior
	Lateral muscles			
	Fibularis (peroneus) brevis		Fibularis (peroneus) brevis	
	Fibularis (peroneus) longus		Fibularis (peroneus) longus	
	Posterior muscles			
	Deep			
	Flexor digitorum longus		Flexor digitorum longus	
	Flexor hallucis longus		Flexor hallucis longus	
	Popliteus		Popliteus	
	Tibialis posterior		Tibialis posterior	
	Superficial			
	Gastrocnemius		Gastrocnemius	
	Plantaris		Plantaris	
	Soleus		Soleus	
				Calcaneal (Achilles)
Ankle/Foot				
Extrinsic — attach to a site in the lower leg as well as a site in the foot with action related to foot movement at the ankle				
	Plantaris		Plantaris	
	Soleus		Soleus	
	Tibialis anterior	Tibialis anterior		
	Tibialis posterior		Tibialis posterior	
Extrinsic — attach to a site in the lower leg as well as a site in the foot with action in the foot related to toe movement				
	Extensor digitorum longus	Extensor digitorum longus		
	Extensor hallucis longus	Extensor hallucis longus		
	Flexor digitorum longus		Flexor digitorum longus	
	Flexor hallucis longus		Flexor hallucis longus	
Intrinsic — found within the ankle/foot only				
	Dorsal muscles			
	Extensor digitorum brevis	Extensor digitorum brevis		
	Extensor hallucis brevis	Extensor hallucis brevis		
	Plantar muscles			
	Abductor digiti minimi		Abductor digiti minimi	
	Abductor hallucis		Abductor hallucis	
	Dorsal interossei	Dorsal interossei	Dorsal interossei	
	Flexor digiti minimi brevis		Flexor digiti minimi brevis	
	Flexor digitorum brevis		Flexor digitorum brevis	
	Flexor hallucis brevis		Flexor hallucis brevis	
	Lumbricals	Lumbricals	Lumbricals	
	Quadratus plantae		Quadratus plantae	
	Plantar interossei	Plantar interossei	Plantar interossei	

Chapter 19. Injury, Poisoning and Certain Other Consequences of External Causes (S00-T88)

NOTE Use secondary code(s) from Chapter 20, External causes of morbidity, to indicate cause of injury. Codes within the T section that include the external cause do not require an additional external cause code.

Use additional code to identify any retained foreign body, if applicable (Z18.-)

EXCLUDES 1 *birth trauma (P10-P15)*
obstetric trauma (O70-O71)

NOTE The chapter uses the S-section for coding different types of injuries related to single body regions and the T-section to cover injuries to unspecified body regions as well as poisoning and certain other consequences of external causes.

AHA: 2016,2Q,3-7; 2015,4Q,35-38; 2015,3Q,37-39,40; 2015,2Q,6; 2015,1Q,3-21

TIP: The specific site of an injury can be determined from the radiology report when authenticated by a radiologist and available at the time of code assignment.

This chapter contains the following blocks:

S00-S09 Injuries to the head
S10-S19 Injuries to the neck
S20-S29 Injuries to the thorax
S30-S39 Injuries to the abdomen, lower back, lumbar spine, pelvis and external genitals
S40-S49 Injuries to the shoulder and upper arm
S50-S59 Injuries to the elbow and forearm
S60-S69 Injuries to the wrist, hand and fingers
S70-S79 Injuries to the hip and thigh
S80-S89 Injuries to the knee and lower leg
S90-S99 Injuries to the ankle and foot
T07 Injuries involving multiple body regions
T14 Injury of unspecified body region
T15-T19 Effects of foreign body entering through natural orifice
T20-T25 Burns and corrosions of external body surface, specified by site
T26-T28 Burns and corrosions confined to eye and internal organs
T30-T32 Burns and corrosions of multiple and unspecified body regions
T33-T34 Frostbite
T36-T50 Poisoning by, adverse effect of and underdosing of drugs, medicaments and biological substances
T51-T65 Toxic effects of substances chiefly nonmedicinal as to source
T66-T78 Other and unspecified effects of external causes
T79 Certain early complications of trauma
T80-T88 Complications of surgical and medical care, not elsewhere classified

Injuries to the head (S00-S09)

INCLUDES injuries of ear
injuries of eye
injuries of face [any part]
injuries of gum
injuries of jaw
injuries of oral cavity
injuries of palate
injuries of periocular area
injuries of scalp
injuries of temporomandibular joint area
injuries of tongue
injuries of tooth

Code also for any associated infection

EXCLUDES 2 *burns and corrosions (T20-T32)*
effects of foreign body in ear (T16)
effects of foreign body in larynx (T17.3)
effects of foreign body in mouth NOS (T18.0)
effects of foreign body in nose (T17.0-T17.1)
effects of foreign body in pharynx (T17.2)
effects of foreign body on external eye (T15.-)
frostbite (T33-T34)
insect bite or sting, venomous (T63.4)

✓4th **S00 Superficial injury of head**

EXCLUDES 1 *diffuse cerebral contusion (S06.2-)*
focal cerebral contusion (S06.3-)
injury of eye and orbit (S05.-)
open wound of head (S01.-)

The appropriate 7th character is to be added to each code from category S00.
A initial encounter
D subsequent encounter
S sequela

✓5th **S00.0 Superficial injury of scalp**
✓x7th **S00.00 Unspecified superficial injury of scalp**
✓x7th **S00.01 Abrasion of scalp**
✓x7th **S00.02 Blister (nonthermal) of scalp**
✓x7th **S00.03 Contusion of scalp** P
Bruise of scalp
Hematoma of scalp
✓x7th **S00.04 External constriction of part of scalp**
✓x7th **S00.05 Superficial foreign body of scalp**
Splinter in the scalp
✓x7th **S00.06 Insect bite (nonvenomous) of scalp**
✓x7th **S00.07 Other superficial bite of scalp**
EXCLUDES 1 *open bite of scalp (S01.05)*

✓5th **S00.1 Contusion of eyelid and periocular area**
Black eye
EXCLUDES 2 *contusion of eyeball and orbital tissues (S05.1-)*
✓x7th **S00.10 Contusion of unspecified eyelid and periocular area**
✓x7th **S00.11 Contusion of right eyelid and periocular area**
✓x7th **S00.12 Contusion of left eyelid and periocular area**

✓5th **S00.2 Other and unspecified superficial injuries of eyelid and periocular area**
EXCLUDES 2 *superficial injury of conjunctiva and cornea (S05.0-)*
✓6th **S00.20 Unspecified superficial injury of eyelid and periocular area**
✓7th **S00.201 Unspecified superficial injury of right eyelid and periocular area**
✓7th **S00.202 Unspecified superficial injury of left eyelid and periocular area**
✓7th **S00.209 Unspecified superficial injury of unspecified eyelid and periocular area**
✓6th **S00.21 Abrasion of eyelid and periocular area**
✓7th **S00.211 Abrasion of right eyelid and periocular area**
✓7th **S00.212 Abrasion of left eyelid and periocular area**
✓7th **S00.219 Abrasion of unspecified eyelid and periocular area**
✓6th **S00.22 Blister (nonthermal) of eyelid and periocular area**
✓7th **S00.221 Blister (nonthermal) of right eyelid and periocular area**
✓7th **S00.222 Blister (nonthermal) of left eyelid and periocular area**
✓7th **S00.229 Blister (nonthermal) of unspecified eyelid and periocular area**
✓6th **S00.24 External constriction of eyelid and periocular area**
✓7th **S00.241 External constriction of right eyelid and periocular area**
✓7th **S00.242 External constriction of left eyelid and periocular area**
✓7th **S00.249 External constriction of unspecified eyelid and periocular area**
✓6th **S00.25 Superficial foreign body of eyelid and periocular area**
Splinter of eyelid and periocular area
EXCLUDES 2 *retained foreign body in eyelid (H02.81-)*
✓7th **S00.251 Superficial foreign body of right eyelid and periocular area**
✓7th **S00.252 Superficial foreign body of left eyelid and periocular area**
✓7th **S00.259 Superficial foreign body of unspecified eyelid and periocular area**
✓6th **S00.26 Insect bite (nonvenomous) of eyelid and periocular area**
✓7th **S00.261 Insect bite (nonvenomous) of right eyelid and periocular area**
✓7th **S00.262 Insect bite (nonvenomous) of left eyelid and periocular area**
✓7th **S00.269 Insect bite (nonvenomous) of unspecified eyelid and periocular area**
✓6th **S00.27 Other superficial bite of eyelid and periocular area**
EXCLUDES 1 *open bite of eyelid and periocular area (S01.15)*
✓7th **S00.271 Other superficial bite of right eyelid and periocular area**
✓7th **S00.272 Other superficial bite of left eyelid and periocular area**
✓7th **S00.279 Other superficial bite of unspecified eyelid and periocular area**

✓5th **S00.3 Superficial injury of nose**
✓x7th **S00.30 Unspecified superficial injury of nose**
✓x7th **S00.31 Abrasion of nose**
✓x7th **S00.32 Blister (nonthermal) of nose**

S00.33 Contusion of nose
Bruise of nose
Hematoma of nose

S00.34 External constriction of nose

S00.35 Superficial foreign body of nose
Splinter in the nose

S00.36 Insect bite (nonvenomous) of nose

S00.37 Other superficial bite of nose
EXCLUDES 1 *open bite of nose (S01.25)*

S00.4 Superficial injury of ear

S00.40 Unspecified superficial injury of ear
S00.401 Unspecified superficial injury of right ear
S00.402 Unspecified superficial injury of left ear
S00.409 Unspecified superficial injury of unspecified ear

S00.41 Abrasion of ear
S00.411 Abrasion of right ear
S00.412 Abrasion of left ear
S00.419 Abrasion of unspecified ear

S00.42 Blister (nonthermal) of ear
S00.421 Blister (nonthermal) of right ear
S00.422 Blister (nonthermal) of left ear
S00.429 Blister (nonthermal) of unspecified ear

S00.43 Contusion of ear
Bruise of ear
Hematoma of ear
S00.431 Contusion of right ear
S00.432 Contusion of left ear
S00.439 Contusion of unspecified ear

S00.44 External constriction of ear
S00.441 External constriction of right ear
S00.442 External constriction of left ear
S00.449 External constriction of unspecified ear

S00.45 Superficial foreign body of ear
Splinter in the ear
S00.451 Superficial foreign body of right ear
S00.452 Superficial foreign body of left ear
S00.459 Superficial foreign body of unspecified ear

S00.46 Insect bite (nonvenomous) of ear
S00.461 Insect bite (nonvenomous) of right ear
S00.462 Insect bite (nonvenomous) of left ear
S00.469 Insect bite (nonvenomous) of unspecified ear

S00.47 Other superficial bite of ear
EXCLUDES 1 *open bite of ear (S01.35)*
S00.471 Other superficial bite of right ear
S00.472 Other superficial bite of left ear
S00.479 Other superficial bite of unspecified ear

S00.5 Superficial injury of lip and oral cavity

S00.50 Unspecified superficial injury of lip and oral cavity
S00.501 Unspecified superficial injury of lip
S00.502 Unspecified superficial injury of oral cavity

S00.51 Abrasion of lip and oral cavity
S00.511 Abrasion of lip
S00.512 Abrasion of oral cavity

S00.52 Blister (nonthermal) of lip and oral cavity
S00.521 Blister (nonthermal) of lip
S00.522 Blister (nonthermal) of oral cavity

S00.53 Contusion of lip and oral cavity
S00.531 Contusion of lip
Bruise of lip
Hematoma of lip
S00.532 Contusion of oral cavity
Bruise of oral cavity
Hematoma of oral cavity

S00.54 External constriction of lip and oral cavity
S00.541 External constriction of lip
S00.542 External constriction of oral cavity

S00.55 Superficial foreign body of lip and oral cavity
S00.551 Superficial foreign body of lip
Splinter of lip and oral cavity
S00.552 Superficial foreign body of oral cavity
Splinter of lip and oral cavity

S00.56 Insect bite (nonvenomous) of lip and oral cavity
S00.561 Insect bite (nonvenomous) of lip
S00.562 Insect bite (nonvenomous) of oral cavity

S00.57 Other superficial bite of lip and oral cavity
S00.571 Other superficial bite of lip
EXCLUDES 1 *open bite of lip (S01.551)*
S00.572 Other superficial bite of oral cavity
EXCLUDES 1 *open bite of oral cavity (S01.552)*

S00.8 Superficial injury of other parts of head
Superficial injuries of face [any part]

S00.80 Unspecified superficial injury of other part of head
S00.81 Abrasion of other part of head
S00.82 Blister (nonthermal) of other part of head
S00.83 Contusion of other part of head
Bruise of other part of head
Hematoma of other part of head
S00.84 External constriction of other part of head
S00.85 Superficial foreign body of other part of head
Splinter in other part of head
S00.86 Insect bite (nonvenomous) of other part of head
S00.87 Other superficial bite of other part of head
EXCLUDES 1 *open bite of other part of head (S01.85)*

S00.9 Superficial injury of unspecified part of head

S00.90 Unspecified superficial injury of unspecified part of head
S00.91 Abrasion of unspecified part of head
S00.92 Blister (nonthermal) of unspecified part of head
S00.93 Contusion of unspecified part of head
Bruise of head
Hematoma of head
S00.94 External constriction of unspecified part of head
S00.95 Superficial foreign body of unspecified part of head
Splinter of head
S00.96 Insect bite (nonvenomous) of unspecified part of head
S00.97 Other superficial bite of unspecified part of head
EXCLUDES 1 *open bite of head (S01.95)*

S01 Open wound of head

Code also any associated:
injury of cranial nerve (S04.-)
injury of muscle and tendon of head (S09.1-)
intracranial injury (S06.-)
wound infection

EXCLUDES 1 *open skull fracture (S02.- with 7th character B)*
EXCLUDES 2 *injury of eye and orbit (S05.-)*
traumatic amputation of part of head (S08.-)

The appropriate 7th character is to be added to each code from category S01.
A initial encounter
D subsequent encounter
S sequela

S01.0 Open wound of scalp
EXCLUDES 1 *avulsion of scalp (S08.0-)*

S01.00 Unspecified open wound of scalp
S01.01 Laceration without foreign body of scalp
S01.02 Laceration with foreign body of scalp
S01.03 Puncture wound without foreign body of scalp
S01.04 Puncture wound with foreign body of scalp
S01.05 Open bite of scalp
Bite of scalp NOS
EXCLUDES 1 *superficial bite of scalp (S00.06, S00.07-)*

S01.1 Open wound of eyelid and periocular area
Open wound of eyelid and periocular area with or without involvement of lacrimal passages
S01.10 Unspecified open wound of eyelid and periocular area
S01.101 Unspecified open wound of right eyelid and periocular area
S01.102 Unspecified open wound of left eyelid and periocular area
S01.109 Unspecified open wound of unspecified eyelid and periocular area
S01.11 Laceration without foreign body of eyelid and periocular area
S01.111 Laceration without foreign body of right eyelid and periocular area
S01.112 Laceration without foreign body of left eyelid and periocular area
S01.119 Laceration without foreign body of unspecified eyelid and periocular area
S01.12 Laceration with foreign body of eyelid and periocular area
S01.121 Laceration with foreign body of right eyelid and periocular area
S01.122 Laceration with foreign body of left eyelid and periocular area
S01.129 Laceration with foreign body of unspecified eyelid and periocular area
S01.13 Puncture wound without foreign body of eyelid and periocular area
S01.131 Puncture wound without foreign body of right eyelid and periocular area
S01.132 Puncture wound without foreign body of left eyelid and periocular area
S01.139 Puncture wound without foreign body of unspecified eyelid and periocular area
S01.14 Puncture wound with foreign body of eyelid and periocular area
S01.141 Puncture wound with foreign body of right eyelid and periocular area
S01.142 Puncture wound with foreign body of left eyelid and periocular area
S01.149 Puncture wound with foreign body of unspecified eyelid and periocular area
S01.15 Open bite of eyelid and periocular area
Bite of eyelid and periocular area NOS
EXCLUDES 1 *superficial bite of eyelid and periocular area (S00.26, S00.27)*
S01.151 Open bite of right eyelid and periocular area
S01.152 Open bite of left eyelid and periocular area
S01.159 Open bite of unspecified eyelid and periocular area
S01.2 Open wound of nose
S01.20 Unspecified open wound of nose
S01.21 Laceration without foreign body of nose
S01.22 Laceration with foreign body of nose
S01.23 Puncture wound without foreign body of nose
S01.24 Puncture wound with foreign body of nose
S01.25 Open bite of nose
Bite of nose NOS
EXCLUDES 1 *superficial bite of nose (S00.36, S00.37)*
S01.3 Open wound of ear
S01.30 Unspecified open wound of ear
S01.301 Unspecified open wound of right ear
S01.302 Unspecified open wound of left ear
S01.309 Unspecified open wound of unspecified ear
S01.31 Laceration without foreign body of ear
S01.311 Laceration without foreign body of right ear
S01.312 Laceration without foreign body of left ear
S01.319 Laceration without foreign body of unspecified ear
S01.32 Laceration with foreign body of ear
S01.321 Laceration with foreign body of right ear
S01.322 Laceration with foreign body of left ear
S01.329 Laceration with foreign body of unspecified ear
S01.33 Puncture wound without foreign body of ear
S01.331 Puncture wound without foreign body of right ear
S01.332 Puncture wound without foreign body of left ear
S01.339 Puncture wound without foreign body of unspecified ear
S01.34 Puncture wound with foreign body of ear
S01.341 Puncture wound with foreign body of right ear
S01.342 Puncture wound with foreign body of left ear
S01.349 Puncture wound with foreign body of unspecified ear
S01.35 Open bite of ear
Bite of ear NOS
EXCLUDES 1 *superficial bite of ear (S00.46, S00.47)*
S01.351 Open bite of right ear
S01.352 Open bite of left ear
S01.359 Open bite of unspecified ear
S01.4 Open wound of cheek and temporomandibular area
S01.40 Unspecified open wound of cheek and temporomandibular area
S01.401 Unspecified open wound of right cheek and temporomandibular area
S01.402 Unspecified open wound of left cheek and temporomandibular area
S01.409 Unspecified open wound of unspecified cheek and temporomandibular area
S01.41 Laceration without foreign body of cheek and temporomandibular area
S01.411 Laceration without foreign body of right cheek and temporomandibular area
S01.412 Laceration without foreign body of left cheek and temporomandibular area
S01.419 Laceration without foreign body of unspecified cheek and temporomandibular area
S01.42 Laceration with foreign body of cheek and temporomandibular area
S01.421 Laceration with foreign body of right cheek and temporomandibular area
S01.422 Laceration with foreign body of left cheek and temporomandibular area
S01.429 Laceration with foreign body of unspecified cheek and temporomandibular area
S01.43 Puncture wound without foreign body of cheek and temporomandibular area
S01.431 Puncture wound without foreign body of right cheek and temporomandibular area
S01.432 Puncture wound without foreign body of left cheek and temporomandibular area
S01.439 Puncture wound without foreign body of unspecified cheek and temporomandibular area
S01.44 Puncture wound with foreign body of cheek and temporomandibular area
S01.441 Puncture wound with foreign body of right cheek and temporomandibular area
S01.442 Puncture wound with foreign body of left cheek and temporomandibular area
S01.449 Puncture wound with foreign body of unspecified cheek and temporomandibular area
S01.45 Open bite of cheek and temporomandibular area
Bite of cheek and temporomandibular area NOS
EXCLUDES 2 *superficial bite of cheek and temporomandibular area (S00.86, S00.87)*
S01.451 Open bite of right cheek and temporomandibular area
S01.452 Open bite of left cheek and temporomandibular area
S01.459 Open bite of unspecified cheek and temporomandibular area

S01.5 Open wound of lip and oral cavity

EXCLUDES 2 *tooth dislocation (S03.2)*
tooth fracture (S02.5)

S01.50 Unspecified open wound of lip and oral cavity

S01.501 Unspecified open wound of lip

S01.502 Unspecified open wound of oral cavity

S01.51 Laceration of lip and oral cavity without foreign body

S01.511 Laceration without foreign body of lip

S01.512 Laceration without foreign body of oral cavity

S01.52 Laceration of lip and oral cavity with foreign body

S01.521 Laceration with foreign body of lip

S01.522 Laceration with foreign body of oral cavity

S01.53 Puncture wound of lip and oral cavity without foreign body

S01.531 Puncture wound without foreign body of lip

S01.532 Puncture wound without foreign body of oral cavity

S01.54 Puncture wound of lip and oral cavity with foreign body

S01.541 Puncture wound with foreign body of lip

S01.542 Puncture wound with foreign body of oral cavity

S01.55 Open bite of lip and oral cavity

S01.551 Open bite of lip

Bite of lip NOS

EXCLUDES 1 *superficial bite of lip (S00.571)*

S01.552 Open bite of oral cavity

Bite of oral cavity NOS

EXCLUDES 1 *superficial bite of oral cavity (S00.572)*

S01.8 Open wound of other parts of head

S01.80 Unspecified open wound of other part of head

S01.81 Laceration without foreign body of other part of head

S01.82 Laceration with foreign body of other part of head

S01.83 Puncture wound without foreign body of other part of head

S01.84 Puncture wound with foreign body of other part of head

S01.85 Open bite of other part of head

Bite of other part of head NOS

EXCLUDES 1 *superficial bite of other part of head (S00.87)*

S01.9 Open wound of unspecified part of head

S01.90 Unspecified open wound of unspecified part of head

S01.91 Laceration without foreign body of unspecified part of head

S01.92 Laceration with foreign body of unspecified part of head

S01.93 Puncture wound without foreign body of unspecified part of head

S01.94 Puncture wound with foreign body of unspecified part of head

S01.95 Open bite of unspecified part of head

Bite of head NOS

EXCLUDES 1 *superficial bite of head NOS (S00.97)*

S02 Fracture of skull and facial bones

NOTE A fracture not indicated as open or closed should be coded to closed.

Code also any associated intracranial injury (S06.-)

AHA: 2021,1Q,6; 2017,1Q,42; 2016,4Q,66-67

The appropriate 7th character is to be added to each code from category S02.
- A initial encounter for closed fracture
- B initial encounter for open fracture
- D subsequent encounter for fracture with routine healing
- G subsequent encounter for fracture with delayed healing
- K subsequent encounter for fracture with nonunion
- S sequela

2 S02.0 Fracture of vault of skull HCC ESR

Fracture of frontal bone
Fracture of parietal bone

S02.1 Fracture of base of skull

EXCLUDES 2 *lateral orbital wall (S02.84-)*
medial orbital wall (S02.83-)
orbital floor (S02.3-)

AHA: 2019,4Q,16-17

S02.10 Unspecified fracture of base of skull

2 S02.101 Fracture of base of skull, right side HCC ESR

2 S02.102 Fracture of base of skull, left side HCC ESR

2 S02.109 Fracture of base of skull, unspecified side HCC ESR

S02.11 Fracture of occiput

2 S02.110 Type I occipital condyle fracture, unspecified side HCC ESR

2 S02.111 Type II occipital condyle fracture, unspecified side HCC ESR

2 S02.112 Type III occipital condyle fracture, unspecified side HCC ESR

2 S02.113 Unspecified occipital condyle fracture HCC ESR

2 S02.118 Other fracture of occiput, unspecified side HCC ESR

2 S02.119 Unspecified fracture of occiput HCC ESR

2 S02.11A Type I occipital condyle fracture, right side HCC ESR

2 S02.11B Type I occipital condyle fracture, left side HCC ESR

2 S02.11C Type II occipital condyle fracture, right side HCC ESR

2 S02.11D Type II occipital condyle fracture, left side HCC ESR

2 S02.11E Type III occipital condyle fracture, right side HCC ESR

2 S02.11F Type III occipital condyle fracture, left side HCC ESR

2 S02.11G Other fracture of occiput, right side HCC ESR

2 S02.11H Other fracture of occiput, left side HCC ESR

S02.12 Fracture of orbital roof

AHA: 2019,4Q,16-17

2 S02.121 Fracture of orbital roof, right side HCC ESR

2 S02.122 Fracture of orbital roof, left side HCC ESR

2 S02.129 Fracture of orbital roof, unspecified side HCC ESR

2 S02.19 Other fracture of base of skull HCC ESR

Fracture of anterior fossa of base of skull
Fracture of ethmoid sinus
Fracture of frontal sinus
Fracture of middle fossa of base of skull
Fracture of posterior fossa of base of skull
Fracture of sphenoid
Fracture of temporal bone

S02.2 Fracture of nasal bones

√5th **SØ2.3 Fracture of orbital floor**
Fracture of inferior orbital wall
EXCLUDES 1 *orbit NOS (SØ2.85)*
EXCLUDES 2 *lateral orbital wall (SØ2.84-)*
medial orbital wall (SØ2.83-)
orbital roof (SØ2.1-)

2 √x7th **SØ2.3Ø Fracture of orbital floor, unspecified side** HCC ESR
2 √x7th **SØ2.31 Fracture of orbital floor, right side** HCC ESR
2 √x7th **SØ2.32 Fracture of orbital floor, left side** HCC ESR

√5th **SØ2.4 Fracture of malar, maxillary and zygoma bones**
Fracture of superior maxilla
Fracture of upper jaw (bone)
Fracture of zygomatic process of temporal bone

√6th **SØ2.4Ø Fracture of malar, maxillary and zygoma bones, unspecified**
2 √7th **SØ2.4ØØ Malar fracture, unspecified side** HCC ESR
2 √7th **SØ2.4Ø1 Maxillary fracture, unspecified side** HCC ESR
2 √7th **SØ2.4Ø2 Zygomatic fracture, unspecified side** HCC ESR
2 √7th **SØ2.4ØA Malar fracture, right side** HCC ESR
2 √7th **SØ2.4ØB Malar fracture, left side** HCC ESR
2 √7th **SØ2.4ØC Maxillary fracture, right side** HCC ESR
2 √7th **SØ2.4ØD Maxillary fracture, left side** HCC ESR
2 √7th **SØ2.4ØE Zygomatic fracture, right side** HCC ESR
2 √7th **SØ2.4ØF Zygomatic fracture, left side** HCC ESR

√6th **SØ2.41 LeFort fracture**
DEF: Named for Rene Le Fort, these fractures describe different combinations of multiple fractures that occur from significant force to the midface. A common denominator in all three types of LeFort fractures is fracture of the pterygoid processes, which are two bony plates resembling wings that extend downward from the sphenoid bone.

LeFort Fracture Types

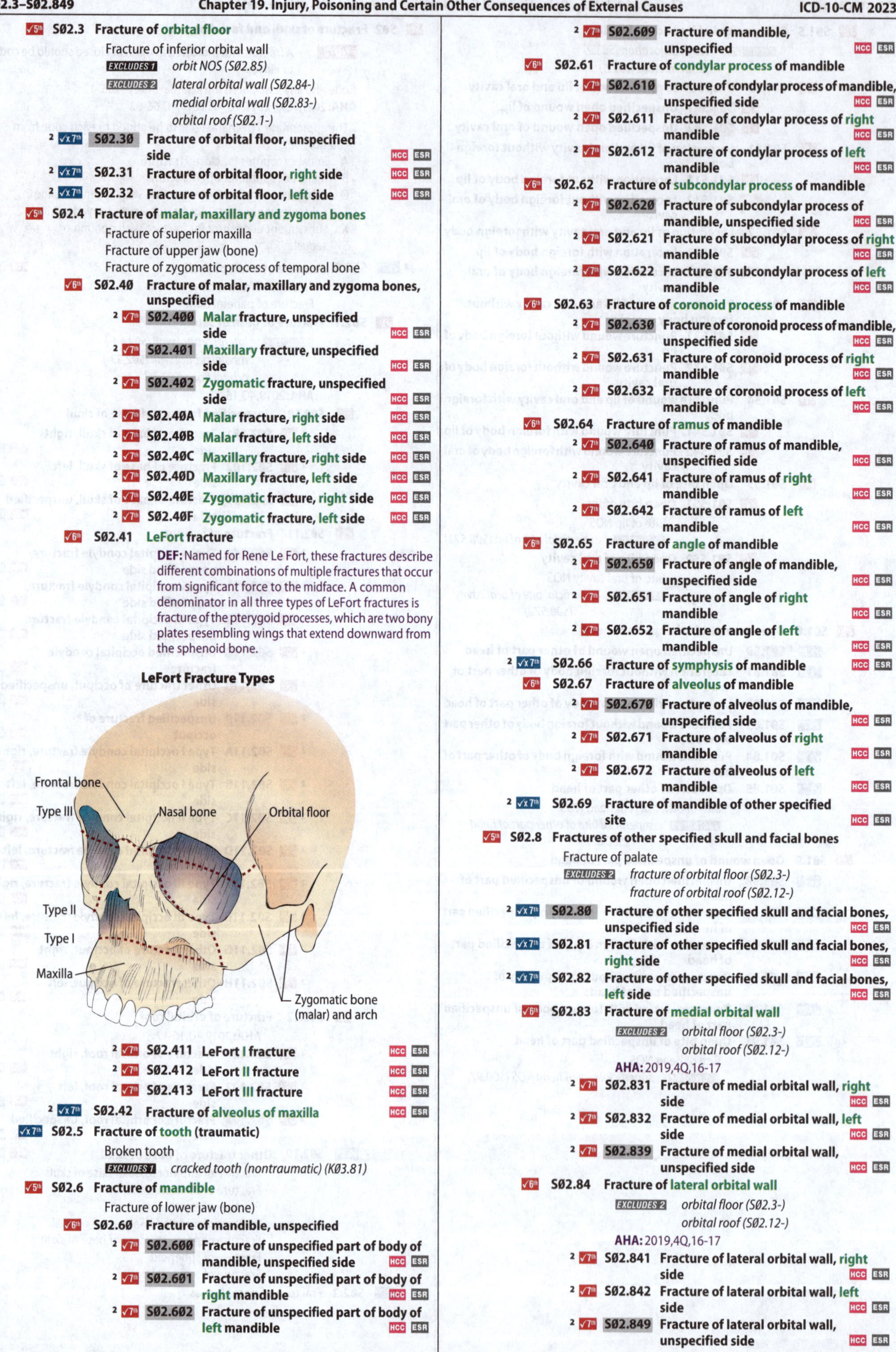

2 √7th **SØ2.411 LeFort I fracture** HCC ESR
2 √7th **SØ2.412 LeFort II fracture** HCC ESR
2 √7th **SØ2.413 LeFort III fracture** HCC ESR

2 √x7th **SØ2.42 Fracture of alveolus of maxilla** HCC ESR

√x7th **SØ2.5 Fracture of tooth (traumatic)**
Broken tooth
EXCLUDES 1 *cracked tooth (nontraumatic) (KØ3.81)*

√5th **SØ2.6 Fracture of mandible**
Fracture of lower jaw (bone)

√6th **SØ2.6Ø Fracture of mandible, unspecified**
2 √7th **SØ2.6ØØ Fracture of unspecified part of body of mandible, unspecified side** HCC ESR
2 √7th **SØ2.6Ø1 Fracture of unspecified part of body of right mandible** HCC ESR
2 √7th **SØ2.6Ø2 Fracture of unspecified part of body of left mandible** HCC ESR
2 √7th **SØ2.6Ø9 Fracture of mandible, unspecified** HCC ESR

√6th **SØ2.61 Fracture of condylar process of mandible**
2 √7th **SØ2.61Ø Fracture of condylar process of mandible, unspecified side** HCC ESR
2 √7th **SØ2.611 Fracture of condylar process of right mandible** HCC ESR
2 √7th **SØ2.612 Fracture of condylar process of left mandible** HCC ESR

√6th **SØ2.62 Fracture of subcondylar process of mandible**
2 √7th **SØ2.62Ø Fracture of subcondylar process of mandible, unspecified side** HCC ESR
2 √7th **SØ2.621 Fracture of subcondylar process of right mandible** HCC ESR
2 √7th **SØ2.622 Fracture of subcondylar process of left mandible** HCC ESR

√6th **SØ2.63 Fracture of coronoid process of mandible**
2 √7th **SØ2.63Ø Fracture of coronoid process of mandible, unspecified side** HCC ESR
2 √7th **SØ2.631 Fracture of coronoid process of right mandible** HCC ESR
2 √7th **SØ2.632 Fracture of coronoid process of left mandible** HCC ESR

√6th **SØ2.64 Fracture of ramus of mandible**
2 √7th **SØ2.64Ø Fracture of ramus of mandible, unspecified side** HCC ESR
2 √7th **SØ2.641 Fracture of ramus of right mandible** HCC ESR
2 √7th **SØ2.642 Fracture of ramus of left mandible** HCC ESR

√6th **SØ2.65 Fracture of angle of mandible**
2 √7th **SØ2.65Ø Fracture of angle of mandible, unspecified side** HCC ESR
2 √7th **SØ2.651 Fracture of angle of right mandible** HCC ESR
2 √7th **SØ2.652 Fracture of angle of left mandible** HCC ESR

2 √x7th **SØ2.66 Fracture of symphysis of mandible** HCC ESR

√6th **SØ2.67 Fracture of alveolus of mandible**
2 √7th **SØ2.67Ø Fracture of alveolus of mandible, unspecified side** HCC ESR
2 √7th **SØ2.671 Fracture of alveolus of right mandible** HCC ESR
2 √7th **SØ2.672 Fracture of alveolus of left mandible** HCC ESR

2 √x7th **SØ2.69 Fracture of mandible of other specified site** HCC ESR

√5th **SØ2.8 Fractures of other specified skull and facial bones**
Fracture of palate
EXCLUDES 2 *fracture of orbital floor (SØ2.3-)*
fracture of orbital roof (SØ2.12-)

2 √x7th **SØ2.8Ø Fracture of other specified skull and facial bones, unspecified side** HCC ESR
2 √x7th **SØ2.81 Fracture of other specified skull and facial bones, right side** HCC ESR
2 √x7th **SØ2.82 Fracture of other specified skull and facial bones, left side** HCC ESR

√6th **SØ2.83 Fracture of medial orbital wall**
EXCLUDES 2 *orbital floor (SØ2.3-)*
orbital roof (SØ2.12-)
AHA: 2019,4Q,16-17
2 √7th **SØ2.831 Fracture of medial orbital wall, right side** HCC ESR
2 √7th **SØ2.832 Fracture of medial orbital wall, left side** HCC ESR
2 √7th **SØ2.839 Fracture of medial orbital wall, unspecified side** HCC ESR

√6th **SØ2.84 Fracture of lateral orbital wall**
EXCLUDES 2 *orbital floor (SØ2.3-)*
orbital roof (SØ2.12-)
AHA: 2019,4Q,16-17
2 √7th **SØ2.841 Fracture of lateral orbital wall, right side** HCC ESR
2 √7th **SØ2.842 Fracture of lateral orbital wall, left side** HCC ESR
2 √7th **SØ2.849 Fracture of lateral orbital wall, unspecified side** HCC ESR

2 √x7th **S02.85 Fracture of orbit, unspecified** HCC ESR
Fracture of orbit NOS
Fracture of orbit wall NOS
EXCLUDES 1 *lateral orbital wall (S02.84-)*
medial orbital wall (S02.83-)
orbital floor (S02.3-)
orbital roof (S02.12-)

√5th **S02.9 Fracture of unspecified skull and facial bones**
2 √x7th **S02.91 Unspecified fracture of skull** HCC ESR
AHA: 2020,2Q,24
2 √x7th **S02.92 Unspecified fracture of facial bones** HCC ESR

√4th **S03 Dislocation and sprain of joints and ligaments of head**
INCLUDES avulsion of joint (capsule) or ligament of head
laceration of cartilage, joint (capsule) or ligament of head
sprain of cartilage, joint (capsule) or ligament of head
traumatic hemarthrosis of joint or ligament of head
traumatic rupture of joint or ligament of head
traumatic subluxation of joint or ligament of head
traumatic tear of joint or ligament of head
Code also any associated open wound
EXCLUDES 2 *strain of muscle or tendon of head (S09.1)*

The appropriate 7th character is to be added to each code from category S03.
A initial encounter
D subsequent encounter
S sequela

√5th **S03.0 Dislocation of jaw**
Dislocation of jaw (cartilage) (meniscus)
Dislocation of mandible
Dislocation of temporomandibular (joint)
AHA: 2016,4Q,67
√x7th **S03.00 Dislocation of jaw, unspecified side**
√x7th **S03.01 Dislocation of jaw, right side**
√x7th **S03.02 Dislocation of jaw, left side**
√x7th **S03.03 Dislocation of jaw, bilateral**
√x7th **S03.1 Dislocation of septal cartilage of nose**
√x7th **S03.2 Dislocation of tooth**
√5th **S03.4 Sprain of jaw**
Sprain of temporomandibular (joint) (ligament)
AHA: 2016,4Q,67
√x7th **S03.40 Sprain of jaw, unspecified side**
√x7th **S03.41 Sprain of jaw, right side**
√x7th **S03.42 Sprain of jaw, left side**
√x7th **S03.43 Sprain of jaw, bilateral**
√x7th **S03.8 Sprain of joints and ligaments of other parts of head**
√x7th **S03.9 Sprain of joints and ligaments of unspecified parts of head**

√4th **S04 Injury of cranial nerve**
The selection of side should be based on the side of the body being affected
Code first any associated intracranial injury (S06.-)
Code also any associated:
open wound of head (S01.-)
skull fracture (S02.-)

The appropriate 7th character is to be added to each code from category S04.
A initial encounter
D subsequent encounter
S sequela

√5th **S04.0 Injury of optic nerve and pathways**
Use additional code to identify any visual field defect or blindness (H53.4-, H54.-)
√6th **S04.01 Injury of optic nerve**
Injury of 2nd cranial nerve
√7th **S04.011 Injury of optic nerve, right eye**
√7th **S04.012 Injury of optic nerve, left eye**
√7th **S04.019 Injury of optic nerve, unspecified eye**
Injury of optic nerve NOS
√x7th **S04.02 Injury of optic chiasm**
√6th **S04.03 Injury of optic tract and pathways**
Injury of optic radiation
√7th **S04.031 Injury of optic tract and pathways, right side**
√7th **S04.032 Injury of optic tract and pathways, left side**
√7th **S04.039 Injury of optic tract and pathways, unspecified side**
Injury of optic tract and pathways NOS
√6th **S04.04 Injury of visual cortex**
√7th **S04.041 Injury of visual cortex, right side**
√7th **S04.042 Injury of visual cortex, left side**
√7th **S04.049 Injury of visual cortex, unspecified side**
Injury of visual cortex NOS
√5th **S04.1 Injury of oculomotor nerve**
Injury of 3rd cranial nerve
√x7th **S04.10 Injury of oculomotor nerve, unspecified side**
√x7th **S04.11 Injury of oculomotor nerve, right side**
√x7th **S04.12 Injury of oculomotor nerve, left side**
√5th **S04.2 Injury of trochlear nerve**
Injury of 4th cranial nerve
√x7th **S04.20 Injury of trochlear nerve, unspecified side**
√x7th **S04.21 Injury of trochlear nerve, right side**
√x7th **S04.22 Injury of trochlear nerve, left side**
√5th **S04.3 Injury of trigeminal nerve**
Injury of 5th cranial nerve
√x7th **S04.30 Injury of trigeminal nerve, unspecified side**
√x7th **S04.31 Injury of trigeminal nerve, right side**
√x7th **S04.32 Injury of trigeminal nerve, left side**
√5th **S04.4 Injury of abducent nerve**
Injury of 6th cranial nerve
√x7th **S04.40 Injury of abducent nerve, unspecified side**
√x7th **S04.41 Injury of abducent nerve, right side**
√x7th **S04.42 Injury of abducent nerve, left side**
√5th **S04.5 Injury of facial nerve**
Injury of 7th cranial nerve
√x7th **S04.50 Injury of facial nerve, unspecified side**
√x7th **S04.51 Injury of facial nerve, right side**
√x7th **S04.52 Injury of facial nerve, left side**
√5th **S04.6 Injury of acoustic nerve**
Injury of auditory nerve
Injury of 8th cranial nerve
√x7th **S04.60 Injury of acoustic nerve, unspecified side**
√x7th **S04.61 Injury of acoustic nerve, right side**
√x7th **S04.62 Injury of acoustic nerve, left side**
√5th **S04.7 Injury of accessory nerve**
Injury of 11th cranial nerve
√x7th **S04.70 Injury of accessory nerve, unspecified side**
√x7th **S04.71 Injury of accessory nerve, right side**
√x7th **S04.72 Injury of accessory nerve, left side**
√5th **S04.8 Injury of other cranial nerves**
√6th **S04.81 Injury of olfactory [1st] nerve**
√7th **S04.811 Injury of olfactory [1st] nerve, right side**
√7th **S04.812 Injury of olfactory [1st] nerve, left side**
√7th **S04.819 Injury of olfactory [1st] nerve, unspecified side**
√6th **S04.89 Injury of other cranial nerves**
Injury of vagus [10th] nerve
√7th **S04.891 Injury of other cranial nerves, right side**
√7th **S04.892 Injury of other cranial nerves, left side**
√7th **S04.899 Injury of other cranial nerves, unspecified side**
√x7th **S04.9 Injury of unspecified cranial nerve**

S05 Injury of eye and orbit

INCLUDES open wound of eye and orbit

EXCLUDES 2 *2nd cranial [optic] nerve injury (S04.0-)*
3rd cranial [oculomotor] nerve injury (S04.1-)
open wound of eyelid and periocular area (S01.1-)
orbital bone fracture (S02.1-, S02.3-, S02.8-)
superficial injury of eyelid (S00.1-S00.2)

The appropriate 7th character is to be added to each code from category S05.
A initial encounter
D subsequent encounter
S sequela

S05.0 Injury of conjunctiva and corneal abrasion without foreign body

EXCLUDES 1 *foreign body in conjunctival sac (T15.1)*
foreign body in cornea (T15.0)

S05.00 Injury of conjunctiva and corneal abrasion without foreign body, unspecified eye

S05.01 Injury of conjunctiva and corneal abrasion without foreign body, right eye

S05.02 Injury of conjunctiva and corneal abrasion without foreign body, left eye

S05.1 Contusion of eyeball and orbital tissues

Traumatic hyphema

EXCLUDES 2 *black eye NOS (S00.1)*
contusion of eyelid and periocular area (S00.1)

S05.10 Contusion of eyeball and orbital tissues, unspecified eye

S05.11 Contusion of eyeball and orbital tissues, right eye

S05.12 Contusion of eyeball and orbital tissues, left eye

S05.2 Ocular laceration and rupture with prolapse or loss of intraocular tissue

S05.20 Ocular laceration and rupture with prolapse or loss of intraocular tissue, unspecified eye

S05.21 Ocular laceration and rupture with prolapse or loss of intraocular tissue, right eye

S05.22 Ocular laceration and rupture with prolapse or loss of intraocular tissue, left eye

S05.3 Ocular laceration without prolapse or loss of intraocular tissue

Laceration of eye NOS

AHA: 2022,1Q,33

DEF: Tear in ocular tissue without displacing structures that is due to blunt trauma. It is characterized by pain, redness, and decreased vision.

S05.30 Ocular laceration without prolapse or loss of intraocular tissue, unspecified eye

S05.31 Ocular laceration without prolapse or loss of intraocular tissue, right eye

S05.32 Ocular laceration without prolapse or loss of intraocular tissue, left eye

S05.4 Penetrating wound of orbit with or without foreign body

EXCLUDES 2 *retained (old) foreign body following penetrating wound in orbit (H05.5-)*

S05.40 Penetrating wound of orbit with or without foreign body, unspecified eye

S05.41 Penetrating wound of orbit with or without foreign body, right eye

S05.42 Penetrating wound of orbit with or without foreign body, left eye

S05.5 Penetrating wound with foreign body of eyeball

EXCLUDES 2 *retained (old) intraocular foreign body (H44.6-, H44.7)*

S05.50 Penetrating wound with foreign body of unspecified eyeball

S05.51 Penetrating wound with foreign body of right eyeball

S05.52 Penetrating wound with foreign body of left eyeball

S05.6 Penetrating wound without foreign body of eyeball

Ocular penetration NOS

S05.60 Penetrating wound without foreign body of unspecified eyeball

S05.61 Penetrating wound without foreign body of right eyeball

S05.62 Penetrating wound without foreign body of left eyeball

S05.7 Avulsion of eye

Traumatic enucleation

S05.70 Avulsion of unspecified eye

S05.71 Avulsion of right eye

S05.72 Avulsion of left eye

S05.8 Other injuries of eye and orbit

Lacrimal duct injury

S05.8X Other injuries of eye and orbit

S05.8X1 Other injuries of right eye and orbit

S05.8X2 Other injuries of left eye and orbit

S05.8X9 Other injuries of unspecified eye and orbit

S05.9 Unspecified injury of eye and orbit

Injury of eye NOS

S05.90 Unspecified injury of unspecified eye and orbit

S05.91 Unspecified injury of right eye and orbit

S05.92 Unspecified injury of left eye and orbit

S06 Intracranial injury

NOTE 7th characters D and S do not apply to codes in category S06 with 6th character 7 – death due to brain injury prior to regaining consciousness, or 8 – death due to other cause prior to regaining consciousness.

INCLUDES traumatic brain injury

Code also any associated:
open wound of head (S01.-)
skull fracture (S02.-)

▶Use additional code, if applicable, to identify mild neurocognitive disorders due to known physiological condition (F06.7-)◀

EXCLUDES 1 *head injury NOS (S09.90)*

AHA: 2017,4Q,25; 2017,1Q,42; 2015,3Q,37

TIP: Do not assign Z87.820 Personal history of traumatic brain injury, when residual conditions persist after an intracranial injury. The codes for the residual conditions should be first listed, followed by a code from category S06 using seventh character S to identify sequelae.

The appropriate 7th character is to be added to each code from category S06.
A initial encounter
D subsequent encounter
S sequela

S06.0 Concussion

Commotio cerebri

EXCLUDES 1 ▶*concussion with other intracranial injuries classified in subcategories S06.1- to S06.6-, and S06.81- to S06.89-, code to specified intracranial injury*◀

AHA: 2016,4Q,67-68

S06.0X Concussion

3 **S06.0X0 Concussion without loss of consciousness** HCC ESR Q

3 **S06.0X1 Concussion with loss of consciousness of 30 minutes or less** HCC ESR Q
▶Concussion with brief loss of consciousness◀

● **S06.0XA Concussion with loss of consciousness status unknown**
Concussion NOS

3 **S06.0X9 Concussion with loss of consciousness of unspecified duration** HCC ESR Q
~~Concussion NOS~~

S06.1 Traumatic cerebral edema

Diffuse traumatic cerebral edema
Focal traumatic cerebral edema

AHA: 2019,3Q,35; 2015,1Q,12-13

S06.1X Traumatic cerebral edema

2 **S06.1X0 Traumatic cerebral edema without loss of consciousness** HCC ESR Q

2 **S06.1X1 Traumatic cerebral edema with loss of consciousness of 30 minutes or less** HCC ESR Q
▶Traumatic cerebral edema with brief loss of consciousness◀

2 **S06.1X2 Traumatic cerebral edema with loss of consciousness of 31 minutes to 59 minutes** HCC ESR Q

S06.1X3 Traumatic cerebral edema with loss of consciousness of 1 hour to 5 hours 59 minutes HCC ESR COM Q

S06.1X4 Traumatic cerebral edema with loss of consciousness of 6 hours to 24 hours HCC ESR COM Q

S06.1X5 Traumatic cerebral edema with loss of consciousness greater than 24 hours with return to pre-existing conscious level HCC ESR COM

S06.1X6 Traumatic cerebral edema with loss of consciousness greater than 24 hours without return to pre-existing conscious level with patient surviving HCC ESR COM

S06.1X7 Traumatic cerebral edema with loss of consciousness of any duration with death due to brain injury prior to regaining consciousness

S06.1X8 Traumatic cerebral edema with loss of consciousness of any duration with death due to other cause prior to regaining consciousness

● S06.1XA Traumatic cerebral edema with loss of consciousness status unknown
Traumatic cerebral edema NOS

S06.1X9 Traumatic cerebral edema with loss of consciousness of unspecified duration HCC ESR Q
~~Traumatic cerebral edema NOS~~

S06.2 Diffuse traumatic brain injury

Diffuse axonal brain injury

Use additional code, if applicable, for traumatic brain compression or herniation (S06.A-)

EXCLUDES 1 *traumatic diffuse cerebral edema (S06.1X-)*

AHA: 2020,3Q,46

S06.2X Diffuse traumatic brain injury

S06.2X0 Diffuse traumatic brain injury without loss of consciousness HCC ESR Q

S06.2X1 Diffuse traumatic brain injury with loss of consciousness of 30 minutes or less HCC ESR Q
▶Diffuse traumatic brain injury with brief loss of consciousness◀

S06.2X2 Diffuse traumatic brain injury with loss of consciousness of 31 minutes to 59 minutes HCC ESR Q

S06.2X3 Diffuse traumatic brain injury with loss of consciousness of 1 hour to 5 hours 59 minutes HCC ESR COM Q

S06.2X4 Diffuse traumatic brain injury with loss of consciousness of 6 hours to 24 hours HCC ESR COM Q

S06.2X5 Diffuse traumatic brain injury with loss of consciousness greater than 24 hours with return to pre-existing conscious levels HCC ESR COM

S06.2X6 Diffuse traumatic brain injury with loss of consciousness greater than 24 hours without return to pre-existing conscious level with patient surviving HCC ESR COM

S06.2X7 Diffuse traumatic brain injury with loss of consciousness of any duration with death due to brain injury prior to regaining consciousness

S06.2X8 Diffuse traumatic brain injury with loss of consciousness of any duration with death due to other cause prior to regaining consciousness

● S06.2XA Diffuse traumatic brain injury with loss of consciousness status unknown
Diffuse traumatic brain injury NOS

S06.2X9 Diffuse traumatic brain injury with loss of consciousness of unspecified duration HCC ESR Q
~~Diffuse traumatic brain injury NOS~~

S06.3 Focal traumatic brain injury

Use additional code, if applicable, for traumatic brain compression or herniation (S06.A-)

EXCLUDES 1 *any condition classifiable to S06.4-S06.6*

EXCLUDES 2 *focal cerebral edema (S06.1)*

AHA: 2020,3Q,46; 2019,3Q,35; 2015,1Q,12-13

S06.30 Unspecified focal traumatic brain injury

S06.300 Unspecified focal traumatic brain injury without loss of consciousness HCC ESR Q

S06.301 Unspecified focal traumatic brain injury with loss of consciousness of 30 minutes or less HCC ESR Q
▶Unspecified focal traumatic brain injury with brief loss of consciousness◀

S06.302 Unspecified focal traumatic brain injury with loss of consciousness of 31 minutes to 59 minutes HCC ESR Q

S06.303 Unspecified focal traumatic brain injury with loss of consciousness of 1 hour to 5 hours 59 minutes HCC ESR COM Q

S06.304 Unspecified focal traumatic brain injury with loss of consciousness of 6 hours to 24 hours HCC ESR COM Q

S06.305 Unspecified focal traumatic brain injury with loss of consciousness greater than 24 hours with return to pre-existing conscious level HCC ESR COM

S06.306 Unspecified focal traumatic brain injury with loss of consciousness greater than 24 hours without return to pre-existing conscious level with patient surviving HCC ESR COM

S06.307 Unspecified focal traumatic brain injury with loss of consciousness of any duration with death due to brain injury prior to regaining consciousness

S06.308 Unspecified focal traumatic brain injury with loss of consciousness of any duration with death due to other cause prior to regaining consciousness

● S06.30A Unspecified focal traumatic brain injury with loss of consciousness status unknown
Unspecified focal traumatic brain injury NOS

S06.309 Unspecified focal traumatic brain injury with loss of consciousness of unspecified duration HCC ESR Q
~~Unspecified focal traumatic brain injury NOS~~

S06.31 Contusion and laceration of right cerebrum

S06.310 Contusion and laceration of right cerebrum without loss of consciousness HCC ESR

S06.311 Contusion and laceration of right cerebrum with loss of consciousness of 30 minutes or less HCC ESR
▶Contusion and laceration of right cerebrum with brief loss of consciousness◀

S06.312 Contusion and laceration of right cerebrum with loss of consciousness of 31 minutes to 59 minutes HCC ESR

S06.313 Contusion and laceration of right cerebrum with loss of consciousness of 1 hour to 5 hours 59 minutes HCC ESR COM

S06.314 Contusion and laceration of right cerebrum with loss of consciousness of 6 hours to 24 hours HCC ESR COM

S06.315 Contusion and laceration of right cerebrum with loss of consciousness greater than 24 hours with return to pre-existing conscious level HCC ESR COM

S06.316 Contusion and laceration of right cerebrum with loss of consciousness greater than 24 hours without return to pre-existing conscious level with patient surviving HCC ESR COM

7th S06.317 **Contusion and laceration of right cerebrum with loss of consciousness of any duration with death due to brain injury prior to regaining consciousness**

7th S06.318 **Contusion and laceration of right cerebrum with loss of consciousness of any duration with death due to other cause prior to regaining consciousness**

● 7th S06.31A **Contusion and laceration of right cerebrum with loss of consciousness status unknown**
Contusion and laceration of right cerebrum NOS

2 7th S06.319 **Contusion and laceration of right cerebrum with loss of consciousness of unspecified duration** HCC ESR
~~Contusion and laceration of right cerebrum NOS~~

6th S06.32 **Contusion and laceration of left cerebrum**

7th S06.320 **Contusion and laceration of left cerebrum without loss of consciousness** HCC ESR

2 7th S06.321 **Contusion and laceration of left cerebrum with loss of consciousness of 30 minutes or less** HCC ESR
▶Contusion and laceration of left cerebrum with brief loss of consciousness◀

2 7th S06.322 **Contusion and laceration of left cerebrum with loss of consciousness of 31 minutes to 59 minutes** HCC ESR

2 7th S06.323 **Contusion and laceration of left cerebrum with loss of consciousness of 1 hour to 5 hours 59 minutes** HCC ESR COM

2 7th S06.324 **Contusion and laceration of left cerebrum with loss of consciousness of 6 hours to 24 hours** HCC ESR COM

2 7th S06.325 **Contusion and laceration of left cerebrum with loss of consciousness greater than 24 hours with return to pre-existing conscious level** HCC ESR COM

2 7th S06.326 **Contusion and laceration of left cerebrum with loss of consciousness greater than 24 hours without return to pre-existing conscious level with patient surviving** HCC ESR COM

7th S06.327 **Contusion and laceration of left cerebrum with loss of consciousness of any duration with death due to brain injury prior to regaining consciousness**

7th S06.328 **Contusion and laceration of left cerebrum with loss of consciousness of any duration with death due to other cause prior to regaining consciousness**

● 7th S06.32A **Contusion and laceration of left cerebrum with loss of consciousness status unknown**
Contusion and laceration of left cerebrum NOS

2 7th S06.329 **Contusion and laceration of left cerebrum with loss of consciousness of unspecified duration** HCC ESR
~~Contusion and laceration of left cerebrum NOS~~

6th S06.33 **Contusion and laceration of cerebrum, unspecified**

2 7th S06.330 **Contusion and laceration of cerebrum, unspecified, without loss of consciousness** HCC ESR

2 7th S06.331 **Contusion and laceration of cerebrum, unspecified, with loss of consciousness of 30 minutes or less** HCC ESR
▶Contusion and laceration of cerebrum, unspecified, with brief loss of consciousness◀

2 7th S06.332 **Contusion and laceration of cerebrum, unspecified, with loss of consciousness of 31 minutes to 59 minutes** HCC ESR

2 7th S06.333 **Contusion and laceration of cerebrum, unspecified, with loss of consciousness of 1 hour to 5 hours 59 minutes** HCC ESR COM

2 7th S06.334 **Contusion and laceration of cerebrum, unspecified, with loss of consciousness of 6 hours to 24 hours** HCC ESR COM

2 7th S06.335 **Contusion and laceration of cerebrum, unspecified, with loss of consciousness greater than 24 hours with return to pre-existing conscious level** HCC ESR COM

2 7th S06.336 **Contusion and laceration of cerebrum, unspecified, with loss of consciousness greater than 24 hours without return to pre-existing conscious level with patient surviving** HCC ESR COM

7th S06.337 **Contusion and laceration of cerebrum, unspecified, with loss of consciousness of any duration with death due to brain injury prior to regaining consciousness**

7th S06.338 **Contusion and laceration of cerebrum, unspecified, with loss of consciousness of any duration with death due to other cause prior to regaining consciousness**

● 7th S06.33A **Contusion and laceration of cerebrum, unspecified, with loss of consciousness status unknown**
Contusion and laceration of cerebrum NOS

2 7th S06.339 **Contusion and laceration of cerebrum, unspecified, with loss of consciousness of unspecified duration** HCC ESR
~~Contusion and laceration of cerebrum NOS~~

6th S06.34 **Traumatic hemorrhage of right cerebrum**
Traumatic intracerebral hemorrhage and hematoma of right cerebrum

2 7th S06.340 **Traumatic hemorrhage of right cerebrum without loss of consciousness** HCC ESR Q

2 7th S06.341 **Traumatic hemorrhage of right cerebrum with loss of consciousness of 30 minutes or less** HCC ESR Q
▶Traumatic hemorrhage of right cerebrum with loss of consciousness◀

2 7th S06.342 **Traumatic hemorrhage of right cerebrum with loss of consciousness of 31 minutes to 59 minutes** HCC ESR Q

2 7th S06.343 **Traumatic hemorrhage of right cerebrum with loss of consciousness of 1 hours to 5 hours 59 minutes** HCC ESR COM Q

2 7th S06.344 **Traumatic hemorrhage of right cerebrum with loss of consciousness of 6 hours to 24 hours** HCC ESR COM Q

2 7th S06.345 **Traumatic hemorrhage of right cerebrum with loss of consciousness greater than 24 hours with return to pre-existing conscious level** HCC ESR COM

2 7th S06.346 **Traumatic hemorrhage of right cerebrum with loss of consciousness greater than 24 hours without return to pre-existing conscious level with patient surviving** HCC ESR COM

7th S06.347 **Traumatic hemorrhage of right cerebrum with loss of consciousness of any duration with death due to brain injury prior to regaining consciousness**

7th S06.348 **Traumatic hemorrhage of right cerebrum with loss of consciousness of any duration with death due to other cause prior to regaining consciousness**

● 7th S06.34A **Traumatic hemorrhage of right cerebrum with loss of consciousness status unknown**
Traumatic hemorrhage of right cerebrum NOS

2 7th S06.349 **Traumatic hemorrhage of right cerebrum with loss of consciousness of unspecified duration** HCC ESR Q
~~Traumatic hemorrhage of right cerebrum NOS~~

6th S06.35 **Traumatic hemorrhage of left cerebrum**
Traumatic intracerebral hemorrhage and hematoma of left cerebrum

2 7th S06.350 **Traumatic hemorrhage of left cerebrum without loss of consciousness** HCC ESR Q

2 7th **S06.351 Traumatic hemorrhage of left cerebrum with loss of consciousness of 30 minutes or less** HCC ESR Q
▶Traumatic hemorrhage of left cerebrum with brief loss of consciousness◀

2 7th **S06.352 Traumatic hemorrhage of left cerebrum with loss of consciousness of 31 minutes to 59 minutes** HCC ESR Q

2 7th **S06.353 Traumatic hemorrhage of left cerebrum with loss of consciousness of 1 hours to 5 hours 59 minutes** HCC ESR COM Q

2 7th **S06.354 Traumatic hemorrhage of left cerebrum with loss of consciousness of 6 hours to 24 hours** HCC ESR COM Q

2 7th **S06.355 Traumatic hemorrhage of left cerebrum with loss of consciousness greater than 24 hours with return to pre-existing conscious level** HCC ESR COM

2 7th **S06.356 Traumatic hemorrhage of left cerebrum with loss of consciousness greater than 24 hours without return to pre-existing conscious level with patient surviving** HCC ESR COM

7th **S06.357 Traumatic hemorrhage of left cerebrum with loss of consciousness of any duration with death due to brain injury prior to regaining consciousness**

7th **S06.358 Traumatic hemorrhage of left cerebrum with loss of consciousness of any duration with death due to other cause prior to regaining consciousness**

● 7th **S06.35A Traumatic hemorrhage of left cerebrum with loss of consciousness status unknown**
Traumatic hemorrhage of left cerebrum NOS

2 7th **S06.359 Traumatic hemorrhage of left cerebrum with loss of consciousness of unspecified duration** HCC ESR Q
~~Traumatic hemorrhage of left cerebrum NOS~~

6th **S06.36 Traumatic hemorrhage of cerebrum, unspecified**
Traumatic intracerebral hemorrhage and hematoma, unspecified

2 7th **S06.360 Traumatic hemorrhage of cerebrum, unspecified, without loss of consciousness** HCC ESR Q

2 7th **S06.361 Traumatic hemorrhage of cerebrum, unspecified, with loss of consciousness of 30 minutes or less** HCC ESR Q
▶Traumatic hemorrhage of cerebrum, unspecified, with brief loss of consciousness◀

2 7th **S06.362 Traumatic hemorrhage of cerebrum, unspecified, with loss of consciousness of 31 minutes to 59 minutes** HCC ESR Q

2 7th **S06.363 Traumatic hemorrhage of cerebrum, unspecified, with loss of consciousness of 1 hours to 5 hours 59 minutes** HCC ESR COM Q

2 7th **S06.364 Traumatic hemorrhage of cerebrum, unspecified, with loss of consciousness of 6 hours to 24 hours** HCC ESR COM Q

2 7th **S06.365 Traumatic hemorrhage of cerebrum, unspecified, with loss of consciousness greater than 24 hours with return to pre-existing conscious level** HCC ESR COM

2 7th **S06.366 Traumatic hemorrhage of cerebrum, unspecified, with loss of consciousness greater than 24 hours without return to pre-existing conscious level with patient surviving** HCC ESR COM

7th **S06.367 Traumatic hemorrhage of cerebrum, unspecified, with loss of consciousness of any duration with death due to brain injury prior to regaining consciousness**

7th **S06.368 Traumatic hemorrhage of cerebrum, unspecified, with loss of consciousness of any duration with death due to other cause prior to regaining consciousness**

● 7th **S06.36A Traumatic hemorrhage of cerebrum, unspecified, with loss of consciousness status unknown**
Traumatic hemorrhage of cerebrum NOS

2 7th **S06.369 Traumatic hemorrhage of cerebrum, unspecified, with loss of consciousness of unspecified duration** HCC ESR Q
~~Traumatic hemorrhage of cerebrum NOS~~

6th **S06.37 Contusion, laceration, and hemorrhage of cerebellum**

2 7th **S06.370 Contusion, laceration, and hemorrhage of cerebellum without loss of consciousness** HCC ESR

2 7th **S06.371 Contusion, laceration, and hemorrhage of cerebellum with loss of consciousness of 30 minutes or less** HCC ESR
▶Contusion, laceration, and hemorrhage of cerebellum with brief loss of consciousness◀

2 7th **S06.372 Contusion, laceration, and hemorrhage of cerebellum with loss of consciousness of 31 minutes to 59 minutes** HCC ESR

2 7th **S06.373 Contusion, laceration, and hemorrhage of cerebellum with loss of consciousness of 1 hour to 5 hours 59 minutes** HCC ESR COM

2 7th **S06.374 Contusion, laceration, and hemorrhage of cerebellum with loss of consciousness of 6 hours to 24 hours** HCC ESR COM

2 7th **S06.375 Contusion, laceration, and hemorrhage of cerebellum with loss of consciousness greater than 24 hours with return to pre-existing conscious level** HCC ESR COM

2 7th **S06.376 Contusion, laceration, and hemorrhage of cerebellum with loss of consciousness greater than 24 hours without return to pre-existing conscious level with patient surviving** HCC ESR COM

7th **S06.377 Contusion, laceration, and hemorrhage of cerebellum with loss of consciousness of any duration with death due to brain injury prior to regaining consciousness**

7th **S06.378 Contusion, laceration, and hemorrhage of cerebellum with loss of consciousness of any duration with death due to other cause prior to regaining consciousness**

● 7th **S06.37A Contusion, laceration, and hemorrhage of cerebellum with loss of consciousness status unknown**
Contusion, laceration, and hemorrhage of cerebellum NOS

2 7th **S06.379 Contusion, laceration, and hemorrhage of cerebellum with loss of consciousness of unspecified duration** HCC ESR
~~Contusion, laceration, and hemorrhage of cerebellum NOS~~

6th **S06.38 Contusion, laceration, and hemorrhage of brainstem**

2 7th **S06.380 Contusion, laceration, and hemorrhage of brainstem without loss of consciousness** HCC ESR

2 7th **S06.381 Contusion, laceration, and hemorrhage of brainstem with loss of consciousness of 30 minutes or less** HCC ESR
▶Contusion, laceration, and hemorrhage of brainstem with brief loss of consciousness◀

2 7th **S06.382 Contusion, laceration, and hemorrhage of brainstem with loss of consciousness of 31 minutes to 59 minutes** HCC ESR

2 7th **S06.383 Contusion, laceration, and hemorrhage of brainstem with loss of consciousness of 1 hour to 5 hours 59 minutes** HCC ESR COM

2 7th **S06.384 Contusion, laceration, and hemorrhage of brainstem with loss of consciousness of 6 hours to 24 hours** HCC ESR COM

2 7th **S06.385 Contusion, laceration, and hemorrhage of brainstem with loss of consciousness greater than 24 hours with return to pre-existing conscious level** HCC ESR COM

2 7th **SØ6.386 Contusion, laceration, and hemorrhage of brainstem with loss of consciousness greater than 24 hours without return to pre-existing conscious level with patient surviving** HCC ESR COM

7th **SØ6.387 Contusion, laceration, and hemorrhage of brainstem with loss of consciousness of any duration with death due to brain injury prior to regaining consciousness**

7th **SØ6.388 Contusion, laceration, and hemorrhage of brainstem with loss of consciousness of any duration with death due to other cause prior to regaining consciousness**

● 7th **SØ6.38A Contusion, laceration, and hemorrhage of brainstem with loss of consciousness status unknown**

Contusion, laceration, and hemorrhage of brainstem NOS

2 7th **SØ6.389 Contusion, laceration, and hemorrhage of brainstem with loss of consciousness of unspecified duration** HCC ESR

~~Contusion, laceration, and hemorrhage of brainstem NOS~~

5th **SØ6.4 Epidural hemorrhage**

Extradural hemorrhage NOS

Extradural hemorrhage (traumatic)

DEF: Epidural space: Space between the endosteum of the cranium (skull) and the dura mater, the outermost layer of a three-layer membrane that covers the brain.

6th **SØ6.4X Epidural hemorrhage**

2 7th **SØ6.4XØ Epidural hemorrhage without loss of consciousness** HCC ESR Q

2 7th **SØ6.4X1 Epidural hemorrhage with loss of consciousness of 3Ø minutes or less** HCC ESR Q

▶Epidural hemorrhage with brief loss of consciousness◀

2 7th **SØ6.4X2 Epidural hemorrhage with loss of consciousness of 31 minutes to 59 minutes** HCC ESR Q

2 7th **SØ6.4X3 Epidural hemorrhage with loss of consciousness of 1 hour to 5 hours 59 minutes** HCC ESR COM Q

2 7th **SØ6.4X4 Epidural hemorrhage with loss of consciousness of 6 hours to 24 hours** HCC ESR COM Q

2 7th **SØ6.4X5 Epidural hemorrhage with loss of consciousness greater than 24 hours with return to pre-existing conscious level** HCC ESR COM

2 7th **SØ6.4X6 Epidural hemorrhage with loss of consciousness greater than 24 hours without return to pre-existing conscious level with patient surviving** HCC ESR COM

7th **SØ6.4X7 Epidural hemorrhage with loss of consciousness of any duration with death due to brain injury prior to regaining consciousness**

7th **SØ6.4X8 Epidural hemorrhage with loss of consciousness of any duration with death due to other causes prior to regaining consciousness**

● 7th **SØ6.4XA Epidural hemorrhage with loss of consciousness status unknown**

Epidural hemorrhage NOS

2 7th **SØ6.4X9 Epidural hemorrhage with loss of consciousness of unspecified duration** HCC ESR Q

~~Epidural hemorrhage NOS~~

5th **SØ6.5 Traumatic subdural hemorrhage**

Use additional code, if applicable, for traumatic brain compression or herniation (SØ6.A-)

AHA: 2021,2Q,5; 2021,1Q,4

DEF: Subdural: Potential space between the dura mater and arachnoid membrane around the brain.

6th **SØ6.5X Traumatic subdural hemorrhage**

2 7th **SØ6.5XØ Traumatic subdural hemorrhage without loss of consciousness** HCC ESR Q

2 7th **SØ6.5X1 Traumatic subdural hemorrhage with loss of consciousness of 3Ø minutes or less** HCC ESR Q

▶Traumatic subdural hemorrhage with brief loss of consciousness◀

2 7th **SØ6.5X2 Traumatic subdural hemorrhage with loss of consciousness of 31 minutes to 59 minutes** HCC ESR Q

2 7th **SØ6.5X3 Traumatic subdural hemorrhage with loss of consciousness of 1 hour to 5 hours 59 minutes** HCC ESR COM Q

2 7th **SØ6.5X4 Traumatic subdural hemorrhage with loss of consciousness of 6 hours to 24 hours** HCC ESR COM Q

2 7th **SØ6.5X5 Traumatic subdural hemorrhage with loss of consciousness greater than 24 hours with return to pre-existing conscious level** HCC ESR COM

2 7th **SØ6.5X6 Traumatic subdural hemorrhage with loss of consciousness greater than 24 hours without return to pre-existing conscious level with patient surviving** HCC ESR COM

7th **SØ6.5X7 Traumatic subdural hemorrhage with loss of consciousness of any duration with death due to brain injury before regaining consciousness**

7th **SØ6.5X8 Traumatic subdural hemorrhage with loss of consciousness of any duration with death due to other cause before regaining consciousness**

● 7th **SØ6.5XA Traumatic subdural hemorrhage with loss of consciousness status unknown**

Traumatic subdural hemorrhage NOS

2 7th **SØ6.5X9 Traumatic subdural hemorrhage with loss of consciousness of unspecified duration** HCC ESR Q

~~Traumatic subdural hemorrhage NOS~~

5th **SØ6.6 Traumatic subarachnoid hemorrhage**

Use additional code, if applicable, for traumatic brain compression or herniation (SØ6.A-)

AHA: 2021,2Q,5; 2021,1Q,4

DEF: Subarachnoid: Space located between the arachnoid membrane and the pia mater that contains cerebrospinal fluid.

6th **SØ6.6X Traumatic subarachnoid hemorrhage**

2 7th **SØ6.6XØ Traumatic subarachnoid hemorrhage without loss of consciousness** HCC ESR Q

2 7th **SØ6.6X1 Traumatic subarachnoid hemorrhage with loss of consciousness of 3Ø minutes or less** HCC ESR Q

▶Traumatic subarachnoid hemorrhage with brief loss of consciousness◀

2 7th **SØ6.6X2 Traumatic subarachnoid hemorrhage with loss of consciousness of 31 minutes to 59 minutes** HCC ESR Q

2 7th **SØ6.6X3 Traumatic subarachnoid hemorrhage with loss of consciousness of 1 hour to 5 hours 59 minutes** HCC ESR COM Q

2 7th **SØ6.6X4 Traumatic subarachnoid hemorrhage with loss of consciousness of 6 hours to 24 hours** HCC ESR COM Q

2 7th **SØ6.6X5 Traumatic subarachnoid hemorrhage with loss of consciousness greater than 24 hours with return to pre-existing conscious level** HCC ESR COM

2 7th **SØ6.6X6 Traumatic subarachnoid hemorrhage with loss of consciousness greater than 24 hours without return to pre-existing conscious level with patient surviving** HCC ESR COM

7th **SØ6.6X7 Traumatic subarachnoid hemorrhage with loss of consciousness of any duration with death due to brain injury prior to regaining consciousness**

7th **SØ6.6X8 Traumatic subarachnoid hemorrhage with loss of consciousness of any duration with death due to other cause prior to regaining consciousness**

● 7th **S06.6XA Traumatic subarachnoid hemorrhage with loss of consciousness status unknown**
Traumatic subarachnoid hemorrhage NOS

2 7th **S06.6X9 Traumatic subarachnoid hemorrhage with loss of consciousness of unspecified duration** HCC ESR Q
~~Traumatic subarachnoid hemorrhage NOS~~

5th **S06.8 Other specified intracranial injuries**

6th **S06.81 Injury of right internal carotid artery, intracranial portion, not elsewhere classified**

2 7th **S06.810 Injury of right internal carotid artery, intracranial portion, not elsewhere classified without loss of consciousness** HCC ESR Q

2 7th **S06.811 Injury of right internal carotid artery, intracranial portion, not elsewhere classified with loss of consciousness of 30 minutes or less** HCC ESR Q
▶Injury of right internal carotid artery, intracranial portion, not elsewhere classified with brief loss of consciousness◀

2 7th **S06.812 Injury of right internal carotid artery, intracranial portion, not elsewhere classified with loss of consciousness of 31 minutes to 59 minutes** HCC ESR Q

2 7th **S06.813 Injury of right internal carotid artery, intracranial portion, not elsewhere classified with loss of consciousness of 1 hour to 5 hours 59 minutes** HCC ESR COM Q

2 7th **S06.814 Injury of right internal carotid artery, intracranial portion, not elsewhere classified with loss of consciousness of 6 hours to 24 hours** HCC ESR COM Q

2 7th **S06.815 Injury of right internal carotid artery, intracranial portion, not elsewhere classified with loss of consciousness greater than 24 hours with return to pre-existing conscious level** HCC ESR COM

2 7th **S06.816 Injury of right internal carotid artery, intracranial portion, not elsewhere classified with loss of consciousness greater than 24 hours without return to pre-existing conscious level with patient surviving** HCC ESR COM

7th **S06.817 Injury of right internal carotid artery, intracranial portion, not elsewhere classified with loss of consciousness of any duration with death due to brain injury prior to regaining consciousness**

7th **S06.818 Injury of right internal carotid artery, intracranial portion, not elsewhere classified with loss of consciousness of any duration with death due to other cause prior to regaining consciousness**

● 7th **S06.81A Injury of right internal carotid artery, intracranial portion, not elsewhere classified with loss of consciousness status unknown**
Injury of right internal carotid artery, intracranial portion, not elsewhere classified NOS

2 7th **S06.819 Injury of right internal carotid artery, intracranial portion, not elsewhere classified with loss of consciousness of unspecified duration** HCC ESR Q
~~Injury of right internal carotid artery, intracranial portion, not elsewhere classified NOS~~

6th **S06.82 Injury of left internal carotid artery, intracranial portion, not elsewhere classified**

2 7th **S06.820 Injury of left internal carotid artery, intracranial portion, not elsewhere classified without loss of consciousness** HCC ESR Q

2 7th **S06.821 Injury of left internal carotid artery, intracranial portion, not elsewhere classified with loss of consciousness of 30 minutes or less** HCC ESR Q
▶Injury of left internal carotid artery, intracranial portion, not elsewhere classified with brief loss of consciousness◀

2 7th **S06.822 Injury of left internal carotid artery, intracranial portion, not elsewhere classified with loss of consciousness of 31 minutes to 59 minutes** HCC ESR Q

2 7th **S06.823 Injury of left internal carotid artery, intracranial portion, not elsewhere classified with loss of consciousness of 1 hour to 5 hours 59 minutes** HCC ESR COM Q

2 7th **S06.824 Injury of left internal carotid artery, intracranial portion, not elsewhere classified with loss of consciousness of 6 hours to 24 hours** HCC ESR COM Q

2 7th **S06.825 Injury of left internal carotid artery, intracranial portion, not elsewhere classified with loss of consciousness greater than 24 hours with return to pre-existing conscious level** HCC ESR COM

2 7th **S06.826 Injury of left internal carotid artery, intracranial portion, not elsewhere classified with loss of consciousness greater than 24 hours without return to pre-existing conscious level with patient surviving** HCC ESR COM

7th **S06.827 Injury of left internal carotid artery, intracranial portion, not elsewhere classified with loss of consciousness of any duration with death due to brain injury prior to regaining consciousness**

7th **S06.828 Injury of left internal carotid artery, intracranial portion, not elsewhere classified with loss of consciousness of any duration with death due to other cause prior to regaining consciousness**

● 7th **S06.82A Injury of left internal carotid artery, intracranial portion, not elsewhere classified with loss of consciousness status unknown**
Injury of left internal carotid artery, intracranial portion, not elsewhere classified NOS

2 7th **S06.829 Injury of left internal carotid artery, intracranial portion, not elsewhere classified with loss of consciousness of unspecified duration** HCC ESR Q
~~Injury of left internal carotid artery, intracranial portion, not elsewhere classified NOS~~

● 6th **S06.8A Primary blast injury of brain, not elsewhere classified**
Code also, if applicable, focal traumatic brain injury (S06.3-)
EXCLUDES 2 *traumatic cerebral edema (S06.1)*

● 7th **S06.8A0 Primary blast injury of brain, not elsewhere classified without loss of consciousness**

● 7th **S06.8A1 Primary blast injury of brain, not elsewhere classified with loss of consciousness of 30 minutes or less**
Primary blast injury of brain, not elsewhere classified with brief loss of consciousness

● 7th **S06.8A2 Primary blast injury of brain, not elsewhere classified with loss of consciousness of 31 minutes to 59 minutes**

● 7th **S06.8A3 Primary blast injury of brain, not elsewhere classified with loss of consciousness of 1 hour to 5 hours 59 minutes**

● 7th **S06.8A4 Primary blast injury of brain, not elsewhere classified with loss of consciousness of 6 hours to 24 hours**

Chapter 19. Injury, Poisoning and Certain Other Consequences of External Causes

● 7th **S06.8A5 Primary blast injury of brain, not elsewhere classified with loss of consciousness greater than 24 hours with return to pre-existing conscious level**

● 7th **S06.8A6 Primary blast injury of brain, not elsewhere classified with loss of consciousness greater than 24 hours without return to pre-existing conscious level with patient surviving**

● 7th **S06.8A7 Primary blast injury of brain, not elsewhere classified with loss of consciousness of any duration with death due to brain injury prior to regaining consciousness**

● 7th **S06.8A8 Primary blast injury of brain, not elsewhere classified with loss of consciousness of any duration with death due to other cause prior to regaining consciousness**

● 7th **S06.8AA Primary blast injury of brain, not elsewhere classified with loss of consciousness status unknown**

Primary blast injury of brain NOS

● 7th **S06.8A9 Primary blast injury of brain, not elsewhere classified with loss of consciousness of unspecified duration**

6th **S06.89 Other specified intracranial injury**

EXCLUDES 1 *concussion (S06.0X-)*

2 7th **S06.890 Other specified intracranial injury without loss of consciousness** HCC ESR Q

2 7th **S06.891 Other specified intracranial injury with loss of consciousness of 30 minutes or less** HCC ESR Q

▶Other specified intracranial injury with brief loss of consciousness◀

2 7th **S06.892 Other specified intracranial injury with loss of consciousness of 31 minutes to 59 minutes** HCC ESR Q

2 7th **S06.893 Other specified intracranial injury with loss of consciousness of 1 hour to 5 hours 59 minutes** HCC ESR COM Q

2 7th **S06.894 Other specified intracranial injury with loss of consciousness of 6 hours to 24 hours** HCC ESR COM Q

2 7th **S06.895 Other specified intracranial injury with loss of consciousness greater than 24 hours with return to pre-existing conscious level** HCC ESR COM

2 7th **S06.896 Other specified intracranial injury with loss of consciousness greater than 24 hours without return to pre-existing conscious level with patient surviving** HCC ESR COM

7th **S06.897 Other specified intracranial injury with loss of consciousness of any duration with death due to brain injury prior to regaining consciousness**

7th **S06.898 Other specified intracranial injury with loss of consciousness of any duration with death due to other cause prior to regaining consciousness**

● 7th **S06.89A Other specified intracranial injury with loss of consciousness status unknown**

2 7th **S06.899 Other specified intracranial injury with loss of consciousness of unspecified duration** HCC ESR Q

5th **S06.9 Unspecified intracranial injury**

Brain injury NOS

Head injury NOS with loss of consciousness

Traumatic brain injury NOS

EXCLUDES 1 *conditions classifiable to S06.0- to S06.8- code to specified intracranial injury*

head injury NOS (S09.90)

AHA: 2020,3Q,46; 2020,2Q,31

6th **S06.9X Unspecified intracranial injury**

2 7th **S06.9X0 Unspecified intracranial injury without loss of consciousness** HCC ESR Q

2 7th **S06.9X1 Unspecified intracranial injury with loss of consciousness of 30 minutes or less** HCC ESR Q

▶Unspecified intracranial injury with brief loss of consciousness◀

2 7th **S06.9X2 Unspecified intracranial injury with loss of consciousness of 31 minutes to 59 minutes** HCC ESR Q

2 7th **S06.9X3 Unspecified intracranial injury with loss of consciousness of 1 hour to 5 hours 59 minutes** HCC ESR COM Q

2 7th **S06.9X4 Unspecified intracranial injury with loss of consciousness of 6 hours to 24 hours** HCC ESR COM Q

2 7th **S06.9X5 Unspecified intracranial injury with loss of consciousness greater than 24 hours with return to pre-existing conscious level** HCC ESR COM

2 7th **S06.9X6 Unspecified intracranial injury with loss of consciousness greater than 24 hours without return to pre-existing conscious level with patient surviving** HCC ESR COM

7th **S06.9X7 Unspecified intracranial injury with loss of consciousness of any duration with death due to brain injury prior to regaining consciousness**

7th **S06.9X8 Unspecified intracranial injury with loss of consciousness of any duration with death due to other cause prior to regaining consciousness**

● 7th **S06.9XA Unspecified intracranial injury with loss of consciousness status unknown**

2 7th **S06.9X9 Unspecified intracranial injury with loss of consciousness of unspecified duration** HCC ESR Q

5th **S06.A Traumatic brain compression and herniation**

Traumatic cerebral compression

Code first the underlying traumatic brain injury, such as:

- diffuse traumatic brain injury (S06.2-)
- focal traumatic brain injury (S06.3-)
- traumatic subdural hemorrhage (S06.5-)
- traumatic subarachnoid hemorrhage (S06.6-)

AHA: 2021,4Q,29

x7th **S06.A0 Traumatic brain compression without herniation** HCC ESR UPD

Traumatic brain compression NOS

Traumatic cerebral compression NOS

x7th **S06.A1 Traumatic brain compression with herniation** HCC ESR UPD

Traumatic brain herniation

Traumatic brainstem compression with herniation

Traumatic cerebellar compression with herniation

Traumatic cerebral compression with herniation

4th **S07 Crushing injury of head**

Use additional code for all associated injuries, such as:

- intracranial injuries (S06.-)
- skull fractures (S02.-)

The appropriate 7th character is to be added to each code from category S07.

A initial encounter
D subsequent encounter
S sequela

x7th **S07.0 Crushing injury of face**

x7th **S07.1 Crushing injury of skull**

x7th **S07.8 Crushing injury of other parts of head**

x7th **S07.9 Crushing injury of head, part unspecified**

4th **S08 Avulsion and traumatic amputation of part of head**

An amputation not identified as partial or complete should be coded to complete

The appropriate 7th character is to be added to each code from category S08.

A initial encounter
D subsequent encounter
S sequela

x7th **S08.0 Avulsion of scalp**

S08.1 Traumatic amputation of ear
S08.11 Complete traumatic amputation of ear
S08.111 Complete traumatic amputation of right ear
S08.112 Complete traumatic amputation of left ear
S08.119 Complete traumatic amputation of unspecified ear
S08.12 Partial traumatic amputation of ear
S08.121 Partial traumatic amputation of right ear
S08.122 Partial traumatic amputation of left ear
S08.129 Partial traumatic amputation of unspecified ear
S08.8 Traumatic amputation of other parts of head
S08.81 Traumatic amputation of nose
S08.811 Complete traumatic amputation of nose
S08.812 Partial traumatic amputation of nose
S08.89 Traumatic amputation of other parts of head

S09 Other and unspecified injuries of head

The appropriate 7th character is to be added to each code from category S09.
A initial encounter
D subsequent encounter
S sequela

S09.0 Injury of blood vessels of head, not elsewhere classified
EXCLUDES 1 *injury of cerebral blood vessels (S06.-)*
injury of precerebral blood vessels (S15.-)
S09.1 Injury of muscle and tendon of head
Code also any associated open wound (S01.-)
EXCLUDES 2 *sprain to joints and ligament of head (S03.9)*
S09.10 Unspecified injury of muscle and tendon of head
Injury of muscle and tendon of head NOS
S09.11 Strain of muscle and tendon of head Q
S09.12 Laceration of muscle and tendon of head
S09.19 Other specified injury of muscle and tendon of head Q
S09.2 Traumatic rupture of ear drum
EXCLUDES 1 *traumatic rupture of ear drum due to blast injury (S09.31-)*
S09.20 Traumatic rupture of unspecified ear drum
S09.21 Traumatic rupture of right ear drum
S09.22 Traumatic rupture of left ear drum
S09.3 Other specified and unspecified injury of middle and inner ear
EXCLUDES 1 *injury to ear NOS (S09.91-)*
EXCLUDES 2 *injury to external ear (S00.4-, S01.3-, S08.1-)*
S09.30 Unspecified injury of middle and inner ear
S09.301 Unspecified injury of right middle and inner ear
S09.302 Unspecified injury of left middle and inner ear
S09.309 Unspecified injury of unspecified middle and inner ear
S09.31 Primary blast injury of ear
Blast injury of ear NOS
S09.311 Primary blast injury of right ear
S09.312 Primary blast injury of left ear
S09.313 Primary blast injury of ear, bilateral
S09.319 Primary blast injury of unspecified ear
S09.39 Other specified injury of middle and inner ear
Secondary blast injury to ear
S09.391 Other specified injury of right middle and inner ear
S09.392 Other specified injury of left middle and inner ear
S09.399 Other specified injury of unspecified middle and inner ear
S09.8 Other specified injuries of head Q
S09.9 Unspecified injury of face and head
S09.90 Unspecified injury of head
Head injury NOS
EXCLUDES 1 *brain injury NOS (S06.9-)*
head injury NOS with loss of consciousness (S06.9-)
intracranial injury NOS (S06.9-)
S09.91 Unspecified injury of ear
Injury of ear NOS
S09.92 Unspecified injury of nose
Injury of nose NOS
S09.93 Unspecified injury of face
Injury of face NOS
AHA: 2019,2Q,23

Injuries to the neck (S10-S19)

INCLUDES injuries of nape
injuries of supraclavicular region
injuries of throat
EXCLUDES 2 *burns and corrosions (T20-T32)*
effects of foreign body in esophagus (T18.1)
effects of foreign body in larynx (T17.3)
effects of foreign body in pharynx (T17.2)
effects of foreign body in trachea (T17.4)
frostbite (T33-T34)
insect bite or sting, venomous (T63.4)

S10 Superficial injury of neck

The appropriate 7th character is to be added to each code from category S10.
A initial encounter
D subsequent encounter
S sequela

S10.0 Contusion of throat
Contusion of cervical esophagus
Contusion of larynx
Contusion of pharynx
Contusion of trachea
S10.1 Other and unspecified superficial injuries of throat
S10.10 Unspecified superficial injuries of throat
S10.11 Abrasion of throat
S10.12 Blister (nonthermal) of throat
S10.14 External constriction of part of throat
S10.15 Superficial foreign body of throat
Splinter in the throat
S10.16 Insect bite (nonvenomous) of throat
S10.17 Other superficial bite of throat
EXCLUDES 1 *open bite of throat (S11.85)*
S10.8 Superficial injury of other specified parts of neck
S10.80 Unspecified superficial injury of other specified part of neck
S10.81 Abrasion of other specified part of neck
S10.82 Blister (nonthermal) of other specified part of neck
S10.83 Contusion of other specified part of neck
S10.84 External constriction of other specified part of neck
S10.85 Superficial foreign body of other specified part of neck
Splinter in other specified part of neck
S10.86 Insect bite of other specified part of neck
S10.87 Other superficial bite of other specified part of neck
EXCLUDES 1 *open bite of other specified parts of neck (S11.85)*
S10.9 Superficial injury of unspecified part of neck
S10.90 Unspecified superficial injury of unspecified part of neck
S10.91 Abrasion of unspecified part of neck
S10.92 Blister (nonthermal) of unspecified part of neck
S10.93 Contusion of unspecified part of neck
S10.94 External constriction of unspecified part of neck
S10.95 Superficial foreign body of unspecified part of neck
S10.96 Insect bite of unspecified part of neck
S10.97 Other superficial bite of unspecified part of neck

S11 Open wound of neck

Code also any associated:
spinal cord injury (S14.0, S14.1-)
wound infection

EXCLUDES 2 *open fracture of vertebra (S12.- with 7th character B)*

The appropriate 7th character is to be added to each code from category S11.
A initial encounter
D subsequent encounter
S sequela

S11.0 Open wound of larynx and trachea

S11.01 Open wound of larynx
EXCLUDES 2 *open wound of vocal cord (S11.03)*
S11.011 Laceration without foreign body of larynx
S11.012 Laceration with foreign body of larynx
S11.013 Puncture wound without foreign body of larynx
S11.014 Puncture wound with foreign body of larynx
S11.015 Open bite of larynx
Bite of larynx NOS
S11.019 Unspecified open wound of larynx

S11.02 Open wound of trachea
Open wound of cervical trachea
Open wound of trachea NOS
EXCLUDES 2 *open wound of thoracic trachea (S27.5-)*
S11.021 Laceration without foreign body of trachea
S11.022 Laceration with foreign body of trachea
S11.023 Puncture wound without foreign body of trachea
S11.024 Puncture wound with foreign body of trachea
S11.025 Open bite of trachea
Bite of trachea NOS
S11.029 Unspecified open wound of trachea

S11.03 Open wound of vocal cord
S11.031 Laceration without foreign body of vocal cord
S11.032 Laceration with foreign body of vocal cord
S11.033 Puncture wound without foreign body of vocal cord
S11.034 Puncture wound with foreign body of vocal cord
S11.035 Open bite of vocal cord
Bite of vocal cord NOS
S11.039 Unspecified open wound of vocal cord

S11.1 Open wound of thyroid gland
S11.10 Unspecified open wound of thyroid gland
S11.11 Laceration without foreign body of thyroid gland
S11.12 Laceration with foreign body of thyroid gland
S11.13 Puncture wound without foreign body of thyroid gland
S11.14 Puncture wound with foreign body of thyroid gland
S11.15 Open bite of thyroid gland
Bite of thyroid gland NOS

S11.2 Open wound of pharynx and cervical esophagus
EXCLUDES 1 *open wound of esophagus NOS (S27.8-)*
S11.20 Unspecified open wound of pharynx and cervical esophagus
S11.21 Laceration without foreign body of pharynx and cervical esophagus
S11.22 Laceration with foreign body of pharynx and cervical esophagus
S11.23 Puncture wound without foreign body of pharynx and cervical esophagus
S11.24 Puncture wound with foreign body of pharynx and cervical esophagus
S11.25 Open bite of pharynx and cervical esophagus
Bite of pharynx and cervical esophagus NOS

S11.8 Open wound of other specified parts of neck
S11.80 Unspecified open wound of other specified part of neck
S11.81 Laceration without foreign body of other specified part of neck
S11.82 Laceration with foreign body of other specified part of neck
S11.83 Puncture wound without foreign body of other specified part of neck
S11.84 Puncture wound with foreign body of other specified part of neck
S11.85 Open bite of other specified part of neck
Bite of other specified part of neck NOS
EXCLUDES 1 *superficial bite of other specified part of neck (S10.87)*
S11.89 Other open wound of other specified part of neck

S11.9 Open wound of unspecified part of neck
S11.90 Unspecified open wound of unspecified part of neck
S11.91 Laceration without foreign body of unspecified part of neck
S11.92 Laceration with foreign body of unspecified part of neck
S11.93 Puncture wound without foreign body of unspecified part of neck
S11.94 Puncture wound with foreign body of unspecified part of neck
S11.95 Open bite of unspecified part of neck
Bite of neck NOS
EXCLUDES 1 *superficial bite of neck (S10.97)*

S12 Fracture of cervical vertebra and other parts of neck

NOTE A fracture not indicated as displaced or nondisplaced should be coded to displaced.
A fracture not indicated as open or closed should be coded to closed.

INCLUDES fracture of cervical neural arch
fracture of cervical spine
fracture of cervical spinous process
fracture of cervical transverse process
fracture of cervical vertebral arch
fracture of neck

Code first any associated cervical spinal cord injury (S14.0, S14.1-)

AHA: 2021,1Q,6; 2018,2Q,12; 2015,3Q,37-39

The appropriate 7th character is to be added to all codes from subcategories S12.0-S12.6.
A initial encounter for closed fracture
B initial encounter for open fracture
D subsequent encounter for fracture with routine healing
G subsequent encounter for fracture with delayed healing
K subsequent encounter for fracture with nonunion
S sequela

S12.0 Fracture of first cervical vertebra
Atlas
S12.00 Unspecified fracture of first cervical vertebra
1 **S12.000 Unspecified displaced fracture of first cervical vertebra** HCC ESR COM Q
1 **S12.001 Unspecified nondisplaced fracture of first cervical vertebra** HCC ESR COM Q
1 **S12.01 Stable burst fracture of first cervical vertebra** HCC ESR COM Q
1 **S12.02 Unstable burst fracture of first cervical vertebra** HCC ESR COM Q
S12.03 Posterior arch fracture of first cervical vertebra
1 **S12.030 Displaced posterior arch fracture of first cervical vertebra** HCC ESR COM Q
1 **S12.031 Nondisplaced posterior arch fracture of first cervical vertebra** HCC ESR COM Q
S12.04 Lateral mass fracture of first cervical vertebra
1 **S12.040 Displaced lateral mass fracture of first cervical vertebra** HCC ESR COM Q
1 **S12.041 Nondisplaced lateral mass fracture of first cervical vertebra** HCC ESR COM Q
S12.09 Other fracture of first cervical vertebra
1 **S12.090 Other displaced fracture of first cervical vertebra** HCC ESR COM Q
1 **S12.091 Other nondisplaced fracture of first cervical vertebra** HCC ESR COM Q

✓5th **S12.1 Fracture of second cervical vertebra**
Axis

✓6th **S12.10 Unspecified fracture of second cervical vertebra**

1 ✓7th **S12.100 Unspecified displaced fracture of second cervical vertebra** HCC ESR COM Q

1 ✓7th **S12.101 Unspecified nondisplaced fracture of second cervical vertebra** HCC ESR COM Q

✓6th **S12.11 Type II dens fracture**

✓7th **S12.110 Anterior displaced Type II dens fracture** HCC ESR COM Q

1 ✓7th **S12.111 Posterior displaced Type II dens fracture** HCC ESR COM Q

1 ✓7th **S12.112 Nondisplaced Type II dens fracture** HCC ESR COM Q

✓6th **S12.12 Other dens fracture**

✓7th **S12.120 Other displaced dens fracture** HCC ESR COM Q

1 ✓7th **S12.121 Other nondisplaced dens fracture** HCC ESR COM Q

✓6th **S12.13 Unspecified traumatic spondylolisthesis of second cervical vertebra**

1 ✓7th **S12.130 Unspecified traumatic displaced spondylolisthesis of second cervical vertebra** HCC ESR COM Q

1 ✓7th **S12.131 Unspecified traumatic nondisplaced spondylolisthesis of second cervical vertebra** HCC ESR COM Q

1 ✓x7th **S12.14 Type III traumatic spondylolisthesis of second cervical vertebra** HCC ESR COM Q

✓6th **S12.15 Other traumatic spondylolisthesis of second cervical vertebra**

1 ✓7th **S12.150 Other traumatic displaced spondylolisthesis of second cervical vertebra** HCC ESR COM Q

1 ✓7th **S12.151 Other traumatic nondisplaced spondylolisthesis of second cervical vertebra** HCC ESR COM Q

✓6th **S12.19 Other fracture of second cervical vertebra**

1 ✓7th **S12.190 Other displaced fracture of second cervical vertebra** HCC ESR COM Q

1 ✓7th **S12.191 Other nondisplaced fracture of second cervical vertebra** HCC ESR COM Q

✓5th **S12.2 Fracture of third cervical vertebra**

✓6th **S12.20 Unspecified fracture of third cervical vertebra**

1 ✓7th **S12.200 Unspecified displaced fracture of third cervical vertebra** HCC ESR COM Q

1 ✓7th **S12.201 Unspecified nondisplaced fracture of third cervical vertebra** HCC ESR COM Q

✓6th **S12.23 Unspecified traumatic spondylolisthesis of third cervical vertebra**

1 ✓7th **S12.230 Unspecified traumatic displaced spondylolisthesis of third cervical vertebra** HCC ESR COM Q

1 ✓7th **S12.231 Unspecified traumatic nondisplaced spondylolisthesis of third cervical vertebra** HCC ESR COM Q

1 ✓x7th **S12.24 Type III traumatic spondylolisthesis of third cervical vertebra** HCC ESR COM Q

✓6th **S12.25 Other traumatic spondylolisthesis of third cervical vertebra**

1 ✓7th **S12.250 Other traumatic displaced spondylolisthesis of third cervical vertebra** HCC ESR COM Q

1 ✓7th **S12.251 Other traumatic nondisplaced spondylolisthesis of third cervical vertebra** HCC ESR COM Q

✓6th **S12.29 Other fracture of third cervical vertebra**

1 ✓7th **S12.290 Other displaced fracture of third cervical vertebra** HCC ESR COM Q

1 ✓7th **S12.291 Other nondisplaced fracture of third cervical vertebra** HCC ESR COM Q

✓5th **S12.3 Fracture of fourth cervical vertebra**

✓6th **S12.30 Unspecified fracture of fourth cervical vertebra**

1 ✓7th **S12.300 Unspecified displaced fracture of fourth cervical vertebra** HCC ESR COM Q

1 ✓7th **S12.301 Unspecified nondisplaced fracture of fourth cervical vertebra** HCC ESR COM Q

✓6th **S12.33 Unspecified traumatic spondylolisthesis of fourth cervical vertebra**

1 ✓7th **S12.330 Unspecified traumatic displaced spondylolisthesis of fourth cervical vertebra** HCC ESR COM Q

1 ✓7th **S12.331 Unspecified traumatic nondisplaced spondylolisthesis of fourth cervical vertebra** HCC ESR COM Q

1 ✓x7th **S12.34 Type III traumatic spondylolisthesis of fourth cervical vertebra** HCC ESR COM Q

✓6th **S12.35 Other traumatic spondylolisthesis of fourth cervical vertebra**

1 ✓7th **S12.350 Other traumatic displaced spondylolisthesis of fourth cervical vertebra** HCC ESR COM Q

1 ✓7th **S12.351 Other traumatic nondisplaced spondylolisthesis of fourth cervical vertebra** HCC ESR COM Q

✓6th **S12.39 Other fracture of fourth cervical vertebra**

1 ✓7th **S12.390 Other displaced fracture of fourth cervical vertebra** HCC ESR COM Q

1 ✓7th **S12.391 Other nondisplaced fracture of fourth cervical vertebra** HCC ESR COM Q

✓5th **S12.4 Fracture of fifth cervical vertebra**

✓6th **S12.40 Unspecified fracture of fifth cervical vertebra**

1 ✓7th **S12.400 Unspecified displaced fracture of fifth cervical vertebra** HCC ESR COM Q

1 ✓7th **S12.401 Unspecified nondisplaced fracture of fifth cervical vertebra** HCC ESR COM Q

✓6th **S12.43 Unspecified traumatic spondylolisthesis of fifth cervical vertebra**

1 ✓7th **S12.430 Unspecified traumatic displaced spondylolisthesis of fifth cervical vertebra** HCC ESR COM Q

1 ✓7th **S12.431 Unspecified traumatic nondisplaced spondylolisthesis of fifth cervical vertebra** HCC ESR COM Q

1 ✓x7th **S12.44 Type III traumatic spondylolisthesis of fifth cervical vertebra** HCC ESR COM Q

✓6th **S12.45 Other traumatic spondylolisthesis of fifth cervical vertebra**

1 ✓7th **S12.450 Other traumatic displaced spondylolisthesis of fifth cervical vertebra** HCC ESR COM Q

1 ✓7th **S12.451 Other traumatic nondisplaced spondylolisthesis of fifth cervical vertebra** HCC ESR COM Q

✓6th **S12.49 Other fracture of fifth cervical vertebra**

1 ✓7th **S12.490 Other displaced fracture of fifth cervical vertebra** HCC ESR COM Q

1 ✓7th **S12.491 Other nondisplaced fracture of fifth cervical vertebra** HCC ESR COM Q

✓5th **S12.5 Fracture of sixth cervical vertebra**

✓6th **S12.50 Unspecified fracture of sixth cervical vertebra**

1 ✓7th **S12.500 Unspecified displaced fracture of sixth cervical vertebra** HCC ESR COM Q

1 ✓7th **S12.501 Unspecified nondisplaced fracture of sixth cervical vertebra** HCC ESR COM Q

✓6th **S12.53 Unspecified traumatic spondylolisthesis of sixth cervical vertebra**

1 ✓7th **S12.530 Unspecified traumatic displaced spondylolisthesis of sixth cervical vertebra** HCC ESR COM Q

1 ✓7th **S12.531 Unspecified traumatic nondisplaced spondylolisthesis of sixth cervical vertebra** HCC ESR COM Q

1 ✓x7th **S12.54 Type III traumatic spondylolisthesis of sixth cervical vertebra** HCC ESR COM Q

✓6th **S12.55 Other traumatic spondylolisthesis of sixth cervical vertebra**

1 ✓7th **S12.550 Other traumatic displaced spondylolisthesis of sixth cervical vertebra** HCC ESR COM Q

1 ✓7th **S12.551 Other traumatic nondisplaced spondylolisthesis of sixth cervical vertebra** HCC ESR COM Q

✓6th **S12.59 Other fracture of sixth cervical vertebra**

1 ✓7th **S12.590 Other displaced fracture of sixth cervical vertebra** HCC ESR COM Q

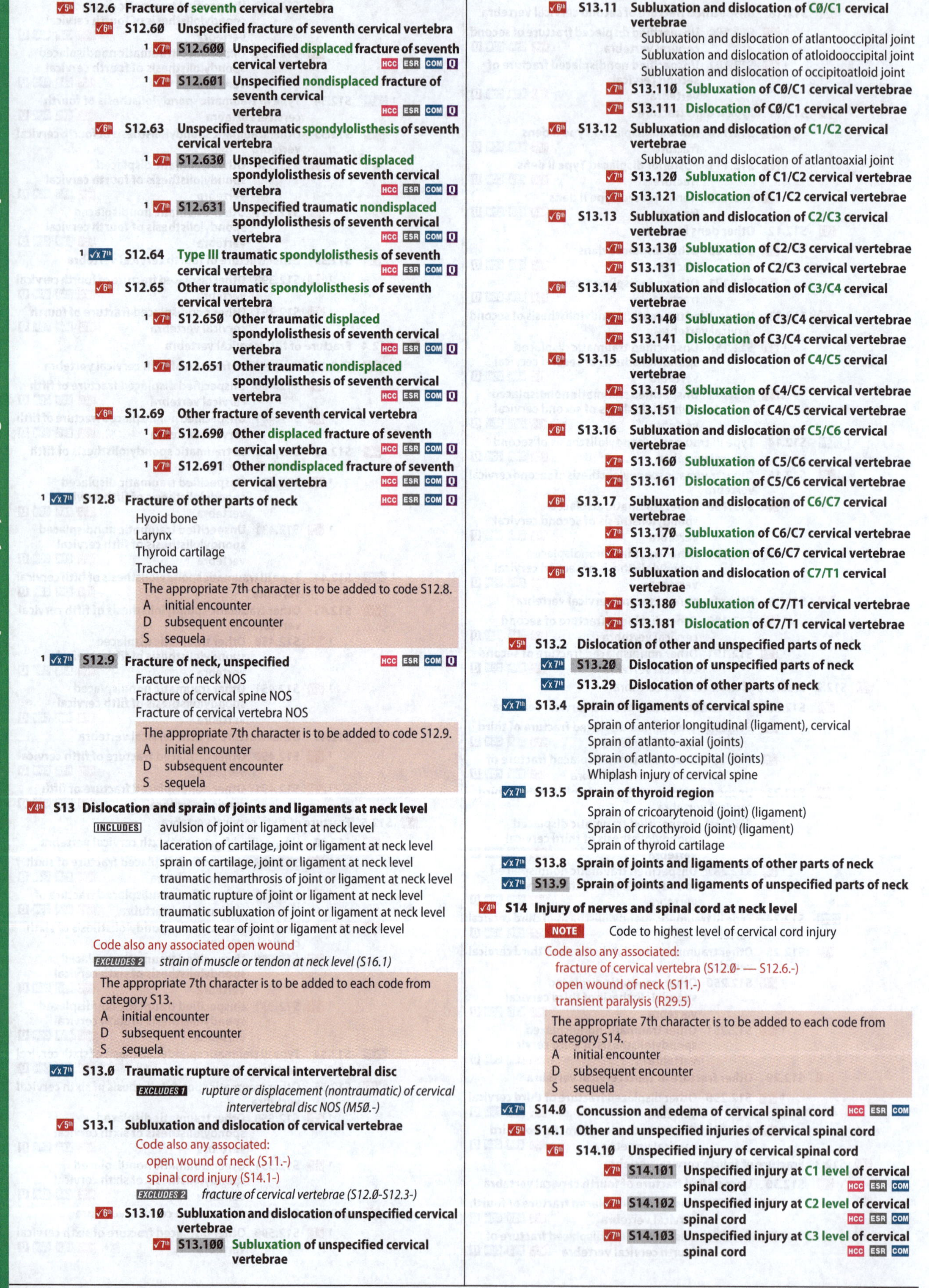

1 ✓7th **S12.591 Other nondisplaced fracture of sixth cervical vertebra** HCC ESR COM Q

✓5th **S12.6 Fracture of seventh cervical vertebra**

✓6th **S12.6Ø Unspecified fracture of seventh cervical vertebra**

1 ✓7th **S12.6ØØ Unspecified displaced fracture of seventh cervical vertebra** HCC ESR COM Q

1 ✓7th **S12.6Ø1 Unspecified nondisplaced fracture of seventh cervical vertebra** HCC ESR COM Q

✓6th **S12.63 Unspecified traumatic spondylolisthesis of seventh cervical vertebra**

1 ✓7th **S12.63Ø Unspecified traumatic displaced spondylolisthesis of seventh cervical vertebra** HCC ESR COM Q

1 ✓7th **S12.631 Unspecified traumatic nondisplaced spondylolisthesis of seventh cervical vertebra** HCC ESR COM Q

1 ✓x7th **S12.64 Type III traumatic spondylolisthesis of seventh cervical vertebra** HCC ESR COM Q

✓6th **S12.65 Other traumatic spondylolisthesis of seventh cervical vertebra**

1 ✓7th **S12.65Ø Other traumatic displaced spondylolisthesis of seventh cervical vertebra** HCC ESR COM Q

1 ✓7th **S12.651 Other traumatic nondisplaced spondylolisthesis of seventh cervical vertebra** HCC ESR COM Q

✓6th **S12.69 Other fracture of seventh cervical vertebra**

1 ✓7th **S12.69Ø Other displaced fracture of seventh cervical vertebra** HCC ESR COM Q

1 ✓7th **S12.691 Other nondisplaced fracture of seventh cervical vertebra** HCC ESR COM Q

1 ✓x7th **S12.8 Fracture of other parts of neck** HCC ESR COM Q

Hyoid bone
Larynx
Thyroid cartilage
Trachea

The appropriate 7th character is to be added to code S12.8.
A initial encounter
D subsequent encounter
S sequela

1 ✓x7th **S12.9 Fracture of neck, unspecified** HCC ESR COM Q

Fracture of neck NOS
Fracture of cervical spine NOS
Fracture of cervical vertebra NOS

The appropriate 7th character is to be added to code S12.9.
A initial encounter
D subsequent encounter
S sequela

✓4th **S13 Dislocation and sprain of joints and ligaments at neck level**

INCLUDES avulsion of joint or ligament at neck level
laceration of cartilage, joint or ligament at neck level
sprain of cartilage, joint or ligament at neck level
traumatic hemarthrosis of joint or ligament at neck level
traumatic rupture of joint or ligament at neck level
traumatic subluxation of joint or ligament at neck level
traumatic tear of joint or ligament at neck level

Code also any associated open wound

EXCLUDES 2 *strain of muscle or tendon at neck level (S16.1)*

The appropriate 7th character is to be added to each code from category S13.
A initial encounter
D subsequent encounter
S sequela

✓x7th **S13.Ø Traumatic rupture of cervical intervertebral disc**

EXCLUDES 1 *rupture or displacement (nontraumatic) of cervical intervertebral disc NOS (M5Ø.-)*

✓5th **S13.1 Subluxation and dislocation of cervical vertebrae**

Code also any associated:
open wound of neck (S11.-)
spinal cord injury (S14.1-)

EXCLUDES 2 *fracture of cervical vertebrae (S12.Ø-S12.3-)*

✓6th **S13.1Ø Subluxation and dislocation of unspecified cervical vertebrae**

✓7th **S13.1ØØ Subluxation of unspecified cervical vertebrae**

✓7th **S13.1Ø1 Dislocation of unspecified cervical vertebrae**

✓6th **S13.11 Subluxation and dislocation of CØ/C1 cervical vertebrae**

Subluxation and dislocation of atlantooccipital joint
Subluxation and dislocation of atloidooccipital joint
Subluxation and dislocation of occipitoatloid joint

✓7th **S13.11Ø Subluxation of CØ/C1 cervical vertebrae**

✓7th **S13.111 Dislocation of CØ/C1 cervical vertebrae**

✓6th **S13.12 Subluxation and dislocation of C1/C2 cervical vertebrae**

Subluxation and dislocation of atlantoaxial joint

✓7th **S13.12Ø Subluxation of C1/C2 cervical vertebrae**

✓7th **S13.121 Dislocation of C1/C2 cervical vertebrae**

✓6th **S13.13 Subluxation and dislocation of C2/C3 cervical vertebrae**

✓7th **S13.13Ø Subluxation of C2/C3 cervical vertebrae**

✓7th **S13.131 Dislocation of C2/C3 cervical vertebrae**

✓6th **S13.14 Subluxation and dislocation of C3/C4 cervical vertebrae**

✓7th **S13.14Ø Subluxation of C3/C4 cervical vertebrae**

✓7th **S13.141 Dislocation of C3/C4 cervical vertebrae**

✓6th **S13.15 Subluxation and dislocation of C4/C5 cervical vertebrae**

✓7th **S13.15Ø Subluxation of C4/C5 cervical vertebrae**

✓7th **S13.151 Dislocation of C4/C5 cervical vertebrae**

✓6th **S13.16 Subluxation and dislocation of C5/C6 cervical vertebrae**

✓7th **S13.16Ø Subluxation of C5/C6 cervical vertebrae**

✓7th **S13.161 Dislocation of C5/C6 cervical vertebrae**

✓6th **S13.17 Subluxation and dislocation of C6/C7 cervical vertebrae**

✓7th **S13.17Ø Subluxation of C6/C7 cervical vertebrae**

✓7th **S13.171 Dislocation of C6/C7 cervical vertebrae**

✓6th **S13.18 Subluxation and dislocation of C7/T1 cervical vertebrae**

✓7th **S13.18Ø Subluxation of C7/T1 cervical vertebrae**

✓7th **S13.181 Dislocation of C7/T1 cervical vertebrae**

✓5th **S13.2 Dislocation of other and unspecified parts of neck**

✓x7th **S13.2Ø Dislocation of unspecified parts of neck**

✓x7th **S13.29 Dislocation of other parts of neck**

✓x7th **S13.4 Sprain of ligaments of cervical spine**

Sprain of anterior longitudinal (ligament), cervical
Sprain of atlanto-axial (joints)
Sprain of atlanto-occipital (joints)
Whiplash injury of cervical spine

✓x7th **S13.5 Sprain of thyroid region**

Sprain of cricoarytenoid (joint) (ligament)
Sprain of cricothyroid (joint) (ligament)
Sprain of thyroid cartilage

✓x7th **S13.8 Sprain of joints and ligaments of other parts of neck**

✓x7th **S13.9 Sprain of joints and ligaments of unspecified parts of neck**

✓4th **S14 Injury of nerves and spinal cord at neck level**

NOTE Code to highest level of cervical cord injury

Code also any associated:
fracture of cervical vertebra (S12.Ø- — S12.6.-)
open wound of neck (S11.-)
transient paralysis (R29.5)

The appropriate 7th character is to be added to each code from category S14.
A initial encounter
D subsequent encounter
S sequela

✓x7th **S14.Ø Concussion and edema of cervical spinal cord** HCC ESR COM

✓5th **S14.1 Other and unspecified injuries of cervical spinal cord**

✓6th **S14.1Ø Unspecified injury of cervical spinal cord**

✓7th **S14.1Ø1 Unspecified injury at C1 level of cervical spinal cord** HCC ESR COM

✓7th **S14.1Ø2 Unspecified injury at C2 level of cervical spinal cord** HCC ESR COM

✓7th **S14.1Ø3 Unspecified injury at C3 level of cervical spinal cord** HCC ESR COM

S14.104 Unspecified injury at C4 level of cervical spinal cord HCC ESR COM
S14.105 Unspecified injury at C5 level of cervical spinal cord HCC ESR COM
S14.106 Unspecified injury at C6 level of cervical spinal cord HCC ESR COM
S14.107 Unspecified injury at C7 level of cervical spinal cord HCC ESR COM
S14.108 Unspecified injury at C8 level of cervical spinal cord HCC ESR COM
S14.109 Unspecified injury at unspecified level of cervical spinal cord HCC ESR COM
Injury of cervical spinal cord NOS

S14.11 Complete lesion of cervical spinal cord
S14.111 Complete lesion at C1 level of cervical spinal cord HCC ESR COM
S14.112 Complete lesion at C2 level of cervical spinal cord HCC ESR COM
S14.113 Complete lesion at C3 level of cervical spinal cord HCC ESR COM
S14.114 Complete lesion at C4 level of cervical spinal cord HCC ESR COM
S14.115 Complete lesion at C5 level of cervical spinal cord HCC ESR COM
S14.116 Complete lesion at C6 level of cervical spinal cord HCC ESR COM
S14.117 Complete lesion at C7 level of cervical spinal cord HCC ESR COM
S14.118 Complete lesion at C8 level of cervical spinal cord HCC ESR COM
S14.119 Complete lesion at unspecified level of cervical spinal cord HCC ESR COM

S14.12 Central cord syndrome of cervical spinal cord
S14.121 Central cord syndrome at C1 level of cervical spinal cord HCC ESR COM
S14.122 Central cord syndrome at C2 level of cervical spinal cord HCC ESR COM
S14.123 Central cord syndrome at C3 level of cervical spinal cord HCC ESR COM
S14.124 Central cord syndrome at C4 level of cervical spinal cord HCC ESR COM
S14.125 Central cord syndrome at C5 level of cervical spinal cord HCC ESR COM
S14.126 Central cord syndrome at C6 level of cervical spinal cord HCC ESR COM
S14.127 Central cord syndrome at C7 level of cervical spinal cord HCC ESR COM
S14.128 Central cord syndrome at C8 level of cervical spinal cord HCC ESR COM
S14.129 Central cord syndrome at unspecified level of cervical spinal cord HCC ESR COM

S14.13 Anterior cord syndrome of cervical spinal cord
S14.131 Anterior cord syndrome at C1 level of cervical spinal cord HCC ESR COM
S14.132 Anterior cord syndrome at C2 level of cervical spinal cord HCC ESR COM
S14.133 Anterior cord syndrome at C3 level of cervical spinal cord HCC ESR COM
S14.134 Anterior cord syndrome at C4 level of cervical spinal cord HCC ESR COM
S14.135 Anterior cord syndrome at C5 level of cervical spinal cord HCC ESR COM
S14.136 Anterior cord syndrome at C6 level of cervical spinal cord HCC ESR COM
S14.137 Anterior cord syndrome at C7 level of cervical spinal cord HCC ESR COM
S14.138 Anterior cord syndrome at C8 level of cervical spinal cord HCC ESR COM
S14.139 Anterior cord syndrome at unspecified level of cervical spinal cord HCC ESR COM

S14.14 Brown-Séquard syndrome of cervical spinal cord
S14.141 Brown-Séquard syndrome at C1 level of cervical spinal cord HCC ESR COM
S14.142 Brown-Séquard syndrome at C2 level of cervical spinal cord HCC ESR COM
S14.143 Brown-Séquard syndrome at C3 level of cervical spinal cord HCC ESR COM
S14.144 Brown-Séquard syndrome at C4 level of cervical spinal cord HCC ESR COM
S14.145 Brown-Séquard syndrome at C5 level of cervical spinal cord HCC ESR COM
S14.146 Brown-Séquard syndrome at C6 level of cervical spinal cord HCC ESR COM
S14.147 Brown-Séquard syndrome at C7 level of cervical spinal cord HCC ESR COM
S14.148 Brown-Séquard syndrome at C8 level of cervical spinal cord HCC ESR COM
S14.149 Brown-Séquard syndrome at unspecified level of cervical spinal cord HCC ESR COM

S14.15 Other incomplete lesions of cervical spinal cord
Incomplete lesion of cervical spinal cord NOS
Posterior cord syndrome of cervical spinal cord
S14.151 Other incomplete lesion at C1 level of cervical spinal cord HCC ESR COM
S14.152 Other incomplete lesion at C2 level of cervical spinal cord HCC ESR COM
S14.153 Other incomplete lesion at C3 level of cervical spinal cord HCC ESR COM
S14.154 Other incomplete lesion at C4 level of cervical spinal cord HCC ESR COM
S14.155 Other incomplete lesion at C5 level of cervical spinal cord HCC ESR COM
S14.156 Other incomplete lesion at C6 level of cervical spinal cord HCC ESR COM
S14.157 Other incomplete lesion at C7 level of cervical spinal cord HCC ESR COM
S14.158 Other incomplete lesion at C8 level of cervical spinal cord HCC ESR COM
S14.159 Other incomplete lesion at unspecified level of cervical spinal cord HCC ESR COM

S14.2 Injury of nerve root of cervical spine
S14.3 Injury of brachial plexus
S14.4 Injury of peripheral nerves of neck
S14.5 Injury of cervical sympathetic nerves
S14.8 Injury of other specified nerves of neck
S14.9 Injury of unspecified nerves of neck

S15 Injury of blood vessels at neck level

Code also any associated open wound (S11.-)

The appropriate 7th character is to be added to each code from category S15.
A initial encounter
D subsequent encounter
S sequela

S15.0 Injury of carotid artery of neck
Injury of carotid artery (common) (external) (internal, extracranial portion)
Injury of carotid artery NOS
EXCLUDES 1 *injury of internal carotid artery, intracranial portion (S06.8)*

S15.00 Unspecified injury of carotid artery
S15.001 Unspecified injury of right carotid artery
S15.002 Unspecified injury of left carotid artery
S15.009 Unspecified injury of unspecified carotid artery

S15.01 Minor laceration of carotid artery
Incomplete transection of carotid artery
Laceration of carotid artery NOS
Superficial laceration of carotid artery
S15.011 Minor laceration of right carotid artery
S15.012 Minor laceration of left carotid artery
S15.019 Minor laceration of unspecified carotid artery

S15.02 Major laceration of carotid artery
Complete transection of carotid artery
Traumatic rupture of carotid artery
S15.021 Major laceration of right carotid artery
S15.022 Major laceration of left carotid artery
S15.029 Major laceration of unspecified carotid artery

Additional Character Required · Placeholder Alert · Manifestation · Unspecified Dx · QPP · UPD Unacceptable PDx

6th S15.09 Other specified injury of carotid artery
7th S15.091 Other specified injury of right carotid artery
7th S15.092 Other specified injury of left carotid artery
7th S15.099 Other specified injury of unspecified carotid artery

5th S15.1 Injury of vertebral artery
6th S15.10 Unspecified injury of vertebral artery
7th S15.101 Unspecified injury of right vertebral artery
7th S15.102 Unspecified injury of left vertebral artery
7th S15.109 Unspecified injury of unspecified vertebral artery

6th S15.11 Minor laceration of vertebral artery
Incomplete transection of vertebral artery
Laceration of vertebral artery NOS
Superficial laceration of vertebral artery
7th S15.111 Minor laceration of right vertebral artery
7th S15.112 Minor laceration of left vertebral artery
7th S15.119 Minor laceration of unspecified vertebral artery

6th S15.12 Major laceration of vertebral artery
Complete transection of vertebral artery
Traumatic rupture of vertebral artery
7th S15.121 Major laceration of right vertebral artery
7th S15.122 Major laceration of left vertebral artery
7th S15.129 Major laceration of unspecified vertebral artery

6th S15.19 Other specified injury of vertebral artery
7th S15.191 Other specified injury of right vertebral artery
7th S15.192 Other specified injury of left vertebral artery
7th S15.199 Other specified injury of unspecified vertebral artery

5th S15.2 Injury of external jugular vein
6th S15.20 Unspecified injury of external jugular vein
7th S15.201 Unspecified injury of right external jugular vein
7th S15.202 Unspecified injury of left external jugular vein
7th S15.209 Unspecified injury of unspecified external jugular vein

6th S15.21 Minor laceration of external jugular vein
Incomplete transection of external jugular vein
Laceration of external jugular vein NOS
Superficial laceration of external jugular vein
7th S15.211 Minor laceration of right external jugular vein
7th S15.212 Minor laceration of left external jugular vein
7th S15.219 Minor laceration of unspecified external jugular vein

6th S15.22 Major laceration of external jugular vein
Complete transection of external jugular vein
Traumatic rupture of external jugular vein
7th S15.221 Major laceration of right external jugular vein
7th S15.222 Major laceration of left external jugular vein
7th S15.229 Major laceration of unspecified external jugular vein

6th S15.29 Other specified injury of external jugular vein
7th S15.291 Other specified injury of right external jugular vein
7th S15.292 Other specified injury of left external jugular vein
7th S15.299 Other specified injury of unspecified external jugular vein

5th S15.3 Injury of internal jugular vein
6th S15.30 Unspecified injury of internal jugular vein
7th S15.301 Unspecified injury of right internal jugular vein
7th S15.302 Unspecified injury of left internal jugular vein
7th S15.309 Unspecified injury of unspecified internal jugular vein

6th S15.31 Minor laceration of internal jugular vein
Incomplete transection of internal jugular vein
Laceration of internal jugular vein NOS
Superficial laceration of internal jugular vein
7th S15.311 Minor laceration of right internal jugular vein
7th S15.312 Minor laceration of left internal jugular vein
7th S15.319 Minor laceration of unspecified internal jugular vein

6th S15.32 Major laceration of internal jugular vein
Complete transection of internal jugular vein
Traumatic rupture of internal jugular vein
7th S15.321 Major laceration of right internal jugular vein
7th S15.322 Major laceration of left internal jugular vein
7th S15.329 Major laceration of unspecified internal jugular vein

6th S15.39 Other specified injury of internal jugular vein
7th S15.391 Other specified injury of right internal jugular vein
7th S15.392 Other specified injury of left internal jugular vein
7th S15.399 Other specified injury of unspecified internal jugular vein

x7th S15.8 Injury of other specified blood vessels at neck level
x7th S15.9 Injury of unspecified blood vessel at neck level

4th S16 Injury of muscle, fascia and tendon at neck level
Code also any associated open wound (S11.-)
EXCLUDES 2 *sprain of joint or ligament at neck level (S13.9)*

The appropriate 7th character is to be added to each code from category S16.
A initial encounter
D subsequent encounter
S sequela

x7th S16.1 Strain of muscle, fascia and tendon at neck level
x7th S16.2 Laceration of muscle, fascia and tendon at neck level
x7th S16.8 Other specified injury of muscle, fascia and tendon at neck level
x7th S16.9 Unspecified injury of muscle, fascia and tendon at neck level

4th S17 Crushing injury of neck
Use additional code for all associated injuries, such as:
injury of blood vessels (S15.-)
open wound of neck (S11.-)
spinal cord injury (S14.0, S14.1-)
vertebral fracture (S12.0- — S12.3-)

The appropriate 7th character is to be added to each code from category S17.
A initial encounter
D subsequent encounter
S sequela

x7th S17.0 Crushing injury of larynx and trachea
x7th S17.8 Crushing injury of other specified parts of neck
x7th S17.9 Crushing injury of neck, part unspecified

4th S19 Other specified and unspecified injuries of neck

The appropriate 7th character is to be added to each code from category S19.
A initial encounter
D subsequent encounter
S sequela

5th S19.8 Other specified injuries of neck
x7th S19.80 Other specified injuries of unspecified part of neck
x7th S19.81 Other specified injuries of larynx
x7th S19.82 Other specified injuries of cervical trachea
EXCLUDES 2 *other specified injury of thoracic trachea (S27.5-)*
x7th S19.83 Other specified injuries of vocal cord
x7th S19.84 Other specified injuries of thyroid gland
x7th S19.85 Other specified injuries of pharynx and cervical esophagus
AHA: 2022,1Q,27

√x7th **S19.89 Other specified injuries of other specified part of neck**

√x7th **S19.9 Unspecified injury of neck**

Injuries to the thorax (S20-S29)

INCLUDES injuries of breast
injuries of chest (wall)
injuries of interscapular area

EXCLUDES 2 *burns and corrosions (T20-T32)*
effects of foreign body in bronchus (T17.5)
effects of foreign body in esophagus (T18.1)
effects of foreign body in lung (T17.8)
effects of foreign body in trachea (T17.4)
frostbite (T33-T34)
injuries of axilla
injuries of clavicle
injuries of scapular region
injuries of shoulder
insect bite or sting, venomous (T63.4)

√4th **S20 Superficial injury of thorax**

AHA: 2020,4Q,39

The appropriate 7th character is to be added to each code from category S20.
A initial encounter
D subsequent encounter
S sequela

√5th **S20.0 Contusion of breast**

√x7th **S20.00 Contusion of breast, unspecified breast**

√x7th **S20.01 Contusion of right breast**

√x7th **S20.02 Contusion of left breast**

√5th **S20.1 Other and unspecified superficial injuries of breast**

√6th **S20.10 Unspecified superficial injuries of breast**

√7th **S20.101 Unspecified superficial injuries of breast, right breast**

√7th **S20.102 Unspecified superficial injuries of breast, left breast**

√7th **S20.109 Unspecified superficial injuries of breast, unspecified breast**

√6th **S20.11 Abrasion of breast**

√7th **S20.111 Abrasion of breast, right breast**

√7th **S20.112 Abrasion of breast, left breast**

√7th **S20.119 Abrasion of breast, unspecified breast**

√6th **S20.12 Blister (nonthermal) of breast**

√7th **S20.121 Blister (nonthermal) of breast, right breast**

√7th **S20.122 Blister (nonthermal) of breast, left breast**

√7th **S20.129 Blister (nonthermal) of breast, unspecified breast**

√6th **S20.14 External constriction of part of breast**

√7th **S20.141 External constriction of part of breast, right breast**

√7th **S20.142 External constriction of part of breast, left breast**

√7th **S20.149 External constriction of part of breast, unspecified breast**

√6th **S20.15 Superficial foreign body of breast**

Splinter in the breast

√7th **S20.151 Superficial foreign body of breast, right breast**

√7th **S20.152 Superficial foreign body of breast, left breast**

√7th **S20.159 Superficial foreign body of breast, unspecified breast**

√6th **S20.16 Insect bite (nonvenomous) of breast**

√7th **S20.161 Insect bite (nonvenomous) of breast, right breast**

√7th **S20.162 Insect bite (nonvenomous) of breast, left breast**

√7th **S20.169 Insect bite (nonvenomous) of breast, unspecified breast**

√6th **S20.17 Other superficial bite of breast**

EXCLUDES 1 *open bite of breast (S21.05-)*

√7th **S20.171 Other superficial bite of breast, right breast**

√7th **S20.172 Other superficial bite of breast, left breast**

√7th **S20.179 Other superficial bite of breast, unspecified breast**

√5th **S20.2 Contusion of thorax**

√x7th **S20.20 Contusion of thorax, unspecified**

√6th **S20.21 Contusion of front wall of thorax**

√7th **S20.211 Contusion of right front wall of thorax**

√7th **S20.212 Contusion of left front wall of thorax**

√7th **S20.213 Contusion of bilateral front wall of thorax**

√7th **S20.214 Contusion of middle front wall of thorax**

√7th **S20.219 Contusion of unspecified front wall of thorax**

√6th **S20.22 Contusion of back wall of thorax**

√7th **S20.221 Contusion of right back wall of thorax**

√7th **S20.222 Contusion of left back wall of thorax**

√7th **S20.223 Contusion of bilateral back wall of thorax**

√7th **S20.224 Contusion of middle back wall of thorax**

√7th **S20.229 Contusion of unspecified back wall of thorax**

√5th **S20.3 Other and unspecified superficial injuries of front wall of thorax**

√6th **S20.30 Unspecified superficial injuries of front wall of thorax**

√7th **S20.301 Unspecified superficial injuries of right front wall of thorax**

√7th **S20.302 Unspecified superficial injuries of left front wall of thorax**

√7th **S20.303 Unspecified superficial injuries of bilateral front wall of thorax**

√7th **S20.304 Unspecified superficial injuries of middle front wall of thorax**

√7th **S20.309 Unspecified superficial injuries of unspecified front wall of thorax**

√6th **S20.31 Abrasion of front wall of thorax**

√7th **S20.311 Abrasion of right front wall of thorax**

√7th **S20.312 Abrasion of left front wall of thorax**

√7th **S20.313 Abrasion of bilateral front wall of thorax**

√7th **S20.314 Abrasion of middle front wall of thorax**

√7th **S20.319 Abrasion of unspecified front wall of thorax**

√6th **S20.32 Blister (nonthermal) of front wall of thorax**

√7th **S20.321 Blister (nonthermal) of right front wall of thorax**

√7th **S20.322 Blister (nonthermal) of left front wall of thorax**

√7th **S20.323 Blister (nonthermal) of bilateral front wall of thorax**

√7th **S20.324 Blister (nonthermal) of middle front wall of thorax**

√7th **S20.329 Blister (nonthermal) of unspecified front wall of thorax**

√6th **S20.34 External constriction of front wall of thorax**

√7th **S20.341 External constriction of right front wall of thorax**

√7th **S20.342 External constriction of left front wall of thorax**

√7th **S20.343 External constriction of bilateral front wall of thorax**

√7th **S20.344 External constriction of middle front wall of thorax**

√7th **S20.349 External constriction of unspecified front wall of thorax**

√6th **S20.35 Superficial foreign body of front wall of thorax**

Splinter in front wall of thorax

√7th **S20.351 Superficial foreign body of right front wall of thorax**

√7th **S20.352 Superficial foreign body of left front wall of thorax**

√7th **S20.353 Superficial foreign body of bilateral front wall of thorax**

√7th **S20.354 Superficial foreign body of middle front wall of thorax**

√7th **S20.359 Superficial foreign body of unspecified front wall of thorax**

√6th **S20.36 Insect bite (nonvenomous) of front wall of thorax**

√7th **S20.361 Insect bite (nonvenomous) of right front wall of thorax**

✓7th **S20.362 Insect bite (nonvenomous) of left front wall of thorax**
✓7th **S20.363 Insect bite (nonvenomous) of bilateral front wall of thorax**
✓7th **S20.364 Insect bite (nonvenomous) of middle front wall of thorax**
✓7th **S20.369 Insect bite (nonvenomous) of unspecified front wall of thorax**
✓6th **S20.37 Other superficial bite of front wall of thorax**
EXCLUDES 1 *open bite of front wall of thorax (S21.15)*
✓7th **S20.371 Other superficial bite of right front wall of thorax**
✓7th **S20.372 Other superficial bite of left front wall of thorax**
✓7th **S20.373 Other superficial bite of bilateral front wall of thorax**
✓7th **S20.374 Other superficial bite of middle front wall of thorax**
✓7th **S20.379 Other superficial bite of unspecified front wall of thorax**
✓5th **S20.4 Other and unspecified superficial injuries of back wall of thorax**
✓6th **S20.40 Unspecified superficial injuries of back wall of thorax**
✓7th **S20.401 Unspecified superficial injuries of right back wall of thorax**
✓7th **S20.402 Unspecified superficial injuries of left back wall of thorax**
✓7th **S20.409 Unspecified superficial injuries of unspecified back wall of thorax**
✓6th **S20.41 Abrasion of back wall of thorax**
✓7th **S20.411 Abrasion of right back wall of thorax**
✓7th **S20.412 Abrasion of left back wall of thorax**
✓7th **S20.419 Abrasion of unspecified back wall of thorax**
✓6th **S20.42 Blister (nonthermal) of back wall of thorax**
✓7th **S20.421 Blister (nonthermal) of right back wall of thorax**
✓7th **S20.422 Blister (nonthermal) of left back wall of thorax**
✓7th **S20.429 Blister (nonthermal) of unspecified back wall of thorax**
✓6th **S20.44 External constriction of back wall of thorax**
✓7th **S20.441 External constriction of right back wall of thorax**
✓7th **S20.442 External constriction of left back wall of thorax**
✓7th **S20.449 External constriction of unspecified back wall of thorax**
✓6th **S20.45 Superficial foreign body of back wall of thorax**
Splinter of back wall of thorax
✓7th **S20.451 Superficial foreign body of right back wall of thorax**
✓7th **S20.452 Superficial foreign body of left back wall of thorax**
✓7th **S20.459 Superficial foreign body of unspecified back wall of thorax**
✓6th **S20.46 Insect bite (nonvenomous) of back wall of thorax**
✓7th **S20.461 Insect bite (nonvenomous) of right back wall of thorax**
✓7th **S20.462 Insect bite (nonvenomous) of left back wall of thorax**
✓7th **S20.469 Insect bite (nonvenomous) of unspecified back wall of thorax**
✓6th **S20.47 Other superficial bite of back wall of thorax**
EXCLUDES 1 *open bite of back wall of thorax (S21.25)*
✓7th **S20.471 Other superficial bite of right back wall of thorax**
✓7th **S20.472 Other superficial bite of left back wall of thorax**
✓7th **S20.479 Other superficial bite of unspecified back wall of thorax**
✓5th **S20.9 Superficial injury of unspecified parts of thorax**
EXCLUDES 1 *contusion of thorax NOS (S20.20)*
✓x7th **S20.90 Unspecified superficial injury of unspecified parts of thorax**
Superficial injury of thoracic wall NOS
✓x7th **S20.91 Abrasion of unspecified parts of thorax**
✓x7th **S20.92 Blister (nonthermal) of unspecified parts of thorax**
✓x7th **S20.94 External constriction of unspecified parts of thorax**
✓x7th **S20.95 Superficial foreign body of unspecified parts of thorax**
Splinter in thorax NOS
✓x7th **S20.96 Insect bite (nonvenomous) of unspecified parts of thorax**
✓x7th **S20.97 Other superficial bite of unspecified parts of thorax**
EXCLUDES 1 *open bite of thorax NOS (S21.95)*

✓4th **S21 Open wound of thorax**

Code also any associated injury, such as:
- injury of heart (S26.-)
- injury of intrathoracic organs (S27.-)
- rib fracture (S22.3-, S22.4-)
- spinal cord injury (S24.0-, S24.1-)
- traumatic hemopneumothorax (S27.3)
- traumatic hemothorax (S27.1)
- traumatic pneumothorax (S27.0)
- wound infection

EXCLUDES 1 *traumatic amputation (partial) of thorax (S28.1)*

The appropriate 7th character is to be added to each code from category S21.
A initial encounter
D subsequent encounter
S sequela

✓5th **S21.0 Open wound of breast**
✓6th **S21.00 Unspecified open wound of breast**
✓7th **S21.001 Unspecified open wound of right breast**
✓7th **S21.002 Unspecified open wound of left breast**
✓7th **S21.009 Unspecified open wound of unspecified breast**
✓6th **S21.01 Laceration without foreign body of breast**
✓7th **S21.011 Laceration without foreign body of right breast**
✓7th **S21.012 Laceration without foreign body of left breast**
✓7th **S21.019 Laceration without foreign body of unspecified breast**
✓6th **S21.02 Laceration with foreign body of breast**
✓7th **S21.021 Laceration with foreign body of right breast**
✓7th **S21.022 Laceration with foreign body of left breast**
✓7th **S21.029 Laceration with foreign body of unspecified breast**
✓6th **S21.03 Puncture wound without foreign body of breast**
✓7th **S21.031 Puncture wound without foreign body of right breast**
✓7th **S21.032 Puncture wound without foreign body of left breast**
✓7th **S21.039 Puncture wound without foreign body of unspecified breast**
✓6th **S21.04 Puncture wound with foreign body of breast**
✓7th **S21.041 Puncture wound with foreign body of right breast**
✓7th **S21.042 Puncture wound with foreign body of left breast**
✓7th **S21.049 Puncture wound with foreign body of unspecified breast**
✓6th **S21.05 Open bite of breast**
Bite of breast NOS
EXCLUDES 1 *superficial bite of breast (S20.17)*
✓7th **S21.051 Open bite of right breast**
✓7th **S21.052 Open bite of left breast**
✓7th **S21.059 Open bite of unspecified breast**
✓5th **S21.1 Open wound of front wall of thorax without penetration into thoracic cavity**
Open wound of chest without penetration into thoracic cavity
✓6th **S21.10 Unspecified open wound of front wall of thorax without penetration into thoracic cavity**
✓7th **S21.101 Unspecified open wound of right front wall of thorax without penetration into thoracic cavity**
✓7th **S21.102 Unspecified open wound of left front wall of thorax without penetration into thoracic cavity**

7th **S21.109** **Unspecified open wound of unspecified front wall of thorax without penetration into thoracic cavity**

6th **S21.11** **Laceration without foreign body of front wall of thorax without penetration into thoracic cavity**

7th **S21.111** **Laceration without foreign body of right front wall of thorax without penetration into thoracic cavity**

7th **S21.112** **Laceration without foreign body of left front wall of thorax without penetration into thoracic cavity**

7th **S21.119** **Laceration without foreign body of unspecified front wall of thorax without penetration into thoracic cavity**

6th **S21.12** **Laceration with foreign body of front wall of thorax without penetration into thoracic cavity**

7th **S21.121** **Laceration with foreign body of right front wall of thorax without penetration into thoracic cavity**

7th **S21.122** **Laceration with foreign body of left front wall of thorax without penetration into thoracic cavity**

7th **S21.129** **Laceration with foreign body of unspecified front wall of thorax without penetration into thoracic cavity**

6th **S21.13** **Puncture wound without foreign body of front wall of thorax without penetration into thoracic cavity**

7th **S21.131** **Puncture wound without foreign body of right front wall of thorax without penetration into thoracic cavity**

7th **S21.132** **Puncture wound without foreign body of left front wall of thorax without penetration into thoracic cavity**

7th **S21.139** **Puncture wound without foreign body of unspecified front wall of thorax without penetration into thoracic cavity**

6th **S21.14** **Puncture wound with foreign body of front wall of thorax without penetration into thoracic cavity**

7th **S21.141** **Puncture wound with foreign body of right front wall of thorax without penetration into thoracic cavity**

7th **S21.142** **Puncture wound with foreign body of left front wall of thorax without penetration into thoracic cavity**

7th **S21.149** **Puncture wound with foreign body of unspecified front wall of thorax without penetration into thoracic cavity**

6th **S21.15** **Open bite of front wall of thorax without penetration into thoracic cavity**

Bite of front wall of thorax NOS

EXCLUDES 1 *superficial bite of front wall of thorax (S20.37)*

7th **S21.151** **Open bite of right front wall of thorax without penetration into thoracic cavity**

7th **S21.152** **Open bite of left front wall of thorax without penetration into thoracic cavity**

7th **S21.159** **Open bite of unspecified front wall of thorax without penetration into thoracic cavity**

5th **S21.2** **Open wound of back wall of thorax without penetration into thoracic cavity**

6th **S21.20** **Unspecified open wound of back wall of thorax without penetration into thoracic cavity**

7th **S21.201** **Unspecified open wound of right back wall of thorax without penetration into thoracic cavity**

7th **S21.202** **Unspecified open wound of left back wall of thorax without penetration into thoracic cavity**

7th **S21.209** **Unspecified open wound of unspecified back wall of thorax without penetration into thoracic cavity**

6th **S21.21** **Laceration without foreign body of back wall of thorax without penetration into thoracic cavity**

7th **S21.211** **Laceration without foreign body of right back wall of thorax without penetration into thoracic cavity**

7th **S21.212** **Laceration without foreign body of left back wall of thorax without penetration into thoracic cavity**

7th **S21.219** **Laceration without foreign body of unspecified back wall of thorax without penetration into thoracic cavity**

6th **S21.22** **Laceration with foreign body of back wall of thorax without penetration into thoracic cavity**

7th **S21.221** **Laceration with foreign body of right back wall of thorax without penetration into thoracic cavity**

7th **S21.222** **Laceration with foreign body of left back wall of thorax without penetration into thoracic cavity**

7th **S21.229** **Laceration with foreign body of unspecified back wall of thorax without penetration into thoracic cavity**

6th **S21.23** **Puncture wound without foreign body of back wall of thorax without penetration into thoracic cavity**

7th **S21.231** **Puncture wound without foreign body of right back wall of thorax without penetration into thoracic cavity**

7th **S21.232** **Puncture wound without foreign body of left back wall of thorax without penetration into thoracic cavity**

7th **S21.239** **Puncture wound without foreign body of unspecified back wall of thorax without penetration into thoracic cavity**

6th **S21.24** **Puncture wound with foreign body of back wall of thorax without penetration into thoracic cavity**

7th **S21.241** **Puncture wound with foreign body of right back wall of thorax without penetration into thoracic cavity**

7th **S21.242** **Puncture wound with foreign body of left back wall of thorax without penetration into thoracic cavity**

7th **S21.249** **Puncture wound with foreign body of unspecified back wall of thorax without penetration into thoracic cavity**

6th **S21.25** **Open bite of back wall of thorax without penetration into thoracic cavity**

Bite of back wall of thorax NOS

EXCLUDES 1 *superficial bite of back wall of thorax (S20.47)*

7th **S21.251** **Open bite of right back wall of thorax without penetration into thoracic cavity**

7th **S21.252** **Open bite of left back wall of thorax without penetration into thoracic cavity**

7th **S21.259** **Open bite of unspecified back wall of thorax without penetration into thoracic cavity**

5th **S21.3** **Open wound of front wall of thorax with penetration into thoracic cavity**

Open wound of chest with penetration into thoracic cavity

6th **S21.30** **Unspecified open wound of front wall of thorax with penetration into thoracic cavity**

7th **S21.301** **Unspecified open wound of right front wall of thorax with penetration into thoracic cavity**

7th **S21.302** **Unspecified open wound of left front wall of thorax with penetration into thoracic cavity**

7th **S21.309** **Unspecified open wound of unspecified front wall of thorax with penetration into thoracic cavity**

6th **S21.31** **Laceration without foreign body of front wall of thorax with penetration into thoracic cavity**

7th **S21.311** **Laceration without foreign body of right front wall of thorax with penetration into thoracic cavity**

7th **S21.312** **Laceration without foreign body of left front wall of thorax with penetration into thoracic cavity**

7th **S21.319** **Laceration without foreign body of unspecified front wall of thorax with penetration into thoracic cavity**

6th **S21.32** **Laceration with foreign body of front wall of thorax with penetration into thoracic cavity**

7th **S21.321** **Laceration with foreign body of right front wall of thorax with penetration into thoracic cavity**

7th **S21.322** **Laceration with foreign body of left front wall of thorax with penetration into thoracic cavity**

7th **S21.329** **Laceration with foreign body of unspecified front wall of thorax with penetration into thoracic cavity**

6th **S21.33** **Puncture wound without foreign body of front wall of thorax with penetration into thoracic cavity**

7th **S21.331** **Puncture wound without foreign body of right front wall of thorax with penetration into thoracic cavity**

7th **S21.332** **Puncture wound without foreign body of left front wall of thorax with penetration into thoracic cavity**

7th **S21.339** **Puncture wound without foreign body of unspecified front wall of thorax with penetration into thoracic cavity**

6th **S21.34** **Puncture wound with foreign body of front wall of thorax with penetration into thoracic cavity**

7th **S21.341** **Puncture wound with foreign body of right front wall of thorax with penetration into thoracic cavity**

7th **S21.342** **Puncture wound with foreign body of left front wall of thorax with penetration into thoracic cavity**

7th **S21.349** **Puncture wound with foreign body of unspecified front wall of thorax with penetration into thoracic cavity**

6th **S21.35** **Open bite of front wall of thorax with penetration into thoracic cavity**

EXCLUDES 1 *superficial bite of front wall of thorax (S20.37)*

7th **S21.351** **Open bite of right front wall of thorax with penetration into thoracic cavity**

7th **S21.352** **Open bite of left front wall of thorax with penetration into thoracic cavity**

7th **S21.359** **Open bite of unspecified front wall of thorax with penetration into thoracic cavity**

5th **S21.4** **Open wound of back wall of thorax with penetration into thoracic cavity**

6th **S21.40** **Unspecified open wound of back wall of thorax with penetration into thoracic cavity**

7th **S21.401** **Unspecified open wound of right back wall of thorax with penetration into thoracic cavity**

7th **S21.402** **Unspecified open wound of left back wall of thorax with penetration into thoracic cavity**

7th **S21.409** **Unspecified open wound of unspecified back wall of thorax with penetration into thoracic cavity**

6th **S21.41** **Laceration without foreign body of back wall of thorax with penetration into thoracic cavity**

7th **S21.411** **Laceration without foreign body of right back wall of thorax with penetration into thoracic cavity**

7th **S21.412** **Laceration without foreign body of left back wall of thorax with penetration into thoracic cavity**

7th **S21.419** **Laceration without foreign body of unspecified back wall of thorax with penetration into thoracic cavity**

6th **S21.42** **Laceration with foreign body of back wall of thorax with penetration into thoracic cavity**

7th **S21.421** **Laceration with foreign body of right back wall of thorax with penetration into thoracic cavity**

7th **S21.422** **Laceration with foreign body of left back wall of thorax with penetration into thoracic cavity**

7th **S21.429** **Laceration with foreign body of unspecified back wall of thorax with penetration into thoracic cavity**

6th **S21.43** **Puncture wound without foreign body of back wall of thorax with penetration into thoracic cavity**

7th **S21.431** **Puncture wound without foreign body of right back wall of thorax with penetration into thoracic cavity**

7th **S21.432** **Puncture wound without foreign body of left back wall of thorax with penetration into thoracic cavity**

7th **S21.439** **Puncture wound without foreign body of unspecified back wall of thorax with penetration into thoracic cavity**

6th **S21.44** **Puncture wound with foreign body of back wall of thorax with penetration into thoracic cavity**

7th **S21.441** **Puncture wound with foreign body of right back wall of thorax with penetration into thoracic cavity**

7th **S21.442** **Puncture wound with foreign body of left back wall of thorax with penetration into thoracic cavity**

7th **S21.449** **Puncture wound with foreign body of unspecified back wall of thorax with penetration into thoracic cavity**

6th **S21.45** **Open bite of back wall of thorax with penetration into thoracic cavity**

Bite of back wall of thorax NOS

EXCLUDES 1 *superficial bite of back wall of thorax (S20.47)*

7th **S21.451** **Open bite of right back wall of thorax with penetration into thoracic cavity**

7th **S21.452** **Open bite of left back wall of thorax with penetration into thoracic cavity**

7th **S21.459** **Open bite of unspecified back wall of thorax with penetration into thoracic cavity**

5th **S21.9** **Open wound of unspecified part of thorax**

Open wound of thoracic wall NOS

x7th **S21.90** **Unspecified open wound of unspecified part of thorax**

x7th **S21.91** **Laceration without foreign body of unspecified part of thorax**

x7th **S21.92** **Laceration with foreign body of unspecified part of thorax**

x7th **S21.93** **Puncture wound without foreign body of unspecified part of thorax**

x7th **S21.94** **Puncture wound with foreign body of unspecified part of thorax**

x7th **S21.95** **Open bite of unspecified part of thorax**

EXCLUDES 1 *superficial bite of thorax (S20.97)*

4th **S22** **Fracture of rib(s), sternum and thoracic spine**

NOTE A fracture not indicated as displaced or nondisplaced should be coded to displaced

A fracture not indicated as open or closed should be coded to closed

INCLUDES fracture of thoracic neural arch
fracture of thoracic spinous process
fracture of thoracic transverse process
fracture of thoracic vertebra
fracture of thoracic vertebral arch

Code first any associated:
injury of intrathoracic organ (S27.-)
spinal cord injury (S24.0-, S24.1-)

EXCLUDES 1 *transection of thorax (S28.1)*

EXCLUDES 2 *fracture of clavicle (S42.0-)*
fracture of scapula (S42.1-)

AHA: 2021,1Q,6; 2018,2Q,12; 2015,3Q,37-39

The appropriate 7th character is to be added to each code from category S22.
A initial encounter for closed fracture
B initial encounter for open fracture
D subsequent encounter for fracture with routine healing
G subsequent encounter for fracture with delayed healing
K subsequent encounter for fracture with nonunion
S sequela

5th **S22.0** **Fracture of thoracic vertebra**

6th **S22.00** **Fracture of unspecified thoracic vertebra**

1 7th **S22.000** **Wedge compression fracture of unspecified thoracic vertebra** HCC ESR COM Q

1 7th **S22.001** **Stable burst fracture of unspecified thoracic vertebra** HCC ESR COM Q

1 7th **S22.002** **Unstable burst fracture of unspecified thoracic vertebra** HCC ESR COM Q

1 7th **S22.008** **Other fracture of unspecified thoracic vertebra** HCC ESR COM Q

1 7th **S22.009** **Unspecified fracture of unspecified thoracic vertebra** HCC ESR COM Q

6th **S22.01** **Fracture of first thoracic vertebra**

1 7th **S22.010** **Wedge compression fracture of first thoracic vertebra** HCC ESR COM Q

1 7th **S22.011** **Stable burst fracture of first thoracic vertebra** HCC ESR COM Q

1 7th **S22.012** **Unstable burst fracture of first thoracic vertebra** HCC ESR COM Q

S22.018 Other fracture of first thoracic vertebra HCC ESR COM Q

S22.019 Unspecified fracture of first thoracic vertebra HCC ESR COM Q

S22.02 Fracture of second thoracic vertebra

S22.020 Wedge compression fracture of second thoracic vertebra HCC ESR COM Q

S22.021 Stable burst fracture of second thoracic vertebra HCC ESR COM Q

S22.022 Unstable burst fracture of second thoracic vertebra HCC ESR COM Q

S22.028 Other fracture of second thoracic vertebra HCC ESR COM Q

S22.029 Unspecified fracture of second thoracic vertebra HCC ESR COM Q

S22.03 Fracture of third thoracic vertebra

S22.030 Wedge compression fracture of third thoracic vertebra HCC ESR COM Q

S22.031 Stable burst fracture of third thoracic vertebra HCC ESR COM Q

S22.032 Unstable burst fracture of third thoracic vertebra HCC ESR COM Q

S22.038 Other fracture of third thoracic vertebra HCC ESR COM Q

S22.039 Unspecified fracture of third thoracic vertebra HCC ESR COM Q

S22.04 Fracture of fourth thoracic vertebra

S22.040 Wedge compression fracture of fourth thoracic vertebra HCC ESR COM Q

S22.041 Stable burst fracture of fourth thoracic vertebra HCC ESR COM Q

S22.042 Unstable burst fracture of fourth thoracic vertebra HCC ESR COM Q

S22.048 Other fracture of fourth thoracic vertebra HCC ESR COM Q

S22.049 Unspecified fracture of fourth thoracic vertebra HCC ESR COM Q

S22.05 Fracture of T5-T6 vertebra

S22.050 Wedge compression fracture of T5-T6 vertebra HCC ESR COM Q

S22.051 Stable burst fracture of T5-T6 vertebra HCC ESR COM Q

S22.052 Unstable burst fracture of T5-T6 vertebra HCC ESR COM Q

S22.058 Other fracture of T5-T6 vertebra HCC ESR COM Q

S22.059 Unspecified fracture of T5-T6 vertebra HCC ESR COM Q

S22.06 Fracture of T7-T8 vertebra

S22.060 Wedge compression fracture of T7-T8 vertebra HCC ESR COM Q

S22.061 Stable burst fracture of T7-T8 vertebra HCC ESR COM Q

S22.062 Unstable burst fracture of T7-T8 vertebra HCC ESR COM Q

S22.068 Other fracture of T7-T8 thoracic vertebra HCC ESR COM Q

S22.069 Unspecified fracture of T7-T8 vertebra HCC ESR COM Q

S22.07 Fracture of T9-T10 vertebra

S22.070 Wedge compression fracture of T9-T10 vertebra HCC ESR COM Q

S22.071 Stable burst fracture of T9-T10 vertebra HCC ESR COM Q

S22.072 Unstable burst fracture of T9-T10 vertebra HCC ESR COM Q

S22.078 Other fracture of T9-T10 vertebra HCC ESR COM Q

S22.079 Unspecified fracture of T9-T10 vertebra HCC ESR COM Q

S22.08 Fracture of T11-T12 vertebra

S22.080 Wedge compression fracture of T11-T12 vertebra HCC ESR COM Q

S22.081 Stable burst fracture of T11-T12 vertebra HCC ESR COM Q

S22.082 Unstable burst fracture of T11-T12 vertebra HCC ESR COM Q

S22.088 Other fracture of T11-T12 vertebra HCC ESR COM Q

S22.089 Unspecified fracture of T11-T12 vertebra HCC ESR COM Q

S22.2 Fracture of sternum

DEF: Break in flat bone (breast bone) in the anterior thorax caused by blunt trauma to the anterior chest.

S22.20 Unspecified fracture of sternum Q

S22.21 Fracture of manubrium Q

S22.22 Fracture of body of sternum Q

S22.23 Sternal manubrial dissociation Q

S22.24 Fracture of xiphoid process Q

S22.3 Fracture of one rib

AHA: 2021,1Q,5

S22.31 Fracture of one rib, right side Q

S22.32 Fracture of one rib, left side Q

S22.39 Fracture of one rib, unspecified side Q

S22.4 Multiple fractures of ribs

Fractures of two or more ribs

EXCLUDES 1 *flail chest (S22.5-)*

AHA: 2021,1Q,5

S22.41 Multiple fractures of ribs, right side Q

S22.42 Multiple fractures of ribs, left side Q

S22.43 Multiple fractures of ribs, bilateral Q

S22.49 Multiple fractures of ribs, unspecified side Q

S22.5 Flail chest Q

S22.9 Fracture of bony thorax, part unspecified Q

S23 Dislocation and sprain of joints and ligaments of thorax

INCLUDES avulsion of joint or ligament of thorax
laceration of cartilage, joint or ligament of thorax
sprain of cartilage, joint or ligament of thorax
traumatic hemarthrosis of joint or ligament of thorax
traumatic rupture of joint or ligament of thorax
traumatic subluxation of joint or ligament of thorax
traumatic tear of joint or ligament of thorax

Code also any associated open wound

EXCLUDES 2 *dislocation, sprain of sternoclavicular joint (S43.2, S43.6)*
strain of muscle or tendon of thorax (S29.01-)

The appropriate 7th character is to be added to each code from category S23.
A initial encounter
D subsequent encounter
S sequela

S23.0 Traumatic rupture of thoracic intervertebral disc

EXCLUDES 1 *rupture or displacement (nontraumatic) of thoracic intervertebral disc NOS (M51.- with fifth character 4)*

S23.1 Subluxation and dislocation of thoracic vertebra

Code also any associated:
open wound of thorax (S21.-)
spinal cord injury (S24.0-, S24.1-)

EXCLUDES 2 *fracture of thoracic vertebrae (S22.0-)*

S23.10 Subluxation and dislocation of unspecified thoracic vertebra

S23.100 Subluxation of unspecified thoracic vertebra

S23.101 Dislocation of unspecified thoracic vertebra

S23.11 Subluxation and dislocation of T1/T2 thoracic vertebra

S23.110 Subluxation of T1/T2 thoracic vertebra

S23.111 Dislocation of T1/T2 thoracic vertebra

S23.12 Subluxation and dislocation of T2/T3-T3/T4 thoracic vertebra

S23.120 Subluxation of T2/T3 thoracic vertebra

S23.121 Dislocation of T2/T3 thoracic vertebra

S23.122 Subluxation of T3/T4 thoracic vertebra

S23.123 Dislocation of T3/T4 thoracic vertebra

S23.13 Subluxation and dislocation of T4/T5-T5/T6 thoracic vertebra

S23.130 Subluxation of T4/T5 thoracic vertebra

S23.131 Dislocation of T4/T5 thoracic vertebra

S23.132 **Subluxation** of T5/T6 thoracic vertebra
S23.133 **Dislocation** of T5/T6 thoracic vertebra
S23.14 Subluxation and dislocation of **T6/T7-T7/T8** thoracic vertebra
S23.14Ø **Subluxation** of T6/T7 thoracic vertebra
S23.141 **Dislocation** of T6/T7 thoracic vertebra
S23.142 **Subluxation** of T7/T8 thoracic vertebra
S23.143 **Dislocation** of T7/T8 thoracic vertebra
S23.15 Subluxation and dislocation of **T8/T9-T9/T1Ø** thoracic vertebra
S23.15Ø **Subluxation** of T8/T9 thoracic vertebra
S23.151 **Dislocation** of T8/T9 thoracic vertebra
S23.152 **Subluxation** of T9/T1Ø thoracic vertebra
S23.153 **Dislocation** of T9/T1Ø thoracic vertebra
S23.16 Subluxation and dislocation of **T1Ø/T11-T11/T12** thoracic vertebra
S23.16Ø **Subluxation** of T1Ø/T11 thoracic vertebra
S23.161 **Dislocation** of T1Ø/T11 thoracic vertebra
S23.162 **Subluxation** of T11/T12 thoracic vertebra
S23.163 **Dislocation** of T11/T12 thoracic vertebra
S23.17 Subluxation and dislocation of **T12/L1** thoracic vertebra
S23.17Ø **Subluxation** of T12/L1 thoracic vertebra
S23.171 **Dislocation** of T12/L1 thoracic vertebra
S23.2 Dislocation of other and unspecified parts of thorax
S23.2Ø Dislocation of unspecified part of thorax
S23.29 Dislocation of other parts of thorax
S23.3 Sprain of ligaments of thoracic spine
S23.4 Sprain of ribs and sternum
S23.41 Sprain of ribs
S23.42 Sprain of sternum
S23.42Ø Sprain of sternoclavicular (joint) (ligament)
S23.421 Sprain of chondrosternal joint
S23.428 Other sprain of sternum
S23.429 Unspecified sprain of sternum
S23.8 Sprain of other specified parts of thorax
S23.9 Sprain of unspecified parts of thorax

S24 Injury of nerves and spinal cord at thorax level

NOTE Code to highest level of thoracic spinal cord injury.
Injuries to the spinal cord (S24.Ø and S24.1) refer to the cord level and not bone level injury, and can affect nerve roots at and below the level given.

Code also any associated:
fracture of thoracic vertebra (S22.Ø-)
open wound of thorax (S21.-)
transient paralysis (R29.5)

EXCLUDES 2 *injury of brachial plexus (S14.3)*

The appropriate 7th character is to be added to each code from category S24.
A initial encounter
D subsequent encounter
S sequela

S24.Ø Concussion and edema of thoracic spinal cord HCC ESR COM
S24.1 Other and unspecified injuries of thoracic spinal cord
S24.1Ø Unspecified injury of thoracic spinal cord
S24.1Ø1 Unspecified injury at **T1** level of thoracic spinal cord HCC ESR COM
S24.1Ø2 Unspecified injury at **T2-T6** level of thoracic spinal cord HCC ESR COM
S24.1Ø3 Unspecified injury at **T7-T1Ø** level of thoracic spinal cord HCC ESR COM
S24.1Ø4 Unspecified injury at **T11-T12** level of thoracic spinal cord HCC ESR COM
S24.1Ø9 Unspecified injury at unspecified level of thoracic spinal cord HCC ESR COM
Injury of thoracic spinal cord NOS
S24.11 **Complete lesion** of thoracic spinal cord
S24.111 Complete lesion at **T1** level of thoracic spinal cord HCC ESR COM
S24.112 Complete lesion at **T2-T6** level of thoracic spinal cord HCC ESR COM
S24.113 Complete lesion at **T7-T1Ø** level of thoracic spinal cord HCC ESR COM
S24.114 Complete lesion at **T11-T12** level of thoracic spinal cord HCC ESR COM
S24.119 Complete lesion at unspecified level of thoracic spinal cord HCC ESR COM
S24.13 **Anterior cord syndrome** of thoracic spinal cord
S24.131 Anterior cord syndrome at **T1** level of thoracic spinal cord HCC ESR COM
S24.132 Anterior cord syndrome at **T2-T6** level of thoracic spinal cord HCC ESR COM
S24.133 Anterior cord syndrome at **T7-T1Ø** level of thoracic spinal cord HCC ESR COM
S24.134 Anterior cord syndrome at **T11-T12** level of thoracic spinal cord HCC ESR COM
S24.139 Anterior cord syndrome at unspecified level of thoracic spinal cord HCC ESR COM
S24.14 **Brown-Séquard syndrome** of thoracic spinal cord
S24.141 Brown-Séquard syndrome at **T1** level of thoracic spinal cord HCC ESR COM
S24.142 Brown-Séquard syndrome at **T2-T6** level of thoracic spinal cord HCC ESR COM
S24.143 Brown-Séquard syndrome at **T7-T1Ø** level of thoracic spinal cord HCC ESR COM
S24.144 Brown-Séquard syndrome at **T11-T12** level of thoracic spinal cord HCC ESR COM
S24.149 Brown-Séquard syndrome at unspecified level of thoracic spinal cord HCC ESR COM
S24.15 Other **incomplete lesions** of thoracic spinal cord
Incomplete lesion of thoracic spinal cord NOS
Posterior cord syndrome of thoracic spinal cord
S24.151 Other incomplete lesion at **T1** level of thoracic spinal cord HCC ESR COM
S24.152 Other incomplete lesion at **T2-T6** level of thoracic spinal cord HCC ESR COM
S24.153 Other incomplete lesion at **T7-T1Ø** level of thoracic spinal cord HCC ESR COM
S24.154 Other incomplete lesion at **T11-T12** level of thoracic spinal cord HCC ESR COM
S24.159 Other incomplete lesion at unspecified level of thoracic spinal cord HCC ESR COM
S24.2 Injury of nerve root of thoracic spine
S24.3 Injury of peripheral nerves of thorax
S24.4 Injury of thoracic sympathetic nervous system
Injury of cardiac plexus
Injury of esophageal plexus
Injury of pulmonary plexus
Injury of stellate ganglion
Injury of thoracic sympathetic ganglion
S24.8 Injury of other specified nerves of thorax
S24.9 Injury of unspecified nerve of thorax

S25 Injury of blood vessels of thorax

Code also any associated open wound (S21.-)

The appropriate 7th character is to be added to each code from category S25.
A initial encounter
D subsequent encounter
S sequela

S25.Ø Injury of **thoracic aorta**
Injury of aorta NOS
S25.ØØ Unspecified injury of thoracic aorta
S25.Ø1 **Minor laceration** of thoracic aorta
Incomplete transection of thoracic aorta
Laceration of thoracic aorta NOS
Superficial laceration of thoracic aorta
S25.Ø2 **Major laceration** of thoracic aorta
Complete transection of thoracic aorta
Traumatic rupture of thoracic aorta
S25.Ø9 Other specified injury of thoracic aorta

✓5th **S25.1 Injury of innominate or subclavian artery**

✓6th **S25.10 Unspecified injury of innominate or subclavian artery**

✓7th **S25.101 Unspecified injury of right innominate or subclavian artery**

✓7th **S25.102 Unspecified injury of left innominate or subclavian artery**

✓7th **S25.109 Unspecified injury of unspecified innominate or subclavian artery**

✓6th **S25.11 Minor laceration of innominate or subclavian artery**

Incomplete transection of innominate or subclavian artery

Laceration of innominate or subclavian artery NOS

Superficial laceration of innominate or subclavian artery

✓7th **S25.111 Minor laceration of right innominate or subclavian artery**

✓7th **S25.112 Minor laceration of left innominate or subclavian artery**

✓7th **S25.119 Minor laceration of unspecified innominate or subclavian artery**

✓6th **S25.12 Major laceration of innominate or subclavian artery**

Complete transection of innominate or subclavian artery

Traumatic rupture of innominate or subclavian artery

✓7th **S25.121 Major laceration of right innominate or subclavian artery**

✓7th **S25.122 Major laceration of left innominate or subclavian artery**

✓7th **S25.129 Major laceration of unspecified innominate or subclavian artery**

✓6th **S25.19 Other specified injury of innominate or subclavian artery**

✓7th **S25.191 Other specified injury of right innominate or subclavian artery**

✓7th **S25.192 Other specified injury of left innominate or subclavian artery**

✓7th **S25.199 Other specified injury of unspecified innominate or subclavian artery**

✓5th **S25.2 Injury of superior vena cava**

Injury of vena cava NOS

✓x7th **S25.20 Unspecified injury of superior vena cava**

✓x7th **S25.21 Minor laceration of superior vena cava**

Incomplete transection of superior vena cava

Laceration of superior vena cava NOS

Superficial laceration of superior vena cava

✓x7th **S25.22 Major laceration of superior vena cava**

Complete transection of superior vena cava

Traumatic rupture of superior vena cava

✓x7th **S25.29 Other specified injury of superior vena cava**

✓5th **S25.3 Injury of innominate or subclavian vein**

✓6th **S25.30 Unspecified injury of innominate or subclavian vein**

✓7th **S25.301 Unspecified injury of right innominate or subclavian vein**

✓7th **S25.302 Unspecified injury of left innominate or subclavian vein**

✓7th **S25.309 Unspecified injury of unspecified innominate or subclavian vein**

✓6th **S25.31 Minor laceration of innominate or subclavian vein**

Incomplete transection of innominate or subclavian vein

Laceration of innominate or subclavian vein NOS

Superficial laceration of innominate or subclavian vein

✓7th **S25.311 Minor laceration of right innominate or subclavian vein**

✓7th **S25.312 Minor laceration of left innominate or subclavian vein**

✓7th **S25.319 Minor laceration of unspecified innominate or subclavian vein**

✓6th **S25.32 Major laceration of innominate or subclavian vein**

Complete transection of innominate or subclavian vein

Traumatic rupture of innominate or subclavian vein

✓7th **S25.321 Major laceration of right innominate or subclavian vein**

✓7th **S25.322 Major laceration of left innominate or subclavian vein**

✓7th **S25.329 Major laceration of unspecified innominate or subclavian vein**

✓6th **S25.39 Other specified injury of innominate or subclavian vein**

✓7th **S25.391 Other specified injury of right innominate or subclavian vein**

✓7th **S25.392 Other specified injury of left innominate or subclavian vein**

✓7th **S25.399 Other specified injury of unspecified innominate or subclavian vein**

✓5th **S25.4 Injury of pulmonary blood vessels**

✓6th **S25.40 Unspecified injury of pulmonary blood vessels**

✓7th **S25.401 Unspecified injury of right pulmonary blood vessels**

✓7th **S25.402 Unspecified injury of left pulmonary blood vessels**

✓7th **S25.409 Unspecified injury of unspecified pulmonary blood vessels**

✓6th **S25.41 Minor laceration of pulmonary blood vessels**

Incomplete transection of pulmonary blood vessels

Laceration of pulmonary blood vessels NOS

Superficial laceration of pulmonary blood vessels

✓7th **S25.411 Minor laceration of right pulmonary blood vessels**

✓7th **S25.412 Minor laceration of left pulmonary blood vessels**

✓7th **S25.419 Minor laceration of unspecified pulmonary blood vessels**

✓6th **S25.42 Major laceration of pulmonary blood vessels**

Complete transection of pulmonary blood vessels

Traumatic rupture of pulmonary blood vessels

✓7th **S25.421 Major laceration of right pulmonary blood vessels**

✓7th **S25.422 Major laceration of left pulmonary blood vessels**

✓7th **S25.429 Major laceration of unspecified pulmonary blood vessels**

✓6th **S25.49 Other specified injury of pulmonary blood vessels**

✓7th **S25.491 Other specified injury of right pulmonary blood vessels**

✓7th **S25.492 Other specified injury of left pulmonary blood vessels**

✓7th **S25.499 Other specified injury of unspecified pulmonary blood vessels**

✓5th **S25.5 Injury of intercostal blood vessels**

✓6th **S25.50 Unspecified injury of intercostal blood vessels**

✓7th **S25.501 Unspecified injury of intercostal blood vessels, right side**

✓7th **S25.502 Unspecified injury of intercostal blood vessels, left side**

✓7th **S25.509 Unspecified injury of intercostal blood vessels, unspecified side**

✓6th **S25.51 Laceration of intercostal blood vessels**

✓7th **S25.511 Laceration of intercostal blood vessels, right side**

✓7th **S25.512 Laceration of intercostal blood vessels, left side**

✓7th **S25.519 Laceration of intercostal blood vessels, unspecified side**

✓6th **S25.59 Other specified injury of intercostal blood vessels**

✓7th **S25.591 Other specified injury of intercostal blood vessels, right side**

✓7th **S25.592 Other specified injury of intercostal blood vessels, left side**

✓7th **S25.599 Other specified injury of intercostal blood vessels, unspecified side**

✓5th **S25.8 Injury of other blood vessels of thorax**

Injury of azygos vein

Injury of mammary artery or vein

✓6th **S25.80 Unspecified injury of other blood vessels of thorax**

✓7th **S25.801 Unspecified injury of other blood vessels of thorax, right side**

✓7th **S25.802 Unspecified injury of other blood vessels of thorax, left side**

✓7th **S25.809 Unspecified injury of other blood vessels of thorax, unspecified side**

✓6th **S25.81 Laceration of other blood vessels of thorax**

✓7th **S25.811 Laceration of other blood vessels of thorax, right side**

Chapter 19. Injury, Poisoning and Certain Other Consequences of External Causes

S25.1–S25.811

S25.812 Laceration of other blood vessels of thorax, left side

S25.819 Laceration of other blood vessels of thorax, unspecified side

S25.89 Other specified injury of other blood vessels of thorax

S25.891 Other specified injury of other blood vessels of thorax, right side

S25.892 Other specified injury of other blood vessels of thorax, left side

S25.899 Other specified injury of other blood vessels of thorax, unspecified side

S25.9 Injury of unspecified blood vessel of thorax

S25.90 Unspecified injury of unspecified blood vessel of thorax

S25.91 Laceration of unspecified blood vessel of thorax

S25.99 Other specified injury of unspecified blood vessel of thorax

S26 Injury of heart

Code also any associated:
open wound of thorax (S21.-)
traumatic hemopneumothorax (S27.2)
traumatic hemothorax (S27.1)
traumatic pneumothorax (S27.Ø)

The appropriate 7th character is to be added to each code from category S26.
A initial encounter
D subsequent encounter
S sequela

S26.Ø Injury of heart with hemopericardium

S26.ØØ Unspecified injury of heart with hemopericardium

S26.Ø1 Contusion of heart with hemopericardium

S26.Ø2 Laceration of heart with hemopericardium

S26.Ø2Ø Mild laceration of heart with hemopericardium
Laceration of heart without penetration of heart chamber

S26.Ø21 Moderate laceration of heart with hemopericardium
Laceration of heart with penetration of heart chamber

S26.Ø22 Major laceration of heart with hemopericardium
Laceration of heart with penetration of multiple heart chambers

S26.Ø9 Other injury of heart with hemopericardium

S26.1 Injury of heart without hemopericardium

S26.1Ø Unspecified injury of heart without hemopericardium

S26.11 Contusion of heart without hemopericardium

S26.12 Laceration of heart without hemopericardium

S26.19 Other injury of heart without hemopericardium

S26.9 Injury of heart, unspecified with or without hemopericardium

S26.9Ø Unspecified injury of heart, unspecified with or without hemopericardium

S26.91 Contusion of heart, unspecified with or without hemopericardium
DEF: Bruising within the heart muscle, with no mention of an open wound, usually caused by blunt chest trauma in motor vehicle accidents, falling from great heights, or receiving CPR.

S26.92 Laceration of heart, unspecified with or without hemopericardium
Laceration of heart NOS
AHA: 2019,2Q,24

S26.99 Other injury of heart, unspecified with or without hemopericardium

S27 Injury of other and unspecified intrathoracic organs

Code also any associated open wound of thorax (S21.-)

EXCLUDES 2 *injury of cervical esophagus (S1Ø-S19)*
injury of trachea (cervical) (S1Ø-S19)

The appropriate 7th character is to be added to each code from category S27.
A initial encounter
D subsequent encounter
S sequela

S27.Ø Traumatic pneumothorax
EXCLUDES 1 *spontaneous pneumothorax (J93.-)*

S27.1 Traumatic hemothorax

S27.2 Traumatic hemopneumothorax

S27.3 Other and unspecified injuries of lung

S27.3Ø Unspecified injury of lung

S27.3Ø1 Unspecified injury of lung, unilateral

S27.3Ø2 Unspecified injury of lung, bilateral

S27.3Ø9 Unspecified injury of lung, unspecified

S27.31 Primary blast injury of lung
Blast injury of lung NOS

S27.311 Primary blast injury of lung, unilateral

S27.312 Primary blast injury of lung, bilateral

S27.319 Primary blast injury of lung, unspecified

S27.32 Contusion of lung
DEF: Bruising of the lung without mention of an open wound.

S27.321 Contusion of lung, unilateral

S27.322 Contusion of lung, bilateral

S27.329 Contusion of lung, unspecified

S27.33 Laceration of lung

S27.331 Laceration of lung, unilateral

S27.332 Laceration of lung, bilateral

S27.339 Laceration of lung, unspecified

S27.39 Other injuries of lung
Secondary blast injury of lung

S27.391 Other injuries of lung, unilateral

S27.392 Other injuries of lung, bilateral

S27.399 Other injuries of lung, unspecified

S27.4 Injury of bronchus

S27.4Ø Unspecified injury of bronchus

S27.4Ø1 Unspecified injury of bronchus, unilateral

S27.4Ø2 Unspecified injury of bronchus, bilateral

S27.4Ø9 Unspecified injury of bronchus, unspecified

S27.41 Primary blast injury of bronchus
Blast injury of bronchus NOS

S27.411 Primary blast injury of bronchus, unilateral

S27.412 Primary blast injury of bronchus, bilateral

S27.419 Primary blast injury of bronchus, unspecified

S27.42 Contusion of bronchus

S27.421 Contusion of bronchus, unilateral

S27.422 Contusion of bronchus, bilateral

S27.429 Contusion of bronchus, unspecified

S27.43 Laceration of bronchus

S27.431 Laceration of bronchus, unilateral

S27.432 Laceration of bronchus, bilateral

S27.439 Laceration of bronchus, unspecified

S27.49 Other injury of bronchus
Secondary blast injury of bronchus

S27.491 Other injury of bronchus, unilateral

S27.492 Other injury of bronchus, bilateral

S27.499 Other injury of bronchus, unspecified

S27.5 Injury of thoracic trachea

S27.5Ø Unspecified injury of thoracic trachea

S27.51 Primary blast injury of thoracic trachea
Blast injury of thoracic trachea NOS

S27.52 Contusion of thoracic trachea

S27.53 Laceration of thoracic trachea

S27.59 Other injury of thoracic trachea
Secondary blast injury of thoracic trachea

S27.6 Injury of pleura

S27.60 Unspecified injury of pleura

S27.63 Laceration of pleura

S27.69 Other injury of pleura

S27.8 Injury of other specified intrathoracic organs

S27.80 Injury of diaphragm

S27.802 Contusion of diaphragm

S27.803 Laceration of diaphragm

S27.808 Other injury of diaphragm

S27.809 Unspecified injury of diaphragm

S27.81 Injury of esophagus (thoracic part)

S27.812 Contusion of esophagus (thoracic part)

S27.813 Laceration of esophagus (thoracic part)

S27.818 Other injury of esophagus (thoracic part)

S27.819 Unspecified injury of esophagus (thoracic part)

S27.89 Injury of other specified intrathoracic organs
Injury of lymphatic thoracic duct
Injury of thymus gland

S27.892 Contusion of other specified intrathoracic organs

S27.893 Laceration of other specified intrathoracic organs

S27.898 Other injury of other specified intrathoracic organs

S27.899 Unspecified injury of other specified intrathoracic organs

S27.9 Injury of unspecified intrathoracic organ

S28 Crushing injury of thorax, and traumatic amputation of part of thorax

The appropriate 7th character is to be added to each code from category S28.
A initial encounter
D subsequent encounter
S sequela

S28.0 Crushed chest
Use additional code for all associated injuries
EXCLUDES 1 *flail chest (S22.5)*

S28.1 Traumatic amputation (partial) of part of thorax, except breast

S28.2 Traumatic amputation of breast

S28.21 Complete traumatic amputation of breast
Traumatic amputation of breast NOS

S28.211 Complete traumatic amputation of right breast

S28.212 Complete traumatic amputation of left breast

S28.219 Complete traumatic amputation of unspecified breast

S28.22 Partial traumatic amputation of breast

S28.221 Partial traumatic amputation of right breast

S28.222 Partial traumatic amputation of left breast

S28.229 Partial traumatic amputation of unspecified breast

S29 Other and unspecified injuries of thorax
Code also any associated open wound (S21.-)

The appropriate 7th character is to be added to each code from category S29.
A initial encounter
D subsequent encounter
S sequela

S29.0 Injury of muscle and tendon at thorax level

S29.00 Unspecified injury of muscle and tendon of thorax

S29.001 Unspecified injury of muscle and tendon of front wall of thorax

S29.002 Unspecified injury of muscle and tendon of back wall of thorax

S29.009 Unspecified injury of muscle and tendon of unspecified wall of thorax

S29.01 Strain of muscle and tendon of thorax

S29.011 Strain of muscle and tendon of front wall of thorax

S29.012 Strain of muscle and tendon of back wall of thorax

S29.019 Strain of muscle and tendon of unspecified wall of thorax

S29.02 Laceration of muscle and tendon of thorax

S29.021 Laceration of muscle and tendon of front wall of thorax

S29.022 Laceration of muscle and tendon of back wall of thorax

S29.029 Laceration of muscle and tendon of unspecified wall of thorax

S29.09 Other injury of muscle and tendon of thorax

S29.091 Other injury of muscle and tendon of front wall of thorax

S29.092 Other injury of muscle and tendon of back wall of thorax

S29.099 Other injury of muscle and tendon of unspecified wall of thorax

S29.8 Other specified injuries of thorax

S29.9 Unspecified injury of thorax

Injuries to the abdomen, lower back, lumbar spine, pelvis and external genitals (S30-S39)

INCLUDES injuries to the abdominal wall
injuries to the anus
injuries to the buttock
injuries to the external genitalia
injuries to the flank
injuries to the groin

EXCLUDES 2 *burns and corrosions (T20-T32)*
effects of foreign body in anus and rectum (T18.5)
effects of foreign body in genitourinary tract (T19.-)
effects of foreign body in stomach, small intestine and colon (T18.2-T18.4)
frostbite (T33-T34)
insect bite or sting, venomous (T63.4)

S30 Superficial injury of abdomen, lower back, pelvis and external genitals
EXCLUDES 2 *superficial injury of hip (S70.-)*

The appropriate 7th character is to be added to each code from category S30.
A initial encounter
D subsequent encounter
S sequela

S30.0 Contusion of lower back and pelvis
Contusion of buttock

S30.1 Contusion of abdominal wall
Contusion of flank
Contusion of groin

S30.2 Contusion of external genital organs

S30.20 Contusion of unspecified external genital organ

S30.201 Contusion of unspecified external genital organ, male ♂

S30.202 Contusion of unspecified external genital organ, female ♀

S30.21 Contusion of penis ♂

S30.22 Contusion of scrotum and testes ♂

S30.23 Contusion of vagina and vulva ♀

S30.3 Contusion of anus

S30.8 Other superficial injuries of abdomen, lower back, pelvis and external genitals

S30.81 Abrasion of abdomen, lower back, pelvis and external genitals

S30.810 Abrasion of lower back and pelvis

S30.811 Abrasion of abdominal wall

S30.812 Abrasion of penis ♂

S30.813 Abrasion of scrotum and testes ♂

S30.814 Abrasion of vagina and vulva ♀

S30.815 Abrasion of unspecified external genital organs, male ♂

- S3Ø.816 Abrasion of unspecified external genital organs, female ♀
- S3Ø.817 Abrasion of anus
- S3Ø.82 Blister (nonthermal) of abdomen, lower back, pelvis and external genitals
  - S3Ø.82Ø Blister (nonthermal) of lower back and pelvis
  - S3Ø.821 Blister (nonthermal) of abdominal wall
  - S3Ø.822 Blister (nonthermal) of penis ♂
  - S3Ø.823 Blister (nonthermal) of scrotum and testes ♂
  - S3Ø.824 Blister (nonthermal) of vagina and vulva ♀
  - S3Ø.825 Blister (nonthermal) of unspecified external genital organs, male ♂
  - S3Ø.826 Blister (nonthermal) of unspecified external genital organs, female ♀
  - S3Ø.827 Blister (nonthermal) of anus
- S3Ø.84 External constriction of abdomen, lower back, pelvis and external genitals
  - S3Ø.84Ø External constriction of lower back and pelvis
  - S3Ø.841 External constriction of abdominal wall
  - S3Ø.842 External constriction of penis ♂
    - Hair tourniquet syndrome of penis
    - Use additional cause code to identify the constricting item (W49.Ø-)
  - S3Ø.843 External constriction of scrotum and testes ♂
  - S3Ø.844 External constriction of vagina and vulva ♀
  - S3Ø.845 External constriction of unspecified external genital organs, male ♂
  - S3Ø.846 External constriction of unspecified external genital organs, female ♀
- S3Ø.85 Superficial foreign body of abdomen, lower back, pelvis and external genitals
  - Splinter in the abdomen, lower back, pelvis and external genitals
  - S3Ø.85Ø Superficial foreign body of lower back and pelvis
  - S3Ø.851 Superficial foreign body of abdominal wall
  - S3Ø.852 Superficial foreign body of penis ♂
  - S3Ø.853 Superficial foreign body of scrotum and testes ♂
  - S3Ø.854 Superficial foreign body of vagina and vulva ♀
  - S3Ø.855 Superficial foreign body of unspecified external genital organs, male ♂
  - S3Ø.856 Superficial foreign body of unspecified external genital organs, female ♀
  - S3Ø.857 Superficial foreign body of anus
- S3Ø.86 Insect bite (nonvenomous) of abdomen, lower back, pelvis and external genitals
  - S3Ø.86Ø Insect bite (nonvenomous) of lower back and pelvis
  - S3Ø.861 Insect bite (nonvenomous) of abdominal wall
  - S3Ø.862 Insect bite (nonvenomous) of penis ♂
  - S3Ø.863 Insect bite (nonvenomous) of scrotum and testes ♂
  - S3Ø.864 Insect bite (nonvenomous) of vagina and vulva ♀
  - S3Ø.865 Insect bite (nonvenomous) of unspecified external genital organs, male ♂
  - S3Ø.866 Insect bite (nonvenomous) of unspecified external genital organs, female ♀
  - S3Ø.867 Insect bite (nonvenomous) of anus
- S3Ø.87 Other superficial bite of abdomen, lower back, pelvis and external genitals
  - EXCLUDES 1 *open bite of abdomen, lower back, pelvis and external genitals (S31.Ø5, S31.15, S31.25, S31.35, S31.45, S31.55)*
  - S3Ø.87Ø Other superficial bite of lower back and pelvis
  - S3Ø.871 Other superficial bite of abdominal wall
  - S3Ø.872 Other superficial bite of penis ♂
  - S3Ø.873 Other superficial bite of scrotum and testes ♂
  - S3Ø.874 Other superficial bite of vagina and vulva ♀
  - S3Ø.875 Other superficial bite of unspecified external genital organs, male ♂
  - S3Ø.876 Other superficial bite of unspecified external genital organs, female ♀
  - S3Ø.877 Other superficial bite of anus
- S3Ø.9 Unspecified superficial injury of abdomen, lower back, pelvis and external genitals
  - S3Ø.91 Unspecified superficial injury of lower back and pelvis
  - S3Ø.92 Unspecified superficial injury of abdominal wall
  - S3Ø.93 Unspecified superficial injury of penis ♂
  - S3Ø.94 Unspecified superficial injury of scrotum and testes ♂
  - S3Ø.95 Unspecified superficial injury of vagina and vulva ♀
  - S3Ø.96 Unspecified superficial injury of unspecified external genital organs, male ♂
  - S3Ø.97 Unspecified superficial injury of unspecified external genital organs, female ♀
  - S3Ø.98 Unspecified superficial injury of anus

S31 Open wound of abdomen, lower back, pelvis and external genitals

Code also any associated:
- spinal cord injury (S24.Ø, S24.1-, S34.Ø-, S34.1-)
- wound infection

EXCLUDES 1 *traumatic amputation of part of abdomen, lower back and pelvis (S38.2-, S38.3)*

EXCLUDES 2 *open wound of hip (S71.ØØ-S71.Ø2)*
open fracture of pelvis (S32.1- - S32.9 with 7th character B)

The appropriate 7th character is to be added to each code from category S31.
- A initial encounter
- D subsequent encounter
- S sequela

- S31.Ø Open wound of lower back and pelvis
  - S31.ØØ Unspecified open wound of lower back and pelvis
    - S31.ØØØ Unspecified open wound of lower back and pelvis without penetration into retroperitoneum
      - Unspecified open wound of lower back and pelvis NOS
    - S31.ØØ1 Unspecified open wound of lower back and pelvis with penetration into retroperitoneum
  - S31.Ø1 Laceration without foreign body of lower back and pelvis
    - S31.Ø1Ø Laceration without foreign body of lower back and pelvis without penetration into retroperitoneum
      - Laceration without foreign body of lower back and pelvis NOS
    - S31.Ø11 Laceration without foreign body of lower back and pelvis with penetration into retroperitoneum
  - S31.Ø2 Laceration with foreign body of lower back and pelvis
    - S31.Ø2Ø Laceration with foreign body of lower back and pelvis without penetration into retroperitoneum
      - Laceration with foreign body of lower back and pelvis NOS
    - S31.Ø21 Laceration with foreign body of lower back and pelvis with penetration into retroperitoneum
  - S31.Ø3 Puncture wound without foreign body of lower back and pelvis
    - S31.Ø3Ø Puncture wound without foreign body of lower back and pelvis without penetration into retroperitoneum
      - Puncture wound without foreign body of lower back and pelvis NOS
    - S31.Ø31 Puncture wound without foreign body of lower back and pelvis with penetration into retroperitoneum

6th S31.Ø4 Puncture wound with foreign body of lower back and pelvis

7th S31.Ø4Ø Puncture wound with foreign body of lower back and pelvis without penetration into retroperitoneum
Puncture wound with foreign body of lower back and pelvis NOS

7th S31.Ø41 Puncture wound with foreign body of lower back and pelvis with penetration into retroperitoneum

6th S31.Ø5 Open bite of lower back and pelvis
Bite of lower back and pelvis NOS
EXCLUDES 1 *superficial bite of lower back and pelvis (S3Ø.86Ø, S3Ø.87Ø)*

7th S31.Ø5Ø Open bite of lower back and pelvis without penetration into retroperitoneum
Open bite of lower back and pelvis NOS

7th S31.Ø51 Open bite of lower back and pelvis with penetration into retroperitoneum

5th S31.1 Open wound of abdominal wall without penetration into peritoneal cavity
Open wound of abdominal wall NOS
EXCLUDES 2 *open wound of abdominal wall with penetration into peritoneal cavity (S31.6-)*

6th S31.1Ø Unspecified open wound of abdominal wall without penetration into peritoneal cavity

7th S31.1ØØ Unspecified open wound of abdominal wall, right upper quadrant without penetration into peritoneal cavity

7th S31.1Ø1 Unspecified open wound of abdominal wall, left upper quadrant without penetration into peritoneal cavity

7th S31.1Ø2 Unspecified open wound of abdominal wall, epigastric region without penetration into peritoneal cavity

7th S31.1Ø3 Unspecified open wound of abdominal wall, right lower quadrant without penetration into peritoneal cavity

7th S31.1Ø4 Unspecified open wound of abdominal wall, left lower quadrant without penetration into peritoneal cavity

7th S31.1Ø5 Unspecified open wound of abdominal wall, periumbilic region without penetration into peritoneal cavity

7th S31.1Ø9 Unspecified open wound of abdominal wall, unspecified quadrant without penetration into peritoneal cavity
Unspecified open wound of abdominal wall NOS

6th S31.11 Laceration without foreign body of abdominal wall without penetration into peritoneal cavity

7th S31.11Ø Laceration without foreign body of abdominal wall, right upper quadrant without penetration into peritoneal cavity

7th S31.111 Laceration without foreign body of abdominal wall, left upper quadrant without penetration into peritoneal cavity

7th S31.112 Laceration without foreign body of abdominal wall, epigastric region without penetration into peritoneal cavity

7th S31.113 Laceration without foreign body of abdominal wall, right lower quadrant without penetration into peritoneal cavity

7th S31.114 Laceration without foreign body of abdominal wall, left lower quadrant without penetration into peritoneal cavity

7th S31.115 Laceration without foreign body of abdominal wall, periumbilic region without penetration into peritoneal cavity

7th S31.119 Laceration without foreign body of abdominal wall, unspecified quadrant without penetration into peritoneal cavity

6th S31.12 Laceration with foreign body of abdominal wall without penetration into peritoneal cavity

7th S31.12Ø Laceration of abdominal wall with foreign body, right upper quadrant without penetration into peritoneal cavity

7th S31.121 Laceration of abdominal wall with foreign body, left upper quadrant without penetration into peritoneal cavity

7th S31.122 Laceration of abdominal wall with foreign body, epigastric region without penetration into peritoneal cavity

7th S31.123 Laceration of abdominal wall with foreign body, right lower quadrant without penetration into peritoneal cavity

7th S31.124 Laceration of abdominal wall with foreign body, left lower quadrant without penetration into peritoneal cavity

7th S31.125 Laceration of abdominal wall with foreign body, periumbilic region without penetration into peritoneal cavity

7th S31.129 Laceration of abdominal wall with foreign body, unspecified quadrant without penetration into peritoneal cavity

6th S31.13 Puncture wound of abdominal wall without foreign body without penetration into peritoneal cavity

7th S31.13Ø Puncture wound of abdominal wall without foreign body, right upper quadrant without penetration into peritoneal cavity

7th S31.131 Puncture wound of abdominal wall without foreign body, left upper quadrant without penetration into peritoneal cavity

7th S31.132 Puncture wound of abdominal wall without foreign body, epigastric region without penetration into peritoneal cavity

7th S31.133 Puncture wound of abdominal wall without foreign body, right lower quadrant without penetration into peritoneal cavity

7th S31.134 Puncture wound of abdominal wall without foreign body, left lower quadrant without penetration into peritoneal cavity

7th S31.135 Puncture wound of abdominal wall without foreign body, periumbilic region without penetration into peritoneal cavity

7th S31.139 Puncture wound of abdominal wall without foreign body, unspecified quadrant without penetration into peritoneal cavity

6th S31.14 Puncture wound of abdominal wall with foreign body without penetration into peritoneal cavity

7th S31.14Ø Puncture wound of abdominal wall with foreign body, right upper quadrant without penetration into peritoneal cavity

7th S31.141 Puncture wound of abdominal wall with foreign body, left upper quadrant without penetration into peritoneal cavity

7th S31.142 Puncture wound of abdominal wall with foreign body, epigastric region without penetration into peritoneal cavity

7th S31.143 Puncture wound of abdominal wall with foreign body, right lower quadrant without penetration into peritoneal cavity

7th S31.144 Puncture wound of abdominal wall with foreign body, left lower quadrant without penetration into peritoneal cavity

7th S31.145 Puncture wound of abdominal wall with foreign body, periumbilic region without penetration into peritoneal cavity

7th S31.149 Puncture wound of abdominal wall with foreign body, unspecified quadrant without penetration into peritoneal cavity

6th S31.15 Open bite of abdominal wall without penetration into peritoneal cavity
Bite of abdominal wall NOS
EXCLUDES 1 *superficial bite of abdominal wall (S3Ø.871)*

7th S31.15Ø Open bite of abdominal wall, right upper quadrant without penetration into peritoneal cavity

S31.151 Open bite of abdominal wall, left upper quadrant without penetration into peritoneal cavity

S31.152 Open bite of abdominal wall, epigastric region without penetration into peritoneal cavity

S31.153 Open bite of abdominal wall, right lower quadrant without penetration into peritoneal cavity

S31.154 Open bite of abdominal wall, left lower quadrant without penetration into peritoneal cavity

S31.155 Open bite of abdominal wall, periumbilic region without penetration into peritoneal cavity

S31.159 Open bite of abdominal wall, unspecified quadrant without penetration into peritoneal cavity

S31.2 Open wound of penis

S31.20 Unspecified open wound of penis ♂

S31.21 Laceration without foreign body of penis ♂

S31.22 Laceration with foreign body of penis ♂

S31.23 Puncture wound without foreign body of penis ♂

S31.24 Puncture wound with foreign body of penis ♂

S31.25 Open bite of penis ♂
Bite of penis NOS
EXCLUDES 1 *superficial bite of penis (S30.862, S30.872)*

S31.3 Open wound of scrotum and testes

S31.30 Unspecified open wound of scrotum and testes ♂

S31.31 Laceration without foreign body of scrotum and testes ♂

S31.32 Laceration with foreign body of scrotum and testes ♂

S31.33 Puncture wound without foreign body of scrotum and testes ♂

S31.34 Puncture wound with foreign body of scrotum and testes ♂

S31.35 Open bite of scrotum and testes ♂
Bite of scrotum and testes NOS
EXCLUDES 1 *superficial bite of scrotum and testes (S30.863, S30.873)*

S31.4 Open wound of vagina and vulva
EXCLUDES 1 *injury to vagina and vulva during delivery (O70.-, O71.4)*

S31.40 Unspecified open wound of vagina and vulva ♀

S31.41 Laceration without foreign body of vagina and vulva ♀

S31.42 Laceration with foreign body of vagina and vulva ♀

S31.43 Puncture wound without foreign body of vagina and vulva ♀

S31.44 Puncture wound with foreign body of vagina and vulva ♀

S31.45 Open bite of vagina and vulva ♀
Bite of vagina and vulva NOS
EXCLUDES 1 *superficial bite of vagina and vulva (S30.864, S30.874)*

S31.5 Open wound of unspecified external genital organs
EXCLUDES 1 *traumatic amputation of external genital organs (S38.21, S38.22)*

S31.50 Unspecified open wound of unspecified external genital organs

S31.501 Unspecified open wound of unspecified external genital organs, male ♂

S31.502 Unspecified open wound of unspecified external genital organs, female ♀

S31.51 Laceration without foreign body of unspecified external genital organs

S31.511 Laceration without foreign body of unspecified external genital organs, male ♂

S31.512 Laceration without foreign body of unspecified external genital organs, female ♀

S31.52 Laceration with foreign body of unspecified external genital organs

S31.521 Laceration with foreign body of unspecified external genital organs, male ♂

S31.522 Laceration with foreign body of unspecified external genital organs, female ♀

S31.53 Puncture wound without foreign body of unspecified external genital organs

S31.531 Puncture wound without foreign body of unspecified external genital organs, male ♂

S31.532 Puncture wound without foreign body of unspecified external genital organs, female ♀

S31.54 Puncture wound with foreign body of unspecified external genital organs

S31.541 Puncture wound with foreign body of unspecified external genital organs, male ♂

S31.542 Puncture wound with foreign body of unspecified external genital organs, female ♀

S31.55 Open bite of unspecified external genital organs
Bite of unspecified external genital organs NOS
EXCLUDES 1 *superficial bite of unspecified external genital organs (S30.865, S30.866, S30.875, S30.876)*

S31.551 Open bite of unspecified external genital organs, male ♂

S31.552 Open bite of unspecified external genital organs, female ♀

S31.6 Open wound of abdominal wall with penetration into peritoneal cavity

S31.60 Unspecified open wound of abdominal wall with penetration into peritoneal cavity

S31.600 Unspecified open wound of abdominal wall, right upper quadrant with penetration into peritoneal cavity

S31.601 Unspecified open wound of abdominal wall, left upper quadrant with penetration into peritoneal cavity

S31.602 Unspecified open wound of abdominal wall, epigastric region with penetration into peritoneal cavity

S31.603 Unspecified open wound of abdominal wall, right lower quadrant with penetration into peritoneal cavity

S31.604 Unspecified open wound of abdominal wall, left lower quadrant with penetration into peritoneal cavity

S31.605 Unspecified open wound of abdominal wall, periumbilic region with penetration into peritoneal cavity

S31.609 Unspecified open wound of abdominal wall, unspecified quadrant with penetration into peritoneal cavity

S31.61 Laceration without foreign body of abdominal wall with penetration into peritoneal cavity

S31.610 Laceration without foreign body of abdominal wall, right upper quadrant with penetration into peritoneal cavity

S31.611 Laceration without foreign body of abdominal wall, left upper quadrant with penetration into peritoneal cavity

S31.612 Laceration without foreign body of abdominal wall, epigastric region with penetration into peritoneal cavity

S31.613 Laceration without foreign body of abdominal wall, right lower quadrant with penetration into peritoneal cavity

S31.614 Laceration without foreign body of abdominal wall, left lower quadrant with penetration into peritoneal cavity

S31.615 Laceration without foreign body of abdominal wall, periumbilic region with penetration into peritoneal cavity

S31.619 Laceration without foreign body of abdominal wall, unspecified quadrant with penetration into peritoneal cavity

S31.62 Laceration with foreign body of abdominal wall with penetration into peritoneal cavity
S31.620 Laceration with foreign body of abdominal wall, right upper quadrant with penetration into peritoneal cavity
S31.621 Laceration with foreign body of abdominal wall, left upper quadrant with penetration into peritoneal cavity
S31.622 Laceration with foreign body of abdominal wall, epigastric region with penetration into peritoneal cavity
S31.623 Laceration with foreign body of abdominal wall, right lower quadrant with penetration into peritoneal cavity
S31.624 Laceration with foreign body of abdominal wall, left lower quadrant with penetration into peritoneal cavity
S31.625 Laceration with foreign body of abdominal wall, periumbilic region with penetration into peritoneal cavity
S31.629 Laceration with foreign body of abdominal wall, unspecified quadrant with penetration into peritoneal cavity
S31.63 Puncture wound without foreign body of abdominal wall with penetration into peritoneal cavity
S31.630 Puncture wound without foreign body of abdominal wall, right upper quadrant with penetration into peritoneal cavity
S31.631 Puncture wound without foreign body of abdominal wall, left upper quadrant with penetration into peritoneal cavity
S31.632 Puncture wound without foreign body of abdominal wall, epigastric region with penetration into peritoneal cavity
S31.633 Puncture wound without foreign body of abdominal wall, right lower quadrant with penetration into peritoneal cavity
S31.634 Puncture wound without foreign body of abdominal wall, left lower quadrant with penetration into peritoneal cavity
S31.635 Puncture wound without foreign body of abdominal wall, periumbilic region with penetration into peritoneal cavity
S31.639 Puncture wound without foreign body of abdominal wall, unspecified quadrant with penetration into peritoneal cavity
S31.64 Puncture wound with foreign body of abdominal wall with penetration into peritoneal cavity
S31.640 Puncture wound with foreign body of abdominal wall, right upper quadrant with penetration into peritoneal cavity
S31.641 Puncture wound with foreign body of abdominal wall, left upper quadrant with penetration into peritoneal cavity
S31.642 Puncture wound with foreign body of abdominal wall, epigastric region with penetration into peritoneal cavity
S31.643 Puncture wound with foreign body of abdominal wall, right lower quadrant with penetration into peritoneal cavity
S31.644 Puncture wound with foreign body of abdominal wall, left lower quadrant with penetration into peritoneal cavity
S31.645 Puncture wound with foreign body of abdominal wall, periumbilic region with penetration into peritoneal cavity
S31.649 Puncture wound with foreign body of abdominal wall, unspecified quadrant with penetration into peritoneal cavity
S31.65 Open bite of abdominal wall with penetration into peritoneal cavity
EXCLUDES 1 *superficial bite of abdominal wall (S30.861, S30.871)*
S31.650 Open bite of abdominal wall, right upper quadrant with penetration into peritoneal cavity
S31.651 Open bite of abdominal wall, left upper quadrant with penetration into peritoneal cavity
S31.652 Open bite of abdominal wall, epigastric region with penetration into peritoneal cavity
S31.653 Open bite of abdominal wall, right lower quadrant with penetration into peritoneal cavity
S31.654 Open bite of abdominal wall, left lower quadrant with penetration into peritoneal cavity
S31.655 Open bite of abdominal wall, periumbilic region with penetration into peritoneal cavity
S31.659 Open bite of abdominal wall, unspecified quadrant with penetration into peritoneal cavity
S31.8 Open wound of other parts of abdomen, lower back and pelvis
S31.80 Open wound of unspecified buttock
S31.801 Laceration without foreign body of unspecified buttock
S31.802 Laceration with foreign body of unspecified buttock
S31.803 Puncture wound without foreign body of unspecified buttock
S31.804 Puncture wound with foreign body of unspecified buttock
S31.805 Open bite of unspecified buttock
Bite of buttock NOS
EXCLUDES 1 *superficial bite of buttock (S30.870)*
S31.809 Unspecified open wound of unspecified buttock
S31.81 Open wound of right buttock
S31.811 Laceration without foreign body of right buttock
S31.812 Laceration with foreign body of right buttock
S31.813 Puncture wound without foreign body of right buttock
S31.814 Puncture wound with foreign body of right buttock
S31.815 Open bite of right buttock
Bite of right buttock NOS
EXCLUDES 1 *superficial bite of buttock (S30.870)*
S31.819 Unspecified open wound of right buttock
S31.82 Open wound of left buttock
S31.821 Laceration without foreign body of left buttock
S31.822 Laceration with foreign body of left buttock
S31.823 Puncture wound without foreign body of left buttock
S31.824 Puncture wound with foreign body of left buttock
S31.825 Open bite of left buttock
Bite of left buttock NOS
EXCLUDES 1 *superficial bite of buttock (S30.870)*
S31.829 Unspecified open wound of left buttock
S31.83 Open wound of anus
S31.831 Laceration without foreign body of anus
S31.832 Laceration with foreign body of anus
S31.833 Puncture wound without foreign body of anus
S31.834 Puncture wound with foreign body of anus
S31.835 Open bite of anus
Bite of anus NOS
EXCLUDES 1 *superficial bite of anus (S30.877)*
S31.839 Unspecified open wound of anus

✓4th S32 Fracture of lumbar spine and pelvis

NOTE A fracture not indicated as displaced or nondisplaced should be coded to displaced.

A fracture not indicated as opened or closed should be coded to closed.

INCLUDES fracture of lumbosacral neural arch
fracture of lumbosacral spinous process
fracture of lumbosacral transverse process
fracture of lumbosacral vertebra
fracture of lumbosacral vertebral arch

Code first any associated spinal cord and spinal nerve injury (S34.-)

EXCLUDES 1 *transection of abdomen (S38.3)*

EXCLUDES 2 *fracture of hip NOS (S72.Ø-)*

AHA: 2021,1Q,6; 2018,2Q,12; 2015,3Q,37-39; 2012,4Q,93

The appropriate 7th character is to be added to each code from category S32.
A initial encounter for closed fracture
B initial encounter for open fracture
D subsequent encounter for fracture with routine healing
G subsequent encounter for fracture with delayed healing
K subsequent encounter for fracture with nonunion
S sequela

✓5th S32.Ø Fracture of lumbar vertebra
Fracture of lumbar spine NOS

✓6th S32.ØØ Fracture of unspecified lumbar vertebra
1 ✓7th **S32.ØØØ Wedge compression fracture of unspecified lumbar vertebra** HCC ESR COM Q
1 ✓7th **S32.ØØ1 Stable burst fracture of unspecified lumbar vertebra** HCC ESR COM Q
1 ✓7th **S32.ØØ2 Unstable burst fracture of unspecified lumbar vertebra** HCC ESR COM Q
1 ✓7th **S32.ØØ8 Other fracture of unspecified lumbar vertebra** HCC ESR COM Q
1 ✓7th **S32.ØØ9 Unspecified fracture of unspecified lumbar vertebra** HCC ESR COM Q

✓6th S32.Ø1 Fracture of first lumbar vertebra
1 ✓7th **S32.Ø1Ø Wedge compression fracture of first lumbar vertebra** HCC ESR COM Q
1 ✓7th **S32.Ø11 Stable burst fracture of first lumbar vertebra** HCC ESR COM Q
1 ✓7th **S32.Ø12 Unstable burst fracture of first lumbar vertebra** HCC ESR COM Q
1 ✓7th **S32.Ø18 Other fracture of first lumbar vertebra** HCC ESR COM Q
1 ✓7th **S32.Ø19 Unspecified fracture of first lumbar vertebra** HCC ESR COM Q

✓6th S32.Ø2 Fracture of second lumbar vertebra
1 ✓7th **S32.Ø2Ø Wedge compression fracture of second lumbar vertebra** HCC ESR COM Q
1 ✓7th **S32.Ø21 Stable burst fracture of second lumbar vertebra** HCC ESR COM Q
1 ✓7th **S32.Ø22 Unstable burst fracture of second lumbar vertebra** HCC ESR COM Q
1 ✓7th **S32.Ø28 Other fracture of second lumbar vertebra** HCC ESR COM Q
1 ✓7th **S32.Ø29 Unspecified fracture of second lumbar vertebra** HCC ESR COM Q

✓6th S32.Ø3 Fracture of third lumbar vertebra
1 ✓7th **S32.Ø3Ø Wedge compression fracture of third lumbar vertebra** HCC ESR COM Q
1 ✓7th **S32.Ø31 Stable burst fracture of third lumbar vertebra** HCC ESR COM Q
1 ✓7th **S32.Ø32 Unstable burst fracture of third lumbar vertebra** HCC ESR COM Q
1 ✓7th **S32.Ø38 Other fracture of third lumbar vertebra** HCC ESR COM Q
1 ✓7th **S32.Ø39 Unspecified fracture of third lumbar vertebra** HCC ESR COM Q

✓6th S32.Ø4 Fracture of fourth lumbar vertebra
1 ✓7th **S32.Ø4Ø Wedge compression fracture of fourth lumbar vertebra** HCC ESR COM Q
1 ✓7th **S32.Ø41 Stable burst fracture of fourth lumbar vertebra** HCC ESR COM Q
1 ✓7th **S32.Ø42 Unstable burst fracture of fourth lumbar vertebra** HCC ESR COM Q
1 ✓7th **S32.Ø48 Other fracture of fourth lumbar vertebra** HCC ESR COM Q
1 ✓7th **S32.Ø49 Unspecified fracture of fourth lumbar vertebra** HCC ESR COM Q

✓6th S32.Ø5 Fracture of fifth lumbar vertebra
1 ✓7th **S32.Ø5Ø Wedge compression fracture of fifth lumbar vertebra** HCC ESR COM Q
1 ✓7th **S32.Ø51 Stable burst fracture of fifth lumbar vertebra** HCC ESR COM Q
1 ✓7th **S32.Ø52 Unstable burst fracture of fifth lumbar vertebra** HCC ESR COM Q
1 ✓7th **S32.Ø58 Other fracture of fifth lumbar vertebra** HCC ESR COM Q
1 ✓7th **S32.Ø59 Unspecified fracture of fifth lumbar vertebra** HCC ESR COM Q

✓5th S32.1 Fracture of sacrum

NOTE For vertical fractures, code to most medial fracture extension

Use two codes if both a vertical and transverse fracture are present

Code also any associated fracture of pelvic ring (S32.8-)

1 ✓x7th **S32.1Ø Unspecified fracture of sacrum** HCC ESR COM Q

✓6th S32.11 Zone I fracture of sacrum
Vertical sacral ala fracture of sacrum

Vertical Sacral Fracture Zones

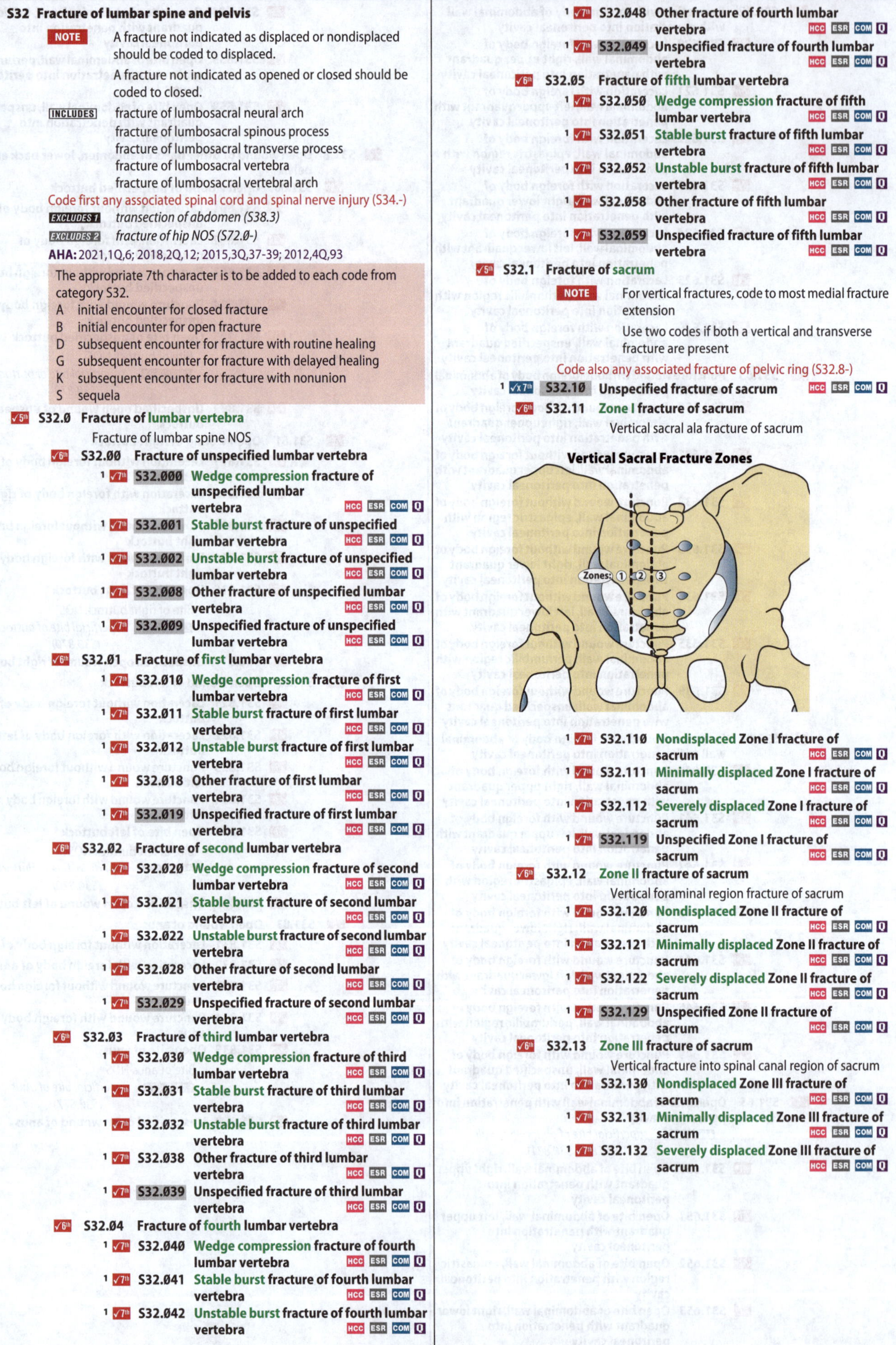

1 ✓7th **S32.11Ø Nondisplaced Zone I fracture of sacrum** HCC ESR COM Q
1 ✓7th **S32.111 Minimally displaced Zone I fracture of sacrum** HCC ESR COM Q
1 ✓7th **S32.112 Severely displaced Zone I fracture of sacrum** HCC ESR COM Q
1 ✓7th **S32.119 Unspecified Zone I fracture of sacrum** HCC ESR COM Q

✓6th S32.12 Zone II fracture of sacrum
Vertical foraminal region fracture of sacrum
1 ✓7th **S32.12Ø Nondisplaced Zone II fracture of sacrum** HCC ESR COM Q
1 ✓7th **S32.121 Minimally displaced Zone II fracture of sacrum** HCC ESR COM Q
1 ✓7th **S32.122 Severely displaced Zone II fracture of sacrum** HCC ESR COM Q
1 ✓7th **S32.129 Unspecified Zone II fracture of sacrum** HCC ESR COM Q

✓6th S32.13 Zone III fracture of sacrum
Vertical fracture into spinal canal region of sacrum
1 ✓7th **S32.13Ø Nondisplaced Zone III fracture of sacrum** HCC ESR COM Q
1 ✓7th **S32.131 Minimally displaced Zone III fracture of sacrum** HCC ESR COM Q
1 ✓7th **S32.132 Severely displaced Zone III fracture of sacrum** HCC ESR COM Q

1 ✓7th **S32.139** Unspecified Zone III fracture of sacrum HCC ESR COM Q

Transverse Sacral Fracture Types

Type 1 Type 2 Type 3 Type 4

1 ✓x7th **S32.14** Type 1 fracture of sacrum HCC ESR COM Q
Transverse flexion fracture of sacrum without displacement

1 ✓x7th **S32.15** Type 2 fracture of sacrum HCC ESR COM Q
Transverse flexion fracture of sacrum with posterior displacement

1 ✓x7th **S32.16** Type 3 fracture of sacrum HCC ESR COM Q
Transverse extension fracture of sacrum with anterior displacement

1 ✓x7th **S32.17** Type 4 fracture of sacrum HCC ESR COM Q
Transverse segmental comminution of upper sacrum

1 ✓x7th **S32.19** Other fracture of sacrum HCC ESR COM Q

1 ✓x7th **S32.2** Fracture of coccyx HCC ESR COM Q

✓5th **S32.3** Fracture of ilium

EXCLUDES 1 *fracture of ilium with associated disruption of pelvic ring (S32.8-)*

✓6th **S32.30** Unspecified fracture of ilium

1 ✓7th **S32.301** Unspecified fracture of right ilium HCC ESR COM Q

1 ✓7th **S32.302** Unspecified fracture of left ilium HCC ESR COM Q

1 ✓7th **S32.309** Unspecified fracture of unspecified ilium HCC ESR COM Q

✓6th **S32.31** Avulsion fracture of ilium

1 ✓7th **S32.311** Displaced avulsion fracture of right ilium HCC ESR COM Q

1 ✓7th **S32.312** Displaced avulsion fracture of left ilium HCC ESR COM Q

1 ✓7th **S32.313** Displaced avulsion fracture of unspecified ilium HCC ESR COM Q

1 ✓7th **S32.314** Nondisplaced avulsion fracture of right ilium HCC ESR COM Q

1 ✓7th **S32.315** Nondisplaced avulsion fracture of left ilium HCC ESR COM Q

1 ✓7th **S32.316** Nondisplaced avulsion fracture of unspecified ilium HCC ESR COM Q

✓6th **S32.39** Other fracture of ilium

1 ✓7th **S32.391** Other fracture of right ilium HCC ESR COM Q

1 ✓7th **S32.392** Other fracture of left ilium HCC ESR COM Q

1 ✓7th **S32.399** Other fracture of unspecified ilium HCC ESR COM Q

✓5th **S32.4** Fracture of acetabulum

Code also any associated fracture of pelvic ring (S32.8-)

AHA: 2016,3Q,16

✓6th **S32.40** Unspecified fracture of acetabulum

1 ✓7th **S32.401** Unspecified fracture of right acetabulum HCC ESR COM Q

1 ✓7th **S32.402** Unspecified fracture of left acetabulum HCC ESR COM Q

1 ✓7th **S32.409** Unspecified fracture of unspecified acetabulum HCC ESR COM Q

✓6th **S32.41** Fracture of anterior wall of acetabulum

1 ✓7th **S32.411** Displaced fracture of anterior wall of right acetabulum HCC ESR COM Q

1 ✓7th **S32.412** Displaced fracture of anterior wall of left acetabulum HCC ESR COM Q

1 ✓7th **S32.413** Displaced fracture of anterior wall of unspecified acetabulum HCC ESR COM Q

1 ✓7th **S32.414** Nondisplaced fracture of anterior wall of right acetabulum HCC ESR COM Q

1 ✓7th **S32.415** Nondisplaced fracture of anterior wall of left acetabulum HCC ESR COM Q

1 ✓7th **S32.416** Nondisplaced fracture of anterior wall of unspecified acetabulum HCC ESR COM Q

✓6th **S32.42** Fracture of posterior wall of acetabulum

1 ✓7th **S32.421** Displaced fracture of posterior wall of right acetabulum HCC ESR COM Q

1 ✓7th **S32.422** Displaced fracture of posterior wall of left acetabulum HCC ESR COM Q

1 ✓7th **S32.423** Displaced fracture of posterior wall of unspecified acetabulum HCC ESR COM Q

1 ✓7th **S32.424** Nondisplaced fracture of posterior wall of right acetabulum HCC ESR COM Q

1 ✓7th **S32.425** Nondisplaced fracture of posterior wall of left acetabulum HCC ESR COM Q

1 ✓7th **S32.426** Nondisplaced fracture of posterior wall of unspecified acetabulum HCC ESR COM Q

✓6th **S32.43** Fracture of anterior column [iliopubic] of acetabulum

1 ✓7th **S32.431** Displaced fracture of anterior column [iliopubic] of right acetabulum HCC ESR COM Q

1 ✓7th **S32.432** Displaced fracture of anterior column [iliopubic] of left acetabulum HCC ESR COM Q

1 ✓7th **S32.433** Displaced fracture of anterior column [iliopubic] of unspecified acetabulum HCC ESR COM Q

1 ✓7th **S32.434** Nondisplaced fracture of anterior column [iliopubic] of right acetabulum HCC ESR COM Q

1 ✓7th **S32.435** Nondisplaced fracture of anterior column [iliopubic] of left acetabulum HCC ESR COM Q

1 ✓7th **S32.436** Nondisplaced fracture of anterior column [iliopubic] of unspecified acetabulum HCC ESR COM Q

✓6th **S32.44** Fracture of posterior column [ilioischial] of acetabulum

1 ✓7th **S32.441** Displaced fracture of posterior column [ilioischial] of right acetabulum HCC ESR COM Q

1 ✓7th **S32.442** Displaced fracture of posterior column [ilioischial] of left acetabulum HCC ESR COM Q

1 ✓7th **S32.443** Displaced fracture of posterior column [ilioischial] of unspecified acetabulum HCC ESR COM Q

1 ✓7th **S32.444** Nondisplaced fracture of posterior column [ilioischial] of right acetabulum HCC ESR COM Q

1 ✓7th **S32.445** Nondisplaced fracture of posterior column [ilioischial] of left acetabulum HCC ESR COM Q

1 ✓7th **S32.446** Nondisplaced fracture of posterior column [ilioischial] of unspecified acetabulum HCC ESR COM Q

✓6th **S32.45** Transverse fracture of acetabulum

1 ✓7th **S32.451** Displaced transverse fracture of right acetabulum HCC ESR COM Q

1 ✓7th **S32.452** Displaced transverse fracture of left acetabulum HCC ESR COM Q

1 ✓7th **S32.453** Displaced transverse fracture of unspecified acetabulum HCC ESR COM Q

1 ✓7th **S32.454** Nondisplaced transverse fracture of right acetabulum HCC ESR COM Q

1 ✓7th **S32.455** Nondisplaced transverse fracture of left acetabulum HCC ESR COM Q

1 ✓7th **S32.456** Nondisplaced transverse fracture of unspecified acetabulum HCC ESR COM Q

√6th **S32.46 Associated transverse-posterior fracture of acetabulum**

1 √7th **S32.461 Displaced associated transverse-posterior fracture of right acetabulum** HCC ESR COM Q

1 √7th **S32.462 Displaced associated transverse-posterior fracture of left acetabulum** HCC ESR COM Q

1 √7th **S32.463 Displaced associated transverse-posterior fracture of unspecified acetabulum** HCC ESR COM Q

1 √7th **S32.464 Nondisplaced associated transverse-posterior fracture of right acetabulum** HCC ESR COM Q

1 √7th **S32.465 Nondisplaced associated transverse-posterior fracture of left acetabulum** HCC ESR COM Q

1 √7th **S32.466 Nondisplaced associated transverse-posterior fracture of unspecified acetabulum** HCC ESR COM Q

√6th **S32.47 Fracture of medial wall of acetabulum**

1 √7th **S32.471 Displaced fracture of medial wall of right acetabulum** HCC ESR COM Q

1 √7th **S32.472 Displaced fracture of medial wall of left acetabulum** HCC ESR COM Q

1 √7th **S32.473 Displaced fracture of medial wall of unspecified acetabulum** HCC ESR COM Q

1 √7th **S32.474 Nondisplaced fracture of medial wall of right acetabulum** HCC ESR COM Q

1 √7th **S32.475 Nondisplaced fracture of medial wall of left acetabulum** HCC ESR COM Q

1 √7th **S32.476 Nondisplaced fracture of medial wall of unspecified acetabulum** HCC ESR COM Q

√6th **S32.48 Dome fracture of acetabulum**

1 √7th **S32.481 Displaced dome fracture of right acetabulum** HCC ESR COM Q

1 √7th **S32.482 Displaced dome fracture of left acetabulum** HCC ESR COM Q

1 √7th **S32.483 Displaced dome fracture of unspecified acetabulum** HCC ESR COM Q

1 √7th **S32.484 Nondisplaced dome fracture of right acetabulum** HCC ESR COM Q

1 √7th **S32.485 Nondisplaced dome fracture of left acetabulum** HCC ESR COM Q

1 √7th **S32.486 Nondisplaced dome fracture of unspecified acetabulum** HCC ESR COM Q

√6th **S32.49 Other specified fracture of acetabulum**

1 √7th **S32.491 Other specified fracture of right acetabulum** HCC ESR COM Q

1 √7th **S32.492 Other specified fracture of left acetabulum** HCC ESR COM Q

1 √7th **S32.499 Other specified fracture of unspecified acetabulum** HCC ESR COM Q

√5th **S32.5 Fracture of pubis**

EXCLUDES 1 *fracture of pubis with associated disruption of pelvic ring (S32.8-)*

√6th **S32.50 Unspecified fracture of pubis**

1 √7th **S32.501 Unspecified fracture of right pubis** HCC ESR COM Q

1 √7th **S32.502 Unspecified fracture of left pubis** HCC ESR COM Q

1 √7th **S32.509 Unspecified fracture of unspecified pubis** HCC ESR COM Q

√6th **S32.51 Fracture of superior rim of pubis**

1 √7th **S32.511 Fracture of superior rim of right pubis** HCC ESR COM Q

1 √7th **S32.512 Fracture of superior rim of left pubis** HCC ESR COM Q

1 √7th **S32.519 Fracture of superior rim of unspecified pubis** HCC ESR COM Q

√6th **S32.59 Other specified fracture of pubis**

1 √7th **S32.591 Other specified fracture of right pubis** HCC ESR COM Q

1 √7th **S32.592 Other specified fracture of left pubis** HCC ESR COM Q

1 √7th **S32.599 Other specified fracture of unspecified pubis** HCC ESR COM Q

√5th **S32.6 Fracture of ischium**

EXCLUDES 1 *fracture of ischium with associated disruption of pelvic ring (S32.8-)*

√6th **S32.60 Unspecified fracture of ischium**

1 √7th **S32.601 Unspecified fracture of right ischium** HCC ESR COM Q

1 √7th **S32.602 Unspecified fracture of left ischium** HCC ESR COM Q

1 √7th **S32.609 Unspecified fracture of unspecified ischium** HCC ESR COM Q

√6th **S32.61 Avulsion fracture of ischium**

1 √7th **S32.611 Displaced avulsion fracture of right ischium** HCC ESR COM Q

1 √7th **S32.612 Displaced avulsion fracture of left ischium** HCC ESR COM Q

1 √7th **S32.613 Displaced avulsion fracture of unspecified ischium** HCC ESR COM Q

1 √7th **S32.614 Nondisplaced avulsion fracture of right ischium** HCC ESR COM Q

1 √7th **S32.615 Nondisplaced avulsion fracture of left ischium** HCC ESR COM Q

1 √7th **S32.616 Nondisplaced avulsion fracture of unspecified ischium** HCC ESR COM Q

√6th **S32.69 Other specified fracture of ischium**

1 √7th **S32.691 Other specified fracture of right ischium** HCC ESR COM Q

1 √7th **S32.692 Other specified fracture of left ischium** HCC ESR COM Q

1 √7th **S32.699 Other specified fracture of unspecified ischium** HCC ESR COM Q

√5th **S32.8 Fracture of other parts of pelvis**

Code also any associated:
fracture of acetabulum (S32.4-)
sacral fracture (S32.1-)

Fractures Disrupting Pelvic Circle

√6th **S32.81 Multiple fractures of pelvis with disruption of pelvic ring**

Multiple pelvic fractures with disruption of pelvic circle

1 √7th **S32.810 Multiple fractures of pelvis with stable disruption of pelvic ring** HCC ESR COM Q

1 √7th **S32.811 Multiple fractures of pelvis with unstable disruption of pelvic ring** HCC ESR COM Q

1 √x7th **S32.82 Multiple fractures of pelvis without disruption of pelvic ring** HCC ESR COM Q

Multiple pelvic fractures without disruption of pelvic circle

1 √x7th **S32.89 Fracture of other parts of pelvis** HCC ESR COM Q

1 √x7th **S32.9 Fracture of unspecified parts of lumbosacral spine and pelvis** HCC ESR COM Q

Fracture of lumbosacral spine NOS
Fracture of pelvis NOS
AHA: 2012,4Q,93

S33 Dislocation and sprain of joints and ligaments of lumbar spine and pelvis

INCLUDES avulsion of joint or ligament of lumbar spine and pelvis
laceration of cartilage, joint or ligament of lumbar spine and pelvis
sprain of cartilage, joint or ligament of lumbar spine and pelvis
traumatic hemarthrosis of joint or ligament of lumbar spine and pelvis
traumatic rupture of joint or ligament of lumbar spine and pelvis
traumatic subluxation of joint or ligament of lumbar spine and pelvis
traumatic tear of joint or ligament of lumbar spine and pelvis

Code also any associated open wound

EXCLUDES 1 *nontraumatic rupture or displacement of lumbar intervertebral disc NOS (M51.-)*
obstetric damage to pelvic joints and ligaments (O71.6)

EXCLUDES 2 *dislocation and sprain of joints and ligaments of hip (S73.-)*
strain of muscle of lower back and pelvis (S39.01-)

The appropriate 7th character is to be added to each code from category S33.
A initial encounter
D subsequent encounter
S sequela

S33.0 Traumatic rupture of lumbar intervertebral disc

EXCLUDES 1 *rupture or displacement (nontraumatic) of lumbar intervertebral disc NOS (M51.- with fifth character 6)*

S33.1 Subluxation and dislocation of lumbar vertebra

Code also any associated:
open wound of abdomen, lower back and pelvis (S31)
spinal cord injury (S24.0, S24.1-, S34.0-, S34.1-)

EXCLUDES 2 *fracture of lumbar vertebrae (S32.0-)*

S33.10 Subluxation and dislocation of unspecified lumbar vertebra
S33.100 Subluxation of unspecified lumbar vertebra
S33.101 Dislocation of unspecified lumbar vertebra
S33.11 Subluxation and dislocation of L1/L2 lumbar vertebra
S33.110 Subluxation of L1/L2 lumbar vertebra
S33.111 Dislocation of L1/L2 lumbar vertebra
S33.12 Subluxation and dislocation of L2/L3 lumbar vertebra
S33.120 Subluxation of L2/L3 lumbar vertebra
S33.121 Dislocation of L2/L3 lumbar vertebra
S33.13 Subluxation and dislocation of L3/L4 lumbar vertebra
S33.130 Subluxation of L3/L4 lumbar vertebra
S33.131 Dislocation of L3/L4 lumbar vertebra
S33.14 Subluxation and dislocation of L4/L5 lumbar vertebra
S33.140 Subluxation of L4/L5 lumbar vertebra
S33.141 Dislocation of L4/L5 lumbar vertebra
S33.2 Dislocation of sacroiliac and sacrococcygeal joint
S33.3 Dislocation of other and unspecified parts of lumbar spine and pelvis
S33.30 Dislocation of unspecified parts of lumbar spine and pelvis
S33.39 Dislocation of other parts of lumbar spine and pelvis
S33.4 Traumatic rupture of symphysis pubis
S33.5 Sprain of ligaments of lumbar spine
S33.6 Sprain of sacroiliac joint
S33.8 Sprain of other parts of lumbar spine and pelvis
S33.9 Sprain of unspecified parts of lumbar spine and pelvis

S34 Injury of lumbar and sacral spinal cord and nerves at abdomen, lower back and pelvis level

NOTE Code to highest level of lumbar cord injury.
Injuries to the spinal cord (S34.0 and S34.1) refer to the cord level and not bone level injury, and can affect nerve roots at and below the level given.

Code also any associated:
fracture of vertebra (S22.0-, S32.0-)
open wound of abdomen, lower back and pelvis (S31.-)
transient paralysis (R29.5)

The appropriate 7th character is to be added to each code from category S34.
A initial encounter
D subsequent encounter
S sequela

S34.0 Concussion and edema of lumbar and sacral spinal cord
S34.01 Concussion and edema of lumbar spinal cord HCC ESR COM
S34.02 Concussion and edema of sacral spinal cord HCC ESR COM
Concussion and edema of conus medullaris
S34.1 Other and unspecified injury of lumbar and sacral spinal cord
S34.10 Unspecified injury to lumbar spinal cord
S34.101 Unspecified injury to L1 level of lumbar spinal cord HCC ESR COM
Unspecified injury to lumbar spinal cord level 1
S34.102 Unspecified injury to L2 level of lumbar spinal cord HCC ESR COM
Unspecified injury to lumbar spinal cord level 2
S34.103 Unspecified injury to L3 level of lumbar spinal cord HCC ESR COM
Unspecified injury to lumbar spinal cord level 3
S34.104 Unspecified injury to L4 level of lumbar spinal cord HCC ESR COM
Unspecified injury to lumbar spinal cord level 4
S34.105 Unspecified injury to L5 level of lumbar spinal cord HCC ESR COM
Unspecified injury to lumbar spinal cord level 5
S34.109 Unspecified injury to unspecified level of lumbar spinal cord HCC ESR COM
S34.11 Complete lesion of lumbar spinal cord
S34.111 Complete lesion of L1 level of lumbar spinal cord HCC ESR COM
Complete lesion of lumbar spinal cord level 1
S34.112 Complete lesion of L2 level of lumbar spinal cord HCC ESR COM
Complete lesion of lumbar spinal cord level 2
S34.113 Complete lesion of L3 level of lumbar spinal cord HCC ESR COM
Complete lesion of lumbar spinal cord level 3
S34.114 Complete lesion of L4 level of lumbar spinal cord HCC ESR COM
Complete lesion of lumbar spinal cord level 4
S34.115 Complete lesion of L5 level of lumbar spinal cord HCC ESR COM
Complete lesion of lumbar spinal cord level 5
S34.119 Complete lesion of unspecified level of lumbar spinal cord HCC ESR COM
S34.12 Incomplete lesion of lumbar spinal cord
S34.121 Incomplete lesion of L1 level of lumbar spinal cord HCC ESR COM
Incomplete lesion of lumbar spinal cord level 1

S34.122 Incomplete lesion of L2 level of lumbar spinal cord HCC ESR COM
Incomplete lesion of lumbar spinal cord level 2

S34.123 Incomplete lesion of L3 level of lumbar spinal cord HCC ESR COM
Incomplete lesion of lumbar spinal cord level 3

S34.124 Incomplete lesion of L4 level of lumbar spinal cord HCC ESR COM
Incomplete lesion of lumbar spinal cord level 4

S34.125 Incomplete lesion of L5 level of lumbar spinal cord HCC ESR COM
Incomplete lesion of lumbar spinal cord level 5

S34.129 Incomplete lesion of unspecified level of lumbar spinal cord HCC ESR COM

S34.13 Other and unspecified injury to sacral spinal cord
Other injury to conus medullaris

S34.131 Complete lesion of sacral spinal cord HCC ESR COM
Complete lesion of conus medullaris

S34.132 Incomplete lesion of sacral spinal cord HCC ESR COM
Incomplete lesion of conus medullaris

S34.139 Unspecified injury to sacral spinal cord HCC ESR COM
Unspecified injury of conus medullaris

S34.2 Injury of nerve root of lumbar and sacral spine

S34.21 Injury of nerve root of lumbar spine

S34.22 Injury of nerve root of sacral spine

1 **S34.3 Injury of cauda equina** HCC ESR COM

S34.4 Injury of lumbosacral plexus

S34.5 Injury of lumbar, sacral and pelvic sympathetic nerves
Injury of celiac ganglion or plexus
Injury of hypogastric plexus
Injury of mesenteric plexus (inferior) (superior)
Injury of splanchnic nerve

S34.6 Injury of peripheral nerve(s) at abdomen, lower back and pelvis level

S34.8 Injury of other nerves at abdomen, lower back and pelvis level

S34.9 Injury of unspecified nerves at abdomen, lower back and pelvis level

S35 Injury of blood vessels at abdomen, lower back and pelvis level
Code also any associated open wound (S31.-)

The appropriate 7th character is to be added to each code from category S35.
A initial encounter
D subsequent encounter
S sequela

S35.0 Injury of abdominal aorta
EXCLUDES 1 *injury of aorta NOS (S25.0)*

S35.00 Unspecified injury of abdominal aorta

S35.01 Minor laceration of abdominal aorta
Incomplete transection of abdominal aorta
Laceration of abdominal aorta NOS
Superficial laceration of abdominal aorta

S35.02 Major laceration of abdominal aorta
Complete transection of abdominal aorta
Traumatic rupture of abdominal aorta

S35.09 Other injury of abdominal aorta

S35.1 Injury of inferior vena cava
Injury of hepatic vein
EXCLUDES 1 *injury of vena cava NOS (S25.2)*

S35.10 Unspecified injury of inferior vena cava

S35.11 Minor laceration of inferior vena cava
Incomplete transection of inferior vena cava
Laceration of inferior vena cava NOS
Superficial laceration of inferior vena cava

S35.12 Major laceration of inferior vena cava
Complete transection of inferior vena cava
Traumatic rupture of inferior vena cava

S35.19 Other injury of inferior vena cava

S35.2 Injury of celiac or mesenteric artery and branches

S35.21 Injury of celiac artery

S35.211 Minor laceration of celiac artery
Incomplete transection of celiac artery
Laceration of celiac artery NOS
Superficial laceration of celiac artery

S35.212 Major laceration of celiac artery
Complete transection of celiac artery
Traumatic rupture of celiac artery

S35.218 Other injury of celiac artery

S35.219 Unspecified injury of celiac artery

S35.22 Injury of superior mesenteric artery

S35.221 Minor laceration of superior mesenteric artery
Incomplete transection of superior mesenteric artery
Laceration of superior mesenteric artery NOS
Superficial laceration of superior mesenteric artery

S35.222 Major laceration of superior mesenteric artery
Complete transection of superior mesenteric artery
Traumatic rupture of superior mesenteric artery

S35.228 Other injury of superior mesenteric artery

S35.229 Unspecified injury of superior mesenteric artery

S35.23 Injury of inferior mesenteric artery

S35.231 Minor laceration of inferior mesenteric artery
Incomplete transection of inferior mesenteric artery
Laceration of inferior mesenteric artery NOS
Superficial laceration of inferior mesenteric artery

S35.232 Major laceration of inferior mesenteric artery
Complete transection of inferior mesenteric artery
Traumatic rupture of inferior mesenteric artery

S35.238 Other injury of inferior mesenteric artery

S35.239 Unspecified injury of inferior mesenteric artery

S35.29 Injury of branches of celiac and mesenteric artery
Injury of gastric artery
Injury of gastroduodenal artery
Injury of hepatic artery
Injury of splenic artery

S35.291 Minor laceration of branches of celiac and mesenteric artery
Incomplete transection of branches of celiac and mesenteric artery
Laceration of branches of celiac and mesenteric artery NOS
Superficial laceration of branches of celiac and mesenteric artery

S35.292 Major laceration of branches of celiac and mesenteric artery
Complete transection of branches of celiac and mesenteric artery
Traumatic rupture of branches of celiac and mesenteric artery

S35.298 Other injury of branches of celiac and mesenteric artery

S35.299 Unspecified injury of branches of celiac and mesenteric artery

5th **S35.3 Injury of portal or splenic vein and branches**

6th **S35.31 Injury of portal vein**

7th **S35.311 Laceration of portal vein**

7th **S35.318 Other specified injury of portal vein**

7th **S35.319 Unspecified injury of portal vein**

6th **S35.32 Injury of splenic vein**

7th **S35.321 Laceration of splenic vein**

7th **S35.328 Other specified injury of splenic vein**

7th **S35.329 Unspecified injury of splenic vein**

6th **S35.33 Injury of superior mesenteric vein**

7th **S35.331 Laceration of superior mesenteric vein**

7th **S35.338 Other specified injury of superior mesenteric vein**

7th **S35.339 Unspecified injury of superior mesenteric vein**

6th **S35.34 Injury of inferior mesenteric vein**

7th **S35.341 Laceration of inferior mesenteric vein**

7th **S35.348 Other specified injury of inferior mesenteric vein**

7th **S35.349 Unspecified injury of inferior mesenteric vein**

5th **S35.4 Injury of renal blood vessels**

6th **S35.40 Unspecified injury of renal blood vessel**

7th **S35.401 Unspecified injury of right renal artery**

7th **S35.402 Unspecified injury of left renal artery**

7th **S35.403 Unspecified injury of unspecified renal artery**

7th **S35.404 Unspecified injury of right renal vein**

7th **S35.405 Unspecified injury of left renal vein**

7th **S35.406 Unspecified injury of unspecified renal vein**

6th **S35.41 Laceration of renal blood vessel**

7th **S35.411 Laceration of right renal artery**

7th **S35.412 Laceration of left renal artery**

7th **S35.413 Laceration of unspecified renal artery**

7th **S35.414 Laceration of right renal vein**

7th **S35.415 Laceration of left renal vein**

7th **S35.416 Laceration of unspecified renal vein**

6th **S35.49 Other specified injury of renal blood vessel**

7th **S35.491 Other specified injury of right renal artery**

7th **S35.492 Other specified injury of left renal artery**

7th **S35.493 Other specified injury of unspecified renal artery**

7th **S35.494 Other specified injury of right renal vein**

7th **S35.495 Other specified injury of left renal vein**

7th **S35.496 Other specified injury of unspecified renal vein**

5th **S35.5 Injury of iliac blood vessels**

x7th **S35.50 Injury of unspecified iliac blood vessel(s)**

6th **S35.51 Injury of iliac artery or vein**

Injury of hypogastric artery or vein

7th **S35.511 Injury of right iliac artery**

7th **S35.512 Injury of left iliac artery**

7th **S35.513 Injury of unspecified iliac artery**

7th **S35.514 Injury of right iliac vein**

7th **S35.515 Injury of left iliac vein**

7th **S35.516 Injury of unspecified iliac vein**

6th **S35.53 Injury of uterine artery or vein**

7th **S35.531 Injury of right uterine artery** ♀

7th **S35.532 Injury of left uterine artery** ♀

7th **S35.533 Injury of unspecified uterine artery** ♀

7th **S35.534 Injury of right uterine vein** ♀

7th **S35.535 Injury of left uterine vein** ♀

7th **S35.536 Injury of unspecified uterine vein** ♀

x7th **S35.59 Injury of other iliac blood vessels**

5th **S35.8 Injury of other blood vessels at abdomen, lower back and pelvis level**

Injury of ovarian artery or vein

6th **S35.8X Injury of other blood vessels at abdomen, lower back and pelvis level**

7th **S35.8X1 Laceration of other blood vessels at abdomen, lower back and pelvis level**

7th **S35.8X8 Other specified injury of other blood vessels at abdomen, lower back and pelvis level**

7th **S35.8X9 Unspecified injury of other blood vessels at abdomen, lower back and pelvis level**

5th **S35.9 Injury of unspecified blood vessel at abdomen, lower back and pelvis level**

x7th **S35.90 Unspecified injury of unspecified blood vessel at abdomen, lower back and pelvis level**

x7th **S35.91 Laceration of unspecified blood vessel at abdomen, lower back and pelvis level**

x7th **S35.99 Other specified injury of unspecified blood vessel at abdomen, lower back and pelvis level**

4th **S36 Injury of intra-abdominal organs**

Code also any associated open wound (S31.-)

The appropriate 7th character is to be added to each code from category S36.
A initial encounter
D subsequent encounter
S sequela

5th **S36.0 Injury of spleen**

AHA: 2015,2Q,36; 2015,1Q,10

x7th **S36.00 Unspecified injury of spleen**

6th **S36.02 Contusion of spleen**

7th **S36.020 Minor contusion of spleen**

Contusion of spleen less than 2 cm

7th **S36.021 Major contusion of spleen**

Contusion of spleen greater than 2 cm

7th **S36.029 Unspecified contusion of spleen**

6th **S36.03 Laceration of spleen**

7th **S36.030 Superficial (capsular) laceration of spleen**

Laceration of spleen less than 1 cm
Minor laceration of spleen

7th **S36.031 Moderate laceration of spleen**

Laceration of spleen 1 to 3 cm

7th **S36.032 Major laceration of spleen**

Avulsion of spleen
Laceration of spleen greater than 3 cm
Massive laceration of spleen
Multiple moderate lacerations of spleen
Stellate laceration of spleen

7th **S36.039 Unspecified laceration of spleen**

x7th **S36.09 Other injury of spleen**

5th **S36.1 Injury of liver and gallbladder and bile duct**

6th **S36.11 Injury of liver**

7th **S36.112 Contusion of liver**

7th **S36.113 Laceration of liver, unspecified degree**

7th **S36.114 Minor laceration of liver**

Laceration involving capsule only, or, without significant involvement of hepatic parenchyma [i.e., less than 1 cm deep]

7th **S36.115 Moderate laceration of liver**

Laceration involving parenchyma but without major disruption of parenchyma [i.e., less than 10 cm long and less than 3 cm deep]

7th **S36.116 Major laceration of liver**

Laceration with significant disruption of hepatic parenchyma [i.e., greater than 10 cm long and 3 cm deep]
Multiple moderate lacerations, with or without hematoma
Stellate laceration of liver

7th **S36.118 Other injury of liver**

7th **S36.119 Unspecified injury of liver**

S36.12 Injury of gallbladder
S36.122 Contusion of gallbladder
S36.123 Laceration of gallbladder
S36.128 Other injury of gallbladder
S36.129 Unspecified injury of gallbladder
S36.13 Injury of bile duct
S36.2 Injury of pancreas
S36.20 Unspecified injury of pancreas
S36.200 Unspecified injury of head of pancreas
S36.201 Unspecified injury of body of pancreas
S36.202 Unspecified injury of tail of pancreas
S36.209 Unspecified injury of unspecified part of pancreas
S36.22 Contusion of pancreas
S36.220 Contusion of head of pancreas
S36.221 Contusion of body of pancreas
S36.222 Contusion of tail of pancreas
S36.229 Contusion of unspecified part of pancreas
S36.23 Laceration of pancreas, unspecified degree
S36.230 Laceration of head of pancreas, unspecified degree
S36.231 Laceration of body of pancreas, unspecified degree
S36.232 Laceration of tail of pancreas, unspecified degree
S36.239 Laceration of unspecified part of pancreas, unspecified degree
S36.24 Minor laceration of pancreas
S36.240 Minor laceration of head of pancreas
S36.241 Minor laceration of body of pancreas
S36.242 Minor laceration of tail of pancreas
S36.249 Minor laceration of unspecified part of pancreas
S36.25 Moderate laceration of pancreas
S36.250 Moderate laceration of head of pancreas
S36.251 Moderate laceration of body of pancreas
S36.252 Moderate laceration of tail of pancreas
S36.259 Moderate laceration of unspecified part of pancreas
S36.26 Major laceration of pancreas
S36.260 Major laceration of head of pancreas
S36.261 Major laceration of body of pancreas
S36.262 Major laceration of tail of pancreas
S36.269 Major laceration of unspecified part of pancreas
S36.29 Other injury of pancreas
S36.290 Other injury of head of pancreas
S36.291 Other injury of body of pancreas
S36.292 Other injury of tail of pancreas
S36.299 Other injury of unspecified part of pancreas
S36.3 Injury of stomach
S36.30 Unspecified injury of stomach
S36.32 Contusion of stomach
S36.33 Laceration of stomach
S36.39 Other injury of stomach
S36.4 Injury of small intestine
S36.40 Unspecified injury of small intestine
S36.400 Unspecified injury of duodenum
S36.408 Unspecified injury of other part of small intestine
S36.409 Unspecified injury of unspecified part of small intestine
S36.41 Primary blast injury of small intestine
Blast injury of small intestine NOS
S36.410 Primary blast injury of duodenum
S36.418 Primary blast injury of other part of small intestine
S36.419 Primary blast injury of unspecified part of small intestine
S36.42 Contusion of small intestine
S36.420 Contusion of duodenum
S36.428 Contusion of other part of small intestine
S36.429 Contusion of unspecified part of small intestine
S36.43 Laceration of small intestine
S36.430 Laceration of duodenum
S36.438 Laceration of other part of small intestine
S36.439 Laceration of unspecified part of small intestine
S36.49 Other injury of small intestine
S36.490 Other injury of duodenum
S36.498 Other injury of other part of small intestine
S36.499 Other injury of unspecified part of small intestine
S36.5 Injury of colon
EXCLUDES 2 *injury of rectum (S36.6-)*
S36.50 Unspecified injury of colon
S36.500 Unspecified injury of ascending [right] colon
S36.501 Unspecified injury of transverse colon
S36.502 Unspecified injury of descending [left] colon
S36.503 Unspecified injury of sigmoid colon
S36.508 Unspecified injury of other part of colon
S36.509 Unspecified injury of unspecified part of colon
S36.51 Primary blast injury of colon
Blast injury of colon NOS
S36.510 Primary blast injury of ascending [right] colon
S36.511 Primary blast injury of transverse colon
S36.512 Primary blast injury of descending [left] colon
S36.513 Primary blast injury of sigmoid colon
S36.518 Primary blast injury of other part of colon
S36.519 Primary blast injury of unspecified part of colon
S36.52 Contusion of colon
S36.520 Contusion of ascending [right] colon
S36.521 Contusion of transverse colon
S36.522 Contusion of descending [left] colon
S36.523 Contusion of sigmoid colon
S36.528 Contusion of other part of colon
S36.529 Contusion of unspecified part of colon
S36.53 Laceration of colon
S36.530 Laceration of ascending [right] colon
S36.531 Laceration of transverse colon
S36.532 Laceration of descending [left] colon
S36.533 Laceration of sigmoid colon
S36.538 Laceration of other part of colon
S36.539 Laceration of unspecified part of colon
S36.59 Other injury of colon
Secondary blast injury of colon
S36.590 Other injury of ascending [right] colon
S36.591 Other injury of transverse colon
S36.592 Other injury of descending [left] colon
S36.593 Other injury of sigmoid colon
S36.598 Other injury of other part of colon
S36.599 Other injury of unspecified part of colon
S36.6 Injury of rectum
S36.60 Unspecified injury of rectum
S36.61 Primary blast injury of rectum
Blast injury of rectum NOS
S36.62 Contusion of rectum
S36.63 Laceration of rectum
S36.69 Other injury of rectum
Secondary blast injury of rectum

S36.8 Injury of other intra-abdominal organs
S36.81 Injury of peritoneum
S36.89 Injury of other intra-abdominal organs
Injury of retroperitoneum
S36.892 Contusion of other intra-abdominal organs
S36.893 Laceration of other intra-abdominal organs
S36.898 Other injury of other intra-abdominal organs
S36.899 Unspecified injury of other intra-abdominal organs
S36.9 Injury of unspecified intra-abdominal organ
S36.90 Unspecified injury of unspecified intra-abdominal organ
S36.92 Contusion of unspecified intra-abdominal organ
S36.93 Laceration of unspecified intra-abdominal organ
S36.99 Other injury of unspecified intra-abdominal organ

S37 Injury of urinary and pelvic organs
Code also any associated open wound (S31.-)
EXCLUDES 1 *obstetric trauma to pelvic organs (O71.-)*
EXCLUDES 2 *injury of peritoneum (S36.81)*
injury of retroperitoneum (S36.89-)

The appropriate 7th character is to be added to each code from category S37.
A initial encounter
D subsequent encounter
S sequela

S37.0 Injury of kidney
EXCLUDES 2 *acute kidney injury (nontraumatic) (N17.9)*
S37.00 Unspecified injury of kidney
S37.001 Unspecified injury of right kidney
S37.002 Unspecified injury of left kidney
S37.009 Unspecified injury of unspecified kidney
S37.01 Minor contusion of kidney
Contusion of kidney less than 2 cm
Contusion of kidney NOS
S37.011 Minor contusion of right kidney
S37.012 Minor contusion of left kidney
S37.019 Minor contusion of unspecified kidney
S37.02 Major contusion of kidney
Contusion of kidney greater than 2 cm
S37.021 Major contusion of right kidney
S37.022 Major contusion of left kidney
S37.029 Major contusion of unspecified kidney
S37.03 Laceration of kidney, unspecified degree
S37.031 Laceration of right kidney, unspecified degree
S37.032 Laceration of left kidney, unspecified degree
S37.039 Laceration of unspecified kidney, unspecified degree
S37.04 Minor laceration of kidney
Laceration of kidney less than 1 cm
S37.041 Minor laceration of right kidney
S37.042 Minor laceration of left kidney
S37.049 Minor laceration of unspecified kidney
S37.05 Moderate laceration of kidney
Laceration of kidney 1 to 3 cm
S37.051 Moderate laceration of right kidney
S37.052 Moderate laceration of left kidney
S37.059 Moderate laceration of unspecified kidney
S37.06 Major laceration of kidney
Avulsion of kidney
Laceration of kidney greater than 3 cm
Massive laceration of kidney
Multiple moderate lacerations of kidney
Stellate laceration of kidney
S37.061 Major laceration of right kidney
S37.062 Major laceration of left kidney
S37.069 Major laceration of unspecified kidney
S37.09 Other injury of kidney
S37.091 Other injury of right kidney
S37.092 Other injury of left kidney
S37.099 Other injury of unspecified kidney
S37.1 Injury of ureter
S37.10 Unspecified injury of ureter
S37.12 Contusion of ureter
S37.13 Laceration of ureter
S37.19 Other injury of ureter
S37.2 Injury of bladder
S37.20 Unspecified injury of bladder
S37.22 Contusion of bladder
S37.23 Laceration of bladder
S37.29 Other injury of bladder
S37.3 Injury of urethra
S37.30 Unspecified injury of urethra
S37.32 Contusion of urethra
S37.33 Laceration of urethra
S37.39 Other injury of urethra
S37.4 Injury of ovary
S37.40 Unspecified injury of ovary
S37.401 Unspecified injury of ovary, unilateral ♀
S37.402 Unspecified injury of ovary, bilateral ♀
S37.409 Unspecified injury of ovary, unspecified ♀
S37.42 Contusion of ovary
S37.421 Contusion of ovary, unilateral ♀
S37.422 Contusion of ovary, bilateral ♀
S37.429 Contusion of ovary, unspecified ♀
S37.43 Laceration of ovary
S37.431 Laceration of ovary, unilateral ♀
S37.432 Laceration of ovary, bilateral ♀
S37.439 Laceration of ovary, unspecified ♀
S37.49 Other injury of ovary
S37.491 Other injury of ovary, unilateral ♀
S37.492 Other injury of ovary, bilateral ♀
S37.499 Other injury of ovary, unspecified ♀
S37.5 Injury of fallopian tube
S37.50 Unspecified injury of fallopian tube
S37.501 Unspecified injury of fallopian tube, unilateral ♀
S37.502 Unspecified injury of fallopian tube, bilateral ♀
S37.509 Unspecified injury of fallopian tube, unspecified ♀
S37.51 Primary blast injury of fallopian tube
Blast injury of fallopian tube NOS
S37.511 Primary blast injury of fallopian tube, unilateral ♀
S37.512 Primary blast injury of fallopian tube, bilateral ♀
S37.519 Primary blast injury of fallopian tube, unspecified ♀
S37.52 Contusion of fallopian tube
S37.521 Contusion of fallopian tube, unilateral ♀
S37.522 Contusion of fallopian tube, bilateral ♀
S37.529 Contusion of fallopian tube, unspecified ♀
S37.53 Laceration of fallopian tube
S37.531 Laceration of fallopian tube, unilateral ♀
S37.532 Laceration of fallopian tube, bilateral ♀
S37.539 Laceration of fallopian tube, unspecified ♀

✓6th **S37.59 Other injury of fallopian tube**
Secondary blast injury of fallopian tube
✓7th **S37.591 Other injury of fallopian tube, unilateral** ♀
✓7th **S37.592 Other injury of fallopian tube, bilateral** ♀
✓7th **S37.599 Other injury of fallopian tube, unspecified** ♀
✓5th **S37.6 Injury of uterus**
EXCLUDES 1 *injury to gravid uterus (O9A.2-)*
injury to uterus during delivery (O71.-)
✓x7th **S37.60 Unspecified injury of uterus** ♀
✓x7th **S37.62 Contusion of uterus** ♀
✓x7th **S37.63 Laceration of uterus** ♀
✓x7th **S37.69 Other injury of uterus** ♀
✓5th **S37.8 Injury of other urinary and pelvic organs**
✓6th **S37.81 Injury of adrenal gland**
✓7th **S37.812 Contusion of adrenal gland**
✓7th **S37.813 Laceration of adrenal gland**
✓7th **S37.818 Other injury of adrenal gland**
✓7th **S37.819 Unspecified injury of adrenal gland**
✓6th **S37.82 Injury of prostate**
✓7th **S37.822 Contusion of prostate** ♂
✓7th **S37.823 Laceration of prostate** ♂
✓7th **S37.828 Other injury of prostate** ♂
✓7th **S37.829 Unspecified injury of prostate** ♂
✓6th **S37.89 Injury of other urinary and pelvic organ**
✓7th **S37.892 Contusion of other urinary and pelvic organ**
✓7th **S37.893 Laceration of other urinary and pelvic organ**
✓7th **S37.898 Other injury of other urinary and pelvic organ**
✓7th **S37.899 Unspecified injury of other urinary and pelvic organ**
✓5th **S37.9 Injury of unspecified urinary and pelvic organ**
✓x7th **S37.90 Unspecified injury of unspecified urinary and pelvic organ**
✓x7th **S37.92 Contusion of unspecified urinary and pelvic organ**
✓x7th **S37.93 Laceration of unspecified urinary and pelvic organ**
✓x7th **S37.99 Other injury of unspecified urinary and pelvic organ**
✓4th **S38 Crushing injury and traumatic amputation of abdomen, lower back, pelvis and external genitals**
NOTE An amputation not identified as partial or complete should be coded to complete

The appropriate 7th character is to be added to each code from category S38.
A initial encounter
D subsequent encounter
S sequela

✓5th **S38.0 Crushing injury of external genital organs**
Use additional code for any associated injuries
✓6th **S38.00 Crushing injury of unspecified external genital organs**
✓7th **S38.001 Crushing injury of unspecified external genital organs, male** ♂
✓7th **S38.002 Crushing injury of unspecified external genital organs, female** ♀
✓x7th **S38.01 Crushing injury of penis** ♂
✓x7th **S38.02 Crushing injury of scrotum and testis** ♂
✓x7th **S38.03 Crushing injury of vulva** ♀
✓x7th **S38.1 Crushing injury of abdomen, lower back, and pelvis**
Use additional code for all associated injuries, such as:
fracture of thoracic or lumbar spine and pelvis (S22.0-, S32.-)
injury to intra-abdominal organs (S36.-)
injury to urinary and pelvic organs (S37.-)
open wound of abdominal wall (S31.-)
spinal cord injury (S34.0, S34.1-)
EXCLUDES 2 *crushing injury of external genital organs (S38.0-)*
✓5th **S38.2 Traumatic amputation of external genital organs**
✓6th **S38.21 Traumatic amputation of female external genital organs**
Traumatic amputation of clitoris
Traumatic amputation of labium (majus) (minus)
Traumatic amputation of vulva
✓7th **S38.211 Complete traumatic amputation of female external genital organs** ♀
✓7th **S38.212 Partial traumatic amputation of female external genital organs** ♀
✓6th **S38.22 Traumatic amputation of penis**
✓7th **S38.221 Complete traumatic amputation of penis** ♂
✓7th **S38.222 Partial traumatic amputation of penis** ♂
✓6th **S38.23 Traumatic amputation of scrotum and testis**
✓7th **S38.231 Complete traumatic amputation of scrotum and testis** ♂
✓7th **S38.232 Partial traumatic amputation of scrotum and testis** ♂
✓x7th **S38.3 Transection (partial) of abdomen**
✓4th **S39 Other and unspecified injuries of abdomen, lower back, pelvis and external genitals**
Code also any associated open wound (S31.-)
EXCLUDES 2 *sprain of joints and ligaments of lumbar spine and pelvis (S33.-)*

The appropriate 7th character is to be added to each code from category S39.
A initial encounter
D subsequent encounter
S sequela

✓5th **S39.0 Injury of muscle, fascia and tendon of abdomen, lower back and pelvis**
✓6th **S39.00 Unspecified injury of muscle, fascia and tendon of abdomen, lower back and pelvis**
✓7th **S39.001 Unspecified injury of muscle, fascia and tendon of abdomen**
✓7th **S39.002 Unspecified injury of muscle, fascia and tendon of lower back**
✓7th **S39.003 Unspecified injury of muscle, fascia and tendon of pelvis**
✓6th **S39.01 Strain of muscle, fascia and tendon of abdomen, lower back and pelvis**
✓7th **S39.011 Strain of muscle, fascia and tendon of abdomen**
✓7th **S39.012 Strain of muscle, fascia and tendon of lower back**
✓7th **S39.013 Strain of muscle, fascia and tendon of pelvis**
✓6th **S39.02 Laceration of muscle, fascia and tendon of abdomen, lower back and pelvis**
✓7th **S39.021 Laceration of muscle, fascia and tendon of abdomen**
✓7th **S39.022 Laceration of muscle, fascia and tendon of lower back**
✓7th **S39.023 Laceration of muscle, fascia and tendon of pelvis**
✓6th **S39.09 Other injury of muscle, fascia and tendon of abdomen, lower back and pelvis**
✓7th **S39.091 Other injury of muscle, fascia and tendon of abdomen**
✓7th **S39.092 Other injury of muscle, fascia and tendon of lower back**
✓7th **S39.093 Other injury of muscle, fascia and tendon of pelvis**
✓5th **S39.8 Other specified injuries of abdomen, lower back, pelvis and external genitals**
✓x7th **S39.81 Other specified injuries of abdomen**
✓x7th **S39.82 Other specified injuries of lower back**
✓x7th **S39.83 Other specified injuries of pelvis**
✓6th **S39.84 Other specified injuries of external genitals**
✓7th **S39.840 Fracture of corpus cavernosum penis** ♂
✓7th **S39.848 Other specified injuries of external genitals**
✓5th **S39.9 Unspecified injury of abdomen, lower back, pelvis and external genitals**
✓x7th **S39.91 Unspecified injury of abdomen**

√x7th **S39.92 Unspecified injury of lower back**

√x7th **S39.93 Unspecified injury of pelvis**

√x7th **S39.94 Unspecified injury of external genitals**

Injuries to the shoulder and upper arm (S4Ø-S49)

INCLUDES injuries of axilla
injuries of scapular region

EXCLUDES 2 *burns and corrosions (T2Ø-T32)*
frostbite (T33-T34)
injuries of elbow (S5Ø-S59)
insect bite or sting, venomous (T63.4)

√4th **S4Ø Superficial injury of shoulder and upper arm**

The appropriate 7th character is to be added to each code from category S4Ø.
A initial encounter
D subsequent encounter
S sequela

√5th **S4Ø.Ø Contusion of shoulder and upper arm**
√6th **S4Ø.Ø1 Contusion of shoulder**
√7th **S4Ø.Ø11 Contusion of right shoulder**
√7th **S4Ø.Ø12 Contusion of left shoulder**
√7th **S4Ø.Ø19 Contusion of unspecified shoulder**
√6th **S4Ø.Ø2 Contusion of upper arm**
√7th **S4Ø.Ø21 Contusion of right upper arm**
√7th **S4Ø.Ø22 Contusion of left upper arm**
√7th **S4Ø.Ø29 Contusion of unspecified upper arm**

√5th **S4Ø.2 Other superficial injuries of shoulder**
√6th **S4Ø.21 Abrasion of shoulder**
√7th **S4Ø.211 Abrasion of right shoulder**
√7th **S4Ø.212 Abrasion of left shoulder**
√7th **S4Ø.219 Abrasion of unspecified shoulder**
√6th **S4Ø.22 Blister (nonthermal) of shoulder**
√7th **S4Ø.221 Blister (nonthermal) of right shoulder**
√7th **S4Ø.222 Blister (nonthermal) of left shoulder**
√7th **S4Ø.229 Blister (nonthermal) of unspecified shoulder**
√6th **S4Ø.24 External constriction of shoulder**
√7th **S4Ø.241 External constriction of right shoulder**
√7th **S4Ø.242 External constriction of left shoulder**
√7th **S4Ø.249 External constriction of unspecified shoulder**
√6th **S4Ø.25 Superficial foreign body of shoulder**
Splinter in the shoulder
√7th **S4Ø.251 Superficial foreign body of right shoulder**
√7th **S4Ø.252 Superficial foreign body of left shoulder**
√7th **S4Ø.259 Superficial foreign body of unspecified shoulder**
√6th **S4Ø.26 Insect bite (nonvenomous) of shoulder**
√7th **S4Ø.261 Insect bite (nonvenomous) of right shoulder**
√7th **S4Ø.262 Insect bite (nonvenomous) of left shoulder**
√7th **S4Ø.269 Insect bite (nonvenomous) of unspecified shoulder**
√6th **S4Ø.27 Other superficial bite of shoulder**
EXCLUDES 1 *open bite of shoulder (S41.Ø5)*
√7th **S4Ø.271 Other superficial bite of right shoulder**
√7th **S4Ø.272 Other superficial bite of left shoulder**
√7th **S4Ø.279 Other superficial bite of unspecified shoulder**

√5th **S4Ø.8 Other superficial injuries of upper arm**
√6th **S4Ø.81 Abrasion of upper arm**
√7th **S4Ø.811 Abrasion of right upper arm**
√7th **S4Ø.812 Abrasion of left upper arm**
√7th **S4Ø.819 Abrasion of unspecified upper arm**
√6th **S4Ø.82 Blister (nonthermal) of upper arm**
√7th **S4Ø.821 Blister (nonthermal) of right upper arm**
√7th **S4Ø.822 Blister (nonthermal) of left upper arm**
√7th **S4Ø.829 Blister (nonthermal) of unspecified upper arm**
√6th **S4Ø.84 External constriction of upper arm**
√7th **S4Ø.841 External constriction of right upper arm**
√7th **S4Ø.842 External constriction of left upper arm**
√7th **S4Ø.849 External constriction of unspecified upper arm**
√6th **S4Ø.85 Superficial foreign body of upper arm**
Splinter in the upper arm
√7th **S4Ø.851 Superficial foreign body of right upper arm**
√7th **S4Ø.852 Superficial foreign body of left upper arm**
√7th **S4Ø.859 Superficial foreign body of unspecified upper arm**
√6th **S4Ø.86 Insect bite (nonvenomous) of upper arm**
√7th **S4Ø.861 Insect bite (nonvenomous) of right upper arm**
√7th **S4Ø.862 Insect bite (nonvenomous) of left upper arm**
√7th **S4Ø.869 Insect bite (nonvenomous) of unspecified upper arm**
√6th **S4Ø.87 Other superficial bite of upper arm**
EXCLUDES 1 *open bite of upper arm (S41.14)*
EXCLUDES 2 *other superficial bite of shoulder (S4Ø.27-)*
√7th **S4Ø.871 Other superficial bite of right upper arm**
√7th **S4Ø.872 Other superficial bite of left upper arm**
√7th **S4Ø.879 Other superficial bite of unspecified upper arm**

√5th **S4Ø.9 Unspecified superficial injury of shoulder and upper arm**
√6th **S4Ø.91 Unspecified superficial injury of shoulder**
√7th **S4Ø.911 Unspecified superficial injury of right shoulder**
√7th **S4Ø.912 Unspecified superficial injury of left shoulder**
√7th **S4Ø.919 Unspecified superficial injury of unspecified shoulder**
√6th **S4Ø.92 Unspecified superficial injury of upper arm**
√7th **S4Ø.921 Unspecified superficial injury of right upper arm**
√7th **S4Ø.922 Unspecified superficial injury of left upper arm**
√7th **S4Ø.929 Unspecified superficial injury of unspecified upper arm**

√4th **S41 Open wound of shoulder and upper arm**
Code also any associated wound infection
EXCLUDES 1 *traumatic amputation of shoulder and upper arm (S48.-)*
EXCLUDES 2 *open fracture of shoulder and upper arm (S42.- with 7th character B or C)*

The appropriate 7th character is to be added to each code from category S41.
A initial encounter
D subsequent encounter
S sequela

√5th **S41.Ø Open wound of shoulder**
√6th **S41.ØØ Unspecified open wound of shoulder**
√7th **S41.ØØ1 Unspecified open wound of right shoulder**
√7th **S41.ØØ2 Unspecified open wound of left shoulder**
√7th **S41.ØØ9 Unspecified open wound of unspecified shoulder**
√6th **S41.Ø1 Laceration without foreign body of shoulder**
√7th **S41.Ø11 Laceration without foreign body of right shoulder**
√7th **S41.Ø12 Laceration without foreign body of left shoulder**
√7th **S41.Ø19 Laceration without foreign body of unspecified shoulder**
√6th **S41.Ø2 Laceration with foreign body of shoulder**
√7th **S41.Ø21 Laceration with foreign body of right shoulder**
√7th **S41.Ø22 Laceration with foreign body of left shoulder**
√7th **S41.Ø29 Laceration with foreign body of unspecified shoulder**
√6th **S41.Ø3 Puncture wound without foreign body of shoulder**
√7th **S41.Ø31 Puncture wound without foreign body of right shoulder**

7th **S41.032 Puncture wound without foreign body of left shoulder**

7th **S41.039 Puncture wound without foreign body of unspecified shoulder**

6th **S41.04 Puncture wound with foreign body of shoulder**

7th **S41.041 Puncture wound with foreign body of right shoulder**

7th **S41.042 Puncture wound with foreign body of left shoulder**

7th **S41.049 Puncture wound with foreign body of unspecified shoulder**

6th **S41.05 Open bite of shoulder**

Bite of shoulder NOS

EXCLUDES 1 *superficial bite of shoulder (S40.27)*

7th **S41.051 Open bite of right shoulder**

7th **S41.052 Open bite of left shoulder**

7th **S41.059 Open bite of unspecified shoulder**

5th **S41.1 Open wound of upper arm**

6th **S41.10 Unspecified open wound of upper arm**

AHA: 2016,3Q,24

7th **S41.101 Unspecified open wound of right upper arm**

7th **S41.102 Unspecified open wound of left upper arm**

7th **S41.109 Unspecified open wound of unspecified upper arm**

6th **S41.11 Laceration without foreign body of upper arm**

7th **S41.111 Laceration without foreign body of right upper arm**

7th **S41.112 Laceration without foreign body of left upper arm**

7th **S41.119 Laceration without foreign body of unspecified upper arm**

6th **S41.12 Laceration with foreign body of upper arm**

7th **S41.121 Laceration with foreign body of right upper arm**

7th **S41.122 Laceration with foreign body of left upper arm**

7th **S41.129 Laceration with foreign body of unspecified upper arm**

6th **S41.13 Puncture wound without foreign body of upper arm**

AHA: 2016,3Q,24

7th **S41.131 Puncture wound without foreign body of right upper arm**

7th **S41.132 Puncture wound without foreign body of left upper arm**

7th **S41.139 Puncture wound without foreign body of unspecified upper arm**

6th **S41.14 Puncture wound with foreign body of upper arm**

AHA: 2016,3Q,24

7th **S41.141 Puncture wound with foreign body of right upper arm**

7th **S41.142 Puncture wound with foreign body of left upper arm**

7th **S41.149 Puncture wound with foreign body of unspecified upper arm**

6th **S41.15 Open bite of upper arm**

Bite of upper arm NOS

EXCLUDES 1 *superficial bite of upper arm (S40.87)*

7th **S41.151 Open bite of right upper arm**

7th **S41.152 Open bite of left upper arm**

7th **S41.159 Open bite of unspecified upper arm**

4th **S42 Fracture of shoulder and upper arm**

NOTE A fracture not indicated as displaced or nondisplaced should be coded to displaced

A fracture not indicated as open or closed should be coded to closed

EXCLUDES 1 *traumatic amputation of shoulder and upper arm (S48.-)*

AHA: 2018,2Q,12; 2015,3Q,37-39

DEF: Diaphysis: Central shaft of a long bone.

DEF: Epiphysis: Proximal and distal rounded ends of a long bone, communicates with the joint.

DEF: Metaphysis: Section of a long bone located between the epiphysis and diaphysis at the proximal and distal ends.

DEF: Physis (growth plate): Narrow zone of cartilaginous tissue between the epiphysis and metaphysis at each end of a long bone. In childhood, proliferation of cells in this zone lengthens the bone. As the bone matures, this area thins, ossification eventually fusing into solid bone and growth stops. ***Synonym(s):*** *Epiphyseal plate.*

The appropriate 7th character is to be added to all codes from category S42 [unless otherwise indicated].

- A initial encounter for closed fracture
- B initial encounter for open fracture
- D subsequent encounter for fracture with routine healing
- G subsequent encounter for fracture with delayed healing
- K subsequent encounter for fracture with nonunion
- P subsequent encounter for fracture with malunion
- S sequela

5th **S42.0 Fracture of clavicle**

6th **S42.00 Fracture of unspecified part of clavicle**

7th **S42.001 Fracture of unspecified part of right clavicle** Q

7th **S42.002 Fracture of unspecified part of left clavicle** Q

7th **S42.009 Fracture of unspecified part of unspecified clavicle** Q

AHA: 2012,4Q,93

6th **S42.01 Fracture of sternal end of clavicle**

7th **S42.011 Anterior displaced fracture of sternal end of right clavicle** Q

7th **S42.012 Anterior displaced fracture of sternal end of left clavicle** Q

7th **S42.013 Anterior displaced fracture of sternal end of unspecified clavicle** Q

Displaced fracture of sternal end of clavicle NOS

7th **S42.014 Posterior displaced fracture of sternal end of right clavicle** Q

7th **S42.015 Posterior displaced fracture of sternal end of left clavicle** Q

7th **S42.016 Posterior displaced fracture of sternal end of unspecified clavicle** Q

7th **S42.017 Nondisplaced fracture of sternal end of right clavicle** Q

7th **S42.018 Nondisplaced fracture of sternal end of left clavicle** Q

7th **S42.019 Nondisplaced fracture of sternal end of unspecified clavicle** Q

6th **S42.02 Fracture of shaft of clavicle**

7th **S42.021 Displaced fracture of shaft of right clavicle** Q

7th **S42.022 Displaced fracture of shaft of left clavicle** Q

7th **S42.023 Displaced fracture of shaft of unspecified clavicle** Q

7th **S42.024 Nondisplaced fracture of shaft of right clavicle** Q

7th **S42.025 Nondisplaced fracture of shaft of left clavicle** Q

7th **S42.026 Nondisplaced fracture of shaft of unspecified clavicle** Q

6th **S42.03 Fracture of lateral end of clavicle**

Fracture of acromial end of clavicle

7th **S42.031 Displaced fracture of lateral end of right clavicle** Q

7th **S42.032 Displaced fracture of lateral end of left clavicle** Q

7th **S42.033 Displaced fracture of lateral end of unspecified clavicle** Q

S42.Ø34 Nondisplaced fracture of lateral end of right clavicle
S42.Ø35 Nondisplaced fracture of lateral end of left clavicle
S42.Ø36 Nondisplaced fracture of lateral end of unspecified clavicle

S42.1 Fracture of scapula

S42.1Ø Fracture of unspecified part of scapula
S42.1Ø1 Fracture of unspecified part of scapula, right shoulder
S42.1Ø2 Fracture of unspecified part of scapula, left shoulder
S42.1Ø9 Fracture of unspecified part of scapula, unspecified shoulder

S42.11 Fracture of body of scapula
S42.111 Displaced fracture of body of scapula, right shoulder
S42.112 Displaced fracture of body of scapula, left shoulder
S42.113 Displaced fracture of body of scapula, unspecified shoulder
S42.114 Nondisplaced fracture of body of scapula, right shoulder
S42.115 Nondisplaced fracture of body of scapula, left shoulder
S42.116 Nondisplaced fracture of body of scapula, unspecified shoulder

S42.12 Fracture of acromial process
S42.121 Displaced fracture of acromial process, right shoulder
S42.122 Displaced fracture of acromial process, left shoulder
S42.123 Displaced fracture of acromial process, unspecified shoulder
S42.124 Nondisplaced fracture of acromial process, right shoulder
S42.125 Nondisplaced fracture of acromial process, left shoulder
S42.126 Nondisplaced fracture of acromial process, unspecified shoulder

S42.13 Fracture of coracoid process
S42.131 Displaced fracture of coracoid process, right shoulder
S42.132 Displaced fracture of coracoid process, left shoulder
S42.133 Displaced fracture of coracoid process, unspecified shoulder
S42.134 Nondisplaced fracture of coracoid process, right shoulder
S42.135 Nondisplaced fracture of coracoid process, left shoulder
S42.136 Nondisplaced fracture of coracoid process, unspecified shoulder

S42.14 Fracture of glenoid cavity of scapula
S42.141 Displaced fracture of glenoid cavity of scapula, right shoulder
S42.142 Displaced fracture of glenoid cavity of scapula, left shoulder
S42.143 Displaced fracture of glenoid cavity of scapula, unspecified shoulder
S42.144 Nondisplaced fracture of glenoid cavity of scapula, right shoulder
S42.145 Nondisplaced fracture of glenoid cavity of scapula, left shoulder
S42.146 Nondisplaced fracture of glenoid cavity of scapula, unspecified shoulder

S42.15 Fracture of neck of scapula
S42.151 Displaced fracture of neck of scapula, right shoulder
S42.152 Displaced fracture of neck of scapula, left shoulder
S42.153 Displaced fracture of neck of scapula, unspecified shoulder
S42.154 Nondisplaced fracture of neck of scapula, right shoulder
S42.155 Nondisplaced fracture of neck of scapula, left shoulder
S42.156 Nondisplaced fracture of neck of scapula, unspecified shoulder

S42.19 Fracture of other part of scapula
S42.191 Fracture of other part of scapula, right shoulder
S42.192 Fracture of other part of scapula, left shoulder
S42.199 Fracture of other part of scapula, unspecified shoulder

S42.2 Fracture of upper end of humerus
Fracture of proximal end of humerus
EXCLUDES 2 *fracture of shaft of humerus (S42.3-)*
physeal fracture of upper end of humerus (S49.Ø-)

S42.2Ø Unspecified fracture of upper end of humerus
S42.2Ø1 Unspecified fracture of upper end of right humerus
S42.2Ø2 Unspecified fracture of upper end of left humerus
S42.2Ø9 Unspecified fracture of upper end of unspecified humerus

S42.21 Unspecified fracture of surgical neck of humerus
Fracture of neck of humerus NOS
S42.211 Unspecified displaced fracture of surgical neck of right humerus
S42.212 Unspecified displaced fracture of surgical neck of left humerus
S42.213 Unspecified displaced fracture of surgical neck of unspecified humerus
S42.214 Unspecified nondisplaced fracture of surgical neck of right humerus
S42.215 Unspecified nondisplaced fracture of surgical neck of left humerus
S42.216 Unspecified nondisplaced fracture of surgical neck of unspecified humerus

S42.22 2-part fracture of surgical neck of humerus
S42.221 2-part displaced fracture of surgical neck of right humerus
S42.222 2-part displaced fracture of surgical neck of left humerus
S42.223 2-part displaced fracture of surgical neck of unspecified humerus
S42.224 2-part nondisplaced fracture of surgical neck of right humerus
S42.225 2-part nondisplaced fracture of surgical neck of left humerus
S42.226 2-part nondisplaced fracture of surgical neck of unspecified humerus

S42.23 3-part fracture of surgical neck of humerus
S42.231 3-part fracture of surgical neck of right humerus
S42.232 3-part fracture of surgical neck of left humerus
S42.239 3-part fracture of surgical neck of unspecified humerus

S42.24 4-part fracture of surgical neck of humerus
S42.241 4-part fracture of surgical neck of right humerus
S42.242 4-part fracture of surgical neck of left humerus
S42.249 4-part fracture of surgical neck of unspecified humerus

S42.25 Fracture of greater tuberosity of humerus
S42.251 Displaced fracture of greater tuberosity of right humerus
S42.252 Displaced fracture of greater tuberosity of left humerus
S42.253 Displaced fracture of greater tuberosity of unspecified humerus
S42.254 Nondisplaced fracture of greater tuberosity of right humerus
S42.255 Nondisplaced fracture of greater tuberosity of left humerus
S42.256 Nondisplaced fracture of greater tuberosity of unspecified humerus

S42.26 Fracture of lesser tuberosity of humerus
S42.261 Displaced fracture of lesser tuberosity of right humerus
S42.262 Displaced fracture of lesser tuberosity of left humerus

Additional Character Required | Placeholder Alert | Manifestation | Unspecified Dx | QPP | Unacceptable PDx

7th **S42.263** Displaced fracture of lesser tuberosity of unspecified humerus Q
7th **S42.264** Nondisplaced fracture of lesser tuberosity of right humerus Q
7th **S42.265** Nondisplaced fracture of lesser tuberosity of left humerus Q
7th **S42.266** Nondisplaced fracture of lesser tuberosity of unspecified humerus Q

6th **S42.27 Torus fracture of upper end of humerus**

The appropriate 7th character is to be added to all codes in subcategory S42.27
A initial encounter for closed fracture
D subsequent encounter for fracture with routine healing
G subsequent encounter for fracture with delayed healing
K subsequent encounter for fracture with nonunion
P subsequent encounter for fracture with malunion
S sequela

7th **S42.271** Torus fracture of upper end of right humerus Q
7th **S42.272** Torus fracture of upper end of left humerus Q
7th **S42.279** Torus fracture of upper end of unspecified humerus Q

6th **S42.29 Other fracture of upper end of humerus**
Fracture of anatomical neck of humerus
Fracture of articular head of humerus
AHA: 2019,1Q,18

7th **S42.291** Other displaced fracture of upper end of right humerus Q
7th **S42.292** Other displaced fracture of upper end of left humerus Q
7th **S42.293** Other displaced fracture of upper end of unspecified humerus Q
7th **S42.294** Other nondisplaced fracture of upper end of right humerus Q
7th **S42.295** Other nondisplaced fracture of upper end of left humerus Q
7th **S42.296** Other nondisplaced fracture of upper end of unspecified humerus Q

5th **S42.3 Fracture of shaft of humerus**
Fracture of humerus NOS
Fracture of upper arm NOS
EXCLUDES 2 *physeal fractures of upper end of humerus (S49.Ø-)*
physeal fractures of lower end of humerus (S49.1-)

6th **S42.3Ø Unspecified fracture of shaft of humerus**
7th **S42.3Ø1** Unspecified fracture of shaft of humerus, right arm Q
7th **S42.3Ø2** Unspecified fracture of shaft of humerus, left arm Q
7th **S42.3Ø9** Unspecified fracture of shaft of humerus, unspecified arm Q

6th **S42.31 Greenstick fracture of shaft of humerus**

The appropriate 7th character is to be added to all codes in subcategory S42.31
A initial encounter for closed fracture
D subsequent encounter for fracture with routine healing
G subsequent encounter for fracture with delayed healing
K subsequent encounter for fracture with nonunion
P subsequent encounter for fracture with malunion
S sequela

7th **S42.311** Greenstick fracture of shaft of humerus, right arm Q
7th **S42.312** Greenstick fracture of shaft of humerus, left arm Q
7th **S42.319** Greenstick fracture of shaft of humerus, unspecified arm Q

6th **S42.32 Transverse fracture of shaft of humerus**
7th **S42.321** Displaced transverse fracture of shaft of humerus, right arm Q
7th **S42.322** Displaced transverse fracture of shaft of humerus, left arm Q
7th **S42.323** Displaced transverse fracture of shaft of humerus, unspecified arm Q
7th **S42.324** Nondisplaced transverse fracture of shaft of humerus, right arm Q
7th **S42.325** Nondisplaced transverse fracture of shaft of humerus, left arm Q
7th **S42.326** Nondisplaced transverse fracture of shaft of humerus, unspecified arm Q

6th **S42.33 Oblique fracture of shaft of humerus**
7th **S42.331** Displaced oblique fracture of shaft of humerus, right arm Q
7th **S42.332** Displaced oblique fracture of shaft of humerus, left arm Q
7th **S42.333** Displaced oblique fracture of shaft of humerus, unspecified arm Q
7th **S42.334** Nondisplaced oblique fracture of shaft of humerus, right arm Q
7th **S42.335** Nondisplaced oblique fracture of shaft of humerus, left arm Q
7th **S42.336** Nondisplaced oblique fracture of shaft of humerus, unspecified arm Q

6th **S42.34 Spiral fracture of shaft of humerus**
7th **S42.341** Displaced spiral fracture of shaft of humerus, right arm Q
7th **S42.342** Displaced spiral fracture of shaft of humerus, left arm Q
7th **S42.343** Displaced spiral fracture of shaft of humerus, unspecified arm Q
7th **S42.344** Nondisplaced spiral fracture of shaft of humerus, right arm Q
7th **S42.345** Nondisplaced spiral fracture of shaft of humerus, left arm Q
7th **S42.346** Nondisplaced spiral fracture of shaft of humerus, unspecified arm Q

6th **S42.35 Comminuted fracture of shaft of humerus**
7th **S42.351** Displaced comminuted fracture of shaft of humerus, right arm Q
7th **S42.352** Displaced comminuted fracture of shaft of humerus, left arm Q
7th **S42.353** Displaced comminuted fracture of shaft of humerus, unspecified arm Q
7th **S42.354** Nondisplaced comminuted fracture of shaft of humerus, right arm Q
7th **S42.355** Nondisplaced comminuted fracture of shaft of humerus, left arm Q
7th **S42.356** Nondisplaced comminuted fracture of shaft of humerus, unspecified arm Q

6th **S42.36 Segmental fracture of shaft of humerus**
7th **S42.361** Displaced segmental fracture of shaft of humerus, right arm Q
7th **S42.362** Displaced segmental fracture of shaft of humerus, left arm Q
7th **S42.363** Displaced segmental fracture of shaft of humerus, unspecified arm Q
7th **S42.364** Nondisplaced segmental fracture of shaft of humerus, right arm Q
7th **S42.365** Nondisplaced segmental fracture of shaft of humerus, left arm Q
7th **S42.366** Nondisplaced segmental fracture of shaft of humerus, unspecified arm Q

6th **S42.39 Other fracture of shaft of humerus**
7th **S42.391** Other fracture of shaft of right humerus Q
7th **S42.392** Other fracture of shaft of left humerus Q
7th **S42.399** Other fracture of shaft of unspecified humerus Q

5th **S42.4 Fracture of lower end of humerus**
Fracture of distal end of humerus
EXCLUDES 2 *fracture of shaft of humerus (S42.3-)*
physeal fracture of lower end of humerus (S49.1-)

6th **S42.4Ø Unspecified fracture of lower end of humerus**
Fracture of elbow NOS
7th **S42.4Ø1** Unspecified fracture of lower end of right humerus Q
7th **S42.4Ø2** Unspecified fracture of lower end of left humerus Q

S42.409 Unspecified fracture of lower end of unspecified humerus

S42.41 Simple supracondylar fracture without intercondylar fracture of humerus

S42.411 Displaced simple supracondylar fracture without intercondylar fracture of right humerus

S42.412 Displaced simple supracondylar fracture without intercondylar fracture of left humerus

S42.413 Displaced simple supracondylar fracture without intercondylar fracture of unspecified humerus

S42.414 Nondisplaced simple supracondylar fracture without intercondylar fracture of right humerus

S42.415 Nondisplaced simple supracondylar fracture without intercondylar fracture of left humerus

S42.416 Nondisplaced simple supracondylar fracture without intercondylar fracture of unspecified humerus

S42.42 Comminuted supracondylar fracture without intercondylar fracture of humerus

S42.421 Displaced comminuted supracondylar fracture without intercondylar fracture of right humerus

S42.422 Displaced comminuted supracondylar fracture without intercondylar fracture of left humerus

S42.423 Displaced comminuted supracondylar fracture without intercondylar fracture of unspecified humerus

S42.424 Nondisplaced comminuted supracondylar fracture without intercondylar fracture of right humerus

S42.425 Nondisplaced comminuted supracondylar fracture without intercondylar fracture of left humerus

S42.426 Nondisplaced comminuted supracondylar fracture without intercondylar fracture of unspecified humerus

S42.43 Fracture (avulsion) of lateral epicondyle of humerus

S42.431 Displaced fracture (avulsion) of lateral epicondyle of right humerus

S42.432 Displaced fracture (avulsion) of lateral epicondyle of left humerus

S42.433 Displaced fracture (avulsion) of lateral epicondyle of unspecified humerus

S42.434 Nondisplaced fracture (avulsion) of lateral epicondyle of right humerus

S42.435 Nondisplaced fracture (avulsion) of lateral epicondyle of left humerus

S42.436 Nondisplaced fracture (avulsion) of lateral epicondyle of unspecified humerus

S42.44 Fracture (avulsion) of medial epicondyle of humerus

S42.441 Displaced fracture (avulsion) of medial epicondyle of right humerus

S42.442 Displaced fracture (avulsion) of medial epicondyle of left humerus

S42.443 Displaced fracture (avulsion) of medial epicondyle of unspecified humerus

S42.444 Nondisplaced fracture (avulsion) of medial epicondyle of right humerus

S42.445 Nondisplaced fracture (avulsion) of medial epicondyle of left humerus

S42.446 Nondisplaced fracture (avulsion) of medial epicondyle of unspecified humerus

S42.447 Incarcerated fracture (avulsion) of medial epicondyle of right humerus

S42.448 Incarcerated fracture (avulsion) of medial epicondyle of left humerus

S42.449 Incarcerated fracture (avulsion) of medial epicondyle of unspecified humerus

S42.45 Fracture of lateral condyle of humerus

Fracture of capitellum of humerus

S42.451 Displaced fracture of lateral condyle of right humerus

S42.452 Displaced fracture of lateral condyle of left humerus

S42.453 Displaced fracture of lateral condyle of unspecified humerus

S42.454 Nondisplaced fracture of lateral condyle of right humerus

S42.455 Nondisplaced fracture of lateral condyle of left humerus

S42.456 Nondisplaced fracture of lateral condyle of unspecified humerus

S42.46 Fracture of medial condyle of humerus

Trochlea fracture of humerus

S42.461 Displaced fracture of medial condyle of right humerus

S42.462 Displaced fracture of medial condyle of left humerus

S42.463 Displaced fracture of medial condyle of unspecified humerus

S42.464 Nondisplaced fracture of medial condyle of right humerus

S42.465 Nondisplaced fracture of medial condyle of left humerus

S42.466 Nondisplaced fracture of medial condyle of unspecified humerus

S42.47 Transcondylar fracture of humerus

S42.471 Displaced transcondylar fracture of right humerus

S42.472 Displaced transcondylar fracture of left humerus

S42.473 Displaced transcondylar fracture of unspecified humerus

S42.474 Nondisplaced transcondylar fracture of right humerus

S42.475 Nondisplaced transcondylar fracture of left humerus

S42.476 Nondisplaced transcondylar fracture of unspecified humerus

S42.48 Torus fracture of lower end of humerus

The appropriate 7th character is to be added to all codes in subcategory S42.48.

- A initial encounter for closed fracture
- D subsequent encounter for fracture with routine healing
- G subsequent encounter for fracture with delayed healing
- K subsequent encounter for fracture with nonunion
- P subsequent encounter for fracture with malunion
- S sequela

S42.481 Torus fracture of lower end of right humerus

S42.482 Torus fracture of lower end of left humerus

S42.489 Torus fracture of lower end of unspecified humerus

S42.49 Other fracture of lower end of humerus

S42.491 Other displaced fracture of lower end of right humerus

S42.492 Other displaced fracture of lower end of left humerus

S42.493 Other displaced fracture of lower end of unspecified humerus

S42.494 Other nondisplaced fracture of lower end of right humerus

S42.495 Other nondisplaced fracture of lower end of left humerus

S42.496 Other nondisplaced fracture of lower end of unspecified humerus

S42.9 Fracture of shoulder girdle, part unspecified

Fracture of shoulder NOS

S42.90 Fracture of unspecified shoulder girdle, part unspecified

S42.91 Fracture of right shoulder girdle, part unspecified

S42.92 Fracture of left shoulder girdle, part unspecified

4th **S43 Dislocation and sprain of joints and ligaments of shoulder girdle**

INCLUDES avulsion of joint or ligament of shoulder girdle
laceration of cartilage, joint or ligament of shoulder girdle
sprain of cartilage, joint or ligament of shoulder girdle
traumatic hemarthrosis of joint or ligament of shoulder girdle
traumatic rupture of joint or ligament of shoulder girdle
traumatic subluxation of joint or ligament of shoulder girdle
traumatic tear of joint or ligament of shoulder girdle

Code also any associated open wound

EXCLUDES 2 *strain of muscle, fascia and tendon of shoulder and upper arm (S46.-)*

The appropriate 7th character is to be added to each code from category S43.
A initial encounter
D subsequent encounter
S sequela

5th **S43.0 Subluxation and dislocation of shoulder joint**
Dislocation of glenohumeral joint
Subluxation of glenohumeral joint

6th **S43.00 Unspecified subluxation and dislocation of shoulder joint**
Dislocation of humerus NOS
Subluxation of humerus NOS

7th **S43.001 Unspecified subluxation of right shoulder joint**
7th **S43.002 Unspecified subluxation of left shoulder joint**
7th **S43.003 Unspecified subluxation of unspecified shoulder joint**
7th **S43.004 Unspecified dislocation of right shoulder joint**
7th **S43.005 Unspecified dislocation of left shoulder joint**
7th **S43.006 Unspecified dislocation of unspecified shoulder joint**

6th **S43.01 Anterior subluxation and dislocation of humerus**
7th **S43.011 Anterior subluxation of right humerus**
7th **S43.012 Anterior subluxation of left humerus**
7th **S43.013 Anterior subluxation of unspecified humerus**
7th **S43.014 Anterior dislocation of right humerus**
7th **S43.015 Anterior dislocation of left humerus**
7th **S43.016 Anterior dislocation of unspecified humerus**

6th **S43.02 Posterior subluxation and dislocation of humerus**
7th **S43.021 Posterior subluxation of right humerus**
7th **S43.022 Posterior subluxation of left humerus**
7th **S43.023 Posterior subluxation of unspecified humerus**
7th **S43.024 Posterior dislocation of right humerus**
7th **S43.025 Posterior dislocation of left humerus**
7th **S43.026 Posterior dislocation of unspecified humerus**

6th **S43.03 Inferior subluxation and dislocation of humerus**
7th **S43.031 Inferior subluxation of right humerus**
7th **S43.032 Inferior subluxation of left humerus**
7th **S43.033 Inferior subluxation of unspecified humerus**
7th **S43.034 Inferior dislocation of right humerus**
7th **S43.035 Inferior dislocation of left humerus**
7th **S43.036 Inferior dislocation of unspecified humerus**

6th **S43.08 Other subluxation and dislocation of shoulder joint**
7th **S43.081 Other subluxation of right shoulder joint**
7th **S43.082 Other subluxation of left shoulder joint**
7th **S43.083 Other subluxation of unspecified shoulder joint**
7th **S43.084 Other dislocation of right shoulder joint**
7th **S43.085 Other dislocation of left shoulder joint**
7th **S43.086 Other dislocation of unspecified shoulder joint**

5th **S43.1 Subluxation and dislocation of acromioclavicular joint**

6th **S43.10 Unspecified dislocation of acromioclavicular joint**
7th **S43.101 Unspecified dislocation of right acromioclavicular joint**
7th **S43.102 Unspecified dislocation of left acromioclavicular joint**
7th **S43.109 Unspecified dislocation of unspecified acromioclavicular joint**

6th **S43.11 Subluxation of acromioclavicular joint**
7th **S43.111 Subluxation of right acromioclavicular joint**
7th **S43.112 Subluxation of left acromioclavicular joint**
7th **S43.119 Subluxation of unspecified acromioclavicular joint**

6th **S43.12 Dislocation of acromioclavicular joint, 100%-200% displacement**
7th **S43.121 Dislocation of right acromioclavicular joint, 100%-200% displacement**
7th **S43.122 Dislocation of left acromioclavicular joint, 100%-200% displacement**
7th **S43.129 Dislocation of unspecified acromioclavicular joint, 100%-200% displacement**

6th **S43.13 Dislocation of acromioclavicular joint, greater than 200% displacement**
7th **S43.131 Dislocation of right acromioclavicular joint, greater than 200% displacement**
7th **S43.132 Dislocation of left acromioclavicular joint, greater than 200% displacement**
7th **S43.139 Dislocation of unspecified acromioclavicular joint, greater than 200% displacement**

6th **S43.14 Inferior dislocation of acromioclavicular joint**
7th **S43.141 Inferior dislocation of right acromioclavicular joint**
7th **S43.142 Inferior dislocation of left acromioclavicular joint**
7th **S43.149 Inferior dislocation of unspecified acromioclavicular joint**

6th **S43.15 Posterior dislocation of acromioclavicular joint**
7th **S43.151 Posterior dislocation of right acromioclavicular joint**
7th **S43.152 Posterior dislocation of left acromioclavicular joint**
7th **S43.159 Posterior dislocation of unspecified acromioclavicular joint**

5th **S43.2 Subluxation and dislocation of sternoclavicular joint**

6th **S43.20 Unspecified subluxation and dislocation of sternoclavicular joint**
7th **S43.201 Unspecified subluxation of right sternoclavicular joint**
7th **S43.202 Unspecified subluxation of left sternoclavicular joint**
7th **S43.203 Unspecified subluxation of unspecified sternoclavicular joint**
7th **S43.204 Unspecified dislocation of right sternoclavicular joint**
7th **S43.205 Unspecified dislocation of left sternoclavicular joint**
7th **S43.206 Unspecified dislocation of unspecified sternoclavicular joint**

6th **S43.21 Anterior subluxation and dislocation of sternoclavicular joint**
7th **S43.211 Anterior subluxation of right sternoclavicular joint**
7th **S43.212 Anterior subluxation of left sternoclavicular joint**
7th **S43.213 Anterior subluxation of unspecified sternoclavicular joint**
7th **S43.214 Anterior dislocation of right sternoclavicular joint**
7th **S43.215 Anterior dislocation of left sternoclavicular joint**
7th **S43.216 Anterior dislocation of unspecified sternoclavicular joint**

6th **S43.22 Posterior subluxation and dislocation of sternoclavicular joint**
7th **S43.221 Posterior subluxation of right sternoclavicular joint**
7th **S43.222 Posterior subluxation of left sternoclavicular joint**

7th **S43.223** **Posterior subluxation of unspecified sternoclavicular joint**
7th **S43.224** **Posterior dislocation of right sternoclavicular joint**
7th **S43.225** **Posterior dislocation of left sternoclavicular joint**
7th **S43.226** **Posterior dislocation of unspecified sternoclavicular joint**

5th **S43.3** **Subluxation and dislocation of other and unspecified parts of shoulder girdle**

6th **S43.30** **Subluxation and dislocation of unspecified parts of shoulder girdle**
Dislocation of shoulder girdle NOS
Subluxation of shoulder girdle NOS
7th **S43.301** **Subluxation of unspecified parts of right shoulder girdle**
7th **S43.302** **Subluxation of unspecified parts of left shoulder girdle**
7th **S43.303** **Subluxation of unspecified parts of unspecified shoulder girdle**
7th **S43.304** **Dislocation of unspecified parts of right shoulder girdle**
7th **S43.305** **Dislocation of unspecified parts of left shoulder girdle**
7th **S43.306** **Dislocation of unspecified parts of unspecified shoulder girdle**

6th **S43.31** **Subluxation and dislocation of scapula**
7th **S43.311** **Subluxation of right scapula**
7th **S43.312** **Subluxation of left scapula**
7th **S43.313** **Subluxation of unspecified scapula**
7th **S43.314** **Dislocation of right scapula**
7th **S43.315** **Dislocation of left scapula**
7th **S43.316** **Dislocation of unspecified scapula**

6th **S43.39** **Subluxation and dislocation of other parts of shoulder girdle**
7th **S43.391** **Subluxation of other parts of right shoulder girdle**
7th **S43.392** **Subluxation of other parts of left shoulder girdle**
7th **S43.393** **Subluxation of other parts of unspecified shoulder girdle**
7th **S43.394** **Dislocation of other parts of right shoulder girdle**
7th **S43.395** **Dislocation of other parts of left shoulder girdle**
7th **S43.396** **Dislocation of other parts of unspecified shoulder girdle**

5th **S43.4** **Sprain of shoulder joint**

6th **S43.40** **Unspecified sprain of shoulder joint**
7th **S43.401** **Unspecified sprain of right shoulder joint**
7th **S43.402** **Unspecified sprain of left shoulder joint**
7th **S43.409** **Unspecified sprain of unspecified shoulder joint**

6th **S43.41** **Sprain of coracohumeral (ligament)**
7th **S43.411** **Sprain of right coracohumeral (ligament)**
7th **S43.412** **Sprain of left coracohumeral (ligament)**
7th **S43.419** **Sprain of unspecified coracohumeral (ligament)**

6th **S43.42** **Sprain of rotator cuff capsule**
EXCLUDES 1 *rotator cuff syndrome (complete) (incomplete), not specified as traumatic (M75.1-)*
EXCLUDES 2 *injury of tendon of rotator cuff (S46.0-)*
7th **S43.421** **Sprain of right rotator cuff capsule**
7th **S43.422** **Sprain of left rotator cuff capsule**
7th **S43.429** **Sprain of unspecified rotator cuff capsule**

6th **S43.43** **Superior glenoid labrum lesion**
SLAP lesion
AHA: 2019,2Q,26
DEF: Detachment injury of the superior aspect of the glenoid labrum, which is the ring of fibrocartilage attached to the rim of the glenoid cavity of the scapula.
7th **S43.431** **Superior glenoid labrum lesion of right shoulder**
7th **S43.432** **Superior glenoid labrum lesion of left shoulder**
7th **S43.439** **Superior glenoid labrum lesion of unspecified shoulder**

6th **S43.49** **Other sprain of shoulder joint**
7th **S43.491** **Other sprain of right shoulder joint**
7th **S43.492** **Other sprain of left shoulder joint**
7th **S43.499** **Other sprain of unspecified shoulder joint**

5th **S43.5** **Sprain of acromioclavicular joint**
Sprain of acromioclavicular ligament
x7th **S43.50** **Sprain of unspecified acromioclavicular joint**
x7th **S43.51** **Sprain of right acromioclavicular joint**
x7th **S43.52** **Sprain of left acromioclavicular joint**

5th **S43.6** **Sprain of sternoclavicular joint**
x7th **S43.60** **Sprain of unspecified sternoclavicular joint**
x7th **S43.61** **Sprain of right sternoclavicular joint**
x7th **S43.62** **Sprain of left sternoclavicular joint**

5th **S43.8** **Sprain of other specified parts of shoulder girdle**
x7th **S43.80** **Sprain of other specified parts of unspecified shoulder girdle**
x7th **S43.81** **Sprain of other specified parts of right shoulder girdle**
x7th **S43.82** **Sprain of other specified parts of left shoulder girdle**

5th **S43.9** **Sprain of unspecified parts of shoulder girdle**
x7th **S43.90** **Sprain of unspecified parts of unspecified shoulder girdle**
Sprain of shoulder girdle NOS
x7th **S43.91** **Sprain of unspecified parts of right shoulder girdle**
x7th **S43.92** **Sprain of unspecified parts of left shoulder girdle**

4th **S44** **Injury of nerves at shoulder and upper arm level**
Code also any associated open wound (S41.-)
EXCLUDES 2 *injury of brachial plexus (S14.3-)*

The appropriate 7th character is to be added to each code from category S44.
A initial encounter
D subsequent encounter
S sequela

5th **S44.0** **Injury of ulnar nerve at upper arm level**
EXCLUDES 1 *ulnar nerve NOS (S54.0)*
x7th **S44.00** **Injury of ulnar nerve at upper arm level, unspecified arm**
x7th **S44.01** **Injury of ulnar nerve at upper arm level, right arm**
x7th **S44.02** **Injury of ulnar nerve at upper arm level, left arm**

5th **S44.1** **Injury of median nerve at upper arm level**
EXCLUDES 1 *median nerve NOS (S54.1)*
x7th **S44.10** **Injury of median nerve at upper arm level, unspecified arm**
x7th **S44.11** **Injury of median nerve at upper arm level, right arm**
x7th **S44.12** **Injury of median nerve at upper arm level, left arm**

5th **S44.2** **Injury of radial nerve at upper arm level**
EXCLUDES 1 *radial nerve NOS (S54.2)*
x7th **S44.20** **Injury of radial nerve at upper arm level, unspecified arm**
x7th **S44.21** **Injury of radial nerve at upper arm level, right arm**
x7th **S44.22** **Injury of radial nerve at upper arm level, left arm**

5th **S44.3** **Injury of axillary nerve**
x7th **S44.30** **Injury of axillary nerve, unspecified arm**
x7th **S44.31** **Injury of axillary nerve, right arm**
x7th **S44.32** **Injury of axillary nerve, left arm**

5th **S44.4** **Injury of musculocutaneous nerve**
x7th **S44.40** **Injury of musculocutaneous nerve, unspecified arm**
x7th **S44.41** **Injury of musculocutaneous nerve, right arm**
x7th **S44.42** **Injury of musculocutaneous nerve, left arm**

5th **S44.5** **Injury of cutaneous sensory nerve at shoulder and upper arm level**
x7th **S44.50** **Injury of cutaneous sensory nerve at shoulder and upper arm level, unspecified arm**
x7th **S44.51** **Injury of cutaneous sensory nerve at shoulder and upper arm level, right arm**
x7th **S44.52** **Injury of cutaneous sensory nerve at shoulder and upper arm level, left arm**

5th S44.8 **Injury of other nerves at shoulder and upper arm level**

6th S44.8X **Injury of other nerves at shoulder and upper arm level**

7th S44.8X1 **Injury of other nerves at shoulder and upper arm level, right arm**

7th S44.8X2 **Injury of other nerves at shoulder and upper arm level, left arm**

7th S44.8X9 **Injury of other nerves at shoulder and upper arm level, unspecified arm**

5th S44.9 **Injury of unspecified nerve at shoulder and upper arm level**

✓7th S44.90 **Injury of unspecified nerve at shoulder and upper arm level, unspecified arm**

✓7th S44.91 **Injury of unspecified nerve at shoulder and upper arm level, right arm**

✓7th S44.92 **Injury of unspecified nerve at shoulder and upper arm level, left arm**

4th **S45 Injury of blood vessels at shoulder and upper arm level**

Code also any associated open wound (S41.-)

EXCLUDES 2 *injury of subclavian artery (S25.1)*
injury of subclavian vein (S25.3)

The appropriate 7th character is to be added to each code from category S45.
A initial encounter
D subsequent encounter
S sequela

5th S45.0 **Injury of axillary artery**

6th S45.00 **Unspecified injury of axillary artery**

7th S45.001 **Unspecified injury of axillary artery, right side**

7th S45.002 **Unspecified injury of axillary artery, left side**

7th S45.009 **Unspecified injury of axillary artery, unspecified side**

6th S45.01 **Laceration of axillary artery**

7th S45.011 **Laceration of axillary artery, right side**

7th S45.012 **Laceration of axillary artery, left side**

7th S45.019 **Laceration of axillary artery, unspecified side**

6th S45.09 **Other specified injury of axillary artery**

7th S45.091 **Other specified injury of axillary artery, right side**

7th S45.092 **Other specified injury of axillary artery, left side**

7th S45.099 **Other specified injury of axillary artery, unspecified side**

5th S45.1 **Injury of brachial artery**

6th S45.10 **Unspecified injury of brachial artery**

7th S45.101 **Unspecified injury of brachial artery, right side**

7th S45.102 **Unspecified injury of brachial artery, left side**

7th S45.109 **Unspecified injury of brachial artery, unspecified side**

6th S45.11 **Laceration of brachial artery**

7th S45.111 **Laceration of brachial artery, right side**

7th S45.112 **Laceration of brachial artery, left side**

7th S45.119 **Laceration of brachial artery, unspecified side**

6th S45.19 **Other specified injury of brachial artery**

7th S45.191 **Other specified injury of brachial artery, right side**

7th S45.192 **Other specified injury of brachial artery, left side**

7th S45.199 **Other specified injury of brachial artery, unspecified side**

5th S45.2 **Injury of axillary or brachial vein**

6th S45.20 **Unspecified injury of axillary or brachial vein**

7th S45.201 **Unspecified injury of axillary or brachial vein, right side**

7th S45.202 **Unspecified injury of axillary or brachial vein, left side**

7th S45.209 **Unspecified injury of axillary or brachial vein, unspecified side**

6th S45.21 **Laceration of axillary or brachial vein**

7th S45.211 **Laceration of axillary or brachial vein, right side**

7th S45.212 **Laceration of axillary or brachial vein, left side**

7th S45.219 **Laceration of axillary or brachial vein, unspecified side**

6th S45.29 **Other specified injury of axillary or brachial vein**

7th S45.291 **Other specified injury of axillary or brachial vein, right side**

7th S45.292 **Other specified injury of axillary or brachial vein, left side**

7th S45.299 **Other specified injury of axillary or brachial vein, unspecified side**

5th S45.3 **Injury of superficial vein at shoulder and upper arm level**

6th S45.30 **Unspecified injury of superficial vein at shoulder and upper arm level**

7th S45.301 **Unspecified injury of superficial vein at shoulder and upper arm level, right arm**

7th S45.302 **Unspecified injury of superficial vein at shoulder and upper arm level, left arm**

7th S45.309 **Unspecified injury of superficial vein at shoulder and upper arm level, unspecified arm**

6th S45.31 **Laceration of superficial vein at shoulder and upper arm level**

7th S45.311 **Laceration of superficial vein at shoulder and upper arm level, right arm**

7th S45.312 **Laceration of superficial vein at shoulder and upper arm level, left arm**

7th S45.319 **Laceration of superficial vein at shoulder and upper arm level, unspecified arm**

6th S45.39 **Other specified injury of superficial vein at shoulder and upper arm level**

7th S45.391 **Other specified injury of superficial vein at shoulder and upper arm level, right arm**

7th S45.392 **Other specified injury of superficial vein at shoulder and upper arm level, left arm**

7th S45.399 **Other specified injury of superficial vein at shoulder and upper arm level, unspecified arm**

5th S45.8 **Injury of other specified blood vessels at shoulder and upper arm level**

6th S45.80 **Unspecified injury of other specified blood vessels at shoulder and upper arm level**

7th S45.801 **Unspecified injury of other specified blood vessels at shoulder and upper arm level, right arm**

7th S45.802 **Unspecified injury of other specified blood vessels at shoulder and upper arm level, left arm**

7th S45.809 **Unspecified injury of other specified blood vessels at shoulder and upper arm level, unspecified arm**

6th S45.81 **Laceration of other specified blood vessels at shoulder and upper arm level**

7th S45.811 **Laceration of other specified blood vessels at shoulder and upper arm level, right arm**

7th S45.812 **Laceration of other specified blood vessels at shoulder and upper arm level, left arm**

7th S45.819 **Laceration of other specified blood vessels at shoulder and upper arm level, unspecified arm**

6th S45.89 **Other specified injury of other specified blood vessels at shoulder and upper arm level**

7th S45.891 **Other specified injury of other specified blood vessels at shoulder and upper arm level, right arm**

7th S45.892 **Other specified injury of other specified blood vessels at shoulder and upper arm level, left arm**

7th S45.899 **Other specified injury of other specified blood vessels at shoulder and upper arm level, unspecified arm**

5th S45.9 **Injury of unspecified blood vessel at shoulder and upper arm level**

6th S45.90 **Unspecified injury of unspecified blood vessel at shoulder and upper arm level**

7th S45.901 **Unspecified injury of unspecified blood vessel at shoulder and upper arm level, right arm**

S45.902 Unspecified injury of unspecified blood vessel at shoulder and upper arm level, left arm

S45.909 Unspecified injury of unspecified blood vessel at shoulder and upper arm level, unspecified arm

S45.91 Laceration of unspecified blood vessel at shoulder and upper arm level

S45.911 Laceration of unspecified blood vessel at shoulder and upper arm level, right arm

S45.912 Laceration of unspecified blood vessel at shoulder and upper arm level, left arm

S45.919 Laceration of unspecified blood vessel at shoulder and upper arm level, unspecified arm

S45.99 Other specified injury of unspecified blood vessel at shoulder and upper arm level

S45.991 Other specified injury of unspecified blood vessel at shoulder and upper arm level, right arm

S45.992 Other specified injury of unspecified blood vessel at shoulder and upper arm level, left arm

S45.999 Other specified injury of unspecified blood vessel at shoulder and upper arm level, unspecified arm

S46 Injury of muscle, fascia and tendon at shoulder and upper arm level

Code also any associated open wound (S41.-)

EXCLUDES 2 *injury of muscle, fascia and tendon at elbow (S56.-)*
sprain of joints and ligaments of shoulder girdle (S43.9)

TIP: Refer to the Muscle/Tendon table at the beginning of this chapter.

The appropriate 7th character is to be added to each code from category S46.
A initial encounter
D subsequent encounter
S sequela

S46.0 Injury of muscle(s) and tendon(s) of the rotator cuff of shoulder

S46.00 Unspecified injury of muscle(s) and tendon(s) of the rotator cuff of shoulder

S46.001 Unspecified injury of muscle(s) and tendon(s) of the rotator cuff of right shoulder

S46.002 Unspecified injury of muscle(s) and tendon(s) of the rotator cuff of left shoulder

S46.009 Unspecified injury of muscle(s) and tendon(s) of the rotator cuff of unspecified shoulder

S46.01 Strain of muscle(s) and tendon(s) of the rotator cuff of shoulder

S46.011 Strain of muscle(s) and tendon(s) of the rotator cuff of right shoulder

S46.012 Strain of muscle(s) and tendon(s) of the rotator cuff of left shoulder

S46.019 Strain of muscle(s) and tendon(s) of the rotator cuff of unspecified shoulder

S46.02 Laceration of muscle(s) and tendon(s) of the rotator cuff of shoulder

S46.021 Laceration of muscle(s) and tendon(s) of the rotator cuff of right shoulder

S46.022 Laceration of muscle(s) and tendon(s) of the rotator cuff of left shoulder

S46.029 Laceration of muscle(s) and tendon(s) of the rotator cuff of unspecified shoulder

S46.09 Other injury of muscle(s) and tendon(s) of the rotator cuff of shoulder

S46.091 Other injury of muscle(s) and tendon(s) of the rotator cuff of right shoulder

S46.092 Other injury of muscle(s) and tendon(s) of the rotator cuff of left shoulder

S46.099 Other injury of muscle(s) and tendon(s) of the rotator cuff of unspecified shoulder

S46.1 Injury of muscle, fascia and tendon of long head of biceps

S46.10 Unspecified injury of muscle, fascia and tendon of long head of biceps

S46.101 Unspecified injury of muscle, fascia and tendon of long head of biceps, right arm

S46.102 Unspecified injury of muscle, fascia and tendon of long head of biceps, left arm

S46.109 Unspecified injury of muscle, fascia and tendon of long head of biceps, unspecified arm

S46.11 Strain of muscle, fascia and tendon of long head of biceps

AHA: 2020,1Q,38; 2019,2Q,27

S46.111 Strain of muscle, fascia and tendon of long head of biceps, right arm

S46.112 Strain of muscle, fascia and tendon of long head of biceps, left arm

S46.119 Strain of muscle, fascia and tendon of long head of biceps, unspecified arm

S46.12 Laceration of muscle, fascia and tendon of long head of biceps

S46.121 Laceration of muscle, fascia and tendon of long head of biceps, right arm

S46.122 Laceration of muscle, fascia and tendon of long head of biceps, left arm

S46.129 Laceration of muscle, fascia and tendon of long head of biceps, unspecified arm

S46.19 Other injury of muscle, fascia and tendon of long head of biceps

S46.191 Other injury of muscle, fascia and tendon of long head of biceps, right arm

S46.192 Other injury of muscle, fascia and tendon of long head of biceps, left arm

S46.199 Other injury of muscle, fascia and tendon of long head of biceps, unspecified arm

S46.2 Injury of muscle, fascia and tendon of other parts of biceps

S46.20 Unspecified injury of muscle, fascia and tendon of other parts of biceps

S46.201 Unspecified injury of muscle, fascia and tendon of other parts of biceps, right arm

S46.202 Unspecified injury of muscle, fascia and tendon of other parts of biceps, left arm

S46.209 Unspecified injury of muscle, fascia and tendon of other parts of biceps, unspecified arm

S46.21 Strain of muscle, fascia and tendon of other parts of biceps

S46.211 Strain of muscle, fascia and tendon of other parts of biceps, right arm

S46.212 Strain of muscle, fascia and tendon of other parts of biceps, left arm

S46.219 Strain of muscle, fascia and tendon of other parts of biceps, unspecified arm

S46.22 Laceration of muscle, fascia and tendon of other parts of biceps

S46.221 Laceration of muscle, fascia and tendon of other parts of biceps, right arm

S46.222 Laceration of muscle, fascia and tendon of other parts of biceps, left arm

S46.229 Laceration of muscle, fascia and tendon of other parts of biceps, unspecified arm

S46.29 Other injury of muscle, fascia and tendon of other parts of biceps

S46.291 Other injury of muscle, fascia and tendon of other parts of biceps, right arm

S46.292 Other injury of muscle, fascia and tendon of other parts of biceps, left arm

S46.299 Other injury of muscle, fascia and tendon of other parts of biceps, unspecified arm

S46.3 Injury of muscle, fascia and tendon of triceps

S46.30 Unspecified injury of muscle, fascia and tendon of triceps

S46.301 Unspecified injury of muscle, fascia and tendon of triceps, right arm

S46.302 Unspecified injury of muscle, fascia and tendon of triceps, left arm

S46.309 Unspecified injury of muscle, fascia and tendon of triceps, unspecified arm

S46.31 Strain of muscle, fascia and tendon of triceps

S46.311 Strain of muscle, fascia and tendon of triceps, right arm

S46.312 Strain of muscle, fascia and tendon of triceps, left arm

S46.319 Strain of muscle, fascia and tendon of triceps, unspecified arm

S46.32 Laceration of muscle, fascia and tendon of triceps

S46.321 Laceration of muscle, fascia and tendon of triceps, right arm

√7th **S46.322** Laceration of muscle, fascia and tendon of triceps, left arm

√7th **S46.329** Laceration of muscle, fascia and tendon of triceps, unspecified arm

√6th **S46.39** Other injury of muscle, fascia and tendon of triceps

√7th **S46.391** Other injury of muscle, fascia and tendon of triceps, right arm

√7th **S46.392** Other injury of muscle, fascia and tendon of triceps, left arm

√7th **S46.399** Other injury of muscle, fascia and tendon of triceps, unspecified arm

√5th **S46.8** Injury of other muscles, fascia and tendons at shoulder and upper arm level

√6th **S46.80** Unspecified injury of other muscles, fascia and tendons at shoulder and upper arm level

√7th **S46.801** Unspecified injury of other muscles, fascia and tendons at shoulder and upper arm level, right arm

√7th **S46.802** Unspecified injury of other muscles, fascia and tendons at shoulder and upper arm level, left arm

√7th **S46.809** Unspecified injury of other muscles, fascia and tendons at shoulder and upper arm level, unspecified arm

√6th **S46.81** Strain of other muscles, fascia and tendons at shoulder and upper arm level

√7th **S46.811** Strain of other muscles, fascia and tendons at shoulder and upper arm level, right arm

√7th **S46.812** Strain of other muscles, fascia and tendons at shoulder and upper arm level, left arm

√7th **S46.819** Strain of other muscles, fascia and tendons at shoulder and upper arm level, unspecified arm

√6th **S46.82** Laceration of other muscles, fascia and tendons at shoulder and upper arm level

√7th **S46.821** Laceration of other muscles, fascia and tendons at shoulder and upper arm level, right arm

√7th **S46.822** Laceration of other muscles, fascia and tendons at shoulder and upper arm level, left arm

√7th **S46.829** Laceration of other muscles, fascia and tendons at shoulder and upper arm level, unspecified arm

√6th **S46.89** Other injury of other muscles, fascia and tendons at shoulder and upper arm level

√7th **S46.891** Other injury of other muscles, fascia and tendons at shoulder and upper arm level, right arm

√7th **S46.892** Other injury of other muscles, fascia and tendons at shoulder and upper arm level, left arm

√7th **S46.899** Other injury of other muscles, fascia and tendons at shoulder and upper arm level, unspecified arm

√5th **S46.9** Injury of unspecified muscle, fascia and tendon at shoulder and upper arm level

√6th **S46.90** Unspecified injury of unspecified muscle, fascia and tendon at shoulder and upper arm level

√7th **S46.901** Unspecified injury of unspecified muscle, fascia and tendon at shoulder and upper arm level, right arm

√7th **S46.902** Unspecified injury of unspecified muscle, fascia and tendon at shoulder and upper arm level, left arm

√7th **S46.909** Unspecified injury of unspecified muscle, fascia and tendon at shoulder and upper arm level, unspecified arm

√6th **S46.91** Strain of unspecified muscle, fascia and tendon at shoulder and upper arm level

√7th **S46.911** Strain of unspecified muscle, fascia and tendon at shoulder and upper arm level, right arm

√7th **S46.912** Strain of unspecified muscle, fascia and tendon at shoulder and upper arm level, left arm

√7th **S46.919** Strain of unspecified muscle, fascia and tendon at shoulder and upper arm level, unspecified arm

√6th **S46.92** Laceration of unspecified muscle, fascia and tendon at shoulder and upper arm level

√7th **S46.921** Laceration of unspecified muscle, fascia and tendon at shoulder and upper arm level, right arm

√7th **S46.922** Laceration of unspecified muscle, fascia and tendon at shoulder and upper arm level, left arm

√7th **S46.929** Laceration of unspecified muscle, fascia and tendon at shoulder and upper arm level, unspecified arm

√6th **S46.99** Other injury of unspecified muscle, fascia and tendon at shoulder and upper arm level

√7th **S46.991** Other injury of unspecified muscle, fascia and tendon at shoulder and upper arm level, right arm

√7th **S46.992** Other injury of unspecified muscle, fascia and tendon at shoulder and upper arm level, left arm

√7th **S46.999** Other injury of unspecified muscle, fascia and tendon at shoulder and upper arm level, unspecified arm

√4th **S47 Crushing injury of shoulder and upper arm**

Use additional code for all associated injuries

EXCLUDES 2 *crushing injury of elbow (S57.0-)*

The appropriate 7th character is to be added to each code from category S47.
A initial encounter
D subsequent encounter
S sequela

√x7th **S47.1** Crushing injury of right shoulder and upper arm

√x7th **S47.2** Crushing injury of left shoulder and upper arm

√x7th **S47.9** Crushing injury of shoulder and upper arm, unspecified arm

√4th **S48 Traumatic amputation of shoulder and upper arm**

An amputation not identified as partial or complete should be coded to complete

EXCLUDES 1 *traumatic amputation at elbow level (S58.0)*

The appropriate 7th character is to be added to each code from category S48.
A initial encounter
D subsequent encounter
S sequela

√5th **S48.0** Traumatic amputation at shoulder joint

√6th **S48.01** Complete traumatic amputation at shoulder joint

2 √7th **S48.011** Complete traumatic amputation at right shoulder joint HCC ESR COM

2 √7th **S48.012** Complete traumatic amputation at left shoulder joint HCC ESR COM

2 √7th **S48.019** Complete traumatic amputation at unspecified shoulder joint HCC ESR COM

√6th **S48.02** Partial traumatic amputation at shoulder joint

2 √7th **S48.021** Partial traumatic amputation at right shoulder joint HCC ESR COM

2 √7th **S48.022** Partial traumatic amputation at left shoulder joint HCC ESR COM

2 √7th **S48.029** Partial traumatic amputation at unspecified shoulder joint HCC ESR COM

√5th **S48.1** Traumatic amputation at level between shoulder and elbow

√6th **S48.11** Complete traumatic amputation at level between shoulder and elbow

2 √7th **S48.111** Complete traumatic amputation at level between right shoulder and elbow HCC ESR COM

2 √7th **S48.112** Complete traumatic amputation at level between left shoulder and elbow HCC ESR COM

2 √7th **S48.119** Complete traumatic amputation at level between unspecified shoulder and elbow HCC ESR COM

√6th **S48.12** Partial traumatic amputation at level between shoulder and elbow

2 √7th **S48.121** Partial traumatic amputation at level between right shoulder and elbow HCC ESR COM

2 √7th **S48.122** Partial traumatic amputation at level between left shoulder and elbow HCC ESR COM

2 ✓7th **S48.129** **Partial traumatic amputation at level between unspecified shoulder and elbow** HCC ESR COM

✓5th **S48.9** **Traumatic amputation of shoulder and upper arm, level unspecified**

✓6th **S48.91** **Complete traumatic amputation of shoulder and upper arm, level unspecified**

2 ✓7th **S48.911** **Complete traumatic amputation of right shoulder and upper arm, level unspecified** HCC ESR COM

2 ✓7th **S48.912** **Complete traumatic amputation of left shoulder and upper arm, level unspecified** HCC ESR COM

2 ✓7th **S48.919** **Complete traumatic amputation of unspecified shoulder and upper arm, level unspecified** HCC ESR COM

✓6th **S48.92** **Partial traumatic amputation of shoulder and upper arm, level unspecified**

2 ✓7th **S48.921** **Partial traumatic amputation of right shoulder and upper arm, level unspecified** HCC ESR COM

2 ✓7th **S48.922** **Partial traumatic amputation of left shoulder and upper arm, level unspecified** HCC ESR COM

2 ✓7th **S48.929** **Partial traumatic amputation of unspecified shoulder and upper arm, level unspecified** HCC ESR COM

✓4th **S49** **Other and unspecified injuries of shoulder and upper arm**

AHA: 2018,2Q,12; 2018,1Q,3

The appropriate 7th character is to be added to each code from subcategories S49.Ø and S49.1.
- A initial encounter for closed fracture
- D subsequent encounter for fracture with routine healing
- G subsequent encounter for fracture with delayed healing
- K subsequent encounter for fracture with nonunion
- P subsequent encounter for fracture with malunion
- S sequela

✓5th **S49.Ø** **Physeal fracture of upper end of humerus**

AHA: 2019,4Q,56

✓6th **S49.ØØ** **Unspecified physeal fracture of upper end of humerus**

✓7th **S49.ØØ1** **Unspecified physeal fracture of upper end of humerus, right arm** Q

✓7th **S49.ØØ2** **Unspecified physeal fracture of upper end of humerus, left arm** Q

✓7th **S49.ØØ9** **Unspecified physeal fracture of upper end of humerus, unspecified arm** Q

✓6th **S49.Ø1** **Salter-Harris Type I physeal fracture of upper end of humerus**

✓7th **S49.Ø11** **Salter-Harris Type I physeal fracture of upper end of humerus, right arm** Q

✓7th **S49.Ø12** **Salter-Harris Type I physeal fracture of upper end of humerus, left arm** Q

✓7th **S49.Ø19** **Salter-Harris Type I physeal fracture of upper end of humerus, unspecified arm** Q

✓6th **S49.Ø2** **Salter-Harris Type II physeal fracture of upper end of humerus**

✓7th **S49.Ø21** **Salter-Harris Type II physeal fracture of upper end of humerus, right arm** Q

✓7th **S49.Ø22** **Salter-Harris Type II physeal fracture of upper end of humerus, left arm** Q

✓7th **S49.Ø29** **Salter-Harris Type II physeal fracture of upper end of humerus, unspecified arm** Q

✓6th **S49.Ø3** **Salter-Harris Type III physeal fracture of upper end of humerus**

✓7th **S49.Ø31** **Salter-Harris Type III physeal fracture of upper end of humerus, right arm** Q

✓7th **S49.Ø32** **Salter-Harris Type III physeal fracture of upper end of humerus, left arm** Q

✓7th **S49.Ø39** **Salter-Harris Type III physeal fracture of upper end of humerus, unspecified arm** Q

✓6th **S49.Ø4** **Salter-Harris Type IV physeal fracture of upper end of humerus**

✓7th **S49.Ø41** **Salter-Harris Type IV physeal fracture of upper end of humerus, right arm** Q

✓7th **S49.Ø42** **Salter-Harris Type IV physeal fracture of upper end of humerus, left arm** Q

✓7th **S49.Ø49** **Salter-Harris Type IV physeal fracture of upper end of humerus, unspecified arm** Q

✓6th **S49.Ø9** **Other physeal fracture of upper end of humerus**

✓7th **S49.Ø91** **Other physeal fracture of upper end of humerus, right arm** Q

✓7th **S49.Ø92** **Other physeal fracture of upper end of humerus, left arm** Q

✓7th **S49.Ø99** **Other physeal fracture of upper end of humerus, unspecified arm** Q

✓5th **S49.1** **Physeal fracture of lower end of humerus**

AHA: 2019,4Q,56

✓6th **S49.1Ø** **Unspecified physeal fracture of lower end of humerus**

✓7th **S49.1Ø1** **Unspecified physeal fracture of lower end of humerus, right arm** Q

✓7th **S49.1Ø2** **Unspecified physeal fracture of lower end of humerus, left arm** Q

✓7th **S49.1Ø9** **Unspecified physeal fracture of lower end of humerus, unspecified arm** Q

✓6th **S49.11** **Salter-Harris Type I physeal fracture of lower end of humerus**

✓7th **S49.111** **Salter-Harris Type I physeal fracture of lower end of humerus, right arm** Q

✓7th **S49.112** **Salter-Harris Type I physeal fracture of lower end of humerus, left arm** Q

✓7th **S49.119** **Salter-Harris Type I physeal fracture of lower end of humerus, unspecified arm** Q

✓6th **S49.12** **Salter-Harris Type II physeal fracture of lower end of humerus**

✓7th **S49.121** **Salter-Harris Type II physeal fracture of lower end of humerus, right arm** Q

✓7th **S49.122** **Salter-Harris Type II physeal fracture of lower end of humerus, left arm** Q

✓7th **S49.129** **Salter-Harris Type II physeal fracture of lower end of humerus, unspecified arm** Q

✓6th **S49.13** **Salter-Harris Type III physeal fracture of lower end of humerus**

✓7th **S49.131** **Salter-Harris Type III physeal fracture of lower end of humerus, right arm** Q

✓7th **S49.132** **Salter-Harris Type III physeal fracture of lower end of humerus, left arm** Q

✓7th **S49.139** **Salter-Harris Type III physeal fracture of lower end of humerus, unspecified arm** Q

✓6th **S49.14** **Salter-Harris Type IV physeal fracture of lower end of humerus**

✓7th **S49.141** **Salter-Harris Type IV physeal fracture of lower end of humerus, right arm** Q

✓7th **S49.142** **Salter-Harris Type IV physeal fracture of lower end of humerus, left arm** Q

✓7th **S49.149** **Salter-Harris Type IV physeal fracture of lower end of humerus, unspecified arm** Q

✓6th **S49.19** **Other physeal fracture of lower end of humerus**

✓7th **S49.191** **Other physeal fracture of lower end of humerus, right arm** Q

✓7th **S49.192** **Other physeal fracture of lower end of humerus, left arm** Q

✓7th **S49.199** **Other physeal fracture of lower end of humerus, unspecified arm** Q

✓5th **S49.8** **Other specified injuries of shoulder and upper arm**

The appropriate 7th character is to be added to each code in subcategory S49.8.
- A initial encounter
- D subsequent encounter
- S sequela

✓x7th **S49.8Ø** **Other specified injuries of shoulder and upper arm, unspecified arm**

✓x7th **S49.81** **Other specified injuries of right shoulder and upper arm**

✓x7th **S49.82** **Other specified injuries of left shoulder and upper arm**

S49.9 **Unspecified injury of shoulder and upper arm**

The appropriate 7th character is to be added to each code in subcategory S49.9.
A initial encounter
D subsequent encounter
S sequela

S49.90 **Unspecified injury of shoulder and upper arm, unspecified arm**
S49.91 **Unspecified injury of right shoulder and upper arm**
S49.92 **Unspecified injury of left shoulder and upper arm**

Injuries to the elbow and forearm (S50-S59)

EXCLUDES 2 *burns and corrosions (T20-T32)*
frostbite (T33-T34)
injuries of wrist and hand (S60-S69)
insect bite or sting, venomous (T63.4)

S50 **Superficial injury of elbow and forearm**

EXCLUDES 2 *superficial injury of wrist and hand (S60.-)*

The appropriate 7th character is to be added to each code from category S50.
A initial encounter
D subsequent encounter
S sequela

S50.0 **Contusion of elbow**
S50.00 **Contusion of unspecified elbow**
S50.01 **Contusion of right elbow**
S50.02 **Contusion of left elbow**
S50.1 **Contusion of forearm**
S50.10 **Contusion of unspecified forearm**
S50.11 **Contusion of right forearm**
S50.12 **Contusion of left forearm**
S50.3 **Other superficial injuries of elbow**
S50.31 **Abrasion of elbow**
S50.311 **Abrasion of right elbow**
S50.312 **Abrasion of left elbow**
S50.319 **Abrasion of unspecified elbow**
S50.32 **Blister (nonthermal) of elbow**
S50.321 **Blister (nonthermal) of right elbow**
S50.322 **Blister (nonthermal) of left elbow**
S50.329 **Blister (nonthermal) of unspecified elbow**
S50.34 **External constriction of elbow**
S50.341 **External constriction of right elbow**
S50.342 **External constriction of left elbow**
S50.349 **External constriction of unspecified elbow**
S50.35 **Superficial foreign body of elbow**
Splinter in the elbow
S50.351 **Superficial foreign body of right elbow**
S50.352 **Superficial foreign body of left elbow**
S50.359 **Superficial foreign body of unspecified elbow**
S50.36 **Insect bite (nonvenomous) of elbow**
S50.361 **Insect bite (nonvenomous) of right elbow**
S50.362 **Insect bite (nonvenomous) of left elbow**
S50.369 **Insect bite (nonvenomous) of unspecified elbow**
S50.37 **Other superficial bite of elbow**
EXCLUDES 1 *open bite of elbow (S51.05)*
S50.371 **Other superficial bite of right elbow**
S50.372 **Other superficial bite of left elbow**
S50.379 **Other superficial bite of unspecified elbow**
S50.8 **Other superficial injuries of forearm**
S50.81 **Abrasion of forearm**
S50.811 **Abrasion of right forearm**
S50.812 **Abrasion of left forearm**
S50.819 **Abrasion of unspecified forearm**
S50.82 **Blister (nonthermal) of forearm**
S50.821 **Blister (nonthermal) of right forearm**
S50.822 **Blister (nonthermal) of left forearm**
S50.829 **Blister (nonthermal) of unspecified forearm**
S50.84 **External constriction of forearm**
S50.841 **External constriction of right forearm**
S50.842 **External constriction of left forearm**
S50.849 **External constriction of unspecified forearm**
S50.85 **Superficial foreign body of forearm**
Splinter in the forearm
S50.851 **Superficial foreign body of right forearm**
S50.852 **Superficial foreign body of left forearm**
S50.859 **Superficial foreign body of unspecified forearm**
S50.86 **Insect bite (nonvenomous) of forearm**
S50.861 **Insect bite (nonvenomous) of right forearm**
S50.862 **Insect bite (nonvenomous) of left forearm**
S50.869 **Insect bite (nonvenomous) of unspecified forearm**
S50.87 **Other superficial bite of forearm**
EXCLUDES 1 *open bite of forearm (S51.85)*
S50.871 **Other superficial bite of right forearm**
S50.872 **Other superficial bite of left forearm**
S50.879 **Other superficial bite of unspecified forearm**
S50.9 **Unspecified superficial injury of elbow and forearm**
S50.90 **Unspecified superficial injury of elbow**
S50.901 **Unspecified superficial injury of right elbow**
S50.902 **Unspecified superficial injury of left elbow**
S50.909 **Unspecified superficial injury of unspecified elbow**
S50.91 **Unspecified superficial injury of forearm**
S50.911 **Unspecified superficial injury of right forearm**
S50.912 **Unspecified superficial injury of left forearm**
S50.919 **Unspecified superficial injury of unspecified forearm**

S51 **Open wound of elbow and forearm**

Code also any associated wound infection

EXCLUDES 1 *open fracture of elbow and forearm (S52.- with open fracture 7th character)*
traumatic amputation of elbow and forearm (S58.-)

EXCLUDES 2 *open wound of wrist and hand (S61.-)*

The appropriate 7th character is to be added to each code from category S51.
A initial encounter
D subsequent encounter
S sequela

S51.0 **Open wound of elbow**
S51.00 **Unspecified open wound of elbow**
S51.001 **Unspecified open wound of right elbow**
AHA: 2012,4Q,108
S51.002 **Unspecified open wound of left elbow**
S51.009 **Unspecified open wound of unspecified elbow**
Open wound of elbow NOS
S51.01 **Laceration without foreign body of elbow**
S51.011 **Laceration without foreign body of right elbow**
S51.012 **Laceration without foreign body of left elbow**
S51.019 **Laceration without foreign body of unspecified elbow**
S51.02 **Laceration with foreign body of elbow**
S51.021 **Laceration with foreign body of right elbow**
S51.022 **Laceration with foreign body of left elbow**
S51.029 **Laceration with foreign body of unspecified elbow**

Chapter 19. Injury, Poisoning and Certain Other Consequences of External Causes
S49.9–S51.029

S51.03 Puncture wound without foreign body of elbow
- S51.031 Puncture wound without foreign body of right elbow
- S51.032 Puncture wound without foreign body of left elbow
- S51.039 Puncture wound without foreign body of unspecified elbow

S51.04 Puncture wound with foreign body of elbow
- S51.041 Puncture wound with foreign body of right elbow
- S51.042 Puncture wound with foreign body of left elbow
- S51.049 Puncture wound with foreign body of unspecified elbow

S51.05 Open bite of elbow

Bite of elbow NOS

EXCLUDES 1 *superficial bite of elbow (S50.36, S50.37)*

- S51.051 Open bite, right elbow
- S51.052 Open bite, left elbow
- S51.059 Open bite, unspecified elbow

S51.8 Open wound of forearm

EXCLUDES 2 *open wound of elbow (S51.0-)*

S51.80 Unspecified open wound of forearm

AHA: 2016,3Q,24

- S51.801 Unspecified open wound of right forearm
- S51.802 Unspecified open wound of left forearm
- S51.809 Unspecified open wound of unspecified forearm
  - Open wound of forearm NOS

S51.81 Laceration without foreign body of forearm
- S51.811 Laceration without foreign body of right forearm
- S51.812 Laceration without foreign body of left forearm
- S51.819 Laceration without foreign body of unspecified forearm

S51.82 Laceration with foreign body of forearm
- S51.821 Laceration with foreign body of right forearm
- S51.822 Laceration with foreign body of left forearm
- S51.829 Laceration with foreign body of unspecified forearm

S51.83 Puncture wound without foreign body of forearm

AHA: 2016,3Q,24

- S51.831 Puncture wound without foreign body of right forearm
- S51.832 Puncture wound without foreign body of left forearm
- S51.839 Puncture wound without foreign body of unspecified forearm

S51.84 Puncture wound with foreign body of forearm

AHA: 2016,3Q,24

- S51.841 Puncture wound with foreign body of right forearm
- S51.842 Puncture wound with foreign body of left forearm
- S51.849 Puncture wound with foreign body of unspecified forearm

S51.85 Open bite of forearm

Bite of forearm NOS

EXCLUDES 1 *superficial bite of forearm (S50.86, S50.87)*

- S51.851 Open bite of right forearm
- S51.852 Open bite of left forearm
- S51.859 Open bite of unspecified forearm

S52 Fracture of forearm

NOTE A fracture not indicated as displaced or nondisplaced should be coded to displaced.

A fracture not indicated as open or closed should be coded to closed.

The open fracture designations are based on the Gustilo open fracture classification.

EXCLUDES 1 *traumatic amputation of forearm (S58.-)*

EXCLUDES 2 *fracture at wrist and hand level (S62.-)*

AHA: 2018,2Q,12; 2016,1Q,33; 2015,3Q,37-39

DEF: Diaphysis: Central shaft of a long bone.

DEF: Epiphysis: Proximal and distal rounded ends of a long bone, communicates with the joint.

DEF: Metaphysis: Section of a long bone located between the epiphysis and diaphysis at the proximal and distal ends.

DEF: Physis (growth plate): Narrow zone of cartilaginous tissue between the epiphysis and metaphysis at each end of a long bone. In childhood, proliferation of cells in this zone lengthens the bone. As the bone matures, this area thins, ossification eventually fusing into solid bone and growth stops. ***Synonym(s):*** *Epiphyseal plate.*

The appropriate 7th character is to be added to all codes from category S52 [unless otherwise indicated].
- A initial encounter for closed fracture
- B initial encounter for open fracture type I or II initial encounter for open fracture NOS
- C initial encounter for open fracture type IIIA, IIIB, or IIIC
- D subsequent encounter for closed fracture with routine healing
- E subsequent encounter for open fracture type I or II with routine healing
- F subsequent encounter for open fracture type IIIA, IIIB, or IIIC with routine healing
- G subsequent encounter for closed fracture with delayed healing
- H subsequent encounter for open fracture type I or II with delayed healing
- J subsequent encounter for open fracture type IIIA, IIIB, or IIIC with delayed healing
- K subsequent encounter for closed fracture with nonunion
- M subsequent encounter for open fracture type I or II with nonunion
- N subsequent encounter for open fracture type IIIA, IIIB, or IIIC with nonunion
- P subsequent encounter for closed fracture with malunion
- Q subsequent encounter for open fracture type I or II with malunion
- R subsequent encounter for open fracture type IIIA, IIIB, or IIIC with malunion
- S sequela

S52.0 Fracture of upper end of ulna

Fracture of proximal end of ulna

EXCLUDES 2 *fracture of elbow NOS (S42.40-)*
fractures of shaft of ulna (S52.2-)

S52.00 Unspecified fracture of upper end of ulna
- S52.001 Unspecified fracture of upper end of right ulna Q
- S52.002 Unspecified fracture of upper end of left ulna Q
- S52.009 Unspecified fracture of upper end of unspecified ulna Q

S52.01 Torus fracture of upper end of ulna

The appropriate 7th character is to be added to all codes in subcategory S52.01
- A initial encounter for closed fracture
- D subsequent encounter for fracture with routine healing
- G subsequent encounter for fracture with delayed healing
- K subsequent encounter for fracture with nonunion
- P subsequent encounter for fracture with malunion
- S sequela

- S52.011 Torus fracture of upper end of right ulna Q
- S52.012 Torus fracture of upper end of left ulna Q
- S52.019 Torus fracture of upper end of unspecified ulna Q

6th **S52.02** Fracture of olecranon process without intraarticular extension of ulna

7th **S52.021** Displaced fracture of olecranon process without intraarticular extension of right ulna

7th **S52.022** Displaced fracture of olecranon process without intraarticular extension of left ulna

7th **S52.023** Displaced fracture of olecranon process without intraarticular extension of unspecified ulna

7th **S52.024** Nondisplaced fracture of olecranon process without intraarticular extension of right ulna

7th **S52.025** Nondisplaced fracture of olecranon process without intraarticular extension of left ulna

7th **S52.026** Nondisplaced fracture of olecranon process without intraarticular extension of unspecified ulna

6th **S52.03** Fracture of olecranon process with intraarticular extension of ulna

7th **S52.031** Displaced fracture of olecranon process with intraarticular extension of right ulna

7th **S52.032** Displaced fracture of olecranon process with intraarticular extension of left ulna

7th **S52.033** Displaced fracture of olecranon process with intraarticular extension of unspecified ulna

7th **S52.034** Nondisplaced fracture of olecranon process with intraarticular extension of right ulna

7th **S52.035** Nondisplaced fracture of olecranon process with intraarticular extension of left ulna

7th **S52.036** Nondisplaced fracture of olecranon process with intraarticular extension of unspecified ulna

6th **S52.04** Fracture of coronoid process of ulna

7th **S52.041** Displaced fracture of coronoid process of right ulna

7th **S52.042** Displaced fracture of coronoid process of left ulna

7th **S52.043** Displaced fracture of coronoid process of unspecified ulna

7th **S52.044** Nondisplaced fracture of coronoid process of right ulna

7th **S52.045** Nondisplaced fracture of coronoid process of left ulna

7th **S52.046** Nondisplaced fracture of coronoid process of unspecified ulna

6th **S52.09** Other fracture of upper end of ulna

7th **S52.091** Other fracture of upper end of right ulna

7th **S52.092** Other fracture of upper end of left ulna

7th **S52.099** Other fracture of upper end of unspecified ulna

5th **S52.1** Fracture of upper end of radius

Fracture of proximal end of radius

EXCLUDES 2 *physeal fractures of upper end of radius (S59.2-)*
fracture of shaft of radius (S52.3-)

6th **S52.10** Unspecified fracture of upper end of radius

7th **S52.101** Unspecified fracture of upper end of right radius

7th **S52.102** Unspecified fracture of upper end of left radius

7th **S52.109** Unspecified fracture of upper end of unspecified radius

6th **S52.11** Torus fracture of upper end of radius

The appropriate 7th character is to be added to all codes in subcategory S52.11
- A initial encounter for closed fracture
- D subsequent encounter for fracture with routine healing
- G subsequent encounter for fracture with delayed healing
- K subsequent encounter for fracture with nonunion
- P subsequent encounter for fracture with malunion
- S sequela

7th **S52.111** Torus fracture of upper end of right radius

7th **S52.112** Torus fracture of upper end of left radius

7th **S52.119** Torus fracture of upper end of unspecified radius

6th **S52.12** Fracture of head of radius

7th **S52.121** Displaced fracture of head of right radius

7th **S52.122** Displaced fracture of head of left radius

7th **S52.123** Displaced fracture of head of unspecified radius

7th **S52.124** Nondisplaced fracture of head of right radius

7th **S52.125** Nondisplaced fracture of head of left radius

7th **S52.126** Nondisplaced fracture of head of unspecified radius

6th **S52.13** Fracture of neck of radius

7th **S52.131** Displaced fracture of neck of right radius

7th **S52.132** Displaced fracture of neck of left radius

7th **S52.133** Displaced fracture of neck of unspecified radius

7th **S52.134** Nondisplaced fracture of neck of right radius

7th **S52.135** Nondisplaced fracture of neck of left radius

7th **S52.136** Nondisplaced fracture of neck of unspecified radius

6th **S52.18** Other fracture of upper end of radius

7th **S52.181** Other fracture of upper end of right radius

7th **S52.182** Other fracture of upper end of left radius

7th **S52.189** Other fracture of upper end of unspecified radius

5th **S52.2** Fracture of shaft of ulna

6th **S52.20** Unspecified fracture of shaft of ulna

Fracture of ulna NOS

7th **S52.201** Unspecified fracture of shaft of right ulna

7th **S52.202** Unspecified fracture of shaft of left ulna

7th **S52.209** Unspecified fracture of shaft of unspecified ulna

6th **S52.21** Greenstick fracture of shaft of ulna

The appropriate 7th character is to be added to all codes in subcategory S52.21
- A initial encounter for closed fracture
- D subsequent encounter for fracture with routine healing
- G subsequent encounter for fracture with delayed healing
- K subsequent encounter for fracture with nonunion
- P subsequent encounter for fracture with malunion
- S sequela

7th **S52.211** Greenstick fracture of shaft of right ulna

7th **S52.212** Greenstick fracture of shaft of left ulna

S52.219 Greenstick fracture of shaft of unspecified ulna

S52.22 Transverse fracture of shaft of ulna

S52.221 Displaced transverse fracture of shaft of right ulna

S52.222 Displaced transverse fracture of shaft of left ulna

S52.223 Displaced transverse fracture of shaft of unspecified ulna

S52.224 Nondisplaced transverse fracture of shaft of right ulna

S52.225 Nondisplaced transverse fracture of shaft of left ulna

S52.226 Nondisplaced transverse fracture of shaft of unspecified ulna

S52.23 Oblique fracture of shaft of ulna

S52.231 Displaced oblique fracture of shaft of right ulna

S52.232 Displaced oblique fracture of shaft of left ulna

S52.233 Displaced oblique fracture of shaft of unspecified ulna

S52.234 Nondisplaced oblique fracture of shaft of right ulna

S52.235 Nondisplaced oblique fracture of shaft of left ulna

S52.236 Nondisplaced oblique fracture of shaft of unspecified ulna

S52.24 Spiral fracture of shaft of ulna

S52.241 Displaced spiral fracture of shaft of ulna, right arm

S52.242 Displaced spiral fracture of shaft of ulna, left arm

S52.243 Displaced spiral fracture of shaft of ulna, unspecified arm

S52.244 Nondisplaced spiral fracture of shaft of ulna, right arm

S52.245 Nondisplaced spiral fracture of shaft of ulna, left arm

S52.246 Nondisplaced spiral fracture of shaft of ulna, unspecified arm

S52.25 Comminuted fracture of shaft of ulna

S52.251 Displaced comminuted fracture of shaft of ulna, right arm

S52.252 Displaced comminuted fracture of shaft of ulna, left arm

S52.253 Displaced comminuted fracture of shaft of ulna, unspecified arm

S52.254 Nondisplaced comminuted fracture of shaft of ulna, right arm

S52.255 Nondisplaced comminuted fracture of shaft of ulna, left arm

S52.256 Nondisplaced comminuted fracture of shaft of ulna, unspecified arm

S52.26 Segmental fracture of shaft of ulna

S52.261 Displaced segmental fracture of shaft of ulna, right arm

S52.262 Displaced segmental fracture of shaft of ulna, left arm

S52.263 Displaced segmental fracture of shaft of ulna, unspecified arm

S52.264 Nondisplaced segmental fracture of shaft of ulna, right arm

S52.265 Nondisplaced segmental fracture of shaft of ulna, left arm

S52.266 Nondisplaced segmental fracture of shaft of ulna, unspecified arm

S52.27 Monteggia's fracture of ulna

Fracture of upper shaft of ulna with dislocation of radial head

S52.271 Monteggia's fracture of right ulna

S52.272 Monteggia's fracture of left ulna

S52.279 Monteggia's fracture of unspecified ulna

S52.28 Bent bone of ulna

S52.281 Bent bone of right ulna

S52.282 Bent bone of left ulna

S52.283 Bent bone of unspecified ulna

S52.29 Other fracture of shaft of ulna

S52.291 Other fracture of shaft of right ulna

S52.292 Other fracture of shaft of left ulna

S52.299 Other fracture of shaft of unspecified ulna

S52.3 Fracture of shaft of radius

S52.30 Unspecified fracture of shaft of radius

S52.301 Unspecified fracture of shaft of right radius

S52.302 Unspecified fracture of shaft of left radius

S52.309 Unspecified fracture of shaft of unspecified radius

S52.31 Greenstick fracture of shaft of radius

The appropriate 7th character is to be added to all codes in subcategory S52.31.
- A initial encounter for closed fracture
- D subsequent encounter for fracture with routine healing
- G subsequent encounter for fracture with delayed healing
- K subsequent encounter for fracture with nonunion
- P subsequent encounter for fracture with malunion
- S sequela

S52.311 Greenstick fracture of shaft of radius, right arm

S52.312 Greenstick fracture of shaft of radius, left arm

S52.319 Greenstick fracture of shaft of radius, unspecified arm

S52.32 Transverse fracture of shaft of radius

S52.321 Displaced transverse fracture of shaft of right radius

S52.322 Displaced transverse fracture of shaft of left radius

S52.323 Displaced transverse fracture of shaft of unspecified radius

S52.324 Nondisplaced transverse fracture of shaft of right radius

S52.325 Nondisplaced transverse fracture of shaft of left radius

S52.326 Nondisplaced transverse fracture of shaft of unspecified radius

S52.33 Oblique fracture of shaft of radius

S52.331 Displaced oblique fracture of shaft of right radius

S52.332 Displaced oblique fracture of shaft of left radius

S52.333 Displaced oblique fracture of shaft of unspecified radius

S52.334 Nondisplaced oblique fracture of shaft of right radius

S52.335 Nondisplaced oblique fracture of shaft of left radius

S52.336 Nondisplaced oblique fracture of shaft of unspecified radius

S52.34 Spiral fracture of shaft of radius

S52.341 Displaced spiral fracture of shaft of radius, right arm

S52.342 Displaced spiral fracture of shaft of radius, left arm

S52.343 Displaced spiral fracture of shaft of radius, unspecified arm

S52.344 Nondisplaced spiral fracture of shaft of radius, right arm

S52.345 Nondisplaced spiral fracture of shaft of radius, left arm

S52.346 Nondisplaced spiral fracture of shaft of radius, unspecified arm

S52.35 Comminuted fracture of shaft of radius

S52.351 Displaced comminuted fracture of shaft of radius, right arm

S52.352 Displaced comminuted fracture of shaft of radius, left arm

S52.353 Displaced comminuted fracture of shaft of radius, unspecified arm

✓7th S52.354 Nondisplaced comminuted fracture of shaft of radius, right arm Q

✓7th S52.355 Nondisplaced comminuted fracture of shaft of radius, left arm Q

✓7th S52.356 Nondisplaced comminuted fracture of shaft of radius, unspecified arm Q

✓6th S52.36 Segmental fracture of shaft of radius

✓7th S52.361 Displaced segmental fracture of shaft of radius, right arm Q

✓7th S52.362 Displaced segmental fracture of shaft of radius, left arm Q

✓7th S52.363 Displaced segmental fracture of shaft of radius, unspecified arm Q

✓7th S52.364 Nondisplaced segmental fracture of shaft of radius, right arm Q

✓7th S52.365 Nondisplaced segmental fracture of shaft of radius, left arm Q

✓7th S52.366 Nondisplaced segmental fracture of shaft of radius, unspecified arm Q

✓6th S52.37 Galeazzi's fracture

Fracture of lower shaft of radius with radioulnar joint dislocation

✓7th S52.371 Galeazzi's fracture of right radius Q

✓7th S52.372 Galeazzi's fracture of left radius Q

✓7th S52.379 Galeazzi's fracture of unspecified radius Q

✓6th S52.38 Bent bone of radius

✓7th S52.381 Bent bone of right radius Q

✓7th S52.382 Bent bone of left radius Q

✓7th S52.389 Bent bone of unspecified radius Q

✓6th S52.39 Other fracture of shaft of radius

✓7th S52.391 Other fracture of shaft of radius, right arm Q

✓7th S52.392 Other fracture of shaft of radius, left arm Q

✓7th S52.399 Other fracture of shaft of radius, unspecified arm Q

✓5th S52.5 Fracture of lower end of radius

Fracture of distal end of radius

EXCLUDES 2 *physeal fractures of lower end of radius (S59.2-)*

DEF: Fracture of the distal end of the radius above the wrist, most commonly caused by a fall onto an outstretched hand.

✓6th S52.50 Unspecified fracture of the lower end of radius

✓7th S52.501 Unspecified fracture of the lower end of right radius Q

✓7th S52.502 Unspecified fracture of the lower end of left radius Q

✓7th S52.509 Unspecified fracture of the lower end of unspecified radius Q

✓6th S52.51 Fracture of radial styloid process

✓7th S52.511 Displaced fracture of right radial styloid process Q

✓7th S52.512 Displaced fracture of left radial styloid process Q

✓7th S52.513 Displaced fracture of unspecified radial styloid process Q

✓7th S52.514 Nondisplaced fracture of right radial styloid process Q

✓7th S52.515 Nondisplaced fracture of left radial styloid process Q

✓7th S52.516 Nondisplaced fracture of unspecified radial styloid process Q

✓6th S52.52 Torus fracture of lower end of radius

The appropriate 7th character is to be added to all codes in subcategory S52.52.

A initial encounter for closed fracture

D subsequent encounter for fracture with routine healing

G subsequent encounter for fracture with delayed healing

K subsequent encounter for fracture with nonunion

P subsequent encounter for fracture with malunion

S sequela

✓7th S52.521 Torus fracture of lower end of right radius Q

✓7th S52.522 Torus fracture of lower end of left radius Q

✓7th S52.529 Torus fracture of lower end of unspecified radius Q

✓6th S52.53 Colles' fracture

AHA: 2016,2Q,4

DEF: Fracture of the radius at the wrist in which the distal fragment is pushed posteriorly. The dorsal angulation of the fragment results in the wrist cocking up.

✓7th S52.531 Colles' fracture of right radius Q

✓7th S52.532 Colles' fracture of left radius Q

✓7th S52.539 Colles' fracture of unspecified radius Q

✓6th S52.54 Smith's fracture

✓7th S52.541 Smith's fracture of right radius Q

✓7th S52.542 Smith's fracture of left radius Q

✓7th S52.549 Smith's fracture of unspecified radius Q

✓6th S52.55 Other extraarticular fracture of lower end of radius

✓7th S52.551 Other extraarticular fracture of lower end of right radius Q

✓7th S52.552 Other extraarticular fracture of lower end of left radius Q

✓7th S52.559 Other extraarticular fracture of lower end of unspecified radius Q

✓6th S52.56 Barton's fracture

✓7th S52.561 Barton's fracture of right radius Q

✓7th S52.562 Barton's fracture of left radius Q

✓7th S52.569 Barton's fracture of unspecified radius Q

✓6th S52.57 Other intraarticular fracture of lower end of radius

✓7th S52.571 Other intraarticular fracture of lower end of right radius Q

✓7th S52.572 Other intraarticular fracture of lower end of left radius Q

✓7th S52.579 Other intraarticular fracture of lower end of unspecified radius Q

✓6th S52.59 Other fractures of lower end of radius

AHA: 2019,3Q,9

✓7th S52.591 Other fractures of lower end of right radius Q

✓7th S52.592 Other fractures of lower end of left radius Q

✓7th S52.599 Other fractures of lower end of unspecified radius Q

✓5th S52.6 Fracture of lower end of ulna

✓6th S52.60 Unspecified fracture of lower end of ulna

✓7th S52.601 Unspecified fracture of lower end of right ulna Q

✓7th S52.602 Unspecified fracture of lower end of left ulna Q

✓7th S52.609 Unspecified fracture of lower end of unspecified ulna Q

✓6th S52.61 Fracture of ulna styloid process

✓7th S52.611 Displaced fracture of right ulna styloid process Q

✓7th S52.612 Displaced fracture of left ulna styloid process Q

✓7th S52.613 Displaced fracture of unspecified ulna styloid process Q

✓7th S52.614 Nondisplaced fracture of right ulna styloid process Q

✓7th S52.615 Nondisplaced fracture of left ulna styloid process Q

✓7th S52.616 Nondisplaced fracture of unspecified ulna styloid process Q

S52.62 Torus fracture of lower end of ulna

The appropriate 7th character is to be added to all codes in subcategory S52.62.
A initial encounter for closed fracture
D subsequent encounter for fracture with routine healing
G subsequent encounter for fracture with delayed healing
K subsequent encounter for fracture with nonunion
P subsequent encounter for fracture with malunion
S sequela

S52.621 Torus fracture of lower end of right ulna Q
S52.622 Torus fracture of lower end of left ulna Q
S52.629 Torus fracture of lower end of unspecified ulna Q

S52.69 Other fracture of lower end of ulna
AHA: 2019,3Q,9
S52.691 Other fracture of lower end of right ulna Q
S52.692 Other fracture of lower end of left ulna Q
S52.699 Other fracture of lower end of unspecified ulna Q

S52.9 Unspecified fracture of forearm
S52.90 Unspecified fracture of unspecified forearm Q
S52.91 Unspecified fracture of right forearm Q
S52.92 Unspecified fracture of left forearm Q

S53 Dislocation and sprain of joints and ligaments of elbow

INCLUDES avulsion of joint or ligament of elbow
laceration of cartilage, joint or ligament of elbow
sprain of cartilage, joint or ligament of elbow
traumatic hemarthrosis of joint or ligament of elbow
traumatic rupture of joint or ligament of elbow
traumatic subluxation of joint or ligament of elbow
traumatic tear of joint or ligament of elbow

Code also any associated open wound

EXCLUDES 2 *strain of muscle, fascia and tendon at forearm level (S56.-)*

The appropriate 7th character is to be added to each code from category S53.
A initial encounter
D subsequent encounter
S sequela

S53.0 Subluxation and dislocation of radial head
Dislocation of radiohumeral joint
Subluxation of radiohumeral joint
EXCLUDES 1 *Monteggia's fracture-dislocation (S52.27-)*

S53.00 Unspecified subluxation and dislocation of radial head
S53.001 Unspecified subluxation of right radial head
S53.002 Unspecified subluxation of left radial head
S53.003 Unspecified subluxation of unspecified radial head
S53.004 Unspecified dislocation of right radial head
S53.005 Unspecified dislocation of left radial head
S53.006 Unspecified dislocation of unspecified radial head

S53.01 Anterior subluxation and dislocation of radial head
Anteriomedial subluxation and dislocation of radial head
S53.011 Anterior subluxation of right radial head
S53.012 Anterior subluxation of left radial head
S53.013 Anterior subluxation of unspecified radial head
S53.014 Anterior dislocation of right radial head
S53.015 Anterior dislocation of left radial head
S53.016 Anterior dislocation of unspecified radial head

S53.02 Posterior subluxation and dislocation of radial head
Posteriolateral subluxation and dislocation of radial head
S53.021 Posterior subluxation of right radial head
S53.022 Posterior subluxation of left radial head
S53.023 Posterior subluxation of unspecified radial head
S53.024 Posterior dislocation of right radial head
S53.025 Posterior dislocation of left radial head
S53.026 Posterior dislocation of unspecified radial head

S53.03 Nursemaid's elbow
S53.031 Nursemaid's elbow, right elbow
S53.032 Nursemaid's elbow, left elbow
S53.033 Nursemaid's elbow, unspecified elbow

S53.09 Other subluxation and dislocation of radial head
S53.091 Other subluxation of right radial head
S53.092 Other subluxation of left radial head
S53.093 Other subluxation of unspecified radial head
S53.094 Other dislocation of right radial head
S53.095 Other dislocation of left radial head
S53.096 Other dislocation of unspecified radial head

S53.1 Subluxation and dislocation of ulnohumeral joint
Subluxation and dislocation of elbow NOS
EXCLUDES 1 *dislocation of radial head alone (S53.0-)*

S53.10 Unspecified subluxation and dislocation of ulnohumeral joint
S53.101 Unspecified subluxation of right ulnohumeral joint
S53.102 Unspecified subluxation of left ulnohumeral joint
S53.103 Unspecified subluxation of unspecified ulnohumeral joint
S53.104 Unspecified dislocation of right ulnohumeral joint
S53.105 Unspecified dislocation of left ulnohumeral joint
S53.106 Unspecified dislocation of unspecified ulnohumeral joint

S53.11 Anterior subluxation and dislocation of ulnohumeral joint
S53.111 Anterior subluxation of right ulnohumeral joint
S53.112 Anterior subluxation of left ulnohumeral joint
S53.113 Anterior subluxation of unspecified ulnohumeral joint
S53.114 Anterior dislocation of right ulnohumeral joint
AHA: 2012,4Q,108
S53.115 Anterior dislocation of left ulnohumeral joint
S53.116 Anterior dislocation of unspecified ulnohumeral joint

S53.12 Posterior subluxation and dislocation of ulnohumeral joint
S53.121 Posterior subluxation of right ulnohumeral joint
S53.122 Posterior subluxation of left ulnohumeral joint
S53.123 Posterior subluxation of unspecified ulnohumeral joint
S53.124 Posterior dislocation of right ulnohumeral joint
S53.125 Posterior dislocation of left ulnohumeral joint
S53.126 Posterior dislocation of unspecified ulnohumeral joint

S53.13 Medial subluxation and dislocation of ulnohumeral joint
S53.131 Medial subluxation of right ulnohumeral joint
S53.132 Medial subluxation of left ulnohumeral joint
S53.133 Medial subluxation of unspecified ulnohumeral joint

✓7th S53.134 Medial dislocation of right ulnohumeral joint
✓7th S53.135 Medial dislocation of left ulnohumeral joint
✓7th S53.136 Medial dislocation of unspecified ulnohumeral joint
✓6th S53.14 Lateral subluxation and dislocation of ulnohumeral joint
✓7th S53.141 Lateral subluxation of right ulnohumeral joint
✓7th S53.142 Lateral subluxation of left ulnohumeral joint
✓7th S53.143 Lateral subluxation of unspecified ulnohumeral joint
✓7th S53.144 Lateral dislocation of right ulnohumeral joint
✓7th S53.145 Lateral dislocation of left ulnohumeral joint
✓7th S53.146 Lateral dislocation of unspecified ulnohumeral joint
✓6th S53.19 Other subluxation and dislocation of ulnohumeral joint
✓7th S53.191 Other subluxation of right ulnohumeral joint
✓7th S53.192 Other subluxation of left ulnohumeral joint
✓7th S53.193 Other subluxation of unspecified ulnohumeral joint
✓7th S53.194 Other dislocation of right ulnohumeral joint
✓7th S53.195 Other dislocation of left ulnohumeral joint
✓7th S53.196 Other dislocation of unspecified ulnohumeral joint
✓5th S53.2 Traumatic rupture of radial collateral ligament
EXCLUDES 1 *sprain of radial collateral ligament NOS (S53.43-)*
✓x7th S53.20 Traumatic rupture of unspecified radial collateral ligament
✓x7th S53.21 Traumatic rupture of right radial collateral ligament
✓x7th S53.22 Traumatic rupture of left radial collateral ligament
✓5th S53.3 Traumatic rupture of ulnar collateral ligament
EXCLUDES 1 *sprain of ulnar collateral ligament (S53.44-)*
✓x7th S53.30 Traumatic rupture of unspecified ulnar collateral ligament
✓x7th S53.31 Traumatic rupture of right ulnar collateral ligament
✓x7th S53.32 Traumatic rupture of left ulnar collateral ligament
✓5th S53.4 Sprain of elbow
EXCLUDES 2 *traumatic rupture of radial collateral ligament (S53.2-)*
traumatic rupture of ulnar collateral ligament (S53.3-)
✓6th S53.40 Unspecified sprain of elbow
✓7th S53.401 Unspecified sprain of right elbow
✓7th S53.402 Unspecified sprain of left elbow
✓7th S53.409 Unspecified sprain of unspecified elbow
Sprain of elbow NOS
✓6th S53.41 Radiohumeral (joint) sprain
✓7th S53.411 Radiohumeral (joint) sprain of right elbow
✓7th S53.412 Radiohumeral (joint) sprain of left elbow
✓7th S53.419 Radiohumeral (joint) sprain of unspecified elbow
✓6th S53.42 Ulnohumeral (joint) sprain
✓7th S53.421 Ulnohumeral (joint) sprain of right elbow
✓7th S53.422 Ulnohumeral (joint) sprain of left elbow
✓7th S53.429 Ulnohumeral (joint) sprain of unspecified elbow
✓6th S53.43 Radial collateral ligament sprain
✓7th S53.431 Radial collateral ligament sprain of right elbow
✓7th S53.432 Radial collateral ligament sprain of left elbow
✓7th S53.439 Radial collateral ligament sprain of unspecified elbow
✓6th S53.44 Ulnar collateral ligament sprain
✓7th S53.441 Ulnar collateral ligament sprain of right elbow
✓7th S53.442 Ulnar collateral ligament sprain of left elbow
✓7th S53.449 Ulnar collateral ligament sprain of unspecified elbow
✓6th S53.49 Other sprain of elbow
✓7th S53.491 Other sprain of right elbow
✓7th S53.492 Other sprain of left elbow
✓7th S53.499 Other sprain of unspecified elbow

✓4th **S54 Injury of nerves at forearm level**
Code also any associated open wound (S51.-)
EXCLUDES 2 *injury of nerves at wrist and hand level (S64.-)*

The appropriate 7th character is to be added to each code from category S54.
A initial encounter
D subsequent encounter
S sequela

✓5th S54.0 Injury of ulnar nerve at forearm level
Injury of ulnar nerve NOS
✓x7th S54.00 Injury of ulnar nerve at forearm level, unspecified arm
✓x7th S54.01 Injury of ulnar nerve at forearm level, right arm
✓x7th S54.02 Injury of ulnar nerve at forearm level, left arm
✓5th S54.1 Injury of median nerve at forearm level
Injury of median nerve NOS
✓x7th S54.10 Injury of median nerve at forearm level, unspecified arm
✓x7th S54.11 Injury of median nerve at forearm level, right arm
✓x7th S54.12 Injury of median nerve at forearm level, left arm
✓5th S54.2 Injury of radial nerve at forearm level
Injury of radial nerve NOS
✓x7th S54.20 Injury of radial nerve at forearm level, unspecified arm
✓x7th S54.21 Injury of radial nerve at forearm level, right arm
✓x7th S54.22 Injury of radial nerve at forearm level, left arm
✓5th S54.3 Injury of cutaneous sensory nerve at forearm level
✓x7th S54.30 Injury of cutaneous sensory nerve at forearm level, unspecified arm
✓x7th S54.31 Injury of cutaneous sensory nerve at forearm level, right arm
✓x7th S54.32 Injury of cutaneous sensory nerve at forearm level, left arm
✓5th S54.8 Injury of other nerves at forearm level
✓6th S54.8X Injury of other nerves at forearm level
✓7th S54.8X1 Injury of other nerves at forearm level, right arm
✓7th S54.8X2 Injury of other nerves at forearm level, left arm
✓7th S54.8X9 Injury of other nerves at forearm level, unspecified arm
✓5th S54.9 Injury of unspecified nerve at forearm level
✓x7th S54.90 Injury of unspecified nerve at forearm level, unspecified arm
✓x7th S54.91 Injury of unspecified nerve at forearm level, right arm
✓x7th S54.92 Injury of unspecified nerve at forearm level, left arm

✓4th **S55 Injury of blood vessels at forearm level**
Code also any associated open wound (S51.-)
EXCLUDES 2 *injury of blood vessels at wrist and hand level (S65.-)*
injury of brachial vessels (S45.1-S45.2)

The appropriate 7th character is to be added to each code from category S55.
A initial encounter
D subsequent encounter
S sequela

✓5th S55.0 Injury of ulnar artery at forearm level
✓6th S55.00 Unspecified injury of ulnar artery at forearm level
✓7th S55.001 Unspecified injury of ulnar artery at forearm level, right arm
✓7th S55.002 Unspecified injury of ulnar artery at forearm level, left arm
✓7th S55.009 Unspecified injury of ulnar artery at forearm level, unspecified arm

Chapter 19. Injury, Poisoning and Certain Other Consequences of External Causes
S53.134–S55.009

S55.Ø1 Laceration of ulnar artery at forearm level
S55.Ø11 Laceration of ulnar artery at forearm level, right arm
S55.Ø12 Laceration of ulnar artery at forearm level, left arm
S55.Ø19 Laceration of ulnar artery at forearm level, unspecified arm
S55.Ø9 Other specified injury of ulnar artery at forearm level
S55.Ø91 Other specified injury of ulnar artery at forearm level, right arm
S55.Ø92 Other specified injury of ulnar artery at forearm level, left arm
S55.Ø99 Other specified injury of ulnar artery at forearm level, unspecified arm
S55.1 Injury of radial artery at forearm level
S55.1Ø Unspecified injury of radial artery at forearm level
S55.1Ø1 Unspecified injury of radial artery at forearm level, right arm
S55.1Ø2 Unspecified injury of radial artery at forearm level, left arm
S55.1Ø9 Unspecified injury of radial artery at forearm level, unspecified arm
S55.11 Laceration of radial artery at forearm level
S55.111 Laceration of radial artery at forearm level, right arm
S55.112 Laceration of radial artery at forearm level, left arm
S55.119 Laceration of radial artery at forearm level, unspecified arm
S55.19 Other specified injury of radial artery at forearm level
S55.191 Other specified injury of radial artery at forearm level, right arm
S55.192 Other specified injury of radial artery at forearm level, left arm
S55.199 Other specified injury of radial artery at forearm level, unspecified arm
S55.2 Injury of vein at forearm level
S55.2Ø Unspecified injury of vein at forearm level
S55.2Ø1 Unspecified injury of vein at forearm level, right arm
S55.2Ø2 Unspecified injury of vein at forearm level, left arm
S55.2Ø9 Unspecified injury of vein at forearm level, unspecified arm
S55.21 Laceration of vein at forearm level
S55.211 Laceration of vein at forearm level, right arm
S55.212 Laceration of vein at forearm level, left arm
S55.219 Laceration of vein at forearm level, unspecified arm
S55.29 Other specified injury of vein at forearm level
S55.291 Other specified injury of vein at forearm level, right arm
S55.292 Other specified injury of vein at forearm level, left arm
S55.299 Other specified injury of vein at forearm level, unspecified arm
S55.8 Injury of other blood vessels at forearm level
S55.8Ø Unspecified injury of other blood vessels at forearm level
S55.8Ø1 Unspecified injury of other blood vessels at forearm level, right arm
S55.8Ø2 Unspecified injury of other blood vessels at forearm level, left arm
S55.8Ø9 Unspecified injury of other blood vessels at forearm level, unspecified arm
S55.81 Laceration of other blood vessels at forearm level
S55.811 Laceration of other blood vessels at forearm level, right arm
S55.812 Laceration of other blood vessels at forearm level, left arm
S55.819 Laceration of other blood vessels at forearm level, unspecified arm
S55.89 Other specified injury of other blood vessels at forearm level
S55.891 Other specified injury of other blood vessels at forearm level, right arm
S55.892 Other specified injury of other blood vessels at forearm level, left arm
S55.899 Other specified injury of other blood vessels at forearm level, unspecified arm
S55.9 Injury of unspecified blood vessel at forearm level
S55.9Ø Unspecified injury of unspecified blood vessel at forearm level
S55.9Ø1 Unspecified injury of unspecified blood vessel at forearm level, right arm
S55.9Ø2 Unspecified injury of unspecified blood vessel at forearm level, left arm
S55.9Ø9 Unspecified injury of unspecified blood vessel at forearm level, unspecified arm
S55.91 Laceration of unspecified blood vessel at forearm level
S55.911 Laceration of unspecified blood vessel at forearm level, right arm
S55.912 Laceration of unspecified blood vessel at forearm level, left arm
S55.919 Laceration of unspecified blood vessel at forearm level, unspecified arm
S55.99 Other specified injury of unspecified blood vessel at forearm level
S55.991 Other specified injury of unspecified blood vessel at forearm level, right arm
S55.992 Other specified injury of unspecified blood vessel at forearm level, left arm
S55.999 Other specified injury of unspecified blood vessel at forearm level, unspecified arm

S56 Injury of muscle, fascia and tendon at forearm level

Code also any associated open wound (S51.-)

EXCLUDES 2 *injury of muscle, fascia and tendon at or below wrist (S66.-)*
sprain of joints and ligaments of elbow (S53.4-)

TIP: Refer to the Muscle/Tendon table at the beginning of this chapter

The appropriate 7th character is to be added to each code from category S56.
A initial encounter
D subsequent encounter
S sequela

S56.Ø Injury of flexor muscle, fascia and tendon of thumb at forearm level
S56.ØØ Unspecified injury of flexor muscle, fascia and tendon of thumb at forearm level
S56.ØØ1 Unspecified injury of flexor muscle, fascia and tendon of right thumb at forearm level
S56.ØØ2 Unspecified injury of flexor muscle, fascia and tendon of left thumb at forearm level
S56.ØØ9 Unspecified injury of flexor muscle, fascia and tendon of unspecified thumb at forearm level
S56.Ø1 Strain of flexor muscle, fascia and tendon of thumb at forearm level
S56.Ø11 Strain of flexor muscle, fascia and tendon of right thumb at forearm level
S56.Ø12 Strain of flexor muscle, fascia and tendon of left thumb at forearm level
S56.Ø19 Strain of flexor muscle, fascia and tendon of unspecified thumb at forearm level
S56.Ø2 Laceration of flexor muscle, fascia and tendon of thumb at forearm level
S56.Ø21 Laceration of flexor muscle, fascia and tendon of right thumb at forearm level
S56.Ø22 Laceration of flexor muscle, fascia and tendon of left thumb at forearm level
S56.Ø29 Laceration of flexor muscle, fascia and tendon of unspecified thumb at forearm level
S56.Ø9 Other injury of flexor muscle, fascia and tendon of thumb at forearm level
S56.Ø91 Other injury of flexor muscle, fascia and tendon of right thumb at forearm level
S56.Ø92 Other injury of flexor muscle, fascia and tendon of left thumb at forearm level
S56.Ø99 Other injury of flexor muscle, fascia and tendon of unspecified thumb at forearm level

S56.1 Injury of flexor muscle, fascia and tendon of other and unspecified finger at forearm level

S56.10 Unspecified injury of flexor muscle, fascia and tendon of other and unspecified finger at forearm level

S56.101 Unspecified injury of flexor muscle, fascia and tendon of right index finger at forearm level

S56.102 Unspecified injury of flexor muscle, fascia and tendon of left index finger at forearm level

S56.103 Unspecified injury of flexor muscle, fascia and tendon of right middle finger at forearm level

S56.104 Unspecified injury of flexor muscle, fascia and tendon of left middle finger at forearm level

S56.105 Unspecified injury of flexor muscle, fascia and tendon of right ring finger at forearm level

S56.106 Unspecified injury of flexor muscle, fascia and tendon of left ring finger at forearm level

S56.107 Unspecified injury of flexor muscle, fascia and tendon of right little finger at forearm level

S56.108 Unspecified injury of flexor muscle, fascia and tendon of left little finger at forearm level

S56.109 Unspecified injury of flexor muscle, fascia and tendon of unspecified finger at forearm level

S56.11 Strain of flexor muscle, fascia and tendon of other and unspecified finger at forearm level

S56.111 Strain of flexor muscle, fascia and tendon of right index finger at forearm level

S56.112 Strain of flexor muscle, fascia and tendon of left index finger at forearm level

S56.113 Strain of flexor muscle, fascia and tendon of right middle finger at forearm level

S56.114 Strain of flexor muscle, fascia and tendon of left middle finger at forearm level

S56.115 Strain of flexor muscle, fascia and tendon of right ring finger at forearm level

S56.116 Strain of flexor muscle, fascia and tendon of left ring finger at forearm level

S56.117 Strain of flexor muscle, fascia and tendon of right little finger at forearm level

S56.118 Strain of flexor muscle, fascia and tendon of left little finger at forearm level

S56.119 Strain of flexor muscle, fascia and tendon of finger of unspecified finger at forearm level

S56.12 Laceration of flexor muscle, fascia and tendon of other and unspecified finger at forearm level

S56.121 Laceration of flexor muscle, fascia and tendon of right index finger at forearm level

S56.122 Laceration of flexor muscle, fascia and tendon of left index finger at forearm level

S56.123 Laceration of flexor muscle, fascia and tendon of right middle finger at forearm level

S56.124 Laceration of flexor muscle, fascia and tendon of left middle finger at forearm level

S56.125 Laceration of flexor muscle, fascia and tendon of right ring finger at forearm level

S56.126 Laceration of flexor muscle, fascia and tendon of left ring finger at forearm level

S56.127 Laceration of flexor muscle, fascia and tendon of right little finger at forearm level

S56.128 Laceration of flexor muscle, fascia and tendon of left little finger at forearm level

S56.129 Laceration of flexor muscle, fascia and tendon of unspecified finger at forearm level

S56.19 Other injury of flexor muscle, fascia and tendon of other and unspecified finger at forearm level

S56.191 Other injury of flexor muscle, fascia and tendon of right index finger at forearm level

S56.192 Other injury of flexor muscle, fascia and tendon of left index finger at forearm level

S56.193 Other injury of flexor muscle, fascia and tendon of right middle finger at forearm level

S56.194 Other injury of flexor muscle, fascia and tendon of left middle finger at forearm level

S56.195 Other injury of flexor muscle, fascia and tendon of right ring finger at forearm level

S56.196 Other injury of flexor muscle, fascia and tendon of left ring finger at forearm level

S56.197 Other injury of flexor muscle, fascia and tendon of right little finger at forearm level

S56.198 Other injury of flexor muscle, fascia and tendon of left little finger at forearm level

S56.199 Other injury of flexor muscle, fascia and tendon of unspecified finger at forearm level

S56.2 Injury of other flexor muscle, fascia and tendon at forearm level

S56.20 Unspecified injury of other flexor muscle, fascia and tendon at forearm level

S56.201 Unspecified injury of other flexor muscle, fascia and tendon at forearm level, right arm

S56.202 Unspecified injury of other flexor muscle, fascia and tendon at forearm level, left arm

S56.209 Unspecified injury of other flexor muscle, fascia and tendon at forearm level, unspecified arm

S56.21 Strain of other flexor muscle, fascia and tendon at forearm level

S56.211 Strain of other flexor muscle, fascia and tendon at forearm level, right arm

S56.212 Strain of other flexor muscle, fascia and tendon at forearm level, left arm

S56.219 Strain of other flexor muscle, fascia and tendon at forearm level, unspecified arm

S56.22 Laceration of other flexor muscle, fascia and tendon at forearm level

S56.221 Laceration of other flexor muscle, fascia and tendon at forearm level, right arm

S56.222 Laceration of other flexor muscle, fascia and tendon at forearm level, left arm

S56.229 Laceration of other flexor muscle, fascia and tendon at forearm level, unspecified arm

S56.29 Other injury of other flexor muscle, fascia and tendon at forearm level

S56.291 Other injury of other flexor muscle, fascia and tendon at forearm level, right arm

S56.292 Other injury of other flexor muscle, fascia and tendon at forearm level, left arm

S56.299 Other injury of other flexor muscle, fascia and tendon at forearm level, unspecified arm

S56.3 Injury of extensor or abductor muscles, fascia and tendons of thumb at forearm level

S56.30 Unspecified injury of extensor or abductor muscles, fascia and tendons of thumb at forearm level

S56.301 Unspecified injury of extensor or abductor muscles, fascia and tendons of right thumb at forearm level

S56.302 Unspecified injury of extensor or abductor muscles, fascia and tendons of left thumb at forearm level

S56.309 Unspecified injury of extensor or abductor muscles, fascia and tendons of unspecified thumb at forearm level

S56.31 Strain of extensor or abductor muscles, fascia and tendons of thumb at forearm level

S56.311 Strain of extensor or abductor muscles, fascia and tendons of right thumb at forearm level

S56.312 Strain of extensor or abductor muscles, fascia and tendons of left thumb at forearm level

S56.319 Strain of extensor or abductor muscles, fascia and tendons of unspecified thumb at forearm level

S56.32 Laceration of extensor or abductor muscles, fascia and tendons of thumb at forearm level

S56.321 Laceration of extensor or abductor muscles, fascia and tendons of right thumb at forearm level

S56.322 Laceration of extensor or abductor muscles, fascia and tendons of left thumb at forearm level

S56.329 Laceration of extensor or abductor muscles, fascia and tendons of unspecified thumb at forearm level

S56.39 Other injury of extensor or abductor muscles, fascia and tendons of thumb at forearm level

S56.391 Other injury of extensor or abductor muscles, fascia and tendons of right thumb at forearm level

S56.392 Other injury of extensor or abductor muscles, fascia and tendons of left thumb at forearm level

S56.399 Other injury of extensor or abductor muscles, fascia and tendons of unspecified thumb at forearm level

S56.4 Injury of extensor muscle, fascia and tendon of other and unspecified finger at forearm level

S56.40 Unspecified injury of extensor muscle, fascia and tendon of other and unspecified finger at forearm level

S56.401 Unspecified injury of extensor muscle, fascia and tendon of right index finger at forearm level

S56.402 Unspecified injury of extensor muscle, fascia and tendon of left index finger at forearm level

S56.403 Unspecified injury of extensor muscle, fascia and tendon of right middle finger at forearm level

S56.404 Unspecified injury of extensor muscle, fascia and tendon of left middle finger at forearm level

S56.405 Unspecified injury of extensor muscle, fascia and tendon of right ring finger at forearm level

S56.406 Unspecified injury of extensor muscle, fascia and tendon of left ring finger at forearm level

S56.407 Unspecified injury of extensor muscle, fascia and tendon of right little finger at forearm level

S56.408 Unspecified injury of extensor muscle, fascia and tendon of left little finger at forearm level

S56.409 Unspecified injury of extensor muscle, fascia and tendon of unspecified finger at forearm level

S56.41 Strain of extensor muscle, fascia and tendon of other and unspecified finger at forearm level

S56.411 Strain of extensor muscle, fascia and tendon of right index finger at forearm level

S56.412 Strain of extensor muscle, fascia and tendon of left index finger at forearm level

S56.413 Strain of extensor muscle, fascia and tendon of right middle finger at forearm level

S56.414 Strain of extensor muscle, fascia and tendon of left middle finger at forearm level

S56.415 Strain of extensor muscle, fascia and tendon of right ring finger at forearm level

S56.416 Strain of extensor muscle, fascia and tendon of left ring finger at forearm level

S56.417 Strain of extensor muscle, fascia and tendon of right little finger at forearm level

S56.418 Strain of extensor muscle, fascia and tendon of left little finger at forearm level

S56.419 Strain of extensor muscle, fascia and tendon of finger, unspecified finger at forearm level

S56.42 Laceration of extensor muscle, fascia and tendon of other and unspecified finger at forearm level

S56.421 Laceration of extensor muscle, fascia and tendon of right index finger at forearm level

S56.422 Laceration of extensor muscle, fascia and tendon of left index finger at forearm level

S56.423 Laceration of extensor muscle, fascia and tendon of right middle finger at forearm level

S56.424 Laceration of extensor muscle, fascia and tendon of left middle finger at forearm level

S56.425 Laceration of extensor muscle, fascia and tendon of right ring finger at forearm level

S56.426 Laceration of extensor muscle, fascia and tendon of left ring finger at forearm level

S56.427 Laceration of extensor muscle, fascia and tendon of right little finger at forearm level

S56.428 Laceration of extensor muscle, fascia and tendon of left little finger at forearm level

S56.429 Laceration of extensor muscle, fascia and tendon of unspecified finger at forearm level

S56.49 Other injury of extensor muscle, fascia and tendon of other and unspecified finger at forearm level

S56.491 Other injury of extensor muscle, fascia and tendon of right index finger at forearm level

S56.492 Other injury of extensor muscle, fascia and tendon of left index finger at forearm level

S56.493 Other injury of extensor muscle, fascia and tendon of right middle finger at forearm level

S56.494 Other injury of extensor muscle, fascia and tendon of left middle finger at forearm level

S56.495 Other injury of extensor muscle, fascia and tendon of right ring finger at forearm level

S56.496 Other injury of extensor muscle, fascia and tendon of left ring finger at forearm level

S56.497 Other injury of extensor muscle, fascia and tendon of right little finger at forearm level

S56.498 Other injury of extensor muscle, fascia and tendon of left little finger at forearm level

S56.499 Other injury of extensor muscle, fascia and tendon of unspecified finger at forearm level

S56.5 Injury of other extensor muscle, fascia and tendon at forearm level

S56.50 Unspecified injury of other extensor muscle, fascia and tendon at forearm level

S56.501 Unspecified injury of other extensor muscle, fascia and tendon at forearm level, right arm

S56.502 Unspecified injury of other extensor muscle, fascia and tendon at forearm level, left arm

S56.509 Unspecified injury of other extensor muscle, fascia and tendon at forearm level, unspecified arm

S56.51 Strain of other extensor muscle, fascia and tendon at forearm level

S56.511 Strain of other extensor muscle, fascia and tendon at forearm level, right arm

S56.512 Strain of other extensor muscle, fascia and tendon at forearm level, left arm

S56.519 Strain of other extensor muscle, fascia and tendon at forearm level, unspecified arm

S56.52 Laceration of other extensor muscle, fascia and tendon at forearm level

S56.521 Laceration of other extensor muscle, fascia and tendon at forearm level, right arm

S56.522 Laceration of other extensor muscle, fascia and tendon at forearm level, left arm

S56.529 Laceration of other extensor muscle, fascia and tendon at forearm level, unspecified arm

S56.59 Other injury of other extensor muscle, fascia and tendon at forearm level

S56.591 Other injury of other extensor muscle, fascia and tendon at forearm level, right arm

S56.592 Other injury of other extensor muscle, fascia and tendon at forearm level, left arm

S56.599 Other injury of other extensor muscle, fascia and tendon at forearm level, unspecified arm

S56.8 Injury of other muscles, fascia and tendons at forearm level

S56.80 Unspecified injury of other muscles, fascia and tendons at forearm level

S56.801 Unspecified injury of other muscles, fascia and tendons at forearm level, right arm

S56.802 Unspecified injury of other muscles, fascia and tendons at forearm level, left arm

S56.809 Unspecified injury of other muscles, fascia and tendons at forearm level, unspecified arm

S56.81 Strain of other muscles, fascia and tendons at forearm level

S56.811 Strain of other muscles, fascia and tendons at forearm level, right arm

S56.812 Strain of other muscles, fascia and tendons at forearm level, left arm

S56.819 Strain of other muscles, fascia and tendons at forearm level, unspecified arm

S56.82 Laceration of other muscles, fascia and tendons at forearm level

S56.821 Laceration of other muscles, fascia and tendons at forearm level, right arm

S56.822 Laceration of other muscles, fascia and tendons at forearm level, left arm

S56.829 Laceration of other muscles, fascia and tendons at forearm level, unspecified arm

S56.89 Other injury of other muscles, fascia and tendons at forearm level

S56.891 Other injury of other muscles, fascia and tendons at forearm level, right arm

S56.892 Other injury of other muscles, fascia and tendons at forearm level, left arm

S56.899 Other injury of other muscles, fascia and tendons at forearm level, unspecified arm

S56.9 Injury of unspecified muscles, fascia and tendons at forearm level

S56.90 Unspecified injury of unspecified muscles, fascia and tendons at forearm level

S56.901 Unspecified injury of unspecified muscles, fascia and tendons at forearm level, right arm

S56.902 Unspecified injury of unspecified muscles, fascia and tendons at forearm level, left arm

S56.909 Unspecified injury of unspecified muscles, fascia and tendons at forearm level, unspecified arm

S56.91 Strain of unspecified muscles, fascia and tendons at forearm level

S56.911 Strain of unspecified muscles, fascia and tendons at forearm level, right arm

S56.912 Strain of unspecified muscles, fascia and tendons at forearm level, left arm

S56.919 Strain of unspecified muscles, fascia and tendons at forearm level, unspecified arm

S56.92 Laceration of unspecified muscles, fascia and tendons at forearm level

S56.921 Laceration of unspecified muscles, fascia and tendons at forearm level, right arm

S56.922 Laceration of unspecified muscles, fascia and tendons at forearm level, left arm

S56.929 Laceration of unspecified muscles, fascia and tendons at forearm level, unspecified arm

S56.99 Other injury of unspecified muscles, fascia and tendons at forearm level

S56.991 Other injury of unspecified muscles, fascia and tendons at forearm level, right arm

S56.992 Other injury of unspecified muscles, fascia and tendons at forearm level, left arm

S56.999 Other injury of unspecified muscles, fascia and tendons at forearm level, unspecified arm

S57 Crushing injury of elbow and forearm

Use additional code(s) for all associated injuries

EXCLUDES 2 *crushing injury of wrist and hand (S67.-)*

The appropriate 7th character is to be added to each code from category S57.
A initial encounter
D subsequent encounter
S sequela

S57.0 Crushing injury of elbow

S57.00 Crushing injury of unspecified elbow

S57.01 Crushing injury of right elbow

S57.02 Crushing injury of left elbow

S57.8 Crushing injury of forearm

S57.80 Crushing injury of unspecified forearm

S57.81 Crushing injury of right forearm

S57.82 Crushing injury of left forearm

S58 Traumatic amputation of elbow and forearm

An amputation not identified as partial or complete should be coded to complete

EXCLUDES 1 *traumatic amputation of wrist and hand (S68.-)*

The appropriate 7th character is to be added to each code from category S58.
A initial encounter
D subsequent encounter
S sequela

S58.0 Traumatic amputation at elbow level

S58.01 Complete traumatic amputation at elbow level

2 S58.011 Complete traumatic amputation at elbow level, right arm HCC ESR COM

2 S58.012 Complete traumatic amputation at elbow level, left arm HCC ESR COM

2 S58.019 Complete traumatic amputation at elbow level, unspecified arm HCC ESR COM

S58.02 Partial traumatic amputation at elbow level

2 S58.021 Partial traumatic amputation at elbow level, right arm HCC ESR COM

2 S58.022 Partial traumatic amputation at elbow level, left arm HCC ESR COM

2 S58.029 Partial traumatic amputation at elbow level, unspecified arm HCC ESR COM

S58.1 Traumatic amputation at level between elbow and wrist

S58.11 Complete traumatic amputation at level between elbow and wrist

2 S58.111 Complete traumatic amputation at level between elbow and wrist, right arm HCC ESR COM

2 S58.112 Complete traumatic amputation at level between elbow and wrist, left arm HCC ESR COM

2 S58.119 Complete traumatic amputation at level between elbow and wrist, unspecified arm HCC ESR COM

S58.12 Partial traumatic amputation at level between elbow and wrist

2 S58.121 Partial traumatic amputation at level between elbow and wrist, right arm HCC ESR COM

2 S58.122 Partial traumatic amputation at level between elbow and wrist, left arm HCC ESR COM

2 S58.129 Partial traumatic amputation at level between elbow and wrist, unspecified arm HCC ESR COM

S58.9 Traumatic amputation of forearm, level unspecified

EXCLUDES 1 *traumatic amputation of wrist (S68.-)*

S58.91 Complete traumatic amputation of forearm, level unspecified

- [2] **S58.911** Complete traumatic amputation of right forearm, level unspecified HCC ESR COM
- [2] **S58.912** Complete traumatic amputation of left forearm, level unspecified HCC ESR COM
- [2] **S58.919** Complete traumatic amputation of unspecified forearm, level unspecified HCC ESR COM

S58.92 Partial traumatic amputation of forearm, level unspecified

- [2] **S58.921** Partial traumatic amputation of right forearm, level unspecified HCC ESR COM
- [2] **S58.922** Partial traumatic amputation of left forearm, level unspecified HCC ESR COM
- [2] **S58.929** Partial traumatic amputation of unspecified forearm, level unspecified HCC ESR COM

S59 Other and unspecified injuries of elbow and forearm

EXCLUDES 2 *other and unspecified injuries of wrist and hand (S69.-)*

AHA: 2018,2Q,12; 2018,1Q,3; 2015,3Q,37-39

The appropriate 7th character is to be added to each code from subcategories S59.Ø, S59.1, and S59.2.

- A initial encounter for closed fracture
- D subsequent encounter for fracture with routine healing
- G subsequent encounter for fracture with delayed healing
- K subsequent encounter for fracture with nonunion
- P subsequent encounter for fracture with malunion
- S sequela

S59.Ø Physeal fracture of lower end of ulna

AHA: 2019,4Q,56

S59.ØØ Unspecified physeal fracture of lower end of ulna

- **S59.ØØ1** Unspecified physeal fracture of lower end of ulna, right arm Q
- **S59.ØØ2** Unspecified physeal fracture of lower end of ulna, left arm Q
- **S59.ØØ9** Unspecified physeal fracture of lower end of ulna, unspecified arm Q

S59.Ø1 Salter-Harris Type I physeal fracture of lower end of ulna

- **S59.Ø11** Salter-Harris Type I physeal fracture of lower end of ulna, right arm Q
- **S59.Ø12** Salter-Harris Type I physeal fracture of lower end of ulna, left arm Q
- **S59.Ø19** Salter-Harris Type I physeal fracture of lower end of ulna, unspecified arm Q

S59.Ø2 Salter-Harris Type II physeal fracture of lower end of ulna

- **S59.Ø21** Salter-Harris Type II physeal fracture of lower end of ulna, right arm Q
- **S59.Ø22** Salter-Harris Type II physeal fracture of lower end of ulna, left arm Q
- **S59.Ø29** Salter-Harris Type II physeal fracture of lower end of ulna, unspecified arm Q

S59.Ø3 Salter-Harris Type III physeal fracture of lower end of ulna

- **S59.Ø31** Salter-Harris Type III physeal fracture of lower end of ulna, right arm Q
- **S59.Ø32** Salter-Harris Type III physeal fracture of lower end of ulna, left arm Q
- **S59.Ø39** Salter-Harris Type III physeal fracture of lower end of ulna, unspecified arm Q

S59.Ø4 Salter-Harris Type IV physeal fracture of lower end of ulna

- **S59.Ø41** Salter-Harris Type IV physeal fracture of lower end of ulna, right arm Q
- **S59.Ø42** Salter-Harris Type IV physeal fracture of lower end of ulna, left arm Q
- **S59.Ø49** Salter-Harris Type IV physeal fracture of lower end of ulna, unspecified arm Q

S59.Ø9 Other physeal fracture of lower end of ulna

- **S59.Ø91** Other physeal fracture of lower end of ulna, right arm Q
- **S59.Ø92** Other physeal fracture of lower end of ulna, left arm Q
- **S59.Ø99** Other physeal fracture of lower end of ulna, unspecified arm Q

S59.1 Physeal fracture of upper end of radius

AHA: 2019,4Q,56

S59.1Ø Unspecified physeal fracture of upper end of radius

- **S59.1Ø1** Unspecified physeal fracture of upper end of radius, right arm Q
- **S59.1Ø2** Unspecified physeal fracture of upper end of radius, left arm Q
- **S59.1Ø9** Unspecified physeal fracture of upper end of radius, unspecified arm Q

S59.11 Salter-Harris Type I physeal fracture of upper end of radius

- **S59.111** Salter-Harris Type I physeal fracture of upper end of radius, right arm Q
- **S59.112** Salter-Harris Type I physeal fracture of upper end of radius, left arm Q
- **S59.119** Salter-Harris Type I physeal fracture of upper end of radius, unspecified arm Q

S59.12 Salter-Harris Type II physeal fracture of upper end of radius

- **S59.121** Salter-Harris Type II physeal fracture of upper end of radius, right arm Q
- **S59.122** Salter-Harris Type II physeal fracture of upper end of radius, left arm Q
- **S59.129** Salter-Harris Type II physeal fracture of upper end of radius, unspecified arm Q

S59.13 Salter-Harris Type III physeal fracture of upper end of radius

- **S59.131** Salter-Harris Type III physeal fracture of upper end of radius, right arm Q
- **S59.132** Salter-Harris Type III physeal fracture of upper end of radius, left arm Q
- **S59.139** Salter-Harris Type III physeal fracture of upper end of radius, unspecified arm Q

S59.14 Salter-Harris Type IV physeal fracture of upper end of radius

- **S59.141** Salter-Harris Type IV physeal fracture of upper end of radius, right arm Q
- **S59.142** Salter-Harris Type IV physeal fracture of upper end of radius, left arm Q
- **S59.149** Salter-Harris Type IV physeal fracture of upper end of radius, unspecified arm Q

S59.19 Other physeal fracture of upper end of radius

- **S59.191** Other physeal fracture of upper end of radius, right arm Q
- **S59.192** Other physeal fracture of upper end of radius, left arm Q
- **S59.199** Other physeal fracture of upper end of radius, unspecified arm Q

S59.2 Physeal fracture of lower end of radius

AHA: 2019,4Q,56

S59.2Ø Unspecified physeal fracture of lower end of radius

- **S59.2Ø1** Unspecified physeal fracture of lower end of radius, right arm Q
- **S59.2Ø2** Unspecified physeal fracture of lower end of radius, left arm Q
- **S59.2Ø9** Unspecified physeal fracture of lower end of radius, unspecified arm Q

S59.21 Salter-Harris Type I physeal fracture of lower end of radius

- **S59.211** Salter-Harris Type I physeal fracture of lower end of radius, right arm Q
- **S59.212** Salter-Harris Type I physeal fracture of lower end of radius, left arm Q
- **S59.219** Salter-Harris Type I physeal fracture of lower end of radius, unspecified arm Q

S59.22 Salter-Harris Type II physeal fracture of lower end of radius

- **S59.221** Salter-Harris Type II physeal fracture of lower end of radius, right arm Q
- **S59.222** Salter-Harris Type II physeal fracture of lower end of radius, left arm Q
- **S59.229** Salter-Harris Type II physeal fracture of lower end of radius, unspecified arm Q

6th **S59.23 Salter-Harris Type III physeal fracture of lower end of radius**

7th **S59.231 Salter-Harris Type III physeal fracture of lower end of radius, right arm** Q

7th **S59.232 Salter-Harris Type III physeal fracture of lower end of radius, left arm** Q

7th **S59.239 Salter-Harris Type III physeal fracture of lower end of radius, unspecified arm** Q

6th **S59.24 Salter-Harris Type IV physeal fracture of lower end of radius**

7th **S59.241 Salter-Harris Type IV physeal fracture of lower end of radius, right arm** Q

7th **S59.242 Salter-Harris Type IV physeal fracture of lower end of radius, left arm** Q

7th **S59.249 Salter-Harris Type IV physeal fracture of lower end of radius, unspecified arm** Q

6th **S59.29 Other physeal fracture of lower end of radius**

7th **S59.291 Other physeal fracture of lower end of radius, right arm** Q

7th **S59.292 Other physeal fracture of lower end of radius, left arm** Q

7th **S59.299 Other physeal fracture of lower end of radius, unspecified arm** Q

5th **S59.8 Other specified injuries of elbow and forearm**

The appropriate 7th character is to be added to each code in subcategory S59.8.
A initial encounter
D subsequent encounter
S sequela

6th **S59.80 Other specified injuries of elbow**

7th **S59.801 Other specified injuries of right elbow**

7th **S59.802 Other specified injuries of left elbow**

7th **S59.809 Other specified injuries of unspecified elbow**

6th **S59.81 Other specified injuries of forearm**

7th **S59.811 Other specified injuries right forearm**

7th **S59.812 Other specified injuries left forearm**

7th **S59.819 Other specified injuries unspecified forearm**

5th **S59.9 Unspecified injury of elbow and forearm**

The appropriate 7th character is to be added to each code in subcategory S59.9.
A initial encounter
D subsequent encounter
S sequela

6th **S59.90 Unspecified injury of elbow**

7th **S59.901 Unspecified injury of right elbow**

7th **S59.902 Unspecified injury of left elbow**

7th **S59.909 Unspecified injury of unspecified elbow**

6th **S59.91 Unspecified injury of forearm**

7th **S59.911 Unspecified injury of right forearm**

7th **S59.912 Unspecified injury of left forearm**

7th **S59.919 Unspecified injury of unspecified forearm**

Injuries to the wrist, hand and fingers (S60-S69)

EXCLUDES 2 *burns and corrosions (T20-T32)*
frostbite (T33-T34)
insect bite or sting, venomous (T63.4)

4th **S60 Superficial injury of wrist, hand and fingers**

The appropriate 7th character is to be added to each code from category S60.
A initial encounter
D subsequent encounter
S sequela

5th **S60.0 Contusion of finger without damage to nail**

EXCLUDES 1 *contusion involving nail (matrix) (S60.1)*

x7th **S60.00 Contusion of unspecified finger without damage to nail**
Contusion of finger(s) NOS

6th **S60.01 Contusion of thumb without damage to nail**

7th **S60.011 Contusion of right thumb without damage to nail**

7th **S60.012 Contusion of left thumb without damage to nail**

7th **S60.019 Contusion of unspecified thumb without damage to nail**

6th **S60.02 Contusion of index finger without damage to nail**

7th **S60.021 Contusion of right index finger without damage to nail**

7th **S60.022 Contusion of left index finger without damage to nail**

7th **S60.029 Contusion of unspecified index finger without damage to nail**

6th **S60.03 Contusion of middle finger without damage to nail**

7th **S60.031 Contusion of right middle finger without damage to nail**

7th **S60.032 Contusion of left middle finger without damage to nail**

7th **S60.039 Contusion of unspecified middle finger without damage to nail**

6th **S60.04 Contusion of ring finger without damage to nail**

7th **S60.041 Contusion of right ring finger without damage to nail**

7th **S60.042 Contusion of left ring finger without damage to nail**

7th **S60.049 Contusion of unspecified ring finger without damage to nail**

6th **S60.05 Contusion of little finger without damage to nail**

7th **S60.051 Contusion of right little finger without damage to nail**

7th **S60.052 Contusion of left little finger without damage to nail**

7th **S60.059 Contusion of unspecified little finger without damage to nail**

5th **S60.1 Contusion of finger with damage to nail**

x7th **S60.10 Contusion of unspecified finger with damage to nail**

6th **S60.11 Contusion of thumb with damage to nail**

7th **S60.111 Contusion of right thumb with damage to nail**

7th **S60.112 Contusion of left thumb with damage to nail**

7th **S60.119 Contusion of unspecified thumb with damage to nail**

6th **S60.12 Contusion of index finger with damage to nail**

7th **S60.121 Contusion of right index finger with damage to nail**

7th **S60.122 Contusion of left index finger with damage to nail**

7th **S60.129 Contusion of unspecified index finger with damage to nail**

6th **S60.13 Contusion of middle finger with damage to nail**

7th **S60.131 Contusion of right middle finger with damage to nail**

7th **S60.132 Contusion of left middle finger with damage to nail**

7th **S60.139 Contusion of unspecified middle finger with damage to nail**

6th **S60.14 Contusion of ring finger with damage to nail**

7th **S60.141 Contusion of right ring finger with damage to nail**

7th **S60.142 Contusion of left ring finger with damage to nail**

7th **S60.149 Contusion of unspecified ring finger with damage to nail**

6th **S60.15 Contusion of little finger with damage to nail**

7th **S60.151 Contusion of right little finger with damage to nail**

7th **S60.152 Contusion of left little finger with damage to nail**

7th **S60.159 Contusion of unspecified little finger with damage to nail**

5th **S60.2 Contusion of wrist and hand**

EXCLUDES 2 *contusion of fingers (S60.0-, S60.1-)*

6th **S60.21 Contusion of wrist**

7th **S60.211 Contusion of right wrist**

7th **S60.212 Contusion of left wrist**

7th **S60.219 Contusion of unspecified wrist**

6th **S60.22 Contusion of hand**

7th **S60.221 Contusion of right hand**

S60.222 Contusion of left hand
S60.229 Contusion of unspecified hand

S60.3 Other superficial injuries of thumb

S60.31 Abrasion of thumb
S60.311 Abrasion of right thumb
S60.312 Abrasion of left thumb
S60.319 Abrasion of unspecified thumb

S60.32 Blister (nonthermal) of thumb
S60.321 Blister (nonthermal) of right thumb
S60.322 Blister (nonthermal) of left thumb
S60.329 Blister (nonthermal) of unspecified thumb

S60.34 External constriction of thumb
Hair tourniquet syndrome of thumb
Use additional cause code to identify the constricting item (W49.0-)
S60.341 External constriction of right thumb
S60.342 External constriction of left thumb
S60.349 External constriction of unspecified thumb

S60.35 Superficial foreign body of thumb
Splinter in the thumb
S60.351 Superficial foreign body of right thumb
S60.352 Superficial foreign body of left thumb
S60.359 Superficial foreign body of unspecified thumb

S60.36 Insect bite (nonvenomous) of thumb
S60.361 Insect bite (nonvenomous) of right thumb
S60.362 Insect bite (nonvenomous) of left thumb
S60.369 Insect bite (nonvenomous) of unspecified thumb

S60.37 Other superficial bite of thumb
EXCLUDES 1 *open bite of thumb (S61.05-, S61.15-)*
S60.371 Other superficial bite of right thumb
S60.372 Other superficial bite of left thumb
S60.379 Other superficial bite of unspecified thumb

S60.39 Other superficial injuries of thumb
S60.391 Other superficial injuries of right thumb
S60.392 Other superficial injuries of left thumb
S60.399 Other superficial injuries of unspecified thumb

S60.4 Other superficial injuries of other fingers

S60.41 Abrasion of fingers
S60.410 Abrasion of right index finger
S60.411 Abrasion of left index finger
S60.412 Abrasion of right middle finger
S60.413 Abrasion of left middle finger
S60.414 Abrasion of right ring finger
S60.415 Abrasion of left ring finger
S60.416 Abrasion of right little finger
S60.417 Abrasion of left little finger
S60.418 Abrasion of other finger
Abrasion of specified finger with unspecified laterality
S60.419 Abrasion of unspecified finger

S60.42 Blister (nonthermal) of fingers
S60.420 Blister (nonthermal) of right index finger
S60.421 Blister (nonthermal) of left index finger
S60.422 Blister (nonthermal) of right middle finger
S60.423 Blister (nonthermal) of left middle finger
S60.424 Blister (nonthermal) of right ring finger
S60.425 Blister (nonthermal) of left ring finger
S60.426 Blister (nonthermal) of right little finger
S60.427 Blister (nonthermal) of left little finger
S60.428 Blister (nonthermal) of other finger
Blister (nonthermal) of specified finger with unspecified laterality
S60.429 Blister (nonthermal) of unspecified finger

S60.44 External constriction of fingers
Hair tourniquet syndrome of finger
Use additional cause code to identify the constricting item (W49.0-)
S60.440 External constriction of right index finger
S60.441 External constriction of left index finger
S60.442 External constriction of right middle finger
S60.443 External constriction of left middle finger
S60.444 External constriction of right ring finger
S60.445 External constriction of left ring finger
S60.446 External constriction of right little finger
S60.447 External constriction of left little finger
S60.448 External constriction of other finger
External constriction of specified finger with unspecified laterality
S60.449 External constriction of unspecified finger

S60.45 Superficial foreign body of fingers
Splinter in the finger(s)
S60.450 Superficial foreign body of right index finger
S60.451 Superficial foreign body of left index finger
S60.452 Superficial foreign body of right middle finger
S60.453 Superficial foreign body of left middle finger
S60.454 Superficial foreign body of right ring finger
S60.455 Superficial foreign body of left ring finger
S60.456 Superficial foreign body of right little finger
S60.457 Superficial foreign body of left little finger
S60.458 Superficial foreign body of other finger
Superficial foreign body of specified finger with unspecified laterality
S60.459 Superficial foreign body of unspecified finger

S60.46 Insect bite (nonvenomous) of fingers
S60.460 Insect bite (nonvenomous) of right index finger
S60.461 Insect bite (nonvenomous) of left index finger
S60.462 Insect bite (nonvenomous) of right middle finger
S60.463 Insect bite (nonvenomous) of left middle finger
S60.464 Insect bite (nonvenomous) of right ring finger
S60.465 Insect bite (nonvenomous) of left ring finger
S60.466 Insect bite (nonvenomous) of right little finger
S60.467 Insect bite (nonvenomous) of left little finger
S60.468 Insect bite (nonvenomous) of other finger
Insect bite (nonvenomous) of specified finger with unspecified laterality
S60.469 Insect bite (nonvenomous) of unspecified finger

S60.47 Other superficial bite of fingers
EXCLUDES 1 *open bite of fingers (S61.25-, S61.35-)*
S60.470 Other superficial bite of right index finger
S60.471 Other superficial bite of left index finger
S60.472 Other superficial bite of right middle finger
S60.473 Other superficial bite of left middle finger
S60.474 Other superficial bite of right ring finger
S60.475 Other superficial bite of left ring finger
S60.476 Other superficial bite of right little finger
S60.477 Other superficial bite of left little finger
S60.478 Other superficial bite of other finger
Other superficial bite of specified finger with unspecified laterality

S60.479 Other superficial bite of unspecified finger

S60.5 Other superficial injuries of hand

EXCLUDES 2 *superficial injuries of fingers (S60.3-, S60.4-)*

S60.51 Abrasion of hand

S60.511 Abrasion of right hand

S60.512 Abrasion of left hand

S60.519 Abrasion of unspecified hand

S60.52 Blister (nonthermal) of hand

S60.521 Blister (nonthermal) of right hand

S60.522 Blister (nonthermal) of left hand

S60.529 Blister (nonthermal) of unspecified hand

S60.54 External constriction of hand

S60.541 External constriction of right hand

S60.542 External constriction of left hand

S60.549 External constriction of unspecified hand

S60.55 Superficial foreign body of hand

Splinter in the hand

S60.551 Superficial foreign body of right hand

S60.552 Superficial foreign body of left hand

S60.559 Superficial foreign body of unspecified hand

S60.56 Insect bite (nonvenomous) of hand

S60.561 Insect bite (nonvenomous) of right hand

S60.562 Insect bite (nonvenomous) of left hand

S60.569 Insect bite (nonvenomous) of unspecified hand

S60.57 Other superficial bite of hand

EXCLUDES 1 *open bite of hand (S61.45-)*

S60.571 Other superficial bite of hand of right hand

S60.572 Other superficial bite of hand of left hand

S60.579 Other superficial bite of hand of unspecified hand

S60.8 Other superficial injuries of wrist

S60.81 Abrasion of wrist

S60.811 Abrasion of right wrist

S60.812 Abrasion of left wrist

S60.819 Abrasion of unspecified wrist

S60.82 Blister (nonthermal) of wrist

S60.821 Blister (nonthermal) of right wrist

S60.822 Blister (nonthermal) of left wrist

S60.829 Blister (nonthermal) of unspecified wrist

S60.84 External constriction of wrist

S60.841 External constriction of right wrist

S60.842 External constriction of left wrist

S60.849 External constriction of unspecified wrist

S60.85 Superficial foreign body of wrist

Splinter in the wrist

S60.851 Superficial foreign body of right wrist

S60.852 Superficial foreign body of left wrist

S60.859 Superficial foreign body of unspecified wrist

S60.86 Insect bite (nonvenomous) of wrist

S60.861 Insect bite (nonvenomous) of right wrist

S60.862 Insect bite (nonvenomous) of left wrist

S60.869 Insect bite (nonvenomous) of unspecified wrist

S60.87 Other superficial bite of wrist

EXCLUDES 1 *open bite of wrist (S61.55)*

S60.871 Other superficial bite of right wrist

S60.872 Other superficial bite of left wrist

S60.879 Other superficial bite of unspecified wrist

S60.9 Unspecified superficial injury of wrist, hand and fingers

S60.91 Unspecified superficial injury of wrist

S60.911 Unspecified superficial injury of right wrist

S60.912 Unspecified superficial injury of left wrist

S60.919 Unspecified superficial injury of unspecified wrist

S60.92 Unspecified superficial injury of hand

S60.921 Unspecified superficial injury of right hand

S60.922 Unspecified superficial injury of left hand

S60.929 Unspecified superficial injury of unspecified hand

S60.93 Unspecified superficial injury of thumb

S60.931 Unspecified superficial injury of right thumb

S60.932 Unspecified superficial injury of left thumb

S60.939 Unspecified superficial injury of unspecified thumb

S60.94 Unspecified superficial injury of other fingers

S60.940 Unspecified superficial injury of right index finger

S60.941 Unspecified superficial injury of left index finger

S60.942 Unspecified superficial injury of right middle finger

S60.943 Unspecified superficial injury of left middle finger

S60.944 Unspecified superficial injury of right ring finger

S60.945 Unspecified superficial injury of left ring finger

S60.946 Unspecified superficial injury of right little finger

S60.947 Unspecified superficial injury of left little finger

S60.948 Unspecified superficial injury of other finger

Unspecified superficial injury of specified finger with unspecified laterality

S60.949 Unspecified superficial injury of unspecified finger

S61 Open wound of wrist, hand and fingers

Code also any associated wound infection

EXCLUDES 1 *open fracture of wrist, hand and finger (S62.- with 7th character B)*

traumatic amputation of wrist and hand (S68.-)

The appropriate 7th character is to be added to each code from category S61.

A initial encounter
D subsequent encounter
S sequela

S61.0 Open wound of thumb without damage to nail

EXCLUDES 1 *open wound of thumb with damage to nail (S61.1-)*

S61.00 Unspecified open wound of thumb without damage to nail

S61.001 Unspecified open wound of right thumb without damage to nail

S61.002 Unspecified open wound of left thumb without damage to nail

S61.009 Unspecified open wound of unspecified thumb without damage to nail

S61.01 Laceration without foreign body of thumb without damage to nail

S61.011 Laceration without foreign body of right thumb without damage to nail

S61.012 Laceration without foreign body of left thumb without damage to nail

S61.019 Laceration without foreign body of unspecified thumb without damage to nail

S61.02 Laceration with foreign body of thumb without damage to nail

S61.021 Laceration with foreign body of right thumb without damage to nail

S61.022 Laceration with foreign body of left thumb without damage to nail

S61.029 Laceration with foreign body of unspecified thumb without damage to nail

S61.03 Puncture wound without foreign body of thumb without damage to nail

S61.031 Puncture wound without foreign body of right thumb without damage to nail

S61.032 Puncture wound without foreign body of left thumb without damage to nail

7th **S61.039 Puncture wound without foreign body of unspecified thumb without damage to nail**

6th **S61.04 Puncture wound with foreign body of thumb without damage to nail**

7th **S61.041 Puncture wound with foreign body of right thumb without damage to nail**

7th **S61.042 Puncture wound with foreign body of left thumb without damage to nail**

7th **S61.049 Puncture wound with foreign body of unspecified thumb without damage to nail**

6th **S61.05 Open bite of thumb without damage to nail**

Bite of thumb NOS

EXCLUDES 1 *superficial bite of thumb (S60.36-, S60.37-)*

7th **S61.051 Open bite of right thumb without damage to nail**

7th **S61.052 Open bite of left thumb without damage to nail**

7th **S61.059 Open bite of unspecified thumb without damage to nail**

5th **S61.1 Open wound of thumb with damage to nail**

6th **S61.10 Unspecified open wound of thumb with damage to nail**

7th **S61.101 Unspecified open wound of right thumb with damage to nail**

7th **S61.102 Unspecified open wound of left thumb with damage to nail**

7th **S61.109 Unspecified open wound of unspecified thumb with damage to nail**

6th **S61.11 Laceration without foreign body of thumb with damage to nail**

7th **S61.111 Laceration without foreign body of right thumb with damage to nail**

7th **S61.112 Laceration without foreign body of left thumb with damage to nail**

7th **S61.119 Laceration without foreign body of unspecified thumb with damage to nail**

6th **S61.12 Laceration with foreign body of thumb with damage to nail**

7th **S61.121 Laceration with foreign body of right thumb with damage to nail**

7th **S61.122 Laceration with foreign body of left thumb with damage to nail**

7th **S61.129 Laceration with foreign body of unspecified thumb with damage to nail**

6th **S61.13 Puncture wound without foreign body of thumb with damage to nail**

7th **S61.131 Puncture wound without foreign body of right thumb with damage to nail**

7th **S61.132 Puncture wound without foreign body of left thumb with damage to nail**

7th **S61.139 Puncture wound without foreign body of unspecified thumb with damage to nail**

6th **S61.14 Puncture wound with foreign body of thumb with damage to nail**

7th **S61.141 Puncture wound with foreign body of right thumb with damage to nail**

7th **S61.142 Puncture wound with foreign body of left thumb with damage to nail**

7th **S61.149 Puncture wound with foreign body of unspecified thumb with damage to nail**

6th **S61.15 Open bite of thumb with damage to nail**

Bite of thumb with damage to nail NOS

EXCLUDES 1 *superficial bite of thumb (S60.36-, S60.37-)*

7th **S61.151 Open bite of right thumb with damage to nail**

7th **S61.152 Open bite of left thumb with damage to nail**

7th **S61.159 Open bite of unspecified thumb with damage to nail**

5th **S61.2 Open wound of other finger without damage to nail**

EXCLUDES 1 *open wound of finger involving nail (matrix) (S61.3-)*

EXCLUDES 2 *open wound of thumb without damage to nail (S61.0-)*

6th **S61.20 Unspecified open wound of other finger without damage to nail**

7th **S61.200 Unspecified open wound of right index finger without damage to nail**

7th **S61.201 Unspecified open wound of left index finger without damage to nail**

7th **S61.202 Unspecified open wound of right middle finger without damage to nail**

7th **S61.203 Unspecified open wound of left middle finger without damage to nail**

7th **S61.204 Unspecified open wound of right ring finger without damage to nail**

7th **S61.205 Unspecified open wound of left ring finger without damage to nail**

7th **S61.206 Unspecified open wound of right little finger without damage to nail**

7th **S61.207 Unspecified open wound of left little finger without damage to nail**

7th **S61.208 Unspecified open wound of other finger without damage to nail**

Unspecified open wound of specified finger with unspecified laterality without damage to nail

7th **S61.209 Unspecified open wound of unspecified finger without damage to nail**

6th **S61.21 Laceration without foreign body of finger without damage to nail**

7th **S61.210 Laceration without foreign body of right index finger without damage to nail**

7th **S61.211 Laceration without foreign body of left index finger without damage to nail**

7th **S61.212 Laceration without foreign body of right middle finger without damage to nail**

7th **S61.213 Laceration without foreign body of left middle finger without damage to nail**

7th **S61.214 Laceration without foreign body of right ring finger without damage to nail**

7th **S61.215 Laceration without foreign body of left ring finger without damage to nail**

7th **S61.216 Laceration without foreign body of right little finger without damage to nail**

7th **S61.217 Laceration without foreign body of left little finger without damage to nail**

7th **S61.218 Laceration without foreign body of other finger without damage to nail**

Laceration without foreign body of specified finger with unspecified laterality without damage to nail

7th **S61.219 Laceration without foreign body of unspecified finger without damage to nail**

6th **S61.22 Laceration with foreign body of finger without damage to nail**

7th **S61.220 Laceration with foreign body of right index finger without damage to nail**

7th **S61.221 Laceration with foreign body of left index finger without damage to nail**

7th **S61.222 Laceration with foreign body of right middle finger without damage to nail**

7th **S61.223 Laceration with foreign body of left middle finger without damage to nail**

7th **S61.224 Laceration with foreign body of right ring finger without damage to nail**

7th **S61.225 Laceration with foreign body of left ring finger without damage to nail**

7th **S61.226 Laceration with foreign body of right little finger without damage to nail**

7th **S61.227 Laceration with foreign body of left little finger without damage to nail**

7th **S61.228 Laceration with foreign body of other finger without damage to nail**

Laceration with foreign body of specified finger with unspecified laterality without damage to nail

7th **S61.229 Laceration with foreign body of unspecified finger without damage to nail**

6th **S61.23 Puncture wound without foreign body of finger without damage to nail**

7th **S61.230 Puncture wound without foreign body of right index finger without damage to nail**

7th **S61.231 Puncture wound without foreign body of left index finger without damage to nail**

7th **S61.232 Puncture wound without foreign body of right middle finger without damage to nail**

7th **S61.233 Puncture wound without foreign body of left middle finger without damage to nail**

7th **S61.234 Puncture wound without foreign body of right ring finger without damage to nail**

7th **S61.235 Puncture wound without foreign body of left ring finger without damage to nail**

7th **S61.236 Puncture wound without foreign body of right little finger without damage to nail**

7th **S61.237 Puncture wound without foreign body of left little finger without damage to nail**

7th **S61.238 Puncture wound without foreign body of other finger without damage to nail**

Puncture wound without foreign body of specified finger with unspecified laterality without damage to nail

7th **S61.239 Puncture wound without foreign body of unspecified finger without damage to nail**

6th **S61.24 Puncture wound with foreign body of finger without damage to nail**

7th **S61.240 Puncture wound with foreign body of right index finger without damage to nail**

7th **S61.241 Puncture wound with foreign body of left index finger without damage to nail**

7th **S61.242 Puncture wound with foreign body of right middle finger without damage to nail**

7th **S61.243 Puncture wound with foreign body of left middle finger without damage to nail**

7th **S61.244 Puncture wound with foreign body of right ring finger without damage to nail**

7th **S61.245 Puncture wound with foreign body of left ring finger without damage to nail**

7th **S61.246 Puncture wound with foreign body of right little finger without damage to nail**

7th **S61.247 Puncture wound with foreign body of left little finger without damage to nail**

7th **S61.248 Puncture wound with foreign body of other finger without damage to nail**

Puncture wound with foreign body of specified finger with unspecified laterality without damage to nail

7th **S61.249 Puncture wound with foreign body of unspecified finger without damage to nail**

6th **S61.25 Open bite of finger without damage to nail**

Bite of finger without damage to nail NOS

EXCLUDES 1 *superficial bite of finger (S6Ø.46-, S6Ø.47-)*

7th **S61.25Ø Open bite of right index finger without damage to nail**

7th **S61.251 Open bite of left index finger without damage to nail**

7th **S61.252 Open bite of right middle finger without damage to nail**

7th **S61.253 Open bite of left middle finger without damage to nail**

7th **S61.254 Open bite of right ring finger without damage to nail**

7th **S61.255 Open bite of left ring finger without damage to nail**

7th **S61.256 Open bite of right little finger without damage to nail**

7th **S61.257 Open bite of left little finger without damage to nail**

7th **S61.258 Open bite of other finger without damage to nail**

Open bite of specified finger with unspecified laterality without damage to nail

7th **S61.259 Open bite of unspecified finger without damage to nail**

5th **S61.3 Open wound of other finger with damage to nail**

6th **S61.3Ø Unspecified open wound of finger with damage to nail**

7th **S61.3ØØ Unspecified open wound of right index finger with damage to nail**

7th **S61.3Ø1 Unspecified open wound of left index finger with damage to nail**

7th **S61.3Ø2 Unspecified open wound of right middle finger with damage to nail**

7th **S61.3Ø3 Unspecified open wound of left middle finger with damage to nail**

7th **S61.3Ø4 Unspecified open wound of right ring finger with damage to nail**

7th **S61.3Ø5 Unspecified open wound of left ring finger with damage to nail**

7th **S61.3Ø6 Unspecified open wound of right little finger with damage to nail**

7th **S61.3Ø7 Unspecified open wound of left little finger with damage to nail**

7th **S61.3Ø8 Unspecified open wound of other finger with damage to nail**

Unspecified open wound of specified finger with unspecified laterality with damage to nail

7th **S61.3Ø9 Unspecified open wound of unspecified finger with damage to nail**

6th **S61.31 Laceration without foreign body of finger with damage to nail**

7th **S61.31Ø Laceration without foreign body of right index finger with damage to nail**

7th **S61.311 Laceration without foreign body of left index finger with damage to nail**

7th **S61.312 Laceration without foreign body of right middle finger with damage to nail**

7th **S61.313 Laceration without foreign body of left middle finger with damage to nail**

7th **S61.314 Laceration without foreign body of right ring finger with damage to nail**

7th **S61.315 Laceration without foreign body of left ring finger with damage to nail**

7th **S61.316 Laceration without foreign body of right little finger with damage to nail**

7th **S61.317 Laceration without foreign body of left little finger with damage to nail**

7th **S61.318 Laceration without foreign body of other finger with damage to nail**

Laceration without foreign body of specified finger with unspecified laterality with damage to nail

7th **S61.319 Laceration without foreign body of unspecified finger with damage to nail**

6th **S61.32 Laceration with foreign body of finger with damage to nail**

7th **S61.32Ø Laceration with foreign body of right index finger with damage to nail**

7th **S61.321 Laceration with foreign body of left index finger with damage to nail**

7th **S61.322 Laceration with foreign body of right middle finger with damage to nail**

7th **S61.323 Laceration with foreign body of left middle finger with damage to nail**

7th **S61.324 Laceration with foreign body of right ring finger with damage to nail**

7th **S61.325 Laceration with foreign body of left ring finger with damage to nail**

7th **S61.326 Laceration with foreign body of right little finger with damage to nail**

7th **S61.327 Laceration with foreign body of left little finger with damage to nail**

7th **S61.328 Laceration with foreign body of other finger with damage to nail**

Laceration with foreign body of specified finger with unspecified laterality with damage to nail

7th **S61.329 Laceration with foreign body of unspecified finger with damage to nail**

6th **S61.33 Puncture wound without foreign body of finger with damage to nail**

7th **S61.33Ø Puncture wound without foreign body of right index finger with damage to nail**

7th **S61.331 Puncture wound without foreign body of left index finger with damage to nail**

7th **S61.332 Puncture wound without foreign body of right middle finger with damage to nail**

7th **S61.333 Puncture wound without foreign body of left middle finger with damage to nail**

7th **S61.334 Puncture wound without foreign body of right ring finger with damage to nail**

7th **S61.335 Puncture wound without foreign body of left ring finger with damage to nail**

7th **S61.336 Puncture wound without foreign body of right little finger with damage to nail**

7th **S61.337 Puncture wound without foreign body of left little finger with damage to nail**

S61.338 **Puncture wound without foreign body of other finger with damage to nail**
Puncture wound without foreign body of specified finger with unspecified laterality with damage to nail

S61.339 **Puncture wound without foreign body of unspecified finger with damage to nail**

S61.34 **Puncture wound with foreign body of finger with damage to nail**

S61.340 **Puncture wound with foreign body of right index finger with damage to nail**

S61.341 **Puncture wound with foreign body of left index finger with damage to nail**

S61.342 **Puncture wound with foreign body of right middle finger with damage to nail**

S61.343 **Puncture wound with foreign body of left middle finger with damage to nail**

S61.344 **Puncture wound with foreign body of right ring finger with damage to nail**

S61.345 **Puncture wound with foreign body of left ring finger with damage to nail**

S61.346 **Puncture wound with foreign body of right little finger with damage to nail**

S61.347 **Puncture wound with foreign body of left little finger with damage to nail**

S61.348 **Puncture wound with foreign body of other finger with damage to nail**
Puncture wound with foreign body of specified finger with unspecified laterality with damage to nail

S61.349 **Puncture wound with foreign body of unspecified finger with damage to nail**

S61.35 **Open bite of finger with damage to nail**
Bite of finger with damage to nail NOS
EXCLUDES 1 *superficial bite of finger (S60.46-, S60.47-)*

S61.350 **Open bite of right index finger with damage to nail**

S61.351 **Open bite of left index finger with damage to nail**

S61.352 **Open bite of right middle finger with damage to nail**

S61.353 **Open bite of left middle finger with damage to nail**

S61.354 **Open bite of right ring finger with damage to nail**

S61.355 **Open bite of left ring finger with damage to nail**

S61.356 **Open bite of right little finger with damage to nail**

S61.357 **Open bite of left little finger with damage to nail**

S61.358 **Open bite of other finger with damage to nail**
Open bite of specified finger with unspecified laterality with damage to nail

S61.359 **Open bite of unspecified finger with damage to nail**

S61.4 **Open wound of hand**

S61.40 **Unspecified open wound of hand**

S61.401 **Unspecified open wound of right hand**

S61.402 **Unspecified open wound of left hand**

S61.409 **Unspecified open wound of unspecified hand**

S61.41 **Laceration without foreign body of hand**

S61.411 **Laceration without foreign body of right hand**

S61.412 **Laceration without foreign body of left hand**

S61.419 **Laceration without foreign body of unspecified hand**

S61.42 **Laceration with foreign body of hand**

S61.421 **Laceration with foreign body of right hand**

S61.422 **Laceration with foreign body of left hand**

S61.429 **Laceration with foreign body of unspecified hand**

S61.43 **Puncture wound without foreign body of hand**

S61.431 **Puncture wound without foreign body of right hand**

S61.432 **Puncture wound without foreign body of left hand**

S61.439 **Puncture wound without foreign body of unspecified hand**

S61.44 **Puncture wound with foreign body of hand**

S61.441 **Puncture wound with foreign body of right hand**

S61.442 **Puncture wound with foreign body of left hand**

S61.449 **Puncture wound with foreign body of unspecified hand**

S61.45 **Open bite of hand**
Bite of hand NOS
EXCLUDES 1 *superficial bite of hand (S60.56-, S60.57-)*

S61.451 **Open bite of right hand**

S61.452 **Open bite of left hand**

S61.459 **Open bite of unspecified hand**

S61.5 **Open wound of wrist**

S61.50 **Unspecified open wound of wrist**

S61.501 **Unspecified open wound of right wrist**

S61.502 **Unspecified open wound of left wrist**

S61.509 **Unspecified open wound of unspecified wrist**

S61.51 **Laceration without foreign body of wrist**

S61.511 **Laceration without foreign body of right wrist**

S61.512 **Laceration without foreign body of left wrist**

S61.519 **Laceration without foreign body of unspecified wrist**

S61.52 **Laceration with foreign body of wrist**

S61.521 **Laceration with foreign body of right wrist**

S61.522 **Laceration with foreign body of left wrist**

S61.529 **Laceration with foreign body of unspecified wrist**

S61.53 **Puncture wound without foreign body of wrist**

S61.531 **Puncture wound without foreign body of right wrist**

S61.532 **Puncture wound without foreign body of left wrist**

S61.539 **Puncture wound without foreign body of unspecified wrist**

S61.54 **Puncture wound with foreign body of wrist**

S61.541 **Puncture wound with foreign body of right wrist**

S61.542 **Puncture wound with foreign body of left wrist**

S61.549 **Puncture wound with foreign body of unspecified wrist**

S61.55 **Open bite of wrist**
Bite of wrist NOS
EXCLUDES 1 *superficial bite of wrist (S60.86-, S60.87-)*

S61.551 **Open bite of right wrist**

S61.552 **Open bite of left wrist**

S61.559 **Open bite of unspecified wrist**

Chapter 19. Injury, Poisoning and Certain Other Consequences of External Causes
S61.338–S61.559

S62 Fracture at wrist and hand level

NOTE A fracture not indicated as displaced or nondisplaced should be coded to displaced

A fracture not indicated as open or closed should be coded to closed

EXCLUDES 1 *traumatic amputation of wrist and hand (S68.-)*

EXCLUDES 2 *fracture of distal parts of ulna and radius (S52.-)*

AHA: 2018,2Q,12; 2015,3Q,37-39

The appropriate 7th character is to be added to each code from category S62.
- A initial encounter for closed fracture
- B initial encounter for open fracture
- D subsequent encounter for fracture with routine healing
- G subsequent encounter for fracture with delayed healing
- K subsequent encounter for fracture with nonunion
- P subsequent encounter for fracture with malunion
- S sequela

S62.0 Fracture of navicular [scaphoid] bone of wrist

S62.00 Unspecified fracture of navicular [scaphoid] bone of wrist

S62.001 Unspecified fracture of navicular [scaphoid] bone of right wrist

S62.002 Unspecified fracture of navicular [scaphoid] bone of left wrist

AHA: 2012,4Q,106

S62.009 Unspecified fracture of navicular [scaphoid] bone of unspecified wrist

S62.01 Fracture of distal pole of navicular [scaphoid] bone of wrist

Fracture of volar tuberosity of navicular [scaphoid] bone of wrist

S62.011 Displaced fracture of distal pole of navicular [scaphoid] bone of right wrist

S62.012 Displaced fracture of distal pole of navicular [scaphoid] bone of left wrist

S62.013 Displaced fracture of distal pole of navicular [scaphoid] bone of unspecified wrist

S62.014 Nondisplaced fracture of distal pole of navicular [scaphoid] bone of right wrist

S62.015 Nondisplaced fracture of distal pole of navicular [scaphoid] bone of left wrist

S62.016 Nondisplaced fracture of distal pole of navicular [scaphoid] bone of unspecified wrist

S62.02 Fracture of middle third of navicular [scaphoid] bone of wrist

S62.021 Displaced fracture of middle third of navicular [scaphoid] bone of right wrist

S62.022 Displaced fracture of middle third of navicular [scaphoid] bone of left wrist

S62.023 Displaced fracture of middle third of navicular [scaphoid] bone of unspecified wrist

S62.024 Nondisplaced fracture of middle third of navicular [scaphoid] bone of right wrist

S62.025 Nondisplaced fracture of middle third of navicular [scaphoid] bone of left wrist

S62.026 Nondisplaced fracture of middle third of navicular [scaphoid] bone of unspecified wrist

S62.03 Fracture of proximal third of navicular [scaphoid] bone of wrist

S62.031 Displaced fracture of proximal third of navicular [scaphoid] bone of right wrist

S62.032 Displaced fracture of proximal third of navicular [scaphoid] bone of left wrist

S62.033 Displaced fracture of proximal third of navicular [scaphoid] bone of unspecified wrist

S62.034 Nondisplaced fracture of proximal third of navicular [scaphoid] bone of right wrist

S62.035 Nondisplaced fracture of proximal third of navicular [scaphoid] bone of left wrist

S62.036 Nondisplaced fracture of proximal third of navicular [scaphoid] bone of unspecified wrist

S62.1 Fracture of other and unspecified carpal bone(s)

EXCLUDES 2 *fracture of scaphoid of wrist (S62.0-)*

S62.10 Fracture of unspecified carpal bone

Fracture of wrist NOS

S62.101 Fracture of unspecified carpal bone, right wrist

S62.102 Fracture of unspecified carpal bone, left wrist

AHA: 2012,4Q,95

S62.109 Fracture of unspecified carpal bone, unspecified wrist

S62.11 Fracture of triquetrum [cuneiform] bone of wrist

S62.111 Displaced fracture of triquetrum [cuneiform] bone, right wrist

S62.112 Displaced fracture of triquetrum [cuneiform] bone, left wrist

S62.113 Displaced fracture of triquetrum [cuneiform] bone, unspecified wrist

S62.114 Nondisplaced fracture of triquetrum [cuneiform] bone, right wrist

S62.115 Nondisplaced fracture of triquetrum [cuneiform] bone, left wrist

S62.116 Nondisplaced fracture of triquetrum [cuneiform] bone, unspecified wrist

S62.12 Fracture of lunate [semilunar]

S62.121 Displaced fracture of lunate [semilunar], right wrist

S62.122 Displaced fracture of lunate [semilunar], left wrist

S62.123 Displaced fracture of lunate [semilunar], unspecified wrist

S62.124 Nondisplaced fracture of lunate [semilunar], right wrist

S62.125 Nondisplaced fracture of lunate [semilunar], left wrist

S62.126 Nondisplaced fracture of lunate [semilunar], unspecified wrist

S62.13 Fracture of capitate [os magnum] bone

S62.131 Displaced fracture of capitate [os magnum] bone, right wrist

S62.132 Displaced fracture of capitate [os magnum] bone, left wrist

S62.133 Displaced fracture of capitate [os magnum] bone, unspecified wrist

S62.134 Nondisplaced fracture of capitate [os magnum] bone, right wrist

S62.135 Nondisplaced fracture of capitate [os magnum] bone, left wrist

S62.136 Nondisplaced fracture of capitate [os magnum] bone, unspecified wrist

S62.14 Fracture of body of hamate [unciform] bone

Fracture of hamate [unciform] bone NOS

S62.141 Displaced fracture of body of hamate [unciform] bone, right wrist

S62.142 Displaced fracture of body of hamate [unciform] bone, left wrist

S62.143 Displaced fracture of body of hamate [unciform] bone, unspecified wrist

S62.144 Nondisplaced fracture of body of hamate [unciform] bone, right wrist

S62.145 Nondisplaced fracture of body of hamate [unciform] bone, left wrist

S62.146 Nondisplaced fracture of body of hamate [unciform] bone, unspecified wrist

S62.15 Fracture of hook process of hamate [unciform] bone
Fracture of unciform process of hamate [unciform] bone
- **S62.151 Displaced fracture of hook process of hamate [unciform] bone, right wrist**
- **S62.152 Displaced fracture of hook process of hamate [unciform] bone, left wrist**
- **S62.153 Displaced fracture of hook process of hamate [unciform] bone, unspecified wrist**
- **S62.154 Nondisplaced fracture of hook process of hamate [unciform] bone, right wrist**
- **S62.155 Nondisplaced fracture of hook process of hamate [unciform] bone, left wrist**
- **S62.156 Nondisplaced fracture of hook process of hamate [unciform] bone, unspecified wrist**

S62.16 Fracture of pisiform
- **S62.161 Displaced fracture of pisiform, right wrist**
- **S62.162 Displaced fracture of pisiform, left wrist**
- **S62.163 Displaced fracture of pisiform, unspecified wrist**
- **S62.164 Nondisplaced fracture of pisiform, right wrist**
- **S62.165 Nondisplaced fracture of pisiform, left wrist**
- **S62.166 Nondisplaced fracture of pisiform, unspecified wrist**

S62.17 Fracture of trapezium [larger multangular]
- **S62.171 Displaced fracture of trapezium [larger multangular], right wrist**
- **S62.172 Displaced fracture of trapezium [larger multangular], left wrist**
- **S62.173 Displaced fracture of trapezium [larger multangular], unspecified wrist**
- **S62.174 Nondisplaced fracture of trapezium [larger multangular], right wrist**
- **S62.175 Nondisplaced fracture of trapezium [larger multangular], left wrist**
- **S62.176 Nondisplaced fracture of trapezium [larger multangular], unspecified wrist**

S62.18 Fracture of trapezoid [smaller multangular]
- **S62.181 Displaced fracture of trapezoid [smaller multangular], right wrist**
- **S62.182 Displaced fracture of trapezoid [smaller multangular], left wrist**
- **S62.183 Displaced fracture of trapezoid [smaller multangular], unspecified wrist**
- **S62.184 Nondisplaced fracture of trapezoid [smaller multangular], right wrist**
- **S62.185 Nondisplaced fracture of trapezoid [smaller multangular], left wrist**
- **S62.186 Nondisplaced fracture of trapezoid [smaller multangular], unspecified wrist**

S62.2 Fracture of first metacarpal bone

S62.20 Unspecified fracture of first metacarpal bone
- **S62.201 Unspecified fracture of first metacarpal bone, right hand**
- **S62.202 Unspecified fracture of first metacarpal bone, left hand**
- **S62.209 Unspecified fracture of first metacarpal bone, unspecified hand**

S62.21 Bennett's fracture
DEF: Intra-articular, two-part fracture at the base of the first metacarpal bone (thumb) on the ulnar side at the carpometacarpal (CMC) joint.
- **S62.211 Bennett's fracture, right hand**
- **S62.212 Bennett's fracture, left hand**
- **S62.213 Bennett's fracture, unspecified hand**

S62.22 Rolando's fracture
DEF: Comminuted, three part intra-articular fracture at the base of the thumb metacarpal.
- **S62.221 Displaced Rolando's fracture, right hand**
- **S62.222 Displaced Rolando's fracture, left hand**
- **S62.223 Displaced Rolando's fracture, unspecified hand**
- **S62.224 Nondisplaced Rolando's fracture, right hand**
- **S62.225 Nondisplaced Rolando's fracture, left hand**
- **S62.226 Nondisplaced Rolando's fracture, unspecified hand**

S62.23 Other fracture of base of first metacarpal bone
- **S62.231 Other displaced fracture of base of first metacarpal bone, right hand**
- **S62.232 Other displaced fracture of base of first metacarpal bone, left hand**
- **S62.233 Other displaced fracture of base of first metacarpal bone, unspecified hand**
- **S62.234 Other nondisplaced fracture of base of first metacarpal bone, right hand**
- **S62.235 Other nondisplaced fracture of base of first metacarpal bone, left hand**
- **S62.236 Other nondisplaced fracture of base of first metacarpal bone, unspecified hand**

S62.24 Fracture of shaft of first metacarpal bone
- **S62.241 Displaced fracture of shaft of first metacarpal bone, right hand**
- **S62.242 Displaced fracture of shaft of first metacarpal bone, left hand**
- **S62.243 Displaced fracture of shaft of first metacarpal bone, unspecified hand**
- **S62.244 Nondisplaced fracture of shaft of first metacarpal bone, right hand**
- **S62.245 Nondisplaced fracture of shaft of first metacarpal bone, left hand**
- **S62.246 Nondisplaced fracture of shaft of first metacarpal bone, unspecified hand**

S62.25 Fracture of neck of first metacarpal bone
- **S62.251 Displaced fracture of neck of first metacarpal bone, right hand**
- **S62.252 Displaced fracture of neck of first metacarpal bone, left hand**
- **S62.253 Displaced fracture of neck of first metacarpal bone, unspecified hand**
- **S62.254 Nondisplaced fracture of neck of first metacarpal bone, right hand**
- **S62.255 Nondisplaced fracture of neck of first metacarpal bone, left hand**
- **S62.256 Nondisplaced fracture of neck of first metacarpal bone, unspecified hand**

S62.29 Other fracture of first metacarpal bone
- **S62.291 Other fracture of first metacarpal bone, right hand**
- **S62.292 Other fracture of first metacarpal bone, left hand**
- **S62.299 Other fracture of first metacarpal bone, unspecified hand**

S62.3 Fracture of other and unspecified metacarpal bone
EXCLUDES 2 *fracture of first metacarpal bone (S62.2-)*

S62.30 Unspecified fracture of other metacarpal bone
- **S62.300 Unspecified fracture of second metacarpal bone, right hand**
- **S62.301 Unspecified fracture of second metacarpal bone, left hand**
- **S62.302 Unspecified fracture of third metacarpal bone, right hand**
- **S62.303 Unspecified fracture of third metacarpal bone, left hand**
- **S62.304 Unspecified fracture of fourth metacarpal bone, right hand**
- **S62.305 Unspecified fracture of fourth metacarpal bone, left hand**
- **S62.306 Unspecified fracture of fifth metacarpal bone, right hand**
- **S62.307 Unspecified fracture of fifth metacarpal bone, left hand**

S62.308 Unspecified fracture of other metacarpal bone
Unspecified fracture of specified metacarpal bone with unspecified laterality

S62.309 Unspecified fracture of unspecified metacarpal bone

S62.31 Displaced fracture of base of other metacarpal bone

S62.310 Displaced fracture of base of second metacarpal bone, right hand

S62.311 Displaced fracture of base of second metacarpal bone, left hand

S62.312 Displaced fracture of base of third metacarpal bone, right hand

S62.313 Displaced fracture of base of third metacarpal bone, left hand

S62.314 Displaced fracture of base of fourth metacarpal bone, right hand

S62.315 Displaced fracture of base of fourth metacarpal bone, left hand

S62.316 Displaced fracture of base of fifth metacarpal bone, right hand

S62.317 Displaced fracture of base of fifth metacarpal bone, left hand

S62.318 Displaced fracture of base of other metacarpal bone
Displaced fracture of base of specified metacarpal bone with unspecified laterality

S62.319 Displaced fracture of base of unspecified metacarpal bone

S62.32 Displaced fracture of shaft of other metacarpal bone

S62.320 Displaced fracture of shaft of second metacarpal bone, right hand

S62.321 Displaced fracture of shaft of second metacarpal bone, left hand

S62.322 Displaced fracture of shaft of third metacarpal bone, right hand

S62.323 Displaced fracture of shaft of third metacarpal bone, left hand

S62.324 Displaced fracture of shaft of fourth metacarpal bone, right hand

S62.325 Displaced fracture of shaft of fourth metacarpal bone, left hand

S62.326 Displaced fracture of shaft of fifth metacarpal bone, right hand

S62.327 Displaced fracture of shaft of fifth metacarpal bone, left hand

S62.328 Displaced fracture of shaft of other metacarpal bone
Displaced fracture of shaft of specified metacarpal bone with unspecified laterality

S62.329 Displaced fracture of shaft of unspecified metacarpal bone

S62.33 Displaced fracture of neck of other metacarpal bone

S62.330 Displaced fracture of neck of second metacarpal bone, right hand

S62.331 Displaced fracture of neck of second metacarpal bone, left hand

S62.332 Displaced fracture of neck of third metacarpal bone, right hand

S62.333 Displaced fracture of neck of third metacarpal bone, left hand

S62.334 Displaced fracture of neck of fourth metacarpal bone, right hand

S62.335 Displaced fracture of neck of fourth metacarpal bone, left hand

S62.336 Displaced fracture of neck of fifth metacarpal bone, right hand

S62.337 Displaced fracture of neck of fifth metacarpal bone, left hand

S62.338 Displaced fracture of neck of other metacarpal bone
Displaced fracture of neck of specified metacarpal bone with unspecified laterality

S62.339 Displaced fracture of neck of unspecified metacarpal bone

S62.34 Nondisplaced fracture of base of other metacarpal bone

S62.340 Nondisplaced fracture of base of second metacarpal bone, right hand

S62.341 Nondisplaced fracture of base of second metacarpal bone, left hand

S62.342 Nondisplaced fracture of base of third metacarpal bone, right hand

S62.343 Nondisplaced fracture of base of third metacarpal bone, left hand

S62.344 Nondisplaced fracture of base of fourth metacarpal bone, right hand

S62.345 Nondisplaced fracture of base of fourth metacarpal bone, left hand

S62.346 Nondisplaced fracture of base of fifth metacarpal bone, right hand

S62.347 Nondisplaced fracture of base of fifth metacarpal bone, left hand

S62.348 Nondisplaced fracture of base of other metacarpal bone
Nondisplaced fracture of base of specified metacarpal bone with unspecified laterality

S62.349 Nondisplaced fracture of base of unspecified metacarpal bone

S62.35 Nondisplaced fracture of shaft of other metacarpal bone

S62.350 Nondisplaced fracture of shaft of second metacarpal bone, right hand

S62.351 Nondisplaced fracture of shaft of second metacarpal bone, left hand

S62.352 Nondisplaced fracture of shaft of third metacarpal bone, right hand

S62.353 Nondisplaced fracture of shaft of third metacarpal bone, left hand

S62.354 Nondisplaced fracture of shaft of fourth metacarpal bone, right hand

S62.355 Nondisplaced fracture of shaft of fourth metacarpal bone, left hand

S62.356 Nondisplaced fracture of shaft of fifth metacarpal bone, right hand

S62.357 Nondisplaced fracture of shaft of fifth metacarpal bone, left hand

S62.358 Nondisplaced fracture of shaft of other metacarpal bone
Nondisplaced fracture of shaft of specified metacarpal bone with unspecified laterality

S62.359 Nondisplaced fracture of shaft of unspecified metacarpal bone

S62.36 Nondisplaced fracture of neck of other metacarpal bone

S62.360 Nondisplaced fracture of neck of second metacarpal bone, right hand

S62.361 Nondisplaced fracture of neck of second metacarpal bone, left hand

S62.362 Nondisplaced fracture of neck of third metacarpal bone, right hand

S62.363 Nondisplaced fracture of neck of third metacarpal bone, left hand

S62.364 Nondisplaced fracture of neck of fourth metacarpal bone, right hand

S62.365 Nondisplaced fracture of neck of fourth metacarpal bone, left hand

S62.366 Nondisplaced fracture of neck of fifth metacarpal bone, right hand

S62.367 Nondisplaced fracture of neck of fifth metacarpal bone, left hand

S62.368 Nondisplaced fracture of neck of other metacarpal bone
Nondisplaced fracture of neck of specified metacarpal bone with unspecified laterality

S62.369 Nondisplaced fracture of neck of unspecified metacarpal bone

S62.39 Other fracture of other metacarpal bone

S62.390 Other fracture of second metacarpal bone, right hand

S62.391 Other fracture of second metacarpal bone, left hand

S62.392 Other fracture of third metacarpal bone, right hand

S62.393 Other fracture of third metacarpal bone, left hand

S62.394 Other fracture of fourth metacarpal bone, right hand

S62.395 Other fracture of fourth metacarpal bone, left hand

S62.396 Other fracture of fifth metacarpal bone, right hand

S62.397 Other fracture of fifth metacarpal bone, left hand

S62.398 Other fracture of other metacarpal bone
Other fracture of specified metacarpal bone with unspecified laterality

S62.399 Other fracture of unspecified metacarpal bone

S62.5 Fracture of thumb

S62.50 Fracture of unspecified phalanx of thumb

S62.501 Fracture of unspecified phalanx of right thumb

S62.502 Fracture of unspecified phalanx of left thumb

S62.509 Fracture of unspecified phalanx of unspecified thumb

S62.51 Fracture of proximal phalanx of thumb

S62.511 Displaced fracture of proximal phalanx of right thumb

S62.512 Displaced fracture of proximal phalanx of left thumb

S62.513 Displaced fracture of proximal phalanx of unspecified thumb

S62.514 Nondisplaced fracture of proximal phalanx of right thumb

S62.515 Nondisplaced fracture of proximal phalanx of left thumb

S62.516 Nondisplaced fracture of proximal phalanx of unspecified thumb

S62.52 Fracture of distal phalanx of thumb

S62.521 Displaced fracture of distal phalanx of right thumb

S62.522 Displaced fracture of distal phalanx of left thumb

S62.523 Displaced fracture of distal phalanx of unspecified thumb

S62.524 Nondisplaced fracture of distal phalanx of right thumb

S62.525 Nondisplaced fracture of distal phalanx of left thumb

S62.526 Nondisplaced fracture of distal phalanx of unspecified thumb

S62.6 Fracture of other and unspecified finger(s)

EXCLUDES 2 *fracture of thumb (S62.5-)*

S62.60 Fracture of unspecified phalanx of finger

S62.600 Fracture of unspecified phalanx of right index finger

S62.601 Fracture of unspecified phalanx of left index finger

S62.602 Fracture of unspecified phalanx of right middle finger

S62.603 Fracture of unspecified phalanx of left middle finger

S62.604 Fracture of unspecified phalanx of right ring finger

S62.605 Fracture of unspecified phalanx of left ring finger

S62.606 Fracture of unspecified phalanx of right little finger

S62.607 Fracture of unspecified phalanx of left little finger

S62.608 Fracture of unspecified phalanx of other finger
Fracture of unspecified phalanx of specified finger with unspecified laterality

S62.609 Fracture of unspecified phalanx of unspecified finger

S62.61 Displaced fracture of proximal phalanx of finger

S62.610 Displaced fracture of proximal phalanx of right index finger

S62.611 Displaced fracture of proximal phalanx of left index finger

S62.612 Displaced fracture of proximal phalanx of right middle finger

S62.613 Displaced fracture of proximal phalanx of left middle finger

S62.614 Displaced fracture of proximal phalanx of right ring finger

S62.615 Displaced fracture of proximal phalanx of left ring finger

S62.616 Displaced fracture of proximal phalanx of right little finger

S62.617 Displaced fracture of proximal phalanx of left little finger

S62.618 Displaced fracture of proximal phalanx of other finger
Displaced fracture of proximal phalanx of specified finger with unspecified laterality

S62.619 Displaced fracture of proximal phalanx of unspecified finger

S62.62 Displaced fracture of middle phalanx of finger

S62.620 Displaced fracture of middle phalanx of right index finger

S62.621 Displaced fracture of middle phalanx of left index finger

S62.622 Displaced fracture of middle phalanx of right middle finger

S62.623 Displaced fracture of middle phalanx of left middle finger

S62.624 Displaced fracture of middle phalanx of right ring finger

S62.625 Displaced fracture of middle phalanx of left ring finger

S62.626 Displaced fracture of middle phalanx of right little finger

S62.627 Displaced fracture of middle phalanx of left little finger

S62.628 Displaced fracture of middle phalanx of other finger
Displaced fracture of middle phalanx of specified finger with unspecified laterality

S62.629 Displaced fracture of middle phalanx of unspecified finger

S62.63 Displaced fracture of distal phalanx of finger

S62.630 Displaced fracture of distal phalanx of right index finger

S62.631 Displaced fracture of distal phalanx of left index finger

S62.632 Displaced fracture of distal phalanx of right middle finger

S62.633 Displaced fracture of distal phalanx of left middle finger

S62.634 Displaced fracture of distal phalanx of right ring finger

S62.635 Displaced fracture of distal phalanx of left ring finger

S62.636 Displaced fracture of distal phalanx of right little finger

S62.637 Displaced fracture of distal phalanx of left little finger

S62.638 Displaced fracture of distal phalanx of other finger
Displaced fracture of distal phalanx of specified finger with unspecified laterality

S62.639 Displaced fracture of distal phalanx of unspecified finger

S62.64 Nondisplaced fracture of proximal phalanx of finger

S62.640 Nondisplaced fracture of proximal phalanx of right index finger

S62.641 Nondisplaced fracture of proximal phalanx of left index finger

S62.642 Nondisplaced fracture of proximal phalanx of right middle finger

S62.643 Nondisplaced fracture of proximal phalanx of left middle finger

S62.644 **Nondisplaced fracture of proximal phalanx of right ring finger**

S62.645 **Nondisplaced fracture of proximal phalanx of left ring finger**

S62.646 **Nondisplaced fracture of proximal phalanx of right little finger**

S62.647 **Nondisplaced fracture of proximal phalanx of left little finger**

S62.648 **Nondisplaced fracture of proximal phalanx of other finger**

Nondisplaced fracture of proximal phalanx of specified finger with unspecified laterality

S62.649 **Nondisplaced fracture of proximal phalanx of unspecified finger**

S62.65 **Nondisplaced fracture of middle phalanx of finger**

S62.650 **Nondisplaced fracture of middle phalanx of right index finger**

S62.651 **Nondisplaced fracture of middle phalanx of left index finger**

S62.652 **Nondisplaced fracture of middle phalanx of right middle finger**

S62.653 **Nondisplaced fracture of middle phalanx of left middle finger**

S62.654 **Nondisplaced fracture of middle phalanx of right ring finger**

S62.655 **Nondisplaced fracture of middle phalanx of left ring finger**

S62.656 **Nondisplaced fracture of middle phalanx of right little finger**

S62.657 **Nondisplaced fracture of middle phalanx of left little finger**

S62.658 **Nondisplaced fracture of middle phalanx of other finger**

Nondisplaced fracture of middle phalanx of specified finger with unspecified laterality

S62.659 **Nondisplaced fracture of middle phalanx of unspecified finger**

S62.66 **Nondisplaced fracture of distal phalanx of finger**

S62.660 **Nondisplaced fracture of distal phalanx of right index finger**

S62.661 **Nondisplaced fracture of distal phalanx of left index finger**

S62.662 **Nondisplaced fracture of distal phalanx of right middle finger**

S62.663 **Nondisplaced fracture of distal phalanx of left middle finger**

S62.664 **Nondisplaced fracture of distal phalanx of right ring finger**

S62.665 **Nondisplaced fracture of distal phalanx of left ring finger**

S62.666 **Nondisplaced fracture of distal phalanx of right little finger**

S62.667 **Nondisplaced fracture of distal phalanx of left little finger**

S62.668 **Nondisplaced fracture of distal phalanx of other finger**

Nondisplaced fracture of distal phalanx of specified finger with unspecified laterality

S62.669 **Nondisplaced fracture of distal phalanx of unspecified finger**

S62.9 **Unspecified fracture of wrist and hand**

S62.90 **Unspecified fracture of unspecified wrist and hand** Q

S62.91 **Unspecified fracture of right wrist and hand** Q

S62.92 **Unspecified fracture of left wrist and hand** Q

S63 Dislocation and sprain of joints and ligaments at wrist and hand level

INCLUDES avulsion of joint or ligament at wrist and hand level
laceration of cartilage, joint or ligament at wrist and hand level
sprain of cartilage, joint or ligament at wrist and hand level
traumatic hemarthrosis of joint or ligament at wrist and hand level
traumatic rupture of joint or ligament at wrist and hand level
traumatic subluxation of joint or ligament at wrist and hand level
traumatic tear of joint or ligament at wrist and hand level

Code also any associated open wound

EXCLUDES 2 *strain of muscle, fascia and tendon of wrist and hand (S66.-)*

The appropriate 7th character is to be added to each code from category S63.
A initial encounter
D subsequent encounter
S sequela

S63.0 **Subluxation and dislocation of wrist and hand joints**

S63.00 **Unspecified subluxation and dislocation of wrist and hand**

Dislocation of carpal bone NOS
Dislocation of distal end of radius NOS
Subluxation of carpal bone NOS
Subluxation of distal end of radius NOS

S63.001 **Unspecified subluxation of right wrist and hand**

S63.002 **Unspecified subluxation of left wrist and hand**

S63.003 **Unspecified subluxation of unspecified wrist and hand**

S63.004 **Unspecified dislocation of right wrist and hand**

S63.005 **Unspecified dislocation of left wrist and hand**

S63.006 **Unspecified dislocation of unspecified wrist and hand**

S63.01 **Subluxation and dislocation of distal radioulnar joint**

S63.011 **Subluxation of distal radioulnar joint of right wrist**

S63.012 **Subluxation of distal radioulnar joint of left wrist**

S63.013 **Subluxation of distal radioulnar joint of unspecified wrist**

S63.014 **Dislocation of distal radioulnar joint of right wrist**

S63.015 **Dislocation of distal radioulnar joint of left wrist**

S63.016 **Dislocation of distal radioulnar joint of unspecified wrist**

S63.02 **Subluxation and dislocation of radiocarpal joint**

S63.021 **Subluxation of radiocarpal joint of right wrist**

S63.022 **Subluxation of radiocarpal joint of left wrist**

S63.023 **Subluxation of radiocarpal joint of unspecified wrist**

S63.024 **Dislocation of radiocarpal joint of right wrist**

S63.025 **Dislocation of radiocarpal joint of left wrist**

S63.026 **Dislocation of radiocarpal joint of unspecified wrist**

S63.03 **Subluxation and dislocation of midcarpal joint**

S63.031 **Subluxation of midcarpal joint of right wrist**

S63.032 **Subluxation of midcarpal joint of left wrist**

S63.033 **Subluxation of midcarpal joint of unspecified wrist**

S63.034 **Dislocation of midcarpal joint of right wrist**

S63.035 **Dislocation of midcarpal joint of left wrist**

S63.036 **Dislocation of midcarpal joint of unspecified wrist**

S63.04 Subluxation and dislocation of carpometacarpal joint of thumb
EXCLUDES 2 *interphalangeal subluxation and dislocation of thumb (S63.1-)*
S63.041 Subluxation of carpometacarpal joint of right thumb
S63.042 Subluxation of carpometacarpal joint of left thumb
S63.043 Subluxation of carpometacarpal joint of unspecified thumb
S63.044 Dislocation of carpometacarpal joint of right thumb
S63.045 Dislocation of carpometacarpal joint of left thumb
S63.046 Dislocation of carpometacarpal joint of unspecified thumb
S63.05 Subluxation and dislocation of other carpometacarpal joint
EXCLUDES 2 *subluxation and dislocation of carpometacarpal joint of thumb (S63.04-)*
S63.051 Subluxation of other carpometacarpal joint of right hand
S63.052 Subluxation of other carpometacarpal joint of left hand
S63.053 Subluxation of other carpometacarpal joint of unspecified hand
S63.054 Dislocation of other carpometacarpal joint of right hand
S63.055 Dislocation of other carpometacarpal joint of left hand
S63.056 Dislocation of other carpometacarpal joint of unspecified hand
S63.06 Subluxation and dislocation of metacarpal (bone), proximal end
S63.061 Subluxation of metacarpal (bone), proximal end of right hand
S63.062 Subluxation of metacarpal (bone), proximal end of left hand
S63.063 Subluxation of metacarpal (bone), proximal end of unspecified hand
S63.064 Dislocation of metacarpal (bone), proximal end of right hand
S63.065 Dislocation of metacarpal (bone), proximal end of left hand
S63.066 Dislocation of metacarpal (bone), proximal end of unspecified hand
S63.07 Subluxation and dislocation of distal end of ulna
S63.071 Subluxation of distal end of right ulna
S63.072 Subluxation of distal end of left ulna
S63.073 Subluxation of distal end of unspecified ulna
S63.074 Dislocation of distal end of right ulna
S63.075 Dislocation of distal end of left ulna
S63.076 Dislocation of distal end of unspecified ulna
S63.09 Other subluxation and dislocation of wrist and hand
S63.091 Other subluxation of right wrist and hand
S63.092 Other subluxation of left wrist and hand
S63.093 Other subluxation of unspecified wrist and hand
S63.094 Other dislocation of right wrist and hand
S63.095 Other dislocation of left wrist and hand
S63.096 Other dislocation of unspecified wrist and hand
S63.1 Subluxation and dislocation of thumb
S63.10 Unspecified subluxation and dislocation of thumb
S63.101 Unspecified subluxation of right thumb
S63.102 Unspecified subluxation of left thumb
S63.103 Unspecified subluxation of unspecified thumb
S63.104 Unspecified dislocation of right thumb
S63.105 Unspecified dislocation of left thumb
S63.106 Unspecified dislocation of unspecified thumb
S63.11 Subluxation and dislocation of metacarpophalangeal joint of thumb
S63.111 Subluxation of metacarpophalangeal joint of right thumb
S63.112 Subluxation of metacarpophalangeal joint of left thumb
S63.113 Subluxation of metacarpophalangeal joint of unspecified thumb
S63.114 Dislocation of metacarpophalangeal joint of right thumb
S63.115 Dislocation of metacarpophalangeal joint of left thumb
S63.116 Dislocation of metacarpophalangeal joint of unspecified thumb
S63.12 Subluxation and dislocation of interphalangeal joint of thumb
S63.121 Subluxation of interphalangeal joint of right thumb
S63.122 Subluxation of interphalangeal joint of left thumb
S63.123 Subluxation of interphalangeal joint of unspecified thumb
S63.124 Dislocation of interphalangeal joint of right thumb
S63.125 Dislocation of interphalangeal joint of left thumb
S63.126 Dislocation of interphalangeal joint of unspecified thumb
S63.2 Subluxation and dislocation of other finger(s)
EXCLUDES 2 *subluxation and dislocation of thumb (S63.1-)*
S63.20 Unspecified subluxation of other finger
S63.200 Unspecified subluxation of right index finger
S63.201 Unspecified subluxation of left index finger
S63.202 Unspecified subluxation of right middle finger
S63.203 Unspecified subluxation of left middle finger
S63.204 Unspecified subluxation of right ring finger
S63.205 Unspecified subluxation of left ring finger
S63.206 Unspecified subluxation of right little finger
S63.207 Unspecified subluxation of left little finger
S63.208 Unspecified subluxation of other finger
Unspecified subluxation of specified finger with unspecified laterality
S63.209 Unspecified subluxation of unspecified finger
S63.21 Subluxation of metacarpophalangeal joint of finger
S63.210 Subluxation of metacarpophalangeal joint of right index finger
S63.211 Subluxation of metacarpophalangeal joint of left index finger
S63.212 Subluxation of metacarpophalangeal joint of right middle finger
S63.213 Subluxation of metacarpophalangeal joint of left middle finger
S63.214 Subluxation of metacarpophalangeal joint of right ring finger
S63.215 Subluxation of metacarpophalangeal joint of left ring finger
S63.216 Subluxation of metacarpophalangeal joint of right little finger
S63.217 Subluxation of metacarpophalangeal joint of left little finger
S63.218 Subluxation of metacarpophalangeal joint of other finger
Subluxation of metacarpophalangeal joint of specified finger with unspecified laterality
S63.219 Subluxation of metacarpophalangeal joint of unspecified finger
S63.22 Subluxation of unspecified interphalangeal joint of finger
S63.220 Subluxation of unspecified interphalangeal joint of right index finger
S63.221 Subluxation of unspecified interphalangeal joint of left index finger
S63.222 Subluxation of unspecified interphalangeal joint of right middle finger
S63.223 Subluxation of unspecified interphalangeal joint of left middle finger

Chapter 19. Injury, Poisoning and Certain Other Consequences of External Causes S63.04–S63.223

√7th **S63.224 Subluxation of unspecified interphalangeal joint of right ring finger**

√7th **S63.225 Subluxation of unspecified interphalangeal joint of left ring finger**

√7th **S63.226 Subluxation of unspecified interphalangeal joint of right little finger**

√7th **S63.227 Subluxation of unspecified interphalangeal joint of left little finger**

√7th **S63.228 Subluxation of unspecified interphalangeal joint of other finger**

Subluxation of unspecified interphalangeal joint of specified finger with unspecified laterality

√7th **S63.229 Subluxation of unspecified interphalangeal joint of unspecified finger**

√6th **S63.23 Subluxation of proximal interphalangeal joint of finger**

√7th **S63.230 Subluxation of proximal interphalangeal joint of right index finger**

√7th **S63.231 Subluxation of proximal interphalangeal joint of left index finger**

√7th **S63.232 Subluxation of proximal interphalangeal joint of right middle finger**

√7th **S63.233 Subluxation of proximal interphalangeal joint of left middle finger**

√7th **S63.234 Subluxation of proximal interphalangeal joint of right ring finger**

√7th **S63.235 Subluxation of proximal interphalangeal joint of left ring finger**

√7th **S63.236 Subluxation of proximal interphalangeal joint of right little finger**

√7th **S63.237 Subluxation of proximal interphalangeal joint of left little finger**

√7th **S63.238 Subluxation of proximal interphalangeal joint of other finger**

Subluxation of proximal interphalangeal joint of specified finger with unspecified laterality

√7th **S63.239 Subluxation of proximal interphalangeal joint of unspecified finger**

√6th **S63.24 Subluxation of distal interphalangeal joint of finger**

√7th **S63.240 Subluxation of distal interphalangeal joint of right index finger**

√7th **S63.241 Subluxation of distal interphalangeal joint of left index finger**

√7th **S63.242 Subluxation of distal interphalangeal joint of right middle finger**

√7th **S63.243 Subluxation of distal interphalangeal joint of left middle finger**

√7th **S63.244 Subluxation of distal interphalangeal joint of right ring finger**

√7th **S63.245 Subluxation of distal interphalangeal joint of left ring finger**

√7th **S63.246 Subluxation of distal interphalangeal joint of right little finger**

√7th **S63.247 Subluxation of distal interphalangeal joint of left little finger**

√7th **S63.248 Subluxation of distal interphalangeal joint of other finger**

Subluxation of distal interphalangeal joint of specified finger with unspecified laterality

√7th **S63.249 Subluxation of distal interphalangeal joint of unspecified finger**

√6th **S63.25 Unspecified dislocation of other finger**

√7th **S63.250 Unspecified dislocation of right index finger**

√7th **S63.251 Unspecified dislocation of left index finger**

√7th **S63.252 Unspecified dislocation of right middle finger**

√7th **S63.253 Unspecified dislocation of left middle finger**

√7th **S63.254 Unspecified dislocation of right ring finger**

√7th **S63.255 Unspecified dislocation of left ring finger**

√7th **S63.256 Unspecified dislocation of right little finger**

√7th **S63.257 Unspecified dislocation of left little finger**

√7th **S63.258 Unspecified dislocation of other finger**

Unspecified dislocation of specified finger with unspecified laterality

√7th **S63.259 Unspecified dislocation of unspecified finger**

Unspecified dislocation of unspecified finger with unspecified laterality

√6th **S63.26 Dislocation of metacarpophalangeal joint of finger**

√7th **S63.260 Dislocation of metacarpophalangeal joint of right index finger**

√7th **S63.261 Dislocation of metacarpophalangeal joint of left index finger**

√7th **S63.262 Dislocation of metacarpophalangeal joint of right middle finger**

√7th **S63.263 Dislocation of metacarpophalangeal joint of left middle finger**

√7th **S63.264 Dislocation of metacarpophalangeal joint of right ring finger**

√7th **S63.265 Dislocation of metacarpophalangeal joint of left ring finger**

√7th **S63.266 Dislocation of metacarpophalangeal joint of right little finger**

√7th **S63.267 Dislocation of metacarpophalangeal joint of left little finger**

√7th **S63.268 Dislocation of metacarpophalangeal joint of other finger**

Dislocation of metacarpophalangeal joint of specified finger with unspecified laterality

√7th **S63.269 Dislocation of metacarpophalangeal joint of unspecified finger**

√6th **S63.27 Dislocation of unspecified interphalangeal joint of finger**

√7th **S63.270 Dislocation of unspecified interphalangeal joint of right index finger**

√7th **S63.271 Dislocation of unspecified interphalangeal joint of left index finger**

√7th **S63.272 Dislocation of unspecified interphalangeal joint of right middle finger**

√7th **S63.273 Dislocation of unspecified interphalangeal joint of left middle finger**

√7th **S63.274 Dislocation of unspecified interphalangeal joint of right ring finger**

√7th **S63.275 Dislocation of unspecified interphalangeal joint of left ring finger**

√7th **S63.276 Dislocation of unspecified interphalangeal joint of right little finger**

√7th **S63.277 Dislocation of unspecified interphalangeal joint of left little finger**

√7th **S63.278 Dislocation of unspecified interphalangeal joint of other finger**

Dislocation of unspecified interphalangeal joint of specified finger with unspecified laterality

√7th **S63.279 Dislocation of unspecified interphalangeal joint of unspecified finger**

Dislocation of unspecified interphalangeal joint of unspecified finger without specified laterality

√6th **S63.28 Dislocation of proximal interphalangeal joint of finger**

√7th **S63.280 Dislocation of proximal interphalangeal joint of right index finger**

√7th **S63.281 Dislocation of proximal interphalangeal joint of left index finger**

√7th **S63.282 Dislocation of proximal interphalangeal joint of right middle finger**

√7th **S63.283 Dislocation of proximal interphalangeal joint of left middle finger**

√7th **S63.284 Dislocation of proximal interphalangeal joint of right ring finger**

√7th **S63.285 Dislocation of proximal interphalangeal joint of left ring finger**

√7th **S63.286 Dislocation of proximal interphalangeal joint of right little finger**

√7th **S63.287 Dislocation of proximal interphalangeal joint of left little finger**

S63.288 Dislocation of proximal interphalangeal joint of other finger
Dislocation of proximal interphalangeal joint of specified finger with unspecified laterality

S63.289 Dislocation of proximal interphalangeal joint of unspecified finger

S63.29 Dislocation of distal interphalangeal joint of finger

S63.290 Dislocation of distal interphalangeal joint of right index finger

S63.291 Dislocation of distal interphalangeal joint of left index finger

S63.292 Dislocation of distal interphalangeal joint of right middle finger

S63.293 Dislocation of distal interphalangeal joint of left middle finger

S63.294 Dislocation of distal interphalangeal joint of right ring finger

S63.295 Dislocation of distal interphalangeal joint of left ring finger

S63.296 Dislocation of distal interphalangeal joint of right little finger

S63.297 Dislocation of distal interphalangeal joint of left little finger

S63.298 Dislocation of distal interphalangeal joint of other finger
Dislocation of distal interphalangeal joint of specified finger with unspecified laterality

S63.299 Dislocation of distal interphalangeal joint of unspecified finger

S63.3 Traumatic rupture of ligament of wrist

S63.30 Traumatic rupture of unspecified ligament of wrist

S63.301 Traumatic rupture of unspecified ligament of right wrist

S63.302 Traumatic rupture of unspecified ligament of left wrist

S63.309 Traumatic rupture of unspecified ligament of unspecified wrist

S63.31 Traumatic rupture of collateral ligament of wrist

S63.311 Traumatic rupture of collateral ligament of right wrist

S63.312 Traumatic rupture of collateral ligament of left wrist

S63.319 Traumatic rupture of collateral ligament of unspecified wrist

S63.32 Traumatic rupture of radiocarpal ligament

S63.321 Traumatic rupture of right radiocarpal ligament

S63.322 Traumatic rupture of left radiocarpal ligament

S63.329 Traumatic rupture of unspecified radiocarpal ligament

S63.33 Traumatic rupture of ulnocarpal (palmar) ligament

S63.331 Traumatic rupture of right ulnocarpal (palmar) ligament

S63.332 Traumatic rupture of left ulnocarpal (palmar) ligament

S63.339 Traumatic rupture of unspecified ulnocarpal (palmar) ligament

S63.39 Traumatic rupture of other ligament of wrist

S63.391 Traumatic rupture of other ligament of right wrist

S63.392 Traumatic rupture of other ligament of left wrist

S63.399 Traumatic rupture of other ligament of unspecified wrist

S63.4 Traumatic rupture of ligament of finger at metacarpophalangeal and interphalangeal joint(s)

S63.40 Traumatic rupture of unspecified ligament of finger at metacarpophalangeal and interphalangeal joint

S63.400 Traumatic rupture of unspecified ligament of right index finger at metacarpophalangeal and interphalangeal joint

S63.401 Traumatic rupture of unspecified ligament of left index finger at metacarpophalangeal and interphalangeal joint

S63.402 Traumatic rupture of unspecified ligament of right middle finger at metacarpophalangeal and interphalangeal joint

S63.403 Traumatic rupture of unspecified ligament of left middle finger at metacarpophalangeal and interphalangeal joint

S63.404 Traumatic rupture of unspecified ligament of right ring finger at metacarpophalangeal and interphalangeal joint

S63.405 Traumatic rupture of unspecified ligament of left ring finger at metacarpophalangeal and interphalangeal joint

S63.406 Traumatic rupture of unspecified ligament of right little finger at metacarpophalangeal and interphalangeal joint

S63.407 Traumatic rupture of unspecified ligament of left little finger at metacarpophalangeal and interphalangeal joint

S63.408 Traumatic rupture of unspecified ligament of other finger at metacarpophalangeal and interphalangeal joint
Traumatic rupture of unspecified ligament of specified finger with unspecified laterality at metacarpophalangeal and interphalangeal joint

S63.409 Traumatic rupture of unspecified ligament of unspecified finger at metacarpophalangeal and interphalangeal joint

S63.41 Traumatic rupture of collateral ligament of finger at metacarpophalangeal and interphalangeal joint

S63.410 Traumatic rupture of collateral ligament of right index finger at metacarpophalangeal and interphalangeal joint

S63.411 Traumatic rupture of collateral ligament of left index finger at metacarpophalangeal and interphalangeal joint

S63.412 Traumatic rupture of collateral ligament of right middle finger at metacarpophalangeal and interphalangeal joint

S63.413 Traumatic rupture of collateral ligament of left middle finger at metacarpophalangeal and interphalangeal joint

S63.414 Traumatic rupture of collateral ligament of right ring finger at metacarpophalangeal and interphalangeal joint

S63.415 Traumatic rupture of collateral ligament of left ring finger at metacarpophalangeal and interphalangeal joint

S63.416 Traumatic rupture of collateral ligament of right little finger at metacarpophalangeal and interphalangeal joint

S63.417 Traumatic rupture of collateral ligament of left little finger at metacarpophalangeal and interphalangeal joint

S63.418 Traumatic rupture of collateral ligament of other finger at metacarpophalangeal and interphalangeal joint
Traumatic rupture of collateral ligament of specified finger with unspecified laterality at metacarpophalangeal and interphalangeal joint

S63.419 Traumatic rupture of collateral ligament of unspecified finger at metacarpophalangeal and interphalangeal joint

6th **S63.42 Traumatic rupture of palmar ligament of finger at metacarpophalangeal and interphalangeal joint**

7th **S63.420 Traumatic rupture of palmar ligament of right index finger at metacarpophalangeal and interphalangeal joint**

7th **S63.421 Traumatic rupture of palmar ligament of left index finger at metacarpophalangeal and interphalangeal joint**

7th **S63.422 Traumatic rupture of palmar ligament of right middle finger at metacarpophalangeal and interphalangeal joint**

7th **S63.423 Traumatic rupture of palmar ligament of left middle finger at metacarpophalangeal and interphalangeal joint**

7th **S63.424 Traumatic rupture of palmar ligament of right ring finger at metacarpophalangeal and interphalangeal joint**

7th **S63.425 Traumatic rupture of palmar ligament of left ring finger at metacarpophalangeal and interphalangeal joint**

7th **S63.426 Traumatic rupture of palmar ligament of right little finger at metacarpophalangeal and interphalangeal joint**

7th **S63.427 Traumatic rupture of palmar ligament of left little finger at metacarpophalangeal and interphalangeal joint**

7th **S63.428 Traumatic rupture of palmar ligament of other finger at metacarpophalangeal and interphalangeal joint**

Traumatic rupture of palmar ligament of specified finger with unspecified laterality at metacarpophalangeal and interphalangeal joint

7th **S63.429 Traumatic rupture of palmar ligament of unspecified finger at metacarpophalangeal and interphalangeal joint**

6th **S63.43 Traumatic rupture of volar plate of finger at metacarpophalangeal and interphalangeal joint**

7th **S63.430 Traumatic rupture of volar plate of right index finger at metacarpophalangeal and interphalangeal joint**

7th **S63.431 Traumatic rupture of volar plate of left index finger at metacarpophalangeal and interphalangeal joint**

7th **S63.432 Traumatic rupture of volar plate of right middle finger at metacarpophalangeal and interphalangeal joint**

7th **S63.433 Traumatic rupture of volar plate of left middle finger at metacarpophalangeal and interphalangeal joint**

7th **S63.434 Traumatic rupture of volar plate of right ring finger at metacarpophalangeal and interphalangeal joint**

7th **S63.435 Traumatic rupture of volar plate of left ring finger at metacarpophalangeal and interphalangeal joint**

7th **S63.436 Traumatic rupture of volar plate of right little finger at metacarpophalangeal and interphalangeal joint**

7th **S63.437 Traumatic rupture of volar plate of left little finger at metacarpophalangeal and interphalangeal joint**

7th **S63.438 Traumatic rupture of volar plate of other finger at metacarpophalangeal and interphalangeal joint**

Traumatic rupture of volar plate of specified finger with unspecified laterality at metacarpophalangeal and interphalangeal joint

7th **S63.439 Traumatic rupture of volar plate of unspecified finger at metacarpophalangeal and interphalangeal joint**

6th **S63.49 Traumatic rupture of other ligament of finger at metacarpophalangeal and interphalangeal joint**

7th **S63.490 Traumatic rupture of other ligament of right index finger at metacarpophalangeal and interphalangeal joint**

7th **S63.491 Traumatic rupture of other ligament of left index finger at metacarpophalangeal and interphalangeal joint**

7th **S63.492 Traumatic rupture of other ligament of right middle finger at metacarpophalangeal and interphalangeal joint**

7th **S63.493 Traumatic rupture of other ligament of left middle finger at metacarpophalangeal and interphalangeal joint**

7th **S63.494 Traumatic rupture of other ligament of right ring finger at metacarpophalangeal and interphalangeal joint**

7th **S63.495 Traumatic rupture of other ligament of left ring finger at metacarpophalangeal and interphalangeal joint**

7th **S63.496 Traumatic rupture of other ligament of right little finger at metacarpophalangeal and interphalangeal joint**

7th **S63.497 Traumatic rupture of other ligament of left little finger at metacarpophalangeal and interphalangeal joint**

7th **S63.498 Traumatic rupture of other ligament of other finger at metacarpophalangeal and interphalangeal joint**

Traumatic rupture of ligament of specified finger with unspecified laterality at metacarpophalangeal and interphalangeal joint

7th **S63.499 Traumatic rupture of other ligament of unspecified finger at metacarpophalangeal and interphalangeal joint**

5th **S63.5 Other and unspecified sprain of wrist**

6th **S63.50 Unspecified sprain of wrist**

7th **S63.501 Unspecified sprain of right wrist**

7th **S63.502 Unspecified sprain of left wrist**

7th **S63.509 Unspecified sprain of unspecified wrist**

6th **S63.51 Sprain of carpal (joint)**

7th **S63.511 Sprain of carpal joint of right wrist**

7th **S63.512 Sprain of carpal joint of left wrist**

7th **S63.519 Sprain of carpal joint of unspecified wrist**

6th **S63.52 Sprain of radiocarpal joint**

EXCLUDES 1 *traumatic rupture of radiocarpal ligament (S63.32-)*

7th **S63.521 Sprain of radiocarpal joint of right wrist**

7th **S63.522 Sprain of radiocarpal joint of left wrist**

7th **S63.529 Sprain of radiocarpal joint of unspecified wrist**

6th **S63.59 Other specified sprain of wrist**

7th **S63.591 Other specified sprain of right wrist**

7th **S63.592 Other specified sprain of left wrist**

7th **S63.599 Other specified sprain of unspecified wrist**

5th **S63.6 Other and unspecified sprain of finger(s)**

EXCLUDES 1 *traumatic rupture of ligament of finger at metacarpophalangeal and interphalangeal joint(s) (S63.4-)*

6th **S63.60 Unspecified sprain of thumb**

7th **S63.601 Unspecified sprain of right thumb**

7th **S63.602 Unspecified sprain of left thumb**

7th **S63.609 Unspecified sprain of unspecified thumb**

6th **S63.61 Unspecified sprain of other and unspecified finger(s)**

7th **S63.610 Unspecified sprain of right index finger**

7th **S63.611 Unspecified sprain of left index finger**

7th **S63.612 Unspecified sprain of right middle finger**

7th **S63.613 Unspecified sprain of left middle finger**

7th **S63.614 Unspecified sprain of right ring finger**

7th **S63.615 Unspecified sprain of left ring finger**

7th **S63.616 Unspecified sprain of right little finger**

7th **S63.617 Unspecified sprain of left little finger**

S63.618 Unspecified sprain of other finger
Unspecified sprain of specified finger with unspecified laterality
S63.619 Unspecified sprain of unspecified finger
S63.62 Sprain of interphalangeal joint of thumb
S63.621 Sprain of interphalangeal joint of right thumb
S63.622 Sprain of interphalangeal joint of left thumb
S63.629 Sprain of interphalangeal joint of unspecified thumb
S63.63 Sprain of interphalangeal joint of other and unspecified finger(s)
S63.630 Sprain of interphalangeal joint of right index finger
S63.631 Sprain of interphalangeal joint of left index finger
S63.632 Sprain of interphalangeal joint of right middle finger
S63.633 Sprain of interphalangeal joint of left middle finger
S63.634 Sprain of interphalangeal joint of right ring finger
S63.635 Sprain of interphalangeal joint of left ring finger
S63.636 Sprain of interphalangeal joint of right little finger
S63.637 Sprain of interphalangeal joint of left little finger
S63.638 Sprain of interphalangeal joint of other finger
S63.639 Sprain of interphalangeal joint of unspecified finger
S63.64 Sprain of metacarpophalangeal joint of thumb
S63.641 Sprain of metacarpophalangeal joint of right thumb
S63.642 Sprain of metacarpophalangeal joint of left thumb
S63.649 Sprain of metacarpophalangeal joint of unspecified thumb
S63.65 Sprain of metacarpophalangeal joint of other and unspecified finger(s)
S63.650 Sprain of metacarpophalangeal joint of right index finger
S63.651 Sprain of metacarpophalangeal joint of left index finger
S63.652 Sprain of metacarpophalangeal joint of right middle finger
S63.653 Sprain of metacarpophalangeal joint of left middle finger
S63.654 Sprain of metacarpophalangeal joint of right ring finger
S63.655 Sprain of metacarpophalangeal joint of left ring finger
S63.656 Sprain of metacarpophalangeal joint of right little finger
S63.657 Sprain of metacarpophalangeal joint of left little finger
S63.658 Sprain of metacarpophalangeal joint of other finger
Sprain of metacarpophalangeal joint of specified finger with unspecified laterality
S63.659 Sprain of metacarpophalangeal joint of unspecified finger
S63.68 Other sprain of thumb
S63.681 Other sprain of right thumb
S63.682 Other sprain of left thumb
S63.689 Other sprain of unspecified thumb
S63.69 Other sprain of other and unspecified finger(s)
S63.690 Other sprain of right index finger
S63.691 Other sprain of left index finger
S63.692 Other sprain of right middle finger
S63.693 Other sprain of left middle finger
S63.694 Other sprain of right ring finger
S63.695 Other sprain of left ring finger
S63.696 Other sprain of right little finger
S63.697 Other sprain of left little finger
S63.698 Other sprain of other finger
Other sprain of specified finger with unspecified laterality
S63.699 Other sprain of unspecified finger
S63.8 Sprain of other part of wrist and hand
S63.8X Sprain of other part of wrist and hand
S63.8X1 Sprain of other part of right wrist and hand
S63.8X2 Sprain of other part of left wrist and hand
S63.8X9 Sprain of other part of unspecified wrist and hand
S63.9 Sprain of unspecified part of wrist and hand
S63.90 Sprain of unspecified part of unspecified wrist and hand
S63.91 Sprain of unspecified part of right wrist and hand
S63.92 Sprain of unspecified part of left wrist and hand

S64 Injury of nerves at wrist and hand level

Code also any associated open wound (S61.-)

The appropriate 7th character is to be added to each code from category S64.
A initial encounter
D subsequent encounter
S sequela

S64.0 Injury of ulnar nerve at wrist and hand level
S64.00 Injury of ulnar nerve at wrist and hand level of unspecified arm
S64.01 Injury of ulnar nerve at wrist and hand level of right arm
S64.02 Injury of ulnar nerve at wrist and hand level of left arm
S64.1 Injury of median nerve at wrist and hand level
S64.10 Injury of median nerve at wrist and hand level of unspecified arm
S64.11 Injury of median nerve at wrist and hand level of right arm
S64.12 Injury of median nerve at wrist and hand level of left arm
S64.2 Injury of radial nerve at wrist and hand level
S64.20 Injury of radial nerve at wrist and hand level of unspecified arm
S64.21 Injury of radial nerve at wrist and hand level of right arm
S64.22 Injury of radial nerve at wrist and hand level of left arm
S64.3 Injury of digital nerve of thumb
S64.30 Injury of digital nerve of unspecified thumb
S64.31 Injury of digital nerve of right thumb
S64.32 Injury of digital nerve of left thumb
S64.4 Injury of digital nerve of other and unspecified finger
S64.40 Injury of digital nerve of unspecified finger
S64.49 Injury of digital nerve of other finger
S64.490 Injury of digital nerve of right index finger
S64.491 Injury of digital nerve of left index finger
S64.492 Injury of digital nerve of right middle finger
S64.493 Injury of digital nerve of left middle finger
S64.494 Injury of digital nerve of right ring finger
S64.495 Injury of digital nerve of left ring finger
S64.496 Injury of digital nerve of right little finger
S64.497 Injury of digital nerve of left little finger
S64.498 Injury of digital nerve of other finger
Injury of digital nerve of specified finger with unspecified laterality
S64.8 Injury of other nerves at wrist and hand level
S64.8X Injury of other nerves at wrist and hand level
S64.8X1 Injury of other nerves at wrist and hand level of right arm
S64.8X2 Injury of other nerves at wrist and hand level of left arm
S64.8X9 Injury of other nerves at wrist and hand level of unspecified arm

✓5th **S64.9 Injury of unspecified nerve at wrist and hand level**

✓x7th **S64.90 Injury of unspecified nerve at wrist and hand level of unspecified arm**

✓x7th **S64.91 Injury of unspecified nerve at wrist and hand level of right arm**

✓x7th **S64.92 Injury of unspecified nerve at wrist and hand level of left arm**

✓4th **S65 Injury of blood vessels at wrist and hand level**

Code also any associated open wound (S61.-)

The appropriate 7th character is to be added to each code from category S65.
A initial encounter
D subsequent encounter
S sequela

✓5th **S65.Ø Injury of ulnar artery at wrist and hand level**

✓6th **S65.ØØ Unspecified injury of ulnar artery at wrist and hand level**

✓7th **S65.ØØ1 Unspecified injury of ulnar artery at wrist and hand level of right arm**

✓7th **S65.ØØ2 Unspecified injury of ulnar artery at wrist and hand level of left arm**

✓7th **S65.ØØ9 Unspecified injury of ulnar artery at wrist and hand level of unspecified arm**

✓6th **S65.Ø1 Laceration of ulnar artery at wrist and hand level**

✓7th **S65.Ø11 Laceration of ulnar artery at wrist and hand level of right arm**

✓7th **S65.Ø12 Laceration of ulnar artery at wrist and hand level of left arm**

✓7th **S65.Ø19 Laceration of ulnar artery at wrist and hand level of unspecified arm**

✓6th **S65.Ø9 Other specified injury of ulnar artery at wrist and hand level**

✓7th **S65.Ø91 Other specified injury of ulnar artery at wrist and hand level of right arm**

✓7th **S65.Ø92 Other specified injury of ulnar artery at wrist and hand level of left arm**

✓7th **S65.Ø99 Other specified injury of ulnar artery at wrist and hand level of unspecified arm**

✓5th **S65.1 Injury of radial artery at wrist and hand level**

✓6th **S65.1Ø Unspecified injury of radial artery at wrist and hand level**

✓7th **S65.1Ø1 Unspecified injury of radial artery at wrist and hand level of right arm**

✓7th **S65.1Ø2 Unspecified injury of radial artery at wrist and hand level of left arm**

✓7th **S65.1Ø9 Unspecified injury of radial artery at wrist and hand level of unspecified arm**

✓6th **S65.11 Laceration of radial artery at wrist and hand level**

✓7th **S65.111 Laceration of radial artery at wrist and hand level of right arm**

✓7th **S65.112 Laceration of radial artery at wrist and hand level of left arm**

✓7th **S65.119 Laceration of radial artery at wrist and hand level of unspecified arm**

✓6th **S65.19 Other specified injury of radial artery at wrist and hand level**

✓7th **S65.191 Other specified injury of radial artery at wrist and hand level of right arm**

✓7th **S65.192 Other specified injury of radial artery at wrist and hand level of left arm**

✓7th **S65.199 Other specified injury of radial artery at wrist and hand level of unspecified arm**

✓5th **S65.2 Injury of superficial palmar arch**

✓6th **S65.2Ø Unspecified injury of superficial palmar arch**

✓7th **S65.2Ø1 Unspecified injury of superficial palmar arch of right hand**

✓7th **S65.2Ø2 Unspecified injury of superficial palmar arch of left hand**

✓7th **S65.2Ø9 Unspecified injury of superficial palmar arch of unspecified hand**

✓6th **S65.21 Laceration of superficial palmar arch**

✓7th **S65.211 Laceration of superficial palmar arch of right hand**

✓7th **S65.212 Laceration of superficial palmar arch of left hand**

✓7th **S65.219 Laceration of superficial palmar arch of unspecified hand**

✓6th **S65.29 Other specified injury of superficial palmar arch**

✓7th **S65.291 Other specified injury of superficial palmar arch of right hand**

✓7th **S65.292 Other specified injury of superficial palmar arch of left hand**

✓7th **S65.299 Other specified injury of superficial palmar arch of unspecified hand**

✓5th **S65.3 Injury of deep palmar arch**

✓6th **S65.3Ø Unspecified injury of deep palmar arch**

✓7th **S65.3Ø1 Unspecified injury of deep palmar arch of right hand**

✓7th **S65.3Ø2 Unspecified injury of deep palmar arch of left hand**

✓7th **S65.3Ø9 Unspecified injury of deep palmar arch of unspecified hand**

✓6th **S65.31 Laceration of deep palmar arch**

✓7th **S65.311 Laceration of deep palmar arch of right hand**

✓7th **S65.312 Laceration of deep palmar arch of left hand**

✓7th **S65.319 Laceration of deep palmar arch of unspecified hand**

✓6th **S65.39 Other specified injury of deep palmar arch**

✓7th **S65.391 Other specified injury of deep palmar arch of right hand**

✓7th **S65.392 Other specified injury of deep palmar arch of left hand**

✓7th **S65.399 Other specified injury of deep palmar arch of unspecified hand**

✓5th **S65.4 Injury of blood vessel of thumb**

✓6th **S65.4Ø Unspecified injury of blood vessel of thumb**

✓7th **S65.4Ø1 Unspecified injury of blood vessel of right thumb**

✓7th **S65.4Ø2 Unspecified injury of blood vessel of left thumb**

✓7th **S65.4Ø9 Unspecified injury of blood vessel of unspecified thumb**

✓6th **S65.41 Laceration of blood vessel of thumb**

✓7th **S65.411 Laceration of blood vessel of right thumb**

✓7th **S65.412 Laceration of blood vessel of left thumb**

✓7th **S65.419 Laceration of blood vessel of unspecified thumb**

✓6th **S65.49 Other specified injury of blood vessel of thumb**

✓7th **S65.491 Other specified injury of blood vessel of right thumb**

✓7th **S65.492 Other specified injury of blood vessel of left thumb**

✓7th **S65.499 Other specified injury of blood vessel of unspecified thumb**

✓5th **S65.5 Injury of blood vessel of other and unspecified finger**

✓6th **S65.5Ø Unspecified injury of blood vessel of other and unspecified finger**

✓7th **S65.5ØØ Unspecified injury of blood vessel of right index finger**

✓7th **S65.5Ø1 Unspecified injury of blood vessel of left index finger**

✓7th **S65.5Ø2 Unspecified injury of blood vessel of right middle finger**

✓7th **S65.5Ø3 Unspecified injury of blood vessel of left middle finger**

✓7th **S65.5Ø4 Unspecified injury of blood vessel of right ring finger**

✓7th **S65.5Ø5 Unspecified injury of blood vessel of left ring finger**

✓7th **S65.5Ø6 Unspecified injury of blood vessel of right little finger**

✓7th **S65.5Ø7 Unspecified injury of blood vessel of left little finger**

✓7th **S65.5Ø8 Unspecified injury of blood vessel of other finger**

Unspecified injury of blood vessel of specified finger with unspecified laterality

✓7th **S65.5Ø9 Unspecified injury of blood vessel of unspecified finger**

✓6th **S65.51 Laceration of blood vessel of other and unspecified finger**

✓7th **S65.51Ø Laceration of blood vessel of right index finger**

Chapter 19. Injury, Poisoning and Certain Other Consequences of External Causes
S64.9–S65.51Ø

7th S65.511 Laceration of blood vessel of left index finger

7th S65.512 Laceration of blood vessel of right middle finger

7th S65.513 Laceration of blood vessel of left middle finger

7th S65.514 Laceration of blood vessel of right ring finger

7th S65.515 Laceration of blood vessel of left ring finger

7th S65.516 Laceration of blood vessel of right little finger

7th S65.517 Laceration of blood vessel of left little finger

7th S65.518 Laceration of blood vessel of other finger

Laceration of blood vessel of specified finger with unspecified laterality

7th S65.519 Laceration of blood vessel of unspecified finger

6th S65.59 Other specified injury of blood vessel of other and unspecified finger

7th S65.590 Other specified injury of blood vessel of right index finger

7th S65.591 Other specified injury of blood vessel of left index finger

7th S65.592 Other specified injury of blood vessel of right middle finger

7th S65.593 Other specified injury of blood vessel of left middle finger

7th S65.594 Other specified injury of blood vessel of right ring finger

7th S65.595 Other specified injury of blood vessel of left ring finger

7th S65.596 Other specified injury of blood vessel of right little finger

7th S65.597 Other specified injury of blood vessel of left little finger

7th S65.598 Other specified injury of blood vessel of other finger

Other specified injury of blood vessel of specified finger with unspecified laterality

7th S65.599 Other specified injury of blood vessel of unspecified finger

5th S65.8 Injury of other blood vessels at wrist and hand level

6th S65.80 Unspecified injury of other blood vessels at wrist and hand level

7th S65.801 Unspecified injury of other blood vessels at wrist and hand level of right arm

7th S65.802 Unspecified injury of other blood vessels at wrist and hand level of left arm

7th S65.809 Unspecified injury of other blood vessels at wrist and hand level of unspecified arm

6th S65.81 Laceration of other blood vessels at wrist and hand level

7th S65.811 Laceration of other blood vessels at wrist and hand level of right arm

7th S65.812 Laceration of other blood vessels at wrist and hand level of left arm

7th S65.819 Laceration of other blood vessels at wrist and hand level of unspecified arm

6th S65.89 Other specified injury of other blood vessels at wrist and hand level

7th S65.891 Other specified injury of other blood vessels at wrist and hand level of right arm

7th S65.892 Other specified injury of other blood vessels at wrist and hand level of left arm

7th S65.899 Other specified injury of other blood vessels at wrist and hand level of unspecified arm

5th S65.9 Injury of unspecified blood vessel at wrist and hand level

6th S65.90 Unspecified injury of unspecified blood vessel at wrist and hand level

7th S65.901 Unspecified injury of unspecified blood vessel at wrist and hand level of right arm

7th S65.902 Unspecified injury of unspecified blood vessel at wrist and hand level of left arm

7th S65.909 Unspecified injury of unspecified blood vessel at wrist and hand level of unspecified arm

6th S65.91 Laceration of unspecified blood vessel at wrist and hand level

7th S65.911 Laceration of unspecified blood vessel at wrist and hand level of right arm

7th S65.912 Laceration of unspecified blood vessel at wrist and hand level of left arm

7th S65.919 Laceration of unspecified blood vessel at wrist and hand level of unspecified arm

6th S65.99 Other specified injury of unspecified blood vessel at wrist and hand level

7th S65.991 Other specified injury of unspecified blood vessel at wrist and hand of right arm

7th S65.992 Other specified injury of unspecified blood vessel at wrist and hand of left arm

7th S65.999 Other specified injury of unspecified blood vessel at wrist and hand of unspecified arm

4th S66 Injury of muscle, fascia and tendon at wrist and hand level

Code also any associated open wound (S61.-)

EXCLUDES 2 *sprain of joints and ligaments of wrist and hand (S63.-)*

TIP: Refer to the Muscle/Tendon table at the beginning of this chapter.

The appropriate 7th character is to be added to each code from category S66.
- A initial encounter
- D subsequent encounter
- S sequela

5th S66.0 Injury of long flexor muscle, fascia and tendon of thumb at wrist and hand level

6th S66.00 Unspecified injury of long flexor muscle, fascia and tendon of thumb at wrist and hand level

7th S66.001 Unspecified injury of long flexor muscle, fascia and tendon of right thumb at wrist and hand level

7th S66.002 Unspecified injury of long flexor muscle, fascia and tendon of left thumb at wrist and hand level

7th S66.009 Unspecified injury of long flexor muscle, fascia and tendon of unspecified thumb at wrist and hand level

6th S66.01 Strain of long flexor muscle, fascia and tendon of thumb at wrist and hand level

7th S66.011 Strain of long flexor muscle, fascia and tendon of right thumb at wrist and hand level

7th S66.012 Strain of long flexor muscle, fascia and tendon of left thumb at wrist and hand level

7th S66.019 Strain of long flexor muscle, fascia and tendon of unspecified thumb at wrist and hand level

6th S66.02 Laceration of long flexor muscle, fascia and tendon of thumb at wrist and hand level

7th S66.021 Laceration of long flexor muscle, fascia and tendon of right thumb at wrist and hand level

7th S66.022 Laceration of long flexor muscle, fascia and tendon of left thumb at wrist and hand level

7th S66.029 Laceration of long flexor muscle, fascia and tendon of unspecified thumb at wrist and hand level

6th S66.09 Other specified injury of long flexor muscle, fascia and tendon of thumb at wrist and hand level

7th S66.091 Other specified injury of long flexor muscle, fascia and tendon of right thumb at wrist and hand level

7th S66.092 Other specified injury of long flexor muscle, fascia and tendon of left thumb at wrist and hand level

7th S66.099 Other specified injury of long flexor muscle, fascia and tendon of unspecified thumb at wrist and hand level

5th S66.1 Injury of flexor muscle, fascia and tendon of other and unspecified finger at wrist and hand level

EXCLUDES 2 *injury of long flexor muscle, fascia and tendon of thumb at wrist and hand level (S66.0-)*

6th S66.10 Unspecified injury of flexor muscle, fascia and tendon of other and unspecified finger at wrist and hand level

7th S66.100 Unspecified injury of flexor muscle, fascia and tendon of right index finger at wrist and hand level

7th **S66.101** **Unspecified injury of flexor muscle, fascia and tendon of left index finger at wrist and hand level**

7th **S66.102** **Unspecified injury of flexor muscle, fascia and tendon of right middle finger at wrist and hand level**

7th **S66.103** **Unspecified injury of flexor muscle, fascia and tendon of left middle finger at wrist and hand level**

7th **S66.104** **Unspecified injury of flexor muscle, fascia and tendon of right ring finger at wrist and hand level**

7th **S66.105** **Unspecified injury of flexor muscle, fascia and tendon of left ring finger at wrist and hand level**

7th **S66.106** **Unspecified injury of flexor muscle, fascia and tendon of right little finger at wrist and hand level**

7th **S66.107** **Unspecified injury of flexor muscle, fascia and tendon of left little finger at wrist and hand level**

7th **S66.108** **Unspecified injury of flexor muscle, fascia and tendon of other finger at wrist and hand level**

Unspecified injury of flexor muscle, fascia and tendon of specified finger with unspecified laterality at wrist and hand level

7th **S66.109** **Unspecified injury of flexor muscle, fascia and tendon of unspecified finger at wrist and hand level**

6th **S66.11** **Strain of flexor muscle, fascia and tendon of other and unspecified finger at wrist and hand level**

7th **S66.110** **Strain of flexor muscle, fascia and tendon of right index finger at wrist and hand level**

7th **S66.111** **Strain of flexor muscle, fascia and tendon of left index finger at wrist and hand level**

7th **S66.112** **Strain of flexor muscle, fascia and tendon of right middle finger at wrist and hand level**

7th **S66.113** **Strain of flexor muscle, fascia and tendon of left middle finger at wrist and hand level**

7th **S66.114** **Strain of flexor muscle, fascia and tendon of right ring finger at wrist and hand level**

7th **S66.115** **Strain of flexor muscle, fascia and tendon of left ring finger at wrist and hand level**

7th **S66.116** **Strain of flexor muscle, fascia and tendon of right little finger at wrist and hand level**

7th **S66.117** **Strain of flexor muscle, fascia and tendon of left little finger at wrist and hand level**

7th **S66.118** **Strain of flexor muscle, fascia and tendon of other finger at wrist and hand level**

Strain of flexor muscle, fascia and tendon of specified finger with unspecified laterality at wrist and hand level

7th **S66.119** **Strain of flexor muscle, fascia and tendon of unspecified finger at wrist and hand level**

6th **S66.12** **Laceration of flexor muscle, fascia and tendon of other and unspecified finger at wrist and hand level**

7th **S66.120** **Laceration of flexor muscle, fascia and tendon of right index finger at wrist and hand level**

7th **S66.121** **Laceration of flexor muscle, fascia and tendon of left index finger at wrist and hand level**

7th **S66.122** **Laceration of flexor muscle, fascia and tendon of right middle finger at wrist and hand level**

7th **S66.123** **Laceration of flexor muscle, fascia and tendon of left middle finger at wrist and hand level**

7th **S66.124** **Laceration of flexor muscle, fascia and tendon of right ring finger at wrist and hand level**

7th **S66.125** **Laceration of flexor muscle, fascia and tendon of left ring finger at wrist and hand level**

7th **S66.126** **Laceration of flexor muscle, fascia and tendon of right little finger at wrist and hand level**

7th **S66.127** **Laceration of flexor muscle, fascia and tendon of left little finger at wrist and hand level**

7th **S66.128** **Laceration of flexor muscle, fascia and tendon of other finger at wrist and hand level**

Laceration of flexor muscle, fascia and tendon of specified finger with unspecified laterality at wrist and hand level

7th **S66.129** **Laceration of flexor muscle, fascia and tendon of unspecified finger at wrist and hand level**

6th **S66.19** **Other injury of flexor muscle, fascia and tendon of other and unspecified finger at wrist and hand level**

7th **S66.190** **Other injury of flexor muscle, fascia and tendon of right index finger at wrist and hand level**

7th **S66.191** **Other injury of flexor muscle, fascia and tendon of left index finger at wrist and hand level**

7th **S66.192** **Other injury of flexor muscle, fascia and tendon of right middle finger at wrist and hand level**

7th **S66.193** **Other injury of flexor muscle, fascia and tendon of left middle finger at wrist and hand level**

7th **S66.194** **Other injury of flexor muscle, fascia and tendon of right ring finger at wrist and hand level**

7th **S66.195** **Other injury of flexor muscle, fascia and tendon of left ring finger at wrist and hand level**

7th **S66.196** **Other injury of flexor muscle, fascia and tendon of right little finger at wrist and hand level**

7th **S66.197** **Other injury of flexor muscle, fascia and tendon of left little finger at wrist and hand level**

7th **S66.198** **Other injury of flexor muscle, fascia and tendon of other finger at wrist and hand level**

Other injury of flexor muscle, fascia and tendon of specified finger with unspecified laterality at wrist and hand level

7th **S66.199** **Other injury of flexor muscle, fascia and tendon of unspecified finger at wrist and hand level**

5th **S66.2** **Injury of extensor muscle, fascia and tendon of thumb at wrist and hand level**

6th **S66.20** **Unspecified injury of extensor muscle, fascia and tendon of thumb at wrist and hand level**

7th **S66.201** **Unspecified injury of extensor muscle, fascia and tendon of right thumb at wrist and hand level**

7th **S66.202** **Unspecified injury of extensor muscle, fascia and tendon of left thumb at wrist and hand level**

7th **S66.209** **Unspecified injury of extensor muscle, fascia and tendon of unspecified thumb at wrist and hand level**

6th **S66.21** **Strain of extensor muscle, fascia and tendon of thumb at wrist and hand level**

7th **S66.211** **Strain of extensor muscle, fascia and tendon of right thumb at wrist and hand level**

7th **S66.212** **Strain of extensor muscle, fascia and tendon of left thumb at wrist and hand level**

7th **S66.219** **Strain of extensor muscle, fascia and tendon of unspecified thumb at wrist and hand level**

6th **S66.22** **Laceration of extensor muscle, fascia and tendon of thumb at wrist and hand level**

7th **S66.221** **Laceration of extensor muscle, fascia and tendon of right thumb at wrist and hand level**

7th **S66.222** **Laceration of extensor muscle, fascia and tendon of left thumb at wrist and hand level**

7th **S66.229** **Laceration of extensor muscle, fascia and tendon of unspecified thumb at wrist and hand level**

6th S66.29 **Other specified injury of extensor muscle, fascia and tendon of thumb at wrist and hand level**
7th S66.291 **Other specified injury of extensor muscle, fascia and tendon of right thumb at wrist and hand level**
7th S66.292 **Other specified injury of extensor muscle, fascia and tendon of left thumb at wrist and hand level**
7th S66.299 **Other specified injury of extensor muscle, fascia and tendon of unspecified thumb at wrist and hand level**

5th S66.3 **Injury of extensor muscle, fascia and tendon of other and unspecified finger at wrist and hand level**
EXCLUDES 2 *injury of extensor muscle, fascia and tendon of thumb at wrist and hand level (S66.2-)*

6th S66.30 **Unspecified injury of extensor muscle, fascia and tendon of other and unspecified finger at wrist and hand level**
7th S66.300 **Unspecified injury of extensor muscle, fascia and tendon of right index finger at wrist and hand level**
7th S66.301 **Unspecified injury of extensor muscle, fascia and tendon of left index finger at wrist and hand level**
7th S66.302 **Unspecified injury of extensor muscle, fascia and tendon of right middle finger at wrist and hand level**
7th S66.303 **Unspecified injury of extensor muscle, fascia and tendon of left middle finger at wrist and hand level**
7th S66.304 **Unspecified injury of extensor muscle, fascia and tendon of right ring finger at wrist and hand level**
7th S66.305 **Unspecified injury of extensor muscle, fascia and tendon of left ring finger at wrist and hand level**
7th S66.306 **Unspecified injury of extensor muscle, fascia and tendon of right little finger at wrist and hand level**
7th S66.307 **Unspecified injury of extensor muscle, fascia and tendon of left little finger at wrist and hand level**
7th S66.308 **Unspecified injury of extensor muscle, fascia and tendon of other finger at wrist and hand level**
Unspecified injury of extensor muscle, fascia and tendon of specified finger with unspecified laterality at wrist and hand level
7th S66.309 **Unspecified injury of extensor muscle, fascia and tendon of unspecified finger at wrist and hand level**

6th S66.31 **Strain of extensor muscle, fascia and tendon of other and unspecified finger at wrist and hand level**
7th S66.310 **Strain of extensor muscle, fascia and tendon of right index finger at wrist and hand level**
7th S66.311 **Strain of extensor muscle, fascia and tendon of left index finger at wrist and hand level**
7th S66.312 **Strain of extensor muscle, fascia and tendon of right middle finger at wrist and hand level**
7th S66.313 **Strain of extensor muscle, fascia and tendon of left middle finger at wrist and hand level**
7th S66.314 **Strain of extensor muscle, fascia and tendon of right ring finger at wrist and hand level**
7th S66.315 **Strain of extensor muscle, fascia and tendon of left ring finger at wrist and hand level**
7th S66.316 **Strain of extensor muscle, fascia and tendon of right little finger at wrist and hand level**
7th S66.317 **Strain of extensor muscle, fascia and tendon of left little finger at wrist and hand level**
7th S66.318 **Strain of extensor muscle, fascia and tendon of other finger at wrist and hand level**
Strain of extensor muscle, fascia and tendon of specified finger with unspecified laterality at wrist and hand level
7th S66.319 **Strain of extensor muscle, fascia and tendon of unspecified finger at wrist and hand level**

6th S66.32 **Laceration of extensor muscle, fascia and tendon of other and unspecified finger at wrist and hand level**
7th S66.320 **Laceration of extensor muscle, fascia and tendon of right index finger at wrist and hand level**
7th S66.321 **Laceration of extensor muscle, fascia and tendon of left index finger at wrist and hand level**
7th S66.322 **Laceration of extensor muscle, fascia and tendon of right middle finger at wrist and hand level**
7th S66.323 **Laceration of extensor muscle, fascia and tendon of left middle finger at wrist and hand level**
7th S66.324 **Laceration of extensor muscle, fascia and tendon of right ring finger at wrist and hand level**
7th S66.325 **Laceration of extensor muscle, fascia and tendon of left ring finger at wrist and hand level**
7th S66.326 **Laceration of extensor muscle, fascia and tendon of right little finger at wrist and hand level**
7th S66.327 **Laceration of extensor muscle, fascia and tendon of left little finger at wrist and hand level**
7th S66.328 **Laceration of extensor muscle, fascia and tendon of other finger at wrist and hand level**
Laceration of extensor muscle, fascia and tendon of specified finger with unspecified laterality at wrist and hand level
7th S66.329 **Laceration of extensor muscle, fascia and tendon of unspecified finger at wrist and hand level**

6th S66.39 **Other injury of extensor muscle, fascia and tendon of other and unspecified finger at wrist and hand level**
7th S66.390 **Other injury of extensor muscle, fascia and tendon of right index finger at wrist and hand level**
7th S66.391 **Other injury of extensor muscle, fascia and tendon of left index finger at wrist and hand level**
7th S66.392 **Other injury of extensor muscle, fascia and tendon of right middle finger at wrist and hand level**
7th S66.393 **Other injury of extensor muscle, fascia and tendon of left middle finger at wrist and hand level**
7th S66.394 **Other injury of extensor muscle, fascia and tendon of right ring finger at wrist and hand level**
7th S66.395 **Other injury of extensor muscle, fascia and tendon of left ring finger at wrist and hand level**
7th S66.396 **Other injury of extensor muscle, fascia and tendon of right little finger at wrist and hand level**
7th S66.397 **Other injury of extensor muscle, fascia and tendon of left little finger at wrist and hand level**
7th S66.398 **Other injury of extensor muscle, fascia and tendon of other finger at wrist and hand level**
Other injury of extensor muscle, fascia and tendon of specified finger with unspecified laterality at wrist and hand level
7th S66.399 **Other injury of extensor muscle, fascia and tendon of unspecified finger at wrist and hand level**

S66.4 Injury of intrinsic muscle, fascia and tendon of thumb at wrist and hand level

S66.40 Unspecified injury of intrinsic muscle, fascia and tendon of thumb at wrist and hand level

S66.401 Unspecified injury of intrinsic muscle, fascia and tendon of right thumb at wrist and hand level

S66.402 Unspecified injury of intrinsic muscle, fascia and tendon of left thumb at wrist and hand level

S66.409 Unspecified injury of intrinsic muscle, fascia and tendon of unspecified thumb at wrist and hand level

S66.41 Strain of intrinsic muscle, fascia and tendon of thumb at wrist and hand level

S66.411 Strain of intrinsic muscle, fascia and tendon of right thumb at wrist and hand level

S66.412 Strain of intrinsic muscle, fascia and tendon of left thumb at wrist and hand level

S66.419 Strain of intrinsic muscle, fascia and tendon of unspecified thumb at wrist and hand level

S66.42 Laceration of intrinsic muscle, fascia and tendon of thumb at wrist and hand level

S66.421 Laceration of intrinsic muscle, fascia and tendon of right thumb at wrist and hand level

S66.422 Laceration of intrinsic muscle, fascia and tendon of left thumb at wrist and hand level

S66.429 Laceration of intrinsic muscle, fascia and tendon of unspecified thumb at wrist and hand level

S66.49 Other specified injury of intrinsic muscle, fascia and tendon of thumb at wrist and hand level

S66.491 Other specified injury of intrinsic muscle, fascia and tendon of right thumb at wrist and hand level

S66.492 Other specified injury of intrinsic muscle, fascia and tendon of left thumb at wrist and hand level

S66.499 Other specified injury of intrinsic muscle, fascia and tendon of unspecified thumb at wrist and hand level

S66.5 Injury of intrinsic muscle, fascia and tendon of other and unspecified finger at wrist and hand level

EXCLUDES 2 *injury of intrinsic muscle, fascia and tendon of thumb at wrist and hand level (S66.4-)*

S66.50 Unspecified injury of intrinsic muscle, fascia and tendon of other and unspecified finger at wrist and hand level

S66.500 Unspecified injury of intrinsic muscle, fascia and tendon of right index finger at wrist and hand level

S66.501 Unspecified injury of intrinsic muscle, fascia and tendon of left index finger at wrist and hand level

S66.502 Unspecified injury of intrinsic muscle, fascia and tendon of right middle finger at wrist and hand level

S66.503 Unspecified injury of intrinsic muscle, fascia and tendon of left middle finger at wrist and hand level

S66.504 Unspecified injury of intrinsic muscle, fascia and tendon of right ring finger at wrist and hand level

S66.505 Unspecified injury of intrinsic muscle, fascia and tendon of left ring finger at wrist and hand level

S66.506 Unspecified injury of intrinsic muscle, fascia and tendon of right little finger at wrist and hand level

S66.507 Unspecified injury of intrinsic muscle, fascia and tendon of left little finger at wrist and hand level

S66.508 Unspecified injury of intrinsic muscle, fascia and tendon of other finger at wrist and hand level

Unspecified injury of intrinsic muscle, fascia and tendon of specified finger with unspecified laterality at wrist and hand level

S66.509 Unspecified injury of intrinsic muscle, fascia and tendon of unspecified finger at wrist and hand level

S66.51 Strain of intrinsic muscle, fascia and tendon of other and unspecified finger at wrist and hand level

S66.510 Strain of intrinsic muscle, fascia and tendon of right index finger at wrist and hand level

S66.511 Strain of intrinsic muscle, fascia and tendon of left index finger at wrist and hand level

S66.512 Strain of intrinsic muscle, fascia and tendon of right middle finger at wrist and hand level

S66.513 Strain of intrinsic muscle, fascia and tendon of left middle finger at wrist and hand level

S66.514 Strain of intrinsic muscle, fascia and tendon of right ring finger at wrist and hand level

S66.515 Strain of intrinsic muscle, fascia and tendon of left ring finger at wrist and hand level

S66.516 Strain of intrinsic muscle, fascia and tendon of right little finger at wrist and hand level

S66.517 Strain of intrinsic muscle, fascia and tendon of left little finger at wrist and hand level

S66.518 Strain of intrinsic muscle, fascia and tendon of other finger at wrist and hand level

Strain of intrinsic muscle, fascia and tendon of specified finger with unspecified laterality at wrist and hand level

S66.519 Strain of intrinsic muscle, fascia and tendon of unspecified finger at wrist and hand level

S66.52 Laceration of intrinsic muscle, fascia and tendon of other and unspecified finger at wrist and hand level

S66.520 Laceration of intrinsic muscle, fascia and tendon of right index finger at wrist and hand level

S66.521 Laceration of intrinsic muscle, fascia and tendon of left index finger at wrist and hand level

S66.522 Laceration of intrinsic muscle, fascia and tendon of right middle finger at wrist and hand level

S66.523 Laceration of intrinsic muscle, fascia and tendon of left middle finger at wrist and hand level

S66.524 Laceration of intrinsic muscle, fascia and tendon of right ring finger at wrist and hand level

S66.525 Laceration of intrinsic muscle, fascia and tendon of left ring finger at wrist and hand level

S66.526 Laceration of intrinsic muscle, fascia and tendon of right little finger at wrist and hand level

S66.527 Laceration of intrinsic muscle, fascia and tendon of left little finger at wrist and hand level

S66.528 Laceration of intrinsic muscle, fascia and tendon of other finger at wrist and hand level

Laceration of intrinsic muscle, fascia and tendon of specified finger with unspecified laterality at wrist and hand level

S66.529 Laceration of intrinsic muscle, fascia and tendon of unspecified finger at wrist and hand level

S66.59 Other injury of intrinsic muscle, fascia and tendon of other and unspecified finger at wrist and hand level
S66.59Ø Other injury of intrinsic muscle, fascia and tendon of right index finger at wrist and hand level
S66.591 Other injury of intrinsic muscle, fascia and tendon of left index finger at wrist and hand level
S66.592 Other injury of intrinsic muscle, fascia and tendon of right middle finger at wrist and hand level
S66.593 Other injury of intrinsic muscle, fascia and tendon of left middle finger at wrist and hand level
S66.594 Other injury of intrinsic muscle, fascia and tendon of right ring finger at wrist and hand level
S66.595 Other injury of intrinsic muscle, fascia and tendon of left ring finger at wrist and hand level
S66.596 Other injury of intrinsic muscle, fascia and tendon of right little finger at wrist and hand level
S66.597 Other injury of intrinsic muscle, fascia and tendon of left little finger at wrist and hand level
S66.598 Other injury of intrinsic muscle, fascia and tendon of other finger at wrist and hand level
Other injury of intrinsic muscle, fascia and tendon of specified finger with unspecified laterality at wrist and hand level
S66.599 Other injury of intrinsic muscle, fascia and tendon of unspecified finger at wrist and hand level
S66.8 Injury of other specified muscles, fascia and tendons at wrist and hand level
S66.8Ø Unspecified injury of other specified muscles, fascia and tendons at wrist and hand level
S66.8Ø1 Unspecified injury of other specified muscles, fascia and tendons at wrist and hand level, right hand
S66.8Ø2 Unspecified injury of other specified muscles, fascia and tendons at wrist and hand level, left hand
S66.8Ø9 Unspecified injury of other specified muscles, fascia and tendons at wrist and hand level, unspecified hand
S66.81 Strain of other specified muscles, fascia and tendons at wrist and hand level
S66.811 Strain of other specified muscles, fascia and tendons at wrist and hand level, right hand
S66.812 Strain of other specified muscles, fascia and tendons at wrist and hand level, left hand
S66.819 Strain of other specified muscles, fascia and tendons at wrist and hand level, unspecified hand
S66.82 Laceration of other specified muscles, fascia and tendons at wrist and hand level
S66.821 Laceration of other specified muscles, fascia and tendons at wrist and hand level, right hand
S66.822 Laceration of other specified muscles, fascia and tendons at wrist and hand level, left hand
S66.829 Laceration of other specified muscles, fascia and tendons at wrist and hand level, unspecified hand
S66.89 Other injury of other specified muscles, fascia and tendons at wrist and hand level
S66.891 Other injury of other specified muscles, fascia and tendons at wrist and hand level, right hand
S66.892 Other injury of other specified muscles, fascia and tendons at wrist and hand level, left hand
S66.899 Other injury of other specified muscles, fascia and tendons at wrist and hand level, unspecified hand
S66.9 Injury of unspecified muscle, fascia and tendon at wrist and hand level
S66.9Ø Unspecified injury of unspecified muscle, fascia and tendon at wrist and hand level
S66.9Ø1 Unspecified injury of unspecified muscle, fascia and tendon at wrist and hand level, right hand
S66.9Ø2 Unspecified injury of unspecified muscle, fascia and tendon at wrist and hand level, left hand
S66.9Ø9 Unspecified injury of unspecified muscle, fascia and tendon at wrist and hand level, unspecified hand
S66.91 Strain of unspecified muscle, fascia and tendon at wrist and hand level
S66.911 Strain of unspecified muscle, fascia and tendon at wrist and hand level, right hand
S66.912 Strain of unspecified muscle, fascia and tendon at wrist and hand level, left hand
S66.919 Strain of unspecified muscle, fascia and tendon at wrist and hand level, unspecified hand
S66.92 Laceration of unspecified muscle, fascia and tendon at wrist and hand level
S66.921 Laceration of unspecified muscle, fascia and tendon at wrist and hand level, right hand
S66.922 Laceration of unspecified muscle, fascia and tendon at wrist and hand level, left hand
S66.929 Laceration of unspecified muscle, fascia and tendon at wrist and hand level, unspecified hand
S66.99 Other injury of unspecified muscle, fascia and tendon at wrist and hand level
S66.991 Other injury of unspecified muscle, fascia and tendon at wrist and hand level, right hand
S66.992 Other injury of unspecified muscle, fascia and tendon at wrist and hand level, left hand
S66.999 Other injury of unspecified muscle, fascia and tendon at wrist and hand level, unspecified hand

S67 Crushing injury of wrist, hand and fingers

Use additional code for all associated injuries, such as:
fracture of wrist and hand (S62.-)
open wound of wrist and hand (S61.-)

The appropriate 7th character is to be added to each code from category S67.
A initial encounter
D subsequent encounter
S sequela

S67.Ø Crushing injury of thumb
S67.ØØ Crushing injury of unspecified thumb
S67.Ø1 Crushing injury of right thumb
S67.Ø2 Crushing injury of left thumb
S67.1 Crushing injury of other and unspecified finger(s)
EXCLUDES 2 *crushing injury of thumb (S67.Ø-)*
S67.1Ø Crushing injury of unspecified finger(s)
S67.19 Crushing injury of other finger(s)
S67.19Ø Crushing injury of right index finger
S67.191 Crushing injury of left index finger
S67.192 Crushing injury of right middle finger
S67.193 Crushing injury of left middle finger
S67.194 Crushing injury of right ring finger
S67.195 Crushing injury of left ring finger
S67.196 Crushing injury of right little finger
S67.197 Crushing injury of left little finger
S67.198 Crushing injury of other finger
Crushing injury of specified finger with unspecified laterality
S67.2 Crushing injury of hand
EXCLUDES 2 *crushing injury of fingers (S67.1-)*
crushing injury of thumb (S67.Ø-)
S67.2Ø Crushing injury of unspecified hand

√x7th **S67.21 Crushing injury of right hand**

√x7th **S67.22 Crushing injury of left hand**

√5th **S67.3 Crushing injury of wrist**

√x7th **S67.30 Crushing injury of unspecified wrist**

√x7th **S67.31 Crushing injury of right wrist**

√x7th **S67.32 Crushing injury of left wrist**

√5th **S67.4 Crushing injury of wrist and hand**

EXCLUDES 1 *crushing injury of hand alone (S67.2-)*
crushing injury of wrist alone (S67.3-)

EXCLUDES 2 *crushing injury of fingers (S67.1-)*
crushing injury of thumb (S67.Ø-)

√x7th **S67.40 Crushing injury of unspecified wrist and hand**

√x7th **S67.41 Crushing injury of right wrist and hand**

√x7th **S67.42 Crushing injury of left wrist and hand**

√5th **S67.9 Crushing injury of unspecified part(s) of wrist, hand and fingers**

√x7th **S67.90 Crushing injury of unspecified part(s) of unspecified wrist, hand and fingers**

√x7th **S67.91 Crushing injury of unspecified part(s) of right wrist, hand and fingers**

√x7th **S67.92 Crushing injury of unspecified part(s) of left wrist, hand and fingers**

√4th **S68 Traumatic amputation of wrist, hand and fingers**

An amputation not identified as partial or complete should be coded to complete.

The appropriate 7th character is to be added to each code from category S68.
A initial encounter
D subsequent encounter
S sequela

√5th **S68.Ø Traumatic metacarpophalangeal amputation of thumb**

Traumatic amputation of thumb NOS

√6th **S68.Ø1 Complete traumatic metacarpophalangeal amputation of thumb**

3 √7th **S68.Ø11 Complete traumatic metacarpophalangeal amputation of right thumb** HCC ESR

3 √7th **S68.Ø12 Complete traumatic metacarpophalangeal amputation of left thumb** HCC ESR

3 √7th **S68.Ø19 Complete traumatic metacarpophalangeal amputation of unspecified thumb** HCC ESR

√6th **S68.Ø2 Partial traumatic metacarpophalangeal amputation of thumb**

3 √7th **S68.Ø21 Partial traumatic metacarpophalangeal amputation of right thumb** HCC ESR

3 √7th **S68.Ø22 Partial traumatic metacarpophalangeal amputation of left thumb** HCC ESR

3 √7th **S68.Ø29 Partial traumatic metacarpophalangeal amputation of unspecified thumb** HCC ESR

√5th **S68.1 Traumatic metacarpophalangeal amputation of other and unspecified finger**

Traumatic amputation of finger NOS

EXCLUDES 2 *traumatic metacarpophalangeal amputation of thumb (S68.Ø-)*

√6th **S68.11 Complete traumatic metacarpophalangeal amputation of other and unspecified finger**

3 √7th **S68.11Ø Complete traumatic metacarpophalangeal amputation of right index finger** HCC ESR

3 √7th **S68.111 Complete traumatic metacarpophalangeal amputation of left index finger** HCC ESR

3 √7th **S68.112 Complete traumatic metacarpophalangeal amputation of right middle finger** HCC ESR

3 √7th **S68.113 Complete traumatic metacarpophalangeal amputation of left middle finger** HCC ESR

3 √7th **S68.114 Complete traumatic metacarpophalangeal amputation of right ring finger** HCC ESR

3 √7th **S68.115 Complete traumatic metacarpophalangeal amputation of left ring finger** HCC ESR

3 √7th **S68.116 Complete traumatic metacarpophalangeal amputation of right little finger** HCC ESR

3 √7th **S68.117 Complete traumatic metacarpophalangeal amputation of left little finger** HCC ESR

3 √7th **S68.118 Complete traumatic metacarpophalangeal amputation of other finger** HCC ESR

Complete traumatic metacarpophalangeal amputation of specified finger with unspecified laterality

3 √7th **S68.119 Complete traumatic metacarpophalangeal amputation of unspecified finger** HCC ESR

√6th **S68.12 Partial traumatic metacarpophalangeal amputation of other and unspecified finger**

3 √7th **S68.12Ø Partial traumatic metacarpophalangeal amputation of right index finger** HCC ESR

3 √7th **S68.121 Partial traumatic metacarpophalangeal amputation of left index finger** HCC ESR

3 √7th **S68.122 Partial traumatic metacarpophalangeal amputation of right middle finger** HCC ESR

3 √7th **S68.123 Partial traumatic metacarpophalangeal amputation of left middle finger** HCC ESR

3 √7th **S68.124 Partial traumatic metacarpophalangeal amputation of right ring finger** HCC ESR

3 √7th **S68.125 Partial traumatic metacarpophalangeal amputation of left ring finger** HCC ESR

3 √7th **S68.126 Partial traumatic metacarpophalangeal amputation of right little finger** HCC ESR

3 √7th **S68.127 Partial traumatic metacarpophalangeal amputation of left little finger** HCC ESR

3 √7th **S68.128 Partial traumatic metacarpophalangeal amputation of other finger** HCC ESR

Partial traumatic metacarpophalangeal amputation of specified finger with unspecified laterality

3 √7th **S68.129 Partial traumatic metacarpophalangeal amputation of unspecified finger** HCC ESR

√5th **S68.4 Traumatic amputation of hand at wrist level**

Traumatic amputation of hand NOS
Traumatic amputation of wrist

√6th **S68.41 Complete traumatic amputation of hand at wrist level**

2 √7th **S68.411 Complete traumatic amputation of right hand at wrist level** HCC ESR COM

2 √7th **S68.412 Complete traumatic amputation of left hand at wrist level** HCC ESR COM

2 √7th **S68.419 Complete traumatic amputation of unspecified hand at wrist level** HCC ESR COM

√6th **S68.42 Partial traumatic amputation of hand at wrist level**

2 √7th **S68.421 Partial traumatic amputation of right hand at wrist level** HCC ESR COM

2 √7th **S68.422 Partial traumatic amputation of left hand at wrist level** HCC ESR COM

2 √7th **S68.429 Partial traumatic amputation of unspecified hand at wrist level** HCC ESR COM

√5th **S68.5 Traumatic transphalangeal amputation of thumb**

Traumatic interphalangeal joint amputation of thumb

√6th **S68.51 Complete traumatic transphalangeal amputation of thumb**

3 √7th **S68.511 Complete traumatic transphalangeal amputation of right thumb** HCC ESR

3 √7th **S68.512 Complete traumatic transphalangeal amputation of left thumb** HCC ESR

3 √7th **S68.519 Complete traumatic transphalangeal amputation of unspecified thumb** HCC ESR

S68.52 Partial traumatic transphalangeal amputation of thumb
- S68.521 Partial traumatic transphalangeal amputation of right thumb HCC ESR
- S68.522 Partial traumatic transphalangeal amputation of left thumb HCC ESR
- S68.529 Partial traumatic transphalangeal amputation of unspecified thumb HCC ESR

S68.6 Traumatic transphalangeal amputation of other and unspecified finger

S68.61 Complete traumatic transphalangeal amputation of other and unspecified finger(s)
- S68.610 Complete traumatic transphalangeal amputation of right index finger HCC ESR
- S68.611 Complete traumatic transphalangeal amputation of left index finger HCC ESR
- S68.612 Complete traumatic transphalangeal amputation of right middle finger HCC ESR
- S68.613 Complete traumatic transphalangeal amputation of left middle finger HCC ESR
- S68.614 Complete traumatic transphalangeal amputation of right ring finger HCC ESR
- S68.615 Complete traumatic transphalangeal amputation of left ring finger HCC ESR
- S68.616 Complete traumatic transphalangeal amputation of right little finger HCC ESR
- S68.617 Complete traumatic transphalangeal amputation of left little finger HCC ESR
- S68.618 Complete traumatic transphalangeal amputation of other finger HCC ESR
  Complete traumatic transphalangeal amputation of specified finger with unspecified laterality
- S68.619 Complete traumatic transphalangeal amputation of unspecified finger HCC ESR

S68.62 Partial traumatic transphalangeal amputation of other and unspecified finger
- S68.620 Partial traumatic transphalangeal amputation of right index finger HCC ESR
- S68.621 Partial traumatic transphalangeal amputation of left index finger HCC ESR
- S68.622 Partial traumatic transphalangeal amputation of right middle finger HCC ESR
- S68.623 Partial traumatic transphalangeal amputation of left middle finger HCC ESR
- S68.624 Partial traumatic transphalangeal amputation of right ring finger HCC ESR
- S68.625 Partial traumatic transphalangeal amputation of left ring finger HCC ESR
- S68.626 Partial traumatic transphalangeal amputation of right little finger HCC ESR
- S68.627 Partial traumatic transphalangeal amputation of left little finger HCC ESR
- S68.628 Partial traumatic transphalangeal amputation of other finger HCC ESR
  Partial traumatic transphalangeal amputation of specified finger with unspecified laterality
- S68.629 Partial traumatic transphalangeal amputation of unspecified finger HCC ESR

S68.7 Traumatic transmetacarpal amputation of hand

S68.71 Complete traumatic transmetacarpal amputation of hand
- S68.711 Complete traumatic transmetacarpal amputation of right hand HCC ESR COM
- S68.712 Complete traumatic transmetacarpal amputation of left hand HCC ESR COM
- S68.719 Complete traumatic transmetacarpal amputation of unspecified hand HCC ESR COM

S68.72 Partial traumatic transmetacarpal amputation of hand
- S68.721 Partial traumatic transmetacarpal amputation of right hand HCC ESR COM
- S68.722 Partial traumatic transmetacarpal amputation of left hand HCC ESR COM
- S68.729 Partial traumatic transmetacarpal amputation of unspecified hand HCC ESR COM

S69 Other and unspecified injuries of wrist, hand and finger(s)

The appropriate 7th character is to be added to each code from category S69.
- A initial encounter
- D subsequent encounter
- S sequela

S69.8 Other specified injuries of wrist, hand and finger(s)
- S69.80 Other specified injuries of unspecified wrist, hand and finger(s)
- S69.81 Other specified injuries of right wrist, hand and finger(s)
- S69.82 Other specified injuries of left wrist, hand and finger(s)

S69.9 Unspecified injury of wrist, hand and finger(s)
- S69.90 Unspecified injury of unspecified wrist, hand and finger(s)
- S69.91 Unspecified injury of right wrist, hand and finger(s)
- S69.92 Unspecified injury of left wrist, hand and finger(s)

Injuries to the hip and thigh (S70-S79)

EXCLUDES 2 *burns and corrosions (T20-T32)*
frostbite (T33-T34)
snake bite (T63.0-)
venomous insect bite or sting (T63.4-)

S70 Superficial injury of hip and thigh

The appropriate 7th character is to be added to each code from category S70.
- A initial encounter
- D subsequent encounter
- S sequela

S70.0 Contusion of hip
- S70.00 Contusion of unspecified hip
- S70.01 Contusion of right hip
- S70.02 Contusion of left hip

S70.1 Contusion of thigh
- S70.10 Contusion of unspecified thigh
- S70.11 Contusion of right thigh
- S70.12 Contusion of left thigh

S70.2 Other superficial injuries of hip

S70.21 Abrasion of hip
- S70.211 Abrasion, right hip
- S70.212 Abrasion, left hip
- S70.219 Abrasion, unspecified hip

S70.22 Blister (nonthermal) of hip
- S70.221 Blister (nonthermal), right hip
- S70.222 Blister (nonthermal), left hip
- S70.229 Blister (nonthermal), unspecified hip

S70.24 External constriction of hip
- S70.241 External constriction, right hip
- S70.242 External constriction, left hip
- S70.249 External constriction, unspecified hip

S70.25 Superficial foreign body of hip
  Splinter in the hip
- S70.251 Superficial foreign body, right hip
- S70.252 Superficial foreign body, left hip
- S70.259 Superficial foreign body, unspecified hip

- ✓6th **S7Ø.26 Insect bite (nonvenomous) of hip**
  - ✓7th **S7Ø.261 Insect bite (nonvenomous), right hip**
  - ✓7th **S7Ø.262 Insect bite (nonvenomous), left hip**
  - ✓7th **S7Ø.269 Insect bite (nonvenomous), unspecified hip**
- ✓6th **S7Ø.27 Other superficial bite of hip**
  - EXCLUDES 1 *open bite of hip (S71.Ø5-)*
  - ✓7th **S7Ø.271 Other superficial bite of hip, right hip**
  - ✓7th **S7Ø.272 Other superficial bite of hip, left hip**
  - ✓7th **S7Ø.279 Other superficial bite of hip, unspecified hip**
- ✓5th **S7Ø.3 Other superficial injuries of thigh**
  - ✓6th **S7Ø.31 Abrasion of thigh**
    - ✓7th **S7Ø.311 Abrasion, right thigh**
    - ✓7th **S7Ø.312 Abrasion, left thigh**
    - ✓7th **S7Ø.319 Abrasion, unspecified thigh**
  - ✓6th **S7Ø.32 Blister (nonthermal) of thigh**
    - ✓7th **S7Ø.321 Blister (nonthermal), right thigh**
    - ✓7th **S7Ø.322 Blister (nonthermal), left thigh**
    - ✓7th **S7Ø.329 Blister (nonthermal), unspecified thigh**
  - ✓6th **S7Ø.34 External constriction of thigh**
    - ✓7th **S7Ø.341 External constriction, right thigh**
    - ✓7th **S7Ø.342 External constriction, left thigh**
    - ✓7th **S7Ø.349 External constriction, unspecified thigh**
  - ✓6th **S7Ø.35 Superficial foreign body of thigh**
    - Splinter in the thigh
    - ✓7th **S7Ø.351 Superficial foreign body, right thigh**
    - ✓7th **S7Ø.352 Superficial foreign body, left thigh**
    - ✓7th **S7Ø.359 Superficial foreign body, unspecified thigh**
  - ✓6th **S7Ø.36 Insect bite (nonvenomous) of thigh**
    - ✓7th **S7Ø.361 Insect bite (nonvenomous), right thigh**
    - ✓7th **S7Ø.362 Insect bite (nonvenomous), left thigh**
    - ✓7th **S7Ø.369 Insect bite (nonvenomous), unspecified thigh**
  - ✓6th **S7Ø.37 Other superficial bite of thigh**
    - EXCLUDES 1 *open bite of thigh (S71.15)*
    - ✓7th **S7Ø.371 Other superficial bite of right thigh**
    - ✓7th **S7Ø.372 Other superficial bite of left thigh**
    - ✓7th **S7Ø.379 Other superficial bite of unspecified thigh**
- ✓5th **S7Ø.9 Unspecified superficial injury of hip and thigh**
  - ✓6th **S7Ø.91 Unspecified superficial injury of hip**
    - ✓7th **S7Ø.911 Unspecified superficial injury of right hip**
    - ✓7th **S7Ø.912 Unspecified superficial injury of left hip**
    - ✓7th **S7Ø.919 Unspecified superficial injury of unspecified hip**
  - ✓6th **S7Ø.92 Unspecified superficial injury of thigh**
    - ✓7th **S7Ø.921 Unspecified superficial injury of right thigh**
    - ✓7th **S7Ø.922 Unspecified superficial injury of left thigh**
    - ✓7th **S7Ø.929 Unspecified superficial injury of unspecified thigh**

✓4th **S71 Open wound of hip and thigh**

Code also any associated wound infection

EXCLUDES 1 *open fracture of hip and thigh (S72.-)*
traumatic amputation of hip and thigh (S78.-)

EXCLUDES 2 *bite of venomous animal (T63.-)*
open wound of ankle, foot and toes (S91.-)
open wound of knee and lower leg (S81.-)

> The appropriate 7th character is to be added to each code from category S71.
> A initial encounter
> D subsequent encounter
> S sequela

- ✓5th **S71.Ø Open wound of hip**
  - ✓6th **S71.ØØ Unspecified open wound of hip**
    - ✓7th **S71.ØØ1 Unspecified open wound, right hip**
    - ✓7th **S71.ØØ2 Unspecified open wound, left hip**
    - ✓7th **S71.ØØ9 Unspecified open wound, unspecified hip**
  - ✓6th **S71.Ø1 Laceration without foreign body of hip**
    - ✓7th **S71.Ø11 Laceration without foreign body, right hip**
    - ✓7th **S71.Ø12 Laceration without foreign body, left hip**
    - ✓7th **S71.Ø19 Laceration without foreign body, unspecified hip**
  - ✓6th **S71.Ø2 Laceration with foreign body of hip**
    - ✓7th **S71.Ø21 Laceration with foreign body, right hip**
    - ✓7th **S71.Ø22 Laceration with foreign body, left hip**
    - ✓7th **S71.Ø29 Laceration with foreign body, unspecified hip**
  - ✓6th **S71.Ø3 Puncture wound without foreign body of hip**
    - ✓7th **S71.Ø31 Puncture wound without foreign body, right hip**
    - ✓7th **S71.Ø32 Puncture wound without foreign body, left hip**
    - ✓7th **S71.Ø39 Puncture wound without foreign body, unspecified hip**
  - ✓6th **S71.Ø4 Puncture wound with foreign body of hip**
    - ✓7th **S71.Ø41 Puncture wound with foreign body, right hip**
    - ✓7th **S71.Ø42 Puncture wound with foreign body, left hip**
    - ✓7th **S71.Ø49 Puncture wound with foreign body, unspecified hip**
  - ✓6th **S71.Ø5 Open bite of hip**
    - Bite of hip NOS
    - EXCLUDES 1 *superficial bite of hip (S7Ø.26, S7Ø.27)*
    - ✓7th **S71.Ø51 Open bite, right hip**
    - ✓7th **S71.Ø52 Open bite, left hip**
    - ✓7th **S71.Ø59 Open bite, unspecified hip**
- ✓5th **S71.1 Open wound of thigh**
  - ✓6th **S71.1Ø Unspecified open wound of thigh**
    - AHA: 2016,3Q,24
    - ✓7th **S71.1Ø1 Unspecified open wound, right thigh**
    - ✓7th **S71.1Ø2 Unspecified open wound, left thigh**
    - ✓7th **S71.1Ø9 Unspecified open wound, unspecified thigh**
  - ✓6th **S71.11 Laceration without foreign body of thigh**
    - ✓7th **S71.111 Laceration without foreign body, right thigh**
    - ✓7th **S71.112 Laceration without foreign body, left thigh**
    - ✓7th **S71.119 Laceration without foreign body, unspecified thigh**
  - ✓6th **S71.12 Laceration with foreign body of thigh**
    - ✓7th **S71.121 Laceration with foreign body, right thigh**
    - ✓7th **S71.122 Laceration with foreign body, left thigh**
    - ✓7th **S71.129 Laceration with foreign body, unspecified thigh**
  - ✓6th **S71.13 Puncture wound without foreign body of thigh**
    - AHA: 2016,3Q,24
    - ✓7th **S71.131 Puncture wound without foreign body, right thigh**
    - ✓7th **S71.132 Puncture wound without foreign body, left thigh**
    - ✓7th **S71.139 Puncture wound without foreign body, unspecified thigh**
  - ✓6th **S71.14 Puncture wound with foreign body of thigh**
    - AHA: 2016,3Q,24
    - ✓7th **S71.141 Puncture wound with foreign body, right thigh**
    - ✓7th **S71.142 Puncture wound with foreign body, left thigh**
    - ✓7th **S71.149 Puncture wound with foreign body, unspecified thigh**
  - ✓6th **S71.15 Open bite of thigh**
    - Bite of thigh NOS
    - EXCLUDES 1 *superficial bite of thigh (S7Ø.37-)*
    - ✓7th **S71.151 Open bite, right thigh**
    - ✓7th **S71.152 Open bite, left thigh**
    - ✓7th **S71.159 Open bite, unspecified thigh**

S72 Fracture of femur

NOTE A fracture not indicated as displaced or nondisplaced should be coded to displaced.

A fracture not indicated as open or closed should be coded to closed.

The open fracture designations are based on the Gustilo open fracture classification.

EXCLUDES 1 *traumatic amputation of hip and thigh (S78.-)*

EXCLUDES 2 *fracture of lower leg and ankle (S82.-)*

fracture of foot (S92.-)

periprosthetic fracture of prosthetic implant of hip (M97.Ø-)

AHA: 2018,2Q,12; 2016,1Q,33; 2015,3Q,37-39; 2015,1Q,17; 2013,4Q,128

DEF: Diaphysis: Central shaft of a long bone.

DEF: Epiphysis: Proximal and distal rounded ends of a long bone communicates with the joint.

DEF: Metaphysis: Section of a long bone located between the epiphysis and diaphysis at the proximal and distal ends.

DEF: Physis (growth plate): Narrow zone of cartilaginous tissue between the epiphysis and metaphysis at each end of a long bone. In childhood, proliferation of cells in this zone lengthens the bone. As the bone matures, this area thins, ossification eventually fusing into solid bone and growth stops. ***Synonym(s):*** *Epiphyseal plate.*

The appropriate 7th character is to be added to all codes from category S72 [unless otherwise indicated].

- A initial encounter for closed fracture
- B initial encounter for open fracture type I or II; initial encounter for open fracture NOS
- C initial encounter for open fracture type IIIA, IIIB, or IIIC
- D subsequent encounter for closed fracture with routine healing
- E subsequent encounter for open fracture type I or II with routine healing
- F subsequent encounter for open fracture type IIIA, IIIB, or IIIC with routine healing
- G subsequent encounter for closed fracture with delayed healing
- H subsequent encounter for open fracture type I or II with delayed healing
- J subsequent encounter for open fracture type IIIA, IIIB, or IIIC with delayed healing
- K subsequent encounter for closed fracture with nonunion
- M subsequent encounter for open fracture type I or II with nonunion
- N subsequent encounter for open fracture type IIIA, IIIB, or IIIC with nonunion
- P subsequent encounter for closed fracture with malunion
- Q subsequent encounter for open fracture type I or II with malunion
- R subsequent encounter for open fracture type IIIA, IIIB, or IIIC with malunion
- S sequela

S72.Ø Fracture of head and neck of femur

EXCLUDES 2 *physeal fracture of upper end of femur (S79.Ø-)*

AHA: 2016,3Q,16

S72.ØØ Fracture of unspecified part of neck of femur

Fracture of hip NOS

Fracture of neck of femur NOS

1 **S72.ØØ1 Fracture of unspecified part of neck of right femur** HCC ESR COM Q

1 **S72.ØØ2 Fracture of unspecified part of neck of left femur** HCC ESR COM Q

1 **S72.ØØ9 Fracture of unspecified part of neck of unspecified femur** HCC ESR COM Q

S72.Ø1 Unspecified intracapsular fracture of femur

Subcapital fracture of femur

1 **S72.Ø11 Unspecified intracapsular fracture of right femur** HCC ESR COM Q

1 **S72.Ø12 Unspecified intracapsular fracture of left femur** HCC ESR COM Q

1 **S72.Ø19 Unspecified intracapsular fracture of unspecified femur** HCC ESR COM Q

S72.Ø2 Fracture of epiphysis (separation) (upper) of femur

Transepiphyseal fracture of femur

EXCLUDES 1 *capital femoral epiphyseal fracture (pediatric) of femur (S79.Ø1-)*

Salter-Harris Type I physeal fracture of upper end of femur (S79.Ø1-)

1 **S72.Ø21 Displaced fracture of epiphysis (separation) (upper) of right femur** HCC ESR COM Q

1 **S72.Ø22 Displaced fracture of epiphysis (separation) (upper) of left femur** HCC ESR COM Q

1 **S72.Ø23 Displaced fracture of epiphysis (separation) (upper) of unspecified femur** HCC ESR COM Q

1 **S72.Ø24 Nondisplaced fracture of epiphysis (separation) (upper) of right femur** HCC ESR COM Q

1 **S72.Ø25 Nondisplaced fracture of epiphysis (separation) (upper) of left femur** HCC ESR COM Q

1 **S72.Ø26 Nondisplaced fracture of epiphysis (separation) (upper) of unspecified femur** HCC ESR COM Q

S72.Ø3 Midcervical fracture of femur

Transcervical fracture of femur NOS

1 **S72.Ø31 Displaced midcervical fracture of right femur** HCC ESR COM Q

1 **S72.Ø32 Displaced midcervical fracture of left femur** HCC ESR COM Q

1 **S72.Ø33 Displaced midcervical fracture of unspecified femur** HCC ESR COM Q

1 **S72.Ø34 Nondisplaced midcervical fracture of right femur** HCC ESR COM Q

1 **S72.Ø35 Nondisplaced midcervical fracture of left femur** HCC ESR COM Q

1 **S72.Ø36 Nondisplaced midcervical fracture of unspecified femur** HCC ESR COM Q

S72.Ø4 Fracture of base of neck of femur

Cervicotrochanteric fracture of femur

1 **S72.Ø41 Displaced fracture of base of neck of right femur** HCC ESR COM Q

1 **S72.Ø42 Displaced fracture of base of neck of left femur** HCC ESR COM Q

1 **S72.Ø43 Displaced fracture of base of neck of unspecified femur** HCC ESR COM Q

1 **S72.Ø44 Nondisplaced fracture of base of neck of right femur** HCC ESR COM Q

1 **S72.Ø45 Nondisplaced fracture of base of neck of left femur** HCC ESR COM Q

1 **S72.Ø46 Nondisplaced fracture of base of neck of unspecified femur** HCC ESR COM Q

S72.Ø5 Unspecified fracture of head of femur

Fracture of head of femur NOS

1 **S72.Ø51 Unspecified fracture of head of right femur** HCC ESR COM Q

1 **S72.Ø52 Unspecified fracture of head of left femur** HCC ESR COM Q

1 **S72.Ø59 Unspecified fracture of head of unspecified femur** HCC ESR COM Q

S72.Ø6 Articular fracture of head of femur

1 **S72.Ø61 Displaced articular fracture of head of right femur** HCC ESR COM Q

1 **S72.Ø62 Displaced articular fracture of head of left femur** HCC ESR COM Q

1 **S72.Ø63 Displaced articular fracture of head of unspecified femur** HCC ESR COM Q

1 **S72.Ø64 Nondisplaced articular fracture of head of right femur** HCC ESR COM Q

1 **S72.Ø65 Nondisplaced articular fracture of head of left femur** HCC ESR COM Q

1 **S72.Ø66 Nondisplaced articular fracture of head of unspecified femur** HCC ESR COM Q

S72.Ø9 Other fracture of head and neck of femur

1 **S72.Ø91 Other fracture of head and neck of right femur** HCC ESR COM Q

1 **S72.Ø92 Other fracture of head and neck of left femur** HCC ESR COM Q

1 **S72.Ø99 Other fracture of head and neck of unspecified femur** HCC ESR COM Q

S72.1 Pertrochanteric fracture

AHA: 2016,3Q,16

S72.1Ø Unspecified trochanteric fracture of femur

Fracture of trochanter NOS

1 **S72.1Ø1 Unspecified trochanteric fracture of right femur** HCC ESR COM Q

1 **S72.1Ø2 Unspecified trochanteric fracture of left femur** HCC ESR COM Q

1 ✓7th S72.109 Unspecified trochanteric fracture of unspecified femur HCC ESR COM Q

✓6th S72.11 Fracture of greater trochanter of femur

1 ✓7th S72.111 Displaced fracture of greater trochanter of right femur HCC ESR COM Q

1 ✓7th S72.112 Displaced fracture of greater trochanter of left femur HCC ESR COM Q

1 ✓7th S72.113 Displaced fracture of greater trochanter of unspecified femur HCC ESR COM Q

1 ✓7th S72.114 Nondisplaced fracture of greater trochanter of right femur HCC ESR COM Q

1 ✓7th S72.115 Nondisplaced fracture of greater trochanter of left femur HCC ESR COM Q

1 ✓7th S72.116 Nondisplaced fracture of greater trochanter of unspecified femur HCC ESR COM Q

✓6th S72.12 Fracture of lesser trochanter of femur

1 ✓7th S72.121 Displaced fracture of lesser trochanter of right femur HCC ESR COM Q

1 ✓7th S72.122 Displaced fracture of lesser trochanter of left femur HCC ESR COM Q

1 ✓7th S72.123 Displaced fracture of lesser trochanter of unspecified femur HCC ESR COM Q

1 ✓7th S72.124 Nondisplaced fracture of lesser trochanter of right femur HCC ESR COM Q

1 ✓7th S72.125 Nondisplaced fracture of lesser trochanter of left femur HCC ESR COM Q

1 ✓7th S72.126 Nondisplaced fracture of lesser trochanter of unspecified femur HCC ESR COM Q

✓6th S72.13 Apophyseal fracture of femur

EXCLUDES 1 *chronic (nontraumatic) slipped upper femoral epiphysis (M93.Ø-)*

1 ✓7th S72.131 Displaced apophyseal fracture of right femur HCC ESR COM Q

1 ✓7th S72.132 Displaced apophyseal fracture of left femur HCC ESR COM Q

1 ✓7th S72.133 Displaced apophyseal fracture of unspecified femur HCC ESR COM Q

1 ✓7th S72.134 Nondisplaced apophyseal fracture of right femur HCC ESR COM Q

1 ✓7th S72.135 Nondisplaced apophyseal fracture of left femur HCC ESR COM Q

1 ✓7th S72.136 Nondisplaced apophyseal fracture of unspecified femur HCC ESR COM Q

✓6th S72.14 Intertrochanteric fracture of femur

1 ✓7th S72.141 Displaced intertrochanteric fracture of right femur HCC ESR COM Q

1 ✓7th S72.142 Displaced intertrochanteric fracture of left femur HCC ESR COM Q

1 ✓7th S72.143 Displaced intertrochanteric fracture of unspecified femur HCC ESR COM Q

1 ✓7th S72.144 Nondisplaced intertrochanteric fracture of right femur HCC ESR COM Q

1 ✓7th S72.145 Nondisplaced intertrochanteric fracture of left femur HCC ESR COM Q

1 ✓7th S72.146 Nondisplaced intertrochanteric fracture of unspecified femur HCC ESR COM Q

✓5th S72.2 Subtrochanteric fracture of femur

1 ✓x7th S72.21 Displaced subtrochanteric fracture of right femur HCC ESR COM Q

1 ✓x7th S72.22 Displaced subtrochanteric fracture of left femur HCC ESR COM Q

1 ✓x7th S72.23 Displaced subtrochanteric fracture of unspecified femur HCC ESR COM Q

1 ✓x7th S72.24 Nondisplaced subtrochanteric fracture of right femur HCC ESR COM Q

1 ✓x7th S72.25 Nondisplaced subtrochanteric fracture of left femur HCC ESR COM Q

1 ✓x7th S72.26 Nondisplaced subtrochanteric fracture of unspecified femur HCC ESR COM Q

✓5th S72.3 Fracture of shaft of femur

✓6th S72.30 Unspecified fracture of shaft of femur

1 ✓7th S72.301 Unspecified fracture of shaft of right femur HCC ESR Q

1 ✓7th S72.302 Unspecified fracture of shaft of left femur HCC ESR Q

1 ✓7th S72.309 Unspecified fracture of shaft of unspecified femur HCC ESR Q

✓6th S72.32 Transverse fracture of shaft of femur

1 ✓7th S72.321 Displaced transverse fracture of shaft of right femur HCC ESR Q

1 ✓7th S72.322 Displaced transverse fracture of shaft of left femur HCC ESR Q

1 ✓7th S72.323 Displaced transverse fracture of shaft of unspecified femur HCC ESR Q

1 ✓7th S72.324 Nondisplaced transverse fracture of shaft of right femur HCC ESR Q

1 ✓7th S72.325 Nondisplaced transverse fracture of shaft of left femur HCC ESR Q

1 ✓7th S72.326 Nondisplaced transverse fracture of shaft of unspecified femur HCC ESR Q

✓6th S72.33 Oblique fracture of shaft of femur

1 ✓7th S72.331 Displaced oblique fracture of shaft of right femur HCC ESR Q

1 ✓7th S72.332 Displaced oblique fracture of shaft of left femur HCC ESR Q

1 ✓7th S72.333 Displaced oblique fracture of shaft of unspecified femur HCC ESR Q

1 ✓7th S72.334 Nondisplaced oblique fracture of shaft of right femur HCC ESR Q

1 ✓7th S72.335 Nondisplaced oblique fracture of shaft of left femur HCC ESR Q

1 ✓7th S72.336 Nondisplaced oblique fracture of shaft of unspecified femur HCC ESR Q

✓6th S72.34 Spiral fracture of shaft of femur

1 ✓7th S72.341 Displaced spiral fracture of shaft of right femur HCC ESR Q

1 ✓7th S72.342 Displaced spiral fracture of shaft of left femur HCC ESR Q

1 ✓7th S72.343 Displaced spiral fracture of shaft of unspecified femur HCC ESR Q

1 ✓7th S72.344 Nondisplaced spiral fracture of shaft of right femur HCC ESR Q

1 ✓7th S72.345 Nondisplaced spiral fracture of shaft of left femur HCC ESR Q

1 ✓7th S72.346 Nondisplaced spiral fracture of shaft of unspecified femur HCC ESR Q

✓6th S72.35 Comminuted fracture of shaft of femur

1 ✓7th S72.351 Displaced comminuted fracture of shaft of right femur HCC ESR Q

1 ✓7th S72.352 Displaced comminuted fracture of shaft of left femur HCC ESR Q

1 ✓7th S72.353 Displaced comminuted fracture of shaft of unspecified femur HCC ESR Q

1 ✓7th S72.354 Nondisplaced comminuted fracture of shaft of right femur HCC ESR Q

1 ✓7th S72.355 Nondisplaced comminuted fracture of shaft of left femur HCC ESR Q

1 ✓7th S72.356 Nondisplaced comminuted fracture of shaft of unspecified femur HCC ESR Q

✓6th S72.36 Segmental fracture of shaft of femur

1 ✓7th S72.361 Displaced segmental fracture of shaft of right femur HCC ESR Q

1 ✓7th S72.362 Displaced segmental fracture of shaft of left femur HCC ESR Q

1 ✓7th S72.363 Displaced segmental fracture of shaft of unspecified femur HCC ESR Q

1 ✓7th S72.364 Nondisplaced segmental fracture of shaft of right femur HCC ESR Q

1 ✓7th S72.365 Nondisplaced segmental fracture of shaft of left femur HCC ESR Q

1 ✓7th S72.366 Nondisplaced segmental fracture of shaft of unspecified femur HCC ESR Q

✓6th S72.39 Other fracture of shaft of femur

1 ✓7th S72.391 Other fracture of shaft of right femur HCC ESR Q

1 ✓7th S72.392 Other fracture of shaft of left femur HCC ESR Q

1 ✓7th S72.399 Other fracture of shaft of unspecified femur HCC ESR Q

S72.4 Fracture of lower end of femur
Fracture of distal end of femur
EXCLUDES 2 fracture of shaft of femur (S72.3-)
physeal fracture of lower end of femur (S79.1-)
AHA: 2016,4Q,42

S72.40 Unspecified fracture of lower end of femur
AHA: 2018,1Q,21; 2016,4Q,42
1 S72.401 Unspecified fracture of lower end of right femur HCC ESR Q
1 S72.402 Unspecified fracture of lower end of left femur HCC ESR Q
1 S72.409 Unspecified fracture of lower end of unspecified femur HCC ESR Q

S72.41 Unspecified condyle fracture of lower end of femur
Condyle fracture of femur NOS
1 S72.411 Displaced unspecified condyle fracture of lower end of right femur HCC ESR Q
1 S72.412 Displaced unspecified condyle fracture of lower end of left femur HCC ESR Q
1 S72.413 Displaced unspecified condyle fracture of lower end of unspecified femur HCC ESR Q
1 S72.414 Nondisplaced unspecified condyle fracture of lower end of right femur HCC ESR Q
1 S72.415 Nondisplaced unspecified condyle fracture of lower end of left femur HCC ESR Q
1 S72.416 Nondisplaced unspecified condyle fracture of lower end of unspecified femur HCC ESR Q

S72.42 Fracture of lateral condyle of femur
1 S72.421 Displaced fracture of lateral condyle of right femur HCC ESR Q
1 S72.422 Displaced fracture of lateral condyle of left femur HCC ESR Q
1 S72.423 Displaced fracture of lateral condyle of unspecified femur HCC ESR Q
1 S72.424 Nondisplaced fracture of lateral condyle of right femur HCC ESR Q
1 S72.425 Nondisplaced fracture of lateral condyle of left femur HCC ESR Q
1 S72.426 Nondisplaced fracture of lateral condyle of unspecified femur HCC ESR Q

S72.43 Fracture of medial condyle of femur
1 S72.431 Displaced fracture of medial condyle of right femur HCC ESR Q
1 S72.432 Displaced fracture of medial condyle of left femur HCC ESR Q
1 S72.433 Displaced fracture of medial condyle of unspecified femur HCC ESR Q
1 S72.434 Nondisplaced fracture of medial condyle of right femur HCC ESR Q
1 S72.435 Nondisplaced fracture of medial condyle of left femur HCC ESR Q
1 S72.436 Nondisplaced fracture of medial condyle of unspecified femur HCC ESR Q

S72.44 Fracture of lower epiphysis (separation) of femur
EXCLUDES 1 Salter-Harris Type I physeal fracture of lower end of femur (S79.11-)
1 S72.441 Displaced fracture of lower epiphysis (separation) of right femur HCC ESR Q
1 S72.442 Displaced fracture of lower epiphysis (separation) of left femur HCC ESR Q
1 S72.443 Displaced fracture of lower epiphysis (separation) of unspecified femur HCC ESR Q
1 S72.444 Nondisplaced fracture of lower epiphysis (separation) of right femur HCC ESR Q
1 S72.445 Nondisplaced fracture of lower epiphysis (separation) of left femur HCC ESR Q
1 S72.446 Nondisplaced fracture of lower epiphysis (separation) of unspecified femur HCC ESR Q

S72.45 Supracondylar fracture without intracondylar extension of lower end of femur
Supracondylar fracture of lower end of femur NOS
EXCLUDES 1 supracondylar fracture with intracondylar extension of lower end of femur (S72.46-)
1 S72.451 Displaced supracondylar fracture without intracondylar extension of lower end of right femur HCC ESR Q
1 S72.452 Displaced supracondylar fracture without intracondylar extension of lower end of left femur HCC ESR Q
1 S72.453 Displaced supracondylar fracture without intracondylar extension of lower end of unspecified femur HCC ESR Q
1 S72.454 Nondisplaced supracondylar fracture without intracondylar extension of lower end of right femur HCC ESR Q
1 S72.455 Nondisplaced supracondylar fracture without intracondylar extension of lower end of left femur HCC ESR Q
1 S72.456 Nondisplaced supracondylar fracture without intracondylar extension of lower end of unspecified femur HCC ESR Q

S72.46 Supracondylar fracture with intracondylar extension of lower end of femur
EXCLUDES 1 supracondylar fracture without intracondylar extension of lower end of femur (S72.45-)
1 S72.461 Displaced supracondylar fracture with intracondylar extension of lower end of right femur HCC ESR Q
1 S72.462 Displaced supracondylar fracture with intracondylar extension of lower end of left femur HCC ESR Q
1 S72.463 Displaced supracondylar fracture with intracondylar extension of lower end of unspecified femur HCC ESR Q
1 S72.464 Nondisplaced supracondylar fracture with intracondylar extension of lower end of right femur HCC ESR Q
1 S72.465 Nondisplaced supracondylar fracture with intracondylar extension of lower end of left femur HCC ESR Q
1 S72.466 Nondisplaced supracondylar fracture with intracondylar extension of lower end of unspecified femur HCC ESR Q

S72.47 Torus fracture of lower end of femur

The appropriate 7th character is to be added to all codes in subcategory S72.47.
A initial encounter for closed fracture
D subsequent encounter for fracture with routine healing
G subsequent encounter for fracture with delayed healing
K subsequent encounter for fracture with nonunion
P subsequent encounter for fracture with malunion
S sequela

1 S72.471 Torus fracture of lower end of right femur HCC ESR Q
1 S72.472 Torus fracture of lower end of left femur HCC ESR Q
1 S72.479 Torus fracture of lower end of unspecified femur HCC ESR Q

S72.49 Other fracture of lower end of femur
1 S72.491 Other fracture of lower end of right femur HCC ESR Q
1 S72.492 Other fracture of lower end of left femur HCC ESR Q
1 S72.499 Other fracture of lower end of unspecified femur HCC ESR Q

S72.8 Other fracture of femur
S72.8X Other fracture of femur
1 S72.8X1 Other fracture of right femur HCC ESR Q
1 S72.8X2 Other fracture of left femur HCC ESR Q

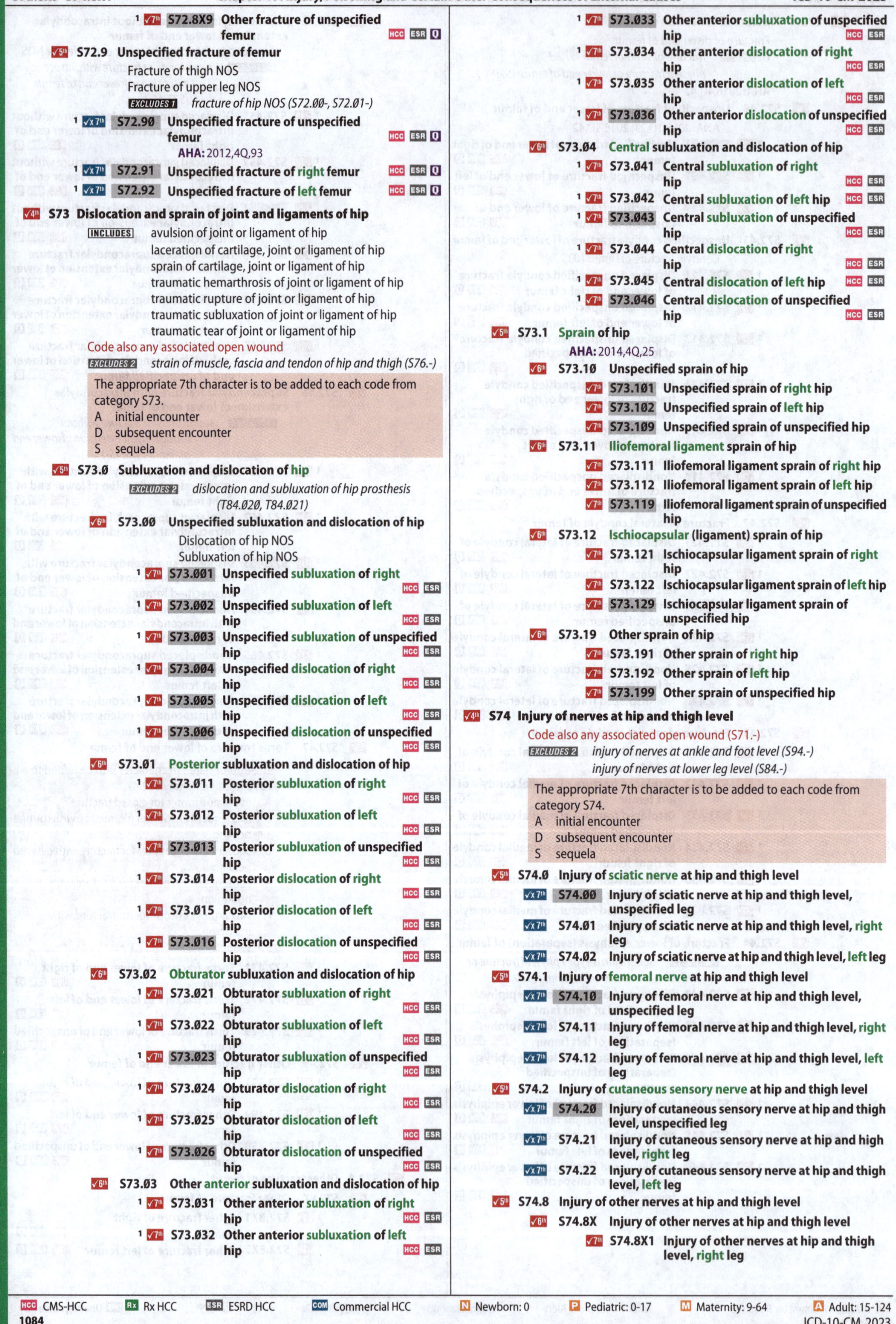

1 √7th S72.8X9 Other fracture of unspecified femur HCC ESR Q

√5th S72.9 Unspecified fracture of femur
Fracture of thigh NOS
Fracture of upper leg NOS
EXCLUDES 1 *fracture of hip NOS (S72.00-, S72.01-)*

1 √x7th S72.90 Unspecified fracture of unspecified femur HCC ESR Q
AHA: 2012,4Q,93

1 √x7th S72.91 Unspecified fracture of right femur HCC ESR Q

1 √x7th S72.92 Unspecified fracture of left femur HCC ESR Q

√4th **S73 Dislocation and sprain of joint and ligaments of hip**
INCLUDES avulsion of joint or ligament of hip
laceration of cartilage, joint or ligament of hip
sprain of cartilage, joint or ligament of hip
traumatic hemarthrosis of joint or ligament of hip
traumatic rupture of joint or ligament of hip
traumatic subluxation of joint or ligament of hip
traumatic tear of joint or ligament of hip
Code also any associated open wound
EXCLUDES 2 *strain of muscle, fascia and tendon of hip and thigh (S76.-)*

The appropriate 7th character is to be added to each code from category S73.
A initial encounter
D subsequent encounter
S sequela

√5th S73.0 Subluxation and dislocation of hip
EXCLUDES 2 *dislocation and subluxation of hip prosthesis (T84.020, T84.021)*

√6th S73.00 Unspecified subluxation and dislocation of hip
Dislocation of hip NOS
Subluxation of hip NOS

1 √7th S73.001 Unspecified subluxation of right hip HCC ESR

1 √7th S73.002 Unspecified subluxation of left hip HCC ESR

1 √7th S73.003 Unspecified subluxation of unspecified hip HCC ESR

1 √7th S73.004 Unspecified dislocation of right hip HCC ESR

1 √7th S73.005 Unspecified dislocation of left hip HCC ESR

1 √7th S73.006 Unspecified dislocation of unspecified hip HCC ESR

√6th S73.01 Posterior subluxation and dislocation of hip

1 √7th S73.011 Posterior subluxation of right hip HCC ESR

1 √7th S73.012 Posterior subluxation of left hip HCC ESR

1 √7th S73.013 Posterior subluxation of unspecified hip HCC ESR

1 √7th S73.014 Posterior dislocation of right hip HCC ESR

1 √7th S73.015 Posterior dislocation of left hip HCC ESR

1 √7th S73.016 Posterior dislocation of unspecified hip HCC ESR

√6th S73.02 Obturator subluxation and dislocation of hip

1 √7th S73.021 Obturator subluxation of right hip HCC ESR

1 √7th S73.022 Obturator subluxation of left hip HCC ESR

1 √7th S73.023 Obturator subluxation of unspecified hip HCC ESR

1 √7th S73.024 Obturator dislocation of right hip HCC ESR

1 √7th S73.025 Obturator dislocation of left hip HCC ESR

1 √7th S73.026 Obturator dislocation of unspecified hip HCC ESR

√6th S73.03 Other anterior subluxation and dislocation of hip

1 √7th S73.031 Other anterior subluxation of right hip HCC ESR

1 √7th S73.032 Other anterior subluxation of left hip HCC ESR

1 √7th S73.033 Other anterior subluxation of unspecified hip HCC ESR

1 √7th S73.034 Other anterior dislocation of right hip HCC ESR

1 √7th S73.035 Other anterior dislocation of left hip HCC ESR

1 √7th S73.036 Other anterior dislocation of unspecified hip HCC ESR

√6th S73.04 Central subluxation and dislocation of hip

1 √7th S73.041 Central subluxation of right hip HCC ESR

1 √7th S73.042 Central subluxation of left hip HCC ESR

1 √7th S73.043 Central subluxation of unspecified hip HCC ESR

1 √7th S73.044 Central dislocation of right hip HCC ESR

1 √7th S73.045 Central dislocation of left hip HCC ESR

1 √7th S73.046 Central dislocation of unspecified hip HCC ESR

√5th S73.1 Sprain of hip
AHA: 2014,4Q,25

√6th S73.10 Unspecified sprain of hip

√7th S73.101 Unspecified sprain of right hip

√7th S73.102 Unspecified sprain of left hip

√7th S73.109 Unspecified sprain of unspecified hip

√6th S73.11 Iliofemoral ligament sprain of hip

√7th S73.111 Iliofemoral ligament sprain of right hip

√7th S73.112 Iliofemoral ligament sprain of left hip

√7th S73.119 Iliofemoral ligament sprain of unspecified hip

√6th S73.12 Ischiocapsular (ligament) sprain of hip

√7th S73.121 Ischiocapsular ligament sprain of right hip

√7th S73.122 Ischiocapsular ligament sprain of left hip

√7th S73.129 Ischiocapsular ligament sprain of unspecified hip

√6th S73.19 Other sprain of hip

√7th S73.191 Other sprain of right hip

√7th S73.192 Other sprain of left hip

√7th S73.199 Other sprain of unspecified hip

√4th **S74 Injury of nerves at hip and thigh level**
Code also any associated open wound (S71.-)
EXCLUDES 2 *injury of nerves at ankle and foot level (S94.-)*
injury of nerves at lower leg level (S84.-)

The appropriate 7th character is to be added to each code from category S74.
A initial encounter
D subsequent encounter
S sequela

√5th S74.0 Injury of sciatic nerve at hip and thigh level

√x7th S74.00 Injury of sciatic nerve at hip and thigh level, unspecified leg

√x7th S74.01 Injury of sciatic nerve at hip and thigh level, right leg

√x7th S74.02 Injury of sciatic nerve at hip and thigh level, left leg

√5th S74.1 Injury of femoral nerve at hip and thigh level

√x7th S74.10 Injury of femoral nerve at hip and thigh level, unspecified leg

√x7th S74.11 Injury of femoral nerve at hip and thigh level, right leg

√x7th S74.12 Injury of femoral nerve at hip and thigh level, left leg

√5th S74.2 Injury of cutaneous sensory nerve at hip and thigh level

√x7th S74.20 Injury of cutaneous sensory nerve at hip and thigh level, unspecified leg

√x7th S74.21 Injury of cutaneous sensory nerve at hip and high level, right leg

√x7th S74.22 Injury of cutaneous sensory nerve at hip and thigh level, left leg

√5th S74.8 Injury of other nerves at hip and thigh level

√6th S74.8X Injury of other nerves at hip and thigh level

√7th S74.8X1 Injury of other nerves at hip and thigh level, right leg

S74.8X2 Injury of other nerves at hip and thigh level, left leg
S74.8X9 Injury of other nerves at hip and thigh level, unspecified leg
S74.9 Injury of unspecified nerve at hip and thigh level
S74.90 Injury of unspecified nerve at hip and thigh level, unspecified leg
S74.91 Injury of unspecified nerve at hip and thigh level, right leg
S74.92 Injury of unspecified nerve at hip and thigh level, left leg

S75 Injury of blood vessels at hip and thigh level
Code also any associated open wound (S71.-)
EXCLUDES 2 *injury of blood vessels at lower leg level (S85.-)*
injury of popliteal artery (S85.0)

The appropriate 7th character is to be added to each code from category S75.
A initial encounter
D subsequent encounter
S sequela

S75.0 Injury of femoral artery
S75.00 Unspecified injury of femoral artery
S75.001 Unspecified injury of femoral artery, right leg
S75.002 Unspecified injury of femoral artery, left leg
S75.009 Unspecified injury of femoral artery, unspecified leg
S75.01 Minor laceration of femoral artery
Incomplete transection of femoral artery
Laceration of femoral artery NOS
Superficial laceration of femoral artery
S75.011 Minor laceration of femoral artery, right leg
S75.012 Minor laceration of femoral artery, left leg
S75.019 Minor laceration of femoral artery, unspecified leg
S75.02 Major laceration of femoral artery
Complete transection of femoral artery
Traumatic rupture of femoral artery
S75.021 Major laceration of femoral artery, right leg
S75.022 Major laceration of femoral artery, left leg
S75.029 Major laceration of femoral artery, unspecified leg
S75.09 Other specified injury of femoral artery
S75.091 Other specified injury of femoral artery, right leg
S75.092 Other specified injury of femoral artery, left leg
S75.099 Other specified injury of femoral artery, unspecified leg
S75.1 Injury of femoral vein at hip and thigh level
S75.10 Unspecified injury of femoral vein at hip and thigh level
S75.101 Unspecified injury of femoral vein at hip and thigh level, right leg
S75.102 Unspecified injury of femoral vein at hip and thigh level, left leg
S75.109 Unspecified injury of femoral vein at hip and thigh level, unspecified leg
S75.11 Minor laceration of femoral vein at hip and thigh level
Incomplete transection of femoral vein at hip and thigh level
Laceration of femoral vein at hip and thigh level NOS
Superficial laceration of femoral vein at hip and thigh level
S75.111 Minor laceration of femoral vein at hip and thigh level, right leg
S75.112 Minor laceration of femoral vein at hip and thigh level, left leg
S75.119 Minor laceration of femoral vein at hip and thigh level, unspecified leg
S75.12 Major laceration of femoral vein at hip and thigh level
Complete transection of femoral vein at hip and thigh level
Traumatic rupture of femoral vein at hip and thigh level
S75.121 Major laceration of femoral vein at hip and thigh level, right leg
S75.122 Major laceration of femoral vein at hip and thigh level, left leg
S75.129 Major laceration of femoral vein at hip and thigh level, unspecified leg
S75.19 Other specified injury of femoral vein at hip and thigh level
S75.191 Other specified injury of femoral vein at hip and thigh level, right leg
S75.192 Other specified injury of femoral vein at hip and thigh level, left leg
S75.199 Other specified injury of femoral vein at hip and thigh level, unspecified leg
S75.2 Injury of greater saphenous vein at hip and thigh level
EXCLUDES 1 *greater saphenous vein NOS (S85.3)*
S75.20 Unspecified injury of greater saphenous vein at hip and thigh level
S75.201 Unspecified injury of greater saphenous vein at hip and thigh level, right leg
S75.202 Unspecified injury of greater saphenous vein at hip and thigh level, left leg
S75.209 Unspecified injury of greater saphenous vein at hip and thigh level, unspecified leg
S75.21 Minor laceration of greater saphenous vein at hip and thigh level
Incomplete transection of greater saphenous vein at hip and thigh level
Laceration of greater saphenous vein at hip and thigh level NOS
Superficial laceration of greater saphenous vein at hip and thigh level
S75.211 Minor laceration of greater saphenous vein at hip and thigh level, right leg
S75.212 Minor laceration of greater saphenous vein at hip and thigh level, left leg
S75.219 Minor laceration of greater saphenous vein at hip and thigh level, unspecified leg
S75.22 Major laceration of greater saphenous vein at hip and thigh level
Complete transection of greater saphenous vein at hip and thigh level
Traumatic rupture of greater saphenous vein at hip and thigh level
S75.221 Major laceration of greater saphenous vein at hip and thigh level, right leg
S75.222 Major laceration of greater saphenous vein at hip and thigh level, left leg
S75.229 Major laceration of greater saphenous vein at hip and thigh level, unspecified leg
S75.29 Other specified injury of greater saphenous vein at hip and thigh level
S75.291 Other specified injury of greater saphenous vein at hip and thigh level, right leg
S75.292 Other specified injury of greater saphenous vein at hip and thigh level, left leg
S75.299 Other specified injury of greater saphenous vein at hip and thigh level, unspecified leg
S75.8 Injury of other blood vessels at hip and thigh level
S75.80 Unspecified injury of other blood vessels at hip and thigh level
S75.801 Unspecified injury of other blood vessels at hip and thigh level, right leg
S75.802 Unspecified injury of other blood vessels at hip and thigh level, left leg
S75.809 Unspecified injury of other blood vessels at hip and thigh level, unspecified leg

6th S75.81 **Laceration of other blood vessels at hip and thigh level**
7th S75.811 Laceration of other blood vessels at hip and thigh level, right leg
7th S75.812 Laceration of other blood vessels at hip and thigh level, left leg
7th S75.819 Laceration of other blood vessels at hip and thigh level, unspecified leg
6th S75.89 Other specified injury of other blood vessels at hip and thigh level
7th S75.891 Other specified injury of other blood vessels at hip and thigh level, right leg
7th S75.892 Other specified injury of other blood vessels at hip and thigh level, left leg
7th S75.899 Other specified injury of other blood vessels at hip and thigh level, unspecified leg
5th S75.9 Injury of unspecified blood vessel at hip and thigh level
6th S75.90 Unspecified injury of unspecified blood vessel at hip and thigh level
7th S75.901 Unspecified injury of unspecified blood vessel at hip and thigh level, right leg
7th S75.902 Unspecified injury of unspecified blood vessel at hip and thigh level, left leg
7th S75.909 Unspecified injury of unspecified blood vessel at hip and thigh level, unspecified leg
6th S75.91 Laceration of unspecified blood vessel at hip and thigh level
7th S75.911 Laceration of unspecified blood vessel at hip and thigh level, right leg
7th S75.912 Laceration of unspecified blood vessel at hip and thigh level, left leg
7th S75.919 Laceration of unspecified blood vessel at hip and thigh level, unspecified leg
6th S75.99 Other specified injury of unspecified blood vessel at hip and thigh level
7th S75.991 Other specified injury of unspecified blood vessel at hip and thigh level, right leg
7th S75.992 Other specified injury of unspecified blood vessel at hip and thigh level, left leg
7th S75.999 Other specified injury of unspecified blood vessel at hip and thigh level, unspecified leg

4th **S76 Injury of muscle, fascia and tendon at hip and thigh level**

Code also any associated open wound (S71.-)

EXCLUDES 2 *injury of muscle, fascia and tendon at lower leg level (S86)*
sprain of joint and ligament of hip (S73.1)

TIP: Refer to the Muscle/Tendon table at the beginning of this chapter.

The appropriate 7th character is to be added to each code from category S76.
A initial encounter
D subsequent encounter
S sequela

5th S76.0 Injury of muscle, fascia and tendon of hip
6th S76.00 Unspecified injury of muscle, fascia and tendon of hip
7th S76.001 Unspecified injury of muscle, fascia and tendon of right hip
7th S76.002 Unspecified injury of muscle, fascia and tendon of left hip
7th S76.009 Unspecified injury of muscle, fascia and tendon of unspecified hip
6th S76.01 Strain of muscle, fascia and tendon of hip
7th S76.011 Strain of muscle, fascia and tendon of right hip
7th S76.012 Strain of muscle, fascia and tendon of left hip
7th S76.019 Strain of muscle, fascia and tendon of unspecified hip
6th S76.02 Laceration of muscle, fascia and tendon of hip
7th S76.021 Laceration of muscle, fascia and tendon of right hip
7th S76.022 Laceration of muscle, fascia and tendon of left hip
7th S76.029 Laceration of muscle, fascia and tendon of unspecified hip
6th S76.09 Other specified injury of muscle, fascia and tendon of hip
7th S76.091 Other specified injury of muscle, fascia and tendon of right hip
7th S76.092 Other specified injury of muscle, fascia and tendon of left hip
7th S76.099 Other specified injury of muscle, fascia and tendon of unspecified hip
5th S76.1 Injury of quadriceps muscle, fascia and tendon
Injury of patellar ligament (tendon)
6th S76.10 Unspecified injury of quadriceps muscle, fascia and tendon
7th S76.101 Unspecified injury of right quadriceps muscle, fascia and tendon
7th S76.102 Unspecified injury of left quadriceps muscle, fascia and tendon
7th S76.109 Unspecified injury of unspecified quadriceps muscle, fascia and tendon
6th S76.11 Strain of quadriceps muscle, fascia and tendon
7th S76.111 Strain of right quadriceps muscle, fascia and tendon
7th S76.112 Strain of left quadriceps muscle, fascia and tendon
7th S76.119 Strain of unspecified quadriceps muscle, fascia and tendon
6th S76.12 Laceration of quadriceps muscle, fascia and tendon
7th S76.121 Laceration of right quadriceps muscle, fascia and tendon
7th S76.122 Laceration of left quadriceps muscle, fascia and tendon
7th S76.129 Laceration of unspecified quadriceps muscle, fascia and tendon
6th S76.19 Other specified injury of quadriceps muscle, fascia and tendon
7th S76.191 Other specified injury of right quadriceps muscle, fascia and tendon
7th S76.192 Other specified injury of left quadriceps muscle, fascia and tendon
7th S76.199 Other specified injury of unspecified quadriceps muscle, fascia and tendon
5th S76.2 Injury of adductor muscle, fascia and tendon of thigh
6th S76.20 Unspecified injury of adductor muscle, fascia and tendon of thigh
7th S76.201 Unspecified injury of adductor muscle, fascia and tendon of right thigh
7th S76.202 Unspecified injury of adductor muscle, fascia and tendon of left thigh
7th S76.209 Unspecified injury of adductor muscle, fascia and tendon of unspecified thigh
6th S76.21 Strain of adductor muscle, fascia and tendon of thigh
7th S76.211 Strain of adductor muscle, fascia and tendon of right thigh
7th S76.212 Strain of adductor muscle, fascia and tendon of left thigh
7th S76.219 Strain of adductor muscle, fascia and tendon of unspecified thigh
6th S76.22 Laceration of adductor muscle, fascia and tendon of thigh
7th S76.221 Laceration of adductor muscle, fascia and tendon of right thigh
7th S76.222 Laceration of adductor muscle, fascia and tendon of left thigh
7th S76.229 Laceration of adductor muscle, fascia and tendon of unspecified thigh
6th S76.29 Other injury of adductor muscle, fascia and tendon of thigh
7th S76.291 Other injury of adductor muscle, fascia and tendon of right thigh
7th S76.292 Other injury of adductor muscle, fascia and tendon of left thigh
7th S76.299 Other injury of adductor muscle, fascia and tendon of unspecified thigh
5th S76.3 Injury of muscle, fascia and tendon of the posterior muscle group at thigh level
6th S76.30 Unspecified injury of muscle, fascia and tendon of the posterior muscle group at thigh level
7th S76.301 Unspecified injury of muscle, fascia and tendon of the posterior muscle group at thigh level, right thigh

S76.302 Unspecified injury of muscle, fascia and tendon of the posterior muscle group at thigh level, left thigh
S76.309 Unspecified injury of muscle, fascia and tendon of the posterior muscle group at thigh level, unspecified thigh
S76.31 Strain of muscle, fascia and tendon of the posterior muscle group at thigh level
S76.311 Strain of muscle, fascia and tendon of the posterior muscle group at thigh level, right thigh
S76.312 Strain of muscle, fascia and tendon of the posterior muscle group at thigh level, left thigh
S76.319 Strain of muscle, fascia and tendon of the posterior muscle group at thigh level, unspecified thigh
S76.32 Laceration of muscle, fascia and tendon of the posterior muscle group at thigh level
S76.321 Laceration of muscle, fascia and tendon of the posterior muscle group at thigh level, right thigh
S76.322 Laceration of muscle, fascia and tendon of the posterior muscle group at thigh level, left thigh
S76.329 Laceration of muscle, fascia and tendon of the posterior muscle group at thigh level, unspecified thigh
S76.39 Other specified injury of muscle, fascia and tendon of the posterior muscle group at thigh level
S76.391 Other specified injury of muscle, fascia and tendon of the posterior muscle group at thigh level, right thigh
S76.392 Other specified injury of muscle, fascia and tendon of the posterior muscle group at thigh level, left thigh
S76.399 Other specified injury of muscle, fascia and tendon of the posterior muscle group at thigh level, unspecified thigh
S76.8 Injury of other specified muscles, fascia and tendons at thigh level
S76.80 Unspecified injury of other specified muscles, fascia and tendons at thigh level
S76.801 Unspecified injury of other specified muscles, fascia and tendons at thigh level, right thigh
S76.802 Unspecified injury of other specified muscles, fascia and tendons at thigh level, left thigh
S76.809 Unspecified injury of other specified muscles, fascia and tendons at thigh level, unspecified thigh
S76.81 Strain of other specified muscles, fascia and tendons at thigh level
S76.811 Strain of other specified muscles, fascia and tendons at thigh level, right thigh
S76.812 Strain of other specified muscles, fascia and tendons at thigh level, left thigh
S76.819 Strain of other specified muscles, fascia and tendons at thigh level, unspecified thigh
S76.82 Laceration of other specified muscles, fascia and tendons at thigh level
S76.821 Laceration of other specified muscles, fascia and tendons at thigh level, right thigh
S76.822 Laceration of other specified muscles, fascia and tendons at thigh level, left thigh
S76.829 Laceration of other specified muscles, fascia and tendons at thigh level, unspecified thigh
S76.89 Other injury of other specified muscles, fascia and tendons at thigh level
S76.891 Other injury of other specified muscles, fascia and tendons at thigh level, right thigh
S76.892 Other injury of other specified muscles, fascia and tendons at thigh level, left thigh
S76.899 Other injury of other specified muscles, fascia and tendons at thigh level, unspecified thigh
S76.9 Injury of unspecified muscles, fascia and tendons at thigh level
S76.90 Unspecified injury of unspecified muscles, fascia and tendons at thigh level
S76.901 Unspecified injury of unspecified muscles, fascia and tendons at thigh level, right thigh
S76.902 Unspecified injury of unspecified muscles, fascia and tendons at thigh level, left thigh
S76.909 Unspecified injury of unspecified muscles, fascia and tendons at thigh level, unspecified thigh
S76.91 Strain of unspecified muscles, fascia and tendons at thigh level
S76.911 Strain of unspecified muscles, fascia and tendons at thigh level, right thigh
S76.912 Strain of unspecified muscles, fascia and tendons at thigh level, left thigh
S76.919 Strain of unspecified muscles, fascia and tendons at thigh level, unspecified thigh
S76.92 Laceration of unspecified muscles, fascia and tendons at thigh level
S76.921 Laceration of unspecified muscles, fascia and tendons at thigh level, right thigh
S76.922 Laceration of unspecified muscles, fascia and tendons at thigh level, left thigh
S76.929 Laceration of unspecified muscles, fascia and tendons at thigh level, unspecified thigh
S76.99 Other specified injury of unspecified muscles, fascia and tendons at thigh level
S76.991 Other specified injury of unspecified muscles, fascia and tendons at thigh level, right thigh
S76.992 Other specified injury of unspecified muscles, fascia and tendons at thigh level, left thigh
S76.999 Other specified injury of unspecified muscles, fascia and tendons at thigh level, unspecified thigh

S77 Crushing injury of hip and thigh

Use additional code(s) for all associated injuries

EXCLUDES 2 *crushing injury of ankle and foot (S97.-)*
crushing injury of lower leg (S87.-)

The appropriate 7th character is to be added to each code from category S77.
A initial encounter
D subsequent encounter
S sequela

S77.0 Crushing injury of hip
S77.00 Crushing injury of unspecified hip
S77.01 Crushing injury of right hip
S77.02 Crushing injury of left hip
S77.1 Crushing injury of thigh
S77.10 Crushing injury of unspecified thigh
S77.11 Crushing injury of right thigh
S77.12 Crushing injury of left thigh
S77.2 Crushing injury of hip with thigh
S77.20 Crushing injury of unspecified hip with thigh
S77.21 Crushing injury of right hip with thigh
S77.22 Crushing injury of left hip with thigh

S78 Traumatic amputation of hip and thigh

An amputation not identified as partial or complete should be coded to complete

EXCLUDES 1 *traumatic amputation of knee (S88.0-)*

The appropriate 7th character is to be added to each code from category S78.
A initial encounter
D subsequent encounter
S sequela

S78.0 Traumatic amputation at hip joint
S78.01 Complete traumatic amputation at hip joint
S78.011 Complete traumatic amputation at right hip joint HCC ESR COM

Additional Character Required | Placeholder Alert | Manifestation | Unspecified Dx | Q QPP | UPD Unacceptable PDx

✓7th **S78.012 Complete traumatic amputation at left hip joint** HCC ESR COM

✓7th **S78.019 Complete traumatic amputation at unspecified hip joint** HCC ESR COM

✓6th **S78.02 Partial traumatic amputation at hip joint**

✓7th **S78.021 Partial traumatic amputation at right hip joint** HCC ESR COM

✓7th **S78.022 Partial traumatic amputation at left hip joint** HCC ESR COM

✓7th **S78.029 Partial traumatic amputation at unspecified hip joint** HCC ESR COM

✓5th **S78.1 Traumatic amputation at level between hip and knee**

EXCLUDES 1 *traumatic amputation of knee (S88.Ø-)*

✓6th **S78.11 Complete traumatic amputation at level between hip and knee**

✓7th **S78.111 Complete traumatic amputation at level between right hip and knee** HCC ESR COM

✓7th **S78.112 Complete traumatic amputation at level between left hip and knee** HCC ESR COM

✓7th **S78.119 Complete traumatic amputation at level between unspecified hip and knee** HCC ESR COM

✓6th **S78.12 Partial traumatic amputation at level between hip and knee**

✓7th **S78.121 Partial traumatic amputation at level between right hip and knee** HCC ESR COM

✓7th **S78.122 Partial traumatic amputation at level between left hip and knee** HCC ESR COM

✓7th **S78.129 Partial traumatic amputation at level between unspecified hip and knee** HCC ESR COM

✓5th **S78.9 Traumatic amputation of hip and thigh, level unspecified**

✓6th **S78.91 Complete traumatic amputation of hip and thigh, level unspecified**

✓7th **S78.911 Complete traumatic amputation of right hip and thigh, level unspecified** HCC ESR COM

✓7th **S78.912 Complete traumatic amputation of left hip and thigh, level unspecified** HCC ESR COM

✓7th **S78.919 Complete traumatic amputation of unspecified hip and thigh, level unspecified** HCC ESR COM

✓6th **S78.92 Partial traumatic amputation of hip and thigh, level unspecified**

✓7th **S78.921 Partial traumatic amputation of right hip and thigh, level unspecified** HCC ESR COM

✓7th **S78.922 Partial traumatic amputation of left hip and thigh, level unspecified** HCC ESR COM

✓7th **S78.929 Partial traumatic amputation of unspecified hip and thigh, level unspecified** HCC ESR COM

✓4th **S79 Other and unspecified injuries of hip and thigh**

NOTE A fracture not indicated as open or closed should be coded to closed

AHA: 2018,2Q,12; 2018,1Q,3; 2015,3Q,37-39

The appropriate 7th character is to be added to each code from subcategories S79.Ø and S79.1.
- A initial encounter for closed fracture
- D subsequent encounter for fracture with routine healing
- G subsequent encounter for fracture with delayed healing
- K subsequent encounter for fracture with nonunion
- P subsequent encounter for fracture with malunion
- S sequela

✓5th **S79.Ø Physeal fracture of upper end of femur**

EXCLUDES 1 *apophyseal fracture of upper end of femur (S72.13-)*
nontraumatic slipped upper femoral epiphysis (M93.Ø-)

AHA: 2019,4Q,56

✓6th **S79.ØØ Unspecified physeal fracture of upper end of femur**

1 ✓7th **S79.ØØ1 Unspecified physeal fracture of upper end of right femur** HCC ESR COM Q

1 ✓7th **S79.ØØ2 Unspecified physeal fracture of upper end of left femur** HCC ESR COM Q

1 ✓7th **S79.ØØ9 Unspecified physeal fracture of upper end of unspecified femur** HCC ESR COM Q

✓6th **S79.Ø1 Salter-Harris Type I physeal fracture of upper end of femur**

Acute on chronic slipped capital femoral epiphysis (traumatic)
Acute slipped capital femoral epiphysis (traumatic)
Capital femoral epiphyseal fracture

EXCLUDES 1 *chronic slipped upper femoral epiphysis (nontraumatic) (M93.Ø2-)*

1 ✓7th **S79.Ø11 Salter-Harris Type I physeal fracture of upper end of right femur** HCC ESR COM Q

1 ✓7th **S79.Ø12 Salter-Harris Type I physeal fracture of upper end of left femur** HCC ESR COM Q

1 ✓7th **S79.Ø19 Salter-Harris Type I physeal fracture of upper end of unspecified femur** HCC ESR COM Q

✓6th **S79.Ø9 Other physeal fracture of upper end of femur**

1 ✓7th **S79.Ø91 Other physeal fracture of upper end of right femur** HCC ESR COM Q

1 ✓7th **S79.Ø92 Other physeal fracture of upper end of left femur** HCC ESR COM Q

1 ✓7th **S79.Ø99 Other physeal fracture of upper end of unspecified femur** HCC ESR COM Q

✓5th **S79.1 Physeal fracture of lower end of femur**

AHA: 2019,4Q,56

✓6th **S79.1Ø Unspecified physeal fracture of lower end of femur**

1 ✓7th **S79.1Ø1 Unspecified physeal fracture of lower end of right femur** HCC ESR Q

1 ✓7th **S79.1Ø2 Unspecified physeal fracture of lower end of left femur** HCC ESR Q

1 ✓7th **S79.1Ø9 Unspecified physeal fracture of lower end of unspecified femur** HCC ESR Q

✓6th **S79.11 Salter-Harris Type I physeal fracture of lower end of femur**

1 ✓7th **S79.111 Salter-Harris Type I physeal fracture of lower end of right femur** HCC ESR Q

1 ✓7th **S79.112 Salter-Harris Type I physeal fracture of lower end of left femur** HCC ESR Q

1 ✓7th **S79.119 Salter-Harris Type I physeal fracture of lower end of unspecified femur** HCC ESR Q

✓6th **S79.12 Salter-Harris Type II physeal fracture of lower end of femur**

1 ✓7th **S79.121 Salter-Harris Type II physeal fracture of lower end of right femur** HCC ESR Q

1 ✓7th **S79.122 Salter-Harris Type II physeal fracture of lower end of left femur** HCC ESR Q

1 ✓7th **S79.129 Salter-Harris Type II physeal fracture of lower end of unspecified femur** HCC ESR Q

✓6th **S79.13 Salter-Harris Type III physeal fracture of lower end of femur**

1 ✓7th **S79.131 Salter-Harris Type III physeal fracture of lower end of right femur** HCC ESR Q

1 ✓7th **S79.132 Salter-Harris Type III physeal fracture of lower end of left femur** HCC ESR Q

1 ✓7th **S79.139 Salter-Harris Type III physeal fracture of lower end of unspecified femur** HCC ESR Q

✓6th **S79.14 Salter-Harris Type IV physeal fracture of lower end of femur**

1 ✓7th **S79.141 Salter-Harris Type IV physeal fracture of lower end of right femur** HCC ESR Q

1 ✓7th **S79.142 Salter-Harris Type IV physeal fracture of lower end of left femur** HCC ESR Q

1 ✓7th **S79.149 Salter-Harris Type IV physeal fracture of lower end of unspecified femur** HCC ESR Q

✓6th **S79.19 Other physeal fracture of lower end of femur**

1 ✓7th **S79.191 Other physeal fracture of lower end of right femur** HCC ESR Q

1 ✓7th **S79.192 Other physeal fracture of lower end of left femur** HCC ESR Q

1 ✓7th **S79.199 Other physeal fracture of lower end of unspecified femur** HCC ESR Q

S79.8 Other specified injuries of hip and thigh

The appropriate 7th character is to be added to each code in subcategory S79.8.
A initial encounter
D subsequent encounter
S sequela

S79.81 Other specified injuries of hip
S79.811 Other specified injuries of right hip
S79.812 Other specified injuries of left hip
S79.819 Other specified injuries of unspecified hip
S79.82 Other specified injuries of thigh
S79.821 Other specified injuries of right thigh
S79.822 Other specified injuries of left thigh
S79.829 Other specified injuries of unspecified thigh

S79.9 Unspecified injury of hip and thigh

The appropriate 7th character is to be added to each code in subcategory S79.9.
A initial encounter
D subsequent encounter
S sequela

S79.91 Unspecified injury of hip
S79.911 Unspecified injury of right hip
S79.912 Unspecified injury of left hip
S79.919 Unspecified injury of unspecified hip
S79.92 Unspecified injury of thigh
S79.921 Unspecified injury of right thigh
S79.922 Unspecified injury of left thigh
S79.929 Unspecified injury of unspecified thigh

Injuries to the knee and lower leg (S80-S89)

EXCLUDES 2 *burns and corrosions (T20-T32)*
frostbite (T33-T34)
injuries of ankle and foot, except fracture of ankle and malleolus (S90-S99)
insect bite or sting, venomous (T63.4)

S80 Superficial injury of knee and lower leg

EXCLUDES 2 *superficial injury of ankle and foot (S90.-)*

The appropriate 7th character is to be added to each code from category S80.
A initial encounter
D subsequent encounter
S sequela

S80.0 Contusion of knee
S80.00 Contusion of unspecified knee
S80.01 Contusion of right knee
S80.02 Contusion of left knee
S80.1 Contusion of lower leg
S80.10 Contusion of unspecified lower leg
S80.11 Contusion of right lower leg
S80.12 Contusion of left lower leg
S80.2 Other superficial injuries of knee
S80.21 Abrasion of knee
S80.211 Abrasion, right knee
S80.212 Abrasion, left knee
S80.219 Abrasion, unspecified knee
S80.22 Blister (nonthermal) of knee
S80.221 Blister (nonthermal), right knee
S80.222 Blister (nonthermal), left knee
S80.229 Blister (nonthermal), unspecified knee
S80.24 External constriction of knee
S80.241 External constriction, right knee
S80.242 External constriction, left knee
S80.249 External constriction, unspecified knee
S80.25 Superficial foreign body of knee
Splinter in the knee
S80.251 Superficial foreign body, right knee
S80.252 Superficial foreign body, left knee
S80.259 Superficial foreign body, unspecified knee
S80.26 Insect bite (nonvenomous) of knee
S80.261 Insect bite (nonvenomous), right knee
S80.262 Insect bite (nonvenomous), left knee
S80.269 Insect bite (nonvenomous), unspecified knee
S80.27 Other superficial bite of knee
EXCLUDES 1 *open bite of knee (S81.05-)*
S80.271 Other superficial bite of right knee
S80.272 Other superficial bite of left knee
S80.279 Other superficial bite of unspecified knee
S80.8 Other superficial injuries of lower leg
S80.81 Abrasion of lower leg
S80.811 Abrasion, right lower leg
S80.812 Abrasion, left lower leg
S80.819 Abrasion, unspecified lower leg
S80.82 Blister (nonthermal) of lower leg
S80.821 Blister (nonthermal), right lower leg
S80.822 Blister (nonthermal), left lower leg
S80.829 Blister (nonthermal), unspecified lower leg
S80.84 External constriction of lower leg
S80.841 External constriction, right lower leg
S80.842 External constriction, left lower leg
S80.849 External constriction, unspecified lower leg
S80.85 Superficial foreign body of lower leg
Splinter in the lower leg
S80.851 Superficial foreign body, right lower leg
S80.852 Superficial foreign body, left lower leg
S80.859 Superficial foreign body, unspecified lower leg
S80.86 Insect bite (nonvenomous) of lower leg
S80.861 Insect bite (nonvenomous), right lower leg
S80.862 Insect bite (nonvenomous), left lower leg
S80.869 Insect bite (nonvenomous), unspecified lower leg
S80.87 Other superficial bite of lower leg
EXCLUDES 1 *open bite of lower leg (S81.85-)*
S80.871 Other superficial bite, right lower leg
S80.872 Other superficial bite, left lower leg
S80.879 Other superficial bite, unspecified lower leg
S80.9 Unspecified superficial injury of knee and lower leg
S80.91 Unspecified superficial injury of knee
S80.911 Unspecified superficial injury of right knee
S80.912 Unspecified superficial injury of left knee
S80.919 Unspecified superficial injury of unspecified knee
S80.92 Unspecified superficial injury of lower leg
S80.921 Unspecified superficial injury of right lower leg
S80.922 Unspecified superficial injury of left lower leg
S80.929 Unspecified superficial injury of unspecified lower leg

S81 Open wound of knee and lower leg

Code also any associated wound infection

EXCLUDES 1 *open fracture of knee and lower leg (S82.-)*
traumatic amputation of lower leg (S88.-)
EXCLUDES 2 *open wound of ankle and foot (S91.-)*

The appropriate 7th character is to be added to each code from category S81.
A initial encounter
D subsequent encounter
S sequela

S81.0 Open wound of knee
S81.00 Unspecified open wound of knee
S81.001 Unspecified open wound, right knee

7th S81.002 Unspecified open wound, left knee
7th S81.009 Unspecified open wound, unspecified knee
6th S81.01 Laceration without foreign body of knee
7th S81.011 Laceration without foreign body, right knee
7th S81.012 Laceration without foreign body, left knee
7th S81.019 Laceration without foreign body, unspecified knee
6th S81.02 Laceration with foreign body of knee
7th S81.021 Laceration with foreign body, right knee
7th S81.022 Laceration with foreign body, left knee
7th S81.029 Laceration with foreign body, unspecified knee
6th S81.03 Puncture wound without foreign body of knee
7th S81.031 Puncture wound without foreign body, right knee
7th S81.032 Puncture wound without foreign body, left knee
7th S81.039 Puncture wound without foreign body, unspecified knee
6th S81.04 Puncture wound with foreign body of knee
7th S81.041 Puncture wound with foreign body, right knee
7th S81.042 Puncture wound with foreign body, left knee
7th S81.049 Puncture wound with foreign body, unspecified knee
6th S81.05 Open bite of knee
Bite of knee NOS
EXCLUDES 1 *superficial bite of knee (S80.27-)*
7th S81.051 Open bite, right knee
7th S81.052 Open bite, left knee
7th S81.059 Open bite, unspecified knee
5th S81.8 Open wound of lower leg
6th S81.80 Unspecified open wound of lower leg
AHA: 2016,3Q,24
7th S81.801 Unspecified open wound, right lower leg
7th S81.802 Unspecified open wound, left lower leg
7th S81.809 Unspecified open wound, unspecified lower leg
6th S81.81 Laceration without foreign body of lower leg
7th S81.811 Laceration without foreign body, right lower leg
7th S81.812 Laceration without foreign body, left lower leg
7th S81.819 Laceration without foreign body, unspecified lower leg
6th S81.82 Laceration with foreign body of lower leg
7th S81.821 Laceration with foreign body, right lower leg
7th S81.822 Laceration with foreign body, left lower leg
7th S81.829 Laceration with foreign body, unspecified lower leg
6th S81.83 Puncture wound without foreign body of lower leg
AHA: 2016,3Q,24
7th S81.831 Puncture wound without foreign body, right lower leg
7th S81.832 Puncture wound without foreign body, left lower leg
7th S81.839 Puncture wound without foreign body, unspecified lower leg
6th S81.84 Puncture wound with foreign body of lower leg
AHA: 2016,3Q,24
7th S81.841 Puncture wound with foreign body, right lower leg
7th S81.842 Puncture wound with foreign body, left lower leg
7th S81.849 Puncture wound with foreign body, unspecified lower leg
6th S81.85 Open bite of lower leg
Bite of lower leg NOS
EXCLUDES 1 *superficial bite of lower leg (S80.86-, S80.87-)*
7th S81.851 Open bite, right lower leg
7th S81.852 Open bite, left lower leg
7th S81.859 Open bite, unspecified lower leg

4th **S82 Fracture of lower leg, including ankle**

NOTE A fracture not indicated as displaced or nondisplaced should be coded to displaced

A fracture not indicated as open or closed should be coded to closed

The open fracture designations are based on the Gustilo open fracture classification.

INCLUDES fracture of malleolus
EXCLUDES 1 *traumatic amputation of lower leg (S88.-)*
EXCLUDES 2 *fracture of foot, except ankle (S92.-)*
periprosthetic fracture around internal prosthetic implant of knee joint (M97.1-)

AHA: 2018,2Q,12; 2016,1Q,33; 2015,3Q,37-39
DEF: Diaphysis: Central shaft of a long bone.
DEF: Epiphysis: Proximal and distal rounded ends of a long bone, communicates with the joint.
DEF: Metaphysis: Section of a long bone located between the epiphysis and diaphysis at the proximal and distal ends.
DEF: Physis (growth plate): Narrow zone of cartilaginous tissue between the epiphysis and metaphysis at each end of a long bone. In childhood, proliferation of cells in this zone lengthens the bone. As the bone matures, this area thins, ossification eventually fusing into solid bone and growth stops. ***Synonym(s):*** *Epiphyseal plate.*

The appropriate 7th character is to be added to all codes from category S82 [unless otherwise indicated].

A initial encounter for closed fracture
B initial encounter for open fracture type I or II
initial encounter for open fracture NOS
C initial encounter for open fracture type IIIA, IIIB, or IIIC
D subsequent encounter for closed fracture with routine healing
E subsequent encounter for open fracture type I or II with routine healing
F subsequent encounter for open fracture type IIIA, IIIB, or IIIC with routine healing
G subsequent encounter for closed fracture with delayed healing
H subsequent encounter for open fracture type I or II with delayed healing
J subsequent encounter for open fracture type IIIA, IIIB, or IIIC with delayed healing
K subsequent encounter for closed fracture with nonunion
M subsequent encounter for open fracture type I or II with nonunion
N subsequent encounter for open fracture type IIIA, IIIB, or IIIC with nonunion
P subsequent encounter for closed fracture with malunion
Q subsequent encounter for open fracture type I or II with malunion
R subsequent encounter for open fracture type IIIA, IIIB, or IIIC with malunion
S sequela

5th S82.0 Fracture of patella
Knee cap
6th S82.00 Unspecified fracture of patella
7th S82.001 Unspecified fracture of right patella Q
7th S82.002 Unspecified fracture of left patella Q
7th S82.009 Unspecified fracture of unspecified patella Q
6th S82.01 Osteochondral fracture of patella
7th S82.011 Displaced osteochondral fracture of right patella Q
7th S82.012 Displaced osteochondral fracture of left patella Q
7th S82.013 Displaced osteochondral fracture of unspecified patella Q
7th S82.014 Nondisplaced osteochondral fracture of right patella Q
7th S82.015 Nondisplaced osteochondral fracture of left patella Q
7th S82.016 Nondisplaced osteochondral fracture of unspecified patella Q
6th S82.02 Longitudinal fracture of patella
7th S82.021 Displaced longitudinal fracture of right patella Q
7th S82.022 Displaced longitudinal fracture of left patella Q

S82.023 Displaced longitudinal fracture of unspecified patella Q
S82.024 Nondisplaced longitudinal fracture of right patella Q
S82.025 Nondisplaced longitudinal fracture of left patella Q
S82.026 Nondisplaced longitudinal fracture of unspecified patella Q

S82.03 Transverse fracture of patella
S82.031 Displaced transverse fracture of right patella Q
S82.032 Displaced transverse fracture of left patella Q
S82.033 Displaced transverse fracture of unspecified patella Q
S82.034 Nondisplaced transverse fracture of right patella Q
S82.035 Nondisplaced transverse fracture of left patella Q
S82.036 Nondisplaced transverse fracture of unspecified patella Q

S82.04 Comminuted fracture of patella
S82.041 Displaced comminuted fracture of right patella Q
S82.042 Displaced comminuted fracture of left patella Q
S82.043 Displaced comminuted fracture of unspecified patella Q
S82.044 Nondisplaced comminuted fracture of right patella Q
S82.045 Nondisplaced comminuted fracture of left patella Q
S82.046 Nondisplaced comminuted fracture of unspecified patella Q

S82.09 Other fracture of patella
S82.091 Other fracture of right patella Q
S82.092 Other fracture of left patella Q
S82.099 Other fracture of unspecified patella Q

S82.1 Fracture of upper end of tibia
Fracture of proximal end of tibia
EXCLUDES 2 *fracture of shaft of tibia (S82.2-)*
physeal fracture of upper end of tibia (S89.0-)

S82.10 Unspecified fracture of upper end of tibia
S82.101 Unspecified fracture of upper end of right tibia Q
S82.102 Unspecified fracture of upper end of left tibia Q
S82.109 Unspecified fracture of upper end of unspecified tibia Q

S82.11 Fracture of tibial spine
S82.111 Displaced fracture of right tibial spine Q
S82.112 Displaced fracture of left tibial spine Q
S82.113 Displaced fracture of unspecified tibial spine Q
S82.114 Nondisplaced fracture of right tibial spine Q
S82.115 Nondisplaced fracture of left tibial spine Q
S82.116 Nondisplaced fracture of unspecified tibial spine Q

S82.12 Fracture of lateral condyle of tibia
S82.121 Displaced fracture of lateral condyle of right tibia Q
S82.122 Displaced fracture of lateral condyle of left tibia Q
S82.123 Displaced fracture of lateral condyle of unspecified tibia Q
S82.124 Nondisplaced fracture of lateral condyle of right tibia Q
S82.125 Nondisplaced fracture of lateral condyle of left tibia Q
S82.126 Nondisplaced fracture of lateral condyle of unspecified tibia Q

S82.13 Fracture of medial condyle of tibia
S82.131 Displaced fracture of medial condyle of right tibia Q
S82.132 Displaced fracture of medial condyle of left tibia Q
S82.133 Displaced fracture of medial condyle of unspecified tibia Q
S82.134 Nondisplaced fracture of medial condyle of right tibia Q
S82.135 Nondisplaced fracture of medial condyle of left tibia Q
S82.136 Nondisplaced fracture of medial condyle of unspecified tibia Q

S82.14 Bicondylar fracture of tibia
Fracture of tibial plateau NOS
S82.141 Displaced bicondylar fracture of right tibia Q
S82.142 Displaced bicondylar fracture of left tibia Q
S82.143 Displaced bicondylar fracture of unspecified tibia Q
S82.144 Nondisplaced bicondylar fracture of right tibia Q
S82.145 Nondisplaced bicondylar fracture of left tibia Q
S82.146 Nondisplaced bicondylar fracture of unspecified tibia Q

S82.15 Fracture of tibial tuberosity
S82.151 Displaced fracture of right tibial tuberosity Q
S82.152 Displaced fracture of left tibial tuberosity Q
S82.153 Displaced fracture of unspecified tibial tuberosity Q
S82.154 Nondisplaced fracture of right tibial tuberosity Q
S82.155 Nondisplaced fracture of left tibial tuberosity Q
S82.156 Nondisplaced fracture of unspecified tibial tuberosity Q

S82.16 Torus fracture of upper end of tibia

The appropriate 7th character is to be added to all codes in subcategory S82.16.
A initial encounter for closed fracture
D subsequent encounter for fracture with routine healing
G subsequent encounter for fracture with delayed healing
K subsequent encounter for fracture with nonunion
P subsequent encounter for fracture with malunion
S sequela

S82.161 Torus fracture of upper end of right tibia Q
S82.162 Torus fracture of upper end of left tibia Q
S82.169 Torus fracture of upper end of unspecified tibia Q

S82.19 Other fracture of upper end of tibia
S82.191 Other fracture of upper end of right tibia Q
S82.192 Other fracture of upper end of left tibia Q
S82.199 Other fracture of upper end of unspecified tibia Q

S82.2 Fracture of shaft of tibia

S82.20 Unspecified fracture of shaft of tibia
Fracture of tibia NOS
S82.201 Unspecified fracture of shaft of right tibia Q
S82.202 Unspecified fracture of shaft of left tibia Q
S82.209 Unspecified fracture of shaft of unspecified tibia Q

S82.22 Transverse fracture of shaft of tibia
S82.221 Displaced transverse fracture of shaft of right tibia Q

S82.222 Displaced transverse fracture of shaft of left tibia
S82.223 Displaced transverse fracture of shaft of unspecified tibia
S82.224 Nondisplaced transverse fracture of shaft of right tibia
S82.225 Nondisplaced transverse fracture of shaft of left tibia
S82.226 Nondisplaced transverse fracture of shaft of unspecified tibia

S82.23 Oblique fracture of shaft of tibia
S82.231 Displaced oblique fracture of shaft of right tibia
S82.232 Displaced oblique fracture of shaft of left tibia
S82.233 Displaced oblique fracture of shaft of unspecified tibia
S82.234 Nondisplaced oblique fracture of shaft of right tibia
S82.235 Nondisplaced oblique fracture of shaft of left tibia
S82.236 Nondisplaced oblique fracture of shaft of unspecified tibia

S82.24 Spiral fracture of shaft of tibia
Toddler fracture
S82.241 Displaced spiral fracture of shaft of right tibia
S82.242 Displaced spiral fracture of shaft of left tibia
S82.243 Displaced spiral fracture of shaft of unspecified tibia
S82.244 Nondisplaced spiral fracture of shaft of right tibia
S82.245 Nondisplaced spiral fracture of shaft of left tibia
S82.246 Nondisplaced spiral fracture of shaft of unspecified tibia

S82.25 Comminuted fracture of shaft of tibia
S82.251 Displaced comminuted fracture of shaft of right tibia
S82.252 Displaced comminuted fracture of shaft of left tibia
S82.253 Displaced comminuted fracture of shaft of unspecified tibia
S82.254 Nondisplaced comminuted fracture of shaft of right tibia
S82.255 Nondisplaced comminuted fracture of shaft of left tibia
S82.256 Nondisplaced comminuted fracture of shaft of unspecified tibia

S82.26 Segmental fracture of shaft of tibia
S82.261 Displaced segmental fracture of shaft of right tibia
S82.262 Displaced segmental fracture of shaft of left tibia
S82.263 Displaced segmental fracture of shaft of unspecified tibia
S82.264 Nondisplaced segmental fracture of shaft of right tibia
S82.265 Nondisplaced segmental fracture of shaft of left tibia
S82.266 Nondisplaced segmental fracture of shaft of unspecified tibia

S82.29 Other fracture of shaft of tibia
S82.291 Other fracture of shaft of right tibia
S82.292 Other fracture of shaft of left tibia
S82.299 Other fracture of shaft of unspecified tibia

S82.3 Fracture of lower end of tibia
EXCLUDES 1 *bimalleolar fracture of lower leg (S82.84-)*
fracture of medial malleolus alone (S82.5-)
Maisonneuve's fracture (S82.86-)
pilon fracture of distal tibia (S82.87-)
trimalleolar fractures of lower leg (S82.85-)

S82.30 Unspecified fracture of lower end of tibia
S82.301 Unspecified fracture of lower end of right tibia
S82.302 Unspecified fracture of lower end of left tibia
S82.309 Unspecified fracture of lower end of unspecified tibia

S82.31 Torus fracture of lower end of tibia

The appropriate 7th character is to be added to all codes in subcategory S82.31.
A initial encounter for closed fracture
D subsequent encounter for fracture with routine healing
G subsequent encounter for fracture with delayed healing
K subsequent encounter for fracture with nonunion
P subsequent encounter for fracture with malunion
S sequela

S82.311 Torus fracture of lower end of right tibia
S82.312 Torus fracture of lower end of left tibia
S82.319 Torus fracture of lower end of unspecified tibia

S82.39 Other fracture of lower end of tibia
AHA: 2015,1Q,25
S82.391 Other fracture of lower end of right tibia
S82.392 Other fracture of lower end of left tibia
S82.399 Other fracture of lower end of unspecified tibia

S82.4 Fracture of shaft of fibula
EXCLUDES 2 *fracture of lateral malleolus alone (S82.6-)*

S82.40 Unspecified fracture of shaft of fibula
S82.401 Unspecified fracture of shaft of right fibula
S82.402 Unspecified fracture of shaft of left fibula
S82.409 Unspecified fracture of shaft of unspecified fibula

S82.42 Transverse fracture of shaft of fibula
S82.421 Displaced transverse fracture of shaft of right fibula
S82.422 Displaced transverse fracture of shaft of left fibula
S82.423 Displaced transverse fracture of shaft of unspecified fibula
S82.424 Nondisplaced transverse fracture of shaft of right fibula
S82.425 Nondisplaced transverse fracture of shaft of left fibula
S82.426 Nondisplaced transverse fracture of shaft of unspecified fibula

S82.43 Oblique fracture of shaft of fibula
S82.431 Displaced oblique fracture of shaft of right fibula
S82.432 Displaced oblique fracture of shaft of left fibula
S82.433 Displaced oblique fracture of shaft of unspecified fibula
S82.434 Nondisplaced oblique fracture of shaft of right fibula
S82.435 Nondisplaced oblique fracture of shaft of left fibula
S82.436 Nondisplaced oblique fracture of shaft of unspecified fibula

S82.44 Spiral fracture of shaft of fibula
S82.441 Displaced spiral fracture of shaft of right fibula
S82.442 Displaced spiral fracture of shaft of left fibula
S82.443 Displaced spiral fracture of shaft of unspecified fibula
S82.444 Nondisplaced spiral fracture of shaft of right fibula
S82.445 Nondisplaced spiral fracture of shaft of left fibula

7th S82.446 **Nondisplaced spiral fracture of shaft of unspecified fibula** Q

6th **S82.45 Comminuted fracture of shaft of fibula**

7th S82.451 Displaced comminuted fracture of shaft of right fibula Q

7th S82.452 Displaced comminuted fracture of shaft of left fibula Q

7th S82.453 Displaced comminuted fracture of shaft of unspecified fibula Q

7th S82.454 Nondisplaced comminuted fracture of shaft of right fibula Q

7th S82.455 Nondisplaced comminuted fracture of shaft of left fibula Q

7th S82.456 Nondisplaced comminuted fracture of shaft of unspecified fibula Q

6th **S82.46 Segmental fracture of shaft of fibula**

7th S82.461 Displaced segmental fracture of shaft of right fibula Q

7th S82.462 Displaced segmental fracture of shaft of left fibula Q

7th S82.463 Displaced segmental fracture of shaft of unspecified fibula Q

7th S82.464 Nondisplaced segmental fracture of shaft of right fibula Q

7th S82.465 Nondisplaced segmental fracture of shaft of left fibula Q

7th S82.466 Nondisplaced segmental fracture of shaft of unspecified fibula Q

6th **S82.49 Other fracture of shaft of fibula**

7th S82.491 Other fracture of shaft of right fibula Q

7th S82.492 Other fracture of shaft of left fibula Q

7th S82.499 Other fracture of shaft of unspecified fibula Q

5th **S82.5 Fracture of medial malleolus**

EXCLUDES 1 *pilon fracture of distal tibia (S82.87-)*
Salter-Harris type III of lower end of tibia (S89.13-)
Salter-Harris type IV of lower end of tibia (S89.14-)

x7th S82.51 Displaced fracture of medial malleolus of right tibia Q

x7th S82.52 Displaced fracture of medial malleolus of left tibia Q

x7th S82.53 Displaced fracture of medial malleolus of unspecified tibia Q

x7th S82.54 Nondisplaced fracture of medial malleolus of right tibia Q

x7th S82.55 Nondisplaced fracture of medial malleolus of left tibia Q

x7th S82.56 Nondisplaced fracture of medial malleolus of unspecified tibia Q

5th **S82.6 Fracture of lateral malleolus**

EXCLUDES 1 *pilon fracture of distal tibia (S82.87-)*

x7th S82.61 Displaced fracture of lateral malleolus of right fibula Q

x7th S82.62 Displaced fracture of lateral malleolus of left fibula Q

x7th S82.63 Displaced fracture of lateral malleolus of unspecified fibula Q

x7th S82.64 Nondisplaced fracture of lateral malleolus of right fibula Q

x7th S82.65 Nondisplaced fracture of lateral malleolus of left fibula Q

x7th S82.66 Nondisplaced fracture of lateral malleolus of unspecified fibula Q

5th **S82.8 Other fractures of lower leg**

6th **S82.81 Torus fracture of upper end of fibula**

The appropriate 7th character is to be added to all codes in subcategory S82.81
- A initial encounter for closed fracture
- D subsequent encounter for fracture with routine healing
- G subsequent encounter for fracture with delayed healing
- K subsequent encounter for fracture with nonunion
- P subsequent encounter for fracture with malunion
- S sequela

7th S82.811 Torus fracture of upper end of right fibula Q

7th S82.812 Torus fracture of upper end of left fibula Q

7th S82.819 Torus fracture of upper end of unspecified fibula Q

6th **S82.82 Torus fracture of lower end of fibula**

The appropriate 7th character is to be added to all codes in subcategory S82.82.
- A initial encounter for closed fracture
- D subsequent encounter for fracture with routine healing
- G subsequent encounter for fracture with delayed healing
- K subsequent encounter for fracture with nonunion
- P subsequent encounter for fracture with malunion
- S sequela

7th S82.821 Torus fracture of lower end of right fibula Q

7th S82.822 Torus fracture of lower end of left fibula Q

7th S82.829 Torus fracture of lower end of unspecified fibula Q

6th **S82.83 Other fracture of upper and lower end of fibula**

AHA: 2015,1Q,25

7th S82.831 Other fracture of upper and lower end of right fibula Q

7th S82.832 Other fracture of upper and lower end of left fibula Q

7th S82.839 Other fracture of upper and lower end of unspecified fibula Q

6th **S82.84 Bimalleolar fracture of lower leg**

Right Bimalleolar Fracture

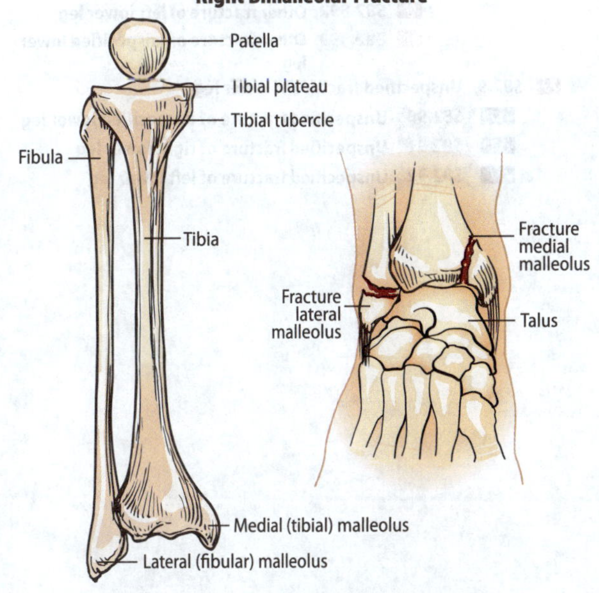

7th S82.841 Displaced bimalleolar fracture of right lower leg Q

- **S82.842 Displaced bimalleolar fracture of left lower leg** Q
- **S82.843 Displaced bimalleolar fracture of unspecified lower leg** Q
- **S82.844 Nondisplaced bimalleolar fracture of right lower leg** Q
- **S82.845 Nondisplaced bimalleolar fracture of left lower leg** Q
- **S82.846 Nondisplaced bimalleolar fracture of unspecified lower leg** Q

S82.85 Trimalleolar fracture of lower leg

- **S82.851 Displaced trimalleolar fracture of right lower leg** Q
- **S82.852 Displaced trimalleolar fracture of left lower leg** Q
- **S82.853 Displaced trimalleolar fracture of unspecified lower leg** Q
- **S82.854 Nondisplaced trimalleolar fracture of right lower leg** Q
- **S82.855 Nondisplaced trimalleolar fracture of left lower leg** Q
- **S82.856 Nondisplaced trimalleolar fracture of unspecified lower leg** Q

S82.86 Maisonneuve's fracture

- **S82.861 Displaced Maisonneuve's fracture of right leg** Q
- **S82.862 Displaced Maisonneuve's fracture of left leg** Q
- **S82.863 Displaced Maisonneuve's fracture of unspecified leg** Q
- **S82.864 Nondisplaced Maisonneuve's fracture of right leg** Q
- **S82.865 Nondisplaced Maisonneuve's fracture of left leg** Q
- **S82.866 Nondisplaced Maisonneuve's fracture of unspecified leg** Q

S82.87 Pilon fracture of tibia

- **S82.871 Displaced pilon fracture of right tibia** Q
- **S82.872 Displaced pilon fracture of left tibia** Q
- **S82.873 Displaced pilon fracture of unspecified tibia** Q
- **S82.874 Nondisplaced pilon fracture of right tibia** Q
- **S82.875 Nondisplaced pilon fracture of left tibia** Q
- **S82.876 Nondisplaced pilon fracture of unspecified tibia** Q

S82.89 Other fractures of lower leg

Fracture of ankle NOS

- **S82.891 Other fracture of right lower leg** Q
- **S82.892 Other fracture of left lower leg** Q
- **S82.899 Other fracture of unspecified lower leg** Q

S82.9 Unspecified fracture of lower leg

- **S82.90 Unspecified fracture of unspecified lower leg** Q
- **S82.91 Unspecified fracture of right lower leg** Q
- **S82.92 Unspecified fracture of left lower leg** Q

S83 Dislocation and sprain of joints and ligaments of knee

INCLUDES avulsion of joint or ligament of knee
laceration of cartilage, joint or ligament of knee
sprain of cartilage, joint or ligament of knee
traumatic hemarthrosis of joint or ligament of knee
traumatic rupture of joint or ligament of knee
traumatic subluxation of joint or ligament of knee
traumatic tear of joint or ligament of knee

Code also any associated open wound

EXCLUDES 2 *derangement of patella (M22.0-M22.3)*
injury of patellar ligament (tendon) (S76.1-)
internal derangement of knee (M23.-)
old dislocation of knee (M24.36)
pathological dislocation of knee (M24.36)
recurrent dislocation of knee (M22.0)
strain of muscle, fascia and tendon of lower leg (S86.-)

The appropriate 7th character is to be added to each code from category S83.
A initial encounter
D subsequent encounter
S sequela

S83.0 Subluxation and dislocation of patella

S83.00 Unspecified subluxation and dislocation of patella

- **S83.001 Unspecified subluxation of right patella**
- **S83.002 Unspecified subluxation of left patella**
- **S83.003 Unspecified subluxation of unspecified patella**
- **S83.004 Unspecified dislocation of right patella**
- **S83.005 Unspecified dislocation of left patella**
- **S83.006 Unspecified dislocation of unspecified patella**

S83.01 Lateral subluxation and dislocation of patella

- **S83.011 Lateral subluxation of right patella**
- **S83.012 Lateral subluxation of left patella**
- **S83.013 Lateral subluxation of unspecified patella**
- **S83.014 Lateral dislocation of right patella**
- **S83.015 Lateral dislocation of left patella**
- **S83.016 Lateral dislocation of unspecified patella**

S83.09 Other subluxation and dislocation of patella

- **S83.091 Other subluxation of right patella**
- **S83.092 Other subluxation of left patella**
- **S83.093 Other subluxation of unspecified patella**
- **S83.094 Other dislocation of right patella**
- **S83.095 Other dislocation of left patella**
- **S83.096 Other dislocation of unspecified patella**

S83.1 Subluxation and dislocation of knee

EXCLUDES 2 *instability of knee prosthesis (T84.022, T84.023)*

S83.10 Unspecified subluxation and dislocation of knee

- **S83.101 Unspecified subluxation of right knee**
- **S83.102 Unspecified subluxation of left knee**
- **S83.103 Unspecified subluxation of unspecified knee**
- **S83.104 Unspecified dislocation of right knee**
- **S83.105 Unspecified dislocation of left knee**
- **S83.106 Unspecified dislocation of unspecified knee**

S83.11 Anterior subluxation and dislocation of proximal end of tibia

Posterior subluxation and dislocation of distal end of femur

- **S83.111 Anterior subluxation of proximal end of tibia, right knee**
- **S83.112 Anterior subluxation of proximal end of tibia, left knee**
- **S83.113 Anterior subluxation of proximal end of tibia, unspecified knee**
- **S83.114 Anterior dislocation of proximal end of tibia, right knee**
- **S83.115 Anterior dislocation of proximal end of tibia, left knee**
- **S83.116 Anterior dislocation of proximal end of tibia, unspecified knee**

S83.12 Posterior subluxation and dislocation of proximal end of tibia
Anterior dislocation of distal end of femur
- **S83.121 Posterior subluxation of proximal end of tibia, right knee**
- **S83.122 Posterior subluxation of proximal end of tibia, left knee**
- **S83.123 Posterior subluxation of proximal end of tibia, unspecified knee**
- **S83.124 Posterior dislocation of proximal end of tibia, right knee**
- **S83.125 Posterior dislocation of proximal end of tibia, left knee**
- **S83.126 Posterior dislocation of proximal end of tibia, unspecified knee**

S83.13 Medial subluxation and dislocation of proximal end of tibia
- **S83.131 Medial subluxation of proximal end of tibia, right knee**
- **S83.132 Medial subluxation of proximal end of tibia, left knee**
- **S83.133 Medial subluxation of proximal end of tibia, unspecified knee**
- **S83.134 Medial dislocation of proximal end of tibia, right knee**
- **S83.135 Medial dislocation of proximal end of tibia, left knee**
- **S83.136 Medial dislocation of proximal end of tibia, unspecified knee**

S83.14 Lateral subluxation and dislocation of proximal end of tibia
- **S83.141 Lateral subluxation of proximal end of tibia, right knee**
- **S83.142 Lateral subluxation of proximal end of tibia, left knee**
- **S83.143 Lateral subluxation of proximal end of tibia, unspecified knee**
- **S83.144 Lateral dislocation of proximal end of tibia, right knee**
- **S83.145 Lateral dislocation of proximal end of tibia, left knee**
- **S83.146 Lateral dislocation of proximal end of tibia, unspecified knee**

S83.19 Other subluxation and dislocation of knee
- **S83.191 Other subluxation of right knee**
- **S83.192 Other subluxation of left knee**
- **S83.193 Other subluxation of unspecified knee**
- **S83.194 Other dislocation of right knee**
- **S83.195 Other dislocation of left knee**
- **S83.196 Other dislocation of unspecified knee**

S83.2 Tear of meniscus, current injury
EXCLUDES 1 *old bucket-handle tear (M23.2)*
AHA: 2019,2Q,26

S83.20 Tear of unspecified meniscus, current injury
Tear of meniscus of knee NOS
- **S83.200 Bucket-handle tear of unspecified meniscus, current injury, right knee**
- **S83.201 Bucket-handle tear of unspecified meniscus, current injury, left knee**
- **S83.202 Bucket-handle tear of unspecified meniscus, current injury, unspecified knee**
- **S83.203 Other tear of unspecified meniscus, current injury, right knee**
- **S83.204 Other tear of unspecified meniscus, current injury, left knee**
- **S83.205 Other tear of unspecified meniscus, current injury, unspecified knee**
- **S83.206 Unspecified tear of unspecified meniscus, current injury, right knee**
- **S83.207 Unspecified tear of unspecified meniscus, current injury, left knee**
- **S83.209 Unspecified tear of unspecified meniscus, current injury, unspecified knee**

S83.21 Bucket-handle tear of medial meniscus, current injury
- **S83.211 Bucket-handle tear of medial meniscus, current injury, right knee**
- **S83.212 Bucket-handle tear of medial meniscus, current injury, left knee**
- **S83.219 Bucket-handle tear of medial meniscus, current injury, unspecified knee**

S83.22 Peripheral tear of medial meniscus, current injury
- **S83.221 Peripheral tear of medial meniscus, current injury, right knee**
- **S83.222 Peripheral tear of medial meniscus, current injury, left knee**
- **S83.229 Peripheral tear of medial meniscus, current injury, unspecified knee**

S83.23 Complex tear of medial meniscus, current injury
- **S83.231 Complex tear of medial meniscus, current injury, right knee**
- **S83.232 Complex tear of medial meniscus, current injury, left knee**
- **S83.239 Complex tear of medial meniscus, current injury, unspecified knee**

S83.24 Other tear of medial meniscus, current injury
- **S83.241 Other tear of medial meniscus, current injury, right knee**
- **S83.242 Other tear of medial meniscus, current injury, left knee**
- **S83.249 Other tear of medial meniscus, current injury, unspecified knee**

S83.25 Bucket-handle tear of lateral meniscus, current injury
- **S83.251 Bucket-handle tear of lateral meniscus, current injury, right knee**
- **S83.252 Bucket-handle tear of lateral meniscus, current injury, left knee**
- **S83.259 Bucket-handle tear of lateral meniscus, current injury, unspecified knee**

S83.26 Peripheral tear of lateral meniscus, current injury
- **S83.261 Peripheral tear of lateral meniscus, current injury, right knee**
- **S83.262 Peripheral tear of lateral meniscus, current injury, left knee**
- **S83.269 Peripheral tear of lateral meniscus, current injury, unspecified knee**

S83.27 Complex tear of lateral meniscus, current injury
- **S83.271 Complex tear of lateral meniscus, current injury, right knee**
- **S83.272 Complex tear of lateral meniscus, current injury, left knee**
- **S83.279 Complex tear of lateral meniscus, current injury, unspecified knee**

S83.28 Other tear of lateral meniscus, current injury
- **S83.281 Other tear of lateral meniscus, current injury, right knee**
- **S83.282 Other tear of lateral meniscus, current injury, left knee**
- **S83.289 Other tear of lateral meniscus, current injury, unspecified knee**

S83.3 Tear of articular cartilage of knee, current
- **S83.30 Tear of articular cartilage of unspecified knee, current**
- **S83.31 Tear of articular cartilage of right knee, current**
- **S83.32 Tear of articular cartilage of left knee, current**

S83.4 Sprain of collateral ligament of knee

S83.40 Sprain of unspecified collateral ligament of knee
- **S83.401 Sprain of unspecified collateral ligament of right knee**
- **S83.402 Sprain of unspecified collateral ligament of left knee**
- **S83.409 Sprain of unspecified collateral ligament of unspecified knee**

S83.41 Sprain of medial collateral ligament of knee
Sprain of tibial collateral ligament
- **S83.411 Sprain of medial collateral ligament of right knee**
- **S83.412 Sprain of medial collateral ligament of left knee**
- **S83.419 Sprain of medial collateral ligament of unspecified knee**

S83.42 Sprain of lateral collateral ligament of knee
Sprain of fibular collateral ligament
- **S83.421 Sprain of lateral collateral ligament of right knee**
- **S83.422 Sprain of lateral collateral ligament of left knee**

7th **S83.429** **Sprain of lateral collateral ligament of unspecified knee**

5th **S83.5** **Sprain of cruciate ligament of knee**

AHA: 2016,2Q,3

6th **S83.50** **Sprain of unspecified cruciate ligament of knee**

7th **S83.501** **Sprain of unspecified cruciate ligament of right knee**

7th **S83.502** **Sprain of unspecified cruciate ligament of left knee**

7th **S83.509** **Sprain of unspecified cruciate ligament of unspecified knee**

6th **S83.51** **Sprain of anterior cruciate ligament of knee**

7th **S83.511** **Sprain of anterior cruciate ligament of right knee**

7th **S83.512** **Sprain of anterior cruciate ligament of left knee**

7th **S83.519** **Sprain of anterior cruciate ligament of unspecified knee**

6th **S83.52** **Sprain of posterior cruciate ligament of knee**

7th **S83.521** **Sprain of posterior cruciate ligament of right knee**

7th **S83.522** **Sprain of posterior cruciate ligament of left knee**

7th **S83.529** **Sprain of posterior cruciate ligament of unspecified knee**

5th **S83.6** **Sprain of the superior tibiofibular joint and ligament**

x7th **S83.60** **Sprain of the superior tibiofibular joint and ligament, unspecified knee**

x7th **S83.61** **Sprain of the superior tibiofibular joint and ligament, right knee**

x7th **S83.62** **Sprain of the superior tibiofibular joint and ligament, left knee**

5th **S83.8** **Sprain of other specified parts of knee**

6th **S83.8X** **Sprain of other specified parts of knee**

7th **S83.8X1** **Sprain of other specified parts of right knee**

7th **S83.8X2** **Sprain of other specified parts of left knee**

7th **S83.8X9** **Sprain of other specified parts of unspecified knee**

5th **S83.9** **Sprain of unspecified site of knee**

x7th **S83.90** **Sprain of unspecified site of unspecified knee**

x7th **S83.91** **Sprain of unspecified site of right knee**

x7th **S83.92** **Sprain of unspecified site of left knee**

4th **S84** **Injury of nerves at lower leg level**

Code also any associated open wound (S81.-)

EXCLUDES 2 *injury of nerves at ankle and foot level (S94.-)*

The appropriate 7th character is to be added to each code from category S84.
A initial encounter
D subsequent encounter
S sequela

5th **S84.0** **Injury of tibial nerve at lower leg level**

x7th **S84.00** **Injury of tibial nerve at lower leg level, unspecified leg**

x7th **S84.01** **Injury of tibial nerve at lower leg level, right leg**

x7th **S84.02** **Injury of tibial nerve at lower leg level, left leg**

5th **S84.1** **Injury of peroneal nerve at lower leg level**

x7th **S84.10** **Injury of peroneal nerve at lower leg level, unspecified leg**

x7th **S84.11** **Injury of peroneal nerve at lower leg level, right leg**

x7th **S84.12** **Injury of peroneal nerve at lower leg level, left leg**

5th **S84.2** **Injury of cutaneous sensory nerve at lower leg level**

x7th **S84.20** **Injury of cutaneous sensory nerve at lower leg level, unspecified leg**

x7th **S84.21** **Injury of cutaneous sensory nerve at lower leg level, right leg**

x7th **S84.22** **Injury of cutaneous sensory nerve at lower leg level, left leg**

5th **S84.8** **Injury of other nerves at lower leg level**

6th **S84.80** **Injury of other nerves at lower leg level**

7th **S84.801** **Injury of other nerves at lower leg level, right leg**

7th **S84.802** **Injury of other nerves at lower leg level, left leg**

7th **S84.809** **Injury of other nerves at lower leg level, unspecified leg**

5th **S84.9** **Injury of unspecified nerve at lower leg level**

x7th **S84.90** **Injury of unspecified nerve at lower leg level, unspecified leg**

x7th **S84.91** **Injury of unspecified nerve at lower leg level, right leg**

x7th **S84.92** **Injury of unspecified nerve at lower leg level, left leg**

4th **S85** **Injury of blood vessels at lower leg level**

Code also any associated open wound (S81.-)

EXCLUDES 2 *injury of blood vessels at ankle and foot level (S95.-)*

The appropriate 7th character is to be added to each code from category S85.
A initial encounter
D subsequent encounter
S sequela

5th **S85.0** **Injury of popliteal artery**

6th **S85.00** **Unspecified injury of popliteal artery**

7th **S85.001** **Unspecified injury of popliteal artery, right leg**

7th **S85.002** **Unspecified injury of popliteal artery, left leg**

7th **S85.009** **Unspecified injury of popliteal artery, unspecified leg**

6th **S85.01** **Laceration of popliteal artery**

7th **S85.011** **Laceration of popliteal artery, right leg**

7th **S85.012** **Laceration of popliteal artery, left leg**

7th **S85.019** **Laceration of popliteal artery, unspecified leg**

6th **S85.09** **Other specified injury of popliteal artery**

7th **S85.091** **Other specified injury of popliteal artery, right leg**

7th **S85.092** **Other specified injury of popliteal artery, left leg**

7th **S85.099** **Other specified injury of popliteal artery, unspecified leg**

5th **S85.1** **Injury of tibial artery**

6th **S85.10** **Unspecified injury of unspecified tibial artery**

Injury of tibial artery NOS

7th **S85.101** **Unspecified injury of unspecified tibial artery, right leg**

7th **S85.102** **Unspecified injury of unspecified tibial artery, left leg**

7th **S85.109** **Unspecified injury of unspecified tibial artery, unspecified leg**

6th **S85.11** **Laceration of unspecified tibial artery**

7th **S85.111** **Laceration of unspecified tibial artery, right leg**

7th **S85.112** **Laceration of unspecified tibial artery, left leg**

7th **S85.119** **Laceration of unspecified tibial artery, unspecified leg**

6th **S85.12** **Other specified injury of unspecified tibial artery**

7th **S85.121** **Other specified injury of unspecified tibial artery, right leg**

7th **S85.122** **Other specified injury of unspecified tibial artery, left leg**

7th **S85.129** **Other specified injury of unspecified tibial artery, unspecified leg**

6th **S85.13** **Unspecified injury of anterior tibial artery**

7th **S85.131** **Unspecified injury of anterior tibial artery, right leg**

7th **S85.132** **Unspecified injury of anterior tibial artery, left leg**

7th **S85.139** **Unspecified injury of anterior tibial artery, unspecified leg**

6th **S85.14** **Laceration of anterior tibial artery**

7th **S85.141** **Laceration of anterior tibial artery, right leg**

7th **S85.142** **Laceration of anterior tibial artery, left leg**

7th **S85.149** **Laceration of anterior tibial artery, unspecified leg**

6th **S85.15** **Other specified injury of anterior tibial artery**

7th **S85.151** **Other specified injury of anterior tibial artery, right leg**

S85.152 Other specified injury of anterior tibial artery, left leg
S85.159 Other specified injury of anterior tibial artery, unspecified leg
S85.16 Unspecified injury of posterior tibial artery
S85.161 Unspecified injury of posterior tibial artery, right leg
S85.162 Unspecified injury of posterior tibial artery, left leg
S85.169 Unspecified injury of posterior tibial artery, unspecified leg
S85.17 Laceration of posterior tibial artery
S85.171 Laceration of posterior tibial artery, right leg
S85.172 Laceration of posterior tibial artery, left leg
S85.179 Laceration of posterior tibial artery, unspecified leg
S85.18 Other specified injury of posterior tibial artery
S85.181 Other specified injury of posterior tibial artery, right leg
S85.182 Other specified injury of posterior tibial artery, left leg
S85.189 Other specified injury of posterior tibial artery, unspecified leg
S85.2 Injury of peroneal artery
S85.20 Unspecified injury of peroneal artery
S85.201 Unspecified injury of peroneal artery, right leg
S85.202 Unspecified injury of peroneal artery, left leg
S85.209 Unspecified injury of peroneal artery, unspecified leg
S85.21 Laceration of peroneal artery
S85.211 Laceration of peroneal artery, right leg
S85.212 Laceration of peroneal artery, left leg
S85.219 Laceration of peroneal artery, unspecified leg
S85.29 Other specified injury of peroneal artery
S85.291 Other specified injury of peroneal artery, right leg
S85.292 Other specified injury of peroneal artery, left leg
S85.299 Other specified injury of peroneal artery, unspecified leg
S85.3 Injury of greater saphenous vein at lower leg level
Injury of greater saphenous vein NOS
Injury of saphenous vein NOS
S85.30 Unspecified injury of greater saphenous vein at lower leg level
S85.301 Unspecified injury of greater saphenous vein at lower leg level, right leg
S85.302 Unspecified injury of greater saphenous vein at lower leg level, left leg
S85.309 Unspecified injury of greater saphenous vein at lower leg level, unspecified leg
S85.31 Laceration of greater saphenous vein at lower leg level
S85.311 Laceration of greater saphenous vein at lower leg level, right leg
S85.312 Laceration of greater saphenous vein at lower leg level, left leg
S85.319 Laceration of greater saphenous vein at lower leg level, unspecified leg
S85.39 Other specified injury of greater saphenous vein at lower leg level
S85.391 Other specified injury of greater saphenous vein at lower leg level, right leg
S85.392 Other specified injury of greater saphenous vein at lower leg level, left leg
S85.399 Other specified injury of greater saphenous vein at lower leg level, unspecified leg
S85.4 Injury of lesser saphenous vein at lower leg level
S85.40 Unspecified injury of lesser saphenous vein at lower leg level
S85.401 Unspecified injury of lesser saphenous vein at lower leg level, right leg
S85.402 Unspecified injury of lesser saphenous vein at lower leg level, left leg
S85.409 Unspecified injury of lesser saphenous vein at lower leg level, unspecified leg
S85.41 Laceration of lesser saphenous vein at lower leg level
S85.411 Laceration of lesser saphenous vein at lower leg level, right leg
S85.412 Laceration of lesser saphenous vein at lower leg level, left leg
S85.419 Laceration of lesser saphenous vein at lower leg level, unspecified leg
S85.49 Other specified injury of lesser saphenous vein at lower leg level
S85.491 Other specified injury of lesser saphenous vein at lower leg level, right leg
S85.492 Other specified injury of lesser saphenous vein at lower leg level, left leg
S85.499 Other specified injury of lesser saphenous vein at lower leg level, unspecified leg
S85.5 Injury of popliteal vein
S85.50 Unspecified injury of popliteal vein
S85.501 Unspecified injury of popliteal vein, right leg
S85.502 Unspecified injury of popliteal vein, left leg
S85.509 Unspecified injury of popliteal vein, unspecified leg
S85.51 Laceration of popliteal vein
S85.511 Laceration of popliteal vein, right leg
S85.512 Laceration of popliteal vein, left leg
S85.519 Laceration of popliteal vein, unspecified leg
S85.59 Other specified injury of popliteal vein
S85.591 Other specified injury of popliteal vein, right leg
S85.592 Other specified injury of popliteal vein, left leg
S85.599 Other specified injury of popliteal vein, unspecified leg
S85.8 Injury of other blood vessels at lower leg level
S85.80 Unspecified injury of other blood vessels at lower leg level
S85.801 Unspecified injury of other blood vessels at lower leg level, right leg
S85.802 Unspecified injury of other blood vessels at lower leg level, left leg
S85.809 Unspecified injury of other blood vessels at lower leg level, unspecified leg
S85.81 Laceration of other blood vessels at lower leg level
S85.811 Laceration of other blood vessels at lower leg level, right leg
S85.812 Laceration of other blood vessels at lower leg level, left leg
S85.819 Laceration of other blood vessels at lower leg level, unspecified leg
S85.89 Other specified injury of other blood vessels at lower leg level
S85.891 Other specified injury of other blood vessels at lower leg level, right leg
S85.892 Other specified injury of other blood vessels at lower leg level, left leg
S85.899 Other specified injury of other blood vessels at lower leg level, unspecified leg
S85.9 Injury of unspecified blood vessel at lower leg level
S85.90 Unspecified injury of unspecified blood vessel at lower leg level
S85.901 Unspecified injury of unspecified blood vessel at lower leg level, right leg
S85.902 Unspecified injury of unspecified blood vessel at lower leg level, left leg
S85.909 Unspecified injury of unspecified blood vessel at lower leg level, unspecified leg
S85.91 Laceration of unspecified blood vessel at lower leg level
S85.911 Laceration of unspecified blood vessel at lower leg level, right leg
S85.912 Laceration of unspecified blood vessel at lower leg level, left leg
S85.919 Laceration of unspecified blood vessel at lower leg level, unspecified leg

- 6th **S85.99 Other specified injury of unspecified blood vessel at lower leg level**
  - 7th **S85.991 Other specified injury of unspecified blood vessel at lower leg level, right leg**
  - 7th **S85.992 Other specified injury of unspecified blood vessel at lower leg level, left leg**
  - 7th **S85.999 Other specified injury of unspecified blood vessel at lower leg level, unspecified leg**

4th **S86 Injury of muscle, fascia and tendon at lower leg level**

Code also any associated open wound (S81.-)

EXCLUDES 2 *injury of muscle, fascia and tendon at ankle (S96.-)*
injury of patellar ligament (tendon) (S76.1-)
sprain of joints and ligaments of knee (S83.-)

TIP: Refer to the Muscle/Tendon table at the beginning of this chapter.

The appropriate 7th character is to be added to each code from category S86.
A initial encounter
D subsequent encounter
S sequela

- 5th **S86.0 Injury of Achilles tendon**
  - 6th **S86.00 Unspecified injury of Achilles tendon**
    - 7th **S86.001 Unspecified injury of right Achilles tendon**
    - 7th **S86.002 Unspecified injury of left Achilles tendon**
    - 7th **S86.009 Unspecified injury of unspecified Achilles tendon**
  - 6th **S86.01 Strain of Achilles tendon**
    - 7th **S86.011 Strain of right Achilles tendon**
    - 7th **S86.012 Strain of left Achilles tendon**
    - 7th **S86.019 Strain of unspecified Achilles tendon**
  - 6th **S86.02 Laceration of Achilles tendon**
    - 7th **S86.021 Laceration of right Achilles tendon**
    - 7th **S86.022 Laceration of left Achilles tendon**
    - 7th **S86.029 Laceration of unspecified Achilles tendon**
  - 6th **S86.09 Other specified injury of Achilles tendon**
    - 7th **S86.091 Other specified injury of right Achilles tendon**
    - 7th **S86.092 Other specified injury of left Achilles tendon**
    - 7th **S86.099 Other specified injury of unspecified Achilles tendon**
- 5th **S86.1 Injury of other muscle(s) and tendon(s) of posterior muscle group at lower leg level**
  - 6th **S86.10 Unspecified injury of other muscle(s) and tendon(s) of posterior muscle group at lower leg level**
    - 7th **S86.101 Unspecified injury of other muscle(s) and tendon(s) of posterior muscle group at lower leg level, right leg**
    - 7th **S86.102 Unspecified injury of other muscle(s) and tendon(s) of posterior muscle group at lower leg level, left leg**
    - 7th **S86.109 Unspecified injury of other muscle(s) and tendon(s) of posterior muscle group at lower leg level, unspecified leg**
  - 6th **S86.11 Strain of other muscle(s) and tendon(s) of posterior muscle group at lower leg level**
    - 7th **S86.111 Strain of other muscle(s) and tendon(s) of posterior muscle group at lower leg level, right leg**
    - 7th **S86.112 Strain of other muscle(s) and tendon(s) of posterior muscle group at lower leg level, left leg**
    - 7th **S86.119 Strain of other muscle(s) and tendon(s) of posterior muscle group at lower leg level, unspecified leg**
  - 6th **S86.12 Laceration of other muscle(s) and tendon(s) of posterior muscle group at lower leg level**
    - 7th **S86.121 Laceration of other muscle(s) and tendon(s) of posterior muscle group at lower leg level, right leg**
    - 7th **S86.122 Laceration of other muscle(s) and tendon(s) of posterior muscle group at lower leg level, left leg**
    - 7th **S86.129 Laceration of other muscle(s) and tendon(s) of posterior muscle group at lower leg level, unspecified leg**
  - 6th **S86.19 Other injury of other muscle(s) and tendon(s) of posterior muscle group at lower leg level**
    - 7th **S86.191 Other injury of other muscle(s) and tendon(s) of posterior muscle group at lower leg level, right leg**
    - 7th **S86.192 Other injury of other muscle(s) and tendon(s) of posterior muscle group at lower leg level, left leg**
    - 7th **S86.199 Other injury of other muscle(s) and tendon(s) of posterior muscle group at lower leg level, unspecified leg**
- 5th **S86.2 Injury of muscle(s) and tendon(s) of anterior muscle group at lower leg level**
  - 6th **S86.20 Unspecified injury of muscle(s) and tendon(s) of anterior muscle group at lower leg level**
    - 7th **S86.201 Unspecified injury of muscle(s) and tendon(s) of anterior muscle group at lower leg level, right leg**
    - 7th **S86.202 Unspecified injury of muscle(s) and tendon(s) of anterior muscle group at lower leg level, left leg**
    - 7th **S86.209 Unspecified injury of muscle(s) and tendon(s) of anterior muscle group at lower leg level, unspecified leg**
  - 6th **S86.21 Strain of muscle(s) and tendon(s) of anterior muscle group at lower leg level**
    - 7th **S86.211 Strain of muscle(s) and tendon(s) of anterior muscle group at lower leg level, right leg**
    - 7th **S86.212 Strain of muscle(s) and tendon(s) of anterior muscle group at lower leg level, left leg**
    - 7th **S86.219 Strain of muscle(s) and tendon(s) of anterior muscle group at lower leg level, unspecified leg**
  - 6th **S86.22 Laceration of muscle(s) and tendon(s) of anterior muscle group at lower leg level**
    - 7th **S86.221 Laceration of muscle(s) and tendon(s) of anterior muscle group at lower leg level, right leg**
    - 7th **S86.222 Laceration of muscle(s) and tendon(s) of anterior muscle group at lower leg level, left leg**
    - 7th **S86.229 Laceration of muscle(s) and tendon(s) of anterior muscle group at lower leg level, unspecified leg**
  - 6th **S86.29 Other injury of muscle(s) and tendon(s) of anterior muscle group at lower leg level**
    - 7th **S86.291 Other injury of muscle(s) and tendon(s) of anterior muscle group at lower leg level, right leg**
    - 7th **S86.292 Other injury of muscle(s) and tendon(s) of anterior muscle group at lower leg level, left leg**
    - 7th **S86.299 Other injury of muscle(s) and tendon(s) of anterior muscle group at lower leg level, unspecified leg**
- 5th **S86.3 Injury of muscle(s) and tendon(s) of peroneal muscle group at lower leg level**
  - 6th **S86.30 Unspecified injury of muscle(s) and tendon(s) of peroneal muscle group at lower leg level**
    - 7th **S86.301 Unspecified injury of muscle(s) and tendon(s) of peroneal muscle group at lower leg level, right leg**
    - 7th **S86.302 Unspecified injury of muscle(s) and tendon(s) of peroneal muscle group at lower leg level, left leg**
    - 7th **S86.309 Unspecified injury of muscle(s) and tendon(s) of peroneal muscle group at lower leg level, unspecified leg**
  - 6th **S86.31 Strain of muscle(s) and tendon(s) of peroneal muscle group at lower leg level**
    - 7th **S86.311 Strain of muscle(s) and tendon(s) of peroneal muscle group at lower leg level, right leg**
    - 7th **S86.312 Strain of muscle(s) and tendon(s) of peroneal muscle group at lower leg level, left leg**
    - 7th **S86.319 Strain of muscle(s) and tendon(s) of peroneal muscle group at lower leg level, unspecified leg**

S86.32 Laceration of muscle(s) and tendon(s) of peroneal muscle group at lower leg level
S86.321 Laceration of muscle(s) and tendon(s) of peroneal muscle group at lower leg level, right leg
S86.322 Laceration of muscle(s) and tendon(s) of peroneal muscle group at lower leg level, left leg
S86.329 Laceration of muscle(s) and tendon(s) of peroneal muscle group at lower leg level, unspecified leg
S86.39 Other injury of muscle(s) and tendon(s) of peroneal muscle group at lower leg level
S86.391 Other injury of muscle(s) and tendon(s) of peroneal muscle group at lower leg level, right leg
S86.392 Other injury of muscle(s) and tendon(s) of peroneal muscle group at lower leg level, left leg
S86.399 Other injury of muscle(s) and tendon(s) of peroneal muscle group at lower leg level, unspecified leg
S86.8 Injury of other muscles and tendons at lower leg level
S86.80 Unspecified injury of other muscles and tendons at lower leg level
S86.801 Unspecified injury of other muscle(s) and tendon(s) at lower leg level, right leg
S86.802 Unspecified injury of other muscle(s) and tendon(s) at lower leg level, left leg
S86.809 Unspecified injury of other muscle(s) and tendon(s) at lower leg level, unspecified leg
S86.81 Strain of other muscles and tendons at lower leg level
S86.811 Strain of other muscle(s) and tendon(s) at lower leg level, right leg
S86.812 Strain of other muscle(s) and tendon(s) at lower leg level, left leg
S86.819 Strain of other muscle(s) and tendon(s) at lower leg level, unspecified leg
S86.82 Laceration of other muscles and tendons at lower leg level
S86.821 Laceration of other muscle(s) and tendon(s) at lower leg level, right leg
S86.822 Laceration of other muscle(s) and tendon(s) at lower leg level, left leg
S86.829 Laceration of other muscle(s) and tendon(s) at lower leg level, unspecified leg
S86.89 Other injury of other muscles and tendons at lower leg level
S86.891 Other injury of other muscle(s) and tendon(s) at lower leg level, right leg
S86.892 Other injury of other muscle(s) and tendon(s) at lower leg level, left leg
S86.899 Other injury of other muscle(s) and tendon(s) at lower leg level, unspecified leg
S86.9 Injury of unspecified muscle and tendon at lower leg level
S86.90 Unspecified injury of unspecified muscle and tendon at lower leg level
S86.901 Unspecified injury of unspecified muscle(s) and tendon(s) at lower leg level, right leg
S86.902 Unspecified injury of unspecified muscle(s) and tendon(s) at lower leg level, left leg
S86.909 Unspecified injury of unspecified muscle(s) and tendon(s) at lower leg level, unspecified leg
S86.91 Strain of unspecified muscle and tendon at lower leg level
S86.911 Strain of unspecified muscle(s) and tendon(s) at lower leg level, right leg
S86.912 Strain of unspecified muscle(s) and tendon(s) at lower leg level, left leg
S86.919 Strain of unspecified muscle(s) and tendon(s) at lower leg level, unspecified leg
S86.92 Laceration of unspecified muscle and tendon at lower leg level
S86.921 Laceration of unspecified muscle(s) and tendon(s) at lower leg level, right leg
S86.922 Laceration of unspecified muscle(s) and tendon(s) at lower leg level, left leg
S86.929 Laceration of unspecified muscle(s) and tendon(s) at lower leg level, unspecified leg
S86.99 Other injury of unspecified muscle and tendon at lower leg level
S86.991 Other injury of unspecified muscle(s) and tendon(s) at lower leg level, right leg
S86.992 Other injury of unspecified muscle(s) and tendon(s) at lower leg level, left leg
S86.999 Other injury of unspecified muscle(s) and tendon(s) at lower leg level, unspecified leg

S87 Crushing injury of lower leg
Use additional code(s) for all associated injuries
EXCLUDES 2 *crushing injury of ankle and foot (S97.-)*

The appropriate 7th character is to be added to each code from category S87.
A initial encounter
D subsequent encounter
S sequela

S87.0 Crushing injury of knee
S87.00 Crushing injury of unspecified knee
S87.01 Crushing injury of right knee
S87.02 Crushing injury of left knee
S87.8 Crushing injury of lower leg
S87.80 Crushing injury of unspecified lower leg
S87.81 Crushing injury of right lower leg
S87.82 Crushing injury of left lower leg

S88 Traumatic amputation of lower leg
An amputation not identified as partial or complete should be coded to complete
EXCLUDES 1 *traumatic amputation of ankle and foot (S98.-)*

The appropriate 7th character is to be added to each code from category S88.
A initial encounter
D subsequent encounter
S sequela

S88.0 Traumatic amputation at knee level
S88.01 Complete traumatic amputation at knee level
S88.011 Complete traumatic amputation at knee level, right lower leg HCC ESR COM
S88.012 Complete traumatic amputation at knee level, left lower leg HCC ESR COM
S88.019 Complete traumatic amputation at knee level, unspecified lower leg HCC ESR COM
S88.02 Partial traumatic amputation at knee level
S88.021 Partial traumatic amputation at knee level, right lower leg HCC ESR COM
S88.022 Partial traumatic amputation at knee level, left lower leg HCC ESR COM
S88.029 Partial traumatic amputation at knee level, unspecified lower leg HCC ESR COM
S88.1 Traumatic amputation at level between knee and ankle
S88.11 Complete traumatic amputation at level between knee and ankle
S88.111 Complete traumatic amputation at level between knee and ankle, right lower leg HCC ESR COM
S88.112 Complete traumatic amputation at level between knee and ankle, left lower leg HCC ESR COM
S88.119 Complete traumatic amputation at level between knee and ankle, unspecified lower leg HCC ESR COM
S88.12 Partial traumatic amputation at level between knee and ankle
S88.121 Partial traumatic amputation at level between knee and ankle, right lower leg HCC ESR COM
S88.122 Partial traumatic amputation at level between knee and ankle, left lower leg HCC ESR COM

✓7th **S88.129 Partial traumatic amputation at level between knee and ankle, unspecified lower leg** HCC ESR COM

✓5th **S88.9 Traumatic amputation of lower leg, level unspecified**

✓6th **S88.91 Complete traumatic amputation of lower leg, level unspecified**

✓7th **S88.911 Complete traumatic amputation of right lower leg, level unspecified** HCC ESR COM

✓7th **S88.912 Complete traumatic amputation of left lower leg, level unspecified** HCC ESR COM

✓7th **S88.919 Complete traumatic amputation of unspecified lower leg, level unspecified** HCC ESR COM

✓6th **S88.92 Partial traumatic amputation of lower leg, level unspecified**

✓7th **S88.921 Partial traumatic amputation of right lower leg, level unspecified** HCC ESR COM

✓7th **S88.922 Partial traumatic amputation of left lower leg, level unspecified** HCC ESR COM

✓7th **S88.929 Partial traumatic amputation of unspecified lower leg, level unspecified** HCC ESR COM

✓4th **S89 Other and unspecified injuries of lower leg**

NOTE A fracture not indicated as open or closed should be coded to closed.

EXCLUDES 2 *other and unspecified injuries of ankle and foot (S99.-)*

AHA: 2018,2Q,12; 2018,1Q,3; 2015,3Q,37-39

The appropriate 7th character is to be added to each code from subcategories S89.Ø, S89.1, S89.2, and S89.3.

- A initial encounter for closed fracture
- D subsequent encounter for fracture with routine healing
- G subsequent encounter for fracture with delayed healing
- K subsequent encounter for fracture with nonunion
- P subsequent encounter for fracture with malunion
- S sequela

✓5th **S89.Ø Physeal fracture of upper end of tibia**

AHA: 2019,4Q,56

✓6th **S89.ØØ Unspecified physeal fracture of upper end of tibia**

✓7th **S89.ØØ1 Unspecified physeal fracture of upper end of right tibia** [Q]

✓7th **S89.ØØ2 Unspecified physeal fracture of upper end of left tibia** [Q]

✓7th **S89.ØØ9 Unspecified physeal fracture of upper end of unspecified tibia** [Q]

✓6th **S89.Ø1 Salter-Harris Type I physeal fracture of upper end of tibia**

✓7th **S89.Ø11 Salter-Harris Type I physeal fracture of upper end of right tibia** [Q]

✓7th **S89.Ø12 Salter-Harris Type I physeal fracture of upper end of left tibia** [Q]

✓7th **S89.Ø19 Salter-Harris Type I physeal fracture of upper end of unspecified tibia** [Q]

✓6th **S89.Ø2 Salter-Harris Type II physeal fracture of upper end of tibia**

✓7th **S89.Ø21 Salter-Harris Type II physeal fracture of upper end of right tibia** [Q]

✓7th **S89.Ø22 Salter-Harris Type II physeal fracture of upper end of left tibia** [Q]

✓7th **S89.Ø29 Salter-Harris Type II physeal fracture of upper end of unspecified tibia** [Q]

✓6th **S89.Ø3 Salter-Harris Type III physeal fracture of upper end of tibia**

✓7th **S89.Ø31 Salter-Harris Type III physeal fracture of upper end of right tibia** [Q]

✓7th **S89.Ø32 Salter-Harris Type III physeal fracture of upper end of left tibia** [Q]

✓7th **S89.Ø39 Salter-Harris Type III physeal fracture of upper end of unspecified tibia** [Q]

✓6th **S89.Ø4 Salter-Harris Type IV physeal fracture of upper end of tibia**

✓7th **S89.Ø41 Salter-Harris Type IV physeal fracture of upper end of right tibia** [Q]

✓7th **S89.Ø42 Salter-Harris Type IV physeal fracture of upper end of left tibia** [Q]

✓7th **S89.Ø49 Salter-Harris Type IV physeal fracture of upper end of unspecified tibia** [Q]

✓6th **S89.Ø9 Other physeal fracture of upper end of tibia**

✓7th **S89.Ø91 Other physeal fracture of upper end of right tibia** [Q]

✓7th **S89.Ø92 Other physeal fracture of upper end of left tibia** [Q]

✓7th **S89.Ø99 Other physeal fracture of upper end of unspecified tibia** [Q]

✓5th **S89.1 Physeal fracture of lower end of tibia**

AHA: 2019,4Q,56

✓6th **S89.1Ø Unspecified physeal fracture of lower end of tibia**

✓7th **S89.1Ø1 Unspecified physeal fracture of lower end of right tibia** [Q]

✓7th **S89.1Ø2 Unspecified physeal fracture of lower end of left tibia** [Q]

✓7th **S89.1Ø9 Unspecified physeal fracture of lower end of unspecified tibia** [Q]

✓6th **S89.11 Salter-Harris Type I physeal fracture of lower end of tibia**

✓7th **S89.111 Salter-Harris Type I physeal fracture of lower end of right tibia** [Q]

✓7th **S89.112 Salter-Harris Type I physeal fracture of lower end of left tibia** [Q]

✓7th **S89.119 Salter-Harris Type I physeal fracture of lower end of unspecified tibia** [Q]

✓6th **S89.12 Salter-Harris Type II physeal fracture of lower end of tibia**

✓7th **S89.121 Salter-Harris Type II physeal fracture of lower end of right tibia** [Q]

✓7th **S89.122 Salter-Harris Type II physeal fracture of lower end of left tibia** [Q]

✓7th **S89.129 Salter-Harris Type II physeal fracture of lower end of unspecified tibia** [Q]

✓6th **S89.13 Salter-Harris Type III physeal fracture of lower end of tibia**

EXCLUDES 1 *fracture of medial malleolus (adult) (S82.5-)*

✓7th **S89.131 Salter-Harris Type III physeal fracture of lower end of right tibia** [Q]

✓7th **S89.132 Salter-Harris Type III physeal fracture of lower end of left tibia** [Q]

✓7th **S89.139 Salter-Harris Type III physeal fracture of lower end of unspecified tibia** [Q]

✓6th **S89.14 Salter-Harris Type IV physeal fracture of lower end of tibia**

EXCLUDES 1 *fracture of medial malleolus (adult) (S82.5-)*

✓7th **S89.141 Salter-Harris Type IV physeal fracture of lower end of right tibia** [Q]

✓7th **S89.142 Salter-Harris Type IV physeal fracture of lower end of left tibia** [Q]

✓7th **S89.149 Salter-Harris Type IV physeal fracture of lower end of unspecified tibia** [Q]

✓6th **S89.19 Other physeal fracture of lower end of tibia**

✓7th **S89.191 Other physeal fracture of lower end of right tibia** [Q]

✓7th **S89.192 Other physeal fracture of lower end of left tibia** [Q]

✓7th **S89.199 Other physeal fracture of lower end of unspecified tibia** [Q]

✓5th **S89.2 Physeal fracture of upper end of fibula**

AHA: 2019,4Q,56

✓6th **S89.2Ø Unspecified physeal fracture of upper end of fibula**

✓7th **S89.2Ø1 Unspecified physeal fracture of upper end of right fibula** [Q]

✓7th **S89.2Ø2 Unspecified physeal fracture of upper end of left fibula** [Q]

✓7th **S89.2Ø9 Unspecified physeal fracture of upper end of unspecified fibula** [Q]

✓6th **S89.21 Salter-Harris Type I physeal fracture of upper end of fibula**

✓7th **S89.211 Salter-Harris Type I physeal fracture of upper end of right fibula** [Q]

✓7th **S89.212 Salter-Harris Type I physeal fracture of upper end of left fibula** [Q]

✓7th **S89.219 Salter-Harris Type I physeal fracture of upper end of unspecified fibula** [Q]

✓6th **S89.22 Salter-Harris Type II physeal fracture of upper end of fibula**

✓7th **S89.221 Salter-Harris Type II physeal fracture of upper end of right fibula** [Q]

S89.222 Salter-Harris Type II physeal fracture of upper end of left fibula Q
S89.229 Salter-Harris Type II physeal fracture of upper end of unspecified fibula Q
S89.29 Other physeal fracture of upper end of fibula
S89.291 Other physeal fracture of upper end of right fibula Q
S89.292 Other physeal fracture of upper end of left fibula Q
S89.299 Other physeal fracture of upper end of unspecified fibula Q
S89.3 Physeal fracture of lower end of fibula
AHA: 2019,4Q,56
S89.30 Unspecified physeal fracture of lower end of fibula
S89.301 Unspecified physeal fracture of lower end of right fibula Q
S89.302 Unspecified physeal fracture of lower end of left fibula Q
S89.309 Unspecified physeal fracture of lower end of unspecified fibula Q
S89.31 Salter-Harris Type I physeal fracture of lower end of fibula
S89.311 Salter-Harris Type I physeal fracture of lower end of right fibula Q
S89.312 Salter-Harris Type I physeal fracture of lower end of left fibula Q
S89.319 Salter-Harris Type I physeal fracture of lower end of unspecified fibula Q
S89.32 Salter-Harris Type II physeal fracture of lower end of fibula
S89.321 Salter-Harris Type II physeal fracture of lower end of right fibula Q
S89.322 Salter-Harris Type II physeal fracture of lower end of left fibula Q
S89.329 Salter-Harris Type II physeal fracture of lower end of unspecified fibula Q
S89.39 Other physeal fracture of lower end of fibula
S89.391 Other physeal fracture of lower end of right fibula Q
S89.392 Other physeal fracture of lower end of left fibula Q
S89.399 Other physeal fracture of lower end of unspecified fibula Q
S89.8 Other specified injuries of lower leg

The appropriate 7th character is to be added to each code in subcategory S89.8.
A initial encounter
D subsequent encounter
S sequela

S89.80 Other specified injuries of unspecified lower leg
S89.81 Other specified injuries of right lower leg
S89.82 Other specified injuries of left lower leg
S89.9 Unspecified injury of lower leg

The appropriate 7th character is to be added to each code in subcategory S89.9.
A initial encounter
D subsequent encounter
S sequela

S89.90 Unspecified injury of unspecified lower leg
S89.91 Unspecified injury of right lower leg
S89.92 Unspecified injury of left lower leg

Injuries to the ankle and foot (S90-S99)

EXCLUDES 2 *burns and corrosions (T20-T32)*
fracture of ankle and malleolus (S82.-)
frostbite (T33-T34)
insect bite or sting, venomous (T63.4)

S90 Superficial injury of ankle, foot and toes

The appropriate 7th character is to be added to each code from category S90.
A initial encounter
D subsequent encounter
S sequela

S90.0 Contusion of ankle
S90.00 Contusion of unspecified ankle
S90.01 Contusion of right ankle
S90.02 Contusion of left ankle
S90.1 Contusion of toe without damage to nail
S90.11 Contusion of great toe without damage to nail
S90.111 Contusion of right great toe without damage to nail
S90.112 Contusion of left great toe without damage to nail
S90.119 Contusion of unspecified great toe without damage to nail
S90.12 Contusion of lesser toe without damage to nail
S90.121 Contusion of right lesser toe(s) without damage to nail
S90.122 Contusion of left lesser toe(s) without damage to nail
S90.129 Contusion of unspecified lesser toe(s) without damage to nail
Contusion of toe NOS
S90.2 Contusion of toe with damage to nail
S90.21 Contusion of great toe with damage to nail
S90.211 Contusion of right great toe with damage to nail
S90.212 Contusion of left great toe with damage to nail
S90.219 Contusion of unspecified great toe with damage to nail
S90.22 Contusion of lesser toe with damage to nail
S90.221 Contusion of right lesser toe(s) with damage to nail
S90.222 Contusion of left lesser toe(s) with damage to nail
S90.229 Contusion of unspecified lesser toe(s) with damage to nail
S90.3 Contusion of foot
EXCLUDES 2 *contusion of toes (S90.1-, S90.2-)*
S90.30 Contusion of unspecified foot
Contusion of foot NOS
S90.31 Contusion of right foot
S90.32 Contusion of left foot
S90.4 Other superficial injuries of toe
S90.41 Abrasion of toe
S90.411 Abrasion, right great toe
S90.412 Abrasion, left great toe
S90.413 Abrasion, unspecified great toe
S90.414 Abrasion, right lesser toe(s)
S90.415 Abrasion, left lesser toe(s)
S90.416 Abrasion, unspecified lesser toe(s)
S90.42 Blister (nonthermal) of toe
S90.421 Blister (nonthermal), right great toe
S90.422 Blister (nonthermal), left great toe
S90.423 Blister (nonthermal), unspecified great toe
S90.424 Blister (nonthermal), right lesser toe(s)
S90.425 Blister (nonthermal), left lesser toe(s)
S90.426 Blister (nonthermal), unspecified lesser toe(s)
S90.44 External constriction of toe
Hair tourniquet syndrome of toe
S90.441 External constriction, right great toe
S90.442 External constriction, left great toe
S90.443 External constriction, unspecified great toe
S90.444 External constriction, right lesser toe(s)
S90.445 External constriction, left lesser toe(s)
S90.446 External constriction, unspecified lesser toe(s)
S90.45 Superficial foreign body of toe
Splinter in the toe
S90.451 Superficial foreign body, right great toe
S90.452 Superficial foreign body, left great toe
S90.453 Superficial foreign body, unspecified great toe
S90.454 Superficial foreign body, right lesser toe(s)

7th S90.455 Superficial foreign body, left lesser toe(s)
7th S90.456 Superficial foreign body, unspecified lesser toe(s)
6th S90.46 Insect bite (nonvenomous) of toe
7th S90.461 Insect bite (nonvenomous), right great toe
7th S90.462 Insect bite (nonvenomous), left great toe
7th S90.463 Insect bite (nonvenomous), unspecified great toe
7th S90.464 Insect bite (nonvenomous), right lesser toe(s)
7th S90.465 Insect bite (nonvenomous), left lesser toe(s)
7th S90.466 Insect bite (nonvenomous), unspecified lesser toe(s)
6th S90.47 Other superficial bite of toe
EXCLUDES 1 *open bite of toe (S91.15-, S91.25-)*
7th S90.471 Other superficial bite of right great toe
7th S90.472 Other superficial bite of left great toe
7th S90.473 Other superficial bite of unspecified great toe
7th S90.474 Other superficial bite of right lesser toe(s)
7th S90.475 Other superficial bite of left lesser toe(s)
7th S90.476 Other superficial bite of unspecified lesser toe(s)
5th S90.5 Other superficial injuries of ankle
6th S90.51 Abrasion of ankle
7th S90.511 Abrasion, right ankle
7th S90.512 Abrasion, left ankle
7th S90.519 Abrasion, unspecified ankle
6th S90.52 Blister (nonthermal) of ankle
7th S90.521 Blister (nonthermal), right ankle
7th S90.522 Blister (nonthermal), left ankle
7th S90.529 Blister (nonthermal), unspecified ankle
6th S90.54 External constriction of ankle
7th S90.541 External constriction, right ankle
7th S90.542 External constriction, left ankle
7th S90.549 External constriction, unspecified ankle
6th S90.55 Superficial foreign body of ankle
Splinter in the ankle
7th S90.551 Superficial foreign body, right ankle
7th S90.552 Superficial foreign body, left ankle
7th S90.559 Superficial foreign body, unspecified ankle
6th S90.56 Insect bite (nonvenomous) of ankle
7th S90.561 Insect bite (nonvenomous), right ankle
7th S90.562 Insect bite (nonvenomous), left ankle
7th S90.569 Insect bite (nonvenomous), unspecified ankle
6th S90.57 Other superficial bite of ankle
EXCLUDES 1 *open bite of ankle (S91.05-)*
7th S90.571 Other superficial bite of ankle, right ankle
7th S90.572 Other superficial bite of ankle, left ankle
7th S90.579 Other superficial bite of ankle, unspecified ankle
5th S90.8 Other superficial injuries of foot
6th S90.81 Abrasion of foot
7th S90.811 Abrasion, right foot
7th S90.812 Abrasion, left foot
7th S90.819 Abrasion, unspecified foot
6th S90.82 Blister (nonthermal) of foot
7th S90.821 Blister (nonthermal), right foot
7th S90.822 Blister (nonthermal), left foot
7th S90.829 Blister (nonthermal), unspecified foot
6th S90.84 External constriction of foot
7th S90.841 External constriction, right foot
7th S90.842 External constriction, left foot
7th S90.849 External constriction, unspecified foot
6th S90.85 Superficial foreign body of foot
Splinter in the foot
7th S90.851 Superficial foreign body, right foot
7th S90.852 Superficial foreign body, left foot
7th S90.859 Superficial foreign body, unspecified foot
6th S90.86 Insect bite (nonvenomous) of foot
7th S90.861 Insect bite (nonvenomous), right foot
7th S90.862 Insect bite (nonvenomous), left foot
7th S90.869 Insect bite (nonvenomous), unspecified foot
6th S90.87 Other superficial bite of foot
EXCLUDES 1 *open bite of foot (S91.35-)*
7th S90.871 Other superficial bite of right foot
7th S90.872 Other superficial bite of left foot
7th S90.879 Other superficial bite of unspecified foot
5th S90.9 Unspecified superficial injury of ankle, foot and toe
6th S90.91 Unspecified superficial injury of ankle
7th S90.911 Unspecified superficial injury of right ankle
7th S90.912 Unspecified superficial injury of left ankle
7th S90.919 Unspecified superficial injury of unspecified ankle
6th S90.92 Unspecified superficial injury of foot
7th S90.921 Unspecified superficial injury of right foot
7th S90.922 Unspecified superficial injury of left foot
7th S90.929 Unspecified superficial injury of unspecified foot
6th S90.93 Unspecified superficial injury of toes
7th S90.931 Unspecified superficial injury of right great toe
7th S90.932 Unspecified superficial injury of left great toe
7th S90.933 Unspecified superficial injury of unspecified great toe
7th S90.934 Unspecified superficial injury of right lesser toe(s)
7th S90.935 Unspecified superficial injury of left lesser toe(s)
7th S90.936 Unspecified superficial injury of unspecified lesser toe(s)

4th **S91 Open wound of ankle, foot and toes**
Code also any associated wound infection
EXCLUDES 1 *open fracture of ankle, foot and toes (S92.- with 7th character B)*
traumatic amputation of ankle and foot (S98.-)
AHA: 2021,1Q,7

The appropriate 7th character is to be added to each code from category S91.
A initial encounter
D subsequent encounter
S sequela

5th S91.0 Open wound of ankle
6th S91.00 Unspecified open wound of ankle
7th S91.001 Unspecified open wound, right ankle
7th S91.002 Unspecified open wound, left ankle
7th S91.009 Unspecified open wound, unspecified ankle
6th S91.01 Laceration without foreign body of ankle
7th S91.011 Laceration without foreign body, right ankle
7th S91.012 Laceration without foreign body, left ankle
7th S91.019 Laceration without foreign body, unspecified ankle
6th S91.02 Laceration with foreign body of ankle
7th S91.021 Laceration with foreign body, right ankle
7th S91.022 Laceration with foreign body, left ankle
7th S91.029 Laceration with foreign body, unspecified ankle
6th S91.03 Puncture wound without foreign body of ankle
7th S91.031 Puncture wound without foreign body, right ankle
7th S91.032 Puncture wound without foreign body, left ankle
7th S91.039 Puncture wound without foreign body, unspecified ankle

S91.04 Puncture wound with foreign body of ankle
S91.041 Puncture wound with foreign body, right ankle
S91.042 Puncture wound with foreign body, left ankle
S91.049 Puncture wound with foreign body, unspecified ankle
S91.05 Open bite of ankle
EXCLUDES 1 *superficial bite of ankle (S90.56-, S90.57-)*
S91.051 Open bite, right ankle
S91.052 Open bite, left ankle
S91.059 Open bite, unspecified ankle
S91.1 Open wound of toe without damage to nail
S91.10 Unspecified open wound of toe without damage to nail
S91.101 Unspecified open wound of right great toe without damage to nail
S91.102 Unspecified open wound of left great toe without damage to nail
S91.103 Unspecified open wound of unspecified great toe without damage to nail
S91.104 Unspecified open wound of right lesser toe(s) without damage to nail
S91.105 Unspecified open wound of left lesser toe(s) without damage to nail
S91.106 Unspecified open wound of unspecified lesser toe(s) without damage to nail
S91.109 Unspecified open wound of unspecified toe(s) without damage to nail
S91.11 Laceration without foreign body of toe without damage to nail
S91.111 Laceration without foreign body of right great toe without damage to nail
S91.112 Laceration without foreign body of left great toe without damage to nail
S91.113 Laceration without foreign body of unspecified great toe without damage to nail
S91.114 Laceration without foreign body of right lesser toe(s) without damage to nail
S91.115 Laceration without foreign body of left lesser toe(s) without damage to nail
S91.116 Laceration without foreign body of unspecified lesser toe(s) without damage to nail
S91.119 Laceration without foreign body of unspecified toe without damage to nail
S91.12 Laceration with foreign body of toe without damage to nail
S91.121 Laceration with foreign body of right great toe without damage to nail
S91.122 Laceration with foreign body of left great toe without damage to nail
S91.123 Laceration with foreign body of unspecified great toe without damage to nail
S91.124 Laceration with foreign body of right lesser toe(s) without damage to nail
S91.125 Laceration with foreign body of left lesser toe(s) without damage to nail
S91.126 Laceration with foreign body of unspecified lesser toe(s) without damage to nail
S91.129 Laceration with foreign body of unspecified toe(s) without damage to nail
S91.13 Puncture wound without foreign body of toe without damage to nail
S91.131 Puncture wound without foreign body of right great toe without damage to nail
S91.132 Puncture wound without foreign body of left great toe without damage to nail
S91.133 Puncture wound without foreign body of unspecified great toe without damage to nail
S91.134 Puncture wound without foreign body of right lesser toe(s) without damage to nail
S91.135 Puncture wound without foreign body of left lesser toe(s) without damage to nail
S91.136 Puncture wound without foreign body of unspecified lesser toe(s) without damage to nail
S91.139 Puncture wound without foreign body of unspecified toe(s) without damage to nail
S91.14 Puncture wound with foreign body of toe without damage to nail
S91.141 Puncture wound with foreign body of right great toe without damage to nail
S91.142 Puncture wound with foreign body of left great toe without damage to nail
S91.143 Puncture wound with foreign body of unspecified great toe without damage to nail
S91.144 Puncture wound with foreign body of right lesser toe(s) without damage to nail
S91.145 Puncture wound with foreign body of left lesser toe(s) without damage to nail
S91.146 Puncture wound with foreign body of unspecified lesser toe(s) without damage to nail
S91.149 Puncture wound with foreign body of unspecified toe(s) without damage to nail
S91.15 Open bite of toe without damage to nail
Bite of toe NOS
EXCLUDES 1 *superficial bite of toe (S90.46-, S90.47-)*
S91.151 Open bite of right great toe without damage to nail
S91.152 Open bite of left great toe without damage to nail
S91.153 Open bite of unspecified great toe without damage to nail
S91.154 Open bite of right lesser toe(s) without damage to nail
S91.155 Open bite of left lesser toe(s) without damage to nail
S91.156 Open bite of unspecified lesser toe(s) without damage to nail
S91.159 Open bite of unspecified toe(s) without damage to nail
S91.2 Open wound of toe with damage to nail
S91.20 Unspecified open wound of toe with damage to nail
S91.201 Unspecified open wound of right great toe with damage to nail
S91.202 Unspecified open wound of left great toe with damage to nail
S91.203 Unspecified open wound of unspecified great toe with damage to nail
S91.204 Unspecified open wound of right lesser toe(s) with damage to nail
S91.205 Unspecified open wound of left lesser toe(s) with damage to nail
S91.206 Unspecified open wound of unspecified lesser toe(s) with damage to nail
S91.209 Unspecified open wound of unspecified toe(s) with damage to nail
S91.21 Laceration without foreign body of toe with damage to nail
S91.211 Laceration without foreign body of right great toe with damage to nail
S91.212 Laceration without foreign body of left great toe with damage to nail
S91.213 Laceration without foreign body of unspecified great toe with damage to nail
S91.214 Laceration without foreign body of right lesser toe(s) with damage to nail
S91.215 Laceration without foreign body of left lesser toe(s) with damage to nail
S91.216 Laceration without foreign body of unspecified lesser toe(s) with damage to nail
S91.219 Laceration without foreign body of unspecified toe(s) with damage to nail
S91.22 Laceration with foreign body of toe with damage to nail
S91.221 Laceration with foreign body of right great toe with damage to nail
S91.222 Laceration with foreign body of left great toe with damage to nail
S91.223 Laceration with foreign body of unspecified great toe with damage to nail
S91.224 Laceration with foreign body of right lesser toe(s) with damage to nail
S91.225 Laceration with foreign body of left lesser toe(s) with damage to nail

7th **S91.226** Laceration with foreign body of unspecified lesser toe(s) with damage to nail

7th **S91.229** Laceration with foreign body of unspecified toe(s) with damage to nail

6th **S91.23 Puncture wound without foreign body of toe with damage to nail**

7th **S91.231** Puncture wound without foreign body of right great toe with damage to nail

7th **S91.232** Puncture wound without foreign body of left great toe with damage to nail

7th **S91.233** Puncture wound without foreign body of unspecified great toe with damage to nail

7th **S91.234** Puncture wound without foreign body of right lesser toe(s) with damage to nail

7th **S91.235** Puncture wound without foreign body of left lesser toe(s) with damage to nail

7th **S91.236** Puncture wound without foreign body of unspecified lesser toe(s) with damage to nail

7th **S91.239** Puncture wound without foreign body of unspecified toe(s) with damage to nail

6th **S91.24 Puncture wound with foreign body of toe with damage to nail**

7th **S91.241** Puncture wound with foreign body of right great toe with damage to nail

7th **S91.242** Puncture wound with foreign body of left great toe with damage to nail

7th **S91.243** Puncture wound with foreign body of unspecified great toe with damage to nail

7th **S91.244** Puncture wound with foreign body of right lesser toe(s) with damage to nail

7th **S91.245** Puncture wound with foreign body of left lesser toe(s) with damage to nail

7th **S91.246** Puncture wound with foreign body of unspecified lesser toe(s) with damage to nail

7th **S91.249** Puncture wound with foreign body of unspecified toe(s) with damage to nail

6th **S91.25 Open bite of toe with damage to nail**

Bite of toe with damage to nail NOS

EXCLUDES 1 *superficial bite of toe (S90.46-, S90.47-)*

7th **S91.251** Open bite of right great toe with damage to nail

7th **S91.252** Open bite of left great toe with damage to nail

7th **S91.253** Open bite of unspecified great toe with damage to nail

7th **S91.254** Open bite of right lesser toe(s) with damage to nail

7th **S91.255** Open bite of left lesser toe(s) with damage to nail

7th **S91.256** Open bite of unspecified lesser toe(s) with damage to nail

7th **S91.259** Open bite of unspecified toe(s) with damage to nail

5th **S91.3 Open wound of foot**

6th **S91.30 Unspecified open wound of foot**

7th **S91.301** Unspecified open wound, right foot

7th **S91.302** Unspecified open wound, left foot

7th **S91.309** Unspecified open wound, unspecified foot

6th **S91.31 Laceration without foreign body of foot**

7th **S91.311** Laceration without foreign body, right foot

7th **S91.312** Laceration without foreign body, left foot

7th **S91.319** Laceration without foreign body, unspecified foot

6th **S91.32 Laceration with foreign body of foot**

7th **S91.321** Laceration with foreign body, right foot

7th **S91.322** Laceration with foreign body, left foot

7th **S91.329** Laceration with foreign body, unspecified foot

6th **S91.33 Puncture wound without foreign body of foot**

7th **S91.331** Puncture wound without foreign body, right foot

7th **S91.332** Puncture wound without foreign body, left foot

7th **S91.339** Puncture wound without foreign body, unspecified foot

6th **S91.34 Puncture wound with foreign body of foot**

7th **S91.341** Puncture wound with foreign body, right foot

7th **S91.342** Puncture wound with foreign body, left foot

7th **S91.349** Puncture wound with foreign body, unspecified foot

6th **S91.35 Open bite of foot**

EXCLUDES 1 *superficial bite of foot (S90.86-, S90.87-)*

7th **S91.351** Open bite, right foot

7th **S91.352** Open bite, left foot

7th **S91.359** Open bite, unspecified foot

4th **S92 Fracture of foot and toe, except ankle**

NOTE A fracture not indicated as displaced or nondisplaced should be coded to displaced

A fracture not indicated as open or closed should be coded to closed.

EXCLUDES 2 *fracture of ankle (S82.-)*
fracture of malleolus (S82.-)
traumatic amputation of ankle and foot (S98.-)

AHA: 2018,2Q,12; 2015,3Q,37-39

The appropriate 7th character is to be added to each code from category S92.

A initial encounter for closed fracture
B initial encounter for open fracture
D subsequent encounter for fracture with routine healing
G subsequent encounter for fracture with delayed healing
K subsequent encounter for fracture with nonunion
P subsequent encounter for fracture with malunion
S sequela

5th **S92.0 Fracture of calcaneus**

Heel bone
Os calcis

EXCLUDES 2 *physeal fracture of calcaneus (S99.0-)*

6th **S92.00 Unspecified fracture of calcaneus**

7th **S92.001** Unspecified fracture of right calcaneus Q

7th **S92.002** Unspecified fracture of left calcaneus Q

7th **S92.009** Unspecified fracture of unspecified calcaneus Q

6th **S92.01 Fracture of body of calcaneus**

7th **S92.011** Displaced fracture of body of right calcaneus Q

7th **S92.012** Displaced fracture of body of left calcaneus Q

7th **S92.013** Displaced fracture of body of unspecified calcaneus Q

7th **S92.014** Nondisplaced fracture of body of right calcaneus Q

7th **S92.015** Nondisplaced fracture of body of left calcaneus Q

7th **S92.016** Nondisplaced fracture of body of unspecified calcaneus Q

6th **S92.02 Fracture of anterior process of calcaneus**

7th **S92.021** Displaced fracture of anterior process of right calcaneus Q

7th **S92.022** Displaced fracture of anterior process of left calcaneus Q

7th **S92.023** Displaced fracture of anterior process of unspecified calcaneus Q

7th **S92.024** Nondisplaced fracture of anterior process of right calcaneus Q

7th **S92.025** Nondisplaced fracture of anterior process of left calcaneus Q

7th **S92.026** Nondisplaced fracture of anterior process of unspecified calcaneus Q

6th **S92.03 Avulsion fracture of tuberosity of calcaneus**

7th **S92.031** Displaced avulsion fracture of tuberosity of right calcaneus Q

7th **S92.032** Displaced avulsion fracture of tuberosity of left calcaneus Q

7th **S92.033** Displaced avulsion fracture of tuberosity of unspecified calcaneus Q

7th **S92.034** Nondisplaced avulsion fracture of tuberosity of right calcaneus Q

S92.Ø35 Nondisplaced avulsion fracture of tuberosity of left calcaneus Q
S92.Ø36 Nondisplaced avulsion fracture of tuberosity of unspecified calcaneus Q
S92.Ø4 Other fracture of tuberosity of calcaneus
S92.Ø41 Displaced other fracture of tuberosity of right calcaneus Q
S92.Ø42 Displaced other fracture of tuberosity of left calcaneus Q
S92.Ø43 Displaced other fracture of tuberosity of unspecified calcaneus Q
S92.Ø44 Nondisplaced other fracture of tuberosity of right calcaneus Q
S92.Ø45 Nondisplaced other fracture of tuberosity of left calcaneus Q
S92.Ø46 Nondisplaced other fracture of tuberosity of unspecified calcaneus Q
S92.Ø5 Other extraarticular fracture of calcaneus
S92.Ø51 Displaced other extraarticular fracture of right calcaneus Q
S92.Ø52 Displaced other extraarticular fracture of left calcaneus Q
S92.Ø53 Displaced other extraarticular fracture of unspecified calcaneus Q
S92.Ø54 Nondisplaced other extraarticular fracture of right calcaneus Q
S92.Ø55 Nondisplaced other extraarticular fracture of left calcaneus Q
S92.Ø56 Nondisplaced other extraarticular fracture of unspecified calcaneus Q
S92.Ø6 Intraarticular fracture of calcaneus
S92.Ø61 Displaced intraarticular fracture of right calcaneus Q
S92.Ø62 Displaced intraarticular fracture of left calcaneus Q
S92.Ø63 Displaced intraarticular fracture of unspecified calcaneus Q
S92.Ø64 Nondisplaced intraarticular fracture of right calcaneus Q
S92.Ø65 Nondisplaced intraarticular fracture of left calcaneus Q
S92.Ø66 Nondisplaced intraarticular fracture of unspecified calcaneus Q
S92.1 Fracture of talus
Astragalus
S92.1Ø Unspecified fracture of talus
S92.1Ø1 Unspecified fracture of right talus Q
S92.1Ø2 Unspecified fracture of left talus Q
S92.1Ø9 Unspecified fracture of unspecified talus Q
S92.11 Fracture of neck of talus
S92.111 Displaced fracture of neck of right talus Q
S92.112 Displaced fracture of neck of left talus Q
S92.113 Displaced fracture of neck of unspecified talus Q
S92.114 Nondisplaced fracture of neck of right talus Q
S92.115 Nondisplaced fracture of neck of left talus Q
S92.116 Nondisplaced fracture of neck of unspecified talus Q
S92.12 Fracture of body of talus
S92.121 Displaced fracture of body of right talus Q
S92.122 Displaced fracture of body of left talus Q
S92.123 Displaced fracture of body of unspecified talus Q
S92.124 Nondisplaced fracture of body of right talus Q
S92.125 Nondisplaced fracture of body of left talus Q
S92.126 Nondisplaced fracture of body of unspecified talus Q
S92.13 Fracture of posterior process of talus
S92.131 Displaced fracture of posterior process of right talus Q
S92.132 Displaced fracture of posterior process of left talus Q
S92.133 Displaced fracture of posterior process of unspecified talus Q
S92.134 Nondisplaced fracture of posterior process of right talus Q
S92.135 Nondisplaced fracture of posterior process of left talus Q
S92.136 Nondisplaced fracture of posterior process of unspecified talus Q
S92.14 Dome fracture of talus
EXCLUDES 1 *osteochondritis dissecans (M93.2)*
S92.141 Displaced dome fracture of right talus Q
S92.142 Displaced dome fracture of left talus Q
S92.143 Displaced dome fracture of unspecified talus Q
S92.144 Nondisplaced dome fracture of right talus Q
S92.145 Nondisplaced dome fracture of left talus Q
S92.146 Nondisplaced dome fracture of unspecified talus Q
S92.15 Avulsion fracture (chip fracture) of talus
S92.151 Displaced avulsion fracture (chip fracture) of right talus Q
S92.152 Displaced avulsion fracture (chip fracture) of left talus Q
S92.153 Displaced avulsion fracture (chip fracture) of unspecified talus Q
S92.154 Nondisplaced avulsion fracture (chip fracture) of right talus Q
S92.155 Nondisplaced avulsion fracture (chip fracture) of left talus Q
S92.156 Nondisplaced avulsion fracture (chip fracture) of unspecified talus Q
S92.19 Other fracture of talus
S92.191 Other fracture of right talus Q
S92.192 Other fracture of left talus Q
S92.199 Other fracture of unspecified talus Q
S92.2 Fracture of other and unspecified tarsal bone(s)
S92.2Ø Fracture of unspecified tarsal bone(s)
S92.2Ø1 Fracture of unspecified tarsal bone(s) of right foot Q
S92.2Ø2 Fracture of unspecified tarsal bone(s) of left foot Q
S92.2Ø9 Fracture of unspecified tarsal bone(s) of unspecified foot Q
S92.21 Fracture of cuboid bone
S92.211 Displaced fracture of cuboid bone of right foot Q
S92.212 Displaced fracture of cuboid bone of left foot Q
S92.213 Displaced fracture of cuboid bone of unspecified foot Q
S92.214 Nondisplaced fracture of cuboid bone of right foot Q
S92.215 Nondisplaced fracture of cuboid bone of left foot Q
S92.216 Nondisplaced fracture of cuboid bone of unspecified foot Q
S92.22 Fracture of lateral cuneiform
S92.221 Displaced fracture of lateral cuneiform of right foot Q
S92.222 Displaced fracture of lateral cuneiform of left foot Q
S92.223 Displaced fracture of lateral cuneiform of unspecified foot Q
S92.224 Nondisplaced fracture of lateral cuneiform of right foot Q
S92.225 Nondisplaced fracture of lateral cuneiform of left foot Q
S92.226 Nondisplaced fracture of lateral cuneiform of unspecified foot Q
S92.23 Fracture of intermediate cuneiform
S92.231 Displaced fracture of intermediate cuneiform of right foot Q

√7th S92.232 Displaced fracture of intermediate cuneiform of left foot
√7th S92.233 Displaced fracture of intermediate cuneiform of unspecified foot
√7th S92.234 Nondisplaced fracture of intermediate cuneiform of right foot
√7th S92.235 Nondisplaced fracture of intermediate cuneiform of left foot
√7th S92.236 Nondisplaced fracture of intermediate cuneiform of unspecified foot

√6th S92.24 Fracture of medial cuneiform
√7th S92.241 Displaced fracture of medial cuneiform of right foot
√7th S92.242 Displaced fracture of medial cuneiform of left foot
√7th S92.243 Displaced fracture of medial cuneiform of unspecified foot
√7th S92.244 Nondisplaced fracture of medial cuneiform of right foot
√7th S92.245 Nondisplaced fracture of medial cuneiform of left foot
√7th S92.246 Nondisplaced fracture of medial cuneiform of unspecified foot

√6th S92.25 Fracture of navicular [scaphoid] of foot
√7th S92.251 Displaced fracture of navicular [scaphoid] of right foot
√7th S92.252 Displaced fracture of navicular [scaphoid] of left foot
√7th S92.253 Displaced fracture of navicular [scaphoid] of unspecified foot
√7th S92.254 Nondisplaced fracture of navicular [scaphoid] of right foot
√7th S92.255 Nondisplaced fracture of navicular [scaphoid] of left foot
√7th S92.256 Nondisplaced fracture of navicular [scaphoid] of unspecified foot

√5th S92.3 Fracture of metatarsal bone(s)

EXCLUDES 2 *physeal fracture of metatarsal (S99.1-)*

AHA: 2018,1Q,3

√6th S92.30 Fracture of unspecified metatarsal bone(s)
√7th S92.301 Fracture of unspecified metatarsal bone(s), right foot
√7th S92.302 Fracture of unspecified metatarsal bone(s), left foot
√7th S92.309 Fracture of unspecified metatarsal bone(s), unspecified foot

√6th S92.31 Fracture of first metatarsal bone
√7th S92.311 Displaced fracture of first metatarsal bone, right foot
√7th S92.312 Displaced fracture of first metatarsal bone, left foot
√7th S92.313 Displaced fracture of first metatarsal bone, unspecified foot
√7th S92.314 Nondisplaced fracture of first metatarsal bone, right foot
√7th S92.315 Nondisplaced fracture of first metatarsal bone, left foot
√7th S92.316 Nondisplaced fracture of first metatarsal bone, unspecified foot

√6th S92.32 Fracture of second metatarsal bone
√7th S92.321 Displaced fracture of second metatarsal bone, right foot
√7th S92.322 Displaced fracture of second metatarsal bone, left foot
√7th S92.323 Displaced fracture of second metatarsal bone, unspecified foot
√7th S92.324 Nondisplaced fracture of second metatarsal bone, right foot
√7th S92.325 Nondisplaced fracture of second metatarsal bone, left foot
√7th S92.326 Nondisplaced fracture of second metatarsal bone, unspecified foot

√6th S92.33 Fracture of third metatarsal bone
√7th S92.331 Displaced fracture of third metatarsal bone, right foot
√7th S92.332 Displaced fracture of third metatarsal bone, left foot
√7th S92.333 Displaced fracture of third metatarsal bone, unspecified foot
√7th S92.334 Nondisplaced fracture of third metatarsal bone, right foot
√7th S92.335 Nondisplaced fracture of third metatarsal bone, left foot
√7th S92.336 Nondisplaced fracture of third metatarsal bone, unspecified foot

√6th S92.34 Fracture of fourth metatarsal bone
√7th S92.341 Displaced fracture of fourth metatarsal bone, right foot
√7th S92.342 Displaced fracture of fourth metatarsal bone, left foot
√7th S92.343 Displaced fracture of fourth metatarsal bone, unspecified foot
√7th S92.344 Nondisplaced fracture of fourth metatarsal bone, right foot
√7th S92.345 Nondisplaced fracture of fourth metatarsal bone, left foot
√7th S92.346 Nondisplaced fracture of fourth metatarsal bone, unspecified foot

√6th S92.35 Fracture of fifth metatarsal bone
√7th S92.351 Displaced fracture of fifth metatarsal bone, right foot
√7th S92.352 Displaced fracture of fifth metatarsal bone, left foot
√7th S92.353 Displaced fracture of fifth metatarsal bone, unspecified foot
√7th S92.354 Nondisplaced fracture of fifth metatarsal bone, right foot
√7th S92.355 Nondisplaced fracture of fifth metatarsal bone, left foot
√7th S92.356 Nondisplaced fracture of fifth metatarsal bone, unspecified foot

√5th S92.4 Fracture of great toe

EXCLUDES 2 *physeal fracture of phalanx of toe (S99.2-)*

√6th S92.40 Unspecified fracture of great toe
√7th S92.401 Displaced unspecified fracture of right great toe
√7th S92.402 Displaced unspecified fracture of left great toe
√7th S92.403 Displaced unspecified fracture of unspecified great toe
√7th S92.404 Nondisplaced unspecified fracture of right great toe
√7th S92.405 Nondisplaced unspecified fracture of left great toe
√7th S92.406 Nondisplaced unspecified fracture of unspecified great toe

√6th S92.41 Fracture of proximal phalanx of great toe
√7th S92.411 Displaced fracture of proximal phalanx of right great toe
√7th S92.412 Displaced fracture of proximal phalanx of left great toe
√7th S92.413 Displaced fracture of proximal phalanx of unspecified great toe
√7th S92.414 Nondisplaced fracture of proximal phalanx of right great toe
√7th S92.415 Nondisplaced fracture of proximal phalanx of left great toe
√7th S92.416 Nondisplaced fracture of proximal phalanx of unspecified great toe

√6th S92.42 Fracture of distal phalanx of great toe
√7th S92.421 Displaced fracture of distal phalanx of right great toe
√7th S92.422 Displaced fracture of distal phalanx of left great toe
√7th S92.423 Displaced fracture of distal phalanx of unspecified great toe
√7th S92.424 Nondisplaced fracture of distal phalanx of right great toe
√7th S92.425 Nondisplaced fracture of distal phalanx of left great toe
√7th S92.426 Nondisplaced fracture of distal phalanx of unspecified great toe

√6th S92.49 Other fracture of great toe
√7th S92.491 Other fracture of right great toe
√7th S92.492 Other fracture of left great toe
√7th S92.499 Other fracture of unspecified great toe

S92.5 Fracture of lesser toe(s)

EXCLUDES 2 *physeal fracture of phalanx of toe (S99.2-)*

S92.50 Unspecified fracture of lesser toe(s)

S92.501 Displaced unspecified fracture of right lesser toe(s)

S92.502 Displaced unspecified fracture of left lesser toe(s)

S92.503 Displaced unspecified fracture of unspecified lesser toe(s)

S92.504 Nondisplaced unspecified fracture of right lesser toe(s)

S92.505 Nondisplaced unspecified fracture of left lesser toe(s)

S92.506 Nondisplaced unspecified fracture of unspecified lesser toe(s)

S92.51 Fracture of proximal phalanx of lesser toe(s)

S92.511 Displaced fracture of proximal phalanx of right lesser toe(s)

S92.512 Displaced fracture of proximal phalanx of left lesser toe(s)

S92.513 Displaced fracture of proximal phalanx of unspecified lesser toe(s)

S92.514 Nondisplaced fracture of proximal phalanx of right lesser toe(s)

S92.515 Nondisplaced fracture of proximal phalanx of left lesser toe(s)

S92.516 Nondisplaced fracture of proximal phalanx of unspecified lesser toe(s)

S92.52 Fracture of middle phalanx of lesser toe(s)

S92.521 Displaced fracture of middle phalanx of right lesser toe(s)

S92.522 Displaced fracture of middle phalanx of left lesser toe(s)

S92.523 Displaced fracture of middle phalanx of unspecified lesser toe(s)

S92.524 Nondisplaced fracture of middle phalanx of right lesser toe(s)

S92.525 Nondisplaced fracture of middle phalanx of left lesser toe(s)

S92.526 Nondisplaced fracture of middle phalanx of unspecified lesser toe(s)

S92.53 Fracture of distal phalanx of lesser toe(s)

S92.531 Displaced fracture of distal phalanx of right lesser toe(s)

S92.532 Displaced fracture of distal phalanx of left lesser toe(s)

S92.533 Displaced fracture of distal phalanx of unspecified lesser toe(s)

S92.534 Nondisplaced fracture of distal phalanx of right lesser toe(s)

S92.535 Nondisplaced fracture of distal phalanx of left lesser toe(s)

S92.536 Nondisplaced fracture of distal phalanx of unspecified lesser toe(s)

S92.59 Other fracture of lesser toe(s)

S92.591 Other fracture of right lesser toe(s)

S92.592 Other fracture of left lesser toe(s)

S92.599 Other fracture of unspecified lesser toe(s)

S92.8 Other fracture of foot, except ankle

S92.81 Other fracture of foot

Sesamoid fracture of foot

AHA: 2016,4Q,68

S92.811 Other fracture of right foot Q

S92.812 Other fracture of left foot Q

S92.819 Other fracture of unspecified foot Q

S92.9 Unspecified fracture of foot and toe

S92.90 Unspecified fracture of foot

S92.901 Unspecified fracture of right foot Q

S92.902 Unspecified fracture of left foot Q

S92.909 Unspecified fracture of unspecified foot Q

S92.91 Unspecified fracture of toe

S92.911 Unspecified fracture of right toe(s)

S92.912 Unspecified fracture of left toe(s)

S92.919 Unspecified fracture of unspecified toe(s)

S93 Dislocation and sprain of joints and ligaments at ankle, foot and toe level

INCLUDES avulsion of joint or ligament of ankle, foot and toe
laceration of cartilage, joint or ligament of ankle, foot and toe
sprain of cartilage, joint or ligament of ankle, foot and toe
traumatic hemarthrosis of joint or ligament of ankle, foot and toe
traumatic rupture of joint or ligament of ankle, foot and toe
traumatic subluxation of joint or ligament of ankle, foot and toe
traumatic tear of joint or ligament of ankle, foot and toe

Code also any associated open wound

EXCLUDES 2 *strain of muscle and tendon of ankle and foot (S96.-)*

The appropriate 7th character is to be added to each code from category S93.
A initial encounter
D subsequent encounter
S sequela

S93.0 Subluxation and dislocation of ankle joint

Subluxation and dislocation of astragalus
Subluxation and dislocation of fibula, lower end
Subluxation and dislocation of talus
Subluxation and dislocation of tibia, lower end

S93.01 Subluxation of right ankle joint

S93.02 Subluxation of left ankle joint

S93.03 Subluxation of unspecified ankle joint

S93.04 Dislocation of right ankle joint

S93.05 Dislocation of left ankle joint

S93.06 Dislocation of unspecified ankle joint

S93.1 Subluxation and dislocation of toe

S93.10 Unspecified subluxation and dislocation of toe

Dislocation of toe NOS
Subluxation of toe NOS

S93.101 Unspecified subluxation of right toe(s)

S93.102 Unspecified subluxation of left toe(s)

S93.103 Unspecified subluxation of unspecified toe(s)

S93.104 Unspecified dislocation of right toe(s)

S93.105 Unspecified dislocation of left toe(s)

S93.106 Unspecified dislocation of unspecified toe(s)

S93.11 Dislocation of interphalangeal joint

S93.111 Dislocation of interphalangeal joint of right great toe

S93.112 Dislocation of interphalangeal joint of left great toe

S93.113 Dislocation of interphalangeal joint of unspecified great toe

S93.114 Dislocation of interphalangeal joint of right lesser toe(s)

S93.115 Dislocation of interphalangeal joint of left lesser toe(s)

S93.116 Dislocation of interphalangeal joint of unspecified lesser toe(s)

S93.119 Dislocation of interphalangeal joint of unspecified toe(s)

S93.12 Dislocation of metatarsophalangeal joint

S93.121 Dislocation of metatarsophalangeal joint of right great toe

S93.122 Dislocation of metatarsophalangeal joint of left great toe

S93.123 Dislocation of metatarsophalangeal joint of unspecified great toe

S93.124 Dislocation of metatarsophalangeal joint of right lesser toe(s)

S93.125 Dislocation of metatarsophalangeal joint of left lesser toe(s)

S93.126 Dislocation of metatarsophalangeal joint of unspecified lesser toe(s)

S93.129 Dislocation of metatarsophalangeal joint of unspecified toe(s)

S93.13 Subluxation of interphalangeal joint

S93.131 Subluxation of interphalangeal joint of right great toe

S93.132 Subluxation of interphalangeal joint of left great toe
S93.133 Subluxation of interphalangeal joint of unspecified great toe
S93.134 Subluxation of interphalangeal joint of right lesser toe(s)
S93.135 Subluxation of interphalangeal joint of left lesser toe(s)
S93.136 Subluxation of interphalangeal joint of unspecified lesser toe(s)
S93.139 Subluxation of interphalangeal joint of unspecified toe(s)

S93.14 Subluxation of metatarsophalangeal joint
S93.141 Subluxation of metatarsophalangeal joint of right great toe
S93.142 Subluxation of metatarsophalangeal joint of left great toe
S93.143 Subluxation of metatarsophalangeal joint of unspecified great toe
S93.144 Subluxation of metatarsophalangeal joint of right lesser toe(s)
S93.145 Subluxation of metatarsophalangeal joint of left lesser toe(s)
S93.146 Subluxation of metatarsophalangeal joint of unspecified lesser toe(s)
S93.149 Subluxation of metatarsophalangeal joint of unspecified toe(s)

S93.3 Subluxation and dislocation of foot
EXCLUDES 2 *dislocation of toe (S93.1-)*

S93.30 Unspecified subluxation and dislocation of foot
Dislocation of foot NOS
Subluxation of foot NOS
S93.301 Unspecified subluxation of right foot
S93.302 Unspecified subluxation of left foot
S93.303 Unspecified subluxation of unspecified foot
S93.304 Unspecified dislocation of right foot
S93.305 Unspecified dislocation of left foot
S93.306 Unspecified dislocation of unspecified foot

S93.31 Subluxation and dislocation of tarsal joint
S93.311 Subluxation of tarsal joint of right foot
S93.312 Subluxation of tarsal joint of left foot
S93.313 Subluxation of tarsal joint of unspecified foot
S93.314 Dislocation of tarsal joint of right foot
S93.315 Dislocation of tarsal joint of left foot
S93.316 Dislocation of tarsal joint of unspecified foot

S93.32 Subluxation and dislocation of tarsometatarsal joint
S93.321 Subluxation of tarsometatarsal joint of right foot
S93.322 Subluxation of tarsometatarsal joint of left foot
S93.323 Subluxation of tarsometatarsal joint of unspecified foot
S93.324 Dislocation of tarsometatarsal joint of right foot
S93.325 Dislocation of tarsometatarsal joint of left foot
S93.326 Dislocation of tarsometatarsal joint of unspecified foot

S93.33 Other subluxation and dislocation of foot
S93.331 Other subluxation of right foot
S93.332 Other subluxation of left foot
S93.333 Other subluxation of unspecified foot
S93.334 Other dislocation of right foot
S93.335 Other dislocation of left foot
S93.336 Other dislocation of unspecified foot

S93.4 Sprain of ankle
EXCLUDES 2 *injury of Achilles tendon (S86.0-)*

S93.40 Sprain of unspecified ligament of ankle
Sprain of ankle NOS
Sprained ankle NOS
S93.401 Sprain of unspecified ligament of right ankle
S93.402 Sprain of unspecified ligament of left ankle
S93.409 Sprain of unspecified ligament of unspecified ankle

S93.41 Sprain of calcaneofibular ligament
S93.411 Sprain of calcaneofibular ligament of right ankle
S93.412 Sprain of calcaneofibular ligament of left ankle
S93.419 Sprain of calcaneofibular ligament of unspecified ankle

S93.42 Sprain of deltoid ligament
S93.421 Sprain of deltoid ligament of right ankle
S93.422 Sprain of deltoid ligament of left ankle
S93.429 Sprain of deltoid ligament of unspecified ankle

S93.43 Sprain of tibiofibular ligament
S93.431 Sprain of tibiofibular ligament of right ankle
S93.432 Sprain of tibiofibular ligament of left ankle
S93.439 Sprain of tibiofibular ligament of unspecified ankle

S93.49 Sprain of other ligament of ankle
Sprain of internal collateral ligament
Sprain of talofibular ligament
S93.491 Sprain of other ligament of right ankle
S93.492 Sprain of other ligament of left ankle
S93.499 Sprain of other ligament of unspecified ankle

S93.5 Sprain of toe

S93.50 Unspecified sprain of toe
S93.501 Unspecified sprain of right great toe
S93.502 Unspecified sprain of left great toe
S93.503 Unspecified sprain of unspecified great toe
S93.504 Unspecified sprain of right lesser toe(s)
S93.505 Unspecified sprain of left lesser toe(s)
S93.506 Unspecified sprain of unspecified lesser toe(s)
S93.509 Unspecified sprain of unspecified toe(s)

S93.51 Sprain of interphalangeal joint of toe
S93.511 Sprain of interphalangeal joint of right great toe
S93.512 Sprain of interphalangeal joint of left great toe
S93.513 Sprain of interphalangeal joint of unspecified great toe
S93.514 Sprain of interphalangeal joint of right lesser toe(s)
S93.515 Sprain of interphalangeal joint of left lesser toe(s)
S93.516 Sprain of interphalangeal joint of unspecified lesser toe(s)
S93.519 Sprain of interphalangeal joint of unspecified toe(s)

S93.52 Sprain of metatarsophalangeal joint of toe
S93.521 Sprain of metatarsophalangeal joint of right great toe
S93.522 Sprain of metatarsophalangeal joint of left great toe
S93.523 Sprain of metatarsophalangeal joint of unspecified great toe
S93.524 Sprain of metatarsophalangeal joint of right lesser toe(s)
S93.525 Sprain of metatarsophalangeal joint of left lesser toe(s)
S93.526 Sprain of metatarsophalangeal joint of unspecified lesser toe(s)
S93.529 Sprain of metatarsophalangeal joint of unspecified toe(s)

S93.6 Sprain of foot
EXCLUDES 2 *sprain of metatarsophalangeal joint of toe (S93.52-)*
sprain of toe (S93.5-)

S93.60 Unspecified sprain of foot
S93.601 Unspecified sprain of right foot
S93.602 Unspecified sprain of left foot

S93.609 Unspecified sprain of unspecified foot

S93.61 Sprain of tarsal ligament of foot
S93.611 Sprain of tarsal ligament of right foot
S93.612 Sprain of tarsal ligament of left foot
S93.619 Sprain of tarsal ligament of unspecified foot

S93.62 Sprain of tarsometatarsal ligament of foot
S93.621 Sprain of tarsometatarsal ligament of right foot
S93.622 Sprain of tarsometatarsal ligament of left foot
S93.629 Sprain of tarsometatarsal ligament of unspecified foot

S93.69 Other sprain of foot
S93.691 Other sprain of right foot
S93.692 Other sprain of left foot
S93.699 Other sprain of unspecified foot

S94 Injury of nerves at ankle and foot level

Code also any associated open wound (S91.-)

The appropriate 7th character is to be added to each code from category S94.
A initial encounter
D subsequent encounter
S sequela

S94.0 Injury of lateral plantar nerve
S94.00 Injury of lateral plantar nerve, unspecified leg
S94.01 Injury of lateral plantar nerve, right leg
S94.02 Injury of lateral plantar nerve, left leg

S94.1 Injury of medial plantar nerve
S94.10 Injury of medial plantar nerve, unspecified leg
S94.11 Injury of medial plantar nerve, right leg
S94.12 Injury of medial plantar nerve, left leg

S94.2 Injury of deep peroneal nerve at ankle and foot level
Injury of terminal, lateral branch of deep peroneal nerve
S94.20 Injury of deep peroneal nerve at ankle and foot level, unspecified leg
S94.21 Injury of deep peroneal nerve at ankle and foot level, right leg
S94.22 Injury of deep peroneal nerve at ankle and foot level, left leg

S94.3 Injury of cutaneous sensory nerve at ankle and foot level
S94.30 Injury of cutaneous sensory nerve at ankle and foot level, unspecified leg
S94.31 Injury of cutaneous sensory nerve at ankle and foot level, right leg
S94.32 Injury of cutaneous sensory nerve at ankle and foot level, left leg

S94.8 Injury of other nerves at ankle and foot level
S94.8X Injury of other nerves at ankle and foot level
S94.8X1 Injury of other nerves at ankle and foot level, right leg
S94.8X2 Injury of other nerves at ankle and foot level, left leg
S94.8X9 Injury of other nerves at ankle and foot level, unspecified leg

S94.9 Injury of unspecified nerve at ankle and foot level
S94.90 Injury of unspecified nerve at ankle and foot level, unspecified leg
S94.91 Injury of unspecified nerve at ankle and foot level, right leg
S94.92 Injury of unspecified nerve at ankle and foot level, left leg

S95 Injury of blood vessels at ankle and foot level

Code also any associated open wound (S91.-)

EXCLUDES 2 *injury of posterior tibial artery and vein (S85.1-, S85.8-)*

The appropriate 7th character is to be added to each code from category S95.
A initial encounter
D subsequent encounter
S sequela

S95.0 Injury of dorsal artery of foot
S95.00 Unspecified injury of dorsal artery of foot
S95.001 Unspecified injury of dorsal artery of right foot
S95.002 Unspecified injury of dorsal artery of left foot
S95.009 Unspecified injury of dorsal artery of unspecified foot
S95.01 Laceration of dorsal artery of foot
S95.011 Laceration of dorsal artery of right foot
S95.012 Laceration of dorsal artery of left foot
S95.019 Laceration of dorsal artery of unspecified foot
S95.09 Other specified injury of dorsal artery of foot
S95.091 Other specified injury of dorsal artery of right foot
S95.092 Other specified injury of dorsal artery of left foot
S95.099 Other specified injury of dorsal artery of unspecified foot

S95.1 Injury of plantar artery of foot
S95.10 Unspecified injury of plantar artery of foot
S95.101 Unspecified injury of plantar artery of right foot
S95.102 Unspecified injury of plantar artery of left foot
S95.109 Unspecified injury of plantar artery of unspecified foot
S95.11 Laceration of plantar artery of foot
S95.111 Laceration of plantar artery of right foot
S95.112 Laceration of plantar artery of left foot
S95.119 Laceration of plantar artery of unspecified foot
S95.19 Other specified injury of plantar artery of foot
S95.191 Other specified injury of plantar artery of right foot
S95.192 Other specified injury of plantar artery of left foot
S95.199 Other specified injury of plantar artery of unspecified foot

S95.2 Injury of dorsal vein of foot
S95.20 Unspecified injury of dorsal vein of foot
S95.201 Unspecified injury of dorsal vein of right foot
S95.202 Unspecified injury of dorsal vein of left foot
S95.209 Unspecified injury of dorsal vein of unspecified foot
S95.21 Laceration of dorsal vein of foot
S95.211 Laceration of dorsal vein of right foot
S95.212 Laceration of dorsal vein of left foot
S95.219 Laceration of dorsal vein of unspecified foot
S95.29 Other specified injury of dorsal vein of foot
S95.291 Other specified injury of dorsal vein of right foot
S95.292 Other specified injury of dorsal vein of left foot
S95.299 Other specified injury of dorsal vein of unspecified foot

S95.8 Injury of other blood vessels at ankle and foot level
S95.80 Unspecified injury of other blood vessels at ankle and foot level
S95.801 Unspecified injury of other blood vessels at ankle and foot level, right leg
S95.802 Unspecified injury of other blood vessels at ankle and foot level, left leg
S95.809 Unspecified injury of other blood vessels at ankle and foot level, unspecified leg

S95.81 Laceration of other blood vessels at ankle and foot level
S95.811 Laceration of other blood vessels at ankle and foot level, right leg
S95.812 Laceration of other blood vessels at ankle and foot level, left leg
S95.819 Laceration of other blood vessels at ankle and foot level, unspecified leg
S95.89 Other specified injury of other blood vessels at ankle and foot level
S95.891 Other specified injury of other blood vessels at ankle and foot level, right leg
S95.892 Other specified injury of other blood vessels at ankle and foot level, left leg
S95.899 Other specified injury of other blood vessels at ankle and foot level, unspecified leg
S95.9 Injury of unspecified blood vessel at ankle and foot level
S95.90 Unspecified injury of unspecified blood vessel at ankle and foot level
S95.901 Unspecified injury of unspecified blood vessel at ankle and foot level, right leg
S95.902 Unspecified injury of unspecified blood vessel at ankle and foot level, left leg
S95.909 Unspecified injury of unspecified blood vessel at ankle and foot level, unspecified leg
S95.91 Laceration of unspecified blood vessel at ankle and foot level
S95.911 Laceration of unspecified blood vessel at ankle and foot level, right leg
S95.912 Laceration of unspecified blood vessel at ankle and foot level, left leg
S95.919 Laceration of unspecified blood vessel at ankle and foot level, unspecified leg
S95.99 Other specified injury of unspecified blood vessel at ankle and foot level
S95.991 Other specified injury of unspecified blood vessel at ankle and foot level, right leg
S95.992 Other specified injury of unspecified blood vessel at ankle and foot level, left leg
S95.999 Other specified injury of unspecified blood vessel at ankle and foot level, unspecified leg

S96 Injury of muscle and tendon at ankle and foot level

Code also any associated open wound (S91.-)

EXCLUDES 2 *injury of Achilles tendon (S86.0-)*
sprain of joints and ligaments of ankle and foot (S93.-)

TIP: Refer to the Muscle/Tendon table at the beginning of this chapter.

The appropriate 7th character is to be added to each code from category S96.
A initial encounter
D subsequent encounter
S sequela

S96.0 Injury of muscle and tendon of long flexor muscle of toe at ankle and foot level
S96.00 Unspecified injury of muscle and tendon of long flexor muscle of toe at ankle and foot level
S96.001 Unspecified injury of muscle and tendon of long flexor muscle of toe at ankle and foot level, right foot
S96.002 Unspecified injury of muscle and tendon of long flexor muscle of toe at ankle and foot level, left foot
S96.009 Unspecified injury of muscle and tendon of long flexor muscle of toe at ankle and foot level, unspecified foot
S96.01 Strain of muscle and tendon of long flexor muscle of toe at ankle and foot level
S96.011 Strain of muscle and tendon of long flexor muscle of toe at ankle and foot level, right foot
S96.012 Strain of muscle and tendon of long flexor muscle of toe at ankle and foot level, left foot
S96.019 Strain of muscle and tendon of long flexor muscle of toe at ankle and foot level, unspecified foot
S96.02 Laceration of muscle and tendon of long flexor muscle of toe at ankle and foot level
S96.021 Laceration of muscle and tendon of long flexor muscle of toe at ankle and foot level, right foot
S96.022 Laceration of muscle and tendon of long flexor muscle of toe at ankle and foot level, left foot
S96.029 Laceration of muscle and tendon of long flexor muscle of toe at ankle and foot level, unspecified foot
S96.09 Other injury of muscle and tendon of long flexor muscle of toe at ankle and foot level
S96.091 Other injury of muscle and tendon of long flexor muscle of toe at ankle and foot level, right foot
S96.092 Other injury of muscle and tendon of long flexor muscle of toe at ankle and foot level, left foot
S96.099 Other injury of muscle and tendon of long flexor muscle of toe at ankle and foot level, unspecified foot
S96.1 Injury of muscle and tendon of long extensor muscle of toe at ankle and foot level
S96.10 Unspecified injury of muscle and tendon of long extensor muscle of toe at ankle and foot level
S96.101 Unspecified injury of muscle and tendon of long extensor muscle of toe at ankle and foot level, right foot
S96.102 Unspecified injury of muscle and tendon of long extensor muscle of toe at ankle and foot level, left foot
S96.109 Unspecified injury of muscle and tendon of long extensor muscle of toe at ankle and foot level, unspecified foot
S96.11 Strain of muscle and tendon of long extensor muscle of toe at ankle and foot level
S96.111 Strain of muscle and tendon of long extensor muscle of toe at ankle and foot level, right foot
S96.112 Strain of muscle and tendon of long extensor muscle of toe at ankle and foot level, left foot
S96.119 Strain of muscle and tendon of long extensor muscle of toe at ankle and foot level, unspecified foot
S96.12 Laceration of muscle and tendon of long extensor muscle of toe at ankle and foot level
S96.121 Laceration of muscle and tendon of long extensor muscle of toe at ankle and foot level, right foot
S96.122 Laceration of muscle and tendon of long extensor muscle of toe at ankle and foot level, left foot
S96.129 Laceration of muscle and tendon of long extensor muscle of toe at ankle and foot level, unspecified foot
S96.19 Other specified injury of muscle and tendon of long extensor muscle of toe at ankle and foot level
S96.191 Other specified injury of muscle and tendon of long extensor muscle of toe at ankle and foot level, right foot
S96.192 Other specified injury of muscle and tendon of long extensor muscle of toe at ankle and foot level, left foot
S96.199 Other specified injury of muscle and tendon of long extensor muscle of toe at ankle and foot level, unspecified foot
S96.2 Injury of intrinsic muscle and tendon at ankle and foot level
S96.20 Unspecified injury of intrinsic muscle and tendon at ankle and foot level
S96.201 Unspecified injury of intrinsic muscle and tendon at ankle and foot level, right foot
S96.202 Unspecified injury of intrinsic muscle and tendon at ankle and foot level, left foot
S96.209 Unspecified injury of intrinsic muscle and tendon at ankle and foot level, unspecified foot
S96.21 Strain of intrinsic muscle and tendon at ankle and foot level
S96.211 Strain of intrinsic muscle and tendon at ankle and foot level, right foot
S96.212 Strain of intrinsic muscle and tendon at ankle and foot level, left foot

7th S96.219 Strain of intrinsic muscle and tendon at ankle and foot level, unspecified foot

6th S96.22 Laceration of intrinsic muscle and tendon at ankle and foot level

7th S96.221 Laceration of intrinsic muscle and tendon at ankle and foot level, right foot

7th S96.222 Laceration of intrinsic muscle and tendon at ankle and foot level, left foot

7th S96.229 Laceration of intrinsic muscle and tendon at ankle and foot level, unspecified foot

6th S96.29 Other specified injury of intrinsic muscle and tendon at ankle and foot level

7th S96.291 Other specified injury of intrinsic muscle and tendon at ankle and foot level, right foot

7th S96.292 Other specified injury of intrinsic muscle and tendon at ankle and foot level, left foot

7th S96.299 Other specified injury of intrinsic muscle and tendon at ankle and foot level, unspecified foot

5th S96.8 Injury of other specified muscles and tendons at ankle and foot level

6th S96.80 Unspecified injury of other specified muscles and tendons at ankle and foot level

7th S96.801 Unspecified injury of other specified muscles and tendons at ankle and foot level, right foot

7th S96.802 Unspecified injury of other specified muscles and tendons at ankle and foot level, left foot

7th S96.809 Unspecified injury of other specified muscles and tendons at ankle and foot level, unspecified foot

6th S96.81 Strain of other specified muscles and tendons at ankle and foot level

7th S96.811 Strain of other specified muscles and tendons at ankle and foot level, right foot

7th S96.812 Strain of other specified muscles and tendons at ankle and foot level, left foot

7th S96.819 Strain of other specified muscles and tendons at ankle and foot level, unspecified foot

6th S96.82 Laceration of other specified muscles and tendons at ankle and foot level

7th S96.821 Laceration of other specified muscles and tendons at ankle and foot level, right foot

7th S96.822 Laceration of other specified muscles and tendons at ankle and foot level, left foot

7th S96.829 Laceration of other specified muscles and tendons at ankle and foot level, unspecified foot

6th S96.89 Other specified injury of other specified muscles and tendons at ankle and foot level

7th S96.891 Other specified injury of other specified muscles and tendons at ankle and foot level, right foot

7th S96.892 Other specified injury of other specified muscles and tendons at ankle and foot level, left foot

7th S96.899 Other specified injury of other specified muscles and tendons at ankle and foot level, unspecified foot

5th S96.9 Injury of unspecified muscle and tendon at ankle and foot level

6th S96.90 Unspecified injury of unspecified muscle and tendon at ankle and foot level

7th S96.901 Unspecified injury of unspecified muscle and tendon at ankle and foot level, right foot

7th S96.902 Unspecified injury of unspecified muscle and tendon at ankle and foot level, left foot

7th S96.909 Unspecified injury of unspecified muscle and tendon at ankle and foot level, unspecified foot

6th S96.91 Strain of unspecified muscle and tendon at ankle and foot level

7th S96.911 Strain of unspecified muscle and tendon at ankle and foot level, right foot

7th S96.912 Strain of unspecified muscle and tendon at ankle and foot level, left foot

7th S96.919 Strain of unspecified muscle and tendon at ankle and foot level, unspecified foot

6th S96.92 Laceration of unspecified muscle and tendon at ankle and foot level

7th S96.921 Laceration of unspecified muscle and tendon at ankle and foot level, right foot

7th S96.922 Laceration of unspecified muscle and tendon at ankle and foot level, left foot

7th S96.929 Laceration of unspecified muscle and tendon at ankle and foot level, unspecified foot

6th S96.99 Other specified injury of unspecified muscle and tendon at ankle and foot level

7th S96.991 Other specified injury of unspecified muscle and tendon at ankle and foot level, right foot

7th S96.992 Other specified injury of unspecified muscle and tendon at ankle and foot level, left foot

7th S96.999 Other specified injury of unspecified muscle and tendon at ankle and foot level, unspecified foot

4th **S97 Crushing injury of ankle and foot**

Use additional code(s) for all associated injuries

The appropriate 7th character is to be added to each code from category S97.
A initial encounter
D subsequent encounter
S sequela

5th S97.0 Crushing injury of ankle

x7th S97.00 Crushing injury of unspecified ankle

x7th S97.01 Crushing injury of right ankle

x7th S97.02 Crushing injury of left ankle

5th S97.1 Crushing injury of toe

6th S97.10 Crushing injury of unspecified toe(s)

7th S97.101 Crushing injury of unspecified right toe(s)

7th S97.102 Crushing injury of unspecified left toe(s)

7th S97.109 Crushing injury of unspecified toe(s)
Crushing injury of toe NOS

6th S97.11 Crushing injury of great toe

7th S97.111 Crushing injury of right great toe

7th S97.112 Crushing injury of left great toe

7th S97.119 Crushing injury of unspecified great toe

6th S97.12 Crushing injury of lesser toe(s)

7th S97.121 Crushing injury of right lesser toe(s)

7th S97.122 Crushing injury of left lesser toe(s)

7th S97.129 Crushing injury of unspecified lesser toe(s)

5th S97.8 Crushing injury of foot

x7th S97.80 Crushing injury of unspecified foot
Crushing injury of foot NOS

x7th S97.81 Crushing injury of right foot

x7th S97.82 Crushing injury of left foot

4th **S98 Traumatic amputation of ankle and foot**

An amputation not identified as partial or complete should be coded to complete

The appropriate 7th character is to be added to each code from category S98.
A initial encounter
D subsequent encounter
S sequela

5th S98.0 Traumatic amputation of foot at ankle level

6th S98.01 Complete traumatic amputation of foot at ankle level

7th S98.011 Complete traumatic amputation of right foot at ankle level HCC ESR COM

7th S98.012 Complete traumatic amputation of left foot at ankle level HCC ESR COM

7th S98.019 Complete traumatic amputation of unspecified foot at ankle level HCC ESR COM

6th S98.02 Partial traumatic amputation of foot at ankle level

7th S98.021 Partial traumatic amputation of right foot at ankle level HCC ESR COM

7th S98.022 Partial traumatic amputation of left foot at ankle level HCC ESR COM

7th S98.029 Partial traumatic amputation of unspecified foot at ankle level HCC ESR COM

5th S98.1 Traumatic amputation of one toe

6th S98.11 Complete traumatic amputation of great toe

7th S98.111 Complete traumatic amputation of right great toe HCC ESR

7th S98.112 Complete traumatic amputation of left great toe HCC ESR

7th S98.119 Complete traumatic amputation of unspecified great toe HCC ESR

6th S98.12 Partial traumatic amputation of great toe

7th S98.121 Partial traumatic amputation of right great toe HCC ESR

7th S98.122 Partial traumatic amputation of left great toe HCC ESR

7th S98.129 Partial traumatic amputation of unspecified great toe HCC ESR

6th S98.13 Complete traumatic amputation of one lesser toe

Traumatic amputation of toe NOS

7th S98.131 Complete traumatic amputation of one right lesser toe HCC ESR

7th S98.132 Complete traumatic amputation of one left lesser toe HCC ESR

7th S98.139 Complete traumatic amputation of one unspecified lesser toe HCC ESR

6th S98.14 Partial traumatic amputation of one lesser toe

7th S98.141 Partial traumatic amputation of one right lesser toe HCC ESR

7th S98.142 Partial traumatic amputation of one left lesser toe HCC ESR

7th S98.149 Partial traumatic amputation of one unspecified lesser toe HCC ESR

5th S98.2 Traumatic amputation of two or more lesser toes

6th S98.21 Complete traumatic amputation of two or more lesser toes

7th S98.211 Complete traumatic amputation of two or more right lesser toes HCC ESR

7th S98.212 Complete traumatic amputation of two or more left lesser toes HCC ESR

7th S98.219 Complete traumatic amputation of two or more unspecified lesser toes HCC ESR

6th S98.22 Partial traumatic amputation of two or more lesser toes

7th S98.221 Partial traumatic amputation of two or more right lesser toes HCC ESR

7th S98.222 Partial traumatic amputation of two or more left lesser toes HCC ESR

7th S98.229 Partial traumatic amputation of two or more unspecified lesser toes HCC ESR

5th S98.3 Traumatic amputation of midfoot

6th S98.31 Complete traumatic amputation of midfoot

7th S98.311 Complete traumatic amputation of right midfoot HCC ESR COM

7th S98.312 Complete traumatic amputation of left midfoot HCC ESR COM

7th S98.319 Complete traumatic amputation of unspecified midfoot HCC ESR COM

6th S98.32 Partial traumatic amputation of midfoot

7th S98.321 Partial traumatic amputation of right midfoot HCC ESR COM

7th S98.322 Partial traumatic amputation of left midfoot HCC ESR COM

7th S98.329 Partial traumatic amputation of unspecified midfoot HCC ESR COM

5th S98.9 Traumatic amputation of foot, level unspecified

6th S98.91 Complete traumatic amputation of foot, level unspecified

7th S98.911 Complete traumatic amputation of right foot, level unspecified HCC ESR COM

7th S98.912 Complete traumatic amputation of left foot, level unspecified HCC ESR COM

7th S98.919 Complete traumatic amputation of unspecified foot, level unspecified HCC ESR COM

6th S98.92 Partial traumatic amputation of foot, level unspecified

7th S98.921 Partial traumatic amputation of right foot, level unspecified HCC ESR COM

7th S98.922 Partial traumatic amputation of left foot, level unspecified HCC ESR COM

7th S98.929 Partial traumatic amputation of unspecified foot, level unspecified HCC ESR COM

4th S99 Other and unspecified injuries of ankle and foot

AHA: 2018,2Q,12; 2018,1Q,3; 2016,4Q,68-69

5th S99.Ø Physeal fracture of calcaneus

AHA: 2019,4Q,56

The appropriate 7th character is to be added to each code from subcategory S99.Ø.
- A initial encounter for closed fracture
- B initial encounter for open fracture
- D subsequent encounter for fracture with routine healing
- G subsequent encounter for fracture with delayed healing
- K subsequent encounter for fracture with nonunion
- P subsequent encounter for fracture with malunion
- S sequela

6th S99.ØØ Unspecified physeal fracture of calcaneus

7th S99.ØØ1 Unspecified physeal fracture of right calcaneus P

7th S99.ØØ2 Unspecified physeal fracture of left calcaneus P

7th S99.ØØ9 Unspecified physeal fracture of unspecified calcaneus P

6th S99.Ø1 Salter-Harris Type I physeal fracture of calcaneus

7th S99.Ø11 Salter-Harris Type I physeal fracture of right calcaneus P

7th S99.Ø12 Salter-Harris Type I physeal fracture of left calcaneus P

7th S99.Ø19 Salter-Harris Type I physeal fracture of unspecified calcaneus P

6th S99.Ø2 Salter-Harris Type II physeal fracture of calcaneus

7th S99.Ø21 Salter-Harris Type II physeal fracture of right calcaneus P

7th S99.Ø22 Salter-Harris Type II physeal fracture of left calcaneus P

7th S99.Ø29 Salter-Harris Type II physeal fracture of unspecified calcaneus P

6th S99.Ø3 Salter-Harris Type III physeal fracture of calcaneus

7th S99.Ø31 Salter-Harris Type III physeal fracture of right calcaneus P

7th S99.Ø32 Salter-Harris Type III physeal fracture of left calcaneus P

7th S99.Ø39 Salter-Harris Type III physeal fracture of unspecified calcaneus P

6th S99.Ø4 Salter-Harris Type IV physeal fracture of calcaneus

7th S99.Ø41 Salter-Harris Type IV physeal fracture of right calcaneus P

7th S99.Ø42 Salter-Harris Type IV physeal fracture of left calcaneus P

7th S99.Ø49 Salter-Harris Type IV physeal fracture of unspecified calcaneus P

6th S99.Ø9 Other physeal fracture of calcaneus

7th S99.Ø91 Other physeal fracture of right calcaneus P

7th S99.Ø92 Other physeal fracture of left calcaneus P

7th S99.Ø99 Other physeal fracture of unspecified calcaneus P

S99.1 Physeal fracture of metatarsal
AHA: 2019,4Q,56

The appropriate 7th character is to be added to each code from subcategory S99.1
- A initial encounter for closed fracture
- B initial encounter for open fracture
- D subsequent encounter for fracture with routine healing
- G subsequent encounter for fracture with delayed healing
- K subsequent encounter for fracture with nonunion
- P subsequent encounter for fracture with malunion
- S sequela

S99.10 Unspecified physeal fracture of metatarsal
- S99.101 Unspecified physeal fracture of right metatarsal Q
- S99.102 Unspecified physeal fracture of left metatarsal Q
- S99.109 Unspecified physeal fracture of unspecified metatarsal Q

S99.11 Salter-Harris Type I physeal fracture of metatarsal
- S99.111 Salter-Harris Type I physeal fracture of right metatarsal Q
- S99.112 Salter-Harris Type I physeal fracture of left metatarsal Q
- S99.119 Salter-Harris Type I physeal fracture of unspecified metatarsal Q

S99.12 Salter-Harris Type II physeal fracture of metatarsal
- S99.121 Salter-Harris Type II physeal fracture of right metatarsal Q
- S99.122 Salter-Harris Type II physeal fracture of left metatarsal Q
- S99.129 Salter-Harris Type II physeal fracture of unspecified metatarsal Q

S99.13 Salter-Harris Type III physeal fracture of metatarsal
- S99.131 Salter-Harris Type III physeal fracture of right metatarsal Q
- S99.132 Salter-Harris Type III physeal fracture of left metatarsal Q
- S99.139 Salter-Harris Type III physeal fracture of unspecified metatarsal Q

S99.14 Salter-Harris Type IV physeal fracture of metatarsal
- S99.141 Salter-Harris Type IV physeal fracture of right metatarsal Q
- S99.142 Salter-Harris Type IV physeal fracture of left metatarsal Q
- S99.149 Salter-Harris Type IV physeal fracture of unspecified metatarsal Q

S99.19 Other physeal fracture of metatarsal
- S99.191 Other physeal fracture of right metatarsal Q
- S99.192 Other physeal fracture of left metatarsal Q
- S99.199 Other physeal fracture of unspecified metatarsal Q

S99.2 Physeal fracture of phalanx of toe
AHA: 2019,4Q,56

The appropriate 7th character is to be added to each code from subcategories S99.2.
- A initial encounter for closed fracture
- B initial encounter for open fracture
- D subsequent encounter for fracture with routine healing
- G subsequent encounter for fracture with delayed healing
- K subsequent encounter for fracture with nonunion
- P subsequent encounter for fracture with malunion
- S sequela

S99.20 Unspecified physeal fracture of phalanx of toe
- S99.201 Unspecified physeal fracture of phalanx of right toe
- S99.202 Unspecified physeal fracture of phalanx of left toe
- S99.209 Unspecified physeal fracture of phalanx of unspecified toe

S99.21 Salter-Harris Type I physeal fracture of phalanx of toe
- S99.211 Salter-Harris Type I physeal fracture of phalanx of right toe
- S99.212 Salter-Harris Type I physeal fracture of phalanx of left toe
- S99.219 Salter-Harris Type I physeal fracture of phalanx of unspecified toe

S99.22 Salter-Harris Type II physeal fracture of phalanx of toe
- S99.221 Salter-Harris Type II physeal fracture of phalanx of right toe
- S99.222 Salter-Harris Type II physeal fracture of phalanx of left toe
- S99.229 Salter-Harris Type II physeal fracture of phalanx of unspecified toe

S99.23 Salter-Harris Type III physeal fracture of phalanx of toe
- S99.231 Salter-Harris Type III physeal fracture of phalanx of right toe
- S99.232 Salter-Harris Type III physeal fracture of phalanx of left toe
- S99.239 Salter-Harris Type III physeal fracture of phalanx of unspecified toe

S99.24 Salter-Harris Type IV physeal fracture of phalanx of toe
- S99.241 Salter-Harris Type IV physeal fracture of phalanx of right toe
- S99.242 Salter-Harris Type IV physeal fracture of phalanx of left toe
- S99.249 Salter-Harris Type IV physeal fracture of phalanx of unspecified toe

S99.29 Other physeal fracture of phalanx of toe
- S99.291 Other physeal fracture of phalanx of right toe
- S99.292 Other physeal fracture of phalanx of left toe
- S99.299 Other physeal fracture of phalanx of unspecified toe

S99.8 Other specified injuries of ankle and foot

The appropriate 7th character is to be added to each code from subcategory S99.8.
- A initial encounter
- D subsequent encounter
- S sequela

S99.81 Other specified injuries of ankle
- S99.811 Other specified injuries of right ankle
- S99.812 Other specified injuries of left ankle
- S99.819 Other specified injuries of unspecified ankle

S99.82 Other specified injuries of foot
- S99.821 Other specified injuries of right foot
- S99.822 Other specified injuries of left foot
- S99.829 Other specified injuries of unspecified foot

S99.9 Unspecified injury of ankle and foot

The appropriate 7th character is to be added to each code from subcategory S99.9.
- A initial encounter
- D subsequent encounter
- S sequela

S99.91 Unspecified injury of ankle
- S99.911 Unspecified injury of right ankle
- S99.912 Unspecified injury of left ankle
- S99.919 Unspecified injury of unspecified ankle

S99.92 Unspecified injury of foot
- S99.921 Unspecified injury of right foot
- S99.922 Unspecified injury of left foot
- S99.929 Unspecified injury of unspecified foot

INJURY, POISONING AND CERTAIN OTHER CONSEQUENCES OF EXTERNAL CAUSES (T07-T88)

Injuries involving multiple body regions (T07)

EXCLUDES 1 *burns and corrosions (T20-T32)*
frostbite (T33-T34)
insect bite or sting, venomous (T63.4)
sunburn (L55.-)

T07 Unspecified multiple injuries

EXCLUDES 1 *injury NOS (T14.90)*

AHA: 2017,4Q,26

The appropriate 7th character is to be added to code T07.
A initial encounter
D subsequent encounter
S sequela

Injury of unspecified body region (T14)

T14 Injury of unspecified body region

EXCLUDES 1 *multiple unspecified injuries (T07)*

AHA: 2017,4Q,26

The appropriate 7th character is to be added to each code from category T14.
A initial encounter
D subsequent encounter
S sequela

T14.8 Other injury of unspecified body region
Abrasion NOS
Contusion NOS
Crush injury NOS
Fracture NOS
Skin injury NOS
Vascular injury NOS
Wound NOS

T14.9 Unspecified injury

T14.90 Injury, unspecified
Injury NOS

T14.91 Suicide attempt HCC Rx ESR COM
Attempted suicide NOS

Effects of foreign body entering through natural orifice (T15-T19)

EXCLUDES 2 *foreign body accidentally left in operation wound (T81.5-)*
foreign body in penetrating wound - see open wound by body region
residual foreign body in soft tissue (M79.5)
splinter, without open wound - see superficial injury by body region

T15 Foreign body on external eye

EXCLUDES 2 *foreign body in penetrating wound of orbit and eye ball (S05.4-, S05.5-)*
open wound of eyelid and periocular area (S01.1-)
retained foreign body in eyelid (H02.8-)
retained (old) foreign body in penetrating wound of orbit and eye ball (H05.5-, H44.6-, H44.7-)
superficial foreign body of eyelid and periocular area (S00.25-)

The appropriate 7th character is to be added to each code from category T15.
A initial encounter
D subsequent encounter
S sequela

T15.0 Foreign body in cornea
T15.00 Foreign body in cornea, unspecified eye
T15.01 Foreign body in cornea, right eye
T15.02 Foreign body in cornea, left eye

T15.1 Foreign body in conjunctival sac
T15.10 Foreign body in conjunctival sac, unspecified eye
T15.11 Foreign body in conjunctival sac, right eye
T15.12 Foreign body in conjunctival sac, left eye

T15.8 Foreign body in other and multiple parts of external eye
Foreign body in lacrimal punctum
T15.80 Foreign body in other and multiple parts of external eye, unspecified eye
T15.81 Foreign body in other and multiple parts of external eye, right eye
T15.82 Foreign body in other and multiple parts of external eye, left eye

T15.9 Foreign body on external eye, part unspecified
T15.90 Foreign body on external eye, part unspecified, unspecified eye
T15.91 Foreign body on external eye, part unspecified, right eye
T15.92 Foreign body on external eye, part unspecified, left eye

T16 Foreign body in ear

INCLUDES foreign body in auditory canal

The appropriate 7th character is to be added to each code from category T16.
A initial encounter
D subsequent encounter
S sequela

T16.1 Foreign body in right ear
T16.2 Foreign body in left ear
T16.9 Foreign body in ear, unspecified ear

T17 Foreign body in respiratory tract

The appropriate 7th character is to be added to each code from category T17.
A initial encounter
D subsequent encounter
S sequela

T17.0 Foreign body in nasal sinus
T17.1 Foreign body in nostril
Foreign body in nose NOS
T17.2 Foreign body in pharynx
Foreign body in nasopharynx
Foreign body in throat NOS
T17.20 Unspecified foreign body in pharynx
T17.200 Unspecified foreign body in pharynx causing asphyxiation
T17.208 Unspecified foreign body in pharynx causing other injury
T17.21 Gastric contents in pharynx
Aspiration of gastric contents into pharynx
Vomitus in pharynx
T17.210 Gastric contents in pharynx causing asphyxiation
T17.218 Gastric contents in pharynx causing other injury
T17.22 Food in pharynx
Bones in pharynx
Seeds in pharynx
T17.220 Food in pharynx causing asphyxiation
T17.228 Food in pharynx causing other injury
T17.29 Other foreign object in pharynx
T17.290 Other foreign object in pharynx causing asphyxiation
T17.298 Other foreign object in pharynx causing other injury
T17.3 Foreign body in larynx
T17.30 Unspecified foreign body in larynx
T17.300 Unspecified foreign body in larynx causing asphyxiation
T17.308 Unspecified foreign body in larynx causing other injury
T17.31 Gastric contents in larynx
Aspiration of gastric contents into larynx
Vomitus in larynx
T17.310 Gastric contents in larynx causing asphyxiation
T17.318 Gastric contents in larynx causing other injury
T17.32 Food in larynx
Bones in larynx
Seeds in larynx
T17.320 Food in larynx causing asphyxiation
T17.328 Food in larynx causing other injury

T17.39 Other foreign object in larynx
T17.390 Other foreign object in larynx causing asphyxiation
T17.398 Other foreign object in larynx causing other injury
T17.4 Foreign body in trachea
T17.40 Unspecified foreign body in trachea
T17.400 Unspecified foreign body in trachea causing asphyxiation
T17.408 Unspecified foreign body in trachea causing other injury
T17.41 Gastric contents in trachea
Aspiration of gastric contents into trachea
Vomitus in trachea
T17.410 Gastric contents in trachea causing asphyxiation
T17.418 Gastric contents in trachea causing other injury
T17.42 Food in trachea
Bones in trachea
Seeds in trachea
T17.420 Food in trachea causing asphyxiation
T17.428 Food in trachea causing other injury
T17.49 Other foreign object in trachea
T17.490 Other foreign object in trachea causing asphyxiation
T17.498 Other foreign object in trachea causing other injury
T17.5 Foreign body in bronchus
T17.50 Unspecified foreign body in bronchus
T17.500 Unspecified foreign body in bronchus causing asphyxiation
T17.508 Unspecified foreign body in bronchus causing other injury
T17.51 Gastric contents in bronchus
Aspiration of gastric contents into bronchus
Vomitus in bronchus
T17.510 Gastric contents in bronchus causing asphyxiation
T17.518 Gastric contents in bronchus causing other injury
T17.52 Food in bronchus
Bones in bronchus
Seeds in bronchus
T17.520 Food in bronchus causing asphyxiation
T17.528 Food in bronchus causing other injury
T17.59 Other foreign object in bronchus
T17.590 Other foreign object in bronchus causing asphyxiation
T17.598 Other foreign object in bronchus causing other injury
T17.8 Foreign body in other parts of respiratory tract
Foreign body in bronchioles
Foreign body in lung
T17.80 Unspecified foreign body in other parts of respiratory tract
T17.800 Unspecified foreign body in other parts of respiratory tract causing asphyxiation
T17.808 Unspecified foreign body in other parts of respiratory tract causing other injury
T17.81 Gastric contents in other parts of respiratory tract
Aspiration of gastric contents into other parts of respiratory tract
Vomitus in other parts of respiratory tract
T17.810 Gastric contents in other parts of respiratory tract causing asphyxiation
T17.818 Gastric contents in other parts of respiratory tract causing other injury
T17.82 Food in other parts of respiratory tract
Bones in other parts of respiratory tract
Seeds in other parts of respiratory tract
T17.820 Food in other parts of respiratory tract causing asphyxiation
T17.828 Food in other parts of respiratory tract causing other injury
T17.89 Other foreign object in other parts of respiratory tract
T17.890 Other foreign object in other parts of respiratory tract causing asphyxiation
T17.898 Other foreign object in other parts of respiratory tract causing other injury
T17.9 Foreign body in respiratory tract, part unspecified
T17.90 Unspecified foreign body in respiratory tract, part unspecified
T17.900 Unspecified foreign body in respiratory tract, part unspecified causing asphyxiation
T17.908 Unspecified foreign body in respiratory tract, part unspecified causing other injury
T17.91 Gastric contents in respiratory tract, part unspecified
Aspiration of gastric contents into respiratory tract, part unspecified
Vomitus in trachea respiratory tract, part unspecified
T17.910 Gastric contents in respiratory tract, part unspecified causing asphyxiation
T17.918 Gastric contents in respiratory tract, part unspecified causing other injury
T17.92 Food in respiratory tract, part unspecified
Bones in respiratory tract, part unspecified
Seeds in respiratory tract, part unspecified
T17.920 Food in respiratory tract, part unspecified causing asphyxiation
T17.928 Food in respiratory tract, part unspecified causing other injury
T17.99 Other foreign object in respiratory tract, part unspecified
T17.990 Other foreign object in respiratory tract, part unspecified in causing asphyxiation
AHA: 2019,3Q,15
T17.998 Other foreign object in respiratory tract, part unspecified causing other injury

T18 Foreign body in alimentary tract

EXCLUDES 2 *foreign body in pharynx (T17.2-)*

The appropriate 7th character is to be added to each code from category T18.
A initial encounter
D subsequent encounter
S sequela

T18.0 Foreign body in mouth
T18.1 Foreign body in esophagus
EXCLUDES 2 *foreign body in respiratory tract (T17.-)*
T18.10 Unspecified foreign body in esophagus
T18.100 Unspecified foreign body in esophagus causing compression of trachea
Unspecified foreign body in esophagus causing obstruction of respiration
T18.108 Unspecified foreign body in esophagus causing other injury
T18.11 Gastric contents in esophagus
Vomitus in esophagus
T18.110 Gastric contents in esophagus causing compression of trachea
Gastric contents in esophagus causing obstruction of respiration
T18.118 Gastric contents in esophagus causing other injury
T18.12 Food in esophagus
Bones in esophagus
Seeds in esophagus
T18.120 Food in esophagus causing compression of trachea
Food in esophagus causing obstruction of respiration
T18.128 Food in esophagus causing other injury

T18.19 Other foreign object in esophagus
AHA: 2022,1Q,27; 2015,1Q,23

T18.190 Other foreign object in esophagus causing compression of trachea
Other foreign body in esophagus causing obstruction of respiration
TIP: Any foreign object lodged in the esophagus requires immediate treatment and is considered an injury. Assign this code when there is respiratory compromise or compression. If no respiratory compromise or compression is documented, assign code T18.198-.

T18.198 Other foreign object in esophagus causing other injury
TIP: Any foreign object lodged in the esophagus requires immediate treatment and is considered an injury. Assign this code when there is no respiratory compromise or compression. If respiratory compromise or compression is documented, assign code T18.190-.

T18.2 Foreign body in stomach
T18.3 Foreign body in small intestine
T18.4 Foreign body in colon
T18.5 Foreign body in anus and rectum
Foreign body in rectosigmoid (junction)
T18.8 Foreign body in other parts of alimentary tract
T18.9 Foreign body of alimentary tract, part unspecified
Foreign body in digestive system NOS
Swallowed foreign body NOS

T19 Foreign body in genitourinary tract
EXCLUDES 2 *complications due to implanted mesh (T83.7-)*
mechanical complications of contraceptive device (intrauterine) (vaginal) (T83.3-)
presence of contraceptive device (intrauterine) (vaginal) (Z97.5)

The appropriate 7th character is to be added to each code from category T19.
A initial encounter
D subsequent encounter
S sequela

T19.0 Foreign body in urethra
T19.1 Foreign body in bladder
T19.2 Foreign body in vulva and vagina ♀
T19.3 Foreign body in uterus ♀
T19.4 Foreign body in penis ♂
T19.8 Foreign body in other parts of genitourinary tract
T19.9 Foreign body in genitourinary tract, part unspecified

BURNS AND CORROSIONS (T20-T32)

INCLUDES burns (thermal) from electrical heating appliances
burns (thermal) from electricity
burns (thermal) from flame
burns (thermal) from friction
burns (thermal) from hot air and hot gases
burns (thermal) from hot objects
burns (thermal) from lightning
burns (thermal) from radiation
chemical burn [corrosion] (external) (internal)
scalds
EXCLUDES 2 *erythema [dermatitis] ab igne (L59.0)*
radiation-related disorders of the skin and subcutaneous tissue (L55-L59)
sunburn (L55.-)
AHA: 2016,2Q,4

Burns and corrosions of external body surface, specified by site (T20-T25)

INCLUDES burns and corrosions of first degree [erythema]
burns and corrosions of second degree [blisters] [epidermal loss]
burns and corrosions of third degree [deep necrosis of underlying tissue] [full-thickness skin loss]
Use additional code from category T31 or T32 to identify extent of body surface involved

T20 Burn and corrosion of head, face, and neck
EXCLUDES 2 *burn and corrosion of ear drum (T28.41, T28.91)*
burn and corrosion of eye and adnexa (T26.-)
burn and corrosion of mouth and pharynx (T28.0)
AHA: 2015,1Q,18-19

The appropriate 7th character is to be added to each code from category T20.
A initial encounter
D subsequent encounter
S sequela

T20.0 Burn of unspecified degree of head, face, and neck
Use additional external cause code to identify the source, place and intent of the burn (X00-X19, X75-X77, X96-X98, Y92)
T20.00 Burn of unspecified degree of head, face, and neck, unspecified site
T20.01 Burn of unspecified degree of ear [any part, except ear drum]
EXCLUDES 2 *burn of ear drum (T28.41-)*
T20.011 Burn of unspecified degree of right ear [any part, except ear drum]
T20.012 Burn of unspecified degree of left ear [any part, except ear drum]
T20.019 Burn of unspecified degree of unspecified ear [any part, except ear drum]
T20.02 Burn of unspecified degree of lip(s)
T20.03 Burn of unspecified degree of chin
T20.04 Burn of unspecified degree of nose (septum)
T20.05 Burn of unspecified degree of scalp [any part]
T20.06 Burn of unspecified degree of forehead and cheek
T20.07 Burn of unspecified degree of neck
T20.09 Burn of unspecified degree of multiple sites of head, face, and neck
T20.1 Burn of first degree of head, face, and neck
Use additional external cause code to identify the source, place and intent of the burn (X00-X19, X75-X77, X96-X98, Y92)
T20.10 Burn of first degree of head, face, and neck, unspecified site
T20.11 Burn of first degree of ear [any part, except ear drum]
EXCLUDES 2 *burn of ear drum (T28.41-)*
T20.111 Burn of first degree of right ear [any part, except ear drum]
T20.112 Burn of first degree of left ear [any part, except ear drum]
T20.119 Burn of first degree of unspecified ear [any part, except ear drum]
T20.12 Burn of first degree of lip(s)
T20.13 Burn of first degree of chin
T20.14 Burn of first degree of nose (septum)
T20.15 Burn of first degree of scalp [any part]
T20.16 Burn of first degree of forehead and cheek

T20.17 Burn of first degree of neck

T20.19 Burn of first degree of multiple sites of head, face, and neck

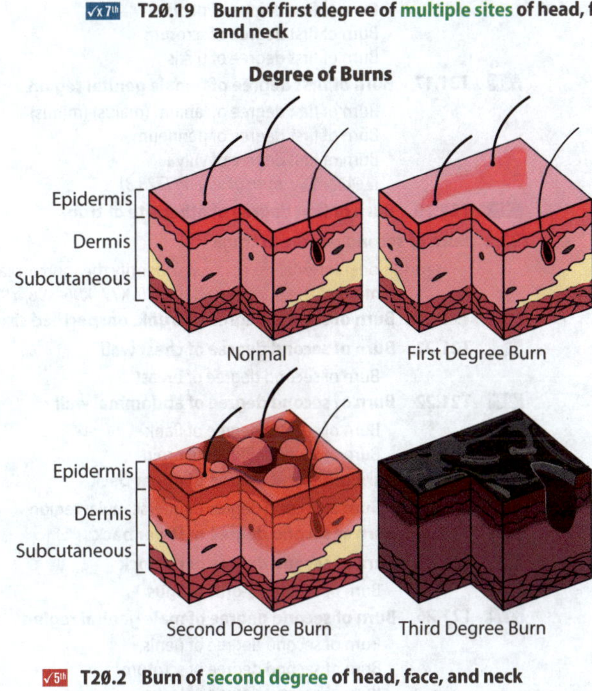

T20.2 Burn of second degree of head, face, and neck

Use additional external cause code to identify the source, place and intent of the burn (X00-X19, X75-X77, X96-X98, Y92)

T20.20 Burn of second degree of head, face, and neck, unspecified site

T20.21 Burn of second degree of ear [any part, except ear drum]

EXCLUDES 2 *burn of ear drum (T28.41-)*

T20.211 Burn of second degree of right ear [any part, except ear drum]

T20.212 Burn of second degree of left ear [any part, except ear drum]

T20.219 Burn of second degree of unspecified ear [any part, except ear drum]

T20.22 Burn of second degree of lip(s)

T20.23 Burn of second degree of chin

T20.24 Burn of second degree of nose (septum)

T20.25 Burn of second degree of scalp [any part]

T20.26 Burn of second degree of forehead and cheek

T20.27 Burn of second degree of neck

T20.29 Burn of second degree of multiple sites of head, face, and neck

T20.3 Burn of third degree of head, face, and neck

Use additional external cause code to identify the source, place and intent of the burn (X00-X19, X75-X77, X96-X98, Y92)

T20.30 Burn of third degree of head, face, and neck, unspecified site COM

T20.31 Burn of third degree of ear [any part, except ear drum]

EXCLUDES 2 *burn of ear drum (T28.41-)*

AHA: 2015,1Q,18

T20.311 Burn of third degree of right ear [any part, except ear drum] COM

T20.312 Burn of third degree of left ear [any part, except ear drum] COM

T20.319 Burn of third degree of unspecified ear [any part, except ear drum] COM

T20.32 Burn of third degree of lip(s) COM

T20.33 Burn of third degree of chin COM

T20.34 Burn of third degree of nose (septum) COM

T20.35 Burn of third degree of scalp [any part] COM

T20.36 Burn of third degree of forehead and cheek COM

T20.37 Burn of third degree of neck COM

T20.39 Burn of third degree of multiple sites of head, face, and neck COM

T20.4 Corrosion of unspecified degree of head, face, and neck

Code first (T51-T65) to identify chemical and intent

Use additional external cause code to identify place (Y92)

T20.40 Corrosion of unspecified degree of head, face, and neck, unspecified site

T20.41 Corrosion of unspecified degree of ear [any part, except ear drum]

EXCLUDES 2 *corrosion of ear drum (T28.91-)*

T20.411 Corrosion of unspecified degree of right ear [any part, except ear drum]

T20.412 Corrosion of unspecified degree of left ear [any part, except ear drum]

T20.419 Corrosion of unspecified degree of unspecified ear [any part, except ear drum]

T20.42 Corrosion of unspecified degree of lip(s)

T20.43 Corrosion of unspecified degree of chin

T20.44 Corrosion of unspecified degree of nose (septum)

T20.45 Corrosion of unspecified degree of scalp [any part]

T20.46 Corrosion of unspecified degree of forehead and cheek

T20.47 Corrosion of unspecified degree of neck

T20.49 Corrosion of unspecified degree of multiple sites of head, face, and neck

T20.5 Corrosion of first degree of head, face, and neck

Code first (T51-T65) to identify chemical and intent

Use additional external cause code to identify place (Y92)

T20.50 Corrosion of first degree of head, face, and neck, unspecified site

T20.51 Corrosion of first degree of ear [any part, except ear drum]

EXCLUDES 2 *corrosion of ear drum (T28.91-)*

T20.511 Corrosion of first degree of right ear [any part, except ear drum]

T20.512 Corrosion of first degree of left ear [any part, except ear drum]

T20.519 Corrosion of first degree of unspecified ear [any part, except ear drum]

T20.52 Corrosion of first degree of lip(s)

T20.53 Corrosion of first degree of chin

T20.54 Corrosion of first degree of nose (septum)

T20.55 Corrosion of first degree of scalp [any part]

T20.56 Corrosion of first degree of forehead and cheek

T20.57 Corrosion of first degree of neck

T20.59 Corrosion of first degree of multiple sites of head, face, and neck

T20.6 Corrosion of second degree of head, face, and neck

Code first (T51-T65) to identify chemical and intent

Use additional external cause code to identify place (Y92)

T20.60 Corrosion of second degree of head, face, and neck, unspecified site

T20.61 Corrosion of second degree of ear [any part, except ear drum]

EXCLUDES 2 *corrosion of ear drum (T28.91-)*

T20.611 Corrosion of second degree of right ear [any part, except ear drum]

T20.612 Corrosion of second degree of left ear [any part, except ear drum]

T20.619 Corrosion of second degree of unspecified ear [any part, except ear drum]

T20.62 Corrosion of second degree of lip(s)

T20.63 Corrosion of second degree of chin

T20.64 Corrosion of second degree of nose (septum)

T20.65 Corrosion of second degree of scalp [any part]

T20.66 Corrosion of second degree of forehead and cheek

T20.67 Corrosion of second degree of neck

T20.69 Corrosion of second degree of multiple sites of head, face, and neck

T20.7 Corrosion of third degree of head, face, and neck

Code first (T51-T65) to identify chemical and intent

Use additional external cause code to identify place (Y92)

T20.70 Corrosion of third degree of head, face, and neck, unspecified site COM

T20.71 **Corrosion of third degree of ear [any part, except ear drum]**
EXCLUDES 2 *corrosion of ear drum (T28.91-)*
T20.711 **Corrosion of third degree of right ear [any part, except ear drum]** COM
T20.712 **Corrosion of third degree of left ear [any part, except ear drum]** COM
T20.719 **Corrosion of third degree of unspecified ear [any part, except ear drum]** COM
T20.72 **Corrosion of third degree of lip(s)** COM
T20.73 **Corrosion of third degree of chin** COM
T20.74 **Corrosion of third degree of nose (septum)** COM
T20.75 **Corrosion of third degree of scalp [any part]** COM
T20.76 **Corrosion of third degree of forehead and cheek** COM
T20.77 **Corrosion of third degree of neck** COM
T20.79 **Corrosion of third degree of multiple sites of head, face, and neck** COM

T21 Burn and corrosion of trunk
INCLUDES burns and corrosion of hip region
EXCLUDES 2 *burns and corrosion of axilla (T22.- with fifth character 4)*
burns and corrosion of scapular region (T22.- with fifth character 6)
burns and corrosion of shoulder (T22.- with fifth character 5)

The appropriate 7th character is to be added to each code from category T21.
A initial encounter
D subsequent encounter
S sequela

T21.0 **Burn of unspecified degree of trunk**
Use additional external cause code to identify the source, place and intent of the burn (X00-X19, X75-X77, X96-X98, Y92)
T21.00 **Burn of unspecified degree of trunk, unspecified site**
T21.01 **Burn of unspecified degree of chest wall**
Burn of unspecified degree of breast
T21.02 **Burn of unspecified degree of abdominal wall**
Burn of unspecified degree of flank
Burn of unspecified degree of groin
T21.03 **Burn of unspecified degree of upper back**
Burn of unspecified degree of interscapular region
T21.04 **Burn of unspecified degree of lower back**
T21.05 **Burn of unspecified degree of buttock**
Burn of unspecified degree of anus
T21.06 **Burn of unspecified degree of male genital region** ♂
Burn of unspecified degree of penis
Burn of unspecified degree of scrotum
Burn of unspecified degree of testis
T21.07 **Burn of unspecified degree of female genital region** ♀
Burn of unspecified degree of labium (majus) (minus)
Burn of unspecified degree of perineum
Burn of unspecified degree of vulva
EXCLUDES 2 *burn of vagina (T28.3)*
T21.09 **Burn of unspecified degree of other site of trunk**

T21.1 **Burn of first degree of trunk**
Use additional external cause code to identify the source, place and intent of the burn (X00-X19, X75-X77, X96-X98, Y92)
T21.10 **Burn of first degree of trunk, unspecified site**
T21.11 **Burn of first degree of chest wall**
Burn of first degree of breast
T21.12 **Burn of first degree of abdominal wall**
Burn of first degree of flank
Burn of first degree of groin
T21.13 **Burn of first degree of upper back**
Burn of first degree of interscapular region
T21.14 **Burn of first degree of lower back**
T21.15 **Burn of first degree of buttock**
Burn of first degree of anus
T21.16 **Burn of first degree of male genital region** ♂
Burn of first degree of penis
Burn of first degree of scrotum
Burn of first degree of testis
T21.17 **Burn of first degree of female genital region** ♀
Burn of first degree of labium (majus) (minus)
Burn of first degree of perineum
Burn of first degree of vulva
EXCLUDES 2 *burn of vagina (T28.3)*
T21.19 **Burn of first degree of other site of trunk**

T21.2 **Burn of second degree of trunk**
Use additional external cause code to identify the source, place and intent of the burn (X00-X19, X75-X77, X96-X98, Y92)
T21.20 **Burn of second degree of trunk, unspecified site**
T21.21 **Burn of second degree of chest wall**
Burn of second degree of breast
T21.22 **Burn of second degree of abdominal wall**
Burn of second degree of flank
Burn of second degree of groin
T21.23 **Burn of second degree of upper back**
Burn of second degree of interscapular region
T21.24 **Burn of second degree of lower back**
T21.25 **Burn of second degree of buttock**
Burn of second degree of anus
T21.26 **Burn of second degree of male genital region** ♂
Burn of second degree of penis
Burn of second degree of scrotum
Burn of second degree of testis
T21.27 **Burn of second degree of female genital region** ♀
Burn of second degree of labium (majus) (minus)
Burn of second degree of perineum
Burn of second degree of vulva
EXCLUDES 2 *burn of vagina (T28.3)*
T21.29 **Burn of second degree of other site of trunk**

T21.3 **Burn of third degree of trunk**
Use additional external cause code to identify the source, place and intent of the burn (X00-X19, X75-X77, X96-X98, Y92)
T21.30 **Burn of third degree of trunk, unspecified site** COM
T21.31 **Burn of third degree of chest wall** COM
Burn of third degree of breast
AHA: 2016,2Q,5
T21.32 **Burn of third degree of abdominal wall** COM
Burn of third degree of flank
Burn of third degree of groin
T21.33 **Burn of third degree of upper back** COM
Burn of third degree of interscapular region
T21.34 **Burn of third degree of lower back** COM
T21.35 **Burn of third degree of buttock** COM
Burn of third degree of anus
T21.36 **Burn of third degree of male genital region** COM ♂
Burn of third degree of penis
Burn of third degree of scrotum
Burn of third degree of testis
T21.37 **Burn of third degree of female genital region** COM ♀
Burn of third degree of labium (majus) (minus)
Burn of third degree of perineum
Burn of third degree of vulva
EXCLUDES 2 *burn of vagina (T28.3)*
T21.39 **Burn of third degree of other site of trunk** COM

T21.4 **Corrosion of unspecified degree of trunk**
Code first (T51-T65) to identify chemical and intent
Use additional external cause code to identify place (Y92)
T21.40 **Corrosion of unspecified degree of trunk, unspecified site**
T21.41 **Corrosion of unspecified degree of chest wall**
Corrosion of unspecified degree of breast

T21.42 Corrosion of unspecified degree of abdominal wall
Corrosion of unspecified degree of flank
Corrosion of unspecified degree of groin

T21.43 Corrosion of unspecified degree of upper back
Corrosion of unspecified degree of interscapular region

T21.44 Corrosion of unspecified degree of lower back

T21.45 Corrosion of unspecified degree of buttock
Corrosion of unspecified degree of anus

T21.46 Corrosion of unspecified degree of male genital region ♂
Corrosion of unspecified degree of penis
Corrosion of unspecified degree of scrotum
Corrosion of unspecified degree of testis

T21.47 Corrosion of unspecified degree of female genital region ♀
Corrosion of unspecified degree of labium (majus) (minus)
Corrosion of unspecified degree of perineum
Corrosion of unspecified degree of vulva
EXCLUDES 2 *corrosion of vagina (T28.8)*

T21.49 Corrosion of unspecified degree of other site of trunk

T21.5 Corrosion of first degree of trunk
Code first (T51-T65) to identify chemical and intent
Use additional external cause code to identify place (Y92)

T21.50 Corrosion of first degree of trunk, unspecified site

T21.51 Corrosion of first degree of chest wall
Corrosion of first degree of breast

T21.52 Corrosion of first degree of abdominal wall
Corrosion of first degree of flank
Corrosion of first degree of groin

T21.53 Corrosion of first degree of upper back
Corrosion of first degree of interscapular region

T21.54 Corrosion of first degree of lower back

T21.55 Corrosion of first degree of buttock
Corrosion of first degree of anus

T21.56 Corrosion of first degree of male genital region ♂
Corrosion of first degree of penis
Corrosion of first degree of scrotum
Corrosion of first degree of testis

T21.57 Corrosion of first degree of female genital region ♀
Corrosion of first degree of labium (majus) (minus)
Corrosion of first degree of perineum
Corrosion of first degree of vulva
EXCLUDES 2 *corrosion of vagina (T28.8)*

T21.59 Corrosion of first degree of other site of trunk

T21.6 Corrosion of second degree of trunk
Code first (T51-T65) to identify chemical and intent
Use additional external cause code to identify place (Y92)

T21.60 Corrosion of second degree of trunk, unspecified site

T21.61 Corrosion of second degree of chest wall
Corrosion of second degree of breast

T21.62 Corrosion of second degree of abdominal wall
Corrosion of second degree of flank
Corrosion of second degree of groin

T21.63 Corrosion of second degree of upper back
Corrosion of second degree of interscapular region

T21.64 Corrosion of second degree of lower back

T21.65 Corrosion of second degree of buttock
Corrosion of second degree of anus

T21.66 Corrosion of second degree of male genital region ♂
Corrosion of second degree of penis
Corrosion of second degree of scrotum
Corrosion of second degree of testis

T21.67 Corrosion of second degree of female genital region ♀
Corrosion of second degree of labium (majus) (minus)
Corrosion of second degree of perineum
Corrosion of second degree of vulva
EXCLUDES 2 *corrosion of vagina (T28.8)*

T21.69 Corrosion of second degree of other site of trunk

T21.7 Corrosion of third degree of trunk
Code first (T51-T65) to identify chemical and intent
Use additional external cause code to identify place (Y92)

T21.70 Corrosion of third degree of trunk, unspecified site COM

T21.71 Corrosion of third degree of chest wall COM
Corrosion of third degree of breast

T21.72 Corrosion of third degree of abdominal wall COM
Corrosion of third degree of flank
Corrosion of third degree of groin

T21.73 Corrosion of third degree of upper back COM
Corrosion of third degree of interscapular region

T21.74 Corrosion of third degree of lower back COM

T21.75 Corrosion of third degree of buttock COM
Corrosion of third degree of anus

T21.76 Corrosion of third degree of male genital region COM ♂
Corrosion of third degree of penis
Corrosion of third degree of scrotum
Corrosion of third degree of testis

T21.77 Corrosion of third degree of female genital region COM ♀
Corrosion of third degree of labium (majus) (minus)
Corrosion of third degree of perineum
Corrosion of third degree of vulva
EXCLUDES 2 *corrosion of vagina (T28.8)*

T21.79 Corrosion of third degree of other site of trunk COM

T22 Burn and corrosion of shoulder and upper limb, except wrist and hand
EXCLUDES 2 *burn and corrosion of interscapular region (T21.-)*
burn and corrosion of wrist and hand (T23.-)

The appropriate 7th character is to be added to each code from category T22.
A initial encounter
D subsequent encounter
S sequela

T22.0 Burn of unspecified degree of shoulder and upper limb, except wrist and hand
Use additional external cause code to identify the source, place and intent of the burn (X00-X19, X75-X77, X96-X98, Y92)

T22.00 Burn of unspecified degree of shoulder and upper limb, except wrist and hand, unspecified site

T22.01 Burn of unspecified degree of forearm

T22.011 Burn of unspecified degree of right forearm

T22.012 Burn of unspecified degree of left forearm

T22.019 Burn of unspecified degree of unspecified forearm

T22.02 Burn of unspecified degree of elbow

T22.021 Burn of unspecified degree of right elbow

T22.022 Burn of unspecified degree of left elbow

T22.029 Burn of unspecified degree of unspecified elbow

T22.03 Burn of unspecified degree of upper arm

T22.031 Burn of unspecified degree of right upper arm

T22.032 Burn of unspecified degree of left upper arm

T22.039 Burn of unspecified degree of unspecified upper arm

T22.04 Burn of unspecified degree of axilla

T22.041 Burn of unspecified degree of right axilla

T22.042 Burn of unspecified degree of left axilla

T22.049 Burn of unspecified degree of unspecified axilla

- T22.05 Burn of unspecified degree of shoulder
  - T22.051 Burn of unspecified degree of right shoulder
  - T22.052 Burn of unspecified degree of left shoulder
  - T22.059 Burn of unspecified degree of unspecified shoulder
- T22.06 Burn of unspecified degree of scapular region
  - T22.061 Burn of unspecified degree of right scapular region
  - T22.062 Burn of unspecified degree of left scapular region
  - T22.069 Burn of unspecified degree of unspecified scapular region
- T22.09 Burn of unspecified degree of multiple sites of shoulder and upper limb, except wrist and hand
  - T22.091 Burn of unspecified degree of multiple sites of right shoulder and upper limb, except wrist and hand
  - T22.092 Burn of unspecified degree of multiple sites of left shoulder and upper limb, except wrist and hand
  - T22.099 Burn of unspecified degree of multiple sites of unspecified shoulder and upper limb, except wrist and hand

T22.1 Burn of first degree of shoulder and upper limb, except wrist and hand

Use additional external cause code to identify the source, place and intent of the burn (X00-X19, X75-X77, X96-X98, Y92)

- T22.10 Burn of first degree of shoulder and upper limb, except wrist and hand, unspecified site
- T22.11 Burn of first degree of forearm
  - T22.111 Burn of first degree of right forearm
  - T22.112 Burn of first degree of left forearm
  - T22.119 Burn of first degree of unspecified forearm
- T22.12 Burn of first degree of elbow
  - T22.121 Burn of first degree of right elbow
  - T22.122 Burn of first degree of left elbow
  - T22.129 Burn of first degree of unspecified elbow
- T22.13 Burn of first degree of upper arm
  - T22.131 Burn of first degree of right upper arm
  - T22.132 Burn of first degree of left upper arm
  - T22.139 Burn of first degree of unspecified upper arm
- T22.14 Burn of first degree of axilla
  - T22.141 Burn of first degree of right axilla
  - T22.142 Burn of first degree of left axilla
  - T22.149 Burn of first degree of unspecified axilla
- T22.15 Burn of first degree of shoulder
  - T22.151 Burn of first degree of right shoulder
  - T22.152 Burn of first degree of left shoulder
  - T22.159 Burn of first degree of unspecified shoulder
- T22.16 Burn of first degree of scapular region
  - T22.161 Burn of first degree of right scapular region
  - T22.162 Burn of first degree of left scapular region
  - T22.169 Burn of first degree of unspecified scapular region
- T22.19 Burn of first degree of multiple sites of shoulder and upper limb, except wrist and hand
  - T22.191 Burn of first degree of multiple sites of right shoulder and upper limb, except wrist and hand
  - T22.192 Burn of first degree of multiple sites of left shoulder and upper limb, except wrist and hand
  - T22.199 Burn of first degree of multiple sites of unspecified shoulder and upper limb, except wrist and hand

T22.2 Burn of second degree of shoulder and upper limb, except wrist and hand

Use additional external cause code to identify the source, place and intent of the burn (X00-X19, X75-X77, X96-X98, Y92)

- T22.20 Burn of second degree of shoulder and upper limb, except wrist and hand, unspecified site
- T22.21 Burn of second degree of forearm
  - T22.211 Burn of second degree of right forearm
  - T22.212 Burn of second degree of left forearm
  - T22.219 Burn of second degree of unspecified forearm
- T22.22 Burn of second degree of elbow
  - T22.221 Burn of second degree of right elbow
  - T22.222 Burn of second degree of left elbow
  - T22.229 Burn of second degree of unspecified elbow
- T22.23 Burn of second degree of upper arm
  - T22.231 Burn of second degree of right upper arm
  - T22.232 Burn of second degree of left upper arm
  - T22.239 Burn of second degree of unspecified upper arm
- T22.24 Burn of second degree of axilla
  - T22.241 Burn of second degree of right axilla
  - T22.242 Burn of second degree of left axilla
  - T22.249 Burn of second degree of unspecified axilla
- T22.25 Burn of second degree of shoulder
  - T22.251 Burn of second degree of right shoulder
  - T22.252 Burn of second degree of left shoulder
  - T22.259 Burn of second degree of unspecified shoulder
- T22.26 Burn of second degree of scapular region
  - T22.261 Burn of second degree of right scapular region
  - T22.262 Burn of second degree of left scapular region
  - T22.269 Burn of second degree of unspecified scapular region
- T22.29 Burn of second degree of multiple sites of shoulder and upper limb, except wrist and hand
  - T22.291 Burn of second degree of multiple sites of right shoulder and upper limb, except wrist and hand
  - T22.292 Burn of second degree of multiple sites of left shoulder and upper limb, except wrist and hand
  - T22.299 Burn of second degree of multiple sites of unspecified shoulder and upper limb, except wrist and hand

T22.3 Burn of third degree of shoulder and upper limb, except wrist and hand

Use additional external cause code to identify the source, place and intent of the burn (X00-X19, X75-X77, X96-X98, Y92)

- T22.30 Burn of third degree of shoulder and upper limb, except wrist and hand, unspecified site COM
- T22.31 Burn of third degree of forearm
  - T22.311 Burn of third degree of right forearm COM
  - T22.312 Burn of third degree of left forearm COM
  - T22.319 Burn of third degree of unspecified forearm COM
- T22.32 Burn of third degree of elbow
  - T22.321 Burn of third degree of right elbow COM
  - T22.322 Burn of third degree of left elbow COM
  - T22.329 Burn of third degree of unspecified elbow COM
- T22.33 Burn of third degree of upper arm
  - T22.331 Burn of third degree of right upper arm COM
  - T22.332 Burn of third degree of left upper arm COM
  - T22.339 Burn of third degree of unspecified upper arm COM
- T22.34 Burn of third degree of axilla
  - T22.341 Burn of third degree of right axilla COM
  - T22.342 Burn of third degree of left axilla COM
  - T22.349 Burn of third degree of unspecified axilla COM

6th T22.35 **Burn of third degree of shoulder**
- 7th T22.351 Burn of third degree of right shoulder COM
- 7th T22.352 Burn of third degree of left shoulder COM
- 7th T22.359 Burn of third degree of unspecified shoulder COM

6th T22.36 **Burn of third degree of scapular region**
- 7th T22.361 Burn of third degree of right scapular region COM
- 7th T22.362 Burn of third degree of left scapular region COM
- 7th T22.369 Burn of third degree of unspecified scapular region COM

6th T22.39 **Burn of third degree of multiple sites of shoulder and upper limb, except wrist and hand**
- 7th T22.391 Burn of third degree of multiple sites of right shoulder and upper limb, except wrist and hand COM
- 7th T22.392 Burn of third degree of multiple sites of left shoulder and upper limb, except wrist and hand COM
- 7th T22.399 Burn of third degree of multiple sites of unspecified shoulder and upper limb, except wrist and hand COM

5th T22.4 **Corrosion of unspecified degree of shoulder and upper limb, except wrist and hand**

Code first (T51-T65) to identify chemical and intent

Use additional external cause code to identify place (Y92)

x7th T22.40 **Corrosion of unspecified degree of shoulder and upper limb, except wrist and hand, unspecified site**

6th T22.41 **Corrosion of unspecified degree of forearm**
- 7th T22.411 Corrosion of unspecified degree of right forearm
- 7th T22.412 Corrosion of unspecified degree of left forearm
- 7th T22.419 Corrosion of unspecified degree of unspecified forearm

6th T22.42 **Corrosion of unspecified degree of elbow**
- 7th T22.421 Corrosion of unspecified degree of right elbow
- 7th T22.422 Corrosion of unspecified degree of left elbow
- 7th T22.429 Corrosion of unspecified degree of unspecified elbow

6th T22.43 **Corrosion of unspecified degree of upper arm**
- 7th T22.431 Corrosion of unspecified degree of right upper arm
- 7th T22.432 Corrosion of unspecified degree of left upper arm
- 7th T22.439 Corrosion of unspecified degree of unspecified upper arm

6th T22.44 **Corrosion of unspecified degree of axilla**
- 7th T22.441 Corrosion of unspecified degree of right axilla
- 7th T22.442 Corrosion of unspecified degree of left axilla
- 7th T22.449 Corrosion of unspecified degree of unspecified axilla

6th T22.45 **Corrosion of unspecified degree of shoulder**
- 7th T22.451 Corrosion of unspecified degree of right shoulder
- 7th T22.452 Corrosion of unspecified degree of left shoulder
- 7th T22.459 Corrosion of unspecified degree of unspecified shoulder

6th T22.46 **Corrosion of unspecified degree of scapular region**
- 7th T22.461 Corrosion of unspecified degree of right scapular region
- 7th T22.462 Corrosion of unspecified degree of left scapular region
- 7th T22.469 Corrosion of unspecified degree of unspecified scapular region

6th T22.49 **Corrosion of unspecified degree of multiple sites of shoulder and upper limb, except wrist and hand**
- 7th T22.491 Corrosion of unspecified degree of multiple sites of right shoulder and upper limb, except wrist and hand
- 7th T22.492 Corrosion of unspecified degree of multiple sites of left shoulder and upper limb, except wrist and hand
- 7th T22.499 Corrosion of unspecified degree of multiple sites of unspecified shoulder and upper limb, except wrist and hand

5th T22.5 **Corrosion of first degree of shoulder and upper limb, except wrist and hand**

Code first (T51-T65) to identify chemical and intent

Use additional external cause code to identify place (Y92)

x7th T22.50 **Corrosion of first degree of shoulder and upper limb, except wrist and hand unspecified site**

6th T22.51 **Corrosion of first degree of forearm**
- 7th T22.511 Corrosion of first degree of right forearm
- 7th T22.512 Corrosion of first degree of left forearm
- 7th T22.519 Corrosion of first degree of unspecified forearm

6th T22.52 **Corrosion of first degree of elbow**
- 7th T22.521 Corrosion of first degree of right elbow
- 7th T22.522 Corrosion of first degree of left elbow
- 7th T22.529 Corrosion of first degree of unspecified elbow

6th T22.53 **Corrosion of first degree of upper arm**
- 7th T22.531 Corrosion of first degree of right upper arm
- 7th T22.532 Corrosion of first degree of left upper arm
- 7th T22.539 Corrosion of first degree of unspecified upper arm

6th T22.54 **Corrosion of first degree of axilla**
- 7th T22.541 Corrosion of first degree of right axilla
- 7th T22.542 Corrosion of first degree of left axilla
- 7th T22.549 Corrosion of first degree of unspecified axilla

6th T22.55 **Corrosion of first degree of shoulder**
- 7th T22.551 Corrosion of first degree of right shoulder
- 7th T22.552 Corrosion of first degree of left shoulder
- 7th T22.559 Corrosion of first degree of unspecified shoulder

6th T22.56 **Corrosion of first degree of scapular region**
- 7th T22.561 Corrosion of first degree of right scapular region
- 7th T22.562 Corrosion of first degree of left scapular region
- 7th T22.569 Corrosion of first degree of unspecified scapular region

6th T22.59 **Corrosion of first degree of multiple sites of shoulder and upper limb, except wrist and hand**
- 7th T22.591 Corrosion of first degree of multiple sites of right shoulder and upper limb, except wrist and hand
- 7th T22.592 Corrosion of first degree of multiple sites of left shoulder and upper limb, except wrist and hand
- 7th T22.599 Corrosion of first degree of multiple sites of unspecified shoulder and upper limb, except wrist and hand

5th T22.6 **Corrosion of second degree of shoulder and upper limb, except wrist and hand**

Code first (T51-T65) to identify chemical and intent

Use additional external cause code to identify place (Y92)

x7th T22.60 **Corrosion of second degree of shoulder and upper limb, except wrist and hand, unspecified site**

6th T22.61 **Corrosion of second degree of forearm**
- 7th T22.611 Corrosion of second degree of right forearm
- 7th T22.612 Corrosion of second degree of left forearm
- 7th T22.619 Corrosion of second degree of unspecified forearm

6th T22.62 **Corrosion of second degree of elbow**
- 7th T22.621 Corrosion of second degree of right elbow
- 7th T22.622 Corrosion of second degree of left elbow
- 7th T22.629 Corrosion of second degree of unspecified elbow

6th T22.63 **Corrosion of second degree of upper arm**
- 7th T22.631 Corrosion of second degree of right upper arm

T22.632 Corrosion of second degree of left upper arm

T22.639 Corrosion of second degree of unspecified upper arm

T22.64 Corrosion of second degree of axilla

T22.641 Corrosion of second degree of right axilla

T22.642 Corrosion of second degree of left axilla

T22.649 Corrosion of second degree of unspecified axilla

T22.65 Corrosion of second degree of shoulder

T22.651 Corrosion of second degree of right shoulder

T22.652 Corrosion of second degree of left shoulder

T22.659 Corrosion of second degree of unspecified shoulder

T22.66 Corrosion of second degree of scapular region

T22.661 Corrosion of second degree of right scapular region

T22.662 Corrosion of second degree of left scapular region

T22.669 Corrosion of second degree of unspecified scapular region

T22.69 Corrosion of second degree of multiple sites of shoulder and upper limb, except wrist and hand

T22.691 Corrosion of second degree of multiple sites of right shoulder and upper limb, except wrist and hand

T22.692 Corrosion of second degree of multiple sites of left shoulder and upper limb, except wrist and hand

T22.699 Corrosion of second degree of multiple sites of unspecified shoulder and upper limb, except wrist and hand

T22.7 Corrosion of third degree of shoulder and upper limb, except wrist and hand

Code first (T51-T65) to identify chemical and intent

Use additional external cause code to identify place (Y92)

T22.70 Corrosion of third degree of shoulder and upper limb, except wrist and hand, unspecified site COM

T22.71 Corrosion of third degree of forearm

T22.711 Corrosion of third degree of right forearm COM

T22.712 Corrosion of third degree of left forearm COM

T22.719 Corrosion of third degree of unspecified forearm COM

T22.72 Corrosion of third degree of elbow

T22.721 Corrosion of third degree of right elbow COM

T22.722 Corrosion of third degree of left elbow COM

T22.729 Corrosion of third degree of unspecified elbow COM

T22.73 Corrosion of third degree of upper arm

T22.731 Corrosion of third degree of right upper arm COM

T22.732 Corrosion of third degree of left upper arm COM

T22.739 Corrosion of third degree of unspecified upper arm COM

T22.74 Corrosion of third degree of axilla

T22.741 Corrosion of third degree of right axilla COM

T22.742 Corrosion of third degree of left axilla COM

T22.749 Corrosion of third degree of unspecified axilla COM

T22.75 Corrosion of third degree of shoulder

T22.751 Corrosion of third degree of right shoulder COM

T22.752 Corrosion of third degree of left shoulder COM

T22.759 Corrosion of third degree of unspecified shoulder COM

T22.76 Corrosion of third degree of scapular region

T22.761 Corrosion of third degree of right scapular region COM

T22.762 Corrosion of third degree of left scapular region COM

T22.769 Corrosion of third degree of unspecified scapular region COM

T22.79 Corrosion of third degree of multiple sites of shoulder and upper limb, except wrist and hand

T22.791 Corrosion of third degree of multiple sites of right shoulder and upper limb, except wrist and hand COM

T22.792 Corrosion of third degree of multiple sites of left shoulder and upper limb, except wrist and hand COM

T22.799 Corrosion of third degree of multiple sites of unspecified shoulder and upper limb, except wrist and hand COM

T23 Burn and corrosion of wrist and hand

AHA: 2015,1Q,19

The appropriate 7th character is to be added to each code from category T23.
- A initial encounter
- D subsequent encounter
- S sequela

T23.0 Burn of unspecified degree of wrist and hand

Use additional external cause code to identify the source, place and intent of the burn (X00-X19, X75-X77, X96-X98, Y92)

T23.00 Burn of unspecified degree of hand, unspecified site

T23.001 Burn of unspecified degree of right hand, unspecified site

T23.002 Burn of unspecified degree of left hand, unspecified site

T23.009 Burn of unspecified degree of unspecified hand, unspecified site

T23.01 Burn of unspecified degree of thumb (nail)

T23.011 Burn of unspecified degree of right thumb (nail)

T23.012 Burn of unspecified degree of left thumb (nail)

T23.019 Burn of unspecified degree of unspecified thumb (nail)

T23.02 Burn of unspecified degree of single finger (nail) except thumb

T23.021 Burn of unspecified degree of single right finger (nail) except thumb

T23.022 Burn of unspecified degree of single left finger (nail) except thumb

T23.029 Burn of unspecified degree of unspecified single finger (nail) except thumb

T23.03 Burn of unspecified degree of multiple fingers (nail), not including thumb

T23.031 Burn of unspecified degree of multiple right fingers (nail), not including thumb

T23.032 Burn of unspecified degree of multiple left fingers (nail), not including thumb

T23.039 Burn of unspecified degree of unspecified multiple fingers (nail), not including thumb

T23.04 Burn of unspecified degree of multiple fingers (nail), including thumb

T23.041 Burn of unspecified degree of multiple right fingers (nail), including thumb

T23.042 Burn of unspecified degree of multiple left fingers (nail), including thumb

T23.049 Burn of unspecified degree of unspecified multiple fingers (nail), including thumb

T23.05 Burn of unspecified degree of palm

T23.051 Burn of unspecified degree of right palm

T23.052 Burn of unspecified degree of left palm

T23.059 Burn of unspecified degree of unspecified palm

T23.06 Burn of unspecified degree of back of hand

T23.061 Burn of unspecified degree of back of right hand

T23.062 Burn of unspecified degree of back of left hand

T23.069 Burn of unspecified degree of back of unspecified hand

T23.07 Burn of unspecified degree of wrist

T23.071 Burn of unspecified degree of right wrist

T23.072 Burn of unspecified degree of left wrist
T23.079 Burn of unspecified degree of unspecified wrist
T23.09 Burn of unspecified degree of multiple sites of wrist and hand
T23.091 Burn of unspecified degree of multiple sites of right wrist and hand
T23.092 Burn of unspecified degree of multiple sites of left wrist and hand
T23.099 Burn of unspecified degree of multiple sites of unspecified wrist and hand
T23.1 Burn of first degree of wrist and hand
Use additional external cause code to identify the source, place and intent of the burn (XØØ-X19, X75-X77, X96-X98, Y92)
T23.1Ø Burn of first degree of hand, unspecified site
T23.1Ø1 Burn of first degree of right hand, unspecified site
T23.1Ø2 Burn of first degree of left hand, unspecified site
T23.1Ø9 Burn of first degree of unspecified hand, unspecified site
T23.11 Burn of first degree of thumb (nail)
T23.111 Burn of first degree of right thumb (nail)
T23.112 Burn of first degree of left thumb (nail)
T23.119 Burn of first degree of unspecified thumb (nail)
T23.12 Burn of first degree of single finger (nail) except thumb
T23.121 Burn of first degree of single right finger (nail) except thumb
T23.122 Burn of first degree of single left finger (nail) except thumb
T23.129 Burn of first degree of unspecified single finger (nail) except thumb
T23.13 Burn of first degree of multiple fingers (nail), not including thumb
T23.131 Burn of first degree of multiple right fingers (nail), not including thumb
T23.132 Burn of first degree of multiple left fingers (nail), not including thumb
T23.139 Burn of first degree of unspecified multiple fingers (nail), not including thumb
T23.14 Burn of first degree of multiple fingers (nail), including thumb
T23.141 Burn of first degree of multiple right fingers (nail), including thumb
T23.142 Burn of first degree of multiple left fingers (nail), including thumb
T23.149 Burn of first degree of unspecified multiple fingers (nail), including thumb
T23.15 Burn of first degree of palm
T23.151 Burn of first degree of right palm
T23.152 Burn of first degree of left palm
T23.159 Burn of first degree of unspecified palm
T23.16 Burn of first degree of back of hand
T23.161 Burn of first degree of back of right hand
T23.162 Burn of first degree of back of left hand
T23.169 Burn of first degree of back of unspecified hand
T23.17 Burn of first degree of wrist
T23.171 Burn of first degree of right wrist
T23.172 Burn of first degree of left wrist
T23.179 Burn of first degree of unspecified wrist
T23.19 Burn of first degree of multiple sites of wrist and hand
T23.191 Burn of first degree of multiple sites of right wrist and hand
T23.192 Burn of first degree of multiple sites of left wrist and hand
T23.199 Burn of first degree of multiple sites of unspecified wrist and hand
T23.2 Burn of second degree of wrist and hand
Use additional external cause code to identify the source, place and intent of the burn (XØØ-X19, X75-X77, X96-X98, Y92)
T23.2Ø Burn of second degree of hand, unspecified site
T23.2Ø1 Burn of second degree of right hand, unspecified site
T23.2Ø2 Burn of second degree of left hand, unspecified site
T23.2Ø9 Burn of second degree of unspecified hand, unspecified site
T23.21 Burn of second degree of thumb (nail)
T23.211 Burn of second degree of right thumb (nail)
T23.212 Burn of second degree of left thumb (nail)
T23.219 Burn of second degree of unspecified thumb (nail)
T23.22 Burn of second degree of single finger (nail) except thumb
T23.221 Burn of second degree of single right finger (nail) except thumb
T23.222 Burn of second degree of single left finger (nail) except thumb
T23.229 Burn of second degree of unspecified single finger (nail) except thumb
T23.23 Burn of second degree of multiple fingers (nail), not including thumb
T23.231 Burn of second degree of multiple right fingers (nail), not including thumb
T23.232 Burn of second degree of multiple left fingers (nail), not including thumb
T23.239 Burn of second degree of unspecified multiple fingers (nail), not including thumb
T23.24 Burn of second degree of multiple fingers (nail), including thumb
T23.241 Burn of second degree of multiple right fingers (nail), including thumb
T23.242 Burn of second degree of multiple left fingers (nail), including thumb
T23.249 Burn of second degree of unspecified multiple fingers (nail), including thumb
T23.25 Burn of second degree of palm
T23.251 Burn of second degree of right palm
T23.252 Burn of second degree of left palm
T23.259 Burn of second degree of unspecified palm
T23.26 Burn of second degree of back of hand
T23.261 Burn of second degree of back of right hand
T23.262 Burn of second degree of back of left hand
T23.269 Burn of second degree of back of unspecified hand
T23.27 Burn of second degree of wrist
T23.271 Burn of second degree of right wrist
T23.272 Burn of second degree of left wrist
T23.279 Burn of second degree of unspecified wrist
T23.29 Burn of second degree of multiple sites of wrist and hand
T23.291 Burn of second degree of multiple sites of right wrist and hand
T23.292 Burn of second degree of multiple sites of left wrist and hand
T23.299 Burn of second degree of multiple sites of unspecified wrist and hand
T23.3 Burn of third degree of wrist and hand
Use additional external cause code to identify the source, place and intent of the burn (XØØ-X19, X75-X77, X96-X98, Y92)
T23.3Ø Burn of third degree of hand, unspecified site
AHA: 2016,2Q,5
T23.3Ø1 Burn of third degree of right hand, unspecified site COM
T23.3Ø2 Burn of third degree of left hand, unspecified site COM
T23.3Ø9 Burn of third degree of unspecified hand, unspecified site COM
T23.31 Burn of third degree of thumb (nail)
T23.311 Burn of third degree of right thumb (nail) COM
T23.312 Burn of third degree of left thumb (nail) COM
T23.319 Burn of third degree of unspecified thumb (nail) COM

6th T23.32 **Burn of third degree of single finger (nail) except thumb**

7th T23.321 Burn of third degree of single right finger (nail) except thumb COM

7th T23.322 Burn of third degree of single left finger (nail) except thumb COM

7th T23.329 Burn of third degree of unspecified single finger (nail) except thumb COM

6th T23.33 **Burn of third degree of multiple fingers (nail), not including thumb**

7th T23.331 Burn of third degree of multiple right fingers (nail), not including thumb COM

7th T23.332 Burn of third degree of multiple left fingers (nail), not including thumb COM

7th T23.339 Burn of third degree of unspecified multiple fingers (nail), not including thumb COM

6th T23.34 **Burn of third degree of multiple fingers (nail), including thumb**

7th T23.341 Burn of third degree of multiple right fingers (nail), including thumb COM

7th T23.342 Burn of third degree of multiple left fingers (nail), including thumb COM

7th T23.349 Burn of third degree of unspecified multiple fingers (nail), including thumb COM

6th T23.35 **Burn of third degree of palm**

7th T23.351 Burn of third degree of right palm COM

7th T23.352 Burn of third degree of left palm COM

7th T23.359 Burn of third degree of unspecified palm COM

6th T23.36 **Burn of third degree of back of hand**

7th T23.361 Burn of third degree of back of right hand COM

7th T23.362 Burn of third degree of back of left hand COM

7th T23.369 Burn of third degree of back of unspecified hand COM

6th T23.37 **Burn of third degree of wrist**

7th T23.371 Burn of third degree of right wrist COM

7th T23.372 Burn of third degree of left wrist COM

7th T23.379 Burn of third degree of unspecified wrist COM

6th T23.39 **Burn of third degree of multiple sites of wrist and hand**

7th T23.391 Burn of third degree of multiple sites of right wrist and hand COM

7th T23.392 Burn of third degree of multiple sites of left wrist and hand COM

7th T23.399 Burn of third degree of multiple sites of unspecified wrist and hand COM

5th **T23.4 Corrosion of unspecified degree of wrist and hand**

Code first (T51-T65) to identify chemical and intent

Use additional external cause code to identify place (Y92)

6th T23.40 **Corrosion of unspecified degree of hand, unspecified site**

7th T23.401 Corrosion of unspecified degree of right hand, unspecified site

7th T23.402 Corrosion of unspecified degree of left hand, unspecified site

7th T23.409 Corrosion of unspecified degree of unspecified hand, unspecified site

6th T23.41 **Corrosion of unspecified degree of thumb (nail)**

7th T23.411 Corrosion of unspecified degree of right thumb (nail)

7th T23.412 Corrosion of unspecified degree of left thumb (nail)

7th T23.419 Corrosion of unspecified degree of unspecified thumb (nail)

6th T23.42 **Corrosion of unspecified degree of single finger (nail) except thumb**

7th T23.421 Corrosion of unspecified degree of single right finger (nail) except thumb

7th T23.422 Corrosion of unspecified degree of single left finger (nail) except thumb

7th T23.429 Corrosion of unspecified degree of unspecified single finger (nail) except thumb

6th T23.43 **Corrosion of unspecified degree of multiple fingers (nail), not including thumb**

7th T23.431 Corrosion of unspecified degree of multiple right fingers (nail), not including thumb

7th T23.432 Corrosion of unspecified degree of multiple left fingers (nail), not including thumb

7th T23.439 Corrosion of unspecified degree of unspecified multiple fingers (nail), not including thumb

6th T23.44 **Corrosion of unspecified degree of multiple fingers (nail), including thumb**

7th T23.441 Corrosion of unspecified degree of multiple right fingers (nail), including thumb

7th T23.442 Corrosion of unspecified degree of multiple left fingers (nail), including thumb

7th T23.449 Corrosion of unspecified degree of unspecified multiple fingers (nail), including thumb

6th T23.45 **Corrosion of unspecified degree of palm**

7th T23.451 Corrosion of unspecified degree of right palm

7th T23.452 Corrosion of unspecified degree of left palm

7th T23.459 Corrosion of unspecified degree of unspecified palm

6th T23.46 **Corrosion of unspecified degree of back of hand**

7th T23.461 Corrosion of unspecified degree of back of right hand

7th T23.462 Corrosion of unspecified degree of back of left hand

7th T23.469 Corrosion of unspecified degree of back of unspecified hand

6th T23.47 **Corrosion of unspecified degree of wrist**

7th T23.471 Corrosion of unspecified degree of right wrist

7th T23.472 Corrosion of unspecified degree of left wrist

7th T23.479 Corrosion of unspecified degree of unspecified wrist

6th T23.49 **Corrosion of unspecified degree of multiple sites of wrist and hand**

7th T23.491 Corrosion of unspecified degree of multiple sites of right wrist and hand

7th T23.492 Corrosion of unspecified degree of multiple sites of left wrist and hand

7th T23.499 Corrosion of unspecified degree of multiple sites of unspecified wrist and hand

5th **T23.5 Corrosion of first degree of wrist and hand**

Code first (T51-T65) to identify chemical and intent

Use additional external cause code to identify place (Y92)

6th T23.50 **Corrosion of first degree of hand, unspecified site**

7th T23.501 Corrosion of first degree of right hand, unspecified site

7th T23.502 Corrosion of first degree of left hand, unspecified site

7th T23.509 Corrosion of first degree of unspecified hand, unspecified site

6th T23.51 **Corrosion of first degree of thumb (nail)**

7th T23.511 Corrosion of first degree of right thumb (nail)

7th T23.512 Corrosion of first degree of left thumb (nail)

7th T23.519 Corrosion of first degree of unspecified thumb (nail)

6th T23.52 **Corrosion of first degree of single finger (nail) except thumb**

7th T23.521 Corrosion of first degree of single right finger (nail) except thumb

7th T23.522 Corrosion of first degree of single left finger (nail) except thumb

7th T23.529 Corrosion of first degree of unspecified single finger (nail) except thumb

6th T23.53 **Corrosion of first degree of multiple fingers (nail), not including thumb**

7th T23.531 Corrosion of first degree of multiple right fingers (nail), not including thumb

T23.532 Corrosion of first degree of multiple left fingers (nail), not including thumb
T23.539 Corrosion of first degree of unspecified multiple fingers (nail), not including thumb
T23.54 Corrosion of first degree of multiple fingers (nail), including thumb
T23.541 Corrosion of first degree of multiple right fingers (nail), including thumb
T23.542 Corrosion of first degree of multiple left fingers (nail), including thumb
T23.549 Corrosion of first degree of unspecified multiple fingers (nail), including thumb
T23.55 Corrosion of first degree of palm
T23.551 Corrosion of first degree of right palm
T23.552 Corrosion of first degree of left palm
T23.559 Corrosion of first degree of unspecified palm
T23.56 Corrosion of first degree of back of hand
T23.561 Corrosion of first degree of back of right hand
T23.562 Corrosion of first degree of back of left hand
T23.569 Corrosion of first degree of back of unspecified hand
T23.57 Corrosion of first degree of wrist
T23.571 Corrosion of first degree of right wrist
T23.572 Corrosion of first degree of left wrist
T23.579 Corrosion of first degree of unspecified wrist
T23.59 Corrosion of first degree of multiple sites of wrist and hand
T23.591 Corrosion of first degree of multiple sites of right wrist and hand
T23.592 Corrosion of first degree of multiple sites of left wrist and hand
T23.599 Corrosion of first degree of multiple sites of unspecified wrist and hand
T23.6 Corrosion of second degree of wrist and hand
Code first (T51-T65) to identify chemical and intent
Use additional external cause code to identify place (Y92)
T23.60 Corrosion of second degree of hand, unspecified site
T23.601 Corrosion of second degree of right hand, unspecified site
T23.602 Corrosion of second degree of left hand, unspecified site
T23.609 Corrosion of second degree of unspecified hand, unspecified site
T23.61 Corrosion of second degree of thumb (nail)
T23.611 Corrosion of second degree of right thumb (nail)
T23.612 Corrosion of second degree of left thumb (nail)
T23.619 Corrosion of second degree of unspecified thumb (nail)
T23.62 Corrosion of second degree of single finger (nail) except thumb
T23.621 Corrosion of second degree of single right finger (nail) except thumb
T23.622 Corrosion of second degree of single left finger (nail) except thumb
T23.629 Corrosion of second degree of unspecified single finger (nail) except thumb
T23.63 Corrosion of second degree of multiple fingers (nail), not including thumb
T23.631 Corrosion of second degree of multiple right fingers (nail), not including thumb
T23.632 Corrosion of second degree of multiple left fingers (nail), not including thumb
T23.639 Corrosion of second degree of unspecified multiple fingers (nail), not including thumb
T23.64 Corrosion of second degree of multiple fingers (nail), including thumb
T23.641 Corrosion of second degree of multiple right fingers (nail), including thumb
T23.642 Corrosion of second degree of multiple left fingers (nail), including thumb
T23.649 Corrosion of second degree of unspecified multiple fingers (nail), including thumb
T23.65 Corrosion of second degree of palm
T23.651 Corrosion of second degree of right palm
T23.652 Corrosion of second degree of left palm
T23.659 Corrosion of second degree of unspecified palm
T23.66 Corrosion of second degree of back of hand
T23.661 Corrosion of second degree back of right hand
T23.662 Corrosion of second degree back of left hand
T23.669 Corrosion of second degree back of unspecified hand
T23.67 Corrosion of second degree of wrist
T23.671 Corrosion of second degree of right wrist
T23.672 Corrosion of second degree of left wrist
T23.679 Corrosion of second degree of unspecified wrist
T23.69 Corrosion of second degree of multiple sites of wrist and hand
T23.691 Corrosion of second degree of multiple sites of right wrist and hand
T23.692 Corrosion of second degree of multiple sites of left wrist and hand
T23.699 Corrosion of second degree of multiple sites of unspecified wrist and hand
T23.7 Corrosion of third degree of wrist and hand
Code first (T51-T65) to identify chemical and intent
Use additional external cause code to identify place (Y92)
T23.70 Corrosion of third degree of hand, unspecified site
T23.701 Corrosion of third degree of right hand, unspecified site COM
T23.702 Corrosion of third degree of left hand, unspecified site COM
T23.709 Corrosion of third degree of unspecified hand, unspecified site COM
T23.71 Corrosion of third degree of thumb (nail)
T23.711 Corrosion of third degree of right thumb (nail) COM
T23.712 Corrosion of third degree of left thumb (nail) COM
T23.719 Corrosion of third degree of unspecified thumb (nail) COM
T23.72 Corrosion of third degree of single finger (nail) except thumb
T23.721 Corrosion of third degree of single right finger (nail) except thumb COM
T23.722 Corrosion of third degree of single left finger (nail) except thumb COM
T23.729 Corrosion of third degree of unspecified single finger (nail) except thumb COM
T23.73 Corrosion of third degree of multiple fingers (nail), not including thumb
T23.731 Corrosion of third degree of multiple right fingers (nail), not including thumb COM
T23.732 Corrosion of third degree of multiple left fingers (nail), not including thumb COM
T23.739 Corrosion of third degree of unspecified multiple fingers (nail), not including thumb COM
T23.74 Corrosion of third degree of multiple fingers (nail), including thumb
T23.741 Corrosion of third degree of multiple right fingers (nail), including thumb COM
T23.742 Corrosion of third degree of multiple left fingers (nail), including thumb COM
T23.749 Corrosion of third degree of unspecified multiple fingers (nail), including thumb COM
T23.75 Corrosion of third degree of palm
T23.751 Corrosion of third degree of right palm COM
T23.752 Corrosion of third degree of left palm COM
T23.759 Corrosion of third degree of unspecified palm COM

6th **T23.76 Corrosion of third degree of back of hand**

7th **T23.761 Corrosion of third degree of back of right hand** COM

7th **T23.762 Corrosion of third degree of back of left hand** COM

7th **T23.769 Corrosion of third degree back of unspecified hand** COM

6th **T23.77 Corrosion of third degree of wrist**

7th **T23.771 Corrosion of third degree of right wrist** COM

7th **T23.772 Corrosion of third degree of left wrist** COM

7th **T23.779 Corrosion of third degree of unspecified wrist** COM

6th **T23.79 Corrosion of third degree of multiple sites of wrist and hand**

7th **T23.791 Corrosion of third degree of multiple sites of right wrist and hand** COM

7th **T23.792 Corrosion of third degree of multiple sites of left wrist and hand** COM

7th **T23.799 Corrosion of third degree of multiple sites of unspecified wrist and hand** COM

4th **T24 Burn and corrosion of lower limb, except ankle and foot**

EXCLUDES 2 *burn and corrosion of ankle and foot (T25.-)*
burn and corrosion of hip region (T21.-)

The appropriate 7th character is to be added to each code from category T24.
A initial encounter
D subsequent encounter
S sequela

5th **T24.Ø Burn of unspecified degree of lower limb, except ankle and foot**

Use additional external cause code to identify the source, place and intent of the burn (XØØ-X19, X75-X77, X96-X98, Y92)

6th **T24.ØØ Burn of unspecified degree of unspecified site of lower limb, except ankle and foot**

7th **T24.ØØ1 Burn of unspecified degree of unspecified site of right lower limb, except ankle and foot**

7th **T24.ØØ2 Burn of unspecified degree of unspecified site of left lower limb, except ankle and foot**

7th **T24.ØØ9 Burn of unspecified degree of unspecified site of unspecified lower limb, except ankle and foot**

6th **T24.Ø1 Burn of unspecified degree of thigh**

7th **T24.Ø11 Burn of unspecified degree of right thigh**

7th **T24.Ø12 Burn of unspecified degree of left thigh**

7th **T24.Ø19 Burn of unspecified degree of unspecified thigh**

6th **T24.Ø2 Burn of unspecified degree of knee**

7th **T24.Ø21 Burn of unspecified degree of right knee**

7th **T24.Ø22 Burn of unspecified degree of left knee**

7th **T24.Ø29 Burn of unspecified degree of unspecified knee**

6th **T24.Ø3 Burn of unspecified degree of lower leg**

7th **T24.Ø31 Burn of unspecified degree of right lower leg**

7th **T24.Ø32 Burn of unspecified degree of left lower leg**

7th **T24.Ø39 Burn of unspecified degree of unspecified lower leg**

6th **T24.Ø9 Burn of unspecified degree of multiple sites of lower limb, except ankle and foot**

7th **T24.Ø91 Burn of unspecified degree of multiple sites of right lower limb, except ankle and foot**

7th **T24.Ø92 Burn of unspecified degree of multiple sites of left lower limb, except ankle and foot**

7th **T24.Ø99 Burn of unspecified degree of multiple sites of unspecified lower limb, except ankle and foot**

5th **T24.1 Burn of first degree of lower limb, except ankle and foot**

Use additional external cause code to identify the source, place and intent of the burn (XØØ-X19, X75-X77, X96-X98, Y92)

6th **T24.1Ø Burn of first degree of unspecified site of lower limb, except ankle and foot**

7th **T24.1Ø1 Burn of first degree of unspecified site of right lower limb, except ankle and foot**

7th **T24.1Ø2 Burn of first degree of unspecified site of left lower limb, except ankle and foot**

7th **T24.1Ø9 Burn of first degree of unspecified site of unspecified lower limb, except ankle and foot**

6th **T24.11 Burn of first degree of thigh**

7th **T24.111 Burn of first degree of right thigh**

7th **T24.112 Burn of first degree of left thigh**

7th **T24.119 Burn of first degree of unspecified thigh**

6th **T24.12 Burn of first degree of knee**

7th **T24.121 Burn of first degree of right knee**

7th **T24.122 Burn of first degree of left knee**

7th **T24.129 Burn of first degree of unspecified knee**

6th **T24.13 Burn of first degree of lower leg**

7th **T24.131 Burn of first degree of right lower leg**

7th **T24.132 Burn of first degree of left lower leg**

7th **T24.139 Burn of first degree of unspecified lower leg**

6th **T24.19 Burn of first degree of multiple sites of lower limb, except ankle and foot**

7th **T24.191 Burn of first degree of multiple sites of right lower limb, except ankle and foot**

7th **T24.192 Burn of first degree of multiple sites of left lower limb, except ankle and foot**

7th **T24.199 Burn of first degree of multiple sites of unspecified lower limb, except ankle and foot**

5th **T24.2 Burn of second degree of lower limb, except ankle and foot**

Use additional external cause code to identify the source, place and intent of the burn (XØØ-X19, X75-X77, X96-X98, Y92)

6th **T24.2Ø Burn of second degree of unspecified site of lower limb, except ankle and foot**

7th **T24.2Ø1 Burn of second degree of unspecified site of right lower limb, except ankle and foot**

7th **T24.2Ø2 Burn of second degree of unspecified site of left lower limb, except ankle and foot**

7th **T24.2Ø9 Burn of second degree of unspecified site of unspecified lower limb, except ankle and foot**

6th **T24.21 Burn of second degree of thigh**

7th **T24.211 Burn of second degree of right thigh**

7th **T24.212 Burn of second degree of left thigh**

7th **T24.219 Burn of second degree of unspecified thigh**

6th **T24.22 Burn of second degree of knee**

7th **T24.221 Burn of second degree of right knee**

7th **T24.222 Burn of second degree of left knee**

7th **T24.229 Burn of second degree of unspecified knee**

6th **T24.23 Burn of second degree of lower leg**

7th **T24.231 Burn of second degree of right lower leg**

7th **T24.232 Burn of second degree of left lower leg**

7th **T24.239 Burn of second degree of unspecified lower leg**

6th **T24.29 Burn of second degree of multiple sites of lower limb, except ankle and foot**

7th **T24.291 Burn of second degree of multiple sites of right lower limb, except ankle and foot**

7th **T24.292 Burn of second degree of multiple sites of left lower limb, except ankle and foot**

7th **T24.299 Burn of second degree of multiple sites of unspecified lower limb, except ankle and foot**

T24.3 Burn of third degree of lower limb, except ankle and foot
Use additional external cause code to identify the source, place and intent of the burn (X00-X19, X75-X77, X96-X98, Y92)
T24.30 Burn of third degree of unspecified site of lower limb, except ankle and foot
T24.301 Burn of third degree of unspecified site of right lower limb, except ankle and foot COM
T24.302 Burn of third degree of unspecified site of left lower limb, except ankle and foot COM
T24.309 Burn of third degree of unspecified site of unspecified lower limb, except ankle and foot COM
T24.31 Burn of third degree of thigh
T24.311 Burn of third degree of right thigh COM
T24.312 Burn of third degree of left thigh COM
T24.319 Burn of third degree of unspecified thigh COM
T24.32 Burn of third degree of knee
T24.321 Burn of third degree of right knee COM
T24.322 Burn of third degree of left knee COM
T24.329 Burn of third degree of unspecified knee COM
T24.33 Burn of third degree of lower leg
T24.331 Burn of third degree of right lower leg COM
T24.332 Burn of third degree of left lower leg COM
T24.339 Burn of third degree of unspecified lower leg COM
T24.39 Burn of third degree of multiple sites of lower limb, except ankle and foot
AHA: 2016,2Q,4
T24.391 Burn of third degree of multiple sites of right lower limb, except ankle and foot COM
T24.392 Burn of third degree of multiple sites of left lower limb, except ankle and foot COM
T24.399 Burn of third degree of multiple sites of unspecified lower limb, except ankle and foot COM
T24.4 Corrosion of unspecified degree of lower limb, except ankle and foot
Code first (T51-T65) to identify chemical and intent
Use additional external cause code to identify place (Y92)
T24.40 Corrosion of unspecified degree of unspecified site of lower limb, except ankle and foot
T24.401 Corrosion of unspecified degree of unspecified site of right lower limb, except ankle and foot
T24.402 Corrosion of unspecified degree of unspecified site of left lower limb, except ankle and foot
T24.409 Corrosion of unspecified degree of unspecified site of unspecified lower limb, except ankle and foot
T24.41 Corrosion of unspecified degree of thigh
T24.411 Corrosion of unspecified degree of right thigh
T24.412 Corrosion of unspecified degree of left thigh
T24.419 Corrosion of unspecified degree of unspecified thigh
T24.42 Corrosion of unspecified degree of knee
T24.421 Corrosion of unspecified degree of right knee
T24.422 Corrosion of unspecified degree of left knee
T24.429 Corrosion of unspecified degree of unspecified knee
T24.43 Corrosion of unspecified degree of lower leg
T24.431 Corrosion of unspecified degree of right lower leg
T24.432 Corrosion of unspecified degree of left lower leg
T24.439 Corrosion of unspecified degree of unspecified lower leg
T24.49 Corrosion of unspecified degree of multiple sites of lower limb, except ankle and foot
T24.491 Corrosion of unspecified degree of multiple sites of right lower limb, except ankle and foot
T24.492 Corrosion of unspecified degree of multiple sites of left lower limb, except ankle and foot
T24.499 Corrosion of unspecified degree of multiple sites of unspecified lower limb, except ankle and foot
T24.5 Corrosion of first degree of lower limb, except ankle and foot
Code first (T51-T65) to identify chemical and intent
Use additional external cause code to identify place (Y92)
T24.50 Corrosion of first degree of unspecified site of lower limb, except ankle and foot
T24.501 Corrosion of first degree of unspecified site of right lower limb, except ankle and foot
T24.502 Corrosion of first degree of unspecified site of left lower limb, except ankle and foot
T24.509 Corrosion of first degree of unspecified site of unspecified lower limb, except ankle and foot
T24.51 Corrosion of first degree of thigh
T24.511 Corrosion of first degree of right thigh
T24.512 Corrosion of first degree of left thigh
T24.519 Corrosion of first degree of unspecified thigh
T24.52 Corrosion of first degree of knee
T24.521 Corrosion of first degree of right knee
T24.522 Corrosion of first degree of left knee
T24.529 Corrosion of first degree of unspecified knee
T24.53 Corrosion of first degree of lower leg
T24.531 Corrosion of first degree of right lower leg
T24.532 Corrosion of first degree of left lower leg
T24.539 Corrosion of first degree of unspecified lower leg
T24.59 Corrosion of first degree of multiple sites of lower limb, except ankle and foot
T24.591 Corrosion of first degree of multiple sites of right lower limb, except ankle and foot
T24.592 Corrosion of first degree of multiple sites of left lower limb, except ankle and foot
T24.599 Corrosion of first degree of multiple sites of unspecified lower limb, except ankle and foot
T24.6 Corrosion of second degree of lower limb, except ankle and foot
Code first (T51-T65) to identify chemical and intent
Use additional external cause code to identify place (Y92)
T24.60 Corrosion of second degree of unspecified site of lower limb, except ankle and foot
T24.601 Corrosion of second degree of unspecified site of right lower limb, except ankle and foot
T24.602 Corrosion of second degree of unspecified site of left lower limb, except ankle and foot
T24.609 Corrosion of second degree of unspecified site of unspecified lower limb, except ankle and foot
T24.61 Corrosion of second degree of thigh
T24.611 Corrosion of second degree of right thigh
T24.612 Corrosion of second degree of left thigh
T24.619 Corrosion of second degree of unspecified thigh
T24.62 Corrosion of second degree of knee
T24.621 Corrosion of second degree of right knee
T24.622 Corrosion of second degree of left knee
T24.629 Corrosion of second degree of unspecified knee
T24.63 Corrosion of second degree of lower leg
T24.631 Corrosion of second degree of right lower leg

7th **T24.632 Corrosion of second degree of left lower leg**

7th **T24.639 Corrosion of second degree of unspecified lower leg**

6th **T24.69 Corrosion of second degree of multiple sites of lower limb, except ankle and foot**

7th **T24.691 Corrosion of second degree of multiple sites of right lower limb, except ankle and foot**

7th **T24.692 Corrosion of second degree of multiple sites of left lower limb, except ankle and foot**

7th **T24.699 Corrosion of second degree of multiple sites of unspecified lower limb, except ankle and foot**

5th **T24.7 Corrosion of third degree of lower limb, except ankle and foot**

Code first (T51-T65) to identify chemical and intent

Use additional external cause code to identify place (Y92)

6th **T24.70 Corrosion of third degree of unspecified site of lower limb, except ankle and foot**

7th **T24.701 Corrosion of third degree of unspecified site of right lower limb, except ankle and foot** COM

7th **T24.702 Corrosion of third degree of unspecified site of left lower limb, except ankle and foot** COM

7th **T24.709 Corrosion of third degree of unspecified site of unspecified lower limb, except ankle and foot** COM

6th **T24.71 Corrosion of third degree of thigh**

7th **T24.711 Corrosion of third degree of right thigh** COM

7th **T24.712 Corrosion of third degree of left thigh** COM

7th **T24.719 Corrosion of third degree of unspecified thigh** COM

6th **T24.72 Corrosion of third degree of knee**

7th **T24.721 Corrosion of third degree of right knee** COM

7th **T24.722 Corrosion of third degree of left knee** COM

7th **T24.729 Corrosion of third degree of unspecified knee** COM

6th **T24.73 Corrosion of third degree of lower leg**

7th **T24.731 Corrosion of third degree of right lower leg** COM

7th **T24.732 Corrosion of third degree of left lower leg** COM

7th **T24.739 Corrosion of third degree of unspecified lower leg** COM

6th **T24.79 Corrosion of third degree of multiple sites of lower limb, except ankle and foot**

7th **T24.791 Corrosion of third degree of multiple sites of right lower limb, except ankle and foot** COM

7th **T24.792 Corrosion of third degree of multiple sites of left lower limb, except ankle and foot** COM

7th **T24.799 Corrosion of third degree of multiple sites of unspecified lower limb, except ankle and foot** COM

4th **T25 Burn and corrosion of ankle and foot**

The appropriate 7th character is to be added to each code from category T25.

A initial encounter

D subsequent encounter

S sequela

5th **T25.Ø Burn of unspecified degree of ankle and foot**

Use additional external cause code to identify the source, place and intent of the burn (XØØ-X19, X75-X77, X96-X98, Y92)

6th **T25.Ø1 Burn of unspecified degree of ankle**

7th **T25.Ø11 Burn of unspecified degree of right ankle**

7th **T25.Ø12 Burn of unspecified degree of left ankle**

7th **T25.Ø19 Burn of unspecified degree of unspecified ankle**

6th **T25.Ø2 Burn of unspecified degree of foot**

EXCLUDES 2 *burn of unspecified degree of toe(s) (nail) (T25.Ø3-)*

7th **T25.Ø21 Burn of unspecified degree of right foot**

7th **T25.Ø22 Burn of unspecified degree of left foot**

7th **T25.Ø29 Burn of unspecified degree of unspecified foot**

6th **T25.Ø3 Burn of unspecified degree of toe(s) (nail)**

7th **T25.Ø31 Burn of unspecified degree of right toe(s) (nail)**

7th **T25.Ø32 Burn of unspecified degree of left toe(s) (nail)**

7th **T25.Ø39 Burn of unspecified degree of unspecified toe(s) (nail)**

6th **T25.Ø9 Burn of unspecified degree of multiple sites of ankle and foot**

7th **T25.Ø91 Burn of unspecified degree of multiple sites of right ankle and foot**

7th **T25.Ø92 Burn of unspecified degree of multiple sites of left ankle and foot**

7th **T25.Ø99 Burn of unspecified degree of multiple sites of unspecified ankle and foot**

5th **T25.1 Burn of first degree of ankle and foot**

Use additional external cause code to identify the source, place and intent of the burn (XØØ-X19, X75-X77, X96-X98, Y92)

6th **T25.11 Burn of first degree of ankle**

7th **T25.111 Burn of first degree of right ankle**

7th **T25.112 Burn of first degree of left ankle**

7th **T25.119 Burn of first degree of unspecified ankle**

6th **T25.12 Burn of first degree of foot**

EXCLUDES 2 *burn of first degree of toe(s) (nail) (T25.13-)*

7th **T25.121 Burn of first degree of right foot**

7th **T25.122 Burn of first degree of left foot**

7th **T25.129 Burn of first degree of unspecified foot**

6th **T25.13 Burn of first degree of toe(s) (nail)**

7th **T25.131 Burn of first degree of right toe(s) (nail)**

7th **T25.132 Burn of first degree of left toe(s) (nail)**

7th **T25.139 Burn of first degree of unspecified toe(s) (nail)**

6th **T25.19 Burn of first degree of multiple sites of ankle and foot**

7th **T25.191 Burn of first degree of multiple sites of right ankle and foot**

7th **T25.192 Burn of first degree of multiple sites of left ankle and foot**

7th **T25.199 Burn of first degree of multiple sites of unspecified ankle and foot**

5th **T25.2 Burn of second degree of ankle and foot**

Use additional external cause code to identify the source, place and intent of the burn (XØØ-X19, X75-X77, X96-X98, Y92)

6th **T25.21 Burn of second degree of ankle**

7th **T25.211 Burn of second degree of right ankle**

7th **T25.212 Burn of second degree of left ankle**

7th **T25.219 Burn of second degree of unspecified ankle**

6th **T25.22 Burn of second degree of foot**

EXCLUDES 2 *burn of second degree of toe(s) (nail) (T25.23-)*

7th **T25.221 Burn of second degree of right foot**

7th **T25.222 Burn of second degree of left foot**

7th **T25.229 Burn of second degree of unspecified foot**

6th **T25.23 Burn of second degree of toe(s) (nail)**

7th **T25.231 Burn of second degree of right toe(s) (nail)**

7th **T25.232 Burn of second degree of left toe(s) (nail)**

7th **T25.239 Burn of second degree of unspecified toe(s) (nail)**

6th **T25.29 Burn of second degree of multiple sites of ankle and foot**

7th **T25.291 Burn of second degree of multiple sites of right ankle and foot**

7th **T25.292 Burn of second degree of multiple sites of left ankle and foot**

7th **T25.299 Burn of second degree of multiple sites of unspecified ankle and foot**

T25.3 Burn of third degree of ankle and foot
Use additional external cause code to identify the source, place and intent of the burn (XØØ-X19, X75-X77, X96-X98, Y92)
T25.31 Burn of third degree of ankle
T25.311 Burn of third degree of right ankle COM
T25.312 Burn of third degree of left ankle COM
T25.319 Burn of third degree of unspecified ankle COM
T25.32 Burn of third degree of foot
EXCLUDES 2 *burn of third degree of toe(s) (nail) (T25.33-)*
T25.321 Burn of third degree of right foot COM
T25.322 Burn of third degree of left foot COM
T25.329 Burn of third degree of unspecified foot COM
T25.33 Burn of third degree of toe(s) (nail)
T25.331 Burn of third degree of right toe(s) (nail) COM
T25.332 Burn of third degree of left toe(s) (nail) COM
T25.339 Burn of third degree of unspecified toe(s) (nail) COM
T25.39 Burn of third degree of multiple sites of ankle and foot
T25.391 Burn of third degree of multiple sites of right ankle and foot COM
T25.392 Burn of third degree of multiple sites of left ankle and foot COM
T25.399 Burn of third degree of multiple sites of unspecified ankle and foot COM
T25.4 Corrosion of unspecified degree of ankle and foot
Code first (T51-T65) to identify chemical and intent
Use additional external cause code to identify place (Y92)
T25.41 Corrosion of unspecified degree of ankle
T25.411 Corrosion of unspecified degree of right ankle
T25.412 Corrosion of unspecified degree of left ankle
T25.419 Corrosion of unspecified degree of unspecified ankle
T25.42 Corrosion of unspecified degree of foot
EXCLUDES 2 *corrosion of unspecified degree of toe(s) (nail) (T25.43-)*
T25.421 Corrosion of unspecified degree of right foot
T25.422 Corrosion of unspecified degree of left foot
T25.429 Corrosion of unspecified degree of unspecified foot
T25.43 Corrosion of unspecified degree of toe(s) (nail)
T25.431 Corrosion of unspecified degree of right toe(s) (nail)
T25.432 Corrosion of unspecified degree of left toe(s) (nail)
T25.439 Corrosion of unspecified degree of unspecified toe(s) (nail)
T25.49 Corrosion of unspecified degree of multiple sites of ankle and foot
T25.491 Corrosion of unspecified degree of multiple sites of right ankle and foot
T25.492 Corrosion of unspecified degree of multiple sites of left ankle and foot
T25.499 Corrosion of unspecified degree of multiple sites of unspecified ankle and foot
T25.5 Corrosion of first degree of ankle and foot
Code first (T51-T65) to identify chemical and intent
Use additional external cause code to identify place (Y92)
T25.51 Corrosion of first degree of ankle
T25.511 Corrosion of first degree of right ankle
T25.512 Corrosion of first degree of left ankle
T25.519 Corrosion of first degree of unspecified ankle
T25.52 Corrosion of first degree of foot
EXCLUDES 2 *corrosion of first degree of toe(s) (nail) (T25.53-)*
T25.521 Corrosion of first degree of right foot
T25.522 Corrosion of first degree of left foot
T25.529 Corrosion of first degree of unspecified foot
T25.53 Corrosion of first degree of toe(s) (nail)
T25.531 Corrosion of first degree of right toe(s) (nail)
T25.532 Corrosion of first degree of left toe(s) (nail)
T25.539 Corrosion of first degree of unspecified toe(s) (nail)
T25.59 Corrosion of first degree of multiple sites of ankle and foot
T25.591 Corrosion of first degree of multiple sites of right ankle and foot
T25.592 Corrosion of first degree of multiple sites of left ankle and foot
T25.599 Corrosion of first degree of multiple sites of unspecified ankle and foot
T25.6 Corrosion of second degree of ankle and foot
Code first (T51-T65) to identify chemical and intent
Use additional external cause code to identify place (Y92)
T25.61 Corrosion of second degree of ankle
T25.611 Corrosion of second degree of right ankle
T25.612 Corrosion of second degree of left ankle
T25.619 Corrosion of second degree of unspecified ankle
T25.62 Corrosion of second degree of foot
EXCLUDES 2 *corrosion of second degree of toe(s) (nail) (T25.63-)*
T25.621 Corrosion of second degree of right foot
T25.622 Corrosion of second degree of left foot
T25.629 Corrosion of second degree of unspecified foot
T25.63 Corrosion of second degree of toe(s) (nail)
T25.631 Corrosion of second degree of right toe(s) (nail)
T25.632 Corrosion of second degree of left toe(s) (nail)
T25.639 Corrosion of second degree of unspecified toe(s) (nail)
T25.69 Corrosion of second degree of multiple sites of ankle and foot
T25.691 Corrosion of second degree of right ankle and foot
T25.692 Corrosion of second degree of left ankle and foot
T25.699 Corrosion of second degree of unspecified ankle and foot
T25.7 Corrosion of third degree of ankle and foot
Code first (T51-T65) to identify chemical and intent
Use additional external cause code to identify place (Y92)
T25.71 Corrosion of third degree of ankle
T25.711 Corrosion of third degree of right ankle COM
T25.712 Corrosion of third degree of left ankle COM
T25.719 Corrosion of third degree of unspecified ankle COM
T25.72 Corrosion of third degree of foot
EXCLUDES 2 *corrosion of third degree of toe(s) (nail) (T25.73-)*
T25.721 Corrosion of third degree of right foot COM
T25.722 Corrosion of third degree of left foot COM
T25.729 Corrosion of third degree of unspecified foot COM
T25.73 Corrosion of third degree of toe(s) (nail)
T25.731 Corrosion of third degree of right toe(s) (nail) COM
T25.732 Corrosion of third degree of left toe(s) (nail) COM
T25.739 Corrosion of third degree of unspecified toe(s) (nail) COM
T25.79 Corrosion of third degree of multiple sites of ankle and foot
T25.791 Corrosion of third degree of multiple sites of right ankle and foot COM

√7th **T25.792** **Corrosion of third degree of multiple sites of left ankle and foot** COM

√7th **T25.799** **Corrosion of third degree of multiple sites of unspecified ankle and foot** COM

Burns and corrosions confined to eye and internal organs (T26-T28)

√4th **T26 Burn and corrosion confined to eye and adnexa**

The appropriate 7th character is to be added to each code from category T26.
A initial encounter
D subsequent encounter
S sequela

√5th **T26.0 Burn of eyelid and periocular area**
Use additional external cause code to identify the source, place and intent of the burn (X00-X19, X75-X77, X96-X98, Y92)

√x7th **T26.00** **Burn of unspecified eyelid and periocular area**
√x7th **T26.01** **Burn of right eyelid and periocular area**
√x7th **T26.02** **Burn of left eyelid and periocular area**

√5th **T26.1 Burn of cornea and conjunctival sac**
Use additional external cause code to identify the source, place and intent of the burn (X00-X19, X75-X77, X96-X98, Y92)

√x7th **T26.10** **Burn of cornea and conjunctival sac, unspecified eye**
√x7th **T26.11** **Burn of cornea and conjunctival sac, right eye**
√x7th **T26.12** **Burn of cornea and conjunctival sac, left eye**

√5th **T26.2 Burn with resulting rupture and destruction of eyeball**
Use additional external cause code to identify the source, place and intent of the burn (X00-X19, X75-X77, X96-X98, Y92)

√x7th **T26.20** **Burn with resulting rupture and destruction of unspecified eyeball**
√x7th **T26.21** **Burn with resulting rupture and destruction of right eyeball**
√x7th **T26.22** **Burn with resulting rupture and destruction of left eyeball**

√5th **T26.3 Burns of other specified parts of eye and adnexa**
Use additional external cause code to identify the source, place and intent of the burn (X00-X19, X75-X77, X96-X98, Y92)

√x7th **T26.30** **Burns of other specified parts of unspecified eye and adnexa**
√x7th **T26.31** **Burns of other specified parts of right eye and adnexa**
√x7th **T26.32** **Burns of other specified parts of left eye and adnexa**

√5th **T26.4 Burn of eye and adnexa, part unspecified**
Use additional external cause code to identify the source, place and intent of the burn (X00-X19, X75-X77, X96-X98, Y92)

√x7th **T26.40** **Burn of unspecified eye and adnexa, part unspecified**
√x7th **T26.41** **Burn of right eye and adnexa, part unspecified**
√x7th **T26.42** **Burn of left eye and adnexa, part unspecified**

√5th **T26.5 Corrosion of eyelid and periocular area**
Code first (T51-T65) to identify chemical and intent
Use additional external cause code to identify place (Y92)

√x7th **T26.50** **Corrosion of unspecified eyelid and periocular area**
√x7th **T26.51** **Corrosion of right eyelid and periocular area**
√x7th **T26.52** **Corrosion of left eyelid and periocular area**

√5th **T26.6 Corrosion of cornea and conjunctival sac**
Code first (T51-T65) to identify chemical and intent
Use additional external cause code to identify place (Y92)

√x7th **T26.60** **Corrosion of cornea and conjunctival sac, unspecified eye**
√x7th **T26.61** **Corrosion of cornea and conjunctival sac, right eye**
√x7th **T26.62** **Corrosion of cornea and conjunctival sac, left eye**

√5th **T26.7 Corrosion with resulting rupture and destruction of eyeball**
Code first (T51-T65) to identify chemical and intent
Use additional external cause code to identify place (Y92)

√x7th **T26.70** **Corrosion with resulting rupture and destruction of unspecified eyeball**
√x7th **T26.71** **Corrosion with resulting rupture and destruction of right eyeball**
√x7th **T26.72** **Corrosion with resulting rupture and destruction of left eyeball**

√5th **T26.8 Corrosions of other specified parts of eye and adnexa**
Code first (T51-T65) to identify chemical and intent
Use additional external cause code to identify place (Y92)

√x7th **T26.80** **Corrosions of other specified parts of unspecified eye and adnexa**
√x7th **T26.81** **Corrosions of other specified parts of right eye and adnexa**
√x7th **T26.82** **Corrosions of other specified parts of left eye and adnexa**

√5th **T26.9 Corrosion of eye and adnexa, part unspecified**
Code first (T51-T65) to identify chemical and intent
Use additional external cause code to identify place (Y92)

√x7th **T26.90** **Corrosion of unspecified eye and adnexa, part unspecified**
√x7th **T26.91** **Corrosion of right eye and adnexa, part unspecified**
√x7th **T26.92** **Corrosion of left eye and adnexa, part unspecified**

√4th **T27 Burn and corrosion of respiratory tract**
Use additional external cause code to identify the source and intent of the burn (X00-X19, X75-X77, X96-X98)
Use additional external cause code to identify place (Y92)

The appropriate 7th character is to be added to each code from category T27.
A initial encounter
D subsequent encounter
S sequela

√x7th **T27.0** **Burn of larynx and trachea**
√x7th **T27.1** **Burn involving larynx and trachea with lung**
√x7th **T27.2** **Burn of other parts of respiratory tract**
Burn of thoracic cavity
√x7th **T27.3** **Burn of respiratory tract, part unspecified**
√x7th **T27.4** **Corrosion of larynx and trachea**
Code first (T51-T65) to identify chemical and intent
√x7th **T27.5** **Corrosion involving larynx and trachea with lung**
Code first (T51-T65) to identify chemical and intent
√x7th **T27.6** **Corrosion of other parts of respiratory tract**
Code first (T51-T65) to identify chemical and intent
√x7th **T27.7** **Corrosion of respiratory tract, part unspecified**
Code first (T51-T65) to identify chemical and intent

√4th **T28 Burn and corrosion of other internal organs**
Use additional external cause code to identify the source and intent of the burn (X00-X19, X75-X77, X96-X98)
Use additional external cause code to identify place (Y92)

The appropriate 7th character is to be added to each code from category T28.
A initial encounter
D subsequent encounter
S sequela

√x7th **T28.0** **Burn of mouth and pharynx**
√x7th **T28.1** **Burn of esophagus**
√x7th **T28.2** **Burn of other parts of alimentary tract**
√x7th **T28.3** **Burn of internal genitourinary organs**
√5th **T28.4** **Burns of other and unspecified internal organs**
√x7th **T28.40** **Burn of unspecified internal organ**
√6th **T28.41** **Burn of ear drum**
√7th **T28.411** **Burn of right ear drum**
√7th **T28.412** **Burn of left ear drum**
√7th **T28.419** **Burn of unspecified ear drum**
√x7th **T28.49** **Burn of other internal organ**
√x7th **T28.5** **Corrosion of mouth and pharynx**
Code first (T51-T65) to identify chemical and intent
√x7th **T28.6** **Corrosion of esophagus**
Code first (T51-T65) to identify chemical and intent
√x7th **T28.7** **Corrosion of other parts of alimentary tract**
Code first (T51-T65) to identify chemical and intent
√x7th **T28.8** **Corrosion of internal genitourinary organs**
Code first (T51-T65) to identify chemical and intent
√5th **T28.9** **Corrosions of other and unspecified internal organs**
Code first (T51-T65) to identify chemical and intent
√x7th **T28.90** **Corrosions of unspecified internal organs**

T28.91 Corrosions of ear drum

T28.911 Corrosions of right ear drum

T28.912 Corrosions of left ear drum

T28.919 Corrosions of unspecified ear drum

T28.99 Corrosions of other internal organs

Burns and corrosions of multiple and unspecified body regions (T30-T32)

T30 Burn and corrosion, body region unspecified

T30.0 Burn of unspecified body region, unspecified degree

This code is not for inpatient use. Code to specified site and degree of burns

Burn NOS

Multiple burns NOS

T30.4 Corrosion of unspecified body region, unspecified degree

This code is not for inpatient use. Code to specified site and degree of corrosion

Corrosion NOS

Multiple corrosion NOS

T31 Burns classified according to extent of body surface involved

NOTE This category is to be used as the primary code only when the site of the burn is unspecified. It should be used as a supplementary code with categories T20-T25 when the site is specified.

T31.0 Burns involving less than 10% of body surface

T31.1 Burns involving 10-19% of body surface

T31.10 Burns involving 10-19% of body surface with 0% to 9% third degree burns COM

Burns involving 10-19% of body surface NOS

T31.11 Burns involving 10-19% of body surface with 10-19% third degree burns HCC ESR COM

T31.2 Burns involving 20-29% of body surface

T31.20 Burns involving 20-29% of body surface with 0% to 9% third degree burns COM

Burns involving 20-29% of body surface NOS

T31.21 Burns involving 20-29% of body surface with 10-19% third degree burns HCC ESR COM

T31.22 Burns involving 20-29% of body surface with 20-29% third degree burns HCC ESR COM

T31.3 Burns involving 30-39% of body surface

T31.30 Burns involving 30-39% of body surface with 0% to 9% third degree burns COM

Burns involving 30-39% of body surface NOS

T31.31 Burns involving 30-39% of body surface with 10-19% third degree burns HCC ESR COM

T31.32 Burns involving 30-39% of body surface with 20-29% third degree burns HCC ESR COM

T31.33 Burns involving 30-39% of body surface with 30-39% third degree burns HCC ESR COM

T31.4 Burns involving 40-49% of body surface

T31.40 Burns involving 40-49% of body surface with 0% to 9% third degree burns COM

Burns involving 40-49% of body surface NOS

T31.41 Burns involving 40-49% of body surface with 10-19% third degree burns HCC ESR COM

T31.42 Burns involving 40-49% of body surface with 20-29% third degree burns HCC ESR COM

T31.43 Burns involving 40-49% of body surface with 30-39% third degree burns HCC ESR COM

T31.44 Burns involving 40-49% of body surface with 40-49% third degree burns HCC ESR COM

T31.5 Burns involving 50-59% of body surface

T31.50 Burns involving 50-59% of body surface with 0% to 9% third degree burns COM

Burns involving 50-59% of body surface NOS

T31.51 Burns involving 50-59% of body surface with 10-19% third degree burns HCC ESR COM

T31.52 Burns involving 50-59% of body surface with 20-29% third degree burns HCC ESR COM

T31.53 Burns involving 50-59% of body surface with 30-39% third degree burns HCC ESR COM

T31.54 Burns involving 50-59% of body surface with 40-49% third degree burns HCC ESR COM

T31.55 Burns involving 50-59% of body surface with 50-59% third degree burns HCC ESR COM

T31.6 Burns involving 60-69% of body surface

T31.60 Burns involving 60-69% of body surface with 0% to 9% third degree burns COM

Burns involving 60-69% of body surface NOS

T31.61 Burns involving 60-69% of body surface with 10-19% third degree burns HCC ESR COM

T31.62 Burns involving 60-69% of body surface with 20-29% third degree burns HCC ESR COM

T31.63 Burns involving 60-69% of body surface with 30-39% third degree burns HCC ESR COM

T31.64 Burns involving 60-69% of body surface with 40-49% third degree burns HCC ESR COM

T31.65 Burns involving 60-69% of body surface with 50-59% third degree burns HCC ESR COM

T31.66 Burns involving 60-69% of body surface with 60-69% third degree burns HCC ESR COM

T31.7 Burns involving 70-79% of body surface

T31.70 Burns involving 70-79% of body surface with 0% to 9% third degree burns COM

Burns involving 70-79% of body surface NOS

T31.71 Burns involving 70-79% of body surface with 10-19% third degree burns HCC ESR COM

T31.72 Burns involving 70-79% of body surface with 20-29% third degree burns HCC ESR COM

T31.73 Burns involving 70-79% of body surface with 30-39% third degree burns HCC ESR COM

T31.74 Burns involving 70-79% of body surface with 40-49% third degree burns HCC ESR COM

T31.75 Burns involving 70-79% of body surface with 50-59% third degree burns HCC ESR COM

T31.76 Burns involving 70-79% of body surface with 60-69% third degree burns HCC ESR COM

T31.77 Burns involving 70-79% of body surface with 70-79% third degree burns HCC ESR COM

T31.8 Burns involving 80-89% of body surface

T31.80 Burns involving 80-89% of body surface with 0% to 9% third degree burns COM

Burns involving 80-89% of body surface NOS

T31.81 Burns involving 80-89% of body surface with 10-19% third degree burns HCC ESR COM

T31.82 Burns involving 80-89% of body surface with 20-29% third degree burns HCC ESR COM

T31.83 Burns involving 80-89% of body surface with 30-39% third degree burns HCC ESR COM

T31.84 Burns involving 80-89% of body surface with 40-49% third degree burns HCC ESR COM

T31.85 Burns involving 80-89% of body surface with 50-59% third degree burns HCC ESR COM

T31.86 Burns involving 80-89% of body surface with 60-69% third degree burns HCC ESR COM

T31.87 Burns involving 80-89% of body surface with 70-79% third degree burns HCC ESR COM

T31.88 Burns involving 80-89% of body surface with 80-89% third degree burns HCC ESR COM

T31.9 Burns involving 90% or more of body surface

T31.90 Burns involving 90% or more of body surface with 0% to 9% third degree burns COM

Burns involving 90% or more of body surface NOS

T31.91 Burns involving 90% or more of body surface with 10-19% third degree burns HCC ESR COM

T31.92 Burns involving 90% or more of body surface with 20-29% third degree burns HCC ESR COM

T31.93 Burns involving 90% or more of body surface with 30-39% third degree burns HCC ESR COM

T31.94 Burns involving 90% or more of body surface with 40-49% third degree burns HCC ESR COM

T31.95 Burns involving 90% or more of body surface with 50-59% third degree burns HCC ESR COM

T31.96 Burns involving 90% or more of body surface with 60-69% third degree burns HCC ESR COM

T31.97 Burns involving 90% or more of body surface with 70-79% third degree burns HCC ESR COM

T31.98 Burns involving 90% or more of body surface with 80-89% third degree burns HCC ESR COM

T31.99 **Burns involving 9Ø% or more of body surface with 9Ø% or more third degree burns** HCC ESR COM

Rule of Nines Estimation of Total Body Surface Burned

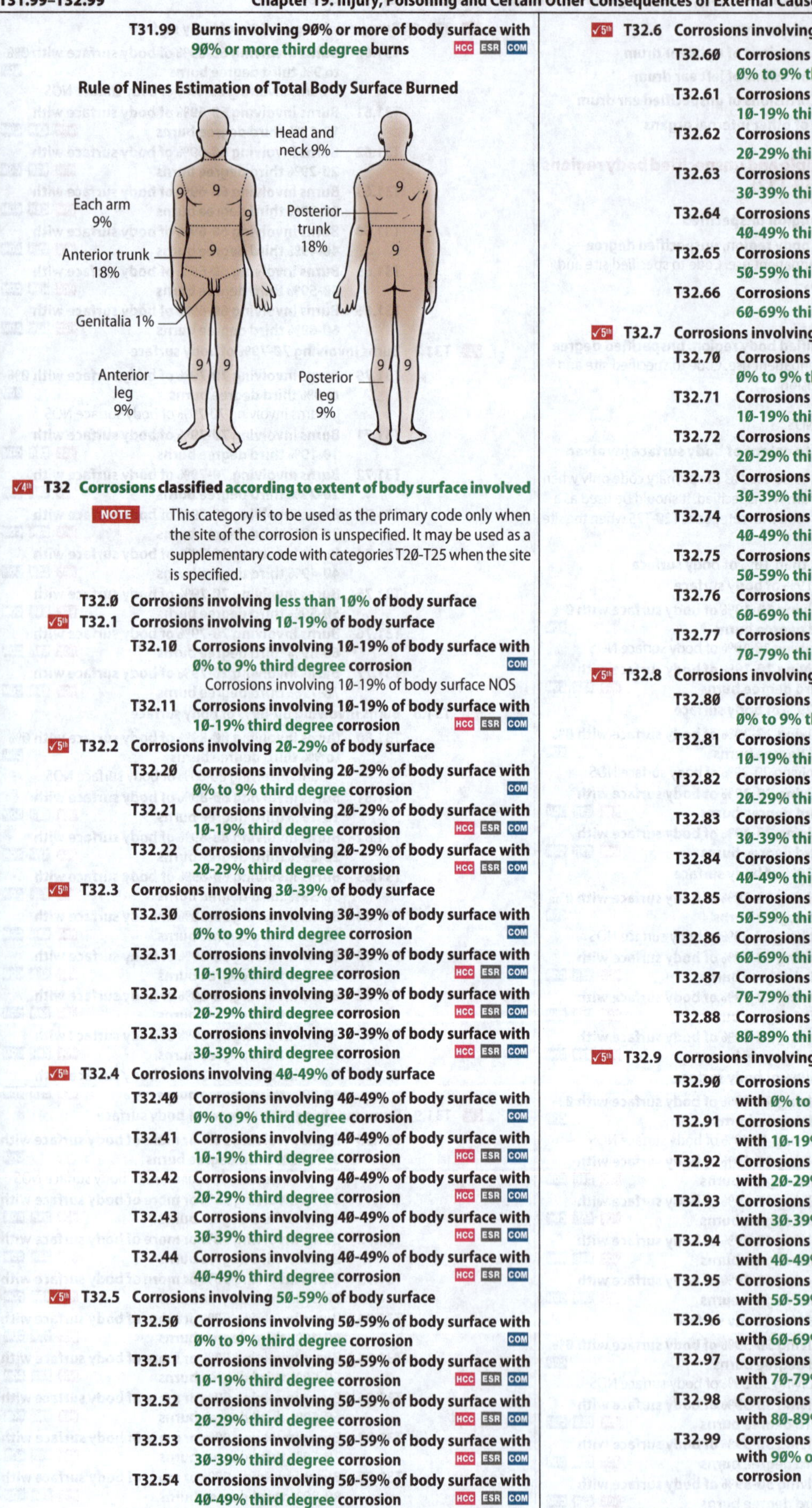

✓4th **T32 Corrosions classified according to extent of body surface involved**

NOTE This category is to be used as the primary code only when the site of the corrosion is unspecified. It may be used as a supplementary code with categories T2Ø-T25 when the site is specified.

T32.Ø **Corrosions involving less than 1Ø% of body surface**

✓5th **T32.1** **Corrosions involving 1Ø-19% of body surface**

T32.1Ø **Corrosions involving 1Ø-19% of body surface with Ø% to 9% third degree corrosion** COM

Corrosions involving 1Ø-19% of body surface NOS

T32.11 **Corrosions involving 1Ø-19% of body surface with 1Ø-19% third degree corrosion** HCC ESR COM

✓5th **T32.2** **Corrosions involving 2Ø-29% of body surface**

T32.2Ø **Corrosions involving 2Ø-29% of body surface with Ø% to 9% third degree corrosion** COM

T32.21 **Corrosions involving 2Ø-29% of body surface with 1Ø-19% third degree corrosion** HCC ESR COM

T32.22 **Corrosions involving 2Ø-29% of body surface with 2Ø-29% third degree corrosion** HCC ESR COM

✓5th **T32.3** **Corrosions involving 3Ø-39% of body surface**

T32.3Ø **Corrosions involving 3Ø-39% of body surface with Ø% to 9% third degree corrosion** COM

T32.31 **Corrosions involving 3Ø-39% of body surface with 1Ø-19% third degree corrosion** HCC ESR COM

T32.32 **Corrosions involving 3Ø-39% of body surface with 2Ø-29% third degree corrosion** HCC ESR COM

T32.33 **Corrosions involving 3Ø-39% of body surface with 3Ø-39% third degree corrosion** HCC ESR COM

✓5th **T32.4** **Corrosions involving 4Ø-49% of body surface**

T32.4Ø **Corrosions involving 4Ø-49% of body surface with Ø% to 9% third degree corrosion** COM

T32.41 **Corrosions involving 4Ø-49% of body surface with 1Ø-19% third degree corrosion** HCC ESR COM

T32.42 **Corrosions involving 4Ø-49% of body surface with 2Ø-29% third degree corrosion** HCC ESR COM

T32.43 **Corrosions involving 4Ø-49% of body surface with 3Ø-39% third degree corrosion** HCC ESR COM

T32.44 **Corrosions involving 4Ø-49% of body surface with 4Ø-49% third degree corrosion** HCC ESR COM

✓5th **T32.5** **Corrosions involving 5Ø-59% of body surface**

T32.5Ø **Corrosions involving 5Ø-59% of body surface with Ø% to 9% third degree corrosion** COM

T32.51 **Corrosions involving 5Ø-59% of body surface with 1Ø-19% third degree corrosion** HCC ESR COM

T32.52 **Corrosions involving 5Ø-59% of body surface with 2Ø-29% third degree corrosion** HCC ESR COM

T32.53 **Corrosions involving 5Ø-59% of body surface with 3Ø-39% third degree corrosion** HCC ESR COM

T32.54 **Corrosions involving 5Ø-59% of body surface with 4Ø-49% third degree corrosion** HCC ESR COM

T32.55 **Corrosions involving 5Ø-59% of body surface with 5Ø-59% third degree corrosion** HCC ESR COM

✓5th **T32.6** **Corrosions involving 6Ø-69% of body surface**

T32.6Ø **Corrosions involving 6Ø-69% of body surface with Ø% to 9% third degree corrosion** COM

T32.61 **Corrosions involving 6Ø-69% of body surface with 1Ø-19% third degree corrosion** HCC ESR COM

T32.62 **Corrosions involving 6Ø-69% of body surface with 2Ø-29% third degree corrosion** HCC ESR COM

T32.63 **Corrosions involving 6Ø-69% of body surface with 3Ø-39% third degree corrosion** HCC ESR COM

T32.64 **Corrosions involving 6Ø-69% of body surface with 4Ø-49% third degree corrosion** HCC ESR COM

T32.65 **Corrosions involving 6Ø-69% of body surface with 5Ø-59% third degree corrosion** HCC ESR COM

T32.66 **Corrosions involving 6Ø-69% of body surface with 6Ø-69% third degree corrosion** HCC ESR COM

✓5th **T32.7** **Corrosions involving 7Ø-79% of body surface**

T32.7Ø **Corrosions involving 7Ø-79% of body surface with Ø% to 9% third degree corrosion** COM

T32.71 **Corrosions involving 7Ø-79% of body surface with 1Ø-19% third degree corrosion** HCC ESR COM

T32.72 **Corrosions involving 7Ø-79% of body surface with 2Ø-29% third degree corrosion** HCC ESR COM

T32.73 **Corrosions involving 7Ø-79% of body surface with 3Ø-39% third degree corrosion** HCC ESR COM

T32.74 **Corrosions involving 7Ø-79% of body surface with 4Ø-49% third degree corrosion** HCC ESR COM

T32.75 **Corrosions involving 7Ø-79% of body surface with 5Ø-59% third degree corrosion** HCC ESR COM

T32.76 **Corrosions involving 7Ø-79% of body surface with 6Ø-69% third degree corrosion** HCC ESR COM

T32.77 **Corrosions involving 7Ø-79% of body surface with 7Ø-79% third degree corrosion** HCC ESR COM

✓5th **T32.8** **Corrosions involving 8Ø-89% of body surface**

T32.8Ø **Corrosions involving 8Ø-89% of body surface with Ø% to 9% third degree corrosion** COM

T32.81 **Corrosions involving 8Ø-89% of body surface with 1Ø-19% third degree corrosion** HCC ESR COM

T32.82 **Corrosions involving 8Ø-89% of body surface with 2Ø-29% third degree corrosion** HCC ESR COM

T32.83 **Corrosions involving 8Ø-89% of body surface with 3Ø-39% third degree corrosion** HCC ESR COM

T32.84 **Corrosions involving 8Ø-89% of body surface with 4Ø-49% third degree corrosion** HCC ESR COM

T32.85 **Corrosions involving 8Ø-89% of body surface with 5Ø-59% third degree corrosion** HCC ESR COM

T32.86 **Corrosions involving 8Ø-89% of body surface with 6Ø-69% third degree corrosion** HCC ESR COM

T32.87 **Corrosions involving 8Ø-89% of body surface with 7Ø-79% third degree corrosion** HCC ESR COM

T32.88 **Corrosions involving 8Ø-89% of body surface with 8Ø-89% third degree corrosion** HCC ESR COM

✓5th **T32.9** **Corrosions involving 9Ø% or more of body surface**

T32.9Ø **Corrosions involving 9Ø% or more of body surface with Ø% to 9% third degree corrosion** COM

T32.91 **Corrosions involving 9Ø% or more of body surface with 1Ø-19% third degree corrosion** HCC ESR COM

T32.92 **Corrosions involving 9Ø% or more of body surface with 2Ø-29% third degree corrosion** HCC ESR COM

T32.93 **Corrosions involving 9Ø% or more of body surface with 3Ø-39% third degree corrosion** HCC ESR COM

T32.94 **Corrosions involving 9Ø% or more of body surface with 4Ø-49% third degree corrosion** HCC ESR COM

T32.95 **Corrosions involving 9Ø% or more of body surface with 5Ø-59% third degree corrosion** HCC ESR COM

T32.96 **Corrosions involving 9Ø% or more of body surface with 6Ø-69% third degree corrosion** HCC ESR COM

T32.97 **Corrosions involving 9Ø% or more of body surface with 7Ø-79% third degree corrosion** HCC ESR COM

T32.98 **Corrosions involving 9Ø% or more of body surface with 8Ø-89% third degree corrosion** HCC ESR COM

T32.99 **Corrosions involving 9Ø% or more of body surface with 9Ø% or more third degree corrosion** HCC ESR COM

Frostbite (T33-T34)

EXCLUDES 2 *hypothermia and other effects of reduced temperature (T68, T69.-)*

T33 Superficial frostbite

INCLUDES frostbite with partial thickness skin loss

The appropriate 7th character is to be added to each code from category T33.
A initial encounter
D subsequent encounter
S sequela

T33.Ø Superficial frostbite of head
T33.Ø1 Superficial frostbite of ear
T33.Ø11 Superficial frostbite of right ear
T33.Ø12 Superficial frostbite of left ear
T33.Ø19 Superficial frostbite of unspecified ear
T33.Ø2 Superficial frostbite of nose
T33.Ø9 Superficial frostbite of other part of head
T33.1 Superficial frostbite of neck
T33.2 Superficial frostbite of thorax
T33.3 Superficial frostbite of abdominal wall, lower back and pelvis
T33.4 Superficial frostbite of arm
EXCLUDES 2 *superficial frostbite of wrist and hand (T33.5-)*
T33.4Ø Superficial frostbite of unspecified arm
T33.41 Superficial frostbite of right arm
T33.42 Superficial frostbite of left arm
T33.5 Superficial frostbite of wrist, hand, and fingers
T33.51 Superficial frostbite of wrist
T33.511 Superficial frostbite of right wrist
T33.512 Superficial frostbite of left wrist
T33.519 Superficial frostbite of unspecified wrist
T33.52 Superficial frostbite of hand
EXCLUDES 2 *superficial frostbite of fingers (T33.53-)*
T33.521 Superficial frostbite of right hand
T33.522 Superficial frostbite of left hand
T33.529 Superficial frostbite of unspecified hand
T33.53 Superficial frostbite of finger(s)
T33.531 Superficial frostbite of right finger(s)
T33.532 Superficial frostbite of left finger(s)
T33.539 Superficial frostbite of unspecified finger(s)
T33.6 Superficial frostbite of hip and thigh
T33.6Ø Superficial frostbite of unspecified hip and thigh
T33.61 Superficial frostbite of right hip and thigh
T33.62 Superficial frostbite of left hip and thigh
T33.7 Superficial frostbite of knee and lower leg
EXCLUDES 2 *superficial frostbite of ankle and foot (T33.8-)*
T33.7Ø Superficial frostbite of unspecified knee and lower leg
T33.71 Superficial frostbite of right knee and lower leg
T33.72 Superficial frostbite of left knee and lower leg
T33.8 Superficial frostbite of ankle, foot, and toe(s)
T33.81 Superficial frostbite of ankle
T33.811 Superficial frostbite of right ankle
T33.812 Superficial frostbite of left ankle
T33.819 Superficial frostbite of unspecified ankle
T33.82 Superficial frostbite of foot
T33.821 Superficial frostbite of right foot
T33.822 Superficial frostbite of left foot
T33.829 Superficial frostbite of unspecified foot
T33.83 Superficial frostbite of toe(s)
T33.831 Superficial frostbite of right toe(s)
T33.832 Superficial frostbite of left toe(s)
T33.839 Superficial frostbite of unspecified toe(s)
T33.9 Superficial frostbite of other and unspecified sites
T33.9Ø Superficial frostbite of unspecified sites
Superficial frostbite NOS
T33.99 Superficial frostbite of other sites
Superficial frostbite of leg NOS
Superficial frostbite of trunk NOS

T34 Frostbite with tissue necrosis

The appropriate 7th character is to be added to each code from category T34.
A initial encounter
D subsequent encounter
S sequela

T34.Ø Frostbite with tissue necrosis of head
T34.Ø1 Frostbite with tissue necrosis of ear
T34.Ø11 Frostbite with tissue necrosis of right ear COM
T34.Ø12 Frostbite with tissue necrosis of left ear COM
T34.Ø19 Frostbite with tissue necrosis of unspecified ear COM
T34.Ø2 Frostbite with tissue necrosis of nose COM
T34.Ø9 Frostbite with tissue necrosis of other part of head COM
T34.1 Frostbite with tissue necrosis of neck COM
T34.2 Frostbite with tissue necrosis of thorax COM
T34.3 Frostbite with tissue necrosis of abdominal wall, lower back and pelvis COM
T34.4 Frostbite with tissue necrosis of arm
EXCLUDES 2 *frostbite with tissue necrosis of wrist and hand (T34.5-)*
T34.4Ø Frostbite with tissue necrosis of unspecified arm COM
T34.41 Frostbite with tissue necrosis of right arm COM
T34.42 Frostbite with tissue necrosis of left arm COM
T34.5 Frostbite with tissue necrosis of wrist, hand, and finger(s)
T34.51 Frostbite with tissue necrosis of wrist
T34.511 Frostbite with tissue necrosis of right wrist COM
T34.512 Frostbite with tissue necrosis of left wrist COM
T34.519 Frostbite with tissue necrosis of unspecified wrist COM
T34.52 Frostbite with tissue necrosis of hand
EXCLUDES 2 *frostbite with tissue necrosis of finger(s) (T34.53-)*
T34.521 Frostbite with tissue necrosis of right hand COM
T34.522 Frostbite with tissue necrosis of left hand COM
T34.529 Frostbite with tissue necrosis of unspecified hand COM
T34.53 Frostbite with tissue necrosis of finger(s)
T34.531 Frostbite with tissue necrosis of right finger(s) COM
T34.532 Frostbite with tissue necrosis of left finger(s) COM
T34.539 Frostbite with tissue necrosis of unspecified finger(s) COM
T34.6 Frostbite with tissue necrosis of hip and thigh
T34.6Ø Frostbite with tissue necrosis of unspecified hip and thigh COM
T34.61 Frostbite with tissue necrosis of right hip and thigh COM
T34.62 Frostbite with tissue necrosis of left hip and thigh COM
T34.7 Frostbite with tissue necrosis of knee and lower leg
EXCLUDES 2 *frostbite with tissue necrosis of ankle and foot (T34.8-)*
T34.7Ø Frostbite with tissue necrosis of unspecified knee and lower leg COM
T34.71 Frostbite with tissue necrosis of right knee and lower leg COM
T34.72 Frostbite with tissue necrosis of left knee and lower leg COM
T34.8 Frostbite with tissue necrosis of ankle, foot, and toe(s)
T34.81 Frostbite with tissue necrosis of ankle
T34.811 Frostbite with tissue necrosis of right ankle COM

Chapter 19. Injury, Poisoning and Certain Other Consequences of External Causes

T33–T34.811

T34.812 **Frostbite with tissue necrosis of left ankle** COM

T34.819 **Frostbite with tissue necrosis of unspecified ankle** COM

T34.82 **Frostbite with tissue necrosis of foot**

T34.821 **Frostbite with tissue necrosis of right foot**

T34.822 **Frostbite with tissue necrosis of left foot**

T34.829 **Frostbite with tissue necrosis of unspecified foot**

T34.83 **Frostbite with tissue necrosis of toe(s)**

T34.831 **Frostbite with tissue necrosis of right toe(s)**

T34.832 **Frostbite with tissue necrosis of left toe(s)**

T34.839 **Frostbite with tissue necrosis of unspecified toe(s)**

T34.9 **Frostbite with tissue necrosis of other and unspecified sites**

T34.90 **Frostbite with tissue necrosis of unspecified sites**

Frostbite with tissue necrosis NOS

T34.99 **Frostbite with tissue necrosis of other sites**

Frostbite with tissue necrosis of leg NOS

Frostbite with tissue necrosis of trunk NOS

Poisoning by, adverse effects of and underdosing of drugs, medicaments and biological substances (T36-T50)

INCLUDES adverse effect of correct substance properly administered
poisoning by overdose of substance
poisoning by wrong substance given or taken in error
underdosing by (inadvertently) (deliberately) taking less substance than prescribed or instructed

Code first, for adverse effects, the nature of the adverse effect, such as:
- adverse effect NOS (T88.7)
- aspirin gastritis (K29.-)
- blood disorders (D56-D76)
- contact dermatitis (L23-L25)
- dermatitis due to substances taken internally (L27.-)
- nephropathy (N14.0-N14.2)

NOTE The drug giving rise to the adverse effect should be identified by use of codes from categories T36-T50 with fifth or sixth character 5.

Use additional code(s) to specify:
- manifestations of poisoning
- underdosing or failure in dosage during medical and surgical care (Y63.6, Y63.8-Y63.9)
- underdosing of medication regimen (Z91.12-, Z91.13-)

EXCLUDES 1 *toxic reaction to local anesthesia in pregnancy (O29.3-)*

EXCLUDES 2 *abuse and dependence of psychoactive substances (F10-F19)*
abuse of non-dependence-producing substances (F55.-)
drug reaction and poisoning affecting newborn (P00-P96)
immunodeficiency due to drugs (D84.821)
pathological drug intoxication (inebriation) (F10-F19)

AHA: 2018,4Q,71; 2016,2Q,8; 2015,3Q,22

T36 **Poisoning by, adverse effect of and underdosing of systemic antibiotics**

EXCLUDES 1 *antineoplastic antibiotics (T45.1-)*
locally applied antibiotic NEC (T49.0)
topically used antibiotic for ear, nose and throat (T49.6)
topically used antibiotic for eye (T49.5)

The appropriate 7th character is to be added to each code from category T36.
- A initial encounter
- D subsequent encounter
- S sequela

T36.0 **Poisoning by, adverse effect of and underdosing of penicillins**

T36.0X **Poisoning by, adverse effect of and underdosing of penicillins**

T36.0X1 **Poisoning by penicillins, accidental (unintentional)**

Poisoning by penicillins NOS

T36.0X2 **Poisoning by penicillins, intentional self-harm** HCC Rx ESR COM

T36.0X3 **Poisoning by penicillins, assault**

T36.0X4 **Poisoning by penicillins, undetermined**

T36.0X5 **Adverse effect of penicillins** UPD

T36.0X6 **Underdosing of penicillins** UPD

T36.1 **Poisoning by, adverse effect of and underdosing of cephalosporins and other beta-lactam antibiotics**

T36.1X **Poisoning by, adverse effect of and underdosing of cephalosporins and other beta-lactam antibiotics**

T36.1X1 **Poisoning by cephalosporins and other beta-lactam antibiotics, accidental (unintentional)**

Poisoning by cephalosporins and other beta-lactam antibiotics NOS

T36.1X2 **Poisoning by cephalosporins and other beta-lactam antibiotics, intentional self-harm** HCC Rx ESR COM

T36.1X3 **Poisoning by cephalosporins and other beta-lactam antibiotics, assault**

T36.1X4 **Poisoning by cephalosporins and other beta-lactam antibiotics, undetermined**

T36.1X5 **Adverse effect of cephalosporins and other beta-lactam antibiotics** UPD

T36.1X6 **Underdosing of cephalosporins and other beta-lactam antibiotics** UPD

T36.2 **Poisoning by, adverse effect of and underdosing of chloramphenicol group**

T36.2X **Poisoning by, adverse effect of and underdosing of chloramphenicol group**

T36.2X1 **Poisoning by chloramphenicol group, accidental (unintentional)**

Poisoning by chloramphenicol group NOS

T36.2X2 **Poisoning by chloramphenicol group, intentional self-harm** HCC Rx ESR COM

T36.2X3 **Poisoning by chloramphenicol group, assault**

T36.2X4 **Poisoning by chloramphenicol group, undetermined**

T36.2X5 **Adverse effect of chloramphenicol group** UPD

T36.2X6 **Underdosing of chloramphenicol group** UPD

T36.3 **Poisoning by, adverse effect of and underdosing of macrolides**

T36.3X **Poisoning by, adverse effect of and underdosing of macrolides**

T36.3X1 **Poisoning by macrolides, accidental (unintentional)**

Poisoning by macrolides NOS

T36.3X2 **Poisoning by macrolides, intentional self-harm** HCC Rx ESR COM

T36.3X3 **Poisoning by macrolides, assault**

T36.3X4 **Poisoning by macrolides, undetermined**

T36.3X5 **Adverse effect of macrolides** UPD

T36.3X6 **Underdosing of macrolides** UPD

T36.4 **Poisoning by, adverse effect of and underdosing of tetracyclines**

T36.4X **Poisoning by, adverse effect of and underdosing of tetracyclines**

T36.4X1 **Poisoning by tetracyclines, accidental (unintentional)**

Poisoning by tetracyclines NOS

T36.4X2 **Poisoning by tetracyclines, intentional self-harm** HCC Rx ESR COM

T36.4X3 **Poisoning by tetracyclines, assault**

T36.4X4 **Poisoning by tetracyclines, undetermined**

T36.4X5 **Adverse effect of tetracyclines** UPD

T36.4X6 **Underdosing of tetracyclines** UPD

T36.5 **Poisoning by, adverse effect of and underdosing of aminoglycosides**

Poisoning by, adverse effect of and underdosing of streptomycin

T36.5X **Poisoning by, adverse effect of and underdosing of aminoglycosides**

T36.5X1 **Poisoning by aminoglycosides, accidental (unintentional)**

Poisoning by aminoglycosides NOS

T36.5X2 **Poisoning by aminoglycosides, intentional self-harm** HCC Rx ESR COM

T36.5X3 **Poisoning by aminoglycosides, assault**

T36.5X4 **Poisoning by aminoglycosides, undetermined**

T36.5X5 **Adverse effect of aminoglycosides** UPD

T36.5X6 **Underdosing of aminoglycosides** UPD

T36.6 Poisoning by, adverse effect of and underdosing of rifampicins

T36.6X Poisoning by, adverse effect of and underdosing of rifampicins

T36.6X1 Poisoning by rifampicins, accidental (unintentional)
Poisoning by rifampicins NOS

2 **T36.6X2 Poisoning by rifampicins, intentional self-harm** HCC Rx ESR COM

T36.6X3 Poisoning by rifampicins, assault

T36.6X4 Poisoning by rifampicins, undetermined

T36.6X5 Adverse effect of rifampicins UPD

T36.6X6 Underdosing of rifampicins UPD

T36.7 Poisoning by, adverse effect of and underdosing of antifungal antibiotics, systemically used

T36.7X Poisoning by, adverse effect of and underdosing of antifungal antibiotics, systemically used

T36.7X1 Poisoning by antifungal antibiotics, systemically used, accidental (unintentional)
Poisoning by antifungal antibiotics, systemically used NOS

2 **T36.7X2 Poisoning by antifungal antibiotics, systemically used, intentional self-harm** HCC Rx ESR COM

T36.7X3 Poisoning by antifungal antibiotics, systemically used, assault

T36.7X4 Poisoning by antifungal antibiotics, systemically used, undetermined

T36.7X5 Adverse effect of antifungal antibiotics, systemically used UPD

T36.7X6 Underdosing of antifungal antibiotics, systemically used UPD

T36.8 Poisoning by, adverse effect of and underdosing of other systemic antibiotics

T36.8X Poisoning by, adverse effect of and underdosing of other systemic antibiotics
AHA: 2017,1Q,39

T36.8X1 Poisoning by other systemic antibiotics, accidental (unintentional)
Poisoning by other systemic antibiotics NOS

2 **T36.8X2 Poisoning by other systemic antibiotics, intentional self-harm** HCC Rx ESR COM

T36.8X3 Poisoning by other systemic antibiotics, assault

T36.8X4 Poisoning by other systemic antibiotics, undetermined

T36.8X5 Adverse effect of other systemic antibiotics UPD

T36.8X6 Underdosing of other systemic antibiotics UPD

T36.9 Poisoning by, adverse effect of and underdosing of unspecified systemic antibiotic

T36.91 Poisoning by unspecified systemic antibiotic, accidental (unintentional)
Poisoning by systemic antibiotic NOS

2 **T36.92 Poisoning by unspecified systemic antibiotic, intentional self-harm** HCC Rx ESR COM

T36.93 Poisoning by unspecified systemic antibiotic, assault

T36.94 Poisoning by unspecified systemic antibiotic, undetermined

T36.95 Adverse effect of unspecified systemic antibiotic UPD

T36.96 Underdosing of unspecified systemic antibiotic UPD

T37 Poisoning by, adverse effect of and underdosing of other systemic anti-infectives and antiparasitics

EXCLUDES 1 *anti-infectives topically used for ear, nose and throat (T49.6-)*
anti-infectives topically used for eye (T49.5-)
locally applied anti-infectives NEC (T49.Ø-)

The appropriate 7th character is to be added to each code from category T37.
A initial encounter
D subsequent encounter
S sequela

T37.Ø Poisoning by, adverse effect of and underdosing of sulfonamides

T37.ØX Poisoning by, adverse effect of and underdosing of sulfonamides

T37.ØX1 Poisoning by sulfonamides, accidental (unintentional)
Poisoning by sulfonamides NOS

2 **T37.ØX2 Poisoning by sulfonamides, intentional self-harm** HCC Rx ESR COM

T37.ØX3 Poisoning by sulfonamides, assault

T37.ØX4 Poisoning by sulfonamides, undetermined

T37.ØX5 Adverse effect of sulfonamides UPD

T37.ØX6 Underdosing of sulfonamides UPD

T37.1 Poisoning by, adverse effect of and underdosing of antimycobacterial drugs

EXCLUDES 1 *rifampicins (T36.6-)*
streptomycin (T36.5-)

T37.1X Poisoning by, adverse effect of and underdosing of antimycobacterial drugs

T37.1X1 Poisoning by antimycobacterial drugs, accidental (unintentional)
Poisoning by antimycobacterial drugs NOS

2 **T37.1X2 Poisoning by antimycobacterial drugs, intentional self-harm** HCC Rx ESR COM

T37.1X3 Poisoning by antimycobacterial drugs, assault

T37.1X4 Poisoning by antimycobacterial drugs, undetermined

T37.1X5 Adverse effect of antimycobacterial drugs UPD

T37.1X6 Underdosing of antimycobacterial drugs UPD

T37.2 Poisoning by, adverse effect of and underdosing of antimalarials and drugs acting on other blood protozoa

EXCLUDES 1 *hydroxyquinoline derivatives (T37.8-)*

T37.2X Poisoning by, adverse effect of and underdosing of antimalarials and drugs acting on other blood protozoa

T37.2X1 Poisoning by antimalarials and drugs acting on other blood protozoa, accidental (unintentional)
Poisoning by antimalarials and drugs acting on other blood protozoa NOS

2 **T37.2X2 Poisoning by antimalarials and drugs acting on other blood protozoa, intentional self-harm** HCC Rx ESR COM

T37.2X3 Poisoning by antimalarials and drugs acting on other blood protozoa, assault

T37.2X4 Poisoning by antimalarials and drugs acting on other blood protozoa, undetermined

T37.2X5 Adverse effect of antimalarials and drugs acting on other blood protozoa UPD

T37.2X6 Underdosing of antimalarials and drugs acting on other blood protozoa UPD

T37.3 Poisoning by, adverse effect of and underdosing of other antiprotozoal drugs

T37.3X Poisoning by, adverse effect of and underdosing of other antiprotozoal drugs

T37.3X1 Poisoning by other antiprotozoal drugs, accidental (unintentional)
Poisoning by other antiprotozoal drugs NOS

2 **T37.3X2 Poisoning by other antiprotozoal drugs, intentional self-harm** HCC Rx ESR COM

T37.3X3 Poisoning by other antiprotozoal drugs, assault

T37.3X4 Poisoning by other antiprotozoal drugs, undetermined

Chapter 19. Injury, Poisoning and Certain Other Consequences of External Causes

T36.6–T37.3X4

7th **T37.3X5 Adverse effect of other antiprotozoal drugs** UPD

7th **T37.3X6 Underdosing of other antiprotozoal drugs** UPD

5th **T37.4 Poisoning by, adverse effect of and underdosing of anthelminthics**

6th **T37.4X Poisoning by, adverse effect of and underdosing of anthelminthics**

7th **T37.4X1 Poisoning by anthelminthics, accidental (unintentional)**
Poisoning by anthelminthics NOS

2 7th **T37.4X2 Poisoning by anthelminthics, intentional self-harm** HCC Rx ESR COM

7th **T37.4X3 Poisoning by anthelminthics, assault**

7th **T37.4X4 Poisoning by anthelminthics, undetermined**

7th **T37.4X5 Adverse effect of anthelminthics** UPD

7th **T37.4X6 Underdosing of anthelminthics** UPD

5th **T37.5 Poisoning by, adverse effect of and underdosing of antiviral drugs**
EXCLUDES 1 *amantadine (T42.8-)*
cytarabine (T45.1-)

6th **T37.5X Poisoning by, adverse effect of and underdosing of antiviral drugs**

7th **T37.5X1 Poisoning by antiviral drugs, accidental (unintentional)**
Poisoning by antiviral drugs NOS

2 7th **T37.5X2 Poisoning by antiviral drugs, intentional self-harm** HCC Rx ESR COM

7th **T37.5X3 Poisoning by antiviral drugs, assault**

7th **T37.5X4 Poisoning by antiviral drugs, undetermined**

7th **T37.5X5 Adverse effect of antiviral drugs** UPD

7th **T37.5X6 Underdosing of antiviral drugs** UPD

5th **T37.8 Poisoning by, adverse effect of and underdosing of other specified systemic anti-infectives and antiparasitics**
Poisoning by, adverse effect of and underdosing of hydroxyquinoline derivatives
EXCLUDES 1 *antimalarial drugs (T37.2-)*

6th **T37.8X Poisoning by, adverse effect of and underdosing of other specified systemic anti-infectives and antiparasitics**

7th **T37.8X1 Poisoning by other specified systemic anti-infectives and antiparasitics, accidental (unintentional)**
Poisoning by other specified systemic anti-infectives and antiparasitics NOS

2 7th **T37.8X2 Poisoning by other specified systemic anti-infectives and antiparasitics, intentional self-harm** HCC Rx ESR COM

7th **T37.8X3 Poisoning by other specified systemic anti-infectives and antiparasitics, assault**

7th **T37.8X4 Poisoning by other specified systemic anti-infectives and antiparasitics, undetermined**

7th **T37.8X5 Adverse effect of other specified systemic anti-infectives and antiparasitics** UPD

7th **T37.8X6 Underdosing of other specified systemic anti-infectives and antiparasitics** UPD

5th **T37.9 Poisoning by, adverse effect of and underdosing of unspecified systemic anti-infective and antiparasitics**

x7th **T37.91 Poisoning by unspecified systemic anti-infective and antiparasitics, accidental (unintentional)**
Poisoning by, adverse effect of and underdosing of systemic anti-infective and antiparasitics NOS

2 x7th **T37.92 Poisoning by unspecified systemic anti-infective and antiparasitics, intentional self-harm** HCC Rx ESR COM

x7th **T37.93 Poisoning by unspecified systemic anti-infective and antiparasitics, assault**

x7th **T37.94 Poisoning by unspecified systemic anti-infective and antiparasitics, undetermined**

x7th **T37.95 Adverse effect of unspecified systemic anti-infective and antiparasitic** UPD

x7th **T37.96 Underdosing of unspecified systemic anti-infectives and antiparasitics** UPD

4th **T38 Poisoning by, adverse effect of and underdosing of hormones and their synthetic substitutes and antagonists, not elsewhere classified**
EXCLUDES 1 *mineralocorticoids and their antagonists (T50.0-)*
oxytocic hormones (T48.0-)
parathyroid hormones and derivatives (T50.9-)

The appropriate 7th character is to be added to each code from category T38.
A initial encounter
D subsequent encounter
S sequela

5th **T38.0 Poisoning by, adverse effect of and underdosing of glucocorticoids and synthetic analogues**
EXCLUDES 1 *glucocorticoids, topically used (T49.-)*

6th **T38.0X Poisoning by, adverse effect of and underdosing of glucocorticoids and synthetic analogues**

7th **T38.0X1 Poisoning by glucocorticoids and synthetic analogues, accidental (unintentional)**
Poisoning by glucocorticoids and synthetic analogues NOS

2 7th **T38.0X2 Poisoning by glucocorticoids and synthetic analogues, intentional self-harm** HCC Rx ESR COM

7th **T38.0X3 Poisoning by glucocorticoids and synthetic analogues, assault**

7th **T38.0X4 Poisoning by glucocorticoids and synthetic analogues, undetermined**

7th **T38.0X5 Adverse effect of glucocorticoids and synthetic analogues** UPD

7th **T38.0X6 Underdosing of glucocorticoids and synthetic analogues** UPD

5th **T38.1 Poisoning by, adverse effect of and underdosing of thyroid hormones and substitutes**

6th **T38.1X Poisoning by, adverse effect of and underdosing of thyroid hormones and substitutes**

7th **T38.1X1 Poisoning by thyroid hormones and substitutes, accidental (unintentional)**
Poisoning by thyroid hormones and substitutes NOS

2 7th **T38.1X2 Poisoning by thyroid hormones and substitutes, intentional self-harm** HCC Rx ESR COM

7th **T38.1X3 Poisoning by thyroid hormones and substitutes, assault**

7th **T38.1X4 Poisoning by thyroid hormones and substitutes, undetermined**

7th **T38.1X5 Adverse effect of thyroid hormones and substitutes** UPD

7th **T38.1X6 Underdosing of thyroid hormones and substitutes** UPD

5th **T38.2 Poisoning by, adverse effect of and underdosing of antithyroid drugs**

6th **T38.2X Poisoning by, adverse effect of and underdosing of antithyroid drugs**

7th **T38.2X1 Poisoning by antithyroid drugs, accidental (unintentional)**
Poisoning by antithyroid drugs NOS

2 7th **T38.2X2 Poisoning by antithyroid drugs, intentional self-harm** HCC Rx ESR COM

7th **T38.2X3 Poisoning by antithyroid drugs, assault**

7th **T38.2X4 Poisoning by antithyroid drugs, undetermined**

7th **T38.2X5 Adverse effect of antithyroid drugs** UPD

7th **T38.2X6 Underdosing of antithyroid drugs** UPD

5th **T38.3 Poisoning by, adverse effect of and underdosing of insulin and oral hypoglycemic [antidiabetic] drugs**

6th **T38.3X Poisoning by, adverse effect of and underdosing of insulin and oral hypoglycemic [antidiabetic] drugs**

7th **T38.3X1 Poisoning by insulin and oral hypoglycemic [antidiabetic] drugs, accidental (unintentional)**
Poisoning by insulin and oral hypoglycemic [antidiabetic] drugs NOS

2 7th **T38.3X2 Poisoning by insulin and oral hypoglycemic [antidiabetic] drugs, intentional self-harm** HCC Rx ESR COM

✓7th **T38.3X3 Poisoning by insulin and oral hypoglycemic [antidiabetic] drugs, assault**

✓7th **T38.3X4 Poisoning by insulin and oral hypoglycemic [antidiabetic] drugs, undetermined**

✓7th **T38.3X5 Adverse effect of insulin and oral hypoglycemic [antidiabetic] drugs** UPD

✓7th **T38.3X6 Underdosing of insulin and oral hypoglycemic [antidiabetic] drugs** UPD

✓5th **T38.4 Poisoning by, adverse effect of and underdosing of oral contraceptives**

Poisoning by, adverse effect of and underdosing of multiple- and single-ingredient oral contraceptive preparations

✓6th **T38.4X Poisoning by, adverse effect of and underdosing of oral contraceptives**

✓7th **T38.4X1 Poisoning by oral contraceptives, accidental (unintentional)**

Poisoning by oral contraceptives NOS

2 ✓7th **T38.4X2 Poisoning by oral contraceptives, intentional self-harm** HCC Rx ESR COM

✓7th **T38.4X3 Poisoning by oral contraceptives, assault**

✓7th **T38.4X4 Poisoning by oral contraceptives, undetermined**

✓7th **T38.4X5 Adverse effect of oral contraceptives** UPD

✓7th **T38.4X6 Underdosing of oral contraceptives** UPD

✓5th **T38.5 Poisoning by, adverse effect of and underdosing of other estrogens and progestogens**

Poisoning by, adverse effect of and underdosing of estrogens and progestogens mixtures and substitutes

✓6th **T38.5X Poisoning by, adverse effect of and underdosing of other estrogens and progestogens**

✓7th **T38.5X1 Poisoning by other estrogens and progestogens, accidental (unintentional)**

Poisoning by other estrogens and progestogens NOS

2 ✓7th **T38.5X2 Poisoning by other estrogens and progestogens, intentional self-harm** HCC Rx ESR COM

✓7th **T38.5X3 Poisoning by other estrogens and progestogens, assault**

✓7th **T38.5X4 Poisoning by other estrogens and progestogens, undetermined**

✓7th **T38.5X5 Adverse effect of other estrogens and progestogens** UPD

✓7th **T38.5X6 Underdosing of other estrogens and progestogens** UPD

✓5th **T38.6 Poisoning by, adverse effect of and underdosing of antigonadotrophins, antiestrogens, antiandrogens, not elsewhere classified**

Poisoning by, adverse effect of and underdosing of tamoxifen

✓6th **T38.6X Poisoning by, adverse effect of and underdosing of antigonadotrophins, antiestrogens, antiandrogens, not elsewhere classified**

✓7th **T38.6X1 Poisoning by antigonadotrophins, antiestrogens, antiandrogens, not elsewhere classified, accidental (unintentional)**

Poisoning by antigonadotrophins, antiestrogens, antiandrogens, not elsewhere classified NOS

2 ✓7th **T38.6X2 Poisoning by antigonadotrophins, antiestrogens, antiandrogens, not elsewhere classified, intentional self-harm** HCC Rx ESR COM

✓7th **T38.6X3 Poisoning by antigonadotrophins, antiestrogens, antiandrogens, not elsewhere classified, assault**

✓7th **T38.6X4 Poisoning by antigonadotrophins, antiestrogens, antiandrogens, not elsewhere classified, undetermined**

✓7th **T38.6X5 Adverse effect of antigonadotrophins, antiestrogens, antiandrogens, not elsewhere classified** UPD

✓7th **T38.6X6 Underdosing of antigonadotrophins, antiestrogens, antiandrogens, not elsewhere classified** UPD

✓5th **T38.7 Poisoning by, adverse effect of and underdosing of androgens and anabolic congeners**

✓6th **T38.7X Poisoning by, adverse effect of and underdosing of androgens and anabolic congeners**

✓7th **T38.7X1 Poisoning by androgens and anabolic congeners, accidental (unintentional)**

Poisoning by androgens and anabolic congeners NOS

2 ✓7th **T38.7X2 Poisoning by androgens and anabolic congeners, intentional self-harm** HCC Rx ESR COM

✓7th **T38.7X3 Poisoning by androgens and anabolic congeners, assault**

✓7th **T38.7X4 Poisoning by androgens and anabolic congeners, undetermined**

✓7th **T38.7X5 Adverse effect of androgens and anabolic congeners** UPD

✓7th **T38.7X6 Underdosing of androgens and anabolic congeners** UPD

✓5th **T38.8 Poisoning by, adverse effect of and underdosing of other and unspecified hormones and synthetic substitutes**

✓6th **T38.80 Poisoning by, adverse effect of and underdosing of unspecified hormones and synthetic substitutes**

✓7th **T38.801 Poisoning by unspecified hormones and synthetic substitutes, accidental (unintentional)**

Poisoning by unspecified hormones and synthetic substitutes NOS

2 ✓7th **T38.802 Poisoning by unspecified hormones and synthetic substitutes, intentional self-harm** HCC Rx ESR COM

✓7th **T38.803 Poisoning by unspecified hormones and synthetic substitutes, assault**

✓7th **T38.804 Poisoning by unspecified hormones and synthetic substitutes, undetermined**

✓7th **T38.805 Adverse effect of unspecified hormones and synthetic substitutes** UPD

✓7th **T38.806 Underdosing of unspecified hormones and synthetic substitutes** UPD

✓6th **T38.81 Poisoning by, adverse effect of and underdosing of anterior pituitary [adenohypophyseal] hormones**

✓7th **T38.811 Poisoning by anterior pituitary [adenohypophyseal] hormones, accidental (unintentional)**

Poisoning by anterior pituitary [adenohypophyseal] hormones NOS

2 ✓7th **T38.812 Poisoning by anterior pituitary [adenohypophyseal] hormones, intentional self-harm** HCC Rx ESR COM

✓7th **T38.813 Poisoning by anterior pituitary [adenohypophyseal] hormones, assault**

✓7th **T38.814 Poisoning by anterior pituitary [adenohypophyseal] hormones, undetermined**

✓7th **T38.815 Adverse effect of anterior pituitary [adenohypophyseal] hormones** UPD

✓7th **T38.816 Underdosing of anterior pituitary [adenohypophyseal] hormones** UPD

✓6th **T38.89 Poisoning by, adverse effect of and underdosing of other hormones and synthetic substitutes**

✓7th **T38.891 Poisoning by other hormones and synthetic substitutes, accidental (unintentional)**

Poisoning by other hormones and synthetic substitutes NOS

2 ✓7th **T38.892 Poisoning by other hormones and synthetic substitutes, intentional self-harm** HCC Rx ESR COM

✓7th **T38.893 Poisoning by other hormones and synthetic substitutes, assault**

✓7th **T38.894 Poisoning by other hormones and synthetic substitutes, undetermined**

✓7th **T38.895 Adverse effect of other hormones and synthetic substitutes** UPD

✓7th **T38.896 Underdosing of other hormones and synthetic substitutes** UPD

✓5th T38.9 **Poisoning by, adverse effect of and underdosing of other and unspecified hormone antagonists**

✓6th T38.90 **Poisoning by, adverse effect of and underdosing of unspecified hormone antagonists**

✓7th T38.901 **Poisoning by unspecified hormone antagonists, accidental (unintentional)**
Poisoning by unspecified hormone antagonists NOS

2 ✓7th T38.902 **Poisoning by unspecified hormone antagonists, intentional self-harm** HCC Rx ESR COM

✓7th T38.903 **Poisoning by unspecified hormone antagonists, assault**

✓7th T38.904 **Poisoning by unspecified hormone antagonists, undetermined**

✓7th T38.905 **Adverse effect of unspecified hormone antagonists** UPD

✓7th T38.906 **Underdosing of unspecified hormone antagonists** UPD

✓6th T38.99 **Poisoning by, adverse effect of and underdosing of other hormone antagonists**

✓7th T38.991 **Poisoning by other hormone antagonists, accidental (unintentional)**
Poisoning by other hormone antagonists NOS

2 ✓7th T38.992 **Poisoning by other hormone antagonists, intentional self-harm** HCC Rx ESR COM

✓7th T38.993 **Poisoning by other hormone antagonists, assault**

✓7th T38.994 **Poisoning by other hormone antagonists, undetermined**

✓7th T38.995 **Adverse effect of other hormone antagonists** UPD

✓7th T38.996 **Underdosing of other hormone antagonists** UPD

✓4th T39 **Poisoning by, adverse effect of and underdosing of nonopioid analgesics, antipyretics and antirheumatics**

The appropriate 7th character is to be added to each code from category T39.
A initial encounter
D subsequent encounter
S sequela

✓5th T39.0 **Poisoning by, adverse effect of and underdosing of salicylates**

✓6th T39.01 **Poisoning by, adverse effect of and underdosing of aspirin**
Poisoning by, adverse effect of and underdosing of acetylsalicylic acid

✓7th T39.011 **Poisoning by aspirin, accidental (unintentional)**

2 ✓7th T39.012 **Poisoning by aspirin, intentional self-harm** HCC Rx ESR COM

✓7th T39.013 **Poisoning by aspirin, assault**

✓7th T39.014 **Poisoning by aspirin, undetermined**

✓7th T39.015 **Adverse effect of aspirin** UPD
AHA: 2016,1Q,15

✓7th T39.016 **Underdosing of aspirin** UPD

✓6th T39.09 **Poisoning by, adverse effect of and underdosing of other salicylates**

✓7th T39.091 **Poisoning by salicylates, accidental (unintentional)**
Poisoning by salicylates NOS

2 ✓7th T39.092 **Poisoning by salicylates, intentional self-harm** HCC Rx ESR COM

✓7th T39.093 **Poisoning by salicylates, assault**

✓7th T39.094 **Poisoning by salicylates, undetermined**

✓7th T39.095 **Adverse effect of salicylates** UPD

✓7th T39.096 **Underdosing of salicylates** UPD

✓5th T39.1 **Poisoning by, adverse effect of and underdosing of 4-Aminophenol derivatives**

✓6th T39.1X **Poisoning by, adverse effect of and underdosing of 4-Aminophenol derivatives**

✓7th T39.1X1 **Poisoning by 4-Aminophenol derivatives, accidental (unintentional)**
Poisoning by 4-Aminophenol derivatives NOS

2 ✓7th T39.1X2 **Poisoning by 4-Aminophenol derivatives, intentional self-harm** HCC Rx ESR COM

✓7th T39.1X3 **Poisoning by 4-Aminophenol derivatives, assault**

✓7th T39.1X4 **Poisoning by 4-Aminophenol derivatives, undetermined**

✓7th T39.1X5 **Adverse effect of 4-Aminophenol derivatives** UPD

✓7th T39.1X6 **Underdosing of 4-Aminophenol derivatives** UPD

✓5th T39.2 **Poisoning by, adverse effect of and underdosing of pyrazolone derivatives**

✓6th T39.2X **Poisoning by, adverse effect of and underdosing of pyrazolone derivatives**

✓7th T39.2X1 **Poisoning by pyrazolone derivatives, accidental (unintentional)**
Poisoning by pyrazolone derivatives NOS

2 ✓7th T39.2X2 **Poisoning by pyrazolone derivatives, intentional self-harm** HCC Rx ESR COM

✓7th T39.2X3 **Poisoning by pyrazolone derivatives, assault**

✓7th T39.2X4 **Poisoning by pyrazolone derivatives, undetermined**

✓7th T39.2X5 **Adverse effect of pyrazolone derivatives** UPD

✓7th T39.2X6 **Underdosing of pyrazolone derivatives** UPD

✓5th T39.3 **Poisoning by, adverse effect of and underdosing of other nonsteroidal anti-inflammatory drugs [NSAID]**

✓6th T39.31 **Poisoning by, adverse effect of and underdosing of propionic acid derivatives**
Poisoning by, adverse effect of and underdosing of fenoprofen
Poisoning by, adverse effect of and underdosing of flurbiprofen
Poisoning by, adverse effect of and underdosing of ibuprofen
Poisoning by, adverse effect of and underdosing of ketoprofen
Poisoning by, adverse effect of and underdosing of naproxen
Poisoning by, adverse effect of and underdosing of oxaprozin

✓7th T39.311 **Poisoning by propionic acid derivatives, accidental (unintentional)**

2 ✓7th T39.312 **Poisoning by propionic acid derivatives, intentional self-harm** HCC Rx ESR COM

✓7th T39.313 **Poisoning by propionic acid derivatives, assault**

✓7th T39.314 **Poisoning by propionic acid derivatives, undetermined**

✓7th T39.315 **Adverse effect of propionic acid derivatives** UPD

✓7th T39.316 **Underdosing of propionic acid derivatives** UPD

✓6th T39.39 **Poisoning by, adverse effect of and underdosing of other nonsteroidal anti-inflammatory drugs [NSAID]**

✓7th T39.391 **Poisoning by other nonsteroidal anti-inflammatory drugs [NSAID], accidental (unintentional)**
Poisoning by other nonsteroidal anti-inflammatory drugs NOS

2 ✓7th T39.392 **Poisoning by other nonsteroidal anti-inflammatory drugs [NSAID], intentional self-harm** HCC Rx ESR COM

✓7th T39.393 **Poisoning by other nonsteroidal anti-inflammatory drugs [NSAID], assault**

✓7th T39.394 **Poisoning by other nonsteroidal anti-inflammatory drugs [NSAID], undetermined**

✓7th T39.395 **Adverse effect of other nonsteroidal anti-inflammatory drugs [NSAID]** UPD

✓7th T39.396 **Underdosing of other nonsteroidal anti-inflammatory drugs [NSAID]** UPD

T39.4 Poisoning by, adverse effect of and underdosing of antirheumatics, not elsewhere classified

EXCLUDES 1 *poisoning by, adverse effect of and underdosing of glucocorticoids (T38.0-)*
poisoning by, adverse effect of and underdosing of salicylates (T39.0-)

T39.4X Poisoning by, adverse effect of and underdosing of antirheumatics, not elsewhere classified

T39.4X1 Poisoning by antirheumatics, not elsewhere classified, accidental (unintentional)
Poisoning by antirheumatics, not elsewhere classified NOS

[2] **T39.4X2 Poisoning by antirheumatics, not elsewhere classified, intentional self-harm** HCC Rx ESR COM

T39.4X3 Poisoning by antirheumatics, not elsewhere classified, assault

T39.4X4 Poisoning by antirheumatics, not elsewhere classified, undetermined

T39.4X5 Adverse effect of antirheumatics, not elsewhere classified UPD

T39.4X6 Underdosing of antirheumatics, not elsewhere classified UPD

T39.8 Poisoning by, adverse effect of and underdosing of other nonopioid analgesics and antipyretics, not elsewhere classified

T39.8X Poisoning by, adverse effect of and underdosing of other nonopioid analgesics and antipyretics, not elsewhere classified

T39.8X1 Poisoning by other nonopioid analgesics and antipyretics, not elsewhere classified, accidental (unintentional)
Poisoning by other nonopioid analgesics and antipyretics, not elsewhere classified NOS

[2] **T39.8X2 Poisoning by other nonopioid analgesics and antipyretics, not elsewhere classified, intentional self-harm** HCC Rx ESR COM

T39.8X3 Poisoning by other nonopioid analgesics and antipyretics, not elsewhere classified, assault

T39.8X4 Poisoning by other nonopioid analgesics and antipyretics, not elsewhere classified, undetermined

T39.8X5 Adverse effect of other nonopioid analgesics and antipyretics, not elsewhere classified UPD

T39.8X6 Underdosing of other nonopioid analgesics and antipyretics, not elsewhere classified UPD

T39.9 Poisoning by, adverse effect of and underdosing of unspecified nonopioid analgesic, antipyretic and antirheumatic

T39.91 Poisoning by unspecified nonopioid analgesic, antipyretic and antirheumatic, accidental (unintentional)
Poisoning by nonopioid analgesic, antipyretic and antirheumatic NOS

[2] **T39.92 Poisoning by unspecified nonopioid analgesic, antipyretic and antirheumatic, intentional self-harm** HCC Rx ESR COM

T39.93 Poisoning by unspecified nonopioid analgesic, antipyretic and antirheumatic, assault

T39.94 Poisoning by unspecified nonopioid analgesic, antipyretic and antirheumatic, undetermined

T39.95 Adverse effect of unspecified nonopioid analgesic, antipyretic and antirheumatic UPD

T39.96 Underdosing of unspecified nonopioid analgesic, antipyretic and antirheumatic UPD

T40 Poisoning by, adverse effect of and underdosing of narcotics and psychodysleptics [hallucinogens]

EXCLUDES 2 *drug dependence and related mental and behavioral disorders due to psychoactive substance use (F10.-F19.-)*

The appropriate 7th character is to be added to each code from category T40.
A initial encounter
D subsequent encounter
S sequela

T40.0 Poisoning by, adverse effect of and underdosing of opium

T40.0X Poisoning by, adverse effect of and underdosing of opium

[1] **T40.0X1 Poisoning by opium, accidental (unintentional)** HCC ESR COM
Poisoning by opium NOS

[2] **T40.0X2 Poisoning by opium, intentional self-harm** HCC Rx ESR COM

T40.0X3 Poisoning by opium, assault

[1] **T40.0X4 Poisoning by opium, undetermined** HCC ESR COM

T40.0X5 Adverse effect of opium UPD

T40.0X6 Underdosing of opium UPD

T40.1 Poisoning by and adverse effect of heroin

T40.1X Poisoning by and adverse effect of heroin

[1] **T40.1X1 Poisoning by heroin, accidental (unintentional)** HCC ESR COM
Poisoning by heroin NOS

[2] **T40.1X2 Poisoning by heroin, intentional self-harm** HCC Rx ESR COM

[1] **T40.1X3 Poisoning by heroin, assault**

[1] **T40.1X4 Poisoning by heroin, undetermined** HCC ESR COM

T40.2 Poisoning by, adverse effect of and underdosing of other opioids

T40.2X Poisoning by, adverse effect of and underdosing of other opioids

[1] **T40.2X1 Poisoning by other opioids, accidental (unintentional)** HCC ESR COM
Poisoning by other opioids NOS

[2] **T40.2X2 Poisoning by other opioids, intentional self-harm** HCC Rx ESR COM

T40.2X3 Poisoning by other opioids, assault

[1] **T40.2X4 Poisoning by other opioids, undetermined** HCC ESR COM

T40.2X5 Adverse effect of other opioids UPD
AHA: 2020,2Q,24

T40.2X6 Underdosing of other opioids UPD

T40.3 Poisoning by, adverse effect of and underdosing of methadone

T40.3X Poisoning by, adverse effect of and underdosing of methadone

[1] **T40.3X1 Poisoning by methadone, accidental (unintentional)** HCC ESR COM
Poisoning by methadone NOS

[2] **T40.3X2 Poisoning by methadone, intentional self-harm** HCC Rx ESR COM

T40.3X3 Poisoning by methadone, assault

T40.3X4 Poisoning by methadone, undetermined HCC ESR COM

T40.3X5 Adverse effect of methadone UPD

T40.3X6 Underdosing of methadone UPD

T40.4 Poisoning by, adverse effect of and underdosing of other synthetic narcotics
AHA: 2020,4Q,40

T40.41 Poisoning by, adverse effect of and underdosing of fentanyl or fentanyl analogs

T40.411 Poisoning by fentanyl or fentanyl analogs, accidental (unintentional) HCC ESR COM

T40.412 Poisoning by fentanyl or fentanyl analogs, intentional self-harm HCC Rx ESR COM

T40.413 Poisoning by fentanyl or fentanyl analogs, assault

T40.414 Poisoning by fentanyl or fentanyl analogs, undetermined HCC ESR COM

T40.415 Adverse effect of fentanyl or fentanyl analogs UPD
T40.416 Underdosing of fentanyl or fentanyl analogs UPD
T40.42 Poisoning by, adverse effect of and underdosing of tramadol
T40.421 Poisoning by tramadol, accidental (unintentional) HCC ESR COM
T40.422 Poisoning by tramadol, intentional self-harm HCC Rx ESR COM
T40.423 Poisoning by tramadol, assault
T40.424 Poisoning by tramadol, undetermined HCC ESR COM
T40.425 Adverse effect of tramadol UPD
T40.426 Underdosing of tramadol UPD
T40.49 Poisoning by, adverse effect of and underdosing of other synthetic narcotics
T40.491 Poisoning by other synthetic narcotics, accidental (unintentional) HCC ESR COM
T40.492 Poisoning by other synthetic narcotics, intentional self-harm HCC Rx ESR COM
T40.493 Poisoning by other synthetic narcotics, assault
T40.494 Poisoning by other synthetic narcotics, undetermined HCC ESR COM
T40.495 Adverse effect of other synthetic narcotics UPD
T40.496 Underdosing of other synthetic narcotics UPD
T40.5 Poisoning by, adverse effect of and underdosing of cocaine
T40.5X Poisoning by, adverse effect of and underdosing of cocaine
1 T40.5X1 Poisoning by cocaine, accidental (unintentional) HCC ESR COM
Poisoning by cocaine NOS
AHA: 2016,2Q,8
2 T40.5X2 Poisoning by cocaine, intentional self-harm HCC Rx ESR COM
T40.5X3 Poisoning by cocaine, assault
1 T40.5X4 Poisoning by cocaine, undetermined HCC ESR COM
T40.5X5 Adverse effect of cocaine UPD
T40.5X6 Underdosing of cocaine UPD
T40.6 Poisoning by, adverse effect of and underdosing of other and unspecified narcotics
T40.60 Poisoning by, adverse effect of and underdosing of unspecified narcotics
1 T40.601 Poisoning by unspecified narcotics, accidental (unintentional) HCC ESR COM
Poisoning by narcotics NOS
2 T40.602 Poisoning by unspecified narcotics, intentional self-harm HCC Rx ESR COM
T40.603 Poisoning by unspecified narcotics, assault
1 T40.604 Poisoning by unspecified narcotics, undetermined HCC ESR COM
T40.605 Adverse effect of unspecified narcotics UPD
T40.606 Underdosing of unspecified narcotics UPD
T40.69 Poisoning by, adverse effect of and underdosing of other narcotics
1 T40.691 Poisoning by other narcotics, accidental (unintentional) HCC ESR COM
Poisoning by other narcotics NOS
2 T40.692 Poisoning by other narcotics, intentional self-harm HCC Rx ESR COM
T40.693 Poisoning by other narcotics, assault
1 T40.694 Poisoning by other narcotics, undetermined HCC ESR COM
T40.695 Adverse effect of other narcotics UPD
T40.696 Underdosing of other narcotics UPD

T40.7 Poisoning by, adverse effect of and underdosing of cannabis (derivatives)
T40.71 Poisoning by, adverse effect of and underdosing of cannabis (derivatives)
AHA: 2021,4Q,30
T40.711 Poisoning by cannabis, accidental (unintentional)
T40.712 Poisoning by cannabis, intentional self-harm HCC Rx ESR COM
T40.713 Poisoning by cannabis, assault
T40.714 Poisoning by cannabis, undetermined
T40.715 Adverse effect of cannabis UPD
T40.716 Underdosing of cannabis UPD
T40.72 Poisoning by, adverse effect of and underdosing of synthetic cannabinoids
AHA: 2021,4Q,30
T40.721 Poisoning by synthetic cannabinoids, accidental (unintentional)
T40.722 Poisoning by synthetic cannabinoids, intentional self-harm HCC Rx ESR COM
T40.723 Poisoning by synthetic cannabinoids, assault
T40.724 Poisoning by synthetic cannabinoids, undetermined
T40.725 Adverse effect of synthetic cannabinoids UPD
T40.726 Underdosing of synthetic cannabinoids UPD
T40.8 Poisoning by and adverse effect of lysergide [LSD]
T40.8X Poisoning by and adverse effect of lysergide [LSD]
1 T40.8X1 Poisoning by lysergide [LSD], accidental (unintentional) HCC ESR COM
Poisoning by lysergide [LSD] NOS
2 T40.8X2 Poisoning by lysergide [LSD], intentional self-harm HCC Rx ESR COM
T40.8X3 Poisoning by lysergide [LSD], assault
1 T40.8X4 Poisoning by lysergide [LSD], undetermined HCC ESR COM
T40.9 Poisoning by, adverse effect of and underdosing of other and unspecified psychodysleptics [hallucinogens]
T40.90 Poisoning by, adverse effect of and underdosing of unspecified psychodysleptics [hallucinogens]
1 T40.901 Poisoning by unspecified psychodysleptics [hallucinogens], accidental (unintentional) HCC ESR COM
2 T40.902 Poisoning by unspecified psychodysleptics [hallucinogens], intentional self-harm HCC Rx ESR COM
T40.903 Poisoning by unspecified psychodysleptics [hallucinogens], assault
1 T40.904 Poisoning by unspecified psychodysleptics [hallucinogens], undetermined HCC ESR COM
T40.905 Adverse effect of unspecified psychodysleptics [hallucinogens] UPD
T40.906 Underdosing of unspecified psychodysleptics [hallucinogens] UPD
T40.99 Poisoning by, adverse effect of and underdosing of other psychodysleptics [hallucinogens]
1 T40.991 Poisoning by other psychodysleptics [hallucinogens], accidental (unintentional) HCC ESR COM
Poisoning by other psychodysleptics [hallucinogens] NOS
2 T40.992 Poisoning by other psychodysleptics [hallucinogens], intentional self-harm HCC Rx ESR COM
T40.993 Poisoning by other psychodysleptics [hallucinogens], assault
1 T40.994 Poisoning by other psychodysleptics [hallucinogens], undetermined HCC ESR COM
T40.995 Adverse effect of other psychodysleptics [hallucinogens] UPD
T40.996 Underdosing of other psychodysleptics [hallucinogens] UPD

HCC CMS-HCC Rx Rx HCC ESR ESRD HCC COM Commercial HCC N Newborn: 0 P Pediatric: 0-17 M Maternity: 9-64 A Adult: 15-124

T41 Poisoning by, adverse effect of and underdosing of anesthetics and therapeutic gases

EXCLUDES 1 *benzodiazepines (T42.4-)*
cocaine (T4Ø.5-)
complications of anesthesia during labor and delivery (O74.-)
complications of anesthesia during pregnancy (O29.-)
complications of anesthesia during the puerperium (O89.-)
opioids (T4Ø.Ø-T4Ø.2-)

The appropriate 7th character is to be added to each code from category T41.
A initial encounter
D subsequent encounter
S sequela

T41.Ø Poisoning by, adverse effect of and underdosing of inhaled anesthetics
EXCLUDES 1 *oxygen (T41.5-)*

T41.ØX Poisoning by, adverse effect of and underdosing of inhaled anesthetics

T41.ØX1 Poisoning by inhaled anesthetics, accidental (unintentional)
Poisoning by inhaled anesthetics NOS

2 **T41.ØX2 Poisoning by inhaled anesthetics, intentional self-harm** HCC Rx ESR COM

T41.ØX3 Poisoning by inhaled anesthetics, assault

T41.ØX4 Poisoning by inhaled anesthetics, undetermined

T41.ØX5 Adverse effect of inhaled anesthetics UPD

T41.ØX6 Underdosing of inhaled anesthetics UPD

T41.1 Poisoning by, adverse effect of and underdosing of intravenous anesthetics
Poisoning by, adverse effect of and underdosing of thiobarbiturates

T41.1X Poisoning by, adverse effect of and underdosing of intravenous anesthetics

T41.1X1 Poisoning by intravenous anesthetics, accidental (unintentional)
Poisoning by intravenous anesthetics NOS

2 **T41.1X2 Poisoning by intravenous anesthetics, intentional self-harm** HCC Rx ESR COM

T41.1X3 Poisoning by intravenous anesthetics, assault

T41.1X4 Poisoning by intravenous anesthetics, undetermined

T41.1X5 Adverse effect of intravenous anesthetics UPD

T41.1X6 Underdosing of intravenous anesthetics UPD

T41.2 Poisoning by, adverse effect of and underdosing of other and unspecified general anesthetics

T41.2Ø Poisoning by, adverse effect of and underdosing of unspecified general anesthetics

T41.2Ø1 Poisoning by unspecified general anesthetics, accidental (unintentional)
Poisoning by general anesthetics NOS

2 **T41.2Ø2 Poisoning by unspecified general anesthetics, intentional self-harm** HCC Rx ESR COM

T41.2Ø3 Poisoning by unspecified general anesthetics, assault

T41.2Ø4 Poisoning by unspecified general anesthetics, undetermined

T41.2Ø5 Adverse effect of unspecified general anesthetics UPD
AHA: 2016,4Q,73

T41.2Ø6 Underdosing of unspecified general anesthetics UPD

T41.29 Poisoning by, adverse effect of and underdosing of other general anesthetics

T41.291 Poisoning by other general anesthetics, accidental (unintentional)
Poisoning by other general anesthetics NOS

2 **T41.292 Poisoning by other general anesthetics, intentional self-harm** HCC Rx ESR COM

T41.293 Poisoning by other general anesthetics, assault

T41.294 Poisoning by other general anesthetics, undetermined

T41.295 Adverse effect of other general anesthetics UPD

T41.296 Underdosing of other general anesthetics UPD

T41.3 Poisoning by, adverse effect of and underdosing of local anesthetics
Cocaine (topical)
EXCLUDES 2 *poisoning by cocaine used as a central nervous system stimulant (T4Ø.5X1-T4Ø.5X4)*

T41.3X Poisoning by, adverse effect of and underdosing of local anesthetics

T41.3X1 Poisoning by local anesthetics, accidental (unintentional)
Poisoning by local anesthetics NOS

2 **T41.3X2 Poisoning by local anesthetics, intentional self-harm** HCC Rx ESR COM

T41.3X3 Poisoning by local anesthetics, assault

T41.3X4 Poisoning by local anesthetics, undetermined

T41.3X5 Adverse effect of local anesthetics UPD

T41.3X6 Underdosing of local anesthetics UPD

T41.4 Poisoning by, adverse effect of and underdosing of unspecified anesthetic

T41.41 Poisoning by unspecified anesthetic, accidental (unintentional)
Poisoning by anesthetic NOS

2 **T41.42 Poisoning by unspecified anesthetic, intentional self-harm** HCC Rx ESR COM

T41.43 Poisoning by unspecified anesthetic, assault

T41.44 Poisoning by unspecified anesthetic, undetermined

T41.45 Adverse effect of unspecified anesthetic UPD

T41.46 Underdosing of unspecified anesthetics UPD

T41.5 Poisoning by, adverse effect of and underdosing of therapeutic gases

T41.5X Poisoning by, adverse effect of and underdosing of therapeutic gases

T41.5X1 Poisoning by therapeutic gases, accidental (unintentional)
Poisoning by therapeutic gases NOS

2 **T41.5X2 Poisoning by therapeutic gases, intentional self-harm** HCC Rx ESR COM

T41.5X3 Poisoning by therapeutic gases, assault

T41.5X4 Poisoning by therapeutic gases, undetermined

T41.5X5 Adverse effect of therapeutic gases UPD

T41.5X6 Underdosing of therapeutic gases UPD

T42 Poisoning by, adverse effect of and underdosing of antiepileptic, sedative- hypnotic and antiparkinsonism drugs

EXCLUDES 2 *drug dependence and related mental and behavioral disorders due to psychoactive substance use (F1Ø.- - F19.-)*

The appropriate 7th character is to be added to each code from category T42.
A initial encounter
D subsequent encounter
S sequela

T42.Ø Poisoning by, adverse effect of and underdosing of hydantoin derivatives

T42.ØX Poisoning by, adverse effect of and underdosing of hydantoin derivatives

T42.ØX1 Poisoning by hydantoin derivatives, accidental (unintentional)
Poisoning by hydantoin derivatives NOS

2 **T42.ØX2 Poisoning by hydantoin derivatives, intentional self-harm** HCC Rx ESR COM

T42.ØX3 Poisoning by hydantoin derivatives, assault

T42.ØX4 Poisoning by hydantoin derivatives, undetermined

T42.ØX5 Adverse effect of hydantoin derivatives UPD

T42.ØX6 Underdosing of hydantoin derivatives UPD

T42.1 Poisoning by, adverse effect of and underdosing of iminostilbenes
Poisoning by, adverse effect of and underdosing of carbamazepine

T42.1X Poisoning by, adverse effect of and underdosing of iminostilbenes

T42.1X1 Poisoning by iminostilbenes, accidental (unintentional)
Poisoning by iminostilbenes NOS

T42.1X2 Poisoning by iminostilbenes, intentional self-harm [2] HCC Rx ESR COM

T42.1X3 Poisoning by iminostilbenes, assault

T42.1X4 Poisoning by iminostilbenes, undetermined

T42.1X5 Adverse effect of iminostilbenes UPD

T42.1X6 Underdosing of iminostilbenes UPD

T42.2 Poisoning by, adverse effect of and underdosing of succinimides and oxazolidinediones

T42.2X Poisoning by, adverse effect of and underdosing of succinimides and oxazolidinediones

T42.2X1 Poisoning by succinimides and oxazolidinediones, accidental (unintentional)
Poisoning by succinimides and oxazolidinediones NOS

T42.2X2 Poisoning by succinimides and oxazolidinediones, intentional self-harm [2] HCC Rx ESR COM

T42.2X3 Poisoning by succinimides and oxazolidinediones, assault

T42.2X4 Poisoning by succinimides and oxazolidinediones, undetermined

T42.2X5 Adverse effect of succinimides and oxazolidinediones UPD

T42.2X6 Underdosing of succinimides and oxazolidinediones UPD

T42.3 Poisoning by, adverse effect of and underdosing of barbiturates
EXCLUDES 1 *poisoning by, adverse effect of and underdosing of thiobarbiturates (T41.1-)*

T42.3X Poisoning by, adverse effect of and underdosing of barbiturates

T42.3X1 Poisoning by barbiturates, accidental (unintentional)
Poisoning by barbiturates NOS

T42.3X2 Poisoning by barbiturates, intentional self-harm [2] HCC Rx ESR COM

T42.3X3 Poisoning by barbiturates, assault

T42.3X4 Poisoning by barbiturates, undetermined

T42.3X5 Adverse effect of barbiturates UPD

T42.3X6 Underdosing of barbiturates UPD

T42.4 Poisoning by, adverse effect of and underdosing of benzodiazepines

T42.4X Poisoning by, adverse effect of and underdosing of benzodiazepines

T42.4X1 Poisoning by benzodiazepines, accidental (unintentional)
Poisoning by benzodiazepines NOS

T42.4X2 Poisoning by benzodiazepines, intentional self-harm [2] HCC Rx ESR COM

T42.4X3 Poisoning by benzodiazepines, assault

T42.4X4 Poisoning by benzodiazepines, undetermined

T42.4X5 Adverse effect of benzodiazepines UPD

T42.4X6 Underdosing of benzodiazepines UPD

T42.5 Poisoning by, adverse effect of and underdosing of mixed antiepileptics

T42.5X Poisoning by, adverse effect of and underdosing of antiepileptics

T42.5X1 Poisoning by mixed antiepileptics, accidental (unintentional)
Poisoning by mixed antiepileptics NOS

T42.5X2 Poisoning by mixed antiepileptics, intentional self-harm [2] HCC Rx ESR COM

T42.5X3 Poisoning by mixed antiepileptics, assault

T42.5X4 Poisoning by mixed antiepileptics, undetermined

T42.5X5 Adverse effect of mixed antiepileptics UPD

T42.5X6 Underdosing of mixed antiepileptics UPD

T42.6 Poisoning by, adverse effect of and underdosing of other antiepileptic and sedative-hypnotic drugs
Poisoning by, adverse effect of and underdosing of methaqualone
Poisoning by, adverse effect of and underdosing of valproic acid
EXCLUDES 1 *poisoning by, adverse effect of and underdosing of carbamazepine (T42.1-)*

T42.6X Poisoning by, adverse effect of and underdosing of other antiepileptic and sedative-hypnotic drugs

T42.6X1 Poisoning by other antiepileptic and sedative-hypnotic drugs, accidental (unintentional)
Poisoning by other antiepileptic and sedative-hypnotic drugs NOS

T42.6X2 Poisoning by other antiepileptic and sedative-hypnotic drugs, intentional self-harm [2] HCC Rx ESR COM

T42.6X3 Poisoning by other antiepileptic and sedative-hypnotic drugs, assault

T42.6X4 Poisoning by other antiepileptic and sedative-hypnotic drugs, undetermined

T42.6X5 Adverse effect of other antiepileptic and sedative-hypnotic drugs UPD

T42.6X6 Underdosing of other antiepileptic and sedative-hypnotic drugs UPD

T42.7 Poisoning by, adverse effect of and underdosing of unspecified antiepileptic and sedative-hypnotic drugs

T42.71 Poisoning by unspecified antiepileptic and sedative-hypnotic drugs, accidental (unintentional)
Poisoning by antiepileptic and sedative-hypnotic drugs NOS

T42.72 Poisoning by unspecified antiepileptic and sedative-hypnotic drugs, intentional self-harm [2] HCC Rx ESR COM

T42.73 Poisoning by unspecified antiepileptic and sedative-hypnotic drugs, assault

T42.74 Poisoning by unspecified antiepileptic and sedative-hypnotic drugs, undetermined

T42.75 Adverse effect of unspecified antiepileptic and sedative-hypnotic drugs UPD

T42.76 Underdosing of unspecified antiepileptic and sedative-hypnotic drugs UPD

T42.8 Poisoning by, adverse effect of and underdosing of antiparkinsonism drugs and other central muscle-tone depressants
Poisoning by, adverse effect of and underdosing of amantadine

T42.8X Poisoning by, adverse effect of and underdosing of antiparkinsonism drugs and other central muscle-tone depressants

T42.8X1 Poisoning by antiparkinsonism drugs and other central muscle-tone depressants, accidental (unintentional)
Poisoning by antiparkinsonism drugs and other central muscle-tone depressants NOS

T42.8X2 Poisoning by antiparkinsonism drugs and other central muscle-tone depressants, intentional self-harm [2] HCC Rx ESR COM

T42.8X3 Poisoning by antiparkinsonism drugs and other central muscle-tone depressants, assault

T42.8X4 Poisoning by antiparkinsonism drugs and other central muscle-tone depressants, undetermined

T42.8X5 Adverse effect of antiparkinsonism drugs and other central muscle-tone depressants UPD

T42.8X6 Underdosing of antiparkinsonism drugs and other central muscle-tone depressants UPD

T43 Poisoning by, adverse effect of and underdosing of psychotropic drugs, not elsewhere classified

EXCLUDES 1 *appetite depressants (T5Ø.5-)*
barbiturates (T42.3-)
benzodiazepines (T42.4-)
methaqualone (T42.6-)
psychodysleptics [hallucinogens] (T4Ø.7-T4Ø.9-)

EXCLUDES 2 *drug dependence and related mental and behavioral disorders due to psychoactive substance use (F1Ø.- – F19.-)*

The appropriate 7th character is to be added to each code from category T43.
A initial encounter
D subsequent encounter
S sequela

T43.Ø Poisoning by, adverse effect of and underdosing of tricyclic and tetracyclic antidepressants

T43.Ø1 Poisoning by, adverse effect of and underdosing of tricyclic antidepressants

T43.Ø11 Poisoning by tricyclic antidepressants, accidental (unintentional)
Poisoning by tricyclic antidepressants NOS

2 **T43.Ø12 Poisoning by tricyclic antidepressants, intentional self-harm** HCC Rx ESR COM

T43.Ø13 Poisoning by tricyclic antidepressants, assault

T43.Ø14 Poisoning by tricyclic antidepressants, undetermined

T43.Ø15 Adverse effect of tricyclic antidepressants UPD

T43.Ø16 Underdosing of tricyclic antidepressants UPD

T43.Ø2 Poisoning by, adverse effect of and underdosing of tetracyclic antidepressants

T43.Ø21 Poisoning by tetracyclic antidepressants, accidental (unintentional)
Poisoning by tetracyclic antidepressants NOS

2 **T43.Ø22 Poisoning by tetracyclic antidepressants, intentional self-harm** HCC Rx ESR COM

T43.Ø23 Poisoning by tetracyclic antidepressants, assault

T43.Ø24 Poisoning by tetracyclic antidepressants, undetermined

T43.Ø25 Adverse effect of tetracyclic antidepressants UPD

T43.Ø26 Underdosing of tetracyclic antidepressants UPD

T43.1 Poisoning by, adverse effect of and underdosing of monoamine-oxidase-inhibitor antidepressants

T43.1X Poisoning by, adverse effect of and underdosing of monoamine-oxidase-inhibitor antidepressants

T43.1X1 Poisoning by monoamine-oxidase-inhibitor antidepressants, accidental (unintentional)
Poisoning by monoamine-oxidase-inhibitor antidepressants NOS

2 **T43.1X2 Poisoning by monoamine-oxidase-inhibitor antidepressants, intentional self-harm** HCC Rx ESR COM

T43.1X3 Poisoning by monoamine-oxidase-inhibitor antidepressants, assault

T43.1X4 Poisoning by monoamine-oxidase-inhibitor antidepressants, undetermined

T43.1X5 Adverse effect of monoamine-oxidase-inhibitor antidepressants UPD

T43.1X6 Underdosing of monoamine-oxidase-inhibitor antidepressants UPD

T43.2 Poisoning by, adverse effect of and underdosing of other and unspecified antidepressants

T43.2Ø Poisoning by, adverse effect of and underdosing of unspecified antidepressants

T43.2Ø1 Poisoning by unspecified antidepressants, accidental (unintentional)
Poisoning by antidepressants NOS

2 **T43.2Ø2 Poisoning by unspecified antidepressants, intentional self-harm** HCC Rx ESR COM

T43.2Ø3 Poisoning by unspecified antidepressants, assault

T43.2Ø4 Poisoning by unspecified antidepressants, undetermined

T43.2Ø5 Adverse effect of unspecified antidepressants UPD
Antidepressant discontinuation syndrome

T43.2Ø6 Underdosing of unspecified antidepressants UPD

T43.21 Poisoning by, adverse effect of and underdosing of selective serotonin and norepinephrine reuptake inhibitors
Poisoning by, adverse effect of and underdosing of SSNRI antidepressants

T43.211 Poisoning by selective serotonin and norepinephrine reuptake inhibitors, accidental (unintentional)

2 **T43.212 Poisoning by selective serotonin and norepinephrine reuptake inhibitors, intentional self-harm** HCC Rx ESR COM

T43.213 Poisoning by selective serotonin and norepinephrine reuptake inhibitors, assault

T43.214 Poisoning by selective serotonin and norepinephrine reuptake inhibitors, undetermined

T43.215 Adverse effect of selective serotonin and norepinephrine reuptake inhibitors UPD

T43.216 Underdosing of selective serotonin and norepinephrine reuptake inhibitors UPD

T43.22 Poisoning by, adverse effect of and underdosing of selective serotonin reuptake inhibitors
Poisoning by, adverse effect of and underdosing of SSRI antidepressants

T43.221 Poisoning by selective serotonin reuptake inhibitors, accidental (unintentional)

2 **T43.222 Poisoning by selective serotonin reuptake inhibitors, intentional self-harm** HCC Rx ESR COM

T43.223 Poisoning by selective serotonin reuptake inhibitors, assault

T43.224 Poisoning by selective serotonin reuptake inhibitors, undetermined

T43.225 Adverse effect of selective serotonin reuptake inhibitors UPD
AHA: 2022,2Q,11

T43.226 Underdosing of selective serotonin reuptake inhibitors UPD

T43.29 Poisoning by, adverse effect of and underdosing of other antidepressants

T43.291 Poisoning by other antidepressants, accidental (unintentional)
Poisoning by other antidepressants NOS

2 **T43.292 Poisoning by other antidepressants, intentional self-harm** HCC Rx ESR COM

T43.293 Poisoning by other antidepressants, assault

T43.294 Poisoning by other antidepressants, undetermined

T43.295 Adverse effect of other antidepressants UPD

T43.296 Underdosing of other antidepressants UPD

5th **T43.3 Poisoning by, adverse effect of and underdosing of phenothiazine antipsychotics and neuroleptics**

6th **T43.3X Poisoning by, adverse effect of and underdosing of phenothiazine antipsychotics and neuroleptics**

7th **T43.3X1 Poisoning by phenothiazine antipsychotics and neuroleptics, accidental (unintentional)**
Poisoning by phenothiazine antipsychotics and neuroleptics NOS

2 7th **T43.3X2 Poisoning by phenothiazine antipsychotics and neuroleptics, intentional self-harm** HCC Rx ESR COM

7th **T43.3X3 Poisoning by phenothiazine antipsychotics and neuroleptics, assault**

7th **T43.3X4 Poisoning by phenothiazine antipsychotics and neuroleptics, undetermined**

7th **T43.3X5 Adverse effect of phenothiazine antipsychotics and neuroleptics** UPD

7th **T43.3X6 Underdosing of phenothiazine antipsychotics and neuroleptics** UPD

5th **T43.4 Poisoning by, adverse effect of and underdosing of butyrophenone and thiothixene neuroleptics**

6th **T43.4X Poisoning by, adverse effect of and underdosing of butyrophenone and thiothixene neuroleptics**

7th **T43.4X1 Poisoning by butyrophenone and thiothixene neuroleptics, accidental (unintentional)**
Poisoning by butyrophenone and thiothixene neuroleptics NOS

2 7th **T43.4X2 Poisoning by butyrophenone and thiothixene neuroleptics, intentional self-harm** HCC Rx ESR COM

7th **T43.4X3 Poisoning by butyrophenone and thiothixene neuroleptics, assault**

7th **T43.4X4 Poisoning by butyrophenone and thiothixene neuroleptics, undetermined**

7th **T43.4X5 Adverse effect of butyrophenone and thiothixene neuroleptics** UPD

7th **T43.4X6 Underdosing of butyrophenone and thiothixene neuroleptics** UPD

5th **T43.5 Poisoning by, adverse effect of and underdosing of other and unspecified antipsychotics and neuroleptics**

EXCLUDES 1 *poisoning by, adverse effect of and underdosing of rauwolfia (T46.5-)*

6th **T43.50 Poisoning by, adverse effect of and underdosing of unspecified antipsychotics and neuroleptics**

7th **T43.501 Poisoning by unspecified antipsychotics and neuroleptics, accidental (unintentional)**
Poisoning by antipsychotics and neuroleptics NOS

2 7th **T43.502 Poisoning by unspecified antipsychotics and neuroleptics, intentional self-harm** HCC Rx ESR COM

7th **T43.503 Poisoning by unspecified antipsychotics and neuroleptics, assault**

7th **T43.504 Poisoning by unspecified antipsychotics and neuroleptics, undetermined**

7th **T43.505 Adverse effect of unspecified antipsychotics and neuroleptics** UPD

7th **T43.506 Underdosing of unspecified antipsychotics and neuroleptics** UPD

6th **T43.59 Poisoning by, adverse effect of and underdosing of other antipsychotics and neuroleptics**
AHA: 2017,1Q,40

7th **T43.591 Poisoning by other antipsychotics and neuroleptics, accidental (unintentional)**
Poisoning by other antipsychotics and neuroleptics NOS

2 7th **T43.592 Poisoning by other antipsychotics and neuroleptics, intentional self-harm** HCC Rx ESR COM

7th **T43.593 Poisoning by other antipsychotics and neuroleptics, assault**

7th **T43.594 Poisoning by other antipsychotics and neuroleptics, undetermined**

7th **T43.595 Adverse effect of other antipsychotics and neuroleptics** UPD
AHA: 2022,2Q,11

7th **T43.596 Underdosing of other antipsychotics and neuroleptics** UPD

5th **T43.6 Poisoning by, adverse effect of and underdosing of psychostimulants**

EXCLUDES 1 *poisoning by, adverse effect of and underdosing of cocaine (T40.5-)*

6th **T43.60 Poisoning by, adverse effect of and underdosing of unspecified psychostimulant**

1 7th **T43.601 Poisoning by unspecified psychostimulants, accidental (unintentional)** HCC ESR COM
Poisoning by psychostimulants NOS

2 7th **T43.602 Poisoning by unspecified psychostimulants, intentional self-harm** HCC Rx ESR COM

7th **T43.603 Poisoning by unspecified psychostimulants, assault**

1 7th **T43.604 Poisoning by unspecified psychostimulants, undetermined** HCC ESR COM

7th **T43.605 Adverse effect of unspecified psychostimulants** UPD

7th **T43.606 Underdosing of unspecified psychostimulants** UPD

6th **T43.61 Poisoning by, adverse effect of and underdosing of caffeine**

1 7th **T43.611 Poisoning by caffeine, accidental (unintentional)** HCC ESR COM
Poisoning by caffeine NOS

2 7th **T43.612 Poisoning by caffeine, intentional self-harm** HCC Rx ESR COM

7th **T43.613 Poisoning by caffeine, assault**

1 7th **T43.614 Poisoning by caffeine, undetermined** HCC ESR COM

7th **T43.615 Adverse effect of caffeine** UPD

7th **T43.616 Underdosing of caffeine** UPD

6th **T43.62 Poisoning by, adverse effect of and underdosing of amphetamines**
Poisoning by, adverse effect of and underdosing of methamphetamines

1 7th **T43.621 Poisoning by amphetamines, accidental (unintentional)** HCC ESR COM
Poisoning by amphetamines NOS
AHA: 2021,3Q,8

2 7th **T43.622 Poisoning by amphetamines, intentional self-harm** HCC Rx ESR COM

7th **T43.623 Poisoning by amphetamines, assault**

1 7th **T43.624 Poisoning by amphetamines, undetermined** HCC ESR COM

7th **T43.625 Adverse effect of amphetamines** UPD

7th **T43.626 Underdosing of amphetamines** UPD

6th **T43.63 Poisoning by, adverse effect of and underdosing of methylphenidate**

1 7th **T43.631 Poisoning by methylphenidate, accidental (unintentional)** HCC ESR COM
Poisoning by methylphenidate NOS

2 7th **T43.632 Poisoning by methylphenidate, intentional self-harm** HCC Rx ESR COM

7th **T43.633 Poisoning by methylphenidate, assault**

1 7th **T43.634 Poisoning by methylphenidate, undetermined** HCC ESR COM

7th **T43.635 Adverse effect of methylphenidate** UPD

7th **T43.636 Underdosing of methylphenidate** UPD

6th **T43.64 Poisoning by ecstasy**
Poisoning by MDMA
Poisoning by 3,4-methylenedioxymethamphetamine
AHA: 2018,4Q,30-31

1 7th **T43.641 Poisoning by ecstasy, accidental (unintentional)** HCC ESR COM
Poisoning by ecstasy NOS

2 7th **T43.642 Poisoning by ecstasy, intentional self-harm** HCC Rx ESR COM

7th **T43.643 Poisoning by ecstasy, assault**

1 7th **T43.644 Poisoning by ecstasy, undetermined** HCC ESR COM

HCC CMS-HCC Rx Rx HCC ESR ESRD HCC COM Commercial HCC N Newborn: 0 P Pediatric: 0-17 M Maternity: 9-64 A Adult: 15-124

● T43.65 Poisoning by, adverse effect of and underdosing of methamphetamines

● T43.651 Poisoning by methamphetamines accidental (unintentional)
Poisoning by methamphetamines NOS

● T43.652 Poisoning by methamphetamines intentional self-harm

● T43.653 Poisoning by methamphetamines, assault

● T43.654 Poisoning by methamphetamines, undetermined

● T43.655 Adverse effect of methamphetamines

● T43.656 Underdosing of methamphetamines

T43.69 Poisoning by, adverse effect of and underdosing of other psychostimulants

T43.691 Poisoning by other psychostimulants, accidental (unintentional) HCC ESR COM
Poisoning by other psychostimulants NOS

T43.692 Poisoning by other psychostimulants, intentional self-harm HCC Rx ESR COM

T43.693 Poisoning by other psychostimulants, assault

T43.694 Poisoning by other psychostimulants, undetermined HCC ESR COM

T43.695 Adverse effect of other psychostimulants UPD

T43.696 Underdosing of other psychostimulants UPD

T43.8 Poisoning by, adverse effect of and underdosing of other psychotropic drugs

T43.8X Poisoning by, adverse effect of and underdosing of other psychotropic drugs

T43.8X1 Poisoning by other psychotropic drugs, accidental (unintentional)
Poisoning by other psychotropic drugs NOS

T43.8X2 Poisoning by other psychotropic drugs, intentional self-harm HCC Rx ESR COM

T43.8X3 Poisoning by other psychotropic drugs, assault

T43.8X4 Poisoning by other psychotropic drugs, undetermined

T43.8X5 Adverse effect of other psychotropic drugs UPD

T43.8X6 Underdosing of other psychotropic drugs UPD

T43.9 Poisoning by, adverse effect of and underdosing of unspecified psychotropic drug

T43.91 Poisoning by unspecified psychotropic drug, accidental (unintentional)
Poisoning by psychotropic drug NOS

T43.92 Poisoning by unspecified psychotropic drug, intentional self-harm HCC Rx ESR COM

T43.93 Poisoning by unspecified psychotropic drug, assault

T43.94 Poisoning by unspecified psychotropic drug, undetermined

T43.95 Adverse effect of unspecified psychotropic drug UPD

T43.96 Underdosing of unspecified psychotropic drug UPD

T44 Poisoning by, adverse effect of and underdosing of drugs primarily affecting the autonomic nervous system

The appropriate 7th character is to be added to each code from category T44.
A initial encounter
D subsequent encounter
S sequela

T44.0 Poisoning by, adverse effect of and underdosing of anticholinesterase agents

T44.0X Poisoning by, adverse effect of and underdosing of anticholinesterase agents

T44.0X1 Poisoning by anticholinesterase agents, accidental (unintentional)
Poisoning by anticholinesterase agents NOS

T44.0X2 Poisoning by anticholinesterase agents, intentional self-harm HCC Rx ESR COM

T44.0X3 Poisoning by anticholinesterase agents, assault

T44.0X4 Poisoning by anticholinesterase agents, undetermined

T44.0X5 Adverse effect of anticholinesterase agents UPD

T44.0X6 Underdosing of anticholinesterase agents UPD

T44.1 Poisoning by, adverse effect of and underdosing of other parasympathomimetics [cholinergics]

T44.1X Poisoning by, adverse effect of and underdosing of other parasympathomimetics [cholinergics]

T44.1X1 Poisoning by other parasympathomimetics [cholinergics], accidental (unintentional)
Poisoning by other parasympathomimetics [cholinergics] NOS

T44.1X2 Poisoning by other parasympathomimetics [cholinergics], intentional self-harm HCC Rx ESR COM

T44.1X3 Poisoning by other parasympathomimetics [cholinergics], assault

T44.1X4 Poisoning by other parasympathomimetics [cholinergics], undetermined

T44.1X5 Adverse effect of other parasympathomimetics [cholinergics] UPD

T44.1X6 Underdosing of other parasympathomimetics [cholinergics] UPD

T44.2 Poisoning by, adverse effect of and underdosing of ganglionic blocking drugs

T44.2X Poisoning by, adverse effect of and underdosing of ganglionic blocking drugs

T44.2X1 Poisoning by ganglionic blocking drugs, accidental (unintentional)
Poisoning by ganglionic blocking drugs NOS

T44.2X2 Poisoning by ganglionic blocking drugs, intentional self-harm HCC Rx ESR COM

T44.2X3 Poisoning by ganglionic blocking drugs, assault

T44.2X4 Poisoning by ganglionic blocking drugs, undetermined

T44.2X5 Adverse effect of ganglionic blocking drugs UPD

T44.2X6 Underdosing of ganglionic blocking drugs UPD

T44.3 Poisoning by, adverse effect of and underdosing of other parasympatholytics [anticholinergics and antimuscarinics] and spasmolytics
Poisoning by, adverse effect of and underdosing of papaverine

T44.3X Poisoning by, adverse effect of and underdosing of other parasympatholytics [anticholinergics and antimuscarinics] and spasmolytics

T44.3X1 Poisoning by other parasympatholytics [anticholinergics and antimuscarinics] and spasmolytics, accidental (unintentional)
Poisoning by other parasympatholytics [anticholinergics and antimuscarinics] and spasmolytics NOS

T44.3X2 Poisoning by other parasympatholytics [anticholinergics and antimuscarinics] and spasmolytics, intentional self-harm HCC Rx ESR COM

T44.3X3 Poisoning by other parasympatholytics [anticholinergics and antimuscarinics] and spasmolytics, assault

T44.3X4 Poisoning by other parasympatholytics [anticholinergics and antimuscarinics] and spasmolytics, undetermined

T44.3X5 Adverse effect of other parasympatholytics [anticholinergics and antimuscarinics] and spasmolytics UPD

T44.3X6 Underdosing of other parasympatholytics [anticholinergics and antimuscarinics] and spasmolytics UPD

✓5th **T44.4 Poisoning by, adverse effect of and underdosing of predominantly alpha-adrenoreceptor agonists**
Poisoning by, adverse effect of and underdosing of metaraminol

✓6th **T44.4X Poisoning by, adverse effect of and underdosing of predominantly alpha-adrenoreceptor agonists**

✓7th **T44.4X1 Poisoning by predominantly alpha-adrenoreceptor agonists, accidental (unintentional)**
Poisoning by predominantly alpha-adrenoreceptor agonists NOS

2 ✓7th **T44.4X2 Poisoning by predominantly alpha-adrenoreceptor agonists, intentional self-harm** HCC Rx ESR COM

✓7th **T44.4X3 Poisoning by predominantly alpha-adrenoreceptor agonists, assault**

✓7th **T44.4X4 Poisoning by predominantly alpha-adrenoreceptor agonists, undetermined**

✓7th **T44.4X5 Adverse effect of predominantly alpha-adrenoreceptor agonists** UPD

✓7th **T44.4X6 Underdosing of predominantly alpha-adrenoreceptor agonists** UPD

✓5th **T44.5 Poisoning by, adverse effect of and underdosing of predominantly beta-adrenoreceptor agonists**
EXCLUDES 1 *poisoning by, adverse effect of and underdosing of beta-adrenoreceptor agonists used in asthma therapy (T48.6-)*

✓6th **T44.5X Poisoning by, adverse effect of and underdosing of predominantly beta-adrenoreceptor agonists**

✓7th **T44.5X1 Poisoning by predominantly beta-adrenoreceptor agonists, accidental (unintentional)**
Poisoning by predominantly beta-adrenoreceptor agonists NOS

2 ✓7th **T44.5X2 Poisoning by predominantly beta-adrenoreceptor agonists, intentional self-harm** HCC Rx ESR COM

✓7th **T44.5X3 Poisoning by predominantly beta-adrenoreceptor agonists, assault**

✓7th **T44.5X4 Poisoning by predominantly beta-adrenoreceptor agonists, undetermined**

✓7th **T44.5X5 Adverse effect of predominantly beta-adrenoreceptor agonists** UPD

✓7th **T44.5X6 Underdosing of predominantly beta-adrenoreceptor agonists** UPD

✓5th **T44.6 Poisoning by, adverse effect of and underdosing of alpha-adrenoreceptor antagonists**
EXCLUDES 1 *poisoning by, adverse effect of and underdosing of ergot alkaloids (T48.0)*

✓6th **T44.6X Poisoning by, adverse effect of and underdosing of alpha-adrenoreceptor antagonists**

✓7th **T44.6X1 Poisoning by alpha-adrenoreceptor antagonists, accidental (unintentional)**
Poisoning by alpha-adrenoreceptor antagonists NOS

2 ✓7th **T44.6X2 Poisoning by alpha-adrenoreceptor antagonists, intentional self-harm** HCC Rx ESR COM

✓7th **T44.6X3 Poisoning by alpha-adrenoreceptor antagonists, assault**

✓7th **T44.6X4 Poisoning by alpha-adrenoreceptor antagonists, undetermined**

✓7th **T44.6X5 Adverse effect of alpha-adrenoreceptor antagonists** UPD

✓7th **T44.6X6 Underdosing of alpha-adrenoreceptor antagonists** UPD

✓5th **T44.7 Poisoning by, adverse effect of and underdosing of beta-adrenoreceptor antagonists**

✓6th **T44.7X Poisoning by, adverse effect of and underdosing of beta-adrenoreceptor antagonists**

✓7th **T44.7X1 Poisoning by beta-adrenoreceptor antagonists, accidental (unintentional)**
Poisoning by beta-adrenoreceptor antagonists NOS

2 ✓7th **T44.7X2 Poisoning by beta-adrenoreceptor antagonists, intentional self-harm** HCC Rx ESR COM

✓7th **T44.7X3 Poisoning by beta-adrenoreceptor antagonists, assault**

✓7th **T44.7X4 Poisoning by beta-adrenoreceptor antagonists, undetermined**

✓7th **T44.7X5 Adverse effect of beta-adrenoreceptor antagonists** UPD

✓7th **T44.7X6 Underdosing of beta-adrenoreceptor antagonists** UPD

✓5th **T44.8 Poisoning by, adverse effect of and underdosing of centrally-acting and adrenergic-neuron- blocking agents**
EXCLUDES 2 *poisoning by, adverse effect of and underdosing of clonidine (T46.5)*
poisoning by, adverse effect of and underdosing of guanethidine (T46.5)

✓6th **T44.8X Poisoning by, adverse effect of and underdosing of centrally-acting and adrenergic-neuron-blocking agents**

✓7th **T44.8X1 Poisoning by centrally-acting and adrenergic-neuron-blocking agents, accidental (unintentional)**
Poisoning by centrally-acting and adrenergic-neuron-blocking agents NOS

2 ✓7th **T44.8X2 Poisoning by centrally-acting and adrenergic-neuron-blocking agents, intentional self-harm** HCC Rx ESR COM

✓7th **T44.8X3 Poisoning by centrally-acting and adrenergic-neuron-blocking agents, assault**

✓7th **T44.8X4 Poisoning by centrally-acting and adrenergic-neuron-blocking agents, undetermined**

✓7th **T44.8X5 Adverse effect of centrally-acting and adrenergic-neuron-blocking agents** UPD

✓7th **T44.8X6 Underdosing of centrally-acting and adrenergic-neuron-blocking agents** UPD

✓5th **T44.9 Poisoning by, adverse effect of and underdosing of other and unspecified drugs primarily affecting the autonomic nervous system**
Poisoning by, adverse effect of and underdosing of drug stimulating both alpha and beta-adrenoreceptors

✓6th **T44.90 Poisoning by, adverse effect of and underdosing of unspecified drugs primarily affecting the autonomic nervous system**

✓7th **T44.901 Poisoning by unspecified drugs primarily affecting the autonomic nervous system, accidental (unintentional)**
Poisoning by unspecified drugs primarily affecting the autonomic nervous system NOS

2 ✓7th **T44.902 Poisoning by unspecified drugs primarily affecting the autonomic nervous system, intentional self-harm** HCC Rx ESR COM

✓7th **T44.903 Poisoning by unspecified drugs primarily affecting the autonomic nervous system, assault**

✓7th **T44.904 Poisoning by unspecified drugs primarily affecting the autonomic nervous system, undetermined**

✓7th **T44.905 Adverse effect of unspecified drugs primarily affecting the autonomic nervous system** UPD

✓7th **T44.906 Underdosing of unspecified drugs primarily affecting the autonomic nervous system** UPD

✓6th **T44.99 Poisoning by, adverse effect of and underdosing of other drugs primarily affecting the autonomic nervous system**

✓7th **T44.991 Poisoning by other drug primarily affecting the autonomic nervous system, accidental (unintentional)**
Poisoning by other drugs primarily affecting the autonomic nervous system NOS

2 ✓7th **T44.992 Poisoning by other drug primarily affecting the autonomic nervous system, intentional self-harm** HCC Rx ESR COM

✓7th **T44.993 Poisoning by other drug primarily affecting the autonomic nervous system, assault**

✓7th **T44.994 Poisoning by other drug primarily affecting the autonomic nervous system, undetermined**

T44.995 Adverse effect of other drug primarily affecting the autonomic nervous system UPD

T44.996 Underdosing of other drug primarily affecting the autonomic nervous system UPD

T45 Poisoning by, adverse effect of and underdosing of primarily systemic and hematological agents, not elsewhere classified

The appropriate 7th character is to be added to each code from category T45.
A initial encounter
D subsequent encounter
S sequela

T45.0 Poisoning by, adverse effect of and underdosing of antiallergic and antiemetic drugs

EXCLUDES 1 *poisoning by, adverse effect of and underdosing of phenothiazine-based neuroleptics (T43.3)*

T45.0X Poisoning by, adverse effect of and underdosing of antiallergic and antiemetic drugs

T45.0X1 Poisoning by antiallergic and antiemetic drugs, accidental (unintentional)
Poisoning by antiallergic and antiemetic drugs NOS

T45.0X2 Poisoning by antiallergic and antiemetic drugs, intentional self-harm [2] HCC Rx ESR COM

T45.0X3 Poisoning by antiallergic and antiemetic drugs, assault

T45.0X4 Poisoning by antiallergic and antiemetic drugs, undetermined

T45.0X5 Adverse effect of antiallergic and antiemetic drugs UPD

T45.0X6 Underdosing of antiallergic and antiemetic drugs UPD

T45.1 Poisoning by, adverse effect of and underdosing of antineoplastic and immunosuppressive drugs

EXCLUDES 1 *poisoning by, adverse effect of and underdosing of tamoxifen (T38.6)*

AHA: 2019,1Q,17,20; 2014,4Q,22

T45.1X Poisoning by, adverse effect of and underdosing of antineoplastic and immunosuppressive drugs

T45.1X1 Poisoning by antineoplastic and immunosuppressive drugs, accidental (unintentional)
Poisoning by antineoplastic and immunosuppressive drugs NOS

T45.1X2 Poisoning by antineoplastic and immunosuppressive drugs, intentional self-harm [2] HCC Rx ESR COM

T45.1X3 Poisoning by antineoplastic and immunosuppressive drugs, assault

T45.1X4 Poisoning by antineoplastic and immunosuppressive drugs, undetermined

T45.1X5 Adverse effect of antineoplastic and immunosuppressive drugs UPD
AHA: 2021,3Q,4; 2020,4Q,11; 2020,3Q,22; 2019,2Q,24,28

T45.1X6 Underdosing of antineoplastic and immunosuppressive drugs UPD

T45.2 Poisoning by, adverse effect of and underdosing of vitamins

EXCLUDES 2 *poisoning by, adverse effect of and underdosing of iron (T45.4)*
poisoning by, adverse effect of and underdosing of nicotinic acid (derivatives) (T46.7)
poisoning by, adverse effect of and underdosing of vitamin K (T45.7)

T45.2X Poisoning by, adverse effect of and underdosing of vitamins

T45.2X1 Poisoning by vitamins, accidental (unintentional)
Poisoning by vitamins NOS

T45.2X2 Poisoning by vitamins, intentional self-harm [2] HCC Rx ESR COM

T45.2X3 Poisoning by vitamins, assault

T45.2X4 Poisoning by vitamins, undetermined

T45.2X5 Adverse effect of vitamins UPD

T45.2X6 Underdosing of vitamins UPD

EXCLUDES 1 *vitamin deficiencies (E50-E56)*

T45.3 Poisoning by, adverse effect of and underdosing of enzymes

T45.3X Poisoning by, adverse effect of and underdosing of enzymes

T45.3X1 Poisoning by enzymes, accidental (unintentional)
Poisoning by enzymes NOS

T45.3X2 Poisoning by enzymes, intentional self-harm [2] HCC Rx ESR COM

T45.3X3 Poisoning by enzymes, assault

T45.3X4 Poisoning by enzymes, undetermined

T45.3X5 Adverse effect of enzymes UPD

T45.3X6 Underdosing of enzymes UPD

T45.4 Poisoning by, adverse effect of and underdosing of iron and its compounds

T45.4X Poisoning by, adverse effect of and underdosing of iron and its compounds

T45.4X1 Poisoning by iron and its compounds, accidental (unintentional)
Poisoning by iron and its compounds NOS

T45.4X2 Poisoning by iron and its compounds, intentional self-harm [2] HCC Rx ESR COM

T45.4X3 Poisoning by iron and its compounds, assault

T45.4X4 Poisoning by iron and its compounds, undetermined

T45.4X5 Adverse effect of iron and its compounds UPD

T45.4X6 Underdosing of iron and its compounds UPD

EXCLUDES 1 *iron deficiency (E61.1)*

T45.5 Poisoning by, adverse effect of and underdosing of anticoagulants and antithrombotic drugs

T45.51 Poisoning by, adverse effect of and underdosing of anticoagulants

T45.511 Poisoning by anticoagulants, accidental (unintentional)
Poisoning by anticoagulants NOS

T45.512 Poisoning by anticoagulants, intentional self-harm [2] HCC Rx ESR COM

T45.513 Poisoning by anticoagulants, assault

T45.514 Poisoning by anticoagulants, undetermined

T45.515 Adverse effect of anticoagulants UPD
AHA: 2021,1Q,4; 2016,1Q,14; 2013,2Q,34

T45.516 Underdosing of anticoagulants UPD

T45.52 Poisoning by, adverse effect of and underdosing of antithrombotic drugs
Poisoning by, adverse effect of and underdosing of antiplatelet drugs

EXCLUDES 2 *poisoning by, adverse effect of and underdosing of aspirin (T39.01-)*
poisoning by, adverse effect of and underdosing of acetylsalicylic acid (T39.01-)

T45.521 Poisoning by antithrombotic drugs, accidental (unintentional)
Poisoning by antithrombotic drug NOS

T45.522 Poisoning by antithrombotic drugs, intentional self-harm [2] HCC Rx ESR COM

T45.523 Poisoning by antithrombotic drugs, assault

T45.524 Poisoning by antithrombotic drugs, undetermined

T45.525 Adverse effect of antithrombotic drugs UPD
AHA: 2016,1Q,15

T45.526 Underdosing of antithrombotic drugs UPD

T45.6 Poisoning by, adverse effect of and underdosing of fibrinolysis-affecting drugs

T45.6Ø Poisoning by, adverse effect of and underdosing of unspecified fibrinolysis-affecting drugs

T45.6Ø1 Poisoning by unspecified fibrinolysis-affecting drugs, accidental (unintentional)
Poisoning by fibrinolysis-affecting drug NOS

2 **T45.6Ø2 Poisoning by unspecified fibrinolysis-affecting drugs, intentional self-harm** HCC Rx ESR COM

T45.6Ø3 Poisoning by unspecified fibrinolysis-affecting drugs, assault

T45.6Ø4 Poisoning by unspecified fibrinolysis-affecting drugs, undetermined

T45.6Ø5 Adverse effect of unspecified fibrinolysis-affecting drugs UPD

T45.6Ø6 Underdosing of unspecified fibrinolysis-affecting drugs UPD

T45.61 Poisoning by, adverse effect of and underdosing of thrombolytic drugs

T45.611 Poisoning by thrombolytic drug, accidental (unintentional)
Poisoning by thrombolytic drug NOS

2 **T45.612 Poisoning by thrombolytic drug, intentional self-harm** HCC Rx ESR COM

T45.613 Poisoning by thrombolytic drug, assault

T45.614 Poisoning by thrombolytic drug, undetermined

T45.615 Adverse effect of thrombolytic drugs UPD
AHA: 2017,2Q,9

T45.616 Underdosing of thrombolytic drugs UPD

T45.62 Poisoning by, adverse effect of and underdosing of hemostatic drugs

T45.621 Poisoning by hemostatic drug, accidental (unintentional)
Poisoning by hemostatic drug NOS

2 **T45.622 Poisoning by hemostatic drug, intentional self-harm** HCC Rx ESR COM

T45.623 Poisoning by hemostatic drug, assault

T45.624 Poisoning by hemostatic drug, undetermined

T45.625 Adverse effect of hemostatic drug UPD

T45.626 Underdosing of hemostatic drugs UPD

T45.69 Poisoning by, adverse effect of and underdosing of other fibrinolysis-affecting drugs

T45.691 Poisoning by other fibrinolysis-affecting drugs, accidental (unintentional)
Poisoning by other fibrinolysis-affecting drug NOS

2 **T45.692 Poisoning by other fibrinolysis-affecting drugs, intentional self-harm** HCC Rx ESR COM

T45.693 Poisoning by other fibrinolysis-affecting drugs, assault

T45.694 Poisoning by other fibrinolysis-affecting drugs, undetermined

T45.695 Adverse effect of other fibrinolysis-affecting drugs UPD

T45.696 Underdosing of other fibrinolysis-affecting drugs UPD

T45.7 Poisoning by, adverse effect of and underdosing of anticoagulant antagonists, vitamin K and other coagulants

T45.7X Poisoning by, adverse effect of and underdosing of anticoagulant antagonists, vitamin K and other coagulants

T45.7X1 Poisoning by anticoagulant antagonists, vitamin K and other coagulants, accidental (unintentional)
Poisoning by anticoagulant antagonists, vitamin K and other coagulants NOS

2 **T45.7X2 Poisoning by anticoagulant antagonists, vitamin K and other coagulants, intentional self-harm** HCC Rx ESR COM

T45.7X3 Poisoning by anticoagulant antagonists, vitamin K and other coagulants, assault

T45.7X4 Poisoning by anticoagulant antagonists, vitamin K and other coagulants, undetermined

T45.7X5 Adverse effect of anticoagulant antagonists, vitamin K and other coagulants UPD

T45.7X6 Underdosing of anticoagulant antagonist, vitamin K and other coagulants UPD
EXCLUDES 1 *vitamin K deficiency (E56.1)*

T45.8 Poisoning by, adverse effect of and underdosing of other primarily systemic and hematological agents
Poisoning by, adverse effect of and underdosing of liver preparations and other antianemic agents
Poisoning by, adverse effect of and underdosing of natural blood and blood products
Poisoning by, adverse effect of and underdosing of plasma substitute
EXCLUDES 2 *poisoning by, adverse effect of and underdosing of immunoglobulin (T5Ø.Z1)*
poisoning by, adverse effect of and underdosing of iron (T45.4)
transfusion reactions (T8Ø.-)

T45.8X Poisoning by, adverse effect of and underdosing of other primarily systemic and hematological agents

T45.8X1 Poisoning by other primarily systemic and hematological agents, accidental (unintentional)
Poisoning by other primarily systemic and hematological agents NOS

2 **T45.8X2 Poisoning by other primarily systemic and hematological agents, intentional self-harm** HCC Rx ESR COM

T45.8X3 Poisoning by other primarily systemic and hematological agents, assault

T45.8X4 Poisoning by other primarily systemic and hematological agents, undetermined

T45.8X5 Adverse effect of other primarily systemic and hematological agents UPD
AHA: 2016,4Q,42

T45.8X6 Underdosing of other primarily systemic and hematological agents UPD

T45.9 Poisoning by, adverse effect of and underdosing of unspecified primarily systemic and hematological agent

T45.91 Poisoning by unspecified primarily systemic and hematological agent, accidental (unintentional)
Poisoning by primarily systemic and hematological agent NOS

2 **T45.92 Poisoning by unspecified primarily systemic and hematological agent, intentional self-harm** HCC Rx ESR COM

T45.93 Poisoning by unspecified primarily systemic and hematological agent, assault

T45.94 Poisoning by unspecified primarily systemic and hematological agent, undetermined

T45.95 Adverse effect of unspecified primarily systemic and hematological agent UPD

T45.96 Underdosing of unspecified primarily systemic and hematological agent UPD

T46 Poisoning by, adverse effect of and underdosing of agents primarily affecting the cardiovascular system
EXCLUDES 1 *poisoning by, adverse effect of and underdosing of metaraminol (T44.4)*

The appropriate 7th character is to be added to each code from category T46.
A initial encounter
D subsequent encounter
S sequela

T46.Ø Poisoning by, adverse effect of and underdosing of cardiac-stimulant glycosides and drugs of similar action

T46.ØX Poisoning by, adverse effect of and underdosing of cardiac-stimulant glycosides and drugs of similar action

T46.ØX1 Poisoning by cardiac-stimulant glycosides and drugs of similar action, accidental (unintentional)
Poisoning by cardiac-stimulant glycosides and drugs of similar action NOS

2 √7th T46.ØX2 Poisoning by cardiac-stimulant glycosides and drugs of similar action, intentional self-harm HCC Rx ESR COM

√7th T46.ØX3 Poisoning by cardiac-stimulant glycosides and drugs of similar action, assault

√7th T46.ØX4 Poisoning by cardiac-stimulant glycosides and drugs of similar action, undetermined

√7th T46.ØX5 Adverse effect of cardiac-stimulant glycosides and drugs of similar action UPD

√7th T46.ØX6 Underdosing of cardiac-stimulant glycosides and drugs of similar action UPD

√5th T46.1 Poisoning by, adverse effect of and underdosing of calcium-channel blockers

√6th T46.1X Poisoning by, adverse effect of and underdosing of calcium-channel blockers

√7th T46.1X1 Poisoning by calcium-channel blockers, accidental (unintentional)

Poisoning by calcium-channel blockers NOS

2 √7th T46.1X2 Poisoning by calcium-channel blockers, intentional self-harm HCC Rx ESR COM

√7th T46.1X3 Poisoning by calcium-channel blockers, assault

√7th T46.1X4 Poisoning by calcium-channel blockers, undetermined

√7th T46.1X5 Adverse effect of calcium-channel blockers UPD

√7th T46.1X6 Underdosing of calcium-channel blockers UPD

√5th T46.2 Poisoning by, adverse effect of and underdosing of other antidysrhythmic drugs, not elsewhere classified

EXCLUDES 1 *poisoning by, adverse effect of and underdosing of beta-adrenoreceptor antagonists (T44.7-)*

√6th T46.2X Poisoning by, adverse effect of and underdosing of other antidysrhythmic drugs

√7th T46.2X1 Poisoning by other antidysrhythmic drugs, accidental (unintentional)

Poisoning by other antidysrhythmic drugs NOS

2 √7th T46.2X2 Poisoning by other antidysrhythmic drugs, intentional self-harm HCC Rx ESR COM

√7th T46.2X3 Poisoning by other antidysrhythmic drugs, assault

√7th T46.2X4 Poisoning by other antidysrhythmic drugs, undetermined

√7th T46.2X5 Adverse effect of other antidysrhythmic drugs UPD

√7th T46.2X6 Underdosing of other antidysrhythmic drugs UPD

√5th T46.3 Poisoning by, adverse effect of and underdosing of coronary vasodilators

Poisoning by, adverse effect of and underdosing of dipyridamole

EXCLUDES 1 *poisoning by, adverse effect of and underdosing of calcium-channel blockers (T46.1)*

√6th T46.3X Poisoning by, adverse effect of and underdosing of coronary vasodilators

√7th T46.3X1 Poisoning by coronary vasodilators, accidental (unintentional)

Poisoning by coronary vasodilators NOS

2 √7th T46.3X2 Poisoning by coronary vasodilators, intentional self-harm HCC Rx ESR COM

√7th T46.3X3 Poisoning by coronary vasodilators, assault

√7th T46.3X4 Poisoning by coronary vasodilators, undetermined

√7th T46.3X5 Adverse effect of coronary vasodilators UPD

√7th T46.3X6 Underdosing of coronary vasodilators UPD

√5th T46.4 Poisoning by, adverse effect of and underdosing of angiotensin-converting-enzyme inhibitors

√6th T46.4X Poisoning by, adverse effect of and underdosing of angiotensin-converting-enzyme inhibitors

√7th T46.4X1 Poisoning by angiotensin-converting-enzyme inhibitors, accidental (unintentional)

Poisoning by angiotensin-converting-enzyme inhibitors NOS

2 √7th T46.4X2 Poisoning by angiotensin-converting-enzyme inhibitors, intentional self-harm HCC Rx ESR COM

√7th T46.4X3 Poisoning by angiotensin-converting-enzyme inhibitors, assault

√7th T46.4X4 Poisoning by angiotensin-converting-enzyme inhibitors, undetermined

√7th T46.4X5 Adverse effect of angiotensin-converting-enzyme inhibitors UPD

√7th T46.4X6 Underdosing of angiotensin-converting-enzyme inhibitors UPD

√5th T46.5 Poisoning by, adverse effect of and underdosing of other antihypertensive drugs

EXCLUDES 2 *poisoning by, adverse effect of and underdosing of beta-adrenoreceptor antagonists (T44.7)*
poisoning by, adverse effect of and underdosing of calcium-channel blockers (T46.1)
poisoning by, adverse effect of and underdosing of diuretics (T5Ø.Ø-T5Ø.2)

√6th T46.5X Poisoning by, adverse effect of and underdosing of other antihypertensive drugs

√7th T46.5X1 Poisoning by other antihypertensive drugs, accidental (unintentional)

Poisoning by other antihypertensive drugs NOS

2 √7th T46.5X2 Poisoning by other antihypertensive drugs, intentional self-harm HCC Rx ESR COM

√7th T46.5X3 Poisoning by other antihypertensive drugs, assault

√7th T46.5X4 Poisoning by other antihypertensive drugs, undetermined

√7th T46.5X5 Adverse effect of other antihypertensive drugs UPD

√7th T46.5X6 Underdosing of other antihypertensive drugs UPD

AHA: 2022,1Q,36

√5th T46.6 Poisoning by, adverse effect of and underdosing of antihyperlipidemic and antiarteriosclerotic drugs

√6th T46.6X Poisoning by, adverse effect of and underdosing of antihyperlipidemic and antiarteriosclerotic drugs

√7th T46.6X1 Poisoning by antihyperlipidemic and antiarteriosclerotic drugs, accidental (unintentional)

Poisoning by antihyperlipidemic and antiarteriosclerotic drugs NOS

2 √7th T46.6X2 Poisoning by antihyperlipidemic and antiarteriosclerotic drugs, intentional self-harm HCC Rx ESR COM

√7th T46.6X3 Poisoning by antihyperlipidemic and antiarteriosclerotic drugs, assault

√7th T46.6X4 Poisoning by antihyperlipidemic and antiarteriosclerotic drugs, undetermined

√7th T46.6X5 Adverse effect of antihyperlipidemic and antiarteriosclerotic drugs UPD

√7th T46.6X6 Underdosing of antihyperlipidemic and antiarteriosclerotic drugs UPD

✓5th **T46.7 Poisoning by, adverse effect of and underdosing of peripheral vasodilators**
Poisoning by, adverse effect of and underdosing of nicotinic acid (derivatives)
EXCLUDES 1 *poisoning by, adverse effect of and underdosing of papaverine (T44.3)*

✓6th **T46.7X Poisoning by, adverse effect of and underdosing of peripheral vasodilators**

✓7th **T46.7X1 Poisoning by peripheral vasodilators, accidental (unintentional)**
Poisoning by peripheral vasodilators NOS

2 ✓7th **T46.7X2 Poisoning by peripheral vasodilators, intentional self-harm** HCC Rx ESR COM

✓7th **T46.7X3 Poisoning by peripheral vasodilators, assault**

✓7th **T46.7X4 Poisoning by peripheral vasodilators, undetermined**

✓7th **T46.7X5 Adverse effect of peripheral vasodilators** UPD

✓7th **T46.7X6 Underdosing of peripheral vasodilators** UPD

✓5th **T46.8 Poisoning by, adverse effect of and underdosing of antivaricose drugs, including sclerosing agents**

✓6th **T46.8X Poisoning by, adverse effect of and underdosing of antivaricose drugs, including sclerosing agents**

✓7th **T46.8X1 Poisoning by antivaricose drugs, including sclerosing agents, accidental (unintentional)**
Poisoning by antivaricose drugs, including sclerosing agents NOS

2 ✓7th **T46.8X2 Poisoning by antivaricose drugs, including sclerosing agents, intentional self-harm** HCC Rx ESR COM

✓7th **T46.8X3 Poisoning by antivaricose drugs, including sclerosing agents, assault**

✓7th **T46.8X4 Poisoning by antivaricose drugs, including sclerosing agents, undetermined**

✓7th **T46.8X5 Adverse effect of antivaricose drugs, including sclerosing agents** UPD

✓7th **T46.8X6 Underdosing of antivaricose drugs, including sclerosing agents** UPD

✓5th **T46.9 Poisoning by, adverse effect of and underdosing of other and unspecified agents primarily affecting the cardiovascular system**

✓6th **T46.9Ø Poisoning by, adverse effect of and underdosing of unspecified agents primarily affecting the cardiovascular system**

✓7th **T46.9Ø1 Poisoning by unspecified agents primarily affecting the cardiovascular system, accidental (unintentional)**

2 ✓7th **T46.9Ø2 Poisoning by unspecified agents primarily affecting the cardiovascular system, intentional self-harm** HCC Rx ESR COM

✓7th **T46.9Ø3 Poisoning by unspecified agents primarily affecting the cardiovascular system, assault**

✓7th **T46.9Ø4 Poisoning by unspecified agents primarily affecting the cardiovascular system, undetermined**

✓7th **T46.9Ø5 Adverse effect of unspecified agents primarily affecting the cardiovascular system** UPD

✓7th **T46.9Ø6 Underdosing of unspecified agents primarily affecting the cardiovascular system** UPD

✓6th **T46.99 Poisoning by, adverse effect of and underdosing of other agents primarily affecting the cardiovascular system**

✓7th **T46.991 Poisoning by other agents primarily affecting the cardiovascular system, accidental (unintentional)**

2 ✓7th **T46.992 Poisoning by other agents primarily affecting the cardiovascular system, intentional self-harm** HCC Rx ESR COM

✓7th **T46.993 Poisoning by other agents primarily affecting the cardiovascular system, assault**

✓7th **T46.994 Poisoning by other agents primarily affecting the cardiovascular system, undetermined**

✓7th **T46.995 Adverse effect of other agents primarily affecting the cardiovascular system** UPD

✓7th **T46.996 Underdosing of other agents primarily affecting the cardiovascular system** UPD

✓4th **T47 Poisoning by, adverse effect of and underdosing of agents primarily affecting the gastrointestinal system**

The appropriate 7th character is to be added to each code from category T47.
A initial encounter
D subsequent encounter
S sequela

✓5th **T47.Ø Poisoning by, adverse effect of and underdosing of histamine H2-receptor blockers**

✓6th **T47.ØX Poisoning by, adverse effect of and underdosing of histamine H2-receptor blockers**

✓7th **T47.ØX1 Poisoning by histamine H2-receptor blockers, accidental (unintentional)**
Poisoning by histamine H2-receptor blockers NOS

2 ✓7th **T47.ØX2 Poisoning by histamine H2-receptor blockers, intentional self-harm** HCC Rx ESR COM

✓7th **T47.ØX3 Poisoning by histamine H2-receptor blockers, assault**

✓7th **T47.ØX4 Poisoning by histamine H2-receptor blockers, undetermined**

✓7th **T47.ØX5 Adverse effect of histamine H2-receptor blockers** UPD

✓7th **T47.ØX6 Underdosing of histamine H2-receptor blockers** UPD

✓5th **T47.1 Poisoning by, adverse effect of and underdosing of other antacids and anti-gastric-secretion drugs**

✓6th **T47.1X Poisoning by, adverse effect of and underdosing of other antacids and anti-gastric-secretion drugs**

✓7th **T47.1X1 Poisoning by other antacids and anti-gastric-secretion drugs, accidental (unintentional)**
Poisoning by other antacids and anti-gastric-secretion drugs NOS

2 ✓7th **T47.1X2 Poisoning by other antacids and anti-gastric-secretion drugs, intentional self-harm** HCC Rx ESR COM

✓7th **T47.1X3 Poisoning by other antacids and anti-gastric-secretion drugs, assault**

✓7th **T47.1X4 Poisoning by other antacids and anti-gastric-secretion drugs, undetermined**

✓7th **T47.1X5 Adverse effect of other antacids and anti-gastric-secretion drugs** UPD

✓7th **T47.1X6 Underdosing of other antacids and anti-gastric-secretion drugs** UPD

✓5th **T47.2 Poisoning by, adverse effect of and underdosing of stimulant laxatives**

✓6th **T47.2X Poisoning by, adverse effect of and underdosing of stimulant laxatives**

✓7th **T47.2X1 Poisoning by stimulant laxatives, accidental (unintentional)**
Poisoning by stimulant laxatives NOS

2 ✓7th **T47.2X2 Poisoning by stimulant laxatives, intentional self-harm** HCC Rx ESR COM

✓7th **T47.2X3 Poisoning by stimulant laxatives, assault**

✓7th **T47.2X4 Poisoning by stimulant laxatives, undetermined**

✓7th **T47.2X5 Adverse effect of stimulant laxatives** UPD

✓7th **T47.2X6 Underdosing of stimulant laxatives** UPD

✓5th **T47.3 Poisoning by, adverse effect of and underdosing of saline and osmotic laxatives**

✓6th **T47.3X Poisoning by and adverse effect of saline and osmotic laxatives**

✓7th **T47.3X1 Poisoning by saline and osmotic laxatives, accidental (unintentional)**
Poisoning by saline and osmotic laxatives NOS

2 ✓7th **T47.3X2 Poisoning by saline and osmotic laxatives, intentional self-harm** HCC Rx ESR COM

T47.3X3 Poisoning by saline and osmotic laxatives, assault

T47.3X4 Poisoning by saline and osmotic laxatives, undetermined

T47.3X5 Adverse effect of saline and osmotic laxatives UPD

T47.3X6 Underdosing of saline and osmotic laxatives UPD

T47.4 Poisoning by, adverse effect of and underdosing of other laxatives

T47.4X Poisoning by, adverse effect of and underdosing of other laxatives

T47.4X1 Poisoning by other laxatives, accidental (unintentional)

Poisoning by other laxatives NOS

2 T47.4X2 Poisoning by other laxatives, intentional self-harm HCC Rx ESR COM

T47.4X3 Poisoning by other laxatives, assault

T47.4X4 Poisoning by other laxatives, undetermined

T47.4X5 Adverse effect of other laxatives UPD

T47.4X6 Underdosing of other laxatives UPD

T47.5 Poisoning by, adverse effect of and underdosing of digestants

T47.5X Poisoning by, adverse effect of and underdosing of digestants

T47.5X1 Poisoning by digestants, accidental (unintentional)

Poisoning by digestants NOS

2 T47.5X2 Poisoning by digestants, intentional self-harm HCC Rx ESR COM

T47.5X3 Poisoning by digestants, assault

T47.5X4 Poisoning by digestants, undetermined

T47.5X5 Adverse effect of digestants UPD

T47.5X6 Underdosing of digestants UPD

T47.6 Poisoning by, adverse effect of and underdosing of antidiarrheal drugs

EXCLUDES 2 *poisoning by, adverse effect of and underdosing of systemic antibiotics and other anti-infectives (T36-T37)*

T47.6X Poisoning by, adverse effect of and underdosing of antidiarrheal drugs

T47.6X1 Poisoning by antidiarrheal drugs, accidental (unintentional)

Poisoning by antidiarrheal drugs NOS

2 T47.6X2 Poisoning by antidiarrheal drugs, intentional self-harm HCC Rx ESR COM

T47.6X3 Poisoning by antidiarrheal drugs, assault

T47.6X4 Poisoning by antidiarrheal drugs, undetermined

T47.6X5 Adverse effect of antidiarrheal drugs UPD

T47.6X6 Underdosing of antidiarrheal drugs UPD

T47.7 Poisoning by, adverse effect of and underdosing of emetics

T47.7X Poisoning by, adverse effect of and underdosing of emetics

T47.7X1 Poisoning by emetics, accidental (unintentional)

Poisoning by emetics NOS

T47.7X2 Poisoning by emetics, intentional self-harm HCC Rx ESR COM

T47.7X3 Poisoning by emetics, assault

T47.7X4 Poisoning by emetics, undetermined

T47.7X5 Adverse effect of emetics UPD

T47.7X6 Underdosing of emetics UPD

T47.8 Poisoning by, adverse effect of and underdosing of other agents primarily affecting gastrointestinal system

T47.8X Poisoning by, adverse effect of and underdosing of other agents primarily affecting gastrointestinal system

T47.8X1 Poisoning by other agents primarily affecting gastrointestinal system, accidental (unintentional)

Poisoning by other agents primarily affecting gastrointestinal system NOS

2 T47.8X2 Poisoning by other agents primarily affecting gastrointestinal system, intentional self-harm HCC Rx ESR COM

T47.8X3 Poisoning by other agents primarily affecting gastrointestinal system, assault

T47.8X4 Poisoning by other agents primarily affecting gastrointestinal system, undetermined

T47.8X5 Adverse effect of other agents primarily affecting gastrointestinal system UPD

T47.8X6 Underdosing of other agents primarily affecting gastrointestinal system UPD

T47.9 Poisoning by, adverse effect of and underdosing of unspecified agents primarily affecting the gastrointestinal system

T47.91 Poisoning by unspecified agents primarily affecting the gastrointestinal system, accidental (unintentional)

Poisoning by agents primarily affecting the gastrointestinal system NOS

2 T47.92 Poisoning by unspecified agents primarily affecting the gastrointestinal system, intentional self-harm HCC Rx ESR COM

T47.93 Poisoning by unspecified agents primarily affecting the gastrointestinal system, assault

T47.94 Poisoning by unspecified agents primarily affecting the gastrointestinal system, undetermined

T47.95 Adverse effect of unspecified agents primarily affecting the gastrointestinal system UPD

T47.96 Underdosing of unspecified agents primarily affecting the gastrointestinal system UPD

T48 Poisoning by, adverse effect of and underdosing of agents primarily acting on smooth and skeletal muscles and the respiratory system

The appropriate 7th character is to be added to each code from category T48.
A initial encounter
D subsequent encounter
S sequela

T48.0 Poisoning by, adverse effect of and underdosing of oxytocic drugs

EXCLUDES 1 *poisoning by, adverse effect of and underdosing of estrogens, progestogens and antagonists (T38.4-T38.6)*

T48.0X Poisoning by, adverse effect of and underdosing of oxytocic drugs

T48.0X1 Poisoning by oxytocic drugs, accidental (unintentional)

Poisoning by oxytocic drugs NOS

2 T48.0X2 Poisoning by oxytocic drugs, intentional self-harm HCC Rx ESR COM

T48.0X3 Poisoning by oxytocic drugs, assault

T48.0X4 Poisoning by oxytocic drugs, undetermined

T48.0X5 Adverse effect of oxytocic drugs UPD

T48.0X6 Underdosing of oxytocic drugs UPD

T48.1 Poisoning by, adverse effect of and underdosing of skeletal muscle relaxants [neuromuscular blocking agents]

T48.1X Poisoning by, adverse effect of and underdosing of skeletal muscle relaxants [neuromuscular blocking agents]

T48.1X1 Poisoning by skeletal muscle relaxants [neuromuscular blocking agents], accidental (unintentional)

Poisoning by skeletal muscle relaxants [neuromuscular blocking agents] NOS

2 T48.1X2 Poisoning by skeletal muscle relaxants [neuromuscular blocking agents], intentional self-harm HCC Rx ESR COM

T48.1X3 Poisoning by skeletal muscle relaxants [neuromuscular blocking agents], assault

T48.1X4 Poisoning by skeletal muscle relaxants [neuromuscular blocking agents], undetermined

T48.1X5 Adverse effect of skeletal muscle relaxants [neuromuscular blocking agents] UPD

T48.1X6 Underdosing of skeletal muscle relaxants [neuromuscular blocking agents] UPD

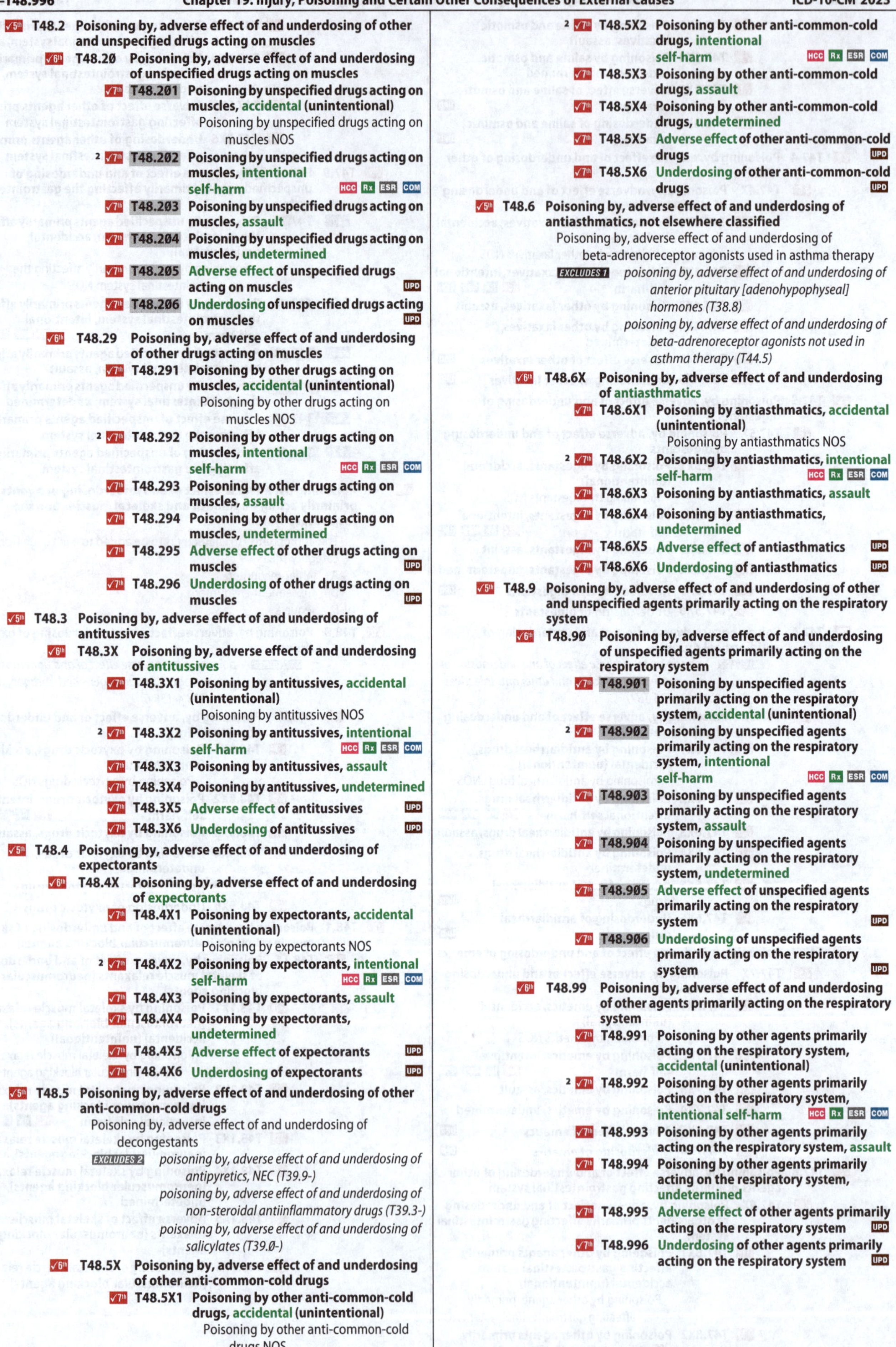

✓5th **T48.2 Poisoning by, adverse effect of and underdosing of other and unspecified drugs acting on muscles**

✓6th **T48.20 Poisoning by, adverse effect of and underdosing of unspecified drugs acting on muscles**

✓7th **T48.201 Poisoning by unspecified drugs acting on muscles, accidental (unintentional)**
Poisoning by unspecified drugs acting on muscles NOS

2 ✓7th **T48.202 Poisoning by unspecified drugs acting on muscles, intentional self-harm** HCC Rx ESR COM

✓7th **T48.203 Poisoning by unspecified drugs acting on muscles, assault**

✓7th **T48.204 Poisoning by unspecified drugs acting on muscles, undetermined**

✓7th **T48.205 Adverse effect of unspecified drugs acting on muscles** UPD

✓7th **T48.206 Underdosing of unspecified drugs acting on muscles** UPD

✓6th **T48.29 Poisoning by, adverse effect of and underdosing of other drugs acting on muscles**

✓7th **T48.291 Poisoning by other drugs acting on muscles, accidental (unintentional)**
Poisoning by other drugs acting on muscles NOS

2 ✓7th **T48.292 Poisoning by other drugs acting on muscles, intentional self-harm** HCC Rx ESR COM

✓7th **T48.293 Poisoning by other drugs acting on muscles, assault**

✓7th **T48.294 Poisoning by other drugs acting on muscles, undetermined**

✓7th **T48.295 Adverse effect of other drugs acting on muscles** UPD

✓7th **T48.296 Underdosing of other drugs acting on muscles** UPD

✓5th **T48.3 Poisoning by, adverse effect of and underdosing of antitussives**

✓6th **T48.3X Poisoning by, adverse effect of and underdosing of antitussives**

✓7th **T48.3X1 Poisoning by antitussives, accidental (unintentional)**
Poisoning by antitussives NOS

2 ✓7th **T48.3X2 Poisoning by antitussives, intentional self-harm** HCC Rx ESR COM

✓7th **T48.3X3 Poisoning by antitussives, assault**

✓7th **T48.3X4 Poisoning by antitussives, undetermined**

✓7th **T48.3X5 Adverse effect of antitussives** UPD

✓7th **T48.3X6 Underdosing of antitussives** UPD

✓5th **T48.4 Poisoning by, adverse effect of and underdosing of expectorants**

✓6th **T48.4X Poisoning by, adverse effect of and underdosing of expectorants**

✓7th **T48.4X1 Poisoning by expectorants, accidental (unintentional)**
Poisoning by expectorants NOS

2 ✓7th **T48.4X2 Poisoning by expectorants, intentional self-harm** HCC Rx ESR COM

✓7th **T48.4X3 Poisoning by expectorants, assault**

✓7th **T48.4X4 Poisoning by expectorants, undetermined**

✓7th **T48.4X5 Adverse effect of expectorants** UPD

✓7th **T48.4X6 Underdosing of expectorants** UPD

✓5th **T48.5 Poisoning by, adverse effect of and underdosing of other anti-common-cold drugs**
Poisoning by, adverse effect of and underdosing of decongestants

EXCLUDES 2 *poisoning by, adverse effect of and underdosing of antipyretics, NEC (T39.9-)*
poisoning by, adverse effect of and underdosing of non-steroidal antiinflammatory drugs (T39.3-)
poisoning by, adverse effect of and underdosing of salicylates (T39.0-)

✓6th **T48.5X Poisoning by, adverse effect of and underdosing of other anti-common-cold drugs**

✓7th **T48.5X1 Poisoning by other anti-common-cold drugs, accidental (unintentional)**
Poisoning by other anti-common-cold drugs NOS

2 ✓7th **T48.5X2 Poisoning by other anti-common-cold drugs, intentional self-harm** HCC Rx ESR COM

✓7th **T48.5X3 Poisoning by other anti-common-cold drugs, assault**

✓7th **T48.5X4 Poisoning by other anti-common-cold drugs, undetermined**

✓7th **T48.5X5 Adverse effect of other anti-common-cold drugs** UPD

✓7th **T48.5X6 Underdosing of other anti-common-cold drugs** UPD

✓5th **T48.6 Poisoning by, adverse effect of and underdosing of antiasthmatics, not elsewhere classified**
Poisoning by, adverse effect of and underdosing of beta-adrenoreceptor agonists used in asthma therapy

EXCLUDES 1 *poisoning by, adverse effect of and underdosing of anterior pituitary [adenohypophyseal] hormones (T38.8)*
poisoning by, adverse effect of and underdosing of beta-adrenoreceptor agonists not used in asthma therapy (T44.5)

✓6th **T48.6X Poisoning by, adverse effect of and underdosing of antiasthmatics**

✓7th **T48.6X1 Poisoning by antiasthmatics, accidental (unintentional)**
Poisoning by antiasthmatics NOS

2 ✓7th **T48.6X2 Poisoning by antiasthmatics, intentional self-harm** HCC Rx ESR COM

✓7th **T48.6X3 Poisoning by antiasthmatics, assault**

✓7th **T48.6X4 Poisoning by antiasthmatics, undetermined**

✓7th **T48.6X5 Adverse effect of antiasthmatics** UPD

✓7th **T48.6X6 Underdosing of antiasthmatics** UPD

✓5th **T48.9 Poisoning by, adverse effect of and underdosing of other and unspecified agents primarily acting on the respiratory system**

✓6th **T48.90 Poisoning by, adverse effect of and underdosing of unspecified agents primarily acting on the respiratory system**

✓7th **T48.901 Poisoning by unspecified agents primarily acting on the respiratory system, accidental (unintentional)**

2 ✓7th **T48.902 Poisoning by unspecified agents primarily acting on the respiratory system, intentional self-harm** HCC Rx ESR COM

✓7th **T48.903 Poisoning by unspecified agents primarily acting on the respiratory system, assault**

✓7th **T48.904 Poisoning by unspecified agents primarily acting on the respiratory system, undetermined**

✓7th **T48.905 Adverse effect of unspecified agents primarily acting on the respiratory system** UPD

✓7th **T48.906 Underdosing of unspecified agents primarily acting on the respiratory system** UPD

✓6th **T48.99 Poisoning by, adverse effect of and underdosing of other agents primarily acting on the respiratory system**

✓7th **T48.991 Poisoning by other agents primarily acting on the respiratory system, accidental (unintentional)**

2 ✓7th **T48.992 Poisoning by other agents primarily acting on the respiratory system, intentional self-harm** HCC Rx ESR COM

✓7th **T48.993 Poisoning by other agents primarily acting on the respiratory system, assault**

✓7th **T48.994 Poisoning by other agents primarily acting on the respiratory system, undetermined**

✓7th **T48.995 Adverse effect of other agents primarily acting on the respiratory system** UPD

✓7th **T48.996 Underdosing of other agents primarily acting on the respiratory system** UPD

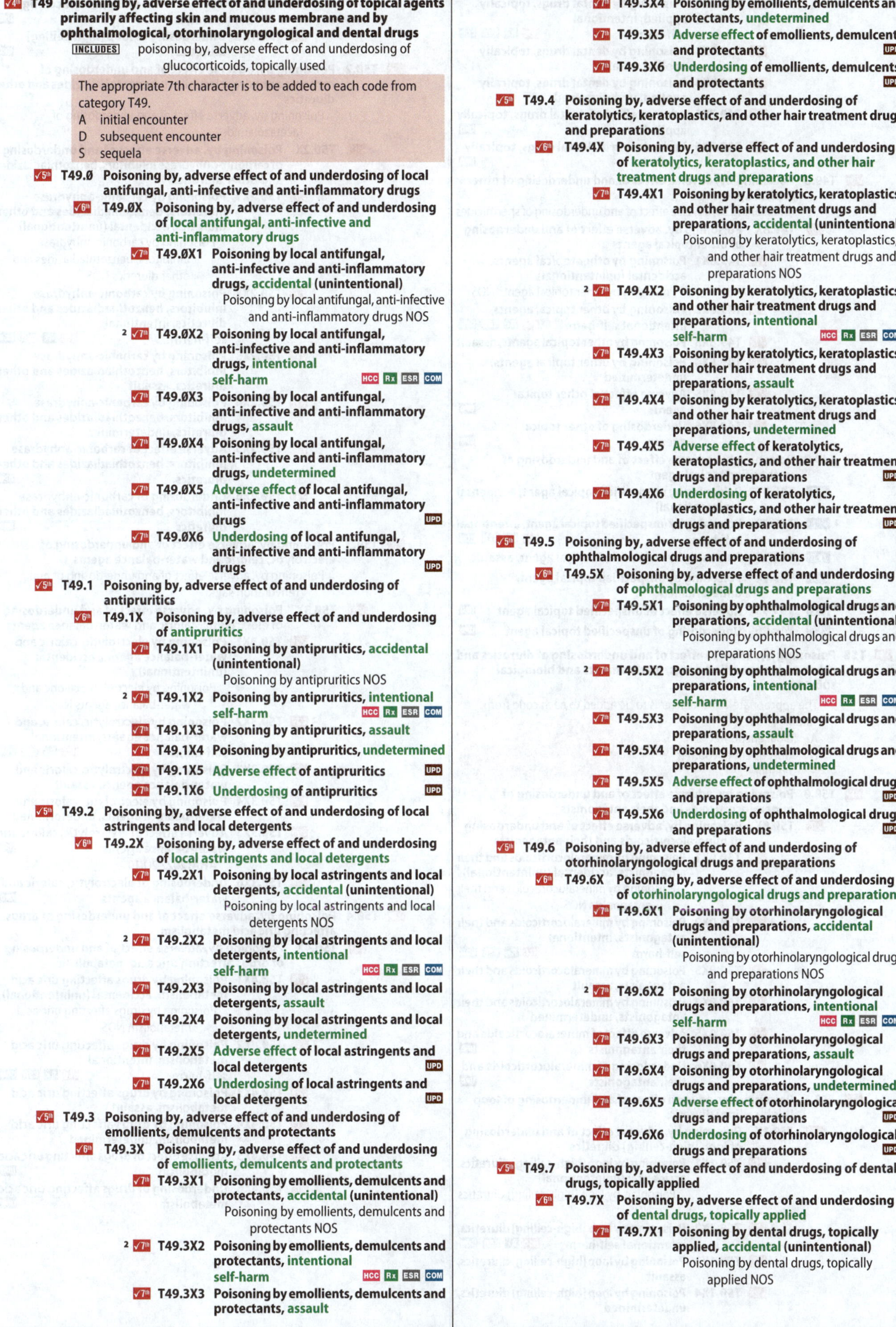

T49 Poisoning by, adverse effect of and underdosing of topical agents primarily affecting skin and mucous membrane and by ophthalmological, otorhinolaryngological and dental drugs

INCLUDES poisoning by, adverse effect of and underdosing of glucocorticoids, topically used

The appropriate 7th character is to be added to each code from category T49.
A initial encounter
D subsequent encounter
S sequela

T49.0 Poisoning by, adverse effect of and underdosing of local antifungal, anti-infective and anti-inflammatory drugs

T49.0X Poisoning by, adverse effect of and underdosing of local antifungal, anti-infective and anti-inflammatory drugs

T49.0X1 Poisoning by local antifungal, anti-infective and anti-inflammatory drugs, accidental (unintentional)
Poisoning by local antifungal, anti-infective and anti-inflammatory drugs NOS

2 **T49.0X2 Poisoning by local antifungal, anti-infective and anti-inflammatory drugs, intentional self-harm** HCC Rx ESR COM

T49.0X3 Poisoning by local antifungal, anti-infective and anti-inflammatory drugs, assault

T49.0X4 Poisoning by local antifungal, anti-infective and anti-inflammatory drugs, undetermined

T49.0X5 Adverse effect of local antifungal, anti-infective and anti-inflammatory drugs UPD

T49.0X6 Underdosing of local antifungal, anti-infective and anti-inflammatory drugs UPD

T49.1 Poisoning by, adverse effect of and underdosing of antipruritics

T49.1X Poisoning by, adverse effect of and underdosing of antipruritics

T49.1X1 Poisoning by antipruritics, accidental (unintentional)
Poisoning by antipruritics NOS

2 **T49.1X2 Poisoning by antipruritics, intentional self-harm** HCC Rx ESR COM

T49.1X3 Poisoning by antipruritics, assault

T49.1X4 Poisoning by antipruritics, undetermined

T49.1X5 Adverse effect of antipruritics UPD

T49.1X6 Underdosing of antipruritics UPD

T49.2 Poisoning by, adverse effect of and underdosing of local astringents and local detergents

T49.2X Poisoning by, adverse effect of and underdosing of local astringents and local detergents

T49.2X1 Poisoning by local astringents and local detergents, accidental (unintentional)
Poisoning by local astringents and local detergents NOS

2 **T49.2X2 Poisoning by local astringents and local detergents, intentional self-harm** HCC Rx ESR COM

T49.2X3 Poisoning by local astringents and local detergents, assault

T49.2X4 Poisoning by local astringents and local detergents, undetermined

T49.2X5 Adverse effect of local astringents and local detergents UPD

T49.2X6 Underdosing of local astringents and local detergents UPD

T49.3 Poisoning by, adverse effect of and underdosing of emollients, demulcents and protectants

T49.3X Poisoning by, adverse effect of and underdosing of emollients, demulcents and protectants

T49.3X1 Poisoning by emollients, demulcents and protectants, accidental (unintentional)
Poisoning by emollients, demulcents and protectants NOS

2 **T49.3X2 Poisoning by emollients, demulcents and protectants, intentional self-harm** HCC Rx ESR COM

T49.3X3 Poisoning by emollients, demulcents and protectants, assault

T49.3X4 Poisoning by emollients, demulcents and protectants, undetermined

T49.3X5 Adverse effect of emollients, demulcents and protectants UPD

T49.3X6 Underdosing of emollients, demulcents and protectants UPD

T49.4 Poisoning by, adverse effect of and underdosing of keratolytics, keratoplastics, and other hair treatment drugs and preparations

T49.4X Poisoning by, adverse effect of and underdosing of keratolytics, keratoplastics, and other hair treatment drugs and preparations

T49.4X1 Poisoning by keratolytics, keratoplastics, and other hair treatment drugs and preparations, accidental (unintentional)
Poisoning by keratolytics, keratoplastics, and other hair treatment drugs and preparations NOS

2 **T49.4X2 Poisoning by keratolytics, keratoplastics, and other hair treatment drugs and preparations, intentional self-harm** HCC Rx ESR COM

T49.4X3 Poisoning by keratolytics, keratoplastics, and other hair treatment drugs and preparations, assault

T49.4X4 Poisoning by keratolytics, keratoplastics, and other hair treatment drugs and preparations, undetermined

T49.4X5 Adverse effect of keratolytics, keratoplastics, and other hair treatment drugs and preparations UPD

T49.4X6 Underdosing of keratolytics, keratoplastics, and other hair treatment drugs and preparations UPD

T49.5 Poisoning by, adverse effect of and underdosing of ophthalmological drugs and preparations

T49.5X Poisoning by, adverse effect of and underdosing of ophthalmological drugs and preparations

T49.5X1 Poisoning by ophthalmological drugs and preparations, accidental (unintentional)
Poisoning by ophthalmological drugs and preparations NOS

2 **T49.5X2 Poisoning by ophthalmological drugs and preparations, intentional self-harm** HCC Rx ESR COM

T49.5X3 Poisoning by ophthalmological drugs and preparations, assault

T49.5X4 Poisoning by ophthalmological drugs and preparations, undetermined

T49.5X5 Adverse effect of ophthalmological drugs and preparations UPD

T49.5X6 Underdosing of ophthalmological drugs and preparations UPD

T49.6 Poisoning by, adverse effect of and underdosing of otorhinolaryngological drugs and preparations

T49.6X Poisoning by, adverse effect of and underdosing of otorhinolaryngological drugs and preparations

T49.6X1 Poisoning by otorhinolaryngological drugs and preparations, accidental (unintentional)
Poisoning by otorhinolaryngological drugs and preparations NOS

2 **T49.6X2 Poisoning by otorhinolaryngological drugs and preparations, intentional self-harm** HCC Rx ESR COM

T49.6X3 Poisoning by otorhinolaryngological drugs and preparations, assault

T49.6X4 Poisoning by otorhinolaryngological drugs and preparations, undetermined

T49.6X5 Adverse effect of otorhinolaryngological drugs and preparations UPD

T49.6X6 Underdosing of otorhinolaryngological drugs and preparations UPD

T49.7 Poisoning by, adverse effect of and underdosing of dental drugs, topically applied

T49.7X Poisoning by, adverse effect of and underdosing of dental drugs, topically applied

T49.7X1 Poisoning by dental drugs, topically applied, accidental (unintentional)
Poisoning by dental drugs, topically applied NOS

Chapter 19. Injury, Poisoning and Certain Other Consequences of External Causes

Additional Character Required | Placeholder Alert | Manifestation | Unspecified Dx | QPP | UPD Unacceptable PDx

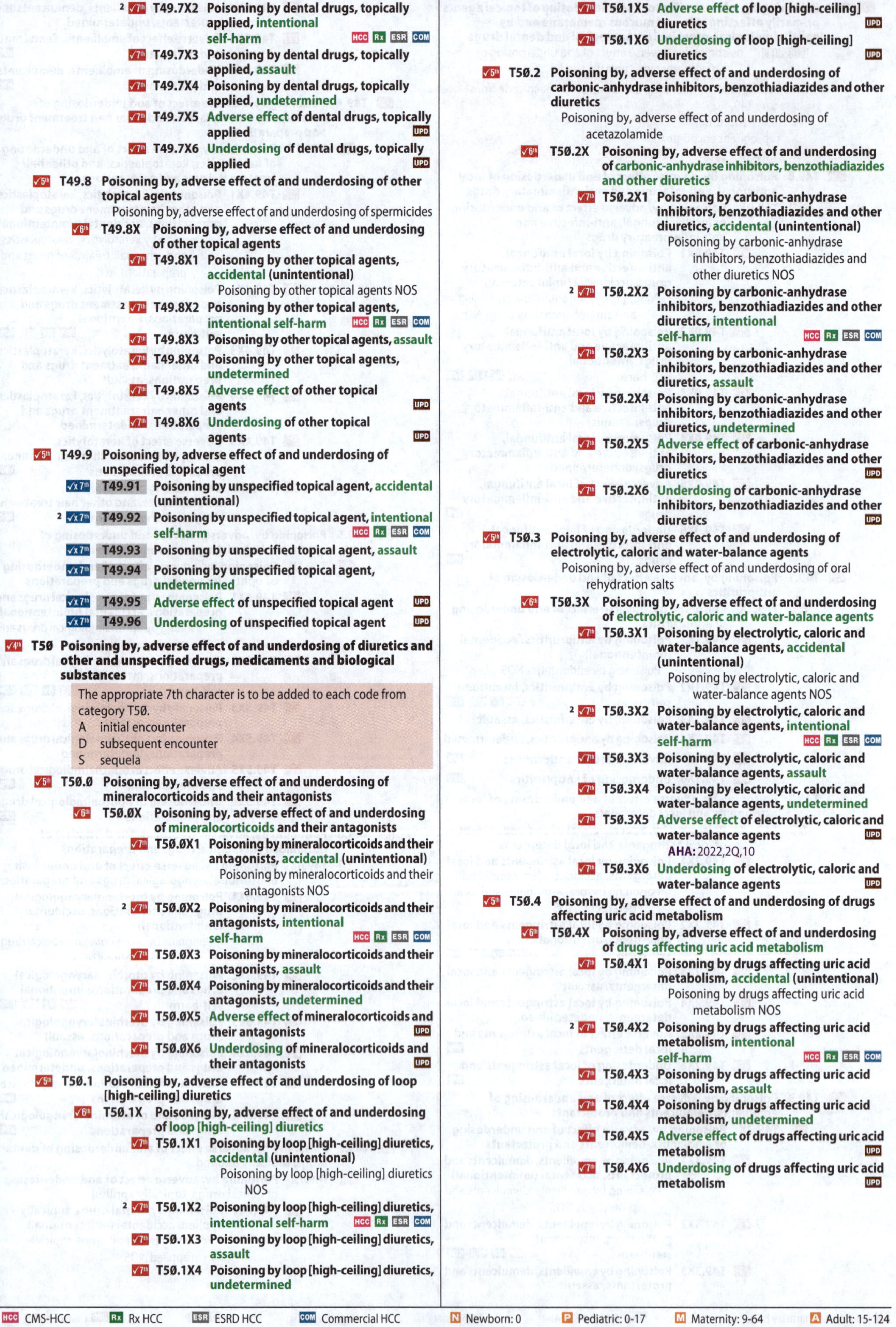

T49.7X2 Poisoning by dental drugs, topically applied, intentional self-harm HCC Rx ESR COM

T49.7X3 Poisoning by dental drugs, topically applied, assault

T49.7X4 Poisoning by dental drugs, topically applied, undetermined

T49.7X5 Adverse effect of dental drugs, topically applied UPD

T49.7X6 Underdosing of dental drugs, topically applied UPD

T49.8 Poisoning by, adverse effect of and underdosing of other topical agents

Poisoning by, adverse effect of and underdosing of spermicides

T49.8X Poisoning by, adverse effect of and underdosing of other topical agents

T49.8X1 Poisoning by other topical agents, accidental (unintentional)

Poisoning by other topical agents NOS

T49.8X2 Poisoning by other topical agents, intentional self-harm HCC Rx ESR COM

T49.8X3 Poisoning by other topical agents, assault

T49.8X4 Poisoning by other topical agents, undetermined

T49.8X5 Adverse effect of other topical agents UPD

T49.8X6 Underdosing of other topical agents UPD

T49.9 Poisoning by, adverse effect of and underdosing of unspecified topical agent

T49.91 Poisoning by unspecified topical agent, accidental (unintentional)

T49.92 Poisoning by unspecified topical agent, intentional self-harm HCC Rx ESR COM

T49.93 Poisoning by unspecified topical agent, assault

T49.94 Poisoning by unspecified topical agent, undetermined

T49.95 Adverse effect of unspecified topical agent UPD

T49.96 Underdosing of unspecified topical agent UPD

T50 Poisoning by, adverse effect of and underdosing of diuretics and other and unspecified drugs, medicaments and biological substances

The appropriate 7th character is to be added to each code from category T50.
- A initial encounter
- D subsequent encounter
- S sequela

T50.0 Poisoning by, adverse effect of and underdosing of mineralocorticoids and their antagonists

T50.0X Poisoning by, adverse effect of and underdosing of mineralocorticoids and their antagonists

T50.0X1 Poisoning by mineralocorticoids and their antagonists, accidental (unintentional)

Poisoning by mineralocorticoids and their antagonists NOS

T50.0X2 Poisoning by mineralocorticoids and their antagonists, intentional self-harm HCC Rx ESR COM

T50.0X3 Poisoning by mineralocorticoids and their antagonists, assault

T50.0X4 Poisoning by mineralocorticoids and their antagonists, undetermined

T50.0X5 Adverse effect of mineralocorticoids and their antagonists UPD

T50.0X6 Underdosing of mineralocorticoids and their antagonists UPD

T50.1 Poisoning by, adverse effect of and underdosing of loop [high-ceiling] diuretics

T50.1X Poisoning by, adverse effect of and underdosing of loop [high-ceiling] diuretics

T50.1X1 Poisoning by loop [high-ceiling] diuretics, accidental (unintentional)

Poisoning by loop [high-ceiling] diuretics NOS

T50.1X2 Poisoning by loop [high-ceiling] diuretics, intentional self-harm HCC Rx ESR COM

T50.1X3 Poisoning by loop [high-ceiling] diuretics, assault

T50.1X4 Poisoning by loop [high-ceiling] diuretics, undetermined

T50.1X5 Adverse effect of loop [high-ceiling] diuretics UPD

T50.1X6 Underdosing of loop [high-ceiling] diuretics UPD

T50.2 Poisoning by, adverse effect of and underdosing of carbonic-anhydrase inhibitors, benzothiadiazides and other diuretics

Poisoning by, adverse effect of and underdosing of acetazolamide

T50.2X Poisoning by, adverse effect of and underdosing of carbonic-anhydrase inhibitors, benzothiadiazides and other diuretics

T50.2X1 Poisoning by carbonic-anhydrase inhibitors, benzothiadiazides and other diuretics, accidental (unintentional)

Poisoning by carbonic-anhydrase inhibitors, benzothiadiazides and other diuretics NOS

T50.2X2 Poisoning by carbonic-anhydrase inhibitors, benzothiadiazides and other diuretics, intentional self-harm HCC Rx ESR COM

T50.2X3 Poisoning by carbonic-anhydrase inhibitors, benzothiadiazides and other diuretics, assault

T50.2X4 Poisoning by carbonic-anhydrase inhibitors, benzothiadiazides and other diuretics, undetermined

T50.2X5 Adverse effect of carbonic-anhydrase inhibitors, benzothiadiazides and other diuretics UPD

T50.2X6 Underdosing of carbonic-anhydrase inhibitors, benzothiadiazides and other diuretics UPD

T50.3 Poisoning by, adverse effect of and underdosing of electrolytic, caloric and water-balance agents

Poisoning by, adverse effect of and underdosing of oral rehydration salts

T50.3X Poisoning by, adverse effect of and underdosing of electrolytic, caloric and water-balance agents

T50.3X1 Poisoning by electrolytic, caloric and water-balance agents, accidental (unintentional)

Poisoning by electrolytic, caloric and water-balance agents NOS

T50.3X2 Poisoning by electrolytic, caloric and water-balance agents, intentional self-harm HCC Rx ESR COM

T50.3X3 Poisoning by electrolytic, caloric and water-balance agents, assault

T50.3X4 Poisoning by electrolytic, caloric and water-balance agents, undetermined

T50.3X5 Adverse effect of electrolytic, caloric and water-balance agents UPD

AHA: 2022,2Q,10

T50.3X6 Underdosing of electrolytic, caloric and water-balance agents UPD

T50.4 Poisoning by, adverse effect of and underdosing of drugs affecting uric acid metabolism

T50.4X Poisoning by, adverse effect of and underdosing of drugs affecting uric acid metabolism

T50.4X1 Poisoning by drugs affecting uric acid metabolism, accidental (unintentional)

Poisoning by drugs affecting uric acid metabolism NOS

T50.4X2 Poisoning by drugs affecting uric acid metabolism, intentional self-harm HCC Rx ESR COM

T50.4X3 Poisoning by drugs affecting uric acid metabolism, assault

T50.4X4 Poisoning by drugs affecting uric acid metabolism, undetermined

T50.4X5 Adverse effect of drugs affecting uric acid metabolism UPD

T50.4X6 Underdosing of drugs affecting uric acid metabolism UPD

T5Ø.5 Poisoning by, adverse effect of and underdosing of appetite depressants

T5Ø.5X Poisoning by, adverse effect of and underdosing of appetite depressants

T5Ø.5X1 Poisoning by appetite depressants, accidental (unintentional)
Poisoning by appetite depressants NOS

2 **T5Ø.5X2 Poisoning by appetite depressants, intentional self-harm** HCC Rx ESR COM

T5Ø.5X3 Poisoning by appetite depressants, assault

T5Ø.5X4 Poisoning by appetite depressants, undetermined

T5Ø.5X5 Adverse effect of appetite depressants UPD

T5Ø.5X6 Underdosing of appetite depressants UPD

T5Ø.6 Poisoning by, adverse effect of and underdosing of antidotes and chelating agents
Poisoning by, adverse effect of and underdosing of alcohol deterrents

T5Ø.6X Poisoning by, adverse effect of and underdosing of antidotes and chelating agents

T5Ø.6X1 Poisoning by antidotes and chelating agents, accidental (unintentional)
Poisoning by antidotes and chelating agents NOS

2 **T5Ø.6X2 Poisoning by antidotes and chelating agents, intentional self-harm** HCC Rx ESR COM

T5Ø.6X3 Poisoning by antidotes and chelating agents, assault

T5Ø.6X4 Poisoning by antidotes and chelating agents, undetermined

T5Ø.6X5 Adverse effect of antidotes and chelating agents UPD

T5Ø.6X6 Underdosing of antidotes and chelating agents UPD

T5Ø.7 Poisoning by, adverse effect of and underdosing of analeptics and opioid receptor antagonists

T5Ø.7X Poisoning by, adverse effect of and underdosing of analeptics and opioid receptor antagonists

T5Ø.7X1 Poisoning by analeptics and opioid receptor antagonists, accidental (unintentional)
Poisoning by analeptics and opioid receptor antagonists NOS

2 **T5Ø.7X2 Poisoning by analeptics and opioid receptor antagonists, intentional self-harm** HCC Rx ESR COM

T5Ø.7X3 Poisoning by analeptics and opioid receptor antagonists, assault

T5Ø.7X4 Poisoning by analeptics and opioid receptor antagonists, undetermined

T5Ø.7X5 Adverse effect of analeptics and opioid receptor antagonists UPD

T5Ø.7X6 Underdosing of analeptics and opioid receptor antagonists UPD

T5Ø.8 Poisoning by, adverse effect of and underdosing of diagnostic agents

T5Ø.8X Poisoning by, adverse effect of and underdosing of diagnostic agents

T5Ø.8X1 Poisoning by diagnostic agents, accidental (unintentional)
Poisoning by diagnostic agents NOS

2 **T5Ø.8X2 Poisoning by diagnostic agents, intentional self-harm** HCC Rx ESR COM

T5Ø.8X3 Poisoning by diagnostic agents, assault

T5Ø.8X4 Poisoning by diagnostic agents, undetermined

T5Ø.8X5 Adverse effect of diagnostic agents UPD
AHA: 2021,3Q,9-10

T5Ø.8X6 Underdosing of diagnostic agents UPD

T5Ø.A Poisoning by, adverse effect of and underdosing of bacterial vaccines

T5Ø.A1 Poisoning by, adverse effect of and underdosing of pertussis vaccine, including combinations with a pertussis component

T5Ø.A11 Poisoning by pertussis vaccine, including combinations with a pertussis component, accidental (unintentional)

2 **T5Ø.A12 Poisoning by pertussis vaccine, including combinations with a pertussis component, intentional self-harm** HCC Rx ESR COM

T5Ø.A13 Poisoning by pertussis vaccine, including combinations with a pertussis component, assault

T5Ø.A14 Poisoning by pertussis vaccine, including combinations with a pertussis component, undetermined

T5Ø.A15 Adverse effect of pertussis vaccine, including combinations with a pertussis component UPD

T5Ø.A16 Underdosing of pertussis vaccine, including combinations with a pertussis component UPD

T5Ø.A2 Poisoning by, adverse effect of and underdosing of mixed bacterial vaccines without a pertussis component

T5Ø.A21 Poisoning by mixed bacterial vaccines without a pertussis component, accidental (unintentional)

2 **T5Ø.A22 Poisoning by mixed bacterial vaccines without a pertussis component, intentional self-harm** HCC Rx ESR COM

T5Ø.A23 Poisoning by mixed bacterial vaccines without a pertussis component, assault

T5Ø.A24 Poisoning by mixed bacterial vaccines without a pertussis component, undetermined

T5Ø.A25 Adverse effect of mixed bacterial vaccines without a pertussis component UPD

T5Ø.A26 Underdosing of mixed bacterial vaccines without a pertussis component UPD

T5Ø.A9 Poisoning by, adverse effect of and underdosing of other bacterial vaccines

T5Ø.A91 Poisoning by other bacterial vaccines, accidental (unintentional)

2 **T5Ø.A92 Poisoning by other bacterial vaccines, intentional self-harm** HCC Rx ESR COM

T5Ø.A93 Poisoning by other bacterial vaccines, assault

T5Ø.A94 Poisoning by other bacterial vaccines, undetermined

T5Ø.A95 Adverse effect of other bacterial vaccines UPD

T5Ø.A96 Underdosing of other bacterial vaccines UPD

T5Ø.B Poisoning by, adverse effect of and underdosing of viral vaccines

T5Ø.B1 Poisoning by, adverse effect of and underdosing of smallpox vaccines

T5Ø.B11 Poisoning by smallpox vaccines, accidental (unintentional)

2 **T5Ø.B12 Poisoning by smallpox vaccines, intentional self-harm** HCC Rx ESR COM

T5Ø.B13 Poisoning by smallpox vaccines, assault

T5Ø.B14 Poisoning by smallpox vaccines, undetermined

T5Ø.B15 Adverse effect of smallpox vaccines UPD

T5Ø.B16 Underdosing of smallpox vaccines UPD

T5Ø.B9 Poisoning by, adverse effect of and underdosing of other viral vaccines

T5Ø.B91 Poisoning by other viral vaccines, accidental (unintentional)

2 **T5Ø.B92 Poisoning by other viral vaccines, intentional self-harm** HCC Rx ESR COM

T5Ø.B93 Poisoning by other viral vaccines, assault

T5Ø.B94 Poisoning by other viral vaccines, undetermined

T5Ø.B95 Adverse effect of other viral vaccines UPD
AHA: 2021,1Q,43

T5Ø.B96 Underdosing of other viral vaccines UPD

T5Ø.Z Poisoning by, adverse effect of and underdosing of other vaccines and biological substances

T5Ø.Z1 Poisoning by, adverse effect of and underdosing of immunoglobulin

T5Ø.Z11 Poisoning by immunoglobulin, accidental (unintentional)

[2] **T50.Z12 Poisoning by immunoglobulin, intentional self-harm** HCC Rx ESR COM

T50.Z13 Poisoning by immunoglobulin, assault

T50.Z14 Poisoning by immunoglobulin, undetermined

T50.Z15 Adverse effect of immunoglobulin UPD

T50.Z16 Underdosing of immunoglobulin UPD

T50.Z9 Poisoning by, adverse effect of and underdosing of other vaccines and biological substances

T50.Z91 Poisoning by other vaccines and biological substances, accidental (unintentional)

[2] **T50.Z92 Poisoning by other vaccines and biological substances, intentional self-harm** HCC Rx ESR COM

T50.Z93 Poisoning by other vaccines and biological substances, assault

T50.Z94 Poisoning by other vaccines and biological substances, undetermined

T50.Z95 Adverse effect of other vaccines and biological substances UPD

AHA: 2020,1Q,18

T50.Z96 Underdosing of other vaccines and biological substances UPD

T50.9 Poisoning by, adverse effect of and underdosing of other and unspecified drugs, medicaments and biological substances

T50.90 Poisoning by, adverse effect of and underdosing of unspecified drugs, medicaments and biological substances

T50.901 Poisoning by unspecified drugs, medicaments and biological substances, accidental (unintentional)

[2] **T50.902 Poisoning by unspecified drugs, medicaments and biological substances, intentional self-harm** HCC Rx ESR COM

T50.903 Poisoning by unspecified drugs, medicaments and biological substances, assault

T50.904 Poisoning by unspecified drugs, medicaments and biological substances, undetermined

T50.905 Adverse effect of unspecified drugs, medicaments and biological substances

T50.906 Underdosing of unspecified drugs, medicaments and biological substances

T50.91 Poisoning by, adverse effect of and underdosing of multiple unspecified drugs, medicaments and biological substances

Multiple drug ingestion NOS

Code also any specific drugs, medicaments and biological substances

T50.911 Poisoning by multiple unspecified drugs, medicaments and biological substances, accidental (unintentional)

[2] **T50.912 Poisoning by multiple unspecified drugs, medicaments and biological substances, intentional self-harm** HCC Rx ESR COM

T50.913 Poisoning by multiple unspecified drugs, medicaments and biological substances, assault

T50.914 Poisoning by multiple unspecified drugs, medicaments and biological substances, undetermined

T50.915 Adverse effect of multiple unspecified drugs, medicaments and biological substances UPD

T50.916 Underdosing of multiple unspecified drugs, medicaments and biological substances UPD

T50.99 Poisoning by, adverse effect of and underdosing of other drugs, medicaments and biological substances

T50.991 Poisoning by other drugs, medicaments and biological substances, accidental (unintentional)

[2] **T50.992 Poisoning by other drugs, medicaments and biological substances, intentional self-harm** HCC Rx ESR COM

T50.993 Poisoning by other drugs, medicaments and biological substances, assault

T50.994 Poisoning by other drugs, medicaments and biological substances, undetermined

T50.995 Adverse effect of other drugs, medicaments and biological substances

T50.996 Underdosing of other drugs, medicaments and biological substances

Toxic effects of substances chiefly nonmedicinal as to source (T51-T65)

NOTE When no intent is indicated code to accidental. Undetermined intent is only for use when there is specific documentation in the record that the intent of the toxic effect cannot be determined.

Use additional code(s) for all associated manifestations of toxic effect, such as:
- personal history of foreign body fully removed (Z87.821)
- respiratory conditions due to external agents (J60-J70)
- to identify any retained foreign body, if applicable (Z18.-)

EXCLUDES 1 *contact with and (suspected) exposure to toxic substances (Z77.-)*

AHA: 2017,1Q,39-40

T51 Toxic effect of alcohol

The appropriate 7th character is to be added to each code from category T51.
- A initial encounter
- D subsequent encounter
- S sequela

T51.0 Toxic effect of ethanol

Toxic effect of ethyl alcohol

EXCLUDES 2 *acute alcohol intoxication or "hangover" effects (F10.129, F10.229, F10.929)*
drunkenness (F10.129, F10.229, F10.929)
pathological alcohol intoxication (F10.129, F10.229, F10.929)

T51.0X Toxic effect of ethanol

[1] **T51.0X1 Toxic effect of ethanol, accidental (unintentional)** HCC ESR

Toxic effect of ethanol NOS

[2] **T51.0X2 Toxic effect of ethanol, intentional self-harm** HCC Rx ESR COM

T51.0X3 Toxic effect of ethanol, assault

[1] **T51.0X4 Toxic effect of ethanol, undetermined** HCC ESR

T51.1 Toxic effect of methanol

Toxic effect of methyl alcohol

T51.1X Toxic effect of methanol

T51.1X1 Toxic effect of methanol, accidental (unintentional)

Toxic effect of methanol NOS

[2] **T51.1X2 Toxic effect of methanol, intentional self-harm** HCC Rx ESR COM

T51.1X3 Toxic effect of methanol, assault

T51.1X4 Toxic effect of methanol, undetermined

T51.2 Toxic effect of 2-Propanol

Toxic effect of isopropyl alcohol

T51.2X Toxic effect of 2-Propanol

T51.2X1 Toxic effect of 2-Propanol, accidental (unintentional)

Toxic effect of 2-Propanol NOS

[2] **T51.2X2 Toxic effect of 2-Propanol, intentional self-harm** HCC Rx ESR COM

T51.2X3 Toxic effect of 2-Propanol, assault

T51.2X4 Toxic effect of 2-Propanol, undetermined

T51.3 Toxic effect of fusel oil

Toxic effect of amyl alcohol

Toxic effect of butyl [1-butanol] alcohol

Toxic effect of propyl [1-propanol] alcohol

T51.3X Toxic effect of fusel oil

T51.3X1 Toxic effect of fusel oil, accidental (unintentional)

Toxic effect of fusel oil NOS

[2] **T51.3X2 Toxic effect of fusel oil, intentional self-harm** HCC Rx ESR COM

T51.3X3 Toxic effect of fusel oil, assault

T51.3X4 Toxic effect of fusel oil, undetermined

√5th T51.8 **Toxic effect of other alcohols**

√6th T51.8X **Toxic effect of other alcohols**

√7th T51.8X1 **Toxic effect of other alcohols, accidental (unintentional)**
Toxic effect of other alcohols NOS

2 √7th T51.8X2 **Toxic effect of other alcohols, intentional self-harm** HCC Rx ESR COM

√7th T51.8X3 **Toxic effect of other alcohols, assault**

√7th T51.8X4 **Toxic effect of other alcohols, undetermined**

√5th T51.9 **Toxic effect of unspecified alcohol**

√x7th T51.91 **Toxic effect of unspecified alcohol, accidental (unintentional)**

2 √x7th T51.92 **Toxic effect of unspecified alcohol, intentional self-harm** HCC Rx ESR COM

√x7th T51.93 **Toxic effect of unspecified alcohol, assault**

√x7th T51.94 **Toxic effect of unspecified alcohol, undetermined**

√4th **T52 Toxic effect of organic solvents**

EXCLUDES 1 *halogen derivatives of aliphatic and aromatic hydrocarbons (T53.-)*

The appropriate 7th character is to be added to each code from category T52.
A initial encounter
D subsequent encounter
S sequela

√5th T52.0 **Toxic effects of petroleum products**
Toxic effects of ether petroleum
Toxic effects of gasoline [petrol]
Toxic effects of kerosene [paraffin oil]
Toxic effects of naphtha petroleum
Toxic effects of paraffin wax
Toxic effects of spirit petroleum

√6th T52.0X **Toxic effects of petroleum products**

√7th T52.0X1 **Toxic effect of petroleum products, accidental (unintentional)**
Toxic effects of petroleum products NOS

2 √7th T52.0X2 **Toxic effect of petroleum products, intentional self-harm** HCC Rx ESR COM

√7th T52.0X3 **Toxic effect of petroleum products, assault**

√7th T52.0X4 **Toxic effect of petroleum products, undetermined**

√5th T52.1 **Toxic effects of benzene**

EXCLUDES 1 *homologues of benzene (T52.2)*
nitroderivatives and aminoderivatives of benzene and its homologues (T65.3)

√6th T52.1X **Toxic effects of benzene**

√7th T52.1X1 **Toxic effect of benzene, accidental (unintentional)**
Toxic effects of benzene NOS

2 √7th T52.1X2 **Toxic effect of benzene, intentional self-harm** HCC Rx ESR COM

√7th T52.1X3 **Toxic effect of benzene, assault**

√7th T52.1X4 **Toxic effect of benzene, undetermined**

√5th T52.2 **Toxic effects of homologues of benzene**
Toxic effects of toluene [methylbenzene]
Toxic effects of xylene [dimethylbenzene]

√6th T52.2X **Toxic effects of homologues of benzene**

√7th T52.2X1 **Toxic effect of homologues of benzene, accidental (unintentional)**
Toxic effects of homologues of benzene NOS

2 √7th T52.2X2 **Toxic effect of homologues of benzene, intentional self-harm** HCC Rx ESR COM

√7th T52.2X3 **Toxic effect of homologues of benzene, assault**

√7th T52.2X4 **Toxic effect of homologues of benzene, undetermined**

√5th T52.3 **Toxic effects of glycols**

√6th T52.3X **Toxic effects of glycols**

√7th T52.3X1 **Toxic effect of glycols, accidental (unintentional)**
Toxic effects of glycols NOS

2 √7th T52.3X2 **Toxic effect of glycols, intentional self-harm** HCC Rx ESR COM

√7th T52.3X3 **Toxic effect of glycols, assault**

√7th T52.3X4 **Toxic effect of glycols, undetermined**

√5th T52.4 **Toxic effects of ketones**

√6th T52.4X **Toxic effects of ketones**

√7th T52.4X1 **Toxic effect of ketones, accidental (unintentional)**
Toxic effects of ketones NOS

2 √7th T52.4X2 **Toxic effect of ketones, intentional self-harm** HCC Rx ESR COM

√7th T52.4X3 **Toxic effect of ketones, assault**

√7th T52.4X4 **Toxic effect of ketones, undetermined**

√5th T52.8 **Toxic effects of other organic solvents**

√6th T52.8X **Toxic effects of other organic solvents**

√7th T52.8X1 **Toxic effect of other organic solvents, accidental (unintentional)**
Toxic effects of other organic solvents NOS

2 √7th T52.8X2 **Toxic effect of other organic solvents, intentional self-harm** HCC Rx ESR COM

√7th T52.8X3 **Toxic effect of other organic solvents, assault**

√7th T52.8X4 **Toxic effect of other organic solvents, undetermined**

√5th T52.9 **Toxic effects of unspecified organic solvent**

√x7th T52.91 **Toxic effect of unspecified organic solvent, accidental (unintentional)**

2 √x7th T52.92 **Toxic effect of unspecified organic solvent, intentional self-harm** HCC Rx ESR COM

√x7th T52.93 **Toxic effect of unspecified organic solvent, assault**

√x7th T52.94 **Toxic effect of unspecified organic solvent, undetermined**

√4th **T53 Toxic effect of halogen derivatives of aliphatic and aromatic hydrocarbons**

The appropriate 7th character is to be added to each code from category T53.
A initial encounter
D subsequent encounter
S sequela

√5th T53.0 **Toxic effects of carbon tetrachloride**
Toxic effects of tetrachloromethane

√6th T53.0X **Toxic effects of carbon tetrachloride**

√7th T53.0X1 **Toxic effect of carbon tetrachloride, accidental (unintentional)**
Toxic effects of carbon tetrachloride NOS

2 √7th T53.0X2 **Toxic effect of carbon tetrachloride, intentional self-harm** HCC Rx ESR COM

√7th T53.0X3 **Toxic effect of carbon tetrachloride, assault**

√7th T53.0X4 **Toxic effect of carbon tetrachloride, undetermined**

√5th T53.1 **Toxic effects of chloroform**
Toxic effects of trichloromethane

√6th T53.1X **Toxic effects of chloroform**

√7th T53.1X1 **Toxic effect of chloroform, accidental (unintentional)**
Toxic effects of chloroform NOS

2 √7th T53.1X2 **Toxic effect of chloroform, intentional self-harm** HCC Rx ESR COM

√7th T53.1X3 **Toxic effect of chloroform, assault**

√7th T53.1X4 **Toxic effect of chloroform, undetermined**

√5th T53.2 **Toxic effects of trichloroethylene**
Toxic effects of trichloroethene

√6th T53.2X **Toxic effects of trichloroethylene**

√7th T53.2X1 **Toxic effect of trichloroethylene, accidental (unintentional)**
Toxic effects of trichloroethylene NOS

2 √7th T53.2X2 **Toxic effect of trichloroethylene, intentional self-harm** HCC Rx ESR COM

√7th T53.2X3 **Toxic effect of trichloroethylene, assault**

√7th T53.2X4 **Toxic effect of trichloroethylene, undetermined**

T53.3 Toxic effects of tetrachloroethylene
Toxic effects of perchloroethylene
Toxic effect of tetrachloroethene

T53.3X Toxic effects of tetrachloroethylene

T53.3X1 Toxic effect of tetrachloroethylene, accidental (unintentional)
Toxic effects of tetrachloroethylene NOS

T53.3X2 Toxic effect of tetrachloroethylene, intentional self-harm HCC Rx ESR COM

T53.3X3 Toxic effect of tetrachloroethylene, assault

T53.3X4 Toxic effect of tetrachloroethylene, undetermined

T53.4 Toxic effects of dichloromethane
Toxic effects of methylene chloride

T53.4X Toxic effects of dichloromethane

T53.4X1 Toxic effect of dichloromethane, accidental (unintentional)
Toxic effects of dichloromethane NOS

T53.4X2 Toxic effect of dichloromethane, intentional self-harm HCC Rx ESR COM

T53.4X3 Toxic effect of dichloromethane, assault

T53.4X4 Toxic effect of dichloromethane, undetermined

T53.5 Toxic effects of chlorofluorocarbons

T53.5X Toxic effects of chlorofluorocarbons

T53.5X1 Toxic effect of chlorofluorocarbons, accidental (unintentional)
Toxic effects of chlorofluorocarbons NOS

T53.5X2 Toxic effect of chlorofluorocarbons, intentional self-harm HCC Rx ESR COM

T53.5X3 Toxic effect of chlorofluorocarbons, assault

T53.5X4 Toxic effect of chlorofluorocarbons, undetermined

T53.6 Toxic effects of other halogen derivatives of aliphatic hydrocarbons

T53.6X Toxic effects of other halogen derivatives of aliphatic hydrocarbons

T53.6X1 Toxic effect of other halogen derivatives of aliphatic hydrocarbons, accidental (unintentional)
Toxic effects of other halogen derivatives of aliphatic hydrocarbons NOS

T53.6X2 Toxic effect of other halogen derivatives of aliphatic hydrocarbons, intentional self-harm HCC Rx ESR COM

T53.6X3 Toxic effect of other halogen derivatives of aliphatic hydrocarbons, assault

T53.6X4 Toxic effect of other halogen derivatives of aliphatic hydrocarbons, undetermined

T53.7 Toxic effects of other halogen derivatives of aromatic hydrocarbons

T53.7X Toxic effects of other halogen derivatives of aromatic hydrocarbons

T53.7X1 Toxic effect of other halogen derivatives of aromatic hydrocarbons, accidental (unintentional)
Toxic effects of other halogen derivatives of aromatic hydrocarbons NOS

T53.7X2 Toxic effect of other halogen derivatives of aromatic hydrocarbons, intentional self-harm HCC Rx ESR COM

T53.7X3 Toxic effect of other halogen derivatives of aromatic hydrocarbons, assault

T53.7X4 Toxic effect of other halogen derivatives of aromatic hydrocarbons, undetermined

T53.9 Toxic effects of unspecified halogen derivatives of aliphatic and aromatic hydrocarbons

T53.91 Toxic effect of unspecified halogen derivatives of aliphatic and aromatic hydrocarbons, accidental (unintentional)

T53.92 Toxic effect of unspecified halogen derivatives of aliphatic and aromatic hydrocarbons, intentional self-harm HCC Rx ESR COM

T53.93 Toxic effect of unspecified halogen derivatives of aliphatic and aromatic hydrocarbons, assault

T53.94 Toxic effect of unspecified halogen derivatives of aliphatic and aromatic hydrocarbons, undetermined

T54 Toxic effect of corrosive substances

The appropriate 7th character is to be added to each code from category T54.
A initial encounter
D subsequent encounter
S sequela

T54.0 Toxic effects of phenol and phenol homologues

T54.0X Toxic effects of phenol and phenol homologues

T54.0X1 Toxic effect of phenol and phenol homologues, accidental (unintentional)
Toxic effects of phenol and phenol homologues NOS

T54.0X2 Toxic effect of phenol and phenol homologues, intentional self-harm HCC Rx ESR COM

T54.0X3 Toxic effect of phenol and phenol homologues, assault

T54.0X4 Toxic effect of phenol and phenol homologues, undetermined

T54.1 Toxic effects of other corrosive organic compounds

T54.1X Toxic effects of other corrosive organic compounds

T54.1X1 Toxic effect of other corrosive organic compounds, accidental (unintentional)
Toxic effects of other corrosive organic compounds NOS

T54.1X2 Toxic effect of other corrosive organic compounds, intentional self-harm HCC Rx ESR COM

T54.1X3 Toxic effect of other corrosive organic compounds, assault

T54.1X4 Toxic effect of other corrosive organic compounds, undetermined

T54.2 Toxic effects of corrosive acids and acid-like substances
Toxic effects of hydrochloric acid
Toxic effects of sulfuric acid

T54.2X Toxic effects of corrosive acids and acid-like substances

T54.2X1 Toxic effect of corrosive acids and acid-like substances, accidental (unintentional)
Toxic effects of corrosive acids and acid-like substances NOS

T54.2X2 Toxic effect of corrosive acids and acid-like substances, intentional self-harm HCC Rx ESR COM

T54.2X3 Toxic effect of corrosive acids and acid-like substances, assault

T54.2X4 Toxic effect of corrosive acids and acid-like substances, undetermined

T54.3 Toxic effects of corrosive alkalis and alkali-like substances
Toxic effects of potassium hydroxide
Toxic effects of sodium hydroxide

T54.3X Toxic effects of corrosive alkalis and alkali-like substances

T54.3X1 Toxic effect of corrosive alkalis and alkali-like substances, accidental (unintentional)
Toxic effects of corrosive alkalis and alkali-like substances NOS

T54.3X2 Toxic effect of corrosive alkalis and alkali-like substances, intentional self-harm HCC Rx ESR COM

T54.3X3 Toxic effect of corrosive alkalis and alkali-like substances, assault

T54.3X4 Toxic effect of corrosive alkalis and alkali-like substances, undetermined

T54.9 Toxic effects of unspecified corrosive substance

T54.91 Toxic effect of unspecified corrosive substance, accidental (unintentional)

T54.92 Toxic effect of unspecified corrosive substance, intentional self-harm HCC Rx ESR COM

T54.93 Toxic effect of unspecified corrosive substance, assault

T54.94 Toxic effect of unspecified corrosive substance, undetermined

HCC CMS-HCC Rx Rx HCC ESR ESRD HCC COM Commercial HCC N Newborn: 0 P Pediatric: 0-17 M Maternity: 9-64 A Adult: 15-124

T55 Toxic effect of soaps and detergents

The appropriate 7th character is to be added to each code from category T55.
A initial encounter
D subsequent encounter
S sequela

T55.Ø Toxic effect of soaps
T55.ØX Toxic effect of soaps
T55.ØX1 Toxic effect of soaps, accidental (unintentional)
Toxic effect of soaps NOS
2 **T55.ØX2 Toxic effect of soaps, intentional self-harm** HCC Rx ESR COM
T55.ØX3 Toxic effect of soaps, assault
T55.ØX4 Toxic effect of soaps, undetermined

T55.1 Toxic effect of detergents
T55.1X Toxic effect of detergents
T55.1X1 Toxic effect of detergents, accidental (unintentional)
Toxic effect of detergents NOS
2 **T55.1X2 Toxic effect of detergents, intentional self-harm** HCC Rx ESR COM
T55.1X3 Toxic effect of detergents, assault
T55.1X4 Toxic effect of detergents, undetermined

T56 Toxic effect of metals

INCLUDES toxic effects of fumes and vapors of metals
toxic effects of metals from all sources, except medicinal substances

Use additional code to identify any retained metal foreign body, if applicable (Z18.Ø-, T18.1-)

EXCLUDES 1 *arsenic and its compounds (T57.Ø)*
manganese and its compounds (T57.2)

The appropriate 7th character is to be added to each code from category T56.
A initial encounter
D subsequent encounter
S sequela

T56.Ø Toxic effects of lead and its compounds
T56.ØX Toxic effects of lead and its compounds
T56.ØX1 Toxic effect of lead and its compounds, accidental (unintentional)
Toxic effects of lead and its compounds NOS
2 **T56.ØX2 Toxic effect of lead and its compounds, intentional self-harm** HCC Rx ESR COM
T56.ØX3 Toxic effect of lead and its compounds, assault
T56.ØX4 Toxic effect of lead and its compounds, undetermined

T56.1 Toxic effects of mercury and its compounds
T56.1X Toxic effects of mercury and its compounds
T56.1X1 Toxic effect of mercury and its compounds, accidental (unintentional)
Toxic effects of mercury and its compounds NOS
2 **T56.1X2 Toxic effect of mercury and its compounds, intentional self-harm** HCC Rx ESR COM
T56.1X3 Toxic effect of mercury and its compounds, assault
T56.1X4 Toxic effect of mercury and its compounds, undetermined

T56.2 Toxic effects of chromium and its compounds
T56.2X Toxic effects of chromium and its compounds
T56.2X1 Toxic effect of chromium and its compounds, accidental (unintentional)
Toxic effects of chromium and its compounds NOS
2 **T56.2X2 Toxic effect of chromium and its compounds, intentional self-harm** HCC Rx ESR COM
T56.2X3 Toxic effect of chromium and its compounds, assault
T56.2X4 Toxic effect of chromium and its compounds, undetermined

T56.3 Toxic effects of cadmium and its compounds
T56.3X Toxic effects of cadmium and its compounds
T56.3X1 Toxic effect of cadmium and its compounds, accidental (unintentional)
Toxic effects of cadmium and its compounds NOS
2 **T56.3X2 Toxic effect of cadmium and its compounds, intentional self-harm** HCC Rx ESR COM
T56.3X3 Toxic effect of cadmium and its compounds, assault
T56.3X4 Toxic effect of cadmium and its compounds, undetermined

T56.4 Toxic effects of copper and its compounds
T56.4X Toxic effects of copper and its compounds
T56.4X1 Toxic effect of copper and its compounds, accidental (unintentional)
Toxic effects of copper and its compounds NOS
2 **T56.4X2 Toxic effect of copper and its compounds, intentional self-harm** HCC Rx ESR COM
T56.4X3 Toxic effect of copper and its compounds, assault
T56.4X4 Toxic effect of copper and its compounds, undetermined

T56.5 Toxic effects of zinc and its compounds
T56.5X Toxic effects of zinc and its compounds
T56.5X1 Toxic effect of zinc and its compounds, accidental (unintentional)
Toxic effects of zinc and its compounds NOS
2 **T56.5X2 Toxic effect of zinc and its compounds, intentional self-harm** HCC Rx ESR COM
T56.5X3 Toxic effect of zinc and its compounds, assault
T56.5X4 Toxic effect of zinc and its compounds, undetermined

T56.6 Toxic effects of tin and its compounds
T56.6X Toxic effects of tin and its compounds
T56.6X1 Toxic effect of tin and its compounds, accidental (unintentional)
Toxic effects of tin and its compounds NOS
2 **T56.6X2 Toxic effect of tin and its compounds, intentional self-harm** HCC Rx ESR COM
T56.6X3 Toxic effect of tin and its compounds, assault
T56.6X4 Toxic effect of tin and its compounds, undetermined

T56.7 Toxic effects of beryllium and its compounds
T56.7X Toxic effects of beryllium and its compounds
T56.7X1 Toxic effect of beryllium and its compounds, accidental (unintentional)
Toxic effects of beryllium and its compounds NOS
2 **T56.7X2 Toxic effect of beryllium and its compounds, intentional self-harm** HCC Rx ESR COM
T56.7X3 Toxic effect of beryllium and its compounds, assault
T56.7X4 Toxic effect of beryllium and its compounds, undetermined

T56.8 Toxic effects of other metals
T56.81 Toxic effect of thallium
T56.811 Toxic effect of thallium, accidental (unintentional)
Toxic effect of thallium NOS
2 **T56.812 Toxic effect of thallium, intentional self-harm** HCC Rx ESR COM
T56.813 Toxic effect of thallium, assault
T56.814 Toxic effect of thallium, undetermined
T56.89 Toxic effects of other metals
T56.891 Toxic effect of other metals, accidental (unintentional)
Toxic effects of other metals NOS
2 **T56.892 Toxic effect of other metals, intentional self-harm** HCC Rx ESR COM
T56.893 Toxic effect of other metals, assault

7th T56.894 Toxic effect of other metals, undetermined

5th T56.9 Toxic effects of unspecified metal

√x7th T56.91 Toxic effect of unspecified metal, accidental (unintentional)

2 √x7th T56.92 Toxic effect of unspecified metal, intentional self-harm HCC Rx ESR COM

√x7th T56.93 Toxic effect of unspecified metal, assault

√x7th T56.94 Toxic effect of unspecified metal, undetermined

4th T57 Toxic effect of other inorganic substances

The appropriate 7th character is to be added to each code from category T57.
A initial encounter
D subsequent encounter
S sequela

5th T57.Ø Toxic effect of arsenic and its compounds

6th T57.ØX Toxic effect of arsenic and its compounds

7th T57.ØX1 Toxic effect of arsenic and its compounds, accidental (unintentional)
Toxic effect of arsenic and its compounds NOS

2 7th T57.ØX2 Toxic effect of arsenic and its compounds, intentional self-harm HCC Rx ESR COM

7th T57.ØX3 Toxic effect of arsenic and its compounds, assault

7th T57.ØX4 Toxic effect of arsenic and its compounds, undetermined

5th T57.1 Toxic effect of phosphorus and its compounds
EXCLUDES 1 *organophosphate insecticides (T6Ø.Ø)*

6th T57.1X Toxic effect of phosphorus and its compounds

7th T57.1X1 Toxic effect of phosphorus and its compounds, accidental (unintentional)
Toxic effect of phosphorus and its compounds NOS

2 7th T57.1X2 Toxic effect of phosphorus and its compounds, intentional self-harm HCC Rx ESR COM

7th T57.1X3 Toxic effect of phosphorus and its compounds, assault

7th T57.1X4 Toxic effect of phosphorus and its compounds, undetermined

5th T57.2 Toxic effect of manganese and its compounds

6th T57.2X Toxic effect of manganese and its compounds

7th T57.2X1 Toxic effect of manganese and its compounds, accidental (unintentional)
Toxic effect of manganese and its compounds NOS

2 7th T57.2X2 Toxic effect of manganese and its compounds, intentional self-harm HCC Rx ESR COM

7th T57.2X3 Toxic effect of manganese and its compounds, assault

7th T57.2X4 Toxic effect of manganese and its compounds, undetermined

5th T57.3 Toxic effect of hydrogen cyanide

6th T57.3X Toxic effect of hydrogen cyanide

7th T57.3X1 Toxic effect of hydrogen cyanide, accidental (unintentional)
Toxic effect of hydrogen cyanide NOS

2 7th T57.3X2 Toxic effect of hydrogen cyanide, intentional self-harm HCC Rx ESR COM

7th T57.3X3 Toxic effect of hydrogen cyanide, assault

7th T57.3X4 Toxic effect of hydrogen cyanide, undetermined

5th T57.8 Toxic effect of other specified inorganic substances

6th T57.8X Toxic effect of other specified inorganic substances

7th T57.8X1 Toxic effect of other specified inorganic substances, accidental (unintentional)
Toxic effect of other specified inorganic substances NOS

2 7th T57.8X2 Toxic effect of other specified inorganic substances, intentional self-harm HCC Rx ESR COM

7th T57.8X3 Toxic effect of other specified inorganic substances, assault

7th T57.8X4 Toxic effect of other specified inorganic substances, undetermined

5th T57.9 Toxic effect of unspecified inorganic substance

√x7th T57.91 Toxic effect of unspecified inorganic substance, accidental (unintentional)

2 √x7th T57.92 Toxic effect of unspecified inorganic substance, intentional self-harm HCC Rx ESR COM

√x7th T57.93 Toxic effect of unspecified inorganic substance, assault

√x7th T57.94 Toxic effect of unspecified inorganic substance, undetermined

4th T58 Toxic effect of carbon monoxide
INCLUDES asphyxiation from carbon monoxide
toxic effect of carbon monoxide from all sources

The appropriate 7th character is to be added to each code from category T58.
A initial encounter
D subsequent encounter
S sequela

5th T58.Ø Toxic effect of carbon monoxide from motor vehicle exhaust
Toxic effect of exhaust gas from gas engine
Toxic effect of exhaust gas from motor pump

√x7th T58.Ø1 Toxic effect of carbon monoxide from motor vehicle exhaust, accidental (unintentional)

2 √x7th T58.Ø2 Toxic effect of carbon monoxide from motor vehicle exhaust, intentional self-harm HCC Rx ESR COM

√x7th T58.Ø3 Toxic effect of carbon monoxide from motor vehicle exhaust, assault

√x7th T58.Ø4 Toxic effect of carbon monoxide from motor vehicle exhaust, undetermined

5th T58.1 Toxic effect of carbon monoxide from utility gas
Toxic effect of acetylene
Toxic effect of gas NOS used for lighting, heating, cooking
Toxic effect of water gas

√x7th T58.11 Toxic effect of carbon monoxide from utility gas, accidental (unintentional)

2 √x7th T58.12 Toxic effect of carbon monoxide from utility gas, intentional self-harm HCC Rx ESR COM

√x7th T58.13 Toxic effect of carbon monoxide from utility gas, assault

√x7th T58.14 Toxic effect of carbon monoxide from utility gas, undetermined

5th T58.2 Toxic effect of carbon monoxide from incomplete combustion of other domestic fuels
Toxic effect of carbon monoxide from incomplete combustion of coal, coke, kerosene, wood

6th T58.2X Toxic effect of carbon monoxide from incomplete combustion of other domestic fuels

7th T58.2X1 Toxic effect of carbon monoxide from incomplete combustion of other domestic fuels, accidental (unintentional)

2 7th T58.2X2 Toxic effect of carbon monoxide from incomplete combustion of other domestic fuels, intentional self-harm HCC Rx ESR COM

7th T58.2X3 Toxic effect of carbon monoxide from incomplete combustion of other domestic fuels, assault

7th T58.2X4 Toxic effect of carbon monoxide from incomplete combustion of other domestic fuels, undetermined

5th T58.8 Toxic effect of carbon monoxide from other source
Toxic effect of carbon monoxide from blast furnace gas
Toxic effect of carbon monoxide from fuels in industrial use
Toxic effect of carbon monoxide from kiln vapor

6th T58.8X Toxic effect of carbon monoxide from other source

7th T58.8X1 Toxic effect of carbon monoxide from other source, accidental (unintentional)

2 7th T58.8X2 Toxic effect of carbon monoxide from other source, intentional self-harm HCC Rx ESR COM

7th T58.8X3 Toxic effect of carbon monoxide from other source, assault

7th T58.8X4 Toxic effect of carbon monoxide from other source, undetermined

5th T58.9 Toxic effect of carbon monoxide from unspecified source

√x7th T58.91 Toxic effect of carbon monoxide from unspecified source, accidental (unintentional)

2 √x7th T58.92 Toxic effect of carbon monoxide from unspecified source, intentional self-harm HCC Rx ESR COM

HCC CMS-HCC Rx Rx HCC ESR ESRD HCC COM Commercial HCC N Newborn: 0 P Pediatric: 0-17 M Maternity: 9-64 A Adult: 15-124

T58.93 Toxic effect of carbon monoxide from unspecified source, assault

T58.94 Toxic effect of carbon monoxide from unspecified source, undetermined

T59 Toxic effect of other gases, fumes and vapors

INCLUDES aerosol propellants

EXCLUDES 1 *chlorofluorocarbons (T53.5)*

The appropriate 7th character is to be added to each code from category T59.
A initial encounter
D subsequent encounter
S sequela

T59.Ø Toxic effect of nitrogen oxides

T59.ØX Toxic effect of nitrogen oxides

T59.ØX1 Toxic effect of nitrogen oxides, accidental (unintentional)
Toxic effect of nitrogen oxides NOS

T59.ØX2 Toxic effect of nitrogen oxides, intentional self-harm [2] HCC Rx ESR COM

T59.ØX3 Toxic effect of nitrogen oxides, assault

T59.ØX4 Toxic effect of nitrogen oxides, undetermined

T59.1 Toxic effect of sulfur dioxide

T59.1X Toxic effect of sulfur dioxide

T59.1X1 Toxic effect of sulfur dioxide, accidental (unintentional)
Toxic effect of sulfur dioxide NOS

T59.1X2 Toxic effect of sulfur dioxide, intentional self-harm [2] HCC Rx ESR COM

T59.1X3 Toxic effect of sulfur dioxide, assault

T59.1X4 Toxic effect of sulfur dioxide, undetermined

T59.2 Toxic effect of formaldehyde

T59.2X Toxic effect of formaldehyde

T59.2X1 Toxic effect of formaldehyde, accidental (unintentional)
Toxic effect of formaldehyde NOS

T59.2X2 Toxic effect of formaldehyde, intentional self-harm [2] HCC Rx ESR COM

T59.2X3 Toxic effect of formaldehyde, assault

T59.2X4 Toxic effect of formaldehyde, undetermined

T59.3 Toxic effect of lacrimogenic gas
Toxic effect of tear gas

T59.3X Toxic effect of lacrimogenic gas

T59.3X1 Toxic effect of lacrimogenic gas, accidental (unintentional)
Toxic effect of lacrimogenic gas NOS

T59.3X2 Toxic effect of lacrimogenic gas, intentional self-harm [2] HCC Rx ESR COM

T59.3X3 Toxic effect of lacrimogenic gas, assault

T59.3X4 Toxic effect of lacrimogenic gas, undetermined

T59.4 Toxic effect of chlorine gas

T59.4X Toxic effect of chlorine gas

T59.4X1 Toxic effect of chlorine gas, accidental (unintentional)
Toxic effect of chlorine gas NOS

T59.4X2 Toxic effect of chlorine gas, intentional self-harm [2] HCC Rx ESR COM

T59.4X3 Toxic effect of chlorine gas, assault

T59.4X4 Toxic effect of chlorine gas, undetermined

T59.5 Toxic effect of fluorine gas and hydrogen fluoride

T59.5X Toxic effect of fluorine gas and hydrogen fluoride

T59.5X1 Toxic effect of fluorine gas and hydrogen fluoride, accidental (unintentional)
Toxic effect of fluorine gas and hydrogen fluoride NOS

T59.5X2 Toxic effect of fluorine gas and hydrogen fluoride, intentional self-harm [2] HCC Rx ESR COM

T59.5X3 Toxic effect of fluorine gas and hydrogen fluoride, assault

T59.5X4 Toxic effect of fluorine gas and hydrogen fluoride, undetermined

T59.6 Toxic effect of hydrogen sulfide

T59.6X Toxic effect of hydrogen sulfide

T59.6X1 Toxic effect of hydrogen sulfide, accidental (unintentional)
Toxic effect of hydrogen sulfide NOS

T59.6X2 Toxic effect of hydrogen sulfide, intentional self-harm [2] HCC Rx ESR COM

T59.6X3 Toxic effect of hydrogen sulfide, assault

T59.6X4 Toxic effect of hydrogen sulfide, undetermined

T59.7 Toxic effect of carbon dioxide

T59.7X Toxic effect of carbon dioxide

T59.7X1 Toxic effect of carbon dioxide, accidental (unintentional)
Toxic effect of carbon dioxide NOS

T59.7X2 Toxic effect of carbon dioxide, intentional self-harm [2] HCC Rx ESR COM

T59.7X3 Toxic effect of carbon dioxide, assault

T59.7X4 Toxic effect of carbon dioxide, undetermined

T59.8 Toxic effect of other specified gases, fumes and vapors

T59.81 Toxic effect of smoke
Smoke inhalation

EXCLUDES 2 *toxic effect of cigarette (tobacco) smoke (T65.22-)*

T59.811 Toxic effect of smoke, accidental (unintentional)
Toxic effect of smoke NOS
AHA: 2013,4Q,121

T59.812 Toxic effect of smoke, intentional self-harm [2] HCC Rx ESR COM

T59.813 Toxic effect of smoke, assault

T59.814 Toxic effect of smoke, undetermined

T59.89 Toxic effect of other specified gases, fumes and vapors

T59.891 Toxic effect of other specified gases, fumes and vapors, accidental (unintentional)

T59.892 Toxic effect of other specified gases, fumes and vapors, intentional self-harm [2] HCC Rx ESR COM

T59.893 Toxic effect of other specified gases, fumes and vapors, assault

T59.894 Toxic effect of other specified gases, fumes and vapors, undetermined

T59.9 Toxic effect of unspecified gases, fumes and vapors

T59.91 Toxic effect of unspecified gases, fumes and vapors, accidental (unintentional)

T59.92 Toxic effect of unspecified gases, fumes and vapors, intentional self-harm [2] HCC Rx ESR COM

T59.93 Toxic effect of unspecified gases, fumes and vapors, assault

T59.94 Toxic effect of unspecified gases, fumes and vapors, undetermined

T6Ø Toxic effect of pesticides

INCLUDES toxic effect of wood preservatives

The appropriate 7th character is to be added to each code from category T6Ø.
A initial encounter
D subsequent encounter
S sequela

T6Ø.Ø Toxic effect of organophosphate and carbamate insecticides

T6Ø.ØX Toxic effect of organophosphate and carbamate insecticides

T6Ø.ØX1 Toxic effect of organophosphate and carbamate insecticides, accidental (unintentional)
Toxic effect of organophosphate and carbamate insecticides NOS

T6Ø.ØX2 Toxic effect of organophosphate and carbamate insecticides, intentional self-harm [2] HCC Rx ESR COM

T6Ø.ØX3 Toxic effect of organophosphate and carbamate insecticides, assault

T6Ø.ØX4 Toxic effect of organophosphate and carbamate insecticides, undetermined

5th **T60.1 Toxic effect of halogenated insecticides**
EXCLUDES 1 *chlorinated hydrocarbon (T53.-)*

6th **T60.1X Toxic effect of halogenated insecticides**
7th **T60.1X1 Toxic effect of halogenated insecticides, accidental (unintentional)**
Toxic effect of halogenated insecticides NOS
2 7th **T60.1X2 Toxic effect of halogenated insecticides, intentional self-harm** HCC Rx ESR COM
7th **T60.1X3 Toxic effect of halogenated insecticides, assault**
7th **T60.1X4 Toxic effect of halogenated insecticides, undetermined**

5th **T60.2 Toxic effect of other insecticides**
6th **T60.2X Toxic effect of other insecticides**
7th **T60.2X1 Toxic effect of other insecticides, accidental (unintentional)**
Toxic effect of other insecticides NOS
2 7th **T60.2X2 Toxic effect of other insecticides, intentional self-harm** HCC Rx ESR COM
7th **T60.2X3 Toxic effect of other insecticides, assault**
7th **T60.2X4 Toxic effect of other insecticides, undetermined**

5th **T60.3 Toxic effect of herbicides and fungicides**
6th **T60.3X Toxic effect of herbicides and fungicides**
7th **T60.3X1 Toxic effect of herbicides and fungicides, accidental (unintentional)**
Toxic effect of herbicides and fungicides NOS
2 7th **T60.3X2 Toxic effect of herbicides and fungicides, intentional self-harm** HCC Rx ESR COM
7th **T60.3X3 Toxic effect of herbicides and fungicides, assault**
7th **T60.3X4 Toxic effect of herbicides and fungicides, undetermined**

5th **T60.4 Toxic effect of rodenticides**
EXCLUDES 1 *strychnine and its salts (T65.1)*
thallium (T56.81-)
6th **T60.4X Toxic effect of rodenticides**
7th **T60.4X1 Toxic effect of rodenticides, accidental (unintentional)**
Toxic effect of rodenticides NOS
2 7th **T60.4X2 Toxic effect of rodenticides, intentional self-harm** HCC Rx ESR COM
7th **T60.4X3 Toxic effect of rodenticides, assault**
7th **T60.4X4 Toxic effect of rodenticides, undetermined**

5th **T60.8 Toxic effect of other pesticides**
6th **T60.8X Toxic effect of other pesticides**
7th **T60.8X1 Toxic effect of other pesticides, accidental (unintentional)**
Toxic effect of other pesticides NOS
2 7th **T60.8X2 Toxic effect of other pesticides, intentional self-harm** HCC Rx ESR COM
7th **T60.8X3 Toxic effect of other pesticides, assault**
7th **T60.8X4 Toxic effect of other pesticides, undetermined**

5th **T60.9 Toxic effect of unspecified pesticide**
x7th **T60.91 Toxic effect of unspecified pesticide, accidental (unintentional)**
2 x7th **T60.92 Toxic effect of unspecified pesticide, intentional self-harm** HCC Rx ESR COM
x7th **T60.93 Toxic effect of unspecified pesticide, assault**
x7th **T60.94 Toxic effect of unspecified pesticide, undetermined**

4th **T61 Toxic effect of noxious substances eaten as seafood**
EXCLUDES 1 *allergic reaction to food, such as:*
anaphylactic reaction or shock due to adverse food reaction (T78.0-)
bacterial foodborne intoxications (A05.-)
dermatitis (L23.6, L25.4, L27.2)
food protein-induced enterocolitis syndrome (K52.21)
food protein-induced enteropathy (K52.22)
gastroenteritis (noninfective) (K52.29)
toxic effect of aflatoxin and other mycotoxins (T64)
toxic effect of cyanides (T65.0-)
toxic effect of harmful algae bloom (T65.82-)
toxic effect of hydrogen cyanide (T57.3-)
toxic effect of mercury (T56.1-)
toxic effect of red tide (T65.82-)

The appropriate 7th character is to be added to each code from category T61.
A initial encounter
D subsequent encounter
S sequela

5th **T61.0 Ciguatera fish poisoning**
x7th **T61.01 Ciguatera fish poisoning, accidental (unintentional)**
2 x7th **T61.02 Ciguatera fish poisoning, intentional self-harm** HCC Rx ESR COM
x7th **T61.03 Ciguatera fish poisoning, assault**
x7th **T61.04 Ciguatera fish poisoning, undetermined**

5th **T61.1 Scombroid fish poisoning**
Histamine-like syndrome
x7th **T61.11 Scombroid fish poisoning, accidental (unintentional)**
2 x7th **T61.12 Scombroid fish poisoning, intentional self-harm** HCC Rx ESR COM
x7th **T61.13 Scombroid fish poisoning, assault**
x7th **T61.14 Scombroid fish poisoning, undetermined**

5th **T61.7 Other fish and shellfish poisoning**
6th **T61.77 Other fish poisoning**
7th **T61.771 Other fish poisoning, accidental (unintentional)**
2 7th **T61.772 Other fish poisoning, intentional self-harm** HCC Rx ESR COM
7th **T61.773 Other fish poisoning, assault**
7th **T61.774 Other fish poisoning, undetermined**
6th **T61.78 Other shellfish poisoning**
7th **T61.781 Other shellfish poisoning, accidental (unintentional)**
2 7th **T61.782 Other shellfish poisoning, intentional self-harm** HCC Rx ESR COM
7th **T61.783 Other shellfish poisoning, assault**
7th **T61.784 Other shellfish poisoning, undetermined**

5th **T61.8 Toxic effect of other seafood**
6th **T61.8X Toxic effect of other seafood**
7th **T61.8X1 Toxic effect of other seafood, accidental (unintentional)**
2 7th **T61.8X2 Toxic effect of other seafood, intentional self-harm** HCC Rx ESR COM
7th **T61.8X3 Toxic effect of other seafood, assault**
7th **T61.8X4 Toxic effect of other seafood, undetermined**

5th **T61.9 Toxic effect of unspecified seafood**
x7th **T61.91 Toxic effect of unspecified seafood, accidental (unintentional)**
2 x7th **T61.92 Toxic effect of unspecified seafood, intentional self-harm** HCC Rx ESR COM
x7th **T61.93 Toxic effect of unspecified seafood, assault**
x7th **T61.94 Toxic effect of unspecified seafood, undetermined**

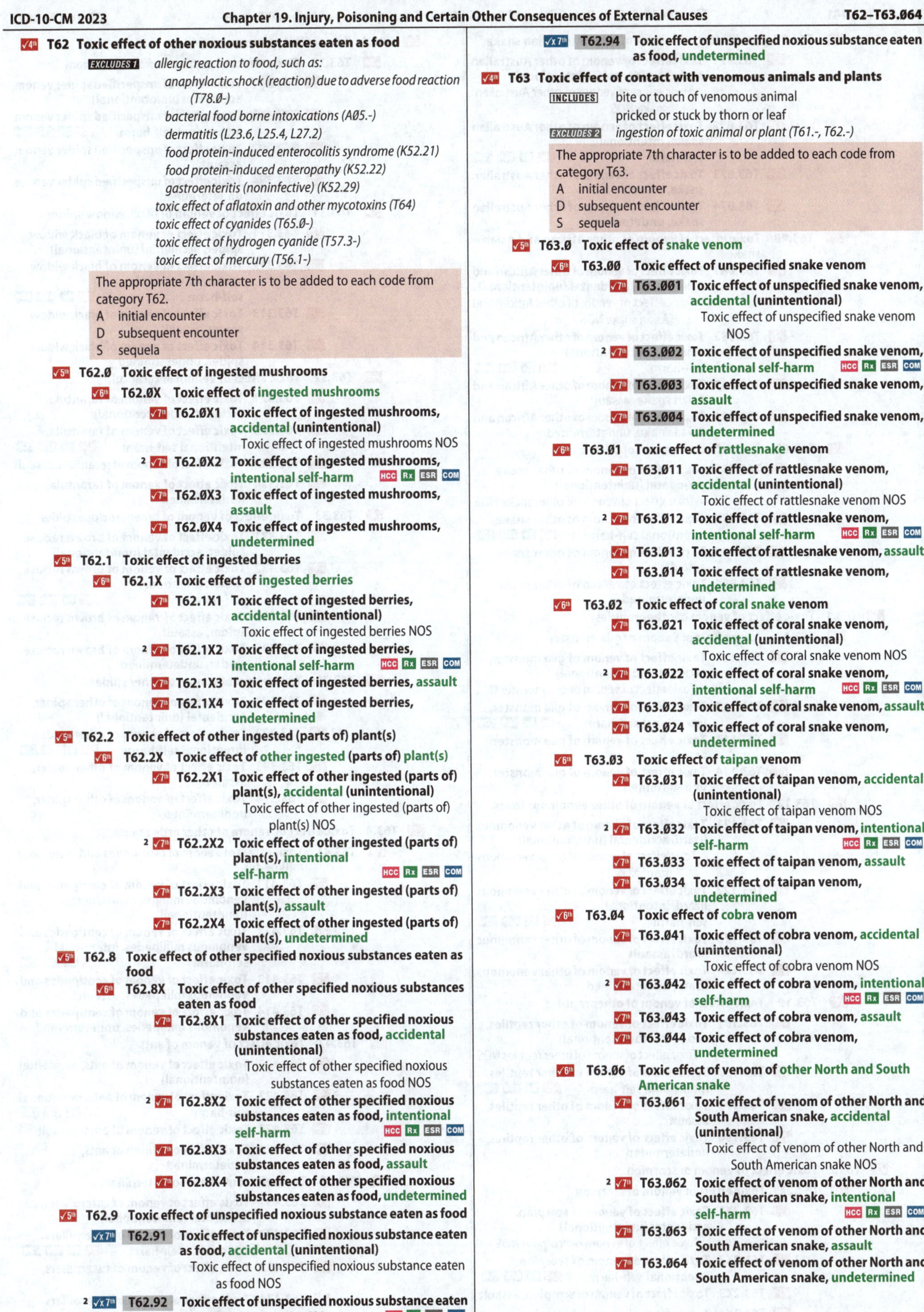

T62 Toxic effect of other noxious substances eaten as food

EXCLUDES 1 *allergic reaction to food, such as:*
anaphylactic shock (reaction) due to adverse food reaction (T78.0-)
bacterial food borne intoxications (A05.-)
dermatitis (L23.6, L25.4, L27.2)
food protein-induced enterocolitis syndrome (K52.21)
food protein-induced enteropathy (K52.22)
gastroenteritis (noninfective) (K52.29)
toxic effect of aflatoxin and other mycotoxins (T64)
toxic effect of cyanides (T65.0-)
toxic effect of hydrogen cyanide (T57.3-)
toxic effect of mercury (T56.1-)

The appropriate 7th character is to be added to each code from category T62.
A initial encounter
D subsequent encounter
S sequela

T62.0 Toxic effect of ingested mushrooms
T62.0X Toxic effect of ingested mushrooms
T62.0X1 Toxic effect of ingested mushrooms, accidental (unintentional)
Toxic effect of ingested mushrooms NOS
2 **T62.0X2 Toxic effect of ingested mushrooms, intentional self-harm** HCC Rx ESR COM
T62.0X3 Toxic effect of ingested mushrooms, assault
T62.0X4 Toxic effect of ingested mushrooms, undetermined

T62.1 Toxic effect of ingested berries
T62.1X Toxic effect of ingested berries
T62.1X1 Toxic effect of ingested berries, accidental (unintentional)
Toxic effect of ingested berries NOS
2 **T62.1X2 Toxic effect of ingested berries, intentional self-harm** HCC Rx ESR COM
T62.1X3 Toxic effect of ingested berries, assault
T62.1X4 Toxic effect of ingested berries, undetermined

T62.2 Toxic effect of other ingested (parts of) plant(s)
T62.2X Toxic effect of other ingested (parts of) plant(s)
T62.2X1 Toxic effect of other ingested (parts of) plant(s), accidental (unintentional)
Toxic effect of other ingested (parts of) plant(s) NOS
2 **T62.2X2 Toxic effect of other ingested (parts of) plant(s), intentional self-harm** HCC Rx ESR COM
T62.2X3 Toxic effect of other ingested (parts of) plant(s), assault
T62.2X4 Toxic effect of other ingested (parts of) plant(s), undetermined

T62.8 Toxic effect of other specified noxious substances eaten as food
T62.8X Toxic effect of other specified noxious substances eaten as food
T62.8X1 Toxic effect of other specified noxious substances eaten as food, accidental (unintentional)
Toxic effect of other specified noxious substances eaten as food NOS
2 **T62.8X2 Toxic effect of other specified noxious substances eaten as food, intentional self-harm** HCC Rx ESR COM
T62.8X3 Toxic effect of other specified noxious substances eaten as food, assault
T62.8X4 Toxic effect of other specified noxious substances eaten as food, undetermined

T62.9 Toxic effect of unspecified noxious substance eaten as food
T62.91 Toxic effect of unspecified noxious substance eaten as food, accidental (unintentional)
Toxic effect of unspecified noxious substance eaten as food NOS
2 **T62.92 Toxic effect of unspecified noxious substance eaten as food, intentional self-harm** HCC Rx ESR COM
T62.93 Toxic effect of unspecified noxious substance eaten as food, assault
T62.94 Toxic effect of unspecified noxious substance eaten as food, undetermined

T63 Toxic effect of contact with venomous animals and plants

INCLUDES bite or touch of venomous animal
pricked or stuck by thorn or leaf

EXCLUDES 2 *ingestion of toxic animal or plant (T61.-, T62.-)*

The appropriate 7th character is to be added to each code from category T63.
A initial encounter
D subsequent encounter
S sequela

T63.0 Toxic effect of snake venom
T63.00 Toxic effect of unspecified snake venom
T63.001 Toxic effect of unspecified snake venom, accidental (unintentional)
Toxic effect of unspecified snake venom NOS
2 **T63.002 Toxic effect of unspecified snake venom, intentional self-harm** HCC Rx ESR COM
T63.003 Toxic effect of unspecified snake venom, assault
T63.004 Toxic effect of unspecified snake venom, undetermined
T63.01 Toxic effect of rattlesnake venom
T63.011 Toxic effect of rattlesnake venom, accidental (unintentional)
Toxic effect of rattlesnake venom NOS
2 **T63.012 Toxic effect of rattlesnake venom, intentional self-harm** HCC Rx ESR COM
T63.013 Toxic effect of rattlesnake venom, assault
T63.014 Toxic effect of rattlesnake venom, undetermined
T63.02 Toxic effect of coral snake venom
T63.021 Toxic effect of coral snake venom, accidental (unintentional)
Toxic effect of coral snake venom NOS
2 **T63.022 Toxic effect of coral snake venom, intentional self-harm** HCC Rx ESR COM
T63.023 Toxic effect of coral snake venom, assault
T63.024 Toxic effect of coral snake venom, undetermined
T63.03 Toxic effect of taipan venom
T63.031 Toxic effect of taipan venom, accidental (unintentional)
Toxic effect of taipan venom NOS
2 **T63.032 Toxic effect of taipan venom, intentional self-harm** HCC Rx ESR COM
T63.033 Toxic effect of taipan venom, assault
T63.034 Toxic effect of taipan venom, undetermined
T63.04 Toxic effect of cobra venom
T63.041 Toxic effect of cobra venom, accidental (unintentional)
Toxic effect of cobra venom NOS
2 **T63.042 Toxic effect of cobra venom, intentional self-harm** HCC Rx ESR COM
T63.043 Toxic effect of cobra venom, assault
T63.044 Toxic effect of cobra venom, undetermined
T63.06 Toxic effect of venom of other North and South American snake
T63.061 Toxic effect of venom of other North and South American snake, accidental (unintentional)
Toxic effect of venom of other North and South American snake NOS
2 **T63.062 Toxic effect of venom of other North and South American snake, intentional self-harm** HCC Rx ESR COM
T63.063 Toxic effect of venom of other North and South American snake, assault
T63.064 Toxic effect of venom of other North and South American snake, undetermined

6th **T63.07 Toxic effect of venom of other Australian snake**

7th **T63.071 Toxic effect of venom of other Australian snake, accidental (unintentional)**
Toxic effect of venom of other Australian snake NOS

[2] 7th **T63.072 Toxic effect of venom of other Australian snake, intentional self-harm** HCC Rx ESR COM

7th **T63.073 Toxic effect of venom of other Australian snake, assault**

7th **T63.074 Toxic effect of venom of other Australian snake, undetermined**

6th **T63.08 Toxic effect of venom of other African and Asian snake**

7th **T63.081 Toxic effect of venom of other African and Asian snake, accidental (unintentional)**
Toxic effect of venom of other African and Asian snake NOS

[2] 7th **T63.082 Toxic effect of venom of other African and Asian snake, intentional self-harm** HCC Rx ESR COM

7th **T63.083 Toxic effect of venom of other African and Asian snake, assault**

7th **T63.084 Toxic effect of venom of other African and Asian snake, undetermined**

6th **T63.09 Toxic effect of venom of other snake**

7th **T63.091 Toxic effect of venom of other snake, accidental (unintentional)**
Toxic effect of venom of other snake NOS

[2] 7th **T63.092 Toxic effect of venom of other snake, intentional self-harm** HCC Rx ESR COM

7th **T63.093 Toxic effect of venom of other snake, assault**

7th **T63.094 Toxic effect of venom of other snake, undetermined**

5th **T63.1 Toxic effect of venom of other reptiles**

6th **T63.11 Toxic effect of venom of gila monster**

7th **T63.111 Toxic effect of venom of gila monster, accidental (unintentional)**
Toxic effect of venom of gila monster NOS

[2] 7th **T63.112 Toxic effect of venom of gila monster, intentional self-harm** HCC Rx ESR COM

7th **T63.113 Toxic effect of venom of gila monster, assault**

7th **T63.114 Toxic effect of venom of gila monster, undetermined**

6th **T63.12 Toxic effect of venom of other venomous lizard**

7th **T63.121 Toxic effect of venom of other venomous lizard, accidental (unintentional)**
Toxic effect of venom of other venomous lizard NOS

[2] 7th **T63.122 Toxic effect of venom of other venomous lizard, intentional self-harm** HCC Rx ESR COM

7th **T63.123 Toxic effect of venom of other venomous lizard, assault**

7th **T63.124 Toxic effect of venom of other venomous lizard, undetermined**

6th **T63.19 Toxic effect of venom of other reptiles**

7th **T63.191 Toxic effect of venom of other reptiles, accidental (unintentional)**
Toxic effect of venom of other reptiles NOS

7th **T63.192 Toxic effect of venom of other reptiles, intentional self-harm** HCC Rx ESR COM

7th **T63.193 Toxic effect of venom of other reptiles, assault**

7th **T63.194 Toxic effect of venom of other reptiles, undetermined**

5th **T63.2 Toxic effect of venom of scorpion**

6th **T63.2X Toxic effect of venom of scorpion**

7th **T63.2X1 Toxic effect of venom of scorpion, accidental (unintentional)**
Toxic effect of venom of scorpion NOS

[2] 7th **T63.2X2 Toxic effect of venom of scorpion, intentional self-harm** HCC Rx ESR COM

7th **T63.2X3 Toxic effect of venom of scorpion, assault**

7th **T63.2X4 Toxic effect of venom of scorpion, undetermined**

5th **T63.3 Toxic effect of venom of spider**

6th **T63.30 Toxic effect of unspecified spider venom**

7th **T63.301 Toxic effect of unspecified spider venom, accidental (unintentional)**

[2] 7th **T63.302 Toxic effect of unspecified spider venom, intentional self-harm** HCC Rx ESR COM

7th **T63.303 Toxic effect of unspecified spider venom, assault**

7th **T63.304 Toxic effect of unspecified spider venom, undetermined**

6th **T63.31 Toxic effect of venom of black widow spider**

7th **T63.311 Toxic effect of venom of black widow spider, accidental (unintentional)**

[2] 7th **T63.312 Toxic effect of venom of black widow spider, intentional self-harm** HCC Rx ESR COM

7th **T63.313 Toxic effect of venom of black widow spider, assault**

7th **T63.314 Toxic effect of venom of black widow spider, undetermined**

6th **T63.32 Toxic effect of venom of tarantula**

7th **T63.321 Toxic effect of venom of tarantula, accidental (unintentional)**

[2] 7th **T63.322 Toxic effect of venom of tarantula, intentional self-harm** HCC Rx ESR COM

7th **T63.323 Toxic effect of venom of tarantula, assault**

7th **T63.324 Toxic effect of venom of tarantula, undetermined**

6th **T63.33 Toxic effect of venom of brown recluse spider**

7th **T63.331 Toxic effect of venom of brown recluse spider, accidental (unintentional)**

[2] 7th **T63.332 Toxic effect of venom of brown recluse spider, intentional self-harm** HCC Rx ESR COM

7th **T63.333 Toxic effect of venom of brown recluse spider, assault**

7th **T63.334 Toxic effect of venom of brown recluse spider, undetermined**

6th **T63.39 Toxic effect of venom of other spider**

7th **T63.391 Toxic effect of venom of other spider, accidental (unintentional)**

[2] 7th **T63.392 Toxic effect of venom of other spider, intentional self-harm** HCC Rx ESR COM

7th **T63.393 Toxic effect of venom of other spider, assault**

7th **T63.394 Toxic effect of venom of other spider, undetermined**

5th **T63.4 Toxic effect of venom of other arthropods**

6th **T63.41 Toxic effect of venom of centipedes and venomous millipedes**

7th **T63.411 Toxic effect of venom of centipedes and venomous millipedes, accidental (unintentional)**

[2] 7th **T63.412 Toxic effect of venom of centipedes and venomous millipedes, intentional self-harm** HCC Rx ESR COM

7th **T63.413 Toxic effect of venom of centipedes and venomous millipedes, assault**

7th **T63.414 Toxic effect of venom of centipedes and venomous millipedes, undetermined**

6th **T63.42 Toxic effect of venom of ants**

7th **T63.421 Toxic effect of venom of ants, accidental (unintentional)**

[2] 7th **T63.422 Toxic effect of venom of ants, intentional self-harm** HCC Rx ESR COM

7th **T63.423 Toxic effect of venom of ants, assault**

7th **T63.424 Toxic effect of venom of ants, undetermined**

6th **T63.43 Toxic effect of venom of caterpillars**

7th **T63.431 Toxic effect of venom of caterpillars, accidental (unintentional)**

[2] 7th **T63.432 Toxic effect of venom of caterpillars, intentional self-harm** HCC Rx ESR COM

7th **T63.433 Toxic effect of venom of caterpillars, assault**

7th **T63.434 Toxic effect of venom of caterpillars, undetermined**

6th **T63.44 Toxic effect of venom of bees**

7th **T63.441 Toxic effect of venom of bees, accidental (unintentional)**

2 7th **T63.442 Toxic effect of venom of bees, intentional self-harm** HCC Rx ESR COM

7th **T63.443 Toxic effect of venom of bees, assault**

7th **T63.444 Toxic effect of venom of bees, undetermined**

6th **T63.45 Toxic effect of venom of hornets**

7th **T63.451 Toxic effect of venom of hornets, accidental (unintentional)**

2 7th **T63.452 Toxic effect of venom of hornets, intentional self-harm** HCC Rx ESR COM

7th **T63.453 Toxic effect of venom of hornets, assault**

7th **T63.454 Toxic effect of venom of hornets, undetermined**

6th **T63.46 Toxic effect of venom of wasps**

Toxic effect of yellow jacket

7th **T63.461 Toxic effect of venom of wasps, accidental (unintentional)**

2 7th **T63.462 Toxic effect of venom of wasps, intentional self-harm** HCC Rx ESR COM

7th **T63.463 Toxic effect of venom of wasps, assault**

7th **T63.464 Toxic effect of venom of wasps, undetermined**

6th **T63.48 Toxic effect of venom of other arthropod**

7th **T63.481 Toxic effect of venom of other arthropod, accidental (unintentional)**

2 7th **T63.482 Toxic effect of venom of other arthropod, intentional self-harm** HCC Rx ESR COM

7th **T63.483 Toxic effect of venom of other arthropod, assault**

7th **T63.484 Toxic effect of venom of other arthropod, undetermined**

5th **T63.5 Toxic effect of contact with venomous fish**

EXCLUDES 2 *poisoning by ingestion of fish (T61.-)*

6th **T63.51 Toxic effect of contact with stingray**

7th **T63.511 Toxic effect of contact with stingray, accidental (unintentional)**

2 7th **T63.512 Toxic effect of contact with stingray, intentional self-harm** HCC Rx ESR COM

7th **T63.513 Toxic effect of contact with stingray, assault**

7th **T63.514 Toxic effect of contact with stingray, undetermined**

6th **T63.59 Toxic effect of contact with other venomous fish**

7th **T63.591 Toxic effect of contact with other venomous fish, accidental (unintentional)**

2 7th **T63.592 Toxic effect of contact with other venomous fish, intentional self-harm** HCC Rx ESR COM

7th **T63.593 Toxic effect of contact with other venomous fish, assault**

7th **T63.594 Toxic effect of contact with other venomous fish, undetermined**

5th **T63.6 Toxic effect of contact with other venomous marine animals**

EXCLUDES 1 *sea-snake venom (T63.Ø9)*

EXCLUDES 2 *poisoning by ingestion of shellfish (T61.78-)*

6th **T63.61 Toxic effect of contact with Portuguese Man-o-war**

Toxic effect of contact with bluebottle

7th **T63.611 Toxic effect of contact with Portuguese Man-o-war, accidental (unintentional)**

2 7th **T63.612 Toxic effect of contact with Portuguese Man-o-war, intentional self-harm** HCC Rx ESR COM

7th **T63.613 Toxic effect of contact with Portuguese Man-o-war, assault**

7th **T63.614 Toxic effect of contact with Portuguese Man-o-war, undetermined**

6th **T63.62 Toxic effect of contact with other jellyfish**

7th **T63.621 Toxic effect of contact with other jellyfish, accidental (unintentional)**

2 7th **T63.622 Toxic effect of contact with other jellyfish, intentional self-harm** HCC Rx ESR COM

7th **T63.623 Toxic effect of contact with other jellyfish, assault**

7th **T63.624 Toxic effect of contact with other jellyfish, undetermined**

6th **T63.63 Toxic effect of contact with sea anemone**

7th **T63.631 Toxic effect of contact with sea anemone, accidental (unintentional)**

2 7th **T63.632 Toxic effect of contact with sea anemone, intentional self-harm** HCC Rx ESR COM

7th **T63.633 Toxic effect of contact with sea anemone, assault**

7th **T63.634 Toxic effect of contact with sea anemone, undetermined**

6th **T63.69 Toxic effect of contact with other venomous marine animals**

7th **T63.691 Toxic effect of contact with other venomous marine animals, accidental (unintentional)**

2 7th **T63.692 Toxic effect of contact with other venomous marine animals, intentional self-harm** HCC Rx ESR COM

7th **T63.693 Toxic effect of contact with other venomous marine animals, assault**

7th **T63.694 Toxic effect of contact with other venomous marine animals, undetermined**

5th **T63.7 Toxic effect of contact with venomous plant**

6th **T63.71 Toxic effect of contact with venomous marine plant**

7th **T63.711 Toxic effect of contact with venomous marine plant, accidental (unintentional)**

2 7th **T63.712 Toxic effect of contact with venomous marine plant, intentional self-harm** HCC Rx ESR COM

7th **T63.713 Toxic effect of contact with venomous marine plant, assault**

7th **T63.714 Toxic effect of contact with venomous marine plant, undetermined**

6th **T63.79 Toxic effect of contact with other venomous plant**

7th **T63.791 Toxic effect of contact with other venomous plant, accidental (unintentional)**

2 7th **T63.792 Toxic effect of contact with other venomous plant, intentional self-harm** HCC Rx ESR COM

7th **T63.793 Toxic effect of contact with other venomous plant, assault**

7th **T63.794 Toxic effect of contact with other venomous plant, undetermined**

5th **T63.8 Toxic effect of contact with other venomous animals**

6th **T63.81 Toxic effect of contact with venomous frog**

EXCLUDES 1 *contact with nonvenomous frog (W62.Ø)*

7th **T63.811 Toxic effect of contact with venomous frog, accidental (unintentional)**

2 7th **T63.812 Toxic effect of contact with venomous frog, intentional self-harm** HCC Rx ESR COM

7th **T63.813 Toxic effect of contact with venomous frog, assault**

7th **T63.814 Toxic effect of contact with venomous frog, undetermined**

6th **T63.82 Toxic effect of contact with venomous toad**

EXCLUDES 1 *contact with nonvenomous toad (W62.1)*

7th **T63.821 Toxic effect of contact with venomous toad, accidental (unintentional)**

2 7th **T63.822 Toxic effect of contact with venomous toad, intentional self-harm** HCC Rx ESR COM

7th **T63.823 Toxic effect of contact with venomous toad, assault**

7th **T63.824 Toxic effect of contact with venomous toad, undetermined**

6th **T63.83 Toxic effect of contact with other venomous amphibian**

EXCLUDES 1 *contact with nonvenomous amphibian (W62.9)*

7th **T63.831 Toxic effect of contact with other venomous amphibian, accidental (unintentional)**

2 7th **T63.832 Toxic effect of contact with other venomous amphibian, intentional self-harm** HCC Rx ESR COM

7th **T63.833 Toxic effect of contact with other venomous amphibian, assault**

7th **T63.834 Toxic effect of contact with other venomous amphibian, undetermined**

6th **T63.89 Toxic effect of contact with other venomous animals**

7th **T63.891 Toxic effect of contact with other venomous animals, accidental (unintentional)**

[2] √7th **T63.892 Toxic effect of contact with other venomous animals, intentional self-harm** HCC Rx ESR COM

√7th **T63.893 Toxic effect of contact with other venomous animals, assault**

√7th **T63.894 Toxic effect of contact with other venomous animals, undetermined**

√5th **T63.9 Toxic effect of contact with unspecified venomous animal**

√x7th **T63.91 Toxic effect of contact with unspecified venomous animal, accidental (unintentional)**

[2] √x7th **T63.92 Toxic effect of contact with unspecified venomous animal, intentional self-harm** HCC Rx ESR COM

√x7th **T63.93 Toxic effect of contact with unspecified venomous animal, assault**

√x7th **T63.94 Toxic effect of contact with unspecified venomous animal, undetermined**

√4th **T64 Toxic effect of aflatoxin and other mycotoxin food contaminants**

The appropriate 7th character is to be added to each code from category T64.
A initial encounter
D subsequent encounter
S sequela

√5th **T64.0 Toxic effect of aflatoxin**

√x7th **T64.01 Toxic effect of aflatoxin, accidental (unintentional)**

[2] √x7th **T64.02 Toxic effect of aflatoxin, intentional self-harm** HCC Rx ESR COM

√x7th **T64.03 Toxic effect of aflatoxin, assault**

√x7th **T64.04 Toxic effect of aflatoxin, undetermined**

√5th **T64.8 Toxic effect of other mycotoxin food contaminants**

√x7th **T64.81 Toxic effect of other mycotoxin food contaminants, accidental (unintentional)**

[2] √x7th **T64.82 Toxic effect of other mycotoxin food contaminants, intentional self-harm** HCC Rx ESR COM

√x7th **T64.83 Toxic effect of other mycotoxin food contaminants, assault**

√x7th **T64.84 Toxic effect of other mycotoxin food contaminants, undetermined**

√4th **T65 Toxic effect of other and unspecified substances**

The appropriate 7th character is to be added to each code from category T65.
A initial encounter
D subsequent encounter
S sequela

√5th **T65.0 Toxic effect of cyanides**

EXCLUDES 1 *hydrogen cyanide (T57.3-)*

√6th **T65.0X Toxic effect of cyanides**

√7th **T65.0X1 Toxic effect of cyanides, accidental (unintentional)**
Toxic effect of cyanides NOS

[2] √7th **T65.0X2 Toxic effect of cyanides, intentional self-harm** HCC Rx ESR COM

√7th **T65.0X3 Toxic effect of cyanides, assault**

√7th **T65.0X4 Toxic effect of cyanides, undetermined**

√5th **T65.1 Toxic effect of strychnine and its salts**

√6th **T65.1X Toxic effect of strychnine and its salts**

√7th **T65.1X1 Toxic effect of strychnine and its salts, accidental (unintentional)**
Toxic effect of strychnine and its salts NOS

[2] √7th **T65.1X2 Toxic effect of strychnine and its salts, intentional self-harm** HCC Rx ESR COM

√7th **T65.1X3 Toxic effect of strychnine and its salts, assault**

√7th **T65.1X4 Toxic effect of strychnine and its salts, undetermined**

√5th **T65.2 Toxic effect of tobacco and nicotine**

EXCLUDES 2 *nicotine dependence (F17.-)*

√6th **T65.21 Toxic effect of chewing tobacco**

√7th **T65.211 Toxic effect of chewing tobacco, accidental (unintentional)**
Toxic effect of chewing tobacco NOS

[2] √7th **T65.212 Toxic effect of chewing tobacco, intentional self-harm** HCC Rx ESR COM

√7th **T65.213 Toxic effect of chewing tobacco, assault**

√7th **T65.214 Toxic effect of chewing tobacco, undetermined**

√6th **T65.22 Toxic effect of tobacco cigarettes**
Toxic effect of tobacco smoke
Use additional code for exposure to second hand tobacco smoke (Z57.31, Z77.22)

√7th **T65.221 Toxic effect of tobacco cigarettes, accidental (unintentional)**
Toxic effect of tobacco cigarettes NOS

[2] √7th **T65.222 Toxic effect of tobacco cigarettes, intentional self-harm** HCC Rx ESR COM

√7th **T65.223 Toxic effect of tobacco cigarettes, assault**

√7th **T65.224 Toxic effect of tobacco cigarettes, undetermined**

√6th **T65.29 Toxic effect of other tobacco and nicotine**

√7th **T65.291 Toxic effect of other tobacco and nicotine, accidental (unintentional)**
Toxic effect of other tobacco and nicotine NOS

[2] √7th **T65.292 Toxic effect of other tobacco and nicotine, intentional self-harm** HCC Rx ESR COM

√7th **T65.293 Toxic effect of other tobacco and nicotine, assault**

√7th **T65.294 Toxic effect of other tobacco and nicotine, undetermined**

√5th **T65.3 Toxic effect of nitroderivatives and aminoderivatives of benzene and its homologues**
Toxic effect of anilin [benzenamine]
Toxic effect of nitrobenzene
Toxic effect of trinitrotoluene

√6th **T65.3X Toxic effect of nitroderivatives and aminoderivatives of benzene and its homologues**

√7th **T65.3X1 Toxic effect of nitroderivatives and aminoderivatives of benzene and its homologues, accidental (unintentional)**
Toxic effect of nitroderivatives and aminoderivatives of benzene and its homologues NOS

[2] √7th **T65.3X2 Toxic effect of nitroderivatives and aminoderivatives of benzene and its homologues, intentional self-harm** HCC Rx ESR COM

√7th **T65.3X3 Toxic effect of nitroderivatives and aminoderivatives of benzene and its homologues, assault**

√7th **T65.3X4 Toxic effect of nitroderivatives and aminoderivatives of benzene and its homologues, undetermined**

√5th **T65.4 Toxic effect of carbon disulfide**

√6th **T65.4X Toxic effect of carbon disulfide**

√7th **T65.4X1 Toxic effect of carbon disulfide, accidental (unintentional)**
Toxic effect of carbon disulfide NOS

[2] √7th **T65.4X2 Toxic effect of carbon disulfide, intentional self-harm** HCC Rx ESR COM

√7th **T65.4X3 Toxic effect of carbon disulfide, assault**

√7th **T65.4X4 Toxic effect of carbon disulfide, undetermined**

√5th **T65.5 Toxic effect of nitroglycerin and other nitric acids and esters**
Toxic effect of 1,2,3-Propanetriol trinitrate

√6th **T65.5X Toxic effect of nitroglycerin and other nitric acids and esters**

√7th **T65.5X1 Toxic effect of nitroglycerin and other nitric acids and esters, accidental (unintentional)**
Toxic effect of nitroglycerin and other nitric acids and esters NOS

[2] √7th **T65.5X2 Toxic effect of nitroglycerin and other nitric acids and esters, intentional self-harm** HCC Rx ESR COM

√7th **T65.5X3 Toxic effect of nitroglycerin and other nitric acids and esters, assault**

√7th **T65.5X4 Toxic effect of nitroglycerin and other nitric acids and esters, undetermined**

√5th **T65.6 Toxic effect of paints and dyes, not elsewhere classified**

√6th **T65.6X Toxic effect of paints and dyes, not elsewhere classified**

√7th **T65.6X1 Toxic effect of paints and dyes, not elsewhere classified, accidental (unintentional)**
Toxic effect of paints and dyes NOS

HCC CMS-HCC Rx Rx HCC ESR ESRD HCC COM Commercial HCC N Newborn: 0 P Pediatric: 0-17 M Maternity: 9-64 A Adult: 15-124

2 ✓7th T65.6X2 **Toxic effect of paints and dyes, not elsewhere classified, intentional self-harm** HCC Rx ESR COM

✓7th T65.6X3 **Toxic effect of paints and dyes, not elsewhere classified, assault**

✓7th T65.6X4 **Toxic effect of paints and dyes, not elsewhere classified, undetermined**

✓5th **T65.8 Toxic effect of other specified substances**

✓6th **T65.81 Toxic effect of latex**

✓7th T65.811 **Toxic effect of latex, accidental (unintentional)**

Toxic effect of latex NOS

2 ✓7th T65.812 **Toxic effect of latex, intentional self-harm** HCC Rx ESR COM

✓7th T65.813 **Toxic effect of latex, assault**

✓7th T65.814 **Toxic effect of latex, undetermined**

✓6th **T65.82 Toxic effect of harmful algae and algae toxins**

Toxic effect of (harmful) algae bloom NOS
Toxic effect of blue-green algae bloom
Toxic effect of brown tide
Toxic effect of cyanobacteria bloom
Toxic effect of Florida red tide
Toxic effect of pfiesteria piscicida
Toxic effect of red tide

✓7th T65.821 **Toxic effect of harmful algae and algae toxins, accidental (unintentional)**

Toxic effect of harmful algae and algae toxins NOS

2 ✓7th T65.822 **Toxic effect of harmful algae and algae toxins, intentional self-harm** HCC Rx ESR COM

✓7th T65.823 **Toxic effect of harmful algae and algae toxins, assault**

✓7th T65.824 **Toxic effect of harmful algae and algae toxins, undetermined**

✓6th **T65.83 Toxic effect of fiberglass**

✓7th T65.831 **Toxic effect of fiberglass, accidental (unintentional)**

Toxic effect of fiberglass NOS

2 ✓7th T65.832 **Toxic effect of fiberglass, intentional self-harm** HCC Rx ESR COM

✓7th T65.833 **Toxic effect of fiberglass, assault**

✓7th T65.834 **Toxic effect of fiberglass, undetermined**

✓6th **T65.89 Toxic effect of other specified substances**

✓7th T65.891 **Toxic effect of other specified substances, accidental (unintentional)**

Toxic effect of other specified substances NOS

AHA: 2018,1Q,5

2 ✓7th T65.892 **Toxic effect of other specified substances, intentional self-harm** HCC Rx ESR COM

✓7th T65.893 **Toxic effect of other specified substances, assault**

✓7th T65.894 **Toxic effect of other specified substances, undetermined**

✓5th **T65.9 Toxic effect of unspecified substance**

✓x7th T65.91 **Toxic effect of unspecified substance, accidental (unintentional)**

Poisoning NOS

2 ✓x7th T65.92 **Toxic effect of unspecified substance, intentional self-harm** HCC Rx ESR COM

✓x7th T65.93 **Toxic effect of unspecified substance, assault**

✓x7th T65.94 **Toxic effect of unspecified substance, undetermined**

Other and unspecified effects of external causes (T66-T78)

✓x7th **T66 Radiation sickness, unspecified**

EXCLUDES 1 *specified adverse effects of radiation, such as:*
burns (T2Ø-T31)
leukemia (C91-C95)
radiation gastroenteritis and colitis (K52.Ø)
radiation pneumonitis (J7Ø.Ø)
radiation related disorders of the skin and subcutaneous tissue (L55-L59)
radiation sunburn (L55.-)

The appropriate 7th character is to be added to code T66.
A initial encounter
D subsequent encounter
S sequela

✓4th **T67 Effects of heat and light**

EXCLUDES 1 *erythema [dermatitis] ab igne (L59.Ø)*
malignant hyperpyrexia due to anesthesia (T88.3)
radiation-related disorders of the skin and subcutaneous tissue (L55-L59)

EXCLUDES 2 *burns (T2Ø-T31)*
sunburn (L55.-)
sweat disorder due to heat (L74-L75)

The appropriate 7th character is to be added to each code from category T67.
A initial encounter
D subsequent encounter
S sequela

✓5th **T67.Ø Heatstroke and sunstroke**

Use additional code(s) to identify any associated complications of heatstroke, such as:
coma and stupor (R4Ø.-)
rhabdomyolysis (M62.82)
systemic inflammatory response syndrome (R65.1-)

AHA: 2019,4Q,17-18

DEF: Headache, vertigo, cramps, and elevated body temperature due to prolonged exposure to high environmental temperatures that requires emergency intervention.

✓x7th T67.Ø1 **Heatstroke and sunstroke**

Heat apoplexy
Heat pyrexia
Siriasis
Thermoplegia

✓x7th T67.Ø2 **Exertional heatstroke**

✓x7th T67.Ø9 **Other heatstroke and sunstroke**

✓x7th **T67.1 Heat syncope**

Heat collapse

✓x7th **T67.2 Heat cramp**

✓x7th **T67.3 Heat exhaustion, anhydrotic**

Heat prostration due to water depletion

EXCLUDES 1 *heat exhaustion due to salt depletion (T67.4)*

✓x7th **T67.4 Heat exhaustion due to salt depletion**

Heat prostration due to salt (and water) depletion

✓x7th **T67.5 Heat exhaustion, unspecified**

Heat prostration NOS

✓x7th **T67.6 Heat fatigue, transient**

✓x7th **T67.7 Heat edema**

✓x7th **T67.8 Other effects of heat and light**

✓x7th **T67.9 Effect of heat and light, unspecified**

√x7th **T68 Hypothermia**
Accidental hypothermia
Hypothermia NOS
Use additional code to identify source of exposure:
exposure to excessive cold of man-made origin (W93)
exposure to excessive cold of natural origin (X31)
EXCLUDES 1 *hypothermia following anesthesia (T88.51)*
hypothermia not associated with low environmental temperature (R68.Ø)
hypothermia of newborn (P8Ø.-)
EXCLUDES 2 *frostbite (T33-T34)*

The appropriate 7th character is to be added to code T68.
A initial encounter
D subsequent encounter
S sequela

√4th **T69 Other effects of reduced temperature**
Use additional code to identify source of exposure:
exposure to excessive cold of man-made origin (W93)
exposure to excessive cold of natural origin (X31)
EXCLUDES 2 *frostbite (T33-T34)*

The appropriate 7th character is to be added to each code from category T69.
A initial encounter
D subsequent encounter
S sequela

√5th **T69.Ø Immersion hand and foot**
√6th **T69.Ø1 Immersion hand**
√7th **T69.Ø11 Immersion hand, right hand**
√7th **T69.Ø12 Immersion hand, left hand**
√7th **T69.Ø19 Immersion hand, unspecified hand**
√6th **T69.Ø2 Immersion foot**
Trench foot
√7th **T69.Ø21 Immersion foot, right foot**
√7th **T69.Ø22 Immersion foot, left foot**
√7th **T69.Ø29 Immersion foot, unspecified foot**
√x7th **T69.1 Chilblains**
DEF: Red, swollen, itchy skin primarily affecting the fingers and toes, nose and ears, and legs. Chilblains follows damp-cold exposure, and can also be associated with pruritus and a burning feeling.
√x7th **T69.8 Other specified effects of reduced temperature**
√x7th **T69.9 Effect of reduced temperature, unspecified**

√4th **T7Ø Effects of air pressure and water pressure**

The appropriate 7th character is to be added to each code from category T7Ø.
A initial encounter
D subsequent encounter
S sequela

√x7th **T7Ø.Ø Otitic barotrauma**
Aero-otitis media
Effects of change in ambient atmospheric pressure or water pressure on ears
√x7th **T7Ø.1 Sinus barotrauma**
Aerosinusitis
Effects of change in ambient atmospheric pressure on sinuses
√5th **T7Ø.2 Other and unspecified effects of high altitude**
EXCLUDES 2 *polycythemia due to high altitude (D75.1)*
√x7th **T7Ø.2Ø Unspecified effects of high altitude**
√x7th **T7Ø.29 Other effects of high altitude**
Alpine sickness
Anoxia due to high altitude
Barotrauma NOS
Hypobaropathy
Mountain sickness
√x7th **T7Ø.3 Caisson disease [decompression sickness]**
Compressed-air disease
Diver's palsy or paralysis
DEF: Rapid reduction in air pressure while breathing compressed air. Symptoms include skin lesions, joint pains, and respiratory and neurological problems.
√x7th **T7Ø.4 Effects of high-pressure fluids**
Hydraulic jet injection (industrial)
Pneumatic jet injection (industrial)
Traumatic jet injection (industrial)
√x7th **T7Ø.8 Other effects of air pressure and water pressure**
√x7th **T7Ø.9 Effect of air pressure and water pressure, unspecified**

√4th **T71 Asphyxiation**
Mechanical suffocation
Traumatic suffocation
EXCLUDES 1 *acute respiratory distress (syndrome) (J8Ø)*
anoxia due to high altitude (T7Ø.2)
asphyxia NOS (RØ9.Ø1)
asphyxia from carbon monoxide (T58.-)
asphyxia from inhalation of food or foreign body (T17.-)
asphyxia from other gases, fumes and vapors (T59.-)
respiratory distress (syndrome) in newborn (P22.-)

The appropriate 7th character is to be added to each code from category T71.
A initial encounter
D subsequent encounter
S sequela

√5th **T71.1 Asphyxiation due to mechanical threat to breathing**
Suffocation due to mechanical threat to breathing
√6th **T71.11 Asphyxiation due to smothering under pillow**
√7th **T71.111 Asphyxiation due to smothering under pillow, accidental**
Asphyxiation due to smothering under pillow NOS
2 √7th **T71.112 Asphyxiation due to smothering under pillow, intentional self-harm** HCC Rx ESR COM
√7th **T71.113 Asphyxiation due to smothering under pillow, assault**
√7th **T71.114 Asphyxiation due to smothering under pillow, undetermined**
√6th **T71.12 Asphyxiation due to plastic bag**
√7th **T71.121 Asphyxiation due to plastic bag, accidental**
Asphyxiation due to plastic bag NOS
2 √7th **T71.122 Asphyxiation due to plastic bag, intentional self-harm** HCC Rx ESR COM
√7th **T71.123 Asphyxiation due to plastic bag, assault**
√7th **T71.124 Asphyxiation due to plastic bag, undetermined**
√6th **T71.13 Asphyxiation due to being trapped in bed linens**
√7th **T71.131 Asphyxiation due to being trapped in bed linens, accidental**
Asphyxiation due to being trapped in bed linens NOS
2 √7th **T71.132 Asphyxiation due to being trapped in bed linens, intentional self-harm** HCC Rx ESR COM
√7th **T71.133 Asphyxiation due to being trapped in bed linens, assault**
√7th **T71.134 Asphyxiation due to being trapped in bed linens, undetermined**
√6th **T71.14 Asphyxiation due to smothering under another person's body (in bed)**
√7th **T71.141 Asphyxiation due to smothering under another person's body (in bed), accidental**
Asphyxiation due to smothering under another person's body (in bed) NOS
√7th **T71.143 Asphyxiation due to smothering under another person's body (in bed), assault**
√7th **T71.144 Asphyxiation due to smothering under another person's body (in bed), undetermined**
√6th **T71.15 Asphyxiation due to smothering in furniture**
√7th **T71.151 Asphyxiation due to smothering in furniture, accidental**
Asphyxiation due to smothering in furniture NOS
2 √7th **T71.152 Asphyxiation due to smothering in furniture, intentional self-harm** HCC Rx ESR COM
√7th **T71.153 Asphyxiation due to smothering in furniture, assault**

T71.154 **Asphyxiation due to smothering in furniture, undetermined**

T71.16 **Asphyxiation due to hanging**

Hanging by window shade cord

Use additional code for any associated injuries, such as:

crushing injury of neck (S17.-)

fracture of cervical vertebrae (S12.Ø-S12.2-)

open wound of neck (S11.-)

T71.161 **Asphyxiation due to hanging, accidental**

Asphyxiation due to hanging NOS

Hanging NOS

2 T71.162 **Asphyxiation due to hanging, intentional self-harm** HCC Rx ESR COM

T71.163 **Asphyxiation due to hanging, assault**

T71.164 **Asphyxiation due to hanging, undetermined**

T71.19 **Asphyxiation due to mechanical threat to breathing due to other causes**

T71.191 **Asphyxiation due to mechanical threat to breathing due to other causes, accidental**

Asphyxiation due to other causes NOS

2 T71.192 **Asphyxiation due to mechanical threat to breathing due to other causes, intentional self-harm** HCC Rx ESR COM

T71.193 **Asphyxiation due to mechanical threat to breathing due to other causes, assault**

T71.194 **Asphyxiation due to mechanical threat to breathing due to other causes, undetermined**

T71.2 **Asphyxiation due to systemic oxygen deficiency due to low oxygen content in ambient air**

Suffocation due to systemic oxygen deficiency due to low oxygen content in ambient air

T71.2Ø **Asphyxiation due to systemic oxygen deficiency due to low oxygen content in ambient air due to unspecified cause**

T71.21 **Asphyxiation due to cave-in or falling earth**

Use additional code for any associated cataclysm (X34-X38)

T71.22 **Asphyxiation due to being trapped in a car trunk**

T71.221 **Asphyxiation due to being trapped in a car trunk, accidental**

2 T71.222 **Asphyxiation due to being trapped in a car trunk, intentional self-harm** HCC Rx ESR COM

T71.223 **Asphyxiation due to being trapped in a car trunk, assault**

T71.224 **Asphyxiation due to being trapped in a car trunk, undetermined**

T71.23 **Asphyxiation due to being trapped in a (discarded) refrigerator**

T71.231 **Asphyxiation due to being trapped in a (discarded) refrigerator, accidental**

2 T71.232 **Asphyxiation due to being trapped in a (discarded) refrigerator, intentional self-harm** HCC Rx ESR COM

T71.233 **Asphyxiation due to being trapped in a (discarded) refrigerator, assault**

T71.234 **Asphyxiation due to being trapped in a (discarded) refrigerator, undetermined**

T71.29 **Asphyxiation due to being trapped in other low oxygen environment**

T71.9 **Asphyxiation due to unspecified cause**

Suffocation (by strangulation) due to unspecified cause

Suffocation NOS

Systemic oxygen deficiency due to low oxygen content in ambient air due to unspecified cause

Systemic oxygen deficiency due to mechanical threat to breathing due to unspecified cause

Traumatic asphyxia NOS

T73 Effects of other deprivation

The appropriate 7th character is to be added to each code from category T73.

A initial encounter

D subsequent encounter

S sequela

T73.Ø **Starvation**

Deprivation of food

T73.1 **Deprivation of water**

T73.2 **Exhaustion due to exposure**

T73.3 **Exhaustion due to excessive exertion**

Exhaustion due to overexertion

T73.8 **Other effects of deprivation**

T73.9 **Effect of deprivation, unspecified**

T74 Adult and child abuse, neglect and other maltreatment, confirmed

Use additional code, if applicable, to identify any associated current injury

Use additional external cause code to identify perpetrator, if known (YØ7.-)

EXCLUDES 1 *abuse and maltreatment in pregnancy (O9A.3-, O9A.4-, O9A.5-)*

adult and child maltreatment, suspected (T76.-)

The appropriate 7th character is to be added to each code from category T74.

A initial encounter

D subsequent encounter

S sequela

T74.Ø **Neglect or abandonment, confirmed**

T74.Ø1 **Adult neglect or abandonment, confirmed** A

T74.Ø2 **Child neglect or abandonment, confirmed** P

T74.1 **Physical abuse, confirmed**

EXCLUDES 2 *sexual abuse (T74.2-)*

T74.11 **Adult physical abuse, confirmed** A

T74.12 **Child physical abuse, confirmed** P

EXCLUDES 2 *shaken infant syndrome (T74.4)*

T74.2 **Sexual abuse, confirmed**

Rape, confirmed

Sexual assault, confirmed

T74.21 **Adult sexual abuse, confirmed** A

T74.22 **Child sexual abuse, confirmed** P

T74.3 **Psychological abuse, confirmed**

Bullying and intimidation, confirmed

Intimidation through social media, confirmed

T74.31 **Adult psychological abuse, confirmed** A

T74.32 **Child psychological abuse, confirmed** P

T74.4 **Shaken infant syndrome** P

T74.5 **Forced sexual exploitation, confirmed**

AHA: 2018,4Q,32-33,65

T74.51 **Adult forced sexual exploitation, confirmed** A

T74.52 **Child sexual exploitation, confirmed** P

T74.6 **Forced labor exploitation, confirmed**

AHA: 2018,4Q,32-33,65

T74.61 **Adult forced labor exploitation, confirmed** A

T74.62 **Child forced labor exploitation, confirmed** P

T74.9 **Unspecified maltreatment, confirmed**

T74.91 **Unspecified adult maltreatment, confirmed** A

T74.92 **Unspecified child maltreatment, confirmed** P

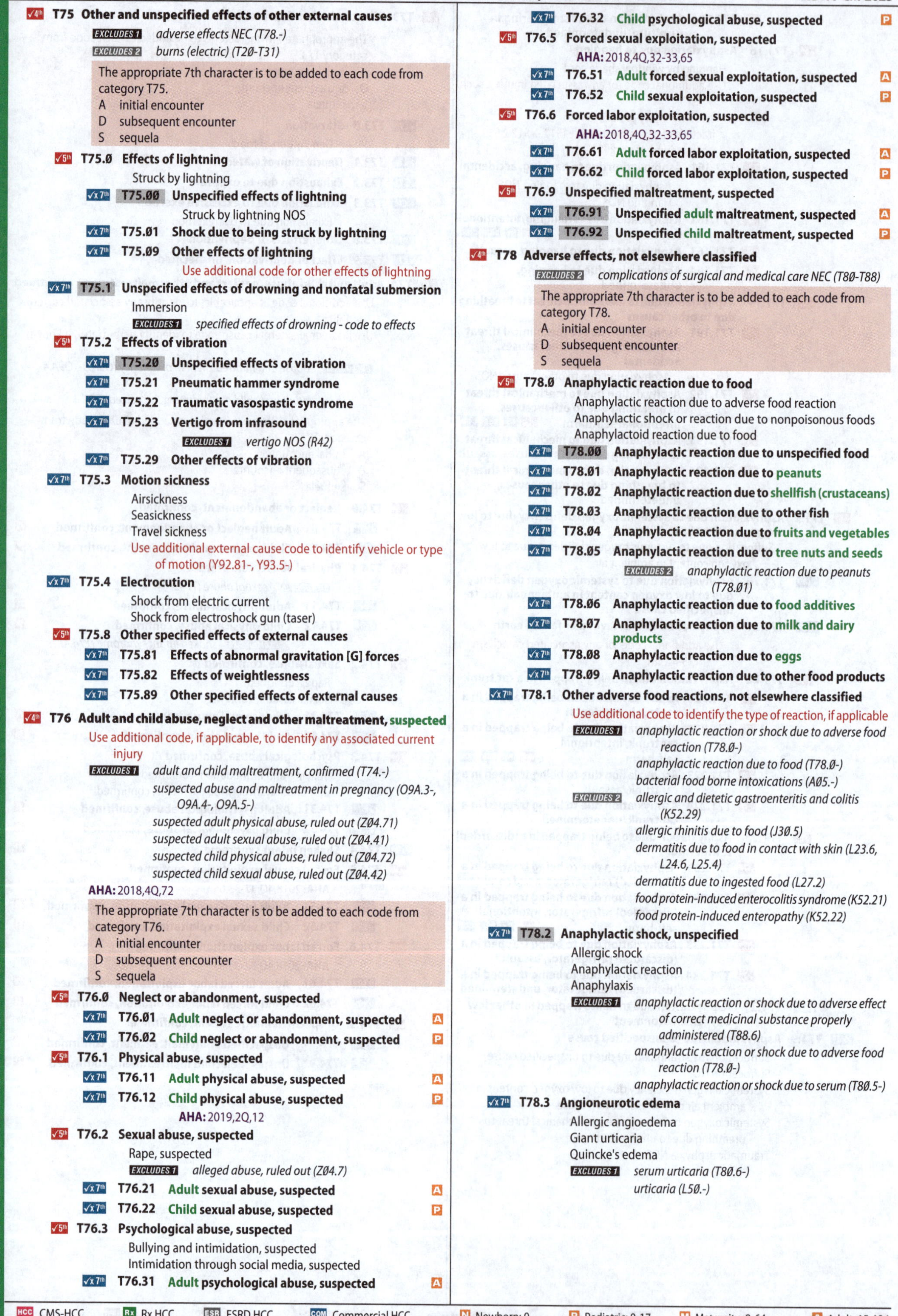

T75 Other and unspecified effects of other external causes

EXCLUDES 1 *adverse effects NEC (T78.-)*

EXCLUDES 2 *burns (electric) (T2Ø-T31)*

The appropriate 7th character is to be added to each code from category T75.
A initial encounter
D subsequent encounter
S sequela

T75.Ø Effects of lightning
Struck by lightning

T75.ØØ Unspecified effects of lightning
Struck by lightning NOS

T75.Ø1 Shock due to being struck by lightning

T75.Ø9 Other effects of lightning
Use additional code for other effects of lightning

T75.1 Unspecified effects of drowning and nonfatal submersion
Immersion
EXCLUDES 1 *specified effects of drowning - code to effects*

T75.2 Effects of vibration

T75.2Ø Unspecified effects of vibration

T75.21 Pneumatic hammer syndrome

T75.22 Traumatic vasospastic syndrome

T75.23 Vertigo from infrasound
EXCLUDES 1 *vertigo NOS (R42)*

T75.29 Other effects of vibration

T75.3 Motion sickness
Airsickness
Seasickness
Travel sickness
Use additional external cause code to identify vehicle or type of motion (Y92.81-, Y93.5-)

T75.4 Electrocution
Shock from electric current
Shock from electroshock gun (taser)

T75.8 Other specified effects of external causes

T75.81 Effects of abnormal gravitation [G] forces

T75.82 Effects of weightlessness

T75.89 Other specified effects of external causes

T76 Adult and child abuse, neglect and other maltreatment, suspected

Use additional code, if applicable, to identify any associated current injury

EXCLUDES 1 *adult and child maltreatment, confirmed (T74.-)*
suspected abuse and maltreatment in pregnancy (O9A.3-, O9A.4-, O9A.5-)
suspected adult physical abuse, ruled out (ZØ4.71)
suspected adult sexual abuse, ruled out (ZØ4.41)
suspected child physical abuse, ruled out (ZØ4.72)
suspected child sexual abuse, ruled out (ZØ4.42)

AHA: 2018,4Q,72

The appropriate 7th character is to be added to each code from category T76.
A initial encounter
D subsequent encounter
S sequela

T76.Ø Neglect or abandonment, suspected

T76.Ø1 Adult neglect or abandonment, suspected A

T76.Ø2 Child neglect or abandonment, suspected P

T76.1 Physical abuse, suspected

T76.11 Adult physical abuse, suspected A

T76.12 Child physical abuse, suspected P
AHA: 2019,2Q,12

T76.2 Sexual abuse, suspected
Rape, suspected
EXCLUDES 1 *alleged abuse, ruled out (ZØ4.7)*

T76.21 Adult sexual abuse, suspected A

T76.22 Child sexual abuse, suspected P

T76.3 Psychological abuse, suspected
Bullying and intimidation, suspected
Intimidation through social media, suspected

T76.31 Adult psychological abuse, suspected A

T76.32 Child psychological abuse, suspected P

T76.5 Forced sexual exploitation, suspected
AHA: 2018,4Q,32-33,65

T76.51 Adult forced sexual exploitation, suspected A

T76.52 Child sexual exploitation, suspected P

T76.6 Forced labor exploitation, suspected
AHA: 2018,4Q,32-33,65

T76.61 Adult forced labor exploitation, suspected A

T76.62 Child forced labor exploitation, suspected P

T76.9 Unspecified maltreatment, suspected

T76.91 Unspecified adult maltreatment, suspected A

T76.92 Unspecified child maltreatment, suspected P

T78 Adverse effects, not elsewhere classified

EXCLUDES 2 *complications of surgical and medical care NEC (T8Ø-T88)*

The appropriate 7th character is to be added to each code from category T78.
A initial encounter
D subsequent encounter
S sequela

T78.Ø Anaphylactic reaction due to food
Anaphylactic reaction due to adverse food reaction
Anaphylactic shock or reaction due to nonpoisonous foods
Anaphylactoid reaction due to food

T78.ØØ Anaphylactic reaction due to unspecified food

T78.Ø1 Anaphylactic reaction due to peanuts

T78.Ø2 Anaphylactic reaction due to shellfish (crustaceans)

T78.Ø3 Anaphylactic reaction due to other fish

T78.Ø4 Anaphylactic reaction due to fruits and vegetables

T78.Ø5 Anaphylactic reaction due to tree nuts and seeds
EXCLUDES 2 *anaphylactic reaction due to peanuts (T78.Ø1)*

T78.Ø6 Anaphylactic reaction due to food additives

T78.Ø7 Anaphylactic reaction due to milk and dairy products

T78.Ø8 Anaphylactic reaction due to eggs

T78.Ø9 Anaphylactic reaction due to other food products

T78.1 Other adverse food reactions, not elsewhere classified
Use additional code to identify the type of reaction, if applicable
EXCLUDES 1 *anaphylactic reaction or shock due to adverse food reaction (T78.Ø-)*
anaphylactic reaction due to food (T78.Ø-)
bacterial food borne intoxications (AØ5.-)
EXCLUDES 2 *allergic and dietetic gastroenteritis and colitis (K52.29)*
allergic rhinitis due to food (J3Ø.5)
dermatitis due to food in contact with skin (L23.6, L24.6, L25.4)
dermatitis due to ingested food (L27.2)
food protein-induced enterocolitis syndrome (K52.21)
food protein-induced enteropathy (K52.22)

T78.2 Anaphylactic shock, unspecified
Allergic shock
Anaphylactic reaction
Anaphylaxis
EXCLUDES 1 *anaphylactic reaction or shock due to adverse effect of correct medicinal substance properly administered (T88.6)*
anaphylactic reaction or shock due to adverse food reaction (T78.Ø-)
anaphylactic reaction or shock due to serum (T8Ø.5-)

T78.3 Angioneurotic edema
Allergic angioedema
Giant urticaria
Quincke's edema
EXCLUDES 1 *serum urticaria (T8Ø.6-)*
urticaria (L5Ø.-)

✓5th **T78.4 Other and unspecified allergy**

EXCLUDES 1 *specified types of allergic reaction such as:*
allergic diarrhea (K52.29)
allergic gastroenteritis and colitis (K52.29)
dermatitis (L23-L25, L27.-)
food protein-induced enterocolitis syndrome (K52.21)
food protein-induced enteropathy (K52.22)
hay fever (J30.1)

✓x7th **T78.40 Allergy, unspecified**
Allergic reaction NOS
Hypersensitivity NOS

✓x7th **T78.41 Arthus phenomenon**
Arthus reaction

✓x7th **T78.49 Other allergy**
AHA: 2021,1Q,42

✓x7th **T78.8 Other adverse effects, not elsewhere classified**

Certain early complications of trauma (T79)

✓4th **T79 Certain early complications of trauma, not elsewhere classified**

EXCLUDES 2 *acute respiratory distress syndrome (J80)*
complications occurring during or following medical procedures (T80-T88)
complications of surgical and medical care NEC (T80-T88)
newborn respiratory distress syndrome (P22.0)

The appropriate 7th character is to be added to each code from category T79.
A initial encounter
D subsequent encounter
S sequela

1 ✓x7th **T79.0 Air embolism (traumatic)** HCC ESR COM

EXCLUDES 1 *air embolism complicating abortion or ectopic or molar pregnancy (O00-O07, O08.2)*
air embolism complicating pregnancy, childbirth and the puerperium (O88.0)
air embolism following infusion, transfusion, and therapeutic injection (T80.0)
air embolism following procedure NEC (T81.7-)

DEF: Arterial or venous obstruction due to the introduction of air bubbles into the blood vessels following surgery or trauma.

1 ✓x7th **T79.1 Fat embolism (traumatic)** HCC ESR COM

EXCLUDES 1 *fat embolism complicating:*
abortion or ectopic or molar pregnancy (O00-O07, O08.2)
pregnancy, childbirth and the puerperium (O88.8)

DEF: Arterial blockage due to the entrance of fat into the circulatory system after a fracture of the large bones or administration of corticosteroids.

1 ✓x7th **T79.2 Traumatic secondary and recurrent hemorrhage and seroma** HCC ESR

1 ✓x7th **T79.4 Traumatic shock** HCC ESR COM
Shock (immediate) (delayed) following injury

EXCLUDES 1 *anaphylactic shock due to adverse food reaction (T78.0-)*
anaphylactic shock due to correct medicinal substance properly administered (T88.6)
anaphylactic shock due to serum (T80.5-)
anaphylactic shock NOS (T78.2)
electric shock (T75.4)
nontraumatic shock NEC (R57.-)
obstetric shock (O75.1)
postprocedural shock (T81.1-)
septic shock (R65.21)
shock complicating abortion or ectopic or molar pregnancy (O00-O07, O08.3)
shock due to anesthesia (T88.2)
shock due to lightning (T75.01)
shock NOS (R57.9)

1 ✓x7th **T79.5 Traumatic anuria** HCC ESR
Crush syndrome
Renal failure following crushing

1 ✓x7th **T79.6 Traumatic ischemia of muscle** HCC ESR
Traumatic rhabdomyolysis
Volkmann's ischemic contracture

EXCLUDES 2 *anterior tibial syndrome (M76.8)*
compartment syndrome (traumatic) (T79.A-)
nontraumatic ischemia of muscle (M62.2-)

AHA: 2019,2Q,12

1 ✓x7th **T79.7 Traumatic subcutaneous emphysema** HCC ESR

EXCLUDES 2 *emphysema NOS (J43)*
emphysema (subcutaneous) resulting from a procedure (T81.82)

✓5th **T79.A Traumatic compartment syndrome**

EXCLUDES 1 *fibromyalgia (M79.7)*
nontraumatic compartment syndrome (M79.A-)

EXCLUDES 2 *traumatic ischemic infarction of muscle (T79.6)*

DEF: Compression of nerves and blood vessels within an enclosed muscle space due to previous trauma, which leads to impaired blood flow and muscle and nerve damage.

1 ✓x7th **T79.A0 Compartment syndrome, unspecified** HCC ESR
Compartment syndrome NOS

✓6th **T79.A1 Traumatic compartment syndrome of upper extremity**
Traumatic compartment syndrome of shoulder, arm, forearm, wrist, hand, and fingers

1 ✓7th **T79.A11 Traumatic compartment syndrome of right upper extremity** HCC ESR

1 ✓7th **T79.A12 Traumatic compartment syndrome of left upper extremity** HCC ESR

1 ✓7th **T79.A19 Traumatic compartment syndrome of unspecified upper extremity** HCC ESR

✓6th **T79.A2 Traumatic compartment syndrome of lower extremity**
Traumatic compartment syndrome of hip, buttock, thigh, leg, foot, and toes

1 ✓7th **T79.A21 Traumatic compartment syndrome of right lower extremity** HCC ESR

1 ✓7th **T79.A22 Traumatic compartment syndrome of left lower extremity** HCC ESR

1 ✓7th **T79.A29 Traumatic compartment syndrome of unspecified lower extremity** HCC ESR

1 ✓x7th **T79.A3 Traumatic compartment syndrome of abdomen** HCC ESR

1 ✓x7th **T79.A9 Traumatic compartment syndrome of other sites** HCC ESR

1 ✓x7th **T79.8 Other early complications of trauma** HCC ESR

1 ✓x7th **T79.9 Unspecified early complication of trauma** HCC ESR

Complications of surgical and medical care, not elsewhere classified (T80-T88)

Use additional code for adverse effect, if applicable, to identify drug (T36-T50 with fifth or sixth character 5)

Use additional code(s) to identify the specified condition resulting from the complication

Use additional code to identify devices involved and details of circumstances (Y62-Y82)

EXCLUDES 2 *any encounters with medical care for postprocedural conditions in which no complications are present, such as:*
- *artificial opening status (Z93.-)*
- *closure of external stoma (Z43.-)*
- *fitting and adjustment of external prosthetic device (Z44.-)*

burns and corrosions from local applications and irradiation (T20-T32)

complications of surgical procedures during pregnancy, childbirth and the puerperium (O00-O9A)

mechanical complication of respirator [ventilator] (J95.850)

poisoning and toxic effects of drugs and chemicals (T36-T65 with fifth or sixth character 1-4 or 6)

postprocedural fever (R50.82)

specified complications classified elsewhere, such as:
- *cerebrospinal fluid leak from spinal puncture (G97.0)*
- *colostomy malfunction (K94.0-)*
- *disorders of fluid and electrolyte imbalance (E86-E87)*
- *functional disturbances following cardiac surgery (I97.0-I97.1)*
- *intraoperative and postprocedural complications of specified body systems (D78.-, E36.-, E89.-, G97.3-, G97.4, H59.3-, H59.-, H95.2-, H95.3, I97.4-, I97.5, J95.6-, J95.7, K91.6-, L76.-, M96.-, N99.-)*
- *ostomy complications (J95.0-, K94.-, N99.5-)*
- *postgastric surgery syndromes (K91.1)*
- *postlaminectomy syndrome NEC (M96.1)*
- *postmastectomy lymphedema syndrome (I97.2)*
- *postsurgical blind-loop syndrome (K91.2)*
- *ventilator associated pneumonia (J95.851)*

AHA: 2015,1Q,15

✓4th T80 Complications following infusion, transfusion and therapeutic injection

INCLUDES complications following perfusion

EXCLUDES 2 *bone marrow transplant rejection (T86.01)*
febrile nonhemolytic transfusion reaction (R50.84)
fluid overload due to transfusion (E87.71)
posttransfusion purpura (D69.51)
transfusion associated circulatory overload (TACO) (E87.71)
transfusion (red blood cell) associated hemochromatosis (E83.111)
transfusion related acute lung injury (TRALI) (J95.84)

The appropriate 7th character is to be added to each code from category T80.
- A initial encounter
- D subsequent encounter
- S sequela

✓x7th T80.0 Air embolism following infusion, transfusion and therapeutic injection

✓x7th T80.1 Vascular complications following infusion, transfusion and therapeutic injection

Use additional code to identify the vascular complication

EXCLUDES 2 *extravasation of vesicant agent (T80.81-)*
infiltration of vesicant agent (T80.81-)
postprocedural vascular complications (T81.7-)
vascular complications specified as due to prosthetic devices, implants and grafts (T82.8-, T83.8-, T84.8-, T85.8-)

✓5th T80.2 Infections following infusion, transfusion and therapeutic injection

Use additional code to identify the specific infection, such as: sepsis (A41.9)

Use additional code (R65.2-) to identify severe sepsis, if applicable

EXCLUDES 2 *infections specified as due to prosthetic devices, implants and grafts (T82.6-T82.7, T83.5-T83.6, T84.5-T84.7, T85.7)*
postprocedural infections (T81.4-)

AHA: 2018,4Q,62

✓6th T80.21 Infection due to central venous catheter

Infection due to pulmonary artery catheter (Swan-Ganz catheter)

AHA: 2019,1Q,13-14

DEF: Central venous catheter: Catheter positioned in the superior vena cava or right atrium and introduced through a large vein, such as the jugular or subclavian, and used to measure venous pressure or administer fluids or medication.

TIP: Code assignment is based on the location of the catheter and not how the catheter is being used; for example, for hemodialysis. Infections resulting from catheters that are not central lines should be coded to T82.7-.

✓7th T80.211 Bloodstream infection due to central venous catheter

Catheter-related bloodstream infection (CRBSI) NOS
Central line-associated bloodstream infection (CLABSI)
Bloodstream infection due to Hickman catheter
Bloodstream infection due to peripherally inserted central catheter (PICC)
Bloodstream infection due to portacath (port-a-cath)
Bloodstream infection due to pulmonary artery catheter
Bloodstream infection due to triple lumen catheter
Bloodstream infection due to umbilical venous catheter

AHA: 2019,1Q,13,14; 2018,4Q,89

✓7th T80.212 Local infection due to central venous catheter

Exit or insertion site infection
Local infection due to Hickman catheter
Local infection due to peripherally inserted central catheter (PICC)
Local infection due to portacath (port-a-cath)
Local infection due to pulmonary artery catheter
Local infection due to triple lumen catheter
Local infection due to umbilical venous catheter
Port or reservoir infection
Tunnel infection

✓7th T80.218 Other infection due to central venous catheter

Other central line-associated infection
Other infection due to Hickman catheter
Other infection due to peripherally inserted central catheter (PICC)
Other infection due to portacath (port-a-cath)
Other infection due to pulmonary artery catheter
Other infection due to triple lumen catheter
Other infection due to umbilical venous catheter

T80.219 Unspecified infection due to central venous catheter
Central line-associated infection NOS
Unspecified infection due to Hickman catheter
Unspecified infection due to peripherally inserted central catheter (PICC)
Unspecified infection due to portacath (port-a-cath)
Unspecified infection due to pulmonary artery catheter
Unspecified infection due to triple lumen catheter
Unspecified infection due to umbilical venous catheter

T80.22 Acute infection following transfusion, infusion, or injection of blood and blood products

T80.29 Infection following other infusion, transfusion and therapeutic injection

T80.3 ABO incompatibility reaction due to transfusion of blood or blood products
EXCLUDES 1 *minor blood group antigens reactions (Duffy) (E) (K) (Kell) (Kidd) (Lewis) (M) (N) (P) (S) (T80.A-)*

T80.30 ABO incompatibility reaction due to transfusion of blood or blood products, unspecified
ABO incompatibility blood transfusion NOS
Reaction to ABO incompatibility from transfusion NOS

T80.31 ABO incompatibility with hemolytic transfusion reaction

T80.310 ABO incompatibility with acute hemolytic transfusion reaction
ABO incompatibility with hemolytic transfusion reaction less than 24 hours after transfusion
Acute hemolytic transfusion reaction (AHTR) due to ABO incompatibility

T80.311 ABO incompatibility with delayed hemolytic transfusion reaction
ABO incompatibility with hemolytic transfusion reaction 24 hours or more after transfusion
Delayed hemolytic transfusion reaction (DHTR) due to ABO incompatibility

T80.319 ABO incompatibility with hemolytic transfusion reaction, unspecified
ABO incompatibility with hemolytic transfusion reaction at unspecified time after transfusion
Hemolytic transfusion reaction (HTR) due to ABO incompatibility NOS

T80.39 Other ABO incompatibility reaction due to transfusion of blood or blood products
Delayed serologic transfusion reaction (DSTR) from ABO incompatibility
Other ABO incompatible blood transfusion
Other reaction to ABO incompatible blood transfusion

T80.4 Rh incompatibility reaction due to transfusion of blood or blood products
Reaction due to incompatibility of Rh antigens (C) (c) (D) (E) (e)

T80.40 Rh incompatibility reaction due to transfusion of blood or blood products, unspecified
Reaction due to Rh factor in transfusion NOS
Rh incompatible blood transfusion NOS

T80.41 Rh incompatibility with hemolytic transfusion reaction

T80.410 Rh incompatibility with acute hemolytic transfusion reaction
Acute hemolytic transfusion reaction (AHTR) due to Rh incompatibility
Rh incompatibility with hemolytic transfusion reaction less than 24 hours after transfusion

T80.411 Rh incompatibility with delayed hemolytic transfusion reaction
Delayed hemolytic transfusion reaction (DHTR) due to Rh incompatibility
Rh incompatibility with hemolytic transfusion reaction 24 hours or more after transfusion

T80.419 Rh incompatibility with hemolytic transfusion reaction, unspecified
Rh incompatibility with hemolytic transfusion reaction at unspecified time after transfusion
Hemolytic transfusion reaction (HTR) due to Rh incompatibility NOS

T80.49 Other Rh incompatibility reaction due to transfusion of blood or blood products
Delayed serologic transfusion reaction (DSTR) from Rh incompatibility
Other reaction to Rh incompatible blood transfusion

T80.A Non-ABO incompatibility reaction due to transfusion of blood or blood products
Reaction due to incompatibility of minor antigens (Duffy) (Kell) (Kidd) (Lewis) (M) (N) (P) (S)

T80.A0 Non-ABO incompatibility reaction due to transfusion of blood or blood products, unspecified
Non-ABO antigen incompatibility reaction from transfusion NOS

T80.A1 Non-ABO incompatibility with hemolytic transfusion reaction

T80.A10 Non-ABO incompatibility with acute hemolytic transfusion reaction
Acute hemolytic transfusion reaction (AHTR) due to non-ABO incompatibility
Non-ABO incompatibility with hemolytic transfusion reaction less than 24 hours after transfusion

T80.A11 Non-ABO incompatibility with delayed hemolytic transfusion reaction
Delayed hemolytic transfusion reaction (DHTR) due to non-ABO incompatibility
Non-ABO incompatibility with hemolytic transfusion reaction 24 or more hours after transfusion

T80.A19 Non-ABO incompatibility with hemolytic transfusion reaction, unspecified
Hemolytic transfusion reaction (HTR) due to non-ABO incompatibility NOS
Non-ABO incompatibility with hemolytic transfusion reaction at unspecified time after transfusion

T80.A9 Other non-ABO incompatibility reaction due to transfusion of blood or blood products
Delayed serologic transfusion reaction (DSTR) from non-ABO incompatibility
Other reaction to non-ABO incompatible blood transfusion

T80.5 Anaphylactic reaction due to serum
Allergic shock due to serum
Anaphylactic shock due to serum
Anaphylactoid reaction due to serum
Anaphylaxis due to serum
EXCLUDES 1 *ABO incompatibility reaction due to transfusion of blood or blood products (T80.3-)*
allergic reaction or shock NOS (T78.2)
anaphylactic reaction or shock NOS (T78.2)
anaphylactic reaction or shock due to adverse effect of correct medicinal substance properly administered (T88.6)
other serum reaction (T80.6-)

DEF: Life-threatening hypersensitivity to a foreign serum causing respiratory distress, vascular collapse, and shock.

T80.51 Anaphylactic reaction due to administration of blood and blood products

T80.52 Anaphylactic reaction due to vaccination
AHA: 2021,1Q,43

T80.59 Anaphylactic reaction due to other serum

T80.6 Other serum reactions
Intoxication by serum
Protein sickness
Serum rash
Serum sickness
Serum urticaria
EXCLUDES 2 *serum hepatitis (B16-B19)*
DEF: Serum sickness: Hypersensitivity to a foreign serum that causes fever, hives, swelling, and lymphadenopathy.

T80.61 Other serum reaction due to administration of blood and blood products

T80.62 Other serum reaction due to vaccination
AHA: 2021,1Q,42

T80.69 Other serum reaction due to other serum
Code also, if applicable, arthropathy in hypersensitivity reactions classified elsewhere (M36.4)

T80.8 Other complications following infusion, transfusion and therapeutic injection

T80.81 Extravasation of vesicant agent
Infiltration of vesicant agent

T80.810 Extravasation of vesicant antineoplastic chemotherapy
Infiltration of vesicant antineoplastic chemotherapy

T80.818 Extravasation of other vesicant agent
Infiltration of other vesicant agent

T80.82 Complication of immune effector cellular therapy
Complication of chimeric antigen receptor (CAR-T) cell therapy
Complication of IEC therapy
Use additional code to identify the specific complication, such as:
cytokine release syndrome (D89.83-)
immune effector cell-associated neurotoxicity syndrome (G92.0-)
EXCLUDES 2 *complication of bone marrow transplant (T86.0)*
complication of stem cell transplant (T86.5)
AHA: 2021,4Q,31

T80.89 Other complications following infusion, transfusion and therapeutic injection
Delayed serologic transfusion reaction (DSTR), unspecified incompatibility
Use additional code to identify graft-versus-host reaction, if applicable, (D89.81-)
AHA: 2020,4Q,14

T80.9 Unspecified complication following infusion, transfusion and therapeutic injection

T80.90 Unspecified complication following infusion and therapeutic injection

T80.91 Hemolytic transfusion reaction, unspecified incompatibility
EXCLUDES 1 *ABO incompatibility with hemolytic transfusion reaction (T80.31-)*
non-ABO incompatibility with hemolytic transfusion reaction (T80.A1-)
Rh incompatibility with hemolytic transfusion reaction (T80.41-)

T80.910 Acute hemolytic transfusion reaction, unspecified incompatibility

T80.911 Delayed hemolytic transfusion reaction, unspecified incompatibility

T80.919 Hemolytic transfusion reaction, unspecified incompatibility, unspecified as acute or delayed
Hemolytic transfusion reaction NOS

T80.92 Unspecified transfusion reaction
Transfusion reaction NOS

T81 Complications of procedures, not elsewhere classified
Use additional code for adverse effect, if applicable, to identify drug (T36-T50 with fifth or sixth character 5)
EXCLUDES 2 *complications following immunization (T88.0-T88.1)*
complications following infusion, transfusion and therapeutic injection (T80.-)
complications of transplanted organs and tissue (T86.-)
specified complications classified elsewhere, such as:
complication of prosthetic devices, implants and grafts (T82-T85)
dermatitis due to drugs and medicaments (L23.3, L24.4, L25.1, L27.0-L27.1)
endosseous dental implant failure (M27.6-)
floppy iris syndrome (IFIS) (intraoperative) (H21.81)
intraoperative and postprocedural complications of specific body system (D78.-, E36.-, E89.-, G97.3-, G97.4, H59.3-, H59.-, H95.2-, H95.3, I97.4-, I97.5, J95, K91.-, L76.-, M96.-, N99.-)
ostomy complications (J95.0-, K94.-, N99.5-)
plateau iris syndrome (post-iridectomy) (postprocedural) H21.82
poisoning and toxic effects of drugs and chemicals (T36-T65 with fifth or sixth character 1-4 or 6)
AHA: 2019,2Q,21

The appropriate 7th character is to be added to each code from category T81.
A initial encounter
D subsequent encounter
S sequela

T81.1 Postprocedural shock
Shock during or resulting from a procedure, not elsewhere classified
EXCLUDES 1 *anaphylactic shock due to correct substance properly administered (T88.6)*
anaphylactic shock due to serum (T80.5-)
anaphylactic shock NOS (T78.2)
electric shock (T75.4)
obstetric shock (O75.1)
septic shock (R65.21)
shock due to anesthesia (T88.2)
shock following abortion or ectopic or molar pregnancy (O00-O07, O08.3)
traumatic shock (T79.4)
AHA: 2021,1Q,13

T81.10 Postprocedural shock unspecified
Collapse NOS during or resulting from a procedure, not elsewhere classified
Postprocedural failure of peripheral circulation
Postprocedural shock NOS

1 **T81.11 Postprocedural cardiogenic shock** HCC ESR

1 **T81.12 Postprocedural septic shock** HCC ESR UPD
Postprocedural endotoxic shock resulting from a procedure, not elsewhere classified
Postprocedural gram-negative shock resulting from a procedure, not elsewhere classified
Code first underlying infection
Use additional code, to identify any associated acute organ dysfunction, if applicable
AHA: 2018,4Q,63

T81.19 Other postprocedural shock
Postprocedural hypovolemic shock

T81.3 Disruption of wound, not elsewhere classified
Disruption of any suture materials or other closure methods
EXCLUDES 1 *breakdown (mechanical) of permanent sutures (T85.612)*
displacement of permanent sutures (T85.622)
disruption of cesarean delivery wound (O90.0)
disruption of perineal obstetric wound (O90.1)
mechanical complication of permanent sutures NEC (T85.692)
AHA: 2014,1Q,23

T81.30 Disruption of wound, unspecified
Disruption of wound NOS

√x7th **T81.31 Disruption of external operation (surgical) wound, not elsewhere classified**
Dehiscence of operation wound NOS
Disruption of operation wound NOS
Disruption or dehiscence of closure of cornea
Disruption or dehiscence of closure of mucosa
Disruption or dehiscence of closure of skin and subcutaneous tissue
Full-thickness skin disruption or dehiscence
Superficial disruption or dehiscence of operation wound
EXCLUDES 1 *dehiscence of amputation stump (T87.81)*

√x7th **T81.32 Disruption of internal operation (surgical) wound, not elsewhere classified**
Deep disruption or dehiscence of operation wound NOS
Disruption or dehiscence of closure of internal organ or other internal tissue
Disruption or dehiscence of closure of muscle or muscle flap
Disruption or dehiscence of closure of ribs or rib cage
Disruption or dehiscence of closure of skull or craniotomy
Disruption or dehiscence of closure of sternum or sternotomy
Disruption or dehiscence of closure of tendon or ligament
Disruption or dehiscence of closure of superficial or muscular fascia
AHA: 2020,2Q,22; 2017,3Q,4

√x7th **T81.33 Disruption of traumatic injury wound repair**
Disruption or dehiscence of closure of traumatic laceration (external) (internal)

√5th **T81.4 Infection following a procedure**
Wound abscess following a procedure
Use additional code to identify infection
Use additional code (R65.2-) to identify severe sepsis, if applicable
EXCLUDES 2 *bleb associated endophthalmitis (H59.4-)*
infection due to infusion, transfusion and therapeutic injection (T80.2-)
infection due to prosthetic devices, implants and grafts (T82.6-T82.7, T83.5-T83.6, T84.5-T84.7, T85.7)
obstetric surgical wound infection (O86.0-)
postprocedural fever NOS (R50.82)
postprocedural retroperitoneal abscess (K68.11)
AHA: 2018,4Q,33-34,62; 2014,1Q,23

√x7th **T81.40 Infection following a procedure, unspecified**

√x7th **T81.41 Infection following a procedure, superficial incisional surgical site**
Subcutaneous abscess following a procedure
Stitch abscess following a procedure

√x7th **T81.42 Infection following a procedure, deep incisional surgical site**
Intra-muscular abscess following a procedure

√x7th **T81.43 Infection following a procedure, organ and space surgical site**
Intra-abdominal abscess following a procedure
Subphrenic abscess following a procedure

1 √x7th **T81.44 Sepsis following a procedure** HCC ESR COM
Use additional code to identify the sepsis

√x7th **T81.49 Infection following a procedure, other surgical site**

√5th **T81.5 Complications of foreign body accidentally left in body following procedure**
AHA: 2014,4Q,24

√6th **T81.50 Unspecified complication of foreign body accidentally left in body following procedure**

√7th **T81.500 Unspecified complication of foreign body accidentally left in body following surgical operation**

√7th **T81.501 Unspecified complication of foreign body accidentally left in body following infusion or transfusion**

√7th **T81.502 Unspecified complication of foreign body accidentally left in body following kidney dialysis** HCC Rx ESR

√7th **T81.503 Unspecified complication of foreign body accidentally left in body following injection or immunization**

√7th **T81.504 Unspecified complication of foreign body accidentally left in body following endoscopic examination**

√7th **T81.505 Unspecified complication of foreign body accidentally left in body following heart catheterization**

√7th **T81.506 Unspecified complication of foreign body accidentally left in body following aspiration, puncture or other catheterization**

√7th **T81.507 Unspecified complication of foreign body accidentally left in body following removal of catheter or packing**

√7th **T81.508 Unspecified complication of foreign body accidentally left in body following other procedure**

√7th **T81.509 Unspecified complication of foreign body accidentally left in body following unspecified procedure**

√6th **T81.51 Adhesions due to foreign body accidentally left in body following procedure**

√7th **T81.510 Adhesions due to foreign body accidentally left in body following surgical operation**

√7th **T81.511 Adhesions due to foreign body accidentally left in body following infusion or transfusion**

√7th **T81.512 Adhesions due to foreign body accidentally left in body following kidney dialysis** HCC Rx ESR

√7th **T81.513 Adhesions due to foreign body accidentally left in body following injection or immunization**

√7th **T81.514 Adhesions due to foreign body accidentally left in body following endoscopic examination**

√7th **T81.515 Adhesions due to foreign body accidentally left in body following heart catheterization**

√7th **T81.516 Adhesions due to foreign body accidentally left in body following aspiration, puncture or other catheterization**

√7th **T81.517 Adhesions due to foreign body accidentally left in body following removal of catheter or packing**

√7th **T81.518 Adhesions due to foreign body accidentally left in body following other procedure**

√7th **T81.519 Adhesions due to foreign body accidentally left in body following unspecified procedure**

√6th **T81.52 Obstruction due to foreign body accidentally left in body following procedure**

√7th **T81.520 Obstruction due to foreign body accidentally left in body following surgical operation**

√7th **T81.521 Obstruction due to foreign body accidentally left in body following infusion or transfusion**

√7th **T81.522 Obstruction due to foreign body accidentally left in body following kidney dialysis** HCC Rx ESR

√7th **T81.523 Obstruction due to foreign body accidentally left in body following injection or immunization**

√7th **T81.524 Obstruction due to foreign body accidentally left in body following endoscopic examination**

√7th **T81.525 Obstruction due to foreign body accidentally left in body following heart catheterization**

√7th **T81.526 Obstruction due to foreign body accidentally left in body following aspiration, puncture or other catheterization**

√7th **T81.527 Obstruction due to foreign body accidentally left in body following removal of catheter or packing**

√7th **T81.528 Obstruction due to foreign body accidentally left in body following other procedure**

7th **T81.529 Obstruction due to foreign body accidentally left in body following unspecified procedure**

6th **T81.53 Perforation due to foreign body accidentally left in body following procedure**

7th **T81.530 Perforation due to foreign body accidentally left in body following surgical operation**

7th **T81.531 Perforation due to foreign body accidentally left in body following infusion or transfusion**

7th **T81.532 Perforation due to foreign body accidentally left in body following kidney dialysis** HCC Rx ESR

7th **T81.533 Perforation due to foreign body accidentally left in body following injection or immunization**

7th **T81.534 Perforation due to foreign body accidentally left in body following endoscopic examination**

7th **T81.535 Perforation due to foreign body accidentally left in body following heart catheterization**

7th **T81.536 Perforation due to foreign body accidentally left in body following aspiration, puncture or other catheterization**

7th **T81.537 Perforation due to foreign body accidentally left in body following removal of catheter or packing**

7th **T81.538 Perforation due to foreign body accidentally left in body following other procedure**

7th **T81.539 Perforation due to foreign body accidentally left in body following unspecified procedure**

6th **T81.59 Other complications of foreign body accidentally left in body following procedure**

EXCLUDES 2 *obstruction or perforation due to prosthetic devices and implants intentionally left in body (T82.Ø-T82.5, T83.Ø-T83.4, T83.7, T84.Ø-T84.4, T85.Ø-T85.6)*

7th **T81.59Ø Other complications of foreign body accidentally left in body following surgical operation**

7th **T81.591 Other complications of foreign body accidentally left in body following infusion or transfusion**

7th **T81.592 Other complications of foreign body accidentally left in body following kidney dialysis** HCC Rx ESR

7th **T81.593 Other complications of foreign body accidentally left in body following injection or immunization**

7th **T81.594 Other complications of foreign body accidentally left in body following endoscopic examination**

7th **T81.595 Other complications of foreign body accidentally left in body following heart catheterization**

7th **T81.596 Other complications of foreign body accidentally left in body following aspiration, puncture or other catheterization**

7th **T81.597 Other complications of foreign body accidentally left in body following removal of catheter or packing**

7th **T81.598 Other complications of foreign body accidentally left in body following other procedure**

7th **T81.599 Other complications of foreign body accidentally left in body following unspecified procedure**

5th **T81.6 Acute reaction to foreign substance accidentally left during a procedure**

EXCLUDES 2 *complications of foreign body accidentally left in body cavity or operation wound following procedure (T81.5-)*

x7th **T81.6Ø Unspecified acute reaction to foreign substance accidentally left during a procedure**

x7th **T81.61 Aseptic peritonitis due to foreign substance accidentally left during a procedure**

Chemical peritonitis

x7th **T81.69 Other acute reaction to foreign substance accidentally left during a procedure**

5th **T81.7 Vascular complications following a procedure, not elsewhere classified**

Air embolism following procedure NEC

Phlebitis or thrombophlebitis resulting from a procedure

EXCLUDES 1 *embolism complicating abortion or ectopic or molar pregnancy (OØØ-OØ7, OØ8.2)*

embolism complicating pregnancy, childbirth and the puerperium (O88.-)

traumatic embolism (T79.Ø)

EXCLUDES 2 *embolism due to prosthetic devices, implants and grafts (T82.8-, T83.81, T84.8-, T85.81-)*

embolism following infusion, transfusion and therapeutic injection (T8Ø.Ø)

AHA: 2019,2Q,22

6th **T81.71 Complication of artery following a procedure, not elsewhere classified**

7th **T81.71Ø Complication of mesenteric artery following a procedure, not elsewhere classified**

7th **T81.711 Complication of renal artery following a procedure, not elsewhere classified**

7th **T81.718 Complication of other artery following a procedure, not elsewhere classified**

AHA: 2019,2Q,21-22

7th **T81.719 Complication of unspecified artery following a procedure, not elsewhere classified**

x7th **T81.72 Complication of vein following a procedure, not elsewhere classified**

5th **T81.8 Other complications of procedures, not elsewhere classified**

EXCLUDES 2 *hypothermia following anesthesia (T88.51)*

malignant hyperpyrexia due to anesthesia (T88.3)

x7th **T81.81 Complication of inhalation therapy**

x7th **T81.82 Emphysema (subcutaneous) resulting from a procedure**

x7th **T81.83 Persistent postprocedural fistula**

AHA: 2017,3Q,3-4

x7th **T81.89 Other complications of procedures, not elsewhere classified**

Use additional code to specify complication, such as: postprocedural delirium (FØ5)

AHA: 2014,1Q,23

x7th **T81.9 Unspecified complication of procedure**

4th **T82 Complications of cardiac and vascular prosthetic devices, implants and grafts**

EXCLUDES 2 *failure and rejection of transplanted organs and tissue (T86.-)*

AHA: 2020,3Q,36-37

The appropriate 7th character is to be added to each code from category T82.
A initial encounter
D subsequent encounter
S sequela

5th **T82.Ø Mechanical complication of heart valve prosthesis**

Mechanical complication of artificial heart valve

EXCLUDES 1 *mechanical complication of biological heart valve graft (T82.22-)*

x7th **T82.Ø1 Breakdown (mechanical) of heart valve prosthesis**

x7th **T82.Ø2 Displacement of heart valve prosthesis**

Malposition of heart valve prosthesis

x7th **T82.Ø3 Leakage of heart valve prosthesis**

x7th **T82.Ø9 Other mechanical complication of heart valve prosthesis**

Obstruction (mechanical) of heart valve prosthesis
Perforation of heart valve prosthesis
Protrusion of heart valve prosthesis

5th **T82.1 Mechanical complication of cardiac electronic device**

6th **T82.11 Breakdown (mechanical) of cardiac electronic device**

7th **T82.11Ø Breakdown (mechanical) of cardiac electrode**

7th **T82.111 Breakdown (mechanical) of cardiac pulse generator (battery)**

T82.118 Breakdown (mechanical) of other cardiac electronic device

T82.119 Breakdown (mechanical) of unspecified cardiac electronic device

T82.12 Displacement of cardiac electronic device
Malposition of cardiac electronic device

T82.120 Displacement of cardiac electrode

T82.121 Displacement of cardiac pulse generator (battery)

T82.128 Displacement of other cardiac electronic device

T82.129 Displacement of unspecified cardiac electronic device

T82.19 Other mechanical complication of cardiac electronic device
Leakage of cardiac electronic device
Obstruction of cardiac electronic device
Perforation of cardiac electronic device
Protrusion of cardiac electronic device

T82.190 Other mechanical complication of cardiac electrode

T82.191 Other mechanical complication of cardiac pulse generator (battery)

T82.198 Other mechanical complication of other cardiac electronic device

T82.199 Other mechanical complication of unspecified cardiac device

T82.2 Mechanical complication of coronary artery bypass graft and biological heart valve graft
EXCLUDES 1 *mechanical complication of artificial heart valve prosthesis (T82.0-)*

T82.21 Mechanical complication of coronary artery bypass graft

T82.211 Breakdown (mechanical) of coronary artery bypass graft

T82.212 Displacement of coronary artery bypass graft
Malposition of coronary artery bypass graft

T82.213 Leakage of coronary artery bypass graft

T82.218 Other mechanical complication of coronary artery bypass graft
Obstruction, mechanical of coronary artery bypass graft
Perforation of coronary artery bypass graft
Protrusion of coronary artery bypass graft

T82.22 Mechanical complication of biological heart valve graft

T82.221 Breakdown (mechanical) of biological heart valve graft

T82.222 Displacement of biological heart valve graft
Malposition of biological heart valve graft

T82.223 Leakage of biological heart valve graft

T82.228 Other mechanical complication of biological heart valve graft
Obstruction of biological heart valve graft
Perforation of biological heart valve graft
Protrusion of biological heart valve graft

T82.3 Mechanical complication of other vascular grafts

T82.31 Breakdown (mechanical) of other vascular grafts

1 T82.310 Breakdown (mechanical) of aortic (bifurcation) graft (replacement) HCC ESR
AHA: 2020,3Q,3-8

1 T82.311 Breakdown (mechanical) of carotid arterial graft (bypass) HCC ESR

1 T82.312 Breakdown (mechanical) of femoral arterial graft (bypass) HCC ESR

1 T82.318 Breakdown (mechanical) of other vascular grafts HCC ESR

1 T82.319 Breakdown (mechanical) of unspecified vascular grafts HCC ESR

T82.32 Displacement of other vascular grafts
Malposition of other vascular grafts

1 T82.320 Displacement of aortic (bifurcation) graft (replacement) HCC ESR

1 T82.321 Displacement of carotid arterial graft (bypass) HCC ESR

1 T82.322 Displacement of femoral arterial graft (bypass) HCC ESR

1 T82.328 Displacement of other vascular grafts HCC ESR

1 T82.329 Displacement of unspecified vascular grafts HCC ESR

T82.33 Leakage of other vascular grafts

1 T82.330 Leakage of aortic (bifurcation) graft (replacement) HCC ESR
AHA: 2020,3Q,3-8

1 T82.331 Leakage of carotid arterial graft (bypass) HCC ESR

1 T82.332 Leakage of femoral arterial graft (bypass) HCC ESR

1 T82.338 Leakage of other vascular grafts HCC ESR

1 T82.339 Leakage of unspecified vascular graft HCC ESR

T82.39 Other mechanical complication of other vascular grafts
Obstruction (mechanical) of other vascular grafts
Perforation of other vascular grafts
Protrusion of other vascular grafts

1 T82.390 Other mechanical complication of aortic (bifurcation) graft (replacement) HCC ESR
AHA: 2020,3Q,3-5

1 T82.391 Other mechanical complication of carotid arterial graft (bypass) HCC ESR

1 T82.392 Other mechanical complication of femoral arterial graft (bypass) HCC ESR

1 T82.398 Other mechanical complication of other vascular grafts HCC ESR

1 T82.399 Other mechanical complication of unspecified vascular grafts HCC ESR

T82.4 Mechanical complication of vascular dialysis catheter
Mechanical complication of hemodialysis catheter
EXCLUDES 1 *mechanical complication of intraperitoneal dialysis catheter (T85.62)*

T82.41 Breakdown (mechanical) of vascular dialysis catheter HCC Rx ESR

T82.42 Displacement of vascular dialysis catheter HCC Rx ESR
Malposition of vascular dialysis catheter

T82.43 Leakage of vascular dialysis catheter HCC Rx ESR

T82.49 Other complication of vascular dialysis catheter HCC Rx ESR
Obstruction (mechanical) of vascular dialysis catheter
Perforation of vascular dialysis catheter
Protrusion of vascular dialysis catheter

T82.5 Mechanical complication of other cardiac and vascular devices and implants
EXCLUDES 2 *mechanical complication of epidural and subdural infusion catheter (T85.61)*

T82.51 Breakdown (mechanical) of other cardiac and vascular devices and implants

1 T82.510 Breakdown (mechanical) of surgically created arteriovenous fistula HCC ESR
AHA: 2020,3Q,36

1 T82.511 Breakdown (mechanical) of surgically created arteriovenous shunt HCC ESR
AHA: 2020,3Q,37

T82.512 Breakdown (mechanical) of artificial heart

1 T82.513 Breakdown (mechanical) of balloon (counterpulsation) device HCC ESR

1 T82.514 Breakdown (mechanical) of infusion catheter HCC ESR

1 T82.515 Breakdown (mechanical) of umbrella device HCC ESR

1 T82.518 Breakdown (mechanical) of other cardiac and vascular devices and implants HCC ESR

T82.519 Breakdown (mechanical) of unspecified cardiac and vascular devices and implants

T82.52 Displacement of other cardiac and vascular devices and implants
Malposition of other cardiac and vascular devices and implants

1 **T82.520 Displacement of surgically created arteriovenous fistula** HCC ESR
AHA: 2020,3Q,36

1 **T82.521 Displacement of surgically created arteriovenous shunt** HCC ESR

T82.522 Displacement of artificial heart

1 **T82.523 Displacement of balloon (counterpulsation) device** HCC ESR

1 **T82.524 Displacement of infusion catheter** HCC ESR
AHA: 2020,2Q,21; 2019,3Q,15

1 **T82.525 Displacement of umbrella device** HCC ESR

1 **T82.528 Displacement of other cardiac and vascular devices and implants** HCC ESR

T82.529 Displacement of unspecified cardiac and vascular devices and implants

T82.53 Leakage of other cardiac and vascular devices and implants

1 **T82.530 Leakage of surgically created arteriovenous fistula** HCC ESR
AHA: 2020,3Q,36

1 **T82.531 Leakage of surgically created arteriovenous shunt** HCC ESR

T82.532 Leakage of artificial heart

1 **T82.533 Leakage of balloon (counterpulsation) device** HCC ESR

1 **T82.534 Leakage of infusion catheter** HCC ESR

1 **T82.535 Leakage of umbrella device** HCC ESR

1 **T82.538 Leakage of other cardiac and vascular devices and implants** HCC ESR

T82.539 Leakage of unspecified cardiac and vascular devices and implants

T82.59 Other mechanical complication of other cardiac and vascular devices and implants
Obstruction (mechanical) of other cardiac and vascular devices and implants
Perforation of other cardiac and vascular devices and implants
Protrusion of other cardiac and vascular devices and implants

1 **T82.590 Other mechanical complication of surgically created arteriovenous fistula** HCC ESR
AHA: 2020,3Q,36

1 **T82.591 Other mechanical complication of surgically created arteriovenous shunt** HCC ESR

T82.592 Other mechanical complication of artificial heart

1 **T82.593 Other mechanical complication of balloon (counterpulsation) device** HCC ESR

1 **T82.594 Other mechanical complication of infusion catheter** HCC ESR

1 **T82.595 Other mechanical complication of umbrella device** HCC ESR

1 **T82.598 Other mechanical complication of other cardiac and vascular devices and implants** HCC ESR

T82.599 Other mechanical complication of unspecified cardiac and vascular devices and implants

1 **T82.6 Infection and inflammatory reaction due to cardiac valve prosthesis** HCC ESR
Use additional code to identify infection

1 **T82.7 Infection and inflammatory reaction due to other cardiac and vascular devices, implants and grafts** HCC ESR
Use additional code to identify infection
AHA: 2019,1Q,13-14
DEF: Midline catheter: Long peripheral catheter introduced via the cephalic, basilic, brachial, or median cubital veins in the upper arm and positioned so that the tip is level or near the level of the axilla and distal to the shoulder. Midline catheters are typically used for IV access, fluid replacement, and medication administration.
TIP: Assign this code for infections and/or cellulitis resulting from catheters that are not centrally placed (e.g., midline catheters).

T82.8 Other specified complications of cardiac and vascular prosthetic devices, implants and grafts
AHA: 2016,4Q,70

T82.81 Embolism due to cardiac and vascular prosthetic devices, implants and grafts

T82.817 Embolism due to cardiac prosthetic devices, implants and grafts

1 **T82.818 Embolism due to vascular prosthetic devices, implants and grafts** HCC ESR

T82.82 Fibrosis due to cardiac and vascular prosthetic devices, implants and grafts

T82.827 Fibrosis due to cardiac prosthetic devices, implants and grafts

1 **T82.828 Fibrosis due vascular prosthetic devices, implants and grafts** HCC ESR

T82.83 Hemorrhage due to cardiac and vascular prosthetic devices, implants and grafts

T82.837 Hemorrhage due to cardiac prosthetic devices, implants and grafts

1 **T82.838 Hemorrhage due to vascular prosthetic devices, implants and grafts** HCC ESR
AHA: 2020,3Q,36-37

T82.84 Pain due to cardiac and vascular prosthetic devices, implants and grafts

T82.847 Pain due to cardiac prosthetic devices, implants and grafts

1 **T82.848 Pain due to vascular prosthetic devices, implants and grafts** HCC ESR

T82.85 Stenosis due to cardiac and vascular prosthetic devices, implants and grafts

T82.855 Stenosis of coronary artery stent
In-stent stenosis (restenosis) of coronary artery stent
Restenosis of coronary artery stent
AHA: 2021,3Q,6-7

1 **T82.856 Stenosis of peripheral vascular stent** HCC ESR
In-stent stenosis (restenosis) of peripheral vascular stent
Restenosis of peripheral vascular stent

T82.857 Stenosis of other cardiac prosthetic devices, implants and grafts

1 **T82.858 Stenosis of other vascular prosthetic devices, implants and grafts** HCC ESR

T82.86 Thrombosis of cardiac and vascular prosthetic devices, implants and grafts

T82.867 Thrombosis due to cardiac prosthetic devices, implants and grafts

1 **T82.868 Thrombosis due to vascular prosthetic devices, implants and grafts** HCC ESR

T82.89 Other specified complication of cardiac and vascular prosthetic devices, implants and grafts

T82.897 Other specified complication of cardiac prosthetic devices, implants and grafts
AHA: 2019,2Q,33

1 **T82.898 Other specified complication of vascular prosthetic devices, implants and grafts** HCC ESR
AHA: 2020,3Q,3-5

T82.9 Unspecified complication of cardiac and vascular prosthetic device, implant and graft

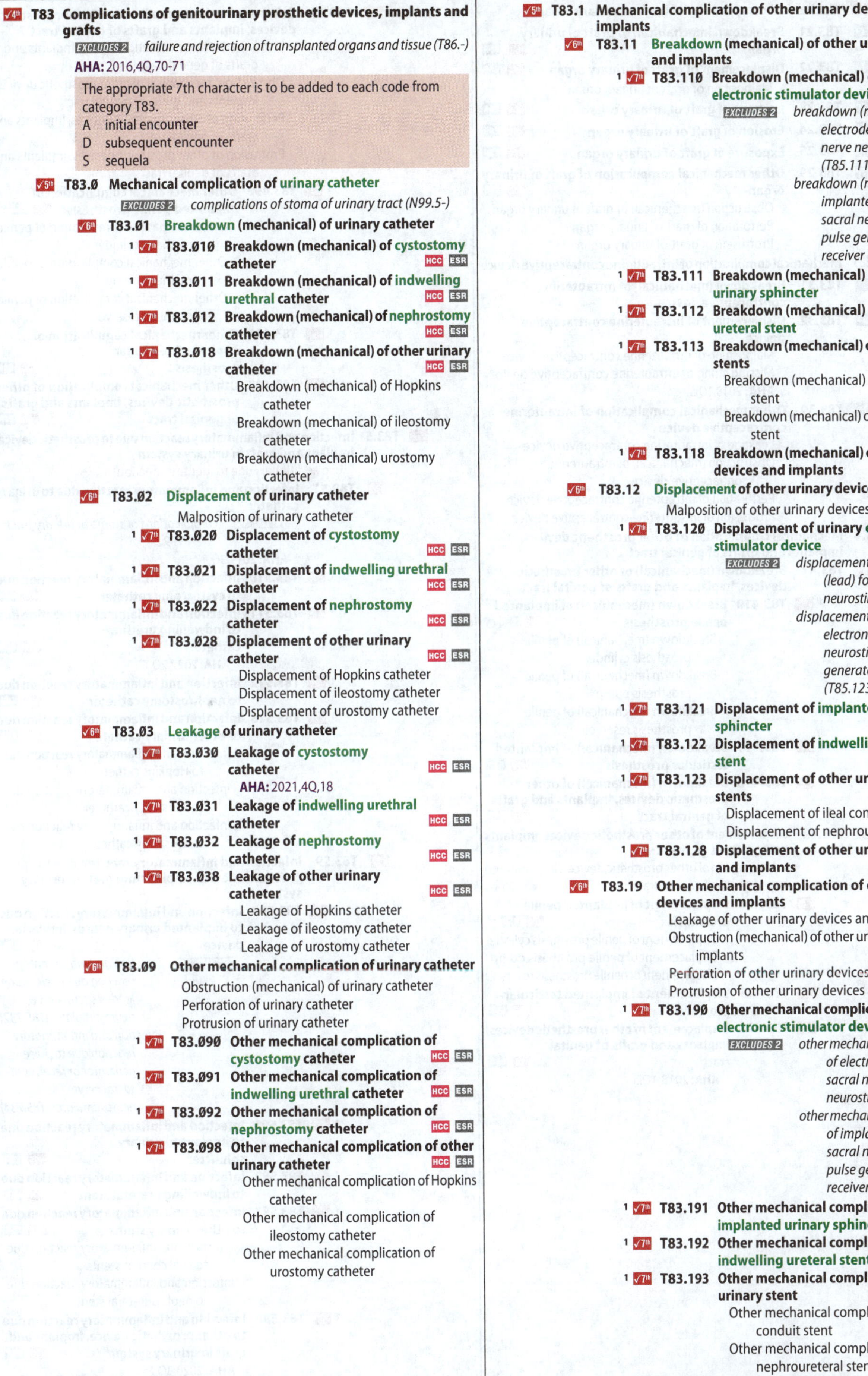

√4th T83 Complications of genitourinary prosthetic devices, implants and grafts

EXCLUDES 2 *failure and rejection of transplanted organs and tissue (T86.-)*

AHA: 2016,4Q,70-71

The appropriate 7th character is to be added to each code from category T83.
- A initial encounter
- D subsequent encounter
- S sequela

√5th T83.0 Mechanical complication of urinary catheter

EXCLUDES 2 *complications of stoma of urinary tract (N99.5-)*

√6th T83.01 Breakdown (mechanical) of urinary catheter

1 √7th **T83.010 Breakdown (mechanical) of cystostomy catheter** HCC ESR

1 √7th **T83.011 Breakdown (mechanical) of indwelling urethral catheter** HCC ESR

1 √7th **T83.012 Breakdown (mechanical) of nephrostomy catheter** HCC ESR

1 √7th **T83.018 Breakdown (mechanical) of other urinary catheter** HCC ESR
- Breakdown (mechanical) of Hopkins catheter
- Breakdown (mechanical) of ileostomy catheter
- Breakdown (mechanical) urostomy catheter

√6th T83.02 Displacement of urinary catheter
- Malposition of urinary catheter

1 √7th **T83.020 Displacement of cystostomy catheter** HCC ESR

1 √7th **T83.021 Displacement of indwelling urethral catheter** HCC ESR

1 √7th **T83.022 Displacement of nephrostomy catheter** HCC ESR

1 √7th **T83.028 Displacement of other urinary catheter** HCC ESR
- Displacement of Hopkins catheter
- Displacement of ileostomy catheter
- Displacement of urostomy catheter

√6th T83.03 Leakage of urinary catheter

1 √7th **T83.030 Leakage of cystostomy catheter** HCC ESR

AHA: 2021,4Q,18

1 √7th **T83.031 Leakage of indwelling urethral catheter** HCC ESR

1 √7th **T83.032 Leakage of nephrostomy catheter** HCC ESR

1 √7th **T83.038 Leakage of other urinary catheter** HCC ESR
- Leakage of Hopkins catheter
- Leakage of ileostomy catheter
- Leakage of urostomy catheter

√6th T83.09 Other mechanical complication of urinary catheter
- Obstruction (mechanical) of urinary catheter
- Perforation of urinary catheter
- Protrusion of urinary catheter

1 √7th **T83.090 Other mechanical complication of cystostomy catheter** HCC ESR

1 √7th **T83.091 Other mechanical complication of indwelling urethral catheter** HCC ESR

1 √7th **T83.092 Other mechanical complication of nephrostomy catheter** HCC ESR

1 √7th **T83.098 Other mechanical complication of other urinary catheter** HCC ESR
- Other mechanical complication of Hopkins catheter
- Other mechanical complication of ileostomy catheter
- Other mechanical complication of urostomy catheter

√5th T83.1 Mechanical complication of other urinary devices and implants

√6th T83.11 Breakdown (mechanical) of other urinary devices and implants

1 √7th **T83.110 Breakdown (mechanical) of urinary electronic stimulator device** HCC ESR

EXCLUDES 2 *breakdown (mechanical) of electrode (lead) for sacral nerve neurostimulator (T85.111)*
breakdown (mechanical) of implanted electronic sacral neurostimulator, pulse generator or receiver (T85.113)

1 √7th **T83.111 Breakdown (mechanical) of implanted urinary sphincter** HCC ESR

1 √7th **T83.112 Breakdown (mechanical) of indwelling ureteral stent** HCC ESR

1 √7th **T83.113 Breakdown (mechanical) of other urinary stents** HCC ESR
- Breakdown (mechanical) of ileal conduit stent
- Breakdown (mechanical) of nephroureteral stent

1 √7th **T83.118 Breakdown (mechanical) of other urinary devices and implants** HCC ESR

√6th T83.12 Displacement of other urinary devices and implants
- Malposition of other urinary devices and implants

1 √7th **T83.120 Displacement of urinary electronic stimulator device** HCC ESR

EXCLUDES 2 *displacement of electrode (lead) for sacral nerve neurostimulator (T85.121)*
displacement of implanted electronic sacral neurostimulator, pulse generator or receiver (T85.123)

1 √7th **T83.121 Displacement of implanted urinary sphincter** HCC ESR

1 √7th **T83.122 Displacement of indwelling ureteral stent** HCC ESR

1 √7th **T83.123 Displacement of other urinary stents** HCC ESR
- Displacement of ileal conduit stent
- Displacement of nephroureteral stent

1 √7th **T83.128 Displacement of other urinary devices and implants** HCC ESR

√6th T83.19 Other mechanical complication of other urinary devices and implants
- Leakage of other urinary devices and implants
- Obstruction (mechanical) of other urinary devices and implants
- Perforation of other urinary devices and implants
- Protrusion of other urinary devices and implants

1 √7th **T83.190 Other mechanical complication of urinary electronic stimulator device** HCC ESR

EXCLUDES 2 *other mechanical complication of electrode (lead) for sacral nerve neurostimulator (T85.191)*
other mechanical complication of implanted electronic sacral neurostimulator, pulse generator or receiver (T85.193)

1 √7th **T83.191 Other mechanical complication of implanted urinary sphincter** HCC ESR

1 √7th **T83.192 Other mechanical complication of indwelling ureteral stent** HCC ESR

1 √7th **T83.193 Other mechanical complication of other urinary stent** HCC ESR
- Other mechanical complication of ileal conduit stent
- Other mechanical complication of nephroureteral stent

1 √7th **T83.198 Other mechanical complication of other urinary devices and implants** HCC ESR

T83.2 Mechanical complication of graft of urinary organ

T83.21 Breakdown (mechanical) of graft of urinary organ HCC ESR

T83.22 Displacement of graft of urinary organ HCC ESR
Malposition of graft of urinary organ

T83.23 Leakage of graft of urinary organ HCC ESR

T83.24 Erosion of graft of urinary organ HCC ESR

T83.25 Exposure of graft of urinary organ HCC ESR

T83.29 Other mechanical complication of graft of urinary organ HCC ESR
Obstruction (mechanical) of graft of urinary organ
Perforation of graft of urinary organ
Protrusion of graft of urinary organ

T83.3 Mechanical complication of intrauterine contraceptive device

T83.31 Breakdown (mechanical) of intrauterine contraceptive device ♀

T83.32 Displacement of intrauterine contraceptive device ♀
Malposition of intrauterine contraceptive device
Missing string of intrauterine contraceptive device
AHA: 2018,1Q,5

T83.39 Other mechanical complication of intrauterine contraceptive device ♀
Leakage of intrauterine contraceptive device
Obstruction (mechanical) of intrauterine contraceptive device
Perforation of intrauterine contraceptive device
Protrusion of intrauterine contraceptive device

T83.4 Mechanical complication of other prosthetic devices, implants and grafts of genital tract

T83.41 Breakdown (mechanical) of other prosthetic devices, implants and grafts of genital tract

T83.410 Breakdown (mechanical) of implanted penile prosthesis HCC ESR ♂
Breakdown (mechanical) of penile prosthesis cylinder
Breakdown (mechanical) of penile prosthesis pump
Breakdown (mechanical) of penile prosthesis reservoir

T83.411 Breakdown (mechanical) of implanted testicular prosthesis HCC ESR

T83.418 Breakdown (mechanical) of other prosthetic devices, implants and grafts of genital tract HCC ESR

T83.42 Displacement of other prosthetic devices, implants and grafts of genital tract
Malposition of other prosthetic devices, implants and grafts of genital tract

T83.420 Displacement of implanted penile prosthesis HCC ESR ♂
Displacement of penile prosthesis cylinder
Displacement of penile prosthesis pump
Displacement of penile prosthesis reservoir

T83.421 Displacement of implanted testicular prosthesis HCC ESR

T83.428 Displacement of other prosthetic devices, implants and grafts of genital tract HCC ESR
AHA: 2018,1Q,5

T83.49 Other mechanical complication of other prosthetic devices, implants and grafts of genital tract
Leakage of other prosthetic devices, implants and grafts of genital tract
Obstruction, mechanical of other prosthetic devices, implants and grafts of genital tract
Perforation of other prosthetic devices, implants and grafts of genital tract
Protrusion of other prosthetic devices, implants and grafts of genital tract

T83.490 Other mechanical complication of implanted penile prosthesis HCC ESR ♂
Other mechanical complication of penile prosthesis cylinder
Other mechanical complication of penile prosthesis pump
Other mechanical complication of penile prosthesis reservoir

T83.491 Other mechanical complication of implanted testicular prosthesis HCC ESR

T83.498 Other mechanical complication of other prosthetic devices, implants and grafts of genital tract HCC ESR

T83.5 Infection and inflammatory reaction due to prosthetic device, implant and graft in urinary system
Use additional code to identify infection

T83.51 Infection and inflammatory reaction due to urinary catheter
EXCLUDES 2 *complications of stoma of urinary tract (N99.5-)*
AHA: 2019,3Q,17

T83.510 Infection and inflammatory reaction due to cystostomy catheter HCC ESR

T83.511 Infection and inflammatory reaction due to indwelling urethral catheter HCC ESR
AHA: 2022,2Q,7

T83.512 Infection and inflammatory reaction due to nephrostomy catheter HCC ESR

T83.518 Infection and inflammatory reaction due to other urinary catheter HCC ESR
Infection and inflammatory reaction due to Hopkins catheter
Infection and inflammatory reaction due to ileostomy catheter
Infection and inflammatory reaction due to urostomy catheter

T83.59 Infection and inflammatory reaction due to prosthetic device, implant and graft in urinary system

T83.590 Infection and inflammatory reaction due to implanted urinary neurostimulation device HCC ESR
EXCLUDES 2 *infection and inflammatory reaction due to electrode lead of sacral nerve neurostimulator (T85.732)*
infection and inflammatory reaction due to pulse generator or receiver of sacral nerve neurostimulator (T85.734)

T83.591 Infection and inflammatory reaction due to implanted urinary sphincter HCC ESR

T83.592 Infection and inflammatory reaction due to indwelling ureteral stent HCC ESR

T83.593 Infection and inflammatory reaction due to other urinary stents HCC ESR
Infection and inflammatory reaction due to ileal conduit stents
Infection and inflammatory reaction due to nephroureteral stent

T83.598 Infection and inflammatory reaction due to other prosthetic device, implant and graft in urinary system HCC ESR
AHA: 2020,3Q,25

T83.6 **Infection and inflammatory reaction due to prosthetic device, implant and graft in genital tract**
Use additional code to identify infection
T83.61 **Infection and inflammatory reaction due to implanted penile prosthesis** HCC ESR
Infection and inflammatory reaction due to penile prosthesis cylinder
Infection and inflammatory reaction due to penile prosthesis pump
Infection and inflammatory reaction due to penile prosthesis reservoir
T83.62 **Infection and inflammatory reaction due to implanted testicular prosthesis** HCC ESR
T83.69 **Infection and inflammatory reaction due to other prosthetic device, implant and graft in genital tract** HCC ESR
T83.7 **Complications due to implanted mesh and other prosthetic materials**
T83.71 **Erosion of implanted mesh and other prosthetic materials**
T83.711 **Erosion of implanted vaginal mesh to surrounding organ or tissue** HCC ESR ♀
Erosion of implanted vaginal mesh into pelvic floor muscles
T83.712 **Erosion of implanted urethral mesh to surrounding organ or tissue** HCC ESR
Erosion of implanted female urethral sling
Erosion of implanted male urethral sling
Erosion of implanted urethral mesh into pelvic floor muscles
T83.713 **Erosion of implanted urethral bulking agent to surrounding organ or tissue** HCC ESR
T83.714 **Erosion of implanted ureteral bulking agent to surrounding organ or tissue** HCC ESR
T83.718 **Erosion of other implanted mesh to organ or tissue** HCC ESR
T83.719 **Erosion of other prosthetic materials to surrounding organ or tissue** HCC ESR
T83.72 **Exposure of implanted mesh and other prosthetic materials into surrounding organ or tissue**
Extrusion of implanted mesh
T83.721 **Exposure of implanted vaginal mesh into vagina** HCC ESR ♀
Exposure of implanted vaginal mesh through vaginal wall
T83.722 **Exposure of implanted urethral mesh into urethra** HCC ESR
Exposure of implanted female urethral sling
Exposure of implanted male urethral sling
Exposure of implanted urethral mesh through urethral wall
T83.723 **Exposure of implanted urethral bulking agent into urethra** HCC ESR
T83.724 **Exposure of implanted ureteral bulking agent into ureter** HCC ESR
T83.728 **Exposure of other implanted mesh into organ or tissue** HCC ESR
T83.729 **Exposure of other prosthetic materials into organ or tissue** HCC ESR
T83.79 **Other specified complications due to other genitourinary prosthetic materials** HCC ESR
T83.8 **Other specified complications of genitourinary prosthetic devices, implants and grafts**
T83.81 **Embolism due to genitourinary prosthetic devices, implants and grafts** HCC ESR
T83.82 **Fibrosis due to genitourinary prosthetic devices, implants and grafts** HCC ESR
T83.83 **Hemorrhage due to genitourinary prosthetic devices, implants and grafts** HCC ESR
T83.84 **Pain due to genitourinary prosthetic devices, implants and grafts** HCC ESR
T83.85 **Stenosis due to genitourinary prosthetic devices, implants and grafts** HCC ESR
T83.86 **Thrombosis due to genitourinary prosthetic devices, implants and grafts** HCC ESR
T83.89 **Other specified complication of genitourinary prosthetic devices, implants and grafts** HCC ESR
AHA: 2016,1Q,19
T83.9 **Unspecified complication of genitourinary prosthetic device, implant and graft** HCC ESR

T84 **Complications of internal orthopedic prosthetic devices, implants and grafts**
EXCLUDES 2 *failure and rejection of transplanted organs and tissues (T86.-)*
fracture of bone following insertion of orthopedic implant, joint prosthesis or bone plate (M96.6)

The appropriate 7th character is to be added to each code from category T84.
A initial encounter
D subsequent encounter
S sequela

T84.0 **Mechanical complication of internal joint prosthesis**
T84.01 **Broken internal joint prosthesis**
Breakage (fracture) of prosthetic joint
Broken prosthetic joint implant
EXCLUDES 1 *periprosthetic joint implant fracture (M97.-)*
AHA: 2016,4Q,42
T84.010 **Broken internal right hip prosthesis** HCC ESR
T84.011 **Broken internal left hip prosthesis** HCC ESR
T84.012 **Broken internal right knee prosthesis** HCC ESR
T84.013 **Broken internal left knee prosthesis** HCC ESR
T84.018 **Broken internal joint prosthesis, other site** HCC ESR
Use additional code to identify the joint (Z96.6-)
T84.019 **Broken internal joint prosthesis, unspecified site** HCC ESR
T84.02 **Dislocation of internal joint prosthesis**
Instability of internal joint prosthesis
Subluxation of internal joint prosthesis
AHA: 2019,2Q,27
T84.020 **Dislocation of internal right hip prosthesis** HCC ESR
T84.021 **Dislocation of internal left hip prosthesis** HCC ESR
T84.022 **Instability of internal right knee prosthesis** HCC ESR
T84.023 **Instability of internal left knee prosthesis** HCC ESR
T84.028 **Dislocation of other internal joint prosthesis** HCC ESR
Use additional code to identify the joint (Z96.6-)
T84.029 **Dislocation of unspecified internal joint prosthesis** HCC ESR
T84.03 **Mechanical loosening of internal prosthetic joint**
Aseptic loosening of prosthetic joint
T84.030 **Mechanical loosening of internal right hip prosthetic joint** HCC ESR
T84.031 **Mechanical loosening of internal left hip prosthetic joint** HCC ESR
T84.032 **Mechanical loosening of internal right knee prosthetic joint** HCC ESR
T84.033 **Mechanical loosening of internal left knee prosthetic joint** HCC ESR
T84.038 **Mechanical loosening of other internal prosthetic joint** HCC ESR
Use additional code to identify the joint (Z96.6-)
T84.039 **Mechanical loosening of unspecified internal prosthetic joint** HCC ESR
T84.05 **Periprosthetic osteolysis of internal prosthetic joint**
Use additional code to identify major osseous defect, if applicable (M89.7-)
T84.050 **Periprosthetic osteolysis of internal prosthetic right hip joint** HCC ESR
T84.051 **Periprosthetic osteolysis of internal prosthetic left hip joint** HCC ESR

1 7th **T84.052 Periprosthetic osteolysis of internal prosthetic right knee joint** HCC ESR

1 7th **T84.053 Periprosthetic osteolysis of internal prosthetic left knee joint** HCC ESR

1 7th **T84.058 Periprosthetic osteolysis of other internal prosthetic joint** HCC ESR

Use additional code to identify the joint (Z96.6-)

1 7th **T84.059 Periprosthetic osteolysis of unspecified internal prosthetic joint** HCC ESR

6th **T84.06 Wear of articular bearing surface of internal prosthetic joint**

1 7th **T84.060 Wear of articular bearing surface of internal prosthetic right hip joint** HCC ESR

1 7th **T84.061 Wear of articular bearing surface of internal prosthetic left hip joint** HCC ESR

1 7th **T84.062 Wear of articular bearing surface of internal prosthetic right knee joint** HCC ESR

1 7th **T84.063 Wear of articular bearing surface of internal prosthetic left knee joint** HCC ESR

1 7th **T84.068 Wear of articular bearing surface of other internal prosthetic joint** HCC ESR

Use additional code to identify the joint (Z96.6-)

1 7th **T84.069 Wear of articular bearing surface of unspecified internal prosthetic joint** HCC ESR

6th **T84.09 Other mechanical complication of internal joint prosthesis**

Prosthetic joint implant failure NOS

AHA: 2019,1Q,20

1 7th **T84.090 Other mechanical complication of internal right hip prosthesis** HCC ESR

1 7th **T84.091 Other mechanical complication of internal left hip prosthesis** HCC ESR

1 7th **T84.092 Other mechanical complication of internal right knee prosthesis** HCC ESR

1 7th **T84.093 Other mechanical complication of internal left knee prosthesis** HCC ESR

1 7th **T84.098 Other mechanical complication of other internal joint prosthesis** HCC ESR

Use additional code to identify the joint (Z96.6-)

1 7th **T84.099 Other mechanical complication of unspecified internal joint prosthesis** HCC ESR

5th **T84.1 Mechanical complication of internal fixation device of bones of limb**

EXCLUDES 2 *mechanical complication of internal fixation device of bones of feet (T84.2-)*

mechanical complication of internal fixation device of bones of fingers (T84.2-)

mechanical complication of internal fixation device of bones of hands (T84.2-)

mechanical complication of internal fixation device of bones of toes (T84.2-)

6th **T84.11 Breakdown (mechanical) of internal fixation device of bones of limb**

1 7th **T84.110 Breakdown (mechanical) of internal fixation device of right humerus** HCC ESR

1 7th **T84.111 Breakdown (mechanical) of internal fixation device of left humerus** HCC ESR

1 7th **T84.112 Breakdown (mechanical) of internal fixation device of bone of right forearm** HCC ESR

1 7th **T84.113 Breakdown (mechanical) of internal fixation device of bone of left forearm** HCC ESR

1 7th **T84.114 Breakdown (mechanical) of internal fixation device of right femur** HCC ESR

1 7th **T84.115 Breakdown (mechanical) of internal fixation device of left femur** HCC ESR

1 7th **T84.116 Breakdown (mechanical) of internal fixation device of bone of right lower leg** HCC ESR

1 7th **T84.117 Breakdown (mechanical) of internal fixation device of bone of left lower leg** HCC ESR

1 7th **T84.119 Breakdown (mechanical) of internal fixation device of unspecified bone of limb** HCC ESR

6th **T84.12 Displacement of internal fixation device of bones of limb**

Malposition of internal fixation device of bones of limb

1 7th **T84.120 Displacement of internal fixation device of right humerus** HCC ESR

1 7th **T84.121 Displacement of internal fixation device of left humerus** HCC ESR

1 7th **T84.122 Displacement of internal fixation device of bone of right forearm** HCC ESR

1 7th **T84.123 Displacement of internal fixation device of bone of left forearm** HCC ESR

1 7th **T84.124 Displacement of internal fixation device of right femur** HCC ESR

1 7th **T84.125 Displacement of internal fixation device of left femur** HCC ESR

1 7th **T84.126 Displacement of internal fixation device of bone of right lower leg** HCC ESR

1 7th **T84.127 Displacement of internal fixation device of bone of left lower leg** HCC ESR

1 7th **T84.129 Displacement of internal fixation device of unspecified bone of limb** HCC ESR

6th **T84.19 Other mechanical complication of internal fixation device of bones of limb**

Obstruction (mechanical) of internal fixation device of bones of limb

Perforation of internal fixation device of bones of limb

Protrusion of internal fixation device of bones of limb

1 7th **T84.190 Other mechanical complication of internal fixation device of right humerus** HCC ESR

1 7th **T84.191 Other mechanical complication of internal fixation device of left humerus** HCC ESR

1 7th **T84.192 Other mechanical complication of internal fixation device of bone of right forearm** HCC ESR

1 7th **T84.193 Other mechanical complication of internal fixation device of bone of left forearm** HCC ESR

1 7th **T84.194 Other mechanical complication of internal fixation device of right femur** HCC ESR

1 7th **T84.195 Other mechanical complication of internal fixation device of left femur** HCC ESR

1 7th **T84.196 Other mechanical complication of internal fixation device of bone of right lower leg** HCC ESR

1 7th **T84.197 Other mechanical complication of internal fixation device of bone of left lower leg** HCC ESR

1 7th **T84.199 Other mechanical complication of internal fixation device of unspecified bone of limb** HCC ESR

5th **T84.2 Mechanical complication of internal fixation device of other bones**

6th **T84.21 Breakdown (mechanical) of internal fixation device of other bones**

1 7th **T84.210 Breakdown (mechanical) of internal fixation device of bones of hand and fingers** HCC ESR

1 7th **T84.213 Breakdown (mechanical) of internal fixation device of bones of foot and toes** HCC ESR

1 7th **T84.216 Breakdown (mechanical) of internal fixation device of vertebrae** HCC ESR

1 7th **T84.218 Breakdown (mechanical) of internal fixation device of other bones** HCC ESR

6th **T84.22 Displacement of internal fixation device of other bones**

Malposition of internal fixation device of other bones

1 7th **T84.220 Displacement of internal fixation device of bones of hand and fingers** HCC ESR

1 ✓7th T84.223 Displacement of internal fixation device of bones of foot and toes HCC ESR

1 ✓7th T84.226 Displacement of internal fixation device of vertebrae HCC ESR

1 ✓7th T84.228 Displacement of internal fixation device of other bones HCC ESR

✓6th T84.29 Other mechanical complication of internal fixation device of other bones
Obstruction (mechanical) of internal fixation device of other bones
Perforation of internal fixation device of other bones
Protrusion of internal fixation device of other bones

1 ✓7th T84.290 Other mechanical complication of internal fixation device of bones of hand and fingers HCC ESR

1 ✓7th T84.293 Other mechanical complication of internal fixation device of bones of foot and toes HCC ESR

1 ✓7th T84.296 Other mechanical complication of internal fixation device of vertebrae HCC ESR

1 ✓7th T84.298 Other mechanical complication of internal fixation device of other bones HCC ESR

✓5th T84.3 Mechanical complication of other bone devices, implants and grafts
EXCLUDES 2 *other complications of bone graft (T86.83-)*

✓6th T84.31 Breakdown (mechanical) of other bone devices, implants and grafts

1 ✓7th T84.310 Breakdown (mechanical) of electronic bone stimulator HCC ESR

1 ✓7th T84.318 Breakdown (mechanical) of other bone devices, implants and grafts HCC ESR

✓6th T84.32 Displacement of other bone devices, implants and grafts
Malposition of other bone devices, implants and grafts

1 ✓7th T84.320 Displacement of electronic bone stimulator HCC ESR

1 ✓7th T84.328 Displacement of other bone devices, implants and grafts HCC ESR
AHA: 2014,4Q,28

✓6th T84.39 Other mechanical complication of other bone devices, implants and grafts
Obstruction (mechanical) of other bone devices, implants and grafts
Perforation of other bone devices, implants and grafts
Protrusion of other bone devices, implants and grafts

1 ✓7th T84.390 Other mechanical complication of electronic bone stimulator HCC ESR

1 ✓7th T84.398 Other mechanical complication of other bone devices, implants and grafts HCC ESR

✓5th T84.4 Mechanical complication of other internal orthopedic devices, implants and grafts

✓6th T84.41 Breakdown (mechanical) of other internal orthopedic devices, implants and grafts

1 ✓7th T84.410 Breakdown (mechanical) of muscle and tendon graft HCC ESR

1 ✓7th T84.418 Breakdown (mechanical) of other internal orthopedic devices, implants and grafts HCC ESR

✓6th T84.42 Displacement of other internal orthopedic devices, implants and grafts
Malposition of other internal orthopedic devices, implants and grafts

1 ✓7th T84.420 Displacement of muscle and tendon graft HCC ESR

1 ✓7th T84.428 Displacement of other internal orthopedic devices, implants and grafts HCC ESR

✓6th T84.49 Other mechanical complication of other internal orthopedic devices, implants and grafts
Mechanical complication of other internal orthopedic devices, implants and grafts NOS
Obstruction (mechanical) of other internal orthopedic devices, implants and grafts
Perforation of other internal orthopedic devices, implants and grafts
Protrusion of other internal orthopedic devices, implants and grafts

1 ✓7th T84.490 Other mechanical complication of muscle and tendon graft HCC ESR

1 ✓7th T84.498 Other mechanical complication of other internal orthopedic devices, implants and grafts HCC ESR

✓5th T84.5 Infection and inflammatory reaction due to internal joint prosthesis
Use additional code to identify infection
AHA: 2019,3Q,16; 2015,1Q,16

1 ✓x7th T84.50 Infection and inflammatory reaction due to unspecified internal joint prosthesis HCC ESR

1 ✓x7th T84.51 Infection and inflammatory reaction due to internal right hip prosthesis HCC ESR

1 ✓x7th T84.52 Infection and inflammatory reaction due to internal left hip prosthesis HCC ESR

1 ✓x7th T84.53 Infection and inflammatory reaction due to internal right knee prosthesis HCC ESR

1 ✓x7th T84.54 Infection and inflammatory reaction due to internal left knee prosthesis HCC ESR

1 ✓x7th T84.59 Infection and inflammatory reaction due to other internal joint prosthesis HCC ESR

✓5th T84.6 Infection and inflammatory reaction due to internal fixation device
Use additional code to identify infection

1 ✓x7th T84.60 Infection and inflammatory reaction due to internal fixation device of unspecified site HCC ESR

✓6th T84.61 Infection and inflammatory reaction due to internal fixation device of arm

1 ✓7th T84.610 Infection and inflammatory reaction due to internal fixation device of right humerus HCC ESR

1 ✓7th T84.611 Infection and inflammatory reaction due to internal fixation device of left humerus HCC ESR

1 ✓7th T84.612 Infection and inflammatory reaction due to internal fixation device of right radius HCC ESR

1 ✓7th T84.613 Infection and inflammatory reaction due to internal fixation device of left radius HCC ESR

1 ✓7th T84.614 Infection and inflammatory reaction due to internal fixation device of right ulna HCC ESR

1 ✓7th T84.615 Infection and inflammatory reaction due to internal fixation device of left ulna HCC ESR

1 ✓7th T84.619 Infection and inflammatory reaction due to internal fixation device of unspecified bone of arm HCC ESR

✓6th T84.62 Infection and inflammatory reaction due to internal fixation device of leg

1 ✓7th T84.620 Infection and inflammatory reaction due to internal fixation device of right femur HCC ESR

1 ✓7th T84.621 Infection and inflammatory reaction due to internal fixation device of left femur HCC ESR

1 ✓7th T84.622 Infection and inflammatory reaction due to internal fixation device of right tibia HCC ESR

1 ✓7th T84.623 Infection and inflammatory reaction due to internal fixation device of left tibia HCC ESR

1 ✓7th T84.624 Infection and inflammatory reaction due to internal fixation device of right fibula HCC ESR

1 ✓7th T84.625 Infection and inflammatory reaction due to internal fixation device of left fibula HCC ESR

1 ✓7th **T84.629 Infection and inflammatory reaction due to internal fixation device of unspecified bone of leg** HCC ESR

1 ✓x7th **T84.63 Infection and inflammatory reaction due to internal fixation device of spine** HCC ESR

1 ✓x7th **T84.69 Infection and inflammatory reaction due to internal fixation device of other site** HCC ESR

1 ✓x7th **T84.7 Infection and inflammatory reaction due to other internal orthopedic prosthetic devices, implants and grafts** HCC ESR

Use additional code to identify infection

✓5th **T84.8 Other specified complications of internal orthopedic prosthetic devices, implants and grafts**

1 ✓x7th **T84.81 Embolism due to internal orthopedic prosthetic devices, implants and grafts** HCC ESR

1 ✓x7th **T84.82 Fibrosis due to internal orthopedic prosthetic devices, implants and grafts** HCC ESR

1 ✓x7th **T84.83 Hemorrhage due to internal orthopedic prosthetic devices, implants and grafts** HCC ESR

1 ✓x7th **T84.84 Pain due to internal orthopedic prosthetic devices, implants and grafts** HCC ESR

1 ✓x7th **T84.85 Stenosis due to internal orthopedic prosthetic devices, implants and grafts** HCC ESR

1 ✓x7th **T84.86 Thrombosis due to internal orthopedic prosthetic devices, implants and grafts** HCC ESR

1 ✓x7th **T84.89 Other specified complication of internal orthopedic prosthetic devices, implants and grafts** HCC ESR

1 ✓x7th **T84.9 Unspecified complication of internal orthopedic prosthetic device, implant and graft** HCC ESR

✓4th **T85 Complications of other internal prosthetic devices, implants and grafts**

EXCLUDES 2 *failure and rejection of transplanted organs and tissue (T86.-)*

AHA: 2016,4Q,71-72

The appropriate 7th character is to be added to each code from category T85.
A initial encounter
D subsequent encounter
S sequela

✓5th **T85.0 Mechanical complication of ventricular intracranial (communicating) shunt**

1 ✓x7th **T85.01 Breakdown (mechanical) of ventricular intracranial (communicating) shunt** HCC ESR

1 ✓x7th **T85.02 Displacement of ventricular intracranial (communicating) shunt** HCC ESR

Malposition of ventricular intracranial (communicating) shunt

1 ✓x7th **T85.03 Leakage of ventricular intracranial (communicating) shunt** HCC ESR

1 ✓x7th **T85.09 Other mechanical complication of ventricular intracranial (communicating) shunt** HCC ESR

Obstruction (mechanical) of ventricular intracranial (communicating) shunt
Perforation of ventricular intracranial (communicating) shunt
Protrusion of ventricular intracranial (communicating) shunt

✓5th **T85.1 Mechanical complication of implanted electronic stimulator of nervous system**

✓6th **T85.11 Breakdown (mechanical) of implanted electronic stimulator of nervous system**

1 ✓7th **T85.110 Breakdown (mechanical) of implanted electronic neurostimulator of brain electrode (lead)** HCC ESR

1 ✓7th **T85.111 Breakdown (mechanical) of implanted electronic neurostimulator of peripheral nerve electrode (lead)** HCC ESR

Breakdown of electrode (lead) for cranial nerve neurostimulators
Breakdown of electrode (lead) for gastric neurostimulator
Breakdown of electrode (lead) for sacral nerve neurostimulator
Breakdown of electrode (lead) for vagal nerve neurostimulators

1 ✓7th **T85.112 Breakdown (mechanical) of implanted electronic neurostimulator of spinal cord electrode (lead)** HCC ESR

1 ✓7th **T85.113 Breakdown (mechanical) of implanted electronic neurostimulator, generator** HCC ESR

Breakdown (mechanical) of implanted electronic neurostimulator generator, brain, peripheral, gastric, spinal
Breakdown (mechanical) of implanted electronic sacral neurostimulator, pulse generator or receiver

1 ✓7th **T85.118 Breakdown (mechanical) of other implanted electronic stimulator of nervous system** HCC ESR

✓6th **T85.12 Displacement of implanted electronic stimulator of nervous system**

Malposition of implanted electronic stimulator of nervous system

1 ✓7th **T85.120 Displacement of implanted electronic neurostimulator of brain electrode (lead)** HCC ESR

1 ✓7th **T85.121 Displacement of implanted electronic neurostimulator of peripheral nerve electrode (lead)** HCC ESR

Displacement of electrode (lead) for cranial nerve neurostimulators
Displacement of electrode (lead) for gastric neurostimulator
Displacement of electrode (lead) for sacral nerve neurostimulator
Displacement of electrode (lead) for vagal nerve neurostimulators

1 ✓7th **T85.122 Displacement of implanted electronic neurostimulator of spinal cord electrode (lead)** HCC ESR

1 ✓7th **T85.123 Displacement of implanted electronic neurostimulator, generator** HCC ESR

Displacement of implanted electronic neurostimulator generator, brain, peripheral, gastric, spinal
Displacement of implanted electronic sacral neurostimulator, pulse generator or receiver

1 ✓7th **T85.128 Displacement of other implanted electronic stimulator of nervous system** HCC ESR

✓6th **T85.19 Other mechanical complication of implanted electronic stimulator of nervous system**

Leakage of implanted electronic stimulator of nervous system
Obstruction (mechanical) of implanted electronic stimulator of nervous system
Perforation of implanted electronic stimulator of nervous system
Protrusion of implanted electronic stimulator of nervous system

1 ✓7th **T85.190 Other mechanical complication of implanted electronic neurostimulator of brain electrode (lead)** HCC ESR

1 ✓7th **T85.191 Other mechanical complication of implanted electronic neurostimulator of peripheral nerve electrode (lead)** HCC ESR

Other mechanical complication of electrode (lead) for cranial nerve neurostimulators
Other mechanical complication of electrode (lead) for gastric neurostimulator
Other mechanical complication of electrode (lead) for sacral nerve neurostimulator
Other mechanical complication of electrode (lead) for vagal nerve neurostimulators

1 ✓7th **T85.192 Other mechanical complication of implanted electronic neurostimulator of spinal cord electrode (lead)** HCC ESR

1 ✓7th **T85.193 Other mechanical complication of implanted electronic neurostimulator, generator** HCC ESR
Other mechanical complication of implanted electronic neurostimulator generator, brain, peripheral, gastric, spinal
Other mechanical complication of implanted electronic sacral neurostimulator, pulse generator or receiver

1 ✓7th **T85.199 Other mechanical complication of other implanted electronic stimulator of nervous system** HCC ESR

✓5th **T85.2 Mechanical complication of intraocular lens**

✓x7th **T85.21 Breakdown (mechanical) of intraocular lens**

✓x7th **T85.22 Displacement of intraocular lens**
Malposition of intraocular lens

✓x7th **T85.29 Other mechanical complication of intraocular lens**
Obstruction (mechanical) of intraocular lens
Perforation of intraocular lens
Protrusion of intraocular lens

✓5th **T85.3 Mechanical complication of other ocular prosthetic devices, implants and grafts**
EXCLUDES 2 *other complications of corneal graft (T86.84-)*

✓6th **T85.31 Breakdown (mechanical) of other ocular prosthetic devices, implants and grafts**

✓7th **T85.310 Breakdown (mechanical) of prosthetic orbit of right eye**

✓7th **T85.311 Breakdown (mechanical) of prosthetic orbit of left eye**

✓7th **T85.318 Breakdown (mechanical) of other ocular prosthetic devices, implants and grafts**

✓6th **T85.32 Displacement of other ocular prosthetic devices, implants and grafts**
Malposition of other ocular prosthetic devices, implants and grafts

✓7th **T85.320 Displacement of prosthetic orbit of right eye**

✓7th **T85.321 Displacement of prosthetic orbit of left eye**

✓7th **T85.328 Displacement of other ocular prosthetic devices, implants and grafts**

✓6th **T85.39 Other mechanical complication of other ocular prosthetic devices, implants and grafts**
Obstruction (mechanical) of other ocular prosthetic devices, implants and grafts
Perforation of other ocular prosthetic devices, implants and grafts
Protrusion of other ocular prosthetic devices, implants and grafts

✓7th **T85.390 Other mechanical complication of prosthetic orbit of right eye**

✓7th **T85.391 Other mechanical complication of prosthetic orbit of left eye**

✓7th **T85.398 Other mechanical complication of other ocular prosthetic devices, implants and grafts**

✓5th **T85.4 Mechanical complication of breast prosthesis and implant**

✓x7th **T85.41 Breakdown (mechanical) of breast prosthesis and implant**

✓x7th **T85.42 Displacement of breast prosthesis and implant**
Malposition of breast prosthesis and implant

✓x7th **T85.43 Leakage of breast prosthesis and implant**

✓x7th **T85.44 Capsular contracture of breast implant**

✓x7th **T85.49 Other mechanical complication of breast prosthesis and implant**
Obstruction (mechanical) of breast prosthesis and implant
Perforation of breast prosthesis and implant
Protrusion of breast prosthesis and implant

✓5th **T85.5 Mechanical complication of gastrointestinal prosthetic devices, implants and grafts**

✓6th **T85.51 Breakdown (mechanical) of gastrointestinal prosthetic devices, implants and grafts**

✓7th **T85.510 Breakdown (mechanical) of bile duct prosthesis**

✓7th **T85.511 Breakdown (mechanical) of esophageal anti-reflux device**

✓7th **T85.518 Breakdown (mechanical) of other gastrointestinal prosthetic devices, implants and grafts**

✓6th **T85.52 Displacement of gastrointestinal prosthetic devices, implants and grafts**
Malposition of gastrointestinal prosthetic devices, implants and grafts

✓7th **T85.520 Displacement of bile duct prosthesis**

✓7th **T85.521 Displacement of esophageal anti-reflux device**

✓7th **T85.528 Displacement of other gastrointestinal prosthetic devices, implants and grafts**

✓6th **T85.59 Other mechanical complication of gastrointestinal prosthetic devices, implants and**
Obstruction, mechanical of gastrointestinal prosthetic devices, implants and grafts
Perforation of gastrointestinal prosthetic devices, implants and grafts
Protrusion of gastrointestinal prosthetic devices, implants and grafts

✓7th **T85.590 Other mechanical complication of bile duct prosthesis**

✓7th **T85.591 Other mechanical complication of esophageal anti-reflux device**

✓7th **T85.598 Other mechanical complication of other gastrointestinal prosthetic devices, implants and grafts**

✓5th **T85.6 Mechanical complication of other specified internal and external prosthetic devices, implants and grafts**

✓6th **T85.61 Breakdown (mechanical) of other specified internal prosthetic devices, implants and grafts**

✓7th **T85.610 Breakdown (mechanical) of cranial or spinal infusion catheter**
Breakdown (mechanical) of epidural infusion catheter
Breakdown (mechanical) of intrathecal infusion catheter
Breakdown (mechanical) of subarachnoid infusion catheter
Breakdown (mechanical) of subdural infusion catheter

✓7th **T85.611 Breakdown (mechanical) of intraperitoneal dialysis catheter** HCC Rx ESR
EXCLUDES 1 *mechanical complication of vascular dialysis catheter (T82.4-)*

✓7th **T85.612 Breakdown (mechanical) of permanent sutures**
EXCLUDES 1 *mechanical complication of permanent (wire) suture used in bone repair (T84.1-T84.2)*

✓7th **T85.613 Breakdown (mechanical) of artificial skin graft and decellularized allodermis**
Failure of artificial skin graft and decellularized allodermis
Non-adherence of artificial skin graft and decellularized allodermis
Poor incorporation of artificial skin graft and decellularized allodermis
Shearing of artificial skin graft and decellularized allodermis

✓7th **T85.614 Breakdown (mechanical) of insulin pump**

1 ✓7th **T85.615 Breakdown (mechanical) of other nervous system device, implant or graft** HCC ESR
Breakdown (mechanical) of intrathecal infusion pump

✓7th **T85.618 Breakdown (mechanical) of other specified internal prosthetic devices, implants and grafts**

√6th **T85.62 Displacement of other specified internal prosthetic devices, implants and grafts**
Malposition of other specified internal prosthetic devices, implants and grafts

√7th **T85.620 Displacement of cranial or spinal infusion catheter**
Displacement of epidural infusion catheter
Displacement of intrathecal infusion catheter
Displacement of subarachnoid infusion catheter
Displacement of subdural infusion catheter

√7th **T85.621 Displacement of intraperitoneal dialysis catheter** HCC Rx ESR
EXCLUDES 1 *mechanical complication of vascular dialysis catheter (T82.4-)*

√7th **T85.622 Displacement of permanent sutures**
EXCLUDES 1 *mechanical complication of permanent (wire) suture used in bone repair (T84.1-T84.2)*

√7th **T85.623 Displacement of artificial skin graft and decellularized allodermis**
Dislodgement of artificial skin graft and decellularized allodermis

√7th **T85.624 Displacement of insulin pump**

1 √7th **T85.625 Displacement of other nervous system device, implant or graft** HCC ESR
Displacement of intrathecal infusion pump

√7th **T85.628 Displacement of other specified internal prosthetic devices, implants and grafts**

√6th **T85.63 Leakage of other specified internal prosthetic devices, implants and grafts**

√7th **T85.630 Leakage of cranial or spinal infusion catheter**
Leakage of epidural infusion catheter
Leakage of intrathecal infusion catheter infusion catheter
Leakage of subdural infusion catheter
Leakage of subarachnoid infusion catheter

√7th **T85.631 Leakage of intraperitoneal dialysis catheter** HCC Rx ESR
EXCLUDES 1 *mechanical complication of vascular dialysis catheter (T82.4)*

√7th **T85.633 Leakage of insulin pump**

1 √7th **T85.635 Leakage of other nervous system device, implant or graft** HCC ESR
Leakage of intrathecal infusion pump

√7th **T85.638 Leakage of other specified internal prosthetic devices, implants and grafts**

√6th **T85.69 Other mechanical complication of other specified internal prosthetic devices, implants and grafts**
Obstruction, mechanical of other specified internal prosthetic devices, implants and grafts
Perforation of other specified internal prosthetic devices, implants and grafts
Protrusion of other specified internal prosthetic devices, implants and grafts

√7th **T85.690 Other mechanical complication of cranial or spinal infusion catheter**
Other mechanical complication of epidural infusion catheter
Other mechanical complication of intrathecal infusion catheter
Other mechanical complication of subarachnoid infusion catheter
Other mechanical complication of subdural infusion catheter

√7th **T85.691 Other mechanical complication of intraperitoneal dialysis catheter** HCC Rx ESR
EXCLUDES 1 *mechanical complication of vascular dialysis catheter (T82.4)*

√7th **T85.692 Other mechanical complication of permanent sutures**
EXCLUDES 1 *mechanical complication of permanent (wire) suture used in bone repair (T84.1-T84.2)*

√7th **T85.693 Other mechanical complication of artificial skin graft and decellularized allodermis**

√7th **T85.694 Other mechanical complication of insulin pump**

1 √7th **T85.695 Other mechanical complication of other nervous system device, implant or graft** HCC ESR
Other mechanical complication of intrathecal infusion pump

√7th **T85.698 Other mechanical complication of other specified internal prosthetic devices, implants and grafts**
Mechanical complication of nonabsorbable surgical material NOS

√5th **T85.7 Infection and inflammatory reaction due to other internal prosthetic devices, implants and grafts**
Use additional code to identify infection

√x7th **T85.71 Infection and inflammatory reaction due to peritoneal dialysis catheter** HCC Rx ESR

1 √x7th **T85.72 Infection and inflammatory reaction due to insulin pump** HCC ESR

√6th **T85.73 Infection and inflammatory reaction due to nervous system devices, implants and graft**

1 √7th **T85.730 Infection and inflammatory reaction due to ventricular intracranial (communicating) shunt** HCC ESR

1 √7th **T85.731 Infection and inflammatory reaction due to implanted electronic neurostimulator of brain, electrode (lead)** HCC ESR

1 √7th **T85.732 Infection and inflammatory reaction due to implanted electronic neurostimulator of peripheral nerve, electrode (lead)** HCC ESR
Infection and inflammatory reaction due to electrode (lead) for cranial nerve neurostimulators
Infection and inflammatory reaction due to electrode (lead) for gastric neurostimulator
Infection and inflammatory reaction due to electrode (lead) for sacral nerve neurostimulator
Infection and inflammatory reaction due to electrode (lead) for vagal nerve neurostimulators

1 √7th **T85.733 Infection and inflammatory reaction due to implanted electronic neurostimulator of spinal cord, electrode (lead)** HCC ESR

1 √7th **T85.734 Infection and inflammatory reaction due to implanted electronic neurostimulator, generator** HCC ESR
Generator pocket infection

1 √7th **T85.735 Infection and inflammatory reaction due to cranial or spinal infusion catheter** HCC ESR
Infection and inflammatory reaction due to epidural catheter
Infection and inflammatory reaction due to intrathecal infusion catheter
Infection and inflammatory reaction due to subarachnoid catheter
Infection and inflammatory reaction due to subdural catheter

1 √7th **T85.738 Infection and inflammatory reaction due to other nervous system device, implant or graft** HCC ESR
Infection and inflammatory reaction due to intrathecal infusion pump

1 √x7th **T85.79 Infection and inflammatory reaction due to other internal prosthetic devices, implants and grafts** HCC ESR
AHA: 2022,2Q,7

√5th **T85.8 Other specified complications of internal prosthetic devices, implants and grafts, not elsewhere classified**

√6th **T85.81 Embolism due to internal prosthetic devices, implants and grafts, not elsewhere classified**

1 √7th **T85.810 Embolism due to nervous system prosthetic devices, implants and grafts** HCC ESR

√7th **T85.818 Embolism due to other internal prosthetic devices, implants and grafts**

√6th **T85.82 Fibrosis due to internal prosthetic devices, implants and grafts, not elsewhere classified**

1 √7th **T85.820 Fibrosis due to nervous system prosthetic devices, implants and grafts** HCC ESR

√7th **T85.828 Fibrosis due to other internal prosthetic devices, implants and grafts**

√6th **T85.83 Hemorrhage due to internal prosthetic devices, implants and grafts, not elsewhere classified**

1 √7th **T85.830 Hemorrhage due to nervous system prosthetic devices, implants and grafts** HCC ESR

√7th **T85.838 Hemorrhage due to other internal prosthetic devices, implants and grafts**

√6th **T85.84 Pain due to internal prosthetic devices, implants and grafts, not elsewhere classified**

1 √7th **T85.840 Pain due to nervous system prosthetic devices, implants and grafts** HCC ESR

√7th **T85.848 Pain due to other internal prosthetic devices, implants and grafts**

√6th **T85.85 Stenosis due to internal prosthetic devices, implants and grafts, not elsewhere classified**

1 √7th **T85.850 Stenosis due to nervous system prosthetic devices, implants and grafts** HCC ESR

√7th **T85.858 Stenosis due to other internal prosthetic devices, implants and grafts**

√6th **T85.86 Thrombosis due to internal prosthetic devices, implants and grafts, not elsewhere classified**

1 √7th **T85.860 Thrombosis due to nervous system prosthetic devices, implants and grafts** HCC ESR

√7th **T85.868 Thrombosis due to other internal prosthetic devices, implants and grafts**

√6th **T85.89 Other specified complication of internal prosthetic devices, implants and grafts, not elsewhere classified**

Erosion or breakdown of subcutaneous device pocket

1 √7th **T85.890 Other specified complication of nervous system prosthetic devices, implants and grafts** HCC ESR

√7th **T85.898 Other specified complication of other internal prosthetic devices, implants and grafts**

√x7th **T85.9 Unspecified complication of internal prosthetic device, implant and graft**

Complication of internal prosthetic device, implant and graft NOS

√4th **T86 Complications of transplanted organs and tissue**

Use additional code to identify other transplant complications, such as:
- graft-versus-host disease (D89.81-)
- malignancy associated with organ transplant (C80.2)
- post-transplant lymphoproliferative disorders (PTLD) (D47.Z1)

AHA: 2020,1Q,18

√5th **T86.0 Complications of bone marrow transplant**

T86.00 Unspecified complication of bone marrow transplant HCC Rx ESR COM

T86.01 Bone marrow transplant rejection HCC Rx ESR COM

T86.02 Bone marrow transplant failure HCC Rx ESR COM

T86.03 Bone marrow transplant infection HCC Rx ESR COM

T86.09 Other complications of bone marrow transplant HCC Rx ESR COM

√5th **T86.1 Complications of kidney transplant**

T86.10 Unspecified complication of kidney transplant Rx COM

T86.11 Kidney transplant rejection Rx COM

T86.12 Kidney transplant failure Rx COM

AHA: 2013,1Q,24

T86.13 Kidney transplant infection Rx COM

Use additional code to specify infection

T86.19 Other complication of kidney transplant Rx COM

AHA: 2019,2Q,7

√5th **T86.2 Complications of heart transplant**

EXCLUDES 1 *complication of:*
- *artificial heart device (T82.5-)*
- *heart-lung transplant (T86.3-)*

T86.20 Unspecified complication of heart transplant HCC Rx ESR COM

T86.21 Heart transplant rejection HCC Rx ESR COM

T86.22 Heart transplant failure HCC Rx ESR COM

T86.23 Heart transplant infection HCC Rx ESR COM

Use additional code to specify infection

√6th **T86.29 Other complications of heart transplant**

T86.290 Cardiac allograft vasculopathy HCC Rx ESR COM

EXCLUDES 1 *atherosclerosis of coronary arteries (I25.75-, I25.76-, I25.81-)*

T86.298 Other complications of heart transplant HCC Rx ESR COM

√5th **T86.3 Complications of heart-lung transplant**

T86.30 Unspecified complication of heart-lung transplant HCC Rx ESR COM

T86.31 Heart-lung transplant rejection HCC Rx ESR COM

T86.32 Heart-lung transplant failure HCC Rx ESR COM

T86.33 Heart-lung transplant infection HCC Rx ESR COM

Use additional code to specify infection

T86.39 Other complications of heart-lung transplant HCC Rx ESR COM

√5th **T86.4 Complications of liver transplant**

T86.40 Unspecified complication of liver transplant HCC Rx ESR COM

T86.41 Liver transplant rejection HCC Rx ESR COM

T86.42 Liver transplant failure HCC Rx ESR COM

T86.43 Liver transplant infection HCC Rx ESR COM

Use additional code to identify infection, such as:
- cytomegalovirus (CMV) infection (B25.-)

T86.49 Other complications of liver transplant HCC Rx ESR COM

T86.5 Complications of stem cell transplant HCC Rx ESR COM

Complications from stem cells from peripheral blood

Complications from stem cells from umbilical cord

AHA: 2020,4Q,14

√5th **T86.8 Complications of other transplanted organs and tissues**

√6th **T86.81 Complications of lung transplant**

EXCLUDES 1 *complication of heart-lung transplant (T86.3-)*

T86.810 Lung transplant rejection HCC Rx ESR COM

T86.811 Lung transplant failure HCC Rx ESR COM

T86.812 Lung transplant infection HCC Rx ESR COM

Use additional code to specify infection

T86.818 Other complications of lung transplant HCC Rx ESR COM

AHA: 2019,2Q,6

T86.819 Unspecified complication of lung transplant HCC Rx ESR COM

√6th **T86.82 Complications of skin graft (allograft) (autograft)**

EXCLUDES 2 *complication of artificial skin graft (T85.693)*

T86.820 Skin graft (allograft) rejection

T86.821 Skin graft (allograft) (autograft) failure

T86.822 Skin graft (allograft) (autograft) infection

Use additional code to specify infection

T86.828 Other complications of skin graft (allograft) (autograft)

T86.829 Unspecified complication of skin graft (allograft) (autograft)

√6th **T86.83 Complications of bone graft**

EXCLUDES 2 *mechanical complications of bone graft (T84.3-)*

T86.830 Bone graft rejection

T86.831 Bone graft failure

Chapter 19. Injury, Poisoning and Certain Other Consequences of External Causes

T85.8–T86.831

T86.832 Bone graft infection
Use additional code to specify infection

T86.838 Other complications of bone graft

T86.839 Unspecified complication of bone graft

✓6th T86.84 Complications of corneal transplant
EXCLUDES 2 *mechanical complications of corneal graft (T85.3-)*
AHA: 2020,4Q,40

✓7th T86.840 Corneal transplant rejection
T86.8401 Corneal transplant rejection, right eye
T86.8402 Corneal transplant rejection, left eye
T86.8403 Corneal transplant rejection, bilateral
T86.8409 Corneal transplant rejection, unspecified eye

✓7th T86.841 Corneal transplant failure
T86.8411 Corneal transplant failure, right eye
T86.8412 Corneal transplant failure, left eye
T86.8413 Corneal transplant failure, bilateral
T86.8419 Corneal transplant failure, unspecified eye

✓7th T86.842 Corneal transplant infection
Use additional code to specify infection
T86.8421 Corneal transplant infection, right eye HCC ESR
T86.8422 Corneal transplant infection, left eye HCC ESR
T86.8423 Corneal transplant infection, bilateral HCC ESR
T86.8429 Corneal transplant infection, unspecified eye HCC ESR

✓7th T86.848 Other complications of corneal transplant
T86.8481 Other complications of corneal transplant, right eye
T86.8482 Other complications of corneal transplant, left eye
T86.8483 Other complications of corneal transplant, bilateral
T86.8489 Other complications of corneal transplant, unspecified eye

✓7th T86.849 Unspecified complication of corneal transplant
T86.8491 Unspecified complication of corneal transplant, right eye
T86.8492 Unspecified complication of corneal transplant, left eye
T86.8493 Unspecified complication of corneal transplant, bilateral
T86.8499 Unspecified complication of corneal transplant, unspecified eye

✓6th T86.85 Complication of intestine transplant
T86.850 Intestine transplant rejection HCC Rx ESR COM
T86.851 Intestine transplant failure HCC Rx ESR COM
T86.852 Intestine transplant infection HCC Rx ESR COM
Use additional code to specify infection
T86.858 Other complications of intestine transplant HCC Rx ESR COM
T86.859 Unspecified complication of intestine transplant HCC Rx ESR COM

✓6th T86.89 Complications of other transplanted tissue
Transplant failure or rejection of pancreas
AHA: 2020,1Q,18
T86.890 Other transplanted tissue rejection
T86.891 Other transplanted tissue failure
T86.892 Other transplanted tissue infection
Use additional code to specify infection
T86.898 Other complications of other transplanted tissue
T86.899 Unspecified complication of other transplanted tissue

✓5th T86.9 Complication of unspecified transplanted organ and tissue
T86.90 Unspecified complication of unspecified transplanted organ and tissue
T86.91 Unspecified transplanted organ and tissue rejection
T86.92 Unspecified transplanted organ and tissue failure
T86.93 Unspecified transplanted organ and tissue infection
Use additional code to specify infection
T86.99 Other complications of unspecified transplanted organ and tissue

✓4th T87 Complications peculiar to reattachment and amputation

✓5th T87.0 Complications of reattached (part of) upper extremity
✓6th T87.0X Complications of reattached (part of) upper extremity
T87.0X1 Complications of reattached (part of) right upper extremity HCC ESR COM
T87.0X2 Complications of reattached (part of) left upper extremity HCC ESR COM
T87.0X9 Complications of reattached (part of) unspecified upper extremity HCC ESR COM

✓5th T87.1 Complications of reattached (part of) lower extremity
✓6th T87.1X Complications of reattached (part of) lower extremity
T87.1X1 Complications of reattached (part of) right lower extremity HCC ESR COM
T87.1X2 Complications of reattached (part of) left lower extremity HCC ESR COM
T87.1X9 Complications of reattached (part of) unspecified lower extremity HCC ESR COM

T87.2 Complications of other reattached body part HCC ESR

✓5th T87.3 Neuroma of amputation stump
DEF: Non-neoplastic tumor generated at the proximal end of severed, partially transected, or injured nerve following amputation.
T87.30 Neuroma of amputation stump, unspecified extremity HCC ESR COM
T87.31 Neuroma of amputation stump, right upper extremity HCC ESR COM
T87.32 Neuroma of amputation stump, left upper extremity HCC ESR COM
T87.33 Neuroma of amputation stump, right lower extremity HCC ESR COM
T87.34 Neuroma of amputation stump, left lower extremity HCC ESR COM

✓5th T87.4 Infection of amputation stump
T87.40 Infection of amputation stump, unspecified extremity HCC ESR COM
T87.41 Infection of amputation stump, right upper extremity HCC ESR COM
T87.42 Infection of amputation stump, left upper extremity HCC ESR COM
T87.43 Infection of amputation stump, right lower extremity HCC ESR COM
T87.44 Infection of amputation stump, left lower extremity HCC ESR COM

✓5th T87.5 Necrosis of amputation stump
T87.50 Necrosis of amputation stump, unspecified extremity HCC ESR COM
T87.51 Necrosis of amputation stump, right upper extremity HCC ESR COM
T87.52 Necrosis of amputation stump, left upper extremity HCC ESR COM
T87.53 Necrosis of amputation stump, right lower extremity HCC ESR COM
T87.54 Necrosis of amputation stump, left lower extremity HCC ESR COM

✓5th T87.8 Other complications of amputation stump
T87.81 Dehiscence of amputation stump HCC ESR COM

HCC CMS-HCC Rx Rx HCC ESR ESRD HCC COM Commercial HCC N Newborn: 0 P Pediatric: 0-17 M Maternity: 9-64 A Adult: 15-124

T87.89 **Other complications of amputation stump** HCC ESR COM
Amputation stump contracture
Amputation stump contracture of next proximal joint
Amputation stump flexion
Amputation stump edema
Amputation stump hematoma
EXCLUDES 2 *phantom limb syndrome (G54.6-G54.7)*

T87.9 **Unspecified complications of amputation stump** HCC ESR COM

✓4th **T88 Other complications of surgical and medical care, not elsewhere classified**
EXCLUDES 2 *complication following infusion, transfusion and therapeutic injection (T8Ø.-)*
complication following procedure NEC (T81.-)
complications of anesthesia in labor and delivery (O74.-)
complications of anesthesia in pregnancy (O29.-)
complications of anesthesia in puerperium (O89.-)
complications of devices, implants and grafts (T82-T85)
complications of obstetric surgery and procedure (O75.4)
dermatitis due to drugs and medicaments (L23.3, L24.4, L25.1, L27.Ø-L27.1)
poisoning and toxic effects of drugs and chemicals (T36-T65 with fifth or sixth character 1-4 or 6)
specified complications classified elsewhere

The appropriate 7th character is to be added to each code from category T88.
A initial encounter
D subsequent encounter
S sequela

√x7th T88.Ø **Infection following immunization**
Sepsis following immunization
AHA: 2018,4Q,62-63

√x7th T88.1 **Other complications following immunization, not elsewhere classified**
Generalized vaccinia
Rash following immunization
EXCLUDES 1 *vaccinia not from vaccine (BØ8.Ø11)*
EXCLUDES 2 *anaphylactic shock due to serum (T8Ø.5-)*
other serum reactions (T8Ø.6-)
postimmunization arthropathy (MØ2.2)
postimmunization encephalitis (GØ4.Ø2)
postimmunization fever (R5Ø.83)

√x7th T88.2 **Shock due to anesthesia**
Use additional code for adverse effect, if applicable, to identify drug (T41.- with fifth or sixth character 5)
EXCLUDES 1 *complications of anesthesia (in):*
labor and delivery (O74.-)
postprocedural shock NOS (T81.1-)
pregnancy (O29.-)
puerperium (O89.-)

√x7th T88.3 **Malignant hyperthermia due to anesthesia**
Use additional code for adverse effect, if applicable, to identify drug (T41.- with fifth or sixth character 5)

√x7th T88.4 **Failed or difficult intubation**

✓5th T88.5 **Other complications of anesthesia**
Use additional code for adverse effect, if applicable, to identify drug (T41.- with fifth or sixth character 5)

√x7th T88.51 **Hypothermia following anesthesia**

√x7th T88.52 **Failed moderate sedation during procedure**
Failed conscious sedation during procedure
EXCLUDES 2 *personal history of failed moderate sedation (Z92.83)*

√x7th T88.53 **Unintended awareness under general anesthesia during procedure**
EXCLUDES 2 *personal history of unintended awareness under general anesthesia (Z92.84)*
AHA: 2016,4Q,72-73

√x7th T88.59 **Other complications of anesthesia**

√x7th T88.6 **Anaphylactic reaction due to adverse effect of correct drug or medicament properly administered**
Anaphylactic shock due to adverse effect of correct drug or medicament properly administered
Anaphylactoid reaction NOS
Use additional code for adverse effect, if applicable, to identify drug (T36-T5Ø with fifth or sixth character 5)
EXCLUDES 1 *anaphylactic reaction due to serum (T8Ø.5-)*
anaphylactic shock or reaction due to adverse food reaction (T78.Ø-)
AHA: 2020,1Q,18

√x7th T88.7 **Unspecified adverse effect of drug or medicament**
Drug hypersensitivity NOS
Drug reaction NOS
Use additional code for adverse effect, if applicable, to identify drug (T36-T5Ø with fifth or sixth character 5)
EXCLUDES 1 *specified adverse effects of drugs and medicaments (AØØ-R94 and T8Ø-T88.6, T88.8)*

√x7th T88.8 **Other specified complications of surgical and medical care, not elsewhere classified**
Use additional code to identify the complication
AHA: 2022,2Q,7

√x7th T88.9 **Complication of surgical and medical care, unspecified**

Chapter 20. External Causes of Morbidity (V00–Y99)

Chapter-specific Guidelines with Coding Examples

The chapter-specific guidelines from the ICD-10-CM Official Guidelines for Coding and Reporting have been provided below. Along with these guidelines are coding examples, contained in the shaded boxes, that have been developed to help illustrate the coding and/or sequencing guidance found in these guidelines.

The external causes of morbidity codes should never be sequenced as the first-listed or principal diagnosis.

External cause codes are intended to provide data for injury research and evaluation of injury prevention strategies. These codes capture how the injury or health condition happened (cause), the intent (unintentional or accidental; or intentional, such as suicide or assault), the place where the event occurred the activity of the patient at the time of the event, and the person's status (e.g., civilian, military).

There is no national requirement for mandatory ICD-10-CM external cause code reporting. Unless a provider is subject to a state-based external cause code reporting mandate or these codes are required by a particular payer, reporting of ICD-10-CM codes in Chapter 20, External Causes of Morbidity, is not required. In the absence of a mandatory reporting requirement, providers are encouraged to voluntarily report external cause codes, as they provide valuable data for injury research and evaluation of injury prevention strategies.

a. General external cause coding guidelines

1) Used with any code in the range of A00.0–T88.9, Z00–Z99

An external cause code may be used with any code in the range of A00.0-T88.9, Z00-Z99, classification that represents a health condition due to an external cause. Though they are most applicable to injuries, they are also valid for use with such things as infections or diseases due to an external source, and other health conditions, such as a heart attack that occurs during strenuous physical activity.

Actinic reticuloid due to tanning bed use

L57.1	**Actinic reticuloid**
W89.1XXA	**Exposure to tanning bed, initial encounter**

Explanation: An external cause code may be used with any code in the range of A00.0–T88.9, Z00–Z99, classifications that describe health conditions due to an external cause. Code W89.1 Exposure to tanning bed requires a seventh character of A to report this initial encounter, with a placeholder X for the fifth and sixth characters.

2) External cause code used for length of treatment

Assign the external cause code, with the appropriate 7th character (initial encounter, subsequent encounter or sequela) for each encounter for which the injury or condition is being treated.

Most categories in chapter 20 have a 7th character requirement for each applicable code. Most categories in this chapter have three 7th character values: A, initial encounter, D, subsequent encounter and S, sequela. While the patient may be seen by a new or different provider over the course of treatment for an injury or condition, assignment of the 7th character for external cause should match the 7th character of the code assigned for the associated injury or condition for the encounter.

3) Use the full range of external cause codes

Use the full range of external cause codes to completely describe the cause, the intent, the place of occurrence, and if applicable, the activity of the patient at the time of the event, and the patient's status, for all injuries, and other health conditions due to an external cause.

4) Assign as many external cause codes as necessary

Assign as many external cause codes as necessary to fully explain each cause. If only one external code can be recorded, assign the code most related to the principal diagnosis.

5) The selection of the appropriate external cause code

The selection of the appropriate external cause code is guided by the Alphabetic Index of External Causes and by Inclusion and Exclusion notes in the Tabular List.

6) External cause code can never be a principal diagnosis

An external cause code can never be a principal (first-listed) diagnosis.

7) Combination external cause codes

Certain of the external cause codes are combination codes that identify sequential events that result in an injury, such as a fall which results in striking against an object. The injury may be due to either event or both. The combination external cause code used should correspond to the sequence of events regardless of which caused the most serious injury.

Toddler tripped and fell while walking and struck his head on an end table, sustaining a scalp contusion

S00.03XA	**Contusion of scalp, initial encounter**
W01.190A	**Fall on same level from slipping, tripping and stumbling with subsequent striking against furniture, initial encounter**

Explanation: Combination external cause codes identify sequential events that result in an injury, such as a fall resulting in striking against an object. The injury may be due to either or both events.

8) No external cause code needed in certain circumstances

No external cause code from Chapter 20 is needed if the external cause and intent are included in a code from another chapter (e.g., T36.0X1-, Poisoning by penicillins, accidental (unintentional)).

b. Place of occurrence guideline

Codes from category Y92, Place of occurrence of the external cause, are secondary codes for use after other external cause codes to identify the location of the patient at the time of injury or other condition.

Generally, a place of occurrence code is assigned only once, at the initial encounter for treatment. However, in the rare instance that a new injury occurs during hospitalization, an additional place of occurrence code may be assigned. No 7th characters are used for Y92.

Do not use place of occurrence code Y92.9 if the place is not stated or is not applicable.

A farmer was working in his barn and sustained a foot contusion when the horse stepped on his left foot

S90.32XA	**Contusion of left foot, initial encounter**
W55.19XA	**Other contact with horse, initial encounter**
Y92.71	**Barn as the place of occurrence of the external cause**

Explanation: A place-of-occurrence code from category Y92 is assigned at the initial encounter to identify the location of the patient at the time the injury occurred.

c. Activity code

Assign a code from category Y93, Activity code, to describe the activity of the patient at the time the injury or other health condition occurred.

An activity code is used only once, at the initial encounter for treatment. Only one code from Y93 should be recorded on a medical record.

The activity codes are not applicable to poisonings, adverse effects, misadventures or sequela.

Do not assign Y93.9, Unspecified activity, if the activity is not stated.

A code from category Y93 is appropriate for use with external cause and intent codes if identifying the activity provides additional information about the event.

Ranch hand who was grooming a horse sustained a foot contusion when the horse stepped on his left foot

S90.32XA	**Contusion of left foot, initial encounter**
W55.19XA	**Other contact with horse, initial encounter**
Y93.K3	**Activity, grooming and shearing an animal**

Explanation: One activity code from category Y93 is assigned at the initial encounter only to describe the activity of the patient at the time the injury occurred.

d. Place of occurrence, activity, and status codes used with other external cause code

When applicable, place of occurrence, activity, and external cause status codes are sequenced after the main external cause code(s). Regardless of the number of external cause codes assigned, generally there should be only one place of occurrence code, one activity code, and one external cause status code assigned to an encounter. However, in the rare instance that a new injury occurs during hospitalization, an additional place of occurrence code may be assigned.

e. If the reporting format limits the number of external cause codes

If the reporting format limits the number of external cause codes that can be used in reporting clinical data, report the code for the cause/intent most related to the principal diagnosis. If the format permits capture of additional external cause codes, the cause/intent, including medical misadventures, of the additional events should be reported rather than the codes for place, activity, or external status.

f. Multiple external cause coding guidelines

More than one external cause code is required to fully describe the external cause of an illness or injury. The assignment of external cause codes should be sequenced in the following priority:

If two or more events cause separate injuries, an external cause code should be assigned for each cause. The first-listed external cause code will be selected in the following order:

External codes for child and adult abuse take priority over all other external cause codes.

See Section I.C.19., Child and Adult abuse guidelines.

External cause codes for terrorism events take priority over all other external cause codes except child and adult abuse.

External cause codes for cataclysmic events take priority over all other external cause codes except child and adult abuse and terrorism.

External cause codes for transport accidents take priority over all other external cause codes except cataclysmic events, child and adult abuse and terrorism.

Activity and external cause status codes are assigned following all causal (intent) external cause codes.

The first-listed external cause code should correspond to the cause of the most serious diagnosis due to an assault, accident, or self-harm, following the order of hierarchy listed above..

30-year-old man accidentally discharged his hunting rifle, sustaining an open gunshot wound, with no retained bullet fragments, to the right thigh, which caused him to fall down the stairs, resulting in closed displaced comminuted fracture of his left radial shaft

S71.131A	**Puncture wound without foreign body, right thigh, initial encounter**
W33.Ø2XA	**Accidental discharge of hunting rifle, initial encounter**
S52.352A	**Displaced comminuted fracture of shaft of radius, left arm, initial encounter for closed fracture**
W1Ø.9XXA	**Fall (on) (from) unspecified stairs and steps, initial encounter**

Explanation: If two or more events cause separate injuries, an external cause code should be assigned for each cause.

g. Child and adult abuse guideline

Adult and child abuse, neglect and maltreatment are classified as assault. Any of the assault codes may be used to indicate the external cause of any injury resulting from the confirmed abuse.

For confirmed cases of abuse, neglect and maltreatment, when the perpetrator is known, a code from YØ7, Perpetrator of maltreatment and neglect, should accompany any other assault codes.

See Section I.C.19. Adult and child abuse, neglect and other maltreatment

h. Unknown or undetermined intent guideline

If the intent (accident, self-harm, assault) of the cause of an injury or other condition is unknown or unspecified, code the intent as accidental intent. All transport accident categories assume accidental intent.

1) Use of undetermined intent

External cause codes for events of undetermined intent are only for use if the documentation in the record specifies that the intent cannot be determined.

i. Sequelae (late effects) of external cause guidelines

1) Sequelae external cause codes

Sequela are reported using the external cause code with the 7th character "S" for sequela. These codes should be used with any report of a late effect or sequela resulting from a previous injury.

See Section I.B.1Ø. Sequela (Late Effects)

2) Sequela external cause code with a related current injury

A sequela external cause code should never be used with a related current nature of injury code.

3) Use of sequela external cause codes for subsequent visits

Use a late effect external cause code for subsequent visits when a late effect of the initial injury is being treated. Do not use a late effect external cause code for subsequent visits for follow-up care (e.g., to assess healing, to receive rehabilitative therapy) of the injury when no late effect of the injury has been documented.

j. Terrorism guidelines

1) Cause of injury identified by the Federal Government (FBI) as terrorism

When the cause of an injury is identified by the Federal Government (FBI) as terrorism, the first-listed external cause code should be a code from category Y38, Terrorism. The definition of terrorism employed by the FBI is found at the inclusion note at the beginning of category Y38. Use additional code for place of occurrence (Y92.-). More than one Y38 code may be assigned if the injury is the result of more than one mechanism of terrorism.

2) Cause of an injury is suspected to be the result of terrorism

When the cause of an injury is suspected to be the result of terrorism a code from category Y38 should not be assigned. Suspected cases should be classified as assault.

3) Code Y38.9, Terrorism, secondary effects

Assign code Y38.9, Terrorism, secondary effects, for conditions occurring subsequent to the terrorist event. This code should not be assigned for conditions that are due to the initial terrorist act.

It is acceptable to assign code Y38.9 with another code from Y38 if there is an injury due to the initial terrorist event and an injury that is a subsequent result of the terrorist event.

k. External cause status

A code from category Y99, External cause status, should be assigned whenever any other external cause code is assigned for an encounter, including an Activity code, except for the events noted below. Assign a code from category Y99, External cause status, to indicate the work status of the person at the time the event occurred. The status code indicates whether the event occurred during military activity, whether a non-military person was at work, whether an individual including a student or volunteer was involved in a non-work activity at the time of the causal event.

A code from Y99, External cause status, should be assigned, when applicable, with other external cause codes, such as transport accidents and falls. The external cause status codes are not applicable to poisonings, adverse effects, misadventures or late effects.

Do not assign a code from category Y99 if no other external cause codes (cause, activity) are applicable for the encounter.

An external cause status code is used only once, at the initial encounter for treatment. Only one code from Y99 should be recorded on a medical record.

Do not assign code Y99.9, Unspecified external cause status, if the status is not stated.

Chapter 20. External Causes of Morbidity (VØØ-Y99)

NOTE This chapter permits the classification of environmental events and circumstances as the cause of injury, and other adverse effects. Where a code from this section is applicable, it is intended that it shall be used secondary to a code from another chapter of the Classification indicating the nature of the condition. Most often, the condition will be classifiable to Chapter 19, Injury, poisoning and certain other consequences of external causes (SØØ-T88). Other conditions that may be stated to be due to external causes are classified in Chapters I to XVIII. For these conditions, codes from Chapter 2Ø should be used to provide additional information as to the cause of the condition.

AHA: 2018,4Q,58-60

This chapter contains the following blocks:

VØØ-X58 Accidents
VØØ-V99 Transport accidents
VØØ-VØ9 Pedestrian injured in transport accident
V1Ø-V19 Pedal cycle rider injured in transport accident
V2Ø-V29 Motorcycle rider injured in transport accident
V3Ø-V39 Occupant of three-wheeled motor vehicle injured in transport accident
V4Ø-V49 Car occupant injured in transport accident
V5Ø-V59 Occupant of pick-up truck or van injured in transport accident
V6Ø-V69 Occupant of heavy transport vehicle injured in transport accident
V7Ø-V79 Bus occupant injured in transport accident
V8Ø-V89 Other land transport accidents
V9Ø-V94 Water transport accidents
V95-V97 Air and space transport accidents
V98-V99 Other and unspecified transport accidents
WØØ-X58 Other external causes of accidental injury
WØØ-W19 Slipping, tripping, stumbling and falls
W2Ø-W49 Exposure to inanimate mechanical forces
W5Ø-W64 Exposure to animate mechanical forces
W65-W74 Accidental non-transport drowning and submersion
W85-W99 Exposure to electric current, radiation and extreme ambient air temperature and pressure
XØØ-XØ8 Exposure to smoke, fire and flames
X1Ø-X19 Contact with heat and hot substances
X3Ø-X39 Exposure to forces of nature
X5Ø Overexertion and strenuous or repetitive movements
X52-X58 Accidental exposure to other specified factors
X71-X83 Intentional self-harm
X92-YØ9 Assault
Y21-Y33 Event of undetermined intent
Y35-Y38 Legal intervention, operations of war, military operations, and terrorism
Y62-Y84 Complications of medical and surgical care
Y62-Y69 Misadventures to patients during surgical and medical care
Y7Ø-Y82 Medical devices associated with adverse incidents in diagnostic and therapeutic use
Y83-Y84 Surgical and other medical procedures as the cause of abnormal reaction of the patient, or of later complication, without mention of misadventure at the time of the procedure
Y9Ø-Y99 Supplementary factors related to causes of morbidity classified elsewhere

ACCIDENTS (VØØ-X58)

AHA: 2018,2Q,7-8

Transport accidents (VØØ-V99)

NOTE This section is structured in 12 groups. Those relating to land transport accidents (VØØ-V89) reflect the victim's mode of transport and are subdivided to identify the victim's 'counterpart' or the type of event. The vehicle of which the injured person is an occupant is identified in the first two characters since it is seen as the most important factor to identify for prevention purposes. A transport accident is one in which the vehicle involved must be moving or running or in use for transport purposes at the time of the accident.

Use additional code to identify:
airbag injury (W22.1)
type of street or road (Y92.4-)
use of cellular telephone and other electronic equipment at the time of the transport accident (Y93.C-)

EXCLUDES 1 *agricultural vehicles in stationary use or maintenance (W31.-)*
assault by crashing of motor vehicle (YØ3.-)
automobile or motor cycle in stationary use or maintenance - code to type of accident
crashing of motor vehicle, undetermined intent (Y32)
intentional self-harm by crashing of motor vehicle (X82)

EXCLUDES 2 *transport accidents due to cataclysm (X34-X38)*

NOTE Definitions related to transport accidents:

(a) A transport accident (VØØ-V99) is any accident involving a device designed primarily for, or used at the time primarily for, conveying persons or good from one place to another.

(b) A public highway [trafficway] or street is the entire width between property lines (or other boundary lines) of land open to the public as a matter of right or custom for purposes of moving persons or property from one place to another. A roadway is that part of the public highway designed, improved and customarily used for vehicular traffic.

(c) A traffic accident is any vehicle accident occurring on the public highway [i.e. originating on, terminating on, or involving a vehicle partially on the highway]. A vehicle accident is assumed to have occurred on the public highway unless another place is specified, except in the case of accidents involving only off-road motor vehicles, which are classified as nontraffic accidents unless the contrary is stated.

(d) A nontraffic accident is any vehicle accident that occurs entirely in any place other than a public highway.

(e) A pedestrian is any person involved in an accident who was not at the time of the accident riding in or on a motor vehicle, railway train, streetcar or animal-drawn or other vehicle, or on a pedal cycle or animal. This includes, a person changing a tire, working on a parked car, or a person on foot. It also includes the user of a pedestrian conveyance such as a baby stroller, ice-skates, skis, sled, roller skates, a skateboard, nonmotorized or motorized wheelchair, motorized mobility scooter, or nonmotorized scooter.

(f) A driver is an occupant of a transport vehicle who is operating or intending to operate it.

(g) A passenger is any occupant of a transport vehicle other than the driver, except a person traveling on the outside of the vehicle.

(h) A person on the outside of a vehicle is any person being transported by a vehicle but not occupying the space normally reserved for the driver or passengers, or the space intended for the transport of property. This includes a person travelling on the bodywork, bumper, fender, roof, running board or step of a vehicle, as well as, hanging on the outside of the vehicle.

(i) A pedal cycle is any land transport vehicle operated solely by nonmotorized pedals including a bicycle or tricycle.

(j) A pedal cyclist is any person riding a pedal cycle or in a sidecar or trailer attached to a pedal cycle.

(k) A motorcycle is a two-wheeled motor vehicle with one or two riding saddles and sometimes with a third wheel for the support of a sidecar. The sidecar is considered part of the motorcycle. This includes a moped, motor scooter, or motorized bicycle.

(l) A motorcycle rider is any person riding a motorcycle or in a sidecar or trailer attached to the motorcycle.

(m) A three-wheeled motor vehicle is a motorized tricycle designed primarily for on-road use. This includes a motor-driven tricycle, a motorized rickshaw, or a three-wheeled motor car.

(n) A car [automobile] is a four-wheeled motor vehicle designed primarily for carrying up to 7 persons. A trailer being towed by the car is considered part of the car. It does not include a van or minivan — see definition (o).

(o) A pick-up truck or van is a four or six-wheeled motor vehicle designed for carrying passengers as well as property or cargo weighing less than the local limit for classification as a heavy goods vehicle, and not requiring a special driver's license. This includes a minivan and a sport-utility vehicle (SUV).

(p) A heavy transport vehicle is a motor vehicle designed primarily for carrying property, meeting local criteria for classification as a heavy goods vehicle in terms of weight and requiring a special driver's license.

(q) A bus (coach) is a motor vehicle designed or adapted primarily for carrying more than 1Ø passengers, and requiring a special driver's license.

(r) A railway train or railway vehicle is any device, with or without freight or passenger cars couple to it, designed for traffic on a railway track. This includes subterranean (subways) or elevated trains.

(s) A streetcar, is a device designed and used primarily for transporting passengers within a municipality, running on rails, usually subject to normal traffic control signals, and operated principally on a right-of-way that forms part of the roadway. This includes a tram or trolley that runs on rails. A trailer being towed by a streetcar is considered part of the streetcar.

(t) A special vehicle mainly used on industrial premises is a motor vehicle designed primarily for use within the buildings and premises of industrial or commercial establishments. This includes battery-powered airport passenger vehicles or baggage/mail trucks, forklifts, coal-cars in a coal mine, logging cars and trucks used in mines or quarries.

(u) A special vehicle mainly used in agriculture is a motor vehicle designed specifically for use in farming and agriculture (horticulture), to work the land, tend and harvest crops and transport materials on the farm. This includes harvesters, farm machinery and tractor and trailers.

(v) A special construction vehicle is a motor vehicle designed specifically for use on construction and demolition sites. This includes bulldozers, diggers, earth levellers, dump trucks, backhoes, front-end loaders, pavers, and mechanical shovels.

(w) A special all-terrain vehicle is a motor vehicle of special design to enable it to negotiate over rough or soft terrain, snow or sand. Examples of special design are high construction, special wheels and tires, tracks, and support on a cushion of air. This includes snow mobiles, All-terrain vehicles (ATV), and dune buggies. It does not include passenger vehicle designated as Sport Utility Vehicles. (SUV)

(x) A watercraft is any device designed for transporting passengers or goods on water. This includes motor or sailboats, ships, and hovercraft.

(y) An aircraft is any device for transporting passengers or goods in the air. This includes hot-air balloons, gliders, helicopters and airplanes.

(z) A military vehicle is any motorized vehicle operating on a public roadway owned by the military and being operated by a member of the military.

Pedestrian injured in transport accident (VØØ-VØ9)

INCLUDES person changing tire on transport vehicle
person examining engine of vehicle broken down in (on side of) road

EXCLUDES 1 *fall due to non-transport collision with other person (WØ3)*
pedestrian on foot falling (slipping) on ice and snow (WØØ.-)
struck or bumped by another person (W51)

The appropriate 7th character is to be added to each code from categories VØØ-VØ9.
A initial encounter
D subsequent encounter
S sequela

4th VØØ Pedestrian conveyance accident

Use additional place of occurrence and activity external cause codes, if known (Y92.-, Y93.-)

EXCLUDES 1 *collision with another person without fall (W51)*
fall due to person on foot colliding with another person on foot (WØ3)
fall from non-moving wheelchair, nonmotorized scooter and motorized mobility scooter without collision (WØ5.-)
pedestrian (conveyance) collision with other land transport vehicle (VØ1-VØ9)
pedestrian on foot falling (slipping) on ice and snow (WØØ.-)

5th VØØ.Ø Pedestrian on foot injured in collision with pedestrian conveyance

x7th VØØ.Ø1 Pedestrian on foot injured in collision with roller-skater

x7th VØØ.Ø2 Pedestrian on foot injured in collision with skateboarder

6th VØØ.Ø3 Pedestrian on foot injured in collision with standing micro-mobility pedestrian conveyance

7th VØØ.Ø31 Pedestrian on foot injured in collision with rider of standing electric scooter

7th VØØ.Ø38 Pedestrian on foot injured in collision with rider of other standing micro-mobility pedestrian conveyance

Pedestrian on foot injured in collision with rider of hoverboard
Pedestrian on foot injured in collision with rider of segway

x7th VØØ.Ø9 Pedestrian on foot injured in collision with other pedestrian conveyance

5th VØØ.1 Rolling-type pedestrian conveyance accident

EXCLUDES 1 *accident with baby stroller (VØØ.82-)*
accident with motorized mobility scooter (VØØ.83-)
accident with wheelchair (powered) (VØØ.81-)

6th VØØ.11 In-line roller-skate accident

7th VØØ.111 Fall from in-line roller-skates

7th VØØ.112 In-line roller-skater colliding with stationary object

7th VØØ.118 Other in-line roller-skate accident

EXCLUDES 1 *roller-skater collision with other land transport vehicle (VØ1-VØ9 with 5th character 1)*

6th VØØ.12 Non-in-line roller-skate accident

7th VØØ.121 Fall from non-in-line roller-skates

7th VØØ.122 Non-in-line roller-skater colliding with stationary object

7th VØØ.128 Other non-in-line roller-skating accident

EXCLUDES 1 *roller-skater collision with other land transport vehicle (VØ1-VØ9 with 5th character 1)*

6th VØØ.13 Skateboard accident

7th VØØ.131 Fall from skateboard

7th VØØ.132 Skateboarder colliding with stationary object

7th VØØ.138 Other skateboard accident

EXCLUDES 1 *skateboarder collision with other land transport vehicle (VØ1-VØ9 with 5th character 2)*

6th VØØ.14 Scooter (nonmotorized) accident

EXCLUDES 1 *motor scooter accident (V2Ø-V29)*

7th VØØ.141 Fall from scooter (nonmotorized)

7th VØØ.142 Scooter (nonmotorized) colliding with stationary object

7th VØØ.148 Other scooter (nonmotorized) accident

EXCLUDES 1 *scooter (nonmotorized) collision with other land transport vehicle (VØ1-VØ9 with fifth character 9)*

6th VØØ.15 Heelies accident

Rolling shoe
Wheeled shoe
Wheelies accident

7th VØØ.151 Fall from heelies

7th VØØ.152 Heelies colliding with stationary object

7th VØØ.158 Other heelies accident

6th VØØ.18 Accident on other rolling-type pedestrian conveyance

7th VØØ.181 Fall from other rolling-type pedestrian conveyance

7th VØØ.182 Pedestrian on other rolling-type pedestrian conveyance colliding with stationary object

7th VØØ.188 Other accident on other rolling-type pedestrian conveyance

5th VØØ.2 Gliding-type pedestrian conveyance accident

6th VØØ.21 Ice-skates accident

7th VØØ.211 Fall from ice-skates

7th VØØ.212 Ice-skater colliding with stationary object

7th VØØ.218 Other ice-skates accident

EXCLUDES 1 *ice-skater collision with other land transport vehicle (VØ1-VØ9 with 5th character 9)*

6th VØØ.22 Sled accident

7th VØØ.221 Fall from sled

7th VØØ.222 Sledder colliding with stationary object

7th VØØ.228 Other sled accident

EXCLUDES 1 *sled collision with other land transport vehicle (VØ1-VØ9 with 5th character 9)*

6th VØØ.28 Other gliding-type pedestrian conveyance accident

7th VØØ.281 Fall from other gliding-type pedestrian conveyance

7th VØØ.282 Pedestrian on other gliding-type pedestrian conveyance colliding with stationary object

7th **V00.288 Other accident on other gliding-type pedestrian conveyance**
EXCLUDES 1 *gliding-type pedestrian conveyance collision with other land transport vehicle (V01-V09 with 5th character 9)*

5th **V00.3 Flat-bottomed pedestrian conveyance accident**

6th **V00.31 Snowboard accident**

7th **V00.311 Fall from snowboard**

7th **V00.312 Snowboarder colliding with stationary object**

7th **V00.318 Other snowboard accident**
EXCLUDES 1 *snowboarder collision with other land transport vehicle (V01-V09 with 5th character 9)*

6th **V00.32 Snow-ski accident**

7th **V00.321 Fall from snow-skis**

7th **V00.322 Snow-skier colliding with stationary object**

7th **V00.328 Other snow-ski accident**
EXCLUDES 1 *snow-skier collision with other land transport vehicle (V01-V09 with 5th character 9)*

6th **V00.38 Other flat-bottomed pedestrian conveyance accident**

7th **V00.381 Fall from other flat-bottomed pedestrian conveyance**

7th **V00.382 Pedestrian on other flat-bottomed pedestrian conveyance colliding with stationary object**

7th **V00.388 Other accident on other flat-bottomed pedestrian conveyance**

5th **V00.8 Accident on other pedestrian conveyance**

6th **V00.81 Accident with wheelchair (powered)**

7th **V00.811 Fall from moving wheelchair (powered)**
EXCLUDES 1 *fall from non-moving wheelchair (W05.0)*

7th **V00.812 Wheelchair (powered) colliding with stationary object**

7th **V00.818 Other accident with wheelchair (powered)**

6th **V00.82 Accident with baby stroller**

7th **V00.821 Fall from baby stroller**

7th **V00.822 Baby stroller colliding with stationary object**

7th **V00.828 Other accident with baby stroller**

6th **V00.83 Accident with motorized mobility scooter**

7th **V00.831 Fall from motorized mobility scooter**
EXCLUDES 1 *fall from non-moving motorized mobility scooter (W05.2)*

7th **V00.832 Motorized mobility scooter colliding with stationary object**

7th **V00.838 Other accident with motorized mobility scooter**

6th **V00.84 Accident with standing micro-mobility pedestrian conveyance**

7th **V00.841 Fall from standing electric scooter**

7th **V00.842 Pedestrian on standing electric scooter colliding with stationary object**

7th **V00.848 Other accident with standing micro-mobility pedestrian conveyance**
Accident with hoverboard
Accident with segway

6th **V00.89 Accident on other pedestrian conveyance**

7th **V00.891 Fall from other pedestrian conveyance**

7th **V00.892 Pedestrian on other pedestrian conveyance colliding with stationary object**

7th **V00.898 Other accident on other pedestrian conveyance**
EXCLUDES 1 *other pedestrian (conveyance) collision with other land transport vehicle (V01-V09 with 5th character 9)*

4th **V01 Pedestrian injured in collision with pedal cycle**

5th **V01.0 Pedestrian injured in collision with pedal cycle in nontraffic accident**

x7th **V01.00 Pedestrian on foot injured in collision with pedal cycle in nontraffic accident**
Pedestrian NOS injured in collision with pedal cycle in nontraffic accident

x7th **V01.01 Pedestrian on roller-skates injured in collision with pedal cycle in nontraffic accident**

x7th **V01.02 Pedestrian on skateboard injured in collision with pedal cycle in nontraffic accident**

6th **V01.03 Pedestrian on standing micro-mobility pedestrian conveyance injured in collision with pedal cycle in nontraffic accident**

7th **V01.031 Pedestrian on standing electric scooter injured in collision with pedal cycle in nontraffic accident**

7th **V01.038 Pedestrian on other standing micro-mobility pedestrian conveyance injured in collision with pedal cycle in nontraffic accident**
Pedestrian on hoverboard injured in collision with pedal cycle in nontraffic accident
Pedestrian on segway injured in collision with pedal cycle in nontraffic accident

x7th **V01.09 Pedestrian with other conveyance injured in collision with pedal cycle in nontraffic accident**
Pedestrian with baby stroller injured in collision with pedal cycle in nontraffic accident
Pedestrian on ice-skates injured in collision with pedal cycle in nontraffic accident
Pedestrian on nonmotorized scooter injured in collision with pedal cycle in nontraffic accident
Pedestrian on sled injured in collision with pedal cycle in nontraffic accident
Pedestrian on snowboard injured in collision with pedal cycle in nontraffic accident
Pedestrian on snow-skis injured in collision with pedal cycle in nontraffic accident
Pedestrian in wheelchair (powered) injured in collision with pedal cycle in nontraffic accident
Pedestrian in motorized mobility scooter injured in collision with pedal cycle in nontraffic accident

5th **V01.1 Pedestrian injured in collision with pedal cycle in traffic accident**

x7th **V01.10 Pedestrian on foot injured in collision with pedal cycle in traffic accident**
Pedestrian NOS injured in collision with pedal cycle in traffic accident

x7th **V01.11 Pedestrian on roller-skates injured in collision with pedal cycle in traffic accident**

x7th **V01.12 Pedestrian on skateboard injured in collision with pedal cycle in traffic accident**

6th **V01.13 Pedestrian on standing micro-mobility pedestrian conveyance injured in collision with pedal cycle in traffic accident**

7th **V01.131 Pedestrian on standing electric scooter injured in collision with pedal cycle in traffic accident**

7th **V01.138 Pedestrian on other standing micro-mobility pedestrian conveyance injured in collision with pedal cycle in traffic accident**
Pedestrian on hoverboard injured in collision with pedal cycle in traffic accident
Pedestrian on segway injured in collision with pedal cycle in traffic accident

V01.19 Pedestrian with other conveyance injured in collision with pedal cycle in traffic accident
Pedestrian with baby stroller injured in collision with pedal cycle in traffic accident
Pedestrian on ice-skates injured in collision with pedal cycle in traffic accident
Pedestrian on nonmotorized scooter injured in collision with pedal cycle in traffic accident
Pedestrian on sled injured in collision with pedal cycle in traffic accident
Pedestrian on snowboard injured in collision with pedal cycle in traffic accident
Pedestrian on snow-skis injured in collision with pedal cycle in traffic accident
Pedestrian in wheelchair (powered) injured in collision with pedal cycle in traffic accident
Pedestrian in motorized mobility scooter injured in collision with pedal cycle in traffic accident

V01.9 Pedestrian injured in collision with pedal cycle, unspecified whether traffic or nontraffic accident

V01.90 Pedestrian on foot injured in collision with pedal cycle, unspecified whether traffic or nontraffic accident
Pedestrian NOS injured in collision with pedal cycle, unspecified whether traffic or nontraffic accident

V01.91 Pedestrian on roller-skates injured in collision with pedal cycle, unspecified whether traffic or nontraffic accident

V01.92 Pedestrian on skateboard injured in collision with pedal cycle, unspecified whether traffic or nontraffic accident

V01.93 Pedestrian on standing micro-mobility pedestrian conveyance injured in collision with pedal cycle, unspecified whether traffic or nontraffic accident

V01.931 Pedestrian on standing electric scooter injured in collision with pedal cycle, unspecified whether traffic or nontraffic accident

V01.938 Pedestrian on other standing micro-mobility pedestrian conveyance injured in collision with pedal cycle, unspecified whether traffic or nontraffic accident
Pedestrian on hoverboard injured in collision with pedal cycle, unspecified whether traffic or nontraffic accident
Pedestrian on segway injured in collision with pedal cycle, unspecified whether traffic or nontraffic accident

V01.99 Pedestrian with other conveyance injured in collision with pedal cycle, unspecified whether traffic or nontraffic accident
Pedestrian with baby stroller injured in collision with pedal cycle, unspecified whether traffic or nontraffic accident
Pedestrian on ice-skates injured in collision with pedal cycle unspecified, whether traffic or nontraffic accident
Pedestrian on nonmotorized scooter injured in collision with pedal cycle, unspecified whether traffic or nontraffic accident
Pedestrian onsled injured in collision with pedal cycle unspecified, whether traffic or nontraffic accident
Pedestrian on snowboard injured in collision with pedal cycle, unspecified whether traffic or nontraffic accident
Pedestrian on snow-skis injured in collision with pedal cycle, unspecified whether traffic or nontraffic accident
Pedestrian in wheelchair (powered) injured in collision with pedal cycle, unspecified whether traffic or nontraffic accident
Pedestrian in motorized mobility scooter injured in collision with pedal cycle, unspecified whether traffic or nontraffic accident

V02 Pedestrian injured in collision with two- or three-wheeled motor vehicle

V02.0 Pedestrian injured in collision with two- or three-wheeled motor vehicle in nontraffic accident

V02.00 Pedestrian on foot injured in collision with two- or three-wheeled motor vehicle in nontraffic accident
Pedestrian NOS injured in collision with two- or three-wheeled motor vehicle in nontraffic accident

V02.01 Pedestrian on roller-skates injured in collision with two- or three-wheeled motor vehicle in nontraffic accident

V02.02 Pedestrian on skateboard injured in collision with two- or three-wheeled motor vehicle in nontraffic accident

V02.03 Pedestrian on standing micro-mobility pedestrian conveyance injured in collision with two- or three-wheeled motor vehicle in nontraffic accident

V02.031 Pedestrian on standing electric scooter injured in collision with two- or three-wheeled motor vehicle in nontraffic accident

V02.038 Pedestrian on other standing micro-mobility pedestrian conveyance injured in collision with two- or three-wheeled motor vehicle in nontraffic accident
Pedestrian on hoverboard injured in collision with two-or three wheeled motor vehicle in nontraffic accident
Pedestrian on segway injured in collision with two- or three-wheeled motor vehicle in nontraffic accident

V02.09 Pedestrian with other conveyance injured in collision with two- or three-wheeled motor vehicle in nontraffic accident
Pedestrian with baby stroller injured in collision with two- or three-wheeled motor vehicle in nontraffic accident
Pedestrian on ice-skates injured in collision with two- or three-wheeled motor vehicle in nontraffic accident
Pedestrian on nonmotorized scooter injured in collision with two- or three-wheeled motor vehicle in nontraffic accident
Pedestrian on sled injured in collision with two- or three-wheeled motor vehicle in nontraffic accident
Pedestrian on snowboard injured in collision with two- or three-wheeled motor vehicle in nontraffic accident
Pedestrian on snow-skis injured in collision with two- or three-wheeled motor vehicle in nontraffic accident
Pedestrian in wheelchair (powered) injured in collision with two- or three-wheeled motor vehicle in nontraffic accident
Pedestrian in motorized mobility scooter injured in collision with two- or three-wheeled motor vehicle in nontraffic accident

V02.1 Pedestrian injured in collision with two- or three-wheeled motor vehicle in traffic accident

V02.10 Pedestrian on foot injured in collision with two- or three-wheeled motor vehicle in traffic accident
Pedestrian NOS injured in collision with two- or three-wheeled motor vehicle in traffic accident

V02.11 Pedestrian on roller-skates injured in collision with two- or three-wheeled motor vehicle in traffic accident

V02.12 Pedestrian on skateboard injured in collision with two- or three-wheeled motor vehicle in traffic accident

V02.13 Pedestrian on standing micro-mobility pedestrian conveyance injured in collision with two- or three-wheeled motor vehicle in traffic accident

V02.131 Pedestrian on standing electric scooter injured in collision with two- or three-wheeled motor vehicle in traffic accident

√7th **V02.138 Pedestrian on other standing micro-mobility pedestrian conveyance injured in collision with two- or three-wheeled motor vehicle in traffic accident**

Pedestrian on hoverboard injured in collision with two-or three wheeled motor vehicle in traffic accident

Pedestrian on segway injured in collision with two- or three-wheeled motor vehicle in traffic accident

√x7th **V02.19 Pedestrian with other conveyance injured in collision with two- or three-wheeled motor vehicle in traffic accident**

Pedestrian with baby stroller injured in collision with two- or three-wheeled motor vehicle in traffic accident

Pedestrian on ice-skates injured in collision with two- or three-wheeled motor vehicle in traffic accident

Pedestrian on nonmotorized scooter injured in collision with two- or three-wheeled motor vehicle in traffic accident

Pedestrian on sled injured in collision with two- or three-wheeled motor vehicle in traffic accident

Pedestrian on snowboard injured in collision with two- or three-wheeled motor vehicle in traffic accident

Pedestrian on snow-skis injured in collision with two- or three-wheeled motor vehicle in traffic accident

Pedestrian in wheelchair (powered) injured in collision with two- or three-wheeled motor vehicle in traffic accident

Pedestrian in motorized mobility scooter injued in collision with two- or three-wheeled motor vehicle in traffic accident

√5th **V02.9 Pedestrian injured in collision with two- or three-wheeled motor vehicle, unspecified whether traffic or nontraffic accident**

√x7th **V02.90 Pedestrian on foot injured in collision with two- or three-wheeled motor vehicle, unspecified whether traffic or nontraffic accident**

Pedestrian NOS injured in collision with two- or three-wheeled motor vehicle, unspecified whether traffic or nontraffic accident

√x7th **V02.91 Pedestrian on roller-skates injured in collision with two- or three-wheeled motor vehicle, unspecified whether traffic or nontraffic accident**

√x7th **V02.92 Pedestrian on skateboard injured in collision with two- or three-wheeled motor vehicle, unspecified whether traffic or nontraffic accident**

√6th **V02.93 Pedestrian on standing micro-mobility pedestrian conveyance injured in collision with two- or three-wheeled motor vehicle, unspecified whether traffic or nontraffic accident**

√7th **V02.931 Pedestrian on standing electric scooter injured in collision with two- or three wheeled motor vehicle, unspecified whether traffic or nontraffic accident**

√7th **V02.938 Pedestrian on other standing micro-mobility pedestrian conveyance injured in collision with two- or three wheeled motor vehicle, unspecified whether traffic or nontraffic accident**

Pedestrian on hoverboard injured in collision with two-three-wheeled motor vehicle, unspecified whether traffic or nontraffic accident

Pedestrian on segway injured in collision with two- or three wheeled motor vehicle, unspecified whether traffic or nontraffic accident

√x7th **V02.99 Pedestrian with other conveyance injured in collision with two- or three-wheeled motor vehicle, unspecified whether traffic or nontraffic accident**

Pedestrian with baby stroller injured in collision with two- or three-wheeled motor vehicle, unspecified whether traffic or nontraffic accident

Pedestrian on ice-skates injured in collision with two- or three-wheeled motor vehicle, unspecified whether traffic or nontraffic accident

Pedestrian on nonmotorized scooter injured in collision with two- or three-wheeled motor vehicle, unspecified whether traffic or nontraffic accident

Pedestrian on sled injured in collision with two- or three-wheeled motor vehicle, unspecified whether traffic or nontraffic accident

Pedestrian on snowboard injured in collision with two- or three-wheeled motor vehicle, unspecified whether traffic or nontraffic accident

Pedestrian on snow-skis injured in collision with two- or three-wheeled motor vehicle, unspecified whether traffic or nontraffic accident

Pedestrian in wheelchair (powered) injured in collision with two- or three-wheeled motor vehicle, unspecified whether traffic or nontraffic accident

Pedestrian in motorized mobility scooter injured in collision with two- or three wheeled motor vehicle, unspecified whether traffic or nontraffic accident

√4th **V03 Pedestrian injured in collision with car, pick-up truck or van**

√5th **V03.0 Pedestrian injured in collision with car, pick-up truck or van in nontraffic accident**

√x7th **V03.00 Pedestrian on foot injured in collision with car, pick-up truck or van in nontraffic accident**

Pedestrian NOS injured in collision with car, pick-up truck or van in nontraffic accident

√x7th **V03.01 Pedestrian on roller-skates injured in collision with car, pick-up truck or van in nontraffic accident**

√x7th **V03.02 Pedestrian on skateboard injured in collision with car, pick-up truck or van in nontraffic accident**

√6th **V03.03 Pedestrian on standing micro-mobility pedestrian conveyance injured in collision with car, pick-up or van in nontraffic accident**

√7th **V03.031 Pedestrian on standing electric scooter injured in collision with car, pick-up or van in nontraffic accident**

√7th **V03.038 Pedestrian on other standing micro-mobility pedestrian conveyance injured in collision with car, pick-up or van in nontraffic accident**

Pedestrian on hoverboard injured in collision with car, pick-up or van in nontraffic accident

Pedestrian on segway injured in collision with car, pick-up or van in nontraffic accident

√x7th **V03.09 Pedestrian with other conveyance injured in collision with car, pick-up truck or van in nontraffic accident**

Pedestrian with baby stroller injured in collision with car, pick-up truck or van in nontraffic accident

Pedestrian on ice-skates injured in collision with car, pick-up truck or van in nontraffic accident

Pedestrian on nonmotorized scooter injured in collision with car, pick-up truck or van in nontraffic accident

Pedestrian on sled injured in collision with car, pick-up truck or van in nontraffic accident

Pedestrian on snowboard injured in collision with car, pick-up truck or van in nontraffic accident

Pedestrian on snow-skis injured in collision with car, pick-up truck or van in nontraffic accident

Pedestrian in wheelchair (powered) injured in collision with car, pick-up truck or van in nontraffic accident

Pedestrian in motorized mobility scooter injured in collision with car, pick-up truck or van in nontraffic accident

√5th **V03.1 Pedestrian injured in collision with car, pick-up truck or van in traffic accident**

√x7th **V03.10 Pedestrian on foot injured in collision with car, pick-up truck or van in traffic accident**
Pedestrian NOS injured in collision with car, pick-up truck or van in traffic accident

√x7th **V03.11 Pedestrian on roller-skates injured in collision with car, pick-up truck or van in traffic accident**

√x7th **V03.12 Pedestrian on skateboard injured in collision with car, pick-up truck or van in traffic accident**

√6th **V03.13 Pedestrian on standing micro-mobility pedestrian conveyance injured in collision with car, pick-up or van in traffic accident**

√7th **V03.131 Pedestrian on standing electric scooter injured in collision with car, pick-up or van in traffic accident**

√7th **V03.138 Pedestrian on other standing micro-mobility pedestrian conveyance injured in collision with car, pick-up or van in traffic accident**
Pedestrian on hoverboard injured in collision with car, pick-up or van in traffic accident
Pedestrian on segway injured in collision with car, pick-up or van in traffic accident

√x7th **V03.19 Pedestrian with other conveyance injured in collision with car, pick-up truck or van in traffic accident**
Pedestrian with baby stroller injured in collision with car, pick-up truck or van in traffic accident
Pedestrian on ice-skates injured in collision with car, pick-up truck or van in traffic accident
Pedestrian on nonmotorized scooter injured in collision with car, pick-up truck or van in nontraffic accident
Pedestrian on sled injured in collision with car, pick-up truck or van in traffic accident
Pedestrian on snowboard injured in collision with car, pick-up truck or van in traffic accident
Pedestrian on snow-skis injured in collision with car, pick-up truck or van in traffic accident
Pedestrian in wheelchair (powered) injured in collision with car, pick-up truck or van in traffic accident
Pedestrian in motorized mobility scooter injured in collision with car, pick-up truck or van in nontraffic accident

√5th **V03.9 Pedestrian injured in collision with car, pick-up truck or van, unspecified whether traffic or nontraffic accident**

√x7th **V03.90 Pedestrian on foot injured in collision with car, pick-up truck or van, unspecified whether traffic or nontraffic accident**
Pedestrian NOS injured in collision with car, pick-up truck or van, unspecified whether traffic or nontraffic accident

√x7th **V03.91 Pedestrian on roller-skates injured in collision with car, pick-up truck or van, unspecified whether traffic or nontraffic accident**

√x7th **V03.92 Pedestrian on skateboard injured in collision with car, pick-up truck or van, unspecified whether traffic or nontraffic accident**

√6th **V03.93 Pedestrian on standing micro-mobility pedestrian conveyance injured in collision with car, pick-up or van, unspecified whether traffic or nontraffic accident**

√7th **V03.931 Pedestrian on standing electric scooter injured in collision with car, pick-up or van, unspecified whether traffic or nontraffic accident**

√7th **V03.938 Pedestrian on other standing micro-mobility pedestrian conveyance injured in collision with car, pick-up or van, unspecified whether traffic or nontraffic accident**
Pedestrian on hoverboard injured in collision with car, pick-up or van, unspecified whether traffic or nontraffic accident
Pedestrian on segway injured in collision with car, pick-up or van, unspecified whether traffic or nontraffic accident

√x7th **V03.99 Pedestrian with other conveyance injured in collision with car, pick-up truck or van, unspecified whether traffic or nontraffic accident**
Pedestrian with baby stroller injured in collision with car, pick-up truck or van, unspecified whether traffic or nontraffic accident
Pedestrian on ice-skates injured in collision with car, pick-up truck or van, unspecified whether traffic or nontraffic accident
Pedestrian on nonmotorized scooter injured in collision with car, pick-up truck or van, unspecified whether traffic or nontraffic accident
Pedestrian on sled injured in collision with car, pick-up truck or van in nontraffic accident
Pedestrian on snowboard injured in collision with car, pick-up truck or van, unspecified whether traffic or nontraffic accident
Pedestrian on snow-skis injured in collision with car, pick-up truck or van, unspecified whether traffic or nontraffic accident
Pedestrian in wheelchair (powered) injured in collision with car, pick-up truck or van, unspecified whether traffic or nontraffic accident
Pedestrian in motorized mobility scooter injured in collision with car, pick-up truck or van, unspecified whether traffic or nontraffic accident

√4th **V04 Pedestrian injured in collision with heavy transport vehicle or bus**

EXCLUDES 1 *pedestrian injured in collision with military vehicle (V09.01, V09.21)*

√5th **V04.0 Pedestrian injured in collision with heavy transport vehicle or bus in nontraffic accident**

√x7th **V04.00 Pedestrian on foot injured in collision with heavy transport vehicle or bus in nontraffic accident**
Pedestrian NOS injured in collision with heavy transport vehicle or bus in nontraffic accident

√x7th **V04.01 Pedestrian on roller-skates injured in collision with heavy transport vehicle or bus in nontraffic accident**

√x7th **V04.02 Pedestrian on skateboard injured in collision with heavy transport vehicle or bus in nontraffic accident**

√6th **V04.03 Pedestrian on standing micro-mobility pedestrian conveyance injured in collision with heavy transport vehicle or bus in nontraffic accident**

√7th **V04.031 Pedestrian on standing electric scooter injured in collision with heavy transport vehicle or bus in nontraffic accident**

√7th **V04.038 Pedestrian on other standing micro-mobility pedestrian conveyance injured in collision with heavy transport vehicle or bus in nontraffic accident**
Pedestrian on hoverboard injured in collision with heavy transport vehicle or bus in nontraffic accident
Pedestrian on segway injured in collision with heavy transport vehicle or bus in nontraffic accident

V04.09 Pedestrian with other conveyance injured in collision with heavy transport vehicle or bus in nontraffic accident
Pedestrian with baby stroller injured in collision with heavy transport vehicle or bus in nontraffic accident
Pedestrian on ice-skates injured in collision with heavy transport vehicle or bus in nontraffic accident
Pedestrian on nonmotorized scooter injured in collision with heavy transport vehicle or bus in nontraffic accident
Pedestrian on sled injured in collision with heavy transport vehicle or bus in nontraffic accident
Pedestrian on snowboard injured in collision with heavy transport vehicle or bus in nontraffic accident
Pedestrian on snow-skis injured in collision with heavy transport vehicle or bus in nontraffic accident
Pedestrian in wheelchair (powered) injured in collision with heavy transport vehicle or bus in nontraffic accident
Pedestrian in motorized mobility scooter injured in collision with heavy transport vehicle or bus in nontraffic accident

V04.1 Pedestrian injured in collision with heavy transport vehicle or bus in traffic accident

V04.10 Pedestrian on foot injured in collision with heavy transport vehicle or bus in traffic accident
Pedestrian NOS injured in collision with heavy transport vehicle or bus in traffic accident

V04.11 Pedestrian on roller-skates injured in collision with heavy transport vehicle or bus in traffic accident

V04.12 Pedestrian on skateboard injured in collision with heavy transport vehicle or bus in traffic accident

V04.13 Pedestrian on standing micro-mobility pedestrian conveyance injured in collision with heavy transport vehicle or bus in traffic accident

V04.131 Pedestrian on standing electric scooter injured in collision with heavy transport vehicle or bus in traffic accident

V04.138 Pedestrian on other standing micro-mobility pedestrian conveyance injured in collision with heavy transport vehicle or bus in traffic accident
Pedestrian on hoverboard injured in collision with heavy transport vehicle or bus in traffic accident
Pedestrian on segway injured in collision with heavy transport vehicle or bus in traffic accident

V04.19 Pedestrian with other conveyance injured in collision with heavy transport vehicle or bus in traffic accident
Pedestrian with baby stroller injured in collision with heavy transport vehicle or bus in traffic accident
Pedestrian on ice-skates injured in collision with heavy transport vehicle or bus in traffic accident
Pedestrian on nonmotorized scooter injured in collision with heavy transport vehicle or bus in traffic accident
Pedestrian on sled injured in collision with heavy transport vehicle or bus in traffic accident
Pedestrian on snowboard injured in collision with heavy transport vehicle or bus in traffic accident
Pedestrian on snow-skis injured in collision with heavy transport vehicle or bus in traffic accident
Pedestrian in wheelchair (powered) injured in collision with heavy transport vehicle or bus in traffic accident
Pedestrian in motorized mobility scooter injured in collision with heavy transport vehicle or bus in traffic accident

V04.9 Pedestrian injured in collision with heavy transport vehicle or bus, unspecified whether traffic or nontraffic accident

V04.90 Pedestrian on foot injured in collision with heavy transport vehicle or bus, unspecified whether traffic or nontraffic accident
Pedestrian NOS injured in collision with heavy transport vehicle or bus, unspecified whether traffic or nontraffic accident

V04.91 Pedestrian on roller-skates injured in collision with heavy transport vehicle or bus, unspecified whether traffic or nontraffic accident

V04.92 Pedestrian on skateboard injured in collision with heavy transport vehicle or bus, unspecified whether traffic or nontraffic accident

V04.93 Pedestrian on standing micro-mobility pedestrian conveyance injured in collision with heavy transport vehicle or bus, unspecified whether traffic or nontraffic accident

V04.931 Pedestrian on standing electric scooter injured in collision with heavy transport vehicle or bus, unspecified whether traffic or nontraffic accident

V04.938 Pedestrian on other standing micro-mobility pedestrian conveyance injured in collision with heavy transport vehicle or bus, unspecified whether traffic or nontraffic accident
Pedestrian on hoverboard injured in collision with heavy transport vehicle or bus, unspecified whether traffic or nontraffic accident
Pedestrian on segway injured in collision with heavy transport vehicle or bus, unspecified whether traffic or nontraffic accident

V04.99 Pedestrian with other conveyance injured in collision with heavy transport vehicle or bus, unspecified whether traffic or nontraffic accident
Pedestrian with baby stroller injured in collision with heavy transport vehicle or bus, unspecified whether traffic or nontraffic accident
Pedestrian on ice-skates injured in collision with heavy transport vehicle or bus, unspecified whether traffic or nontraffic accident
Pedestrian on nonmotorized scooter injured in collision with heavy transport vehicle or bus, unspecified whether traffic or nontraffic accident
Pedestrian on sled injured in collision with heavy transport vehicle or bus, unspecified whether traffic or nontraffic accident
Pedestrian on snowboard injured in collision with heavy transport vehicle or bus, unspecified whether traffic or nontraffic accident
Pedestrian on snow-skis injured in collision with heavy transport vehicle or bus, unspecified whether traffic or nontraffic accident
Pedestrian in wheelchair (powered) injured in collision with heavy transport vehicle or bus, unspecified whether traffic or nontraffic accident
Pedestrian in motorized mobility scooter injured in collision with heavy transport vehicle or bus, unspecified whether traffic or nontraffic accident

V05 Pedestrian injured in collision with railway train or railway vehicle

V05.0 Pedestrian injured in collision with railway train or railway vehicle in nontraffic accident

V05.00 Pedestrian on foot injured in collision with railway train or railway vehicle in nontraffic accident
Pedestrian NOS injured in collision with railway train or railway vehicle in nontraffic accident

V05.01 Pedestrian on roller-skates injured in collision with railway train or railway vehicle in nontraffic accident

V05.02 Pedestrian on skateboard injured in collision with railway train or railway vehicle in nontraffic accident

V05.03 Pedestrian on standing micro-mobility pedestrian conveyance injured in collision with railway train or railway vehicle in nontraffic accident

V05.031 Pedestrian on standing electric scooter injured in collision with railway train or railway vehicle in nontraffic accident

7th **VØ5.Ø38 Pedestrian on other standing micro-mobility pedestrian conveyance injured in collision with railway train or railway vehicle in nontraffic accident**
Pedestrian on hoverboard injured in collision with railway train or railway vehicle in nontraffic accident
Pedestrian on segway injured in collision with railway train or railway vehicle in nontraffic accident

x7th **VØ5.Ø9 Pedestrian with other conveyance injured in collision with railway train or railway vehicle in nontraffic accident**
Pedestrian with baby stroller injured in collision with railway train or railway vehicle in nontraffic accident
Pedestrian on ice-skates injured in collision with railway train or railway vehicle in nontraffic accident
Pedestrian on nonmotorized scooter injured in collision with railway train or railway vehicle in nontraffic accident
Pedestrian on sled injured in collision with railway train or railway vehicle in nontraffic accident
Pedestrian on snowboard injured in collision with railway train or railway vehicle in nontraffic accident
Pedestrian on snow-skis injured in collision with railway train or railway vehicle in nontraffic accident
Pedestrian in wheelchair (powered) injured in collision with railway train or railway vehicle in nontraffic accident
Pedestrian in motorized mobility scooter injured in collision with railway train or railway vehicle in nontraffic accident

5th **VØ5.1 Pedestrian injured in collision with railway train or railway vehicle in traffic accident**

x7th **VØ5.1Ø Pedestrian on foot injured in collision with railway train or railway vehicle in traffic accident**
Pedestrian NOS injured in collision with railway train or railway vehicle in traffic accident

x7th **VØ5.11 Pedestrian on roller-skates injured in collision with railway train or railway vehicle in traffic accident**

x7th **VØ5.12 Pedestrian on skateboard injured in collision with railway train or railway vehicle in traffic accident**

6th **VØ5.13 Pedestrian on standing micro-mobility pedestrian conveyance injured in collision with railway train or railway vehicle in traffic accident**

7th **VØ5.131 Pedestrian on standing electric scooter injured in collision with railway train or railway vehicle in traffic accident**

7th **VØ5.138 Pedestrian on other standing micro-mobility pedestrian conveyance injured in collision with railway train or railway vehicle in traffic accident**
Pedestrian on hoverboard injured in collision with railway train or railway vehicle in traffic accident
Pedestrian on segway injured in collision with railway train or railway vehicle in traffic accident

x7th **VØ5.19 Pedestrian with other conveyance injured in collision with railway train or railway vehicle in traffic accident**
Pedestrian with baby stroller injured in collision with railway train or railway vehicle in traffic accident
Pedestrian on ice-skates injured in collision with railway train or railway vehicle in traffic accident
Pedestrian on nonmotorized scooter injured in collision with railway train or railway vehicle in traffic accident
Pedestrian on sled injured in collision with railway train or railway vehicle in traffic accident
Pedestrian on snowboard injured in collision with railway train or railway vehicle in traffic accident
Pedestrian on snow-skis injured in collision with railway train or railway vehicle in traffic accident
Pedestrian in wheelchair (powered) injured in collision with railway train or railway vehicle in traffic accident
Pedestrian in motorized mobility scooter injured in collision with railway train or railway vehicle in traffic accident

5th **VØ5.9 Pedestrian injured in collision with railway train or railway vehicle, unspecified whether traffic or nontraffic accident**

x7th **VØ5.9Ø Pedestrian on foot injured in collision with railway train or railway vehicle, unspecified whether traffic or nontraffic accident**
Pedestrian NOS injured in collision with railway train or railway vehicle, unspecified whether traffic or nontraffic accident

x7th **VØ5.91 Pedestrian on roller-skates injured in collision with railway train or railway vehicle, unspecified whether traffic or nontraffic accident**

x7th **VØ5.92 Pedestrian on skateboard injured in collision with railway train or railway vehicle, unspecified whether traffic or nontraffic accident**

6th **VØ5.93 Pedestrian on standing micro-mobility pedestrian conveyance injured in collision with railway train or railway vehicle, unspecified whether traffic or nontraffic accident**

7th **VØ5.931 Pedestrian on standing electric scooter injured in collision with railway train or railway vehicle, unspecified whether traffic or nontraffic accident**

7th **VØ5.938 Pedestrian on other standing micro-mobility pedestrian conveyance injured in collision with railway train or railway vehicle, unspecified whether traffic or nontraffic accident**
Pedestrian on hoverboard injured in collision with railway train or railway vehicle, unspecified whether traffic or nontraffic accident
Pedestrian on segway injured in collision with railway train or railway vehicle, unspecified whether traffic or nontraffic accident

√x7th **VØ5.99 Pedestrian with other conveyance injured in collision with railway train or railway vehicle, unspecified whether traffic or nontraffic accident**
Pedestrian with baby stroller injured in collision with railway train or railway vehicle, unspecified whether traffic or nontraffic
Pedestrian on ice-skates injured in collision with railway train or railway vehicle, unspecified whether traffic or nontraffic
Pedestrian on nonmotorized scooter injured in collision with railway train or railway vehicle, unspecified whether traffic or nontraffic
Pedestrian on sled injured in collision with railway train or railway vehicle, unspecified whether traffic or nontraffic
Pedestrian snowboard injured in collision with railway train or railway vehicle, unspecified whether traffic or nontraffic
Pedestrian on snow-skis injured in collision with railway train or railway vehicle, unspecified whether traffic or nontraffic
Pedestrian in wheelchair (powered) injured in collision with railway train or railway vehicle, unspecified whether traffic or nontraffic
Pedestrian in motorized mobility scooter injured in collision with railway train or railway vehicle, unspecified whether traffic or nontraffic

√4th **VØ6 Pedestrian injured in collision with other nonmotor vehicle**
INCLUDES collision with animal-drawn vehicle, animal being ridden, nonpowered streetcar
EXCLUDES 1 *pedestrian injured in collision with pedestrian conveyance (VØØ.Ø-)*

√5th **VØ6.Ø Pedestrian injured in collision with other nonmotor vehicle in nontraffic accident**

√x7th **VØ6.ØØ Pedestrian on foot injured in collision with other nonmotor vehicle in nontraffic accident**
Pedestrian NOS injured in collision with other nonmotor vehicle in nontraffic accident

√x7th **VØ6.Ø1 Pedestrian on roller-skates injured in collision with other nonmotor vehicle in nontraffic accident**

√x7th **VØ6.Ø2 Pedestrian on skateboard injured in collision with other nonmotor vehicle in nontraffic accident**

√6th **VØ6.Ø3 Pedestrian on standing micro-mobility pedestrian conveyance injured in collision with other nonmotor vehicle in nontraffic accident**

√7th **VØ6.Ø31 Pedestrian on standing electric scooter injured in collision with other nonmotor vehicle in nontraffic accident**

√7th **VØ6.Ø38 Pedestrian on other standing micro-mobility pedestrian conveyance injured in collision with other nonmotor vehicle in nontraffic accident**
Pedestrian on hoverboard injured in collision with other nonmotor vehicle in nontraffic accident
Pedestrian on segway injured in collision with other nonmotor vehicle in nontraffic accident

√x7th **VØ6.Ø9 Pedestrian with other conveyance injured in collision with other nonmotor vehicle in nontraffic accident**
Pedestrian with baby stroller injured in collision with other nonmotor vehicle in nontraffic accident
Pedestrian on ice-skates injured in collision with other nonmotor vehicle in nontraffic accident
Pedestrian on nonmotorized scooter injured in collision with other nonmotor vehicle in nontraffic accident
Pedestrian on sled injured in collision with other nonmotor vehicle in nontraffic accident
Pedestrian on snowboard injured in collision with other nonmotor vehicle in nontraffic accident
Pedestrian on snow-skis injured in collision with other nonmotor vehicle in nontraffic accident
Pedestrian in wheelchair (powered) injured in collision with other nonmotor vehicle in nontraffic accident
Pedestrian in motorized mobility scooter injured in collision with other nonmotor vehicle in nontraffic accident

√5th **VØ6.1 Pedestrian injured in collision with other nonmotor vehicle in traffic accident**

√x7th **VØ6.1Ø Pedestrian on foot injured in collision with other nonmotor vehicle in traffic accident**
Pedestrian NOS injured in collision with other nonmotor vehicle in traffic accident

√x7th **VØ6.11 Pedestrian on roller-skates injured in collision with other nonmotor vehicle in traffic accident**

√x7th **VØ6.12 Pedestrian on skateboard injured in collision with other nonmotor vehicle in traffic accident**

√6th **VØ6.13 Pedestrian on standing micro-mobility pedestrian conveyance injured in collision with other nonmotor vehicle in traffic accident**

√7th **VØ6.131 Pedestrian on standing electric scooter injured in collision with other nonmotor vehicle in traffic accident**

√7th **VØ6.138 Pedestrian on other standing micro-mobility pedestrian conveyance injured in collision with other nonmotor vehicle in traffic accident**
Pedestrian on hoverboard injured in collision with other nonmotor vehicle in traffic accident
Pedestrian on segway injured in collision with other nonmotor vehicle in traffic accident

√x7th **VØ6.19 Pedestrian with other conveyance injured in collision with other nonmotor vehicle in traffic accident**
Pedestrian with baby stroller injured in collision with other nonmotor vehicle in traffic accident
Pedestrian on ice-skates injured in collision with other nonmotor vehicle in traffic accident
Pedestrian on nonmotorized scooter injured in collision with other nonmotor vehicle in traffic accident
Pedestrian on sled injured in collision with other nonmotor vehicle in traffic accident
Pedestrian on snowboard injured in collision with other nonmotor vehicle in traffic accident
Pedestrian on snow-skis injured in collision with other nonmotor vehicle in traffic accident
Pedestrian in wheelchair (powered) injured in collision with other nonmotor vehicle in traffic accident
Pedestrian in motorized mobility scooter injured in collision with other nonmotor vehicle in traffic accident

√5th **VØ6.9 Pedestrian injured in collision with other nonmotor vehicle, unspecified whether traffic or nontraffic accident**

√x7th **VØ6.9Ø Pedestrian on foot injured in collision with other nonmotor vehicle, unspecified whether traffic or nontraffic accident**
Pedestrian NOS injured in collision with other nonmotor vehicle, unspecified whether traffic or nontraffic accident

√x7th **VØ6.91 Pedestrian on roller-skates injured in collision with other nonmotor vehicle, unspecified whether traffic or nontraffic accident**

√7th **V06.92 Pedestrian on skateboard injured in collision with other nonmotor vehicle, unspecified whether traffic or nontraffic accident**

√6th **V06.93 Pedestrian on standing micro-mobility pedestrian conveyance injured in collision with other nonmotor vehicle, unspecified whether traffic or nontraffic accident**

√7th **V06.931 Pedestrian on standing electric scooter injured in collision with other nonmotor vehicle, unspecified whether traffic or nontraffic accident**

√7th **V06.938 Pedestrian on other standing micro-mobility pedestrian conveyance injured in collision with other nonmotor vehicle, unspecified whether traffic or nontraffic accident**

Pedestrian on hoverboard injured in collision with other nonmotor, unspecified whether traffic or nontraffic accident

Pedestrian on segway injured in collision with other nonmotor vehicle, unspecified whether traffic or nontraffic accident

√7th **V06.99 Pedestrian with other conveyance injured in collision with other nonmotor vehicle, unspecified whether traffic or nontraffic accident**

Pedestrian with baby stroller injured in collision with other nonmotor vehicle, unspecified whether traffic or nontraffic accident

Pedestrian on ice-skates injured in collision with other nonmotor vehicle, unspecified whether traffic or nontraffic accident

Pedestrian on nonmotorized scooter injured in collision with other nonmotor vehicle, unspecified whether traffic or nontraffic accident

Pedestrian on sled injured in collision with other nonmotor vehicle, unspecified whether traffic or nontraffic accident

Pedestrian on snowboard injured in collision with other nonmotor vehicle, unspecified whether traffic or nontraffic accident

Pedestrian on snow-skis injured in collision with other nonmotor vehicle, unspecified whether traffic or nontraffic accident

Pedestrian in wheelchair (powered) injured in collision with other nonmotor vehicle, unspecified whether traffic or nontraffic accident

Pedestrian in motorized mobility scooter injured in collision with other nonmotorized vehicle, unspecified whether traffic or nontraffic accident

√4th **V09 Pedestrian injured in other and unspecified transport accidents**

√5th **V09.0 Pedestrian injured in nontraffic accident involving other and unspecified motor vehicles**

√7th **V09.00 Pedestrian injured in nontraffic accident involving unspecified motor vehicles**

√7th **V09.01 Pedestrian injured in nontraffic accident involving military vehicle**

√7th **V09.09 Pedestrian injured in nontraffic accident involving other motor vehicles**

Pedestrian injured in nontraffic accident by special vehicle

√7th **V09.1 Pedestrian injured in unspecified nontraffic accident**

√5th **V09.2 Pedestrian injured in traffic accident involving other and unspecified motor vehicles**

√7th **V09.20 Pedestrian injured in traffic accident involving unspecified motor vehicles**

√7th **V09.21 Pedestrian injured in traffic accident involving military vehicle**

√7th **V09.29 Pedestrian injured in traffic accident involving other motor vehicles**

√7th **V09.3 Pedestrian injured in unspecified traffic accident**

√7th **V09.9 Pedestrian injured in unspecified transport accident**

Pedal cycle rider injured in transport accident (V10-V19)

INCLUDES any non-motorized vehicle, excluding an animal-drawn vehicle, or a sidecar or trailer attached to the pedal cycle

EXCLUDES 2 *rupture of pedal cycle tire (W37.0)*

The appropriate 7th character is to be added to each code from categories V10-V19.
A initial encounter
D subsequent encounter
S sequela

√4th **V10 Pedal cycle rider injured in collision with pedestrian or animal**

EXCLUDES 1 *pedal cycle rider collision with animal-drawn vehicle or animal being ridden (V16.-)*

√7th **V10.0 Pedal cycle driver injured in collision with pedestrian or animal in nontraffic accident**

√7th **V10.1 Pedal cycle passenger injured in collision with pedestrian or animal in nontraffic accident**

√7th **V10.2 Unspecified pedal cyclist injured in collision with pedestrian or animal in nontraffic accident**

√7th **V10.3 Person boarding or alighting a pedal cycle injured in collision with pedestrian or animal**

√7th **V10.4 Pedal cycle driver injured in collision with pedestrian or animal in traffic accident**

√7th **V10.5 Pedal cycle passenger injured in collision with pedestrian or animal in traffic accident**

√7th **V10.9 Unspecified pedal cyclist injured in collision with pedestrian or animal in traffic accident**

√4th **V11 Pedal cycle rider injured in collision with other pedal cycle**

√7th **V11.0 Pedal cycle driver injured in collision with other pedal cycle in nontraffic accident**

√7th **V11.1 Pedal cycle passenger injured in collision with other pedal cycle in nontraffic accident**

√7th **V11.2 Unspecified pedal cyclist injured in collision with other pedal cycle in nontraffic accident**

√7th **V11.3 Person boarding or alighting a pedal cycle injured in collision with other pedal cycle**

√7th **V11.4 Pedal cycle driver injured in collision with other pedal cycle in traffic accident**

√7th **V11.5 Pedal cycle passenger injured in collision with other pedal cycle in traffic accident**

√7th **V11.9 Unspecified pedal cyclist injured in collision with other pedal cycle in traffic accident**

√4th **V12 Pedal cycle rider injured in collision with two- or three-wheeled motor vehicle**

√7th **V12.0 Pedal cycle driver injured in collision with two- or three-wheeled motor vehicle in nontraffic accident**

√7th **V12.1 Pedal cycle passenger injured in collision with two- or three-wheeled motor vehicle in nontraffic accident**

√7th **V12.2 Unspecified pedal cyclist injured in collision with two- or three-wheeled motor vehicle in nontraffic accident**

√7th **V12.3 Person boarding or alighting a pedal cycle injured in collision with two- or three-wheeled motor vehicle**

√7th **V12.4 Pedal cycle driver injured in collision with two- or three-wheeled motor vehicle in traffic accident**

√7th **V12.5 Pedal cycle passenger injured in collision with two- or three-wheeled motor vehicle in traffic accident**

√7th **V12.9 Unspecified pedal cyclist injured in collision with two- or three-wheeled motor vehicle in traffic accident**

√4th **V13 Pedal cycle rider injured in collision with car, pick-up truck or van**

√7th **V13.0 Pedal cycle driver injured in collision with car, pick-up truck or van in nontraffic accident**

√7th **V13.1 Pedal cycle passenger injured in collision with car, pick-up truck or van in nontraffic accident**

√7th **V13.2 Unspecified pedal cyclist injured in collision with car, pick-up truck or van in nontraffic accident**

√7th **V13.3 Person boarding or alighting a pedal cycle injured in collision with car, pick-up truck or van**

√7th **V13.4 Pedal cycle driver injured in collision with car, pick-up truck or van in traffic accident**

√7th **V13.5 Pedal cycle passenger injured in collision with car, pick-up truck or van in traffic accident**

√7th **V13.9 Unspecified pedal cyclist injured in collision with car, pick-up truck or van in traffic accident**

√4th **V14 Pedal cycle rider injured in collision with heavy transport vehicle or bus**

EXCLUDES 1 *pedal cycle rider injured in collision with military vehicle (V19.81)*

√7th **V14.0 Pedal cycle driver injured in collision with heavy transport vehicle or bus in nontraffic accident**

√x7th **V14.1 Pedal cycle passenger injured in collision with heavy transport vehicle or bus in nontraffic accident**

√x7th **V14.2 Unspecified pedal cyclist injured in collision with heavy transport vehicle or bus in nontraffic accident**

√x7th **V14.3 Person boarding or alighting a pedal cycle injured in collision with heavy transport vehicle or bus**

√x7th **V14.4 Pedal cycle driver injured in collision with heavy transport vehicle or bus in traffic accident**

√x7th **V14.5 Pedal cycle passenger injured in collision with heavy transport vehicle or bus in traffic accident**

√x7th **V14.9 Unspecified pedal cyclist injured in collision with heavy transport vehicle or bus in traffic accident**

√4th **V15 Pedal cycle rider injured in collision with railway train or railway vehicle**

√x7th **V15.Ø Pedal cycle driver injured in collision with railway train or railway vehicle in nontraffic accident**

√x7th **V15.1 Pedal cycle passenger injured in collision with railway train or railway vehicle in nontraffic accident**

√x7th **V15.2 Unspecified pedal cyclist injured in collision with railway train or railway vehicle in nontraffic accident**

√x7th **V15.3 Person boarding or alighting a pedal cycle injured in collision with railway train or railway vehicle**

√x7th **V15.4 Pedal cycle driver injured in collision with railway train or railway vehicle in traffic accident**

√x7th **V15.5 Pedal cycle passenger injured in collision with railway train or railway vehicle in traffic accident**

√x7th **V15.9 Unspecified pedal cyclist injured in collision with railway train or railway vehicle in traffic accident**

√4th **V16 Pedal cycle rider injured in collision with other nonmotor vehicle**

INCLUDES collision with animal-drawn vehicle, animal being ridden, streetcar

√x7th **V16.Ø Pedal cycle driver injured in collision with other nonmotor vehicle in nontraffic accident**

√x7th **V16.1 Pedal cycle passenger injured in collision with other nonmotor vehicle in nontraffic accident**

√x7th **V16.2 Unspecified pedal cyclist injured in collision with other nonmotor vehicle in nontraffic accident**

√x7th **V16.3 Person boarding or alighting a pedal cycle injured in collision with other nonmotor vehicle in nontraffic accident**

√x7th **V16.4 Pedal cycle driver injured in collision with other nonmotor vehicle in traffic accident**

√x7th **V16.5 Pedal cycle passenger injured in collision with other nonmotor vehicle in traffic accident**

√x7th **V16.9 Unspecified pedal cyclist injured in collision with other nonmotor vehicle in traffic accident**

√4th **V17 Pedal cycle rider injured in collision with fixed or stationary object**

√x7th **V17.Ø Pedal cycle driver injured in collision with fixed or stationary object in nontraffic accident**

√x7th **V17.1 Pedal cycle passenger injured in collision with fixed or stationary object in nontraffic accident**

√x7th **V17.2 Unspecified pedal cyclist injured in collision with fixed or stationary object in nontraffic accident**

√x7th **V17.3 Person boarding or alighting a pedal cycle injured in collision with fixed or stationary object**

√x7th **V17.4 Pedal cycle driver injured in collision with fixed or stationary object in traffic accident**

√x7th **V17.5 Pedal cycle passenger injured in collision with fixed or stationary object in traffic accident**

√x7th **V17.9 Unspecified pedal cyclist injured in collision with fixed or stationary object in traffic accident**

√4th **V18 Pedal cycle rider injured in noncollision transport accident**

INCLUDES fall or thrown from pedal cycle (without antecedent collision)
overturning pedal cycle NOS
overturning pedal cycle without collision

√x7th **V18.Ø Pedal cycle driver injured in noncollision transport accident in nontraffic accident**

√x7th **V18.1 Pedal cycle passenger injured in noncollision transport accident in nontraffic accident**

√x7th **V18.2 Unspecified pedal cyclist injured in noncollision transport accident in nontraffic accident**

√x7th **V18.3 Person boarding or alighting a pedal cycle injured in noncollision transport accident**

√x7th **V18.4 Pedal cycle driver injured in noncollision transport accident in traffic accident**

√x7th **V18.5 Pedal cycle passenger injured in noncollision transport accident in traffic accident**

√x7th **V18.9 Unspecified pedal cyclist injured in noncollision transport accident in traffic accident**

√4th **V19 Pedal cycle rider injured in other and unspecified transport accidents**

√5th **V19.Ø Pedal cycle driver injured in collision with other and unspecified motor vehicles in nontraffic accident**

√x7th **V19.ØØ Pedal cycle driver injured in collision with unspecified motor vehicles in nontraffic accident**

√x7th **V19.Ø9 Pedal cycle driver injured in collision with other motor vehicles in nontraffic accident**

√5th **V19.1 Pedal cycle passenger injured in collision with other and unspecified motor vehicles in nontraffic accident**

√x7th **V19.1Ø Pedal cycle passenger injured in collision with unspecified motor vehicles in nontraffic accident**

√x7th **V19.19 Pedal cycle passenger injured in collision with other motor vehicles in nontraffic accident**

√5th **V19.2 Unspecified pedal cyclist injured in collision with other and unspecified motor vehicles in nontraffic accident**

√x7th **V19.2Ø Unspecified pedal cyclist injured in collision with unspecified motor vehicles in nontraffic accident**
Pedal cycle collision NOS, nontraffic

√x7th **V19.29 Unspecified pedal cyclist injured in collision with other motor vehicles in nontraffic accident**

√x7th **V19.3 Pedal cyclist (driver) (passenger) injured in unspecified nontraffic accident**
Pedal cycle accident NOS, nontraffic
Pedal cyclist injured in nontraffic accident NOS

√5th **V19.4 Pedal cycle driver injured in collision with other and unspecified motor vehicles in traffic accident**

√x7th **V19.4Ø Pedal cycle driver injured in collision with unspecified motor vehicles in traffic accident**

√x7th **V19.49 Pedal cycle driver injured in collision with other motor vehicles in traffic accident**

√5th **V19.5 Pedal cycle passenger injured in collision with other and unspecified motor vehicles in traffic accident**

√x7th **V19.5Ø Pedal cycle passenger injured in collision with unspecified motor vehicles in traffic accident**

√x7th **V19.59 Pedal cycle passenger injured in collision with other motor vehicles in traffic accident**

√5th **V19.6 Unspecified pedal cyclist injured in collision with other and unspecified motor vehicles in traffic accident**

√x7th **V19.6Ø Unspecified pedal cyclist injured in collision with unspecified motor vehicles in traffic accident**
Pedal cycle collision NOS (traffic)

√x7th **V19.69 Unspecified pedal cyclist injured in collision with other motor vehicles in traffic accident**

√5th **V19.8 Pedal cyclist (driver) (passenger) injured in other specified transport accidents**

√x7th **V19.81 Pedal cyclist (driver) (passenger) injured in transport accident with military vehicle**

√x7th **V19.88 Pedal cyclist (driver) (passenger) injured in other specified transport accidents**

√x7th **V19.9 Pedal cyclist (driver) (passenger) injured in unspecified traffic accident**
Pedal cycle accident NOS

Motorcycle rider injured in transport accident (V2Ø-V29)

INCLUDES ▶electric bicycle◀
▶e-bike◀
▶e-bicycle◀
moped
motorcycle with sidecar
motorized bicycle
motor scooter

EXCLUDES 1 *three-wheeled motor vehicle (V3Ø-V39)*

The appropriate 7th character is to be added to each code from categories V2Ø-V29.
A initial encounter
D subsequent encounter
S sequela

√4th **V2Ø Motorcycle rider injured in collision with pedestrian or animal**

EXCLUDES 1 *motorcycle rider collision with animal-drawn vehicle or animal being ridden (V26.-)*

√5th **V2Ø.Ø Motorcycle driver injured in collision with pedestrian or animal in nontraffic accident**

● √x7th **V2Ø.Ø1 Electric (assisted) bicycle driver injured in collision with pedestrian or animal in nontraffic accident**

● √x7th **V2Ø.Ø9 Other motorcycle driver injured in collision with pedestrian or animal in nontraffic accident**

V20.1 Motorcycle passenger injured in collision with pedestrian or animal in nontraffic accident
- V20.11 Electric (assisted) bicycle passenger injured in collision with pedestrian or animal in nontraffic accident
- V20.19 Other motorcycle passenger injured in collision with pedestrian or animal in nontraffic accident

V20.2 Unspecified motorcycle rider injured in collision with pedestrian or animal in nontraffic accident
- V20.21 Unspecified electric (assisted) bicycle rider injured in collision with pedestrian or animal in nontraffic accident
- V20.29 Unspecified rider of other motorcycle injured in collision with pedestrian or animal in nontraffic accident

V20.3 Person boarding or alighting a motorcycle injured in collision with pedestrian or animal
- V20.31 Person boarding or alighting an electric (assisted) bicycle injured in collision with pedestrian or animal
- V20.39 Person boarding or alighting other motorcycle injured in collision with pedestrian or animal

V20.4 Motorcycle driver injured in collision with pedestrian or animal in traffic accident
- V20.41 Electric (assisted) bicycle driver injured in collision with pedestrian or animal in traffic accident
- V20.49 Other motorcycle driver injured in collision with pedestrian or animal in traffic accident

V20.5 Motorcycle passenger injured in collision with pedestrian or animal in traffic accident
- V20.51 Electric (assisted) bicycle passenger injured in collision with pedestrian or animal in traffic accident
- V20.59 Other motorcycle passenger injured in collision with pedestrian or animal in traffic accident

V20.9 Unspecified motorcycle rider injured in collision with pedestrian or animal in traffic accident
- V20.91 Unspecified electric (assisted) bicycle rider injured in collision with pedestrian or animal in traffic accident
- V20.99 Unspecified rider of other motorcycle injured in collision with pedestrian or animal in traffic accident

V21 Motorcycle rider injured in collision with pedal cycle

V21.0 Motorcycle driver injured in collision with pedal cycle in nontraffic accident
- V21.01 Electric (assisted) bicycle driver injured in collision with pedal cycle in nontraffic accident
- V21.09 Other motorcycle driver injured in collision with pedal cycle in nontraffic accident

V21.1 Motorcycle passenger injured in collision with pedal cycle in nontraffic accident
- V21.11 Electric (assisted) bicycle passenger injured in collision with pedal cycle in nontraffic accident
- V21.19 Other motorcycle passenger injured in collision with pedal cycle in nontraffic accident

V21.2 Unspecified motorcycle rider injured in collision with pedal cycle in nontraffic accident
- V21.21 Unspecified electric (assisted) bicycle rider injured in collision with pedal cycle in nontraffic accident
- V21.29 Unspecified rider of other motorcycle injured in collision with pedal cycle in nontraffic accident

V21.3 Person boarding or alighting a motorcycle injured in collision with pedal cycle
- V21.31 Person boarding or alighting an electric (assisted) bicycle injured in collision with pedal cycle
- V21.39 Person boarding or alighting other motorcycle injured in collision with pedal cycle

V21.4 Motorcycle driver injured in collision with pedal cycle in traffic accident
- V21.41 Electric (assisted) bicycle driver injured in collision with pedal cycle in traffic accident
- V21.49 Other motorcycle driver injured in collision with pedal cycle in traffic accident

V21.5 Motorcycle passenger injured in collision with pedal cycle in traffic accident
- V21.51 Electric (assisted) bicycle passenger injured in collision with pedal cycle in traffic accident
- V21.59 Other motorcycle passenger injured in collision with pedal cycle in traffic accident

V21.9 Unspecified motorcycle rider injured in collision with pedal cycle in traffic accident
- V21.91 Unspecified electric (assisted) bicycle rider injured in collision with pedal cycle in traffic accident
- V21.99 Unspecified rider of other motorcycle injured in collision with pedal cycle in traffic accident

V22 Motorcycle rider injured in collision with two- or three-wheeled motor vehicle

V22.0 Motorcycle driver injured in collision with two- or three-wheeled motor vehicle in nontraffic accident
- V22.01 Electric (assisted) bicycle driver injured in collision with two- or three-wheeled motor vehicle in nontraffic accident
- V22.09 Other motorcycle driver injured in collision with two- or three-wheeled motor vehicle in nontraffic accident

V22.1 Motorcycle passenger injured in collision with two- or three-wheeled motor vehicle in nontraffic accident
- V22.11 Electric (assisted) bicycle passenger injured in collision with two- or three-wheeled motor vehicle in nontraffic accident
- V22.19 Other motorcycle passenger injured in collision with two- or three-wheeled motor vehicle in nontraffic accident

V22.2 Unspecified motorcycle rider injured in collision with two- or three-wheeled motor vehicle in nontraffic accident
- V22.21 Unspecified electric (assisted) bicycle rider injured in collision with two- or three-wheeled motor vehicle in nontraffic accident
- V22.29 Unspecified rider of other motorcycle injured in collision with two- or three-wheeled motor vehicle in nontraffic accident

V22.3 Person boarding or alighting a motorcycle injured in collision with two- or three-wheeled motor vehicle
- V22.31 Person boarding or alighting an electric (assisted) bicycle injured in collision with two- or three-wheeled motor vehicle
- V22.39 Person boarding or alighting other motorcycle injured in collision with two- or three-wheeled motor vehicle

V22.4 Motorcycle driver injured in collision with two- or three-wheeled motor vehicle in traffic accident
- V22.41 Electric (assisted) bicycle driver injured in collision with two- or three-wheeled motor vehicle in traffic accident
- V22.49 Other motorcycle driver injured in collision with two- or three-wheeled motor vehicle in traffic accident

V22.5 Motorcycle passenger injured in collision with two- or three-wheeled motor vehicle in traffic accident
- V22.51 Electric (assisted) bicycle passenger injured in collision with two- or three-wheeled motor vehicle in traffic accident
- V22.59 Other motorcycle passenger injured in collision with two- or three-wheeled motor vehicle in traffic accident

V22.9 Unspecified motorcycle rider injured in collision with two- or three-wheeled motor vehicle in traffic accident
- V22.91 Unspecified electric (assisted) bicycle rider injured in collision with two- or three-wheeled motor vehicle in traffic accident
- V22.99 Unspecified rider of other motorcycle injured in collision with two- or three-wheeled motor vehicle in traffic accident

V23 Motorcycle rider injured in collision with car, pick-up truck or van

V23.0 Motorcycle driver injured in collision with car, pick-up truck or van in nontraffic accident
- V23.01 Electric (assisted) bicycle driver injured in collision with car, pick-up truck or van in nontraffic accident
- V23.09 Other motorcycle driver injured in collision with car, pick-up truck or van in nontraffic accident

V23.1 Motorcycle passenger injured in collision with car, pick-up truck or van in nontraffic accident
- V23.11 Electric (assisted) bicycle passenger injured in collision with car, pick-up truck or van in nontraffic accident
- V23.19 Other motorcycle passenger injured in collision with car, pick-up truck or van in nontraffic accident

V23.2 Unspecified motorcycle rider injured in collision with car, pick-up truck or van in nontraffic accident

● V23.21 Unspecified electric (assisted) bicycle rider injured in collision with car, pick-up truck or van in nontraffic accident

● V23.29 Unspecified rider of other motorcycle injured in collision with car, pick-up truck or van in nontraffic accident

V23.3 Person boarding or alighting a motorcycle injured in collision with car, pick-up truck or van

● V23.31 Person boarding or alighting an electric (assisted) bicycle injured in collision with car, pick-up truck or van

● V23.39 Person boarding or alighting other motorcycle injured in collision with car, pick-up truck or van

V23.4 Motorcycle driver injured in collision with car, pick-up truck or van in traffic accident

● V23.41 Electric (assisted) bicycle driver injured in collision with car, pick-up truck or van in traffic accident

● V23.49 Other motorcycle driver injured in collision with car, pick-up truck or van in traffic accident

V23.5 Motorcycle passenger injured in collision with car, pick-up truck or van in traffic accident

● V23.51 Electric (assisted) bicycle passenger injured in collision with car, pick-up truck or van in traffic accident

● V23.59 Other motorcycle passenger injured in collision with car, pick-up truck or van in traffic accident

V23.9 Unspecified motorcycle rider injured in collision with car, pick-up truck or van in traffic accident

● V23.91 Unspecified electric (assisted) bicycle rider injured in collision with car, pick-up truck or van in traffic accident

● V23.99 Unspecified rider of other motorcycle injured in collision with car, pick-up truck or van in traffic accident

V24 Motorcycle rider injured in collision with heavy transport vehicle or bus

EXCLUDES 1 *motorcycle rider injured in collision with military vehicle ►(V29.818)◄*

V24.0 Motorcycle driver injured in collision with heavy transport vehicle or bus in nontraffic accident

● V24.01 Electric (assisted) bicycle driver injured in collision with heavy transport vehicle or bus in nontraffic accident

● V24.09 Other motorcycle driver injured in collision with heavy transport vehicle or bus in nontraffic accident

V24.1 Motorcycle passenger injured in collision with heavy transport vehicle or bus in nontraffic accident

● V24.11 Electric (assisted) bicycle passenger injured in collision with heavy transport vehicle or bus in nontraffic accident

● V24.19 Other motorcycle passenger injured in collision with heavy transport vehicle or bus in nontraffic accident

V24.2 Unspecified motorcycle rider injured in collision with heavy transport vehicle or bus in nontraffic accident

● V24.21 Unspecified electric (assisted) bicycle rider injured in collision with heavy transport vehicle or bus in nontraffic accident

● V24.29 Unspecified rider of other motorcycle injured in collision with heavy transport vehicle or bus in nontraffic accident

V24.3 Person boarding or alighting a motorcycle injured in collision with heavy transport vehicle or bus

● V24.31 Person boarding or alighting an electric (assisted) bicycle injured in collision with heavy transport vehicle or bus

● V24.39 Person boarding or alighting other motorcycle injured in collision with heavy transport vehicle or bus

V24.4 Motorcycle driver injured in collision with heavy transport vehicle or bus in traffic accident

● V24.41 Electric (assisted) bicycle driver injured in collision with heavy transport vehicle or bus in traffic accident

● V24.49 Other motorcycle driver injured in collision with heavy transport vehicle or bus in traffic accident

V24.5 Motorcycle passenger injured in collision with heavy transport vehicle or bus in traffic accident

● V24.51 Electric (assisted) bicycle passenger injured in collision with heavy transport vehicle or bus in traffic accident

● V24.59 Other motorcycle passenger injured in collision with heavy transport vehicle or bus in traffic accident

V24.9 Unspecified motorcycle rider injured in collision with heavy transport vehicle or bus in traffic accident

● V24.91 Unspecified electric (assisted) bicycle rider injured in collision with heavy transport vehicle or bus in traffic accident

● V24.99 Unspecified rider of other motorcycle injured in collision with heavy transport vehicle or bus in traffic accident

V25 Motorcycle rider injured in collision with railway train or railway vehicle

V25.0 Motorcycle driver injured in collision with railway train or railway vehicle in nontraffic accident

● V25.01 Electric (assisted) bicycle driver injured in collision with railway train or railway vehicle in nontraffic accident

● V25.09 Other motorcycle driver injured in collision with railway train or railway vehicle in nontraffic accident

V25.1 Motorcycle passenger injured in collision with railway train or railway vehicle in nontraffic accident

● V25.11 Electric (assisted) bicycle passenger injured in collision with railway train or railway vehicle in nontraffic accident

● V25.19 Other motorcycle passenger injured in collision with railway train or railway vehicle in nontraffic accident

V25.2 Unspecified motorcycle rider injured in collision with railway train or railway vehicle in nontraffic accident

● V25.21 Unspecified electric (assisted) bicycle rider injured in collision with railway train or railway vehicle in nontraffic accident

● V25.29 Unspecified rider of other motorcycle injured in collision with railway train or railway vehicle in nontraffic accident

V25.3 Person boarding or alighting a motorcycle injured in collision with railway train or railway vehicle

● V25.31 Person boarding or alighting an electric (assisted) bicycle injured in collision with railway train or railway vehicle

● V25.39 Person boarding or alighting other motorcycle injured in collision with railway train or railway vehicle

V25.4 Motorcycle driver injured in collision with railway train or railway vehicle in traffic accident

● V25.41 Electric (assisted) bicycle driver injured in collision with railway train or railway vehicle in traffic accident

● V25.49 Other motorcycle driver injured in collision with railway train or railway vehicle in traffic accident

V25.5 Motorcycle passenger injured in collision with railway train or railway vehicle in traffic accident

● V25.51 Electric (assisted) bicycle passenger injured in collision with railway train or railway vehicle in traffic accident

● V25.59 Other motorcycle passenger injured in collision with railway train or railway vehicle in traffic accident

V25.9 Unspecified motorcycle rider injured in collision with railway train or railway vehicle in traffic accident

● V25.91 Unspecified electric (assisted) bicycle rider injured in collision with railway train or railway vehicle in traffic accident

● V25.99 Unspecified rider of other motorcycle injured in collision with railway train or railway vehicle in traffic accident

V26 Motorcycle rider injured in collision with other nonmotor vehicle

INCLUDES collision with animal-drawn vehicle, animal being ridden, streetcar

V26.0 Motorcycle driver injured in collision with other nonmotor vehicle in nontraffic accident

● V26.01 Electric (assisted) bicycle driver injured in collision with other nonmotor vehicle in nontraffic accident

● V26.09 Other motorcycle driver injured in collision with other nonmotor vehicle in nontraffic accident

V26.1 Motorcycle passenger injured in collision with other nonmotor vehicle in nontraffic accident

● V26.11 Electric (assisted) bicycle passenger injured in collision with other nonmotor vehicle in nontraffic accident

Additional Character Required | Placeholder Alert | Manifestation | Unspecified Dx | QPP | Unacceptable PDx

● V26.19 Other motorcycle passenger injured in collision with other nonmotor vehicle in nontraffic accident

V26.2 Unspecified motorcycle rider injured in collision with other nonmotor vehicle in nontraffic accident

● V26.21 Unspecified electric (assisted) bicycle rider injured in collision with other nonmotor vehicle in nontraffic accident

● V26.29 Unspecified rider of other motorcycle injured in collision with other nonmotor vehicle in nontraffic accident

V26.3 Person boarding or alighting a motorcycle injured in collision with other nonmotor vehicle

● V26.31 Person boarding or alighting an electric (assisted) bicycle injured in collision with other nonmotor vehicle

● V26.39 Person boarding or alighting other motorcycle injured in collision with other nonmotor vehicle

V26.4 Motorcycle driver injured in collision with other nonmotor vehicle in traffic accident

● V26.41 Electric (assisted) bicycle driver injured in collision with other nonmotor vehicle in traffic accident

● V26.49 Other motorcycle driver injured in collision with other nonmotor vehicle in traffic accident

V26.5 Motorcycle passenger injured in collision with other nonmotor vehicle in traffic accident

● V26.51 Electric (assisted) bicycle passenger injured in collision with other nonmotor vehicle in traffic accident

● V26.59 Other motorcycle passenger injured in collision with other nonmotor vehicle in traffic accident

V26.9 Unspecified motorcycle rider injured in collision with other nonmotor vehicle in traffic accident

● V26.91 Unspecified electric (assisted) bicycle rider injured in collision with other nonmotor vehicle in traffic accident

● V26.99 Unspecified rider of other motorcycle injured in collision with other nonmotor vehicle in traffic accident

V27 Motorcycle rider injured in collision with fixed or stationary object

V27.Ø Motorcycle driver injured in collision with fixed or stationary object in nontraffic accident

● V27.Ø1 Electric (assisted) bicycle driver injured in collision with fixed or stationary object in nontraffic accident

● V27.Ø9 Other motorcycle driver injured in collision with fixed or stationary object in nontraffic accident

V27.1 Motorcycle passenger injured in collision with fixed or stationary object in nontraffic accident

● V27.11 Electric (assisted) bicycle passenger injured in collision with fixed or stationary object in nontraffic accident

● V27.19 Other motorcycle passenger injured in collision with fixed or stationary object in nontraffic accident

V27.2 Unspecified motorcycle rider injured in collision with fixed or stationary object in nontraffic accident

● V27.21 Unspecified electric (assisted) bicycle rider injured in collision with fixed or stationary object in nontraffic accident

● V27.29 Unspecified rider of other motorcycle injured in collision with fixed or stationary object in nontraffic accident

V27.3 Person boarding or alighting a motorcycle injured in collision with fixed or stationary object

● V27.31 Person boarding or alighting an electric (assisted) bicycle injured in collision with fixed or stationary object

● V27.39 Person boarding or alighting other motorcycle injured in collision with fixed or stationary object

V27.4 Motorcycle driver injured in collision with fixed or stationary object in traffic accident

● V27.41 Electric (assisted) bicycle driver injured in collision with fixed or stationary object in traffic accident

● V27.49 Other motorcycle driver injured in collision with fixed or stationary object in traffic accident

V27.5 Motorcycle passenger injured in collision with fixed or stationary object in traffic accident

● V27.51 Electric (assisted) bicycle passenger injured in collision with fixed or stationary object in traffic accident

● V27.59 Other motorcycle passenger injured in collision with fixed or stationary object in traffic accident

V27.9 Unspecified motorcycle rider injured in collision with fixed or stationary object in traffic accident

● V27.91 Unspecified electric (assisted) bicycle rider injured in collision with fixed or stationary object in traffic accident

● V27.99 Unspecified rider of other motorcycle injured in collision with fixed or stationary object in traffic accident

V28 Motorcycle rider injured in noncollision transport accident

INCLUDES fall or thrown from motorcycle (without antecedent collision)
overturning motorcycle NOS
overturning motorcycle without collision

V28.Ø Motorcycle driver injured in noncollision transport accident in nontraffic accident

● V28.Ø1 Electric (assisted) bicycle driver injured in noncollision transport accident in nontraffic accident

● V28.Ø9 Other motorcycle driver injured in noncollision transport accident in nontraffic accident

V28.1 Motorcycle passenger injured in noncollision transport accident in nontraffic accident

● V28.11 Electric (assisted) bicycle passenger injured in noncollision transport accident in nontraffic accident

● V28.19 Other motorcycle passenger injured in noncollision transport accident in nontraffic accident

V28.2 Unspecified motorcycle rider injured in noncollision transport accident in nontraffic accident

● V28.21 Unspecified electric (assisted) bicycle rider injured in noncollision transport accident in nontraffic accident

● V28.29 Unspecified rider of other motorcycle injured in noncollision transport accident in nontraffic accident

V28.3 Person boarding or alighting a motorcycle injured in noncollision transport accident

● V28.31 Person boarding or alighting an electric (assisted) bicycle injured in noncollision transport accident

● V28.39 Person boarding or alighting other motorcycle injured in noncollision transport accident

V28.4 Motorcycle driver injured in noncollision transport accident in traffic accident

● V28.41 Electric (assisted) bicycle driver injured in noncollision transport accident in traffic accident

● V28.49 Other motorcycle driver injured in noncollision transport accident in traffic accident

V28.5 Motorcycle passenger injured in noncollision transport accident in traffic accident

● V28.51 Electric (assisted) bicycle passenger injured in noncollision transport accident in traffic accident

● V28.59 Other motorcycle passenger injured in noncollision transport accident in traffic accident

V28.9 Unspecified motorcycle rider injured in noncollision transport accident in traffic accident

● V28.91 Unspecified electric (assisted) bicycle rider injured in noncollision transport accident in traffic accident

● V28.99 Unspecified rider of other motorcycle injured in noncollision transport accident in traffic accident

V29 Motorcycle rider injured in other and unspecified transport accidents

V29.Ø Motorcycle driver injured in collision with other and unspecified motor vehicles in nontraffic accident

V29.ØØ Motorcycle driver injured in collision with unspecified motor vehicles in nontraffic accident

● V29.ØØ1 Electric (assisted) bicycle driver injured in collision with unspecified motor vehicles in nontraffic accident

● V29.ØØ8 Other motorcycle driver injured in collision with unspecified motor vehicles in nontraffic accident

V29.Ø9 Motorcycle driver injured in collision with other motor vehicles in nontraffic accident

● V29.Ø91 Electric (assisted) bicycle driver injured in collision with other motor vehicles in nontraffic accident

● V29.Ø98 Other motorcycle driver injured in collision with other motor vehicles in nontraffic accident

V29.1 Motorcycle passenger injured in collision with other and unspecified motor vehicles in nontraffic accident

V29.10 Motorcycle passenger injured in collision with unspecified motor vehicles in nontraffic accident

● V29.101 Electric (assisted) bicycle passenger injured in collision with unspecified motor vehicles in nontraffic accident

● V29.108 Other motorcycle passenger injured in collision with unspecified motor vehicles in nontraffic accident

V29.19 Motorcycle passenger injured in collision with other motor vehicles in nontraffic accident

● V29.191 Electric (assisted) bicycle passenger injured in collision with other motor vehicles in nontraffic accident

● V29.198 Other motorcycle passenger injured in collision with other motor vehicles in nontraffic accident

V29.2 Unspecified motorcycle rider injured in collision with other and unspecified motor vehicles in nontraffic accident

V29.20 Unspecified motorcycle rider injured in collision with unspecified motor vehicles in nontraffic accident
Motorcycle collision NOS, nontraffic

● V29.201 Unspecified electric (assisted) bicycle rider injured in collision with unspecified motor vehicles in nontraffic accident

● V29.208 Unspecified rider of other motorcycle injured in collision with unspecified motor vehicles in nontraffic accident
Motorcycle collision NOS, nontraffic

V29.29 Unspecified motorcycle rider injured in collision with other motor vehicles in nontraffic accident

● V29.291 Unspecified electric (assisted) bicycle rider injured in collision with other motor vehicles in nontraffic accident

● V29.298 Unspecified rider of other motorcycle injured in collision with other motor vehicles in nontraffic accident

V29.3 Motorcycle rider (driver) (passenger) injured in unspecified nontraffic accident
Motorcycle accident NOS, nontraffic
Motorcycle rider injured in nontraffic accident NOS

● V29.31 Electric (assisted) bicycle (driver) (passenger) injured in unspecified nontraffic accident

● V29.39 Other motorcycle (driver) (passenger) injured in unspecified nontraffic accident
Motorcycle accident NOS, nontraffic
Motorcycle rider injured in nontraffic accident NOS

V29.4 Motorcycle driver injured in collision with other and unspecified motor vehicles in traffic accident

V29.40 Motorcycle driver injured in collision with unspecified motor vehicles in traffic accident

● V29.401 Electric (assisted) bicycle driver injured in collision with unspecified motor vehicles in traffic accident

● V29.408 Other motorcycle driver injured in collision with unspecified motor vehicles in traffic accident

V29.49 Motorcycle driver injured in collision with other motor vehicles in traffic accident

● V29.491 Electric (assisted) bicycle driver injured in collision with other motor vehicles in traffic accident

● V29.498 Other motorcycle driver injured in collision with other motor vehicles in traffic accident

V29.5 Motorcycle passenger injured in collision with other and unspecified motor vehicles in traffic accident

V29.50 Motorcycle passenger injured in collision with unspecified motor vehicles in traffic accident

● V29.501 Electric (assisted) bicycle passenger injured in collision with unspecified motor vehicles in traffic accident

● V29.508 Other motorcycle passenger injured in collision with unspecified motor vehicles in traffic accident

V29.59 Motorcycle passenger injured in collision with other motor vehicles in traffic accident

● V29.591 Electric (assisted) bicycle passenger injured in collision with other motor vehicles in traffic accident

● V29.598 Other motorcycle passenger injured in collision with other motor vehicles in traffic accident

V29.6 Unspecified motorcycle rider injured in collision with other and unspecified motor vehicles in traffic accident

V29.60 Unspecified motorcycle rider injured in collision with unspecified motor vehicles in traffic accident
Motorcycle collision NOS (traffic)

● V29.601 Unspecified electric (assisted) bicycle rider injured in collision with unspecified motor vehicles in traffic accident

● V29.608 Unspecified rider of other motorcycle injured in collision with unspecified motor vehicles in traffic accident
Motorcycle collision NOS (traffic)

V29.69 Unspecified motorcycle rider injured in collision with other motor vehicles in traffic accident

● V29.691 Unspecified electric (assisted) bicycle rider injured in collision with other motor vehicles in traffic accident

● V29.698 Unspecified rider of other motorcycle injured in collision with other motor vehicles in traffic accident

V29.8 Motorcycle rider (driver) (passenger) injured in other specified transport accidents

V29.81 Motorcycle rider (driver) (passenger) injured in transport accident with military vehicle

● V29.811 Electric (assisted) bicycle rider (driver) (passenger) injured in transport accident with military vehicle

● V29.818 Rider (driver) (passenger) of other motorcycle injured in transport accident with military vehicle

V29.88 Motorcycle rider (driver) (passenger) injured in other specified transport accidents

● V29.881 Electric (assisted) bicycle rider (driver) (passenger) injured in other specified transport accidents

● V29.888 Rider (driver) (passenger) of other motorcycle injured in other specified transport accidents

V29.9 Motorcycle rider (driver) (passenger) injured in unspecified traffic accident
Motorcycle accident NOS

● V29.91 Electric (assisted) bicycle rider (driver) (passenger) injured in unspecified traffic accident

● V29.99 Rider (driver) (passenger) of other motorcycle injured in unspecified traffic accident
Motorcycle accident NOS

Occupant of three-wheeled motor vehicle injured in transport accident (V30-V39)

INCLUDES motorized tricycle
motorized rickshaw
three-wheeled motor car

EXCLUDES 1 *all-terrain vehicles (V86.-)*
motorcycle with sidecar (V20-V29)
vehicle designed primarily for off-road use (V86.-)

The appropriate 7th character is to be added to each code from categories V30-V39.
A initial encounter
D subsequent encounter
S sequela

V30 Occupant of three-wheeled motor vehicle injured in collision with pedestrian or animal

EXCLUDES 1 *three-wheeled motor vehicle collision with animal-drawn vehicle or animal being ridden (V36.-)*

V30.0 Driver of three-wheeled motor vehicle injured in collision with pedestrian or animal in nontraffic accident

V30.1 Passenger in three-wheeled motor vehicle injured in collision with pedestrian or animal in nontraffic accident

V30.2 Person on outside of three-wheeled motor vehicle injured in collision with pedestrian or animal in nontraffic accident

V30.3 Unspecified occupant of three-wheeled motor vehicle injured in collision with pedestrian or animal in nontraffic accident

V30.4 Person boarding or alighting a three-wheeled motor vehicle injured in collision with pedestrian or animal

V30.5 Driver of three-wheeled motor vehicle injured in collision with pedestrian or animal in traffic accident

V30.6 Passenger in three-wheeled motor vehicle injured in collision with pedestrian or animal in traffic accident x7th V30.7 Person on outside of three-wheeled motor vehicle injured in collision with pedestrian or animal in traffic accident

x7th V30.9 Unspecified occupant of three-wheeled motor vehicle injured in collision with pedestrian or animal in traffic accident

4th **V31 Occupant of three-wheeled motor vehicle injured in collision with pedal cycle**

x7th V31.0 Driver of three-wheeled motor vehicle injured in collision with pedal cycle in nontraffic accident

x7th V31.1 Passenger in three-wheeled motor vehicle injured in collision with pedal cycle in nontraffic accident

x7th V31.2 Person on outside of three-wheeled motor vehicle injured in collision with pedal cycle in nontraffic accident

x7th V31.3 Unspecified occupant of three-wheeled motor vehicle injured in collision with pedal cycle in nontraffic accident

x7th V31.4 Person boarding or alighting a three-wheeled motor vehicle injured in collision with pedal cycle

x7th V31.5 Driver of three-wheeled motor vehicle injured in collision with pedal cycle in traffic accident

x7th V31.6 Passenger in three-wheeled motor vehicle injured in collision with pedal cycle in traffic accident

x7th V31.7 Person on outside of three-wheeled motor vehicle injured in collision with pedal cycle in traffic accident

x7th V31.9 Unspecified occupant of three-wheeled motor vehicle injured in collision with pedal cycle in traffic accident

4th **V32 Occupant of three-wheeled motor vehicle injured in collision with two- or three-wheeled motor vehicle**

x7th V32.0 Driver of three-wheeled motor vehicle injured in collision with two- or three-wheeled motor vehicle in nontraffic accident

x7th V32.1 Passenger in three-wheeled motor vehicle injured in collision with two- or three-wheeled motor vehicle in nontraffic accident

x7th V32.2 Person on outside of three-wheeled motor vehicle injured in collision with two- or three-wheeled motor vehicle in nontraffic accident

x7th V32.3 Unspecified occupant of three-wheeled motor vehicle injured in collision with two- or three-wheeled motor vehicle in nontraffic accident

x7th V32.4 Person boarding or alighting a three-wheeled motor vehicle injured in collision with two- or three-wheeled motor vehicle

x7th V32.5 Driver of three-wheeled motor vehicle injured in collision with two- or three-wheeled motor vehicle in traffic accident

x7th V32.6 Passenger in three-wheeled motor vehicle injured in collision with two- or three-wheeled motor vehicle in traffic accident

x7th V32.7 Person on outside of three-wheeled motor vehicle injured in collision with two- or three-wheeled motor vehicle in traffic accident

x7th V32.9 Unspecified occupant of three-wheeled motor vehicle injured in collision with two- or three-wheeled motor vehicle in traffic accident

4th **V33 Occupant of three-wheeled motor vehicle injured in collision with car, pick-up truck or van**

x7th V33.0 Driver of three-wheeled motor vehicle injured in collision with car, pick-up truck or van in nontraffic accident

x7th V33.1 Passenger in three-wheeled motor vehicle injured in collision with car, pick-up truck or van in nontraffic accident

x7th V33.2 Person on outside of three-wheeled motor vehicle injured in collision with car, pick-up truck or van in nontraffic accident

x7th V33.3 Unspecified occupant of three-wheeled motor vehicle injured in collision with car, pick-up truck or van in nontraffic accident

x7th V33.4 Person boarding or alighting a three-wheeled motor vehicle injured in collision with car, pick-up truck or van

x7th V33.5 Driver of three-wheeled motor vehicle injured in collision with car, pick-up truck or van in traffic accident

x7th V33.6 Passenger in three-wheeled motor vehicle injured in collision with car, pick-up truck or van in traffic accident

x7th V33.7 Person on outside of three-wheeled motor vehicle injured in collision with car, pick-up truck or van in traffic accident

x7th V33.9 Unspecified occupant of three-wheeled motor vehicle injured in collision with car, pick-up truck or van in traffic accident

4th **V34 Occupant of three-wheeled motor vehicle injured in collision with heavy transport vehicle or bus**

EXCLUDES 1 *occupant of three-wheeled motor vehicle injured in collision with military vehicle (V39.81)*

x7th V34.0 Driver of three-wheeled motor vehicle injured in collision with heavy transport vehicle or bus in nontraffic accident

x7th V34.1 Passenger in three-wheeled motor vehicle injured in collision with heavy transport vehicle or bus in nontraffic accident

x7th V34.2 Person on outside of three-wheeled motor vehicle injured in collision with heavy transport vehicle or bus in nontraffic accident

x7th V34.3 Unspecified occupant of three-wheeled motor vehicle injured in collision with heavy transport vehicle or bus in nontraffic accident

x7th V34.4 Person boarding or alighting a three-wheeled motor vehicle injured in collision with heavy transport vehicle or bus

x7th V34.5 Driver of three-wheeled motor vehicle injured in collision with heavy transport vehicle or bus in traffic accident

x7th V34.6 Passenger in three-wheeled motor vehicle injured in collision with heavy transport vehicle or bus in traffic accident

x7th V34.7 Person on outside of three-wheeled motor vehicle injured in collision with heavy transport vehicle or bus in traffic accident

x7th V34.9 Unspecified occupant of three-wheeled motor vehicle injured in collision with heavy transport vehicle or bus in traffic accident

4th **V35 Occupant of three-wheeled motor vehicle injured in collision with railway train or railway vehicle**

x7th V35.0 Driver of three-wheeled motor vehicle injured in collision with railway train or railway vehicle in nontraffic accident

x7th V35.1 Passenger in three-wheeled motor vehicle injured in collision with railway train or railway vehicle in nontraffic accident

x7th V35.2 Person on outside of three-wheeled motor vehicle injured in collision with railway train or railway vehicle in nontraffic accident

x7th V35.3 Unspecified occupant of three-wheeled motor vehicle injured in collision with railway train or railway vehicle in nontraffic accident

x7th V35.4 Person boarding or alighting a three-wheeled motor vehicle injured in collision with railway train or railway vehicle

x7th V35.5 Driver of three-wheeled motor vehicle injured in collision with railway train or railway vehicle in traffic accident

x7th V35.6 Passenger in three-wheeled motor vehicle injured in collision with railway train or railway vehicle in traffic accident

x7th V35.7 Person on outside of three-wheeled motor vehicle injured in collision with railway train or railway vehicle in traffic accident

x7th V35.9 Unspecified occupant of three-wheeled motor vehicle injured in collision with railway train or railway vehicle in traffic accident

4th **V36 Occupant of three-wheeled motor vehicle injured in collision with other nonmotor vehicle**

INCLUDES collision with animal-drawn vehicle, animal being ridden, streetcar

x7th V36.0 Driver of three-wheeled motor vehicle injured in collision with other nonmotor vehicle in nontraffic accident

x7th V36.1 Passenger in three-wheeled motor vehicle injured in collision with other nonmotor vehicle in nontraffic accident

x7th V36.2 Person on outside of three-wheeled motor vehicle injured in collision with other nonmotor vehicle in nontraffic accident

x7th V36.3 Unspecified occupant of three-wheeled motor vehicle injured in collision with other nonmotor vehicle in nontraffic accident

x7th V36.4 Person boarding or alighting a three-wheeled motor vehicle injured in collision with other nonmotor vehicle

x7th V36.5 Driver of three-wheeled motor vehicle injured in collision with other nonmotor vehicle in traffic accident

x7th V36.6 Passenger in three-wheeled motor vehicle injured in collision with other nonmotor vehicle in traffic accident

x7th V36.7 Person on outside of three-wheeled motor vehicle injured in collision with other nonmotor vehicle in traffic accident

x7th V36.9 Unspecified occupant of three-wheeled motor vehicle injured in collision with other nonmotor vehicle in traffic accident

4th **V37 Occupant of three-wheeled motor vehicle injured in collision with fixed or stationary object**

x7th V37.0 Driver of three-wheeled motor vehicle injured in collision with fixed or stationary object in nontraffic accident

x7th V37.1 Passenger in three-wheeled motor vehicle injured in collision with fixed or stationary object in nontraffic accident

x7th V37.2 Person on outside of three-wheeled motor vehicle injured in collision with fixed or stationary object in nontraffic accident

x7th V37.3 Unspecified occupant of three-wheeled motor vehicle injured in collision with fixed or stationary object in nontraffic accident

x7th V37.4 Person boarding or alighting a three-wheeled motor vehicle injured in collision with fixed or stationary object

x7th V37.5 Driver of three-wheeled motor vehicle injured in collision with fixed or stationary object in traffic accident

√x7th V37.6 **Passenger in three-wheeled motor vehicle injured in collision with fixed or stationary object in traffic accident**

√x7th V37.7 **Person on outside of three-wheeled motor vehicle injured in collision with fixed or stationary object in traffic accident**

√x7th V37.9 **Unspecified occupant of three-wheeled motor vehicle injured in collision with fixed or stationary object in traffic accident**

√4th **V38 Occupant of three-wheeled motor vehicle injured in noncollision transport accident**

INCLUDES fall or thrown from three-wheeled motor vehicle
overturning of three-wheeled motor vehicle NOS
overturning of three-wheeled motor vehicle without collision

√x7th V38.Ø **Driver of three-wheeled motor vehicle injured in noncollision transport accident in nontraffic accident**

√x7th V38.1 **Passenger in three-wheeled motor vehicle injured in noncollision transport accident in nontraffic accident**

√x7th V38.2 **Person on outside of three-wheeled motor vehicle injured in noncollision transport accident in nontraffic accident**

√x7th V38.3 **Unspecified occupant of three-wheeled motor vehicle injured in noncollision transport accident in nontraffic accident**

√x7th V38.4 **Person boarding or alighting a three-wheeled motor vehicle injured in noncollision transport accident**

√x7th V38.5 **Driver of three-wheeled motor vehicle injured in noncollision transport accident in traffic accident**

√x7th V38.6 **Passenger in three-wheeled motor vehicle injured in noncollision transport accident in traffic accident**

√x7th V38.7 **Person on outside of three-wheeled motor vehicle injured in noncollision transport accident in traffic accident**

√x7th V38.9 **Unspecified occupant of three-wheeled motor vehicle injured in noncollision transport accident in traffic accident**

√4th **V39 Occupant of three-wheeled motor vehicle injured in other and unspecified transport accidents**

√5th V39.Ø **Driver of three-wheeled motor vehicle injured in collision with other and unspecified motor vehicles in nontraffic accident**

√x7th V39.ØØ **Driver of three-wheeled motor vehicle injured in collision with unspecified motor vehicles in nontraffic accident**

√x7th V39.Ø9 **Driver of three-wheeled motor vehicle injured in collision with other motor vehicles in nontraffic accident**

√5th V39.1 **Passenger in three-wheeled motor vehicle injured in collision with other and unspecified motor vehicles in nontraffic accident**

√x7th V39.1Ø **Passenger in three-wheeled motor vehicle injured in collision with unspecified motor vehicles in nontraffic accident**

√x7th V39.19 **Passenger in three-wheeled motor vehicle injured in collision with other motor vehicles in nontraffic accident**

√5th V39.2 **Unspecified occupant of three-wheeled motor vehicle injured in collision with other and unspecified motor vehicles in nontraffic accident**

√x7th V39.2Ø **Unspecified occupant of three-wheeled motor vehicle injured in collision with unspecified motor vehicles in nontraffic accident**

Collision NOS involving three-wheeled motor vehicle, nontraffic

√x7th V39.29 **Unspecified occupant of three-wheeled motor vehicle injured in collision with other motor vehicles in nontraffic accident**

√x7th V39.3 **Occupant (driver) (passenger) of three-wheeled motor vehicle injured in unspecified nontraffic accident**

Accident NOS involving three-wheeled motor vehicle, nontraffic
Occupant of three-wheeled motor vehicle injured in nontraffic accident NOS

√5th V39.4 **Driver of three-wheeled motor vehicle injured in collision with other and unspecified motor vehicles in traffic accident**

√x7th V39.4Ø **Driver of three-wheeled motor vehicle injured in collision with unspecified motor vehicles in traffic accident**

√x7th V39.49 **Driver of three-wheeled motor vehicle injured in collision with other motor vehicles in traffic accident**

√5th V39.5 **Passenger in three-wheeled motor vehicle injured in collision with other and unspecified motor vehicles in traffic accident**

√x7th V39.5Ø **Passenger in three-wheeled motor vehicle injured in collision with unspecified motor vehicles in traffic accident**

√x7th V39.59 **Passenger in three-wheeled motor vehicle injured in collision with other motor vehicles in traffic accident**

√5th V39.6 **Unspecified occupant of three-wheeled motor vehicle injured in collision with other and unspecified motor vehicles in traffic accident**

√x7th V39.6Ø **Unspecified occupant of three-wheeled motor vehicle injured in collision with unspecified motor vehicles in traffic accident**

Collision NOS involving three-wheeled motor vehicle (traffic)

√x7th V39.69 **Unspecified occupant of three-wheeled motor vehicle injured in collision with other motor vehicles in traffic accident**

√5th V39.8 **Occupant (driver) (passenger) of three-wheeled motor vehicle injured in other specified transport accidents**

√x7th V39.81 **Occupant (driver) (passenger) of three-wheeled motor vehicle injured in transport accident with military vehicle**

√x7th V39.89 **Occupant (driver) (passenger) of three-wheeled motor vehicle injured in other specified transport accidents**

√x7th V39.9 **Occupant (driver) (passenger) of three-wheeled motor vehicle injured in unspecified traffic accident**

Accident NOS involving three-wheeled motor vehicle

Car occupant injured in transport accident (V4Ø-V49)

INCLUDES a four-wheeled motor vehicle designed primarily for carrying passengers
automobile (pulling a trailer or camper)

EXCLUDES 1 *bus (V5Ø-V59)*
minibus (V5Ø-V59)
minivan (V5Ø-V59)
motorcoach (V7Ø-V79)
pick-up truck (V5Ø-V59)
sport utility vehicle (SUV) (V5Ø-V59)

The appropriate 7th character is to be added to each code from categories V4Ø-V49.
A initial encounter
D subsequent encounter
S sequela

√4th **V4Ø Car occupant injured in collision with pedestrian or animal**

EXCLUDES 1 *car collision with animal-drawn vehicle or animal being ridden (V46.-)*

√x7th V4Ø.Ø **Car driver injured in collision with pedestrian or animal in nontraffic accident**

√x7th V4Ø.1 **Car passenger injured in collision with pedestrian or animal in nontraffic accident**

√x7th V4Ø.2 **Person on outside of car injured in collision with pedestrian or animal in nontraffic accident**

√x7th V4Ø.3 **Unspecified car occupant injured in collision with pedestrian or animal in nontraffic accident**

√x7th V4Ø.4 **Person boarding or alighting a car injured in collision with pedestrian or animal**

√x7th V4Ø.5 **Car driver injured in collision with pedestrian or animal in traffic accident**

√x7th V4Ø.6 **Car passenger injured in collision with pedestrian or animal in traffic accident**

√x7th V4Ø.7 **Person on outside of car injured in collision with pedestrian or animal in traffic accident**

√x7th V4Ø.9 **Unspecified car occupant injured in collision with pedestrian or animal in traffic accident**

√4th **V41 Car occupant injured in collision with pedal cycle**

√x7th V41.Ø **Car driver injured in collision with pedal cycle in nontraffic accident**

√x7th V41.1 **Car passenger injured in collision with pedal cycle in nontraffic accident**

√x7th V41.2 **Person on outside of car injured in collision with pedal cycle in nontraffic accident**

√x7th V41.3 **Unspecified car occupant injured in collision with pedal cycle in nontraffic accident**

√x7th V41.4 **Person boarding or alighting a car injured in collision with pedal cycle**

√x7th V41.5 **Car driver injured in collision with pedal cycle in traffic accident**

√x7th V41.6 **Car passenger injured in collision with pedal cycle in traffic accident**

√x7th V41.7 **Person on outside of car injured in collision with pedal cycle in traffic accident**

√x7th V41.9 **Unspecified car occupant injured in collision with pedal cycle in traffic accident**

V42 Car occupant injured in collision with two- or three-wheeled motor vehicle

- V42.Ø Car driver injured in collision with two- or three-wheeled motor vehicle in nontraffic accident
- V42.1 Car passenger injured in collision with two- or three-wheeled motor vehicle in nontraffic accident
- V42.2 Person on outside of car injured in collision with two- or three-wheeled motor vehicle in nontraffic accident
- V42.3 Unspecified car occupant injured in collision with two- or three-wheeled motor vehicle in nontraffic accident
- V42.4 Person boarding or alighting a car injured in collision with two- or three-wheeled motor vehicle
- V42.5 Car driver injured in collision with two- or three-wheeled motor vehicle in traffic accident
- V42.6 Car passenger injured in collision with two- or three-wheeled motor vehicle in traffic accident
- V42.7 Person on outside of car injured in collision with two- or three-wheeled motor vehicle in traffic accident
- V42.9 Unspecified car occupant injured in collision with two- or three-wheeled motor vehicle in traffic accident

V43 Car occupant injured in collision with car, pick-up truck or van

- V43.Ø Car driver injured in collision with car, pick-up truck or van in nontraffic accident
  - V43.Ø1 Car driver injured in collision with sport utility vehicle in nontraffic accident
  - V43.Ø2 Car driver injured in collision with other type car in nontraffic accident
  - V43.Ø3 Car driver injured in collision with pick-up truck in nontraffic accident
  - V43.Ø4 Car driver injured in collision with van in nontraffic accident
- V43.1 Car passenger injured in collision with car, pick-up truck or van in nontraffic accident
  - V43.11 Car passenger injured in collision with sport utility vehicle in nontraffic accident
  - V43.12 Car passenger injured in collision with other type car in nontraffic accident
  - V43.13 Car passenger injured in collision with pick-up truck in nontraffic accident
  - V43.14 Car passenger injured in collision with van in nontraffic accident
- V43.2 Person on outside of car injured in collision with car, pick-up truck or van in nontraffic accident
  - V43.21 Person on outside of car injured in collision with sport utility vehicle in nontraffic accident
  - V43.22 Person on outside of car injured in collision with other type car in nontraffic accident
  - V43.23 Person on outside of car injured in collision with pick-up truck in nontraffic accident
  - V43.24 Person on outside of car injured in collision with van in nontraffic accident
- V43.3 Unspecified car occupant injured in collision with car, pick-up truck or van in nontraffic accident
  - V43.31 Unspecified car occupant injured in collision with sport utility vehicle in nontraffic accident
  - V43.32 Unspecified car occupant injured in collision with other type car in nontraffic accident
  - V43.33 Unspecified car occupant injured in collision with pick-up truck in nontraffic accident
  - V43.34 Unspecified car occupant injured in collision with van in nontraffic accident
- V43.4 Person boarding or alighting a car injured in collision with car, pick-up truck or van
  - V43.41 Person boarding or alighting a car injured in collision with sport utility vehicle
  - V43.42 Person boarding or alighting a car injured in collision with other type car
  - V43.43 Person boarding or alighting a car injured in collision with pick-up truck
  - V43.44 Person boarding or alighting a car injured in collision with van
- V43.5 Car driver injured in collision with car, pick-up truck or van in traffic accident
  - V43.51 Car driver injured in collision with sport utility vehicle in traffic accident
  - V43.52 Car driver injured in collision with other type car in traffic accident
  - V43.53 Car driver injured in collision with pick-up truck in traffic accident
  - V43.54 Car driver injured in collision with van in traffic accident
- V43.6 Car passenger injured in collision with car, pick-up truck or van in traffic accident
  - V43.61 Car passenger injured in collision with sport utility vehicle in traffic accident
  - V43.62 Car passenger injured in collision with other type car in traffic accident
  - V43.63 Car passenger injured in collision with pick-up truck in traffic accident
  - V43.64 Car passenger injured in collision with van in traffic accident
- V43.7 Person on outside of car injured in collision with car, pick-up truck or van in traffic accident
  - V43.71 Person on outside of car injured in collision with sport utility vehicle in traffic accident
  - V43.72 Person on outside of car injured in collision with other type car in traffic accident
  - V43.73 Person on outside of car injured in collision with pick-up truck in traffic accident
  - V43.74 Person on outside of car injured in collision with van in traffic accident
- V43.9 Unspecified car occupant injured in collision with car, pick-up truck or van in traffic accident
  - V43.91 Unspecified car occupant injured in collision with sport utility vehicle in traffic accident
  - V43.92 Unspecified car occupant injured in collision with other type car in traffic accident
  - V43.93 Unspecified car occupant injured in collision with pick-up truck in traffic accident
  - V43.94 Unspecified car occupant injured in collision with van in traffic accident

V44 Car occupant injured in collision with heavy transport vehicle or bus

EXCLUDES 1 *car occupant injured in collision with military vehicle (V49.81)*

- V44.Ø Car driver injured in collision with heavy transport vehicle or bus in nontraffic accident
- V44.1 Car passenger injured in collision with heavy transport vehicle or bus in nontraffic accident
- V44.2 Person on outside of car injured in collision with heavy transport vehicle or bus in nontraffic accident
- V44.3 Unspecified car occupant injured in collision with heavy transport vehicle or bus in nontraffic accident
- V44.4 Person boarding or alighting a car injured in collision with heavy transport vehicle or bus
- V44.5 Car driver injured in collision with heavy transport vehicle or bus in traffic accident
- V44.6 Car passenger injured in collision with heavy transport vehicle or bus in traffic accident
- V44.7 Person on outside of car injured in collision with heavy transport vehicle or bus in traffic accident
- V44.9 Unspecified car occupant injured in collision with heavy transport vehicle or bus in traffic accident

V45 Car occupant injured in collision with railway train or railway vehicle

- V45.Ø Car driver injured in collision with railway train or railway vehicle in nontraffic accident
- V45.1 Car passenger injured in collision with railway train or railway vehicle in nontraffic accident
- V45.2 Person on outside of car injured in collision with railway train or railway vehicle in nontraffic accident
- V45.3 Unspecified car occupant injured in collision with railway train or railway vehicle in nontraffic accident
- V45.4 Person boarding or alighting a car injured in collision with railway train or railway vehicle
- V45.5 Car driver injured in collision with railway train or railway vehicle in traffic accident
- V45.6 Car passenger injured in collision with railway train or railway vehicle in traffic accident
- V45.7 Person on outside of car injured in collision with railway train or railway vehicle in traffic accident
- V45.9 Unspecified car occupant injured in collision with railway train or railway vehicle in traffic accident

V46 Car occupant injured in collision with other nonmotor vehicle

INCLUDES collision with animal-drawn vehicle, animal being ridden, streetcar

- V46.Ø Car driver injured in collision with other nonmotor vehicle in nontraffic accident
- V46.1 Car passenger injured in collision with other nonmotor vehicle in nontraffic accident
- V46.2 Person on outside of car injured in collision with other nonmotor vehicle in nontraffic accident

✓x7th **V46.3** **Unspecified car occupant injured in collision with other nonmotor vehicle in nontraffic accident**

✓x7th **V46.4** **Person boarding or alighting a car injured in collision with other nonmotor vehicle**

✓x7th **V46.5** **Car driver injured in collision with other nonmotor vehicle in traffic accident**

✓x7th **V46.6** **Car passenger injured in collision with other nonmotor vehicle in traffic accident**

✓x7th **V46.7** **Person on outside of car injured in collision with other nonmotor vehicle in traffic accident**

✓x7th **V46.9** **Unspecified car occupant injured in collision with other nonmotor vehicle in traffic accident**

✓4th **V47** **Car occupant injured in collision with fixed or stationary object**

AHA: 2016,4Q,73

✓x7th **V47.0** **Car driver injured in collision with fixed or stationary object in nontraffic accident**

✓x7th **V47.1** **Car passenger injured in collision with fixed or stationary object in nontraffic accident**

✓x7th **V47.2** **Person on outside of car injured in collision with fixed or stationary object in nontraffic accident**

✓x7th **V47.3** **Unspecified car occupant injured in collision with fixed or stationary object in nontraffic accident**

✓x7th **V47.4** **Person boarding or alighting a car injured in collision with fixed or stationary object**

✓x7th **V47.5** **Car driver injured in collision with fixed or stationary object in traffic accident**

✓x7th **V47.6** **Car passenger injured in collision with fixed or stationary object in traffic accident**

✓x7th **V47.7** **Person on outside of car injured in collision with fixed or stationary object in traffic accident**

✓x7th **V47.9** **Unspecified car occupant injured in collision with fixed or stationary object in traffic accident**

✓4th **V48** **Car occupant injured in noncollision transport accident**

INCLUDES overturning car NOS
overturning car without collision

✓x7th **V48.0** **Car driver injured in noncollision transport accident in nontraffic accident**

✓x7th **V48.1** **Car passenger injured in noncollision transport accident in nontraffic accident**

✓x7th **V48.2** **Person on outside of car injured in noncollision transport accident in nontraffic accident**

✓x7th **V48.3** **Unspecified car occupant injured in noncollision transport accident in nontraffic accident**

✓x7th **V48.4** **Person boarding or alighting a car injured in noncollision transport accident**

✓x7th **V48.5** **Car driver injured in noncollision transport accident in traffic accident**

✓x7th **V48.6** **Car passenger injured in noncollision transport accident in traffic accident**

✓x7th **V48.7** **Person on outside of car injured in noncollision transport accident in traffic accident**

✓x7th **V48.9** **Unspecified car occupant injured in noncollision transport accident in traffic accident**

✓4th **V49** **Car occupant injured in other and unspecified transport accidents**

✓5th **V49.0** **Driver injured in collision with other and unspecified motor vehicles in nontraffic accident**

✓x7th **V49.00** **Driver injured in collision with unspecified motor vehicles in nontraffic accident**

✓x7th **V49.09** **Driver injured in collision with other motor vehicles in nontraffic accident**

✓5th **V49.1** **Passenger injured in collision with other and unspecified motor vehicles in nontraffic accident**

✓x7th **V49.10** **Passenger injured in collision with unspecified motor vehicles in nontraffic accident**

✓x7th **V49.19** **Passenger injured in collision with other motor vehicles in nontraffic accident**

✓5th **V49.2** **Unspecified car occupant injured in collision with other and unspecified motor vehicles in nontraffic accident**

✓x7th **V49.20** **Unspecified car occupant injured in collision with unspecified motor vehicles in nontraffic accident**

Car collision NOS, nontraffic

✓x7th **V49.29** **Unspecified car occupant injured in collision with other motor vehicles in nontraffic accident**

✓x7th **V49.3** **Car occupant (driver) (passenger) injured in unspecified nontraffic accident**

Car accident NOS, nontraffic
Car occupant injured in nontraffic accident NOS

✓5th **V49.4** **Driver injured in collision with other and unspecified motor vehicles in traffic accident**

✓x7th **V49.40** **Driver injured in collision with unspecified motor vehicles in traffic accident**

✓x7th **V49.49** **Driver injured in collision with other motor vehicles in traffic accident**

✓5th **V49.5** **Passenger injured in collision with other and unspecified motor vehicles in traffic accident**

✓x7th **V49.50** **Passenger injured in collision with unspecified motor vehicles in traffic accident**

✓x7th **V49.59** **Passenger injured in collision with other motor vehicles in traffic accident**

✓5th **V49.6** **Unspecified car occupant injured in collision with other and unspecified motor vehicles in traffic accident**

✓x7th **V49.60** **Unspecified car occupant injured in collision with unspecified motor vehicles in traffic accident**

Car collision NOS (traffic)

✓x7th **V49.69** **Unspecified car occupant injured in collision with other motor vehicles in traffic accident**

✓5th **V49.8** **Car occupant (driver) (passenger) injured in other specified transport accidents**

✓x7th **V49.81** **Car occupant (driver) (passenger) injured in transport accident with military vehicle**

✓x7th **V49.88** **Car occupant (driver) (passenger) injured in other specified transport accidents**

✓x7th **V49.9** **Car occupant (driver) (passenger) injured in unspecified traffic accident**

Car accident NOS

Occupant of pick-up truck or van injured in transport accident (V50-V59)

INCLUDES a four or six wheel motor vehicle designed primarily for carrying passengers and property but weighing less than the local limit for classification as a heavy goods vehicle
minibus
minivan
sport utility vehicle (SUV)
truck
van

EXCLUDES 1 *heavy transport vehicle (V60-V69)*

The appropriate 7th character is to be added to each code from categories V50-V59.
A initial encounter
D subsequent encounter
S sequela

✓4th **V50** **Occupant of pick-up truck or van injured in collision with pedestrian or animal**

EXCLUDES 1 *pick-up truck or van collision with animal-drawn vehicle or animal being ridden (V56.-)*

✓x7th **V50.0** **Driver of pick-up truck or van injured in collision with pedestrian or animal in nontraffic accident**

✓x7th **V50.1** **Passenger in pick-up truck or van injured in collision with pedestrian or animal in nontraffic accident**

✓x7th **V50.2** **Person on outside of pick-up truck or van injured in collision with pedestrian or animal in nontraffic accident**

✓x7th **V50.3** **Unspecified occupant of pick-up truck or van injured in collision with pedestrian or animal in nontraffic accident**

✓x7th **V50.4** **Person boarding or alighting a pick-up truck or van injured in collision with pedestrian or animal**

✓x7th **V50.5** **Driver of pick-up truck or van injured in collision with pedestrian or animal in traffic accident**

✓x7th **V50.6** **Passenger in pick-up truck or van injured in collision with pedestrian or animal in traffic accident**

✓x7th **V50.7** **Person on outside of pick-up truck or van injured in collision with pedestrian or animal in traffic accident**

✓x7th **V50.9** **Unspecified occupant of pick-up truck or van injured in collision with pedestrian or animal in traffic accident**

✓4th **V51** **Occupant of pick-up truck or van injured in collision with pedal cycle**

✓x7th **V51.0** **Driver of pick-up truck or van injured in collision with pedal cycle in nontraffic accident**

✓x7th **V51.1** **Passenger in pick-up truck or van injured in collision with pedal cycle in nontraffic accident**

✓x7th **V51.2** **Person on outside of pick-up truck or van injured in collision with pedal cycle in nontraffic accident**

✓x7th **V51.3** **Unspecified occupant of pick-up truck or van injured in collision with pedal cycle in nontraffic accident**

✓x7th **V51.4** **Person boarding or alighting a pick-up truck or van injured in collision with pedal cycle**

✓x7th **V51.5** **Driver of pick-up truck or van injured in collision with pedal cycle in traffic accident**

√x7th V51.6 Passenger in pick-up truck or van injured in collision with pedal cycle in traffic accident

√x7th V51.7 Person on outside of pick-up truck or van injured in collision with pedal cycle in traffic accident

√x7th V51.9 Unspecified occupant of pick-up truck or van injured in collision with pedal cycle in traffic accident

√4th **V52 Occupant of pick-up truck or van injured in collision with two- or three-wheeled motor vehicle**

√x7th V52.0 Driver of pick-up truck or van injured in collision with two- or three-wheeled motor vehicle in nontraffic accident

√x7th V52.1 Passenger in pick-up truck or van injured in collision with two- or three-wheeled motor vehicle in nontraffic accident

√x7th V52.2 Person on outside of pick-up truck or van injured in collision with two- or three-wheeled motor vehicle in nontraffic accident

√x7th V52.3 Unspecified occupant of pick-up truck or van injured in collision with two- or three-wheeled motor vehicle in nontraffic accident

√x7th V52.4 Person boarding or alighting a pick-up truck or van injured in collision with two- or three-wheeled motor vehicle

√x7th V52.5 Driver of pick-up truck or van injured in collision with two- or three-wheeled motor vehicle in traffic accident

√x7th V52.6 Passenger in pick-up truck or van injured in collision with two- or three-wheeled motor vehicle in traffic accident

√x7th V52.7 Person on outside of pick-up truck or van injured in collision with two- or three-wheeled motor vehicle in traffic accident

√x7th V52.9 Unspecified occupant of pick-up truck or van injured in collision with two- or three-wheeled motor vehicle in traffic accident

√4th **V53 Occupant of pick-up truck or van injured in collision with car, pick-up truck or van**

√x7th V53.0 Driver of pick-up truck or van injured in collision with car, pick-up truck or van in nontraffic accident

√x7th V53.1 Passenger in pick-up truck or van injured in collision with car, pick-up truck or van in nontraffic accident

√x7th V53.2 Person on outside of pick-up truck or van injured in collision with car, pick-up truck or van in nontraffic accident

√x7th V53.3 Unspecified occupant of pick-up truck or van injured in collision with car, pick-up truck or van in nontraffic accident

√x7th V53.4 Person boarding or alighting a pick-up truck or van injured in collision with car, pick-up truck or van

√x7th V53.5 Driver of pick-up truck or van injured in collision with car, pick-up truck or van in traffic accident

√x7th V53.6 Passenger in pick-up truck or van injured in collision with car, pick-up truck or van in traffic accident

√x7th V53.7 Person on outside of pick-up truck or van injured in collision with car, pick-up truck or van in traffic accident

√x7th V53.9 Unspecified occupant of pick-up truck or van injured in collision with car, pick-up truck or van in traffic accident

√4th **V54 Occupant of pick-up truck or van injured in collision with heavy transport vehicle or bus**

EXCLUDES 1 *occupant of pick-up truck or van injured in collision with military vehicle (V59.81)*

√x7th V54.0 Driver of pick-up truck or van injured in collision with heavy transport vehicle or bus in nontraffic accident

√x7th V54.1 Passenger in pick-up truck or van injured in collision with heavy transport vehicle or bus in nontraffic accident

√x7th V54.2 Person on outside of pick-up truck or van injured in collision with heavy transport vehicle or bus in nontraffic accident

√x7th V54.3 Unspecified occupant of pick-up truck or van injured in collision with heavy transport vehicle or bus in nontraffic accident

√x7th V54.4 Person boarding or alighting a pick-up truck or van injured in collision with heavy transport vehicle or bus

√x7th V54.5 Driver of pick-up truck or van injured in collision with heavy transport vehicle or bus in traffic accident

√x7th V54.6 Passenger in pick-up truck or van injured in collision with heavy transport vehicle or bus in traffic accident

√x7th V54.7 Person on outside of pick-up truck or van injured in collision with heavy transport vehicle or bus in traffic accident

√x7th V54.9 Unspecified occupant of pick-up truck or van injured in collision with heavy transport vehicle or bus in traffic accident

√4th **V55 Occupant of pick-up truck or van injured in collision with railway train or railway vehicle**

√x7th V55.0 Driver of pick-up truck or van injured in collision with railway train or railway vehicle in nontraffic accident

√x7th V55.1 Passenger in pick-up truck or van injured in collision with railway train or railway vehicle in nontraffic accident

√x7th V55.2 Person on outside of pick-up truck or van injured in collision with railway train or railway vehicle in nontraffic accident

√x7th V55.3 Unspecified occupant of pick-up truck or van injured in collision with railway train or railway vehicle in nontraffic accident

√x7th V55.4 Person boarding or alighting a pick-up truck or van injured in collision with railway train or railway vehicle

√x7th V55.5 Driver of pick-up truck or van injured in collision with railway train or railway vehicle in traffic accident

√x7th V55.6 Passenger in pick-up truck or van injured in collision with railway train or railway vehicle in traffic accident

√x7th V55.7 Person on outside of pick-up truck or van injured in collision with railway train or railway vehicle in traffic accident

√x7th V55.9 Unspecified occupant of pick-up truck or van injured in collision with railway train or railway vehicle in traffic accident

√4th **V56 Occupant of pick-up truck or van injured in collision with other nonmotor vehicle**

INCLUDES collision with animal-drawn vehicle, animal being ridden, streetcar

√x7th V56.0 Driver of pick-up truck or van injured in collision with other nonmotor vehicle in nontraffic accident

√x7th V56.1 Passenger in pick-up truck or van injured in collision with other nonmotor vehicle in nontraffic accident

√x7th V56.2 Person on outside of pick-up truck or van injured in collision with other nonmotor vehicle in nontraffic accident

√x7th V56.3 Unspecified occupant of pick-up truck or van injured in collision with other nonmotor vehicle in nontraffic accident

√x7th V56.4 Person boarding or alighting a pick-up truck or van injured in collision with other nonmotor vehicle

√x7th V56.5 Driver of pick-up truck or van injured in collision with other nonmotor vehicle in traffic accident

√x7th V56.6 Passenger in pick-up truck or van injured in collision with other nonmotor vehicle in traffic accident

√x7th V56.7 Person on outside of pick-up truck or van injured in collision with other nonmotor vehicle in traffic accident

√x7th V56.9 Unspecified occupant of pick-up truck or van injured in collision with other nonmotor vehicle in traffic accident

√4th **V57 Occupant of pick-up truck or van injured in collision with fixed or stationary object**

√x7th V57.0 Driver of pick-up truck or van injured in collision with fixed or stationary object in nontraffic accident

√x7th V57.1 Passenger in pick-up truck or van injured in collision with fixed or stationary object in nontraffic accident

√x7th V57.2 Person on outside of pick-up truck or van injured in collision with fixed or stationary object in nontraffic accident

√x7th V57.3 Unspecified occupant of pick-up truck or van injured in collision with fixed or stationary object in nontraffic accident

√x7th V57.4 Person boarding or alighting a pick-up truck or van injured in collision with fixed or stationary object

√x7th V57.5 Driver of pick-up truck or van injured in collision with fixed or stationary object in traffic accident

√x7th V57.6 Passenger in pick-up truck or van injured in collision with fixed or stationary object in traffic accident

√x7th V57.7 Person on outside of pick-up truck or van injured in collision with fixed or stationary object in traffic accident

√x7th V57.9 Unspecified occupant of pick-up truck or van injured in collision with fixed or stationary object in traffic accident

√4th **V58 Occupant of pick-up truck or van injured in noncollision transport accident**

INCLUDES overturning pick-up truck or van NOS
overturning pick-up truck or van without collision

√x7th V58.0 Driver of pick-up truck or van injured in noncollision transport accident in nontraffic accident

√x7th V58.1 Passenger in pick-up truck or van injured in noncollision transport accident in nontraffic accident

√x7th V58.2 Person on outside of pick-up truck or van injured in noncollision transport accident in nontraffic accident

√x7th V58.3 Unspecified occupant of pick-up truck or van injured in noncollision transport accident in nontraffic accident

√x7th V58.4 Person boarding or alighting a pick-up truck or van injured in noncollision transport accident

√x7th V58.5 Driver of pick-up truck or van injured in noncollision transport accident in traffic accident

√x7th V58.6 Passenger in pick-up truck or van injured in noncollision transport accident in traffic accident

√x7th V58.7 Person on outside of pick-up truck or van injured in noncollision transport accident in traffic accident

√x7th V58.9 Unspecified occupant of pick-up truck or van injured in noncollision transport accident in traffic accident

V59 Occupant of pick-up truck or van injured in other and unspecified transport accidents

V59.Ø Driver of pick-up truck or van injured in collision with other and unspecified motor vehicles in nontraffic accident

V59.ØØ Driver of pick-up truck or van injured in collision with unspecified motor vehicles in nontraffic accident

V59.Ø9 Driver of pick-up truck or van injured in collision with other motor vehicles in nontraffic accident

V59.1 Passenger in pick-up truck or van injured in collision with other and unspecified motor vehicles in nontraffic accident

V59.1Ø Passenger in pick-up truck or van injured in collision with unspecified motor vehicles in nontraffic accident

V59.19 Passenger in pick-up truck or van injured in collision with other motor vehicles in nontraffic accident

V59.2 Unspecified occupant of pick-up truck or van injured in collision with other and unspecified motor vehicles in nontraffic accident

V59.2Ø Unspecified occupant of pick-up truck or van injured in collision with unspecified motor vehicles in nontraffic accident

Collision NOS involving pick-up truck or van, nontraffic

V59.29 Unspecified occupant of pick-up truck or van injured in collision with other motor vehicles in nontraffic accident

V59.3 Occupant (driver) (passenger) of pick-up truck or van injured in unspecified nontraffic accident

Accident NOS involving pick-up truck or van, nontraffic

Occupant of pick-up truck or van injured in nontraffic accident NOS

V59.4 Driver of pick-up truck or van injured in collision with other and unspecified motor vehicles in traffic accident

V59.4Ø Driver of pick-up truck or van injured in collision with unspecified motor vehicles in traffic accident

V59.49 Driver of pick-up truck or van injured in collision with other motor vehicles in traffic accident

V59.5 Passenger in pick-up truck or van injured in collision with other and unspecified motor vehicles in traffic accident

V59.5Ø Passenger in pick-up truck or van injured in collision with unspecified motor vehicles in traffic accident

V59.59 Passenger in pick-up truck or van injured in collision with other motor vehicles in traffic accident

V59.6 Unspecified occupant of pick-up truck or van injured in collision with other and unspecified motor vehicles in traffic accident

V59.6Ø Unspecified occupant of pick-up truck or van injured in collision with unspecified motor vehicles in traffic accident

Collision NOS involving pick-up truck or van (traffic)

V59.69 Unspecified occupant of pick-up truck or van injured in collision with other motor vehicles in traffic accident

V59.8 Occupant (driver) (passenger) of pick-up truck or van injured in other specified transport accidents

V59.81 Occupant (driver) (passenger) of pick-up truck or van injured in transport accident with military vehicle

V59.88 Occupant (driver) (passenger) of pick-up truck or van injured in other specified transport accidents

V59.9 Occupant (driver) (passenger) of pick-up truck or van injured in unspecified traffic accident

Accident NOS involving pick-up truck or van

Occupant of heavy transport vehicle injured in transport accident (V6Ø-V69)

INCLUDES 18 wheeler
armored car
panel truck

EXCLUDES1 *bus*
motorcoach

The appropriate 7th character is to be added to each code from categories V6Ø-V69.
A initial encounter
D subsequent encounter
S sequela

V6Ø Occupant of heavy transport vehicle injured in collision with pedestrian or animal

EXCLUDES1 *heavy transport vehicle collision with animal-drawn vehicle or animal being ridden (V66.-)*

V6Ø.Ø Driver of heavy transport vehicle injured in collision with pedestrian or animal in nontraffic accident

V6Ø.1 Passenger in heavy transport vehicle injured in collision with pedestrian or animal in nontraffic accident

V6Ø.2 Person on outside of heavy transport vehicle injured in collision with pedestrian or animal in nontraffic accident

V6Ø.3 Unspecified occupant of heavy transport vehicle injured in collision with pedestrian or animal in nontraffic accident

V6Ø.4 Person boarding or alighting a heavy transport vehicle injured in collision with pedestrian or animal

V6Ø.5 Driver of heavy transport vehicle injured in collision with pedestrian or animal in traffic accident

V6Ø.6 Passenger in heavy transport vehicle injured in collision with pedestrian or animal in traffic accident

V6Ø.7 Person on outside of heavy transport vehicle injured in collision with pedestrian or animal in traffic accident

V6Ø.9 Unspecified occupant of heavy transport vehicle injured in collision with pedestrian or animal in traffic accident

V61 Occupant of heavy transport vehicle injured in collision with pedal cycle

V61.Ø Driver of heavy transport vehicle injured in collision with pedal cycle in nontraffic accident

V61.1 Passenger in heavy transport vehicle injured in collision with pedal cycle in nontraffic accident

V61.2 Person on outside of heavy transport vehicle injured in collision with pedal cycle in nontraffic accident

V61.3 Unspecified occupant of heavy transport vehicle injured in collision with pedal cycle in nontraffic accident

V61.4 Person boarding or alighting a heavy transport vehicle injured in collision with pedal cycle while boarding or alighting

V61.5 Driver of heavy transport vehicle injured in collision with pedal cycle in traffic accident

V61.6 Passenger in heavy transport vehicle injured in collision with pedal cycle in traffic accident

V61.7 Person on outside of heavy transport vehicle injured in collision with pedal cycle in traffic accident

V61.9 Unspecified occupant of heavy transport vehicle injured in collision with pedal cycle in traffic accident

V62 Occupant of heavy transport vehicle injured in collision with two- or three-wheeled motor vehicle

V62.Ø Driver of heavy transport vehicle injured in collision with two- or three-wheeled motor vehicle in nontraffic accident

V62.1 Passenger in heavy transport vehicle injured in collision with two- or three-wheeled motor vehicle in nontraffic accident

V62.2 Person on outside of heavy transport vehicle injured in collision with two- or three-wheeled motor vehicle in nontraffic accident

V62.3 Unspecified occupant of heavy transport vehicle injured in collision with two- or three-wheeled motor vehicle in nontraffic accident

V62.4 Person boarding or alighting a heavy transport vehicle injured in collision with two- or three-wheeled motor vehicle

V62.5 Driver of heavy transport vehicle injured in collision with two- or three-wheeled motor vehicle in traffic accident

V62.6 Passenger in heavy transport vehicle injured in collision with two- or three-wheeled motor vehicle in traffic accident

V62.7 Person on outside of heavy transport vehicle injured in collision with two- or three-wheeled motor vehicle in traffic accident

V62.9 Unspecified occupant of heavy transport vehicle injured in collision with two- or three-wheeled motor vehicle in traffic accident

V63 Occupant of heavy transport vehicle injured in collision with car, pick-up truck or van

- **V63.0** Driver of heavy transport vehicle injured in collision with car, pick-up truck or van in nontraffic accident
- **V63.1** Passenger in heavy transport vehicle injured in collision with car, pick-up truck or van in nontraffic accident
- **V63.2** Person on outside of heavy transport vehicle injured in collision with car, pick-up truck or van in nontraffic accident
- **V63.3** Unspecified occupant of heavy transport vehicle injured in collision with car, pick-up truck or van in nontraffic accident
- **V63.4** Person boarding or alighting a heavy transport vehicle injured in collision with car, pick-up truck or van
- **V63.5** Driver of heavy transport vehicle injured in collision with car, pick-up truck or van in traffic accident
- **V63.6** Passenger in heavy transport vehicle injured in collision with car, pick-up truck or van in traffic accident
- **V63.7** Person on outside of heavy transport vehicle injured in collision with car, pick-up truck or van in traffic accident
- **V63.9** Unspecified occupant of heavy transport vehicle injured in collision with car, pick-up truck or van in traffic accident

V64 Occupant of heavy transport vehicle injured in collision with heavy transport vehicle or bus

EXCLUDES 1 *occupant of heavy transport vehicle injured in collision with military vehicle (V69.81)*

- **V64.0** Driver of heavy transport vehicle injured in collision with heavy transport vehicle or bus in nontraffic accident
- **V64.1** Passenger in heavy transport vehicle injured in collision with heavy transport vehicle or bus in nontraffic accident
- **V64.2** Person on outside of heavy transport vehicle injured in collision with heavy transport vehicle or bus in nontraffic accident
- **V64.3** Unspecified occupant of heavy transport vehicle injured in collision with heavy transport vehicle or bus in nontraffic accident
- **V64.4** Person boarding or alighting a heavy transport vehicle injured in collision with heavy transport vehicle or bus while boarding or alighting
- **V64.5** Driver of heavy transport vehicle injured in collision with heavy transport vehicle or bus in traffic accident
- **V64.6** Passenger in heavy transport vehicle injured in collision with heavy transport vehicle or bus in traffic accident
- **V64.7** Person on outside of heavy transport vehicle injured in collision with heavy transport vehicle or bus in traffic accident
- **V64.9** Unspecified occupant of heavy transport vehicle injured in collision with heavy transport vehicle or bus in traffic accident

V65 Occupant of heavy transport vehicle injured in collision with railway train or railway vehicle

- **V65.0** Driver of heavy transport vehicle injured in collision with railway train or railway vehicle in nontraffic accident
- **V65.1** Passenger in heavy transport vehicle injured in collision with railway train or railway vehicle in nontraffic accident
- **V65.2** Person on outside of heavy transport vehicle injured in collision with railway train or railway vehicle in nontraffic accident
- **V65.3** Unspecified occupant of heavy transport vehicle injured in collision with railway train or railway vehicle in nontraffic accident
- **V65.4** Person boarding or alighting a heavy transport vehicle injured in collision with railway train or railway vehicle
- **V65.5** Driver of heavy transport vehicle injured in collision with railway train or railway vehicle in traffic accident
- **V65.6** Passenger in heavy transport vehicle injured in collision with railway train or railway vehicle in traffic accident
- **V65.7** Person on outside of heavy transport vehicle injured in collision with railway train or railway vehicle in traffic accident
- **V65.9** Unspecified occupant of heavy transport vehicle injured in collision with railway train or railway vehicle in traffic accident

V66 Occupant of heavy transport vehicle injured in collision with other nonmotor vehicle

INCLUDES collision with animal-drawn vehicle, animal being ridden, streetcar

- **V66.0** Driver of heavy transport vehicle injured in collision with other nonmotor vehicle in nontraffic accident
- **V66.1** Passenger in heavy transport vehicle injured in collision with other nonmotor vehicle in nontraffic accident
- **V66.2** Person on outside of heavy transport vehicle injured in collision with other nonmotor vehicle in nontraffic accident
- **V66.3** Unspecified occupant of heavy transport vehicle injured in collision with other nonmotor vehicle in nontraffic accident
- **V66.4** Person boarding or alighting a heavy transport vehicle injured in collision with other nonmotor vehicle
- **V66.5** Driver of heavy transport vehicle injured in collision with other nonmotor vehicle in traffic accident
- **V66.6** Passenger in heavy transport vehicle injured in collision with other nonmotor vehicle in traffic accident
- **V66.7** Person on outside of heavy transport vehicle injured in collision with other nonmotor vehicle in traffic accident
- **V66.9** Unspecified occupant of heavy transport vehicle injured in collision with other nonmotor vehicle in traffic accident

V67 Occupant of heavy transport vehicle injured in collision with fixed or stationary object

- **V67.0** Driver of heavy transport vehicle injured in collision with fixed or stationary object in nontraffic accident
- **V67.1** Passenger in heavy transport vehicle injured in collision with fixed or stationary object in nontraffic accident
- **V67.2** Person on outside of heavy transport vehicle injured in collision with fixed or stationary object in nontraffic accident
- **V67.3** Unspecified occupant of heavy transport vehicle injured in collision with fixed or stationary object in nontraffic accident
- **V67.4** Person boarding or alighting a heavy transport vehicle injured in collision with fixed or stationary object
- **V67.5** Driver of heavy transport vehicle injured in collision with fixed or stationary object in traffic accident
- **V67.6** Passenger in heavy transport vehicle injured in collision with fixed or stationary object in traffic accident
- **V67.7** Person on outside of heavy transport vehicle injured in collision with fixed or stationary object in traffic accident
- **V67.9** Unspecified occupant of heavy transport vehicle injured in collision with fixed or stationary object in traffic accident

V68 Occupant of heavy transport vehicle injured in noncollision transport accident

INCLUDES overturning heavy transport vehicle NOS
overturning heavy transport vehicle without collision

- **V68.0** Driver of heavy transport vehicle injured in noncollision transport accident in nontraffic accident
- **V68.1** Passenger in heavy transport vehicle injured in noncollision transport accident in nontraffic accident
- **V68.2** Person on outside of heavy transport vehicle injured in noncollision transport accident in nontraffic accident
- **V68.3** Unspecified occupant of heavy transport vehicle injured in noncollision transport accident in nontraffic accident
- **V68.4** Person boarding or alighting a heavy transport vehicle injured in noncollision transport accident
- **V68.5** Driver of heavy transport vehicle injured in noncollision transport accident in traffic accident
- **V68.6** Passenger in heavy transport vehicle injured in noncollision transport accident in traffic accident
- **V68.7** Person on outside of heavy transport vehicle injured in noncollision transport accident in traffic accident
- **V68.9** Unspecified occupant of heavy transport vehicle injured in noncollision transport accident in traffic accident

V69 Occupant of heavy transport vehicle injured in other and unspecified transport accidents

- **V69.0** Driver of heavy transport vehicle injured in collision with other and unspecified motor vehicles in nontraffic accident
  - **V69.00** Driver of heavy transport vehicle injured in collision with unspecified motor vehicles in nontraffic accident
  - **V69.09** Driver of heavy transport vehicle injured in collision with other motor vehicles in nontraffic accident
- **V69.1** Passenger in heavy transport vehicle injured in collision with other and unspecified motor vehicles in nontraffic accident
  - **V69.10** Passenger in heavy transport vehicle injured in collision with unspecified motor vehicles in nontraffic accident
  - **V69.19** Passenger in heavy transport vehicle injured in collision with other motor vehicles in nontraffic accident
- **V69.2** Unspecified occupant of heavy transport vehicle injured in collision with other and unspecified motor vehicles in nontraffic accident
  - **V69.20** Unspecified occupant of heavy transport vehicle injured in collision with unspecified motor vehicles in nontraffic accident
    Collision NOS involving heavy transport vehicle, nontraffic

V69.29 Unspecified occupant of heavy transport vehicle injured in collision with other motor vehicles in nontraffic accident

V69.3 Occupant (driver) (passenger) of heavy transport vehicle injured in unspecified nontraffic accident
Accident NOS involving heavy transport vehicle, nontraffic
Occupant of heavy transport vehicle injured in nontraffic accident NOS

V69.4 Driver of heavy transport vehicle injured in collision with other and unspecified motor vehicles in traffic accident
V69.40 Driver of heavy transport vehicle injured in collision with unspecified motor vehicles in traffic accident
V69.49 Driver of heavy transport vehicle injured in collision with other motor vehicles in traffic accident

V69.5 Passenger in heavy transport vehicle injured in collision with other and unspecified motor vehicles in traffic accident
V69.50 Passenger in heavy transport vehicle injured in collision with unspecified motor vehicles in traffic accident
V69.59 Passenger in heavy transport vehicle injured in collision with other motor vehicles in traffic accident

V69.6 Unspecified occupant of heavy transport vehicle injured in collision with other and unspecified motor vehicles in traffic accident
V69.60 Unspecified occupant of heavy transport vehicle injured in collision with unspecified motor vehicles in traffic accident
Collision NOS involving heavy transport vehicle (traffic)
V69.69 Unspecified occupant of heavy transport vehicle injured in collision with other motor vehicles in traffic accident

V69.8 Occupant (driver) (passenger) of heavy transport vehicle injured in other specified transport accidents
V69.81 Occupant (driver) (passenger) of heavy transport vehicle injured in transport accidents with military vehicle
V69.88 Occupant (driver) (passenger) of heavy transport vehicle injured in other specified transport accidents

V69.9 Occupant (driver) (passenger) of heavy transport vehicle injured in unspecified traffic accident
Accident NOS involving heavy transport vehicle

Bus occupant injured in transport accident (V70-V79)

INCLUDES motorcoach
EXCLUDES 1 *minibus (V50-V59)*

The appropriate 7th character is to be added to each code from categories V70-V79.
A initial encounter
D subsequent encounter
S sequela

V70 Bus occupant injured in collision with pedestrian or animal
EXCLUDES 1 *bus collision with animal-drawn vehicle or animal being ridden (V76.-)*
V70.0 Driver of bus injured in collision with pedestrian or animal in nontraffic accident
V70.1 Passenger on bus injured in collision with pedestrian or animal in nontraffic accident
V70.2 Person on outside of bus injured in collision with pedestrian or animal in nontraffic accident
V70.3 Unspecified occupant of bus injured in collision with pedestrian or animal in nontraffic accident
V70.4 Person boarding or alighting from bus injured in collision with pedestrian or animal
V70.5 Driver of bus injured in collision with pedestrian or animal in traffic accident
V70.6 Passenger on bus injured in collision with pedestrian or animal in traffic accident
V70.7 Person on outside of bus injured in collision with pedestrian or animal in traffic accident
V70.9 Unspecified occupant of bus injured in collision with pedestrian or animal in traffic accident

V71 Bus occupant injured in collision with pedal cycle
V71.0 Driver of bus injured in collision with pedal cycle in nontraffic accident
V71.1 Passenger on bus injured in collision with pedal cycle in nontraffic accident
V71.2 Person on outside of bus injured in collision with pedal cycle in nontraffic accident
V71.3 Unspecified occupant of bus injured in collision with pedal cycle in nontraffic accident
V71.4 Person boarding or alighting from bus injured in collision with pedal cycle
V71.5 Driver of bus injured in collision with pedal cycle in traffic accident
V71.6 Passenger on bus injured in collision with pedal cycle in traffic accident
V71.7 Person on outside of bus injured in collision with pedal cycle in traffic accident
V71.9 Unspecified occupant of bus injured in collision with pedal cycle in traffic accident

V72 Bus occupant injured in collision with two- or three-wheeled motor vehicle
V72.0 Driver of bus injured in collision with two- or three-wheeled motor vehicle in nontraffic accident
V72.1 Passenger on bus injured in collision with two- or three-wheeled motor vehicle in nontraffic accident
V72.2 Person on outside of bus injured in collision with two- or three-wheeled motor vehicle in nontraffic accident
V72.3 Unspecified occupant of bus injured in collision with two- or three-wheeled motor vehicle in nontraffic accident
V72.4 Person boarding or alighting from bus injured in collision with two- or three-wheeled motor vehicle
V72.5 Driver of bus injured in collision with two- or three-wheeled motor vehicle in traffic accident
V72.6 Passenger on bus injured in collision with two- or three-wheeled motor vehicle in traffic accident
V72.7 Person on outside of bus injured in collision with two- or three-wheeled motor vehicle in traffic accident
V72.9 Unspecified occupant of bus injured in collision with two- or three-wheeled motor vehicle in traffic accident

V73 Bus occupant injured in collision with car, pick-up truck or van
V73.0 Driver of bus injured in collision with car, pick-up truck or van in nontraffic accident
V73.1 Passenger on bus injured in collision with car, pick-up truck or van in nontraffic accident
V73.2 Person on outside of bus injured in collision with car, pick-up truck or van in nontraffic accident
V73.3 Unspecified occupant of bus injured in collision with car, pick-up truck or van in nontraffic accident
V73.4 Person boarding or alighting from bus injured in collision with car, pick-up truck or van
V73.5 Driver of bus injured in collision with car, pick-up truck or van in traffic accident
V73.6 Passenger on bus injured in collision with car, pick-up truck or van in traffic accident
V73.7 Person on outside of bus injured in collision with car, pick-up truck or van in traffic accident
V73.9 Unspecified occupant of bus injured in collision with car, pick-up truck or van in traffic accident

V74 Bus occupant injured in collision with heavy transport vehicle or bus
EXCLUDES 1 *bus occupant injured in collision with military vehicle (V79.81)*
V74.0 Driver of bus injured in collision with heavy transport vehicle or bus in nontraffic accident
V74.1 Passenger on bus injured in collision with heavy transport vehicle or bus in nontraffic accident
V74.2 Person on outside of bus injured in collision with heavy transport vehicle or bus in nontraffic accident
V74.3 Unspecified occupant of bus injured in collision with heavy transport vehicle or bus in nontraffic accident
V74.4 Person boarding or alighting from bus injured in collision with heavy transport vehicle or bus
V74.5 Driver of bus injured in collision with heavy transport vehicle or bus in traffic accident
V74.6 Passenger on bus injured in collision with heavy transport vehicle or bus in traffic accident
V74.7 Person on outside of bus injured in collision with heavy transport vehicle or bus in traffic accident
V74.9 Unspecified occupant of bus injured in collision with heavy transport vehicle or bus in traffic accident

V75 Bus occupant injured in collision with railway train or railway vehicle
V75.0 Driver of bus injured in collision with railway train or railway vehicle in nontraffic accident
V75.1 Passenger on bus injured in collision with railway train or railway vehicle in nontraffic accident
V75.2 Person on outside of bus injured in collision with railway train or railway vehicle in nontraffic accident

√x7th **V75.3** **Unspecified occupant of bus injured in collision with railway train or railway vehicle in nontraffic accident**

√x7th **V75.4** **Person boarding or alighting from bus injured in collision with railway train or railway vehicle**

√x7th **V75.5** **Driver of bus injured in collision with railway train or railway vehicle in traffic accident**

√x7th **V75.6** **Passenger on bus injured in collision with railway train or railway vehicle in traffic accident**

√x7th **V75.7** **Person on outside of bus injured in collision with railway train or railway vehicle in traffic accident**

√x7th **V75.9** **Unspecified occupant of bus injured in collision with railway train or railway vehicle in traffic accident**

√4th **V76** **Bus occupant injured in collision with other nonmotor vehicle**

INCLUDES collision with animal-drawn vehicle, animal being ridden, streetcar

√x7th **V76.0** **Driver of bus injured in collision with other nonmotor vehicle in nontraffic accident**

√x7th **V76.1** **Passenger on bus injured in collision with other nonmotor vehicle in nontraffic accident**

√x7th **V76.2** **Person on outside of bus injured in collision with other nonmotor vehicle in nontraffic accident**

√x7th **V76.3** **Unspecified occupant of bus injured in collision with other nonmotor vehicle in nontraffic accident**

√x7th **V76.4** **Person boarding or alighting from bus injured in collision with other nonmotor vehicle**

√x7th **V76.5** **Driver of bus injured in collision with other nonmotor vehicle in traffic accident**

√x7th **V76.6** **Passenger on bus injured in collision with other nonmotor vehicle in traffic accident**

√x7th **V76.7** **Person on outside of bus injured in collision with other nonmotor vehicle in traffic accident**

√x7th **V76.9** **Unspecified occupant of bus injured in collision with other nonmotor vehicle in traffic accident**

√4th **V77** **Bus occupant injured in collision with fixed or stationary object**

√x7th **V77.0** **Driver of bus injured in collision with fixed or stationary object in nontraffic accident**

√x7th **V77.1** **Passenger on bus injured in collision with fixed or stationary object in nontraffic accident**

√x7th **V77.2** **Person on outside of bus injured in collision with fixed or stationary object in nontraffic accident**

√x7th **V77.3** **Unspecified occupant of bus injured in collision with fixed or stationary object in nontraffic accident**

√x7th **V77.4** **Person boarding or alighting from bus injured in collision with fixed or stationary object**

√x7th **V77.5** **Driver of bus injured in collision with fixed or stationary object in traffic accident**

√x7th **V77.6** **Passenger on bus injured in collision with fixed or stationary object in traffic accident**

√x7th **V77.7** **Person on outside of bus injured in collision with fixed or stationary object in traffic accident**

√x7th **V77.9** **Unspecified occupant of bus injured in collision with fixed or stationary object in traffic accident**

√4th **V78** **Bus occupant injured in noncollision transport accident**

INCLUDES overturning bus NOS
overturning bus without collision

√x7th **V78.0** **Driver of bus injured in noncollision transport accident in nontraffic accident**

√x7th **V78.1** **Passenger on bus injured in noncollision transport accident in nontraffic accident**

√x7th **V78.2** **Person on outside of bus injured in noncollision transport accident in nontraffic accident**

√x7th **V78.3** **Unspecified occupant of bus injured in noncollision transport accident in nontraffic accident**

√x7th **V78.4** **Person boarding or alighting from bus injured in noncollision transport accident**

√x7th **V78.5** **Driver of bus injured in noncollision transport accident in traffic accident**

√x7th **V78.6** **Passenger on bus injured in noncollision transport accident in traffic accident**

√x7th **V78.7** **Person on outside of bus injured in noncollision transport accident in traffic accident**

√x7th **V78.9** **Unspecified occupant of bus injured in noncollision transport accident in traffic accident**

√4th **V79** **Bus occupant injured in other and unspecified transport accidents**

√5th **V79.0** **Driver of bus injured in collision with other and unspecified motor vehicles in nontraffic accident**

√x7th **V79.00** **Driver of bus injured in collision with unspecified motor vehicles in nontraffic accident**

√x7th **V79.09** **Driver of bus injured in collision with other motor vehicles in nontraffic accident**

√5th **V79.1** **Passenger on bus injured in collision with other and unspecified motor vehicles in nontraffic accident**

√x7th **V79.10** **Passenger on bus injured in collision with unspecified motor vehicles in nontraffic accident**

√x7th **V79.19** **Passenger on bus injured in collision with other motor vehicles in nontraffic accident**

√5th **V79.2** **Unspecified bus occupant injured in collision with other and unspecified motor vehicles in nontraffic accident**

√x7th **V79.20** **Unspecified bus occupant injured in collision with unspecified motor vehicles in nontraffic accident**

Bus collision NOS, nontraffic

√x7th **V79.29** **Unspecified bus occupant injured in collision with other motor vehicles in nontraffic accident**

√x7th **V79.3** **Bus occupant (driver) (passenger) injured in unspecified nontraffic accident**

Bus accident NOS, nontraffic
Bus occupant injured in nontraffic accident NOS

√5th **V79.4** **Driver of bus injured in collision with other and unspecified motor vehicles in traffic accident**

√x7th **V79.40** **Driver of bus injured in collision with unspecified motor vehicles in traffic accident**

√x7th **V79.49** **Driver of bus injured in collision with other motor vehicles in traffic accident**

√5th **V79.5** **Passenger on bus injured in collision with other and unspecified motor vehicles in traffic accident**

√x7th **V79.50** **Passenger on bus injured in collision with unspecified motor vehicles in traffic accident**

√x7th **V79.59** **Passenger on bus injured in collision with other motor vehicles in traffic accident**

√5th **V79.6** **Unspecified bus occupant injured in collision with other and unspecified motor vehicles in traffic accident**

√x7th **V79.60** **Unspecified bus occupant injured in collision with unspecified motor vehicles in traffic accident**

Bus collision NOS (traffic)

√x7th **V79.69** **Unspecified bus occupant injured in collision with other motor vehicles in traffic accident**

√5th **V79.8** **Bus occupant (driver) (passenger) injured in other specified transport accidents**

√x7th **V79.81** **Bus occupant (driver) (passenger) injured in transport accidents with military vehicle**

√x7th **V79.88** **Bus occupant (driver) (passenger) injured in other specified transport accidents**

√x7th **V79.9** **Bus occupant (driver) (passenger) injured in unspecified traffic accident**

Bus accident NOS

Other land transport accidents (V80-V89)

The appropriate 7th character is to be added to each code from categories V80-V89.
A initial encounter
D subsequent encounter
S sequela

√4th **V80** **Animal-rider or occupant of animal-drawn vehicle injured in transport accident**

√5th **V80.0** **Animal-rider or occupant of animal drawn vehicle injured by fall from or being thrown from animal or animal-drawn vehicle in noncollision accident**

√6th **V80.01** **Animal-rider injured by fall from or being thrown from animal in noncollision accident**

√7th **V80.010** **Animal-rider injured by fall from or being thrown from horse in noncollision accident**

√7th **V80.018** **Animal-rider injured by fall from or being thrown from other animal in noncollision accident**

√x7th **V80.02** **Occupant of animal-drawn vehicle injured by fall from or being thrown from animal-drawn vehicle in noncollision accident**

Overturning animal-drawn vehicle NOS
Overturning animal-drawn vehicle without collision

√5th **V80.1** **Animal-rider or occupant of animal-drawn vehicle injured in collision with pedestrian or animal**

EXCLUDES 1 *animal-rider or animal-drawn vehicle collision with animal-drawn vehicle or animal being ridden (V80.7)*

√x7th **V80.11** **Animal-rider injured in collision with pedestrian or animal**

√x7th **V80.12** **Occupant of animal-drawn vehicle injured in collision with pedestrian or animal**

V8Ø.2 Animal-rider or occupant of animal-drawn vehicle injured in collision with pedal cycle
- **V8Ø.21 Animal-rider injured in collision with pedal cycle**
- **V8Ø.22 Occupant of animal-drawn vehicle injured in collision with pedal cycle**

V8Ø.3 Animal-rider or occupant of animal-drawn vehicle injured in collision with two- or three-wheeled motor vehicle
- **V8Ø.31 Animal-rider injured in collision with two- or three-wheeled motor vehicle**
- **V8Ø.32 Occupant of animal-drawn vehicle injured in collision with two- or three-wheeled motor vehicle**

V8Ø.4 Animal-rider or occupant of animal-drawn vehicle injured in collision with car, pick-up truck, van, heavy transport vehicle or bus

EXCLUDES 1 *animal-rider injured in collision with military vehicle (V8Ø.91Ø)*
occupant of animal-drawn vehicle injured in collision with military vehicle (V8Ø.92Ø)

- **V8Ø.41 Animal-rider injured in collision with car, pick-up truck, van, heavy transport vehicle or bus**
- **V8Ø.42 Occupant of animal-drawn vehicle injured in collision with car, pick-up truck, van, heavy transport vehicle or bus**

V8Ø.5 Animal-rider or occupant of animal-drawn vehicle injured in collision with other specified motor vehicle
- **V8Ø.51 Animal-rider injured in collision with other specified motor vehicle**
- **V8Ø.52 Occupant of animal-drawn vehicle injured in collision with other specified motor vehicle**

V8Ø.6 Animal-rider or occupant of animal-drawn vehicle injured in collision with railway train or railway vehicle
- **V8Ø.61 Animal-rider injured in collision with railway train or railway vehicle**
- **V8Ø.62 Occupant of animal-drawn vehicle injured in collision with railway train or railway vehicle**

V8Ø.7 Animal-rider or occupant of animal-drawn vehicle injured in collision with other nonmotor vehicles
- **V8Ø.71 Animal-rider or occupant of animal-drawn vehicle injured in collision with animal being ridden**
  - **V8Ø.71Ø Animal-rider injured in collision with other animal being ridden**
  - **V8Ø.711 Occupant of animal-drawn vehicle injured in collision with animal being ridden**
- **V8Ø.72 Animal-rider or occupant of animal-drawn vehicle injured in collision with other animal-drawn vehicle**
  - **V8Ø.72Ø Animal-rider injured in collision with animal-drawn vehicle**
  - **V8Ø.721 Occupant of animal-drawn vehicle injured in collision with other animal-drawn vehicle**
- **V8Ø.73 Animal-rider or occupant of animal-drawn vehicle injured in collision with streetcar**
  - **V8Ø.73Ø Animal-rider injured in collision with streetcar**
  - **V8Ø.731 Occupant of animal-drawn vehicle injured in collision with streetcar**
- **V8Ø.79 Animal-rider or occupant of animal-drawn vehicle injured in collision with other nonmotor vehicles**
  - **V8Ø.79Ø Animal-rider injured in collision with other nonmotor vehicles**
  - **V8Ø.791 Occupant of animal-drawn vehicle injured in collision with other nonmotor vehicles**

V8Ø.8 Animal-rider or occupant of animal-drawn vehicle injured in collision with fixed or stationary object
- **V8Ø.81 Animal-rider injured in collision with fixed or stationary object**
- **V8Ø.82 Occupant of animal-drawn vehicle injured in collision with fixed or stationary object**

V8Ø.9 Animal-rider or occupant of animal-drawn vehicle injured in other and unspecified transport accidents
- **V8Ø.91 Animal-rider injured in other and unspecified transport accidents**
  - **V8Ø.91Ø Animal-rider injured in transport accident with military vehicle**
  - **V8Ø.918 Animal-rider injured in other transport accident**
  - **V8Ø.919 Animal-rider injured in unspecified transport accident**
    Animal rider accident NOS
- **V8Ø.92 Occupant of animal-drawn vehicle injured in other and unspecified transport accidents**
  - **V8Ø.92Ø Occupant of animal-drawn vehicle injured in transport accident with military vehicle**
  - **V8Ø.928 Occupant of animal-drawn vehicle injured in other transport accident**
  - **V8Ø.929 Occupant of animal-drawn vehicle injured in unspecified transport accident**
    Animal-drawn vehicle accident NOS

V81 Occupant of railway train or railway vehicle injured in transport accident

INCLUDES derailment of railway train or railway vehicle
person on outside of train

EXCLUDES 1 *streetcar (V82.-)*

- **V81.Ø Occupant of railway train or railway vehicle injured in collision with motor vehicle in nontraffic accident**
  EXCLUDES 1 *occupant of railway train or railway vehicle injured due to collision with military vehicle (V81.83)*
- **V81.1 Occupant of railway train or railway vehicle injured in collision with motor vehicle in traffic accident**
  EXCLUDES 1 *occupant of railway train or railway vehicle injured due to collision with military vehicle (V81.83)*
- **V81.2 Occupant of railway train or railway vehicle injured in collision with or hit by rolling stock**
- **V81.3 Occupant of railway train or railway vehicle injured in collision with other object**
  Railway collision NOS
- **V81.4 Person injured while boarding or alighting from railway train or railway vehicle**
- **V81.5 Occupant of railway train or railway vehicle injured by fall in railway train or railway vehicle**
- **V81.6 Occupant of railway train or railway vehicle injured by fall from railway train or railway vehicle**
- **V81.7 Occupant of railway train or railway vehicle injured in derailment without antecedent collision**
- **V81.8 Occupant of railway train or railway vehicle injured in other specified railway accidents**
  - **V81.81 Occupant of railway train or railway vehicle injured due to explosion or fire on train**
  - **V81.82 Occupant of railway train or railway vehicle injured due to object falling onto train**
    Occupant of railway train or railway vehicle injured due to falling earth onto train
    Occupant of railway train or railway vehicle injured due to falling rocks onto train
    Occupant of railway train or railway vehicle injured due to falling snow onto train
    Occupant of railway train or railway vehicle injured due to falling trees onto train
  - **V81.83 Occupant of railway train or railway vehicle injured due to collision with military vehicle**
  - **V81.89 Occupant of railway train or railway vehicle injured due to other specified railway accident**
- **V81.9 Occupant of railway train or railway vehicle injured in unspecified railway accident**
  Railway accident NOS

V82 Occupant of powered streetcar injured in transport accident

INCLUDES interurban electric car
person on outside of streetcar
tram (car)
trolley (car)

EXCLUDES 1 *bus (V7Ø-V79)*
motorcoach (V7Ø-V79)
nonpowered streetcar (V76.-)
train (V81.-)

- **V82.Ø Occupant of streetcar injured in collision with motor vehicle in nontraffic accident**
- **V82.1 Occupant of streetcar injured in collision with motor vehicle in traffic accident**
- **V82.2 Occupant of streetcar injured in collision with or hit by rolling stock**
- **V82.3 Occupant of streetcar injured in collision with other object**
  EXCLUDES 1 *collision with animal-drawn vehicle or animal being ridden (V82.8)*
- **V82.4 Person injured while boarding or alighting from streetcar**

√x7th **V82.5 Occupant of streetcar injured by fall in streetcar**
EXCLUDES 1 *fall in streetcar:*
while boarding or alighting (V82.4)
with antecedent collision (V82.Ø-V82.3)

√x7th **V82.6 Occupant of streetcar injured by fall from streetcar**
EXCLUDES 1 *fall from streetcar:*
while boarding or alighting (V82.4)
with antecedent collision (V82.Ø-V82.3)

√x7th **V82.7 Occupant of streetcar injured in derailment without antecedent collision**
EXCLUDES 1 *occupant of streetcar injured in derailment with antecedent collision (V82.Ø-V82.3)*

√x7th **V82.8 Occupant of streetcar injured in other specified transport accidents**
Streetcar collision with military vehicle
Streetcar collision with train or nonmotor vehicles

√x7th **V82.9 Occupant of streetcar injured in unspecified traffic accident**
Streetcar accident NOS

√4th **V83 Occupant of special vehicle mainly used on industrial premises injured in transport accident**
INCLUDES battery-powered airport passenger vehicle
battery-powered truck (baggage) (mail)
coal-car in mine
forklift (truck)
logging car
self-propelled industrial truck
station baggage truck (powered)
tram, truck, or tub (powered) in mine or quarry
EXCLUDES 1 *special construction vehicles (V85.-)*
special industrial vehicle in stationary use or maintenance (W31.-)

√x7th **V83.Ø Driver of special industrial vehicle injured in traffic accident**
√x7th **V83.1 Passenger of special industrial vehicle injured in traffic accident**
√x7th **V83.2 Person on outside of special industrial vehicle injured in traffic accident**
√x7th **V83.3 Unspecified occupant of special industrial vehicle injured in traffic accident**
√x7th **V83.4 Person injured while boarding or alighting from special industrial vehicle**
√x7th **V83.5 Driver of special industrial vehicle injured in nontraffic accident**
√x7th **V83.6 Passenger of special industrial vehicle injured in nontraffic accident**
√x7th **V83.7 Person on outside of special industrial vehicle injured in nontraffic accident**
√x7th **V83.9 Unspecified occupant of special industrial vehicle injured in nontraffic accident**
Special-industrial-vehicle accident NOS

√4th **V84 Occupant of special vehicle mainly used in agriculture injured in transport accident**
INCLUDES self-propelled farm machinery
tractor (and trailer)
EXCLUDES 1 *animal-powered farm machinery accident (W3Ø.8-)*
contact with combine harvester (W3Ø.Ø)
special agricultural vehicle in stationary use or maintenance (W3Ø.-)

√x7th **V84.Ø Driver of special agricultural vehicle injured in traffic accident**
√x7th **V84.1 Passenger of special agricultural vehicle injured in traffic accident**
√x7th **V84.2 Person on outside of special agricultural vehicle injured in traffic accident**
√x7th **V84.3 Unspecified occupant of special agricultural vehicle injured in traffic accident**
√x7th **V84.4 Person injured while boarding or alighting from special agricultural vehicle**
√x7th **V84.5 Driver of special agricultural vehicle injured in nontraffic accident**
√x7th **V84.6 Passenger of special agricultural vehicle injured in nontraffic accident**
√x7th **V84.7 Person on outside of special agricultural vehicle injured in nontraffic accident**
√x7th **V84.9 Unspecified occupant of special agricultural vehicle injured in nontraffic accident**
Special-agricultural vehicle accident NOS

√4th **V85 Occupant of special construction vehicle injured in transport accident**
INCLUDES bulldozer
digger
dump truck
earth-leveller
mechanical shovel
road-roller
EXCLUDES 1 *special industrial vehicle (V83.-)*
special construction vehicle in stationary use or maintenance (W31.-)

√x7th **V85.Ø Driver of special construction vehicle injured in traffic accident**
√x7th **V85.1 Passenger of special construction vehicle injured in traffic accident**
√x7th **V85.2 Person on outside of special construction vehicle injured in traffic accident**
√x7th **V85.3 Unspecified occupant of special construction vehicle injured in traffic accident**
√x7th **V85.4 Person injured while boarding or alighting from special construction vehicle**
√x7th **V85.5 Driver of special construction vehicle injured in nontraffic accident**
√x7th **V85.6 Passenger of special construction vehicle injured in nontraffic accident**
√x7th **V85.7 Person on outside of special construction vehicle injured in nontraffic accident**
√x7th **V85.9 Unspecified occupant of special construction vehicle injured in nontraffic accident**
Special-construction-vehicle accident NOS

√4th **V86 Occupant of special all-terrain or other off-road motor vehicle, injured in transport accident**
EXCLUDES 1 *special all-terrain vehicle in stationary use or maintenance (W31.-)*
sport-utility vehicle (V5Ø-V59)
three-wheeled motor vehicle designed for on-road use (V3Ø-V39)

AHA: 2017,4Q,26

√5th **V86.Ø Driver of special all-terrain or other off-road motor vehicle injured in traffic accident**
√x7th **V86.Ø1 Driver of ambulance or fire engine injured in traffic accident**
√x7th **V86.Ø2 Driver of snowmobile injured in traffic accident**
√x7th **V86.Ø3 Driver of dune buggy injured in traffic accident**
√x7th **V86.Ø4 Driver of military vehicle injured in traffic accident**
√x7th **V86.Ø5 Driver of 3- or 4- wheeled all-terrain vehicle (ATV) injured in traffic accident**
√x7th **V86.Ø6 Driver of dirt bike or motor/cross bike injured in traffic accident**
√x7th **V86.Ø9 Driver of other special all-terrain or other off-road motor vehicle injured in traffic accident**
Driver of go cart injured in traffic accident
Driver of golf cart injured in traffic accident

√5th **V86.1 Passenger of special all-terrain or other off-road motor vehicle injured in traffic accident**
√x7th **V86.11 Passenger of ambulance or fire engine injured in traffic accident**
√x7th **V86.12 Passenger of snowmobile injured in traffic accident**
√x7th **V86.13 Passenger of dune buggy injured in traffic accident**
√x7th **V86.14 Passenger of military vehicle injured in traffic accident**
√x7th **V86.15 Passenger of 3- or 4- wheeled all-terrain vehicle (ATV) injured in traffic accident**
√x7th **V86.16 Passenger of dirt bike or motor/cross bike injured in traffic accident**
√x7th **V86.19 Passenger of other special all-terrain or other off-road motor vehicle injured in traffic accident**
Passenger of go cart injured in traffic accident
Passenger of golf cart injured in traffic accident

√5th **V86.2 Person on outside of special all-terrain or other off-road motor vehicle injured in traffic accident**
√x7th **V86.21 Person on outside of ambulance or fire engine injured in traffic accident**
√x7th **V86.22 Person on outside of snowmobile injured in traffic accident**
√x7th **V86.23 Person on outside of dune buggy injured in traffic accident**
√x7th **V86.24 Person on outside of military vehicle injured in traffic accident**

x7th **V86.25 Person on outside of 3- or 4- wheeled all-terrain vehicle (ATV) injured in traffic accident**

x7th **V86.26 Person on outside of dirt bike or motor/cross bike injured in traffic accident**

x7th **V86.29 Person on outside of other special all-terrain or other off-road motor vehicle injured in traffic accident**

Person on outside of go cart in traffic accident

Person on outside of golf cart injured in traffic accident

5th **V86.3 Unspecified occupant of special all-terrain or other off-road motor vehicle injured in traffic accident**

x7th **V86.31 Unspecified occupant of ambulance or fire engine injured in traffic accident**

x7th **V86.32 Unspecified occupant of snowmobile injured in traffic accident**

x7th **V86.33 Unspecified occupant of dune buggy injured in traffic accident**

x7th **V86.34 Unspecified occupant of military vehicle injured in traffic accident**

x7th **V86.35 Unspecified occupant of 3- or 4- wheeled all-terrain vehicle (ATV) injured in traffic accident**

x7th **V86.36 Unspecified occupant of dirt bike or motor/cross bike injured in traffic accident**

x7th **V86.39 Unspecified occupant of other special all-terrain or other off-road motor vehicle injured in traffic accident**

Unspecified occupant of go cart injured in traffic accident

Unspecified occupant of golf cart injured in traffic accident

5th **V86.4 Person injured while boarding or alighting from special all-terrain or other off-road motor vehicle**

x7th **V86.41 Person injured while boarding or alighting from ambulance or fire engine**

x7th **V86.42 Person injured while boarding or alighting from snowmobile**

x7th **V86.43 Person injured while boarding or alighting from dune buggy**

x7th **V86.44 Person injured while boarding or alighting from military vehicle**

x7th **V86.45 Person injured while boarding or alighting from a 3- or 4- wheeled all-terrain vehicle (ATV)**

x7th **V86.46 Person injured while boarding or alighting from a dirt bike or motor/cross bike**

x7th **V86.49 Person injured while boarding or alighting from other special all-terrain or other off-road motor vehicle**

Person injured while boarding or alighting from go cart

Person injured while boarding or alighting from golf cart

5th **V86.5 Driver of special all-terrain or other off-road motor vehicle injured in nontraffic accident**

x7th **V86.51 Driver of ambulance or fire engine injured in nontraffic accident**

x7th **V86.52 Driver of snowmobile injured in nontraffic accident**

x7th **V86.53 Driver of dune buggy injured in nontraffic accident**

x7th **V86.54 Driver of military vehicle injured in nontraffic accident**

x7th **V86.55 Driver of 3- or 4- wheeled all-terrain vehicle (ATV) injured in nontraffic accident**

x7th **V86.56 Driver of dirt bike or motor/cross bike injured in nontraffic accident**

x7th **V86.59 Driver of other special all-terrain or other off-road motor vehicle injured in nontraffic accident**

Driver of go cart injured in nontraffic accident

Driver of golf cart injured in nontraffic accident

5th **V86.6 Passenger of special all-terrain or other off-road motor vehicle injured in nontraffic accident**

x7th **V86.61 Passenger of ambulance or fire engine injured in nontraffic accident**

x7th **V86.62 Passenger of snowmobile injured in nontraffic accident**

x7th **V86.63 Passenger of dune buggy injured in nontraffic accident**

x7th **V86.64 Passenger of military vehicle injured in nontraffic accident**

x7th **V86.65 Passenger of 3- or 4- wheeled all-terrain vehicle (ATV) injured in nontraffic accident**

x7th **V86.66 Passenger of dirt bike or motor/cross bike injured in nontraffic accident**

x7th **V86.69 Passenger of other special all-terrain or other off-road motor vehicle injured in nontraffic accident**

Passenger of go cart injured in nontraffic accident

Passenger of golf cart injured in nontraffic accident

5th **V86.7 Person on outside of special all-terrain or other off-road motor vehicle injured in nontraffic accident**

x7th **V86.71 Person on outside of ambulance or fire engine injured in nontraffic accident**

x7th **V86.72 Person on outside of snowmobile injured in nontraffic accident**

x7th **V86.73 Person on outside of dune buggy injured in nontraffic accident**

x7th **V86.74 Person on outside of military vehicle injured in nontraffic accident**

x7th **V86.75 Person on outside of 3- or 4- wheeled all-terrain vehicle (ATV) injured in nontraffic accident**

x7th **V86.76 Person on outside of dirt bike or motor/cross bike injured in nontraffic accident**

x7th **V86.79 Person on outside of other special all-terrain or other off-road motor vehicles injured in nontraffic accident**

Person on outside of go cart injured in nontraffic accident

Person on outside of golf cart injured in nontraffic accident

5th **V86.9 Unspecified occupant of special all-terrain or other off-road motor vehicle injured in nontraffic accident**

x7th **V86.91 Unspecified occupant of ambulance or fire engine injured in nontraffic accident**

x7th **V86.92 Unspecified occupant of snowmobile injured in nontraffic accident**

x7th **V86.93 Unspecified occupant of dune buggy injured in nontraffic accident**

x7th **V86.94 Unspecified occupant of military vehicle injured in nontraffic accident**

x7th **V86.95 Unspecified occupant of 3- or 4- wheeled all-terrain vehicle (ATV) injured in nontraffic accident**

x7th **V86.96 Unspecified occupant of dirt bike or motor/cross bike injured in nontraffic accident**

x7th **V86.99 Unspecified occupant of other special all-terrain or other off-road motor vehicle injured in nontraffic accident**

Off-road motor-vehicle accident NOS

Other motor-vehicle accident NOS

Unspecified occupant of go cart injured in nontraffic accident

Unspecified occupant of golf cart injured in nontraffic accident

4th **V87 Traffic accident of specified type but victim's mode of transport unknown**

EXCLUDES 1 *collision involving:*

pedal cycle (V10-V19)

pedestrian (V01-V09)

x7th **V87.0 Person injured in collision between car and two- or three-wheeled powered vehicle (traffic)**

x7th **V87.1 Person injured in collision between other motor vehicle and two- or three-wheeled motor vehicle (traffic)**

x7th **V87.2 Person injured in collision between car and pick-up truck or van (traffic)**

x7th **V87.3 Person injured in collision between car and bus (traffic)**

x7th **V87.4 Person injured in collision between car and heavy transport vehicle (traffic)**

x7th **V87.5 Person injured in collision between heavy transport vehicle and bus (traffic)**

x7th **V87.6 Person injured in collision between railway train or railway vehicle and car (traffic)**

x7th **V87.7 Person injured in collision between other specified motor vehicles (traffic)**

x7th **V87.8 Person injured in other specified noncollision transport accidents involving motor vehicle (traffic)**

x7th **V87.9 Person injured in other specified (collision)(noncollision) transport accidents involving nonmotor vehicle (traffic)**

✓4th **V88 Nontraffic accident of specified type but victim's mode of transport unknown**

EXCLUDES 1 *collision involving:*
pedal cycle (V10-V19)
pedestrian (V01-V09)

✓x7th **V88.0 Person injured in collision between car and two- or three-wheeled motor vehicle, nontraffic**

✓x7th **V88.1 Person injured in collision between other motor vehicle and two- or three-wheeled motor vehicle, nontraffic**

✓x7th **V88.2 Person injured in collision between car and pick-up truck or van, nontraffic**

✓x7th **V88.3 Person injured in collision between car and bus, nontraffic**

✓x7th **V88.4 Person injured in collision between car and heavy transport vehicle, nontraffic**

✓x7th **V88.5 Person injured in collision between heavy transport vehicle and bus, nontraffic**

✓x7th **V88.6 Person injured in collision between railway train or railway vehicle and car, nontraffic**

✓x7th **V88.7 Person injured in collision between other specified motor vehicle, nontraffic**

✓x7th **V88.8 Person injured in other specified noncollision transport accidents involving motor vehicle, nontraffic**

✓x7th **V88.9 Person injured in other specified (collision)(noncollision) transport accidents involving nonmotor vehicle, nontraffic**

✓4th **V89 Motor- or nonmotor-vehicle accident, type of vehicle unspecified**

✓x7th **V89.0 Person injured in unspecified motor-vehicle accident, nontraffic**
Motor-vehicle accident NOS, nontraffic

✓x7th **V89.1 Person injured in unspecified nonmotor-vehicle accident, nontraffic**
Nonmotor-vehicle accident NOS (nontraffic)

✓x7th **V89.2 Person injured in unspecified motor-vehicle accident, traffic**
Motor-vehicle accident [MVA] NOS
Road (traffic) accident [RTA] NOS

✓x7th **V89.3 Person injured in unspecified nonmotor-vehicle accident, traffic**
Nonmotor-vehicle traffic accident NOS

✓x7th **V89.9 Person injured in unspecified vehicle accident**
Collision NOS

Water transport accidents (V90-V94)

The appropriate 7th character is to be added to each code from categories V90-V94.
A initial encounter
D subsequent encounter
S sequela

✓4th **V90 Drowning and submersion due to accident to watercraft**

EXCLUDES 1 *civilian water transport accident involving military watercraft (V94.81-)*
fall into water not from watercraft (W16.-)
military watercraft accident in military or war operations (Y36.0-, Y37.0-)
water-transport-related drowning or submersion without accident to watercraft (V92.-)

✓5th **V90.0 Drowning and submersion due to watercraft overturning**

✓x7th **V90.00 Drowning and submersion due to merchant ship overturning**

✓x7th **V90.01 Drowning and submersion due to passenger ship overturning**
Drowning and submersion due to Ferry-boat overturning
Drowning and submersion due to Liner overturning

✓x7th **V90.02 Drowning and submersion due to fishing boat overturning**

✓x7th **V90.03 Drowning and submersion due to other powered watercraft overturning**
Drowning and submersion due to Hovercraft (on open water) overturning
Drowning and submersion due to Jet ski overturning

✓x7th **V90.04 Drowning and submersion due to sailboat overturning**

✓x7th **V90.05 Drowning and submersion due to canoe or kayak overturning**

✓x7th **V90.06 Drowning and submersion due to (nonpowered) inflatable craft overturning**

✓x7th **V90.08 Drowning and submersion due to other unpowered watercraft overturning**
Drowning and submersion due to windsurfer overturning

✓x7th **V90.09 Drowning and submersion due to unspecified watercraft overturning**
Drowning and submersion due to boat NOS overturning
Drowning and submersion due to ship NOS overturning
Drowning and submersion due to watercraft NOS overturning

✓5th **V90.1 Drowning and submersion due to watercraft sinking**

✓x7th **V90.10 Drowning and submersion due to merchant ship sinking**

✓x7th **V90.11 Drowning and submersion due to passenger ship sinking**
Drowning and submersion due to Ferry-boat sinking
Drowning and submersion due to Liner sinking

✓x7th **V90.12 Drowning and submersion due to fishing boat sinking**

✓x7th **V90.13 Drowning and submersion due to other powered watercraft sinking**
Drowning and submersion due to Hovercraft (on open water) sinking
Drowning and submersion due to Jet ski sinking

✓x7th **V90.14 Drowning and submersion due to sailboat sinking**

✓x7th **V90.15 Drowning and submersion due to canoe or kayak sinking**

✓x7th **V90.16 Drowning and submersion due to (nonpowered) inflatable craft sinking**

✓x7th **V90.18 Drowning and submersion due to other unpowered watercraft sinking**

✓x7th **V90.19 Drowning and submersion due to unspecified watercraft sinking**
Drowning and submersion due to boat NOS sinking
Drowning and submersion due to ship NOS sinking
Drowning and submersion due to watercraft NOS sinking

✓5th **V90.2 Drowning and submersion due to falling or jumping from burning watercraft**

✓x7th **V90.20 Drowning and submersion due to falling or jumping from burning merchant ship**

✓x7th **V90.21 Drowning and submersion due to falling or jumping from burning passenger ship**
Drowning and submersion due to falling or jumping from burning Ferry-boat
Drowning and submersion due to falling or jumping from burning Liner

✓x7th **V90.22 Drowning and submersion due to falling or jumping from burning fishing boat**

✓x7th **V90.23 Drowning and submersion due to falling or jumping from other burning powered watercraft**
Drowning and submersion due to falling and jumping from burning Hovercraft (on open water)
Drowning and submersion due to falling and jumping from burning Jet ski

✓x7th **V90.24 Drowning and submersion due to falling or jumping from burning sailboat**

✓x7th **V90.25 Drowning and submersion due to falling or jumping from burning canoe or kayak**

✓x7th **V90.26 Drowning and submersion due to falling or jumping from burning (nonpowered) inflatable craft**

✓x7th **V90.27 Drowning and submersion due to falling or jumping from burning water-skis**

✓x7th **V90.28 Drowning and submersion due to falling or jumping from other burning unpowered watercraft**
Drowning and submersion due to falling and jumping from burning surf-board
Drowning and submersion due to falling and jumping from burning windsurfer

✓x7th **V90.29 Drowning and submersion due to falling or jumping from unspecified burning watercraft**
Drowning and submersion due to falling or jumping from burning boat NOS
Drowning and submersion due to falling or jumping from burning ship NOS
Drowning and submersion due to falling or jumping from burning watercraft NOS

V90.3 Drowning and submersion due to falling or jumping from crushed watercraft

V90.30 Drowning and submersion due to falling or jumping from crushed merchant ship

V90.31 Drowning and submersion due to falling or jumping from crushed passenger ship

Drowning and submersion due to falling and jumping from crushed Ferry boat

Drowning and submersion due to falling and jumping from crushed Liner

V90.32 Drowning and submersion due to falling or jumping from crushed fishing boat

V90.33 Drowning and submersion due to falling or jumping from other crushed powered watercraft

Drowning and submersion due to falling and jumping from crushed Hovercraft

Drowning and submersion due to falling and jumping from crushed Jet ski

V90.34 Drowning and submersion due to falling or jumping from crushed sailboat

V90.35 Drowning and submersion due to falling or jumping from crushed canoe or kayak

V90.36 Drowning and submersion due to falling or jumping from crushed (nonpowered) inflatable craft

V90.37 Drowning and submersion due to falling or jumping from crushed water-skis

V90.38 Drowning and submersion due to falling or jumping from other crushed unpowered watercraft

Drowning and submersion due to falling and jumping from crushed surf-board

Drowning and submersion due to falling and jumping from crushed windsurfer

V90.39 Drowning and submersion due to falling or jumping from crushed unspecified watercraft

Drowning and submersion due to falling and jumping from crushed boat NOS

Drowning and submersion due to falling and jumping from crushed ship NOS

Drowning and submersion due to falling and jumping from crushed watercraft NOS

V90.8 Drowning and submersion due to other accident to watercraft

V90.80 Drowning and submersion due to other accident to merchant ship

V90.81 Drowning and submersion due to other accident to passenger ship

Drowning and submersion due to other accident to Ferry-boat

Drowning and submersion due to other accident to Liner

V90.82 Drowning and submersion due to other accident to fishing boat

V90.83 Drowning and submersion due to other accident to other powered watercraft

Drowning and submersion due to other accident to Hovercraft (on open water)

Drowning and submersion due to other accident to Jet ski

V90.84 Drowning and submersion due to other accident to sailboat

V90.85 Drowning and submersion due to other accident to canoe or kayak

V90.86 Drowning and submersion due to other accident to (nonpowered) inflatable craft

V90.87 Drowning and submersion due to other accident to water-skis

V90.88 Drowning and submersion due to other accident to other unpowered watercraft

Drowning and submersion due to other accident to surf-board

Drowning and submersion due to other accident to windsurfer

V90.89 Drowning and submersion due to other accident to unspecified watercraft

Drowning and submersion due to other accident to boat NOS

Drowning and submersion due to other accident to ship NOS

Drowning and submersion due to other accident to watercraft NOS

V91 Other injury due to accident to watercraft

INCLUDES any injury except drowning and submersion as a result of an accident to watercraft

EXCLUDES 1 *civilian water transport accident involving military watercraft (V94.81-)*

military watercraft accident in military or war operations (Y36, Y37.-)

EXCLUDES 2 *drowning and submersion due to accident to watercraft (V90.-)*

V91.0 Burn due to watercraft on fire

EXCLUDES 1 *burn from localized fire or explosion on board ship without accident to watercraft (V93.-)*

V91.00 Burn due to merchant ship on fire

V91.01 Burn due to passenger ship on fire

Burn due to Ferry-boat on fire

Burn due to Liner on fire

V91.02 Burn due to fishing boat on fire

V91.03 Burn due to other powered watercraft on fire

Burn due to Hovercraft (on open water) on fire

Burn due to Jet ski on fire

V91.04 Burn due to sailboat on fire

V91.05 Burn due to canoe or kayak on fire

V91.06 Burn due to (nonpowered) inflatable craft on fire

V91.07 Burn due to water-skis on fire

V91.08 Burn due to other unpowered watercraft on fire

V91.09 Burn due to unspecified watercraft on fire

Burn due to boat NOS on fire

Burn due to ship NOS on fire

Burn due to watercraft NOS on fire

V91.1 Crushed between watercraft and other watercraft or other object due to collision

Crushed by lifeboat after abandoning ship in a collision

NOTE Select the specified type of watercraft that the victim was on at the time of the collision

V91.10 Crushed between merchant ship and other watercraft or other object due to collision

V91.11 Crushed between passenger ship and other watercraft or other object due to collision

Crushed between Ferry-boat and other watercraft or other object due to collision

Crushed between Liner and other watercraft or other object due to collision

V91.12 Crushed between fishing boat and other watercraft or other object due to collision

V91.13 Crushed between other powered watercraft and other watercraft or other object due to collision

Crushed between Hovercraft (on open water) and other watercraft or other object due to collision

Crushed between Jet ski and other watercraft or other object due to collision

V91.14 Crushed between sailboat and other watercraft or other object due to collision

V91.15 Crushed between canoe or kayak and other watercraft or other object due to collision

V91.16 Crushed between (nonpowered) inflatable craft and other watercraft or other object due to collision

V91.18 Crushed between other unpowered watercraft and other watercraft or other object due to collision

Crushed between surfboard and other watercraft or other object due to collision

Crushed between windsurfer and other watercraft or other object due to collision

V91.19 Crushed between unspecified watercraft and other watercraft or other object due to collision
Crushed between boat NOS and other watercraft or other object due to collision
Crushed between ship NOS and other watercraft or other object due to collision
Crushed between watercraft NOS and other watercraft or other object due to collision

V91.2 Fall due to collision between watercraft and other watercraft or other object
Fall while remaining on watercraft after collision
NOTE Select the specified type of watercraft that the victim was on at the time of the collision
EXCLUDES 1 *crushed between watercraft and other watercraft and other object due to collision (V91.1-)*
drowning and submersion due to falling from crushed watercraft (V9Ø.3-)

V91.2Ø Fall due to collision between merchant ship and other watercraft or other object

V91.21 Fall due to collision between passenger ship and other watercraft or other object
Fall due to collision between Ferry-boat and other watercraft or other object
Fall due to collision between Liner and other watercraft or other object

V91.22 Fall due to collision between fishing boat and other watercraft or other object

V91.23 Fall due to collision between other powered watercraft and other watercraft or other object
Fall due to collision between Hovercraft (on open water) and other watercraft or other object
Fall due to collision between Jet ski and other watercraft or other object

V91.24 Fall due to collision between sailboat and other watercraft or other object

V91.25 Fall due to collision between canoe or kayak and other watercraft or other object

V91.26 Fall due to collision between (nonpowered) inflatable craft and other watercraft or other object

V91.29 Fall due to collision between unspecified watercraft and other watercraft or other object
Fall due to collision between boat NOS and other watercraft or other object
Fall due to collision between ship NOS and other watercraft or other object
Fall due to collision between watercraft NOS and other watercraft or other object

V91.3 Hit or struck by falling object due to accident to watercraft
Hit or struck by falling object (part of damaged watercraft or other object) after falling or jumping from damaged watercraft
EXCLUDES 2 *drowning or submersion due to fall or jumping from damaged watercraft (V9Ø.2-, V9Ø.3-)*

V91.3Ø Hit or struck by falling object due to accident to merchant ship

V91.31 Hit or struck by falling object due to accident to passenger ship
Hit or struck by falling object due to accident to Ferry-boat
Hit or struck by falling object due to accident to Liner

V91.32 Hit or struck by falling object due to accident to fishing boat

V91.33 Hit or struck by falling object due to accident to other powered watercraft
Hit or struck by falling object due to accident to Hovercraft (on open water)
Hit or struck by falling object due to accident to Jet ski

V91.34 Hit or struck by falling object due to accident to sailboat

V91.35 Hit or struck by falling object due to accident to canoe or kayak

V91.36 Hit or struck by falling object due to accident to (nonpowered) inflatable craft

V91.37 Hit or struck by falling object due to accident to water-skis
Hit by water-skis after jumping off of waterskis

V91.38 Hit or struck by falling object due to accident to other unpowered watercraft
Hit or struck by surf-board after falling off damaged surf-board
Hit or struck by object after falling off damaged windsurfer

V91.39 Hit or struck by falling object due to accident to unspecified watercraft
Hit or struck by falling object due to accident to boat NOS
Hit or struck by falling object due to accident to ship NOS
Hit or struck by falling object due to accident to watercraft NOS

V91.8 Other injury due to other accident to watercraft

V91.8Ø Other injury due to other accident to merchant ship

V91.81 Other injury due to other accident to passenger ship
Other injury due to other accident to Ferry-boat
Other injury due to other accident to Liner

V91.82 Other injury due to other accident to fishing boat

V91.83 Other injury due to other accident to other powered watercraft
Other injury due to other accident to Hovercraft (on open water)
Other injury due to other accident Jet ski

V91.84 Other injury due to other accident to sailboat

V91.85 Other injury due to other accident to canoe or kayak

V91.86 Other injury due to other accident to (nonpowered) inflatable craft

V91.87 Other injury due to other accident to water-skis

V91.88 Other injury due to other accident to other unpowered watercraft
Other injury due to other accident to surf-board
Other injury due to other accident to windsurfer

V91.89 Other injury due to other accident to unspecified watercraft
Other injury due to other accident to boat NOS
Other injury due to other accident to ship NOS
Other injury due to other accident to watercraft NOS

V92 Drowning and submersion due to accident on board watercraft, without accident to watercraft
EXCLUDES 1 *civilian water transport accident involving military watercraft (V94.81-)*
drowning or submersion due to accident to watercraft (V9Ø-V91)
drowning or submersion of diver who voluntarily jumps from boat not involved in an accident (W16.711, W16.721)
fall into water without watercraft (W16.-)
military watercraft accident in military or war operations (Y36, Y37)

V92.Ø Drowning and submersion due to fall off watercraft
Drowning and submersion due to fall from gangplank of watercraft
Drowning and submersion due to fall overboard watercraft
EXCLUDES 2 *hitting head on object or bottom of body of water due to fall from watercraft (V94.Ø-)*

V92.ØØ Drowning and submersion due to fall off merchant ship

V92.Ø1 Drowning and submersion due to fall off passenger ship
Drowning and submersion due to fall off Ferry-boat
Drowning and submersion due to fall off Liner

V92.Ø2 Drowning and submersion due to fall off fishing boat

V92.Ø3 Drowning and submersion due to fall off other powered watercraft
Drowning and submersion due to fall off Hovercraft (on open water)
Drowning and submersion due to fall off Jet ski

V92.Ø4 Drowning and submersion due to fall off sailboat

V92.Ø5 Drowning and submersion due to fall off canoe or kayak

V92.Ø6 Drowning and submersion due to fall off (nonpowered) inflatable craft

V92.07 **Drowning and submersion due to fall off water-skis**
EXCLUDES 1 *drowning and submersion due to falling off burning water-skis (V90.27)*
drowning and submersion due to falling off crushed water-skis (V90.37)
hit by boat while water-skiing NOS (V94.X)

V92.08 **Drowning and submersion due to fall off other unpowered watercraft**
Drowning and submersion due to fall off surf-board
Drowning and submersion due to fall off windsurfer
EXCLUDES 1 *drowning and submersion due to fall off burning unpowered watercraft (V90.28)*
drowning and submersion due to fall off crushed unpowered watercraft (V90.38)
drowning and submersion due to fall off damaged unpowered watercraft (V90.88)
drowning and submersion due to rider of nonpowered watercraft being hit by other watercraft (V94.-)
other injury due to rider of nonpowered watercraft being hit by other watercraft (V94.-)

V92.09 **Drowning and submersion due to fall off unspecified watercraft**
Drowning and submersion due to fall off boat NOS
Drowning and submersion due to fall off ship
Drowning and submersion due to fall off watercraft NOS

V92.1 **Drowning and submersion due to being thrown overboard by motion of watercraft**
EXCLUDES 1 *drowning and submersion due to fall off surf-board (V92.08)*
drowning and submersion due to fall off water-skis (V92.07)
drowning and submersion due to fall off windsurfer (V92.08)

V92.10 **Drowning and submersion due to being thrown overboard by motion of merchant ship**

V92.11 **Drowning and submersion due to being thrown overboard by motion of passenger ship**
Drowning and submersion due to being thrown overboard by motion of Ferry-boat
Drowning and submersion due to being thrown overboard by motion of Liner

V92.12 **Drowning and submersion due to being thrown overboard by motion of fishing boat**

V92.13 **Drowning and submersion due to being thrown overboard by motion of other powered watercraft**
Drowning and submersion due to being thrown overboard by motion of Hovercraft

V92.14 **Drowning and submersion due to being thrown overboard by motion of sailboat**

V92.15 **Drowning and submersion due to being thrown overboard by motion of canoe or kayak**

V92.16 **Drowning and submersion due to being thrown overboard by motion of (nonpowered) inflatable craft**

V92.19 **Drowning and submersion due to being thrown overboard by motion of unspecified watercraft**
Drowning and submersion due to being thrown overboard by motion of boat NOS
Drowning and submersion due to being thrown overboard by motion of ship NOS
Drowning and submersion due to being thrown overboard by motion of watercraft NOS

V92.2 **Drowning and submersion due to being washed overboard from watercraft**
Code first any associated cataclysm (X37.0-)

V92.20 **Drowning and submersion due to being washed overboard from merchant ship**

V92.21 **Drowning and submersion due to being washed overboard from passenger ship**
Drowning and submersion due to being washed overboard from Ferry-boat
Drowning and submersion due to being washed overboard from Liner

V92.22 **Drowning and submersion due to being washed overboard from fishing boat**

V92.23 **Drowning and submersion due to being washed overboard from other powered watercraft**
Drowning and submersion due to being washed overboard from Hovercraft (on open water)
Drowning and submersion due to being washed overboard from Jet ski

V92.24 **Drowning and submersion due to being washed overboard from sailboat**

V92.25 **Drowning and submersion due to being washed overboard from canoe or kayak**

V92.26 **Drowning and submersion due to being washed overboard from (nonpowered) inflatable craft**

V92.27 **Drowning and submersion due to being washed overboard from water-skis**
EXCLUDES 1 *drowning and submersion due to fall off water-skis (V92.07)*

V92.28 **Drowning and submersion due to being washed overboard from other unpowered watercraft**
Drowning and submersion due to being washed overboard from surf-board
Drowning and submersion due to being washed overboard from windsurfer

V92.29 **Drowning and submersion due to being washed overboard from unspecified watercraft**
Drowning and submersion due to being washed overboard from boat NOS
Drowning and submersion due to being washed overboard from ship NOS
Drowning and submersion due to being washed overboard from watercraft NOS

V93 **Other injury due to accident on board watercraft, without accident to watercraft**
EXCLUDES 1 *civilian water transport accident involving military watercraft (V94.81-)*
other injury due to accident to watercraft (V91.-)
military watercraft accident in military or war operations (Y36, Y37.-)
EXCLUDES 2 *drowning and submersion due to accident on board watercraft, without accident to watercraft (V92.-)*

V93.0 **Burn due to localized fire on board watercraft**
EXCLUDES 1 *burn due to watercraft on fire (V91.0-)*

V93.00 **Burn due to localized fire on board merchant vessel**

V93.01 **Burn due to localized fire on board passenger vessel**
Burn due to localized fire on board Ferry-boat
Burn due to localized fire on board Liner

V93.02 **Burn due to localized fire on board fishing boat**

V93.03 **Burn due to localized fire on board other powered watercraft**
Burn due to localized fire on board Hovercraft
Burn due to localized fire on board Jet ski

V93.04 **Burn due to localized fire on board sailboat**

V93.09 **Burn due to localized fire on board unspecified watercraft**
Burn due to localized fire on board boat NOS
Burn due to localized fire on board ship NOS
Burn due to localized fire on board watercraft NOS

V93.1 **Other burn on board watercraft**
Burn due to source other than fire on board watercraft
EXCLUDES 1 *burn due to watercraft on fire (V91.0-)*

V93.10 **Other burn on board merchant vessel**

V93.11 **Other burn on board passenger vessel**
Other burn on board Ferry-boat
Other burn on board Liner

V93.12 **Other burn on board fishing boat**

V93.13 **Other burn on board other powered watercraft**
Other burn on board Hovercraft
Other burn on board Jet ski

V93.14 **Other burn on board sailboat**

√x7th **V93.19 Other burn on board unspecified watercraft**
Other burn on board boat NOS
Other burn on board ship NOS
Other burn on board watercraft NOS

√5th **V93.2 Heat exposure on board watercraft**
EXCLUDES 1 *exposure to man-made heat not aboard watercraft (W92)*
exposure to natural heat while on board watercraft (X30)
exposure to sunlight while on board watercraft (X32)
EXCLUDES 2 *burn due to fire on board watercraft (V93.0-)*

√x7th **V93.20 Heat exposure on board merchant ship**
√x7th **V93.21 Heat exposure on board passenger ship**
Heat exposure on board Ferry-boat
Heat exposure on board Liner
√x7th **V93.22 Heat exposure on board fishing boat**
√x7th **V93.23 Heat exposure on board other powered watercraft**
Heat exposure on board hovercraft
√x7th **V93.24 Heat exposure on board sailboat**
√x7th **V93.29 Heat exposure on board unspecified watercraft**
Heat exposure on board boat NOS
Heat exposure on board ship NOS
Heat exposure on board watercraft NOS

√5th **V93.3 Fall on board watercraft**
EXCLUDES 1 *fall due to collision of watercraft (V91.2-)*

√x7th **V93.30 Fall on board merchant ship**
√x7th **V93.31 Fall on board passenger ship**
Fall on board Ferry-boat
Fall on board Liner
√x7th **V93.32 Fall on board fishing boat**
√x7th **V93.33 Fall on board other powered watercraft**
Fall on board Hovercraft (on open water)
Fall on board Jet ski
√x7th **V93.34 Fall on board sailboat**
√x7th **V93.35 Fall on board canoe or kayak**
√x7th **V93.36 Fall on board (nonpowered) inflatable craft**
√x7th **V93.38 Fall on board other unpowered watercraft**
√x7th **V93.39 Fall on board unspecified watercraft**
Fall on board boat NOS
Fall on board ship NOS
Fall on board watercraft NOS

√5th **V93.4 Struck by falling object on board watercraft**
Hit by falling object on board watercraft
EXCLUDES 1 *struck by falling object due to accident to watercraft (V91.3)*

√x7th **V93.40 Struck by falling object on merchant ship**
√x7th **V93.41 Struck by falling object on passenger ship**
Struck by falling object on Ferry-boat
Struck by falling object on Liner
√x7th **V93.42 Struck by falling object on fishing boat**
√x7th **V93.43 Struck by falling object on other powered watercraft**
Struck by falling object on Hovercraft
√x7th **V93.44 Struck by falling object on sailboat**
√x7th **V93.48 Struck by falling object on other unpowered watercraft**
√x7th **V93.49 Struck by falling object on unspecified watercraft**

√5th **V93.5 Explosion on board watercraft**
Boiler explosion on steamship
EXCLUDES 2 *fire on board watercraft (V93.0-)*

√x7th **V93.50 Explosion on board merchant ship**
√x7th **V93.51 Explosion on board passenger ship**
Explosion on board Ferry-boat
Explosion on board Liner
√x7th **V93.52 Explosion on board fishing boat**
√x7th **V93.53 Explosion on board other powered watercraft**
Explosion on board Hovercraft
Explosion on board Jet ski
√x7th **V93.54 Explosion on board sailboat**
√x7th **V93.59 Explosion on board unspecified watercraft**
Explosion on board boat NOS
Explosion on board ship NOS
Explosion on board watercraft NOS

√5th **V93.6 Machinery accident on board watercraft**
EXCLUDES 1 *machinery explosion on board watercraft (V93.4-)*
machinery fire on board watercraft (V93.0-)

√x7th **V93.60 Machinery accident on board merchant ship**
√x7th **V93.61 Machinery accident on board passenger ship**
Machinery accident on board Ferry-boat
Machinery accident on board Liner
√x7th **V93.62 Machinery accident on board fishing boat**
√x7th **V93.63 Machinery accident on board other powered watercraft**
Machinery accident on board Hovercraft
√x7th **V93.64 Machinery accident on board sailboat**
√x7th **V93.69 Machinery accident on board unspecified watercraft**
Machinery accident on board boat NOS
Machinery accident on board ship NOS
Machinery accident on board watercraft NOS

√5th **V93.8 Other injury due to other accident on board watercraft**
Accidental poisoning by gases or fumes on watercraft

√x7th **V93.80 Other injury due to other accident on board merchant ship**
√x7th **V93.81 Other injury due to other accident on board passenger ship**
Other injury due to other accident on board Ferry-boat
Other injury due to other accident on board Liner
√x7th **V93.82 Other injury due to other accident on board fishing boat**
√x7th **V93.83 Other injury due to other accident on board other powered watercraft**
Other injury due to other accident on board Hovercraft
Other injury due to other accident on board Jet ski
√x7th **V93.84 Other injury due to other accident on board sailboat**
√x7th **V93.85 Other injury due to other accident on board canoe or kayak**
√x7th **V93.86 Other injury due to other accident on board (nonpowered) inflatable craft**
√x7th **V93.87 Other injury due to other accident on board water-skis**
Hit or struck by object while waterskiing
√x7th **V93.88 Other injury due to other accident on board other unpowered watercraft**
Hit or struck by object while surfing
Hit or struck by object while on board windsurfer
√x7th **V93.89 Other injury due to other accident on board unspecified watercraft**
Other injury due to other accident on board boat NOS
Other injury due to other accident on board ship NOS
Other injury due to other accident on board watercraft NOS

√4th **V94 Other and unspecified water transport accidents**
EXCLUDES 1 *military watercraft accidents in military or war operations (Y36, Y37)*

√x7th **V94.0 Hitting object or bottom of body of water due to fall from watercraft**
EXCLUDES 2 *drowning and submersion due to fall from watercraft (V92.0-)*

√5th **V94.1 Bather struck by watercraft**
Swimmer hit by watercraft

√x7th **V94.11 Bather struck by powered watercraft**
√x7th **V94.12 Bather struck by nonpowered watercraft**

√5th **V94.2 Rider of nonpowered watercraft struck by other watercraft**

√x7th **V94.21 Rider of nonpowered watercraft struck by other nonpowered watercraft**
Canoer hit by other nonpowered watercraft
Surfer hit by other nonpowered watercraft
Windsurfer hit by other nonpowered watercraft

V94.22 **Rider of nonpowered watercraft struck by powered watercraft**
Canoer hit by motorboat
Surfer hit by motorboat
Windsurfer hit by motorboat

V94.3 **Injury to rider of (inflatable) watercraft being pulled behind other watercraft**

V94.31 **Injury to rider of (inflatable) recreational watercraft being pulled behind other watercraft**
Injury to rider of inner-tube pulled behind motor boat

V94.32 **Injury to rider of non-recreational watercraft being pulled behind other watercraft**
Injury to occupant of dingy being pulled behind boat or ship
Injury to occupant of life-raft being pulled behind boat or ship

V94.4 **Injury to barefoot water-skier**
Injury to person being pulled behind boat or ship

V94.8 **Other water transport accident**

V94.81 **Water transport accident involving military watercraft**

V94.810 **Civilian watercraft involved in water transport accident with military watercraft**
Passenger on civilian watercraft injured due to accident with military watercraft

V94.811 **Civilian in water injured by military watercraft**

V94.818 **Other water transport accident involving military watercraft**

V94.89 **Other water transport accident**

V94.9 **Unspecified water transport accident**
Water transport accident NOS

Air and space transport accidents (V95-V97)

EXCLUDES 1 *military aircraft accidents in military or war operations (Y36, Y37)*

The appropriate 7th character is to be added to each code from categories V95-V97.
A initial encounter
D subsequent encounter
S sequela

V95 **Accident to powered aircraft causing injury to occupant**

V95.0 **Helicopter accident injuring occupant**

V95.00 **Unspecified helicopter accident injuring occupant**

V95.01 **Helicopter crash injuring occupant**

V95.02 **Forced landing of helicopter injuring occupant**

V95.03 **Helicopter collision injuring occupant**
Helicopter collision with any object, fixed, movable or moving

V95.04 **Helicopter fire injuring occupant**

V95.05 **Helicopter explosion injuring occupant**

V95.09 **Other helicopter accident injuring occupant**

V95.1 **Ultralight, microlight or powered-glider accident injuring occupant**

V95.10 **Unspecified ultralight, microlight or powered-glider accident injuring occupant**

V95.11 **Ultralight, microlight or powered-glider crash injuring occupant**

V95.12 **Forced landing of ultralight, microlight or powered-glider injuring occupant**

V95.13 **Ultralight, microlight or powered-glider collision injuring occupant**
Ultralight, microlight or powered-glider collision with any object, fixed, movable or moving

V95.14 **Ultralight, microlight or powered-glider fire injuring occupant**

V95.15 **Ultralight, microlight or powered-glider explosion injuring occupant**

V95.19 **Other ultralight, microlight or powered-glider accident injuring occupant**

V95.2 **Other private fixed-wing aircraft accident injuring occupant**

V95.20 **Unspecified accident to other private fixed-wing aircraft, injuring occupant**

V95.21 **Other private fixed-wing aircraft crash injuring occupant**

V95.22 **Forced landing of other private fixed-wing aircraft injuring occupant**

V95.23 **Other private fixed-wing aircraft collision injuring occupant**
Other private fixed-wing aircraft collision with any object, fixed, movable or moving

V95.24 **Other private fixed-wing aircraft fire injuring occupant**

V95.25 **Other private fixed-wing aircraft explosion injuring occupant**

V95.29 **Other accident to other private fixed-wing aircraft injuring occupant**

V95.3 **Commercial fixed-wing aircraft accident injuring occupant**

V95.30 **Unspecified accident to commercial fixed-wing aircraft injuring occupant**

V95.31 **Commercial fixed-wing aircraft crash injuring occupant**

V95.32 **Forced landing of commercial fixed-wing aircraft injuring occupant**

V95.33 **Commercial fixed-wing aircraft collision injuring occupant**
Commercial fixed-wing aircraft collision with any object, fixed, movable or moving

V95.34 **Commercial fixed-wing aircraft fire injuring occupant**

V95.35 **Commercial fixed-wing aircraft explosion injuring occupant**

V95.39 **Other accident to commercial fixed-wing aircraft injuring occupant**

V95.4 **Spacecraft accident injuring occupant**

V95.40 **Unspecified spacecraft accident injuring occupant**

V95.41 **Spacecraft crash injuring occupant**

V95.42 **Forced landing of spacecraft injuring occupant**

V95.43 **Spacecraft collision injuring occupant**
Spacecraft collision with any object, fixed, moveable or moving

V95.44 **Spacecraft fire injuring occupant**

V95.45 **Spacecraft explosion injuring occupant**

V95.49 **Other spacecraft accident injuring occupant**

V95.8 **Other powered aircraft accidents injuring occupant**

V95.9 **Unspecified aircraft accident injuring occupant**
Aircraft accident NOS
Air transport accident NOS

V96 **Accident to nonpowered aircraft causing injury to occupant**

V96.0 **Balloon accident injuring occupant**

V96.00 **Unspecified balloon accident injuring occupant**

V96.01 **Balloon crash injuring occupant**

V96.02 **Forced landing of balloon injuring occupant**

V96.03 **Balloon collision injuring occupant**
Balloon collision with any object, fixed, moveable or moving

V96.04 **Balloon fire injuring occupant**

V96.05 **Balloon explosion injuring occupant**

V96.09 **Other balloon accident injuring occupant**

V96.1 **Hang-glider accident injuring occupant**

V96.10 **Unspecified hang-glider accident injuring occupant**

V96.11 **Hang-glider crash injuring occupant**

V96.12 **Forced landing of hang-glider injuring occupant**

V96.13 **Hang-glider collision injuring occupant**
Hang-glider collision with any object, fixed, moveable or moving

V96.14 **Hang-glider fire injuring occupant**

V96.15 **Hang-glider explosion injuring occupant**

V96.19 **Other hang-glider accident injuring occupant**

V96.2 **Glider (nonpowered) accident injuring occupant**

V96.20 **Unspecified glider (nonpowered) accident injuring occupant**

V96.21 **Glider (nonpowered) crash injuring occupant**

V96.22 **Forced landing of glider (nonpowered) injuring occupant**

Chapter 20. External Causes of Morbidity

√x7th **V96.23 Glider (nonpowered) collision injuring occupant**
Glider (nonpowered) collision with any object, fixed, moveable or moving

√x7th **V96.24 Glider (nonpowered) fire injuring occupant**

√x7th **V96.25 Glider (nonpowered) explosion injuring occupant**

√x7th **V96.29 Other glider (nonpowered) accident injuring occupant**

√x7th **V96.8 Other nonpowered-aircraft accidents injuring occupant**
Kite carrying a person accident injuring occupant

√x7th **V96.9 Unspecified nonpowered-aircraft accident injuring occupant**
Nonpowered-aircraft accident NOS

√4th **V97 Other specified air transport accidents**

√x7th **V97.0 Occupant of aircraft injured in other specified air transport accidents**
Fall in, on or from aircraft in air transport accident
EXCLUDES 1 *accident while boarding or alighting aircraft (V97.1)*

√x7th **V97.1 Person injured while boarding or alighting from aircraft**

√5th **V97.2 Parachutist accident**

√x7th **V97.21 Parachutist entangled in object**
Parachutist landing in tree

√x7th **V97.22 Parachutist injured on landing**

√x7th **V97.29 Other parachutist accident**

√5th **V97.3 Person on ground injured in air transport accident**

√x7th **V97.31 Hit by object falling from aircraft**
Hit by crashing aircraft
Injured by aircraft hitting house
Injured by aircraft hitting car

√x7th **V97.32 Injured by rotating propeller**

√x7th **V97.33 Sucked into jet engine**

√x7th **V97.39 Other injury to person on ground due to air transport accident**

√5th **V97.8 Other air transport accidents, not elsewhere classified**
EXCLUDES 1 *aircraft accident NOS (V95.9)*
exposure to changes in air pressure during ascent or descent (W94.-)

√6th **V97.81 Air transport accident involving military aircraft**

√7th **V97.810 Civilian aircraft involved in air transport accident with military aircraft**
Passenger in civilian aircraft injured due to accident with military aircraft

√7th **V97.811 Civilian injured by military aircraft**

√7th **V97.818 Other air transport accident involving military aircraft**

√x7th **V97.89 Other air transport accidents, not elsewhere classified**
Injury from machinery on aircraft

Other and unspecified transport accidents (V98-V99)

EXCLUDES 1 *vehicle accident, type of vehicle unspecified (V89.-)*

The appropriate 7th character is to be added to each code from categories V98-V99.
A initial encounter
D subsequent encounter
S sequela

√4th **V98 Other specified transport accidents**

√x7th **V98.0 Accident to, on or involving cable-car, not on rails**
Caught or dragged by cable-car, not on rails
Fall or jump from cable-car, not on rails
Object thrown from or in cable-car, not on rails

√x7th **V98.1 Accident to, on or involving land-yacht**

√x7th **V98.2 Accident to, on or involving ice yacht**

√x7th **V98.3 Accident to, on or involving ski lift**
Accident to, on or involving ski chair-lift
Accident to, on or involving ski-lift with gondola

√x7th **V98.8 Other specified transport accidents**

√x7th **V99 Unspecified transport accident**

OTHER EXTERNAL CAUSES OF ACCIDENTAL INJURY (W00-X58)

Slipping, tripping, stumbling and falls (W00-W19)

EXCLUDES 1 *assault involving a fall (Y01-Y02)*
fall from animal (V80.-)
fall (in) (from) machinery (in operation) (W28-W31)
fall (in) (from) transport vehicle (V01-V99)
intentional self-harm involving a fall (X80-X81)
EXCLUDES 2 *at risk for fall (history of fall) Z91.81*
fall (in) (from) burning building (X00.-)
fall into fire (X00-X04, X08)

The appropriate 7th character is to be added to each code from categories W00-W19.
A initial encounter
D subsequent encounter
S sequela

√4th **W00 Fall due to ice and snow**
INCLUDES pedestrian on foot falling (slipping) on ice and snow
EXCLUDES 1 *fall on (from) ice and snow involving pedestrian conveyance (V00.-)*
fall from stairs and steps not due to ice and snow (W10.-)
AHA: 2016,2Q,4

√x7th **W00.0 Fall on same level due to ice and snow**

√x7th **W00.1 Fall from stairs and steps due to ice and snow**

√x7th **W00.2 Other fall from one level to another due to ice and snow**

√x7th **W00.9 Unspecified fall due to ice and snow**

√4th **W01 Fall on same level from slipping, tripping and stumbling**
INCLUDES fall on moving sidewalk
EXCLUDES 1 *fall due to bumping (striking) against object (W18.0-)*
fall in shower or bathtub (W18.2-)
fall on same level NOS (W18.30)
fall on same level from slipping, tripping and stumbling due to ice or snow (W00.0)
fall off or from toilet (W18.1-)
slipping, tripping and stumbling NOS (W18.40)
slipping, tripping and stumbling without falling (W18.4-)

√x7th **W01.0 Fall on same level from slipping, tripping and stumbling without subsequent striking against object**
Falling over animal

√5th **W01.1 Fall on same level from slipping, tripping and stumbling with subsequent striking against object**

√x7th **W01.10 Fall on same level from slipping, tripping and stumbling with subsequent striking against unspecified object**

√6th **W01.11 Fall on same level from slipping, tripping and stumbling with subsequent striking against sharp object**

√7th **W01.110 Fall on same level from slipping, tripping and stumbling with subsequent striking against sharp glass**

√7th **W01.111 Fall on same level from slipping, tripping and stumbling with subsequent striking against power tool or machine**

√7th **W01.118 Fall on same level from slipping, tripping and stumbling with subsequent striking against other sharp object**

√7th **W01.119 Fall on same level from slipping, tripping and stumbling with subsequent striking against unspecified sharp object**

√6th **W01.19 Fall on same level from slipping, tripping and stumbling with subsequent striking against other object**

√7th **W01.190 Fall on same level from slipping, tripping and stumbling with subsequent striking against furniture**

√7th **W01.198 Fall on same level from slipping, tripping and stumbling with subsequent striking against other object**

√x7th **W03 Other fall on same level due to collision with another person**

Fall due to non-transport collision with other person

EXCLUDES 1 *collision with another person without fall (W51)*
crushed or pushed by a crowd or human stampede (W52)
fall involving pedestrian conveyance (V00-V09)
fall due to ice or snow (W00)
fall on same level NOS (W18.30)

AHA: 2012,4Q,108

√x7th **W04 Fall while being carried or supported by other persons**

Accidentally dropped while being carried

√4th **W05 Fall from non-moving wheelchair, nonmotorized scooter and motorized mobility scooter**

EXCLUDES 1 *fall from moving wheelchair (powered) (V00.811)*
fall from moving motorized mobility scooter (V00.831)
fall from nonmotorized scooter (V00.141)

√x7th **W05.0 Fall from non-moving wheelchair**

AHA: 2019,2Q,27

√x7th **W05.1 Fall from non-moving nonmotorized scooter**

√x7th **W05.2 Fall from non-moving motorized mobility scooter**

√x7th **W06 Fall from bed**

√x7th **W07 Fall from chair**

√x7th **W08 Fall from other furniture**

▶Fall from stool◀

√4th **W09 Fall on and from playground equipment**

EXCLUDES 1 *fall involving recreational machinery (W31)*

√x7th **W09.0 Fall on or from playground slide**

√x7th **W09.1 Fall from playground swing**

√x7th **W09.2 Fall on or from jungle gym**

√x7th **W09.8 Fall on or from other playground equipment**

√4th **W10 Fall on and from stairs and steps**

EXCLUDES 1 *Fall from stairs and steps due to ice and snow (W00.1)*

√x7th **W10.0 Fall (on)(from) escalator**

√x7th **W10.1 Fall (on)(from) sidewalk curb**

√x7th **W10.2 Fall (on)(from) incline**

Fall (on) (from) ramp

√x7th **W10.8 Fall (on) (from) other stairs and steps**

√x7th **W10.9 Fall (on) (from) unspecified stairs and steps**

√x7th **W11 Fall on and from ladder**

√x7th **W12 Fall on and from scaffolding**

√4th **W13 Fall from, out of or through building or structure**

√x7th **W13.0 Fall from, out of or through balcony**

Fall from, out of or through railing

√x7th **W13.1 Fall from, out of or through bridge**

√x7th **W13.2 Fall from, out of or through roof**

√x7th **W13.3 Fall through floor**

√x7th **W13.4 Fall from, out of or through window**

EXCLUDES 2 *fall with subsequent striking against sharp glass (W01.110-)*

√x7th **W13.8 Fall from, out of or through other building or structure**

Fall from, out of or through viaduct
Fall from, out of or through wall
Fall from, out of or through flag-pole

√x7th **W13.9 Fall from, out of or through building, not otherwise specified**

EXCLUDES 1 *collapse of a building or structure (W20.-)*
fall or jump from burning building or structure (X00.-)

√x7th **W14 Fall from tree**

√x7th **W15 Fall from cliff**

√4th **W16 Fall, jump or diving into water**

EXCLUDES 1 *accidental non-watercraft drowning and submersion not involving fall (W65-W74)*
effects of air pressure from diving (W94.-)
fall into water from watercraft (V90-V94)
hitting an object or against bottom when falling from watercraft (V94.0)

EXCLUDES 2 *striking or hitting diving board (W21.4)*

√5th **W16.0 Fall into swimming pool**

Fall into swimming pool NOS

EXCLUDES 1 *fall into empty swimming pool (W17.3)*

√6th **W16.01 Fall into swimming pool striking water surface**

√7th **W16.011 Fall into swimming pool striking water surface causing drowning and submersion**

EXCLUDES 1 *drowning and submersion while in swimming pool without fall (W67)*

√7th **W16.012 Fall into swimming pool striking water surface causing other injury**

√6th **W16.02 Fall into swimming pool striking bottom**

√7th **W16.021 Fall into swimming pool striking bottom causing drowning and submersion**

EXCLUDES 1 *drowning and submersion while in swimming pool without fall (W67)*

√7th **W16.022 Fall into swimming pool striking bottom causing other injury**

√6th **W16.03 Fall into swimming pool striking wall**

√7th **W16.031 Fall into swimming pool striking wall causing drowning and submersion**

EXCLUDES 1 *drowning and submersion while in swimming pool without fall (W67)*

√7th **W16.032 Fall into swimming pool striking wall causing other injury**

√5th **W16.1 Fall into natural body of water**

Fall into lake
Fall into open sea
Fall into river
Fall into stream

√6th **W16.11 Fall into natural body of water striking water surface**

√7th **W16.111 Fall into natural body of water striking water surface causing drowning and submersion**

EXCLUDES 1 *drowning and submersion while in natural body of water without fall (W69)*

√7th **W16.112 Fall into natural body of water striking water surface causing other injury**

√6th **W16.12 Fall into natural body of water striking bottom**

√7th **W16.121 Fall into natural body of water striking bottom causing drowning and submersion**

EXCLUDES 1 *drowning and submersion while in natural body of water without fall (W69)*

√7th **W16.122 Fall into natural body of water striking bottom causing other injury**

√6th **W16.13 Fall into natural body of water striking side**

√7th **W16.131 Fall into natural body of water striking side causing drowning and submersion**

EXCLUDES 1 *drowning and submersion while in natural body of water without fall (W69)*

√7th **W16.132 Fall into natural body of water striking side causing other injury**

√5th **W16.2 Fall in (into) filled bathtub or bucket of water**

√6th **W16.21 Fall in (into) filled bathtub**

EXCLUDES 1 *fall into empty bathtub (W18.2)*

√7th **W16.211 Fall in (into) filled bathtub causing drowning and submersion**

EXCLUDES 1 *drowning and submersion while in filled bathtub without fall (W65)*

√7th **W16.212 Fall in (into) filled bathtub causing other injury**

6th **W16.22 Fall in (into) bucket of water**

7th **W16.221 Fall in (into) bucket of water causing drowning and submersion**

7th **W16.222 Fall in (into) bucket of water causing other injury**

5th **W16.3 Fall into other water**

Fall into fountain

Fall into reservoir

6th **W16.31 Fall into other water striking water surface**

7th **W16.311 Fall into other water striking water surface causing drowning and submersion**

EXCLUDES 1 *drowning and submersion while in other water without fall (W73)*

7th **W16.312 Fall into other water striking water surface causing other injury**

6th **W16.32 Fall into other water striking bottom**

7th **W16.321 Fall into other water striking bottom causing drowning and submersion**

EXCLUDES 1 *drowning and submersion while in other water without fall (W73)*

7th **W16.322 Fall into other water striking bottom causing other injury**

6th **W16.33 Fall into other water striking wall**

7th **W16.331 Fall into other water striking wall causing drowning and submersion**

EXCLUDES 1 *drowning and submersion while in other water without fall (W73)*

7th **W16.332 Fall into other water striking wall causing other injury**

5th **W16.4 Fall into unspecified water**

x7th **W16.41 Fall into unspecified water causing drowning and submersion**

x7th **W16.42 Fall into unspecified water causing other injury**

5th **W16.5 Jumping or diving into swimming pool**

6th **W16.51 Jumping or diving into swimming pool striking water surface**

7th **W16.511 Jumping or diving into swimming pool striking water surface causing drowning and submersion**

EXCLUDES 1 *drowning and submersion while in swimming pool without jumping or diving (W67)*

7th **W16.512 Jumping or diving into swimming pool striking water surface causing other injury**

6th **W16.52 Jumping or diving into swimming pool striking bottom**

7th **W16.521 Jumping or diving into swimming pool striking bottom causing drowning and submersion**

EXCLUDES 1 *drowning and submersion while in swimming pool without jumping or diving (W67)*

7th **W16.522 Jumping or diving into swimming pool striking bottom causing other injury**

6th **W16.53 Jumping or diving into swimming pool striking wall**

7th **W16.531 Jumping or diving into swimming pool striking wall causing drowning and submersion**

EXCLUDES 1 *drowning and submersion while in swimming pool without jumping or diving (W67)*

7th **W16.532 Jumping or diving into swimming pool striking wall causing other injury**

5th **W16.6 Jumping or diving into natural body of water**

Jumping or diving into lake

Jumping or diving into open sea

Jumping or diving into river

Jumping or diving into stream

6th **W16.61 Jumping or diving into natural body of water striking water surface**

7th **W16.611 Jumping or diving into natural body of water striking water surface causing drowning and submersion**

EXCLUDES 1 *drowning and submersion while in natural body of water without jumping or diving (W69)*

7th **W16.612 Jumping or diving into natural body of water striking water surface causing other injury**

6th **W16.62 Jumping or diving into natural body of water striking bottom**

7th **W16.621 Jumping or diving into natural body of water striking bottom causing drowning and submersion**

EXCLUDES 1 *drowning and submersion while in natural body of water without jumping or diving (W69)*

7th **W16.622 Jumping or diving into natural body of water striking bottom causing other injury**

5th **W16.7 Jumping or diving from boat**

EXCLUDES 1 *fall from boat into water - see watercraft accident (V90-V94)*

6th **W16.71 Jumping or diving from boat striking water surface**

7th **W16.711 Jumping or diving from boat striking water surface causing drowning and submersion**

7th **W16.712 Jumping or diving from boat striking water surface causing other injury**

6th **W16.72 Jumping or diving from boat striking bottom**

7th **W16.721 Jumping or diving from boat striking bottom causing drowning and submersion**

7th **W16.722 Jumping or diving from boat striking bottom causing other injury**

5th **W16.8 Jumping or diving into other water**

Jumping or diving into fountain

Jumping or diving into reservoir

6th **W16.81 Jumping or diving into other water striking water surface**

7th **W16.811 Jumping or diving into other water striking water surface causing drowning and submersion**

EXCLUDES 1 *drowning and submersion while in other water without jumping or diving (W73)*

7th **W16.812 Jumping or diving into other water striking water surface causing other injury**

6th **W16.82 Jumping or diving into other water striking bottom**

7th **W16.821 Jumping or diving into other water striking bottom causing drowning and submersion**

EXCLUDES 1 *drowning and submersion while in other water without jumping or diving (W73)*

7th **W16.822 Jumping or diving into other water striking bottom causing other injury**

6th **W16.83 Jumping or diving into other water striking wall**

7th **W16.831 Jumping or diving into other water striking wall causing drowning and submersion**

EXCLUDES 1 *drowning and submersion while in other water without jumping or diving (W73)*

7th **W16.832 Jumping or diving into other water striking wall causing other injury**

W16.9 Jumping or diving into unspecified water
W16.91 Jumping or diving into unspecified water causing drowning and submersion
W16.92 Jumping or diving into unspecified water causing other injury

W17 Other fall from one level to another
W17.0 Fall into well
W17.1 Fall into storm drain or manhole
W17.2 Fall into hole
Fall into pit
W17.3 Fall into empty swimming pool
EXCLUDES 1 *fall into filled swimming pool (W16.0-)*
W17.4 Fall from dock
W17.8 Other fall from one level to another
W17.81 Fall down embankment (hill)
W17.82 Fall from (out of) grocery cart
Fall due to grocery cart tipping over
W17.89 Other fall from one level to another
Fall from cherry picker
Fall from lifting device
Fall from mobile elevated work platform [MEWP]
Fall from sky lift
AHA: 2015,2Q,6

W18 Other slipping, tripping and stumbling and falls
W18.0 Fall due to bumping against object
Striking against object with subsequent fall
EXCLUDES 1 *fall on same level due to slipping, tripping, or stumbling with subsequent striking against object (W01.1-)*
W18.00 Striking against unspecified object with subsequent fall
W18.01 Striking against sports equipment with subsequent fall
W18.02 Striking against glass with subsequent fall
W18.09 Striking against other object with subsequent fall
W18.1 Fall from or off toilet
W18.11 Fall from or off toilet without subsequent striking against object
Fall from (off) toilet NOS
W18.12 Fall from or off toilet with subsequent striking against object
W18.2 Fall in (into) shower or empty bathtub
EXCLUDES 1 *fall in full bathtub causing drowning or submersion (W16.21-)*
W18.3 Other and unspecified fall on same level
W18.30 Fall on same level, unspecified
W18.31 Fall on same level due to stepping on an object
Fall on same level due to stepping on an animal
EXCLUDES 1 *slipping, tripping and stumbling without fall due to stepping on animal (W18.41)*
W18.39 Other fall on same level
W18.4 Slipping, tripping and stumbling without falling
EXCLUDES 1 *collision with another person without fall (W51)*
W18.40 Slipping, tripping and stumbling without falling, unspecified
W18.41 Slipping, tripping and stumbling without falling due to stepping on object
Slipping, tripping and stumbling without falling due to stepping on animal
EXCLUDES 1 *slipping, tripping and stumbling with fall due to stepping on animal (W18.31)*
W18.42 Slipping, tripping and stumbling without falling due to stepping into hole or opening
W18.43 Slipping, tripping and stumbling without falling due to stepping from one level to another
W18.49 Other slipping, tripping and stumbling without falling

W19 Unspecified fall
Accidental fall NOS
AHA: 2012,4Q,95

Exposure to inanimate mechanical forces (W20-W49)

EXCLUDES 1 *assault (X92-Y09)*
contact or collision with animals or persons (W50-W64)
exposure to inanimate mechanical forces involving military or war operations (Y36.-, Y37.-)
intentional self-harm (X71-X83)

The appropriate 7th character is to be added to each code from categories W20-W49.
A initial encounter
D subsequent encounter
S sequela

W20 Struck by thrown, projected or falling object
Code first any associated:
cataclysm (X34-X39)
lightning strike (T75.00)
EXCLUDES 1 *falling object in machinery accident (W24, W28-W31)*
falling object in transport accident (V01-V99)
object set in motion by explosion (W35-W40)
object set in motion by firearm (W32-W34)
struck by thrown sports equipment (W21.-)
W20.0 Struck by falling object in cave-in
EXCLUDES 2 *asphyxiation due to cave-in (T71.21)*
W20.1 Struck by object due to collapse of building
EXCLUDES 1 *struck by object due to collapse of burning building (X00.2, X02.2)*
W20.8 Other cause of strike by thrown, projected or falling object
EXCLUDES 1 *struck by thrown sports equipment (W21.-)*

W21 Striking against or struck by sports equipment
EXCLUDES 1 *assault with sports equipment (Y08.0-)*
striking against or struck by sports equipment with subsequent fall (W18.01)
W21.0 Struck by hit or thrown ball
W21.00 Struck by hit or thrown ball, unspecified type
W21.01 Struck by football
W21.02 Struck by soccer ball
W21.03 Struck by baseball
W21.04 Struck by golf ball
W21.05 Struck by basketball
W21.06 Struck by volleyball
W21.07 Struck by softball
W21.09 Struck by other hit or thrown ball
W21.1 Struck by bat, racquet or club
W21.11 Struck by baseball bat
W21.12 Struck by tennis racquet
W21.13 Struck by golf club
W21.19 Struck by other bat, racquet or club
W21.2 Struck by hockey stick or puck
W21.21 Struck by hockey stick
W21.210 Struck by ice hockey stick
W21.211 Struck by field hockey stick
W21.22 Struck by hockey puck
W21.220 Struck by ice hockey puck
W21.221 Struck by field hockey puck
W21.3 Struck by sports foot wear
W21.31 Struck by shoe cleats
Stepped on by shoe cleats
W21.32 Struck by skate blades
Skated over by skate blades
W21.39 Struck by other sports foot wear
W21.4 Striking against diving board
Use additional code for subsequent falling into water, if applicable (W16.-)
W21.8 Striking against or struck by other sports equipment
W21.81 Striking against or struck by football helmet
W21.89 Striking against or struck by other sports equipment
W21.9 Striking against or struck by unspecified sports equipment

4th **W22 Striking against or struck by other objects**

EXCLUDES 1 *striking against or struck by object with subsequent fall (W18.Ø9)*

5th **W22.Ø Striking against stationary object**

EXCLUDES 1 *striking against stationary sports equipment (W21.8)*

√x7th **W22.Ø1 Walked into wall**

√x7th **W22.Ø2 Walked into lamppost**

√x7th **W22.Ø3 Walked into furniture**

6th **W22.Ø4 Striking against wall of swimming pool**

7th **W22.Ø41 Striking against wall of swimming pool causing drowning and submersion**

EXCLUDES 1 *drowning and submersion while swimming without striking against wall (W67)*

7th **W22.Ø42 Striking against wall of swimming pool causing other injury**

√x7th **W22.Ø9 Striking against other stationary object**

5th **W22.1 Striking against or struck by automobile airbag**

√x7th **W22.1Ø Striking against or struck by unspecified automobile airbag**

√x7th **W22.11 Striking against or struck by driver side automobile airbag**

√x7th **W22.12 Striking against or struck by front passenger side automobile airbag**

√x7th **W22.19 Striking against or struck by other automobile airbag**

√x7th **W22.8 Striking against or struck by other objects**

Striking against or struck by object NOS

EXCLUDES 1 *struck by thrown, projected or falling object (W2Ø.-)*

4th **W23 Caught, crushed, jammed or pinched in or between objects**

EXCLUDES 1 *injury caused by cutting or piercing instruments (W25-W27)*
injury caused by firearms malfunction (W32.1, W33.1-, W34.1-)
injury caused by lifting and transmission devices (W24.-)
injury caused by machinery (W28-W31)
injury caused by nonpowered hand tools (W27.-)
injury caused by transport vehicle being used as a means of transportation (VØ1-V99)
injury caused by struck by thrown, projected or falling object (W2Ø.-)

√x7th **W23.Ø Caught, crushed, jammed, or pinched between moving objects**

√x7th **W23.1 Caught, crushed, jammed, or pinched between stationary objects**

● √x7th **W23.2 Caught, crushed, jammed or pinched between a moving and stationary object**

4th **W24 Contact with lifting and transmission devices, not elsewhere classified**

EXCLUDES 1 *transport accidents (VØ1-V99)*

√x7th **W24.Ø Contact with lifting devices, not elsewhere classified**

Contact with chain hoist
Contact with drive belt
Contact with pulley (block)

√x7th **W24.1 Contact with transmission devices, not elsewhere classified**

Contact with transmission belt or cable

√x7th **W25 Contact with sharp glass**

Code first any associated:
injury due to flying glass from explosion or firearm discharge (W32-W4Ø)
transport accident (VØØ-V99)

EXCLUDES 1 *fall on same level due to slipping, tripping and stumbling with subsequent striking against sharp glass (WØ1.11Ø-)*
striking against sharp glass with subsequent fall (W18.Ø2-)

EXCLUDES 2 *glass embedded in skin (W45.-)*

4th **W26 Contact with other sharp objects**

EXCLUDES 2 *sharp object(s) embedded in skin (W45.-)*

AHA: 2016,4Q,73

√x7th **W26.Ø Contact with knife**

EXCLUDES 1 *contact with electric knife (W29.1)*

√x7th **W26.1 Contact with sword or dagger**

√x7th **W26.2 Contact with edge of stiff paper**

Paper cut

√x7th **W26.8 Contact with other sharp object(s), not elsewhere classified**

Contact with tin can lid

√x7th **W26.9 Contact with unspecified sharp object(s)**

4th **W27 Contact with nonpowered hand tool**

√x7th **W27.Ø Contact with workbench tool**

Contact with auger
Contact with axe
Contact with chisel
Contact with handsaw
Contact with screwdriver

√x7th **W27.1 Contact with garden tool**

Contact with hoe
Contact with nonpowered lawn mower
Contact with pitchfork
Contact with rake

√x7th **W27.2 Contact with scissors**

√x7th **W27.3 Contact with needle (sewing)**

EXCLUDES 1 *contact with hypodermic needle (W46.-)*

√x7th **W27.4 Contact with kitchen utensil**

Contact with fork
Contact with ice-pick
Contact with can-opener NOS

√x7th **W27.5 Contact with paper-cutter**

√x7th **W27.8 Contact with other nonpowered hand tool**

Contact with nonpowered sewing machine
Contact with shovel

√x7th **W28 Contact with powered lawn mower**

Powered lawn mower (commercial) (residential)

EXCLUDES 1 *contact with nonpowered lawn mower (W27.1)*

EXCLUDES 2 *exposure to electric current (W86.-)*

4th **W29 Contact with other powered hand tools and household machinery**

EXCLUDES 1 *contact with commercial machinery (W31.82)*
contact with hot household appliance (X15)
contact with nonpowered hand tool (W27.-)
exposure to electric current (W86)

√x7th **W29.Ø Contact with powered kitchen appliance**

Contact with blender
Contact with can-opener
Contact with garbage disposal
Contact with mixer

√x7th **W29.1 Contact with electric knife**

√x7th **W29.2 Contact with other powered household machinery**

Contact with electric fan
Contact with powered dryer (clothes) (powered) (spin)
Contact with washing-machine
Contact with sewing machine

√x7th **W29.3 Contact with powered garden and outdoor hand tools and machinery**

Contact with chainsaw
Contact with edger
Contact with garden cultivator (tiller)
Contact with hedge trimmer
Contact with other powered garden tool

EXCLUDES 1 *contact with powered lawn mower (W28)*

√x7th **W29.4 Contact with nail gun**

√x7th **W29.8 Contact with other powered hand tools and household machinery**

Contact with do-it-yourself tool NOS

4th **W3Ø Contact with agricultural machinery**

INCLUDES animal-powered farm machine

EXCLUDES 1 *agricultural transport vehicle accident (VØ1-V99)*
explosion of grain store (W4Ø.8)
exposure to electric current (W86.-)

√x7th **W3Ø.Ø Contact with combine harvester**

Contact with reaper
Contact with thresher

√x7th **W3Ø.1 Contact with power take-off devices (PTO)**

√x7th **W3Ø.2 Contact with hay derrick**

✓x7th **W30.3 Contact with grain storage elevator**

EXCLUDES 1 *explosion of grain store (W40.8)*

✓5th **W30.8 Contact with other specified agricultural machinery**

✓x7th **W30.81 Contact with agricultural transport vehicle in stationary use**

Contact with agricultural transport vehicle under repair, not on public roadway

EXCLUDES 1 *agricultural transport vehicle accident (V01-V99)*

✓x7th **W30.89 Contact with other specified agricultural machinery**

✓x7th **W30.9 Contact with unspecified agricultural machinery**

Contact with farm machinery NOS

✓4th **W31 Contact with other and unspecified machinery**

EXCLUDES 1 *contact with agricultural machinery (W30.-)*
contact with machinery in transport under own power or being towed by a vehicle (V01-V99)
exposure to electric current (W86)

✓x7th **W31.0 Contact with mining and earth-drilling machinery**

Contact with bore or drill (land) (seabed)
Contact with shaft hoist
Contact with shaft lift
Contact with undercutter

✓x7th **W31.1 Contact with metalworking machines**

Contact with abrasive wheel
Contact with forging machine
Contact with lathe
Contact with mechanical shears
Contact with metal drilling machine
Contact with milling machine
Contact with power press
Contact with rolling-mill
Contact with metal sawing machine

✓x7th **W31.2 Contact with powered woodworking and forming machines**

Contact with band saw
Contact with bench saw
Contact with circular saw
Contact with molding machine
Contact with overhead plane
Contact with powered saw
Contact with radial saw
Contact with sander

EXCLUDES 1 *nonpowered woodworking tools (W27.0)*

✓x7th **W31.3 Contact with prime movers**

Contact with gas turbine
Contact with internal combustion engine
Contact with steam engine
Contact with water driven turbine

✓5th **W31.8 Contact with other specified machinery**

✓x7th **W31.81 Contact with recreational machinery**

Contact with roller coaster

✓x7th **W31.82 Contact with other commercial machinery**

Contact with commercial electric fan
Contact with commercial kitchen appliances
Contact with commercial powered dryer (clothes) (powered) (spin)
Contact with commercial washing-machine
Contact with commercial sewing machine

EXCLUDES 1 *contact with household machinery (W29.-)*
contact with powered lawn mower (W28)

✓x7th **W31.83 Contact with special construction vehicle in stationary use**

Contact with special construction vehicle under repair, not on public roadway

EXCLUDES 1 *special construction vehicle accident (V01-V99)*

✓x7th **W31.89 Contact with other specified machinery**

✓x7th **W31.9 Contact with unspecified machinery**

Contact with machinery NOS

✓4th **W32 Accidental handgun discharge and malfunction**

INCLUDES accidental discharge and malfunction of gun for single hand use
accidental discharge and malfunction of pistol
accidental discharge and malfunction of revolver
handgun discharge and malfunction NOS

EXCLUDES 1 *accidental airgun discharge and malfunction (W34.010, W34.110)*
accidental BB gun discharge and malfunction (W34.010, W34.110)
accidental pellet gun discharge and malfunction (W34.010, W34.110)
accidental shotgun discharge and malfunction (W33.01, W33.11)
assault by handgun discharge (X93)
handgun discharge involving legal intervention (Y35.0-)
handgun discharge involving military or war operations (Y36.4-)
intentional self-harm by handgun discharge (X72)
Very pistol discharge and malfunction (W34.09, W34.19)

✓x7th **W32.0 Accidental handgun discharge**

✓x7th **W32.1 Accidental handgun malfunction**

Injury due to explosion of handgun (parts)
Injury due to malfunction of mechanism or component of handgun
Injury due to recoil of handgun
Powder burn from handgun

✓4th **W33 Accidental rifle, shotgun and larger firearm discharge and malfunction**

INCLUDES rifle, shotgun and larger firearm discharge and malfunction NOS

EXCLUDES 1 *accidental airgun discharge and malfunction (W34.010, W34.110)*
accidental BB gun discharge and malfunction (W34.010, W34.110)
accidental handgun discharge and malfunction (W32.-)
accidental pellet gun discharge and malfunction (W34.010, W34.110)
assault by rifle, shotgun and larger firearm discharge (X94)
firearm discharge involving legal intervention (Y35.0-)
firearm discharge involving military or war operations (Y36.4-)
intentional self-harm by rifle, shotgun and larger firearm discharge (X73)

✓5th **W33.0 Accidental rifle, shotgun and larger firearm discharge**

✓x7th **W33.00 Accidental discharge of unspecified larger firearm**

Discharge of unspecified larger firearm NOS

✓x7th **W33.01 Accidental discharge of shotgun**

Discharge of shotgun NOS

✓x7th **W33.02 Accidental discharge of hunting rifle**

Discharge of hunting rifle NOS

✓x7th **W33.03 Accidental discharge of machine gun**

Discharge of machine gun NOS

✓x7th **W33.09 Accidental discharge of other larger firearm**

Discharge of other larger firearm NOS

✓5th **W33.1 Accidental rifle, shotgun and larger firearm malfunction**

Injury due to explosion of rifle, shotgun and larger firearm (parts)
Injury due to malfunction of mechanism or component of rifle, shotgun and larger firearm
Injury due to piercing, cutting, crushing or pinching due to (by) slide trigger mechanism, scope or other gun part
Injury due to recoil of rifle, shotgun and larger firearm
Powder burn from rifle, shotgun and larger firearm

✓x7th **W33.10 Accidental malfunction of unspecified larger firearm**

Malfunction of unspecified larger firearm NOS

✓x7th **W33.11 Accidental malfunction of shotgun**

Malfunction of shotgun NOS

✓x7th **W33.12 Accidental malfunction of hunting rifle**

Malfunction of hunting rifle NOS

✓x7th **W33.13 Accidental malfunction of machine gun**

Malfunction of machine gun NOS

√x7th **W33.19 Accidental malfunction of other larger firearm**
Malfunction of other larger firearm NOS

√4th **W34 Accidental discharge and malfunction from other and unspecified firearms and guns**

√5th **W34.0 Accidental discharge from other and unspecified firearms and guns**

√x7th **W34.00 Accidental discharge from unspecified firearms or gun**
Discharge from firearm NOS
Gunshot wound NOS
Shot NOS

√6th **W34.01 Accidental discharge of gas, air or spring-operated guns**

√7th **W34.010 Accidental discharge of airgun**
Accidental discharge of BB gun
Accidental discharge of pellet gun

√7th **W34.011 Accidental discharge of paintball gun**
Accidental injury due to paintball discharge

√7th **W34.018 Accidental discharge of other gas, air or spring-operated gun**

√x7th **W34.09 Accidental discharge from other specified firearms**
Accidental discharge from Very pistol [flare]

√5th **W34.1 Accidental malfunction from other and unspecified firearms and guns**

√x7th **W34.10 Accidental malfunction from unspecified firearms or gun**
Firearm malfunction NOS

√6th **W34.11 Accidental malfunction of gas, air or spring-operated guns**

√7th **W34.110 Accidental malfunction of airgun**
Accidental malfunction of BB gun
Accidental malfunction of pellet gun

√7th **W34.111 Accidental malfunction of paintball gun**
Accidental injury due to paintball gun malfunction

√7th **W34.118 Accidental malfunction of other gas, air or spring-operated gun**

√x7th **W34.19 Accidental malfunction from other specified firearms**
Accidental malfunction from Very pistol [flare]

√x7th **W35 Explosion and rupture of boiler**
EXCLUDES 1 *explosion and rupture of boiler on watercraft (V93.4)*

√4th **W36 Explosion and rupture of gas cylinder**

√x7th **W36.1 Explosion and rupture of aerosol can**

√x7th **W36.2 Explosion and rupture of air tank**

√x7th **W36.3 Explosion and rupture of pressurized-gas tank**

√x7th **W36.8 Explosion and rupture of other gas cylinder**

√x7th **W36.9 Explosion and rupture of unspecified gas cylinder**

√4th **W37 Explosion and rupture of pressurized tire, pipe or hose**

√x7th **W37.0 Explosion of bicycle tire**

√x7th **W37.8 Explosion and rupture of other pressurized tire, pipe or hose**

√x7th **W38 Explosion and rupture of other specified pressurized devices**

√x7th **W39 Discharge of firework**

√4th **W40 Explosion of other materials**
EXCLUDES 1 *assault by explosive material (X96)*
explosion involving legal intervention (Y35.1-)
explosion involving military or war operations (Y36.0-, Y36.2-)
intentional self-harm by explosive material (X75)

√x7th **W40.0 Explosion of blasting material**
Explosion of blasting cap
Explosion of detonator
Explosion of dynamite
Explosion of explosive (any) used in blasting operations

√x7th **W40.1 Explosion of explosive gases**
Explosion of acetylene
Explosion of butane
Explosion of coal gas
Explosion in mine NOS
Explosion of explosive gas
Explosion of fire damp
Explosion of gasoline fumes
Explosion of methane
Explosion of propane

√x7th **W40.8 Explosion of other specified explosive materials**
Explosion in dump NOS
Explosion in factory NOS
Explosion in grain store
Explosion in munitions
EXCLUDES 1 *explosion involving legal intervention (Y35.1-)*
explosion involving military or war operations (Y36.0-, Y36.2-)

√x7th **W40.9 Explosion of unspecified explosive materials**
Explosion NOS

√4th **W42 Exposure to noise**

√x7th **W42.0 Exposure to supersonic waves**

√x7th **W42.9 Exposure to other noise**
Exposure to sound waves NOS

√4th **W45 Foreign body or object entering through skin**
INCLUDES foreign body or object embedded in skin
nail embedded in skin
EXCLUDES 2 *contact with hand tools (nonpowered) (powered) (W27-W29)*
contact with other sharp objects (W26.-)
contact with sharp glass (W25.-)
struck by objects (W20-W22)

√x7th **W45.0 Nail entering through skin**

√x7th **W45.8 Other foreign body or object entering through skin**
Splinter in skin NOS

√4th **W46 Contact with hypodermic needle**

√x7th **W46.0 Contact with hypodermic needle**
Hypodermic needle stick NOS

√x7th **W46.1 Contact with contaminated hypodermic needle**

√4th **W49 Exposure to other inanimate mechanical forces**
INCLUDES exposure to abnormal gravitational [G] forces
exposure to inanimate mechanical forces NEC
EXCLUDES 1 *exposure to inanimate mechanical forces involving military or war operations (Y36.-, Y37.-)*

√5th **W49.0 Item causing external constriction**

√x7th **W49.01 Hair causing external constriction**

√x7th **W49.02 String or thread causing external constriction**

√x7th **W49.03 Rubber band causing external constriction**

√x7th **W49.04 Ring or other jewelry causing external constriction**

√x7th **W49.09 Other specified item causing external constriction**

√x7th **W49.9 Exposure to other inanimate mechanical forces**

Exposure to animate mechanical forces (W50-W64)

EXCLUDES 1 *toxic effect of contact with venomous animals and plants (T63.-)*

The appropriate 7th character is to be added to each code from categories W50-W64.
A initial encounter
D subsequent encounter
S sequela

√4th **W50 Accidental hit, strike, kick, twist, bite or scratch by another person**
INCLUDES hit, strike, kick, twist, bite, or scratch by another person NOS
EXCLUDES 1 *assault by bodily force (Y04)*
struck by objects (W20-W22)

√x7th **W50.0 Accidental hit or strike by another person**
Hit or strike by another person NOS

√x7th **W50.1 Accidental kick by another person**
Kick by another person NOS

√x7th **W50.2 Accidental twist by another person**
Twist by another person NOS

W5Ø.3 Accidental bite by another person
Human bite
Bite by another person NOS

W5Ø.4 Accidental scratch by another person
Scratch by another person NOS

W51 Accidental striking against or bumped into by another person
EXCLUDES 1 *assault by striking against or bumping into by another person (YØ4.2)*
fall due to collision with another person (WØ3)

W52 Crushed, pushed or stepped on by crowd or human stampede
Crushed, pushed or stepped on by crowd or human stampede with or without fall

W53 Contact with rodent
INCLUDES contact with saliva, feces or urine of rodent

W53.Ø Contact with mouse
W53.Ø1 Bitten by mouse
W53.Ø9 Other contact with mouse

W53.1 Contact with rat
W53.11 Bitten by rat
W53.19 Other contact with rat

W53.2 Contact with squirrel
W53.21 Bitten by squirrel
W53.29 Other contact with squirrel

W53.8 Contact with other rodent
W53.81 Bitten by other rodent
W53.89 Other contact with other rodent

W54 Contact with dog
INCLUDES contact with saliva, feces or urine of dog

W54.Ø Bitten by dog
W54.1 Struck by dog
Knocked over by dog
W54.8 Other contact with dog

W55 Contact with other mammals
INCLUDES contact with saliva, feces or urine of mammal
EXCLUDES 1 *animal being ridden - see transport accidents*
bitten or struck by dog (W54)
bitten or struck by rodent (W53.-)
contact with marine mammals (W56.-)

W55.Ø Contact with cat
W55.Ø1 Bitten by cat
W55.Ø3 Scratched by cat
W55.Ø9 Other contact with cat

W55.1 Contact with horse
W55.11 Bitten by horse
W55.12 Struck by horse
W55.19 Other contact with horse

W55.2 Contact with cow
Contact with bull
W55.21 Bitten by cow
W55.22 Struck by cow
Gored by bull
W55.29 Other contact with cow

W55.3 Contact with other hoof stock
Contact with goats
Contact with sheep
W55.31 Bitten by other hoof stock
W55.32 Struck by other hoof stock
Gored by goat
Gored by ram
W55.39 Other contact with other hoof stock

W55.4 Contact with pig
W55.41 Bitten by pig
W55.42 Struck by pig
W55.49 Other contact with pig

W55.5 Contact with raccoon
W55.51 Bitten by raccoon
W55.52 Struck by raccoon
W55.59 Other contact with raccoon

W55.8 Contact with other mammals
W55.81 Bitten by other mammals
W55.82 Struck by other mammals
W55.89 Other contact with other mammals

W56 Contact with nonvenomous marine animal
EXCLUDES 1 *contact with venomous marine animal (T63.-)*

W56.Ø Contact with dolphin
W56.Ø1 Bitten by dolphin
W56.Ø2 Struck by dolphin
W56.Ø9 Other contact with dolphin

W56.1 Contact with sea lion
W56.11 Bitten by sea lion
W56.12 Struck by sea lion
W56.19 Other contact with sea lion

W56.2 Contact with orca
Contact with killer whale
W56.21 Bitten by orca
W56.22 Struck by orca
W56.29 Other contact with orca

W56.3 Contact with other marine mammals
W56.31 Bitten by other marine mammals
W56.32 Struck by other marine mammals
W56.39 Other contact with other marine mammals

W56.4 Contact with shark
W56.41 Bitten by shark
W56.42 Struck by shark
W56.49 Other contact with shark

W56.5 Contact with other fish
W56.51 Bitten by other fish
W56.52 Struck by other fish
W56.59 Other contact with other fish

W56.8 Contact with other nonvenomous marine animals
W56.81 Bitten by other nonvenomous marine animals
W56.82 Struck by other nonvenomous marine animals
W56.89 Other contact with other nonvenomous marine animals

W57 Bitten or stung by nonvenomous insect and other nonvenomous arthropods
EXCLUDES 1 *contact with venomous insects and arthropods (T63.2-, T63.3-, T63.4-)*

W58 Contact with crocodile or alligator

W58.Ø Contact with alligator
W58.Ø1 Bitten by alligator
W58.Ø2 Struck by alligator
W58.Ø3 Crushed by alligator
W58.Ø9 Other contact with alligator

W58.1 Contact with crocodile
W58.11 Bitten by crocodile
W58.12 Struck by crocodile
W58.13 Crushed by crocodile
W58.19 Other contact with crocodile

W59 Contact with other nonvenomous reptiles
EXCLUDES 1 *contact with venomous reptile (T63.Ø-, T63.1-)*

W59.Ø Contact with nonvenomous lizards
W59.Ø1 Bitten by nonvenomous lizards
W59.Ø2 Struck by nonvenomous lizards
W59.Ø9 Other contact with nonvenomous lizards
Exposure to nonvenomous lizards

W59.1 Contact with nonvenomous snakes
W59.11 Bitten by nonvenomous snake
W59.12 Struck by nonvenomous snake
W59.13 Crushed by nonvenomous snake
W59.19 Other contact with nonvenomous snake

✓5th **W59.2 Contact with turtles**
EXCLUDES 1 *contact with tortoises (W59.8-)*
✓x7th **W59.21 Bitten by turtle**
✓x7th **W59.22 Struck by turtle**
✓x7th **W59.29 Other contact with turtle**
Exposure to turtles
✓5th **W59.8 Contact with other nonvenomous reptiles**
✓x7th **W59.81 Bitten by other nonvenomous reptiles**
✓x7th **W59.82 Struck by other nonvenomous reptiles**
✓x7th **W59.83 Crushed by other nonvenomous reptiles**
✓x7th **W59.89 Other contact with other nonvenomous reptiles**

✓x7th **W60 Contact with nonvenomous plant thorns and spines and sharp leaves**
EXCLUDES 1 *contact with venomous plants (T63.7-)*

✓4th **W61 Contact with birds (domestic) (wild)**
INCLUDES contact with excreta of birds
✓5th **W61.0 Contact with parrot**
✓x7th **W61.01 Bitten by parrot**
✓x7th **W61.02 Struck by parrot**
✓x7th **W61.09 Other contact with parrot**
Exposure to parrots
✓5th **W61.1 Contact with macaw**
✓x7th **W61.11 Bitten by macaw**
✓x7th **W61.12 Struck by macaw**
✓x7th **W61.19 Other contact with macaw**
Exposure to macaws
✓5th **W61.2 Contact with other psittacines**
✓x7th **W61.21 Bitten by other psittacines**
✓x7th **W61.22 Struck by other psittacines**
✓x7th **W61.29 Other contact with other psittacines**
Exposure to other psittacines
✓5th **W61.3 Contact with chicken**
✓x7th **W61.32 Struck by chicken**
✓x7th **W61.33 Pecked by chicken**
✓x7th **W61.39 Other contact with chicken**
Exposure to chickens
✓5th **W61.4 Contact with turkey**
✓x7th **W61.42 Struck by turkey**
✓x7th **W61.43 Pecked by turkey**
✓x7th **W61.49 Other contact with turkey**
✓5th **W61.5 Contact with goose**
✓x7th **W61.51 Bitten by goose**
✓x7th **W61.52 Struck by goose**
✓x7th **W61.59 Other contact with goose**
✓5th **W61.6 Contact with duck**
✓x7th **W61.61 Bitten by duck**
✓x7th **W61.62 Struck by duck**
✓x7th **W61.69 Other contact with duck**
✓5th **W61.9 Contact with other birds**
✓x7th **W61.91 Bitten by other birds**
✓x7th **W61.92 Struck by other birds**
✓x7th **W61.99 Other contact with other birds**
Contact with bird NOS

✓4th **W62 Contact with nonvenomous amphibians**
EXCLUDES 1 *contact with venomous amphibians (T63.81-R63.83)*
✓x7th **W62.0 Contact with nonvenomous frogs**
✓x7th **W62.1 Contact with nonvenomous toads**
✓x7th **W62.9 Contact with other nonvenomous amphibians**

✓x7th **W64 Exposure to other animate mechanical forces**
INCLUDES exposure to nonvenomous animal NOS
EXCLUDES 1 *contact with venomous animal (T63.-)*

Accidental non-transport drowning and submersion (W65-W74)

EXCLUDES 1 *accidental drowning and submersion due to fall into water (W16.-)*
accidental drowning and submersion due to water transport accident (V90.-, V92.-)
EXCLUDES 2 *accidental drowning and submersion due to cataclysm (X34-X39)*

The appropriate 7th character is to be added to each code from categories W65-W74.
A initial encounter
D subsequent encounter
S sequela

✓x7th **W65 Accidental drowning and submersion while in bath-tub**
EXCLUDES 1 *accidental drowning and submersion due to fall in (into) bathtub (W16.211)*

✓x7th **W67 Accidental drowning and submersion while in swimming-pool**
EXCLUDES 1 *accidental drowning and submersion due to fall into swimming pool (W16.011, W16.021, W16.031)*
accidental drowning and submersion due to striking into wall of swimming pool (W22.041)

✓x7th **W69 Accidental drowning and submersion while in natural water**
Accidental drowning and submersion while in lake
Accidental drowning and submersion while in open sea
Accidental drowning and submersion while in river
Accidental drowning and submersion while in stream
EXCLUDES 1 *accidental drowning and submersion due to fall into natural body of water (W16.111, W16.121, W16.131)*

✓x7th **W73 Other specified cause of accidental non-transport drowning and submersion**
Accidental drowning and submersion while in quenching tank
Accidental drowning and submersion while in reservoir
EXCLUDES 1 *accidental drowning and submersion due to fall into other water (W16.311, W16.321, W16.331)*

✓x7th **W74 Unspecified cause of accidental drowning and submersion**
Drowning NOS

Exposure to electric current, radiation and extreme ambient air temperature and pressure (W85-W99)

EXCLUDES 1 *exposure to:*
failure in dosage of radiation or temperature during surgical and medical care (Y63.2-Y63.5)
lightning (T75.0-)
natural cold (X31)
natural heat (X30)
natural radiation NOS (X39)
radiological procedure and radiotherapy (Y84.2)
sunlight (X32)

AHA: 2018,2Q,7-8

The appropriate 7th character is to be added to each code from categories W85-W99.
A initial encounter
D subsequent encounter
S sequela

✓x7th **W85 Exposure to electric transmission lines**
Broken power line

✓4th **W86 Exposure to other specified electric current**
✓x7th **W86.0 Exposure to domestic wiring and appliances**
✓x7th **W86.1 Exposure to industrial wiring, appliances and electrical machinery**
Exposure to conductors
Exposure to control apparatus
Exposure to electrical equipment and machinery
Exposure to transformers
✓x7th **W86.8 Exposure to other electric current**
Exposure to wiring and appliances in or on farm (not farmhouse)
Exposure to wiring and appliances outdoors
Exposure to wiring and appliances in or on public building
Exposure to wiring and appliances in or on residential institutions
Exposure to wiring and appliances in or on schools

✓4th **W88 Exposure to ionizing radiation**
EXCLUDES 1 *exposure to sunlight (X32)*
✓x7th **W88.0 Exposure to X-rays**
✓x7th **W88.1 Exposure to radioactive isotopes**

W88.8 Exposure to other ionizing radiation

W89 Exposure to man-made visible and ultraviolet light

INCLUDES exposure to welding light (arc)

EXCLUDES 2 *exposure to sunlight (X32)*

W89.0 Exposure to welding light (arc)

W89.1 Exposure to tanning bed

W89.8 Exposure to other man-made visible and ultraviolet light

W89.9 Exposure to unspecified man-made visible and ultraviolet light

W90 Exposure to other nonionizing radiation

EXCLUDES 2 *exposure to sunlight (X32)*

AHA: 2019,1Q,21

W90.0 Exposure to radiofrequency

W90.1 Exposure to infrared radiation

W90.2 Exposure to laser radiation

W90.8 Exposure to other nonionizing radiation

W92 Exposure to excessive heat of man-made origin

W93 Exposure to excessive cold of man-made origin

W93.0 Contact with or inhalation of dry ice

W93.01 Contact with dry ice

W93.02 Inhalation of dry ice

W93.1 Contact with or inhalation of liquid air

W93.11 Contact with liquid air

Contact with liquid hydrogen
Contact with liquid nitrogen

W93.12 Inhalation of liquid air

Inhalation of liquid hydrogen
Inhalation of liquid nitrogen

W93.2 Prolonged exposure in deep freeze unit or refrigerator

W93.8 Exposure to other excessive cold of man-made origin

W94 Exposure to high and low air pressure and changes in air pressure

W94.0 Exposure to prolonged high air pressure

W94.1 Exposure to prolonged low air pressure

W94.11 Exposure to residence or prolonged visit at high altitude

W94.12 Exposure to other prolonged low air pressure

W94.2 Exposure to rapid changes in air pressure during ascent

W94.21 Exposure to reduction in atmospheric pressure while surfacing from deep-water diving

W94.22 Exposure to reduction in atmospheric pressure while surfacing from underground

W94.23 Exposure to sudden change in air pressure in aircraft during ascent

W94.29 Exposure to other rapid changes in air pressure during ascent

W94.3 Exposure to rapid changes in air pressure during descent

W94.31 Exposure to sudden change in air pressure in aircraft during descent

W94.32 Exposure to high air pressure from rapid descent in water

W94.39 Exposure to other rapid changes in air pressure during descent

W99 Exposure to other man-made environmental factors

Exposure to smoke, fire and flames (X00-X08)

EXCLUDES 1 *arson (X97)*

EXCLUDES 2 *explosions (W35-W40)*
lightning (T75.0-)
transport accident (V01-V99)

AHA: 2018,2Q,7-8

The appropriate 7th character is to be added to each code from categories X00-X08.
A initial encounter
D subsequent encounter
S sequela

X00 Exposure to uncontrolled fire in building or structure

INCLUDES conflagration in building or structure

Code first any associated cataclysm

EXCLUDES 2 *exposure to ignition or melting of nightwear (X05)*
exposure to ignition or melting of other clothing and apparel (X06.-)
exposure to other specified smoke, fire and flames (X08.-)

AHA: 2016,2Q,5

X00.0 Exposure to flames in uncontrolled fire in building or structure

X00.1 Exposure to smoke in uncontrolled fire in building or structure

X00.2 Injury due to collapse of burning building or structure in uncontrolled fire

EXCLUDES 1 *injury due to collapse of building not on fire (W20.1)*

X00.3 Fall from burning building or structure in uncontrolled fire

X00.4 Hit by object from burning building or structure in uncontrolled fire

AHA: 2016,2Q,4

X00.5 Jump from burning building or structure in uncontrolled fire

X00.8 Other exposure to uncontrolled fire in building or structure

X01 Exposure to uncontrolled fire, not in building or structure

INCLUDES exposure to forest fire

X01.0 Exposure to flames in uncontrolled fire, not in building or structure

X01.1 Exposure to smoke in uncontrolled fire, not in building or structure

X01.3 Fall due to uncontrolled fire, not in building or structure

X01.4 Hit by object due to uncontrolled fire, not in building or structure

X01.8 Other exposure to uncontrolled fire, not in building or structure

X02 Exposure to controlled fire in building or structure

INCLUDES exposure to fire in fireplace
exposure to fire in stove

X02.0 Exposure to flames in controlled fire in building or structure

X02.1 Exposure to smoke in controlled fire in building or structure

X02.2 Injury due to collapse of burning building or structure in controlled fire

EXCLUDES 1 *Injury due to collapse of building not on fire (W20.1)*

X02.3 Fall from burning building or structure in controlled fire

X02.4 Hit by object from burning building or structure in controlled fire

X02.5 Jump from burning building or structure in controlled fire

X02.8 Other exposure to controlled fire in building or structure

X03 Exposure to controlled fire, not in building or structure

INCLUDES exposure to bon fire
exposure to camp-fire
exposure to trash fire

X03.0 Exposure to flames in controlled fire, not in building or structure

X03.1 Exposure to smoke in controlled fire, not in building or structure

X03.3 Fall due to controlled fire, not in building or structure

X03.4 Hit by object due to controlled fire, not in building or structure

X03.8 Other exposure to controlled fire, not in building or structure

√7th **X04 Exposure to ignition of highly flammable material**
Exposure to ignition of gasoline
Exposure to ignition of kerosene
Exposure to ignition of petrol
EXCLUDES 2 *exposure to ignition or melting of nightwear (X05)*
exposure to ignition or melting of other clothing and apparel (X06)
AHA: 2016,2Q,4

√7th **X05 Exposure to ignition or melting of nightwear**
EXCLUDES 2 *exposure to uncontrolled fire in building or structure (X00.-)*
exposure to uncontrolled fire, not in building or structure (X01.-)
exposure to controlled fire in building or structure (X02.-)
exposure to controlled fire, not in building or structure (X03.-)
exposure to ignition of highly flammable materials (X04.-)

√4th **X06 Exposure to ignition or melting of other clothing and apparel**
EXCLUDES 2 *exposure to uncontrolled fire in building or structure (X00.-)*
exposure to uncontrolled fire, not in building or structure (X01.-)
exposure to controlled fire in building or structure (X02.-)
exposure to controlled fire, not in building or structure (X03.-)
exposure to ignition of highly flammable materials (X04.-)

√7th **X06.0 Exposure to ignition of plastic jewelry**
√7th **X06.1 Exposure to melting of plastic jewelry**
√7th **X06.2 Exposure to ignition of other clothing and apparel**
√7th **X06.3 Exposure to melting of other clothing and apparel**

√4th **X08 Exposure to other specified smoke, fire and flames**
√5th **X08.0 Exposure to bed fire**
Exposure to mattress fire
√7th **X08.00 Exposure to bed fire due to unspecified burning material**
√7th **X08.01 Exposure to bed fire due to burning cigarette**
√7th **X08.09 Exposure to bed fire due to other burning material**
√5th **X08.1 Exposure to sofa fire**
√7th **X08.10 Exposure to sofa fire due to unspecified burning material**
√7th **X08.11 Exposure to sofa fire due to burning cigarette**
√7th **X08.19 Exposure to sofa fire due to other burning material**
√5th **X08.2 Exposure to other furniture fire**
√7th **X08.20 Exposure to other furniture fire due to unspecified burning material**
√7th **X08.21 Exposure to other furniture fire due to burning cigarette**
√7th **X08.29 Exposure to other furniture fire due to other burning material**
√7th **X08.8 Exposure to other specified smoke, fire and flames**

Contact with heat and hot substances (X10-X19)

EXCLUDES 1 *exposure to excessive natural heat (X30)*
exposure to fire and flames (X00-X08)
AHA: 2018,2Q,7-8

The appropriate 7th character is to be added to each code from categories X10-X19.
A initial encounter
D subsequent encounter
S sequela

√4th **X10 Contact with hot drinks, food, fats and cooking oils**
√7th **X10.0 Contact with hot drinks**
√7th **X10.1 Contact with hot food**
√7th **X10.2 Contact with fats and cooking oils**

√4th **X11 Contact with hot tap-water**
INCLUDES contact with boiling tap-water
contact with boiling water NOS
EXCLUDES 1 *contact with water heated on stove (X12)*
√7th **X11.0 Contact with hot water in bath or tub**
EXCLUDES 1 *contact with running hot water in bath or tub (X11.1)*
√7th **X11.1 Contact with running hot water**
Contact with hot water running out of hose
Contact with hot water running out of tap
√7th **X11.8 Contact with other hot tap-water**
Contact with hot water in bucket
Contact with hot tap-water NOS

√7th **X12 Contact with other hot fluids**
Contact with water heated on stove
EXCLUDES 1 *hot (liquid) metals (X18)*

√4th **X13 Contact with steam and other hot vapors**
√7th **X13.0 Inhalation of steam and other hot vapors**
√7th **X13.1 Other contact with steam and other hot vapors**

√4th **X14 Contact with hot air and other hot gases**
√7th **X14.0 Inhalation of hot air and gases**
√7th **X14.1 Other contact with hot air and other hot gases**

√4th **X15 Contact with hot household appliances**
EXCLUDES 1 *contact with heating appliances (X16)*
contact with powered household appliances (W29.-)
exposure to controlled fire in building or structure due to household appliance (X02.8)
exposure to household appliances electrical current (W86.0)
√7th **X15.0 Contact with hot stove (kitchen)**
√7th **X15.1 Contact with hot toaster**
√7th **X15.2 Contact with hotplate**
√7th **X15.3 Contact with hot saucepan or skillet**
▶Contact with hot cooking pan◀
▶Contact with hot cooking pot◀
√7th **X15.8 Contact with other hot household appliances**
Contact with cooker
Contact with kettle
Contact with light bulbs

√7th **X16 Contact with hot heating appliances, radiators and pipes**
EXCLUDES 1 *contact with powered appliances (W29.-)*
exposure to controlled fire in building or structure due to appliance (X02.8)
exposure to industrial appliances electrical current (W86.1)

√7th **X17 Contact with hot engines, machinery and tools**
EXCLUDES 1 *contact with hot heating appliances, radiators and pipes (X16)*
contact with hot household appliances (X15)

√7th **X18 Contact with other hot metals**
Contact with liquid metal

√7th **X19 Contact with other heat and hot substances**
EXCLUDES 1 *objects that are not normally hot, e.g., an object made hot by a house fire (X00-X08)*

Exposure to forces of nature (X30-X39)

AHA: 2018,2Q,7-8

The appropriate 7th character is to be added to each code from categories X30-X39.
A initial encounter
D subsequent encounter
S sequela

√7th **X30 Exposure to excessive natural heat**
Exposure to excessive heat as the cause of sunstroke
Exposure to heat NOS
EXCLUDES 1 *excessive heat of man-made origin (W92)*
exposure to man-made radiation (W89)
exposure to sunlight (X32)
exposure to tanning bed (W89)

√7th **X31 Exposure to excessive natural cold**
Excessive cold as the cause of chilblains NOS
Excessive cold as the cause of immersion foot or hand
Exposure to cold NOS
Exposure to weather conditions
EXCLUDES 1 *cold of man-made origin (W93.-)*
contact with or inhalation of dry ice (W93.-)
contact with or inhalation of liquefied gas (W93.-)

√7th **X32 Exposure to sunlight**
EXCLUDES 1 *man-made radiation (tanning bed) (W89)*
EXCLUDES 2 *radiation-related disorders of the skin and subcutaneous tissue (L55-L59)*

X34 Earthquake

EXCLUDES 2 *tidal wave (tsunami) due to earthquake (X37.41)*

X35 Volcanic eruption

EXCLUDES 2 *tidal wave (tsunami) due to volcanic eruption (X37.41)*

X36 Avalanche, landslide and other earth movements

INCLUDES victim of mudslide of cataclysmic nature

EXCLUDES 1 *earthquake (X34)*

EXCLUDES 2 *transport accident involving collision with avalanche or landslide not in motion (V01-V99)*

X36.0 Collapse of dam or man-made structure causing earth movement

X36.1 Avalanche, landslide, or mudslide

X37 Cataclysmic storm

X37.0 Hurricane

Storm surge
Typhoon

X37.1 Tornado

Cyclone
Twister

X37.2 Blizzard (snow)(ice)

X37.3 Dust storm

X37.4 Tidalwave

X37.41 Tidal wave due to earthquake or volcanic eruption

Tidal wave NOS
Tsunami

X37.42 Tidal wave due to storm

X37.43 Tidal wave due to landslide

X37.8 Other cataclysmic storms

Cloudburst
Torrential rain

EXCLUDES 2 *flood (X38)*

X37.9 Unspecified cataclysmic storm

Storm NOS

EXCLUDES 1 *collapse of dam or man-made structure causing earth movement (X36.0)*

X38 Flood

Flood arising from remote storm
Flood of cataclysmic nature arising from melting snow
Flood resulting directly from storm

EXCLUDES 1 *collapse of dam or man-made structure causing earth movement (X36.0)*
tidal wave NOS (X37.41)
tidal wave caused by storm (X37.42)

X39 Exposure to other forces of nature

X39.0 Exposure to natural radiation

EXCLUDES 1 *contact with and (suspected) exposure to radon and other naturally occurring radiation (Z77.123)*
exposure to man-made radiation (W88-W90)
exposure to sunlight (X32)

X39.01 Exposure to radon

X39.08 Exposure to other natural radiation

X39.8 Other exposure to forces of nature

Overexertion and strenuous or repetitive movements (X50)

X50 Overexertion and strenuous or repetitive movements

AHA: 2018,2Q,7-8; 2016,4Q,73-74

The appropriate 7th character is to be added to each code from category X50.
A initial encounter
D subsequent encounter
S sequela

X50.0 Overexertion from strenuous movement or load

Lifting heavy objects
Lifting weights

X50.1 Overexertion from prolonged static or awkward postures

Prolonged bending
Prolonged kneeling
Prolonged reaching
Prolonged sitting
Prolonged standing
Prolonged twisting
Static bending
Static kneeling
Static reaching
Static sitting
Static standing
Static twisting

X50.3 Overexertion from repetitive movements

Use of hand as hammer

EXCLUDES 2 *overuse from prolonged static or awkward postures (X50.1)*

X50.9 Other and unspecified overexertion or strenuous movements or postures

Contact pressure
Contact stress

Accidental exposure to other specified factors (X52-X58)

AHA: 2018,2Q,7-8

The appropriate 7th character is to be added to each code from categories X52-X58.
A initial encounter
D subsequent encounter
S sequela

X52 Prolonged stay in weightless environment

Weightlessness in spacecraft (simulator)

X58 Exposure to other specified factors

Accident NOS
Exposure NOS

Intentional self-harm (X71-X83)

Purposely self-inflicted injury
Suicide (attempted)

The appropriate 7th character is to be added to each code from categories X71-X83.
A initial encounter
D subsequent encounter
S sequela

X71 Intentional self-harm by drowning and submersion

X71.0 Intentional self-harm by drowning and submersion while in bathtub HCC Rx ESR COM

X71.1 Intentional self-harm by drowning and submersion while in swimming pool HCC Rx ESR COM

X71.2 Intentional self-harm by drowning and submersion after jump into swimming pool HCC Rx ESR COM

X71.3 Intentional self-harm by drowning and submersion in natural water HCC Rx ESR COM

X71.8 Other intentional self-harm by drowning and submersion HCC Rx ESR COM

X71.9 Intentional self-harm by drowning and submersion, unspecified HCC Rx ESR COM

X72 Intentional self-harm by handgun discharge HCC Rx ESR COM

Intentional self-harm by gun for single hand use
Intentional self-harm by pistol
Intentional self-harm by revolver

EXCLUDES 1 *Very pistol (X74.8)*

X73 Intentional self-harm by rifle, shotgun and larger firearm discharge

EXCLUDES 1 *airgun (X74.01)*

X73.0 Intentional self-harm by shotgun discharge HCC Rx ESR COM

X73.1 Intentional self-harm by hunting rifle discharge HCC Rx ESR COM

X73.2 Intentional self-harm by machine gun discharge HCC Rx ESR COM

X73.8 Intentional self-harm by other larger firearm discharge HCC Rx ESR COM

X73.9 Intentional self-harm by unspecified larger firearm discharge HCC Rx ESR COM

X74 Intentional self-harm by other and unspecified firearm and gun discharge

X74.0 Intentional self-harm by gas, air or spring-operated guns

X74.01 Intentional self-harm by airgun HCC Rx ESR COM
Intentional self-harm by BB gun discharge
Intentional self-harm by pellet gun discharge

X74.02 Intentional self-harm by paintball gun HCC Rx ESR COM

X74.09 Intentional self-harm by other gas, air or spring-operated gun HCC Rx ESR COM

X74.8 Intentional self-harm by other firearm discharge HCC Rx ESR COM
Intentional self-harm by Very pistol [flare] discharge

X74.9 Intentional self-harm by unspecified firearm discharge HCC Rx ESR COM

X75 Intentional self-harm by explosive material HCC Rx ESR COM

X76 Intentional self-harm by smoke, fire and flames HCC Rx ESR COM

X77 Intentional self-harm by steam, hot vapors and hot objects

X77.0 Intentional self-harm by steam or hot vapors HCC Rx ESR COM

X77.1 Intentional self-harm by hot tap water HCC Rx ESR COM

X77.2 Intentional self-harm by other hot fluids HCC Rx ESR COM

X77.3 Intentional self-harm by hot household appliances HCC Rx ESR COM

X77.8 Intentional self-harm by other hot objects HCC Rx ESR COM

X77.9 Intentional self-harm by unspecified hot objects HCC Rx ESR COM

X78 Intentional self-harm by sharp object

X78.0 Intentional self-harm by sharp glass HCC Rx ESR COM

X78.1 Intentional self-harm by knife HCC Rx ESR COM

X78.2 Intentional self-harm by sword or dagger HCC Rx ESR COM

X78.8 Intentional self-harm by other sharp object HCC Rx ESR COM
AHA: 2022,1Q,27

X78.9 Intentional self-harm by unspecified sharp object HCC Rx ESR COM

X79 Intentional self-harm by blunt object HCC Rx ESR COM

X80 Intentional self-harm by jumping from a high place HCC Rx ESR COM
Intentional fall from one level to another

X81 Intentional self-harm by jumping or lying in front of moving object

X81.0 Intentional self-harm by jumping or lying in front of motor vehicle HCC Rx ESR COM

X81.1 Intentional self-harm by jumping or lying in front of (subway) train HCC Rx ESR COM

X81.8 Intentional self-harm by jumping or lying in front of other moving object HCC Rx ESR COM

X82 Intentional self-harm by crashing of motor vehicle

X82.0 Intentional collision of motor vehicle with other motor vehicle HCC Rx ESR COM

X82.1 Intentional collision of motor vehicle with train HCC Rx ESR COM

X82.2 Intentional collision of motor vehicle with tree HCC Rx ESR COM

X82.8 Other intentional self-harm by crashing of motor vehicle HCC Rx ESR COM

X83 Intentional self-harm by other specified means
EXCLUDES 1 *intentional self-harm by poisoning or contact with toxic substance - see Table of Drugs and Chemicals*

X83.0 Intentional self-harm by crashing of aircraft HCC Rx ESR COM

X83.1 Intentional self-harm by electrocution HCC Rx ESR COM

X83.2 Intentional self-harm by exposure to extremes of cold HCC Rx ESR COM

X83.8 Intentional self-harm by other specified means HCC Rx ESR COM

Assault (X92-Y09)

INCLUDES homicide
injuries inflicted by another person with intent to injure or kill, by any means

EXCLUDES 1 *injuries due to legal intervention (Y35.-)*
injuries due to operations of war (Y36.-)
injuries due to terrorism (Y38.-)

The appropriate 7th character is to be added to each code from categories X92-Y04 and Y08.
A initial encounter
D subsequent encounter
S sequela

X92 Assault by drowning and submersion

X92.0 Assault by drowning and submersion while in bathtub

X92.1 Assault by drowning and submersion while in swimming pool

X92.2 Assault by drowning and submersion after push into swimming pool

X92.3 Assault by drowning and submersion in natural water

X92.8 Other assault by drowning and submersion

X92.9 Assault by drowning and submersion, unspecified

X93 Assault by handgun discharge
Assault by discharge of gun for single hand use
Assault by discharge of pistol
Assault by discharge of revolver
EXCLUDES 1 *Very pistol (X95.8)*

X94 Assault by rifle, shotgun and larger firearm discharge
EXCLUDES 1 *airgun (X95.01)*

X94.0 Assault by shotgun

X94.1 Assault by hunting rifle

X94.2 Assault by machine gun

X94.8 Assault by other larger firearm discharge

X94.9 Assault by unspecified larger firearm discharge

X95 Assault by other and unspecified firearm and gun discharge

X95.0 Assault by gas, air or spring-operated guns

X95.01 Assault by airgun discharge
Assault by BB gun discharge
Assault by pellet gun discharge

X95.02 Assault by paintball gun discharge

X95.09 Assault by other gas, air or spring-operated gun

X95.8 Assault by other firearm discharge
Assault by Very pistol [flare] discharge

X95.9 Assault by unspecified firearm discharge

X96 Assault by explosive material
EXCLUDES 1 *incendiary device (X97)*
terrorism involving explosive material (Y38.2-)

X96.0 Assault by antipersonnel bomb
EXCLUDES 1 *antipersonnel bomb use in military or war (Y36.2-)*

X96.1 Assault by gasoline bomb

X96.2 Assault by letter bomb

X96.3 Assault by fertilizer bomb

X96.4 Assault by pipe bomb

X96.8 Assault by other specified explosive

X96.9 Assault by unspecified explosive

X97 Assault by smoke, fire and flames
Assault by arson
Assault by cigarettes
Assault by incendiary device

X98 Assault by steam, hot vapors and hot objects

X98.0 Assault by steam or hot vapors

X98.1 Assault by hot tap water

X98.2 Assault by hot fluids

X98.3 Assault by hot household appliances

X98.8 Assault by other hot objects

X98.9 Assault by unspecified hot objects

X99 Assault by sharp object

EXCLUDES 1 *assault by strike by sports equipment (Y08.0-)*

X99.0 Assault by sharp glass

X99.1 Assault by knife

X99.2 Assault by sword or dagger

X99.8 Assault by other sharp object

X99.9 Assault by unspecified sharp object

Assault by stabbing NOS

Y00 Assault by blunt object

EXCLUDES 1 *assault by strike by sports equipment (Y08.0-)*

Y01 Assault by pushing from high place

Y02 Assault by pushing or placing victim in front of moving object

Y02.0 Assault by pushing or placing victim in front of motor vehicle

Y02.1 Assault by pushing or placing victim in front of (subway) train

Y02.8 Assault by pushing or placing victim in front of other moving object

Y03 Assault by crashing of motor vehicle

Y03.0 Assault by being hit or run over by motor vehicle

Y03.8 Other assault by crashing of motor vehicle

Y04 Assault by bodily force

EXCLUDES 1 *assault by:*
submersion (X92.-)
use of weapon (X93-X95, X99, Y00)

Y04.0 Assault by unarmed brawl or fight

Y04.1 Assault by human bite

Y04.2 Assault by strike against or bumped into by another person

Y04.8 Assault by other bodily force

Assault by bodily force NOS

Y07 Perpetrator of assault, maltreatment and neglect

NOTE Codes from this category are for use only in cases of confirmed abuse (T74.-)

Selection of the correct perpetrator code is based on the relationship between the perpetrator and the victim

INCLUDES perpetrator of abandonment
perpetrator of emotional neglect
perpetrator of mental cruelty
perpetrator of physical abuse
perpetrator of physical neglect
perpetrator of sexual abuse
perpetrator of torture

Y07.0 Spouse or partner, perpetrator of maltreatment and neglect

Spouse or partner, perpetrator of maltreatment and neglect against spouse or partner

Y07.01 Husband, perpetrator of maltreatment and neglect

Y07.02 Wife, perpetrator of maltreatment and neglect

Y07.03 Male partner, perpetrator of maltreatment and neglect

Y07.04 Female partner, perpetrator of maltreatment and neglect

Y07.1 Parent (adoptive) (biological), perpetrator of maltreatment and neglect

Y07.11 Biological father, perpetrator of maltreatment and neglect

Y07.12 Biological mother, perpetrator of maltreatment and neglect

Y07.13 Adoptive father, perpetrator of maltreatment and neglect

Y07.14 Adoptive mother, perpetrator of maltreatment and neglect

Y07.4 Other family member, perpetrator of maltreatment and neglect

Y07.41 Sibling, perpetrator of maltreatment and neglect

EXCLUDES 1 *stepsibling, perpetrator of maltreatment and neglect (Y07.435, Y07.436)*

Y07.410 Brother, perpetrator of maltreatment and neglect

Y07.411 Sister, perpetrator of maltreatment and neglect

Y07.42 Foster parent, perpetrator of maltreatment and neglect

Y07.420 Foster father, perpetrator of maltreatment and neglect

Y07.421 Foster mother, perpetrator of maltreatment and neglect

Y07.43 Stepparent or stepsibling, perpetrator of maltreatment and neglect

Y07.430 Stepfather, perpetrator of maltreatment and neglect

Y07.432 Male friend of parent (co-residing in household), perpetrator of maltreatment and neglect

Y07.433 Stepmother, perpetrator of maltreatment and neglect

Y07.434 Female friend of parent (co-residing in household), perpetrator of maltreatment and neglect

Y07.435 Stepbrother, perpetrator or maltreatment and neglect

Y07.436 Stepsister, perpetrator of maltreatment and neglect

Y07.49 Other family member, perpetrator of maltreatment and neglect

Y07.490 Male cousin, perpetrator of maltreatment and neglect

Y07.491 Female cousin, perpetrator of maltreatment and neglect

Y07.499 Other family member, perpetrator of maltreatment and neglect

Y07.5 Non-family member, perpetrator of maltreatment and neglect

Y07.50 Unspecified non-family member, perpetrator of maltreatment and neglect

Y07.51 Daycare provider, perpetrator of maltreatment and neglect

Y07.510 At-home childcare provider, perpetrator of maltreatment and neglect

Y07.511 Daycare center childcare provider, perpetrator of maltreatment and neglect

Y07.512 At-home adultcare provider, perpetrator of maltreatment and neglect

Y07.513 Adultcare center provider, perpetrator of maltreatment and neglect

Y07.519 Unspecified daycare provider, perpetrator of maltreatment and neglect

Y07.52 Healthcare provider, perpetrator of maltreatment and neglect

Y07.521 Mental health provider, perpetrator of maltreatment and neglect

Y07.528 Other therapist or healthcare provider, perpetrator of maltreatment and neglect

Nurse perpetrator of maltreatment and neglect

Occupational therapist perpetrator of maltreatment and neglect

Physical therapist perpetrator of maltreatment and neglect

Speech therapist perpetrator of maltreatment and neglect

Y07.529 Unspecified healthcare provider, perpetrator of maltreatment and neglect

Y07.53 Teacher or instructor, perpetrator of maltreatment and neglect

Coach, perpetrator of maltreatment and neglect

Y07.59 Other non-family member, perpetrator of maltreatment and neglect

Y07.6 Multiple perpetrators of maltreatment and neglect

AHA: 2018,4Q,32

Y07.9 Unspecified perpetrator of maltreatment and neglect

Y08 Assault by other specified means

Y08.0 Assault by strike by sport equipment

Y08.01 Assault by strike by hockey stick

Y08.02 Assault by strike by baseball bat

Y08.09 Assault by strike by other specified type of sport equipment

Y08.8 Assault by other specified means

Y08.81 Assault by crashing of aircraft

Y08.89 Assault by other specified means

Chapter 20. External Causes of Morbidity

X99–Y08.89

Y09 Assault by unspecified means

Assassination (attempted) NOS
Homicide (attempted) NOS
Manslaughter (attempted) NOS
Murder (attempted) NOS

Event of undetermined intent (Y21-Y33)

Undetermined intent is only for use when there is specific documentation in the record that the intent of the injury cannot be determined. If no such documentation is present, code to accidental (unintentional).

The appropriate 7th character is to be added to each code from categories Y21-Y33.
A initial encounter
D subsequent encounter
S sequela

Y21 Drowning and submersion, undetermined intent

- **Y21.0 Drowning and submersion while in bathtub, undetermined intent**
- **Y21.1 Drowning and submersion after fall into bathtub, undetermined intent**
- **Y21.2 Drowning and submersion while in swimming pool, undetermined intent**
- **Y21.3 Drowning and submersion after fall into swimming pool, undetermined intent**
- **Y21.4 Drowning and submersion in natural water, undetermined intent**
- **Y21.8 Other drowning and submersion, undetermined intent**
- **Y21.9 Unspecified drowning and submersion, undetermined intent**

Y22 Handgun discharge, undetermined intent

Discharge of gun for single hand use, undetermined intent
Discharge of pistol, undetermined intent
Discharge of revolver, undetermined intent
EXCLUDES 2 *Very pistol (Y24.8)*

Y23 Rifle, shotgun and larger firearm discharge, undetermined intent

EXCLUDES 2 *airgun (Y24.0)*

- **Y23.0 Shotgun discharge, undetermined intent**
- **Y23.1 Hunting rifle discharge, undetermined intent**
- **Y23.2 Military firearm discharge, undetermined intent**
- **Y23.3 Machine gun discharge, undetermined intent**
- **Y23.8 Other larger firearm discharge, undetermined intent**
- **Y23.9 Unspecified larger firearm discharge, undetermined intent**

Y24 Other and unspecified firearm discharge, undetermined intent

- **Y24.0 Airgun discharge, undetermined intent**
  BB gun discharge, undetermined intent
  Pellet gun discharge, undetermined intent
- **Y24.8 Other firearm discharge, undetermined intent**
  Paintball gun discharge, undetermined intent
  Very pistol [flare] discharge, undetermined intent
- **Y24.9 Unspecified firearm discharge, undetermined intent**

Y25 Contact with explosive material, undetermined intent

Y26 Exposure to smoke, fire and flames, undetermined intent

Y27 Contact with steam, hot vapors and hot objects, undetermined intent

- **Y27.0 Contact with steam and hot vapors, undetermined intent**
- **Y27.1 Contact with hot tap water, undetermined intent**
- **Y27.2 Contact with hot fluids, undetermined intent**
- **Y27.3 Contact with hot household appliance, undetermined intent**
- **Y27.8 Contact with other hot objects, undetermined intent**
- **Y27.9 Contact with unspecified hot objects, undetermined intent**

Y28 Contact with sharp object, undetermined intent

- **Y28.0 Contact with sharp glass, undetermined intent**
- **Y28.1 Contact with knife, undetermined intent**
- **Y28.2 Contact with sword or dagger, undetermined intent**
- **Y28.8 Contact with other sharp object, undetermined intent**
- **Y28.9 Contact with unspecified sharp object, undetermined intent**

Y29 Contact with blunt object, undetermined intent

Y30 Falling, jumping or pushed from a high place, undetermined intent

Victim falling from one level to another, undetermined intent

Y31 Falling, lying or running before or into moving object, undetermined intent

Y32 Crashing of motor vehicle, undetermined intent

Y33 Other specified events, undetermined intent

Legal intervention, operations of war, military operations, and terrorism (Y35-Y38)

The appropriate 7th character is to be added to each code from categories Y35-Y38.
A initial encounter
D subsequent encounter
S sequela

Y35 Legal intervention

INCLUDES any injury sustained as a result of an encounter with any law enforcement official, serving in any capacity at the time of the encounter, whether on-duty or off-duty. Includes injury to law enforcement official, suspect and bystander

AHA: 2019,4Q,18-19

Y35.0 Legal intervention involving firearm discharge

- **Y35.00 Legal intervention involving unspecified firearm discharge**
  Legal intervention involving gunshot wound
  Legal intervention involving shot NOS
  - **Y35.001 Legal intervention involving unspecified firearm discharge, law enforcement official injured**
  - **Y35.002 Legal intervention involving unspecified firearm discharge, bystander injured**
  - **Y35.003 Legal intervention involving unspecified firearm discharge, suspect injured**
  - **Y35.009 Legal intervention involving unspecified firearm discharge, unspecified person injured**
- **Y35.01 Legal intervention involving injury by machine gun**
  - **Y35.011 Legal intervention involving injury by machine gun, law enforcement official injured**
  - **Y35.012 Legal intervention involving injury by machine gun, bystander injured**
  - **Y35.013 Legal intervention involving injury by machine gun, suspect injured**
  - **Y35.019 Legal intervention involving injury by machine gun, unspecified person injured**
- **Y35.02 Legal intervention involving injury by handgun**
  - **Y35.021 Legal intervention involving injury by handgun, law enforcement official injured**
  - **Y35.022 Legal intervention involving injury by handgun, bystander injured**
  - **Y35.023 Legal intervention involving injury by handgun, suspect injured**
  - **Y35.029 Legal intervention involving injury by handgun, unspecified person injured**
- **Y35.03 Legal intervention involving injury by rifle pellet**
  - **Y35.031 Legal intervention involving injury by rifle pellet, law enforcement official injured**
  - **Y35.032 Legal intervention involving injury by rifle pellet, bystander injured**
  - **Y35.033 Legal intervention involving injury by rifle pellet, suspect injured**
  - **Y35.039 Legal intervention involving injury by rifle pellet, unspecified person injured**
- **Y35.04 Legal intervention involving injury by rubber bullet**
  - **Y35.041 Legal intervention involving injury by rubber bullet, law enforcement official injured**
  - **Y35.042 Legal intervention involving injury by rubber bullet, bystander injured**
  - **Y35.043 Legal intervention involving injury by rubber bullet, suspect injured**
  - **Y35.049 Legal intervention involving injury by rubber bullet, unspecified person injured**
- **Y35.09 Legal intervention involving other firearm discharge**
  - **Y35.091 Legal intervention involving other firearm discharge, law enforcement official injured**

Y35.092 Legal intervention involving other firearm discharge, bystander injured

Y35.093 Legal intervention involving other firearm discharge, suspect injured

Y35.099 Legal intervention involving other firearm discharge, unspecified person injured

Y35.1 Legal intervention involving explosives

Y35.10 Legal intervention involving unspecified explosives

Y35.101 Legal intervention involving unspecified explosives, law enforcement official injured

Y35.102 Legal intervention involving unspecified explosives, bystander injured

Y35.103 Legal intervention involving unspecified explosives, suspect injured

Y35.109 Legal intervention involving unspecified explosives, unspecified person injured

Y35.11 Legal intervention involving injury by dynamite

Y35.111 Legal intervention involving injury by dynamite, law enforcement official injured

Y35.112 Legal intervention involving injury by dynamite, bystander injured

Y35.113 Legal intervention involving injury by dynamite, suspect injured

Y35.119 Legal intervention involving injury by dynamite, unspecified person injured

Y35.12 Legal intervention involving injury by explosive shell

Y35.121 Legal intervention involving injury by explosive shell, law enforcement official injured

Y35.122 Legal intervention involving injury by explosive shell, bystander injured

Y35.123 Legal intervention involving injury by explosive shell, suspect injured

Y35.129 Legal intervention involving injury by explosive shell, unspecified person injured

Y35.19 Legal intervention involving other explosives

Legal intervention involving injury by grenade

Legal intervention involving injury by mortar bomb

Y35.191 Legal intervention involving other explosives, law enforcement official injured

Y35.192 Legal intervention involving other explosives, bystander injured

Y35.193 Legal intervention involving other explosives, suspect injured

Y35.199 Legal intervention involving other explosives, unspecified person injured

Y35.2 Legal intervention involving gas

Legal intervention involving asphyxiation by gas

Legal intervention involving poisoning by gas

Y35.20 Legal intervention involving unspecified gas

Y35.201 Legal intervention involving unspecified gas, law enforcement official injured

Y35.202 Legal intervention involving unspecified gas, bystander injured

Y35.203 Legal intervention involving unspecified gas, suspect injured

Y35.209 Legal intervention involving unspecified gas, unspecified person injured

Y35.21 Legal intervention involving injury by tear gas

Y35.211 Legal intervention involving injury by tear gas, law enforcement official injured

Y35.212 Legal intervention involving injury by tear gas, bystander injured

Y35.213 Legal intervention involving injury by tear gas, suspect injured

Y35.219 Legal intervention involving injury by tear gas, unspecified person injured

Y35.29 Legal intervention involving other gas

Y35.291 Legal intervention involving other gas, law enforcement official injured

Y35.292 Legal intervention involving other gas, bystander injured

Y35.293 Legal intervention involving other gas, suspect injured

Y35.299 Legal intervention involving other gas, unspecified person injured

Y35.3 Legal intervention involving blunt objects

Legal intervention involving being hit or struck by blunt object

Y35.30 Legal intervention involving unspecified blunt objects

Y35.301 Legal intervention involving unspecified blunt objects, law enforcement official injured

Y35.302 Legal intervention involving unspecified blunt objects, bystander injured

Y35.303 Legal intervention involving unspecified blunt objects, suspect injured

Y35.309 Legal intervention involving unspecified blunt objects, unspecified person injured

Y35.31 Legal intervention involving baton

Y35.311 Legal intervention involving baton, law enforcement official injured

Y35.312 Legal intervention involving baton, bystander injured

Y35.313 Legal intervention involving baton, suspect injured

Y35.319 Legal intervention involving baton, unspecified person injured

Y35.39 Legal intervention involving other blunt objects

Y35.391 Legal intervention involving other blunt objects, law enforcement official injured

Y35.392 Legal intervention involving other blunt objects, bystander injured

Y35.393 Legal intervention involving other blunt objects, suspect injured

Y35.399 Legal intervention involving other blunt objects, unspecified person injured

Y35.4 Legal intervention involving sharp objects

Legal intervention involving being cut by sharp objects

Legal intervention involving being stabbed by sharp objects

Y35.40 Legal intervention involving unspecified sharp objects

Y35.401 Legal intervention involving unspecified sharp objects, law enforcement official injured

Y35.402 Legal intervention involving unspecified sharp objects, bystander injured

Y35.403 Legal intervention involving unspecified sharp objects, suspect injured

Y35.409 Legal intervention involving unspecified sharp objects, unspecified person injured

Y35.41 Legal intervention involving bayonet

Y35.411 Legal intervention involving bayonet, law enforcement official injured

Y35.412 Legal intervention involving bayonet, bystander injured

Y35.413 Legal intervention involving bayonet, suspect injured

Y35.419 Legal intervention involving bayonet, unspecified person injured

Y35.49 Legal intervention involving other sharp objects

Y35.491 Legal intervention involving other sharp objects, law enforcement official injured

Y35.492 Legal intervention involving other sharp objects, bystander injured

Y35.493 Legal intervention involving other sharp objects, suspect injured

Y35.499 Legal intervention involving other sharp objects, unspecified person injured

Y35.8 Legal intervention involving other specified means

AHA: 2019,4Q,19

Y35.81 Legal intervention involving manhandling

Y35.811 Legal intervention involving manhandling, law enforcement official injured

Y35.812 Legal intervention involving manhandling, bystander injured

Y35.813 Legal intervention involving manhandling, suspect injured

Y35.819 Legal intervention involving manhandling, unspecified person injured

√6th Y35.83 **Legal intervention involving a conducted energy device**
Electroshock device (taser)
Stun gun
√7th Y35.831 **Legal intervention involving a conducted energy device, law enforcement official injured**
√7th Y35.832 **Legal intervention involving a conducted energy device, bystander injured**
√7th Y35.833 **Legal intervention involving a conducted energy device, suspect injured**
√7th Y35.839 **Legal intervention involving a conducted energy device, unspecified person injured**
√6th Y35.89 **Legal intervention involving other specified means**
√7th Y35.891 **Legal intervention involving other specified means, law enforcement official injured**
√7th Y35.892 **Legal intervention involving other specified means, bystander injured**
√7th Y35.893 **Legal intervention involving other specified means, suspect injured**
AHA: 2018,1Q,5
√7th Y35.899 **Legal intervention involving other specified means, unspecified person injured**
√5th Y35.9 **Legal intervention, means unspecified**
√x7th Y35.91 **Legal intervention, means unspecified, law enforcement official injured**
√x7th Y35.92 **Legal intervention, means unspecified, bystander injured**
√x7th Y35.93 **Legal intervention, means unspecified, suspect injured**
√x7th Y35.99 **Legal intervention, means unspecified, unspecified person injured**

√4th **Y36 Operations of war**
INCLUDES injuries to military personnel and civilians caused by war, civil insurrection, and peacekeeping missions
EXCLUDES 1 *injury to military personnel occurring during peacetime military operations (Y37.-)*
military vehicles involved in transport accidents with non-military vehicle during peacetime ►(V09.01, V09.21, V19.81, V29.818, V39.81, V49.81, V59.81, V69.81, V79.81)◄
AHA: 2014,3Q,4
√5th Y36.0 **War operations involving explosion of marine weapons**
√6th Y36.00 **War operations involving explosion of unspecified marine weapon**
War operations involving underwater blast NOS
√7th Y36.000 **War operations involving explosion of unspecified marine weapon, military personnel**
√7th Y36.001 **War operations involving explosion of unspecified marine weapon, civilian**
√6th Y36.01 **War operations involving explosion of depth-charge**
√7th Y36.010 **War operations involving explosion of depth-charge, military personnel**
√7th Y36.011 **War operations involving explosion of depth-charge, civilian**
√6th Y36.02 **War operations involving explosion of marine mine**
War operations involving explosion of marine mine, at sea or in harbor
√7th Y36.020 **War operations involving explosion of marine mine, military personnel**
√7th Y36.021 **War operations involving explosion of marine mine, civilian**
√6th Y36.03 **War operations involving explosion of sea-based artillery shell**
√7th Y36.030 **War operations involving explosion of sea-based artillery shell, military personnel**
√7th Y36.031 **War operations involving explosion of sea-based artillery shell, civilian**
√6th Y36.04 **War operations involving explosion of torpedo**
√7th Y36.040 **War operations involving explosion of torpedo, military personnel**
√7th Y36.041 **War operations involving explosion of torpedo, civilian**
√6th Y36.05 **War operations involving accidental detonation of onboard marine weapons**
√7th Y36.050 **War operations involving accidental detonation of onboard marine weapons, military personnel**
√7th Y36.051 **War operations involving accidental detonation of onboard marine weapons, civilian**
√6th Y36.09 **War operations involving explosion of other marine weapons**
√7th Y36.090 **War operations involving explosion of other marine weapons, military personnel**
√7th Y36.091 **War operations involving explosion of other marine weapons, civilian**
√5th Y36.1 **War operations involving destruction of aircraft**
√6th Y36.10 **War operations involving unspecified destruction of aircraft**
√7th Y36.100 **War operations involving unspecified destruction of aircraft, military personnel**
√7th Y36.101 **War operations involving unspecified destruction of aircraft, civilian**
√6th Y36.11 **War operations involving destruction of aircraft due to enemy fire or explosives**
War operations involving destruction of aircraft due to air to air missile
War operations involving destruction of aircraft due to explosive placed on aircraft
War operations involving destruction of aircraft due to rocket propelled grenade [RPG]
War operations involving destruction of aircraft due to small arms fire
War operations involving destruction of aircraft due to surface to air missile
√7th Y36.110 **War operations involving destruction of aircraft due to enemy fire or explosives, military personnel**
√7th Y36.111 **War operations involving destruction of aircraft due to enemy fire or explosives, civilian**
√6th Y36.12 **War operations involving destruction of aircraft due to collision with other aircraft**
√7th Y36.120 **War operations involving destruction of aircraft due to collision with other aircraft, military personnel**
√7th Y36.121 **War operations involving destruction of aircraft due to collision with other aircraft, civilian**
√6th Y36.13 **War operations involving destruction of aircraft due to onboard fire**
√7th Y36.130 **War operations involving destruction of aircraft due to onboard fire, military personnel**
√7th Y36.131 **War operations involving destruction of aircraft due to onboard fire, civilian**
√6th Y36.14 **War operations involving destruction of aircraft due to accidental detonation of onboard munitions and explosives**
√7th Y36.140 **War operations involving destruction of aircraft due to accidental detonation of onboard munitions and explosives, military personnel**
√7th Y36.141 **War operations involving destruction of aircraft due to accidental detonation of onboard munitions and explosives, civilian**
√6th Y36.19 **War operations involving other destruction of aircraft**
√7th Y36.190 **War operations involving other destruction of aircraft, military personnel**
√7th Y36.191 **War operations involving other destruction of aircraft, civilian**

✓5th **Y36.2 War operations involving other explosions and fragments**

EXCLUDES 1 *war operations involving explosion of aircraft (Y36.1-)*
war operations involving explosion of marine weapons (Y36.Ø-)
war operations involving explosion of nuclear weapons (Y36.5-)
war operations involving explosion occurring after cessation of hostilities (Y36.8-)

✓6th **Y36.2Ø War operations involving unspecified explosion and fragments**
War operations involving air blast NOS
War operations involving blast NOS
War operations involving blast fragments NOS
War operations involving blast wave NOS
War operations involving blast wind NOS
War operations involving explosion NOS
War operations involving explosion of bomb NOS

✓7th **Y36.2ØØ War operations involving unspecified explosion and fragments, military personnel**

✓7th **Y36.2Ø1 War operations involving unspecified explosion and fragments, civilian**

✓6th **Y36.21 War operations involving explosion of aerial bomb**

✓7th **Y36.21Ø War operations involving explosion of aerial bomb, military personnel**

✓7th **Y36.211 War operations involving explosion of aerial bomb, civilian**

✓6th **Y36.22 War operations involving explosion of guided missile**

✓7th **Y36.22Ø War operations involving explosion of guided missile, military personnel**

✓7th **Y36.221 War operations involving explosion of guided missile, civilian**

✓6th **Y36.23 War operations involving explosion of improvised explosive device [IED]**
War operations involving explosion of person-borne improvised explosive device [IED]
War operations involving explosion of vehicle-borne improvised explosive device [IED]
War operations involving explosion of roadside improvised explosive device [IED]

✓7th **Y36.23Ø War operations involving explosion of improvised explosive device [IED], military personnel**

✓7th **Y36.231 War operations involving explosion of improvised explosive device [IED], civilian**

✓6th **Y36.24 War operations involving explosion due to accidental detonation and discharge of own munitions or munitions launch device**

✓7th **Y36.24Ø War operations involving explosion due to accidental detonation and discharge of own munitions or munitions launch device, military personnel**

✓7th **Y36.241 War operations involving explosion due to accidental detonation and discharge of own munitions or munitions launch device, civilian**

✓6th **Y36.25 War operations involving fragments from munitions**

✓7th **Y36.25Ø War operations involving fragments from munitions, military personnel**

✓7th **Y36.251 War operations involving fragments from munitions, civilian**

✓6th **Y36.26 War operations involving fragments of improvised explosive device [IED]**
War operations involving fragments of person-borne improvised explosive device [IED]
War operations involving fragments of vehicle-borne improvised explosive device [IED]
War operations involving fragments of roadside improvised explosive device [IED]

✓7th **Y36.26Ø War operations involving fragments of improvised explosive device [IED], military personnel**

✓7th **Y36.261 War operations involving fragments of improvised explosive device [IED], civilian**

✓6th **Y36.27 War operations involving fragments from weapons**

✓7th **Y36.27Ø War operations involving fragments from weapons, military personnel**

✓7th **Y36.271 War operations involving fragments from weapons, civilian**

✓6th **Y36.29 War operations involving other explosions and fragments**
War operations involving explosion of grenade
War operations involving explosions of land mine
War operations involving shrapnel NOS

✓7th **Y36.29Ø War operations involving other explosions and fragments, military personnel**

✓7th **Y36.291 War operations involving other explosions and fragments, civilian**

✓5th **Y36.3 War operations involving fires, conflagrations and hot substances**
War operations involving smoke, fumes, and heat from fires, conflagrations and hot substances

EXCLUDES 1 *war operations involving fires and conflagrations aboard military aircraft (Y36.1-)*
war operations involving fires and conflagrations aboard military watercraft (Y36.Ø-)
war operations involving fires and conflagrations caused indirectly by conventional weapons (Y36.2-)
war operations involving fires and thermal effects of nuclear weapons (Y36.53-)

✓6th **Y36.3Ø War operations involving unspecified fire, conflagration and hot substance**

✓7th **Y36.3ØØ War operations involving unspecified fire, conflagration and hot substance, military personnel**

✓7th **Y36.3Ø1 War operations involving unspecified fire, conflagration and hot substance, civilian**

✓6th **Y36.31 War operations involving gasoline bomb**
War operations involving incendiary bomb
War operations involving petrol bomb

✓7th **Y36.31Ø War operations involving gasoline bomb, military personnel**

✓7th **Y36.311 War operations involving gasoline bomb, civilian**

✓6th **Y36.32 War operations involving incendiary bullet**

✓7th **Y36.32Ø War operations involving incendiary bullet, military personnel**

✓7th **Y36.321 War operations involving incendiary bullet, civilian**

✓6th **Y36.33 War operations involving flamethrower**

✓7th **Y36.33Ø War operations involving flamethrower, military personnel**

✓7th **Y36.331 War operations involving flamethrower, civilian**

✓6th **Y36.39 War operations involving other fires, conflagrations and hot substances**

✓7th **Y36.39Ø War operations involving other fires, conflagrations and hot substances, military personnel**

✓7th **Y36.391 War operations involving other fires, conflagrations and hot substances, civilian**

✓5th **Y36.4 War operations involving firearm discharge and other forms of conventional warfare**

✓6th **Y36.41 War operations involving rubber bullets**

✓7th **Y36.41Ø War operations involving rubber bullets, military personnel**

✓7th **Y36.411 War operations involving rubber bullets, civilian**

✓6th **Y36.42 War operations involving firearms pellets**

✓7th **Y36.42Ø War operations involving firearms pellets, military personnel**

✓7th **Y36.421 War operations involving firearms pellets, civilian**

✓6th **Y36.43 War operations involving other firearms discharge**
War operations involving bullets NOS

EXCLUDES 1 *war operations involving munitions fragments (Y36.25-)*
war operations involving incendiary bullets (Y36.32-)

✓7th **Y36.43Ø War operations involving other firearms discharge, military personnel**

✓7th **Y36.431 War operations involving other firearms discharge, civilian**

Chapter 20. External Causes of Morbidity

Y36.44 War operations involving unarmed hand to hand combat

EXCLUDES 1 *war operations involving combat using blunt or piercing object (Y36.45-)*
war operations involving intentional restriction of air and airway (Y36.46-)
war operations involving unintentional restriction of air and airway (Y36.47-)

Y36.440 War operations involving unarmed hand to hand combat, military personnel

Y36.441 War operations involving unarmed hand to hand combat, civilian

Y36.45 War operations involving combat using blunt or piercing object

Y36.450 War operations involving combat using blunt or piercing object, military personnel

Y36.451 War operations involving combat using blunt or piercing object, civilian

Y36.46 War operations involving intentional restriction of air and airway

Y36.460 War operations involving intentional restriction of air and airway, military personnel

Y36.461 War operations involving intentional restriction of air and airway, civilian

Y36.47 War operations involving unintentional restriction of air and airway

Y36.470 War operations involving unintentional restriction of air and airway, military personnel

Y36.471 War operations involving unintentional restriction of air and airway, civilian

Y36.49 War operations involving other forms of conventional warfare

Y36.490 War operations involving other forms of conventional warfare, military personnel

Y36.491 War operations involving other forms of conventional warfare, civilian

Y36.5 War operations involving nuclear weapons

War operations involving dirty bomb NOS

Y36.50 War operations involving unspecified effect of nuclear weapon

Y36.500 War operations involving unspecified effect of nuclear weapon, military personnel

Y36.501 War operations involving unspecified effect of nuclear weapon, civilian

Y36.51 War operations involving direct blast effect of nuclear weapon

War operations involving blast pressure of nuclear weapon

Y36.510 War operations involving direct blast effect of nuclear weapon, military personnel

Y36.511 War operations involving direct blast effect of nuclear weapon, civilian

Y36.52 War operations involving indirect blast effect of nuclear weapon

War operations involving being thrown by blast of nuclear weapon

War operations involving being struck or crushed by blast debris of nuclear weapon

Y36.520 War operations involving indirect blast effect of nuclear weapon, military personnel

Y36.521 War operations involving indirect blast effect of nuclear weapon, civilian

Y36.53 War operations involving thermal radiation effect of nuclear weapon

War operations involving direct heat from nuclear weapon

War operation involving fireball effects from nuclear weapon

Y36.530 War operations involving thermal radiation effect of nuclear weapon, military personnel

Y36.531 War operations involving thermal radiation effect of nuclear weapon, civilian

Y36.54 War operation involving nuclear radiation effects of nuclear weapon

War operation involving acute radiation exposure from nuclear weapon

War operation involving exposure to immediate ionizing radiation from nuclear weapon

War operation involving fallout exposure from nuclear weapon

War operation involving secondary effects of nuclear weapons

Y36.540 War operation involving nuclear radiation effects of nuclear weapon, military personnel

Y36.541 War operation involving nuclear radiation effects of nuclear weapon, civilian

Y36.59 War operation involving other effects of nuclear weapons

Y36.590 War operation involving other effects of nuclear weapons, military personnel

Y36.591 War operation involving other effects of nuclear weapons, civilian

Y36.6 War operations involving biological weapons

Y36.6X War operations involving biological weapons

Y36.6X0 War operations involving biological weapons, military personnel

Y36.6X1 War operations involving biological weapons, civilian

Y36.7 War operations involving chemical weapons and other forms of unconventional warfare

EXCLUDES 1 *war operations involving incendiary devices (Y36.3-, Y36.5-)*

Y36.7X War operations involving chemical weapons and other forms of unconventional warfare

Y36.7X0 War operations involving chemical weapons and other forms of unconventional warfare, military personnel

Y36.7X1 War operations involving chemical weapons and other forms of unconventional warfare, civilian

Y36.8 War operations occurring after cessation of hostilities

War operations classifiable to categories Y36.0-Y36.8 but occurring after cessation of hostilities

Y36.81 Explosion of mine placed during war operations but exploding after cessation of hostilities

Y36.810 Explosion of mine placed during war operations but exploding after cessation of hostilities, military personnel

Y36.811 Explosion of mine placed during war operations but exploding after cessation of hostilities, civilian

Y36.82 Explosion of bomb placed during war operations but exploding after cessation of hostilities

Y36.820 Explosion of bomb placed during war operations but exploding after cessation of hostilities, military personnel

Y36.821 Explosion of bomb placed during war operations but exploding after cessation of hostilities, civilian

Y36.88 Other war operations occurring after cessation of hostilities

Y36.880 Other war operations occurring after cessation of hostilities, military personnel

Y36.881 Other war operations occurring after cessation of hostilities, civilian

Y36.89 Unspecified war operations occurring after cessation of hostilities

Y36.890 Unspecified war operations occurring after cessation of hostilities, military personnel

Y36.891 Unspecified war operations occurring after cessation of hostilities, civilian

Y36.9 Other and unspecified war operations

Y36.90 War operations, unspecified

Y36.91 War operations involving unspecified weapon of mass destruction [WMD]

Y36.92 War operations involving friendly fire

Y37 Military operations

INCLUDES injuries to military personnel and civilians occurring during peacetime on military property and during routine military exercises and operations

EXCLUDES 1 *military aircraft involved in aircraft accident with civilian aircraft (V97.81-)*
military vehicles involved in transport accident with civilian vehicle ▶(V09.01, V09.21, V19.81, V29.818, V39.81, V49.81, V59.81, V69.81, V79.81)◀
military watercraft involved in water transport accident with civilian watercraft (V94.81-)
war operations (Y36.-)

Y37.0 Military operations involving explosion of marine weapons

Y37.00 Military operations involving explosion of unspecified marine weapon
Military operations involving underwater blast NOS

Y37.000 Military operations involving explosion of unspecified marine weapon, military personnel

Y37.001 Military operations involving explosion of unspecified marine weapon, civilian

Y37.01 Military operations involving explosion of depth-charge

Y37.010 Military operations involving explosion of depth-charge, military personnel

Y37.011 Military operations involving explosion of depth-charge, civilian

Y37.02 Military operations involving explosion of marine mine
Military operations involving explosion of marine mine, at sea or in harbor

Y37.020 Military operations involving explosion of marine mine, military personnel

Y37.021 Military operations involving explosion of marine mine, civilian

Y37.03 Military operations involving explosion of sea-based artillery shell

Y37.030 Military operations involving explosion of sea-based artillery shell, military personnel

Y37.031 Military operations involving explosion of sea-based artillery shell, civilian

Y37.04 Military operations involving explosion of torpedo

Y37.040 Military operations involving explosion of torpedo, military personnel

Y37.041 Military operations involving explosion of torpedo, civilian

Y37.05 Military operations involving accidental detonation of onboard marine weapons

Y37.050 Military operations involving accidental detonation of onboard marine weapons, military personnel

Y37.051 Military operations involving accidental detonation of onboard marine weapons, civilian

Y37.09 Military operations involving explosion of other marine weapons

Y37.090 Military operations involving explosion of other marine weapons, military personnel

Y37.091 Military operations involving explosion of other marine weapons, civilian

Y37.1 Military operations involving destruction of aircraft

Y37.10 Military operations involving unspecified destruction of aircraft

Y37.100 Military operations involving unspecified destruction of aircraft, military personnel

Y37.101 Military operations involving unspecified destruction of aircraft, civilian

Y37.11 Military operations involving destruction of aircraft due to enemy fire or explosives
Military operations involving destruction of aircraft due to air to air missile
Military operations involving destruction of aircraft due to explosive placed on aircraft
Military operations involving destruction of aircraft due to rocket propelled grenade [RPG]
Military operations involving destruction of aircraft due to small arms fire
Military operations involving destruction of aircraft due to surface to air missile

Y37.110 Military operations involving destruction of aircraft due to enemy fire or explosives, military personnel

Y37.111 Military operations involving destruction of aircraft due to enemy fire or explosives, civilian

Y37.12 Military operations involving destruction of aircraft due to collision with other aircraft

Y37.120 Military operations involving destruction of aircraft due to collision with other aircraft, military personnel

Y37.121 Military operations involving destruction of aircraft due to collision with other aircraft, civilian

Y37.13 Military operations involving destruction of aircraft due to onboard fire

Y37.130 Military operations involving destruction of aircraft due to onboard fire, military personnel

Y37.131 Military operations involving destruction of aircraft due to onboard fire, civilian

Y37.14 Military operations involving destruction of aircraft due to accidental detonation of onboard munitions and explosives

Y37.140 Military operations involving destruction of aircraft due to accidental detonation of onboard munitions and explosives, military personnel

Y37.141 Military operations involving destruction of aircraft due to accidental detonation of onboard munitions and explosives, civilian

Y37.19 Military operations involving other destruction of aircraft

Y37.190 Military operations involving other destruction of aircraft, military personnel

Y37.191 Military operations involving other destruction of aircraft, civilian

Y37.2 Military operations involving other explosions and fragments

EXCLUDES 1 *military operations involving explosion of aircraft (Y37.1-)*
military operations involving explosion of marine weapons (Y37.0-)
military operations involving explosion of nuclear weapons (Y37.5-)

Y37.20 Military operations involving unspecified explosion and fragments
Military operations involving air blast NOS
Military operations involving blast NOS
Military operations involving blast fragments NOS
Military operations involving blast wave NOS
Military operations involving blast wind NOS
Military operations involving explosion NOS
Military operations involving explosion of bomb NOS

Y37.200 Military operations involving unspecified explosion and fragments, military personnel

Y37.201 Military operations involving unspecified explosion and fragments, civilian

Y37.21 Military operations involving explosion of aerial bomb

Y37.210 Military operations involving explosion of aerial bomb, military personnel

Y37.211 Military operations involving explosion of aerial bomb, civilian

Y37.22 Military operations involving explosion of guided missile

Y37.220 Military operations involving explosion of guided missile, military personnel

7th **Y37.221 Military operations involving explosion of guided missile, civilian**

6th **Y37.23 Military operations involving explosion of improvised explosive device [IED]**

Military operations involving explosion of person-borne improvised explosive device [IED]

Military operations involving explosion of vehicle-borne improvised explosive device [IED]

Military operations involving explosion of roadside improvised explosive device [IED]

7th **Y37.230 Military operations involving explosion of improvised explosive device [IED], military personnel**

7th **Y37.231 Military operations involving explosion of improvised explosive device [IED], civilian**

6th **Y37.24 Military operations involving explosion due to accidental detonation and discharge of own munitions or munitions launch device**

7th **Y37.240 Military operations involving explosion due to accidental detonation and discharge of own munitions or munitions launch device, military personnel**

7th **Y37.241 Military operations involving explosion due to accidental detonation and discharge of own munitions or munitions launch device, civilian**

6th **Y37.25 Military operations involving fragments from munitions**

7th **Y37.250 Military operations involving fragments from munitions, military personnel**

7th **Y37.251 Military operations involving fragments from munitions, civilian**

6th **Y37.26 Military operations involving fragments of improvised explosive device [IED]**

Military operations involving fragments of person-borne improvised explosive device [IED]

Military operations involving fragments of vehicle-borne improvised explosive device [IED]

Military operations involving fragments of roadside improvised explosive device [IED]

7th **Y37.260 Military operations involving fragments of improvised explosive device [IED], military personnel**

7th **Y37.261 Military operations involving fragments of improvised explosive device [IED], civilian**

6th **Y37.27 Military operations involving fragments from weapons**

7th **Y37.270 Military operations involving fragments from weapons, military personnel**

7th **Y37.271 Military operations involving fragments from weapons, civilian**

6th **Y37.29 Military operations involving other explosions and fragments**

Military operations involving explosion of grenade

Military operations involving explosions of land mine

Military operations involving shrapnel NOS

7th **Y37.290 Military operations involving other explosions and fragments, military personnel**

7th **Y37.291 Military operations involving other explosions and fragments, civilian**

5th **Y37.3 Military operations involving fires, conflagrations and hot substances**

Military operations involving smoke, fumes, and heat from fires, conflagrations and hot substances

EXCLUDES 1 *military operations involving fires and conflagrations aboard military aircraft (Y37.1-)*

military operations involving fires and conflagrations aboard military watercraft (Y37.0-)

military operations involving fires and conflagrations caused indirectly by conventional weapons (Y37.2-)

military operations involving fires and thermal effects of nuclear weapons (Y36.53-)

6th **Y37.30 Military operations involving unspecified fire, conflagration and hot substance**

7th **Y37.300 Military operations involving unspecified fire, conflagration and hot substance, military personnel**

7th **Y37.301 Military operations involving unspecified fire, conflagration and hot substance, civilian**

6th **Y37.31 Military operations involving gasoline bomb**

Military operations involving incendiary bomb

Military operations involving petrol bomb

7th **Y37.310 Military operations involving gasoline bomb, military personnel**

7th **Y37.311 Military operations involving gasoline bomb, civilian**

6th **Y37.32 Military operations involving incendiary bullet**

7th **Y37.320 Military operations involving incendiary bullet, military personnel**

7th **Y37.321 Military operations involving incendiary bullet, civilian**

6th **Y37.33 Military operations involving flamethrower**

7th **Y37.330 Military operations involving flamethrower, military personnel**

7th **Y37.331 Military operations involving flamethrower, civilian**

6th **Y37.39 Military operations involving other fires, conflagrations and hot substances**

7th **Y37.390 Military operations involving other fires, conflagrations and hot substances, military personnel**

7th **Y37.391 Military operations involving other fires, conflagrations and hot substances, civilian**

5th **Y37.4 Military operations involving firearm discharge and other forms of conventional warfare**

6th **Y37.41 Military operations involving rubber bullets**

7th **Y37.410 Military operations involving rubber bullets, military personnel**

7th **Y37.411 Military operations involving rubber bullets, civilian**

6th **Y37.42 Military operations involving firearms pellets**

7th **Y37.420 Military operations involving firearms pellets, military personnel**

7th **Y37.421 Military operations involving firearms pellets, civilian**

6th **Y37.43 Military operations involving other firearms discharge**

Military operations involving bullets NOS

EXCLUDES 1 *military operations involving munitions fragments (Y37.25-)*

military operations involving incendiary bullets (Y37.32-)

7th **Y37.430 Military operations involving other firearms discharge, military personnel**

7th **Y37.431 Military operations involving other firearms discharge, civilian**

6th **Y37.44 Military operations involving unarmed hand to hand combat**

EXCLUDES 1 *military operations involving combat using blunt or piercing object (Y37.45-)*

military operations involving intentional restriction of air and airway (Y37.46-)

military operations involving unintentional restriction of air and airway (Y37.47-)

7th **Y37.440 Military operations involving unarmed hand to hand combat, military personnel**

7th **Y37.441 Military operations involving unarmed hand to hand combat, civilian**

6th **Y37.45 Military operations involving combat using blunt or piercing object**

7th **Y37.450 Military operations involving combat using blunt or piercing object, military personnel**

7th **Y37.451 Military operations involving combat using blunt or piercing object, civilian**

6th **Y37.46 Military operations involving intentional restriction of air and airway**

7th **Y37.460 Military operations involving intentional restriction of air and airway, military personnel**

7th **Y37.461 Military operations involving intentional restriction of air and airway, civilian**

Y37.47 Military operations involving unintentional restriction of air and airway

Y37.470 Military operations involving unintentional restriction of air and airway, military personnel

Y37.471 Military operations involving unintentional restriction of air and airway, civilian

Y37.49 Military operations involving other forms of conventional warfare

Y37.490 Military operations involving other forms of conventional warfare, military personnel

Y37.491 Military operations involving other forms of conventional warfare, civilian

Y37.5 Military operations involving nuclear weapons

Military operation involving dirty bomb NOS

Y37.50 Military operations involving unspecified effect of nuclear weapon

Y37.500 Military operations involving unspecified effect of nuclear weapon, military personnel

Y37.501 Military operations involving unspecified effect of nuclear weapon, civilian

Y37.51 Military operations involving direct blast effect of nuclear weapon

Military operations involving blast pressure of nuclear weapon

Y37.510 Military operations involving direct blast effect of nuclear weapon, military personnel

Y37.511 Military operations involving direct blast effect of nuclear weapon, civilian

Y37.52 Military operations involving indirect blast effect of nuclear weapon

Military operations involving being thrown by blast of nuclear weapon

Military operations involving being struck or crushed by blast debris of nuclear weapon

Y37.520 Military operations involving indirect blast effect of nuclear weapon, military personnel

Y37.521 Military operations involving indirect blast effect of nuclear weapon, civilian

Y37.53 Military operations involving thermal radiation effect of nuclear weapon

Military operations involving direct heat from nuclear weapon

Military operation involving fireball effects from nuclear weapon

Y37.530 Military operations involving thermal radiation effect of nuclear weapon, military personnel

Y37.531 Military operations involving thermal radiation effect of nuclear weapon, civilian

Y37.54 Military operation involving nuclear radiation effects of nuclear weapon

Military operation involving acute radiation exposure from nuclear weapon

Military operation involving exposure to immediate ionizing radiation from nuclear weapon

Military operation involving fallout exposure from nuclear weapon

Military operation involving secondary effects of nuclear weapons

Y37.540 Military operation involving nuclear radiation effects of nuclear weapon, military personnel

Y37.541 Military operation involving nuclear radiation effects of nuclear weapon, civilian

Y37.59 Military operation involving other effects of nuclear weapons

Y37.590 Military operation involving other effects of nuclear weapons, military personnel

Y37.591 Military operation involving other effects of nuclear weapons, civilian

Y37.6 Military operations involving biological weapons

Y37.6X Military operations involving biological weapons

Y37.6X0 Military operations involving biological weapons, military personnel

Y37.6X1 Military operations involving biological weapons, civilian

Y37.7 Military operations involving chemical weapons and other forms of unconventional warfare

EXCLUDES 1 *military operations involving incendiary devices (Y36.3-, Y36.5-)*

Y37.7X Military operations involving chemical weapons and other forms of unconventional warfare

Y37.7X0 Military operations involving chemical weapons and other forms of unconventional warfare, military personnel

Y37.7X1 Military operations involving chemical weapons and other forms of unconventional warfare, civilian

Y37.9 Other and unspecified military operations

Y37.90 Military operations, unspecified

Y37.91 Military operations involving unspecified weapon of mass destruction [WMD]

Y37.92 Military operations involving friendly fire

Y38 Terrorism

NOTE These codes are for use to identify injuries resulting from the unlawful use of force or violence against persons or property to intimidate or coerce a Government, the civilian population, or any segment thereof, in furtherance of political or social objective

Use additional code for place of occurrence (Y92.-)

Y38.0 Terrorism involving explosion of marine weapons

Terrorism involving depth-charge

Terrorism involving marine mine

Terrorism involving mine NOS, at sea or in harbor

Terrorism involving sea-based artillery shell

Terrorism involving torpedo

Terrorism involving underwater blast

Y38.0X Terrorism involving explosion of marine weapons

Y38.0X1 Terrorism involving explosion of marine weapons, public safety official injured

Y38.0X2 Terrorism involving explosion of marine weapons, civilian injured

Y38.0X3 Terrorism involving explosion of marine weapons, terrorist injured

Y38.1 Terrorism involving destruction of aircraft

Terrorism involving aircraft burned

Terrorism involving aircraft exploded

Terrorism involving aircraft being shot down

Terrorism involving aircraft used as a weapon

Y38.1X Terrorism involving destruction of aircraft

Y38.1X1 Terrorism involving destruction of aircraft, public safety official injured

Y38.1X2 Terrorism involving destruction of aircraft, civilian injured

Y38.1X3 Terrorism involving destruction of aircraft, terrorist injured

Y38.2 Terrorism involving other explosions and fragments

Terrorism involving antipersonnel (fragments) bomb

Terrorism involving blast NOS

Terrorism involving explosion NOS

Terrorism involving explosion of breech block

Terrorism involving explosion of cannon block

Terrorism involving explosion (fragments) of artillery shell

Terrorism involving explosion (fragments) of bomb

Terrorism involving explosion (fragments) of grenade

Terrorism involving explosion (fragments) of guided missile

Terrorism involving explosion (fragments) of land mine

Terrorism involving explosion of mortar bomb

Terrorism involving explosion of munitions

Terrorism involving explosion (fragments) of rocket

Terrorism involving explosion (fragments) of shell

Terrorism involving shrapnel

Terrorism involving mine NOS, on land

EXCLUDES 1 *terrorism involving explosion of nuclear weapon (Y38.5)*

terrorism involving suicide bomber (Y38.81)

Y38.2X Terrorism involving other explosions and fragments

Y38.2X1 Terrorism involving other explosions and fragments, public safety official injured

7th **Y38.2X2 Terrorism involving other explosions and fragments, civilian injured**

7th **Y38.2X3 Terrorism involving other explosions and fragments, terrorist injured**

5th **Y38.3 Terrorism involving fires, conflagration and hot substances**

Terrorism involving conflagration NOS
Terrorism involving fire NOS
Terrorism involving petrol bomb

EXCLUDES 1 *terrorism involving fire or heat of nuclear weapon (Y38.5)*

6th **Y38.3X Terrorism involving fires, conflagration and hot substances**

7th **Y38.3X1 Terrorism involving fires, conflagration and hot substances, public safety official injured**

7th **Y38.3X2 Terrorism involving fires, conflagration and hot substances, civilian injured**

7th **Y38.3X3 Terrorism involving fires, conflagration and hot substances, terrorist injured**

5th **Y38.4 Terrorism involving firearms**

Terrorism involving carbine bullet
Terrorism involving machine gun bullet
Terrorism involving pellets (shotgun)
Terrorism involving pistol bullet
Terrorism involving rifle bullet
Terrorism involving rubber (rifle) bullet

6th **Y38.4X Terrorism involving firearms**

7th **Y38.4X1 Terrorism involving firearms, public safety official injured**

7th **Y38.4X2 Terrorism involving firearms, civilian injured**

7th **Y38.4X3 Terrorism involving firearms, terrorist injured**

5th **Y38.5 Terrorism involving nuclear weapons**

Terrorism involving blast effects of nuclear weapon
Terrorism involving exposure to ionizing radiation from nuclear weapon
Terrorism involving fireball effect of nuclear weapon
Terrorism involving heat from nuclear weapon

6th **Y38.5X Terrorism involving nuclear weapons**

7th **Y38.5X1 Terrorism involving nuclear weapons, public safety official injured**

7th **Y38.5X2 Terrorism involving nuclear weapons, civilian injured**

7th **Y38.5X3 Terrorism involving nuclear weapons, terrorist injured**

5th **Y38.6 Terrorism involving biological weapons**

Terrorism involving anthrax
Terrorism involving cholera
Terrorism involving smallpox

6th **Y38.6X Terrorism involving biological weapons**

7th **Y38.6X1 Terrorism involving biological weapons, public safety official injured**

7th **Y38.6X2 Terrorism involving biological weapons, civilian injured**

7th **Y38.6X3 Terrorism involving biological weapons, terrorist injured**

5th **Y38.7 Terrorism involving chemical weapons**

Terrorism involving gases, fumes, chemicals
Terrorism involving hydrogen cyanide
Terrorism involving phosgene
Terrorism involving sarin

6th **Y38.7X Terrorism involving chemical weapons**

7th **Y38.7X1 Terrorism involving chemical weapons, public safety official injured**

7th **Y38.7X2 Terrorism involving chemical weapons, civilian injured**

7th **Y38.7X3 Terrorism involving chemical weapons, terrorist injured**

5th **Y38.8 Terrorism involving other and unspecified means**

x7th **Y38.8Ø Terrorism involving unspecified means**

Terrorism NOS

6th **Y38.81 Terrorism involving suicide bomber**

7th **Y38.811 Terrorism involving suicide bomber, public safety official injured**

7th **Y38.812 Terrorism involving suicide bomber, civilian injured**

6th **Y38.89 Terrorism involving other means**

Terrorism involving drowning and submersion
Terrorism involving lasers
Terrorism involving piercing or stabbing instruments

7th **Y38.891 Terrorism involving other means, public safety official injured**

7th **Y38.892 Terrorism involving other means, civilian injured**

7th **Y38.893 Terrorism involving other means, terrorist injured**

5th **Y38.9 Terrorism, secondary effects**

NOTE This code is for use to identify conditions occurring subsequent to a terrorist attack not those that are due to the initial terrorist attack

6th **Y38.9X Terrorism, secondary effects**

7th **Y38.9X1 Terrorism, secondary effects, public safety official injured**

7th **Y38.9X2 Terrorism, secondary effects, civilian injured**

COMPLICATIONS OF MEDICAL AND SURGICAL CARE (Y62-Y84)

INCLUDES complications of medical devices
surgical and medical procedures as the cause of abnormal reaction of the patient, or of later complication, without mention of misadventure at the time of the procedure

Misadventures to patients during surgical and medical care (Y62-Y69)

EXCLUDES 1 *surgical and medical procedures as the cause of abnormal reaction of the patient, without mention of misadventure at the time of the procedure (Y83-Y84)*

EXCLUDES 2 *breakdown or malfunctioning of medical device (during procedure) (after implantation) (ongoing use) (Y7Ø-Y82)*

4th **Y62 Failure of sterile precautions during surgical and medical care**

Y62.Ø Failure of sterile precautions during surgical operation

Y62.1 Failure of sterile precautions during infusion or transfusion

Y62.2 Failure of sterile precautions during kidney dialysis and other perfusion HCC Rx ESR

Y62.3 Failure of sterile precautions during injection or immunization

Y62.4 Failure of sterile precautions during endoscopic examination

Y62.5 Failure of sterile precautions during heart catheterization

Y62.6 Failure of sterile precautions during aspiration, puncture and other catheterization

Y62.8 Failure of sterile precautions during other surgical and medical care

Y62.9 Failure of sterile precautions during unspecified surgical and medical care

4th **Y63 Failure in dosage during surgical and medical care**

EXCLUDES 2 *accidental overdose of drug or wrong drug given in error (T36-T5Ø)*

Y63.Ø Excessive amount of blood or other fluid given during transfusion or infusion

Y63.1 Incorrect dilution of fluid used during infusion

Y63.2 Overdose of radiation given during therapy

Y63.3 Inadvertent exposure of patient to radiation during medical care

Y63.4 Failure in dosage in electroshock or insulin-shock therapy

Y63.5 Inappropriate temperature in local application and packing

Y63.6 Underdosing and nonadministration of necessary drug, medicament or biological substance

AHA: 2018,4Q,72

Y63.8 Failure in dosage during other surgical and medical care

AHA: 2018,4Q,72

Y63.9 Failure in dosage during unspecified surgical and medical care

AHA: 2018,4Q,72

4th **Y64 Contaminated medical or biological substances**

Y64.Ø Contaminated medical or biological substance, transfused or infused

Y64.1 Contaminated medical or biological substance, injected or used for immunization

Y64.8 Contaminated medical or biological substance administered by other means

Y64.9 Contaminated medical or biological substance administered by unspecified means
Administered contaminated medical or biological substance NOS

Y65 Other misadventures during surgical and medical care
- **Y65.0 Mismatched blood in transfusion**
- **Y65.1 Wrong fluid used in infusion**
- **Y65.2 Failure in suture or ligature during surgical operation**
- **Y65.3 Endotracheal tube wrongly placed during anesthetic procedure**
- **Y65.4 Failure to introduce or to remove other tube or instrument**
- **Y65.5 Performance of wrong procedure (operation)**
  - **Y65.51 Performance of wrong procedure (operation) on correct patient**
    Wrong device implanted into correct surgical site
    EXCLUDES 1 *performance of correct procedure (operation) on wrong side or body part (Y65.53)*
  - **Y65.52 Performance of procedure (operation) on patient not scheduled for surgery**
    Performance of procedure (operation) intended for another patient
    Performance of procedure (operation) on wrong patient
  - **Y65.53 Performance of correct procedure (operation) on wrong side or body part**
    Performance of correct procedure (operation) on wrong side
    Performance of correct procedure (operation) on wrong site
- **Y65.8 Other specified misadventures during surgical and medical care**
  AHA: 2022,1Q,22; 2019,2Q,23-24

Y66 Nonadministration of surgical and medical care
Premature cessation of surgical and medical care
EXCLUDES 1 *DNR status (Z66)*
palliative care (Z51.5)

Y69 Unspecified misadventure during surgical and medical care

Medical devices associated with adverse incidents in diagnostic and therapeutic use (Y70-Y82)

INCLUDES breakdown or malfunction of medical devices (during use) (after implantation) (ongoing use)

EXCLUDES 2 *later complications following use of medical devices without breakdown or malfunctioning of device (Y83-Y84)*
misadventure to patients during surgical and medical care, classifiable to (Y62-Y69)
surgical and other medical procedures as the cause of abnormal reaction of the patient, or of later complication, without mention of misadventure at the time of the procedure (Y83-Y84)

Y70 Anesthesiology devices associated with adverse incidents
- **Y70.0 Diagnostic and monitoring anesthesiology devices associated with adverse incidents**
- **Y70.1 Therapeutic (nonsurgical) and rehabilitative anesthesiology devices associated with adverse incidents**
- **Y70.2 Prosthetic and other implants, materials and accessory anesthesiology devices associated with adverse incidents**
- **Y70.3 Surgical instruments, materials and anesthesiology devices (including sutures) associated with adverse incidents**
- **Y70.8 Miscellaneous anesthesiology devices associated with adverse incidents, not elsewhere classified**

Y71 Cardiovascular devices associated with adverse incidents
- **Y71.0 Diagnostic and monitoring cardiovascular devices associated with adverse incidents**
- **Y71.1 Therapeutic (nonsurgical) and rehabilitative cardiovascular devices associated with adverse incidents**
- **Y71.2 Prosthetic and other implants, materials and accessory cardiovascular devices associated with adverse incidents**
- **Y71.3 Surgical instruments, materials and cardiovascular devices (including sutures) associated with adverse incidents**
- **Y71.8 Miscellaneous cardiovascular devices associated with adverse incidents, not elsewhere classified**

Y72 Otorhinolaryngological devices associated with adverse incidents
- **Y72.0 Diagnostic and monitoring otorhinolaryngological devices associated with adverse incidents**
- **Y72.1 Therapeutic (nonsurgical) and rehabilitative otorhinolaryngological devices associated with adverse incidents**
- **Y72.2 Prosthetic and other implants, materials and accessory otorhinolaryngological devices associated with adverse incidents**
- **Y72.3 Surgical instruments, materials and otorhinolaryngological devices (including sutures) associated with adverse incidents**
- **Y72.8 Miscellaneous otorhinolaryngological devices associated with adverse incidents, not elsewhere classified**

Y73 Gastroenterology and urology devices associated with adverse incidents
- **Y73.0 Diagnostic and monitoring gastroenterology and urology devices associated with adverse incidents**
- **Y73.1 Therapeutic (nonsurgical) and rehabilitative gastroenterology and urology devices associated with adverse incidents**
- **Y73.2 Prosthetic and other implants, materials and accessory gastroenterology and urology devices associated with adverse incidents**
- **Y73.3 Surgical instruments, materials and gastroenterology and urology devices (including sutures) associated with adverse incidents**
- **Y73.8 Miscellaneous gastroenterology and urology devices associated with adverse incidents, not elsewhere classified**

Y74 General hospital and personal-use devices associated with adverse incidents
- **Y74.0 Diagnostic and monitoring general hospital and personal-use devices associated with adverse incidents**
- **Y74.1 Therapeutic (nonsurgical) and rehabilitative general hospital and personal-use devices associated with adverse incidents**
- **Y74.2 Prosthetic and other implants, materials and accessory general hospital and personal-use devices associated with adverse incidents**
- **Y74.3 Surgical instruments, materials and general hospital and personal-use devices (including sutures) associated with adverse incidents**
- **Y74.8 Miscellaneous general hospital and personal-use devices associated with adverse incidents, not elsewhere classified**

Y75 Neurological devices associated with adverse incidents
- **Y75.0 Diagnostic and monitoring neurological devices associated with adverse incidents**
- **Y75.1 Therapeutic (nonsurgical) and rehabilitative neurological devices associated with adverse incidents**
- **Y75.2 Prosthetic and other implants, materials and neurological devices associated with adverse incidents**
- **Y75.3 Surgical instruments, materials and neurological devices (including sutures) associated with adverse incidents**
- **Y75.8 Miscellaneous neurological devices associated with adverse incidents, not elsewhere classified**

Y76 Obstetric and gynecological devices associated with adverse incidents
- **Y76.0 Diagnostic and monitoring obstetric and gynecological devices associated with adverse incidents** ♀
- **Y76.1 Therapeutic (nonsurgical) and rehabilitative obstetric and gynecological devices associated with adverse incidents** ♀
- **Y76.2 Prosthetic and other implants, materials and accessory obstetric and gynecological devices associated with adverse incidents** ♀
- **Y76.3 Surgical instruments, materials and obstetric and gynecological devices (including sutures) associated with adverse incidents** ♀
- **Y76.8 Miscellaneous obstetric and gynecological devices associated with adverse incidents, not elsewhere classified** ♀

Y77 Ophthalmic devices associated with adverse incidents
- **Y77.0 Diagnostic and monitoring ophthalmic devices associated with adverse incidents**
- **Y77.1 Therapeutic (nonsurgical) and rehabilitative ophthalmic devices associated with adverse incidents**
  AHA: 2020,4Q,41
  - **Y77.11 Contact lens associated with adverse incidents**
    Rigid gas permeable contact lens associated with adverse incidents
    Soft (hydrophilic) contact lens associated with adverse incidents
  - **Y77.19 Other therapeutic (nonsurgical) and rehabilitative ophthalmic devices associated with adverse incidents**
- **Y77.2 Prosthetic and other implants, materials and accessory ophthalmic devices associated with adverse incidents**
- **Y77.3 Surgical instruments, materials and ophthalmic devices (including sutures) associated with adverse incidents**

Y77.8 **Miscellaneous ophthalmic devices associated with adverse incidents, not elsewhere classified**

4th Y78 **Radiological devices associated with adverse incidents**

Y78.0 **Diagnostic and monitoring radiological devices associated with adverse incidents**

Y78.1 **Therapeutic (nonsurgical) and rehabilitative radiological devices associated with adverse incidents**

Y78.2 **Prosthetic and other implants, materials and accessory radiological devices associated with adverse incidents**

Y78.3 **Surgical instruments, materials and radiological devices (including sutures) associated with adverse incidents**

Y78.8 **Miscellaneous radiological devices associated with adverse incidents, not elsewhere classified**

4th Y79 **Orthopedic devices associated with adverse incidents**

Y79.0 **Diagnostic and monitoring orthopedic devices associated with adverse incidents**

Y79.1 **Therapeutic (nonsurgical) and rehabilitative orthopedic devices associated with adverse incidents**

Y79.2 **Prosthetic and other implants, materials and accessory orthopedic devices associated with adverse incidents**

Y79.3 **Surgical instruments, materials and orthopedic devices (including sutures) associated with adverse incidents**

Y79.8 **Miscellaneous orthopedic devices associated with adverse incidents, not elsewhere classified**

4th Y80 **Physical medicine devices associated with adverse incidents**

Y80.0 **Diagnostic and monitoring physical medicine devices associated with adverse incidents**

Y80.1 **Therapeutic (nonsurgical) and rehabilitative physical medicine devices associated with adverse incidents**

Y80.2 **Prosthetic and other implants, materials and accessory physical medicine devices associated with adverse incidents**

Y80.3 **Surgical instruments, materials and physical medicine devices (including sutures) associated with adverse incidents**

Y80.8 **Miscellaneous physical medicine devices associated with adverse incidents, not elsewhere classified**

4th Y81 **General- and plastic-surgery devices associated with adverse incidents**

Y81.0 **Diagnostic and monitoring general- and plastic-surgery devices associated with adverse incidents**

Y81.1 **Therapeutic (nonsurgical) and rehabilitative general- and plastic-surgery devices associated with adverse incidents**

Y81.2 **Prosthetic and other implants, materials and accessory general- and plastic-surgery devices associated with adverse incidents**

Y81.3 **Surgical instruments, materials and general- and plastic-surgery devices (including sutures) associated with adverse incidents**

Y81.8 **Miscellaneous general- and plastic-surgery devices associated with adverse incidents, not elsewhere classified**

4th Y82 **Other and unspecified medical devices associated with adverse incidents**

Y82.8 **Other medical devices associated with adverse incidents**

Y82.9 **Unspecified medical devices associated with adverse incidents**

Surgical and other medical procedures as the cause of abnormal reaction of the patient, or of later complication, without mention of misadventure at the time of the procedure (Y83-Y84)

EXCLUDES 1 *misadventures to patients during surgical and medical care, classifiable to (Y62-Y69)*

EXCLUDES 2 *breakdown or malfunctioning of medical device (during procedure) (after implantation) (ongoing use) (Y70-Y82)*

4th Y83 **Surgical operation and other surgical procedures as the cause of abnormal reaction of the patient, or of later complication, without mention of misadventure at the time of the procedure**

Y83.0 **Surgical operation with transplant of whole organ as the cause of abnormal reaction of the patient, or of later complication, without mention of misadventure at the time of the procedure**

Y83.1 **Surgical operation with implant of artificial internal device as the cause of abnormal reaction of the patient, or of later complication, without mention of misadventure at the time of the procedure**

Y83.2 **Surgical operation with anastomosis, bypass or graft as the cause of abnormal reaction of the patient, or of later complication, without mention of misadventure at the time of the procedure**

Y83.3 **Surgical operation with formation of external stoma as the cause of abnormal reaction of the patient, or of later complication, without mention of misadventure at the time of the procedure**

Y83.4 **Other reconstructive surgery as the cause of abnormal reaction of the patient, or of later complication, without mention of misadventure at the time of the procedure**

Y83.5 **Amputation of limb(s) as the cause of abnormal reaction of the patient, or of later complication, without mention of misadventure at the time of the procedure**

Y83.6 **Removal of other organ (partial) (total) as the cause of abnormal reaction of the patient, or of later complication, without mention of misadventure at the time of the procedure**

Y83.8 **Other surgical procedures as the cause of abnormal reaction of the patient, or of later complication, without mention of misadventure at the time of the procedure**

Y83.9 **Surgical procedure, unspecified as the cause of abnormal reaction of the patient, or of later complication, without mention of misadventure at the time of the procedure**

4th Y84 **Other medical procedures as the cause of abnormal reaction of the patient, or of later complication, without mention of misadventure at the time of the procedure**

Y84.0 **Cardiac catheterization as the cause of abnormal reaction of the patient, or of later complication, without mention of misadventure at the time of the procedure**

Y84.1 **Kidney dialysis as the cause of abnormal reaction of the patient, or of later complication, without mention of misadventure at the time of the procedure**

Y84.2 **Radiological procedure and radiotherapy as the cause of abnormal reaction of the patient, or of later complication, without mention of misadventure at the time of the procedure**

AHA: 2019,1Q,21; 2017,1Q,33

Y84.3 **Shock therapy as the cause of abnormal reaction of the patient, or of later complication, without mention of misadventure at the time of the procedure**

Y84.4 **Aspiration of fluid as the cause of abnormal reaction of the patient, or of later complication, without mention of misadventure at the time of the procedure**

Y84.5 **Insertion of gastric or duodenal sound as the cause of abnormal reaction of the patient, or of later complication, without mention of misadventure at the time of the procedure**

Y84.6 **Urinary catheterization as the cause of abnormal reaction of the patient, or of later complication, without mention of misadventure at the time of the procedure**

Y84.7 **Blood-sampling as the cause of abnormal reaction of the patient, or of later complication, without mention of misadventure at the time of the procedure**

Y84.8 **Other medical procedures as the cause of abnormal reaction of the patient, or of later complication, without mention of misadventure at the time of the procedure**

AHA: 2021,1Q,5; 2014,4Q,24

Y84.9 **Medical procedure, unspecified as the cause of abnormal reaction of the patient, or of later complication, without mention of misadventure at the time of the procedure**

Supplementary factors related to causes of morbidity classified elsewhere (Y90-Y99)

NOTE These categories may be used to provide supplementary information concerning causes of morbidity. They are not to be used for single-condition coding.

4th Y90 **Evidence of alcohol involvement determined by blood alcohol level**

Code first any associated alcohol related disorders (F10)

Y90.0 **Blood alcohol level of less than 20 mg/100 ml**

Y90.1 **Blood alcohol level of 20-39 mg/100 ml**

Y90.2 **Blood alcohol level of 40-59 mg/100 ml**

Y90.3 **Blood alcohol level of 60-79 mg/100 ml**

Y90.4 **Blood alcohol level of 80-99 mg/100 ml**

Y90.5 **Blood alcohol level of 100-119 mg/100 ml**

Y90.6 **Blood alcohol level of 120-199 mg/100 ml**

Y90.7 **Blood alcohol level of 200-239 mg/100 ml**

Y90.8 **Blood alcohol level of 240 mg/100 ml or more**

Y90.9 **Presence of alcohol in blood, level not specified**

✓4th Y92 Place of occurrence of the external cause

The following category is for use, when relevant, to identify the place of occurrence of the external cause. Use in conjunction with an activity code.

Place of occurrence should be recorded only at the initial encounter for treatment

✓5th Y92.Ø Non-institutional (private) residence as the place of occurrence of the external cause

EXCLUDES 1 *abandoned or derelict house (Y92.89)*
home under construction but not yet occupied (Y92.6-)
institutional place of residence (Y92.1-)

✓6th Y92.ØØ Unspecified non-institutional (private) residence as the place of occurrence of the external cause

Y92.ØØØ Kitchen of unspecified non-institutional (private) residence as the place of occurrence of the external cause

Y92.ØØ1 Dining room of unspecified non-institutional (private) residence as the place of occurrence of the external cause

Y92.ØØ2 Bathroom of unspecified non-institutional (private) residence as the place of occurrence of the external cause

Y92.ØØ3 Bedroom of unspecified non-institutional (private) residence as the place of occurrence of the external cause

Y92.ØØ7 Garden or yard of unspecified non-institutional (private) residence as the place of occurrence of the external cause

Y92.ØØ8 Other place in unspecified non-institutional (private) residence as the place of occurrence of the external cause

Y92.ØØ9 Unspecified place in unspecified non-institutional (private) residence as the place of occurrence of the external cause

Home (NOS) as the place of occurrence of the external cause

✓6th Y92.Ø1 Single-family non-institutional (private) house as the place of occurrence of the external cause

Farmhouse as the place of occurrence of the external cause

EXCLUDES 1 *barn (Y92.71)*
chicken coop or hen house (Y92.72)
farm field (Y92.73)
orchard (Y92.74)
single family mobile home or trailer (Y92.Ø2-)
slaughter house (Y92.86)

Y92.Ø1Ø Kitchen of single-family (private) house as the place of occurrence of the external cause

Y92.Ø11 Dining room of single-family (private) house as the place of occurrence of the external cause

Y92.Ø12 Bathroom of single-family (private) house as the place of occurrence of the external cause

Y92.Ø13 Bedroom of single-family (private) house as the place of occurrence of the external cause

Y92.Ø14 Private driveway to single-family (private) house as the place of occurrence of the external cause

Y92.Ø15 Private garage of single-family (private) house as the place of occurrence of the external cause

Y92.Ø16 Swimming-pool in single-family (private) house or garden as the place of occurrence of the external cause

Y92.Ø17 Garden or yard in single-family (private) house as the place of occurrence of the external cause

Y92.Ø18 Other place in single-family (private) house as the place of occurrence of the external cause

Y92.Ø19 Unspecified place in single-family (private) house as the place of occurrence of the external cause

✓6th Y92.Ø2 Mobile home as the place of occurrence of the external cause

Y92.Ø2Ø Kitchen in mobile home as the place of occurrence of the external cause

Y92.Ø21 Dining room in mobile home as the place of occurrence of the external cause

Y92.Ø22 Bathroom in mobile home as the place of occurrence of the external cause

Y92.Ø23 Bedroom in mobile home as the place of occurrence of the external cause

Y92.Ø24 Driveway of mobile home as the place of occurrence of the external cause

Y92.Ø25 Garage of mobile home as the place of occurrence of the external cause

Y92.Ø26 Swimming-pool of mobile home as the place of occurrence of the external cause

Y92.Ø27 Garden or yard of mobile home as the place of occurrence of the external cause

Y92.Ø28 Other place in mobile home as the place of occurrence of the external cause

Y92.Ø29 Unspecified place in mobile home as the place of occurrence of the external cause

✓6th Y92.Ø3 Apartment as the place of occurrence of the external cause

Condominium as the place of occurrence of the external cause

Co-op apartment as the place of occurrence of the external cause

Y92.Ø3Ø Kitchen in apartment as the place of occurrence of the external cause

Y92.Ø31 Bathroom in apartment as the place of occurrence of the external cause

Y92.Ø32 Bedroom in apartment as the place of occurrence of the external cause

Y92.Ø38 Other place in apartment as the place of occurrence of the external cause

Y92.Ø39 Unspecified place in apartment as the place of occurrence of the external cause

✓6th Y92.Ø4 Boarding-house as the place of occurrence of the external cause

Y92.Ø4Ø Kitchen in boarding-house as the place of occurrence of the external cause

Y92.Ø41 Bathroom in boarding-house as the place of occurrence of the external cause

Y92.Ø42 Bedroom in boarding-house as the place of occurrence of the external cause

Y92.Ø43 Driveway of boarding-house as the place of occurrence of the external cause

Y92.Ø44 Garage of boarding-house as the place of occurrence of the external cause

Y92.Ø45 Swimming-pool of boarding-house as the place of occurrence of the external cause

Y92.Ø46 Garden or yard of boarding-house as the place of occurrence of the external cause

Y92.Ø48 Other place in boarding-house as the place of occurrence of the external cause

Y92.Ø49 Unspecified place in boarding-house as the place of occurrence of the external cause

✓6th Y92.Ø9 Other non-institutional residence as the place of occurrence of the external cause

AHA: 2017,2Q,10

Y92.Ø9Ø Kitchen in other non-institutional residence as the place of occurrence of the external cause

Y92.Ø91 Bathroom in other non-institutional residence as the place of occurrence of the external cause

Y92.Ø92 Bedroom in other non-institutional residence as the place of occurrence of the external cause

Y92.Ø93 Driveway of other non-institutional residence as the place of occurrence of the external cause

Y92.Ø94 Garage of other non-institutional residence as the place of occurrence of the external cause

Y92.Ø95 Swimming-pool of other non-institutional residence as the place of occurrence of the external cause

Y92.Ø96 Garden or yard of other non-institutional residence as the place of occurrence of the external cause

Y92.098 **Other place in other non-institutional residence as the place of occurrence of the external cause**

Y92.099 **Unspecified place in other non-institutional residence as the place of occurrence of the external cause**

✓5th **Y92.1** **Institutional (nonprivate) residence as the place of occurrence of the external cause**

Y92.10 **Unspecified residential institution as the place of occurrence of the external cause**

✓6th **Y92.11** **Children's home and orphanage as the place of occurrence of the external cause**

Y92.110 **Kitchen in children's home and orphanage as the place of occurrence of the external cause**

Y92.111 **Bathroom in children's home and orphanage as the place of occurrence of the external cause**

Y92.112 **Bedroom in children's home and orphanage as the place of occurrence of the external cause**

Y92.113 **Driveway of children's home and orphanage as the place of occurrence of the external cause**

Y92.114 **Garage of children's home and orphanage as the place of occurrence of the external cause**

Y92.115 **Swimming-pool of children's home and orphanage as the place of occurrence of the external cause**

Y92.116 **Garden or yard of children's home and orphanage as the place of occurrence of the external cause**

Y92.118 **Other place in children's home and orphanage as the place of occurrence of the external cause**

Y92.119 **Unspecified place in children's home and orphanage as the place of occurrence of the external cause**

✓6th **Y92.12** **Nursing home as the place of occurrence of the external cause**

Home for the sick as the place of occurrence of the external cause

Hospice as the place of occurrence of the external cause

AHA: 2017,2Q,10

Y92.120 **Kitchen in nursing home as the place of occurrence of the external cause**

Y92.121 **Bathroom in nursing home as the place of occurrence of the external cause**

Y92.122 **Bedroom in nursing home as the place of occurrence of the external cause**

Y92.123 **Driveway of nursing home as the place of occurrence of the external cause**

Y92.124 **Garage of nursing home as the place of occurrence of the external cause**

Y92.125 **Swimming-pool of nursing home as the place of occurrence of the external cause**

Y92.126 **Garden or yard of nursing home as the place of occurrence of the external cause**

Y92.128 **Other place in nursing home as the place of occurrence of the external cause**

Y92.129 **Unspecified place in nursing home as the place of occurrence of the external cause**

✓6th **Y92.13** **Military base as the place of occurrence of the external cause**

EXCLUDES 1 *military training grounds (Y92.84)*

Y92.130 **Kitchen on military base as the place of occurrence of the external cause**

Y92.131 **Mess hall on military base as the place of occurrence of the external cause**

Y92.133 **Barracks on military base as the place of occurrence of the external cause**

Y92.135 **Garage on military base as the place of occurrence of the external cause**

Y92.136 **Swimming-pool on military base as the place of occurrence of the external cause**

Y92.137 **Garden or yard on military base as the place of occurrence of the external cause**

Y92.138 **Other place on military base as the place of occurrence of the external cause**

Y92.139 **Unspecified place military base as the place of occurrence of the external cause**

✓6th **Y92.14** **Prison as the place of occurrence of the external cause**

Y92.140 **Kitchen in prison as the place of occurrence of the external cause**

Y92.141 **Dining room in prison as the place of occurrence of the external cause**

Y92.142 **Bathroom in prison as the place of occurrence of the external cause**

Y92.143 **Cell of prison as the place of occurrence of the external cause**

Y92.146 **Swimming-pool of prison as the place of occurrence of the external cause**

Y92.147 **Courtyard of prison as the place of occurrence of the external cause**

Y92.148 **Other place in prison as the place of occurrence of the external cause**

Y92.149 **Unspecified place in prison as the place of occurrence of the external cause**

✓6th **Y92.15** **Reform school as the place of occurrence of the external cause**

Y92.150 **Kitchen in reform school as the place of occurrence of the external cause**

Y92.151 **Dining room in reform school as the place of occurrence of the external cause**

Y92.152 **Bathroom in reform school as the place of occurrence of the external cause**

Y92.153 **Bedroom in reform school as the place of occurrence of the external cause**

Y92.154 **Driveway of reform school as the place of occurrence of the external cause**

Y92.155 **Garage of reform school as the place of occurrence of the external cause**

Y92.156 **Swimming-pool of reform school as the place of occurrence of the external cause**

Y92.157 **Garden or yard of reform school as the place of occurrence of the external cause**

Y92.158 **Other place in reform school as the place of occurrence of the external cause**

Y92.159 **Unspecified place in reform school as the place of occurrence of the external cause**

✓6th **Y92.16** **School dormitory as the place of occurrence of the external cause**

EXCLUDES 1 *reform school as the place of occurrence of the external cause (Y92.15-)*
school buildings and grounds as the place of occurrence of the external cause (Y92.2-)
school sports and athletic areas as the place of occurrence of the external cause (Y92.3-)

Y92.160 **Kitchen in school dormitory as the place of occurrence of the external cause**

Y92.161 **Dining room in school dormitory as the place of occurrence of the external cause**

Y92.162 **Bathroom in school dormitory as the place of occurrence of the external cause**

Y92.163 **Bedroom in school dormitory as the place of occurrence of the external cause**

Y92.168 **Other place in school dormitory as the place of occurrence of the external cause**

Y92.169 **Unspecified place in school dormitory as the place of occurrence of the external cause**

✓6th **Y92.19** **Other specified residential institution as the place of occurrence of the external cause**

AHA: 2017,2Q,10

Y92.190 **Kitchen in other specified residential institution as the place of occurrence of the external cause**

Y92.191 **Dining room in other specified residential institution as the place of occurrence of the external cause**

Y92.192 **Bathroom in other specified residential institution as the place of occurrence of the external cause**

Y92.193 **Bedroom in other specified residential institution as the place of occurrence of the external cause**

Y92.194 **Driveway of other specified residential institution as the place of occurrence of the external cause**

Y92.195 Garage of other specified residential institution as the place of occurrence of the external cause

Y92.196 Pool of other specified residential institution as the place of occurrence of the external cause

Y92.197 Garden or yard of other specified residential institution as the place of occurrence of the external cause

Y92.198 Other place in other specified residential institution as the place of occurrence of the external cause

Y92.199 Unspecified place in other specified residential institution as the place of occurrence of the external cause

5th Y92.2 School, other institution and public administrative area as the place of occurrence of the external cause

Building and adjacent grounds used by the general public or by a particular group of the public

EXCLUDES 1 *building under construction as the place of occurrence of the external cause (Y92.6)*

residential institution as the place of occurrence of the external cause (Y92.1)

school dormitory as the place of occurrence of the external cause (Y92.16-)

sports and athletics area of schools as the place of occurrence of the external cause (Y92.3-)

6th Y92.21 School (private) (public) (state) as the place of occurrence of the external cause

Y92.210 Daycare center as the place of occurrence of the external cause

Y92.211 Elementary school as the place of occurrence of the external cause

Kindergarten as the place of occurrence of the external cause

Y92.212 Middle school as the place of occurrence of the external cause

Y92.213 High school as the place of occurrence of the external cause

AHA: 2012,4Q,108

Y92.214 College as the place of occurrence of the external cause

University as the place of occurrence of the external cause

Y92.215 Trade school as the place of occurrence of the external cause

Y92.218 Other school as the place of occurrence of the external cause

Y92.219 Unspecified school as the place of occurrence of the external cause

Y92.22 Religious institution as the place of occurrence of the external cause

Church as the place of occurrence of the external cause

Mosque as the place of occurrence of the external cause

Synagogue as the place of occurrence of the external cause

6th Y92.23 Hospital as the place of occurrence of the external cause

EXCLUDES 1 *ambulatory (outpatient) health services establishments (Y92.53-)*

home for the sick as the place of occurrence of the external cause (Y92.12-)

hospice as the place of occurrence of the external cause (Y92.12-)

nursing home as the place of occurrence of the external cause (Y92.12-)

Y92.230 Patient room in hospital as the place of occurrence of the external cause

Y92.231 Patient bathroom in hospital as the place of occurrence of the external cause

Y92.232 Corridor of hospital as the place of occurrence of the external cause

Y92.233 Cafeteria of hospital as the place of occurrence of the external cause

Y92.234 Operating room of hospital as the place of occurrence of the external cause

Y92.238 Other place in hospital as the place of occurrence of the external cause

Y92.239 Unspecified place in hospital as the place of occurrence of the external cause

6th Y92.24 Public administrative building as the place of occurrence of the external cause

Y92.240 Courthouse as the place of occurrence of the external cause

Y92.241 Library as the place of occurrence of the external cause

Y92.242 Post office as the place of occurrence of the external cause

Y92.243 City hall as the place of occurrence of the external cause

Y92.248 Other public administrative building as the place of occurrence of the external cause

6th Y92.25 Cultural building as the place of occurrence of the external cause

Y92.250 Art Gallery as the place of occurrence of the external cause

Y92.251 Museum as the place of occurrence of the external cause

Y92.252 Music hall as the place of occurrence of the external cause

Y92.253 Opera house as the place of occurrence of the external cause

Y92.254 Theater (live) as the place of occurrence of the external cause

Y92.258 Other cultural public building as the place of occurrence of the external cause

Y92.26 Movie house or cinema as the place of occurrence of the external cause

Y92.29 Other specified public building as the place of occurrence of the external cause

Assembly hall as the place of occurrence of the external cause

Clubhouse as the place of occurrence of the external cause

6th Y92.3 Sports and athletics area as the place of occurrence of the external cause

6th Y92.31 Athletic court as the place of occurrence of the external cause

EXCLUDES 1 *tennis court in private home or garden (Y92.09)*

Y92.310 Basketball court as the place of occurrence of the external cause

Y92.311 Squash court as the place of occurrence of the external cause

Y92.312 Tennis court as the place of occurrence of the external cause

Y92.318 Other athletic court as the place of occurrence of the external cause

6th Y92.32 Athletic field as the place of occurrence of the external cause

Y92.320 Baseball field as the place of occurrence of the external cause

Y92.321 Football field as the place of occurrence of the external cause

Y92.322 Soccer field as the place of occurrence of the external cause

Y92.328 Other athletic field as the place of occurrence of the external cause

Cricket field as the place of occurrence of the external cause

Hockey field as the place of occurrence of the external cause

6th Y92.33 Skating rink as the place of occurrence of the external cause

Y92.330 Ice skating rink (indoor) (outdoor) as the place of occurrence of the external cause

Y92.331 Roller skating rink as the place of occurrence of the external cause

Y92.34 Swimming pool (public) as the place of occurrence of the external cause

EXCLUDES 1 *swimming pool in private home or garden (Y92.016)*

Y92.39 Other specified sports and athletic area as the place of occurrence of the external cause
Golf-course as the place of occurrence of the external cause
Gymnasium as the place of occurrence of the external cause
Riding-school as the place of occurrence of the external cause
Stadium as the place of occurrence of the external cause

✓5th **Y92.4 Street, highway and other paved roadways as the place of occurrence of the external cause**
EXCLUDES 1 *private driveway of residence (Y92.014, Y92.024, Y92.043, Y92.093, Y92.113, Y92.123, Y92.154, Y92.194)*

✓6th **Y92.41 Street and highway as the place of occurrence of the external cause**
Y92.410 Unspecified street and highway as the place of occurrence of the external cause
Road NOS as the place of occurrence of the external cause
Y92.411 Interstate highway as the place of occurrence of the external cause
Freeway as the place of occurrence of the external cause
Motorway as the place of occurrence of the external cause
Y92.412 Parkway as the place of occurrence of the external cause
Y92.413 State road as the place of occurrence of the external cause
Y92.414 Local residential or business street as the place of occurrence of the external cause
Y92.415 Exit ramp or entrance ramp of street or highway as the place of occurrence of the external cause

✓6th **Y92.48 Other paved roadways as the place of occurrence of the external cause**
Y92.480 Sidewalk as the place of occurrence of the external cause
Y92.481 Parking lot as the place of occurrence of the external cause
Y92.482 Bike path as the place of occurrence of the external cause
Y92.488 Other paved roadways as the place of occurrence of the external cause

✓5th **Y92.5 Trade and service area as the place of occurrence of the external cause**
EXCLUDES 1 *garage in private home (Y92.015)*
schools and other public administration buildings (Y92.2-)

✓6th **Y92.51 Private commercial establishments as the place of occurrence of the external cause**
Y92.510 Bank as the place of occurrence of the external cause
Y92.511 Restaurant or café as the place of occurrence of the external cause
Y92.512 Supermarket, store or market as the place of occurrence of the external cause
Y92.513 Shop (commercial) as the place of occurrence of the external cause

✓6th **Y92.52 Service areas as the place of occurrence of the external cause**
Y92.520 Airport as the place of occurrence of the external cause
Y92.521 Bus station as the place of occurrence of the external cause
Y92.522 Railway station as the place of occurrence of the external cause
Y92.523 Highway rest stop as the place of occurrence of the external cause
Y92.524 Gas station as the place of occurrence of the external cause
Petroleum station as the place of occurrence of the external cause
Service station as the place of occurrence of the external cause

✓6th **Y92.53 Ambulatory health services establishments as the place of occurrence of the external cause**
Y92.530 Ambulatory surgery center as the place of occurrence of the external cause
Outpatient surgery center, including that connected with a hospital as the place of occurrence of the external cause
Same day surgery center, including that connected with a hospital as the place of occurrence of the external cause
Y92.531 Health care provider office as the place of occurrence of the external cause
Physician office as the place of occurrence of the external cause
Y92.532 Urgent care center as the place of occurrence of the external cause
Y92.538 Other ambulatory health services establishments as the place of occurrence of the external cause
AHA: 2019,1Q,21

Y92.59 Other trade areas as the place of occurrence of the external cause
Office building as the place of occurrence of the external cause
Casino as the place of occurrence of the external cause
Garage (commercial) as the place of occurrence of the external cause
Hotel as the place of occurrence of the external cause
Radio or television station as the place of occurrence of the external cause
Shopping mall as the place of occurrence of the external cause
Warehouse as the place of occurrence of the external cause

✓5th **Y92.6 Industrial and construction area as the place of occurrence of the external cause**
Y92.61 Building [any] under construction as the place of occurrence of the external cause
Y92.62 Dock or shipyard as the place of occurrence of the external cause
Dockyard as the place of occurrence of the external cause
Dry dock as the place of occurrence of the external cause
Shipyard as the place of occurrence of the external cause
Y92.63 Factory as the place of occurrence of the external cause
Factory building as the place of occurrence of the external cause
Factory premises as the place of occurrence of the external cause
Industrial yard as the place of occurrence of the external cause
Y92.64 Mine or pit as the place of occurrence of the external cause
Mine as the place of occurrence of the external cause
Y92.65 Oil rig as the place of occurrence of the external cause
Pit (coal) (gravel) (sand) as the place of occurrence of the external cause
Y92.69 Other specified industrial and construction area as the place of occurrence of the external cause
Gasworks as the place of occurrence of the external cause
Power-station (coal) (nuclear) (oil) as the place of occurrence of the external cause
Tunnel under construction as the place of occurrence of the external cause
Workshop as the place of occurrence of the external cause

✓5th **Y92.7 Farm as the place of occurrence of the external cause**
Ranch as the place of occurrence of the external cause
EXCLUDES 1 *farmhouse and home premises of farm (Y92.01-)*
Y92.71 Barn as the place of occurrence of the external cause

Y92.72 **Chicken coop as the place of occurrence of the external cause**
Hen house as the place of occurrence of the external cause

Y92.73 **Farm field as the place of occurrence of the external cause**

Y92.74 **Orchard as the place of occurrence of the external cause**

Y92.79 **Other farm location as the place of occurrence of the external cause**

✓5th Y92.8 **Other places as the place of occurrence of the external cause**

✓6th Y92.81 **Transport vehicle as the place of occurrence of the external cause**
EXCLUDES 1 *transport accidents (VØØ-V99)*

Y92.81Ø **Car as the place of occurrence of the external cause**

Y92.811 **Bus as the place of occurrence of the external cause**

Y92.812 **Truck as the place of occurrence of the external cause**

Y92.813 **Airplane as the place of occurrence of the external cause**

Y92.814 **Boat as the place of occurrence of the external cause**

Y92.815 **Train as the place of occurrence of the external cause**

Y92.816 **Subway car as the place of occurrence of the external cause**

Y92.818 **Other transport vehicle as the place of occurrence of the external cause**

✓6th Y92.82 **Wilderness area**

Y92.82Ø **Desert as the place of occurrence of the external cause**

Y92.821 **Forest as the place of occurrence of the external cause**

Y92.828 **Other wilderness area as the place of occurrence of the external cause**
Swamp as the place of occurrence of the external cause
Mountain as the place of occurrence of the external cause
Marsh as the place of occurrence of the external cause
Prairie as the place of occurrence of the external cause

✓6th Y92.83 **Recreation area as the place of occurrence of the external cause**

Y92.83Ø **Public park as the place of occurrence of the external cause**

Y92.831 **Amusement park as the place of occurrence of the external cause**

Y92.832 **Beach as the place of occurrence of the external cause**
Seashore as the place of occurrence of the external cause

Y92.833 **Campsite as the place of occurrence of the external cause**

Y92.834 **Zoological garden (Zoo) as the place of occurrence of the external cause**

Y92.838 **Other recreation area as the place of occurrence of the external cause**

Y92.84 **Military training ground as the place of occurrence of the external cause**

Y92.85 **Railroad track as the place of occurrence of the external cause**

Y92.86 **Slaughter house as the place of occurrence of the external cause**

Y92.89 **Other specified places as the place of occurrence of the external cause**
Derelict house as the place of occurrence of the external cause

Y92.9 **Unspecified place or not applicable**

✓4th **Y93 Activity codes**

NOTE Category Y93 is provided for use to indicate the activity of the person seeking healthcare for an injury or health condition, such as a heart attack while shoveling snow, which resulted from, or was contributed to, by the activity. These codes are appropriate for use for both acute injuries, such as those from chapter 19, and conditions that are due to the long-term, cumulative effects of an activity, such as those from chapter 13. They are also appropriate for use with external cause codes for cause and intent if identifying the activity provides additional information on the event. These codes should be used in conjunction with codes for external cause status (Y99) and place of occurrence (Y92).

This section contains the following broad activity categories:

Y93.Ø	Activities involving walking and running
Y93.1	Activities involving water and water craft
Y93.2	Activities involving ice and snow
Y93.3	Activities involving climbing, rappelling, and jumping off
Y93.4	Activities involving dancing and other rhythmic movement
Y93.5	Activities involving other sports and athletics played individually
Y93.6	Activities involving other sports and athletics played as a team or group
Y93.7	Activities involving other specified sports and athletics
Y93.A	Activities involving other cardiorespiratory exercise
Y93.B	Activities involving other muscle strengthening exercises
Y93.C	Activities involving computer technology and electronic devices
Y93.D	Activities involving arts and handcrafts
Y93.E	Activities involving personal hygiene and interior property and clothing maintenance
Y93.F	Activities involving caregiving
Y93.G	Activities involving food preparation, cooking and grilling
Y93.H	Activities involving exterior property and land maintenance, building and construction
Y93.I	Activities involving roller coasters and other types of external motion
Y93.J	Activities involving playing musical instrument
Y93.K	Activities involving animal care
Y93.8	Activities, other specified
Y93.9	Activity, unspecified

✓5th Y93.Ø **Activities involving walking and running**
EXCLUDES 1 *activity, walking an animal (Y93.K1)*
activity, walking or running on a treadmill (Y93.A1)

Y93.Ø1 **Activity, walking, marching and hiking**
Activity, walking, marching and hiking on level or elevated terrain
EXCLUDES 1 *activity, mountain climbing (Y93.31)*

Y93.Ø2 **Activity, running**

✓5th Y93.1 **Activities involving water and water craft**
EXCLUDES 1 *activities involving ice (Y93.2-)*

Y93.11 **Activity, swimming**

Y93.12 **Activity, springboard and platform diving**

Y93.13 **Activity, water polo**

Y93.14 **Activity, water aerobics and water exercise**

Y93.15 **Activity, underwater diving and snorkeling**
Activity, SCUBA diving

Y93.16 **Activity, rowing, canoeing, kayaking, rafting and tubing**
Activity, canoeing, kayaking, rafting and tubing in calm and turbulent water

Y93.17 **Activity, water skiing and wake boarding**

Y93.18 **Activity, surfing, windsurfing and boogie boarding**
Activity, water sliding

Y93.19 **Activity, other involving water and watercraft**
Activity involving water NOS
Activity, parasailing
Activity, water survival training and testing

✓5th Y93.2 Activities involving ice and snow
EXCLUDES 1 *activity, shoveling ice and snow (Y93.H1)*
Y93.21 Activity, ice skating
Activity, figure skating (singles) (pairs)
Activity, ice dancing
EXCLUDES 1 *activity, ice hockey (Y93.22)*
Y93.22 Activity, ice hockey
Y93.23 Activity, snow (alpine) (downhill) skiing, snowboarding, sledding, tobogganing and snow tubing
EXCLUDES 1 *activity, cross country skiing (Y93.24)*
Y93.24 Activity, cross country skiing
Activity, nordic skiing
Y93.29 Activity, other involving ice and snow
Activity involving ice and snow NOS

✓5th Y93.3 Activities involving climbing, rappelling and jumping off
EXCLUDES 1 *activity, hiking on level or elevated terrain (Y93.Ø1)*
activity, jumping rope (Y93.56)
activity, trampoline jumping (Y93.44)
Y93.31 Activity, mountain climbing, rock climbing and wall climbing
Y93.32 Activity, rappelling
Y93.33 Activity, BASE jumping
Activity, Building, Antenna, Span, Earth jumping
Y93.34 Activity, bungee jumping
Y93.35 Activity, hang gliding
Y93.39 Activity, other involving climbing, rappelling and jumping off

✓5th Y93.4 Activities involving dancing and other rhythmic movement
EXCLUDES 1 *activity, martial arts (Y93.75)*
Y93.41 Activity, dancing
AHA: 2012,4Q,108
Y93.42 Activity, yoga
Y93.43 Activity, gymnastics
Activity, rhythmic gymnastics
EXCLUDES 1 *activity, trampolining (Y93.44)*
Y93.44 Activity, trampolining
Y93.45 Activity, cheerleading
Y93.49 Activity, other involving dancing and other rhythmic movements

✓5th Y93.5 Activities involving other sports and athletics played individually
EXCLUDES 1 *activity, dancing (Y93.41)*
activity, gymnastic (Y93.43)
activity, trampolining (Y93.44)
activity, yoga (Y93.42)
Y93.51 Activity, roller skating (inline) and skateboarding
Y93.52 Activity, horseback riding
Y93.53 Activity, golf
Y93.54 Activity, bowling
Y93.55 Activity, bike riding
Y93.56 Activity, jumping rope
Y93.57 Activity, non-running track and field events
EXCLUDES 1 *activity, running (any form) (Y93.Ø2)*
Y93.59 Activity, other involving other sports and athletics played individually
EXCLUDES 1 *activities involving climbing, rappelling, and jumping (Y93.3-)*
activities involving ice and snow (Y93.2-)
activities involving walking and running (Y93.Ø-)
activities involving water and watercraft (Y93.1-)

✓5th Y93.6 Activities involving other sports and athletics played as a team or group
EXCLUDES 1 *activity, ice hockey (Y93.22)*
activity, water polo (Y93.13)
Y93.61 Activity, American tackle football
Activity, football NOS
Y93.62 Activity, American flag or touch football
Y93.63 Activity, rugby
Y93.64 Activity, baseball
Activity, softball
Y93.65 Activity, lacrosse and field hockey
Y93.66 Activity, soccer
Y93.67 Activity, basketball
Y93.68 Activity, volleyball (beach) (court)
Y93.6A Activity, physical games generally associated with school recess, summer camp and children
Activity, capture the flag
Activity, dodge ball
Activity, four square
Activity, kickball
Y93.69 Activity, other involving other sports and athletics played as a team or group
Activity, cricket

✓5th Y93.7 Activities involving other specified sports and athletics
Y93.71 Activity, boxing
Y93.72 Activity, wrestling
Y93.73 Activity, racquet and hand sports
Activity, handball
Activity, racquetball
Activity, squash
Activity, tennis
Y93.74 Activity, frisbee
Activity, ultimate frisbee
Y93.75 Activity, martial arts
Activity, combatives
Y93.79 Activity, other specified sports and athletics
EXCLUDES 1 *sports and athletics activities specified in categories Y93.Ø-Y93.6*

✓5th Y93.A Activities involving other cardiorespiratory exercise
Activities involving physical training
Y93.A1 Activity, exercise machines primarily for cardiorespiratory conditioning
Activity, elliptical and stepper machines
Activity, stationary bike
Activity, treadmill
Y93.A2 Activity, calisthenics
Activity, jumping jacks
Activity, warm up and cool down
Y93.A3 Activity, aerobic and step exercise
Y93.A4 Activity, circuit training
Y93.A5 Activity, obstacle course
Activity, challenge course
Activity, confidence course
Y93.A6 Activity, grass drills
Activity, guerilla drills
Y93.A9 Activity, other involving cardiorespiratory exercise
EXCLUDES 1 *activities involving cardiorespiratory exercise specified in categories Y93.Ø-Y93.7*

✓5th Y93.B Activities involving other muscle strengthening exercises
Y93.B1 Activity, exercise machines primarily for muscle strengthening
Y93.B2 Activity, push-ups, pull-ups, sit-ups
Y93.B3 Activity, free weights
Activity, barbells
Activity, dumbbells
Y93.B4 Activity, pilates
Y93.B9 Activity, other involving muscle strengthening exercises
EXCLUDES 1 *activities involving muscle strengthening specified in categories Y93.Ø-Y93.A*

✓5th Y93.C Activities involving computer technology and electronic devices
EXCLUDES 1 *activity, electronic musical keyboard or instruments (Y93.J-)*
Y93.C1 Activity, computer keyboarding
Activity, electronic game playing using keyboard or other stationary device
Y93.C2 Activity, hand held interactive electronic device
Activity, cellular telephone and communication device
Activity, electronic game playing using interactive device
EXCLUDES 1 *activity, electronic game playing using keyboard or other stationary device (Y93.C1)*
Y93.C9 Activity, other involving computer technology and electronic devices

✓5th Y93.D Activities involving arts and handcrafts
EXCLUDES 1 *activities involving playing musical instrument (Y93.J-)*
Y93.D1 Activity, knitting and crocheting

Y93.D2 Activity, sewing

Y93.D3 Activity, furniture building and finishing
Activity, furniture repair

Y93.D9 Activity, other involving arts and handcrafts

√5th **Y93.E Activities involving personal hygiene and interior property and clothing maintenance**
EXCLUDES 1 *activities involving cooking and grilling (Y93.G-)*
activities involving exterior property and land maintenance, building and construction (Y93.H-)
activities involving caregiving (Y93.F-)
activity, dishwashing (Y93.G1)
activity, food preparation (Y93.G1)
activity, gardening (Y93.H2)

Y93.E1 Activity, personal bathing and showering

Y93.E2 Activity, laundry

Y93.E3 Activity, vacuuming

Y93.E4 Activity, ironing

Y93.E5 Activity, floor mopping and cleaning

Y93.E6 Activity, residential relocation
Activity, packing up and unpacking involved in moving to a new residence

Y93.E8 Activity, other personal hygiene

Y93.E9 Activity, other interior property and clothing maintenance

√5th **Y93.F Activities involving caregiving**
Activity involving the provider of caregiving

Y93.F1 Activity, caregiving, bathing

Y93.F2 Activity, caregiving, lifting

Y93.F9 Activity, other caregiving

√5th **Y93.G Activities involving food preparation, cooking and grilling**

Y93.G1 Activity, food preparation and clean up
Activity, dishwashing

Y93.G2 Activity, grilling and smoking food

Y93.G3 Activity, cooking and baking
Activity, use of stove, oven and microwave oven

Y93.G9 Activity, other involving cooking and grilling

√5th **Y93.H Activities involving exterior property and land maintenance, building and construction**

Y93.H1 Activity, digging, shoveling and raking
Activity, dirt digging
Activity, raking leaves
Activity, snow shoveling

Y93.H2 Activity, gardening and landscaping
Activity, pruning, trimming shrubs, weeding

Y93.H3 Activity, building and construction

Y93.H9 Activity, other involving exterior property and land maintenance, building and construction

√5th **Y93.I Activities involving roller coasters and other types of external motion**

Y93.I1 Activity, rollercoaster riding

Y93.I9 Activity, other involving external motion

√5th **Y93.J Activities involving playing musical instrument**
Activity involving playing electric musical instrument

Y93.J1 Activity, piano playing
Activity, musical keyboard (electronic) playing

Y93.J2 Activity, drum and other percussion instrument playing

Y93.J3 Activity, string instrument playing

Y93.J4 Activity, winds and brass instrument playing

√5th **Y93.K Activities involving animal care**
EXCLUDES 1 *activity, horseback riding (Y93.52)*

Y93.K1 Activity, walking an animal

Y93.K2 Activity, milking an animal

Y93.K3 Activity, grooming and shearing an animal

Y93.K9 Activity, other involving animal care

√5th **Y93.8 Activities, other specified**

Y93.81 Activity, refereeing a sports activity

Y93.82 Activity, spectator at an event

Y93.83 Activity, rough housing and horseplay

Y93.84 Activity, sleeping

Y93.85 Activity, choking game
Activity, blackout game
Activity, fainting game
Activity, pass out game
AHA: 2016,4Q,74-76

Y93.89 Activity, other specified

Y93.9 Activity, unspecified

Y95 Nosocomial condition
AHA: 2013,4Q,119

√4th **Y99 External cause status**
NOTE A single code from category Y99 should be used in conjunction with the external cause code(s) assigned to a record to indicate the status of the person at the time the event occurred.

Y99.Ø Civilian activity done for income or pay
Civilian activity done for financial or other compensation
EXCLUDES 1 *military activity (Y99.1)*
volunteer activity (Y99.2)

Y99.1 Military activity
EXCLUDES 1 *activity of off duty military personnel (Y99.8)*

Y99.2 Volunteer activity
EXCLUDES 1 *activity of child or other family member assisting in compensated work of other family member (Y99.8)*

Y99.8 Other external cause status
Activity NEC
Activity of child or other family member assisting in compensated work of other family member
Hobby not done for income
Leisure activity
Off-duty activity of military personnel
Recreation or sport not for income or while a student
Student activity
EXCLUDES 1 *civilian activity done for income or compensation (Y99.Ø)*
military activity (Y99.1)
AHA: 2012,4Q,108

Y99.9 Unspecified external cause status

Chapter 21. Factors Influencing Health Status and Contact with Health Services (Z00–Z99)

Chapter-specific Guidelines with Coding Examples

The chapter-specific guidelines from the ICD-10-CM Official Guidelines for Coding and Reporting have been provided below. Along with these guidelines are coding examples, contained in the shaded boxes, that have been developed to help illustrate the coding and/or sequencing guidance found in these guidelines.

Note: The chapter-specific guidelines provide additional information about the use of Z codes for specified encounters.

a. Use of Z Codes in any healthcare setting

Z codes are for use in any healthcare setting. Z codes may be used as either a first-listed (principal diagnosis code in the inpatient setting) or secondary code, depending on the circumstances of the encounter. Certain Z codes may only be used as first-listed or principal diagnosis.

> Patient with middle lobe lung cancer presents for initiation of chemotherapy
>
> **Z51.11 Encounter for antineoplastic chemotherapy**
>
> **C34.2 Malignant neoplasm of middle lobe, bronchus or lung**
>
> *Explanation:* A Z code can be used as first-listed in this situation based on guidelines in this chapter as well as chapter 2, "Neoplasms."

> Patient has chronic lymphocytic leukemia for which the patient had previous chemotherapy and is now in remission
>
> **C91.11 Chronic lymphocytic leukemia of B-cell type in remission**
>
> **Z92.21 Personal history of antineoplastic chemotherapy**
>
> *Explanation:* The personal history Z code is used to describe a secondary (supplementary) diagnosis to identify that this patient has had chemotherapy in the past.

b. Z Codes indicate a reason for an encounter or provide additional information about a patient encounter

Z codes are not procedure codes. A corresponding procedure code must accompany a Z code to describe any procedure performed.

c. Categories of Z Codes

1) Contact/exposure

Category Z20 indicates contact with, and suspected exposure to, communicable diseases. These codes are for patients who are suspected to have been exposed to a disease by close personal contact with an infected individual or are in an area where a disease is epidemic.

Category Z77, Other contact with and (suspected) exposures hazardous to health, indicates contact with and suspected exposures hazardous to health.

Contact/exposure codes may be used as a first-listed code to explain an encounter for testing, or, more commonly, as a secondary code to identify a potential risk.

2) Inoculations and vaccinations

Code Z23 is for encounters for inoculations and vaccinations. It indicates that a patient is being seen to receive a prophylactic inoculation against a disease. Procedure codes are required to identify the actual administration of the injection and the type(s) of immunizations given. Code Z23 may be used as a secondary code if the inoculation is given as a routine part of preventive health care, such as a well-baby visit.

3) Status

Status codes indicate that a patient is either a carrier of a disease or has the sequelae or residual of a past disease or condition. This includes such things as the presence of prosthetic or mechanical devices resulting from past treatment. A status code is informative, because the status may affect the course of treatment and its outcome. A status code is distinct from a history code. The history code indicates that the patient no longer has the condition.

A status code should not be used with a diagnosis code from one of the body system chapters, if the diagnosis code includes the information provided by the status code. For example, code Z94.1, Heart transplant status, should not be used with a code from subcategory T86.2, Complications of heart transplant. The status code does not provide additional information. The complication code indicates that the patient is a heart transplant patient.

For encounters for weaning from a mechanical ventilator, assign a code from subcategory J96.1, Chronic respiratory failure, followed by code Z99.11, Dependence on respirator [ventilator] status.

The status Z codes/categories are:

Z14 Genetic carrier

Genetic carrier status indicates that a person carries a gene, associated with a particular disease, which may be passed to offspring who may develop that disease. The person does not have the disease and is not at risk of developing the disease.

Z15 Genetic susceptibility to disease

Genetic susceptibility indicates that a person has a gene that increases the risk of that person developing the disease.

Codes from category Z15 should not be used as principal or first-listed codes. If the patient has the condition to which he/she is susceptible, and that condition is the reason for the encounter, the code for the current condition should be sequenced first. If the patient is being seen for follow-up after completed treatment for this condition, and the condition no longer exists, a follow-up code should be sequenced first, followed by the appropriate personal history and genetic susceptibility codes. If the purpose of the encounter is genetic counseling associated with procreative management, code Z31.5, Encounter for genetic counseling, should be assigned as the first-listed code, followed by a code from category Z15. Additional codes should be assigned for any applicable family or personal history.

Z16 Resistance to antimicrobial drugs

This code indicates that a patient has a condition that is resistant to antimicrobial drug treatment. Sequence the infection code first.

Z17 Estrogen receptor status

Z18 Retained foreign body fragments

Z19 Hormone sensitivity malignancy status

Z21 Asymptomatic HIV infection status

This code indicates that a patient has tested positive for HIV but has manifested no signs or symptoms of the disease.

Z22 Carrier of infectious disease

Carrier status indicates that a person harbors the specific organisms of a disease without manifest symptoms and is capable of transmitting the infection.

Z28.3 Underimmunization status

See Section I.B.14. for underimmunization documentation by clinicians other than the patient's provider.

Z33.1 Pregnant state, incidental

This code is a secondary code only for use when the pregnancy is in no way complicating the reason for visit. Otherwise, a code from the obstetric chapter is required.

Z66 Do not resuscitate

This code may be used when it is documented by the provider that a patient is on do not resuscitate status at any time during the stay.

Z67 Blood type

Z68 Body mass index (BMI)

BMI codes should only be assigned when there is an associated, reportable diagnosis (such as obesity). Do not assign BMI codes during pregnancy.

See Section I.B.14. for BMI documentation by clinicians other than the patient's provider.

> Patient seen today for chest pain, noncardiac in nature. Nurses notes identify a BMI of 20.5.
>
> **R07.89 Other chest pain**
>
> *Explanation:* Section I.B.14 stipulates that the BMI can be assigned from documentation of someone other than the patient's provider, such as nursing notes, only when the provider has documented that the diagnosis is associated with the BMI. As there is no supporting documentation from the provider linking the BMI to an associated condition, no code is assigned for the BMI.

Z74.Ø1 Bed confinement status

Z76.82 Awaiting organ transplant status

Z78 Other specified health status

Code Z78.1, Physical restraint status, may be used when it is documented by the provider that a patient has been put in restraints during the current encounter. Please note that this code should not be reported when it is documented by the provider that a patient is temporarily restrained during a procedure.

Z79 Long-term (current) drug therapy

Codes from this category indicate a patient's continuous use of a prescribed drug (including such things as aspirin therapy) for the long-term treatment of a condition or for prophylactic use. It is not for use for patients who have addictions to drugs. This subcategory is not for use of medications for detoxification or maintenance programs to prevent withdrawal symptoms (e.g., methadone maintenance for opiate dependence). Assign the appropriate code for the drug use, abuse, or dependence instead.

Assign a code from Z79 if the patient is receiving a medication for an extended period as a prophylactic measure (such as for the prevention of deep vein thrombosis) or as treatment of a chronic condition (such as arthritis) or a disease requiring a lengthy course of treatment (such as cancer). Do not assign a code from category Z79 for medication being administered for a brief period of time to treat an acute illness or injury (such as a course of antibiotics to treat acute bronchitis).

Z88 Allergy status to drugs, medicaments and biological substances

Except: Z88.9, Allergy status to unspecified drugs, medicaments and biological substances status

Z89 Acquired absence of limb

Z9Ø Acquired absence of organs, not elsewhere classified

Z91.Ø- Allergy status, other than to drugs and biological substances

Z92.82 Status post administration of tPA (rtPA) in a different facility within the last 24 hours prior to admission to a current facility

Assign code Z92.82, Status post administration of tPA (rtPA) in a different facility within the last 24 hours prior to admission to current facility, as a secondary diagnosis when a patient is received by transfer into a facility and documentation indicates they were administered tissue plasminogen activator (tPA) within the last 24 hours prior to admission to the current facility.

This guideline applies even if the patient is still receiving the tPA at the time they are received into the current facility.

The appropriate code for the condition for which the tPA was administered (such as cerebrovascular disease or myocardial infarction) should be assigned first.

Code Z92.82 is only applicable to the receiving facility record and not to the transferring facility record.

Z93 Artificial opening status

Z94 Transplanted organ and tissue status

Z95 Presence of cardiac and vascular implants and grafts

Z96 Presence of other functional implants

Z97 Presence of other devices

Z98 Other postprocedural states

Assign code Z98.85, Transplanted organ removal status, to indicate that a transplanted organ has been previously removed. This code should not be assigned for the encounter in which the transplanted organ is removed. The complication necessitating removal of the transplant organ should be assigned for that encounter.

See section I.C.19. for information on the coding of organ transplant complications.

Z99 Dependence on enabling machines and devices, not elsewhere classified

Note: Categories Z89-Z9Ø and Z93-Z99 are for use only if there are no complications or malfunctions of the organ or tissue replaced, the amputation site or the equipment on which the patient is dependent.

4) History (of)

There are two types of history Z codes, personal and family. Personal history codes explain a patient's past medical condition that no longer exists and is not receiving any treatment, but that has the potential for recurrence, and therefore may require continued monitoring.

Family history codes are for use when a patient has a family member(s) who has had a particular disease that causes the patient to be at higher risk of also contracting the disease.

Personal history codes may be used in conjunction with follow-up codes and family history codes may be used in conjunction with screening codes to explain the need for a test or procedure. History codes are also acceptable on any medical record regardless of the reason for visit. A history of an illness, even if no longer present, is important information that may alter the type of treatment ordered.

The reason for the encounter (for example, screening or counseling) should be sequenced first and the appropriate personal and/or family history code(s) should be assigned as additional diagnos(es).

The history Z code categories are:

Z8Ø Family history of primary malignant neoplasm

Z81 Family history of mental and behavioral disorders

Z82 Family history of certain disabilities and chronic diseases (leading to disablement)

Z83 Family history of other specific disorders

Z84 Family history of other conditions

Z85 Personal history of malignant neoplasm

Z86 Personal history of certain other diseases

Z87 Personal history of other diseases and conditions

Z91.4- Personal history of psychological trauma, not elsewhere classified

Z91.5- Personal history of self-harm

Z91.81 History of falling

Z91.82 Personal history of military deployment

Z92 Personal history of medical treatment

Except: Z92.Ø, Personal history of contraception

Except: Z92.82, Status post administration of tPA (rtPA) in a different facility within the last 24 hours prior to admission to a current facility

5) Screening

Screening is the testing for disease or disease precursors in seemingly well individuals so that early detection and treatment can be provided for those who test positive for the disease (e.g., screening mammogram).

The testing of a person to rule out or confirm a suspected diagnosis because the patient has some sign or symptom is a diagnostic examination, not a screening. In these cases, the sign or symptom is used to explain the reason for the test.

A screening code may be a first-listed code if the reason for the visit is specifically the screening exam. It may also be used as an additional code if the screening is done during an office visit for other health problems. A screening code is not necessary if the screening is inherent to a routine examination, such as a pap smear done during a routine pelvic examination.

Should a condition be discovered during the screening then the code for the condition may be assigned as an additional diagnosis.

Prostate screening of healthy 5Ø-year-old male patient; PSA noted to be elevated but normal digital rectal exam

Z12.5 **Encounter for screening for malignant neoplasm of prostate**

R97.2Ø **Elevated prostate specific antigen [PSA]**

Explanation: The patient had no signs or symptoms of any prostate-related illness prior to coming in for the screening. The screening code is appropriately used as the first-listed code to signify that this was for routine screening. The elevated PSA is reported as a secondary diagnosis to reflect that an abnormal lab value was found as a result of the screening procedure(s).

The Z code indicates that a screening exam is planned. A procedure code is required to confirm that the screening was performed.

The screening Z codes/categories:

Z11 Encounter for screening for infectious and parasitic diseases

Z12 Encounter for screening for malignant neoplasms

Z13 Encounter for screening for other diseases and disorders

Except: Z13.9, Encounter for screening, unspecified

Z36 Encounter for antenatal screening for mother

6) Observation

There are three observation Z code categories. They are for use in very limited circumstances when a person is being observed for a suspected condition that is ruled out. The observation codes are not for use if an injury or illness or any signs or symptoms related to the suspected condition are present. In such cases the diagnosis/symptom code is used with the corresponding external cause code.

The observation codes are primarily to be used as a principal/first-listed diagnosis. An observation code may be assigned as a secondary diagnosis code when the patient is being observed for a condition that is ruled out and is unrelated to the principal/first-listed diagnosis. Also, when the principal diagnosis is required to be a code from category Z38, Liveborn infants according to place of birth and type of delivery. Then a code from category ZØ5, Encounter for observation and evaluation of newborn for suspected diseases and conditions ruled out, is sequenced after the Z38 code. Additional codes may be used in addition to the observation code but only if they are unrelated to the suspected condition being observed.

Codes from subcategory ZØ3.7, Encounter for suspected maternal and fetal conditions ruled out, may either be used as a first-listed or as an additional code assignment depending on the case. They are for use in very limited circumstances on a maternal record when an encounter is for a suspected maternal or fetal condition that is ruled out during that encounter (for example, a maternal or fetal condition may be suspected due to an abnormal test result). These codes should not be used when the condition is confirmed. In those cases, the confirmed condition should be coded. In addition, these codes are not for use if an illness or any signs or symptoms related to the suspected condition or problem are present. In such cases the diagnosis/symptom code is used.

Additional codes may be used in addition to the code from subcategory ZØ3.7, but only if they are unrelated to the suspected condition being evaluated.

Codes from subcategory ZØ3.7 may not be used for encounters for antenatal screening of mother. *See Section I.C.21. Screening.*

For encounters for suspected fetal condition that are inconclusive following testing and evaluation, assign the appropriate code from category O35, O36, O4Ø or O41.

The observation Z code categories:

ZØ3	Encounter for medical observation for suspected diseases and conditions ruled out
ZØ4	Encounter for examination and observation for other reasons
	Except: ZØ4.9, Encounter for examination and observation for unspecified reason
ZØ5	Encounter for observation and evaluation of newborn for suspected diseases and conditions ruled out

7) Aftercare

Aftercare visit codes cover situations when the initial treatment of a disease has been performed and the patient requires continued care during the healing or recovery phase, or for the long-term consequences of the disease. The aftercare Z code should not be used if treatment is directed at a current, acute disease. The diagnosis code is to be used in these cases. Exceptions to this rule are codes Z51.Ø, Encounter for antineoplastic radiation therapy, and codes from subcategory Z51.1, Encounter for antineoplastic chemotherapy and immunotherapy. These codes are to be first listed, followed by the diagnosis code when a patient's encounter is solely to receive radiation therapy, chemotherapy, or immunotherapy for the treatment of a neoplasm. If the reason for the encounter is more than one type of antineoplastic therapy, code Z51.Ø and a code from subcategory Z51.1 may be assigned together, in which case one of these codes would be reported as a secondary diagnosis.

The aftercare Z codes should also not be used for aftercare for injuries. For aftercare of an injury, assign the acute injury code with the appropriate 7th character (for subsequent encounter).

The aftercare codes are generally first listed to explain the specific reason for the encounter. An aftercare code may be used as an additional code when some type of aftercare is provided in addition to the reason for admission and no diagnosis code is applicable. An example of this would be the closure of a colostomy during an encounter for treatment of another condition.

Aftercare codes should be used in conjunction with other aftercare codes or diagnosis codes to provide better detail on the specifics of an aftercare encounter visit, unless otherwise directed by the classification. The sequencing of multiple aftercare codes depends on the circumstances of the encounter.

Patient presents for third round of gemcitabine and first dose of antineoplastic radiation therapy for advanced pancreatic carcinoma

Z51.11	**Encounter for antineoplastic chemotherapy**
Z51.Ø	**Encounter for antineoplastic radiation therapy**
C25.9	**Malignant neoplasm of pancreas, unspecified**

Explanation: Gemcitabine is an antineoplastic chemotherapy. Since the encounter was solely to administer antineoplastic treatment, both forms of treatment are reported and either code can be the first-listed diagnosis, followed by the neoplastic condition code. Aftercare codes are typically not assigned for current treatment of disease; however, Z51.Ø and subcategory Z51.1 are an exception to this standard.

Certain aftercare Z code categories need a secondary diagnosis code to describe the resolving condition or sequelae. For others, the condition is included in the code title.

Additional Z code aftercare category terms include fitting and adjustment, and attention to artificial openings.

Status Z codes may be used with aftercare Z codes to indicate the nature of the aftercare. For example code Z95.1, Presence of aortocoronary bypass graft, may be used with code Z48.812, Encounter for surgical aftercare following surgery on the circulatory system, to indicate the surgery for which the aftercare is being performed. A status code should not be used when the aftercare code indicates the type of status, such as using Z43.Ø, Encounter for attention to tracheostomy, with Z93.Ø, Tracheostomy status.

The aftercare Z category/codes:

Z42	Encounter for plastic and reconstructive surgery following medical procedure or healed injury
Z43	Encounter for attention to artificial openings
Z44	Encounter for fitting and adjustment of external prosthetic device
Z45	Encounter for adjustment and management of implanted device
Z46	Encounter for fitting and adjustment of other devices
Z47	Orthopedic aftercare
Z48	Encounter for other postprocedural aftercare
Z49	Encounter for care involving renal dialysis
Z51	Encounter for other aftercare and medical care

8) Follow-up

The follow-up codes are used to explain continuing surveillance following completed treatment of a disease, condition, or injury. They imply that the condition has been fully treated and no longer exists. They should not be confused with aftercare codes, or injury codes with a 7th character for subsequent encounter, that explain ongoing care of a healing condition or its sequelae. Follow-up codes may be used in conjunction with history codes to provide the full picture of the healed condition and its treatment. The follow-up code is sequenced first, followed by the history code.

A follow-up code may be used to explain multiple visits. Should a condition be found to have recurred on the follow-up visit, then the diagnosis code for the condition should be assigned in place of the follow-up code.

The follow-up Z code categories:

ZØ8	Encounter for follow-up examination after completed treatment for malignant neoplasm
ZØ9	Encounter for follow-up examination after completed treatment for conditions other than malignant neoplasm
Z39	Encounter for maternal postpartum care and examination

Follow-up for patient several months after completing a regime of IV antibiotics for recurrent pneumonia; lungs are clear and pneumonia is resolved

ZØ9	**Encounter for follow-up examination after completed treatment for conditions other than malignant neoplasm**
Z87.Ø1	**Personal history of pneumonia (recurrent)**

Explanation: Code ZØ9 identifies the follow-up visit as being unrelated to a malignant neoplasm, and code Z87 describes the condition that has now resolved.

Follow-up for patient several months after completing a regime of IV antibiotics for recurrent pneumonia; pneumonia has recurred, and a new antibiotic regimen has been prescribed

J18.9 Pneumonia, unspecified organism

Explanation: Since the follow-up exam for pneumonia determined that the pneumonia was not resolved or recurred, code Z09 Encounter for follow-up examination after completed treatment for conditions other than malignant neoplasm, no longer applies. Instead the first-listed code describes the pneumonia.

9) Donor

Codes in category Z52, Donors of organs and tissues, are used for living individuals who are donating blood or other body tissue. These codes are for individuals donating for others, as well as for self-donations. They are not used to identify cadaveric donations.

10)Counseling

Counseling Z codes are used when a patient or family member receives assistance in the aftermath of an illness or injury, or when support is required in coping with family or social problems.

The counseling Z codes/categories:

Z30.Ø-	Encounter for general counseling and advice on contraception
Z31.5	Encounter for procreative genetic counseling
Z31.6-	Encounter for general counseling and advice on procreation
Z32.2	Encounter for childbirth instruction
Z32.3	Encounter for childcare instruction
Z69	Encounter for mental health services for victim and perpetrator of abuse
Z7Ø	Counseling related to sexual attitude, behavior and orientation
Z71	Persons encountering health services for other counseling and medical advice, not elsewhere classified

Note: Code Z71.84, Encounter for health counseling related to travel, is to be used for health risk and safety counseling for future travel purposes.

Code Z71.85, Encounter for immunization safety counseling, is to be used for counseling of the patient or caregiver regarding the safety of a vaccine. This code should not be used for the provision of general information regarding risks and potential side effects during routine encounters for the administration of vaccines.

Code Z71.87, Encounter for pediatric-to-adult transition counseling, should be assigned when pediatric-to-adult transition counseling is the sole reason for the encounter or when this counseling is provided in addition to other services, such as treatment of a chronic condition. If both transition counseling and treatment of a medical condition are provided during the same encounter, the code(s) for the medical condition(s) treated and code Z71.87 should be assigned, with sequencing depending on the circumstances of the encounter.

Z76.81	Expectant mother prebirth pediatrician visit

11)Encounters for obstetrical and reproductive services

See Section I.C.15. Pregnancy, Childbirth, and the Puerperium, for further instruction on the use of these codes.

Z codes for pregnancy are for use in those circumstances when none of the problems or complications included in the codes from the Obstetrics chapter exist (a routine prenatal visit or postpartum care). Codes in category Z34, Encounter for supervision of normal pregnancy, are always first-listed and are not to be used with any other code from the OB chapter.

Codes in category Z3A, Weeks of gestation, may be assigned to provide additional information about the pregnancy. Category Z3A codes should not be assigned for pregnancies with abortive outcomes (categories OØØ-OØ8), elective termination of pregnancy (code Z33.2), nor for postpartum conditions, as category Z3A is not applicable to these conditions. The date of the admission should be used to determine weeks of gestation for inpatient admissions that encompass more than one gestational week.

The outcome of delivery, category Z37, should be included on all maternal delivery records. It is always a secondary code.

Codes in category Z37 should not be used on the newborn record.

Z codes for family planning (contraceptive) or procreative management and counseling should be included on an obstetric record either during the pregnancy or the postpartum stage, if applicable.

Z codes/categories for obstetrical and reproductive services:

Z3Ø	Encounter for contraceptive management
Z31	Encounter for procreative management
Z32.2	Encounter for childbirth instruction
Z32.3	Encounter for childcare instruction
Z33	Pregnant state
Z34	Encounter for supervision of normal pregnancy
Z36	Encounter for antenatal screening of mother
Z3A	Weeks of gestation
Z37	Outcome of delivery
Z39	Encounter for maternal postpartum care and examination
Z76.81	Expectant mother prebirth pediatrician visit

12)Newborns and infants

See Section I.C.16. Newborn (Perinatal) Guidelines, for further instruction on the use of these codes.

Newborn Z codes/categories:

Z76.1	Encounter for health supervision and care of foundling
ZØØ.1-	Encounter for routine child health examination
Z38	Liveborn infants according to place of birth and type of delivery

13)Routine and administrative examinations

The Z codes allow for the description of encounters for routine examinations, such as, a general check-up, or, examinations for administrative purposes, such as, a pre-employment physical. The codes are not to be used if the examination is for diagnosis of a suspected condition or for treatment purposes. In such cases the diagnosis code is used. During a routine exam, should a diagnosis or condition be discovered, it should be coded as an additional code. Pre-existing and chronic conditions and history codes may also be included as additional codes as long as the examination is for administrative purposes and not focused on any particular condition.

Some of the codes for routine health examinations distinguish between "with" and "without" abnormal findings. Code assignment depends on the information that is known at the time the encounter is being coded. For example, if no abnormal findings were found during the examination, but the encounter is being coded before test results are back, it is acceptable to assign the code for "without abnormal findings." When assigning a code for "with abnormal findings," additional code(s) should be assigned to identify the specific abnormal finding(s).

12-month-old boy presented for well-child visit; pediatrician notices some eczema on the child's scalp and back of the knees

ZØØ.121 Encounter for routine child health examination with abnormal findings

L3Ø.9 Dermatitis, unspecified

Explanation: The Z code identifying that this is a routine well-child visit is reported first. Because an abnormal finding (eczema) was documented, a code for this condition may also be appended.

Pre-operative examination and pre-procedural laboratory examination Z codes are for use only in those situations when a patient is being cleared for a procedure or surgery and no treatment is given.

The Z codes/categories for routine and administrative examinations:

ZØØ	Encounter for general examination without complaint, suspected or reported diagnosis
ZØ1	Encounter for other special examination without complaint, suspected or reported diagnosis
ZØ2	Encounter for administrative examination
	Except: ZØ2.9, Encounter for administrative examinations, unspecified
Z32.Ø-	Encounter for pregnancy test

14)Miscellaneous Z codes

The miscellaneous Z codes capture a number of other health care encounters that do not fall into one of the other categories. Some of these codes identify the reason for the encounter; others are for use as additional codes that provide useful information on circumstances that may affect a patient's care and treatment.

Prophylactic organ removal

For encounters specifically for prophylactic removal of an organ (such as prophylactic removal of breasts due to a genetic susceptibility to cancer or a family history of cancer), the principal or first-listed code should be a code from category Z4Ø, Encounter for prophylactic surgery, followed by the appropriate codes to identify the associated risk factor (such as genetic susceptibility or family history).

If the patient has a malignancy of one site and is having prophylactic removal at another site to prevent either a new primary malignancy or metastatic disease, a code for the malignancy should also be assigned in addition to a code from subcategory Z4Ø.Ø, Encounter for prophylactic surgery for risk factors related to malignant neoplasms. A Z4Ø.Ø code should not be assigned if the patient is having organ removal for treatment of a malignancy, such as the removal of the testes for the treatment of prostate cancer.

Miscellaneous Z codes/categories:

- Z28 Immunization not carried out
  Except: Z28.3-, Underimmunization status
- Z29 Encounter for other prophylactic measures
- Z4Ø Encounter for prophylactic surgery
- Z41 Encounter for procedures for purposes other than remedying health state
  Except: Z41.9, Encounter for procedure for purposes other than remedying health state, unspecified
- Z53 Persons encountering health services for specific procedures and treatment, not carried out
- Z72 Problems related to lifestyle
  Note: These codes should be assigned only when the documentation specifies that the patient has an associated problem
- Z73 Problems related to life management difficulty
  Note: These codes should be assigned only when the documentation specifies that the patient has an associated problem.
- Z74 Problems related to care provider dependency
  Except: Z74.Ø1, Bed confinement status
- Z75 Problems related to medical facilities and other health care
- Z76.Ø Encounter for issue of repeat prescription
- Z76.3 Healthy person accompanying sick person
- Z76.4 Other boarder to healthcare facility
- Z76.5 Malingerer [conscious simulation]
- Z91.1- Patient's noncompliance with medical treatment and regimen
- Z91.83 Wandering in diseases classified elsewhere
- Z91.84- Oral health risk factors
- Z91.89 Other specified personal risk factors, not elsewhere classified

See Section I.B.14. for Z55-Z65 Persons with potential health hazards related to socioeconomic and psychosocial circumstances, documentation by clinicians other than the patient's provider

15)Nonspecific Z codes

Certain Z codes are so non-specific, or potentially redundant with other codes in the classification, that there can be little justification for their use in the inpatient setting. Their use in the outpatient setting should be limited to those instances when there is no further documentation to permit more precise coding. Otherwise, any sign or symptom or any other reason for visit that is captured in another code should be used.

Nonspecific Z codes/categories:

- ZØ2.9 Encounter for administrative examinations, unspecified
- ZØ4.9 Encounter for examination and observation for unspecified reason
- Z13.9 Encounter for screening, unspecified
- Z41.9 Encounter for procedure for purposes other than remedying health state, unspecified
- Z52.9 Donor of unspecified organ or tissue
- Z86.59 Personal history of other mental and behavioral disorders
- Z88.9 Allergy status to unspecified drugs, medicaments and biological substances status
- Z92.Ø Personal history of contraception

16)Z codes that may only be principal/first-listed diagnosis

The following Z codes/categories may only be reported as the principal/first-listed diagnosis, except when there are multiple encounters on the same day and the medical records for the encounters are combined:

- ZØØ Encounter for general examination without complaint, suspected or reported diagnosis
  Except: ZØØ.6
- ZØ1 Encounter for other special examination without complaint, suspected or reported diagnosis
- ZØ2 Encounter for administrative examination
- ZØ4 Encounter for examination and observation for other reasons
- Z33.2 Encounter for elective termination of pregnancy
- Z31.81 Encounter for male factor infertility in female patient
- Z31.83 Encounter for assisted reproductive fertility procedure cycle
- Z31.84 Encounter for fertility preservation procedure
- Z34 Encounter for supervision of normal pregnancy
- Z39 Encounter for maternal postpartum care and examination
- Z38 Liveborn infants according to place of birth and type of delivery
- Z4Ø Encounter for prophylactic surgery
- Z42 Encounter for plastic and reconstructive surgery following medical procedure or healed injury
- Z51.Ø Encounter for antineoplastic radiation therapy
- Z51.1- Encounter for antineoplastic chemotherapy and immunotherapy
- Z52 Donors of organs and tissues
  Except: Z52.9, Donor of unspecified organ or tissue
- Z76.1 Encounter for health supervision and care of foundling
- Z76.2 Encounter for health supervision and care of other healthy infant and child
- Z99.12 Encounter for respirator [ventilator] dependence during power failure

Female patient seen at 32 weeks' gestation to check the progress of her first pregnancy

Z34.Ø3 Encounter for supervision of normal first pregnancy, third trimester

Z3A.32 32 weeks gestation of pregnancy

Explanation: Category Z34 is appropriate as a first-listed diagnosis. Category Z3A helps to clarify at which point in the pregnancy the patient was provided supervision.

17)Social determinants of health

Codes describing **problems or risk factors related to** social determinants of health (SDOH) should be assigned when this information is documented. **Assign as many SDOH codes as are necessary to describe all of the problems or risk factors. These codes should be assigned only when the documentation specifies that the patient has an associated problem or risk factor. For example, not every individual living alone would be assigned code Z60.2, Problems related to living alone.**

For social determinants of health, such as information found in categories Z55-Z65, Persons with potential health hazards related to socioeconomic and psychosocial circumstances, code assignment may be based on medical record documentation from clinicians involved in the care of the patient who are not the patient's provider since this information represents social information, rather than medical diagnoses.

For example, coding professionals may utilize documentation of social information from social workers, community health workers, case managers, or nurses, if their documentation is included in the official medical record.

Patient self-reported documentation may be used to assign codes for social determinants of health, as long as the patient self-reported information is signed-off by and incorporated into the medical record by either a clinician or provider.

Social determinants of health codes are located primarily in these Z code categories:

- Z55 Problems related to education and literacy
- Z56 Problems related to employment and unemployment
- Z57 Occupational exposure to risk factors
- Z58 Problems related to physical environment
- Z59 Problems related to housing and economic circumstances
- Z6Ø Problems related to social environment
- Z62 Problems related to upbringing
- Z63 Other problems related to primary support group, including family circumstances
- Z64 Problems related to certain psychosocial circumstances
- Z65 Problems related to other psychosocial circumstances

See Section I.B.14. Documentation by Clinicians Other than the Patient's Provider.

Chapter 21. Factors Influencing Health Status and Contact With Health Services (Z00-Z99)

NOTE Z codes represent reasons for encounters. A corresponding procedure code must accompany a Z code if a procedure is performed. Categories Z00-Z99 are provided for occasions when circumstances other than a disease, injury or external cause classifiable to categories A00-Y89 are recorded as "diagnoses" or "problems." This can arise in two main ways:

(a) When a person who may or may not be sick encounters the health services for some specific purpose, such as to receive limited care or service for a current condition, to donate an organ or tissue, to receive prophylactic vaccination (immunization), or to discuss a problem which is in itself not a disease or injury.

(b) When some circumstance or problem is present which influences the person's health status but is not in itself a current illness or injury.

AHA: 2018,4Q,60-61

This chapter contains the following blocks:

- Z00-Z13 Persons encountering health services for examinations
- Z14-Z15 Genetic carrier and genetic susceptibility to disease
- Z16 Resistance to antimicrobial drugs
- Z17 Estrogen receptor status
- Z18 Retained foreign body fragments
- Z19 Hormone sensitivity malignancy status
- Z20-Z29 Persons with potential health hazards related to communicable diseases
- Z30-Z39 Persons encountering health services in circumstances related to reproduction
- Z40-Z53 Encounters for other specific health care
- Z55-Z65 Persons with potential health hazards related to socioeconomic and psychosocial circumstances
- Z66 Do not resuscitate status
- Z67 Blood type
- Z68 Body mass index (BMI)
- Z69-Z76 Persons encountering health services in other circumstances
- Z77-Z99 Persons with potential health hazards related to family and personal history and certain conditions influencing health status

Persons encountering health services for examinations (Z00-Z13)

NOTE Nonspecific abnormal findings disclosed at the time of these examinations are classified to categories R70-R94.

EXCLUDES 1 *examinations related to pregnancy and reproduction (Z30-Z36, Z39.-)*

✓4th **Z00 Encounter for general examination without complaint, suspected or reported diagnosis**

EXCLUDES 1 *encounter for examination for administrative purposes (Z02.-)*

EXCLUDES 2 *encounter for pre-procedural examinations (Z01.81-)*
special screening examinations (Z11-Z13)

AHA: 2017,4Q,95

✓5th **Z00.0 Encounter for general adult medical examination**

Encounter for adult periodic examination (annual) (physical) and any associated laboratory and radiologic examinations

EXCLUDES 1 *encounter for examination of sign or symptom - code to sign or symptom*
general health check-up of infant or child (Z00.12.-)

Z00.00 Encounter for general adult medical examination without abnormal findings PDx A

Encounter for adult health check-up NOS

AHA: 2016,1Q,36

Z00.01 Encounter for general adult medical examination with abnormal findings PDx A

Use additional code to identify abnormal findings

AHA: 2016,1Q,35-36

✓5th **Z00.1 Encounter for newborn, infant and child health examinations**

✓6th **Z00.11 Newborn health examination**

Health check for child under 29 days old

Use additional code to identify any abnormal findings

EXCLUDES 1 *health check for child over 28 days old (Z00.12-)*

Z00.110 Health examination for newborn under 8 days old PDx N

Health check for newborn under 8 days old

Z00.111 Health examination for newborn 8 to 28 days old PDx N

Health check for newborn 8 to 28 days old

Newborn weight check

✓6th **Z00.12 Encounter for routine child health examination**

Health check (routine) for child over 28 days old

Immunizations appropriate for age

Routine developmental screening of infant or child

Routine vison and hearing testing

EXCLUDES 1 *health check for child under 29 days old (Z00.11-)*
health supervision of foundling or other healthy infant or child (Z76.1-Z76.2)
newborn health examination (Z00.11-)

AHA: 2018,4Q,36

Z00.121 Encounter for routine child health examination with abnormal findings PDx P

Use additional code to identify abnormal findings

AHA: 2016,1Q,34-35

Z00.129 Encounter for routine child health examination without abnormal findings PDx P

Encounter for routine child health examination NOS

AHA: 2016,1Q,34

Z00.2 Encounter for examination for period of rapid growth in childhood PDx P

Z00.3 Encounter for examination for adolescent development state PDx P

Encounter for puberty development state

Z00.5 Encounter for examination of potential donor of organ and tissue PDx

Z00.6 Encounter for examination for normal comparison and control in clinical research program

Examination of participant or control in clinical research program

✓5th **Z00.7 Encounter for examination for period of delayed growth in childhood**

Z00.70 Encounter for examination for period of delayed growth in childhood without abnormal findings PDx P

Z00.71 Encounter for examination for period of delayed growth in childhood with abnormal findings PDx P

Use additional code to identify abnormal findings

Z00.8 Encounter for other general examination PDx

Encounter for health examination in population surveys

✓4th **Z01 Encounter for other special examination without complaint, suspected or reported diagnosis**

INCLUDES routine examination of specific system

NOTE Codes from category Z01 represent the reason for the encounter. A separate procedure code is required to identify any examinations or procedures performed

EXCLUDES 1 *encounter for examination for administrative purposes (Z02.-)*
encounter for examination for suspected conditions, proven not to exist (Z03.-)
encounter for laboratory and radiologic examinations as a component of general medical examinations (Z00.0-)
encounter for laboratory, radiologic and imaging examinations for sign(s) and symptom(s) - code to the sign(s) or symptom(s)

EXCLUDES 2 *screening examinations (Z11-Z13)*

✓5th **Z01.0 Encounter for examination of eyes and vision**

EXCLUDES 1 *examination for driving license (Z02.4)*

Z01.00 Encounter for examination of eyes and vision without abnormal findings PDx

Encounter for examination of eyes and vision NOS

Z01.01 Encounter for examination of eyes and vision with abnormal findings PDx

Use additional code to identify abnormal findings

AHA: 2016,4Q,21

Z01.02 Encounter for examination of eyes and vision following failed vision screening
EXCLUDES 1 *encounter for examination of eyes and vision with abnormal findings (Z01.01)*
encounter for examination of eyes and vision without abnormal findings (Z01.00)
AHA: 2019,4Q,20

Z01.020 Encounter for examination of eyes and vision following failed vision screening without abnormal findings PDx

Z01.021 Encounter for examination of eyes and vision following failed vision screening with abnormal findings PDx
Use additional code to identify abnormal findings

Z01.1 Encounter for examination of ears and hearing

Z01.10 Encounter for examination of ears and hearing without abnormal findings PDx
Encounter for examination of ears and hearing NOS
AHA: 2016,4Q,24

Z01.11 Encounter for examination of ears and hearing with abnormal findings
AHA: 2016,3Q,17-18

Z01.110 Encounter for hearing examination following failed hearing screening PDx

Z01.118 Encounter for examination of ears and hearing with other abnormal findings PDx
Use additional code to identify abnormal findings

Z01.12 Encounter for hearing conservation and treatment PDx

Z01.2 Encounter for dental examination and cleaning

Z01.20 Encounter for dental examination and cleaning without abnormal findings PDx
Encounter for dental examination and cleaning NOS

Z01.21 Encounter for dental examination and cleaning with abnormal findings PDx
Use additional code to identify abnormal findings

Z01.3 Encounter for examination of blood pressure

Z01.30 Encounter for examination of blood pressure without abnormal findings PDx
Encounter for examination of blood pressure NOS

Z01.31 Encounter for examination of blood pressure with abnormal findings PDx
Use additional code to identify abnormal findings

Z01.4 Encounter for gynecological examination
EXCLUDES 2 *pregnancy examination or test (Z32.0-)*
routine examination for contraceptive maintenance (Z30.4-)

Z01.41 Encounter for routine gynecological examination
Encounter for general gynecological examination with or without cervical smear
Encounter for gynecological examination (general) (routine) NOS
Encounter for pelvic examination (annual) (periodic)
Use additional code:
for screening for human papillomavirus, if applicable, (Z11.51)
for screening vaginal pap smear, if applicable (Z12.72)
to identify acquired absence of uterus, if applicable (Z90.71-)
EXCLUDES 1 *gynecologic examination status-post hysterectomy for malignant condition (Z08)*
screening cervical pap smear not a part of a routine gynecological examination (Z12.4)

Z01.411 Encounter for gynecological examination (general) (routine) with abnormal findings PDx ♀
Use additional code to identify abnormal findings

Z01.419 Encounter for gynecological examination (general) (routine) without abnormal findings PDx ♀

Z01.42 Encounter for cervical smear to confirm findings of recent normal smear following initial abnormal smear PDx ♀

Z01.8 Encounter for other specified special examinations

Z01.81 Encounter for preprocedural examinations
Encounter for preoperative examinations
Encounter for radiological and imaging examinations as part of preprocedural examination
TIP: Assign a code for the condition necessitating surgery and any findings as additional diagnoses.

Z01.810 Encounter for preprocedural cardiovascular examination PDx

Z01.811 Encounter for preprocedural respiratory examination PDx

Z01.812 Encounter for preprocedural laboratory examination PDx
Blood and urine tests prior to treatment or procedure
AHA: 2020,3Q,14
TIP: During the COVID-19 pandemic, assign this code followed by code Z20.822 Contact with and (suspected) exposure to COVID-19, when COVID-19 testing is being performed as part of preoperative testing.

Z01.818 Encounter for other preprocedural examination PDx
Encounter for preprocedural examination NOS
Encounter for examinations prior to antineoplastic chemotherapy

Z01.82 Encounter for allergy testing PDx
EXCLUDES 1 *encounter for antibody response examination (Z01.84)*

Z01.83 Encounter for blood typing PDx
Encounter for Rh typing

Z01.84 Encounter for antibody response examination PDx
Encounter for immunity status testing
EXCLUDES 1 *encounter for allergy testing (Z01.82)*
AHA: 2020,2Q,11

Z01.89 Encounter for other specified special examinations PDx

Z02 Encounter for administrative examination

Z02.0 Encounter for examination for admission to educational institution PDx
Encounter for examination for admission to preschool (education)
Encounter for examination for re-admission to school following illness or medical treatment

Z02.1 Encounter for pre-employment examination PDx

Z02.2 Encounter for examination for admission to residential institution PDx
EXCLUDES 1 *examination for admission to prison (Z02.89)*

Z02.3 Encounter for examination for recruitment to armed forces PDx

Z02.4 Encounter for examination for driving license PDx

Z02.5 Encounter for examination for participation in sport PDx
EXCLUDES 1 *blood-alcohol and blood-drug test (Z02.83)*

Z02.6 Encounter for examination for insurance purposes PDx

Z02.7 Encounter for issue of medical certificate
EXCLUDES 1 *encounter for general medical examination (Z00-Z01, Z02.0-Z02.6, Z02.8-Z02.9)*

Z02.71 Encounter for disability determination PDx
Encounter for issue of medical certificate of incapacity
Encounter for issue of medical certificate of invalidity

Z02.79 Encounter for issue of other medical certificate PDx

Z02.8 Encounter for other administrative examinations

Z02.81 Encounter for paternity testing PDx

Z02.82 Encounter for adoption services PDx

Z02.83 Encounter for blood-alcohol and blood-drug test PDx

Use additional code for findings of alcohol or drugs in blood (R78.-)

Z02.89 Encounter for other administrative examinations PDx

Encounter for examination for admission to prison

Encounter for examination for admission to summer camp

Encounter for immigration examination

Encounter for naturalization examination

Encounter for premarital examination

EXCLUDES 1 *health supervision of foundling or other healthy infant or child (Z76.1-Z76.2)*

Z02.9 Encounter for administrative examinations, unspecified PDx

✓4th **Z03 Encounter for medical observation for suspected diseases and conditions ruled out**

This category is to be used when a person without a diagnosis is suspected of having an abnormal condition, without signs or symptoms, which requires study, but after examination and observation, is ruled out. This category is also for use for administrative and legal observation status.

EXCLUDES 1 *contact with and (suspected) exposures hazardous to health (Z77.-)*

encounter for observation and evaluation of newborn for suspected diseases and conditions ruled out (Z05.-)

person with feared complaint in whom no diagnosis is made (Z71.1)

signs or symptoms under study - code to signs or symptoms

AHA: 2020,2Q,8; 2018,2Q,7-8; 2017,4Q,27

Z03.6 Encounter for observation for suspected toxic effect from ingested substance ruled out

Encounter for observation for suspected adverse effect from drug

Encounter for observation for suspected poisoning

✓5th **Z03.7 Encounter for suspected maternal and fetal conditions ruled out**

Encounter for suspected maternal and fetal conditions not found

EXCLUDES 1 *known or suspected fetal anomalies affecting management of mother, not ruled out (O26.-, O35.-, O36.-, O40.-, O41.-)*

Z03.71 Encounter for suspected problem with amniotic cavity and membrane ruled out M ♀

Encounter for suspected oligohydramnios ruled out

Encounter for suspected polyhydramnios ruled out

Z03.72 Encounter for suspected placental problem ruled out M ♀

Z03.73 Encounter for suspected fetal anomaly ruled out M ♀

Z03.74 Encounter for suspected problem with fetal growth ruled out M ♀

Z03.75 Encounter for suspected cervical shortening ruled out M ♀

Z03.79 Encounter for other suspected maternal and fetal conditions ruled out M ♀

✓5th **Z03.8 Encounter for observation for other suspected diseases and conditions ruled out**

✓6th **Z03.81 Encounter for observation for suspected exposure to biological agents ruled out**

Z03.810 Encounter for observation for suspected exposure to anthrax ruled out

Z03.818 Encounter for observation for suspected exposure to other biological agents ruled out

AHA: 2020,2Q,8; 2020,1Q,34-36

TIP: During the COVID-19 pandemic, possible exposure to COVID-19 should be coded using Z20.822 Contact with and (suspected) exposure to COVID-19, even when the COVID-19 infection has been ruled out.

✓6th **Z03.82 Encounter for observation for suspected foreign body ruled out**

EXCLUDES 1 *retained foreign body (Z18.-)*

retained foreign body in eyelid (H02.81)

residual foreign body in soft tissue (M79.5)

EXCLUDES 2 *confirmed foreign body ingestion or aspiration including:*

foreign body in alimentary tract (T18)

foreign body in ear (T16)

foreign body on external eye (T15)

foreign body in respiratory tract (T17)

AHA: 2020,4Q,42

Z03.821 Encounter for observation for suspected ingested foreign body ruled out

Z03.822 Encounter for observation for suspected aspirated (inhaled) foreign body ruled out

Z03.823 Encounter for observation for suspected inserted (injected) foreign body ruled out

Encounter for observation for suspected inserted (injected) foreign body in eye ruled out

Encounter for observation for suspected inserted (injected) foreign body in orifice ruled out

Encounter for observation for suspected inserted (injected) foreign body in skin ruled out

● **Z03.83 Encounter for observation for suspected conditions related to home physiologic monitoring device ruled out**

Encounter for observation for apnea alarm without findings

Encounter for observation for bradycardia alarm without findings

Encounter for observation for malfunction of home cardiorespiratory monitor

Encounter for observation for non-specific findings home physiologic monitoring device

Encounter for observation for pulse oximeter alarm without findings

EXCLUDES 1 *apnea NOS (R06.81)*

neonatal bradycardia (P29.12)

newborn apnea (P28.4-)

primary sleep apnea of newborn (P28.3-)

sleep apnea (G47.3-)

Z03.89 Encounter for observation for other suspected diseases and conditions ruled out

✓4th **Z04 Encounter for examination and observation for other reasons**

INCLUDES encounter for examination for medicolegal reasons

This category is to be used when a person without a diagnosis is suspected of having an abnormal condition, without signs or symptoms, which requires study, but after examination and observation, is ruled-out. This category is also for use for administrative and legal observation status.

AHA: 2018,2Q,7-8

Z04.1 Encounter for examination and observation following transport accident PDx

EXCLUDES 1 *encounter for examination and observation following work accident (Z04.2)*

AHA: 2019,2Q,11; 2018,2Q,8

Z04.2 Encounter for examination and observation following work accident PDx

Z04.3 Encounter for examination and observation following other accident PDx

✓5th **Z04.4 Encounter for examination and observation following alleged rape**

Encounter for examination and observation of victim following alleged rape

Encounter for examination and observation of victim following alleged sexual abuse

Z04.41 Encounter for examination and observation following alleged adult rape PDx A

Suspected adult rape, ruled out

Suspected adult sexual abuse, ruled out

Z04.42 **Encounter for examination and observation following alleged child rape** PDx P
Suspected child rape, ruled out
Suspected child sexual abuse, ruled out

Z04.6 **Encounter for general psychiatric examination, requested by authority** PDx

✓5th Z04.7 **Encounter for examination and observation following alleged physical abuse**

Z04.71 **Encounter for examination and observation following alleged adult physical abuse** PDx A
Suspected adult physical abuse, ruled out
EXCLUDES 1 *confirmed case of adult physical abuse (T74.-)*
encounter for examination and observation following alleged adult sexual abuse (Z04.41)
suspected case of adult physical abuse, not ruled out (T76.-)

Z04.72 **Encounter for examination and observation following alleged child physical abuse** PDx P
Suspected child physical abuse, ruled out
EXCLUDES 1 *confirmed case of child physical abuse (T74.-)*
encounter for examination and observation following alleged child sexual abuse (Z04.42)
suspected case of child physical abuse, not ruled out (T76.-)

✓5th Z04.8 **Encounter for examination and observation for other specified reasons**
Encounter for examination and observation for request for expert evidence
AHA: 2018,4Q,32,35,72

Z04.81 **Encounter for examination and observation of victim following forced sexual exploitation** PDx

Z04.82 **Encounter for examination and observation of victim following forced labor exploitation** PDx

Z04.89 **Encounter for examination and observation for other specified reasons** PDx

Z04.9 **Encounter for examination and observation for unspecified reason** PDx
Encounter for observation NOS

✓4th Z05 **Encounter for observation and evaluation of newborn for suspected diseases and conditions ruled out**
This category is to be used for newborns, within the neonatal period (the first 28 days of life), who are suspected of having an abnormal condition, but without signs or symptoms, and which, after examination and observation, is ruled out.
AHA: 2022,1Q,17-18; 2017,4Q,27; 2016,4Q,77

Z05.0 **Observation and evaluation of newborn for suspected cardiac condition ruled out** N

Z05.1 **Observation and evaluation of newborn for suspected infectious condition ruled out** N
AHA: 2019,2Q,10

Z05.2 **Observation and evaluation of newborn for suspected neurological condition ruled out** N

Z05.3 **Observation and evaluation of newborn for suspected respiratory condition ruled out** N

✓5th Z05.4 **Observation and evaluation of newborn for suspected genetic, metabolic or immunologic condition ruled out**

Z05.41 **Observation and evaluation of newborn for suspected genetic condition ruled out** N
AHA: 2016,4Q,55

Z05.42 **Observation and evaluation of newborn for suspected metabolic condition ruled out** N

Z05.43 **Observation and evaluation of newborn for suspected immunologic condition ruled out** N

Z05.5 **Observation and evaluation of newborn for suspected gastrointestinal condition ruled out** N

Z05.6 **Observation and evaluation of newborn for suspected genitourinary condition ruled out** N

✓5th Z05.7 **Observation and evaluation of newborn for suspected skin, subcutaneous, musculoskeletal and connective tissue condition ruled out**

Z05.71 **Observation and evaluation of newborn for suspected skin and subcutaneous tissue condition ruled out** N

Z05.72 **Observation and evaluation of newborn for suspected musculoskeletal condition ruled out** N

Z05.73 **Observation and evaluation of newborn for suspected connective tissue condition ruled out** N

Z05.8 **Observation and evaluation of newborn for other specified suspected condition ruled out** N
AHA: 2022,1Q,17-18

Z05.9 **Observation and evaluation of newborn for unspecified suspected condition ruled out** N

Z08 **Encounter for follow-up examination after completed treatment for malignant neoplasm**
Medical surveillance following completed treatment
Use additional code to identify any acquired absence of organs (Z90.-)
Use additional code to identify the personal history of malignant neoplasm (Z85.-)
EXCLUDES 1 *aftercare following medical care (Z43-Z49, Z51)*
AHA: 2020,3Q,30

Z09 **Encounter for follow-up examination after completed treatment for conditions other than malignant neoplasm**
Medical surveillance following completed treatment
Use additional code to identify any applicable history of disease code (Z86.-, Z87.-)
EXCLUDES 1 *aftercare following medical care (Z43-Z49, Z51)*
surveillance of contraception (Z30.4-)
surveillance of prosthetic and other medical devices (Z44-Z46)
AHA: 2021,1Q,33; 2020,2Q,10; 2017,1Q,9; 2015,1Q,8

✓4th Z11 **Encounter for screening for infectious and parasitic diseases**
Screening is the testing for disease or disease precursors in asymptomatic individuals so that early detection and treatment can be provided for those who test positive for the disease.
EXCLUDES 1 *encounter for diagnostic examination - code to sign or symptom*

Z11.0 **Encounter for screening for intestinal infectious diseases**

Z11.1 **Encounter for screening for respiratory tuberculosis**
Encounter for screening for active tuberculosis disease

Z11.2 **Encounter for screening for other bacterial diseases**

Z11.3 **Encounter for screening for infections with a predominantly sexual mode of transmission**
EXCLUDES 2 *encounter for screening for human immunodeficiency virus [HIV] (Z11.4)*
encounter for screening for human papillomavirus (Z11.51)

Z11.4 **Encounter for screening for human immunodeficiency virus [HIV]**

✓5th Z11.5 **Encounter for screening for other viral diseases**
EXCLUDES 2 *encounter for screening for viral intestinal disease (Z11.0)*

Z11.51 **Encounter for screening for human papillomavirus (HPV)**

Z11.52 **Encounter for screening for COVID-19**
AHA: 2021,1Q,27,37,41
TIP: This code is not appropriate for use during the pandemic phase of COVID-19. Use Z20.822 Contact with or (suspected) exposure to COVID-19, instead.

Z11.59 **Encounter for screening for other viral diseases**
AHA: 2020,3Q,14

Z11.6 **Encounter for screening for other protozoal diseases and helminthiases**
EXCLUDES 2 *encounter for screening for protozoal intestinal disease (Z11.0)*

Z11.7 **Encounter for testing for latent tuberculosis infection**
AHA: 2019,4Q,20

Z11.8 **Encounter for screening for other infectious and parasitic diseases**
Encounter for screening for chlamydia
Encounter for screening for rickettsial
Encounter for screening for spirochetal
Encounter for screening for mycoses

Z11.9 **Encounter for screening for infectious and parasitic diseases, unspecified**

Z12 Encounter for screening for malignant neoplasms

Screening is the testing for disease or disease precursors in asymptomatic individuals so that early detection and treatment can be provided for those who test positive for the disease.

Use additional code to identify any family history of malignant neoplasm (Z80.-)

EXCLUDES 1 *encounter for diagnostic examination - code to sign or symptom*

Z12.0 Encounter for screening for malignant neoplasm of stomach

Z12.1 Encounter for screening for malignant neoplasm of intestinal tract

AHA: 2017,1Q,8,9

Z12.10 Encounter for screening for malignant neoplasm of intestinal tract, unspecified

Z12.11 Encounter for screening for malignant neoplasm of colon

Encounter for screening colonoscopy NOS

AHA: 2019,1Q,32-33; 2018,1Q,6

TIP: Surveillance colonoscopies are a type of screening exam used to screen for malignancies in those patients with history of polyps and/or cancer (previously removed). If polyps or cancer are removed during the colonoscopy, code the appropriate neoplasm code instead of Z12.11.

Z12.12 Encounter for screening for malignant neoplasm of rectum

AHA: 2018,1Q,6

Z12.13 Encounter for screening for malignant neoplasm of small intestine

Z12.2 Encounter for screening for malignant neoplasm of respiratory organs

Z12.3 Encounter for screening for malignant neoplasm of breast

Z12.31 Encounter for screening mammogram for malignant neoplasm of breast

EXCLUDES 1 *inconclusive mammogram (R92.2)*

AHA: 2015,1Q,24

Z12.39 Encounter for other screening for malignant neoplasm of breast

Z12.4 Encounter for screening for malignant neoplasm of cervix ♀

Encounter for screening pap smear for malignant neoplasm of cervix

EXCLUDES 1 *when screening is part of general gynecological examination (Z01.4-)*

EXCLUDES 2 *encounter for screening for human papillomavirus (Z11.51)*

Z12.5 Encounter for screening for malignant neoplasm of prostate ♂

Z12.6 Encounter for screening for malignant neoplasm of bladder

Z12.7 Encounter for screening for malignant neoplasm of other genitourinary organs

Z12.71 Encounter for screening for malignant neoplasm of testis ♂

Z12.72 Encounter for screening for malignant neoplasm of vagina ♀

Vaginal pap smear status-post hysterectomy for non-malignant condition

Use additional code to identify acquired absence of uterus (Z90.71-)

EXCLUDES 1 *vaginal pap smear status-post hysterectomy for malignant conditions (Z08)*

Z12.73 Encounter for screening for malignant neoplasm of ovary ♀

Z12.79 Encounter for screening for malignant neoplasm of other genitourinary organs

Z12.8 Encounter for screening for malignant neoplasm of other sites

Z12.81 Encounter for screening for malignant neoplasm of oral cavity

Z12.82 Encounter for screening for malignant neoplasm of nervous system

Z12.83 Encounter for screening for malignant neoplasm of skin

Z12.89 Encounter for screening for malignant neoplasm of other sites

AHA: 2021,1Q,14

Z12.9 Encounter for screening for malignant neoplasm, site unspecified

Z13 Encounter for screening for other diseases and disorders

Screening is the testing for disease or disease precursors in asymptomatic individuals so that early detection and treatment can be provided for those who test positive for the disease.

EXCLUDES 1 *encounter for diagnostic examination - code to sign or symptom*

Z13.0 Encounter for screening for diseases of the blood and blood-forming organs and certain disorders involving the immune mechanism

Z13.1 Encounter for screening for diabetes mellitus

Z13.2 Encounter for screening for nutritional, metabolic and other endocrine disorders

Z13.21 Encounter for screening for nutritional disorder

Z13.22 Encounter for screening for metabolic disorder

Z13.220 Encounter for screening for lipoid disorders

Encounter for screening for cholesterol level

Encounter for screening for hypercholesterolemia

Encounter for screening for hyperlipidemia

Z13.228 Encounter for screening for other metabolic disorders

Z13.29 Encounter for screening for other suspected endocrine disorder

EXCLUDES 2 *encounter for screening for diabetes mellitus (Z13.1)*

Z13.3 Encounter for screening examination for mental health and behavioral disorders

AHA: 2018,4Q,35-36

Z13.30 Encounter for screening examination for mental health and behavioral disorders, unspecified

Z13.31 Encounter for screening for depression

Encounter for screening for depression, adult

Encounter for screening for depression for child or adolescent

Z13.32 Encounter for screening for maternal depression ♀

Encounter for screening for perinatal depression

Z13.39 Encounter for screening examination for other mental health and behavioral disorders

Encounter for screening for alcoholism

Encounter for screening for intellectual disabilities

Z13.4 Encounter for screening for certain developmental disorders in childhood

Encounter for development testing of infant or child

Encounter for screening for developmental handicaps in early childhood

EXCLUDES 2 *encounter for routine child health examination (Z00.12-)*

AHA: 2018,4Q,36

Z13.40 Encounter for screening for unspecified developmental delays

Z13.41 Encounter for autism screening

Z13.42 Encounter for screening for global developmental delays (milestones)

Encounter for screening for developmental handicaps in early childhood

Z13.49 Encounter for screening for other developmental delays

Z13.5 Encounter for screening for eye and ear disorders

EXCLUDES 2 *encounter for general hearing examination (Z01.1-)*
encounter for general vision examination (Z01.0-)

AHA: 2016,3Q,17

Z13.6 Encounter for screening for cardiovascular disorders

Z13.7 Encounter for screening for genetic and chromosomal anomalies

EXCLUDES 1 *genetic testing for procreative management (Z31.4-)*

Z13.71 Encounter for nonprocreative screening for genetic disease carrier status

Z13.79 Encounter for other screening for genetic and chromosomal anomalies

Z13.8 Encounter for screening for other specified diseases and disorders

EXCLUDES 2 *screening for malignant neoplasms (Z12.-)*

Z13.81 Encounter for screening for digestive system disorders

Z13.810 Encounter for screening for upper gastrointestinal disorder

Z13.811 **Encounter for screening for lower gastrointestinal disorder**

EXCLUDES 1 *encounter for screening for intestinal infectious disease (Z11.Ø)*

Z13.818 **Encounter for screening for other digestive system disorders**

✓6th Z13.82 **Encounter for screening for musculoskeletal disorder**

Z13.82Ø **Encounter for screening for osteoporosis**

Z13.828 **Encounter for screening for other musculoskeletal disorder**

Z13.83 **Encounter for screening for respiratory disorder NEC**

EXCLUDES 1 *encounter for screening for respiratory tuberculosis (Z11.1)*

Z13.84 **Encounter for screening for dental disorders**

✓6th Z13.85 **Encounter for screening for nervous system disorders**

Z13.85Ø **Encounter for screening for traumatic brain injury**

Z13.858 **Encounter for screening for other nervous system disorders**

Z13.88 **Encounter for screening for disorder due to exposure to contaminants**

EXCLUDES 1 *those exposed to contaminants without suspected disorders (Z57.-, Z77.-)*

Z13.89 **Encounter for screening for other disorder**

Encounter for screening for genitourinary disorders

Z13.9 **Encounter for screening, unspecified**

Genetic carrier and genetic susceptibility to disease (Z14-Z15)

✓4th **Z14 Genetic carrier**

DEF: Individuals carrying a gene mutation associated with a certain disease that typically do not develop the disease but are able to pass the mutated genes to offspring.

✓5th Z14.Ø **Hemophilia A carrier**

Z14.Ø1 **Asymptomatic hemophilia A carrier**

Z14.Ø2 **Symptomatic hemophilia A carrier**

Z14.1 **Cystic fibrosis carrier**

Z14.8 **Genetic carrier of other disease**

✓4th **Z15 Genetic susceptibility to disease**

INCLUDES confirmed abnormal gene

Use additional code, if applicable, for any associated family history of the disease (Z8Ø-Z84)

EXCLUDES 1 *chromosomal anomalies (QØØ-Q99)*

✓5th Z15.Ø **Genetic susceptibility to malignant neoplasm**

Code first, if applicable, any current malignant neoplasm (CØØ-C75, C81-C96)

Use additional code, if applicable, for any personal history of malignant neoplasm (Z85.-)

Z15.Ø1 **Genetic susceptibility to malignant neoplasm of breast**

Z15.Ø2 **Genetic susceptibility to malignant neoplasm of ovary** ♀

Z15.Ø3 **Genetic susceptibility to malignant neoplasm of prostate** ♂

Z15.Ø4 **Genetic susceptibility to malignant neoplasm of endometrium** ♀

Z15.Ø9 **Genetic susceptibility to other malignant neoplasm**

AHA: 2021,1Q,14

✓5th Z15.8 **Genetic susceptibility to other disease**

Z15.81 **Genetic susceptibility to multiple endocrine neoplasia [MEN]**

EXCLUDES 1 *multiple endocrine neoplasia [MEN] syndromes (E31.2-)*

DEF: Group of conditions in which several endocrine glands grow excessively (such as in adenomatous hyperplasia) and/or develop benign or malignant tumors. Tumors and hyperplasia associated with MEN often produce excess hormones, which impede normal physiology. There is no comprehensive cure known for MEN syndrome. Treatment is directed at the hyperplasia or tumors in each individual gland. Tumors are usually surgically removed and oral medications or hormonal injections are used to correct hormone imbalances.

Z15.89 **Genetic susceptibility to other disease**

Resistance to antimicrobial drugs (Z16)

✓4th **Z16 Resistance to antimicrobial drugs**

NOTE The codes in this category are provided for use as additional codes to identify the resistance and non-responsiveness of a condition to antimicrobial drugs.

Code first the infection

EXCLUDES 1 *Methicillin resistant Staphylococcus aureus infection (A49.Ø2)*
Methicillin resistant Staphylococcus aureus pneumonia (J15.212)
sepsis due to Methicillin resistant Staphylococcus aureus (A41.Ø2)

✓5th Z16.1 **Resistance to beta lactam antibiotics**

Z16.1Ø **Resistance to unspecified beta lactam antibiotics** UPD

Z16.11 **Resistance to penicillins** UPD

Resistance to amoxicillin

Resistance to ampicillin

Z16.12 **Extended spectrum beta lactamase (ESBL) resistance** UPD

EXCLUDES 2 *Methicillin resistant Staphylococcus aureus infection in diseases classified elsewhere (B95.62)*

Z16.19 **Resistance to other specified beta lactam antibiotics** UPD

Resistance to cephalosporins

✓5th Z16.2 **Resistance to other antibiotics**

Z16.2Ø **Resistance to unspecified antibiotic** UPD

Resistance to antibiotics NOS

Z16.21 **Resistance to vancomycin** UPD

Z16.22 **Resistance to vancomycin related antibiotics** UPD

Z16.23 **Resistance to quinolones and fluoroquinolones** UPD

Z16.24 **Resistance to multiple antibiotics** UPD

Z16.29 **Resistance to other single specified antibiotic** UPD

Resistance to aminoglycosides

Resistance to macrolides

Resistance to sulfonamides

Resistance to tetracyclines

✓5th Z16.3 **Resistance to other antimicrobial drugs**

EXCLUDES 1 *resistance to antibiotics (Z16.1-, Z16.2-)*

Z16.3Ø **Resistance to unspecified antimicrobial drugs** UPD

Drug resistance NOS

Z16.31 **Resistance to antiparasitic drug(s)** UPD

Resistance to quinine and related compounds

Z16.32 **Resistance to antifungal drug(s)** UPD

Z16.33 **Resistance to antiviral drug(s)** UPD

✓6th Z16.34 **Resistance to antimycobacterial drug(s)**

Resistance to tuberculostatics

Z16.341 **Resistance to single antimycobacterial drug** UPD

Resistance to antimycobacterial drug NOS

Z16.342 **Resistance to multiple antimycobacterial drugs** UPD

Z16.35 **Resistance to multiple antimicrobial drugs** UPD

EXCLUDES 1 *resistance to multiple antibiotics only (Z16.24)*

Z16.39 **Resistance to other specified antimicrobial drug** UPD

Estrogen receptor status (Z17)

✓4th **Z17 Estrogen receptor status**

Code first malignant neoplasm of breast (C5Ø.-)

DEF: Receptor status of breast cancer cells for the hormone estrogen that is used to help determine treatment and evaluate prognosis. ER+ breast cancer responds to hormone therapies while ER- breast cancer does not.

Z17.Ø **Estrogen receptor positive status [ER+]** UPD

Z17.1 **Estrogen receptor negative status [ER-]** UPD

Retained foreign body fragments (Z18)

✓4th Z18 Retained foreign body fragments

INCLUDES embedded fragment (status)
embedded splinter (status)
retained foreign body status

EXCLUDES 1 *artificial joint prosthesis status (Z96.6-)*
foreign body accidentally left during a procedure (T81.5-)
foreign body entering through orifice (T15-T19)
in situ cardiac device (Z95.-)
organ or tissue replaced by means other than transplant (Z96.-, Z97.-)
organ or tissue replaced by transplant (Z94.-)
personal history of retained foreign body fully removed Z87.821
superficial foreign body (non-embedded splinter) - code to superficial foreign body, by site

DEF: Embedded or retained fragment, splinter, or foreign body, natural or synthetic that can cause infection.

✓5th Z18.Ø Retained radioactive fragments

Z18.Ø1 Retained depleted uranium fragments

Z18.Ø9 Other retained radioactive fragments
Other retained depleted isotope fragments
Retained nontherapeutic radioactive fragments

✓5th Z18.1 Retained metal fragments

EXCLUDES 1 *retained radioactive metal fragments (Z18.Ø1-Z18.Ø9)*

Z18.1Ø Retained metal fragments, unspecified
Retained metal fragment NOS

Z18.11 Retained magnetic metal fragments

Z18.12 Retained nonmagnetic metal fragments

Z18.2 Retained plastic fragments
Acrylics fragments
Diethylhexyl phthalates fragments
Isocyanate fragments

✓5th Z18.3 Retained organic fragments

Z18.31 Retained animal quills or spines

Z18.32 Retained tooth

Z18.33 Retained wood fragments

Z18.39 Other retained organic fragments

✓5th Z18.8 Other specified retained foreign body

Z18.81 Retained glass fragments

Z18.83 Retained stone or crystalline fragments
Retained concrete or cement fragments

Z18.89 Other specified retained foreign body fragments

Z18.9 Retained foreign body fragments, unspecified material

Hormone sensitivity malignancy status (Z19)

✓4th Z19 Hormone sensitivity malignancy status

Code first malignant neoplasm — see Table of Neoplasms, by site, malignant

AHA: 2016,4Q,76

Z19.1 Hormone sensitive malignancy status UPD

Z19.2 Hormone resistant malignancy status UPD
Castrate resistant prostate malignancy status

Persons with potential health hazards related to communicable diseases (Z2Ø-Z29)

✓4th Z2Ø Contact with and (suspected) exposure to communicable diseases

EXCLUDES 1 *carrier of infectious disease (Z22.-)*
diagnosed current infectious or parasitic disease - see Alphabetic Index

EXCLUDES 2 *personal history of infectious and parasitic diseases (Z86.1-)*

✓5th Z2Ø.Ø Contact with and (suspected) exposure to intestinal infectious diseases

Z2Ø.Ø1 Contact with and (suspected) exposure to intestinal infectious diseases due to Escherichia coli (E. coli)

Z2Ø.Ø9 Contact with and (suspected) exposure to other intestinal infectious diseases

Z2Ø.1 Contact with and (suspected) exposure to tuberculosis

Z2Ø.2 Contact with and (suspected) exposure to infections with a predominantly sexual mode of transmission

Z2Ø.3 Contact with and (suspected) exposure to rabies

Z2Ø.4 Contact with and (suspected) exposure to rubella

Z2Ø.5 Contact with and (suspected) exposure to viral hepatitis

Z2Ø.6 Contact with and (suspected) exposure to human immunodeficiency virus [HIV]

EXCLUDES 1 *asymptomatic human immunodeficiency virus [HIV] HIV infection status (Z21)*

Z2Ø.7 Contact with and (suspected) exposure to pediculosis, acariasis and other infestations

✓5th Z2Ø.8 Contact with and (suspected) exposure to other communicable diseases

✓6th Z2Ø.81 Contact with and (suspected) exposure to other bacterial communicable diseases

Z2Ø.81Ø Contact with and (suspected) exposure to anthrax

Z2Ø.811 Contact with and (suspected) exposure to meningococcus

Z2Ø.818 Contact with and (suspected) exposure to other bacterial communicable diseases
AHA: 2019,2Q,10

✓6th Z2Ø.82 Contact with and (suspected) exposure to other viral communicable diseases

Z2Ø.82Ø Contact with and (suspected) exposure to varicella

Z2Ø.821 Contact with and (suspected) exposure to Zika virus
AHA: 2018,4Q,35,64

Z2Ø.822 Contact with and (suspected) exposure to COVID-19
Contact with and (suspected) exposure to SARS-CoV-2
AHA: 2022,2Q,28-29; 2021,4Q,109; 2021,1Q,27-29,37-38,41

Z2Ø.828 Contact with and (suspected) exposure to other viral communicable diseases
AHA: 2021,1Q,37-38; 2020,4Q,99; 2020,3Q,14-15; 2020,2Q,4,8; 2020,1Q,34-36

Z2Ø.89 Contact with and (suspected) exposure to other communicable diseases

Z2Ø.9 Contact with and (suspected) exposure to unspecified communicable disease

Z21 Asymptomatic human immunodeficiency virus [HIV] infection status HCC Rx ESR COM
HIV positive NOS

Code first human immunodeficiency virus [HIV] disease complicating pregnancy, childbirth and the puerperium, if applicable (O98.7-)

EXCLUDES 1 *acquired immunodeficiency syndrome (B2Ø)*
contact with human immunodeficiency virus [HIV] (Z2Ø.6)
exposure to human immunodeficiency virus [HIV] (Z2Ø.6)
human immunodeficiency virus [HIV] disease (B2Ø)
inconclusive laboratory evidence of human immunodeficiency virus [HIV] (R75)

AHA: 2022,1Q,36; 2019,1Q,8-11

DEF: Phase of human immunodeficiency virus (HIV) infection with no clinical symptoms. This phase may last for 10 years or more.

✓4th Z22 Carrier of infectious disease

INCLUDES colonization status
suspected carrier

EXCLUDES 2 *carrier of viral hepatitis (B18.-)*

Z22.Ø Carrier of typhoid

Z22.1 Carrier of other intestinal infectious diseases

Z22.2 Carrier of diphtheria

✓5th Z22.3 Carrier of other specified bacterial diseases

Z22.31 Carrier of bacterial disease due to meningococci

✓6th Z22.32 Carrier of bacterial disease due to staphylococci

Z22.321 Carrier or suspected carrier of Methicillin susceptible Staphylococcus aureus
MSSA colonization

Z22.322 Carrier or suspected carrier of Methicillin resistant Staphylococcus aureus
MRSA colonization

DEF: Carriers (colonization) of methicillin resistant *Staphylococcus aureus* (MRSA) have MRSA on their skin or in their body but do not exhibit signs of infection. These individuals are able to pass MRSA on to others who may develop an infection.

Z22.33 Carrier of bacterial disease due to streptococci

Z22.330 Carrier of Group B streptococcus

EXCLUDES 1 *carrier of streptococcus group B (GBS) complicating pregnancy, childbirth and the puerperium (O99.82-)*

Z22.338 Carrier of other streptococcus

Z22.39 Carrier of other specified bacterial diseases

Z22.4 Carrier of infections with a predominantly sexual mode of transmission

Z22.6 Carrier of human T-lymphotropic virus type-1 [HTLV-1] infection

Z22.7 Latent tuberculosis

Latent tuberculosis infection (LTBI)

EXCLUDES 1 *nonspecific reaction to cell mediated immunity measurement of gamma interferon antigen response without active tuberculosis (R76.12)*

nonspecific reaction to tuberculin skin test without active tuberculosis (R76.11)

AHA: 2019,4Q,19

Z22.8 Carrier of other infectious diseases

Z22.9 Carrier of infectious disease, unspecified

Z23 Encounter for immunization

NOTE Procedure codes are required to identify the types of immunizations given

Code first any routine childhood examination

Code also, if applicable, encounter for immunization safety counseling (Z71.85)

Z28 Immunization not carried out and underimmunization status

INCLUDES vaccination not carried out

Code also, if applicable, encounter for immunization safety counseling (Z71.85)

Z28.0 Immunization not carried out because of contraindication

DEF: Contraindication: Situation where a drug, surgery, or other procedure may negatively affect or cause harm to a patient.

Z28.01 Immunization not carried out because of acute illness of patient

Z28.02 Immunization not carried out because of chronic illness or condition of patient

Z28.03 Immunization not carried out because of immune compromised state of patient

Z28.04 Immunization not carried out because of patient allergy to vaccine or component

Z28.09 Immunization not carried out because of other contraindication

Z28.1 Immunization not carried out because of patient decision for reasons of belief or group pressure

Immunization not carried out because of religious belief

Z28.2 Immunization not carried out because of patient decision for other and unspecified reason

Z28.20 Immunization not carried out because of patient decision for unspecified reason

Z28.21 Immunization not carried out because of patient refusal

Z28.29 Immunization not carried out because of patient decision for other reason

▲ Z28.3 Underimmunization status

~~Delinquent immunization status~~

~~Lapsed immunization schedule status~~

▶Use additional code, if applicable, to identify:◀

▶immunization not carried out because of contraindication (Z28.0-)◀

▶immunization not carried out because of patient decision for other and unspecified reason (Z28.2-)◀

▶immunization not carried out because of patient decision for reasons of belief or group pressure (Z28.1)◀

▶immunization not carried out for other reason (Z28.8-)◀

AHA: 2022,1Q,4-5

● Z28.31 Underimmunization for COVID-19 status

NOTE These codes should not be used for individuals who are not eligible for the COVID-19 vaccines, as determined by the healthcare provider.

● Z28.310 Unvaccinated for COVID-19 UPD

● Z28.311 Partially vaccinated for COVID-19 UPD

● Z28.39 Other underimmunization status UPD

Delinquent immunization status

Lapsed immunization schedule status

Z28.8 Immunization not carried out for other reason

Z28.81 Immunization not carried out due to patient having had the disease

Z28.82 Immunization not carried out because of caregiver refusal

Immunization not carried out because of guardian refusal

Immunization not carried out because of parent refusal

EXCLUDES 1 *immunization not carried out because of caregiver refusal because of religious belief (Z28.1)*

Z28.83 Immunization not carried out due to unavailability of vaccine

Delay in delivery of vaccine

Lack of availability of vaccine

Manufacturer delay of vaccine

AHA: 2018,4Q,36

Z28.89 Immunization not carried out for other reason

Z28.9 Immunization not carried out for unspecified reason

Z29 Encounter for other prophylactic measures

EXCLUDES 1 *desensitization to allergens (Z51.6)*

prophylactic surgery (Z40.-)

AHA: 2016,4Q,78-79

Z29.1 Encounter for prophylactic immunotherapy

Encounter for administration of immunoglobulin

Z29.11 Encounter for prophylactic immunotherapy for respiratory syncytial virus (RSV)

Z29.12 Encounter for prophylactic antivenin

Z29.13 Encounter for prophylactic Rho(D) immune globulin

AHA: 2019,3Q,5

Z29.14 Encounter for prophylactic rabies immune globin

Z29.3 Encounter for prophylactic fluoride administration

Z29.8 Encounter for other specified prophylactic measures

AHA: 2022,2Q,27

Z29.9 Encounter for prophylactic measures, unspecified

Persons encountering health services in circumstances related to reproduction (Z30-Z39)

Z30 Encounter for contraceptive management

AHA: 2016,4Q,78

DEF: Contraceptive management to prevent pregnancy. Methods include oral medications, intrauterine devices, and surgical procedures for males and females (sterilization).

Z30.0 Encounter for general counseling and advice on contraception

Z30.01 Encounter for initial prescription of contraceptives

EXCLUDES 1 *encounter for surveillance of contraceptives (Z30.4-)*

Z30.011 Encounter for initial prescription of contraceptive pills ♀

Z30.012 Encounter for prescription of emergency contraception ♀

Encounter for postcoital contraception

Z30.013 Encounter for initial prescription of injectable contraceptive ♀

Z30.014 Encounter for initial prescription of intrauterine contraceptive device ♀

EXCLUDES 1 *encounter for insertion of intrauterine contraceptive device (Z30.430, Z30.432)*

Z30.015 Encounter for initial prescription of vaginal ring hormonal contraceptive ♀

Z30.016 Encounter for initial prescription of transdermal patch hormonal contraceptive device ♀

Z30.017 Encounter for initial prescription of implantable subdermal contraceptive ♀

Z30.018 Encounter for initial prescription of other contraceptives ♀
Encounter for initial prescription of barrier contraception
Encounter for initial prescription of diaphragm

Z30.019 Encounter for initial prescription of contraceptives, unspecified ♀

Z30.02 Counseling and instruction in natural family planning to avoid pregnancy

Z30.09 Encounter for other general counseling and advice on contraception
Encounter for family planning advice NOS

Z30.2 Encounter for sterilization
AHA: 2021,3Q,13

✓5th **Z30.4 Encounter for surveillance of contraceptives**

Z30.40 Encounter for surveillance of contraceptives, unspecified

Z30.41 Encounter for surveillance of contraceptive pills ♀
Encounter for repeat prescription for contraceptive pill

Z30.42 Encounter for surveillance of injectable contraceptive ♀

✓6th **Z30.43 Encounter for surveillance of intrauterine contraceptive device**

Z30.430 Encounter for insertion of intrauterine contraceptive device ♀

Z30.431 Encounter for routine checking of intrauterine contraceptive device ♀

Z30.432 Encounter for removal of intrauterine contraceptive device ♀

Z30.433 Encounter for removal and reinsertion of intrauterine contraceptive device ♀
Encounter for replacement of intrauterine contraceptive device

Z30.44 Encounter for surveillance of vaginal ring hormonal contraceptive device ♀

Z30.45 Encounter for surveillance of transdermal patch hormonal contraceptive device ♀

Z30.46 Encounter for surveillance of implantable subdermal contraceptive ♀
Encounter for checking, reinsertion or removal of implantable subdermal contraceptive

Z30.49 Encounter for surveillance of other contraceptives ♀
Encounter for surveillance of barrier contraception
Encounter for surveillance of diaphragm

Z30.8 Encounter for other contraceptive management
Encounter for postvasectomy sperm count
Encounter for routine examination for contraceptive maintenance
EXCLUDES 1 *sperm count following sterilization reversal (Z31.42)*
sperm count for fertility testing (Z31.41)

Z30.9 Encounter for contraceptive management, unspecified

✓4th **Z31 Encounter for procreative management**
EXCLUDES 2 *complications associated with artificial fertilization (N98.-)*
female infertility (N97.-)
male infertility (N46.-)

Z31.0 Encounter for reversal of previous sterilization

✓5th **Z31.4 Encounter for procreative investigation and testing**
EXCLUDES 1 *postvasectomy sperm count (Z30.8)*

Z31.41 Encounter for fertility testing
Encounter for fallopian tube patency testing
Encounter for sperm count for fertility testing

Z31.42 Aftercare following sterilization reversal
Sperm count following sterilization reversal

✓6th **Z31.43 Encounter for genetic testing of female for procreative management**
Use additional code for recurrent pregnancy loss, if applicable (N96, O26.2-)
EXCLUDES 1 *nonprocreative genetic testing (Z13.7-)*

Z31.430 Encounter of female for testing for genetic disease carrier status for procreative management ♀

Z31.438 Encounter for other genetic testing of female for procreative management ♀

✓6th **Z31.44 Encounter for genetic testing of male for procreative management**
EXCLUDES 1 *nonprocreative genetic testing (Z13.7-)*

Z31.440 Encounter of male for testing for genetic disease carrier status for procreative management ♂

Z31.441 Encounter for testing of male partner of patient with recurrent pregnancy loss A ♂

Z31.448 Encounter for other genetic testing of male for procreative management A ♂

Z31.49 Encounter for other procreative investigation and testing

Z31.5 Encounter for procreative genetic counseling
AHA: 2017,4Q,27

✓5th **Z31.6 Encounter for general counseling and advice on procreation**

Z31.61 Procreative counseling and advice using natural family planning

Z31.62 Encounter for fertility preservation counseling
Encounter for fertility preservation counseling prior to cancer therapy
Encounter for fertility preservation counseling prior to surgical removal of gonads

Z31.69 Encounter for other general counseling and advice on procreation

Z31.7 Encounter for procreative management and counseling for gestational carrier ♀
EXCLUDES 1 *pregnant state, gestational carrier (Z33.3)*
AHA: 2016,4Q,78

✓5th **Z31.8 Encounter for other procreative management**

Z31.81 Encounter for male factor infertility in female patient PDx ♀

Z31.82 Encounter for Rh incompatibility status ♀
AHA: 2015,3Q,40; 2014,4Q,17

Z31.83 Encounter for assisted reproductive fertility procedure cycle PDx ♀
Patient undergoing in vitro fertilization cycle
Use additional code to identify the type of infertility
EXCLUDES 1 *pre-cycle diagnosis and testing - code to reason for encounter*
AHA: 2022,2Q,15-16

Z31.84 Encounter for fertility preservation procedure PDx
Encounter for fertility preservation procedure prior to cancer therapy
Encounter for fertility preservation procedure prior to surgical removal of gonads

Z31.89 Encounter for other procreative management

Z31.9 Encounter for procreative management, unspecified

✓4th **Z32 Encounter for pregnancy test and childbirth and childcare instruction**

✓5th **Z32.0 Encounter for pregnancy test**

Z32.00 Encounter for pregnancy test, result unknown ♀
Encounter for pregnancy test NOS

Z32.01 Encounter for pregnancy test, result positive COM M ♀

Z32.02 Encounter for pregnancy test, result negative ♀

Z32.2 Encounter for childbirth instruction

Z32.3 Encounter for childcare instruction
Encounter for prenatal or postpartum childcare instruction

✓4th **Z33 Pregnant state**

Z33.1 Pregnant state, incidental COM M ♀
Pregnancy NOS
Pregnant state NOS
EXCLUDES 1 *complications of pregnancy (O00-O9A)*
pregnant state, gestational carrier (Z33.3)

Z33.2 Encounter for elective termination of pregnancy PDx M ♀
EXCLUDES 1 *early fetal death with retention of dead fetus (O02.1)*
late fetal death (O36.4)
spontaneous abortion (O03)
AHA: 2022,1Q,20
TIP: Do not assign a code from category Z3A with this code.

Z33.3 Pregnant state, gestational carrier COM M ♀
EXCLUDES 1 *encounter for procreative management and counseling for gestational carrier (Z31.7)*
AHA: 2016,4Q,78

Z34 Encounter for supervision of normal pregnancy
EXCLUDES 1 *any complication of pregnancy (OØØ-O9A)*
encounter for pregnancy test (Z32.Ø-)
encounter for supervision of high risk pregnancy (OØ9.-)
AHA: 2019,3Q,5; 2014,4Q,17

Z34.Ø Encounter for supervision of normal first pregnancy
- **Z34.ØØ Encounter for supervision of normal first pregnancy, unspecified trimester** COM PDx M ♀
- **Z34.Ø1 Encounter for supervision of normal first pregnancy, first trimester** COM PDx M ♀
- **Z34.Ø2 Encounter for supervision of normal first pregnancy, second trimester** COM PDx M ♀
- **Z34.Ø3 Encounter for supervision of normal first pregnancy, third trimester** COM PDx M ♀

Z34.8 Encounter for supervision of other normal pregnancy
- **Z34.8Ø Encounter for supervision of other normal pregnancy, unspecified trimester** COM PDx M ♀
- **Z34.81 Encounter for supervision of other normal pregnancy, first trimester** COM PDx M ♀
- **Z34.82 Encounter for supervision of other normal pregnancy, second trimester** COM PDx M ♀
- **Z34.83 Encounter for supervision of other normal pregnancy, third trimester** COM PDx M ♀

Z34.9 Encounter for supervision of normal pregnancy, unspecified
- **Z34.9Ø Encounter for supervision of normal pregnancy, unspecified, unspecified trimester** COM PDx M ♀
- **Z34.91 Encounter for supervision of normal pregnancy, unspecified, first trimester** COM PDx M ♀
- **Z34.92 Encounter for supervision of normal pregnancy, unspecified, second trimester** COM PDx M ♀
- **Z34.93 Encounter for supervision of normal pregnancy, unspecified, third trimester** COM PDx M ♀

Z36 Encounter for antenatal screening of mother
INCLUDES encounter for placental sample (taken vaginally)
screening is the testing for disease or disease precursors in asymptomatic individuals so that early detection and treatment can be provided for those who test positive for the disease.
EXCLUDES 1 *diagnostic examination - code to sign or symptom*
encounter for suspected maternal and fetal conditions ruled out (ZØ3.7-)
suspected fetal condition affecting management of pregnancy - code to condition in Chapter 15
EXCLUDES 2 *abnormal findings on antenatal screening of mother (O28.-)*
genetic counseling and testing (Z31.43-, Z31.5)
routine prenatal care (Z34)
AHA: 2017,4Q,28

Z36.Ø Encounter for antenatal screening for chromosomal anomalies COM M ♀

Z36.1 Encounter for antenatal screening for raised alphafetoprotein level COM M ♀
Encounter for antenatal screening for elevated maternal serum alphafetoprotein level
DEF: High levels of alpha-fetoprotein (AFP) that may indicate a possibility of spina bifida and other neural tube defects, anencephaly, or omphalocele in the fetus.

Z36.2 Encounter for other antenatal screening follow-up COM M ♀
Non-visualized anatomy on a previous scan

Z36.3 Encounter for antenatal screening for malformations COM M ♀
Screening for a suspected anomaly

Z36.4 Encounter for antenatal screening for fetal growth retardation COM M ♀
Intrauterine growth restriction (IUGR)/small-for-dates

Z36.5 Encounter for antenatal screening for isoimmunization COM M ♀

Z36.8 Encounter for other antenatal screening
- **Z36.81 Encounter for antenatal screening for hydrops fetalis** COM M ♀
  DEF: Hydrops fetalis: Abnormal accumulation of fluid in two or more parts of the fetus, such as ascites, effusion of the pleural or pericardial tissues, or edema.
- **Z36.82 Encounter for antenatal screening for nuchal translucency** COM M ♀
- **Z36.83 Encounter for fetal screening for congenital cardiac abnormalities** COM M ♀
- **Z36.84 Encounter for antenatal screening for fetal lung maturity** COM M ♀
- **Z36.85 Encounter for antenatal screening for Streptococcus B** COM M ♀
- **Z36.86 Encounter for antenatal screening for cervical length** COM M ♀
  Screening for risk of pre-term labor
- **Z36.87 Encounter for antenatal screening for uncertain dates** COM M ♀
- **Z36.88 Encounter for antenatal screening for fetal macrosomia** COM M ♀
  Screening for large-for-dates
- **Z36.89 Encounter for other specified antenatal screening** COM M ♀
- **Z36.8A Encounter for antenatal screening for other genetic defects** COM M ♀

Z36.9 Encounter for antenatal screening, unspecified COM M ♀

Z3A Weeks of gestation
NOTE Codes from category Z3A are for use, only on the maternal record, to indicate the weeks of gestation of the pregnancy, if known.
Code first obstetric condition or encounter for delivery (OØ9-O6Ø, O8Ø-O82)
AHA: 2022,2Q,3; 2019,2Q,11; 2016,2Q,34; 2014,3Q,17; 2014,2Q,9; 2013,2Q,33
TIP: Do not assign a code from this category with codes from categories O00-O08 or code Z33.2.

Z3A.Ø Weeks of gestation of pregnancy, unspecified or less than 1Ø weeks
- **Z3A.ØØ Weeks of gestation of pregnancy not specified** COM UPD M ♀
- **Z3A.Ø1 Less than 8 weeks gestation of pregnancy** COM UPD M ♀
- **Z3A.Ø8 8 weeks gestation of pregnancy** COM UPD M ♀
- **Z3A.Ø9 9 weeks gestation of pregnancy** COM UPD M ♀

Z3A.1 Weeks of gestation of pregnancy, weeks 1Ø-19
- **Z3A.1Ø 1Ø weeks gestation of pregnancy** COM UPD M ♀
- **Z3A.11 11 weeks gestation of pregnancy** COM UPD M ♀
- **Z3A.12 12 weeks gestation of pregnancy** COM UPD M ♀
- **Z3A.13 13 weeks gestation of pregnancy** COM UPD M ♀
- **Z3A.14 14 weeks gestation of pregnancy** COM UPD M ♀
- **Z3A.15 15 weeks gestation of pregnancy** COM UPD M ♀
- **Z3A.16 16 weeks gestation of pregnancy** COM UPD M ♀
- **Z3A.17 17 weeks gestation of pregnancy** COM UPD M ♀
- **Z3A.18 18 weeks gestation of pregnancy** COM UPD M ♀
- **Z3A.19 19 weeks gestation of pregnancy** COM UPD M ♀

Z3A.2 Weeks of gestation of pregnancy, weeks 2Ø-29
- **Z3A.2Ø 2Ø weeks gestation of pregnancy** COM UPD M ♀
- **Z3A.21 21 weeks gestation of pregnancy** COM UPD M ♀
- **Z3A.22 22 weeks gestation of pregnancy** COM UPD M ♀
- **Z3A.23 23 weeks gestation of pregnancy** COM UPD M ♀
- **Z3A.24 24 weeks gestation of pregnancy** COM UPD M ♀
- **Z3A.25 25 weeks gestation of pregnancy** COM UPD M ♀
- **Z3A.26 26 weeks gestation of pregnancy** COM UPD M ♀
- **Z3A.27 27 weeks gestation of pregnancy** COM UPD M ♀
- **Z3A.28 28 weeks gestation of pregnancy** COM UPD M ♀
- **Z3A.29 29 weeks gestation of pregnancy** COM UPD M ♀

Z3A.3 Weeks of gestation of pregnancy, weeks 3Ø-39
- **Z3A.3Ø 3Ø weeks gestation of pregnancy** COM UPD M ♀
- **Z3A.31 31 weeks gestation of pregnancy** COM UPD M ♀
- **Z3A.32 32 weeks gestation of pregnancy** COM UPD M ♀
- **Z3A.33 33 weeks gestation of pregnancy** COM UPD M ♀
- **Z3A.34 34 weeks gestation of pregnancy** COM UPD M ♀
- **Z3A.35 35 weeks gestation of pregnancy** COM UPD M ♀

Z3A.36 36 weeks gestation of pregnancy COM UPD M ♀
Z3A.37 37 weeks gestation of pregnancy COM UPD M ♀
Z3A.38 38 weeks gestation of pregnancy COM UPD M ♀
Z3A.39 39 weeks gestation of pregnancy COM UPD M ♀

5th Z3A.4 **Weeks of gestation of pregnancy, weeks 40 or greater**
AHA: 2014,4Q,23
Z3A.40 40 weeks gestation of pregnancy COM UPD M ♀
Z3A.41 41 weeks gestation of pregnancy COM UPD M ♀
Z3A.42 42 weeks gestation of pregnancy COM UPD M ♀
Z3A.49 Greater than 42 weeks gestation of pregnancy COM UPD M ♀

4th **Z37 Outcome of delivery**
This category is intended for use as an additional code to identify the outcome of delivery on the mother's record. It is not for use on the newborn record.
EXCLUDES 1 *stillbirth (P95)*

Z37.0 Single live birth COM UPD M ♀
AHA: 2016,2Q,34; 2014,2Q,9
Z37.1 Single stillbirth COM UPD M ♀
Z37.2 Twins, both liveborn COM UPD M ♀
Z37.3 Twins, one liveborn and one stillborn COM UPD M ♀
Z37.4 Twins, both stillborn COM UPD M ♀
5th Z37.5 **Other multiple births, all liveborn**
Z37.50 Multiple births, unspecified, all liveborn COM UPD M ♀
Z37.51 Triplets, all liveborn COM UPD M ♀
Z37.52 Quadruplets, all liveborn COM UPD M ♀
Z37.53 Quintuplets, all liveborn COM UPD M ♀
Z37.54 Sextuplets, all liveborn COM UPD M ♀
Z37.59 Other multiple births, all liveborn COM UPD M ♀
5th Z37.6 **Other multiple births, some liveborn**
Z37.60 Multiple births, unspecified, some liveborn COM UPD M ♀
Z37.61 Triplets, some liveborn COM UPD M ♀
Z37.62 Quadruplets, some liveborn COM UPD M ♀
Z37.63 Quintuplets, some liveborn COM UPD M ♀
Z37.64 Sextuplets, some liveborn COM UPD M ♀
Z37.69 Other multiple births, some liveborn COM UPD M ♀
Z37.7 Other multiple births, all stillborn COM UPD M ♀
Z37.9 Outcome of delivery, unspecified COM UPD M ♀
Multiple birth NOS
Single birth NOS

4th **Z38 Liveborn infants according to place of birth and type of delivery**
This category is for use as the principal code on the initial record of a newborn baby. It is to be used for the initial birth record only. It is not to be used on the mother's record.
AHA: 2020,2Q,13; 2017,2Q,5-7; 2016,3Q,18; 2015,2Q,15
TIP: For attending physician services, a code from this category can be reported as first listed every time the physician visits the newborn during the birth admission.

5th Z38.0 **Single liveborn infant, born in hospital**
Single liveborn infant, born in birthing center or other health care facility
Z38.00 Single liveborn infant, delivered vaginally COM PDx N
Z38.01 Single liveborn infant, delivered by cesarean COM PDx N
Z38.1 Single liveborn infant, born outside hospital COM PDx N
Z38.2 Single liveborn infant, unspecified as to place of birth COM PDx N
Single liveborn infant NOS
5th Z38.3 **Twin liveborn infant, born in hospital**
Z38.30 Twin liveborn infant, delivered vaginally COM PDx N
Z38.31 Twin liveborn infant, delivered by cesarean COM PDx N
Z38.4 Twin liveborn infant, born outside hospital COM PDx N
Z38.5 Twin liveborn infant, unspecified as to place of birth COM PDx N
5th Z38.6 **Other multiple liveborn infant, born in hospital**
Z38.61 Triplet liveborn infant, delivered vaginally COM PDx N
Z38.62 Triplet liveborn infant, delivered by cesarean COM PDx N
Z38.63 Quadruplet liveborn infant, delivered vaginally COM PDx N
Z38.64 Quadruplet liveborn infant, delivered by cesarean COM PDx N
Z38.65 Quintuplet liveborn infant, delivered vaginally COM PDx N
Z38.66 Quintuplet liveborn infant, delivered by cesarean COM PDx N
Z38.68 Other multiple liveborn infant, delivered vaginally COM PDx N
Z38.69 Other multiple liveborn infant, delivered by cesarean COM PDx N
Z38.7 Other multiple liveborn infant, born outside hospital COM PDx N
Z38.8 Other multiple liveborn infant, unspecified as to place of birth COM PDx N

4th **Z39 Encounter for maternal postpartum care and examination**
Z39.0 Encounter for care and examination of mother immediately after delivery COM PDx M ♀
Care and observation in uncomplicated cases when the delivery occurs outside a healthcare facility
EXCLUDES 1 *care for postpartum complication - see Alphabetic Index*
AHA: 2021,3Q,13
Z39.1 Encounter for care and examination of lactating mother PDx M ♀
Encounter for supervision of lactation
EXCLUDES 1 *disorders of lactation (O92.-)*
Z39.2 Encounter for routine postpartum follow-up COM PDx M ♀

Encounters for other specific health care (Z40-Z53)

Categories Z40-Z53 are intended for use to indicate a reason for care. They may be used for patients who have already been treated for a disease or injury, but who are receiving aftercare or prophylactic care, or care to consolidate the treatment, or to deal with a residual state
EXCLUDES 2 *follow-up examination for medical surveillance after treatment (Z08-Z09)*

4th **Z40 Encounter for prophylactic surgery**
EXCLUDES 1 *organ donations (Z52.-)*
therapeutic organ removal - code to condition
DEF: Treatment measure intended to prevent or ward off a disease or condition.

5th Z40.0 **Encounter for prophylactic surgery for risk factors related to malignant neoplasms**
Admission for prophylactic organ removal
Use additional code to identify risk factor
AHA: 2017,4Q,28-29
Z40.00 Encounter for prophylactic removal of unspecified organ PDx
Z40.01 Encounter for prophylactic removal of breast PDx
Z40.02 Encounter for prophylactic removal of ovary(s) PDx ♀
Encounter for prophylactic removal of ovary(s) and fallopian tube(s)
Z40.03 Encounter for prophylactic removal of fallopian tube(s) PDx ♀
Z40.09 Encounter for prophylactic removal of other organ PDx
Z40.8 Encounter for other prophylactic surgery PDx
Z40.9 Encounter for prophylactic surgery, unspecified PDx

4th **Z41 Encounter for procedures for purposes other than remedying health state**
Z41.1 Encounter for cosmetic surgery
Encounter for cosmetic breast implant
Encounter for cosmetic procedure
EXCLUDES 1 *encounter for plastic and reconstructive surgery following medical procedure or healed injury (Z42.-)*
encounter for post-mastectomy breast implantation (Z42.1)

Z41.2 Encounter for routine and ritual male circumcision ♂
AHA: 2018,3Q,15
TIP: This code should only be reported when the circumcision is elective (unrelated to a specific diagnosis) and was not performed during the birth admission.

Z41.3 Encounter for ear piercing

Z41.8 Encounter for other procedures for purposes other than remedying health state

Z41.9 Encounter for procedure for purposes other than remedying health state, unspecified

✓4th **Z42** Encounter for plastic and reconstructive surgery following medical procedure or healed injury
EXCLUDES 1 *encounter for cosmetic plastic surgery (Z41.1)*
encounter for plastic surgery for treatment of current injury - code to relevent injury

Z42.1 Encounter for breast reconstruction following mastectomy PDx A
EXCLUDES 1 *deformity and disproportion of reconstructed breast (N65.1-)*

Z42.8 Encounter for other plastic and reconstructive surgery following medical procedure or healed injury PDx
AHA: 2017,1Q,42

✓4th **Z43** Encounter for attention to artificial openings
INCLUDES closure of artificial openings
passage of sounds or bougies through artificial openings
reforming artificial openings
removal of catheter from artificial openings
toilet or cleansing of artificial openings
EXCLUDES 1 *complications of external stoma (J95.Ø-, K94.-, N99.5-)*
EXCLUDES 2 *fitting and adjustment of prosthetic and other devices (Z44-Z46)*
AHA: 2019,2Q,33

Z43.Ø Encounter for attention to tracheostomy HCC ESR COM

Z43.1 Encounter for attention to gastrostomy HCC ESR COM
EXCLUDES 2 *artificial opening status only, without need for care (Z93.-)*

Z43.2 Encounter for attention to ileostomy HCC ESR COM

Z43.3 Encounter for attention to colostomy HCC ESR COM

Z43.4 Encounter for attention to other artificial openings of digestive tract HCC ESR COM

Z43.5 Encounter for attention to cystostomy HCC ESR COM

Z43.6 Encounter for attention to other artificial openings of urinary tract HCC ESR COM
Encounter for attention to nephrostomy
Encounter for attention to ureterostomy
Encounter for attention to urethrostomy

Z43.7 Encounter for attention to artificial vagina

Z43.8 Encounter for attention to other artificial openings HCC ESR COM

Z43.9 Encounter for attention to unspecified artificial opening HCC ESR COM

✓4th **Z44** Encounter for fitting and adjustment of external prosthetic device
INCLUDES removal or replacement of external prosthetic device
EXCLUDES 1 *malfunction or other complications of device - see Alphabetical Index*
presence of prosthetic device (Z97.-)

✓5th **Z44.Ø** Encounter for fitting and adjustment of artificial arm

✓6th **Z44.ØØ** Encounter for fitting and adjustment of unspecified artificial arm

Z44.ØØ1 Encounter for fitting and adjustment of unspecified right artificial arm COM

Z44.ØØ2 Encounter for fitting and adjustment of unspecified left artificial arm COM

Z44.ØØ9 Encounter for fitting and adjustment of unspecified artificial arm, unspecified arm COM

✓6th **Z44.Ø1** Encounter for fitting and adjustment of complete artificial arm

Z44.Ø11 Encounter for fitting and adjustment of complete right artificial arm COM

Z44.Ø12 Encounter for fitting and adjustment of complete left artificial arm COM

Z44.Ø19 Encounter for fitting and adjustment of complete artificial arm, unspecified arm COM

✓6th **Z44.Ø2** Encounter for fitting and adjustment of partial artificial arm

Z44.Ø21 Encounter for fitting and adjustment of partial artificial right arm COM

Z44.Ø22 Encounter for fitting and adjustment of partial artificial left arm COM

Z44.Ø29 Encounter for fitting and adjustment of partial artificial arm, unspecified arm COM

✓5th **Z44.1** Encounter for fitting and adjustment of artificial leg

✓6th **Z44.1Ø** Encounter for fitting and adjustment of unspecified artificial leg

Z44.1Ø1 Encounter for fitting and adjustment of unspecified right artificial leg HCC ESR COM

Z44.1Ø2 Encounter for fitting and adjustment of unspecified left artificial leg HCC ESR COM

Z44.1Ø9 Encounter for fitting and adjustment of unspecified artificial leg, unspecified leg HCC ESR COM

✓6th **Z44.11** Encounter for fitting and adjustment of complete artificial leg

Z44.111 Encounter for fitting and adjustment of complete right artificial leg HCC ESR COM

Z44.112 Encounter for fitting and adjustment of complete left artificial leg HCC ESR COM

Z44.119 Encounter for fitting and adjustment of complete artificial leg, unspecified leg HCC ESR COM

✓6th **Z44.12** Encounter for fitting and adjustment of partial artificial leg

Z44.121 Encounter for fitting and adjustment of partial artificial right leg HCC ESR COM

Z44.122 Encounter for fitting and adjustment of partial artificial left leg HCC ESR COM

Z44.129 Encounter for fitting and adjustment of partial artificial leg, unspecified leg HCC ESR COM

✓5th **Z44.2** Encounter for fitting and adjustment of artificial eye
EXCLUDES 1 *mechanical complication of ocular prosthesis (T85.3)*

Z44.2Ø Encounter for fitting and adjustment of artificial eye, unspecified

Z44.21 Encounter for fitting and adjustment of artificial right eye

Z44.22 Encounter for fitting and adjustment of artificial left eye

✓5th **Z44.3** Encounter for fitting and adjustment of external breast prosthesis
EXCLUDES 1 *complications of breast implant (T85.4-)*
encounter for adjustment or removal of breast implant (Z45.81-)
encounter for initial breast implant insertion for cosmetic breast augmentation (Z41.1)
encounter for breast reconstruction following mastectomy (Z42.1)

Z44.3Ø Encounter for fitting and adjustment of external breast prosthesis, unspecified breast

Z44.31 Encounter for fitting and adjustment of external right breast prosthesis

Z44.32 Encounter for fitting and adjustment of external left breast prosthesis

Z44.8 Encounter for fitting and adjustment of other external prosthetic devices

Z44.9 Encounter for fitting and adjustment of unspecified external prosthetic device

Z45 Encounter for adjustment and management of implanted device

INCLUDES removal or replacement of implanted device

EXCLUDES 1 *malfunction or other complications of device - see Alphabetical Index*

EXCLUDES 2 *encounter for fitting and adjustment of non-implanted device (Z46.-)*

Z45.Ø Encounter for adjustment and management of cardiac device

TIP: Assign an additional code for the associated condition if that condition requires constant intervention from the device, as in cases of sick sinus syndrome. For conditions that do not require constant intervention from the device, as in cases of ventricular fibrillation, an additional code for the associated condition should be assigned only if the patient is experiencing the condition and the device is firing during the current admission.

Z45.Ø1 Encounter for adjustment and management of cardiac pacemaker

Encounter for adjustment and management of cardiac resynchronization therapy pacemaker (CRT-P)

EXCLUDES 1 *encounter for adjustment and management of automatic implantable cardiac defibrillator with synchronous cardiac pacemaker (Z45.Ø2)*

Z45.Ø1Ø Encounter for checking and testing of cardiac pacemaker pulse generator [battery]

Encounter for replacing cardiac pacemaker pulse generator [battery]

Z45.Ø18 Encounter for adjustment and management of other part of cardiac pacemaker

EXCLUDES 1 *presence of other part of cardiac pacemaker (Z95.Ø)*

EXCLUDES 2 *presence of prosthetic and other devices (Z95.1-Z95.5, Z95.811-Z97)*

Z45.Ø2 Encounter for adjustment and management of automatic implantable cardiac defibrillator

Encounter for adjustment and management of automatic implantable cardiac defibrillator with synchronous cardiac pacemaker

Encounter for adjustment and management of cardiac resynchronization therapy defibrillator (CRT-D)

Z45.Ø9 Encounter for adjustment and management of other cardiac device

Z45.1 Encounter for adjustment and management of infusion pump

Z45.2 Encounter for adjustment and management of vascular access device

Encounter for adjustment and management of vascular catheters

EXCLUDES 1 *encounter for adjustment and management of renal dialysis catheter (Z49.Ø1)*

AHA: 2020,2Q,21; 2018,3Q,20

Z45.3 Encounter for adjustment and management of implanted devices of the special senses

Z45.31 Encounter for adjustment and management of implanted visual substitution device

Z45.32 Encounter for adjustment and management of implanted hearing device

EXCLUDES 1 *encounter for fitting and adjustment of hearing aide (Z46.1)*

Z45.32Ø Encounter for adjustment and management of bone conduction device

Z45.321 Encounter for adjustment and management of cochlear device

Z45.328 Encounter for adjustment and management of other implanted hearing device

Z45.4 Encounter for adjustment and management of implanted nervous system device

Z45.41 Encounter for adjustment and management of cerebrospinal fluid drainage device

Encounter for adjustment and management of cerebral ventricular (communicating) shunt

Z45.42 Encounter for adjustment and management of neurostimulator

Encounter for adjustment and management of brain neurostimulator

Encounter for adjustment and management of gastric neurostimulator

Encounter for adjustment and management of peripheral nerve neurostimulator

Encounter for adjustment and management of sacral nerve neurostimulator

Encounter for adjustment and management of spinal cord neurostimulator

Encounter for adjustment and management of vagus nerve neurostimulator

Z45.49 Encounter for adjustment and management of other implanted nervous system device

AHA: 2014,3Q,19

Z45.8 Encounter for adjustment and management of other implanted devices

Z45.81 Encounter for adjustment or removal of breast implant

Encounter for elective implant exchange (different material) (different size)

Encounter for removal of tissue expander with or without synchronous insertion of permanent implant

EXCLUDES 1 *complications of breast implant (T85.4-)*

encounter for initial breast implant insertion for cosmetic breast augmentation (Z41.1)

encounter for breast reconstruction following mastectomy (Z42.1)

Z45.811 Encounter for adjustment or removal of right breast implant

Z45.812 Encounter for adjustment or removal of left breast implant

Z45.819 Encounter for adjustment or removal of unspecified breast implant

Z45.82 Encounter for adjustment or removal of myringotomy device (stent) (tube)

Z45.89 Encounter for adjustment and management of other implanted devices

AHA: 2014,4Q,26-28

Z45.9 Encounter for adjustment and management of unspecified implanted device

Z46 Encounter for fitting and adjustment of other devices

INCLUDES removal or replacement of other device

EXCLUDES 1 *malfunction or other complications of device - see Alphabetical Index*

EXCLUDES 2 *encounter for fitting and management of implanted devices (Z45.-)*

issue of repeat prescription only (Z76.Ø)

presence of prosthetic and other devices (Z95-Z97)

Z46.Ø Encounter for fitting and adjustment of spectacles and contact lenses

Z46.1 Encounter for fitting and adjustment of hearing aid

EXCLUDES 1 *encounter for adjustment and management of implanted hearing device (Z45.32-)*

Z46.2 Encounter for fitting and adjustment of other devices related to nervous system and special senses

EXCLUDES 2 *encounter for adjustment and management of implanted nervous system device (Z45.4-)*

encounter for adjustment and management of implanted visual substitution device (Z45.31)

Z46.3 Encounter for fitting and adjustment of dental prosthetic device

Encounter for fitting and adjustment of dentures

Z46.4 Encounter for fitting and adjustment of orthodontic device

Z46.5 Encounter for fitting and adjustment of other gastrointestinal appliance and device

EXCLUDES 1 *encounter for attention to artificial openings of digestive tract (Z43.1-Z43.4)*

Z46.51 Encounter for fitting and adjustment of gastric lap band

Z46.59 Encounter for fitting and adjustment of other gastrointestinal appliance and device

Z46.6 Encounter for fitting and adjustment of urinary device
EXCLUDES 2 *attention to artificial openings of urinary tract (Z43.5, Z43.6)*

√5th **Z46.8 Encounter for fitting and adjustment of other specified devices**

Z46.81 Encounter for fitting and adjustment of insulin pump
Encounter for insulin pump instruction and training
Encounter for insulin pump titration

Z46.82 Encounter for fitting and adjustment of non-vascular catheter

Z46.89 Encounter for fitting and adjustment of other specified devices
Encounter for fitting and adjustment of wheelchair

Z46.9 Encounter for fitting and adjustment of unspecified device

√4th **Z47 Orthopedic aftercare**
EXCLUDES 1 *aftercare for healing fracture - code to fracture with 7th character D*

Z47.1 Aftercare following joint replacement surgery
Use additional code to identify the joint (Z96.6-)
AHA: 2020,1Q,23

Z47.2 Encounter for removal of internal fixation device
EXCLUDES 1 *encounter for adjustment of internal fixation device for fracture treatment - code to fracture with appropriate 7th character*
encounter for removal of external fixation device - code to fracture with 7th character D
infection or inflammatory reaction to internal fixation device (T84.6-)
mechanical complication of internal fixation device (T84.1-)

√5th **Z47.3 Aftercare following explantation of joint prosthesis**
Aftercare following explantation of joint prosthesis, staged procedure
Encounter for joint prosthesis insertion following prior explantation of joint prosthesis
AHA: 2020,1Q,23; 2015,1Q,16
TIP: For staged removal of elbow joint prosthesis, assign code Z47.1.

Z47.31 Aftercare following explantation of shoulder joint prosthesis
EXCLUDES 1 *acquired absence of shoulder joint following prior explantation of shoulder joint prosthesis (Z89.23-)*
shoulder joint prosthesis explantation status (Z89.23-)

Z47.32 Aftercare following explantation of hip joint prosthesis
EXCLUDES 1 *acquired absence of hip joint following prior explantation of hip joint prosthesis (Z89.62-)*
hip joint prosthesis explantation status (Z89.62-)

Z47.33 Aftercare following explantation of knee joint prosthesis
EXCLUDES 1 *acquired absence of knee joint following prior explantation of knee prosthesis (Z89.52-)*
knee joint prosthesis explantation status (Z89.52-)

√5th **Z47.8 Encounter for other orthopedic aftercare**

Z47.81 Encounter for orthopedic aftercare following surgical amputation
Use additional code to identify the limb amputated (Z89.-)

Z47.82 Encounter for orthopedic aftercare following scoliosis surgery

Z47.89 Encounter for other orthopedic aftercare
AHA: 2015,1Q,8

√4th **Z48 Encounter for other postprocedural aftercare**
EXCLUDES 1 *encounter for aftercare following injury - code to Injury, by site, with appropriate 7th character for subsequent encounter*
encounter for follow-up examination after completed treatment (Z08-Z09)
EXCLUDES 2 *encounter for attention to artificial openings (Z43.-)*
encounter for fitting and adjustment of prosthetic and other devices (Z44-Z46)
AHA: 2015,4Q,38; 2015,1Q,6-7

√5th **Z48.0 Encounter for attention to dressings, sutures and drains**
EXCLUDES 1 *encounter for planned postprocedural wound closure (Z48.1)*

Z48.00 Encounter for change or removal of nonsurgical wound dressing
Encounter for change or removal of wound dressing NOS

Z48.01 Encounter for change or removal of surgical wound dressing
AHA: 2019,2Q,33

Z48.02 Encounter for removal of sutures
Encounter for removal of staples

Z48.03 Encounter for change or removal of drains
AHA: 2019,2Q,33

Z48.1 Encounter for planned postprocedural wound closure
EXCLUDES 1 *encounter for attention to dressings and sutures (Z48.0-)*

√5th **Z48.2 Encounter for aftercare following organ transplant**

Z48.21 Encounter for aftercare following heart transplant HCC Rx ESR COM

Z48.22 Encounter for aftercare following kidney transplant Rx COM

Z48.23 Encounter for aftercare following liver transplant HCC Rx ESR COM

Z48.24 Encounter for aftercare following lung transplant HCC Rx ESR COM

√6th **Z48.28 Encounter for aftercare following multiple organ transplant**

Z48.280 Encounter for aftercare following heart-lung transplant HCC Rx ESR COM

Z48.288 Encounter for aftercare following multiple organ transplant

√6th **Z48.29 Encounter for aftercare following other organ transplant**

Z48.290 Encounter for aftercare following bone marrow transplant HCC Rx ESR COM

Z48.298 Encounter for aftercare following other organ transplant

Z48.3 Aftercare following surgery for neoplasm
Use additional code to identify the neoplasm

√5th **Z48.8 Encounter for other specified postprocedural aftercare**

√6th **Z48.81 Encounter for surgical aftercare following surgery on specified body systems**
These codes identify the body system requiring aftercare. They are for use in conjunction with other aftercare codes to fully explain the aftercare encounter. The condition treated should also be coded if still present.
EXCLUDES 1 *aftercare for injury - code the injury with 7th character D*
aftercare following surgery for neoplasm (Z48.3)
EXCLUDES 2 *aftercare following organ transplant (Z48.2-)*
orthopedic aftercare (Z47.-)
AHA: 2015,4Q,38

Z48.810 Encounter for surgical aftercare following surgery on the sense organs

Z48.811 Encounter for surgical aftercare following surgery on the nervous system
EXCLUDES 2 *encounter for surgical aftercare following surgery on the sense organs (Z48.810)*

Z48.812 Encounter for surgical aftercare following surgery on the circulatory system
AHA: 2012,4Q,96

Z48.813 Encounter for surgical aftercare following surgery on the respiratory system
AHA: 2019,2Q,33
Z48.814 Encounter for surgical aftercare following surgery on the teeth or oral cavity
Z48.815 Encounter for surgical aftercare following surgery on the digestive system
Z48.816 Encounter for surgical aftercare following surgery on the genitourinary system
EXCLUDES 1 encounter for aftercare following sterilization reversal (Z31.42)
Z48.817 Encounter for surgical aftercare following surgery on the skin and subcutaneous tissue
Z48.89 Encounter for other specified surgical aftercare

✓4th Z49 Encounter for care involving renal dialysis
Code also associated end stage renal disease (N18.6)
✓5th Z49.0 Preparatory care for renal dialysis
Encounter for dialysis instruction and training
Z49.01 Encounter for fitting and adjustment of extracorporeal dialysis catheter HCC Rx ESR
Removal or replacement of renal dialysis catheter
Toilet or cleansing of renal dialysis catheter
Z49.02 Encounter for fitting and adjustment of peritoneal dialysis catheter HCC Rx ESR
✓5th Z49.3 Encounter for adequacy testing for dialysis
Z49.31 Encounter for adequacy testing for hemodialysis HCC Rx ESR
Z49.32 Encounter for adequacy testing for peritoneal dialysis HCC Rx ESR
Encounter for peritoneal equilibration test

✓4th Z51 Encounter for other aftercare and medical care
Code also condition requiring care
EXCLUDES 1 follow-up examination after treatment (Z08-Z09)
Z51.0 Encounter for antineoplastic radiation therapy PDx
AHA: 2017,4Q,103
TIP: Do not assign when admission is for insertion/implantation of radioactive elements. Assign a code for the malignancy instead. Any complications related to the radioactive elements should be assigned as secondary diagnoses.
✓5th Z51.1 Encounter for antineoplastic chemotherapy and immunotherapy
EXCLUDES 2 encounter for chemotherapy and immunotherapy for nonneoplastic condition - code to condition
Z51.11 Encounter for antineoplastic chemotherapy PDx
AHA: 2022,1Q,16; 2015,3Q,19
Z51.12 Encounter for antineoplastic immunotherapy PDx
Z51.5 Encounter for palliative care
AHA: 2022,1Q,18; 2020,4Q,98; 2017,1Q,48
Z51.6 Encounter for desensitization to allergens
AHA: 2016,4Q,77
✓5th Z51.8 Encounter for other specified aftercare
EXCLUDES 1 holiday relief care (Z75.5)
Z51.81 Encounter for therapeutic drug level monitoring
Code also any long-term (current) drug therapy (Z79.-)
EXCLUDES 1 encounter for blood-drug test for administrative or medicolegal reasons (Z02.83)
DEF: Drug monitoring: Measurement of the level of a specific drug in the body or measurement of a specific function to assess effectiveness of a drug.
Z51.89 Encounter for other specified aftercare
AHA: 2012,4Q,95-97

✓4th Z52 Donors of organs and tissues
INCLUDES autologous and other living donors
EXCLUDES 1 cadaveric donor - omit code
examination of potential donor (Z00.5)
AHA: 2012,4Q,99
✓5th Z52.0 Blood donor
✓6th Z52.00 Unspecified blood donor
Z52.000 Unspecified donor, whole blood PDx
Z52.001 Unspecified donor, stem cells PDx
Z52.008 Unspecified donor, other blood PDx
✓6th Z52.01 Autologous blood donor
Z52.010 Autologous donor, whole blood PDx
Z52.011 Autologous donor, stem cells PDx
Z52.018 Autologous donor, other blood PDx
✓6th Z52.09 Other blood donor
Volunteer donor
Z52.090 Other blood donor, whole blood PDx
Z52.091 Other blood donor, stem cells PDx
Z52.098 Other blood donor, other blood PDx
✓5th Z52.1 Skin donor
Z52.10 Skin donor, unspecified PDx
Z52.11 Skin donor, autologous PDx
Z52.19 Skin donor, other PDx
✓5th Z52.2 Bone donor
Z52.20 Bone donor, unspecified PDx
Z52.21 Bone donor, autologous PDx
Z52.29 Bone donor, other PDx
Z52.3 Bone marrow donor PDx
Z52.4 Kidney donor PDx
Z52.5 Cornea donor PDx
Z52.6 Liver donor PDx
✓5th Z52.8 Donor of other specified organs or tissues
✓6th Z52.81 Egg (Oocyte) donor
Z52.810 Egg (Oocyte) donor under age 35, anonymous recipient PDx ♀
Egg donor under age 35 NOS
Z52.811 Egg (Oocyte) donor under age 35, designated recipient PDx ♀
Z52.812 Egg (Oocyte) donor age 35 and over, anonymous recipient PDx ♀
Egg donor age 35 and over NOS
Z52.813 Egg (Oocyte) donor age 35 and over, designated recipient PDx ♀
Z52.819 Egg (Oocyte) donor, unspecified PDx ♀
Z52.89 Donor of other specified organs or tissues PDx
Z52.9 Donor of unspecified organ or tissue
Donor NOS

✓4th Z53 Persons encountering health services for specific procedures and treatment, not carried out
✓5th Z53.0 Procedure and treatment not carried out because of contraindication
Z53.01 Procedure and treatment not carried out due to patient smoking
Z53.09 Procedure and treatment not carried out because of other contraindication
Z53.1 Procedure and treatment not carried out because of patient's decision for reasons of belief and group pressure
✓5th Z53.2 Procedure and treatment not carried out because of patient's decision for other and unspecified reasons
Z53.20 Procedure and treatment not carried out because of patient's decision for unspecified reasons
Z53.21 Procedure and treatment not carried out due to patient leaving prior to being seen by health care provider
Z53.29 Procedure and treatment not carried out because of patient's decision for other reasons
✓5th Z53.3 Procedure converted to open procedure
AHA: 2016,4Q,79
Z53.31 Laparoscopic surgical procedure converted to open procedure UPD
Z53.32 Thoracoscopic surgical procedure converted to open procedure UPD
Z53.33 Arthroscopic surgical procedure converted to open procedure UPD
Z53.39 Other specified procedure converted to open procedure UPD
Z53.8 Procedure and treatment not carried out for other reasons
Z53.9 Procedure and treatment not carried out, unspecified reason

Persons with potential health hazards related to socioeconomic and psychosocial circumstances (Z55-Z65)

AHA: 2021,4Q,34-37; 2019,4Q,66; 2018,4Q,58,73; 2018,1Q,18

DEF: Social determinants of health: Socioeconomic factors that can affect a person's health, including both environmental and societal conditions such as education and literacy, employment, health behaviors, housing, lack of adequate food or water, occupational exposure to risk factors, social support, transportation, and violence. Tracking social needs that impact patients allows providers to identify population health trends and to promote the personalized care that addresses the medical and social needs of individual patients. ***Synonym(s):*** *SDOH.*

TIP: Because codes in these categories represent social information rather than medical diagnoses, they can be assigned based on documentation by nonphysician clinicians involved in the care of these patients as well as self-reported documentation from the patient, as long as the approved and incorporated into the medical record by a clinician or provider.

✓4th **Z55 Problems related to education and literacy**
EXCLUDES 1 *disorders of psychological development (F80-F89)*
Z55.0 Illiteracy and low-level literacy
Z55.1 Schooling unavailable and unattainable
Z55.2 Failed school examinations
Z55.3 Underachievement in school
Z55.4 Educational maladjustment and discord with teachers and classmates
Z55.5 Less than a high school diploma UPD
No general equivalence degree (GED)
Z55.8 Other problems related to education and literacy
Problems related to inadequate teaching
Z55.9 Problems related to education and literacy, unspecified
Academic problems NOS

✓4th **Z56 Problems related to employment and unemployment**
EXCLUDES 2 *occupational exposure to risk factors (Z57.-)*
problems related to housing and economic circumstances (Z59.-)
Z56.0 Unemployment, unspecified
Z56.1 Change of job A
Z56.2 Threat of job loss
Z56.3 Stressful work schedule
Z56.4 Discord with boss and workmates
Z56.5 Uncongenial work environment
Difficult conditions at work
Z56.6 Other physical and mental strain related to work
✓5th **Z56.8 Other problems related to employment**
Z56.81 Sexual harassment on the job
Z56.82 Military deployment status
Individual (civilian or military) currently deployed in theater or in support of military war, peacekeeping and humanitarian operations
Z56.89 Other problems related to employment
Z56.9 Unspecified problems related to employment
Occupational problems NOS

✓4th **Z57 Occupational exposure to risk factors**
Z57.0 Occupational exposure to noise
Z57.1 Occupational exposure to radiation
Z57.2 Occupational exposure to dust
✓5th **Z57.3 Occupational exposure to other air contaminants**
Z57.31 Occupational exposure to environmental tobacco smoke
EXCLUDES 2 *exposure to environmental tobacco smoke (Z77.22)*
Z57.39 Occupational exposure to other air contaminants
Z57.4 Occupational exposure to toxic agents in agriculture
Occupational exposure to solids, liquids, gases or vapors in agriculture
Z57.5 Occupational exposure to toxic agents in other industries
Occupational exposure to solids, liquids, gases or vapors in other industries
Z57.6 Occupational exposure to extreme temperature
Z57.7 Occupational exposure to vibration
Z57.8 Occupational exposure to other risk factors
Z57.9 Occupational exposure to unspecified risk factor

✓4th **Z58 Problems related to physical environment**
EXCLUDES 2 *occupational exposure (Z57.-)*
Z58.6 Inadequate drinking-water supply
Lack of safe drinking water
EXCLUDES 2 *deprivation of water (T73.1)*

✓4th **Z59 Problems related to housing and economic circumstances**
EXCLUDES 2 *problems related to upbringing (Z62.-)*
✓5th **Z59.0 Homelessness**
Z59.00 Homelessness unspecified UPD
Z59.01 Sheltered homelessness UPD
Doubled up
Living in a shelter such as: motel, scattered site housing, temporary or transitional living situation
Z59.02 Unsheltered homelessness UPD
Residing in place not meant for human habitation such as: abandoned buildings, cars, parks, sidewalk
Residing on the street
Z59.1 Inadequate housing
Lack of heating
Restriction of space
Technical defects in home preventing adequate care
Unsatisfactory surroundings
EXCLUDES 1 *problems related to the natural and physical environment (Z77.1-)*
Z59.2 Discord with neighbors, lodgers and landlord
Z59.3 Problems related to living in residential institution
Boarding-school resident
EXCLUDES 1 *institutional upbringing (Z62.2)*
✓5th **Z59.4 Lack of adequate food**
EXCLUDES 2 *deprivation of food (T73.0)*
effects of hunger (T73.0)
inappropriate diet or eating habits (Z72.4)
malnutrition (E40-E46)
Z59.41 Food insecurity UPD
Z59.48 Other specified lack of adequate food UPD
Inadequate food
Lack of food
Z59.5 Extreme poverty
Z59.6 Low income
Z59.7 Insufficient social insurance and welfare support
✓5th **Z59.8 Other problems related to housing and economic circumstances**
✓6th **Z59.81 Housing instability, housed**
Foreclosure on home loan
Past due on rent or mortgage
Unwanted multiple moves in the last 12 months
Z59.811 Housing instability, housed, with risk of homelessness UPD
Imminent risk of homelessness
Z59.812 Housing instability, housed, homelessness in past 12 months UPD
Z59.819 Housing instability, housed unspecified UPD
● **Z59.82 Transportation insecurity**
Excessive transportation time
Inaccessible transportation
Inadequate transportation
Lack of transportation
Unaffordable transportation
Unreliable transportation
Unsafe transportation

● **Z59.86 Financial insecurity**
Bankruptcy
Burdensome debt
Economic strain
Financial strain
Money problems
Running out of money
Unable to make ends meet
EXCLUDES 2 *extreme poverty (Z59.5)*
low income (Z59.6)
material hardship, not elsewhere classified (Z59.87)

● **Z59.87 Material hardship**
Material deprivation
Unable to obtain adequate childcare
Unable to obtain adequate clothing
Unable to obtain adequate utilities
Unable to obtain basic needs
EXCLUDES 2 *extreme poverty (Z59.5)*
financial insecurity, not elsewhere classified (Z59.86)
low income (Z59.6)

Z59.89 Other problems related to housing and economic circumstances UPD
Foreclosure on loan
Isolated dwelling
Problems with creditors

Z59.9 Problem related to housing and economic circumstances, unspecified

✓4th **Z60 Problems related to social environment**

Z60.0 Problems of adjustment to life-cycle transitions
Empty nest syndrome
Phase of life problem
Problem with adjustment to retirement [pension]

Z60.2 Problems related to living alone

Z60.3 Acculturation difficulty
Problem with migration
Problem with social transplantation
DEF: Problem adapting to a different culture or environment not based on any coexisting mental disorder.

Z60.4 Social exclusion and rejection
Exclusion and rejection on the basis of personal characteristics, such as unusual physical appearance, illness or behavior.
EXCLUDES 1 *target of adverse discrimination such as for racial or religious reasons (Z60.5)*

Z60.5 Target of (perceived) adverse discrimination and persecution
EXCLUDES 1 *social exclusion and rejection (Z60.4)*

Z60.8 Other problems related to social environment

Z60.9 Problem related to social environment, unspecified

✓4th **Z62 Problems related to upbringing**
INCLUDES current and past negative life events in childhood
current and past problems of a child related to upbringing
EXCLUDES 2 *maltreatment syndrome (T74.-)*
problems related to housing and economic circumstances (Z59.-)

Z62.0 Inadequate parental supervision and control

Z62.1 Parental overprotection

✓5th **Z62.2 Upbringing away from parents**
EXCLUDES 1 *problems with boarding school (Z59.3)*

Z62.21 Child in welfare custody P
Child in care of non-parental family member
Child in foster care
EXCLUDES 2 *problem for parent due to child in welfare custody (Z63.5)*

Z62.22 Institutional upbringing
Child living in orphanage or group home

Z62.29 Other upbringing away from parents

Z62.3 Hostility towards and scapegoating of child P

Z62.6 Inappropriate (excessive) parental pressure

✓5th **Z62.8 Other specified problems related to upbringing**

✓6th **Z62.81 Personal history of abuse in childhood**

Z62.810 Personal history of physical and sexual abuse in childhood
EXCLUDES 1 *current child physical abuse (T74.12, T76.12)*
current child sexual abuse (T74.22, T76.22)

Z62.811 Personal history of psychological abuse in childhood
EXCLUDES 1 *current child psychological abuse (T74.32, T76.32)*

Z62.812 Personal history of neglect in childhood
EXCLUDES 1 *current child neglect (T74.02, T76.02)*

Z62.813 Personal history of forced labor or sexual exploitation in childhood
AHA: 2018,4Q,32,35

Z62.819 Personal history of unspecified abuse in childhood
EXCLUDES 1 *current child abuse NOS (T74.92, T76.92)*

✓6th **Z62.82 Parent-child conflict**

Z62.820 Parent-biological child conflict
Parent-child problem NOS

Z62.821 Parent-adopted child conflict

Z62.822 Parent-foster child conflict

✓6th **Z62.89 Other specified problems related to upbringing**

Z62.890 Parent-child estrangement NEC

Z62.891 Sibling rivalry

Z62.898 Other specified problems related to upbringing

Z62.9 Problem related to upbringing, unspecified

✓4th **Z63 Other problems related to primary support group, including family circumstances**
EXCLUDES 2 *maltreatment syndrome (T74.-, T76)*
parent-child problems (Z62.-)
problems related to negative life events in childhood (Z62.-)
problems related to upbringing (Z62.-)

Z63.0 Problems in relationship with spouse or partner
Relationship distress with spouse or intimate partner
EXCLUDES 1 *counseling for spousal or partner abuse problems (Z69.1)*
counseling related to sexual attitude, behavior, and orientation (Z70.-)

Z63.1 Problems in relationship with in-laws

✓5th **Z63.3 Absence of family member**
EXCLUDES 1 *absence of family member due to disappearance and death (Z63.4)*
absence of family member due to separation and divorce (Z63.5)

Z63.31 Absence of family member due to military deployment
Individual or family affected by other family member being on military deployment
EXCLUDES 1 *family disruption due to return of family member from military deployment (Z63.71)*

Z63.32 Other absence of family member

Z63.4 Disappearance and death of family member
Assumed death of family member
Bereavement
AHA: 2014,1Q,25

Z63.5 Disruption of family by separation and divorce
Marital estrangement

Z63.6 Dependent relative needing care at home

✓5th **Z63.7 Other stressful life events affecting family and household**

Z63.71 Stress on family due to return of family member from military deployment
Individual or family affected by family member having returned from military deployment (current or past conflict)

Z63.72 Alcoholism and drug addiction in family

Z63.79 Other stressful life events affecting family and household
Anxiety (normal) about sick person in family
Health problems within family
Ill or disturbed family member
Isolated family

Z63.8 Other specified problems related to primary support group
Family discord NOS
Family estrangement NOS
High expressed emotional level within family
Inadequate family support NOS
Inadequate or distorted communication within family

Z63.9 Problem related to primary support group, unspecified
Relationship disorder NOS

Z64 Problems related to certain psychosocial circumstances

Z64.0 Problems related to unwanted pregnancy ♀

Z64.1 Problems related to multiparity ♀

Z64.4 Discord with counselors
Discord with probation officer
Discord with social worker

Z65 Problems related to other psychosocial circumstances

Z65.0 Conviction in civil and criminal proceedings without imprisonment

Z65.1 Imprisonment and other incarceration

Z65.2 Problems related to release from prison

Z65.3 Problems related to other legal circumstances
Arrest
Child custody or support proceedings
Litigation
Prosecution

Z65.4 Victim of crime and terrorism
Victim of torture

Z65.5 Exposure to disaster, war and other hostilities
EXCLUDES 1 *target of perceived discrimination or persecution (Z60.5)*

Z65.8 Other specified problems related to psychosocial circumstances
Religious or spiritual problem

Z65.9 Problem related to unspecified psychosocial circumstances

Do not resuscitate status (Z66)

Z66 Do not resuscitate
DNR status
DEF: Medical order written by a physician that instructs others not to perform cardiopulmonary resuscitation (CPR), intubation, or advanced cardiac life support (ACLS). It prevents unnecessary invasive treatment to prolong life should breathing stop or cardiac arrest occur.

Blood type (Z67)

Z67 Blood type
AHA: 2015,3Q,40

Z67.1 Type A blood
Z67.10 Type A blood, Rh positive
Z67.11 Type A blood, Rh negative

Z67.2 Type B blood
Z67.20 Type B blood, Rh positive
Z67.21 Type B blood, Rh negative

Z67.3 Type AB blood
Z67.30 Type AB blood, Rh positive
Z67.31 Type AB blood, Rh negative

Z67.4 Type O blood
Z67.40 Type O blood, Rh positive
Z67.41 Type O blood, Rh negative

Z67.9 Unspecified blood type
Z67.90 Unspecified blood type, Rh positive
Z67.91 Unspecified blood type, Rh negative

Body mass index [BMI] (Z68)

Z68 Body mass index [BMI]
Kilograms per meters squared
NOTE BMI adult codes are for use for persons 20 years of age or older
BMI pediatric codes are for use for persons 2-19 years of age.
These percentiles are based on the growth charts published by the Centers for Disease Control and Prevention (CDC)
AHA: 2019,4Q,19,57; 2018,4Q,73,77-83; 2017,1Q,39
DEF: Index used to help determine whether an individual is underweight, a healthy weight, overweight, or obese.
TIP: A BMI code may be assigned to support an associated condition based on medical record documentation from clinicians who are not the patient's provider.
TIP: In order to assign a BMI code, the associated condition must meet the definition of a reportable diagnosis for outpatient encounters, per section IV.J of the *ICD-10-CM Official Guidelines for Coding and Reporting.*

Z68.1 Body mass index [BMI] 19.9 or less, adult UPD A

Z68.2 Body mass index [BMI] 20-29, adult
Z68.20 Body mass index [BMI] 20.0-20.9, adult UPD A
Z68.21 Body mass index [BMI] 21.0-21.9, adult UPD A
Z68.22 Body mass index [BMI] 22.0-22.9, adult UPD A
Z68.23 Body mass index [BMI] 23.0-23.9, adult UPD A
Z68.24 Body mass index [BMI] 24.0-24.9, adult UPD A
Z68.25 Body mass index [BMI] 25.0-25.9, adult UPD A
Z68.26 Body mass index [BMI] 26.0-26.9, adult UPD A
Z68.27 Body mass index [BMI] 27.0-27.9, adult UPD A
Z68.28 Body mass index [BMI] 28.0-28.9, adult UPD A
Z68.29 Body mass index [BMI] 29.0-29.9, adult UPD A

Z68.3 Body mass index [BMI] 30-39, adult
Z68.30 Body mass index [BMI] 30.0-30.9, adult UPD A
Z68.31 Body mass index [BMI] 31.0-31.9, adult UPD A
Z68.32 Body mass index [BMI] 32.0-32.9, adult UPD A
Z68.33 Body mass index [BMI] 33.0-33.9, adult UPD A
Z68.34 Body mass index [BMI] 34.0-34.9, adult UPD A
Z68.35 Body mass index [BMI] 35.0-35.9, adult UPD A
Z68.36 Body mass index [BMI] 36.0-36.9, adult UPD A
Z68.37 Body mass index [BMI] 37.0-37.9, adult UPD A
Z68.38 Body mass index [BMI] 38.0-38.9, adult UPD A
Z68.39 Body mass index [BMI] 39.0-39.9, adult UPD A

Z68.4 Body mass index [BMI] 40 or greater, adult
Z68.41 Body mass index [BMI] 40.0-44.9, adult HCC ESR UPD A
Z68.42 Body mass index [BMI] 45.0-49.9, adult HCC ESR UPD A
Z68.43 Body mass index [BMI] 50.0-59.9, adult HCC ESR UPD A
Z68.44 Body mass index [BMI] 60.0-69.9, adult HCC ESR UPD A
Z68.45 Body mass index [BMI] 70 or greater, adult HCC ESR UPD A

Z68.5 Body mass index [BMI] pediatric
AHA: 2018,4Q,81-82
Z68.51 Body mass index [BMI] pediatric, less than 5th percentile for age UPD
Z68.52 Body mass index [BMI] pediatric, 5th percentile to less than 85th percentile for age UPD
Z68.53 Body mass index [BMI] pediatric, 85th percentile to less than 95th percentile for age UPD
Z68.54 Body mass index [BMI] pediatric, greater than or equal to 95th percentile for age UPD

Chapter 21. Factors Influencing Health Status and Contact With Health Services

Z63.79–Z68.54

Additional Character Required | Placeholder Alert | Manifestation | Unspecified Dx | QPP | UPD Unacceptable PDx

Persons encountering health services in other circumstances (Z69-Z76)

Z69 Encounter for mental health services for victim and perpetrator of abuse (4th)
INCLUDES counseling for victims and perpetrators of abuse

Z69.Ø Encounter for mental health services for child abuse problems (5th)

Z69.Ø1 Encounter for mental health services for parental child abuse (6th)

Z69.Ø1Ø Encounter for mental health services for victim of parental child abuse P
Encounter for mental health services for victim of child abuse by parent
Encounter for mental health services for victim of child neglect by parent
Encounter for mental health services for victim of child psychological abuse by parent
Encounter for mental health services for victim of child sexual abuse by parent

Z69.Ø11 Encounter for mental health services for perpetrator of parental child abuse
Encounter for mental health services for perpetrator of parental child neglect
Encounter for mental health services for perpetrator of parental child psychological abuse
Encounter for mental health services for perpetrator of parental child sexual abuse
EXCLUDES 1 *encounter for mental health services for non-parental child abuse (Z69.Ø2-)*

Z69.Ø2 Encounter for mental health services for non-parental child abuse (6th)

Z69.Ø2Ø Encounter for mental health services for victim of non-parental child abuse P
Encounter for mental health services for victim of non-parental child neglect
Encounter for mental health services for victim of non-parental child psychological abuse
Encounter for mental health services for victim of non-parental child sexual abuse

Z69.Ø21 Encounter for mental health services for perpetrator of non-parental child abuse
Encounter for mental health services for perpetrator of non-parental child neglect
Encounter for mental health services for perpetrator of non-parental child psychological abuse
Encounter for mental health services for perpetrator of non-parental child sexual abuse

Z69.1 Encounter for mental health services for spousal or partner abuse problems (5th)

Z69.11 Encounter for mental health services for victim of spousal or partner abuse
Encounter for mental health services for victim of spouse or partner neglect
Encounter for mental health services for victim of spouse or partner psychological abuse
Encounter for mental health services for victim of spouse or partner violence, physical

Z69.12 Encounter for mental health services for perpetrator of spousal or partner abuse
Encounter for mental health services for perpetrator of spouse or partner neglect
Encounter for mental health services for perpetrator of spouse or partner psychological abuse
Encounter for mental health services for perpetrator of spouse or partner violence, physical
Encounter for mental health services for perpetrator of spouse or partner violence, sexual

Z69.8 Encounter for mental health services for victim or perpetrator of other abuse (5th)

Z69.81 Encounter for mental health services for victim of other abuse
Encounter for mental health services for victim of non-spousal adult abuse
Encounter for mental health services for victim of spouse or partner violence, sexual
Encounter for rape victim counseling

Z69.82 Encounter for mental health services for perpetrator of other abuse
Encounter for mental health services for perpetrator of non-spousal adult abuse

Z7Ø Counseling related to sexual attitude, behavior and orientation (4th)
INCLUDES encounter for mental health services for sexual attitude, behavior and orientation
EXCLUDES 2 *contraceptive or procreative counseling (Z3Ø-Z31)*

Z7Ø.Ø Counseling related to sexual attitude

Z7Ø.1 Counseling related to patient's sexual behavior and orientation
Patient concerned regarding impotence
Patient concerned regarding non-responsiveness
Patient concerned regarding promiscuity
Patient concerned regarding sexual orientation

Z7Ø.2 Counseling related to sexual behavior and orientation of third party
Advice sought regarding sexual behavior and orientation of child
Advice sought regarding sexual behavior and orientation of partner
Advice sought regarding sexual behavior and orientation of spouse

Z7Ø.3 Counseling related to combined concerns regarding sexual attitude, behavior and orientation

Z7Ø.8 Other sex counseling
Encounter for sex education

Z7Ø.9 Sex counseling, unspecified

Z71 Persons encountering health services for other counseling and medical advice, not elsewhere classified (4th)
EXCLUDES 2 *contraceptive or procreation counseling (Z3Ø-Z31)*
sex counseling (Z7Ø.-)

Z71.Ø Person encountering health services to consult on behalf of another person
Person encountering health services to seek advice or treatment for non-attending third party
EXCLUDES 2 *anxiety (normal) about sick person in family (Z63.7)*
expectant (adoptive) parent(s) pre-birth pediatrician visit (Z76.81)

Z71.1 Person with feared health complaint in whom no diagnosis is made
Person encountering health services with feared condition which was not demonstrated
Person encountering health services in which problem was normal state
"Worried well"
EXCLUDES 1 *medical observation for suspected diseases and conditions proven not to exist (ZØ3.-)*

Z71.2 Person consulting for explanation of examination or test findings

Z71.3 Dietary counseling and surveillance
Use additional code for any associated underlying medical condition
Use additional code to identify body mass index (BMI), if known (Z68.-)

Z71.4 Alcohol abuse counseling and surveillance (5th)
Use additional code for alcohol abuse or dependence (F1Ø.-)

Z71.41 Alcohol abuse counseling and surveillance of alcoholic

Z71.42 Counseling for family member of alcoholic
Counseling for significant other, partner, or friend of alcoholic

Z71.5 Drug abuse counseling and surveillance (5th)
Use additional code for drug abuse or dependence (F11-F16, F18-F19)

Z71.51 Drug abuse counseling and surveillance of drug abuser

Z71.52 Counseling for family member of drug abuser
Counseling for significant other, partner, or friend of drug abuser

Z71.6 Tobacco abuse counseling
Use additional code for nicotine dependence (F17.-)

Z71.7 Human immunodeficiency virus [HIV] counseling

✓5th **Z71.8 Other specified counseling**
EXCLUDES 2 *counseling for contraception (Z30.Ø-)*
AHA: 2017,4Q,27

Z71.81 Spiritual or religious counseling

Z71.82 Exercise counseling

Z71.83 Encounter for nonprocreative genetic counseling
EXCLUDES 1 *counseling for procreative genetics (Z31.5)*
counseling for procreative management (Z31.6)

Z71.84 Encounter for health counseling related to travel
Encounter for health risk and safety counseling for (international) travel
Code also, if applicable, encounter for immunization (Z23)
EXCLUDES 2 *encounter for administrative examination (ZØ2.-)*
encounter for other special examination without complaint, suspected or reported diagnosis (ZØ1.-)
AHA: 2019,4Q,20,57

Z71.85 Encounter for immunization safety counseling
Encounter for vaccine product safety counseling
Code also, if applicable, encounter for immunization (Z23)
Code also, if applicable, immunization not carried out (Z28.-)
EXCLUDES 1 *encounter for health counseling related to travel (Z71.84)*
AHA: 2021,4Q,34

● **Z71.87 Encounter for pediatric-to-adult transition counseling**
Code also chronic condition, if applicable, such as:
autism spectrum disorder (F84.Ø)
congenital malformations of the circulatory system (Q2Ø-Q28)
cystic fibrosis (E84-)
sickle-cell disorder (D57-)

● **Z71.88 Encounter for counseling for socioeconomic factors**

Z71.89 Other specified counseling

Z71.9 Counseling, unspecified
Encounter for medical advice NOS

✓4th **Z72 Problems related to lifestyle**
EXCLUDES 2 *problems related to life-management difficulty (Z73.-)*
problems related to socioeconomic and psychosocial circumstances (Z55-Z65)

Z72.Ø Tobacco use
Tobacco use NOS
EXCLUDES 1 *history of tobacco dependence (Z87.891)*
nicotine dependence (F17.2-)
tobacco dependence (F17.2-)
tobacco use during pregnancy (O99.33-)

Z72.3 Lack of physical exercise

Z72.4 Inappropriate diet and eating habits
EXCLUDES 1 *behavioral eating disorders of infancy or childhood (F98.2-F98.3)*
eating disorders (F5Ø.-)
lack of adequate food (Z59.48)
malnutrition and other nutritional deficiencies (E4Ø-E64)

✓5th **Z72.5 High risk sexual behavior**
Promiscuity
EXCLUDES 1 *paraphilias (F65)*

Z72.51 High risk heterosexual behavior

Z72.52 High risk homosexual behavior

Z72.53 High risk bisexual behavior

Z72.6 Gambling and betting
EXCLUDES 1 *compulsive or pathological gambling (F63.Ø)*

✓5th **Z72.8 Other problems related to lifestyle**

✓6th **Z72.81 Antisocial behavior**
EXCLUDES 1 *conduct disorders (F91.-)*

Z72.81Ø Child and adolescent antisocial behavior P
Antisocial behavior (child) (adolescent) without manifest psychiatric disorder
Delinquency NOS
Group delinquency
Offenses in the context of gang membership
Stealing in company with others
Truancy from school

Z72.811 Adult antisocial behavior A
Adult antisocial behavior without manifest psychiatric disorder

✓6th **Z72.82 Problems related to sleep**

Z72.82Ø Sleep deprivation
Lack of adequate sleep
EXCLUDES 1 *insomnia (G47.Ø-)*

Z72.821 Inadequate sleep hygiene
Bad sleep habits
Irregular sleep habits
Unhealthy sleep wake schedule
EXCLUDES 1 *insomnia (F51.Ø-, G47.Ø-)*

● **Z72.823 Risk of suffocation (smothering) under another while sleeping**
Child-caregiver co-sleeping
Infant bed-sharing

Z72.89 Other problems related to lifestyle
Self-damaging behavior

Z72.9 Problem related to lifestyle, unspecified

✓4th **Z73 Problems related to life management difficulty**
EXCLUDES 2 *problems related to socioeconomic and psychosocial circumstances (Z55-Z65)*
DEF: State of emotional, mental, and physical exhaustion causing difficulties in managing personal, school, or work circumstances. It is usually due to prolonged stress or poor interpersonal relationship skills or parenting skills.

Z73.Ø Burn-out

Z73.1 Type A behavior pattern

Z73.2 Lack of relaxation and leisure

Z73.3 Stress, not elsewhere classified
Physical and mental strain NOS
EXCLUDES 1 *stress related to employment or unemployment (Z56.-)*

Z73.4 Inadequate social skills, not elsewhere classified

Z73.5 Social role conflict, not elsewhere classified

Z73.6 Limitation of activities due to disability
EXCLUDES 1 *care-provider dependency (Z74.-)*

✓5th **Z73.8 Other problems related to life management difficulty**

✓6th **Z73.81 Behavioral insomnia of childhood**
DEF: Behaviors on the part of the child or caregivers that cause negative compliance with a child's sleep schedule resulting in lack of adequate sleep.

Z73.81Ø Behavioral insomnia of childhood, sleep-onset association type P

Z73.811 Behavioral insomnia of childhood, limit setting type P

Z73.812 Behavioral insomnia of childhood, combined type P

Z73.819 Behavioral insomnia of childhood, unspecified type P

Z73.82 Dual sensory impairment

Z73.89 Other problems related to life management difficulty

Z73.9 Problem related to life management difficulty, unspecified

✓4th **Z74 Problems related to care provider dependency**
EXCLUDES 2 *dependence on enabling machines or devices NEC (Z99.-)*

✓5th **Z74.Ø Reduced mobility**

Z74.Ø1 Bed confinement status
Bedridden

Chapter 21. Factors Influencing Health Status and Contact With Health Services

Z71.52–Z74.Ø1

Z74.09 Other reduced mobility
Chair ridden
Reduced mobility NOS
EXCLUDES 2 *wheelchair dependence (Z99.3)*

Z74.1 Need for assistance with personal care

Z74.2 Need for assistance at home and no other household member able to render care

Z74.3 Need for continuous supervision

Z74.8 Other problems related to care provider dependency

Z74.9 Problem related to care provider dependency, unspecified

Z75 Problems related to medical facilities and other health care

Z75.0 Medical services not available in home
EXCLUDES 1 *no other household member able to render care (Z74.2)*

Z75.1 Person awaiting admission to adequate facility elsewhere

Z75.2 Other waiting period for investigation and treatment

Z75.3 Unavailability and inaccessibility of health-care facilities
EXCLUDES 1 *bed unavailable (Z75.1)*

Z75.4 Unavailability and inaccessibility of other helping agencies

Z75.5 Holiday relief care

Z75.8 Other problems related to medical facilities and other health care

Z75.9 Unspecified problem related to medical facilities and other health care

Z76 Persons encountering health services in other circumstances

Z76.0 Encounter for issue of repeat prescription
Encounter for issue of repeat prescription for appliance
Encounter for issue of repeat prescription for medicaments
Encounter for issue of repeat prescription for spectacles
EXCLUDES 2 *issue of medical certificate (Z02.7)*
repeat prescription for contraceptive (Z30.4-)

Z76.1 Encounter for health supervision and care of foundling PDx

Z76.2 Encounter for health supervision and care of other healthy infant and child PDx P
Encounter for medical or nursing care or supervision of healthy infant under circumstances such as adverse socioeconomic conditions at home
Encounter for medical or nursing care or supervision of healthy infant under circumstances such as awaiting foster or adoptive placement
Encounter for medical or nursing care or supervision of healthy infant under circumstances such as maternal illness
Encounter for medical or nursing care or supervision of healthy infant under circumstances such as number of children at home preventing or interfering with normal care

Z76.3 Healthy person accompanying sick person

Z76.4 Other boarder to healthcare facility
EXCLUDES 1 *homelessness (Z59.0-)*

Z76.5 Malingerer [conscious simulation]
Person feigning illness (with obvious motivation)
EXCLUDES 1 *factitious disorder (F68.1-, F68.A)*
peregrinating patient (F68.1-)
DEF: Act of intentionally exaggerating an illness or disability in order to receive personal gain or to avoid punishment or responsibility.

Z76.8 Persons encountering health services in other specified circumstances

Z76.81 Expectant parent(s) prebirth pediatrician visit
Pre-adoption pediatrician visit for adoptive parent(s)

Z76.82 Awaiting organ transplant status
Patient waiting for organ availability

Z76.89 Persons encountering health services in other specified circumstances
Persons encountering health services NOS
AHA: 2014,2Q,10

Persons with potential health hazards related to family and personal history and certain conditions influencing health status (Z77-Z99)

Code also any follow-up examination (Z08-Z09)

Z77 Other contact with and (suspected) exposures hazardous to health
INCLUDES contact with and (suspected) exposures to potential hazards to health
EXCLUDES 2 *contact with and (suspected) exposure to communicable diseases (Z20.-)*
exposure to (parental) (environmental) tobacco smoke in the perinatal period (P96.81)
newborn affected by noxious substances transmitted via placenta or breast milk (P04.-)
occupational exposure to risk factors (Z57.-)
retained foreign body (Z18.-)
retained foreign body fully removed (Z87.821)
toxic effects of substances chiefly nonmedicinal as to source (T51-T65)

Z77.0 Contact with and (suspected) exposure to hazardous, chiefly nonmedicinal, chemicals

Z77.01 Contact with and (suspected) exposure to hazardous metals

Z77.010 Contact with and (suspected) exposure to arsenic

Z77.011 Contact with and (suspected) exposure to lead

Z77.012 Contact with and (suspected) exposure to uranium
EXCLUDES 1 *retained depleted uranium fragments (Z18.01)*

Z77.018 Contact with and (suspected) exposure to other hazardous metals
Contact with and (suspected) exposure to chromium compounds
Contact with and (suspected) exposure to nickel dust

Z77.02 Contact with and (suspected) exposure to hazardous aromatic compounds

Z77.020 Contact with and (suspected) exposure to aromatic amines

Z77.021 Contact with and (suspected) exposure to benzene

Z77.028 Contact with and (suspected) exposure to other hazardous aromatic compounds
Aromatic dyes NOS
Polycyclic aromatic hydrocarbons

Z77.09 Contact with and (suspected) exposure to other hazardous, chiefly nonmedicinal, chemicals

Z77.090 Contact with and (suspected) exposure to asbestos

Z77.098 Contact with and (suspected) exposure to other hazardous, chiefly nonmedicinal, chemicals
Dyes NOS

Z77.1 Contact with and (suspected) exposure to environmental pollution and hazards in the physical environment

Z77.11 Contact with and (suspected) exposure to environmental pollution

Z77.110 Contact with and (suspected) exposure to air pollution

Z77.111 Contact with and (suspected) exposure to water pollution

Z77.112 Contact with and (suspected) exposure to soil pollution

Z77.118 Contact with and (suspected) exposure to other environmental pollution

Z77.12 Contact with and (suspected) exposure to hazards in the physical environment

Z77.120 Contact with and (suspected) exposure to mold (toxic)

Z77.121 Contact with and (suspected) exposure to harmful algae and algae toxins
Contact with and (suspected) exposure to (harmful) algae bloom NOS
Contact with and (suspected) exposure to blue-green algae bloom
Contact with and (suspected) exposure to brown tide
Contact with and (suspected) exposure to cyanobacteria bloom
Contact with and (suspected) exposure to Florida red tide
Contact with and (suspected) exposure to pfiesteria piscicida
Contact with and (suspected) exposure to red tide

Z77.122 Contact with and (suspected) exposure to noise

Z77.123 Contact with and (suspected) exposure to radon and other naturally occurring radiation
EXCLUDES 2 *radiation exposure as the cause of a confirmed condition (W88-W90, X39.0-)*
radiation sickness NOS (T66)

Z77.128 Contact with and (suspected) exposure to other hazards in the physical environment

5th **Z77.2 Contact with and (suspected) exposure to other hazardous substances**

Z77.21 Contact with and (suspected) exposure to potentially hazardous body fluids

Z77.22 Contact with and (suspected) exposure to environmental tobacco smoke (acute) (chronic)
Exposure to second hand tobacco smoke (acute) (chronic)
Passive smoking (acute) (chronic)
EXCLUDES 1 *nicotine dependence (F17.-)*
tobacco use (Z72.0)
EXCLUDES 2 *occupational exposure to environmental tobacco smoke (Z57.31)*

Z77.29 Contact with and (suspected) exposure to other hazardous substances
AHA: 2016,2Q,33

Z77.9 Other contact with and (suspected) exposures hazardous to health

4th **Z78 Other specified health status**
EXCLUDES 2 *asymptomatic human immunodeficiency virus [HIV] infection status (Z21)*
postprocedural status (Z93-Z99)
sex reassignment status (Z87.890)

Z78.0 Asymptomatic menopausal state A ♀
Menopausal state NOS
Postmenopausal status NOS
EXCLUDES 2 *symptomatic menopausal state (N95.1)*

Z78.1 Physical restraint status
EXCLUDES 1 *physical restraint due to a procedure - omit code*
DEF: Application of mechanical restraining devices or manual restraints to limit physical mobility of a patient.

Z78.9 Other specified health status

4th **Z79 Long term (current) drug therapy**
INCLUDES long term (current) drug use for prophylactic purposes
Code also any therapeutic drug level monitoring (Z51.81)
EXCLUDES 2 *drug abuse and dependence (F11-F19)*
drug use complicating pregnancy, childbirth, and the puerperium (O99.32-)
AHA: 2021,1Q,12

5th **Z79.0 Long term (current) use of anticoagulants and antithrombotics/antiplatelets**
EXCLUDES 2 *long term (current) use of aspirin (Z79.82)*

Z79.01 Long term (current) use of anticoagulants
AHA: 2022,2Q,17; 2021,1Q,4; 2020,2Q,20

Z79.02 Long term (current) use of antithrombotics/antiplatelets UPD

Z79.1 Long term (current) use of non-steroidal anti-inflammatories (NSAID) UPD
EXCLUDES 2 *long term (current) use of aspirin (Z79.82)*

Z79.2 Long term (current) use of antibiotics UPD

Z79.3 Long term (current) use of hormonal contraceptives
Long term (current) use of birth control pill or patch

Z79.4 Long term (current) use of insulin HCC Rx ESR COM
EXCLUDES 2 ▶*long-term (current) use of injectable non-insulin antidiabetic drugs (Z79.85)*◀
long term (current) use of oral antidiabetic drugs (Z79.84)
long term (current) use of oral hypoglycemic drugs (Z79.84)
AHA: 2020,3Q,31

5th **Z79.5 Long term (current) use of steroids**

Z79.51 Long term (current) use of inhaled steroids UPD

Z79.52 Long term (current) use of systemic steroids UPD

● 5th **Z79.6 Long term (current) use of immunomodulators and immunosuppressants**
EXCLUDES 2 *long term (current) use of steroids (Z79.5-)*
long term (current) use of agents affecting estrogen receptors and estrogen levels (Z79.81-)

● **Z79.60 Long term (current) use of unspecified immunomodulators and immunosuppressants**

● **Z79.61 Long term (current) use of immunomodulator**
Long term (current) use of apremilast
Long term (current) use of immunomodulatory imide drug
Long term (current) use of lenalidomide
Long term (current) use of pomalidomide

● 6th **Z79.62 Long term (current) use of immunosuppressant**

● **Z79.620 Long term (current) use of immunosuppressive biologic**
Long term (current) use of adalimumab
Long term (current) use of etanercept
Long term (current) use of infliximab
Long term (current) use of monoclonal antibodies

● **Z79.621 Long term (current) use of calcineurin inhibitor**
Long term (current) use of cyclosporine
Long term (current) use of tacrolimus

● **Z79.622 Long term (current) use of Janus kinase inhibitor**
Long term (current) use of tofacitinib

● **Z79.623 Long term (current) use of mammalian target of rapamycin (mTOR) inhibitor**
Long term (current) use of sirolimus

● **Z79.624 Long term (current) use of inhibitors of nucleotide synthesis**
Long term (current) use of azathioprine
Long term (current) use omycophenolate
Long term (current) use of purine synthesis (IMDH) inhibitors

● 6th **Z79.63 Long term (current) use of chemotherapeutic agent**

● **Z79.630 Long term (current) use of alkylating agent**
Long term (current) use of chlorambucil
Long term (current) use of cisplatin
Long term (current) use of cyclophosphamide

● **Z79.631 Long term (current) use of antimetabolite agent**
Long term (current) use of 5-fluorouracil
Long term (current) use of 6-mercaptopurine
Long term (current) use of cytarabine
Long term (current) use of methotrexate

● **Z79.632 Long term (current) use of antitumor antibiotic**
Long term (current) use of bleomycin
Long term (current) use of doxorubicin
Long term (current) use of mitomycin C

● **Z79.633 Long term (current) use of mitotic inhibitor**
Long term (current) use of paclitaxel
Long term (current) use of plant alkaloids
Long term (current) use of vinblastine
Long term (current) use of vincristine

● **Z79.634 Long term (current) use of topoisomerase inhibitor**
Long term (current) use of etoposide
Long term (current) use of irinotecan
Long term (current) use of topotecan

● **Z79.64 Long term (current) use of myelosuppressive agent**
Long term (current) use of hydroxyurea

● **Z79.69 Long term (current) use of other immunomodulators and immunosuppressants**

Z79.8 Other long term (current) drug therapy

Z79.81 Long term (current) use of agents affecting estrogen receptors and estrogen levels
Code first, if applicable:
malignant neoplasm of breast (C5Ø.-)
malignant neoplasm of prostate (C61)
Use additional code, if applicable, to identify:
estrogen receptor positive status (Z17.Ø)
family history of breast cancer (Z8Ø.3)
genetic susceptibility to malignant neoplasm (cancer) (Z15.Ø-)
personal history of breast cancer (Z85.3)
personal history of prostate cancer (Z85.46)
postmenopausal status (Z78.Ø)
EXCLUDES 1 *hormone replacement therapy (Z79.89Ø)*

Z79.81Ø Long term (current) use of selective estrogen receptor modulators (SERMs) UPD
Long term (current) use of raloxifene (Evista)
Long term (current) use of tamoxifen (Nolvadex)
Long term (current) use of toremifene (Fareston)

Z79.811 Long term (current) use of aromatase inhibitors UPD
Long term (current) use of anastrozole (Arimidex)
Long term (current) use of exemestane (Aromasin)
Long term (current) use of letrozole (Femara)

Z79.818 Long term (current) use of other agents affecting estrogen receptors and estrogen levels UPD
Long term (current) use of estrogen receptor downregulators
Long term (current) use of fulvestrant (Faslodex)
Long term (current) use of gonadotropin-releasing hormone (GnRH) agonist
Long term (current) use of goserelin acetate (Zoladex)
Long term (current) use of leuprolide acetate (leuprorelin) (Lupron)
Long term (current) use of megestrol acetate (Megace)

Z79.82 Long term (current) use of aspirin

Z79.83 Long term (current) use of bisphosphonates UPD
AHA: 2016,4Q,42

Z79.84 Long term (current) use of oral hypoglycemic drugs UPD
Long term (current) use of oral antidiabetic drugs
EXCLUDES 2 *▶long-term (current) use of injectable non-insulin antidiabetic drugs (Z79.85)◀*
long term (current) use of insulin (Z79.4)
AHA: 2020,3Q,31; 2016,4Q,76

● **Z79.85 Long-term (current) use of injectable non-insulin antidiabetic drugs**
EXCLUDES 2 *long term (current) use of insulin (Z79.4)*
long term (current) use of oral hypoglycemic drugs (Z79.84)

Z79.89 Other long term (current) drug therapy

Z79.89Ø Hormone replacement therapy UPD

Z79.891 Long term (current) use of opiate analgesic
Long term (current) use of methadone for pain management
EXCLUDES 1 *methodone use NOS (F11.9-)*
use of methodone for treatment of heroin addiction (F11.2-)

Z79.899 Other long term (current) drug therapy
AHA: 2020,4Q,11; 2020,3Q,31; 2020,2Q,14; 2015,4Q,34; 2015,3Q,21

Z8Ø Family history of primary malignant neoplasm

Z8Ø.Ø Family history of malignant neoplasm of digestive organs UPD
Conditions classifiable to C15-C26
AHA: 2018,1Q,6

Z8Ø.1 Family history of malignant neoplasm of trachea, bronchus and lung UPD
Conditions classifiable to C33-C34

Z8Ø.2 Family history of malignant neoplasm of other respiratory and intrathoracic organs UPD
Conditions classifiable to C3Ø-C32, C37-C39

Z8Ø.3 Family history of malignant neoplasm of breast UPD
Conditions classifiable to C5Ø.-

Z8Ø.4 Family history of malignant neoplasm of genital organs
Conditions classifiable to C51-C63

Z8Ø.41 Family history of malignant neoplasm of ovary UPD

Z8Ø.42 Family history of malignant neoplasm of prostate UPD

Z8Ø.43 Family history of malignant neoplasm of testis UPD

Z8Ø.49 Family history of malignant neoplasm of other genital organs UPD

Z8Ø.5 Family history of malignant neoplasm of urinary tract
Conditions classifiable to C64-C68

Z8Ø.51 Family history of malignant neoplasm of kidney UPD

Z8Ø.52 Family history of malignant neoplasm of bladder UPD

Z8Ø.59 Family history of malignant neoplasm of other urinary tract organ UPD

Z8Ø.6 Family history of leukemia UPD
Conditions classifiable to C91-C95

Z8Ø.7 Family history of other malignant neoplasms of lymphoid, hematopoietic and related tissues UPD
Conditions classifiable to C81-C9Ø, C96.-

Z8Ø.8 Family history of malignant neoplasm of other organs or systems UPD
Conditions classifiable to CØØ-C14, C4Ø-C49, C69-C79

Z8Ø.9 Family history of malignant neoplasm, unspecified UPD
Conditions classifiable to C8Ø.1

Z81 Family history of mental and behavioral disorders

Z81.Ø Family history of intellectual disabilities
Conditions classifiable to F7Ø-F79

Z81.1 Family history of alcohol abuse and dependence
Conditions classifiable to F1Ø.-

Z81.2 Family history of tobacco abuse and dependence
Conditions classifiable to F17.-

Z81.3 Family history of other psychoactive substance abuse and dependence
Conditions classifiable to F11-F16, F18-F19

Z81.4 Family history of other substance abuse and dependence
Conditions classifiable to F55

Z81.8 Family history of other mental and behavioral disorders
Conditions classifiable elsewhere in FØ1-F99

Z82 Family history of certain disabilities and chronic diseases (leading to disablement)

Z82.Ø Family history of epilepsy and other diseases of the nervous system UPD
Conditions classifiable to GØØ-G99

Z82.1 Family history of blindness and visual loss UPD
Conditions classifiable to H54.-

Z82.2 Family history of deafness and hearing loss UPD
Conditions classifiable to H9Ø-H91

Z82.3 Family history of stroke UPD
Conditions classifiable to I60-I64

Z82.4 Family history of ischemic heart disease and other diseases of the circulatory system (5th)
Conditions classifiable to I00-I5A, I65-I99

Z82.41 Family history of sudden cardiac death UPD

Z82.49 Family history of ischemic heart disease and other diseases of the circulatory system UPD

Z82.5 Family history of asthma and other chronic lower respiratory diseases UPD
Conditions classifiable to J40-J47
EXCLUDES 2 *family history of other diseases of the respiratory system (Z83.6)*

Z82.6 Family history of arthritis and other diseases of the musculoskeletal system and connective tissue (5th)
Conditions classifiable to M00-M99

Z82.61 Family history of arthritis UPD

Z82.62 Family history of osteoporosis UPD

Z82.69 Family history of other diseases of the musculoskeletal system and connective tissue UPD

Z82.7 Family history of congenital malformations, deformations and chromosomal abnormalities (5th)
Conditions classifiable to Q00-Q99

Z82.71 Family history of polycystic kidney UPD

Z82.79 Family history of other congenital malformations, deformations and chromosomal abnormalities UPD

Z82.8 Family history of other disabilities and chronic diseases leading to disablement, not elsewhere classified UPD

Z83 Family history of other specific disorders (4th)
EXCLUDES 2 *contact with and (suspected) exposure to communicable disease in the family (Z20.-)*

Z83.0 Family history of human immunodeficiency virus [HIV] disease UPD
Conditions classifiable to B20

Z83.1 Family history of other infectious and parasitic diseases UPD
Conditions classifiable to A00-B19, B25-B94, B99

Z83.2 Family history of diseases of the blood and blood-forming organs and certain disorders involving the immune mechanism UPD
Conditions classifiable to D50-D89

Z83.3 Family history of diabetes mellitus UPD
Conditions classifiable to E08-E13

Z83.4 Family history of other endocrine, nutritional and metabolic diseases (5th)
Conditions classifiable to E00-E07, E15-E88

Z83.41 Family history of multiple endocrine neoplasia [MEN] syndrome UPD

Z83.42 Family history of familial hypercholesterolemia UPD
AHA: 2016,4Q,77

Z83.43 Family history of other disorder of lipoprotein metabolism and other lipidemias (6th)
AHA: 2018,4Q,6,35

Z83.430 Family history of elevated lipoprotein(a) UPD
Family history of elevated Lp(a)

Z83.438 Family history of other disorder of lipoprotein metabolism and other lipidemia UPD
Family history of familial combined hyperlipidemia

Z83.49 Family history of other endocrine, nutritional and metabolic diseases UPD

Z83.5 Family history of eye and ear disorders (5th)

Z83.51 Family history of eye disorders (6th)
Conditions classifiable to H00-H53, H55-H59
EXCLUDES 2 *family history of blindness and visual loss (Z82.1)*

Z83.511 Family history of glaucoma UPD

Z83.518 Family history of other specified eye disorder UPD

Z83.52 Family history of ear disorders UPD
Conditions classifiable to H60-H83, H92-H95
EXCLUDES 2 *family history of deafness and hearing loss (Z82.2)*

Z83.6 Family history of other diseases of the respiratory system UPD
Conditions classifiable to J00-J39, J60-J99
EXCLUDES 2 *family history of asthma and other chronic lower respiratory diseases (Z82.5)*

Z83.7 Family history of diseases of the digestive system (5th)
Conditions classifiable to K00-K93

Z83.71 Family history of colonic polyps UPD
EXCLUDES 2 *family history of malignant neoplasm of digestive organs (Z80.0)*
AHA: 2021,1Q,14

Z83.79 Family history of other diseases of the digestive system UPD

Z84 Family history of other conditions (4th)

Z84.0 Family history of diseases of the skin and subcutaneous tissue UPD
Conditions classifiable to L00-L99

Z84.1 Family history of disorders of kidney and ureter UPD
Conditions classifiable to N00-N29

Z84.2 Family history of other diseases of the genitourinary system UPD
Conditions classifiable to N30-N99

Z84.3 Family history of consanguinity UPD

Z84.8 Family history of other specified conditions (5th)

Z84.81 Family history of carrier of genetic disease UPD
AHA: 2021,1Q,14

Z84.82 Family history of sudden infant death syndrome UPD
Family history of SIDS
AHA: 2016,4Q,77

Z84.89 Family history of other specified conditions UPD

Z85 Personal history of malignant neoplasm (4th)
Code first any follow-up examination after treatment of malignant neoplasm (Z08)
Use additional code to identify:
- alcohol use and dependence (F10.-)
- exposure to environmental tobacco smoke (Z77.22)
- history of tobacco dependence (Z87.891)
- occupational exposure to environmental tobacco smoke (Z57.31)
- tobacco dependence (F17.-)
- tobacco use (Z72.0)

EXCLUDES 2 *personal history of benign neoplasm (Z86.01-)*
personal history of carcinoma-in-situ (Z86.00-)
AHA: 2020,3Q,30; 2018,4Q,64

Z85.0 Personal history of malignant neoplasm of digestive organs (5th)
AHA: 2017,1Q,9

Z85.00 Personal history of malignant neoplasm of unspecified digestive organ

Z85.01 Personal history of malignant neoplasm of esophagus
Conditions classifiable to C15

Z85.02 Personal history of malignant neoplasm of stomach (6th)

Z85.020 Personal history of malignant carcinoid tumor of stomach
Conditions classifiable to C7A.092

Z85.028 Personal history of other malignant neoplasm of stomach
Conditions classifiable to C16

Z85.03 Personal history of malignant neoplasm of large intestine (6th)

Z85.030 Personal history of malignant carcinoid tumor of large intestine
Conditions classifiable to C7A.022-C7A.025, C7A.029

Z85.038 Personal history of other malignant neoplasm of large intestine
Conditions classifiable to C18

Z85.04 Personal history of malignant neoplasm of rectum, rectosigmoid junction, and anus (6th)

Z85.040 Personal history of malignant carcinoid tumor of rectum
Conditions classifiable to C7A.026

Z85.048 Personal history of other malignant neoplasm of rectum, rectosigmoid junction, and anus
Conditions classifiable to C19-C21

Z85.05 Personal history of malignant neoplasm of liver
Conditions classifiable to C22

√6th **Z85.06 Personal history of malignant neoplasm of small intestine**

Z85.060 Personal history of malignant carcinoid tumor of small intestine
Conditions classifiable to C7A.01-

Z85.068 Personal history of other malignant neoplasm of small intestine
Conditions classifiable to C17

Z85.07 Personal history of malignant neoplasm of pancreas
Conditions classifiable to C25

Z85.09 Personal history of malignant neoplasm of other digestive organs

√5th **Z85.1 Personal history of malignant neoplasm of trachea, bronchus and lung**

√6th **Z85.11 Personal history of malignant neoplasm of bronchus and lung**

Z85.110 Personal history of malignant carcinoid tumor of bronchus and lung
Conditions classifiable to C7A.090

Z85.118 Personal history of other malignant neoplasm of bronchus and lung
Conditions classifiable to C34

Z85.12 Personal history of malignant neoplasm of trachea
Conditions classifiable to C33

√5th **Z85.2 Personal history of malignant neoplasm of other respiratory and intrathoracic organs**

Z85.20 Personal history of malignant neoplasm of unspecified respiratory organ

Z85.21 Personal history of malignant neoplasm of larynx
Conditions classifiable to C32

Z85.22 Personal history of malignant neoplasm of nasal cavities, middle ear, and accessory sinuses
Conditions classifiable to C30-C31

√6th **Z85.23 Personal history of malignant neoplasm of thymus**

Z85.230 Personal history of malignant carcinoid tumor of thymus
Conditions classifiable to C7A.091

Z85.238 Personal history of other malignant neoplasm of thymus
Conditions classifiable to C37

Z85.29 Personal history of malignant neoplasm of other respiratory and intrathoracic organs

Z85.3 Personal history of malignant neoplasm of breast
Conditions classifiable to C50.-

√5th **Z85.4 Personal history of malignant neoplasm of genital organs**
Conditions classifiable to C51-C63

Z85.40 Personal history of malignant neoplasm of unspecified female genital organ ♀

Z85.41 Personal history of malignant neoplasm of cervix uteri ♀

Z85.42 Personal history of malignant neoplasm of other parts of uterus ♀

Z85.43 Personal history of malignant neoplasm of ovary ♀

Z85.44 Personal history of malignant neoplasm of other female genital organs ♀

Z85.45 Personal history of malignant neoplasm of unspecified male genital organ ♂

Z85.46 Personal history of malignant neoplasm of prostate ♂

Z85.47 Personal history of malignant neoplasm of testis ♂

Z85.48 Personal history of malignant neoplasm of epididymis ♂

Z85.49 Personal history of malignant neoplasm of other male genital organs ♂

√5th **Z85.5 Personal history of malignant neoplasm of urinary tract**
Conditions classifiable to C64-C68

Z85.50 Personal history of malignant neoplasm of unspecified urinary tract organ

Z85.51 Personal history of malignant neoplasm of bladder

√6th **Z85.52 Personal history of malignant neoplasm of kidney**

EXCLUDES 1 *personal history of malignant neoplasm of renal pelvis (Z85.53)*

Z85.520 Personal history of malignant carcinoid tumor of kidney
Conditions classifiable to C7A.093

Z85.528 Personal history of other malignant neoplasm of kidney
Conditions classifiable to C64

Z85.53 Personal history of malignant neoplasm of renal pelvis

Z85.54 Personal history of malignant neoplasm of ureter

Z85.59 Personal history of malignant neoplasm of other urinary tract organ

Z85.6 Personal history of leukemia
Conditions classifiable to C91-C95

EXCLUDES 1 *leukemia in remission C91.0-C95.9 with 5th character 1*

√5th **Z85.7 Personal history of other malignant neoplasms of lymphoid, hematopoietic and related tissues**

Z85.71 Personal history of Hodgkin lymphoma
Conditions classifiable to C81

Z85.72 Personal history of non-Hodgkin lymphomas
Conditions classifiable to C82-C85

Z85.79 Personal history of other malignant neoplasms of lymphoid, hematopoietic and related tissues
Conditions classifiable to C88-C90, C96

EXCLUDES 1 *multiple myeloma in remission (C90.01)*
plasma cell leukemia in remission (C90.11)
plasmacytoma in remission (C90.21)

√5th **Z85.8 Personal history of malignant neoplasms of other organs and systems**
Conditions classifiable to C00-C14, C40-C49, C69-C75, C7A.098, C76-C79

√6th **Z85.81 Personal history of malignant neoplasm of lip, oral cavity, and pharynx**
Conditions classifiable to C00-C14

Z85.810 Personal history of malignant neoplasm of tongue

Z85.818 Personal history of malignant neoplasm of other sites of lip, oral cavity, and pharynx

Z85.819 Personal history of malignant neoplasm of unspecified site of lip, oral cavity, and pharynx

√6th **Z85.82 Personal history of malignant neoplasm of skin**

Z85.820 Personal history of malignant melanoma of skin
Conditions classifiable to C43

Z85.821 Personal history of Merkel cell carcinoma
Conditions classifiable to C4A

Z85.828 Personal history of other malignant neoplasm of skin
Conditions classifiable to C44

√6th **Z85.83 Personal history of malignant neoplasm of bone and soft tissue**
Conditions classifiable to C40-C41; C45-C49

Z85.830 Personal history of malignant neoplasm of bone

Z85.831 Personal history of malignant neoplasm of soft tissue

EXCLUDES 2 *personal history of malignant neoplasm of skin (Z85.82-)*

√6th **Z85.84 Personal history of malignant neoplasm of eye and nervous tissue**
Conditions classifiable to C69-C72

Z85.840 Personal history of malignant neoplasm of eye

Z85.841 Personal history of malignant neoplasm of brain

Z85.848 Personal history of malignant neoplasm of other parts of nervous tissue

√6th **Z85.85 Personal history of malignant neoplasm of endocrine glands**
Conditions classifiable to C73-C75

Z85.850 Personal history of malignant neoplasm of thyroid

Z85.858 Personal history of malignant neoplasm of other endocrine glands

HCC CMS-HCC Rx Rx HCC ESR ESRD HCC COM Commercial HCC PDx Primary Dx Only N Newborn: 0 P Pediatric: 0-17 M Maternity: 9-64 A Adult: 15-124

Z85.89 Personal history of malignant neoplasm of other organs and systems
Conditions classifiable to C7A.Ø98, C76, C77-C79

Z85.9 Personal history of malignant neoplasm, unspecified
Conditions classifiable to C7A.ØØ, C8Ø.1

✓4th Z86 Personal history of certain other diseases
Code first any follow-up examination after treatment (ZØ9)

✓5th Z86.Ø Personal history of in-situ and benign neoplasms and neoplasms of uncertain behavior
EXCLUDES 2 *personal history of malignant neoplasms (Z85.-)*
AHA: 2017,1Q,9

✓6th Z86.ØØ Personal history of in-situ neoplasm
Conditions classifiable to DØØ-DØ9
AHA: 2019,4Q,20

Z86.ØØØ Personal history of in-situ neoplasm of breast
Conditions classifiable to DØ5

Z86.ØØ1 Personal history of in-situ neoplasm of cervix uteri ♀
Conditions classifiable to DØ6
Personal history of cervical intraepithelial neoplasia III [CIN III]

Z86.ØØ2 Personal history of in-situ neoplasm of other and unspecified genital organs
Conditions classifiable to DØ7
Personal history of high-grade prostatic intraepithelial neoplasia III [HGPIN III]
Personal history of vaginal intraepithelial neoplasia III [VAIN III]
Personal history of vulvar intraepithelial neoplasia III [VIN III]

Z86.ØØ3 Personal history of in-situ neoplasm of oral cavity, esophagus and stomach
Conditions classifiable to DØØ

Z86.ØØ4 Personal history of in-situ neoplasm of other and unspecified digestive organs
Conditions classifiable to DØ1
Personal history of anal intraepithelial neoplasia (AIN III)

Z86.ØØ5 Personal history of in-situ neoplasm of middle ear and respiratory system
Conditions classifiable to DØ2

Z86.ØØ6 Personal history of melanoma in-situ
Conditions classifiable to DØ3
EXCLUDES 2 *sites other than skin - code to personal history of in-situ neoplasm of the site*

Z86.ØØ7 Personal history of in-situ neoplasm of skin
Conditions classifiable to DØ4
Personal history of carcinoma in situ of skin

Z86.ØØ8 Personal history of in-situ neoplasm of other site
Conditions classifiable to DØ9

✓6th Z86.Ø1 Personal history of benign neoplasm

Z86.Ø1Ø Personal history of colonic polyps
AHA: 2021,1Q,14; 2017,1Q,14

Z86.Ø11 Personal history of benign neoplasm of the brain

Z86.Ø12 Personal history of benign carcinoid tumor

Z86.Ø18 Personal history of other benign neoplasm
AHA: 2017,1Q,14

Z86.Ø3 Personal history of neoplasm of uncertain behavior

✓5th Z86.1 Personal history of infectious and parasitic diseases
Conditions classifiable to AØØ-B89, B99
EXCLUDES 1 *personal history of infectious diseases specific to a body system*
sequelae of infectious and parasitic diseases (B9Ø-B94)

Z86.11 Personal history of tuberculosis

Z86.12 Personal history of poliomyelitis

Z86.13 Personal history of malaria

Z86.14 Personal history of Methicillin resistant Staphylococcus aureus infection
Personal history of MRSA infection

Z86.15 Personal history of latent tuberculosis infection

Z86.16 Personal history of COVID-19 UPD
EXCLUDES 1 *post COVID-19 condition (UØ9.9)*
AHA: 2021,4Q,107-108; 2021,1Q,28-29,33-35,40-41,44-45

Z86.19 Personal history of other infectious and parasitic diseases
AHA: 2021,1Q,33-34,40; 2020,3Q,13; 2020,2Q,10,12

Z86.2 Personal history of diseases of the blood and blood-forming organs and certain disorders involving the immune mechanism
Conditions classifiable to D5Ø-D89

✓5th Z86.3 Personal history of endocrine, nutritional and metabolic diseases
Conditions classifiable to EØØ-E88

Z86.31 Personal history of diabetic foot ulcer
EXCLUDES 2 *current diabetic foot ulcer (EØ8.621, EØ9.621, E1Ø.621, E11.621, E13.621)*

Z86.32 Personal history of gestational diabetes ♀
Personal history of conditions classifiable to O24.4-
EXCLUDES 1 *gestational diabetes mellitus in current pregnancy (O24.4-)*

Z86.39 Personal history of other endocrine, nutritional and metabolic disease
AHA: 2020,1Q,12

✓5th Z86.5 Personal history of mental and behavioral disorders
Conditions classifiable to F4Ø-F59

Z86.51 Personal history of combat and operational stress reaction A

Z86.59 Personal history of other mental and behavioral disorders

✓5th Z86.6 Personal history of diseases of the nervous system and sense organs
Conditions classifiable to GØØ-G99, HØØ-H95

Z86.61 Personal history of infections of the central nervous system
Personal history of encephalitis
Personal history of meningitis

Z86.69 Personal history of other diseases of the nervous system and sense organs
AHA: 2016,4Q,24

✓5th Z86.7 Personal history of diseases of the circulatory system
Conditions classifiable to IØØ-I99
EXCLUDES 2 *old myocardial infarction (I25.2)*
personal history of anaphylactic shock (Z87.892)
postmyocardial infarction syndrome (I24.1)

✓6th Z86.71 Personal history of venous thrombosis and embolism

Z86.711 Personal history of pulmonary embolism

Z86.718 Personal history of other venous thrombosis and embolism
AHA: 2020,2Q,20

Z86.72 Personal history of thrombophlebitis

Z86.73 Personal history of transient ischemic attack (TIA), and cerebral infarction without residual deficits
Personal history of prolonged reversible ischemic neurological deficit (PRIND)
Personal history of stroke NOS without residual deficits
EXCLUDES 1 *personal history of traumatic brain injury (Z87.82Ø)*
sequelae of cerebrovascular disease (I69.-)
AHA: 2012,4Q,92

Z86.74 Personal history of sudden cardiac arrest
Personal history of sudden cardiac death successfully resuscitated

Z86.79 Personal history of other diseases of the circulatory system
AHA: 2022,2Q,14; 2020,1Q,12

✓4th Z87 Personal history of other diseases and conditions
Code first any follow-up examination after treatment (ZØ9)

✓5th Z87.Ø Personal history of diseases of the respiratory system
Conditions classifiable to JØØ-J99

Z87.Ø1 Personal history of pneumonia (recurrent)

Z87.Ø9 Personal history of other diseases of the respiratory system

✓5th Z87.1 Personal history of diseases of the digestive system
Conditions classifiable to KØØ-K93

Z87.11 Personal history of peptic ulcer disease

Z87.19 **Personal history of other diseases of the digestive system**
AHA: 2017,1Q,14

Z87.2 **Personal history of diseases of the skin and subcutaneous tissue**
Conditions classifiable to LØØ-L99
EXCLUDES 2 *personal history of diabetic foot ulcer (Z86.31)*

5th Z87.3 **Personal history of diseases of the musculoskeletal system and connective tissue**
Conditions classifiable to MØØ-M99
EXCLUDES 2 *personal history of (healed) traumatic fracture (Z87.81)*

6th Z87.31 **Personal history of (healed) nontraumatic fracture**

Z87.31Ø **Personal history of (healed) osteoporosis fracture**
Personal history of (healed) fragility fracture
Personal history of (healed) collapsed vertebra due to osteoporosis
TIP: Assign for history of osteoporosis fractures that have resolved, even when a code from category M80 indicating current osteoporosis fracture is also reported.

Z87.311 **Personal history of (healed) other pathological fracture**
Personal history of (healed) collapsed vertebra NOS
EXCLUDES 2 *personal history of osteoporosis fracture (Z87.31Ø)*

Z87.312 **Personal history of (healed) stress fracture**
Personal history of (healed) fatigue fracture

Z87.39 **Personal history of other diseases of the musculoskeletal system and connective tissue**

5th Z87.4 **Personal history of diseases of the genitourinary system**
Conditions classifiable to NØØ-N99

6th Z87.41 **Personal history of dysplasia of the female genital tract**
EXCLUDES 1 *personal history of intraepithelial neoplasia III of female genital tract (Z86.ØØ1, Z86.ØØ8)*
personal history of malignant neoplasm of female genital tract (Z85.4Ø-Z85.44)

Z87.41Ø **Personal history of cervical dysplasia** ♀

Z87.411 **Personal history of vaginal dysplasia** ♀

Z87.412 **Personal history of vulvar dysplasia** ♀

Z87.42 **Personal history of other diseases of the female genital tract** ♀

6th Z87.43 **Personal history of diseases of the male genital organs**

Z87.43Ø **Personal history of prostatic dysplasia** ♂
EXCLUDES 1 *personal history of malignant neoplasm of prostate (Z85.46)*

Z87.438 **Personal history of other diseases of male genital organs** ♂

6th Z87.44 **Personal history of diseases of the urinary system**
EXCLUDES 1 *personal history of malignant neoplasm of cervix uteri (Z85.41)*

Z87.44Ø **Personal history of urinary (tract) infections**

Z87.441 **Personal history of nephrotic syndrome**

Z87.442 **Personal history of urinary calculi**
Personal history of kidney stones

Z87.448 **Personal history of other diseases of urinary system**

5th Z87.5 **Personal history of complications of pregnancy, childbirth and the puerperium**
Conditions classifiable to OØØ-O9A
EXCLUDES 2 *recurrent pregnancy loss (N96)*

Z87.51 **Personal history of pre-term labor** ♀
EXCLUDES 1 *current pregnancy with history of pre-term labor (OØ9.21-)*

Z87.59 **Personal history of other complications of pregnancy, childbirth and the puerperium** ♀
Personal history of trophoblastic disease

● 5th Z87.6 **Personal history of certain (corrected) conditions arising in the perinatal period**
Conditions classifiable to PØØ-P96
EXCLUDES 1 *personal history of (corrected) congenital malformations (Z87.7-)*

● Z87.61 **Personal history of (corrected) necrotizing enterocolitis of newborn**

● Z87.68 **Personal history of other (corrected) conditions arising in the perinatal period**

5th Z87.7 **Personal history of (corrected) congenital malformations**
Conditions classifiable to QØØ-Q89 that have been repaired or corrected
EXCLUDES 1 ~~*congenital malformations that have been partially corrected or repair but which still require medical treatment - code to condition*~~
EXCLUDES 2 ▸*congenital malformations that have been partially corrected or repaired but which still require medical treatment - code to condition*◂
other postprocedural states (Z98.-)
personal history of medical treatment (Z92.-)
presence of cardiac and vascular implants and grafts (Z95.-)
presence of other devices (Z97.-)
presence of other functional implants (Z96.-)
transplanted organ and tissue status (Z94.-)

6th Z87.71 **Personal history of (corrected) congenital malformations of genitourinary system**

Z87.71Ø **Personal history of (corrected) hypospadias** ♂

Z87.718 **Personal history of other specified (corrected) congenital malformations of genitourinary system**

6th Z87.72 **Personal history of (corrected) congenital malformations of nervous system and sense organs**

Z87.72Ø **Personal history of (corrected) congenital malformations of eye**

Z87.721 **Personal history of (corrected) congenital malformations of ear**

Z87.728 **Personal history of other specified (corrected) congenital malformations of nervous system and sense organs**

6th Z87.73 **Personal history of (corrected) congenital malformations of digestive system**

Z87.73Ø **Personal history of (corrected) cleft lip and palate**

● Z87.731 **Personal history of (corrected) tracheoesophageal fistula or atresia**

● Z87.732 **Personal history of (corrected) persistent cloaca or cloacal malformations**

Z87.738 **Personal history of other specified (corrected) congenital malformations of digestive system**

Z87.74 **Personal history of (corrected) congenital malformations of heart and circulatory system**

Z87.75 **Personal history of (corrected) congenital malformations of respiratory system**

▲ 6th Z87.76 **Personal history of (corrected) congenital malformations of integument, limbs and musculoskeletal system**

● Z87.76Ø **Personal history of (corrected) congenital diaphragmatic hernia or other congenital diaphragm malformations**

● Z87.761 **Personal history of (corrected) gastroschisis**

● Z87.762 **Personal history of (corrected) prune belly malformation**

● Z87.763 **Personal history of other (corrected) congenital abdominal wall malformations**

● Z87.768 **Personal history of other specified (corrected) congenital malformations of integument, limbs and musculoskeletal system**

6th Z87.79 **Personal history of other (corrected) congenital malformations**

Z87.79Ø **Personal history of (corrected) congenital malformations of face and neck**

Z87.798 **Personal history of other (corrected) congenital malformations**

Z87.8 Personal history of other specified conditions

EXCLUDES 2 *personal history of self harm (Z91.5-)*

Z87.81 Personal history of (healed) traumatic fracture

EXCLUDES 2 *personal history of (healed) nontraumatic fracture (Z87.31-)*

Z87.82 Personal history of other (healed) physical injury and trauma

Conditions classifiable to SØØ-T88, except traumatic fractures

Z87.82Ø Personal history of traumatic brain injury

EXCLUDES 1 *personal history of transient ischemic attack (TIA), and cerebral infarction without residual deficits (Z86.73)*

Z87.821 Personal history of retained foreign body fully removed

Z87.828 Personal history of other (healed) physical injury and trauma

Z87.89 Personal history of other specified conditions

Z87.89Ø Personal history of sex reassignment

Z87.891 Personal history of nicotine dependence

EXCLUDES 1 *current nicotine dependence (F17.2-)*

AHA: 2017,2Q,27

Z87.892 Personal history of anaphylaxis

Code also allergy status such as:

allergy status to drugs, medicaments and biological substances (Z88.-)

allergy status, other than to drugs and biological substances (Z91.Ø-)

Z87.898 Personal history of other specified conditions

AHA: 2013,1Q,21

Z88 Allergy status to drugs, medicaments and biological substances

EXCLUDES 2 *allergy status, other than to drugs and biological substances (Z91.Ø-)*

AHA: 2015,3Q,23

Z88.Ø Allergy status to penicillin

Z88.1 Allergy status to other antibiotic agents

Z88.2 Allergy status to sulfonamides

Z88.3 Allergy status to other anti-infective agents

Z88.4 Allergy status to anesthetic agent

Z88.5 Allergy status to narcotic agent

Z88.6 Allergy status to analgesic agent

Z88.7 Allergy status to serum and vaccine

Z88.8 Allergy status to other drugs, medicaments and biological substances

Z88.9 Allergy status to unspecified drugs, medicaments and biological substances

Z89 Acquired absence of limb

INCLUDES amputation status

postprocedural loss of limb

post-traumatic loss of limb

EXCLUDES 1 *acquired deformities of limbs (M2Ø-M21)*

congenital absence of limbs (Q71-Q73)

Z89.Ø Acquired absence of thumb and other finger(s)

Z89.Ø1 Acquired absence of thumb

Z89.Ø11 Acquired absence of right thumb

Z89.Ø12 Acquired absence of left thumb

Z89.Ø19 Acquired absence of unspecified thumb

Z89.Ø2 Acquired absence of other finger(s)

EXCLUDES 2 *acquired absence of thumb (Z89.Ø1-)*

Z89.Ø21 Acquired absence of right finger(s)

Z89.Ø22 Acquired absence of left finger(s)

Z89.Ø29 Acquired absence of unspecified finger(s)

Z89.1 Acquired absence of hand and wrist

Z89.11 Acquired absence of hand

Z89.111 Acquired absence of right hand COM

Z89.112 Acquired absence of left hand COM

Z89.119 Acquired absence of unspecified hand COM

Z89.12 Acquired absence of wrist

Disarticulation at wrist

Z89.121 Acquired absence of right wrist COM

Z89.122 Acquired absence of left wrist COM

Z89.129 Acquired absence of unspecified wrist COM

Z89.2 Acquired absence of upper limb above wrist

Z89.2Ø Acquired absence of upper limb, unspecified level

Z89.2Ø1 Acquired absence of right upper limb, unspecified level COM

Z89.2Ø2 Acquired absence of left upper limb, unspecified level COM

Z89.2Ø9 Acquired absence of unspecified upper limb, unspecified level COM

Acquired absence of arm NOS

Z89.21 Acquired absence of upper limb below elbow

Z89.211 Acquired absence of right upper limb below elbow COM

Z89.212 Acquired absence of left upper limb below elbow COM

Z89.219 Acquired absence of unspecified upper limb below elbow COM

Z89.22 Acquired absence of upper limb above elbow

Disarticulation at elbow

Z89.221 Acquired absence of right upper limb above elbow COM

Z89.222 Acquired absence of left upper limb above elbow COM

Z89.229 Acquired absence of unspecified upper limb above elbow COM

Z89.23 Acquired absence of shoulder

Acquired absence of shoulder joint following explantation of shoulder joint prosthesis, with or without presence of antibiotic-impregnated cement spacer

Z89.231 Acquired absence of right shoulder

Z89.232 Acquired absence of left shoulder

Z89.239 Acquired absence of unspecified shoulder

Z89.4 Acquired absence of toe(s), foot, and ankle

Z89.41 Acquired absence of great toe

Z89.411 Acquired absence of right great toe HCC ESR

Z89.412 Acquired absence of left great toe HCC ESR

Z89.419 Acquired absence of unspecified great toe HCC ESR

Z89.42 Acquired absence of other toe(s)

EXCLUDES 2 *acquired absence of great toe (Z89.41-)*

Z89.421 Acquired absence of other right toe(s) HCC ESR

Z89.422 Acquired absence of other left toe(s) HCC ESR

Z89.429 Acquired absence of other toe(s), unspecified side HCC ESR

Z89.43 Acquired absence of foot

Z89.431 Acquired absence of right foot HCC ESR COM

Z89.432 Acquired absence of left foot HCC ESR COM

Z89.439 Acquired absence of unspecified foot HCC ESR COM

Z89.44 Acquired absence of ankle

Disarticulation of ankle

Z89.441 Acquired absence of right ankle HCC ESR COM

Z89.442 Acquired absence of left ankle HCC ESR COM

Z89.449 Acquired absence of unspecified ankle HCC ESR COM

Z89.5 Acquired absence of leg below knee

Z89.51 Acquired absence of leg below knee

Z89.511 Acquired absence of right leg below knee HCC ESR COM

Z89.512 Acquired absence of left leg below knee HCC ESR COM

Z89.519 Acquired absence of unspecified leg below knee HCC ESR COM

Z89.52 Acquired absence of knee
Acquired absence of knee joint following explantation of knee joint prosthesis, with or without presence of antibiotic-impregnated cement spacer
Z89.521 Acquired absence of right knee
Z89.522 Acquired absence of left knee
Z89.529 Acquired absence of unspecified knee
Z89.6 Acquired absence of leg above knee
Z89.61 Acquired absence of leg above knee
Acquired absence of leg NOS
Disarticulation at knee
Z89.611 Acquired absence of right leg above knee HCC ESR COM
Z89.612 Acquired absence of left leg above knee HCC ESR COM
Z89.619 Acquired absence of unspecified leg above knee HCC ESR COM
Z89.62 Acquired absence of hip
Acquired absence of hip joint following explantation of hip joint prosthesis, with or without presence of antibiotic-impregnated cement spacer
Disarticulation at hip
Z89.621 Acquired absence of right hip joint
Z89.622 Acquired absence of left hip joint
Z89.629 Acquired absence of unspecified hip joint
Z89.9 Acquired absence of limb, unspecified COM

Z90 Acquired absence of organs, not elsewhere classified
INCLUDES postprocedural or post-traumatic loss of body part NEC
EXCLUDES 1 *congenital absence - see Alphabetical Index*
EXCLUDES 2 *postprocedural absence of endocrine glands (E89.-)*
Z90.0 Acquired absence of part of head and neck
Z90.01 Acquired absence of eye
Z90.02 Acquired absence of larynx
Z90.09 Acquired absence of other part of head and neck
Acquired absence of nose
EXCLUDES 2 *teeth (K08.1)*
Z90.1 Acquired absence of breast and nipple
Z90.10 Acquired absence of unspecified breast and nipple
Z90.11 Acquired absence of right breast and nipple
Z90.12 Acquired absence of left breast and nipple
Z90.13 Acquired absence of bilateral breasts and nipples
Z90.2 Acquired absence of lung [part of]
Z90.3 Acquired absence of stomach [part of]
Z90.4 Acquired absence of other specified parts of digestive tract
Z90.41 Acquired absence of pancreas
Code also exocrine pancreatic insufficiency (K86.81)
Use additional code to identify any associated: diabetes mellitus, postpancreatectomy (E13.-) insulin use (Z79.4)
Z90.410 Acquired total absence of pancreas
Acquired absence of pancreas NOS
Z90.411 Acquired partial absence of pancreas
Z90.49 Acquired absence of other specified parts of digestive tract
Z90.5 Acquired absence of kidney
Z90.6 Acquired absence of other parts of urinary tract
Acquired absence of bladder
Z90.7 Acquired absence of genital organ(s)
EXCLUDES 1 *personal history of sex reassignment (Z87.890)*
EXCLUDES 2 *female genital mutilation status (N90.81-)*
Z90.71 Acquired absence of cervix and uterus
Z90.710 Acquired absence of both cervix and uterus ♀
Acquired absence of uterus NOS
Status post total hysterectomy
Z90.711 Acquired absence of uterus with remaining cervical stump ♀
Status post partial hysterectomy with remaining cervical stump
Z90.712 Acquired absence of cervix with remaining uterus ♀
Z90.72 Acquired absence of ovaries
Z90.721 Acquired absence of ovaries, unilateral ♀
Z90.722 Acquired absence of ovaries, bilateral ♀
Z90.79 Acquired absence of other genital organ(s)
Z90.8 Acquired absence of other organs
Z90.81 Acquired absence of spleen
Z90.89 Acquired absence of other organs

Z91 Personal risk factors, not elsewhere classified
EXCLUDES 2 *contact with and (suspected) exposures hazardous to health (Z77.-)*
exposure to pollution and other problems related to physical environment (Z77.1-)
female genital mutilation status (N90.81-)
personal history of physical injury and trauma (Z87.81, Z87.82-)
occupational exposure to risk factors (Z57.-)
Z91.0 Allergy status, other than to drugs and biological substances
EXCLUDES 2 *allergy status to drugs, medicaments, and biological substances (Z88.-)*
Z91.01 Food allergy status
EXCLUDES 2 *food additives allergy status (Z91.02)*
Z91.010 Allergy to peanuts
Z91.011 Allergy to milk products
EXCLUDES 1 *lactose intolerance (E73.-)*
Z91.012 Allergy to eggs
Z91.013 Allergy to seafood
Allergy to shellfish
Allergy to octopus or squid ink
Z91.014 Allergy to mammalian meats
Allergy to beef
Allergy to lamb
Allergy to pork
Allergy to red meats
AHA: 2021,4Q,33
Z91.018 Allergy to other foods
Allergy to nuts other than peanuts
Z91.02 Food additives allergy status
Z91.03 Insect allergy status
Z91.030 Bee allergy status
Z91.038 Other insect allergy status
Z91.04 Nonmedicinal substance allergy status
Z91.040 Latex allergy status
Latex sensitivity status
Z91.041 Radiographic dye allergy status
Allergy status to contrast media used for diagnostic X-ray procedure
Z91.048 Other nonmedicinal substance allergy status
Z91.09 Other allergy status, other than to drugs and biological substances
Z91.1 Patient's noncompliance with medical treatment and regimen
EXCLUDES 2 *▶caregiver noncompliance with patient's medical treatment and regimen (Z91.A-)◀*
▲ Z91.11 Patient's noncompliance with dietary regimen
▶Code also, if applicable, food insecurity (Z59.4-)◀
● Z91.110 Patient's noncompliance with dietary regimen due to financial hardship
● Z91.118 Patient's noncompliance with dietary regimen for other reason
Inability to comply with dietary regimen
● Z91.119 Patient's noncompliance with dietary regimen due to unspecified reason
Z91.12 Patient's intentional underdosing of medication regimen
Code first underdosing of medication (T36-T50) with fifth or sixth character 6
EXCLUDES 1 *adverse effect of prescribed drug taken as directed - code to adverse effect*
poisoning (overdose) - code to poisoning
AHA: 2018,4Q,72
Z91.120 Patient's intentional underdosing of medication regimen due to financial hardship
Z91.128 Patient's intentional underdosing of medication regimen for other reason

Z91.13 Patient's unintentional underdosing of medication regimen
Code first underdosing of medication (T36-T5Ø) with fifth or sixth character 6
EXCLUDES 1 *adverse effect of prescribed drug taken as directed - code to adverse effect*
poisoning (overdose) - code to poisoning
AHA: 2018,4Q,72

Z91.13Ø Patient's unintentional underdosing of medication regimen due to age-related debility

Z91.138 Patient's unintentional underdosing of medication regimen for other reason

Z91.14 Patient's other noncompliance with medication regimen
Patient's underdosing of medication NOS
AHA: 2022,1Q,36; 2018,4Q,72

Z91.15 Patient's noncompliance with renal dialysis HCC Rx ESR

▲ **Z91.19 Patient's noncompliance with other medical treatment and regimen**
▶Patient's nonadherence to medical treatment◀

● **Z91.19Ø Patient's noncompliance with other medical treatment and regimen due to financial hardship**

● **Z91.198 Patient's noncompliance with other medical treatment and regimen for other reason**

● **Z91.199 Patient's noncompliance with other medical treatment and regimen due to unspecified reason**

● **Z91.A Caregiver's noncompliance with patient's medical treatment and regimen**

● **Z91.A1 Caregiver's noncompliance with patient's dietary regimen**
Caregiver's inability to comply with patient's dietary regimen
Code also, if applicable, food insecurity (Z59.4-)

● **Z91.A1Ø Caregiver's noncompliance with patient's dietary regimen due to financial hardship**

● **Z91.A18 Caregiver's noncompliance with patient's dietary regimen for other reason**

● **Z91.A2 Caregiver's intentional underdosing of patient's medication regimen**
Code first underdosing of medication (T36-T5Ø) with fifth or sixth character 6

● **Z91.A2Ø Caregiver's intentional underdosing of patient's medication regimen due to financial hardship**

● **Z91.A28 Caregiver's intentional underdosing of medication regimen for other reason**

● **Z91.A3 Caregiver's unintentional underdosing of patient's medication regimen**
Code first underdosing of medication (T36-T5Ø) with fifth or sixth character 6

● **Z91.A4 Caregiver's other noncompliance with patient's medication regimen**
Caregiver's underdosing of patient's medication NOS

● **Z91.A5 Caregiver's noncompliance with patient's renal dialysis**

● **Z91.A9 Caregiver's noncompliance with patient's other medical treatment and regimen**
Caregiver's nonadherence to patient's medical treatment

Z91.4 Personal history of psychological trauma, not elsewhere classified

Z91.41 Personal history of adult abuse
EXCLUDES 2 *personal history of abuse in childhood (Z62.81-)*

Z91.41Ø Personal history of adult physical and sexual abuse A
EXCLUDES 1 *current adult physical abuse (T74.11, T76.11)*
current adult sexual abuse (T74.21, T76.11)

Z91.411 Personal history of adult psychological abuse A

Z91.412 Personal history of adult neglect A
EXCLUDES 1 *current adult neglect (T74.Ø1, T76.Ø1)*

Z91.419 Personal history of unspecified adult abuse A

Z91.42 Personal history of forced labor or sexual exploitation
AHA: 2018,4Q,32,35

Z91.49 Other personal history of psychological trauma, not elsewhere classified

Z91.5 Personal history of self-harm
Code also mental health disorder, if known
AHA: 2021,4Q,33

Z91.51 Personal history of suicidal behavior UPD
Personal history of parasuicide
Personal history of self-poisoning
Personal history of suicide attempt

Z91.52 Personal history of nonsuicidal self-harm UPD
Personal history of nonsuicidal self-injury
Personal history of self-inflicted injury without suicidal intent
Personal history of self-mutilation

Z91.8 Other specified personal risk factors, not elsewhere classified

Z91.81 History of falling
At risk for falling

Z91.82 Personal history of military deployment A
Individual (civilian or military) with past history of military war, peacekeeping and humanitarian deployment (current or past conflict)
Returned from military deployment

Z91.83 Wandering in diseases classified elsewhere
Code first underlying disorder such as:
Alzheimer's disease (G3Ø.-)
autism or pervasive developmental disorder (F84.-)
intellectual disabilities (F7Ø-F79)
unspecified dementia with behavioral disturbance ▶(FØ3.9-, FØ3.A-, FØ3.B-, FØ3.C-)◀

Z91.84 Oral health risk factors
AHA: 2017,4Q,29

Z91.841 Risk for dental caries, low

Z91.842 Risk for dental caries, moderate

Z91.843 Risk for dental caries, high

Z91.849 Unspecified risk for dental caries

Z91.89 Other specified personal risk factors, not elsewhere classified
AHA: 2017,1Q,45

Z92 Personal history of medical treatment
EXCLUDES 2 *postprocedural states (Z98.-)*

Z92.Ø Personal history of contraception
EXCLUDES 1 *counseling or management of current contraceptive practices (Z3Ø.-)*
long term (current) use of contraception (Z79.3)
presence of (intrauterine) contraceptive device (Z97.5)

Z92.2 Personal history of drug therapy
EXCLUDES 2 *long term (current) drug therapy (Z79.-)*

Z92.21 Personal history of antineoplastic chemotherapy

Z92.22 Personal history of monoclonal drug therapy

Z92.23 Personal history of estrogen therapy

Z92.24 Personal history of steroid therapy

Z92.24Ø Personal history of inhaled steroid therapy

Z92.241 Personal history of systemic steroid therapy
Personal history of steroid therapy NOS

Z92.25 Personal history of immunosuppression therapy
EXCLUDES 2 *personal history of steroid therapy (Z92.24)*

Z92.29 Personal history of other drug therapy

Z92.3 Personal history of irradiation
Personal history of exposure to therapeutic radiation
EXCLUDES 1 *exposure to radiation in the physical environment (Z77.12)*
occupational exposure to radiation (Z57.1)

Z92.8 Personal history of other medical treatment

Z92.81 Personal history of extracorporeal membrane oxygenation (ECMO)

Z92.82 Status post administration of tPA (rtPA) in a different facility within the last 24 hours prior to admission to current facility UPD

Code first condition requiring tPA administration, such as:
acute cerebral infarction (I63.-)
acute myocardial infarction (I21.-, I22.-)

AHA: 2013,4Q,124

Z92.83 Personal history of failed moderate sedation
Personal history of failed conscious sedation
EXCLUDES 2 *failed moderate sedation during procedure (T88.52)*

Z92.84 Personal history of unintended awareness under general anesthesia
EXCLUDES 2 *unintended awareness under general anesthesia during procedure (T88.53)*
AHA: 2016,4Q,72-73,77

6th **Z92.85 Personal history of cellular therapy**
AHA: 2021,4Q,33-34

Z92.85Ø Personal history of Chimeric Antigen Receptor T-cell therapy UPD
Personal history of CAR T-cell therapy

Z92.858 Personal history of other cellular therapy UPD

Z92.859 Personal history of cellular therapy, unspecified UPD

Z92.86 Personal history of gene therapy UPD
AHA: 2021,4Q,33-34

Z92.89 Personal history of other medical treatment
AHA: 2020,1Q,18

4th **Z93 Artificial opening status**
EXCLUDES 1 *artificial openings requiring attention or management (Z43.-)*
complications of external stoma (J95.Ø-, K94.-, N99.5-)

Z93.Ø Tracheostomy status HCC ESR COM
AHA: 2013,4Q,129

Z93.1 Gastrostomy status HCC ESR COM

Z93.2 Ileostomy status HCC ESR COM

Z93.3 Colostomy status HCC ESR COM

Z93.4 Other artificial openings of gastrointestinal tract status HCC ESR COM

5th **Z93.5 Cystostomy status**

Z93.5Ø Unspecified cystostomy status HCC ESR COM

Z93.51 Cutaneous-vesicostomy status HCC ESR COM

Z93.52 Appendico-vesicostomy status HCC ESR COM

Z93.59 Other cystostomy status HCC ESR COM

Z93.6 Other artificial openings of urinary tract status HCC ESR COM
Nephrostomy status
Ureterostomy status
Urethrostomy status

Z93.8 Other artificial opening status HCC ESR COM

Z93.9 Artificial opening status, unspecified HCC ESR COM

4th **Z94 Transplanted organ and tissue status**
INCLUDES organ or tissue replaced by heterogenous or homogenous transplant
EXCLUDES 1 *complications of transplanted organ or tissue - see Alphabetical Index*
EXCLUDES 2 *presence of vascular grafts (Z95.-)*

Z94.Ø Kidney transplant status Rx COM

Z94.1 Heart transplant status HCC Rx ESR COM
EXCLUDES 1 *artificial heart status (Z95.812)*
heart-valve replacement status (Z95.2-Z95.4)

Z94.2 Lung transplant status HCC Rx ESR COM

Z94.3 Heart and lungs transplant status HCC Rx ESR COM

Z94.4 Liver transplant status HCC Rx ESR COM

Z94.5 Skin transplant status
Autogenous skin transplant status

Z94.6 Bone transplant status

Z94.7 Corneal transplant status

5th **Z94.8 Other transplanted organ and tissue status**

Z94.81 Bone marrow transplant status HCC Rx ESR COM

Z94.82 Intestine transplant status HCC Rx ESR COM

Z94.83 Pancreas transplant status HCC Rx ESR COM

Z94.84 Stem cells transplant status HCC Rx ESR COM

Z94.89 Other transplanted organ and tissue status

Z94.9 Transplanted organ and tissue status, unspecified

4th **Z95 Presence of cardiac and vascular implants and grafts**
EXCLUDES 2 *complications of cardiac and vascular devices, implants and grafts (T82.-)*

Z95.Ø Presence of cardiac pacemaker
Presence of cardiac resynchronization therapy (CRT-P) pacemaker
EXCLUDES 1 *adjustment or management of cardiac device (Z45.Ø-)*
adjustment or management of cardiac pacemaker (Z45.Ø)
presence of automatic (implantable) cardiac defibrillator with synchronous cardiac pacemaker (Z95.81Ø)
AHA: 2022,2Q,14; 2019,1Q,33
TIP: Assign an additional code for the associated condition if that condition requires constant intervention from the device, as in cases of sick sinus syndrome. For conditions that do not require constant intervention from the device, as in cases of ventricular fibrillation, an additional code for the associated condition should be assigned only if the patient is experiencing the condition and the device is firing during the current admission.

Z95.1 Presence of aortocoronary bypass graft
Presence of coronary artery bypass graft

Z95.2 Presence of prosthetic heart valve
Presence of heart valve NOS

Z95.3 Presence of xenogenic heart valve

Z95.4 Presence of other heart-valve replacement

Z95.5 Presence of coronary angioplasty implant and graft
EXCLUDES 1 *coronary angioplasty status without implant and graft (Z98.61)*

5th **Z95.8 Presence of other cardiac and vascular implants and grafts**

6th **Z95.81 Presence of other cardiac implants and grafts**

Z95.81Ø Presence of automatic (implantable) cardiac defibrillator
Presence of automatic (implantable) cardiac defibrillator with synchronous cardiac pacemaker
Presence of cardiac resynchronization therapy defibrillator (CRT-D)
Presence of cardioverter-defibrillator (ICD)
AHA: 2022,2Q,14; 2019,1Q,33
TIP: Assign an additional code for the associated condition if that condition requires constant intervention from the device, as in cases of sick sinus syndrome. For conditions that do not require constant intervention from the device, as in cases of ventricular fibrillation, an additional code for the associated condition should be assigned only if the patient is experiencing the condition and the device is firing during the current admission.

Z95.811 Presence of heart assist device HCC ESR COM

Z95.812 Presence of fully implantable artificial heart HCC ESR COM

Z95.818 Presence of other cardiac implants and grafts

6th **Z95.82 Presence of other vascular implants and grafts**

Z95.82Ø Peripheral vascular angioplasty status with implants and grafts
EXCLUDES 1 *peripheral vascular angioplasty without implant and graft (Z98.62)*

Z95.828 Presence of other vascular implants and grafts
Presence of intravascular prosthesis NEC

Z95.9 Presence of cardiac and vascular implant and graft, unspecified

4th **Z96 Presence of other functional implants**
EXCLUDES 2 *complications of internal prosthetic devices, implants and grafts (T82-T85)*
fitting and adjustment of prosthetic and other devices (Z44-Z46)

Z96.Ø Presence of urogenital implants

Z96.1 **Presence of intraocular lens**
Presence of pseudophakia

Z96.2 **Presence of otological and audiological implants**
- **Z96.20** **Presence of otological and audiological implant, unspecified**
- **Z96.21** **Cochlear implant status**
- **Z96.22** **Myringotomy tube(s) status**
- **Z96.29** **Presence of other otological and audiological implants**
  Presence of bone-conduction hearing device
  Presence of eustachian tube stent
  Stapes replacement

Z96.3 **Presence of artificial larynx**

Z96.4 **Presence of endocrine implants**
- **Z96.41** **Presence of insulin pump (external) (internal)**
- **Z96.49** **Presence of other endocrine implants**

Z96.5 **Presence of tooth-root and mandibular implants**

Z96.6 **Presence of orthopedic joint implants**
AHA: 2019,3Q,16
- **Z96.60** **Presence of unspecified orthopedic joint implant**
- **Z96.61** **Presence of artificial shoulder joint**
  - **Z96.611** **Presence of right artificial shoulder joint**
  - **Z96.612** **Presence of left artificial shoulder joint**
  - **Z96.619** **Presence of unspecified artificial shoulder joint**
- **Z96.62** **Presence of artificial elbow joint**
  - **Z96.621** **Presence of right artificial elbow joint**
  - **Z96.622** **Presence of left artificial elbow joint**
  - **Z96.629** **Presence of unspecified artificial elbow joint**
- **Z96.63** **Presence of artificial wrist joint**
  - **Z96.631** **Presence of right artificial wrist joint**
  - **Z96.632** **Presence of left artificial wrist joint**
  - **Z96.639** **Presence of unspecified artificial wrist joint**
- **Z96.64** **Presence of artificial hip joint**
  Hip-joint replacement (partial) (total)
  - **Z96.641** **Presence of right artificial hip joint**
  - **Z96.642** **Presence of left artificial hip joint**
  - **Z96.643** **Presence of artificial hip joint, bilateral**
  - **Z96.649** **Presence of unspecified artificial hip joint**
- **Z96.65** **Presence of artificial knee joint**
  - **Z96.651** **Presence of right artificial knee joint**
  - **Z96.652** **Presence of left artificial knee joint**
  - **Z96.653** **Presence of artificial knee joint, bilateral**
  - **Z96.659** **Presence of unspecified artificial knee joint**
- **Z96.66** **Presence of artificial ankle joint**
  - **Z96.661** **Presence of right artificial ankle joint**
  - **Z96.662** **Presence of left artificial ankle joint**
  - **Z96.669** **Presence of unspecified artificial ankle joint**
- **Z96.69** **Presence of other orthopedic joint implants**
  - **Z96.691** **Finger-joint replacement of right hand**
  - **Z96.692** **Finger-joint replacement of left hand**
  - **Z96.693** **Finger-joint replacement, bilateral**
  - **Z96.698** **Presence of other orthopedic joint implants**

Z96.7 **Presence of other bone and tendon implants**
Presence of skull plate

Z96.8 **Presence of other specified functional implants**
- **Z96.81** **Presence of artificial skin**
- **Z96.82** **Presence of neurostimulator**
  Presence of brain neurostimulator
  Presence of gastric neurostimulator
  Presence of peripheral nerve neurostimulator
  Presence of sacral nerve neurostimulator
  Presence of spinal cord neurostimulator
  Presence of vagus nerve neurostimulator
  AHA: 2019,4Q,19
- **Z96.89** **Presence of other specified functional implants**

Z96.9 **Presence of functional implant, unspecified**

Z97 Presence of other devices

EXCLUDES 1 *complications of internal prosthetic devices, implants and grafts (T82-T85)*

EXCLUDES 2 *fitting and adjustment of prosthetic and other devices (Z44-Z46)*
presence of cerebrospinal fluid drainage device (Z98.2)

Z97.0 **Presence of artificial eye**

Z97.1 **Presence of artificial limb (complete) (partial)**
- **Z97.10** **Presence of artificial limb (complete) (partial), unspecified** COM
- **Z97.11** **Presence of artificial right arm (complete) (partial)** COM
- **Z97.12** **Presence of artificial left arm (complete) (partial)** COM
- **Z97.13** **Presence of artificial right leg (complete) (partial)** COM
- **Z97.14** **Presence of artificial left leg (complete) (partial)** COM
- **Z97.15** **Presence of artificial arms, bilateral (complete) (partial)** COM
- **Z97.16** **Presence of artificial legs, bilateral (complete) (partial)** COM

Z97.2 **Presence of dental prosthetic device (complete) (partial)**
Presence of dentures (complete) (partial)

Z97.3 **Presence of spectacles and contact lenses**

Z97.4 **Presence of external hearing-aid**

Z97.5 **Presence of (intrauterine) contraceptive device** ♀
EXCLUDES 1 *checking, reinsertion or removal of implantable subdermal contraceptive (Z30.46)*
checking, reinsertion or removal of intrauterine contraceptive device (Z30.43-)

Z97.8 **Presence of other specified devices**

Z98 Other postprocedural states

EXCLUDES 2 *aftercare (Z43-Z49, Z51)*
follow-up medical care (Z08-Z09)
postprocedural complication - see Alphabetical Index

Z98.0 **Intestinal bypass and anastomosis status**
EXCLUDES 2 *bariatric surgery status (Z98.84)*
gastric bypass status (Z98.84)
obesity surgery status (Z98.84)

Z98.1 **Arthrodesis status**

Z98.2 **Presence of cerebrospinal fluid drainage device**
Presence of CSF shunt

Z98.3 **Post therapeutic collapse of lung status** UPD
Code first underlying disease

Z98.4 **Cataract extraction status**
Use additional code to identify intraocular lens implant status (Z96.1)
EXCLUDES 1 *aphakia (H27.0)*
- **Z98.41** **Cataract extraction status, right eye**
- **Z98.42** **Cataract extraction status, left eye**
- **Z98.49** **Cataract extraction status, unspecified eye**

Z98.5 **Sterilization status**
EXCLUDES 1 *female infertility (N97.-)*
male infertility (N46.-)
- **Z98.51** **Tubal ligation status** ♀
- **Z98.52** **Vasectomy status** A ♂

Z98.6 **Angioplasty status**
- **Z98.61** **Coronary angioplasty status**
  EXCLUDES 1 *coronary angioplasty status with implant and graft (Z95.5)*
- **Z98.62** **Peripheral vascular angioplasty status**
  EXCLUDES 1 *peripheral vascular angioplasty status with implant and graft (Z95.820)*

Z98.8 **Other specified postprocedural states**
- **Z98.81** **Dental procedure status**
  - **Z98.810** **Dental sealant status**
  - **Z98.811** **Dental restoration status**
    Dental crown status
    Dental fillings status
  - **Z98.818** **Other dental procedure status**
- **Z98.82** **Breast implant status**
  EXCLUDES 1 *breast implant removal status (Z98.86)*

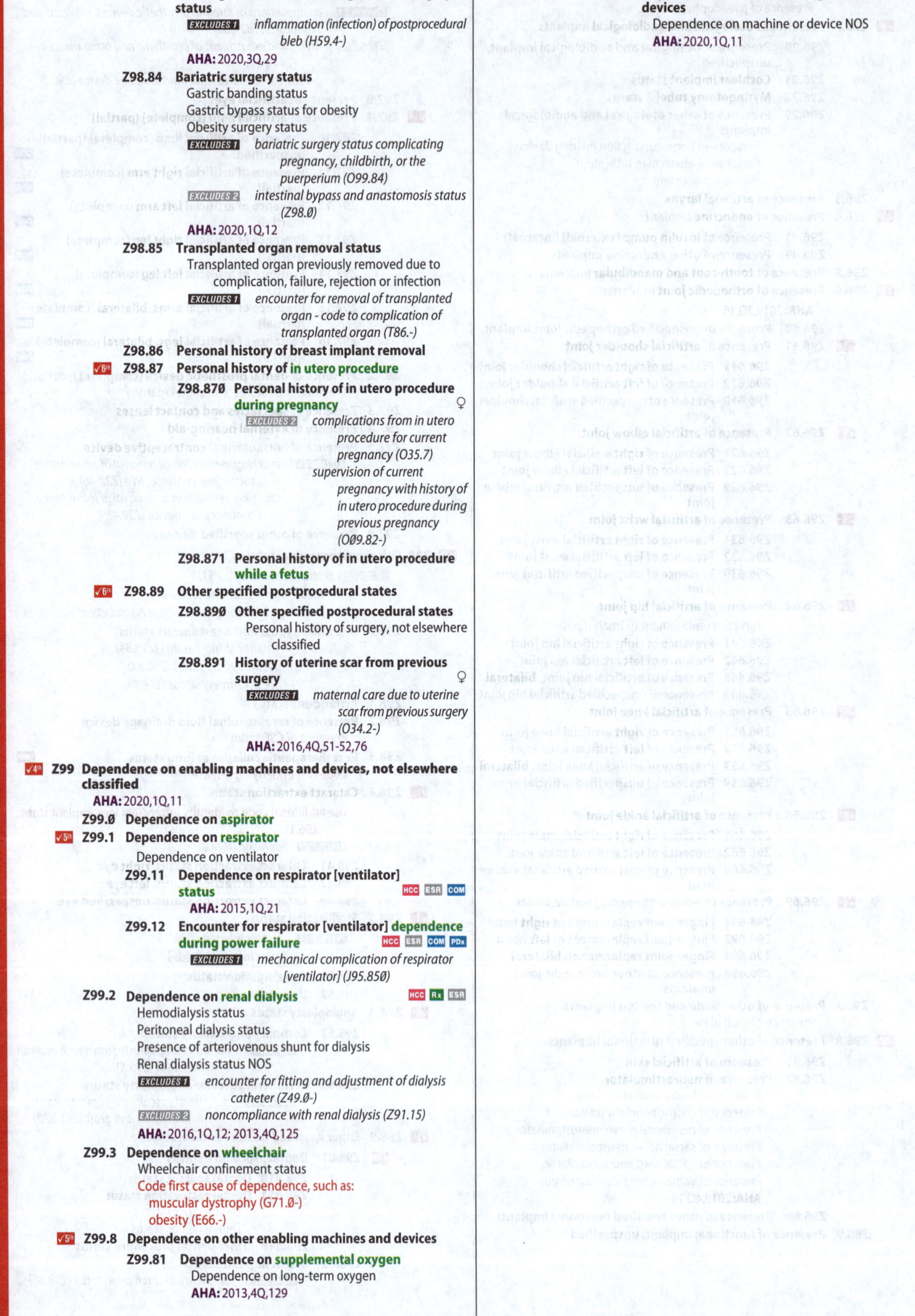

Z98.83 Filtering (vitreous) bleb after glaucoma surgery status
EXCLUDES 1 *inflammation (infection) of postprocedural bleb (H59.4-)*
AHA: 2020,3Q,29

Z98.84 Bariatric surgery status
Gastric banding status
Gastric bypass status for obesity
Obesity surgery status
EXCLUDES 1 *bariatric surgery status complicating pregnancy, childbirth, or the puerperium (O99.84)*
EXCLUDES 2 *intestinal bypass and anastomosis status (Z98.Ø)*
AHA: 2020,1Q,12

Z98.85 Transplanted organ removal status
Transplanted organ previously removed due to complication, failure, rejection or infection
EXCLUDES 1 *encounter for removal of transplanted organ - code to complication of transplanted organ (T86.-)*

Z98.86 Personal history of breast implant removal

✓6th **Z98.87 Personal history of in utero procedure**

Z98.87Ø Personal history of in utero procedure during pregnancy ♀
EXCLUDES 2 *complications from in utero procedure for current pregnancy (O35.7)*
supervision of current pregnancy with history of in utero procedure during previous pregnancy (OØ9.82-)

Z98.871 Personal history of in utero procedure while a fetus

✓6th **Z98.89 Other specified postprocedural states**

Z98.89Ø Other specified postprocedural states
Personal history of surgery, not elsewhere classified

Z98.891 History of uterine scar from previous surgery ♀
EXCLUDES 1 *maternal care due to uterine scar from previous surgery (O34.2-)*
AHA: 2016,4Q,51-52,76

✓4th **Z99 Dependence on enabling machines and devices, not elsewhere classified**
AHA: 2020,1Q,11

Z99.Ø Dependence on aspirator

✓5th **Z99.1 Dependence on respirator**
Dependence on ventilator

Z99.11 Dependence on respirator [ventilator] status HCC ESR COM
AHA: 2015,1Q,21

Z99.12 Encounter for respirator [ventilator] dependence during power failure HCC ESR COM PDx
EXCLUDES 1 *mechanical complication of respirator [ventilator] (J95.85Ø)*

Z99.2 Dependence on renal dialysis HCC Rx ESR
Hemodialysis status
Peritoneal dialysis status
Presence of arteriovenous shunt for dialysis
Renal dialysis status NOS
EXCLUDES 1 *encounter for fitting and adjustment of dialysis catheter (Z49.Ø-)*
EXCLUDES 2 *noncompliance with renal dialysis (Z91.15)*
AHA: 2016,1Q,12; 2013,4Q,125

Z99.3 Dependence on wheelchair
Wheelchair confinement status
Code first cause of dependence, such as:
muscular dystrophy (G71.Ø-)
obesity (E66.-)

✓5th **Z99.8 Dependence on other enabling machines and devices**

Z99.81 Dependence on supplemental oxygen
Dependence on long-term oxygen
AHA: 2013,4Q,129

Z99.89 Dependence on other enabling machines and devices
Dependence on machine or device NOS
AHA: 2020,1Q,11

Chapter 22. Codes for Special Purposes (UØØ–U85)

Chapter-specific Guidelines

UØ7.Ø	Vaping-related disorder (see Section I.C.1Ø.e., Vaping-related disorders)
UØ7.1	COVID-19 (see Section I.C.1.g.1., COVID-19 infection)
UØ9.9	Post COVID-19 condition, unspecified (see Section I.C.1.g.1.m.)

Chapter 22. Codes for Special Purposes (UØØ-U85)

This chapter contains the following blocks:

UØØ-U49 Provisional assignment of new diseases of uncertain etiology or emergency use

Provisional assignment of new diseases of uncertain etiology or emergency use (UØØ-U49)

UØ7 Emergency use of UØ7

UØ7.Ø Vaping-related disorder

Dabbing related lung damage
Dabbing related lung injury
E-cigarette, or vaping, product use associated lung injury [EVALI]
Electronic cigarette related lung damage
Electronic cigarette related lung injury

Use additional code, to identify manifestations, such as:
- abdominal pain (R1Ø.84)
- acute respiratory distress syndrome (J8Ø)
- diarrhea (R19.7)
- drug-induced interstitial lung disorder (J7Ø.4)
- lipoid pneumonia (J69.1)
- weight loss (R63.4)

DEF: Respiratory illness or injury caused by harmful aerosolized substances and chemicals produced by electronic cigarettes, vapes, e-pipes, and other battery-powered vaping devices. Symptoms may include shortness of breath and fever, while some patients experience severe, sometimes fatal, lung damage. ***Synonym(s):*** *e-cigarette and vaping product use-associated lung injury, EVALI.*

UØ7.1 COVID-19

Use additional code to identify pneumonia or other manifestations, such as:
- pneumonia due to COVID-19 (J12.82)

EXCLUDES 2 *coronavirus as the cause of diseases classified elsewhere (B97.2-)*
coronavirus infection, unspecified (B34.2)
pneumonia due to SARS-associated coronavirus (J12.81)

AHA: 2022,2Q,28; 2021,4Q,101,107-108; 2021,1Q,25-30,31-49; 2020,4Q,14,99; 2020,3Q,9-16; 2020,2Q,3-13

DEF: First diagnosed in December 2019 in China, coronavirus disease 2019 (COVID-19) is a respiratory infection caused by a newly identified (novel) virus not previously seen in humans, known as severe acute respiratory syndrome coronavirus 2 (SARS-CoV-2). Symptoms of this lower respiratory illness include fever, dry cough, and tiredness that may progress to include difficulty breathing. Older patients and those with high blood pressure, heart problems, and diabetes are more likely to develop serious symptoms of the illness. ***Synonym(s):*** *SARS-CoV-2, coronavirus disease 2019.*

TIP: Only a confirmed diagnosis of COVID-19 can be coded to UØ7.1; a positive COVID-19 test result or documentation by the provider that the disease is confirmed is sufficient.

TIP: Assign for asymptomatic individuals who test positive for COVID-19. Even though asymptomatic, the individual is considered to have the COVID-19 infection due to the positive test result.

TIP: Assign appropriate codes for presenting signs/symptoms associated with COVID-19 (cough, fever, shortness of breath), instead of UØ7.1, if a definitive diagnosis has not been established.

UØ9 Post COVID-19 condition

UØ9.9 Post COVID-19 condition, unspecified

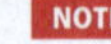
NOTE This code enables establishment of a link with COVID-19.

This code is not to be used in cases that are still presenting with active COVID-19. However, an exception is made in cases of re-infection with COVID-19, occurring with a condition related to prior COVID-19.

~~Post-acute sequela of COVID-19~~

▶Post-acute sequela of COVID-19◀

Code first the specific condition related to COVID-19 if known, such as:
- chronic respiratory failure (J96.1-)
- loss of smell (R43.8)
- loss of taste (R43.8)
- multisystem inflammatory syndrome (M35.81)
- pulmonary embolism (I26.-)
- pulmonary fibrosis (J84.1Ø)

AHA: 2021,4Q,31-32,102-106

Notes

Notes

Notes

Notes

Illustrations

Chapter 3. Diseases of the Blood and Blood-forming Organs and Certain Disorders Involving the Immune Mechanism (D5Ø–D89)

Red Blood Cells

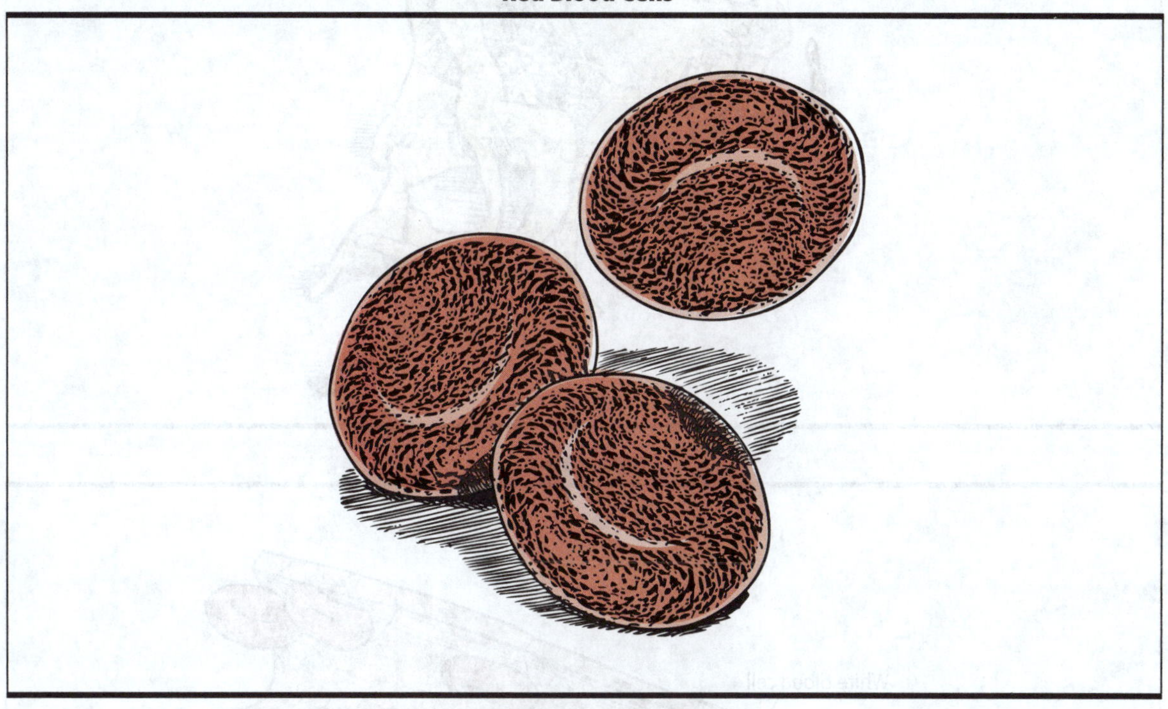

White Blood Cell

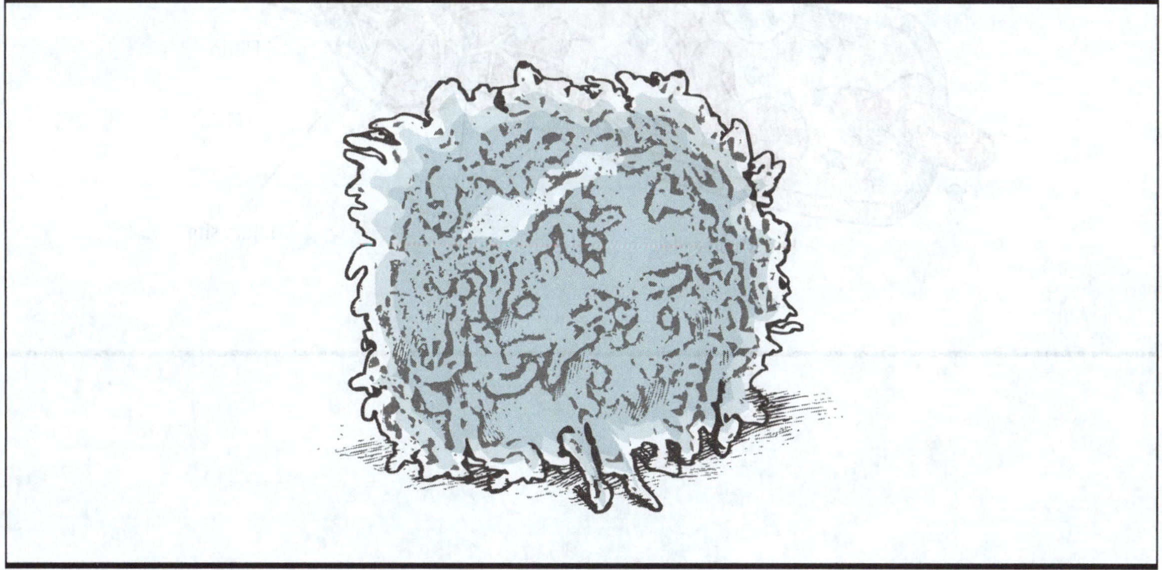

Platelet

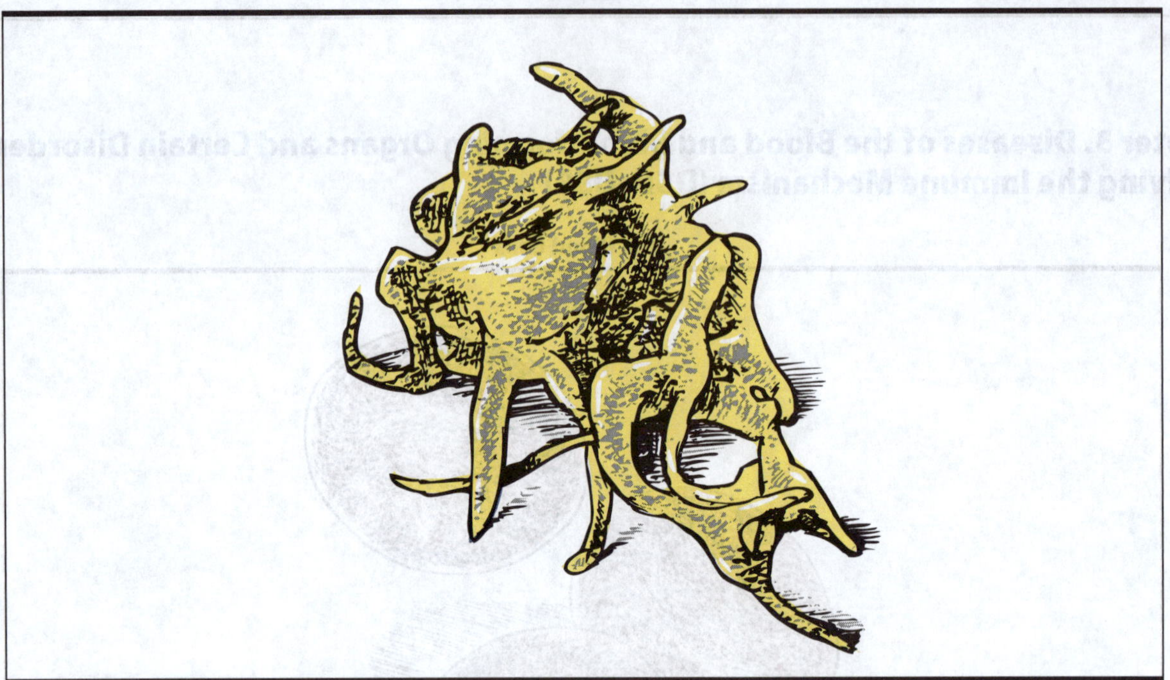

Coagulation

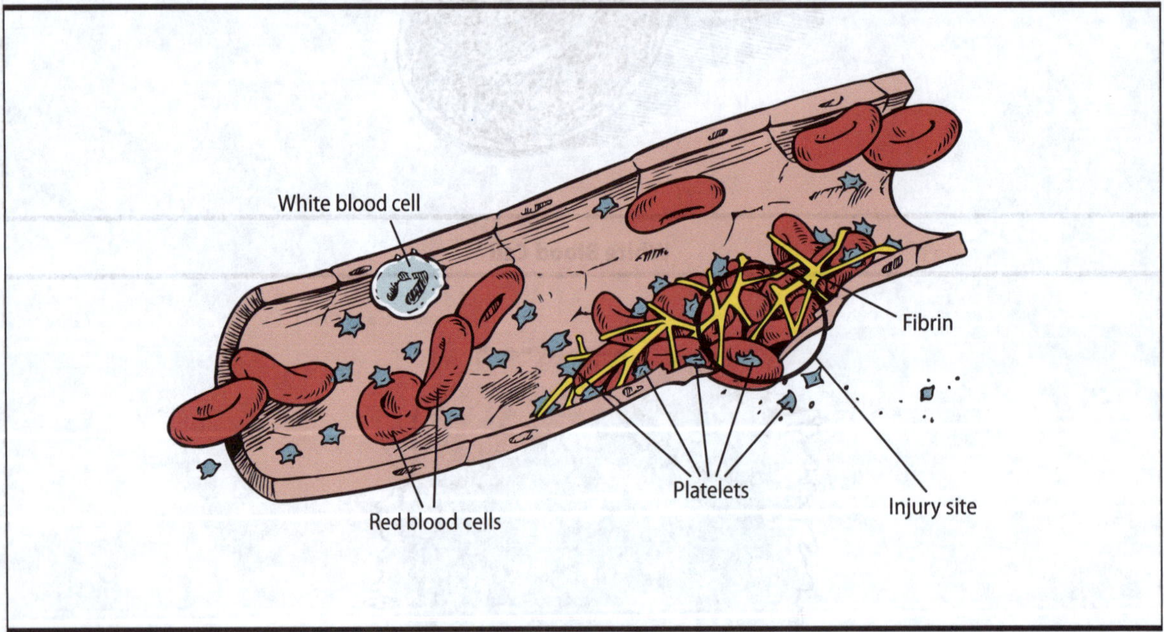

Spleen Anatomical Location and External Structures

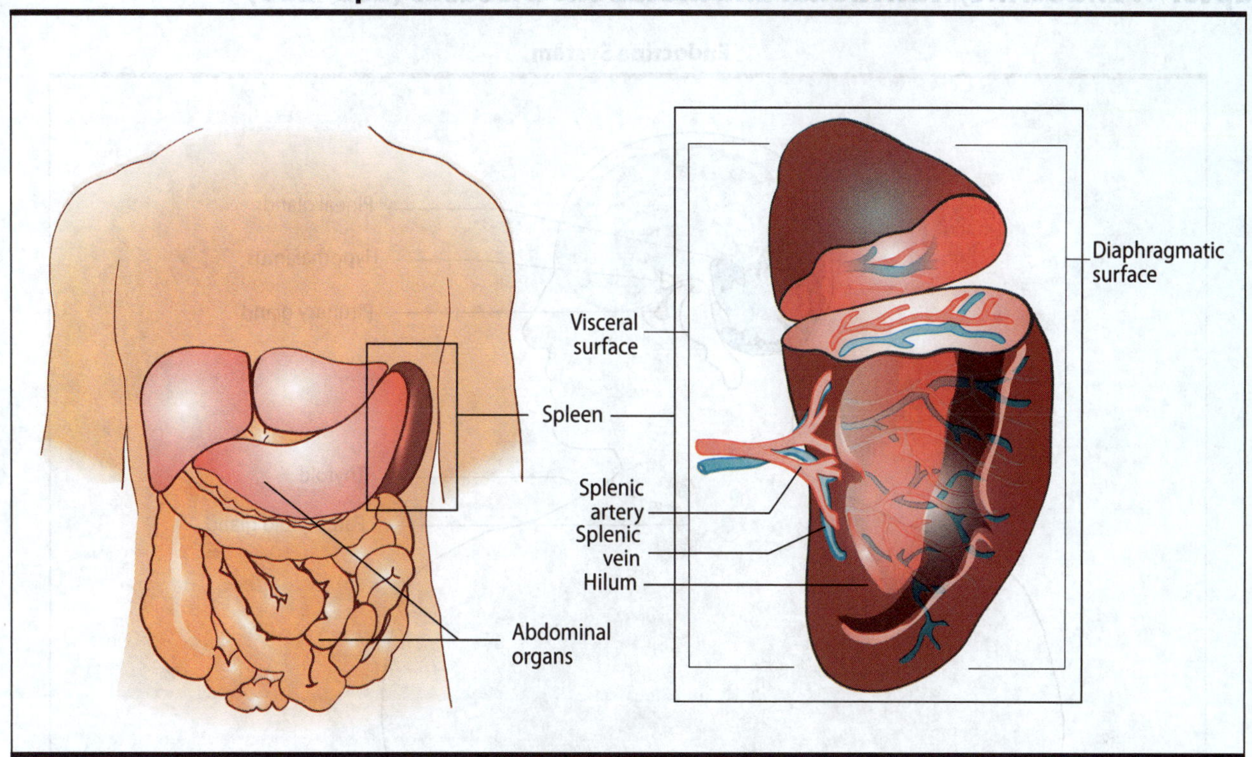

Spleen Interior Structures

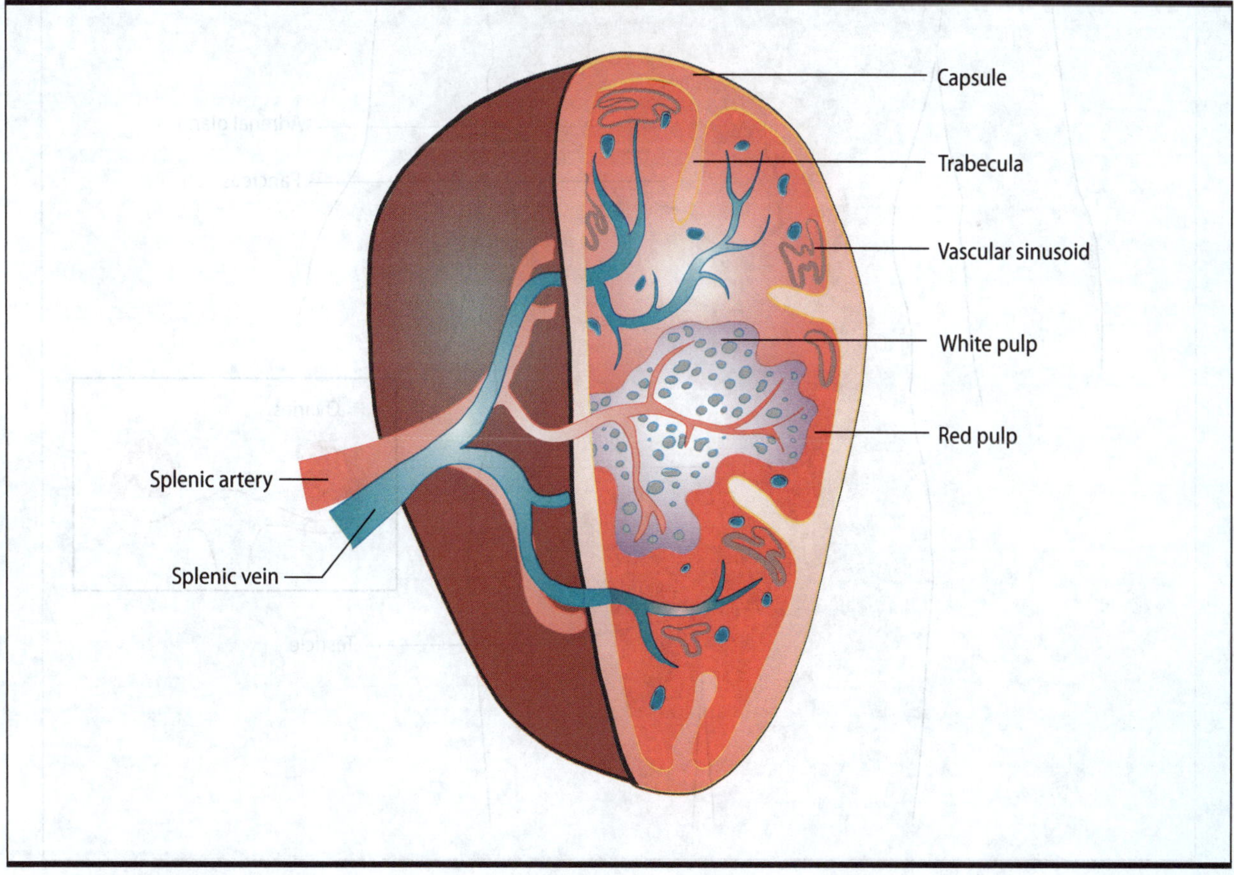

Chapter 4. Endocrine, Nutritional and Metabolic Diseases (EØØ–E89)

Endocrine System

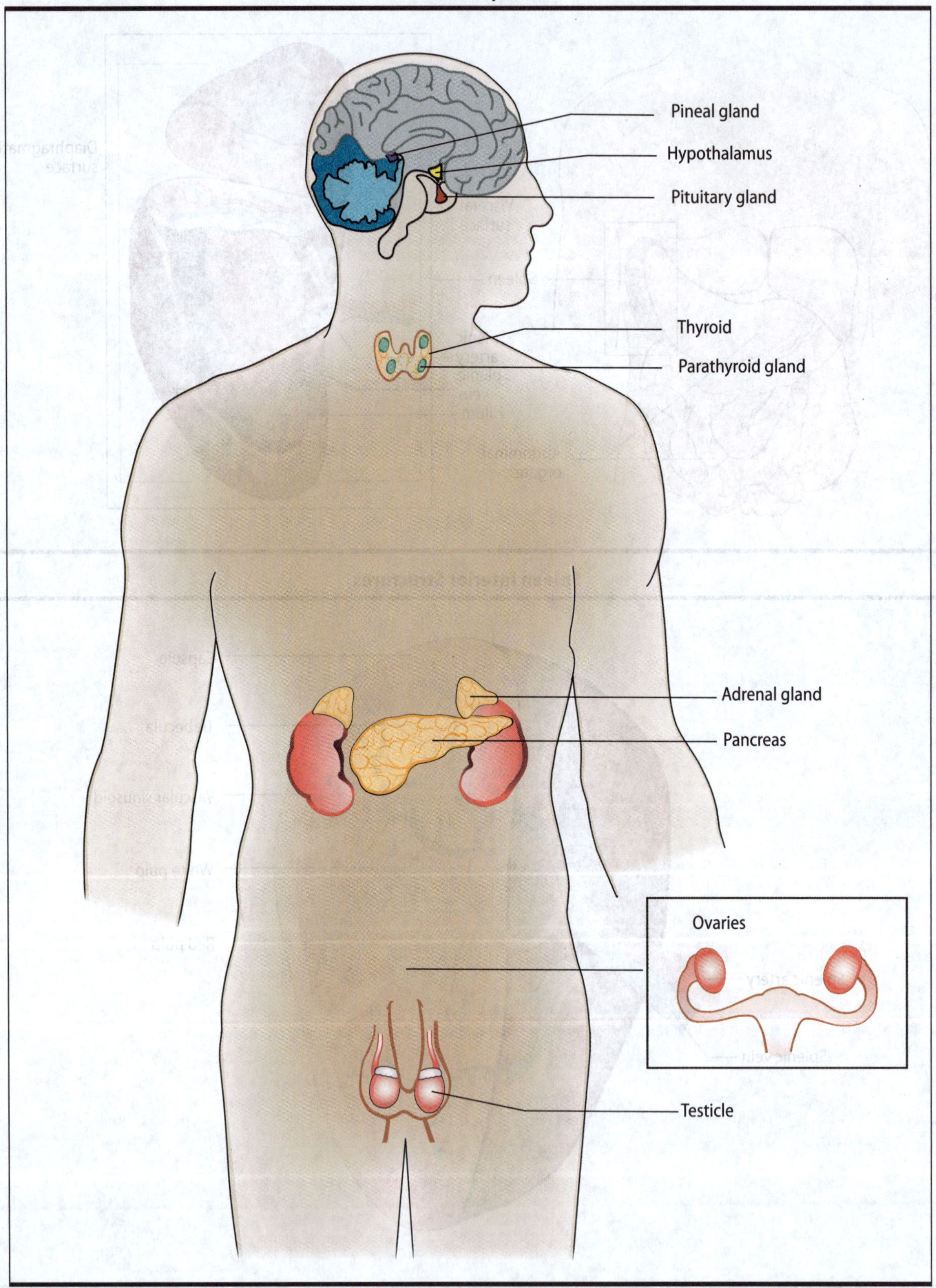

Thyroid

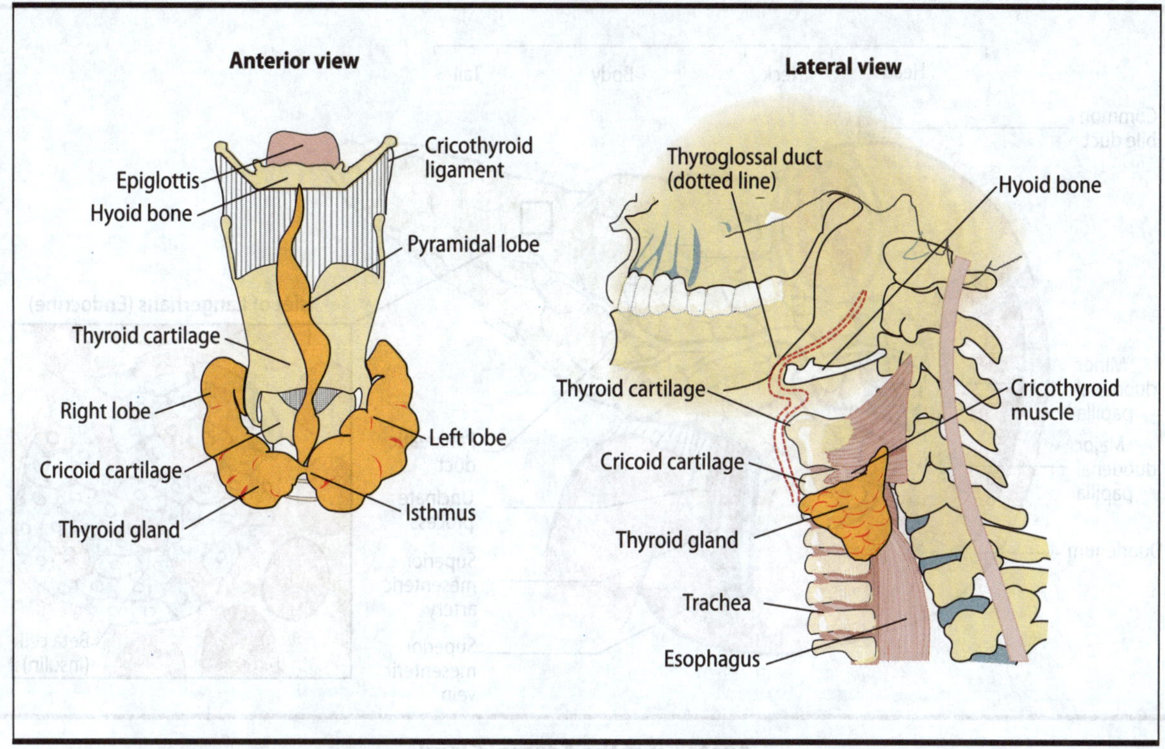

Thyroid and Parathyroid Glands

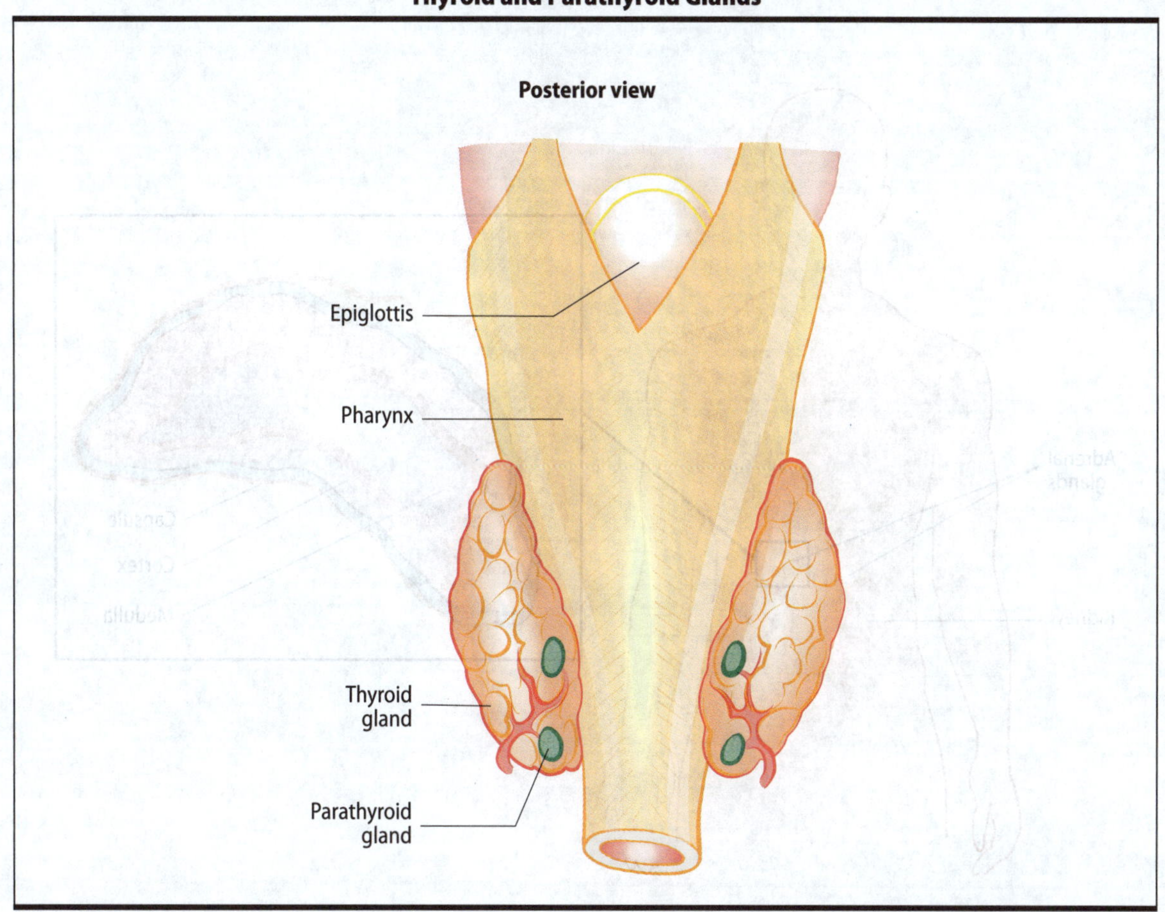

Pancreas

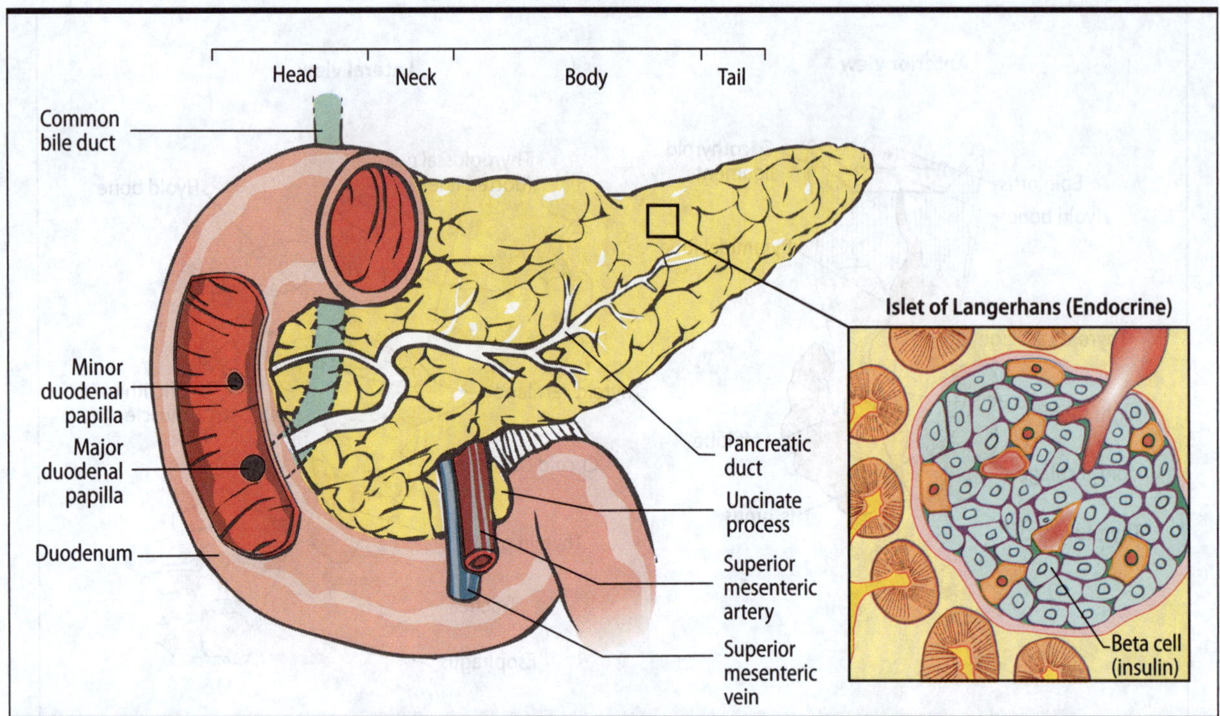

Anatomy of the Adrenal Gland

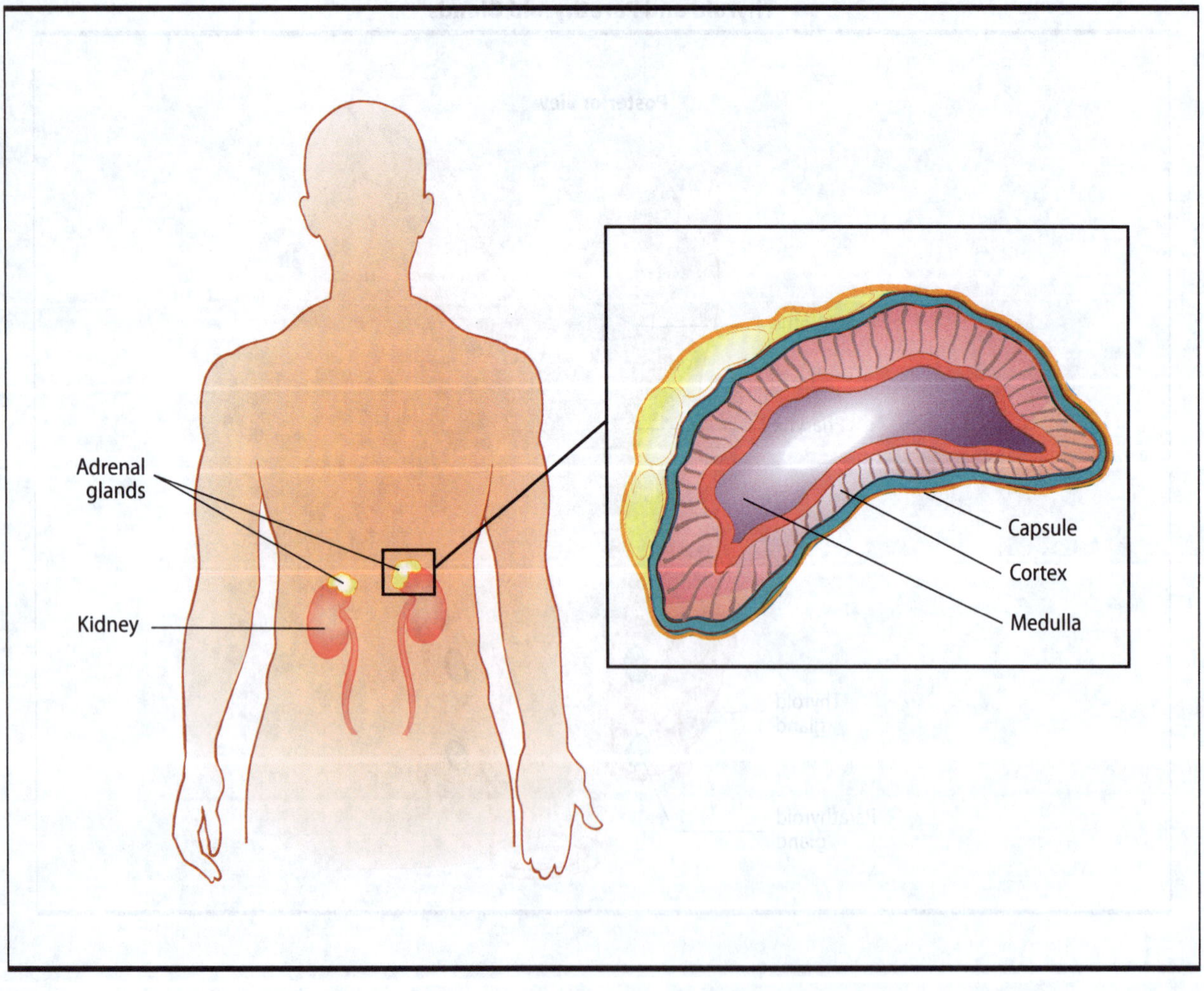

Adrenal glands
Kidney
Capsule
Cortex
Medulla

Structure of an Ovary

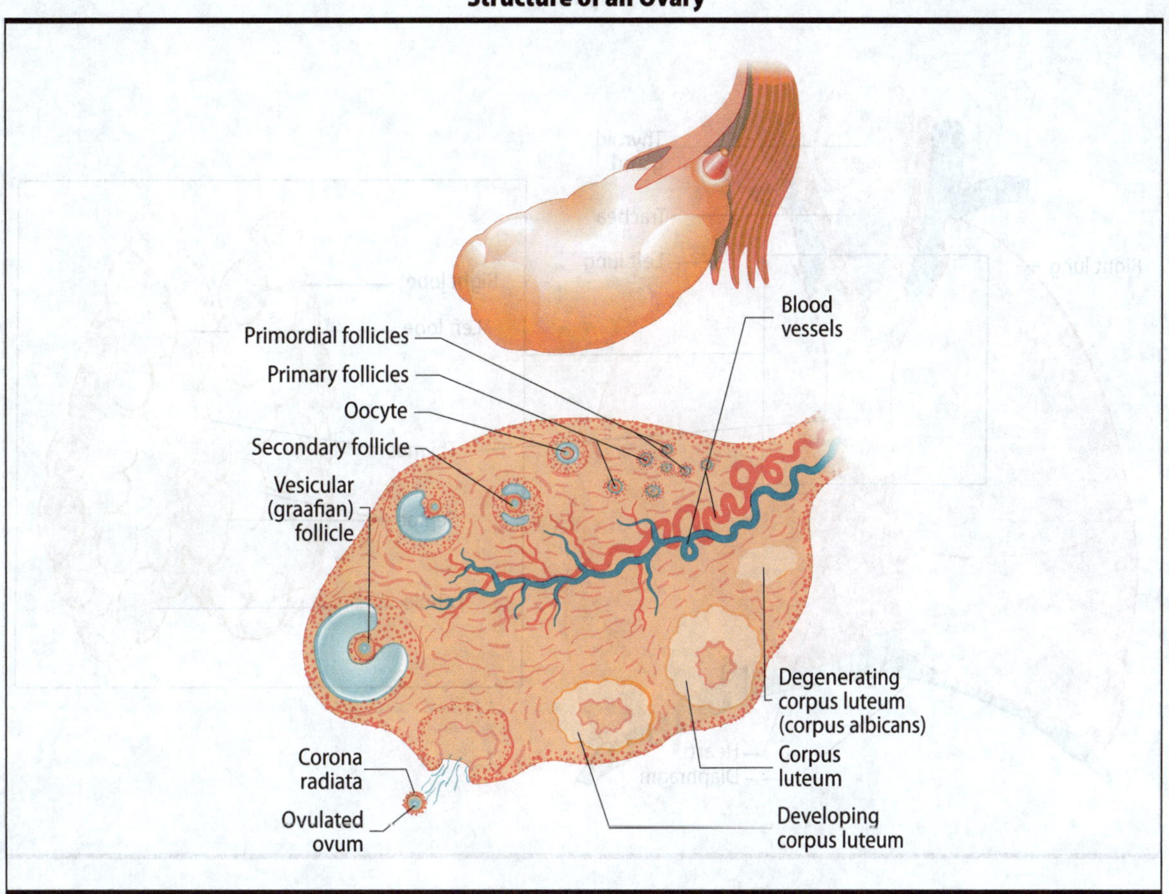

Testis and Associated Structures

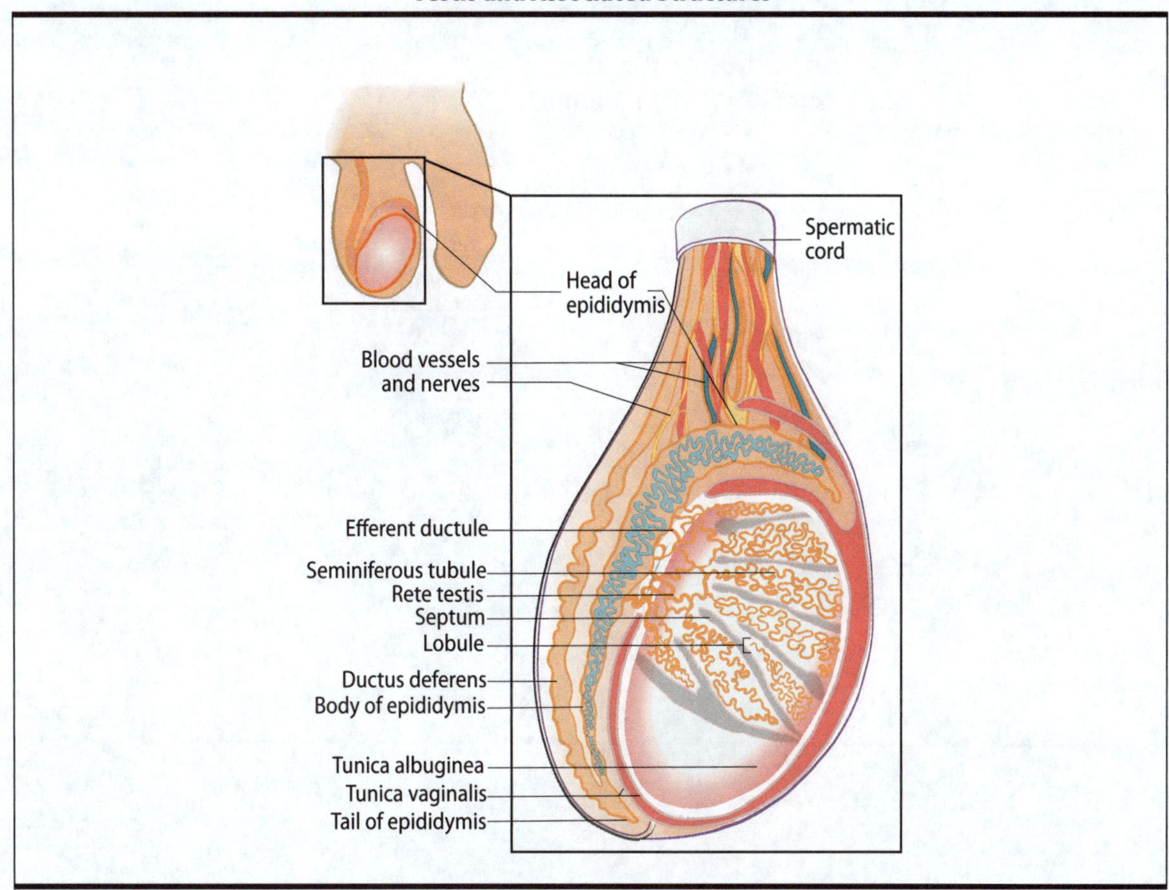

Thymus

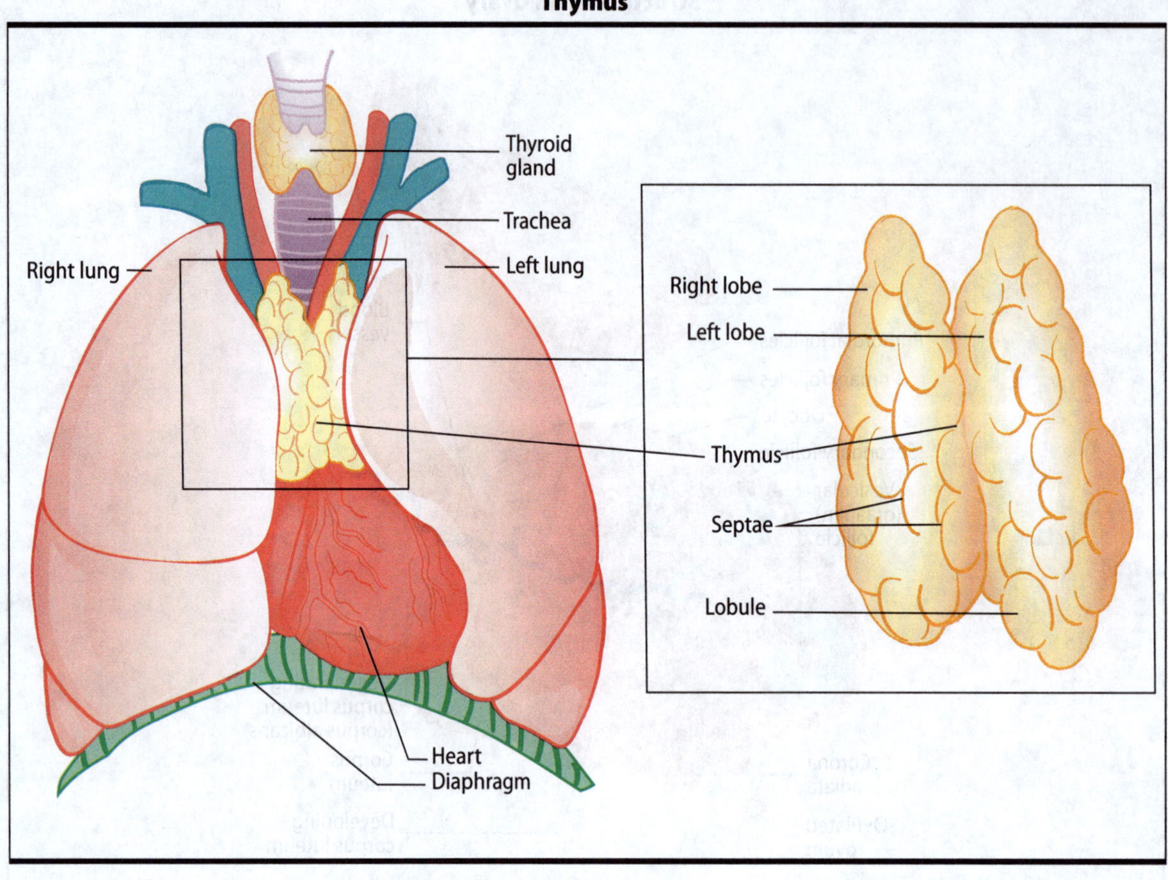

Thyroid gland
Trachea
Right lung
Left lung
Thymus
Heart
Diaphragm
Right lobe
Left lobe
Septae
Lobule

Chapter 6. Diseases of the Nervous System (GØØ–G99)

Brain

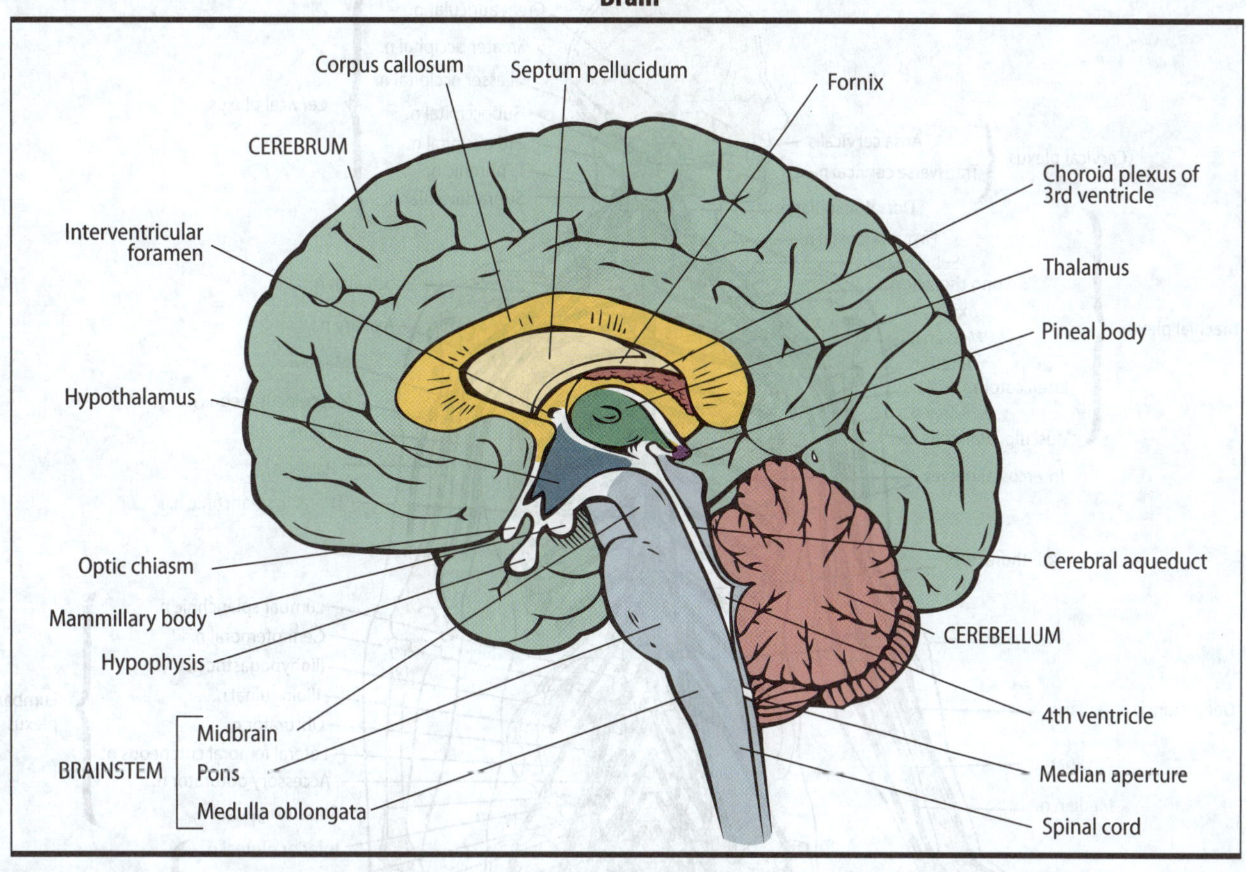

Cranial Nerves

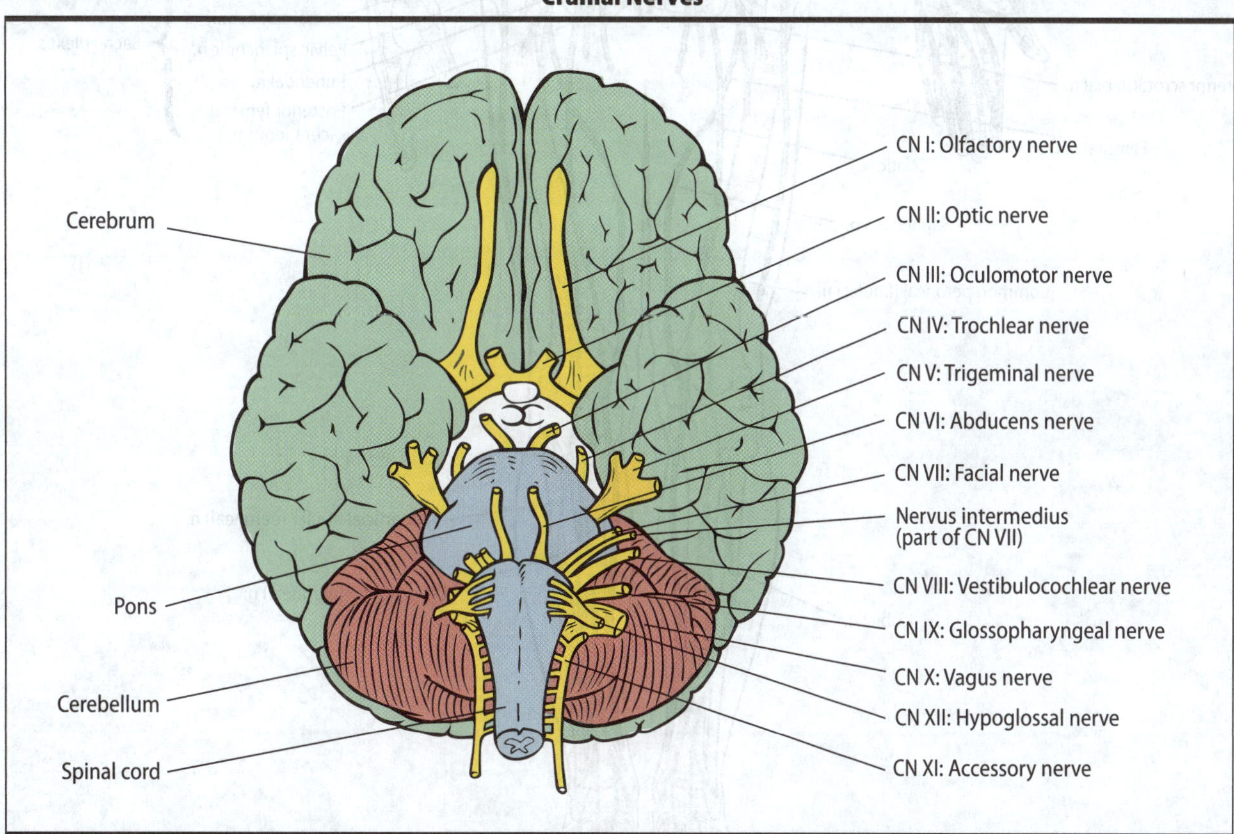

Peripheral Nervous System

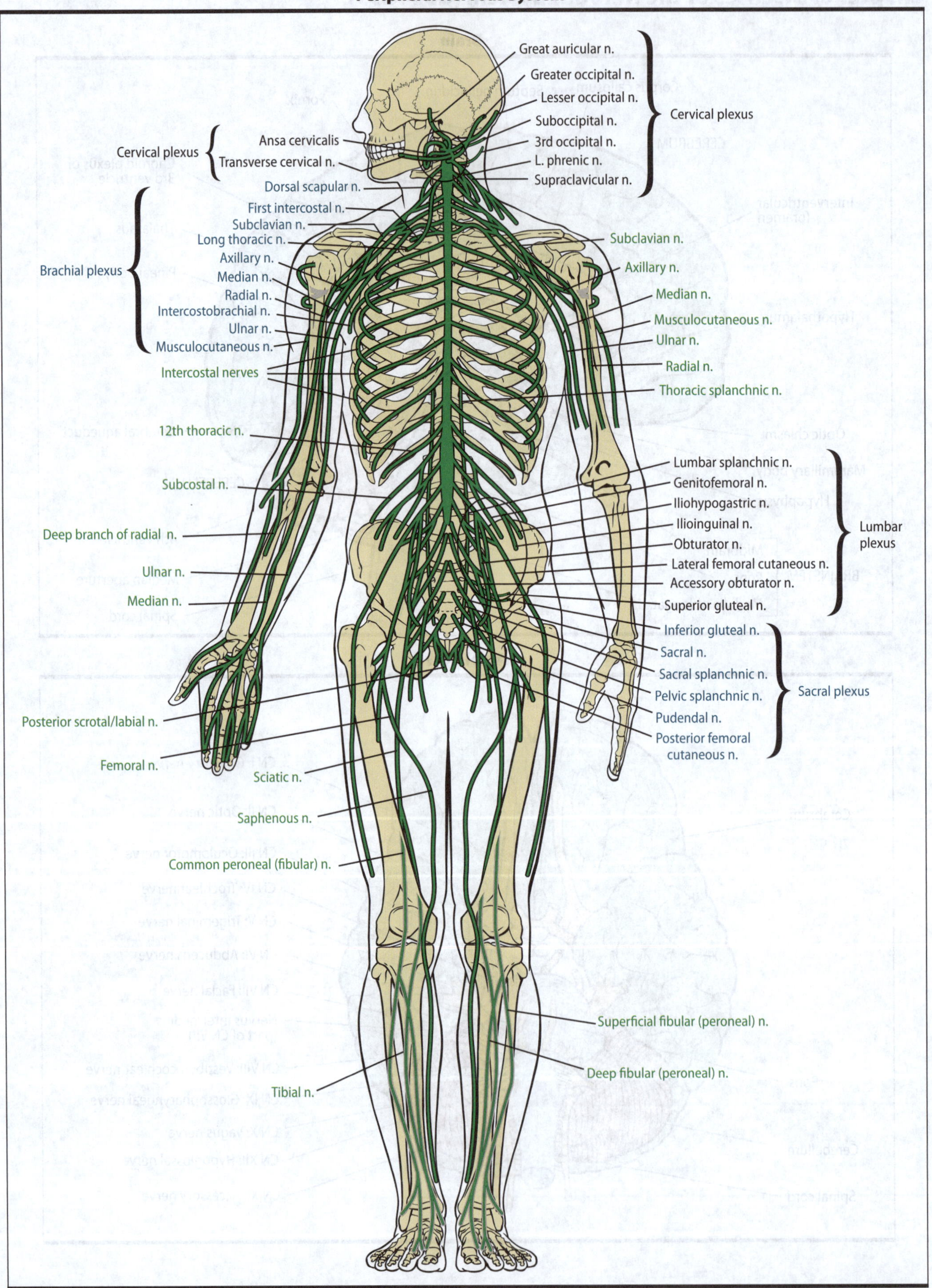

Spinal Cord and Spinal Nerves

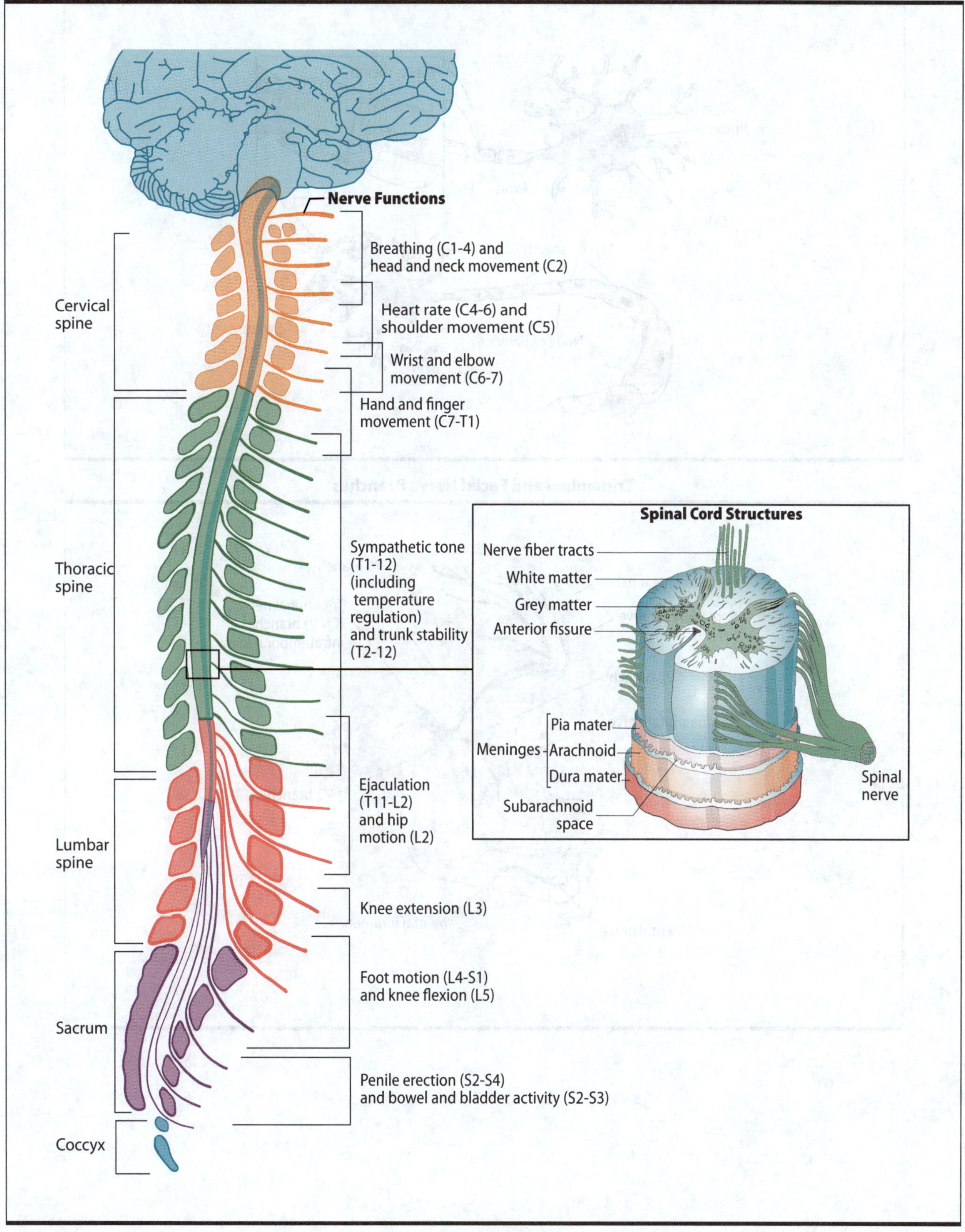

Nerve Cell

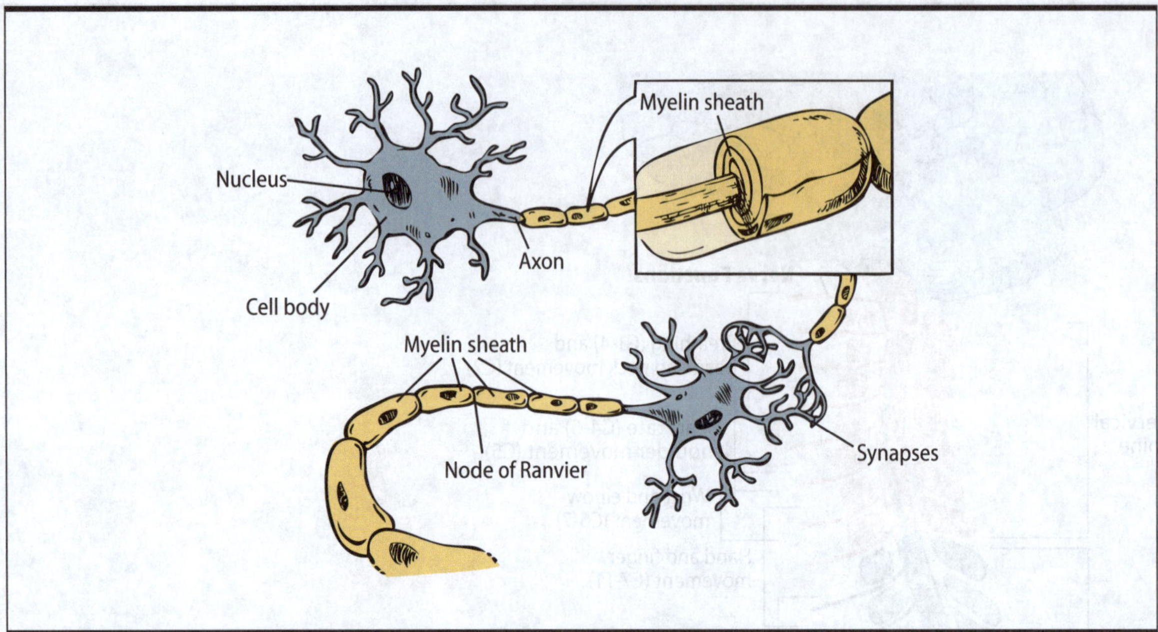

Trigeminal and Facial Nerve Branches

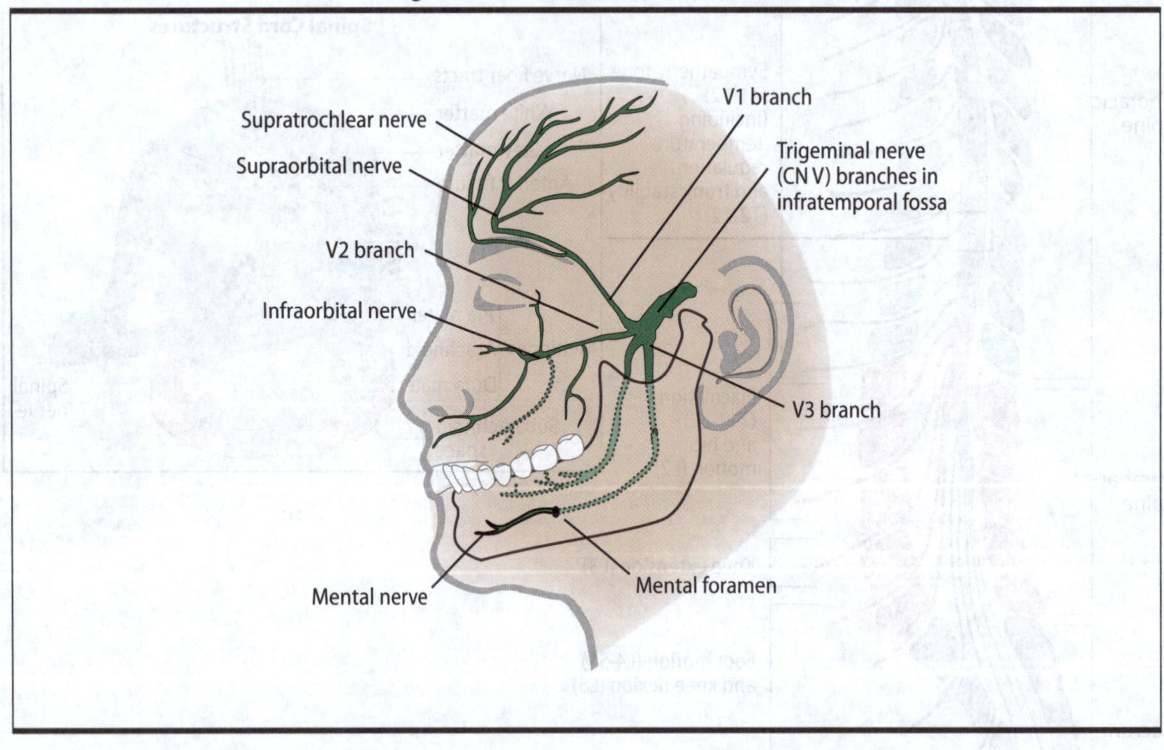

Chapter 7. Diseases of the Eye and Adnexa (HØØ–H59)

Eye

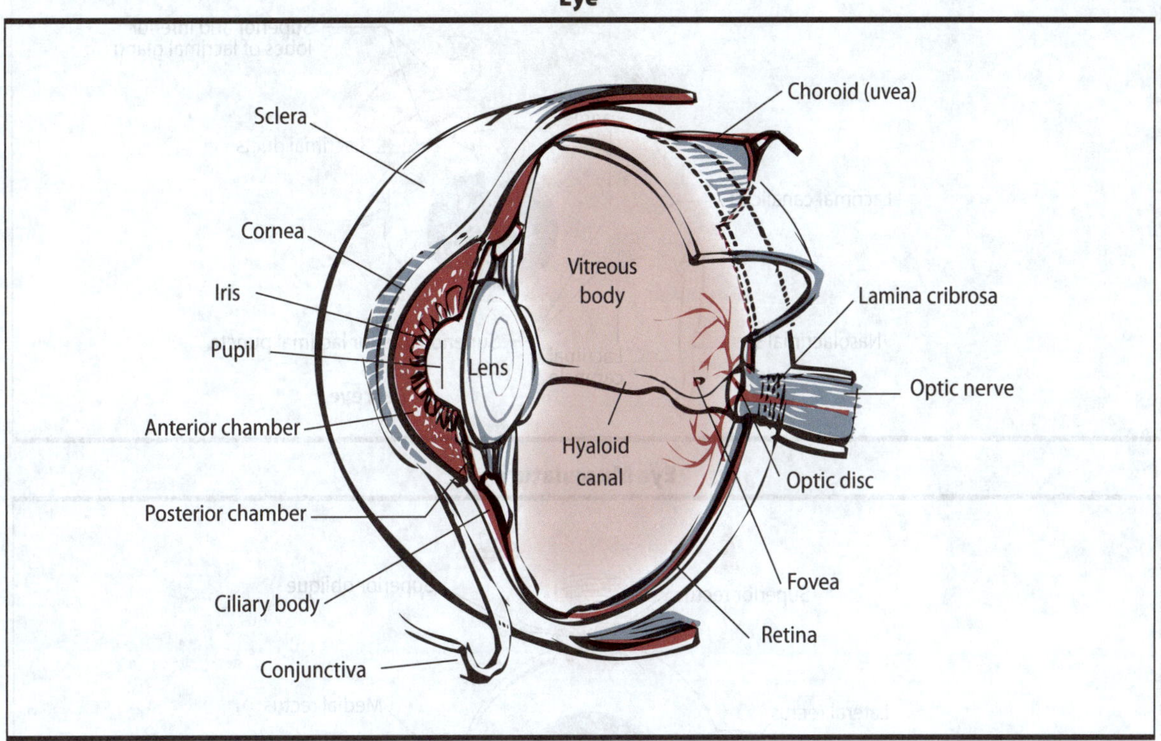

Posterior Pole of Globe/Flow of Aqueous Humor

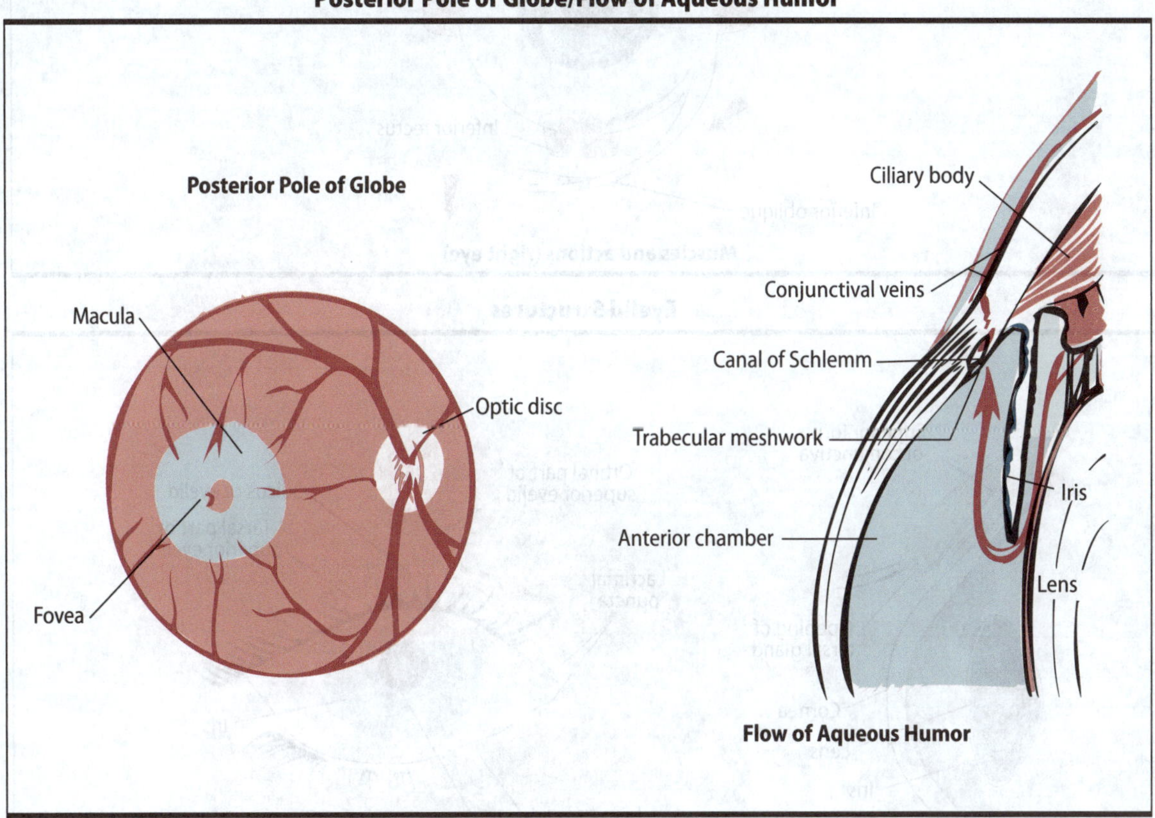

Lacrimal System

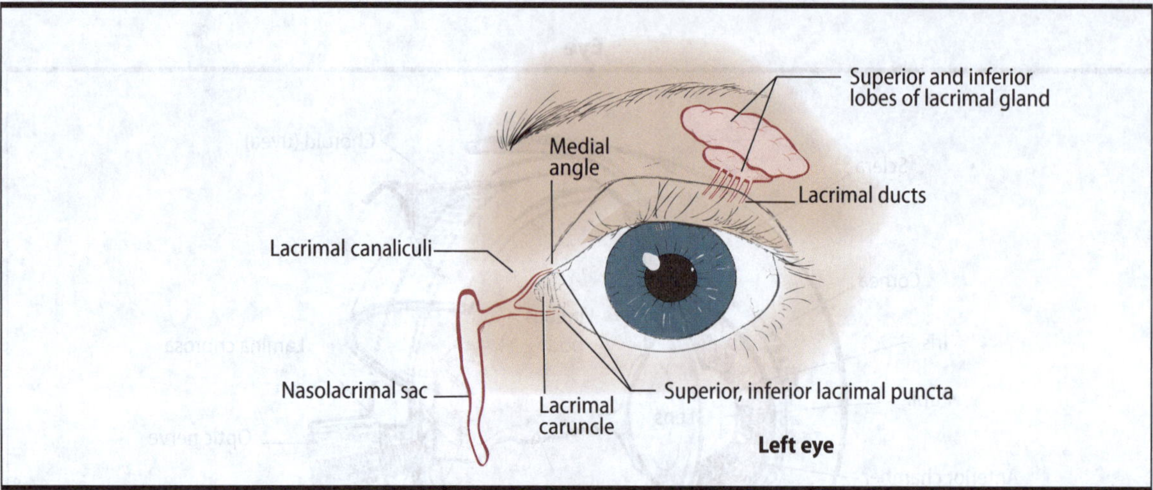

Eye Musculature

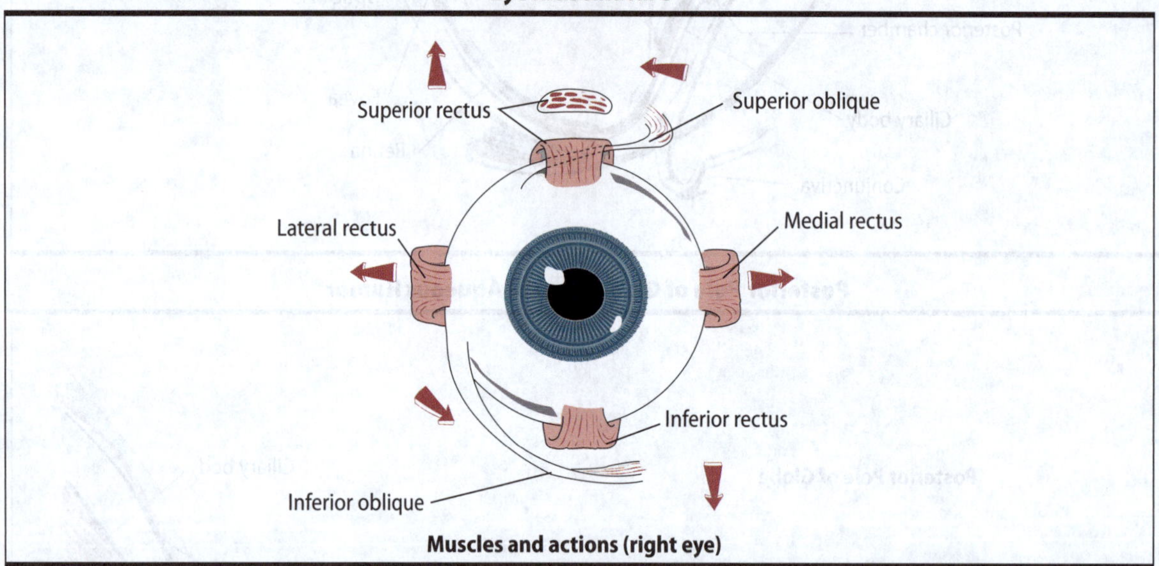

Eyelid Structures

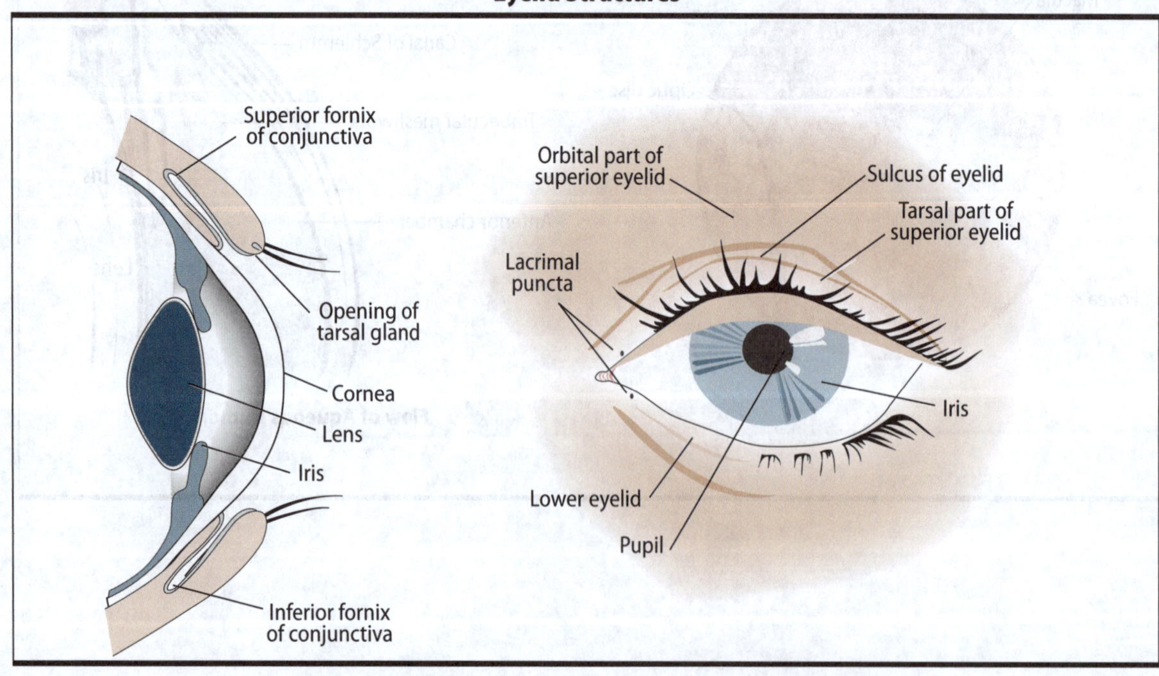

Chapter 8. Diseases of the Ear and Mastoid Process (H6Ø–H95)

Ear Anatomy

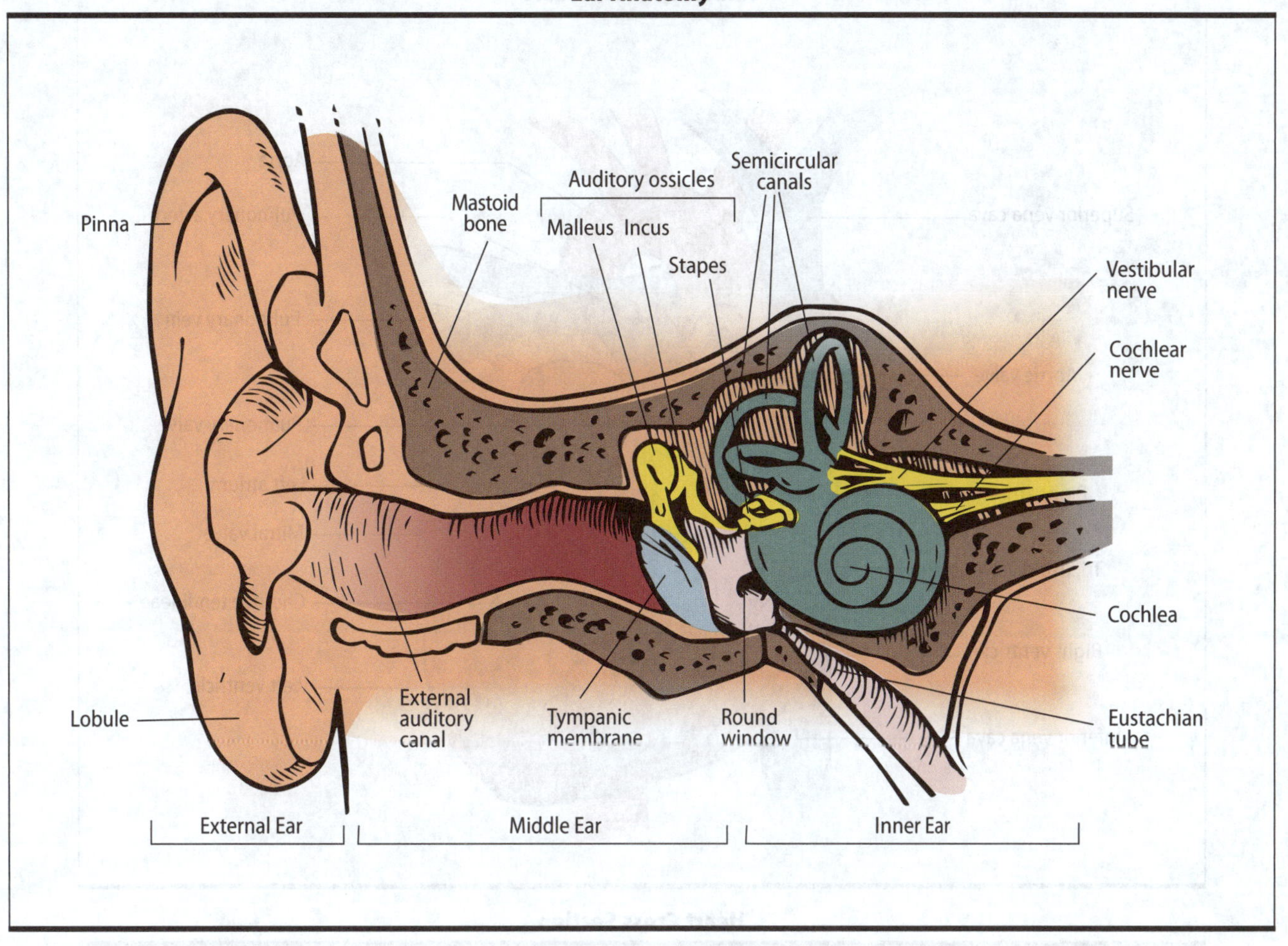

Chapter 9. Diseases of the Circulatory System (I00–I99)

Anatomy of the Heart

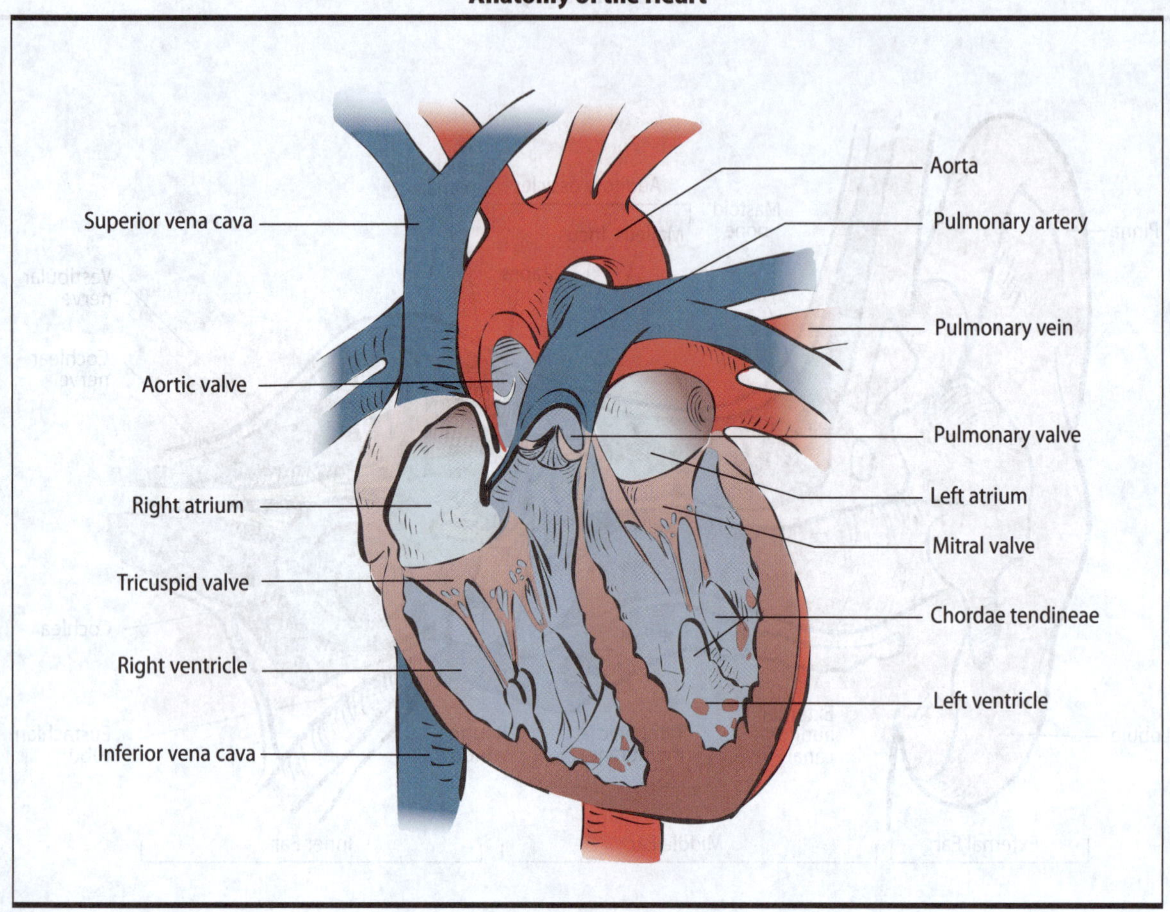

Heart Cross Section

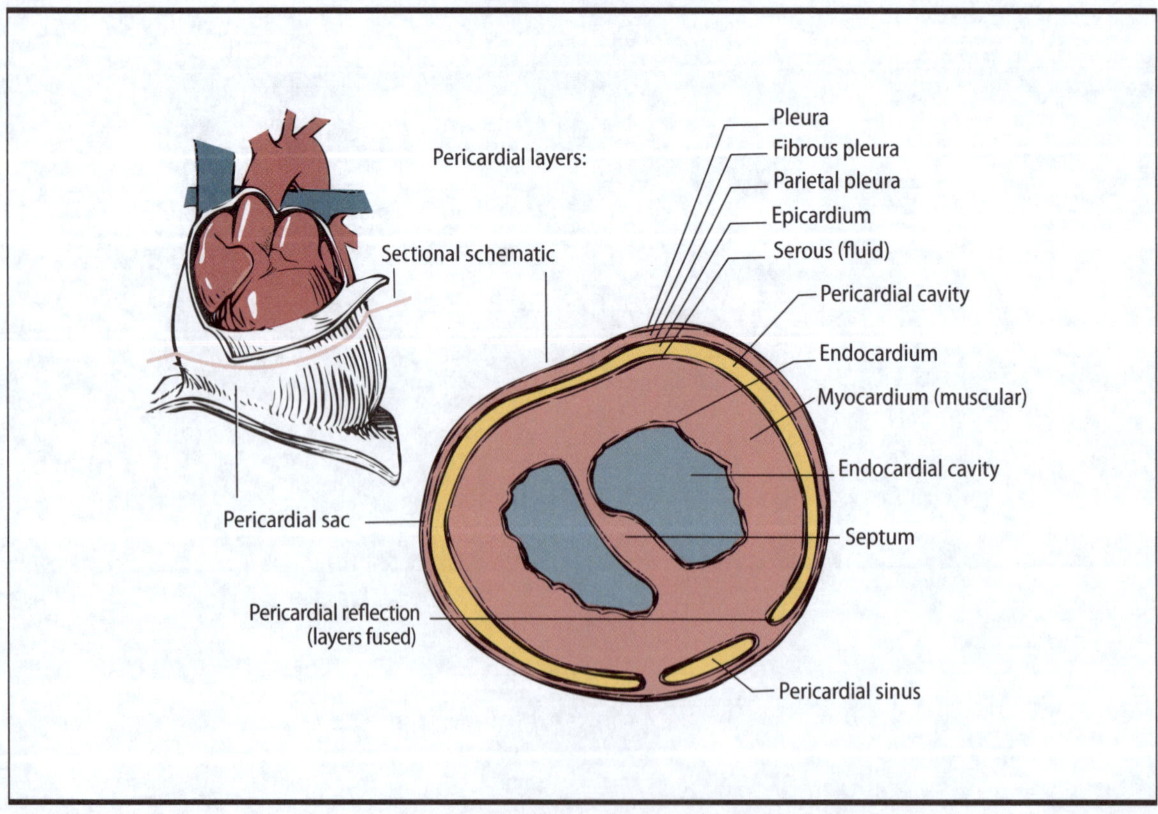

Heart Valves

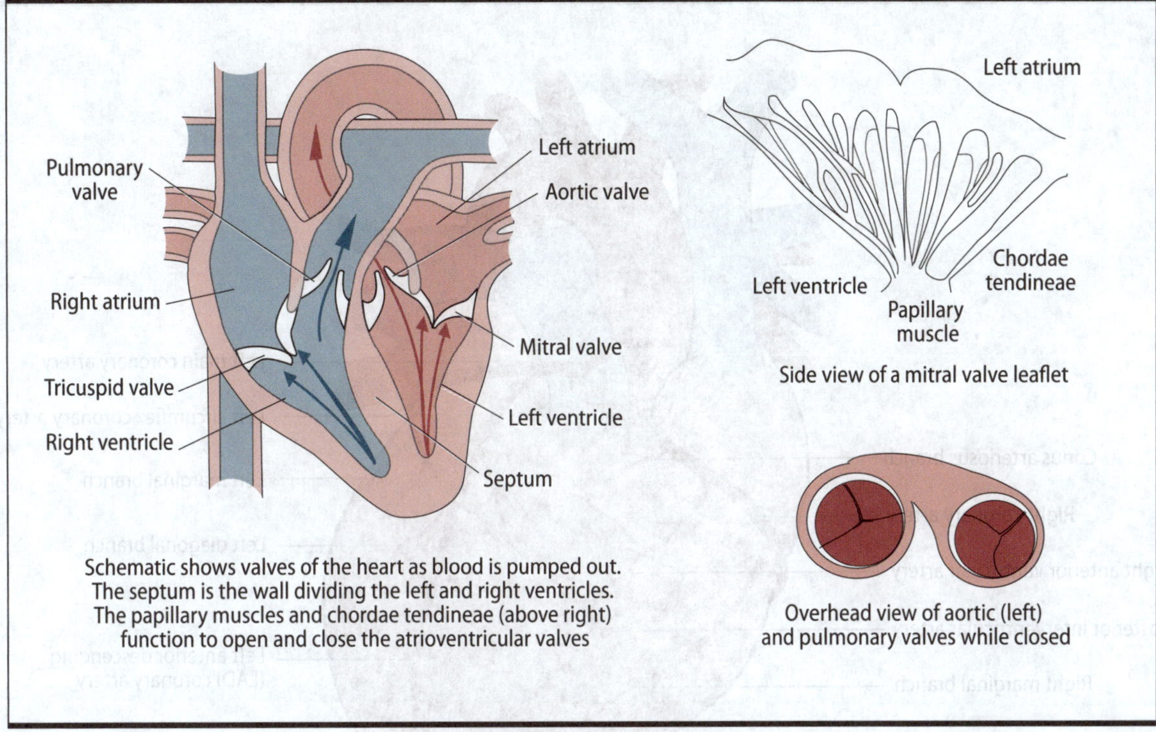

Schematic shows valves of the heart as blood is pumped out. The septum is the wall dividing the left and right ventricles. The papillary muscles and chordae tendineae (above right) function to open and close the atrioventricular valves

Side view of a mitral valve leaflet

Overhead view of aortic (left) and pulmonary valves while closed

Heart Conduction System

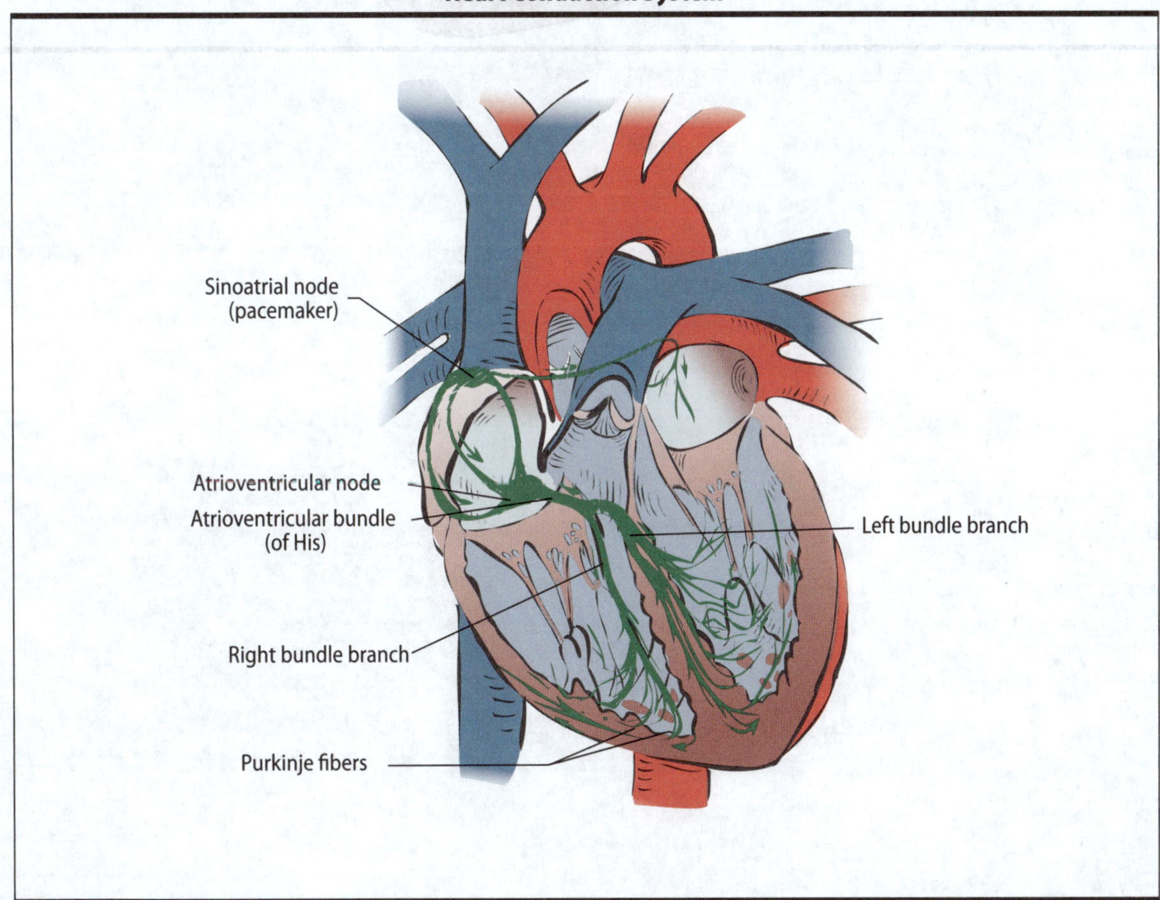

Coronary Arteries

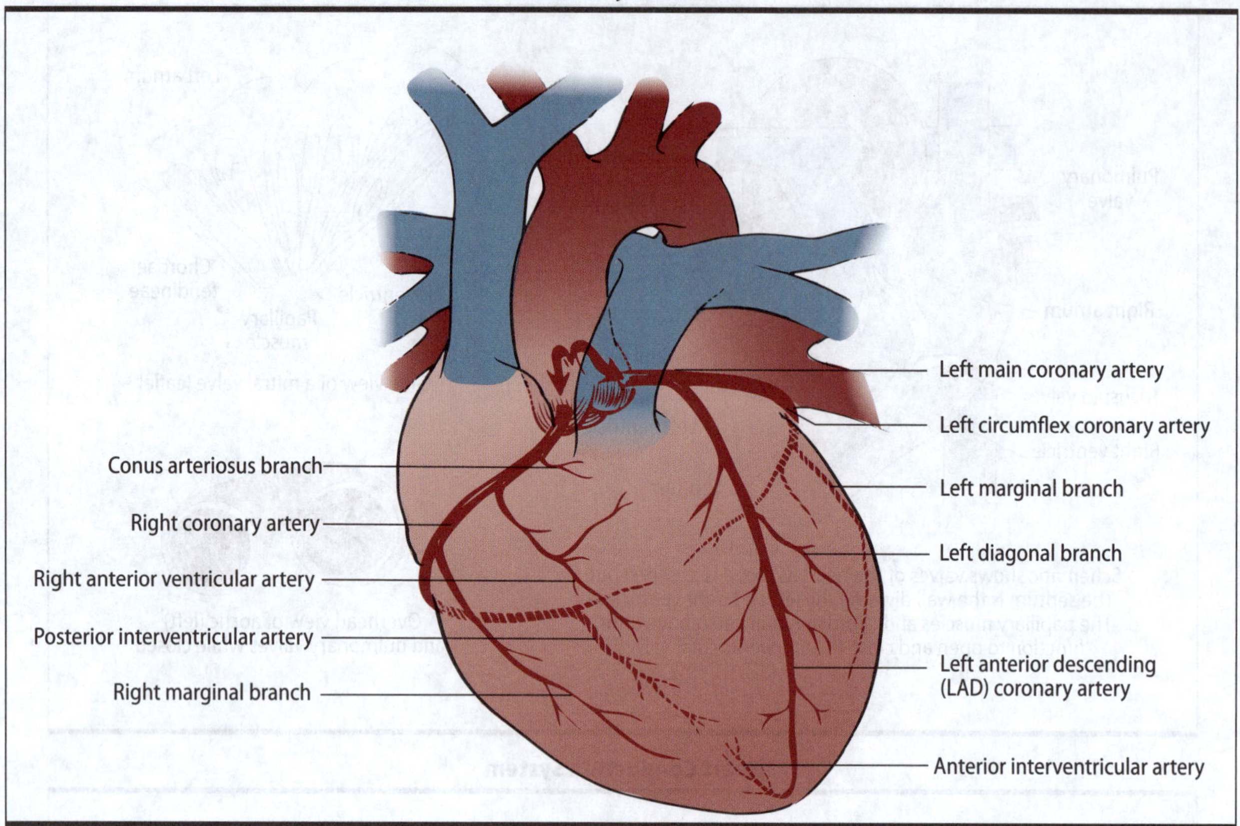

Arteries

Middle temporal a.
Transverse facial a.
Superficial temporal a.
External carotid a.
Internal carotid a.
Common carotid a.
Superior thyroid a.
Vertebral a.
Inferior thyroid a.
Subclavian a.
Innominate a.
Arch of aorta
Ascending aorta
Pulmonary a.
Axillary a.
Internal thoracic a. (mammary)
Descending aorta
Brachial a.
Common hepatic a.
L. gastric a.
Celiac trunk (artery)
Splenic a.
R. gastric a.
Renal a.
Superior mesenteric a.
R. colic a.
Abdominal aorta
L. colic a.
Radial a.
Inferior mesenteric a.
Ulnar a.
Common iliac a.
Internal iliac a.
External iliac a.
Uterine a.
Femoral a.
Popliteal a.
Anterior tibial a.
Peroneal a.
Posterior tibial a.

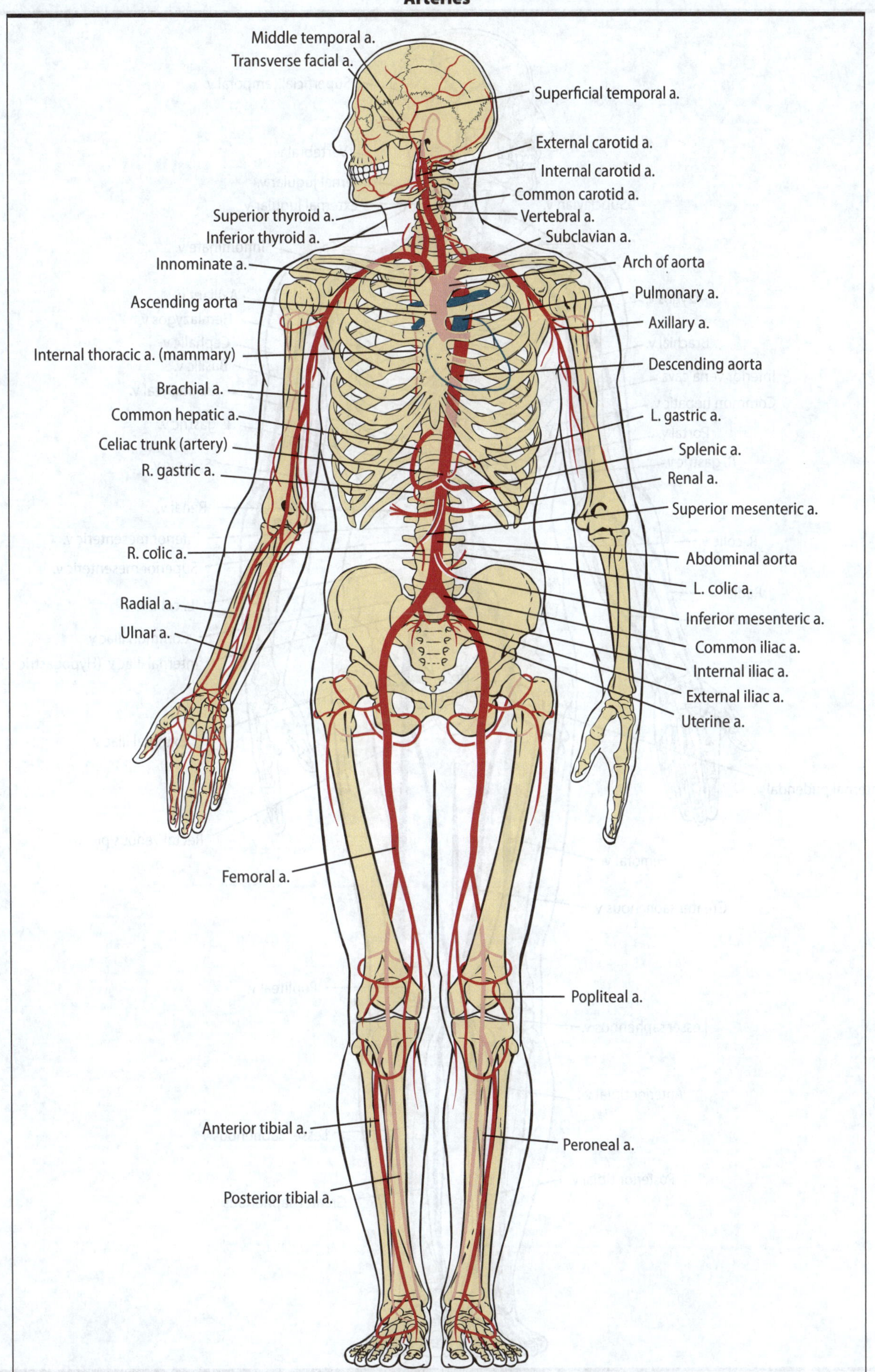

Veins

Superficial temporal v.
Vertebral v.
Internal jugular v.
External jugular v.
Subclavian v.
Innominate v.
Azygos v.
Axillary v.
Hemiazygos v.
Brachial v.
Cephalic v.
Basilic v.
Inferior vena cava
Esophageal v.
Common hepatic v.
L. gastric v.
Portal v.
R. gastric v.
Splenic v.
Renal v.
R. colic v.
Inferior mesenteric v.
Superior mesenteric v.
Radial v.
L. colic v.
Ulnar v.
Common iliac v.
Internal iliac v. (Hypogastric v.)
External iliac v.
Internal pudendal v.
Rectal venous plexus
Femoral v.
Greater saphenous v.
Popliteal v.
Lesser saphenous v.
Anterior tibial v.
Lesser saphenous v.
Posterior tibial v.
Greater saphenous v.

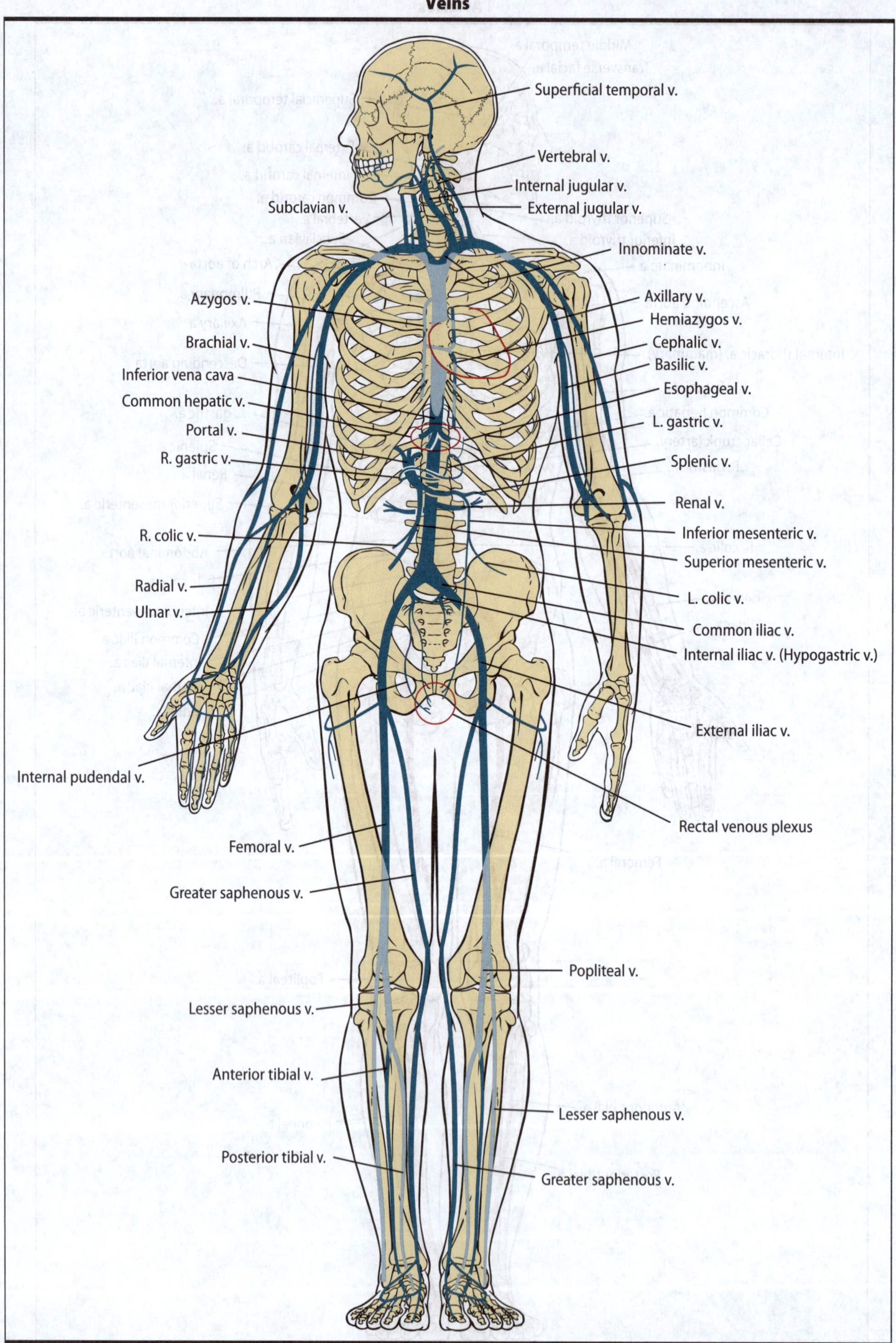

Internal Carotid and Vertebral Arteries and Branches

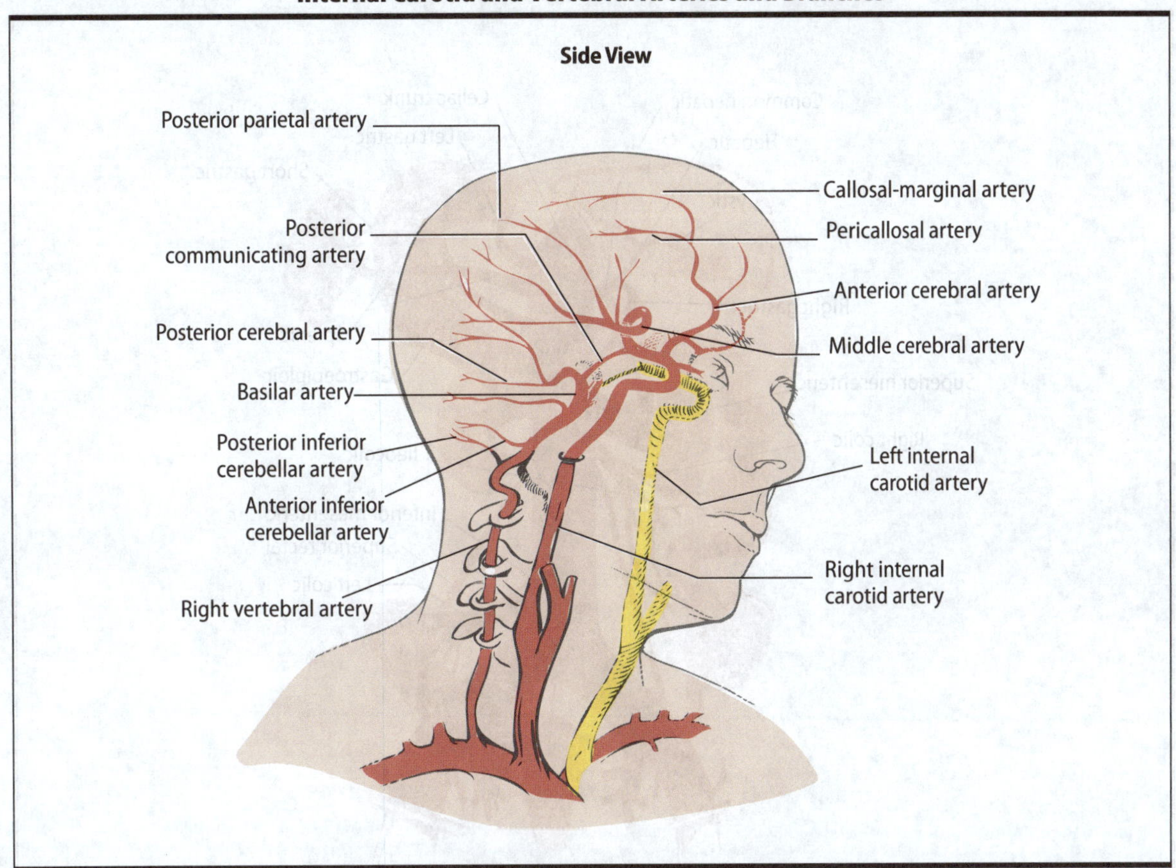

External Carotid Artery and Branches

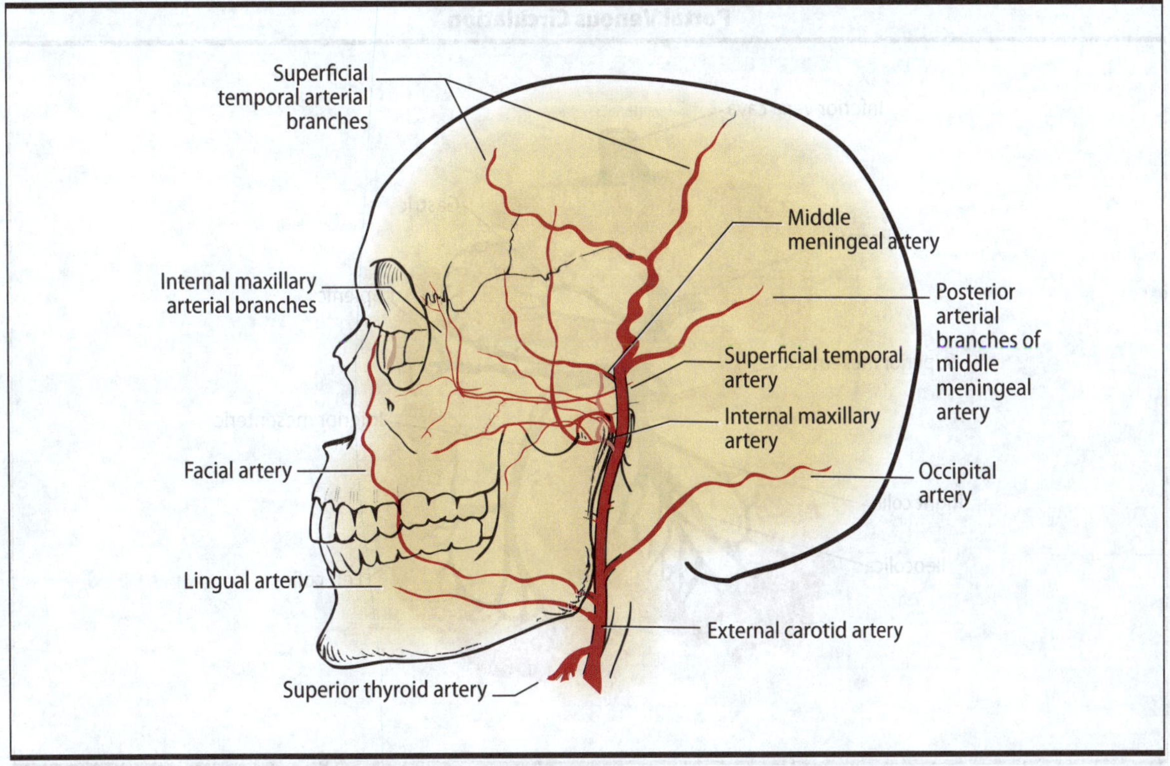

Branches of Abdominal Aorta

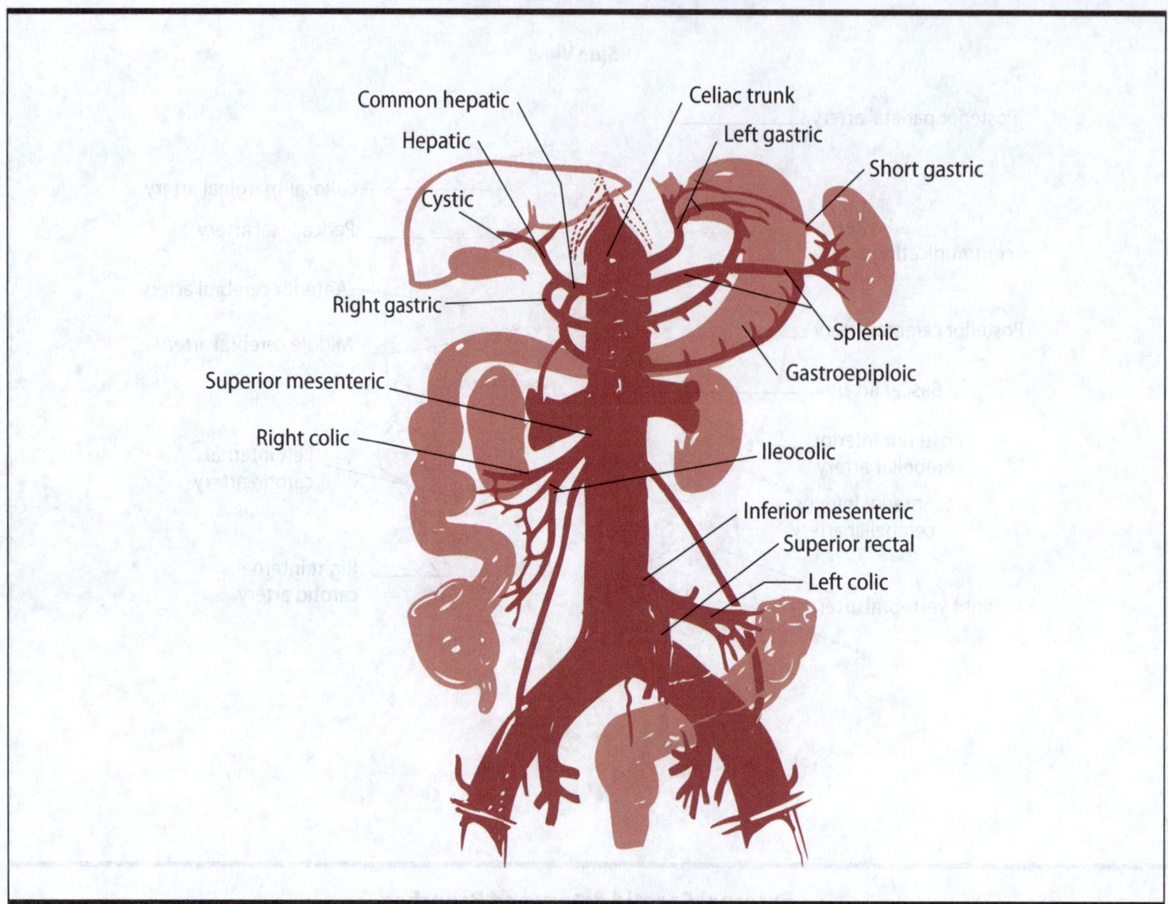

Portal Venous Circulation

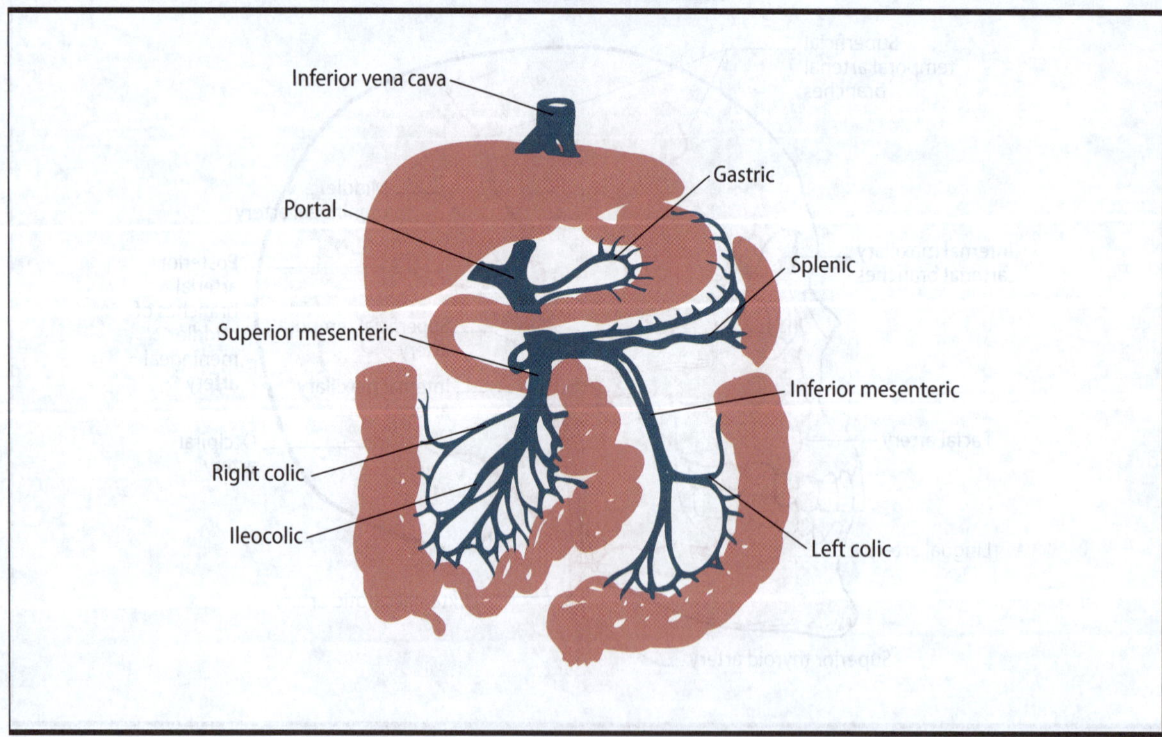

Lymphatic System

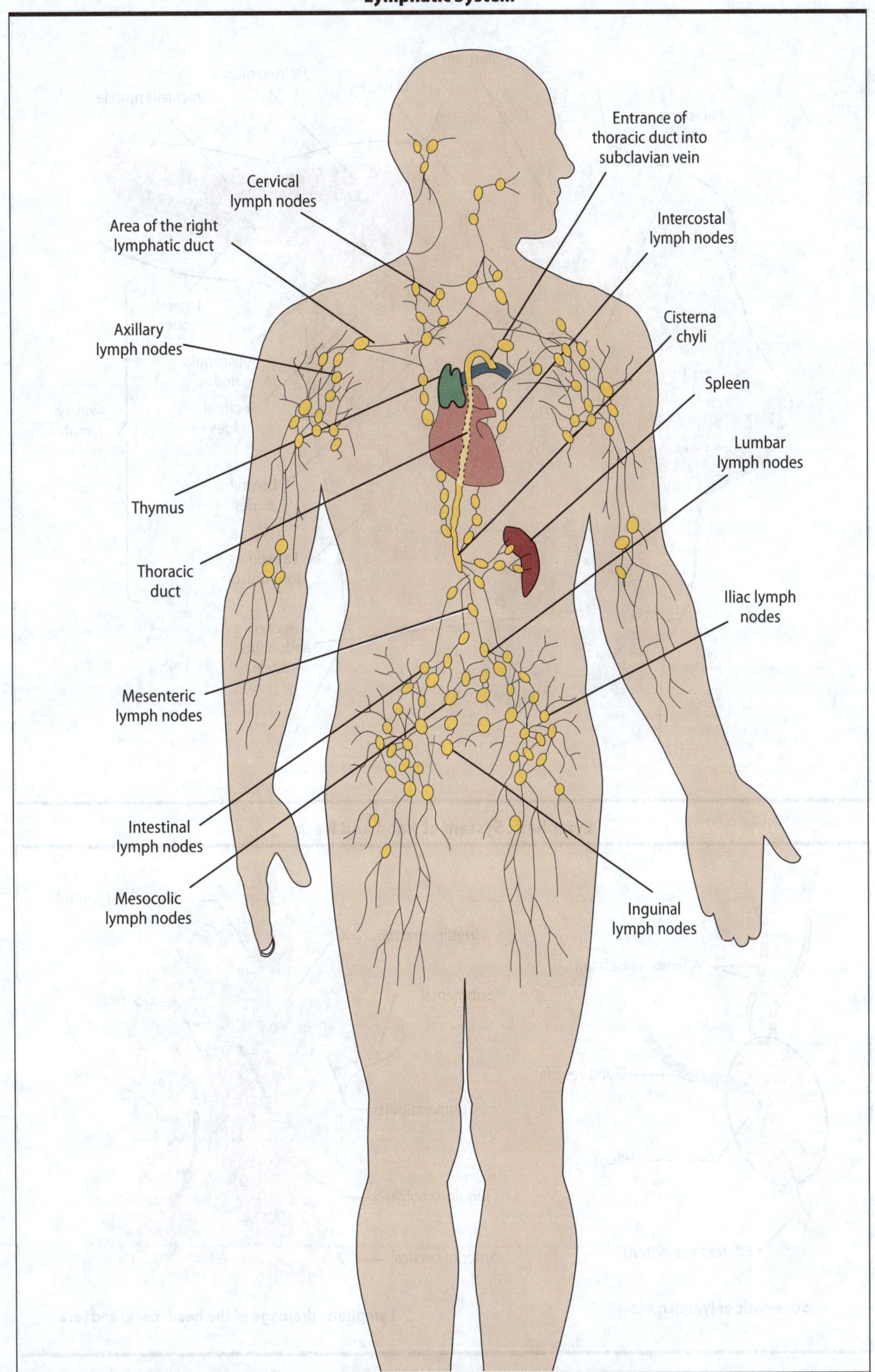

Axillary Lymph Nodes

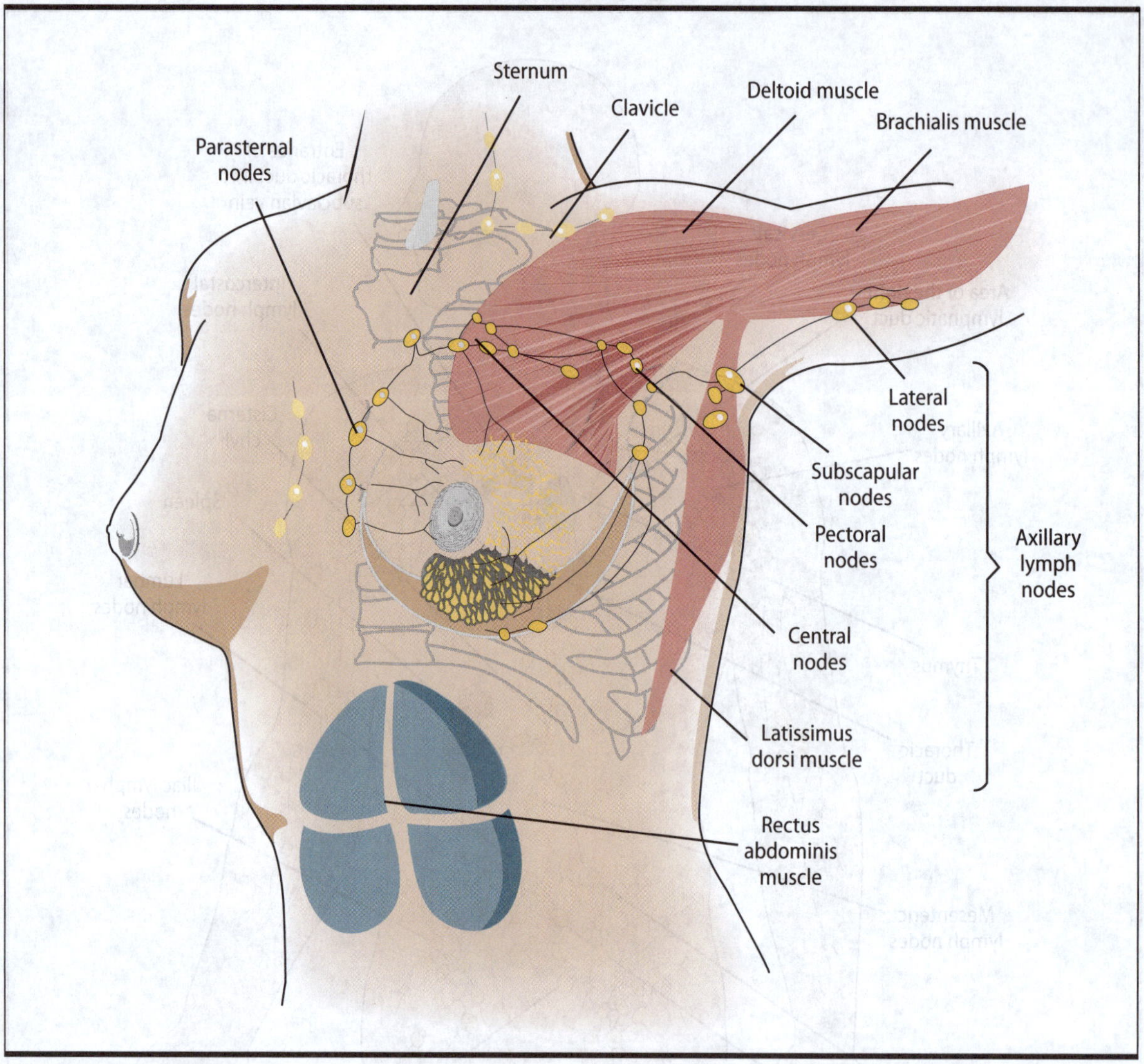

Sternum
Clavicle
Deltoid muscle
Brachialis muscle
Parasternal nodes
Lateral nodes
Subscapular nodes
Pectoral nodes
Axillary lymph nodes
Central nodes
Latissimus dorsi muscle
Rectus abdominis muscle

Lymphatic System of Head and Neck

Afferent vessels (in)
Blood vessels
Hilum
Efferent vessel (out)
Superficial parotid
Jugulodigastric
Submental
Occipital
Submandibular
Jugulo-omohyoid
Anterior cervical

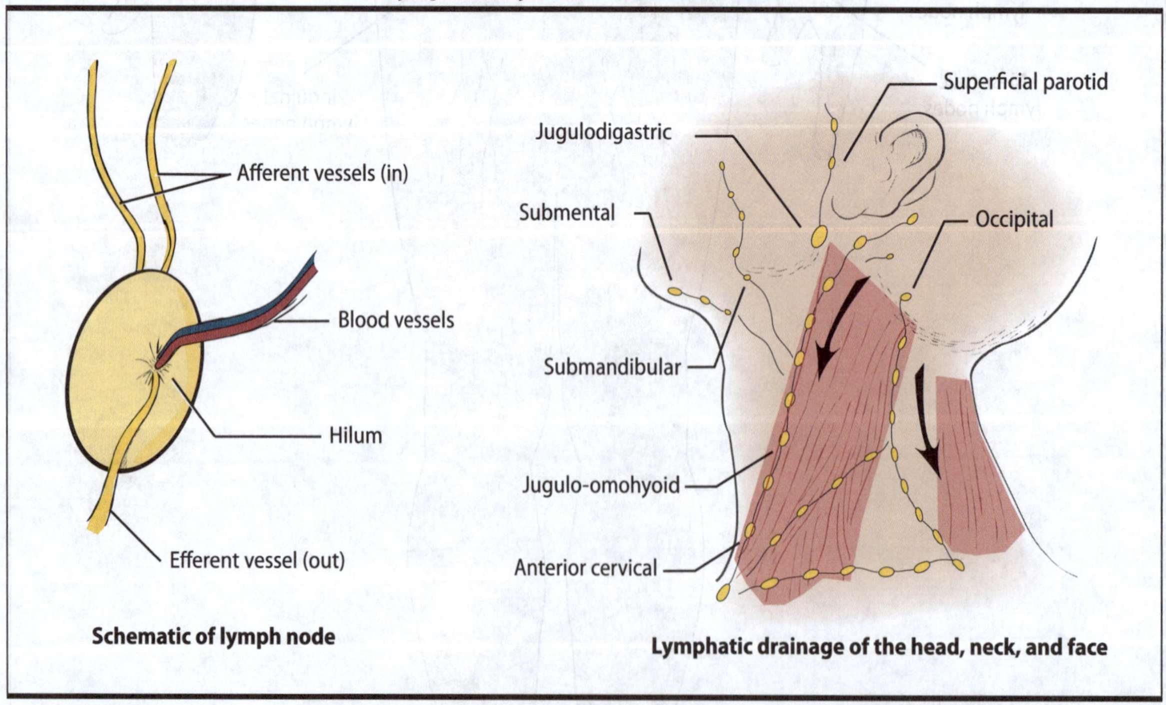

Schematic of lymph node

Lymphatic drainage of the head, neck, and face

Lymphatic Capillaries

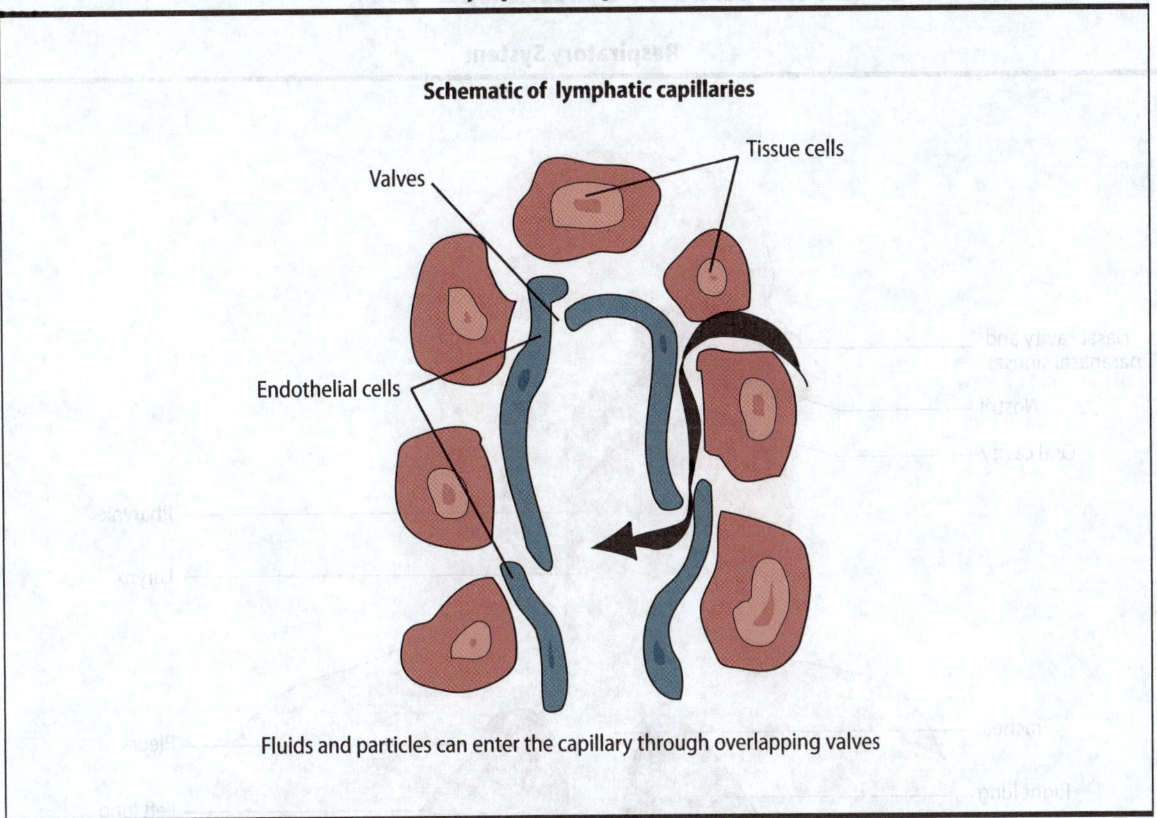

Schematic of lymphatic capillaries
Tissue cells
Valves
Endothelial cells
Fluids and particles can enter the capillary through overlapping valves

Lymphatic Drainage

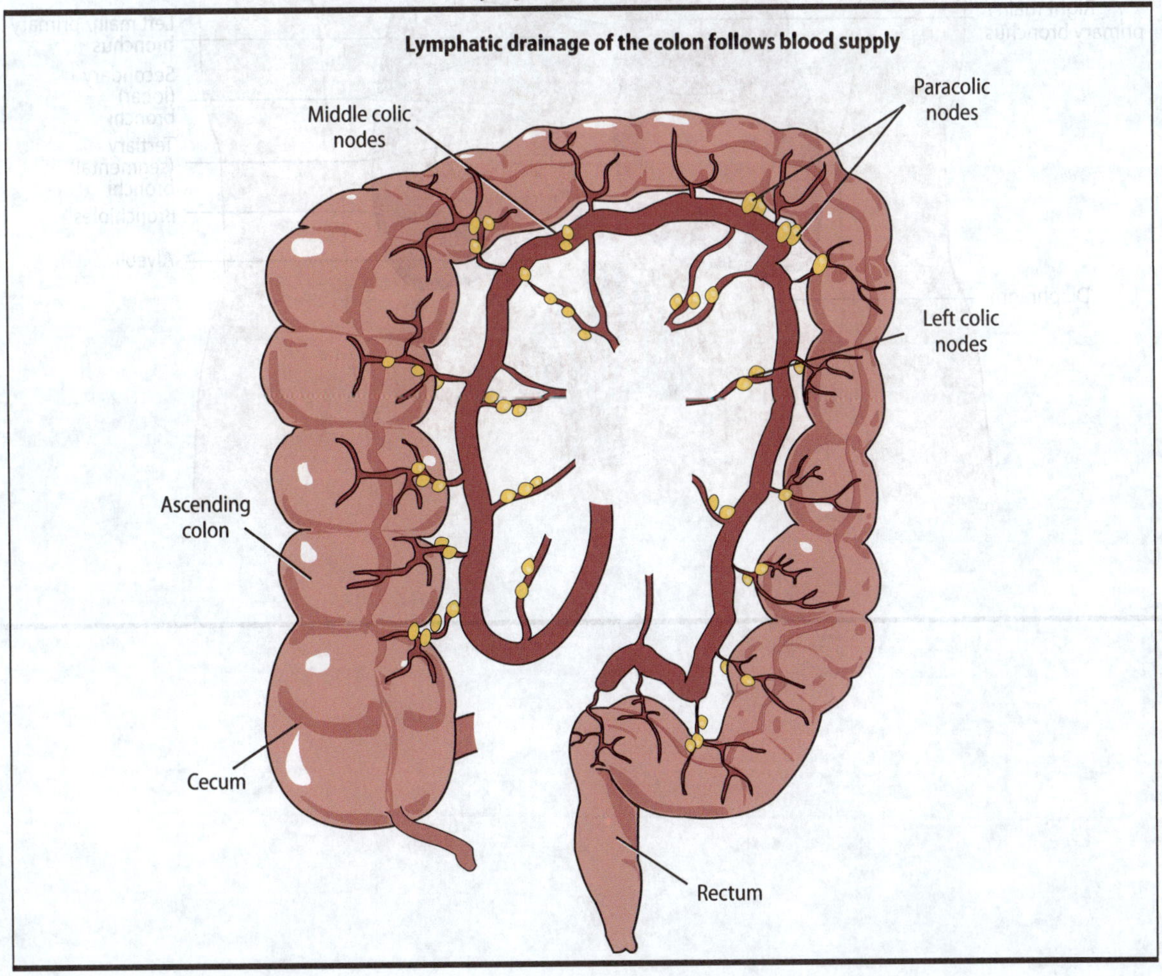

Lymphatic drainage of the colon follows blood supply
Paracolic nodes
Middle colic nodes
Left colic nodes
Ascending colon
Cecum
Rectum

Chapter 10. Diseases of the Respiratory System (JØØ–J99)

Respiratory System

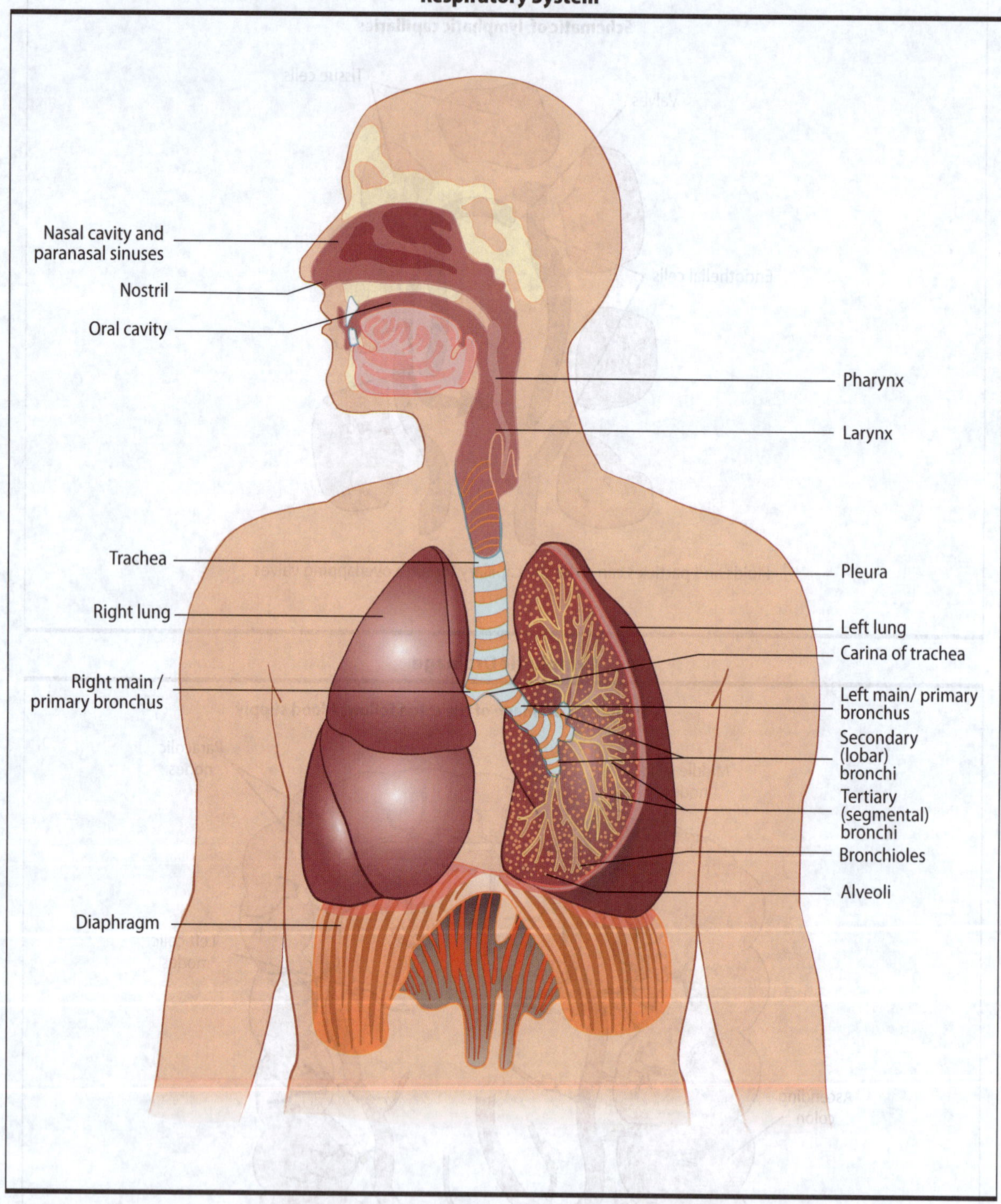

Upper Respiratory System

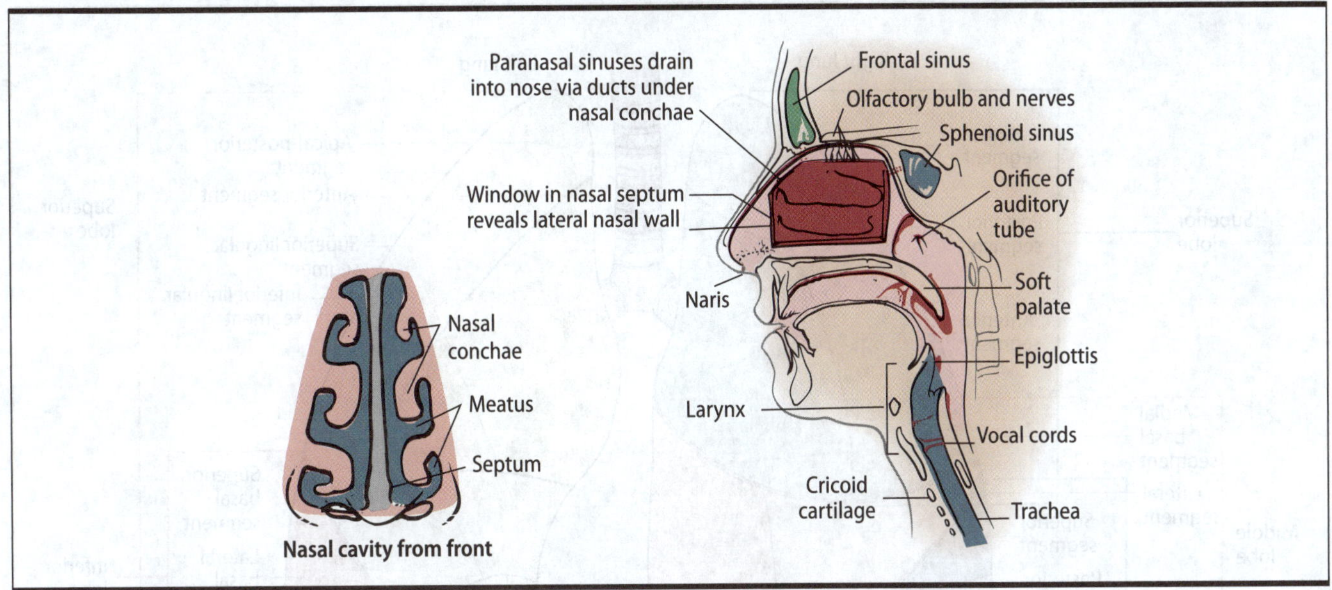

Lower Respiratory System

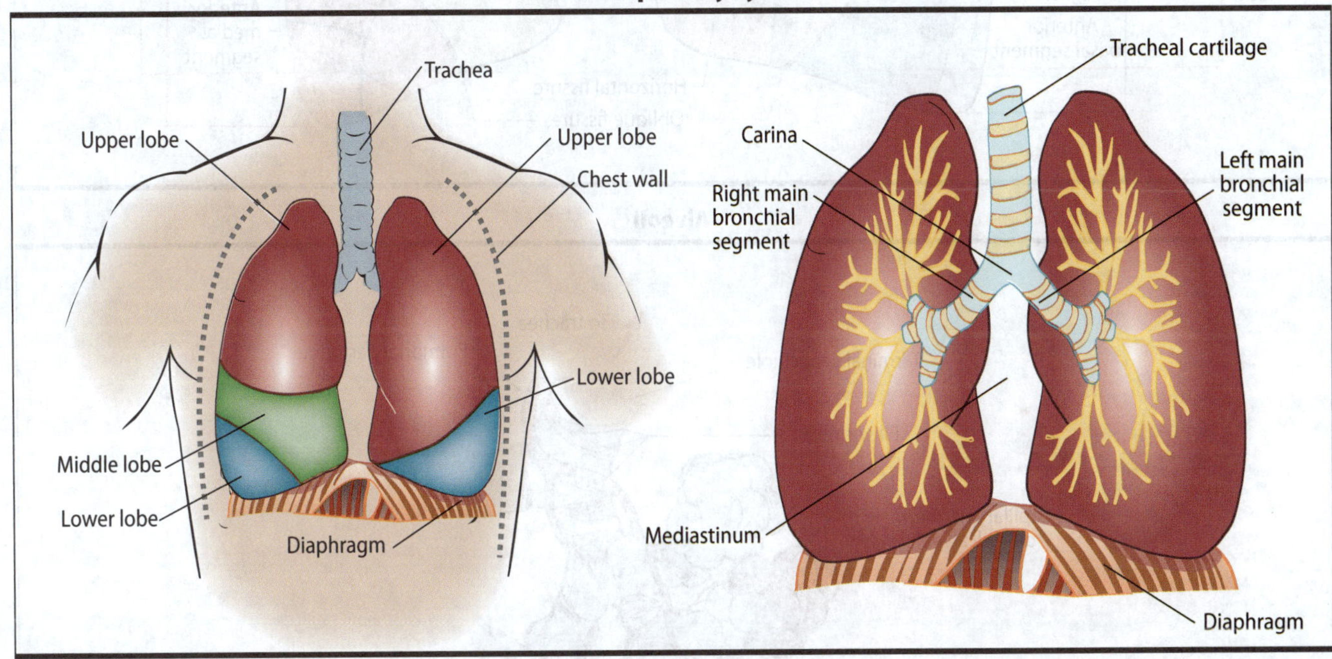

Paranasal Sinuses

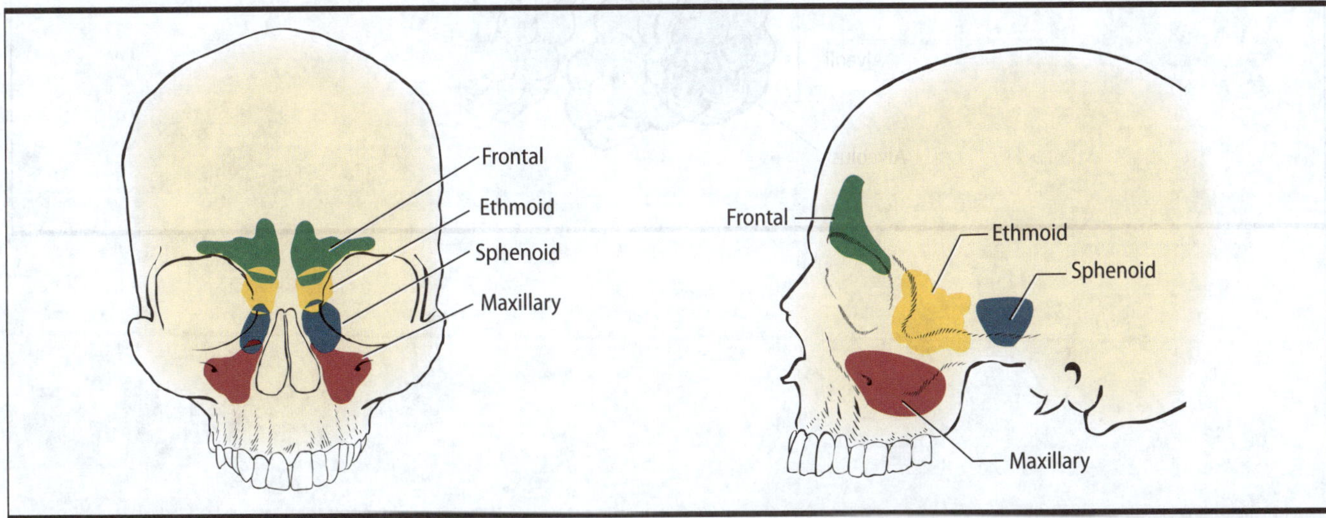

Lung Segments

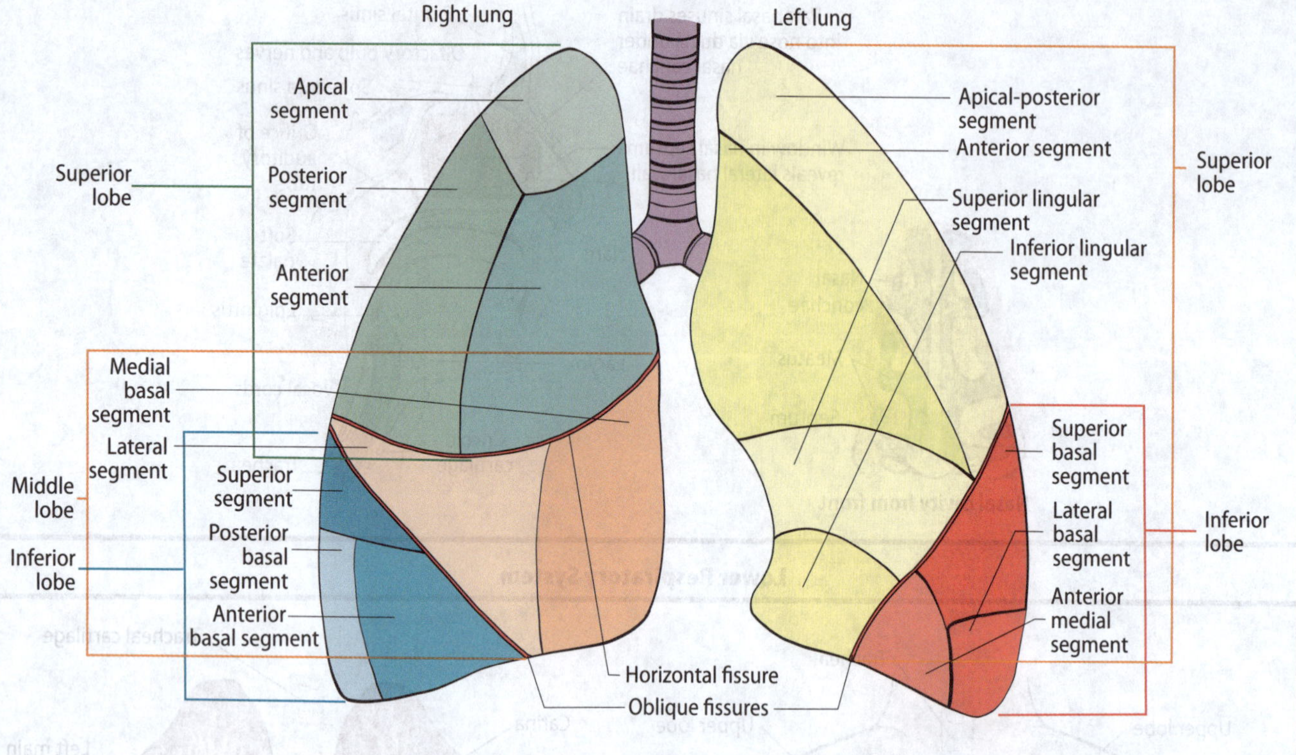

Right lung
Left lung
Apical segment
Posterior segment
Anterior segment
Superior lobe
Medial basal segment
Lateral segment
Middle lobe
Superior segment
Posterior basal segment
Inferior lobe
Anterior basal segment
Apical-posterior segment
Anterior segment
Superior lingular segment
Inferior lingular segment
Superior lobe
Superior basal segment
Lateral basal segment
Inferior lobe
Anterior medial segment
Horizontal fissure
Oblique fissures

Alveoli

To trachea
Terminal bronchiole
Pulmonary arteriole
Elastic fibers
Capillary network over all alveoli
Alveoli
Alveolus

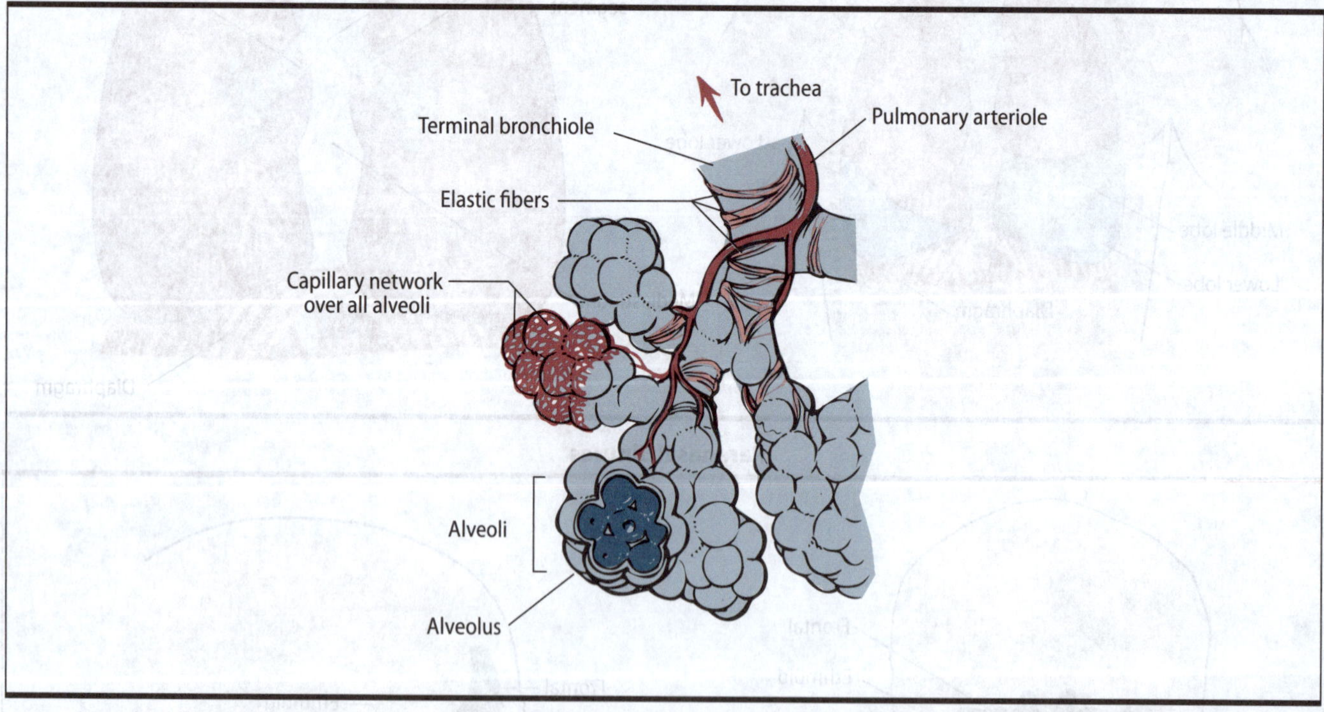

Chapter 11. Diseases of the Digestive System (KØØ–K95)

Digestive System

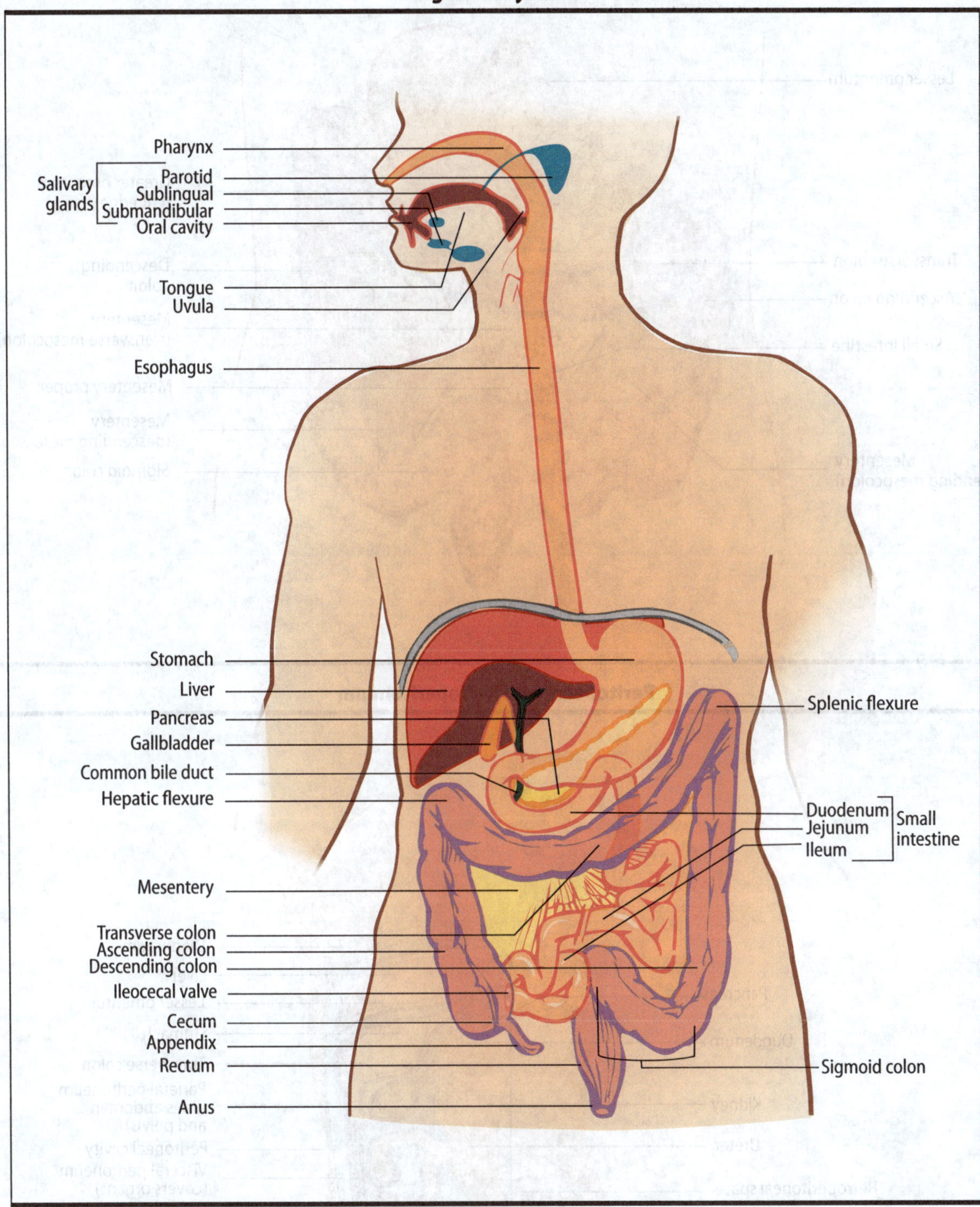

Omentum and Mesentery

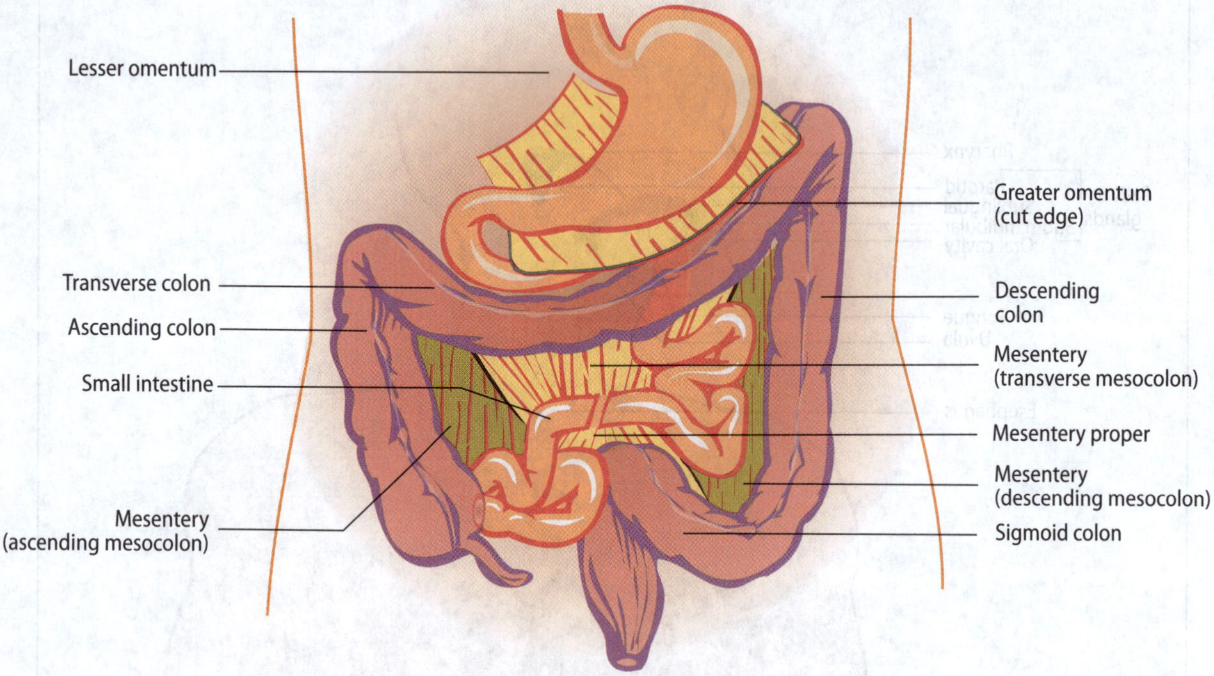

Peritoneum and Retroperitoneum

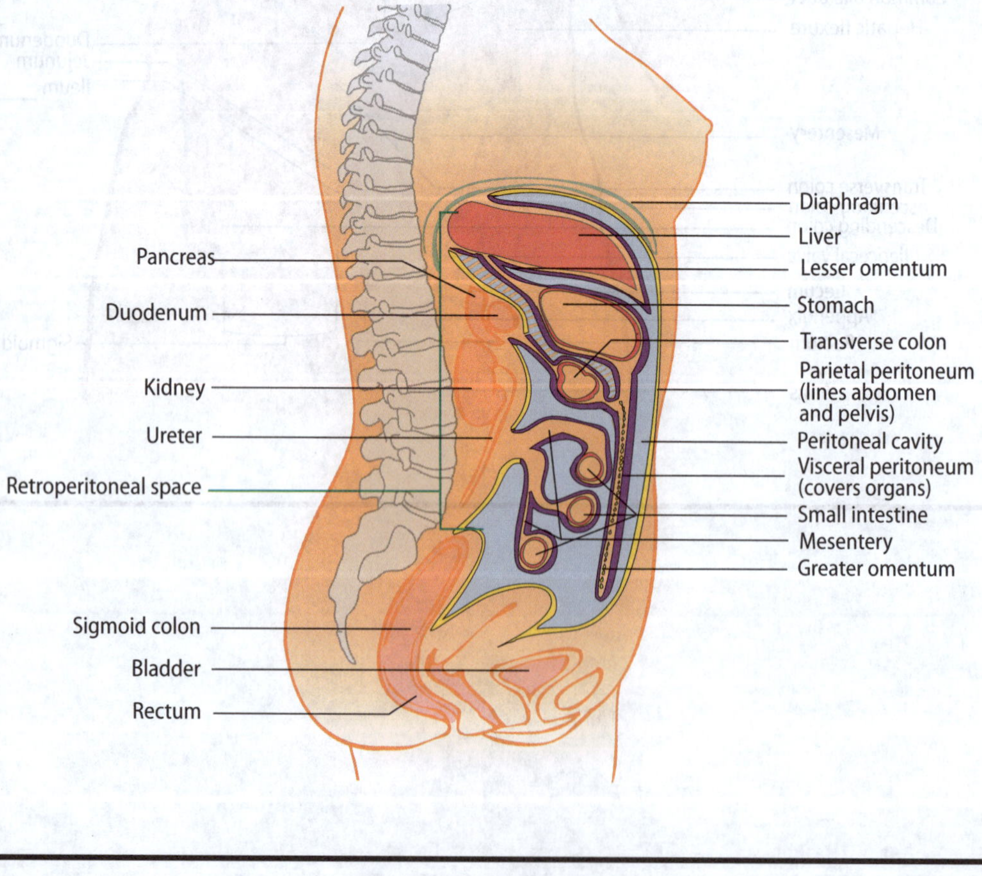

Chapter 12. Diseases of the Skin and Subcutaneous Tissue (LØØ–L99)

Nail Anatomy

Hyponychium
Cuticle
Nail plate
Nail fold
Nail bed
Nail root
Hyponychium
Matrix
Skin
Distal phalanx bone

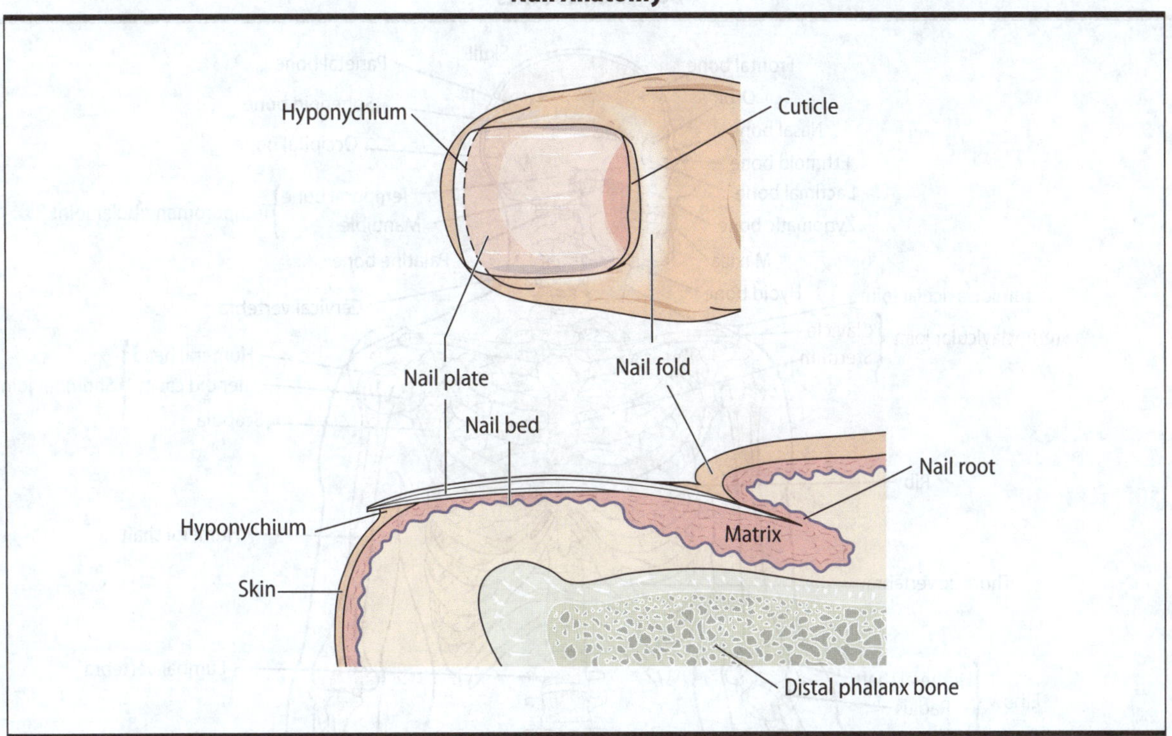

Skin and Subcutaneous Tissue

Hair
Basal layer
Corneal layer (corneum)
Epidermis
Hair shaft
Dermis
Sebaceous gland
Bulb
Hypodermis (subcutaneous layer)
Hair follicles
Sweat (eccrine gland)
Sensory nerve
Adipose tissue
Blood vessels

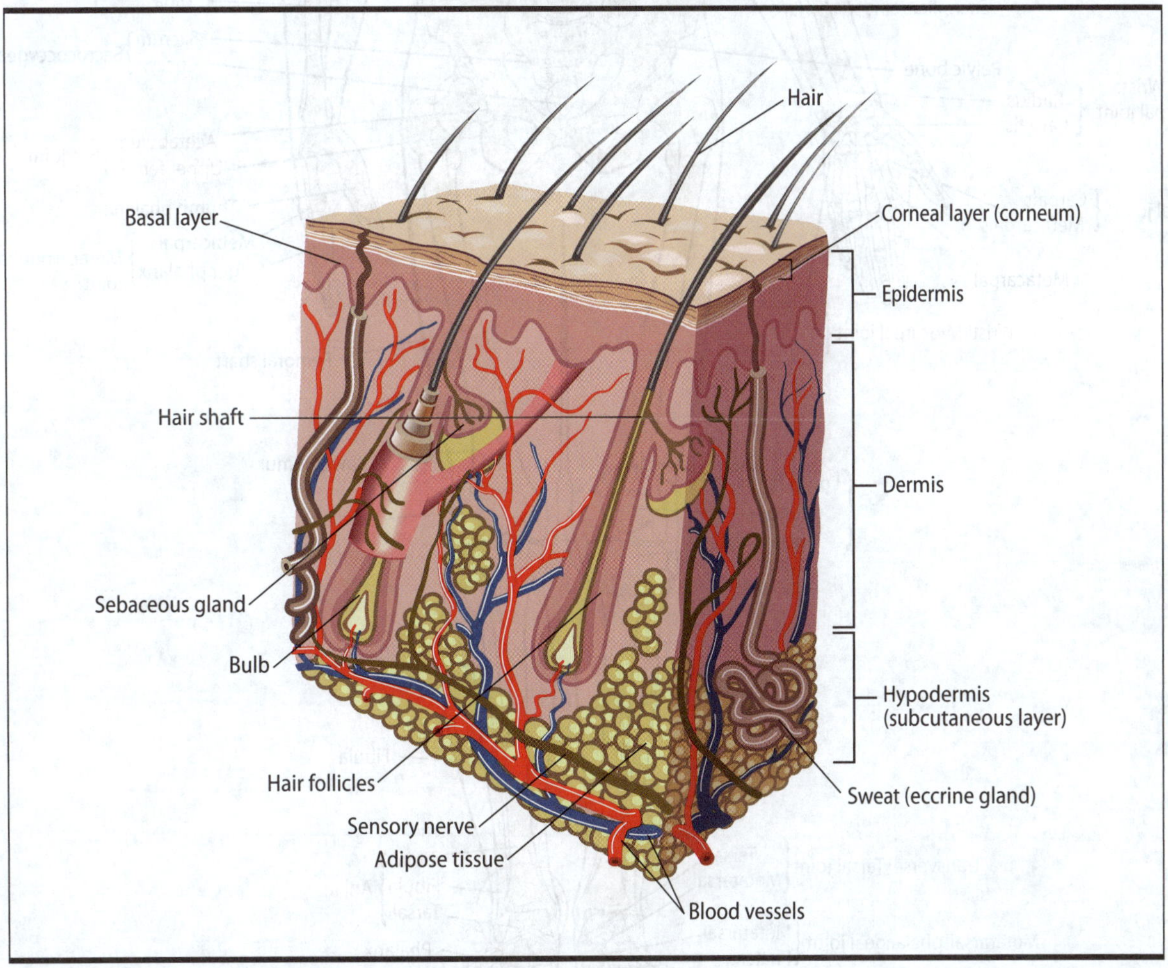

Chapter 13. Diseases of the Musculoskeletal System and Connective Tissue (MØØ–M99)

Bones and Joints

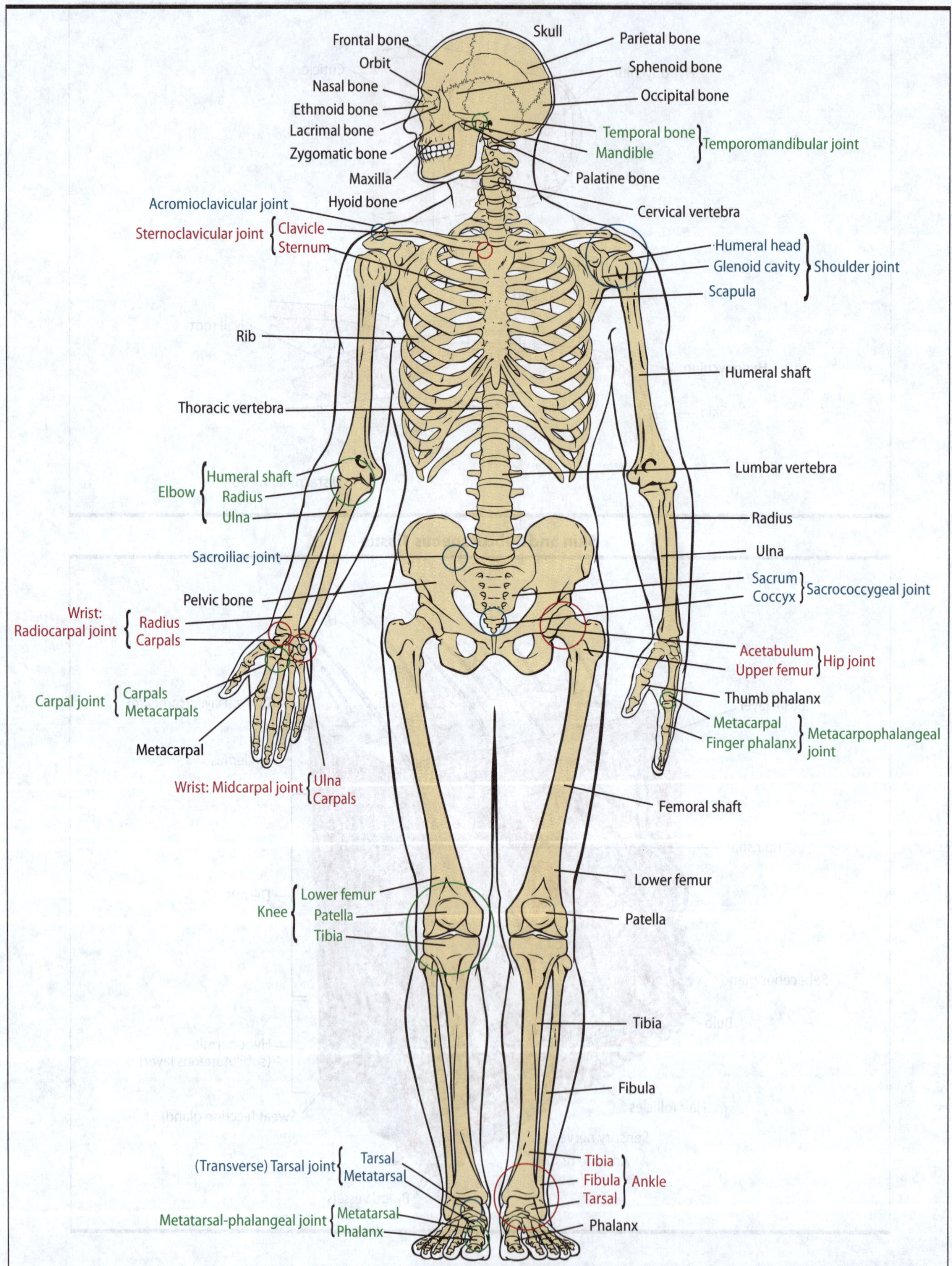

Shoulder Anterior View

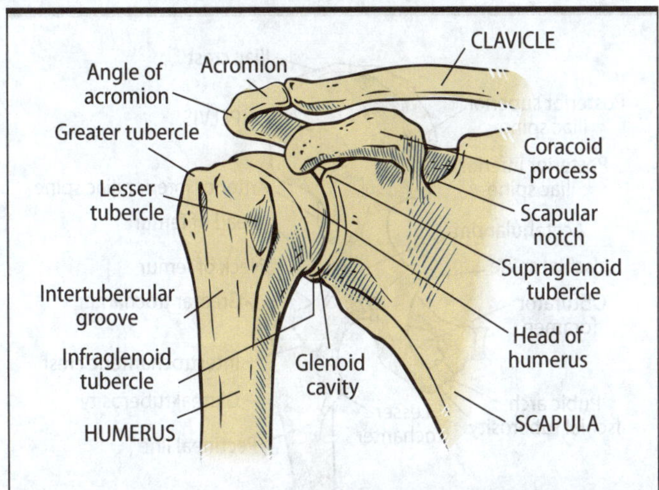

Shoulder Posterior View

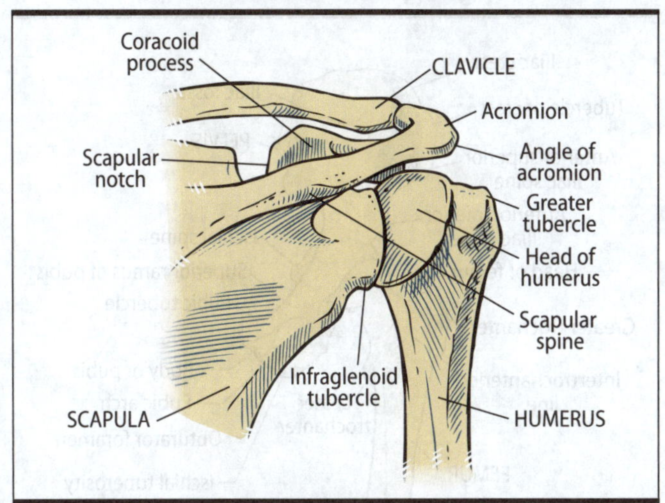

Elbow Anterior View

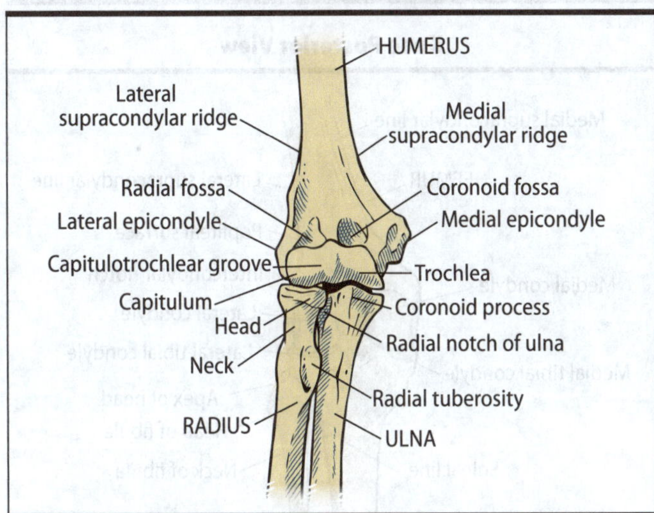

Elbow Posterior View

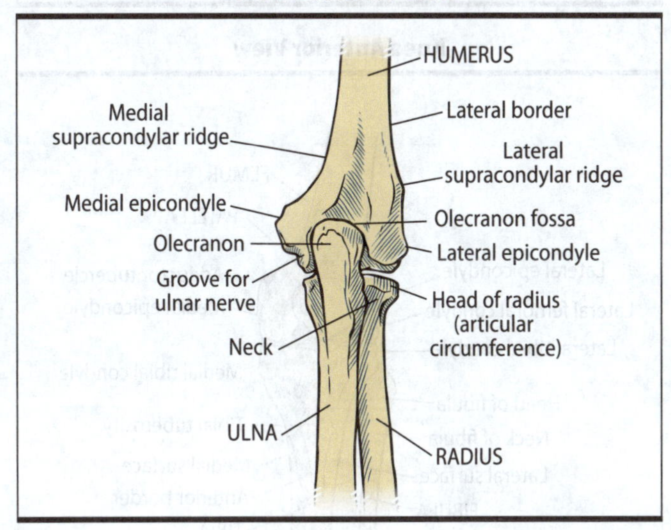

Hand

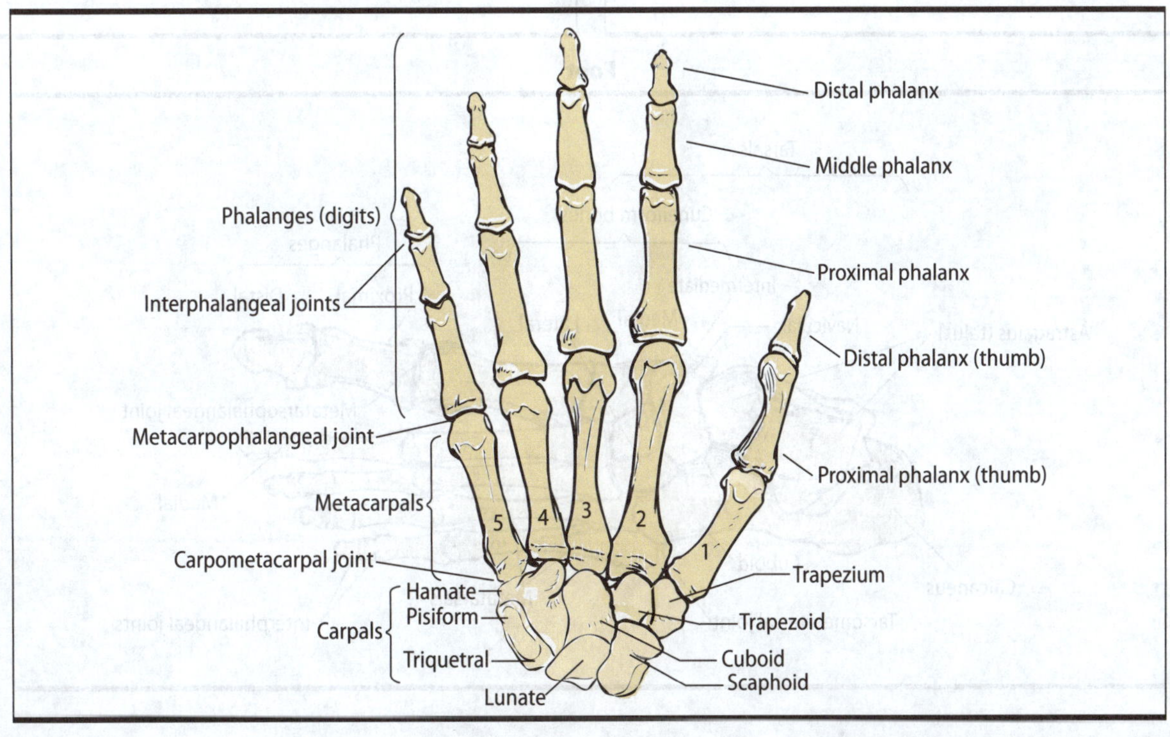

Hip Anterior View

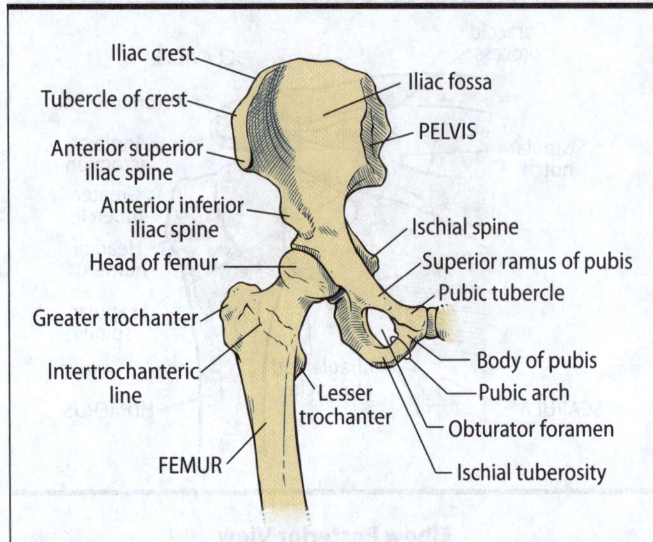

Hip Posterior View

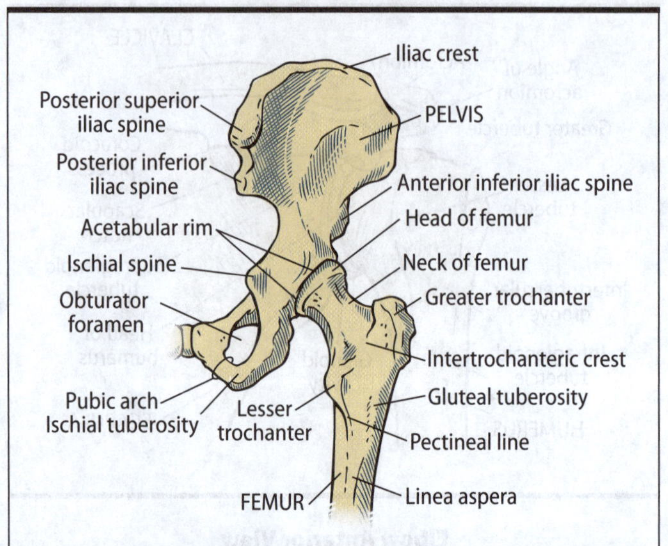

Knee Anterior View

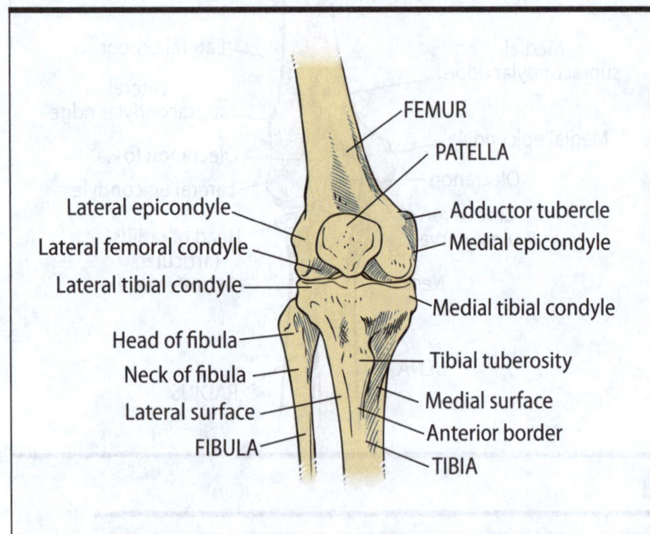

Knee Posterior View

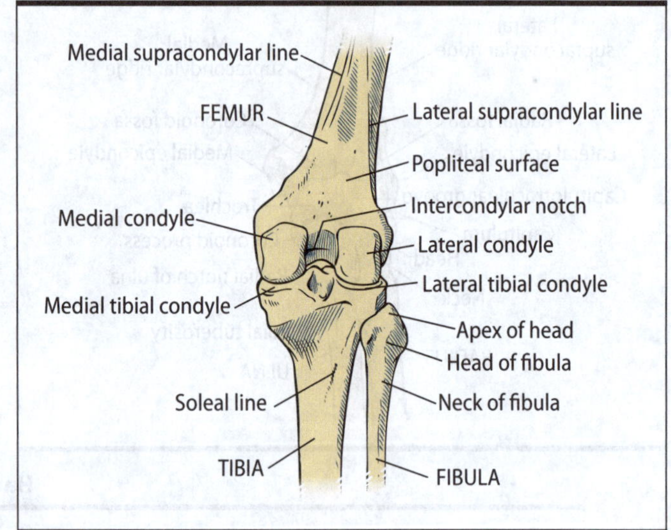

Foot

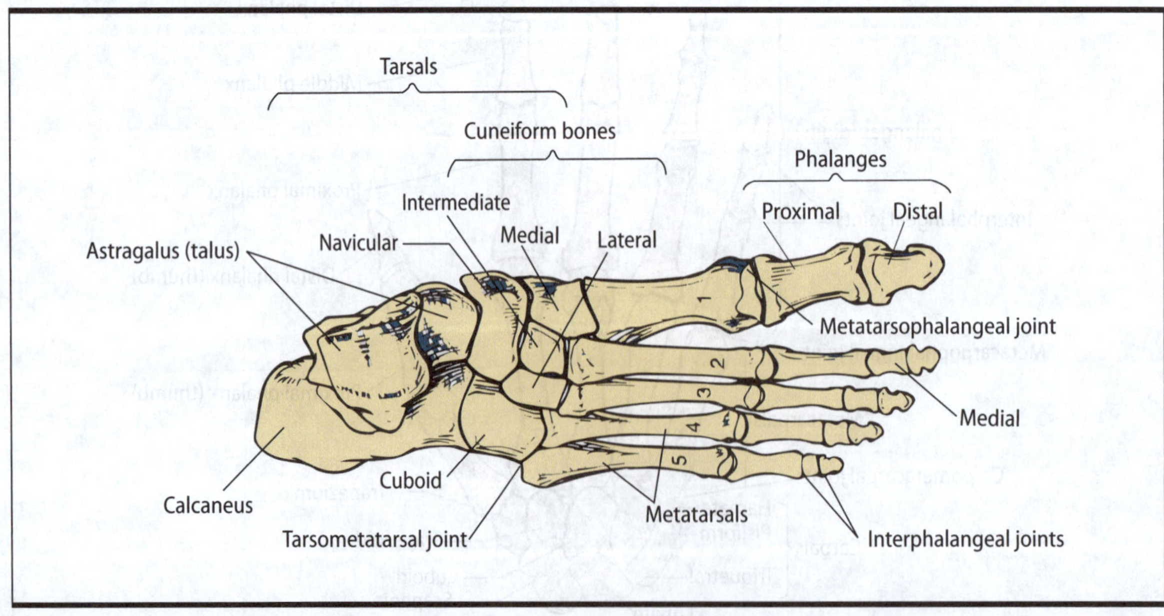

Muscles

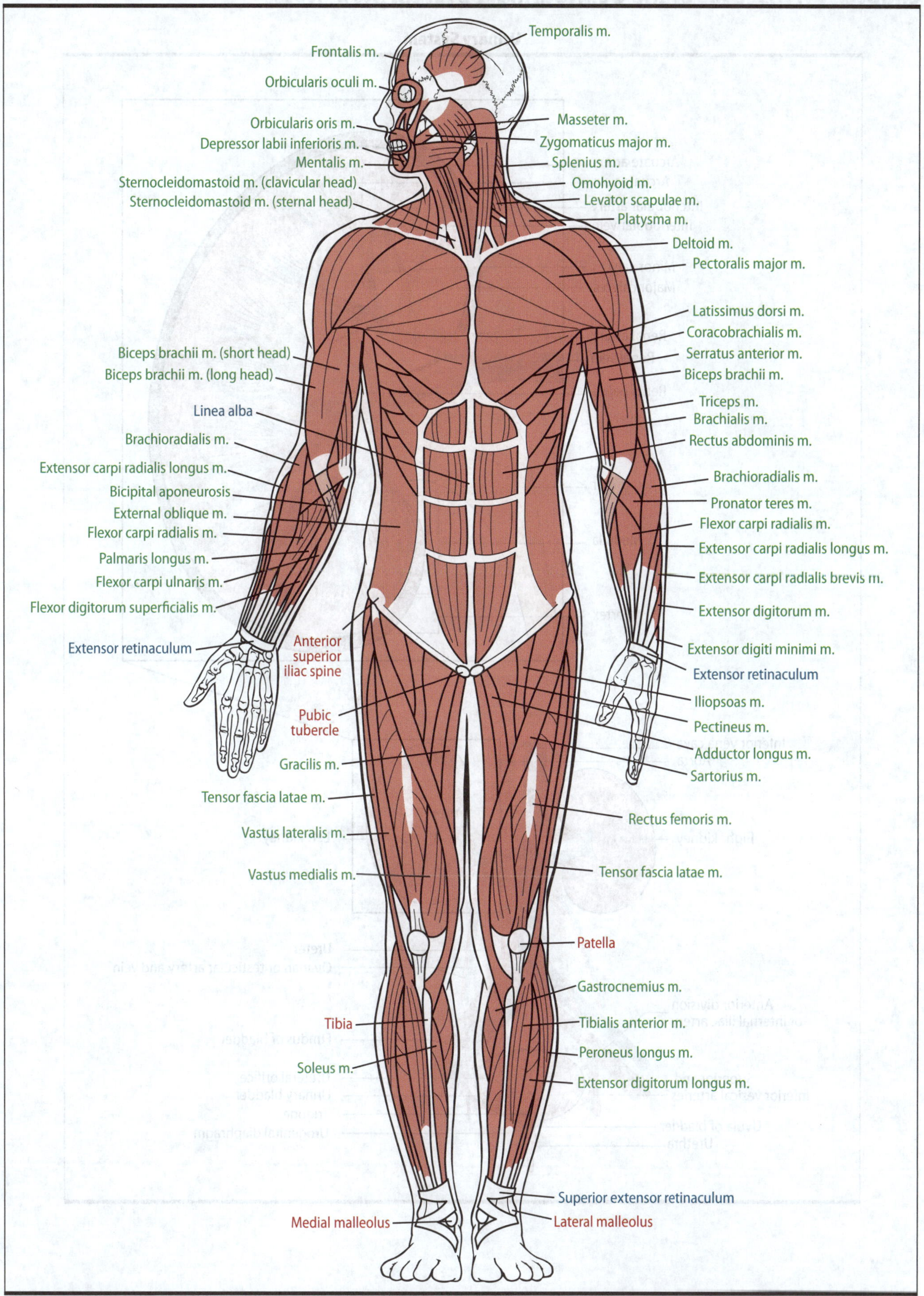

Temporalis m.
Frontalis m.
Orbicularis oculi m.
Orbicularis oris m.
Masseter m.
Depressor labii inferioris m.
Zygomaticus major m.
Mentalis m.
Splenius m.
Sternocleidomastoid m. (clavicular head)
Omohyoid m.
Sternocleidomastoid m. (sternal head)
Levator scapulae m.
Platysma m.
Deltoid m.
Pectoralis major m.
Latissimus dorsi m.
Coracobrachialis m.
Biceps brachii m. (short head)
Serratus anterior m.
Biceps brachii m. (long head)
Biceps brachii m.
Triceps m.
Linea alba
Brachialis m.
Brachioradialis m.
Rectus abdominis m.
Extensor carpi radialis longus m.
Brachioradialis m.
Bicipital aponeurosis
Pronator teres m.
External oblique m.
Flexor carpi radialis m.
Flexor carpi radialis m.
Extensor carpi radialis longus m.
Palmaris longus m.
Flexor carpi ulnaris m.
Extensor carpi radialis brevis m.
Flexor digitorum superficialis m.
Extensor digitorum m.
Extensor retinaculum
Anterior superior iliac spine
Extensor digiti minimi m.
Extensor retinaculum
Iliopsoas m.
Pubic tubercle
Pectineus m.
Adductor longus m.
Gracilis m.
Sartorius m.
Tensor fascia latae m.
Rectus femoris m.
Vastus lateralis m.
Vastus medialis m.
Tensor fascia latae m.
Patella
Gastrocnemius m.
Tibia
Tibialis anterior m.
Peroneus longus m.
Soleus m.
Extensor digitorum longus m.
Superior extensor retinaculum
Medial malleolus
Lateral malleolus

Chapter 14. Diseases of the Genitourinary System (NØØ–N99)

Urinary System

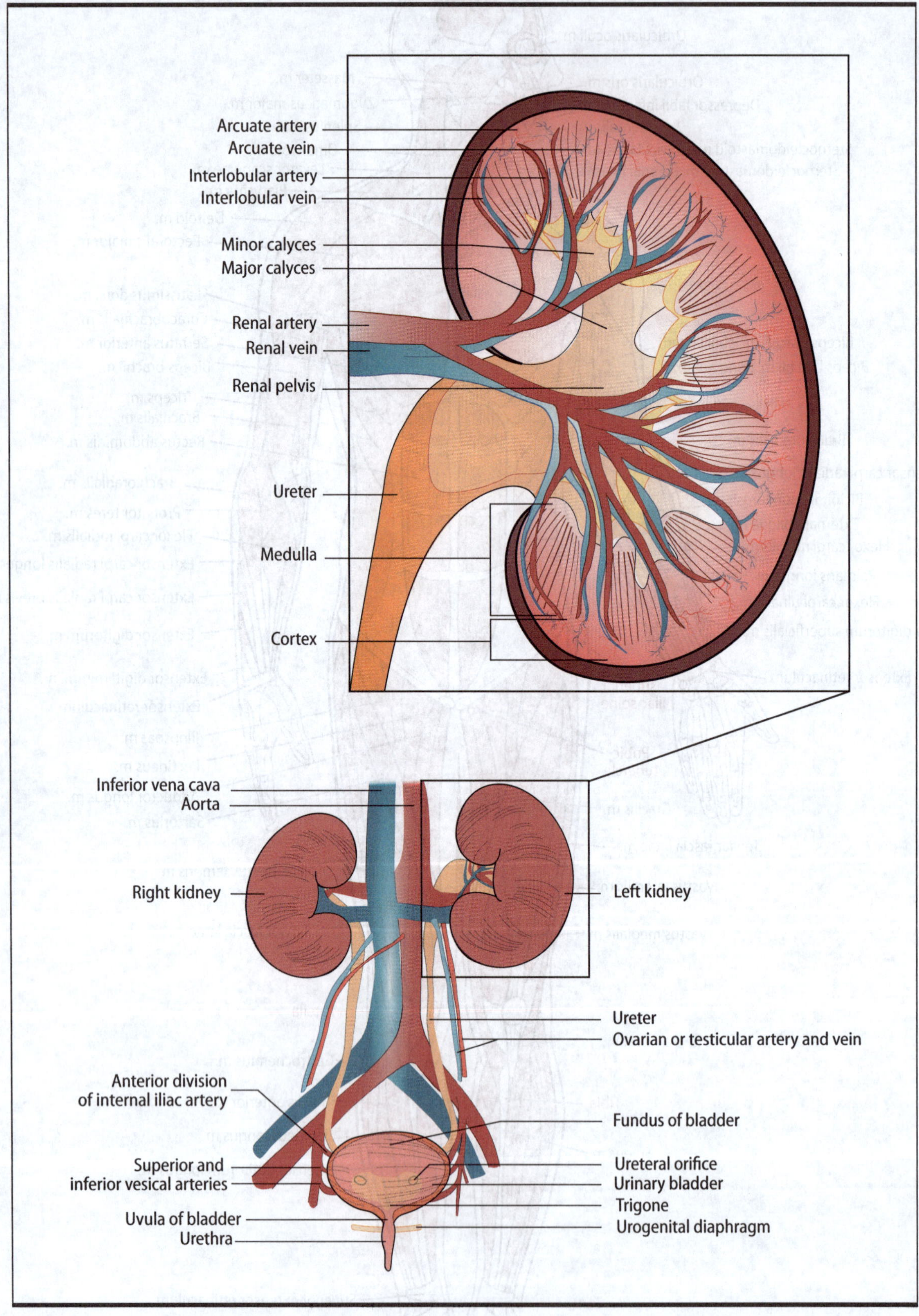

Male Genitourinary System

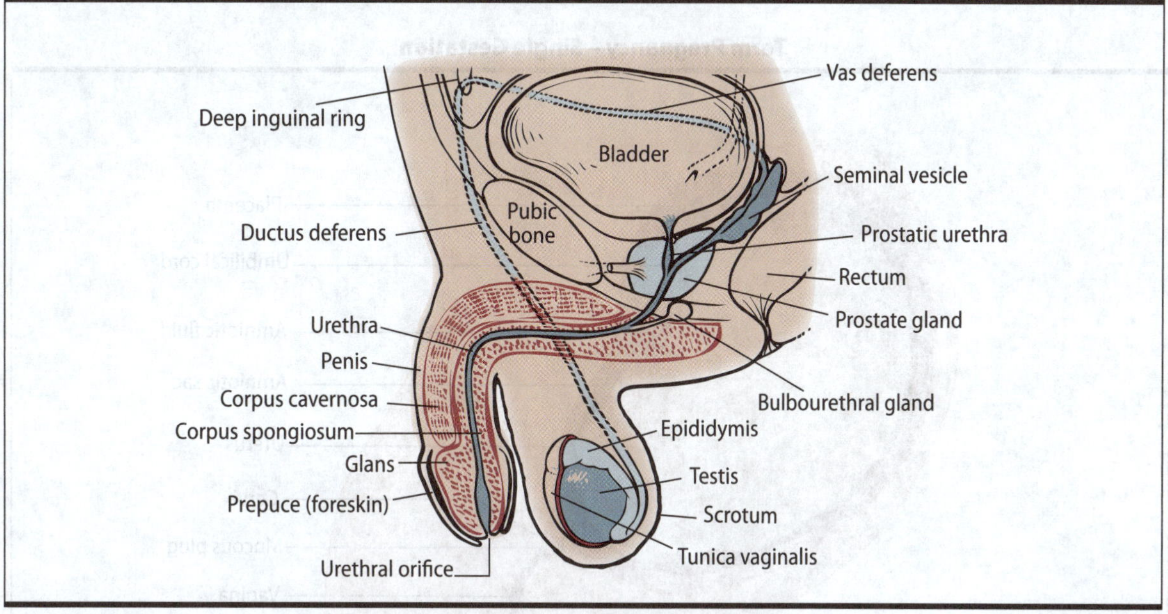

Female Internal Genitalia

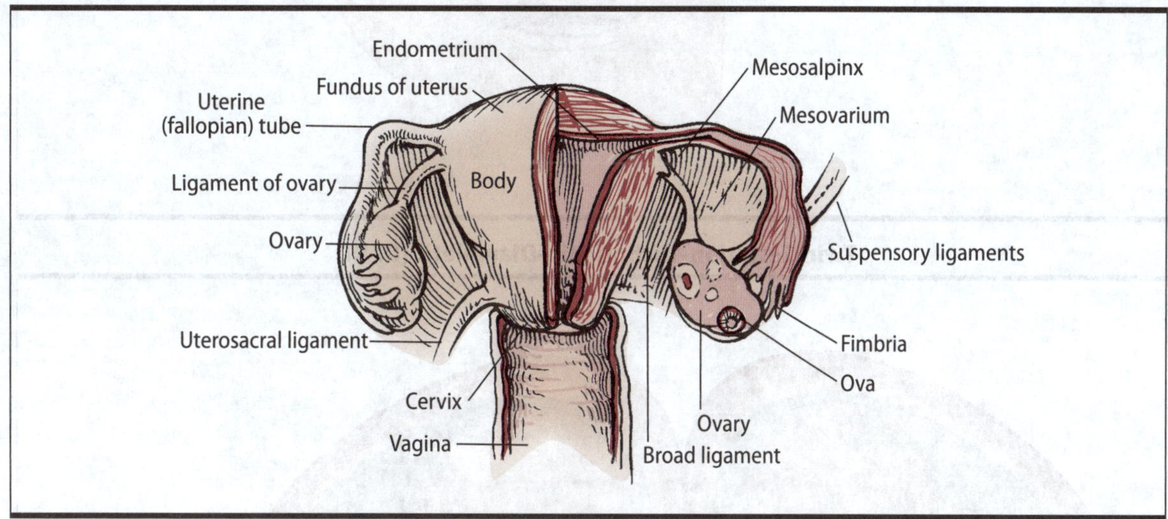

Female Genitourinary Tract Lateral View

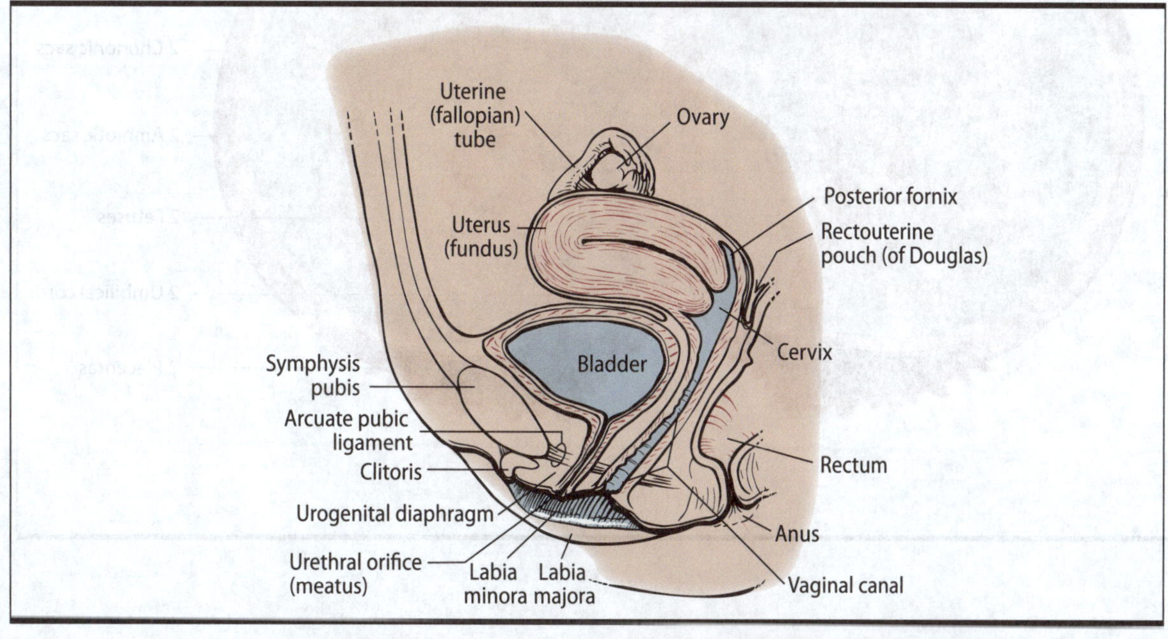

Chapter 15. Pregnancy, Childbirth and the Puerperium (OØØ–O9A)

Term Pregnancy – Single Gestation

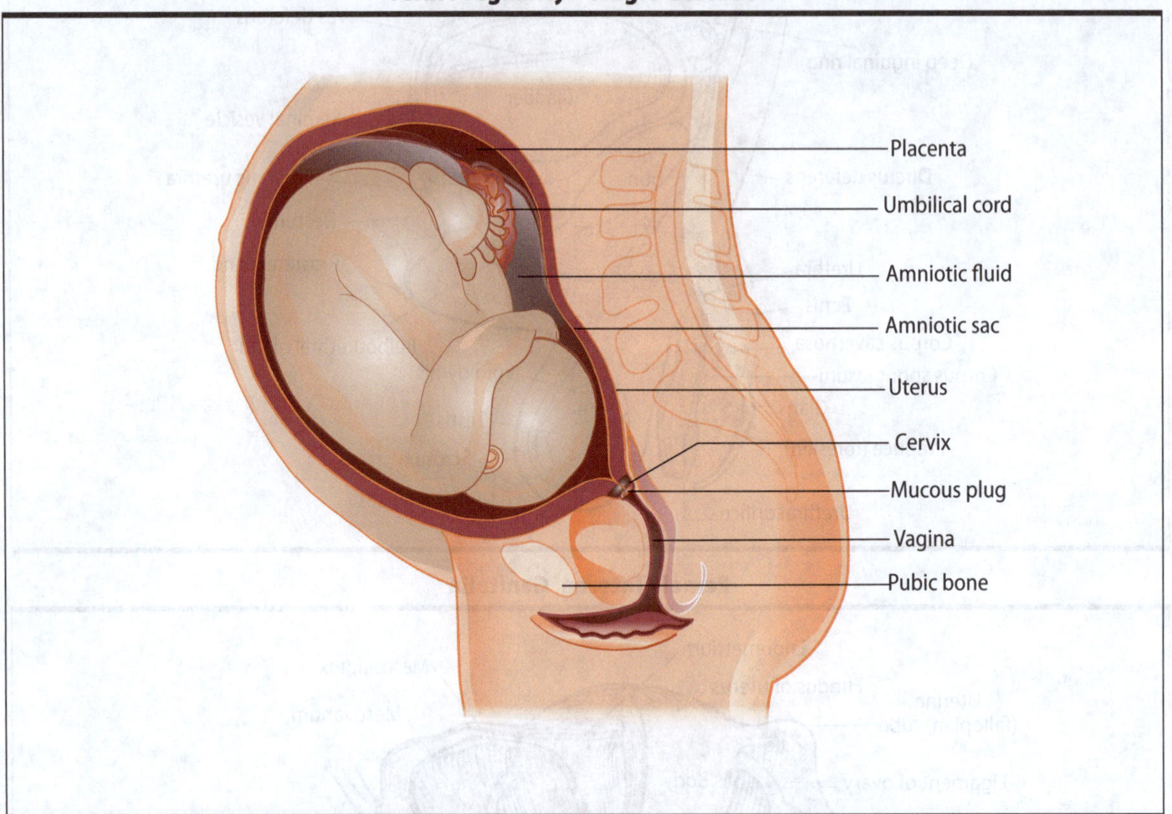

Twin Gestation–Dichorionic–Diamniotic (DI-DI)

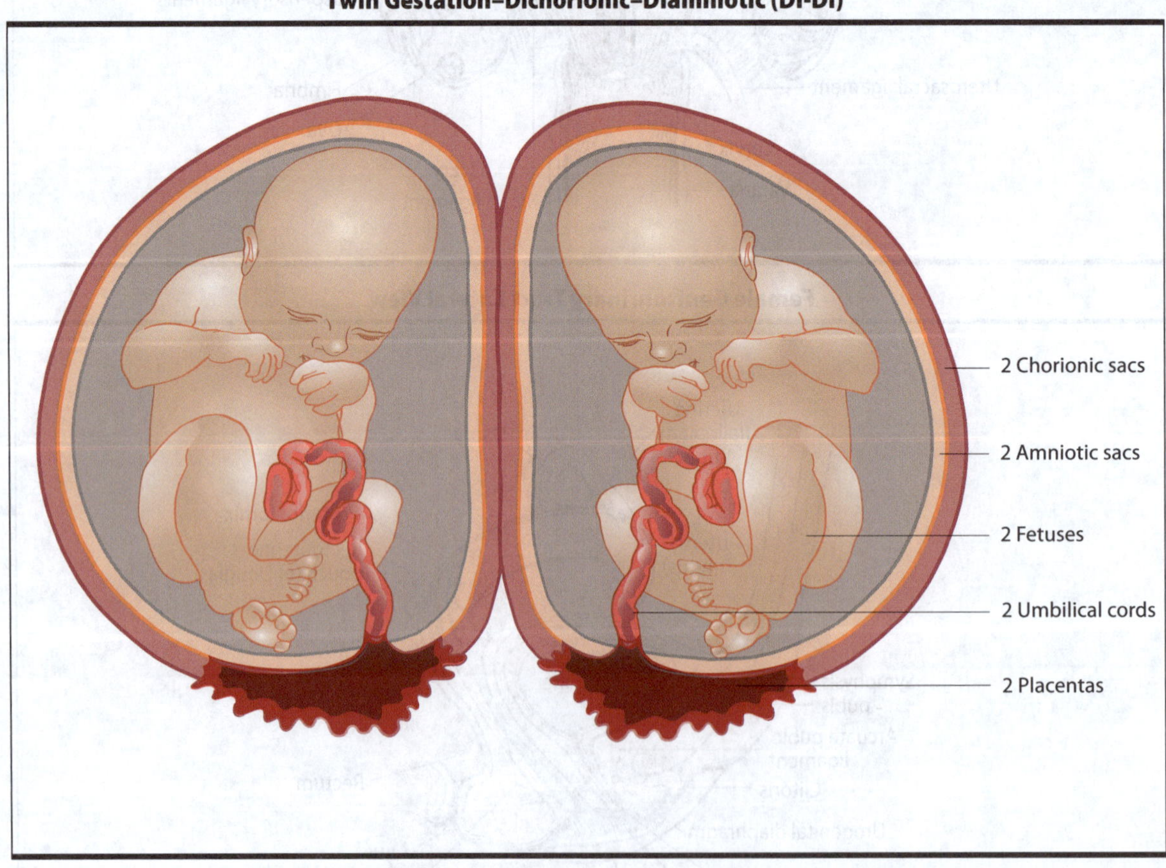

Twin Gestation–Monochorionic–Diamniotic (MO-DI)

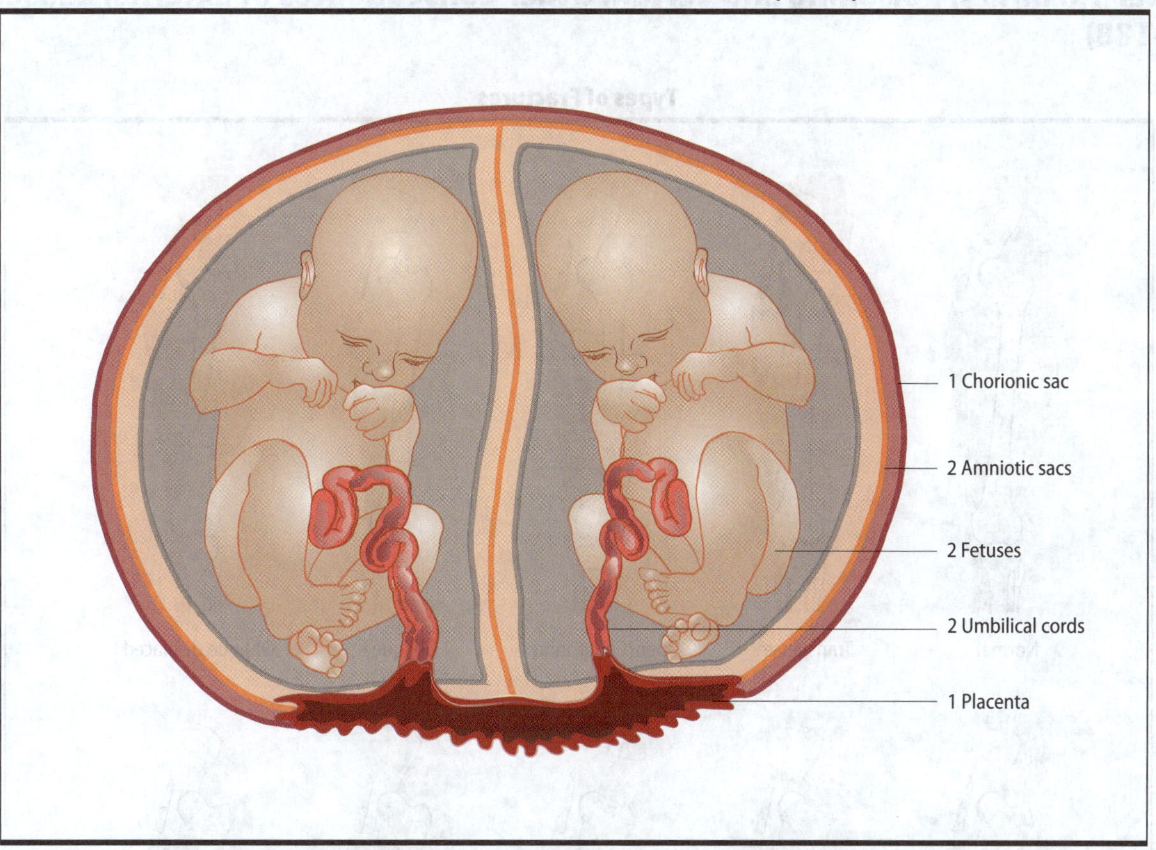

Twin Gestation–Monochorionic–Monoamniotic (MO-MO)

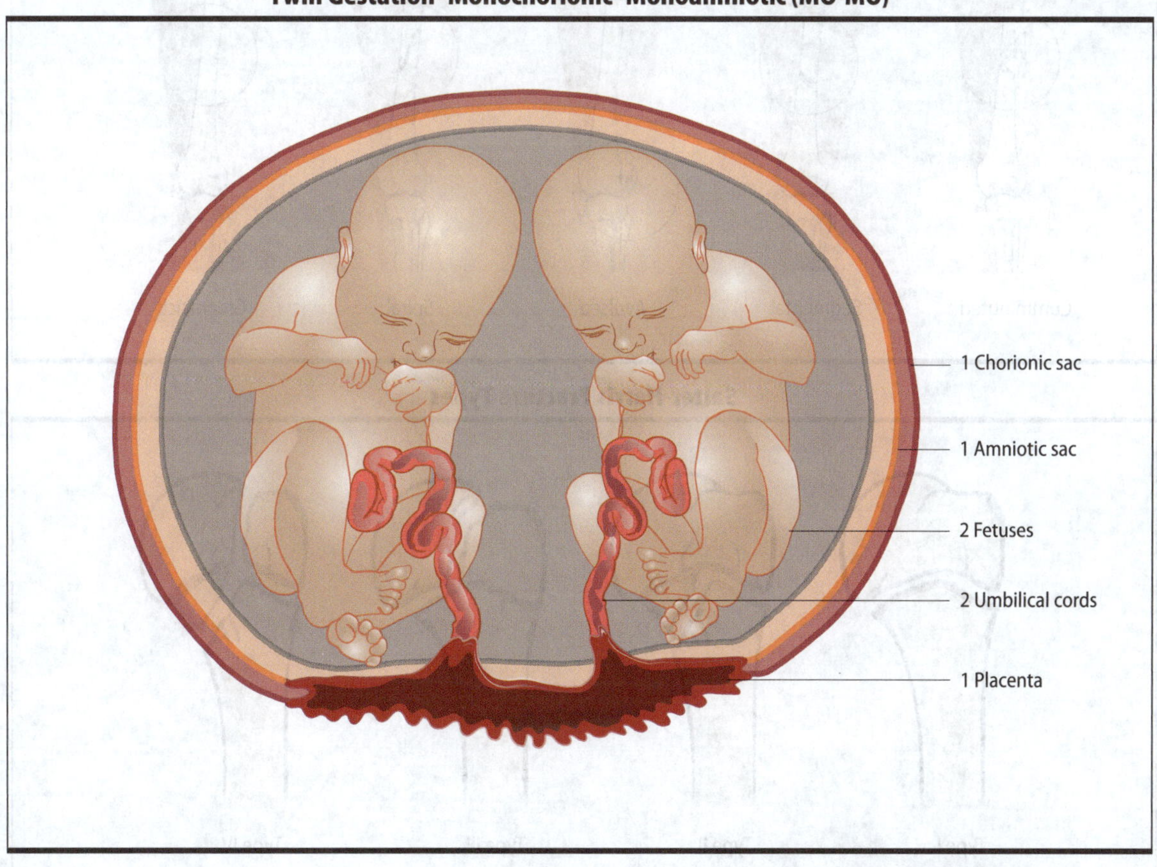

Chapter 19. Injury, Poisoning and Certain Other Consequences of External Causes (SØØ–T88)

Types of Fractures

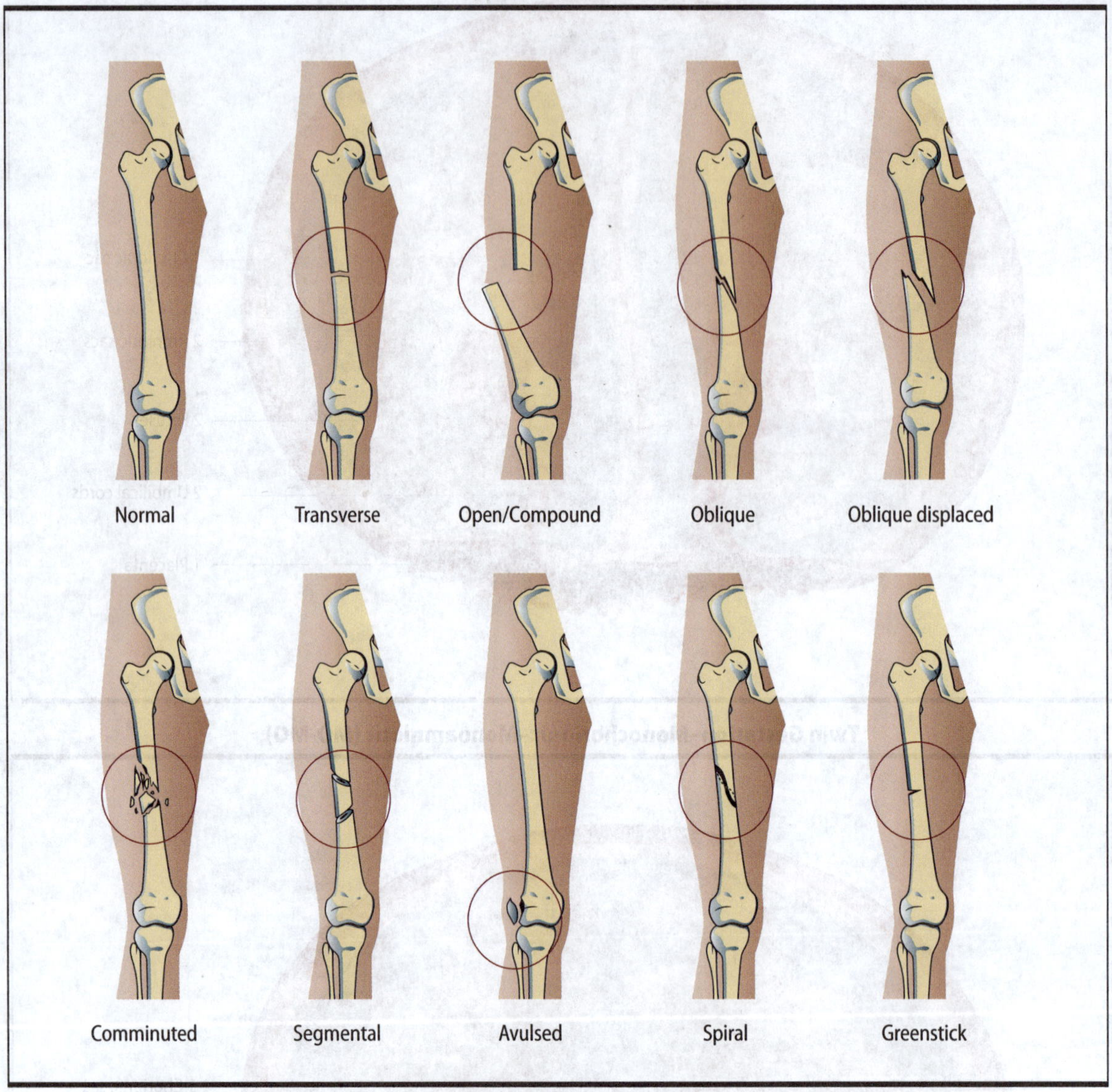

Normal
Transverse
Open/Compound
Oblique
Oblique displaced
Comminuted
Segmental
Avulsed
Spiral
Greenstick

Salter-Harris Fracture Types

Type I
Type II
Type III
Type IV

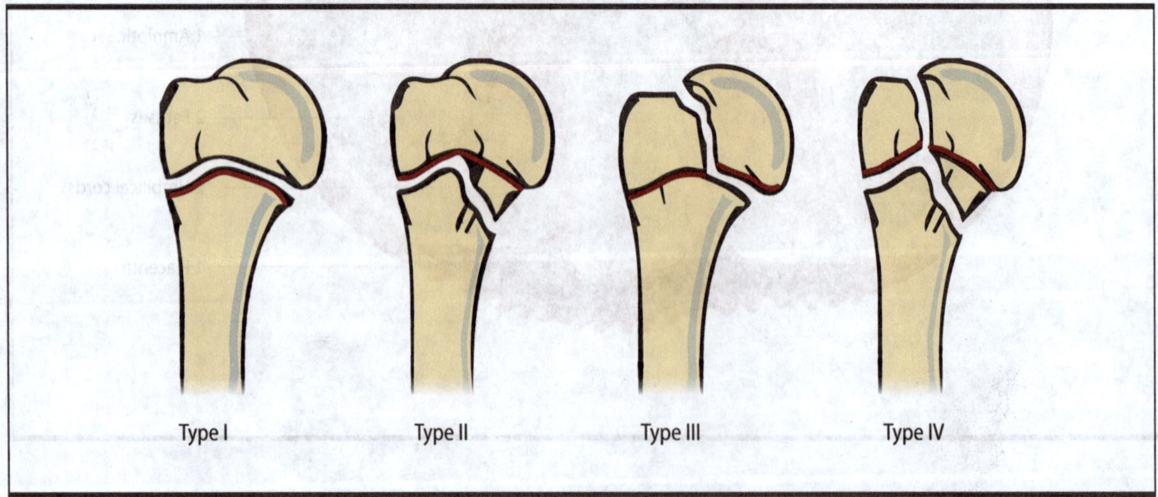